MW00845950

2018

ICD-10-CM Expert for Home Health and Hospice

The complete official code set

Codes valid October 1, 2017, through September 30, 2018

POWER UP YOUR CODING with Optum360, your trusted
coding partner for 32 years. **Visit optum360coding.com.**

Publisher's Notice

The *ICD-10-CM Expert for Home Health and Hospice: The Complete Official Code Set* is designed to be an accurate and authoritative source regarding coding. Every reasonable effort has been made to ensure accuracy and completeness of the content. However, Optum360 makes no guarantee, warranty, or representation that this publication is accurate, complete or without errors. It is understood that Optum360 is not rendering any legal or other professional services or advice in this publication and that Optum360 bears no liability for any results or consequences that may arise from the use of this book.

Please address all correspondence to:
Optum360
2525 Lake Park Blvd.
West Valley City, UT 84120

Acknowledgments

Lauri Gray, RHIT, CPC, AHIMA-approved ICD-10-CM/PCS Trainer, *Product Manager*
Karen Schmidt, BSN, *Technical Director*
Anita Schmidt, BS, RHIT, AHIMA-approved ICD-10-CM/PCS Trainer, *Clinical Technical Editor*
Brandi Whitemyer, RN, COS-C, HCS-D, HCS-O, AHIMA-approved ICD-10-CM/PCS Trainer/Ambassador, *Clinical Technical Editor*
Anne Kenney, BA, MBA, CCA, CCS, *Clinical Technical Editor*
Karen Krawzik, RHIT, CCS, AHIMA-approved ICD-10-CM/PCS Trainer, *Clinical Technical Editor*
Peggy Willard, CCS, AHIMA-approved ICD-10-CM/PCS Trainer, *Clinical Technical Editor*
Leanne Patterson, CPC, *Clinical Technical Editor*
Stacy Perry, *Manager, Desktop Publishing*
Lisa Singley, *Project Manager*
Tracy Betzler, *Senior Desktop Publishing Specialist*
Hope M. Dunn, *Senior Desktop Publishing Specialist*
Katie Russell, *Desktop Publishing Specialist*
Kate Holden, *Editor*

Our Commitment to Accuracy

Optum360 is committed to producing accurate and reliable materials.

To report corrections, please visit www.optum360coding.com/accuracy or email accuracy@optum.com. You can also reach customer service by calling 1.800.464.3649, option 1.

Copyright

Property of Optum360, LLC. Optum360 and the Optum360 logo are trademarks of Optum360, LLC. All other brand or product names are trademarks or registered trademarks of their respective owner.

© 2017 Optum360, LLC. All rights reserved.

Made in the USA
ISBN 978-1-62254-356-4

Anita Schmidt, BS, RHIT, AHIMA-approved ICD-10-CM/PCS Trainer

Ms. Schmidt has expertise in Level I Adult and Pediatric Trauma hospital coding, specializing in ICD-9-CM, ICD-10-CM/PCS, DRG, and CPT coding. Her experience includes analysis of medical record documentation, assignment of ICD-10-CM and PCS codes, DRG validation, as well as CPT code assignments for same-day surgery cases. She has conducted coding training and auditing, including DRG validation, conducted electronic health record training, and worked with clinical documentation specialists to identify documentation needs and potential areas for physician education. Most recently she has been developing content for resource and educational products related to ICD-10-CM and ICD-10-PCS. Ms. Schmidt is an AHIMA-approved ICD-10-CM/PCS trainer, and is an active member of the American Health Information Management Association (AHIMA) and the Minnesota Health Information Management Association (MHIMA).

Brandi Whitemyer, RN, COS-C, HCS-D, HCS-O, AHIMA-approved ICD-10-CM/PCS Trainer/Ambassador

Ms. Whitemyer's expertise is in ICD-10 coding and coding education, along with OASIS and outcomes management. She has more than 16 years of experience in post-acute healthcare as a former owner of a full-service coding and consulting company, along with experience in the development of coding and education resources for post-acute care. Ms. Whitemyer has worked with home health and hospice agencies nationally in providing consulting services, survey compliance, managing medical reviews and appeals of Medicare denials, writing corrective action plans, policy development, developing coding and quality assurance processes, and development of coding education. In recent years, she has both contributed to and created a number of print and electronic product resources focused on coding, billing, quality management, and clinical best practices. Ms. Whitemyer is a member of the American Health Information Management Association (AHIMA) and the Association of Home Health Coders (AHCC).

Contents

Contents

Preface

ICD-10-CM Official Preface

This FY 2018 update of the International Statistical Classification of Diseases and Related Health Problems, 10th revision, Clinical Modification (ICD-10-CM) is being published by the United States government in recognition of its responsibility to promulgate this classification throughout the United States for morbidity coding. The International Statistical Classification of Diseases and Related Health Problems, 10th Revision (ICD-10), published by the World Health Organization (WHO), is the foundation of ICD-10-CM. ICD-10 continues to be the classification used in cause-of-death coding in the United States. The ICD-10-CM is comparable with the ICD-10. The WHO Collaborating Center for the Family of International Classifications in North America, housed at the Centers for Disease Control and Prevention's National Center for Health Statistics (NCHS), has responsibility for the implementation of ICD and other WHO-FIC classifications and serves as a liaison with the WHO, fulfilling international obligations for comparable classifications and the national health data needs of the United States. The historical background of ICD and ICD-10 can be found in the Introduction to the International Classification of Diseases and Related Health Problems (ICD-10), 2010, World Health Organization, Geneva, Switzerland.

ICD-10-CM is the United States' clinical modification of the World Health Organization's ICD-10. The term "clinical" is used to emphasize the modification's intent: to serve as a useful tool in the area of classification of morbidity data for indexing of health records, medical care review, and ambulatory and other health care programs, as well as for basic health statistics. To describe the clinical picture of the patient the codes must be more precise than those needed only for statistical groupings and trend analysis.

Characteristics of ICD-10-CM

ICD-10-CM far exceeds its predecessors in the number of concepts and codes provided. The disease classification has been expanded to include health-related conditions and to provide greater specificity at the sixth and seventh character level. The sixth and seventh characters are not optional and are intended for use in recording the information documented in the clinical record.

ICD-10-CM extensions, interpretations, modifications, addenda, or errata other than those approved by the Centers for Disease Control and Prevention are not to be considered official and should not be utilized. Continuous maintenance of the ICD-10- CM is the responsibility of the aforementioned agencies. However, because the ICD-10- CM represents the best in contemporary thinking of clinicians, nosologists, epidemiologists, and statisticians from both public and private sectors, when future modifications are considered, advice will be sought from all stakeholders.

All official authorized addenda since the last complete update (October 1, 2017) have been included in this revision. For more detailed information please see the complete official authorized addenda to ICD-10-CM, including the "ICD-10-CM Official Guidelines for Coding and Reporting," and a description of the ICD-10-CM updating and maintenance process.

What's New for 2018

Official Updates

The National Center for Health Statistics (NCHS), a section of the Centers for Disease Control and Prevention (CDC), is the agency charged with maintaining and updating ICD-10-CM. The 2018 official addendum was posted to the Centers for Medicare and Medicaid Services (CMS) website on June 13, 2017, identifying the changes to the ICD-10-CM code set for fiscal 2018. A summary of changes is provided below:

- 360 new codes added
- 226 code descriptions revised
- 34 codes changed from valid to invalid

Note: Validity changes are the result of new codes being added to the classification, changing a previously valid code to an invalid code, creating a new subcategory

A04.7	Enterocolitis due to Clostridium difficile
C96.2	Malignant mast cell tumor
D47.0	Histiocytic and mast cell tumors of uncertain behavior
E85.8	Other amyloidosis
H54.0	Blindness, both eyes
H54.11	Blindness, right eye, low vision left eye
H54.12	Blindness, left eye, low vision right eye
H54.2	Low vision, both eyes
H54.41	Blindness, right eye, normal vision left eye
H54.42	Blindness, left eye, normal vision right eye
H54.51	Low vision, right eye, normal vision left eye
H54.52	Low vision, left eye, normal vision right eye
I27.2	Other secondary pulmonary hypertension
K06.0	Gingival recession
K56.5	Intestinal adhesions [bands] with obstruction (postprocedural) (postinfection)
K56.60	Unspecified intestinal obstruction
K56.69	Other intestinal obstruction
K91.3	Postprocedural intestinal obstruction
M48.06	Spinal stenosis, lumbar region
N63	Unspecified lump in breast
O00.10	Tubal pregnancy without intrauterine pregnancy
O00.11	Tubal pregnancy with intrauterine pregnancy
O00.20	Ovarian pregnancy without intrauterine pregnancy
O00.21	Ovarian pregnancy with intrauterine pregnancy
P29.3	Persistent fetal circulation
P83.8	Other specified conditions of integument specific to newborn
P91.8	Other specified disturbances of cerebral status of newborn
Q53.11	Abdominal testis, unilateral
Q53.21	Abdominal testis, bilateral
T07	Unspecified multiple injuries
T14.8	Other injury of unspecified body region
T14.90	Injury, unspecified
T14.91	Suicide attempt
Z36	Encounter for antenatal screening of mother

- 122 codes deleted from the classification

S06.1X7D	Traumatic cerebral edema with loss of consciousness of any duration with death due to brain injury prior to regaining consciousness, subsequent encounter
S06.1X7S	Traumatic cerebral edema with loss of consciousness of any duration with death due to brain injury prior to regaining consciousness, sequela
S06.1X8D	Traumatic cerebral edema with loss of consciousness of any duration with death due to other cause prior to regaining consciousness, subsequent encounter
S06.1X8S	Traumatic cerebral edema with loss of consciousness of any duration with death due to other cause prior to regaining consciousness, sequela
S06.2X7D	Diffuse traumatic brain injury with loss of consciousness of any duration with death due to brain injury prior to regaining consciousness, subsequent encounter
S06.2X7S	Diffuse traumatic brain injury with loss of consciousness of any duration with death due to brain injury prior to regaining consciousness, sequela
S06.2X8D	Diffuse traumatic brain injury with loss of consciousness of any duration with death due to other cause prior to regaining consciousness, subsequent encounter
S06.2X8S	Diffuse traumatic brain injury with loss of consciousness of any duration with death due to other cause prior to regaining consciousness, sequela
S06.307D	Unspecified focal traumatic brain injury with loss of consciousness of any duration with death due to brain injury prior to regaining consciousness, subsequent encounter
S06.307S	Unspecified focal traumatic brain injury with loss of consciousness of any duration with death due to brain injury prior to regaining consciousness, sequela
S06.308D	Unspecified focal traumatic brain injury with loss of consciousness of any duration with death due to other cause prior to regaining consciousness, subsequent encounter
S06.308S	Unspecified focal traumatic brain injury with loss of consciousness of any duration with death due to other cause prior to regaining consciousness, sequela
S06.317D	Contusion and laceration of right cerebrum with loss of consciousness of any duration with death due to brain injury prior to regaining consciousness, subsequent encounter
S06.317S	Contusion and laceration of right cerebrum with loss of consciousness of any duration with death due to brain injury prior to regaining consciousness, sequela
S06.318D	Contusion and laceration of right cerebrum with loss of consciousness of any duration with death due to other cause prior to regaining consciousness, subsequent encounter
S06.318S	Contusion and laceration of right cerebrum with loss of consciousness of any duration with death due to other cause prior to regaining consciousness, sequela
S06.327D	Contusion and laceration of left cerebrum with loss of consciousness of any duration with death due to brain injury prior to regaining consciousness, subsequent encounter
S06.327S	Contusion and laceration of left cerebrum with loss of consciousness of any duration with death due to brain injury prior to regaining consciousness, sequela
S06.328D	Contusion and laceration of left cerebrum with loss of consciousness of any duration with death due to other cause prior to regaining consciousness, subsequent encounter
S06.328S	Contusion and laceration of left cerebrum with loss of consciousness of any duration with death due to other cause prior to regaining consciousness, sequela
S06.337D	Contusion and laceration of cerebrum, unspecified, with loss of consciousness of any duration with death due to brain injury prior to regaining consciousness, subsequent encounter
S06.337S	Contusion and laceration of cerebrum, unspecified, with loss of consciousness of any duration with death due to brain injury prior to regaining consciousness, sequela
S06.338D	Contusion and laceration of cerebrum, unspecified, with loss of consciousness of any duration with death due to other cause prior to regaining consciousness, subsequent encounter
S06.338S	Contusion and laceration of cerebrum, unspecified, with loss of consciousness of any duration with death due to other cause prior to regaining consciousness, sequela
S06.347D	Traumatic hemorrhage of right cerebrum with loss of consciousness of any duration with death due to brain injury prior to regaining consciousness, subsequent encounter

S06.347S Traumatic hemorrhage of right cerebrum with loss of consciousness of any duration with death due to brain injury prior to regaining consciousness, sequela

S06.348D Traumatic hemorrhage of right cerebrum with loss of consciousness of any duration with death due to other cause prior to regaining consciousness, subsequent encounter

S06.348S Traumatic hemorrhage of right cerebrum with loss of consciousness of any duration with death due to other cause prior to regaining consciousness, sequela

S06.357D Traumatic hemorrhage of left cerebrum with loss of consciousness of any duration with death due to brain injury prior to regaining consciousness, subsequent encounter

S06.357S Traumatic hemorrhage of left cerebrum with loss of consciousness of any duration with death due to brain injury prior to regaining consciousness, sequela

S06.358D Traumatic hemorrhage of left cerebrum with loss of consciousness of any duration with death due to other cause prior to regaining consciousness, subsequent encounter

S06.358S Traumatic hemorrhage of left cerebrum with loss of consciousness of any duration with death due to other cause prior to regaining consciousness, sequela

S06.367D Traumatic hemorrhage of cerebrum, unspecified, with loss of consciousness of any duration with death due to brain injury prior to regaining consciousness, subsequent encounter

S06.367S Traumatic hemorrhage of cerebrum, unspecified, with loss of consciousness of any duration with death due to brain injury prior to regaining consciousness, sequela

S06.368D Traumatic hemorrhage of cerebrum, unspecified, with loss of consciousness of any duration with death due to other cause prior to regaining consciousness, subsequent encounter

S06.368S Traumatic hemorrhage of cerebrum, unspecified, with loss of consciousness of any duration with death due to other cause prior to regaining consciousness, sequela

S06.377D Contusion, laceration, and hemorrhage of cerebellum with loss of consciousness of any duration with death due to brain injury prior to regaining consciousness, subsequent encounter

S06.377S Contusion, laceration, and hemorrhage of cerebellum with loss of consciousness of any duration with death due to brain injury prior to regaining consciousness, sequela

S06.378D Contusion, laceration, and hemorrhage of cerebellum with loss of consciousness of any duration with death due to other cause prior to regaining consciousness, subsequent encounter

S06.378S Contusion, laceration, and hemorrhage of cerebellum with loss of consciousness of any duration with death due to other cause prior to regaining consciousness, sequela

S06.387D Contusion, laceration, and hemorrhage of brainstem with loss of consciousness of any duration with death due to brain injury prior to regaining consciousness, subsequent encounter

S06.387S Contusion, laceration, and hemorrhage of brainstem with loss of consciousness of any duration with death due to brain injury prior to regaining consciousness, sequela

S06.388D Contusion, laceration, and hemorrhage of brainstem with loss of consciousness of any duration with death due to other cause prior to regaining consciousness, subsequent encounter

S06.388S Contusion, laceration, and hemorrhage of brainstem with loss of consciousness of any duration with death due to other cause prior to regaining consciousness, sequela

S06.4X7D Epidural hemorrhage with loss of consciousness of any duration with death due to brain injury prior to regaining consciousness, subsequent encounter

S06.4X7S Epidural hemorrhage with loss of consciousness of any duration with death due to brain injury prior to regaining consciousness, sequela

S06.4X8D Epidural hemorrhage with loss of consciousness of any duration with death due to other causes prior to regaining consciousness, subsequent encounter

S06.4X8S Epidural hemorrhage with loss of consciousness of any duration with death due to other causes prior to regaining consciousness, sequela

S06.5X7D Traumatic subdural hemorrhage with loss of consciousness of any duration with death due to brain injury before regaining consciousness, subsequent encounter

S06.5X7S Traumatic subdural hemorrhage with loss of consciousness of any duration with death due to brain injury before regaining consciousness, sequela

S06.5X8D Traumatic subdural hemorrhage with loss of consciousness of any duration with death due to other cause before regaining consciousness, subsequent encounter

S06.5X8S Traumatic subdural hemorrhage with loss of consciousness of any duration with death due to other cause before regaining consciousness, sequela

S06.6X7D Traumatic subarachnoid hemorrhage with loss of consciousness of any duration with death due to brain injury prior to regaining consciousness, subsequent encounter

S06.6X7S Traumatic subarachnoid hemorrhage with loss of consciousness of any duration with death due to brain injury prior to regaining consciousness, sequela

S06.6X8D Traumatic subarachnoid hemorrhage with loss of consciousness of any duration with death due to other cause prior to regaining consciousness, subsequent encounter

S06.6X8S Traumatic subarachnoid hemorrhage with loss of consciousness of any duration with death due to other cause prior to regaining consciousness, sequela

S06.817D Injury of right internal carotid artery, intracranial portion, not elsewhere classified with loss of consciousness of any duration with death due to brain injury prior to regaining consciousness, subsequent encounter

S06.817S Injury of right internal carotid artery, intracranial portion, not elsewhere classified with loss of consciousness of any duration with death due to brain injury prior to regaining consciousness, sequela

S06.818D Injury of right internal carotid artery, intracranial portion, not elsewhere classified with loss of consciousness of any duration with death due to other cause prior to regaining consciousness, subsequent encounter

S06.818S Injury of right internal carotid artery, intracranial portion, not elsewhere classified with loss of consciousness of any duration with death due to other cause prior to regaining consciousness, sequela

S06.827D Injury of left internal carotid artery, intracranial portion, not elsewhere classified with loss of consciousness of any duration with death due to brain injury prior to regaining consciousness, subsequent encounter

S06.827S Injury of left internal carotid artery, intracranial portion, not elsewhere classified with loss of consciousness of any duration with death due to brain injury prior to regaining consciousness, sequela

S06.828D Injury of left internal carotid artery, intracranial portion, not elsewhere classified with loss of consciousness of any duration with death due to other cause prior to regaining consciousness, subsequent encounter

S06.828S Injury of left internal carotid artery, intracranial portion, not elsewhere classified with loss of consciousness of any duration with death due to other cause prior to regaining consciousness, sequela

S06.897D Other specified intracranial injury with loss of consciousness of any duration with death due to brain injury prior to regaining consciousness, subsequent encounter

S06.897S Other specified intracranial injury with loss of consciousness of any duration with death due to brain injury prior to regaining consciousness, sequela

S06.898D Other specified intracranial injury with loss of consciousness of any duration with death due to other cause prior to regaining consciousness, subsequent encounter

S06.898S Other specified intracranial injury with loss of consciousness of any duration with death due to other cause prior to regaining consciousness, sequela

S06.9X7D Unspecified intracranial injury with loss of consciousness of any duration with death due to brain injury prior to regaining consciousness, subsequent encounter

Code	Description
S06.9X7S	Unspecified intracranial injury with loss of consciousness of any duration with death due to brain injury prior to regaining consciousness, sequela
S06.9X8D	Unspecified intracranial injury with loss of consciousness of any duration with death due to other cause prior to regaining consciousness, subsequent encounter
S06.9X8S	Unspecified intracranial injury with loss of consciousness of any duration with death due to other cause prior to regaining consciousness, sequela
S63.13	Subluxation and dislocation of proximal interphalangeal joint of thumb
S63.131	Subluxation of proximal interphalangeal joint of right thumb
S63.131A	Subluxation of proximal interphalangeal joint of right thumb, initial encounter
S63.131D	Subluxation of proximal interphalangeal joint of right thumb, subsequent encounter
S63.131S	Subluxation of proximal interphalangeal joint of right thumb, sequela
S63.132	Subluxation of proximal interphalangeal joint of left thumb
S63.132A	Subluxation of proximal interphalangeal joint of left thumb, initial encounter
S63.132D	Subluxation of proximal interphalangeal joint of left thumb, subsequent encounter
S63.132S	Subluxation of proximal interphalangeal joint of left thumb, sequela
S63.133	Subluxation of proximal interphalangeal joint of unspecified thumb
S63.133A	Subluxation of proximal interphalangeal joint of unspecified thumb, initial encounter
S63.133D	Subluxation of proximal interphalangeal joint of unspecified thumb, subsequent encounter
S63.133S	Subluxation of proximal interphalangeal joint of unspecified thumb, sequela
S63.134	Dislocation of proximal interphalangeal joint of right thumb
S63.134A	Dislocation of proximal interphalangeal joint of right thumb, initial encounter
S63.134D	Dislocation of proximal interphalangeal joint of right thumb, subsequent encounter
S63.134S	Dislocation of proximal interphalangeal joint of right thumb, sequela
S63.135	Dislocation of proximal interphalangeal joint of left thumb
S63.135A	Dislocation of proximal interphalangeal joint of left thumb, initial encounter
S63.135D	Dislocation of proximal interphalangeal joint of left thumb, subsequent encounter
S63.135S	Dislocation of proximal interphalangeal joint of left thumb, sequela
S63.136	Dislocation of proximal interphalangeal joint of unspecified thumb
S63.136A	Dislocation of proximal interphalangeal joint of unspecified thumb, initial encounter
S63.136D	Dislocation of proximal interphalangeal joint of unspecified thumb, subsequent encounter
S63.136S	Dislocation of proximal interphalangeal joint of unspecified thumb, sequela
S63.14	Subluxation and dislocation of distal interphalangeal joint of thumb
S63.141	Subluxation of distal interphalangeal joint of right thumb
S63.141A	Subluxation of distal interphalangeal joint of right thumb, initial encounter
S63.141D	Subluxation of distal interphalangeal joint of right thumb, subsequent encounter
S63.141S	Subluxation of distal interphalangeal joint of right thumb, sequela
S63.142	Subluxation of distal interphalangeal joint of left thumb
S63.142A	Subluxation of distal interphalangeal joint of left thumb, initial encounter
S63.142D	Subluxation of distal interphalangeal joint of left thumb, subsequent encounter S63.142SSubluxation of distal interphalangeal joint of left thumb, sequela
S63.143	Subluxation of distal interphalangeal joint of unspecified thumb
S63.143A	Subluxation of distal interphalangeal joint of unspecified thumb, initial encounter
S63.143D	Subluxation of distal interphalangeal joint of unspecified thumb, subsequent encounter
S63.143S	Subluxation of distal interphalangeal joint of unspecified thumb, sequela
S63.144	Dislocation of distal interphalangeal joint of right thumb
S63.144A	Dislocation of distal interphalangeal joint of right thumb, initial encounter
S63.144D	Dislocation of distal interphalangeal joint of right thumb, subsequent encounter
S63.144S	Dislocation of distal interphalangeal joint of right thumb, sequela
S63.145	Dislocation of distal interphalangeal joint of left thumb
S63.145A	Dislocation of distal interphalangeal joint of left thumb, initial encounter
S63.145D	Dislocation of distal interphalangeal joint of left thumb, subsequent encounter
S63.145S	Dislocation of distal interphalangeal joint of left thumb, sequela
S63.146	Dislocation of distal interphalangeal joint of unspecified thumb
S63.146A	Dislocation of distal interphalangeal joint of unspecified thumb, initial encounter
S63.146D	Dislocation of distal interphalangeal joint of unspecified thumb, subsequent encounter
S63.146S	Dislocation of distal interphalangeal joint of unspecified thumb, sequela

Proprietary Updates

The following proprietary features have also been added:

- 150+ new definitions that describe, in lay terms, a specific condition or disease process

- 50+ new illustrations

- Updated *AHA Coding Clinic* references through second quarter 2017

- Updated pharmacology list

- New tips that identify specific coding or reimbursement nuances in post-acute care settings

- Updated coding examples in the chapter-specific guidelines specific to home health or hospice settings

Introduction

History of ICD-10-CM

The ICD-10-CM classification system was developed by the National Center for Health Statistics (NCHS) as a clinical modification to the ICD-10 system developed by the World Health Organization (WHO), primarily as a unique system for use in the United States for morbidity and mortality reporting. Although ICD-10 replaced ICD-9 for use in coding and classifying mortality data from death certificates beginning January 1, 1999, ICD-10-CM implementation was postponed many years until legislation to replace ICD-9-CM, volumes 1 and 2, with ICD-10-CM was approved.

ICD-10 is the copyrighted product of the World Health Organization (WHO), which has authorized the development of a clinical modification (CM) of ICD-10 for use in the United States. However, all modifications to the ICD-10 must conform to WHO conventions for ICD. The development of ICD-10-CM included comprehensive evaluation by a Technical Advisory Panel and extensive consultation with physician groups, clinical coders, and other industry experts.

The ICD-10-CM and crosswalk between ICD-9-CM and ICD-10-CM were made available on the Centers for Medicare and Medicaid Services (CMS) website for public comment. The initial public comment period extended from December 1997 through February 1998. A field test for ICD-10-CM was conducted in the summer of 2003 jointly by the American Hospital Association (AHA) and the American Health Information Management Association (AHIMA). Public comments and suggestions were reviewed and additional modifications to ICD-10-CM were made. Revisions were made to ICD-10-CM based on the established update process for ICD-10-CM (the ICD-10-CM Coordination and Maintenance Committee) and the World Health Organization's ICD-10 (the Update and Revision Committee).

These revisions to ICD-10-CM have included:

- Information relevant to ambulatory and managed care encounters
- Expanded injury codes
- Creation of combination diagnosis/symptom codes to reduce the number of codes needed to fully describe a condition
- The addition of 6th and 7th character classifications
- Incorporation of common 4th and 5th character classifications
- Classifications specific to laterality
- Classification refinement for increased data granularity

This new structure allows for further expansion than was possible with the ICD-9-CM classification system.

The Department of Health and Human Services (HHS) published the final rule regarding the adoption of both ICD-10-CM and ICD-10-PCS in the January 16, 2009, *Federal Register* (45 CFR part 162 [CMS—0013—F]). The initial compliance date for implementation of ICD-10-CM and ICD-10-PCS as a replacement for ICD-9-CM was set at October 1, 2013. On April 17, 2012, the Department of Health and Human Services (HHS) released a notice to postpone the date by which certain health care entities have to comply with International Classification of Diseases, 10th Revision diagnosis and procedure codes (ICD-10). The compliance date for implementation of ICD-10-CM and ICD-10-PCS as a replacement for ICD-9-CM was changed to October 1, 2014. On April 1, 2014, Congress enacted the Protecting Access to Medicare Act of 2014, which contained a provision to delay the implementation of ICD-10-CM/PCS by at least one year, prohibiting the Department of Health and Human Services (HHS)

from adopting the ICD-10-CM/PCS code sets as the mandatory standard until October 1, 2015. Eventually, the ICD-10-CM/PCS code sets were implemented in their entirety on October 1, 2015, and volumes 1 and 2 of ICD-9-CM were retired.

ICD-10-CM: The Complete Official Code Set

ICD-10-CM: The Complete Official Code Set 2018 edition includes many of the enhancements described below in direct response to requests from our subscribers.

As you review the content, you will find the following:

- Optum360 Exclusive feature — Check Placeholder Alert symbol, indicating the need for one or more "filler" X character assignments in the 5th and/or 6th character position, in order to appropriately assign a required character in the 7th character position
- Optum360 Exclusive feature — Key word differentiation by the use of a green font that highlights the differentiating terms in similar code descriptions in a given category
- Optum360 Exclusive color coding, symbols, and footnotes that alert coders to coding and reimbursement issues, including the majority of the Medicare code edits
- Optum360 Exclusive feature — Exclusive *following* references and Check Additional Character symbol in the indexes. The *following* references (designed and used exclusively by Optum360) help coders locate those alphanumeric codes that are out of sequence in the tabular section.
- Optum360 Exclusive feature — Exclusive shaded guides in the index that help users easily follow the indent levels for the subterms under a main term
- Illustrations throughout the tabular list and at the back of the book that feature anatomy and terminology included in the ICD-10-CM classification system
- Optum360 Exclusive feature—Detailed Muscle/Tendon tables that correspond to codes in chapters 13 and 19
- The complete ICD-10-CM Official Guidelines for Coding and Reporting, published by the U.S. Department of Health and Human Services and approved by the cooperating parties (American Health Information Management Association, National Center for Health Statistics, Centers for Medicare and Medicaid Services, American Hospital Association)
- Optum360 Exclusive feature—Official chapter-specific guidelines with coding examples at the beginning of each chapter
- All the official ICD-10-CM codes, indexes, notes, footnotes, and symbols
- Icons and definitions to differentiate between the two types of Excludes notes
- Check 4th, 5th, 6th, and 7th character symbols that identify codes that require the addition of a 4th, 5th, 6th, or 7th character for code specificity and validity
- Color coding and symbol legend at the bottom of each page

Please review "How to Use *ICD-10-CM Expert for Home Health and Hospices*" in this section to learn about the features that will help you assign and report correct codes, ensuring appropriate reimbursement.

How to Use ICD-10-CM Expert for Home Health and Hospice 2018

This International Classification of Diseases, 10th Revision, Clinical Modification (ICD-10-CM) is being published by the United States Government in recognition of its responsibility to promulgate this classification throughout the United States for morbidity coding. This code book represents an adaptation of ICD-10 that was created specifically for use in the United States. Revisions to ICD-10-CM will be made based on the established update process for ICD-10-CM (the ICD-10-CM Coordination and Maintenance Committee) and the World Health Organization's ICD-10 (the Update and Revision Committee).

Use of Official Sources

The *ICD-10-CM Expert for Home Health and Hospice* contains the official U.S. Department of Health and Human Services, Tenth Revision, Clinical Modification, ICD-10-CM codes, effective for the current year.

Much of the color coding and many of the symbols that identify coding and reimbursement issues are derived from official federal government sources, including the Integrated Outpatient Code Editor (IOCE), version 18.2, and the January 2017 home health prospective payment system (HH PPS) Grouper software.

For the most current IOCE documents and HH PPS Grouper software please refer to the following:

https://www.cms.gov/Medicare/Coding/OutpatientCodeEdit/ OCEQtrReleaseSpecs.html

https://www.cms.gov/Medicare/Medicare-Fee-for-Service-Payment/ HomeHealthPPS/CaseMixGrouperSoftware.html.

Steps to Correct Coding

1. Before beginning to use this code book, review section I.A., "Conventions for the ICD-10-CM," and section I.B., "General Coding Guidelines," of the ICD-10-CM Official Guidelines for Coding and Reporting.

2. Look up the main term in the alphabetic index and scan the subterm entries as appropriate. Review continued lines and additional subterms that may appear in the next column or on the next page.

3. Note all parenthetical terms (nonessential modifiers) that help in code selection but do not affect code assignment. Shaded vertical guidelines in the index are provided to help determine the indentation level for each subterm in relation to the main terms.

4. Pay close attention to the following instructions in the index:

   – "See," "see also," and "see category" cross-references

   – "With"/"without" notes

   – "Omit code" notes

   – "Due to" subterms

   – Other instructions found in note boxes, such as "code by site"

   – *Following* references and Check Additional Character symbol in the indexes. The *following* references (designed and used exclusively by Optum360) help coders locate those alphanumeric codes that are out of sequence in the tabular section.

5. Do not code from the alphabetic index without verifying the accuracy of the code in the tabular list. Locate the code in the alphanumerically arranged tabular list.

6. To determine the appropriateness of the code selection and proper coding, read all instructional material:

   – "Includes" and both types of "Excludes" notes

   – "Use additional code" and "code first underlying disease" instructions

   – "Code also"

   – 4th, 5th, and 6th character requirements and 7th character extension requirements

   – Age and sex symbols

7. Consult the official ICD-10-CM guidelines, which govern the use of specific codes. These guidelines provide both general and chapter-specific coding guidance.

8. Confirm and assign the correct code.

Organization

This book is organized in the following manner:

Introduction

The introductory material in this book includes the ICD-10-CM Official Preface, the history of ICD-10-CM as well as an overview of the classification system.

Official ICD-10-CM Conventions and Guidelines

This section provides an explanation of the conventions and guidelines regulating the appropriate assignment and reporting of ICD-10-CM codes. This coding guidance is presented by the National Center for Health Statistics (NCHS), a governmental agency of the Centers for Disease Control and Prevention (CDC), within the United States Department of Health and Human Services (DHHS).

Alphabetic Index to Diseases

The Alphabetic Index to Diseases is arranged in alphabetic order by disease — by specific illness, injury, eponym, abbreviation, or other descriptive diagnostic term. The index also lists diagnostic terms for other reasons for encounters with health care professionals.

Neoplasm Table

The Neoplasm Table provides the proper code based upon histology of the neoplasm and site.

Table of Drugs and Chemicals

The Table of Drugs and Chemicals lists the drug and the specific codes that identify the drug and the intent. No additional external cause of injury and poisoning code is assigned in ICD-10-CM.

Index to External Causes

The Alphabetic Index to External Causes of Injuries is arranged in alphabetic order by main term indicating the event.

Tabular List of Diseases

ICD-10-CM codes and descriptors are arranged numerically within the tabular list of diseases within 21 separate chapters according to body system or nature of injury and disease. Classifications that were previously considered supplemental to ICD-9-CM (e.g., V codes and E codes) are incorporated into the tabular listing of ICD-10-CM as individual chapters. Chapters 20, "External Causes of Morbidity," and 21, "Factors Influencing

Health Status and Contact with Health Services," include chapter-specific guidelines.

Appendixes

The additional resources described below have been included as appendixes for the *ICD-10-CM Expert for Home Health and Hospice: The Complete Official Code Set*. These resources further instruct the professional coder on the appropriate application of the ICD-10-CM code set.

Appendix A: 10 Steps to Correct Coding

This step-by-step tutorial walks the coder through the process of locating the correct code in the alphabetic index and verifying it in the tabular section while following applicable conventions and guidelines. Detailed examples are provided and explained along with advice for proper sequencing.

Appendix B: Valid 3-character ICD-10-CM Codes

The user may consult this table to confirm that no further specificity, such as the use of 4th, 5th, 6th or 7th characters or placeholders (X), is necessary. All ICD-10-CM codes that are valid at the three-character level are listed.

Appendix C: Pharmacology List 2018

This reference is a comprehensive but not all-inclusive list of pharmacological agents used to treat acute and/or chronic conditions. Drugs are listed in alphabetical order by their brand and/or generic names along with their drug action and indications for which they may commonly be prescribed. Some drugs have also been mapped to their appropriate Z code for long-term drug use.

Appendix D: Z Codes for Long-Term Drug Use with Associated Drugs

This resource correlates Z codes that are used to identify current long-term drug use with a list of drugs that are typically categorized to that class of drug.

Note: These tables are not all-inclusive but list some of the more commonly used drugs.

Appendix E: Z Codes Only as Principal/First-Listed Diagnosis

Chapter 21, Factors Influencing Health Status and Contact with Health Services, provides codes to deal with encounters for circumstances other than a disease or injury. Many of these codes may be reported *only* as the principal/first listed diagnosis. This resource lists all of these codes in one table for quick and easy reference to ensure accurate reporting.

Appendix F: Qualifications for Medicare Coverage of Home Health Services

Medicare coverage for home health services is subject to specific criteria the patient must meet to qualify for coverage. This resource summarizes the coverage requirements provided in the Medicare Benefit Policy Manual (Pub. 100-02), chapter 7, "Home Health Services."

Appendix G: Overview of the Home Health Prospective Payment System

Medicare uses the home health prospective payment system (HH PPS) to pay for home health services under Part A and Part B. This resource provides an overview of how a unit of payment is defined and the elements needed to calculate these payments.

Appendix H: OASIS Diagnosis Guidance

This resource provides guidance for OASIS items that address reporting and coding diagnoses, specifically items M1011, M1017, M1021, M1023, and M1025.

OASIS item M1011 identifies diagnoses for which the patient was actively receiving treatment in an inpatient facility within the past 14 days. Item M1017 identifies changes that may have occurred to the patient's treatment regimen, health care services, or medications within the past 14 days, and confirms the patient's recent history by identifying new diagnoses or diagnoses that have been exacerbated over the past two weeks. Item M1021 reports the patient's primary home health diagnosis, and M1023 reports the secondary home health diagnoses. Item M1023 is optional and may be used to report a resolved underlying condition. The official source for this information is found in the OASIS-C2/ICD-10 Guidance Manual, chapter 3.

Appendix I: Case-Mix Adjustment Variables and Scores

This resource provides two of the three dimensions of case-mix—the case-mix scores and functional dimension scores that along with services utilization dimension classify a case to a specific home health resource group (HHRG).

Appendix J: Case-Mix Groups

Each of the 22 case-mix groups contains specific ICD-10-CM codes. Each ICD-10-CM code is scored based on the group to which it is categorized and whether it is a primary or secondary diagnosis. This resource provides each case-mix group and its corresponding ICD-10-CM codes.

Appendix K: NRS Case-Mix Adjustment Variables and Scores

Nonroutine supply (NRS) case-mix adjustment is based upon a six-group severity level approach. An ICD-10-CM code may qualify a case for NRS case-mix adjustment depending on several factors, including whether it is categorized to one of the six NRS groups and whether it is used as a primary or secondary diagnosis. Scores are given based on these and other criteria and are used to determine the case-mix.

Appendix L: Diagnosis Categories for Nonroutine Supplies Case-Mix Adjustment

This resource identifies the 12 specific NRS groups and their associated ICD-10-CM codes. Along with other case-mix conditional requirements, each code in this table may be eligible for case-mix points depending on the NRS group to which it is classified and whether it describes a primary or secondary diagnosis, when included on the OASIS instrument.

Appendix M: Valid Diagnosis/Etiology Pairings List

The home health prospective payment system (HH PPS) provides case-mix group assignment and/or nonroutine supply (NRS) adjustments for valid etiology and manifestation code pairs. This resource is a complete list of these valid diagnosis/etiology pairs.

Appendix N: Hospice Criteria for Medicare Coverage on Noncancer Hospice Care

This resource provides the requirements that must be met for an individual to be recommended and covered for hospice care; in particular, when a patient does not have a cancer diagnosis.

Appendix O: Hospice Diagnosis and Quality Reporting Guidance

This resource provides an overview of the FY 2017 hospice rule, including a summary of the major provisions regarding diagnosis reporting as well as quality measures and data submission requirements for the Hospice Quality Reporting Program.

Illustrations

This section includes illustrations of normal anatomy with ICD-10-CM specific terminology.

Overview of ICD-10-CM Official Conventions

This is an overview of the ICD-10-CM official conventions, which are general rules for using the classification system, independent of the guidelines. The official conventions and instructions of the classification, which take precedence over the guidelines, are incorporated within the alphabetic index and tabular list as instructional notes and are applicable regardless of the health care setting. For the full version of the official conventions, see the ICD-10-CM Official Guidelines for Coding and Reporting, section I.A., which is included in this book.

Format

ICD-10-CM is divided into two main parts: the index, an alphabetical list of terms and their corresponding code, and the tabular list, a sequential, alphanumeric list of codes divided into chapters based on body system or condition. The index contains the Index to Diseases and Injuries (main index) and the Index to External Causes of Injury. Also included in the main index is the Neoplasm Table and a Table of Drugs and Chemicals.

The tabular list contains categories, subcategories, and valid codes. ICD-10-CM is an alphanumeric classification system. The 1st character of a three-character category is a letter. The 2nd and 3rd characters may be numbers or alpha characters. A three-character category without further subclassification is equivalent to a valid three-character code. Subcategories are either four or five characters. Subcategory characters include either letters or numbers. Codes may be three, four, five, six, or seven characters in length, in which each level of subdivision after a category is a subcategory. The final level of subdivision is a valid code. The final character in a code may be either a letter or a number.

The ICD-10-CM uses the letter "X" as a placeholder. A placeholder "X" is used as a 5th character placeholder at certain six-character codes to allow for future expansion, without disturbing the 6th character structure. For instance, an initial encounter for accidental poisoning by penicillin is coded to T36.0X1A. The "X" in the 5th character position is a placeholder, or filler character.

Similarly, certain categories have applicable 7th character extensions. In these cases, the 7th character extension is required for all codes within the category, or as otherwise instructed in the tabular list notations. 7th character extensions must always be the last character in the data field. If a code is not a full six characters in length, a dummy placeholder "X" must be used to fill in the empty characters when a 7th character extension is required.

Punctuation

[ ]   In the tabular list, brackets are used to enclose synonyms, alternative wording, or explanatory phrases. In the index, brackets are used to identify manifestation codes.

( )   Parentheses are used in both the index and tabular list to enclose nonessential modifiers; supplementary words that may be present or absent in the statement of a disease or procedure without affecting the code number to which it is assigned.

:   Colons are used in the tabular list after an incomplete term that needs one or more of the modifiers following the colon to make it assignable to a given category.

Abbreviations

NEC

The abbreviation NEC, "Not elsewhere classifiable" represents "other specified" in the ICD-10-CM. An index entry that states NEC directs the coder to an "other specified" code in the tabular list. Codes titled "Other" or "Other specified" in the tabular list (usually a code with a 4th or 6th character 8 and 5th character 9) are for use when the information in the medical record provides detail for which a specific code does not exist.

NOS

The abbreviation NOS, "Not otherwise specified," in the tabular list may be interpreted as "unspecified." Codes in the tabular list with "Unspecified" in the title (usually a code with a 4th or 6th character 9 and 5th character 0) are for use when the information in the medical record is insufficient to assign a more specific code.

Typeface

Boldface

Boldface type is used for main term entries in the alphabetic index, and all codes and descriptions in the tabular list.

General Notes

The following conventions and notes appear only in the tabular list of diseases:

Includes Notes

The word INCLUDES appears immediately under certain categories to further define, clarify, or give examples of the content of a code category.

Inclusion Terms

Lists of inclusion terms are included under certain codes. These terms indicate some of the conditions for which that code number may be used. Inclusion terms may be synonyms with the code title, or, in the case of "other specified" codes, the terms may also provide a list of various conditions included within a classification code. The inclusion terms are not exhaustive. The index may provide additional terms that may also be assigned to a given code.

Excludes Notes

ICD-10-CM has two types of excludes notes. Each note has a different definition for use. However, they are similar in that they both indicate that codes excluded from each other are independent of each other.

Excludes 1

An EXCLUDES1 note is a "pure" excludes. It means "NOT CODED HERE!" An Excludes 1 note indicates mutually exclusive codes: two conditions that cannot be reported together. For example, a congenital form of a disease may not be reported with the acquired form of the same condition. The code excluded should never be reported with the applicable codes listed above the excludes notation.

An exception to the Excludes1 definition is the circumstance when the two conditions are unrelated to each other. If it is not clear whether the two conditions involving an Excludes1 note are related or not, query the provider. For example, code F45.8, Other somatoform disorders, has an Excludes1 note for "sleep related teeth grinding (G47.63)," because "teeth grinding" is an inclusion term under F45.8. Only one of these two codes should be assigned for teeth grinding. However psychogenic dysmenorrhea is also an inclusion term under F45.8, and a patient could have both this condition and sleep related teeth grinding. In this case, the two conditions are clearly unrelated to each other, and so it would be appropriate to report F45.8 and G47.63 together.

Excludes 2

An EXCLUDES 2 note means "NOT INCLUDED HERE." An Excludes 2 note indicates that although the excluded condition is not part of the condition it is excluded from, a patient may have both conditions at the same time. Therefore, when an Excludes 2 note appears under a code, it may be acceptable to use both the code and the excluded code together if supported by the medical documentation.

Note

NOTE The term "NOTE" appears as an icon and precedes the instructional information. These notes function as alerts to highlight coding instructions within the text.

Default Codes

In the index, the default code is the code listed next to the main term. The default code represents the condition most commonly associated with the main term. This code may be assigned when documentation does not facilitate reporting a more specific code. Alternatively, it may provide an unspecified code for the condition.

Syndromes

Follow the alphabetic index guidance when coding syndromes. In the absence of index guidance, assign codes for the documented manifestations of the syndrome.

And

When the term "and" is used in a narrative statement or code title it may be interpreted as "and/or."

With

The word "with" or "in" should be interpreted to mean "associated with" or "due to" when it appears in a code title, the Alphabetic Index, or an instructional note in the Tabular List. The classification presumes a causal relationship between the two conditions linked by these terms in the Alphabetic Index or Tabular List. These conditions should be coded as related even in the absence of provider documentation explicitly linking them, unless the documentation clearly states the conditions are unrelated or when another guideline exists that specifically requires a documented linkage between two conditions (e.g., sepsis guideline for "acute organ dysfunction that is not clearly associated with the sepsis"). For conditions not specifically linked by these relational terms in the classification or when a guideline requires that a linkage between two conditions be explicitly documented, provider documentation must link the conditions in order to code them as related.

The word "with" in the Alphabetic Index is sequenced immediately following the main term, not in alphabetical order.

See and See Also

When the instruction "See" follows a main term in the alphabetic index, it indicates that another term must be referenced in order to locate the correct code. The instructional note "See also" simply provides alternative terms that may be useful in determining the correct code but is not necessary to follow if the main term supplies the appropriate code.

Instructional Notes Used in the Tabular List

In the tabular section, the following instructional notes appear in red type for emphasis:

Code First/Use additional code:

These instructional notes provide sequencing instruction. They may appear independently of each other or to designate certain etiology/manifestation paired codes. These instructions signal the coder that an additional code should be reported to provide a more complete picture of that diagnosis.

In etiology/manifestation coding, ICD-10-CM requires the underlying condition to be sequenced first, followed by the manifestation. In these situations, codes with "In diseases classified elsewhere" in the code description are never permitted as a first-listed or principal diagnosis code and must be sequenced following the underlying condition code.

Code Also:

A "code also" note alerts the coder that more than one code may be required to fully describe the condition. The sequencing depends on the circumstances of the encounter. Factors that may determine sequencing include severity and reason for the encounter.

Code Assignment and Clinical Criteria

Diagnosis code assignment must be based on the provider's diagnostic statement that the condition exists and is not based on clinical criteria the provider used to establish the diagnosis. Conflicting documentation must be queried.

Additional Annotations

Code-Level Notations

The tabular section of ICD-10-CM has various colors, symbols, and other tabular annotations that may help in code selection, provide clinical or coding information, or alert the coder to reimbursement issues affected by the diagnosis code assignment. Some codes may have more than one annotation. For quick reference to the meanings of the colors and symbols, look at the color/symbol legend at the bottom of each page in the tabular list.

Italics

Italicized type is used for all exclusion notes and to identify manifestation codes, those codes that should not be reported as first-listed (principal) diagnoses.

Color Coding/Symbols

New Code

This ● icon identifies the codes that are new to the classification system for the current year. The new code icon is to the left of the code.

Revised Code Title

This ▲ icon to the left of a code alerts the user to a change in that code's title. This change may be as simple as adding or removing punctuation, which may or may not change the intent of the code, to adding or removing specific terms from a code description that completely alter the circumstances in which the code would be used.

Revised Text

The revised text ▶◀ "bow ties" alert the user to changes in parenthetical notes for the current year. Revised text may include the following:

* A change in a current parenthetical description

* A change in the code(s) associated with a current parenthetical note

* A change in how a current parenthetical note is classified (e.g., an Excludes 1 note that changed to an Excludes 2 note)

* Addition of a new parenthetical note(s) to a code

Deleted Text

Strikethrough on code description(s) and/or code note(s) indicates a deletion from the classification for the current year.

Examples:

✓4ᵗʰ **N25 Disorders resulting from impaired renal tubular function**
    EXCLUDES 1 ~~metabolic disorders classifiable to E70-E88~~

The strikethrough over the Excludes 1 note indicates that this note was deleted from the classification and is no longer applicable to codes in category N25.

✓7ᵗʰ ~~S63.131   Subluxation of proximal interphalangeal joint of right thumb~~

The strikethrough over the code and the code description indicates that all codes in subcategory S63.131 (S63.131A, S63.131D, and S63.131S) have been deleted from the classification.

Additional Characters Required

✓4ᵗʰ This symbol indicates that the code requires a 4th character.

✓5ᵗʰ This symbol indicates that the code requires a 5th character.

✓6ᵗʰ This symbol indicates that the code requires a 6th character.

✓7ᵗʰ This symbol indicates that the code requires a 7th character.

✓x7ᵗʰ This symbol indicates that the code requires a 7th character following the placeholder "X." Codes with fewer than six characters that require a 7th character must contain placeholder "X" to fill in the empty character(s).

Key Word

Green font is used throughout the Tabular List of Diseases to differentiate the key words that appear in similar code descriptions in a given category or subcategory.

For example, refer to the list of codes below from category C7A:

C7A.020   Malignant carcinoid tumor of the **appendix**

C7A.021   Malignant carcinoid tumor of the **cecum**

C7A.022   Malignant carcinoid tumor of the **ascending colon**

C7A.023   Malignant carcinoid tumor of the **transverse colon**

C7A.024   Malignant carcinoid tumor of the **descending colon**

C7A.025   Malignant carcinoid tumor of the **sigmoid colon**

C7A.026   Malignant carcinoid tumor of the **rectum**

C7A.029   Malignant carcinoid tumor of the large intestine, unspecified portion

The portion of the code description that appears in **green font** in the tabular list assists the coder in quickly identifying the key terms and the correct code. This convention is especially useful when the codes describe laterality, such as the following codes from subcategory H40.22:

H40.221   Chronic angle-closure glaucoma, **right** eye

H40.222   Chronic angle-closure glaucoma, **left** eye

H40.223   Chronic angle-closure glaucoma, **bilateral**

H40.229   Chronic angle-closure glaucoma, unspecified eye

The key word convention is used only in those categories in which there are multiple codes with very similar descriptions with only a few words that differentiate them.

Medicare Code Edits

Medicare Administrative Contractors and many payers use Medicare code edits to check the coding accuracy on claims. The coding edit information in this manual reflects those edits used for outpatient institutional providers, which also include hospitals that are subject to the outpatient prospective payment system (OPPS). These edits have been updated to reflect changes in the Integrated Outpatient Code Editor (IOCE), version 18.2.

Manifestation Code

These codes appear in italic type, with a ***blue color bar*** over the title. A manifestation code cannot be reported as a first-listed or principal diagnosis. By definition, a manifestation code represents a demonstration of some aspect of an underlying disease, which is separately classifiable. In the alphabetic index, these codes are listed as the secondary code in brackets. The underlying disease code is listed first.

Age and Sex Edit

The age and sex edits below are used to detect inconsistencies between the patient's age and/or sex and the patient's diagnosis. The following edit symbols appear in the tabular list to the right of the code description.

Newborn Age: 0   Ⓝ

These diagnoses are intended for newborns and neonates and the patient's age must be 0 years.

Pediatric Age: 0-17   P

These diagnoses are intended for children and the patient's age must be between 0 and 17 years.

Maternity Age: 12-55   M

These diagnoses are intended for childbearing patients between the age of 12 and 55 years.

Adult Age: 15-124   A

These diagnoses are intended for patients between the age of 15 and 124 years.

Male diagnosis only   ♂

Female diagnosis only   ♀

Home Health Prospective Payment System (HH PPS) Edits

Case-Mix Diagnosis

The purple color bar over the code title identifies a diagnosis code that is a clinical condition or comorbidity associated with one of 22 case-mix diagnosis groups. Each case-mix diagnosis group is assigned case-mix points, which are used, along with other variables, to calculate the home health resource group (HHRG).

Note: Not all 7th character designations may allow a case-mix code to be eligible for case-mix adjustment. A footnote superscript is found to the left of the code number, and a definition for that footnote at the bottom of the page identifies the specific 7th character designations applicable to HH PPS.

Nonroutine Supply Symbol   NRS

This symbol identifies diagnoses that generally require high nonroutine medical supply utilization. The nonroutine supply reimbursement is based upon a six-group severity level approach.

Note: Not all 7th character designations may allow an NRS code to be eligible for NRS reimbursement. A footnote superscript is found to the left of the code number, and a definition for that footnote at the bottom of the page identifies the specific 7th character designations applicable to HHPPS.

Other Code-Level Notations

Noncancer Diagnosis   NC Dx

This symbol indicates a noncancer diagnosis that may satisfy the medical necessity criteria for Medicare coverage of hospice care. The diagnosis alone does not support medical necessity but represents one of the many factors that establish medical necessity. For more detailed explanation of the noncancer diagnosis policies for hospice care, please refer to appendix N, "Hospice Criteria for Medicare Coverage on Noncancer Hospice Care," at the back of this book.

Unspecified Code   ▽

Use these codes when neither the diagnostic statement nor the documentation provides enough information to assign a more specific diagnosis code. These codes may be stated as "Unspecified" or "Not otherwise specified (NOS)."

Note: Do not assign these codes when a more specific diagnosis has been determined.

PDx Symbol   PDx

This symbol identifies a Z code that generally is for use as a first-listed (or principal) diagnosis only but may be used as an additional diagnosis if the patient has more than one encounter on the same day or there is more than one reason for the encounter.

The instructions for Z code use contained in the ICD-10-CM official coding guidelines identify those Z codes that can be used only as a PDx. All other Z codes may either be SDx or PDx, depending upon circumstances of the encounter, by meeting the definition of first-listed or principal diagnosis, and by following any specific Z code guidelines in section I.C.21 a-c. The

responsibility of those assigning the Z codes as PDx is to make sure the circumstances of the encounter meet the definition of first-listed or principal diagnosis, follow all coding instructions, and follow the Z code specific guidelines. Optum360 does not include any SDx edit since there is no official source for it and the Z code use is determined by circumstances of the encounter.

Note: Please note that the Z code "principal or first-listed only" designation and the Z codes that may be principal or first-listed diagnoses included in the official coding guidelines (section 1.C.21.c.16) are consistent with reporting guidelines for health care encounters *excluding acute care inpatient admissions*. In addition, hospice claims billed for both inpatient and outpatient hospice services may not assign any Z code as a primary or first-listed diagnosis under any condition. To report hospice services, both inpatient and outpatient, the claim must list as primary or first listed the condition resulting in a terminal diagnosis with life expectancy of six months or less. Hospices may assign Z codes to the claim as secondary codes at their discretion to provide additional information regarding a patient's overall condition.

AHA:

This symbol precedes official citations from AHA's *Coding Clinic for ICD-10-CM/PCS*. Similar to the parenthetical notes, AHA references are placed in a hierarchical pattern at the chapter, code block, category, subcategory, or valid code level. This means that the information found in the reference applies to one or more codes depending on where the citation is placed.

The citations appear in purple type and are listed with the most current citation first. *Coding Clinic* citations included in this edition have been updated through second quarter 2017.

DEF:

This symbol precedes a definition of a condition or disease.

The definition appears in purple type directly under the code.

TIP:

This symbol precedes coding advice that is not readily available within the ICD-10-CM classification. It may relate official coding guidelines, indexing nuances, or advice from *AHA's Coding Clinic for ICD-10-CM/PCS*.

The tip appears in purple type directly under the code.

Footnotes

All footnotes are identified by a numerical superscript that appears to the upper left of the code.

The following list identifies and explains the meaning of the numeric footnotes found in the tabular list:

1   A case-mix diagnosis only when the 7th character signifies a "subsequent" encounter. Appropriate 7th characters may include **D, E, F, G, H, J, K, M, N, P, Q,** or **R.**

2   Case-mix diagnosis only when the 7th character signifies a "subsequent" or "sequela" encounter. Appropriate 7th characters may include **D, E, F, G, H, J, K, M, N, P, Q, R** or **S.**

3   Case-mix diagnosis only when the 7th character signifies a "sequela" encounter. The appropriate 7th character would be **S.**

4   Case-mix diagnosis only when the 7th character signifies an "initial" or "subsequent" encounter. Appropriate 7th characters would be **A** or **D.**

5   NRS supply diagnosis only when the 7th character signifies an "initial" or "subsequent" encounter. The appropriate 7th character would be **A** or **D.**

6   NRS supply diagnosis only when the 7th character signifies a "subsequent" encounter. The appropriate 7th character would be **D.**

7   Hospice noncancer diagnosis only when the 7th character signifies "subsequent" encounter. The appropriate 7th character would be **D.**

8   Hospice questionable admission noncancer diagnosis.

A code identified by this footnote, when used as the admitting diagnosis on a hospice encounter, may be viewed by Medicare as a questionable admission. The code may lack the specificity that would reasonably be contained in the medical record or the code conflicts with official coding guidelines and conventions. The patient's medical record and official coding guidelines should be reviewed carefully to ensure that a more appropriate diagnosis is not warranted.

Chapter-Level Notations

Chapter-Specific Guidelines with Coding Examples
Each chapter begins with the *Official Guidelines for Coding and Reporting* specific to that chapter, where provided. Coding examples specific to post-acute care settings have been provided to illustrate the coding and/or sequencing guidance in these guidelines.

Muscle and Tendon Table
ICD-10-CM categorizes certain muscles and tendons in the upper and lower extremities by their action (e.g., extension or flexion) as well as their anatomical location. The Muscle/Tendon table is provided at the beginning of chapter 13 and chapter 19 to help users when code selection depends on the action of the muscle and/or tendon.

Note: This table is not all-inclusive, and proper code assignment should be based on the provider's documentation.

Index Notations
 Subterms under main terms may continue to next column or page. This warning statement is a reminder to always check for additional subterms and information that may continue onto the next page or column before making a final selection.

Following References
The index includes *following* references to assist in locating "out-of-sequence" codes in the tabular list. "Out-of-sequence" codes contain an alphabetic character (letter) in the 3rd or 4th character position. These codes are placed according to the classification rules — the placement of the codes according to condition — not according to alphabetic or numeric sequencing rules.

Examples:

Carcinoma (malignant) (*see also,* Neoplasm, by site, malignant)
    neuroendocrine (*see also* Tumor, neuroendocrine)
        high grade, any site C7A.1 (*following* C75)
        poorly differentiated, any site C7A.1 (*following* C75)

In the tabular rubric, C7A is included after rubric C75 and before C76.

Gout, chronic (*see also* Gout, gouty) M1A.9
    drug-induced M1A.20 (*following* M08)
        ankle M1A.27-(*following* M08)
        elbow M1A.22-(*following* M08)

In the tabular rubric, M1A is included after rubric M08 and before M10.

ICD-10-CM Official Guidelines for Coding and Reporting

Narrative changes appear in **bold** text

Items <u>underlined</u> have been moved within the guidelines since the FY 2017 version

Italics are used to indicate revisions to heading changes

The Centers for Medicare and Medicaid Services (CMS) and the National Center for Health Statistics (NCHS), two departments within the U.S. Federal Government's Department of Health and Human Services (DHHS) provide the following guidelines for coding and reporting using the International Classification of Diseases, 10th Revision, Clinical Modification (ICD-10-CM). These guidelines should be used as a companion document to the official version of the ICD-10-CM as published on the NCHS website. The ICD-10-CM is a morbidity classification published by the United States for classifying diagnoses and reason for visits in all health care settings. The ICD-10-CM is based on the ICD-10, the statistical classification of disease published by the World Health Organization (WHO).

These guidelines have been approved by the four organizations that make up the Cooperating Parties for the ICD-10-CM: the American Hospital Association (AHA), the American Health Information Management Association (AHIMA), CMS, and NCHS.

These guidelines are a set of rules that have been developed to accompany and complement the official conventions and instructions provided within the ICD-10-CM itself. The instructions and conventions of the classification take precedence over guidelines. These guidelines are based on the coding and sequencing instructions in the Tabular List and Alphabetic Index of ICD-10-CM, but provide additional instruction. Adherence to these guidelines when assigning ICD-10-CM diagnosis codes is required under the Health Insurance Portability and Accountability Act (HIPAA). The diagnosis codes (Tabular List and Alphabetic Index) have been adopted under HIPAA for all healthcare settings. A joint effort between the healthcare provider and the coder is essential to achieve complete and accurate documentation, code assignment, and reporting of diagnoses and procedures. These guidelines have been developed to assist both the healthcare provider and the coder in identifying those diagnoses that are to be reported. The importance of consistent, complete documentation in the medical record cannot be overemphasized. Without such documentation accurate coding cannot be achieved. The entire record should be reviewed to determine the specific reason for the encounter and the conditions treated.

The term encounter is used for all settings, including hospital admissions. In the context of these guidelines, the term provider is used throughout the guidelines to mean physician or any qualified health care practitioner who is legally accountable for establishing the patient's diagnosis. Only this set of guidelines, approved by the Cooperating Parties, is official.

The guidelines are organized into sections. Section I includes the structure and conventions of the classification and general guidelines that apply to the entire classification, and chapter-specific guidelines that correspond to the chapters as they are arranged in the classification. Section II includes guidelines for selection of principal diagnosis for non-outpatient settings. Section III includes guidelines for reporting additional diagnoses in non-outpatient settings. Section IV is for outpatient coding and reporting. It is necessary to review all sections of the guidelines to fully understand all of the rules and instructions needed to code properly.

Section I. Conventions, general coding guidelines and chapter specific guidelines

The conventions, general guidelines and chapter-specific guidelines are applicable to all health care settings unless otherwise indicated. The conventions and instructions of the classification take precedence over guidelines.

A. Conventions for the ICD-10-CM

The conventions for the ICD-10-CM are the general rules for use of the classification independent of the guidelines. These conventions are incorporated within the Alphabetic Index and Tabular List of the ICD-10-CM as instructional notes.

1. **The Alphabetic Index and Tabular List**
   The ICD-10-CM is divided into the Alphabetic Index, an alphabetical list of terms and their corresponding code, and the Tabular List, a structured list of codes divided into chapters based on body system or condition. The Alphabetic Index consists of the following parts: the Index of Diseases and Injury, the Index of External Causes of Injury, the Table of Neoplasms and the Table of Drugs and Chemicals.

   See Section I.C2. General guidelines

   See Section I.C.19. Adverse effects, poisoning, underdosing and toxic effects

2. **Format and Structure:**
   The ICD-10-CM Tabular List contains categories, subcategories and codes. Characters for categories, subcategories and codes may be either a letter or a number. All categories are 3 characters. A three-character category that has no further subdivision is equivalent to a code. Subcategories are either 4 or 5 characters. Codes may be 3, 4, 5, 6 or 7 characters. That is, each level of subdivision after a category is a subcategory. The final level of subdivision is a code. Codes that have applicable 7th characters are still referred to as codes, not subcategories. A code that has an applicable 7th character is considered invalid without the 7th character.

   The ICD-10-CM uses an indented format for ease in reference.

3. **Use of codes for reporting purposes**
   For reporting purposes only codes are permissible, not categories or subcategories, and any applicable 7th character is required.

4. **Placeholder character**
   The ICD-10-CM utilizes a placeholder character "X". The "X" is used as a placeholder at certain codes to allow for future expansion. An example of this is at the poisoning, adverse effect and underdosing codes, categories T36-T50.

   Where a placeholder exists, the X must be used in order for the code to be considered a valid code.

5. **7th Characters**
   Certain ICD-10-CM categories have applicable 7th characters. The applicable 7th character is required for all codes within the category, or as the notes in the Tabular List instruct. The 7th character must always be the 7th character in the data field. If a code that requires a 7th character is not 6 characters, a placeholder X must be used to fill in the empty characters.

6. **Abbreviations**
   a. **Alphabetic Index abbreviations**
      NEC "Not elsewhere classifiable"

      This abbreviation in the Alphabetic Index represents "other specified." When a specific code is not available for a condition, the Alphabetic Index directs the coder to the "other specified" code in the Tabular List.

      NOS "Not otherwise specified"

      This abbreviation is the equivalent of unspecified.

   b. **Tabular List abbreviations**
      NEC "Not elsewhere classifiable"

      This abbreviation in the Tabular List represents "other specified". When a specific code is not available for a condition, the Tabular List

includes an NEC entry under a code to identify the code as the "other specified" code.

NOS "Not otherwise specified"

This abbreviation is the equivalent of unspecified.

7. **Punctuation**
   [ ] Brackets are used in the Tabular List to enclose synonyms, alternative wording or explanatory phrases. Brackets are used in the Alphabetic Index to identify manifestation codes.

   ( ) Parentheses are used in both the Alphabetic Index and Tabular List to enclose supplementary words that may be present or absent in the statement of a disease or procedure without affecting the code number to which it is assigned. The terms within the parentheses are referred to as nonessential modifiers. The nonessential modifiers in the Alphabetic Index to Diseases apply to subterms following a main term except when a nonessential modifier and a subentry are mutually exclusive, the subentry takes precedence. For example, in the ICD-10-CM Alphabetic Index under the main term Enteritis, "acute" is a nonessential modifier and "chronic" is a subentry. In this case, the nonessential modifier "acute" does not apply to the subentry "chronic".

   : Colons are used in the Tabular List after an incomplete term which needs one or more of the modifiers following the colon to make it assignable to a given category.

8. **Use of "and".**
   See Section I.A.14. Use of the term "And"

9. **Other and Unspecified codes**
   a. **"Other" codes**
      Codes titled "other" or "other specified" are for use when the information in the medical record provides detail for which a specific code does not exist. Alphabetic Index entries with NEC in the line designate "other" codes in the Tabular List. These Alphabetic Index entries represent specific disease entities for which no specific code exists so the term is included within an "other" code.

   b. **"Unspecified" codes**
      Codes titled "unspecified" are for use when the information in the medical record is insufficient to assign a more specific code. For those categories for which an unspecified code is not provided, the "other specified" code may represent both other and unspecified.

      See Section I.B.18 Use of Signs/Symptom/Unspecified Codes

10. **Includes Notes**
    This note appears immediately under a three character code title to further define, or give examples of, the content of the category.

11. **Inclusion terms**
    List of terms is included under some codes. These terms are the conditions for which that code is to be used. The terms may be synonyms of the code title, or, in the case of "other specified" codes, the terms are a list of the various conditions assigned to that code. The inclusion terms are not necessarily exhaustive. Additional terms found only in the Alphabetic Index may also be assigned to a code.

12. **Excludes Notes**
    The ICD-10-CM has two types of excludes notes. Each type of note has a different definition for use but they are all similar in that they indicate that codes excluded from each other are independent of each other.

    a. **Excludes1**
       A type 1 Excludes note is a pure excludes note. It means "NOT CODED HERE!" An Excludes1 note indicates that the code excluded should never be used at the same time as the code above the Excludes1 note. An Excludes1 is used when two conditions cannot occur together, such as a congenital form versus an acquired form of the same condition.

       An exception to the Excludes1 definition is the circumstance when the two conditions are unrelated to each other. If it is not clear whether the two conditions involving an Excludes1 note are related or not, query the provider. For example, code F45.8, Other somatoform disorders, has an Excludes1 note for "sleep related teeth grinding (G47.63)," because "teeth grinding" is an inclusion term under F45.8. Only one of these two codes should be assigned for teeth grinding. However psychogenic dysmenorrhea is also an inclusion term under F45.8, and a patient could have both this condition and sleep related teeth grinding. In this case, the two conditions are clearly unrelated to each other, and so it would be appropriate to report F45.8 and G47.63 together.

b. **Excludes2**

A type 2 Excludes note represents "Not included here." An excludes2 note indicates that the condition excluded is not part of the condition represented by the code, but a patient may have both conditions at the same time. When an Excludes2 note appears under a code, it is acceptable to use both the code and the excluded code together, when appropriate.

13. **Etiology/manifestation convention ("code first", "use additional code" and "in diseases classified elsewhere" notes)**

Certain conditions have both an underlying etiology and multiple body system manifestations due to the underlying etiology. For such conditions, the ICD-10-CM has a coding convention that requires the underlying condition be sequenced first, if applicable, followed by the manifestation. Wherever such a combination exists, there is a "use additional code" note at the etiology code, and a "code first" note at the manifestation code. These instructional notes indicate the proper sequencing order of the codes, etiology followed by manifestation.

In most cases the manifestation codes will have in the code title, "in diseases classified elsewhere." Codes with this title are a component of the etiology/ manifestation convention. The code title indicates that it is a manifestation code. "In diseases classified elsewhere" codes are never permitted to be used as first-listed or principal diagnosis codes. They must be used in conjunction with an underlying condition code and they must be listed following the underlying condition. See category F02, Dementia in other diseases classified elsewhere, for an example of this convention.

There are manifestation codes that do not have "in diseases classified elsewhere" in the title. For such codes, there is a "use additional code" note at the etiology code and a "code first" note at the manifestation code, and the rules for sequencing apply.

In addition to the notes in the Tabular List, these conditions also have a specific Alphabetic Index entry structure. In the Alphabetic Index both conditions are listed together with the etiology code first followed by the manifestation codes in brackets. The code in brackets is always to be sequenced second.

An example of the etiology/manifestation convention is dementia in Parkinson's disease. In the Alphabetic Index, code G20 is listed first, followed by code F02.80 or F02.81 in brackets. Code G20 represents the underlying etiology, Parkinson's disease, and must be sequenced first, whereas code F02.80 and F02.81 represent the manifestation of dementia in diseases classified elsewhere, with or without behavioral disturbance.

"Code first" and "Use additional code" notes are also used as sequencing rules in the classification for certain codes that are not part of an etiology/ manifestation combination.

See Section I.B.7. Multiple coding for a single condition.

14. **"And"**

The word "and" should be interpreted to mean either "and" or "or" when it appears in a title.

For example, cases of "tuberculosis of bones", "tuberculosis of joints" and "tuberculosis of bones and joints" are classified to subcategory A18.0, Tuberculosis of bones and joints.

15. **"With"**

The word "with" **or "in"** should be interpreted to mean "associated with" or "due to" when it appears in a code title, the Alphabetic Index, or an instructional note in the Tabular List. The classification presumes a causal relationship between the two conditions linked by these terms in the Alphabetic Index or Tabular List. These conditions should be coded as related even in the absence of provider documentation explicitly linking them, unless the documentation clearly states the conditions are unrelated **or when another guideline exists that specifically requires a documented linkage between two conditions (e.g., sepsis guideline for "acute organ dysfunction that is not clearly associated with the sepsis").**

For conditions not specifically linked by these relational terms in the classification **or when a guideline requires that a linkage between two conditions be explicitly documented,** provider documentation must link the conditions in order to code them as related.

The word "with" in the Alphabetic Index is sequenced immediately following the main term, not in alphabetical order.

16. **"See" and "See Also"**

The "see" instruction following a main term in the Alphabetic Index indicates that another term should be referenced. It is necessary to go to the main term referenced with the "see" note to locate the correct code.

A "see also" instruction following a main term in the Alphabetic Index instructs that there is another main term that may also be referenced that may provide additional Alphabetic Index entries that may be useful. It is not necessary to follow the "see also" note when the original main term provides the necessary code.

17. **"Code also" note**

A "code also" note instructs that two codes may be required to fully describe a condition, but this note does not provide sequencing direction. **The sequencing depends on the circumstances of the encounter.**

18. **Default codes**

A code listed next to a main term in the ICD-10-CM Alphabetic Index is referred to as a default code. The default code represents that condition that is most commonly associated with the main term, or is the unspecified code for the condition. If a condition is documented in a medical record (for example, appendicitis) without any additional information, such as acute or chronic, the default code should be assigned.

19. **Code assignment and Clinical Criteria**

The assignment of a diagnosis code is based on the provider's diagnostic statement that the condition exists. The provider's statement that the patient has a particular condition is sufficient. Code assignment is not based on clinical criteria used by the provider to establish the diagnosis.

B. General Coding Guidelines

1. **Locating a code in the ICD-10-CM**

To select a code in the classification that corresponds to a diagnosis or reason for visit documented in a medical record, first locate the term in the Alphabetic Index, and then verify the code in the Tabular List. Read and be guided by instructional notations that appear in both the Alphabetic Index and the Tabular List.

It is essential to use both the Alphabetic Index and Tabular List when locating and assigning a code. The Alphabetic Index does not always provide the full code. Selection of the full code, including laterality and any applicable 7th character can only be done in the Tabular List. A dash (-) at the end of an Alphabetic Index entry indicates that additional characters are required. Even if a dash is not included at the Alphabetic Index entry, it is necessary to refer to the Tabular List to verify that no 7th character is required.

2. **Level of Detail in Coding**

Diagnosis codes are to be used and reported at their highest number of characters available.

ICD-10-CM diagnosis codes are composed of codes with 3, 4, 5, 6 or 7 characters. Codes with three characters are included in ICD-10-CM as the heading of a category of codes that may be further subdivided by the use of fourth and/or fifth characters and/or sixth characters, which provide greater detail.

A three-character code is to be used only if it is not further subdivided. A code is invalid if it has not been coded to the full number of characters required for that code, including the 7th character, if applicable.

3. **Code or codes from A00.0 through T88.9, Z00-Z99.8**

The appropriate code or codes from A00.0 through T88.9, Z00-Z99.8 must be used to identify diagnoses, symptoms, conditions, problems, complaints or other reason(s) for the encounter/visit.

4. **Signs and symptoms**

Codes that describe symptoms and signs, as opposed to diagnoses, are acceptable for reporting purposes when a related definitive diagnosis has not been established (confirmed) by the provider. Chapter 18 of ICD-10-CM, Symptoms, Signs, and Abnormal Clinical and Laboratory Findings, Not Elsewhere Classified (codes R00.0 - R99) contains many, but not all, codes for symptoms.

See Section I.B.18 Use of Signs/Symptom/Unspecified Codes

5. **Conditions that are an integral part of a disease process**

Signs and symptoms that are associated routinely with a disease process should not be assigned as additional codes, unless otherwise instructed by the classification.

6. Conditions that are not an integral part of a disease process

Additional signs and symptoms that may not be associated routinely with a disease process should be coded when present.

7. Multiple coding for a single condition

In addition to the etiology/manifestation convention that requires two codes to fully describe a single condition that affects multiple body systems, there are other single conditions that also require more than one code. "Use additional code" notes are found in the Tabular List at codes that are not part of an etiology/manifestation pair where a secondary code is useful to fully describe a condition. The sequencing rule is the same as the etiology/manifestation pair, "use additional code" indicates that a secondary code should be added, **if known.**

For example, for bacterial infections that are not included in chapter 1, a secondary code from category B95, Streptococcus, Staphylococcus, and Enterococcus, as the cause of diseases classified elsewhere, or B96, Other bacterial agents as the cause of diseases classified elsewhere, may be required to identify the bacterial organism causing the infection. A "use additional code" note will normally be found at the infectious disease code, indicating a need for the organism code to be added as a secondary code.

"Code first" notes are also under certain codes that are not specifically manifestation codes but may be due to an underlying cause. When there is a "code first" note and an underlying condition is present, the underlying condition should be sequenced first, **if known.**

"Code, if applicable, any causal condition first" notes indicate that this code may be assigned as a principal diagnosis when the causal condition is unknown or not applicable. If a causal condition is known, then the code for that condition should be sequenced as the principal or first-listed diagnosis.

Multiple codes may be needed for sequela, complication codes and obstetric codes to more fully describe a condition. See the specific guidelines for these conditions for further instruction.

8. Acute and Chronic Conditions

If the same condition is described as both acute (subacute) and chronic, and separate subentries exist in the Alphabetic Index at the same indentation level, code both and sequence the acute (subacute) code first.

9. Combination Code

A combination code is a single code used to classify:

    Two diagnoses, or

    A diagnosis with an associated secondary process (manifestation)

    A diagnosis with an associated complication

Combination codes are identified by referring to subterm entries in the Alphabetic Index and by reading the inclusion and exclusion notes in the Tabular List.

Assign only the combination code when that code fully identifies the diagnostic conditions involved or when the Alphabetic Index so directs. Multiple coding should not be used when the classification provides a combination code that clearly identifies all of the elements documented in the diagnosis. When the combination code lacks necessary specificity in describing the manifestation or complication, an additional code should be used as a secondary code.

10. Sequela (Late Effects)

A sequela is the residual effect (condition produced) after the acute phase of an illness or injury has terminated. There is no time limit on when a sequela code can be used. The residual may be apparent early, such as in cerebral infarction, or it may occur months or years later, such as that due to a previous injury. Examples of sequela include: scar formation resulting from a burn, deviated septum due to a nasal fracture, and infertility due to tubal occlusion from old tuberculosis. Coding of sequela generally requires two codes sequenced in the following order: the condition or nature of the sequela is sequenced first. The sequela code is sequenced second.

An exception to the above guidelines are those instances where the code for the sequela is followed by a manifestation code identified in the Tabular List and title, or the sequela code has been expanded (at the fourth, fifth or sixth character levels) to include the manifestation(s). The code for the acute phase of an illness or injury that led to the sequela is never used with a code for the late effect.

See Section I.C.9. Sequelae of cerebrovascular disease

See Section I.C.15. Sequelae of complication of pregnancy, childbirth and the puerperium

See Section I.C.19. Application of 7th characters for Chapter 19

11. Impending or Threatened Condition

Code any condition described at the time of discharge as "impending" or "threatened" as follows:

    If it did occur, code as confirmed diagnosis.

    If it did not occur, reference the Alphabetic Index to determine if the condition has a subentry term for "impending" or "threatened" and also reference main term entries for "Impending" and for "Threatened."

    If the subterms are listed, assign the given code.

    If the subterms are not listed, code the existing underlying condition(s) and not the condition described as impending or threatened.

12. Reporting Same Diagnosis Code more than Once

Each unique ICD-10-CM diagnosis code may be reported only once for an encounter. This applies to bilateral conditions when there are no distinct codes identifying laterality or two different conditions classified to the same ICD-10-CM diagnosis code.

13. Laterality

Some ICD-10-CM codes indicate laterality, specifying whether the condition occurs on the left, right or is bilateral. If no bilateral code is provided and the condition is bilateral, assign separate codes for both the left and right side. If the side is not identified in the medical record, assign the code for the unspecified side.

When a patient has a bilateral condition and each side is treated during separate encounters, assign the "bilateral" code (as the condition still exists on both sides), including for the encounter to treat the first side. For the second encounter for treatment after one side has previously been treated and the condition no longer exists on that side, assign the appropriate unilateral code for the side where the condition still exists (e.g., cataract surgery performed on each eye in separate encounters). The bilateral code would not be assigned for the subsequent encounter, as the patient no longer has the condition in the previously-treated site. If the treatment on the first side did not completely resolve the condition, then the bilateral code would still be appropriate.

14. Documentation for BMI, Depth of Non-pressure ulcers, Pressure Ulcer Stages, Coma Scale, and NIH Stroke Scale

For the Body Mass Index (BMI), depth of non-pressure chronic ulcers, pressure ulcer stage, coma scale, and NIH stroke scale (NIHSS) codes, code assignment may be based on medical record documentation from clinicians who are not the patient's provider (i.e., physician or other qualified healthcare practitioner legally accountable for establishing the patient's diagnosis), since this information is typically documented by other clinicians involved in the care of the patient (e.g., a dietitian often documents the BMI, a nurse often documents the pressure ulcer stages, and an emergency medical technician often documents the coma scale). However, the associated diagnosis (such as overweight, obesity, acute stroke, or pressure ulcer) must be documented by the patient's provider. If there is conflicting medical record documentation, either from the same clinician or different clinicians, the patient's attending provider should be queried for clarification.

The BMI, coma scale, and NIHSS codes should only be reported as secondary diagnoses.

15. Syndromes

Follow the Alphabetic Index guidance when coding syndromes. In the absence of Alphabetic Index guidance, assign codes for the documented manifestations of the syndrome. Additional codes for manifestations that are not an integral part of the disease process may also be assigned when the condition does not have a unique code.

16. Documentation of Complications of Care

Code assignment is based on the provider's documentation of the relationship between the condition and the care or procedure, unless otherwise instructed by the classification. The guideline extends to any complications of care, regardless of the chapter the code is located in. It is important to note that not all conditions that occur during or following medical care or surgery are classified as complications. There must be a cause-and-effect relationship between the care provided and the condition, and an indication in the documentation that it is a complication. Query the provider for clarification, if the complication is not clearly documented.

17. Borderline Diagnosis

If the provider documents a "borderline" diagnosis at the time of discharge, the diagnosis is coded as confirmed, unless the classification provides a specific entry (e.g., borderline diabetes). If a borderline condition has a specific index entry in ICD-10-CM, it should be coded as such. Since borderline conditions are not uncertain diagnoses, no distinction is made between the care setting (inpatient versus outpatient). Whenever the documentation is unclear regarding a borderline condition, coders are encouraged to query for clarification.

18. Use of Sign/Symptom/Unspecified Codes

Sign/symptom and "unspecified" codes have acceptable, even necessary, uses. While specific diagnosis codes should be reported when they are supported by the available medical record documentation and clinical knowledge of the patient's health condition, there are instances when signs/symptoms or unspecified codes are the best choices for accurately reflecting the healthcare encounter. Each healthcare encounter should be coded to the level of certainty known for that encounter.

If a definitive diagnosis has not been established by the end of the encounter, it is appropriate to report codes for sign(s) and/or symptom(s) in lieu of a definitive diagnosis. When sufficient clinical information isn't known or available about a particular health condition to assign a more specific code, it is acceptable to report the appropriate "unspecified" code (e.g., a diagnosis of pneumonia has been determined, but not the specific type). Unspecified codes should be reported when they are the codes that most accurately reflect what is known about the patient's condition at the time of that particular encounter. It would be inappropriate to select a specific code that is not supported by the medical record documentation or conduct medically unnecessary diagnostic testing in order to determine a more specific code.

C. Chapter-Specific Coding Guidelines

In addition to general coding guidelines, there are guidelines for specific diagnoses and/or conditions in the classification. Unless otherwise indicated, these guidelines apply to all health care settings. Please refer to Section II for guidelines on the selection of principal diagnosis.

1. Chapter 1: Certain Infectious and Parasitic Diseases (A00-B99)

a. Human Immunodeficiency Virus (HIV) Infections

1) Code only confirmed cases

Code only confirmed cases of HIV infection/illness. This is an exception to the hospital inpatient guideline Section II, H.

In this context, "confirmation" does not require documentation of positive serology or culture for HIV; the provider's diagnostic statement that the patient is HIV positive, or has an HIV-related illness is sufficient.

2) Selection and sequencing of HIV codes

(a) Patient admitted for HIV-related condition

If a patient is admitted for an HIV-related condition, the principal diagnosis should be B20, Human immunodeficiency virus [HIV] disease followed by additional diagnosis codes for all reported HIV-related conditions.

(b) Patient with HIV disease admitted for unrelated condition

If a patient with HIV disease is admitted for an unrelated condition (such as a traumatic injury), the code for the unrelated condition (e.g., the nature of injury code) should be the principal diagnosis. Other diagnoses would be B20 followed by additional diagnosis codes for all reported HIV-related conditions.

(c) Whether the patient is newly diagnosed

Whether the patient is newly diagnosed or has had previous admissions/encounters for HIV conditions is irrelevant to the sequencing decision.

(d) Asymptomatic human immunodeficiency virus

Z21, Asymptomatic human immunodeficiency virus [HIV] infection status, is to be applied when the patient without any documentation of symptoms is listed as being "HIV positive," "known HIV," "HIV test positive," or similar terminology. Do not use this code if the term "AIDS" is used

or if the patient is treated for any HIV-related illness or is described as having any condition(s) resulting from his/her HIV positive status; use B20 in these cases.

(e) Patients with inconclusive HIV serology

Patients with inconclusive HIV serology, but no definitive diagnosis or manifestations of the illness, may be assigned code R75, Inconclusive laboratory evidence of human immunodeficiency virus [HIV].

(f) Previously diagnosed HIV-related illness

Patients with any known prior diagnosis of an HIV-related illness should be coded to B20. Once a patient has developed an HIV-related illness, the patient should always be assigned code B20 on every subsequent admission/encounter. Patients previously diagnosed with any HIV illness (B20) should never be assigned to R75 or Z21, Asymptomatic human immunodeficiency virus [HIV] infection status.

(g) HIV Infection in Pregnancy, Childbirth and the Puerperium

During pregnancy, childbirth or the puerperium, a patient admitted (or presenting for a health care encounter) because of an HIV-related illness should receive a principal diagnosis code of O98.7-, Human immunodeficiency [HIV] disease complicating pregnancy, childbirth and the puerperium, followed by B20 and the code(s) for the HIV-related illness(es). Codes from Chapter 15 always take sequencing priority.

Patients with asymptomatic HIV infection status admitted (or presenting for a health care encounter) during pregnancy, childbirth, or the puerperium should receive codes of O98.7- and Z21.

(h) Encounters for testing for HIV

If a patient is being seen to determine his/her HIV status, use code Z11.4, Encounter for screening for human immunodeficiency virus [HIV]. Use additional codes for any associated high risk behavior.

If a patient with signs or symptoms is being seen for HIV testing, code the signs and symptoms. An additional counseling code Z71.7, Human immunodeficiency virus [HIV] counseling, may be used if counseling is provided during the encounter for the test.

When a patient returns to be informed of his/her HIV test results and the test result is negative, use code Z71.7, Human immunodeficiency virus [HIV] counseling.

If the results are positive, see previous guidelines and assign codes as appropriate.

b. Infectious agents as the cause of diseases classified to other chapters

Certain infections are classified in chapters other than Chapter 1 and no organism is identified as part of the infection code. In these instances, it is necessary to use an additional code from Chapter 1 to identify the organism. A code from category B95, Streptococcus, Staphylococcus, and Enterococcus as the cause of diseases classified to other chapters, B96, Other bacterial agents as the cause of diseases classified to other chapters, or B97, Viral agents as the cause of diseases classified to other chapters, is to be used as an additional code to identify the organism. An instructional note will be found at the infection code advising that an additional organism code is required.

c. Infections resistant to antibiotics

Many bacterial infections are resistant to current antibiotics. It is necessary to identify all infections documented as antibiotic resistant. Assign a code from category Z16, Resistance to antimicrobial drugs, following the infection code only if the infection code does not identify drug resistance.

d. Sepsis, Severe Sepsis, and Septic Shock

1) Coding of Sepsis and Severe Sepsis

(a) Sepsis

For a diagnosis of sepsis, assign the appropriate code for the underlying systemic infection. If the type of infection or causal organism is not further specified, assign code A41.9, Sepsis, unspecified organism.

A code from subcategory R65.2, Severe sepsis, should not be assigned unless severe sepsis or an associated acute organ dysfunction is documented.

(i) Negative or inconclusive blood cultures and sepsis

Negative or inconclusive blood cultures do not preclude a diagnosis of sepsis in patients with clinical evidence of the condition; however, the provider should be queried.

(ii) Urosepsis

The term urosepsis is a nonspecific term. It is not to be considered synonymous with sepsis. It has no default code in the Alphabetic Index. Should a provider use this term, he/she must be queried for clarification.

(iii) Sepsis with organ dysfunction

If a patient has sepsis and associated acute organ dysfunction or multiple organ dysfunction (MOD), follow the instructions for coding severe sepsis.

(iv) Acute organ dysfunction that is not clearly associated with the sepsis

If a patient has sepsis and an acute organ dysfunction, but the medical record documentation indicates that the acute organ dysfunction is related to a medical condition other than the sepsis, do not assign a code from subcategory R65.2, Severe sepsis. An acute organ dysfunction must be associated with the sepsis in order to assign the severe sepsis code. If the documentation is not clear as to whether an acute organ dysfunction is related to the sepsis or another medical condition, query the provider.

(b) Severe sepsis

The coding of severe sepsis requires a minimum of 2 codes: first a code for the underlying systemic infection, followed by a code from subcategory R65.2, Severe sepsis. If the causal organism is not documented, assign code A41.9, Sepsis, unspecified organism, for the infection. Additional code(s) for the associated acute organ dysfunction are also required.

Due to the complex nature of severe sepsis, some cases may require querying the provider prior to assignment of the codes.

2) Septic shock

(a) Septic shock generally refers to circulatory failure associated with severe sepsis, and therefore, it represents a type of acute organ dysfunction.

For cases of septic shock, the code for the systemic infection should be sequenced first, followed by code R65.21, Severe sepsis with septic shock or code T81.12, Postprocedural septic shock. Any additional codes for the other acute organ dysfunctions should also be assigned. As noted in the sequencing instructions in the Tabular List, the code for septic shock cannot be assigned as a principal diagnosis.

3) Sequencing of severe sepsis

If severe sepsis is present on admission, and meets the definition of principal diagnosis, the underlying systemic infection should be assigned as principal diagnosis followed by the appropriate code from subcategory R65.2 as required by the sequencing rules in the Tabular List. A code from subcategory R65.2 can never be assigned as a principal diagnosis.

When severe sepsis develops during an encounter (it was not present on admission), the underlying systemic infection and the appropriate code from subcategory R65.2 should be assigned as secondary diagnoses.

Severe sepsis may be present on admission, but the diagnosis may not be confirmed until sometime after admission. If the documentation is not clear whether severe sepsis was present on admission, the provider should be queried.

4) Sepsis and severe sepsis with a localized infection

If the reason for admission is both sepsis or severe sepsis and a localized infection, such as pneumonia or cellulitis, a code(s) for the underlying systemic infection should be assigned first and the code for the localized infection should be assigned as a secondary diagnosis. If the patient has severe sepsis, a code from subcategory R65.2 should also be assigned as a secondary diagnosis. If the patient is admitted with a localized infection, such as pneumonia, and sepsis/severe sepsis doesn't develop until after admission, the localized infection should be assigned first, followed by the appropriate sepsis/severe sepsis codes.

5) Sepsis due to a postprocedural infection

(a) Documentation of causal relationship

As with all postprocedural complications, code assignment is based on the provider's documentation of the relationship between the infection and the procedure.

(b) Sepsis due to a postprocedural infection

For such cases, the postprocedural infection code, such as T80.2, Infections following infusion, transfusion, and therapeutic injection, T81.4, Infection following a procedure, T88.0, Infection following immunization, or O86.0, Infection of obstetric surgical wound, should be coded first, followed by the code for the specific infection. If the patient has severe sepsis, the appropriate code from subcategory R65.2 should also be assigned with the additional code(s) for any acute organ dysfunction.

(c) Postprocedural infection and postprocedural septic shock

In cases where a postprocedural infection has occurred and has resulted in severe sepsis the code for the precipitating complication such as code T81.4, Infection following a procedure, or O86.0, Infection of obstetrical surgical wound should be coded first followed by code R65.20, Severe sepsis without septic shock. A code for the systemic infection should also be assigned.

If a postprocedural infection has resulted in postprocedural septic shock, the code for the precipitating complication such as code T81.4, Infection following a procedure, or O86.0, Infection of obstetrical surgical wound should be coded first followed by code T81.12-, Postprocedural septic shock. A code for the systemic infection should also be assigned.

6) Sepsis and severe sepsis associated with a noninfectious process (condition)

In some cases a noninfectious process (condition), such as trauma, may lead to an infection which can result in sepsis or severe sepsis. If sepsis or severe sepsis is documented as associated with a noninfectious condition, such as a burn or serious injury, and this condition meets the definition for principal diagnosis, the code for the noninfectious condition should be sequenced first, followed by the code for the resulting infection. If severe sepsis is present, a code from subcategory R65.2 should also be assigned with any associated organ dysfunction(s) codes. It is not necessary to assign a code from subcategory R65.1, Systemic inflammatory response syndrome (SIRS) of non-infectious origin, for these cases.

If the infection meets the definition of principal diagnosis, it should be sequenced before the non-infectious condition. When both the associated non-infectious condition and the infection meet the definition of principal diagnosis, either may be assigned as principal diagnosis.

Only one code from category R65, Symptoms and signs specifically associated with systemic inflammation and infection, should be assigned. Therefore, when a non-infectious condition leads to an infection resulting in severe sepsis, assign the appropriate code from subcategory R65.2, Severe sepsis. Do not additionally assign a code from subcategory R65.1, Systemic inflammatory response syndrome (SIRS) of non-infectious origin.

See Section I.C.18. SIRS due to non-infectious process

7) Sepsis and septic shock complicating abortion, pregnancy, childbirth, and the puerperium

See Section I.C.15. Sepsis and septic shock complicating abortion, pregnancy, childbirth and the puerperium

8) Newborn sepsis

See Section I.C.16. f. Bacterial sepsis of Newborn

ICD-10-CM Official Guidelines for Coding and Reporting 2018

e. Methicillin Resistant Staphylococcus aureus (MRSA) Conditions

1) Selection and sequencing of MRSA codes

(a) Combination codes for MRSA infection

When a patient is diagnosed with an infection that is due to methicillin resistant *Staphylococcus aureus* (MRSA), and that infection has a combination code that includes the causal organism (e.g., sepsis, pneumonia) assign the appropriate combination code for the condition (e.g., code A41.02, Sepsis due to Methicillin resistant Staphylococcus aureus or code J15.212, Pneumonia due to Methicillin resistant Staphylococcus aureus). Do not assign code B95.62, Methicillin resistant Staphylococcus aureus infection as the cause of diseases classified elsewhere, as an additional code, because the combination code includes the type of infection and the MRSA organism. Do not assign a code from subcategory Z16.11, Resistance to penicillins, as an additional diagnosis.

See Section C.1. for instructions on coding and sequencing of sepsis and severe sepsis.

(b) Other codes for MRSA infection

When there is documentation of a current infection (e.g., wound infection, stitch abscess, urinary tract infection) due to MRSA, and that infection does not have a combination code that includes the causal organism, assign the appropriate code to identify the condition along with code B95.62, Methicillin resistant Staphylococcus aureus infection as the cause of diseases classified elsewhere for the MRSA infection. Do not assign a code from subcategory Z16.11, Resistance to penicillins.

(c) Methicillin susceptible Staphylococcus aureus (MSSA) and MRSA colonization

The condition or state of being colonized or carrying MSSA or MRSA is called colonization or carriage, while an individual person is described as being colonized or being a carrier. Colonization means that MSSA or MSRA is present on or in the body without necessarily causing illness. A positive MRSA colonization test might be documented by the provider as "MRSA screen positive" or "MRSA nasal swab positive".

Assign code Z22.322, Carrier or suspected carrier of Methicillin resistant Staphylococcus aureus, for patients documented as having MRSA colonization. Assign code Z22.321, Carrier or suspected carrier of Methicillin susceptible Staphylococcus aureus, for patient documented as having MSSA colonization. Colonization is not necessarily indicative of a disease process or as the cause of a specific condition the patient may have unless documented as such by the provider.

(d) MRSA colonization and infection

If a patient is documented as having both MRSA colonization and infection during a hospital admission, code Z22.322, Carrier or suspected carrier of Methicillin resistant Staphylococcus aureus, and a code for the MRSA infection may both be assigned.

f. Zika virus infections

1) Code only confirmed cases

Code only a confirmed diagnosis of Zika virus (A92.5, Zika virus disease) as documented by the provider. This is an exception to the hospital inpatient guideline Section II, H. In this context, "confirmation" does not require documentation of the type of test performed; the physician's diagnostic statement that the condition is confirmed is sufficient. This code should be assigned regardless of the stated mode of transmission.

If the provider documents "suspected", "possible" or "probable" Zika, do not assign code A92.5. Assign a code(s) explaining the reason for encounter (such as fever, rash, or joint pain) or Z20.828, Contact with and (suspected) exposure to other viral communicable diseases.

2. Chapter 2: Neoplasms (C00-D49)
General guidelines

Chapter 2 of the ICD-10-CM contains the codes for most benign and all malignant neoplasms. Certain benign neoplasms, such as prostatic adenomas, may be found in the specific body system chapters. To properly code a neoplasm it is necessary to determine from the record if the neoplasm is benign, in-situ, malignant, or of uncertain histologic behavior. If malignant, any secondary (metastatic) sites should also be determined.

Primary malignant neoplasms overlapping site boundaries

A primary malignant neoplasm that overlaps two or more contiguous (next to each other) sites should be classified to the subcategory/code .8 ('overlapping lesion'), unless the combination is specifically indexed elsewhere. For multiple neoplasms of the same site that are not contiguous such as tumors in different quadrants of the same breast, codes for each site should be assigned.

Malignant neoplasm of ectopic tissue

Malignant neoplasms of ectopic tissue are to be coded to the site of origin mentioned, e.g., ectopic pancreatic malignant neoplasms involving the stomach are coded to **malignant neoplasm of** pancreas, unspecified (C25.9).

The neoplasm table in the Alphabetic Index should be referenced first. However, if the histological term is documented, that term should be referenced first, rather than going immediately to the Neoplasm Table, in order to determine which column in the Neoplasm Table is appropriate. For example, if the documentation indicates "adenoma," refer to the term in the Alphabetic Index to review the entries under this term and the instructional note to "see also neoplasm, by site, benign." The table provides the proper code based on the type of neoplasm and the site. It is important to select the proper column in the table that corresponds to the type of neoplasm. The Tabular List should then be referenced to verify that the correct code has been selected from the table and that a more specific site code does not exist.

See Section I.C.21. Factors influencing health status and contact with health services, Status, for information regarding Z15.0, codes for genetic susceptibility to cancer.

a. Treatment directed at the malignancy

If the treatment is directed at the malignancy, designate the malignancy as the principal diagnosis.

The only exception to this guideline is if a patient admission/encounter is solely for the administration of chemotherapy, immunotherapy or **external beam** radiation therapy, assign the appropriate Z51.-- code as the first-listed or principal diagnosis, and the diagnosis or problem for which the service is being performed as a secondary diagnosis.

b. Treatment of secondary site

When a patient is admitted because of a primary neoplasm with metastasis and treatment is directed toward the secondary site only, the secondary neoplasm is designated as the principal diagnosis even though the primary malignancy is still present.

c. Coding and sequencing of complications

Coding and sequencing of complications associated with the malignancies or with the therapy thereof are subject to the following guidelines:

1) Anemia associated with malignancy

When admission/encounter is for management of an anemia associated with the malignancy, and the treatment is only for anemia, the appropriate code for the malignancy is sequenced as the principal or first-listed diagnosis followed by the appropriate code for the anemia (such as code D63.0, Anemia in neoplastic disease**).**

2) Anemia associated with chemotherapy, immunotherapy and radiation therapy

When the admission/encounter is for management of an anemia associated with an adverse effect of the administration of chemotherapy or immunotherapy and the only treatment is for the anemia, the anemia code is sequenced first followed by the appropriate codes for the neoplasm and the adverse effect (T45.1X5-, Adverse effect of antineoplastic and immunosuppressive drugs).

When the admission/encounter is for management of an anemia associated with an adverse effect of radiotherapy, the anemia code should be sequenced first, followed by the appropriate neoplasm code and code Y84.2, Radiological procedure and radiotherapy as the cause of abnormal reaction of the patient, or of later complication, without mention of misadventure at the time of the procedure.

3) **Management of dehydration due to the malignancy**
When the admission/encounter is for management of dehydration due to the malignancy and only the dehydration is being treated (intravenous rehydration), the dehydration is sequenced first, followed by the code(s) for the malignancy.

4) **Treatment of a complication resulting from a surgical procedure**
When the admission/encounter is for treatment of a complication resulting from a surgical procedure, designate the complication as the principal or first-listed diagnosis if treatment is directed at resolving the complication.

d. **Primary malignancy previously excised**
When a primary malignancy has been previously excised or eradicated from its site and there is no further treatment directed to that site and there is no evidence of any existing primary malignancy, a code from category Z85, Personal history of malignant neoplasm, should be used to indicate the former site of the malignancy. Any mention of extension, invasion, or metastasis to another site is coded as a secondary malignant neoplasm to that site. The secondary site may be the principal or first-listed with the Z85 code used as a secondary code.

e. **Admissions/Encounters involving chemotherapy, immunotherapy and radiation therapy**

1) **Episode of care involves surgical removal of neoplasm**
When an episode of care involves the surgical removal of a neoplasm, primary or secondary site, followed by adjunct chemotherapy or radiation treatment during the same episode of care, the code for the neoplasm should be assigned as principal or first-listed diagnosis.

2) **Patient admission/encounter solely for administration of chemotherapy, immunotherapy and radiation therapy**
If a patient admission/encounter is solely for the administration of chemotherapy, immunotherapy or **external beam** radiation therapy assign code Z51.0, Encounter for antineoplastic radiation therapy, or Z51.11, Encounter for antineoplastic chemotherapy, or Z51.12, Encounter for antineoplastic immunotherapy as the first-listed or principal diagnosis. If a patient receives more than one of these therapies during the same admission more than one of these codes may be assigned, in any sequence.

The malignancy for which the therapy is being administered should be assigned as a secondary diagnosis.

If a patient admission/encounter is for the insertion or implantation of radioactive elements (e.g., brachytherapy) the appropriate code for the malignancy is sequenced as the principal or first-listed diagnosis. Code Z51.0 should not be assigned.

3) **Patient admitted for radiation therapy, chemotherapy or immunotherapy and develops complications**
When a patient is admitted for the purpose of **external beam** radiotherapy, immunotherapy or chemotherapy and develops complications such as uncontrolled nausea and vomiting or dehydration, the principal or first-listed diagnosis is Z51.0, Encounter for antineoplastic radiation therapy, or Z51.11, Encounter for antineoplastic chemotherapy, or Z51.12, Encounter for antineoplastic immunotherapy followed by any codes for the complications.

When a patient is admitted for the purpose of insertion or implantation of radioactive elements (e.g., brachytherapy) and develops complications such as uncontrolled nausea and vomiting or dehydration, the principal or first-listed diagnosis is the appropriate code for the malignancy followed by any codes for the complications.

f. **Admission/encounter to determine extent of malignancy**
When the reason for admission/encounter is to determine the extent of the malignancy, or for a procedure such as paracentesis or thoracentesis, the primary malignancy or appropriate metastatic site is designated as the principal or first-listed diagnosis, even though chemotherapy or radiotherapy is administered.

g. **Symptoms, signs, and abnormal findings listed in Chapter 18 associated with neoplasms**
Symptoms, signs, and ill-defined conditions listed in Chapter 18 characteristic of, or associated with, an existing primary or

secondary site malignancy cannot be used to replace the malignancy as principal or first-listed diagnosis, regardless of the number of admissions or encounters for treatment and care of the neoplasm.

See section I.C.21. Factors influencing health status and contact with health services, Encounter for prophylactic organ removal.

h. **Admission/encounter for pain control/management**
See Section I.C.6. for information on coding admission/encounter for pain control/management.

i. **Malignancy in two or more noncontiguous sites**
A patient may have more than one malignant tumor in the same organ. These tumors may represent different primaries or metastatic disease, depending on the site. Should the documentation be unclear, the provider should be queried as to the status of each tumor so that the correct codes can be assigned.

j. **Disseminated malignant neoplasm, unspecified**
Code C80.0, Disseminated malignant neoplasm, unspecified, is for use only in those cases where the patient has advanced metastatic disease and no known primary or secondary sites are specified. It should not be used in place of assigning codes for the primary site and all known secondary sites.

k. **Malignant neoplasm without specification of site**
Code C80.1, Malignant (primary) neoplasm, unspecified, equates to Cancer, unspecified. This code should only be used when no determination can be made as to the primary site of a malignancy. This code should rarely be used in the inpatient setting.

l. **Sequencing of neoplasm codes**

1) **Encounter for treatment of primary malignancy**
If the reason for the encounter is for treatment of a primary malignancy, assign the malignancy as the principal/first-listed diagnosis. The primary site is to be sequenced first, followed by any metastatic sites.

2) **Encounter for treatment of secondary malignancy**
When an encounter is for a primary malignancy with metastasis and treatment is directed toward the metastatic (secondary) site(s) only, the metastatic site(s) is designated as the principal/first-listed diagnosis. The primary malignancy is coded as an additional code.

3) **Malignant neoplasm in a pregnant patient**
When a pregnant woman has a malignant neoplasm, a code from subcategory O9A.1-, Malignant neoplasm complicating pregnancy, childbirth, and the puerperium, should be sequenced first, followed by the appropriate code from Chapter 2 to indicate the type of neoplasm.

4) **Encounter for complication associated with a neoplasm**
When an encounter is for management of a complication associated with a neoplasm, such as dehydration, and the treatment is only for the complication, the complication is coded first, followed by the appropriate code(s) for the neoplasm.

The exception to this guideline is anemia. When the admission/encounter is for management of an anemia associated with the malignancy, and the treatment is only for anemia, the appropriate code for the malignancy is sequenced as the principal or first-listed diagnosis followed by code D63.0, Anemia in neoplastic disease.

5) **Complication from surgical procedure for treatment of a neoplasm**
When an encounter is for treatment of a complication resulting from a surgical procedure performed for the treatment of the neoplasm, designate the complication as the principal/first-listed diagnosis. See guideline regarding the coding of a current malignancy versus personal history to determine if the code for the neoplasm should also be assigned.

6) **Pathologic fracture due to a neoplasm**
When an encounter is for a pathological fracture due to a neoplasm, and the focus of treatment is the fracture, a code from subcategory M84.5, Pathological fracture in neoplastic disease, should be sequenced first, followed by the code for the neoplasm.

If the focus of treatment is the neoplasm with an associated pathological fracture, the neoplasm code should be sequenced first, followed by a code from M84.5 for the pathological fracture.

m. Current malignancy versus personal history of malignancy
When a primary malignancy has been excised but further treatment, such as an additional surgery for the malignancy, radiation therapy or chemotherapy is directed to that site, the primary malignancy code should be used until treatment is completed.

When a primary malignancy has been previously excised or eradicated from its site, there is no further treatment (of the malignancy) directed to that site, and there is no evidence of any existing primary malignancy, a code from category Z85, Personal history of malignant neoplasm, should be used to indicate the former site of the malignancy.

See Section I.C.21. Factors influencing health status and contact with health services, History (of)

n. Leukemia, Multiple Myeloma, and Malignant Plasma Cell Neoplasms in remission versus personal history
The categories for leukemia, and category C90, Multiple myeloma and malignant plasma cell neoplasms, have codes indicating whether or not the leukemia has achieved remission. There are also codes Z85.6, Personal history of leukemia, and Z85.79, Personal history of other malignant neoplasms of lymphoid, hematopoietic and related tissues. If the documentation is unclear as to whether the leukemia has achieved remission, the provider should be queried.

See Section I.C.21. Factors influencing health status and contact with health services, History (of)

o. Aftercare following surgery for neoplasm
See Section I.C.21. Factors influencing health status and contact with health services, Aftercare

p. Follow-up care for completed treatment of a malignancy
See Section I.C.21. Factors influencing health status and contact with health services, Follow-up

q. Prophylactic organ removal for prevention of malignancy
See Section I.C. 21, Factors influencing health status and contact with health services, Prophylactic organ removal

r. Malignant neoplasm associated with transplanted organ
A malignant neoplasm of a transplanted organ should be coded as a transplant complication. Assign first the appropriate code from category T86.-, Complications of transplanted organs and tissue, followed by code C80.2, Malignant neoplasm associated with transplanted organ. Use an additional code for the specific malignancy.

3. Chapter 3: Disease of the blood and blood-forming organs and certain disorders involving the immune mechanism (D50-D89)
Reserved for future guideline expansion

4. Chapter 4: Endocrine, Nutritional, and Metabolic Diseases (E00-E89)

a. Diabetes mellitus
The diabetes mellitus codes are combination codes that include the type of diabetes mellitus, the body system affected, and the complications affecting that body system. As many codes within a particular category as are necessary to describe all of the complications of the disease may be used. They should be sequenced based on the reason for a particular encounter. Assign as many codes from categories E08 – E13 as needed to identify all of the associated conditions that the patient has.

1) Type of diabetes
The age of a patient is not the sole determining factor, though most type 1 diabetics develop the condition before reaching puberty. For this reason type 1 diabetes mellitus is also referred to as juvenile diabetes.

2) Type of diabetes mellitus not documented
If the type of diabetes mellitus is not documented in the medical record the default is E11.-, Type 2 diabetes mellitus.

3) Diabetes mellitus and the use of insulin and oral hypoglycemics
If the documentation in a medical record does not indicate the type of diabetes but does indicate that the patient uses insulin, code E11-, Type 2 diabetes mellitus, should be assigned. **An additional code should be assigned from category Z79 to**

identify the long-term (current) use of insulin or oral hypoglycemic drugs. If the patient is treated with both oral medications and insulin, only the code for long-term (current) use of insulin should be assigned. Code Z79.4 should not be assigned if insulin is given temporarily to bring a type 2 patient's blood sugar under control during an encounter.

4) Diabetes mellitus in pregnancy and gestational diabetes
See Section I.C.15. Diabetes mellitus in pregnancy.

See Section I.C.15. Gestational (pregnancy induced) diabetes

5) Complications due to insulin pump malfunction

(a) Underdose of insulin due to insulin pump failure
An underdose of insulin due to an insulin pump failure should be assigned to a code from subcategory T85.6, Mechanical complication of other specified internal and external prosthetic devices, implants and grafts, that specifies the type of pump malfunction, as the principal or first-listed code, followed by code T38.3X6-, Underdosing of insulin and oral hypoglycemic [antidiabetic] drugs. Additional codes for the type of diabetes mellitus and any associated complications due to the underdosing should also be assigned.

(b) Overdose of insulin due to insulin pump failure
The principal or first-listed code for an encounter due to an insulin pump malfunction resulting in an overdose of insulin, should also be T85.6-, Mechanical complication of other specified internal and external prosthetic devices, implants and grafts, followed by code T38.3X1-, Poisoning by insulin and oral hypoglycemic [antidiabetic] drugs, accidental (unintentional).

6) Secondary diabetes mellitus
Codes under categories E08, Diabetes mellitus due to underlying condition, E09, Drug or chemical induced diabetes mellitus, and E13, Other specified diabetes mellitus, identify complications/manifestations associated with secondary diabetes mellitus. Secondary diabetes is always caused by another condition or event (e.g., cystic fibrosis, malignant neoplasm of pancreas, pancreatectomy, adverse effect of drug, or poisoning).

(a) Secondary diabetes mellitus and the use of insulin or *oral* hypoglycemic drugs
For patients with secondary diabetes mellitus who routinely use insulin or oral hypoglycemic drugs, an additional code from category Z79 should be assigned to identify the long-term (current) use of insulin or oral hypoglycemic drugs. If the patient is treated with both oral medications and insulin, only the code for long-term (current) use of insulin should be assigned. Code Z79.4 should not be assigned if insulin is given temporarily to bring a type 2 patient's blood sugar under control during an encounter.

(b) Assigning and sequencing secondary diabetes codes and its causes
The sequencing of the secondary diabetes codes in relationship to codes for the cause of the diabetes is based on the Tabular List instructions for categories E08, E09 and E13.

(i) Secondary diabetes mellitus due to pancreatectomy
For postpancreatectomy diabetes mellitus (lack of insulin due to the surgical removal of all or part of the pancreas), assign code E89.1, Postprocedural hypoinsulinemia. Assign a code from category E13 and a code from subcategory Z90.41, Acquired absence of pancreas, as additional codes.

(ii) Secondary diabetes due to drugs
Secondary diabetes may be caused by an adverse effect of correctly administered medications, poisoning or sequela of poisoning.
See section I.C.19.e for coding of adverse effects and poisoning, and section I.C.20 for external cause code reporting.

5. **Chapter 5: Mental, Behavioral and Neurodevelopmental disorders (F01 – F99)**
   a. **Pain disorders related to psychological factors**

   Assign code F45.41, for pain that is exclusively related to psychological disorders. As indicated by the Excludes 1 note under category G89, a code from category G89 should not be assigned with code F45.41.

   Code F45.42, Pain disorders with related psychological factors, should be used with a code from category G89, Pain, not elsewhere classified, if there is documentation of a psychological component for a patient with acute or chronic pain.

   See Section I.C.6. Pain

   b. **Mental and behavioral disorders due to psychoactive substance use**
      1) **In Remission**

      Selection of codes for "in remission" for categories F10-F19, Mental and behavioral disorders due to psychoactive substance use (categories F10-F19 with **-11**, -.21) requires the provider's clinical judgment. The appropriate codes for "in remission" are assigned only on the basis of provider documentation (as defined in the Official Guidelines for Coding and Reporting)**, unless otherwise instructed by the classification.**

      Mild substance use disorders in early or sustained remission are classified to the appropriate codes for substance abuse in remission, and moderate or severe substance use disorders in early or sustained remission are classified to the appropriate codes for substance dependence in remission.

      2) **Psychoactive Substance Use, Abuse and Dependence**

      When the provider documentation refers to use, abuse and dependence of the same substance (e.g. alcohol, opioid, cannabis, etc.), only one code should be assigned to identify the pattern of use based on the following hierarchy:

      - If both use and abuse are documented, assign only the code for abuse
      - If both abuse and dependence are documented, assign only the code for dependence
      - If use, abuse and dependence are all documented, assign only the code for dependence
      - If both use and dependence are documented, assign only the code for dependence.

      3) **Psychoactive Substance Use** *Disorders*

      As with all other diagnoses, the codes for psychoactive substance use **disorders** (F10.9-, F11.9-, F12.9-, F13.9-, F14.9-, F15.9-, F16.9-) should only be assigned based on provider documentation and when they meet the definition of a reportable diagnosis (see Section III, Reporting Additional Diagnoses). The codes are to be used only when the psychoactive substance use is associated with a **physical,** mental or behavioral disorder, and such a relationship is documented by the provider.

6. **Chapter 6: Diseases of the Nervous System (G00-G99)**
   a. **Dominant/nondominant side**

   Codes from category G81, Hemiplegia and hemiparesis, and subcategories G83.1, Monoplegia of lower limb, G83.2, Monoplegia of upper limb, and G83.3, Monoplegia, unspecified, identify whether the dominant or nondominant side is affected. Should the affected side be documented, but not specified as dominant or nondominant, and the classification system does not indicate a default, code selection is as follows:

   - For ambidextrous patients, the default should be dominant.
   - If the left side is affected, the default is non-dominant.
   - If the right side is affected, the default is dominant.

   b. **Pain - Category G89**
      1) **General coding information**

      Codes in category G89, Pain, not elsewhere classified, may be used in conjunction with codes from other categories and chapters to provide more detail about acute or chronic pain and neoplasm-related pain, unless otherwise indicated below.

      If the pain is not specified as acute or chronic, post-thoracotomy, postprocedural, or neoplasm-related, do not assign codes from category G89.

A code from category G89 should not be assigned if the underlying (definitive) diagnosis is known, unless the reason for the encounter is pain control/ management and not management of the underlying condition.

When an admission or encounter is for a procedure aimed at treating the underlying condition (e.g., spinal fusion, kyphoplasty), a code for the underlying condition (e.g., vertebral fracture, spinal stenosis) should be assigned as the principal diagnosis. No code from category G89 should be assigned.

   (a) **Category G89 Codes as Principal or First-Listed Diagnosis**

   Category G89 codes are acceptable as principal diagnosis or the first-listed code:

   - When pain control or pain management is the reason for the admission/encounter (e.g., a patient with displaced intervertebral disc, nerve impingement and severe back pain presents for injection of steroid into the spinal canal). The underlying cause of the pain should be reported as an additional diagnosis, if known.

   - When a patient is admitted for the insertion of a neurostimulator for pain control, assign the appropriate pain code as the principal or first-listed diagnosis. When an admission or encounter is for a procedure aimed at treating the underlying condition and a neurostimulator is inserted for pain control during the same admission/encounter, a code for the underlying condition should be assigned as the principal diagnosis and the appropriate pain code should be assigned as a secondary diagnosis.

   (b) **Use of Category G89 Codes in Conjunction with Site Specific Pain Codes**
      (i) **Assigning Category G89 and Site-Specific Pain Codes**

      Codes from category G89 may be used in conjunction with codes that identify the site of pain (including codes from chapter 18) if the category G89 code provides additional information. For example, if the code describes the site of the pain, but does not fully describe whether the pain is acute or chronic, then both codes should be assigned.

      (ii) **Sequencing of Category G89 Codes with Site-Specific Pain Codes**

      The sequencing of category G89 codes with site-specific pain codes (including chapter 18 codes), is dependent on the circumstances of the encounter/admission as follows:

      - If the encounter is for pain control or pain management, assign the code from category G89 followed by the code identifying the specific site of pain (e.g., encounter for pain management for acute neck pain from trauma is assigned code G89.11, Acute pain due to trauma, followed by code M54.2, Cervicalgia, to identify the site of pain).

      - If the encounter is for any other reason except pain control or pain management, and a related definitive diagnosis has not been established (confirmed) by the provider, assign the code for the specific site of pain first, followed by the appropriate code from category G89.

   2) **Pain due to devices, implants and grafts**
   See Section I.C.19. Pain due to medical devices

   3) **Postoperative Pain**

   The provider's documentation should be used to guide the coding of postoperative pain, as well as *Section III. Reporting Additional Diagnoses and Section IV. Diagnostic Coding and Reporting in the Outpatient Setting.*

   The default for post-thoracotomy and other postoperative pain not specified as acute or chronic is the code for the acute form.

   Routine or expected postoperative pain immediately after surgery should not be coded.

(a) **Postoperative pain not associated with specific postoperative complication**

Postoperative pain not associated with a specific postoperative complication is assigned to the appropriate postoperative pain code in category G89.

(b) **Postoperative pain associated with specific postoperative complication**

Postoperative pain associated with a specific postoperative complication (such as painful wire sutures) is assigned to the appropriate code(s) found in Chapter 19, Injury, poisoning, and certain other consequences of external causes. If appropriate, use additional code(s) from category G89 to identify acute or chronic pain (G89.18 or G89.28).

4) **Chronic pain**

Chronic pain is classified to subcategory G89.2. There is no time frame defining when pain becomes chronic pain. The provider's documentation should be used to guide use of these codes.

5) **Neoplasm Related Pain**

Code G89.3 is assigned to pain documented as being related, associated or due to cancer, primary or secondary malignancy, or tumor. This code is assigned regardless of whether the pain is acute or chronic.

This code may be assigned as the principal or first-listed code when the stated reason for the admission/encounter is documented as pain control/pain management. The underlying neoplasm should be reported as an additional diagnosis.

When the reason for the admission/encounter is management of the neoplasm and the pain associated with the neoplasm is also documented, code G89.3 may be assigned as an additional diagnosis. It is not necessary to assign an additional code for the site of the pain.

See Section I.C.2 for instructions on the sequencing of neoplasms for all other stated reasons for the admission/encounter (except for pain control/pain management).

6) **Chronic pain syndrome**

Central pain syndrome (G89.0) and chronic pain syndrome (G89.4) are different than the term "chronic pain," and therefore codes should only be used when the provider has specifically documented this condition.

See Section I.C.5. Pain disorders related to psychological factors

7. **Chapter 7: Diseases of the Eye and Adnexa (H00-H59)**
   a. **Glaucoma**
   1) **Assigning Glaucoma Codes**

   Assign as many codes from category H40, Glaucoma, as needed to identify the type of glaucoma, the affected eye, and the glaucoma stage.

   2) **Bilateral glaucoma with same type and stage**

   When a patient has bilateral glaucoma and both eyes are documented as being the same type and stage, and there is a code for bilateral glaucoma, report only the code for the type of glaucoma, bilateral, with the seventh character for the stage.

   When a patient has bilateral glaucoma and both eyes are documented as being the same type and stage, and the classification does not provide a code for bilateral glaucoma (i.e. subcategories H40.10, H40.11 and H40.20) report only one code for the type of glaucoma with the appropriate seventh character for the stage.

   3) **Bilateral glaucoma stage with different types or stages**

   When a patient has bilateral glaucoma and each eye is documented as having a different type or stage, and the classification distinguishes laterality, assign the appropriate code for each eye rather than the code for bilateral glaucoma.

   When a patient has bilateral glaucoma and each eye is documented as having a different type, and the classification does not distinguish laterality (i.e. subcategories H40.10, H40.11 and H40.20), assign one code for each type of glaucoma with the appropriate seventh character for the stage.

   When a patient has bilateral glaucoma and each eye is documented as having the same type, but different stage, and the classification does not distinguish laterality (i.e. subcategories H40.10, H40.11 and H40.20), assign a code for

the type of glaucoma for each eye with the seventh character for the specific glaucoma stage documented for each eye.

4) **Patient admitted with glaucoma and stage evolves during the admission**

If a patient is admitted with glaucoma and the stage progresses during the admission, assign the code for highest stage documented.

5) **Indeterminate stage glaucoma**

Assignment of the seventh character "4" for "indeterminate stage" should be based on the clinical documentation. The seventh character "4" is used for glaucomas whose stage cannot be clinically determined. This seventh character should not be confused with the seventh character "0", unspecified, which should be assigned when there is no documentation regarding the stage of the glaucoma.

b. **Blindness**

If "blindness" or "low vision" of both eyes is documented but the visual impairment category is not documented, assign code H54.3, Unqualified visual loss, both eyes. If "blindness" or "low vision" in one eye is documented but the visual impairment category is not documented, assign a code from H54.6-, Unqualified visual loss, one eye. If "blindness" or "visual loss" is documented without any information about whether one or both eyes are affected, assign code H54.7, Unspecified visual loss.

8. **Chapter 8: Diseases of the Ear and Mastoid Process (H60-H95)**
   Reserved for future guideline expansion

9. **Chapter 9: Diseases of the Circulatory System (I00-I99)**
   a. **Hypertension**

   The classification presumes a causal relationship between hypertension and heart involvement and between hypertension and kidney involvement, as the two conditions are linked by the term "with" in the Alphabetic Index. These conditions should be coded as related even in the absence of provider documentation explicitly linking them, unless the documentation clearly states the conditions are unrelated.

   For hypertension and conditions not specifically linked by relational terms such as "with," "associated with" or "due to" in the classification, provider documentation must link the conditions in order to code them as related.

   1) **Hypertension with Heart Disease**

   Hypertension with heart conditions classified to I50.- or I51.4-I51.9, are assigned to a code from category I11, Hypertensive heart disease. Use additional code(s) from category I50, Heart failure, to identify the type(s) of heart failure in those patients with heart failure.

   The same heart conditions (I50.-, I51.4-I51.9) with hypertension are coded separately if the provider has specifically documented a different cause. Sequence according to the circumstances of the admission/encounter.

   2) **Hypertensive Chronic Kidney Disease**

   Assign codes from category I12, Hypertensive chronic kidney disease, when both hypertension and a condition classifiable to category N18, Chronic kidney disease (CKD), are present. CKD should not be coded as hypertensive if the physician has specifically documented a different cause.

   The appropriate code from category N18 should be used as a secondary code with a code from category I12 to identify the stage of chronic kidney disease.

   See Section I.C.14. Chronic kidney disease.

   If a patient has hypertensive chronic kidney disease and acute renal failure, an additional code for the acute renal failure is required.

   3) **Hypertensive Heart and Chronic Kidney Disease**

   Assign codes from combination category I13, Hypertensive heart and chronic kidney disease, when there is hypertension with both heart and kidney involvement. If heart failure is present, assign an additional code from category I50 to identify the type of heart failure.

   The appropriate code from category N18, Chronic kidney disease, should be used as a secondary code with a code from category I13 to identify the stage of chronic kidney disease.

See Section I.C.14. Chronic kidney disease.

The codes in category I13, Hypertensive heart and chronic kidney disease, are combination codes that include hypertension, heart disease and chronic kidney disease. The Includes note at I13 specifies that the conditions included at I11 and I12 are included together in I13. If a patient has hypertension, heart disease and chronic kidney disease, then a code from I13 should be used, not individual codes for hypertension, heart disease and chronic kidney disease, or codes from I11 or I12.

For patients with both acute renal failure and chronic kidney disease, an additional code for acute renal failure is required.

4) Hypertensive Cerebrovascular Disease
For hypertensive cerebrovascular disease, first assign the appropriate code from categories I60-I69, followed by the appropriate hypertension code.

5) Hypertensive Retinopathy
Subcategory H35.0, Background retinopathy and retinal vascular changes, should be used with a code from category I10-I15, Hypertensive disease to include the systemic hypertension. The sequencing is based on the reason for the encounter.

6) Hypertension, Secondary
Secondary hypertension is due to an underlying condition. Two codes are required: one to identify the underlying etiology and one from category I15 to identify the hypertension. Sequencing of codes is determined by the reason for admission/encounter.

7) Hypertension, Transient
Assign code R03.0, Elevated blood pressure reading without diagnosis of hypertension, unless patient has an established diagnosis of hypertension. Assign code O13.-, Gestational [pregnancy-induced] hypertension without significant proteinuria, or O14.-, Pre-eclampsia, for transient hypertension of pregnancy.

8) Hypertension, Controlled
This diagnostic statement usually refers to an existing state of hypertension under control by therapy. Assign the appropriate code from categories I10-I15, Hypertensive diseases.

9) Hypertension, Uncontrolled
Uncontrolled hypertension may refer to untreated hypertension or hypertension not responding to current therapeutic regimen. In either case, assign the appropriate code from categories I10-I15, Hypertensive diseases.

10) Hypertensive Crisis
Assign a code from category I16, Hypertensive crisis, for documented hypertensive urgency, hypertensive emergency or unspecified hypertensive crisis. Code also any identified hypertensive disease (I10-I15). The sequencing is based on the reason for the encounter.

10) Pulmonary Hypertension
Pulmonary hypertension is classified to category I27, Other pulmonary heart diseases. For secondary pulmonary hypertension (I27.1, I27.2-), code also any associated conditions or adverse effects of drugs or toxins. The sequencing is based on the reason for the encounter.

b. Atherosclerotic Coronary Artery Disease and Angina
ICD-10-CM has combination codes for atherosclerotic heart disease with angina pectoris. The subcategories for these codes are I25.11, Atherosclerotic heart disease of native coronary artery with angina pectoris and I25.7, Atherosclerosis of coronary artery bypass graft(s) and coronary artery of transplanted heart with angina pectoris.

When using one of these combination codes it is not necessary to use an additional code for angina pectoris. A causal relationship can be assumed in a patient with both atherosclerosis and angina pectoris, unless the documentation indicates the angina is due to something other than the atherosclerosis.

If a patient with coronary artery disease is admitted due to an acute myocardial infarction (AMI), the AMI should be sequenced before the coronary artery disease.

See Section I.C.9. Acute myocardial infarction (AMI)

c. Intraoperative and Postprocedural Cerebrovascular Accident
Medical record documentation should clearly specify the cause-and-effect relationship between the medical intervention and the cerebrovascular accident in order to assign a code for intraoperative or postprocedural cerebrovascular accident.

Proper code assignment depends on whether it was an infarction or hemorrhage and whether it occurred intraoperatively or postoperatively. If it was a cerebral hemorrhage, code assignment depends on the type of procedure performed.

d. Sequelae of Cerebrovascular Disease

1) Category I69, Sequelae of Cerebrovascular disease
Category I69 is used to indicate conditions classifiable to categories I60-I67 as the causes of sequela (neurologic deficits), themselves classified elsewhere. These "late effects" include neurologic deficits that persist after initial onset of conditions classifiable to categories I60-I67. The neurologic deficits caused by cerebrovascular disease may be present from the onset or may arise at any time after the onset of the condition classifiable to categories I60-I67.

Codes from category I69, Sequelae of cerebrovascular disease, that specify hemiplegia, hemiparesis and monoplegia identify whether the dominant or nondominant side is affected. Should the affected side be documented, but not specified as dominant or nondominant, and the classification system does not indicate a default, code selection is as follows:

- For ambidextrous patients, the default should be dominant.
- If the left side is affected, the default is non-dominant.
- If the right side is affected, the default is dominant.

2) Codes from category I69 with codes from I60-I67
Codes from category I69 may be assigned on a health care record with codes from I60-I67, if the patient has a current cerebrovascular disease and deficits from an old cerebrovascular disease.

3) Codes from category I69 and Personal history of transient ischemic attack (TIA) and cerebral infarction (Z86.73)
Codes from category I69 should not be assigned if the patient does not have neurologic deficits.

See Section I.C.21. 4. History (of) for use of personal history codes

e. Acute myocardial infarction (AMI)

1) Type 1 ST elevation myocardial infarction (STEMI) and non-ST elevation myocardial infarction (NSTEMI)
The ICD-10-CM codes for **type 1** acute myocardial infarction (AMI) identify the site, such as anterolateral wall or true posterior wall. Subcategories I21.0-I21.2 and code I21.3 are used for **type 1** ST elevation myocardial infarction (STEMI). Code I21.4, Non-ST elevation (NSTEMI) myocardial infarction, is used for **type 1** non ST elevation myocardial infarction (NSTEMI) and nontransmural MIs.

If **a type 1** NSTEMI evolves to STEMI, assign the STEMI code. If **a type 1** STEMI converts to NSTEMI due to thrombolytic therapy, it is still coded as STEMI.

For encounters occurring while the myocardial infarction is equal to, or less than, four weeks old, including transfers to another acute setting or a postacute setting, and the myocardial infarction meets the definition for "other diagnoses" (see Section III, Reporting Additional Diagnoses), codes from category I21 may continue to be reported. For encounters after the 4 week time frame and the patient is still receiving care related to the myocardial infarction, the appropriate aftercare code should be assigned, rather than a code from category I21. For old or healed myocardial infarctions not requiring further care, code I25.2, Old myocardial infarction, may be assigned.

2) Acute myocardial infarction, unspecified
Code **I21.9, Acute myocardial infarction, unspecified,** is the default for unspecified acute myocardial infarction **or unspecified type**. If only **type 1** STEMI or transmural MI without the site is documented, assign code I21.3, **ST elevation (STEMI) myocardial infarction of unspecified site**.

3) AMI documented as nontransmural or subendocardial but site provided
If an AMI is documented as nontransmural or subendocardial, but the site is provided, it is still coded as a subendocardial AMI.

See Section I.C.21.3 for information on coding status post administration of tPA in a different facility within the last 24 hours.

4) Subsequent acute myocardial infarction
A code from category I22, Subsequent ST elevation (STEMI) and non-ST elevation (NSTEMI) myocardial infarction, is to be used when a patient who has suffered **a type 1 or unspecified** AMI has a new AMI within the 4 week time frame of the initial AMI. A code from category I22 must be used in conjunction with a code from category I21. The sequencing of the I22 and I21 codes depends on the circumstances of the encounter.

Do not assign code I22 for subsequent myocardial infarctions other than type 1 or unspecified. For subsequent type 2 AMI assign only code I21.A1. For subsequent type 4 or type 5 AMI, assign only code I21.A9.

5) Other Types of Myocardial Infarction
The ICD-10-CM provides codes for different types of myocardial infarction. Type 1 myocardial infarctions are assigned to codes I21.0-I21.4.

Type 2 myocardial infarction, and myocardial infarction due to demand ischemia or secondary to ischemic balance, is assigned to code I21.A1, Myocardial infarction type 2 with a code for the underlying cause. Do not assign code I24.8, Other forms of acute ischemic heart disease for the demand ischemia. Sequencing of type 2 AMI or the underlying cause is dependent on the circumstances of admission. When a type 2 AMI code is described as NSTEMI or STEMI, only assign code I21.A1. Codes I21.01-I21.4 should only be assigned for type 1 AMIs.

Acute myocardial infarctions type 3, 4a, 4b, 4c and 5 are assigned to code I21.A9, Other myocardial infarction type.

The "Code also" and "Code first" notes should be followed related to complications, and for coding of postprocedural myocardial infarctions during or following cardiac surgery.

10. Chapter 10: Diseases of the Respiratory System (J00-J99)
a. Chronic Obstructive Pulmonary Disease [COPD] and Asthma
1) Acute exacerbation of chronic obstructive bronchitis and asthma
The codes in categories J44 and J45 distinguish between uncomplicated cases and those in acute exacerbation. An acute exacerbation is a worsening or a decompensation of a chronic condition. An acute exacerbation is not equivalent to an infection superimposed on a chronic condition, though an exacerbation may be triggered by an infection.

b. Acute Respiratory Failure
1) Acute respiratory failure as principal diagnosis
A code from subcategory J96.0, Acute respiratory failure, or subcategory J96.2, Acute and chronic respiratory failure, may be assigned as a principal diagnosis when it is the condition established after study to be chiefly responsible for occasioning the admission to the hospital, and the selection is supported by the Alphabetic Index and Tabular List. However, chapter-specific coding guidelines (such as obstetrics, poisoning, HIV, newborn) that provide sequencing direction take precedence.

2) Acute respiratory failure as secondary diagnosis
Respiratory failure may be listed as a secondary diagnosis if it occurs after admission, or if it is present on admission, but does not meet the definition of principal diagnosis.

3) Sequencing of acute respiratory failure and another acute condition
When a patient is admitted with respiratory failure and another acute condition, (e.g., myocardial infarction, cerebrovascular accident, aspiration pneumonia), the principal diagnosis will not be the same in every situation. This applies whether the other acute condition is a respiratory or nonrespiratory condition. Selection of the principal diagnosis will be dependent on the circumstances of admission. If both the respiratory failure and the other acute condition are equally responsible for occasioning the admission to the hospital, and there are no chapter-specific sequencing rules, the guideline regarding two or more diagnoses that equally meet the definition for principal diagnosis *(Section II, C.)* may be applied in these situations.

If the documentation is not clear as to whether acute respiratory failure and another condition are equally responsible for occasioning the admission, query the provider for clarification.

c. Influenza due to certain identified influenza viruses
Code only confirmed cases of influenza due to certain identified influenza viruses (category J09), and due to other identified influenza virus (category J10). This is an exception to the hospital inpatient guideline Section II, H. (Uncertain Diagnosis).

In this context, "confirmation" does not require documentation of positive laboratory testing specific for avian or other novel influenza A or other identified influenza virus. However, coding should be based on the provider's diagnostic statement that the patient has avian influenza, or other novel influenza A, for category J09, or has another particular identified strain of influenza, such as H1N1 or H3N2, but not identified as novel or variant, for category J10.

If the provider records "suspected" or "possible" or "probable" avian influenza, or novel influenza, or other identified influenza, then the appropriate influenza code from category J11, Influenza due to unidentified influenza virus, should be assigned. A code from category J09, Influenza due to certain identified influenza viruses, should not be assigned nor should a code from category J10, Influenza due to other identified influenza virus.

d. Ventilator associated Pneumonia
1) Documentation of Ventilator associated Pneumonia
As with all procedural or postprocedural complications, code assignment is based on the provider's documentation of the relationship between the condition and the procedure.

Code J95.851, Ventilator associated pneumonia, should be assigned only when the provider has documented ventilator associated pneumonia (VAP). An additional code to identify the organism (e.g., Pseudomonas aeruginosa, code B96.5) should also be assigned. Do not assign an additional code from categories J12-J18 to identify the type of pneumonia.

Code J95.851 should not be assigned for cases where the patient has pneumonia and is on a mechanical ventilator and the provider has not specifically stated that the pneumonia is ventilator-associated pneumonia. If the documentation is unclear as to whether the patient has a pneumonia that is a complication attributable to the mechanical ventilator, query the provider.

2) Ventilator associated Pneumonia Develops after Admission
A patient may be admitted with one type of pneumonia (e.g., code J13, Pneumonia due to Streptococcus pneumonia) and subsequently develop VAP. In this instance, the principal diagnosis would be the appropriate code from categories J12-J18 for the pneumonia diagnosed at the time of admission. Code J95.851, Ventilator associated pneumonia, would be assigned as an additional diagnosis when the provider has also documented the presence of ventilator associated pneumonia.

11. Chapter 11: Diseases of the Digestive System (K00-K95)
Reserved for future guideline expansion

12. Chapter 12: Diseases of the Skin and Subcutaneous Tissue (L00-L99)
a. Pressure ulcer stage codes
1) Pressure ulcer stages
Codes from category L89, Pressure ulcer, identify the site of the pressure ulcer as well as the stage of the ulcer.

The ICD-10-CM classifies pressure ulcer stages based on severity, which is designated by stages 1-4, unspecified stage and unstageable.

Assign as many codes from category L89 as needed to identify all the pressure ulcers the patient has, if applicable.

2) Unstageable pressure ulcers
Assignment of the code for unstageable pressure ulcer (L89.--0) should be based on the clinical documentation. These codes are used for pressure ulcers whose stage cannot be clinically determined (e.g., the ulcer is covered by eschar or has been treated with a skin or muscle graft) and pressure ulcers that are documented as deep tissue injury but not documented as due to trauma. This code should not be confused with the codes for unspecified stage (L89.--9). When there is no documentation

regarding the stage of the pressure ulcer, assign the appropriate code for unspecified stage (L89.--9).

3) Documented pressure ulcer stage
Assignment of the pressure ulcer stage code should be guided by clinical documentation of the stage or documentation of the terms found in the Alphabetic Index. For clinical terms describing the stage that are not found in the Alphabetic Index, and there is no documentation of the stage, the provider should be queried.

4) Patients admitted with pressure ulcers documented as healed
No code is assigned if the documentation states that the pressure ulcer is completely healed.

5) Patients admitted with pressure ulcers documented as healing
Pressure ulcers described as healing should be assigned the appropriate pressure ulcer stage code based on the documentation in the medical record. If the documentation does not provide information about the stage of the healing pressure ulcer, assign the appropriate code for unspecified stage.

If the documentation is unclear as to whether the patient has a current (new) pressure ulcer or if the patient is being treated for a healing pressure ulcer, query the provider.

For ulcers that were present on admission but healed at the time of discharge, assign the code for the site and stage of the pressure ulcer at the time of admission.

6) Patient admitted with pressure ulcer evolving into another stage during the admission
If a patient is admitted **to an inpatient hospital** with a pressure ulcer at one stage and it progresses to a higher stage, two separate codes should be assigned: one code for the site and stage of the ulcer on admission and a second code for the same ulcer site and the highest stage reported during the stay.

b. Non-Pressure Chronic Ulcers

1) Patients admitted with non-pressure ulcers documented as healed
No code is assigned if the documentation states that the non-pressure ulcer is completely healed.

2) Patients admitted with non-pressure ulcers documented as healing
Non-pressure ulcers described as healing should be assigned the appropriate non-pressure ulcer code based on the documentation in the medical record. If the documentation does not provide information about the severity of the healing non-pressure ulcer, assign the appropriate code for unspecified severity.

If the documentation is unclear as to whether the patient has a current (new) non-pressure ulcer or if the patient is being treated for a healing non-pressure ulcer, query the provider.

For ulcers that were present on admission but healed at the time of discharge, assign the code for the site and severity of the non-pressure ulcer at the time of admission.

3) Patient admitted with non-pressure ulcer that progresses to another severity level during the admission
If a patient is admitted to an inpatient hospital with a non-pressure ulcer at one severity level and it progresses to a higher severity level, two separate codes should be assigned: one code for the site and severity level of the ulcer on admission and a second code for the same ulcer site and the highest severity level reported during the stay.

13. Chapter 13: Diseases of the Musculoskeletal System and Connective Tissue (M00-M99)
a. Site and laterality
Most of the codes within Chapter 13 have site and laterality designations. The site represents the bone, joint or the muscle involved. For some conditions where more than one bone, joint or muscle is usually involved, such as osteoarthritis, there is a "multiple sites" code available. For categories where no multiple site code is provided and more than one bone, joint or muscle is involved,

multiple codes should be used to indicate the different sites involved.

1) Bone versus joint
For certain conditions, the bone may be affected at the upper or lower end, (e.g., avascular necrosis of bone, M87, Osteoporosis, M80, M81). Though the portion of the bone affected may be at the joint, the site designation will be the bone, not the joint.

b. Acute traumatic versus chronic or recurrent musculoskeletal conditions
Many musculoskeletal conditions are a result of previous injury or trauma to a site, or are recurrent conditions. Bone, joint or muscle conditions that are the result of a healed injury are usually found in chapter 13. Recurrent bone, joint or muscle conditions are also usually found in chapter 13. Any current, acute injury should be coded to the appropriate injury code from chapter 19. Chronic or recurrent conditions should generally be coded with a code from chapter 13. If it is difficult to determine from the documentation in the record which code is best to describe a condition, query the provider.

c. Coding of Pathologic Fractures
7th character A is for use as long as the patient is receiving active treatment for the fracture. While the patient may be seen by a new or different provider over the course of treatment for a pathological fracture, assignment of the 7th character is based on whether the patient is undergoing active treatment and not whether the provider is seeing the patient for the first time.

7th character D is to be used for encounters after the patient has completed active treatment **for the fracture and is receiving routine care for the fracture during the healing or recovery phase.** The other 7th characters, listed under each subcategory in the Tabular List, are to be used for subsequent encounters for treatment of problems associated with the healing, such as malunions, nonunions, and sequelae.

Care for complications of surgical treatment for fracture repairs during the healing or recovery phase should be coded with the appropriate complication codes.

See Section I.C.19. Coding of traumatic fractures.

d. Osteoporosis
Osteoporosis is a systemic condition, meaning that all bones of the musculoskeletal system are affected. Therefore, site is not a component of the codes under category M81, Osteoporosis without current pathological fracture. The site codes under category M80, Osteoporosis with current pathological fracture, identify the site of the fracture, not the osteoporosis.

1) Osteoporosis without pathological fracture
Category M81, Osteoporosis without current pathological fracture, is for use for patients with osteoporosis who do not currently have a pathologic fracture due to the osteoporosis, even if they have had a fracture in the past. For patients with a history of osteoporosis fractures, status code Z87.310, Personal history of (healed) osteoporosis fracture, should follow the code from M81.

2) Osteoporosis with current pathological fracture
Category M80, Osteoporosis with current pathological fracture, is for patients who have a current pathologic fracture at the time of an encounter. The codes under M80 identify the site of the fracture. A code from category M80, not a traumatic fracture code, should be used for any patient with known osteoporosis who suffers a fracture, even if the patient had a minor fall or trauma, if that fall or trauma would not usually break a normal, healthy bone.

14. Chapter 14: Diseases of Genitourinary System (N00-N99)
a. Chronic kidney disease
1) Stages of chronic kidney disease (CKD)
The ICD-10-CM classifies CKD based on severity. The severity of CKD is designated by stages 1-5. Stage 2, code N18.2, equates to mild CKD; stage 3, code N18.3, equates to moderate CKD; and stage 4, code N18.4, equates to severe CKD. Code N18.6, End stage renal disease (ESRD), is assigned when the provider has documented end-stage-renal disease (ESRD).

If both a stage of CKD and ESRD are documented, assign code N18.6 only.

ICD-10-CM Official Guidelines for Coding and Reporting 2018

2) Chronic kidney disease and kidney transplant status

Patients who have undergone kidney transplant may still have some form of chronic kidney disease (CKD) because the kidney transplant may not fully restore kidney function. Therefore, the presence of CKD alone does not constitute a transplant complication. Assign the appropriate N18 code for the patient's stage of CKD and code Z94.0, Kidney transplant status. If a transplant complication such as failure or rejection or other transplant complication is documented, see section I.C.19.g for information on coding complications of a kidney transplant. If the documentation is unclear as to whether the patient has a complication of the transplant, query the provider.

3) Chronic kidney disease with other conditions

Patients with CKD may also suffer from other serious conditions, most commonly diabetes mellitus and hypertension. The sequencing of the CKD code in relationship to codes for other contributing conditions is based on the conventions in the Tabular List.

See I.C.9. Hypertensive chronic kidney disease.

See I.C.19. Chronic kidney disease and kidney transplant complications.

15. Chapter 15: Pregnancy, Childbirth, and the Puerperium (O00-O9A)

a. General Rules for Obstetric Cases

1) Codes from chapter 15 and sequencing priority

Obstetric cases require codes from chapter 15, codes in the range O00-O9A, Pregnancy, Childbirth, and the Puerperium. Chapter 15 codes have sequencing priority over codes from other chapters. Additional codes from other chapters may be used in conjunction with chapter 15 codes to further specify conditions. Should the provider document that the pregnancy is incidental to the encounter, then code Z33.1, Pregnant state, incidental, should be used in place of any chapter 15 codes. It is the provider's responsibility to state that the condition being treated is not affecting the pregnancy.

2) Chapter 15 codes used only on the maternal record

Chapter 15 codes are to be used only on the maternal record, never on the record of the newborn.

3) Final character for trimester

The majority of codes in Chapter 15 have a final character indicating the trimester of pregnancy. The timeframes for the trimesters are indicated at the beginning of the chapter. If trimester is not a component of a code, it is because the condition always occurs in a specific trimester, or the concept of trimester of pregnancy is not applicable. Certain codes have characters for only certain trimesters because the condition does not occur in all trimesters, but it may occur in more than just one.

Assignment of the final character for trimester should be based on the provider's documentation of the trimester (or number of weeks) for the current admission/encounter. This applies to the assignment of trimester for pre-existing conditions as well as those that develop during or are due to the pregnancy. The provider's documentation of the number of weeks may be used to assign the appropriate code identifying the trimester.

Whenever delivery occurs during the current admission, and there is an "in childbirth" option for the obstetric complication being coded, the "in childbirth" code should be assigned.

4) Selection of trimester for inpatient admissions that encompass more than one trimester

In instances when a patient is admitted to a hospital for complications of pregnancy during one trimester and remains in the hospital into a subsequent trimester, the trimester character for the antepartum complication code should be assigned on the basis of the trimester when the complication developed, not the trimester of the discharge. If the condition developed prior to the current admission/encounter or represents a pre-existing condition, the trimester character for the trimester at the time of the admission/encounter should be assigned.

5) Unspecified trimester

Each category that includes codes for trimester has a code for "unspecified trimester." The "unspecified trimester" code should rarely be used, such as when the documentation in the record is insufficient to determine the trimester and it is not possible to obtain clarification.

6) 7th character for Fetus Identification

Where applicable, a 7th character is to be assigned for certain categories (O31, O32, O33.3 - O33.6, O35, O36, O40, O41, O60.1, O60.2, O64, and O69) to identify the fetus for which the complication code applies.

Assign 7th character "0":

- For single gestations
- When the documentation in the record is insufficient to determine the fetus affected and it is not possible to obtain clarification.
- When it is not possible to clinically determine which fetus is affected.

b. Selection of OB Principal or First-listed Diagnosis

1) Routine outpatient prenatal visits

For routine outpatient prenatal visits when no complications are present, a code from category Z34, Encounter for supervision of normal pregnancy, should be used as the first-listed diagnosis. These codes should not be used in conjunction with chapter 15 codes.

2) Supervision of High-Risk Pregnancy

Codes from category O09, Supervision of high-risk pregnancy, are intended for use only during the prenatal period. For complications during the labor or delivery episode as a result of a high-risk pregnancy, assign the applicable complication codes from Chapter 15. If there are no complications during the labor or delivery episode, assign code O80, Encounter for full-term uncomplicated delivery.

For routine prenatal outpatient visits for patients with high-risk pregnancies, a code from category O09, Supervision of high-risk pregnancy, should be used as the first-listed diagnosis. Secondary chapter 15 codes may be used in conjunction with these codes if appropriate.

3) Episodes when no delivery occurs

In episodes when no delivery occurs, the principal diagnosis should correspond to the principal complication of the pregnancy which necessitated the encounter. Should more than one complication exist, all of which are treated or monitored, any of the complications codes may be sequenced first.

4) When a delivery occurs

When an obstetric patient is admitted and delivers during that admission, the condition that prompted the admission should be sequenced as the principal diagnosis. If multiple conditions prompted the admission, sequence the one most related to the delivery as the principal diagnosis. A code for any complication of the delivery should be assigned as an additional diagnosis. In cases of cesarean delivery, if the patient was admitted with a condition that resulted in the performance of a cesarean procedure, that condition should be selected as the principal diagnosis. If the reason for the admission was unrelated to the condition resulting in the cesarean delivery, the condition related to the reason for the admission should be selected as the principal diagnosis.

5) Outcome of delivery

A code from category Z37, Outcome of delivery, should be included on every maternal record when a delivery has occurred. These codes are not to be used on subsequent records or on the newborn record.

c. Pre-existing conditions versus conditions due to the pregnancy

Certain categories in Chapter 15 distinguish between conditions of the mother that existed prior to pregnancy (pre-existing) and those that are a direct result of pregnancy. When assigning codes from Chapter 15, it is important to assess if a condition was pre-existing prior to pregnancy or developed during or due to the pregnancy in order to assign the correct code.

Categories that do not distinguish between pre-existing and pregnancy-related conditions may be used for either. It is acceptable to use codes specifically for the puerperium with codes complicating pregnancy and childbirth if a condition arises postpartum during the delivery encounter.

d. **Pre-existing hypertension in pregnancy**
Category O10, Pre-existing hypertension complicating pregnancy, childbirth and the puerperium, includes codes for hypertensive heart and hypertensive chronic kidney disease. When assigning one of the O10 codes that includes hypertensive heart disease or hypertensive chronic kidney disease, it is necessary to add a secondary code from the appropriate hypertension category to specify the type of heart failure or chronic kidney disease.
See Section I.C.9. Hypertension.

e. **Fetal Conditions Affecting the Management of the Mother**
1) **Codes from categories O35 and O36**
Codes from categories O35, Maternal care for known or suspected fetal abnormality and damage, and O36, Maternal care for other fetal problems, are assigned only when the fetal condition is actually responsible for modifying the management of the mother, i.e., by requiring diagnostic studies, additional observation, special care, or termination of pregnancy. The fact that the fetal condition exists does not justify assigning a code from this series to the mother's record.

2) **In utero surgery**
In cases when surgery is performed on the fetus, a diagnosis code from category O35, Maternal care for known or suspected fetal abnormality and damage, should be assigned identifying the fetal condition. Assign the appropriate procedure code for the procedure performed.

No code from Chapter 16, the perinatal codes, should be used on the mother's record to identify fetal conditions. Surgery performed in utero on a fetus is still to be coded as an obstetric encounter.

f. **HIV Infection in Pregnancy, Childbirth and the Puerperium**
During pregnancy, childbirth or the puerperium, a patient admitted because of an HIV-related illness should receive a principal diagnosis from subcategory O98.7-, Human immunodeficiency [HIV] disease complicating pregnancy, childbirth and the puerperium, followed by the code(s) for the HIV-related illness(es).

Patients with asymptomatic HIV infection status admitted during pregnancy, childbirth, or the puerperium should receive codes of O98.7- and Z21, Asymptomatic human immunodeficiency virus [HIV] infection status.

g. **Diabetes mellitus in pregnancy**
Diabetes mellitus is a significant complicating factor in pregnancy. Pregnant women who are diabetic should be assigned a code from category O24, Diabetes mellitus in pregnancy, childbirth, and the puerperium, first, followed by the appropriate diabetes code(s) (E08-E13) from Chapter 4.

h. **Long term use of insulin and oral hypoglycemics**
See section I.C.4.a.3 for information on the long term use of insulin and oral hypoglycemic.

i. **Gestational (pregnancy induced) diabetes**
Gestational (pregnancy induced) diabetes can occur during the second and third trimester of pregnancy in women who were not diabetic prior to pregnancy. Gestational diabetes can cause complications in the pregnancy similar to those of pre-existing diabetes mellitus. It also puts the woman at greater risk of developing diabetes after the pregnancy. Codes for gestational diabetes are in subcategory O24.4, Gestational diabetes mellitus. No other code from category O24, Diabetes mellitus in pregnancy, childbirth, and the puerperium, should be used with a code from O24.4.

The codes under subcategory O24.4 include diet controlled, insulin controlled, and controlled by oral hypoglycemic drugs. If a patient with gestational diabetes is treated with both diet and insulin, only the code for insulin-controlled is required. If a patient with gestational diabetes is treated with both diet and oral hypoglycemic medications, only the code for "controlled by oral hypoglycemic drugs" is required. Code Z79.4, Long-term (current) use of insulin or code Z79.84, Long-term (current) use of oral hypoglycemic drugs, should not be assigned with codes from subcategory O24.4.

An abnormal glucose tolerance in pregnancy is assigned a code from subcategory O99.81, Abnormal glucose complicating pregnancy, childbirth, and the puerperium.

j. **Sepsis and septic shock complicating abortion, pregnancy, childbirth and the puerperium**
When assigning a chapter 15 code for sepsis complicating abortion, pregnancy, childbirth, and the puerperium, a code for the specific type of infection should be assigned as an additional diagnosis. If severe sepsis is present, a code from subcategory R65.2, Severe sepsis, and code(s) for associated organ dysfunction(s) should also be assigned as additional diagnoses.

k. **Puerperal sepsis**
Code O85, Puerperal sepsis, should be assigned with a secondary code to identify the causal organism (e.g., for a bacterial infection, assign a code from category B95-B96, Bacterial infections in conditions classified elsewhere). A code from category A40, Streptococcal sepsis, or A41, Other sepsis, should not be used for puerperal sepsis. If applicable, use additional codes to identify severe sepsis (R65.2-) and any associated acute organ dysfunction.

l. **Alcohol and tobacco use during pregnancy, childbirth and the puerperium**
1) **Alcohol use during pregnancy, childbirth and the puerperium**
Codes under subcategory O99.31, Alcohol use complicating pregnancy, childbirth, and the puerperium, should be assigned for any pregnancy case when a mother uses alcohol during the pregnancy or postpartum. A secondary code from category F10, Alcohol related disorders, should also be assigned to identify manifestations of the alcohol use.

2) **Tobacco use during pregnancy, childbirth and the puerperium**
Codes under subcategory O99.33, Smoking (tobacco) complicating pregnancy, childbirth, and the puerperium, should be assigned for any pregnancy case when a mother uses any type of tobacco product during the pregnancy or postpartum. A secondary code from category F17, Nicotine dependence, should also be assigned to identify the type of nicotine dependence.

m. **Poisoning, toxic effects, adverse effects and underdosing in a pregnant patient**
A code from subcategory O9A.2, Injury, poisoning and certain other consequences of external causes complicating pregnancy, childbirth, and the puerperium, should be sequenced first, followed by the appropriate injury, poisoning, toxic effect, adverse effect or underdosing code, and then the additional code(s) that specifies the condition caused by the poisoning, toxic effect, adverse effect or underdosing.
See Section I.C.19. Adverse effects, poisoning, underdosing and toxic effects.

n. **Normal Delivery, Code O80**
1) **Encounter for full term uncomplicated delivery**
Code O80 should be assigned when a woman is admitted for a full-term normal delivery and delivers a single, healthy infant without any complications antepartum, during the delivery, or postpartum during the delivery episode. Code O80 is always a principal diagnosis. It is not to be used if any other code from chapter 15 is needed to describe a current complication of the antenatal, delivery, or perinatal period. Additional codes from other chapters may be used with code O80 if they are not related to or are in any way complicating the pregnancy.

2) **Uncomplicated delivery with resolved antepartum complication**
Code O80 may be used if the patient had a complication at some point during the pregnancy, but the complication is not present at the time of the admission for delivery.

3) **Outcome of delivery for O80**
Z37.0, Single live birth, is the only outcome of delivery code appropriate for use with O80.

o. **The Peripartum and Postpartum Periods**
1) **Peripartum and Postpartum periods**
The postpartum period begins immediately after delivery and continues for six weeks following delivery. The peripartum period is defined as the last month of pregnancy to five months postpartum.

ICD-10-CM Official Guidelines for Coding and Reporting 2018

2) Peripartum and postpartum complication
A postpartum complication is any complication occurring within the six-week period.

3) Pregnancy-related complications after 6 week period
Chapter 15 codes may also be used to describe pregnancy-related complications after the peripartum or postpartum period if the provider documents that a condition is pregnancy related.

4) Admission for routine postpartum care following delivery outside hospital
When the mother delivers outside the hospital prior to admission and is admitted for routine postpartum care and no complications are noted, code Z39.0, Encounter for care and examination of mother immediately after delivery, should be assigned as the principal diagnosis.

5) Pregnancy associated cardiomyopathy
Pregnancy associated cardiomyopathy, code O90.3, is unique in that it may be diagnosed in the third trimester of pregnancy but may continue to progress months after delivery. For this reason, it is referred to as peripartum cardiomyopathy. Code O90.3 is only for use when the cardiomyopathy develops as a result of pregnancy in a woman who did not have pre-existing heart disease.

p. Code O94, Sequelae of complication of pregnancy, childbirth, and the puerperium

1) Code O94
Code O94, Sequelae of complication of pregnancy, childbirth, and the puerperium, is for use in those cases when an initial complication of a pregnancy develops a sequelae requiring care or treatment at a future date.

2) After the initial postpartum period
This code may be used at any time after the initial postpartum period.

3) Sequencing of Code O94
This code, like all sequela codes, is to be sequenced following the code describing the sequelae of the complication.

q. Termination of Pregnancy and Spontaneous abortions

1) Abortion with Liveborn Fetus
When an attempted termination of pregnancy results in a liveborn fetus, assign code Z33.2, Encounter for elective termination of pregnancy and a code from category Z37, Outcome of Delivery.

2) Retained Products of Conception following an abortion
Subsequent encounters for retained products of conception following a spontaneous abortion or elective termination of pregnancy, **without complications** are assigned O03.**4, Incomplete spontaneous,** abortion **without complication,** or codes O07.4, Failed attempted termination of pregnancy without complication. This advice is appropriate even when the patient was discharged previously with a discharge diagnosis of complete abortion. **If the patient has a specific complication associated with the spontaneous abortion or elective termination of pregnancy in addition to retained products of conception, assign the appropriate complication in category O03 or O07 instead of code O03.4 or O07.4**

3) Complications leading to abortion
Codes from Chapter 15 may be used as additional codes to identify any documented complications of the pregnancy in conjunction with codes in categories in **O04,** O07 and O08.

r. Abuse in a pregnant patient
For suspected or confirmed cases of abuse of a pregnant patient, a code(s) from subcategories O9A.3, Physical abuse complicating pregnancy, childbirth, and the puerperium, O9A.4, Sexual abuse complicating pregnancy, childbirth, and the puerperium, and O9A.5, Psychological abuse complicating pregnancy, childbirth, and the puerperium, should be sequenced first, followed by the appropriate codes (if applicable) to identify any associated current injury due to physical abuse, sexual abuse, and the perpetrator of abuse.

See Section I.C.19. Adult and child abuse, neglect and other maltreatment.

16. Chapter 16: Certain Conditions Originating in the Perinatal Period (P00-P96)
For coding and reporting purposes the perinatal period is defined as before birth through the 28th day following birth. The following guidelines are provided for reporting purposes.

a. General Perinatal Rules

1) Use of Chapter 16 Codes
Codes in this chapter are never for use on the maternal record. Codes from Chapter 15, the obstetric chapter, are never permitted on the newborn record. Chapter 16 codes may be used throughout the life of the patient if the condition is still present.

2) Principal Diagnosis for Birth Record
When coding the birth episode in a newborn record, assign a code from category Z38, Liveborn infants according to place of birth and type of delivery, as the principal diagnosis. A code from category Z38 is assigned only once, to a newborn at the time of birth. If a newborn is transferred to another institution, a code from category Z38 should not be used at the receiving hospital.

A code from category Z38 is used only on the newborn record, not on the mother's record.

3) Use of Codes from other Chapters with Codes from Chapter 16
Codes from other chapters may be used with codes from chapter 16 if the codes from the other chapters provide more specific detail. Codes for signs and symptoms may be assigned when a definitive diagnosis has not been established. If the reason for the encounter is a perinatal condition, the code from chapter 16 should be sequenced first.

4) Use of Chapter 16 Codes after the Perinatal Period
Should a condition originate in the perinatal period, and continue throughout the life of the patient, the perinatal code should continue to be used regardless of the patient's age.

5) Birth process or community acquired conditions
If a newborn has a condition that may be either due to the birth process or community acquired and the documentation does not indicate which it is, the default is due to the birth process and the code from Chapter 16 should be used. If the condition is community-acquired, a code from Chapter 16 should not be assigned.

6) Code all clinically significant conditions
All clinically significant conditions noted on routine newborn examination should be coded. A condition is clinically significant if it requires:

- clinical evaluation; or
- therapeutic treatment; or
- diagnostic procedures; or
- extended length of hospital stay; or
- increased nursing care and/or monitoring; or
- has implications for future health care needs

Note: The perinatal guidelines listed above are the same as the general coding guidelines for "additional diagnoses", except for the final point regarding implications for future health care needs. Codes should be assigned for conditions that have been specified by the provider as having implications for future health care needs.

b. Observation and Evaluation of Newborns for Suspected Conditions not Found

1) *Use of Z05 codes*
Assign a code from category Z05, Observation and evaluation of newborns and infants for suspected conditions ruled out, to identify those instances when a healthy newborn is evaluated for a suspected condition that is determined after study not to be present. Do not use a code from category Z05 when the patient has identified signs or symptoms of a suspected problem; in such cases code the sign or symptom.

2) *Z05 on Other than the Birth Record*
A code from category Z05 may also be assigned as a principal or first-listed code for readmissions or encounters when the code from category Z38 code no longer applies. Codes from category

Z05 are for use only for healthy newborns and infants for which no condition after study is found to be present.

3) **Z05 on a birth record**
A code from category Z05 is to be used as a secondary code after the code from category Z38, Liveborn infants according to place of birth and type of delivery.

c. **Coding Additional Perinatal Diagnoses**
1) **Assigning codes for conditions that require treatment**
Assign codes for conditions that require treatment or further investigation, prolong the length of stay, or require resource utilization.

2) **Codes for conditions specified as having implications for future health care needs**
Assign codes for conditions that have been specified by the provider as having implications for future health care needs.

Note: This guideline should not be used for adult patients.

d. **Prematurity and Fetal Growth Retardation**
Providers utilize different criteria in determining prematurity. A code for prematurity should not be assigned unless it is documented. Assignment of codes in categories P05, Disorders of newborn related to slow fetal growth and fetal malnutrition, and P07, Disorders of newborn related to short gestation and low birth weight, not elsewhere classified, should be based on the recorded birth weight and estimated gestational age.

When both birth weight and gestational age are available, two codes from category P07 should be assigned, with the code for birth weight sequenced before the code for gestational age.

e. **Low birth weight and immaturity status**
Codes from category P07, Disorders of newborn related to short gestation and low birth weight, not elsewhere classified, are for use for a child or adult who was premature or had a low birth weight as a newborn and this is affecting the patient's current health status.

See Section I.C.21. Factors influencing health status and contact with health services, Status.

f. **Bacterial Sepsis of Newborn**
Category P36, Bacterial sepsis of newborn, includes congenital sepsis. If a perinate is documented as having sepsis without documentation of congenital or community acquired, the default is congenital and a code from category P36 should be assigned. If the P36 code includes the causal organism, an additional code from category B95, Streptococcus, Staphylococcus, and Enterococcus as the cause of diseases classified elsewhere, or B96, Other bacterial agents as the cause of diseases classified elsewhere, should not be assigned. If the P36 code does not include the causal organism, assign an additional code from category B96. If applicable, use additional codes to identify severe sepsis (R65.2-) and any associated acute organ dysfunction.

g. **Stillbirth**
Code P95, Stillbirth, is only for use in institutions that maintain separate records for stillbirths. No other code should be used with P95. Code P95 should not be used on the mother's record.

17. **Chapter 17: Congenital malformations, deformations, and chromosomal abnormalities (Q00-Q99)**
Assign an appropriate code(s) from categories Q00-Q99, Congenital malformations, deformations, and chromosomal abnormalities when a malformation/deformation or chromosomal abnormality is documented. A malformation/deformation/or chromosomal abnormality may be the principal/first-listed diagnosis on a record or a secondary diagnosis.

When a malformation/deformation or chromosomal abnormality does not have a unique code assignment, assign additional code(s) for any manifestations that may be present.

When the code assignment specifically identifies the malformation/deformation or chromosomal abnormality, manifestations that are an inherent component of the anomaly should not be coded separately. Additional codes should be assigned for manifestations that are not an inherent component.

Codes from Chapter 17 may be used throughout the life of the patient. If a congenital malformation or deformity has been corrected, a personal history code should be used to identify the history of the malformation or deformity. Although present at birth, malformation/deformation/or chromosomal abnormality may not be identified until later in life.

Whenever the condition is diagnosed by the physician, it is appropriate to assign a code from codes Q00-Q99.For the birth admission, the appropriate code from category Z38, Liveborn infants, according to place of birth and type of delivery, should be sequenced as the principal diagnosis, followed by any congenital anomaly codes, Q00- Q99.

18. **Chapter 18: Symptoms, signs, and abnormal clinical and laboratory findings, not elsewhere classified (R00-R99)**
Chapter 18 includes symptoms, signs, abnormal results of clinical or other investigative procedures, and ill-defined conditions regarding which no diagnosis classifiable elsewhere is recorded. Signs and symptoms that point to a specific diagnosis have been assigned to a category in other chapters of the classification.

a. **Use of symptom codes**
Codes that describe symptoms and signs are acceptable for reporting purposes when a related definitive diagnosis has not been established (confirmed) by the provider.

b. **Use of a symptom code with a definitive diagnosis code**
Codes for signs and symptoms may be reported in addition to a related definitive diagnosis when the sign or symptom is not routinely associated with that diagnosis, such as the various signs and symptoms associated with complex syndromes. The definitive diagnosis code should be sequenced before the symptom code.

Signs or symptoms that are associated routinely with a disease process should not be assigned as additional codes, unless otherwise instructed by the classification.

c. **Combination codes that include symptoms**
ICD-10-CM contains a number of combination codes that identify both the definitive diagnosis and common symptoms of that diagnosis.

When using one of these combination codes, an additional code should not be assigned for the symptom.

d. **Repeated falls**
Code R29.6, Repeated falls, is for use for encounters when a patient has recently fallen and the reason for the fall is being investigated.

Code Z91.81, History of falling, is for use when a patient has fallen in the past and is at risk for future falls. When appropriate, both codes R29.6 and Z91.81 may be assigned together.

e. **Coma scale**
The coma scale codes (R40.2-) can be used in conjunction with traumatic brain injury codes, acute cerebrovascular disease or sequelae of cerebrovascular disease codes. These codes are primarily for use by trauma registries, but they may be used in any setting where this information is collected. The coma scale may also be used to assess the status of the central nervous system for other non-trauma conditions, such as monitoring patients in the intensive care unit regardless of medical condition. The coma scale codes should be sequenced after the diagnosis code(s).

These codes, one from each subcategory, are needed to complete the scale. The 7th character indicates when the scale was recorded. The 7th character should match for all three codes.

At a minimum, report the initial score documented on presentation at your facility. This may be a score from the emergency medicine technician (EMT) or in the emergency department. If desired, a facility may choose to capture multiple coma scale scores.

Assign code R40.24, Glasgow coma scale, total score, when only the total score is documented in the medical record and not the individual score(s).

f. **Functional quadriplegia**
GUIDELINE HAS BEEN DELETED EFFECTIVE OCTOBER 1, 2017

g. **SIRS due to Non-Infectious Process**
The systemic inflammatory response syndrome (SIRS) can develop as a result of certain non-infectious disease processes, such as trauma, malignant neoplasm, or pancreatitis. When SIRS is documented with a noninfectious condition, and no subsequent infection is documented, the code for the underlying condition, such as an injury, should be assigned, followed by code R65.10, Systemic inflammatory response syndrome (SIRS) of non-infectious origin without acute organ dysfunction, or code R65.11, Systemic inflammatory response syndrome (SIRS) of non-infectious origin with acute organ dysfunction. If an associated acute organ dysfunction is documented, the appropriate code(s) for the specific type of organ dysfunction(s) should be assigned in addition to code

R65.11. If acute organ dysfunction is documented, but it cannot be determined if the acute organ dysfunction is associated with SIRS or due to another condition (e.g., directly due to the trauma), the provider should be queried.

h.   Death NOS

Code R99, Ill-defined and unknown cause of mortality, is only for use in the very limited circumstance when a patient who has already died is brought into an emergency department or other healthcare facility and is pronounced dead upon arrival. It does not represent the discharge disposition of death.

i.   NIHSS Stroke Scale

The NIH stroke scale (NIHSS) codes (R29.7- -) can be used in conjunction with acute stroke codes (I63) to identify the patient's neurological status and the severity of the stroke. The stroke scale codes should be sequenced after the acute stroke diagnosis code(s).

At a minimum, report the initial score documented. If desired, a facility may choose to capture multiple stroke scale scores.

See Section I.B.14. for information concerning the medical record documentation that may be used for assignment of the NIHSS codes.

19. Chapter 19: Injury, poisoning, and certain other consequences of external causes (S00-T88)

a.   Application of 7th Characters in Chapter 19

Most categories in chapter 19 have a 7th character requirement for each applicable code. Most categories in this chapter have three 7th character values (with the exception of fractures): A, initial encounter, D, subsequent encounter and S, sequela. Categories for traumatic fractures have additional 7th character values. While the patient may be seen by a new or different provider over the course of treatment for an injury, assignment of the 7th character is based on whether the patient is undergoing active treatment and not whether the provider is seeing the patient for the first time.

For complication codes, active treatment refers to treatment for the condition described by the code, even though it may be related to an earlier precipitating problem. For example, code T84.50XA, Infection and inflammatory reaction due to unspecified internal joint prosthesis, initial encounter, is used when active treatment is provided for the infection, even though the condition relates to the prosthetic device, implant or graft that was placed at a previous encounter.

7th character "A", initial encounter is used for each encounter where the patient is receiving active treatment for the condition.

7th character "D" subsequent encounter is used for encounters after the patient has completed active treatment of the condition and is receiving routine care for the condition during the healing or recovery phase.

The aftercare Z codes should not be used for aftercare for conditions such as injuries or poisonings, where 7th characters are provided to identify subsequent care. For example, for aftercare of an injury, assign the acute injury code with the 7th character "D" (subsequent encounter).

7th character "S", sequela, is for use for complications or conditions that arise as a direct result of a condition, such as scar formation after a burn. The scars are sequelae of the burn. When using 7th character "S", it is necessary to use both the injury code that precipitated the sequela and the code for the sequela itself. The "S" is added only to the injury code, not the sequela code. The 7th character "S" identifies the injury responsible for the sequela. The specific type of sequela (e.g. scar) is sequenced first, followed by the injury code.

See Section I.B.10 Sequelae, (Late Effects)

b.   Coding of Injuries

When coding injuries, assign separate codes for each injury unless a combination code is provided, in which case the combination code is assigned. **Codes from category T07,** Unspecified multiple injuries should not be assigned in the inpatient setting unless information for a more specific code is not available. Traumatic injury codes (S00-T14.9) are not to be used for normal, healing surgical wounds or to identify complications of surgical wounds.

The code for the most serious injury, as determined by the provider and the focus of treatment, is sequenced first.

1)   Superficial injuries

Superficial injuries such as abrasions or contusions are not coded when associated with more severe injuries of the same site.

2)   Primary injury with damage to nerves/blood vessels

When a primary injury results in minor damage to peripheral nerves or blood vessels, the primary injury is sequenced first with additional code(s) for injuries to nerves and spinal cord (such as category S04), and/or injury to blood vessels (such as category S15). When the primary injury is to the blood vessels or nerves, that injury should be sequenced first.

c.   Coding of Traumatic Fractures

The principles of multiple coding of injuries should be followed in coding fractures. Fractures of specified sites are coded individually by site in accordance with both the provisions within categories S02, S12, S22, S32, S42, S49, S52, S59, S62, S72, S79, S82, S89, S92 and the level of detail furnished by medical record content.

A fracture not indicated as open or closed should be coded to closed. A fracture not indicated whether displaced or not displaced should be coded to displaced.

More specific guidelines are as follows:

1)   Initial vs. Subsequent Encounter for Fractures

Traumatic fractures are coded using the appropriate 7th character for initial encounter (A, B, C) for each encounter where the patient is receiving active treatment for the fracture. The appropriate 7th character for initial encounter should also be assigned for a patient who delayed seeking treatment for the fracture or nonunion.

Fractures are coded using the appropriate 7th character for subsequent care for encounters after the patient has completed active treatment of the fracture and is receiving routine care for the fracture during the healing or recovery phase.

Care for complications of surgical treatment for fracture repairs during the healing or recovery phase should be coded with the appropriate complication codes.

Care of complications of fractures, such as malunion and nonunion, should be reported with the appropriate 7th character for subsequent care with nonunion (K, M, N,) or subsequent care with malunion (P, Q, R).

Malunion/nonunion: The appropriate 7th character for initial encounter should also be assigned for a patient who delayed seeking treatment for the fracture or nonunion.

The open fracture designations in the assignment of the 7th character for fractures of the forearm, femur and lower leg, including ankle are based on the Gustilo open fracture classification. When the Gustilo classification type is not specified for an open fracture, the 7th character for open fracture type I or II should be assigned (B, E, H, M, Q).

A code from category M80, not a traumatic fracture code, should be used for any patient with known osteoporosis who suffers a fracture, even if the patient had a minor fall or trauma, if that fall or trauma would not usually break a normal, healthy bone.

See Section I.C.13. Osteoporosis.

The aftercare Z codes should not be used for aftercare for traumatic fractures. For aftercare of a traumatic fracture, assign the acute fracture code with the appropriate 7th character.

2)   Multiple fractures sequencing

Multiple fractures are sequenced in accordance with the severity of the fracture.

d.   Coding of Burns and Corrosions

The ICD-10-CM makes a distinction between burns and corrosions. The burn codes are for thermal burns, except sunburns, that come from a heat source, such as a fire or hot appliance. The burn codes are also for burns resulting from electricity and radiation. Corrosions are burns due to chemicals. The guidelines are the same for burns and corrosions.

Current burns (T20-T25) are classified by depth, extent and by agent (X code). Burns are classified by depth as first degree (erythema), second degree (blistering), and third degree (full-thickness involvement). Burns of the eye and internal organs (T26-T28) are classified by site, but not by degree.

1) **Sequencing of burn and related condition codes**
Sequence first the code that reflects the highest degree of burn when more than one burn is present.

   a. When the reason for the admission or encounter is for treatment of external multiple burns, sequence first the code that reflects the burn of the highest degree.

   b. When a patient has both internal and external burns, the circumstances of admission govern the selection of the principal diagnosis or first-listed diagnosis.

   c. When a patient is admitted for burn injuries and other related conditions such as smoke inhalation and/or respiratory failure, the circumstances of admission govern the selection of the principal or first-listed diagnosis.

2) **Burns of the same local site**
Classify burns of the same local site (three-character category level, T20-T28) but of different degrees to the subcategory identifying the highest degree recorded in the diagnosis.

3) **Non-healing burns**
Non-healing burns are coded as acute burns.

   Necrosis of burned skin should be coded as a non-healed burn.

4) **Infected Burn**
For any documented infected burn site, use an additional code for the infection.

5) **Assign separate codes for each burn site**
When coding burns, assign separate codes for each burn site. Category T30, Burn and corrosion, body region unspecified is extremely vague and should rarely be used.

6) **Burns and Corrosions Classified According to Extent of Body Surface Involved**
Assign codes from category T31, Burns classified according to extent of body surface involved, or T32, Corrosions classified according to extent of body surface involved, when the site of the burn is not specified or when there is a need for additional data. It is advisable to use category T31 as additional coding when needed to provide data for evaluating burn mortality, such as that needed by burn units. It is also advisable to use category T31 as an additional code for reporting purposes when there is mention of a third-degree burn involving 20 percent or more of the body surface.

   Categories T31 and T32 are based on the classic "rule of nines" in estimating body surface involved: head and neck are assigned nine percent, each arm nine percent, each leg 18 percent, the anterior trunk 18 percent, posterior trunk 18 percent, and genitalia one percent. Providers may change these percentage assignments where necessary to accommodate infants and children who have proportionally larger heads than adults, and patients who have large buttocks, thighs, or abdomen that involve burns.

7) **Encounters for treatment of sequela of burns**
Encounters for the treatment of the late effects of burns or corrosions (i.e., scars or joint contractures) should be coded with a burn or corrosion code with the 7th character "S" for sequela.

8) **Sequelae with a late effect code and current burn**
When appropriate, both a code for a current burn or corrosion with 7th character "A" or "D" and a burn or corrosion code with 7th character "S" may be assigned on the same record (when both a current burn and sequelae of an old burn exist). Burns and corrosions do not heal at the same rate and a current healing wound may still exist with sequela of a healed burn or corrosion.

   See Section I.B.10 Sequela (Late Effects)

9) **Use of an external cause code with burns and corrosions**
An external cause code should be used with burns and corrosions to identify the source and intent of the burn, as well as the place where it occurred.

e. **Adverse Effects, Poisoning, Underdosing and Toxic Effects**
Codes in categories T36-T65 are combination codes that include the substance that was taken as well as the intent. No additional external cause code is required for poisonings, toxic effects, adverse effects and underdosing codes.

1) **Do not code directly from the Table of Drugs**
Do not code directly from the Table of Drugs and Chemicals. Always refer back to the Tabular List.

2) **Use as many codes as necessary to describe**
Use as many codes as necessary to describe completely all drugs, medicinal or biological substances.

3) **If the same code would describe the causative agent**
If the same code would describe the causative agent for more than one adverse reaction, poisoning, toxic effect or underdosing, assign the code only once.

4) **If two or more drugs, medicinal or biological substances**
If two or more drugs, medicinal or biological substances are reported, code each individually unless a combination code is listed in the Table of Drugs and Chemicals.

5) **The occurrence of drug toxicity is classified in ICD-10-CM as follows:**

   (a) **Adverse Effect**
   When coding an adverse effect of a drug that has been correctly prescribed and properly administered, assign the appropriate code for the nature of the adverse effect followed by the appropriate code for the adverse effect of the drug (T36-T50). The code for the drug should have a 5th or 6th character "5" (for example T36.0X5-) Examples of the nature of an adverse effect are tachycardia, delirium, gastrointestinal hemorrhaging, vomiting, hypokalemia, hepatitis, renal failure, or respiratory failure.

   (b) **Poisoning**
   When coding a poisoning or reaction to the improper use of a medication (e.g., overdose, wrong substance given or taken in error, wrong route of administration), first assign the appropriate code from categories T36-T50. The poisoning codes have an associated intent as their 5th or 6th character (accidental, intentional self-harm, assault and undetermined. If the intent of the poisoning is unknown or unspecified, code the intent as accidental intent. The undetermined intent is only for use if the documentation in the record specifies that the intent cannot be determined. Use additional code(s) for all manifestations of poisonings.

   If there is also a diagnosis of abuse or dependence of the substance, the abuse or dependence is assigned as an additional code.

   Examples of poisoning include:

   (i) Error was made in drug prescription
   Errors made in drug prescription or in the administration of the drug by provider, nurse, patient, or other person.

   (ii) Overdose of a drug intentionally taken
   If an overdose of a drug was intentionally taken or administered and resulted in drug toxicity, it would be coded as a poisoning.

   (iii) Nonprescribed drug taken with correctly prescribed and properly administered drug
   If a nonprescribed drug or medicinal agent was taken in combination with a correctly prescribed and properly administered drug, any drug toxicity or other reaction resulting from the interaction of the two drugs would be classified as a poisoning.

   (iv) Interaction of drug(s) and alcohol
   When a reaction results from the interaction of a drug(s) and alcohol, this would be classified as poisoning.

   See Section I.C.4. if poisoning is the result of insulin pump malfunctions.

   (c) **Underdosing**
   Underdosing refers to taking less of a medication than is prescribed by a provider or a manufacturer's instruction. For underdosing, assign the code from categories T36-T50 (fifth or sixth character "6").

   Codes for underdosing should never be assigned as principal or first-listed codes. If a patient has a relapse or exacerbation of the medical condition for which the drug is prescribed because of the reduction in dose, then the medical condition itself should be coded.

Noncompliance (Z91.12-, Z91.13-) or complication of care (Y63.6-Y63.9) codes are to be used with an underdosing code to indicate intent, if known.

(d) Toxic Effects

When a harmful substance is ingested or comes in contact with a person, this is classified as a toxic effect. The toxic effect codes are in categories T51-T65.

Toxic effect codes have an associated intent: accidental, intentional self-harm, assault and undetermined.

f. Adult and child abuse, neglect and other maltreatment

Sequence first the appropriate code from categories T74, Adult and child abuse, neglect and other maltreatment, confirmed) or T76, Adult and child abuse, neglect and other maltreatment, suspected) for abuse, neglect and other maltreatment, followed by any accompanying mental health or injury code(s).

If the documentation in the medical record states abuse or neglect it is coded as confirmed (T74.-). It is coded as suspected if it is documented as suspected (T76.-).

For cases of confirmed abuse or neglect an external cause code from the assault section (X92-Y09) should be added to identify the cause of any physical injuries. A perpetrator code (Y07) should be added when the perpetrator of the abuse is known. For suspected cases of abuse or neglect, do not report external cause or perpetrator code.

If a suspected case of abuse, neglect or mistreatment is ruled out during an encounter code Z04.71, Encounter for examination and observation following alleged physical adult abuse, ruled out, or code Z04.72, Encounter for examination and observation following alleged child physical abuse, ruled out, should be used, not a code from T76.

If a suspected case of alleged rape or sexual abuse is ruled out during an encounter code Z04.41, Encounter for examination and observation following alleged adult rape or code Z04.42, Encounter for examination and observation following alleged child rape, should be used, not a code from T76.

See Section I.C.15. Abuse in a pregnant patient.

g. Complications of care

1) General guidelines for complications of care

(a) Documentation of complications of care

See Section I.B.16. for information on documentation of complications of care.

2) Pain due to medical devices

Pain associated with devices, implants or grafts left in a surgical site (for example painful hip prosthesis) is assigned to the appropriate code(s) found in Chapter 19, Injury, poisoning, and certain other consequences of external causes. Specific codes for pain due to medical devices are found in the T code section of the ICD-10-CM. Use additional code(s) from category G89 to identify acute or chronic pain due to presence of the device, implant or graft (G89.18 or G89.28).

3) Transplant complications

(a) Transplant complications other than kidney

Codes under category T86, Complications of transplanted organs and tissues, are for use for both complications and rejection of transplanted organs. A transplant complication code is only assigned if the complication affects the function of the transplanted organ. Two codes are required to fully describe a transplant complication: the appropriate code from category T86 and a secondary code that identifies the complication.

Pre-existing conditions or conditions that develop after the transplant are not coded as complications unless they affect the function of the transplanted organs.

See I.C.21. for transplant organ removal status

See I.C.2. for malignant neoplasm associated with transplanted organ.

(b) Kidney transplant complications

Patients who have undergone kidney transplant may still have some form of chronic kidney disease (CKD) because the kidney transplant may not fully restore kidney function.

Code T86.1- should be assigned for documented complications of a kidney transplant, such as transplant failure or rejection or other transplant complication. Code T86.1- should not be assigned for post kidney transplant patients who have chronic kidney (CKD) unless a transplant complication such as transplant failure or rejection is documented. If the documentation is unclear as to whether the patient has a complication of the transplant, query the provider.

Conditions that affect the function of the transplanted kidney, other than CKD, should be assigned a code from subcategory T86.1, Complications of transplanted organ, Kidney, and a secondary code that identifies the complication.

For patients with CKD following a kidney transplant, but who do not have a complication such as failure or rejection, *see section I.C.14. Chronic kidney disease and kidney transplant status.*

4) Complication codes that include the external cause

As with certain other T codes, some of the complications of care codes have the external cause included in the code. The code includes the nature of the complication as well as the type of procedure that caused the complication. No external cause code indicating the type of procedure is necessary for these codes.

5) Complications of care codes within the body system chapters

Intraoperative and postprocedural complication codes are found within the body system chapters with codes specific to the organs and structures of that body system. These codes should be sequenced first, followed by a code(s) for the specific complication, if applicable.

20. Chapter 20: External Causes of Morbidity (V00-Y99)

The external causes of morbidity codes should never be sequenced as the first-listed or principal diagnosis.

External cause codes are intended to provide data for injury research and evaluation of injury prevention strategies. These codes capture how the injury or health condition happened (cause), the intent (unintentional or accidental; or intentional, such as suicide or assault), the place where the event occurred the activity of the patient at the time of the event, and the person's status (e.g., civilian, military).

There is no national requirement for mandatory ICD-10-CM external cause code reporting. Unless a provider is subject to a state-based external cause code reporting mandate or these codes are required by a particular payer, reporting of ICD-10-CM codes in Chapter 20, External Causes of Morbidity, is not required. In the absence of a mandatory reporting requirement, providers are encouraged to voluntarily report external cause codes, as they provide valuable data for injury research and evaluation of injury prevention strategies.

a. General External Cause Coding Guidelines

1) Used with any code in the range of A00.0-T88.9 Z00-Z99

An external cause code may be used with any code in the range of A00.0-T88.9, Z00-Z99, classification that represents a health condition due to an external cause. Though they are most applicable to injuries, they are also valid for use with such things as infections or diseases due to an external source, and other health conditions, such as a heart attack that occurs during strenuous physical activity.

2) External cause code used for length of treatment

Assign the external cause code, with the appropriate 7th character (initial encounter, subsequent encounter or sequela) for each encounter for which the injury or condition is being treated.

Most categories in chapter 20 have a 7th character requirement for each applicable code. Most categories in this chapter have three 7th character values: A, initial encounter, D, subsequent encounter and S, sequela. While the patient may be seen by a new or different provider over the course of treatment for an injury or condition, assignment of the 7th character for external cause should match the 7th character of the code assigned for the associated injury or condition for the encounter.

3) Use the full range of external cause codes
Use the full range of external cause codes to completely describe the cause, the intent, the place of occurrence, and if applicable, the activity of the patient at the time of the event, and the patient's status, for all injuries, and other health conditions due to an external cause.

4) Assign as many external cause codes as necessary
Assign as many external cause codes as necessary to fully explain each cause. If only one external code can be recorded, assign the code most related to the principal diagnosis.

5) The selection of the appropriate external cause code
The selection of the appropriate external cause code is guided by the Alphabetic Index of External Causes and by Inclusion and Exclusion notes in the Tabular List.

6) External cause code can never be a principal diagnosis
An external cause code can never be a principal (first-listed) diagnosis.

7) Combination external cause codes
Certain of the external cause codes are combination codes that identify sequential events that result in an injury, such as a fall which results in striking against an object. The injury may be due to either event or both. The combination external cause code used should correspond to the sequence of events regardless of which caused the most serious injury.

8) No external cause code needed in certain circumstances
No external cause code from Chapter 20 is needed if the external cause and intent are included in a code from another chapter (e.g. T36.0X1- Poisoning by penicillins, accidental (unintentional)).

b. Place of Occurrence Guideline
Codes from category Y92, Place of occurrence of the external cause, are secondary codes for use after other external cause codes to identify the location of the patient at the time of injury or other condition.

Generally, a place of occurrence code is assigned only once, at the initial encounter for treatment. However, in the rare instance that a new injury occurs during hospitalization, an additional place of occurrence code may be assigned. No 7th characters are used for Y92.

Do not use place of occurrence code Y92.9 if the place is not stated or is not applicable.

c. Activity Code
Assign a code from category Y93, Activity code, to describe the activity of the patient at the time the injury or other health condition occurred.

An activity code is used only once, at the initial encounter for treatment. Only one code from Y93 should be recorded on a medical record.

The activity codes are not applicable to poisonings, adverse effects, misadventures or sequela.

Do not assign Y93.9, Unspecified activity, if the activity is not stated.

A code from category Y93 is appropriate for use with external cause and intent codes if identifying the activity provides additional information about the event.

d. Place of Occurrence, Activity, and Status Codes Used with other External Cause Code
When applicable, place of occurrence, activity, and external cause status codes are sequenced after the main external cause code(s). Regardless of the number of external cause codes assigned, generally there should be only one place of occurrence code, one activity code, and one external cause status code assigned to an encounter. However, in the rare instance that a new injury occurs during hospitalization, an additional place of occurrence code may be assigned.

e. If the Reporting Format Limits the Number of External Cause Codes
If the reporting format limits the number of external cause codes that can be used in reporting clinical data, report the code for the cause/intent most related to the principal diagnosis. If the format permits capture of additional external cause codes, the cause/intent, including medical misadventures, of the additional

events should be reported rather than the codes for place, activity, or external status.

f. Multiple External Cause Coding Guidelines
More than one external cause code is required to fully describe the external cause of an illness or injury. The assignment of external cause codes should be sequenced in the following priority:

If two or more events cause separate injuries, an external cause code should be assigned for each cause. The first-listed external cause code will be selected in the following order:

External codes for child and adult abuse take priority over all other external cause codes.

See Section I.C.19., Child and Adult abuse guidelines.

External cause codes for terrorism events take priority over all other external cause codes except child and adult abuse.

External cause codes for cataclysmic events take priority over all other external cause codes except child and adult abuse and terrorism.

External cause codes for transport accidents take priority over all other external cause codes except cataclysmic events, child and adult abuse and terrorism.

Activity and external cause status codes are assigned following all causal (intent) external cause codes.

The first-listed external cause code should correspond to the cause of the most serious diagnosis due to an assault, accident, or self-harm, following the order of hierarchy listed above.

g. Child and Adult Abuse Guideline
Adult and child abuse, neglect and maltreatment are classified as assault. Any of the assault codes may be used to indicate the external cause of any injury resulting from the confirmed abuse.

For confirmed cases of abuse, neglect and maltreatment, when the perpetrator is known, a code from Y07, Perpetrator of maltreatment and neglect, should accompany any other assault codes.

See Section I.C.19. Adult and child abuse, neglect and other maltreatment

h. Unknown or Undetermined Intent Guideline
If the intent (accident, self-harm, assault) of the cause of an injury or other condition is unknown or unspecified, code the intent as accidental intent. All transport accident categories assume accidental intent.

1) Use of undetermined intent
External cause codes for events of undetermined intent are only for use if the documentation in the record specifies that the intent cannot be determined.

i. Sequelae (Late Effects) of External Cause Guidelines
1) Sequelae external cause codes
Sequela are reported using the external cause code with the 7th character "S" for sequela. These codes should be used with any report of a late effect or sequela resulting from a previous injury.

See Section I.B.10 Sequela (Late Effects)

2) Sequela external cause code with a related current injury
A sequela external cause code should never be used with a related current nature of injury code.

3) Use of sequela external cause codes for subsequent visits
Use a late effect external cause code for subsequent visits when a late effect of the initial injury is being treated. Do not use a late effect external cause code for subsequent visits for follow-up care (e.g., to assess healing, to receive rehabilitative therapy) of the injury when no late effect of the injury has been documented.

j. Terrorism Guidelines
1) Cause of injury identified by the Federal Government (FBI) as terrorism
When the cause of an injury is identified by the Federal Government (FBI) as terrorism, the first-listed external cause code should be a code from category Y38, Terrorism. The definition of terrorism employed by the FBI is found at the inclusion note at the beginning of category Y38. Use additional code for place of occurrence (Y92.-). More than one Y38 code

may be assigned if the injury is the result of more than one mechanism of terrorism.

2) **Cause of an injury is suspected to be the result of terrorism**
When the cause of an injury is suspected to be the result of terrorism a code from category Y38 should not be assigned. Suspected cases should be classified as assault.

3) **Code Y38.9, Terrorism, secondary effects**
Assign code Y38.9, Terrorism, secondary effects, for conditions occurring subsequent to the terrorist event. This code should not be assigned for conditions that are due to the initial terrorist act.

It is acceptable to assign code Y38.9 with another code from Y38 if there is an injury due to the initial terrorist event and an injury that is a subsequent result of the terrorist event.

k. **External cause status**
A code from category Y99, External cause status, should be assigned whenever any other external cause code is assigned for an encounter, including an Activity code, except for the events noted below. Assign a code from category Y99, External cause status, to indicate the work status of the person at the time the event occurred. The status code indicates whether the event occurred during military activity, whether a non-military person was at work, whether an individual including a student or volunteer was involved in a non-work activity at the time of the causal event.

A code from Y99, External cause status, should be assigned, when applicable, with other external cause codes, such as transport accidents and falls. The external cause status codes are not applicable to poisonings, adverse effects, misadventures or late effects.

Do not assign a code from category Y99 if no other external cause codes (cause, activity) are applicable for the encounter.

An external cause status code is used only once, at the initial encounter for treatment. Only one code from Y99 should be recorded on a medical record.

Do not assign code Y99.9, Unspecified external cause status, if the status is not stated.

21. **Chapter 21: Factors influencing health status and contact with health services (Z00-Z99)**
Note: The chapter specific guidelines provide additional information about the use of Z codes for specified encounters.

a. **Use of Z codes in any healthcare setting**
Z codes are for use in any healthcare setting. Z codes may be used as either a first-listed (principal diagnosis code in the inpatient setting) or secondary code, depending on the circumstances of the encounter. Certain Z codes may only be used as first-listed or principal diagnosis.

b. **Z Codes indicate a reason for an encounter**
Z codes are not procedure codes. A corresponding procedure code must accompany a Z code to describe any procedure performed.

c. **Categories of Z Codes**
1) **Contact/Exposure**
Category Z20 indicates contact with, and suspected exposure to, communicable diseases. These codes are for patients who do not show any sign or symptom of a disease but are suspected to have been exposed to it by close personal contact with an infected individual or are in an area where a disease is epidemic.

Category Z77, Other contact with and (suspected) exposures hazardous to health, indicates contact with and suspected exposures hazardous to health.

Contact/exposure codes may be used as a first-listed code to explain an encounter for testing, or, more commonly, as a secondary code to identify a potential risk.

2) **Inoculations and vaccinations**
Code Z23 is for encounters for inoculations and vaccinations. It indicates that a patient is being seen to receive a prophylactic inoculation against a disease. Procedure codes are required to identify the actual administration of the injection and the type(s) of immunizations given. Code Z23 may be used as a secondary code if the inoculation is given as a routine part of preventive health care, such as a well-baby visit.

3) **Status**
Status codes indicate that a patient is either a carrier of a disease or has the sequelae or residual of a past disease or condition. This includes such things as the presence of prosthetic or mechanical devices resulting from past treatment. A status code is informative, because the status may affect the course of treatment and its outcome. A status code is distinct from a history code. The history code indicates that the patient no longer has the condition.

A status code should not be used with a diagnosis code from one of the body system chapters, if the diagnosis code includes the information provided by the status code. For example, code Z94.1, Heart transplant status, should not be used with a code from subcategory T86.2, Complications of heart transplant. The status code does not provide additional information. The complication code indicates that the patient is a heart transplant patient.

For encounters for weaning from a mechanical ventilator, assign a code from subcategory J96.1, Chronic respiratory failure, followed by code Z99.11, Dependence on respirator [ventilator] status.

The status Z codes/categories are:

Z14 Genetic carrier

Genetic carrier status indicates that a person carries a gene, associated with a particular disease, which may be passed to offspring who may develop that disease. The person does not have the disease and is not at risk of developing the disease.

Z15 Genetic susceptibility to disease

Genetic susceptibility indicates that a person has a gene that increases the risk of that person developing the disease.

Codes from category Z15 should not be used as principal or first-listed codes. If the patient has the condition to which he/she is susceptible, and that condition is the reason for the encounter, the code for the current condition should be sequenced first. If the patient is being seen for follow-up after completed treatment for this condition, and the condition no longer exists, a follow-up code should be sequenced first, followed by the appropriate personal history and genetic susceptibility codes. If the purpose of the encounter is genetic counseling associated with procreative management, code Z31.5, Encounter for genetic counseling, should be assigned as the first-listed code, followed by a code from category Z15. Additional codes should be assigned for any applicable family or personal history.

Z16 Resistance to antimicrobial drugs

This code indicates that a patient has a condition that is resistant to antimicrobial drug treatment. Sequence the infection code first.

Z17 Estrogen receptor status

Z18 Retained foreign body fragments

Z19 Hormone sensitivity malignancy status

Z21 Asymptomatic HIV infection status

This code indicates that a patient has tested positive for HIV but has manifested no signs or symptoms of the disease.

Z22 Carrier of infectious disease

Carrier status indicates that a person harbors the specific organisms of a disease without manifest symptoms and is capable of transmitting the infection.

Z28.3 Underimmunization status

Z33.1 Pregnant state, incidental

This code is a secondary code only for use when the pregnancy is in no way complicating the reason for visit. Otherwise, a code from the obstetric chapter is required.

Z66 Do not resuscitate

This code may be used when it is documented by the provider that a patient is on do not resuscitate status at any time during the stay.

Z67   Blood type

Z68   Body mass index (BMI)

As with all other secondary diagnosis codes, the BMI codes should only be assigned when they meet the definition of a reportable diagnosis (see Section III, Reporting Additional Diagnoses).

Z74.01 Bed confinement status

Z76.82 Awaiting organ transplant status

Z78   Other specified health status

Code Z78.1, Physical restraint status, may be used when it is documented by the provider that a patient has been put in restraints during the current encounter. Please note that this code should not be reported when it is documented by the provider that a patient is temporarily restrained during a procedure.

Z79   Long-term (current) drug therapy

Codes from this category indicate a patient's continuous use of a prescribed drug (including such things as aspirin therapy) for the long-term treatment of a condition or for prophylactic use. It is not for use for patients who have addictions to drugs. This subcategory is not for use of medications for detoxification or maintenance programs to prevent withdrawal symptoms in patients with drug dependence (e.g., methadone maintenance for opiate dependence). Assign the appropriate code for the drug dependence instead.

Assign a code from Z79 if the patient is receiving a medication for an extended period as a prophylactic measure (such as for the prevention of deep vein thrombosis) or as treatment of a chronic condition (such as arthritis) or a disease requiring a lengthy course of treatment (such as cancer). Do not assign a code from category Z79 for medication being administered for a brief period of time to treat an acute illness or injury (such as a course of antibiotics to treat acute bronchitis).

Z88   Allergy status to drugs, medicaments and biological substances

Except: Z88.9, Allergy status to unspecified drugs, medicaments and biological substances status

Z89   Acquired absence of limb

Z90   Acquired absence of organs, not elsewhere classified

Z91.0- Allergy status, other than to drugs and biological substances

Z92.82 Status post administration of tPA (rtPA) in a different facility within the last 24 hours prior to admission to a current facility

Assign code Z92.82, Status post administration of tPA (rtPA) in a different facility within the last 24 hours prior to admission to current facility, as a secondary diagnosis when a patient is received by transfer into a facility and documentation indicates they were administered tissue plasminogen activator (tPA) within the last 24 hours prior to admission to the current facility.

This guideline applies even if the patient is still receiving the tPA at the time they are received into the current facility.

The appropriate code for the condition for which the tPA was administered (such as cerebrovascular disease or myocardial infarction) should be assigned first.

Code Z92.82 is only applicable to the receiving facility record and not to the transferring facility record.

Z93   Artificial opening status

Z94   Transplanted organ and tissue status

Z95   Presence of cardiac and vascular implants and grafts

Z96   Presence of other functional implants

Z97   Presence of other devices

Z98   Other postprocedural states

Assign code Z98.85, Transplanted organ removal status, to indicate that a transplanted organ has been previously removed. This code should not be assigned for the encounter in which the transplanted organ is removed. The complication necessitating removal of the transplant organ should be assigned for that encounter.

See section I.C19. for information on the coding of organ transplant complications.

Z99   Dependence on enabling machines and devices, not elsewhere classified

Note: Categories Z89-Z90 and Z93-Z99 are for use only if there are no complications or malfunctions of the organ or tissue replaced, the amputation site or the equipment on which the patient is dependent.

4) **History (of)**
There are two types of history Z codes, personal and family. Personal history codes explain a patient's past medical condition that no longer exists and is not receiving any treatment, but that has the potential for recurrence, and therefore may require continued monitoring.

Family history codes are for use when a patient has a family member(s) who has had a particular disease that causes the patient to be at higher risk of also contracting the disease.

Personal history codes may be used in conjunction with follow-up codes and family history codes may be used in conjunction with screening codes to explain the need for a test or procedure. History codes are also acceptable on any medical record regardless of the reason for visit. A history of an illness, even if no longer present, is important information that may alter the type of treatment ordered.

The history Z code categories are:

Z80   Family history of primary malignant neoplasm

Z81   Family history of mental and behavioral disorders

Z82   Family history of certain disabilities and chronic diseases (leading to disablement)

Z83   Family history of other specific disorders

Z84   Family history of other conditions

Z85   Personal history of malignant neoplasm

Z86   Personal history of certain other diseases

Z87   Personal history of other diseases and conditions

Z91.4- Personal history of psychological trauma, not elsewhere classified

Z91.5   Personal history of self-harm

Z91.81 History of falling

Z91.82 Personal history of military deployment

Z92   Personal history of medical treatment

Except: Z92.0, Personal history of contraception

Except: Z92.82, Status post administration of tPA (rtPA) in a different facility within the last 24 hours prior to admission to a current facility

5) **Screening**
Screening is the testing for disease or disease precursors in seemingly well individuals so that early detection and treatment can be provided for those who test positive for the disease (e.g., screening mammogram).

The testing of a person to rule out or confirm a suspected diagnosis because the patient has some sign or symptom is a diagnostic examination, not a screening. In these cases, the sign or symptom is used to explain the reason for the test.

A screening code may be a first-listed code if the reason for the visit is specifically the screening exam. It may also be used as an additional code if the screening is done during an office visit for other health problems. A screening code is not necessary if the screening is inherent to a routine examination, such as a pap smear done during a routine pelvic examination.

Should a condition be discovered during the screening then the code for the condition may be assigned as an additional diagnosis.

The Z code indicates that a screening exam is planned. A procedure code is required to confirm that the screening was performed.

The screening Z codes/categories:

Z11   Encounter for screening for infectious and parasitic diseases

Z12   Encounter for screening for malignant neoplasms

Z13   Encounter for screening for other diseases and disorders

Except: Z13.9, Encounter for screening, unspecified

Z36   Encounter for antenatal screening for mother

6) Observation

There are three observation Z code categories. They are for use in very limited circumstances when a person is being observed for a suspected condition that is ruled out. The observation codes are not for use if an injury or illness or any signs or symptoms related to the suspected condition are present. In such cases the diagnosis/symptom code is used with the corresponding external cause code.

The observation codes are to be used as principal diagnosis only. The only exception to this is when the principal diagnosis is required to be a code from category Z38, Liveborn infants according to place of birth and type of delivery. Then a code from category Z05, Encounter for observation and evaluation of newborn for suspected diseases and conditions ruled out, is sequenced after the Z38 code. Additional codes may be used in addition to the observation code, but only if they are unrelated to the suspected condition being observed.

Codes from subcategory Z03.7, Encounter for suspected maternal and fetal conditions ruled out, may either be used as a first-listed or as an additional code assignment depending on the case. They are for use in very limited circumstances on a maternal record when an encounter is for a suspected maternal or fetal condition that is ruled out during that encounter (for example, a maternal or fetal condition may be suspected due to an abnormal test result). These codes should not be used when the condition is confirmed. In those cases, the confirmed condition should be coded. In addition, these codes are not for use if an illness or any signs or symptoms related to the suspected condition or problem are present. In such cases the diagnosis/symptom code is used.

Additional codes may be used in addition to the code from subcategory Z03.7, but only if they are unrelated to the suspected condition being evaluated.

Codes from subcategory Z03.7 may not be used for encounters for antenatal screening of mother. *See Section I.C.21. Screening.*

For encounters for suspected fetal condition that are inconclusive following testing and evaluation, assign the appropriate code from category O35, O36, O40 or O41.

The observation Z code categories:

Z03   Encounter for medical observation for suspected diseases and conditions ruled out

Z04   Encounter for examination and observation for other reasons

Except: Z04.9, Encounter for examination and observation for unspecified reason

Z05   Encounter for observation and evaluation of newborn for suspected diseases and conditions ruled out

7) Aftercare

Aftercare visit codes cover situations when the initial treatment of a disease has been performed and the patient requires continued care during the healing or recovery phase, or for the long-term consequences of the disease. The aftercare Z code should not be used if treatment is directed at a current, acute disease. The diagnosis code is to be used in these cases. Exceptions to this rule are codes Z51.0, Encounter for antineoplastic radiation therapy, and codes from subcategory Z51.1, Encounter for antineoplastic chemotherapy and

immunotherapy. These codes are to be first-listed, followed by the diagnosis code when a patient's encounter is solely to receive radiation therapy, chemotherapy, or immunotherapy for the treatment of a neoplasm. If the reason for the encounter is more than one type of antineoplastic therapy, code Z51.0 and a code from subcategory Z51.1 may be assigned together, in which case one of these codes would be reported as a secondary diagnosis.

The aftercare Z codes should also not be used for aftercare for injuries. For aftercare of an injury, assign the acute injury code with the appropriate 7th character (for subsequent encounter).

The aftercare codes are generally first-listed to explain the specific reason for the encounter. An aftercare code may be used as an additional code when some type of aftercare is provided in addition to the reason for admission and no diagnosis code is applicable. An example of this would be the closure of a colostomy during an encounter for treatment of another condition.

Aftercare codes should be used in conjunction with other aftercare codes or diagnosis codes to provide better detail on the specifics of an aftercare encounter visit, unless otherwise directed by the classification. Should a patient receive multiple types of antineoplastic therapy during the same encounter, code Z51.0, Encounter for antineoplastic radiation therapy, and codes from subcategory Z51.1, Encounter for antineoplastic chemotherapy and immunotherapy, may be used together on a record. The sequencing of multiple aftercare codes depends on the circumstances of the encounter.

Certain aftercare Z code categories need a secondary diagnosis code to describe the resolving condition or sequelae. For others, the condition is included in the code title.

Additional Z code aftercare category terms include fitting and adjustment, and attention to artificial openings.

Status Z codes may be used with aftercare Z codes to indicate the nature of the aftercare. For example code Z95.1, Presence of aortocoronary bypass graft, may be used with code Z48.812, Encounter for surgical aftercare following surgery on the circulatory system, to indicate the surgery for which the aftercare is being performed. A status code should not be used when the aftercare code indicates the type of status, such as using Z43.0, Encounter for attention to tracheostomy, with Z93.0, Tracheostomy status.

The aftercare Z category/codes:

Z42   Encounter for plastic and reconstructive surgery following medical procedure or healed injury

Z43   Encounter for attention to artificial openings

Z44   Encounter for fitting and adjustment of external prosthetic device

Z45   Encounter for adjustment and management of implanted device

Z46   Encounter for fitting and adjustment of other devices

Z47   Orthopedic aftercare

Z48   Encounter for other postprocedural aftercare

Z49   Encounter for care involving renal dialysis

Z51   Encounter for other aftercare and medical care

8) Follow-up

The follow-up codes are used to explain continuing surveillance following completed treatment of a disease, condition, or injury. They imply that the condition has been fully treated and no longer exists. They should not be confused with aftercare codes, or injury codes with a 7th character for subsequent encounter, that explain ongoing care of a healing condition or its sequelae. Follow-up codes may be used in conjunction with history codes to provide the full picture of the healed condition and its treatment. The follow-up code is sequenced first, followed by the history code.

A follow-up code may be used to explain multiple visits. Should a condition be found to have recurred on the follow-up visit, then the diagnosis code for the condition should be assigned in place of the follow-up code.

The follow-up Z code categories:

Z08   Encounter for follow-up examination after completed treatment for malignant neoplasm

Z09   Encounter for follow-up examination after completed treatment for conditions other than malignant neoplasm

Z39   Encounter for maternal postpartum care and examination

9) **Donor**
Codes in category Z52, Donors of organs and tissues, are used for living individuals who are donating blood or other body tissue. These codes are only for individuals donating for others, not for self-donations. They are not used to identify cadaveric donations.

10) **Counseling**
Counseling Z codes are used when a patient or family member receives assistance in the aftermath of an illness or injury, or when support is required in coping with family or social problems.

The counseling Z codes/categories:

Z30.0- Encounter for general counseling and advice on contraception

Z31.5   Encounter for **procreative** genetic counseling

Z31.6- Encounter for general counseling and advice on procreation

Z32.2   Encounter for childbirth instruction

Z32.3   Encounter for childcare instruction

Z69   Encounter for mental health services for victim and perpetrator of abuse

Z70   Counseling related to sexual attitude, behavior and orientation

Z71   Persons encountering health services for other counseling and medical advice, not elsewhere classified

Z76.81 Expectant mother prebirth pediatrician visit

11) **Encounters for Obstetrical and Reproductive Services**
See Section I.C.15. Pregnancy, Childbirth, and the Puerperium, for further instruction on the use of these codes.

Z codes for pregnancy are for use in those circumstances when none of the problems or complications included in the codes from the Obstetrics chapter exist (a routine prenatal visit or postpartum care). Codes in category Z34, Encounter for supervision of normal pregnancy, are always first-listed and are not to be used with any other code from the OB chapter.

Codes in category Z3A, Weeks of gestation, may be assigned to provide additional information about the pregnancy. Category Z3A codes should not be assigned for pregnancies with abortive outcomes (categories O00-O08), elective termination of pregnancy (code **Z33.2**), nor for postpartum conditions, as category Z3A is not applicable to these conditions. The date of the admission should be used to determine weeks of gestation for inpatient admissions that encompass more than one gestational week.

The outcome of delivery, category Z37, should be included on all maternal delivery records. It is always a secondary code. Codes in category Z37 should not be used on the newborn record.

Z codes for family planning (contraceptive) or procreative management and counseling should be included on an obstetric record either during the pregnancy or the postpartum stage, if applicable.

Z codes/categories for obstetrical and reproductive services:

Z30   Encounter for contraceptive management

Z31   Encounter for procreative management

Z32.2 Encounter for childbirth instruction

Z32.3 Encounter for childcare instruction

Z33   Pregnant state

Z34   Encounter for supervision of normal pregnancy

Z36   Encounter for antenatal screening of mother

Z3A   Weeks of gestation

Z37   Outcome of delivery

Z39   Encounter for maternal postpartum care and examination

Z76.81 Expectant mother prebirth pediatrician visit

12) **Newborns and Infants**
See Section I.C.16. Newborn (Perinatal) Guidelines, for further instruction on the use of these codes.

Newborn Z codes/categories:

Z76.1 Encounter for health supervision and care of foundling

Z00.1- Encounter for routine child health examination

Z38'   Liveborn infants according to place of birth and type of delivery

13) **Routine and administrative examinations**
The Z codes allow for the description of encounters for routine examinations, such as, a general check-up, or, examinations for administrative purposes, such as, a pre-employment physical. The codes are not to be used if the examination is for diagnosis of a suspected condition or for treatment purposes. In such cases the diagnosis code is used. During a routine exam, should a diagnosis or condition be discovered, it should be coded as an additional code. Pre-existing and chronic conditions and history codes may also be included as additional codes as long as the examination is for administrative purposes and not focused on any particular condition.

Some of the codes for routine health examinations distinguish between "with" and "without" abnormal findings. Code assignment depends on the information that is known at the time the encounter is being coded. For example, if no abnormal findings were found during the examination, but the encounter is being coded before test results are back, it is acceptable to assign the code for "without abnormal findings." When assigning a code for "with abnormal findings," additional code(s) should be assigned to identify the specific abnormal finding(s).

Pre-operative examination and pre-procedural laboratory examination Z codes are for use only in those situations when a patient is being cleared for a procedure or surgery and no treatment is given.

The Z codes/categories for routine and administrative examinations:

Z00   Encounter for general examination without complaint, suspected or reported diagnosis

Z01   Encounter for other special examination without complaint, suspected or reported diagnosis

Z02   Encounter for administrative examination
       Except: Z02.9, Encounter for administrative examinations, unspecified

Z32.0- Encounter for pregnancy test

14) **Miscellaneous Z codes**
The miscellaneous Z codes capture a number of other health care encounters that do not fall into one of the other categories.

Certain of these codes identify the reason for the encounter; others are for use as additional codes that provide useful information on circumstances that may affect a patient's care and treatment.

Prophylactic Organ Removal

For encounters specifically for prophylactic removal of an organ (such as prophylactic removal of breasts due to a genetic susceptibility to cancer or a family history of cancer), the principal or first-listed code should be a code from category Z40, Encounter for prophylactic surgery, followed by the appropriate codes to identify the associated risk factor (such as genetic susceptibility or family history).

If the patient has a malignancy of one site and is having prophylactic removal at another site to prevent either a new primary malignancy or metastatic disease, a code for the malignancy should also be assigned in addition to a code from subcategory Z40.0, Encounter for prophylactic surgery for risk factors related to malignant neoplasms. A Z40.0 code should not be assigned if the patient is having organ removal for treatment of a malignancy, such as the removal of the testes for the treatment of prostate cancer.

Miscellaneous Z codes/categories:

Z28   Immunization not carried out

    Except: Z28.3, Underimmunization status

Z29   Encounter for other prophylactic measures

Z40   Encounter for prophylactic surgery

Z41   Encounter for procedures for purposes other than remedying health state

    Except: Z41.9, Encounter for procedure for purposes other than remedying health state, unspecified

Z53   Persons encountering health services for specific procedures and treatment, not carried out

Z55   Problems related to education and literacy

Z56   Problems related to employment and unemployment

Z57   Occupational exposure to risk factors

Z58   Problems related to physical environment

Z59   Problems related to housing and economic circumstances

Z60   Problems related to social environment

Z62   Problems related to upbringing

Z63   Other problems related to primary support group, including family circumstances

Z64   Problems related to certain psychosocial circumstances

Z65   Problems related to other psychosocial circumstances

Z72   Problems related to lifestyle

    Note: These codes should be assigned only when the documentation specifies that the patient has an associated problem

Z73   Problems related to life management difficulty

Z74   Problems related to care provider dependency

    Except: Z74.01, Bed confinement status

Z75   Problems related to medical facilities and other health care

Z76.0 Encounter for issue of repeat prescription

Z76.3 Healthy person accompanying sick person

Z76.4 Other boarder to healthcare facility

Z76.5 Malingerer [conscious simulation]

Z91.1- Patient's noncompliance with medical treatment and regimen

Z91.83 Wandering in diseases classified elsewhere

Z91.84-Oral health risk factors

Z91.89 Other specified personal risk factors, not elsewhere classified

15) Nonspecific Z codes

Certain Z codes are so non-specific, or potentially redundant with other codes in the classification, that there can be little justification for their use in the inpatient setting. Their use in the outpatient setting should be limited to those instances when there is no further documentation to permit more precise coding. Otherwise, any sign or symptom or any other reason for visit that is captured in another code should be used.

Nonspecific Z codes/categories:

Z02.9 Encounter for administrative examinations, unspecified

Z04.9 Encounter for examination and observation for unspecified reason

Z13.9 Encounter for screening, unspecified

Z41.9 Encounter for procedure for purposes other than remedying health state, unspecified

Z52.9 Donor of unspecified organ or tissue

Z86.59 Personal history of other mental and behavioral disorders

Z88.9 Allergy status to unspecified drugs, medicaments and biological substances status

Z92.0 Personal history of contraception

16) Z Codes That May Only be Principal/First-Listed Diagnosis

The following Z codes/categories may only be reported as the principal/first-listed diagnosis, except when there are multiple encounters on the same day and the medical records for the encounters are combined:

Z00   Encounter for general examination without complaint, suspected or reported diagnosis

    Except: Z00.6

Z01   Encounter for other special examination without complaint, suspected or reported diagnosis

Z02   Encounter for administrative examination

Z03   Encounter for medical observation for suspected diseases and conditions ruled out

Z04   Encounter for examination and observation for other reasons

Z33.2 Encounter for elective termination of pregnancy

Z31.81 Encounter for male factor infertility in female patient

Z31.83 Encounter for assisted reproductive fertility procedure cycle

Z31.84 Encounter for fertility preservation procedure

Z34   Encounter for supervision of normal pregnancy

Z39   Encounter for maternal postpartum care and examination

Z38   Liveborn infants according to place of birth and type of delivery

Z40   Encounter for prophylactic surgery

Z42   Encounter for plastic and reconstructive surgery following medical procedure or healed injury

Z51.0 Encounter for antineoplastic radiation therapy

Z51.1- Encounter for antineoplastic chemotherapy and immunotherapy

Z52   Donors of organs and tissues

    Except: Z52.9, Donor of unspecified organ or tissue

Z76.1 Encounter for health supervision and care of foundling

Z76.2 Encounter for health supervision and care of other healthy infant and child

Z99.12 Encounter for respirator [ventilator] dependence during power failure

Section II. Selection of Principal Diagnosis

The circumstances of inpatient admission always govern the selection of principal diagnosis. The principal diagnosis is defined in the Uniform Hospital Discharge Data Set (UHDDS) as "that condition established after study to be chiefly responsible for occasioning the admission of the patient to the hospital for care."

The UHDDS definitions are used by hospitals to report inpatient data elements in a standardized manner. These data elements and their definitions can be found in the July 31, 1985, Federal Register (Vol. 50, No, 147), pp. 31038-40.

Since that time the application of the UHDDS definitions has been expanded to include all non-outpatient settings (acute care, short term, long term care and psychiatric hospitals; home health agencies; rehab facilities; nursing homes, etc). The UHDDS definitions also apply to hospice services (all levels of care).

In determining principal diagnosis, coding conventions in the ICD-10-CM, the Tabular List and Alphabetic Index take precedence over these official coding guidelines.

(See Section I.A., Conventions for the ICD-10-CM)

The importance of consistent, complete documentation in the medical record cannot be overemphasized. Without such documentation the application of all coding guidelines is a difficult, if not impossible, task.

A. Codes for symptoms, signs, and ill-defined conditions

Codes for symptoms, signs, and ill-defined conditions from Chapter 18 are not to be used as principal diagnosis when a related definitive diagnosis has been established.

B. Two or more interrelated conditions, each potentially meeting the definition for principal diagnosis.

When there are two or more interrelated conditions (such as diseases in the same ICD-10-CM chapter or manifestations characteristically associated with a certain disease) potentially meeting the definition of principal diagnosis, either condition may be sequenced first, unless the circumstances of the admission, the therapy provided, the Tabular List, or the Alphabetic Index indicate otherwise.

C. Two or more diagnoses that equally meet the definition for principal diagnosis

In the unusual instance when two or more diagnoses equally meet the criteria for principal diagnosis as determined by the circumstances of admission, diagnostic workup and/or therapy provided, and the Alphabetic Index, Tabular List, or another coding guidelines does not provide sequencing direction, any one of the diagnoses may be sequenced first.

D. Two or more comparative or contrasting conditions

In those rare instances when two or more contrasting or comparative diagnoses are documented as "either/or" (or similar terminology), they are coded as if the diagnoses were confirmed and the diagnoses are sequenced according to the circumstances of the admission. If no further determination can be made as to which diagnosis should be principal, either diagnosis may be sequenced first.

E. A symptom(s) followed by contrasting/comparative diagnoses

GUIDELINE HAS BEEN DELETED EFFECTIVE OCTOBER 1, 2014

F. Original treatment plan not carried out

Sequence as the principal diagnosis the condition, which after study occasioned the admission to the hospital, even though treatment may not have been carried out due to unforeseen circumstances.

G. Complications of surgery and other medical care

When the admission is for treatment of a complication resulting from surgery or other medical care, the complication code is sequenced as the principal diagnosis. If the complication is classified to the T80-T88 series and the code lacks the necessary specificity in describing the complication, an additional code for the specific complication should be assigned.

H. Uncertain Diagnosis

If the diagnosis documented at the time of discharge is qualified as "probable", "suspected", "likely", "questionable", "possible", or "still to be ruled out", or other similar terms indicating uncertainty, code the condition as if it existed or was established. The bases for these guidelines are the diagnostic workup, arrangements for further workup or observation, and initial therapeutic approach that correspond most closely with the established diagnosis.

Note: This guideline is applicable only to inpatient admissions to short-term, acute, long-term care and psychiatric hospitals.

I. Admission from Observation Unit

1. Admission Following Medical Observation

When a patient is admitted to an observation unit for a medical condition, which either worsens or does not improve, and is subsequently admitted as an inpatient of the same hospital for this same medical condition, the principal diagnosis would be the medical condition which led to the hospital admission.

2. Admission Following Post-Operative Observation

When a patient is admitted to an observation unit to monitor a condition (or complication) that develops following outpatient surgery, and then is subsequently admitted as an inpatient of the same hospital, hospitals should apply the Uniform Hospital Discharge Data Set (UHDDS) definition of principal diagnosis as "that condition established after study to be chiefly responsible for occasioning the admission of the patient to the hospital for care."

J. Admission from Outpatient Surgery

When a patient receives surgery in the hospital's outpatient surgery department and is subsequently admitted for continuing inpatient care at the same hospital, the following guidelines should be followed in selecting the principal diagnosis for the inpatient admission:

- If the reason for the inpatient admission is a complication, assign the complication as the principal diagnosis.

- If no complication, or other condition, is documented as the reason for the inpatient admission, assign the reason for the outpatient surgery as the principal diagnosis.

- If the reason for the inpatient admission is another condition unrelated to the surgery, assign the unrelated condition as the principal diagnosis.

K. Admissions/Encounters for Rehabilitation

When the purpose for the admission/encounter is rehabilitation, sequence first the code for the condition for which the service is being performed. For example, for an admission/encounter for rehabilitation for right-sided dominant hemiplegia following a cerebrovascular infarction, report code I69.351, Hemiplegia and hemiparesis following cerebral infarction affecting right dominant side, as the first-listed or principal diagnosis.

If the condition for which the rehabilitation service is no longer present, report the appropriate aftercare code **as the first-listed or principal diagnosis, unless the rehabilitation service is being provided following an injury. For rehabilitation services following active treatment of an injury, assign the injury code with the appropriate seventh character for subsequent encounter** as the first-listed or principal diagnosis. For example, if a patient with severe degenerative osteoarthritis of the hip, underwent hip replacement and the current encounter/admission is for rehabilitation, report code Z47.1, Aftercare following joint replacement surgery, as the first-listed or principal diagnosis. **If the patient requires rehabilitation post hip replacement for right intertrochanteric femur fracture, report code S72.141D, Displaced intertrochanteric fracture of right femur, subsequent encounter for closed fracture with routine healing, as the first-listed or principal diagnosis.**

See Section I.C.21.c.7, Factors influencing health states and contact with health services, Aftercare.

See Section I.C.19.a for additional information about the use of 7th characters for injury codes.

Section III. Reporting Additional Diagnoses

GENERAL RULES FOR OTHER (ADDITIONAL) DIAGNOSES

For reporting purposes the definition for "other diagnoses" is interpreted as additional conditions that affect patient care in terms of requiring:

clinical evaluation; or

therapeutic treatment; or

diagnostic procedures; or

extended length of hospital stay; or

increased nursing care and/or monitoring.

The UHDDS item #11-b defines Other Diagnoses as "all conditions that coexist at the time of admission, that develop subsequently, or that affect the treatment received and/or the length of stay. Diagnoses that relate to an earlier episode which have no bearing on the current hospital stay are to be excluded." UHDDS definitions apply to inpatients in acute care, short-term, long term care and psychiatric hospital setting. The UHDDS definitions are used by acute care short-term hospitals to report inpatient data elements in a standardized manner. These data elements and their definitions can be found in the July 31, 1985, Federal Register (Vol. 50, No, 147), pp. 31038-40.

Since that time the application of the UHDDS definitions has been expanded to include all non-outpatient settings (acute care, short term, long term care and psychiatric hospitals; home health agencies; rehab facilities; nursing homes, etc). The UHDDS definitions also apply to hospice services (all levels of care).

The following guidelines are to be applied in designating "other diagnoses" when neither the Alphabetic Index nor the Tabular List in ICD-10-CM provide direction. The listing of the diagnoses in the patient record is the responsibility of the attending provider.

A. Previous conditions

If the provider has included a diagnosis in the final diagnostic statement, such as the discharge summary or the face sheet, it should ordinarily be coded. Some providers include in the diagnostic statement resolved conditions or diagnoses and status-post procedures from previous admission that have no bearing on the current stay. Such conditions are not to be reported and are coded only if required by hospital policy.

However, history codes (categories Z80-Z87) may be used as secondary codes if the historical condition or family history has an impact on current care or influences treatment.

B. Abnormal findings

Abnormal findings (laboratory, x-ray, pathologic, and other diagnostic results) are not coded and reported unless the provider indicates their clinical significance. If the findings are outside the normal range and the attending provider has ordered other tests to evaluate the condition or prescribed treatment, it is appropriate to ask the provider whether the abnormal finding should be added.

Please note: This differs from the coding practices in the outpatient setting for coding encounters for diagnostic tests that have been interpreted by a provider.

C. Uncertain Diagnosis

If the diagnosis documented at the time of discharge is qualified as "probable", "suspected", "likely", "questionable", "possible", or "still to be ruled out" or other similar terms indicating uncertainty, code the condition as if it existed or was established. The bases for these guidelines are the diagnostic workup, arrangements for further workup or observation, and initial therapeutic approach that correspond most closely with the established diagnosis.

Note: This guideline is applicable only to inpatient admissions to short-term, acute, long-term care and psychiatric hospitals.

Section IV.Diagnostic Coding and Reporting Guidelines for Outpatient Services

These coding guidelines for outpatient diagnoses have been approved for use by hospitals/ providers in coding and reporting hospital-based outpatient services and provider-based office visits. Guidelines in Section I, Conventions, general coding guidelines and chapter-specific guidelines, should also be applied for outpatient services and office visits.

Information about the use of certain abbreviations, punctuation, symbols, and other conventions used in the ICD-10-CM Tabular List (code numbers and titles), can be found in Section IA of these guidelines, under "Conventions Used in the Tabular List." Section I.B. contains general guidelines that apply to the entire classification. Section I.C. contains chapter-specific guidelines that correspond to the chapters as they are arranged in the classification. Information about the correct sequence to use in finding a code is also described in Section I.

The terms encounter and visit are often used interchangeably in describing outpatient service contacts and, therefore, appear together in these guidelines without distinguishing one from the other.

Though the conventions and general guidelines apply to all settings, coding guidelines for outpatient and provider reporting of diagnoses will vary in a number of instances from those for inpatient diagnoses, recognizing that:

The Uniform Hospital Discharge Data Set (UHDDS) definition of principal diagnosis does not apply to hospital-based outpatient services and provider-based office visits.

Coding guidelines for inconclusive diagnoses (probable, suspected, rule out, etc.) were developed for inpatient reporting and do not apply to outpatients.

A. Selection of first-listed condition

In the outpatient setting, the term first-listed diagnosis is used in lieu of principal diagnosis.

In determining the first-listed diagnosis the coding conventions of ICD-10-CM, as well as the general and disease specific guidelines take precedence over the outpatient guidelines.

Diagnoses often are not established at the time of the initial encounter/visit. It may take two or more visits before the diagnosis is confirmed.

The most critical rule involves beginning the search for the correct code assignment through the Alphabetic Index. Never begin searching initially in the Tabular List as this will lead to coding errors.

1. Outpatient Surgery

When a patient presents for outpatient surgery (same day surgery), code the reason for the surgery as the first-listed diagnosis (reason for the encounter), even if the surgery is not performed due to a contraindication.

2. Observation Stay

When a patient is admitted for observation for a medical condition, assign a code for the medical condition as the first-listed diagnosis.

When a patient presents for outpatient surgery and develops complications requiring admission to observation, code the reason for the surgery as the first reported diagnosis (reason for the encounter), followed by codes for the complications as secondary diagnoses.

B. Codes from A00.0 through T88.9, Z00-Z99

The appropriate code(s) from A00.0 through T88.9, Z00-Z99 must be used to identify diagnoses, symptoms, conditions, problems, complaints, or other reason(s) for the encounter/visit.

C. Accurate reporting of ICD-10-CM diagnosis codes

For accurate reporting of ICD-10-CM diagnosis codes, the documentation should describe the patient's condition, using terminology which includes specific diagnoses as well as symptoms, problems, or reasons for the encounter. There are ICD-10-CM codes to describe all of these.

D. Codes that describe symptoms and signs

Codes that describe symptoms and signs, as opposed to diagnoses, are acceptable for reporting purposes when a diagnosis has not been established (confirmed) by the provider. Chapter 18 of ICD-10-CM, Symptoms, Signs, and Abnormal Clinical and Laboratory Findings Not Elsewhere Classified (codes R00-R99) contain many, but not all codes for symptoms.

E. Encounters for circumstances other than a disease or injury

ICD-10-CM provides codes to deal with encounters for circumstances other than a disease or injury. The Factors Influencing Health Status and Contact with Health Services codes (Z00-Z99) are provided to deal with occasions when circumstances other than a disease or injury are recorded as diagnosis or problems.

See Section I.C.21. Factors influencing health status and contact with health services.

F. Level of Detail in Coding

1. ICD-10-CM codes with 3, 4, 5, 6 or 7 characters

ICD-10-CM is composed of codes with 3, 4, 5, 6 or 7 characters. Codes with three characters are included in ICD-10-CM as the heading of a category of codes that may be further subdivided by the use of fourth, fifth, sixth or seventh characters to provide greater specificity.

2. Use of full number of characters required for a code

A three-character code is to be used only if it is not further subdivided. A code is invalid if it has not been coded to the full number of characters required for that code, including the 7th character, if applicable.

G. ICD-10-CM code for the diagnosis, condition, problem, or other reason for encounter/visit

List first the ICD-10-CM code for the diagnosis, condition, problem, or other reason for encounter/visit shown in the medical record to be chiefly responsible for the services provided. List additional codes that describe any coexisting conditions. In some cases the first-listed diagnosis may be a symptom when a diagnosis has not been established (confirmed) by the physician.

H. Uncertain diagnosis

Do not code diagnoses documented as "probable", "suspected," "questionable," "rule out," or "working diagnosis" or other similar terms indicating uncertainty. Rather, code the condition(s) to the highest degree of certainty for that encounter/visit, such as symptoms, signs, abnormal test results, or other reason for the visit.

Please note: This differs from the coding practices used by short-term, acute care, long-term care and psychiatric hospitals.

I. Chronic diseases

Chronic diseases treated on an ongoing basis may be coded and reported as many times as the patient receives treatment and care for the condition(s)

J. Code all documented conditions that coexist

Code all documented conditions that coexist at the time of the encounter/visit, and require or affect patient care treatment or management. Do not code conditions that were previously treated and no longer exist. However, history codes (categories Z80-Z87) may be used as secondary codes if the historical condition or family history has an impact on current care or influences treatment.

K. Patients receiving diagnostic services only

For patients receiving diagnostic services only during an encounter/visit, sequence first the diagnosis, condition, problem, or other reason for encounter/visit shown in the medical record to be chiefly responsible for the outpatient services provided during the encounter/visit. Codes for other diagnoses (e.g., chronic conditions) may be sequenced as additional diagnoses.

For encounters for routine laboratory/radiology testing in the absence of any signs, symptoms, or associated diagnosis, assign Z01.89, Encounter for other specified special examinations. If routine testing is performed during the same encounter as a test to evaluate a sign, symptom, or diagnosis, it is appropriate to assign both the Z code and the code describing the reason for the non-routine test.

For outpatient encounters for diagnostic tests that have been interpreted by a physician, and the final report is available at the time of coding, code any confirmed or definitive diagnosis(es) documented in the interpretation. Do not code related signs and symptoms as additional diagnoses.

Please note: This differs from the coding practice in the hospital inpatient setting regarding abnormal findings on test results.

L. Patients receiving therapeutic services only

For patients receiving therapeutic services only during an encounter/visit, sequence first the diagnosis, condition, problem, or other reason for encounter/visit shown in the medical record to be chiefly responsible for the outpatient services provided during the encounter/visit. Codes for other diagnoses (e.g., chronic conditions) may be sequenced as additional diagnoses.

The only exception to this rule is that when the primary reason for the admission/encounter is chemotherapy or radiation therapy, the appropriate Z code for the service is listed first, and the diagnosis or problem for which the service is being performed listed second.

M. Patients receiving preoperative evaluations only

For patients receiving preoperative evaluations only, sequence first a code from subcategory Z01.81, Encounter for pre-procedural examinations, to describe the pre-op consultations. Assign a code for the condition to describe the reason for the surgery as an additional diagnosis. Code also any findings related to the pre-op evaluation.

N. Ambulatory surgery

For ambulatory surgery, code the diagnosis for which the surgery was performed. If the postoperative diagnosis is known to be different from the preoperative diagnosis at the time the diagnosis is confirmed, select the postoperative diagnosis for coding, since it is the most definitive.

O. Routine outpatient prenatal visits

See Section I.C.15. Routine outpatient prenatal visits.

P. Encounters for general medical examinations with abnormal findings

The subcategories for encounters for general medical examinations, Z00.0- **and encounter for routine child health examination, Z00.12-**, provide codes for with and without abnormal findings. Should a general medical examination result in an abnormal finding, the code for general medical examination with abnormal finding should be assigned as the first-listed diagnosis. An examination with abnormal findings refers to a condition/diagnosis that is newly identified or a change in severity of a chronic condition (such as uncontrolled hypertension, or an acute exacerbation of chronic obstructive pulmonary disease) during a routine physical examination. A secondary code for the abnormal finding should also be coded.

Q. Encounters for routine health screenings

See Section I.C.21. Factors influencing health status and contact with health services, Screening

Appendix I. Present on Admission Reporting Guidelines

Introduction

These guidelines are to be used as a supplement to the *ICD-10-CM Official Guidelines for Coding and Reporting* to facilitate the assignment of the Present on Admission (POA) indicator for each diagnosis and external cause of injury code reported on claim forms (UB-04 and 837 Institutional).

These guidelines are not intended to replace any guidelines in the main body of the *ICD-10-CM Official Guidelines for Coding and Reporting*. The POA guidelines are not intended to provide guidance on when a condition should

be coded, but rather, how to apply the POA indicator to the final set of diagnosis codes that have been assigned in accordance with Sections I, II, and III of the official coding guidelines. Subsequent to the assignment of the ICD-10-CM codes, the POA indicator should then be assigned to those conditions that have been coded.

As stated in the Introduction to the ICD-10-CM Official Guidelines for Coding and Reporting, a joint effort between the healthcare provider and the coder is essential to achieve complete and accurate documentation, code assignment, and reporting of diagnoses and procedures. The importance of consistent, complete documentation in the medical record cannot be overemphasized. Medical record documentation from any provider involved in the care and treatment of the patient may be used to support the determination of whether a condition was present on admission or not. In the context of the official coding guidelines, the term "provider" means a physician or any qualified healthcare practitioner who is legally accountable for establishing the patient's diagnosis.

These guidelines are not a substitute for the provider's clinical judgment as to the determination of whether a condition was/was not present on admission. The provider should be queried regarding issues related to the linking of signs/symptoms, timing of test results, and the timing of findings.

Please see the CDC website for the detailed list of ICD-10-CM codes that do not require the use of a POA indicator (https://www.cdc.gov/nchs/icd/icd10cm.htm) (https://www.cms.gov/Medicare/Coding/ICD10/2018-ICD-10-CM-and-GEMs.html). The **codes and categories** on this exempt list **are** for circumstances regarding the healthcare encounter or factors influencing health status that do not represent a current disease or injury or **that describe conditions that** are always present on admission.

General Reporting Requirements

All claims involving inpatient admissions to general acute care hospitals or other facilities that are subject to a law or regulation mandating collection of present on admission information.

Present on admission is defined as present at the time the order for inpatient admission occurs -- conditions that develop during an outpatient encounter, including emergency department, observation, or outpatient surgery, are considered as present on admission.

POA indicator is assigned to principal and secondary diagnoses (as defined in Section II of the Official Guidelines for Coding and Reporting) and the external cause of injury codes.

Issues related to inconsistent, missing, conflicting or unclear documentation must still be resolved by the provider.

If a condition would not be coded and reported based on UHDDS definitions and current official coding guidelines, then the POA indicator would not be reported.

Reporting Options

    Y - Yes

    N - No

    U - Unknown

    W – Clinically undetermined

Unreported/Not used – (Exempt from POA reporting)

Reporting Definitions

    Y = present at the time of inpatient admission

    N = not present at the time of inpatient admission

    U = documentation is insufficient to determine if condition is present on admission

    W = provider is unable to clinically determine whether condition was present on admission or not

Timeframe for POA Identification and Documentation

There is no required timeframe as to when a provider (per the definition of "provider" used in these guidelines) must identify or document a condition to be present on admission. In some clinical situations, it may not be possible for a provider to make a definitive diagnosis (or a condition may not be recognized or reported by the patient) for a period of time after admission. In some cases it may be several days before the provider arrives at a definitive diagnosis. This does not mean that the condition was not present on admission. Determination of whether the condition was present on admission or not will be based on the applicable POA guideline as identified in this document, or on the provider's best clinical judgment.

If at the time of code assignment the documentation is unclear as to whether a condition was present on admission or not, it is appropriate to query the provider for clarification.

Assigning the POA Indicator

Condition is on the "Exempt from Reporting" list

Leave the "present on admission" field blank if the condition is on the list of ICD-10-CM codes for which this field is not applicable. This is the only circumstance in which the field may be left blank.

POA Explicitly Documented

Assign Y for any condition the provider explicitly documents as being present on admission.

Assign N for any condition the provider explicitly documents as not present at the time of admission.

Conditions diagnosed prior to inpatient admission

Assign "Y" for conditions that were diagnosed prior to admission (example: hypertension, diabetes mellitus, asthma)

Conditions diagnosed during the admission but clearly present before admission

Assign "Y" for conditions diagnosed during the admission that were clearly present but not diagnosed until after admission occurred.

Diagnoses subsequently confirmed after admission are considered present on admission if at the time of admission they are documented as suspected, possible, rule out, differential diagnosis, or constitute an underlying cause of a symptom that is present at the time of admission.

Condition develops during outpatient encounter prior to inpatient admission

Assign Y for any condition that develops during an outpatient encounter prior to a written order for inpatient admission.

Documentation does not indicate whether condition was present on admission

Assign "U" when the medical record documentation is unclear as to whether the condition was present on admission. "U" should not be routinely assigned and used only in very limited circumstances. Coders are encouraged to query the providers when the documentation is unclear.

Documentation states that it cannot be determined whether the condition was or was not present on admission

Assign "W" when the medical record documentation indicates that it cannot be clinically determined whether or not the condition was present on admission.

Chronic condition with acute exacerbation during the admission

If a single code identifies both the chronic condition and the acute exacerbation, see POA guidelines pertaining to codes that contain multiple clinical concepts.

If a single code only identifies the chronic condition and not the acute exacerbation (e.g., acute exacerbation of chronic leukemia), assign "Y."

Conditions documented as possible, probable, suspected, or rule out at the time of discharge

If the final diagnosis contains a possible, probable, suspected, or rule out diagnosis, and this diagnosis was based on signs, symptoms or clinical findings suspected at the time of inpatient admission, assign "Y."

If the final diagnosis contains a possible, probable, suspected, or rule out diagnosis, and this diagnosis was based on signs, symptoms or clinical findings that were not present on admission, assign "N."

Conditions documented as impending or threatened at the time of discharge

If the final diagnosis contains an impending or threatened diagnosis, and this diagnosis is based on symptoms or clinical findings that were present on admission, assign "Y."

If the final diagnosis contains an impending or threatened diagnosis, and this diagnosis is based on symptoms or clinical findings that were not present on admission, assign "N."

Acute and Chronic Conditions

Assign "Y" for acute conditions that are present at time of admission and N for acute conditions that are not present at time of admission.

Assign "Y" for chronic conditions, even though the condition may not be diagnosed until after admission.

If a single code identifies both an acute and chronic condition, see the POA guidelines for codes that contain multiple clinical concepts.

Codes That Contain Multiple Clinical Concepts

Assign "N" if at least one of the clinical concepts included in the code was not present on admission (e.g., COPD with acute exacerbation and the exacerbation was not present on admission; gastric ulcer that does not start bleeding until after admission; asthma patient develops status asthmaticus after admission).

Assign "Y" if all of the clinical concepts included in the code were present on admission (e.g., duodenal ulcer that perforates prior to admission).

For infection codes that include the causal organism, assign "Y" if the infection (or signs of the infection) were present on admission, even though the culture results may not be known until after admission (e.g., patient is admitted with pneumonia and the provider documents Pseudomonas as the causal organism a few days later).

Same Diagnosis Code for Two or More Conditions

When the same ICD-10-CM diagnosis code applies to two or more conditions during the same encounter (e.g. two separate conditions classified to the same ICD-10-CM diagnosis code):

Assign "Y" if all conditions represented by the single ICD-10-CM code were present on admission (e.g. bilateral unspecified age-related cataracts).

Assign "N" if any of the conditions represented by the single ICD-10-CM code was not present on admission (e.g. traumatic secondary and recurrent hemorrhage and seroma is assigned to a single code T79.2, but only one of the conditions was present on admission).

Obstetrical conditions

Whether or not the patient delivers during the current hospitalization does not affect assignment of the POA indicator. The determining factor for POA assignment is whether the pregnancy complication or obstetrical condition described by the code was present at the time of admission or not.

If the pregnancy complication or obstetrical condition was present on admission (e.g., patient admitted in preterm labor), assign "Y".

If the pregnancy complication or obstetrical condition was not present on admission (e.g., 2nd degree laceration during delivery, postpartum hemorrhage that occurred during current hospitalization, fetal distress develops after admission), assign "N".

If the obstetrical code includes more than one diagnosis and any of the diagnoses identified by the code were not present on admission assign "N". (e.g., Category O11, Pre-existing hypertension with pre-eclampsia)

Perinatal conditions

Newborns are not considered to be admitted until after birth. Therefore, any condition present at birth or that developed in utero is considered present at admission and should be assigned "Y". This includes conditions that occur during delivery (e.g., injury during delivery, meconium aspiration, exposure to streptococcus B in the vaginal canal).

Congenital conditions and anomalies

Assign "Y" for congenital conditions and anomalies except for categories Q00-Q99, Congenital anomalies, which are on the exempt list. Congenital conditions are always considered present on admission.

External cause of injury codes

Assign "Y" for any external cause code representing an external cause of morbidity that occurred prior to inpatient admission (e.g., patient fell out of bed at home, patient fell out of bed in emergency room prior to admission)

Assign "N" for any external cause code representing an external cause of morbidity that occurred during inpatient hospitalization (e.g., patient fell out of hospital bed during hospital stay, patient experienced an adverse reaction to a medication administered after inpatient admission)

A

Aarskog's syndrome Q87.1
Abandonment — *see* Maltreatment
Abasia (-astasia) (hysterical) F44.4
Abderhalden-Kaufmann-Lignac syndrome (cystinosis) E72.04
Abdomen, abdominal (*see also* condition)
  acute R10.0
  angina K55.1
  muscle deficiency syndrome Q79.4
Abdominalgia — *see* Pain, abdominal
Abduction contracture, hip or other joint — *see* Contraction, joint
Aberrant (congenital) (*see also* Malposition, congenital)
  adrenal gland Q89.1
  artery (peripheral) Q27.8
   basilar NEC Q28.1
   cerebral Q28.3
   coronary Q24.5
   digestive system Q27.8
   eye Q15.8
   lower limb Q27.8
   precerebral Q28.1
   pulmonary Q25.79
   renal Q27.2
   retina Q14.1
   specified site NEC Q27.8
   subclavian Q27.8
   upper limb Q27.8
   vertebral Q28.1
  breast Q83.8
  endocrine gland NEC Q89.2
  hepatic duct Q44.5
  pancreas Q45.3
  parathyroid gland Q89.2
  pituitary gland Q89.2
  sebaceous glands, mucous membrane, mouth, congenital Q38.6
  spleen Q89.09
  subclavian artery Q27.8
  thymus (gland) Q89.2
  thyroid gland Q89.2
  vein (peripheral) NEC Q27.8
   cerebral Q28.3
   digestive system Q27.8
   lower limb Q27.8
   precerebral Q28.1
   specified site NEC Q27.8
   upper limb Q27.8
Aberration
  distantal — *see* Disturbance, visual
  mental F99
Abetalipoproteinemia E78.6
Abiotrophy R68.89
Ablatio, ablation
  retinae — *see* Detachment, retina
Ablepharia, ablepharon Q10.3
Abnormal, abnormality, abnormalities (*see also* Anomaly)
  acid-base balance (mixed) E87.4
  albumin R77.0
  alphafetoprotein R77.2
  alveolar ridge K08.9
  anatomical relationship Q89.9
  apertures, congenital, diaphragm Q79.1
  auditory perception H93.29- ☑
   diplacusis — *see* Diplacusis
   hyperacusis — *see* Hyperacusis
   recruitment — *see* Recruitment, auditory
   threshold shift — *see* Shift, auditory threshold
  autosomes Q99.9
   fragile site Q95.5
  basal metabolic rate R94.8
  biosynthesis, testicular androgen E29.1
  bleeding time R79.1
  blood level (of)
   cobalt R79.0
   copper R79.0
   iron R79.0
   lithium R78.89
   magnesium R79.0

Abnormal, abnormality, abnormalities — *continued*
  blood level — *continued*
   mineral NEC R79.0
   zinc R79.0
  blood pressure
   elevated R03.0
   low reading (nonspecific) R03.1
  blood sugar R73.09
  blood-gas level R79.81
  bowel sounds R19.15
   absent R19.11
   hyperactive R19.12
  brain scan R94.02
  breathing R06.9
  caloric test R94.138
  cerebrospinal fluid R83.9
   cytology R83.6
   drug level R83.2
   enzyme level R83.0
   hormones R83.1
   immunology R83.4
   microbiology R83.5
   nonmedicinal level R83.3
   specified type NEC R83.8
  chemistry, blood R79.9
   C-reactive protein R79.82
   drugs — *see* Findings, abnormal, in blood
   gas level R79.81
   minerals R79.0
   pancytopenia D61.818
   PTT R79.1
   specified NEC R79.89
   toxins — *see* Findings, abnormal, in blood
  chest sounds (friction) (rales) R09.89
  chromosome, chromosomal Q99.9
   with more than three X chromosomes, female Q97.1
   analysis result R89.8
    bronchial washings R84.8
    cerebrospinal fluid R83.8
    cervix uteri NEC R87.89
    nasal secretions R84.8
    nipple discharge R89.8
    peritoneal fluid R85.89
    pleural fluid R84.8
    prostatic secretions R86.8
    saliva R85.89
    seminal fluid R86.8
    sputum R84.8
    synovial fluid R89.8
    throat scrapings R84.8
    vagina R87.89
    vulva R87.89
    wound secretions R89.8
   dicentric replacement Q93.2
   ring replacement Q93.2
   sex Q99.8
    female phenotype Q97.9
     specified NEC Q97.8
    male phenotype Q98.9
     specified NEC Q98.8
    structural male Q98.6
   specified NEC Q99.8
  clinical findings NEC R68.89
  coagulation D68.9
   newborn, transient P61.6
   profile R79.1
   time R79.1
  communication — *see* Fistula
  conjunctiva, vascular H11.41- ☑
  coronary artery Q24.5
  cortisol-binding globulin E27.8
  course, eustachian tube Q17.8
  creatinine clearance R94.4
  cytology
   anus R85.619
    atypical squamous cells cannot exclude high grade squamous intraepithelial lesion (ASC-H) R85.611
    atypical squamous cells of undetermined significance (ASC-US) R85.610
    cytologic evidence of malignancy R85.614

Abnormal, abnormality, abnormalities — *continued*
  cytology — *continued*
   anus — *continued*
    high grade squamous intraepithelial lesion (HGSIL) R85.613
    human papillomavirus (HPV) DNA test
     high risk positive R85.81
     low risk postive R85.82
    inadequate smear R85.615
    low grade squamous intraepithelial lesion (LGSIL) R85.612
    satisfactory anal smear but lacking transformation zone R85.616
    specified NEC R85.618
    unsatisfactory smear R85.615
   female genital organs — *see* Abnormal, Papanicolaou (smear)
  dark adaptation curve H53.61
  dentofacial NEC — *see* Anomaly, dentofacial
  development, developmental Q89.9
   central nervous system Q07.9
  diagnostic imaging
   abdomen, abdominal region NEC R93.5
   biliary tract R93.2
   bladder R93.41
   breast R92.8
   central nervous system NEC R90.89
   cerebrovascular NEC R90.89
   coronary circulation R93.1
   digestive tract NEC R93.3
   gastrointestinal (tract) R93.3
   genitourinary organs R93.8
   head R93.0
   heart R93.1
   intrathoracic organ NEC R93.8
   kidney R93.42- ☑
   limbs R93.6
   liver R93.2
   lung (field) R91.8
   musculoskeletal system NEC R93.7
   renal pelvis R93.41
   retroperitoneum R93.5
   site specified NEC R93.8
   skin and subcutaneous tissue R93.8
   skull R93.0
   ureter R93.41
   urinary organs specified NEC R93.49
  direction, teeth, fully erupted M26.30
  ear ossicles, acquired NEC H74.39- ☑
   ankylosis — *see* Ankylosis, ear ossicles
   discontinuity — *see* Discontinuity, ossicles, ear
   partial loss — *see* Loss, ossicles, ear (partial)
  Ebstein Q22.5
  echocardiogram R93.1
  echoencephalogram R90.81
  echogram — *see* Abnormal, diagnostic imaging
  electrocardiogram [ECG] [EKG] R94.31
  electroencephalogram [EEG] R94.01
  electrolyte — *see* Imbalance, electrolyte
  electromyogram [EMG] R94.131
  electro-oculogram [EOG] R94.110
  electrophysiological intracardiac studies R94.39
  electroretinogram [ERG] R94.111
  erythrocytes
   congenital, with perinatal jaundice D58.9
  feces (color) (contents) (mucus) R19.5
  finding — *see* Findings, abnormal, without diagnosis
  fluid
   amniotic — *see* Abnormal, specimen, specified
   cerebrospinal — *see* Abnormal, cerebrospinal fluid
   peritoneal — *see* Abnormal, specimen, digestive organs
   pleural — *see* Abnormal, specimen, respiratory organs
   synovial — *see* Abnormal, specimen, specified
   thorax (bronchial washings) (pleural fluid) — *see* Abnormal, specimen, respiratory organs
   vaginal — *see* Abnormal, specimen, female genital organs
  form
   teeth K00.2
   uterus — *see* Anomaly, uterus

Abnormal, abnormality, abnormalities —
　　continued
　function studies
　　auditory R94.120
　　bladder R94.8
　　brain R94.09
　　cardiovascular R94.30
　　ear R94.128
　　endocrine NEC R94.7
　　eye NEC R94.118
　　kidney R94.4
　　liver R94.5
　　nervous system
　　　central NEC R94.09
　　　peripheral NEC R94.138
　　pancreas R94.8
　　placenta R94.8
　　pulmonary R94.2
　　special senses NEC R94.128
　　spleen R94.8
　　thyroid R94.6
　　vestibular R94.121
　gait — see Gait
　　hysterical F44.4
　gastrin secretion E16.4
　globulin R77.1
　　cortisol-binding E27.8
　　thyroid-binding E07.89
　glomerular, minor (see also N00-N07 with fourth
　　character .0) N05.0
　glucagon secretion E16.3
　glucose tolerance (test) (non-fasting) R73.09
　gravitational (G) forces or states (effect of) T75.81 ☑
　hair (color) (shaft) L67.9
　　specified NEC L67.8
　hard tissue formation in pulp (dental) K04.3
　head movement R25.0
　heart
　　rate R00.9
　　　specified NEC R00.8
　　shadow R93.1
　　sounds NEC R01.2
　hemoglobin (disease) (see also Disease, hemoglobin)
　　D58.2
　　trait — see Trait, hemoglobin, abnormal
　histology NEC R89.7
　immunological findings R89.4
　　in serum R76.9
　　　specified NEC R76.8
　increase in appetite R63.2
　involuntary movement — see Abnormal, movement,
　　involuntary
　jaw closure M26.51
　karyotype R89.8
　kidney function test R94.4
　knee jerk R29.2
　leukocyte (cell) (differential) NEC D72.9
　liver function test R94.5
　loss of
　　height R29.890
　　weight R63.4
　mammogram NEC R92.8
　　calcification (calculus) R92.1
　　microcalcification R92.0
　Mantoux test R76.11
　movement (disorder) (see also Disorder, movement)
　　head R25.0
　　involuntary R25.9
　　　fasciculation R25.3
　　　of head R25.0
　　　spasm R25.2
　　　specified type NEC R25.8
　　　tremor R25.1
　myoglobin (Aberdeen) (Annapolis) R89.7
　neonatal screening P09
　oculomotor study R94.113
　palmar creases Q82.8
　Papanicolaou (smear)
　　anus R85.619
　　　atypical squamous cells cannot exclude high
　　　　grade squamous intraepithelial lesion
　　　　(ASC-H) R85.611
　　　atypical squamous cells of undetermined signif-
　　　　icance (ASC-US) R85.610
　　　cytologic evidence of malignancy R85.614
　　　high grade squamous intraepithelial lesion
　　　　(HGSIL) R85.613
　　　human papillomavirus (HPV) DNA test
　　　　high risk positive R85.81

Abnormal, abnormality, abnormalities —
　　continued
　Papanicolaou — continued
　　anus — continued
　　　human papillomavirus DNA test — contin-
　　　　ued
　　　　low risk postive R85.82
　　　inadequate smear R85.615
　　　low grade squamous intraepithelial lesion
　　　　(LGSIL) R85.612
　　　satisfactory anal smear but lacking transforma-
　　　　tion zone R85.616
　　　specified NEC R85.618
　　　unsatisfactory smear R85.615
　　bronchial washings R84.6
　　cerebrospinal fluid R83.6
　　cervix R87.619
　　　atypical squamous cells cannot exclude high
　　　　grade squamous intraepithelial lesion
　　　　(ASC-H) R87.611
　　　atypical squamous cells of undetermined signif-
　　　　icance (ASC-US) R87.610
　　　cytologic evidence of malignancy R87.614
　　　high grade squamous intraepithelial lesion
　　　　(HGSIL) R87.613
　　　inadequate smear R87.615
　　　low grade squamous intraepithelial lesion
　　　　(LGSIL) R87.612
　　　non-atypical endometrial cells R87.618
　　　satisfactory cervical smear but lacking transfor-
　　　　mation zone R87.616
　　　specified NEC R87.618
　　　thin preparaton R87.619
　　　unsatisfactory smear R87.615
　　nasal secretions R84.6
　　nipple discharge R89.6
　　peritoneal fluid R85.69
　　pleural fluid R84.6
　　prostatic secretions R86.6
　　saliva R85.69
　　seminal fluid R86.6
　　sites NEC R89.6
　　sputum R84.6
　　synovial fluid R89.6
　　throat scrapings R84.6
　　vagina R87.629
　　　atypical squamous cells cannot exclude high
　　　　grade squamous intraepithelial lesion
　　　　(ASC-H) R87.621
　　　atypical squamous cells of undetermined signif-
　　　　icance (ASC-US) R87.620
　　　cytologic evidence of malignancy R87.624
　　　high grade squamous intraepithelial lesion
　　　　(HGSIL) R87.623
　　　inadequate smear R87.625
　　　low grade squamous intraepithelial lesion
　　　　(LGSIL) R87.622
　　　specified NEC R87.628
　　　thin preparation R87.629
　　　unsatisfactory smear R87.625
　　vulva R87.69
　　wound secretions R89.6
　partial thromboplastin time (PTT) R79.1
　pelvis (bony) — see Deformity, pelvis
　percussion, chest (tympany) R09.89
　periods (grossly) — see Menstruation
　phonocardiogram R94.39
　plantar reflex R29.2
　plasma
　　protein R77.9
　　　specified NEC R77.8
　　viscosity R70.1
　pleural (folds) Q34.0
　posture R29.3
　product of conception O02.9
　　specified type NEC O02.89
　prothrombin time (PT) R79.1
　pulmonary
　　artery, congenital Q25.79
　　function, newborn P28.89
　　test results R94.2
　pulsations in neck R00.2
　pupillary H21.56- ☑
　　function (reaction) (reflex) — see Anomaly, pupil,
　　　function
　radiological examination — see Abnormal, diagnostic
　　imaging
　red blood cell(s) (morphology) (volume) R71.8
　reflex — see Reflex

Abnormal, abnormality, abnormalities —
　　continued
　renal function test R94.4
　response to nerve stimulation R94.130
　retinal correspondence H53.31
　retinal function study R94.111
　rhythm, heart (see also Arrhythmia)
　saliva — see Abnormal, specimen, digestive organs
　scan
　　kidney R94.4
　　liver R93.2
　　thyroid R94.6
　secretion
　　gastrin E16.4
　　glucagon E16.3
　semen, seminal fluid — see Abnormal, specimen, male
　　genital organs
　serum level (of)
　　acid phosphatase R74.8
　　alkaline phosphatase R74.8
　　amylase R74.8
　　enzymes R74.9
　　　specified NEC R74.8
　　lipase R74.8
　　triacylglycerol lipase R74.8
　shape
　　gravid uterus — see Anomaly, uterus
　sinus venosus Q21.1
　size, tooth, teeth K00.2
　spacing, tooth, teeth, fully erupted M26.30
　specimen
　　digestive organs (peritoneal fluid) (saliva) R85.9
　　　cytology R85.69
　　　drug level R85.2
　　　enzyme level R85.0
　　　histology R85.7
　　　hormones R85.1
　　　immunology R85.4
　　　microbiology R85.5
　　　nonmedicinal level R85.3
　　　specified type NEC R85.89
　　female genital organs (secretions) (smears) R87.9
　　　cytology R87.69
　　　　cervix R87.619
　　　　　human papillomavirus (HPV) DNA test
　　　　　　high risk positive R87.810
　　　　　　low risk positive R87.820
　　　　　inadequate (unsatisfactory) smear
　　　　　　R87.615
　　　　　non-atypical endometrial cells R87.618
　　　　　specified NEC R87.618
　　　　vagina R87.629
　　　　　human papillomavirus (HPV) DNA test
　　　　　　high risk positive R87.811
　　　　　　low risk positive R87.821
　　　　　inadequate (unsatisfactory) smear
　　　　　　R87.625
　　　　vulva R87.69
　　　drug level R87.2
　　　enzyme level R87.0
　　　histological R87.7
　　　hormones R87.1
　　　immunology R87.4
　　　microbiology R87.5
　　　nonmedicinal level R87.3
　　　specified type NEC R87.89
　　male genital organs (prostatic secretions) (semen)
　　　R86.9
　　　cytology R86.6
　　　drug level R86.2
　　　enzyme level R86.0
　　　histological R86.7
　　　hormones R86.1
　　　immunology R86.4
　　　microbiology R86.5
　　　nonmedicinal level R86.3
　　　specified type NEC R86.8
　　nipple discharge — see Abnormal, specimen,
　　　specified
　　respiratory organs (bronchial washings) (nasal se-
　　　cretions) (pleural fluid) (sputum) R84.9
　　　cytology R84.6
　　　drug level R84.2
　　　enzyme level R84.0
　　　histology R84.7
　　　hormones R84.1
　　　immunology R84.4
　　　microbiology R84.5
　　　nonmedicinal level R84.3

Abnormal, abnormality, abnormalities — *continued*
  specimen — *continued*
    respiratory organs — *continued*
      specified type NEC R84.8
    specified organ, system and tissue NOS R89.9
      cytology R89.6
      drug level R89.2
      enzyme level R89.Ø
      histology R89.7
      hormones R89.1
      immunology R89.4
      microbiology R89.5
      nonmedicinal level R89.3
      specified type NEC R89.8
    synovial fluid — *see* Abnormal, specimen, specified
    thorax (bronchial washings) (pleural fluids) — *see* Abnormal, specimen, respiratory organs
    vagina (secretion) (smear) R87.629
    vulva (secretion) (smear) R87.69
    wound secretion — *see* Abnormal, specimen, specified
  spermatozoa — *see* Abnormal, specimen, male genital organs
  sputum (amount) (color) (odor) RØ9.3
  stool (color) (contents) (mucus) R19.5
    bloody K92.1
    guaiac positive R19.5
  synchondrosis Q78.8
  thermography (*see also* Abnormal, diagnostic imaging) R93.8
  thyroid-binding globulin EØ7.89
  tooth, teeth (form) (size) KØØ.2
  toxicology (findings) R78.9
  transport protein E88.Ø9
  tumor marker NEC R97.8
  ultrasound results — *see* Abnormal, diagnostic imaging
  umbilical cord complicating delivery O69.9 ☑
  urination NEC R39.198
  urine (constituents) R82.9Ø
    bile R82.2
    cytological examination R82.8
    drugs R82.5
    fat R82.Ø
    glucose R81
    heavy metals R82.6
    hemoglobin R82.3
    histological examination R82.8
    ketones R82.4
    microbiological examination (culture) R82.79
    myoglobin R82.1
    positive culture R82.79
    protein — *see* Proteinuria
    specified substance NEC R82.99
      chromoabnormality NEC R82.91
    substances nonmedical R82.6
  uterine hemorrhage — *see* Hemorrhage, uterus
  vectorcardiogram R94.39
  visually evoked potential (VEP) R94.112
  white blood cells D72.9
    specified NEC D72.89
  X-ray examination — *see* Abnormal, diagnostic imaging
Abnormity (any organ or part) — *see* Anomaly
Abocclusion M26.29
  hemolytic disease (newborn) P55.1
  incompatibility reaction ABO — *see* Complication(s), transfusion, incompatibility reaction, ABO
Abolition, language R48.8
Aborter, habitual or recurrent — *see* Loss (of), pregnancy, recurrent
Abortion (complete) (spontaneous) OØ3.9
  with
    retained products of conception — *see* Abortion, incomplete
  attempted (elective) (failed) OØ7.4
    complicated by OØ7.3Ø
      afibrinogenemia OØ7.1
      cardiac arrest OØ7.36
      chemical damage of pelvic organ(s) OØ7.34
      circulatory collapse OØ7.31
      cystitis OØ7.38
      defibrination syndrome OØ7.1
      electrolyte imbalance OØ7.33
      embolism (air) (amniotic fluid) (blood clot) (fat) (pulmonary) (septic) (soap) OØ7.2
      endometritis OØ7.Ø

Abortion — *continued*
  attempted — *continued*
    complicated by — *continued*
      genital tract and pelvic infection OØ7.Ø
      hemolysis OØ7.1
      hemorrhage (delayed) (excessive) OØ7.1
      infection
        genital tract or pelvic OØ7.Ø
        urinary tract tract OØ7.38
      intravascular coagulation OØ7.1
      laceration of pelvic organ(s) OØ7.34
      metabolic disorder OØ7.33
      oliguria OØ7.32
      oophoritis OØ7.Ø
      parametritis OØ7.Ø
      pelvic peritonitis OØ7.Ø
      perforation of pelvic organ(s) OØ7.34
      renal failure or shutdown OØ7.32
      salpingitis or salpingo-oophoritis OØ7.Ø
      sepsis OØ7.37
      shock OØ7.31
      specified condition NEC OØ7.39
      tubular necrosis (renal) OØ7.32
      uremia OØ7.32
      urinary tract infection OØ7.38
      venous complication NEC OØ7.35
        embolism (air) (amniotic fluid) (blood clot) (fat) (pulmonary) (septic) (soap) OØ7.2
  complicated (by) (following) OØ3.8Ø
    afibrinogenemia OØ3.6
    cardiac arrest OØ3.86
    chemical damage of pelvic organ(s) OØ3.84
    circulatory collapse OØ3.81
    cystitis OØ3.88
    defibrination syndrome OØ3.6
    electrolyte imbalance OØ3.83
    embolism (air) (amniotic fluid) (blood clot) (fat) (pulmonary) (septic) (soap) OØ3.7
    endometritis OØ3.5
    genital tract and pelvic infection OØ3.5
    hemolysis OØ3.6
    hemorrhage (delayed) (excessive) OØ3.6
    infection
      genital tract or pelvic OØ3.5
      urinary tract OØ3.88
    intravascular coagulation OØ3.6
    laceration of pelvic organ(s) OØ3.84
    metabolic disorder OØ3.83
    oliguria OØ3.82
    oophoritis OØ3.5
    parametritis OØ3.5
    pelvic peritonitis OØ3.5
    perforation of pelvic organ(s) OØ3.84
    renal failure or shutdown OØ3.82
    salpingitis or salpingo-oophoritis OØ3.5
    sepsis OØ3.87
    shock OØ3.81
    specified condition NEC OØ3.89
    tubular necrosis (renal) OØ3.82
    uremia OØ3.82
    urinary tract infection OØ3.88
    venous complication NEC OØ3.85
      embolism (air) (amniotic fluid) (blood clot) (fat) (pulmonary) (septic) (soap) OØ3.7
  failed — *see* Abortion, attempted
  habitual or recurrent N96
    with current abortion — *see* categories OØ3-OØ4
    without current pregnancy N96
      care in current pregnancy O26.2- ☑
  incomplete (spontaneous) OØ3.4
    complicated (by) (following) OØ3.3Ø
      afibrinogenemia OØ3.1
      cardiac arrest OØ3.36
      chemical damage of pelvic organ(s) OØ3.34
      circulatory collapse OØ3.31
      cystitis OØ3.38
      defibrination syndrome OØ3.1
      electrolyte imbalance OØ3.33
      embolism (air) (amniotic fluid) (blood clot) (fat) (pulmonary) (septic) (soap) OØ3.2
      endometritis OØ3.Ø
      genital tract and pelvic infection OØ3.Ø
      hemolysis OØ3.1
      hemorrhage (delayed) (excessive) OØ3.1
      infection
        genital tract or pelvic OØ3.Ø
        urinary tract OØ3.38
      intravascular coagulation OØ3.1
      laceration of pelvic organ(s) OØ3.34

Abortion — *continued*
  incomplete — *continued*
    complicated — *continued*
      metabolic disorder OØ3.33
      oliguria OØ3.32
      oophoritis OØ3.Ø
      parametritis OØ3.Ø
      pelvic peritonitis OØ3.Ø
      perforation of pelvic organ(s) OØ3.34
      renal failure or shutdown OØ3.32
      salpingitis or salpingo-oophoritis OØ3.Ø
      sepsis OØ3.37
      shock OØ3.31
      specified condition NEC OØ3.39
      tubular necrosis (renal) OØ3.32
      uremia OØ3.32
      urinary infection OØ3.38
      venous complication NEC OØ3.35
        embolism (air) (amniotic fluid) (blood clot) (fat) (pulmonary) (septic) (soap) OØ3.2
  induced (encounter for) Z33.2
    complicated by OØ4.8Ø
      afibrinogenemia OØ4.6
      cardiac arrest OØ4.86
      chemical damage of pelvic organ(s) OØ4.84
      circulatory collapse OØ4.81
      cystitis OØ4.88
      defibrination syndrome OØ4.6
      electrolyte imbalance OØ4.83
      embolism (air) (amniotic fluid) (blood clot) (fat) (pulmonary) (septic) (soap) OØ4.7
      endometritis OØ4.5
      genital tract and pelvic infection OØ4.5
      hemolysis OØ4.6
      hemorrhage (delayed) (excessive) OØ4.6
      infection
        genital tract or pelvic OØ4.5
        urinary tract OØ4.88
      intravascular coagulation OØ4.6
      laceration of pelvic organ(s) OØ4.84
      metabolic disorder OØ4.83
      oliguria OØ4.82
      oophoritis OØ4.5
      parametritis OØ4.5
      pelvic peritonitis OØ4.5
      perforation of pelvic organ(s) OØ4.84
      renal failure or shutdown OØ4.82
      salpingitis or salpingo-oophoritis OØ4.5
      sepsis OØ4.87
      shock OØ4.81
      specified condition NEC OØ4.89
      tubular necrosis (renal) OØ4.82
      uremia OØ4.82
      urinary tract infection OØ4.88
      venous complication NEC OØ4.85
        embolism (air) (amniotic fluid) (blood clot) (fat) (pulmonary) (septic) (soap) OØ4.7
  missed OØ2.1
  spontaneous — *see* Abortion (complete) (spontaneous)
    threatened O2Ø.Ø
  threatened (spontaneous) O2Ø.Ø
  tubal OØØ.1Ø- ☑
    with intrauterine pregnancy OØØ.11- ☑
Abortus fever A23.1
Aboulomania F6Ø.7
Abrami's disease D59.8
Abramov-Fiedler myocarditis (acute isolated myocarditis) I4Ø.1
Abrasion T14.8 ☑
  abdomen, abdominal (wall) S3Ø.811 ☑
  alveolar process SØØ.512 ☑
  ankle S9Ø.51- ☑
  antecubital space — *see* Abrasion, elbow
  anus S3Ø.817 ☑
  arm (upper) S4Ø.81- ☑
  auditory canal — *see* Abrasion, ear
  auricle — *see* Abrasion, ear
  axilla — *see* Abrasion, arm
  back, lower S3Ø.81Ø ☑
  breast S2Ø.11- ☑
  brow SØØ.81 ☑
  buttock S3Ø.81Ø ☑
  calf — *see* Abrasion, leg
  canthus — *see* Abrasion, eyelid
  cheek SØØ.81 ☑
    internal SØØ.512 ☑
  chest wall — *see* Abrasion, thorax

Index

Abrasion — Abscess

Abrasion — *continued*
- chin S00.81 ☑
- clitoris S30.814 ☑
- cornea S05.0- ☑
- costal region — *see* Abrasion, thorax
- dental K03.1
- digit(s)
  - foot — *see* Abrasion, toe
  - hand — *see* Abrasion, finger
- ear S00.41- ☑
- elbow S50.31- ☑
- epididymis S30.813 ☑
- epigastric region S30.811 ☑
- epiglottis S10.11 ☑
- esophagus (thoracic) S27.818 ☑
  - cervical S10.11 ☑
- eyebrow — *see* Abrasion, eyelid
- eyelid S00.21- ☑
- face S00.81 ☑
- finger(s) S60.41- ☑
  - index S60.41- ☑
  - little S60.41- ☑
  - middle S60.41- ☑
  - ring S60.41- ☑
- flank S30.811 ☑
- foot (except toe(s) alone) S90.81- ☑
  - toe — *see* Abrasion, toe
- forearm S50.81- ☑
  - elbow only — *see* Abrasion, elbow
- forehead S00.81 ☑
- genital organs, external
  - female S30.816 ☑
  - male S30.815 ☑
- groin S30.811 ☑
- gum S00.512 ☑
- hand S60.51- ☑
- head S00.91 ☑
  - ear — *see* Abrasion, ear
  - eyelid — *see* Abrasion, eyelid
  - lip S00.511 ☑
  - nose S00.31 ☑
  - oral cavity S00.512 ☑
  - scalp S00.01 ☑
  - specified site NEC S00.81 ☑
- heel — *see* Abrasion, foot
- hip S70.21- ☑
- inguinal region S30.811 ☑
- interscapular region S20.419 ☑
- jaw S00.81 ☑
- knee S80.21- ☑
- labium (majus) (minus) S30.814 ☑
- larynx S10.11 ☑
- leg (lower) S80.81- ☑
  - knee — *see* Abrasion, knee
  - upper — *see* Abrasion, thigh
- lip S00.511 ☑
- lower back S30.810 ☑
- lumbar region S30.810 ☑
- malar region S00.81 ☑
- mammary — *see* Abrasion, breast
- mastoid region S00.81 ☑
- mouth S00.512 ☑
- nail
  - finger — *see* Abrasion, finger
  - toe — *see* Abrasion, toe
- nape S10.81 ☑
- nasal S00.31 ☑
- neck S10.91 ☑
  - specified site NEC S10.81 ☑
  - throat S10.11 ☑
- nose S00.31 ☑
- occipital region S00.01 ☑
- oral cavity S00.512 ☑
- orbital region — *see* Abrasion, eyelid
- palate S00.512 ☑
- palm — *see* Abrasion, hand
- parietal region S00.01 ☑
- pelvis S30.810 ☑
- penis S30.812 ☑
- perineum
  - female S30.814 ☑
  - male S30.810 ☑
- periocular area — *see* Abrasion, eyelid
- phalanges
  - finger — *see* Abrasion, finger
  - toe — *see* Abrasion, toe

Abrasion — *continued*
- pharynx S10.11 ☑
- pinna — *see* Abrasion, ear
- popliteal space — *see* Abrasion, knee
- prepuce S30.812 ☑
- pubic region S30.810 ☑
- pudendum
  - female S30.816 ☑
  - male S30.815 ☑
- sacral region S30.810 ☑
- scalp S00.01 ☑
- scapular region — *see* Abrasion, shoulder
- scrotum S30.813 ☑
- shin — *see* Abrasion, leg
- shoulder S40.21- ☑
- skin NEC T14.8 ☑
- sternal region S20.319 ☑
- submaxillary region S00.81 ☑
- submental region S00.81 ☑
- subungual
  - finger(s) — *see* Abrasion, finger
  - toe(s) — *see* Abrasion, toe
- supraclavicular fossa S10.81 ☑
- supraorbital S00.81 ☑
- temple S00.81 ☑
- temporal region S00.81 ☑
- testis S30.813 ☑
- thigh S70.31- ☑
- thorax, thoracic (wall) S20.91 ☑
  - back S20.41- ☑
  - front S20.31- ☑
- throat S10.11 ☑
- thumb S60.31- ☑
- toe(s) (lesser) S90.416 ☑
  - great S90.41- ☑
- tongue S00.512 ☑
- tooth, teeth (dentifrice) (habitual) (hard tissues) (occupational) (ritual) (traditional) K03.1
- trachea S10.11 ☑
- tunica vaginalis S30.813 ☑
- tympanum, tympanic membrane — *see* Abrasion, ear
- uvula S00.512 ☑
- vagina S30.814 ☑
- vocal cords S10.11 ☑
- vulva S30.814 ☑
- wrist S60.81- ☑

Abrism — *see* Poisoning, food, noxious, plant
Abruptio placentae O45.9- ☑
- with
  - afibrinogenemia O45.01- ☑
  - coagulation defect O45.00- ☑
    - specified NEC O45.09- ☑
  - disseminated intravascular coagulation O45.02- ☑
  - hypofibrinogenemia O45.01- ☑
- specified NEC O45.8- ☑

Abruption, placenta — *see* Abruptio placentae
Abscess (connective tissue) (embolic) (fistulous) (infective) (metastatic) (multiple) (pernicious) (pyogenic) (septic) L02.91
- with
  - diverticular disease (intestine) K57.80
    - with bleeding K57.81
    - large intestine K57.20
      - with
        - bleeding K57.21
        - small intestine K57.40
          - with bleeding K57.41
    - small intestine K57.00
      - with
        - bleeding K57.01
        - large intestine K57.40
          - with bleeding K57.41
  - lymphangitis — *code by* site under Abscess
- abdomen, abdominal
  - cavity K65.1
  - wall L02.211
- abdominopelvic K65.1
- accessory sinus — *see* Sinusitis
- adrenal (capsule) (gland) E27.8
- alveolar K04.7
  - with sinus K04.6
- amebic A06.4
  - brain (and liver or lung abscess) A06.6
  - genitourinary tract A06.82
  - liver (without mention of brain or lung abscess) A06.4

Abscess — *continued*
- amebic — *continued*
  - lung (and liver) (without mention of brain abscess) A06.5
  - specified site NEC A06.89
  - spleen A06.89
- anerobic A48.0
- ankle — *see* Abscess, lower limb
- anorectal K61.2
- antecubital space — *see* Abscess, upper limb
- antrum (chronic) (Highmore) — *see* Sinusitis, maxillary
- anus K61.0
- apical (tooth) K04.7
  - with sinus (alveolar) K04.6
- appendix K35.3
- areola (acute) (chronic) (nonpuerperal) N61.1
  - puerperal, postpartum or gestational — *see* Infection, nipple
- arm (any part) — *see* Abscess, upper limb
- artery (wall) I77.89
- atheromatous I77.2
- auricle, ear — *see* Abscess, ear, external
- axilla (region) L02.41- ☑
  - lymph gland or node L04.2
- back (any part, except buttock) L02.212
- Bartholin's gland N75.1
  - with
    - abortion — *see* Abortion, by type complicated by, sepsis
    - ectopic or molar pregnancy O08.0
  - following ectopic or molar pregnancy O08.0
- Bezold's — *see* Mastoiditis, acute
- bilharziasis B65.1
- bladder (wall) — *see* Cystitis, specified type NEC
- bone (subperiosteal) (*see also* Osteomyelitis, specified type NEC)
  - accessory sinus (chronic) — *see* Sinusitis
  - chronic or old — *see* Osteomyelitis, chronic
  - jaw (lower) (upper) M27.2
  - mastoid — *see* Mastoiditis, acute, subperiosteal
  - petrous — *see* Petrositis
  - spinal (tuberculous) A18.01
    - nontuberculous — *see* Osteomyelitis, vertebra
- bowel K63.0
- brain (any part) (cystic) (otogenic) G06.0
  - amebic (with abscess of any other site) A06.6
  - gonococcal A54.82
  - pheomycotic (chromomycotic) B43.1
  - tuberculous A17.81
- breast (acute) (chronic) (nonpuerperal) N61.1
  - newborn P39.0
  - puerperal, postpartum, gestational — *see* Mastitis, obstetric, purulent
- broad ligament N73.2
  - acute N73.0
  - chronic N73.1
- Brodie's (localized) (chronic) M86.8X- ☑
- bronchi J98.09
- buccal cavity K12.2
- bulbourethral gland N34.0
- bursa M71.00
  - ankle M71.07- ☑
  - elbow M71.02- ☑
  - foot M71.07- ☑
  - hand M71.04- ☑
  - hip M71.05- ☑
  - knee M71.06- ☑
  - multiple sites M71.09
  - pharyngeal J39.1
  - shoulder M71.01- ☑
  - specified site NEC M71.08
  - wrist M71.03- ☑
- buttock L02.31
- canthus — *see* Blepharoconjunctivitis
- cartilage — *see* Disorder, cartilage, specified type NEC
- cecum K35.3
- cerebellum, cerebellar G06.0
  - sequelae G09
- cerebral (embolic) G06.0
  - sequelae G09
- cervical (meaning neck) L02.11
  - lymph gland or node L04.0
- cervix (stump) (uteri) — *see* Cervicitis
- cheek (external) L02.01
  - inner K12.2
- chest J86.9
  - with fistula J86.0
  - wall L02.213

☑ **Additional Character Required** — Refer to the Tabular List for Character Selection   Subterms under main terms may continue to next column or page

Abscess — *continued*
chin L02.01
choroid — *see* Inflammation, chorioretinal
circumtonsillar J36
cold (lung) (tuberculous) (*see also* Tuberculosis, abscess, lung)
    articular — *see* Tuberculosis, joint
colon (wall) K63.0
colostomy K94.02
conjunctiva — *see* Conjunctivitis, acute
cornea H16.31- ☑
corpus
    cavernosum N48.21
    luteum — *see* Oophoritis
Cowper's gland N34.0
cranium G06.0
cul-de-sac (Douglas') (posterior) — *see* Peritonitis, pelvic, female
cutaneous — *see* Abscess, by site
dental K04.7
    with sinus (alveolar) K04.6
dentoalveolar K04.7
    with sinus K04.6
diaphragm, diaphragmatic K65.1
Douglas' cul-de-sac or pouch — *see* Peritonitis, pelvic, female
Dubois A50.59
ear (middle) (*see also* Otitis, media, suppurative)
    acute — *see* Otitis, media, suppurative, acute
    external H60.0- ☑
entamebic — *see* Abscess, amebic
enterostomy K94.12
epididymis N45.4
epidural G06.2
    brain G06.0
    spinal cord G06.1
epiglottis J38.7
epiploon, epiploic K65.1
erysipelatous — *see* Erysipelas
esophagus K20.8
ethmoid (bone) (chronic) (sinus) J32.2
external auditory canal — *see* Abscess, ear, external
extradural G06.2
    brain G06.0
        sequelae G09
    spinal cord G06.1
extraperitoneal K68.19
eye — *see* Endophthalmitis, purulent
eyelid H00.03- ☑
face (any part, except ear, eye and nose) L02.01
fallopian tube — *see* Salpingitis
fascia M72.8
fauces J39.1
fecal K63.0
femoral (region) — *see* Abscess, lower limb
filaria, filarial — *see* Infestation, filarial
finger (any) (*see also* Abscess, hand)
    nail — *see* Cellulitis, finger
foot L02.61- ☑
forehead L02.01
frontal sinus (chronic) J32.1
gallbladder K81.0
genital organ or tract
    female (external) N76.4
    male N49.9
        multiple sites N49.8
        specified NEC N49.8
gestational mammary O91.11- ☑
gestational subareolar O91.11- ☑
gingival — *see* Peridontitis, aggressive, localized
gland, glandular (lymph) (acute) — *see* Lymphadenitis, acute
gluteal (region) L02.31
gonorrheal — *see* Gonococcus
groin L02.214
gum — *see* Peridontitis, aggressive, localized
hand L02.51- ☑
head NEC L02.811
    face (any part, except ear, eye and nose) L02.01
heart — *see* Carditis
heel — *see* Abscess, foot
helminthic — *see* Infestation, helminth
hepatic (cholangitic) (hematogenic) (lymphogenic) (pylephlebitic) K75.0
    amebic A06.4
hip (region) — *see* Abscess, lower limb
ileocecal K35.3
ileostomy (bud) K94.12

Abscess — *continued*
iliac (region) L02.214
    fossa K35.3
infraclavicular (fossa) — *see* Abscess, upper limb
inguinal (region) L02.214
    lymph gland or node L04.1
intestine, intestinal NEC K63.0
    rectal K61.1
intra-abdominal (*see also* Abscess, peritoneum) K65.1
    postprocedural T81.4 ☑
        retroperitoneal K68.11
intracranial G06.0
intramammary — *see* Abscess, breast
intraorbital — *see* Abscess, orbit
intraperitoneal K65.1
intrasphincteric (anus) K61.4
intraspinal G06.1
intratonsillar J36
ischiorectal (fossa) K61.3
jaw (bone) (lower) (upper) M27.2
joint — *see* Arthritis, pyogenic or pyemic
    spine (tuberculous) A18.01
        nontuberculous — *see* Spondylopathy, infective
kidney N15.1
    with calculus N20.0
        with hydronephrosis N13.6
    puerperal (postpartum) O86.21
knee (*see also* Abscess, lower limb)
    joint M00.9
labium (majus) (minus) N76.4
lacrimal
    caruncle — *see* Inflammation, lacrimal, passages, acute
    gland — *see* Dacryoadenitis
    passages (duct) (sac) — *see* Inflammation, lacrimal, passages, acute
lacunar N34.0
larynx J38.7
lateral (alveolar) K04.7
    with sinus K04.6
leg (any part) — *see* Abscess, lower limb
lens H27.8
lingual K14.0
    tonsil J36
lip K13.0
Littre's gland N34.0
liver (cholangitic) (hematogenic) (lymphogenic) (pylephlebitic) (pyogenic) K75.0
    amebic (due to Entamoeba histolytica) (dysenteric) (tropical) A06.4
        with
            brain abscess (and liver or lung abscess) A06.6
            lung abscess A06.5
loin (region) L02.211
lower limb L02.41- ☑
lumbar (tuberculous) A18.01
    nontuberculous L02.212
lung (miliary) (putrid) J85.2
    with pneumonia J85.1
        due to specified organism (see Pneumonia, in (due to))
    amebic (with liver abscess) A06.5
        with
            brain abscess A06.6
            pneumonia A06.5
lymph, lymphatic, gland or node (acute) (*see also* Lymphadenitis, acute)
    mesentery I88.0
malar M27.2
mammary gland — *see* Abscess, breast
marginal, anus K61.0
mastoid — *see* Mastoiditis, acute
maxilla, maxillary M27.2
    molar (tooth) K04.7
        with sinus K04.6
    premolar K04.7
    sinus (chronic) J32.0
mediastinum J85.3
meibomian gland — *see* Hordeolum
meninges G06.2
mesentery, mesenteric K65.1
mesosalpinx — *see* Salpingitis
mons pubis L02.215
mouth (floor) K12.2
muscle — *see* Myositis, infective
myocardium I40.0

Abscess — *continued*
nabothian (follicle) — *see* Cervicitis
nasal J32.9
nasopharyngeal J39.1
navel L02.216
    newborn P38.9
        with mild hemorrhage P38.1
        without hemorrhage P38.9
neck (region) L02.11
    lymph gland or node L04.0
nephritic — *see* Abscess, kidney
nipple N61.1
    associated with
        lactation — *see* Pregnancy, complicated by
        pregnancy — *see* Pregnancy, complicated by
nose (external) (fossa) (septum) J34.0
    sinus (chronic) — *see* Sinusitis
omentum K65.1
operative wound T81.4 ☑
orbit, orbital — *see* Cellulitis, orbit
otogenic G06.0
ovary, ovarian (corpus luteum) — *see* Oophoritis
oviduct — *see* Oophoritis
palate (soft) K12.2
    hard M27.2
palmar (space) — *see* Abscess, hand
pancreas (duct) — *see* Pancreatitis, acute
parafrenal N48.21
parametric, parametrium N73.2
    acute N73.0
    chronic N73.1
paranephric N15.1
parapancreatic — *see* Pancreatitis, acute
parapharyngeal J39.0
pararectal K61.1
parasinus — *see* Sinusitis
parauterine (*see also* Disease, pelvis, inflammatory) N73.2
paravaginal — *see* Vaginitis
parietal region (scalp) L02.811
parodontal — *see* Peridontitis, aggressive, localized
parotid (duct) (gland) K11.3
    region K12.2
pectoral (region) L02.213
pelvis, pelvic
    female — *see* Disease, pelvis, inflammatory
    male, peritoneal K65.1
penis N48.21
    gonococcal (accessory gland) (periurethral) A54.1
perianal K61.0
periapical K04.7
    with sinus (alveolar) K04.6
periappendicular K35.3
pericardial I30.1
pericecal K35.3
pericemental — *see* Peridontitis, aggressive, localized
pericholecystic — *see* Cholecystitis, acute
pericoronal — *see* Peridontitis, aggressive, localized
peridental — *see* Peridontitis, aggressive, localized
perimetric (*see also* Disease, pelvis, inflammatory) N73.2
perinephric, perinephritic — *see* Abscess, kidney
perineum, perineal (superficial) L02.215
    urethra N34.0
periodontal (parietal) — *see* Peridontitis, aggressive, localized
    apical K04.7
periosteum, periosteal (*see also* Osteomyelitis, specified type NEC)
    with osteomyelitis (*see also* Osteomyelitis, specified type NEC)
        acute — *see* Osteomyelitis, acute
        chronic — *see* Osteomyelitis, chronic
peripharyngeal J39.0
peripleuritic J86.9
    with fistula J86.0
periprostatic N41.2
perirectal K61.1
perirenal (tissue) — *see* Abscess, kidney
perisinuous (nose) — *see* Sinusitis
peritoneum, peritoneal (perforated) (ruptured) K65.1
    with appendicitis K35.3
    pelvic
        female — *see* Peritonitis, pelvic, female
        male K65.1
    postoperative T81.4 ☑
    puerperal, postpartum, childbirth O85
    tuberculous A18.31

Abscess — *continued*
 peritonsillar J36
 perityphlic K35.3
 periureteral N28.89
 periurethral N34.0
  gonococcal (accessory gland) (periurethral) A54.1
 periuterine (*see also* Disease, pelvis, inflammatory) N73.2
 perivesical — *see* Cystitis, specified type NEC
 petrous bone — *see* Petrositis
 phagedenic NOS L02.91
  chancroid A57
 pharynx, pharyngeal (lateral) J39.1
 pilonidal L05.01
 pituitary (gland) E23.6
 pleura J86.9
  with fistula J86.0
 popliteal — *see* Abscess, lower limb
 postcecal K35.3
 postlaryngeal J38.7
 postnasal J34.0
 postoperative (any site) T81.4 ☑
  retroperitoneal K68.11
 postpharyngeal J39.0
 posttonsillar J36
 post-typhoid A01.09
 pouch of Douglas — *see* Peritonitis, pelvic, female
 premammary — *see* Abscess, breast
 prepatellar — *see* Abscess, lower limb
 prostate N41.2
  gonococcal (acute) (chronic) A54.22
 psoas muscle K68.12
 puerperal — *code by* site under Puerperal, abscess
 pulmonary — *see* Abscess, lung
 pulp, pulpal (dental) K04.01
  irreversible K04.02
  reversible K04.01
 rectovaginal septum K63.0
 rectovesical — *see* Cystitis, specified type NEC
 rectum K61.1
 renal — *see* Abscess, kidney
 retina — *see* Inflammation, chorioretinal
 retrobulbar — *see* Abscess, orbit
 retrocecal K65.1
 retrolaryngeal J38.7
 retromammary — *see* Abscess, breast
 retroperitoneal NEC K68.19
  postprocedural K68.11
 retropharyngeal J39.0
 retrouterine — *see* Peritonitis, pelvic, female
 retrovesical — *see* Cystitis, specified type NEC
 root, tooth K04.7
  with sinus (alveolar) K04.6
 round ligament (*see also* Disease, pelvis, inflammatory) N73.2
 rupture (spontaneous) NOS L02.91
 sacrum (tuberculous) A18.01
  nontuberculous M46.28
 salivary (duct) (gland) K11.3
 scalp (any part) L02.811
 scapular — *see* Osteomyelitis, specified type NEC
 sclera — *see* Scleritis
 scrofulous (tuberculous) A18.2
 scrotum N49.2
 seminal vesicle N49.0
 septal, dental K04.7
  with sinus (alveolar) K04.6
 serous — *see* Periostitis
 shoulder (region) — *see* Abscess, upper limb
 sigmoid K63.0
 sinus (accessory) (chronic) (nasal) (*see also* Sinusitis)
  intracranial venous (any) G06.0
 Skene's duct or gland N34.0
 skin — *see* Abscess, by site
 specified site NEC L02.818
 spermatic cord N49.1
 sphenoidal (sinus) (chronic) J32.3
 spinal cord (any part) (staphylococcal) G06.1
  tuberculous A17.81
 spine (column) (tuberculous) A18.01
  epidural G06.1
  nontuberculous — *see* Osteomyelitis, vertebra
 spleen D73.3
  amebic A06.89
 stitch T81.4 ☑
 subarachnoid G06.2
  brain G06.0
  spinal cord G06.1

Abscess — *continued*
 subareolar — *see* Abscess, breast
 subcecal K35.3
 subcutaneous (*see also* Abscess, by site)
  pheomycotic (chromomycotic) B43.2
 subdiaphragmatic K65.1
 subdural G06.2
  brain G06.0
   sequelae G09
  spinal cord G06.1
 subgaleal L02.811
 subhepatic K65.1
 sublingual K12.2
  gland K11.3
 submammary — *see* Abscess, breast
 submandibular (region) (space) (triangle) K12.2
  gland K11.3
 submaxillary (region) L02.01
  gland K11.3
 submental L02.01
  gland K11.3
 subperiosteal — *see* Osteomyelitis, specified type NEC
 subphrenic K65.1
  postoperative T81.4 ☑
 suburethral N34.0
 sudoriparous L75.8
 supraclavicular (fossa) — *see* Abscess, upper limb
 suprapelvic, acute N73.0
 suprarenal (capsule) (gland) E27.8
 sweat gland L74.8
 tear duct — *see* Inflammation, lacrimal, passages, acute
 temple L02.01
 temporal region L02.01
 temporosphenoidal G06.0
 tendon (sheath) M65.00
  ankle M65.07- ☑
  foot M65.07- ☑
  forearm M65.03- ☑
  hand M65.04- ☑
  lower leg M65.06- ☑
  pelvic region M65.05- ☑
  shoulder region M65.01- ☑
  specified site NEC M65.08
  thigh M65.05- ☑
  upper arm M65.02- ☑
 testis N45.4
 thigh — *see* Abscess, lower limb
 thorax J86.9
  with fistula J86.0
 throat J39.1
 thumb (*see also* Abscess, hand)
  nail — *see* Cellulitis, finger
 thymus (gland) E32.1
 thyroid (gland) E06.0
 toe (any) (*see also* Abscess, foot)
  nail — *see* Cellulitis, toe
 tongue (staphylococcal) K14.0
 tonsil(s) (lingual) J36
 tonsillopharyngeal J36
 tooth, teeth (root) K04.7
  with sinus (alveolar) K04.6
  supporting structures NEC — *see* Peridontitis, aggressive, localized
 trachea J39.8
 trunk L02.219
  abdominal wall L02.211
  back L02.212
  chest wall L02.213
  groin L02.214
  perineum L02.215
  umbilicus L02.216
 tubal — *see* Salpingitis
 tuberculous — *see* Tuberculosis, abscess
 tubo-ovarian — *see* Salpingo-oophoritis
 tunica vaginalis N49.1
 umbilicus L02.216
 upper
  limb L02.41- ☑
  respiratory J39.8
 urethral (gland) N34.0
 urinary N34.0
 uterus, uterine (wall) (*see also* Endometritis)
  ligament (*see also* Disease, pelvis, inflammatory) N73.2
  neck — *see* Cervicitis
 uvula K12.2
 vagina (wall) — *see* Vaginitis

Abscess — *continued*
 vaginorectal — *see* Vaginitis
 vas deferens N49.1
 vermiform appendix K35.3
 vertebra (column) (tuberculous) A18.01
  nontuberculous — *see* Osteomyelitis, vertebra
 vesical — *see* Cystitis, specified type NEC
 vesico-uterine pouch — *see* Peritonitis, pelvic, female
 vitreous (humor) — *see* Endophthalmitis, purulent
 vocal cord J38.3
 von Bezold's — *see* Mastoiditis, acute
 vulva N76.4
 vulvovaginal gland N75.1
 web space — *see* Abscess, hand
 wound T81.4 ☑
 wrist — *see* Abscess, upper limb
Absence (of) (organ or part) (complete or partial)
 adrenal (gland) (congenital) Q89.1
  acquired E89.6
 albumin in blood E88.09
 alimentary tract (congenital) Q45.8
  upper Q40.8
 alveolar process (acquired) — *see* Anomaly, alveolar
 ankle (acquired) Z89.44- ☑
 anus (congenital) Q42.3
  with fistula Q42.2
 aorta (congenital) Q25.41
 appendix, congenital Q42.8
 arm (acquired) Z89.20- ☑
  above elbow Z89.22- ☑
   congenital (with hand present) — *see* Agenesis, arm, with hand present
   and hand — *see* Agenesis, forearm, and hand
  below elbow Z89.21- ☑
   congenital (with hand present) — *see* Agenesis, arm, with hand present
   and hand — *see* Agenesis, forearm, and hand
  congenital — *see* Defect, reduction, upper limb
  shoulder (following explantation of shoulder joint prosthesis) (joint) (with or without presence of antibiotic-impregnated cement spacer) Z89.23- ☑
   congenital (with hand present) — *see* Agenesis, arm, with hand present
 artery (congenital) (peripheral) Q27.8
  brain Q28.3
  coronary Q24.5
  pulmonary Q25.79
  specified NEC Q27.8
  umbilical Q27.0
 atrial septum (congenital) Q21.1
 auditory canal (congenital) (external) Q16.1
 auricle (ear), congenital Q16.0
 bile, biliary duct, congenital Q44.5
 bladder (acquired) Z90.6
  congenital Q64.5
 bowel sounds R19.11
 brain Q00.0
  part of Q04.3
 breast(s) (and nipple(s)) (acquired) Z90.1- ☑
  congenital Q83.8
 broad ligament Q50.6
 bronchus (congenital) Q32.4
 canaliculus lacrimalis, congenital Q10.4
 cerebellum (vermis) Q04.3
 cervix (acquired) (with uterus) Z90.710
  with remaining uterus Z90.712
  congenital Q51.5
 chin, congenital Q18.8
 cilia (congenital) Q10.3
  acquired — *see* Madarosis
 clitoris (congenital) Q52.6
 coccyx, congenital Q76.49
 cold sense R20.8
 congenital
  lumen — *see* Atresia
  organ or site NEC — *see* Agenesis
  septum — *see* Imperfect, closure
 corpus callosum Q04.0
 cricoid cartilage, congenital Q31.8
 diaphragm (with hernia), congenital Q79.1
 digestive organ(s) or tract, congenital Q45.8
  acquired NEC Z90.49
  upper Q40.8
 ductus arteriosus Q28.8
 duodenum (acquired) Z90.49

☑ Additional Character Required — Refer to the Tabular List for Character Selection

▽ Subterms under main terms may continue to next column or page

Absence — *continued*
duodenum — *continued*
congenital Q41.0
ear, congenital Q16.9
acquired H93.8- ☑
auricle Q16.0
external Q16.0
inner Q16.5
lobe, lobule Q17.8
middle, except ossicles Q16.4
ossicles Q16.3
ossicles Q16.3
ejaculatory duct (congenital) Q55.4
endocrine gland (congenital) NEC Q89.2
acquired E89.89
epididymis (congenital) Q55.4
acquired Z90.79
epiglottis, congenital Q31.8
esophagus (congenital) Q39.8
acquired (partial) Z90.49
eustachian tube (congenital) Q16.2
extremity (acquired) Z89.9
congenital Q73.0
knee (following explantation of knee joint prosthesis) (joint) (with or without presence of antibiotic-impregnated cement spacer) Z89.52- ☑
lower (above knee) Z89.619
below knee Z89.51- ☑
upper — *see* Absence, arm
eye (acquired) Z90.01
congenital Q11.1
muscle (congenital) Q10.3
eyeball (acquired) Z90.01
eyelid (fold) (congenital) Q10.3
acquired Z90.01
face, specified part NEC Q18.8
fallopian tube(s) (acquired) Z90.79
congenital Q50.6
family member (causing problem in home) NEC (*see also* Disruption, family) Z63.32
femur, congenital — *see* Defect, reduction, lower limb, longitudinal, femur
fibrinogen (congenital) D68.2
acquired D65
finger(s) (acquired) Z89.02- ☑
congenital — *see* Agenesis, hand
foot (acquired) Z89.43- ☑
congenital — *see* Agenesis, foot
forearm (acquired) — *see* Absence, arm, below elbow
gallbladder (acquired) Z90.49
congenital Q44.0
gamma globulin in blood D80.1
hereditary D80.0
genital organs
acquired (female) (male) Z90.79
female, congenital Q52.8
external Q52.71
internal NEC Q52.8
male, congenital Q55.8
genitourinary organs, congenital NEC
female Q52.8
male Q55.8
globe (acquired) Z90.01
congenital Q11.1
glottis, congenital Q31.8
hand and wrist (acquired) Z89.11- ☑
congenital — *see* Agenesis, hand
head, part (acquired) NEC Z90.09
heat sense R20.8
hip (following explantation of hip joint prosthesis) (joint) (with or without presence of antibiotic-impregnated cement spacer) Z89.62- ☑
hymen (congenital) Q52.4
ileum (acquired) Z90.49
congenital Q41.2
immunoglobulin, isolated NEC D80.3
IgA D80.2
IgG D80.3
IgM D80.4
incus (acquired) — *see* Loss, ossicles, ear
congenital Q16.3
inner ear, congenital Q16.5
intestine (acquired) (small) Z90.49
congenital Q41.9
specified NEC Q41.8
large Z90.49
congenital Q42.9

Absence — *continued*
intestine — *continued*
large — *continued*
congenital — *continued*
specified NEC Q42.8
iris, congenital Q13.1
jejunum (acquired) Z90.49
congenital Q41.1
joint
acquired
hip (following explantation of hip joint prosthesis) (with or without presence of antibiotic-impregnated cement spacer) Z89.62- ☑
knee (following explantation of knee joint prosthesis) (with or without presence of antibiotic-impregnated cement spacer) Z89.52- ☑
shoulder (following explantation of shoulder joint prosthesis) (with or without presence of antibiotic-impregnated cement spacer) Z89.23- ☑
congenital NEC Q74.8
kidney(s) (acquired) Z90.5
congenital Q60.2
bilateral Q60.1
unilateral Q60.0
knee (following explantation of knee joint prosthesis) (joint) (with or without presence of antibiotic-impregnated cement spacer) Z89.52- ☑
labyrinth, membranous Q16.5
larynx (congenital) Q31.8
acquired Z90.02
leg (acquired) (above knee) Z89.61- ☑
below knee (acquired) Z89.51- ☑
congenital — *see* Defect, reduction, lower limb
lens (acquired) (*see also* Aphakia)
congenital Q12.3
post cataract extraction Z98.4- ☑
limb (acquired) — *see* Absence, extremity
lip Q38.6
liver (congenital) Q44.7
lung (fissure) (lobe) (bilateral) (unilateral) (congenital) Q33.3
acquired (any part) Z90.2
menstruation — *see* Amenorrhea
muscle (congenital) (pectoral) Q79.8
ocular Q10.3
neck, part Q18.8
neutrophil — *see* Agranulocytosis
nipple(s) (with breast(s)) (acquired) Z90.1- ☑
congenital Q83.2
nose (congenital) Q30.1
acquired Z90.09
organ
of Corti, congenital Q16.5
or site, congenital NEC Q89.8
acquired NEC Z90.89
osseous meatus (ear) Q16.4
ovary (acquired)
bilateral Z90.722
congenital
bilateral Q50.02
unilateral Q50.01
unilateral Z90.721
oviduct (acquired)
bilateral Z90.722
congenital Q50.6
unilateral Z90.721
pancreas (congenital) Q45.0
acquired Z90.410
complete Z90.410
partial Z90.411
total Z90.410
parathyroid gland (acquired) E89.2
congenital Q89.2
patella, congenital Q74.1
penis (congenital) Q55.5
acquired Z90.79
pericardium (congenital) Q24.8
pituitary gland (congenital) Q89.2
acquired E89.3
prostate (acquired) Z90.79
congenital Q55.4
pulmonary valve Q22.0
punctum lacrimale (congenital) Q10.4
radius, congenital — *see* Defect, reduction, upper limb, longitudinal, radius

Absence — *continued*
rectum (congenital) Q42.1
with fistula Q42.0
acquired Z90.49
respiratory organ NOS Q34.9
rib (acquired) Z90.89
congenital Q76.6
sacrum, congenital Q76.49
salivary gland(s), congenital Q38.4
scrotum, congenital Q55.29
seminal vesicles (congenital) Q55.4
acquired Z90.79
septum
atrial (congenital) Q21.1
between aorta and pulmonary artery Q21.4
ventricular (congenital) Q20.4
sex chromosome
female phenotype Q97.8
male phenotype Q98.8
skull bone (congenital) Q75.8
with
anencephaly Q00.0
encephalocele — *see* Encephalocele
hydrocephalus Q03.9
with spina bifida — *see* Spina bifida, by site, with hydrocephalus
microcephaly Q02
spermatic cord, congenital Q55.4
spine, congenital Q76.49
spleen (congenital) Q89.01
acquired Z90.81
sternum, congenital Q76.7
stomach (acquired) (partial) Z90.3
congenital Q40.2
superior vena cava, congenital Q26.8
teeth, tooth (congenital) K00.0
acquired (complete) K08.109
class I K08.101
class II K08.102
class III K08.103
class IV K08.104
due to
caries K08.139
class I K08.131
class II K08.132
class III K08.133
class IV K08.134
periodontal disease K08.129
class I K08.121
class II K08.122
class III K08.123
class IV K08.124
specified NEC K08.199
class I K08.191
class II K08.192
class III K08.193
class IV K08.194
trauma K08.119
class I K08.111
class II K08.112
class III K08.113
class IV K08.114
partial K08.409
class I K08.401
class II K08.402
class III K08.403
class IV K08.404
due to
caries K08.439
class I K08.431
class II K08.432
class III K08.433
class IV K08.434
periodontal disease K08.429
class I K08.421
class II K08.422
class III K08.423
class IV K08.424
specified NEC K08.499
class I K08.491
class II K08.492
class III K08.493
class IV K08.494
trauma K08.419
class I K08.411
class II K08.412
class III K08.413
class IV K08.414
tendon (congenital) Q79.8

Index

Absence — Abuse

Absence — *continued*
- testis (congenital) Q55.0
  - acquired Z90.79
- thumb (acquired) Z89.01- ☑
  - congenital — *see* Agenesis, hand
- thymus gland Q89.2
- thyroid (gland) (acquired) E89.0
  - cartilage, congenital Q31.8
  - congenital E03.1
- toe(s) (acquired) Z89.42- ☑
  - with foot — *see* Absence, foot and ankle
  - congenital — *see* Agenesis, foot
  - great Z89.41- ☑
- tongue, congenital Q38.3
- trachea (cartilage), congenital Q32.1
- transverse aortic arch, congenital Q25.49
- tricuspid valve Q22.4
- umbilical artery, congenital Q27.0
- upper arm and forearm with hand present, congenital — *see* Agenesis, arm, with hand present
- ureter (congenital) Q62.4
  - acquired Z90.6
- urethra, congenital Q64.5
- uterus (acquired) Z90.710
  - with cervix Z90.710
  - with remaining cervical stump Z90.711
  - congenital Q51.0
- uvula, congenital Q38.5
- vagina, congenital Q52.0
- vas deferens (congenital) Q55.4
  - acquired Z90.79
- vein (peripheral) congenital NEC Q27.8
  - cerebral Q28.3
  - digestive system Q27.8
  - great Q26.8
  - lower limb Q27.8
  - portal Q26.5
  - precerebral Q28.1
  - specified site NEC Q27.8
  - upper limb Q27.8
- vena cava (inferior) (superior), congenital Q26.8
- ventricular septum Q20.4
- vertebra, congenital Q76.49
- vulva, congenital Q52.71
- wrist (acquired) Z89.12- ☑

Absorbent system disease I87.8

Absorption
- carbohydrate, disturbance K90.49
- chemical — *see* Table of Drugs and Chemicals
  - through placenta (newborn) P04.9
    - environmental substance P04.6
    - nutritional substance P04.5
    - obstetric anesthetic or analgesic drug P04.0
- drug NEC — *see* Table of Drugs and Chemicals
  - addictive
    - through placenta (newborn) P04.49
      - cocaine P04.41
  - medicinal
    - through placenta (newborn) P04.1
    - through placenta (newborn) P04.1
      - obstetric anesthetic or analgesic drug P04.0
- fat, disturbance K90.49
  - pancreatic K90.3
- noxious substance — *see* Table of Drugs and Chemicals
- protein, disturbance K90.49
- starch, disturbance K90.49
- toxic substance — *see* Table of Drugs and Chemicals
- uremic — *see* Uremia

Abstinence symptoms, syndrome
- alcohol F10.239
  - with delirium F10.231
- cocaine F14.23
- neonatal P96.1
- nicotine — *see* Dependence, drug, nicotine, with, withdrawal
- opioid F11.93
  - with dependence F11.23
- psychoactive NEC F19.939
  - with
    - delirium F19.931
    - dependence F19.239
      - with
        - delirium F19.231
        - perceptual disturbance F19.232
      - uncomplicated F19.230
    - perceptual disturbance F19.932
  - uncomplicated F19.930

Abstinence symptoms, syndrome — *continued*
- sedative F13.939
  - with
    - delirium F13.931
    - dependence F13.239
      - with
        - delirium F13.231
        - perceptual disturbance F13.232
      - uncomplicated F13.230
    - perceptual disturbance F13.932
  - uncomplicated F13.930
- stimulant NEC F15.93
  - with dependence F15.23

Abulia R68.89

Abulomania F60.7

Abuse
- adult — *see* Maltreatment, adult
  - as reason for
    - couple seeking advice (including offender) Z63.0
- alcohol (non-dependent) F10.10
  - with
    - anxiety disorder F10.180
    - intoxication F10.129
      - with delirium F10.121
      - uncomplicated F10.120
    - mood disorder F10.14
    - other specified disorder F10.188
    - psychosis F10.159
      - delusions F10.150
      - hallucinations F10.151
    - sexual dysfunction F10.181
    - sleep disorder F10.182
    - unspecified disorder F10.19
  - counseling and surveillance Z71.41
  - in remission (early) (sustained) F10.11
- amphetamine (or related substance) — *see* Abuse, drug, stimulant NEC
- analgesics (non-prescribed) (over the counter) F55.8
- antacids F55.0
- antidepressants — *see* Abuse, drug, psychoactive NEC
- anxiolytic — *see* Abuse, drug, sedative
- barbiturates — *see* Abuse, drug, sedative
- caffeine — *see* Abuse, drug, stimulant NEC
- cannabis, cannabinoids — *see* Abuse, drug, cannabis
- child — *see* Maltreatment, child
- cocaine — *see* Abuse, drug, cocaine
- drug NEC (non-dependent) F19.10
  - with sleep disorder F19.182
  - amphetamine type — *see* Abuse, drug, stimulant NEC
  - analgesics (non-prescribed) (over the counter) F55.8
  - antacids F55.0
  - antidepressants — *see* Abuse, drug, psychoactive NEC
  - anxiolytics — *see* Abuse, drug, sedative
  - barbiturates — *see* Abuse, drug, sedative
  - caffeine — *see* Abuse, drug, stimulant NEC
  - cannabis F12.10
    - with
      - anxiety disorder F12.180
      - intoxication F12.129
        - with
          - delirium F12.121
          - perceptual disturbance F12.122
        - uncomplicated F12.120
      - other specified disorder F12.188
      - psychosis F12.159
        - delusions F12.150
        - hallucinations F12.151
      - unspecified disorder F12.19
    - in remission (early) (sustained) F12.11
  - cocaine F14.10
    - with
      - anxiety disorder F14.180
      - intoxication F14.129
        - with
          - delirium F14.121
          - perceptual disturbance F14.122
        - uncomplicated F14.120
      - mood disorder F14.14
      - other specified disorder F14.188
      - psychosis F14.159
        - delusions F14.150
        - hallucinations F14.151
      - sexual dysfunction F14.181
      - sleep disorder F14.182

Abuse — *continued*
- drug — *continued*
  - cocaine — *continued*
    - with — *continued*
      - unspecified disorder F14.19
    - in remission (early) (sustained) F14.11
  - counseling and surveillance Z71.51
  - hallucinogen F16.10
    - with
      - anxiety disorder F16.180
      - flashbacks F16.183
      - intoxication F16.129
        - with
          - delirium F16.121
          - perceptual disturbance F16.122
        - uncomplicated F16.120
      - mood disorder F16.14
      - other specified disorder F16.188
      - perception disorder, persisting F16.183
      - psychosis F16.159
        - delusions F16.150
        - hallucinations F16.151
      - unspecified disorder F16.19
    - in remission (early) (sustained) F16.11
  - hashish — *see* Abuse, drug, cannabis
  - herbal or folk remedies F55.1
  - hormones F55.3
  - hypnotics — *see* Abuse, drug, sedative
  - in remission (early) (sustained) F19.11
  - inhalant F18.10
    - with
      - anxiety disorder F18.180
      - dementia, persisting F18.17
      - intoxication F18.129
        - with delirium F18.121
        - uncomplicated F18.120
      - mood disorder F18.14
      - other specified disorder F18.188
      - psychosis F18.159
        - delusions F18.150
        - hallucinations F18.151
      - unspecified disorder F18.19
    - in remission (early) (sustained) F18.11
  - laxatives F55.2
  - LSD — *see* Abuse, drug, hallucinogen
  - marihuana — *see* Abuse, drug, cannabis
  - morphine type (opioids) — *see* Abuse, drug, opioid
  - opioid F11.10
    - with
      - intoxication F11.129
        - with
          - delirium F11.121
          - perceptual disturbance F11.122
        - uncomplicated F11.120
      - mood disorder F11.14
      - other specified disorder F11.188
      - psychosis F11.159
        - delusions F11.150
        - hallucinations F11.151
      - sexual dysfunction F11.181
      - sleep disorder F11.182
      - unspecified disorder F11.19
    - in remission (early) (sustained) F11.11
  - PCP (phencyclidine) (or related substance) — *see* Abuse, drug, hallucinogen
  - psychoactive NEC F19.10
    - with
      - amnestic disorder F19.16
      - anxiety disorder F19.180
      - dementia F19.17
      - intoxication F19.129
        - with
          - delirium F19.121
          - perceptual disturbance F19.122
        - uncomplicated F19.120
      - mood disorder F19.14
      - other specified disorder F19.188
      - psychosis F19.159
        - delusions F19.150
        - hallucinations F19.151
      - sexual dysfunction F19.181
      - sleep disorder F19.182
      - unspecified disorder F19.19
  - sedative, hypnotic or anxiolytic F13.10
    - with
      - anxiety disorder F13.180
      - intoxication F13.129
        - with delirium F13.121
        - uncomplicated F13.120

☑ Additional Character Required — Refer to the Tabular List for Character Selection ▽ Subterms under main terms may continue to next column or page

Abuse — *continued*
  drug — *continued*
    sedative, hypnotic or anxiolytic — *continued*
      with — *continued*
        mood disorder F13.14
        other specified disorder F13.188
        psychosis F13.159
          delusions F13.150
          hallucinations F13.151
        sexual dysfunction F13.181
        sleep disorder F13.182
        unspecified disorder F13.19
      in remission (early) (sustained) F13.11
    solvent — *see* Abuse, drug, inhalant
    steroids F55.3
    stimulant NEC F15.10
      with
        anxiety disorder F15.180
        intoxication F15.129
          with
            delirium F15.121
            perceptual disturbance F15.122
          uncomplicated F15.120
        mood disorder F15.14
        other specified disorder F15.188
        psychosis F15.159
          delusions F15.150
          hallucinations F15.151
        sexual dysfunction F15.181
        sleep disorder F15.182
        unspecified disorder F15.19
      in remission (early) (sustained) F15.11
    tranquilizers — *see* Abuse, drug, sedative
    vitamins F55.4
  hallucinogens — *see* Abuse, drug, hallucinogen
  hashish — *see* Abuse, drug, cannabis
  herbal or folk remedies F55.1
  hormones F55.3
  hypnotic — *see* Abuse, drug, sedative
  inhalant — *see* Abuse, drug, inhalant
  laxatives F55.2
  LSD — *see* Abuse, drug, hallucinogen
  marihuana — *see* Abuse, drug, cannabis
  morphine type (opioids) — *see* Abuse, drug, opioid
  non-psychoactive substance NEC F55.8
    antacids F55.0
    folk remedies F55.1
    herbal remedies F55.1
    hormones F55.3
    laxatives F55.2
    steroids F55.3
    vitamins F55.4
  opioids — *see* Abuse, drug, opioid
  PCP (phencyclidine) (or related substance) — *see* Abuse, drug, hallucinogen
  physical (adult) (child) — *see* Maltreatment
  psychoactive substance — *see* Abuse, drug, psychoactive NEC
  psychological (adult) (child) — *see* Maltreatment
  sedative — *see* Abuse, drug, sedative
  sexual — *see* Maltreatment
  solvent — *see* Abuse, drug, inhalant
  steroids F55.3
  vitamins F55.4
Acalculia R48.8
  developmental F81.2
Acanthamebiasis (with) B60.10
  conjunctiva B60.12
  keratoconjunctivitis B60.13
  meningoencephalitis B60.11
  other specified B60.19
Acanthocephaliasis B83.8
Acanthocheilonemiasis B74.4
Acanthocytosis E78.6
Acantholysis L11.9
Acanthosis (acquired) (nigricans) L83
  benign Q82.8
  congenital Q82.8
  seborrheic L82.1
    inflamed L82.0
  tongue K14.3
Acapnia E87.3
Acarbia E87.2
Acardia, acardius Q89.8
Acardiacus amorphus Q89.8
Acardiotrophia I51.4
Acariasis B88.0
  scabies B86

Acarodermatitis (urticarioides) B88.0
Acarophobia F40.218
Acatalasemia, acatalasia E80.3
Acathisia (drug induced) G25.71
Accelerated atrioventricular conduction I45.6
Accentuation of personality traits (type A) Z73.1
Accessory (congenital)
  adrenal gland Q89.1
  anus Q43.4
  appendix Q43.4
  atrioventricular conduction I45.6
  auditory ossicles Q16.3
  auricle (ear) Q17.0
  biliary duct or passage Q44.5
  bladder Q64.79
  blood vessels NEC Q27.9
    coronary Q24.5
  bone NEC Q79.8
  breast tissue, axilla Q83.1
  carpal bones Q74.0
  cecum Q43.4
  chromosome(s) NEC (nonsex) Q92.9
    with complex rearrangements NEC Q92.5
      seen only at prometaphase Q92.8
    13 — *see* Trisomy, 13
    18 — *see* Trisomy, 18
    21 — *see* Trisomy, 21
    partial Q92.9
    sex
      female phenotype Q97.8
  coronary artery Q24.5
  cusp(s), heart valve NEC Q24.8
    pulmonary Q22.3
  cystic duct Q44.5
  digit(s) Q69.9
  ear (auricle) (lobe) Q17.0
  endocrine gland NEC Q89.2
  eye muscle Q10.3
  eyelid Q10.3
  face bone(s) Q75.8
  fallopian tube (fimbria) (ostium) Q50.6
  finger(s) Q69.0
  foreskin N47.8
  frontonasal process Q75.8
  gallbladder Q44.1
  genital organ(s)
    female Q52.8
      external Q52.79
      internal NEC Q52.8
    male Q55.8
  genitourinary organs NEC Q89.8
    female Q52.8
    male Q55.8
  hallux Q69.2
  heart Q24.8
    valve NEC Q24.8
      pulmonary Q22.3
  hepatic ducts Q44.5
  hymen Q52.4
  intestine (large) (small) Q43.4
  kidney Q63.0
  lacrimal canal Q10.6
  leaflet, heart valve NEC Q24.8
  ligament, broad Q50.6
  liver Q44.7
    duct Q44.5
  lobule (ear) Q17.0
  lung (lobe) Q33.1
  muscle Q79.8
  navicular of carpus Q74.0
  nervous system, part NEC Q07.8
  nipple Q83.3
  nose Q30.8
  organ or site not listed — *see* Anomaly, by site
  ovary Q50.31
  oviduct Q50.6
  pancreas Q45.3
  parathyroid gland Q89.2
  parotid gland (and duct) Q38.4
  pituitary gland Q89.2
  preauricular appendage Q17.0
  prepuce N47.8
  renal arteries (multiple) Q27.2
  rib Q76.6
    cervical Q76.5
  roots (teeth) K00.2
  salivary gland Q38.4
  sesamoid bones Q74.8

Accessory — *continued*
  sesamoid bones — *continued*
    foot Q74.2
    hand Q74.0
  skin tags Q82.8
  spleen Q89.09
  sternum Q76.7
  submaxillary gland Q38.4
  tarsal bones Q74.2
  teeth, tooth K00.1
  tendon Q79.8
  thumb Q69.1
  thymus gland Q89.2
  thyroid gland Q89.2
  toes Q69.2
  tongue Q38.3
  tooth, teeth K00.1
  tragus Q17.0
  ureter Q62.5
  urethra Q64.79
  urinary organ or tract NEC Q64.8
  uterus Q51.2
  vagina Q52.10
  valve, heart NEC Q24.8
    pulmonary Q22.3
  vertebra Q76.49
  vocal cords Q31.8
  vulva Q52.79
Accident
  birth — *see* Birth, injury
  cardiac — *see* Infarct, myocardium
  cerebral I63.9
  cerebrovascular (embolic) (ischemic) (thrombotic) I63.9
    aborted I63.9
    hemorrhagic — *see* Hemorrhage, intracranial, intracerebral
    old (without sequelae) Z86.73
      with sequelae (of) — *see* Sequelae, infarction, cerebral
  coronary — *see* Infarct, myocardium
  craniovascular I63.9
  vascular, brain I63.9
Accidental — *see* condition
Accommodation (disorder) (*see also* condition)
  hysterical paralysis of F44.89
  insufficiency of H52.4
  paresis — *see* Paresis, of accommodation
  spasm — *see* Spasm, of accommodation
Accouchement — *see* Delivery
Accreta placenta O43.21- ☑
Accretio cordis (nonrheumatic) I31.0
Accretions, tooth, teeth K03.6
Acculturation difficulty Z60.3
Accumulation secretion, prostate N42.89
Acephalia, acephalism, acephalus, acephaly Q00.0
Acephalobrachia monster Q89.8
Acephalochirus monster Q89.8
Acephalogaster Q89.8
Acephalostomus monster Q89.8
Acephalothorax Q89.8
Acerophobia F40.298
Acetonemia R79.89
  in Type 1 diabetes E10.10
    with coma E10.11
Acetonuria R82.4
Achalasia (cardia) (esophagus) K22.0
  congenital Q39.5
  pylorus Q40.0
  sphincteral NEC K59.8
Ache(s) — *see* Pain
Acheilia Q38.6
Achillobursitis — *see* Tendinitis, Achilles
Achillodynia — *see* Tendinitis, Achilles
Achlorhydria, achlorhydric (neurogenic) K31.83
  anemia D50.8
  diarrhea K31.83
  psychogenic F45.8
  secondary to vagotomy K91.1
Achluophobia F40.228
Acholia K82.8
Acholuric jaundice (familial) (splenomegalic) (*see also* Spherocytosis)
  acquired D59.8
Achondrogenesis Q77.0
Achondroplasia (osteosclerosis congenita) Q77.4
Achroma, cutis L80

Achromat (ism), achromatopsia (acquired) (congenital) H53.51
Achromia, congenital — see Albinism
Achromia parasitica B36.0
Achylia gastrica K31.89
  psychogenic F45.8
Acid
  burn — see Corrosion
  deficiency
    amide nicotinic E52
    ascorbic E54
    folic E53.8
    nicotinic E52
    pantothenic E53.8
  intoxication E87.2
  peptic disease K30
  phosphatase deficiency E83.39
  stomach K30
    psychogenic F45.8
Acidemia E87.2
  argininosuccinic E72.22
  isovaleric E71.110
  metabolic (newborn) P19.9
    first noted before onset of labor P19.0
    first noted during labor P19.1
    noted at birth P19.2
  methylmalonic E71.120
  pipecolic E72.3
  propionic E71.121
Acidity, gastric (high) K30
  psychogenic F45.8
Acidocytopenia — see Agranulocytosis
Acidocytosis D72.1
Acidopenia — see Agranulocytosis
Acidosis (lactic) (respiratory) E87.2
  in Type 1 diabetes E10.10
    with coma E10.11
  kidney, tubular N25.89
  lactic E87.2
  metabolic NEC E87.2
    with respiratory acidosis E87.4
    late, of newborn P74.0
  mixed metabolic and respiratory, newborn P84
  newborn P84
  renal (hyperchloremic) (tubular) N25.89
  respiratory E87.2
    complicated by
      metabolic
        acidosis E87.4
        alkalosis E87.4
Aciduria
  argininosuccinic E72.22
  glutaric (type I) E72.3
    type II E71.313
    type III E71.5- ☑
  orotic (congenital) (hereditary) (pyrimidine deficiency) E79.8
    anemia D53.0
Acladiosis (skin) B36.0
Aclasis, diaphyseal Q78.6
Acleistocardia Q21.1
Aclusion — see Anomaly, dentofacial, malocclusion
Acne L70.9
  artificialis L70.8
  atrophica L70.2
  cachecticorum (Hebra) L70.8
  conglobata L70.1
  cystic L70.0
  decalvans L66.2
  excoriée (des jeunes filles) L70.5
  frontalis L70.2
  indurata L70.0
  infantile L70.4
  keloid L73.0
  lupoid L70.2
  necrotic, necrotica (miliaris) L70.2
  neonatal L70.4
  nodular L70.0
  occupational L70.8
  picker's L70.5
  pustular L70.0
  rodens L70.2
  rosacea L71.9
  specified NEC L70.8
  tropica L70.3
  varioliformis L70.2
  vulgaris L70.0
Acnitis (primary) A18.4

Acosta's disease T70.29 ☑
Acoustic — see condition
Acousticophobia F40.298
Acquired (see also condition)
  immunodeficiency syndrome (AIDS) B20
Acrania Q00.0
Acroangiodermatitis I78.9
Acroasphyxia, chronic I73.89
Acrobystitis N47.7
Acrocephalopolysyndactyly Q87.0
Acrocephalosyndactyly Q87.0
Acrocephaly Q75.0
Acrochondrohyperplasia — see Syndrome, Marfan's
Acrocyanosis I73.8 ☑
  newborn P28.2
    meaning transient blue hands and feet — omit code
Acrodermatitis L30.8
  atrophicans (chronica) L90.4
  continua (Hallopeau) L40.2
  enteropathica (hereditary) E83.2
  Hallopeau's L40.2
  infantile papular L44.4
  perstans L40.2
  pustulosa continua L40.2
  recalcitrant pustular L40.2
Acrodynia — see Poisoning, mercury
Acromegaly, acromegalia E22.0
Acromelalgia I73.81
Acromicria, acromikria Q79.8
Acronyx L60.0
Acropachy, thyroid — see Thyrotoxicosis
Acroparesthesia (simple) (vasomotor) I73.89
Acropathy, thyroid — see Thyrotoxicosis
Acrophobia F40.241
Acroposthitis N47.7
Acroscleriasis, acroscleroderma, acrosclerosis — see Sclerosis, systemic
Acrosphacelus I96
Acrospiroma, eccrine — see Neoplasm, skin, benign
Acrostealgia — see Osteochondropathy
Acrotrophodynia — see Immersion
ACTH ectopic syndrome E24.3
Actinic — see condition
Actinobacillosis, actinobacillus A28.8
  mallei A24.0
  muris A25.1
Actinomyces israelii (infection) — see Actinomycosis
Actinomycetoma (foot) B47.1
Actinomycosis, actinomycotic A42.9
  with pneumonia A42.0
  abdominal A42.1
  cervicofacial A42.2
  cutaneous A42.89
  gastrointestinal A42.1
  pulmonary A42.0
  sepsis A42.7
  specified site NEC A42.89
Actinoneuritis G62.82
Action, heart
  disorder I49.9
  irregular I49.9
    psychogenic F45.8
Activated protein C resistance D68.51
Activation
  mast cell (disorder) (syndrome) D89.40
    idiopathic D89.42
    monoclonal D89.41
    secondary D89.43
    specified type NEC D89.49
Active — see condition
Acute (see also condition)
  abdomen R10.0
  gallbladder — see Cholecystitis, acute
Acyanotic heart disease (congenital) Q24.9
Acystia Q64.5
Adair-Dighton syndrome (brittle bones and blue sclera, deafness) Q78.0
Adamantinoblastoma — see Ameloblastoma
Adamantinoma (see also Cyst, calcifying odontogenic)
  long bones C40.90
    lower limb C40.2- ☑
    upper limb C40.0- ☑
  malignant C41.1
    jaw (bone) (lower) C41.1
      upper C41.0
  tibial C40.2- ☑

Adamantoblastoma — see Ameloblastoma
Adams-Stokes (-Morgagni) disease or syndrome I45.9
Adaption reaction — see Disorder, adjustment
Addiction (see also Dependence) F19.20
  alcohol, alcoholic (ethyl) (methyl) (wood) (without remission) F10.20
    with remission F10.21
  drug — see Dependence, drug
  ethyl alcohol (without remission) F10.20
    with remission F10.21
  heroin — see Dependence, drug, opioid
  methyl alcohol (without remission) F10.20
    with remission F10.21
  methylated spirit (without remission) F10.20
    with remission F10.21
  morphine (-like substances) — see Dependence, drug, opioid
  nicotine — see Dependence, drug, nicotine
  opium and opioids — see Dependence, drug, opioid
  tobacco — see Dependence, drug, nicotine
Addison-Biermer anemia (pernicious) D51.0
Addisonian crisis E27.2
Addison's
  anemia (pernicious) D51.0
  disease (bronze) or syndrome E27.1
    tuberculous A18.7
  keloid L94.0
Addison-Schilder complex E71.528
Additional (see also Accessory)
  chromosome(s) Q99.8
    21 — see Trisomy, 21
    sex — see Abnormal, chromosome, sex
Adduction contracture, hip or other joint — see Contraction, joint
Adenitis (see also Lymphadenitis)
  acute, unspecified site L04.9
  axillary I88.9
    acute L04.2
    chronic or subacute I88.1
  Bartholin's gland N75.8
  bulbourethral gland — see Urethritis
  cervical I88.9
    acute L04.0
    chronic or subacute I88.1
  chancroid (Hemophilus ducreyi) A57
  chronic, unspecified site I88.1
  Cowper's gland — see Urethritis
  due to Pasteurella multocida (P. septica) A28.0
  epidemic, acute B27.09
  gangrenous L04.9
  gonorrheal NEC A54.89
  groin I88.9
    acute L04.1
    chronic or subacute I88.1
  infectious (acute) (epidemic) B27.09
  inguinal I88.9
    acute L04.1
    chronic or subacute I88.1
  lymph gland or node, except mesenteric I88.9
    acute — see Lymphadenitis, acute
    chronic or subacute I88.1
  mesenteric (acute) (chronic) (nonspecific) (subacute) I88.0
  parotid gland (suppurative) — see Sialoadenitis
  salivary gland (any) (suppurative) — see Sialoadenitis
  scrofulous (tuberculous) A18.2
  Skene's duct or gland — see Urethritis
  strumous, tuberculous A18.2
  subacute, unspecified site I88.1
  sublingual gland (suppurative) — see Sialoadenitis
  submandibular gland (suppurative) — see Sialoadenitis
  submaxillary gland (suppurative) — see Sialoadenitis
  tuberculous — see Tuberculosis, lymph gland
  urethral gland — see Urethritis
  Wharton's duct — see Sialoadenitis
Adenoacanthoma — see Neoplasm, malignant, by site
Adenoameloblastoma — see Cyst, calcifying odontogenic
Adenocarcinoid (tumor) — see Neoplasm, malignant, by site
Adenocarcinoma (see also Neoplasm, malignant, by site)
  acidophil
    specified site — see Neoplasm, by site, malignant
    unspecified site C75.1
  adrenal cortical C74.0- ☑
  alveolar — see Neoplasm, lung, malignant

☑ Additional Character Required — Refer to the Tabular List for Character Selection   ▽ Subterms under main terms may continue to next column or page

Adenocarcinoma — *continued*
  apocrine
    breast — *see* Neoplasm, breast, malignant
    in situ
      breast D05.8- ☑
      specified site NEC — *see* Neoplasm, skin, in situ
      unspecified site D04.9
    specified site NEC — *see* Neoplasm, skin, malignant
    unspecified site C44.99
  basal cell
    specified site — *see* Neoplasm, skin, malignant
    unspecified site C08.9
  basophil
    specified site — *see* Neoplasm, malignant, by site
    unspecified site C75.1
  bile duct type C22.1
    liver C22.1
    specified site NEC — *see* Neoplasm, malignant, by site
    unspecified site C22.1
  bronchiolar — *see* Neoplasm, lung, malignant
  bronchioloalveolar — *see* Neoplasm, lung, malignant
  ceruminous C44.29- ☑
  cervix, in situ (*see also* Carcinoma, cervix uteri, in situ) D06.9
  chromophobe
    specified site — *see* Neoplasm, malignant, by site
    unspecified site C75.1
  diffuse type
    specified site — *see* Neoplasm, malignant, by site
    unspecified site C16.9
  duct
    infiltrating
      with Paget's disease — *see* Neoplasm, breast, malignant
      specified site — *see* Neoplasm, malignant, by site
      unspecified site (female) C50.91- ☑
        male C50.92- ☑
    specified site — *see* Neoplasm, malignant, by site
    unspecified site
      female C56.9
      male C61
  eosinophil
    specified site — *see* Neoplasm, malignant, by site
    unspecified site C75.1
  follicular
    with papillary C73
    moderately differentiated C73
    specified site — *see* Neoplasm, malignant, by site
    trabecular C73
    unspecified site C73
    well differentiated C73
  Hurthle cell C73
  in
    adenomatous
      polyposis coli C18.9
  infiltrating duct
    with Paget's disease — *see* Neoplasm, breast, malignant
    specified site — *see* Neoplasm, by site, malignant
    unspecified site (female) C50.91- ☑
      male C50.92- ☑
  inflammatory
    specified site — *see* Neoplasm, by site, malignant
    unspecified site (female) C50.91- ☑
      male C50.92- ☑
  intestinal type
    specified site — *see* Neoplasm, by site, malignant
    unspecified site C16.9
  intracystic papillary
  intraductal
    breast D05.1- ☑
    noninfiltrating
      breast D05.1- ☑
      papillary
        with invasion
          specified site — *see* Neoplasm, by site, malignant
          unspecified site (female) C50.91- ☑
            male C50.92- ☑
        breast D05.1- ☑
        specified site NEC — *see* Neoplasm, in situ, by site
        unspecified site D05.1- ☑
      specified site NEC — *see* Neoplasm, in situ, by site

Adenocarcinoma — *continued*
  intraductal — *continued*
    noninfiltrating — *continued*
      unspecified site D05.1- ☑
    papillary
      with invasion
        specified site — *see* Neoplasm, malignant, by site
        unspecified site (female) C50.91- ☑
          male C50.92- ☑
      breast D05.1- ☑
      specified site — *see* Neoplasm, in situ, by site
      unspecified site D05.1- ☑
    specified site NEC — *see* Neoplasm, in situ, by site
    unspecified site D05.1- ☑
  islet cell
    with exocrine, mixed
      specified site — *see* Neoplasm, malignant, by site
      unspecified site C25.9
    pancreas C25.4
    specified site NEC — *see* Neoplasm, malignant, by site
    unspecified site C25.4
  lobular
    in situ
      breast D05.0- ☑
      specified site NEC — *see* Neoplasm, in situ, by site
      unspecified site D05.0- ☑
    specified site — *see* Neoplasm, malignant, by site
    unspecified site (female) C50.91- ☑
      male C50.92- ☑
  mucoid (*see also* Neoplasm, malignant, by site)
    cell
      specified site — *see* Neoplasm, malignant, by site
      unspecified site C75.1
  nonencapsulated sclerosing C73
  papillary
    with follicular C73
    follicular variant C73
    intraductal (noninfiltrating)
      with invasion
        specified site — *see* Neoplasm, malignant, by site
        unspecified site (female) C50.91- ☑
          male C50.92- ☑
      breast D05.1- ☑
      specified site NEC — *see* Neoplasm, in situ, by site
      unspecified site D05.1- ☑
    serous
      specified site — *see* Neoplasm, malignant, by site
      unspecified site C56.9
  papillocystic
    specified site — *see* Neoplasm, malignant, by site
    unspecified site C56.9
  pseudomucinous
    specified site — *see* Neoplasm, malignant, by site
    unspecified site C56.9
  renal cell C64- ☑
  sebaceous — *see* Neoplasm, skin, malignant
  serous (*see also* Neoplasm, malignant, by site)
    papillary
      specified site — *see* Neoplasm, malignant, by site
      unspecified site C56.9
  sweat gland — *see* Neoplasm, skin, malignant
  water-clear cell C75.0
Adenocarcinoma-in-situ (*see also* Neoplasm, in situ, by site)
  breast D05.9- ☑
Adenofibroma
  clear cell — *see* Neoplasm, benign, by site
  endometrioid D27.9
    borderline malignancy D39.10
    malignant C56- ☑
  mucinous
    specified site — *see* Neoplasm, benign, by site
    unspecified site D27.9
  papillary
    specified site — *see* Neoplasm, benign, by site
    unspecified site D27.9
  prostate — *see* Enlargement, enlarged, prostate

Adenofibroma — *continued*
  serous
    specified site — *see* Neoplasm, benign, by site
    unspecified site D27.9
  specified site — *see* Neoplasm, benign, by site
  unspecified site D27.9
Adenofibrosis
  breast — *see* Fibroadenosis, breast
  endometrioid N80.0
Adenoiditis (chronic) J35.02
  with tonsillitis J35.03
  acute J03.90
    recurrent J03.91
    specified organism NEC J03.80
      recurrent J03.81
    staphylococcal J03.80
      recurrent J03.81
    streptococcal J03.00
      recurrent J03.01
Adenoids — *see* condition
Adenolipoma — *see* Neoplasm, benign, by site
Adenolipomatosis, Launois-Bensaude E88.89
Adenolymphoma
  specified site — *see* Neoplasm, benign, by site
  unspecified site D11.9
Adenoma (*see also* Neoplasm, benign, by site)
  acidophil
    specified site — *see* Neoplasm, benign, by site
    unspecified site D35.2
  acidophil-basophil, mixed
    specified site — *see* Neoplasm, benign, by site
    unspecified site D35.2
  adrenal (cortical) D35.00
    clear cell D35.00
    compact cell D35.00
    glomerulosa cell D35.00
    heavily pigmented variant D35.00
    mixed cell D35.00
  alpha-cell
    pancreas D13.7
    specified site NEC — *see* Neoplasm, benign, by site
    unspecified site D13.7
  alveolar D14.30
  apocrine
    breast D24- ☑
    specified site NEC — *see* Neoplasm, skin, benign, by site
    unspecified site D23.9
  basal cell D11.9
  basophil
    specified site — *see* Neoplasm, benign, by site
    unspecified site D35.2
  basophil-acidophil, mixed
    specified site — *see* Neoplasm, benign, by site
    unspecified site D35.2
  beta-cell
    pancreas D13.7
    specified site NEC — *see* Neoplasm, benign, by site
    unspecified site D13.7
  bile duct D13.4
    common D13.5
    extrahepatic D13.5
    intrahepatic D13.4
    specified site NEC — *see* Neoplasm, benign, by site
    unspecified site D13.4
  black D35.00
  bronchial D38.1
    cylindroid type — *see* Neoplasm, lung, malignant
  ceruminous D23.2- ☑
  chief cell D35.1
  chromophobe
    specified site — *see* Neoplasm, benign, by site
    unspecified site D35.2
  colloid
    specified site — *see* Neoplasm, benign, by site
    unspecified site D34
  duct
  eccrine, papillary — *see* Neoplasm, skin, benign
  endocrine, multiple
    single specified site — *see* Neoplasm, uncertain behavior, by site
    two or more specified sites D44- ☑
    unspecified site D44.9
  endometrioid (*see also* Neoplasm, benign)
    borderline malignancy — *see* Neoplasm, uncertain behavior, by site
  eosinophil
    specified site — *see* Neoplasm, benign, by site

⬚ **Subterms under main terms may continue to next column or page**   ☑ **Additional Character Required — Refer to the Tabular List for Character Selection**   **11**

Adenocarcinoma — Adenoma

Index

Adenoma — Adhesions, adhesive

Adenoma — *continued*
eosinophil — *continued*
unspecified site D35.2
fetal
specified site — *see* Neoplasm, benign, by site
unspecified site D34
follicular
specified site — *see* Neoplasm, benign, by site
unspecified site D34
hepatocellular D13.4
Hurthle cell D34
islet cell
pancreas D13.7
specified site NEC — *see* Neoplasm, benign, by site
unspecified site D13.7
liver cell D13.4
macrofollicular
specified site — *see* Neoplasm, benign, by site
unspecified site D34
malignant, malignum — *see* Neoplasm, malignant, by site
microcystic
pancreas D13.6
specified site NEC — *see* Neoplasm, benign, by site
unspecified site D13.6
microfollicular
specified site — *see* Neoplasm, benign, by site
unspecified site D34
mucoid cell
specified site — *see* Neoplasm, benign, by site
unspecified site D35.2
multiple endocrine
single specified site — *see* Neoplasm, uncertain behavior, by site
two or more specified sites D44- ☑
unspecified site D44.9
nipple D24- ☑
papillary (*see also* Neoplasm, benign, by site)
eccrine — *see* Neoplasm, skin, benign, by site
Pick's tubular
specified site — *see* Neoplasm, benign, by site
unspecified site
female D27.9
male D29.20
pleomorphic
carcinoma in — *see* Neoplasm, salivary gland, malignant
specified site — *see* Neoplasm, malignant, by site
unspecified site C08.9
polypoid (*see also* Neoplasm, benign)
adenocarcinoma in — *see* Neoplasm, malignant, by site
adenocarcinoma in situ — *see* Neoplasm, in situ, by site
prostate — *see* Neoplasm, benign, prostate
rete cell D29.20
sebaceous — *see* Neoplasm, skin, benign
Sertoli cell
specified site — *see* Neoplasm, benign, by site
unspecified site
female D27.9
male D29.20
skin appendage — *see* Neoplasm, skin, benign
sudoriferous gland — *see* Neoplasm, skin, benign
sweat gland — *see* Neoplasm, skin, benign
testicular
specified site — *see* Neoplasm, benign, by site
unspecified site
female D27.9
male D29.20
tubular (*see also* Neoplasm, benign, by site)
adenocarcinoma in — *see* Neoplasm, malignant, by site
adenocarcinoma in situ — *see* Neoplasm, in situ, by site
Pick's
specified site — *see* Neoplasm, benign, by site
unspecified site
female D27.9
male D29.20
tubulovillous (*see also* Neoplasm, benign, by site)
adenocarcinoma in — *see* Neoplasm, malignant, by site
adenocarcinoma in situ — *see* Neoplasm, in situ, by site
villous — *see* Neoplasm, uncertain behavior, by site

Adenoma — *continued*
villous — *see* Neoplasm, uncertain behavior, by site — *continued*
adenocarcinoma in — *see* Neoplasm, malignant, by site
adenocarcinoma in situ — *see* Neoplasm, in situ, by site
water-clear cell D35.1
Adenomatosis
endocrine (multiple) E31.20
single specified site — *see* Neoplasm, uncertain behavior, by site
erosive of nipple D24- ☑
pluriendocrine — *see* Adenomatosis, endocrine
pulmonary D38.1
malignant — *see* Neoplasm, lung, malignant
specified site — *see* Neoplasm, benign, by site
unspecified site D12.6
Adenomatous
goiter (nontoxic) E04.9
with hyperthyroidism — *see* Hyperthyroidism, with, goiter, nodular
toxic — *see* Hyperthyroidism, with, goiter, nodular
Adenomyoma (*see also* Neoplasm, benign, by site)
prostate — *see* Enlarged, prostate
Adenomyometritis N80.0
Adenomyosis N80.0
Adenopathy (lymph gland) R59.9
generalized R59.1
inguinal R59.0
localized R59.0
mediastinal R59.0
mesentery R59.0
syphilitic (secondary) A51.49
tracheobronchial R59.0
tuberculous A15.4
primary (progressive) A15.7
tuberculous (*see also* Tuberculosis, lymph gland)
tracheobronchial A15.4
primary (progressive) A15.7
Adenosalpingitis — *see* Salpingitis
Adenosarcoma — *see* Neoplasm, malignant, by site
Adenosclerosis I88.8
Adenosis (sclerosing) breast — *see* Fibroadenosis, breast
Adenovirus, as cause of disease classified elsewhere B97.0
Adentia (complete) (partial) — *see* Absence, teeth
Adherent (*see also* Adhesions)
labia (minora) N90.89
pericardium (nonrheumatic) I31.0
rheumatic I09.2
placenta (with hemorrhage) O72.0
without hemorrhage O73.0
prepuce, newborn N47.0
scar (skin) L90.5
tendon in scar L90.5
Adhesions, adhesive (postinfective) K66.0
with intestinal obstruction K56.50
complete K56.52
incomplete K56.51
partial K56.51
abdominal (wall) — *see* Adhesions, peritoneum
appendix K38.8
bile duct (common) (hepatic) K83.8
bladder (sphincter) N32.89
bowel — *see* Adhesions, peritoneum
cardiac I31.0
rheumatic I09.2
cecum — *see* Adhesions, peritoneum
cervicovaginal N88.1
congenital Q52.8
postpartal O90.89
old N88.1
cervix N88.1
ciliary body NEC — *see* Adhesions, iris
clitoris N90.89
colon — *see* Adhesions, peritoneum
common duct K83.8
congenital (*see also* Anomaly, by site)
fingers — *see* Syndactylism, complex, fingers
omental, anomalous Q43.3
peritoneal Q43.3
tongue (to gum or roof of mouth) Q38.3
conjunctiva (acquired) H11.21- ☑
congenital Q15.8
cystic duct K82.8
diaphragm — *see* Adhesions, peritoneum
due to foreign body — *see* Foreign body

Adhesions, adhesive — *continued*
duodenum — *see* Adhesions, peritoneum
ear
middle H74.1- ☑
epididymis N50.89
epidural — *see* Adhesions, meninges
epiglottis J38.7
eyelid H02.59
female pelvis N73.6
gallbladder K82.8
globe H44.89
heart I31.0
rheumatic I09.2
ileocecal (coil) — *see* Adhesions, peritoneum
ileum — *see* Adhesions, peritoneum
intestine (*see also* Adhesions, peritoneum)
with obstruction K56.50
complete K56.52
incomplete K56.51
partial K56.51
intra-abdominal — *see* Adhesions, peritoneum
iris H21.50- ☑
anterior H21.51- ☑
goniosynechiae H21.52- ☑
posterior H21.54- ☑
to corneal graft T85.898 ☑
joint — *see* Ankylosis
knee M23.8X ☑
temporomandibular M26.61- ☑
labium (majus) (minus), congenital Q52.5
liver — *see* Adhesions, peritoneum
lung J98.4
mediastinum J98.59
meninges (cerebral) (spinal) G96.12
congenital Q07.8
tuberculous (cerebral) (spinal) A17.0
mesenteric — *see* Adhesions, peritoneum
nasal (septum) (to turbinates) J34.89
ocular muscle — *see* Strabismus, mechanical
omentum — *see* Adhesions, peritoneum
ovary N73.6
congenital (to cecum, kidney or omentum) Q50.39
paraovarian N73.6
pelvic (peritoneal)
female N73.6
postprocedural N99.4
male — *see* Adhesions, peritoneum
postpartal (old) N73.6
tuberculous A18.17
penis to scrotum (congenital) Q55.8
periappendiceal (*see also* Adhesions, peritoneum)
pericardium (nonrheumatic) I31.0
focal I31.8
rheumatic I09.2
tuberculous A18.84
pericholecystic K82.8
perigastric — *see* Adhesions, peritoneum
periovarian N73.6
periprostatic N42.89
perirectal — *see* Adhesions, peritoneum
perirenal N28.89
peritoneum, peritoneal (postinfective)
with obstruction (intestinal) K56.50
complete K56.52
incomplete K56.51
partial K56.51
congenital Q43.3
pelvic, female N73.6
postprocedural N99.4
postpartal, pelvic N73.6
postprocedural K66.0
to uterus N73.6
peritubal N73.6
periureteral N28.89
periuterine N73.6
perivesical N32.89
perivesicular (seminal vesicle) N50.89
pleura, pleuritic J94.8
tuberculous NEC A15.6
pleuropericardial J94.8
postoperative (gastrointestinal tract) K66.0
with obstruction (*see also* Obstruction, intestine, postoperative) K91.30
due to foreign body accidentally left in wound — *see* Foreign body, accidentally left during a procedure
pelvic peritoneal N99.4
urethra — *see* Stricture, urethra, postprocedural

☑ **Additional Character Required — Refer to the Tabular List for Character Selection**   ▽ **Subterms under main terms may continue to next column or page**

Adhesions, adhesive — *continued*
  postoperative — *continued*
    vagina N99.2
  postpartal, old (vulva or perineum) N90.89
  preputial, prepuce N47.5
  pulmonary J98.4
  pylorus — *see* Adhesions, peritoneum
  sciatic nerve — *see* Lesion, nerve, sciatic
  seminal vesicle N50.89
  shoulder (joint) — *see* Capsulitis, adhesive
  sigmoid flexure — *see* Adhesions, peritoneum
  spermatic cord (acquired) N50.89
    congenital Q55.4
  spinal canal G96.12
  stomach — *see* Adhesions, peritoneum
  subscapular — *see* Capsulitis, adhesive
  temporomandibular M26.61- ☑
  tendinitis (*see also* Tenosynovitis, specified type NEC)
    shoulder — *see* Capsulitis, adhesive
  testis N44.8
  tongue, congenital (to gum or roof of mouth) Q38.3
    acquired K14.8
  trachea J39.8
  tubo-ovarian N73.6
  tunica vaginalis N44.8
  uterus N73.6
    internal N85.6
    to abdominal wall N73.6
  vagina (chronic) N89.5
    postoperative N99.2
  vitreomacular H43.82- ☑
  vitreous H43.89
  vulva N90.89
Adiaspiromycosis B48.8
Adie (-Holmes) **pupil or syndrome** — *see* Anomaly, pupil, function, tonic pupil
Adiponecrosis neonatorum P83.88
Adiposis (*see also* Obesity)
  cerebralis E23.6
  dolorosa E88.2
Adiposity (*see also* Obesity)
  heart — *see* Degeneration, myocardial
  localized E65
Adiposogenital dystrophy E23.6
Adjustment
  disorder — *see* Disorder, adjustment
  implanted device — *see* Encounter (for), adjustment (of)
  prosthesis, external — *see* Fitting
  reaction — *see* Disorder, adjustment
Administration of tPA (rtPA) in a different facility within the last 24 hours prior to admission to current facility Z92.82
Admission (for) (*see also* Encounter (for))
  adjustment (of)
    artificial
      arm Z44.00- ☑
        complete Z44.01- ☑
        partial Z44.02- ☑
      eye Z44.2 ☑
      leg Z44.10- ☑
        complete Z44.11- ☑
        partial Z44.12- ☑
    brain neuropacemaker Z46.2
      implanted Z45.42
    breast
      implant Z45.81 ☑
      prosthesis (external) Z44.3 ☑
    colostomy belt Z46.89
    contact lenses Z46.0
    cystostomy device Z46.6
    dental prosthesis Z46.3
    device NEC
      abdominal Z46.89
      implanted Z45.89
        cardiac Z45.09
          defibrillator (with synchronous cardiace pacemaker) Z45.02
          pacemaker (cardiac resynchronization therapy (CRT-P)) Z45.018
          pulse generator Z45.010
          resynchronization therapy defibrillator (CRT-D) Z45.02
        hearing device Z45.328
          bone conduction Z45.320
          cochlear Z45.321
        infusion pump Z45.1
        nervous system Z45.49

Admission — *continued*
  adjustment — *continued*
    device — *continued*
      implanted — *continued*
        nervous system — *continued*
          CSF drainage Z45.41
          hearing device — *see* Admission, adjustment, device, implanted, hearing device
          neuropacemaker Z45.42
          visual substitution Z45.31
        specified NEC Z45.89
        vascular access Z45.2
        visual substitution Z45.31
      nervous system Z46.2
        implanted — *see* Admission, adjustment, device, implanted, nervous system
      orthodontic Z46.4
      prosthetic Z44.9
        arm — *see* Admission, adjustment, artificial, arm
        breast Z44.3 ☑
        dental Z46.3
        eye Z44.2 ☑
        leg — *see* Admission, adjustment, artificial, leg
        specified type NEC Z44.8
      substitution
        auditory Z46.2
          implanted — *see* Admission, adjustment, device, implanted, hearing device
        nervous system Z46.2
          implanted — *see* Admission, adjustment, device, implanted, nervous system
        visual Z46.2
          implanted Z45.31
      urinary Z46.6
    hearing aid Z46.1
      implanted — *see* Admission, adjustment, device, implanted, hearing device
    ileostomy device Z46.89
    intestinal appliance or device NEC Z46.89
    neuropacemaker (brain) (peripheral nerve) (spinal cord) Z46.2
      implanted Z45.42
    orthodontic device Z46.4
    orthopedic (brace) (cast) (device) (shoes) Z46.89
    pacemaker (cardiac resynchronization therapy (CRT-P))
      cardiac Z45.018
        pulse generator Z45.010
      nervous system Z46.2
        implanted Z45.42
    portacath (port-a-cath) Z45.2
    prosthesis Z44.9
      arm — *see* Admission, adjustment, artificial, arm
      breast Z44.3 ☑
      dental Z46.3
      eye Z44.2 ☑
      leg — *see* Admission, adjustment, artificial, leg
      specified NEC Z44.8
    spectacles Z46.0
  aftercare (*see also* Aftercare) Z51.89
    postpartum
      immediately after delivery Z39.0
      routine follow-up Z39.2
    radiation therapy (antineoplastic) Z51.0
  attention to artificial opening (of) Z43.9
    artificial vagina Z43.7
    colostomy Z43.3
    cystostomy Z43.5
    enterostomy Z43.4
    gastrostomy Z43.1
    ileostomy Z43.2
    jejunostomy Z43.4
    nephrostomy Z43.6
    specified site NEC Z43.8
      intestinal tract Z43.4
      urinary tract Z43.6
    tracheostomy Z43.0
    ureterostomy Z43.6
    urethrostomy Z43.6
  breast augmentation or reduction Z41.1
  breast reconstruction following mastectomy Z42.1

Admission — *continued*
  change of
    dressing (nonsurgical) Z48.00
    neuropacemaker device (brain) (peripheral nerve) (spinal cord) Z46.2
      implanted Z45.42
    surgical dressing Z48.01
  circumcision, ritual or routine (in absence of diagnosis) Z41.2
  clinical research investigation (control) (normal comparison) (participant) Z00.6
  contraceptive management Z30.9
  cosmetic surgery NEC Z41.1
  counseling (*see also* Counseling)
    dietary Z71.3
    gestational carrier Z31.7
    HIV Z71.7
    human immunodeficiency virus Z71.7
    nonattending third party Z71.0
    procreative management NEC Z31.69
  delivery, full-term, uncomplicated O80
    cesarean, without indication O82
  desensitization to allergens Z51.6
  dietary surveillance and counseling Z71.3
  ear piercing Z41.3
  examination at health care facility (adult) (*see also* Examination) Z00.00
    with abnormal findings Z00.01
    clinical research investigation (control) (normal comparison) (participant) Z00.6
    dental Z01.20
      with abnormal findings Z01.21
    donor (potential) Z00.5
    ear Z01.10
      with abnormal findings NEC Z01.118
    eye Z01.00
      with abnormal findings Z01.01
    general, specified reason NEC Z00.8
    hearing Z01.10
      with abnormal findings NEC Z01.118
    postpartum checkup Z39.2
    psychiatric (general) Z00.8
      requested by authority Z04.6
    vision Z01.00
      with abnormal findings Z01.01
  fitting (of)
    artificial
      arm — *see* Admission, adjustment, artificial, arm
      eye Z44.2 ☑
      leg — *see* Admission, adjustment, artificial, leg
    brain neuropacemaker Z46.2
      implanted Z45.42
    breast prosthesis (external) Z44.3 ☑
    colostomy belt Z46.89
    contact lenses Z46.0
    cystostomy device Z46.6
    dental prosthesis Z46.3
    dentures Z46.3
    device NEC
      abdominal Z46.89
      nervous system Z46.2
        implanted — *see* Admission, adjustment, device, implanted, nervous system
      orthodontic Z46.4
      prosthetic Z44.9
        breast Z44.3 ☑
        dental Z46.3
        eye Z44.2 ☑
      substitution
        auditory Z46.2
          implanted — *see* Admission, adjustment, device, implanted, hearing device
        nervous system Z46.2
          implanted — *see* Admission, adjustment, device, implanted, nervous system
        visual Z46.2
          implanted Z45.31
    hearing aid Z46.1
    ileostomy device Z46.89
    intestinal appliance or device NEC Z46.89
    neuropacemaker (brain) (peripheral nerve) (spinal cord) Z46.2
      implanted Z45.42
    orthodontic device Z46.4
    orthopedic device (brace) (cast) (shoes) Z46.89

Index

Admission — Agenesis

Admission — continued
  fitting — continued
    prosthesis Z44.9
      arm — see Admission, adjustment, artificial,
        arm
      breast Z44.3 ☑
      dental Z46.3
      eye Z44.2 ☑
      leg — see Admission, adjustment, artificial, leg
      specified type NEC Z44.8
      spectacles Z46.0
  follow-up examination Z09
  intrauterine device management Z30.431
    initial prescription Z30.014
  mental health evaluation Z00.8
    requested by authority Z04.6
  observation — see Observation
  Papanicolaou smear, cervix Z12.4
    for suspected malignant neoplasm Z12.4
  plastic and reconstructive surgery following medical procedure or healed injury NEC Z42.8
  plastic surgery, cosmetic NEC Z41.1
  postpartum observation
    immediately after delivery Z39.0
    routine follow-up Z39.2
  poststerilization (for restoration) Z31.0
    aftercare Z31.42
  procreative management Z31.9
  prophylactic (measure) — (see also Encounter, prophylactic measures)
    organ removal Z40.00
      breast Z40.01
      fallopian tube(s) Z40.03
        with ovary(s) Z40.02
      ovary(s) Z40.02
      specified organ NEC Z40.09
      testes Z40.09
    vaccination Z23
  psychiatric examination (general) Z00.8
    requested by authority Z04.6
  radiation therapy (antineoplastic) Z51.0
  reconstructive surgery following medical procedure or healed injury NEC Z42.8
  removal of
    cystostomy catheter Z43.5
    drains Z48.03
    dressing (nonsurgical) Z48.00
    implantable subdermal contraceptive Z30.46
    intrauterine contraceptive device Z30.432
    neuropacemaker (brain) (peripheral nerve) (spinal cord) Z46.2
      implanted Z45.42
    staples Z48.02
    surgical dressing Z48.01
    sutures Z48.02
    ureteral stent Z46.6
  respirator [ventilator] use during power failure Z99.12
  restoration of organ continuity (poststerilization) Z31.0
    aftercare Z31.42
  sensitivity test (see also Test, skin)
    allergy NEC Z01.82
    Mantoux Z11.1
  tuboplasty following previous sterilization Z31.0
    aftercare Z31.42
  vasoplasty following previous sterilization Z31.0
    aftercare Z31.42
  vision examination Z01.00
    with abnormal findings Z01.01
  waiting period for admission to other facility Z75.1
Adnexitis (suppurative) — see Salpingo-oophoritis
Adolescent X-linked adrenoleukodystrophy E71.521
Adrenal (gland) — see condition
Adrenalism, tuberculous A18.7
Adrenalitis, adrenitis E27.8
  autoimmune E27.1
  meningococcal, hemorrhagic A39.1
Adrenarche, premature E27.0
Adrenocortical syndrome — see Cushing's, syndrome
Adrenogenital syndrome E25.9
  acquired E25.8
  congenital E25.0
  salt loss E25.0
Adrenogenitalism, congenital E25.0
Adrenoleukodystrophy E71.529
  neonatal E71.511
  X-linked E71.529
    Addison only phenotype E71.528
    Addison-Schilder E71.528

Adrenoleukodystrophy — continued
  X-linked — continued
    adolescent E71.521
    adrenomyeloneuropathy E71.522
    childhood cerebral E71.520
    other specified E71.528
Adrenomyeloneuropathy E71.522
Adventitious bursa — see Bursopathy, specified type NEC
Adverse effect — see Table of Drugs and Chemicals, categories T36-T50, with 6th character 5
Advice — see Counseling
Adynamia (episodica) (hereditary) (periodic) G72.3
Aeration lung imperfect, newborn — see Atelectasis
Aerobullosis T70.3 ☑
Aerocele — see Embolism, air
Aerodermectasia
  subcutaneous (traumatic) T79.7 ☑
Aerodontalgia T70.29 ☑
Aeroembolism T70.3 ☑
Aerogenes capsulatus infection A48.0
Aero-otitis media T70.0 ☑
Aerophagy, aerophagia (psychogenic) F45.8
Aerophobia F40.228
Aerosinusitis T70.1 ☑
Aerotitis T70.0 ☑
Affection — see Disease
Afibrinogenemia (see also Defect, coagulation) D68.8
  acquired D65
  congenital D68.2
  following ectopic or molar pregnancy O08.1
  in abortion — see Abortion, by type, complicated by, afibrinogenemia
  puerperal O72.3
African
  sleeping sickness B56.9
  tick fever A68.1
  trypanosomiasis B56.9
    gambian B56.0
    rhodesian B56.1
Aftercare (see also Care) Z51.89
  following surgery (for) (on)
    amputation Z47.81
    attention to
      drains Z48.03
      dressings (nonsurgical) Z48.00
        surgical Z48.01
      sutures Z48.02
    circulatory system Z48.812
    delayed (planned) wound closure Z48.1
    digestive system Z48.815
    explantation of joint prosthesis (staged procedure)
      hip Z47.32
      knee Z47.33
      shoulder Z47.31
    genitourinary system Z48.816
    joint replacement Z47.1
    neoplasm Z48.3
    nervous system Z48.811
    oral cavity Z48.814
    organ transplant
      bone marrow Z48.290
      heart Z48.21
      heart-lung Z48.280
      kidney Z48.22
      liver Z48.23
      lung Z48.24
      multiple organs NEC Z48.288
      specified NEC Z48.298
    orthopedic NEC Z47.89
    planned wound closure Z48.1
    removal of internal fixation device Z47.2
    respiratory system Z48.813
    scoliosis Z47.82
    sense organs Z48.810
    skin and subcutaneous tissue Z48.817
    specified body system
      circulatory Z48.812
      digestive Z48.815
      genitourinary Z48.816
      nervous Z48.811
      oral cavity Z48.814
      respiratory Z48.813
      sense organs Z48.810
      skin and subcutaneous tissue Z48.817
      teeth Z48.814
    specified NEC Z48.89
    spinal Z47.89

Aftercare — continued
  following surgery — continued
    teeth Z48.814
  fracture — code to fracture with seventh character D
  involving
    removal of
      drains Z48.03
      dressings (nonsurgical) Z48.00
      staples Z48.02
      surgical dressings Z48.01
      sutures Z48.02
  neuropacemaker (brain) (peripheral nerve) (spinal cord) Z46.2
    implanted Z45.42
  orthopedic NEC Z47.89
  postprocedural — see Aftercare, following surgery
After-cataract — see Cataract, secondary
Agalactia (primary) O92.3
  elective, secondary or therapeutic O92.5
Agammaglobulinemia (acquired (secondary) (nonfamilial) D80.1
  with
    immunoglobulin-bearing B-lymphocytes D80.1
    lymphopenia D81.9
  autosomal recessive (Swiss type) D80.0
  Bruton's X-linked D80.0
  common variable (CVAgamma) D80.1
  congenital sex-linked D80.0
  hereditary D80.0
  lymphopenic D81.9
  Swiss type (autosomal recessive) D80.0
  X-linked (with growth hormone deficiency) (Bruton) D80.0
Aganglionosis (bowel) (colon) Q43.1
Age (old) — see Senility
Agenesis
  adrenal (gland) Q89.1
  alimentary tract (complete) (partial) NEC Q45.8
    upper Q40.8
  anus, anal (canal) Q42.3
    with fistula Q42.2
  aorta Q25.41
  appendix Q42.8
  arm (complete) Q71.0- ☑
    with hand present Q71.1- ☑
  artery (peripheral) Q27.9
    brain Q28.3
    coronary Q24.5
    pulmonary Q25.79
    specified NEC Q27.8
    umbilical Q27.0
  auditory (canal) (external) Q16.1
  auricle (ear) Q16.0
  bile duct or passage Q44.5
  bladder Q64.5
  bone Q79.9
  brain Q00.0
    part of Q04.3
  breast (with nipple present) Q83.8
    with absent nipple Q83.0
  bronchus Q32.4
  canaliculus lacrimalis Q10.4
  carpus — see Agenesis, hand
  cartilage Q79.9
  cecum Q42.8
  cerebellum Q04.3
  cervix Q51.5
  chin Q18.8
  cilia Q10.3
  circulatory system, part NOS Q28.9
  clavicle Q74.0
  clitoris Q52.6
  coccyx Q76.49
  colon Q42.9
    specified NEC Q42.8
  corpus callosum Q04.0
  cricoid cartilage Q31.8
  diaphragm (with hernia) Q79.1
  digestive organ(s) or tract (complete) (partial) NEC Q45.8
    upper Q40.8
  ductus arteriosus Q28.8
  duodenum Q41.0
  ear Q16.9
    auricle Q16.0
    lobe Q17.8
  ejaculatory duct Q55.4
  endocrine (gland) NEC Q89.2

☑ **Additional Character Required** — Refer to the Tabular List for Character Selection   ▽ **Subterms under main terms may continue to next column or page**

Agenesis — continued
  epiglottis Q31.8
  esophagus Q39.8
  eustachian tube Q16.2
  eye Q11.1
    adnexa Q15.8
  eyelid (fold) Q10.3
  face
    bones NEC Q75.8
    specified part NEC Q18.8
  fallopian tube Q50.6
  femur — see Defect, reduction, lower limb, longitudinal, femur
  fibula — see Defect, reduction, lower limb, longitudinal, fibula
  finger (complete) (partial) — see Agenesis, hand
  foot (and toes) (complete) (partial) Q72.3- ☑
  forearm (with hand present) — see Agenesis, arm, with hand present
    and hand Q71.2- ☑
  gallbladder Q44.0
  gastric Q40.2
  genitalia, genital (organ(s))
    female Q52.8
      external Q52.71
      internal NEC Q52.8
    male Q55.8
  glottis Q31.8
  hair Q84.0
  hand (and fingers) (complete) (partial) Q71.3- ☑
  heart Q24.8
    valve NEC Q24.8
      pulmonary Q22.0
  hepatic Q44.7
  humerus — see Defect, reduction, upper limb
  hymen Q52.4
  ileum Q41.2
  incus Q16.3
  intestine (small) Q41.9
    large Q42.9
      specified NEC Q42.8
  iris (dilator fibers) Q13.1
  jaw M26.09
  jejunum Q41.1
  kidney(s) (partial) Q60.2
    bilateral Q60.1
    unilateral Q60.0
  labium (majus) (minus) Q52.71
  labyrinth, membranous Q16.5
  lacrimal apparatus Q10.4
  larynx Q31.8
  leg (complete) Q72.0- ☑
    with foot present Q72.1- ☑
    lower leg (with foot present) — see Agenesis, leg, with foot present
      and foot Q72.2- ☑
  lens Q12.3
  limb (complete) Q73.0
    lower — see Agenesis, leg
    upper — see Agenesis, arm
  lip Q38.0
  liver Q44.7
  lung (fissure) (lobe) (bilateral) (unilateral) Q33.3
  mandible, maxilla M26.09
  metacarpus — see Agenesis, hand
  metatarsus — see Agenesis, foot
  muscle Q79.8
    eyelid Q10.3
    ocular Q15.8
  musculoskeletal system NEC Q79.8
  nail(s) Q84.3
  neck, part Q18.8
  nerve Q07.8
  nervous system, part NEC Q07.8
  nipple Q83.2
  nose Q30.1
  nuclear Q07.8
  organ
    of Corti Q16.5
    or site not listed — see Anomaly, by site
  osseous meatus (ear) Q16.1
  ovary
    bilateral Q50.02
    unilateral Q50.01
  oviduct Q50.6
  pancreas Q45.0
  parathyroid (gland) Q89.2
  parotid gland(s) Q38.4

Agenesis — continued
  patella Q74.1
  pelvic girdle (complete) (partial) Q74.2
  penis Q55.5
  pericardium Q24.8
  pituitary (gland) Q89.2
  prostate Q55.4
  punctum lacrimale Q10.4
  radioulnar — see Defect, reduction, upper limb
  radius — see Defect, reduction, upper limb, longitudinal, radius
  rectum Q42.1
    with fistula Q42.0
  renal Q60.2
    bilateral Q60.1
    unilateral Q60.0
  respiratory organ NEC Q34.8
  rib Q76.6
  roof of orbit Q75.8
  round ligament Q52.8
  sacrum Q76.49
  salivary gland Q38.4
  scapula Q74.0
  scrotum Q55.29
  seminal vesicles Q55.4
  septum
    atrial Q21.1
    between aorta and pulmonary artery Q21.4
    ventricular Q20.4
  shoulder girdle (complete) (partial) Q74.0
  skull (bone) Q75.8
    with
      anencephaly Q00.0
      encephalocele — see Encephalocele
      hydrocephalus Q03.9
        with spina bifida — see Spina bifida, by site, with hydrocephalus
      microcephaly Q02
  spermatic cord Q55.4
  spinal cord Q06.0
  spine Q76.49
  spleen Q89.01
  sternum Q76.7
  stomach Q40.2
  submaxillary gland(s) (congenital) Q38.4
  tarsus — see Agenesis, foot
  tendon Q79.8
  testicle Q55.0
  thymus (gland) Q89.2
  thyroid (gland) E03.1
    cartilage Q31.8
  tibia — see Defect, reduction, lower limb, longitudinal, tibia
  tibiofibular — see Defect, reduction, lower limb, specified type NEC
  toe (and foot) (complete) (partial) — see Agenesis, foot
  tongue Q38.3
  trachea (cartilage) Q32.1
  ulna — see Defect, reduction, upper limb, longitudinal, ulna
  upper limb — see Agenesis, arm
  ureter Q62.4
  urethra Q64.5
  urinary tract NEC Q64.8
  uterus Q51.0
  uvula Q38.5
  vagina Q52.0
  vas deferens Q55.4
  vein(s) (peripheral) Q27.9
    brain Q28.3
    great NEC Q26.8
    portal Q26.5
    vena cava (inferior) (superior) Q26.8
  vermis of cerebellum Q04.3
  vertebra Q76.49
  vulva Q52.71
Ageusia R43.2
Agitated — see condition
Agitation R45.1
Aglossia (congenital) Q38.3
Aglossia-adactylia syndrome Q87.0
Aglycogenosis E74.00
Agnosia (body image) (other senses) (tactile) R48.1
  developmental F88
  verbal R48.1
    auditory R48.1
      developmental F80.2

Agnosia — continued
  verbal — continued
    developmental F80.2
  visual (object) R48.3
Agoraphobia F40.00
  with panic disorder F40.01
  without panic disorder F40.02
Agrammatism R48.8
Agranulocytopenia — see Agranulocytosis
Agranulocytosis (chronic) (cyclical) (genetic) (infantile) (periodic) (pernicious) (see also Neutropenia) D70.9
  congenital D70.0
  cytoreductive cancer chemotherapy sequela D70.1
  drug-induced D70.2
    due to cytoreductive cancer chemotherapy D70.1
  due to infection D70.3
  secondary D70.4
    drug-induced D70.2
      due to cytoreductive cancer chemotherapy D70.1
Agraphia (absolute) R48.8
  with alexia R48.0
  developmental F81.81
Ague (dumb) — see Malaria
Agyria Q04.3
Ahumada-del Castillo syndrome E23.0
Aichomophobia F40.298
AIDS (related complex) B20
Ailment heart — see Disease, heart
Ailurophobia F40.218
AIN — see Neoplasia, intraepithelial, anal
Ainhum (disease) L94.6
AIPHI (acute idiopathic pulmonary hemorrhage in infants (over 28 days old)) R04.81
Air
  anterior mediastinum J98.2
  compressed, disease T70.3 ☑
  conditioner lung or pneumonitis J67.7
  embolism (artery) (cerebral) (any site) T79.0 ☑
    with ectopic or molar pregnancy O08.2
    due to implanted device NEC — see Complications, by site and type, specified NEC
    following
      abortion — see Abortion by type, complicated by, embolism
      ectopic or molar pregnancy O08.2
    infusion, therapeutic injection or transfusion T80.0 ☑
    in pregnancy, childbirth or puerperium — see Embolism, obstetric
    traumatic T79.0 ☑
  hunger, psychogenic F45.8
  rarefied, effects of — see Effect, adverse, high altitude
  sickness T75.3 ☑
Airplane sickness T75.3 ☑
Akathisia (drug-induced) (treatment-induced) G25.71
  neuroleptic induced (acute) G25.71
  tardive G25.71
Akinesia R29.898
Akinetic mutism R41.89
Akureyri's disease G93.3
Alactasia, congenital E73.0
Alagille's syndrome Q44.7
Alastrim B03
Albers-Schönberg syndrome Q78.2
Albert's syndrome — see Tendinitis, Achilles
Albinism, albino E70.30
  with hematologic abnormality E70.339
    Chédiak-Higashi syndrome E70.330
    Hermansky-Pudlak syndrome E70.331
    other specified E70.338
  I E70.320
  II E70.321
  ocular E70.319
    autosomal recessive E70.311
    other specified E70.318
    X-linked E70.310
  oculocutaneous E70.329
    other specified E70.328
    tyrosinase (ty) negative E70.320
    tyrosinase (ty) positive E70.321
  other specified E70.39
Albinismus E70.30
Albright (-McCune)(-Sternberg) syndrome Q78.1
Albuminous — see condition
Albuminuria, albuminuric (acute) (chronic) (subacute) (see also Proteinuria) R80.9

Index

Albuminuria, albuminuric — Alpine sickness

Albuminuria, albuminuric — continued
 complicating pregnancy — see Proteinuria, gestational
  with
   gestational hypertension — see Pre-eclampsia
   pre-existing hypertension — see Hypertension,
    complicating pregnancy, pre-existing,
    with, pre-eclampsia
  gestational — see Proteinuria, gestational
  with
   gestational hypertension — see Pre-eclampsia
   pre-existing hypertension — see Hypertension,
    complicating pregnancy, pre-existing,
    with, pre-eclampsia
 orthostatic R80.2
 postural R80.2
 pre-eclamptic — see Pre-eclampsia
 scarlatinal A38.8
Albuminurophobia F40.298
Alcaptonuria E70.29
Alcohol, alcoholic, alcohol-induced
 addiction (without remission) F10.20
  with remission F10.21
 amnestic disorder, persisting F10.96
  with dependence F10.26
 anxiety disorder F10.980
 bipolar and related disorder F10.94
 brain syndrome, chronic F10.97
  with dependence F10.27
 cardiopathy I42.6
 counseling and surveillance Z71.41
  family member Z71.42
 delirium (acute) (tremens) (withdrawal) F10.231
  with intoxication F10.921
   in
    abuse F10.121
    dependence F10.221
 dementia F10.97
  with dependence F10.27
 depressive disorder F10.94
 deterioration F10.97
  with dependence F10.27
 hallucinosis (acute) F10.951
  in
   abuse F10.151
   dependence F10.251
 insanity F10.959
 intoxication (acute) (without dependence) F10.129
  with
   delirium F10.121
   dependence F10.229
    with delirium F10.221
    uncomplicated F10.220
   uncomplicated F10.120
 jealousy F10.988
 Korsakoff's, Korsakov's, Korsakow's F10.26
 liver K70.9
  acute — see Disease, liver, alcoholic, hepatitis
 major neurocognitive disorder, amnestic-confabulatory type F10.96
 major neurocognitive disorder, nonamnestic-confabulatory type F10.97
 mania (acute) (chronic) F10.959
 mild neurocognitive disorder F10.988
 paranoia, paranoid (type) psychosis F10.950
 pellagra E52
 poisoning, accidental (acute) NEC — see Table of Drugs
  and Chemicals, alcohol, poisoning
 psychosis — see Psychosis, alcoholic
 psychotic disorder F10.959
 sexual dysfunction F10.981
 sleep disorder F10.982
 withdrawal (without convulsions) F10.239
  with delirium F10.231
Alcoholism (chronic) (without remission) F10.20
 with
  psychosis — see Psychosis, alcoholic
  remission F10.21
 Korsakov's F10.96
  with dependence F10.26
Alder (-Reilly) **anomaly or syndrome** (leukocyte granulation) D72.0
Aldosteronism E26.9
 familial (type I) E26.02
 glucocorticoid-remediable E26.02
 primary (due to (bilateral) adrenal hyperplasia) E26.09
 primary NEC E26.09
 secondary E26.1
 specified NEC E26.89

Aldosteronoma D44.10
Aldrich (-Wiskott) **syndrome** (eczema-thrombocytopenia) D82.0
Alektorophobia F40.218
Aleppo boil B55.1
Aleukemic — see condition
Aleukia
 congenital D70.0
 hemorrhagica D61.9
  congenital D61.09
 splenica D73.1
Alexia R48.0
 developmental F81.0
 secondary to organic lesion R48.0
Algoneurodystrophy M89.00
 ankle M89.07- ☑
 foot M89.07- ☑
 forearm M89.03- ☑
 hand M89.04- ☑
 lower leg M89.06- ☑
 multiple sites M89.0- ☑
 shoulder M89.01- ☑
 specified site NEC M89.08
 thigh M89.05- ☑
 upper arm M89.02- ☑
Algophobia F40.298
Alienation, mental — see Psychosis
Alkalemia E87.3
Alkalosis E87.3
 metabolic E87.3
  with respiratory acidosis E87.4
 respiratory E87.3
Alkaptonuria E70.29
Allen-Masters syndrome N83.8
Allergy, allergic (reaction) (to) T78.40 ☑
 air-borne substance NEC (rhinitis) J30.89
 alveolitis (extrinsic) J67.9
  due to
   Aspergillus clavatus J67.4
   Cryptostroma corticale J67.6
   organisms (fungal, thermophilic actinomycete)
    growing in ventilation (air conditioning)
    systems J67.7
  specified type NEC J67.8
 anaphylactic reaction or shock T78.2 ☑
 angioneurotic edema T78.3 ☑
 animal (dander) (epidermal) (hair) (rhinitis) J30.81
 bee sting (anaphylactic shock) — see Toxicity, venom,
  arthropod, bee
 biological — see Allergy, drug
 colitis (see also Colitis, allergic) K52.29
 dander (animal) (rhinitis) J30.81
 dandruff (rhinitis) J30.81
 dental restorative material (existing) K08.55
 dermatitis — see Dermatitis, contact, allergic
 diathesis — see History, allergy
 drug, medicament & biological (any) (external) (internal) T78.40 ☑
  correct substance properly administered — see
   Table of Drugs and Chemicals, by drug, adverse effect
  wrong substance given or taken NEC (by accident)
   — see Table of Drugs and Chemicals, by
   drug, poisoning
 due to pollen J30.1
 dust (house) (stock) (rhinitis) J30.89
  with asthma — see Asthma, allergic extrinsic
 eczema — see Dermatitis, contact, allergic
 epidermal (animal) (rhinitis) J30.81
 feathers (rhinitis) J30.89
 food (any) (ingested) NEC T78.1 ☑
  anaphylactic shock — see Shock, anaphylactic, due
   to food
  dermatitis — see Dermatitis, due to, food
  dietary counseling and surveillance Z71.3
  in contact with skin L23.6
  rhinitis J30.5
  status (without reaction) Z91.018
   eggs Z91.012
   milk products Z91.011
   peanuts Z91.010
   seafood Z91.013
   specified NEC Z91.018
 gastrointestinal — see also specific type of allergic
  reaction
  meaning colitis (see also Colitis, allergic) K52.29

Allergy, allergic — continued
 gastrointestinal — see also specific type of allergic reaction — continued
  meaning gastroenteritis (see also Gastroenteritis,
   allergic) K52.29
  meaning other adverse food reaction not elsewhere classified T78.1 ☑
 grain J30.1
 grass (hay fever) (pollen) J30.1
  asthma — see Asthma, allergic extrinsic
 hair (animal) (rhinitis) J30.81
 history (of) — see History, allergy
 horse serum — see Allergy, serum
 inhalant (rhinitis) J30.89
  pollen J30.1
 kapok (rhinitis) J30.89
 medicine — see Allergy, drug
 milk protein (see also Allergy, food) Z91.011
  anaphylactic reaction T78.07 ☑
  dermatitis L27.2
  enterocolitis syndrome K52.21
  enteropathy K52.22
  gastroenteritis K52.29
  gastroesophageal reflux (see also Reaction, adverse,
   food) K21.9
   with esophagitis K21.0
  proctocolitis K52.82
 nasal, seasonal due to pollen J30.1
 pneumonia J82
 pollen (any) (hay fever) J30.1
  asthma — see Asthma, allergic extrinsic
 primrose J30.1
 primula J30.1
 proctocolitis K52.82
 purpura D69.0
 ragweed (hay fever) (pollen) J30.1
  asthma — see Asthma, allergic extrinsic
 rose (pollen) J30.1
 seasonal NEC J30.2
 Senecio jacobae (pollen) J30.1
 serum (see also Reaction, serum) T80.69 ☑
  anaphylactic shock T80.59 ☑
 shock (anaphylactic) T78.2 ☑
  due to
   administration of blood and blood products
    T80.51 ☑
   adverse effect of correct medicinal substance
    properly administered T88.6 ☑
   immunization T80.52 ☑
   serum NEC T80.59 ☑
   vaccination T80.52 ☑
 specific NEC T78.49 ☑
 tree (any) (hay fever) (pollen) J30.1
  asthma — see Asthma, allergic extrinsic
 upper respiratory J30.9
 urticaria L50.0
 vaccine — see Allergy, serum
 wheat — see Allergy, food
Allescheriasis B48.2
Alligator skin disease Q80.9
Allocheiria, allochiria R20.8
Almeida's disease — see Paracoccidioidomycosis
Alopecia (hereditaria) (seborrheica) L65.9
 androgenic L64.9
  drug-induced L64.0
  specified NEC L64.8
 areata L63.9
  ophiasis L63.2
  specified NEC L63.8
  totalis L63.0
  universalis L63.1
 cicatricial L66.9
  specified NEC L66.8
 circumscripta L63.9
 congenital, congenitalis Q84.0
 due to cytotoxic drugs NEC L65.8
 mucinosa L65.2
 postinfective NEC L65.8
 postpartum L65.0
 premature L64.8
 specific (syphilitic) A51.32
 specified NEC L65.8
 syphilitic (secondary) A51.32
 totalis (capitis) L63.0
 universalis (entire body) L63.1
 X-ray L58.1
Alpers' disease G31.81
Alpine sickness T70.29 ☑

Alport syndrome Q87.81
ALTE (apparent life threatening event) **in newborn and infant** R68.13
Alteration (of), **Altered**
  awareness
    transient R40.4
    unintended under general anesthesia, during procedure T88.53 ☑
  mental status R41.82
  pattern of family relationships affecting child Z62.898
  sensation
    following
      cerebrovascular disease I69.998
        cerebral infarction I69.398
        intracerebral hemorrhage I69.198
        nontraumatic intracranial hemorrhage NEC I69.298
        specified disease NEC I69.898
        subarachnoid hemorrhage I69.098
Alternating — see condition
Altitude, high (effects) — see Effect, adverse, high altitude
Aluminosis (of lung) J63.0
Alveolitis
  allergic (extrinsic) — see Pneumonitis, hypersensitivity
  due to
    Aspergillus clavatus J67.4
    Cryptostroma corticale J67.6
  fibrosing (cryptogenic) (idiopathic) J84.112
  jaw M27.3
  sicca dolorosa M27.3
Alveolus, alveolar — see condition
Alymphocytosis D72.810
  thymic (with immunodeficiency) D82.1
Alymphoplasia, thymic D82.1
Alzheimer's disease or sclerosis — see Disease, Alzheimer's
Amastia (with nipple present) Q83.8
  with absent nipple Q83.0
Amathophobia F40.228
Amaurosis (acquired) (congenital) (see also Blindness)
  fugax G45.3
  hysterical F44.6
  Leber's congenital H35.50
  uremic — see Uremia
Amaurotic idiocy (infantile) (juvenile) (late) E75.4
Amaxophobia F40.248
Ambiguous genitalia Q56.4
Amblyopia (congenital) (ex anopsia) (partial) (suppression) H53.00- ☑
  anisometropic — see Amblyopia, refractive
  deprivation H53.01- ☑
  hysterical F44.6
  nocturnal (see also Blindness, night)
    vitamin A deficiency E50.5
  refractive H53.02- ☑
  strabismic H53.03- ☑
  suspect H53.04- ☑
  tobacco H53.8
  toxic NEC H53.8
  uremic — see Uremia
Ameba, amebic (histolytica) (see also Amebiasis)
  abscess (liver) A06.4
Amebiasis A06.9
  with abscess — see Abscess, amebic
  acute A06.0
  chronic (intestine) A06.1
    with abscess — see Abscess, amebic
  cutaneous A06.7
  cutis A06.7
  cystitis A06.81
  genitourinary tract NEC A06.82
  hepatic — see Abscess, liver, amebic
  intestine A06.0
  nondysenteric colitis A06.2
  skin A06.7
  specified site NEC A06.89
Ameboma (of intestine) A06.3
Amelia Q73.0
  lower limb — see Agenesis, leg
  upper limb — see Agenesis, arm
Ameloblastoma (see also Cyst, calcifying odontogenic)
  long bones C40.9- ☑
    lower limb C40.2- ☑
    upper limb C40.0- ☑
  malignant C41.1
    jaw (bone) (lower) C41.1

Ameloblastoma — continued
  malignant — continued
    jaw — continued
      upper C41.0
    tibial C40.2- ☑
Amelogenesis imperfecta K00.5
  nonhereditaria (segmentalis) K00.4
Amenorrhea N91.2
  hyperhormonal E28.8
  primary N91.0
  secondary N91.1
Amentia — see Disability, intellectual
  Meynert's (nonalcoholic) F04
American
  leishmaniasis B55.2
  mountain tick fever A93.2
Ametropia — see Disorder, refraction
AMH (asymptomatic microscopic hematuria) R31.21
Amianthosis J61
Amimia R48.8
Amino-acid disorder E72.9
  anemia D53.0
Aminoacidopathy E72.9
Aminoaciduria E72.9
Amnesia R41.3
  anterograde R41.1
  auditory R48.8
  dissociative F44.0
    with dissociative fugue F44.1
  hysterical F44.0
  postictal in epilepsy — see Epilepsy
  psychogenic F44.0
  retrograde R41.2
  transient global G45.4
Amnes(t)ic syndrome (post-traumatic) F04
  induced by
    alcohol F10.96
      with dependence F10.26
    psychoactive NEC F19.96
      with
        abuse F19.16
        dependence F19.26
    sedative F13.96
      with dependence F13.26
Amnion, amniotic — see condition
Amnionitis — see Pregnancy, complicated by
Amok F68.8
Amoral traits F60.89
Amphetamine (or other stimulant) **-induced**
  anxiety disorder F15.980
  bipolar and related disorder F15.94
  delirium F15.921
  depressive disorder F15.94
  obsessive-compulsive and related disorder F15.988
  psychotic disorder F15.959
  sexual dysfunction F15.981
  sleep disorder F15.982
  stimulant withdrawal F15.23
Ampulla
  lower esophagus K22.8
  phrenic K22.8
Amputation (see also Absence, by site, acquired)
  neuroma (postoperative) (traumatic) — see Complications, amputation stump, neuroma
  stump (surgical)
    abnormal, painful, or with complication (late) — see Complications, amputation stump
    healed or old NOS Z89.9
  traumatic (complete) (partial)
    arm (upper) (complete) S48.91- ☑
      at
        elbow S58.01- ☑
          partial S58.02- ☑
        shoulder joint (complete) S48.01- ☑
          partial S48.02- ☑
      between
        elbow and wrist (complete) S58.11- ☑
          partial S58.12- ☑
        shoulder and elbow (complete) S48.11- ☑
          partial S48.12- ☑
      partial S48.92- ☑
    breast (complete) S28.21- ☑
      partial S28.22- ☑
    clitoris (complete) S38.211 ☑
      partial S38.212 ☑
    ear (complete) S08.11- ☑
      partial S08.12- ☑

Amputation — continued
  traumatic — continued
    finger (complete) (metacarpophalangeal)
      S68.11- ☑
      index S68.11- ☑
      little S68.11- ☑
      middle S68.11- ☑
      partial S68.12- ☑
        index S68.12- ☑
        little S68.12- ☑
        middle S68.12- ☑
        ring S68.12- ☑
      ring S68.11- ☑
      thumb — see Amputation, traumatic, thumb
      transphalangeal (complete) S68.61- ☑
        index S68.61- ☑
        little S68.61- ☑
        middle S68.61- ☑
        partial S68.62- ☑
          index S68.62- ☑
          little S68.62- ☑
          middle S68.62- ☑
          ring S68.62- ☑
        ring S68.61- ☑
    foot (complete) S98.91- ☑
      at ankle level S98.01- ☑
        partial S98.02- ☑
      midfoot S98.31- ☑
        partial S98.32- ☑
      partial S98.92- ☑
    forearm (complete) S58.91- ☑
      at elbow level (complete) S58.01- ☑
        partial S58.02- ☑
      between elbow and wrist (complete) S58.11- ☑
        partial S58.12- ☑
      partial S58.92- ☑
    genital organ(s) (external)
      female (complete) S38.211 ☑
        partial S38.212 ☑
      male
        penis (complete) S38.221 ☑
          partial S38.222 ☑
        scrotum (complete) S38.231 ☑
          partial S38.232 ☑
        testes (complete) S38.231 ☑
          partial S38.232 ☑
    hand (complete) (wrist level) S68.41- ☑
      finger(s) alone — see Amputation, traumatic, finger
      partial S68.42- ☑
      thumb alone — see Amputation, traumatic, thumb
      transmetacarpal (complete) S68.71- ☑
        partial S68.72- ☑
    head
      ear — see Amputation, traumatic, ear
      nose (partial) S08.812 ☑
        complete S08.811 ☑
      part S08.89 ☑
        scalp S08.0 ☑
    hip (and thigh) (complete) S78.91- ☑
      at hip joint (complete) S78.01- ☑
        partial S78.02- ☑
      between hip and knee (complete) S78.11- ☑
        partial S78.12- ☑
      partial S78.92- ☑
    labium (majus) (minus) (complete) S38.21- ☑
      partial S38.21- ☑
    leg (lower) S88.91- ☑
      at knee level S88.01- ☑
        partial S88.02- ☑
      between knee and ankle S88.11- ☑
        partial S88.12- ☑
      partial S88.92- ☑
    nose (partial) S08.812 ☑
      complete S08.811 ☑
    penis (complete) S38.221 ☑
      partial S38.222 ☑
    scrotum (complete) S38.231 ☑
      partial S38.232 ☑
    shoulder — see Amputation, traumatic, arm
      at shoulder joint — see Amputation, traumatic, arm, at shoulder joint
    testes (complete) S38.231 ☑
      partial S38.232 ☑
    thigh — see Amputation, traumatic, hip

Index

Amputation — *continued*
traumatic — *continued*
thorax, part of S28.1 ☑
breast — *see* Amputation, traumatic, breast
thumb (complete) (metacarpophalangeal)
S68.Ø1- ☑
partial S68.Ø2- ☑
transphalangeal (complete) S68.51- ☑
partial S68.52- ☑
toe (lesser) S98.13- ☑
great S98.11- ☑
partial S98.12- ☑
more than one S98.21- ☑
partial S98.22- ☑
partial S98.14- ☑
vulva (complete) S38.211 ☑
partial S38.212 ☑
Amputee (bilateral) (old) Z89.9
Amsterdam dwarfism Q87.1
Amusia R48.8
developmental F8Ø.89
Amyelencephalus, amyelencephaly QØØ.Ø
Amyelia QØ6.Ø
Amygdalitis — *see* Tonsillitis
Amygdalolith J35.8
Amyloid heart (disease) E85.4 [I43]
Amyloidosis (generalized) (primary) E85.9
with lung involvement E85.4 [J99]
familial E85.2
genetic E85.2
heart E85.4 [I43]
hemodialysis-associated E85.3
light chain (AL) E85.81
liver E85.4 [K77]
localized E85.4
neuropathic heredofamilial E85.1
non-neuropathic heredofamilial E85.Ø
organ limited E85.4
Portuguese E85.1
pulmonary E85.4 [J99]
secondary systemic E85.3
senile systemic (SSA) E85.82
skin (lichen) (macular) E85.4 [L99]
specified NEC E85.89
subglottic E85.4 [J99]
wild-type transthyretin-related (ATTR) E85.82
Amylopectinosis (brancher enzyme deficiency) E74.Ø3
Amylophagia — *see* Pica
Amyoplasia congenita Q79.8
Amyotonia M62.89
congenita G7Ø.2
Amyotrophia, amyotrophy, amyotrophic G71.8
congenita Q79.8
diabetic — *see* Diabetes, amyotrophy
lateral sclerosis G12.21
neuralgic G54.5
spinal progressive G12.25
Anacidity, gastric K31.83
psychogenic F45.8
Anaerosis of newborn P28.89
Analbuminemia E88.Ø9
Analgesia — *see* Anesthesia
Analphalipoproteinemia E78.6
Anaphylactic
purpura D69.Ø
shock or reaction — *see* Shock, anaphylactic
Anaphylactoid shock or reaction — *see* Shock, anaphylactic
Anaphylactoid syndrome of pregnancy O88.Ø1- ☑
Anaphylaxis — *see* Shock, anaphylactic
Anaplasia cervix (*see also* Dysplasia, cervix) N87.9
Anaplasmosis, human A77.49
Anarthria R47.1
Anasarca R6Ø.1
cardiac — *see* Failure, heart, congestive
lung J18.2
newborn P83.2
nutritional E43
pulmonary J18.2
renal NØ4.9
Anastomosis
aneurysmal — *see* Aneurysm
arteriovenous ruptured brain I6Ø.8
intestinal K63.89
complicated NEC K91.89
involving urinary tract N99.89
retinal and choroidal vessels (congenital) Q14.8

Anatomical narrow angle H4Ø.Ø3- ☑
Ancylostoma, ancylostomiasis (braziliense) (caninum) (ceylanicum) (duodenale) B76.Ø
Necator americanus B76.1
Andersen's disease (glycogen storage) E74.Ø9
Anderson-Fabry disease E75.21
Andes disease T7Ø.29
Andrews' disease (bacterid) LØ8.89
Androblastoma
benign
specified site — *see* Neoplasm, benign, by site
unspecified site
female D27.9
male D29.2Ø
malignant
specified site — *see* Neoplasm, malignant, by site
unspecified site
female C56.9
male C62.9Ø
specified site — *see* Neoplasm, uncertain behavior, by site
tubular
with lipid storage
specified site — *see* Neoplasm, benign, by site
unspecified site
female D27.9
male D29.2Ø
specified site — *see* Neoplasm, benign, by site
unspecified site
female D27.9
male D29.2Ø
unspecified site
female D39.1Ø
male D4Ø.1Ø
Androgen insensitivity syndrome (*see also* Syndrome, androgen insensitivity) E34.5Ø
Androgen resistance syndrome (*see also* Syndrome, androgen insensitivity) E34.5Ø
Android pelvis Q74.2
with disproportion (fetopelvic) O33.3 ☑
causing obstructed labor O65.3
Androphobia F4Ø.29Ø
Anectasis, pulmonary (newborn) — *see* Atelectasis
Anemia (essential) (general) (hemoglobin deficiency) (infantile) (primary) (profound) D64.9
with (due to) (in)
disorder of
anaerobic glycolysis D55.2
pentose phosphate pathway D55.1
koilonychia D5Ø.9
achlorhydric D5Ø.8
achrestic D53.1
Addison (-Biermer) (pernicious) D51.Ø
agranulocytic — *see* Agranulocytosis
amino-acid-deficiency D53.Ø
aplastic D61.9
congenital D61.Ø9
drug-induced D61.1
due to
drugs D61.1
external agents NEC D61.2
infection D61.2
radiation D61.2
idiopathic D61.3
red cell (pure) D6Ø.9
chronic D6Ø.Ø
congenital D61.Ø1
specified type NEC D6Ø.8
transient D6Ø.1
specified type NEC D61.89
toxic D61.2
aregenerative
congenital D61.Ø9
asiderotic D5Ø.9
atypical (primary) D64.9
Baghdad spring D55.Ø
Balantidium coli AØ7.Ø
Biermer's (pernicious) D51.Ø
blood loss (chronic) D5Ø.Ø
acute D62
bothriocephalus B7Ø.Ø [D63.8]
brickmaker's B76.9 [D63.8]
cerebral I67.89
childhood D58.9
chlorotic D5Ø.8
chronic
blood loss D5Ø.Ø
hemolytic D58.9

Anemia — *continued*
chronic — *continued*
hemolytic — *continued*
idiopathic D59.9
simple D53.9
chronica congenita aregenerativa D61.Ø9
combined system disease NEC D51.Ø [G32.Ø]
due to dietary vitamin B12 deficiency D51.3 [G32.Ø]
complicating pregnancy, childbirth or puerperium — *see* Pregnancy, complicated by (management affected by), anemia
congenital P61.4
aplastic D61.Ø9
due to isoimmunization NOS P55.9
dyserythropoietic, dyshematopoietic D64.4
following fetal blood loss P61.3
Heinz body D58.2
hereditary hemolytic NOS D58.9
pernicious D51.Ø
spherocytic D58.Ø
Cooley's (erythroblastic) D56.1
cytogenic D51.Ø
deficiency D53.9
6-PGD D55.1
2, 3 diphosphoglycurate mutase D55.2
2, 3 PG D55.2
6 phosphogluconate dehydrogenase D55.1
amino-acid D53.Ø
combined B12 and folate D53.1
enzyme D55.9
drug-induced (hemolytic) D59.2
glucose-6-phosphate dehydrogenase (G6PD) D55.Ø
glycolytic D55.2
nucleotide metabolism D55.3
related to hexose monophosphate (HMP) shunt pathway NEC D55.1
specified type NEC D55.8
erythrocytic glutathione D55.1
folate D52.9
dietary D52.Ø
drug-induced D52.1
folic acid D52.9
dietary D52.Ø
drug-induced D52.1
G SH D55.1
G6PD D55.Ø
GGS-R D55.1
glucose-6-phosphate dehydrogenase D55.Ø
glutathione reductase D55.1
glyceraldehyde phosphate dehydrogenase D55.2
hexokinase D55.2
iron D5Ø.9
secondary to blood loss (chronic) D5Ø.Ø
nutritional D53.9
with
poor iron absorption D5Ø.8
specified deficiency NEC D53.8
phosphofructo-aldolase D55.2
phosphoglycerate kinase D55.2
PK D55.2
protein D53.Ø
pyruvate kinase D55.2
transcobalamin II D51.2
triose-phosphate isomerase D55.2
vitamin B12 NOS D51.9
dietary D51.3
due to
intrinsic factor deficiency D51.Ø
selective vitamin B12 malabsorption with proteinuria D51.1
pernicious D51.Ø
specified type NEC D51.8
Diamond-Blackfan (congenital hypoplastic) D61.Ø1
dibothriocephalus B7Ø.Ø [D63.8]
dimorphic D53.1
diphasic D53.1
Diphyllobothrium (Dibothriocephalus) B7Ø.Ø [D63.8]
due to (in) (with)
antineoplastic chemotherapy D64.81
blood loss (chronic) D5Ø.Ø
acute D62
chemotherapy, antineoplastic D64.81
chronic disease classified elsewhere NEC D63.8
chronic kidney disease D63.1
deficiency
amino-acid D53.Ø
copper D53.8
folate (folic acid) D52.9

Amputation — Anemia

Anemia — *continued*
  due to — *continued*
    deficiency — *continued*
      folate — *continued*
        dietary D52.0
        drug-induced D52.1
      molybdenum D53.8
      protein D53.0
      zinc D53.8
    dietary vitamin B12 deficiency D51.3
    disorder of
      glutathione metabolism D55.1
      nucleotide metabolism D55.3
    drug — *see* Anemia, by type (*see also* Table of Drugs and Chemicals)
    end stage renal disease D63.1
    enzyme disorder D55.9
    fetal blood loss P61.3
    fish tapeworm (D.latum) infestation B70.0 [D63.8]
    hemorrhage (chronic) D50.0
      acute D62
    impaired absorption D50.9
    loss of blood (chronic) D50.0
      acute D62
    myxedema E03.9 [D63.8]
    Necator americanus B76.1 [D63.8]
    prematurity P61.2
    selective vitamin B12 malabsorption with proteinuria D51.1
    transcobalamin II deficiency D51.2
  Dyke-Young type (secondary) (symptomatic) D59.1
  dyserythropoietic (congenital) D64.4
  dyshematopoietic (congenital) D64.4
  Egyptian B76.9 [D63.8]
  elliptocytosis — *see* Elliptocytosis
  enzyme-deficiency, drug-induced D59.2
  epidemic (*see also* Ancylostomiasis) B76.9 [D63.8]
  erythroblastic
    familial D56.1
    newborn (*see also* Disease, hemolytic) P55.9
      of childhood D56.1
  erythrocytic glutathione deficiency D55.1
  erythropoietin-resistant anemia (EPO resistant anemia) D63.1
  Faber's (achlorhydric anemia) D50.9
  factitious (self-induced blood letting) D50.0
  familial erythroblastic D56.1
  Fanconi's (congenital pancytopenia) D61.09
  favism D55.0
  fish tapeworm (D. latum) infestation B70.0 [D63.8]
  folate (folic acid) deficiency D52.9
  glucose-6-phosphate dehydrogenase (G6PD) deficiency D55.0
  glutathione-reductase deficiency D55.1
  goat's milk D52.0
  granulocytic — *see* Agranulocytosis
  Heinz body, congenital D58.2
  hemolytic D58.9
    acquired D59.9
      with hemoglobinuria NEC D59.6
      autoimmune NEC D59.1
      infectious D59.4
      specified type NEC D59.8
      toxic D59.4
    acute D59.9
      due to enzyme deficiency specified type NEC D55.8
      Lederer's D59.1
    autoimmune D59.1
      drug-induced D59.0
    chronic D58.9
      idiopathic D59.9
    cold type (secondary) (symptomatic) D59.1
    congenital (spherocytic) — *see* Spherocytosis
    due to
      cardiac conditions D59.4
      drugs (nonautoimmune) D59.2
        autoimmune D59.0
      enzyme disorder D55.9
        drug-induced D59.2
      presence of shunt or other internal prosthetic device D59.4
    familial D58.9
    hereditary D58.9
      due to enzyme disorder D55.9
        specified type NEC D55.8
      specified type NEC D58.8
    idiopathic (chronic) D59.9
    mechanical D59.4

Anemia — *continued*
  hemolytic — *continued*
    microangiopathic D59.4
    nonautoimmune D59.4
      drug-induced D59.2
    nonspherocytic
      congenital or hereditary NEC D55.8
        glucose-6-phosphate dehydrogenase deficiency D55.0
        pyruvate kinase deficiency D55.2
        type
          I D55.1
          II D55.2
      type
        I D55.1
        II D55.2
    secondary D59.4
      autoimmune D59.1
    specified (hereditary) type NEC D58.8
    Stransky-Regala type (*see also* Hemoglobinopathy) D58.8
    symptomatic D59.4
      autoimmune D59.1
    toxic D59.4
    warm type (secondary) (symptomatic) D59.1
  hemorrhagic (chronic) D50.0
    acute D62
  Herrick's D57.1
  hexokinase deficiency D55.2
  hookworm B76.9 [D63.8]
  hypochromic (idiopathic) (microcytic) (normoblastic) D50.9
    due to blood loss (chronic) D50.0
      acute D62
    familial sex-linked D64.0
    pyridoxine-responsive D64.3
    sideroblastic, sex-linked D64.0
  hypoplasia, red blood cells D61.9
    congenital or familial D61.01
  hypoplastic (idiopathic) D61.9
    congenital or familial (of childhood) D61.01
  hypoproliferative (refractive) D61.9
  idiopathic D64.9
    aplastic D61.3
    hemolytic, chronic D59.9
  in (due to) (with)
    chronic kidney disease D63.1
    end stage renal disease D63.1
    failure, kidney (renal) D63.1
    neoplastic disease (*see also* Neoplasm) D63.0
  intertropical (*see also* Ancylostomiasis) D63.8
  iron deficiency D50.9
    secondary to blood loss (chronic) D50.0
      acute D62
    specified type NEC D50.8
  Joseph-Diamond-Blackfan (congenital hypoplastic) D61.01
  Lederer's (hemolytic) D59.1
  leukoerythroblastic D61.82
  macrocytic D53.9
    nutritional D52.0
    tropical D52.8
  malarial (*see also* Malaria) B54 [D63.8]
  malignant (progressive) D51.0
  malnutrition D53.9
  marsh (*see also* Malaria) B54 [D63.8]
  Mediterranean (with other hemoglobinopathy) D56.9
  megaloblastic D53.1
    combined B12 and folate deficiency D53.1
    hereditary D51.1
    nutritional D52.0
    orotic aciduria D53.0
    refractory D53.1
    specified type NEC D53.1
  megalocytic D53.1
  microcytic (hypochromic) D50.9
    due to blood loss (chronic) D50.0
      acute D62
    familial D56.8
  microdrepanocytosis D57.40
  microelliptopoikilocytic (Rietti-Greppi- Micheli) D56.9
  miner's B76.9 [D63.8]
  myelodysplastic D46.9
  myelofibrosis D75.81
  myelogenous D64.89
  myelopathic D64.89
  myelophthisic D61.82
  myeloproliferative D47.Z9 (*following* D47.4)
  newborn P61.4

Anemia — *continued*
  newborn — *continued*
    due to
      ABO (antibodies, isoimmunization, maternal/fetal incompatibility) P55.1
      Rh (antibodies, isoimmunization, maternal/fetal incompatibility) P55.0
      following fetal blood loss P61.3
      posthemorrhagic (fetal) P61.3
    nonspherocytic hemolytic — *see* Anemia, hemolytic, nonspherocytic
    normocytic (infectional) D64.9
      due to blood loss (chronic) D50.0
        acute D62
      myelophthisic D61.82
    nutritional (deficiency) D53.9
      with
        poor iron absorption D50.8
        specified deficiency NEC D53.8
      megaloblastic D52.0
    of prematurity P61.2
    orotaciduric (congenital) (hereditary) D53.0
    osteosclerotic D64.89
    ovalocytosis (hereditary) — *see* Elliptocytosis
    paludal (*see also* Malaria) B54 [D63.8]
    pernicious (congenital) (malignant) (progressive) D51.0
    pleochromic D64.89
      of sprue D52.8
    posthemorrhagic (chronic) D50.0
      acute D62
      newborn P61.3
    postoperative (postprocedural)
      due to (acute) blood loss D62
        chronic blood loss D50.0
      specified NEC D64.9
    postpartum O90.81
    pressure D64.89
    progressive D64.9
      malignant D51.0
      pernicious D51.0
    protein-deficiency D53.0
    pseudoleukemica infantum D64.89
    pure red cell D60.9
      congenital D61.01
    pyridoxine-responsive D64.3
    pyruvate kinase deficiency D55.2
    refractory D46.4
      with
        excess of blasts D46.20
          1 (RAEB 1) D46.21
          2 (RAEB 2) D46.22
          in transformation (RAEB T) — *see* Leukemia, acute myeloblastic
        hemochromatosis D46.1
        sideroblasts (ring) (RARS) D46.1
      without ring sideroblasts, so stated D46.0
      without sideroblasts without excess of blasts D46.0
      megaloblastic D53.1
      sideroblastic D46.1
      sideropenic D50.9
    Rietti-Greppi-Micheli D56.9
    scorbutic D53.2
    secondary to
      blood loss (chronic) D50.0
        acute D62
      hemorrhage (chronic) D50.0
        acute D62
    semiplastic D61.89
    sickle-cell — *see* Disease, sickle-cell
    sideroblastic D64.3
      hereditary D64.0
      hypochromic, sex-linked D64.0
      pyridoxine-responsive NEC D64.3
      refractory D46.1
      secondary (due to)
        disease D64.1
        drugs and toxins D64.2
        specified type NEC D64.3
    sideropenic (refractory) D50.9
      due to blood loss (chronic) D50.0
        acute D62
    simple chronic D53.9
    specified type NEC D64.89
    spherocytic (hereditary) — *see* Spherocytosis
    splenic D64.89
    splenomegalic D64.89
    stomatocytosis D58.8
    syphilitic (acquired) (late) A52.79 [D63.8]
    target cell D64.89

Anemia — *continued*
  thalassemia D56.9
  thrombocytopenic — *see* Thrombocytopenia
  toxic D61.2
  tropical B76.9 [D63.8]
    macrocytic D52.8
  tuberculous A18.89 [D63.8]
  vegan D51.3
  vitamin
    B6-responsive D64.3
    B12 deficiency (dietary) pernicious D51.0
  von Jaksch's D64.89
  Witts' (achlorhydric anemia) D50.8
Anemophobia F40.228
Anencephalus, anencephaly Q00.0
Anergasia — *see* Psychosis, organic
Anesthesia, anesthetic R20.0
  complication or reaction NEC (*see also* Complications, anesthesia) T88.59 ☑
    due to
      correct substance properly administered — *see* Table of Drugs and Chemicals, by drug, adverse effect
      overdose or wrong substance given — *see* Table of Drugs and Chemicals, by drug, poisoning
    unintended awareness under general anesthesia during procedure T88.53 ☑
      personal history of Z92.84
  cornea H18.81- ☑
  dissociative F44.6
  functional (hysterical) F44.6
  hyperesthetic, thalamic G89.0
  hysterical F44.6
  local skin lesion R20.0
  sexual (psychogenic) F52.1
  shock (due to) T88.2 ☑
  skin R20.0
  testicular N50.9
Anetoderma (maculosum) (of) L90.8
  Jadassohn-Pellizzari L90.2
  Schweniger-Buzzi L90.1
Aneurin deficiency E51.9
Aneurysm (anastomotic) (artery) (cirsoid) (diffuse) (false) (fusiform) (multiple) (saccular) I72.9
  abdominal (aorta) I71.4
    ruptured I71.3
    syphilitic A52.01
  aorta, aortic (nonsyphilitic) I71.9
    abdominal I71.4
      ruptured I71.3
    arch I71.2
      ruptured I71.1
    arteriosclerotic I71.9
      ruptured I71.8
    ascending I71.2
      ruptured I71.1
    congenital Q25.43
    descending I71.9
      abdominal I71.4
        ruptured I71.3
      ruptured I71.8
      thoracic I71.2
        ruptured I71.1
    root Q25.43
    ruptured I71.8
    sinus, congenital Q25.43
    syphilitic A52.01
    thoracic I71.2
      ruptured I71.1
    thoracoabdominal I71.6
      ruptured I71.5
    thorax, thoracic (arch) I71.2
      ruptured I71.1
    transverse I71.2
      ruptured I71.1
    valve (heart) (*see also* Endocarditis, aortic) I35.8
  arteriosclerotic I72.9
    cerebral I67.1
      ruptured — *see* Hemorrhage, intracranial, subarachnoid
    arteriovenous (congenital) (*see also* Malformation, arteriovenous)
      acquired I77.0
        brain I67.1
        coronary I25.41
        pulmonary I28.0
      brain Q28.2

Aneurysm — *continued*
  arteriovenous (*see also* Malformation, arteriovenous) — *continued*
    brain — *continued*
      ruptured I60.8
    peripheral — *see* Malformation, arteriovenous, peripheral
    precerebral vessels Q28.0
    specified site NEC (*see also* Malformation, arteriovenous)
      acquired I77.0
  basal — *see* Aneurysm, brain
  basilar (trunk) I72.5
  berry (congenital) (nonruptured) I67.1
    ruptured I60.7
  brain I67.1
    arteriosclerotic I67.1
      ruptured — *see* Hemorrhage, intracranial, subarachnoid
    arteriovenous (congenital) (nonruptured) Q28.2
      acquired I67.1
        ruptured I60.8
      ruptured I60.8
    berry (congenital) (nonruptured) I67.1
      ruptured (*see also* Hemorrhage, intracranial, subarachnoid) I60.7
    congenital Q28.3
      ruptured I60.7
    meninges I67.1
      ruptured I60.8
    miliary (congenital) (nonruptured) I67.1
      ruptured (*see also* Hemorrhage, intracranial, subarachnoid) I60.7
    mycotic I33.0
    ruptured — *see* Hemorrhage, intracranial, subarachnoid
    syphilitic (hemorrhage) A52.05
  cardiac (false) (*see also* Aneurysm, heart) I25.3
  carotid artery (common) (external) I72.0
    internal (intracranial) I67.1
      extracranial portion I72.0
    ruptured into brain I60.0- ☑
    syphilitic A52.09
      intracranial A52.05
  cavernous sinus I67.1
    arteriovenous (congenital) (nonruptured) Q28.3
      ruptured I60.8
  celiac I72.8
  central nervous system, syphilitic A52.05
  cerebral — *see* Aneurysm, brain
  chest — *see* Aneurysm, thorax
  circle of Willis I67.1
    congenital Q28.3
      ruptured I60.6
    ruptured I60.6
  common iliac artery I72.3
  congenital (peripheral) Q27.8
    aorta (root) (sinus) Q25.43
    brain Q28.3
      ruptured I60.7
    coronary Q24.5
    digestive system Q27.8
    lower limb Q27.8
    pulmonary Q25.79
    retina Q14.1
    specified site NEC Q27.8
    upper limb Q27.8
  conjunctiva — *see* Abnormality, conjunctiva, vascular
  conus arteriosus — *see* Aneurysm, heart
  coronary (arteriosclerotic) (artery) I25.41
    arteriovenous, congenital Q24.5
    congenital Q24.5
    ruptured — *see* Infarct, myocardium
    syphilitic A52.06
    vein I25.89
  cylindroid (aorta) I71.9
    ruptured I71.8
    syphilitic A52.01
  ductus arteriosus Q25.0
  endocardial, infective (any valve) I33.0
  femoral (artery) (ruptured) I72.4
  gastroduodenal I72.8
  gastroepiploic I72.8
  heart (wall) (chronic or with a stated duration of over 4 weeks) I25.3
    valve — *see* Endocarditis
  hepatic I72.8
  iliac (common) (artery) (ruptured) I72.3

Aneurysm — *continued*
  infective I72.9
    endocardial (any valve) I33.0
  innominate (nonsyphilitic) I72.8
    syphilitic A52.09
  interauricular septum — *see* Aneurysm, heart
  interventricular septum — *see* Aneurysm, heart
  intrathoracic (nonsyphilitic) I71.2
    ruptured I71.1
    syphilitic A52.01
  lower limb I72.4
  lung (pulmonary artery) I28.1
  mediastinal (nonsyphilitic) I72.8
    syphilitic A52.09
  miliary (congenital) I67.1
    ruptured — *see* Hemorrhage, intracerebral, subarachnoid, intracranial
  mitral (heart) (valve) I34.8
  mural — *see* Aneurysm, heart
  mycotic I72.9
    endocardial (any valve) I33.0
    ruptured, brain — *see* Hemorrhage, intracerebral, subarachnoid
  myocardium — *see* Aneurysm, heart
  neck I72.0
  pancreaticoduodenal I72.8
  patent ductus arteriosus Q25.0
  peripheral NEC I72.8
    congenital Q27.8
      digestive system Q27.8
      lower limb Q27.8
      specified site NEC Q27.8
      upper limb Q27.8
  popliteal (artery) (ruptured) I72.4
  precerebral
    congenital (nonruptured) Q28.1
    specified site, NEC I72.5
  pulmonary I28.1
    arteriovenous Q25.72
      acquired I28.0
    syphilitic A52.09
    valve (heart) — *see* Endocarditis, pulmonary
  racemose (peripheral) I72.9
    congenital — *see* Aneurysm, congenital
  radial I72.1
  Rasmussen NEC A15.0
  renal (artery) I72.2
  retina (*see also* Disorder, retina, microaneurysms)
    congenital Q14.1
    diabetic — *see* Diabetes, microaneurysms, retinal
  sinus of Valsalva Q25.49
  specified NEC I72.8
  spinal (cord) I72.8
    syphilitic (hemorrhage) A52.09
  splenic I72.8
  subclavian (artery) (ruptured) I72.8
    syphilitic A52.09
  superior mesenteric I72.8
  syphilitic (aorta) A52.01
    central nervous system A52.05
    congenital (late) A50.54 [I79.0]
    spine, spinal A52.09
  thoracoabdominal (aorta) I71.6
    ruptured I71.5
    syphilitic A52.01
  thorax, thoracic (aorta) (arch) (nonsyphilitic) I71.2
    ruptured I71.1
    syphilitic A52.01
  traumatic (complication) (early), specified site — *see* Injury, blood vessel
  tricuspid (heart) (valve) I07.8
  ulnar I72.1
  upper limb (ruptured) I72.1
  valve, valvular — *see* Endocarditis
  venous (*see also* Varix) I86.8
    congenital Q27.8
      digestive system Q27.8
      lower limb Q27.8
      specified site NEC Q27.8
      upper limb Q27.8
  ventricle — *see* Aneurysm, heart
  vertebral artery I72.6
  visceral NEC I72.8
Angelman syndrome Q93.5
Anger R45.4
Angiectasis, angiectopia I99.8
Angiitis I77.6
  allergic granulomatous M30.1

Angiitis — *continued*
 hypersensitivity M31.0
 necrotizing M31.9
  specified NEC M31.8
 nervous system, granulomatous I67.7
Angina (attack) (cardiac) (chest) (heart) (pectoris) (syndrome) (vasomotor) I20.9
 with
  atherosclerotic heart disease — *see* Arteriosclerosis, coronary (artery),
  documented spasm I20.1
 abdominal K55.1
 accelerated — *see* Angina, unstable
 agranulocytic — *see* Agranulocytosis
 angiospastic — *see* Angina, with documented spasm
 aphthous B08.5
 crescendo — *see* Angina, unstable
 croupous J05.0
 cruris I73.9
 de novo effort — *see* Angina, unstable
 diphtheritic, membranous A36.0
 equivalent I20.8
 exudative, chronic J37.0
 following acute myocardial infarction I23.7
 gangrenous diphtheritic A36.0
 intestinal K55.1
 Ludovici K12.2
 Ludwig's K12.2
 malignant diphtheritic A36.0
 membranous J05.0
  diphtheritic A36.0
  Vincent's A69.1
 mesenteric K55.1
 monocytic — *see* Mononucleosis, infectious
 of effort — *see* Angina, specified NEC
 phlegmonous J36
  diphtheritic A36.0
 post-infarctional I23.7
 pre-infarctional — *see* Angina, unstable
 Prinzmetal — *see* Angina, with documented spasm
 progressive — *see* Angina, unstable
 pseudomembranous A69.1
 pultaceous, diphtheritic A36.0
 spasm-induced — *see* Angina, with documented spasm
 specified NEC I20.8
 stable I20.8
 stenocardia — *see* Angina, specified NEC
 stridulous, diphtheritic A36.2
 tonsil J36
 trachealis J05.0
 unstable I20.0
 variant — *see* Angina, with documented spasm
 Vincent's A69.1
 worsening effort — *see* Angina, unstable
Angioblastoma — *see* Neoplasm, connective tissue, uncertain behavior
Angiocholecystitis — *see* Cholecystitis, acute
Angiocholitis (*see also* Cholecystitis, acute) K83.0
Angiodysgenesis spinalis G95.19
Angiodysplasia (cecum) (colon) K55.20
 with bleeding K55.21
 duodenum (and stomach) K31.819
  with bleeding K31.811
 stomach (and duodenum) K31.819
  with bleeding K31.811
Angioedema (allergic) (any site) (with urticaria) T78.3 ✓
 hereditary D84.1
Angioendothelioma — *see* Neoplasm, uncertain behavior, by site
 benign D18.00
  intra-abdominal D18.03
  intracranial D18.02
  skin D18.01
  specified site NEC D18.09
 bone — *see* Neoplasm, bone, malignant
 Ewing's — *see* Neoplasm, bone, malignant
Angioendotheliomatosis C85.8- ✓
Angiofibroma (*see also* Neoplasm, benign, by site)
 juvenile
  specified site — *see* Neoplasm, benign, by site
  unspecified site D10.6
Angiohemophilia (A) (B) D68.0
Angioid streaks (choroid) (macula) (retina) H35.33
Angiokeratoma — *see* Neoplasm, skin, benign
 corporis diffusum E75.21
Angioleiomyoma — *see* Neoplasm, connective tissue, benign

Angiolipoma (*see also* Lipoma)
 infiltrating — *see* Lipoma
Angioma (*see also* Hemangioma, by site)
 capillary I78.1
 hemorrhagicum hereditaria I78.0
 intra-abdominal D18.03
 intracranial D18.02
 malignant — *see* Neoplasm, connective tissue, malignant
 plexiform D18.00
  intra-abdominal D18.03
  intracranial D18.02
  skin D18.01
  specified site NEC D18.09
 senile I78.1
 serpiginosum L81.7
 skin D18.01
 specified site NEC D18.09
 spider I78.1
 stellate I78.1
 venous Q28.3
Angiomatosis Q82.8
 bacillary A79.89
 encephalotrigeminal Q85.8
 hemorrhagic familial I78.0
 hereditary familial I78.0
 liver K76.4
Angiomyolipoma — *see* Lipoma
Angiomyoliposarcoma — *see* Neoplasm, connective tissue, malignant
Angiomyoma — *see* Neoplasm, connective tissue, benign
Angiomyosarcoma — *see* Neoplasm, connective tissue, malignant
Angiomyxoma — *see* Neoplasm, connective tissue, uncertain behavior
Angioneurosis F45.8
Angioneurotic edema (allergic) (any site) (with urticaria) T78.3 ✓
 hereditary D84.1
Angiopathia, angiopathy I99.9
 cerebral I67.9
  amyloid E85.4 [I68.0]
 diabetic (peripheral) — *see* Diabetes, angiopathy
 peripheral I73.9
  diabetic — *see* Diabetes, angiopathy
  specified type NEC I73.89
 retinae syphilitica A52.05
 retinalis (juvenilis)
  diabetic — *see* Diabetes, retinopathy
  proliferative — *see* Retinopathy, proliferative
Angiosarcoma (*see also* Neoplasm, connective tissue, malignant)
 liver C22.3
Angiosclerosis — *see* Arteriosclerosis
Angiospasm (peripheral) (traumatic) (vessel) I73.9
 brachial plexus G54.0
 cerebral G45.9
 cervical plexus G54.2
 nerve
  arm — *see* Mononeuropathy, upper limb
   axillary G54.0
   median — *see* Lesion, nerve, median
   ulnar — *see* Lesion, nerve, ulnar
  axillary G54.0
  leg — *see* Mononeuropathy, lower limb
  median — *see* Lesion, nerve, median
  plantar — *see* Lesion, nerve, plantar
  ulnar — *see* Lesion, nerve, ulnar
Angiospastic disease or edema I73.9
Angiostrongyliasis
 due to
  Parastrongylus
   cantonensis B83.2
   costaricensis B81.3
  intestinal B81.3
Anguillulosis — *see* Strongyloidiasis
Angulation
 cecum — *see* Obstruction, intestine
 coccyx (acquired) (*see also* subcategory) M43.8 ✓
  congenital NEC Q76.49
 femur (acquired) (*see also* Deformity, limb, specified type NEC, thigh)
  congenital Q74.2
 intestine (large) (small) — *see* Obstruction, intestine
 sacrum (acquired) (*see also* subcategory) M43.8 ✓
  congenital NEC Q76.49
 sigmoid (flexure) — *see* Obstruction, intestine

Angulation — *continued*
 spine — *see* Dorsopathy, deforming, specified NEC
 tibia (acquired) (*see also* Deformity, limb, specified type NEC, lower leg)
  congenital Q74.2
 ureter N13.5
  with infection N13.6
 wrist (acquired) (*see also* Deformity, limb, specified type NEC, forearm)
  congenital Q74.0
Angulus infectiosus (lips) K13.0
Anhedonia R45.84
 sexual F52.0
Anhidrosis L74.4
Anhydration E86.0
Anhydremia E86.0
Anidrosis L74.4
Aniridia (congenital) Q13.1
Anisakiasis (infection) (infestation) B81.0
Anisakis larvae infestation B81.0
Aniseikonia H52.32
Anisocoria (pupil) H57.02
 congenital Q13.2
Anisocytosis R71.8
Anisometropia (congenital) H52.31
Ankle — *see* condition
Ankyloblepharon (eyelid) (acquired) (*see also* Blepharophimosis)
 filiforme (adnatum) (congenital) Q10.3
 total Q10.3
Ankyloglossia Q38.1
Ankylosis (fibrous) (osseous) (joint) M24.60
 ankle M24.67- ✓
 arthrodesis status Z98.1
 cricoarytenoid (cartilage) (joint) (larynx) J38.7
 dental K03.5
 ear ossicles H74.31- ✓
 elbow M24.62- ✓
 foot M24.67- ✓
 hand M24.64- ✓
 hip M24.65- ✓
 incostapedial joint (infectional) — *see* Ankylosis, ear ossicles
 jaw (temporomandibular) M26.61- ✓
 knee M24.66- ✓
 lumbosacral (joint) M43.27
 postoperative (status) Z98.1
 produced by surgical fusion, status Z98.1
 sacro-iliac (joint) M43.28
 shoulder M24.61- ✓
 spine (joint) (*see also* Fusion, spine)
  spondylitic — *see* Spondylitis, ankylosing
 surgical Z98.1
 temporomandibular M26.61- ✓
 tooth, teeth (hard tissues) K03.5
 wrist M24.63- ✓
Ankylostoma — *see* Ancylostoma
Ankylostomiasis — *see* Ancylostomiasis
Ankylurethria — *see* Stricture, urethra
Annular (*see also* condition)
 detachment, cervix N88.8
 organ or site, congenital NEC — *see* Distortion
 pancreas (congenital) Q45.1
Anodontia (complete) (partial) (vera) K00.0
 acquired K08.10 ✓
Anomaly, anomalous (congenital) (unspecified type) Q89.9
 abdominal wall NEC Q79.59
 acoustic nerve Q07.8
 adrenal (gland) Q89.1
 Alder (-Reilly) (leukocyte granulation) D72.0
 alimentary tract Q45.9
  upper Q40.9
 alveolar M26.70
  hyperplasia M26.79
   mandibular M26.72
   maxillary M26.71
  hypoplasia M26.79
   mandibular M26.74
   maxillary M26.73
  ridge (process) M26.79
  specified NEC M26.79
 ankle (joint) Q74.2
 anus Q43.9
 aorta (arch) NEC Q25.40
  coarctation (preductal) (postductal) Q25.1
 aortic cusp or valve Q23.9

Anomaly, anomalous — *continued*
appendix Q43.8
apple peel syndrome Q41.1
aqueduct of Sylvius Q03.0
   with spina bifida — *see* Spina bifida, with hydro-
      cephalus
arm Q74.0
arteriovenous NEC
   coronary Q24.5
   gastrointestinal Q27.33
      acquired — *see* Angiodysplasia
artery (peripheral) Q27.9
   basilar NEC Q28.1
   cerebral Q28.3
   coronary Q24.5
   digestive system Q27.8
   eye Q15.8
   great Q25.9
      specified NEC Q25.8
   lower limb Q27.8
   peripheral Q27.9
      specified NEC Q27.8
   pulmonary NEC Q25.79
   renal Q27.2
   retina Q14.1
   specified site NEC Q27.8
   subclavian Q27.8
      origin Q25.48
   umbilical Q27.0
   upper limb Q27.8
   vertebral NEC Q28.1
aryteno-epiglottic folds Q31.8
atrial
   bands or folds Q20.8
   septa Q21.1
atrioventricular
   excitation I45.6
   septum Q21.0
auditory canal Q17.8
auricle
   ear Q17.8
      causing impairment of hearing Q16.9
   heart Q20.8
Axenfeld's Q15.0
back Q89.9
band
   atrial Q20.8
   heart Q24.8
   ventricular Q24.8
Bartholin's duct Q38.4
biliary duct or passage Q44.5
bladder Q64.70
   absence Q64.5
   diverticulum Q64.6
   exstrophy Q64.10
      cloacal Q64.12
      extroversion Q64.19
      specified type NEC Q64.19
      supravesical fissure Q64.11
   neck obstruction Q64.31
   specified type NEC Q64.79
bone Q79.9
   arm Q74.0
   face Q75.9
   leg Q74.2
   pelvic girdle Q74.2
   shoulder girdle Q74.0
   skull Q75.9
      with
         anencephaly Q00.0
         encephalocele — *see* Encephalocele
         hydrocephalus Q03.9
            with spina bifida — *see* Spina bifida, by
               site, with hydrocephalus
         microcephaly Q02
brain (multiple) Q04.9
   vessel Q28.3
breast Q83.9
broad ligament Q50.6
bronchus Q32.4
bulbus cordis Q21.9
bursa Q79.9
canal of Nuck Q52.4
canthus Q10.3
capillary Q27.9
cardiac Q24.9
   chambers Q20.9
      specified NEC Q20.8
   septal closure Q21.9

Anomaly, anomalous — *continued*
cardiac — *continued*
   septal closure — *continued*
      specified NEC Q21.8
   valve NEC Q24.8
      pulmonary Q22.3
cardiovascular system Q28.8
carpus Q74.0
caruncle, lacrimal Q10.6
cascade stomach Q40.2
cauda equina Q06.3
cecum Q43.9
cerebral Q04.9
   vessels Q28.3
cervix Q51.9
Chédiak-Higashi (-Steinbrinck) (congenital gigantism
      of peroxidase granules) E70.330
cheek Q18.9
chest wall Q67.8
   bones Q76.9
chin Q18.9
chordae tendineae Q24.8
choroid Q14.3
   plexus Q07.8
chromosomes, chromosomal Q99.9
   D (1) — *see* condition, chromosome 13
   E (3) — *see* condition, chromosome 18
   G — *see* condition, chromosome 21
   sex
      female phenotype Q97.8
      gonadal dysgenesis (pure) Q99.1
      Klinefelter's Q98.4
      male phenotype Q98.9
      Turner's Q96.9
   specified NEC Q99.8
cilia Q10.3
circulatory system Q28.9
clavicle Q74.0
clitoris Q52.6
coccyx Q76.49
colon Q43.9
common duct Q44.5
communication
   coronary artery Q24.5
   left ventricle with right atrium Q21.0
concha (ear) Q17.3
connection
   portal vein Q26.5
   pulmonary venous Q26.4
      partial Q26.3
      total Q26.2
   renal artery with kidney Q27.2
cornea (shape) Q13.4
coronary artery or vein Q24.5
cranium — *see* Anomaly, skull
cricoid cartilage Q31.8
cystic duct Q44.5
dental
   alveolar — *see* Anomaly, alveolar
   arch relationship M26.20
      specified NEC M26.29
dentofacial M26.9
   alveolar — *see* Anomaly, alveolar
   dental arch relationship M26.20
      specified NEC M26.29
   functional M26.50
      specified NEC M26.59
   jaw size M26.00
      macrogenia M26.05
      mandibular
         hyperplasia M26.03
         hypoplasia M26.04
      maxillary
         hyperplasia M26.01
         hypoplasia M26.02
      microgenia M26.06
      specified type NEC M26.09
   jaw-cranial base relationship M26.10
      asymmetry M26.12
         maxillary M26.11
      specified type NEC M26.19
   malocclusion M26.4
      dental arch relationship NEC M26.29
      jaw size — *see* Anomaly, dentofacial, jaw size
      jaw-cranial base relationship — *see* Anomaly,
         dentofacial, jaw-cranial base relationship
   specified type NEC M26.89
   temporomandibular joint M26.60- ☑

Anomaly, anomalous — *continued*
dentofacial — *continued*
   temporomandibular joint — *continued*
      adhesions M26.61- ☑
      ankylosis M26.61- ☑
      arthralgia M26.62- ☑
      articular disc M26.63- ☑
      specified type NEC M26.69
   tooth position, fully erupted M26.30
      specified NEC M26.39
dermatoglyphic Q82.8
diaphragm (apertures) NEC Q79.1
digestive organ(s) or tract Q45.9
   lower Q43.9
   upper Q40.9
distance, interarch (excessive) (inadequate) M26.25
distribution, coronary artery Q24.5
ductus
   arteriosus Q25.0
   botalli Q25.0
duodenum Q43.9
dura (brain) Q04.9
   spinal cord Q06.9
ear (external) Q17.9
   causing impairment of hearing Q16.9
   inner Q16.5
   middle (causing impairment of hearing) Q16.4
      ossicles Q16.3
Ebstein's (heart) (tricuspid valve) Q22.5
ectodermal Q82.9
Eisenmenger's (ventricular septal defect) Q21.8
ejaculatory duct Q55.4
elbow Q74.0
endocrine gland NEC Q89.2
epididymis Q55.4
epiglottis Q31.8
esophagus Q39.9
eustachian tube Q17.8
eye Q15.9
   anterior segment Q13.9
      specified NEC Q13.89
   posterior segment Q14.9
      specified NEC Q14.8
   ptosis (eyelid) Q10.0
   specified NEC Q15.8
eyebrow Q18.8
eyelid Q10.3
   ptosis Q10.0
face Q18.9
   bone(s) Q75.9
fallopian tube Q50.6
fascia Q79.9
femur NEC Q74.2
fibula NEC Q74.2
finger Q74.0
fixation, intestine Q43.3
flexion (joint) NOS Q74.9
   hip or thigh Q65.89
foot NEC Q74.2
   varus (congenital) Q66.3
foramen
   Botalli Q21.1
   ovale Q21.1
forearm Q74.0
forehead Q75.8
form, teeth K00.2
fovea centralis Q14.1
frontal bone — *see* Anomaly, skull
gallbladder (position) (shape) (size) Q44.1
Gartner's duct Q52.4
gastrointestinal tract Q45.9
genitalia, genital organ(s) or system
   female Q52.9
      external Q52.70
      internal NOS Q52.9
   male Q55.9
      hydrocele P83.5
      specified NEC Q55.8
genitourinary NEC
   female Q52.9
   male Q55.9
Gerbode Q21.0
glottis Q31.8
granulation or granulocyte, genetic (constitutional)
      (leukocyte) D72.0
gum Q38.6
gyri Q07.9
hair Q84.2
hand Q74.0

☑ **Additional Character Required** — Refer to the Tabular List for Character Selection   ▽ Subterms under main terms may continue to next column or page

Anomaly, anomalous — *continued*
  hard tissue formation in pulp K04.3
  head — *see* Anomaly, skull
  heart Q24.9
    auricle Q20.8
    bands or folds Q24.8
    fibroelastosis cordis I42.4
    obstructive NEC Q22.6
    patent ductus arteriosus (Botalli) Q25.0
    septum Q21.9
      auricular Q21.1
      interatrial Q21.1
      interventricular Q21.0
        with pulmonary stenosis or atresia, dextra-
          position of aorta and hypertrophy of
          right ventricle Q21.3
      specified NEC Q21.8
      ventricular Q21.0
        with pulmonary stenosis or atresia, dextra-
          position of aorta and hypertrophy of
          right ventricle Q21.3
    tetralogy of Fallot Q21.3
    valve NEC Q24.8
      aortic
        bicuspid valve Q23.1
        insufficiency Q23.1
        stenosis Q23.0
          subaortic Q24.4
      mitral
        insufficiency Q23.3
        stenosis Q23.2
      pulmonary Q22.3
        atresia Q22.0
        insufficiency Q22.2
        stenosis Q22.1
          infundibular Q24.3
          subvalvular Q24.3
      tricuspid
        atresia Q22.4
        stenosis Q22.4
    ventricle Q20.8
  heel NEC Q74.2
  Hegglin's D72.0
  hemianencephaly Q00.0
  hemicephaly Q00.0
  hemicrania Q00.0
  hepatic duct Q44.5
  hip NEC Q74.2
  hourglass stomach Q40.2
  humerus Q74.0
  hydatid of Morgagni
    female Q50.5
    male (epididymal) Q55.4
      testicular Q55.29
  hymen Q52.4
  hypersegmentation of neutrophils, hereditary D72.0
  hypophyseal Q89.2
  ileocecal (coil) (valve) Q43.9
  ileum Q43.9
  ilium NEC Q74.2
  integument Q84.9
    specified NEC Q84.8
  interarch distance (excessive) (inadequate) M26.25
  intervertebral cartilage or disc Q76.49
  intestine (large) (small) Q43.9
    with anomalous adhesions, fixation or malrotation
      Q43.3
  iris Q13.2
  ischium NEC Q74.2
  jaw — *see* Anomaly, dentofacial
    alveolar — *see* Anomaly, alveolar
  jaw-cranial base relationship — *see* Anomaly, dento-
    facial, jaw-cranial base relationship
  jejunum Q43.8
  joint Q74.9
    specified NEC Q74.8
  Jordan's D72.0
  kidney(s) (calyx) (pelvis) Q63.9
    artery Q27.2
    specified NEC Q63.8
  Klippel-Feil (brevicollis) Q76.1
  knee Q74.1
  labium (majus) (minus) Q52.70
  labyrinth, membranous Q16.5
  lacrimal apparatus or duct Q10.6
  larynx, laryngeal (muscle) Q31.9
    web (bed) Q31.0
  lens Q12.9
  leukocytes, genetic D72.0

Anomaly, anomalous — *continued*
  leukocytes, genetic — *continued*
    granulation (constitutional) D72.0
  lid (fold) Q10.3
  ligament Q79.9
    broad Q50.6
    round Q52.8
  limb Q74.9
    lower NEC Q74.2
      reduction deformity — *see* Defect, reduction,
        lower limb
    upper Q74.0
  lip Q38.0
  liver Q44.7
    duct Q44.5
  lower limb NEC Q74.2
  lumbosacral (joint) (region) Q76.49
    kyphosis — *see* Kyphosis, congenital
    lordosis — *see* Lordosis, congenital
  lung (fissure) (lobe) Q33.9
  mandible — *see* Anomaly, dentofacial
  maxilla — *see* Anomaly, dentofacial
  May (-Hegglin) D72.0
  meatus urinarius NEC Q64.79
  meningeal bands or folds Q07.9
    constriction of Q07.8
    spinal Q06.9
  meninges Q07.9
    cerebral Q04.8
    spinal Q06.9
  meningocele Q05.9
  mesentery Q45.9
  metacarpus Q74.0
  metatarsus NEC Q74.2
  middle ear Q16.4
    ossicles Q16.3
  mitral (leaflets) (valve) Q23.9
    insufficiency Q23.3
    specified NEC Q23.8
    stenosis Q23.2
  mouth Q38.6
  Müllerian (*see also* Anomaly, by site)
    uterus NEC Q51.818
  multiple NEC Q89.7
  muscle Q79.9
    eyelid Q10.3
  musculoskeletal system, except limbs Q79.9
  myocardium Q24.8
  nail Q84.6
  narrowness, eyelid Q10.3
  nasal sinus (wall) Q30.8
  neck (any part) Q18.9
  nerve Q07.9
    acoustic Q07.8
    optic Q07.8
  nervous system (central) Q07.9
  nipple Q83.9
  nose, nasal (bones) (cartilage) (septum) (sinus) Q30.9
    specified NEC Q30.8
  ocular muscle Q15.8
  omphalomesenteric duct Q43.0
  opening, pulmonary veins Q26.4
  optic
    disc Q14.2
    nerve Q07.8
  opticociliary vessels Q13.2
  orbit (eye) Q10.7
  organ Q89.9
    of Corti Q16.5
  origin
    artery
      innominate Q25.8
      pulmonary Q25.79
      renal Q27.2
      subclavian Q25.48
  osseous meatus (ear) Q16.1
  ovary Q50.39
  oviduct Q50.6
  palate (hard) (soft) NEC Q38.5
  pancreas or pancreatic duct Q45.3
  papillary muscles Q24.8
  parathyroid gland Q89.2
  paraurethral ducts Q64.79
  parotid (gland) Q38.4
  patella Q74.1
  Pelger-Huët (hereditary hyposegmentation) D72.0
  pelvic girdle NEC Q74.2
  pelvis (bony) NEC Q74.2
    rachitic E64.3

Anomaly, anomalous — *continued*
  penis (glans) Q55.69
  pericardium Q24.8
  peripheral vascular system Q27.9
  Peter's Q13.4
  pharynx Q38.8
  pigmentation L81.9
    congenital Q82.8
  pituitary (gland) Q89.2
  pleural (folds) Q34.0
  portal vein Q26.5
    connection Q26.5
  position, tooth, teeth, fully erupted M26.30
    specified NEC M26.39
  precerebral vessel Q28.1
  prepuce Q55.69
  prostate Q55.4
  pulmonary Q33.9
    artery NEC Q25.79
    valve Q22.3
      atresia Q22.0
      insufficiency Q22.2
      specified type NEC Q22.3
      stenosis Q22.1
        infundibular Q24.3
        subvalvular Q24.3
    venous connection Q26.4
      partial Q26.3
      total Q26.2
  pupil Q13.2
    function H57.00
      anisocoria H57.02
      Argyll Robertson pupil H57.01
      miosis H57.03
      mydriasis H57.04
      specified type NEC H57.09
      tonic pupil H57.05- ✓
  pylorus Q40.3
  radius Q74.0
  rectum Q43.9
  reduction (extremity) (limb)
    femur (longitudinal) — *see* Defect, reduction,
      lower limb, longitudinal, femur
    fibula (longitudinal) — *see* Defect, reduction, lower
      limb, longitudinal, fibula
    lower limb — *see* Defect, reduction, lower limb
    radius (longitudinal) — *see* Defect, reduction, up-
      per limb, longitudinal, radius
    tibia (longitudinal) — *see* Defect, reduction, lower
      limb, longitudinal, tibia
    ulna (longitudinal) — *see* Defect, reduction, upper
      limb, longitudinal, ulna
    upper limb — *see* Defect, reduction, upper limb
  refraction — *see* Disorder, refraction
  renal Q63.9
    artery Q27.2
    pelvis Q63.9
      specified NEC Q63.8
  respiratory system Q34.9
    specified NEC Q34.8
  retina Q14.1
  rib Q76.6
    cervical Q76.5
  Rieger's Q13.81
  rotation — *see* Malrotation
    hip or thigh Q65.89
  round ligament Q52.8
  sacroiliac (joint) NEC Q74.2
  sacrum NEC Q76.49
    kyphosis — *see* Kyphosis, congenital
    lordosis — *see* Lordosis, congenital
  saddle nose, syphilitic A50.57
  salivary duct or gland Q38.4
  scapula Q74.0
  scrotum — *see* Malformation, testis and scrotum
  sebaceous gland Q82.9
  seminal vesicles Q55.4
  sense organs NEC Q07.8
  sex chromosomes NEC (*see also* Anomaly, chromo-
    somes)
    female phenotype Q97.8
    male phenotype Q98.9
  shoulder (girdle) (joint) Q74.0
  sigmoid (flexure) Q43.9
  simian crease Q82.8
  sinus of Valsalva Q25.49
  skeleton generalized Q78.9
  skin (appendage) Q82.9

Anomaly, anomalous — continued
skull Q75.9
with
anencephaly Q00.0
encephalocele — see Encephalocele
hydrocephalus Q03.9
with spina bifida — see Spina bifida, by site,
with hydrocephalus
microcephaly Q02
specified organ or site NEC Q89.8
spermatic cord Q55.4
spine, spinal NEC Q76.49
column NEC Q76.49
kyphosis — see Kyphosis, congenital
lordosis — see Lordosis, congenital
cord Q06.9
nerve root Q07.8
spleen Q89.09
agenesis Q89.01
stenonian duct Q38.4
sternum NEC Q76.7
stomach Q40.3
submaxillary gland Q38.4
tarsus NEC Q74.2
tendon Q79.9
testis — see Malformation, testis and scrotum
thigh NEC Q74.2
thorax (wall) Q67.8
bony Q76.9
throat Q38.8
thumb Q74.0
thymus gland Q89.2
thyroid (gland) Q89.2
cartilage Q31.8
tibia NEC Q74.2
saber A50.56
toe Q74.2
tongue Q38.3
tooth, teeth K00.9
eruption K00.6
position, fully erupted M26.30
spacing, fully erupted M26.30
trachea (cartilage) Q32.1
tragus Q17.9
tricuspid (leaflet) (valve) Q22.9
atresia or stenosis Q22.4
Ebstein's Q22.5
Uhl's (hypoplasia of myocardium, right ventricle) Q24.8
ulna Q74.0
umbilical artery Q27.0
union
cricoid cartilage and thyroid cartilage Q31.8
thyroid cartilage and hyoid bone Q31.8
trachea with larynx Q31.8
upper limb Q74.0
urachus Q64.4
ureter Q62.8
obstructive NEC Q62.39
cecoureterocele Q62.32
orthotopic ureterocele Q62.31
urethra Q64.70
absence Q64.5
double Q64.74
fistula to rectum Q64.73
obstructive Q64.39
stricture Q64.32
prolapse Q64.71
specified type NEC Q64.79
urinary tract Q64.9
uterus Q51.9
with only one functioning horn Q51.4
uvula Q38.5
vagina Q52.4
valleculae Q31.8
valve (heart) NEC Q24.8
coronary sinus Q24.5
inferior vena cava Q24.8
pulmonary Q22.3
sinus coronario Q24.5
venae cavae inferioris Q24.8
vas deferens Q55.4
vascular Q27.9
brain Q28.3
ring Q25.45
vein(s) (peripheral) Q27.9
brain Q28.3
cerebral Q28.3
coronary Q24.5
developmental Q28.3

Anomaly, anomalous — continued
vein(s) — continued
great Q26.9
specified NEC Q26.8
vena cava (inferior) (superior) Q26.9
venous — see Anomaly, vein(s)
venous return Q26.8
ventricular
bands or folds Q24.8
septa Q21.0
vertebra Q76.49
kyphosis — see Kyphosis, congenital
lordosis — see Lordosis, congenital
vesicourethral orifice Q64.79
vessel(s) Q27.9
optic papilla Q14.2
precerebral Q28.1
vitelline duct Q43.0
vitreous body or humor Q14.0
vulva Q52.70
wrist (joint) Q74.0
Anomia R48.8
Anonychia (congenital) Q84.3
acquired L60.8
Anophthalmos, anophthalmus (congenital) (globe)
Q11.1
acquired Z90.01
Anopia, anopsia H53.46- ☑
quadrant H53.46- ☑
Anorchia, anorchism, anorchidism Q55.0
Anorexia R63.0
hysterical F44.89
nervosa F50.00
atypical F50.9
binge-eating type F50.2
with purging F50.02
restricting type F50.01
Anorgasmy, psychogenic (female) F52.31
male F52.32
Anosmia R43.0
hysterical F44.6
postinfectional J39.8
Anosognosia R41.89
Anosteoplasia Q78.9
Anovulatory cycle N97.0
Anoxemia R09.02
newborn P84
Anoxia (pathological) R09.02
altitude T70.29 ☑
cerebral G93.1
complicating
anesthesia (general) (local) or other sedation
T88.59 ☑
in labor and delivery O74.3
in pregnancy O29.21- ☑
postpartum, puerperal O89.2
delivery (cesarean) (instrumental) O75.4
during a procedure G97.81
newborn P84
resulting from a procedure G97.82
due to
drowning T75.1 ☑
high altitude T70.29 ☑
heart — see Insufficiency, coronary
intrauterine P84
myocardial — see Insufficiency, coronary
newborn P84
spinal cord G95.11
systemic (by suffocation) (low content in atmosphere)
— see Asphyxia, traumatic
Anteflexion — see Anteversion
Antenatal
care (normal pregnancy) Z34.90
screening (encounter for) of mother (see also Encounter, antenatal screening) Z36.9
Antepartum — see condition
Anterior — see condition
Antero-occlusion M26.220
Anteversion
cervix — see Anteversion, uterus
femur (neck), congenital Q65.89
uterus, uterine (cervix) (postinfectional) (postpartal,
old) N85.4
congenital Q51.818
in pregnancy or childbirth — see Pregnancy,
complicated by
Anthophobia F40.228
Anthracosilicosis J60

Anthracosis (lung) (occupational) J60
lingua K14.3
Anthrax A22.9
with pneumonia A22.1
cerebral A22.8
colitis A22.2
cutaneous A22.0
gastrointestinal A22.2
inhalation A22.1
intestinal A22.2
meningitis A22.8
pulmonary A22.1
respiratory A22.1
sepsis A22.7
specified manifestation NEC A22.8
Anthropoid pelvis Q74.2
with disproportion (fetopelvic) O33.0
Anthropophobia F40.10
generalized F40.11
Antibodies, maternal (blood group) — see Isoimmunization, affecting management of pregnancy
anti-D — see Isoimmunization, affecting management
of pregnancy, Rh
newborn P55.0
Antibody
anticardiolipin R76.0
with
hemorrhagic disorder D68.312
hypercoagulable state D68.61
antiphosphatidylglycerol R76.0
with
hemorrhagic disorder D68.312
hypercoagulable state D68.61
antiphosphatidylinositol R76.0
with
hemorrhagic disorder D68.312
hypercoagulable state D68.61
antiphosphatidylserine R76.0
with
hemorrhagic disorder D68.312
hypercoagulable state D68.61
antiphospholipid R76.0
with
hemorrhagic disorder D68.312
hypercoagulable state D68.61
Anticardiolipin syndrome D68.61
Anticoagulant, circulating (intrinsic) (see also Disorder,
hemorrhagic) D68.318
drug-induced (extrinsic) (see also Disorder, hemorrhagic) D68.32
iatrogenic D68.32
Antidiuretic hormone syndrome E22.2
Antimonial cholera — see Poisoning, antimony
Antiphospholipid
antibody
with hemorrhagic disorder D68.312
syndrome D68.61
Antisocial personality F60.2
Antithrombinemia — see Circulating anticoagulants
Antithromboplastinemia D68.318
Antithromboplastinogenemia D68.318
Antitoxin complication or reaction — see Complications, vaccination
Antlophobia F40.228
Antritis J32.0
maxilla J32.0
acute J01.00
recurrent J01.01
stomach K29.60
with bleeding K29.61
Antrum, antral — see condition
Anuria R34
calculus (impacted) (recurrent) (see also Calculus,
urinary) N20.9
following
abortion — see Abortion by type complicated by,
renal failure
ectopic or molar pregnancy O08.4
newborn P96.0
postprocedural N99.0
postrenal N13.8
traumatic (following crushing) T79.5 ☑
Anus, anal — see condition
Anusitis K62.89
Anxiety F41.9
depression F41.8
episodic paroxysmal F41.0
generalized F41.1

☑ Additional Character Required — Refer to the Tabular List for Character Selection   Subterms under main terms may continue to next column or page

Anxiety — *continued*
  hysteria F41.8
  neurosis F41.1
  panic type F41.0
  reaction F41.1
  separation, abnormal (of childhood) F93.0
  specified NEC F41.8
  state F41.1
Aorta, aortic — *see* condition
Aortectasia — *see* Ectasia, aorta
  with aneurysm — *see* Aneurysm, aorta
Aortitis (nonsyphilitic) (calcific) I77.6
  arteriosclerotic I70.0
  Doehle-Heller A52.02
  luetic A52.02
  rheumatic — *see* Endocarditis, acute, rheumatic
  specific (syphilitic) A52.02
  syphilitic A52.02
    congenital A50.54 [I79.1]
Apathetic thyroid storm — *see* Thyrotoxicosis
Apathy R45.3
Apeirophobia F40.228
Apepsia K30
  psychogenic F45.8
Aperistalsis, esophagus K22.0
Apertognathia M26.29
Apert's syndrome Q87.0
Aphagia R13.0
  psychogenic F50.9
Aphakia (acquired) (postoperative) H27.0- ☑
  congenital Q12.3
Aphasia (amnestic) (global) (nominal) (semantic) (syntactic) R47.01
  acquired, with epilepsy (Landau-Kleffner syndrome) — *see* Epilepsy, specified NEC
  auditory (developmental) F80.2
  developmental (receptive type) F80.2
    expressive type F80.1
    Wernicke's F80.2
  following
    cerebrovascular disease I69.920
      cerebral infarction I69.320
      intracerebral hemorrhage I69.120
      nontraumatic intracranial hemorrhage NEC I69.220
      specified disease NEC I69.820
      subarachnoid hemorrhage I69.020
  primary progressive G31.01 [F02.80]
    with behavioral disturbance G31.01 [F02.81]
  progressive isolated G31.01 [F02.80]
    with behavioral disturbance G31.01 [F02.81]
  sensory F80.2
  syphilis, tertiary A52.19
  Wernicke's (developmental) F80.2
Aphonia (organic) R49.1
  hysterical F44.4
  psychogenic F44.4
Aphthae, aphthous (*see also* condition)
  Bednar's K12.0
  cachectic K14.0
  epizootic B08.8
  fever B08.8
  oral (recurrent) K12.0
  stomatitis (major) (minor) K12.0
  thrush B37.0
  ulcer (oral) (recurrent) K12.0
    genital organ(s) NEC
      female N76.6
      male N50.89
    larynx J38.7
Apical — *see* condition
Apiphobia F40.218
Aplasia (*see also* Agenesis)
  abdominal muscle syndrome Q79.4
  alveolar process (acquired) — *see* Anomaly, alveolar
    congenital Q38.6
  aorta (congenital) Q25.41
  axialis extracorticalis (congenita) E75.29
  bone marrow (myeloid) D61.9
    congenital D61.01
  brain Q00.0
    part of Q04.3
  bronchus Q32.4
  cementum K00.4
  cerebellum Q04.3
  cervix (congenital) Q51.5
  congenital pure red cell D61.01
  corpus callosum Q04.0

Aplasia — *continued*
  cutis congenita Q84.8
  erythrocyte congenital D61.01
  extracortical axial E75.29
  eye Q11.1
  fovea centralis (congenital) Q14.1
  gallbladder, congenital Q44.0
  iris Q13.1
  labyrinth, membranous Q16.5
  limb (congenital) Q73.8
    lower — *see* Defect, reduction, lower limb
    upper — *see* Agenesis, arm
  lung, congenital (bilateral) (unilateral) Q33.3
  pancreas Q45.0
  parathyroid-thymic D82.1
  Pelizaeus-Merzbacher E75.29
  penis Q55.5
  prostate Q55.4
  red cell (with thymoma) D60.9
    acquired D60.9
      due to drugs D60.9
    adult D60.9
    chronic D60.0
    congenital D61.01
    constitutional D61.01
    due to drugs D60.9
    hereditary D61.01
    of infants D61.01
    primary D61.01
    pure D61.01
      due to drugs D60.9
    specified type NEC D60.8
    transient D60.1
  round ligament Q52.8
  skin Q84.8
  spermatic cord Q55.4
  spleen Q89.01
  testicle Q55.0
  thymic, with immunodeficiency D82.1
  thyroid (congenital) (with myxedema) E03.1
  uterus Q51.0
  ventral horn cell Q06.1
Apnea, apneic (of) (spells) R06.81
  newborn NEC P28.4
    obstructive P28.4
    sleep (central) (obstructive) (primary) P28.3
  prematurity P28.4
  sleep G47.30
    central (primary) G47.31
      idiopathic G47.31
      in conditions classified elsewhere G47.37
    obstructive (adult) (pediatric) G47.33
      hypopnea G47.33
    primary central G47.31
    specified NEC G47.39
Apneumatosis, newborn P28.0
Apocrine metaplasia (breast) — *see* Dysplasia, mammary, specified type NEC
Apophysitis (bone) (*see also* Osteochondropathy)
  calcaneus M92.8
  juvenile M92.9
Apoplectiform convulsions (cerebral ischemia) I67.82
Apoplexia, apoplexy, apoplectic
  adrenal A39.1
  heart (auricle) (ventricle) — *see* Infarct, myocardium
  heat T67.0 ☑
  hemorrhagic (stroke) — *see* Hemorrhage, intracranial
  meninges, hemorrhagic — *see* Hemorrhage, intracranial, subarachnoid
  uremic N18.9 [I68.8]
Appearance
  bizarre R46.1
  specified NEC R46.89
  very low level of personal hygiene R46.0
Appendage
  epididymal (organ of Morgagni) Q55.4
  intestine (epiploic) Q43.8
  preauricular Q17.0
  testicular (organ of Morgagni) Q55.29
Appendicitis (pneumococcal) (retrocecal) K37
  with
    perforation or rupture K35.2
    peritoneal abscess K35.3
    peritonitis NEC K35.3
      generalized (with perforation or rupture) K35.2
      localized (with perforation or rupture) K35.3
  acute (catarrhal) (fulminating) (gangrenous) (obstructive) (retrocecal) (suppurative) K35.80

Appendicitis — *continued*
  acute — *continued*
    with
      peritoneal abscess K35.3
      peritonitis NEC K35.3
        generalized (with perforation or rupture) K35.2
        localized (with perforation or rupture) K35.3
    specified NEC K35.89
  amebic A06.89
  chronic (recurrent) K36
  exacerbation — *see* Appendicitis, acute
  gangrenous — *see* Appendicitis, acute
  healed (obliterative) K36
  interval K36
  neurogenic K36
  obstructive K36
  recurrent K36
  relapsing K36
  subacute (adhesive) K36
  subsiding K36
  suppurative — *see* Appendicitis, acute
  tuberculous A18.32
Appendicopathia oxyurica B80
Appendix, appendicular (*see also* condition)
  epididymis Q55.4
  Morgagni
    female Q50.5
    male (epididymal) Q55.4
      testicular Q55.29
  testis Q55.29
Appetite
  depraved — *see* Pica
  excessive R63.2
  lack or loss (*see also* Anorexia) R63.0
    nonorganic origin F50.89
    psychogenic F50.89
  perverted (hysterical) — *see* Pica
Apple peel syndrome Q41.1
Apprehension state F41.1
Apprehensiveness, abnormal F41.9
Approximal wear K03.0
Apraxia (classic) (ideational) (ideokinetic) (ideomotor) (motor) (verbal) R48.2
  following
    cerebrovascular disease I69.990
      cerebral infarction I69.390
      intracerebral hemorrhage I69.190
      nontraumatic intracranial hemorrhage NEC I69.290
      specified disease NEC I69.890
      subarachnoid hemorrhage I69.090
  oculomotor, congenital H51.8
Aptyalism K11.7
Apudoma — *see* Neoplasm, uncertain behavior, by site
Aqueous misdirection H40.83- ☑
Arabicum elephantiasis — *see* Infestation, filarial
Arachnitis — *see* Meningitis
Arachnodactyly — *see* Syndrome, Marfan's
Arachnoiditis (acute) (adhesive) (basal) (brain) (cerebrospinal) — *see* Meningitis
Arachnophobia F40.210
Arboencephalitis, Australian A83.4
Arborization block (heart) I45.5
ARC (AIDS-related complex) B20
Arch
  aortic Q25.49
  bovine Q25.49
Arches — *see* condition
Arcuate uterus Q51.810
Arcuatus uterus Q51.810
Arcus (cornea) senilis — *see* Degeneration, cornea, senile
Arc-welder's lung J63.4
Areflexia R29.2
Areola — *see* condition
Argentaffinoma (*see also* Neoplasm, uncertain behavior, by site)
  malignant — *see* Neoplasm, malignant, by site
  syndrome E34.0
Argininemia E72.21
Arginosuccinic aciduria E72.22
Argyll Robertson phenomenon, pupil or syndrome (syphilitic) A52.19
  atypical H57.09
  nonsyphilitic H57.09
Argyria, argyriasis
  conjunctival H11.13- ☑

Argyria, argyriasis — *continued*
  from drug or medicament — *see* Table of Drugs and Chemicals, by substance
Argyrosis, conjunctival H11.13- ☑
Arhinencephaly Q04.1
Ariboflavinosis E53.0
Arm — *see* condition
Arnold-Chiari disease, obstruction or syndrome (type II) Q07.00
  with
    hydrocephalus Q07.02
      with spina bifida Q07.03
    spina bifida Q07.01
      with hydrocephalus Q07.03
    type III — *see* Encephalocele
    type IV Q04.8
Aromatic amino-acid metabolism disorder E70.9
  specified NEC E70.8
Arousals, confusional G47.51
Arrest, arrested
  cardiac I46.9
    complicating
      abortion — *see* Abortion, by type, complicated by, cardiac arrest
      anesthesia (general) (local) or other sedation — *see* Table of Drugs and Chemicals, by drug
        in labor and delivery O74.2
        in pregnancy O29.11-
        postpartum, puerperal O89.1
      delivery (cesarean) (instrumental) O75.4
    due to
      cardiac condition I46.2
      specified condition NEC I46.8
    intraoperative I97.71- ☑
    newborn P29.81
    personal history, successfully resuscitated Z86.74
    postprocedural I97.12- ☑
      obstetric procedure O75.4
  cardiorespiratory — *see* Arrest, cardiac
  circulatory — *see* Arrest, cardiac
  deep transverse O64.0 ☑
  development or growth
    bone — *see* Disorder, bone, development or growth
    child R62.50
    tracheal rings Q32.1
  epiphyseal
    complete
      femur M89.15- ☑
      humerus M89.12- ☑
      tibia M89.16- ☑
      ulna M89.13- ☑
      forearm M89.13- ☑
        specified NEC M89.13- ☑
        ulna — *see* Arrest, epiphyseal, by type, ulna
      lower leg M89.16- ☑
        specified NEC M89.168
        tibia — *see* Arrest, epiphyseal, by type, tibia
    partial
      femur M89.15- ☑
      humerus M89.12- ☑
      tibia M89.16- ☑
      ulna M89.13- ☑
      specified NEC M89.18
  granulopoiesis — *see* Agranulocytosis
  growth plate — *see* Arrest, epiphyseal
  heart — *see* Arrest, cardiac
  legal, anxiety concerning Z65.3
  physeal — *see* Arrest, epiphyseal
  respiratory R09.2
    newborn P28.81
  sinus I45.5
  spermatogenesis (complete) — *see* Azoospermia
    incomplete — *see* Oligospermia
  transverse (deep) O64.0 ☑
Arrhenoblastoma
  benign
    specified site — *see* Neoplasm, benign, by site
    unspecified site
      female D27.9
      male D29.20
  malignant
    specified site — *see* Neoplasm, malignant, by site
    unspecified site
      female C56.9
      male C62.90

Arrhenoblastoma — *continued*
    specified site — *see* Neoplasm, uncertain behavior, by site
  unspecified site
    female D39.10
    male D40.10
Arrhythmia (auricle) (cardiac) (juvenile) (nodal) (reflex) (sinus) (supraventricular) (transitory) (ventricle) I49.9
  block I45.9
  extrasystolic I49.49
  newborn
    bradycardia P29.12
    occurring before birth P03.819
      before onset of labor P03.810
      during labor P03.811
    tachycardia P29.11
  psychogenic F45.8
  specified NEC I49.8
  vagal R55
  ventricular re-entry I47.0
Arrillaga-Ayerza syndrome (pulmonary sclerosis with pulmonary hypertension) I27.0
Arsenical pigmentation L81.8
  from drug or medicament — *see* Table of Drugs and Chemicals
Arsenism — *see* Poisoning, arsenic
Arterial — *see* condition
Arteriofibrosis — *see* Arteriosclerosis
Arteriolar sclerosis — *see* Arteriosclerosis
Arteriolith — *see* Arteriosclerosis
Arteriolitis I77.6
  necrotizing, kidney I77.5
  renal — *see* Hypertension, kidney
Arteriolosclerosis — *see* Arteriosclerosis
Arterionephrosclerosis — *see* Hypertension, kidney
Arteriopathy I77.9
Arteriosclerosis, arteriosclerotic (diffuse) (obliterans) (of) (senile) (with calcification) I70.90
  aorta I70.0
  arteries of extremities — *see* Arteriosclerosis, extremities
  brain I67.2
  bypass graft
    coronary — *see* Arteriosclerosis, coronary, bypass graft
    extremities — *see* Arteriosclerosis, extremities, bypass graft
  cardiac — *see* Disease, heart, ischemic, atherosclerotic
  cardiopathy — *see* Disease, heart, ischemic, atherosclerotic
  cardiorenal — *see* Hypertension, cardiorenal
  cardiovascular — *see* Disease, heart, ischemic, atherosclerotic
  carotid (*see also* Occlusion, artery, carotid) I65.2- ☑
  central nervous system I67.2
  cerebral I67.2
  cerebrovascular I67.2
  coronary (artery) I25.10
    bypass graft I25.810
      with
        angina pectoris I25.709
          with documented spasm I25.701
          specified type NEC I25.708
          unstable I25.700
        ischemic chest pain I25.709
      autologous artery I25.810
        with
          angina pectoris I25.729
            with documented spasm I25.721
            specified type I25.728
            unstable I25.720
          ischemic chest pain I25.729
      autologous vein I25.810
        with
          angina pectoris I25.719
            with documented spasm I25.711
            specified type I25.718
            unstable I25.710
          ischemic chest pain I25.719
      nonautologous biological I25.810
        with
          angina pectoris I25.739
            with documented spasm I25.731
            specified type I25.738
            unstable I25.730
          ischemic chest pain I25.739
      specified type NEC I25.810

Arteriosclerosis, arteriosclerotic — *continued*
  coronary — *continued*
    bypass graft — *continued*
      specified type — *continued*
        with
          angina pectoris I25.799
            with documented spasm I25.791
            specified type I25.798
            unstable I25.790
          ischemic chest pain I25.799
      due to
        calcified coronary lesion (severely) I25.84
        lipid rich plaque I25.83
      native vessel
        with
          angina pectoris I25.119
            with documented spasm I25.111
            specified type NEC I25.118
            unstable I25.110
          ischemic chest pain I25.119
    transplanted heart I25.811
      bypass graft I25.812
        with
          angina pectoris I25.769
            with documented spasm I25.761
            specified type I25.768
            unstable I25.760
          ischemic chest pain I25.769
      native coronary artery I25.811
        with
          angina pectoris I25.759
            with documented spasm I25.751
            specified type I25.758
            unstable I25.750
          ischemic chest pain I25.759
  extremities (native arteries) I70.209
    bypass graft I70.309
      autologous vein graft I70.409
        leg I70.409
          with
            gangrene (and intermittent claudication, rest pain and ulcer) I70.469
            intermittent claudication I70.419
            rest pain (and intermittent claudication) I70.429
          bilateral I70.403
            with
              gangrene (and intermittent claudication, rest pain and ulcer) I70.463
              intermittent claudication I70.463
              rest pain (and intermittent claudication) I70.423
              specified type NEC I70.493
          left I70.402
            with
              gangrene (and intermittent claudication, rest pain and ulcer) I70.462
              intermittent claudication I70.412
              rest pain (and intermittent claudication) I70.422
              ulceration (and intermittent claudication and rest pain) I70.449
                ankle I70.443
                calf I70.442
                foot site NEC I70.445
                heel I70.444
                lower leg NEC I70.448
                midfoot I70.444
                thigh I70.441
              specified type NEC I70.492
          right I70.401
            with
              gangrene (and intermittent claudication, rest pain and ulcer) I70.461
              intermittent claudication I70.411
              rest pain (and intermittent claudication) I70.421
              ulceration (and intermittent claudication and rest pain) I70.439
                ankle I70.433
                calf I70.432
                foot site NEC I70.435
                heel I70.434

☑ Additional Character Required — Refer to the Tabular List for Character Selection   Subterms under main terms may continue to next column or page

Arteriosclerosis, arteriosclerotic — *continued*
  extremities — *continued*
    bypass graft — *continued*
      autologous vein graft — *continued*
        leg — *continued*
          right — *continued*
            with — *continued*
              ulceration — *continued*
                lower leg NEC I70.438
                midfoot I70.434
                thigh I70.431
              specified type NEC I70.491
          specified type NEC I70.499
        specified NEC I70.408
          with
            gangrene (and intermittent claudication, rest pain and ulcer) I70.468
            intermittent claudication I70.418
            rest pain (and intermittent claudication) I70.428
            ulceration (and intermittent claudication and rest pain) I70.45
          specified type NEC I70.498
      leg I70.309
        with
          gangrene (and intermittent claudication, rest pain and ulcer) I70.369
          intermittent claudication I70.319
          rest pain (and intermittent claudication) I70.329
        bilateral I70.303
          with
            gangrene (and intermittent claudication, rest pain and ulcer) I70.363
            intermittent claudication I70.313
            rest pain (and intermittent claudication) I70.323
          specified type NEC I70.393
        left I70.302
          with
            gangrene (and intermittent claudication, rest pain and ulcer) I70.362
            intermittent claudication I70.312
            rest pain (and intermittent claudication) I70.322
            ulceration (and intermittent claudication and rest pain) I70.349
              ankle I70.343
              calf I70.342
              foot site NEC I70.345
              heel I70.344
              lower leg NEC I70.348
              midfoot I70.344
              thigh I70.341
          specified type NEC I70.392
        right I70.301
          with
            gangrene (and intermittent claudication, rest pain and ulcer) I70.361
            intermittent claudication I70.311
            rest pain (and intermittent claudication) I70.321
            ulceration (and intermittent claudication and rest pain) I70.339
              ankle I70.333
              calf I70.332
              foot site NEC I70.335
              heel I70.334
              lower leg NEC I70.338
              midfoot I70.334
              thigh I70.331
          specified type NEC I70.391
        specified type NEC I70.399
      nonautologous biological graft I70.509
        leg I70.509
          with
            gangrene (and intermittent claudication, rest pain and ulcer) I70.569
            intermittent claudication I70.519
            rest pain (and intermittent claudication) I70.529
          bilateral I70.503

Arteriosclerosis, arteriosclerotic — *continued*
  extremities — *continued*
    bypass graft — *continued*
      nonautologous biological graft — *continued*
        leg — *continued*
          bilateral — *continued*
            with
              gangrene (and intermittent claudication, rest pain and ulcer) I70.563
              intermittent claudication I70.513
              rest pain (and intermittent claudication) I70.523
            specified type NEC I70.593
          left I70.502
            with
              gangrene (and intermittent claudication, rest pain and ulcer) I70.562
              intermittent claudication I70.512
              rest pain (and intermittent claudication) I70.522
              ulceration (and intermittent claudication and rest pain) I70.549
                ankle I70.543
                calf I70.542
                foot site NEC I70.545
                heel I70.544
                lower leg NEC I70.548
                midfoot I70.544
                thigh I70.541
            specified type NEC I70.592
          right I70.501
            with
              gangrene (and intermittent claudication, rest pain and ulcer) I70.561
              intermittent claudication I70.511
              rest pain (and intermittent claudication) I70.521
              ulceration (and intermittent claudication and rest pain) I70.539
                ankle I70.533
                calf I70.532
                foot site NEC I70.535
                heel I70.534
                lower leg NEC I70.538
                midfoot I70.534
                thigh I70.531
            specified type NEC I70.591
          specified type NEC I70.599
        specified NEC I70.508
          with
            gangrene (and intermittent claudication, rest pain and ulcer) I70.568
            intermittent claudication I70.518
            rest pain (and intermittent claudication) I70.528
            ulceration (and intermittent claudication and rest pain) I70.55
          specified type NEC I70.598
      nonbiological graft I70.609
        leg I70.609
          with
            gangrene (and intermittent claudication, rest pain and ulcer) I70.669
            intermittent claudication I70.619
            rest pain (and intermittent claudication) I70.629
          bilateral I70.603
            with
              gangrene (and intermittent claudication, rest pain and ulcer) I70.663
              intermittent claudication I70.613
              rest pain (and intermittent claudication) I70.623
            specified type NEC I70.693
          left I70.602
            with
              gangrene (and intermittent claudication, rest pain and ulcer) I70.662
              intermittent claudication I70.612

Arteriosclerosis, arteriosclerotic — *continued*
  extremities — *continued*
    bypass graft — *continued*
      nonbiological graft — *continued*
        leg — *continued*
          left — *continued*
            with — *continued*
              rest pain (and intermittent claudication) I70.622
              ulceration (and intermittent claudication and rest pain) I70.649
                ankle I70.643
                calf I70.642
                foot site NEC I70.645
                heel I70.644
                lower leg NEC I70.648
                midfoot I70.644
                thigh I70.641
            specified type NEC I70.692
          right I70.601
            with
              gangrene (and intermittent claudication, rest pain and ulcer) I70.661
              intermittent claudication I70.611
              rest pain (and intermittent claudication) I70.621
              ulceration (and intermittent claudication and rest pain) I70.639
                ankle I70.633
                calf I70.632
                foot site NEC I70.635
                heel I70.634
                lower leg NEC I70.638
                midfoot I70.634
                thigh I70.631
            specified type NEC I70.691
          specified NEC I70.608
            with
              gangrene (and intermittent claudication, rest pain and ulcer) I70.668
              intermittent claudication I70.618
              rest pain (and intermittent claudication) I70.628
              ulceration (and intermittent claudication and rest pain) I70.65
            specified type NEC I70.698
      specified graft NEC I70.709
        leg I70.709
          with
            gangrene (and intermittent claudication, rest pain and ulcer) I70.769
            intermittent claudication I70.719
            rest pain (and intermittent claudication) I70.729
          bilateral I70.703
            with
              gangrene (and intermittent claudication, rest pain and ulcer) I70.763
              intermittent claudication I70.713
              rest pain (and intermittent claudication) I70.723
            specified type NEC I70.793
          left I70.702
            with
              gangrene (and intermittent claudication, rest pain and ulcer) I70.762
              intermittent claudication I70.712
              rest pain (and intermittent claudication) I70.722
              ulceration (and intermittent claudication and rest pain) I70.749
                ankle I70.743
                calf I70.742
                foot site NEC I70.745
                heel I70.744
                lower leg NEC I70.748
                midfoot I70.744
                thigh I70.741
            specified type NEC I70.792
          right I70.701

☑ Additional Character Required — Refer to the Tabular List for Character Selection

Index

Arteriosclerosis, arteriosclerotic — Arthritis, arthritic

Arteriosclerosis, arteriosclerotic — *continued*
  extremities — *continued*
    bypass graft — *continued*
      specified graft — *continued*
        leg — *continued*
          right — *continued*
            with
              gangrene (and intermittent claudication, rest pain and ulcer) I70.761
              intermittent claudication I70.711
              rest pain (and Intermittent claudication) I70.721
              ulceration (and intermittent claudication and rest pain) I70.739
                ankle I70.733
                calf I70.732
                foot site NEC I70.735
                heel I70.734
                lower leg NEC I70.738
                midfoot I70.734
                thigh I70.731
            specified type NEC I70.791
        specified type NEC I70.799
    specified NEC I70.708
      with
        gangrene (and intermittent claudication, rest pain and ulcer) I70.768
        intermittent claudication I70.718
        rest pain (and intermittent claudication) I70.728
        ulceration (and intermittent claudication and rest pain) I70.75
      specified type NEC I70.798
  specified NEC I70.308
    with
      gangrene (and intermittent claudication, rest pain and ulcer) I70.368
      intermittent claudication I70.318
      rest pain (and intermittent claudication) I70.328
      ulceration (and intermittent claudication and rest pain) I70.35
    specifiec type NEC I70.398
  leg I70.209
    with
      gangrene (and intermittent claudication, rest pain and ulcer) I70.269
      intermittent claudication I70.219
      rest pain (and intermittent claudication) I70.229
    bilateral I70.203
      with
        gangrene (and intermittent claudication, rest pain and ulcer) I70.263
        intermittent claudication I70.213
        rest pain (and intermittent claudication) I70.223
      specified type NEC I70.293
    left I70.202
      with
        gangrene (and intermittent claudication, rest pain and ulcer) I70.262
        intermittent claudication I70.212
        rest pain (and intermittent claudication) I70.222
        ulceration (and intermittent claudication and rest pain) I70.249
          ankle I70.243
          calf I70.242
          foot site NEC I70.245
          heel I70.244
          lower leg NEC I70.248
          midfoot I70.244
          thigh I70.241
      specified type NEC I70.292
    right I70.201
      with
        gangrene (and intermittent claudication, rest pain and ulcer) I70.261
        intermittent claudication I70.211
        rest pain (and intermittent claudication) I70.221
        ulceration (and intermittent claudication and rest pain) I70.239
          ankle I70.233
          calf I70.232

Arteriosclerosis, arteriosclerotic — *continued*
  extremities — *continued*
    leg — *continued*
      right — *continued*
        with — *continued*
          ulceration — *continued*
            foot site NEC I70.235
            heel I70.234
            lower leg NEC I70.238
            midfoot I70.234
            thigh I70.231
          specified type NEC I70.291
        specified type NEC I70.299
    specified site NEC I70.208
      with
        gangrene (and intermittent claudication, rest pain and ulcer) I70.268
        intermittent claudication I70.218
        rest pain (and intermittent claudication) I70.228
        ulceration (and intermittent claudication and rest pain) I70.25
      specified type NEC I70.298
  generalized I70.91
  heart (disease) — *see* Arteriosclerosis, coronary (artery),
  kidney — *see* Hypertension, kidney
  medial — *see* Arteriosclerosis, extremities
  mesenteric (artery) K55.1
  Mönckeberg's — *see* Arteriosclerosis, extremities
  myocarditis I51.4
  peripheral (of extremities) — *see* Arteriosclerosis, extremities
  pulmonary (idiopathic) I27.0
  renal (arterioles) (*see also* Hypertension, kidney)
    artery I70.1
  retina (vascular) I70.8 [H35.0-] ☑
  specified artery NEC I70.8
  spinal (cord) G95.19
  vertebral (artery) I67.2
Arteriospasm I73.9
Arteriovenous — *see* condition
Arteritis I77.6
  allergic M31.0
  aorta (nonsyphilitic) I77.6
    syphilitic A52.02
  aortic arch M31.4
  brachiocephalic M31.4
  brain I67.7
    syphilitic A52.04
  cerebral I67.7
    in systemic lupus erythematosus M32.19
    listerial A32.89
    syphilitic A52.04
    tuberculous A18.89
  coronary (artery) I25.89
    rheumatic I01.8
      chronic I09.89
    syphilitic A52.06
  cranial (left) (right), giant cell M31.6
  deformans — *see* Arteriosclerosis
  giant cell NEC M31.6
    with polymyalgia rheumatica M31.5
  necrosing or necrotizing M31.9
    specified NEC M31.8
  nodosa M30.0
  obliterans — *see* Arteriosclerosis
  pulmonary I28.8
  rheumatic — *see* Fever, rheumatic
  senile — *see* Arteriosclerosis
  suppurative I77.2
  syphilitic (general) A52.09
    brain A52.04
    coronary A52.06
    spinal A52.09
  temporal, giant cell M31.6
  young female aortic arch syndrome M31.4
Artery, arterial (*see also* condition)
  abscess I77.89
  single umbilical Q27.0
Arthralgia (allergic) (*see also* Pain, joint)
  in caisson disease T70.3 ☑
  temporomandibular M26.62- ☑
Arthritis, arthritic (acute) (chronic) (nonpyogenic) (subacute) M19.90
  allergic — *see* Arthritis, specified form NEC
  ankylosing (crippling) (spine) (*see also* Spondylitis, ankylosing)

Arthritis, arthritic — *continued*
  ankylosing (*see also* Spondylitis, ankylosing) — *continued*
    sites other than spine — *see* Arthritis, specified form NEC
  atrophic — *see* Osteoarthritis
    spine — *see* Spondylitis, ankylosing
  back — *see* Spondylopathy, inflammatory
  blennorrhagic (gonococcal) A54.42
  Charcot's — *see* Arthropathy, neuropathic
    diabetic — *see* Diabetes, arthropathy, neuropathic
    syringomyelic G95.0
  chylous (filarial) (*see also* category M01) B74.9
  climacteric (any site) NEC — *see* Arthritis, specified form NEC
  crystal (-induced) — *see* Arthritis, in, crystals
  deformans — *see* Osteoarthritis
  degenerative — *see* Osteoarthritis
  due to or associated with
    acromegaly E22.0
    brucellosis — *see* Brucellosis
    caisson disease T70.3 ☑
    diabetes — *see* Diabetes, arthropathy
    dracontiasis (*see also* category M01) B72
    enteritis NEC
      regional — *see* Enteritis, regional
    erysipelas (*see also* category M01) A46
    erythema
      epidemic A25.1
      nodosum L52
    filariasis NOS B74.9
    glanders A24.0
    helminthiasis (*see also* category M01) B83.9
    hemophilia D66 [M36.2]
    Henoch- (Schönlein) purpura D69.0 [M36.4]
    human parvovirus (*see also* category M01) B97.6
    infectious disease NEC M01 ☑
    leprosy (*see also* category M01) (*see also* Leprosy) A30.9
    Lyme disease A69.23
    mycobacteria (*see also* category M01) A31.8
    parasitic disease NEC (*see also* category M01) B89
    paratyphoid fever (see also category M01) (*see also* Fever, paratyphoid) A01.4
    rat bite fever (*see also* category M01) A25.1
    regional enteritis — *see* Enteritis, regional
    respiratory disorder NOS J98.9
    serum sickness (*see also* Reaction, serum) T80.69 ☑
    syringomyelia G95.0
    typhoid fever A01.04
  epidemic erythema A25.1
  febrile — *see* Fever, rheumatic
  gonococcal A54.42
  gouty (acute) — *see* Gout
  in (due to)
    acromegaly (*see also* subcategory M14.8-) E22.0
    amyloidosis (*see also* subcategory M14.8-) E85.4
    bacterial disease (*see also* subcategory M01) A49.9
    Behçet's syndrome M35.2
    caisson disease (*see also* subcategory M14.8-) T70.3 ☑
    coliform bacilli (Escherichia coli) — *see* Arthritis, in, pyogenic organism NEC
    crystals M11.9
      dicalcium phosphate — *see* Arthritis, in, crystals, specified type NEC
      hydroxyapatite M11.0- ☑
      pyrophosphate — *see* Arthritis, in, crystals, specified type NEC
      specified type NEC M11.80
        ankle M11.87- ☑
        elbow M11.82- ☑
        foot joint M11.87- ☑
        hand joint M11.84- ☑
        hip M11.85- ☑
        knee M11.86- ☑
        multiple sites M11.8- ☑
        shoulder M11.81- ☑
        vertebrae M11.88
        wrist M11.83- ☑
    dermatoarthritis, lipoid E78.81
    dracontiasis (dracunculiasis) (*see also* category M01) B72
    endocrine disorder NEC (*see also* subcategory M14.8-) E34.9
    enteritis, infectious NEC (*see also* category M01) A09

Arthritis, arthritic — *continued*
  in — *continued*
    enteritis, infectious (*see also* category M01) —
      continued
      specified organism NEC (*see also* category M01)
        A08.8
    erythema
      multiforme (*see also* subcategory M14.8-) L51.9
      nodosum (*see also* subcategory M14.8-) L52
    gout — *see* Gout
    helminthiasis NEC (*see also* category M01) B83.9
    hemochromatosis (*see also* subcategory M14.8-)
      E83.118
    hemoglobinopathy NEC D58.2 [M36.3]
    hemophilia NEC D66 [M36.2]
    Hemophilus influenzae M00.8- ☑ [B96.3]
    Henoch (-Schönlein) purpura D69.0 [M36.4]
    hyperparathyroidism NEC (*see also* subcategory
      M14.8-) E21.3
    hypersensitivity reaction NEC T78.49 ☑ [M36.4]
    hypogammaglobulinemia (*see also* subcategory
      M14.8-) D80.1
    hypothyroidism NEC (*see also* subcategory M14.8-)
      E03.9
    infection — *see* Arthritis, pyogenic or pyemic
      spine — *see* Spondylopathy, infective
    infectious disease NEC M01 ☑
    leprosy (*see also* category M01) A30.9
    leukemia NEC C95.9- ☑ [M36.1]
    lipoid dermatoarthritis E78.81
    Lyme disease A69.23
    Mediterranean fever, familial (*see also* subcategory
      M14.8-) M04.1
    Meningococcus A39.83
    metabolic disorder NEC (*see also* subcategory
      M14.8-) E88.9
    multiple myelomatosis C90.0- ☑ [M36.1]
    mumps B26.85
    mycosis NEC (*see also* category M01) B49
    myelomatosis (multiple) C90.0- ☑ [M36.1]
    neurological disorder NEC G98.0
    ochronosis (*see also* subcategory M14.8-) E70.29
    O'nyong-nyong (*see also* category M01) A92.1
    parasitic disease NEC (*see also* category M01) B89
    paratyphoid fever (*see also* category M01) A01.4
    Pseudomonas — *see* Arthritis, pyogenic, bacterial
      NEC
    psoriasis L40.50
    pyogenic organism NEC — *see* Arthritis, pyogenic,
      bacterial NEC
    Reiter's disease — *see* Reiter's disease
    respiratory disorder NEC (*see also* subcategory
      M14.8-) J98.9
    reticulosis, malignant (*see also* subcategory M14.8-
) C86.0
    rubella B06.82
    Salmonella (arizonae) (cholerae-suis) (enteritidis)
      (typhimurium) A02.23
    sarcoidosis D86.86
    specified bacteria NEC — *see* Arthritis, pyogenic,
      bacterial NEC
    sporotrichosis B42.82
    syringomyelia G95.0
    thalassemia NEC D56.9 [M36.3]
    tuberculosis — *see* Tuberculosis, arthritis
    typhoid fever A01.04
    urethritis, Reiter's — *see* Reiter's disease
    viral disease NEC (*see also* category M01) B34.9
  infectious or infective (*see also* Arthritis, pyogenic or
    pyemic)
    spine — *see* Spondylopathy, infective
  juvenile M08.90
    with systemic onset — *see* Still's disease
    ankle M08.97- ☑
    elbow M08.92- ☑
    foot joint M08.97- ☑
    hand joint M08.94- ☑
    hip M08.95- ☑
    knee M08.96- ☑
    multiple site M08.99
    pauciarticular M08.40
      ankle M08.47- ☑
      elbow M08.42- ☑
      foot joint M08.47- ☑
      hand joint M08.44- ☑
      hip M08.45- ☑
      knee M08.46- ☑

Arthritis, arthritic — *continued*
  juvenile — *continued*
    pauciarticular — *continued*
      shoulder M08.41- ☑
      vertebrae M08.48
      wrist M08.43- ☑
    psoriatic L40.54
    rheumatoid — *see* Arthritis, rheumatoid, juvenile
    shoulder M08.91- ☑
    specified type NEC M08.80
      ankle M08.87- ☑
      elbow M08.82- ☑
      foot joint M08.87- ☑
      hand joint M08.84- ☑
      hip M08.85- ☑
      knee M08.86- ☑
      multiple site M08.89
      shoulder M08.81- ☑
      specified joint NEC M08.88
      vertebrae M08.88
      wrist M08.83- ☑
    wrist M08.93- ☑
  meaning osteoarthritis — *see* Osteoarthritis
  meningococcal A39.83
  menopausal (any site) NEC — *see* Arthritis, specified
    form NEC
  mutilans (psoriatic) L40.52
  mycotic NEC (*see also* category M01) B49
  neuropathic (Charcot) — *see* Arthropathy, neuropathic
    diabetic — *see* Diabetes, arthropathy, neuropathic
    nonsyphilitic NEC G98.0
    syringomyelic G95.0
  ochronotic (*see also* subcategory M14.8-) E70.29
  palindromic (any site) — *see* Rheumatism, palindromic
  pneumococcal M00.10
    ankle M00.17- ☑
    elbow M00.12- ☑
    foot joint — *see* Arthritis, pneumococcal, ankle
    hand joint M00.14- ☑
    hip M00.15- ☑
    knee M00.16- ☑
    multiple site M00.19
    shoulder M00.11- ☑
    vertebra M00.18
    wrist M00.13- ☑
  postdysenteric — *see* Arthropathy, postdysenteric
  postmeningococcal A39.84
  postrheumatic, chronic — *see* Arthropathy,
    postrheumatic, chronic
  primary progressive (*see also* Arthritis, specified form
    NEC)
    spine — *see* Spondylitis, ankylosing
  psoriatic L40.50
  purulent (any site except spine) — *see* Arthritis, pyo-
    genic or pyemic
    spine — *see* Spondylopathy, infective
  pyogenic or pyemic (any site except spine) M00.9
    bacterial NEC M00.80
      ankle M00.87- ☑
      elbow M00.82- ☑
      foot joint — *see* Arthritis, pyogenic, bacterial
        NEC, ankle
      hand joint M00.84- ☑
      hip M00.85- ☑
      knee M00.86- ☑
      multiple site M00.89
      shoulder M00.81- ☑
      vertebra M00.88
      wrist M00.83- ☑
    pneumococcal — *see* Arthritis, pneumococcal
    spine — *see* Spondylopathy, infective
    staphylococcal — *see* Arthritis, staphylococcal
    streptococcal — *see* Arthritis, streptococcal NEC
      pneumococcal — *see* Arthritis, pneumococcal
  reactive — *see* Reiter's disease
  rheumatic (*see also* Arthritis, rheumatoid)
    acute or subacute — *see* Fever, rheumatic
  rheumatoid M06.9
    with
      carditis — *see* Rheumatoid, carditis
      endocarditis — *see* Rheumatoid, carditis
      heart involvement NEC — *see* Rheumatoid,
        carditis
      lung involvement — *see* Rheumatoid, lung
      myocarditis — *see* Rheumatoid, carditis
      myopathy — *see* Rheumatoid, myopathy
      pericarditis — *see* Rheumatoid, carditis

Arthritis, arthritic — *continued*
  rheumatoid — *continued*
    with — *continued*
      polyneuropathy — *see* Rheumatoid, polyneu-
        ropathy
      rheumatoid factor — *see* Arthritis, rheumatoid,
        seropositive
      splenoadenomegaly and leukopenia — *see*
        Felty's syndrome
      vasculitis — *see* Rheumatoid, vasculitis
      visceral involvement NEC — *see* Rheumatoid,
        arthritis, with involvement of organs NEC
    juvenile (with or without rheumatoid factor)
      M08.00
      ankle M08.07- ☑
      elbow M08.02- ☑
      foot joint M08.07- ☑
      hand joint M08.04- ☑
      hip M08.05- ☑
      knee M08.06- ☑
      multiple site M08.09
      shoulder M08.01- ☑
      vertebra M08.08
      wrist M08.03- ☑
    seronegative M06.00
      ankle M06.07- ☑
      elbow M06.02- ☑
      foot joint M06.07- ☑
      hand joint M06.04- ☑
      hip M06.05- ☑
      knee M06.06- ☑
      multiple site M06.09
      shoulder M06.01- ☑
      vertebra M06.08
      wrist M06.03- ☑
    seropositive M05.9
      without organ involvement M05.70
        ankle M05.77- ☑
        elbow M05.72- ☑
        foot joint M05.77- ☑
        hand joint M05.74- ☑
        hip M05.75- ☑
        knee M05.76- ☑
        multiple sites M05.79
        shoulder M05.71- ☑
        vertebra — *see* Spondylitis, ankylosing
        wrist M05.73- ☑
      specified NEC M05.80
        ankle M05.87- ☑
        elbow M05.82- ☑
        foot joint M05.87- ☑
        hand joint M05.84- ☑
        hip M05.85- ☑
        knee M05.86- ☑
        multiple sites M05.89
        shoulder M05.81- ☑
        vertebra — *see* Spondylitis, ankylosing
        wrist M05.83- ☑
    specified type NEC M06.80
      ankle M06.87- ☑
      elbow M06.82- ☑
      foot joint M06.87- ☑
      hand joint M06.84- ☑
      hip M06.85- ☑
      knee M06.86- ☑
      multiple site M06.89
      shoulder M06.81- ☑
      vertebra M06.88
      wrist M06.83- ☑
    spine — *see* Spondylitis, ankylosing
  rubella B06.82
  scorbutic (*see also* subcategory M14.8-) E54
  senile or senescent — *see* Osteoarthritis
  septic (any site except spine) — *see* Arthritis, pyogenic
    or pyemic
    spine — *see* Spondylopathy, infective
  serum (nontherapeutic) (therapeutic) — *see*
    Arthropathy, postimmunization
  specified form NEC M13.80
    ankle M13.87- ☑
    elbow M13.82- ☑
    foot joint M13.87- ☑
    hand joint M13.84- ☑
    hip M13.85- ☑
    knee M13.86- ☑
    multiple site M13.89

Index

Arthritis, arthritic — Artificial

Arthritis, arthritic — *continued*
 specified form — *continued*
  shoulder M13.81- ☑
  specified joint NEC M13.88
  wrist M13.83- ☑
 spine (*see also* Spondylopathy, inflammatory)
  infectious or infective NEC — *see* Spondylopathy,
   infective
  Marie-Strümpell — *see* Spondylitis, ankylosing
  pyogenic — *see* Spondylopathy, infective
  rheumatoid — *see* Spondylitis, ankylosing
  traumatic (old) — *see* Spondylopathy, traumatic
  tuberculous A18.01
 staphylococcal M00.00
  ankle M00.07- ☑
  elbow M00.02- ☑
  foot joint — *see* Arthritis, staphylococcal, ankle
  hand joint M00.04- ☑
  hip M00.05- ☑
  knee M00.06- ☑
  multiple site M00.09
  shoulder M00.01- ☑
  vertebra M00.08
  wrist M00.03- ☑
 streptococcal NEC M00.20
  ankle M00.27- ☑
  elbow M00.22- ☑
  foot joint — *see* Arthritis, streptococcal, ankle
  hand joint M00.24- ☑
  hip M00.25- ☑
  knee M00.26- ☑
  multiple site M00.29
  shoulder M00.21- ☑
  vertebra M00.28
  wrist M00.23- ☑
 suppurative — *see* Arthritis, pyogenic or pyemic
 syphilitic (late) A52.16
  congenital A50.55 [M12.80]
 syphilitica deformans (Charcot) A52.16
 temporomandibular M26.69
 toxic of menopause (any site) — *see* Arthritis, specified
   form NEC
 transient — *see* Arthropathy, specified form NEC
 traumatic (chronic) — *see* Arthropathy, traumatic
 tuberculous A18.02
  spine A18.01
 uratic — *see* Gout
 urethritica (Reiter's) — *see* Reiter's disease
 vertebral — *see* Spondylopathy, inflammatory
 villous (any site) — *see* Arthropathy, specified form
   NEC
Arthrocele — *see* Effusion, joint
Arthrodesis status Z98.1
Arthrodynia (*see also* Pain, joint)
Arthrodysplasia Q74.9
Arthrofibrosis, joint — *see* Ankylosis
Arthrogryposis (congenital) Q68.8
 multiplex congenita Q74.3
Arthrokatadysis M24.7
Arthropathy (*see also* Arthritis) M12.9
 Charcot's — *see* Arthropathy, neuropathic
  diabetic — *see* Diabetes, arthropathy, neuropathic
  syringomyelic G95.0
 cricoarytenoid J38.7
 crystal (-induced) — *see* Arthritis, in, crystals
 diabetic NEC — *see* Diabetes, arthropathy
 distal interphalangeal, psoriatic L40.51
 enteropathic M07.60
  ankle M07.67- ☑
  elbow M07.62- ☑
  foot joint M07.67- ☑
  hand joint M07.64- ☑
  hip M07.65- ☑
  knee M07.66- ☑
  multiple site M07.69
  shoulder M07.61- ☑
  vertebra M07.68
  wrist M07.63- ☑
 following intestinal bypass M02.00
  ankle M02.07- ☑
  elbow M02.02- ☑
  foot joint M02.07- ☑
  hand joint M02.04- ☑
  hip M02.05- ☑
  knee M02.06- ☑
  multiple site M02.09
  shoulder M02.01- ☑

Arthropathy — *continued*
 following intestinal bypass — *continued*
  vertebra M02.08
  wrist M02.03- ☑
 gouty (*see also* Gout)
  in (due to)
   Lesch-Nyhan syndrome E79.1 [M14.8-] ☑
   sickle-cell disorders D57- ☑ [M14.8-] ☑
 hemophilic NEC D66 [M36.2]
  in (due to)
   hyperparathyroidism NEC E21.3 [M14.8-] ☑
   metabolic disease NOS E88.9 [M14.8-] ☑
 in (due to)
  acromegaly E22.0 [M14.8-] ☑
  amyloidosis E85.4 [M14.8-] ☑
  blood disorder NOS D75.9 [M36.3]
  diabetes — *see* Diabetes, arthropathy
  endocrine disease NOS E34.9 [M14.8-] ☑
  erythema
   multiforme L51.9 [M14.8-] ☑
   nodosum L52 [M14.8-] ☑
  hemochromatosis E83.118 [M14.8-] ☑
  hemoglobinopathy NEC D58.2 [M36.3]
  hemophilia NEC D66 [M36.2]
  Henoch-Schönlein purpura D69.0 [M36.4]
  hyperthyroidism E05.90 [M14.8-] ☑
  hypothyroidism E03.9 [M14.8-] ☑
  infective endocarditis I33.0 [M12.80]
  leukemia NEC C95.9- ☑ [M36.1]
  malignant histiocytosis C96.A [M36.1]
  metabolic disease NOS E88.9 [M14.8-] ☑
  multiple myeloma C90.0- ☑ [M36.1]
  neoplastic disease NOS (*see also* Neoplasm)
   D49.9 [M36.1]
  nutritional deficiency (*see also* subcategory
   M14.8-) E63.9
  psoriasis NOS L40.50
  sarcoidosis D86.86
  syphilis (late) A52.77
   congenital A50.55 [M12.80]
  thyrotoxicosis (*see also* subcategory M14.8-) E05.90
  ulcerative colitis K51.90 [M07.60]
  viral hepatitis (postinfectious) NEC B19.9 [M12.80]
  Whipple's disease (*see also* subcategory M14.8-)
   K90.81
 Jaccoud — *see* Arthropathy, postrheumatic, chronic
 juvenile — *see* Arthritis, juvenile
  psoriatic L40.54
 mutilans (psoriatic) L40.52
 neuropathic (Charcot) M14.60
  ankle M14.67- ☑
  diabetic — *see* Diabetes, arthropathy, neuropathic
  elbow M14.62- ☑
  foot joint M14.67- ☑
  hand joint M14.64- ☑
  hip M14.65- ☑
  knee M14.66- ☑
  multiple site M14.69
  nonsyphilitic NEC G98.0
  shoulder M14.61- ☑
  syringomyelic G95.0
  vertebra M14.68
  wrist M14.63- ☑
 osteopulmonary — *see* Osteoarthropathy, hypertrophic, specified NEC
 postdysenteric M02.10
  ankle M02.17- ☑
  elbow M02.12- ☑
  foot joint M02.17- ☑
  hand joint M02.14- ☑
  hip M02.15- ☑
  knee M02.16- ☑
  multiple site M02.19
  shoulder M02.11- ☑
  vertebra M02.18
  wrist M02.13- ☑
 postimmunization M02.20
  ankle M02.27- ☑
  elbow M02.22- ☑
  foot joint M02.27- ☑
  hand joint M02.24- ☑
  hip M02.25- ☑
  knee M02.26- ☑
  multiple site M02.29
  shoulder M02.21- ☑
  vertebra M02.28
  wrist M02.23- ☑

Arthropathy — *continued*
 postinfectious NEC B99 ☑ [M12.80]
  in (due to)
   enteritis due to Yersinia enterocolitica
    A04.6 [M12.80]
   syphilis A52.77
   viral hepatitis NEC B19.9 [M12.80]
 postrheumatic, chronic (Jaccoud) M12.00
  ankle M12.07- ☑
  elbow M12.02- ☑
  foot joint M12.07- ☑
  hand joint M12.04- ☑
  hip M12.05- ☑
  knee M12.06- ☑
  multiple site M12.09
  shoulder M12.01- ☑
  specified joint NEC M12.08
  vertebrae M12.08
  wrist M12.03- ☑
 psoriatic NEC L40.59
  interphalangeal, distal L40.51
 reactive M02.9
  in (due to)
   infective endocarditis I33.0 [M02.9]
   specified type NEC M02.80
    ankle M02.87- ☑
    elbow M02.82- ☑
    foot joint M02.87- ☑
    hand joint M02.84- ☑
    hip M02.85- ☑
    knee M02.86- ☑
    multiple site M02.89
    shoulder M02.81- ☑
    vertebra M02.88
    wrist M02.83- ☑
 specified form NEC M12.80
  ankle M12.87- ☑
  elbow M12.82- ☑
  foot joint M12.87- ☑
  hand joint M12.84- ☑
  hip M12.85- ☑
  knee M12.86- ☑
  multiple site M12.89
  shoulder M12.81- ☑
  specified joint NEC M12.88
  vertebrae M12.88
  wrist M12.83- ☑
 syringomyelic G95.0
 tabes dorsalis A52.16
 tabetic A52.16
 transient — *see* Arthropathy, specified form NEC
 traumatic M12.50
  ankle M12.57- ☑
  elbow M12.52- ☑
  foot joint M12.57- ☑
  hand joint M12.54- ☑
  hip M12.55- ☑
  knee M12.56- ☑
  multiple site M12.59
  shoulder M12.51- ☑
  specified joint NEC M12.58
  vertebrae M12.58
  wrist M12.53- ☑
Arthropyosis — *see* Arthritis, pyogenic or pyemic
Arthrosis (deformans) (degenerative) (localized) (*see also*
  Osteoarthritis) M19.90
 spine — *see* Spondylosis
Arthus' phenomenon or reaction T78.41 ☑
 due to
  drug — *see* Table of Drugs and Chemicals, by drug
Articular — *see* condition
Articulation, reverse (teeth) M26.24
Artificial
 insemination complication — *see* Complications, artificial, fertilization
 opening status (functioning) (without complication)
   Z93.9
  anus (colostomy) Z93.3
  colostomy Z93.3
  cystostomy Z93.50
   appendico-vesicostomy Z93.52
   cutaneous Z93.51
   specified NEC Z93.59
  enterostomy Z93.4
  gastrostomy Z93.1
  ileostomy Z93.2
  intestinal tract NEC Z93.4

☑ **Additional Character Required** — Refer to the Tabular List for Character Selection   ⬧ Subterms under main terms may continue to next column or page

Artificial — continued
  opening status — continued
    jejunostomy Z93.4
    nephrostomy Z93.6
    specified site NEC Z93.8
    tracheostomy Z93.0
    ureterostomy Z93.6
    urethrostomy Z93.6
    urinary tract NEC Z93.6
    vagina Z93.8
  vagina status Z93.8
Arytenoid — see condition
Asbestosis (occupational) J61
Ascariasis B77.9
  with
    complications NEC B77.89
    intestinal complications B77.0
    pneumonia, pneumonitis B77.81
Ascaridosis, ascariasis — see Ascariasis
Ascaris (infection) (infestation) (lumbricoides) — see
  Ascariasis
Ascending — see condition
ASC-H (atypical squamous cells cannot exclude high
  grade squamous intraepithelial lesion on cytologic
  smear)
  anus R85.611
  cervix R87.611
  vagina R87.621
Aschoff's bodies — see Myocarditis, rheumatic
Ascites (abdominal) R18.8
  cardiac (see also Failure, heart, right) I50.810
  chylous (nonfilarial) I89.8
    filarial — see Infestation, filarial
  due to
    cirrhosis, alcoholic K70.31
    hepatitis
      alcoholic K70.11
      chronic active K71.51
    S. japonicum B65.2
  heart (see also Failure, heart, right) I50.810
  malignant R18.0
  pseudochylous R18.8
  syphilitic A52.74
  tuberculous A18.31
ASC-US (atypical squamous cells of undetermined signif-
  icance on cytologic smear)
  anus R85.610
  cervix R87.610
  vagina R87.620
Aseptic — see condition
Asherman's syndrome N85.6
Asialia K11.7
Asiatic cholera — see Cholera
Asimultagnosia (simultanagnosia) R48.3
Askin's tumor — see Neoplasm, connective tissue, malignant
Asocial personality F60.2
Asomatognosia R41.4
Aspartylglucosaminuria E77.1
Asperger's disease or syndrome F84.5
Aspergilloma — see Aspergillosis
Aspergillosis (with pneumonia) B44.9
  bronchopulmonary, allergic B44.81
  disseminated B44.7
  generalized B44.7
  pulmonary NEC B44.1
    allergic B44.81
    invasive B44.0
  specified NEC B44.89
  tonsillar B44.2
Aspergillus (flavus) (fumigatus) (infection) (terreus) —
  see Aspergillosis
Aspermatogenesis — see Azoospermia
Aspermia (testis) — see Azoospermia
Asphyxia, asphyxiation (by) R09.01
  antenatal P84
  birth P84
  bunny bag — see Asphyxia, due to, mechanical threat
    to breathing, trapped in bed clothes
  crushing S28.0 ☑
  drowning T75.1 ☑
  gas, fumes, or vapor — see Table of Drugs and Chem-
    icals
  inhalation — see Inhalation
  intrauterine P84
  local I73.00
    with gangrene I73.01

Asphyxia, asphyxiation — continued
  mucus (see also Foreign body, respiratory tract, causing
    asphyxia)
  newborn P84
  pathological R09.01
  postnatal P84
    mechanical — see Asphyxia, due to, mechanical
      threat to breathing
  prenatal P84
  reticularis R23.1
  strangulation — see Asphyxia, due to, mechanical
    threat to breathing
  submersion T75.1 ☑
  traumatic T71.9 ☑
    due to
      crushed chest S28.0 ☑
      foreign body (in) — see Foreign body, respira-
        tory tract, causing asphyxia
      low oxygen content of ambient air T71.20 ☑
        due to
          being trapped in
            low oxygen environment T71.29 ☑
            in car trunk T71.221 ☑
              circumstances undetermined
                T71.224 ☑
              done with intent to harm by
                another person T71.223 ☑
                self T71.222 ☑
            in refrigerator T71.231 ☑
              circumstances undetermined
                T71.234 ☑
              done with intent to harm by
                another person T71.233 ☑
                self T71.232 ☑
        cave-in T71.21 ☑
      mechanical threat to breathing (accidental)
        T71.191 ☑
        circumstances undetermined T71.194 ☑
        done with intent to harm by
          another person T71.193 ☑
          self T71.192 ☑
        hanging T71.161 ☑
          circumstances undetermined T71.164 ☑
          done with intent to harm by
            another person T71.163 ☑
            self T71.162 ☑
        plastic bag T71.121 ☑
          circumstances undetermined T71.124 ☑
          done with intent to harm by
            another person T71.123 ☑
            self T71.122 ☑
        smothering
          in furniture T71.151 ☑
            circumstances undetermined
              T71.154 ☑
            done with intent to harm by
              another person T71.153 ☑
              self T71.152 ☑
          under
            another person's body T71.141 ☑
              circumstances undetermined
                T71.144 ☑
              done with intent to harm
                T71.143 ☑
            pillow T71.111 ☑
              circumstances undetermined
                T71.114 ☑
              done with intent to harm by
                another person T71.113 ☑
                self T71.112 ☑
        trapped in bed clothes T71.131 ☑
          circumstances undetermined T71.134 ☑
          done with intent to harm by
            another person T71.133 ☑
            self T71.132 ☑
  vomiting, vomitus — see Foreign body, respiratory
    tract, causing asphyxia
Aspiration
  amniotic (clear) fluid (newborn) P24.10
    with
      pneumonia (pneumonitis) P24.11
      respiratory symptoms P24.11
  blood
    newborn (without respiratory symptoms) P24.20
      with
        pneumonia (pneumonitis) P24.21
        respiratory symptoms P24.21

Aspiration — continued
  blood — continued
    specified age NEC — see Foreign body, respiratory
      tract
  bronchitis J69.0
  food or foreign body (with asphyxiation) — see Asphyx-
    ia, food
  liquor (amnii) (newborn) P24.10
    with
      pneumonia (pneumonitis) P24.11
      respiratory symptoms P24.11
  meconium (newborn) (without respiratory symptoms)
    P24.00
    with
      pneumonitis (pneumonitis) P24.01
      respiratory symptoms P24.01
  milk (newborn) (without respiratory symptoms) P24.30
    with
      pneumonia (pneumonitis) P24.31
      respiratory symptoms P24.31
    specified age NEC — see Foreign body, respiratory
      tract
  mucus (see also Foreign body, by site, causing asphyx-
    ia)
    newborn P24.10
      with
        pneumonia (pneumonitis) P24.11
        respiratory symptoms P24.11
  neonatal P24.9
    specific NEC (without respiratory symptoms) P24.80
      with
        pneumonia (pneumonitis) P24.81
        respiratory symptoms P24.81
  newborn P24.9
    specific NEC (without respiratory symptoms) P24.80
      with
        pneumonia (pneumonitis) P24.81
        respiratory symptoms P24.81
  pneumonia J69.0
  pneumonitis J69.0
  syndrome of newborn — see Aspiration, by substance,
    with pneumonia
  vernix caseosa (newborn) P24.80
    with
      pneumonia (pneumonitis) P24.81
      respiratory symptoms P24.81
  vomitus (see also Foreign body, respiratory tract)
    newborn (without respiratory symptoms) P24.30
      with
        pneumonia (pneumonitis) P24.31
        respiratory symptoms P24.31
Asplenia (congenital) Q89.01
  postsurgical Z90.81
Assam fever B55.0
Assault, sexual — see Maltreatment
Assmann's focus NEC A15.0
Astasia (-abasia) (hysterical) F44.4
Asteatosis cutis L85.3
Astereognosia, astereognosis R48.1
Asterixis R27.8
  in liver disease K71.3
Asteroid hyalitis — see Deposit, crystalline
Asthenia, asthenic R53.1
  cardiac (see also Failure, heart) I50.9
    psychogenic F45.8
  cardiovascular (see also Failure, heart) I50.9
    psychogenic F45.8
  heart (see also Failure, heart) I50.9
    psychogenic F45.8
  hysterical F44.4
  myocardial (see also Failure, heart) I50.9
    psychogenic F45.8
  nervous F48.8
  neurocirculatory F45.8
  neurotic F48.8
  psychogenic F48.8
  psychoneurotic F48.8
  psychophysiologic F48.8
  reaction (psychophysiologic) F48.8
  senile R54
Asthenopia (see also Discomfort, visual)
  hysterical F44.6
  psychogenic F44.6
Asthenospermia — see Abnormal, specimen, male
  genital organs
Asthma, asthmatic (bronchial) (catarrh) (spasmodic)
  J45.909

Index

Asthma, asthmatic — Atheroma, atheromatous

Asthma, asthmatic — *continued*
  with
    chronic obstructive bronchitis J44.9
      with
        acute lower respiratory infection J44.0
        exacerbation (acute) J44.1
    chronic obstructive pulmonary disease J44.9
      with
        acute lower respiratory infection J44.0
        exacerbation (acute) J44.1
    exacerbation (acute) J45.901
    hay fever — *see* Asthma, allergic extrinsic
    rhinitis, allergic — *see* Asthma, allergic extrinsic
    status asthmaticus J45.902
  allergic extrinsic J45.909
    with
      exacerbation (acute) J45.901
      status asthmaticus J45.902
  atopic — *see* Asthma, allergic extrinsic
  cardiac — *see* Failure, ventricular, left
  cardiobronchial I50.1
  childhood J45.909
    with
      exacerbation (acute) J45.901
      status asthmaticus J45.902
  chronic obstructive J44.9
    with
      acute lower respiratory infection J44.0
      exacerbation (acute) J44.1
  collier's J60
  cough variant J45.991
  detergent J69.8
  due to
    detergent J69.8
    inhalation of fumes J68.3
  eosinophilic J82
  extrinsic, allergic — *see* Asthma, allergic extrinsic
  grinder's J62.8
  hay — *see* Asthma, allergic extrinsic
  heart I50.1
  idiosyncratic — *see* Asthma, nonallergic
  intermittent (mild) J45.20
    with
      exacerbation (acute) J45.21
      status asthmaticus J45.22
  intrinsic, nonallergic — *see* Asthma, nonallergic
  Kopp's E32.8
  late-onset J45.909
    with
      exacerbation (acute) J45.901
      status asthmaticus J45.902
  mild intermittent J45.20
    with
      exacerbation (acute) J45.21
      status asthmaticus J45.22
  mild persistent J45.30
    with
      exacerbation (acute) J45.31
      status asthmaticus J45.32
  Millar's (laryngismus stridulus) J38.5
  miner's J60
  mixed J45.909
    with
      exacerbation (acute) J45.901
      status asthmaticus J45.902
  moderate persistent J45.40
    with
      exacerbation (acute) J45.41
      status asthmaticus J45.42
  nervous — *see* Asthma, nonallergic
  nonallergic (intrinsic) J45.909
    with
      exacerbation (acute) J45.901
      status asthmaticus J45.902
  persistent
    mild J45.30
      with
        exacerbation (acute) J45.31
        status asthmaticus J45.32
    moderate J45.40
      with
        exacerbation (acute) J45.41
        status asthmaticus J45.42
    severe J45.50
      with
        exacerbation (acute) J45.51
        status asthmaticus J45.52
  platinum J45.998

Asthma, asthmatic — *continued*
  pneumoconiotic NEC J64
  potter's J62.8
  predominantly allergic J45.909
  psychogenic F54
  pulmonary eosinophilic J82
  red cedar J67.8
  Rostan's I50.1
  sandblaster's J62.8
  sequoiosis J67.8
  severe persistent J45.50
    with
      exacerbation (acute) J45.51
      status asthmaticus J45.52
  specified NEC J45.998
  stonemason's J62.8
  thymic E32.8
  tuberculous — *see* Tuberculosis, pulmonary
  Wichmann's (laryngismus stridulus) J38.5
  wood J67.8
Astigmatism (compound) (congenital) H52.20- ☑
  irregular H52.21- ☑
  regular H52.22- ☑
Astraphobia F40.220
Astroblastoma
  specified site — *see* Neoplasm, malignant, by site
  unspecified site C71.9
Astrocytoma (cystic)
  anaplastic
    specified site — *see* Neoplasm, malignant, by site
    unspecified site C71.9
  fibrillary
    specified site — *see* Neoplasm, malignant, by site
    unspecified site C71.9
  fibrous
    specified site — *see* Neoplasm, malignant, by site
    unspecified site C71.9
  gemistocytic
    specified site — *see* Neoplasm, malignant, by site
    unspecified site C71.9
  juvenile
    specified site — *see* Neoplasm, malignant, by site
    unspecified site C71.9
  pilocytic
    specified site — *see* Neoplasm, malignant, by site
    unspecified site C71.9
  piloid
    specified site — *see* Neoplasm, malignant, by site
    unspecified site C71.9
  protoplasmic
    specified site — *see* Neoplasm, malignant, by site
    unspecified site C71.9
  specified site NEC — *see* Neoplasm, malignant, by site
  subependymal D43.2
    giant cell
      specified site — *see* Neoplasm, uncertain be-havior, by site
      unspecified site D43.2
    specified site — *see* Neoplasm, uncertain behavior, by site
    unspecified site D43.2
  unspecified site C71.9
Astroglioma
  specified site — *see* Neoplasm, malignant, by site
  unspecified site C71.9
Asymbolia R48.8
Asymmetry (*see also* Distortion)
  between native and reconstructed breast N65.1
  face Q67.0
  jaw (lower) — *see* Anomaly, dentofacial, jaw-cranial base relationship, asymmetry
Asynergia, asynergy R27.8
  ventricular I51.89
Asystole (heart) — *see* Arrest, cardiac
At risk
  for
    dental caries Z91.849
      high Z91.843
      low Z91.841
      moderate Z91.842
    falling Z91.81
Ataxia, ataxy, ataxic R27.0
  acute R27.8
  brain (hereditary) G11.9
  cerebellar (hereditary) G11.9
    with defective DNA repair G11.3
    alcoholic G31.2
    early-onset G11.1

Ataxia, ataxy, ataxic — *continued*
  cerebellar — *continued*
    in
      alcoholism G31.2
      myxedema E03.9 [G13.2]
      neoplastic disease (*see also* Neoplasm) D49.9 [G32.81]
      specified disease NEC G32.81
    late-onset (Marie's) G11.2
  cerebral (hereditary) G11.9
  congenital nonprogressive G11.0
  family, familial — *see* Ataxia, hereditary
  following
    cerebrovascular disease I69.993
      cerebral infarction I69.393
      intracerebral hemorrhage I69.193
      nontraumatic intracranial hemorrhage NEC I69.293
      specified disease NEC I69.893
      subarachnoid hemorrhage I69.093
  Friedreich's (heredofamilial) (cerebellar) (spinal) G11.1
  gait R26.0
    hysterical F44.4
  general R27.8
  gluten M35.9 [G32.81]
    with celiac disease K90.0 [G32.81]
  hereditary G11.9
    with neuropathy G60.2
    cerebellar — *see* Ataxia, cerebellar
    spastic G11.4
    specified NEC G11.8
    spinal (Friedreich's) G11.1
  heredofamilial — *see* Ataxia, hereditary
  Hunt's G11.1
  hysterical F44.4
  locomotor (progressive) (syphilitic) (partial) (spastic) A52.11
    diabetic — *see* Diabetes, ataxia
  Marie's (cerebellar) (heredofamilial) (late- onset) G11.2
  nonorganic origin F44.4
  nonprogressive, congenital G11.0
  psychogenic F44.4
  Roussy-Lévy G60.0
  Sanger-Brown's (hereditary) G11.2
  spastic hereditary G11.4
  spinal
    hereditary (Friedreich's) G11.1
    progressive (syphilitic) A52.11
  spinocerebellar, X-linked recessive G11.1
  telangiectasia (Louis-Bar) G11.3
Ataxia-telangiectasia (Louis-Bar) G11.3
Atelectasis (massive) (partial) (pressure) (pulmonary) J98.11
  newborn P28.10
    due to resorption P28.11
    partial P28.19
    primary P28.0
    secondary P28.19
  primary (newborn) P28.0
  tuberculous — *see* Tuberculosis, pulmonary
Atelocardia Q24.9
Atelomyelia Q06.1
Atheroembolism
  of
    extremities
      lower I75.02- ☑
      upper I75.01- ☑
    kidney I75.81
    specified NEC I75.89
Atheroma, atheromatous (*see also* Arteriosclerosis) I70.90
  aorta, aortic I70.0
    valve (*see also* Endocarditis, aortic) I35.8
  aorto-iliac I70.0
  artery — *see* Arteriosclerosis
  basilar (artery) I67.2
  carotid (artery) (common) (internal) I67.2
  cerebral (arteries) I67.2
  coronary (artery) I25.10
    with angina pectoris — *see* Arteriosclerosis, coro-nary (artery),
  degeneration — *see* Arteriosclerosis
  heart, cardiac — *see* Disease, heart, ischemic, atherosclerotic
  mitral (valve) I34.8
  myocardium, myocardial — *see* Disease, heart, is-chemic, atherosclerotic

☑ **Additional Character Required — Refer to the Tabular List for Character Selection** ▽ **Subterms under main terms may continue to next column or page**

Atheroma, atheromatous — *continued*
  pulmonary valve (heart) (*see also* Endocarditis, pulmonary) I37.8
  tricuspid (heart) (valve) I36.8
  valve, valvular — *see* Endocarditis
  vertebral (artery) I67.2
Atheromatosis — *see* Arteriosclerosis
Atherosclerosis (*see also* Arteriosclerosis)
  coronary
    artery I25.10
     with angina pectoris — *see* Arteriosclerosis, coronary (artery),
     due to
      calcified coronary lesion (severely) I25.84
      lipid rich plaque I25.83
    transplanted heart I25.811
     bypass graft I25.812
      with angina pectoris — *see* Arteriosclerosis, coronary (artery),
     native coronary artery I25.811
      with angina pectoris — *see* Arteriosclerosis, coronary (artery),
Athetosis (acquired) R25.8
  bilateral (congenital) G80.3
  congenital (bilateral) (double) G80.3
  double (congenital) G80.3
  unilateral R25.8
Athlete's
  foot B35.3
  heart I51.7
Athrepsia E41
Athyrea (acquired) (*see also* Hypothyroidism)
  congenital E03.1
Atonia, atony, atonic
  bladder (sphincter) (neurogenic) N31.2
  capillary I78.8
  cecum K59.8
    psychogenic F45.8
  colon — *see* Atony, intestine
  congenital P94.2
  esophagus K22.8
  intestine K59.8
    psychogenic F45.8
  stomach K31.89
    neurotic or psychogenic F45.8
  uterus (during labor) O62.2
    with hemorrhage (postpartum) O72.1
    postpartum (with hemorrhage) O72.1
     without hemorrhage O75.89
Atopy — *see* History, allergy
Atransferrinemia, congenital E88.09
Atresia, atretic
  alimentary organ or tract NEC Q45.8
    upper Q40.8
  ani, anus, anal (canal) Q42.3
    with fistula Q42.2
  aorta (ring) Q25.29
  aortic (orifice) (valve) Q23.0
    arch Q25.21
    congenital with hypoplasia of ascending aorta and defective development of left ventricle (with mitral stenosis) Q23.4
    in hypoplastic left heart syndrome Q23.4
  aqueduct of Sylvius Q03.0
    with spina bifida — *see* Spina bifida, with hydrocephalus
  artery NEC Q27.8
    cerebral Q28.3
    coronary Q24.5
    digestive system Q27.8
    eye Q15.8
    lower limb Q27.8
    pulmonary Q25.5
    specified site NEC Q27.8
    umbilical Q27.0
    upper limb Q27.8
  auditory canal (external) Q16.1
  bile duct (common) (congenital) (hepatic) Q44.2
    acquired — *see* Obstruction, bile duct
  bladder (neck) Q64.39
    obstruction Q64.31
  bronchus Q32.4
  cecum Q42.8
  cervix (acquired) N88.2
    congenital Q51.828
    in pregnancy or childbirth — *see* Anomaly, cervix, in pregnancy or childbirth
     causing obstructed labor O65.5

Atresia, atretic — *continued*
  choana Q30.0
  colon Q42.9
    specified NEC Q42.8
  common duct Q44.2
  cricoid cartilage Q31.8
  cystic duct Q44.2
    acquired K82.8
     with obstruction K82.0
  digestive organs NEC Q45.8
  duodenum Q41.0
  ear canal Q16.1
  ejaculatory duct Q55.4
  epiglottis Q31.8
  esophagus Q39.0
    with tracheoesophageal fistula Q39.1
  eustachian tube Q17.8
  fallopian tube (congenital) Q50.6
    acquired N97.1
  follicular cyst N83.0- ☑
  foramen of
    Luschka Q03.1
     with spina bifida — *see* Spina bifida, with hydrocephalus
    Magendie Q03.1
     with spina bifida — *see* Spina bifida, with hydrocephalus
  gallbladder Q44.1
  genital organ
    external
     female Q52.79
     male Q55.8
    internal
     female Q52.8
     male Q55.8
  glottis Q31.8
  gullet Q39.0
    with tracheoesophageal fistula Q39.1
  heart valve NEC Q24.8
    pulmonary Q22.0
    tricuspid Q22.4
  hymen Q52.3
    acquired (postinfective) N89.6
  ileum Q41.2
  intestine (small) Q41.9
    large Q42.9
     specified NEC Q42.8
  iris, filtration angle Q15.0
  jejunum Q41.1
  lacrimal apparatus Q10.4
  larynx Q31.8
  meatus urinarius Q64.33
  mitral valve Q23.2
    in hypoplastic left heart syndrome Q23.4
  nares (anterior) (posterior) Q30.0
  nasopharynx Q34.8
  nose, nostril Q30.0
    acquired J34.89
  organ or site NEC Q89.8
  osseous meatus (ear) Q16.1
  oviduct (congenital) Q50.6
    acquired N97.1
  parotid duct Q38.4
    acquired K11.8
  pulmonary (artery) Q25.5
    valve Q22.0
  pulmonic Q22.0
  pupil Q13.2
  rectum Q42.1
    with fistula Q42.0
  salivary duct Q38.4
    acquired K11.8
  sublingual duct Q38.4
    acquired K11.8
  submandibular duct Q38.4
    acquired K11.8
  submaxillary duct Q38.4
    acquired K11.8
  thyroid cartilage Q31.8
  trachea Q32.1
  tricuspid valve Q22.4
  ureter Q62.10
    pelvic junction Q62.11
    vesical orifice Q62.12
  ureteropelvic junction Q62.11
  ureterovesical orifice Q62.12
  urethra (valvular) Q64.39
    stricture Q64.32
  urinary tract NEC Q64.8

Atresia, atretic — *continued*
  uterus Q51.818
    acquired N85.8
  vagina (congenital) Q52.4
    acquired (postinfectional) (senile) N89.5
  vas deferens Q55.3
  vascular NEC Q27.8
    cerebral Q28.3
    digestive system Q27.8
    lower limb Q27.8
    specified site NEC Q27.8
    upper limb Q27.8
    vein NEC Q27.8
     digestive system Q27.8
     great Q26.8
     lower limb Q27.8
     portal Q26.5
     pulmonary Q26.4
      partial Q26.3
      total Q26.2
     specified site NEC Q27.8
     upper limb Q27.8
    vena cava (inferior) (superior) Q26.8
  vesicourethral orifice Q64.31
  vulva Q52.79
    acquired N90.5
Atrichia, atrichosis — *see* Alopecia
Atrophia (*see also* Atrophy)
  cutis senilis L90.8
    due to radiation L57.8
  gyrata of choroid and retina H31.23
  senilis R54
    dermatological L90.8
     due to radiation (nonionizing) (solar) L57.8
  unguium L60.3
    congenita Q84.6
Atrophie blanche (en plaque) (de Milian) L95.0
Atrophoderma, atrophodermia (of) L90.9
  diffusum (idiopathic) L90.4
  maculatum L90.8
    et striatum L90.8
     due to syphilis A52.79
    syphilitic A51.39
  neuriticum L90.8
  Pasini and Pierini L90.3
  pigmentosum Q82.1
  reticulatum symmetricum faciei L66.4
  senile L90.8
    due to radiation (nonionizing) (solar) L57.8
  vermiculata (cheeks) L66.4
Atrophy, atrophic (of)
  adrenal (capsule) (gland) E27.49
    primary (autoimmune) E27.1
  alveolar process or ridge (edentulous) K08.20
  anal sphincter (disuse) N81.84
  appendix K38.8
  arteriosclerotic — *see* Arteriosclerosis
  bile duct (common) (hepatic) K83.8
  bladder N32.89
    neurogenic N31.8
  blanche (en plaque) (of Milian) L95.0
  bone (senile) NEC (*see also* Disorder, bone, specified type NEC)
    due to
     tabes dorsalis (neurogenic) A52.11
  brain (cortex) (progressive) G31.9
    frontotemporal circumscribed G31.01 [F02.80]
     with behavioral disturbance G31.01 [F02.81]
    senile NEC G31.1
  breast N64.2
    obstetric — *see* Disorder, breast, specified type NEC
  buccal cavity K13.79
  cardiac — *see* Degeneration, myocardial
  cartilage (infectional) (joint) — *see* Disorder, cartilage, specified NEC
  cerebellar — *see* Atrophy, brain
  cerebral — *see* Atrophy, brain
  cervix (mucosa) (senile) (uteri) N88.8
    menopausal N95.8
  Charcot-Marie-Tooth G60.0
  choroid (central) (macular) (myopic) (retina) H31.10- ☑
    diffuse secondary H31.12- ☑
    gyrate H31.23
    senile H31.11- ☑
  ciliary body — *see* Atrophy, iris
  conjunctiva (senile) H11.89
  corpus cavernosum N48.89

Atrophy, atrophic — *continued*
  cortical — *see* Atrophy, brain
  cystic duct K82.8
  Déjérine-Thomas G23.8
  disuse NEC — *see* Atrophy, muscle
  Duchenne-Aran G12.21
  ear H93.8- ☑
  edentulous alveolar ridge K08.20
  endometrium (senile) N85.8
      cervix N88.8
  enteric K63.89
  epididymis N50.89
  eyeball — *see* Disorder, globe, degenerated condition, atrophy
  eyelid (senile) — *see* Disorder, eyelid, degenerative
  facial (skin) L90.9
  fallopian tube (senile) N83.32- ☑
      with ovary N83.33- ☑
  fascioscapulohumeral (Landouzy- Déjérine) G71.0
  fatty, thymus (gland) E32.8
  gallbladder K82.8
  gastric K29.40
      with bleeding K29.41
  gastrointestinal K63.89
  glandular I89.8
  globe H44.52- ☑
  gum — *see* Recession, gingival
  hair L67.8
  heart (brown) — *see* Degeneration, myocardial
  hemifacial Q67.4
      Romberg G51.8
  infantile E41
      paralysis, acute — *see* Poliomyelitis, paralytic
  intestine K63.89
  iris (essential) (progressive) H21.26- ☑
      specified NEC H21.29
  kidney (senile) (terminal) (*see also* Sclerosis, renal) N26.1
      congenital or infantile Q60.5
          bilateral Q60.4
          unilateral Q60.3
      hydronephrotic — *see* Hydronephrosis
  lacrimal gland (primary) H04.14- ☑
      secondary H04.15- ☑
  Landouzy-Déjérine G71.0
  laryngitis, infective J37.0
  larynx J38.7
  Leber's optic (hereditary) H47.22
  lip K13.0
  liver (yellow) K72.90
      with coma K72.91
      acute, subacute K72.00
          with coma K72.01
      chronic K72.10
          with coma K72.11
  lung (senile) J98.4
  macular (dermatological) L90.8
      syphilitic, skin A51.39
          striated A52.79
  mandible (edentulous) K08.20
      minimal K08.21
      moderate K08.22
      severe K08.23
  maxilla K08.20
      minimal K08.24
      moderate K08.25
      severe K08.26
  muscle, muscular (diffuse) (general) (idiopathic) (primary) M62.50
      ankle M62.57- ☑
      Duchenne-Aran G12.21
      foot M62.57- ☑
      forearm M62.53- ☑
      hand M62.54- ☑
      infantile spinal G12.0
      lower leg M62.56- ☑
      multiple sites M62.59
      myelopathic — *see* Atrophy, muscle, spinal
      myotonic G71.11
      neuritic G58.9
      neuropathic (peroneal) (progressive) G60.0
      pelvic (disuse) N81.84
      peroneal G60.0
      progressive (bulbar) G12.21
          adult G12.1
          infantile (spinal) G12.0
          spinal G12.25
              adult G12.1

Atrophy, atrophic — *continued*
  muscle, muscular — *continued*
      progressive — *continued*
          spinal — *continued*
              infantile G12.0
          pseudohypertrophic G71.0
      shoulder region M62.51- ☑
      specified site NEC M62.58
      spinal G12.9
          adult form G12.1
          Aran-Duchenne G12.21
          childhood form, type II G12.1
          distal G12.1
          hereditary NEC G12.1
          infantile, type I (Werdnig-Hoffmann) G12.0
          juvenile form, type III (Kugelberg- Welander) G12.1
          progressive G12.25
          scapuloperoneal form G12.1
          specified NEC G12.8
      syphilitic A52.78
      thigh M62.55- ☑
      upper arm M62.52- ☑
  myocardium — *see* Degeneration, myocardial
  myometrium (senile) N85.8
      cervix N88.8
  myopathic NEC — *see* Atrophy, muscle
  myotonia G71.11
  nail L60.3
  nasopharynx J31.1
  nerve (*see also* Disorder, nerve)
      abducens — *see* Strabismus, paralytic, sixth nerve
      accessory G52.8
      acoustic or auditory H93.3 ☑
      cranial G52.9
          eighth (auditory) H93.3 ☑
          eleventh (accessory) G52.8
          fifth (trigeminal) G50.8
          first (olfactory) G52.0
          fourth (trochlear) — *see* Strabismus, paralytic, fourth nerve
          second (optic) H47.20
          sixth (abducens) — *see* Strabismus, paralytic, sixth nerve
          tenth (pneumogastric) (vagus) G52.2
          third (oculomotor) — *see* Strabismus, paralytic, third nerve
          twelfth (hypoglossal) G52.3
      hypoglossal G52.3
      oculomotor — *see* Strabismus, paralytic, third nerve
      olfactory G52.0
      optic (papillomacular bundle)
          syphilitic (late) A52.15
              congenital A50.44
      pneumogastric G52.2
      trigeminal G50.8
      trochlear — *see* Strabismus, paralytic, fourth nerve
      vagus (pneumogastric) G52.2
  neurogenic, bone, tabetic A52.11
  nutritional E41
  old age R54
  olivopontocerebellar G23.8
  optic (nerve) H47.20
      glaucomatous H47.23- ☑
      hereditary H47.22
      primary H47.21- ☑
      specified type NEC H47.29- ☑
      syphilitic (late) A52.15
          congenital A50.44
  orbit H05.31- ☑
  ovary (senile) N83.31- ☑
      with fallopian tube N83.33- ☑
  oviduct (senile) — *see* Atrophy, fallopian tube
  palsy, diffuse (progressive) G12.22
  pancreas (duct) (senile) K86.89
  parotid gland K11.0
  pelvic muscle N81.84
  penis N48.89
  pharynx J39.2
  pluriglandular E31.8
      autoimmune E31.0
  polyarthritis M15.9
  prostate N42.89
  pseudohypertrophic (muscle) G71.0
  renal (*see also* Sclerosis, renal) N26.1
  retina, retinal (postinfectional) H35.89
  rhinitis J31.0

Atrophy, atrophic — *continued*
  salivary gland K11.0
  scar L90.5
  sclerosis, lobar (of brain) G31.09 [F02.80]
      with behavioral disturbance G31.09 [F02.81]
  scrotum N50.89
  seminal vesicle N50.89
  senile R54
      due to radiation (nonionizing) (solar) L57.8
  skin (patches) (spots) L90.9
      degenerative (senile) L90.8
      due to radiation (nonionizing) (solar) L57.8
      senile L90.8
  spermatic cord N50.89
  spinal (acute) (cord) G95.89
      muscular — *see* Atrophy, muscle, spinal
      paralysis G12.20
          acute — *see* Poliomyelitis, paralytic
          meaning progressive muscular atrophy G12.21
  spine (column) — *see* Spondylopathy, specified NEC
  spleen (senile) D73.0
  stomach K29.40
      with bleeding K29.41
  striate (skin) L90.6
      syphilitic A52.79
  subcutaneous L90.9
  sublingual gland K11.0
  submandibular gland K11.0
  submaxillary gland K11.0
  Sudeck's — *see* Algoneurodystrophy
  suprarenal (capsule) (gland) E27.49
      primary E27.1
  systemic affecting central nervous system
      in
          myxedema E03.9 [G13.2]
          neoplastic disease (*see also* Neoplasm) D49.9 [G13.1]
          specified disease NEC G13.8
  tarso-orbital fascia, congenital Q10.3
  testis N50.0
  thenar, partial — *see* Syndrome, carpal tunnel
  thymus (fatty) E32.8
  thyroid (gland) (acquired) E03.4
      with cretinism E03.1
      congenital (with myxedema) E03.1
  tongue (senile) K14.8
      papillae K14.4
  trachea J39.8
  tunica vaginalis N50.89
  turbinate J34.89
  tympanic membrane (nonflaccid) H73.82- ☑
      flaccid H73.81- ☑
  upper respiratory tract J39.8
  uterus, uterine (senile) N85.8
      cervix N88.8
      due to radiation (intended effect) N85.8
          adverse effect or misadventure N99.89
  vagina (senile) N95.2
  vas deferens N50.89
  vascular I99.8
  vertebra (senile) — *see* Spondylopathy, specified NEC
  vulva (senile) N90.5
  Werdnig-Hoffmann G12.0
  yellow — *see* Failure, hepatic
Attack, attacks
  with alteration of consciousness (with automatisms) — *see* Epilepsy, localization-related, symptomatic, with complex partial seizures
  without alteration of consciousness — *see* Epilepsy, localization-related, symptomatic, with simple partial seizures
  Adams-Stokes I45.9
  akinetic — *see* Epilepsy, generalized, specified NEC
  angina — *see* Angina
  atonic — *see* Epilepsy, generalized, specified NEC
  benign shuddering G25.83
  cataleptic — *see* Catalepsy
  coronary — *see* Infarct, myocardium
  cyanotic, newborn P28.2
  drop NEC R55
  epileptic — *see* Epilepsy
  heart — *see* infarct, myocardium
  hysterical F44.9
  jacksonian — *see* Epilepsy, localization-related, symptomatic, with simple partial seizures
  myocardium, myocardial — *see* Infarct, myocardium
  myoclonic — *see* Epilepsy, generalized, specified NEC
  panic F41.0

☑ **Additional Character Required — Refer to the Tabular List for Character Selection**   🔽 **Subterms under main terms may continue to next column or page**

Attack, attacks — *continued*
  psychomotor — *see* Epilepsy, localization-related, symptomatic, with complex partial seizures
  salaam — *see* Epilepsy, spasms
  schizophreniform, brief F23
  shuddering, benign G25.83
  Stokes-Adams I45.9
  syncope R55
  transient ischemic (TIA) G45.9
    specified NEC G45.8
  unconsciousness R55
    hysterical F44.89
  vasomotor R55
  vasovagal (paroxysmal) (idiopathic) R55
Attention (to)
  artificial
    opening (of) Z43.9
      digestive tract NEC Z43.4
        colon Z43.3
        ilium Z43.2
        stomach Z43.1
      specified NEC Z43.8
      trachea Z43.0
      urinary tract NEC Z43.6
        cystostomy Z43.5
        nephrostomy Z43.6
        ureterostomy Z43.6
        urethrostomy Z43.6
      vagina Z43.7
    colostomy Z43.3
    cystostomy Z43.5
    deficit disorder or syndrome F98.8
      with hyperactivity — *see* Disorder, attention-deficit hyperactivity
    gastrostomy Z43.1
    ileostomy Z43.2
    jejunostomy Z43.4
    nephrostomy Z43.6
    surgical dressings Z48.01
    sutures Z48.02
    tracheostomy Z43.0
    ureterostomy Z43.6
    urethrostomy Z43.6
Attrition
  gum — *see* Recession, gingival
  tooth, teeth (excessive) (hard tissues) K03.0
Atypical, atypism (*see also* condition)
  cells (on cytoglacial smear) (endocervical) (endometrial) (glandular)
    cervix R87.619
    vagina R87.629
  cervical N87.9
  endometrium N85.9
    hyperplasia N85.00
  parenting situation Z62.9
Auditory — *see* condition
Aujeszky's disease B33.8
Aurantiasis, cutis E67.1
Auricle, auricular (*see also* condition)
  cervical Q18.2
Auriculotemporal syndrome G50.8
Austin Flint murmur (aortic insufficiency) I35.1
Australian
  Q fever A78
  X disease A83.4
Autism, autistic (childhood) (infantile) F84.0
  atypical F84.9
  spectrum disorder F84.0
Autodigestion R68.89
Autoerythrocyte sensitization (syndrome) D69.2
Autographism L50.3
Autoimmune
  disease (systemic) M35.9
  inhibitors to clotting factors D68.311
  lymphoproliferative syndrome [ALPS] D89.82
  thyroiditis E06.3
Autointoxication R68.89
Automatism G93.89
  with temporal sclerosis G93.81
  epileptic — *see* Epilepsy, localization-related, symptomatic, with complex partial seizures
  paroxysmal, idiopathic — *see* Epilepsy, localization-related, symptomatic, with complex partial seizures
Autonomic, autonomous
  bladder (neurogenic) N31.2
  hysteria seizure F44.5
Autosensitivity, erythrocyte D69.2

Autosensitization, cutaneous L30.2
Autosome — *see* condition by chromosome involved
Autotopagnosia R48.1
Autotoxemia R68.89
Autumn — *see* condition
Avellis' syndrome G46.8
Aversion
  oral R63.3
    newborn P92.- ☑
    nonorganic origin F98.2 ☑
  sexual F52.1
Aviator's
  disease or sickness — *see* Effect, adverse, high altitude
  ear T70.0 ☑
Avitaminosis (multiple) (*see also* Deficiency, vitamin)
  E56.9
  B E53.9
    with
      beriberi E51.11
      pellagra E52
  B2 E53.0
  B6 E53.1
  B12 E53.8
  D E55.9
    with rickets E55.0
  G E53.0
  K E56.1
  nicotinic acid E52
AVNRT (atrioventricular nodal re-entrant tachycardia) I47.1
AVRT (atrioventricular nodal re-entrant tachycardia) I47.1
Avulsion (traumatic)
  blood vessel — *see* Injury, blood vessel
  bone — *see* Fracture, by site
  cartilage (*see also* Dislocation, by site)
    symphyseal (inner), complicating delivery O71.6
  external site other than limb — *see* Wound, open, by site
  eye S05.7- ☑
  head (intracranial)
    external site NEC S08.89 ☑
    scalp S08.0 ☑
  internal organ or site — *see* Injury, by site
  joint (*see also* Dislocation, by site)
    capsule — *see* Sprain, by site
  kidney S37.06- ☑
  ligament — *see* Sprain, by site
  limb (*see also* Amputation, traumatic, by site)
    skin and subcutaneous tissue — *see* Wound, open, by site
  muscle — *see* Injury, muscle
  nerve (root) — *see* Injury, nerve
  scalp S08.0 ☑
  skin and subcutaneous tissue — *see* Wound, open, by site
  spleen S36.032 ☑
  symphyseal cartilage (inner), complicating delivery O71.6
  tendon — *see* Injury, muscle
  tooth S03.2 ☑
Awareness of heart beat R00.2
Axenfeld's
  anomaly or syndrome Q15.0
  degeneration (calcareous) Q13.4
Axilla, axillary (*see also* condition)
  breast Q83.1
Axonotmesis — *see* Injury, nerve
Ayerza's disease or syndrome (pulmonary artery sclerosis with pulmonary hypertension) I27.0
Azoospermia (organic) N46.01
  due to
    drug therapy N46.021
    efferent duct obstruction N46.023
    infection N46.022
    radiation N46.024
    specified cause NEC N46.029
    systemic disease N46.025
Azotemia R79.89
  meaning uremia N19
Aztec ear Q17.3
Azygos
  continuation inferior vena cava Q26.8
  lobe (lung) Q33.1

B

Baastrup's disease — *see* Kissing spine

Babesiosis B60.0
Babington's disease (familial hemorrhagic telangiectasia) I78.0
Babinski's syndrome A52.79
Baby
  crying constantly R68.11
  floppy (syndrome) P94.2
Bacillary — *see* condition
Bacilluria R82.71
Bacillus (*see also* Infection, bacillus)
  abortus infection A23.1
  anthracis infection A22.9
  coli infection (*see also* Escherichia coli) B96.20
  Flexner's A03.1
  mallei infection A24.0
  Shiga's A03.0
  suipestifer infection — *see* Infection, salmonella
Back — *see* condition
Backache (postural) M54.9
  sacroiliac M53.3
  specified NEC M54.89
Backflow — *see* Reflux
Backward reading (dyslexia) F81.0
Bacteremia R78.81
  with sepsis — *see* Sepsis
Bactericholia — *see* Cholecystitis, acute
Bacterid, bacteride (pustular) L40.3
Bacterium, bacteria, bacterial
  agent NEC, as cause of disease classified elsewhere B96.89
  in blood — *see* Bacteremia
  in urine — *see* Bacteriuria
Bacteriuria, bacteruria R82.71
  asymptomatic R82.71
Bacteroides
  fragilis, as cause of disease classified elsewhere B96.6
Bad
  heart — *see* Disease, heart
  trip
    due to drug abuse — *see* Abuse, drug, hallucinogen
    due to drug dependence — *see* Dependence, drug, hallucinogen
Baelz's disease (cheilitis glandularis apostematosa) K13.0
Baerensprung's disease (eczema marginatum) B35.6
Bagasse disease or pneumonitis J67.1
Bagassosis J67.1
Baker's cyst — *see* Cyst, Baker's
Bakwin-Krida syndrome (metaphyseal dysplasia) Q78.5
Balancing side interference M26.56
Balanitis (circinata) (erosiva) (gangrenosa) (phagedenic) (vulgaris) N48.1
  amebic A06.82
  candidal B37.42
  due to Haemophilus ducreyi A57
  gonococcal (acute) (chronic) A54.09
  xerotica obliterans N48.0
Balanoposthitis N47.6
  gonococcal (acute) (chronic) A54.09
  ulcerative (specific) A63.8
Balanorrhagia — *see* Balanitis
Balantidiasis, balantidiosis A07.0
Bald tongue K14.4
Baldness (*see also* Alopecia)
  male-pattern — *see* Alopecia, androgenic
Balkan grippe A78
Balloon disease — *see* Effect, adverse, high altitude
Balo's disease (concentric sclerosis) G37.5
Bamberger-Marie disease — *see* Osteoarthropathy, hypertrophic, specified type NEC
Bancroft's filariasis B74.0
Band(s)
  adhesive — *see* Adhesions, peritoneum
  anomalous or congenital (*see also* Anomaly, by site)
    heart (atrial) (ventricular) Q24.8
    intestine Q43.3
    omentum Q43.3
  cervix N88.1
  constricting, congenital Q79.8
  gallbladder (congenital) Q44.1
  intestinal (adhesive) — *see* Adhesions, peritoneum
  obstructive
    intestine K56.50
      complete K56.52
      incomplete K56.51
      partial K56.51
    peritoneum K56.50

Index

Band — Bilharziasis

Band(s) — *continued*
obstructive — *continued*
peritoneum — *continued*
complete K56.52
incomplete K56.51
partial K56.51
periappendiceal, congenital Q43.3
peritoneal (adhesive) — *see* Adhesions, peritoneum
uterus N73.6
internal N85.6
vagina N89.5
Bandemia D72.825
Bandl's ring (contraction), complicating delivery O62.4
Bangkok hemorrhagic fever A91
Bang's disease (brucella abortus) A23.1
Bankruptcy, anxiety concerning Z59.8
Bannister's disease T78.3 ☑
hereditary D84.1
Banti's disease or syndrome (with cirrhosis) (with portal hypertension) K76.6
Bar, median, prostate — *see* Enlargement, enlarged, prostate
Barcoo disease or rot — *see* Ulcer, skin
Barlow's disease E54
Barodontalgia T70.29 ☑
Baron Münchausen syndrome — *see* Disorder, factitious
Barosinusitis T70.1 ☑
Barotitis T70.0 ☑
Barotrauma T70.29 ☑
odontalgia T70.29 ☑
otitic T70.0 ☑
sinus T70.1 ☑
Barraquer (-Simons) **disease or syndrome** (progressive lipodystrophy) E88.1
Barré-Guillain disease or syndrome G61.0
Barrel chest M95.4
Barré-Liéou syndrome (posterior cervical sympathetic) M53.0
Barrett's
disease — *see* Barrett's, esophagus
esophagus K22.70
with dysplasia K22.719
high grade K22.711
low grade K22.710
without dysplasia K22.70
syndrome — *see* Barrett's, esophagus
ulcer K22.10
with bleeding K22.11
without bleeding K22.10
Bársony (-Polgár) (-Teschendorf) **syndrome** (corkscrew esophagus) K22.4
Barth syndrome E78.71
Bartholinitis (suppurating) N75.8
gonococcal (acute) (chronic) (with abscess) A54.1
Bartonellosis A44.9
cutaneous A44.1
mucocutaneous A44.1
specified NEC A44.8
systemic A44.0
Barton's fracture S52.56- ☑
Bartter's syndrome E26.81
Basal — *see* condition
Basan's (hidrotic) ectodermal dysplasia Q82.4
Baseball finger — *see* Dislocation, finger
Basedow's disease (exophthalmic goiter) — *see* Hyperthyroidism, with, goiter
Basic — *see* condition
Basilar — *see* condition
Bason's (hidrotic) ectodermal dysplasia Q82.4
Basopenia — *see* Agranulocytosis
Basophilia D72.824
Basophilism (cortico-adrenal) (Cushing's) (pituitary) E24.0
Bassen-Kornzweig disease or syndrome E78.6
Bat ear Q17.5
Bateman's
disease B08.1
purpura (senile) D69.2
Bathing cramp T75.1 ☑
Bathophobia F40.248
Batten (-Mayou) **disease** E75.4
retina E75.4 [H36]
Batten-Steinert syndrome G71.11
Battered — *see* Maltreatment
Battey Mycobacterium infection A31.0
Battle exhaustion F43.0

Battledore placenta O43.19- ☑
Baumgarten-Cruveilhier cirrhosis, disease or syndrome K74.69
Bauxite fibrosis (of lung) J63.1
Bayle's disease (general paresis) A52.17
Bazin's disease (primary) (tuberculous) A18.4
Beach ear — *see* Swimmer's, ear
Beaded hair (congenital) Q84.1
Béal conjunctivitis or syndrome B30.2
Beard's disease (neurasthenia) F48.8
Beat(s)
atrial, premature I49.1
ectopic I49.49
elbow — *see* Bursitis, elbow
escaped, heart I49.49
hand — *see* Bursitis, hand
knee — *see* Bursitis, knee
premature I49.40
atrial I49.1
auricular I49.1
supraventricular I49.1
Beau's
disease or syndrome — *see* Degeneration, myocardial
lines (transverse furrows on fingernails) L60.4
Bechterev's syndrome — *see* Spondylitis, ankylosing
Becker's
cardiomyopathy I42.8
disease
idiopathic mural endomyocardial disease I42.3
myotonia congenita, recessive form G71.12
dystrophy G71.0
pigmented hairy nevus D22.5
Beck's syndrome (anterior spinal artery occlusion) I65.8
Beckwith-Wiedemann syndrome Q87.3
Bed confinement status Z74.01
Bed sore — *see* Ulcer, pressure, by site
Bedbug bite(s) — *see* Bite(s), by site, superficial, insect
Bedclothes, asphyxiation or suffocation by — *see* Asphyxia, traumatic, due to, mechanical, trapped
Bednar's
aphthae K12.0
tumor — *see* Neoplasm, malignant, by site
Bedridden Z74.01
Bedsore — *see* Ulcer, pressure, by site
Bedwetting — *see* Enuresis
Bee sting (with allergic or anaphylactic shock) — *see* Toxicity, venom, arthropod, bee
Beer drinker's heart (disease) I42.6
Begbie's disease (exophthalmic goiter) — *see* Hyperthyroidism, with, goiter
Behavior
antisocial
adult Z72.811
child or adolescent Z72.810
disorder, disturbance — *see* Disorder, conduct
disruptive — *see* Disorder, conduct
drug seeking Z76.5
inexplicable R46.2
marked evasiveness R46.5
obsessive-compulsive R46.81
overactivity R46.3
poor responsiveness R46.4
self-damaging (life-style) Z72.89
sleep-incompatible Z72.821
slowness R46.4
specified NEC R46.89
strange (and inexplicable) R46.2
suspiciousness R46.5
type A pattern Z73.1
undue concern or preoccupation with stressful events R46.6
verbosity and circumstantial detail obscuring reason for contact R46.7
Behçet's disease or syndrome M35.2
Behr's disease — *see* Degeneration, macula
Beigel's disease or morbus (white piedra) B36.2
Bejel A65
Bekhterev's syndrome — *see* Spondylitis, ankylosing
Belching — *see* Eructation
Bell's
mania F30.8
palsy, paralysis G51.0
infant or newborn P11.3
spasm G51.3
Bence Jones albuminuria or proteinuria NEC R80.3
Bends T70.3 ☑
Benedikt's paralysis or syndrome G46.3

Benign (*see also* condition)
prostatic hyperplasia — *see* Hyperplasia, prostate
Bennett's fracture (displaced) S62.21- ☑
Benson's disease — *see* Deposit, crystalline
Bent
back (hysterical) F44.4
nose M95.0
congenital Q67.4
Bereavement (uncomplicated) Z63.4
Bergeron's disease (hysterical chorea) F44.4
Berger's disease — *see* Nephropathy, IgA
Beriberi (dry) E51.11
heart (disease) E51.12
polyneuropathy E51.11
wet E51.12
involving circulatory system E51.11
Berlin's disease or edema (traumatic) S05.8X- ☑
Berlock (berloque) **dermatitis** L56.2
Bernard-Horner syndrome G90.2
Bernard-Soulier disease or thrombopathia D69.1
Bernhardt (-Roth) **disease** — *see* Mononeuropathy, lower limb, meralgia paresthetica
Bernheim's syndrome — *see* Failure, heart, right
Bertielliasis B71.8
Berylliosis (lung) J63.2
Besnier-Boeck (-Schaumann) **disease** — *see* Sarcoidosis
Besnier's
lupus pernio D86.3
prurigo L20.0
Bestiality F65.89
Best's disease H35.50
Betalipoproteinemia, broad or floating E78.2
Beta-mercaptolactate-cysteine disulfiduria E72.09
Betting and gambling Z72.6
pathological (compulsive) F63.0
Bezoar T18.9 ☑
intestine T18.3 ☑
stomach T18.2 ☑
Bezold's abscess — *see* Mastoiditis, acute
Bianchi's syndrome R48.8
Bicornate or bicornis uterus Q51.3
in pregnancy or childbirth O34.00
causing obstructed labor O65.5
Bicuspid aortic valve Q23.1
Biedl-Bardet syndrome Q87.89
Bielschowsky (-Jansky) disease E75.4
Biermer's (pernicious) anemia or disease D51.0
Biett's disease L93.0
Bifid (congenital)
apex, heart Q24.8
clitoris Q52.6
kidney Q63.8
nose Q30.2
patella Q74.1
scrotum Q55.29
toe NEC Q74.2
tongue Q38.3
ureter Q62.8
uterus Q51.3
uvula Q35.7
Biforis uterus (suprasimplex) Q51.3
Bifurcation (congenital)
gallbladder Q44.1
kidney pelvis Q63.8
renal pelvis Q63.8
rib Q76.6
tongue, congenital Q38.3
trachea Q32.1
ureter Q62.8
urethra Q64.74
vertebra Q76.49
Big spleen syndrome D73.1
Bigeminal pulse R00.8
Bilateral — *see* condition
Bile
duct — *see* condition
pigments in urine R82.2
Bilharziasis (*see also* Schistosomiasis)
chyluria B65.0
cutaneous B65.3
galactura B65.0
hematochyluria B65.0
intestinal B65.1
lipemia B65.9
lipuria B65.9
oriental B65.2
piarhemia B65.9

☑ Additional Character Required — Refer to the Tabular List for Character Selection   ▽ Subterms under main terms may continue to next column or page

Bilharziasis — *continued*
  pulmonary NOS B65.9 [J99]
    pneumonia B65.9 [J17]
  tropical hematuria B65.0
  vesical B65.0
Biliary — *see* condition
Bilirubin metabolism disorder E80.7
  specified NEC E80.6
Bilirubinemia, familial nonhemolytic E80.4
Bilirubinuria R82.2
Biliuria R82.2
Bilocular stomach K31.2
Binswanger's disease I67.3
Biparta, bipartite
  carpal scaphoid Q74.0
  patella Q74.1
  vagina Q52.10
Bird
  face Q75.8
  fancier's disease or lung J67.2
Birth
  complications in mother — *see* Delivery, complicated
  compression during NOS P15.9
  defect — *see* Anomaly
  immature (less than 37 completed weeks) — *see* Preterm, newborn
    extremely (less than 28 completed weeks) — *see* Immaturity, extreme
  inattention, at or after — *see* Maltreatment, child, neglect
  injury NOS P15.9
    basal ganglia P11.1
    brachial plexus NEC P14.3
    brain (compression) (pressure) P11.2
    central nervous system NOS P11.9
    cerebellum P11.1
    cerebral hemorrhage P10.1
    external genitalia P15.5
    eye P15.3
    face P15.4
    fracture
      bone P13.9
        specified NEC P13.8
      clavicle P13.4
      femur P13.2
      humerus P13.3
      long bone, except femur P13.3
      radius and ulna P13.3
      skull P13.0
      spine P11.5
      tibia and fibula P13.3
    intracranial P11.2
      laceration or hemorrhage P10.9
        specified NEC P10.8
    intraventricular hemorrhage P10.2
    laceration
      brain P10.1
      by scalpel P15.8
      peripheral nerve P14.9
    liver P15.0
    meninges
      brain P11.1
      spinal cord P11.5
    nerve
      brachial plexus P14.3
      cranial NEC (except facial) P11.4
      facial P11.3
      peripheral P14.9
      phrenic (paralysis) P14.2
    paralysis
      facial nerve P11.3
      spinal P11.5
    penis P15.5
    rupture
      spinal cord P11.5
    scalp P12.9
    scalpel wound P15.8
    scrotum P15.5
    skull NEC P13.1
      fracture P13.0
    specified type NEC P15.8
    spinal cord P11.5
    spine P11.5
    spleen P15.1
    sternomastoid (hematoma) P15.2
    subarachnoid hemorrhage P10.3
    subcutaneous fat necrosis P15.6
    subdural hemorrhage P10.0

Birth — *continued*
  injury — *continued*
    tentorial tear P10.4
    testes P15.5
    vulva P15.5
  lack of care, at or after — *see* Maltreatment, child, neglect
  neglect, at or after — *see* Maltreatment, child, neglect
  palsy or paralysis, newborn, NOS (birth injury) P14.9
  premature (infant) — *see* Preterm, newborn
  shock, newborn P96.89
  trauma — *see* Birth, injury
  weight
    4000 grams to 4499 grams P08.1
    4500 grams or more P08.0
    low (2499 grams or less) — *see* Low, birthweight
      extremely (999 grams or less) — *see* Low, birthweight, extreme
Birthmark Q82.5
Birt-Hogg-Dube syndrome Q87.89
Bisalbuminemia E88.09
Biskra's button B55.1
Bite(s) (animal) (human)
  abdomen, abdominal
    wall S31.159 ☑
      with penetration into peritoneal cavity S31.659 ☑
      epigastric region S31.152 ☑
        with penetration into peritoneal cavity S31.652 ☑
      left
        lower quadrant S31.154 ☑
          with penetration into peritoneal cavity S31.654 ☑
        upper quadrant S31.151 ☑
          with penetration into peritoneal cavity S31.651 ☑
      periumbilic region S31.155 ☑
        with penetration into peritoneal cavity S31.655 ☑
      right
        lower quadrant S31.153 ☑
          with penetration into peritoneal cavity S31.653 ☑
        upper quadrant S31.150 ☑
          with penetration into peritoneal cavity S31.650 ☑
      superficial NEC S30.871 ☑
        insect S30.861 ☑
  alveolar (process) — *see* Bite, oral cavity
  amphibian (venomous) — *see* Venom, bite, amphibian
  animal (*see also* Bite, by site)
    venomous — *see* Venom
  ankle S91.05- ☑
    superficial NEC S90.57- ☑
      insect S90.56- ☑
  antecubital space — *see* Bite, elbow
  anus S31.835 ☑
    superficial NEC S30.877 ☑
      insect S30.867 ☑
  arm (upper) S41.15- ☑
    lower — *see* Bite, forearm
    superficial NEC S40.87- ☑
      insect S40.86- ☑
  arthropod NEC — *see* Venom, bite, arthropod
  auditory canal (external) (meatus) — *see* Bite, ear
  auricle, ear — *see* Bite, ear
  axilla — *see* Bite, arm
  back (*see also* Bite, thorax, back)
    lower S31.050 ☑
      with penetration into retroperitoneal space S31.051 ☑
      superficial NEC S30.870 ☑
        insect S30.860 ☑
  bedbug — *see* Bite(s), by site, superficial, insect
  breast S21.05- ☑
    superficial NEC S20.17- ☑
      insect S20.16- ☑
  brow — *see* Bite, head, specified site NEC
  buttock S31.805 ☑
    left S31.825 ☑
    right S31.815 ☑
    superficial NEC S30.870 ☑
      insect S30.860 ☑
  calf — *see* Bite, leg
  canaliculus lacrimalis — *see* Bite, eyelid

Bite(s) — *continued*
  canthus, eye — *see* Bite, eyelid
  centipede — *see* Toxicity, venom, arthropod, centipede
  cheek (external) S01.45- ☑
    internal — *see* Bite, oral cavity
    superficial NEC S00.87 ☑
      insect S00.86 ☑
  chest wall — *see* Bite, thorax
  chigger B88.0
  chin — *see* Bite, head, specified site NEC
  clitoris — *see* Bite, vulva
  costal region — *see* Bite, thorax
  digit(s)
    hand — *see* Bite, finger
    toe — *see* Bite, toe
  ear (canal) (external) S01.35- ☑
    superficial NEC S00.47- ☑
      insect S00.46- ☑
  elbow S51.05- ☑
    superficial NEC S50.37- ☑
      insect S50.36- ☑
  epididymis — *see* Bite, testis
  epigastric region — *see* Bite, abdomen
  epiglottis — *see* Bite, neck, specified site NEC
  esophagus, cervical S11.25 ☑
    superficial NEC S10.17 ☑
      insect S10.16 ☑
  eyebrow — *see* Bite, eyelid
  eyelid S01.15- ☑
    superficial NEC S00.27- ☑
      insect S00.26- ☑
  face NEC — *see* Bite, head, specified site NEC
  finger(s) S61.259 ☑
    with
      damage to nail S61.359 ☑
    index S61.258 ☑
      with
        damage to nail S61.358 ☑
        left S61.251 ☑
          with
            damage to nail S61.351 ☑
        right S61.250 ☑
          with
            damage to nail S61.350 ☑
      superficial NEC S60.478 ☑
        insect S60.46- ☑
    little S61.25- ☑
      with
        damage to nail S61.35- ☑
      superficial NEC S60.47- ☑
        insect S60.46- ☑
    middle S61.25- ☑
      with
        damage to nail S61.35- ☑
      superficial NEC S60.47- ☑
        insect S60.46- ☑
    ring S61.25- ☑
      with
        damage to nail S61.35- ☑
      superficial NEC S60.47- ☑
        insect S60.46- ☑
    superficial NEC S60.479 ☑
      insect S60.469 ☑
    thumb — *see* Bite, thumb
  flank — *see* Bite, abdomen, wall
  flea — *see* Bite, by site, superficial, insect
  foot (except toe(s) alone) S91.35- ☑
    superficial NEC S90.87- ☑
      insect S90.86- ☑
    toe — *see* Bite, toe
  forearm S51.85- ☑
    elbow only — *see* Bite, elbow
    superficial NEC S50.87- ☑
      insect S50.86- ☑
  forehead — *see* Bite, head, specified site NEC
  genital organs, external
    female S31.552 ☑
      superficial NEC S30.876 ☑
        insect S30.866 ☑
      vagina and vulva — *see* Bite, vulva
    male S31.551 ☑
      penis — *see* Bite, penis
      scrotum — *see* Bite, scrotum
      superficial NEC S30.875 ☑
        insect S30.865 ☑

Bite(s) — *continued*
  genital organs, external — *continued*
    male — *continued*
      testes — *see* Bite, testis
  groin — *see* Bite, abdomen, wall
  gum — *see* Bite, oral cavity
  hand S61.45-☑
    finger — *see* Bite, finger
    superficial NEC S60.57-☑
      insect S60.56-☑
    thumb — *see* Bite, thumb
  head S01.95☑
    cheek — *see* Bite, cheek
    ear — *see* Bite, ear
    eyelid — *see* Bite, eyelid
    lip — *see* Bite, lip
    nose — *see* Bite, nose
    oral cavity — *see* Bite, oral cavity
    scalp — *see* Bite, scalp
    specified site NEC S01.85☑
      superficial NEC S00.87☑
        insect S00.86☑
    superficial NEC S00.97☑
      insect S00.96☑
    temporomandibular area — *see* Bite, cheek
  heel — *see* Bite, foot
  hip S71.05-☑
    superficial NEC S70.27-☑
      insect S70.26-☑
  hymen S31.45☑
  hypochondrium — *see* Bite, abdomen, wall
  hypogastric region — *see* Bite, abdomen, wall
  inguinal region — *see* Bite, abdomen, wall
  insect — *see* Bite, by site, superficial, insect
  instep — *see* Bite, foot
  interscapular region — *see* Bite, thorax, back
  jaw — *see* Bite, head, specified site NEC
  knee S81.05-☑
    superficial NEC S80.27-☑
      insect S80.26-☑
  labium (majus) (minus) — *see* Bite, vulva
  lacrimal duct — *see* Bite, eyelid
  larynx S11.015☑
    superficial NEC S10.17☑
      insect S10.16☑
  leg (lower) S81.85-☑
    ankle — *see* Bite, ankle
    foot — *see* Bite, foot
    knee — *see* Bite, knee
    superficial NEC S80.87-☑
      insect S80.86-☑
    toe — *see* Bite, toe
    upper — *see* Bite, thigh
  lip S01.551☑
    superficial NEC S00.571☑
      insect S00.561☑
  lizard (venomous) — *see* Venom, bite, reptile
  loin — *see* Bite, abdomen, wall
  lower back — *see* Bite, back, lower
  lumbar region — *see* Bite, back, lower
  malar region — *see* Bite, head, specified site NEC
  mammary — *see* Bite, breast
  marine animals (venomous) — *see* Toxicity, venom, marine animal
  mastoid region — *see* Bite, head, specified site NEC
  mouth — *see* Bite, oral cavity
  nail
    finger — *see* Bite, finger
    toe — *see* Bite, toe
  nape — *see* Bite, neck, specified site NEC
  nasal (septum) (sinus) — *see* Bite, nose
  nasopharynx — *see* Bite, head, specified site NEC
  neck S11.95☑
    involving
      cervical esophagus — *see* Bite, esophagus, cervical
      larynx — *see* Bite, larynx
      pharynx — *see* Bite, pharynx
      thyroid gland S11.15☑
      trachea — *see* Bite, trachea
    specified site NEC S11.85☑
      superficial NEC S10.87☑
        insect S10.86☑
    superficial NEC S10.97☑
      insect S10.96☑
    throat S11.85☑

Bite(s) — *continued*
  neck — *continued*
    throat — *continued*
      superficial NEC S10.17☑
        insect S10.16☑
  nose (septum) (sinus) S01.25☑
    superficial NEC S00.37☑
      insect S00.36☑
  occipital region — *see* Bite, scalp
  oral cavity S01.552☑
    superficial NEC S00.572☑
      insect S00.562☑
  orbital region — *see* Bite, eyelid
  palate — *see* Bite, oral cavity
  palm — *see* Bite, hand
  parietal region — *see* Bite, scalp
  pelvis S31.050☑
    with penetration into retroperitoneal space S31.051☑
    superficial NEC S30.870☑
      insect S30.860☑
  penis S31.25☑
    superficial NEC S30.872☑
      insect S30.862☑
  perineum
    female — *see* Bite, vulva
    male — *see* Bite, pelvis
  periocular area (with or without lacrimal passages) — *see* Bite, eyelid
  phalanges
    finger — *see* Bite, finger
    toe — *see* Bite, toe
  pharynx S11.25☑
    superficial NEC S10.17☑
      insect S10.16☑
  pinna — *see* Bite, ear
  poisonous — *see* Venom
  popliteal space — *see* Bite, knee
  prepuce — *see* Bite, penis
  pubic region — *see* Bite, abdomen, wall
  rectovaginal septum — *see* Bite, vulva
  red bug B88.0
  reptile NEC (*see also* Venom, bite, reptile)
    nonvenomous — *see* Bite, by site
    snake — *see* Venom, bite, snake
  sacral region — *see* Bite, back, lower
  sacroiliac region — *see* Bite, back, lower
  salivary gland — *see* Bite, oral cavity
  scalp S01.05☑
    superficial NEC S00.07☑
      insect S00.06☑
  scapular region — *see* Bite, shoulder
  scrotum S31.35☑
    superficial NEC S30.873☑
      insect S30.863☑
  sea-snake (venomous) — *see* Toxicity, venom, snake, sea snake
  shin — *see* Bite, leg
  shoulder S41.05-☑
    superficial NEC S40.27-☑
      insect S40.26-☑
  snake (*see also* Venom, bite, snake)
    nonvenomous — *see* Bite, by site
  spermatic cord — *see* Bite, testis
  spider (venomous) — *see* Toxicity, venom, spider
    nonvenomous — *see* Bite, by site, superficial, insect
  sternal region — *see* Bite, thorax, front
  submaxillary region — *see* Bite, head, specified site NEC
  submental region — *see* Bite, head, specified site NEC
  subungual
    finger(s) — *see* Bite, finger
    toe — *see* Bite, toe
  superficial — *see* Bite, by site, superficial
  supraclavicular fossa S11.85☑
  supraorbital — *see* Bite, head, specified site NEC
  temple, temporal region — *see* Bite, head, specified site NEC
  temporomandibular area — *see* Bite, cheek
  testis S31.35☑
    superficial NEC S30.873☑
      insect S30.863☑
  thigh S71.15-☑
    superficial NEC S70.37-☑
      insect S70.36-☑
  thorax, thoracic (wall) S21.95☑

Bite(s) — *continued*
  thorax, thoracic — *continued*
    back S21.25-☑
      with penetration into thoracic cavity S21.45-☑
    breast — *see* Bite, breast
    front S21.15-☑
      with penetration into thoracic cavity S21.35-☑
    superficial NEC S20.97☑
      back S20.47-☑
      front S20.37-☑
      insect S20.96☑
        back S20.46-☑
        front S20.36☑
  throat — *see* Bite, neck, throat
  thumb S61.05-☑
    with
      damage to nail S61.15-☑
    superficial NEC S60.37-☑
      insect S60.36-☑
  thyroid S11.15☑
    superficial NEC S10.87☑
      insect S10.86☑
  toe(s) S91.15-☑
    with
      damage to nail S91.25-☑
    great S91.15-☑
      with
        damage to nail S91.25-☑
    lesser S91.15-☑
      with
        damage to nail S91.25-☑
    superficial NEC S90.47-☑
      great S90.47-☑
      insect S90.46-☑
        great S90.46-☑
  tongue S01.552☑
  trachea S11.025☑
    superficial NEC S10.17☑
      insect S10.16☑
  tunica vaginalis — *see* Bite, testis
  tympanum, tympanic membrane — *see* Bite, ear
  umbilical region S31.155☑
  uvula — *see* Bite, oral cavity
  vagina — *see* Bite, vulva
  venomous — *see* Venom
  vocal cords S11.035☑
    superficial NEC S10.17☑
      insect S10.16☑
  vulva S31.45☑
    superficial NEC S30.874☑
      insect S30.864☑
  wrist S61.55-☑
    superficial NEC S60.87-☑
      insect S60.86-☑
Biting, cheek or lip K13.1
Biventricular failure (heart) I50.82
Björck (-Thorson) **syndrome** (malignant carcinoid) E34.0
Black
  death A20.9
  eye S00.1-☑
  hairy tongue K14.3
  heel (foot) S90.3-☑
  lung (disease) J60
  palm (hand) S60.22-☑
Blackfan-Diamond anemia or syndrome (congenital hypoplastic anemia) D61.01
Blackhead L70.0
Blackout R55
Bladder — *see* condition
Blast (air) (hydraulic) (immersion) (underwater)
  blindness S05.8X-☑
  injury
    abdomen or thorax — *see* Injury, by site
    ear (acoustic nerve trauma) — *see* Injury, nerve, acoustic, specified type NEC
  syndrome NEC T70.8
Blastoma — *see* Neoplasm, malignant, by site
  pulmonary — *see* Neoplasm, lung, malignant
Blastomycosis, blastomycotic B40.9
  Brazilian — *see* Paracoccidioidomycosis
  cutaneous B40.3
  disseminated B40.7
  European — *see* Cryptococcosis
  generalized B40.7
  keloidal B48.0
  North American B40.9

Blastomycosis, blastomycotic — *continued*
  primary pulmonary B40.0
  pulmonary B40.2
    acute B40.0
    chronic B40.1
  skin B40.3
  South American — *see* Paracoccidioidomycosis
  specified NEC B40.89
Bleb(s) R23.8
  emphysematous (lung) (solitary) J43.9
  endophthalmitis H59.43
  filtering (vitreous), after glaucoma surgery Z98.83
  inflamed (infected), postprocedural H59.40
    stage 1 H59.41
    stage 2 H59.42
    stage 3 H59.43
  lung (ruptured) J43.9
    congenital — *see* Atelectasis
    newborn P25.8
  subpleural (emphysematous) J43.9
Blebitis, postprocedural H59.40
  stage 1 H59.41
  stage 2 H59.42
  stage 3 H59.43
Bleeder (familial) (hereditary) — *see* Hemophilia
Bleeding (*see also* Hemorrhage)
  anal K62.5
  anovulatory N97.0
  atonic, following delivery O72.1
  capillary I78.8
    puerperal O72.2
  contact (postcoital) N93.0
  due to uterine subinvolution N85.3
  ear — *see* Otorrhagia
  excessive, associated with menopausal onset N92.4
  familial — *see* Defect, coagulation
  following intercourse N93.0
  gastrointestinal K92.2
  hemorrhoids — *see* Hemorrhoids
  intermenstrual (regular) N92.3
    irregular N92.1
  intraoperative — *see* Complication, intraoperative, hemorrhage
  irregular N92.6
  menopausal N92.4
  newborn, intraventricular — *see* Newborn, affected by, hemorrhage, intraventricular
  nipple N64.59
  nose R04.0
  ovulation N92.3
  postclimacteric N95.0
  postcoital N93.0
  postmenopausal N95.0
  postoperative — *see* Complication, postprocedural, hemorrhage
  preclimacteric N92.4
  pre-pubertal vaginal N93.1
  puberty (excessive, with onset of menstrual periods) N92.2
  rectum, rectal K62.5
    newborn P54.2
  tendencies — *see* Defect, coagulation
  throat R04.1
  tooth socket (post-extraction) K91.840
  umbilical stump P51.9
  uterus, uterine NEC N93.9
    climacteric N92.4
    dysfunctional or functional N93.8
    menopausal N92.4
    preclimacteric or premenopausal N92.4
    unrelated to menstrual cycle N93.9
  vagina, vaginal (abnormal) N93.9
    dysfunctional or functional N93.8
    newborn P54.6
    pre-pubertal N93.1
  vicarious N94.89
Blennorrhagia, blennorrhagic — *see* Gonorrhea
Blennorrhea (acute) (chronic) (*see also* Gonorrhea)
  inclusion (neonatal) (newborn) P39.1
  lower genitourinary tract (gonococcal) A54.00
  neonatorum (gonococcal ophthalmia) A54.31
Blepharelosis — *see* Entropion
Blepharitis (angularis) (ciliaris) (eyelid) (marginal) (nonulcerative) H01.009
  herpes zoster B02.39
  left H01.006
    lower H01.005
    upper H01.004

Blepharitis — *continued*
  right H01.003
    lower H01.002
    upper H01.001
  squamous H01.029
    left H01.026
      lower H01.025
      upper H01.024
    right H01.023
      lower H01.022
      upper H01.021
  ulcerative H01.019
    left H01.016
      lower H01.015
      upper H01.014
    right H01.013
      lower H01.012
      upper H01.011
Blepharochalasis H02.30
  congenital Q10.0
  left H02.36
    lower H02.35
    upper H02.34
  right H02.33
    lower H02.32
    upper H02.31
Blepharoclonus H02.59
Blepharoconjunctivitis H10.50- ☑
  angular H10.52- ☑
  contact H10.53- ☑
  ligneous H10.51- ☑
Blepharophimosis (eyelid) H02.529
  congenital Q10.3
  left H02.526
    lower H02.525
    upper H02.524
  right H02.523
    lower H02.522
    upper H02.521
Blepharoptosis H02.40- ☑
  congenital Q10.0
  mechanical H02.41- ☑
  myogenic H02.42- ☑
  neurogenic H02.43- ☑
  paralytic H02.43- ☑
Blepharopyorrhea, gonococcal A54.39
Blepharospasm G24.5
  drug induced G24.01
Blighted ovum O02.0
Blind (*see also* Blindness)
  bronchus (congenital) Q32.4
  loop syndrome K90.2
    congenital Q43.8
  sac, fallopian tube (congenital) Q50.6
  spot, enlarged — *see* Defect, visual field, localized, scotoma, blind spot area
  tract or tube, congenital NEC — *see* Atresia, by site
Blindness (acquired) (congenital) (both eyes) H54.0X- ☑
  blast S05.8X- ☑
  color — *see* Deficiency, color vision
  concussion S05.8X- ☑
  cortical H47.619
    left brain H47.612
    right brain H47.611
  day H53.11
  due to injury (current episode) S05.9- ☑
    sequelae — *code to* injury with seventh character S
  eclipse (total) — *see* Retinopathy, solar
  emotional (hysterical) F44.6
  face H53.16
  hysterical F44.6
  legal (both eyes) (USA definition) H54.8
  mind R48.8
  night H53.60
    abnormal dark adaptation curve H53.61
    acquired H53.62
    congenital H53.63
    specified type NEC H53.69
    vitamin A deficiency E50.5
  one eye (other eye normal) H54.40
    left (normal vision on right) H54.42- ☑
      low vision on right H54.12- ☑
    low vision, other eye H54.10
    right (normal vision on left) H54.41- ☑
      low vision on left H54.11- ☑
  psychic R48.8
  river B73.01

Blindness — *continued*
  snow — *see* Photokeratitis
  sun, solar — *see* Retinopathy, solar
  transient — *see* Disturbance, vision, subjective, loss, transient
  traumatic (current episode) S05.9- ☑
  word (developmental) F81.0
    acquired R48.0
    secondary to organic lesion R48.0
Blister (nonthermal)
  abdominal wall S30.821 ☑
  alveolar process S00.522 ☑
  ankle S90.52- ☑
  antecubital space — *see* Blister, elbow
  anus S30.827 ☑
  arm (upper) S40.82- ☑
  auditory canal — *see* Blister, ear
  auricle — *see* Blister, ear
  axilla — *see* Blister, arm
  back, lower S30.820 ☑
  beetle dermatitis L24.89
  breast S20.12- ☑
  brow S00.82 ☑
  calf — *see* Blister, leg
  canthus — *see* Blister, eyelid
  cheek S00.82 ☑
    internal S00.522 ☑
  chest wall — *see* Blister, thorax
  chin S00.82 ☑
  costal region — *see* Blister, thorax
  digit(s)
    foot — *see* Blister, toe
    hand — *see* Blister, finger
  due to burn — *see* Burn, by site, second degree
  ear S00.42- ☑
  elbow S50.32- ☑
  epiglottis S10.12 ☑
  esophagus, cervical S10.12 ☑
  eyebrow — *see* Blister, eyelid
  eyelid S00.22- ☑
  face S00.82 ☑
  fever B00.1
  finger(s) S60.429 ☑
    index S60.42- ☑
    little S60.42- ☑
    middle S60.42- ☑
    ring S60.42- ☑
  foot (except toe(s) alone) S90.82- ☑
    toe — *see* Blister, toe
  forearm S50.82- ☑
    elbow only — *see* Blister, elbow
  forehead S00.82 ☑
  fracture — *omit code*
  genital organ
    female S30.826 ☑
    male S30.825 ☑
  gum S00.522 ☑
  hand S60.52- ☑
  head S00.92 ☑
    ear — *see* Blister, ear
    eyelid — *see* Blister, eyelid
    lip S00.521 ☑
    nose S00.32 ☑
    oral cavity S00.522 ☑
    scalp S00.02 ☑
    specified site NEC S00.82 ☑
  heel — *see* Blister, foot
  hip S70.22- ☑
  interscapular region S20.429 ☑
  jaw S00.82 ☑
  knee S80.22- ☑
  larynx S10.12 ☑
  leg (lower) S80.82- ☑
    knee — *see* Blister, knee
    upper — *see* Blister, thigh
  lip S00.521 ☑
  malar region S00.82 ☑
  mammary — *see* Blister, breast
  mastoid region S00.82 ☑
  mouth S00.522 ☑
  multiple, skin, nontraumatic R23.8
  nail
    finger — *see* Blister, finger
    toe — *see* Blister, toe
  nasal S00.32 ☑
  neck S10.92 ☑

Subterms under main terms may continue to next column or page

Blister — *continued*
  neck — *continued*
    specified site NEC S10.82 ☑
      throat S10.12 ☑
    nose S00.32 ☑
    occipital region S00.02 ☑
    oral cavity S00.522 ☑
    orbital region — *see* Blister, eyelid
    palate S00.522 ☑
    palm — *see* Blister, hand
    parietal region S00.02 ☑
    pelvis S30.820 ☑
    penis S30.822 ☑
    periocular area — *see* Blister, eyelid
    phalanges
      finger — *see* Blister, finger
      toe — *see* Blister, toe
    pharynx S10.12 ☑
    pinna — *see* Blister, ear
    popliteal space — *see* Blister, knee
    scalp S00.02 ☑
    scapular region — *see* Blister, shoulder
    scrotum S30.823 ☑
    shin — *see* Blister, leg
    shoulder S40.22- ☑
    sternal region S20.329 ☑
    submaxillary region S00.82 ☑
    submental region S00.82 ☑
    subungual
      finger(s) — *see* Blister, finger
      toe(s) — *see* Blister, toe
    supraclavicular fossa S10.82 ☑
    supraorbital S00.82 ☑
    temple S00.82 ☑
    temporal region S00.82 ☑
    testis S30.823 ☑
    thermal — *see* Burn, second degree, by site
    thigh S70.32- ☑
    thorax, thoracic (wall) S20.92 ☑
      back S20.42- ☑
      front S20.32- ☑
    throat S10.12 ☑
    thumb S60.32- ☑
    toe(s) S90.42- ☑
      great S90.42- ☑
    tongue S00.522 ☑
    trachea S10.12 ☑
    tympanum, tympanic membrane — *see* Blister, ear
    upper arm — *see* Blister, arm (upper)
    uvula S00.522 ☑
    vagina S30.824 ☑
    vocal cords S10.12 ☑
    vulva S30.824 ☑
    wrist S60.82- ☑
Bloating R14.0
Bloch-Sulzberger disease or syndrome Q82.3
Block, blocked
  alveolocapillary J84.10
  arborization (heart) I45.5
  arrhythmic I45.9
  atrioventricular (incomplete) (partial) I44.30
    with atrioventricular dissociation I44.2
    complete I44.2
      congenital Q24.6
    congenital Q24.6
    first degree I44.0
    second degree (types I and II) I44.1
    specified NEC I44.39
    third degree I44.2
    types I and II I44.1
  auriculoventricular — *see* Block, atrioventricular
  bifascicular (cardiac) I45.2
  bundle-branch (complete) (false) (incomplete) I45.4
    bilateral I45.2
    left I44.7
      with right bundle branch block I45.2
      hemiblock I44.60
        anterior I44.4
        posterior I44.5
      incomplete I44.7
        with right bundle branch block I45.2
    right I45.10
      with
        left bundle branch block I45.2
        left fascicular block I45.2
      specified NEC I45.19
    Wilson's type I45.19

Block, blocked — *continued*
  cardiac I45.9
  conduction I45.9
    complete I44.2
  fascicular (left) I44.60
    anterior I44.4
    posterior I44.5
    right I45.0
    specified NEC I44.69
  foramen Magendie (acquired) G91.1
    congenital Q03.1
      with spina bifida — *see* Spina bifida, by site,
        with hydrocephalus
  heart I45.9
    bundle branch I45.4
      bilateral I45.2
    complete (atrioventricular) I44.2
    congenital Q24.6
    first degree (atrioventricular) I44.0
    second degree (atrioventricular) I44.1
    specified type NEC I45.5
    third degree (atrioventricular) I44.2
  hepatic vein I82.0
  intraventricular (nonspecific) I45.4
    bundle branch
      bilateral I45.2
  kidney N28.9
    postcystoscopic or postprocedural N99.0
  Mobitz (types I and II) I44.1
  myocardial — *see* Block, heart
  nodal I45.5
  organ or site, congenital NEC — *see* Atresia, by site
  portal (vein) I81
  second degree (types I and II) I44.1
  sinoatrial I45.5
  sinoauricular I45.5
  third degree I44.2
  trifascicular I45.3
  tubal N97.1
  vein NOS I82.90
  Wenckebach (types I and II) I44.1
Blockage — *see* Obstruction
Blocq's disease F44.4
Blood
  constituents, abnormal R78.9
  disease D75.9
  donor — *see* Donor, blood
  dyscrasia D75.9
    with
      abortion — *see* Abortion, by type, complicated
        by, hemorrhage
      ectopic pregnancy O08.1
      molar pregnancy O08.1
    following ectopic or molar pregnancy O08.1
    newborn P61.9
    puerperal, postpartum O72.3
  flukes NEC — *see* Schistosomiasis
  in
    feces K92.1
      occult R19.5
    urine — *see* Hematuria
  mole O02.0
  occult in feces R19.5
  pressure
    decreased, due to shock following injury T79.4 ☑
    examination only Z01.30
    fluctuating I99.8
    high — *see* Hypertension
      borderline R03.0
      incidental reading, without diagnosis of hyper-
        tension R03.0
    low (*see also* Hypotension)
      incidental reading, without diagnosis of hy-
        potension R03.1
  spitting — *see* Hemoptysis
  staining cornea — *see* Pigmentation, cornea, stromal
  transfusion
    reaction or complication — *see* Complications,
      transfusion
  type
    A (Rh positive) Z67.10
      Rh negative Z67.11
    AB (Rh positive) Z67.30
      Rh negative Z67.31
    B (Rh positive) Z67.20
      Rh negative Z67.21
    O (Rh positive) Z67.40
      Rh negative Z67.41

Blood — *continued*
  type — *continued*
    Rh (positive) Z67.90
      negative Z67.91
  vessel rupture — *see* Hemorrhage
  vomiting — *see* Hematemesis
Blood-forming organs, disease D75.9
Bloodgood's disease — *see* Mastopathy, cystic
Bloom (-Machacek)(-Torre) **syndrome** Q82.8
Blount's disease or osteochondrosis — *see* Osteochon-
    drosis, juvenile, tibia
Blue
  baby Q24.9
  diaper syndrome E72.09
  dome cyst (breast) — *see* Cyst, breast
  dot cataract Q12.0
  nevus D22.9
  sclera Q13.5
    with fragility of bone and deafness Q78.0
  toe syndrome I75.02- ☑
Blueness — *see* Cyanosis
Blues, postpartal O90.6
  baby O90.6
Blurring, visual H53.8
Blushing (abnormal) (excessive) R23.2
BMI — *see* Body, mass index
Boarder, hospital NEC Z76.4
  accompanying sick person Z76.3
  healthy infant or child Z76.2
    foundling Z76.1
Bockhart's impetigo L01.02
Bodechtel-Guttman disease (subacute sclerosing pa-
    nencephalitis) A81.1
Boder-Sedgwick syndrome (ataxia-telangiectasia)
    G11.3
Body, bodies
  Aschoff's — *see* Myocarditis, rheumatic
  asteroid, vitreous — *see* Deposit, crystalline
  cytoid (retina) — *see* Occlusion, artery, retina
  drusen (degenerative) (macula) (retinal) (*see also* De-
    generation, macula, drusen)
    optic disc — *see* Drusen, optic disc
  foreign — *see* Foreign body
  loose
    joint, except knee — *see* Loose, body, joint
      knee M23.4- ☑
    sheath, tendon — *see* Disorder, tendon, specified
      type NEC
  mass index (BMI)
    adult
      19.9 or less Z68.1
      20.0-20.9 Z68.20
      21.0-21.9 Z68.21
      22.0-22.9 Z68.22
      23.0-23.9 Z68.23
      24.0-24.9 Z68.24
      25.0-25.9 Z68.25
      26.0-26.9 Z68.26
      27.0-27.9 Z68.27
      28.0-28.9 Z68.28
      29.0-29.9 Z68.29
      30.0-30.9 Z68.30
      31.0-31.9 Z68.31
      32.0-32.9 Z68.32
      33.0-33.9 Z68.33
      34.0-34.9 Z68.34
      35.0-35.9 Z68.35
      36.0-36.9 Z68.36
      37.0-37.9 Z68.37
      38.0-38.9 Z68.38
      39.0-39.9 Z68.39
      40.0-44.9 Z68.41
      45.0-49.9 Z68.42
      50.0-59.9 Z68.43
      60.0-69.9 Z68.44
      70 and over Z68.45
    pediatric
      5th percentile to less than 85th percentile for
        age Z68.52
      85th percentile to less than 95th percentile for
        age Z68.53
      less than fifth percentile for age Z68.51
      greater than or equal to ninety-fifth percentile
        for age Z68.54
  Mooser's A75.2
  rice (*see also* Loose, body, joint)
    knee M23.4- ☑
  rocking F98.4

Boeck's
   disease or sarcoid — *see* Sarcoidosis
   lupoid (miliary) D86.3
Boerhaave's syndrome (spontaneous esophageal rupture) K22.3
Boggy
   cervix N88.8
   uterus N85.8
Boil (*see also* Furuncle, by site)
   Aleppo B55.1
   Baghdad B55.1
   Delhi B55.1
   lacrimal
      gland — *see* Dacryoadenitis
      passages (duct) (sac) — *see* Inflammation, lacrimal, passages, acute
   Natal B55.1
   orbit, orbital — *see* Abscess, orbit
   tropical B55.1
Bold hives — *see* Urticaria
Bombé, iris — *see* Membrane, pupillary
Bone — *see* condition
Bonnevie-Ullrich syndrome (*see also* Turner's syndrome) Q87.1
Bonnier's syndrome H81.8 ☑
Bonvale dam fever T73.3 ☑
Bony block of joint — *see* Ankylosis
BOOP (bronchiolitis obliterans organized pneumonia) J84.89
Borderline
   diabetes mellitus R73.03
   hypertension R03.0
   osteopenia M85.8- ☑
   pelvis, with obstruction during labor O65.1
   personality F60.3
Borna disease A83.9
Bornholm disease B33.0
Boston exanthem A88.0
Botalli, ductus (patent) (persistent) Q25.0
Bothriocephalus latus infestation B70.0
Botulism (foodborne intoxication) A05.1
   infant A48.51
   non-foodborne A48.52
   wound A48.52
Bouba — *see* Yaws
Bouchard's nodes (with arthropathy) M15.2
Bouffée délirante F23
Bouillaud's disease or syndrome (rheumatic heart disease) I01.9
Bourneville's disease Q85.1
Boutonniere deformity (finger) — *see* Deformity, finger, boutonniere
Bouveret (-Hoffmann) **syndrome** (paroxysmal tachycardia) I47.9
Bovine heart — *see* Hypertrophy, cardiac
Bowel — *see* condition
Bowen's
   dermatosis (precancerous) — *see* Neoplasm, skin, in situ
   disease — *see* Neoplasm, skin, in situ
   epithelioma — *see* Neoplasm, skin, in situ
   type
      epidermoid carcinoma-in-situ — *see* Neoplasm, skin, in situ
      intraepidermal squamous cell carcinoma — *see* Neoplasm, skin, in situ
Bowing
   femur (*see also* Deformity, limb, specified type NEC, thigh)
      congenital Q68.3
   fibula (*see also* Deformity, limb, specified type NEC, lower leg)
      congenital Q68.4
   forearm — *see* Deformity, limb, specified type NEC, forearm
   leg(s), long bones, congenital Q68.5
   radius — *see* Deformity, limb, specified type NEC, forearm
   tibia (*see also* Deformity, limb, specified type NEC, lower leg)
      congenital Q68.4
Bowleg(s) (acquired) M21.16- ☑
   congenital Q68.5
   rachitic E64.3
Boyd's dysentery A03.2
Brachial — *see* condition
Brachycardia R00.1

Brachycephaly Q75.0
Bradley's disease A08.19
Bradyarrhythmia, cardiac I49.8
Bradycardia (sinoatrial) (sinus) (vagal) R00.1
   neonatal P29.12
   reflex G90.09
   tachycardia syndrome I49.5
Bradykinesia R25.8
Bradypnea R06.89
Bradytachycardia I49.5
Brailsford's disease or osteochondrosis — *see* Osteochondrosis, juvenile, radius
Brain (*see also* condition)
   death G93.82
   syndrome — *see* Syndrome, brain
Branched-chain amino-acid disorder E71.2
Branchial — *see* condition
   cartilage, congenital Q18.2
Branchiogenic remnant (in neck) Q18.0
Brandt's syndrome (acrodermatitis enteropathica) E83.2
Brash (water) R12
Bravais-jacksonian epilepsy — *see* Epilepsy, localization-related, symptomatic, with simple partial seizures
Braxton Hicks contractions — *see* False, labor
Brazilian leishmaniasis B55.2
BRBPR K62.5
Break, retina (without detachment) H33.30- ☑
   with retinal detachment — *see* Detachment, retina
   horseshoe tear H33.31- ☑
   multiple H33.33- ☑
   round hole H33.32- ☑
Breakdown
   device, graft or implant (*see also* Complications, by site and type, mechanical) T85.618 ☑
      arterial graft NEC — *see* Complication, cardiovascular device, mechanical, vascular
      breast (implant) T85.41 ☑
      catheter NEC T85.618 ☑
         cystostomy T83.010 ☑
         dialysis (renal) T82.41 ☑
            intraperitoneal T85.611 ☑
         Hopkins T83.018 ☑
         ileostomy T83.018 ☑
         infusion NEC T82.514 ☑
            cranial T85.610- ☑
            epidural T85.610 ☑
            intrathecal T85.610 ☑
            spinal T85.610 ☑
            subarachnoid T85.610 ☑
            subdural T85.610 ☑
         nephrostomy T83.012 ☑
         urethral indwelling T83.011 ☑
         urinary NEC T83.018 ☑
         urostomy T83.018 ☑
      electronic (electrode) (pulse generator) (stimulator)
         bone T84.310 ☑
         cardiac T82.119 ☑
            electrode T82.110 ☑
            pulse generator T82.111 ☑
            specified type NEC T82.118 ☑
         nervous system — *see* Complication, prosthetic device, mechanical, electronic nervous system stimulator
         urinary — *see* Complication, genitourinary, device, urinary, mechanical
      fixation, internal (orthopedic) NEC — *see* Complication, fixation device, mechanical
      gastrointestinal — *see* Complications, prosthetic device, mechanical, gastrointestinal device
      genital NEC T83.418 ☑
         intrauterine contraceptive device T83.31 ☑
         penile prosthesis (cylinder) (implanted) (pump) (resevoir) T83.410 ☑
         testicular prosthesis T83.411 ☑
      heart NEC — *see* Complication, cardiovascular device, mechanical
      intrathecal infusion pump T85.615 ☑
      joint prosthesis — *see* Complications..., joint prosthesis,internal, mechanical, by site
      nervous system, specified device NEC T85.615 ☑
      ocular NEC — *see* Complications, prosthetic device, mechanical, ocular device
      orthopedic NEC — *see* Complication, orthopedic, device, mechanical
      specified NEC T85.618 ☑

Breakdown — *continued*
   device, graft or implant (*see also* Complications, by site and type, mechanical) — *continued*
      subcutaneous device pocket
         nervous system prosthetic device, implant, or graft T85.890 ☑
         other internal prosthetic device, implant, or graft T85.898 ☑
      sutures, permanent T85.612 ☑
         used in bone repair — *see* Complications, fixation device, internal (orthopedic), mechanical
      urinary NEC T83.118 ☑
         graft T83.21 ☑
         sphincter, implanted T83.111 ☑
         stent (ileal conduit) (nephroureteral) T83.113 ☑
            ureteral indwelling T83.112 ☑
      vascular NEC — *see* Complication, cardiovascular device, mechanical
      ventricular intracranial shunt T85.01 ☑
   nervous F48.8
   perineum O90.1
   respirator J95.850
      specified NEC J95.859
   ventilator J95.850
      specified NEC J95.859
Breast (*see also* condition)
   buds E30.1
      in newborn P96.89
   dense R92.2
   nodule (*see also* Lump, breast) N63.0
Breath
   foul R19.6
   holder, child R06.89
   holding spell R06.89
   shortness R06.02
Breathing
   labored — *see* Hyperventilation
   mouth R06.5
      causing malocclusion M26.5 ☑
   periodic R06.3
      high altitude G47.32
Breathlessness R06.81
Breda's disease — *see* Yaws
Breech presentation (mother) O32.1 ☑
   causing obstructed labor O64.1 ☑
   footling O32.8 ☑
      causing obstructed labor O64.8 ☑
   incomplete O32.8 ☑
      causing obstructed labor O64.8 ☑
Breisky's disease N90.4
Brennemann's syndrome I88.0
Brenner
   tumor (benign) D27.9
      borderline malignancy D39.1- ☑
      malignant C56
      proliferating D39.1- ☑
Bretonneau's disease or angina A36.0
Breus' mole O02.0
Brevicollis Q76.49
Brickmakers' anemia B76.9 [D63.8]
Bridge, myocardial Q24.5
Bright red blood per rectum (BRBPR) K62.5
Bright's disease (*see also* Nephritis)
   arteriosclerotic — *see* Hypertension, kidney
Brill (-Zinsser) **disease** (recrudescent typhus) A75.1
   flea-borne A75.2
   louse-borne A75.1
Brill-Symmers' disease C82.90
Brion-Kayser disease — *see* Fever, parathyroid
Briquet's disorder or syndrome F45.0
Brissaud's
   infantilism or dwarfism E23.0
   motor-verbal tic F95.2
Brittle
   bones disease Q78.0
   nails L60.3
      congenital Q84.6
Broad (*see also* condition)
   beta disease E78.2
   ligament laceration syndrome N83.8
Broad- or floating-betalipoproteinemia E78.2
Brock's syndrome (atelectasis due to enlarged lymph nodes) J98.19
Brocq-Duhring disease (dermatitis herpetiformis) L13.0
Brodie's abscess or disease M86.8X- ☑

Broken
arches (see also Deformity, limb, flat foot)
arm (meaning upper limb) — see Fracture, arm
back — see Fracture, vertebra
bone — see Fracture
implant or internal device — see Complications, by
    site and type, mechanical
leg (meaning lower limb) — see Fracture, leg
nose S02.2 ☑
tooth, teeth — see Fracture, tooth
Bromhidrosis, bromidrosis L75.0
Bromidism, bromism G92
chronic (dependence) F13.20
due to
    correct substance properly administered — see
        Table of Drugs and Chemicals, by drug, ad-
        verse effect
    overdose or wrong substance given or taken —
        see Table of Drugs and Chemicals, by drug,
        poisoning
Bromidrosiphobia F40.298
Bronchi, bronchial — see condition
Bronchiectasis (cylindrical) (diffuse) (fusiform) (localized)
    (saccular) J47.9
with
    acute
        bronchitis J47.0
        lower respiratory infection J47.0
    exacerbation (acute) J47.1
congenital Q33.4
tuberculous NEC — see Tuberculosis, pulmonary
Bronchiolectasis — see Bronchiectasis
Bronchiolitis (acute) (infective) (subacute) J21.9
with
    bronchospasm or obstruction J21.9
    influenza, flu or grippe — see Influenza, with, res-
        piratory manifestations NEC
chemical (chronic) J68.4
    acute J68.0
chronic (fibrosing) (obliterative) J44.9
due to
    external agent — see Bronchitis, acute, due to
    human metapneumovirus J21.1
    respiratory syncytial virus J21.0
    specified organism NEC J21.8
fibrosa obliterans J44.9
influenzal — see Influenza, with, respiratory manifes-
    tations NEC
obliterans J42
    with organizing pneumonia (BOOP) J84.89
obliterative (chronic) (subacute) J44.9
    due to chemicals, gases, fumes or vapors (inhala-
        tion) J68.4
    due to fumes or vapors J68.4
respiratory, interstitial lung disease J84.115
Bronchitis (diffuse) (fibrinous) (hypostatic) (infective)
    (membranous) J40
with
    influenza, flu or grippe — see Influenza, with, res-
        piratory manifestations NEC
    obstruction (airway) (lung) J44.9
    tracheitis (l5 years of age and above) J40
        acute or subacute J20.9
        chronic J42
        under l5 years of age J20.9
acute or subacute (with bronchospasm or obstruction)
    J20.9
    with
        bronchiectasis J47.0
        chronic obstructive pulmonary disease J44.9
    chemical (due to gases, fumes or vapors) J68.0
    due to
        fumes or vapors J68.0
        Haemophilus influenzae J20.1
        Mycoplasma pneumoniae J20.0
        radiation J70.0
        specified organism NEC J20.8
        Streptococcus J20.2
        virus
            coxsackie J20.3
            echovirus J20.7
            parainfluenzae J20.4
            respiratory syncytial J20.5
            rhinovirus J20.6
        viral NEC J20.8
allergic (acute) J45.909
    with
        exacerbation (acute) J45.901

Bronchitis — continued
allergic — continued
    with — continued
        status asthmaticus J45.902
    arachidic T17.528 ☑
    aspiration (due to fumes or vapors) J68.0
    asthmatic J45.9 ☑
        chronic J44.9
            with
                acute lower respiratory infection J44.0
                exacerbation (acute) J44.1
    capillary — see Pneumonia, broncho
    caseous (tuberculous) A15.5
    Castellani's A69.8
    catarrhal (l5 years of age and above) J40
        acute — see Bronchitis, acute
        chronic J41.0
        under l5 years of age J20.9
    chemical (acute) (subacute) J68.0
        chronic J68.4
        due to fumes or vapors J68.0
            chronic J68.4
    chronic J42
        with
            airways obstruction J44.9
            tracheitis (chronic) J42
        asthmatic (obstructive) J44.9
        catarrhal J41.0
        chemical (due to fumes or vapors) J68.4
        due to
            chemicals, gases, fumes or vapors (inhalation)
                J68.4
            radiation J70.1
            tobacco smoking J41.0
        emphysematous J44.9
        mucopurulent J41.1
        non-obstructive J41.0
        obliterans J44.9
        obstructive J44.9
        purulent J41.1
        simple J41.0
    croupous — see Bronchitis, acute
    due to gases, fumes or vapors (chemical) J68.0
    emphysematous (obstructive) J44.9
    exudative — see Bronchitis, acute
    fetid J41.1
    grippal — see Influenza, with, respiratory manifesta-
        tions NEC
    in those under l5 years age — see Bronchitis, acute
        chronic — see Bronchitis, chronic
    influenzal — see Influenza, with, respiratory manifes-
        tations NEC
    mixed simple and mucopurulent J41.8
    moulder's J62.8
    mucopurulent (chronic) (recurrent) J41.1
        acute or subacute J20.9
        simple (mixed) J41.8
    obliterans (chronic) J44.9
    obstructive (chronic) (diffuse) J44.9
    pituitous J41.1
    pneumococcal, acute or subacute J20.2
    pseudomembranous, acute or subacute — see Bron-
        chitis, acute
    purulent (chronic) (recurrent) J41.1
        acute or subacute — see Bronchitis, acute
    putrid J41.1
    senile (chronic) J42
    simple and mucopurulent (mixed) J41.8
    smokers' J41.0
    spirochetal NEC A69.8
    subacute — see Bronchitis, acute
    suppurative (chronic) J41.1
        acute or subacute — see Bronchitis, acute
    tuberculous A15.5
    under l5 years of age — see Bronchitis, acute
        chronic — see Bronchitis, chronic
    viral NEC, acute or subacute (see also Bronchitis, acute)
        J20.8
Bronchoalveolitis J18.0
Bronchoaspergillosis B44.1
Bronchocele meaning goiter E04.0
Broncholithiasis J98.09
    tuberculous NEC A15.5
Bronchomalacia J98.09
    congenital Q32.2
Bronchomycosis NOS B49 [J99]
    candidal B37.1
Bronchopleuropneumonia — see Pneumonia, broncho

Bronchopneumonia — see Pneumonia, broncho
Bronchopneumonitis — see Pneumonia, broncho
Bronchopulmonary — see condition
Bronchopulmonitis — see Pneumonia, broncho
Bronchorrhagia (see Hemoptysis)
Bronchorrhea J98.09
    acute J20.9
    chronic (infective) (purulent) J42
Bronchospasm (acute) J98.01
with
    bronchiolitis, acute J21.9
    bronchitis, acute (conditions in J20) — see Bronchi-
        tis, acute
    due to external agent — see condition, respiratory,
        acute, due to
    exercise induced J45.990
Bronchospirochetosis A69.8
    Castellani A69.8
Bronchostenosis J98.09
Bronchus — see condition
Brontophobia F40.220
Bronze baby syndrome P83.88
Brooke's tumor — see Neoplasm, skin, benign
Brown enamel of teeth (hereditary) K00.5
Brown's sheath syndrome H50.61- ☑
Brown-Séquard disease, paralysis or syndrome
    G83.81
Bruce sepsis A23.0
Brucellosis (infection) A23.9
    abortus A23.1
    canis A23.3
    dermatitis A23.9
    melitensis A23.0
    mixed A23.8
    sepsis A23.9
        melitensis A23.0
        specified NEC A23.8
    suis A23.2
Bruck-de Lange disease Q87.1
Bruck's disease — see Deformity, limb
BRUE (brief resolved unexplained event) R68.13
Brugsch's syndrome Q82.8
Bruise (skin surface intact) (see also Contusion)
with
    open wound — see Wound, open
    internal organ — see Injury, by site
    newborn P54.5
    scalp, due to birth injury, newborn P12.3
    umbilical cord O69.5 ☑
Bruit (arterial) R09.89
    cardiac R01.1
Brush burn — see Abrasion, by site
Bruton's X-linked agammaglobulinemia D80.0
Bruxism
    psychogenic F45.8
    sleep related G47.63
Bubbly lung syndrome P27.0
Bubo I88.8
    blennorrhagic (gonococcal) A54.89
    chancroidal A57
    climatic A55
    due to Haemophilus ducreyi A57
    gonococcal A54.89
    indolent (nonspecific) I88.8
    inguinal (nonspecific) I88.8
        chancroidal A57
        climatic A55
        due to H. ducreyi A57
        infective I88.8
    scrofulous (tuberculous) A18.2
    soft chancre A57
    suppurating — see Lymphadenitis, acute
    syphilitic (primary) A51.0
        congenital A50.07
    tropical A55
    virulent (chancroidal) A57
Bubonic plague A20.0
Bubonocele — see Hernia, inguinal
Buccal — see condition
Buchanan's disease or osteochondrosis M91.0
Buchem's syndrome (hyperostosis corticalis) M85.2
Bucket-handle fracture or tear (semilunar cartilage)
    — see Tear, meniscus
Budd-Chiari syndrome (hepatic vein thrombosis) I82.0
Budgerigar fancier's disease or lung J67.2
Buds
    breast E30.1

Buds — *continued*
  breast — *continued*
    in newborn P96.89
Buerger's disease (thromboangiitis obliterans) I73.1
Bulbar — *see* condition
Bulbus cordis (left ventricle) (persistent) Q21.8
Bulimia (nervosa) F50.2
  atypical F50.9
  normal weight F50.9
Bulky
  stools R19.5
  uterus N85.2
Bulla (e) R23.8
  lung (emphysematous) (solitary) J43.9
    newborn P25.8
Bullet wound (*see also* Wound, open)
  fracture — *code as* Fracture, by site
  internal organ — *see* Injury, by site
Bundle
  branch block (complete) (false) (incomplete) — *see* Block, bundle-branch
  of His — *see* condition
Bunion M21.61- ☑
  tailor's M21.62- ☑
Bunionette M21.62- ☑
Buphthalmia, buphthalmos (congenital) Q15.0
Burdwan fever B55.0
Bürger-Grütz disease or syndrome E78.3
Buried
  penis (congenital) Q55.64
    acquired N48.83
  roots K08.3
Burke's syndrome K86.89
Burkitt
  cell leukemia C91.0- ☑
  lymphoma (malignant) C83.7- ☑
    small noncleaved, diffuse C83.7- ☑
    spleen C83.77
    undifferentiated C83.7- ☑
  tumor C83.7- ☑
  type
    acute lymphoblastic leukemia C91.0- ☑
    undifferentiated C83.7- ☑
Burn (electricity) (flame) (hot gas, liquid or hot object) (radiation) (steam) (thermal) T30.0
  abdomen, abdominal (muscle) (wall) T21.02 ☑
    first degree T21.12 ☑
    second degree T21.22 ☑
    third degree T21.32 ☑
  above elbow T22.039 ☑
    first degree T22.139 ☑
    left T22.032 ☑
      first degree T22.132 ☑
      second degree T22.232 ☑
      third degree T22.332 ☑
    right T22.031 ☑
      first degree T22.131 ☑
      second degree T22.231 ☑
      third degree T22.331 ☑
    second degree T22.239 ☑
    third degree T22.339 ☑
  acid (caustic) (internal) — *see* Corrosion, by site
  alimentary tract NEC T28.2 ☑
    esophagus T28.1 ☑
    mouth T28.0 ☑
    pharynx T28.0 ☑
  alkaline (caustic) (external) (internal) — *see* Corrosion, by site
  ankle T25.019 ☑
    first degree T25.119 ☑
    left T25.012 ☑
      first degree T25.112 ☑
      second degree T25.212 ☑
      third degree T25.312 ☑
    multiple with foot — *see* Burn, lower, limb, multiple, ankle and foot
    right T25.011 ☑
      first degree T25.111 ☑
      second degree T25.211 ☑
      third degree T25.311 ☑
    second degree T25.219 ☑
    third degree T25.319 ☑
  anus — *see* Burn, buttock
  arm (lower) (upper) — *see* Burn, upper, limb
  axilla T22.049 ☑

Burn — *continued*
  axilla — *continued*
    first degree T22.149 ☑
    left T22.042 ☑
      first degree T22.142 ☑
      second degree T22.242 ☑
      third degree T22.342 ☑
    right T22.041 ☑
      first degree T22.141 ☑
      second degree T22.241 ☑
      third degree T22.341 ☑
    second degree T22.249 ☑
    third degree T22.349 ☑
  back (lower) T21.04 ☑
    first degree T21.14 ☑
    second degree T21.24 ☑
    third degree T21.34 ☑
    upper T21.03 ☑
      first degree T21.13 ☑
      second degree T21.23 ☑
      third degree T21.33 ☑
  blisters — *code as* Burn, second degree, by site
  breast(s) — *see* Burn, chest wall
  buttock(s) T21.05 ☑
    first degree T21.15 ☑
    second degree T21.25 ☑
    third degree T21.35 ☑
  calf T24.039 ☑
    first degree T24.139 ☑
    left T24.032 ☑
      first degree T24.132 ☑
      second degree T24.232 ☑
      third degree T24.332 ☑
    right T24.031 ☑
      first degree T24.131 ☑
      second degree T24.231 ☑
      third degree T24.331 ☑
    second degree T24.239 ☑
    third degree T24.339 ☑
  canthus (eye) — *see* Burn, eyelid
  caustic acid or alkaline — *see* Corrosion, by site
  cervix T28.3 ☑
  cheek T20.06 ☑
    first degree T20.16 ☑
    second degree T20.26 ☑
    third degree T20.36 ☑
  chemical (acids) (alkalines) (caustics) (external) (internal) — *see* Corrosion, by site
  chest wall T21.01 ☑
    first degree T21.11 ☑
    second degree T21.21 ☑
    third degree T21.31 ☑
  chin T20.03 ☑
    first degree T20.13 ☑
    second degree T20.23 ☑
    third degree T20.33 ☑
  colon T28.2 ☑
  conjunctiva (and cornea) — *see* Burn, cornea
  cornea (and conjunctiva) T26.1- ☑
    chemical — *see* Corrosion, cornea
  corrosion (external) (internal) — *see* Corrosion, by site
  deep necrosis of underlying tissue — *code as* Burn, third degree, by site
  dorsum of hand T23.069 ☑
    first degree T23.169 ☑
    left T23.062 ☑
      first degree T23.162 ☑
      second degree T23.262 ☑
      third degree T23.362 ☑
    right T23.061 ☑
      first degree T23.161 ☑
      second degree T23.261 ☑
      third degree T23.361 ☑
    second degree T23.269 ☑
    third degree T23.369 ☑
  due to ingested chemical agent — *see* Corrosion, by site
  ear (auricle) (external) (canal) T20.01 ☑
    first degree T20.11 ☑
    second degree T20.21 ☑
    third degree T20.31 ☑
  elbow T22.029 ☑
    first degree T22.129 ☑
    left T22.022 ☑
      first degree T22.122 ☑
      second degree T22.222 ☑

Burn — *continued*
  elbow — *continued*
    left — *continued*
      third degree T22.322 ☑
    right T22.021 ☑
      first degree T22.121 ☑
      second degree T22.221 ☑
      third degree T22.321 ☑
    second degree T22.229 ☑
    third degree T22.329 ☑
  epidermal loss — *code as* Burn, second degree, by site
  erythema, erythematous — *code as* Burn, first degree, by site
  esophagus T28.1 ☑
  extent (percentage of body surface)
    less than 10 percent T31.0
    10-19 percent T31.10
      with 0-9 percent third degree burns T31.10
      with 10-19 percent third degree burns T31.11
    20-29 percent T31.20
      with 0-9 percent third degree burns T31.20
      with 10-19 percent third degree burns T31.21
      with 20-29 percent third degree burns T31.22
    30-39 percent T31.30
      with 0-9 percent third degree burns T31.30
      with 10-19 percent third degree burns T31.31
      with 20-29 percent third degree burns T31.32
      with 30-39 percent third degree burns T31.33
    40-49 percent T31.40
      with 0-9 percent third degree burns T31.40
      with 10-19 percent third degree burns T31.41
      with 20-29 percent third degree burns T31.42
      with 30-39 percent third degree burns T31.43
      with 40-49 percent third degree burns T31.44
    50-59 percent T31.50
      with 0-9 percent third degree burns T31.50
      with 10-19 percent third degree burns T31.51
      with 20-29 percent third degree burns T31.52
      with 30-39 percent third degree burns T31.53
      with 40-49 percent third degree burns T31.54
      with 50-59 percent third degree burns T31.55
    60-69 percent T31.60
      with 0-9 percent third degree burns T31.60
      with 10-19 percent third degree burns T31.61
      with 20-29 percent third degree burns T31.62
      with 30-39 percent third degree burns T31.63
      with 40-49 percent third degree burns T31.64
      with 50-59 percent third degree burns T31.65
      with 60-69 percent third degree burns T31.66
    70-79 percent T31.70
      with 0-9 percent third degree burns T31.70
      with 10-19 percent third degree burns T31.71
      with 20-29 percent third degree burns T31.72
      with 30-39 percent third degree burns T31.73
      with 40-49 percent third degree burns T31.74
      with 50-59 percent third degree burns T31.75
      with 60-69 percent third degree burns T31.76
      with 70-79 percent third degree burns T31.77
    80-89 percent T31.80
      with 0-9 percent third degree burns T31.80
      with 10-19 percent third degree burns T31.81
      with 20-29 percent third degree burns T31.82
      with 30-39 percent third degree burns T31.83
      with 40-49 percent third degree burns T31.84
      with 50-59 percent third degree burns T31.85
      with 60-69 percent third degree burns T31.86
      with 70-79 percent third degree burns T31.87
      with 80-89 percent third degree burns T31.88
    90 percent or more T31.90
      with 0-9 percent third degree burns T31.90
      with 10-19 percent third degree burns T31.91
      with 20-29 percent third degree burns T31.92
      with 30-39 percent third degree burns T31.93
      with 40-49 percent third degree burns T31.94
      with 50-59 percent third degree burns T31.95
      with 60-69 percent third degree burns T31.96
      with 70-79 percent third degree burns T31.97
      with 80-89 percent third degree burns T31.98
      with 90 percent or more third degree burns T31.99
  extremity — *see* Burn, limb
  eye(s) and adnexa T26.4- ☑
    with resulting rupture and destruction of eyeball T26.2- ☑
    conjunctival sac — *see* Burn, cornea
    cornea — *see* Burn, cornea
    lid — *see* Burn, eyelid
    periocular area — *see* Burn, eyelid

Burn — *continued*
  eye(s) and adnexa — *continued*
    specified site NEC T26.3- ☑
  eyeball — *see* Burn, eye
  eyelid(s) T26.0- ☑
    chemical — *see* Corrosion, eyelid
  face — *see* Burn, head
  finger T23.029 ☑
    first degree T23.129 ☑
    left T23.022 ☑
      first degree T23.122 ☑
      second degree T23.222 ☑
      third degree T23.322 ☑
    multiple sites (without thumb) T23.039 ☑
      with thumb T23.049 ☑
        first degree T23.149 ☑
        left T23.042 ☑
          first degree T23.142 ☑
          second degree T23.242 ☑
          third degree T23.342 ☑
        right T23.041 ☑
          first degree T23.141 ☑
          second degree T23.241 ☑
          third degree T23.341 ☑
      second degree T23.249 ☑
      third degree T23.349 ☑
    first degree T23.139 ☑
    left T23.032 ☑
      first degree T23.132 ☑
      second degree T23.232 ☑
      third degree T23.332 ☑
    right T23.031 ☑
      first degree T23.131 ☑
      second degree T23.231 ☑
      third degree T23.331 ☑
    second degree T23.239 ☑
    third degree T23.339 ☑
    right T23.021 ☑
      first degree T23.121 ☑
      second degree T23.221 ☑
      third degree T23.321 ☑
    second degree T23.229 ☑
    third degree T23.329 ☑
  flank — *see* Burn, abdominal wall
  foot T25.029 ☑
    first degree T25.129 ☑
    left T25.022 ☑
      first degree T25.122 ☑
      second degree T25.222 ☑
      third degree T25.322 ☑
    multiple with ankle — *see* Burn, lower, limb, multiple, ankle and foot
    right T25.021 ☑
      first degree T25.121 ☑
      second degree T25.221 ☑
      third degree T25.321 ☑
    second degree T25.229 ☑
    third degree T25.329 ☑
  forearm T22.019 ☑
    first degree T22.119 ☑
    left T22.012 ☑
      first degree T22.112 ☑
      second degree T22.212 ☑
      third degree T22.312 ☑
    right T22.011 ☑
      first degree T22.111 ☑
      second degree T22.211 ☑
      third degree T22.311 ☑
    second degree T22.219 ☑
    third degree T22.319 ☑
  forehead T20.06 ☑
    first degree T20.16 ☑
    second degree T20.26 ☑
    third degree T20.36 ☑
  fourth degree — *code as* Burn, third degree, by site
  friction — *see* Burn, by site
  from swallowing caustic or corrosive substance NEC — *see* Corrosion, by site
  full thickness skin loss — *code as* Burn, third degree, by site
  gastrointestinal tract NEC T28.2 ☑
    from swallowing caustic or corrosive substance T28.7 ☑
  genital organs
    external
      female T21.07 ☑

Burn — *continued*
  genital organs — *continued*
    external — *continued*
      female — *continued*
        first degree T21.17 ☑
        second degree T21.27 ☑
        third degree T21.37 ☑
      male T21.06 ☑
        first degree T21.16 ☑
        second degree T21.26 ☑
        third degree T21.36 ☑
    internal T28.3 ☑
    from caustic or corrosive substance T28.8 ☑
  groin — *see* Burn, abdominal wall
  hand(s) T23.009 ☑
    back — *see* Burn, dorsum of hand
    finger — *see* Burn, finger
    first degree T23.109 ☑
    left T23.002 ☑
      first degree T23.102 ☑
      second degree T23.202 ☑
      third degree T23.302 ☑
    multiple sites with wrist T23.099 ☑
      first degree T23.199 ☑
      left T23.092 ☑
        first degree T23.192 ☑
        second degree T23.292 ☑
        third degree T23.392 ☑
      right T23.091 ☑
        first degree T23.191 ☑
        second degree T23.291 ☑
        third degree T23.391 ☑
      second degree T23.299 ☑
      third degree T23.399 ☑
    palm — *see* Burn, palm
    right T23.001 ☑
      first degree T23.101 ☑
      second degree T23.201 ☑
      third degree T23.301 ☑
    second degree T23.209 ☑
    third degree T23.309 ☑
    thumb — *see* Burn, thumb
  head (and face) (and neck) T20.00 ☑
    cheek — *see* Burn, cheek
    chin — *see* Burn, chin
    ear — *see* Burn, ear
    eye(s) only — *see* Burn, eye
    first degree T20.10 ☑
    forehead — *see* Burn, forehead
    lip — *see* Burn, lip
    multiple sites T20.09 ☑
      first degree T20.19 ☑
      second degree T20.29 ☑
      third degree T20.39 ☑
    neck — *see* Burn, neck
    nose — *see* Burn, nose
    scalp — *see* Burn, scalp
    second degree T20.20 ☑
    third degree T20.30 ☑
  hip(s) — *see* Burn, thigh
  inhalation — *see* Burn, respiratory tract
    caustic or corrosive substance (fumes) — *see* Corrosion, respiratory tract
  internal organ(s) T28.40 ☑
    alimentary tract T28.2 ☑
      esophagus T28.1 ☑
    eardrum T28.41 ☑
    esophagus T28.1 ☑
    from caustic or corrosive substance (swallowing) NEC — *see* Corrosion, by site
    genitourinary T28.3 ☑
    mouth T28.0 ☑
    pharynx T28.0 ☑
    respiratory tract — *see* Burn, respiratory tract
    specified organ NEC T28.49 ☑
  interscapular region — *see* Burn, back, upper
  intestine (large) (small) T28.2 ☑
  knee T24.029 ☑
    first degree T24.129 ☑
    left T24.022 ☑
      first degree T24.122 ☑
      second degree T24.222 ☑
      third degree T24.322 ☑
    right T24.021 ☑
      first degree T24.121 ☑
      second degree T24.221 ☑

Burn — *continued*
  knee — *continued*
    right — *continued*
      third degree T24.321 ☑
    second degree T24.229 ☑
    third degree T24.329 ☑
  labium (majus) (minus) — *see* Burn, genital organs, external, female
  lacrimal apparatus, duct, gland or sac — *see* Burn, eye, specified site NEC
  larynx T27.0 ☑
    with lung T27.1 ☑
  leg(s) (lower) (upper) — *see* Burn, lower, limb
  lightning — *see* Burn, by site
  limb(s)
    lower (except ankle or foot alone) — *see* Burn, lower, limb
    upper — *see* Burn, upper limb
  lip(s) T20.02 ☑
    first degree T20.12 ☑
    second degree T20.22 ☑
    third degree T20.32 ☑
  lower
    back — *see* Burn, back
    limb T24.009 ☑
      ankle — *see* Burn, ankle
      calf — *see* Burn, calf
      first degree T24.109 ☑
      foot — *see* Burn, foot
      hip — *see* Burn, thigh
      knee — *see* Burn, knee
      left T24.002 ☑
        first degree T24.102 ☑
        second degree T24.202 ☑
        third degree T24.302 ☑
      multiple sites, except ankle and foot T24.099 ☑
        ankle and foot T25.099 ☑
          first degree T25.199 ☑
          left T25.092 ☑
            first degree T25.192 ☑
            second degree T25.292 ☑
            third degree T25.392 ☑
          right T25.091 ☑
            first degree T25.191 ☑
            second degree T25.291 ☑
            third degree T25.391 ☑
          second degree T25.299 ☑
          third degree T25.399 ☑
        first degree T24.199 ☑
        left T24.092 ☑
          first degree T24.192 ☑
          second degree T24.292 ☑
          third degree T24.392 ☑
        right T24.091 ☑
          first degree T24.191 ☑
          second degree T24.291 ☑
          third degree T24.391 ☑
        second degree T24.299 ☑
        third degree T24.399 ☑
      right T24.001 ☑
        first degree T24.101 ☑
        second degree T24.201 ☑
        third degree T24.301 ☑
      second degree T24.209 ☑
      thigh — *see* Burn, thigh
      third degree T24.309 ☑
      toe — *see* Burn, toe
  lung (with larynx and trachea) T27.1 ☑
  mouth T28.0 ☑
  neck T20.07 ☑
    first degree T20.17 ☑
    second degree T20.27 ☑
    third degree T20.37 ☑
  nose (septum) T20.04 ☑
    first degree T20.14 ☑
    second degree T20.24 ☑
    third degree T20.34 ☑
  ocular adnexa — *see* Burn, eye
  orbit region — *see* Burn, eyelid
  palm T23.059 ☑
    first degree T23.159 ☑
    left T23.052 ☑
      first degree T23.152 ☑
      second degree T23.252 ☑
      third degree T23.352 ☑
    right T23.051 ☑

☑ Additional Character Required — Refer to the Tabular List for Character Selection   ▽ Subterms under main terms may continue to next column or page

Burn — *continued*
  palm — *continued*
    right — *continued*
      first degree T23.151 ☑
      second degree T23.251 ☑
      third degree T23.351 ☑
    second degree T23.259 ☑
    third degree T23.359 ☑
  partial thickness — *code as* Burn, unspecified degree, by site
  pelvis — *see* Burn, trunk
  penis — *see* Burn, genital organs, external, male
  perineum
    female — *see* Burn, genital organs, external, female
    male — *see* Burn, genital organs, external, male
  periocular area — *see* Burn, eyelid
  pharynx T28.0 ☑
  rectum T28.2 ☑
  respiratory tract T27.3 ☑
    larynx — *see* Burn, larynx
    specified part NEC T27.2 ☑
    trachea — *see* Burn, trachea
  sac, lacrimal — *see* Burn, eye, specified site NEC
  scalp T20.05 ☑
    first degree T20.15 ☑
    second degree T20.25 ☑
    third degree T20.35 ☑
  scapular region T22.069 ☑
    first degree T22.169 ☑
    left T22.062 ☑
      first degree T22.162 ☑
      second degree T22.262 ☑
      third degree T22.362 ☑
    right T22.061 ☑
      first degree T22.161 ☑
      second degree T22.261 ☑
      third degree T22.361 ☑
    second degree T22.269 ☑
    third degree T22.369 ☑
  sclera — *see* Burn, eye, specified site NEC
  scrotum — *see* Burn, genital organs, external, male
  shoulder T22.059 ☑
    first degree T22.159 ☑
    left T22.052 ☑
      first degree T22.152 ☑
      second degree T22.252 ☑
      third degree T22.352 ☑
    right T22.051 ☑
      first degree T22.151 ☑
      second degree T22.251 ☑
      third degree T22.351 ☑
    second degree T22.259 ☑
    third degree T22.359 ☑
  stomach T28.2 ☑
  temple — *see* Burn, head
  testis — *see* Burn, genital organs, external, male
  thigh T24.019 ☑
    first degree T24.119 ☑
    left T24.012 ☑
      first degree T24.112 ☑
      second degree T24.212 ☑
      third degree T24.312 ☑
    right T24.011 ☑
      first degree T24.111 ☑
      second degree T24.211 ☑
      third degree T24.311 ☑
    second degree T24.219 ☑
    third degree T24.319 ☑
  thorax (external) — *see* Burn, trunk
  throat (meaning pharynx) T28.0 ☑
  thumb(s) T23.019 ☑
    first degree T23.119 ☑
    left T23.012 ☑
      first degree T23.112 ☑
      second degree T23.212 ☑
      third degree T23.312 ☑
    multiple sites with fingers T23.049 ☑
      first degree T23.149 ☑
      left T23.042 ☑
        first degree T23.142 ☑
        second degree T23.242 ☑
        third degree T23.342 ☑
      right T23.041 ☑
        first degree T23.141 ☑
        second degree T23.241 ☑
        third degree T23.341 ☑

Burn — *continued*
  thumb(s) — *continued*
    multiple sites with fingers — *continued*
      second degree T23.249 ☑
      third degree T23.349 ☑
    right T23.011 ☑
      first degree T23.111 ☑
      second degree T23.211 ☑
      third degree T23.311 ☑
    second degree T23.219 ☑
    third degree T23.319 ☑
  toe T25.039 ☑
    first degree T25.139 ☑
    left T25.032 ☑
      first degree T25.132 ☑
      second degree T25.232 ☑
      third degree T25.332 ☑
    right T25.031 ☑
      first degree T25.131 ☑
      second degree T25.231 ☑
      third degree T25.331 ☑
    second degree T25.239 ☑
    third degree T25.339 ☑
  tongue T28.0 ☑
  tonsil(s) T28.0 ☑
  trachea T27.0 ☑
    with lung T27.1 ☑
  trunk T21.00 ☑
    abdominal wall — *see* Burn, abdominal wall
    anus — *see* Burn, buttock
    axilla — *see* Burn, upper limb
    back — *see* Burn, back
    breast — *see* Burn, chest wall
    buttock — *see* Burn, buttock
    chest wall — *see* Burn, chest wall
    first degree T21.10 ☑
    flank — *see* Burn, abdominal wall
    genital
      female — *see* Burn, genital organs, external, female
      male — *see* Burn, genital organs, external, male
    groin — *see* Burn, abdominal wall
    interscapular region — *see* Burn, back, upper
    labia — *see* Burn, genital organs, external, female
    lower back — *see* Burn, back
    penis — *see* Burn, genital organs, external, male
    perineum
      female — *see* Burn, genital organs, external, female
      male — *see* Burn, genital organs, external, male
    scapula region — *see* Burn, scapular region
    scrotum — *see* Burn, genital organs, external, male
    second degree T21.20 ☑
    specified site NEC T21.09 ☑
      first degree T21.19 ☑
      second degree T21.29 ☑
      third degree T21.39 ☑
    testes — *see* Burn, genital organs, external, male
    third degree T21.30 ☑
    upper back — *see* Burn, back, upper
    vulva — *see* Burn, genital organs, external, female
  unspecified site with extent of body surface involved specified
    less than 10 percent T31.0
    10-19 percent (0-9 percent third degree) T31.10
      with 10-19 percent third degree T31.11
    20-29 percent (0-9 percent third degree) T31.20
      with
        10-19 percent third degree T31.21
        20-29 percent third degree T31.22
    30-39 percent (0-9 percent third degree) T31.30
      with
        10-19 percent third degree T31.31
        20-29 percent third degree T31.32
        30-39 percent third degree T31.33
    40-49 percent (0-9 percent third degree) T31.40
      with
        10-19 percent third degree T31.41
        20-29 percent third degree T31.42
        30-39 percent third degree T31.43
        40-49 percent third degree T31.44
    50-59 percent (0-9 percent third degree) T31.50
      with
        10-19 percent third degree T31.51
        20-29 percent third degree T31.52
        30-39 percent third degree T31.53
        40-49 percent third degree T31.54

Burn — *continued*
  unspecified site with extent of body surface involved specified — *continued*
    50-59 percent — *continued*
      with — *continued*
        50-59 percent third degree T31.55
    60-69 percent (0-9 percent third degree) T31.60
      with
        10-19 percent third degree T31.61
        20-29 percent third degree T31.62
        30-39 percent third degree T31.63
        40-49 percent third degree T31.64
        50-59 percent third degree T31.65
        60-69 percent third degree T31.66
    70-79 percent (0-9 percent third degree) T31.70
      with
        10-19 percent third degree T31.71
        20-29 percent third degree T31.72
        30-39 percent third degree T31.73
        40-49 percent third degree T31.74
        50-59 percent third degree T31.75
        60-69 percent third degree T31.76
        70-79 percent third degree T31.77
    80-89 percent (0-9 percent third degree) T31.80
      with
        10-19 percent third degree T31.81
        20-29 percent third degree T31.82
        30-39 percent third degree T31.83
        40-49 percent third degree T31.84
        50-59 percent third degree T31.85
        60-69 percent third degree T31.86
        70-79 percent third degree T31.87
        80-89 percent third degree T31.88
    90 percent or more (0-9 percent third degree) T31.90
      with
        10-19 percent third degree T31.91
        20-29 percent third degree T31.92
        30-39 percent third degree T31.93
        40-49 percent third degree T31.94
        50-59 percent third degree T31.95
        60-69 percent third degree T31.96
        70-79 percent third degree T31.97
        80-89 percent third degree T31.98
        90-99 percent third degree T31.99
  upper limb T22.00 ☑
    above elbow — *see* Burn, above elbow
    axilla — *see* Burn, axilla
    elbow — *see* Burn, elbow
    first degree T22.10 ☑
    forearm — *see* Burn, forearm
    hand — *see* Burn, hand
    interscapular region — *see* Burn, back, upper
    multiple sites T22.099 ☑
      first degree T22.199 ☑
      left T22.092 ☑
        first degree T22.192 ☑
        second degree T22.292 ☑
        third degree T22.392 ☑
      right T22.091 ☑
        first degree T22.191 ☑
        second degree T22.291 ☑
        third degree T22.391 ☑
      second degree T22.299 ☑
      third degree T22.399 ☑
    scapular region — *see* Burn, scapular region
    second degree T22.20 ☑
    shoulder — *see* Burn, shoulder
    third degree T22.30 ☑
    wrist — *see* Burn, wrist
  uterus T28.3 ☑
  vagina T28.3 ☑
  vulva — *see* Burn, genital organs, external, female
  wrist T23.079 ☑
    first degree T23.179 ☑
    left T23.072 ☑
      first degree T23.172 ☑
      second degree T23.272 ☑
      third degree T23.372 ☑
    multiple sites with hand T23.099 ☑
      first degree T23.199 ☑
      left T23.092 ☑
        first degree T23.192 ☑
        second degree T23.292 ☑
        third degree T23.392 ☑
      right T23.091 ☑
        first degree T23.191 ☑

☜ Subterms under main terms may continue to next column or page   ☑ Additional Character Required — Refer to the Tabular List for Character Selection   45

Burn — Burn

Index

Burn — Calcification

Burn — *continued*
wrist — *continued*
multiple sites with hand — *continued*
right — *continued*
second degree T23.291 ☑
third degree T23.391 ☑
second degree T23.299 ☑
third degree T23.399 ☑
right T23.071 ☑
first degree T23.171 ☑
second degree T23.271 ☑
third degree T23.371 ☑
second degree T23.279 ☑
third degree T23.379 ☑
Burnett's syndrome E83.52
Burning
feet syndrome E53.9
sensation R20.8
tongue K14.6
Burn-out (state) Z73.0
Burns' disease or osteochondrosis — *see* Osteochondrosis, juvenile, ulna
Bursa — *see* condition
Bursitis M71.9
Achilles — *see* Tendinitis, Achilles
adhesive — *see* Bursitis, specified NEC
ankle — *see* Enthesopathy, lower limb, ankle, specified type NEC
calcaneal — *see* Enthesopathy, foot, specified type NEC
collateral ligament, tibial — *see* Bursitis, tibial collateral
due to use, overuse, pressure (*see also* Disorder, soft tissue, due to use, specified type NEC)
specified NEC — *see* Disorder, soft tissue, due to use, specified NEC
Duplay's M75.0 ☑
elbow NEC M70.3- ☑
olecranon M70.2- ☑
finger — *see* Disorder, soft tissue, due to use, specified type NEC, hand
foot — *see* Enthesopathy, foot, specified type NEC
gonococcal A54.49
gouty — *see* Gout
hand M70.1- ☑
hip NEC M70.7- ☑
trochanteric M70.6- ☑
infective NEC M71.10
abscess — *see* Abscess, bursa
ankle M71.17- ☑
elbow M71.12- ☑
foot M71.17- ☑
hand M71.14- ☑
hip M71.15- ☑
knee M71.16- ☑
multiple sites M71.19
shoulder M71.11- ☑
specified site NEC M71.18
wrist M71.13- ☑
ischial — *see* Bursitis, hip
knee NEC M70.5- ☑
prepatellar M70.4- ☑
occupational NEC (*see also* Disorder, soft tissue, due to, use)
olecranon — *see* Bursitis, elbow, olecranon
pharyngeal J39.1
popliteal — *see* Bursitis, knee
prepatellar M70.4- ☑
radiohumeral M77.8
rheumatoid M06.20
ankle M06.27- ☑
elbow M06.22- ☑
foot joint M06.27- ☑
hand joint M06.24- ☑
hip M06.25- ☑
knee M06.26- ☑
multiple site M06.29
shoulder M06.21- ☑
vertebra M06.28
wrist M06.23- ☑
scapulohumeral — *see* Bursitis, shoulder
semimembranous muscle (knee) — *see* Bursitis, knee
shoulder M75.5- ☑
adhesive — *see* Capsulitis, adhesive
specified NEC M71.50
ankle M71.57- ☑

Bursitis — *continued*
specified — *continued*
due to use, overuse or pressure — *see* Disorder, soft tissue, due to, use
elbow M71.52- ☑
foot M71.57- ☑
hand M71.54- ☑
hip M71.55- ☑
knee M71.56- ☑
shoulder — *see* Bursitis, shoulder
specified site NEC M71.58
tibial collateral M76.4- ☑
wrist M71.53- ☑
subacromial — *see* Bursitis, shoulder
subcoracoid — *see* Bursitis, shoulder
subdeltoid — *see* Bursitis, shoulder
syphilitic A52.78
Thornwaldt, Tornwaldt J39.2
tibial collateral M76.4- ☑
toe — *see* Enthesopathy, foot, specified type NEC
trochanteric (area) — *see* Bursitis, hip, trochanteric
wrist — *see* Bursitis, hand
Bursopathy M71.9
specified type NEC M71.80
ankle M71.87- ☑
elbow M71.82- ☑
foot M71.87- ☑
hand M71.84- ☑
hip M71.85- ☑
knee M71.86- ☑
multiple sites M71.89
shoulder M71.81- ☑
specified site NEC M71.88
wrist M71.83- ☑
Burst stitches or sutures (complication of surgery) T81.31 ☑
external operation wound T81.31 ☑
internal operation wound T81.32 ☑
Buruli ulcer A31.1
Bury's disease L95.1
Buschke's
disease B45.3
scleredema — *see* Sclerosis, systemic
Busse-Buschke disease B45.3
Buttock — *see* condition
Button
Biskra B55.1
Delhi B55.1
oriental B55.1
Buttonhole deformity (finger) — *see* Deformity, finger, boutonniere
Bwamba fever A92.8
Byssinosis J66.0
Bywaters' syndrome T79.5 ☑

C

Cachexia R64
cancerous R64
cardiac — *see* Disease, heart
dehydration E86.0
due to malnutrition R64
exophthalmic — *see* Hyperthyroidism
heart — *see* Disease, heart
hypophyseal E23.0
hypopituitary E23.0
lead — *see* Poisoning, lead
malignant R64
marsh — *see* Malaria
nervous F48.8
old age R54
paludal — *see* Malaria
pituitary E23.0
renal N28.9
saturnine — *see* Poisoning, lead
senile R54
Simmonds' E23.0
splenica D73.0
strumipriva E03.4
tuberculous NEC — *see* Tuberculosis
Café, au lait spots L81.3
Caffeine-induced
anxiety disorder F15.980
sleep disorder F15.982
Caffey's syndrome Q78.8
Caisson disease T70.3 ☑
Cake kidney Q63.1

Caked breast (puerperal, postpartum) O92.79
Calabar swelling B74.3
Calcaneal spur — *see* Spur, bone, calcaneal
Calcaneo-apophysitis M92.8
Calcareous — *see* condition
Calcicosis J62.8
Calciferol (vitamin D) deficiency E55.9
with rickets E55.0
Calcification
adrenal (capsule) (gland) E27.49
tuberculous E35 [B90.8]
aorta I70.0
artery (annular) — *see* Arteriosclerosis
auricle (ear) — *see* Disorder, pinna, specified type NEC
basal ganglia G23.8
bladder N32.89
due to Schistosoma hematobium B65.0
brain (cortex) — *see* Calcification, cerebral
bronchus J98.09
bursa M71.40
ankle M71.47- ☑
elbow M71.42- ☑
foot M71.47- ☑
hand M71.44- ☑
hip M71.45- ☑
knee M71.46- ☑
multiple sites M71.49
shoulder M75.3- ☑
specified site NEC M71.48
wrist M71.43- ☑
cardiac — *see* Degeneration, myocardial
cerebral (cortex) G93.89
artery I67.2
cervix (uteri) N88.8
choroid plexus G93.89
conjunctiva — *see* Concretion, conjunctiva
corpora cavernosa (penis) N48.89
cortex (brain) — *see* Calcification, cerebral
dental pulp (nodular) K04.2
dentinal papilla K00.4
fallopian tube N83.8
falx cerebri G96.19
gallbladder K82.8
general E83.59
heart (*see also* Degeneration, myocardial)
valve — *see* Endocarditis
idiopathic infantile arterial (IIAC) Q28.8
intervertebral cartilage or disc (postinfective) — *see* Disorder, disc, specified NEC
intracranial — *see* Calcification, cerebral
joint — *see* Disorder, joint, specified type NEC
kidney N28.89
tuberculous N29 [B90.1]
larynx (senile) J38.7
lens — *see* Cataract, specified NEC
lung (active) (postinfectional) J98.4
tuberculous B90.9
lymph gland or node (postinfectional) I89.8
tuberculous (*see also* Tuberculosis, lymph gland) B90.8
mammographic R92.1
massive (paraplegic) — *see* Myositis, ossificans, in, quadriplegia
medial — *see* Arteriosclerosis, extremities
meninges (cerebral) (spinal) G96.19
metastatic E83.59
Mönckeberg's — *see* Arteriosclerosis, extremities
muscle M61.9
due to burns — *see* Myositis, ossificans, in, burns
paralytic — *see* Myositis, ossificans, in, quadriplegia
specified type NEC M61.40
ankle M61.47- ☑
foot M61.47- ☑
forearm M61.43- ☑
hand M61.44- ☑
lower leg M61.46- ☑
multiple sites M61.49
pelvic region M61.45- ☑
shoulder region M61.41- ☑
specified site NEC M61.48
thigh M61.45- ☑
upper arm M61.42- ☑
myocardium, myocardial — *see* Degeneration, myocardial
ovary N83.8
pancreas K86.89
penis N48.89

Calcification — continued
- periarticular — see Disorder, joint, specified type NEC
- pericardium (see also Pericarditis) I31.1
- pineal gland E34.8
- pleura J94.8
  - postinfectional J94.8
  - tuberculous NEC B90.9
- pulpal (dental) (nodular) K04.2
- sclera H15.89
- spleen D73.89
- subcutaneous L94.2
- suprarenal (capsule) (gland) E27.49
- tendon (sheath) (see also Tenosynovitis, specified type NEC)
  - with bursitis, synovitis or tenosynovitis — see Tendinitis, calcific
- trachea J39.8
- ureter N28.89
- uterus N85.8
- vitreous — see Deposit, crystalline

Calcified — see Calcification

Calcinosis (interstitial) (tumoral) (universalis) E83.59
- with Raynaud's phenomenon, esophageal dysfunction, sclerodactyly, telangiectasia (CREST syndrome) M34.1
- circumscripta (skin) L94.2
- cutis L94.2

Calciphylaxis (see also Calcification, by site) E83.59

Calcium
- deposits — see Calcification, by site
- metabolism disorder E83.50
- salts or soaps in vitreous — see Deposit, crystalline

Calciuria R82.99

Calculi — see Calculus

Calculosis, intrahepatic — see Calculus, bile duct

Calculus, calculi, calculous
- ampulla of Vater — see Calculus, bile duct
- anuria (impacted) (recurrent) (see also Calculus, urinary) N20.9
- appendix K38.1
- bile duct (common) (hepatic) K80.50
  - with
    - calculus of gallbladder — see Calculus, gallbladder and bile duct
    - cholangitis K80.30
      - with
        - cholecystitis — see Calculus, bile duct, with cholecystitis
        - obstruction K80.31
      - acute K80.32
        - with
          - chronic cholangitis K80.36
            - with obstruction K80.37
          - obstruction K80.33
      - chronic K80.34
        - with
          - acute cholangitis K80.36
            - with obstruction K80.37
          - obstruction K80.35
    - cholecystitis (with cholangitis) K80.40
      - with obstruction K80.41
      - acute K80.42
        - with
          - chronic cholecystitis K80.46
            - with obstruction K80.47
          - obstruction K80.43
      - chronic K80.44
        - with
          - acute cholecystitis K80.46
            - with obstruction K80.47
          - obstruction K80.45
- biliary (see also Calculus, gallbladder)
  - specified NEC K80.80
    - with obstruction K80.81
- bilirubin, multiple — see Calculus, gallbladder
- bladder (encysted) (impacted) (urinary) (diverticulum) N21.0
- bronchus J98.09
- calyx (kidney) (renal) — see Calculus, kidney
- cholesterol (pure) (solitary) — see Calculus, gallbladder
- common duct (bile) — see Calculus, bile duct
- conjunctiva — see Concretion, conjunctiva
- cystic N21.0
  - duct — see Calculus, gallbladder
- dental (subgingival) (supragingival) K03.6
- diverticulum
  - bladder N21.0
  - kidney N20.0

Calculus, calculi, calculous — continued
- epididymis N50.89
- gallbladder K80.20
  - with
    - bile duct calculus — see Calculus, gallbladder and bile duct
    - cholecystitis K80.10
      - with obstruction K80.11
      - acute K80.00
        - with
          - chronic cholecystitis K80.12
            - with obstruction K80.13
          - obstruction K80.01
      - chronic K80.10
        - with
          - acute cholecystitis K80.12
            - with obstruction K80.13
          - obstruction K80.11
    - specified NEC K80.18
      - with obstruction K80.19
    - obstruction K80.21
- gallbladder and bile duct K80.70
  - with
    - cholecystitis K80.60
      - with obstruction K80.61
      - acute K80.62
        - with
          - chronic cholecystitis K80.66
            - with obstruction K80.67
          - obstruction K80.63
      - chronic K80.64
        - with
          - acute cholecystitis K80.66
            - with obstruction K80.67
          - obstruction K80.65
    - obstruction K80.71
- hepatic (duct) — see Calculus, bile duct
- ileal conduit N21.8
- intestinal (impaction) (obstruction) K56.49
- kidney (impacted) (multiple) (pelvis) (recurrent) (staghorn) N20.0
  - with calculus, ureter N20.2
  - congenital Q63.8
- lacrimal passages — see Dacryolith
- liver (impacted) — see Calculus, bile duct
- lung J98.4
- mammographic R92.1
- nephritic (impacted) (recurrent) — see Calculus, kidney
- nose J34.89
- pancreas (duct) K86.89
- parotid duct or gland K11.5
- pelvis, encysted — see Calculus, kidney
- prostate N42.0
- pulmonary J98.4
- pyelitis (impacted) (recurrent) N20.0
  - with hydronephrosis N13.2
- pyelonephritis (impacted) (recurrent) N20 ☑
  - with hydronephrosis N13.2
- renal (impacted) (recurrent) — see Calculus, kidney
- salivary (duct) (gland) K11.5
- seminal vesicle N50.89
- staghorn — see Calculus, kidney
- Stensen's duct K11.5
- stomach K31.89
- sublingual duct or gland K11.5
  - congenital Q38.4
- submandibular duct, gland or region K11.5
- submaxillary duct, gland or region K11.5
- suburethral N21.8
- tonsil J35.8
- tooth, teeth (subgingival) (supragingival) K03.6
- tunica vaginalis N50.89
- ureter (impacted) (recurrent) N20.1
  - with calculus, kidney N20.2
    - with hydronephrosis N13.2
      - with infection N13.6
- urethra (impacted) N21.1
- urinary (duct) (impacted) (passage) (tract) N20.9
  - with hydronephrosis N13.2
    - with infection N13.6
  - in (due to)
  - lower N21.9
    - specified NEC N21.8
- vagina N89.8
- vesical (impacted) N21.0
- Wharton's duct K11.5
- xanthine E79.8 [N22]

Calicectasis N28.89

Caliectasis N28.89

California
- disease B38.9
- encephalitis A83.5

Caligo cornea — see Opacity, cornea, central

Callositas, callosity (infected) L84

Callus (infected) L84
- bone — see Osteophyte
  - excessive, following fracture — code as Sequelae of fracture

CALME (childhood asymmetric labium majus enlargement) N90.61

Calorie deficiency or malnutrition (see also Malnutrition) E46

Calvé-Perthes disease — see Legg-Calvé-Perthes disease

Calvé's disease — see Osteochondrosis, juvenile, spine

Calvities — see Alopecia, androgenic

Cameroon fever — see Malaria

Camptocormia (hysterical) F44.4

Camurati-Engelmann syndrome Q78.3

Canal (see also condition)
- atrioventricular common Q21.2

Canaliculitis (lacrimal) (acute) (subacute) H04.33- ☑
- Actinomyces A42.89
- chronic H04.42- ☑

Canavan's disease E75.29

Canceled procedure (surgical) Z53.9
- because of
  - contraindication Z53.09
    - smoking Z53.01
  - left against medical advice (AMA) Z53.21
  - patient's decision Z53.20
    - for reasons of belief or group pressure Z53.1
    - specified reason NEC Z53.29
  - specified reason NEC Z53.8

Cancer (see also Neoplasm, by site, malignant)
- bile duct type liver C22.1
- blood — see Leukemia
- breast (see also Neoplasm, breast, malignant) C50.91- ☑
- hepatocellular C22.0
- lung (see also Neoplasm, lung, malignant) C34.90
- ovarian (see also Neoplasm ovary, malignant) C56.9
- unspecified site (primary) C80.1

Cancer (o)**phobia** F45.29

Cancerous — see Neoplasm, malignant, by site

Cancrum oris A69.0

Candidiasis, candidal B37.9
- balanitis B37.42
- bronchitis B37.1
- cheilitis B37.83
- congenital P37.5
- cystitis B37.41
- disseminated B37.7
- endocarditis B37.6
- enteritis B37.82
- esophagitis B37.81
- intertrigo B37.2
- lung B37.1
- meningitis B37.5
- mouth B37.0
- nails B37.2
- neonatal P37.5
- onychia B37.2
- oral B37.0
- osteomyelitis B37.89
- otitis externa B37.84
- paronychia B37.2
- perionyxis B37.2
- pneumonia B37.1
- proctitis B37.82
- pulmonary B37.1
- pyelonephritis B37.49
- sepsis B37.7
- skin B37.2
- specified site NEC B37.89
- stomatitis B37.0
- systemic B37.7
- urethritis B37.41
- urogenital site NEC B37.49
- vagina B37.3
- vulva B37.3
- vulvovaginitis B37.3

Candidid L30.2

Candidosis — see Candidiasis

Candiru infection or infestation B88.8

Canities (premature) L67.1

Canities — *continued*
congenital Q84.2
Canker (mouth) (sore) K12.Ø
rash A38.9
Cannabinosis J66.2
Cannabis induced
anxiety disorder F12.98Ø
psychotic disorder F12.959
sleep disorder F12.988
Canton fever A75.9
Cantrell's syndrome Q87.89
Capillariasis (intestinal) B81.1
hepatic B83.8
Capillary — *see* condition
Caplan's syndrome — *see* Rheumatoid, lung
Capsule — *see* condition
Capsulitis (joint) (*see also* Enthesopathy)
adhesive (shoulder) M75.Ø- ☑
hepatic K65.8
labyrinthine — *see* Otosclerosis, specified NEC
thyroid EØ6.9
Caput
crepitus Q75.8
medusae I86.8
succedaneum P12.81
Car sickness T75.3 ☑
Carapata (disease) A68.Ø
Carate — *see* Pinta
Carbon lung J6Ø
Carbuncle LØ2.93
abdominal wall LØ2.231
anus K61.Ø
auditory canal, external — *see* Abscess, ear, external
auricle ear — *see* Abscess, ear, external
axilla LØ2.43- ☑
back (any part) LØ2.232
breast N61.1
buttock LØ2.33
cheek (external) LØ2.Ø3
chest wall LØ2.233
chin LØ2.Ø3
corpus cavernosum N48.21
ear (any part) (external) (middle) — *see* Abscess, ear, external
external auditory canal — *see* Abscess, ear, external
eyelid — *see* Abscess, eyelid
face NEC LØ2.Ø3
femoral (region) — *see* Carbuncle, lower limb
finger — *see* Carbuncle, hand
flank LØ2.231
foot LØ2.63- ☑
forehead LØ2.Ø3
genital — *see* Abscess, genital
gluteal (region) LØ2.33
groin LØ2.234
hand LØ2.53- ☑
head NEC LØ2.831
heel — *see* Carbuncle, foot
hip — *see* Carbuncle, lower limb
kidney — *see* Abscess, kidney
knee — *see* Carbuncle, lower limb
labium (majus) (minus) N76.4
lacrimal
gland — *see* Dacryoadenitis
passages (duct) (sac) — *see* Inflammation, lacrimal, passages, acute
leg — *see* Carbuncle, lower limb
lower limb LØ2.43- ☑
malignant A22.Ø
navel LØ2.236
neck LØ2.13
nose (external) (septum) J34.Ø
orbit, orbital — *see* Abscess, orbit
palmar (space) — *see* Carbuncle, hand
partes posteriores LØ2.33
pectoral region LØ2.233
penis N48.21
perineum LØ2.235
pinna — *see* Abscess, ear, external
popliteal — *see* Carbuncle, lower limb
scalp LØ2.831
seminal vesicle N49.Ø
shoulder — *see* Carbuncle, upper limb
specified site NEC LØ2.838
temple (region) LØ2.Ø3
thumb — *see* Carbuncle, hand
toe — *see* Carbuncle, foot

Carbuncle — *continued*
trunk LØ2.239
abdominal wall LØ2.231
back LØ2.232
chest wall LØ2.233
groin LØ2.234
perineum LØ2.235
umbilicus LØ2.236
umbilicus LØ2.236
upper limb LØ2.43- ☑
urethra N34.Ø
vulva N76.4
Carbunculus — *see* Carbuncle
Carcinoid (tumor) — *see* Tumor, carcinoid
Carcinoidosis E34.Ø
Carcinoma (malignant) (*see also* Neoplasm, by site, malignant)
acidophil
specified site — *see* Neoplasm, malignant, by site
unspecified site C75.1
acidophil-basophil, mixed
specified site — *see* Neoplasm, malignant, by site
unspecified site C75.1
adnexal (skin) — *see* Neoplasm, skin, malignant
adrenal cortical C74.Ø- ☑
alveolar — *see* Neoplasm, lung, malignant
cell — *see* Neoplasm, lung, malignant
ameloblastic C41.1
upper jaw (bone) C41.Ø
apocrine
breast — *see* Neoplasm, breast, malignant
specified site NEC — *see* Neoplasm, skin, malignant
unspecified site C44.99
basal cell (pigmented) (*see also* Neoplasm, skin, malignant) C44.91
fibro-epithelial — *see* Neoplasm, skin, malignant
morphea — *see* Neoplasm, skin, malignant
multicentric — *see* Neoplasm, skin, malignant
basaloid
basal-squamous cell, mixed — *see* Neoplasm, skin, malignant
basophil
specified site — *see* Neoplasm, malignant, by site
unspecified site C75.1
basophil-acidophil, mixed
specified site — *see* Neoplasm, malignant, by site
unspecified site C75.1
basosquamous — *see* Neoplasm, skin, malignant
bile duct
with hepatocellular, mixed C22.Ø
liver C22.1
specified site NEC — *see* Neoplasm, malignant, by site
unspecified site C22.1
branchial or branchiogenic C1Ø.4
bronchial or bronchogenic — *see* Neoplasm, lung, malignant
bronchiolar — *see* Neoplasm, lung, malignant
bronchioloalveolar — *see* Neoplasm, lung, malignant
C cell
specified site — *see* Neoplasm, malignant, by site
unspecified site C73
ceruminous C44.29- ☑
cervix uteri
in situ DØ6.9
endocervix DØ6.Ø
exocervix DØ6.1
specified site NEC DØ6.7
chorionic
specified site — *see* Neoplasm, malignant, by site
unspecified site
female C58
male C62.9Ø
chromophobe
specified site — *see* Neoplasm, malignant, by site
unspecified site C75.1
cloacogenic
specified site — *see* Neoplasm, malignant, by site
unspecified site C21.2
diffuse type
specified site — *see* Neoplasm, malignant, by site
unspecified site C16.9
duct (cell)
with Paget's disease — *see* Neoplasm, breast, malignant

Carcinoma — *continued*
duct — *continued*
infiltrating
with lobular carcinoma (in situ)
specified site — *see* Neoplasm, malignant, by site
unspecified site (female) C5Ø.91- ☑
male C5Ø.92- ☑
specified site — *see* Neoplasm, malignant, by site
unspecified site (female) C5Ø.91- ☑
male C5Ø.92- ☑
ductal
with lobular
specified site — *see* Neoplasm, malignant, by site
unspecified site (female) C5Ø.91- ☑
male C5Ø.92- ☑
ductular, infiltrating
specified site — *see* Neoplasm, malignant, by site
unspecified site (female) C5Ø.91- ☑
male C5Ø.92- ☑
embryonal
liver C22.7
endometrioid
specified site — *see* Neoplasm, malignant, by site
unspecified site
female C56.9
male C61
eosinophil
specified site — *see* Neoplasm, malignant, by site
unspecified site C75.1
epidermoid (*see also* Neoplasm, skin, malignant)
in situ, Bowen's type — *see* Neoplasm, skin, in situ
fibroepithelial, basal cell — *see* Neoplasm, skin, malignant
follicular
with papillary (mixed) C73
moderately differentiated C73
pure follicle C73
specified site — *see* Neoplasm, malignant, by site
trabecular C73
unspecified site C73
well differentiated C73
generalized, with unspecified primary site C8Ø.Ø
glycogen-rich — *see* Neoplasm, breast, malignant
granulosa cell C56- ☑
hepatic cell C22.Ø
hepatocellular C22.Ø
with bile duct, mixed C22.Ø
fibrolamellar C22.Ø
hepatocholangiolitic C22.Ø
Hurthle cell C73
in
adenomatous
polyposis coli C18.9
pleomorphic adenoma — *see* Neoplasm, salivary glands, malignant
situ — *see* Carcinoma-in-situ
infiltrating
duct
with lobular
specified site — *see* Neoplasm, malignant, by site
unspecified site (female) C5Ø.91- ☑
male C5Ø.92- ☑
with Paget's disease — *see* Neoplasm, breast, malignant
specified site — *see* Neoplasm, malignant
unspecified site (female) C5Ø.91- ☑
male C5Ø.92- ☑
ductular
specified site — *see* Neoplasm, malignant
unspecified site (female) C5Ø.91- ☑
male C5Ø.92- ☑
lobular
specified site — *see* Neoplasm, malignant
unspecified site (female) C5Ø.91- ☑
male C5Ø.92- ☑
inflammatory
specified site — *see* Neoplasm, malignant
unspecified site (female) C5Ø.91- ☑
male C5Ø.92- ☑
intestinal type
specified site — *see* Neoplasm, malignant, by site
unspecified site C16.9

Carcinoma — *continued*
  intracystic
    noninfiltrating — *see* Neoplasm, in situ, by site
  intraductal (noninfiltrating)
    with Paget's disease — *see* Neoplasm, breast, malignant
    breast D05.1- ☑
    papillary
      with invasion
        specified site — *see* Neoplasm, malignant, by site
        unspecified site (female) C50.91- ☑
          male C50.92- ☑
      breast D05.1- ☑
      specified site NEC — *see* Neoplasm, in situ, by site
      unspecified site (female) D05.1- ☑
    specified site NEC — *see* Neoplasm, in situ, by site
    unspecified site (female) D05.1- ☑
  intraepidermal — *see* Neoplasm, in situ
    squamous cell, Bowen's type — *see* Neoplasm, skin, in situ
  intraepithelial — *see* Neoplasm, in situ, by site
    squamous cell — *see* Neoplasm, in situ, by site
  intraosseous C41.1
    upper jaw (bone) C41.0
  islet cell
    with exocrine, mixed
      specified site — *see* Neoplasm, malignant, by site
      unspecified site C25.9
    pancreas C25.4
    specified site NEC — *see* Neoplasm, malignant, by site
    unspecified site C25.4
  juvenile, breast — *see* Neoplasm, breast, malignant
  large cell
    small cell
      specified site — *see* Neoplasm, malignant, by site
      unspecified site C34.90
  Leydig cell (testis)
    specified site — *see* Neoplasm, malignant, by site
    unspecified site
      female C56.9
      male C62.90
  lipid-rich (female) C50.91- ☑
    male C50.92- ☑
  liver cell C22.0
  liver NEC C22.7
  lobular (infiltrating)
    with intraductal
      specified site — *see* Neoplasm, malignant, by site
      unspecified site (female) C50.91- ☑
        male C50.92- ☑
    noninfiltrating
      breast D05.0- ☑
      specified site NEC — *see* Neoplasm, in situ, by site
      unspecified site D05.0- ☑
    specified site — *see* Neoplasm, malignant, by site
    unspecified site (female) C50.91- ☑
      male C50.92- ☑
  medullary
    with
      amyloid stroma
        specified site — *see* Neoplasm, malignant, by site
        unspecified site C73
      lymphoid stroma
        specified site — *see* Neoplasm, malignant, by site
        unspecified site (female) C50.91- ☑
          male C50.92- ☑
  Merkel cell C4A.9 (*following* C43)
    anal margin C4A.51 (*following* C43)
    anal skin C4A.51 (*following* C43)
    canthus C4A.1- ☑ (*following* C43)
    ear and external auricular canal C4A.2- ☑ (*following* C43)
    external auricular canal C4A.2- ☑ (*following* C43)
    eyelid, including canthus C4A.1- ☑ (*following* C43)
    face C4A.30 (*following* C43)
      specified NEC C4A.39 (*following* C43)
    hip C4A.7- ☑ (*following* C43)
    lip C4A.0 (*following* C43)

Carcinoma — *continued*
  Merkel cell — *continued*
    lower limb, including hip C4A.7- ☑ (*following* C43)
    neck C4A.4 (*following* C43)
    nodal presentation C7B.1 (*following* C75)
    nose C4A.31 (*following* C43)
    overlapping sites C4A.8 (*following* C43)
    perianal skin C4A.51 (*following* C43)
    scalp C4A.4 (*following* C43)
    secondary C7B.1 (*following* C75)
    shoulder C4A.6- ☑ (*following* C43)
    skin of breast C4A.52 (*following* C43)
    trunk NEC C4A.59 (*following* C43)
    upper limb, including shoulder C4A.6- ☑ (*following* C43)
    visceral metastatic C7B.1 (*following* C75)
  metastatic — *see* Neoplasm, secondary, by site
  metatypical — *see* Neoplasm, skin, malignant
  morphea, basal cell — *see* Neoplasm, skin, malignant
  mucoid
    cell
      specified site — *see* Neoplasm, malignant, by site
      unspecified site C75.1
  neuroendocrine (*see also* Tumor, neuroendocrine)
    high grade, any site C7A.1 (*following* C75)
    poorly differentiated, any site C7A.1 (*following* C75)
  nonencapsulated sclerosing C73
  noninfiltrating
    intracystic — *see* Neoplasm, in situ, by site
    intraductal
      breast D05.1- ☑
      papillary
        breast D05.1- ☑
        specified site NEC — *see* Neoplasm, in situ, by site
        unspecified site D05.1- ☑
      specified site — *see* Neoplasm, in situ, by site
      unspecified site D05.1- ☑
    lobular
      breast D05.0- ☑
      specified site NEC — *see* Neoplasm, in situ, by site
      unspecified site (female) D05.0- ☑
  oat cell
    specified site — *see* Neoplasm, malignant, by site
    unspecified site C34.90
  odontogenic C41.1
    upper jaw (bone) C41.0
  papillary
    with follicular (mixed) C73
    follicular variant C73
    intraductal (noninfiltrating)
      with invasion
        specified site — *see* Neoplasm, malignant, by site
        unspecified site (female) C50.91- ☑
          male C50.92- ☑
      breast D05.1- ☑
      specified site NEC — *see* Neoplasm, in situ, by site
      unspecified site D05.1- ☑
    serous
      specified site — *see* Neoplasm, malignant, by site
      surface
        specified site — *see* Neoplasm, malignant, by site
        unspecified site C56.9
      unspecified site C56.9
  papillocystic
    specified site — *see* Neoplasm, malignant, by site
    unspecified site C56.9
  parafollicular cell
    specified site — *see* Neoplasm, malignant, by site
    unspecified site C73
  pilomatrix — *see* Neoplasm, skin, malignant
  pseudomucinous
    specified site — *see* Neoplasm, malignant, by site
    unspecified site C56.9
  renal cell C64- ☑
  Schmincke — *see* Neoplasm, nasopharynx, malignant
  Schneiderian
    specified site — *see* Neoplasm, malignant, by site
    unspecified site C30.0
  sebaceous — *see* Neoplasm, skin, malignant

Carcinoma — *continued*
  secondary (*see also* Neoplasm, secondary, by site)
    Merkel cell C7B.1 (*following* C75)
  secretory, breast — *see* Neoplasm, breast, malignant
  serous
    papillary
      specified site — *see* Neoplasm, malignant, by site
      unspecified site C56.9
    surface, papillary
      specified site — *see* Neoplasm, malignant, by site
      unspecified site C56.9
  Sertoli cell
    specified site — *see* Neoplasm, malignant, by site
    unspecified site C62.90
      female C56.9
      male C62.90
  skin appendage — *see* Neoplasm, skin, malignant
  small cell
    fusiform cell
      specified site — *see* Neoplasm, malignant, by site
      unspecified site C34.90
    intermediate cell
      specified site — *see* Neoplasm, malignant, by site
      unspecified site C34.90
    large cell
      specified site — *see* Neoplasm, malignant, by site
      unspecified site C34.90
  solid
    with amyloid stroma
      specified site — *see* Neoplasm, malignant, by site
      unspecified site C73
    microinvasive
      specified site — *see* Neoplasm, malignant, by site
      unspecified site C53.9
  sweat gland — *see* Neoplasm, skin, malignant
  theca cell C56.- ☑
  thymic C37
  unspecified site (primary) C80.1
  water-clear cell C75.0
Carcinoma-in-situ (*see also* Neoplasm, in situ, by site)
  breast NOS D05.9- ☑
    specified type NEC D05.8- ☑
  epidermoid (*see also* Neoplasm, in situ, by site)
    with questionable stromal invasion
      cervix D06.9
      specified site NEC — *see* Neoplasm, in situ, by site
      unspecified site D06.9
    Bowen's type — *see* Neoplasm, skin, in situ
  intraductal
    breast D05.1- ☑
    specified site NEC — *see* Neoplasm, in situ, by site
    unspecified site D05.1- ☑
  lobular
    with
      infiltrating duct
        breast (female) C50.91- ☑
          male C50.92- ☑
        specified site NEC — *see* Neoplasm, malignant
        unspecified site (female) C50.91- ☑
          male C50.92- ☑
      intraductal
        breast D05.8- ☑
        specified site NEC — *see* Neoplasm, in situ, by site
        unspecified site (female) D05.8- ☑
    breast D05.0- ☑
    specified site NEC — *see* Neoplasm, in situ, by site
    unspecified site D05.0- ☑
  squamous cell (*see also* Neoplasm, in situ, by site)
    with questionable stromal invasion
      cervix D06.9
      specified site NEC — *see* Neoplasm, in situ, by site
      unspecified site D06.9
Carcinomaphobia F45.29
Carcinomatosis C80.0
  peritonei C78.6

▽ Subterms under main terms may continue to next column or page   ☑ Additional Character Required — Refer to the Tabular List for Character Selection   49

Carcinoma — Carcinomatosis

Carcinomatosis — *continued*
  unspecified site (primary) (secondary) C80.0
Carcinosarcoma — *see* Neoplasm, malignant, by site
  embryonal — *see* Neoplasm, malignant, by site
Cardia, cardial — *see* condition
Cardiac (*see also* condition)
  death, sudden — *see* Arrest, cardiac
  pacemaker
    in situ Z95.0
    management or adjustment Z45.018
  tamponade I31.4
Cardialgia — *see* Pain, precordial
Cardiectasis — *see* Hypertrophy, cardiac
Cardiochalasia K21.9
Cardiomalacia I51.5
Cardiomegalia glycogenica diffusa E74.02 [I43]
Cardiomegaly (*see also* Hypertrophy, cardiac)
  congenital Q24.8
  glycogen E74.02 [I43]
  idiopathic I51.7
Cardiomyoliposis I51.5
Cardiomyopathy (familial) (idiopathic) I42.9
  alcoholic I42.6
  amyloid E85.4 [I43]
    transthyretin-related (ATTR) familial E85.4
  arteriosclerotic — *see* Disease, heart, ischemic, atherosclerotic
  beriberi E51.12
  cobalt-beer I42.6
  congenital I42.4
  congestive I42.0
  constrictive NOS I42.5
  dilated I42.0
  due to
    alcohol I42.6
    beriberi E51.12
    cardiac glycogenosis E74.02 [I43]
    drugs I42.7
    external agents NEC I42.7
    Friedreich's ataxia G11.1
    myotonia atrophica G71.11 [I43]
    progressive muscular dystrophy G71.0 [I43]
  glycogen storage E74.02 [I43]
  hypertensive — *see* Hypertension, heart
  hypertrophic (nonobstructive) I42.2
    obstructive I42.1
      congenital Q24.8
  in
    Chagas' disease (chronic) B57.2
      acute B57.0
    sarcoidosis D86.85
  ischemic I25.5
  metabolic E88.9 [I43]
    thyrotoxic E05.90 [I43]
      with thyroid storm E05.91 [I43]
  newborn I42.8
    congenital I42.4
  nutritional E63.9 [I43]
    beriberi E51.12
  obscure of Africa I42.8
  peripartum O90.3
  postpartum O90.3
  restrictive NEC I42.5
  rheumatic I09.0
  secondary I42.9
  stress induced I51.81
  takotsubo I51.81
  thyrotoxic E05.90 [I43]
    with thyroid storm E05.91 [I43]
  toxic NEC I42.7
  transthyretin-related (ATTR) familial amyloid E85.4
  tuberculous A18.84
  viral B33.24
Cardionephritis — *see* Hypertension, cardiorenal
Cardionephropathy — *see* Hypertension, cardiorenal
Cardionephrosis — *see* Hypertension, cardiorenal
Cardiopathia nigra I27.0
Cardiopathy (*see also* Disease, heart) I51.9
  idiopathic I42.9
  mucopolysaccharidosis E76.3 [I52]
Cardiopericarditis — *see* Pericarditis
Cardiophobia F45.29
Cardiorenal — *see* condition
Cardiorrhexis — *see* Infarct, myocardium
Cardiosclerosis — *see* Disease, heart, ischemic, atherosclerotic
Cardiosis — *see* Disease, heart
Cardiospasm (esophagus) (reflex) (stomach) K22.0

Cardiospasm — *continued*
  congenital Q39.5
    with megaesophagus Q39.5
Cardiostenosis — *see* Disease, heart
Cardiosymphysis I31.0
Cardiovascular — *see* condition
Carditis (acute) (bacterial) (chronic) (subacute) I51.89
  meningococcal A39.50
  rheumatic — *see* Disease, heart, rheumatic
  rheumatoid — *see* Rheumatoid, carditis
  viral B33.20
Care (of) (for) (following)
  child (routine) Z76.2
  family member (handicapped) (sick)
    creating problem for family Z63.6
    provided away from home for holiday relief Z75.5
    unavailable, due to
      absence (person rendering care) (sufferer) Z74.2
      inability (any reason) of person rendering care Z74.2
  foundling Z76.1
  holiday relief Z75.5
  improper — *see* Maltreatment
  lack of (at or after birth) (infant) — *see* Maltreatment, child, neglect
  lactating mother Z39.1
  palliative Z51.5
  postpartum
    immediately after delivery Z39.0
    routine follow-up Z39.2
  respite Z75.5
  unavailable, due to
    absence of person rendering care Z74.2
    inability (any reason) of person rendering care Z74.2
  well-baby Z76.2
Caries
  bone NEC A18.03
  dental (dentino enamel junction) (early childhood) (of dentine) (pre-eruptive) (recurrent) (to the pulp) K02.9
    arrested (coronal) (root) K02.3
    chewing surface
      limited to enamel K02.51
      penetrating into dentin K02.52
      penetrating into pulp K02.53
    coronal surface
      chewing surface
        limited to enamel K02.51
        penetrating into dentin K02.52
        penetrating into pulp K02.53
      pit and fissure surface
        limited to enamel K02.51
        penetrating into dentin K02.52
        penetrating into pulp K02.53
      smooth surface
        limited to enamel K02.61
        penetrating into dentin K02.62
        penetrating into pulp K02.63
    pit and fissure surface
      limited to enamel K02.51
      penetrating into dentin K02.52
      penetrating into pulp K02.53
    primary, cervical origin K02.52
    root K02.7
    smooth surface
      limited to enamel K02.61
      penetrating into dentin K02.62
      penetrating into pulp K02.63
  external meatus — *see* Disorder, ear, external, specified type NEC
  hip (tuberculous) A18.02
  initial (tooth)
    chewing surface K02.51
    pit and fissure surface K02.51
    smooth surface K02.61
  knee (tuberculous) A18.02
  labyrinth H83.8 ✓
  limb NEC (tuberculous) A18.03
  mastoid process (chronic) — *see* Mastoiditis, chronic
    tuberculous A18.03
  middle ear H74.8 ✓
  nose (tuberculous) A18.03
  orbit (tuberculous) A18.03
  ossicles, ear — *see* Abnormal, ear ossicles
  petrous bone — *see* Petrositis
  root (dental) (tooth) K02.7
  sacrum (tuberculous) A18.01

Caries — *continued*
  spine, spinal (column) (tuberculous) A18.01
  syphilitic A52.77
    congenital (early) A50.02 [M90.80]
  tooth, teeth — *see* Caries, dental
  tuberculous A18.03
  vertebra (column) (tuberculous) A18.01
Carious teeth — *see* Caries, dental
Carneous mole O02.0
Carnitine insufficiency E71.40
Carotid body or sinus syndrome G90.01
Carotidynia G90.01
Carotinemia (dietary) E67.1
Carotinosis (cutis) (skin) E67.1
Carpal tunnel syndrome — *see* Syndrome, carpal tunnel
Carpenter's syndrome Q87.0
Carpopedal spasm — *see* Tetany
Carr-Barr-Plunkett syndrome Q97.1
Carrier (suspected) of
  amebiasis Z22.1
  bacterial disease NEC Z22.39
    diphtheria Z22.2
    intestinal infectious NEC Z22.1
      typhoid Z22.0
    meningococcal Z22.31
    sexually transmitted Z22.4
    specified NEC Z22.39
    staphylococcal (Methicillin susceptible) Z22.321
      Methicillin resistant Z22.322
    streptococcal Z22.338
      group B Z22.330
        complicating pregnancy or delivery O99.82- ✓
    typhoid Z22.0
  cholera Z22.1
  diphtheria Z22.2
  gastrointestinal pathogens NEC Z22.1
  genetic Z14.8
    cystic fibrosis Z14.1
    hemophilia A (asymptomatic) Z14.01
      symptomatic Z14.02
  gestational, pregnant Z33.1
  gonorrhea Z22.4
  HAA (hepatitis Australian-antigen) B18.8
  HB (c)(s)-AG B18.1
  hepatitis (viral) B18.9
    Australia-antigen (HAA) B18.8
    B surface antigen (HBsAg) B18.1
      with acute delta- (super)infection B17.0
    C B18.2
    specified NEC B18.8
  human T-cell lymphotropic virus type-1 (HTLV-1) infection Z22.6
  infectious organism Z22.9
    specified NEC Z22.8
  meningococci Z22.31
  Salmonella typhosa Z22.0
  serum hepatitis — *see* Carrier, hepatitis
  staphylococci (Methicillin susceptible) Z22.321
    Methicillin resistant Z22.322
  streptococci Z22.338
    group B Z22.330
      complicating pregnancy or delivery O99.82- ✓
  syphilis Z22.4
  typhoid Z22.0
  venereal disease NEC Z22.4
Carrion's disease A44.0
Carter's relapsing fever (Asiatic) A68.1
Cartilage — *see* condition
Caruncle (inflamed)
  conjunctiva (acute) — *see* Conjunctivitis, acute
  labium (majus) (minus) N90.89
  lacrimal — *see* Inflammation, lacrimal, passages
  myrtiform N89.8
  urethral (benign) N36.2
Cascade stomach K31.2
Caseation lymphatic gland (tuberculous) A18.2
Cassidy (-Scholte) syndrome (malignant carcinoid) E34.0
Castellani's disease A69.8
Castration, traumatic, male S38.231 ✓
Casts in urine R82.99
Cat
  cry syndrome Q93.4
  ear Q17.3
  eye syndrome Q92.8
Catabolism, senile R54
Catalepsy (hysterical) F44.2
  schizophrenic F20.2

Cataplexy (idiopathic) — *see* Narcolepsy
Cataract (cortical) (immature) (incipient) H26.9
  with
    neovascularization — *see* Cataract, complicated
  age-related — *see* Cataract, senile
  anterior
    and posterior axial embryonal Q12.0
    pyramidal Q12.0
  associated with
    galactosemia E74.21 [H28]
    myotonic disorders G71.19 [H28]
  blue Q12.0
  central Q12.0
  cerulean Q12.0
  complicated H26.20
    with
      neovascularization H26.21- ☑
      ocular disorder H26.22- ☑
      glaucomatous flecks H26.23- ☑
  congenital Q12.0
  coraliform Q12.0
  coronary Q12.0
  crystalline Q12.0
  diabetic — *see* Diabetes, cataract
  drug-induced H26.3- ☑
  due to
    ocular disorder — *see* Cataract, complicated
    radiation H26.8
  electric H26.8
  extraction status Z98.4- ☑
  glass-blower's H26.8
  heat ray H26.8
  heterochromic — *see* Cataract, complicated
  hypermature — *see* Cataract, senile, morgagnian type
  in (due to)
    chronic iridocyclitis — *see* Cataract, complicated
    diabetes — *see* Diabetes, cataract
    endocrine disease E34.9 [H28]
    eye disease — *see* Cataract, complicated
    hypoparathyroidism E20.9 [H28]
    malnutrition-dehydration E46 [H28]
    metabolic disease E88.9 [H28]
    myotonic disorders G71.19 [H28]
    nutritional disease E63.9 [H28]
  infantile — *see* Cataract, presenile
  irradiational — *see* Cataract, specified NEC
  juvenile — *see* Cataract, presenile
  malnutrition-dehydration E46 [H28]
  morgagnian — *see* Cataract, senile, morgagnian type
  myotonic G71.19 [H28]
  myxedema E03.9 [H28]
  nuclear
    embryonal Q12.0
    sclerosis — *see* Cataract, senile, nuclear
  presenile H26.00- ☑
    combined forms H26.06- ☑
    cortical H26.01- ☑
    lamellar — *see* Cataract, presenile, cortical
    nuclear H26.03- ☑
    specified NEC H26.09
    subcapsular polar (anterior) H26.04- ☑
      posterior H26.05- ☑
    zonular — *see* Cataract, presenile, cortical
  secondary H26.40
    Soemmering's ring H26.41- ☑
    specified NEC H26.49- ☑
    to eye disease — *see* Cataract, complicated
  senile H25.9
    brunescens — *see* Cataract, senile, nuclear
    combined forms H25.81- ☑
    coronary — *see* Cataract, senile, incipient
    cortical H25.01- ☑
    hypermature — *see* Cataract, senile, morgagnian type
    incipient (mature) (total) H25.09- ☑
      cortical — *see* Cataract, senile, cortical
      subcapsular — *see* Cataract, senile, subcapsular
    morgagnian type (hypermature) H25.2- ☑
    nuclear (sclerosis) H25.1- ☑
    polar subcapsular (anterior) (posterior) — *see* Cataract, senile, incipient
    punctate — *see* Cataract, senile, incipient
    specified NEC H25.89
    subcapsular polar (anterior) H25.03- ☑
      posterior H25.04- ☑
  snowflake — *see* Diabetes, cataract
  specified NEC H26.8

Cataract — *continued*
  toxic — *see* Cataract, drug-induced
  traumatic H26.10- ☑
    localized H26.11- ☑
    partially resolved H26.12- ☑
    total H26.13- ☑
  zonular (perinuclear) Q12.0
Cataracta (*see also* Cataract)
  brunescens — *see* Cataract, senile, nuclear
  centralis pulverulenta Q12.0
  cerulea Q12.0
  complicata — *see* Cataract, complicated
  congenita Q12.0
  coralliformis Q12.0
  coronaria Q12.0
  diabetic — *see* Diabetes, cataract
  membranacea
    accreta — *see* Cataract, secondary
    congenita Q12.0
  nigra — *see* Cataract, senile, nuclear
  sunflower — *see* Cataract, complicated
Catarrh, catarrhal (acute) (febrile) (infectious) (inflammation) (*see also* condition) J00
  bronchial — *see* Bronchitis
  chest — *see* Bronchitis
  chronic J31.0
  due to congenital syphilis A50.03
  enteric — *see* Enteritis
  eustachian H68.009
  fauces — *see* Pharyngitis
  gastrointestinal — *see* Enteritis
  gingivitis K05.00
    nonplaque induced K05.01
    plaque induced K05.00
  hay — *see* Fever, hay
  intestinal — *see* Enteritis
  larynx, chronic J37.0
  liver B15.9
    with hepatic coma B15.0
  lung — *see* Bronchitis
  middle ear, chronic — *see* Otitis, media, nonsuppurative, chronic, serous
  mouth K12.1
  nasal (chronic) — *see* Rhinitis
  nasobronchial J31.1
  nasopharyngeal (chronic) J31.1
    acute J00
  pulmonary — *see* Bronchitis
  spring (eye) (vernal) — *see* Conjunctivitis, acute, atopic
  summer (hay) — *see* Fever, hay
  throat J31.2
  tubotympanal (*see also* Otitis, media, nonsuppurative)
    chronic — *see* Otitis, media, nonsuppurative, chronic, serous
Catatonia (schizophrenic) F20.2
Catatonic
  disorder due to known physiologic condition F06.1
  schizophrenia F20.2
  stupor R40.1
Cat-scratch (*see also* Abrasion)
  disease or fever A28.1
Cauda equina — *see* condition
Cauliflower ear M95.1- ☑
Causalgia (upper limb) G56.4- ☑
  lower limb G57.7- ☑
Cause
  external, general effects T75.89 ☑
Caustic burn — *see* Corrosion, by site
Cavare's disease (familial periodic paralysis) G72.3
Cave-in, injury
  crushing (severe) — *see* Crush
  suffocation — *see* Asphyxia, traumatic, due to low oxygen, due to cave-in
Cavernitis (penis) N48.29
Cavernositis N48.29
Cavernous — *see* condition
Cavitation of lung (*see also* Tuberculosis, pulmonary)
  nontuberculous J98.4
Cavities, dental — *see* Caries, dental
Cavity
  lung — *see* Cavitation of lung
  optic papilla Q14.2
  pulmonary — *see* Cavitation of lung
Cavovarus foot, congenital Q66.1
Cavus foot (congenital) Q66.7
  acquired — *see* Deformity, limb, foot, specified NEC
Cazenave's disease L10.2

Cecitis K52.9
  with perforation, peritonitis, or rupture K65.8
Cecum — *see* condition
Celiac
  artery compression syndrome I77.4
  disease (with steatorrhea) K90.0
  infantilism K90.0
Cell(s), **cellular** (*see also* condition)
  in urine R82.99
Cellulitis (diffuse) (phlegmonous) (septic) (suppurative) L03.90
  abdominal wall L03.311
  anaerobic A48.0
  ankle — *see* Cellulitis, lower limb
  anus K61.0
  arm — *see* Cellulitis, upper limb
  auricle (ear) — *see* Cellulitis, ear
  axilla L03.11- ☑
  back (any part) L03.312
  breast (acute) (nonpuerperal) (subacute) N61.0
    nipple N61.0
  broad ligament
    acute N73.0
  buttock L03.317
  cervical (meaning neck) L03.221
  cervix (uteri) — *see* Cervicitis
  cheek (external) L03.211
    internal K12.2
  chest wall L03.313
  chronic L03.90
  clostridial A48.0
  corpus cavernosum N48.22
  digit
    finger — *see* Cellulitis, finger
    toe — *see* Cellulitis, toe
  Douglas' cul-de-sac or pouch
    acute N73.0
  drainage site (following operation) T81.4 ☑
  ear (external) H60.1- ☑
  eosinophilic (granulomatous) L98.3
  erysipelatous — *see* Erysipelas
  external auditory canal — *see* Cellulitis, ear
  eyelid — *see* Abscess, eyelid
  face NEC L03.211
  finger (intrathecal) (periosteal) (subcutaneous) (subcuticular) L03.01- ☑
  foot — *see* Cellulitis, lower limb
  gangrenous — *see* Gangrene
  genital organ NEC
    female (external) N76.4
    male N49.9
      multiple sites N49.8
      specified NEC N49.8
  gluteal (region) L03.317
  gonococcal A54.89
  groin L03.314
  hand — *see* Cellulitis, upper limb
  head NEC L03.811
    face (any part, except ear, eye and nose) L03.211
  heel — *see* Cellulitis, lower limb
  hip — *see* Cellulitis, lower limb
  jaw (region) L03.211
  knee — *see* Cellulitis, lower limb
  labium (majus) (minus) — *see* Vulvitis
  lacrimal passages — *see* Inflammation, lacrimal, passages
  larynx J38.7
  leg — *see* Cellulitis, lower limb
  lip K13.0
  lower limb L03.11- ☑
    toe — *see* Cellulitis, toe
  mouth (floor) K12.2
  multiple sites, so stated L03.90
  nasopharynx J39.1
  navel L03.316
    newborn P38.9
      with mild hemorrhage P38.1
      without hemorrhage P38.9
  neck (region) L03.221
  nipple (acute) (nonpuerperal) (subacute) N61.0
  nose (septum) (external) J34.0
  orbit, orbital H05.01- ☑
  palate (soft) K12.2
  pectoral (region) L03.313
  pelvis, pelvic (chronic)
    female (*see also* Disease, pelvis, inflammatory) N73.2
      acute N73.0

Cellulitis — *continued*
pelvis, pelvic — *continued*
following ectopic or molar pregnancy O08.0
male K65.0
penis N48.22
perineal, perineum L03.315
periorbital L03.213
perirectal K61.1
peritonsillar J36
periurethral N34.0
periuterine (*see also* Disease, pelvis, inflammatory) N73.2
acute N73.0
pharynx J39.1
preseptal L03.213
rectum K61.1
retroperitoneal K68.9
round ligament
acute N73.0
scalp (any part) L03.811
scrotum N49.2
seminal vesicle N49.0
shoulder — *see* Cellulitis, upper limb
specified site NEC L03.818
submandibular (region) (space) (triangle) K12.2
gland K11.3
submaxillary (region) K12.2
gland K11.3
thigh — *see* Cellulitis, lower limb
thumb (intrathecal) (periosteal) (subcutaneous) (subcuticular) — *see* Cellulitis, finger
toe (intrathecal) (periosteal) (subcutaneous) (subcuticular) L03.03- ☑
tonsil J36
trunk L03.319
abdominal wall L03.311
back (any part) L03.312
buttock L03.317
chest wall L03.313
groin L03.314
perineal, perineum L03.315
umbilicus L03.316
tuberculous (primary) A18.4
umbilicus L03.316
upper limb L03.11- ☑
axilla — *see* Cellulitis, axilla
finger — *see* Cellulitis, finger
thumb — *see* Cellulitis, finger
vaccinal T88.0 ☑
vocal cord J38.3
vulva — *see* Vulvitis
wrist — *see* Cellulitis, upper limb
Cementoblastoma, benign — *see* Cyst, calcifying odontogenic
Cementoma — *see* Cyst, calcifying odontogenic
Cementoperiostitis — *see* Periodontitis
Cementosis K03.4
Central auditory processing disorder H93.25
Central pain syndrome G89.0
Cephalematocele, cephal (o)hematocele
newborn P52.8
birth injury P10.8
traumatic — *see* Hematoma, brain
Cephalematoma, cephalhematoma (calcified)
newborn (birth injury) P12.0
traumatic — *see* Hematoma, brain
Cephalgia, cephalalgia (*see also* Headache)
histamine G44.009
intractable G44.001
not intractable G44.009
trigeminal autonomic (TAC) NEC G44.099
intractable G44.091
not intractable G44.099
Cephalic — *see* condition
Cephalitis — *see* Encephalitis
Cephalocele — *see* Encephalocele
Cephalomenia N94.89
Cephalopelvic — *see* condition
Cerclage (with cervical incompetence) in pregnancy — *see* Incompetence, cervix, in pregnancy
Cerebellitis — *see* Encephalitis
Cerebellum, cerebellar — *see* condition
Cerebral — *see* condition
Cerebritis — *see* Encephalitis
Cerebro-hepato-renal syndrome Q87.89
Cerebromalacia — *see* Softening, brain
sequelae of cerebrovascular disease I69.398
Cerebroside lipidosis E75.22

Cerebrospasticity (congenital) G80.1
Cerebrospinal — *see* condition
Cerebrum — *see* condition
Ceroid-lipofuscinosis, neuronal E75.4 ☑
Cerumen (accumulation) (impacted) H61.2- ☑
Cervical (*see also* condition)
auricle Q18.2
dysplasia in pregnancy — *see* Abnormal, cervix, in pregnancy or childbirth
erosion in pregnancy — *see* Abnormal, cervix, in pregnancy or childbirth
fibrosis in pregnancy — *see* Abnormal, cervix, in pregnancy or childbirth
fusion syndrome Q76.1
rib Q76.5
shortening (complicating pregnancy) O26.87- ☑
Cervicalgia M54.2
Cervicitis (acute) (chronic) (nonvenereal) (senile (atrophic)) (subacute) (with ulceration) N72
with
abortion — *see* Abortion, by type complicated by genital tract and pelvic infection
ectopic pregnancy O08.0
molar pregnancy O08.0
chlamydial A56.09
gonococcal A54.03
herpesviral A60.03
puerperal (postpartum) O86.11
syphilitic A52.76
trichomonal A59.09
tuberculous A18.16
Cervicocolpitis (emphysematosa) (see also Cervicitis) N72
Cervix — *see* condition
Cesarean delivery, previous, affecting management of pregnancy O34.219
classical (vertical) scar O34.212
low transverse scar O34.211
Céstan (-Chenais) paralysis or syndrome G46.3
Céstan-Raymond syndrome I65.8
Cestode infestation B71.9
specified type NEC B71.8
Cestodiasis B71.9
Chabert's disease A22.9
Chacaleh E53.8
Chafing L30.4
Chagas' (-Mazza) disease (chronic) B57.2
with
cardiovascular involvement NEC B57.2
digestive system involvement B57.30
megacolon B57.32
megaesophagus B57.31
other specified B57.39
megacolon B57.32
megaesophagus B57.31
myocarditis B57.2
nervous system involvement B57.40
meningitis B57.41
meningoencephalitis B57.42
other specified B57.49
specified organ involvement NEC B57.5
acute (with) B57.1
cardiovascular NEC B57.0
myocarditis B57.0
Chagres fever B50.9
Chairridden Z74.09
Chalasia (cardiac sphincter) K21.9
Chalazion H00.19
left H00.16
lower H00.15
upper H00.14
right H00.13
lower H00.12
upper H00.11
Chalcosis (*see also* Disorder, globe, degenerative, chalcosis)
cornea — *see* Deposit, cornea
crystalline lens — *see* Cataract, complicated
retina H35.89
Chalicosis (pulmonum) J62.8
Chancre (any genital site) (hard) (hunterian) (mixed) (primary) (seronegative) (seropositive) (syphilitic) A51.0
congenital A50.07
conjunctiva NEC A51.2
Ducrey's A57
extragenital A51.2
eyelid A51.2

Chancre — *continued*
lip A51.2
nipple A51.2
Nisbet's A57
of
carate A67.0
pinta A67.0
yaws A66.0
palate, soft A51.2
phagedenic A57
simple A57
soft A57
bubo A57
palate A51.2
urethra A51.0
yaws A66.0
Chancroid (anus) (genital) (penis) (perineum) (rectum) (urethra) (vulva) A57
Chandler's disease (osteochondritis dissecans, hip) — *see* Osteochondritis, dissecans, hip
Change(s) (in) (of) (*see also* Removal)
arteriosclerotic — *see* Arteriosclerosis
bone (*see also* Disorder, bone)
diabetic — *see* Diabetes, bone change
bowel habit R19.4
cardiorenal (vascular) — *see* Hypertension, cardiorenal
cardiovascular — *see* Disease, cardiovascular
circulatory I99.9
cognitive (mild) (organic) R41.89
color, tooth, teeth
during formation K00.8
posteruptive K03.7
contraceptive device Z30.433
corneal membrane H18.30
Bowman's membrane fold or rupture H18.31- ☑
Descemet's membrane
fold H18.32- ☑
rupture H18.33- ☑
coronary — *see* Disease, heart, ischemic
degenerative, spine or vertebra — *see* Spondylosis
dental pulp, regressive K04.2
dressing (nonsurgical) Z48.00
surgical Z48.01
heart — *see* Disease, heart
hip joint — *see* Derangement, joint, hip
hyperplastic larynx J38.7
hypertrophic
nasal sinus J34.89
turbinate, nasal J34.3
upper respiratory tract J39.8
indwelling catheter Z46.6
inflammatory (*see also* Inflammation)
sacroiliac M46.1
job, anxiety concerning Z56.1
joint — *see* Derangement, joint
life — *see* Menopause
mental status R41.82
minimal (glomerular) (*see also* N00-N07 with fourth character .0) N05.0
myocardium, myocardial — *see* Degeneration, myocardial
of life — *see* Menopause
pacemaker Z45.018
pulse generator Z45.010
personality (enduring) F68.8
due to (secondary to)
general medical condition F07.0
secondary (nonspecific) F60.89
regressive, dental pulp K04.2
renal — *see* Disease, renal
retina H35.9
myopic (*see also* Myopia, degenerative) H44.2- ☑
sacroiliac joint M53.3
senile (*see also* condition) R54
sensory R20.8
skin R23.9
acute, due to ultraviolet radiation L56.9
specified NEC L56.8
chronic, due to nonionizing radiation L57.9
specified NEC L57.8
cyanosis R23.0
flushing R23.2
pallor R23.1
petechiae R23.3
specified change NEC R23.8
swelling — *see* Mass, localized
texture R23.4

▽ Subterms under main terms may continue to next column or page   ☑ Additional Character Required — Refer to the Tabular List for Character Selection   **53**

Index   Change — Chondritis

Chondritis — *continued*
  aural H61.03- ☑
  costal (Tietze's) M94.0
  external ear H61.03- ☑
  patella, posttraumatic — *see* Chondromalacia, patella
  pinna H61.03- ☑
  purulent M94.8X- ☑
  tuberculous NEC A18.02
    intervertebral A18.01
Chondroblastoma (*see also* Neoplasm, bone, benign)
  malignant — *see* Neoplasm, bone, malignant
Chondrocalcinosis M11.20
  ankle M11.27- ☑
  elbow M11.22- ☑
  familial M11.10
    ankle M11.17- ☑
    elbow M11.12- ☑
    foot joint M11.17- ☑
    hand joint M11.14- ☑
    hip M11.15- ☑
    knee M11.16- ☑
    multiple site M11.19
    shoulder M11.11- ☑
    vertebrae M11.18
    wrist M11.13- ☑
  foot joint M11.27- ☑
  hand joint M11.24- ☑
  hip M11.25- ☑
  knee M11.26- ☑
  multiple site M11.29
  shoulder M11.21- ☑
  specified type NEC M11.20
    ankle M11.27- ☑
    elbow M11.22- ☑
    foot joint M11.27- ☑
    hand joint M11.24- ☑
    hip M11.25- ☑
    knee M11.26- ☑
    multiple site M11.29
    shoulder M11.21- ☑
    vertebrae M11.28
    wrist M11.23- ☑
  vertebrae M11.28
  wrist M11.23- ☑
Chondrodermatitis nodularis helicis or anthelicis
  — *see* Perichondritis, ear
Chondrodysplasia Q78.9
  with hemangioma Q78.4
  calcificans congenita Q77.3
  fetalis Q77.4
  metaphyseal (Jansen's) (McKusick's) (Schmid's) Q78.8
  punctata Q77.3
Chondrodystrophy, chondrodystrophia (familial)
    (fetalis) (hypoplastic) Q78.9
  calcificans congenita Q77.3
  myotonic (congenital) G71.13
  punctata Q77.3
Chondroectodermal dysplasia Q77.6
Chondrogenesis imperfecta Q77.4
Chondrolysis M94.35-
Chondroma (*see also* Neoplasm, cartilage, benign)
  juxtacortical — *see* Neoplasm, bone, benign
  periosteal — *see* Neoplasm, bone, benign
Chondromalacia (systemic) M94.20
  acromioclavicular joint M94.21- ☑
  ankle M94.27- ☑
  elbow M94.22- ☑
  foot joint M94.27- ☑
  glenohumeral joint M94.21- ☑
  hand joint M94.24- ☑
  hip M94.25- ☑
  knee M94.26- ☑
    patella M22.4- ☑
  multiple sites M94.29
  patella M22.4- ☑
  rib M94.28
  sacroiliac joint M94.259
  shoulder M94.21- ☑
  sternoclavicular joint M94.21- ☑
  vertebral joint M94.28
  wrist M94.23- ☑
Chondromatosis (*see also* Neoplasm, cartilage, uncertain
    behavior)
  internal Q78.4
Chondromyxosarcoma — *see* Neoplasm, cartilage,
    malignant

Chondro-osteodysplasia (Morquio-Brailsford type)
    E76.219
Chondro-osteodystrophy E76.29
Chondro-osteoma — *see* Neoplasm, bone, benign
Chondropathia tuberosa M94.0
Chondrosarcoma — *see* Neoplasm, cartilage, malignant
  juxtacortical — *see* Neoplasm, bone, malignant
  mesenchymal — *see* Neoplasm, connective tissue,
    malignant
  myxoid — *see* Neoplasm, cartilage, malignant
Chordee (nonvenereal) N48.89
  congenital Q54.4
  gonococcal A54.09
Chorditis (fibrinous) (nodosa) (tuberosa) J38.2
Chordoma — *see* Neoplasm, vertebral (column), malig-
    nant
Chorea (chronic) (gravis) (posthemiplegic) (senile)
    (spasmodic) G25.5
  with
    heart involvement I02.0
      active or acute (conditions in I01-) I02.0
      rheumatic I02.9
        with valvular disorder I02.0
      rheumatic heart disease (chronic) (inactive)(quies-
        cent) — *code to* rheumatic heart condition
        involved
  drug-induced G25.4
  habit F95.8
  hereditary G10
  Huntington's G10
  hysterical F44.4
  minor I02.9
    with heart involvement I02.0
  progressive G25.5
    hereditary G10
  rheumatic (chronic) I02.9
    with heart involvement I02.0
  Sydenham's I02.9
    with heart involvement — *see* Chorea, with
      rheumatic heart disease
  nonrheumatic G25.5
Choreoathetosis (paroxysmal) G25.5
Chorioadenoma (destruens) D39.2
Chorioamnionitis O41.12- ☑
Chorioangioma D26.7
Choriocarcinoma — *see* Neoplasm, malignant, by site
  combined with
    embryonal carcinoma — *see* Neoplasm, malignant,
      by site
    other germ cell elements — *see* Neoplasm, malig-
      nant, by site
    teratoma — *see* Neoplasm, malignant, by site
  specified site — *see* Neoplasm, malignant, by site
  unspecified site
    female C58
    male C62.90
Chorioencephalitis (acute) (lymphocytic) (serous) A87.2
Chorioepithelioma — *see* Choriocarcinoma
Choriomeningitis (acute) (lymphocytic) (serous) A87.2
Chorionepithelioma — *see* Choriocarcinoma
Chorioretinitis (*see also* Inflammation, chorioretinal)
  disseminated (*see also* Inflammation, chorioretinal,
    disseminated)
    in neurosyphilis A52.19
  Egyptian B76.9 [D63.8]
  focal (*see also* Inflammation, chorioretinal, focal)
  histoplasmic B39.9 [H32]
  in (due to)
    histoplasmosis B39.9 [H32]
    syphilis (secondary) A51.43
      late A52.71
    toxoplasmosis (acquired) B58.01
      congenital (active) P37.1 [H32]
    tuberculosis A18.53
  juxtapapillary, juxtapapillaris — *see* Inflammation,
    chorioretinal, focal, juxtapapillary
  leprous A30.9 [H32]
  miner's B76.9 [D63.8]
  progressive myopia (degeneration) (*see also* Myopia,
    degenerative) H44.2- ☑
  syphilitic (secondary) A51.43
    congenital (early) A50.01 [H32]
      late A50.32
    late A52.71
  tuberculous A18.53
Chorioretinopathy, central serous H35.71- ☑
Choroid — *see* condition
Choroideremia H31.21

Choroiditis — *see* Chorioretinitis
Choroidopathy — *see* Disorder, choroid
Choroidoretinitis — *see* Chorioretinitis
Choroidoretinopathy, central serous — *see* Chori-
    oretinopathy, central serous
Christian-Weber disease M35.6
Christmas disease D67
Chromaffinoma (*see also* Neoplasm, benign, by site)
  malignant — *see* Neoplasm, malignant, by site
Chromatopsia — *see* Deficiency, color vision
Chromhidrosis, chromidrosis L75.1
Chromoblastomycosis — *see* Chromomycosis
Chromoconversion R82.91
Chromomycosis B43.9
  brain abscess B43.1
  cerebral B43.1
  cutaneous B43.0
  skin B43.0
  specified NEC B43.8
  subcutaneous abscess or cyst B43.2
Chromophytosis B36.0
Chromosome — *see* Anomaly, by chromosome involved
  D (1) — *see* Anomaly, chromosome 13
  E (3) — *see* Anomaly, chromosome 18
  G — *see* Anomaly, chromosome 21
Chromotrichomycosis B36.8
Chronic — *see* condition
  fracture — *see* Fracture, pathological
Churg-Strauss syndrome M30.1
Chyle cyst, mesentery I89.8
Chylocele (nonfilarial) I89.8
  filarial (*see also* Infestation, filarial) B74.9 [N51]
  tunica vaginalis N50.89
    filarial (*see also* Infestation, filarial) B74.9 [N51]
Chylomicronemia (fasting) (with hyperprebetalipopro-
    teinemia) E78.3
Chylopericardium I31.3
  acute I30.9
Chylothorax (nonfilarial) I89.8
  filarial (*see also* Infestation, filarial) B74.9 [J91.8]
Chylous — *see* condition
Chyluria (nonfilarial) R82.0
  due to
    bilharziasis B65.0
    Brugia (malayi) B74.1
      timori B74.2
    schistosomiasis (bilharziasis) B65.0
    Wuchereria (bancrofti) B74.0
  filarial — *see* Infestation, filarial
Cicatricial (deformity) — *see* Cicatrix
Cicatrix (adherent) (contracted) (painful) (vicious) (*see
    also* Scar) L90.5
  adenoid (and tonsil) J35.8
  alveolar process M26.79
  anus K62.89
  auricle — *see* Disorder, pinna, specified type NEC
  bile duct (common) (hepatic) K83.8
  bladder N32.89
  bone — *see* Disorder, bone, specified type NEC
  brain G93.89
  cervix (postoperative) (postpartal) N88.1
  common duct K83.8
  cornea H17.9
    tuberculous A18.59
  duodenum (bulb), obstructive K31.5
  esophagus K22.2
  eyelid — *see* Disorder, eyelid function
  hypopharynx J39.2
  lacrimal passages — *see* Obstruction, lacrimal
  larynx J38.7
  lung J98.4
  middle ear H74.8 ☑
  mouth K13.79
  muscle M62.89
    with contracture — *see* Contraction, muscle NEC
  nasopharynx J39.2
  palate (soft) K13.79
  penis N48.89
  pharynx J39.2
  prostate N42.89
  rectum K62.89
  retina — *see* Scar, chorioretinal
  semilunar cartilage — *see* Derangement, meniscus
  seminal vesicle N50.89
  skin L90.5
    infected L08.89
    postinfective L90.5

Chondritis — Cicatrix

54   ☑ **Additional Character Required** — Refer to the Tabular List for Character Selection   ▽ Subterms under main terms may continue to next column or page

Cicatrix — *continued*
  skin — *continued*
    tuberculous B90.8
  specified site NEC L90.5
  throat J39.2
  tongue K14.8
  tonsil (and adenoid) J35.8
  trachea J39.8
  tuberculous NEC B90.9
  urethra N36.8
  uterus N85.8
  vagina N89.8
    postoperative N99.2
  vocal cord J38.3
  wrist, constricting (annular) L90.5
CIDP (chronic inflammatory demyelinating polyneuropathy) G61.81
CIN — *see* Neoplasia, intraepithelial, cervix
CINCA (chronic infantile neurological, cutaneous and articular syndrome) M04.2
Cinchonism — *see* Deafness, ototoxic
  correct substance properly administered — *see* Table of Drugs and Chemicals, by drug, adverse effect
  overdose or wrong substance given or taken — *see* Table of Drugs and Chemicals, by drug, poisoning
Circle of Willis — *see* condition
Circular — *see* condition
Circulating anticoagulants (*see also* Disorder, hemorrhagic) D68.318
  due to drugs (*see also* Disorder, hemorrhagic) D68.32
  following childbirth O72.3
Circulation
  collateral, any site I99.8
  defective (lower extremity) I99.9
    congenital Q28.9
  embryonic Q28.9
  failure (peripheral) R57.9
    newborn P29.89
  fetal, persistent P29.38
  heart, incomplete Q28.9
Circulatory system — *see* condition
Circulus senilis (cornea) — *see* Degeneration, cornea, senile
Circumcision (in absence of medical indication) (ritual) (routine) Z41.2
Circumscribed — *see* condition
Circumvallate placenta O43.11- ☑
Cirrhosis, cirrhotic (hepatic) (liver) K74.60
  alcoholic K70.30
    with ascites K70.31
  atrophic — *see* Cirrhosis, liver
  Baumgarten-Cruveilhier K74.69
  biliary (cholangiolitic) (cholangitic) (hypertrophic) (obstructive) (pericholangiolitic) K74.5
    due to
      Clonorchiasis B66.1
      flukes B66.3
    primary K74.3
    secondary K74.4
  cardiac (of liver) K76.1
  Charcot's K74.3
  cholangiolitic, cholangitic, cholostatic (primary) K74.3
  congestive K76.1
  Cruveilhier-Baumgarten K74.69
  cryptogenic (liver) K74.69
  due to
    hepatolenticular degeneration E83.01
    Wilson's disease E83.01
    xanthomatosis E78.2
  fatty K76.0
    alcoholic K70.0
  Hanot's (hypertrophic) K74.3
  hepatic — *see* Cirrhosis, liver
  hypertrophic K74.3
  Indian childhood K74.69
  kidney — *see* Sclerosis, renal
  Laennec's K70.30
    with ascites K70.31
    alcoholic K70.30
      with ascites K70.31
    nonalcoholic K74.69
  liver K74.60
    alcoholic K70.30
      with ascites K70.31
      fatty K70.0
    congenital P78.81
    syphilitic A52.74

Cirrhosis, cirrhotic — *continued*
  lung (chronic) J84.10
  macronodular K74.69
    alcoholic K70.30
      with ascites K70.31
  micronodular K74.69
    alcoholic K70.30
      with ascites K70.31
  mixed type K74.69
  monolobular K74.3
  nephritis — *see* Sclerosis, renal
  nutritional K74.69
    alcoholic K70.30
      with ascites K70.31
  obstructive — *see* Cirrhosis, biliary
  ovarian N83.8
  pancreas (duct) K86.89
  pigmentary E83.110
  portal K74.69
    alcoholic K70.30
      with ascites K70.31
  postnecrotic K74.69
    alcoholic K70.30
      with ascites K70.31
  pulmonary J84.10
  renal — *see* Sclerosis, renal
  spleen D73.2
  stasis K76.1
  Todd's K74.3
  unilobar K74.3
  xanthomatous (biliary) K74.5
    due to xanthomatosis (familial) (metabolic) (primary) E78.2
Cistern, subarachnoid R93.0
Citrullinemia E72.23
Citrullinuria E72.23
Civatte's disease or poikiloderma L57.3
Clam digger's itch B65.3
Clammy skin R23.1
Clap — *see* Gonorrhea
Clarke-Hadfield syndrome (pancreatic infantilism) K86.89
Clark's paralysis G80.9
Clastothrix L67.8
Claude Bernard-Horner syndrome G90.2
  traumatic — *see* Injury, nerve, cervical sympathetic
Claude's disease or syndrome G46.3
Claudicatio venosa intermittens I87.8
Claudication (intermittent) I73.9
  cerebral (artery) G45.9
  spinal cord (arteriosclerotic) G95.19
    syphilitic A52.09
  venous (axillary) I87.8
Claustrophobia F40.240
Clavus (infected) L84
Clawfoot (congenital) Q66.89
  acquired — *see* Deformity, limb, clawfoot
Clawhand (acquired) (*see also* Deformity, limb, clawhand)
  congenital Q68.1
Clawtoe (congenital) Q66.89
  acquired — *see* Deformity, toe, specified NEC
Clay eating — *see* Pica
Cleansing of artificial opening — *see* Attention to, artificial, opening
Cleft (congenital) — *see also* Imperfect, closure
  alveolar process M26.79
  branchial (persistent) Q18.2
    cyst Q18.0
      fistula Q18.0
      sinus Q18.0
  cricoid cartilage, posterior Q31.8
  cyst Q18.0
    fistula Q18.0
    sinus Q18.0
  foot Q72.7 ☑
  hand Q71.6 ☑
  lip (unilateral) Q36.9
    with cleft palate Q37.9
      hard Q37.1
        with soft Q37.5
      soft Q37.3
        with hard Q37.5
    bilateral Q36.0
      with cleft palate Q37.8
        hard Q37.0
          with soft Q37.4
        soft Q37.2
          with hard Q37.4

Cleft — *continued*
  lip — *continued*
    median Q36.1
  nose Q30.2
  palate Q35.9
    with cleft lip (unilateral) Q37.9
      bilateral Q37.8
    hard Q35.1
      with
        cleft lip (unilateral) Q37.1
          bilateral Q37.0
        soft Q35.5
          with cleft lip (unilateral) Q37.5
            bilateral Q37.4
    medial Q35.5
    soft Q35.3
      with
        cleft lip (unilateral) Q37.3
          bilateral Q37.2
        hard Q35.5
          with cleft lip (unilateral) Q37.5
            bilateral Q37.4
  penis Q55.69
  scrotum Q55.29
  thyroid cartilage Q31.8
  uvula Q35.7
Cleidocranial dysostosis Q74.0
Cleptomania F63.2
Clicking hip (newborn) R29.4
Climacteric (female) (*see also* Menopause)
  arthritis (any site) NEC — *see* Arthritis, specified form NEC
  depression (single episode) F32.89
    recurrent episode F33.8
  male (symptoms) (syndrome) NEC N50.89
  melancholia (single episode) F32.89
    recurrent episode F33.8
  paranoid state F22
  polyarthritis NEC — *see* Arthritis, specified form NEC
  symptoms (female) N95.1
Clinical research investigation (clinical trial) (control subject) (normal comparison) (participant) Z00.6
Clitoris — *see* condition
Cloaca (persistent) Q43.7
Clonorchiasis, clonorchis infection (liver) B66.1
Clonus R25.8
Closed bite M26.29
Clostridium (C.) **perfringens, as cause of disease classified elsewhere** B96.7
Closure
  congenital, nose Q30.0
  cranial sutures, premature Q75.0
  defective or imperfect NEC — *see* Imperfect, closure
  fistula, delayed — *see* Fistula
  foramen ovale, imperfect Q21.1
  hymen N89.6
  interauricular septum, defective Q21.1
  interventricular septum, defective Q21.0
  lacrimal duct (*see also* Stenosis, lacrimal, duct)
    congenital Q10.5
  nose (congenital) Q30.0
    acquired M95.0
  of artificial opening — *see* Attention to, artificial, opening
  vagina N89.5
  valve — *see* Endocarditis
  vulva N90.5
Clot (blood) (*see also* Embolism)
  artery (obstruction) (occlusion) — *see* Embolism
  bladder N32.89
  brain (intradural or extradural) — *see* Occlusion, artery, cerebral
  circulation I74.9
  heart (*see also* Infarct, myocardium)
    not resulting in infarction I51.3
  vein — *see* Thrombosis
Clouded state R40.1
  epileptic — *see* Epilepsy, specified NEC
  paroxysmal — *see* Epilepsy, specified NEC
Cloudy antrum, antra J32.0
Clouston's (hidrotic) **ectodermal dysplasia** Q82.4
Clubbed nail pachydermoperiostosis M89.40 [L62]
Clubbing of finger(s) (nails) R68.3
Clubfinger R68.3
  congenital Q68.1
Clubfoot (congenital) Q66.89
  acquired — *see* Deformity, limb, clubfoot
  equinovarus Q66.0

Clubfoot — *continued*
  paralytic — *see* Deformity, limb, clubfoot
Clubhand (congenital) (radial) Q71.4- ☑
  acquired — *see* Deformity, limb, clubhand
Clubnail R68.3
  congenital Q84.6
Clump, kidney Q63.1
Clumsiness, clumsy child syndrome F82
Cluttering F80.81
Clutton's joints A50.51 [M12.80]
Coagulation, intravascular (diffuse) (disseminated)
  (*see also* Defibrination syndrome)
  complicating abortion — *see* Abortion, by type, complicated by, intravascular coagulation
  following ectopic or molar pregnancy O08.1
Coagulopathy (*see also* Defect, coagulation)
  consumption D65
  intravascular D65
    newborn P60
Coalition
  calcaneo-scaphoid Q66.89
  tarsal Q66.89
Coalminer's
  elbow — *see* Bursitis, elbow, olecranon
  lung or pneumoconiosis J60
Coalworker's lung or pneumoconiosis J60
Coarctation
  aorta (preductal) (postductal) Q25.1
  pulmonary artery Q25.71
Coated tongue K14.3
Coats' disease (exudative retinopathy) — *see* Retinopathy, exudative
Cocaine-induced
  anxiety disorder F14.980
  bipolar and related disorder F14.94
  depressive disorder F14.94
  obsessive-compulsive and related disorder F14.988
  psychotic disorder F14.959
  sexual dysfunction F14.981
  sleep disorder F14.982
Cocainism — *see* Disorder, cocaine use
Coccidioidomycosis B38.9
  cutaneous B38.3
  disseminated B38.7
  generalized B38.7
  meninges B38.4
  prostate B38.81
  pulmonary B38.2
    acute B38.0
    chronic B38.1
  skin B38.3
  specified NEC B38.89
Coccidioidosis — *see* Coccidioidomycosis
Coccidiosis (intestinal) A07.3
Coccydynia, coccygodynia M53.3
Coccyx — *see* condition
Cochin-China diarrhea K90.1
Cockayne's syndrome Q87.1
Cocked up toe — *see* Deformity, toe, specified NEC
Cock's peculiar tumor L72.3
Codman's tumor — *see* Neoplasm, bone, benign
Coenurosis B71.8
Coffee-worker's lung J67.8
Cogan's syndrome H16.32- ☑
  oculomotor apraxia H51.8
Coitus, painful (female) N94.10
  male N53.12
  psychogenic F52.6
Cold J00
  with influenza, flu, or grippe — *see* Influenza, with, respiratory manifestations NEC
  agglutinin disease or hemoglobinuria (chronic) D59.1
  bronchial — *see* Bronchitis
  chest — *see* Bronchitis
  common (head) J00
  effects of T69.9 ☑
    specified effect NEC T69.8 ☑
  excessive, effects of T69.9 ☑
    specified effect NEC T69.8 ☑
  exhaustion from T69.8 ☑
  exposure to T69.9 ☑
    specified effect NEC T69.8 ☑
  head J00
  injury syndrome (newborn) P80.0
  on lung — *see* Bronchitis
  rose J30.1
  sensitivity, auto-immune D59.1

Cold — *continued*
  symptoms J00
  virus J00
Coldsore B00.1
Colibacillosis A49.8
  as the cause of other disease (*see also* Escherichia coli) B96.20
  generalized A41.50
Colic (bilious) (infantile) (intestinal) (recurrent) (spasmodic) R10.83
  abdomen R10.83
    psychogenic F45.8
  appendix, appendicular K38.8
  bile duct — *see* Calculus, bile duct
  biliary — *see* Calculus, bile duct
  common duct — *see* Calculus, bile duct
  cystic duct — *see* Calculus, gallbladder
  Devonshire NEC — *see* Poisoning, lead
  gallbladder — *see* Calculus, gallbladder
  gallstone — *see* Calculus, gallbladder
    gallbladder or cystic duct — *see* Calculus, gallbladder
  hepatic (duct) — *see* Calculus, bile duct
  hysterical F45.8
  kidney N23
  lead NEC — *see* Poisoning, lead
  mucous K58.9
    with diarrhea K58.0
    psychogenic F54
  nephritic N23
  painter's NEC — *see* Poisoning, lead
  pancreas K86.89
  psychogenic F45.8
  renal N23
  saturnine NEC — *see* Poisoning, lead
  ureter N23
  urethral N36.8
    due to calculus N21.1
  uterus NEC N94.89
    menstrual — *see* Dysmenorrhea
  worm NOS B83.9
Colicystitis — *see* Cystitis
Colitis (acute) (catarrhal) (chronic) (noninfective) (hemorrhagic) (*see also* Enteritis) K52.9
  allergic K52.29
    with
      food protein-induced enterocolitis syndrome K52.21
      proctocolitis K52.82
  amebic (acute) (*see also* Amebiasis) A06.0
    nondysenteric A06.2
  anthrax A22.2
  bacillary — *see* Infection, Shigella
  balantidial A07.0
  Clostridium difficile
    not specified as recurrent A04.72
    recurrent A04.71
  coccidial A07.3
  collagenous K52.831
  cystica superficialis K52.89
  dietary counseling and surveillance (for) Z71.3
  dietetic (*see also* Colitis, allergic) K52.29
  drug-induced K52.1
  due to radiation K52.0
  eosinophilic K52.82
  food hypersensitivity (*see also* Colitis, allergic) K52.29
  giardial A07.1
  granulomatous — *see* Enteritis, regional, large intestine
  indeterminate, so stated K52.3
  infectious — *see* Enteritis, infectious
  ischemic K55.9
    acute (subacute) (*see also* Ischemia, intestine, acute) K55.039
    chronic K55.1
    due to mesenteric artery insufficiency K55.1
    fulminant (acute) (*see also* Ischemia, intestine, acute) K55.039
  left sided K51.50
    with
      abscess K51.514
      complication K51.519
        specified NEC K51.518
      fistula K51.513
      obstruction K51.512
      rectal bleeding K51.511
  lymphocytic K52.832

Colitis — *continued*
  membranous
    psychogenic F54
  microscopic K52.839
    specified NEC K52.838
  mucous — *see* Syndrome, irritable, bowel
    psychogenic F54
  noninfective K52.9
    specified NEC K52.89
  polyposa — *see* Polyp, colon, inflammatory
  protozoal A07.9
  pseudomembranous
    not specified as recurrent A04.72
    recurrent A04.71
  pseudomucinous — *see* Syndrome, irritable, bowel
  regional — *see* Enteritis, regional, large intestine
    infectious A09
  segmental — *see* Enteritis, regional, large intestine
  septic — *see* Enteritis, infectious
  spastic K58.9
    with diarrhea K58.0
    psychogenic F54
  staphylococcal A04.8
    foodborne A05.0
  subacute ischemic (*see also* Ischemia, intestine, acute) K55.039
  thromboulcerative (*see also* Ischemia, intestine, acute) K55.039
  toxic NEC K52.1
    due to Clostridium difficile
      not specified as recurrent A04.72
      recurrent A04.71
  transmural — *see* Enteritis, regional, large intestine
  trichomonal A07.8
  tuberculous (ulcerative) A18.32
  ulcerative (chronic) K51.90
    with
      complication K51.919
        abscess K51.914
        fistula K51.913
        obstruction K51.912
        rectal bleeding K51.911
        specified complication NEC K51.918
    enterocolitis — *see* Enterocolitis, ulcerative
    ileocolitis — *see* Ileocolitis, ulcerative
    mucosal proctocolitis — *see* Proctocolitis, mucosal
    proctitis — *see* Proctitis, ulcerative
    pseudopolyposis — *see* Polyp, colon, inflammatory
    psychogenic F54
    rectosigmoiditis — *see* Rectosigmoiditis, ulcerative
    specified type NEC K51.80
      with
        complication K51.819
          abscess K51.814
          fistula K51.813
          obstruction K51.812
          rectal bleeding K51.811
          specified complication NEC K51.818
Collagenosis, collagen disease (nonvascular) (vascular) M35.9
  cardiovascular I42.8
  reactive perforating L87.1
  specified NEC M35.8
Collapse R55
  adrenal E27.2
  cardiorespiratory R57.0
  cardiovascular R57.0
    newborn P29.89
  circulatory (peripheral) R57.9
    during or after labor and delivery O75.1
    following ectopic or molar pregnancy O08.3
    newborn P29.89
  during or
    after labor and delivery O75.1
    resulting from a procedure, not elsewhere classified T81.10 ☑
  external ear canal — *see* Stenosis, external ear canal
  general R55
  heart — *see* Disease, heart
  heat T67.1 ☑
  hysterical F44.89
  labyrinth, membranous (congenital) Q16.5
  lung (massive) (*see also* Atelectasis) J98.19
    pressure due to anesthesia (general) (local) or other sedation T88.2 ☑
      during labor and delivery O74.1
      in pregnancy O29.02- ☑
      postpartum, puerperal O89.09

☑ **Additional Character Required** — Refer to the Tabular List for Character Selection   ▽ Subterms under main terms may continue to next column or page

Collapse — *continued*
- myocardial — *see* Disease, heart
- nervous F48.8
- neurocirculatory F45.8
- nose M95.0
- postoperative T81.10 ☑
- pulmonary (*see also* Atelectasis) J98.19
  - newborn — *see* Atelectasis
- trachea J39.8
- tracheobronchial J98.09
- valvular — *see* Endocarditis
- vascular (peripheral) R57.9
  - during or after labor and delivery O75.1
  - following ectopic or molar pregnancy O08.3
  - newborn P29.89
- vertebra M48.50- ☑
  - cervical region M48.52- ☑
  - cervicothoracic region M48.53- ☑
  - in (due to)
    - metastasis — *see* Collapse, vertebra, in, specified disease NEC
    - osteoporosis (*see also* Osteoporosis) M80.88 ☑
      - cervical region M80.88 ☑
      - cervicothoracic region M80.88 ☑
      - lumbar region M80.88 ☑
      - lumbosacral region M80.88 ☑
      - multiple sites M80.88 ☑
      - occipito-atlanto-axial region M80.88 ☑
      - sacrococcygeal region M80.88 ☑
      - thoracic region M80.88 ☑
      - thoracolumbar region M80.88 ☑
    - specified disease NEC M48.50- ☑
      - cervical region M48.52- ☑
      - cervicothoracic region M48.53- ☑
      - lumbar region M48.56- ☑
      - lumbosacral region M48.57- ☑
      - occipito-atlanto-axial region M48.51- ☑
      - sacrococcygeal region M48.58- ☑
      - thoracic region M48.54- ☑
      - thoracolumbar region M48.55- ☑
  - lumbar region M48.56- ☑
  - lumbosacral region M48.57- ☑
  - occipito-atlanto-axial region M48.51- ☑
  - sacrococcygeal region M48.58- ☑
  - thoracic region M48.54- ☑
  - thoracolumbar region M48.55- ☑

Collateral (*see also* condition)
- circulation (venous) I87.8
- dilation, veins I87.8

Colles' fracture S52.53- ☑
Collet (-Sicard) syndrome G52.7
Collier's asthma or lung J60
Collodion baby Q80.2
Colloid nodule (of thyroid) (cystic) E04.1
Coloboma (iris) Q13.0
- eyelid Q10.3
- fundus Q14.8
- lens Q12.2
- optic disc (congenital) Q14.2
  - acquired H47.31- ☑

Coloenteritis — *see* Enteritis
Colon — *see* condition
Colonization
- MRSA (Methicillin resistant Staphylococcus aureus) Z22.322
- MSSA (Methicillin susceptible Staphylococcus aureus) Z22.321
- status — *see* Carrier (suspected) of

Coloptosis K63.4
Color blindness — *see* Deficiency, color vision
Colostomy
- attention to Z43.3
- fitting or adjustment Z46.89
- malfunctioning K94.03
- status Z93.3

Colpitis (acute) — *see* Vaginitis
Colpocele N81.5
Colpocystitis — *see* Vaginitis
Colpospasm N94.2
Column, spinal, vertebral — *see* condition
Coma R40.20
- with
  - motor response (none) R40.231 ☑
    - abnormal extensor posturing to pain or noxious stimuli (< 2 years of age) R40.232 ☑
    - abnormal flexure posturing to pain or noxious stimuli (0-5 years of age) R40.233 ☑

Coma — *continued*
- with — *continued*
  - motor response — *continued*
    - extensor posturing to pain or noxious stimuli (2-5 years of age) R40.232 ☑
    - flexion/decorticate posturing (< 2 years of age) R40.233 ☑
    - localizes pain (2-5 years of age) R40.235 ☑
    - normal or spontaneous movement (< 2 years of age) R40.236 ☑
    - obeys commands (2-5 years of age) R40.236 ☑
    - withdraws from pain or noxious stimuli (0-5 years of age) R40.234 ☑
    - withdraws to touch (< 2 years of age) R40.235 ☑
  - opening of eyes (never) R40.211 ☑
    - in response to
      - pain R40.212 ☑
      - sound R40.213 ☑
    - spontaneous R40.214 ☑
  - verbal response (none) R40.221 ☑
    - confused conversation R40.224 ☑
    - cooing or babbling or crying appropriately (< 2 years of age) R40.225 ☑
    - inappropriate crying or screaming (< 2 years of age) R40.223 ☑
    - inappropriate words (2-5 years of age) R40.224 ☑
    - incomprehensible sounds (2-5 years of age) R40.222 ☑
    - incomprehensible words R40.222 ☑
    - irritable cries (< 2 years of age) R40.224 ☑
    - moans/grunts to pain; restless (< 2 years old) R40.222 ☑
    - oriented R40.225 ☑
    - screaming (2-5 years of age) R40.223 ☑
    - uses appropriate words (2-5 years of age) R40.225 ☑
- eclamptic — *see* Eclampsia
- epileptic — *see* Epilepsy
- Glasgow, scale score — *see* Glasgow coma scale
- hepatic — *see* Failure, hepatic, by type, with coma
- hyperglycemic (diabetic) — *see* Diabetes, by type, with hyperosmolarity, with coma
- hyperosmolar (diabetic) — *see* Diabetes, by type, with hyperosmolarity, with coma
- hypoglycemic (diabetic) — *see* Diabetes, by type, with hypoglycemia, with coma
  - nondiabetic E15
- in diabetes — *see* Diabetes, coma
- insulin-induced — *see* Coma, hypoglycemic
- ketoacidotic (diabetic) — *see* Diabetes, by type, with ketoacidosis, with coma
- myxedematous E03.5
- newborn P91.5
- persistent vegetative state R40.3
- specified NEC, without documented Glasgow coma scale score, or with partial Glasgow coma scale score reported R40.244 ☑

Comatose — *see* Coma
Combat fatigue F43.0
Combined — *see* condition
Comedo, comedones (giant) L70.0
Comedocarcinoma (*see also* Neoplasm, breast, malignant)
- noninfiltrating
  - breast D05.8- ☑
  - specified site — *see* Neoplasm, in situ, by site
  - unspecified site D05.8- ☑

Comedomastitis — *see* Ectasia, mammary duct
Comminuted fracture — *code as* Fracture, closed
Common
- arterial trunk Q20.0
- atrioventricular canal Q21.2
- atrium Q21.1
- cold (head) J00
- truncus (arteriosus) Q20.0
- variable immunodeficiency — *see* Immunodeficiency, common variable
- ventricle Q20.4

Commotio, commotion (current)
- brain — *see* Injury, intracranial, concussion
- cerebri — *see* Injury, intracranial, concussion
- retinae S05.8X-
- spinal cord — *see* Injury, spinal cord, by region
- spinalis — *see* Injury, spinal cord, by region

Communication
- between
  - base of aorta and pulmonary artery Q21.4
  - left ventricle and right atrium Q20.5
  - pericardial sac and pleural sac Q34.8
  - pulmonary artery and pulmonary vein, congenital Q25.72
- congenital between uterus and digestive or urinary tract Q51.7

Compartment syndrome (deep) (posterior) (traumatic) T79.A0 ☑ (*following* T79.7)
- abdomen T79.A3 ☑ (*following* T79.7)
- lower extremity (hip, buttock, thigh, leg, foot, toes) T79.A2 ☑ (*following* T79.7)
- nontraumatic
  - abdomen M79.A3 (*following* M79.7)
  - lower extremity (hip, buttock, thigh, leg, foot, toes) M79.A2- ☑ (*following* M79.7)
  - specified site NEC M79.A9 (*following* M79.7)
  - upper extremity (shoulder, arm, forearm, wrist, hand, fingers) M79.A1- ☑ (*following* M79.7)
- specified site NEC T79.A9 ☑ (*following* T79.7)
- upper extremity (shoulder, arm, forearm, wrist, hand, fingers) T79.A1- ☑ (*following* T79.7)

Compensation
- failure — *see* Disease, heart
- neurosis, psychoneurosis — *see* Disorder, factitious

Complaint (*see also* Disease)
- bowel, functional K59.9
  - psychogenic F45.8
- intestine, functional K59.9
  - psychogenic F45.8
- kidney — *see* Disease, renal
- miners' J60

Complete — *see* condition
Complex
- Addison-Schilder E71.528
- cardiorenal — *see* Hypertension, cardiorenal
- Costen's M26.69
- disseminated mycobacterium avium- intracellulare (DMAC) A31.2
- Eisenmenger's (ventricular septal defect) I27.83
- hypersexual F52.8
- jumped process, spine — *see* Dislocation, vertebra
- primary, tuberculous A15.7
- Schilder-Addison E71.528
- subluxation (vertebral) M99.19
  - abdomen M99.19
  - acromioclavicular M99.17
  - cervical region M99.11
  - cervicothoracic M99.11
  - costochondral M99.18
  - costovertebral M99.18
  - head region M99.10
  - hip M99.15
  - lower extremity M99.16
  - lumbar region M99.13
  - lumbosacral M99.13
  - occipitocervical M99.10
  - pelvic region M99.15
  - pubic M99.15
  - rib cage M99.18
  - sacral region M99.14
  - sacrococcygeal M99.14
  - sacroiliac M99.14
  - specified NEC M99.19
  - sternochondral M99.18
  - sternoclavicular M99.17
  - thoracic region M99.12
  - thoracolumbar M99.12
  - upper extremity M99.17
- Taussig-Bing (transposition, aorta and overriding pulmonary artery) Q20.1

Complication(s) (from) (of)
- accidental puncture or laceration during a procedure (of) — *see* Complications, intraoperative (intraprocedural), puncture or laceration
- amputation stump (surgical) (late) NEC T87.9
  - dehiscence T87.81
  - infection or inflammation T87.40
    - lower limb T87.4- ☑
    - upper limb T87.4- ☑
  - necrosis T87.50
    - lower limb T87.5- ☑
    - upper limb T87.5- ☑
  - neuroma T87.30
    - lower limb T87.3- ☑
    - upper limb T87.3- ☑

Index

Complication — Complication

Complication(s) — *continued*
  amputation stump — *continued*
    specified type NEC T87.89
  anastomosis (and bypass) (*see also* Complications, prosthetic device or implant)
    intestinal (internal) NEC K91.89
      involving urinary tract N99.89
    urinary tract (involving intestinal tract) N99.89
    vascular — *see* Complications, cardiovascular device or implant
  anesthesia, anesthetic (*see also* Anesthesia, complication) T88.59
    brain, postpartum, puerperal O89.2
    cardiac
      in
        labor and delivery O74.2
          pregnancy O29.19- ☑
      postpartum, puerperal O89.1
    central nervous system
      in
        labor and delivery O74.3
          pregnancy O29.29- ☑
      postpartum, puerperal O89.2
    difficult or failed intubation T88.4 ☑
      in pregnancy O29.6- ☑
    failed sedation (conscious) (moderate) during procedure T88.52 ☑
    general, unintended awareness during procedure T88.53 ☑
    hyperthermia, malignant T88.3 ☑
    hypothermia T88.51 ☑
    intubation failure T88.4 ☑
    malignant hyperthermia T88.3 ☑
    pulmonary
      in
        labor and delivery O74.1
          pregnancy NEC O29.09- ☑
      postpartum, puerperal O89.09
    shock T88.2 ☑
    spinal and epidural
      in
        labor and delivery NEC O74.6
          headache O74.5
          pregnancy NEC O29.5X- ☑
      postpartum, puerperal NEC O89.5
        headache O89.4
    unintended awareness under general anesthesia during procedure T88.53 ☑
  anti-reflux device — *see* Complications, esophageal anti-reflux device
  aortic (bifurcation) graft — *see* Complications, graft, vascular
  aortocoronary (bypass) graft — *see* Complications, coronary artery (bypass) graft
  aortofemoral (bypass) graft — *see* Complications, extremity artery (bypass) graft
  arteriovenous
    fistula, surgically created T82.9 ☑
      embolism T82.818 ☑
      fibrosis T82.828 ☑
      hemorrhage T82.838 ☑
      infection or inflammation T82.7 ☑
      mechanical
        breakdown T82.510 ☑
        displacement T82.520 ☑
        leakage T82.530 ☑
        malposition T82.520 ☑
        obstruction T82.590 ☑
        perforation T82.590 ☑
        protrusion T82.590 ☑
      pain T82.848 ☑
      specified type NEC T82.898 ☑
      stenosis T82.858 ☑
      thrombosis T82.868 ☑
    shunt, surgically created T82.9 ☑
      embolism T82.818 ☑
      fibrosis T82.828 ☑
      hemorrhage T82.838 ☑
      infection or inflammation T82.7 ☑
      mechanical
        breakdown T82.511 ☑
        displacement T82.521 ☑
        leakage T82.531 ☑
        malposition T82.521 ☑
        obstruction T82.591 ☑
        perforation T82.591 ☑
        protrusion T82.591 ☑

Complication(s) — *continued*
  arteriovenous — *continued*
    shunt, surgically created — *continued*
      pain T82.848 ☑
      specified type NEC T82.898 ☑
      stenosis T82.858 ☑
      thrombosis T82.868 ☑
  arthroplasty — *see* Complications, joint prosthesis
  artificial
    fertilization or insemination N98.9
      attempted introduction (of)
        embryo in embryo transfer N98.3
        ovum following in vitro fertilization N98.2
      hyperstimulation of ovaries N98.1
      infection N98.0
      specified NEC N98.8
    heart T82.9 ☑
      embolism T82.817 ☑
      fibrosis T82.827 ☑
      hemorrhage T82.837 ☑
      infection or inflammation T82.7 ☑
      mechanical
        breakdown T82.512 ☑
        displacement T82.522 ☑
        leakage T82.532 ☑
        malposition T82.522 ☑
        obstruction T82.592 ☑
        perforation T82.592 ☑
        protrusion T82.592 ☑
      pain T82.847 ☑
      specified type NEC T82.897 ☑
      stenosis T82.857 ☑
      thrombosis T82.867 ☑
    opening
      cecostomy — *see* Complications, colostomy
      colostomy — *see* Complications, colostomy
      cystostomy — *see* Complications, cystostomy
      enterostomy — *see* Complications, enterostomy
      gastrostomy — *see* Complications, gastrostomy
      ileostomy — *see* Complications, enterostomy
      jejunostomy — *see* Complications, enterostomy
      nephrostomy — *see* Complications, stoma, urinary tract
      tracheostomy — *see* Complications, tracheostomy
      ureterostomy — *see* Complications, stoma, urinary tract
      urethrostomy — *see* Complications, stoma, urinary tract
  balloon implant or device
    gastrointestinal T85.9 ☑
      embolism T85.818 ☑
      fibrosis T85.828 ☑
      hemorrhage T85.838 ☑
      infection and inflammation T85.79 ☑
      pain T85.848 ☑
      specified type NEC T85.898 ☑
      stenosis T85.858 ☑
      thrombosis T85.868 ☑
    vascular (counterpulsation) T82.9 ☑
      embolism T82.818 ☑
      fibrosis T82.828 ☑
      hemorrhage T82.838 ☑
      infection or inflammation T82.7 ☑
      mechanical
        breakdown T82.513 ☑
        displacement T82.523 ☑
        leakage T82.533 ☑
        malposition T82.523 ☑
        obstruction T82.593 ☑
        perforation T82.593 ☑
        protrusion T82.593 ☑
      pain T82.848 ☑
      specified type NEC T82.898 ☑
      stenosis T82.858 ☑
      thrombosis T82.868 ☑
  bariatric procedure
    gastric band procedure K95.09
      infection K95.01
    specified procedure NEC K95.89
      infection K95.81
  bile duct implant (prosthetic) T85.9 ☑
    embolism T85.818 ☑
    fibrosis T85.828 ☑
    hemorrhage T85.838 ☑

Complication(s) — *continued*
  bile duct implant — *continued*
    infection and inflammation T85.79 ☑
    mechanical
      breakdown T85.510 ☑
      displacement T85.520 ☑
      malfunction T85.510 ☑
      malposition T85.520 ☑
      obstruction T85.590 ☑
      perforation T85.590 ☑
      protrusion T85.590 ☑
      specified NEC T85.590 ☑
    pain T85.848 ☑
    specified type NEC T85.898 ☑
    stenosis T85.858 ☑
    thrombosis T85.868 ☑
  bladder device (auxiliary) — *see* Complications, genitourinary, device or implant, urinary system
  bleeding (postoperative) — *see* Complication, postoperative, hemorrhage
    intraoperative — *see* Complication, intraoperative, hemorrhage
  blood vessel graft — *see* Complications, graft, vascular
  bone
    device NEC T84.9 ☑
      embolism T84.81 ☑
      fibrosis T84.82 ☑
      hemorrhage T84.83 ☑
      infection or inflammation T84.7 ☑
      mechanical
        breakdown T84.318 ☑
        displacement T84.328 ☑
        malposition T84.328 ☑
        obstruction T84.398 ☑
        perforation T84.398 ☑
        protrusion T84.398 ☑
      pain T84.84 ☑
      specified type NEC T84.89 ☑
      stenosis T84.85 ☑
      thrombosis T84.86 ☑
    graft — *see* Complications, graft, bone
    growth stimulator (electrode) — *see* Complications, electronic stimulator device, bone
    marrow transplant — *see* Complications, transplant, bone, marrow
  brain neurostimulator (electrode) — *see* Complications, electronic stimulator device, brain
  breast implant (prosthetic) T85.9 ☑
    capsular contracture T85.44 ☑
    embolism T85.818 ☑
    fibrosis T85.828 ☑
    hemorrhage T85.838 ☑
    infection and inflammation T85.79 ☑
    mechanical
      breakdown T85.41 ☑
      displacement T85.42 ☑
      leakage T85.43 ☑
      malposition T85.42 ☑
      obstruction T85.49 ☑
      perforation T85.49 ☑
      protrusion T85.49 ☑
      specified NEC T85.49 ☑
    pain T85.848 ☑
    specified type NEC T85.898 ☑
    stenosis T85.858 ☑
    thrombosis T85.868 ☑
  bypass (*see also* Complications, prosthetic device or implant)
    aortocoronary — *see* Complications, coronary artery (bypass) graft
    arterial (*see also* Complications, graft, vascular)
      extremity — *see* Complications, extremity artery (bypass) graft
  cardiac (*see also* Disease, heart)
    device, implant or graft T82.9 ☑
      embolism T82.817 ☑
      fibrosis T82.827 ☑
      hemorrhage T82.837 ☑
      infection or inflammation T82.7 ☑
        valve prosthesis T82.6 ☑
      mechanical
        breakdown T82.519 ☑
          specified device NEC T82.518 ☑
        displacement T82.529 ☑
          specified device NEC T82.528 ☑
        leakage T82.539 ☑

Complication(s) — *continued*
  cardiac (*see also* Disease, heart) — *continued*
    device, implant or graft — *continued*
      mechanical — *continued*
        leakage — *continued*
          specified device NEC T82.538 ☑
        malposition T82.529 ☑
          specified device NEC T82.528 ☑
        obstruction T82.599 ☑
          specified device NEC T82.598 ☑
        perforation T82.599 ☑
          specified device NEC T82.598 ☑
        protrusion T82.599 ☑
          specified device NEC T82.598 ☑
      pain T82.847 ☑
      specified type NEC T82.897 ☑
      stenosis T82.857 ☑
      thrombosis T82.867 ☑
  cardiovascular device, graft or implant T82.9 ☑
    aortic graft — *see* Complications, graft, vascular
    arteriovenous
      fistula, artificial — *see* Complication, arteriovenous, fistula, surgically created
      shunt — *see* Complication, arteriovenous, shunt, surgically created
    artificial heart — *see* Complication, artificial, heart
    balloon (counterpulsation) device — *see* Complication, balloon implant, vascular
    carotid artery graft — *see* Complications, graft, vascular
    coronary bypass graft — *see* Complication, coronary artery (bypass) graft
    dialysis catheter (vascular) — *see* Complication, catheter, dialysis
    electronic T82.9 ☑
      electrode T82.9 ☑
        embolism T82.817 ☑
        fibrosis T82.827 ☑
        hemorrhage T82.837 ☑
        infection T82.7 ☑
        mechanical
          breakdown T82.110 ☑
          displacement T82.120 ☑
          leakage T82.190 ☑
          obstruction T82.190 ☑
          perforation T82.190 ☑
          protrusion T82.190 ☑
          specified type NEC T82.190 ☑
        pain T82.847 ☑
        specified NEC T82.897 ☑
        stenosis T82.857 ☑
        thrombosis T82.867 ☑
      embolism T82.817 ☑
      fibrosis T82.827 ☑
      hemorrhage T82.837 ☑
      infection T82.7 ☑
      mechanical
        breakdown T82.119 ☑
        displacement T82.129 ☑
        leakage T82.199 ☑
        obstruction T82.199 ☑
        perforation T82.199 ☑
        protrusion T82.199 ☑
        specified type NEC T82.199 ☑
      pain T82.847 ☑
      pulse generator T82.9 ☑
        embolism T82.817 ☑
        fibrosis T82.827 ☑
        hemorrhage T82.837 ☑
        infection T82.7 ☑
        mechanical
          breakdown T82.111 ☑
          displacement T82.121 ☑
          leakage T82.191 ☑
          obstruction T82.191 ☑
          perforation T82.191 ☑
          protrusion T82.191 ☑
          specified type NEC T82.191 ☑
        pain T82.847 ☑
        specified NEC T82.897 ☑
        stenosis T82.857 ☑
        thrombosis T82.867 ☑
      specified condition NEC T82.897 ☑
      specified device NEC T82.9 ☑
        embolism T82.817 ☑
        fibrosis T82.827 ☑

Complication(s) — *continued*
  cardiovascular device, graft or implant — *continued*
    electronic — *continued*
      specified device — *continued*
        hemorrhage T82.837 ☑
        infection T82.7 ☑
        mechanical
          breakdown T82.118 ☑
          displacement T82.128 ☑
          leakage T82.198 ☑
          obstruction T82.198 ☑
          perforation T82.198 ☑
          protrusion T82.198 ☑
          specified type NEC T82.198 ☑
        pain T82.847 ☑
        specified NEC T82.897 ☑
        stenosis T82.857 ☑
        thrombosis T82.867 ☑
      stenosis T82.857 ☑
      thrombosis T82.867 ☑
    extremity artery graft — *see* Complication, extremity artery (bypass) graft
    femoral artery graft — *see* Complication, extremity artery (bypass) graft
    heart
      transplant — *see* Complication, transplant, heart
      valve — *see* Complication, prosthetic device, heart valve
      graft — *see* Complication, heart, valve, graft
    heart-lung transplant — *see* Complication, transplant, heart, with lung
    infection or inflammation T82.7 ☑
    umbrella device — *see* Complication, umbrella device, vascular
    vascular graft (or anastomosis) — *see* Complication, graft, vascular
  carotid artery (bypass) graft — *see* Complications, graft, vascular
  catheter (device) NEC (*see also* Complications, prosthetic device or implant)
    cranial infusion
      infection and inflammation T85.735 ☑
      mechanical
        breakdown T85.610 ☑
        displacement T85.620 ☑
        leakage T85.630 ☑
        malfunction T85.690 ☑
        malposition T85.620 ☑
        obstruction T85.690 ☑
        perforation T85.690 ☑
        protrusion T85.690 ☑
        specified NEC T85.690 ☑
    cystostomy T83.9 ☑
      embolism T83.81 ☑
      fibrosis T83.82 ☑
      hemorrhage T83.83 ☑
      infection and inflammation T83.510 ☑
      mechanical
        breakdown T83.010 ☑
        displacement T83.020 ☑
        leakage T83.030 ☑
        malposition T83.020 ☑
        obstruction T83.090 ☑
        perforation T83.090 ☑
        protrusion T83.090 ☑
        specified NEC T83.090 ☑
      pain T83.84 ☑
      specified type NEC T83.89 ☑
      stenosis T83.85 ☑
      thrombosis T83.86 ☑
    dialysis (vascular) T82.9 ☑
      embolism T82.818 ☑
      fibrosis T82.828 ☑
      hemorrhage T82.838 ☑
      infection and inflammation T82.7 ☑
      intraperitoneal — *see* Complications, catheter, intraperitoneal
      mechanical
        breakdown T82.41 ☑
        displacement T82.42 ☑
        leakage T82.43 ☑
        malposition T82.42 ☑
        obstruction T82.49 ☑
        perforation T82.49 ☑

Complication(s) — *continued*
  catheter (*see also* Complications, prosthetic device or implant) — *continued*
    dialysis — *continued*
      mechanical — *continued*
        protrusion T82.49 ☑
      pain T82.848 ☑
      specified type NEC T82.898 ☑
      stenosis T82.858 ☑
      thrombosis T82.868 ☑
    epidural infusion T85.9 ☑
      embolism T85.810 ☑
      fibrosis T85.820 ☑
      hemorrhage T85.830 ☑
      infection and inflammation T85.735 ☑
      mechanical
        breakdown T85.610 ☑
        displacement T85.620 ☑
        leakage T85.630 ☑
        malfunction T85.610 ☑
        malposition T85.620 ☑
        obstruction T85.690 ☑
        perforation T85.690 ☑
        protrusion T85.690 ☑
        specified NEC T85.690 ☑
      pain T85.840 ☑
      specified type NEC T85.890 ☑
      stenosis T85.850 ☑
      thrombosis T85.860 ☑
    intraperitoneal dialysis T85.9 ☑
      embolism T85.818 ☑
      fibrosis T85.828 ☑
      hemorrhage T85.838 ☑
      infection and inflammation T85.71 ☑
      mechanical
        breakdown T85.611 ☑
        displacement T85.621 ☑
        leakage T85.631 ☑
        malfunction T85.611 ☑
        malposition T85.621 ☑
        obstruction T85.691 ☑
        perforation T85.691 ☑
        protrusion T85.691 ☑
        specified NEC T85.691 ☑
      pain T85.848 ☑
      specified type NEC T85.898 ☑
      stenosis T85.858 ☑
      thrombosis T85.868 ☑
    intrathecal infusion
      infection and inflammation T85.735 ☑
      mechanical
        breakdown T85.610 ☑
        displacement T85.620 ☑
        leakage T85.630 ☑
        malfunction T85.690 ☑
        malposition T85.620 ☑
        obstruction T85.690 ☑
        perforation T85.690 ☑
        protrusion T85.690 ☑
        specified NEC T85.690 ☑
    intravenous infusion T82.9 ☑
      embolism T82.818 ☑
      fibrosis T82.828 ☑
      hemorrhage T82.838 ☑
      infection or inflammation T82.7 ☑
      mechanical
        breakdown T82.514 ☑
        displacement T82.524 ☑
        leakage T82.534 ☑
        malposition T82.524 ☑
        obstruction T82.594 ☑
        perforation T82.594 ☑
        protrusion T82.594 ☑
      pain T82.848 ☑
      specified type NEC T82.898 ☑
      stenosis T82.858 ☑
      thrombosis T82.868 ☑
    spinal infusion
      infection and inflammation T85.735 ☑
      mechanical
        breakdown T85.610 ☑
        displacement T85.620 ☑
        leakage T85.630 ☑
        malfunction T85.690 ☑
        malposition T85.620 ☑
        obstruction T85.690 ☑

Complication(s) — continued
catheter (see also Complications, prosthetic device or
implant) — continued
spinal infusion — continued
mechanical — continued
perforation T85.690 ☑
protrusion T85.690 ☑
specified NEC T85.690 ☑
subarachnoid infusion
infection and inflammation T85.735 ☑
mechanical
breakdown T85.610 ☑
displacement T85.620 ☑
leakage T85.630 ☑
malfunction T85.690 ☑
malposition T85.620 ☑
obstruction T85.690 ☑
perforation T85.690 ☑
protrusion T85.690 ☑
specified NEC T85.690 ☑
subdural infusion T85.9 ☑
embolism T85.810 ☑
fibrosis T85.820 ☑
hemorrhage T85.830 ☑
infection and inflammation T85.735 ☑
mechanical
breakdown T85.610 ☑
displacement T85.620 ☑
leakage T85.630 ☑
malfunction T85.610 ☑
malposition T85.620 ☑
obstruction T85.690 ☑
perforation T85.690 ☑
protrusion T85.690 ☑
specified NEC T85.690 ☑
pain T85.840 ☑
specified type NEC T85.890 ☑
stenosis T85.850 ☑
thrombosis T85.860 ☑
urethral T83.9 ☑
displacement T83.028 ☑
embolism T83.81 ☑
fibrosis T83.82 ☑
hemorrhage T83.83 ☑
indwelling
breakdown T83.011 ☑
displacement T83.021 ☑
infection and inflammation T83.511 ☑
leakage T83.031 ☑
specified complication NEC T83.091 ☑
infection and inflammation T83.511 ☑
leakage T83.038 ☑
malposition T83.028 ☑
mechanical
breakdown T83.011 ☑
obstruction (mechanical) T83.091 ☑
pain T83.84 ☑
perforation T83.091 ☑
protrusion T83.091 ☑
specified type NEC T83.091 ☑
stenosis T83.85 ☑
thrombosis T83.86 ☑
urinary NEC
breakdown T83.018 ☑
displacement T83.028 ☑
infection and inflammation T83.518 ☑
leakage T83.038 ☑
specified complication NEC T83.098 ☑
cecostomy (stoma) — see Complications, colostomy
cesarean delivery wound NEC O90.89
disruption O90.0
hematoma O90.2
infection (following delivery) O86.0
chemotherapy (antineoplastic) NEC T88.7 ☑
chin implant (prosthetic) — see Complication, prosthetic device or implant, specified NEC
circulatory system I99.8
intraoperative I97.88
postprocedural I97.89
following cardiac surgery (see also Infarct, myocardium, associated with revascularization procedure) I97.19- ☑
postcardiotomy syndrome I97.0
hypertension I97.3
lymphedema after mastectomy I97.2
postcardiotomy syndrome I97.0

Complication(s) — continued
circulatory system — continued
postprocedural — continued
specified NEC I97.89
colostomy (stoma) K94.00
hemorrhage K94.01
infection K94.02
malfunction K94.03
mechanical K94.03
specified complication NEC K94.09
contraceptive device, intrauterine — see Complications, intrauterine, contraceptive device
cord (umbilical) — see Complications, umbilical cord
corneal graft — see Complications, graft, cornea
coronary artery (bypass) graft T82.9 ☑
atherosclerosis — see Arteriosclerosis, coronary
(artery),
embolism T82.818 ☑
fibrosis T82.828 ☑
hemorrhage T82.838 ☑
infection and inflammation T82.7 ☑
mechanical
breakdown T82.211 ☑
displacement T82.212 ☑
leakage T82.213 ☑
malposition T82.212 ☑
obstruction T82.218 ☑
perforation T82.218 ☑
protrusion T82.218 ☑
specified NEC T82.218 ☑
pain T82.848 ☑
specified type NEC T82.898 ☑
stenosis T82.858 ☑
thrombosis T82.868 ☑
counterpulsation device (balloon), intra- aortic — see
Complications, balloon implant, vascular
cystostomy (stoma) N99.518
catheter — see Complications, catheter, cystostomy
hemorrhage N99.510
infection N99.511
malfunction N99.512
specified type NEC N99.518
delivery (see also Complications, obstetric) O75.9
procedure (instrumental) (manual) (surgical) O75.4
specified NEC O75.89
dialysis (peritoneal) (renal) (see also Complications,
infusion)
catheter (vascular) — see Complication, catheter,
dialysis
peritoneal, intraperitoneal — see Complications, catheter, intraperitoneal
dorsal column (spinal) neurostimulator — see Complications, electronic stimulator device, spinal cord
drug NEC T88.7 ☑
ear procedure (see also Disorder, ear)
intraoperative H95.88
hematoma — see Complications, intraoperative, hemorrhage (hematoma) (of), ear
hemorrhage — see Complications, intraoperative, hemorrhage (hematoma) (of), ear
laceration — see Complications, intraoperative,
puncture or laceration..., ear
specified NEC H95.88
postoperative H95.89
external ear canal stenosis H95.81- ☑
hematoma — see Complications, postprocedural, hematoma (of), ear
hemorrhage — see Complications, postprocedural, hemorrhage (of), ear
postmastoidectomy — see Complications,
postmastoidectomy
seroma — see Complications, postprocedural,
seroma (of), mastoid process
specified NEC H95.89
ectopic pregnancy O08.9
damage to pelvic organs O08.6
embolism O08.2
genital infection O08.0
hemorrhage (delayed) (excessive) O08.1
metabolic disorder O08.5
renal failure O08.4
shock O08.3
specified type NEC O08.0
venous complication NEC O08.7

Complication(s) — continued
electronic stimulator device
bladder (urinary) — see Complications, electronic
stimulator device, urinary
bone T84.9 ☑
breakdown T84.310 ☑
displacement T84.320 ☑
embolism T84.81 ☑
fibrosis T84.82 ☑
hemorrhage T84.83 ☑
infection or inflammation T84.7 ☑
malfunction T84.310 ☑
malposition T84.320 ☑
mechanical NEC T84.390 ☑
obstruction T84.390 ☑
pain T84.84 ☑
perforation T84.390 ☑
protrusion T84.390 ☑
specified type NEC T84.89 ☑
stenosis T84.85 ☑
thrombosis T84.86 ☑
brain T85.9 ☑
embolism T85.810 ☑
fibrosis T85.820 ☑
hemorrhage T85.830 ☑
infection and inflammation T85.731 ☑
mechanical
breakdown T85.110 ☑
displacement T85.120 ☑
leakage T85.190 ☑
malposition T85.120 ☑
obstruction T85.190 ☑
perforation T85.190 ☑
protrusion T85.190 ☑
specified NEC T85.190 ☑
pain T85.840 ☑
specified type NEC T85.890 ☑
stenosis T85.850 ☑
thrombosis T85.860 ☑
cardiac (defibrillator) (pacemaker) — see Complications, cardiovascular device or implant,
electronic
generator (brain) (gastric) (peripheral) (sacral)
(spinal)
breakdown T85.113 ☑
displacement T85.123 ☑
leakage T85.193 ☑
malposition T85.123 ☑
obstruction T85.193 ☑
perforation T85.193 ☑
protrusion T85.193 ☑
specified type NEC T85.193 ☑
muscle T84.9 ☑
breakdown T84.418 ☑
displacement T84.428 ☑
embolism T84.81 ☑
fibrosis T84.82 ☑
hemorrhage T84.83 ☑
infection or inflammation T84.7 ☑
mechanical NEC T84.498 ☑
pain T84.84 ☑
specified type NEC T84.89 ☑
stenosis T84.85 ☑
thrombosis T84.86 ☑
nervous system T85.9 ☑
brain — see Complications, electronic stimulator device, brain
cranial nerve — see Complications, electronic
stimulator device, peripheral nerve
embolism T85.810 ☑
fibrosis T85.820 ☑
gastric nerve — see Complications, electronic
stimulator device, peripheral nerve
hemorrhage T85.830 ☑
infection and inflammation T85.738 ☑
mechanical
breakdown T85.118 ☑
displacement T85.128 ☑
leakage T85.199 ☑
malposition T85.128 ☑
obstruction T85.199 ☑
perforation T85.199 ☑
protrusion T85.199 ☑
specified NEC T85.199 ☑
pain T85.840 ☑

Complication(s) — *continued*
  electronic stimulator device — *continued*
    nervous system — *continued*
      peripheral nerve — *see* Complications, electronic stimulator device, peripheral nerve
      sacral nerve — *see* Complications, electronic stimulator device, peripheral nerve
      specified type NEC T85.890 ☑
      spinal cord — *see* Complications, electronic stimulator device, spinal cord
      stenosis T85.850 ☑
      thrombosis T85.860 ☑
      vagal nerve — *see* Complications, electronic stimulator device, peripheral nerve
    peripheral nerve T85.9 ☑
      embolism T85.810 ☑
      fibrosis T85.820 ☑
      hemorrhage T85.830 ☑
      infection and inflammation T85.732 ☑
      mechanical
        breakdown T85.111 ☑
        displacement T85.121 ☑
        leakage T85.191 ☑
        malposition T85.121 ☑
        obstruction T85.191 ☑
        perforation T85.191 ☑
        protrusion T85.191 ☑
        specified NEC T85.191 ☑
      pain T85.840 ☑
      specified type NEC T85.890 ☑
      stenosis T85.850 ☑
      thrombosis T85.860 ☑
    spinal cord T85.9 ☑
      embolism T85.810 ☑
      fibrosis T85.820 ☑
      hemorrhage T85.830 ☑
      infection and inflammation T85.733 ☑
      mechanical
        breakdown T85.112 ☑
        displacement T85.122 ☑
        leakage T85.192 ☑
        malposition T85.122 ☑
        obstruction T85.192 ☑
        perforation T85.192 ☑
        protrusion T85.192 ☑
        specified NEC T85.192 ☑
      pain T85.840 ☑
      specified type NEC T85.890 ☑
      stenosis T85.850 ☑
      thrombosis T85.860 ☑
    urinary T83.9 ☑
      embolism T83.81 ☑
      fibrosis T83.82 ☑
      hemorrhage T83.83 ☑
      infection and inflammation T83.598 ☑
      mechanical
        breakdown T83.110 ☑
        displacement T83.120 ☑
        malposition T83.120 ☑
        perforation T83.190 ☑
        protrusion T83.190 ☑
        specified NEC T83.190 ☑
      pain T83.84 ☑
      specified type NEC T83.89 ☑
      stenosis T83.85 ☑
      thrombosis T83.86 ☑
  electroshock therapy T88.9 ☑
    specified NEC T88.8 ☑
  endocrine E34.9
    postprocedural
      adrenal hypofunction E89.6
      hypoinsulinemia E89.1
      hypoparathyroidism E89.2
      hypopituitarism E89.3
      hypothyroidism E89.0
      ovarian failure E89.40
        asymptomatic E89.40
        symptomatic E89.41
      specified NEC E89.89
      testicular hypofunction E89.5
  endodontic treatment NEC M27.59
  enterostomy (stoma) K94.10
    hemorrhage K94.11
    infection K94.12
    malfunction K94.13
    mechanical K94.13

Complication(s) — *continued*
  enterostomy — *continued*
    specified complication NEC K94.19
  episiotomy, disruption O90.1
  esophageal anti-reflux device T85.9 ☑
    embolism T85.818 ☑
    fibrosis T85.828 ☑
    hemorrhage T85.838 ☑
    infection and inflammation T85.79 ☑
    mechanical
      breakdown T85.511 ☑
      displacement T85.521 ☑
      malfunction T85.511 ☑
      malposition T85.521 ☑
      obstruction T85.591 ☑
      perforation T85.591 ☑
      protrusion T85.591 ☑
      specified NEC T85.591 ☑
    pain T85.848 ☑
    specified type NEC T85.898 ☑
    stenosis T85.858 ☑
    thrombosis T85.868 ☑
  esophagostomy K94.30
    hemorrhage K94.31
    infection K94.32
    malfunction K94.33
    mechanical K94.33
    specified complication NEC K94.39
  extracorporeal circulation T80.90 ☑
  extremity artery (bypass) graft T82.9 ☑
    arteriosclerosis — *see* Arteriosclerosis, extremities, bypass graft
    embolism T82.818 ☑
    fibrosis T82.828 ☑
    hemorrhage T82.838 ☑
    infection and inflammation T82.7 ☑
    mechanical
      breakdown T82.318 ☑
        femoral artery T82.312 ☑
      displacement T82.328 ☑
        femoral artery T82.322 ☑
      leakage T82.338 ☑
        femoral artery T82.332 ☑
      malposition T82.328 ☑
        femoral artery T82.322 ☑
      obstruction T82.398 ☑
        femoral artery T82.392 ☑
      perforation T82.398 ☑
        femoral artery T82.392 ☑
      protrusion T82.398 ☑
        femoral artery T82.392 ☑
    pain T82.848 ☑
    specified type NEC T82.898 ☑
    stenosis T82.858 ☑
    thrombosis T82.868 ☑
  eye H57.9
    corneal graft — *see* Complications, graft, cornea
    implant (prosthetic) T85.9 ☑
      embolism T85.818 ☑
      fibrosis T85.828 ☑
      hemorrhage T85.838 ☑
      infection and inflammation T85.79 ☑
      mechanical
        breakdown T85.318 ☑
        displacement T85.328 ☑
        leakage T85.398 ☑
        malposition T85.328 ☑
        obstruction T85.398 ☑
        perforation T85.398 ☑
        protrusion T85.398 ☑
        specified NEC T85.398 ☑
      pain T85.848 ☑
      specified type NEC T85.898 ☑
      stenosis T85.858 ☑
      thrombosis T85.868 ☑
    intraocular lens — *see* Complications, intraocular lens
    orbital prosthesis — *see* Complications, orbital prosthesis
  female genital N94.9
    device, implant or graft NEC — *see* Complications, genitourinary, device or implant, genital tract
  femoral artery (bypass) graft — *see* Complication, extremity artery (bypass) graft
  fixation device, internal (orthopedic) T84.9 ☑
    infection and inflammation T84.60 ☑

Complication(s) — *continued*
  fixation device, internal — *continued*
    infection and inflammation — *continued*
      arm T84.61- ☑
        humerus T84.61- ☑
        radius T84.61- ☑
        ulna T84.61- ☑
      leg T84.629 ☑
        femur T84.62- ☑
        fibula T84.62- ☑
        tibia T84.62- ☑
      specified site NEC T84.89 ☑
      spine T84.63 ☑
    mechanical
      breakdown
        limb T84.119 ☑
          carpal T84.210 ☑
          femur T84.11- ☑
          fibula T84.11- ☑
          humerus T84.11- ☑
          metacarpal T84.210 ☑
          metatarsal T84.213 ☑
          phalanx
            foot T84.213 ☑
            hand T84.210 ☑
          radius T84.11- ☑
          tarsal T84.213 ☑
          tibia T84.11- ☑
          ulna T84.11- ☑
        specified bone NEC T84.218 ☑
        spine T84.216 ☑
      displacement
        limb T84.129 ☑
          carpal T84.220 ☑
          femur T84.12- ☑
          fibula T84.12- ☑
          humerus T84.12- ☑
          metacarpal T84.220 ☑
          metatarsal T84.223 ☑
          phalanx
            foot T84.223 ☑
            hand T84.220 ☑
          radius T84.12- ☑
          tarsal T84.223 ☑
          tibia T84.12- ☑
          ulna T84.12- ☑
        specified bone NEC T84.228 ☑
        spine T84.226 ☑
      malposition — *see* Complications, fixation device, internal, mechanical, displacement
      obstruction — *see* Complications, fixation device, internal, mechanical, specified type NEC
      perforation — *see* Complications, fixation device, internal, mechanical, specified type NEC
      protrusion — *see* Complications, fixation device, internal, mechanical, specified type NEC
      specified type NEC
        limb T84.199 ☑
          carpal T84.290 ☑
          femur T84.19- ☑
          fibula T84.19- ☑
          humerus T84.19- ☑
          metacarpal T84.290 ☑
          metatarsal T84.293 ☑
          phalanx
            foot T84.293 ☑
            hand T84.290 ☑
          radius T84.19- ☑
          tarsal T84.293 ☑
          tibia T84.19- ☑
          ulna T84.19- ☑
        specified bone NEC T84.298 ☑
        vertebra T84.296 ☑
    specified type NEC T84.89 ☑
      embolism T84.81 ☑
      fibrosis T84.82 ☑
      hemorrhage T84.83 ☑
      pain T84.84 ☑
      specified complication NEC T84.89 ☑
      stenosis T84.85 ☑
      thrombosis T84.86 ☑
  following
    acute myocardial infarction NEC I23.8

Complication(s) — *continued*
  following — *continued*
    acute myocardial infarction — *continued*
      aneurysm (false) (of cardiac wall) (of heart wall)
        (ruptured) I23.3
      angina I23.7
      atrial
        septal defect I23.1
        thrombosis I23.6
      cardiac wall rupture I23.3
      chordae tendinae rupture I23.4
      defect
        septal
          atrial (heart) I23.1
          ventricular (heart) I23.2
      hemopericardium I23.0
      papillary muscle rupture I23.5
      rupture
        cardiac wall I23.3
          with hemopericardium I23.0
        chordae tendineae I23.4
        papillary muscle I23.5
      specified NEC I23.8
      thrombosis
        atrium I23.6
        auricular appendage I23.6
        ventricle (heart) I23.6
      ventricular
        septal defect I23.2
        thrombosis I23.6
    ectopic or molar pregnancy O08.9
      cardiac arrest O08.81
      sepsis O08.82
      specified type NEC O08.89
      urinary tract infection O08.83
    termination of pregnancy — *see* Abortion
  gastrointestinal K92.9
    bile duct prosthesis — *see* Complications, bile duct
      implant
    esophageal anti-reflux device — *see* Complications,
      esophageal anti-reflux device
    postoperative
      colostomy — *see* Complications, colostomy
      dumping syndrome K91.1
      enterostomy — *see* Complications, enterosto-
        my
      gastrostomy — *see* Complications, gastrostomy
      malabsorption NEC K91.2
      obstruction (*see also* Obstruction, intestine,
        postoperative) K91.30
      postcholecystectomy syndrome K91.5
      specified NEC K91.89
      vomiting after GI surgery K91.0
    prosthetic device or implant
      bile duct prosthesis — *see* Complications, bile
        duct implant
      esophageal anti-reflux device — *see* Complica-
        tions, esophageal anti-reflux device
      specified type NEC
        embolism T85.818 ☑
        fibrosis T85.828 ☑
        hemorrhage T85.838 ☑
        mechanical
          breakdown T85.518 ☑
          displacement T85.528 ☑
          malfunction T85.518 ☑
          malposition T85.528 ☑
          obstruction T85.598 ☑
          perforation T85.598 ☑
          protrusion T85.598 ☑
          specified NEC T85.598 ☑
        pain T85.848 ☑
        specified complication NEC T85.898 ☑
        stenosis T85.858 ☑
        thrombosis T85.868 ☑
  gastrostomy (stoma) K94.20
    hemorrhage K94.21
    infection K94.22
    malfunction K94.23
    mechanical K94.23
    specified complication NEC K94.29
  genitourinary
    device or implant T83.9 ☑
      genital tract T83.9 ☑
        infection or inflammation T83.69 ☑
        intrauterine contraceptive device — *see*
          Complications, intrauterine, contra-
          ceptive device

Complication(s) — *continued*
  genitourinary — *continued*
    device or implant — *continued*
      genital tract — *continued*
        mechanical — *see* Complications, by device,
          mechanical
        mesh — *see* Complications, mesh
        penile prosthesis — *see* Complications,
          prosthetic device, penile
        specified type NEC T83.89 ☑
          embolism T83.81 ☑
          fibrosis T83.82 ☑
          hemorrhage T83.83 ☑
          pain T83.84 ☑
          specified complication NEC T83.89 ☑
          stenosis T83.85 ☑
          thrombosis T83.86 ☑
        vaginal mesh — *see* Complications, mesh
      urinary system T83.9 ☑
        cystostomy catheter — *see* Complication,
          catheter, cystostomy
        electronic stimulator — *see* Complications,
          electronic stimulator device, urinary
        indwelling urethral catheter — *see* Compli-
          cations, catheter, urethral, indwelling
        infection or inflammation T83.598 ☑
          indwelling urethral catheter T83.511 ☑
        kidney transplant — *see* Complication,
          transplant, kidney
        organ graft — *see* Complication, graft, uri-
          nary organ
        specified type NEC T83.89 ☑
          embolism T83.81 ☑
          fibrosis T83.82 ☑
          hemorrhage T83.83 ☑
          mechanical T83.198 ☑
            breakdown T83.118 ☑
            displacement T83.128 ☑
            malfunction T83.118 ☑
            malposition T83.128 ☑
            obstruction T83.198 ☑
            perforation T83.198 ☑
            protrusion T83.198 ☑
            specified NEC T83.198 ☑
        sphincter implant — *see* Complications,
          implant, urinary sphincter
        sphincter, implanted T83.191 ☑
        stent (ileal conduit) (nephroureteral)
          T83.193 ☑
        pain T83.84 ☑
        specified complication NEC T83.89 ☑
        stenosis T83.85 ☑
        thrombosis T83.86 ☑
        ureteral indwelling T83.192 ☑
    postprocedural
      pelvic peritoneal adhesions N99.4
      renal failure N99.0
      specified NEC N99.89
      stoma — *see* Complications, stoma, urinary
        tract
      urethral stricture — *see* Stricture, urethra,
        postprocedural
      vaginal
        adhesions N99.2
        vault prolapse N99.3
  graft (bypass) (patch) (*see also* Complications, prosthet-
    ic device or implant)
    aorta — *see* Complications, graft, vascular
    arterial — *see* Complication, graft, vascular
    bone T86.839
      failure T86.831
      infection T86.832
      mechanical T84.318 ☑
        breakdown T84.318 ☑
        displacement T84.328 ☑
        protrusion T84.398 ☑
        specified type NEC T84.398 ☑
      rejection T86.830
      specified type NEC T86.838
    carotid artery — *see* Complications, graft, vascular
    cornea T86.849
      failure T86.841
      infection T86.842
      mechanical T85.398 ☑
        breakdown T85.318 ☑
        displacement T85.328 ☑
        protrusion T85.398 ☑

Complication(s) — *continued*
  graft (*see also* Complications, prosthetic device or im-
    plant) — *continued*
    cornea — *continued*
      mechanical — *continued*
        specified type NEC T85.398 ☑
      rejection T86.840
      retroprosthetic membrane T85.398 ☑
      specified type NEC T86.848
    femoral artery (bypass) — *see* Complication, ex-
      tremity artery (bypass) graft
    genital organ or tract — *see* Complications, geni-
      tourinary, device or implant, genital tract
    muscle T84.9 ☑
      breakdown T84.410 ☑
      displacement T84.420 ☑
      embolism T84.81 ☑
      fibrosis T84.82 ☑
      hemorrhage T84.83 ☑
      infection and inflammation T84.7 ☑
      mechanical NEC T84.490 ☑
      pain T84.84 ☑
      specified type NEC T84.89 ☑
      stenosis T84.85 ☑
      thrombosis T84.86 ☑
    nerve — *see* Complication, prosthetic device or
      implant, specified NEC
    skin — *see* Complications, prosthetic device or
      implant, skin graft
    tendon T84.9 ☑
      breakdown T84.410 ☑
      displacement T84.420 ☑
      embolism T84.81 ☑
      fibrosis T84.82 ☑
      hemorrhage T84.83 ☑
      infection and inflammation T84.7 ☑
      mechanical NEC T84.490 ☑
      pain T84.84 ☑
      specified type NEC T84.89 ☑
      stenosis T84.85 ☑
      thrombosis T84.86 ☑
    urinary organ T83.9 ☑
      embolism T83.81 ☑
      fibrosis T83.82 ☑
      hemorrhage T83.83 ☑
      infection and inflammation T83.598 ☑
        indwelling urethral catheter T83.511 ☑
      mechanical
        breakdown T83.21 ☑
        displacement T83.22 ☑
        erosion T83.24 ☑
        exposure T83.25 ☑
        leakage T83.23 ☑
        malposition T83.22 ☑
        obstruction T83.29 ☑
        perforation T83.29 ☑
        protrusion T83.29 ☑
        specified NEC T83.29 ☑
      pain T83.84 ☑
      specified type NEC T83.89 ☑
      stenosis T83.85 ☑
      thrombosis T83.86 ☑
    vascular T82.9 ☑
      embolism T82.818 ☑
      femoral artery — *see* Complication, extremity
        artery (bypass) graft
      fibrosis T82.828 ☑
      hemorrhage T82.838 ☑
      mechanical
        breakdown T82.319 ☑
          aorta (bifurcation) T82.310 ☑
          carotid artery T82.311 ☑
          specified vessel NEC T82.318 ☑
        displacement T82.329 ☑
          aorta (bifurcation) T82.320 ☑
          carotid artery T82.321 ☑
          specified vessel NEC T82.328 ☑
        leakage T82.339 ☑
          aorta (bifurcation) T82.330 ☑
          carotid artery T82.331 ☑
          specified vessel NEC T82.338 ☑
        malposition T82.329 ☑
          aorta (bifurcation) T82.320 ☑
          carotid artery T82.321 ☑
          specified vessel NEC T82.328 ☑
        obstruction T82.399 ☑

Complication(s) — *continued*
　graft (*see also* Complications, prosthetic device or implant) — *continued*
　　vascular — *continued*
　　　mechanical — *continued*
　　　　obstruction — *continued*
　　　　　aorta (bifurcation) T82.390 ☑
　　　　　carotid artery T82.391 ☑
　　　　　specified vessel NEC T82.398 ☑
　　　　perforation T82.399 ☑
　　　　　aorta (bifurcation) T82.390 ☑
　　　　　carotid artery T82.391 ☑
　　　　　specified vessel NEC T82.398 ☑
　　　　protrusion T82.399 ☑
　　　　　aorta (bifurcation) T82.390 ☑
　　　　　carotid artery T82.391 ☑
　　　　　specified vessel NEC T82.398 ☑
　　　pain T82.848 ☑
　　　specified complication NEC T82.898 ☑
　　　stenosis T82.858 ☑
　　　thrombosis T82.868 ☑
　heart I51.9
　　assist device
　　　infection and inflammation T82.7 ☑
　　following acute myocardial infarction — *see* Complications, following, acute myocardial infarction
　　postoperative — *see* Complications, circulatory system
　　transplant — *see* Complication, transplant, heart
　　and lung(s) — *see* Complications, transplant, heart, with lung
　　valve
　　　graft (biological) T82.9 ☑
　　　　embolism T82.817 ☑
　　　　fibrosis T82.827 ☑
　　　　hemorrhage T82.837 ☑
　　　　infection and inflammation T82.7 ☑
　　　　mechanical T82.228 ☑
　　　　　breakdown T82.221 ☑
　　　　　displacement T82.222 ☑
　　　　　leakage T82.223 ☑
　　　　　malposition T82.222 ☑
　　　　　obstruction T82.228 ☑
　　　　　perforation T82.228 ☑
　　　　　protrusion T82.228 ☑
　　　　pain T82.847 ☑
　　　　specified type NEC T82.897 ☑
　　　　stenosis T82.857 ☑
　　　　thrombosis T82.867 ☑
　　　prosthesis T82.9 ☑
　　　　embolism T82.817 ☑
　　　　fibrosis T82.827 ☑
　　　　hemorrhage T82.837 ☑
　　　　infection or inflammation T82.6 ☑
　　　　mechanical T82.09 ☑
　　　　　breakdown T82.01 ☑
　　　　　displacement T82.02 ☑
　　　　　leakage T82.03 ☑
　　　　　malposition T82.02 ☑
　　　　　obstruction T82.09 ☑
　　　　　perforation T82.09 ☑
　　　　　protrusion T82.09 ☑
　　　　pain T82.847 ☑
　　　　specified type NEC T82.897 ☑
　　　　　mechanical T82.09 ☑
　　　　stenosis T82.857 ☑
　　　　thrombosis T82.867 ☑
　hematoma
　　intraoperative — *see* Complication, intraoperative, hemorrhage
　　postprocedural — *see* Complication, postprocedural, hematoma
　hemodialysis — *see* Complications, dialysis
　hemorrhage
　　intraoperative — *see* Complication, intraoperative, hemorrhage
　　postprocedural — *see* Complication, postprocedural, hemorrhage
　ileostomy (stoma) — *see* Complications, enterostomy
　immunization (procedure) — *see* Complications, vaccination
　implant (*see also* Complications, by site and type)
　　urinary sphincter T83.9 ☑
　　　embolism T83.81 ☑
　　　fibrosis T83.82 ☑

Complication(s) — *continued*
　implant (*see also* Complications, by site and type) — *continued*
　　urinary sphincter — *continued*
　　　hemorrhage T83.83 ☑
　　　infection and inflammation T83.591 ☑
　　　mechanical
　　　　breakdown T83.111 ☑
　　　　displacement T83.121 ☑
　　　　leakage T83.191 ☑
　　　　malposition T83.121 ☑
　　　　obstruction T83.191 ☑
　　　　perforation T83.191 ☑
　　　　protrusion T83.191 ☑
　　　　specified NEC T83.191 ☑
　　　pain T83.84 ☑
　　　specified type NEC T83.89 ☑
　　　stenosis T83.85 ☑
　　　thrombosis T83.86 ☑
　infusion (procedure) T80.90 ☑
　　air embolism T80.0 ☑
　　blood — *see* Complications, transfusion
　　catheter — *see* Complications, catheter
　　infection T80.29 ☑
　　pump — *see* Complications, cardiovascular, device or implant
　　sepsis T80.29 ☑
　　serum reaction (*see also* Reaction, serum) T80.69 ☑
　　　anaphylactic shock (*see also* Shock, anaphylactic) T80.59 ☑
　　specified type NEC T80.89 ☑
　inhalation therapy NEC T81.81 ☑
　injection (procedure) T80.90 ☑
　　drug reaction — *see* Reaction, drug
　　infection T80.29 ☑
　　sepsis T80.29 ☑
　　serum (prophylactic) (therapeutic) — *see* Complications, vaccination
　　specified type NEC T80.89 ☑
　　vaccine (any) — *see* Complications, vaccination
　inoculation (any) — *see* Complications, vaccination
　insulin pump
　　infection and inflammation T85.72 ☑
　　mechanical
　　　breakdown T85.614 ☑
　　　displacement T85.624 ☑
　　　leakage T85.633 ☑
　　　malposition T85.624 ☑
　　　obstruction T85.694 ☑
　　　perforation T85.694 ☑
　　　protrusion T85.694 ☑
　　　specified NEC T85.694 ☑
　intestinal pouch NEC K91.858
　intraocular lens (prosthetic) T85.9 ☑
　　embolism T85.818 ☑
　　fibrosis T85.828 ☑
　　hemorrhage T85.838 ☑
　　infection and inflammation T85.79 ☑
　　mechanical
　　　breakdown T85.21 ☑
　　　displacement T85.22 ☑
　　　malposition T85.22 ☑
　　　obstruction T85.29 ☑
　　　perforation T85.29 ☑
　　　protrusion T85.29 ☑
　　　specified NEC T85.29 ☑
　　pain T85.848 ☑
　　specified type NEC T85.898 ☑
　　stenosis T85.858 ☑
　　thrombosis T85.868 ☑
　intraoperative (intraprocedural)
　　cardiac arrest (*see also* Infarct, myocardium, associated with revascularization procedure)
　　　during cardiac surgery I97.710
　　　during other surgery I97.711
　　cardiac functional disturbance NEC (*see also* Infarct, myocardium, associated with revascularization procedure)
　　　during cardiac surgery I97.790
　　　during other surgery I97.791
　　hemorrhage (hematoma) (of)
　　　circulatory system organ or structure
　　　　during cardiac bypass I97.411
　　　　during cardiac catheterization I97.410
　　　　during other circulatory system procedure I97.418

Complication(s) — *continued*
　intraoperative — *continued*
　　hemorrhage — *continued*
　　　circulatory system organ or structure — *continued*
　　　　during other procedure I97.42
　　　digestive system organ
　　　　during procedure on digestive system K91.61
　　　　during procedure on other organ K91.62
　　　ear
　　　　during procedure on ear and mastoid process H95.21
　　　　during procedure on other organ H95.22
　　　endocrine system organ or structure
　　　　during procedure on endocrine system organ or structure E36.01
　　　　during procedure on other organ E36.02
　　　eye and adnexa
　　　　during ophthalmic procedure H59.11- ☑
　　　　during other procedure H59.12- ☑
　　　genitourinary organ or structure
　　　　during procedure on genitourinary organ or structure N99.61
　　　　during procedure on other organ N99.62
　　　mastoid process
　　　　during procedure on ear and mastoid process H95.21
　　　　during procedure on other organ H95.22
　　　musculoskeletal structure
　　　　during musculoskeletal surgery M96.810
　　　　during non-orthopedic surgery M96.811
　　　　during orthopedic surgery M96.810
　　　nervous system
　　　　during a nervous system procedure G97.31
　　　　during other procedure G97.32
　　　respiratory system
　　　　during other procedure J95.62
　　　　during procedure on respiratory system organ or structure J95.61
　　　skin and subcutaneous tissue
　　　　during a dermatologic procedure L76.01
　　　　during a procedure on other organ L76.02
　　　spleen
　　　　during a procedure on other organ D78.02
　　　　during a procedure on the spleen D78.01
　　puncture or laceration (accidental) (unintentional) (of)
　　　brain
　　　　during a nervous system procedure G97.48
　　　　during other procedure G97.49
　　　circulatory system organ or structure
　　　　during circulatory system procedure I97.51
　　　　during other procedure I97.52
　　　digestive system
　　　　during procedure on digestive system K91.71
　　　　during procedure on other organ K91.72
　　　ear
　　　　during procedure on ear and mastoid process H95.31
　　　　during procedure on other organ H95.32
　　　endocrine system organ or structure
　　　　during procedure on endocrine system organ or structure E36.11
　　　　during procedure on other organ E36.12
　　　eye and adnexa
　　　　during ophthalmic procedure H59.21- ☑
　　　　during other procedure H59.22- ☑
　　　genitourinary organ or structure
　　　　during procedure on genitourinary organ or structure N99.71
　　　　during procedure on other organ N99.72
　　　mastoid process
　　　　during procedure on ear and mastoid process H95.31
　　　　during procedure on other organ H95.32
　　　musculoskeletal structure
　　　　during musculoskeletal surgery M96.820
　　　　during non-orthopedic surgery M96.821
　　　　during orthopedic surgery M96.820
　　　nervous system
　　　　during a nervous system procedure G97.48
　　　　during other procedure G97.49
　　　respiratory system
　　　　during other procedure J95.72
　　　　during procedure on respiratory system organ or structure J95.71

Complication(s) — *continued*
  intraoperative — *continued*
    puncture or laceration — *continued*
      skin and subcutaneous tissue
        during a dermatologic procedure L76.11
        during a procedure on other organ L76.12
      spleen
        during a procedure on other organ D78.12
        during a procedure on the spleen D78.11
    specified NEC
      circulatory system I97.88
      digestive system K91.81
      ear H95.88
      endocrine system E36.8
      eye and adnexa H59.88
      genitourinary system N99.81
      mastoid process H95.88
      musculoskeletal structure M96.89
      nervous system G97.81
      respiratory system J95.88
      skin and subcutaneous tissue L76.81
      spleen D78.81
  intraperitoneal catheter (dialysis) (infusion) — *see* Complications, catheter, intraperitoneal
  intrathecal infusion pump
    infection and inflammation T85.738 ☑
    mechanical
      breakdown T85.615 ☑
      displacement T85.625 ☑
      leakage T85.635 ☑
      malfunction T85.695 ☑
      malposition T85.625 ☑
      obstruction T85.695 ☑
      perforation T85.695 ☑
      protrusion T85.695 ☑
      specified NEC T85.695 ☑
  intrauterine
    contraceptive device
      embolism T83.81 ☑
      fibrosis T83.82 ☑
      hemorrhage T83.83 ☑
      infection and inflammation T83.69 ☑
      mechanical
        breakdown T83.31 ☑
        displacement T83.32 ☑
        malposition T83.32 ☑
        obstruction T83.39 ☑
        perforation T83.39 ☑
        protrusion T83.39 ☑
        specified NEC T83.39 ☑
      pain T83.84 ☑
      specified type NEC T83.89 ☑
      stenosis T83.85 ☑
      thrombosis T83.86 ☑
    procedure (fetal), to newborn P96.5
  jejunostomy (stoma) — *see* Complications, enterostomy
  joint prosthesis, internal T84.9 ☑
    breakage (fracture) T84.01- ☑
    dislocation T84.02- ☑
    fracture T84.01- ☑
    infection or inflammation T84.50 ☑
      hip T84.5- ☑
      knee T84.5- ☑
      specified joint NEC T84.59 ☑
    instability T84.02- ☑
    malposition — *see* Complications, joint prosthesis, mechanical, displacement
    mechanical
      breakage, broken T84.01- ☑
      dislocation T84.02- ☑
      fracture T84.01- ☑
      instability T84.02- ☑
      leakage — *see* Complications, joint prosthesis, mechanical, specified NEC
      loosening T84.039 ☑
        hip T84.03- ☑
        knee T84.03- ☑
        specified joint NEC T84.038 ☑
      obstruction — *see* Complications, joint prosthesis, mechanical, specified NEC
      perforation — *see* Complications, joint prosthesis, mechanical, specified NEC
      osteolysis T84.059 ☑
        hip T84.05- ☑
        knee T84.05- ☑
        other specified joint T84.058 ☑

Complication(s) — *continued*
  joint prosthesis, internal — *continued*
    mechanical — *continued*
      protrusion — *see* Complications, joint prosthesis, mechanical, specified NEC
      specified complication NEC T84.099 ☑
        hip T84.09- ☑
        knee T84.09- ☑
        other specified joint T84.098 ☑
      subluxation T84.02- ☑
      wear of articular bearing surface T84.069 ☑
        hip T84.06- ☑
        knee T84.06- ☑
        other specified joint T84.068 ☑
    specified joint NEC T84.89 ☑
      embolism T84.81 ☑
      fibrosis T84.82 ☑
      hemorrhage T84.83 ☑
      pain T84.84 ☑
      specified complication NEC T84.89 ☑
      stenosis T84.85 ☑
      thrombosis T84.86 ☑
    subluxation T84.02- ☑
  kidney transplant — *see* Complications, transplant, kidney
  labor O75.9
    specified NEC O75.89
  liver transplant (immune or nonimmune) — *see* Complications, transplant, liver
  lumbar puncture G97.1
    cerebrospinal fluid leak G97.0
    headache or reaction G97.1
  lung transplant — *see* Complications, transplant, lung
    and heart — *see* Complications, transplant, lung, with heart
  male genital N50.9
    device, implant or graft — *see* Complications, genitourinary, device or implant, genital tract
    postprocedural or postoperative — *see* Complications, genitourinary, postprocedural
    specified NEC N99.89
  mastoid (process) procedure
    intraoperative H95.88
      hematoma — *see* Complications, intraoperative, hemorrhage (hematoma) (of), mastoid process
      hemorrhage — *see* Complications, intraoperative, hemorrhage (hematoma) (of), mastoid process
      laceration — *see* Complications, intraoperative, puncture or laceration, mastoid process
      specified NEC H95.88
    postmastoidectomy — *see* Complications, postmastoidectomy
    postoperative H95.89
      external ear canal stenosis H95.81 ☑
      hematoma — *see* Complications, postprocedural, hematoma (of), mastoid process
      hemorrhage — *see* Complications, postprocedural, hemorrhage (of), mastoid process
      postmastoidectomy — *see* Complications, postmastoidectomy
      seroma — *see* Complications, postprocedural, seroma (of), mastoid process
      specified NEC H95.89
  mastoidectomy cavity — *see* Complications, postmastoidectomy
  mechanical — *see* Complications, by site and type, mechanical
  medical procedures (*see also* Complication(s), intraoperative) T88.9 ☑
  metabolic E88.9
    postoperative E89.89
    specified NEC E89.89
  molar pregnancy NOS O08.9
    damage to pelvic organs O08.6
    embolism O08.2
    genital infection O08.0
    hemorrhage (delayed) (excessive) O08.1
    metabolic disorder O08.5
    renal failure O08.4
    shock O08.3
    specified type NEC O08.0
    venous complication NEC O08.7

Complication(s) — *continued*
  musculoskeletal system (*see also* Complication, intraoperative (intraprocedural), by site)
    device, implant or graft NEC — *see* Complications, orthopedic, device or implant
      internal fixation (nail) (plate) (rod) — *see* Complications, fixation device, internal
      joint prosthesis — *see* Complications, joint prosthesis
    post radiation M96.89
      kyphosis M96.2
      scoliosis M96.5
      specified complication NEC M96.89
    postoperative (postprocedural) M96.89
      with osteoporosis — *see* Osteoporosis
      fracture following insertion of device — *see* Fracture, following insertion of orthopedic implant, joint prosthesis or bone plate
      joint instability after prosthesis removal M96.89
      lordosis M96.4
      postlaminectomy syndrome NEC M96.1
        kyphosis M96.3
      pseudarthrosis M96.0
      specified complication NEC M96.89
  nephrostomy (stoma) — *see* Complications, stoma, urinary tract, external NEC
  nervous system G98.8
    central G96.9
    device, implant or graft (*see also* Complication, prosthetic device or implant, specified NEC)
      electronic stimulator (electrode(s)) — *see* Complications, electronic stimulator device
      specified NEC
        infection and inflammation T85.738 ☑
        mechanical T85.695 ☑
          breakdown T85.615 ☑
          displacement T85.625 ☑
          leakage T85.635 ☑
          malfunction T85.695 ☑
          malposition T85.625 ☑
          obstruction T85.695 ☑
          perforation T85.695 ☑
          protrusion T85.695 ☑
          specified NEC T85.695 ☑
      ventricular shunt — *see* Complications, ventricular shunt
    electronic stimulator (electrode(s)) — *see* Complications, electronic stimulator device
    postprocedural G97.82
      intracranial hypotension G97.2
      specified NEC G97.82
      spinal fluid leak G97.0
  newborn, due to intrauterine (fetal) procedure P96.5
  nonabsorbable (permanent) sutures — *see* Complication, sutures, permanent
  obstetric O75.9
    procedure (instrumental) (manual) (surgical)
      specified NEC O75.4
    specified NEC O75.89
    surgical wound NEC O90.89
      hematoma O90.2
      infection O86.0
  ocular lens implant — *see* Complications, intraocular lens
  ophthalmologic
    postprocedural bleb — *see* Blebitis
  orbital prosthesis T85.9 ☑
    embolism T85.818 ☑
    fibrosis T85.828 ☑
    hemorrhage T85.838 ☑
    infection and inflammation T85.79 ☑
    mechanical
      breakdown T85.31- ☑
      displacement T85.32- ☑
      malposition T85.32- ☑
      obstruction T85.39- ☑
      perforation T85.39- ☑
      protrusion T85.39- ☑
      specified NEC T85.39- ☑
    pain T85.848 ☑
    specified type NEC T85.898 ☑
    stenosis T85.858 ☑
    thrombosis T85.868 ☑
  organ or tissue transplant (partial) (total) — *see* Complications, transplant

Complication(s) — *continued*
  orthopedic (*see also* Disorder, soft tissue)

    device or implant T84.9 ☑
      bone
        device or implant — *see* Complication,
          bone, device NEC
        graft — *see* Complication, graft, bone
      breakdown T84.418 ☑
      displacement T84.428 ☑
      electronic bone stimulator — *see* Complica-
        tions, electronic stimulator device, bone
      embolism T84.81 ☑
      fibrosis T84.82 ☑
      fixation device — *see* Complication, fixation
        device, internal
      hemorrhage T84.83 ☑
      infection or inflammation T84.7 ☑
      joint prosthesis — *see* Complication, joint
        prosthesis, internal
      malfunction T84.418 ☑
      malposition T84.428 ☑
      mechanical NEC T84.498 ☑
      muscle graft — *see* Complications, graft, muscle
      obstruction T84.498 ☑
      pain T84.84 ☑
      perforation T84.498 ☑
      protrusion T84.498 ☑
      specified complication NEC T84.89 ☑
      stenosis T84.85 ☑
      tendon graft — *see* Complications, graft, ten-
        don
      thrombosis T84.86 ☑
    fracture (following insertion of device) — *see*
      Fracture, following insertion of orthopedic
      implant, joint prosthesis or bone plate
    postprocedural M96.89
      fracture — *see* Fracture, following insertion of
        orthopedic implant, joint prosthesis or
        bone plate
      postlaminectomy syndrome NEC M96.1
        kyphosis M96.3
        lordosis M96.4
      postradiation
        kyphosis M96.2
        scoliosis M96.5
      pseudarthrosis post-fusion M96.0
      specified type NEC M96.89
  pacemaker (cardiac) — *see* Complications, cardiovas-
    cular device or implant, electronic
  pancreas transplant — *see* Complications, transplant,
    pancreas
  penile prosthesis (implant) — *see* Complications,
    prosthetic device, penile
  perfusion NEC T80.90 ☑
  perineal repair (obstetrical) NEC O90.89
    disruption O90.1
    hematoma O90.2
    infection (following delivery) O86.0
  phototherapy T88.9 ☑
    specified NEC T88.8 ☑
  postmastoidectomy NEC H95.19- ☑
    cyst, mucosal H95.13- ☑
    granulation H95.12- ☑
    inflammation, chronic H95.11- ☑
    recurrent cholesteatoma H95.0- ☑
  postoperative — *see* Complications, postprocedural
    circulatory — *see* Complications, circulatory system
    ear — *see* Complications, ear
    endocrine — *see* Complications, endocrine
    eye — *see* Complications, eye
    lumbar puncture G97.1
      cerebrospinal fluid leak G97.0
    nervous system (central) (peripheral) — *see* Com-
      plications, nervous system
    respiratory system — *see* Complications, respirato-
      ry system
  postprocedural (*see also* Complications, surgical pro-
    cedure)
    cardiac arrest (*see also* Infarct, myocardium, associ-
      ated with revascularization procedure)
      following cardiac surgery I97.120
      following other surgery I97.121
    cardiac functional disturbance NEC (*see also* Infarct,
      myocardium, associated with revasculariza-
      tion procedure)
      following cardiac surgery I97.190

Complication(s) — *continued*
  postprocedural (*see also* Complications, surgical pro-
    cedure) — *continued*
    cardiac functional disturbance (*see also* Infarct,
      myocardium, associated with revasculariza-
      tion procedure) — *continued*
      following other surgery I97.191
    cardiac insufficiency
      following cardiac surgery I97.110
      following other surgery I97.111
    chorioretinal scars following retinal surgery
      H59.81-
    following cataract surgery
      cataract (lens) fragments H59.02- ☑
      cystoid macular edema H59.03- ☑
      specified NEC H59.09- ☑
      vitreous (touch) syndrome H59.01- ☑
    heart failure
      following cardiac surgery I97.130
      following other surgery I97.131
    hematoma (of)
      circulatory system organ or structure
        following cardiac bypass I97.631
        following cardiac catheterization I97.630
        following other circulatory system proce-
          dure I97.638
        following other procedure I97.621
      digestive system
        following procedure on digestive system
          K91.870
        following procedure on other organ K91.871
      ear
        following other procedure H95.52
        following procedure on ear and mastoid
          process H95.51
      endocrine system
        following endocrine system procedure
          E89.820
        following other procedure E89.821
      eye and adnexa
        following ophthalmic procedure H59.33- ☑
        following other procedure H59.34- ☑
      genitourinary organ or structure
        following procedure on genitourinary organ
          or structure N99.840
        following procedure on other organ
          N99.841
      mastoid process
        following other procedure H95.52
        following procedure on ear and mastoid
          process H95.51
      musculoskeletal structure
        following musculoskeletal surgery M96.840
        following non-orthopedic surgery M96.841
        following orthopedic surgery M96.840
      nervous system
        following nervous system procedure G97.61
        following other procedure G97.62
      respiratory system
        following other procedure J95.861
        following procedure on respiratory system
          organ or structure J95.860
      skin and subcutaneous tissue
        following dermatologic procedure L76.31
        following procedure on other organ L76.32
      spleen
        following procedure on other organ D78.32
        following procedure on the spleen D78.31
    hemorrhage (of)
      circulatory system organ or structure
        following cardiac bypass I97.611
        following cardiac catheterization I97.610
        following other circulatory system proce-
          dure I97.618
        following other procedure I97.620
      digestive system
        following procedure on digestive system
          K91.840
        following procedure on other organ K91.841
      ear
        following other procedure H95.42
        following procedure on ear and mastoid
          process H95.41
      endocrine system
        following endocrine system procedure
          E89.810
        following other procedure E89.811

Complication(s) — *continued*
  postprocedural (*see also* Complications, surgical pro-
    cedure) — *continued*
    hemorrhage — *continued*
      eye and adnexa
        following ophthalmic procedure H59.31- ☑
        following other procedure H59.32- ☑
      genitourinary organ or structure
        following procedure on genitourinary organ
          or structure N99.820
        following procedure on other organ
          N99.821
      mastoid process
        following other procedure H95.42
        following procedure on ear and mastoid
          process H95.41
      musculoskeletal structure
        following musculoskeletal surgery M96.830
        following non-orthopedic surgery M96.831
        following orthopedic surgery M96.830
      nervous system
        following nervous system procedure G97.51
        following other procedure G97.52
      respiratory system
        following a respiratory system procedure
          J95.830
        following other procedure J95.831
      skin and subcutaneous tissue
        following a procedure on other organ
          L76.22
        following dermatologic procedure L76.21
      spleen
        following procedure on other organ D78.22
        following procedure on the spleen D78.21
    seroma (of)
      circulatory system organ or structure
        following cardiac bypass I97.641
        following cardiac catheterization I97.640
        following other circulatory system proce-
          dure I97.648
        following other procedure I97.622
      digestive system
        following procedure on digestive system
          K91.872
        following procedure on other organ K91.873
      ear
        following other procedure H95.54
        following procedure on ear and mastoid
          process H95.53
      endocrine system
        following endocrine system procedure
          E89.822
        following other procedure E89.823
      eye and adnexa
        following ophthalmic procedure H59.35- ☑
        following other procedure H59.36- ☑
      genitourinary organ or structure
        following procedure on genitourinary organ
          or structure N99.842
        following procedure on other organ
          N99.843
      mastoid process
        following other procedure H95.54
        following procedure on ear and mastoid
          process H95.53
      musculoskeletal structure
        following musculoskeletal surgery M96.842
        following non-orthopedic surgery M96.843
        following orthopedic surgery M96.842
      nervous system
        following nervous system procedure G97.63
        following other procedure G97.64
      respiratory system
        following other procedure J95.863
        following procedure on respiratory system
          organ or structure J95.862
      skin and subcutaneous tissue
        following dermatologic procedure L76.33
        following procedure on other organ L76.34
      spleen
        following procedure on other organ D78.34
        following procedure on the spleen D78.33
    specified NEC
      circulatory system I97.89
      digestive K91.89
      ear H95.89
      endocrine E89.89
      eye and adnexa H59.89
      genitourinary N99.89

Complication(s) — *continued*
  postprocedural (*see also* Complications, surgical procedure) — *continued*
    specified — *continued*
      mastoid process H95.89
      metabolic E89.89
      musculoskeletal structure M96.89
      nervous system G97.82
      respiratory system J95.89
      skin and subcutaneous tissue L76.82
      spleen D78.89
  pregnancy NEC — *see* Pregnancy, complicated by
  prosthetic device or implant T85.9 ☑
    bile duct — *see* Complications, bile duct implant
    breast — *see* Complications, breast implant
    bulking agent
      ureteral
        erosion T83.714 ☑
        exposure T83.724 ☑
      urethral
        erosion T83.713 ☑
        exposure T83.723 ☑
    cardiac and vascular NEC — *see* Complications, cardiovascular device or implant
    corneal transplant — *see* Complications, graft, cornea
    electronic nervous system stimulator — *see* Complications, electronic stimulator device
    epidural infusion catheter — *see* Complications, catheter, epidural
    esophageal anti-reflux device — *see* Complications, esophageal anti-reflux device
    genital organ or tract — *see* Complications, genitourinary, device or implant, genital tract
      specified NEC T83.79- ☑
    heart valve — *see* Complications, heart, valve, prosthesis
    infection or inflammation T85.79 ☑
      intestine transplant T86.892
      liver transplant T86.43
      lung transplant T86.812
      pancreas transplant T86.892
      skin graft T86.822
    intraocular lens — *see* Complications, intraocular lens
    intraperitoneal (dialysis) catheter — *see* Complications, catheter, intraperitoneal
    joint — *see* Complications, joint prosthesis, internal
    mechanical NEC T85.698 ☑
      dialysis catheter (vascular) (*see also* Complication, catheter, dialysis, mechanical)
        peritoneal — *see* Complication, catheter, intraperitoneal, mechanical
      gastrointestinal device T85.598 ☑
      ocular device T85.398 ☑
      subdural (infusion) catheter T85.690 ☑
      suture, permanent T85.692 ☑
        that for bone repair — *see* Complications, fixation device, internal (orthopedic), mechanical
      ventricular shunt
        breakdown T85.01 ☑
        displacement T85.02 ☑
        leakage T85.03 ☑
        malposition T85.02 ☑
        obstruction T85.09 ☑
        perforation T85.09 ☑
        protrusion T85.09 ☑
        specified NEC T85.09 ☑
    mesh
      erosion (to surrounding organ or tissue) T83.718 ☑
        urethral (into pelvic floor muscles) T83.712 ☑
        vaginal (into pelvic floor muscles) T83.711 ☑
      exposure (into surrounding organ or tissue) T83.728 ☑
        urethral (through urethral wall) T83.722 ☑
        vaginal (into vagina) (through vaginal wall) T83.721 ☑
    orbital — *see* Complications, orbital prosthesis
    penile T83.9 ☑
      embolism T83.81 ☑
      fibrosis T83.82 ☑
      hemorrhage T83.83 ☑
      infection and inflammation T83.61 ☑

Complication(s) — *continued*
  prosthetic device or implant — *continued*
    penile — *continued*
      mechanical
        breakdown T83.410 ☑
        displacement T83.420 ☑
        leakage T83.490 ☑
        malposition T83.420 ☑
        obstruction T83.490 ☑
        perforation T83.490 ☑
        protrusion T83.490 ☑
        specified NEC T83.490 ☑
      pain T83.84 ☑
      specified type NEC T83.89 ☑
      stenosis T83.85 ☑
      thrombosis T83.86 ☑
    prosthetic materials NEC
      erosion (to surrounding organ or tissue) T83.718 ☑
      exposure (into surrounding organ or tissue) T83.728 ☑
    skin graft T86.829
      artificial skin or decellularized allodermis
        embolism T85.818 ☑
        fibrosis T85.828 ☑
        hemorrhage T85.838 ☑
        infection and inflammation T85.79 ☑
        mechanical
          breakdown T85.613 ☑
          displacement T85.623 ☑
          malfunction T85.613 ☑
          malposition T85.623 ☑
          obstruction T85.693 ☑
          perforation T85.693 ☑
          protrusion T85.693 ☑
          specified NEC T85.693 ☑
        pain T85.848 ☑
        specified type NEC T85.898 ☑
        stenosis T85.858 ☑
        thrombosis T85.868 ☑
      failure T86.821
      infection T86.822
      rejection T86.820
      specified NEC T86.828
    sling
      urethral (female) (male)
        erosion T83.712 ☑
        exposure T83.722 ☑
    specified NEC T85.9 ☑
      embolism T85.818 ☑
      fibrosis T85.828 ☑
      hemorrhage T85.838 ☑
      infection and inflammation T85.79 ☑
      mechanical
        breakdown T85.618 ☑
        displacement T85.628 ☑
        leakage T85.638 ☑
        malfunction T85.618 ☑
        malposition T85.628 ☑
        obstruction T85.698 ☑
        perforation T85.698 ☑
        protrusion T85.698 ☑
        specified NEC T85.698 ☑
      pain T85.848 ☑
      specified type NEC T85.898 ☑
      stenosis T85.858 ☑
      thrombosis T85.868 ☑
    subdural infusion catheter — *see* Complications, catheter, subdural
    sutures — *see* Complications, sutures
    urinary organ or tract NEC — *see* Complications, genitourinary, device or implant, urinary system
    vascular — *see* Complications, cardiovascular device or implant
    ventricular shunt — *see* Complications, ventricular shunt (device)
  puerperium — *see* Puerperal
  puncture, spinal G97.1
    cerebrospinal fluid leak G97.0
    headache or reaction G97.1
  pyelogram N99.89
  radiation
    kyphosis M96.2
    scoliosis M96.5

Complication(s) — *continued*
  reattached
    extremity (infection) (rejection)
      lower T87.1X- ☑
      upper T87.0X- ☑
    specified body part NEC T87.2
  reconstructed breast
    asymmetry between native and reconstructed breast N65.1
    deformity N65.0
    disproportion between native and reconstructed breast N65.1
    excess tissue N65.0
    misshappen N65.0
  reimplant NEC (*see also* Complications, prosthetic device or implant)
    limb (infection) (rejection) — *see* Complications, reattached, extremity
    organ (partial) (total) — *see* Complications, transplant
    prosthetic device NEC — *see* Complications, prosthetic device
  renal N28.9
    allograft — *see* Complications, transplant, kidney
    dialysis — *see* Complications, dialysis
  respirator
    mechanical J95.850
    specified NEC J95.859
  respiratory system J98.9
    device, implant or graft — *see* Complication, prosthetic device or implant, specified NEC
    lung transplant — *see* Complications, prosthetic device or implant, lung transplant
    postoperative J95.89
      air leak J95.812
      Mendelson's syndrome (chemical pneumonitis) J95.4
      pneumothorax J95.811
      pulmonary insufficiency (acute) (after nonthoracic surgery) J95.2
        chronic J95.3
        following thoracic surgery J95.1
      respiratory failure (acute) J95.821
        acute and chronic J95.822
      specified NEC J95.89
      subglottic stenosis J95.5
      tracheostomy complication — *see* Complications, tracheostomy
    therapy T81.89 ☑
  sedation during labor and delivery O74.9
    cardiac O74.2
    central nervous system O74.3
    pulmonary NEC O74.1
  shunt (*see also* Complications, prosthetic device or implant)
    arteriovenous — *see* Complications, arteriovenous, shunt
    ventricular (communicating) — *see* Complications, ventricular shunt
  skin
    graft T86.829
      failure T86.821
      infection T86.822
      rejection T86.820
      specified type NEC T86.828
  spinal
    anesthesia — *see* Complications, anesthesia, spinal
    catheter (epidural) (subdural) — *see* Complications, catheter
    puncture or tap G97.1
      cerebrospinal fluid leak G97.0
      headache or reaction G97.1
  stent
    bile duct — *see* Complications, bile duct prosthesis
    ureteral indwelling
      breakdown T83.112 ☑
      displacement T83.122 ☑
      leakage T83.192 ☑
      malposition T83.122 ☑
      obstruction T83.192 ☑
      perforation T83.192 ☑
      protrusion T83.192 ☑
      specified NEC T83.192 ☑
    urinary NEC (ileal conduit) (nephroureteral) T83.193 ☑
      embolism T83.81 ☑
      fibrosis T83.82 ☑
      hemorrhage T83.83 ☑

Complication(s) — continued
  stent — continued
    urinary — continued
      infection and inflammation T83.593 ☑
      mechanical
        breakdown T83.113 ☑
        displacement T83.123 ☑
        leakage T83.193 ☑
        malposition T83.123 ☑
        obstruction T83.193 ☑
        perforation T83.193 ☑
        protrusion T83.193 ☑
        specified NEC T83.193 ☑
      pain T83.84 ☑
      specified type NEC T83.89 ☑
      stenosis T83.85 ☑
      thrombosis T83.86 ☑
    vascular
      end stent stenosis — see Restenosis, stent
      in stent stenosis — see Restenosis, stent
  stoma
    digestive tract
      colostomy — see Complications, colostomy
      enterostomy — see Complications, enterosto-
        my
      esophagostomy — see Complications,
        esophagostomy
      gastrostomy — see Complications, gastrostomy
    urinary tract N99.528
      continent N99.538
        hemorrhage N99.530
        herniation N99.533
        infection N99.531
        malfunction N99.532
        specified type NEC N99.538
        stenosis N99.534
      cystostomy — see Complications, cystostomy
      external NOS N99.528
      hemorrhage N99.520
      herniation N99.523
      incontinent N99.528
        hemorrhage N99.520
        herniation N99.523
        infection N99.521
        malfunction N99.522
        specified type NEC N99.528
        stenosis N99.524
      infection N99.521
      malfunction N99.522
      specified type NEC N99.528
      stenosis N99.524
  stomach banding — see Complication(s), bariatric
    procedure
  stomach stapling — see Complication(s), bariatric
    procedure
  surgical material, nonabsorbable — see Complication,
    suture, permanent
  surgical procedure (on) T81.9 ☑
    amputation stump (late) — see Complications,
      amputation stump
    cardiac — see Complications, circulatory system
    cholesteatoma, recurrent — see Complications,
      postmastoidectomy, recurrent
      cholesteatoma
    circulatory (early) — see Complications, circulatory
      system
    digestive system — see Complications, gastroin-
      testinal
    dumping syndrome (postgastrectomy) K91.1
    ear — see Complications, ear
    elephantiasis or lymphedema I97.89
      postmastectomy I97.2
    emphysema (surgical) T81.82 ☑
    endocrine — see Complications, endocrine
    eye — see Complications, eye
    fistula (persistent postoperative) T81.83 ☑
    foreign body inadvertently left in wound (sponge)
      (suture) (swab) — see Foreign body, acciden-
      tally left during a procedure
    gastrointestinal — see Complications, gastrointesti-
      nal
    genitourinary NEC N99.89
    hematoma
      intraoperative — see Complication, intraopera-
        tive, hemorrhage
      postprocedural — see Complication, postpro-
        cedural, hematoma

Complication(s) — continued
  surgical procedure — continued
    hemorrhage
      intraoperative — see Complication, intraopera-
        tive, hemorrhage
      postprocedural — see Complication, postpro-
        cedural, hemorrhage
    hepatic failure K91.82
    hyperglycemia (postpancreatectomy) E89.1
    hypoinsulinemia (postpancreatectomy) E89.1
    hypoparathyroidism (postparathyroidectomy)
      E89.2
    hypopituitarism (posthypophysectomy) E89.3
    hypothyroidism (post-thyroidectomy) E89.0
    intestinal obstruction (see also Obstruction, intes-
      tine, postoperative) K91.30
    intracranial hypotension following ventricular
      shunting (ventriculostomy) G97.2
    lymphedema I97.89
      postmastectomy I97.2
    malabsorption (postsurgical) NEC K91.2
      osteoporosis — see Osteoporosis, postsurgical
        malabsorption
    mastoidectomy cavity NEC — see Complications,
      postmastoidectomy
    metabolic E89.89
      specified NEC E89.89
    musculoskeletal — see Complications, muscu-
      loskeletal system
    nervous system (central) (peripheral) — see Com-
      plications, nervous system
    ovarian failure E89.40
      asymptomatic E89.40
      symptomatic E89.41
    peripheral vascular — see Complications, surgical
      procedure, vascular
    postcardiotomy syndrome I97.0
    postcholecystectomy syndrome K91.5
    postcommissurotomy syndrome I97.0
    postgastrectomy dumping syndrome K91.1
    postlaminectomy syndrome NEC M96.1
      kyphosis M96.3
    postmastectomy lymphedema syndrome I97.2
    postmastoidectomy cholesteatoma — see Compli-
      cations, postmastoidectomy, recurrent
      cholesteatoma
    postvagotomy syndrome K91.1
    postvalvulotomy syndrome I97.0
    pulmonary insufficiency (acute) J95.2
      chronic J95.3
      following thoracic surgery J95.1
    reattached body part — see Complications, reat-
      tached
    respiratory — see Complications, respiratory sys-
      tem
    shock (hypovolemic) T81.19 ☑
    spleen (postoperative) D78.89
      intraoperative D78.81
    stitch abscess T81.4 ☑
    subglottic stenosis (postsurgical) J95.5
    testicular hypofunction E89.5
    transplant — see Complications, organ or tissue
      transplant
    urinary NEC N99.89
    vaginal vault prolapse (posthysterectomy) N99.3
    vascular (peripheral)
      artery T81.719 ☑
        mesenteric T81.710 ☑
        renal T81.711 ☑
        specified NEC T81.718 ☑
      vein T81.72 ☑
    wound infection T81.4 ☑
  suture, permanent (wire) NEC T85.9 ☑
    with repair of bone — see Complications, fixation
      device, internal
    embolism T85.818 ☑
    fibrosis T85.828 ☑
    hemorrhage T85.838 ☑
    infection and inflammation T85.79 ☑
    mechanical
      breakdown T85.612 ☑
      displacement T85.622 ☑
      malfunction T85.612 ☑
      malposition T85.622 ☑
      obstruction T85.692 ☑
      perforation T85.692 ☑
      protrusion T85.692 ☑

Complication(s) — continued
  suture, permanent — continued
    mechanical — continued
      specified NEC T85.692 ☑
    pain T85.848 ☑
    specified type NEC T85.898 ☑
    stenosis T85.858 ☑
    thrombosis T85.868 ☑
  tracheostomy J95.00
    granuloma J95.09
    hemorrhage J95.01
    infection J95.02
    malfunction J95.03
    mechanical J95.03
    obstruction J95.03
    specified type NEC J95.09
    tracheo-esophageal fistula J95.04
  transfusion (blood) (lymphocytes) (plasma) T80.92 ☑
    air emblism T80.0 ☑
    circulatory overload E87.71
    febrile nonhemolytic transfusion reaction R50.84
    hemochromatosis E83.111
    hemolysis T80.89 ☑
    hemolytic reaction (antigen unspecified)
      T80.919 ☑
    incompatibility reaction (antigen unspecified)
      T80.919 ☑
      ABO T80.30 ☑
        delayed serologic (DSTR) T80.39 ☑
        hemolytic transfusion reaction (HTR) (un-
          specified time after transfusion)
          T80.319 ☑
          acute (AHTR) (less than 24 hours after
            transfusion) T80.310 ☑
          delayed (DHTR) (24 hours or more after
            transfusion) T80.311 ☑
        specified NEC T80.39 ☑
      acute (antigen unspecified) T80.910 ☑
      delayed (antigen unspecified) T80.911 ☑
      delayed serologic (DSTR) T80.89 ☑
      non-ABO (minor antigens (Duffy) (Kell) (Kidd)
        (Lewis) (M) (N) (P) (S)) T80.A0 ☑ (follow-
        ing T80.4)
        delayed serologic (DSTR) T80.A9 ☑ (follow-
          ing T80.4)
        hemolytic transfusion reaction (HTR) (un-
          specified time after transfusion)
          T80.A19 ☑ (following T80.4)
          acute (AHTR) (less than 24 hours after
            transfusion) T80.A10 ☑ (following
            T80.4)
          delayed (DHTR) (24 hours or more after
            transfusion) T80.A11 ☑ (following
            T80.4)
        specified NEC T80.A9 ☑ (following T80.4)
      Rh (antigens (C) (c) (D) (E) (e)) (factor) T80.40 ☑
        delayed serologic (DSTR) T80.49 ☑
        hemolytic transfusion reaction (HTR) (un-
          specified time after transfusion)
          T80.419 ☑
          acute (AHTR) (less than 24 hours after
            transfusion) T80.410 ☑
          delayed (DHTR) (24 hours or more after
            transfusion) T80.411 ☑
        specified NEC T80.49 ☑
    infection T80.29 ☑
      acute T80.22- ☑
    reaction NEC T80.89 ☑
    sepsis T80.29 ☑
    shock T80.89 ☑
  transplant T86.90
    bone T86.839
      failure T86.831
      infection T86.832
      rejection T86.830
      specified type NEC T86.838
    bone marrow T86.00
      failure T86.02
      infection T86.03
      rejection T86.01
      specified type NEC T86.09
    cornea T86.849
      failure T86.841
      infection T86.842
      rejection T86.840
      specified type NEC T86.848
    failure T86.92

Complication(s) — continued
  transplant — continued
    heart T86.20
      with lung T86.30
        cardiac allograft vasculopathy T86.290
        failure T86.32
        infection T86.33
        rejection T86.31
        specified type NEC T86.39
      failure T86.22
      infection T86.23
      rejection T86.21
      specified type NEC T86.298
    infection T86.93
    intestine T86.859
      failure T86.851
      infection T86.852
      rejection T86.850
      specified type NEC T86.858
    kidney T86.10
      failure T86.12
      infection T86.13
      rejection T86.11
      specified type NEC T86.19
    liver T86.40
      failure T86.42
      infection T86.43
      rejection T86.41
      specified type NEC T86.49
    lung T86.819
      with heart T86.30
        failure T86.32
        infection T86.33
        rejection T86.31
        specified type NEC T86.39
      failure T86.811
      infection T86.812
      rejection T86.810
      specified type NEC T86.818
    malignant neoplasm C80.2
    pancreas T86.899
      failure T86.891
      infection T86.892
      rejection T86.890
      specified type NEC T86.898
    peripheral blood stem cells T86.5
    post-transplant lymphoproliferative disorder (PTLD) D47.Z1 (following D47.4)
    rejection T86.91
    skin T86.829
      failure T86.821
      infection T86.822
      rejection T86.820
      specified type NEC T86.828
    specified
      tissue T86.899
        failure T86.891
        infection T86.892
        rejection T86.890
        specified type NEC T86.898
      type NEC T86.99
    stem cell (from peripheral blood) (from umbilical cord) T86.5
    umbilical cord stem cells T86.5
  trauma (early) T79.9 ☑
    specified NEC T79.8 ☑
  ultrasound therapy NEC T88.9 ☑
  umbilical cord NEC
    complicating delivery O69.9 ☑
    specified NEC O69.89 ☑
  umbrella device, vascular T82.9 ☑
    embolism T82.818 ☑
    fibrosis T82.828 ☑
    hemorrhage T82.838 ☑
    infection or inflammation T82.7 ☑
    mechanical
      breakdown T82.515 ☑
      displacement T82.525 ☑
      leakage T82.535 ☑
      malposition T82.525 ☑
      obstruction T82.595 ☑
      perforation T82.595 ☑
      protrusion T82.595 ☑
    pain T82.848 ☑
    specified type NEC T82.898 ☑
    stenosis T82.858 ☑
    thrombosis T82.868 ☑

Complication(s) — continued
  urethral catheter — see Complications, catheter, urethral, indwelling
  vaccination T88.1 ☑
    anaphylaxis NEC T80.52 ☑
    arthropathy — see Arthropathy, postimmunization
    cellulitis T88.0 ☑
    encephalitis or encephalomyelitis G04.02
    infection (general) (local) NEC T88.0 ☑
    meningitis G03.8
    myelitis G04.02
    protein sickness T80.62 ☑
    rash T88.1 ☑
    reaction (allergic) T88.1 ☑
      serum T80.62 ☑
    sepsis T88.0 ☑
    serum intoxication, sickness, rash, or other serum reaction NEC T80.62 ☑
      anaphylactic shock T80.52 ☑
    shock (allergic) (anaphylactic) T80.52 ☑
    vaccinia (generalized) (localized) T88.1 ☑
  vas deferens device or implant — see Complications, genitourinary, device or implant, genital tract
  vascular I99.9
    device or implant T82.9 ☑
      embolism T82.818 ☑
      fibrosis T82.828 ☑
      hemorrhage T82.838 ☑
      infection or inflammation T82.7 ☑
      mechanical
        breakdown T82.519 ☑
          specified device NEC T82.518 ☑
        displacement T82.529 ☑
          specified device NEC T82.528 ☑
        leakage T82.539 ☑
          specified device NEC T82.538 ☑
        malposition T82.529 ☑
          specified device NEC T82.528 ☑
        obstruction T82.599 ☑
          specified device NEC T82.598 ☑
        perforation T82.599 ☑
          specified device NEC T82.598 ☑
        protrusion T82.599 ☑
          specified device NEC T82.598 ☑
      pain T82.848 ☑
      specified type NEC T82.898 ☑
      stenosis T82.858 ☑
      thrombosis T82.868 ☑
    dialysis catheter — see Complication, catheter, dialysis
    following infusion, therapeutic injection or transfusion T80.1 ☑
    graft T82.9 ☑
      embolism T82.818 ☑
      fibrosis T82.828 ☑
      hemorrhage T82.838 ☑
      mechanical
        breakdown T82.319 ☑
          aorta (bifurcation) T82.310 ☑
          carotid artery T82.311 ☑
          specified vessel NEC T82.318 ☑
        displacement T82.329 ☑
          aorta (bifurcation) T82.320 ☑
          carotid artery T82.321 ☑
          specified vessel NEC T82.328 ☑
        leakage T82.339 ☑
          aorta (bifurcation) T82.330 ☑
          carotid artery T82.331 ☑
          specified vessel NEC T82.338 ☑
        malposition T82.329 ☑
          aorta (bifurcation) T82.320 ☑
          carotid artery T82.321 ☑
          specified vessel NEC T82.328 ☑
        obstruction T82.399 ☑
          aorta (bifurcation) T82.390 ☑
          carotid artery T82.391 ☑
          specified vessel NEC T82.398 ☑
        perforation T82.399 ☑
          aorta (bifurcation) T82.390 ☑
          carotid artery T82.391 ☑
          specified vessel NEC T82.398 ☑
        protrusion T82.399 ☑
          aorta (bifurcation) T82.390 ☑
          carotid artery T82.391 ☑
          specified vessel NEC T82.398 ☑
      pain T82.848 ☑

Complication(s) — continued
  vascular — continued
    graft — continued
      specified complication NEC T82.898 ☑
      stenosis T82.858 ☑
      thrombosis T82.868 ☑
    postoperative — see Complications, postoperative, circulatory
  vena cava device (filter) (sieve) (umbrella) — see Complications, umbrella device, vascular
  ventilation therapy NEC T81.81 ☑
  ventilator
    mechanical J95.850
      specified NEC J95.859
  ventricular (communicating) shunt (device) T85.9 ☑
    embolism T85.810 ☑
    fibrosis T85.820 ☑
    hemorrhage T85.830 ☑
    infection and inflammation T85.730 ☑
    mechanical
      breakdown T85.01 ☑
      displacement T85.02 ☑
      leakage T85.03 ☑
      malposition T85.02 ☑
      obstruction T85.09 ☑
      perforation T85.09 ☑
      protrusion T85.09 ☑
      specified NEC T85.09 ☑
    pain T85.840 ☑
    specified type NEC T85.890 ☑
    stenosis T85.850 ☑
    thrombosis T85.860 ☑
  wire suture, permanent (implanted) — see Complications, suture, permanent
Compressed air disease T70.3 ☑
Compression
  with injury — code by Nature of injury
  artery I77.1
    celiac, syndrome I77.4
  brachial plexus G54.0
  brain (stem) G93.5
    due to
      contusion (diffuse) — see Injury, intracranial, diffuse
        focal — see Injury, intracranial, focal
      injury NEC — see Injury, intracranial, diffuse
      traumatic — see Injury, intracranial, diffuse
  bronchus J98.09
  cauda equina G83.4
  celiac (artery) (axis) I77.4
  cerebral — see Compression, brain
  cervical plexus G54.2
  cord
    spinal — see Compression, spinal
    umbilical — see Compression, umbilical cord
  cranial nerve G52.9
    eighth H93.3 ☑
    eleventh G52.8
    fifth G50.8
    first G52.0
    fourth — see Strabismus, paralytic, fourth nerve
    ninth G52.1
    second — see Disorder, nerve, optic
    seventh G51.8
    sixth — see Strabismus, paralytic, sixth nerve
    tenth G52.2
    third — see Strabismus, paralytic, third nerve
    twelfth G52.3
  diver's squeeze T70.3 ☑
  during birth (newborn) P15.9
  esophagus K22.2
  eustachian tube — see Obstruction, eustachian tube, cartilaginous
  facies Q67.1
  fracture
    nontraumatic NOS — see Collapse, vertebra
    pathological — see Fracture, pathological
    traumatic — see Fracture, traumatic
  heart — see Disease, heart
  intestine — see Obstruction, intestine
  laryngeal nerve, recurrent G52.2
    with paralysis of vocal cords and larynx J38.00
      bilateral J38.02
      unilateral J38.01
  lumbosacral plexus G54.1
  lung J98.4
  lymphatic vessel I89.0

☑ Additional Character Required — Refer to the Tabular List for Character Selection   Ⓥ Subterms under main terms may continue to next column or page

Compression — *continued*
  medulla — *see* Compression, brain
  nerve (*see also* Disorder, nerve) G58.9
    arm NEC — *see* Mononeuropathy, upper limb
    axillary G54.0
    cranial — *see* Compression, cranial nerve
    leg NEC — *see* Mononeuropathy, lower limb
    median (in carpal tunnel) — *see* Syndrome, carpal tunnel
    optic — *see* Disorder, nerve, optic
    plantar — *see* Lesion, nerve, plantar
    posterior tibial (in tarsal tunnel) — *see* Syndrome, tarsal tunnel
    root or plexus NOS (in) G54.9
      intervertebral disc disorder NEC — *see* Disorder, disc, with, radiculopathy
      with myelopathy — *see* Disorder, disc, with, myelopathy
      neoplastic disease (*see also* Neoplasm) D49.9 [G55]
      spondylosis — *see* Spondylosis, with radiculopathy
    sciatic (acute) — *see* Lesion, nerve, sciatic
    sympathetic G90.8
    traumatic — *see* Injury, nerve
    ulnar — *see* Lesion, nerve, ulnar
    upper extremity NEC — *see* Mononeuropathy, upper limb
  spinal (cord) G95.20
    by displacement of intervertebral disc NEC (*see also* Disorder, disc, with, myelopathy)
    nerve root NOS G54.9
      due to displacement of intervertebral disc NEC — *see* Disorder, disc, with, radiculopathy
      with myelopathy — *see* Disorder, disc, with, myelopathy
    specified NEC G95.29
    spondylogenic (cervical) (lumbar, lumbosacral) (thoracic) — *see* Spondylosis, with myelopathy NEC
    anterior — *see* Syndrome, anterior, spinal artery, compression
    traumatic — *see* Injury, spinal cord, by region
  subcostal nerve (syndrome) — *see* Mononeuropathy, upper limb, specified NEC
  sympathetic nerve NEC G90.8
  syndrome T79.5 ☑
  trachea J39.8
  ulnar nerve (by scar tissue) — *see* Lesion, nerve, ulnar
  umbilical cord
    complicating delivery O69.2 ☑
      cord around neck O69.1 ☑
      prolapse O69.0 ☑
      specified NEC O69.2 ☑
  ureter N13.5
  vein I87.1
  vena cava (inferior) (superior) I87.1
Compulsion, compulsive
  gambling F63.0
  neurosis F42.8
  personality F60.5
  states F42.8
  swearing F42.8
    in Gilles de la Tourette's syndrome F95.2
  tics and spasms F95.9
Concato's disease (pericardial polyserositis) A19.9
  nontubercular I31.1
  pleural — *see* Pleurisy, with effusion
Concavity chest wall M95.4
Concealed penis Q55.69
Concern (normal) **about sick person in family** Z63.6
Concrescence (teeth) K00.2
Concretio cordis I31.1
  rheumatic I09.2
Concretion (*see also* Calculus)
  appendicular K38.1
  canaliculus — *see* Dacryolith
  clitoris N90.89
  conjunctiva H11.12- ☑
  eyelid — *see* Disorder, eyelid, specified type NEC
  lacrimal passages — *see* Dacryolith
  prepuce (male) N47.8
  salivary gland (any) K11.5
  seminal vesicle N50.89
  tonsil J35.8
Concussion (brain) (cerebral) (current) S06.0X9 ☑

Concussion — *continued*
  with
    loss of consciousness of 30 minutes or less S06.0X1 ☑
    loss of consciousness of unspecified duration S06.0X9 ☑
    without loss of consciousness S06.0X0 ☑
  blast (air) (hydraulic) (immersion) (underwater)
    abdomen or thorax — *see* Injury, blast, by site
    ear with acoustic nerve injury — *see* Injury, nerve, acoustic, specified type NEC
  cauda equina S34.3 ☑
  conus medullaris S34.02 ☑
  ocular S05.8X- ☑
  spinal (cord)
    cervical S14.0 ☑
    lumbar S34.01 ☑
    sacral S34.02 ☑
    thoracic S24.0 ☑
  syndrome F07.81
Condition — *see* Disease
Conditions arising in the perinatal period — *see* Newborn, affected by
Conduct disorder — *see* Disorder, conduct
Condyloma A63.0
  acuminatum A63.0
  gonorrheal A54.09
  latum A51.31
  syphilitic A51.31
    congenital A50.07
  venereal, syphilitic A51.31
Conflagration (*see also* Burn)
  asphyxia (by inhalation of gases, fumes or vapors) (*see also* Table of Drugs and Chemicals) T59.9- ☑
Conflict (with) (*see also* Discord)
  family Z73.9
  marital Z63.0
    involving divorce or estrangement Z63.5
  parent-child Z62.820
    parent-adopted child Z62.821
    parent-biological child Z62.820
    parent-foster child Z62.822
  social role NEC Z73.5
Confluent — *see* condition
Confusion, confused R41.0
  epileptic F05
  mental state (psychogenic) F44.89
  psychogenic F44.89
  reactive (from emotional stress, psychological trauma) F44.89
Confusional arousals G47.51
Congelation T69.9 ☑
Congenital (*see also* condition)
  aortic septum Q25.49
  intrinsic factor deficiency D51.0
  malformation — *see* Anomaly
Congestion, congestive
  bladder N32.89
  bowel K63.89
  brain G93.89
  breast N64.59
  bronchial J98.09
  catarrhal J31.0
  chest R09.89
  chill, malarial — *see* Malaria
  circulatory NEC I99.8
  duodenum K31.89
  eye — *see* Hyperemia, conjunctiva
  facial, due to birth injury P15.4
  general R68.89
  glottis J37.0
  heart — *see* Failure, heart, congestive
  hepatic K76.1
  hypostatic (lung) — *see* Edema, lung
  intestine K63.89
  kidney N28.89
  labyrinth H83.8 ☑
  larynx J37.0
  liver K76.1
  lung R09.89
    active or acute — *see* Pneumonia
  malaria, malarial — *see* Malaria
  nasal R09.81
  nose R09.81
  orbit, orbital (*see also* Exophthalmos)
    inflammatory (chronic) — *see* Inflammation, orbit
  ovary N83.8

Congestion, congestive — *continued*
  pancreas K86.89
  pelvic, female N94.89
  pleural J94.8
  prostate (active) N42.1
  pulmonary — *see* Congestion, lung
  renal N28.89
  retina H35.81
  seminal vesicle N50.1
  spinal cord G95.19
  spleen (chronic) D73.2
  stomach K31.89
  trachea — *see* Tracheitis
  urethra N36.8
  uterus N85.8
    with subinvolution N85.3
  venous (passive) I87.8
  viscera R68.89
Congestive — *see* Congestion
Conical
  cervix (hypertrophic elongation) N88.4
  cornea — *see* Keratoconus
  teeth K00.2
Conjoined twins Q89.4
Conjugal maladjustment Z63.0
  involving divorce or estrangement Z63.5
Conjunctiva — *see* condition
Conjunctivitis (staphylococcal) (streptococcal) NOS H10.9
  Acanthamoeba B60.12
  acute H10.3- ☑
    atopic H10.1- ☑
    chemical (*see also* Corrosion, cornea) H10.21- ☑
    mucopurulent H10.02- ☑
      follicular H10.01- ☑
    pseudomembranous H10.22- ☑
    serous except viral H10.23- ☑
    viral — *see* Conjunctivitis, viral
    toxic H10.21- ☑
  adenoviral (acute) (follicular) B30.1
  allergic (acute) — *see* Conjunctivitis, acute, atopic
    chronic H10.45
    vernal H10.44
  anaphylactic — *see* Conjunctivitis, acute, atopic
  Apollo B30.3
  atopic (acute) — *see* Conjunctivitis, acute, atopic
  Béal's B30.2
  blennorrhagic (gonococcal) (neonatorum) A54.31
  chemical (acute) (*see also* Corrosion, cornea) H10.21- ☑
  chlamydial A74.0
    due to trachoma A71.1
    neonatal P39.1
  chronic (nodosa) (petrificans) (phlyctenular) H10.40- ☑
    allergic H10.45
    vernal H10.44
    follicular H10.43- ☑
    giant papillary H10.41- ☑
    simple H10.42- ☑
    vernal H10.44
  coxsackievirus 24 B30.3
  diphtheritic A36.86
  due to
    dust — *see* Conjunctivitis, acute, atopic
    filariasis B74.9
    mucocutaneous leishmaniasis B55.2
  enterovirus type 70 (hemorrhagic) B30.3
  epidemic (viral) B30.9
    hemorrhagic B30.3
  gonococcal (neonatorum) A54.31
  granular (trachomatous) A71.1
    sequelae (late effect) B94.0
  hemorrhagic (acute) (epidemic) B30.3
  herpes zoster B02.31
  in (due to)
    Acanthamoeba B60.12
    adenovirus (acute) (follicular) B30.1
    Chlamydia A74.0
    coxsackievirus 24 B30.3
    diphtheria A36.86
    enterovirus type 70 (hemorrhagic) B30.3
    filariasis B74.9
    gonococci A54.31
    herpes (simplex) virus B00.53
      zoster B02.31
    infectious disease NEC B99 ☑
    meningococci A39.89
    mucocutaneous leishmaniasis B55.2

Index

Conjunctivitis — continued
- in — continued
  - rosacea L71.9
  - syphilis (late) A52.71
  - zoster B02.31
- inclusion A74.0
- infantile P39.1
  - gonococcal A54.31
- Koch-Weeks' — see Conjunctivitis, acute, mucopurulent
- light — see Conjunctivitis, acute, atopic
- ligneous — see Blepharoconjunctivitis, ligneous
- meningococcal A39.89
- mucopurulent — see Conjunctivitis, acute, mucopurulent
- neonatal P39.1
  - gonococcal A54.31
- Newcastle B30.8
- of Béal B30.2
- parasitic
  - filariasis B74.9
  - mucocutaneous leishmaniasis B55.2
- Parinaud's H10.89
- petrificans H10.89
- rosacea L71.9
- specified NEC H10.89
- swimming-pool B30.1
- trachomatous A71.1
  - acute A71.0
  - sequelae (late effect) B94.0
- traumatic NEC H10.89
- tuberculous A18.59
- tularemic A21.1
- tularensis A21.1
- viral B30.9
  - due to
    - adenovirus B30.1
    - enterovirus B30.3
  - specified NEC B30.8

Conjunctivochalasis H11.82- ☑
Connective tissue — see condition
Conn's syndrome E26.01
Conradi (-Hunermann) **disease** Q77.3
Consanguinity Z84.3
- counseling Z71.89
Conscious simulation (of illness) Z76.5
Consecutive — see condition
Consolidation lung (base) — see Pneumonia, lobar
Constipation (atonic) (neurogenic) (simple) (spastic) K59.00
- chronic K59.09
  - idiopathic K59.04
- drug-induced K59.03
- functional K59.04
- outlet dysfunction K59.02
- psychogenic F45.8
- slow transit K59.01
- specified NEC K59.09
Constitutional (see also condition)
- substandard F60.7
Constitutionally substandard F60.7
Constriction (see also Stricture)
- auditory canal — see Stenosis, external ear canal
- bronchial J98.09
- duodenum K31.5
- esophagus K22.2
- external
  - abdomen, abdominal (wall) S30.841 ☑
  - alveolar process S00.542 ☑
  - ankle S90.54- ☑
  - antecubital space — see Constriction, external, forearm
  - arm (upper) S40.84- ☑
  - auricle — see Constriction, external, ear
  - axilla — see Constriction, external, arm
  - back, lower S30.840 ☑
  - breast S20.14- ☑
  - brow S00.84 ☑
  - buttock S30.840 ☑
  - calf — see Constriction, external, leg
  - canthus — see Constriction, external, eyelid
  - cheek S00.84 ☑
    - internal S00.542 ☑
  - chest wall — see Constriction, external, thorax
  - chin S00.84 ☑
  - clitoris S30.844 ☑
  - costal region — see Constriction, external, thorax

Constriction — continued
- external — continued
  - digit(s)
    - foot — see Constriction, external, toe
    - hand — see Constriction, external, finger
  - ear S00.44- ☑
  - elbow S50.34- ☑
  - epididymis S30.843 ☑
  - epigastric region S30.841 ☑
  - esophagus, cervical S10.14 ☑
  - eyebrow — see Constriction, external, eyelid
  - eyelid S00.24- ☑
  - face S00.84 ☑
  - finger(s) S60.44- ☑
    - index S60.44- ☑
    - little S60.44- ☑
    - middle S60.44- ☑
    - ring S60.44- ☑
  - flank S30.841 ☑
  - foot (except toe(s) alone) S90.84- ☑
    - toe — see Constriction, external, toe
  - forearm S50.84- ☑
    - elbow only — see Constriction, external, elbow
  - forehead S00.84 ☑
  - genital organs, external
    - female S30.846 ☑
    - male S30.845 ☑
  - groin S30.841 ☑
  - gum S00.542 ☑
  - hand S60.54- ☑
  - head S00.94 ☑
    - ear — see Constriction, external, ear
    - eyelid — see Constriction, external, eyelid
    - lip S00.541 ☑
    - nose S00.34 ☑
    - oral cavity S00.542 ☑
    - scalp S00.04 ☑
    - specified site NEC S00.84 ☑
  - heel — see Constriction, external, foot
  - hip S70.24- ☑
  - inguinal region S30.841 ☑
  - interscapular region S20.449 ☑
  - jaw S00.84 ☑
  - knee S80.24- ☑
  - labium (majus) (minus) S30.844 ☑
  - larynx S10.14 ☑
  - leg (lower) S80.84- ☑
    - knee — see Constriction, external, knee
    - upper — see Constriction, external, thigh
  - lip S00.541 ☑
  - lower back S30.840 ☑
  - lumbar region S30.840 ☑
  - malar region S00.84 ☑
  - mammary — see Constriction, external, breast
  - mastoid region S00.84 ☑
  - mouth S00.542 ☑
  - nail
    - finger — see Constriction, external, finger
    - toe — see Constriction, external, toe
  - nasal S00.34 ☑
  - neck S10.94 ☑
    - specified site NEC S10.84 ☑
    - throat S10.14 ☑
  - nose S00.34 ☑
  - occipital region S00.04 ☑
  - oral cavity S00.542 ☑
  - orbital region — see Constriction, external, eyelid
  - palate S00.542 ☑
  - palm — see Constriction, external, hand
  - parietal region S00.04 ☑
  - pelvis S30.840 ☑
  - penis S30.842 ☑
  - perineum
    - female S30.844 ☑
    - male S30.840 ☑
  - periocular area — see Constriction, external, eyelid
  - phalanges
    - finger — see Constriction, external, finger
    - toe — see Constriction, external, toe
  - pharynx S10.14 ☑
  - pinna — see Constriction, external, ear
  - popliteal space — see Constriction, external, knee
  - prepuce S30.842 ☑
  - pubic region S30.840 ☑
  - pudendum
    - female S30.846 ☑

Constriction — continued
- external — continued
  - pudendum — continued
    - male S30.845 ☑
  - sacral region S30.840 ☑
  - scalp S00.04 ☑
  - scapular region — see Constriction, external, shoulder
  - scrotum S30.843 ☑
  - shin — see Constriction, external, leg
  - shoulder S40.24- ☑
  - sternal region S20.349 ☑
  - submaxillary region S00.84 ☑
  - submental region S00.84 ☑
  - subungual
    - finger(s) — see Constriction, external, finger
    - toe(s) — see Constriction, external, toe
  - supraclavicular fossa S10.84 ☑
  - supraorbital S00.84 ☑
  - temple S00.84 ☑
  - temporal region S00.84 ☑
  - testis S30.843 ☑
  - thigh S70.34- ☑
  - thorax, thoracic (wall) S20.94 ☑
    - back S20.44- ☑
    - front S20.34- ☑
  - throat S10.14 ☑
  - thumb S60.34- ☑
  - toe(s) (lesser) S90.44- ☑
    - great S90.44- ☑
  - tongue S00.542 ☑
  - trachea S10.14 ☑
  - tunica vaginalis S30.843 ☑
  - uvula S00.542 ☑
  - vagina S30.844 ☑
  - vulva S30.844 ☑
  - wrist S60.84- ☑
- gallbladder — see Obstruction, gallbladder
- intestine — see Obstruction, intestine
- larynx J38.6
  - congenital Q31.8
    - specified NEC Q31.8
    - subglottic Q31.1
- organ or site, congenital NEC — see Atresia, by site
- prepuce (acquired) (congenital) N47.1
- pylorus (adult hypertrophic) K31.1
  - congenital or infantile Q40.0
  - newborn Q40.0
- ring dystocia (uterus) O62.4
- spastic (see also Spasm)
  - ureter N13.5
- ureter N13.5
  - with infection N13.6
- urethra — see Stricture, urethra
- visual field (peripheral) (functional) — see Defect, visual field
Constrictive — see condition
Consultation
- without complaint or sickness Z71.9
  - feared complaint unfounded Z71.1
  - specified reason NEC Z71.89
- medical — see Counseling, medical
- religious Z71.81
- specified reason NEC Z71.89
- spiritual Z71.81
Consumption — see Tuberculosis
Contact (with) (see also Exposure (to))
- acariasis Z20.7
- AIDS virus Z20.6
- air pollution Z77.110
- algae and algae toxins Z77.121
- algae bloom Z77.121
- anthrax Z20.810
- aromatic amines Z77.020
- aromatic (hazardous) compounds NEC Z77.028
- aromatic dyes NOS Z77.028
- arsenic Z77.010
- asbestos Z77.090
- bacterial disease NEC Z20.818
- benzene Z77.021
- blue-green algae bloom Z77.121
- body fluids (potentially hazardous) Z77.21
- brown tide Z77.121
- chemicals (chiefly nonmedicinal) (hazardous) NEC Z77.098
- cholera Z20.09
- chromium compounds Z77.018

☑ **Additional Character Required** — Refer to the Tabular List for Character Selection   ⬇ Subterms under main terms may continue to next column or page

Conjunctivitis — Contact

Contusion — *continued*
- throat S10.0 ☑
- thumb S60.01- ☑
  - with damage to nail S60.11- ☑
- toe(s) (lesser) S90.12- ☑
  - with damage to nail S90.22- ☑
  - great S90.11- ☑
    - with damage to nail S90.21- ☑
- tongue S00.532 ☑
- trachea (cervical) S10.0 ☑
  - thoracic S27.52 ☑
- tunica vaginalis S30.22 ☑
- tympanum, tympanic membrane — *see* Contusion, ear
- ureter S37.12 ☑
- urethra S37.32 ☑
- urinary organ NEC S37.892 ☑
- uterus S37.62 ☑
- uvula S00.532 ☑
- vagina S30.23 ☑
- vas deferens S37.892 ☑
- vesical S37.22 ☑
- vocal cord(s) S10.0 ☑
- vulva S30.23 ☑
- wrist S60.21- ☑

Conus (congenital) (any type) Q14.8
- cornea — *see* Keratoconus
- medullaris syndrome G95.81

Conversion hysteria, neurosis or reaction F44.9
Converter, tuberculosis (test reaction) R76.11
Conviction (legal), **anxiety concerning** Z65.0
- with imprisonment Z65.1

Convulsions (idiopathic) (*see also* Seizure(s)) R56.9
- apoplectiform (cerebral ischemia) I67.82
- dissociative F44.5
- epileptic — *see* Epilepsy
- epileptiform, epileptoid — *see* Seizure, epileptiform
- ether (anesthetic) — *see* Table of Drugs and Chemicals, by drug
- febrile R56.00
  - with status epilepticus G40.901
  - complex R56.01
    - with status epilepticus G40.901
  - simple R56.00
- hysterical F44.5
- infantile P90
  - epilepsy — *see* Epilepsy
- jacksonian — *see* Epilepsy, localization-related, symptomatic, with simple partial seizures
- myoclonic G25.3
- newborn P90
- obstetrical (nephritic) (uremic) — *see* Eclampsia
- paretic A52.17
- post traumatic R56.1
- psychomotor — *see* Epilepsy, localization-related, symptomatic, with complex partial seizures
- recurrent R56.9
- reflex R25.8
- scarlatinal A38.8
- tetanus, tetanic — *see* Tetanus
- thymic E32.8

Convulsive (*see also* Convulsions)
Cooley's anemia D56.1
Coolie itch B76.9
Cooper's
- disease — *see* Mastopathy, cystic
- hernia — *see* Hernia, abdomen, specified site NEC

Copra itch B88.0
Coprophagy F50.89
Coprophobia F40.298
Coproporphyria, hereditary E80.29
Cor
- biloculare Q20.8
- bovis, bovinum — *see* Hypertrophy, cardiac
- pulmonale (chronic) I27.81
  - acute I26.09
- triatriatum, triatrium Q24.2
- triloculare Q20.8
  - biatrium Q20.4
  - biventriculare Q21.1

Corbus' disease (gangrenous balanitis) N48.1
Cord (*see also* condition)
- around neck
  - complicating delivery O69.81 ☑
    - with compression O69.1 ☑
- bladder G95.89
  - tabetic A52.19

Cordis ectopia Q24.8
Corditis (spermatic) N49.1
Corectopia Q13.2
Cori's disease (glycogen storage) E74.03
Corkhandler's disease or lung J67.3
Corkscrew esophagus K22.4
Corkworker's disease or lung J67.3
Corn (infected) L84
Cornea (*see also* condition)
- donor Z52.5
- plana Q13.4

Cornelia de Lange syndrome Q87.1
Cornu cutaneum L85.8
Cornual gestation or pregnancy O00.80
- with intrauterine pregnancy O00.81

Coronary (artery) — *see* condition
Coronavirus, as cause of disease classified elsewhere B97.29
- SARS-associated B97.21

Corpora (*see also* condition)
- amylacea, prostate N42.89
- cavernosa — *see* condition

Corpulence — *see* Obesity
Corpus — *see* condition
Corrected transposition Q20.5
Corrosion (injury) (acid) (caustic) (chemical) (lime) (external) (internal) T30.4
- abdomen, abdominal (muscle) (wall) T21.42 ☑
  - first degree T21.52 ☑
  - second degree T21.62 ☑
  - third degree T21.72 ☑
- above elbow T22.439 ☑
  - first degree T22.539 ☑
  - left T22.432 ☑
    - first degree T22.532 ☑
    - second degree T22.632 ☑
    - third degree T22.732 ☑
  - right T22.431 ☑
    - first degree T22.531 ☑
    - second degree T22.631 ☑
    - third degree T22.731 ☑
  - second degree T22.639 ☑
  - third degree T22.739 ☑
- alimentary tract NEC T28.7 ☑
- ankle T25.419 ☑
  - first degree T25.519 ☑
  - left T25.412 ☑
    - first degree T25.512 ☑
    - second degree T25.612 ☑
    - third degree T25.712 ☑
  - multiple with foot — *see* Corrosion, lower, limb, multiple, ankle and foot
  - right T25.411 ☑
    - first degree T25.511 ☑
    - second degree T25.611 ☑
    - third degree T25.711 ☑
  - second degree T25.619 ☑
  - third degree T25.719 ☑
- anus — *see* Corrosion, buttock
- arm(s) (meaning upper limb(s)) — *see* Corrosion, upper limb
- axilla T22.449 ☑
  - first degree T22.549 ☑
  - left T22.442 ☑
    - first degree T22.542 ☑
    - second degree T22.642 ☑
    - third degree T22.742 ☑
  - right T22.441 ☑
    - first degree T22.541 ☑
    - second degree T22.641 ☑
    - third degree T22.741 ☑
  - second degree T22.649 ☑
  - third degree T22.749 ☑
- back (lower) T21.44 ☑
  - first degree T21.54 ☑
  - second degree T21.64 ☑
  - third degree T21.74 ☑
  - upper T21.43 ☑
    - first degree T21.53 ☑
    - second degree T21.63 ☑
    - third degree T21.73 ☑
- blisters — *code as* Corrosion, second degree, by site
- breast(s) — *see* Corrosion, chest wall
- buttock(s) T21.45 ☑
  - first degree T21.55 ☑
  - second degree T21.65 ☑

Corrosion — *continued*
- buttock(s) — *continued*
  - third degree T21.75 ☑
- calf T24.439 ☑
  - first degree T24.539 ☑
  - left T24.432 ☑
    - first degree T24.532 ☑
    - second degree T24.632 ☑
    - third degree T24.732 ☑
  - right T24.431 ☑
    - first degree T24.531 ☑
    - second degree T24.631 ☑
    - third degree T24.731 ☑
  - second degree T24.639 ☑
  - third degree T24.739 ☑
- canthus (eye) — *see* Corrosion, eyelid
- cervix T28.8 ☑
- cheek T20.46 ☑
  - first degree T20.56 ☑
  - second degree T20.66 ☑
  - third degree T20.76 ☑
- chest wall T21.41 ☑
  - first degree T21.51 ☑
  - second degree T21.61 ☑
  - third degree T21.71 ☑
- chin T20.43 ☑
  - first degree T20.53 ☑
  - second degree T20.63 ☑
  - third degree T20.73 ☑
- colon T28.7 ☑
- conjunctiva (and cornea) — *see* Corrosion, cornea
- cornea (and conjunctiva) T26.6- ☑
- deep necrosis of underlying tissue — *code as* Corrosion, third degree, by site
- dorsum of hand T23.469 ☑
  - first degree T23.569 ☑
  - left T23.462 ☑
    - first degree T23.562 ☑
    - second degree T23.662 ☑
    - third degree T23.762 ☑
  - right T23.461 ☑
    - first degree T23.561 ☑
    - second degree T23.661 ☑
    - third degree T23.761- ☑
  - second degree T23.669 ☑
  - third degree T23.769 ☑
- ear (auricle) (external) (canal) T20.41 ☑
  - drum T28.91 ☑
  - first degree T20.51 ☑
  - second degree T20.61 ☑
  - third degree T20.71 ☑
- elbow T22.429 ☑
  - first degree T22.529 ☑
  - left T22.422 ☑
    - first degree T22.522 ☑
    - second degree T22.622 ☑
    - third degree T22.722 ☑
  - right T22.421 ☑
    - first degree T22.521 ☑
    - second degree T22.621 ☑
    - third degree T22.721 ☑
  - second degree T22.629 ☑
  - third degree T22.729 ☑
- entire body — *see* Corrosion, multiple body regions
- epidermal loss — *code as* Corrosion, second degree, by site
- epiglottis T27.4 ☑
- erythema, erythematous — *code as* Corrosion, first degree, by site
- esophagus T28.6 ☑
- extent (percentage of body surface)
  - less than 10 percent T32.0
  - 10-19 percent (0-9 percent third degree) T32.10
    - with 10-19 percent third degree T32.11
  - 20-29 percent (0-9 percent third degree) T32.20
    - with
      - 10-19 percent third degree T32.21
      - 20-29 percent third degree T32.22
  - 30-39 percent (0-9 percent third degree) T32.30
    - with
      - 10-19 percent third degree T32.31
      - 20-29 percent third degree T32.32
      - 30-39 percent third degree T32.33
  - 40-49 percent (0-9 percent third degree) T32.40
    - with
      - 10-19 percent third degree T32.41

◤ Subterms under main terms may continue to next column or page   ☑ Additional Character Required — Refer to the Tabular List for Character Selection   73

Contusion — Corrosion

Index

Corrosion — Corrosion

Corrosion — *continued*
  extent — *continued*
    40-49 percent — *continued*
      with — *continued*
        20-29 percent third degree T32.42
        30-39 percent third degree T32.43
        40-49 percent third degree T32.44
    50-59 percent (0-9 percent third degree) T32.50
      with
        10-19 percent third degree T32.51
        20-29 percent third degree T32.52
        30-39 percent third degree T32.53
        40-49 percent third degree T32.54
        50-59 percent third degree T32.55
    60-69 percent (0-9 percent third degree) T32.60
      with
        10-19 percent third degree T32.61
        20-29 percent third degree T32.62
        30-39 percent third degree T32.63
        40-49 percent third degree T32.64
        50-59 percent third degree T32.65
        60-69 percent third degree T32.66
    70-79 percent (0-9 percent third degree) T32.70
      with
        10-19 percent third degree T32.71
        20-29 percent third degree T32.72
        30-39 percent third degree T32.73
        40-49 percent third degree T32.74
        50-59 percent third degree T32.75
        60-69 percent third degree T32.76
        70-79 percent third degree T32.77
    80-89 percent (0-9 percent third degree) T32.80
      with
        10-19 percent third degree T32.81
        20-29 percent third degree T32.82
        30-39 percent third degree T32.83
        40-49 percent third degree T32.84
        50-59 percent third degree T32.85
        60-69 percent third degree T32.86
        70-79 percent third degree T32.87
        80-89 percent third degree T32.88
    90 percent or more (0-9 percent third degree) T32.90
      with
        10-19 percent third degree T32.91
        20-29 percent third degree T32.92
        30-39 percent third degree T32.93
        40-49 percent third degree T32.94
        50-59 percent third degree T32.95
        60-69 percent third degree T32.96
        70-79 percent third degree T32.97
        80-89 percent third degree T32.98
        90-99 percent third degree T32.99
  extremity — *see* Corrosion, limb
  eye(s) and adnexa T26.9- ☑
    with resulting rupture and destruction of eyeball T26.7- ☑
    conjunctival sac — *see* Corrosion, cornea
    cornea — *see* Corrosion, cornea
    lid — *see* Corrosion, eyelid
    periocular area — *see* Corrosion eyelid
    specified site NEC T26.8- ☑
  eyeball — *see* Corrosion, eye
  eyelid(s) T26.5- ☑
  face — *see* Corrosion, head
  finger T23.429 ☑
    first degree T23.529 ☑
    left T23.422 ☑
      first degree T23.522 ☑
      second degree T23.622 ☑
      third degree T23.722 ☑
      multiple sites (without thumb) T23.439 ☑
        with thumb T23.449 ☑
          first degree T23.549 ☑
          left T23.442 ☑
            first degree T23.542 ☑
            second degree T23.642 ☑
            third degree T23.742 ☑
          right T23.441 ☑
            first degree T23.541 ☑
            second degree T23.641 ☑
            third degree T23.741 ☑
          second degree T23.649 ☑
          third degree T23.749 ☑
      first degree T23.539 ☑
      left T23.432 ☑
        first degree T23.532 ☑

Corrosion — *continued*
  finger — *continued*
    multiple sites — *continued*
      left — *continued*
        second degree T23.632 ☑
        third degree T23.732 ☑
      right T23.431 ☑
        first degree T23.531 ☑
        second degree T23.631 ☑
        third degree T23.731 ☑
      second degree T23.639 ☑
      third degree T23.739 ☑
    right T23.421 ☑
      first degree T23.521 ☑
      second degree T23.621 ☑
      third degree T23.721 ☑
    second degree T23.629 ☑
    third degree T23.729 ☑
  flank — *see* Corrosion, abdomen
  foot T25.429 ☑
    first degree T25.529 ☑
    left T25.422 ☑
      first degree T25.522 ☑
      second degree T25.622 ☑
      third degree T25.722 ☑
    multiple with ankle — *see* Corrosion, lower, limb, multiple, ankle and foot
    right T25.421 ☑
      first degree T25.521 ☑
      second degree T25.621 ☑
      third degree T25.721 ☑
    second degree T25.629 ☑
    third degree T25.729 ☑
  forearm T22.419 ☑
    first degree T22.519 ☑
    left T22.412 ☑
      first degree T22.512 ☑
      second degree T22.612 ☑
      third degree T22.712 ☑
    right T22.411 ☑
      first degree T22.511 ☑
      second degree T22.611 ☑
      third degree T22.711 ☑
    second degree T22.619 ☑
    third degree T22.719 ☑
  forehead T20.46 ☑
    first degree T20.56 ☑
    second degree T20.66 ☑
    third degree T20.76 ☑
  fourth degree — *code as* Corrosion, third degree, by site
  full thickness skin loss — *code as* Corrosion, third degree, by site
  gastrointestinal tract NEC T28.7 ☑
  genital organs
    external
      female T21.47 ☑
        first degree T21.57 ☑
        second degree T21.67 ☑
        third degree T21.77 ☑
      male T21.46 ☑
        first degree T21.56 ☑
        second degree T21.66 ☑
        third degree T21.76 ☑
    internal T28.8 ☑
  groin — *see* Corrosion, abdominal wall
  hand(s) T23.409 ☑
    back — *see* Corrosion, dorsum of hand
    finger — *see* Corrosion, finger
    first degree T23.509 ☑
    left T23.402 ☑
      first degree T23.502 ☑
      second degree T23.602 ☑
      third degree T23.702 ☑
    multiple sites with wrist T23.499 ☑
      first degree T23.599 ☑
      left T23.492 ☑
        first degree T23.592 ☑
        second degree T23.692 ☑
        third degree T23.792 ☑
      right T23.491 ☑
        first degree T23.591 ☑
        second degree T23.691 ☑
        third degree T23.791 ☑
      second degree T23.699 ☑
      third degree T23.799 ☑

Corrosion — *continued*
  hand(s) — *continued*
    palm — *see* Corrosion, palm
    right T23.401 ☑
      first degree T23.501 ☑
      second degree T23.601 ☑
      third degree T23.701 ☑
    second degree T23.609 ☑
    third degree T23.709 ☑
    thumb — *see* Corrosion, thumb
  head (and face) (and neck) T20.40 ☑
    cheek — *see* Corrosion, cheek
    chin — *see* Corrosion, chin
    ear — *see* Corrosion, ear
    eye(s) only — *see* Corrosion, eye
    first degree T20.50 ☑
    forehead — *see* Corrosion, forehead
    lip — *see* Corrosion, lip
    multiple sites T20.49 ☑
      first degree T20.59 ☑
      second degree T20.69 ☑
      third degree T20.79 ☑
    neck — *see* Corrosion, neck
    nose — *see* Corrosion, nose
    scalp — *see* Corrosion, scalp
    second degree T20.60 ☑
    third degree T20.70 ☑
  hip(s) — *see* Corrosion, lower, limb
  inhalation — *see* Corrosion, respiratory tract
  internal organ(s) (*see also* Corrosion, by site) T28.90 ☑
    alimentary tract T28.7 ☑
      esophagus T28.6 ☑
    esophagus T28.6 ☑
    genitourinary T28.8 ☑
    mouth T28.5 ☑
    pharynx T28.5 ☑
    specified organ NEC T28.99 ☑
  interscapular region — *see* Corrosion, back, upper
  intestine (large) (small) T28.7 ☑
  knee T24.429 ☑
    first degree T24.529 ☑
    left T24.422 ☑
      first degree T24.522 ☑
      second degree T24.622 ☑
      third degree T24.722 ☑
    right T24.421 ☑
      first degree T24.521 ☑
      second degree T24.621 ☑
      third degree T24.721 ☑
    second degree T24.629 ☑
    third degree T24.729 ☑
  labium (majus) (minus) — *see* Corrosion, genital organs, external, female
  lacrimal apparatus, duct, gland or sac — *see* Corrosion, eye, specified site NEC
  larynx T27.4 ☑
    with lung T27.5 ☑
  leg(s) (meaning lower limb(s)) — *see* Corrosion, lower limb
  limb(s)
    lower — *see* Corrosion, lower, limb
    upper — *see* Corrosion, upper limb
  lip(s) T20.42 ☑
    first degree T20.52 ☑
    second degree T20.62 ☑
    third degree T20.72 ☑
  lower
    back — *see* Corrosion, back
    limb T24.409 ☑
      ankle — *see* Corrosion, ankle
      calf — *see* Corrosion, calf
      first degree T24.509 ☑
      foot — *see* Corrosion, foot
      knee — *see* Corrosion, knee
      left T24.402 ☑
        first degree T24.502 ☑
        second degree T24.602 ☑
        third degree T24.702 ☑
      multiple sites, except ankle and foot T24.499 ☑
        ankle and foot T25.499 ☑
          first degree T25.599 ☑
          left T25.492 ☑
            first degree T25.592 ☑
            second degree T25.692 ☑
            third degree T25.792 ☑
          right T25.491 ☑

☑ **Additional Character Required** — Refer to the Tabular List for Character Selection   ☜ **Subterms under main terms may continue to next column or page**

Corrosion — *continued*
  lower — *continued*
    limb — *continued*
      multiple sites, except ankle and foot — *continued*
        ankle and foot — *continued*
          right — *continued*
            first degree T25.591 ☑
            second degree T25.691 ☑
            third degree T25.791 ☑
          second degree T25.699 ☑
          third degree T25.799 ☑
        first degree T24.599 ☑
        left T24.492 ☑
          first degree T24.592 ☑
          second degree T24.692 ☑
          third degree T24.792 ☑
        right T24.491 ☑
          first degree T24.591 ☑
          second degree T24.691 ☑
          third degree T24.791 ☑
        second degree T24.699 ☑
        third degree T24.799 ☑
      right T24.401 ☑
        first degree T24.501 ☑
        second degree T24.601 ☑
        third degree T24.701 ☑
      second degree T24.609 ☑
      thigh — *see* Corrosion, thigh
      third degree T24.709 ☑
  lung (with larynx and trachea) T27.5 ☑
  mouth T28.5 ☑
  neck T20.47 ☑
    first degree T20.57 ☑
    second degree T20.67 ☑
    third degree T20.77 ☑
  nose (septum) T20.44 ☑
    first degree T20.54 ☑
    second degree T20.64 ☑
    third degree T20.74 ☑
  ocular adnexa — *see* Corrosion, eye
  orbit region — *see* Corrosion, eyelid
  palm T23.459 ☑
    first degree T23.559 ☑
    left T23.452 ☑
      first degree T23.552 ☑
      second degree T23.652 ☑
      third degree T23.752 ☑
    right T23.451 ☑
      first degree T23.551 ☑
      second degree T23.651 ☑
      third degree T23.751 ☑
    second degree T23.659 ☑
    third degree T23.759 ☑
  partial thickness — *code as* Corrosion, unspecified degree, by site
  pelvis — *see* Corrosion, trunk
  penis — *see* Corrosion, genital organs, external, male
  perineum
    female — *see* Corrosion, genital organs, external, female
    male — *see* Corrosion, genital organs, external, male
  periocular area — *see* Corrosion, eyelid
  pharynx T28.5 ☑
  rectum T28.7 ☑
  respiratory tract T27.7 ☑
    larynx — *see* Corrosion, larynx
    specified part NEC T27.6 ☑
    trachea — *see* Corrosion, larynx
  sac, lacrimal — *see* Corrosion, eye, specified site NEC
  scalp T20.45 ☑
    first degree T20.55 ☑
    second degree T20.65 ☑
    third degree T20.75 ☑
  scapular region T22.469 ☑
    first degree T22.569 ☑
    left T22.462 ☑
      first degree T22.562 ☑
      second degree T22.662 ☑
      third degree T22.762 ☑
    right T22.461 ☑
      first degree T22.561 ☑
      second degree T22.661 ☑
      third degree T22.761 ☑
    second degree T22.669 ☑

Corrosion — *continued*
  scapular region — *continued*
    third degree T22.769 ☑
  sclera — *see* Corrosion, eye, specified site NEC
  scrotum — *see* Corrosion, genital organs, external, male
  shoulder T22.459 ☑
    first degree T22.559 ☑
    left T22.452 ☑
      first degree T22.552 ☑
      second degree T22.652 ☑
      third degree T22.752 ☑
    right T22.451 ☑
      first degree T22.551 ☑
      second degree T22.651 ☑
      third degree T22.751 ☑
    second degree T22.659 ☑
    third degree T22.759 ☑
  stomach T28.7 ☑
  temple — *see* Corrosion, head
  testis — *see* Corrosion, genital organs, external, male
  thigh T24.419 ☑
    first degree T24.519 ☑
    left T24.412 ☑
      first degree T24.512 ☑
      second degree T24.612 ☑
      third degree T24.712 ☑
    right T24.411 ☑
      first degree T24.511 ☑
      second degree T24.611 ☑
      third degree T24.711 ☑
    second degree T24.619 ☑
    third degree T24.719 ☑
  thorax (external) — *see* Corrosion, trunk
  throat (meaning pharynx) T28.5 ☑
  thumb(s) T23.419 ☑
    first degree T23.519 ☑
    left T23.412 ☑
      first degree T23.512 ☑
      second degree T23.612 ☑
      third degree T23.712 ☑
    multiple sites with fingers T23.449 ☑
      first degree T23.549 ☑
      left T23.442 ☑
        first degree T23.542 ☑
        second degree T23.642 ☑
        third degree T23.742 ☑
      right T23.441 ☑
        first degree T23.541 ☑
        second degree T23.641 ☑
        third degree T23.741 ☑
      second degree T23.649 ☑
      third degree T23.749 ☑
    right T23.411 ☑
      first degree T23.511 ☑
      second degree T23.611 ☑
      third degree T23.711 ☑
    second degree T23.619 ☑
    third degree T23.719 ☑
  toe T25.439 ☑
    first degree T25.539 ☑
    left T25.432 ☑
      first degree T25.532 ☑
      second degree T25.632 ☑
      third degree T25.732 ☑
    right T25.431 ☑
      first degree T25.531 ☑
      second degree T25.631 ☑
      third degree T25.731 ☑
    second degree T25.639 ☑
    third degree T25.739 ☑
  tongue T28.5 ☑
  tonsil(s) T28.5 ☑
  total body — *see* Corrosion, multiple body regions
  trachea T27.4 ☑
    with lung T27.5 ☑
  trunk T21.40 ☑
    abdominal wall — *see* Corrosion, abdominal wall
    anus — *see* Corrosion, buttock
    axilla — *see* Corrosion, upper limb
    back — *see* Corrosion, back
    breast — *see* Corrosion, chest wall
    buttock — *see* Corrosion, buttock
    chest wall — *see* Corrosion, chest wall
      first degree T21.50 ☑
    flank — *see* Corrosion, abdominal wall

Corrosion — *continued*
  trunk — *continued*
    genital
      female — *see* Corrosion, genital organs, external, female
      male — *see* Corrosion, genital organs, external, male
    groin — *see* Corrosion, abdominal wall
    interscapular region — *see* Corrosion, back, upper
    labia — *see* Corrosion, genital organs, external, female
    lower back — *see* Corrosion, back
    penis — *see* Corrosion, genital organs, external, male
    perineum
      female — *see* Corrosion, genital organs, external, female
      male — *see* Corrosion, genital organs, external, male
    scapular region — *see* Corrosion, upper limb
    scrotum — *see* Corrosion, genital organs, external, male
    second degree T21.60 ☑
    shoulder — *see* Corrosion, upper limb
    specified site NEC T21.49 ☑
      first degree T21.59 ☑
      second degree T21.69 ☑
      third degree T21.79 ☑
    testes — *see* Corrosion, genital organs, external, male
    third degree T21.70 ☑
    upper back — *see* Corrosion, back, upper
    vagina T28.8 ☑
    vulva — *see* Corrosion, genital organs, external, female
  unspecified site with extent of body surface involved specified
    less than 10 percent T32.0
    10-19 percent (0-9 percent third degree) T32.10
      with 10-19 percent third degree T32.11
    20-29 percent (0-9 percent third degree) T32.20
      with
        10-19 percent third degree T32.21
        20-29 percent third degree T32.22
    30-39 percent (0-9 percent third degree) T32.30
      with
        10-19 percent third degree T32.31
        20-29 percent third degree T32.32
        30-39 percent third degree T32.33
    40-49 percent (0-9 percent third degree) T32.40
      with
        10-19 percent third degree T32.41
        20-29 percent third degree T32.42
        30-39 percent third degree T32.43
        40-49 percent third degree T32.44
    50-59 percent (0-9 percent third degree) T32.50
      with
        10-19 percent third degree T32.51
        20-29 percent third degree T32.52
        30-39 percent third degree T32.53
        40-49 percent third degree T32.54
        50-59 percent third degree T32.55
    60-69 percent (0-9 percent third degree) T32.60
      with
        10-19 percent third degree T32.61
        20-29 percent third degree T32.62
        30-39 percent third degree T32.63
        40-49 percent third degree T32.64
        50-59 percent third degree T32.65
        60-69 percent third degree T32.66
    70-79 percent (0-9 percent third degree) T32.70
      with
        10-19 percent third degree T32.71
        20-29 percent third degree T32.72
        30-39 percent third degree T32.73
        40-49 percent third degree T32.74
        50-59 percent third degree T32.75
        60-69 percent third degree T32.76
        70-79 percent third degree T32.77
    80-89 percent (0-9 percent third degree) T32.80
      with
        10-19 percent third degree T32.81
        20-29 percent third degree T32.82
        30-39 percent third degree T32.83
        40-49 percent third degree T32.84
        50-59 percent third degree T32.85
        60-69 percent third degree T32.86
        70-79 percent third degree T32.87

Corrosion — *continued*
  unspecified site with extent of body surface involved
    specified — *continued*
      80-89 percent — *continued*
        with — *continued*
          80-89 percent third degree T32.88
      90 percent or more (0-9 percent third degree)
        T32.90
        with
          10-19 percent third degree T32.91
          20-29 percent third degree T32.92
          30-39 percent third degree I32.93
          40-49 percent third degree T32.94
          50-59 percent third degree T32.95
          60-69 percent third degree T32.96
          70-79 percent third degree T32.97
          80-89 percent third degree T32.98
          90-99 percent third degree T32.99
  upper limb (axilla) (scapular region) T22.40 ☑
    above elbow — *see* Corrosion, above elbow
    axilla — *see* Corrosion, axilla
    elbow — *see* Corrosion, elbow
    first degree T22.50 ☑
    forearm — *see* Corrosion, forearm
    hand — *see* Corrosion, hand
    interscapular region — *see* Corrosion, back, upper
    multiple sites T22.499 ☑
      first degree T22.599 ☑
      left T22.492 ☑
        first degree T22.592 ☑
        second degree T22.692 ☑
        third degree T22.792 ☑
      right T22.491 ☑
        first degree T22.591 ☑
        second degree T22.691 ☑
        third degree T22.791 ☑
      second degree T22.699 ☑
      third degree T22.799 ☑
    scapular region — *see* Corrosion, scapular region
    second degree T22.60 ☑
    shoulder — *see* Corrosion, shoulder
    third degree T22.70 ☑
    wrist — *see* Corrosion, hand
  uterus T28.8 ☑
  vagina T28.8 ☑
  vulva — *see* Corrosion, genital organs, external, female
  wrist T23.479 ☑
    first degree T23.579 ☑
    left T23.472 ☑
      first degree T23.572 ☑
      second degree T23.672 ☑
      third degree T23.772 ☑
    multiple sites with hand T23.499 ☑
      first degree T23.599 ☑
      left T23.492 ☑
        first degree T23.592 ☑
        second degree T23.692 ☑
        third degree T23.792 ☑
      right T23.491 ☑
        first degree T23.591 ☑
        second degree T23.691 ☑
        third degree T23.791 ☑
      second degree T23.699 ☑
      third degree T23.799 ☑
    right T23.471 ☑
      first degree T23.571 ☑
      second degree T23.671 ☑
      third degree T23.771 ☑
    second degree T23.679 ☑
    third degree T23.779 ☑
Corrosive burn — *see* Corrosion
Corsican fever — *see* Malaria
Cortical — *see* condition
Cortico-adrenal — *see* condition
Coryza (acute) J00
  with grippe or influenza — *see* Influenza, with, respi-
    ratory manifestations NEC
  syphilitic
    congenital (chronic) A50.05
Costen's syndrome or complex M26.69
Costiveness — *see* Constipation
Costochondritis M94.0
Cot death R99
Cotard's syndrome F22
Cotia virus B08.8
Cotton wool spots (retinal) H35.81

Cotungo's disease — *see* Sciatica
Cough (affected) (chronic) (epidemic) (nervous) R05
  with hemorrhage — *see* Hemoptysis
  bronchial R05
    with grippe or influenza — *see* Influenza, with,
      respiratory manifestations NEC
  functional F45.8
  hysterical F45.8
  laryngeal, spasmodic R05
  psychogenic F45.8
  smokers' J41.0
  tea taster's B49
Counseling (for) Z71.9
  abuse NEC
    perpetrator Z69.82
    victim Z69.81
  alcohol abuser Z71.41
    family Z71.42
  child abuse
    nonparental
      perpetrator Z69.021
      victim Z69.020
    parental
      perpetrator Z69.011
      victim Z69.010
  consanguinity Z71.89
  contraceptive Z30.09
  dietary Z71.3
  drug abuser Z71.51
    family member Z71.52
  exercise Z71.82
  family Z71.89
  fertility preservation (prior to cancer therapy) (prior
    to removal of gonads) Z31.62
  for non-attending third party Z71.0
    related to sexual behavior or orientation Z70.2
  genetic
    nonprocreative Z71.83
    procreative NEC Z31.5
  gestational carrier Z31.7
  health (advice) (education) (instruction) — *see* Coun-
    seling, medical
  human immunodeficiency virus (HIV) Z71.7
  impotence Z70.1
  insulin pump use Z46.81
  medical (for) Z71.9
    boarding school resident Z59.3
    consanguinity Z71.89
    feared complaint and no disease found Z71.1
    human immunodeficiency virus (HIV) Z71.7
    institutional resident Z59.3
    on behalf of another Z71.0
      related to sexual behavior or orientation Z70.2
    person living alone Z60.2
    specified reason NEC Z71.89
  natural family planning
    procreative Z31.61
    to avoid pregnancy Z30.02
  perpetrator (of)
    abuse NEC Z69.82
    child abuse
      non-parental Z69.021
      parental Z69.011
    rape NEC Z69.82
    spousal abuse Z69.12
  procreative NEC Z31.69
    fertility preservation (prior to cancer therapy) (prior
      to removal of gonads) Z31.62
    using natural family planning Z31.61
  promiscuity Z70.1
  rape victim Z69.81
  religious Z71.81
  sex, sexual (related to) Z70.9
    attitude(s) Z70.0
    behavior or orientation Z70.1
    combined concerns Z70.3
    non-responsiveness Z70.1
    on behalf of third party Z70.2
    specified reason NEC Z70.8
  specified reason NEC Z71.89
  spiritual Z71.81
  spousal abuse (perpetrator) Z69.12
    victim Z69.11
  substance abuse Z71.89
    alcohol Z71.41
    drug Z71.51
    tobacco Z71.6
  tobacco use Z71.6

Counseling — *continued*
  use (of)
    insulin pump Z46.81
  victim (of)
    abuse Z69.81
    child abuse
      by parent Z69.010
      non-parental Z69.020
    rape NEC Z69.81
Coupled rhythm R00.8
Couvelaire syndrome or uterus (complicating delivery)
  O45.8X- ☑
Cowperitis — *see* Urethritis
Cowper's gland — *see* condition
Cowpox B08.010
  due to vaccination T88.1 ☑
Coxa
  magna M91.4- ☑
  plana M91.2- ☑
  valga (acquired) (*see also* Deformity, limb, specified
    type NEC, thigh)
    congenital Q65.81
    sequelae (late effect) of rickets E64.3
  vara (acquired) (*see also* Deformity, limb, specified
    type NEC, thigh)
    congenital Q65.82
    sequelae (late effect) of rickets E64.3
Coxalgia, coxalgic (nontuberculous) (*see also* Pain, joint,
  hip)
  tuberculous A18.02
Coxitis — *see* Monoarthritis, hip
Coxsackie (virus) (infection) B34.1
  as cause of disease classified elsewhere B97.11
  carditis B33.20
  central nervous system NEC A88.8
  endocarditis B33.21
  enteritis A08.39
  meningitis (aseptic) A87.0
  myocarditis B33.22
  pericarditis B33.23
  pharyngitis B08.5
  pleurodynia B33.0
  specific disease NEC B33.8
Crabs, meaning pubic lice B85.3
Crack baby P04.41
Cracked nipple N64.0
  associated with
    lactation O92.13
    pregnancy O92.11- ☑
    puerperium O92.12
Cracked tooth K03.81
Cradle cap L21.0
Craft neurosis F48.8
Cramp(s) R25.2
  abdominal — *see* Pain, abdominal
  bathing T75.1 ☑
  colic R10.83
    psychogenic F45.8
  due to immersion T75.1 ☑
  fireman T67.2 ☑
  heat T67.2 ☑
  immersion T75.1 ☑
  intestinal — *see* Pain, abdominal
    psychogenic F45.8
  leg, sleep related G47.62
  limb (lower) (upper) NEC R25.2
    sleep related G47.62
  linotypist's F48.8
    organic G25.89
  muscle (limb) (general) R25.2
    due to immersion T75.1 ☑
    psychogenic F45.8
  occupational (hand) F48.8
    organic G25.89
  salt-depletion E87.1
  sleep related, leg G47.62
  stoker's T67.2 ☑
  swimmer's T75.1 ☑
  telegrapher's F48.8
    organic G25.89
  typist's F48.8
    organic G25.89
  uterus N94.89
    menstrual — *see* Dysmenorrhea
  writer's F48.8
    organic G25.89
Cranial — *see* condition

76

☑ Additional Character Required — Refer to the Tabular List for Character Selection   ⬮ Subterms under main terms may continue to next column or page

Craniocleidodysostosis Q74.0
Craniofenestria (skull) Q75.8
Craniolacunia (skull) Q75.8
Craniopagus Q89.4
Craniopathy, metabolic M85.2
Craniopharyngeal — see condition
Craniopharyngioma D44.4
Craniorachischisis (totalis) Q00.1
Cranioschisis Q75.8
Craniostenosis Q75.0
Craniosynostosis Q75.0
Craniotabes (cause unknown) M83.8
  neonatal P96.3
  rachitic E64.3
  syphilitic A50.56
Cranium — see condition
Craw-craw — see Onchocerciasis
Creaking joint — see Derangement, joint, specified type
  NEC
Creeping
  eruption B76.9
  palsy or paralysis G12.22
Crenated tongue K14.8
Creotoxism A05.9
Crepitus
  caput Q75.8
  joint — see Derangement, joint, specified type NEC
Crescent or conus choroid, congenital Q14.3
CREST syndrome M34.1
Cretin, cretinism (congenital) (endemic) (nongoitrous)
  (sporadic) E00.9
  pelvis
    with disproportion (fetopelvic) O33.0
      causing obstructed labor O65.0
  type
    hypothyroid E00.1
    mixed E00.2
    myxedematous E00.1
    neurological E00.0
Creutzfeldt-Jakob disease or syndrome (with dementia) A81.00
  familial A81.09
  iatrogenic A81.09
  specified NEC A81.09
  sporadic A81.09
  variant (vCJD) A81.01
Crib death R99
Cribriform hymen Q52.3
Cri-du-chat syndrome Q93.4
Crigler-Najjar disease or syndrome E80.5
Crime, victim of Z65.4
Crimean hemorrhagic fever A98.0
Criminalism F60.2
Crisis
  abdomen R10.0
  acute reaction F43.0
  addisonian E27.2
  adrenal (cortical) E27.2
  celiac K90.0
  Dietl's N13.8
  emotional (see also Disorder, adjustment)
    acute reaction to stress F43.0
    specific to childhood and adolescence F93.8
  glaucomatocyclitic — see Glaucoma, secondary, inflammation
  heart — see Failure, heart
  nitritoid I95.2
    correct substance properly administered — see Table of Drugs and Chemicals, by drug, adverse effect
    overdose or wrong substance given or taken — see Table of Drugs and Chemicals, by drug, poisoning
  oculogyric H51.8
    psychogenic F45.8
  Pel's (tabetic) A52.11
  psychosexual identity F64.2
  renal N28.0
  sickle-cell D57.00
    with
      acute chest syndrome D57.01
      splenic sequestration D57.02
  state (acute reaction) F43.0
  tabetic A52.11
  thyroid — see Thyrotoxicosis with thyroid storm
  thyrotoxic — see Thyrotoxicosis with thyroid storm
Crocq's disease (acrocyanosis) I73.89

Crohn's disease — see Enteritis, regional
Crooked septum, nasal J34.2
Cross syndrome E70.328
Crossbite (anterior) (posterior) M26.24
Cross-eye — see Strabismus, convergent concomitant
Croup, croupous (catarrhal) (infectious) (inflammatory) (nondiphtheritic) J05.0
  bronchial J20.9
  diphtheritic A36.2
  false J38.5
  spasmodic J38.5
    diphtheritic A36.2
  stridulous J38.5
    diphtheritic A36.2
Crouzon's disease Q75.1
Crowding, tooth, teeth, fully erupted M26.31
CRST syndrome M34.1
Cruchet's disease A85.8
Cruelty in children (see also Disorder, conduct)
Crural ulcer — see Ulcer, lower limb
Crush, crushed, crushing T14.8 ☑
  abdomen S38.1 ☑
  ankle S97.0- ☑
  arm (upper) (and shoulder) S47.- ☑
  axilla — see Crush, arm
  back, lower S38.1 ☑
  buttock S38.1 ☑
  cheek S07.0 ☑
  chest S28.0 ☑
  cranium S07.1 ☑
  ear S07.0 ☑
  elbow S57.0- ☑
  extremity
    lower
      ankle — see Crush, ankle
      below knee — see Crush, leg
      foot — see Crush, foot
      hip — see Crush, hip
      knee — see Crush, knee
      thigh — see Crush, thigh
      toe — see Crush, toe
    upper
      below elbow S67.9- ☑
      elbow — see Crush, elbow
      finger — see Crush, finger
      forearm — see Crush, forearm
      hand — see Crush, hand
      thumb — see Crush, thumb
      upper arm — see Crush, arm
      wrist — see Crush, wrist
  face S07.0 ☑
  finger(s) S67.1- ☑
    with hand (and wrist) — see Crush, hand, specified site NEC
    index S67.19- ☑
    little S67.19- ☑
    middle S67.19- ☑
    ring S67.19- ☑
    thumb — see Crush, thumb
  foot S97.8- ☑
    toe — see Crush, toe
  forearm S57.8- ☑
  genitalia, external
    female S38.002 ☑
      vagina S38.03 ☑
      vulva S38.03 ☑
    male S38.001 ☑
      penis S38.01 ☑
      scrotum S38.02 ☑
      testis S38.02 ☑
  hand (except fingers alone) S67.2- ☑
    with wrist S67.4- ☑
  head S07.9 ☑
    specified NEC S07.8 ☑
  heel — see Crush, foot
  hip S77.0- ☑
    with thigh S77.2- ☑
  internal organ (abdomen, chest, or pelvis) NEC T14.8 ☑
  knee S87.0- ☑
  labium (majus) (minus) S38.03 ☑
  larynx S17.0 ☑
  leg (lower) S87.8- ☑
    knee — see Crush, knee
  lip S07.0 ☑

Crush, crushed, crushing — continued
  lower
    back S38.1 ☑
    leg — see Crush, leg
  neck S17.9 ☑
  nerve — see Injury, nerve
  nose S07.0 ☑
  pelvis S38.1 ☑
  penis S38.01 ☑
  scalp S07.8 ☑
  scapular region — see Crush, arm
  scrotum S38.02 ☑
  severe, unspecified site T14.8 ☑
  shoulder (and upper arm) — see Crush, arm
  skull S07.1 ☑
  syndrome (complication of trauma) T79.5 ☑
  testis S38.02 ☑
  thigh S77.1- ☑
    with hip S77.2- ☑
  throat S17.8 ☑
  thumb S67.0- ☑
    with hand (and wrist) — see Crush, hand, specified site NEC
  toe(s) S97.10- ☑
    great S97.11- ☑
    lesser S97.12- ☑
  trachea S17.0 ☑
  vagina S38.03 ☑
  vulva S38.03 ☑
  wrist S67.3- ☑
    with hand S67.4- ☑
Crusta lactea L21.0
Crusts R23.4
Crutch paralysis — see Injury, brachial plexus
Cruveilhier-Baumgarten cirrhosis, disease or syndrome K74.69
Cruveilhier's atrophy or disease G12.8
Crying (constant) (continuous) (excessive)
  child, adolescent, or adult R45.83
  infant (baby) (newborn) R68.11
Cryofibrinogenemia D89.2
Cryoglobulinemia (essential) (idiopathic) (mixed) (primary) (purpura) (secondary) (vasculitis) D89.1
  with lung involvement D89.1 [J99]
Cryptitis (anal) (rectal) K62.89
Cryptococcosis, cryptococcus (infection) (neoformans) B45.9
  bone B45.3
  cerebral B45.1
  cutaneous B45.2
  disseminated B45.7
  generalized B45.7
  meningitis B45.1
  meningocerebralis B45.1
  osseous B45.3
  pulmonary B45.0
  skin B45.2
  specified NEC B45.8
Cryptopapillitis (anus) K62.89
Cryptophthalmos Q11.2
  syndrome Q87.0
Cryptorchid, cryptorchism, cryptorchidism Q53.9
  bilateral Q53.20
    abdominal Q53.211
    perineal Q53.22
  unilateral Q53.10
    abdominal Q53.111
    perineal Q53.12
Cryptosporidiosis A07.2
  hepatobiliary B88.8
  respiratory B88.8
Cryptostromosis J67.6
Crystalluria R82.99
Cubitus
  congenital Q68.8
  valgus (acquired) M21.0- ☑
    congenital Q68.8
    sequelae (late effect) of rickets E64.3
  varus (acquired) M21.1- ☑
    congenital Q68.8
    sequelae (late effect) of rickets E64.3
Cultural deprivation or shock Z60.3
Curling esophagus K22.4
Curling's ulcer — see Ulcer, peptic, acute
Curschmann (-Batten) (-Steinert) **disease or syndrome** G71.11
Curse, Ondine's — see Apnea, sleep

Curvature

Curvature
- organ or site, congenital NEC — *see* Distortion
- penis (lateral) Q55.61
- Pott's (spinal) A18.01
- radius, idiopathic, progressive (congenital) Q74.0
- spine (acquired) (angular) (idiopathic) (incorrect) (postural) — *see* Dorsopathy, deforming
  - congenital Q67.5
  - due to or associated with
    - Charcot-Marie-Tooth disease (*see also* subcategory M49.8) G60.0
    - osteitis
      - deformans M88.88
      - fibrosa cystica (*see also* subcategory M49.8) E21.0
    - tuberculosis (Pott's curvature) A18.01
  - sequelae (late effect) of rickets E64.3
  - tuberculous A18.01

Cushingoid due to steroid therapy E24.2
- correct substance properly administered — *see* Table of Drugs and Chemicals, by drug, adverse effect
- overdose or wrong substance given or taken — *see* Table of Drugs and Chemicals, by drug, poisoning

Cushing's
- syndrome or disease E24.9
  - drug-induced E24.2
  - iatrogenic E24.2
  - pituitary-dependent E24.0
  - specified NEC E24.8
- ulcer — *see* Ulcer, peptic, acute

Cusp, Carabelli — *omit code*

Cut (external) (*see also* Laceration)
- muscle — *see* Injury, muscle

Cutaneous (*see also* condition)
- hemorrhage R23.3
- larva migrans B76.9

Cutis (*see also* condition)
- hyperelastica Q82.8
  - acquired L57.4
- laxa (hyperelastica) — *see* Dermatolysis
- marmorata R23.8
- osteosis L94.2
- pendula — *see* Dermatolysis
- rhomboidalis nuchae L57.2
- verticis gyrata Q82.8
  - acquired L91.8

Cyanosis R23.0
- due to
  - patent foramen botalli Q21.1
  - persistent foramen ovale Q21.1
- enterogenous D74.8
- paroxysmal digital — *see* Raynaud's disease
  - with gangrene I73.01
- retina, retinal H35.89

Cyanotic heart disease I24.9
- congenital Q24.9

Cycle
- anovulatory N97.0
- menstrual, irregular N92.6

Cyclencephaly Q04.9

Cyclical vomiting (*see also* Vomiting, cyclical) G43.A0 (*following* G43.7)
- psychogenic F50.89

Cyclitis (*see also* Iridocyclitis) H20.9
- chronic — *see* Iridocyclitis, chronic
- Fuchs' heterochromic H20.81- ☑
- granulomatous — *see* Iridocyclitis, chronic
- lens-induced — *see* Iridocyclitis, lens-induced
- posterior H30.2- ☑

Cycloid personality F34.0

Cyclophoria H50.54

Cyclopia, cyclops Q87.0

Cyclopism Q87.0

Cyclosporiasis A07.4

Cyclothymia F34.0

Cyclothymic personality F34.0

Cyclotropia H50.41- ☑

Cylindroma (*see also* Neoplasm, malignant, by site)
- eccrine dermal — *see* Neoplasm, skin, benign
- skin — *see* Neoplasm, skin, benign

Cylindruria R82.99

Cynanche
- diphtheritic A36.2
- tonsillaris J36

Cynophobia F40.218

Cynorexia R63.2

Cyphosis — *see* Kyphosis

Cyprus fever — *see* Brucellosis

Cyst (colloid) (mucous) (simple) (retention)
- adenoid (infected) J35.8
- adrenal gland E27.8
  - congenital Q89.1
- air, lung J98.4
- allantoic Q64.4
- alveolar process (jaw bone) M27.40
- amnion, amniotic O41.8X- ☑
- aneurysmal M27.49
- anterior
  - chamber (eye) — *see* Cyst, iris
  - nasopalatine K09.1
- antrum J34.1
- anus K62.89
- apical (tooth) (periodontal) K04.8
- appendix K38.8
- arachnoid, brain (acquired) G93.0
  - congenital Q04.6
- arytenoid J38.7
- Baker's M71.2- ☑
  - ruptured M66.0
  - tuberculous A18.02
- Bartholin's gland N75.0
- bile duct (common) (hepatic) K83.5
- bladder (multiple) (trigone) N32.89
- blue dome (breast) — *see* Cyst, breast
- bone (local) NEC M85.60
  - aneurysmal M85.50
    - ankle M85.57- ☑
    - foot M85.57- ☑
    - forearm M85.53- ☑
    - hand M85.54- ☑
    - jaw M27.49
    - lower leg M85.56- ☑
    - multiple site M85.59
    - neck M85.58
    - rib M85.58
    - shoulder M85.51- ☑
    - skull M85.58
    - specified site NEC M85.58
    - thigh M85.55- ☑
    - toe M85.57- ☑
    - upper arm M85.52- ☑
    - vertebra M85.58
  - solitary M85.40
    - ankle M85.47- ☑
    - fibula M85.46- ☑
    - foot M85.47- ☑
    - hand M85.44- ☑
    - humerus M85.42- ☑
    - jaw M27.49
    - neck M85.48
    - pelvis M85.45- ☑
    - radius M85.43- ☑
    - rib M85.48
    - shoulder M85.41- ☑
    - skull M85.48
    - specified site NEC M85.48
    - tibia M85.46- ☑
    - toe M85.47- ☑
    - ulna M85.43- ☑
    - vertebra M85.48
  - specified type NEC M85.60
    - ankle M85.67- ☑
    - foot M85.67- ☑
    - forearm M85.63- ☑
    - hand M85.64- ☑
    - jaw M27.40
      - developmental (nonodontogenic) K09.1
      - odontogenic K09.0
      - latent M27.0
    - lower leg M85.66- ☑
    - multiple site M85.69
    - neck M85.68
    - rib M85.68
    - shoulder M85.61- ☑
    - skull M85.68
    - specified site NEC M85.68
    - thigh M85.65- ☑
    - toe M85.67- ☑
    - upper arm M85.62- ☑
    - vertebra M85.68
- brain (acquired) G93.0
  - congenital Q04.6
  - hydatid B67.99 [G94]

Cyst — *continued*
- brain — *continued*
  - third ventricle (colloid), congenital Q04.6
- branchial (cleft) Q18.0
- branchiogenic Q18.0
- breast (benign) (blue dome) (pedunculated) (solitary) N60.0- ☑
  - involution — *see* Dysplasia, mammary, specified type NEC
  - sebaceous — *see* Dysplasia, mammary, specified type NEC
- broad ligament (benign) N83.8
- bronchogenic (mediastinal) (sequestration) J98.4
  - congenital Q33.0
- buccal K09.8
- bulbourethral gland N36.8
- bursa, bursal NEC M71.30
  - with rupture — *see* Rupture, synovium
  - ankle M71.37- ☑
  - elbow M71.32- ☑
  - foot M71.37- ☑
  - hand M71.34- ☑
  - hip M71.35- ☑
  - multiple sites M71.39
  - pharyngeal J39.2
  - popliteal space — *see* Cyst, Baker's
  - shoulder M71.31- ☑
  - specified site NEC M71.38
  - wrist M71.33- ☑
- calcifying odontogenic D16.5
  - upper jaw (bone) (maxilla) D16.4
- canal of Nuck (female) N94.89
  - congenital Q52.4
- canthus — *see* Cyst, conjunctiva
- carcinomatous — *see* Neoplasm, malignant, by site
- cauda equina G95.89
- cavum septi pellucidi — *see* Cyst, brain
- celomic (pericardium) Q24.8
- cerebellopontine (angle) — *see* Cyst, brain
- cerebellum — *see* Cyst, brain
- cerebral — *see* Cyst, brain
- cervical lateral Q18.0
- cervix NEC N88.8
  - embryonic Q51.6
  - nabothian N88.8
- chiasmal optic NEC — *see* Disorder, optic, chiasm
- chocolate (ovary) N80.1
- choledochus, congenital Q44.4
- chorion O41.8X- ☑
- choroid plexus G93.0
- ciliary body — *see* Cyst, iris
- clitoris N90.7
- colon K63.89
- common (bile) duct K83.5
- congenital NEC Q89.8
  - adrenal gland Q89.1
  - epiglottis Q31.8
  - esophagus Q39.8
  - fallopian tube Q50.4
  - kidney Q61.00
    - more than one (multiple) Q61.02
      - specified as polycystic Q61.3
        - adult type Q61.2
        - infantile type NEC Q61.19
          - collecting duct dilation Q61.11
    - solitary Q61.01
  - larynx Q31.8
  - liver Q44.6
  - lung Q33.0
  - mediastinum Q34.1
  - ovary Q50.1
  - oviduct Q50.4
  - periurethral (tissue) Q64.79
  - prepuce Q55.69
  - salivary gland (any) Q38.4
  - sublingual Q38.6
  - submaxillary gland Q38.6
  - thymus (gland) Q89.2
  - tongue Q38.3
  - ureterovesical orifice Q62.8
  - vulva Q52.79
- conjunctiva H11.44- ☑
- cornea H18.89- ☑
- corpora quadrigemina G93.0
- corpus
  - albicans N83.29- ☑
  - luteum (hemorrhagic) (ruptured) N83.1- ☑
- Cowper's gland (benign) (infected) N36.8

Cyst — *continued*
  cranial meninges G93.0
  craniobuccal pouch E23.6
  craniopharyngeal pouch E23.6
  cystic duct K82.8
  Cysticercus — *see* Cysticercosis
  Dandy-Walker Q03.1
    with spina bifida — *see* Spina bifida
  dental (root) K04.8
    developmental K09.0
    eruption K09.0
    primordial K09.0
  dentigerous (mandible) (maxilla) K09.0
  dermoid — *see* Neoplasm, benign, by site
    with malignant transformation C56.- ☑
    implantation
      external area or site (skin) NEC L72.0
      iris — *see* Cyst, iris, implantation
      vagina N89.8
      vulva N90.7
    mouth K09.8
    oral soft tissue K09.8
    sacrococcygeal — *see* Cyst, pilonidal
  developmental K09.1
    odontogenic K09.0
    oral region (nonodontogenic) K09.1
    ovary, ovarian Q50.1
  dura (cerebral) G93.0
    spinal G96.19
  ear (external) Q18.1
  echinococcal — *see* Echinococcus
  embryonic
    cervix uteri Q51.6
    fallopian tube Q50.4
    vagina Q52.4
  endometrium, endometrial (uterus) N85.8
    ectopic — *see* Endometriosis
  enterogenous Q43.8
  epidermal, epidermoid (inclusion) (*see also* Cyst, skin)
        L72.0
    mouth K09.8
    oral soft tissue K09.8
  epididymis N50.3
  epiglottis J38.7
  epiphysis cerebri E34.8
  epithelial (inclusion) L72.0
  epoophoron Q50.5
  eruption K09.0
  esophagus K22.8
  ethmoid sinus J34.1
  external female genital organs NEC N90.7
  eyelid (sebaceous) H02.829
    infected — *see* Hordeolum
    left H02.826
      lower H02.825
      upper H02.824
    right H02.823
      lower H02.822
      upper H02.821
  eye NEC H57.8
    congenital Q15.8
  fallopian tube N83.8
    congenital Q50.4
  fimbrial (twisted) Q50.4
  fissural (oral region) K09.1
  follicle (graafian) (hemorrhagic) N83.0- ☑
    nabothian N88.8
  follicular (atretic) (hemorrhagic) (ovarian) N83.0- ☑
    dentigerous K09.0
    odontogenic K09.0
    skin L72.9
      specified NEC L72.8
  frontal sinus J34.1
  gallbladder K82.8
  ganglion — *see* Ganglion
  Gartner's duct Q52.4
  gingiva K09.0
  gland of Moll — *see* Cyst, eyelid
  globulomaxillary K09.1
  graafian follicle (hemorrhagic) N83.0- ☑
  granulosal lutein (hemorrhagic) N83.1- ☑
  hemangiomatous D18.00
    intra-abdominal D18.03
    intracranial D18.02
    skin D18.01
    specified site NEC D18.09
  hemorrhagic M27.49
  hydatid (*see also* Echinococcus) B67.90

Cyst — *continued*
  hydatid (*see also* Echinococcus) — *continued*
    brain B67.99 [G94]
    liver (*see also* Cyst, liver, hydatid) B67.8
    lung NEC B67.99 [J99]
    Morgagni
      female Q50.5
      male (epididymal) Q55.4
        testicular Q55.29
    specified site NEC B67.99
  hymen N89.8
    embryonic Q52.4
  hypopharynx J39.2
  hypophysis, hypophyseal (duct) (recurrent) E23.6
    cerebri E23.6
  implantation (dermoid)
    external area or site (skin) NEC L72.0
    iris — *see* Cyst, iris, implantation
    vagina N89.8
    vulva N90.7
  incisive canal K09.1
  inclusion (epidermal) (epithelial) (epidermoid) (squamous) L72.0
    not of skin — *code under* Cyst, by site
  intestine (large) (small) K63.89
  intracranial — *see* Cyst, brain
  intraligamentous (*see also* Disorder, ligament)
    knee — *see* Derangement, knee
  intrasellar E23.6
  iris H21.309
    exudative H21.31- ☑
    idiopathic H21.30- ☑
    implantation H21.32- ☑
    parasitic H21.33- ☑
    pars plana (primary) H21.34- ☑
      exudative H21.35- ☑
  jaw (bone) M27.40
    aneurysmal M27.49
    developmental (odontogenic) K09.0
    fissural K09.1
    hemorrhagic M27.49
    traumatic M27.49
  joint NEC — *see* Disorder, joint, specified type NEC
  kidney (acquired) N28.1
    calyceal — *see* Hydronephrosis
    congenital Q61.00
    more than one (multiple) Q61.02
      specified as polycystic Q61.3
        adult type (autosomal dominant) Q61.2
        infantile type (autosomal recessive) NEC
          Q61.19
          collecting duct dilation Q61.11
    pyelogenic — *see* Hydronephrosis
    simple N28.1
    solitary (single) Q61.01
      acquired N28.1
  labium (majus) (minus) N90.7
    sebaceous N90.7
  lacrimal (*see also* Disorder, lacrimal system, specified
        NEC)
    gland H04.13- ☑
    passages or sac — *see* Disorder, lacrimal system,
        specified NEC
  larynx J38.7
  lateral periodontal K09.0
  lens H27.8
    congenital Q12.8
  lip (gland) K13.0
  liver (idiopathic) (simple) K76.89
    congenital Q44.6
    hydatid B67.8
      granulosus B67.0
      multilocularis B67.5
  lung J98.4
    congenital Q33.0
    giant bullous J43.9
  lutein N83.1- ☑
  lymphangiomatous D18.1
  lymphoepithelial, oral soft tissue K09.8
  macula — *see* Degeneration, macula, hole
  malignant — *see* Neoplasm, malignant, by site
  mammary gland — *see* Cyst, breast
  mandible M27.40
    dentigerous K09.0
    radicular K04.8
  maxilla M27.40
    dentigerous K09.0
    radicular K04.8

Cyst — *continued*
  medial, face and neck Q18.8
  median
    anterior maxillary K09.1
    palatal K09.1
  mediastinum, congenital Q34.1
  meibomian (gland) — *see* Chalazion
    infected — *see* Hordeolum
  membrane, brain G93.0
  meninges (cerebral) G93.0
    spinal G96.19
  meniscus, knee — *see* Derangement, knee, meniscus,
      cystic
  mesentery, mesenteric K66.8
    chyle I89.8
  mesonephric duct
    female Q50.5
    male Q55.4
  milk N64.89
  Morgagni (hydatid)
    female Q50.5
    male (epididymal) Q55.4
      testicular Q55.29
  mouth K09.8
  Müllerian duct Q50.4
    appendix testis Q55.29
    cervix Q51.6
    fallopian tube Q50.4
    female Q50.4
    male Q55.29
    prostatic utricle Q55.4
    vagina (embryonal) Q52.4
  multilocular (ovary) D39.10
    benign — *see* Neoplasm, benign, by site
  myometrium N85.8
  nabothian (follicle) (ruptured) N88.8
  nasoalveolar K09.1
  nasolabial K09.1
  nasopalatine (anterior) (duct) K09.1
  nasopharynx J39.2
  neoplastic — *see* Neoplasm, uncertain behavior, by
      site
    benign — *see* Neoplasm, benign, by site
  nervous system NEC G96.8
  neuroenteric (congenital) Q06.8
  nipple — *see* Cyst, breast
  nose (turbinates) J34.1
    sinus J34.1
  odontogenic, developmental K09.0
  omentum (lesser) K66.8
    congenital Q45.8
  ora serrata — *see* Cyst, retina, ora serrata
  oral
    region K09.9
      developmental (nonodontogenic) K09.1
        specified NEC K09.8
    soft tissue K09.9
      specified NEC K09.8
  orbit H05.81- ☑
  ovary, ovarian (twisted) N83.20- ☑
    adherent N83.20- ☑
    chocolate N80.1
    corpus
      albicans N83.29- ☑
      luteum (hemorrhagic) N83.1- ☑
    dermoid D27.9
    developmental Q50.1
    due to failure of involution NEC N83.20- ☑
    endometrial N80.1
    follicular (graafian) (hemorrhagic) N83.0- ☑
    hemorrhagic N83.20- ☑
    in pregnancy or childbirth O34.8- ☑
      with obstructed labor O65.5
    multilocular D39.10
    pseudomucinous D27.9
    retention N83.29- ☑
    serous N83.20- ☑
    specified NEC N83.29- ☑
    theca lutein (hemorrhagic) N83.1- ☑
    tuberculous A18.18
  oviduct N83.8
  palate (median) (fissural) K09.1
  palatine papilla (jaw) K09.1
  pancreas, pancreatic (hemorrhagic) (true) K86.2
    congenital Q45.2
    false K86.3
  paralabral
    hip M24.85- ☑

Index

Cyst — Cystadenoma

Cyst — *continued*
  paralabral — *continued*
    shoulder S43.43- ☑
  paramesonephric duct Q50.4
    female Q50.4
    male Q55.29
  paranephric N28.1
  paraphysis, cerebri, congenital Q04.6
  parasitic B89
  parathyroid (gland) E21.4
  paratubal N83.8
  paraurethral duct N36.8
  paroophoron Q50.5
  parotid gland K11.6
  parovarian Q50.5
  pelvis, female N94.89
    in pregnancy or childbirth O34.8- ☑
      causing obstructed labor O65.5
  penis (sebaceous) N48.89
  periapical K04.8
  pericardial (congenital) Q24.8
    acquired (secondary) I31.8
  pericoronal K09.0
  periodontal K04.8
    lateral K09.0
  peripelvic (lymphatic) N28.1
  peritoneum K66.8
    chylous I89.8
  periventricular, acquired, newborn P91.1
  pharynx (wall) J39.2
  pilar L72.11
  pilonidal (infected) (rectum) L05.91
    with abscess L05.01
    malignant C44.59- ☑
  pituitary (duct) (gland) E23.6
  placenta O43.19- ☑
  pleura J94.8
  popliteal — *see* Cyst, Baker's
  porencephalic Q04.6
    acquired G93.0
  postanal (infected) — *see* Cyst, pilonidal
  postmastoidectomy cavity (mucosal) — *see* Complications, postmastoidectomy, cyst
  preauricular Q18.1
  prepuce N47.4
    congenital Q55.69
  primordial (jaw) K09.0
  prostate N42.83
  pseudomucinous (ovary) D27.9
  pupillary, miotic H21.27- ☑
  radicular (residual) K04.8
  radiculodental K04.8
  ranular K11.8
  Rathke's pouch E23.6
  rectum (epithelium) (mucous) K62.89
  renal — *see* Cyst, kidney
  residual (radicular) K04.8
  retention (ovary) N83.29- ☑
    salivary gland K11.6
  retina H33.19- ☑
    ora serrata H33.11- ☑
    parasitic H33.12- ☑
  retroperitoneal K68.9
  sacrococcygeal (dermoid) — *see* Cyst, pilonidal
  salivary gland or duct (mucous extravasation or retention) K11.6
  Sampson's N80.1
  sclera H15.89
  scrotum L72.9
    sebaceous L72.3
  sebaceous (duct) (gland) L72.3
    breast — *see* Dysplasia, mammary, specified type NEC
    eyelid — *see* Cyst, eyelid
    genital organ NEC
      female N94.89
      male N50.89
    scrotum L72.3
  semilunar cartilage (knee) (multiple) — *see* Derangement, knee, meniscus, cystic
  seminal vesicle N50.89
  serous (ovary) N83.20- ☑
  sinus (accessory) (nasal) J34.1
  Skene's gland N36.8
  skin L72.9
    breast — *see* Dysplasia, mammary, specified type NEC
    epidermal, epidermoid L72.0

Cyst — *continued*
  skin — *continued*
    epithelial L72.0
    eyelid — *see* Cyst, eyelid
    genital organ NEC
      female N90.7
      male N50.89
    inclusion L72.0
    scrotum L72.9
    sebaceous L72.3
    sweat gland or duct L74.8
  solitary
    bone — *see* Cyst, bone, solitary
    jaw M27.40
    kidney N28.1
  spermatic cord N50.89
  sphenoid sinus J34.1
  spinal meninges G96.19
  spleen NEC D73.4
    congenital Q89.09
    hydatid (*see also* Echinococcus) B67.99 [D77]
  Stafne's M27.0
  subarachnoid intrasellar R93.0
  subcutaneous, pheomycotic (chromomycotic) B43.2
  subdural (cerebral) G93.0
    spinal cord G96.19
  sublingual gland K11.6
  submandibular gland K11.6
  submaxillary gland K11.6
  suburethral N36.8
  suprarenal gland E27.8
  suprasellar — *see* Cyst, brain
  sweat gland or duct L74.8
  synovial (*see also* Cyst, bursa)
    ruptured — *see* Rupture, synovium
  tarsal — *see* Chalazion
  tendon (sheath) — *see* Disorder, tendon, specified type NEC
  testis N44.2
    tunica albuginea N44.1
  theca lutein (ovary) N83.1- ☑
  Thornwaldt's J39.2
  thymus (gland) E32.8
  thyroglossal duct (infected) (persistent) Q89.2
  thyroid (gland) E04.1
  thyrolingual duct (infected) (persistent) Q89.2
  tongue K14.8
  tonsil J35.8
  tooth — *see* Cyst, dental
  Tornwaldt's J39.2
  trichilemmal (proliferating) L72.12
  trichodermal L72.12
  tubal (fallopian) N83.8
    inflammatory — *see* Salpingitis, chronic
  tubo-ovarian N83.8
    inflammatory N70.13
  tunica
    albuginea testis N44.1
    vaginalis N50.89
  turbinate (nose) J34.1
  Tyson's gland N48.89
  urachus, congenital Q64.4
  ureter N28.89
  ureterovesical orifice N28.89
  urethra, urethral (gland) N36.8
  uterine ligament N83.8
  uterus (body) (corpus) (recurrent) N85.8
    embryonic Q51.818
      cervix Q51.6
  vagina, vaginal (implantation) (inclusion) (squamous cell) (wall) N89.8
    embryonic Q52.4
  vallecula, vallecular (epiglottis) J38.7
  vesical (orifice) N32.89
  vitreous body H43.89
  vulva (implantation) (inclusion) N90.7
    congenital Q52.79
    sebaceous gland N90.7
  vulvovaginal gland N90.7
  wolffian
    female Q50.5
    male Q55.4

Cystadenocarcinoma — *see* Neoplasm, malignant, by site
  bile duct C22.1
  endometrioid — *see* Neoplasm, malignant, by site
    specified site — *see* Neoplasm, malignant, by site

Cystadenocarcinoma — *continued*
  endometrioid — *see* Neoplasm, malignant, by site — *continued*
    unspecified site
      female C56.9
      male C61
  mucinous
    papillary
      specified site — *see* Neoplasm, malignant, by site
      unspecified site C56.9
    specified site — *see* Neoplasm, malignant, by site
    unspecified site C56.9
  papillary
    mucinous
      specified site — *see* Neoplasm, malignant, by site
      unspecified site C56.9
    pseudomucinous
      specified site — *see* Neoplasm, malignant, by site
      unspecified site C56.9
    serous
      specified site — *see* Neoplasm, malignant, by site
      unspecified site C56.9
    specified site — *see* Neoplasm, malignant, by site
    unspecified site C56.9
  pseudomucinous
    papillary
      specified site — *see* Neoplasm, malignant, by site
      unspecified site C56.9
    specified site — *see* Neoplasm, malignant, by site
    unspecified site C56.9
  serous
    papillary
      specified site — *see* Neoplasm, malignant, by site
      unspecified site C56.9
    specified site — *see* Neoplasm, malignant, by site
    unspecified site C56.9

Cystadenofibroma
  clear cell — *see* Neoplasm, benign, by site
  endometrioid D27.9
    borderline malignancy D39.1- ☑
    malignant C56.- ☑
  mucinous
    specified site — *see* Neoplasm, benign, by site
    unspecified site D27.9
  serous
    specified site — *see* Neoplasm, benign, by site
    unspecified site D27.9
  specified site — *see* Neoplasm, benign, by site
  unspecified site D27.9

Cystadenoma (*see also* Neoplasm, benign, by site)
  bile duct D13.4
  endometrioid — *see* Neoplasm, benign, by site
    borderline malignancy — *see* Neoplasm, uncertain behavior, by site
  malignant — *see* Neoplasm, malignant, by site
  mucinous
    borderline malignancy
      ovary C56.- ☑
      specified site NEC — *see* Neoplasm, uncertain behavior, by site
      unspecified site C56.9
    papillary
      borderline malignancy
        ovary C56.- ☑
        specified site NEC — *see* Neoplasm, uncertain behavior, by site
        unspecified site C56.9
      specified site — *see* Neoplasm, benign, by site
      unspecified site D27.9
    specified site — *see* Neoplasm, benign, by site
    unspecified site D27.9
  papillary
    borderline malignancy
      ovary C56.- ☑
      specified site NEC — *see* Neoplasm, uncertain behavior, by site
      unspecified site C56.9
    lymphomatosum
      specified site — *see* Neoplasm, benign, by site
      unspecified site D11.9

☑ **Additional Character Required** — Refer to the Tabular List for Character Selection   ⏎ Subterms under main terms may continue to next column or page

Cystadenoma — *continued*
  papillary — *continued*
    mucinous
      borderline malignancy
        ovary C56.- ☑
        specified site NEC — *see* Neoplasm, uncertain behavior, by site
        unspecified site C56.9
      specified site — *see* Neoplasm, benign, by site
      unspecified site D27.9
    pseudomucinous
      borderline malignancy
        ovary C56.- ☑
        specified site NEC — *see* Neoplasm, uncertain behavior, by site
        unspecified site C56.9
      specified site — *see* Neoplasm, benign, by site
      unspecified site D27.9
    serous
      borderline malignancy
        ovary C56.- ☑
        specified site NEC — *see* Neoplasm, uncertain behavior, by site
        unspecified site C56.9
      specified site — *see* Neoplasm, benign, by site
      unspecified site D27.9
  pseudomucinous
    borderline malignancy
      ovary C56.- ☑
      specified site NEC — *see* Neoplasm, uncertain behavior, by site
      unspecified site C56.9
    papillary
      borderline malignancy
        ovary C56.- ☑
        specified site NEC — *see* Neoplasm, uncertain behavior, by site
        unspecified site C56.9
      specified site — *see* Neoplasm, benign, by site
      unspecified site D27.9
    specified site — *see* Neoplasm, benign, by site
    unspecified site D27.9
  serous
    borderline malignancy
      ovary C56.- ☑
      specified site NEC — *see* Neoplasm, uncertain behavior, by site
      unspecified site C56.9
    papillary
      borderline malignancy
        ovary C56.- ☑
        specified site NEC — *see* Neoplasm, uncertain behavior, by site
        unspecified site C56.9
      specified site — *see* Neoplasm, benign, by site
      unspecified site D27.9
    specified site — *see* Neoplasm, benign, by site
    unspecified site D27.9

Cystathionine synthase deficiency E72.11
Cystathioninemia E72.19
Cystathioninuria E72.19
Cystic (*see also* condition)
  breast (chronic) — *see* Mastopathy, cystic
  corpora lutea (hemorrhagic) N83.1- ☑
  duct — *see* condition
  eyeball (congenital) Q11.0
  fibrosis — *see* Fibrosis, cystic
  kidney (congenital) Q61.9

Cystic — *continued*
  kidney — *continued*
    adult type Q61.2
    infantile type NEC Q61.19
      collecting duct dilatation Q61.11
    medullary Q61.5
  liver, congenital Q44.6
  lung disease J98.4
    congenital Q33.0
  mastitis, chronic — *see* Mastopathy, cystic
  medullary, kidney Q61.5
  meniscus — *see* Derangement, knee, meniscus, cystic
  ovary N83.20- ☑
Cysticercosis, cysticerciasis B69.9
  with
    epileptiform fits B69.0
    myositis B69.81
  brain B69.0
  central nervous system B69.0
  cerebral B69.0
  ocular B69.1
  specified NEC B69.89
Cysticercus cellulose infestation — *see* Cysticercosis
Cystinosis (malignant) E72.04
Cystinuria E72.01
Cystitis (exudative) (hemorrhagic) (septic) (suppurative) N30.90
  with
    fibrosis — *see* Cystitis, chronic, interstitial
    hematuria N30.91
    leukoplakia — *see* Cystitis, chronic, interstitial
    malakoplakia — *see* Cystitis, chronic, interstitial
    metaplasia — *see* Cystitis, chronic, interstitial
    prostatitis N41.3
  acute N30.00
    with hematuria N30.01
    of trigone N30.30
      with hematuria N30.31
  allergic — *see* Cystitis, specified type NEC
  amebic A06.81
  bilharzial B65.9 [N33]
  blennorrhagic (gonococcal) A54.01
  bullous — *see* Cystitis, specified type NEC
  calculous N21.0
  chlamydial A56.01
  chronic N30.20
    with hematuria N30.21
    interstitial N30.10
      with hematuria N30.11
    of trigone N30.30
      with hematuria N30.31
    specified NEC N30.20
      with hematuria N30.21
  cystic (a) — *see* Cystitis, specified type NEC
  diphtheritic A36.85
  echinococcal
    granulosus B67.39
    multilocularis B67.69
  emphysematous — *see* Cystitis, specified type NEC
  encysted — *see* Cystitis, specified type NEC
  eosinophilic — *see* Cystitis, specified type NEC
  follicular — *see* Cystitis, of trigone
  gangrenous — *see* Cystitis, specified type NEC
  glandularis — *see* Cystitis, specified type NEC
  gonococcal A54.01
  incrusted — *see* Cystitis, specified type NEC
  interstitial (chronic) — *see* Cystitis, chronic, interstitial
  irradiation N30.40
    with hematuria N30.41
  irritation — *see* Cystitis, specified type NEC

Cystitis — *continued*
  malignant — *see* Cystitis, specified type NEC
  of trigone N30.30
    with hematuria N30.31
  panmural — *see* Cystitis, chronic, interstitial
  polyposa — *see* Cystitis, specified type NEC
  prostatic N41.3
  puerperal (postpartum) O86.22
  radiation — *see* Cystitis, irradiation
  specified type NEC N30.80
    with hematuria N30.81
  subacute — *see* Cystitis, chronic
  submucous — *see* Cystitis, chronic, interstitial
  syphilitic (late) A52.76
  trichomonal A59.03
  tuberculous A18.12
  ulcerative — *see* Cystitis, chronic, interstitial
Cystocele (-urethrocele)
  female N81.10
    with prolapse of uterus — *see* Prolapse, uterus
    lateral N81.12
    midline N81.11
    paravaginal N81.12
  in pregnancy or childbirth O34.8- ☑
    causing obstructed labor O65.5
  male N32.89
Cystolithiasis N21.0
Cystoma (*see also* Neoplasm, benign, by site)
  endometrial, ovary N80.1
  mucinous
    specified site — *see* Neoplasm, benign, by site
    unspecified site D27.9
  serous
    specified site — *see* Neoplasm, benign, by site
    unspecified site D27.9
  simple (ovary) N83.29- ☑
Cystoplegia N31.2
Cystoptosis N32.89
Cystopyelitis — *see* Pyelonephritis
Cystorrhagia N32.89
Cystosarcoma phyllodes D48.6- ☑
  benign D24- ☑
  malignant — *see* Neoplasm, breast, malignant
Cystostomy
  attention to Z43.5
  complication — *see* Complications, cystostomy
  status Z93.50
    appendico-vesicostomy Z93.52
    cutaneous Z93.51
    specified NEC Z93.59
Cystourethritis — *see* Urethritis
Cystourethrocele (*see also* Cystocele)
  female N81.10
    with uterine prolapse — *see* Prolapse, uterus
    lateral N81.12
    midline N81.11
    paravaginal N81.12
  male N32.89
Cytomegalic inclusion disease
  congenital P35.1
Cytomegalovirus infection B25.9
Cytomycosis (reticuloendothelial) B39.4
Cytopenia D75.9
  refractory
    with multilineage dysplasia D46.A (*following* D46.2)
      and ring sideroblasts (RCMD RS) D46.B (*following* D46.2)
Czerny's disease (periodic hydrarthrosis of the knee) — *see* Effusion, joint, knee

⛛ Subterms under main terms may continue to next column or page   ☑ Additional Character Required — Refer to the Tabular List for Character Selection   81

Cystadenoma — Czerny's disease

D

Da Costa's syndrome F45.8
Daae (-Finsen) **disease** (epidemic pleurodynia) B33.Ø
Dabney's grip B33.Ø
Dacryoadenitis, dacryadenitis HØ4.ØØ- ☑
   acute HØ4.Ø1- ☑
   chronic HØ4.Ø2- ☑
Dacryocystitis HØ4.3Ø- ☑
   acute HØ4.32- ☑
   chronic HØ4.41- ☑
   neonatal P39.1
   phlegmonous HØ4.31- ☑
   syphilitic A52.71
      congenital (early) A5Ø.Ø1
   trachomatous, active A71.1
      sequelae (late effect) B94.Ø
Dacryocystoblenorrhea — see Inflammation, lacrimal,
   passages, chronic
Dacryocystocele — see Disorder, lacrimal system,
   changes
Dacryolith, dacryolithiasis HØ4.51- ☑
Dacryoma — see Disorder, lacrimal system, changes
Dacryopericystitis — see Dacryocystitis
Dacryops HØ4.11- ☑
Dacryostenosis (see also Stenosis, lacrimal)
   congenital Q1Ø.5
Dactylitis
   bone — see Osteomyelitis
   sickle-cell D57.ØØ
      Hb C D57.219
      Hb SS D57.ØØ
      specified NEC D57.819
   skin LØ8.9
   syphilitic A52.77
   tuberculous A18.Ø3
Dactylolysis spontanea (ainhum) L94.6
Dactylosymphysis Q7Ø.9
   fingers — see Syndactylism, complex, fingers
   toes — see Syndactylism, complex, toes
Damage
   arteriosclerotic — see Arteriosclerosis
   brain (nontraumatic) G93.9
      anoxic, hypoxic G93.1
         resulting from a procedure G97.82
      child NEC G8Ø.9
      due to birth injury P11.2
   cardiorenal (vascular) — see Hypertension, cardiorenal
   cerebral NEC — see Damage, brain
   coccyx, complicating delivery O71.6
   coronary — see Disease, heart, ischemic
   eye, birth injury P15.3
   liver (nontraumatic) K76.9
      alcoholic K7Ø.9
      due to drugs — see Disease, liver, toxic
      toxic — see Disease, liver, toxic
   medication T88.7 ☑
   pelvic
      joint or ligament, during delivery O71.6
      organ NEC
         during delivery O71.5
         following ectopic or molar pregnancy OØ8.6
   renal — see Disease, renal
   subendocardium, subendocardial — see Degeneration,
      myocardial
   vascular I99.9
Dana-Putnam syndrome (subacute combined sclerosis
   with pernicious anemia) — see Degeneration,
   combined
Danbolt (-Cross) **syndrome** (acrodermatitis enteropathica) E83.2
Dandruff L21.Ø
Dandy-Walker syndrome QØ3.1
   with spina bifida — see Spina bifida
Danlos' syndrome Q79.6
Darier (-White) **disease** (congenital) Q82.8
   meaning erythema annulare centrifugum L53.1
Darier-Roussy sarcoid D86.3
Darling's disease or histoplasmosis B39.4
Darwin's tubercle Q17.8
Dawson's (inclusion body) **encephalitis** A81.1

De Beurmann (-Gougerot) **disease** B42.1
De la Tourette's syndrome F95.2
De Lange's syndrome Q87.1
De Morgan's spots (senile angiomas) I78.1
De Quervain's
   disease (tendon sheath) M65.4
   syndrome E34.51
   thyroiditis (subacute granulomatous thyroiditis) EØ6.1
De Toni-Fanconi (-Debré) **syndrome** E72.Ø9
   with cystinosis E72.Ø4
Dead
   fetus, retained (mother) O36.4 ☑
      early pregnancy OØ2.1
   labyrinth H83.2 ☑
   ovum, retained OØ2.Ø
Deaf nonspeaking NEC H91.3
Deafmutism (acquired) (congenital) NEC H91.3
   hysterical F44.6
   syphilitic, congenital (see also subcategory) H94.8
      A5Ø.Ø9
Deafness (acquired) (complete) (hereditary) (partial)
   H91.9- ☑
   with blue sclera and fragility of bone Q78.Ø
   auditory fatigue — see Deafness, specified type NEC
   aviation T7Ø.Ø ☑
      nerve injury — see Injury, nerve, acoustic, specified
         type NEC
   boilermaker's H83.3 ☑
   central — see Deafness, sensorineural
   conductive H9Ø.2
      and sensorineural
         mixed H9Ø.8
            bilateral H9Ø.6
         bilateral H9Ø.Ø
         unilateral H9Ø.1- ☑
            with restricted hearing on the contralateral side
               H9Ø.A- ☑
   congenital H9Ø.5
      with blue sclera and fragility of bone Q78.Ø
   due to toxic agents — see Deafness, ototoxic
   emotional (hysterical) F44.6
   functional (hysterical) F44.6
   high frequency H91.9- ☑
   hysterical F44.6
   low frequency H91.9- ☑
   mental R48.8
   mixed conductive and sensorineural H9Ø.8
      bilateral H9Ø.6
      unilateral H9Ø.7- ☑
   nerve — see Deafness, sensorineural
   neural — see Deafness, sensorineural
   noise-induced (see also subcategory) H83.3 ☑
      nerve injury — see Injury, nerve, acoustic, specified
         type NEC
   nonspeaking H91.3
   ototoxic H91.Ø ☑
   perceptive — see Deafness, sensorineural
   psychogenic (hysterical) F44.6
   sensorineural H9Ø.5
      and conductive
         bilateral H9Ø.6
         mixed H9Ø.8
            bilateral H9Ø.6
      bilateral H9Ø.3
      unilateral H9Ø.4- ☑
         with restricted hearing on the contralateral side
            H9Ø.A- ☑
   sensory — see Deafness, sensorineural
   specified type NEC H91.8 ☑
   sudden (idiopathic) H91.2- ☑
   syphilitic A52.15
   transient ischemic H93.Ø1- ☑
   traumatic — see Injury, nerve, acoustic, specified type
      NEC
   word (developmental) H93.25
Death (cause unknown) (of) (unexplained) (unspecified
   cause) R99
   brain G93.82
   cardiac (sudden) (with successful resuscitation) —
      code to underlying disease
      family history of Z82.41
      personal history of Z86.74

Death — continued
   family member (assumed) Z63.4
Debility (chronic) (general) (nervous) R53.81
   congenital or neonatal NOS P96.9
   nervous R53.81
   old age R54
   senile R54
Débove's disease (splenomegaly) R16.1
Decalcification
   bone — see Osteoporosis
   teeth KØ3.89
Decapsulation, kidney N28.89
Decay
   dental — see Caries, dental
   senile R54
   tooth, teeth — see Caries, dental
Deciduitis (acute)
   following ectopic or molar pregnancy OØ8.Ø
Decline (general) — see Debility
   cognitive, age-associated R41.81
Decompensation
   cardiac (acute) (chronic) — see Disease, heart
   cardiovascular — see Disease, cardiovascular
   heart — see Disease, heart
   hepatic — see Failure, hepatic
   myocardial (acute) (chronic) — see Disease, heart
   respiratory J98.8
Decompression sickness T7Ø.3 ☑
Decrease (d)
   absolute neutrophile count — see Neutropenia
   blood
      platelets — see Thrombocytopenia
      pressure RØ3.1
         due to shock following
            injury T79.4 ☑
            operation T81.19 ☑
   estrogen E28.39
      postablative E89.4Ø
         asymptomatic E89.4Ø
         symptomatic E89.41
   fragility of erythrocytes D58.8
   function
      lipase (pancreatic) K9Ø.3
      ovary in hypopituitarism E23.Ø
      parenchyma of pancreas K86.89
      pituitary (gland) (anterior) (lobe) E23.Ø
         posterior (lobe) E23.Ø
   functional activity R68.89
   glucose R73.Ø9
   hematocrit R71.Ø
   hemoglobin R71.Ø
   leukocytes D72.819
      specified NEC D72.818
   libido R68.82
   lymphocytes D72.81Ø
   platelets D69.6
   respiration, due to shock following injury T79.4 ☑
   sexual desire R68.82
   tear secretion NEC — see Syndrome, dry eye
   tolerance
      fat K9Ø.49
      glucose R73.Ø9
      pancreatic K9Ø.3
      salt and water E87.8
   vision NEC H54.7
   white blood cell count D72.819
      specified NEC D72.818
Decubitus (ulcer) — see Ulcer, pressure, by site
   cervix N86
Deepening acetabulum — see Derangement, joint,
   specified type NEC, hip
Defect, defective Q89.9
   3-beta-hydroxysteroid dehydrogenase E25.Ø
   11-hydroxylase E25.Ø
   21-hydroxylase E25.Ø
   abdominal wall, congenital Q79.59
   antibody immunodeficiency D8Ø.9
   aorticopulmonary septum Q21.4
   atrial septal (ostium secundum type) Q21.1
      following acute myocardial infarction (current
         complication) I23.1
      ostium primum type Q21.2

☑ Additional Character Required — Refer to the Tabular List for Character Selection

🔻 Subterms under main terms may continue to next column or page

Da Costa's syndrome — Defect, defective

Defect, defective — *continued*
- atrioventricular
  - canal Q21.2
  - septum Q21.2
- auricular septal Q21.1
- bilirubin excretion NEC E80.6
- biosynthesis, androgen (testicular) E29.1
- bulbar septum Q21.0
- catalase E80.3
- cell membrane receptor complex (CR3) D71
- circulation I99.9
  - congenital Q28.9
  - newborn Q28.9
- coagulation (factor) (*see also* Deficiency, factor) D68.9
  - with
    - ectopic pregnancy O08.1
    - molar pregnancy O08.1
  - acquired D68.4
  - antepartum with hemorrhage — *see* Hemorrhage, antepartum, with coagulation defect
  - due to
    - liver disease D68.4
    - vitamin K deficiency D68.4
  - hereditary NEC D68.2
  - intrapartum O67.0
  - newborn, transient P61.6
  - postpartum O99.13
    - with hemorrhage O72.3
  - specified type NEC D68.8
- complement system D84.1
- conduction (heart) I45.9
  - bone — *see* Deafness, conductive
- congenital, organ or site not listed — *see* Anomaly, by site
- coronary sinus Q21.1
- cushion, endocardial Q21.2
- degradation, glycoprotein E77.1
- dental bridge, crown, fillings — *see* Defect, dental restoration
- dental restoration K08.50
  - specified NEC K08.59
- dentin (hereditary) K00.5
- Descemet's membrane, congenital Q13.89
- developmental (*see also* Anomaly)
  - cauda equina Q06.3
- diaphragm
  - with elevation, eventration or hernia — *see* Hernia, diaphragm
  - congenital Q79.1
    - with hernia Q79.0
    - gross (with hernia) Q79.0
- ectodermal, congenital Q82.9
- Eisenmenger's Q21.8
- enzyme
  - catalase E80.3
  - peroxidase E80.3
- esophagus, congenital Q39.9
- extensor retinaculum M62.89
- fibrin polymerization D68.2
- filling
  - bladder R93.41
  - kidney R93.42- ☑
  - renal pelvis R93.41
  - stomach R93.3
  - ureter R93.41
  - urinary organs, specified NEC R93.49
- Gerbode Q21.0
- glycoprotein degradation E77.1
- Hageman (factor) D68.2
- hearing — *see* Deafness
- high grade F70
- interatrial septal Q21.1
- interauricular septal Q21.1
- interventricular septal Q21.0
  - with dextroposition of aorta, pulmonary stenosis and hypertrophy of right ventricle Q21.3
  - in tetralogy of Fallot Q21.3
- learning (specific) — *see* Disorder, learning
- lymphocyte function antigen-1 (LFA-1) D84.0
- lysosomal enzyme, post-translational modification E77.0
- major osseous M89.70
  - ankle M89.77- ☑
  - carpus M89.74- ☑
  - clavicle M89.71- ☑
  - femur M89.75- ☑
  - fibula M89.76- ☑
  - fingers M89.74- ☑

Defect, defective — *continued*
- major osseous — *continued*
  - foot M89.77- ☑
  - forearm M89.73- ☑
  - hand M89.74- ☑
  - humerus M89.72- ☑
  - lower leg M89.76- ☑
  - metacarpus M89.74- ☑
  - metatarsus M89.77- ☑
  - multiple sites M89.79
  - pelvic region M89.75- ☑
  - pelvis M89.75-
  - radius M89.73- ☑
  - scapula M89.71- ☑
  - shoulder region M89.71- ☑
  - specified NEC M89.78
  - tarsus M89.77- ☑
  - thigh M89.75- ☑
  - tibia M89.76- ☑
  - toes M89.77- ☑
  - ulna M89.73- ☑
- mental — *see* Disability, intellectual
- modification, lysosomal enzymes, post-translational E77.0
- obstructive, congenital
  - renal pelvis Q62.39
  - ureter Q62.39
    - atresia — *see* Atresia, ureter
    - cecoureterocele Q62.32
    - megaureter Q62.2
    - orthotopic ureterocele Q62.31
- osseous, major M89.70
  - ankle M89.77- ☑
  - carpus M89.74- ☑
  - clavicle M89.71- ☑
  - femur M89.75- ☑
  - fibula M89.76- ☑
  - fingers M89.74- ☑
  - foot M89.77- ☑
  - forearm M89.73- ☑
  - hand M89.74- ☑
  - humerus M89.72- ☑
  - lower leg M89.76- ☑
  - metacarpus M89.74- ☑
  - metatarsus M89.77- ☑
  - multiple sites M89.9
  - pelvic region M89.75- ☑
  - pelvis M89.75-
  - radius M89.73- ☑
  - scapula M89.71- ☑
  - shoulder region M89.71- ☑
  - specified NEC M89.78
  - tarsus M89.77- ☑
  - thigh M89.75- ☑
  - tibia M89.76- ☑
  - toes M89.77- ☑
  - ulna M89.73- ☑
- osteochondral NEC (*see also* Deformity) M95.8
- ostium
  - primum Q21.2
  - secundum Q21.1
- peroxidase E80.3
- placental blood supply — *see* Insufficiency, placental
- platelets, qualitative D69.1
  - constitutional D68.0
- postural NEC, spine — *see* Dorsopathy, deforming
- reduction
  - limb Q73.8
    - lower Q72.9- ☑
      - absence — *see* Agenesis, leg
        - foot — *see* Agenesis, foot
      - longitudinal
        - femur Q72.4- ☑
        - fibula Q72.6- ☑
        - tibia Q72.5- ☑
      - specified type NEC Q72.89- ☑
      - split foot Q72.7- ☑
    - specified type NEC Q73.8
    - upper Q71.9- ☑
      - absence — *see* Agenesis, arm
        - forearm — *see* Agenesis, forearm
        - hand — *see* Agenesis, hand
      - lobster-claw hand Q71.6- ☑
      - longitudinal
        - radius Q71.4- ☑
        - ulna Q71.5- ☑

Defect, defective — *continued*
- reduction — *continued*
  - limb — *continued*
    - upper — *continued*
      - specified type NEC Q71.89- ☑
- renal pelvis Q63.8
  - obstructive Q62.39
- respiratory system, congenital Q34.9
- restoration, dental K08.50
  - specified NEC K08.59
- retinal nerve bundle fibers H35.89
- septal (heart) NOS Q21.9
  - acquired (atrial) (auricular) (ventricular) (old) I51.0
  - atrial Q21.1
    - concurrent with acute myocardial infarction — *see* Infarct, myocardium
    - following acute myocardial infarction (current complication) I23.1
  - ventricular (*see also* Defect, ventricular septal) Q21.0
- sinus venosus Q21.1
- speech R47.9
  - developmental F80.9
  - specified NEC R47.89
- Taussig-Bing (aortic transposition and overriding pulmonary artery) Q20.1
- teeth, wedge K03.1
- vascular (local) I99.9
  - congenital Q27.9
- ventricular septal Q21.0
  - concurrent with acute myocardial infarction — *see* Infarct, myocardium
  - following acute myocardial infarction (current complication) I23.2
  - in tetralogy of Fallot Q21.3
- vision NEC H54.7
- visual field H53.40
  - bilateral
    - heteronymous H53.47
    - homonymous H53.46- ☑
  - generalized contraction H53.48- ☑
  - localized
    - arcuate H53.43- ☑
    - scotoma (central area) H53.41- ☑
      - blind spot area H53.42- ☑
    - sector H53.43- ☑
  - specified type NEC H53.45- ☑
- voice R49.9
  - specified NEC R49.8
- wedge, tooth, teeth (abrasion) K03.1

Deferentitis N49.1
- gonorrheal (acute) (chronic) A54.23

Defibrination (syndrome) D65
- antepartum — *see* Hemorrhage, antepartum, with coagulation defect, disseminated intravascular coagulation
- following ectopic or molar pregnancy O08.1
- intrapartum O67.0
- newborn P60
- postpartum O72.3

Deficiency, deficient
- 3-beta hydroxysteroid dehydrogenase E25.0
- 5-alpha reductase (with male pseudo-hermaphroditism) E29.1
- 11-hydroxylase E25.0
- 21-hydroxylase E25.0
- abdominal muscle syndrome Q79.4
- AC globulin (congenital) (hereditary) D68.2
  - acquired D68.4
- accelerator globulin (Ac G) (blood) D68.2
- acid phosphatase E83.39
- activating factor (blood) D68.2
- adenosine deaminase (ADA) D81.3
- aldolase (hereditary) E74.19
- alpha-1-antitrypsin E88.01
- amino-acids E72.9
- anemia — *see* Anemia
- aneurin E51.9
- antibody with
  - hyperimmunoglobulinemia D80.6
  - near-normal immunoglobins D80.6
- antidiuretic hormone E23.2
- anti-hemophilic
  - factor (A) D66
    - B D67
    - C D68.1
  - globulin (AHG) NEC D66
- antithrombin (antithrombin III) D68.59

Deficiency, deficient — *continued*
ascorbic acid E54
attention (disorder) (syndrome) F98.8
    with hyperactivity — *see* Disorder, attention-deficit
        hyperactivity
autoprothrombin
    C D68.2
    I D68.2
    II D67
beta-glucuronidase E76.29
biotin E53.8
biotin-dependent carboxylase D81.819
biotinidase D81.810
brancher enzyme (amylopectinosis) E74.03
C1 esterase inhibitor (C1-INH) D84.1
calciferol E55.9
    with
        adult osteomalacia M83.8
        rickets — *see* Rickets
calcium (dietary) E58
calorie, severe E43
    with marasmus E41
        and kwashiorkor E42
cardiac — *see* Insufficiency, myocardial
carnitine E71.40
    due to
        hemodialysis E71.43
        inborn errors of metabolism E71.42
        Valproic acid therapy E71.43
    iatrogenic E71.43
    muscle palmityltransferase E71.314
    primary E71.41
    secondary E71.448
carotene E50.9
central nervous system G96.8
ceruloplasmin (Wilson) E83.01
choline E53.8
Christmas factor D67
chromium E61.4
clotting (blood) (*see also* Deficiency, coagulation factor) D68.9
clotting factor NEC (hereditary) (*see also* Deficiency, factor) D68.2
coagulation NOS D68.9
    with
        ectopic pregnancy O08.1
        molar pregnancy O08.1
    acquired (any) D68.4
    antepartum hemorrhage — *see* Hemorrhage, antepartum, with coagulation defect
    clotting factor NEC (*see also* Deficiency, factor) D68.2
    due to
        hyperprothrombinemia D68.4
        liver disease D68.4
        vitamin K deficiency D68.4
    newborn, transient P61.6
    postpartum O72.3
    specified NEC D68.8
cognitive F09
color vision H53.50
    achromatopsia H53.51
    acquired H53.52
    deuteranomaly H53.53
    protanomaly H53.54
    specified type NEC H53.59
    tritanomaly H53.55
combined glucocorticoid and mineralocorticoid E27.49
contact factor D68.2
copper (nutritional) E61.0
corticoadrenal E27.40
    primary E27.1
craniofacial axis Q75.0
cyanocobalamin E53.8
debrancher enzyme (limit dextrinosis) E74.03
dehydrogenase
    long chain/very long chain acyl CoA E71.310
    medium chain acyl CoA E71.311
    short chain acyl CoA E71.312
diet E63.9
dihydropyrimidine dehydrogenase (DPD) E88.89
disaccharidase E73.9
edema — *see* Malnutrition, severe
endocrine E34.9
energy-supply — *see* Malnutrition
enzymes, circulating NEC E88.09
ergosterol E55.9

Deficiency, deficient — *continued*
ergosterol — *continued*
    with
        adult osteomalacia M83.8
        rickets — *see* Rickets
essential fatty acid (EFA) E63.0
factor (*see also* Deficiency, coagulation)
    Hageman D68.2
    I (congenital) (hereditary) D68.2
    II (congenital) (hereditary) D68.2
    IX (congenital) (functional) (hereditary) (with functional defect) D67
    multiple (congenital) D68.8
        acquired D68.4
    V (congenital) (hereditary) D68.2
    VII (congenital) (hereditary) D68.2
    VIII (congenital) (functional) (hereditary) (with functional defect) D66
        with vascular defect D68.0
    X (congenital) (hereditary) D68.2
    XI (congenital) (hereditary) D68.1
    XII (congenital) (hereditary) D68.2
    XIII (congenital) (hereditary) D68.2
femoral, proximal focal (congenital) — *see* Defect, reduction, lower limb, longitudinal, femur
fibrinase D68.2
fibrinogen (congenital) (hereditary) D68.2
    acquired D65
fibrin-stabilizing factor (congenital) (hereditary) D68.2
    acquired D68.4
folate E53.8
folic acid E53.8
foreskin N47.3
fructokinase E74.11
fructose 1,6-diphosphatase E74.19
fructose-1-phosphate aldolase E74.19
galactokinase E74.29
galactose-1-phosphate uridyl transferase E74.29
gammaglobulin in blood D80.1
    hereditary D80.0
glass factor D68.2
glucocorticoid E27.49
    mineralocorticoid E27.49
glucose-6-phosphatase E74.01
glucose-6-phosphate dehydrogenase anemia D55.0
glucuronyl transferase E80.5
glycogen synthetase E74.09
gonadotropin (isolated) E23.0
growth hormone (idiopathic) (isolated) E23.0
Hageman factor D68.2
hemoglobin D64.9
hepatophosphorylase E74.09
homogentisate 1,2-dioxygenase E70.29
hormone
    anterior pituitary (partial) NEC E23.0
        growth E23.0
    growth (isolated) E23.0
    pituitary E23.0
    testicular E29.1
hypoxanthine- (guanine)-phosphoribosyltransferase (HG- PRT) (total H-PRT) E79.1
immunity D84.9
    cell-mediated D84.8
        with thrombocytopenia and eczema D82.0
    combined D81.9
    humoral D80.9
    IgA (secretory) D80.2
    IgG D80.3
    IgM D80.4
immuno — *see* Immunodeficiency
immunoglobulin, selective
    A (IgA) D80.2
    G (IgG) (subclasses) D80.3
    M (IgM) D80.4
inositol (B complex) E53.8
intrinsic
    factor (congenital) D51.0
    sphincter N36.42
        with urethral hypermobility N36.43
iodine E61.8
    congenital syndrome — *see* Syndrome, iodine-deficiency, congenital
iron E61.1
    anemia D50.9
kalium E87.6
kappa-light chain D80.8
labile factor (congenital) (hereditary) D68.2
    acquired D68.4

Deficiency, deficient — *continued*
lacrimal fluid (acquired) (*see also* Syndrome, dry eye)
    congenital Q10.6
lactase
    congenital E73.0
    secondary E73.1
Laki-Lorand factor D68.2
lecithin cholesterol acyltransferase E78.6
lipocaic K86.89
lipoprotein (familial) (high density) E78.6
liver phosphorylase E74.09
lysosomal alpha-1, 4 glucosidase E74.02
magnesium E61.2
major histocompatibility complex
    class I D81.6
    class II D81.7
manganese E61.3
menadione (vitamin K) E56.1
    newborn P53
mental (familial) (hereditary) — *see* Disability, intellectual
methylenetetrahydrofolate reductase (MTHFR) E72.12
mevalonate kinase M04.1
mineralocorticoid E27.49
    with glucocorticoid E27.49
mineral NEC E61.8
molybdenum (nutritional) E61.5
moral F60.2
multiple nutrient elements E61.7
muscle
    carnitine (palmityltransferase) E71.314
    phosphofructokinase E74.09
myoadenylate deaminase E79.2
myocardial — *see* Insufficiency, myocardial
myophosphorylase E74.04
NADH diaphorase or reductase (congenital) D74.0
NADH-methemoglobin reductase (congenital) D74.0
natrium E87.1
niacin (amide) (-tryptophan) E52
nicotinamide E52
nicotinic acid E52
number of teeth — *see* Anodontia
nutrient element E61.9
    multiple E61.7
    specified NEC E61.8
nutrition, nutritional E63.9
    sequelae — *see* Sequelae, nutritional deficiency
    specified NEC E63.8
of interleukin 1 receptor antagonist [DIRA] M04.8
ornithine transcarbamylase E72.4
ovarian E28.39
oxygen — *see* Anoxia
pantothenic acid E53.8
parathyroid (gland) E20.9
perineum (female) N81.89
phenylalanine hydroxylase E70.1
phosphoenolpyruvate carboxykinase E74.4
phosphofructokinase E74.19
phosphomannomutuse E74.8
phosphomannose isomerase E74.8
phosphomannosyl mutase E74.8
phosphorylase kinase, liver E74.09
pituitary hormone (isolated) E23.0
plasma thromboplastin
    antecedent (PTA) D68.1
    component (PTC) D67
platelet NEC D69.1
    constitutional D68.0
polyglandular E31.8
    autoimmune E31.0
potassium (K) E87.6
prepuce N47.3
proaccelerin (congenital) (hereditary) D68.2
    acquired D68.4
proconvertin factor (congenital) (hereditary) D68.2
    acquired D68.4
protein (*see also* Malnutrition) E46
    anemia D53.0
    C D68.59
    S D68.59
prothrombin (congenital) (hereditary) D68.2
    acquired D68.4
Prower factor D68.2
pseudocholinesterase E88.09
PTA (plasma thromboplastin antecedent) D68.1
PTC (plasma thromboplastin component) D67
purine nucleoside phosphorylase (PNP) D81.5

☑ **Additional Character Required — Refer to the Tabular List for Character Selection**

⚐ Subterms under main terms may continue to next column or page

Deficiency, deficient — Deficiency, deficient

Deficiency, deficient — *continued*
  pyracin (alpha) (beta) E53.1
  pyridoxal E53.1
  pyridoxamine E53.1
  pyridoxine (derivatives) E53.1
  pyruvate
    carboxylase E74.4
    dehydrogenase E74.4
  riboflavin (vitamin B2) E53.Ø
  salt E87.1
  secretion
    ovary E28.39
    salivary gland (any) K11.7
    urine R34
  selenium (dietary) E59
  serum antitrypsin, familial E88.Ø1
  short stature homeobox gene (SHOX)
    with
      dyschondrosteosis Q78.8
      short stature (idiopathic) E34.3
      Turner's syndrome Q96.9
  sodium (Na) E87.1
  SPCA (factor VII) D68.2
  sphincter, intrinsic N36.42
    with urethral hypermobility N36.43
  stable factor (congenital) (hereditary) D68.2
    acquired D68.4
  Stuart-Prower (factor X) D68.2
  sucrase E74.39
  sulfatase E75.29
  sulfite oxidase E72.19
  thiamin, thiaminic (chloride) E51.9
    beriberi (dry) E51.11
      wet E51.12
  thrombokinase D68.2
    newborn P53
  thyroid (gland) — *see* Hypothyroidism
  tocopherol E56.Ø
  tooth bud KØØ.Ø
  transcobalamine II (anemia) D51.2
  vanadium E61.6
  vascular I99.9
  vasopressin E23.2
  vertical ridge KØ6.8
  viosterol — *see* Deficiency, calciferol
  vitamin (multiple) NOS E56.9
    A E5Ø.9
      with
        Bitot's spot (corneal) E5Ø.1
        follicular keratosis E5Ø.8
        keratomalacia E5Ø.4
        manifestations NEC E5Ø.8
        night blindness E5Ø.5
        scar of cornea, xerophthalmic E5Ø.6
        xeroderma E5Ø.8
        xerophthalmia E5Ø.7
        xerosis
          conjunctival E5Ø.Ø
            and Bitot's spot E5Ø.1
          cornea E5Ø.2
            and ulceration E5Ø.3
      sequelae E64.1
    B (complex) NOS E53.9
      with
        beriberi (dry) E51.11
          wet E51.12
        pellagra E52
    B1 NOS E51.9
      beriberi (dry) E51.11
        with circulatory system manifestations E51.11
        wet E51.12
    B2 (riboflavin) E53.Ø
    B6 E53.1
    B12 E53.8
    C E54
      sequelae E64.2
    D E55.9
      with
        adult osteomalacia M83.8
        rickets — *see* Rickets
      25-hydroxylase E83.32
    E E56.Ø
    folic acid E53.8
    G E53.Ø
    group B E53.9
      specified NEC E53.8
    H (biotin) E53.8
    K E56.1

Deficiency, deficient — *continued*
  vitamin — *continued*
    K — *continued*
      of newborn P53
    nicotinic E52
    P E56.8
    PP (pellagra-preventing) E52
    specified NEC E56.8
    thiamin E51.9
      beriberi — *see* Beriberi
  zinc, dietary E6Ø
Deficit (*see also* Deficiency)
  attention and concentration R41.84Ø
    disorder — *see* Attention, deficit
    following
      cerebral infarction I69.31Ø
      cerebrovascular disease I69.91Ø
        specified disease NEC I69.81Ø
      nontraumatic
        intracerebral hemorrhage I69.11Ø
        specified intracranial hemorrhage NEC I69.21Ø
        subarachnoid hemorrhage I69.Ø1Ø
  cognitive
    communication R41.841
    emotional
      following
        cerebral infarction I69.315
        cerebrovascular disease I69.915
          specified disease NEC I69.815
        nontraumatic
          intracerebral hemorrhage I69.115
          specified intracranial hemorrhage NEC I69.215
          subarachnoid hemorrhage I69.Ø15
    following
      cerebral infarction I69.319
      cerebrovascular disease I69.919
        specified disease NEC I69.819
      nontraumatic
        intracerebral hemorrhage I69.119
        specified intracranial hemorrhage NEC I69.219
        subarachnoid hemorrhage I69.Ø19
    social
      following
        cerebral infarction I69.315
        cerebrovascular disease I69.915
          specified disease NEC I69.815
        nontraumatic
          intracerebral hemorrhage I69.115
          specified intracranial hemorrhage NEC I69.215
          subarachnoid hemorrhage I69.Ø15
  cognitive NEC R41.89
    following
      cerebral infarction I69.318
      cerebrovascular disease I69.918
        specified disease NEC I69.818
      nontraumatic
        intracerebral hemorrhage I69.118
        specified intracranial hemorrhage NEC I69.218
        subarachnoid hemorrhage I69.Ø18
  concentration R41.84Ø
  executive function R41.844
    following
      cerebral infarction I69.314
      cerebrovascular disease I69.914
        specified disease NEC I69.814
      nontraumatic
        intracerebral hemorrhage I69.114
        specified intracranial hemorrhage NEC I69.214
        subarachnoid hemorrhage I69.Ø14
  frontal lobe R41.844
    following
      cerebral infarction I69.314
      cerebrovascular disease I69.914
        specified disease NEC I69.814
      nontraumatic
        intracerebral hemorrhage I69.114
        specified intracranial hemorrhage NEC I69.214
        subarachnoid hemorrhage I69.Ø14
  memory
    following
      cerebral infarction I69.311
      cerebrovascular disease I69.911

Deficit — *continued*
  memory — *continued*
    following — *continued*
      cerebrovascular disease — *continued*
        specified disease NEC I69.811
      nontraumatic
        intracerebral hemorrhage I69.111
        specified intracranial hemorrhage NEC I69.211
        subarachnoid hemorrhage I69.Ø11
  neurologic NEC R29.818
    ischemic
      reversible (RIND) I63.9
        prolonged (PRIND) I63.9
  oxygen RØ9.Ø2
  prolonged reversible ischemic neurologic (PRIND) I63.9
  psychomotor R41.843
    following
      cerebral infarction I69.313
      cerebrovascular disease I69.913
        specified disease NEC I69.813
      nontraumatic
        intracerebral hemorrhage I69.113
        specified intracranial hemorrhage NEC I69.213
        subarachnoid hemorrhage I69.Ø13
  visuospatial R41.842
    following
      cerebral infarction I69.312
      cerebrovascular disease I69.912
        specified disease NEC I69.812
      nontraumatic
        intracerebral hemorrhage I69.112
        specified intracranial hemorrhage NEC I69.212
        subarachnoid hemorrhage I69.Ø12
Deflection
  radius — *see* Deformity, limb, specified type NEC, forearm
  septum (acquired) (nasal) (nose) J34.2
  spine — *see* Curvature, spine
  turbinate (nose) J34.2
Defluvium
  capillorum — *see* Alopecia
  cilicorum — *see* Madarosis
  unguium L6Ø.8
Deformity Q89.9
  abdomen, congenital Q89.9
  abdominal wall
    acquired M95.8
    congenital Q79.59
  acquired (unspecified site) M95.9
  adrenal gland Q89.1
  alimentary tract, congenital Q45.9
    upper Q4Ø.9
  ankle (joint) (acquired) (*see also* Deformity, limb, lower leg)
    abduction — *see* Contraction, joint, ankle
    congenital Q68.8
    contraction — *see* Contraction, joint, ankle
    specified type NEC — *see* Deformity, limb, foot, specified NEC
  anus (acquired) K62.89
    congenital Q43.9
  aorta (arch) (congenital) Q25.4Ø
    acquired I77.89
  aortic
    arch, acquired I77.89
    cusp or valve (congenital) Q23.8
      acquired (*see also* Endocarditis, aortic) I35.8
  arm (acquired) (upper) (*see also* Deformity, limb, upper arm)
    congenital Q68.8
    forearm — *see* Deformity, limb, forearm
  artery (congenital) (peripheral) NOS Q27.9
    acquired I77.89
    coronary (acquired) I25.9
      congenital Q24.5
    umbilical Q27.Ø
  atrial septal Q21.1
  auditory canal (external) (congenital) (*see also* Malformation, ear, external)
    acquired — *see* Disorder, ear, external, specified type NEC
  auricle
    ear (congenital) (*see also* Malformation, ear, external)
      acquired — *see* Disorder, pinna, deformity

Deformity — *continued*
  back — *see* Dorsopathy, deforming
  bile duct (common) (congenital) (hepatic) Q44.5
    acquired K83.8
  biliary duct or passage (congenital) Q44.5
    acquired K83.8
  bladder (neck) (trigone) (sphincter) (acquired) N32.89
    congenital Q64.79
  bone (acquired) NOS M95.9
    congenital Q79.9
    turbinate M95.0
  brain (congenital) Q04.9
    acquired G93.89
    reduction Q04.3
  breast (acquired) N64.89
    congenital Q83.9
    reconstructed N65.0
  bronchus (congenital) Q32.4
    acquired NEC J98.09
  bursa, congenital Q79.9
  canaliculi (lacrimalis) (acquired) (*see also* Disorder, lacrimal system, changes)
    congenital Q10.6
  canthus, acquired — *see* Disorder, eyelid, specified type NEC
  capillary (acquired) I78.8
  cardiovascular system, congenital Q28.9
  caruncle, lacrimal (acquired) (*see also* Disorder, lacrimal system, changes)
    congenital Q10.6
  cascade, stomach K31.2
  cecum (congenital) Q43.9
    acquired K63.89
  cerebral, acquired G93.89
    congenital Q04.9
  cervix (uterus) (acquired) NEC N88.8
    congenital Q51.9
  cheek (acquired) M95.2
    congenital Q18.9
  chest (acquired) (wall) M95.4
    congenital Q67.8
    sequelae (late effect) of rickets E64.3
  chin (acquired) M95.2
    congenital Q18.9
  choroid (congenital) Q14.3
    acquired H31.8
    plexus Q07.8
      acquired G96.19
  cicatricial — *see* Cicatrix
  cilia, acquired — *see* Disorder, eyelid, specified type NEC
  clavicle (acquired) M95.8
    congenital Q68.8
  clitoris (congenital) Q52.6
    acquired N90.89
  clubfoot — *see* Clubfoot
  coccyx (acquired) — *see* subcategory M43.8 ☑
  colon (congenital) Q43.9
    acquired K63.89
  concha (ear), congenital (*see also* Malformation, ear, external)
    acquired — *see* Disorder, pinna, deformity
  cornea (acquired) H18.70
    congenital Q13.4
    descemetocele — *see* Descemetocele
    ectasia — *see* Ectasia, cornea
    specified NEC H18.79- ☑
    staphyloma — *see* Staphyloma, cornea
  coronary artery (acquired) I25.9
    congenital Q24.5
  cranium (acquired) — *see* Deformity, skull
  cricoid cartilage (congenital) Q31.8
    acquired J38.7
  cystic duct (congenital) Q44.5
    acquired K82.8
  Dandy-Walker Q03.1
    with spina bifida — *see* Spina bifida
  diaphragm (congenital) Q79.1
    acquired J98.6
  digestive organ NOS Q45.9
  ductus arteriosus Q25.0
  duodenal bulb K31.89
  duodenum (congenital) Q43.9
    acquired K31.89
  dura — *see* Deformity, meninges
  ear (acquired) (*see also* Disorder, pinna, deformity)
    congenital (external) Q17.9
      internal Q16.5

Deformity — *continued*
  ear (*see also* Disorder, pinna, deformity) — *continued*
    congenital — *continued*
      middle Q16.4
        ossicles Q16.3
      ossicles Q16.3
  ectodermal (congenital) NEC Q84.9
  ejaculatory duct (congenital) Q55.4
    acquired N50.89
  elbow (joint) (acquired) (*see also* Deformity, limb, upper arm)
    congenital Q68.8
    contraction — *see* Contraction, joint, elbow
  endocrine gland NEC Q89.2
  epididymis (congenital) Q55.4
    acquired N50.89
  epiglottis (congenital) Q31.8
    acquired J38.7
  esophagus (congenital) Q39.9
    acquired K22.8
  eustachian tube (congenital) NEC Q17.8
  eye, congenital Q15.9
  eyebrow (congenital) Q18.8
  eyelid (acquired) (*see also* Disorder, eyelid, specified type NEC)
    congenital Q10.3
  face (acquired) M95.2
    congenital Q18.9
  fallopian tube, acquired N83.8
  femur (acquired) — *see* Deformity, limb, specified type NEC, thigh
  fetal
    with fetopelvic disproportion O33.7 ☑
    causing obstructed labor O66.3
  finger (acquired) M20.00- ☑
    boutonniere M20.02- ☑
    congenital Q68.1
    flexion contracture — *see* Contraction, joint, hand
    mallet finger M20.01- ☑
    specified NEC M20.09- ☑
    swan-neck M20.03- ☑
  flexion (joint) (acquired) (*see also* Deformity, limb, flexion) M21.20
    congenital NOS Q74.9
      hip Q65.89
  foot (acquired) (*see also* Deformity, limb, lower leg)
    cavovarus (congenital) Q66.1
    congenital NOS Q66.9
      specified type NEC Q66.89
    specified type NEC — *see* Deformity, limb, foot, specified NEC
    valgus (congenital) Q66.6
      acquired — *see* Deformity, valgus, ankle
    varus (congenital) Q66.3
      acquired — *see* Deformity, varus, ankle
  forearm (acquired) (*see also* Deformity, limb, forearm)
    congenital Q68.8
  forehead (acquired) M95.2
    congenital Q75.8
  frontal bone (acquired) M95.2
    congenital Q75.8
  gallbladder (congenital) Q44.1
    acquired K82.8
  gastrointestinal tract (congenital) NOS Q45.9
    acquired K63.89
  genitalia, genital organ(s) or system NEC
    female (congenital) Q52.9
      acquired N94.89
      external Q52.70
    male (congenital) Q55.9
      acquired N50.89
  globe (eye) (congenital) Q15.8
    acquired H44.89
  gum, acquired NEC K06.8
  hand (acquired) — *see* Deformity, limb, hand
    congenital Q68.1
  head (acquired) M95.2
    congenital Q75.8
  heart (congenital) Q24.9
    septum Q21.9
      auricular Q21.1
      ventricular Q21.0
    valve (congenital) NEC Q24.8
      acquired — *see* Endocarditis
  heel (acquired) — *see* Deformity, foot
  hepatic duct (congenital) Q44.5
    acquired K83.8

Deformity — *continued*
  hip (joint) (acquired) (*see also* Deformity, limb, thigh)
    congenital Q65.9
    due to (previous) juvenile osteochondrosis — *see* Coxa, plana
    flexion — *see* Contraction, joint, hip
  hourglass — *see* Contraction, hourglass
  humerus (acquired) M21.82- ☑
    congenital Q74.0
  hypophyseal (congenital) Q89.2
  ileocecal (coil) (valve) (acquired) K63.89
    congenital Q43.9
  ileum (congenital) Q43.9
    acquired K63.89
  ilium (acquired) M95.5
    congenital Q74.2
  integument (congenital) Q84.9
  intervertebral cartilage or disc (acquired) — *see* Disorder, disc, specified NEC
  intestine (large) (small) (congenital) NOS Q43.9
    acquired K63.89
  intrinsic minus or plus (hand) — *see* Deformity, limb, specified type NEC, forearm
  iris (acquired) H21.89
    congenital Q13.2
  ischium (acquired) M95.5
    congenital Q74.2
  jaw (acquired) (congenital) M26.9
  joint (acquired) NEC M21.90
    congenital Q68.8
    elbow M21.92- ☑
    hand M21.94- ☑
    hip M21.95- ☑
    knee M21.96- ☑
    shoulder M21.92- ☑
    wrist M21.93- ☑
  kidney(s) (calyx) (pelvis) (congenital) Q63.9
    acquired N28.89
    artery (congenital) Q27.2
      acquired I77.89
  Klippel-Feil (brevicollis) Q76.1
  knee (acquired) NEC (*see also* Deformity, limb, lower leg)
    congenital Q68.2
  labium (majus) (minus) (congenital) Q52.79
    acquired N90.89
  lacrimal passages or duct (congenital) NEC Q10.6
    acquired — *see* Disorder, lacrimal system, changes
  larynx (muscle) (congenital) Q31.8
    acquired J38.7
    web (glottic) Q31.0
  leg (upper) (acquired) NEC (*see also* Deformity, limb, thigh)
    congenital Q68.8
    lower — *see* Deformity, limb, lower leg
  lens (acquired) H27.8
    congenital Q12.9
  lid (fold) (acquired) (*see also* Disorder, eyelid, specified type NEC)
    congenital Q10.3
  ligament (acquired) — *see* Disorder, ligament
    congenital Q79.9
  limb (acquired) M21.90
    clawfoot M21.53- ☑
    clawhand M21.51- ☑
    clubfoot M21.54- ☑
    clubhand M21.52- ☑
    congenital, except reduction deformity Q74.9
    flat foot M21.4- ☑
    flexion M21.20
      ankle M21.27- ☑
      elbow M21.22- ☑
      finger M21.24- ☑
      hip M21.25- ☑
      knee M21.26- ☑
      shoulder M21.21- ☑
      toe M21.27- ☑
      wrist M21.23- ☑
    foot
      claw — *see* Deformity, limb, clawfoot
      club — *see* Deformity, limb, clubfoot
      drop M21.37- ☑
      flat — *see* Deformity, limb, flat foot
      specified NEC M21.6X- ☑
    forearm M21.93- ☑
    hand M21.94- ☑
    lower leg M21.96- ☑

☑ **Additional Character Required — Refer to the Tabular List for Character Selection**   ▽ **Subterms under main terms may continue to next column or page**

Deformity — continued
  limb — continued
    specified type NEC M21.80
      forearm M21.83- ☑
      lower leg M21.86- ☑
      thigh M21.85- ☑
      upper arm M21.82- ☑
    thigh M21.95- ☑
    unequal length M21.70
      short site is
        femur M21.75- ☑
        fibula M21.76- ☑
        humerus M21.72- ☑
        radius M21.73- ☑
        tibia M21.76- ☑
        ulna M21.73- ☑
      upper arm M21.92- ☑
    valgus — see Deformity, valgus
    varus — see Deformity, varus
    wrist drop M21.33- ☑
  lip (acquired) NEC K13.0
    congenital Q38.0
  liver (congenital) Q44.7
    acquired K76.89
  lumbosacral (congenital) (joint) (region) Q76.49
    acquired — see subcategory M43.8 ☑
    kyphosis — see Kyphosis, congenital
    lordosis — see Lordosis, congenital
  lung (congenital) Q33.9
    acquired J98.4
  lymphatic system, congenital Q89.9
  Madelung's (radius) Q74.0
  mandible (acquired) (congenital) M26.9
  maxilla (acquired) (congenital) M26.9
  meninges or membrane (congenital) Q07.9
    cerebral Q04.8
      acquired G96.19
    spinal cord (congenital) G96.19
      acquired G96.19
  metacarpus (acquired) — see Deformity, limb, forearm
    congenital Q74.0
  metatarsus (acquired) — see Deformity, foot
    congenital Q66.9
  middle ear (congenital) Q16.4
    ossicles Q16.3
  mitral (leaflets) (valve) I05.8
    parachute Q23.2
    stenosis, congenital Q23.2
  mouth (acquired) K13.79
    congenital Q38.6
  multiple, congenital NEC Q89.7
  muscle (acquired) M62.89
    congenital Q79.9
      sternocleidomastoid Q68.0
  musculoskeletal system (acquired) M95.9
    congenital Q79.9
    specified NEC M95.8
  nail (acquired) L60.8
    congenital Q84.6
  nasal — see Deformity, nose
  neck (acquired) M95.3
    congenital Q18.9
      sternocleidomastoid Q68.0
  nervous system (congenital) Q07.9
  nipple (congenital) Q83.9
    acquired N64.89
  nose (acquired) (cartilage) M95.0
    bone (turbinate) M95.0
    congenital Q30.9
      bent or squashed Q67.4
    saddle M95.0
      syphilitic A50.57
    septum (acquired) J34.2
      congenital Q30.8
    sinus (wall) (congenital) Q30.8
      acquired M95.0
    syphilitic (congenital) A50.57
      late A52.73
  ocular muscle (congenital) Q10.3
    acquired — see Strabismus, mechanical
  opticociliary vessels (congenital) Q13.2
  orbit (eye) (acquired) H05.30
    atrophy — see Atrophy, orbit
    congenital Q10.7
    due to
      bone disease NEC H05.32- ☑
      trauma or surgery H05.33- ☑
    enlargement — see Enlargement, orbit

Deformity — continued
  orbit — continued
    exostosis — see Exostosis, orbit
  organ of Corti (congenital) Q16.5
  ovary (congenital) Q50.39
    acquired N83.8
  oviduct, acquired N83.8
  palate (congenital) Q38.5
    acquired M27.8
    cleft (congenital) — see Cleft, palate
  pancreas (congenital) Q45.3
    acquired K86.89
  parathyroid (gland) Q89.2
  parotid (gland) (congenital) Q38.4
    acquired K11.8
  patella (acquired) — see Disorder, patella, specified
    NEC
  pelvis, pelvic (acquired) (bony) M95.5
    with disproportion (fetopelvic) O33.0
      causing obstructed labor O65.0
    congenital Q74.2
    rachitic sequelae (late effect) E64.3
  penis (glans) (congenital) Q55.69
    acquired N48.89
  pericardium (congenital) Q24.8
    acquired — see Pericarditis
  pharynx (congenital) Q38.8
    acquired J39.2
  pinna, acquired (see also Disorder, pinna, deformity)
    congenital Q17.9
  pituitary (congenital) Q89.2
  posture — see Dorsopathy, deforming
  prepuce (congenital) Q55.69
    acquired N47.8
  prostate (congenital) Q55.4
    acquired N42.89
  pupil (congenital) Q13.2
    acquired — see Abnormality, pupillary
  pylorus (congenital) Q40.3
    acquired K31.89
  rachitic (acquired), old or healed E64.3
  radius (acquired) (see also Deformity, limb, forearm)
    congenital Q68.8
  rectum (congenital) Q43.9
    acquired K62.89
  reduction (extremity) (limb), congenital (see also con-
    dition and site) Q73.8
    brain Q04.3
    lower — see Defect, reduction, lower limb
    upper — see Defect, reduction, upper limb
  renal — see Deformity, kidney
  respiratory system (congenital) Q34.9
  rib (acquired) M95.4
    congenital Q76.6
      cervical Q76.5
  rotation (joint) (acquired) — see Deformity, limb,
    specified site NEC
    congenital Q74.9
    hip — see Deformity, limb, specified type NEC,
      thigh
      congenital Q65.89
  sacroiliac joint (congenital) — see subcategory Q74.2
    acquired — see subcategory M43.8 ☑
  sacrum (acquired) — see subcategory M43.8 ☑
  saddle
    back — see Lordosis
    nose M95.0
      syphilitic A50.57
  salivary gland or duct (congenital) Q38.4
    acquired K11.8
  scapula (acquired) M95.8
    congenital Q68.8
  scrotum (congenital) (see also Malformation, testis
    and scrotum)
    acquired N50.89
  seminal vesicles (congenital) Q55.4
    acquired N50.89
  septum, nasal (acquired) J34.2
  shoulder (joint) (acquired) — see Deformity, limb,
    upper arm
    congenital Q74.0
    contraction — see Contraction, joint, shoulder
  sigmoid (flexure) (congenital) Q43.9
    acquired K63.89
  skin (congenital) Q82.9
  skull (acquired) M95.2
    congenital Q75.8

Deformity — continued
  skull — continued
    congenital — continued
      with
        anencephaly Q00.0
        encephalocele — see Encephalocele
        hydrocephalus Q03.9
          with spina bifida — see Spina bifida, by
            site, with hydrocephalus
        microcephaly Q02
  soft parts, organs or tissues (of pelvis)
    in pregnancy or childbirth NEC O34.8- ☑
      causing obstructed labor O65.5
  spermatic cord (congenital) Q55.4
    acquired N50.89
    torsion — see Torsion, spermatic cord
  spinal — see Dorsopathy, deforming
    column (acquired) — see Dorsopathy, deforming
    congenital Q67.5
    cord (congenital) Q06.9
      acquired G95.89
    nerve root (congenital) Q07.9
  spine (acquired) (see also Dorsopathy, deforming)
    congenital Q67.5
    rachitic E64.3
    specified NEC — see Dorsopathy, deforming,
      specified NEC
  spleen
    acquired D73.89
    congenital Q89.09
  Sprengel's (congenital) Q74.0
  sternocleidomastoid (muscle), congenital Q68.0
  sternum (acquired) M95.4
    congenital NEC Q76.7
  stomach (congenital) Q40.3
    acquired K31.89
  submandibular gland (congenital) Q38.4
  submaxillary gland (congenital) Q38.4
    acquired K11.8
  talipes — see Talipes
  testis (congenital) (see also Malformation, testis and
    scrotum)
    acquired N44.8
    torsion — see Torsion, testis
  thigh (acquired) (see also Deformity, limb, thigh)
    congenital NEC Q68.8
  thorax (acquired) (wall) M95.4
    congenital Q67.8
    sequelae of rickets E64.3
  thumb (acquired) (see also Deformity, finger)
    congenital NEC Q68.1
  thymus (tissue) (congenital) Q89.2
  thyroid (gland) (congenital) Q89.2
    cartilage Q31.8
    acquired J38.7
  tibia (acquired) (see also Deformity, limb, specified
    type NEC, lower leg)
    congenital NEC Q68.8
    saber (syphilitic) A50.56
  toe (acquired) M20.6- ☑
    congenital Q66.9
    hallux rigidus M20.2- ☑
    hallux valgus M20.1- ☑
    hallux varus M20.3- ☑
    hammer toe M20.4- ☑
    specified NEC M20.5X- ☑
  tongue (congenital) Q38.3
    acquired K14.8
  tooth, teeth K00.2
  trachea (rings) (congenital) Q32.1
    acquired J39.8
  transverse aortic arch (congenital) Q25.49
  tricuspid (leaflets) (valve) I07.8
    atresia or stenosis Q22.4
    Ebstein's Q22.5
  trunk (acquired) M95.8
    congenital Q89.9
  ulna (acquired) (see also Deformity, limb, forearm)
    congenital NEC Q68.8
  urachus, congenital Q64.4
  ureter (opening) (congenital) Q62.8
    acquired N28.89
  urethra (congenital) Q64.79
    acquired N36.8
  urinary tract (congenital) Q64.9
    urachus Q64.4
  uterus (congenital) Q51.9
    acquired N85.8

▽ Subterms under main terms may continue to next column or page   ☑ Additional Character Required — Refer to the Tabular List for Character Selection   87

Deformity — Deformity

Deformity — continued
uvula (congenital) Q38.5
vagina (acquired) N89.8
congenital Q52.4
valgus NEC M21.00
ankle M21.07- ☑
elbow M21.02- ☑
hip M21.05- ☑
knee M21.06- ☑
valve, valvular (congenital) (heart) Q24.8
acquired — see Endocarditis
varus NEC M21.10
ankle M21.17- ☑
elbow M21.12- ☑
hip M21.15 ☑
knee M21.16- ☑
tibia — see Osteochondrosis, juvenile, tibia
vas deferens (congenital) Q55.4
acquired N50.89
vein (congenital) Q27.9
great Q26.9
vertebra — see Dorsopathy, deforming
vertical talus (congenital) Q66.80
left foot Q66.82
right foot Q66.81
vesicourethral orifice (acquired) N32.89
congenital NEC Q64.79
vessels of optic papilla (congenital) Q14.2
visual field (contraction) — see Defect, visual field
vitreous body, acquired H43.89
vulva (congenital) Q52.79
acquired N90.89
wrist (joint) (acquired) (see also Deformity, limb, forearm)
congenital Q68.8
contraction — see Contraction, joint, wrist

Degeneration, degenerative
adrenal (capsule) (fatty) (gland) (hyaline) (infectional) E27.8
amyloid (see also Amyloidosis) E85.9
anterior cornua, spinal cord G12.29
anterior labral S43.49- ☑
aorta, aortic I70.0
fatty I77.89
aortic valve (heart) — see Endocarditis, aortic
arteriovascular — see Arteriosclerosis
artery, arterial (atheromatous) (calcareous) (see also Arteriosclerosis)
cerebral, amyloid E85.4 [I68.0]
medial — see Arteriosclerosis, extremities
articular cartilage NEC — see Derangement, joint, articular cartilage, by site
atheromatous — see Arteriosclerosis
basal nuclei or ganglia G23.9
specified NEC G23.8
bone NEC — see Disorder, bone, specified type NEC
brachial plexus G54.0
brain (cortical) (progressive) G31.9
alcoholic G31.2
arteriosclerotic I67.2
childhood G31.9
specified NEC G31.89
cystic G31.89
congenital Q04.6
in
alcoholism G31.2
beriberi E51.2
cerebrovascular disease I67.9
congenital hydrocephalus Q03.9
with spina bifida (see also Spina bifida)
Fabry-Anderson disease E75.21
Gaucher's disease E75.22
Hunter's syndrome E76.1
lipidosis
cerebral E75.4
generalized E75.6
mucopolysaccharidosis — see Mucopolysaccharidosis
myxedema E03.9 [G32.89]
neoplastic disease (see also Neoplasm) D49.6 [G32.89]
Niemann-Pick disease E75.249 [G32.89]
sphingolipidosis E75.3 [G32.89]
vitamin B12 deficiency E53.8 [G32.89]
senile NEC G31.1
breast N64.89
Bruch's membrane — see Degeneration, choroid
capillaries (fatty) I78.8

Degeneration, degenerative — continued
capillaries — continued
amyloid E85.89 [I79.8]
cardiac (see also Degeneration, myocardial)
valve, valvular — see Endocarditis
cardiorenal — see Hypertension, cardiorenal
cardiovascular (see also Disease, cardiovascular)
renal — see Hypertension, cardiorenal
cerebellar NOS G31.9
alcoholic G31.2
primary (hereditary) (sporadic) G11.9
cerebral — see Degeneration, brain
cerebrovascular I67.9
due to hypertension I67.4
cervical plexus G54.2
cervix N88.8
due to radiation (intended effect) N88.8
adverse effect or misadventure N99.89
chamber angle H21.21- ☑
changes, spine or vertebra — see Spondylosis
chorioretinal (see also Degeneration, choroid)
hereditary H31.20
choroid (colloid) (drusen) H31.10- ☑
atrophy — see Atrophy, choroidal
hereditary — see Dystrophy, choroidal, hereditary
ciliary body H21.22- ☑
cochlear — see subcategory H83.8 ☑
combined (spinal cord) (subacute) E53.8 [G32.0]
with anemia (pernicious) D51.0 [G32.0]
due to dietary vitamin B12 deficiency D51.3 [G32.0]
in (due to)
vitamin B12 deficiency E53.8 [G32.0]
anemia D51.9 [G32.0]
conjunctiva H11.10
concretions — see Concretion, conjunctiva
deposits — see Deposit, conjunctiva
pigmentations — see Pigmentation, conjunctiva
pinguecula — see Pinguecula
xerosis — see Xerosis, conjunctiva
cornea H18.40
calcerous H18.43
band keratopathy H18.42- ☑
familial, hereditary — see Dystrophy, cornea
hyaline (of old scars) H18.49
keratomalacia — see Keratomalacia
nodular H18.45- ☑
peripheral H18.46- ☑
senile H18.41- ☑
specified type NEC H18.49
cortical (cerebellar) (parenchymatous) G31.89
alcoholic G31.2
diffuse, due to arteriopathy I67.2
corticobasal G31.85
cutis L98.8
amyloid E85.4 [L99]
dental pulp K04.2
disc disease — see Degeneration, intervertebral disc NEC
dorsolateral (spinal cord) — see Degeneration, combined
extrapyramidal G25.9
eye, macular (see also Degeneration, macula)
congenital or hereditary — see Dystrophy, retina
facet joints — see Spondylosis
fatty
liver NEC K76.0
alcoholic K70.0
grey matter (brain) (Alpers') G31.81
heart (see also Degeneration, myocardial)
amyloid E85.4 [I43]
atheromatous — see Disease, heart, ischemic, atherosclerotic
ischemic — see Disease, heart, ischemic
hepatolenticular (Wilson's) E83.01
hepatorenal K76.7
hyaline (diffuse) (generalized)
localized — see Degeneration, by site
infrapatellar fat pad M79.4
intervertebral disc NOS
with
myelopathy — see Disorder, disc, with, myelopathy
radiculitis or radiculopathy — see Disorder, disc, with, radiculopathy
cervical, cervicothoracic — see Disorder, disc, cervical, degeneration

Degeneration, degenerative — continued
intervertebral disc — continued
cervical, cervicothoracic — see Disorder, disc, cervical, degeneration — continued
with
myelopathy — see Disorder, disc, cervical, with myelopathy
neuritis, radiculitis or radiculopathy — see Disorder, disc, cervical, with neuritis
lumbar region M51.36
with
myelopathy M51.06
neuritis, radiculitis, radiculopathy or sciatica M51.16
lumbosacral region M51.37
with
neuritis, radiculitis, radiculopathy or sciatica M51.17
sacrococcygeal region M53.3
thoracic region M51.34
with
myelopathy M51.04
neuritis, radiculitis, radiculopathy M51.14
thoracolumbar region M51.35
with
myelopathy M51.05
neuritis, radiculitis, radiculopathy M51.15
intestine, amyloid E85.4
iris (pigmentary) H21.23- ☑
ischemic — see Ischemia
joint disease — see Osteoarthritis
kidney N28.89
amyloid E85.4 [N29]
cystic, congenital Q61.9
fatty N28.89
polycystic Q61.3
adult type (autosomal dominant) Q61.2
infantile type (autosomal recessive) NEC Q61.19
collecting duct dilatation Q61.11
Kuhnt-Junius (see also Degeneration, macula) H35.32- ☑
lens — see Cataract
lenticular (familial) (progressive) (Wilson's) (with cirrhosis of liver) E83.01
liver (diffuse) NEC K76.89
amyloid E85.4 [K77]
cystic K76.89
congenital Q44.6
fatty NEC K76.0
alcoholic K70.0
hypertrophic K76.89
parenchymatous, acute or subacute K72.00
with coma K72.01
pigmentary K76.89
toxic (acute) K71.9
lung J98.4
lymph gland I89.8
hyaline I89.8
macula, macular (acquired) (age-related) (senile) H35.30
angioid streaks H35.33
atrophic age-related H35.31- ☑
congenital or hereditary — see Dystrophy, retina
cystoid H35.35- ☑
drusen H35.36- ☑
dry age-related H35.31- ☑
exudative H35.32- ☑
hole H35.34- ☑
nonexudative H35.31- ☑
puckering H35.37- ☑
toxic H35.38- ☑
wet age-related H35.32- ☑
membranous labyrinth, congenital (causing impairment of hearing) Q16.5
meniscus — see Derangement, meniscus
mitral — see Insufficiency, mitral
Mönckeberg's — see Arteriosclerosis, extremities
motor centers, senile G31.1
multi-system G90.3
mural — see Degeneration, myocardial
muscle (fatty) (fibrous) (hyaline) (progressive) M62.89
heart — see Degeneration, myocardial
myelin, central nervous system G37.9
myocardial, myocardium (fatty) (hyaline) (senile) I51.5
with rheumatic fever (conditions in I00) I09.0
active, acute or subacute I01.2
with chorea I02.0
inactive or quiescent (with chorea) I09.0

Degeneration, degenerative — *continued*
  myocardial, myocardium — *continued*
    hypertensive — *see* Hypertension, heart
    rheumatic — *see* Degeneration, myocardial, with
      rheumatic fever
    syphilitic A52.06
  nasal sinus (mucosa) J32.9
    frontal J32.1
    maxillary J32.0
  nerve — *see* Disorder, nerve
  nervous system G31.9
    alcoholic G31.2
    amyloid E85.4 [G99.8]
    autonomic G90.9
    fatty G31.89
    specified NEC G31.89
  nipple N64.89
  olivopontocerebellar (hereditary) (familial) G23.8
  osseous labyrinth — *see* subcategory H83.8 ☑
  ovary N83.8
    cystic N83.20- ☑
    microcystic N83.20- ☑
  pallidal pigmentary (progressive) G23.0
  pancreas K86.89
    tuberculous A18.83
  penis N48.89
  pigmentary (diffuse) (general)
    localized — *see* Degeneration, by site
    pallidal (progressive) G23.0
  pineal gland E34.8
  pituitary (gland) E23.6
  popliteal fat pad M79.4
  posterolateral (spinal cord) — *see* Degeneration,
    combined
  pulmonary valve (heart) I37.8
  pulp (tooth) K04.2
  pupillary margin H21.24- ☑
  renal — *see* Degeneration, kidney
  retina H35.9
    hereditary (cerebroretinal) (congenital) (juvenile)
      (macula) (peripheral) (pigmentary) — *see*
      Dystrophy, retina
    Kuhnt-Junius (*see also* Degeneration, macula)
      H35.32- ☑
    macula (cystic) (exudative) (hole) (nonexudative)
      (pseudohole) (senile) (toxic) — *see* Degener-
      ation, macula
    peripheral H35.40
      lattice H35.41- ☑
      microcystoid H35.42- ☑
      paving stone H35.43- ☑
      secondary
        pigmentary H35.45- ☑
        vitreoretinal H35.46- ☑
      senile reticular H35.44- ☑
    pigmentary (primary) (*see also* Dystrophy, retina)
      secondary — *see* Degeneration, retina, periph-
      eral, secondary
    posterior pole — *see* Degeneration, macula
  saccule, congenital (causing impairment of hearing)
    Q16.5
  senile R54
    brain G31.1
    cardiac, heart or myocardium — *see* Degeneration,
      myocardial
    motor centers G31.1
    vascular — *see* Arteriosclerosis
  sinus (cystic) (*see also* Sinusitis)
    polypoid J33.1
  skin L98.8
    amyloid E85.4 [L99]
    colloid L98.8
  spinal (cord) G31.89
    amyloid E85.4 [G32.89]
    combined (subacute) — *see* Degeneration, com-
      bined
    dorsolateral — *see* Degeneration, combined
    familial NEC G31.89
    fatty G31.89
    funicular — *see* Degeneration, combined
    posterolateral — *see* Degeneration, combined
    subacute combined — *see* Degeneration, com-
      bined
    tuberculous A17.81
  spleen D73.0
    amyloid E85.4 [D77]
  stomach K31.89
  striatonigral G23.2

Degeneration, degenerative — *continued*
  suprarenal (capsule) (gland) E27.8
  synovial membrane (pulpy) — *see* Disorder, synovium,
    specified type NEC
  tapetoretinal — *see* Dystrophy, retina
  thymus (gland) E32.8
    fatty E32.8
  thyroid (gland) E07.89
  tricuspid (heart) (valve) I07.9
  tuberculous NEC — *see* Tuberculosis
  turbinate J34.89
  uterus (cystic) N85.8
  vascular (senile) — *see* Arteriosclerosis
    hypertensive — *see* Hypertension
  vitreoretinal, secondary — *see* Degeneration, retina,
    peripheral, secondary, vitreoretinal
  vitreous (body) H43.81- ☑
  Wallerian — *see* Disorder, nerve
  Wilson's hepatolenticular E83.01
Deglutition
  paralysis R13.0
    hysterical F44.4
  pneumonia J69.0
Degos' disease I77.89
Dehiscence (of)
  amputation stump T87.81
  cesarean wound O90.0
  closure of
    cornea T81.31 ☑
    craniotomy T81.32 ☑
    fascia (muscular) (superficial) T81.32 ☑
    internal organ or tissue T81.32 ☑
    laceration (external) (internal) T81.33 ☑
    ligament T81.32 ☑
    mucosa T81.31 ☑
    muscle or muscle flap T81.32 ☑
    ribs or rib cage T81.32 ☑
    skin and subcutaneous tissue (full-thickness) (su-
      perficial) T81.31 ☑
    skull T81.32 ☑
    sternum (sternotomy) T81.32 ☑
    tendon T81.32 ☑
    traumatic laceration (external) (internal) T81.33 ☑
  episiotomy O90.1
  operation wound NEC T81.31 ☑
    external operation wound (superficial) T81.31 ☑
    internal operation wound (deep) T81.32 ☑
  perineal wound (postpartum) O90.1
  traumatic injury wound repair T81.33 ☑
  wound T81.30 ☑
    traumatic repair T81.33 ☑
Dehydration E86.0
  newborn P74.1
Déjérine-Roussy syndrome G89.0
Déjérine-Sottas disease or neuropathy (hypertrophic)
  G60.0
Déjérine-Thomas atrophy G23.8
Delay, delayed
  any plane in pelvis
    complicating delivery O66.9
  birth or delivery NOS O63.9
  closure, ductus arteriosus (Botalli) P29.38
  coagulation — *see* Defect, coagulation
  conduction (cardiac) (ventricular) I45.9
  delivery, second twin, triplet, etc O63.2
  development R62.50
    global F88
    intellectual (specific) F81.9
    language F80.9
      due to hearing loss F80.4
    learning F81.9
    pervasive F84.9
    physiological R62.50
      specified stage NEC R62.0
    reading F81.0
    sexual E30.0
    speech F80.9
      due to hearing loss F80.4
    spelling F81.81
  ejaculation F52.32
  gastric emptying K30
  menarche E30.0
  menstruation (cause unknown) N91.0
  milestone R62.0
  passage of meconium (newborn) P76.0
  primary respiration P28.9
  puberty (constitutional) E30.0

Delay, delayed — *continued*
  separation of umbilical cord P96.82
  sexual maturation, female E30.0
  sleep phase syndrome G47.21
  union, fracture — *see* Fracture, by site
  vaccination Z28.9
Deletion(s)
  autosome Q93.9
    identified by fluorescence in situ hybridization
      (FISH) Q93.89
    identified by in situ hybridization (ISH) Q93.89
  chromosome
    with complex rearrangements NEC Q93.7
    part of NEC Q93.5
    seen only at prometaphase Q93.89
    short arm
      22q11.2 Q93.81
      4 Q93.3
      5p Q93.4
    specified NEC Q93.89
  long arm chromosome 18 or 21 Q93.89
    with complex rearrangements NEC Q93.7
  microdeletions NEC Q93.88
Delhi boil or button B55.1
Delinquency (juvenile) (neurotic) F91.8
  group Z72.810
Delinquent immunization status Z28.3
Delirium, delirious (acute or subacute) (not alcohol- or
  drug-induced) (with dementia) R41.0
  alcoholic (acute) (tremens) (withdrawal) F10.921
    with intoxication F10.921
      in
        abuse F10.121
        dependence F10.221
  due to (secondary to)
    alcohol
      intoxication F10.921
        in
          abuse F10.121
          dependence F10.221
      withdrawal F10.231
    amphetamine intoxication F15.921
      in
        abuse F15.121
        dependence F15.221
    anxiolytic
      intoxication F13.921
        in
          abuse F13.121
          dependence F13.221
      withdrawal F13.231
    cannabis intoxication (acute) F12.921
      in
        abuse F12.121
        dependence F12.221
    cocaine intoxication (acute) F14.921
      in
        abuse F14.121
        dependence F14.221
    general medical condition F05
    hallucinogen intoxication F16.921
      in
        abuse F16.121
        dependence F16.221
    hypnotic
      intoxication F13.921
        in
          abuse F13.121
          dependence F13.221
      withdrawal F13.231
    inhalant intoxication (acute) F18.921
      in
        abuse F18.121
        dependence F18.221
    multiple etiologies F05
    opioid intoxication (acute) F11.921
      in
        abuse F11.121
        dependence F11.221
    other (or unknown) substance F19.921
    phencyclidine intoxication (acute) F16.921
      in
        abuse F16.121
        dependence F16.221
    psychoactive substance NEC intoxication (acute)
      F19.921
      in
        abuse F19.121
        dependence F19.221

Delirium, delirious — *continued*
  due to — *continued*
    sedative
      intoxication F13.921
        in
          abuse F13.121
          dependence F13.221
      withdrawal F13.231
    unknown etiology F05
  exhaustion F43.0
  hysterical F44.89
  postprocedural (postoperative) F05
  puerperal F05
  thyroid — *see* Thyrotoxicosis with thyroid storm
  traumatic — *see* Injury, intracranial
  tremens (alcohol-induced) F10.231
    sedative-induced F13.231
Delivery (childbirth) (labor)
  arrested active phase O62.1
  cesarean (for)
    without indication O82
    abnormal
      pelvis (bony) (deformity) (major) NEC with disproportion (fetopelvic) O33.0
        with obstructed labor O65.0
      presentation or position O32.9 ☑
    abruptio placentae (*see also* Abruptio placentae) O45.9- ☑
    acromion presentation O32.2 ☑
    atony, uterus O62.2
    breech presentation O32.1 ☑
      incomplete O32.8 ☑
    brow presentation O32.3 ☑
    cephalopelvic disproportion O33.9
    cerclage O34.3- ☑
    chin presentation O32.3 ☑
    cicatrix of cervix O34.4- ☑
    contracted pelvis (general)
      inlet O33.2
      outlet O33.3 ☑
    cord presentation or prolapse O69.0 ☑
    cystocele O34.8- ☑
    deformity (acquired) (congenital)
      pelvic organs or tissues NEC O34.8- ☑
      pelvis (bony) NEC O33.0
    disproportion NOS O33.9
    eclampsia — *see* Eclampsia
    face presentation O32.3 ☑
    failed
      forceps O66.5
      induction of labor O61.9
        instrumental O61.1
        mechanical O61.1
        medical O61.0
        specified NEC O61.8
        surgical O61.1
      trial of labor NOS O66.40
        following previous cesarean delivery O66.41
      vacuum extraction O66.5
      ventouse O66.5
    fetal-maternal hemorrhage O43.01- ☑
    hemorrhage (intrapartum) O67.9
      with coagulation defect O67.0
      specified cause NEC O67.8
    high head at term O32.4 ☑
    hydrocephalic fetus O33.6 ☑
    incarceration of uterus O34.51- ☑
    incoordinate uterine action O62.4
    increased size, fetus O33.5 ☑
    inertia, uterus O62.2
      primary O62.0
      secondary O62.1
    lateroversion, uterus O34.59- ☑
    mal lie O32.9 ☑
    malposition
      fetus O32.9 ☑
      pelvic organs or tissues NEC O34.8- ☑
      uterus NEC O34.59- ☑
    malpresentation NOS O32.9 ☑
    oblique presentation O32.2 ☑
    occurring after 37 completed weeks of gestation but before 39 completed weeks gestation due to (spontaneous) onset of labor O75.82
    oversize fetus O33.5 ☑
    pelvic tumor NEC O34.8- ☑
    placenta previa O44.0- ☑
      complete O44.0- ☑

Delivery — *continued*
  cesarean — *continued*
    placenta previa — *continued*
      complete — *continued*
        with hemorrhage O44.1- ☑
      placental insufficiency O36.51- ☑
      planned, occurring after 37 completed weeks of gestation but before 39 completed weeks gestation due to (spontaneous) onset of labor O75.82
    polyp, cervix O34.4- ☑
      causing obstructed labor O65.5
    poor dilatation, cervix O62.0
    pre-eclampsia O14.94
      mild O14.04
      moderate O14.04
      severe O14.14
        with hemolysis, elevated liver enzymes and low platelet count (HELLP) O14.24
    previous
      cesarean delivery O34.219
        classical (vertical) scar O34.212
        low transverse scar O34.211
      surgery (to)
        cervix O34.4- ☑
        gynecological NEC O34.8- ☑
        rectum O34.7- ☑
        uterus O34.29
        vagina O34.6- ☑
    prolapse
      arm or hand O32.2 ☑
      uterus O34.52- ☑
    prolonged labor NOS O63.9
    rectocele O34.8- ☑
    retroversion
      uterus O34.53- ☑
    rigid
      cervix O34.4- ☑
      pelvic floor O34.8- ☑
      perineum O34.7- ☑
      vagina O34.6- ☑
      vulva O34.7- ☑
    sacculation, pregnant uterus O34.59- ☑
    scar(s)
      cervix O34.4- ☑
      cesarean delivery O34.219
        classical (vertical) O34.212
        low transverse O34.211
      transmural uterine O34.29
      uterus O34.29
    Shirodkar suture in situ O34.3- ☑
    shoulder presentation O32.2 ☑
    stenosis or stricture, cervix O34.4- ☑
    streptococcus group B (GBS) carrier state O99.824
    transmural uterine scar O34.29
    transverse presentation or lie O32.2 ☑
    tumor, pelvic organs or tissues NEC O34.8- ☑
      cervix O34.4- ☑
    umbilical cord presentation or prolapse O69.0 ☑
  completely normal case O80
  complicated O75.9
    by
      abnormal, abnormality (of)
        forces of labor O62.9
          specified type NEC O62.8
        glucose O99.814
        uterine contractions NOS O62.9
      abruptio placentae (*see also* Abruptio placentae) O45.9- ☑
      abuse
        physical O9A.32 (*following* O99)
        psychological O9A.52 (*following* O99)
        sexual O9A.42 (*following* O99)
      adherent placenta O72.0
        without hemorrhage O73.0
      alcohol use O99.314
      anemia (pre-existing) O99.02
      anesthetic death O74.8
      annular detachment of cervix O71.3
      atony, uterus O62.2
      attempted vacuum extraction and forceps O66.5
      Bandl's ring O62.4
      bariatric surgery status O99.844
      biliary tract disorder O26.62
      bleeding — *see* Delivery, complicated by, hemorrhage
      blood disorder NEC O99.12

Delivery — *continued*
  complicated — *continued*
    by — *continued*
      cervical dystocia (hypotonic) O62.2
        primary O62.0
        secondary O62.1
      circulatory system disorder O99.42
      compression of cord (umbilical) NEC O69.2 ☑
      condition NEC O99.89
      contraction, contracted ring O62.4
      cord (umbilical)
        around neck
          with compression O69.1 ☑
          without compression O69.81 ☑
        bruising O69.5 ☑
        complication O69.9 ☑
          specified NEC O69.89 ☑
        compression NEC O69.2 ☑
        entanglement O69.2 ☑
          without compression O69.82 ☑
        hematoma O69.5 ☑
        presentation O69.0 ☑
        prolapse O69.0 ☑
        short O69.3 ☑
        thrombosis (vessels) O69.5 ☑
        vascular lesion O69.5 ☑
      Couvelaire uterus O45.8X- ☑
      damage to (injury to) NEC
        perineum O71.82
        periurethral tissue O71.82
        vulva O71.82
      delay following rupture of membranes (spontaneous) — *see* Pregnancy, complicated by, premature rupture of membranes
      depressed fetal heart tones O76
      diabetes O24.92
        gestational O24.429
          diet controlled O24.420
          insulin controlled O24.424
          oral drug controlled (antidiabetic) (hypoglycemic) O24.425
        pre-existing O24.32
          specified NEC O24.82
          type 1 O24.02
          type 2 O24.12
      diastasis recti (abdominis) O71.89
      dilatation
        bladder O66.8
        cervix incomplete, poor or slow O62.0
      disease NEC O99.89
      disruptio uteri — *see* Delivery, complicated by, rupture, uterus
      drug use O99.324
      dysfunction, uterus NOS O62.9
        hypertonic O62.4
        hypotonic O62.2
          primary O62.0
          secondary O62.1
        incoordinate O62.4
      eclampsia O15.1
      embolism (pulmonary) — *see* Embolism, obstetric
      endocrine, nutritional or metabolic disease NEC O99.284
      failed
        attempted vaginal birth after previous cesarean delivery O66.41
        induction of labor O61.9
          instrumental O61.1
          mechanical O61.1
          medical O61.0
          specified NEC O61.8
          surgical O61.1
        trial of labor O66.40
      female genital mutilation O65.5
      fetal
        abnormal acid-base balance O68
        acidemia O68
        acidosis O68
        alkalosis O68
        death, early O02.1
        deformity O66.3
        heart rate or rhythm (abnormal) (non-reassuring) O76
        hypoxia O77.8
        stress O77.9
          due to drug administration O77.1
          electrocardiographic evidence of O77.8

☑ **Additional Character Required — Refer to the Tabular List for Character Selection**   ▼ Subterms under main terms may continue to next column or page

Delivery — *continued*
  complicated — *continued*
    by — *continued*
      fetal — *continued*
        stress — *continued*
          specified NEC O77.8
          ultrasound evidence of O77.8
      fever during labor O75.2
      gastric banding status O99.844
      gastric bypass status O99.844
      gastrointestinal disease NEC O99.62
      gestational
        diabetes O24.429
          diet controlled O24.420
          insulin (and diet) controlled O24.424
          oral drug controlled (antidiabetic) (hypo-
            glycemic) O24.425
        edema O12.04
          with proteinuria O12.24
        proteinuria O12.14
      gonorrhea O98.22
      hematoma O71.7
        ischial spine O71.7
        pelvic O71.7
        vagina O71.7
        vulva or perineum O71.7
      hemorrhage (uterine) O67.9
        associated with
          afibrinogenemia O67.0
          coagulation defect O67.0
          hyperfibrinolysis O67.0
          hypofibrinogenemia O67.0
        due to
          low implantation of placenta O44.5- ☑
          low-lying placenta O44.5- ☑
          placenta previa O44.1- ☑
            marginal O44.3- ☑
            partial O44.3- ☑
          premature separation of placenta (nor-
            mally implanted) (*see also* Abrup-
            tio placentae) O45.9- ☑
          retained placenta O72.0
          uterine leiomyoma O67.8
        placenta NEC O67.8
        postpartum NEC (atonic) (immediate) O72.1
          with retained or trapped placenta O72.0
          delayed O72.2
          secondary O72.2
          third stage O72.0
      hourglass contraction, uterus O62.4
      hypertension, hypertensive (pre-existing) —
        see Hypertension, complicated by, child-
        birth (labor)
      hypotension O26.5- ☑
      incomplete dilatation (cervix) O62.0
      incoordinate uterus contractions O62.4
      inertia, uterus O62.2
        during latent phase of labor O62.0
        primary O62.0
        secondary O62.1
      infection (maternal) O98.92
        carrier state NEC O99.834
        gonorrhea O98.22
        human immunodeficiency virus (HIV)
          O98.72
        sexually transmitted NEC O98.32
        specified NEC O98.82
        syphilis O98.12
        tuberculosis O98.02
        viral hepatitis O98.42
        viral NEC O98.52
      injury (to mother) (*see also* Delivery, complicat-
        ed, by, damage to) O71.9
        nonobstetric O9A.22 (*following* O99)
          caused by abuse — *see* Delivery, compli-
            cated by, abuse
      intrauterine fetal death, early O02.1
      inversion, uterus O71.2
      laceration (perineal) O70.9
        anus (sphincter) O70.4
          with third degree laceration (*see also*
            Delivery, complicated, by, lacera-
            tion, perineum, third degree)
            O70.20
            with mucosa O70.3
          without third degree laceration O70.2 ☑
        bladder (urinary) O71.5
        bowel O71.5

Delivery — *continued*
  complicated — *continued*
    by — *continued*
      laceration — *continued*
        cervix (uteri) O71.3
        fourchette O70.0
        hymen O70.0
        labia O70.0
        pelvic
          floor O70.1
          organ NEC O71.5
        perineum, perineal O70.9
          first degree O70.0
          fourth degree O70.3
          muscles O70.1
          second degree O70.1
          skin O70.0
          slight O70.0
          third degree O70.20
            with
              less than 50% of external anal
                sphincter (EAS) thickness
                torn (IIIa) O70.21
              both external anal sphincter (EAS)
                and internal anal sphincter
                (IAS) torn (IIIc) O70.23
              more than 50% external anal
                sphincter (EAS) thickness
                torn (IIIb) O70.22
            IIIa O70.21
            IIIb O70.22
            IIIc O70.23
        peritoneum (pelvic) O71.5
        rectovaginal (septum) (without perineal
          laceration) O71.4
          with perineum (*see also* Delivery, compli-
            cated, by, laceration, perineum,
            third degree) O70.20
          with anal or rectal mucosa O70.3
        specified NEC O71.89
        sphincter ani — *see* Delivery, complicated,
          by, laceration, anus (sphincter)
        urethra O71.5
        uterus O71.81
          before labor O71.81
        vagina, vaginal (deep) (high) (without per-
          ineal laceration) O71.4
          with perineum O70.0
          muscles, with perineum O70.1
        vulva O70.0
      liver disorder O26.62
      malignancy O9A.12 (*following* O99)
      malnutrition O25.2
      malposition, malpresentation
        without obstruction (*see also* Delivery,
          complicated by, obstruction) O32.9 ☑
          breech O32.1 ☑
          compound O32.6 ☑
          face (brow) (chin) O32.3 ☑
          footling O32.8 ☑
          high head O32.4 ☑
          oblique O32.2 ☑
          specified NEC O32.8 ☑
          transverse O32.2 ☑
          unstable lie O32.0 ☑
        placenta O44.0- ☑
          with hemorrhage O44.1- ☑
        uterus or cervix O65.5
      meconium in amniotic fluid O77.0
      mental disorder NEC O99.344
      metrorrhexis — *see* Delivery, complicated by,
        rupture, uterus
      nervous system disorder O99.354
      obesity (pre-existing) O99.214
      obesity surgery status O99.844
      obstetric trauma O71.9
        specified NEC O71.89
      obstructed labor
        due to
          breech (complete) (frank) presentation
            O64.1 ☑
            incomplete O64.8 ☑
          brow presenation O64.3 ☑
          buttock presentation O64.1 ☑
          chin presentation O64.2 ☑
          compound presentation O64.5 ☑
          contracted pelvis O65.1
          deep transverse arrest O64.0 ☑

Delivery — *continued*
  complicated — *continued*
    by — *continued*
      obstructed labor — *continued*
        due to — *continued*
          deformed pelvis O65.0
          dystocia (fetal) O66.9
            due to
              conjoined twins O66.3
              fetal
                abnormality NEC O66.3
                ascites O66.3
                hydrops O66.3
                meningomyelocele O66.3
                sacral teratoma O66.3
                tumor O66.3
              hydrocephalic fetus O66.3
          shoulder O66.0
          face presentation O64.2 ☑
          fetopelvic disproportion O65.4
          footling presentation O64.8 ☑
          impacted shoulders O66.0
          incomplete rotation of fetal head
            O64.0 ☑
          large fetus O66.2
          locked twins O66.1
          malposition O64.9 ☑
            specified NEC O64.8 ☑
          malpresentation O64.9 ☑
            specified NEC O64.8 ☑
          multiple fetuses NEC O66.6
          pelvic
            abnormality (maternal) O65.9
              organ O65.5
              specified NEC O65.8
            contraction
              inlet O65.2
              mid-cavity O65.3
              outlet O65.3
          persistent (position)
            occipitoiliac O64.0 ☑
            occipitoposterior O64.0 ☑
            occipitosacral O64.0 ☑
            occipitotransverse O64.0 ☑
          prolapsed arm O64.4 ☑
          shoulder presentation O64.4 ☑
        specified NEC O66.8
      pathological retraction ring, uterus O62.4
      penetration, pregnant uterus by instrument
        O71.1
      perforation — *see* Delivery, complicated by,
        laceration
      placenta, placental
        ablatio (*see also* Abruptio placentae)
          O45.9- ☑
        abnormality O43.9- ☑
          specified NEC O43.89- ☑
        abruptio (*see also* Abruptio placentae)
          O45.9- ☑
        accreta O43.21- ☑
        adherent (with hemorrhage) O72.0
          without hemorrhage O73.0
        detachment (premature) (*see also* Abruptio
          placentae) O45.9- ☑
        disorder O43.9- ☑
          specified NEC O43.89- ☑
        hemorrhage NEC O67.8
        increta O43.22- ☑
        low (implantation) (lying) O44.4- ☑
          with hemorrhage O44.5- ☑
        malformation O43.10- ☑
        malposition O44.0- ☑
          without hemorrhage O44.1- ☑
        percreta O43.23- ☑
        previa (central) (complete) (lateral) (total)
          O44.0- ☑
          with hemorrhage O44.1- ☑
          marginal O44.2- ☑
            with hemorrhage O44.3- ☑
          partial O44.2- ☑
            with hemorrhage O44.3- ☑
        retained (with hemorrhage) O72.0
          without hemorrhage O73.0
        separation (premature) O45.9- ☑
          specified NEC O45.8X- ☑
        vicious insertion O44.1- ☑
      precipitate labor O62.3

Delivery — *continued*
  complicated — *continued*
    by — *continued*
      premature rupture, membranes (*see also* Pregnancy, complicated by, premature rupture of membranes) O42.90
      prolapse
        arm or hand O32.2 ☑
        cord (umbilical) O69.0 ☑
        foot or leg O32.8 ☑
        uterus O34.52-
      prolonged labor O63.9
        first stage O63.0
        second stage O63.1
      protozoal disease (maternal) O98.62
      respiratory disease NEC O99.52
      retained membranes or portions of placenta O72.2
        without hemorrhage O73.1
      retarded birth O63.9
      retention of secundines (with hemorrhage) O72.0
        without hemorrhage O73.0
        partial O72.2
          without hemorrhage O73.1
      rupture
        bladder (urinary) O71.5
        cervix O71.3
        pelvic organ NEC O71.5
        urethra O71.5
        uterus (during or after labor) O71.1
          before labor O71.0- ☑
      separation, pubic bone (symphysis pubis) O71.6
      shock O75.1
      shoulder presentation O64.4 ☑
      skin disorder NEC O99.72
      spasm, cervix O62.4
      stenosis or stricture, cervix O65.5
      streptococcus group B (GBS) carrier state O99.824
      subluxation of symphysis (pubis) O26.72
      syphilis (maternal) O98.12
      tear — *see* Delivery, complicated by, laceration
      tetanic uterus O62.4
      trauma (obstetrical) (*see also* Delivery, complicated, by, damage to) O71.9
        non-obstetric O9A.22 (*following* O99)
        periurethral O71.82
        specified NEC O71.89
      tuberculosis (maternal) O98.02
      tumor, pelvic organs or tissues NEC O65.5
      umbilical cord around neck
        with compression O69.1 ☑
        without compression O69.81 ☑
      uterine inertia O62.2
        during latent phase of labor O62.0
        primary O62.0
        secondary O62.1
      vasa previa O69.4 ☑
      velamentous insertion of cord O43.12- ☑
    specified complication NEC O75.89
  delayed NOS O63.9
    following rupture of membranes
      artificial O75.5
    second twin, triplet, etc. O63.2
  forceps, low following failed vacuum extraction O66.5
  missed (at or near term) O36.4 ☑
  normal O80
  obstructed — *see* Delivery, complicated by, obstructed labor
  precipitate O62.3
  preterm (*see also* Pregnancy, complicated by, preterm labor) O60.10 ☑
  spontaneous O80
  term pregnancy NOS O80
  uncomplicated O80
  vaginal, following previous cesarean delivery O34.219
    classical (vertical) scar O34.212
    low transverse scar O34.211
Delusions (paranoid) — *see* Disorder, delusional
Dementia (degenerative (primary)) (old age) (persisting) F03.90
  with
    aggressive behavior F03.91
    behavioral disturbance F03.91
    combative behavior F03.91
    Lewy bodies G31.83 [F02.80]
      with behavioral disturbance G31.83 [F02.81]

Dementia — *continued*
  with — *continued*
    Parkinsonism G31.83 [F02.80]
      with behavioral disturbance G31.83 [F02.81]
    Parkinson's disease G20 [F02.80]
      with behavioral disturbance G20 [F02.81]
    violent behavior F03.91
  alcoholic F10.97
    with dependence F10.27
  Alzheimer's type — *see* Disease, Alzheimer's
  arteriosclerotic — *see* Dementia, vascular
  atypical, Alzheimer's type — *see* Disease, Alzheimer's, specified NEC
  congenital — *see* Disability, intellectual
  frontal (lobe) G31.09 [F02.80]
    with behavioral disturbance G31.09 [F02.81]
  frontotemporal G31.09 [F02.80]
    with behavioral disturbance G31.09 [F02.81]
    specified NEC G31.09 [F02.80]
      with behavioral disturbance G31.09 [F02.81]
  Huntington's disease or chorea G10
    with dementia G10 [F02.80]
  in (due to)
    with behavioral disturbance G31.83 [F02.81]
    alcohol F10.97
      with dependence F10.27
    Alzheimer's disease — *see* Disease, Alzheimer's
    arteriosclerotic brain disease — *see* Dementia, vascular
    cerebral lipidoses E75.- ☑ [F02.80]
      with behavioral disturbance E75.- ☑ [F02.81]
    Creutzfeldt-Jakob disease (*see also* Creutzfeldt-Jakob disease or syndrome (with dementia)) A81.00
    epilepsy G40.- ☑ [F02.80]
      with behavioral disturbance G40.- ☑ [F02.81]
    hepatolenticular degeneration E83.01 [F02.80]
      with behavioral disturbance E83.01 [F02.81]
    human immunodeficiency virus (HIV) disease B20 [F02.80]
      with behavioral disturbance B20 [F02.81]
    Huntington's disease or chorea G10 [F02.80]
      with behavioral disturbance G10 [F02.81]
    hypercalcemia E83.52 [F02.80]
      with behavioral disturbance E83.52 [F02.81]
    hypothyroidism, acquired E03.9 [F02.80]
      with behavioral disturbance E03.9 [F02.81]
      due to iodine deficiency E01.8 [F02.80]
        with behavioral disturbance E01.8 [F02.81]
    inhalants F18.97
      with dependence F18.27
    multiple
      etiologies F03 ☑
      sclerosis G35 [F02.80]
        with behavioral disturbance G35 [F02.81]
    neurosyphilis A52.17 [F02.80]
      with behavioral disturbance A52.17 [F02.81]
      juvenile A50.49 [F02.80]
        with behavioral disturbance A50.49 [F02.81]
    niacin deficiency E52 [F02.80]
      with behavioral disturbance E52 [F02.81]
    paralysis agitans G20 [F02.80]
      with behavioral disturbance G20 [F02.81]
    Parkinson's disease G20 [F02.80]
    pellagra E52 [F02.80]
      with behavioral disturbance E52 [F02.81]
    Pick's G31.01 [F02.80]
      with behavioral disturbance G31.01 [F02.81]
    polyarteritis nodosa M30.0 [F02.80]
      with behavioral disturbance M30.0 [F02.81]
    psychoactive drug F19.97
      with dependence F19.27
      inhalants F18.97
        with dependence F18.27
      sedatives, hypnotics or anxiolytics F13.97
        with dependence F13.27
    sedatives, hypnotics or anxiolytics F13.97
      with dependence F13.27
    systemic lupus erythematosus M32.- ☑ [F02.80]
      with behavioral disturbance M32.- ☑ [F02.81]
    trypanosomiasis
      African B56.9 [F02.80]
        with behavioral disturbance B56.9 [F02.81]
    unknown etiology F03 ☑
    vitamin B12 deficiency E53.8 [F02.80]
      with behavioral disturbance E53.8 [F02.81]
    volatile solvents F18.97
      with dependence F18.27

Dementia — *continued*
  infantile, infantilis F84.3
  Lewy body G31.83 [F02.80]
    with behavioral disturbance G31.83 [F02.81]
  multi-infarct — *see* Dementia, vascular
  paralytica, paralytic (syphilitic) A52.17 [F02.80]
    with behavioral disturbance A52.17 [F02.81]
    juvenilis A50.45
  paretic A52.17
  praecox — *see* Schizophrenia
  presenile F03 ☑
    Alzheimer's type — *see* Disease, Alzheimer's, early onset
  primary degenerative F03 ☑
  progressive, syphilitic A52.17
  senile F03 ☑
    with acute confusional state F05
    Alzheimer's type — *see* Disease, Alzheimer's, late onset
    depressed or paranoid type F03 ☑
  vascular (acute onset) (mixed) (multi-infarct) (subcortical) F01.50
    with behavioral disturbance F01.51
Demineralization, bone — *see* Osteoporosis
Demodex folliculorum (infestation) B88.0
Demophobia F40.248
Demoralization R45.3
Demyelination, demyelinization
  central nervous system G37.9
    specified NEC G37.8
  corpus callosum (central) G37.1
  disseminated, acute G36.9
    specified NEC G36.8
  global G35
  in optic neuritis G36.0
Dengue (classical) (fever) A90
  hemorrhagic A91
  sandfly A93.1
Dennie-Marfan syphilitic syndrome A50.45
Dens evaginatus, in dente or invaginatus K00.2
Dense breasts R92.2
Density
  increased, bone (disseminated) (generalized) (spotted) — *see* Disorder, bone, density and structure, specified type NEC
  lung (nodular) J98.4
Dental (*see also* condition)
  examination Z01.20
    with abnormal findings Z01.21
  restoration
    aesthetically inadequate or displeasing K08.56
    defective K08.50
      specified NEC K08.59
    failure of marginal integrity K08.51
    failure of periodontal anatomical integrity K08.54
Dentia praecox K00.6
Denticles (pulp) K04.2
Dentigerous cyst K09.0
Dentin
  irregular (in pulp) K04.3
  opalescent K00.5
  secondary (in pulp) K04.3
  sensitive K03.89
Dentinogenesis imperfecta K00.5
Dentinoma — *see* Cyst, calcifying odontogenic
Dentition (syndrome) K00.7
  delayed K00.6
  difficult K00.7
  precocious K00.6
  premature K00.6
  retarded K00.6
Dependence (on) (syndrome) F19.20
  with remission F19.21
  alcohol (ethyl) (methyl) (without remission) F10.20
    with
      amnestic disorder, persisting F10.26
      anxiety disorder F10.280
      dementia, persisting F10.27
      intoxication F10.229
        with delirium F10.221
        uncomplicated F10.220
      mood disorder F10.24
      psychotic disorder F10.259
        with
          delusions F10.250
          hallucinations F10.251
      remission F10.21
      sexual dysfunction F10.281

☑ **Additional Character Required** — Refer to the Tabular List for Character Selection   ⬇ Subterms under main terms may continue to next column or page

Dependence — *continued*
  alcohol — *continued*
    with — *continued*
      sleep disorder F10.282
      specified disorder NEC F10.288
      withdrawal F10.239
        with
          delirium F10.231
          perceptual disturbance F10.232
        uncomplicated F10.230
      counseling and surveillance Z71.41
  amobarbital — *see* Dependence, drug, sedative
  amphetamine(s) (type) — *see* Dependence, drug, stimulant NEC
  amytal (sodium) — *see* Dependence, drug, sedative
  analgesic NEC F55.8
  anesthetic (agent) (gas) (general) (local) NEC — *see* Dependence, drug, psychoactive NEC
  anxiolytic NEC — *see* Dependence, drug, sedative
  barbital(s) — *see* Dependence, drug, sedative
  barbiturate(s) (compounds) (drugs classifiable to T42) — *see* Dependence, drug, sedative
  benzedrine — *see* Dependence, drug, stimulant NEC
  bhang — *see* Dependence, drug, cannabis
  bromide(s) NEC — *see* Dependence, drug, sedative
  caffeine — *see* Dependence, drug, stimulant NEC
  cannabis (sativa) (indica) (resin) (derivatives) (type) — *see* Dependence, drug, cannabis
  chloral (betaine) (hydrate) — *see* Dependence, drug, sedative
  chlordiazepoxide — *see* Dependence, drug, sedative
  coca (leaf) (derivatives) — *see* Dependence, drug, cocaine
  cocaine — *see* Dependence, drug, cocaine
  codeine — *see* Dependence, drug, opioid
  combinations of drugs F19.20
  dagga — *see* Dependence, drug, cannabis
  demerol — *see* Dependence, drug, opioid
  dexamphetamine — *see* Dependence, drug, stimulant NEC
  dexedrine — *see* Dependence, drug, stimulant NEC
  dextromethorphan — *see* Dependence, drug, opioid
  dextromoramide — *see* Dependence, drug, opioid
  dextro-nor-pseudo-ephedrine — *see* Dependence, drug, stimulant NEC
  dextrorphan — *see* Dependence, drug, opioid
  diazepam — *see* Dependence, drug, sedative
  dilaudid — *see* Dependence, drug, opioid
  D-lysergic acid diethylamide — *see* Dependence, drug, hallucinogen
  drug NEC F19.20
    with sleep disorder F19.282
    cannabis F12.20
      with
        anxiety disorder F12.280
        intoxication F12.229
          with
            delirium F12.221
            perceptual disturbance F12.222
          uncomplicated F12.220
        other specified disorder F12.288
        psychosis F12.259
          delusions F12.250
          hallucinations F12.251
        unspecified disorder F12.29
      in remission F12.21
    cocaine F14.20
      with
        anxiety disorder F14.280
        intoxication F14.229
          with
            delirium F14.221
            perceptual disturbance F14.222
          uncomplicated F14.220
        mood disorder F14.24
        other specified disorder F14.288
        psychosis F14.259
          delusions F14.250
          hallucinations F14.251
        sexual dysfunction F14.281
        sleep disorder F14.282
        unspecified disorder F14.29
        withdrawal F14.23
      in remission F14.21
      withdrawal symptoms in newborn P96.1
    counseling and surveillance Z71.51
    hallucinogen F16.20

Dependence — *continued*
  drug — *continued*
    hallucinogen — *continued*
      with
        anxiety disorder F16.280
        flashbacks F16.283
        intoxication F16.229
          with delirium F16.221
          uncomplicated F16.220
        mood disorder F16.24
        other specified disorder F16.288
        perception disorder, persisting F16.283
        psychosis F16.259
          delusions F16.250
          hallucinations F16.251
        unspecified disorder F16.29
      in remission F16.21
    in remission F19.21
    inhalant F18.20
      with
        anxiety disorder F18.280
        dementia, persisting F18.27
        intoxication F18.229
          with delirium F18.221
          uncomplicated F18.220
        mood disorder F18.24
        other specified disorder F18.288
        psychosis F18.259
          delusions F18.250
          hallucinations F18.251
        unspecified disorder F18.29
      in remission F18.21
    nicotine F17.200
      with disorder F17.209
        in remission F17.201
        specified disorder NEC F17.208
        withdrawal F17.203
      chewing tobacco F17.220
        with disorder F17.229
          in remission F17.221
          specified disorder NEC F17.228
          withdrawal F17.223
      cigarettes F17.210
        with disorder F17.219
          in remission F17.211
          specified disorder NEC F17.218
          withdrawal F17.213
      specified product NEC F17.290
        with disorder F17.299
          remission F17.291
          specified disorder NEC F17.298
          withdrawal F17.293
    opioid F11.20
      with
        intoxication F11.229
          with
            delirium F11.221
            perceptual disturbance F11.222
          uncomplicated F11.220
        mood disorder F11.24
        other specified disorder F11.288
        psychosis F11.259
          delusions F11.250
          hallucinations F11.251
        sexual dysfunction F11.281
        sleep disorder F11.282
        unspecified disorder F11.29
        withdrawal F11.23
      in remission F11.21
    psychoactive NEC F19.20
      with
        amnestic disorder F19.26
        anxiety disorder F19.280
        dementia F19.27
        intoxication F19.229
          with
            delirium F19.221
            perceptual disturbance F19.222
          uncomplicated F19.220
        mood disorder F19.24
        other specified disorder F19.288
        psychosis F19.259
          delusions F19.250
          hallucinations F19.251
        sexual dysfunction F19.281
        sleep disorder F19.282
        unspecified disorder F19.29
        withdrawal F19.239

Dependence — *continued*
  drug — *continued*
    psychoactive — *continued*
      with — *continued*
        withdrawal — *continued*
          with
            delirium F19.231
            perceptual disturbance F19.232
          uncomplicated F19.230
    sedative, hypnotic or anxiolytic F13.20
      with
        amnestic disorder F13.26
        anxiety disorder F13.280
        dementia, persisting F13.27
        intoxication F13.229
          with delirium F13.221
          uncomplicated F13.220
        mood disorder F13.24
        other specified disorder F13.288
        psychosis F13.259
          delusions F13.250
          hallucinations F13.251
        sexual dysfunction F13.281
        sleep disorder F13.282
        unspecified disorder F13.29
        withdrawal F13.239
          with
            delirium F13.231
            perceptual disturbance F13.232
          uncomplicated F13.230
      in remission F13.21
    stimulant NEC F15.20
      with
        anxiety disorder F15.280
        intoxication F15.229
          with
            delirium F15.221
            perceptual disturbance F15.222
          uncomplicated F15.220
        mood disorder F15.24
        other specified disorder F15.288
        psychosis F15.259
          delusions F15.250
          hallucinations F15.251
        sexual dysfunction F15.281
        sleep disorder F15.282
        unspecified disorder F15.29
        withdrawal F15.23
      in remission F15.21
  ethyl
    alcohol (without remission) F10.20
      with remission F10.21
    bromide — *see* Dependence, drug, sedative
    carbamate F19.20
    chloride F19.20
    morphine — *see* Dependence, drug, opioid
  ganja — *see* Dependence, drug, cannabis
  glue (airplane) (sniffing) — *see* Dependence, drug, inhalant
  glutethimide — *see* Dependence, drug, sedative
  hallucinogenics — *see* Dependence, drug, hallucinogen
  hashish — *see* Dependence, drug, cannabis
  hemp — *see* Dependence, drug, cannabis
  heroin (salt) (any) — *see* Dependence, drug, opioid
  hypnotic NEC — *see* Dependence, drug, sedative
  Indian hemp — *see* Dependence, drug, cannabis
  inhalants — *see* Dependence, drug, inhalant
  khat — *see* Dependence, drug, stimulant NEC
  laudanum — *see* Dependence, drug, opioid
  LSD (-25) (derivatives) — *see* Dependence, drug, hallucinogen
  luminal — *see* Dependence, drug, sedative
  lysergic acid — *see* Dependence, drug, hallucinogen
  maconha — *see* Dependence, drug, cannabis
  marihuana — *see* Dependence, drug, cannabis
  meprobamate — *see* Dependence, drug, sedative
  mescaline — *see* Dependence, drug, hallucinogen
  methadone — *see* Dependence, drug, opioid
  methamphetamine(s) — *see* Dependence, drug, stimulant NEC
  methaqualone — *see* Dependence, drug, sedative
  methyl
    alcohol (without remission) F10.20
      with remission F10.21
    bromide — *see* Dependence, drug, sedative
    morphine — *see* Dependence, drug, opioid

Index

Dependence — Derangement

Dependence — continued
  methyl — continued
    phenidate — see Dependence, drug, stimulant NEC
    sulfonal — see Dependence, drug, sedative
  morphine (sulfate) (sulfite) (type) — see Dependence, drug, opioid
  narcotic (drug) NEC — see Dependence, drug, opioid
  nembutal — see Dependence, drug, sedative
  neraval — see Dependence, drug, sedative
  neravan — see Dependence, drug, sedative
  neurobarb — see Dependence, drug, sedative
  nicotine — see Dependence, drug, nicotine
  nitrous oxide F19.20
  nonbarbiturate sedatives and tranquilizers with similar effect — see Dependence, drug, sedative
  on
    artificial heart (fully implantable) (mechanical) Z95.812
    aspirator Z99.0
    care provider (because of) Z74.9
      impaired mobility Z74.09
      need for
        assistance with personal care Z74.1
        continuous supervision Z74.3
      no other household member able to render care Z74.2
      specified reason NEC Z74.8
    machine Z99.89
      enabling NEC Z99.89
      specified type NEC Z99.89
    renal dialysis (hemodialysis) (peritoneal) Z99.2
    respirator Z99.11
    ventilator Z99.11
    wheelchair Z99.3
  opiate — see Dependence, drug, opioid
  opioids — see Dependence, drug, opioid
  opium (alkaloids) (derivatives) (tincture) — see Dependence, drug, opioid
  oxygen (long-term) (supplemental) Z99.81
  paraldehyde — see Dependence, drug, sedative
  paregoric — see Dependence, drug, opioid
  PCP (phencyclidine) (or related substance) — see Dependence, drug, hallucinogen
  pentobarbital — see Dependence, drug, sedative
  pentobarbitone (sodium) — see Dependence, drug, sedative
  pentothal — see Dependence, drug, sedative
  peyote — see Dependence, drug, hallucinogen
  phencyclidine (PCP) (or related substance) — see Dependence, drug, hallucinogen
  phenmetrazine — see Dependence, drug, stimulant NEC
  phenobarbital — see Dependence, drug, sedative
  polysubstance F19.20
  psilocibin, psilocin, psilocyn, psilocyline — see Dependence, drug, hallucinogen
  psychostimulant NEC — see Dependence, drug, stimulant NEC
  psychostimulant NEC — see Dependence, drug, stimulant NEC
  secobarbital — see Dependence, drug, sedative
  seconal — see Dependence, drug, sedative
  sedative NEC — see Dependence, drug, sedative
  specified drug NEC — see Dependence, drug
  stimulant NEC — see Dependence, drug, stimulant NEC
  substance NEC — see Dependence, drug
  supplemental oxygen Z99.81
  tobacco — see Dependence, drug, nicotine
    counseling and surveillance Z71.6
  tranquilizer NEC — see Dependence, drug, sedative
  vitamin B6 E53.1
  volatile solvents — see Dependence, drug, inhalant
Dependency
  care-provider Z74.9
  passive F60.7
  reactions (persistent) F60.7
Depersonalization (in neurotic state) (neurotic) (syndrome) F48.1
Depletion
  extracellular fluid E86.9
  plasma E86.1
  potassium E87.6
    nephropathy N25.89
  salt or sodium E87.1
    causing heat exhaustion or prostration T67.4 ☑
    nephropathy N28.9
  volume NOS E86.9

Deployment (current) (military) status Z56.82
  in theater or in support of military war, peacekeeping and humanitarian operations Z56.82
  personal history of Z91.82
    military war, peacekeeping and humanitarian deployment (current or past conflict) Z91.82
  returned from Z91.82
Depolarization, premature I49.40
  atrial I49.1
  junctional I49.2
  specified NEC I49.49
  ventricular I49.3
Deposit
  bone in Boeck's sarcoid D86.89
  calcareous, calcium — see Calcification
  cholesterol
    retina H35.89
    vitreous (body) (humor) — see Deposit, crystalline
  conjunctiva H11.11- ☑
  cornea H18.00- ☑
    argentous H18.02- ☑
    due to metabolic disorder H18.03- ☑
    Kayser-Fleischer ring H18.04- ☑
    pigmentation — see Pigmentation, cornea
  crystalline, vitreous (body) (humor) H43.2- ☑
  hemosiderin in old scars of cornea — see Pigmentation, cornea, stromal
  metallic in lens — see Cataract, specified NEC
  skin R23.8
  tooth, teeth (betel) (black) (green) (materia alba) (orange) (tobacco) K03.6
  urate, kidney — see Calculus, kidney
Depraved appetite — see Pica
Depressed
  HDL cholesterol E78.6
Depression (acute) (mental) F32.9
  agitated (single episode) F32.2
  anaclitic — see Disorder, adjustment
  anxiety F41.8
    persistent F34.1
  arches (see also Deformity, limb, flat foot)
  atypical (single episode) F32.89
    recurrent episode F33.8
  basal metabolic rate R94.8
  bone marrow D75.89
  central nervous system R09.2
  cerebral R29.818
    newborn P91.4
  cerebrovascular I67.9
  chest wall M95.4
  climacteric (single episode) F32.89
    recurrent episode F33.8
  endogenous (without psychotic symptoms) F33.2
    with psychotic symptoms F33.3
  functional activity R68.89
  hysterical F44.89
  involutional (single episode) F32.89
    recurrent episode F33.8
  major F32.9
    with psychotic symptoms F32.3
    recurrent — see Disorder, depressive, recurrent
  manic-depressive — see Disorder, depressive, recurrent
  masked (single episode) F32.89
  medullary G93.89
  menopausal (single episode) F32.89
    recurrent episode F33.8
  metatarsus — see Depression, arches
  monopolar F33.9
  nervous F34.1
  neurotic F34.1
  nose M95.0
  postnatal F53
  postpartum F53
  post-psychotic of schizophrenia F32.89
  post-schizophrenic F32.89
  psychogenic (reactive) (single episode) F32.9
  psychoneurotic F34.1
  psychotic (single episode) F32.3
    recurrent F33.3
  reactive (psychogenic) (single episode) F32.9
    psychotic (single episode) F32.3
  recurrent — see Disorder, depressive, recurrent
  respiratory center G93.89
  seasonal — see Disorder, depressive, recurrent
  senile F03 ☑
  severe, single episode F32.2
  situational F43.21

Depression — continued
  skull Q67.4
  specified NEC (single episode) F32.89
  sternum M95.4
  visual field — see Defect, visual field
  vital (recurrent) (without psychotic symptoms) F33.2
    with psychotic symptoms F33.3
    single episode F32.2
Deprivation
  cultural Z60.3
  effects NOS T73.9 ☑
    specified NEC T73.8 ☑
  emotional NEC Z65.8
    affecting infant or child — see Maltreatment, child, psychological
  food T73.0 ☑
  protein — see Malnutrition
  sleep Z72.820
  social Z60.4
    affecting infant or child — see Maltreatment, child, psychological
  specified NEC T73.8 ☑
  vitamins — see Deficiency, vitamin
  water T73.1 ☑
Derangement
  ankle (internal) — see Derangement, joint, ankle
  cartilage (articular) NEC — see Derangement, joint, articular cartilage, by site
    recurrent — see Dislocation, recurrent
  cruciate ligament, anterior, current injury — see Sprain, knee, cruciate, anterior
  elbow (internal) — see Derangement, joint, elbow
  hip (joint) (internal) (old) — see Derangement, joint, hip
  joint (internal) M24.9
    ankylosis — see Ankylosis
    articular cartilage M24.10
      ankle M24.17- ☑
      elbow M24.12- ☑
      foot M24.17- ☑
      hand M24.14- ☑
      hip M24.15- ☑
      knee NEC M23.9- ☑
      loose body — see Loose, body
      shoulder M24.11- ☑
      wrist M24.13- ☑
    contracture — see Contraction, joint
    current injury (see also Dislocation)
      knee, meniscus or cartilage — see Tear, meniscus
    dislocation
      pathological — see Dislocation, pathological
      recurrent — see Dislocation, recurrent
    knee — see Derangement, knee
    ligament — see Disorder, ligament
    loose body — see Loose, body
    recurrent — see Dislocation, recurrent
    specified type NEC M24.80
      ankle M24.87- ☑
      elbow M24.82- ☑
      foot joint M24.87- ☑
      hand joint M24.84- ☑
      hip M24.85- ☑
      shoulder M24.81- ☑
      wrist M24.83- ☑
    temporomandibular M26.69
  knee (recurrent) M23.9- ☑
    ligament disruption, spontaneous M23.60- ☑
      anterior cruciate M23.61- ☑
      capsular M23.67- ☑
      instability, chronic M23.5- ☑
      lateral collateral M23.64- ☑
      medial collateral M23.63- ☑
      posterior cruciate M23.62- ☑
    loose body M23.4- ☑
    meniscus M23.30- ☑
      cystic M23.00- ☑
        lateral M23.002
          anterior horn M23.04- ☑
          posterior horn M23.05- ☑
          specified NEC M23.06- ☑
        medial M23.005
          anterior horn M23.01- ☑
          posterior horn M23.02- ☑
          specified NEC M23.03- ☑

☑ Additional Character Required — Refer to the Tabular List for Character Selection   ▽ Subterms under main terms may continue to next column or page

Derangement — *continued*
  knee — *continued*
    meniscus — *continued*
      degenerate — *see* Derangement, knee, meniscus, specified NEC
      detached — *see* Derangement, knee, meniscus, specified NEC
      due to old tear or injury M23.20- ☑
        lateral M23.20- ☑
          anterior horn M23.24- ☑
          posterior horn M23.25- ☑
          specified NEC M23.26- ☑
        medial M23.20- ☑
          anterior horn M23.21- ☑
          posterior horn M23.22- ☑
          specified NEC M23.23- ☑
      retained — *see* Derangement, knee, meniscus, specified NEC
      specified NEC M23.30- ☑
        lateral M23.30- ☑
          anterior horn M23.34- ☑
          posterior horn M23.35- ☑
          specified NEC M23.36- ☑
        medial M23.30- ☑
          anterior horn M23.31- ☑
          posterior horn M23.32- ☑
          specified NEC M23.33- ☑
    old M23.8X- ☑
    specified NEC — *see* subcategory M23.8
  low back NEC — *see* Dorsopathy, specified NEC
  meniscus — *see* Derangement, knee, meniscus
  mental — *see* Psychosis
  patella, specified NEC — *see* Disorder, patella, derangement NEC
  semilunar cartilage (knee) — *see* Derangement, knee, meniscus, specified NEC
  shoulder (internal) — *see* Derangement, joint, shoulder

Dercum's disease E88.2
Derealization (neurotic) F48.1
Dermal — *see* condition
Dermaphytid — *see* Dermatophytosis
Dermatitis (eczematous) L30.9
  ab igne L59.0
  acarine B88.0
  actinic (due to sun) L57.8
    other than from sun L59.8
  allergic — *see* Dermatitis, contact, allergic
  ambustionis, due to burn or scald — *see* Burn
  amebic A06.7
  ammonia L22
  arsenical (ingested) L27.8
  artefacta L98.1
    psychogenic F54
  atopic L20.9
    psychogenic F54
    specified NEC L20.89
  autoimmune progesterone L30.8
  berlock, berloque L56.2
  blastomycotic B40.3
  blister beetle L24.89
  bullous, bullosa L13.9
    mucosynechial, atrophic L12.1
    seasonal L30.8
    specified NEC L13.8
  calorica L59.0
    due to burn or scald — *see* Burn
  caterpillar L24.89
  cercarial B65.3
  combustionis L59.0
    due to burn or scald — *see* Burn
  congelationis T69.1 ☑
  contact (occupational) L25.9
    allergic L23.9
      due to
        adhesives L23.1
        cement L23.5
        chemical products NEC L23.5
        chromium L23.0
        cosmetics L23.2
        dander (cat) (dog) L23.81
        drugs in contact with skin L23.3
        dyes L23.4
        food in contact with skin L23.6
        hair (cat) (dog) L23.81
        insecticide L23.5
        metals L23.0

Dermatitis — *continued*
  contact — *continued*
    allergic — *continued*
      due to — *continued*
        nickel L23.0
        plants, non-food L23.7
        plastic L23.5
        rubber L23.5
        specified agent NEC L23.89
      due to
        cement L25.3
        chemical products NEC L25.3
        cosmetics L25.0
        dander (cat) (dog) L23.81
        drugs in contact with skin L25.1
        dyes L25.2
        food in contact with skin L25.4
        hair (cat) (dog) L23.81
        plants, non-food L25.5
        specified agent NEC L25.8
    irritant L24.9
      due to
        cement L24.5
        chemical products NEC L24.5
        cosmetics L24.3
        detergents L24.0
        drugs in contact with skin L24.4
        food in contact with skin L24.6
        oils and greases L24.1
        plants, non-food L24.7
        solvents L24.2
        specified agent NEC L24.89
  contusiformis L52
  diabetic — *see* E08-E13 with .620
  diaper L22
  diphtheritica A36.3
  dry skin L85.3
  due to
    acetone (contact) (irritant) L24.2
    acids (contact) (irritant) L24.5
    adhesive(s) (allergic) (contact) (plaster) L23.1
      irritant L24.5
    alcohol (irritant) (skin contact) (substances in category T51) L24.2
      taken internally L27.8
    alkalis (contact) (irritant) L24.5
    arsenic (ingested) L27.8
    carbon disulfide (contact) (irritant) L24.2
    caustics (contact) (irritant) L24.5
    cement (contact) L25.3
    cereal (ingested) L27.2
    chemical(s) NEC L25.3
      taken internally L27.8
    chlorocompounds L24.2
    chromium (contact) (irritant) L24.81
    coffee (ingested) L27.2
    cold weather L30.8
    cosmetics (contact) L25.0
      allergic L23.2
      irritant L24.3
    cyclohexanes L24.2
    dander (cat) (dog) L23.81
    Demodex species B88.0
    Dermanyssus gallinae B88.0
    detergents (contact) (irritant) L24.0
    dichromate L24.81
    drugs and medicaments (generalized) (internal use) L27.0
      external — *see* Dermatitis, due to, drugs, in contact with skin
      in contact with skin L25.1
        allergic L23.3
        irritant L24.4
      localized skin eruption L27.1
      specified substance — *see* Table of Drugs and Chemicals
    dyes (contact) L25.2
      allergic L23.4
      irritant L24.89
    epidermophytosis — *see* Dermatophytosis
    esters L24.2
    external irritant NEC L24.9
    fish (ingested) L27.2
    flour (ingested) L27.2
    food (ingested) L27.2
      in contact with skin L25.4
    fruit (ingested) L27.2
    furs (allergic) (contact) L23.81
    glues — *see* Dermatitis, due to, adhesives

Dermatitis — *continued*
  due to — *continued*
    glycols L24.2
    greases NEC (contact) (irritant) L24.1
    hair (cat) (dog) L23.81
    hot
      objects and materials — *see* Burn
      weather or places L59.0
    hydrocarbons L24.2
    infrared rays L59.8
    ingestion, ingested substance L27.9
      chemical NEC L27.8
      drugs and medicaments — *see* Dermatitis, due to, drugs
      food L27.2
      specified NEC L27.8
    insecticide in contact with skin L24.5
    internal agent L27.9
      drugs and medicaments (generalized) — *see* Dermatitis, due to, drugs
      food L27.2
    irradiation — *see* Dermatitis, due to, radioactive substance
    ketones L24.2
    lacquer tree (allergic) (contact) L23.7
    light (sun) NEC L57.8
      acute L56.8
      other L59.8
    Liponyssoides sanguineus B88.0
    low temperature L30.8
    meat (ingested) L27.2
    metals, metal salts (contact) (irritant) L24.81
    milk (ingested) L27.2
    nickel (contact) (irritant) L24.81
    nylon (contact) (irritant) L24.5
    oils NEC (contact) (irritant) L24.1
    paint solvent (contact) (irritant) L24.2
    petroleum products (contact) (irritant) (substances in T52.0) L24.2
    plants NEC (contact) L25.5
      allergic L23.7
      irritant L24.7
    plasters (adhesive) (any) (allergic) (contact) L23.1
      irritant L24.5
    plastic (contact) L25.3
    preservatives (contact) — *see* Dermatitis, due to, chemical, in contact with skin
    primrose (allergic) (contact) L23.7
    primula (allergic) (contact) L23.7
    radiation L59.8
      nonionizing (chronic exposure) L57.8
      sun NEC L57.8
        acute L56.8
    radioactive substance L58.9
      acute L58.0
      chronic L58.1
    radium L58.9
      acute L58.0
      chronic L58.1
    ragweed (allergic) (contact) L23.7
    Rhus (allergic) (contact) (diversiloba) (radicans) (toxicodendron) (venenata) (verniciflua) L23.7
    rubber (contact) L24.5
    Senecio jacobaea (allergic) (contact) L23.7
    solvents (contact) (irritant) (substances in category T52) L24.2
    specified agent NEC (contact) L25.8
      allergic L23.89
      irritant L24.89
    sunshine NEC L57.8
      acute L56.8
    tetrachlorethylene (contact) (irritant) L24.2
    toluene (contact) (irritant) L24.2
    turpentine (contact) L24.2
    ultraviolet rays (sun NEC) (chronic exposure) L57.8
      acute L56.8
    vaccine or vaccination L27.0
      specified substance — *see* Table of Drugs and Chemicals
    varicose veins — *see* Varix, leg, with, inflammation
    X-rays L58.9
      acute L58.0
      chronic L58.1
  dyshydrotic L30.1
  dysmenorrheica N94.6
  escharotica — *see* Burn
  exfoliative, exfoliativa (generalized) L26

Dermatitis — *continued*
  exfoliative, exfoliativa — *continued*
    neonatorum L00
  eyelid (*see also* Dermatosis, eyelid)
    allergic H01.119
      left H01.116
        lower H01.115
        upper H01.114
      right H01.113
        lower H01.112
        upper H01.111
    contact — *see* Dermatitis, eyelid, allergic
    due to
      Demodex species B88.0
      herpes (zoster) B02.39
        simplex B00.59
    eczematous H01.139
      left H01.136
        lower H01.135
        upper H01.134
      right H01.133
        lower H01.132
        upper H01.131
  facta, factitia, factitial L98.1
    psychogenic F54
  flexural NEC L20.82
  friction L30.4
  fungus B36.9
    specified type NEC B36.8
  gangrenosa, gangrenous infantum L08.0
  harvest mite B88.0
  heat L59.0
  herpesviral, vesicular (ear) (lip) B00.1
  herpetiformis (bullous) (erythematous) (pustular)
      (vesicular) L13.0
    juvenile L12.2
    senile L12.0
  hiemalis L30.8
  hypostatic, hypostatica — *see* Varix, leg, with, inflam-
      mation
  infectious eczematoid L30.3
  infective L30.3
  irritant — *see* Dermatitis, contact, irritant
  Jacquet's (diaper dermatitis) L22
  Leptus B88.0
  lichenified NEC L28.0
  medicamentosa (generalized) (internal use) — *see*
      Dermatitis, due to drugs
  mite B88.0
  multiformis L13.0
    juvenile L12.2
  napkin L22
  neurotica L13.0
  nummular L30.0
  papillaris capillitii L73.0
  pellagrous E52
  perioral L71.0
  photocontact L56.2
  polymorpha dolorosa L13.0
  pruriginosa L13.0
  pruritic NEC L30.8
  psychogenic F54
  purulent L08.0
  pustular
    contagious B08.02
    subcorneal L13.1
  pyococcal L08.0
  pyogenica L08.0
  repens L40.2
  Ritter's (exfoliativa) L00
  Schamberg's L81.7
  schistosome B65.3
  seasonal bullous L30.8
  seborrheic L21.9
    infantile L21.1
    specified NEC L21.8
  sensitization NOS L23.9
  septic L08.0
  solare L57.8
  specified NEC L30.8
  stasis I87.2
    with
      varicose ulcer — *see* Varix, leg, with ulcer, with
        inflammation
      varicose veins — *see* Varix, leg, with, inflamma-
        tion
    due to postthrombotic syndrome — *see* Syndrome,
        postthrombotic

Dermatitis — *continued*
  suppurative L08.0
  traumatic NEC L30.4
  trophoneurotica L13.0
  ultraviolet (sun) (chronic exposure) L57.8
    acute L56.8
  varicose — *see* Varix, leg, with, inflammation
  vegetans L10.1
  verrucosa B43.0
  vesicular, herpesviral B00.1
Dermatoarthritis, lipoid E78.81
Dermatochalasis, eyelid H02.839
  left H02.836
    lower H02.835
    upper H02.834
  right H02.833
    lower H02.832
    upper H02.831
Dermatofibroma (lenticulare) — *see* Neoplasm, skin,
    benign
  protuberans — *see* Neoplasm, skin, uncertain behavior
Dermatofibrosarcoma (pigmented) (protuberans) —
    see Neoplasm, skin, malignant
Dermatographia L50.3
Dermatolysis (exfoliativa) (congenital) Q82.8
  acquired L57.4
  eyelids — *see* Blepharochalasis
  palpebrarum — *see* Blepharochalasis
  senile L57.4
Dermatomegaly NEC Q82.8
Dermatomucosomyositis M33.10
  with
    myopathy M33.12
    respiratory involvement M33.11
    specified organ involvement NEC M33.19
Dermatomycosis B36.9
  furfuracea B36.0
  specified type NEC B36.8
Dermatomyositis (acute) (chronic) (*see also* Der-
    matopolymyositis)
  adult (*see also* Dermatomyositis, specified NEC) M33.10
  in (due to) neoplastic disease (*see also* Neoplasm)
      D49.9 [M36.0]
  juvenile M33.00
    with
      myopathy M33.02
      respiratory involvement M33.01
      specified organ involvement NEC M33.09
    without myopathy M33.03
  specified NEC M33.10
    with
      myopathy M33.12
      respiratory involvement M33.11
      specified organ involvement NEC M33.19
    without myopathy M33.13
Dermatoneuritis of children — *see* Poisoning, mercury
Dermatophilosis A48.8
Dermatophytid L30.2
Dermatophytide — *see* Dermatophytosis
Dermatophytosis (epidermophyton) (infection) (Mi-
    crosporum) (tinea) (Trichophyton) B35.9
  beard B35.0
  body B35.4
  capitis B35.0
  corporis B35.4
  deep-seated B35.8
  disseminated B35.8
  foot B35.3
  granulomatous B35.8
  groin B35.6
  hand B35.2
  nail B35.1
  perianal (area) B35.6
  scalp B35.0
  specified NEC B35.8
Dermatopolymyositis M33.90
  with
    myopathy M33.92
    respiratory involvement M33.91
    specified organ involvement NEC M33.99
  without myopathy M33.93
  in neoplastic disease (*see also* Neoplasm)
      D49.9 [M36.0]
  juvenile M33.00
    with
      myopathy M33.02
      respiratory involvement M33.01
      specified organ involvement NEC M33.09

Dermatopolymyositis — *continued*
  specified NEC M33.10
    myopathy M33.12
    respiratory involvement M33.11
    specified organ involvement NEC M33.19
Dermatopolyneuritis — *see* Poisoning, mercury
Dermatorrhexis Q79.6
  acquired L57.4
Dermatosclerosis (*see also* Scleroderma)
  localized L94.0
Dermatosis L98.9
  Andrews' L08.89
  Bowen's — *see* Neoplasm, skin, in situ
  bullous L13.9
    specified NEC L13.8
  exfoliativa L26
  eyelid (noninfectious)
    dermatitis — *see* Dermatitis, eyelid
    discoid lupus erythematosus — *see* Lupus, erythe-
        matosus, eyelid
    xeroderma — *see* Xeroderma, acquired, eyelid
  factitial L98.1
  febrile neutrophilic L98.2
  gonococcal A54.89
  herpetiformis L13.0
    juvenile L12.2
  linear IgA L13.8
  menstrual NEC L98.8
  neutrophilic, febrile L98.2
  occupational — *see* Dermatitis, contact
  papulosa nigra L82.1
  pigmentary L81.9
    progressive L81.7
    Schamberg's L81.7
  psychogenic F54
  purpuric, pigmented L81.7
  pustular, subcorneal L13.1
  transient acantholytic L11.1
Dermographia, dermographism L50.3
Dermoid (cyst) (*see also* Neoplasm, benign, by site)
  with malignant transformation C56- ☑
  due to radiation (nonionizing) L57.8
Dermopathy
  infiltrative with thyrotoxicosis — *see* Thyrotoxicosis
  nephrogenic fibrosing L90.8
Dermophytosis — *see* Dermatophytosis
Descemetocele H18.73- ☑
Descemet's membrane — *see* condition
Descending — *see* condition
Descensus uteri — *see* Prolapse, uterus
Desert
  rheumatism B38.0
  sore — *see* Ulcer, skin
Desertion (newborn) — *see* Maltreatment
Desmoid (extra-abdominal) (tumor) — *see* Neoplasm,
    connective tissue, uncertain behavior
  abdominal D48.1
Despondency F32.9
Desquamation, skin R23.4
Destruction, destructive (*see also* Damage)
  articular facet (*see also* Derangement, joint, specified
      type NEC)
    knee M23.8X- ☑
    vertebra — *see* Spondylosis
  bone (*see also* Disorder, bone, specified type NEC)
    syphilitic A52.77
  joint (*see also* Derangement, joint, specified type NEC)
    sacroiliac M53.3
  rectal sphincter K62.89
  septum (nasal) J34.89
  tuberculous NEC — *see* Tuberculosis
  tympanum, tympanic membrane (nontraumatic) —
      see Disorder, tympanic membrane, specified
      NEC
  vertebral disc — *see* Degeneration, intervertebral disc
Destructiveness (*see also* Disorder, conduct)
  adjustment reaction — *see* Disorder, adjustment
Desultory labor O62.2
Detachment
  cartilage — *see* Sprain
  cervix, annular N88.8
    complicating delivery O71.3
  choroid (old) (postinfectional) (simple) (spontaneous)
      H31.40- ☑
    hemorrhagic H31.41- ☑
    serous H31.42- ☑
  ligament — *see* Sprain

☑ **Additional Character Required — Refer to the Tabular List for Character Selection**   ▽ **Subterms under main terms may continue to next column or page**

Detachment — *continued*
  meniscus (knee) (*see also* Derangement, knee, meniscus, specified NEC)
    current injury — *see* Tear, meniscus
    due to old tear or injury — *see* Derangement, knee, meniscus, due to old tear
  retina (without retinal break) (serous) H33.2- ☑
    with retinal:
      break H33.00- ☑
        giant H33.03- ☑
        multiple H33.02- ☑
        single H33.01- ☑
      dialysis H33.04- ☑
    pigment epithelium — *see* Degeneration, retina, separation of layers, pigment epithelium detachment
    rhegmatogenous — *see* Detachment, retina, with retinal, break
    specified NEC H33.8
    total H33.05- ☑
    traction H33.4- ☑
  vitreous (body) H43.81 ☑
Detergent asthma J69.8
Deterioration
  epileptic F06.8
  general physical R53.81
  heart, cardiac — *see* Degeneration, myocardial
  mental — *see* Psychosis
  myocardial, myocardium — *see* Degeneration, myocardial
  senile (simple) R54
Deuteranomaly (anomalous trichromat) H53.53
Deuteranopia (complete) (incomplete) H53.53
Development
  abnormal, bone Q79.9
  arrested R62.50
    bone — *see* Arrest, development or growth, bone
    child R62.50
    due to malnutrition E45
  defective, congenital (*see also* Anomaly, by site)
    cauda equina Q06.3
    left ventricle Q24.8
      in hypoplastic left heart syndrome Q23.4
    valve Q24.8
      pulmonary Q22.3
  delayed (*see also* Delay, development) R62.50
    arithmetical skills F81.2
    language (skills) (expressive) F80.1
    learning skill F81.9
    mixed skills F88
    motor coordination F82
    reading F81.0
    specified learning skill NEC F81.89
    speech F80.9
    spelling F81.81
    written expression F81.81
  imperfect, congenital (*see also* Anomaly, by site)
    heart Q24.9
    lungs Q33.6
  incomplete
    bronchial tree Q32.4
    organ or site not listed — *see* Hypoplasia, by site
    respiratory system Q34.9
  sexual, precocious NEC E30.1
  tardy, mental (*see also* Disability, intellectual) F79
Developmental — *see* condition
  testing, infant or child — *see* Examination, child
Devergie's disease (pityriasis rubra pilaris) L44.0
Deviation (in)
  conjugate palsy (eye) (spastic) H51.0
  esophagus (acquired) K22.8
  eye, skew H51.8
  midline (jaw) (teeth) (dental arch) M26.29
    specified site NEC — *see* Malposition
  nasal septum J34.2
    congenital Q67.4
  opening and closing of the mandible M26.53
  organ or site, congenital NEC — *see* Malposition, congenital
  septum (nasal) (acquired) J34.2
    congenital Q67.4
  sexual F65.9
    bestiality F65.89
    erotomania F52.8
    exhibitionism F65.2
    fetishism, fetishistic F65.0
      transvestism F65.1
    frotteurism F65.81

Deviation — *continued*
  sexual — *continued*
    masochism F65.51
    multiple F65.89
    necrophilia F65.89
    nymphomania F52.8
    pederosis F65.4
    pedophilia F65.4
    sadism, sadomasochism F65.52
    satyriasis F52.8
    specified type NEC F65.89
    transvestism F64.1
    voyeurism F65.3
  teeth, midline M26.29
  trachea J39.8
  ureter, congenital Q62.61
Device
  cerebral ventricle (communicating) in situ Z98.2
  contraceptive — *see* Contraceptive, device
  drainage, cerebrospinal fluid, in situ Z98.2
Devic's disease G36.0
Devil's
  grip B33.0
  pinches (purpura simplex) D69.2
Devitalized tooth K04.99
Devonshire colic — *see* Poisoning, lead
Dextraposition, aorta Q20.3
  in tetralogy of Fallot Q21.3
Dextrinosis, limit (debrancher enzyme deficiency) E74.03
Dextrocardia (true) Q24.0
  with
    complete transposition of viscera Q89.3
    situs inversus Q89.3
Dextrotransposition, aorta Q20.3
d-glycericacidemia E72.59
Dhat syndrome F48.8
Dhobi itch B35.6
Di George's syndrome D82.1
Di Guglielmo's disease C94.0- ☑
Diabetes, diabetic (mellitus) (sugar) E11.9
  with
    amyotrophy E11.44
    arthropathy NEC E11.618
    autonomic (poly)neuropathy E11.43
    cataract E11.36
    Charcot's joints E11.610
    chronic kidney disease E11.22
    circulatory complication NEC E11.59
    complication E11.8
      specified NEC E11.69
    dermatitis E11.620
    foot ulcer E11.621
    gangrene E11.52
    gastroparalysis E11.43
    gastroparesis E11.43
    glomerulonephrosis, intracapillary E11.21
    glomerulosclerosis, intercapillary E11.21
    hyperglycemia E11.65
    hyperosmolarity E11.00
      with coma E11.01
    hypoglycemia E11.649
      with coma E11.641
    ketoacidosis E11.10
      with coma E11.11
    kidney complications NEC E11.29
    Kimmelstiel-Wilson disease E11.21
    loss of protective sensation (LOPS) — *see* Diabetes, by type, with neuropathy
    mononeuropathy E11.41
    myasthenia E11.44
    necrobiosis lipoidica E11.620
    nephropathy E11.21
    neuralgia E11.42
    neurologic complication NEC E11.49
    neuropathic arthropathy E11.610
    neuropathy E11.40
    ophthalmic complication NEC E11.39
    oral complication NEC E11.638
    osteomyelitis E11.69
    periodontal disease E11.630
    peripheral angiopathy E11.51
      with gangrene E11.52
    polyneuropathy E11.42
    renal complication NEC E11.29
    renal tubular degeneration E11.29
    retinopathy E11.319
      with macular edema E11.311

Diabetes, diabetic — *continued*
  with — *continued*
    retinopathy — *continued*
      with macular edema — *continued*
        resolved following treatment E11.37 ☑
      nonproliferative E11.329 ☑
        with macular edema E11.321 ☑
        mild E11.329 ☑
          with macular edema E11.321 ☑
        moderate E11.339 ☑
          with macular edema E11.331 ☑
        severe E11.349 ☑
          with macular edema E11.341 ☑
      proliferative E11.359 ☑
        with
          combined traction retinal detachment and rhegmatogenous retinal detachment E11.354 ☑
          macular edema E11.351 ☑
          stable proliferative diabetic retinopathy E11.355 ☑
          traction retinal detachment involving the macula E11.352 ☑
          traction retinal detachment not involving the macula E11.353 ☑
    skin complication NEC E11.628
    skin ulcer NEC E11.622
  brittle — *see* Diabetes, type 1
  bronzed E83.110
  complicating pregnancy — *see* Pregnancy, complicated by, diabetes
  dietary counseling and surveillance Z71.3
  due to
    autoimmune process — *see* Diabetes, type 1
    immune mediated pancreatic islet beta-cell destruction — *see* Diabetes, type 1
  due to drug or chemical E09.9
    with
      amyotrophy E09.44
      arthropathy NEC E09.618
      autonomic (poly)neuropathy E09.43
      cataract E09.36
      Charcot's joints E09.610
      chronic kidney disease E09.22
      circulatory complication NEC E09.59
      complication E09.8
        specified NEC E09.69
      dermatitis E09.620
      foot ulcer E09.621
      gangrene E09.52
      gastroparalysis E09.43
      gastroparesis E09.43
      glomerulonephrosis, intracapillary E09.21
      glomerulosclerosis, intercapillary E09.21
      hyperglycemia E09.65
      hyperosmolarity E09.00
        with coma E09.01
      hypoglycemia E09.649
        with coma E09.641
      ketoacidosis E09.10
        with coma E09.11
      kidney complications NEC E09.29
      Kimmelstiel-Wilson disease E09.21
      mononeuropathy E09.41
      myasthenia E09.44
      necrobiosis lipoidica E09.620
      nephropathy E09.21
      neuralgia E09.42
      neurologic complication NEC E09.49
      neuropathic arthropathy E09.610
      neuropathy E09.40
      ophthalmic complication NEC E09.39
      oral complication NEC E09.638
      periodontal disease E09.630
      peripheral angiopathy E09.51
        with gangrene E09.52
      polyneuropathy E09.42
      renal complication NEC E09.29
      renal tubular degeneration E09.29
      retinopathy E09.319
        with macular edema E09.311
        nonproliferative E09.329 ☑
          with macular edema E09.321 ☑
          mild E09.329 ☑
            with macular edema E09.321 ☑
          moderate E09.339 ☑
            with macular edema E09.331 ☑
          severe E09.349 ☑

Diabetes, diabetic — *continued*
  due to drug or chemical — *continued*
    with — *continued*
      retinopathy — *continued*
        nonproliferative — *continued*
          severe — *continued*
            with macular edema E09.341 ☑
        proliferative E09.359 ☑
          with
            combined traction retinal detachment and rhegmatogenous retinal detachment E09.354 ☑
            macular edema E09.351 ☑
            stable proliferative diabetic retinopathy E09.355 ☑
            traction retinal detachment involving the macula E09.352 ☑
            traction retinal detachment not involving the macula E09.353 ☑
        resolved following treatment E09.37 ☑
      skin complication NEC E09.628
      skin ulcer NEC E09.622
  due to underlying condition E08.9
    with
      amyotrophy E08.44
      arthropathy NEC E08.618
      autonomic (poly)neuropathy E08.43
      cataract E08.36
      Charcot's joints E08.610
      chronic kidney disease E08.22
      circulatory complication NEC E08.59
      complication E08.8
        specified NEC E08.69
      dermatitis E08.620
      foot ulcer E08.621
      gangrene E08.52
      gastroparalysis E08.43
      gastroparesis E08.43
      glomerulonephrosis, intracapillary E08.21
      glomerulosclerosis, intercapillary E08.21
      hyperglycemia E08.65
      hyperosmolarity E08.00
        with coma E08.01
      hypoglycemia E08.649
        with coma E08.641
      ketoacidosis E08.10
        with coma E08.11
      kidney complications NEC E08.29
      Kimmelsteil-Wilson disease E08.21
      mononeuropathy E08.41
      myasthenia E08.44
      necrobiosis lipoidica E08.620
      nephropathy E08.21
      neuralgia E08.42
      neurologic complication NEC E08.49
      neuropathic arthropathy E08.610
      neuropathy E08.40
      ophthalmic complication NEC E08.39
      oral complication NEC E08.638
      periodontal disease E08.630
      peripheral angiopathy E08.51
        with gangrene E08.52
      polyneuropathy E08.42
      renal complication NEC E08.29
      renal tubular degeneration E08.29
      retinopathy E08.319
        with macular edema E08.311
        nonproliferative E08.329 ☑
          with macular edema E08.321 ☑
          mild E08.329 ☑
            with macular edema E08.321 ☑
          moderate E08.339 ☑
            with macular edema E08.331 ☑
          severe E08.349 ☑
            with macular edema E08.341 ☑
        proliferative E08.359 ☑
          with
            combined traction retinal detachment and rhegmatogenous retinal detachment E08.354 ☑
            macular edema E08.351 ☑
            stable proliferative diabetic retinopathy E08.355 ☑
            traction retinal detachment involving the macula E08.352 ☑
            traction retinal detachment not involving the macula E08.353 ☑
        resolved following treatment E08.37 ☑

Diabetes, diabetic — *continued*
  due to underlying condition — *continued*
    with — *continued*
      skin complication NEC E08.628
      skin ulcer NEC E08.622
  gestational (in pregnancy) O24.419
    affecting newborn P70.0
    diet controlled O24.410
    in childbirth O24.429
      diet controlled O24.420
      insulin (and diet) controlled O24.424
      oral drug controlled (antidiabetic) (hypoglycemic) O24.425
    insulin (and diet) controlled O24.414
    oral drug controlled (antidiabetic) (hypoglycemic) O24.415
    puerperal O24.439
      diet controlled O24.430
      insulin (and diet) controlled O24.434
      oral drug controlled (antidiabetic) (hypoglycemic) O24.435
  hepatogenous E13.9
  idiopathic — *see* Diabetes, type 1
  inadequately controlled — *code to* Diabetes, by type, with hyperglycemia
  insipidus E23.2
    nephrogenic N25.1
    pituitary E23.2
    vasopressin resistant N25.1
  insulin dependent — *code to* type of diabetes
  juvenile-onset — *see* Diabetes, type 1
  ketosis-prone — *see* Diabetes, type 1
  latent R73.03
  neonatal (transient) P70.2
  non-insulin dependent — *code to* type of diabetes
  out of control — *code to* Diabetes, by type, with hyperglycemia
  phosphate E83.39
  poorly controlled — *code to* Diabetes, by type, with hyperglycemia
  postpancreatectomy — *see* Diabetes, specified type NEC
  postprocedural — *see* Diabetes, specified type NEC
  secondary diabetes mellitus NEC — *see* Diabetes, specified type NEC
  specified type NEC E13.9
    with
      amyotrophy E13.44
      arthropathy NEC E13.618
      autonomic (poly)neuropathy E13.43
      cataract E13.36
      Charcot's joints E13.610
      chronic kidney disease E13.22
      circulatory complication NEC E13.59
      complication E13.8
        specified NEC E13.69
      dermatitis E13.620
      foot ulcer E13.621
      gangrene E13.52
      gastroparalysis E13.43
      gastroparesis E13.43
      glomerulonephrosis, intracapillary E13.21
      glomerulosclerosis, intercapillary E13.21
      hyperglycemia E13.65
      hyperosmolarity E13.00
        with coma E13.01
      hypoglycemia E13.649
        with coma E13.641
      ketoacidosis E13.10
        with coma E13.11
      kidney complications NEC E13.29
      Kimmelsteil-Wilson disease E13.21
      mononeuropathy E13.41
      myasthenia E13.44
      necrobiosis lipoidica E13.620
      nephropathy E13.21
      neuralgia E13.42
      neurologic complication NEC E13.49
      neuropathic arthropathy E13.610
      neuropathy E13.40
      ophthalmic complication NEC E13.39
      oral complication NEC E13.638
      periodontal disease E13.630
      peripheral angiopathy E13.51
        with gangrene E13.52
      polyneuropathy E13.42
      renal complication NEC E13.29
      renal tubular degeneration E13.29

Diabetes, diabetic — *continued*
  specified type — *continued*
    with — *continued*
      retinopathy E13.319
        with macular edema E13.311
        nonproliferative E13.329 ☑
          with macular edema E13.321 ☑
          mild E13.329 ☑
            with macular edema E13.321 ☑
          moderate E13.339 ☑
            with macular edema E13.331 ☑
          severe E13.349 ☑
            with macular edema E13.341 ☑
        proliferative E13.359 ☑
          with
            combined traction retinal detachment and rhegmatogenous retinal detachment E13.354 ☑
            macular edema E13.351 ☑
            stable proliferative diabetic retinopathy E13.355 ☑
            traction retinal detachment involving the macula E13.352 ☑
            traction retinal detachment not involving the macula E13.353 ☑
        resolved following treatment E13.37 ☑
      skin complication NEC E13.628
      skin ulcer NEC E13.622
  steroid-induced — *see* Diabetes, due to, drug or chemical
  type 1 E10.9
    with
      amyotrophy E10.44
      arthropathy NEC E10.618
      autonomic (poly)neuropathy E10.43
      cataract E10.36
      Charcot's joints E10.610
      chronic kidney disease E10.22
      circulatory complication NEC E10.59
      complication E10.8
        specified NEC E10.69
      dermatitis E10.620
      foot ulcer E10.621
      gangrene E10.52
      gastroparalysis E10.43
      gastroparesis E10.43
      glomerulonephrosis, intracapillary E10.21
      glomerulosclerosis, intercapillary E10.21
      hyperglycemia E10.65
      hypoglycemia E10.649
        with coma E10.641
      ketoacidosis E10.10
        with coma E10.11
      kidney complications NEC E10.29
      Kimmelsteil-Wilson disease E10.21
      mononeuropathy E10.41
      myasthenia E10.44
      necrobiosis lipoidica E10.620
      nephropathy E10.21
      neuralgia E10.42
      neurologic complication NEC E10.49
      neuropathic arthropathy E10.610
      neuropathy E10.40
      ophthalmic complication NEC E10.39
      oral complication NEC E10.638
      osteomyelitis E10.69
      periodontal disease E10.630
      peripheral angiopathy E10.51
        with gangrene E10.52
      polyneuropathy E10.42
      renal complication NEC E10.29
      renal tubular degeneration E10.29
      retinopathy E10.319
        with macular edema E10.311
        nonproliferative E10.329 ☑
          with macular edema E10.321 ☑
          mild E10.329 ☑
            with macular edema E10.321 ☑
          moderate E10.339 ☑
            with macular edema E10.331 ☑
          severe E10.349 ☑
            with macular edema E10.341 ☑
        proliferative E10.359 ☑
          with
            combined traction retinal detachment and rhegmatogenous retinal detachment E10.354 ☑
            macular edema E10.351 ☑

☑ Additional Character Required — Refer to the Tabular List for Character Selection   ▽ Subterms under main terms may continue to next column or page

Diabetes, diabetic — *continued*
  type 1 — *continued*
    with — *continued*
      retinopathy — *continued*
        proliferative — *continued*
          with — *continued*
            stable proliferative diabetic
              retinopathy E10.355 ☑
            traction retinal detachment involving
              the macula E10.352 ☑
            traction retinal detachment not in-
              volving the macula E10.353 ☑
        resolved following treatment E10.37 ☑
      skin complication NEC E10.628
      skin ulcer NEC E10.622
  type 2 E11.9
    with
      amyotrophy E11.44
      arthropathy NEC E11.618
      autonomic (poly)neuropathy E11.43
      cataract E11.36
      Charcot's joints E11.610
      chronic kidney disease E11.22
      circulatory complication NEC E11.59
      complication E11.8
        specified NEC E11.69
      dermatitis E11.620
      foot ulcer E11.621
      gangrene E11.52
      gastroparalysis E11.43
      gastroparesis E11.43
      glomerulonephrosis, intracapillary E11.21
      glomerulosclerosis, intercapillary E11.21
      hyperglycemia E11.65
      hyperosmolarity E11.00
        with coma E11.01
      hypoglycemia E11.649
        with coma E11.641
      ketoacidosis E11.10
        with coma E11.11
      kidney complications NEC E11.29
      Kimmelstiel-Wilson disease E11.21
      mononeuropathy E11.41
      myasthenia E11.44
      necrobiosis lipoidica E11.620
      nephropathy E11.21
      neuralgia E11.42
      neurologic complication NEC E11.49
      neuropathic arthropathy E11.610
      neuropathy E11.40
      ophthalmic complication NEC E11.39
      oral complication NEC E11.638
      osteomyelitis E11.69
      periodontal disease E11.630
      peripheral angiopathy E11.51
        with gangrene E11.52
      polyneuropathy E11.42
      renal complication NEC E11.29
      renal tubular degeneration E11.29
      retinopathy E11.319
        with macular edema E11.311
        nonproliferative E11.329 ☑
          with macular edema E11.321 ☑
          mild E11.329 ☑
            with macular edema E11.321 ☑
          moderate E11.339 ☑
            with macular edema E11.331 ☑
          severe E11.349 ☑
            with macular edema E11.341 ☑
        proliferative E11.359 ☑
          with
            combined traction retinal detach-
              ment and rhegmatogenous
              retinal detachment E11.354 ☑
            macular edema E11.351 ☑
            stable proliferative diabetic
              retinopathy E11.355 ☑
            traction retinal detachment involving
              the macula E11.352 ☑
            traction retinal detachment not in-
              volving the macula E11.353 ☑
        resolved following treatment E11.37 ☑
      skin complication NEC E11.628
      skin ulcer NEC E11.622
  uncontrolled
    meaning
      hyperglycemia — *see* Diabetes, by type, with,
        hyperglycemia

Diabetes, diabetic — *continued*
  uncontrolled — *continued*
    meaning — *continued*
      hypoglycemia — *see* Diabetes, by type, with,
        hypoglycemia
Diacyclothrombopathia D69.1
Diagnosis deferred R69
Dialysis (intermittent) (treatment)
  noncompliance (with) Z91.15
  renal (hemodialysis) (peritoneal), status Z99.2
  retina, retinal — *see* Detachment, retina, with retinal,
    dialysis
Diamond-Blackfan anemia (congenital hypoplastic)
  D61.01
Diamond-Gardener syndrome (autoerythrocyte sensi-
  tization) D69.2
Diaper rash L22
Diaphoresis (excessive) R61
Diaphragm — *see* condition
Diaphragmalgia R07.1
Diaphragmatitis, diaphragmitis J98.6
Diaphysial aclasis Q78.6
Diaphysitis — *see* Osteomyelitis, specified type NEC
Diarrhea, diarrheal (disease) (infantile) (inflammatory)
  R19.7
  achlorhydric K31.83
  allergic K52.29
    due to
      colitis — *see* Colitis, allergic
      enteritis — *see* Enteritis, allergic
  amebic (*see also* Amebiasis) A06.0
    with abscess — *see* Abscess, amebic
    acute A06.0
    chronic A06.1
    nondysenteric A06.2
  bacillary — *see* Dysentery, bacillary
  balantidial A07.0
  cachectic NEC K52.89
  Chilomastix A07.8
  choleriformis A00.1
  chronic (noninfectious) K52.9
  coccidial A07.3
  Cochin-China K90.1
    strongyloidiasis B78.0
  Dientamoeba A07.8
  dietetic (*see also* Diarrhea, allergic) K52.29
  drug-induced K52.1
  due to
    bacteria A04.9
      specified NEC A04.8
    Campylobacter A04.5
    Capillaria philippinensis B81.1
    Clostridium difficile
      not specified as recurrent A04.72
      recurrent A04.71
    Clostridium perfringens (C) (F) A04.8
    Cryptosporidium A07.2
    drugs K52.1
    Escherichia coli A04.4
      enteroaggregative A04.4
      enterohemorrhagic A04.3
      enteroinvasive A04.2
      enteropathogenic A04.0
      enterotoxigenic A04.1
      specified NEC A04.4
    food hypersensitivity (*see also* Diarrhea, allergic)
      K52.29
    Necator americanus B76.1
    S. japonicum B65.2
    specified organism NEC A08.8
      bacterial A04.8
      viral A08.39
    Staphylococcus A04.8
    Trichuris trichiuria B79
    virus — *see* Enteritis, viral
    Yersinia enterocolitica A04.6
  dysenteric A09
  endemic A09
  epidemic A09
  flagellate A07.9
  Flexner's (ulcerative) A03.1
  functional K59.1
    following gastrointestinal surgery K91.89
    psychogenic F45.8
  Giardia lamblia A07.1
  giardial A07.1
  hill K90.1
  infectious A09

Diarrhea, diarrheal — *continued*
  malarial — *see* Malaria
  mite B88.0
  mycotic NEC B49
  neonatal (noninfectious) P78.3
  nervous F45.8
  neurogenic K59.1
  noninfectious K52.9
  postgastrectomy K91.1
  postvagotomy K91.1
  protozoal A07.9
    specified NEC A07.8
  psychogenic F45.8
  specified
    bacterium NEC A04.8
    virus NEC A08.39
  strongyloidiasis B78.0
  toxic K52.1
  trichomonal A07.8
  tropical K90.1
  tuberculous A18.32
  viral — *see* Enteritis, viral
Diastasis
  cranial bones M84.88
    congenital NEC Q75.8
  joint (traumatic) — *see* Dislocation
  muscle M62.00
    ankle M62.07- ☑
    congenital Q79.8
    foot M62.07- ☑
    forearm M62.03- ☑
    hand M62.04- ☑
    lower leg M62.06- ☑
    pelvic region M62.05- ☑
    shoulder region M62.01- ☑
    specified site NEC M62.08
    thigh M62.05- ☑
    upper arm M62.02- ☑
  recti (abdomen)
    complicating delivery O71.89
    congenital Q79.59
Diastema, tooth, teeth, fully erupted M26.32
Diastematomyelia Q06.2
Diataxia, cerebral G80.4
Diathesis
  allergic — *see* History, allergy
  bleeding (familial) D69.9
  cystine (familial) E72.00
  gouty — *see* Gout
  hemorrhagic (familial) D69.9
    newborn NEC P53
  spasmophilic R29.0
Diaz's disease or osteochondrosis (juvenile) (talus) —
  see Osteochondrosis, juvenile, tarsus
Dibothriocephalus, dibothriocephaliasis (latus) (infection) (infestation) B70.0
  larval B70.1
Dicephalus, dicephaly Q89.4
Dichotomy, teeth K00.2
Dichromat, dichromatopsia (congenital) — *see* Deficiency, color vision
Dichuchwa A65
Dicroceliasis B66.2
Didelphia, didelphys — *see* Double uterus
Didymytis N45.1
  with orchitis N45.3
Dietary
  inadequacy or deficiency E63.9
  surveillance and counseling Z71.3
Dietl's crisis N13.8
Dieulafoy lesion (hemorrhagic)
  duodenum K31.82
  esophagus K22.8
  intestine (colon) K63.81
  stomach K31.82
Difficult, difficulty (in)
  acculturation Z60.3
  feeding R63.3
    newborn P92.9
      breast P92.5
      specified NEC P92.8
    nonorganic (infant or child) F98.29
  intubation, in anesthesia T88.4 ☑
  mechanical, gastroduodenal stoma K91.89
    causing obstruction (*see also* Obstruction, intestine,
      postoperative) K91.30
  micturition
    need to immediately re-void R39.191

Index

Difficult, difficulty — Disease, diseased

Difficult, difficulty — continued
  micturition — continued
    position dependent R39.192
    specified NEC R39.198
  reading (developmental) F81.0
    secondary to emotional disorders F93.9
  spelling (specific) F81.81
    with reading disorder F81.89
    due to inadequate teaching Z55.8
  swallowing — see Dysphagia
  walking R26.2
  work
    conditions NEC Z56.5
    schedule Z56.3
Diffuse — see condition
Digestive — see condition
Dihydropyrimidine dehydrogenase disease (DPD) E88.89
Diktyoma — see Neoplasm, malignant, by site
Dilaceration, tooth K00.4
Dilatation
  anus K59.8
    venule — see Hemorrhoids
  aorta (focal) (general) — see Ectasia, aorta
    with aneuysm — see Aneurysm, aorta
    congenital Q25.44
  artery — see Aneurysm
  bladder (sphincter) N32.89
    congenital Q64.79
  blood vessel I99.8
  bronchial J47.9
    with
      exacerbation (acute) J47.1
      lower respiratory infection J47.0
  calyx (due to obstruction) — see Hydronephrosis
  capillaries I78.8
  cardiac (acute) (chronic) (see also Hypertrophy, cardiac)
    congenital Q24.8
      valve NEC Q24.8
        pulmonary Q22.3
    valve — see Endocarditis
  cavum septi pellucidi Q06.8
  cervix (uteri) (see also Incompetency, cervix)
    incomplete, poor, slow complicating delivery O62.0
  colon K59.39
    congenital Q43.1
    psychogenic F45.8
    toxic K59.31
  common duct (acquired) K83.8
    congenital Q44.5
  cystic duct (acquired) K82.8
    congenital Q44.5
  duct, mammary — see Ectasia, mammary duct
  duodenum K59.8
  esophagus K22.8
    congenital Q39.5
    due to achalasia K22.0
  eustachian tube, congenital Q17.8
  gallbladder K82.8
  gastric — see Dilatation, stomach
  heart (acute) (chronic) (see also Hypertrophy, cardiac)
    congenital Q24.8
    valve — see Endocarditis
  ileum K59.8
    psychogenic F45.8
  jejunum K59.8
    psychogenic F45.8
  kidney (calyx) (collecting structures) (cystic) (parenchyma) (pelvis) (idiopathic) N28.89
  lacrimal passages or duct — see Disorder, lacrimal system, changes
  lymphatic vessel I89.8
  mammary duct — see Ectasia, mammary duct
  Meckel's diverticulum (congenital) Q43.0
    malignant — see Table of Neoplasms, small intestine, malignant
  myocardium (acute) (chronic) — see Hypertrophy, cardiac
  organ or site, congenital NEC — see Distortion
  pancreatic duct K86.89
  pericardium — see Pericarditis
  pharynx J39.2
  prostate N42.89
  pulmonary
    artery (idiopathic) I28.8
    valve, congenital Q22.3
  pupil H57.04
  rectum K59.39

Dilatation — continued
  saccule, congenital Q16.5
  salivary gland (duct) K11.8
  sphincter ani K62.89
  stomach K31.89
    acute K31.0
    psychogenic F45.8
  submaxillary duct K11.8
  trachea, congenital Q32.1
  ureter (idiopathic) N28.82
    congenital Q62.2
    due to obstruction N13.4
  urethra (acquired) N36.8
  vasomotor I73.9
  vein I86.8
  ventricular, ventricle (acute) (chronic) (see also Hypertrophy, cardiac)
    cerebral, congenital Q04.8
  venule NEC I86.8
  vesical orifice N32.89
Dilated, dilation — see Dilatation
Diminished, diminution
  hearing (acuity) — see Deafness
  sense or sensation (cold) (heat) (tactile) (vibratory) R20.8
  vision NEC H54.7
  vital capacity R94.2
Diminuta taenia B71.0
Dimitri-Sturge-Weber disease Q85.8
Dimple
  congenital sacral Q82.6
  parasacral Q82.6
  pilonidal or postanal — see Cyst, pilonidal
Dioctophyme renalis (infection) (infestation) B83.8
Dipetalonemiasis B74.4
Diphallus Q55.69
Diphtheria, diphtheritic (gangrenous) (hemorrhagic) A36.9
  carrier (suspected) Z22.2
  cutaneous A36.3
  faucial A36.0
  infection of wound A36.3
  laryngeal A36.2
  myocarditis A36.81
  nasal, anterior A36.89
  nasopharyngeal A36.1
  neurological complication A36.89
  pharyngeal A36.0
  specified site NEC A36.89
  tonsillar A36.0
Diphyllobothriasis (intestine) B70.0
  larval B70.1
Diplacusis H93.22- ☑
Diplegia (upper limbs) G83.0
  congenital (cerebral) G80.8
  facial G51.0
  lower limbs G82.20
  spastic G80.1
Diplococcus, diplococcal — see condition
Diplopia H53.2
Dipsomania F10.20
  with
    psychosis — see Psychosis, alcoholic
    remission F10.21
Dipylidiasis B71.1
DIRA (deficiency of interleukin 1 receptor antagonist) M04.8
Direction, teeth, abnormal, fully erupted M26.30
Dirofilariasis B74.8
Dirt-eating child F98.3
Disability, disabilities
  heart — see Disease, heart
  intellectual F79
    with
      autistic features F84.9
    mild (I.Q. 50-69) F70
    moderate (I.Q. 35-49) F71
    profound (I.Q. under 20) F73
    severe (I.Q. 20-34) F72
    specified level NEC F78
  knowledge acquisition F81.9
  learning F81.9
  limiting activities Z73.6
  spelling, specific F81.81
Disappearance of family member Z63.4
Disarticulation — see Amputation
  meaning traumatic amputation — see Amputation, traumatic

Discharge (from)
  abnormal finding in — see Abnormal, specimen
  breast (female) (male) N64.52
  diencephalic autonomic idiopathic — see Epilepsy, specified NEC
  ear (see also Otorrhea)
    blood — see Otorrhagia
  excessive urine R35.8
  nipple N64.52
  penile R36.9
  postnasal R09.82
  prison, anxiety concerning Z65.2
  urethral R36.9
    without blood R36.0
    hematospermia R36.1
  vaginal N89.8
Discitis, diskitis M46.40
  cervical region M46.42
  cervicothoracic region M46.43
  lumbar region M46.46
  lumbosacral region M46.47
  multiple sites M46.49
  occipito-atlanto-axial region M46.41
  pyogenic — see Infection, intervertebral disc, pyogenic
  sacrococcygeal region M46.48
  thoracic region M46.44
  thoracolumbar region M46.45
Discoid
  meniscus (congenital) Q68.6
  semilunar cartilage (congenital) — see Derangement, knee, meniscus, specified NEC
Discoloration
  nails L60.8
  teeth (posteruptive) K03.7
    during formation K00.8
Discomfort
  chest R07.89
  visual H53.14- ☑
Discontinuity, ossicles, ear H74.2- ☑
Discord (with)
  boss Z56.4
  classmates Z55.4
  counselor Z64.4
  employer Z56.4
  family Z63.8
  fellow employees Z56.4
  in-laws Z63.1
  landlord Z59.2
  lodgers Z59.2
  neighbors Z59.2
  probation officer Z64.4
  social worker Z64.4
  teachers Z55.4
  workmates Z56.4
Discordant connection
  atrioventricular (congenital) Q20.5
  ventriculoarterial Q20.3
Discrepancy
  centric occlusion maximum intercuspation M26.55
  leg length (acquired) — see Deformity, limb, unequal length
    congenital — see Defect, reduction, lower limb
  uterine size date O26.84- ☑
Discrimination
  ethnic Z60.5
  political Z60.5
  racial Z60.5
  religious Z60.5
  sex Z60.5
Disease, diseased (see also Syndrome)
  absorbent system I87.8
  acid-peptic K30
  Acosta's T70.29 ☑
  Adams-Stokes (-Morgagni) (syncope with heart block) I45.9
  Addison's anemia (pernicious) D51.0
  adenoids (and tonsils) J35.9
  adrenal (capsule) (cortex) (gland) (medullary) E27.9
    hyperfunction E27.0
    specified NEC E27.8
  ainhum L94.6
  airway
    obstructive, chronic J44.9
      due to
        cotton dust J66.0
        specific organic dusts NEC J66.8
    reactive — see Asthma
  akamushi (scrub typhus) A75.3

Disease, diseased — continued
Albers-Schönberg (marble bones) Q78.2
Albert's — see Tendinitis, Achilles
alimentary canal K63.9
alligator-skin Q80.9
    acquired L85.0
alpha heavy chain C88.3
alpine T70.29 ☑
altitude T70.20 ☑
alveolar ridge
    edentulous K06.9
        specified NEC K06.8
alveoli, teeth K08.9
Alzheimer's G30.9 [F02.80]
    with behavioral disturbance G30.9 [F02.81]
    early onset G30.0 [F02.80]
        with behavioral disturbance G30.0 [F02.81]
    late onset G30.1 [F02.80]
        with behavioral disturbance G30.1 [F02.81]
    specified NEC G30.8 [F02.80]
        with behavioral disturbance G30.8 [F02.81]
amyloid — see Amyloidosis
Andersen's (glycogenosis IV) E74.09
Andes T70.29 ☑
Andrews' (bacterid) L08.89
angiospastic I73.9
    cerebral G45.9
    vein I87.8
anterior
    chamber H21.9
    horn cell G12.29
antiglomerular basement membrane (anti- GBM) anti-
        body M31.0
    tubulo-interstitial nephritis N12
antral — see Sinusitis, maxillary
anus K62.9
    specified NEC K62.89
aorta (nonsyphilitic) I77.9
    syphilitic NEC A52.02
aortic (heart) (valve) I35.9
    rheumatic I06.9
Apollo B30.3
aponeuroses — see Enthesopathy
appendix K38.9
    specified NEC K38.8
aqueous (chamber) H21.9
Arnold-Chiari — see Arnold-Chiari disease
arterial I77.9
    occlusive — see Occlusion, by site
        due to stricture or stenosis I77.1
arteriocardiorenal — see Hypertension, cardiorenal
arteriolar (generalized) (obliterative) I77.9
arteriorenal — see Hypertension, kidney
arteriosclerotic (see also Arteriosclerosis)
    cardiovascular — see Disease, heart, ischemic,
        atherosclerotic
    coronary (artery) — see Disease, heart, ischemic,
        atherosclerotic
    heart — see Disease, heart, ischemic, atherosclerot-
        ic
artery I77.9
    cerebral I67.9
    coronary I25.10
        with angina pectoris — see Arteriosclerosis,
            coronary (artery)
arthropod-borne NOS (viral) A94
    specified type NEC A93.8
atticoantral, chronic H66.20
    left H66.22
        with right H66.23
    right H66.21
        with left H66.23
auditory canal — see Disorder, ear, external
auricle, ear NEC — see Disorder, pinna
Australian X A83.4
autoimmune (systemic) NOS M35.9
    hemolytic (cold type) (warm type) D59.1
        drug-induced D59.0
    thyroid E06.3
aviator's — see Effect, adverse, high altitude
Ayerza's (pulmonary artery sclerosis with pulmonary
        hypertension) I27.0
Babington's (familial hemorrhagic telangiectasia) I78.0
bacterial A49.9
    specified NEC A48.8
    zoonotic A28.9
        specified type NEC A28.8
Baelz's (cheilitis glandularis apostematosa) K13.0

Disease, diseased — continued
bagasse J67.1
balloon — see Effect, adverse, high altitude
Bang's (brucella abortus) A23.1
Bannister's T78.3 ☑
barometer makers' — see Poisoning, mercury
Barraquer (-Simons') (progressive lipodystrophy) E88.1
Barrett's — see Barrett's, esophagus
Bartholin's gland N75.9
basal ganglia G25.9
    degenerative G23.9
        specified NEC G23.8
    specified NEC G25.89
Basedow's (exophthalmic goiter) — see Hyperthy-
        roidism, with, goiter (diffuse)
Bateman's B08.1
Batten-Steinert G71.11
Battey A31.0
Beard's (neurasthenia) F48.8
Becker
    idiopathic mural endomyocardial I42.3
    myotonia congenita G71.12
Begbie's (exophthalmic goiter) — see Hyperthy-
        roidism, with, goiter (diffuse)
behavioral, organic F07.9
Beigel's (white piedra) B36.2
Benson's — see Deposit, crystalline
Bernard-Soulier (thrombopathy) D69.1
Bernhardt (-Roth) — see Mononeuropathy, lower limb,
        meralgia paresthetica
Biermer's (pernicious anemia) D51.0
bile duct (common) (hepatic) K83.9
    with calculus, stones — see Calculus, bile duct
        specified NEC K83.8
biliary (tract) K83.9
    specified NEC K83.8
Billroth's — see Spina bifida
bird fancier's J67.2
black lung J60
bladder N32.9
    in (due to)
        schistosomiasis (bilharziasis) B65.0 [N33]
    specified NEC N32.89
bleeder's D66
blood D75.9
    forming organs D75.9
    vessel I99.9
Bloodgood's — see Mastopathy, cystic
Bodechtel-Guttmann (subacute sclerosing panen-
        cephalitis) A81.1
bone (see also Disorder, bone)
    aluminum M83.4
    fibrocystic NEC
        jaw M27.49
bone-marrow D75.9
Borna A83.9
Bornholm (epidemic pleurodynia) B33.0
Bouchard's (myopathic dilatation of the stomach)
        K31.0
Bourneville (-Brissaud) (tuberous sclerosis) Q85.1
Bouveret (-Hoffmann) (paroxysmal tachycardia) I47.9
bowel K63.9
    functional K59.9
        psychogenic F45.8
brain G93.9
    arterial, artery I67.9
    arteriosclerotic I67.2
    congenital Q04.9
    degenerative — see Degeneration, brain
    inflammatory — see Encephalitis
    organic G93.9
        arteriosclerotic I67.2
    parasitic NEC B71.9 [G94]
    senile NEC G31.1
    specified NEC G93.89
breast (see also Disorder, breast) N64.9
    cystic (chronic) — see Mastopathy, cystic
    fibrocystic — see Mastopathy, cystic
    Paget's
        female, unspecified side C50.91- ☑
        male, unspecified side C50.92- ☑
    specified NEC N64.89
Breda's — see Yaws
Bretonneau's (diphtheritic malignant angina) A36.0
Bright's — see Nephritis
    arteriosclerotic — see Hypertension, kidney
Brill's (recrudescent typhus) A75.1

Disease, diseased — continued
Brill-Zinsser (recrudescent typhus) A75.1
Brion-Kayser — see Fever, paratyphoid
broad
    beta E78.2
    ligament (noninflammatory) N83.9
        inflammatory — see Disease, pelvis, inflamma-
            tory
        specified NEC N83.8
Brocq-Duhring (dermatitis herpetiformis) L13.0
Brocq's
    meaning
        dermatitis herpetiformis L13.0
        prurigo L28.2
bronchopulmonary J98.4
bronchus NEC J98.09
bronze Addison's E27.1
    tuberculous A18.7
budgerigar fancier's J67.2
Buerger's (thromboangiitis obliterans) I73.1
bullous L13.9
    chronic of childhood L12.2
    specified NEC L13.8
Bürger-Grütz (essential familial hyperlipemia) E78.3
bursa — see Bursopathy
caisson T70.3 ☑
California — see Coccidioidomycosis
capillaries I78.9
    specified NEC I78.8
Carapata A68.0
cardiac — see Disease, heart
cardiopulmonary, chronic I27.9
cardiorenal (hepatic) (hypertensive) (vascular) — see
        Hypertension, cardiorenal
cardiovascular (atherosclerotic) I25.10
    with angina pectoris — see Arteriosclerosis, coro-
        nary (artery),
    congenital Q28.9
    hypertensive — see Hypertension, heart
    newborn P29.9
        specified NEC P29.89
    renal (hypertensive) — see Hypertension, cardiore-
        nal
    syphilitic (asymptomatic) A52.00
cartilage — see Disorder, cartilage
Castellani's A69.8
Castleman (unicentric) (multicentric) D47.Z2
    HHV-8-associated (see also Herpesvirus, human, 8)
        D47.Z2
cat-scratch A28.1
Cavare's (familial periodic paralysis) G72.3
cecum K63.9
celiac (adult) (infantile) (with steatorrhea) K90.0
cellular tissue L98.9
central core G71.2
cerebellar, cerebellum — see Disease, brain
cerebral (see also Disease, brain)
    degenerative — see Degeneration, brain
cerebrospinal G96.9
cerebrovascular I67.9
    acute I67.89
        embolic I63.4- ☑
        thrombotic I63.3- ☑
    arteriosclerotic I67.2
    specified NEC I67.89
cervix (uteri) (noninflammatory) N88.9
    inflammatory — see Cervicitis
    specified NEC N88.8
Chabert's A22.9
Chandler's (osteochondritis dissecans, hip) — see Os-
        teochondritis, dissecans, hip
Charlouis — see Yaws
Chédiak-Steinbrinck (-Higashi) (congenital gigantism
        of peroxidase granules) E70.330
chest J98.9
Chiari's (hepatic vein thrombosis) I82.0
Chicago B40.9
Chignon B36.8
chigo, chigoe B88.1
childhood granulomatous D71
Chinese liver fluke B66.1
chlamydial A74.9
    specified NEC A74.89
cholecystic K82.9
choroid H31.9
    specified NEC H31.8
Christmas D67
chronic bullous of childhood L12.2

Index

Disease, diseased — Disease, diseased

Disease, diseased — *continued*
- chylomicron retention E78.3
- ciliary body H21.9
  - specified NEC H21.89
- circulatory (system) NEC I99.8
  - newborn P29.9
  - syphilitic A52.00
    - congenital A50.54
- coagulation factor deficiency (congenital) — *see* Defect, coagulation
- coccidioidal — *see* Coccidioidomycosis
- cold
  - agglutinin or hemoglobinuria D59.1
    - paroxysmal D59.6
  - hemagglutinin (chronic) D59.1
- collagen NOS (nonvascular) (vascular) M35.9
  - specified NEC M35.8
- colon K63.9
  - functional K59.9
    - congenital Q43.2
  - ischemic (*see also* Ischemia, intestine, acute) K55.039
- colonic inflammatory bowel, unclassified (IBDU) K52.3
- combined system — *see* Degeneration, combined
- compressed air T70.3 ☑
- Concato's (pericardial polyserositis) A19.9
  - nontubercular I31.1
  - pleural — *see* Pleurisy, with effusion
- conjunctiva H11.9
  - chlamydial A74.0
  - specified NEC H11.89
  - viral B30.9
    - specified NEC B30.8
- connective tissue, systemic (diffuse) M35.9
  - in (due to)
    - hypogammaglobulinemia D80.1 [M36.8]
    - ochronosis E70.29 [M36.8]
  - specified NEC M35.8
- Conor and Bruch's (boutonneuse fever) A77.1
- Cooper's — *see* Mastopathy, cystic
- Cori's (glycogenosis III) E74.03
- corkhandler's or corkworker's J67.3
- cornea H18.9
  - specified NEC H18.89- ☑
- coronary (artery) — *see* Disease, heart, ischemic, atherosclerotic
  - congenital Q24.5
  - ostial, syphilitic (aortic) (mitral) (pulmonary) A52.03
- corpus cavernosum N48.9
  - specified NEC N48.89
- Cotugno's — *see* Sciatica
- coxsackie (virus) NEC B34.1
- cranial nerve NOS G52.9
- Creutzfeldt-Jakob — *see* Creutzfeldt-Jakob disease or syndrome
- Crocq's (acrocyanosis) I73.89
- Crohn's — *see* Enteritis, regional
- Curschmann G71.11
- cystic
  - breast (chronic) — *see* Mastopathy, cystic
  - kidney, congenital Q61.9
  - liver, congenital Q44.6
  - lung J98.4
    - congenital Q33.0
- cytomegalic inclusion (generalized) B25.9
  - with pneumonia B25.0
  - congenital P35.1
- cytomegaloviral B25.9
  - specified NEC B25.8
- Czerny's (periodic hydrarthrosis of the knee) — *see* Effusion, joint, knee
- Daae (-Finsen) (epidemic pleurodynia) B33.0
- Darling's — *see* Histoplasmosis capsulati
- de Quervain's (tendon sheath) M65.4
  - thyroid (subacute granulomatous thyroiditis) E06.1
- Débove's (splenomegaly) R16.1
- deer fly — *see* Tularemia
- Degos' I77.89
- demyelinating, demyelinizating (nervous system) G37.9
  - multiple sclerosis G35
  - specified NEC G37.8
- dense deposit (*see also* N00-N07 with fourth character .6) N05.6
- deposition, hydroxyapatite — *see* Disease, hydroxyapatite deposition
- Devergie's (pityriasis rubra pilaris) L44.0
- Devic's G36.0

Disease, diseased — *continued*
- diaphorase deficiency D74.0
- diaphragm J98.6
- diarrheal, infectious NEC A09
- digestive system K92.9
  - specified NEC K92.89
- disc, degenerative — *see* Degeneration, intervertebral disc
- discogenic (*see also* Displacement, intervertebral disc NEC)
  - with myelopathy — *see* Disorder, disc, with, myelopathy
- diverticular — *see* Diverticula
- Dubois (thymus) A50.59 [E35]
- Duchenne-Griesinger G71.0
- Duchenne's
  - muscular dystrophy G71.0
  - pseudohypertrophy, muscles G71.0
- ductless glands E34.9
- Duhring's (dermatitis herpetiformis) L13.0
- duodenum K31.9
  - specified NEC K31.89
- Dupré's (meningism) R29.1
- Dupuytren's (muscle contracture) M72.0
- Durand-Nicholas-Favre (climatic bubo) A55
- Duroziez's (congenital mitral stenosis) Q23.2
- ear — *see* Disorder, ear
- Eberth's — *see* Fever, typhoid
- Ebola (virus) A98.4
- Ebstein's heart Q22.5
- echinococcus — *see* Echinococcus
- echovirus NEC B34.1
- Eddowes' (brittle bones and blue sclera) Q78.0
- edentulous (alveolar) ridge K06.9
  - specified NEC K06.8
- Edsall's T67.2 ☑
- Eichstedt's (pityriasis versicolor) B36.0
- Eisenmenger's (irreversible) I27.83
- Ellis-van Creveld (chondroectodermal dysplasia) Q77.6
- end stage renal (ESRD) N18.6
  - due to hypertension I12.0
- endocrine glands or system NEC E34.9
- endomyocardial (eosinophilic) I42.3
- English (rickets) E55.0
- enteroviral, enterovirus NEC B34.1
  - central nervous system NEC A88.8
- epidemic B99.9
  - specified NEC B99.8
- epididymis N50.9
- Erb (-Landouzy) G71.0
- Erdheim-Chester (ECD) E88.89
- esophagus K22.9
  - functional K22.4
  - psychogenic F45.8
  - specified NEC K22.8
- Eulenburg's (congenital paramyotonia) G71.19
- eustachian tube — *see* Disorder, eustachian tube
- external
  - auditory canal — *see* Disorder, ear, external
  - ear — *see* Disorder, ear, external
- extrapyramidal G25.9
  - specified NEC G25.89
- eye H57.9
  - anterior chamber H21.9
  - inflammatory NEC H57.8
  - muscle (external) — *see* Strabismus
  - specified NEC H57.8
  - syphilitic — *see* Oculopathy, syphilitic
- eyeball H44.9
  - specified NEC H44.89
- eyelid — *see* Disorder, eyelid
  - specified NEC — *see* Disorder, eyelid, specified type NEC
- eyeworm of Africa B74.3
- facial nerve (seventh) G51.9
  - newborn (birth injury) P11.3
- Fahr (of brain) G23.8
- Fahr Volhard (of kidney) I12.- ☑
- fallopian tube (noninflammatory) N83.9
  - inflammatory — *see* Salpingo-oophoritis
  - specified NEC N83.8
- familial periodic paralysis G72.3
- Fanconi's (congenital pancytopenia) D61.09
- fascia NEC — *see* Disorder, muscle
  - inflammatory — *see* Myositis
  - specified NEC M62.89
- Fauchard's (periodontitis) — *see* Periodontitis
- Favre-Durand-Nicolas (climatic bubo) A55

Disease, diseased — *continued*
- Fede's K14.0
- Feer's — *see* Poisoning, mercury
- female pelvic inflammatory (*see also* Disease, pelvis, inflammatory) N73.9
  - syphilitic (secondary) A51.42
  - tuberculous A18.17
- Fernels' (aortic aneurysm) I71.9
- fibrocaseous of lung — *see* Tuberculosis, pulmonary
- fibrocystic — *see* Fibrocystic disease
- Fiedler's (leptospiral jaundice) A27.0
- fifth B08.3
- file-cutter's — *see* Poisoning, lead
- fish-skin Q80.9
  - acquired L85.0
- Flajani (-Basedow) (exophthalmic goiter) — *see* Hyperthyroidism, with, goiter (diffuse)
- flax-dresser's J66.1
- fluke — *see* Infestation, fluke
- foot and mouth B08.8
- foot process N04.9
- Forbes' (glycogenosis III) E74.03
- Fordyce-Fox (apocrine miliaria) L75.2
- Fordyce's (ectopic sebaceous glands) (mouth) Q38.6
- Forestier's (rhizomelic pseudopolyarthritis) M35.3
  - meaning ankylosing hyperostosis — *see* Hyperostosis, ankylosing
- Fothergill's
  - neuralgia — *see* Neuralgia, trigeminal
  - scarlatina anginosa A38.9
- Fournier (gangrene) N49.3
  - female N76.89
- fourth B08.8
- Fox (-Fordyce) (apocrine miliaria) L75.2
- Francis' — *see* Tularemia
- Franklin C88.2
- Frei's (climatic bubo) A55
- Friedreich's
  - combined systemic or ataxia G11.1
  - myoclonia G25.3
- frontal sinus — *see* Sinusitis, frontal
- fungus NEC B49
- Gaisböck's (polycythemia hypertonica) D75.1
- gallbladder K82.9
  - calculus — *see* Calculus, gallbladder
  - cholecystitis — *see* Cholecystitis
  - cholesterolosis K82.4
  - fistula — *see* Fistula, gallbladder
  - hydrops K82.1
  - obstruction — *see* Obstruction, gallbladder
  - perforation K82.2
  - specified NEC K82.8
- gamma heavy chain C88.2
- Gamna's (siderotic splenomegaly) D73.2
- Gamstorp's (adynamia episodica hereditaria) G72.3
- Gandy-Nanta (siderotic splenomegaly) D73.2
- ganister J62.8
- gastric — *see* Disease, stomach
- gastroesophageal reflux (GERD) K21.9
  - with esophagitis K21.0
- gastrointestinal (tract) K92.9
  - amyloid E85.4
  - functional K59.9
    - psychogenic F45.8
  - specified NEC K92.89
- Gee (-Herter) (-Heubner) (-Thaysen) (nontropical sprue) K90.0
- genital organs
  - female N94.9
  - male N50.9
- Gerhardt's (erythromelalgia) I73.81
- Gibert's (pityriasis rosea) L42
- Gierke's (glycogenosis I) E74.01
- Gilles de la Tourette's (motor-verbal tic) F95.2
- gingiva K06.9
  - plaque induced K05.00
  - specified NEC K06.8
- gland (lymph) I89.9
- Glanzmann's (hereditary hemorrhagic thrombasthenia) D69.1
- glass-blower's (cataract) — *see* Cataract, specified NEC
  - salivary gland hypertrophy K11.1
- Glisson's — *see* Rickets
- globe H44.9
  - specified NEC H44.89
- glomerular (*see also* Glomerulonephritis)
  - with edema — *see* Nephrosis
  - acute — *see* Nephritis, acute

☑ **Additional Character Required** — Refer to the Tabular List for Character Selection ⓦ **Subterms under main terms may continue to next column or page**

Disease, diseased — *continued*

glomerular (*see also* Glomerulonephritis) — *continued*

  chronic — *see* Nephritis, chronic

  minimal change N05.0

  rapidly progressive N01.9

glycogen storage E74.00

  Andersen's E74.09

  Cori's E74.03

  Forbes' E74.03

  generalized E74.00

  glucose-6-phosphatase deficiency E74.01

  heart E74.02 [I43]

  hepatorenal E74.09

  Hers' E74.09

  liver and kidney E74.09

  McArdle's E74.04

  muscle phosphofructokinase E74.09

  myocardium E74.02 [I43]

  Pompe's E74.02

  Tauri's E74.09

  type 0 E74.09

  type I E74.01

  type II E74.02

  type III E74.03

  type IV E74.09

  type V E74.04

  type VI-XI E74.09

  Von Gierke's E74.01

Goldstein's (familial hemorrhagic telangiectasia) I78.0

gonococcal NOS A54.9

graft-versus-host (GVH) D89.813

  acute D89.810

  acute on chronic D89.812

  chronic D89.811

grainhandler's J67.8

granulomatous (childhood) (chronic) D71

Graves' (exophthalmic goiter) — *see* Hyperthyroidism, with, goiter (diffuse)

Griesinger's — *see* Ancylostomiasis

Grisel's M43.6

Gruby's (tinea tonsurans) B35.0

Guillain-Barré G61.0

Guinon's (motor-verbal tic) F95.2

gum K06.9

gynecological N94.9

H (Hartnup's) E72.02

Haff — *see* Poisoning, mercury

Hageman (congenital factor XII deficiency) D68.2

hair (color) (shaft) L67.9

  follicles L73.9

    specified NEC L73.8

Hamman's (spontaneous mediastinal emphysema) J98.2

hand, foot and mouth B08.4

Hansen's — *see* Leprosy

Hantavirus, with pulmonary manifestations B33.4

  with renal manifestations A98.5

Harada's H30.81- ☑

Hartnup (pellagra-cerebellar ataxia-renal aminoaciduria) E72.02

Hart's (pellagra-cerebellar ataxia-renal aminoaciduria) E72.02

Hashimoto's (struma lymphomatosa) E06.3

Hb — *see* Disease, hemoglobin

heart (organic) I51.9

  with

    pulmonary edema (acute) (*see also* Failure, ventricular, left) I50.1

    rheumatic fever (conditions in I00)

      active I01.9

        with chorea I02.0

        specified NEC I01.8

      inactive or quiescent (with chorea) I09.9

        specified NEC I09.89

  amyloid E85.4 [I43]

  aortic (valve) I35.9

  arteriosclerotic or sclerotic (senile) — *see* Disease, heart, ischemic, atherosclerotic

  artery, arterial — *see* Disease, heart, ischemic, atherosclerotic

  beer drinkers' I42.6

  beriberi (wet) E51.12

  black I27.0

  congenital Q24.9

    cyanotic Q24.9

    specified NEC Q24.8

  coronary — *see* Disease, heart, ischemic

Disease, diseased — *continued*

heart — *continued*

  cryptogenic I51.9

  fibroid — *see* Myocarditis

  functional I51.89

    psychogenic F45.8

  glycogen storage E74.02 [I43]

  gonococcal A54.83

  hypertensive — *see* Hypertension, heart

  hyperthyroid (*see also* Hyperthyroidism)

    E05.90 [I43]

    with thyroid storm E05.91 [I43]

  ischemic (chronic or with a stated duration of over 4 weeks) I25.9

    atherosclerotic (of) I25.10

      with angina pectoris — *see* Arteriosclerosis, coronary (artery)

      coronary artery bypass graft — *see* Arteriosclerosis, coronary (artery),

      cardiomyopathy I25.5

      diagnosed on ECG or other special investigation, but currently presenting no symptoms I25.6

    silent I25.6

    specified form NEC I25.89

  kyphoscoliotic I27.1

  meningococcal A39.50

    endocarditis A39.51

    myocarditis A39.52

    pericarditis A39.53

  mitral I05.9

    specified NEC I05.8

  muscular — *see* Degeneration, myocardial

  psychogenic (functional) F45.8

  pulmonary (chronic) I27.9

    in schistosomiasis B65.9 [I52]

    specified NEC I27.89

  rheumatic (chronic) (inactive) (old) (quiescent) (with chorea) I09.9

    active or acute I01.9

      with chorea (acute) (rheumatic) (Sydenham's) I02.0

    specified NEC I09.89

  senile — *see* Myocarditis

  syphilitic A52.06

    aortic A52.03

      aneurysm A52.01

    congenital A50.54 [I52]

  thyrotoxic (*see also* Thyrotoxicosis) E05.90 [I43]

    with thyroid storm E05.91 [I43]

  valve, valvular (obstructive) (regurgitant) (*see also* Endocarditis)

    congenital NEC Q24.8

    pulmonary Q22.3

  vascular — *see* Disease, cardiovascular

heavy chain NEC C88.2

  alpha C88.3

  gamma C88.2

  mu C88.2

Hebra's

  pityriasis

    maculata et circinata L42

    rubra pilaris L44.0

  prurigo L28.2

hematopoietic organs D75.9

hemoglobin or Hb

  abnormal (mixed) NEC D58.2

    with thalassemia D56.9

  AS genotype D57.3

  Bart's D56.0

  C (Hb-C) D58.2

    with other abnormal hemoglobin NEC D58.2

    elliptocytosis D58.1

    Hb-S D57.2- ☑

    sickle-cell D57.2- ☑

    thalassemia D56.8

  Constant Spring D58.2

  D (Hb-D) D58.2

  E (Hb-E) D58.2

  E-beta thalassemia D56.5

  elliptocytosis D58.1

  H (Hb-H) (thalassemia) D56.0

    with other abnormal hemoglobin NEC D56.9

    Constant Spring D56.0

  I thalassemia D56.9

  M D74.0

  S or SS D57.1

  SC D57.2- ☑

Disease, diseased — *continued*

hemoglobin or Hb — *continued*

    SD D57.8- ☑

    SE D57.8- ☑

  spherocytosis D58.0

  unstable, hemolytic D58.2

hemolytic (newborn) P55.9

  autoimmune (cold type) (warm type) D59.1

  drug-induced D59.0

  due to or with

    incompatibility

      ABO (blood group) P55.1

      blood (group) (Duffy) (K(ell)) (Kidd) (Lewis) (M) (S) NEC P55.8

      Rh (blood group) (factor) P55.0

    Rh negative mother P55.0

  specified type NEC P55.8

  unstable hemoglobin D58.2

hemorrhagic D69.9

  newborn P53

Henoch (-Schönlein) (purpura nervosa) D69.0

hepatic — *see* Disease, liver

hepatolenticular E83.01

heredodegenerative NEC

  spinal cord G95.89

herpesviral, disseminated B00.7

Hers' (glycogenosis VI) E74.09

Herter (-Gee) (-Heubner) (nontropical sprue) K90.0

Heubner-Herter (nontropical sprue) K90.0

high fetal gene or hemoglobin thalassemia D56.9

Hildenbrand's — *see* Typhus

hip (joint) M25.9

  congenital Q65.89

  suppurative M00.9

  tuberculous A18.02

His (-Werner) (trench fever) A79.0

Hodgson's I71.2

  ruptured I71.1

Holla — *see* Spherocytosis

hookworm B76.9

  specified NEC B76.8

host-versus-graft D89.813

  acute D89.810

  acute on chronic D89.812

  chronic D89.811

human immunodeficiency virus (HIV) B20

Huntington's G10

  with dementia G10 [F02.80]

Hutchinson's (cheiropompholyx) — *see* Hutchinson's disease

hyaline (diffuse) (generalized)

  membrane (lung) (newborn) P22.0

    adult J80

hydatid — *see* Echinococcus

hydroxyapatite deposition M11.00

  ankle M11.07- ☑

  elbow M11.02- ☑

  foot joint M11.07- ☑

  hand joint M11.04- ☑

  hip M11.05- ☑

  knee M11.06- ☑

  multiple site M11.09

  shoulder M11.01- ☑

  vertebra M11.08

  wrist M11.03- ☑

hyperkinetic — *see* Hyperkinesia

hypertensive — *see* Hypertension

hypophysis E23.7

Iceland G93.3

I-cell E77.0

immune D89.9

immunoproliferative (malignant) C88.9

  small intestinal C88.3

  specified NEC C88.8

inclusion B25.9

  salivary gland B25.9

infectious, infective B99.9

  congenital P37.9

    specified NEC P37.8

    viral P35.9

      specified type NEC P35.8

  specified NEC B99.8

inflammatory

  penis N48.29

    abscess N48.21

    cellulitis N48.22

  prepuce N47.7

    balanoposthitis N47.6

Disease, diseased — *continued*
inflammatory — *continued*
tubo-ovarian — *see* Salpingo-oophoritis
intervertebral disc (*see also* Disorder, disc)
with myelopathy — *see* Disorder, disc, with, myelopathy
cervical, cervicothoracic — *see* Disorder, disc, cervical
with
myelopathy — *see* Disorder, disc, cervical, with myelopathy
neuritis, radiculitis or radiculopathy — *see* Disorder, disc, cervical, with neuritis
specified NEC — *see* Disorder, disc, cervical, specified type NEC
lumbar (with)
myelopathy M51.06
neuritis, radiculitis, radiculopathy or sciatica M51.16
specified NEC M51.86
lumbosacral (with)
neuritis, radiculitis, radiculopathy or sciatica M51.17
specified NEC M51.87
specified NEC — *see* Disorder, disc, specified NEC
thoracic (with)
myelopathy M51.04
neuritis, radiculitis or radiculopathy M51.14
specified NEC M51.84
thoracolumbar (with)
myelopathy M51.05
neuritis, radiculitis or radiculopathy M51.15
specified NEC M51.85
intestine K63.9
functional K59.9
psychogenic F45.8
specified NEC K59.8
organic K63.9
protozoal A07.9
specified NEC K63.89
iris H21.9
specified NEC H21.89
iron metabolism or storage E83.10
island (scrub typhus) A75.3
itai-itai — *see* Poisoning, cadmium
Jakob-Creutzfeldt — *see* Creutzfeldt-Jakob disease or syndrome
jaw M27.9
fibrocystic M27.49
specified NEC M27.8
jigger B88.1
joint (*see also* Disorder, joint)
Charcot's — *see* Arthropathy, neuropathic (Charcot)
degenerative — *see* Osteoarthritis
multiple M15.9
spine — *see* Spondylosis
hypertrophic — *see* Osteoarthritis
sacroiliac M53.3
specified NEC — *see* Disorder, joint, specified type NEC
spine NEC — *see* Dorsopathy
suppurative — *see* Arthritis, pyogenic or pyemic
Jourdain's (acute gingivitis) K05.00
nonplaque induced K05.01
plaque induced K05.00
Kaschin-Beck (endemic polyarthritis) M12.10
ankle M12.17- ☑
elbow M12.12- ☑
foot joint M12.17- ☑
hand joint M12.14- ☑
hip M12.15- ☑
knee M12.16- ☑
multiple site M12.19
shoulder M12.11- ☑
vertebra M12.18
wrist M12.13- ☑
Katayama B65.2
Kedani (scrub typhus) A75.3
Keshan E59
kidney (functional) (pelvis) N28.9
chronic N18.9
hypertensive — *see* Hypertension, kidney
stage 1 N18.1
stage 2 (mild) N18.2
stage 3 (moderate) N18.3
stage 4 (severe) N18.4
stage 5 N18.5

Disease, diseased — *continued*
kidney — *continued*
complicating pregnancy — *see* Pregnancy, complicated by, renal disease
cystic (congenital) Q61.9
fibrocystic (congenital) Q61.8
hypertensive — *see* Hypertension, kidney
in (due to)
schistosomiasis (bilharziasis) B65.9 [N29]
multicystic Q61.4
polycystic Q61.3
adult type Q61.2
childhood type NEC Q61.19
collecting duct dilatation Q61.11
Kimmelstiel (-Wilson) (intercapillary polycystic (congenital) glomerulosclerosis) — *see* E08-E13 with .21
Kinnier Wilson's (hepatolenticular degeneration) E83.01
kissing — *see* Mononucleosis, infectious
Klebs' (*see also* Glomerulonephritis) N05- ☑
Klippel-Feil (brevicollis) Q76.1
Köhler-Pellegrini-Stieda (calcification, knee joint) — *see* Bursitis, tibial collateral
Kok Q89.8
König's (osteochondritis dissecans) — *see* Osteochondritis, dissecans
Korsakoff's (nonalcoholic) F04
alcoholic F10.96
with dependence F10.26
Kostmann's (infantile genetic agranulocytosis) D70.0
kuru A81.81
Kyasanur Forest A98.2
labyrinth, ear — *see* Disorder, ear, inner
lacrimal system — *see* Disorder, lacrimal system
Lafora's — *see* Epilepsy, generalized, idiopathic
Lancereaux-Mathieu (leptospiral jaundice) A27.0
Landry's G61.0
Larrey-Weil (leptospiral jaundice) A27.0
larynx J38.7
legionnaires' A48.1
nonpneumonic A48.2
Lenegre's I44.2
lens H27.9
specified NEC H27.8
Lev's (acquired complete heart block) I44.2
Lewy body (dementia) G31.83 [F02.80]
with behavioral disturbance G31.83 [F02.81]
Lichtheim's (subacute combined sclerosis with pernicious anemia) D51.0
Lightwood's (renal tubular acidosis) N25.89
Lignac's (cystinosis) E72.04
lip K13.0
lipid-storage E75.6
specified NEC E75.5
Lipschütz's N76.6
liver (chronic) (organic) K76.9
alcoholic (chronic) K70.9
acute — *see* Disease, liver, alcoholic, hepatitis
cirrhosis K70.30
with ascites K70.31
failure K70.40
with coma K70.41
fatty liver K70.0
fibrosis K70.2
hepatitis K70.10
with ascites K70.11
sclerosis K70.2
cystic, congenital Q44.6
drug-induced (idiosyncratic) (toxic) (predictable) (unpredictable) — *see* Disease, liver, toxic
end stage K72.90
due to hepatitis — *see* Hepatitis
fatty, nonalcoholic (NAFLD) K76.0
alcoholic K70.0
fibrocystic (congenital) Q44.6
fluke
Chinese B66.1
oriental B66.1
sheep B66.3
gestational alloimmune (GALD) P78.84
glycogen storage E74.09 [K77]
in (due to)
schistosomiasis (bilharziasis) B65.9 [K77]
inflammatory K75.9
alcoholic K70.1 ☑
specified NEC K75.89
polycystic (congenital) Q44.6

Disease, diseased — *continued*
liver — *continued*
toxic K71.9
with
cholestasis K71.0
cirrhosis (liver) K71.7
fibrosis (liver) K71.7
focal nodular hyperplasia K71.8
hepatic granuloma K71.8
hepatic necrosis K71.10
with coma K71.11
hepatitis NEC K71.6
acute K71.2
chronic
active K71.50
with ascites K71.51
lobular K71.4
persistent K71.3
lupoid K71.50
with ascites K71.51
peliosis hepatis K71.8
veno-occlusive disease (VOD) of liver K71.8
veno-occlusive K76.5
Lobo's (keloid blastomycosis) B48.0
Lobstein's (brittle bones and blue sclera) Q78.0
Ludwig's (submaxillary cellulitis) K12.2
lumbosacral region M53.87
lung J98.4
black J60
congenital Q33.9
cystic J98.4
congenital Q33.0
fibroid (chronic) — *see* Fibrosis, lung
fluke B66.4
oriental B66.4
in
amyloidosis E85.4 [J99]
sarcoidosis D86.0
Sjögren's syndrome M35.02
systemic
lupus erythematosus M32.13
sclerosis M34.81
interstitial J84.9
of childhood, specified NEC J84.848
respiratory bronchiolitis J84.115
specified NEC J84.89
obstructive (chronic) J44.9
with
acute
bronchitis J44.0
exacerbation NEC J44.1
lower respiratory infection J44.0
alveolitis, allergic J67.9
asthma J44.9
bronchiectasis J47.9
with
exacerbation (acute) J47.1
lower respiratory infection J47.0
bronchitis J44.9
with
exacerbation (acute) J44.1
lower respiratory infection J44.0
emphysema J43.9
hypersensitivity pneumonitis J67.9
decompensated J44.1
with
exacerbation (acute) J44.1
polycystic J98.4
congenital Q33.0
rheumatoid (diffuse) (interstitial) — *see* Rheumatoid, lung
Lutembacher's (atrial septal defect with mitral stenosis) Q21.1
Lyme A69.20
lymphatic (gland) (system) (channel) (vessel) I89.9
lymphoproliferative D47.9
specified NEC D47.Z9 (*following* D47.4)
T-gamma D47.Z9 (*following* D47.4)
X-linked D82.3
Magitot's M27.2
malarial — *see* Malaria
malignant (*see also* Neoplasm, malignant, by site)
Manson's B65.1
maple bark J67.6
maple-syrup-urine E71.0
Marburg (virus) A98.3
Marion's (bladder neck obstruction) N32.0
Marsh's (exophthalmic goiter) — *see* Hyperthyroidism, with, goiter (diffuse)

Disease, diseased — *continued*
- mastoid (process) — *see* Disorder, ear, middle
- Mathieu's (leptospiral jaundice) A27.0
- Maxcy's A75.2
- McArdle (-Schmid-Pearson) (glycogenosis V) E74.04
- mediastinum J98.59
- medullary center (idiopathic) (respiratory) G93.89
- Meige's (chronic hereditary edema) Q82.0
- meningococcal — *see* Infection, meningococcal
- mental F99
  - organic F09
- mesenchymal M35.9
- mesenteric embolic (*see also* Ischemia, intestine, acute) K55.039
- metabolic, metabolism E88.9
  - bilirubin E80.7
- metal-polisher's J62.8
- metastatic (*see also* Neoplasm, secondary, by site) C79.9
- microvascular - code to condition
- microvillus
  - atrophy Q43.8
  - inclusion (MVD) Q43.8
- middle ear — *see* Disorder, ear, middle
- Mikulicz' (dryness of mouth, absent or decreased lacrimation) K11.8
- Milroy's (chronic hereditary edema) Q82.0
- Minamata — *see* Poisoning, mercury
- minicore G71.2
- Minor's G95.19
- Minot's (hemorrhagic disease, newborn) P53
- Minot-von Willebrand-Jürgens (angiohemophilia) D68.0
- Mitchell's (erythromelalgia) I73.81
- mitral (valve) I05.9
  - nonrheumatic I34.9
- mixed connective tissue M35.1
- moldy hay J67.0
- Monge's T70.29 ☑
- Morgagni-Adams-Stokes (syncope with heart block) I45.9
- Morgagni's (syndrome) (hyperostosis frontalis interna) M85.2
- Morton's (with metatarsalgia) — *see* Lesion, nerve, plantar
- Morvan's G60.8
- motor neuron (bulbar) (mixed type) (spinal) G12.20
  - amyotrophic lateral sclerosis G12.21
    - familial G12.24
  - progressive bulbar palsy G12.22
  - specified NEC G12.29
- moyamoya I67.5
- mu heavy chain disease C88.2
- multicore G71.2
- muscle (*see also* Disorder, muscle)
  - inflammatory — *see* Myositis
  - ocular (external) — *see* Strabismus
- musculoskeletal system, soft tissue — *see* also Disorder, soft tissue
  - specified NEC — *see* Disorder, soft tissue, specified type NEC
- mushroom workers' J67.5
- mycotic B49
- myelodysplastic, not classified C94.6
- myeloproliferative, not classified C94.6
  - chronic D47.1
- myocardium, myocardial (*see also* Degeneration, myocardial) I51.5
  - primary (idiopathic) I42.9
- myoneural G70.9
- Naegeli's D69.1
- nails L60.9
  - specified NEC L60.8
- Nairobi (sheep virus) A93.8
- nasal J34.9
- nemaline body G71.2
- nerve — *see* Disorder, nerve
- nervous system G98.8
  - autonomic G90.9
  - central G96.9
    - specified NEC G96.8
  - congenital Q07.9
  - parasympathetic G90.9
  - specified NEC G98.8
  - sympathetic G90.9
  - vegetative G90.9
- neuromuscular system G70.9
- Newcastle B30.8

Disease, diseased — *continued*
- Nicolas (-Durand)-Favre (climatic bubo) A55
- nipple N64.9
  - Paget's C50.01- ☑
    - female C50.01- ☑
    - male C50.02- ☑
- Nishimoto (-Takeuchi) I67.5
- nonarthropod-borne NOS (viral) B34.9
  - enterovirus NEC B34.1
- nonautoimmune hemolytic D59.4
  - drug-induced D59.2
- Nonne-Milroy-Meige (chronic hereditary edema) Q82.0
- nose J34.9
- nucleus pulposus — *see* Disorder, disc
- nutritional E63.9
- oast-house-urine E72.19
  - ocular
    - herpesviral B00.50
    - zoster B02.30
- obliterative vascular I77.1
- Ohara's — *see* Tularemia
- Opitz's (congestive splenomegaly) D73.2
- Oppenheim-Urbach (necrobiosis lipoidica diabetico-rum) — *see* E08-E13 with .620
- optic nerve NEC — *see* Disorder, nerve, optic
- orbit — *see* Disorder, orbit
- Oriental liver fluke B66.1
- Oriental lung fluke B66.4
- Ormond's N13.5
- Oropouche virus A93.0
- Osler-Rendu (familial hemorrhagic telangiectasia) I78.0
- osteofibrocystic E21.0
- Otto's M24.7
- outer ear — *see* Disorder, ear, external
- ovary (noninflammatory) N83.9
  - cystic N83.20- ☑
  - inflammatory — *see* Salpingo-oophoritis
  - polycystic E28.2
  - specified NEC N83.8
- Owren's (congenital) — *see* Defect, coagulation
- pancreas K86.9
  - cystic K86.2
  - fibrocystic E84.9
  - specified NEC K86.89
- panvalvular I08.9
  - specified NEC I08.8
- parametrium (noninflammatory) N83.9
- parasitic B89
  - cerebral NEC B71.9 [G94]
  - intestinal NOS B82.9
  - mouth B37.0
  - skin NOS B88.9
  - specified type — *see* Infestation
  - tongue B37.0
- parathyroid (gland) E21.5
  - specified NEC E21.4
- Parkinson's G20
- parodontal K05.6
- Parrot's (syphilitic osteochondritis) A50.02
- Parry's (exophthalmic goiter) — *see* Hyperthyroidism, with, goiter (diffuse)
- Parson's (exophthalmic goiter) — *see* Hyperthyroidism, with, goiter (diffuse)
- Paxton's (white piedra) B36.2
- pearl-worker's — *see* Osteomyelitis, specified type NEC
- Pellegrini-Stieda (calcification, knee joint) — *see* Bursitis, tibial collateral
- pelvis, pelvic
  - female NOS N94.9
    - specified NEC N94.89
  - gonococcal (acute) (chronic) A54.24
  - inflammatory (female) N73.9
    - acute N73.0
    - chlamydial A56.11
    - chronic N73.1
    - specified NEC N73.8
    - syphilitic (secondary) A51.42
      - late A52.76
    - tuberculous A18.17
  - organ, female N94.9
  - peritoneum, female NEC N94.89
- penis N48.9
  - inflammatory N48.29
    - abscess N48.21
    - cellulitis N48.22
  - specified NEC N48.89
- periapical tissues NOS K04.90

Disease, diseased — *continued*
- periodontal K05.6
  - specified NEC K05.5
- periosteum — *see* Disorder, bone, specified type NEC
- peripheral
  - arterial I73.9
  - autonomic nervous system G90.9
  - nerves — *see* Polyneuropathy
  - vascular NOS I73.9
- peritoneum K66.9
  - pelvic, female NEC N94.89
  - specified NEC K66.8
- persistent mucosal (middle ear) H66.20
  - left H66.22
    - with right H66.23
  - right H66.21
    - with left H66.23
- Petit's — *see* Hernia, abdomen, specified site NEC
- pharynx J39.2
  - specified NEC J39.2
- Phocas' — *see* Mastopathy, cystic
- photochromogenic (acid-fast bacilli) (pulmonary) A31.0
  - nonpulmonary A31.9
- Pick's G31.01 [F02.80]
  - with behavioral disturbance G31.01 [F02.81]
    - brain G31.01 [F02.80]
      - with behavioral disturbance G31.01 [F02.81]
  - of pericardium (pericardial pseudocirrhosis of liver) I31.1
- pigeon fancier's J67.2
- pineal gland E34.8
- pink — *see* Poisoning, mercury
- Pinkus' (lichen nitidus) L44.1
- pinworm B80
- Piry virus A93.8
- pituitary (gland) E23.7
- pituitary-snuff-taker's J67.8
- pleura (cavity) J94.9
  - specified NEC J94.8
- pneumatic drill (hammer) T75.21 ☑
- Pollitzer's (hidradenitis suppurativa) L73.2
- polycystic
  - kidney or renal Q61.3
    - adult type Q61.2
    - childhood type NEC Q61.19
      - collecting duct dilatation Q61.11
  - liver or hepatic Q44.6
  - lung or pulmonary J98.4
    - congenital Q33.0
  - ovary, ovaries E28.2
  - spleen Q89.09
- polyethylene T84.05- ☑
- Pompe's (glycogenosis II) E74.02
- Posadas-Wernicke B38.9
- Potain's (pulmonary edema) — *see* Edema, lung
- prepuce N47.8
  - inflammatory N47.7
    - balanoposthitis N47.6
- Pringle's (tuberous sclerosis) Q85.1
- prion, central nervous system A81.9
  - specified NEC A81.89
- prostate N42.9
  - specified NEC N42.89
- protozoal B64
  - acanthamebiasis — *see* Acanthamebiasis
  - African trypanosomiasis — *see* African trypanosomiasis
  - babesiosis B60.0
  - Chagas disease — *see* Chagas disease
  - intestine, intestinal A07.9
  - leishmaniasis — *see* Leishmaniasis
  - malaria — *see* Malaria
  - naegleriasis B60.2
  - pneumocystosis B59
  - specified organism NEC B60.8
  - toxoplasmosis — *see* Toxoplasmosis
- pseudo-Hurler's E77.0
- psychiatric F99
- psychotic — *see* Psychosis
- Puente's (simple glandular cheilitis) K13.0
- puerperal (*see also* Puerperal) O90.89
- pulmonary (*see also* Disease, lung)
  - artery I28.9
  - chronic obstructive J44.9
    - with
      - acute bronchitis J44.0
      - exacerbation (acute) J44.1

Disease, diseased ICD-10-CM 2018

Index

Disease, diseased — Disease, diseased

Disease, diseased — continued
pulmonary (see also Disease, lung) — continued
chronic obstructive — continued
with — continued
lower respiratory infection (acute) J44.0
decompensated J44.1
with
exacerbation (acute) J44.1
heart I27.9
specified NEC I27.89
hypertensive (vascular) (see also Hypertension, pulmonary) I27.20
primary (idiopathic) I27.0
NEC I27.2 ☑
valve I37.9
rheumatic I09.89
pulp (dental) NOS K04.90
pulseless M31.4
Putnam's (subacute combined sclerosis with pernicious anemia) D51.0
Pyle (-Cohn) (metaphyseal dysplasia) Q78.5
ragpicker's or ragsorter's A22.1
Raynaud's — see Raynaud's disease
reactive airway — see Asthma
Reclus' (cystic) — see Mastopathy, cystic
rectum K62.9
specified NEC K62.89
Refsum's (heredopathia atactica polyneuritiformis) G60.1
renal (functional) (pelvis) (see also Disease, kidney) N28.9
with
edema — see Nephrosis
glomerular lesion — see Glomerulonephritis
with edema — see Nephrosis
interstitial nephritis N12
acute N28.9
chronic (see also Disease, kidney, chronic) N18.9
cystic, congenital Q61.9
diabetic — see E08-E13 with .22
end-stage (failure) N18.6
due to hypertension I12.0
fibrocystic (congenital) Q61.8
hypertensive — see Hypertension, kidney
lupus M32.14
phosphate-losing (tubular) N25.0
polycystic (congenital) Q61.3
adult type Q61.2
childhood type NEC Q61.19
collecting duct dilatation Q61.11
rapidly progressive N01.9
subacute N01.9
Rendu-Osler-Weber (familial hemorrhagic telangiectasia) I78.0
renovascular (arteriosclerotic) — see Hypertension, kidney
respiratory (tract) J98.9
acute or subacute NOS J06.9
due to
chemicals, gases, fumes or vapors (inhalation) J68.3
external agent J70.9
specified NEC J70.8
radiation J70.0
smoke inhalation J70.5
noninfectious J39.8
chronic NOS J98.9
due to
chemicals, gases, fumes or vapors J68.4
external agent J70.9
specified NEC J70.8
radiation J70.1
newborn P27.9
specified NEC P27.8
due to
chemicals, gases, fumes or vapors J68.9
acute or subacute NEC J68.3
chronic J68.4
external agent J70.9
specified NEC J70.8
newborn P28.9
specified type NEC P28.89
upper J39.9
acute or subacute J06.9
noninfectious NEC J39.8
specified NEC J39.8
streptococcal J06.9
retina, retinal H35.9

Disease, diseased — continued
retina, retinal — continued
Batten's or Batten-Mayou E75.4 [H36]
specified NEC H35.89
rheumatoid — see Arthritis, rheumatoid
rickettsial NOS A79.9
specified type NEC A79.89
Riga (-Fede) (cachectic aphthae) K14.0
Riggs' (compound periodontitis) — see Periodontitis
Ritter's L00
Rivalta's (cervicofacial actinomycosis) A42.2
Robles' (onchocerciasis) B73.01
Roger's (congenital interventricular septal defect) Q21.0
Rosenthal's (factor XI deficiency) D68.1
Ross River B33.1
Rossbach's (hyperchlorhydria) K30
Rotes Quérol — see Hyperostosis, ankylosing
Roth (-Bernhardt) — see Mononeuropathy, lower limb, meralgia paresthetica
Runeberg's (progressive pernicious anemia) D51.0
sacroiliac NEC M53.3
salivary gland or duct K11.9
inclusion B25.9
specified NEC K11.8
virus B25.9
sandworm B76.9
Schimmelbusch's — see Mastopathy, cystic
Schmorl's — see Schmorl's disease or nodes
Schönlein (-Henoch) (purpura rheumatica) D69.0
Schottmüller's — see Fever, paratyphoid
Schultz's (agranulocytosis) — see Agranulocytosis
Schwalbe-Ziehen-Oppenheim G24.1
Schwartz-Jampel G71.13
sclera H15.9
specified NEC H15.89
scrofulous (tuberculous) A18.2
scrotum N50.9
sebaceous glands L73.9
semilunar cartilage, cystic (see also Derangement, knee, meniscus, cystic)
seminal vesicle N50.9
serum NEC (see also Reaction, serum) T80.69 ☑
sexually transmitted A64
anogenital
herpesviral infection — see Herpes, anogenital
warts A63.0
chancroid A57
chlamydial infection — see Chlamydia
gonorrhea — see Gonorrhea
granuloma inguinale A58
specified organism NEC A63.8
syphilis — see Syphilis
trichomoniasis — see Trichomoniasis
Sézary C84.1- ☑
shimamushi (scrub typhus) A75.3
shipyard B30.0
sickle-cell D57.1
with crisis (vasoocclusive pain) D57.00
with
acute chest syndrome D57.01
splenic sequestration D57.02
elliptocytosis D57.8- ☑
Hb-C D57.20
with crisis (vasoocclusive pain) D57.219
with
acute chest syndrome D57.211
splenic sequestration D57.212
without crisis D57.20
Hb-SD D57.80
with crisis D57.819
with
acute chest syndrome D57.811
splenic sequestration D57.812
Hb-SE D57.80
with crisis D57.819
with
acute chest syndrome D57.811
splenic sequestration D57.812
specified D57.80
with crisis D57.819
with
acute chest syndrome D57.811
splenic sequestration D57.812
spherocytosis D57.80
with crisis D57.819
with
acute chest syndrome D57.811

Disease, diseased — continued
sickle-cell — continued
spherocytosis — continued
with crisis — continued
with — continued
splenic sequestration D57.812
thalassemia D57.40
with crisis (vasoocclusive pain) D57.419
with
acute chest syndrome D57.411
splenic sequestration D57.412
without crisis D57.40
silo-filler's J68.8
bronchitis J68.0
pneumonitis J68.0
pulmonary edema J68.1
simian B B00.4
Simons' (progressive lipodystrophy) E88.1
sin nombre virus B33.4
sinus — see Sinusitis
Sirkari's B55.0
sixth B08.20
due to human herpesvirus 6 B08.21
due to human herpesvirus 7 B08.22
skin L98.9
due to metabolic disorder NEC E88.9 [L99]
specified NEC L98.8
slim (HIV) B20
small vessel I73.9
Sneddon-Wilkinson (subcorneal pustular dermatosis) L13.1
South African creeping B88.0
spinal (cord) G95.9
congenital Q06.9
specified NEC G95.89
spine (see also Spondylopathy)
joint — see Dorsopathy
tuberculous A18.01
spinocerebellar (hereditary) G11.9
specified NEC G11.8
spleen D73.9
amyloid E85.4 [D77]
organic D73.9
polycystic Q89.09
postinfectional D73.89
sponge-diver's — see Toxicity, venom, marine animal, sea anemone
Startle Q89.8
Steinert's G71.11
Sticker's (erythema infectiosum) B08.3
Stieda's (calcification, knee joint) — see Bursitis, tibial collateral
Stokes' (exophthalmic goiter) — see Hyperthyroidism, with, goiter (diffuse)
Stokes-Adams (syncope with heart block) I45.9
stomach K31.9
functional, psychogenic F45.8
specified NEC K31.89
stonemason's J62.8
storage
glycogen — see Disease, glycogen storage
mucopolysaccharide — see Mucopolysaccharidosis
striatopallidal system NEC G25.89
Stuart-Prower (congenital factor X deficiency) D68.2
Stuart's (congenital factor X deficiency) D68.2
subcutaneous tissue — see Disease, skin
supporting structures of teeth K08.9
specified NEC K08.89
suprarenal (capsule) (gland) E27.9
hyperfunction E27.0
specified NEC E27.8
sweat glands L74.9
specified NEC L74.8
Sweeley-Klionsky E75.21
Swift (-Feer) — see Poisoning, mercury
swimming-pool granuloma A31.1
Sylvest's (epidemic pleurodynia) B33.0
sympathetic nervous system G90.9
synovium — see Disorder, synovium
syphilitic — see Syphilis
systemic tissue mast cell C96.20
tanapox (virus) B08.71
Tangier E78.6
Tarral-Besnier (pityriasis rubra pilaris) L44.0
Tauri's E74.09
tear duct — see Disorder, lacrimal system
tendon, tendinous (see also Disorder, tendon)
nodular — see Trigger finger

☑ Additional Character Required — Refer to the Tabular List for Character Selection ▽ Subterms under main terms may continue to next column or page

Disease, diseased — *continued*
  terminal vessel I73.9
  testis N50.9
  thalassemia Hb-S — *see* Disease, sickle-cell, thalassemia
  Thaysen-Gee (nontropical sprue) K90.0
  Thomsen G71.12
  throat J39.2
    septic J02.0
  thromboembolic — *see* Embolism
  thymus (gland) E32.9
    specified NEC E32.8
  thyroid (gland) E07.9
    heart (*see also* Hyperthyroidism) E05.90 [I43]
      with thyroid storm E05.91 [I43]
    specified NEC E07.89
  Tietze's M94.0
  tongue K14.9
    specified NEC K14.8
  tonsils, tonsillar (and adenoids) J35.9
  tooth, teeth K08.9
    hard tissues K03.9
      specified NEC K03.89
    pulp NEC K04.99
    specified NEC K08.89
  Tourette's F95.2
  trachea NEC J39.8
  tricuspid I07.9
    nonrheumatic I36.9
  triglyceride-storage E75.5
  trophoblastic — *see* Mole, hydatidiform
  tsutsugamushi A75.3
  tube (fallopian) (noninflammatory) N83.9
    inflammatory — *see* Salpingitis
    specified NEC N83.8
  tuberculous NEC — *see* Tuberculosis
  tubo-ovarian (noninflammatory) N83.9
    inflammatory — *see* Salpingo-oophoritis
    specified NEC N83.8
  tubotympanic, chronic — *see* Otitis, media, suppurative, chronic, tubotympanic
  tubulo-interstitial N15.9
    specified NEC N15.8
  tympanum — *see* Disorder, tympanic membrane
  Uhl's Q24.8
  Underwood's (sclerema neonatorum) P83.0
  Unverricht (-Lundborg) — *see* Epilepsy, generalized, idiopathic
  Urbach-Oppenheim (necrobiosis lipoidica diabeticorum) — *see* E08-E13 with .620
  ureter N28.9
    in (due to)
      schistosomiasis (bilharziasis) B65.0 [N29]
  urethra N36.9
    specified NEC N36.8
  urinary (tract) N39.9
    bladder N32.9
      specified NEC N32.89
    specified NEC N39.8
  uterus (noninflammatory) N85.9
    infective — *see* Endometritis
    inflammatory — *see* Endometritis
    specified NEC N85.8
  uveal tract (anterior) H21.9
    posterior H31.9
  vagabond's B85.1
  vagina, vaginal (noninflammatory) N89.9
    inflammatory NEC N76.89
    specified NEC N89.8
  valve, valvular I38
    multiple I08.9
      specified NEC I08.8
  van Creveld-von Gierke (glycogenosis I) E74.01
  vas deferens N50.9
  vascular I99.9
    arteriosclerotic — *see* Arteriosclerosis
    ciliary body NEC — *see* Disorder, iris, vascular
    hypertensive — *see* Hypertension
    iris NEC — *see* Disorder, iris, vascular
    obliterative I77.1
      peripheral I73.9
    occlusive I99.8
    peripheral (occlusive) I73.9
      in diabetes mellitus — *see* E08-E13 with .51
  vasomotor I73.9
  vasospastic I73.9
  vein I87.9
  venereal (*see also* Disease, sexually transmitted) A64

Disease, diseased — *continued*
  venereal (*see also* Disease, sexually transmitted) — *continued*
    chlamydial NEC A56.8
      anus A56.3
      genitourinary NOS A56.2
      pharynx A56.4
      rectum A56.3
    fifth A55
    sixth A55
    specified nature or type NEC A63.8
  vertebra, vertebral (*see also* Spondylopathy)
    disc — *see* Disorder, disc
  vibration — *see* Vibration, adverse effects
  viral, virus (*see also* Disease, by type of virus) B34.9
    arbovirus NOS A94
    arthropod-borne NOS A94
    congenital P35.9
      specified NEC P35.8
    Hanta (with renal manifestations) (Dobrava) (Puumala) (Seoul) A98.5
      with pulmonary manifestations (Andes) (Bayou) (Bermejo) (Black Creek Canal) (Choclo) (Juquitiba) (Laguna negra) (Lechiguanas) (New York) (Oran) (Sin nombre) B33.4
    Hantaan (Korean hemorrhagic fever) A98.5
    human immunodeficiency (HIV) B20
    Kunjin A83.4
    nonarthropod-borne NOS B34.9
    Powassan A84.8
    Rocio (encephalitis) A83.6
    Sin nombre (Hantavirus) (cardio)-pulmonary syndrome) B33.4
    Tahyna B33.8
    vesicular stomatitis A93.8
  vitreous H43.9
    specified NEC H43.89
  vocal cord J38.3
  Volkmann's, acquired T79.6 ☑
  von Eulenburg's (congenital paramyotonia) G71.19
  von Gierke's (glycogenosis I) E74.01
  von Graefe's — *see* Strabismus, paralytic, ophthalmoplegia, progressive
  von Willebrand (-Jürgens) (angiohemophilia) D68.0
  Vrolik's (osteogenesis imperfecta) Q78.0
  vulva (noninflammatory) N90.9
    inflammatory NEC N76.89
    specified NEC N90.89
  Wallgren's (obstruction of splenic vein with collateral circulation) I87.8
  Wassilieff's (leptospiral jaundice) A27.0
  wasting NEC R64
    due to malnutrition E41
  Waterhouse-Friderichsen A39.1
  Wegner's (syphilitic osteochondritis) A50.02
  Weil's (leptospiral jaundice of lung) A27.0
  Weir Mitchell's (erythromelalgia) I73.81
  Werdnig-Hoffmann G12.0
  Wermer's E31.21
  Werner-His (trench fever) A79.0
  Werner-Schultz (neutropenic splenomegaly) D73.81
  Wernicke-Posadas B38.9
  whipworm B79
  white blood cells D72.9
    specified NEC D72.89
  white matter R90.82
  white-spot, meaning lichen sclerosus et atrophicus L90.0
    penis N48.0
    vulva N90.4
  Wilkie's K55.1
  Wilkinson-Sneddon (subcorneal pustular dermatosis) L13.1
  Willis' — *see* Diabetes
  Wilson's (hepatolenticular degeneration) E83.01
  woolsorter's A22.1
  yaba monkey tumor B08.72
  yaba pox (virus) B08.72
  Zika virus A92.5
  zoonotic, bacterial A28.9
    specified type NEC A28.8
Disfigurement (due to scar) L90.5
Disgerminoma — *see* Dysgerminoma
DISH (diffuse idiopathic skeletal hyperostosis) — *see* Hyperostosis, ankylosing
Disinsertion, retina — *see* Detachment, retina
Dislocatable hip, congenital Q65.6

Dislocation (articular)
  with fracture — *see* Fracture
  acromioclavicular (joint) S43.10- ☑
    with displacement
      100%-200% S43.12- ☑
      more than 200% S43.13- ☑
    inferior S43.14- ☑
    posterior S43.15- ☑
  ankle S93.0- ☑
  astragalus — *see* Dislocation, ankle
  atlantoaxial S13.121 ☑
  atlantooccipital S13.111 ☑
  atloidooccipital S13.111 ☑
  breast bone S23.29 ☑
  capsule, joint — *code by* site under Dislocation
  carpal (bone) — *see* Dislocation, wrist
  carpometacarpal (joint) NEC S63.05- ☑
    thumb S63.04- ☑
  cartilage (joint) — *code by* site under Dislocation
  cervical spine (vertebra) — *see* Dislocation, vertebra, cervical
  chronic — *see* Dislocation, recurrent
  clavicle — *see* Dislocation, acromioclavicular joint
  coccyx S33.2 ☑
  congenital NEC Q68.8
  coracoid — *see* Dislocation, shoulder
  costal cartilage S23.29 ☑
  costochondral S23.29 ☑
  cricoarytenoid articulation S13.29 ☑
  cricothyroid articulation S13.29 ☑
  dorsal vertebra — *see* Dislocation, vertebra, thoracic
  ear ossicle — *see* Discontinuity, ossicles, ear
  elbow S53.10- ☑
    congenital Q68.8
    pathological — *see* Dislocation, pathological NEC, elbow
    radial head alone — *see* Dislocation, radial head
    recurrent — *see* Dislocation, recurrent, elbow
    traumatic S53.10- ☑
      anterior S53.11- ☑
      lateral S53.14- ☑
      medial S53.13- ☑
      posterior S53.12- ☑
      specified type NEC S53.19- ☑
  eye, nontraumatic — *see* Luxation, globe
  eyeball, nontraumatic — *see* Luxation, globe
  femur
    distal end — *see* Dislocation, knee
    proximal end — *see* Dislocation, hip
  fibula
    distal end — *see* Dislocation, ankle
    proximal end — *see* Dislocation, knee
  finger S63.25- ☑
    index S63.25- ☑
    interphalangeal S63.27- ☑
      distal S63.29- ☑
        index S63.29- ☑
        little S63.29- ☑
        middle S63.29- ☑
        ring S63.29- ☑
      index S63.27- ☑
      little S63.27- ☑
      middle S63.27- ☑
      proximal S63.28- ☑
        index S63.28- ☑
        little S63.28- ☑
        middle S63.28- ☑
        ring S63.28- ☑
      ring S63.27- ☑
    little S63.25- ☑
    metacarpophalangeal S63.26- ☑
      index S63.26- ☑
      little S63.26- ☑
      middle S63.26- ☑
      ring S63.26- ☑
    middle S63.25- ☑
    recurrent — *see* Dislocation, recurrent, finger
    ring S63.25- ☑
    thumb — *see* Dislocation, thumb
  foot S93.30- ☑
    recurrent — *see* Dislocation, recurrent, foot
    specified site NEC S93.33- ☑
    tarsal joint S93.31- ☑
    tarsometatarsal joint S93.32- ☑
    toe — *see* Dislocation, toe
  fracture — *see* Fracture

Dislocation — *continued*
  vertebra — *continued*
    lumbar — *continued*
      joint between — *continued*
        L2 and L3 S33.121 ☑
        L3 and L4 S33.131 ☑
        L4 and L5 S33.141 ☑
      nontraumatic — *see* Displacement, intervertebral
        disc
      partial — *see* Subluxation, by site
      recurrent NEC — *see* subcategory M43.5 ☑
    thoracic S23.101 ☑
      joint between
        T1 and T2 S23.111 ☑
        T2 and T3 S23.121 ☑
        T3 and T4 S23.123 ☑
        T4 and T5 S23.131 ☑
        T5 and T6 S23.133 ☑
        T6 and T7 S23.141 ☑
        T7 and T8 S23.143 ☑
        T8 and T9 S23.151 ☑
        T9 and T10 S23.153 ☑
        T10 and T11 S23.161 ☑
        T11 and T12 S23.163 ☑
        T12 and L1 S23.171 ☑
  wrist (carpal bone) S63.006 ☑
    carpometacarpal joint — *see* Dislocation, car-
      pometacarpal (joint)
    distal radioulnar joint — *see* Dislocation, radioulnar
      (joint), distal
    metacarpal bone, proximal — *see* Dislocation,
      metacarpal (bone), proximal end
    midcarpal — *see* Dislocation, midcarpal (joint)
    radiocarpal joint — *see* Dislocation, radiocarpal
      (joint)
    recurrent — *see* Dislocation, recurrent, wrist
    specified site NEC S63.09- ☑
    ulna — *see* Dislocation, ulna, distal end
  xiphoid cartilage S23.29 ☑
Disorder (of) (*see also* Disease)
  acantholytic L11.9
    specified NEC L11.8
  acute
    psychotic — *see* Psychosis, acute
    stress F43.0
  adjustment (grief) F43.20
    with
      anxiety F43.22
        with depressed mood F43.23
      conduct disturbance F43.24
        with emotional disturbance F43.25
      depressed mood F43.21
        with anxiety F43.23
      other specified symptom F43.29
  adrenal (capsule) (gland) (medullary) E27.9
    specified NEC E27.8
  adrenogenital E25.9
    drug-induced E25.8
    iatrogenic E25.8
    idiopathic E25.8
  adult personality (and behavior) F69
    specified NEC F68.8
  affective (mood) — *see* Disorder, mood
  aggressive, unsocialized F91.1
  alcohol use
    mild F10.10
      with
        alcohol intoxication F10.129
          delirium F10.121
        alcohol-induced
          anxiety disorder F10.180
          bipolar and related disorder F10.14
          depressive disorder F10.14
          psychotic disorder F10.159
          sexual dysfunction F10.181
          sleep disorder F10.182
      in remission (early) (sustained) F10.11
    moderate or severe F10.20
      with
        alcohol intoxication F10.229
          delirium F10.221
        alcohol-induced
          anxiety disorder F10.280
          bipolar and related disorder F10.24
          depressive disorder F10.24
          major neurocognitive disorder, amnes-
            tic-confabulatory type F10.26

Disorder — *continued*
  alcohol use — *continued*
    moderate or severe — *continued*
      with
        alcohol-induced — *continued*
          major neurocognitive disorder, non-
            amnestic-confabulatory type
            F10.27
          mild neurocognitive disorder F10.288
          psychotic disorder F10.259
          sexual dysfunction F10.281
          sleep disorder F10.282
      in remission (early) (sustained) F10.21
  alcohol-related F10.99
    with
      amnestic disorder, persisting F10.96
      anxiety disorder F10.980
      dementia, persisting F10.97
      intoxication F10.929
        with delirium F10.921
        uncomplicated F10.920
      mood disorder F10.94
      other specified F10.988
      psychotic disorder F10.959
        with
          delusions F10.950
          hallucinations F10.951
      sexual dysfunction F10.981
      sleep disorder F10.982
  allergic — *see* Allergy
  alveolar NEC J84.09
  amino-acid
    cystathioninuria E72.19
    cystinosis E72.04
    cystinuria E72.01
    glycinuria E72.09
    homocystinuria E72.11
    metabolism — *see* Disturbance, metabolism,
      amino-acid
      specified NEC E72.8
    neonatal, transitory P74.8
    renal transport NEC E72.09
    transport NEC E72.09
  amnesic, amnestic
    alcohol-induced F10.96
      with dependence F10.26
    due to (secondary to) general medical condition
      F04
    psychoactive NEC-induced F19.96
      with
        abuse F19.16
        dependence F19.26
    sedative, hypnotic or anxiolytic-induced F13.96
      with dependence F13.26
  amphetamine (or other stimulant) use
    mild
      with
        amphetamine, cocaine, or other stimulant
          intoxication
          with perceptual disturbances F15.122
          without perceptual disturbances F15.129
        amphetamine (or other stimulant) -induced
          anxiety disorder F15.180
          bipolar and related disorder F15.14
          depressive disorder F15.14
          obsessive-compulsive and related disor-
            der F15.188
          psychotic disorder F15.159
          sexual dysfunction F15.181
        intoxication delirium F15.121
    moderate or severe
      with
        amphetamine, cocaine, or other stimulant
          intoxication
          with perceptual disturbances F15.222
          without perceptual disturbances F15.229
        amphetamine (or other stimulant) -induced
          anxiety disorder F15.280
          bipolar and related disorder F15.24
          depressive disorder F15.24
          obsessive-compulsive and related disor-
            der F15.288
          psychotic disorder F15.259
          sexual dysfunction F15.281
        intoxication delirium F15.221
  amphetamine-type substance use
    mild F15.10
      in remission (early) (sustained) F15.11
    moderate F15.20

Disorder — *continued*
  amphetamine-type substance use — *continued*
    moderate — *continued*
      in remission (early) (sustained) F15.21
    severe F15.20
      in remission (early) (sustained) F15.21
  anaerobic glycolysis with anemia D55.2
  anxiety F41.9
    due to (secondary to)
      alcohol F10.980
        in
          abuse F10.180
          dependence F10.280
      amphetamine F15.980
        in
          abuse F15.180
          dependence F15.280
      anxiolytic F13.980
        in
          abuse F13.180
          dependence F13.280
      caffeine F15.980
        in
          abuse F15.180
          dependence F15.280
      cannabis F12.980
        in
          abuse F12.180
          dependence F12.280
      cocaine F14.980
        in
          abuse F14.180
          dependence F14.180
      general medical condition F06.4
      hallucinogen F16.980
        in
          abuse F16.180
          dependence F16.280
      hypnotic F13.980
        in
          abuse F13.180
          dependence F13.280
      inhalant F18.980
        in
          abuse F18.180
          dependence F18.280
      phencyclidine F16.980
        in
          abuse F16.180
          dependence F16.280
      psychoactive substance NEC F19.980
        in
          abuse F19.180
          dependence F19.280
      sedative F13.980
        in
          abuse F13.180
          dependence F13.280
      volatile solvents F18.980
        in
          abuse F18.180
          dependence F18.280
    generalized F41.1
    illness F45.21
    mixed
      with depression (mild) F41.8
      specified NEC F41.3
    organic F06.4
    phobic F40.9
      of childhood F40.8
    specified NEC F41.8
  aortic valve — *see* Endocarditis, aortic
  aromatic amino-acid metabolism E70.9
    specified NEC E70.8
  arteriole NEC I77.89
  artery NEC I77.89
  articulation — *see* Disorder, joint
  attachment (childhood)
    disinhibited F94.2
    reactive F94.1
  attention-deficit hyperactivity (adolescent) (adult)
    (child) F90.9
    combined
      presentation F90.2
      type F90.2
    hyperactive
      impulsive presentation F90.1
      type F90.1

Disorder — *continued*
  attention-deficit hyperactivity — *continued*
    inattentive
      presentation F90.0
      type F90.0
    specified type NEC F90.8
  attention-deficit without hyperactivity (adolescent) (adult) (child) F98.8
  auditory processing (central) H93.25
  autism spectrum F84.0
  autistic F84.0
  autoimmune D89.89
  autonomic nervous system G90.9
    specified NEC G90.8
  avoidant
    child or adolescent F40.10
    restrictive food intake F50.82
  balance
    acid-base E87.8
      mixed E87.4
    electrolyte E87.8
    fluid NEC E87.8
  behavioral (disruptive) — *see* Disorder, conduct
  beta-amino-acid metabolism E72.8
  bile acid and cholesterol metabolism E78.70
    Barth syndrome E78.71
    other specified E78.79
    Smith-Lemli-Opitz syndrome E78.72
  bilirubin excretion E80.6
  binge eating F50.81
  binocular
    movement H51.9
      convergence
        excess H51.12
        insufficiency H51.11
      internuclear ophthalmoplegia — *see* Ophthalmoplegia, internuclear
      palsy of conjugate gaze H51.0
      specified type NEC H51.8
    vision NEC — *see* Disorder, vision, binocular
  bipolar (I) (type I) F31.9
    and related due to a known physiological condition
      with
        manic features F06.33
        manic- or hypomanic-like episodes F06.33
        mixed features F06.34
    current (or most recent) episode
      depressed F31.9
        with psychotic features F31.5
        without psychotic features F31.30
          mild F31.31
          moderate F31.32
          severe (without psychotic features) F31.4
            with psychotic features F31.5
      hypomanic F31.0
      manic F31.9
        with psychotic features F31.2
        without psychotic features F31.10
          mild F31.11
          moderate F31.12
          severe (without psychotic features) F31.13
            with psychotic features F31.2
      mixed F31.60
        mild F31.61
        moderate F31.62
        severe (without psychotic features) F31.63
          with psychotic features F31.64
        severe depression (without psychotic features) F31.4
          with psychotic features F31.5
    in remission (currently) F31.70
      in full remission
        most recent episode
          depressed F31.76
          hypomanic F31.72
          manic F31.74
          mixed F31.78
      in partial remission
        most recent episode
          depressed F31.75
          hypomanic F31.71
          manic F31.73
          mixed F31.77
    organic F06.30
    single manic episode F30.9
      mild F30.11
      moderate F30.12
      severe (without psychotic symptoms) F30.13

Disorder — *continued*
  bipolar — *continued*
    single manic episode — *continued*
      severe — *continued*
        with psychotic symptoms F30.2
      specified NEC F31.89
  bipolar II (type 2) F31.81
  bladder N32.9
    functional NEC N31.9
    in schistosomiasis B65.0 [N33]
    specified NEC N32.89
  bleeding D68.9
  blood D75.9
    in congenital early syphilis A50.09 [D77]
  body dysmorphic F45.22
  bone M89.9
    continuity M84.9
      specified type NEC M84.80
        ankle M84.87- ☑
        fibula M84.86- ☑
        foot M84.87- ☑
        hand M84.84- ☑
        humerus M84.82- ☑
        neck M84.88
        pelvis M84.859
        radius M84.83- ☑
        rib M84.88
        shoulder M84.81- ☑
        skull M84.88
        thigh M84.85- ☑
        tibia M84.86- ☑
        ulna M84.83- ☑
        vertebra M84.88
    density and structure M85.9
      cyst (*see also* Cyst, bone, specified type NEC)
        aneurysmal — *see* Cyst, bone, aneurysmal
        solitary — *see* Cyst, bone, solitary
      diffuse idiopathic skeletal hyperostosis — *see* Hyperostosis, ankylosing
      fibrous dysplasia (monostotic) — *see* Dysplasia, fibrous, bone
      fluorosis — *see* Fluorosis, skeletal
      hyperostosis of skull M85.2
      osteitis condensans — *see* Osteitis, condensans
      specified type NEC M85.8- ☑
        ankle M85.87- ☑
        foot M85.87- ☑
        forearm M85.83- ☑
        hand M85.84- ☑
        lower leg M85.86- ☑
        multiple sites M85.89
        neck M85.88
        rib M85.88
        shoulder M85.81- ☑
        skull M85.88
        thigh M85.85- ☑
        upper arm M85.82- ☑
        vertebra M85.88
    development and growth NEC M89.20
      carpus M89.24- ☑
      clavicle M89.21- ☑
      femur M89.25- ☑
      fibula M89.26- ☑
      finger M89.24- ☑
      humerus M89.22- ☑
      ilium M89.259
      ischium M89.259
      metacarpus M89.24- ☑
      metatarsus M89.27- ☑
      multiple sites M89.29
      neck M89.28
      radius M89.23- ☑
      rib M89.28
      scapula M89.21- ☑
      skull M89.28
      tarsus M89.27- ☑
      tibia M89.26- ☑
      toe M89.27- ☑
      ulna M89.23- ☑
      vertebra M89.28
    specified type NEC M89.8X- ☑
  brachial plexus G54.0
  branched-chain amino-acid metabolism E71.2
    specified NEC E71.19
  breast N64.9
    agalactia — *see* Agalactia

Disorder — *continued*
  breast — *continued*
    associated with
      lactation O92.70
        specified NEC O92.79
      pregnancy O92.20
        specified NEC O92.29
      puerperium O92.20
        specified NEC O92.29
    cracked nipple — *see* Cracked nipple
    galactorrhea — *see* Galactorrhea
    hypogalactia O92.4
    lactation disorder NEC O92.79
    mastitis — *see* Mastitis
    nipple infection — *see* Infection, nipple
    retracted nipple — *see* Retraction, nipple
    specified type NEC N64.89
  Briquet's F45.0
  bullous, in diseases classified elsewhere L14
  caffeine use
    mild
      with
        caffeine-induced
          anxiety disorder F15.180
          sleep disorder F15.182
    moderate or severe
      with
        caffeine-induced
          anxiety disorder F15.280
          sleep disorder F15.282
  cannabis use
    mild F12.10
      with
        cannabis intoxication delirium F12.121
          with perceptual disturbances F12.122
          without perceptual disturbances F12.129
        cannabis-induced
          anxiety disorder F12.180
          psychotic disorder F12.159
          sleep disorder F12.188
      in remission (early) (sustained) F12.11
    moderate or severe F12.20
      with
        cannabis intoxication
          with perceptual disturbances F12.222
          without perceptual disturbances F12.229
        cannabis-induced
          anxiety disorder F12.280
          psychotic disorder F12.259
          sleep disorder F12.288
        delirium F12.221
      in remission (early) (sustained) F12.21
  carbohydrate
    absorption, intestinal NEC E74.39
    metabolism (congenital) E74.9
      specified NEC E74.8
  cardiac, functional I51.89
  carnitine metabolism E71.40
  cartilage M94.9
    articular NEC — *see* Derangement, joint, articular cartilage
    chondrocalcinosis — *see* Chondrocalcinosis
    specified type NEC M94.8X- ☑
      articular — *see* Derangement, joint, articular cartilage
      multiple sites M94.8X0
  catatonia (due to known physiological condition) (with another mental disorder) F06.1
  catatonic
    due to (secondary to) known physiological condition F06.1
    organic F06.1
  central auditory processing H93.25
  cervical
    region NEC M53.82
    root (nerve) NEC G54.2
  character NOS F60.9
  childhood disintegrative NEC F84.3
  cholesterol and bile acid metabolism E78.70
    Barth syndrome E78.71
    other specified E78.79
    Smith-Lemli-Opitz syndrome E78.72
  choroid H31.9
    atrophy — *see* Atrophy, choroid
    degeneration — *see* Degeneration, choroid
    detachment — *see* Detachment, choroid
    dystrophy — *see* Dystrophy, choroid
    hemorrhage — *see* Hemorrhage, choroid

☑ **Additional Character Required** — Refer to the Tabular List for Character Selection   ⚐ Subterms under main terms may continue to next column or page

Disorder — *continued*
  choroid — *continued*
    rupture — *see* Rupture, choroid
    scar — *see* Scar, chorioretinal
    solar retinopathy — *see* Retinopathy, solar
    specified type NEC H31.8
  ciliary body — *see* Disorder, iris
    degeneration — *see* Degeneration, ciliary body
  coagulation (factor) (*see also* Defect, coagulation)
    D68.9
    newborn, transient P61.6
  cocaine use
    mild F14.10
      with
        amphetamine, cocaine, or other stimulant
          intoxication
            with perceptual disturbances F14.122
            without perceptual disturbances F14.129
        cocaine intoxication delirium F14.121
        cocaine-induced
          anxiety disorder F14.180
          bipolar and related disorder F14.14
          depressive disorder F14.14
          obsessive-compulsive and related disor-
            der F14.188
          psychotic disorder F14.159
          sexual dysfunction F14.181
          sleep disorder F14.182
      in remission (early) (sustained) F14.11
    moderate or severe F14.20
      with
        amphetamine, cocaine, or other stimulant
          intoxication
            with perceptual disturbances F14.222
            without perceptual disturbances F14.229
        cocaine intoxication delirium F14.221
        cocaine-induced
          anxiety disorder F14.280
          bipolar and related disorder F14.24
          depressive disorder F14.24
          obsessive-compulsive and related disor-
            der F14.288
          psychotic disorder F14.259
          sexual dysfunction F14.281
          sleep disorder F14.282
      in remission (early) (sustained) F14.21
  coccyx NEC M53.3
  cognitive F09
    due to (secondary to) general medical condition
      F09
    persisting R41.89
      due to
        alcohol F10.97
          with dependence F10.27
        anxiolytics F13.97
          with dependence F13.27
        hypnotics F13.97
          with dependence F13.27
        sedatives F13.97
          with dependence F13.27
        specified substance NEC F19.97
          with
            abuse F19.17
            dependence F19.27
  communication F80.9
    social pragmatic F80.82
  conduct (childhood) F91.9
    adjustment reaction — *see* Disorder, adjustment
    adolescent onset type F91.2
    childhood onset type F91.1
    compulsive F63.9
    confined to family context F91.0
    depressive F91.8
    group type F91.2
    hyperkinetic — *see* Disorder, attention-deficit hy-
      peractivity
    oppositional defiance F91.3
    socialized F91.2
    solitary aggressive type F91.1
    specified NEC F91.8
    unsocialized (aggressive) F91.1
  conduction, heart I45.9
  congenital glycosylation (CDG) E74.8
  conjunctiva H11.9
    infection — *see* Conjunctivitis
  connective tissue, localized L94.9
    specified NEC L94.8

Disorder — *continued*
  conversion (functional neurological symptom disorder)
    with
      abnormal movement F44.4
      anesthesia or sensory loss F44.6
      attacks or seizures F44.5
      mixed symptoms F44.7
      special sensory symptoms F44.6
      speech symptoms F44.4
      swallowing symptoms F44.4
      weakness or paralysis F44.4
  convulsive (secondary) — *see* Convulsions
  cornea H18.9
    deformity — *see* Deformity, cornea
    degeneration — *see* Degeneration, cornea
    deposits — *see* Deposit, cornea
    due to contact lens H18.82- ☑
      specified as edema — *see* Edema, cornea
    edema — *see* Edema, cornea
    keratitis — *see* Keratitis
    keratoconjunctivitis — *see* Keratoconjunctivitis
    membrane change — *see* Change, corneal mem-
      brane
    neovascularization — *see* Neovascularization,
      cornea
    scar — *see* Opacity, cornea
    specified type NEC H18.89- ☑
    ulcer — *see* Ulcer, cornea
  corpus cavernosum N48.9
  cranial nerve — *see* Disorder, nerve, cranial
  cyclothymic F34.0
  defiant oppositional F91.3
  delusional (persistent) (systematized) F22
    induced F24
  depersonalization F48.1
  depressive F32.9
    due to known physiological condition
      with
        depressive features F06.31
        major depressive-like episode F06.32
        mixed features F06.34
    major F32.9
      with psychotic symptoms F32.3
      in remission (full) F32.5
        partial F32.4
      recurrent F33.9
        with psychotic features F33.3
      single episode F32.9
        mild F32.0
        moderate F32.1
        severe (without psychotic symptoms) F32.2
          with psychotic symptoms F32.3
    organic F06.31
    persistent F34.1
    recurrent F33.9
      current episode
        mild F33.0
        moderate F33.1
        severe (without psychotic symptoms) F33.2
          with psychotic symptoms F33.3
      in remission F33.40
        full F33.42
        partial F33.41
      specified NEC F33.8
    single episode — *see* Episode, depressive
    specified NEC F32.89
  developmental F89
    arithmetical skills F81.2
    coordination (motor) F82
    expressive writing F81.81
    language F80.9
      expressive F80.1
      mixed receptive and expressive F80.2
      receptive type F80.2
      specified NEC F80.89
    learning F81.9
      arithmetical F81.2
      reading F81.0
    mixed F88
    motor coordination or function F82
    pervasive F84.9
      specified NEC F84.8
    phonological F80.0
    reading F81.0
    scholastic skills (*see also* Disorder, learning)
      mixed F81.89
    specified NEC F88
    speech F80.9

Disorder — *continued*
  developmental — *continued*
    speech — *continued*
      articulation F80.0
      specified NEC F80.89
    written expression F81.81
  diaphragm J98.6
  digestive (system) K92.9
    newborn P78.9
      specified NEC P78.89
    postprocedural — *see* Complication, gastrointesti-
      nal
    psychogenic F45.8
  disc (intervertebral) M51.9
    with
      myelopathy
        cervical region M50.00
        cervicothoracic region M50.03
        high cervical region M50.01
        lumbar region M51.06
        mid-cervical region M50.020
        sacrococcygeal region M53.3
        thoracic region M51.04
        thoracolumbar region M51.05
      radiculopathy
        cervical region M50.10
        cervicothoracic region M50.13
        high cervical region M50.11
        lumbar region M51.16
        lumbosacral region M51.17
        mid-cervical region M50.120
        sacrococcygeal region M53.3
        thoracic region M51.14
        thoracolumbar region M51.15
    cervical M50.90
      with
        myelopathy M50.00
          C2-C3 M50.01
          C3-C4 M50.01
          C4-C5 M50.021
          C5-C6 M50.022
          C6-C7 M50.023
          C7-T1 M50.03
          cervicothoracic region M50.03
          high cervical region M50.01
          mid-cervical region M50.020
        neuritis, radiculitis or radiculopathy M50.10
          C2-C3 M50.11
          C3-C4 M50.11
          C4-C5 M50.121
          C5-C6 M50.122
          C6-C7 M50.123
          C7-T1 M50.13
          cervicothoracic region M50.13
          high cervical region M50.11
          mid-cervical region M50.120
        C2-C3 M50.91
        C3-C4 M50.91
        C4-C5 M50.921
        C5-C6 M50.922
        C6-C7 M50.923
        C7-T1 M50.93
        cervicothoracic region M50.93
        degeneration M50.30
          C2-C3 M50.31
          C3-C4 M50.31
          C4-C5 M50.321
          C5-C6 M50.322
          C6-C7 M50.323
          C7-T1 M50.33
          cervicothoracic region M50.33
          high cervical region M50.31
          mid-cervical region M50.320
        displacement M50.20
          C2-C3 M50.21
          C3-C4 M50.21
          C4-C5 M50.221
          C5-C6 M50.222
          C6-C7 M50.223
          C7-T1 M50.23
          cervicothoracic region M50.23
          high cervical region M50.21
          mid-cervical region M50.220
        high cervical region M50.91
        mid-cervical region M50.920
        specified type NEC M50.80
          C2-C3 M50.81
          C3 C4 M50.81
          C4-C5 M50.821

▽ Subterms under main terms may continue to next column or page   ☑ Additional Character Required — Refer to the Tabular List for Character Selection   111

Disorder — Disorder

Disorder — *continued*
  disc — *continued*
    cervical — *continued*
      specified type — *continued*
        C5-C6 M50.822
        C6-C7 M50.823
        C7-T1 M50.83
        cervicothoracic region M50.83
        high cervical region M50.81
        mid-cervical region M50.820
      specified NEC
        lumbar region M51.86
        lumbosacral region M51.87
        sacrococcygeal region M53.3
        thoracic region M51.84
        thoracolumbar region M51.85
  disinhibited attachment (childhood) F94.2
  disintegrative, childhood NEC F84.3
  disruptive F91.9
    mood dysregulation F34.81
    specified NEC F91.8
  disruptive behavior — *see* Disorder, conduct
  dissocial personality F60.2
  dissociative F44.9
    affecting
      motor function F44.4
        and sensation F44.7
      sensation F44.6
        and motor function F44.7
    brief reactive F43.0
    due to (secondary to) general medical condition F06.8
    mixed F44.7
    organic F06.8
    other specified NEC F44.89
  double heterozygous sickling — *see* Disease, sickle-cell
  dream anxiety F51.5
  drug induced hemorrhagic D68.32
  drug related F19.99
    abuse — *see* Abuse, drug
    dependence — *see* Dependence, drug
  dysmorphic body F45.22
  dysthymic F34.1
  ear H93.9- ☑
    bleeding — *see* Otorrhagia
    deafness — *see* Deafness
    degenerative H93.09- ☑
    discharge — *see* Otorrhea
    external H61.9- ☑
      auditory canal stenosis — *see* Stenosis, external ear canal
      exostosis — *see* Exostosis, external ear canal
      impacted cerumen — *see* Impaction, cerumen
      otitis — *see* Otitis, externa
      perichondritis — *see* Perichondritis, ear
      pinna — *see* Disorder, pinna
      specified type NEC H61.89- ☑
    inner H83.9- ☑
      vestibular dysfunction — *see* Disorder, vestibular function
    middle H74.9- ☑
      adhesive H74.1- ☑
      ossicle — *see* Abnormal, ear ossicles
      polyp — *see* Polyp, ear (middle)
      specified NEC, in diseases classified elsewhere H75.8- ☑
    postprocedural — *see* Complications, ear, procedure
    specified NEC, in diseases classified elsewhere H94.8- ☑
  eating (adult) (psychogenic) F50.9
    anorexia — *see* Anorexia
    binge F50.81
    bulimia F50.2
    child F98.29
      pica F98.3
      rumination disorder F98.21
    pica F50.89
      childhood F98.3
  electrolyte (balance) NEC E87.8
    with
      abortion — *see* Abortion by type complicated by specified condition NEC
      ectopic pregnancy O08.5
      molar pregnancy O08.5
    acidosis (metabolic) (respiratory) E87.2
    alkalosis (metabolic) (respiratory) E87.3

Disorder — *continued*
  elimination, transepidermal L87.9
    specified NEC L87.8
  emotional (persistent) F34.9
    of childhood F93.9
      specified NEC F93.8
  endocrine E34.9
    postprocedural E89.89
      specified NEC E89.89
  erectile (male) (organic) (*see also* Dysfunction, sexual, male, erectile) N52.9
    nonorganic F52.21
  erythematous — *see* Erythema
  esophagus K22.9
    functional K22.4
    psychogenic F45.8
  eustachian tube H69.9- ☑
    infection — *see* Salpingitis, eustachian
    obstruction — *see* Obstruction, eustachian tube
    patulous — *see* Patulous, eustachian tube
    specified NEC H69.8- ☑
  exhibitionistic F65.2
  extrapyramidal G25.9
    in deseases classified elsewhere — *see* category G26
    specified type NEC G25.89
  eye H57.9
    postprocedural — *see* Complication, postprocedural, eye
  eyelid H02.9
    cyst — *see* Cyst, eyelid
    degenerative H02.70
      chloasma — *see* Chloasma, eyelid
      madarosis — *see* Madarosis
      specified type NEC H02.79
      vitiligo — *see* Vitiligo, eyelid
      xanthelasma — *see* Xanthelasma
    dermatochalasis — *see* Dermatochalasis
    edema — *see* Edema, eyelid
    elephantiasis — *see* Elephantiasis, eyelid
    foreign body, retained — *see* Foreign body, retained, eyelid
    function H02.59
      abnormal innervation syndrome — *see* Syndrome, abnormal innervation
      blepharochalasis — *see* Blepharochalasis
      blepharoclonus — *see* Blepharoclonus
      blepharophimosis — *see* Blepharophimosis
      blepharoptosis — *see* Blepharoptosis
      lagophthalmos — *see* Lagophthalmos
      lid retraction — *see* Retraction, lid
    hypertrichosis — *see* Hypertrichosis, eyelid
    specified type NEC H02.89
    vascular H02.879
      left H02.876
        lower H02.875
        upper H02.874
      right H02.873
        lower H02.872
        upper H02.871
  factitious F68.10
    with predominantly
      physical symptoms F68.12
        with psychological symptoms F68.13
      psychological symptoms F68.11
        with physical symptoms F68.13
  factor, coagulation — *see* Defect, coagulation
  fatty acid
    metabolism E71.30
      specified NEC E71.39
    oxidation
      LCAD E71.310
      MCAD E71.311
      SCAD E71.312
      specified deficiency NEC E71.318
  feeding (infant or child) (*see also* Disorder, eating) R63.3
    or eating disorder F50.9
    specified NEC F50.9
  feigned (with obvious motivation) Z76.5
    without obvious motivation — *see* Disorder, factitious
  female
    hypoactive sexual desire F52.0
    orgasmic F52.31
    sexual interest/arousal F52.22
  fetishistic F65.0
  fibroblastic M72.9

Disorder — *continued*
  fibroblastic — *continued*
    specified NEC M72.8
  fluency
    adult onset F98.5
    childhood onset F80.81
    following
      cerebral infarction I69.323
      cerebrovascular disease I69.923
        specified disease NEC I69.823
      intracerebral hemorrhage I69.123
      nontraumatic intracranial hemorrhage NEC I69.223
      subarachnoid hemorrhage I69.023
    in conditions classified elsewhere R47.82
  fluid balance E87.8
  follicular (skin) L73.9
    specified NEC L73.8
  frotteuristic F65.81
  fructose metabolism E74.10
    essential fructosuria E74.11
    fructokinase deficiency E74.11
    fructose-1, 6-diphosphatase deficiency E74.19
    hereditary fructose intolerance E74.12
    other specified E74.19
  functional polymorphonuclear neutrophils D71
  gallbladder, biliary tract and pancreas in diseases classified elsewhere K87
  gambling F63.0
  gamma-glutamyl cycle E72.8
  gastric (functional) K31.9
    motility K30
    psychogenic F45.8
    secretion K30
  gastrointestinal (functional) NOS K92.9
    newborn P78.9
    psychogenic F45.8
  gender-identity or -role F64.9
    childhood F64.2
    effect on relationship F66
    of adolescence or adulthood F64.0
      nontranssexual F64.8
    specified NEC F64.8
    uncertainty F66
  genito-pelvic pain penetration F52.6
  genitourinary system
    female N94.9
    male N50.9
    psychogenic F45.8
  globe H44.9
    degenerated condition H44.50
      absolute glaucoma H44.51- ☑
      atrophy H44.52- ☑
      leucocoria H44.53- ☑
    degenerative H44.30
      chalcosis H44.31- ☑
      myopia (*see also* Myopia, degenerative) H44.2- ☑
      siderosis H44.32- ☑
      specified type NEC H44.39- ☑
    endophthalmitis — *see* Endophthalmitis
    foreign body, retained — *see* Foreign body, intraocular, old, retained
    hemophthalmos — *see* Hemophthalmos
    hypotony H44.40
      due to
        ocular fistula H44.42- ☑
        specified disorder NEC H44.43- ☑
      flat anterior chamber H44.41- ☑
      primary H44.44- ☑
    luxation — *see* Luxation, globe
    specified type NEC H44.89
  glomerular (in) N05.9
    amyloidosis E85.4 [N08]
    cryoglobulinemia D89.1 [N08]
    disseminated intravascular coagulation D65 [N08]
    Fabry's disease E75.21 [N08]
    familial lecithin cholesterol acyltransferase deficiency E78.6 [N08]
    Goodpasture's syndrome M31.0
    hemolytic-uremic syndrome D59.3
    Henoch (-Schönlein) purpura D69.0 [N08]
    malariae malaria B52.0
    microscopic polyangiitis M31.7 [N08]
    multiple myeloma C90.0- ☑ [N08]
    mumps B26.83
    schistosomiasis B65.9 [N08]
    sepsis NEC A41.- ☑ [N08]

Disorder — *continued*
  glomerular — *continued*
    sepsis — *continued*
      streptococcal A40.- ☑ [N08]
    sickle-cell disorders D57.- ☑ [N08]
    strongyloidiasis B78.9 [N08]
    subacute bacterial endocarditis I33.0 [N08]
    syphilis A52.75
    systemic lupus erythematosus M32.14
    thrombotic thrombocytopenic purpura
      M31.1 [N08]
    Waldenström macroglobulinemia C88.0 [N08]
    Wegener's granulomatosis M31.31
  gluconeogenesis E74.4
  glucosaminoglycan metabolism — *see* Disorder,
    metabolism, glucosaminoglycan
  glycine metabolism E72.50
    d-glycericacidemia E72.59
    hyperhydroxyprolinemia E72.59
    hyperoxaluria E72.53
    hyperprolinemia E72.59
    non-ketotic hyperglycinemia E72.51
    oxalosis E72.53
    oxaluria E72.53
    sarcosinemia E72.59
    trimethylaminuria E72.52
  glycoprotein metabolism E77.9
    specified NEC E77.8
  habit (and impulse) F63.9
    involving sexual behavior NEC F65.9
    specified NEC F63.89
  hallucinogen use
    mild F16.10
      with
        hallucinogen intoxication delirium F16.121
        hallucinogen-induced
          anxiety disorder F16.180
          bipolar and related disorder F16.14
          depressive disorder F16.14
          psychotic disorder F16.159
        other hallucinogen intoxication F16.129
      in remission (early) (sustained) F16.11
    moderate or severe F16.20
      with
        hallucinogen intoxication delirium F16.221
        hallucinogen-induced
          anxiety disorder F16.280
          bipolar and related disorder F16.24
          depressive disorder F16.24
          psychotic disorder F16.259
        other hallucinogen intoxication F16.229
      in remission (early) (sustained) F16.21
  heart action I49.9
  hematological D75.9
    newborn (transient) P61.9
      specified NEC P61.8
  hematopoietic organs D75.9
  hemorrhagic NEC D69.9
    drug-induced D68.32
    due to
      extrinsic circulating anticoagulants D68.32
      increase in
        anti-IIa D68.32
        anti-Xa D68.32
      intrinsic
        circulating anticoagulants D68.318
        increase in
          anti-IXa D68.318
          antithrombin D68.318
          anti-VIIIa D68.318
          anti-XIa D68.318
    following childbirth O72.3
  hemostasis — *see* Defect, coagulation
  histidine metabolism E70.40
    histidinemia E70.41
    other specified E70.49
  hoarding F42.3
  hyperkinetic — *see* Disorder, attention-deficit hyper-
    activity
  hyperleucine-isoleucinemia E71.19
  hypervalinemia E71.19
  hypoactive sexual desire F52.0
  hypochondriacal F45.20
    body dysmorphic F45.22
    neurosis F45.21
    other specified F45.29
  identity
    dissociative F44.81
    illness anxiety F45.21

Disorder — *continued*
  identity — *continued*
    of childhood F93.8
  immune mechanism (immunity) D89.9
    specified type NEC D89.89
  impaired renal tubular function N25.9
    specified NEC N25.89
  impulse (control) F63.9
  inflammatory
    pelvic, in diseases classified elsewhere — *see* cate-
      gory N74
    penis N48.29
      abscess N48.21
      cellulitis N48.22
  inhalant use
    mild F18.10
      with
        inhalant intoxication F18.129
        inhalant intoxication delirium F18.121
        inhalant-induced
          anxiety disorder F18.180
          depressive disorder F18.14
          major neurocognitive disorder F18.17
          mild neurocognitive disorder F18.188
          psychotic disorder F18.159
      in remission (early) (sustained) F18.11
    moderate or severe F18.20
      with
        inhalant intoxication F18.229
        inhalant intoxication delirium F18.221
        inhalant-induced
          anxiety disorder F18.280
          depressive disorder F18.24
          major neurocognitive disorder F18.27
          mild neurocognitive disorder F18.288
          psychotic disorder F18.259
      in remission (early) (sustained) F18.21
  integument, newborn P83.9
    specified NEC P83.88
  intermittent explosive F63.81
  internal secretion pancreas — *see* Increased, secretion,
    pancreas, endocrine
  intestine, intestinal
    carbohydrate absorption NEC E74.39
      postoperative K91.2
    functional NEC K59.9
      postoperative K91.89
    psychogenic F45.8
    vascular K55.9
      chronic K55.1
      specified NEC K55.8
  intraoperative (intraprocedural) — *see* Complications,
    intraoperative
  involuntary emotional expression (IEED) F07.89
  iris H21.9
    adhesions — *see* Adhesions, iris
    atrophy — *see* Atrophy, iris
    chamber angle recession — *see* Recession, cham-
      ber angle
    cyst — *see* Cyst, iris
    degeneration — *see* Degeneration, iris
    in diseases classified elsewhere H22
    iridodialysis — *see* Iridodialysis
    iridoschisis — *see* Iridoschisis
    miotic pupillary cyst — *see* Cyst, pupillary
    pupillary
      abnormality — *see* Abnormality, pupillary
      membrane — *see* Membrane, pupillary
    specified type NEC H21.89
    vascular NEC H21.1X- ☑
  iron metabolism E83.10
    specified NEC E83.19
  isovaleric acidemia E71.110
  jaw, developmental M27.0
    temporomandibular (*see also* Anomaly, dentofacial,
      temporomandibular joint) M26.60- ☑
  joint M25.9
    derangement — *see* Derangement, joint
    effusion — *see* Effusion, joint
    fistula — *see* Fistula, joint
    hemarthrosis — *see* Hemarthrosis
    instability — *see* Instability, joint
    osteophyte — *see* Osteophyte
    pain — *see* Pain, joint
    psychogenic F45.8
    specified type NEC M25.80
      ankle M25.87- ☑
      elbow M25.82- ☑

Disorder — *continued*
  joint — *continued*
    specified type — *continued*
      foot joint M25.87- ☑
      hand joint M25.84- ☑
      hip M25.85- ☑
      knee M25.86- ☑
      shoulder M25.81- ☑
      wrist M25.83- ☑
    stiffness — *see* Stiffness, joint
  ketone metabolism E71.32
  kidney N28.9
    functional (tubular) N25.9
    in
      schistosomiasis B65.9 [N29]
    tubular function N25.9
      specified NEC N25.89
  lacrimal system H04.9
    changes H04.69
      fistula — *see* Fistula, lacrimal
    gland H04.19
      atrophy — *see* Atrophy, lacrimal gland
      cyst — *see* Cyst, lacrimal, gland
      dacryops — *see* Dacryops
      dislocation — *see* Dislocation, lacrimal gland
      dry eye syndrome — *see* Syndrome, dry eye
      infection — *see* Dacryoadenitis
    granuloma — *see* Granuloma, lacrimal
    inflammation — *see* Inflammation, lacrimal
    obstruction — *see* Obstruction, lacrimal
    specified NEC H04.89
  lactation NEC O92.79
  language (developmental) F80.9
    expressive F80.1
    mixed receptive and expressive F80.2
    receptive F80.2
  late luteal phase dysphoric N94.89
  learning (specific) F81.9
    acalculia R48.8
    alexia R48.0
    mathematics F81.2
    reading F81.0
    specified
      with impairment in
        mathematics F81.2
        reading F81.0
        written expression F81.81
    specified NEC F81.89
    spelling F81.81
    written expression F81.81
  lens H27.9
    aphakia — *see* Aphakia
    cataract — *see* Cataract
    dislocation — *see* Dislocation, lens
    specified type NEC H27.8
  ligament M24.20
    ankle M24.27- ☑
    attachment, spine — *see* Enthesopathy, spinal
    elbow M24.22- ☑
    foot joint M24.27- ☑
    hand joint M24.24- ☑
    hip M24.25- ☑
    knee — *see* Derangement, knee, specified NEC
    shoulder M24.21- ☑
    vertebra M24.28
    wrist M24.23- ☑
  ligamentous attachments (*see also* Enthesopathy)
    spine — *see* Enthesopathy, spinal
  lipid
    metabolism, congenital E78.9
    storage E75.6
      specified NEC E75.5
  lipoprotein
    deficiency (familial) E78.6
    metabolism E78.9
      specified NEC E78.89
  liver K76.9
    malarial B54 [K77]
  low back (*see also* Dorsopathy, specified NEC)
  lumbosacral
    plexus G54.1
    root (nerve) NEC G54.4
  lung, interstitial, drug-induced J70.4
    acute J70.2
    chronic J70.3
  lymphoproliferative, post-transplant (PTLD) D47.Z1
    (*following* D47.4)
  lysine and hydroxylysine metabolism E72.3

⚐ Subterms under main terms may continue to next column or page   ☑ Additional Character Required — Refer to the Tabular List for Character Selection   **113**

Disorder — Disorder

Disorder — *continued*
- major neurocognitive — *see* Dementia, in (due to)
- male
  - erectile (organic) (*see also* Dysfunction, sexual, male, erectile) N52.9
    - nonorganic F52.21
  - hypoactive sexual desire F52.0
  - orgasmic F52.32
- manic F30.9
  - organic F06.33
- mast cell activation — *see* Activation, mast cell
- mastoid (*see also* Disorder, ear, middle)
  - postprocedural — *see* Complications, ear, procedure
- meniscus — *see* Derangement, knee, meniscus
- menopausal N95.9
  - specified NEC N95.8
- menstrual N92.6
  - psychogenic F45.8
  - specified NEC N92.5
- mental (or behavioral) (nonpsychotic) F99
  - due to (secondary to)
    - amphetamine
      - due to drug abuse — *see* Abuse, drug, stimulant
      - due to drug dependence — *see* Dependence, drug, stimulant
    - brain disease, damage and dysfunction F09
    - caffeine use
      - due to drug abuse — *see* Abuse, drug, stimulant
      - due to drug dependence — *see* Dependence, drug, stimulant
    - cannabis use
      - due to drug abuse — *see* Abuse, drug, cannabis
      - due to drug dependence — *see* Dependence, drug, cannabis
    - general medical condition F09
    - sedative or hypnotic use
      - due to drug abuse — *see* Abuse, drug, sedative
      - due to drug dependence — *see* Dependence, drug, sedative
    - tobacco (nicotine) use — *see* Dependence, drug, nicotine
  - following organic brain damage F07.9
    - frontal lobe syndrome F07.0
    - personality change F07.0
    - postconcussional syndrome F07.81
    - specified NEC F07.89
  - infancy, childhood or adolescence F98.9
  - neurotic — *see* Neurosis
  - organic or symptomatic F09
  - presenile, psychotic F03 ☑
  - problem NEC
  - psychoneurotic — *see* Neurosis
  - psychotic — *see* Psychosis
  - puerperal F53
  - senile, psychotic NEC F03 ☑
- metabolic, amino acid, transitory, newborn P74.8
- metabolism NOS E88.9
  - amino-acid E72.9
    - aromatic E70.9
      - albinism — *see* Albinism
      - histidine E70.40
        - histidinemia E70.41
        - other specified E70.49
      - hyperphenylalaninemia E70.1
        - classical phenylketonuria E70.0
      - other specified E70.8
      - tryptophan E70.5
      - tyrosine E70.20
        - hypertyrosinemia E70.21
        - other specified E70.29
    - branched chain E71.2
      - 3-methylglutaconic aciduria E71.111
      - hyperleucine-isoleucinemia E71.19
      - hypervalinemia E71.19
      - isovaleric acidemia E71.110
      - maple syrup urine disease E71.0
      - methylmalonic acidemia E71.120
      - organic aciduria NEC E71.118
      - other specified E71.19
      - propionate NEC E71.128
      - propionic acidemia E71.121
    - glycine E72.50
      - d-glycericacidemia E72.59

Disorder — *continued*
- metabolism — *continued*
  - amino-acid — *continued*
    - glycine — *continued*
      - hyperhydroxyprolinemia E72.59
      - hyperoxaluria E72.53
      - hyperprolinemia E72.59
      - non-ketotic hyperglycinemia E72.51
      - other specified E72.59
      - sarcosinemia E72.59
      - trimethylaminuria E72.52
    - hydroxylysine E72.3
    - lysine E72.3
    - ornithine E72.4
    - other specified E72.8
      - beta-amino acid E72.8
      - gamma-glutamyl cycle E72.8
      - straight-chain E72.8
      - sulfur-bearing E72.10
        - homocystinuria E72.11
        - methylenetetrahydrofolate reductase deficiency E72.12
        - other specified E72.19
  - bile acid and cholesterol metabolism E78.70
  - bilirubin E80.7
    - specified NEC E80.6
  - calcium E83.50
    - hypercalcemia E83.52
    - hypocalcemia E83.51
    - other specified E83.59
  - carbohydrate E74.9
    - specified NEC E74.8
  - cholesterol and bile acid metabolism E78.70
  - congenital E88.9
  - copper E83.00
    - specified type NEC E83.09
    - Wilson's disease E83.01
  - cystinuria E72.01
  - fructose E74.10
  - galactose E74.20
  - glucosaminoglycan E76.9
    - mucopolysaccharidosis — *see* Mucopolysaccharidosis
    - specified NEC E76.8
  - glutamine E72.8
  - glycine E72.50
  - glycogen storage (hepatorenal) E74.09
  - glycoprotein E77.9
    - specified NEC E77.8
  - glycosaminoglycan E76.9
    - specified NEC E76.8
  - in labor and delivery O75.89
  - iron E83.10
  - isoleucine E71.19
  - leucine E71.19
  - lipoid E78.9
  - lipoprotein E78.9
    - specified NEC E78.89
  - magnesium E83.40
    - hypermagnesemia E83.41
    - hypomagnesemia E83.42
    - other specified E83.49
  - mineral E83.9
    - specified NEC E83.89
  - mitochondrial E88.40
    - MELAS syndrome E88.41
    - MERRF syndrome (myoclonic epilepsy associated with ragged-red fibers) E88.42
    - other specified E88.49
  - ornithine E72.4
  - phosphatases E83.30
  - phosphorus E83.30
    - acid phosphatase deficiency E83.39
    - hypophosphatasia E83.39
    - hypophosphatemia E83.39
      - familial E83.31
    - other specified E83.39
    - pseudovitamin D deficiency E83.32
  - plasma protein NEC E88.09
  - porphyrin — *see* Porphyria
  - postprocedural E89.89
    - specified NEC E89.89
  - purine E79.9
    - specified NEC E79.8
  - pyrimidine E79.9
    - specified NEC E79.8
  - pyruvate E74.4
  - serine E72.8
  - sodium E87.8

Disorder — *continued*
- metabolism — *continued*
  - specified NEC E88.89
  - threonine E72.8
  - valine E71.19
  - zinc E83.2
- methylmalonic acidemia E71.120
- micturition NEC (*see also* Difficulty, micturition) R39.198
  - feeling of incomplete emptying R39.14
  - hesitancy R39.11
  - poor stream R39.12
  - psychogenic F45.8
  - split stream R39.13
  - straining R39.16
  - urgency R39.15
- mild neurocognitive G31.84
- mitochondrial metabolism E88.40
- mitral (valve) — *see* Endocarditis, mitral
- mixed
  - anxiety and depressive F41.8
  - of scholastic skills (developmental) F81.89
  - receptive expressive language F80.2
- mood F39
  - bipolar — *see* Disorder, bipolar
  - depressive — *see* Disorder, depressive
  - due to (secondary to)
    - alcohol F10.94
    - amphetamine F15.94
      - in
        - abuse F15.14
        - dependence F15.24
    - anxiolytic F13.94
      - in
        - abuse F13.14
        - dependence F13.24
    - cocaine F14.94
      - in
        - abuse F14.14
        - dependence F14.24
    - general medical condition F06.30
    - hallucinogen F16.94
      - in
        - abuse F16.14
        - dependence F16.24
    - hypnotic F13.94
      - in
        - abuse F13.14
        - dependence F13.24
    - inhalant F18.94
      - in
        - abuse F18.14
        - dependence F18.24
    - opioid F11.94
      - in
        - abuse F11.14
        - dependence F11.24
    - phencyclidine (PCP) F16.94
      - in
        - abuse F16.14
        - dependence F16.24
    - physiological condition F06.30
      - with
        - depressive features F06.31
        - major depressive-like episode F06.32
        - manic features F06.33
        - mixed features F06.34
    - psychoactive substance NEC F19.94
      - in
        - abuse F19.14
        - dependence F19.24
    - sedative F13.94
      - in
        - abuse F13.14
        - dependence F13.24
    - volatile solvents F18.94
      - in
        - abuse F18.14
        - dependence F18.24
  - manic episode F30.9
    - with psychotic symptoms F30.2
    - without psychotic symptoms F30.10
      - mild F30.11
      - moderate F30.12
      - severe F30.13
    - in remission (full) F30.4
      - partial F30.3
    - specified type NEC F30.8
  - organic F06.30

Disorder — *continued*
  mood — *continued*
    organic — *continued*
      right hemisphere F07.89
    persistent F34.9
      cyclothymia F34.0
      dysthymia F34.1
      specified type NEC F34.89
    recurrent F39
    right hemisphere organic F07.89
  movement G25.9
    drug-induced G25.70
      akathisia G25.71
      specified NEC G25.79
    hysterical F44.4
    in diseases classified elsewhere — *see* category G26
    periodic limb G47.61
      sleep related G47.61
    sleep related NEC G47.69
    specified NEC G25.89
    stereotyped F98.4
    treatment-induced G25.9
  multiple personality F44.81
  muscle M62.9
    attachment, spine — *see* Enthesopathy, spinal
    in trichinellosis — *see* Trichinellosis, with muscle disorder
    psychogenic F45.8
    specified type NEC M62.89
    tone, newborn P94.9
      specified NEC P94.8
  muscular
    attachments (*see also* Enthesopathy)
      spine — *see* Enthesopathy, spinal
    urethra N36.44
  musculoskeletal system, soft tissue — *see* Disorder, soft tissue
    postprocedural M96.89
    psychogenic F45.8
  myoneural G70.9
    due to lead G70.1
    specified NEC G70.89
    toxic G70.1
  myotonic NEC G71.19
  nail, in diseases classified elsewhere L62
  neck region NEC — *see* Dorsopathy, specified NEC
  neonatal onset multisystemic inflammatory (NOMID) M04.2
  nerve G58.9
    abducent NEC — *see* Strabismus, paralytic, sixth nerve
    accessory G52.8
    acoustic — *see* subcategory H93.3 ☑
    auditory — *see* subcategory H93.3 ☑
    auriculotemporal G50.8
    axillary G54.0
    cerebral — *see* Disorder, nerve, cranial
    cranial G52.9
      eighth — *see* subcategory H93.3 ☑
      eleventh G52.8
      fifth G50.9
      first G52.0
      fourth NEC — *see* Strabismus, paralytic, fourth nerve
      multiple G52.7
      ninth G52.1
      second NEC — *see* Disorder, nerve, optic
      seventh NEC G51.8
      sixth NEC — *see* Strabismus, paralytic, sixth nerve
      specified NEC G52.8
      tenth G52.2
      third NEC — *see* Strabismus, paralytic, third nerve
      twelfth G52.3
    entrapment — *see* Neuropathy, entrapment
    facial G51.9
      specified NEC G51.8
    femoral — *see* Lesion, nerve, femoral
    glossopharyngeal NEC G52.1
    hypoglossal G52.3
    intercostal G58.0
    lateral
      cutaneous of thigh — *see* Mononeuropathy, lower limb, meralgia paresthetica
      popliteal — *see* Lesion, nerve, popliteal
    lower limb — *see* Mononeuropathy, lower limb

Disorder — *continued*
  nerve — *continued*
    medial popliteal — *see* Lesion, nerve, popliteal, medial
    median NEC — *see* Lesion, nerve, median
    multiple G58.7
    oculomotor NEC — *see* Strabismus, paralytic, third nerve
    olfactory G52.0
    optic NEC H47.09- ☑
      hemorrhage into sheath — *see* Hemorrhage, optic nerve
      ischemic H47.01- ☑
    peroneal — *see* Lesion, nerve, popliteal
    phrenic G58.8
    plantar — *see* Lesion, nerve, plantar
    pneumogastric G52.2
    posterior tibial — *see* Syndrome, tarsal tunnel
    radial — *see* Lesion, nerve, radial
    recurrent laryngeal G52.2
    root G54.9
      cervical G54.2
      lumbosacral G54.1
      specified NEC G54.8
      thoracic G54.3
    sciatic NEC — *see* Lesion, nerve, sciatic
    specified NEC G58.8
      lower limb — *see* Mononeuropathy, lower limb, specified NEC
      upper limb — *see* Mononeuropathy, upper limb, specified NEC
    sympathetic G90.9
    tibial — *see* Lesion, nerve, popliteal, medial
    trigeminal G50.9
      specified NEC G50.8
    trochlear NEC — *see* Strabismus, paralytic, fourth nerve
    ulnar — *see* Lesion, nerve, ulnar
    upper limb — *see* Mononeuropathy, upper limb
    vagus G52.2
  nervous system G98.8
    autonomic (peripheral) G90.9
      specified NEC G90.8
    central G96.9
      specified NEC G96.8
    parasympathetic G90.9
    specified NEC G98.8
    sympathetic G90.9
    vegetative G90.9
  neurocognitive R41.9
    major
      with
        aggressive behavior F01.51
        combative behavior F01.51
        violent behavior F01.51
      without behavioral disturbance F01.50
      due to vascular disease, with behavioral disturbance F01.51
      in (due to) (other diseases classified elsewhere) (*see also* Dementia, in (due to)) F02.80
        with
          aggressive behavior F02.81
          combative behavior F02.81
          violent behavior F02.81
    mild G31.84
  neurodevelopmental F89
    specified NEC F88
  neurohypophysis NEC E23.3
  neurological NEC R29.818
  neuromuscular G70.9
    hereditary NEC G71.9
    specified NEC G70.89
    toxic G70.1
  neurotic F48.9
    specified NEC F48.8
  neutrophil, polymorphonuclear D71
  nicotine use — *see* Dependence, drug, nicotine
  nightmare F51.5
  non-rapid eye movement sleep arousal
    sleep terror type F51.4
    sleepwalking type F51.3
  nose J34.9
    specified NEC J34.89
  obsessive-compulsive F42.9
    and related disorder due to a known physiological condition F06.8
  odontogenesis NOS K00.9

Disorder — *continued*
  opioid use
    with
      opioid-induced psychotic disorder F11.959
        with
          delusions F11.950
          hallucinations F11.951
      due to drug abuse — *see* Abuse, drug, opioid
      due to drug dependence — *see* Dependence, drug, opioid
    mild F11.10
      with
        opioid intoxication
          with perceptual disturbances F11.122
          without perceptual disturbances F11.129
          delirium F11.121
        opioid-induced
          anxiety disorder F11.188
          depressive disorder F11.14
          sexual dysfunction F11.181
      in remission (early) (sustained) F11.11
    moderate or severe F11.20
      with
        opioid intoxication
          with perceptual disturbances F11.222
          without perceptual disturbances F11.229
          delirium F11.221
        opioid-induced
          anxiety disorder F11.288
          anxiety disorder F11.988
          depressive disorder F11.24
          depressive disorder F11.94
          sexual dysfunction F11.281
          sexual dysfunction F11.981
      in remission (early) (sustained) F11.21
  oppositional defiant F91.3
  optic
    chiasm H47.49
      due to
        inflammatory disorder H47.41
        neoplasm H47.42
        vascular disorder H47.43
    disc H47.39- ☑
      coloboma — *see* Coloboma, optic disc
      drusen — *see* Drusen, optic disc
      pseudopapilledema — *see* Pseudopapilledema
    radiations — *see* Disorder, visual, pathway
    tracts — *see* Disorder, visual, pathway
  orbit H05.9
    cyst — *see* Cyst, orbit
    deformity — *see* Deformity, orbit
    edema — *see* Edema, orbit
    enophthalmos — *see* Enophthalmos
    exophthalmos — *see* Exophthalmos
    hemorrhage — *see* Hemorrhage, orbit
    inflammation — *see* Inflammation, orbit
    myopathy — *see* Myopathy, extraocular muscles
    retained foreign body — *see* Foreign body, orbit, old
    specified type NEC H05.89
  organic
    anxiety F06.4
    catatonic F06.1
    delusional F06.2
    dissociative F06.8
    emotionally labile (asthenic) F06.8
    mood (affective) F06.30
    schizophrenia-like F06.2
  orgasmic (female) F52.31
    male F52.32
  ornithine metabolism E72.4
  overanxious F41.1
    of childhood F93.8
  pain
    with related psychological factors F45.42
    exclusively related to psychological factors F45.41
    genito-pelvic penetration disorder F52.6
  pancreatic internal secretion E16.9
    specified NEC E16.8
  panic F41.0
    with agoraphobia F40.01
  papulosquamous L44.9
    in diseases classified elsewhere L45
    specified NEC L44.8
  paranoid F22
    induced F24
    shared F24
  paraphilic F65.9

Disorder — *continued*
  paraphilic — *continued*
    specified NEC F65.89
  parathyroid (gland) E21.5
    specified NEC E21.4
  parietoalveolar NEC J84.09
  paroxysmal, mixed R56.9
  patella M22.9- ☑
    chondromalacia — *see* Chondromalacia, patella
    derangement NEC M22.3X- ☑
    recurrent
      dislocation — *see* Dislocation, patella, recurrent
      subluxation — *see* Dislocation, patella, recurrent, incomplete
    specified NEC M22.8X- ☑
  patellofemoral M22.2X- ☑
  pedophilic F65.4
  pentose phosphate pathway with anemia D55.1
  perception, due to hallucinogens F16.983
    in
      abuse F16.183
      dependence F16.283
  peripheral nervous system NEC G64
  peroxisomal E71.50
    biogenesis
      neonatal adrenoleukodystrophy E71.511
      specified disorder NEC E71.518
      Zellweger syndrome E71.510
    rhizomelic chondrodysplasia punctata E71.540
    specified form NEC E71.548
      group 1 E71.518
      group 2 E71.53
      group 3 E71.542
    X-linked adrenoleukodystrophy E71.529
      adolescent E71.521
      adrenomyeloneuropathy E71.522
      childhood E71.520
      specified form NEC E71.528
    Zellweger-like syndrome E71.541
  persistent
    (somatoform) pain F45.41
    affective (mood) F34.9
  personality (*see also* Personality) F60.9
    affective F34.0
    aggressive F60.3
    amoral F60.2
    anankastic F60.5
    antisocial F60.2
    anxious F60.6
    asocial F60.2
    asthenic F60.7
    avoidant F60.6
    borderline F60.3
    change (secondary) due to general medical condition F07.0
    compulsive F60.5
    cyclothymic F34.0
    dependent (passive) F60.7
    depressive F34.1
    dissocial F60.2
    emotional instability F60.3
    expansive paranoid F60.0
    explosive F60.3
    following organic brain damage F07.9
    histrionic F60.4
    hyperthymic F34.0
    hypothymic F34.1
    hysterical F60.4
    immature F60.89
    inadequate F60.7
    labile F60.3
    mixed (nonspecific) F60.89
    moral deficiency F60.2
    narcissistic F60.81
    negativistic F60.89
    obsessional F60.5
    obsessive (-compulsive) F60.5
    organic F07.9
    overconscientious F60.5
    paranoid F60.0
    passive (-dependent) F60.7
    passive-aggressive F60.89
    pathological NEC F60.9
    pseudosocial F60.2
    psychopathic F60.2
    schizoid F60.1
    schizotypal F21
    self-defeating F60.7

Disorder — *continued*
  personality (*see also* Personality) — *continued*
    specified NEC F60.89
    type A F60.5
    unstable (emotional) F60.3
  pervasive, developmental F84.9
  phencyclidine use
    mild F16.10
      with
        phencyclidine intoxication F16.129
        phencyclidine intoxication delirium F16.121
        phencyclidine-induced
          anxiety disorder F16.180
          bipolar and related disorder F16.14
          depressive disorder F16.14
          psychotic disorder F16.159
      in remission (early) (sustained) F16.11
    moderate or severe F16.20
      with
        phencyclidine intoxication F16.229
        phencyclidine intoxication delirium F16.221
        phencyclidine-induced
          anxiety disorder F16.280
          bipolar and related disorder F16.14
          depressive disorder F16.24
          psychotic disorder F16.259
      in remission (early) (sustained) F16.21
  phobic anxiety, childhood F40.8
  phosphate-losing tubular N25.0
  pigmentation L81.9
    choroid, congenital Q14.3
    diminished melanin formation L81.6
    iron L81.8
    specified NEC L81.8
  pinna (noninfective) H61.10- ☑
    deformity, acquired H61.11- ☑
    hematoma H61.12- ☑
    perichondritis — *see* Perichondritis, ear
    specified type NEC H61.19- ☑
  pituitary gland E23.7
    iatrogenic (postprocedural) E89.3
    specified NEC E23.6
  platelets D69.1
  plexus G54.9
    specified NEC G54.8
  polymorphonuclear neutrophils D71
  porphyrin metabolism — *see* Porphyria
  postconcussional F07.81
  posthallucinogen perception F16.983
    in
      abuse F16.183
      dependence F16.283
  postmenopausal N95.9
    specified NEC N95.8
  postprocedural (postoperative) — *see* Complications, postprocedural
  post-transplant lymphoproliferative D47.Z1 (*following* D47.4)
  post-traumatic stress (PTSD) F43.10
    acute F43.11
    chronic F43.12
  premenstrual dysphoric (PMDD) F32.81
  prepuce N47.8
  propionic acidemia E71.121
  prostate N42.9
    specified NEC N42.89
  psychogenic NOS (*see also* condition) F45.9
    anxiety F41.8
    appetite F50.9
    asthenic F48.8
    cardiovascular (system) F45.8
    compulsive F42.8
    cutaneous F54
    depressive F32.9
    digestive (system) F45.8
    dysmenorrheic F45.8
    dyspneic F45.8
    endocrine (system) F54
    eye NEC F45.8
    feeding — *see* Disorder, eating
    functional NEC F45.8
    gastric F45.8
    gastrointestinal (system) F45.8
    genitourinary (system) F45.8
    heart (function) (rhythm) F45.8
    hyperventilatory F45.8
    hypochondriacal — *see* Disorder, hypochondriacal
    intestinal F45.8

Disorder — *continued*
  psychogenic (*see also* condition) — *continued*
    joint F45.8
    learning F81.9
    limb F45.8
    lymphatic (system) F45.8
    menstrual F45.8
    micturition F45.8
    monoplegic NEC F44.4
    motor F44.4
    muscle F45.8
    musculoskeletal F45.8
    neurocirculatory F45.8
    obsessive F42.8
    occupational F48.8
    organ or part of body NEC F45.8
    paralytic NEC F44.4
    phobic F40.9
    physical NEC F45.8
    rectal F45.8
    respiratory (system) F45.8
    rheumatic F45.8
    sexual (function) F52.9
    skin (allergic) (eczematous) F54
    sleep F51.9
    specified part of body NEC F45.8
    stomach F45.8
  psychological F99
    associated with
      disease classified elsewhere F54
      sexual
        development F66
        relationship F66
      uncertainty about gender identity F64.9
  psychomotor NEC F44.4
    hysterical F44.4
  psychoneurotic (*see also* Neurosis)
    mixed NEC F48.8
  psychophysiologic — *see* Disorder, somatoform
  psychosexual F65.9
    development F66
    identity of childhood F64.2
  psychosomatic NOS — *see* Disorder, somatoform
    multiple F45.0
    undifferentiated F45.1
  psychotic — *see* Psychosis
    transient (acute) F23
  puberty E30.9
    specified NEC E30.8
  pulmonary (valve) — *see* Endocarditis, pulmonary
  purine metabolism E79.9
  pyrimidine metabolism E79.9
  pyruvate metabolism E74.4
  reactive attachment (childhood) F94.1
  reading R48.0
    developmental (specific) F81.0
  receptive language F80.2
  receptor, hormonal, peripheral (*see also* Syndrome, androgen insensitivity) E34.50
  recurrent brief depressive F33.8
  reflex R29.2
  refraction H52.7
    aniseikonia H52.32
    anisometropia H52.31
    astigmatism — *see* Astigmatism
    hypermetropia — *see* Hypermetropia
    myopia — *see* Myopia
    presbyopia H52.4
    specified NEC H52.6
  relationship F68.8
    due to sexual orientation F66
  REM sleep behavior G47.52
  renal function, impaired (tubular) N25.9
  resonance R49.9
    specified NEC R49.8
  respiratory function, impaired (*see also* Failure, respiration)
    postprocedural — *see* Complication, postoperative, respiratory system
    psychogenic F45.8
  retina H35.9
    angioid streaks H35.33
    changes in vascular appearance H35.01- ☑
    degeneration — *see* Degeneration, retina
    dystrophy (hereditary) — *see* Dystrophy, retina
    edema H35.81
    hemorrhage — *see* Hemorrhage, retina
    ischemia H35.82

☑ Additional Character Required — Refer to the Tabular List for Character Selection   ▧ Subterms under main terms may continue to next column or page

Disorder — *continued*
  retina — *continued*
    macular degeneration — *see* Degeneration, macula
    microaneurysms H35.04- ☑
    microvascular abnormality NEC H35.09
    neovascularization — *see* Neovascularization, retina
    retinopathy — *see* Retinopathy
    separation of layers H35.70
      central serous chorioretinopathy H35.71- ☑
      pigment epithelium detachment (serous) H35.72- ☑
        hemorrhagic H35.73- ☑
      specified type NEC H35.89
    telangiectasis — *see* Telangiectasis, retina
    vasculitis — *see* Vasculitis, retina
  retroperitoneal K68.9
  right hemisphere organic affective F07.89
  rumination (infant or child) F98.21
  sacrum, sacrococcygeal NEC M53.3
  schizoaffective F25.9
    bipolar type F25.0
    depressive type F25.1
    manic type F25.0
    mixed type F25.0
    specified NEC F25.8
  schizoid of childhood F84.5
  schizophrenia spectrum and other psychotic disorder F29
    specified NEC F28
  schizophreniform F20.81
    brief F23
  schizotypal (personality) F21
  secretion, thyrocalcitonin E07.0
  sedative, hypnotic, or anxiolytic use
    mild F13.10
      with
        sedative, hypnotic, or anxiolytic intoxication F13.129
        sedative, hypnotic, or anxiolytic intoxication delirium F13.121
        sedative, hypnotic, or anxiolytic-induced
          anxiety disorder F13.180
          bipolar and related disorder F13.14
          depressive disorder F13.14
          psychotic disorder F13.159
          sexual dysfunction F13.181
      in remission (early) (sustained) F13.11
    moderate or severe F13.20
      with
        sedative, hypnotic, or anxiolytic intoxication F13.229
        sedative, hypnotic, or anxiolytic intoxication delirium F13.221
        sedative, hypnotic, or anxiolytic-induced
          anxiety disorder F13.280
          bipolar and related disorder F13.24
          depressive disorder F13.24
          major neurocognitive disorder F13.27
          mild neurocognitive disorder F13.288
          psychotic disorder F13.259
          sexual dysfunction F13.281
      in remission (early) (sustained) F13.21
  seizure (*see also* Epilepsy) G40.909
    intractable G40.919
      with status epilepticus G40.911
  semantic pragmatic F80.89
    with autism F84.0
  sense of smell R43.1
    psychogenic F45.8
  separation anxiety, of childhood F93.0
  sexual
    aversion F52.1
    function, psychogenic F52.9
    interest/arousal, female F52.22
    masochism F65.51
    maturation F66
    nonorganic F52.9
    preference (*see also* Deviation, sexual) F65.9
      fetishistic transvestism F65.1
    relationship F66
    sadism F65.52
  shyness, of childhood and adolescence F40.10
  sibling rivalry F93.8
  sickle-cell (sickling) (homozygous) — *see* Disease, sickle-cell
    heterozygous D57.3
    specified type NEC D57.8- ☑

Disorder — *continued*
  sickle-cell — *see* Disease, sickle-cell — *continued*
    trait D57.3
  sinus (nasal) J34.9
    specified NEC J34.89
  skin L98.9
    atrophic L90.9
      specified NEC L90.8
    granulomatous L92.9
      specified NEC L92.8
    hypertrophic L91.9
      specified NEC L91.8
    infiltrative NEC L98.6
    newborn P83.9
      specified NEC P83.88
    picking F42.4
    psychogenic (allergic) (eczematous) F54
  sleep G47.9
    breathing-related — *see* Apnea, sleep
    circadian rhythm G47.20
      advance sleep phase type G47.22
      delayed sleep phase type G47.21
      due to
        alcohol
          abuse F10.182
          dependence F10.282
          use F10.982
        amphetamines
          abuse F15.182
          dependence F15.282
          use F15.982
        caffeine
          abuse F15.182
          dependence F15.282
          use F15.982
        cocaine
          abuse F14.182
          dependence F14.282
          use F14.982
        drug NEC
          abuse F19.182
          dependence F19.282
          use F19.982
        opioid
          abuse F11.182
          dependence F11.282
          use F11.982
        psychoactive substance NEC
          abuse F19.182
          dependence F19.282
          use F19.982
        sedative, hypnotic, or anxiolytic
          abuse F13.182
          dependence F13.282
          use F13.982
        stimulant NEC
          abuse F15.182
          dependence F15.282
          use F15.982
      free running type G47.24
      in conditions classified elsewhere G47.27
      irregular sleep wake type G47.23
      jet lag type G47.25
      non-24-hour sleep-wake type G47.24
      shift work type G47.26
      specified NEC G47.29
    due to
      alcohol
        abuse F10.182
        dependence F10.282
        use F10.982
      amphetamine
        abuse F15.182
        dependence F15.282
        use F15.982
      anxiolytic
        abuse F13.182
        dependence F13.282
        use F13.982
      caffeine
        abuse F15.182
        dependence F15.282
        use F15.982
      cocaine
        abuse F14.182
        dependence F14.282
        use F14.982
      drug NEC
        abuse F19.182

Disorder — *continued*
  sleep — *continued*
    due to — *continued*
      drug — *continued*
        dependence F19.282
        use F19.982
      hypnotic
        abuse F13.182
        dependence F13.282
        use F13.982
      opioid
        abuse F11.182
        dependence F11.282
        use F11.982
      psychoactive substance NEC
        abuse F19.182
        dependence F19.282
        use F19.982
      sedative
        abuse F13.182
        dependence F13.282
        use F13.982
      stimulant NEC
        abuse F15.182
        dependence F15.282
        use F15.982
    emotional F51.9
    excessive somnolence — *see* Hypersomnia
    hypersomnia type — *see* Hypersomnia
    initiating or maintaining — *see* Insomnia
    nightmares F51.5
    nonorganic F51.9
      specified NEC F51.8
    parasomnia type G47.50
    specified NEC G47.8
    terrors F51.4
    walking F51.3
  sleep-wake pattern or schedule (*see also* Disorder, sleep, circadian rhythm) G47.9
    specified NEC G47.8
  social
    anxiety (of childhood) F40.10
      generalized F40.11
    functioning in childhood F94.9
      specified NEC F94.8
    pragmatic F80.82
  soft tissue M79.9
    ankle M79.9
    due to use, overuse and pressure M70.90
      ankle M70.97- ☑
      bursitis — *see* Bursitis
      foot M70.97- ☑
      forearm M70.93- ☑
      hand M70.94- ☑
      lower leg M70.96- ☑
      multiple sites M70.99
      pelvic region M70.95- ☑
      shoulder region M70.91- ☑
      specified site NEC M70.98
      specified type NEC M70.80
        ankle M70.87- ☑
        foot M70.87- ☑
        forearm M70.83- ☑
        hand M70.84- ☑
        lower leg M70.86- ☑
        multiple sites M70.89
        pelvic region M70.85- ☑
        shoulder region M70.81- ☑
        specified site NEC M70.88
        thigh M70.85- ☑
        upper arm M70.82- ☑
      thigh M70.95- ☑
      upper arm M70.92- ☑
    foot M79.9
    forearm M79.9
    hand M79.9
    lower leg M79.9
    multiple sites M79.9
    occupational — *see* Disorder, soft tissue, due to use, overuse and pressure
    pelvic region M79.9
    shoulder region M79.9
    specified type NEC M79.89
    thigh M79.9
    upper arm M79.9
  somatic symptom F45.1
  somatization F45.0
  somatoform F45.9

Index

Disorder — Displacement, displaced

Disorder — *continued*
somatoform — *continued*
pain (persistent) F45.41
somatization (multiple) (long-lasting) F45.0
specified NEC F45.8
undifferentiated F45.1
somnolence, excessive — *see* Hypersomnia
specific
arithmetical F81.2
developmental, of motor F82
reading F81.0
speech and language F80.9
spelling F81.81
written expression F81.81
speech R47.9
articulation (functional) (specific) F80.0
developmental F80.9
specified NEC R47.89
speech-sound F80.0
spelling (specific) F81.81
spine (*see also* Dorsopathy)
ligamentous or muscular attachments, peripheral
— *see* Enthesopathy, spinal
specified NEC — *see* Dorsopathy, specified NEC
stereotyped, habit or movement F98.4
stimulant use (other) (unspecified)
mild F15.10
in remission (early) (sustained) F15.11
moderate or severe F15.20
in remission (early) (sustained) F15.21
stomach (functional) — *see* Disorder, gastric
stress F43.9
acute F43.0
post-traumatic F43.10
acute F43.11
chronic F43.12
substance use (other) (unknown)
mild F19.10
with substance-induced
anxiety disorder F19.180
bipolar and related disorder F19.14
depressive disorder F19.14
major neurocognitive disorder F19.17
mild neurocognitive disorder F19.188
obsessive-compulsive and related disorder
F19.188
sexual dysfunction F19.181
substance intoxication F19.129
substance intoxication delirium F19.121
moderate or severe F19.20
with substance-induced
anxiety disorder F19.280
bipolar and related disorder F19.24
depressive disorder F19.24
major neurocognitive disorder F19.27
mild neurocognitive disorder F19.288
obsessive-compulsive and related disorder
F19.288
sexual dysfunction F19.281
in remission (early) (sustained) F19.21
substance intoxication F19.229
substance intoxication delirium F19.221
sulfur-bearing amino-acid metabolism E72.10
sweat gland (eccrine) L74.9
apocrine L75.9
specified NEC L75.8
specified NEC L74.8
synovium M67.90
acromioclavicular M67.91- ☑
ankle M67.97- ☑
elbow M67.92- ☑
foot M67.97- ☑
forearm M67.93- ☑
hand M67.94- ☑
hip M67.95- ☑
knee M67.96- ☑
multiple sites M67.99
rupture — *see* Rupture, synovium
shoulder M67.91- ☑
specified type NEC M67.80
acromioclavicular M67.81- ☑
ankle M67.87- ☑
elbow M67.82- ☑
foot M67.87- ☑
hand M67.84- ☑
hip M67.85- ☑
knee M67.86- ☑
multiple sites M67.89

Disorder — *continued*
synovium — *continued*
specified type — *continued*
wrist M67.83- ☑
synovitis — *see* Synovitis
upper arm M67.92- ☑
wrist M67.93- ☑
temperature regulation, newborn P81.9
specified NEC P81.8
temporomandibular joint M26.60- ☑
tendon M67.90
acromioclavicular M67.91- ☑
ankle M67.97- ☑
contracture — *see* Contracture, tendon
elbow M67.92- ☑
foot M67.97- ☑
forearm M67.93- ☑
hand M67.94- ☑
hip M67.95- ☑
knee M67.96- ☑
multiple sites M67.99
rupture — *see* Rupture, tendon
shoulder M67.91- ☑
specified type NEC M67.80
acromioclavicular M67.81- ☑
ankle M67.87- ☑
elbow M67.82- ☑
foot M67.87- ☑
hand M67.84- ☑
hip M67.85- ☑
knee M67.86- ☑
multiple sites M67.89
trunk M67.88
wrist M67.83- ☑
synovitis — *see* Synovitis
tendinitis — *see* Tendinitis
tenosynovitis — *see* Tenosynovitis
trunk M67.98
upper arm M67.92- ☑
wrist M67.93- ☑
thoracic root (nerve) NEC G54.3
thyrocalcitonin hypersecretion E07.0
thyroid (gland) E07.9
function NEC, neonatal, transitory P72.2
iodine-deficiency related E01.8
specified NEC E07.89
tic — *see* Tic
tobacco use
chewing tobacco (mild) (moderate) (severe)
in remission (early) (sustained) F17.221
cigarettes (mild) (moderate) (severe)
in remission (early) (sustained) F17.211
mild Z72.0
in remission (early) (sustained) F17.201
moderate F17.200
in remission (early) (sustained) F17.201
severe F17.200
in remission (early) (sustained) F17.201
specified product NEC (mild) (moderate) (severe)
in remission (early) (sustained) F17.291
tooth K08.9
development K00.9
specified NEC K00.8
eruption K00.6
Tourette's F95.2
trance and possession F44.89
transvestic F65.1
trauma and stressor-related F43.9
other specified F43.8
tricuspid (valve) — *see* Endocarditis, tricuspid
tryptophan metabolism E70.5
tubular, phosphate-losing N25.0
tubulo-interstitial (in)
brucellosis A23.9 [N16]
cystinosis E72.04
diphtheria A36.84
glycogen storage disease E74.00 [N16]
leukemia NEC C95.9- ☑ [N16]
lymphoma NEC C85.9- ☑ [N16]
mixed cryoglobulinemia D89.1 [N16]
multiple myeloma C90.0- ☑ [N16]
Salmonella infection A02.25
sarcoidosis D86.84
sepsis A41.9 [N16]
streptococcal A40.9 [N16]
systemic lupus erythematosus M32.15
toxoplasmosis B58.83

Disorder — *continued*
tubulo-interstitial — *continued*
transplant rejection T86.91 [N16]
Wilson's disease E83.01 [N16]
tubulo-renal function, impaired N25.9
specified NEC N25.89
tympanic membrane H73.9- ☑
atrophy — *see* Atrophy, tympanic membrane
infection — *see* Myringitis
perforation — *see* Perforation, tympanum
specified NEC H73.89- ☑
unsocialized aggressive F91.1
urea cycle metabolism E72.20
argininemia E72.21
arginosuccinic aciduria E72.22
citrullinemia E72.23
ornithine transcarbamylase deficiency E72.4
other specified E72.29
ureter (in) N28.9
schistosomiasis B65.0 [N29]
tuberculosis A18.11
urethra N36.9
specified NEC N36.8
urinary system N39.9
specified NEC N39.8
valve, heart
aortic — *see* Endocarditis, aortic
mitral — *see* Endocarditis, mitral
pulmonary — *see* Endocarditis, pulmonary
rheumatic
aortic — *see* Endocarditis, aortic, rheumatic
mitral — *see* Endocarditis, mitral
pulmonary — *see* Endocarditis, pulmonary,
rheumatic
tricuspid — *see* Endocarditis, tricuspid
tricuspid — *see* Endocarditis, tricuspid
vestibular function H81.9- ☑
specified NEC — *see* subcategory H81.8 ☑
in diseases classified elsewhere H82.- ☑
vertigo — *see* Vertigo
vision, binocular H53.30
abnormal retinal correspondence H53.31
diplopia H53.2
fusion with defective stereopsis H53.32
simultaneous perception H53.33
suppression H53.34
visual
cortex
blindness H47.619
left brain H47.612
right brain H47.611
due to
inflammatory disorder H47.629
left brain H47.622
right brain H47.621
neoplasm H47.639
left brain H47.632
right brain H47.631
vascular disorder H47.649
left brain H47.642
right brain H47.641
pathway H47.9
due to
inflammatory disorder H47.51- ☑
neoplasm H47.52- ☑
vascular disorder H47.53- ☑
optic chiasm — *see* Disorder, optic, chiasm
vitreous body H43.9
crystalline deposits — *see* Deposit, crystalline
degeneration — *see* Degeneration, vitreous
hemorrhage — *see* Hemorrhage, vitreous
opacities — *see* Opacity, vitreous
prolapse — *see* Prolapse, vitreous
specified type NEC H43.89
voice R49.9
specified type NEC R49.8
volatile solvent use
due to drug abuse — *see* Abuse, drug, inhalant
due to drug dependence — *see* Dependence, drug,
inhalant
voyeuristic F65.3
white blood cells D72.9
specified NEC D72.89
withdrawing, child or adolescent F40.10
Disorientation R41.0
Displacement, displaced
acquired traumatic of bone, cartilage, joint, tendon
NEC — *see* Dislocation

☑ Additional Character Required — Refer to the Tabular List for Character Selection

⋲ Subterms under main terms may continue to next column or page

Displacement, displaced — *continued*
- adrenal gland (congenital) Q89.1
- appendix, retrocecal (congenital) Q43.8
- auricle (congenital) Q17.4
- bladder (acquired) N32.89
  - congenital Q64.19
- brachial plexus (congenital) Q07.8
- brain stem, caudal (congenital) Q04.8
- canaliculus (lacrimalis), congenital Q10.6
- cardia through esophageal hiatus (congenital) Q40.1
- cerebellum, caudal (congenital) Q04.8
- cervix — *see* Malposition, uterus
- colon (congenital) Q43.3
- device, implant or graft (*see also* Complications, by site and type, mechanical) T85.628 ☑
  - arterial graft NEC — *see* Complication, cardiovascular device, mechanical, vascular
  - breast (implant) T85.42 ☑
  - catheter NEC T85.628 ☑
    - dialysis (renal) T82.42 ☑
      - intraperitoneal T85.621 ☑
    - infusion NEC T82.524 ☑
      - spinal (epidural) (subdural) T85.620 ☑
    - urinary
      - cystostomy T83.020 ☑
      - Hopkins T83.028 ☑
      - ileostomy T83.028 ☑
      - indwelling T83.021 ☑
      - nephrostomy T83.022 ☑
      - specified NEC T83.028 ☑
      - urostomy T83.028 ☑
  - electronic (electrode) (pulse generator) (stimulator) — *see* Complication, electronic stimulator
  - fixation, internal (orthopedic) NEC — *see* Complication, fixation device, mechanical
  - gastrointestinal — *see* Complications, prosthetic device, mechanical, gastrointestinal device
  - genital NEC T83.428 ☑
    - intrauterine contraceptive device (string) T83.32 ☑
    - penile prosthesis (cylinder) (implanted) (pump) (reservoir) T83.420 ☑
    - testicular prosthesis T83.421 ☑
  - heart NEC — *see* Complication, cardiovascular device, mechanical
  - joint prosthesis — *see* Complications, joint prosthesis, mechanical
  - ocular — *see* Complications, prosthetic device, mechanical, ocular device
  - orthopedic NEC — *see* Complication, orthopedic, device or graft, mechanical
  - specified NEC T85.628 ☑
  - urinary NEC T83.128 ☑
    - graft T83.22 ☑
    - sphincter, implanted T83.121 ☑
    - stent (ileal conduit) (nephroureteral) T83.123 ☑
    - ureteral indwelling T83.122 ☑
  - vascular NEC — *see* Complication, cardiovascular device, mechanical
  - ventricular intracranial shunt T85.02 ☑
- electronic stimulator
  - bone T84.320 ☑
  - cardiac — *see* Complications, cardiac device, electronic
  - nervous system — *see* Complication, prosthetic device, mechanical, electronic nervous system stimulator
  - urinary — *see* Complications, electronic stimulator, urinary
- esophageal mucosa into cardia of stomach, congenital Q39.8
- esophagus (acquired) K22.8
  - congenital Q39.8
- eyeball (acquired) (lateral) (old) — *see* Displacement, globe
  - congenital Q15.8
  - current — *see* Avulsion, eye
- fallopian tube (acquired) N83.4- ☑
  - congenital Q50.6
  - opening (congenital) Q50.6
- gallbladder (congenital) Q44.1
- gastric mucosa (congenital) Q40.2
- globe (acquired) (old) (lateral) H05.21- ☑
  - current — *see* Avulsion, eye
- heart (congenital) Q24.8
  - acquired I51.89
- hymen (upward) (congenital) Q52.4

Displacement, displaced — *continued*
- intervertebral disc NEC
  - with myelopathy — *see* Disorder, disc, with, myelopathy
  - cervical, cervicothoracic (with) M50.20
    - myelopathy — *see* Disorder, disc, cervical, with myelopathy
    - neuritis, radiculitis or radiculopathy — *see* Disorder, disc, cervical, with neuritis
  - due to trauma — *see* Dislocation, vertebra
  - lumbar region M51.26
    - with
      - myelopathy M51.06
      - neuritis, radiculitis, radiculopathy or sciatica M51.16
  - lumbosacral region M51.27
    - with
      - neuritis, radiculitis, radiculopathy or sciatica M51.17
  - sacrococcygeal region M53.3
  - thoracic region M51.24
    - with
      - myelopathy M51.04
      - neuritis, radiculitis, radiculopathy M51.14
  - thoracolumbar region M51.25
    - with
      - myelopathy M51.05
      - neuritis, radiculitis, radiculopathy M51.15
- intrauterine device (string) T83.32 ☑
- kidney (acquired) N28.83
  - congenital Q63.2
- lachrymal, lacrimal apparatus or duct (congenital) Q10.6
- lens, congenital Q12.1
- macula (congenital) Q14.1
- Meckel's diverticulum Q43.0
  - malignant — *see* Table of Neoplasms, small intestine, malignant
- nail (congenital) Q84.6
  - acquired L60.8
- opening of Wharton's duct in mouth Q38.4
- organ or site, congenital NEC — *see* Malposition, congenital
- ovary (acquired) N83.4- ☑
  - congenital Q50.39
    - free in peritoneal cavity (congenital) Q50.39
    - into hernial sac N83.4- ☑
- oviduct (acquired) N83.4- ☑
  - congenital Q50.6
- parathyroid (gland) E21.4
- parotid gland (congenital) Q38.4
- punctum lacrimale (congenital) Q10.6
- sacro-iliac (joint) (congenital) Q74.2
  - current injury S33.2 ☑
  - old — *see* subcategory M53.2 ☑
- salivary gland (any) (congenital) Q38.4
- spleen (congenital) Q89.09
- stomach, congenital Q40.2
- sublingual duct Q38.4
- tongue (downward) (congenital) Q38.3
- tooth, teeth, fully erupted M26.30
  - horizontal M26.33
  - vertical M26.34
- trachea (congenital) Q32.1
- ureter or ureteric opening or orifice (congenital) Q62.62
- uterine opening of oviducts or fallopian tubes Q50.6
- uterus, uterine — *see* Malposition, uterus
- ventricular septum Q21.0
  - with rudimentary ventricle Q20.4

Disproportion
- between native and reconstructed breast N65.1
- fiber-type G71.2

Disruptio uteri — *see* Rupture, uterus
Disruption (of)
- ciliary body NEC H21.89
- closure of
  - cornea T81.31 ☑
  - craniotomy T81.32 ☑
  - fascia (muscular) (superficial) T81.32 ☑
  - internal organ or tissue T81.32 ☑
  - laceration (external) (internal) T81.33 ☑
  - ligament T81.32 ☑
  - mucosa T81.31 ☑
  - muscle or muscle flap T81.32 ☑
  - ribs or rib cage T81.32 ☑
  - skin and subcutaneous tissue (full-thickness) (superficial) T81.31 ☑

Disruption — *continued*
- closure of — *continued*
  - skull T81.32 ☑
  - sternum (sternotomy) T81.32 ☑
  - tendon T81.32 ☑
  - traumatic laceration (external) (internal) T81.33 ☑
- family Z63.8
  - due to
    - absence of family member due to military deployment Z63.31
    - absence of family member NEC Z63.32
    - alcoholism and drug addiction in family Z63.72
    - bereavement Z63.4
    - death (assumed) or disappearance of family member Z63.4
    - divorce or separation Z63.5
    - drug addiction in family Z63.72
    - return of family member from military deployment (current or past conflict) Z63.71
    - stressful life events NEC Z63.79
- iris NEC H21.89
- ligament(s) (*see also* Sprain)
  - knee
    - current injury — *see* Dislocation, knee
    - old (chronic) — *see* Derangement, knee, instability
    - spontaneous NEC — *see* Derangement, knee, disruption ligament
- ossicular chain — *see* Discontinuity, ossicles, ear
- pelvic ring (stable) S32.810 ☑
  - unstable S32.811 ☑
- traumatic injury wound repair T81.33 ☑
- wound T81.30 ☑
  - episiotomy O90.1
  - operation T81.31 ☑
    - cesarean O90.0
    - external operation wound (superficial) T81.31 ☑
    - internal operation wound (deep) T81.32 ☑
  - perineal (obstetric) O90.1
  - traumatic injury repair T81.33 ☑

Dissatisfaction with
- employment Z56.9
- school environment Z55.4

Dissecting — *see* condition
Dissection
- aorta I71.00
  - abdominal I71.02
  - thoracic I71.01
  - thoracoabdominal I71.03
- artery I77.70
  - basilar (trunk) I77.75
  - carotid I77.71
  - cerebral (nonruptured) I67.0
    - ruptured — *see* Hemorrhage, intracranial, subarachnoid
  - coronary I25.42
  - extremity
    - lower I77.77
    - upper I77.76
  - iliac I77.72
  - precerebral
    - congenital (nonruptured) Q28.1
    - specified site NEC I77.75
  - renal I77.73
  - specified NEC I77.79
  - vertebral I77.74
- precerebral artery, congenital (nonruptured) Q28.1
- Heartland A93.8
- traumatic — *see* Wound, open, by site
- vascular I99.8
- wound — *see* Wound, open

Disseminated — *see* condition
Dissociation
- auriculoventricular or atrioventricular (AV) (any degree) (isorhythmic) I45.89
  - with heart block I44.2
  - interference I45.89

Dissociative reaction, state F44.9
Dissolution, vertebra — *see* Osteoporosis
Distension, distention
- abdomen R14.0
- bladder N32.89
- cecum K63.89
- colon K63.89
- gallbladder K82.8
- intestine K63.89
- kidney N28.89

Distension, distention — *continued*
liver K76.89
seminal vesicle N50.89
stomach K31.89
acute K31.0
psychogenic F45.8
ureter — *see* Dilatation, ureter
uterus N85.8
Distoma hepaticum infestation B66.3
Distomiasis B66.9
bile passages B66.3
hemic B65.9
hepatic B66.3
due to Clonorchis sinensis B66.1
intestinal B66.5
liver B66.3
due to Clonorchis sinensis B66.1
lung B66.4
pulmonary B66.4
Distomolar (fourth molar) K00.1
Disto-occlusion (Division I) (Division II) M26.212
Distortion(s) (congenital)
adrenal (gland) Q89.1
arm NEC Q68.8
bile duct or passage Q44.5
bladder Q64.79
brain Q04.9
cervix (uteri) Q51.9
chest (wall) Q67.8
bones Q76.8
clavicle Q74.0
clitoris Q52.6
coccyx Q76.49
common duct Q44.5
coronary Q24.5
cystic duct Q44.5
ear (auricle) (external) Q17.3
inner Q16.5
middle Q16.4
ossicles Q16.3
endocrine NEC Q89.2
eustachian tube Q17.8
eye (adnexa) Q15.8
face bone(s) NEC Q75.8
fallopian tube Q50.6
femur NEC Q68.8
fibula NEC Q68.8
finger(s) Q68.1
foot Q66.9
genitalia, genital organ(s)
female Q52.8
external Q52.79
internal NEC Q52.8
gyri Q04.8
hand bone(s) Q68.1
heart (auricle) (ventricle) Q24.8
valve (cusp) Q24.8
hepatic duct Q44.5
humerus NEC Q68.8
hymen Q52.4
intrafamilial communications Z63.8
jaw NEC M26.89
labium (majus) (minus) Q52.79
leg NEC Q68.8
lens Q12.8
liver Q44.7
lumbar spine Q76.49
with disproportion O33.8
causing obstructed labor O65.0
lumbosacral (joint) (region) Q76.49
kyphosis — *see* Kyphosis, congenital
lordosis — *see* Lordosis, congenital
nerve Q07.8
nose Q30.8
organ
of Corti Q16.5
or site not listed — *see* Anomaly, by site
ossicles, ear Q16.3
oviduct Q50.6
pancreas Q45.3
parathyroid (gland) Q89.2
pituitary (gland) Q89.2
radius NEC Q68.8
sacroiliac joint Q74.2
sacrum Q76.49
scapula Q74.0
shoulder girdle Q74.0
skull bone(s) NEC Q75.8

Distortion(s) — *continued*
skull bone(s) — *continued*
with
anencephalus Q00.0
encephalocele — *see* Encephalocele
hydrocephalus Q03.9
with spina bifida — *see* Spina bifida, with
hydrocephalus
microcephaly Q02
spinal cord Q06.8
spine Q76.49
kyphosis — *see* Kyphosis, congenital
lordosis — *see* Lordosis, congenital
spleen Q89.09
sternum NEC Q76.7
thorax (wall) Q67.8
bony Q76.8
thymus (gland) Q89.2
thyroid (gland) Q89.2
tibia NEC Q68.8
toe(s) Q66.9
tongue Q38.3
trachea (cartilage) Q32.1
ulna NEC Q68.8
ureter Q62.8
urethra Q64.79
causing obstruction Q64.39
uterus Q51.9
vagina Q52.4
vertebra Q76.49
kyphosis — *see* Kyphosis, congenital
lordosis — *see* Lordosis, congenital
visual (*see also* Disturbance, vision)
shape and size H53.15
vulva Q52.79
wrist (bones) (joint) Q68.8
Distress
abdomen — *see* Pain, abdominal
acute respiratory R06.03
syndrome (adult) (child) J80
epigastric R10.13
fetal P84
complicating pregnancy — *see* Stress, fetal
gastrointestinal (functional) K30
psychogenic F45.8
intestinal (functional) NOS K59.9
psychogenic F45.8
maternal, during labor and delivery O75.0
relationship, with spouse or intimate partner Z63.0
respiratory (adult) (child) R06.03
newborn P22.9
specified NEC P22.8
orthopnea R06.01
psychogenic F45.8
shortness of breath R06.02
specified type NEC R06.09
Distribution vessel, atypical Q27.9
coronary artery Q24.5
precerebral Q28.1
Districhiasis L68.8
Disturbance(s) (*see also* Disease)
absorption K90.9
calcium E58
carbohydrate K90.49
fat K90.49
pancreatic K90.3
protein K90.49
starch K90.49
vitamin — *see* Deficiency, vitamin
acid-base equilibrium E87.8
mixed E87.4
activity and attention (with hyperkinesis) — *see* Disorder, attention-deficit hyperactivity
amino acid transport E72.00
assimilation, food K90.9
auditory nerve, except deafness — *see* subcategory
H93.3 ☑
behavior — *see* Disorder, conduct
blood clotting (mechanism) (*see also* Defect, coagulation) D68.9
cerebral
nerve — *see* Disorder, nerve, cranial
status, newborn P91.9
specified NEC P91.88
circulatory I99.9
conduct (*see also* Disorder, conduct) F91.9
adjustment reaction — *see* Disorder, adjustment
compulsive F63.9

Disturbance(s) — *continued*
conduct (*see also* Disorder, conduct) — *continued*
disruptive F91.9
hyperkinetic — *see* Disorder, attention-deficit hyperactivity
socialized F91.2
specified NEC F91.8
unsocialized F91.1
coordination R27.8
cranial nerve — *see* Disorder, nerve, cranial
deep sensibility — *see* Disturbance, sensation
digestive K30
psychogenic F45.8
electrolyte (*see also* Imbalance, electrolyte)
newborn, transitory P74.4
hyperammonemia P74.6
potassium balance P74.3
sodium balance P74.2
specified type NEC P74.4
emotions specific to childhood and adolescence F93.9
with
anxiety and fearfulness NEC F93.8
elective mutism F94.0
oppositional disorder F91.3
sensitivity (withdrawal) F40.10
shyness F40.10
social withdrawal F40.10
involving relationship problems F93.8
mixed F93.8
specified NEC F93.8
endocrine (gland) E34.9
neonatal, transitory P72.9
specified NEC P72.8
equilibrium R42
fructose metabolism E74.10
gait — *see* Gait
hysterical F44.4
psychogenic F44.4
gastrointestinal (functional) K30
psychogenic F45.8
habit, child F98.9
hearing, except deafness and tinnitus — *see* Abnormal,
auditory perception
heart, functional (conditions in I44-I50)
due to presence of (cardiac) prosthesis I97.19- ☑
postoperative I97.89
cardiac surgery (*see also* Infarct, myocardium,
associated with revascularization procedure) I97.19- ☑
hormones E34.9
innervation uterus (parasympathetic) (sympathetic)
N85.8
keratinization NEC
gingiva K05.10
nonplaque induced K05.11
plaque induced K05.10
lip K13.0
oral (mucosa) (soft tissue) K13.29
tongue K13.29
learning (specific) — *see* Disorder, learning
memory — *see* Amnesia
mild, following organic brain damage F06.8
mental F99
associated with diseases classified elsewhere F54
metabolism E88.9
with
abortion — *see* Abortion, by type with other
specified complication
ectopic pregnancy O08.5
molar pregnancy O08.5
amino-acid E72.9
aromatic E70.9
branched-chain E71.2
straight-chain E72.8
sulfur-bearing E72.10
ammonia E72.20
arginine E72.21
arginosuccinic acid E72.22
carbohydrate E74.9
cholesterol E78.9
citrulline E72.23
cystathionine E72.19
general E88.9
glutamine E72.8
histidine E70.40
homocystine E72.19
hydroxylysine E72.3
in labor or delivery O75.89

☑ Additional Character Required — Refer to the Tabular List for Character Selection   Subterms under main terms may continue to next column or page

Disturbance(s) — *continued*
  metabolism — *continued*
    iron E83.10
    lipoid E78.9
    lysine E72.3
    methionine E72.19
    neonatal, transitory P74.9
      calcium and magnesium P71.9
        specified type NEC P71.8
      carbohydrate metabolism P70.9
        specified type NEC P70.8
      specified NEC P74.8
    ornithine E72.4
    phosphate E83.39
    sodium NEC E87.8
    threonine E72.8
    tryptophan E70.5
    tyrosine E70.20
    urea cycle E72.20
  motor R29.2
  nervous, functional R45.0
  neuromuscular mechanism (eye), due to syphilis A52.15
  nutritional E63.9
    nail L60.3
  ocular motion H51.9
    psychogenic F45.8
  oculogyric H51.8
    psychogenic F45.8
  oculomotor H51.9
    psychogenic F45.8
  olfactory nerve R43.1
  optic nerve NEC — *see* Disorder, nerve, optic
  oral epithelium, including tongue NEC K13.29
  perceptual due to
    alcohol withdrawal F10.232
    amphetamine intoxication F15.922
      in
        abuse F15.122
        dependence F15.222
    anxiolytic withdrawal F13.232
    cannabis intoxication (acute) F12.922
      in
        abuse F12.122
        dependence F12.222
    cocaine intoxication (acute) F14.922
      in
        abuse F14.122
        dependence F14.222
    hypnotic withdrawal F13.232
    opioid intoxication (acute) F11.922
      in
        abuse F11.122
        dependence F11.222
    phencyclidine intoxication (acute) F16.122
    sedative withdrawal F13.232
  personality (pattern) (trait) (*see also* Disorder, personality) F60.9
  following organic brain damage F07.9
  polyglandular E31.9
    specified NEC E31.8
  potassium balance, newborn P74.3
  psychogenic F45.9
  psychomotor F44.4
  psychophysical visual H53.16
  pupillary — *see* Anomaly, pupil, function
  reflex R29.2
  rhythm, heart I49.9
  salivary secretion K11.7
  sensation (cold) (heat) (localization) (tactile discrimination) (texture) (vibratory) NEC R20.9
    hysterical F44.6
    skin R20.9
      anesthesia R20.0
      hyperesthesia R20.3
      hypoesthesia R20.1
      paresthesia R20.2
      specified type NEC R20.8
    smell R43.9
      and taste (mixed) R43.8
      anosmia R43.0
      parosmia R43.1
      specified NEC R43.8
    taste R43.9
      and smell (mixed) R43.8
      parageusia R43.2
      specified NEC R43.8
  sensory — *see* Disturbance, sensation

Disturbance(s) — *continued*
  situational (transient) (*see also* Disorder, adjustment)
    acute F43.0
  sleep G47.9
    nonorganic origin F51.9
  smell — *see* Disturbance, sensation, smell
  sociopathic F60.2
  sodium balance, newborn P74.2
  speech R47.9
    developmental F80.9
    specified NEC R47.89
  stomach (functional) K31.9
  sympathetic (nerve) G90.9
  taste — *see* Disturbance, sensation, taste
  temperature
    regulation, newborn P81.9
      specified NEC P81.8
    sense R20.8
      hysterical F44.6
  tooth
    eruption K00.6
    formation K00.4
    structure, hereditary NEC K00.5
  touch — *see* Disturbance, sensation
  vascular I99.9
    arteriosclerotic — *see* Arteriosclerosis
  vasomotor I73.9
  vasospastic I73.9
  vision, visual H53.9
    following
      cerebral infarction I69.398
      cerebrovascular disease I69.998
        specified NEC I69.898
      intracerebral hemorrhage I69.198
      nontraumatic intracranial hemorrhage NEC I69.298
      specified disease NEC I69.898
      subarachnoid hemorrhage I69.098
    psychophysical H53.16
    specified NEC H53.8
    subjective H53.10
      day blindness H53.11
      discomfort H53.14- ☑
      distortions of shape and size H53.15
      loss
        sudden H53.13- ☑
        transient H53.12- ☑
      specified type NEC H53.19
  voice R49.9
    psychogenic F44.4
    specified NEC R49.8
Diuresis R35.8
Diver's palsy, paralysis or squeeze T70.3 ☑
Diverticulitis (acute) K57.92
  bladder — *see* Cystitis
  ileum — *see* Diverticulitis, intestine, small
  intestine K57.92
    with
      abscess, perforation or peritonitis K57.80
        with bleeding K57.81
      bleeding K57.93
    congenital Q43.8
    large K57.32
      with
        abscess, perforation or peritonitis K57.20
          with bleeding K57.21
        bleeding K57.33
        small intestine K57.52
          with
            abscess, perforation or peritonitis K57.40
              with bleeding K57.41
            bleeding K57.53
    small K57.12
      with
        abscess, perforation or peritonitis K57.00
          with bleeding K57.01
        bleeding K57.13
        large intestine K57.52
          with
            abscess, perforation or peritonitis K57.40
              with bleeding K57.41
            bleeding K57.53
Diverticulosis K57.90
  with bleeding K57.91
  large intestine K57.30

Diverticulosis — *continued*
  large intestine — *continued*
    with
      bleeding K57.31
      small intestine K57.50
        with bleeding K57.51
  small intestine K57.10
    with
      bleeding K57.11
      large intestine K57.50
        with bleeding K57.51
Diverticulum, diverticula (multiple) K57.90
  appendix (noninflammatory) K38.2
  bladder (sphincter) N32.3
    congenital Q64.6
  bronchus (congenital) Q32.4
    acquired J98.09
  calyx, calyceal (kidney) N28.89
  cardia (stomach) K31.4
  cecum — *see* Diverticulosis, intestine, large
    congenital Q43.8
  colon — *see* Diverticulosis, intestine, large
    congenital Q43.8
  duodenum — *see* Diverticulosis, intestine, small
    congenital Q43.8
  epiphrenic (esophagus) K22.5
  esophagus (congenital) Q39.6
    acquired (epiphrenic) (pulsion) (traction) K22.5
  eustachian tube — *see* Disorder, eustachian tube, specified NEC
  fallopian tube N83.8
  gastric K31.4
  heart (congenital) Q24.8
  ileum — *see* Diverticulosis, intestine, small
  jejunum — *see* Diverticulosis, intestine, small
  kidney (pelvis) (calyces) N28.89
    with calculus — *see* Calculus, kidney
  Meckel's (displaced) (hypertrophic) Q43.0
    malignant — *see* Table of Neoplasms, small intestine, malignant
  midthoracic K22.5
  organ or site, congenital NEC — *see* Distortion
  pericardium (congenital) (cyst) Q24.8
    acquired I31.8
  pharyngoesophageal (congenital) Q39.6
    acquired K22.5
  pharynx (congenital) Q38.7
  rectosigmoid — *see* Diverticulosis, intestine, large
    congenital Q43.8
  rectum — *see* Diverticulosis, intestine, large
  Rokitansky's K22.5
  seminal vesicle N50.89
  sigmoid — *see* Diverticulosis, intestine, large
    congenital Q43.8
  stomach (acquired) K31.4
    congenital Q40.2
  trachea (acquired) J39.8
  ureter (acquired) N28.89
    congenital Q62.8
  ureterovesical orifice N28.89
  urethra (acquired) N36.1
    congenital Q64.79
  ventricle, left (congenital) Q24.8
  vesical N32.3
    congenital Q64.6
  Zenker's (esophagus) K22.5
Division
  cervix uteri (acquired) N88.8
  glans penis Q55.69
  labia minora (congenital) Q52.79
  ligament (partial or complete) (current) (*see also* Sprain)
    with open wound — *see* Wound, open
  muscle (partial or complete) (current) (*see also* Injury, muscle)
    with open wound — *see* Wound, open
  nerve (traumatic) — *see* Injury, nerve
  spinal cord — *see* Injury, spinal cord, by region
  vein I87.8
Divorce, causing family disruption Z63.5
Dix-Hallpike neurolabyrinthitis — *see* Neuronitis, vestibular
Dizziness R42
  hysterical F44.89
  psychogenic F45.8
DMAC (disseminated mycobacterium avium- intracellulare complex) A31.2
DNR (do not resuscitate) Z66

Index

Doan-Wiseman syndrome — Dwarfism

Doan-Wiseman syndrome (primary splenic neutropenia) — see Agranulocytosis
Doehle-Heller aortitis A52.02
Dog bite — see Bite
Dohle body panmyelopathic syndrome D72.0
Dolichocephaly Q67.2
Dolichocolon Q43.8
Dolichostenomelia — see Syndrome, Marfan's
Donohue's syndrome E34.8
Donor (organ or tissue) Z52.9
  blood (whole) Z52.000
    autologous Z52.010
    specified component (lymphocytes) (platelets) NEC Z52.008
      autologous Z52.018
      specified donor NEC Z52.098
    specified donor NEC Z52.090
    stem cells Z52.001
      autologous Z52.011
      specified donor NEC Z52.091
  bone Z52.20
    autologous Z52.21
    marrow Z52.3
    specified type NEC Z52.29
  cornea Z52.5
  egg (Oocyte) Z52.819
    age 35 and over Z52.812
      anonymous recipient Z52.812
      designated recipient Z52.813
    under age 35 Z52.810
      anonymous recipient Z52.810
      designated recipient Z52.811
  kidney Z52.4
  liver Z52.6
  lung Z52.89
  lymphocyte — see Donor, blood, specified components NEC
  Oocyte — see Donor, egg
  platelets Z52.008
  potential, examination of Z00.5
  semen Z52.89
  skin Z52.10
    autologous Z52.11
    specified type NEC Z52.19
  specified organ or tissue NEC Z52.89
  sperm Z52.89
Donovanosis A58
Dorsalgia M54.9
  psychogenic F45.41
  specified NEC M54.89
Dorsopathy M53.9
  deforming M43.9
    specified NEC — see subcategory M43.8 ☑
  specified NEC M53.80
    cervical region M53.82
    cervicothoracic region M53.83
    lumbar region M53.86
    lumbosacral region M53.87
    occipito-atlanto-axial region M53.81
    sacrococcygeal region M53.88
    thoracic region M53.84
    thoracolumbar region M53.85
Double
  albumin E88.09
  aortic arch Q25.45
  auditory canal Q17.8
  auricle (heart) Q20.8
  bladder Q64.79
  cervix Q51.820
    with doubling of uterus (and vagina) Q51.10
      with obstruction Q51.11
  inlet ventricle Q20.4
  kidney with double pelvis (renal) Q63.0
  meatus urinarius Q64.75
  monster Q89.4
  outlet
    left ventricle Q20.2
    right ventricle Q20.1
  pelvis (renal) with double ureter Q62.5
  tongue Q38.3
  ureter (one or both sides) Q62.5
    with double pelvis (renal) Q62.5
  urethra Q64.74
  urinary meatus Q64.75
  uterus Q51.2
    with
      doubling of cervix (and vagina) Q51.10
        with obstruction Q51.11

Double — continued
  uterus — continued
    in pregnancy or childbirth O34.59- ☑
      causing obstructed labor O65.5
  vagina Q52.10
    with doubling of uterus (and cervix) Q51.10
      with obstruction Q51.11
  vision H53.2
  vulva Q52.79
Douglas' pouch, cul-de-sac — see condition
Down syndrome Q90.9
  meiotic nondisjunction Q90.0
  mitotic nondisjunction Q90.1
  mosaicism Q90.1
  translocation Q90.2
DPD (dihydropyrimidine dehydrogenase deficiency) E88.89
Dracontiasis B72
Dracunculiasis, dracunculosis B72
Dream state, hysterical F44.89
Drepanocytic anemia — see Disease, sickle-cell
Dresbach's syndrome (elliptocytosis) D58.1
Dreschlera (hawaiiensis) (infection) B43.8
Dressler's syndrome I24.1
Drift, ulnar — see Deformity, limb, specified type NEC, forearm
Drinking (alcohol)
  excessive, to excess NEC (without dependence) F10.10
    habitual (continual) (without remission) F10.20
      with remission F10.21
Drip, postnasal (chronic) R09.82
  due to
    allergic rhinitis — see Rhinitis, allergic
    common cold J00
    gastroesophageal reflux — see Reflux, gastroesophageal
    nasopharyngitis — see Nasopharyngitis
    other known condition — code to condition
    sinusitis — see Sinusitis
Droop
  facial R29.810
    cerebrovascular disease I69.992
      cerebral infarction I69.392
      intracerebral hemorrhage I69.192
      nontraumatic intracranial hemorrhage NEC I69.292
      specified disease NEC I69.892
      subarachnoid hemorrhage I69.092
Drop (in)
  attack NEC R55
  finger — see Deformity, finger
  foot — see Deformity, limb, foot, drop
  hematocrit (precipitous) R71.0
  hemoglobin R71.0
  toe — see Deformity, toe, specified NEC
  wrist — see Deformity, limb, wrist drop
Dropped heart beats I45.9
Dropsy, dropsical (see also Hydrops)
  abdomen R18.8
  brain — see Hydrocephalus
  cardiac, heart — see Failure, heart, congestive
  gangrenous — see Gangrene
  heart — see Failure, heart, congestive
  kidney — see Nephrosis
  lung — see Edema, lung
  newborn due to isoimmunization P56.0
  pericardium — see Pericarditis
Drowned, drowning (near) T75.1 ☑
Drowsiness R40.0
Drug
  abuse counseling and surveillance Z71.51
  addiction — see Dependence
  dependence — see Dependence
  habit — see Dependence
  harmful use — see Abuse, drug
  induced fever R50.2
  overdose — see Table of Drugs and Chemicals, by drug, poisoning
  poisoning — see Table of Drugs and Chemicals, by drug, poisoning
  resistant organism infection (see also Resistant, organism, to, drug) Z16.30
  therapy
    long term (current) (prophylactic) — see Therapy, drug long-term (current) (prophylactic)

Drug — continued
  therapy — continued
    short term — omit code
  wrong substance given or taken in error — see Table of Drugs and Chemicals, by drug, poisoning
Drunkenness (without dependence) F10.129
  acute in alcoholism F10.229
  chronic (without remission) F10.20
    with remission F10.21
  pathological (without dependence) F10.129
    with dependence F10.229
  sleep F51.9
Drusen
  macula (degenerative) (retina) — see Degeneration, macula, drusen
  optic disc H47.32- ☑
Dry, dryness (see also condition)
  larynx J38.7
  mouth R68.2
    due to dehydration E86.0
  nose J34.89
  socket (teeth) M27.3
  throat J39.2
DSAP L56.5
Duane's syndrome H50.81- ☑
Dubin-Johnson disease or syndrome E80.6
Dubois' disease (thymus gland) A50.59 [E35]
Dubowitz' syndrome Q87.1
Duchenne-Aran muscular atrophy G12.21
Duchenne-Griesinger disease G71.0
Duchenne's
  disease or syndrome
    motor neuron disease G12.22
    muscular dystrophy G71.0
  locomotor ataxia (syphilitic) A52.11
  paralysis
    birth injury P14.0
    due to or associated with
      motor neuron disease G12.22
      muscular dystrophy G71.0
Ducrey's chancre A57
Duct, ductus — see condition
Duhring's disease (dermatitis herpetiformis) L13.0
Dullness, cardiac (decreased) (increased) R01.2
Dumb ague — see Malaria
Dumbness — see Aphasia
Dumdum fever B55.0
Dumping syndrome (postgastrectomy) K91.1
Duodenitis (nonspecific) (peptic) K29.80
  with bleeding K29.81
Duodenocholangitis — see Cholangitis
Duodenum, duodenal — see condition
Duplay's bursitis or periarthritis — see Tendinitis, calcific, shoulder
Duplication, duplex (see also Accessory)
  alimentary tract Q45.8
  anus Q43.4
  appendix (and cecum) Q43.4
  biliary duct (any) Q44.5
  bladder Q64.79
  cecum (and appendix) Q43.4
  cervix Q51.820
  chromosome NEC
    with complex rearrangements NEC Q92.5
    seen only at prometaphase Q92.8
  cystic duct Q44.5
  digestive organs Q45.8
  esophagus Q39.8
  frontonasal process Q75.8
  intestine (large) (small) Q43.4
  kidney Q63.0
  liver Q44.7
  pancreas Q45.3
  penis Q55.69
  respiratory organs NEC Q34.8
  salivary duct Q38.4
  spinal cord (incomplete) Q06.2
  stomach Q40.2
Dupré's disease (meningism) R29.1
Dupuytren's contraction or disease M72.0
Durand-Nicolas-Favre disease A55
Durotomy (inadvertent) (incidental) G97.41
Duroziez's disease (congenital mitral stenosis) Q23.2
Dutton's relapsing fever (West African) A68.1
Dwarfism E34.3
  achondroplastic Q77.4
  congenital E34.3
  constitutional E34.3

☑ Additional Character Required — Refer to the Tabular List for Character Selection   ▽ Subterms under main terms may continue to next column or page

Dwarfism — *continued*
  hypochondroplastic Q77.4
  hypophyseal E23.0
  infantile E34.3
  Laron-type E34.3
  Lorain (-Levi) type E23.0
  metatropic Q77.8
  nephrotic-glycosuric (with hypophosphatemic rickets) E72.09
  nutritional E45
  pancreatic K86.89
  pituitary E23.0
  renal N25.0
  thanatophoric Q77.1
Dyke-Young anemia (secondary) (symptomatic) D59.1
Dysacusis — *see* Abnormal, auditory perception
Dysadrenocortism E27.9
  hyperfunction E27.0
Dysarthria R47.1
  following
    cerebral infarction I69.322
    cerebrovascular disease I69.922
      specified disease NEC I69.822
    intracerebral hemorrhage I69.122
    nontraumatic intracranial hemorrhage NEC I69.222
    subarachnoid hemorrhage I69.022
Dysautonomia (familial) G90.1
Dysbarism T70.3 ☑
Dysbasia R26.2
  angiosclerotica intermittens I73.9
  hysterical F44.4
  lordotica (progressiva) G24.1
  nonorganic origin F44.4
  psychogenic F44.4
Dysbetalipoproteinemia (familial) E78.2
Dyscalculia R48.8
  developmental F81.2
Dyschezia K59.00
Dyschondroplasia (with hemangiomata) Q78.4
Dyschromia (skin) L81.9
Dyscollagenosis M35.9
Dyscranio-pygo-phalangy Q87.0
Dyscrasia
  blood (with) D75.9
    antepartum hemorrhage — *see* Hemorrhage, antepartum, with coagulation defect
    intrapartum hemorrhage O67.0
    newborn P61.9
      specified type NEC P61.8
    puerperal, postpartum O72.3
  polyglandular, pluriglandular E31.9
Dysendocrinism E34.9
Dysentery, dysenteric (catarrhal) (diarrhea) (epidemic) (hemorrhagic) (infectious) (sporadic) (tropical) A09
  abscess, liver A06.4
  amebic (*see also* Amebiasis) A06.0
    with abscess — *see* Abscess, amebic
    acute A06.0
    chronic A06.1
  arthritis (*see also* category M01) A09
    bacillary (*see also* category M01) A03.9
  bacillary A03.9
    arthritis (*see also* category M01) A03.9
    Boyd A03.2
    Flexner A03.1
    Schmitz (-Stutzer) A03.0
    Shiga (-Kruse) A03.0
    Shigella A03.9
      boydii A03.2
      dysenteriae A03.0
      flexneri A03.1
      group A A03.0
      group B A03.1
      group C A03.2
      group D A03.3
      sonnei A03.3
      specified type NEC A03.8
    Sonne A03.3
    specified type NEC A03.8
  balantidial A07.0
  Balantidium coli A07.0
  Boyd's A03.2
  candidal B37.82
  Chilomastix A07.8
  Chinese A03.9
  coccidial A07.3
  Dientamoeba (fragilis) A07.8
  Embadomonas A07.8

Dysentery, dysenteric — *continued*
  Entamoeba, entambic — *see* Dysentery, amebic
  Flexner-Boyd A03.2
  Flexner's A03.1
  Giardia lamblia A07.1
  Hiss-Russell A03.1
  Lamblia A07.1
  leishmanial B55.0
  malarial — *see* Malaria
  metazoal B82.0
  monilial B37.0
  protozoal A07.9
  Salmonella A02.0
  schistosomal B65.1
  Schmitz (-Stutzer) A03.0
  Shiga (-Kruse) A03.0
  Shigella NOS — *see* Dysentery, bacillary
  Sonne A03.3
  strongyloidiasis B78.0
  trichomonal A07.8
  viral (*see also* Enteritis, viral) A08.4
Dysequilibrium R42
Dysesthesia R20.8
  hysterical F44.6
Dysfibrinogenemia (congenital) D68.2
Dysfunction
  adrenal E27.9
    hyperfunction E27.0
  autonomic
    due to alcohol G31.2
    somatoform F45.8
  bladder N31.9
    neurogenic NOS — *see* Dysfunction, bladder, neuromuscular
    neuromuscular NOS N31.9
      atonic (motor) (sensory) N31.2
      autonomous N31.2
      flaccid N31.2
      nonreflex N31.2
      reflex N31.1
      specified NEC N31.8
      uninhibited N31.0
  bleeding, uterus N93.8
  cerebral G93.89
  colon K59.9
    psychogenic F45.8
  colostomy K94.03
  cystic duct K82.8
  cystostomy (stoma) — *see* Complications, cystostomy
  ejaculatory N53.19
    anejaculatory orgasm N53.13
    painful N53.12
    premature F52.4
    retarded N53.11
  endocrine NOS E34.9
  endometrium N85.8
  enterostomy K94.13
  erectile — *see* Dysfunction, sexual, male, erectile
  gallbladder K82.8
  gastrostomy (stoma) K94.23
  gland, glandular NOS E34.9
  heart I51.89
  hemoglobin D75.89
  hepatic K76.89
  hypophysis E23.7
  hypothalamic NEC E23.3
  ileostomy (stoma) K94.13
  jejunostomy (stoma) K94.13
  kidney — *see* Disease, renal
  labyrinthine — *see* subcategory H83.2 ☑
  left ventricular, following sudden emotional stress I51.81
  liver K76.89
  male — *see* Dysfunction, sexual, male
  orgasmic (female) F52.31
    male F52.32
  ovary E28.9
    specified NEC E28.8
  papillary muscle I51.89
  parathyroid E21.4
  physiological NEC R68.89
    psychogenic F59
  pineal gland E34.8
  pituitary (gland) E23.3
  platelets D69.1
  polyglandular E31.9
    specified NEC E31.8
  psychophysiologic F59

Dysfunction — *continued*
  psychosexual F52.9
    with
      dyspareunia F52.6
      premature ejaculation F52.4
      vaginismus F52.5
  pylorus K31.9
  rectum K59.9
    psychogenic F45.8
  reflex (sympathetic) — *see* Syndrome, pain, complex regional I
  segmental — *see* Dysfunction, somatic
  senile R54
  sexual (due to) R37
    alcohol F10.981
    amphetamine F15.981
      in
        abuse F15.181
        dependence F15.281
    anxiolytic F13.981
      in
        abuse F13.181
        dependence F13.281
    cocaine F14.981
      in
        abuse F14.181
        dependence F14.281
    excessive sexual drive F52.8
    failure of genital response (male) F52.21
      female F52.22
    female N94.9
      aversion F52.1
      dyspareunia N94.10
        psychogenic F52.6
      frigidity F52.22
      nymphomania F52.8
      orgasmic F52.31
      psychogenic F52.9
        aversion F52.1
        dyspareunia F52.6
        frigidity F52.22
        nymphomania F52.8
        orgasmic F52.31
        vaginismus F52.5
      vaginismus N94.2
        psychogenic F52.5
    hypnotic F13.981
      in
        abuse F13.181
        dependence F13.281
    inhibited orgasm (female) F52.31
      male F52.32
    lack
      of sexual enjoyment F52.1
      or loss of sexual desire F52.0
    male N53.9
      anejaculatory orgasm N53.13
      ejaculatory N53.19
        painful N53.12
        premature F52.4
        retarded N53.11
      erectile N52.9
        drug induced N52.2
        due to
          disease classified elsewhere N52.1
          drug N52.2
        postoperative (postprocedural) N52.39
          following
            cryotherapy N52.37
            interstitial seed therapy N52.36
            prostate ablative therapy N52.37
            prostatectomy N52.34
              radical N52.31
            radiation therapy N52.35
            radical cystectomy N52.32
            ultrasound ablative therapy N52.37
            urethral surgery N52.33
        psychogenic F52.21
        specified cause NEC N52.8
        vasculogenic
          arterial insufficiency N52.01
            with corporo-venous occlusive N52.03
          corporo-venous occlusive N52.02
            with arterial insufficiency N52.03
      impotence — *see* Dysfunction, sexual, male, erectile
      psychogenic F52.9
        aversion F52.1

Dysfunction — continued
  sexual — continued
    male — continued
      psychogenic — continued
        erectile F52.21
        orgasmic F52.32
        premature ejaculation F52.4
        satyriasis F52.8
        specified type NEC F52.8
      specified type NEC N53.8
    nonorganic F52.9
      specified NEC F52.8
    opioid F11.981
      in
        abuse F11.181
        dependence F11.281
    orgasmic dysfunction (female) F52.31
      male F52.32
    premature ejaculation F52.4
    psychoactive substances NEC F19.981
      in
        abuse F19.181
        dependence F19.281
    psychogenic F52.9
    sedative F13.981
      in
        abuse F13.181
        dependence F13.281
    sexual aversion F52.1
    vaginismus (nonorganic) (psychogenic) F52.5
  sinoatrial node I49.5
  somatic M99.09
    abdomen M99.09
    acromioclavicular M99.07
    cervical region M99.01
    cervicothoracic M99.01
    costochondral M99.08
    costovertebral M99.08
    head region M99.00
    hip M99.05
    lower extremity M99.06
    lumbar region M99.03
    lumbosacral M99.03
    occipitocervical M99.00
    pelvic region M99.05
    pubic M99.05
    rib cage M99.08
    sacral region M99.04
    sacrococcygeal M99.04
    sacroiliac M99.04
    specified NEC M99.09
    sternochondral M99.08
    sternoclavicular M99.07
    thoracic region M99.02
    thoracolumbar M99.02
    upper extremity M99.07
  somatoform autonomic F45.8
  stomach K31.89
    psychogenic F45.8
  suprarenal E27.9
    hyperfunction E27.0
  symbolic R48.9
    specified type NEC R48.8
  temporomandibular (joint) M26.69
    joint-pain syndrome M26.62- ☑
  testicular (endocrine) E29.9
    specified NEC E29.8
  thymus E32.9
  thyroid E07.9
  ureterostomy (stoma) — see Complications, stoma, urinary tract
  urethrostomy (stoma) — see Complications, stoma, urinary tract
  uterus, complicating delivery O62.9
    hypertonic O62.4
    hypotonic O62.2
      primary O62.0
      secondary O62.1
  ventricular I51.9
    with congestive heart failure (see also Failure, heart) I50.9
    left, reversible, following sudden emotional stress I51.81

Dysgenesis
  gonadal (due to chromosomal anomaly) Q96.9
    pure Q99.1
  renal Q60.5
    bilateral Q60.4
    unilateral Q60.3

Dysgenesis — continued
  reticular D72.0
  tidal platelet D69.3
Dysgerminoma
  specified site — see Neoplasm, malignant, by site
  unspecified site
    female C56.9
    male C62.90
Dysgeusia R43.2
Dysgraphia R27.8
Dyshidrosis, dysidrosis L30.1
Dyskaryotic cervical smear R87.619
Dyskeratosis L85.8
  cervix — see Dysplasia, cervix
  congenital Q82.8
  uterus NEC N85.8
Dyskinesia G24.9
  biliary (cystic duct or gallbladder) K82.8
  drug induced
    orofacial G24.01
  esophagus K22.4
  hysterical F44.4
  intestinal K59.8
  nonorganic origin F44.4
  orofacial (idiopathic) G24.4
    drug induced G24.01
  psychogenic F44.4
  subacute, drug induced G24.01
  tardive G24.01
    neuroleptic induced G24.01
  trachea J39.8
  tracheobronchial J98.09
Dyslalia (developmental) F80.0
Dyslexia R48.0
  developmental F81.0
Dyslipidemia E78.5
  depressed HDL cholesterol E78.6
  elevated fasting triglycerides E78.1
Dysmaturity (see also Light for dates)
  pulmonary (newborn) (Wilson-Mikity) P27.0
Dysmenorrhea (essential) (exfoliative) N94.6
  congestive (syndrome) N94.6
  primary N94.4
  psychogenic F45.8
  secondary N94.5
Dysmetabolic syndrome X E88.81
Dysmetria R27.8
Dysmorphism (due to)
  alcohol Q86.0
  exogenous cause NEC Q86.8
  hydantoin Q86.1
  warfarin Q86.2
Dysmorphophobia (nondelusional) F45.22
  delusional F22
Dysnomia R47.01
Dysorexia R63.0
  psychogenic F50.89
Dysostosis
  cleidocranial, cleidocranialis Q74.0
  craniofacial Q75.1
  Fairbank's (idiopathic familial generalized osteophytosis) Q78.9
  mandibulofacial (incomplete) Q75.4
  multiplex E76.01
  oculomandibular Q75.5
Dyspareunia (female) N94.10
  deep N94.12
  male N53.12
  nonorganic F52.6
  psychogenic F52.6
  secondary N94.19
  specified NEC N94.19
  superficial (introital) N94.11
Dyspepsia R10.13
  atonic K30
  functional (allergic) (congenital) (gastrointestinal) (occupational) (reflex) K30
  intestinal K59.8
  nervous F45.8
  neurotic F45.8
  psychogenic F45.8
Dysphagia R13.10
  cervical R13.19
  following
    cerebral infarction I69.391
    cerebrovascular disease I69.991
      specified NEC I69.891
    intracerebral hemorrhage I69.191

Dysphagia — continued
  following — continued
    nontraumatic intracranial hemorrhage NEC I69.291
    specified disease NEC I69.891
    subarachnoid hemorrhage I69.091
  functional (hysterical) F45.8
  hysterical F45.8
  nervous (hysterical) F45.8
  neurogenic R13.19
  oral phase R13.11
  oropharyngeal phase R13.12
  pharyngeal phase R13.13
  pharyngoesophageal phase R13.14
  psychogenic F45.8
  sideropenic D50.1
  spastica K22.4
  specified NEC R13.19
Dysphagocytosis, congenital D71
Dysphasia R47.02
  developmental
    expressive type F80.1
    receptive type F80.2
  following
    cerebrovascular disease I69.921
      cerebral infarction I69.321
      intracerebral hemorrhage I69.121
      nontraumatic intracranial hemorrhage NEC I69.221
      specified disease NEC I69.821
      subarachnoid hemorrhage I69.021
Dysphonia R49.0
  functional F44.4
  hysterical F44.4
  psychogenic F44.4
  spastica J38.3
Dysphoria
  gender F64.9
    in
      adolescence and adulthood F64.0
      children F64.2
    specified NEC F64.8
  postpartal O90.6
Dyspituitarism E23.3
Dysplasia (see also Anomaly)
  acetabular, congenital Q65.89
  alveolar capillary, with vein misalignment J84.843
  anus (histologically confirmed) (mild) (moderate) K62.82
    severe D01.3
  arrhythmogenic right ventricular I42.8
  arterial, fibromuscular I77.3
  asphyxiating thoracic (congenital) Q77.2
  brain Q07.9
  bronchopulmonary, perinatal P27.1
  cervix (uteri) N87.9
    mild N87.0
    moderate N87.1
    severe D06.9
  chondroectodermal Q77.6
  colon D12.6
  craniometaphyseal Q78.8
  dentinal K00.5
  diaphyseal, progressive Q78.3
  dystrophic Q77.5
  ectodermal (anhidrotic) (congenital) (hereditary) Q82.4
    hydrotic Q82.8
  epithelial, uterine cervix — see Dysplasia, cervix
  eye (congenital) Q11.2
  fibrous
    bone NEC (monostotic) M85.00
      ankle M85.07- ☑
      foot M85.07- ☑
      forearm M85.03- ☑
      hand M85.04- ☑
      lower leg M85.06- ☑
      multiple site M85.09
      neck M85.08
      rib M85.08
      shoulder M85.01- ☑
      skull M85.08
      specified site NEC M85.08
      thigh M85.05- ☑
      toe M85.07- ☑
      upper arm M85.02- ☑
      vertebra M85.08
  diaphyseal, progressive Q78.3
  jaw M27.8
  polyostotic Q78.1

Dysplasia — continued

florid osseous (*see also* Cyst, calcifying odontogenic)
high grade, focal D12.6
hip, congenital Q65.89
joint, congenital Q74.8
kidney Q61.4
    multicystic Q61.4
leg Q74.2
lung, congenital (not associated with short gestation) Q33.6
mammary (gland) (benign) N60.9- ☑
    cyst (solitary) — *see* Cyst, breast
    cystic — *see* Mastopathy, cystic
    duct ectasia — *see* Ectasia, mammary duct
    fibroadenosis — *see* Fibroadenosis, breast
    fibrosclerosis — *see* Fibrosclerosis, breast
    specified type NEC N60.8- ☑
metaphyseal Q78.5
muscle Q79.8
oculodentodigital Q87.0
periapical (cemental) (cemento-osseous) — *see* Cyst, calcifying odontogenic
periosteum — *see* Disorder, bone, specified type NEC
polyostotic fibrous Q78.1
prostate (*see also* Neoplasia, intraepithelial, prostate) N42.30
    severe D07.5
    specified NEC N42.39
renal Q61.4
    multicystic Q61.4
retinal, congenital Q14.1
right ventricular, arrhythmogenic I42.8
septo-optic Q04.4
skin L98.8
spinal cord Q06.1
spondyloepiphyseal Q77.7
thymic, with immunodeficiency D82.1
vagina N89.3
    mild N89.0
    moderate N89.1
    severe NEC D07.2
vulva N90.3
    mild N90.0
    moderate N90.1
    severe NEC D07.1

Dyspnea (nocturnal) (paroxysmal) R06.00

asthmatic (bronchial) J45.909
    with
        bronchitis J45.909
            with
                exacerbation (acute) J45.901
                status asthmaticus J45.902
            chronic J44.9
        exacerbation (acute) J45.901
        status asthmaticus J45.902
    cardiac — *see* Failure, ventricular, left
cardiac — *see* Failure, ventricular, left
functional F45.8
hyperventilation R06.4
hysterical F45.8
newborn P28.89
orthopnea R06.01
psychogenic F45.8
shortness of breath R06.02
specified type NEC R06.09

Dyspraxia R27.8
    developmental (syndrome) F82
Dysproteinemia E88.09
Dysreflexia, autonomic G90.4
Dysrhythmia
cardiac I49.9
    newborn
        bradycardia P29.12
        occurring before birth P03.819
            before onset of labor P03.810
            during labor P03.811
        tachycardia P29.11
        postoperative I97.89
cerebral or cortical — *see* Epilepsy
Dyssomnia — *see* Disorder, sleep
Dyssynergia
biliary K83.8
bladder sphincter N36.44
cerebellaris myoclonica (Hunt's ataxia) G11.1
Dysthymia F34.1
Dysthyroidism E07.9
Dystocia O66.9
affecting newborn P03.1

Dystocia — continued

cervical (hypotonic) O62.2
    affecting newborn P03.6
    primary O62.0
    secondary O62.1
contraction ring O62.4
fetal O66.9
    abnormality NEC O66.3
    conjoined twins O66.3
    oversize O66.2
maternal O66.9
positional O64.9 ☑
shoulder (girdle) O66.0
    causing obstructed labor O66.0
uterine NEC O62.4

Dystonia G24.9

deformans progressiva G24.1
drug induced NEC G24.09
    acute G24.02
    specified NEC G24.09
familial G24.1
idiopathic G24.1
    familial G24.1
    nonfamilial G24.2
    orofacial G24.4
lenticularis G24.8
musculorum deformans G24.1
neuroleptic induced (acute) G24.02
orofacial (idiopathic) G24.4
oromandibular G24.4
    due to drug G24.01
specified NEC G24.8
torsion (familial) (idiopathic) G24.1
    acquired G24.8
    genetic G24.1
    symptomatic (nonfamilial) G24.2

Dystonic movements R25.8

Dystrophy, dystrophia

adiposogenital E23.6
Becker's type G71.0
cervical sympathetic G90.2
choroid (hereditary) H31.20
    central areolar H31.22
    choroideremia H31.21
    gyrate atrophy H31.23
    specified type NEC H31.29
cornea (hereditary) H18.50
    endothelial H18.51
    epithelial H18.52
    granular H18.53
    lattice H18.54
    macular H18.55
    specified type NEC H18.59
Duchenne's type G71.0
due to malnutrition E45
Erb's G71.0
Fuchs' H18.51
Gower's muscular G71.0
hair L67.8
infantile neuraxonal G31.89
Landouzy-Déjérine G71.0
Leyden-Möbius G71.0
muscular G71.0
    benign (Becker type) G71.0
    congenital (hereditary) (progressive) (with specific morphological abnormalities of the muscle fiber) G71.0
        myotonic G71.11
    distal G71.0
    Duchenne type G71.0
    Emery-Dreifuss G71.0
    Erb type G71.0
    facioscapulohumeral G71.0
    Gower's G71.0
    hereditary (progressive) G71.0
    Landouzy-Déjérine type G71.0
    limb-girdle G71.0
    myotonic G71.11
    progressive (hereditary) G71.0
        Charcot-Marie (-Tooth) type G60.0
    pseudohypertrophic (infantile) G71.0
    severe (Duchenne type) G71.0
myocardium, myocardial — *see* Degeneration, myocardial
nail L60.3
    congenital Q84.6
nutritional E45
ocular G71.0
oculocerebrorenal E72.03

Dystrophy, dystrophia — continued

oculopharyngeal G71.0
ovarian N83.8
polyglandular E31.8
reflex (neuromuscular) (sympathetic) — *see* Syndrome, pain, complex regional I
retinal (hereditary) H35.50
    in
        lipid storage disorders E75.6 [H36]
        systemic lipidoses E75.6 [H36]
    involving
        pigment epithelium H35.54
        sensory area H35.53
    pigmentary H35.52
    vitreoretinal H35.51
Salzmann's nodular — *see* Degeneration, cornea, nodular
scapuloperoneal G71.0
skin NEC L98.8
sympathetic (reflex) — *see* Syndrome, pain, complex regional I
    cervical G90.2
tapetoretinal H35.54
thoracic, asphyxiating Q77.2
unguium L60.3
    congenital Q84.6
vitreoretinal H35.51
vulva N90.4
yellow (liver) — *see* Failure, hepatic

Dysuria R30.0
psychogenic F45.8

E

Eales' disease H35.06- ☑
Ear (*see also* condition)
piercing Z41.3
tropical NEC B36.9 [H62.40]
    in
        aspergillosis B44.89
        candidiasis B37.84
        moniliasis B37.84
wax (impacted) H61.20
    left H61.22
        with right H61.23
    right H61.21
        with left H61.23
Earache — *see* subcategory H92.0 ☑
Early satiety R68.81
Eaton-Lambert syndrome — *see* Syndrome, Lambert-Eaton
Eberth's disease (typhoid fever) A01.00
Ebola virus disease A98.4
Ebstein's anomaly or syndrome (heart) Q22.5
Eccentro-osteochondrodysplasia E76.29
Ecchondroma — *see* Neoplasm, bone, benign
Ecchondrosis D48.0
Ecchymosis R58
conjunctiva — *see* Hemorrhage, conjunctiva
eye (traumatic) — *see* Contusion, eyeball
eyelid (traumatic) — *see* Contusion, eyelid
newborn P54.5
spontaneous R23.3
traumatic — *see* Contusion
Echinococciasis — *see* Echinococcus
Echinococcosis — *see* Echinococcus
Echinococcus (infection) B67.90
granulosus B67.4
    bone B67.2
    liver B67.0
    lung B67.1
    multiple sites B67.32
    specified site NEC B67.39
    thyroid B67.31
liver NOS B67.8
    granulosus B67.0
    multilocularis B67.5
lung NEC B67.99
    granulosus B67.1
    multilocularis B67.69
multilocularis B67.7
    liver B67.5
    multiple sites B67.61
    specified site NEC B67.69
specified site NEC B67.99
    granulosus B67.39
    multilocularis B67.69
thyroid NEC B67.99

Echinococcus — continued
  thyroid — continued
    granulosus B67.31
    multilocularis B67.69 [E35]
Echinorhynchiasis B83.8
Echinostomiasis B66.8
Echolalia R48.8
Echovirus, as cause of disease classified elsewhere
  B97.12
Eclampsia, eclamptic (coma) (convulsions) (delirium)
  (with hypertension) NEC O15.9
  complicating
    labor and delivery O15.1
    postpartum O15.2
    pregnancy O15.0- ☑
    puerperium O15.2
Economic circumstances affecting care Z59.9
Economo's disease A85.8
Ectasia, ectasis
  annuloaortic I35.8
  aorta I77.819
    with aneurysm — see Aneurysm, aorta
    abdominal I77.811
    thoracic I77.810
    thoracoabdominal I77.812
  breast — see Ectasia, mammary duct
  capillary I78.8
  cornea H18.71- ☑
  gastric antral vascular (GAVE) K31.819
    with hemorrhage K31.811
    without hemorrhage K31.819
  mammary duct N60.4- ☑
  salivary gland (duct) K11.8
  sclera — see Sclerectasia
Ecthyma L08.0
  contagiosum B08.02
  gangrenosum L08.0
  infectiosum B08.02
Ectocardia Q24.8
Ectodermal dysplasia (anhidrotic) Q82.4
Ectodermosis erosiva pluriorificialis L51.1
Ectopic, ectopia (congenital)
  abdominal viscera Q45.8
    due to defect in anterior abdominal wall Q79.59
  ACTH syndrome E24.3
  adrenal gland Q89.1
  anus Q43.5
  atrial beats I49.1
  beats I49.49
    atrial I49.1
    ventricular I49.3
  bladder Q64.10
  bone and cartilage in lung Q33.5
  brain Q04.8
  breast tissue Q83.8
  cardiac Q24.8
  cerebral Q04.8
  cordis Q24.8
  endometrium — see Endometriosis
  gastric mucosa Q40.2
  gestation — see Pregnancy, by site
  heart Q24.8
  hormone secretion NEC E34.2
  kidney (crossed) (pelvis) Q63.2
  lens, lentis Q12.1
  mole — see Pregnancy, by site
  organ or site NEC — see Malposition, congenital
  pancreas Q45.3
  pregnancy — see Pregnancy, ectopic
  pupil — see Abnormality, pupillary
  renal Q63.2
  sebaceous glands of mouth Q38.6
  spleen Q89.09
  testis Q53.00
    bilateral Q53.02
    unilateral Q53.01
  thyroid Q89.2
  tissue in lung Q33.5
  ureter Q62.63
  ventricular beats I49.3
  vesicae Q64.10
Ectromelia Q73.8
  lower limb — see Defect, reduction, limb, lower,
    specified type NEC
  upper limb — see Defect, reduction, limb, upper,
    specified type NEC
Ectropion H02.109
  cervix N86

Ectropion — continued
  cervix — continued
    with cervicitis N72
  congenital Q10.1
  eyelid (paralytic) H02.109
    cicatricial H02.119
      left H02.116
        lower H02.115
        upper H02.114
      right H02.113
        lower H02.112
        upper H02.111
    congenital Q10.1
    left H02.106
      lower H02.105
      upper H02.104
    mechanical H02.129
      left H02.126
        lower H02.125
        upper H02.124
      right H02.123
        lower H02.122
        upper H02.121
    right H02.103
      lower H02.102
      upper H02.101
    senile H02.139
      left H02.136
        lower H02.135
        upper H02.134
      right H02.133
        lower H02.132
        upper H02.131
    spastic H02.149
      left H02.146
        lower H02.145
        upper H02.144
      right H02.143
        lower H02.142
        upper H02.141
  iris H21.89
  lip (acquired) K13.0
    congenital Q38.0
  urethra N36.8
  uvea H21.89
Eczema (acute) (chronic) (erythematous) (fissum)
  (rubrum) (squamous) (see also Dermatitis) L30.9
  contact — see Dermatitis, contact
  dyshydrotic L30.1
  external ear — see Otitis, externa, acute, eczematoid
  flexural L20.82
  herpeticum B00.0
  hypertrophicum L28.0
  hypostatic — see Varix, leg, with, inflammation
  impetiginous L01.1
  infantile (due to any substance) L20.83
    intertriginous L21.1
    seborrheic L21.1
  intertriginous NEC L30.4
    infantile L21.1
  intrinsic (allergic) L20.84
  lichenified NEC L28.0
  marginatum (hebrae) B35.6
  pustular L30.3
  stasis I87.2
    with varicose veins — see Varix, leg, with, inflam-
      mation
  vaccination, vaccinatum T88.1 ☑
  varicose — see Varix, leg, with, inflammation
Eczematid L30.2
Eddowes (-Spurway) **syndrome** Q78.0
Edema, edematous (infectious) (pitting) (toxic) R60.9
  with nephritis — see Nephrosis
  allergic T78.3 ☑
  amputation stump (surgical) (sequelae) (late effect))
    T87.89
  angioneurotic (allergic) (any site) (with urticaria)
    T78.3 ☑
    hereditary D84.1
  angiospastic I73.9
  Berlin's (traumatic) S05.8X- ☑
  brain (cytotoxic) (vasogenic) G93.6
    due to birth injury P11.0
    newborn (anoxia or hypoxia) P52.4
      birth injury P11.0
    traumatic — see Injury, intracranial, cerebral edema
  cardiac — see Failure, heart, congestive
  cardiovascular — see Failure, heart, congestive

Edema, edematous — continued
  cerebral — see Edema, brain
  cerebrospinal — see Edema, brain
  cervix (uteri) (acute) N88.8
    puerperal, postpartum O90.89
  chronic hereditary Q82.0
  circumscribed, acute T78.3 ☑
    hereditary D84.1
  conjunctiva H11.42- ☑
  cornea H18.2- ☑
    idiopathic H18.22- ☑
    secondary H18.23- ☑
      due to contact lens H18.21- ☑
  due to
    lymphatic obstruction I89.0
    salt retention E87.0
  epiglottis — see Edema, glottis
  essential, acute T78.3 ☑
    hereditary D84.1
  extremities, lower — see Edema, legs
  eyelid NEC H02.849
    left H02.846
      lower H02.845
      upper H02.844
    right H02.843
      lower H02.842
      upper H02.841
  familial, hereditary Q82.0
  famine — see Malnutrition, severe
  generalized R60.1
  glottis, glottic, glottidis (obstructive) (passive) J38.4
    allergic T78.3 ☑
      hereditary D84.1
  heart — see Failure, heart, congestive
  heat T67.7 ☑
  hereditary Q82.0
  inanition — see Malnutrition, severe
  intracranial G93.6
  iris H21.89
  joint — see Effusion, joint
  larynx — see Edema, glottis
  legs R60.0
    due to venous obstruction I87.1
    hereditary Q82.0
  localized R60.0
    due to venous obstruction I87.1
  lower limbs — see Edema, legs
  lung J81.1
    with heart condition or failure — see Failure, ven-
      tricular, left
    acute J81.0
      chemical (acute) J68.1
        chronic J68.1
    chronic J81.1
      due to
        chemicals, gases, fumes or vapors (inhala-
          tion) J68.1
        external agent J70.9
          specified NEC J70.8
        radiation J70.1
    due to
      chemicals, fumes or vapors (inhalation) J68.1
      external agent J70.9
        specified NEC J70.8
      high altitude T70.29 ☑
      near drowning T75.1 ☑
      radiation J70.0
    meaning failure, left ventricle I50.1
  lymphatic I89.0
    due to mastectomy I97.2
  macula H35.81
    cystoid, following cataract surgery — see Compli-
      cations, postprocedural, following cataract
      surgery
    diabetic — see Diabetes, by type, with, retinopathy,
      with macular edema
  malignant — see Gangrene, gas
  Milroy's Q82.0
  nasopharynx J39.2
  newborn P83.30
    hydrops fetalis — see Hydrops, fetalis
    specified NEC P83.39
  nutritional (see also Malnutrition, severe)
    with dyspigmentation, skin and hair E40
  optic disc or nerve — see Papilledema
  orbit H05.22- ☑
  pancreas K86.89
  papilla, optic — see Papilledema

☑ **Additional Character Required** — **Refer to the Tabular List for Character Selection**   �om **Subterms under main terms may continue to next column or page**

Edema, edematous — continued
  penis N48.89
  periodic T78.3 ☑
    hereditary D84.1
  pharynx J39.2
  pulmonary — see Edema, lung
  Quincke's T78.3 ☑
    hereditary D84.1
  renal — see Nephrosis
  retina H35.81
    diabetic — see Diabetes, by type, with, retinopathy, with macular edema
  salt E87.0
  scrotum N50.89
  seminal vesicle N50.89
  spermatic cord N50.89
  spinal (cord) (vascular) (nontraumatic) G95.19
  starvation — see Malnutrition, severe
  stasis — see Hypertension, venous, (chronic)
  subglottic — see Edema, glottis
  supraglottic — see Edema, glottis
  testis N44.8
  tunica vaginalis N50.89
  vas deferens N50.89
  vulva (acute) N90.89
Edentulism — see Absence, teeth, acquired
Edsall's disease T67.2 ☑
Educational handicap Z55.9
  specified NEC Z55.8
Edward's syndrome — see Trisomy, 18
Effect(s) (of) (from) — see Effect, adverse NEC
Effect, adverse
  abnormal gravitational (G) forces or states T75.81 ☑
  abuse — see Maltreatment
  air pressure T70.9 ☑
    specified NEC T70.8 ☑
  altitude (high) — see Effect, adverse, high altitude
  anesthesia (see also Anesthesia) T88.59 ☑
    in labor and delivery O74.9
    local, toxic
      in labor and delivery O74.4
      in pregnancy NEC O29.3- ☑
      postpartum, puerperal O89.3
    postpartum, puerperal O89.9
    specified NEC T88.59 ☑
      in labor and delivery O74.8
      postpartum, puerperal O89.8
    spinal and epidural T88.59 ☑
      headache T88.59 ☑
        in labor and delivery O74.5
        postpartum, puerperal O89.4
      specified NEC
        in labor and delivery O74.6
        postpartum, puerperal O89.5
  antitoxin — see Complications, vaccination
  atmospheric pressure T70.9 ☑
    due to explosion T70.8 ☑
    high T70.3 ☑
    low — see Effect, adverse, high altitude
    specified effect NEC T70.8 ☑
  biological, correct substance properly administered — see Effect, adverse, drug
  blood (derivatives) (serum) (transfusion) — see Complications, transfusion
  chemical substance — see Table of Drugs and Chemicals
  cold (temperature) (weather) T69.9 ☑
    chilblains T69.1 ☑
    frostbite — see Frostbite
    specified effect NEC T69.8 ☑
  drugs and medicaments T88.7 ☑
    specified drug — see Table of Drugs and Chemicals, by drug, adverse effect
    specified effect — see code to condition
  electric current, electricity (shock) T75.4 ☑
    burn — see Burn
  exertion (excessive) T73.3 ☑
  exposure — see Exposure
  external cause NEC T75.89 ☑
  foodstuffs T78.1 ☑
    allergic reaction — see Allergy, food
      causing anaphylaxis — see Shock, anaphylactic, due to food
    noxious — see Poisoning, food, noxious
  gases, fumes, or vapors T59.9- ☑
    specified agent — see Table of Drugs and Chemicals

Effect, adverse — continued
  glue (airplane) sniffing
    due to drug abuse — see Abuse, drug, inhalant
    due to drug dependence — see Dependence, drug, inhalant
  heat — see Heat
  high altitude NEC T70.29 ☑
    anoxia T70.29 ☑
    on
      ears T70.0 ☑
      sinuses T70.1 ☑
    polycythemia D75.1
  high pressure fluids T70.4 ☑
  hot weather — see Heat
  hunger T73.0 ☑
  immersion, foot — see Immersion
  immunization — see Complications, vaccination
  immunological agents — see Complications, vaccination
  infrared (radiation) (rays) NOS T66 ☑
    dermatitis or eczema L59.8
  infusion — see Complications, infusion
  lack of care of infants — see Maltreatment, child
  lightning — see Lightning
  medical care T88.9 ☑
    specified NEC T88.8 ☑
  medicinal substance, correct, properly administered — see Effect, adverse, drug
  motion T75.3 ☑
  noise, on inner ear — see subcategory H83.3 ☑
  overheated places — see Heat
  psychosocial, of work environment Z56.5
  radiation (diagnostic) (infrared) (natural source) (therapeutic) (ultraviolet) (X-ray) NOS T66 ☑
    dermatitis or eczema — see Dermatitis, due to, radiation
    fibrosis of lung J70.1
    pneumonitis J70.0
    pulmonary manifestations
      acute J70.0
      chronic J70.1
    skin L59.9
  radioactive substance NOS
    dermatitis or eczema — see Radiodermatitis
  reduced temperature T69.9 ☑
    immersion foot or hand — see Immersion
    specified effect NEC T69.8 ☑
  serum NEC (see also Reaction, serum) T80.69 ☑
  specified NEC T78.8 ☑
    external cause NEC T75.89 ☑
  strangulation — see Asphyxia, traumatic
  submersion T75.1 ☑
  thirst T73.1 ☑
  toxic — see Toxicity
  transfusion — see Complications, transfusion
  ultraviolet (radiation) (rays) NOS T66 ☑
    burn — see Burn
    dermatitis or eczema — see Dermatitis, due to, ultraviolet rays
      acute L56.8
  vaccine (any) — see Complications, vaccination
  vibration — see Vibration, adverse effects
  water pressure NEC T70.9 ☑
    specified NEC T70.8 ☑
  weightlessness T75.82 ☑
  whole blood — see Complications, transfusion
  work environment Z56.5
Effects, late — see Sequelae
Effluvium
  anagen L65.1
  telogen L65.0
Effort syndrome (psychogenic) F45.8
Effusion
  amniotic fluid — see Pregnancy, complicated by, premature rupture of membranes
  brain (serous) G93.6
  bronchial — see Bronchitis
  cerebral G93.6
  cerebrospinal (see also Meningitis)
    vessel G93.6
  chest — see Effusion, pleura
  chylous, chyliform (pleura) J94.0
  intracranial G93.6
  joint M25.40
    ankle M25.47- ☑
    elbow M25.42- ☑
    foot joint M25.47- ☑

Effusion — continued
  joint — continued
    hand joint M25.44- ☑
    hip M25.45- ☑
    knee M25.46- ☑
    shoulder M25.41- ☑
    specified joint NEC M25.48
    wrist M25.43- ☑
  malignant pleural J91.0
  meninges — see Meningitis
  pericardium, pericardial (noninflammatory) I31.3
    acute — see Pericarditis, acute
  peritoneal (chronic) R18.8
  pleura, pleurisy, pleuritic, pleuropericardial J90
    chylous, chyliform J94.0
    due to systemic lupus erythematosis M32.13
    in conditions classified elsewhere J91.8
    influenzal — see Influenza, with, respiratory manifestations NEC
    malignant J91.0
    newborn P28.89
    tuberculous NEC A15.6
      primary (progressive) A15.7
  spinal — see Meningitis
  thorax, thoracic — see Effusion, pleura
Egg shell nails L60.3
  congenital Q84.6
Egyptian splenomegaly B65.1
Ehlers-Danlos syndrome Q79.6
Ehrlichiosis A77.40
  due to
    E. chafeensis A77.41
    E. sennetsu A79.81
    specified organism NEC A77.49
Eichstedt's disease B36.0
Eisenmenger's
  complex or syndrome I27.83
  defect Q21.8
Ejaculation
  delayed F52.32
  painful N53.12
  premature F52.4
  retarded N53.11
  retrograde N53.14
  semen, painful N53.12
  psychogenic F52.6
Ekbom's syndrome (restless legs) G25.81
Ekman's syndrome (brittle bones and blue sclera) Q78.0
Elastic skin Q82.8
  acquired L57.4
Elastofibroma — see Neoplasm, connective tissue, benign
Elastoma (juvenile) Q82.8
  Miescher's L87.2
Elastomyofibrosis I42.4
Elastosis
  actinic, solar L57.8
  atrophicans (senile) L57.4
  perforans serpiginosa L87.2
  senilis L57.4
Elbow — see condition
Electric current, electricity, effects (concussion) (fatal) (nonfatal) (shock) T75.4 ☑
  burn — see Burn
Electric feet syndrome E53.8
Electrocution T75.4 ☑
  from electroshock gun (taser) T75.4 ☑
Electrolyte imbalance E87.8
  with
    abortion — see Abortion by type, complicated by, electrolyte imbalance
    ectopic pregnancy O08.5
    molar pregnancy O08.5
Elephantiasis (nonfilarial) I89.0
  arabicum — see Infestation, filarial
  bancroftian B74.0
  congenital (any site) (hereditary) Q82.0
  due to
    Brugia (malayi) B74.1
      timori B74.2
    mastectomy I97.2
    Wuchereria (bancrofti) B74.0
  eyelid H02.859
    left H02.856
      lower H02.855
      upper H02.854
    right H02.853
      lower H02.852

Elephantiasis — *continued*
  eyelid — *continued*
    right — *continued*
      upper H02.851
  filarial, filariensis — *see* Infestation, filarial
  glandular I89.0
  graecorum A30.9
  lymphangiectatic I89.0
  lymphatic vessel I89.0
    due to mastectomy I97.2
  scrotum (nonfilarial) I89.0
  streptococcal I89.0
  surgical I97.89
    postmastectomy I97.2
  telangiectodes I89.0
  vulva (nonfilarial) N90.89
Elevated, elevation
  antibody titer R76.0
  basal metabolic rate R94.8
  blood pressure (*see also* Hypertension)
    reading (incidental) (isolated) (nonspecific), no di-
      agnosis of hypertension R03.0
  blood sugar R73.9
  body temperature (of unknown origin) R50.9
  cancer antigen 125 [CA 125] R97.1
  carcinoembryonic antigen [CEA] R97.0
  cholesterol E78.00
    with high triglycerides E78.2
  conjugate, eye H51.0
  C-reactive protein (CRP) R79.82
  diaphragm, congenital Q79.1
  erythrocyte sedimentation rate R70.0
  fasting glucose R73.01
  fasting triglycerides E78.1
  finding on laboratory examination — *see* Findings,
    abnormal, inconclusive, without diagnosis, by
    type of exam
  GFR (glomerular filtration rate) — *see* Findings, abnor-
    mal, inconclusive, without diagnosis, by type of
    exam
  glucose tolerance (oral) R73.02
  immunoglobulin level R76.8
  indoleacetic acid R82.5
  lactic acid dehydrogenase (LDH) level R74.0
  leukocytes D72.829
  lipoprotein a level E78.8 ☑
  liver function
    study R94.5
    test R79.89
      alkaline phosphatase R74.8
      aminotransferase R74.0
      bilirubin R17
      hepatic enzyme R74.8
      lactate dehydrogenase R74.0
  lymphocytes D72.820
  prostate specific antigen [PSA] R97.20
  Rh titer — *see* Complication(s), transfusion, incompat-
    ibility reaction, Rh (factor)
  scapula, congenital Q74.0
  sedimentation rate R70.0
  SGOT R74.0
  SGPT R74.0
  transaminase level R74.0
  triglycerides E78.1
    with high cholesterol E78.2
  tumor associated antigens [TAA] NEC R97.8
  tumor specific antigens [TSA] NEC R97.8
  urine level of
    17-ketosteroids R82.5
    catecholamine R82.5
    indoleacetic acid R82.5
    steroids R82.5
    vanillylmandelic acid (VMA) R82.5
  venous pressure I87.8
  white blood cell count D72.829
    specified NEC D72.828
Elliptocytosis (congenital) (hereditary) D58.1
  Hb C (disease) D58.1
  hemoglobin disease D58.1
  sickle-cell (disease) D57.8- ☑
    trait D57.3
Ellison-Zollinger syndrome E16.4
Ellis-van Creveld syndrome (chondroectodermal dysplasia) Q77.6
Elongated, elongation (congenital) (*see also* Distortion)
  bone Q79.9
  cervix (uteri) Q51.828
    acquired N88.4

Elongated, elongation — *continued*
  cervix — *continued*
    hypertrophic N88.4
  colon Q43.8
  common bile duct Q44.5
  cystic duct Q44.5
  frenulum, penis Q55.69
  labia minora (acquired) N90.69
  ligamentum patellae Q74.1
  petiolus (epiglottidis) Q31.8
  tooth, teeth K00.2
  uvula Q38.6
Eltor cholera A00.1
Emaciation (due to malnutrition) E41
Embadomoniasis A07.8
Embedded tooth, teeth K01.0
  root only K08.3
Embolic — *see* condition
Embolism (multiple) (paradoxical) I74.9
  air (any site) (traumatic) T79.0 ☑
    following
      abortion — *see* Abortion by type complicated
        by embolism
      ectopic pregnancy O08.2
      infusion, therapeutic injection or transfusion
        T80.0 ☑
      molar pregnancy O08.2
      procedure NEC
        artery T81.719 ☑
          mesenteric T81.710 ☑
          renal T81.711 ☑
          specified NEC T81.718 ☑
        vein T81.72 ☑
    in pregnancy, childbirth or puerperium — *see*
      Embolism, obstetric
  amniotic fluid (pulmonary) (*see also* Embolism, obstet-
    ric)
    following
      abortion — *see* Abortion by type complicated
        by embolism
      ectopic pregnancy O08.2
      molar pregnancy O08.2
  aorta, aortic I74.10
    abdominal I74.09
      saddle I74.01
    bifurcation I74.09
    saddle I74.01
    thoracic I74.11
  artery I74.9
    auditory, internal I65.8
    basilar — *see* Occlusion, artery, basilar
    carotid (common) (internal) — *see* Occlusion,
      artery, carotid
    cerebellar (anterior inferior) (posterior inferior)
      (superior) I66.3
    cerebral — *see* Occlusion, artery, cerebral
    choroidal (anterior) I65.8
    communicating posterior I65.8
    coronary (*see also* Infarct, myocardium)
      not resulting in infarction I24.0
    extremity I74.4
      lower I74.3
      upper I74.2
    hypophyseal I65.8
    iliac I74.5
    limb I74.4
      lower I74.3
      upper I74.2
    mesenteric (with gangrene) (*see also* Ischemia, in-
      testine, acute) K55.059
    ophthalmic — *see* Occlusion, artery, retina
    peripheral I74.4
    pontine I65.8
    precerebral — *see* Occlusion, artery, precerebral
    pulmonary — *see* Embolism, pulmonary
    renal N28.0
    retinal — *see* Occlusion, artery, retina
    septic I76
    specified NEC I74.8
    vertebral — *see* Occlusion, artery, vertebral
  basilar (artery) I65.1
  blood clot
    following
      abortion — *see* Abortion by type complicated
        by embolism
      ectopic or molar pregnancy O08.2
    in pregnancy, childbirth or puerperium — *see*
      Embolism, obstetric

Embolism — *continued*
  brain (*see also* Occlusion, artery, cerebral)
    following
      abortion — *see* Abortion by type complicated
        by embolism
      ectopic or molar pregnancy O08.2
    puerperal, postpartum, childbirth — *see* Embolism,
      obstetric
  capillary I78.8
  cardiac (*see also* Infarct, myocardium)
    not resulting in infarction I51.3
  carotid (artery) (common) (internal) — *see* Occlusion,
    artery, carotid
  cavernous sinus (venous) — *see* Embolism, intracranial
    venous sinus
  cerebral — *see* Occlusion, artery, cerebral
  cholesterol — *see* Atheroembolism
  coronary (artery or vein) (systemic) — *see* Occlusion,
    coronary
  due to device, implant or graft (*see also* Complications,
    by site and type, specified NEC)
    arterial graft NEC T82.818 ☑
    breast (implant) T85.818 ☑
    catheter NEC T85.818 ☑
      dialysis (renal) T82.818 ☑
        intraperitoneal T85.818 ☑
      infusion NEC T82.818 ☑
        spinal (epidural) (subdural) T85.810 ☑
      urinary (indwelling) T83.81 ☑
    electronic (electrode) (pulse generator) (stimulator)
      bone T84.81 ☑
      cardiac T82.817 ☑
      nervous system (brain) (peripheral nerve)
        (spinal) T85.810 ☑
      urinary T83.81 ☑
    fixation, internal (orthopedic) NEC T84.81 ☑
    gastrointestinal (bile duct) (esophagus) T85.818 ☑
    genital NEC T83.81 ☑
    heart (graft) (valve) T82.817 ☑
    joint prosthesis T84.81 ☑
    ocular (corneal graft) (orbital implant) T85.818 ☑
    orthopedic (bone graft) NEC T86.838
    specified NEC T85.818 ☑
    urinary (graft) NEC T83.81 ☑
    vascular NEC T82.818 ☑
    ventricular intracranial shunt T85.810 ☑
  extremities
    lower — *see* Embolism, vein, lower extremity
      arterial I74.3
    upper I74.2
  eye H34.9
  fat (cerebral) (pulmonary) (systemic) T79.1 ☑
    complicating delivery — *see* Embolism, obstetric
    following
      abortion — *see* Abortion by type complicated
        by embolism
      ectopic or molar pregnancy O08.2
  following
    abortion — *see* Abortion by type complicated by
      embolism
    ectopic or molar pregnancy O08.2
    infusion, therapeutic injection or transfusion
      air T80.0 ☑
  heart (fatty) (*see also* Infarct, myocardium)
    not resulting in infarction I51.3
  hepatic (vein) I82.0
  in pregnancy, childbirth or puerperium — *see* Em-
    bolism, obstetric
  intestine (artery) (vein) (with gangrene) (*see also* Is-
    chemia, intestine, acute) K55.039
  intracranial (*see also* Occlusion, artery, cerebral)
    venous sinus (any) G08
      nonpyogenic I67.6
  intraspinal venous sinuses or veins G08
    nonpyogenic G95.19
  kidney (artery) N28.0
  lateral sinus (venous) — *see* Embolism, intracranial,
    venous sinus
  leg — *see* Embolism, vein, lower extremity
    arterial I74.3
  longitudinal sinus (venous) — *see* Embolism, intracra-
    nial, venous sinus
  lung (massive) — *see* Embolism, pulmonary
  meninges I66.8
  mesenteric (artery) (vein) (with gangrene) (*see also*
    Ischemia, intestine, acute) K55.059

Embolism — continued
- obstetric (in) (pulmonary)
  - childbirth O88.22
    - air O88.02
    - amniotic fluid O88.12
    - blood clot O88.22
    - fat O88.82
    - pyemic O88.32
    - septic O88.32
    - specified type NEC O88.82
  - pregnancy O88.21- ☑
    - air O88.01- ☑
    - amniotic fluid O88.11- ☑
    - blood clot O88.21- ☑
    - fat O88.81- ☑
    - pyemic O88.31- ☑
    - septic O88.31- ☑
    - specified type NEC O88.81- ☑
  - puerperal O88.23
    - air O88.03
    - amniotic fluid O88.13
    - blood clot O88.23
    - fat O88.83
    - pyemic O88.33
    - septic O88.33
    - specified type NEC O88.83
- ophthalmic — see Occlusion, artery, retina
- penis N48.81
- peripheral artery NOS I74.4
- pituitary E23.6
- popliteal (artery) I74.3
- portal (vein) I81
- postoperative, postprocedural
  - artery T81.719 ☑
    - mesenteric T81.710 ☑
    - renal T81.711 ☑
    - specified NEC T81.718 ☑
  - vein T81.72 ☑
- precerebral artery — see Occlusion, artery, precerebral
- puerperal — see Embolism, obstetric
- pulmonary (acute) (artery) (vein) I26.99
  - with acute cor pulmonale I26.09
  - chronic I27.82
  - following
    - abortion — see Abortion by type complicated by embolism
    - ectopic or molar pregnancy O08.2
  - healed or old Z86.711
  - in pregnancy, childbirth or puerperium — see Embolism, obstetric
  - personal history of Z86.711
  - saddle I26.92
    - with acute cor pulmonale I26.02
  - septic I26.90
    - with acute cor pulmonale I26.01
- pyemic (multiple) I76
  - following
    - abortion — see Abortion by type complicated by embolism
    - ectopic or molar pregnancy O08.2
  - Hemophilus influenzae A41.3
  - pneumococcal A40.3
    - with pneumonia J13
  - puerperal, postpartum, childbirth (any organism) — see Embolism, obstetric
  - specified organism NEC A41.89
  - staphylococcal A41.2
  - streptococcal A40.9
- renal (artery) N28.0
  - vein I82.3
- retina, retinal — see Occlusion, artery, retina
- saddle
  - abdominal aorta I74.01
  - pulmonary artery I26.92
    - with acute cor pulmonale I26.02
- septic (arterial) I76
  - complicating abortion — see Abortion, by type, complicated by, embolism
- sinus — see Embolism, intracranial, venous sinus
- soap complicating abortion — see Abortion, by type, complicated by, embolism
- spinal cord G95.19
  - pyogenic origin G06.1
- spleen, splenic (artery) I74.8
- upper extremity I74.2
- vein (acute) I82.90
  - antecubital I82.61- ☑
    - chronic I82.71- ☑

Embolism — continued
- vein — continued
  - axillary I82.A1- ☑ (following I82.7)
    - chronic I82.A2- ☑ (following I82.7)
  - basilic I82.61- ☑
    - chronic I82.71- ☑
  - brachial I82.62- ☑
    - chronic I82.72- ☑
  - brachiocephalic (innominate) I82.290
    - chronic I82.291
  - cephalic I82.61- ☑
    - chronic I82.71- ☑
  - chronic I82.91
  - deep (DVT) I82.40- ☑
    - calf I82.4Z- ☑
      - chronic I82.5Z- ☑
    - lower leg I82.4Z- ☑
      - chronic I82.5Z- ☑
    - thigh I82.4Y- ☑
      - chronic I82.5Y- ☑
    - upper leg I82.4Y ☑
      - chronic I82.5Y-
  - femoral I82.41- ☑
    - chronic I82.51- ☑
  - iliac (iliofemoral) I82.42- ☑
    - chronic I82.52- ☑
  - innominate I82.290
    - chronic I82.291
  - internal jugular I82.C1- ☑ (following I82.7)
    - chronic I82.C2- ☑ (following I82.7)
  - lower extremity
    - deep I82.40- ☑
      - chronic I82.50- ☑
      - specified NEC I82.49- ☑
        - chronic NEC I82.59- ☑
    - distal
      - deep I82.4Z- ☑
    - proximal
      - deep I82.4Y- ☑
        - chronic I82.5Y- ☑
    - superficial I82.81- ☑
  - popliteal I82.43- ☑
    - chronic I82.53- ☑
  - radial I82.62- ☑
    - chronic I82.72- ☑
  - renal I82.3
  - saphenous (greater) (lesser) I82.81- ☑
  - specified NEC I82.890
    - chronic NEC I82.891
  - subclavian I82.B1- ☑ (following I82.7)
    - chronic I82.B2- ☑ (following I82.7)
  - thoracic NEC I82.290
    - chronic I82.291
  - tibial I82.44- ☑
    - chronic I82.54- ☑
  - ulnar I82.62- ☑
    - chronic I82.72- ☑
  - upper extremity I82.60- ☑
    - chronic I82.70- ☑
    - deep I82.62- ☑
      - chronic I82.72- ☑
    - superficial I82.61- ☑
      - chronic I82.71- ☑
  - vena cava
    - inferior (acute) I82.220
      - chronic I82.221
    - superior (acute) I82.210
      - chronic I82.211
  - venous sinus G08
  - vessels of brain — see Occlusion, artery, cerebral
Embolus — see Embolism
Embryoma (see also Neoplasm, uncertain behavior, by site)
- benign — see Neoplasm, benign, by site
- kidney C64.- ☑
- liver C22.0
- malignant (see also Neoplasm, malignant, by site)
  - kidney C64.- ☑
  - liver C22.0
  - testis C62.9- ☑
    - descended (scrotal) C62.1- ☑
    - undescended C62.0- ☑
- testis C62.9- ☑
  - descended (scrotal) C62.1- ☑
  - undescended C62.0- ☑

Embryonic
- circulation Q28.9
- heart Q28.9
- vas deferens Q55.4
Embryopathia NOS Q89.9
Embryotoxon Q13.4
Emesis — see Vomiting
Emotional lability R45.86
Emotionality, pathological F60.3
Emotogenic disease — see Disorder, psychogenic
Emphysema (atrophic) (bullous) (chronic) (interlobular) (lung) (obstructive) (pulmonary) (senile) (vesicular) J43.9
- cellular tissue (traumatic) T79.7 ☑
  - surgical T81.82 ☑
- centrilobular J43.2
- compensatory J98.3
- congenital (interstitial) P25.0
- conjunctiva H11.89
- connective tissue (traumatic) T79.7 ☑
  - surgical T81.82 ☑
- due to chemicals, gases, fumes or vapors J68.4
- eyelid(s) — see Disorder, eyelid, specified type NEC
  - surgical T81.82 ☑
  - traumatic T79.7 ☑
- interstitial J98.2
  - congenital P25.0
  - perinatal period P25.0
- laminated tissue T79.7 ☑
  - surgical T81.82 ☑
- mediastinal J98.2
  - newborn P25.2
- orbit, orbital — see Disorder, orbit, specified type NEC
- panacinar J43.1
- panlobular J43.1
- specified NEC J43.8
- subcutaneous (traumatic) T79.7 ☑
  - nontraumatic J98.2
  - postprocedural T81.82 ☑
  - surgical T81.82 ☑
- surgical T81.82 ☑
- thymus (gland) (congenital) E32.8
- traumatic (subcutaneous) T79.7 ☑
- unilateral J43.0
Empty nest syndrome Z60.0
Empyema (acute) (chest) (double) (pleura) (supradiaphragmatic) (thorax) J86.9
- with fistula J86.0
- accessory sinus (chronic) — see Sinusitis
- antrum (chronic) — see Sinusitis, maxillary
- brain (any part) — see Abscess, brain
- ethmoidal (chronic) (sinus) — see Sinusitis, ethmoidal
- extradural — see Abscess, extradural
- frontal (chronic) (sinus) — see Sinusitis, frontal
- gallbladder K81.0
- mastoid (process) (acute) — see Mastoiditis, acute
- maxilla, maxillary M27.2
  - sinus (chronic) — see Sinusitis, maxillary
- nasal sinus (chronic) — see Sinusitis
- sinus (accessory) (chronic) (nasal) — see Sinusitis
- sphenoidal (sinus) (chronic) — see Sinusitis, sphenoidal
- subarachnoid — see Abscess, extradural
- subdural — see Abscess, subdural
- tuberculous A15.6
- ureter — see Ureteritis
- ventricular — see Abscess, brain
En coup de sabre lesion L94.1
Enamel pearls K00.2
Enameloma K00.2
Enanthema, viral B09
Encephalitis (chronic) (hemorrhagic) (idiopathic) (nonepidemic) (spurious) (subacute) G04.90
- acute (see also Encephalitis, viral) A86
  - disseminated G04.00
    - infectious G04.01
    - noninfectious G04.81
    - postimmunization (postvaccination) G04.02
    - postinfectious G04.01
  - inclusion body A85.8
  - necrotizing hemorrhagic G04.30
    - postimmunization G04.32
    - postinfectious G04.31
    - specified NEC G04.39
- arboviral, arbovirus NEC A85.2
- arthropod-borne NEC (viral) A85.2
- Australian A83.4

Encephalitis — *continued*
California (virus) A83.5
Central European (tick-borne) A84.1
Czechoslovakian A84.1
Dawson's (inclusion body) A81.1
diffuse sclerosing A81.1
disseminated, acute G04.00
due to
cat scratch disease A28.1
human immunodeficiency virus (HIV) disease
B20 [G05.3]
malaria — *see* Malaria
rickettsiosis — *see* Rickettsiosis
smallpox inoculation G04.02
typhus — *see* Typhus
Eastern equine A83.2
endemic (viral) A86
epidemic NEC (viral) A86
equine (acute) (infectious) (viral) A83.9
Eastern A83.2
Venezuelan A92.2
Western A83.1
Far Eastern (tick-borne) A84.0
following vaccination or other immunization procedure G04.02
herpes zoster B02.0
herpesviral B00.4
due to herpesvirus 6 B10.01
due to herpesvirus 7 B10.09
specified NEC B10.09
Ilheus (virus) A83.8
in (due to)
actinomycosis A42.82
adenovirus A85.1
African trypanosomiasis B56.9 [G05.3]
Chagas' disease (chronic) B57.42
cytomegalovirus B25.8
enterovirus A85.0
herpes (simplex) virus B00.4
due to herpesvirus 6 B10.01
due to herpesvirus 7 B10.09
specified NEC B10.09
infectious disease NEC B99 ☑ [G05.3]
influenza — *see* Influenza, with, encephalopathy
listeriosis A32.12
measles B05.0
mumps B26.2
naegleriasis B60.2
parasitic disease NEC B89 [G05.3]
poliovirus A80.9 [G05.3]
rubella B06.01
syphilis
congenital A50.42
late A52.14
systemic lupus erythematosus M32.19
toxoplasmosis (acquired) B58.2
congenital P37.1
tuberculosis A17.82
zoster B02.0
inclusion body A81.1
infectious (acute) (virus) NEC A86
Japanese (B type) A83.0
La Crosse A83.5
lead — *see* Poisoning, lead
lethargica (acute) (infectious) A85.8
louping ill A84.8
lupus erythematosus, systemic M32.19
lymphatica A87.2
Mengo A85.8
meningococcal A39.81
Murray Valley A83.4
otitic NEC H66.40 [G05.3]
parasitic NOS B71.9
periaxial G37.0
periaxialis (concentrica) (diffuse) G37.5
postchickenpox B01.11
postexanthematous NEC B09
postimmunization G04.02
postinfectious NEC G04.01
postmeasles B05.0
postvaccinal G04.02
postvaricella B01.11
postviral NEC A86
Powassan A84.8
Rasmussen G04.81
Rio Bravo A85.8
Russian
autumnal A83.0
spring-summer (taiga) A84.0

Encephalitis — *continued*
saturnine — *see* Poisoning, lead
specified NEC G04.81
St. Louis A83.3
subacute sclerosing A81.1
summer A83.0
suppurative G04.81
tick-borne A84.9
Torula, torular (cryptococcal) B45.1
toxic NEC G92
trichinosis B75 [G05.3]
type
B A83.0
C A83.3
van Bogaert's A81.1
Venezuelan equine A92.2
Vienna A85.8
viral, virus A86
arthropod-borne NEC A85.2
mosquito-borne A83.9
Australian X disease A83.4
California virus A83.5
Eastern equine A83.2
Japanese (B type) A83.0
Murray Valley A83.4
specified NEC A83.8
St. Louis A83.3
type B A83.0
type C A83.3
Western equine A83.1
tick-borne A84.9
biundulant A84.1
central European A84.1
Czechoslovakian A84.1
diphasic meningoencephalitis A84.1
Far Eastern A84.0
Russian spring-summer (taiga) A84.0
specified NEC A84.8
specified type NEC A85.8
Western equine A83.1
Encephalocele Q01.9
frontal Q01.0
nasofrontal Q01.1
occipital Q01.2
specified NEC Q01.8
Encephalocystocele — *see* Encephalocele
Encephaloduroarteriomyosynangiosis (EDAMS) I67.5
Encephalomalacia (brain) (cerebellar) (cerebral) — *see* Softening, brain
Encephalomeningitis — *see* Meningoencephalitis
Encephalomeningocele — *see* Encephalocele
Encephalomeningomyelitis — *see* Meningoencephali-tis
Encephalomyelitis (*see also* Encephalitis) G04.90
acute disseminated G04.00
infectious G04.01
noninfectious G04.81
postimmunization G04.02
postinfectious G04.01
acute necrotizing hemorrhagic G04.30
postimmunization G04.32
postinfectious G04.31
specified NEC G04.39
benign myalgic G93.3
equine A83.9
Eastern A83.2
Venezuelan A92.2
Western A83.1
in diseases classified elsewhere G05.3
myalgic, benign G93.3
postchickenpox B01.11
postinfectious NEC G04.01
postmeasles B05.0
postvaccinal G04.02
postvaricella B01.11
rubella B06.01
specified NEC G04.81
Venezuelan equine A92.2
Encephalomyelocele — *see* Encephalocele
Encephalomyelomeningitis — *see* Meningoencephali-tis
Encephalomyelopathy G96.9
Encephalomyeloradiculitis (acute) G61.0
Encephalomyeloradiculoneuritis (acute) (Guillain-Barré) G61.0
Encephalomyeloradiculopathy G96.9
Encephalopathia hyperbilirubinemica, newborn P57.9

Encephalopathia hyperbilirubinemica, newborn — *continued*
due to isoimmunization (conditions in P55) P57.0
Encephalopathy (acute) G93.40
acute necrotizing hemorrhagic G04.30
postimmunization G04.32
postinfectious G04.31
specified NEC G04.39
alcoholic G31.2
anoxic — *see* Damage, brain, anoxic
arteriosclerotic I67.2
centrolobar progressive (Schilder) G37.0
congenital Q07.9
degenerative, in specified disease NEC G32.89
demyelinating callosal G37.1
due to
drugs (*see also* Table of Drugs and Chemicals) G92
hepatic — *see* Failure, hepatic
hyperbilirubinemic, newborn P57.9
due to isoimmunization (conditions in P55) P57.0
hypertensive I67.4
hypoglycemic E16.2
hypoxic — *see* Damage, brain, anoxic
hypoxic ischemic P91.60
mild P91.61
moderate P91.62
severe P91.63
in (due to) (with)
birth injury P11.1
hyperinsulinism E16.1 [G94]
influenza — *see* Influenza, with, encephalopathy
lack of vitamin (*see also* Deficiency, vitamin) E56.9 [G32.89]
neoplastic disease (*see also* Neoplasm) D49.9 [G13.1]
serum (*see also* Reaction, serum) T80.69 ☑
syphilis A52.17
trauma (postconcussional) F07.81
current injury — *see* Injury, intracranial
vaccination G04.02
lead — *see* Poisoning, lead
metabolic G93.41
drug induced G92
toxic G92
myoclonic, early, symptomatic — *see* Epilepsy, gener-alized, specified NEC
necrotizing, subacute (Leigh) G31.82
neonatal P91.819
in diseases classified elsewhere P91.811
pellagrous E52 [G32.89]
portosystemic — *see* Failure, hepatic
postcontusional F07.81
current injury — *see* Injury, intracranial, diffuse
posthypoglycemic (coma) E16.1 [G94]
postradiation G93.89
saturnine — *see* Poisoning, lead
septic G93.41
specified NEC G93.49
spongioform, subacute (viral) A81.09
toxic G92
metabolic G92
traumatic (postconcussional) F07.81
current injury — *see* Injury, intracranial
vitamin B deficiency NEC E53.9 [G32.89]
vitamin B1 E51.2
Wernicke's E51.2
Encephalorrhagia — *see* Hemorrhage, intracranial, in-tracerebral
Encephalosis, posttraumatic F07.81
Enchondroma (*see also* Neoplasm, bone, benign)
Enchondromatosis (cartilaginous) (multiple) Q78.4
Encopresis R15.9
functional F98.1
nonorganic origin F98.1
psychogenic F98.1
Encounter (with health service) (for) Z76.89
adjustment and management (of)
breast implant Z45.81 ☑
implanted device NEC Z45.89
myringotomy device (stent) (tube) Z45.82
administrative purpose only Z02.9
examination for
adoption Z02.82
armed forces Z02.3
disability determination Z02.71
driving license Z02.4
employment Z02.1
insurance Z02.6

☑ Additional Character Required — Refer to the Tabular List for Character Selection   ▽ Subterms under main terms may continue to next column or page

Encounter — *continued*
administrative purpose only — *continued*
examination for — *continued*
medical certificate NEC Z02.79
paternity testing Z02.81
residential institution admission Z02.2
school admission Z02.0
sports Z02.5
specified reason NEC Z02.89
aftercare — *see* Aftercare
antenatal screening Z36.9
cervical length Z36.86
chromosomal anomalies Z36.0
congenital cardiac abnormalities Z36.83
elevated maternal serum alphafetoprotein Z36.1
fetal growth retardation Z36.4
fetal lung maturity Z36.84
fetal macrosomia Z36.88
hydrops fetalis Z36.81
intrauterine growth restriction (IUGR) /small-for-dates Z36.4
isoimmunization Z36.5
large-for-dates Z36.88
malformations Z36.3
non-visualized anatomy on a previous scan Z36.2
nuchal translucency Z36.82
raised alphafetoprotein level Z36.1
risk of pre-term labor Z36.86
specified follow-up NEC Z36.2
specified genetic defects NEC Z36.8A
specified type NEC Z36.89
Streptococcus B Z36.85
suspected anomaly Z36.3
uncertain dates Z36.87
assisted reproductive fertility procedure cycle Z31.83
blood typing Z01.83
Rh typing Z01.83
breast augmentation or reduction Z41.1
breast implant exchange (different material) (different size) Z45.81 ☑
breast reconstruction following mastectomy Z42.1
check-up — *see* Examination
chemotherapy for neoplasm Z51.11
colonoscopy, screening Z12.11
counseling — *see* Counseling
delivery, full-term, uncomplicated O80
cesarean, without indication O82
desensitization to allergens Z51.6
ear piercing Z41.3
examination — *see* Examination
expectant parent(s) (adoptive) pre-birth pediatrician visit Z76.81
fertility preservation procedure (prior to cancer therapy) (prior to removal of gonads) Z31.84
fitting (of) — *see* Fitting (and adjustment) (of)
genetic
counseling
nonprocreative Z71.83
procreative Z31.5
testing — *see* Test, genetic
hearing conservation and treatment Z01.12
immunotherapy for neoplasm Z51.12
in vitro fertilization cycle Z31.83
instruction (in)
child care (postpartal) (prenatal) Z32.3
childbirth Z32.2
natural family planning
procreative Z31.61
to avoid pregnancy Z30.02
insulin pump titration Z46.81
joint prosthesis insertion following prior explantation of joint prosthesis (staged procedure)
hip Z47.32
knee Z47.33
shoulder Z47.31
laboratory (as part of a general medical examination) Z00.00
with abnormal findings Z00.01
mental health services (for)
abuse NEC
perpetrator Z69.82
victim Z69.81
child abuse
nonparental
perpetrator Z69.021
victim Z69.020
parental
perpetrator Z69.011

Encounter — *continued*
mental health services — *continued*
child abuse — *continued*
parental — *continued*
victim Z69.010
child neglect
nonparental
perpetrator Z69.021
victim Z69.020
parental
perpetrator Z69.011
victim Z69.010
child psychological abuse
nonparental
perpetrator Z69.021
victim Z69.020
parental
perpetrator Z69.011
victim Z69.010
child sexual abuse
nonparental
perpetrator Z69.021
victim Z69.020
parental
perpetrator Z69.011
victim Z69.010
non-spousal adult abuse (perpetrator) (victim) Z69.81
spousal or partner
abuse
perpetrator Z69.12
victim Z69.11
neglect
perpetrator Z69.12
victim Z69.11
psychological abuse
perpetrator Z69.12
victim Z69.11
violence
perpetrator (physical) (sexual) Z69.12
victim (physical) Z69.11
sexual Z69.81
observation (for) (ruled out)
exposure to (suspected)
anthrax Z03.810
biological agent NEC Z03.818
pediatrician visit, by expectant parent(s) (adoptive) Z76.81
placental sample (taken vaginally) (*see also* Encounter, antenatal screening) Z36.9
plastic and reconstructive surgery following medical procedure or healed injury NEC Z42.8
pregnancy
supervision of — *see* Pregnancy, supervision of
test Z32.00
result negative Z32.02
result positive Z32.01
procreative management and counseling for gestational carrier Z31.7
prophylactic measures Z29.9
antivenin Z29.12
fluoride administration Z29.3
immunotherapy for respiratory syncytial virus (RSV) Z29.11
rabies immune globin Z29.14
Rho (D) immune globulin Z29.13
specified NEC Z29.8
radiation therapy (antineoplastic) Z51.0
radiological (as part of a general medical examination) Z00.00
with abnormal findings Z00.01
reconstructive surgery following medical procedure or healed injury NEC Z42.8
removal (of) (*see also* Removal)
artificial
arm Z44.00- ☑
complete Z44.01- ☑
partial Z44.02- ☑
eye Z44.2- ☑
leg Z44.10- ☑
complete Z44.11- ☑
partial Z44.12- ☑
breast implant Z45.81 ☑
tissue expander (without synchronous insertion of permanent implant) Z45.81 ☑
device Z46.9
specified NEC Z46.89

Encounter — *continued*
removal (*see also* Removal) — *continued*
external
fixation device — *code to* fracture with seventh character D
prosthesis, prosthetic device Z44.9
breast Z44.3- ☑
specified NEC Z44.8
implanted device NEC Z45.89
insulin pump Z46.81
internal fixation device Z47.2
myringotomy device (stent) (tube) Z45.82
nervous system device NEC Z46.2
brain neuropacemaker Z46.2
visual substitution device Z46.2
implanted Z45.31
non-vascular catheter Z46.82
orthodontic device Z46.4
stent
ureteral Z46.6
urinary device Z46.6
repeat cervical smear to confirm findings of recent normal smear following initial abnormal smear Z01.42
respirator [ventilator] use during power failure Z99.12
Rh typing Z01.83
screening — *see* Screening
specified NEC Z76.89
sterilization Z30.2
suspected condition, ruled out
amniotic cavity and membrane Z03.71
cervical shortening Z03.75
fetal anomaly Z03.73
fetal growth Z03.74
maternal and fetal conditions NEC Z03.79
oligohydramnios Z03.71
placental problem Z03.72
polyhydramnios Z03.71
suspected exposure (to), ruled out
anthrax Z03.810
biological agents NEC Z03.818
termination of pregnancy, elective Z33.2
testing — *see* Test
therapeutic drug level monitoring Z51.81
titration, insulin pump Z46.81
to determine fetal viability of pregnancy O36.80 ☑
training
insulin pump Z46.81
X-ray of chest (as part of a general medical examination) Z00.00
with abnormal findings Z00.01
Encystment — *see* Cyst
Endarteritis (bacterial, subacute) (infective) I77.6
brain I67.7
cerebral or cerebrospinal I67.7
deformans — *see* Arteriosclerosis
embolic — *see* Embolism
obliterans (*see also* Arteriosclerosis)
pulmonary I28.8
pulmonary I28.8
retina — *see* Vasculitis, retina
senile — *see* Arteriosclerosis
syphilitic A52.09
brain or cerebral A52.04
congenital A50.54 [I79.8]
tuberculous A18.89
Endemic — *see* condition
Endocarditis (chronic) (marantic) (nonbacterial) (thrombotic) (valvular) I38
with rheumatic fever (conditions in I00)
active — *see* Endocarditis, acute, rheumatic
inactive or quiescent (with chorea) I09.1
acute or subacute I33.9
infective I33.0
rheumatic (aortic) (mitral) (pulmonary) (tricuspid) I01.1
with chorea (acute) (rheumatic) (Sydenham's) I02.0
aortic (heart) (nonrheumatic) (valve) I35.8
with
mitral disease I08.0
with tricuspid (valve) disease I08.3
active or acute I01.1
with chorea (acute) (rheumatic) (Sydenham's) I02.0
rheumatic fever (conditions in I00)
active — *see* Endocarditis, acute, rheumatic
inactive or quiescent (with chorea) I06.9

Index

Endocarditis — Enlargement, enlarged

Endocarditis — *continued*
- aortic — *continued*
  - with — *continued*
    - tricuspid (valve) disease I08.2
      - with mitral (valve) disease I08.3
  - acute or subacute I33.9
  - arteriosclerotic I35.8
  - rheumatic I06.9
    - with mitral disease I08.0
      - with tricuspid (valve) disease I08.3
        - active or acute I01.1
          - with chorea (acute) (rheumatic) (Sydenham's) I02.0
      - active or acute I01.1
        - with chorea (acute) (rheumatic) (Sydenham's) I02.0
    - specified NEC I06.8
  - specified cause NEC I35.8
  - syphilitic A52.03
- arteriosclerotic I38
- atypical verrucous (Libman-Sacks) M32.11
- bacterial (acute) (any valve) (subacute) I33.0
- candidal B37.6
- congenital Q24.8
- constrictive I33.0
- Coxiella burnetii A78 [I39]
- Coxsackie B33.21
- due to
  - prosthetic cardiac valve T82.6 ☑
  - Q fever A78 [I39]
  - Serratia marcescens I33.0
  - typhoid (fever) A01.02
- gonococcal A54.83
- infectious or infective (acute) (any valve) (subacute) I33.0
- lenta (acute) (any valve) (subacute) I33.0
- Libman-Sacks M32.11
- listerial A32.82
- Löffler's I42.3
- malignant (acute) (any valve) (subacute) I33.0
- meningococcal A39.51
- mitral (chronic) (double) (fibroid) (heart) (inactive) (valve) (with chorea) I05.9
  - with
    - aortic (valve) disease I08.0
      - with tricuspid (valve) disease I08.3
        - active or acute I01.1
          - with chorea (acute) (rheumatic) (Sydenham's) I02.0
      - rheumatic fever (conditions in I00)
        - active — *see* Endocarditis, acute, rheumatic
        - inactive or quiescent (with chorea) I05.9
      - tricuspid (valve) disease I08.1
        - with aortic (valve) disease I08.3
    - active or acute I01.1
      - with chorea (acute) (rheumatic) (Sydenham's) I02.0
    - bacterial I33.0
  - arteriosclerotic I34.8
  - nonrheumatic I34.8
    - acute or subacute I33.9
  - specified NEC I05.8
- monilial B37.6
- multiple valves I08.9
  - specified disorders I08.8
- mycotic (acute) (any valve) (subacute) I33.0
- pneumococcal (acute) (any valve) (subacute) I33.0
- pulmonary (chronic) (heart) (valve) I37.8
  - with rheumatic fever (conditions in I00)
    - active — *see* Endocarditis, acute, rheumatic
    - inactive or quiescent (with chorea) I09.89
      - with aortic, mitral or tricuspid disease I08.8
  - acute or subacute I33.9
    - rheumatic I01.1
      - with chorea (acute) (rheumatic) (Sydenham's) I02.0
  - arteriosclerotic I37.8
  - congenital Q22.2
  - rheumatic (chronic) (inactive) (with chorea) I09.89
    - active or acute I01.1
      - with chorea (acute) (rheumatic) (Sydenham's) I02.0
  - syphilitic A52.03
- purulent (acute) (any valve) (subacute) I33.0
- Q fever A78 [I39]
- rheumatic (chronic) (inactive) (with chorea) I09.1
  - active or acute (aortic) (mitral) (pulmonary) (tricuspid) I01.1

Endocarditis — *continued*
- rheumatic — *continued*
  - active or acute — *continued*
    - with chorea (acute) (rheumatic) (Sydenham's) I02.0
- rheumatoid — *see* Rheumatoid, carditis
- septic (acute) (any valve) (subacute) I33.0
- streptococcal (acute) (any valve) (subacute) I33.0
- subacute — *see* Endocarditis, acute
- suppurative (acute) (any valve) (subacute) I33.0
- syphilitic A52.03
- toxic I33.9
- tricuspid (chronic) (heart) (inactive) (rheumatic) (valve) (with chorea) I07.9
  - with
    - aortic (valve) disease I08.2
      - mitral (valve) disease I08.3
    - mitral (valve) disease I08.1
      - aortic (valve) disease I08.3
    - rheumatic fever (conditions in I00)
      - active — *see* Endocarditis, acute, rheumatic
      - inactive or quiescent (with chorea) I07.8
  - active or acute I01.1
    - with chorea (acute) (rheumatic) (Sydenham's) I02.0
  - arteriosclerotic I36.8
  - nonrheumatic I36.8
    - acute or subacute I33.9
  - specified cause, except rheumatic I36.8
- tuberculous — *see* Tuberculosis, endocarditis
- typhoid A01.02
- ulcerative (acute) (any valve) (subacute) I33.0
- vegetative (acute) (any valve) (subacute) I33.0
- verrucous (atypical) (nonbacterial) (nonrheumatic) M32.11

Endocardium, endocardial (*see also* condition)
- cushion defect Q21.2

Endocervicitis (*see also* Cervicitis)
- due to intrauterine (contraceptive) device T83.69 ☑
- hyperplastic N72

Endocrine — *see* condition

Endocrinopathy, pluriglandular E31.9

Endodontic
- overfill M27.52
- underfill M27.53

Endodontitis K04.01
- irreversible K04.02
- reversible K04.01

Endomastoiditis — *see* Mastoiditis

Endometrioma N80.9

Endometriosis N80.9
- appendix N80.5
- bladder N80.8
- bowel N80.5
- broad ligament N80.3
- cervix N80.0
- colon N80.5
- cul-de-sac (Douglas') N80.3
- exocervix N80.0
- fallopian tube N80.2
- female genital organ NEC N80.8
- gallbladder N80.8
- in scar of skin N80.6
- internal N80.0
- intestine N80.5
- lung N80.8
- myometrium N80.0
- ovary N80.1
- parametrium N80.3
- pelvic peritoneum N80.3
- peritoneal (pelvic) N80.3
- rectovaginal septum N80.4
- rectum N80.5
- round ligament N80.3
- skin (scar) N80.6
- specified site NEC N80.8
- stromal D39.0
- thorax N80.8
- umbilicus N80.8
- uterus (internal) N80.0
- vagina N80.4
- vulva N80.8

Endometritis (decidual) (nonspecific) (purulent) (senile) (atrophic) (suppurative) N71.9
- with ectopic pregnancy O08.0
- acute N71.0
- blenorrhagic (gonococcal) (acute) (chronic) A54.24

Endometritis — *continued*
- cervix, cervical (with erosion or ectropion) (*see also* Cervicitis)
  - hyperplastic N72
- chlamydial A56.11
- chronic N71.1
- following
  - abortion — *see* Abortion by type complicated by genital infection
  - ectopic or molar pregnancy O08.0
- gonococcal, gonorrheal (acute) (chronic) A54.24
- hyperplastic (*see also* Hyperplasia, endometrial) N85.00
  - cervix N72
- puerperal, postpartum, childbirth O86.12
- subacute N71.0
- tuberculous A18.17

Endometrium — *see* condition

Endomyocardiopathy, South African I42.3

Endomyocarditis — *see* Endocarditis

Endomyofibrosis I42.3

Endomyometritis — *see* Endometritis

Endopericarditis — *see* Endocarditis

Endoperineuritis — *see* Disorder, nerve

Endophlebitis — *see* Phlebitis

Endophthalmia — *see* Endophthalmitis, purulent

Endophthalmitis (acute) (infective) (metastatic) (subacute) H44.009
- bleb associated (*see also* Bleb, inflamed (infected), postprocedural H59.4 ☑
- gonorrheal A54.39
- in (due to)
  - cysticercosis B69.1
  - onchocerciasis B73.01
  - toxocariasis B83.0
- panuveitis — *see* Panuveitis
- parasitic H44.12- ☑
- purulent H44.00- ☑
  - panophthalmitis — *see* Panophthalmitis
  - vitreous abscess H44.02- ☑
- specified NEC H44.19
- sympathetic — *see* Uveitis, sympathetic

Endosalpingioma D28.2

Endosalpingiosis N94.89

Endosteitis — *see* Osteomyelitis

Endothelioma, bone — *see* Neoplasm, bone, malignant

Endotheliosis (hemorrhagic infectional) D69.8

Endotoxemia — code to condition

Endotrachelitis — *see* Cervicitis

Engelmann (-Camurati) **syndrome** Q78.3

English disease — *see* Rickets

Engman's disease L30.3

Engorgement
- breast N64.59
  - newborn P83.4
  - puerperal, postpartum O92.79
- lung (passive) — *see* Edema, lung
- pulmonary (passive) — *see* Edema, lung
- stomach K31.89
- venous, retina — *see* Occlusion, retina, vein, engorgement

Enlargement, enlarged (*see also* Hypertrophy)
- adenoids J35.2
  - with tonsils J35.3
- alveolar ridge K08.89
  - congenital — *see* Anomaly, alveolar
- apertures of diaphragm (congenital) Q79.1
- gingival K06.1
- heart, cardiac — *see* Hypertrophy, cardiac
- labium majus, childhood asymmetric (CALME) N90.61
- lacrimal gland, chronic H04.03- ☑
- liver — *see* Hypertrophy, liver
- lymph gland or node R59.9
  - generalized R59.1
  - localized R59.0
- orbit H05.34- ☑
- organ or site, congenital NEC — *see* Anomaly, by site
- parathyroid (gland) E21.0
- pituitary fossa R93.0
- prostate N40.0
  - with lower urinary tract symptoms (LUTS) N40.1
  - without lower urinary tract symtpoms (LUTS) N40.0
- sella turcica R93.0
- spleen — *see* Splenomegaly
- thymus (gland) (congenital) E32.0
- thyroid (gland) — *see* Goiter
- tongue K14.8
- tonsils J35.1

☑ **Additional Character Required — Refer to the Tabular List for Character Selection**   Subterms under main terms may continue to next column or page

Enlargement, enlarged — continued
- tonsils — continued
  - with adenoids J35.3
- uterus N85.2
- vestibular aqueduct Q16.5

Enophthalmos H05.40- ☑
- due to
  - orbital tissue atrophy H05.41- ☑
  - trauma or surgery H05.42- ☑

Enostosis M27.8

Entamebic, entamebiasis — see Amebiasis

Entanglement
- umbilical cord(s) O69.82 ☑
  - with compression O69.2 ☑
  - without compression O69.82 ☑
  - around neck (with compression) O69.81 ☑
    - with compression O69.1 ☑
    - without compression O69.81 ☑
  - of twins in monoamniotic sac O69.2 ☑

Enteralgia — see Pain, abdominal

Enteric — see condition

Enteritis (acute) (diarrheal) (hemorrhagic) (noninfective) K52.9
- adenovirus A08.2
- aertrycke infection A02.0
- allergic K52.29
  - with
    - eosinophilic gastritis or gastroenteritis K52.81
    - food protein-induced enterocolitis syndrome K52.21
    - food protein-induced enteropathy K52.22
- amebic (acute) A06.0
  - with abscess — see Abscess, amebic
  - chronic A06.1
    - with abscess — see Abscess, amebic
    - nondysenteric A06.2
  - nondysenteric A06.2
- astrovirus A08.32
- bacillary NOS A03.9
- bacterial A04.9
  - specified NEC A04.8
- calicivirus A08.31
- candidal B37.82
- Chilomastix A07.8
- choleriformis A00.1
- chronic (noninfectious) K52.9
  - ulcerative — see Colitis, ulcerative
- cicatrizing (chronic) — see Enteritis, regional, small intestine
- Clostridium
  - botulinum (food poisoning) A05.1
  - difficile
    - not specified as recurrent A04.72
    - recurrent A04.71
- coccidial A07.3
- coxsackie virus A08.39
- dietetic (see also Enteritis, allergic) K52.29
- drug-induced K52.1
- due to
  - astrovirus A08.32
  - calicivirus A08.31
  - coxsackie virus A08.39
  - drugs K52.1
  - echovirus A08.39
  - enterovirus NEC A08.39
  - food hypersensitivity (see also Enteritis, allergic) K52.29
  - infectious organism (bacterial) (viral) — see Enteritis, infectious
  - torovirus A08.39
  - Yersinia enterocolitica A04.6
- echovirus A08.39
- eltor A00.1
- enterovirus NEC A08.39
- eosinophilic K52.81
- epidemic (infectious) A09
- fulminant (see also Ischemia, intestine, acute) K55.019
- gangrenous — see Enteritis, infectious
- giardial A07.1
- infectious NOS A09
  - due to
    - adenovirus A08.2
    - Aerobacter aerogenes A04.8
    - Arizona (bacillus) A02.0
    - bacteria NOS A04.9
      - specified NEC A04.8
    - Campylobacter A04.5

Enteritis — continued
- infectious — continued
  - due to — continued
    - Clostridium difficile
      - not specified as recurrent A04.72
      - recurrent A04.71
    - Clostridium perfringens A04.8
    - Enterobacter aerogenes A04.8
    - enterovirus A08.39
    - Escherichia coli A04.4
      - enteroaggregative A04.4
      - enterohemorrhagic A04.3
      - enteroinvasive A04.2
      - enteropathogenic A04.0
      - enterotoxigenic A04.1
      - specified NEC A04.4
    - specified
      - bacteria NEC A04.8
      - virus NEC A08.39
    - Staphylococcus A04.8
    - virus NEC A08.4
      - specified type NEC A08.39
    - Yersinia enterocolitica A04.6
  - specified organism NEC A08.8
- influenzal — see Influenza, with, digestive manifestations
- ischemic K55.9
  - acute (see also Ischemia, intestine, acute) K55.019
  - chronic K55.1
- microsporidial A07.8
- mucomembranous, myxomembranous — see Syndrome, irritable bowel
- mucous — see Syndrome, irritable bowel
- necroticans A05.2
- necrotizing of newborn — see Enterocolitis, necrotizing, in newborn
- neurogenic — see Syndrome, irritable bowel
- newborn necrotizing — see Enterocolitis, necrotizing, in newborn
- noninfectious K52.9
- norovirus A08.11
- parasitic NEC B82.9
- paratyphoid (fever) — see Fever, paratyphoid
- protozoal A07.9
  - specified NEC A07.8
- radiation K52.0
- regional (of) K50.90
  - with
    - complication K50.919
      - abscess K50.914
      - fistula K50.913
      - intestinal obstruction K50.912
      - rectal bleeding K50.911
      - specified complication NEC K50.918
  - colon — see Enteritis, regional, large intestine
  - duodenum — see Enteritis, regional, small intestine
  - ileum — see Enteritis, regional, small intestine
  - jejunum — see Enteritis, regional, small intestine
  - large bowel — see Enteritis, regional, large intestine
  - large intestine (colon) (rectum) K50.10
    - with
      - complication K50.119
        - abscess K50.114
        - fistula K50.113
        - intestinal obstruction K50.112
        - rectal bleeding K50.111
        - small intestine (duodenum) (ileum) (jejunum) involvement K50.80
          - with
            - complication K50.819
              - abscess K50.814
              - fistula K50.813
              - intestinal obstruction K50.812
              - rectal bleeding K50.811
              - specified complication NEC K50.818
        - specified complication NEC K50.118
  - rectum — see Enteritis, regional, large intestine
  - small intestine (duodenum) (ileum) (jejunum) K50.00
    - with
      - complication K50.019
        - abscess K50.014
        - fistula K50.013
        - intestinal obstruction K50.012
        - large intestine (colon) (rectum) involvement K50.80

Enteritis — continued
- regional — continued
  - small intestine — continued
    - with — continued
      - complication — continued
        - large intestine involvement — continued
          - with
            - complication K50.819
              - abscess K50.814
              - fistula K50.813
              - intestinal obstruction K50.812
              - rectal bleeding K50.811
              - specified complication NEC K50.818
            - rectal bleeding K50.011
            - specified complication NEC K50.018
- rotaviral A08.0
- Salmonella, salmonellosis (arizonae) (cholerae-suis) (enteritidis) (typhimurium) A02.0
- segmental — see Enteritis, regional
- septic A09
- Shigella — see Infection, Shigella
- small round structured NEC A08.19
- spasmodic, spastic — see Syndrome, irritable bowel
- staphylococcal A04.8
  - due to food A05.0
- torovirus A08.39
- toxic NEC K52.1
  - due to Clostridium difficile
    - not specified as recurrent A04.72
    - recurrent A04.71
- trichomonal A07.8
- tuberculous A18.32
- typhosa A01.00
- ulcerative (chronic) — see Colitis, ulcerative
- viral A08.4
  - adenovirus A08.2
  - enterovirus A08.39
  - Rotavirus A08.0
  - small round structured NEC A08.19
  - specified NEC A08.39
  - virus specified NEC A08.39

Enterobiasis B80

Enterobius vermicularis (infection) (infestation) B80

Enterocele (see also Hernia, abdomen)
- pelvic, pelvis (acquired) (congenital) N81.5
- vagina, vaginal (acquired) (congenital) NEC N81.5

Enterocolitis (see also Enteritis) K52.9
- due to Clostridium difficile
  - not specified as recurrent A04.72
  - recurrent A04.71
- fulminant ischemic (see also Ischemia, intestine, acute) K55.059
- granulomatous — see Enteritis, regional
- hemorrhagic (acute) (see also Ischemia, intestine, acute) K55.059
  - chronic K55.1
- infectious NEC A09
- ischemic K55.9
- necrotizing K55.30
  - with
    - perforation K55.33
    - pneumatosis K55.32
      - and perforation K55.33
  - without pneumatosis or perforation K55.31
  - due to Clostridium difficile
    - not specified as recurrent A04.72
    - recurrent A04.71
  - in newborn P77.9
    - stage 1 (without pneumatosis, without perforation) P77.1
    - stage 2 (with pneumatosis, without perforation) P77.2
    - stage 3 (with pneumatosis, with perforation) P77.3
  - in non-newborn K55.30
    - stage 1 (without pneumatosis, without perforation) K55.31
    - stage 2 (with pneumatosis, without perforation) K55.32
    - stage 3 (with pneumatosis, with perforation) K55.33
- noninfectious K52.9
  - newborn — see Enterocolitis, necrotizing, in newborn
- pseudomembranous (newborn)
  - not specified as recurrent A04.72

Enterocolitis — *continued*
  pseudomembranous — *continued*
    recurrent A04.71
  radiation K52.0
    newborn — *see* Enterocolitis, necrotizing, in new-
      born
  ulcerative (chronic) — *see* Pancolitis, ulcerative
    (chronic)
Enterogastritis — *see* Enteritis
Enteropathy K63.9
  celiac-gluten-sensitive K90.0
    non-celiac K90.41
  food protein-induced enterocolitis K52.22
  hemorrhagic, terminal (*see also* Ischemia, intestine,
    acute) K55.059
  protein-losing K90.49
Enteroperitonitis — *see* Peritonitis
Enteroptosis K63.4
Enterorrhagia K92.2
Enterospasm (*see also* Syndrome, irritable, bowel)
  psychogenic F45.8
Enterostenosis (*see also* Obstruction, intestine, specified
  NEC) K56.699
Enterostomy
  complication — *see* Complication, enterostomy
  status Z93.4
Enterovirus, as cause of disease classified elsewhere
  B97.10
  coxsackievirus B97.11
  echovirus B97.12
  other specified B97.19
Enthesopathy (peripheral) M77.9
  Achilles tendinitis — *see* Tendinitis, Achilles
  ankle and tarsus M77.9
    specified type NEC — *see* Enthesopathy, foot,
      specified type NEC
  anterior tibial syndrome M76.81- ☑
  calcaneal spur — *see* Spur, bone, calcaneal
  elbow region M77.8
    lateral epicondylitis — *see* Epicondylitis, lateral
    medial epicondylitis — *see* Epicondylitis, medial
  foot NEC M77.9
    metatarsalgia — *see* Metatarsalgia
    specified type NEC M77.5- ☑
  forearm M77.9
  gluteal tendinitis — *see* Tendinitis, gluteal
  hand M77.9
  hip — *see* Enthesopathy, lower limb, specified type
    NEC
  iliac crest spur — *see* Spur, bone, iliac crest
  iliotibial band syndrome — *see* Syndrome, iliotibial
    band
  knee — *see* Enthesopathy, lower limb, lower leg,
    specified type NEC
  lateral epicondylitis — *see* Epicondylitis, lateral
  lower limb (excluding foot) M76.9
    Achilles tendinitis — *see* Tendinitis, Achilles
    anterior tibial syndrome M76.81- ☑
    gluteal tendinitis — *see* Tendinitis, gluteal
    iliac crest spur — *see* Spur, bone, iliac crest
    iliotibial band syndrome — *see* Syndrome, iliotibial
      band
    patellar tendinitis — *see* Tendinitis, patellar
    pelvic region — *see* Enthesopathy, lower limb,
      specified type NEC
    peroneal tendinitis — *see* Tendinitis, peroneal
    posterior tibial syndrome M76.82- ☑
    psoas tendinitis — *see* Tendinitis, psoas
    shoulder M77.9
    specified type NEC M76.89- ☑
    tibial collateral bursitis — *see* Bursitis, tibial collat-
      eral
  medial epicondylitis — *see* Epicondylitis, medial
  metatarsalgia — *see* Metatarsalgia
  multiple sites M77.9
  patellar tendinitis — *see* Tendinitis, patellar
  pelvis M77.9
  periarthritis of wrist — *see* Periarthritis, wrist
  peroneal tendinitis — *see* Tendinitis, peroneal
  posterior tibial syndrome M76.82- ☑
  psoas tendinitis — *see* Tendinitis, psoas
  shoulder region — *see* Lesion, shoulder
  specified site NEC M77.9
  specified type NEC M77.8
  spinal M46.00
    cervical region M46.02
    cervicothoracic region M46.03

Enthesopathy — *continued*
  spinal — *continued*
    lumbar region M46.06
    lumbosacral region M46.07
    multiple sites M46.09
    occipito-atlanto-axial region M46.01
    sacrococcygeal region M46.08
    thoracic region M46.04
    thoracolumbar region M46.05
  tibial collateral bursitis — *see* Bursitis, tibial collateral
  upper arm M77.9
  wrist and carpus NEC M77.8
    calcaneal spur — *see* Spur, bone, calcaneal
    periarthritis of wrist — *see* Periarthritis, wrist
Entomophobia F40.218
Entomophthoromycosis B46.8
Entrance, air into vein — *see* Embolism, air
Entrapment, nerve — *see* Neuropathy, entrapment
Entropion (eyelid) (paralytic) H02.009
  cicatricial H02.019
    left H02.016
      lower H02.015
      upper H02.014
    right H02.013
      lower H02.012
      upper H02.011
  congenital Q10.2
  left H02.006
    lower H02.005
    upper H02.004
  mechanical H02.029
    left H02.026
      lower H02.025
      upper H02.024
    right H02.023
      lower H02.022
      upper H02.021
  right H02.003
    lower H02.002
    upper H02.001
  senile H02.039
    left H02.036
      lower H02.035
      upper H02.034
    right H02.033
      lower H02.032
      upper H02.031
  spastic H02.049
    left H02.046
      lower H02.045
      upper H02.044
    right H02.043
      lower H02.042
      upper H02.041
Enucleated eye (traumatic, current) S05.7- ☑
Enuresis R32
  functional F98.0
  habit disturbance F98.0
  nocturnal N39.44
    psychogenic F98.0
  nonorganic origin F98.0
  psychogenic F98.0
Eosinopenia — *see* Agranulocytosis
Eosinophilia (allergic) (hereditary) (idiopathic) (secondary) D72.1
  with
    angiolymphoid hyperplasia (ALHE) D18.01
  infiltrative J82
  Löffler's J82
  peritoneal — *see* Peritonitis, eosinophilic
  pulmonary NEC J82
  tropical (pulmonary) J82
Eosinophilia-myalgia syndrome M35.8
Ependymitis (acute) (cerebral) (chronic) (granular) —
  see Encephalomyelitis
Ependymoblastoma
  specified site — *see* Neoplasm, malignant, by site
  unspecified site C71.9
Ependymoma (epithelial) (malignant)
  anaplastic
    specified site — *see* Neoplasm, malignant, by site
    unspecified site C71.9
  benign
    specified site — *see* Neoplasm, benign, by site
    unspecified site D33.2
  myxopapillary D43.2
    specified site — *see* Neoplasm, uncertain behavior,
      by site

Ependymoma — *continued*
  myxopapillary — *continued*
    unspecified site D43.2
  papillary D43.2
    specified site — *see* Neoplasm, uncertain behavior,
      by site
    unspecified site D43.2
  specified site — *see* Neoplasm, malignant, by site
  unspecified site C71.9
Ependymopathy G93.89
Ephelis, ephelides L81.2
Epiblepharon (congenital) Q10.3
Epicanthus, epicanthic fold (eyelid) (congenital) Q10.3
Epicondylitis (elbow)
  lateral M77.1- ☑
  medial M77.0- ☑
Epicystitis — *see* Cystitis
Epidemic — *see* condition
Epidermidalization, cervix — *see* Dysplasia, cervix
Epidermis, epidermal — *see* condition
Epidermodysplasia verruciformis B07.8
Epidermolysis
  bullosa (congenital) Q81.9
    acquired L12.30
      drug-induced L12.31
        specified cause NEC L12.35
    dystrophica Q81.2
    letalis Q81.1
    simplex Q81.0
    specified NEC Q81.8
  necroticans combustiformis L51.2
    due to drug — *see* Table of Drugs and Chemicals,
      by drug
Epidermophytid — *see* Dermatophytosis
Epidermophytosis (infected) — *see* Dermatophytosis
Epididymis — *see* condition
Epididymitis (acute) (nonvenereal) (recurrent) (residual)
  N45.1
  with orchitis N45.3
  blennorrhagic (gonococcal) A54.23
  caseous (tuberculous) A18.15
  chlamydial A56.19
  filarial (*see also* Infestation, filarial) B74.9 [N51]
  gonococcal A54.23
  syphilitic A52.76
  tuberculous A18.15
Epididymo-orchitis (*see also* Epididymitis) N45.3
Epidural — *see* condition
Epigastrium, epigastric — *see* condition
Epigastrocele — *see* Hernia, ventral
Epiglottis — *see* condition
Epiglottitis, epiglottiditis (acute) J05.10
  with obstruction J05.11
  chronic J37.0
Epignathus Q89.4
Epilepsia partialis continua (*see also* Kozhevnikof's
  epilepsy) G40.1- ☑
Epilepsy, epileptic, epilepsia (attack) (cerebral) (con-
  vulsion) (fit) (seizure) G40.909

> *Note: the following terms are to be considered
> equivalent to intractable: pharmacoresistant
> (pharmacologically resistant), treatment resistant,
> refractory (medically) and poorly controlled*

  with
    complex partial seizures — *see* Epilepsy, localiza-
      tion-related, symptomatic, with complex
      partial seizures
    grand mal seizures on awakening — *see* Epilepsy,
      generalized, specified NEC
    myoclonic absences — *see* Epilepsy, generalized,
      specified NEC
    myoclonic-astatic seizures — *see* Epilepsy, gener-
      alized, specified NEC
    simple partial seizures — *see* Epilepsy, localization-
      related, symptomatic, with simple partial
      seizures
  akinetic — *see* Epilepsy, generalized, specified NEC
  benign childhood with centrotemporal EEG spikes —
    see Epilepsy, localization-related, idiopathic
  benign myoclonic in infancy G40.80- ☑
  Bravais-jacksonian — *see* Epilepsy, localization-related,
    symptomatic, with simple partial seizures
  childhood
    with occipital EEG paroxysms — *see* Epilepsy, local-
      ization-related, idiopathic
    absence G40.A09 (*following* G40.3)

Epilepsy, epileptic, epilepsia — *continued*
  childhood — *continued*
    absence — *continued*
      intractable G40.A19 (*following G40.3*)
        with status epilepticus G40.A11 (*following G40.3*)
        without status epilepticus G40.A19 (*following G40.3*)
      not intractable G40.A09 (*following G40.3*)
        with status epilepticus G40.A01 (*following G40.3*)
        without status epilepticus G40.A09 (*following G40.3*)
  climacteric — *see* Epilepsy, specified NEC
  cysticercosis B69.0
  deterioration (mental) F06.8
  due to syphilis A52.19
  focal — *see* Epilepsy, localization-related, symptomatic, with simple partial seizures
  generalized
    idiopathic G40.309
      intractable G40.319
        with status epilepticus G40.311
        without status epilepticus G40.319
      not intractable G40.309
        with status epilepticus G40.301
        without status epilepticus G40.309
    specified NEC G40.409
      intractable G40.419
        with status epilepticus G40.411
        without status epilepticus G40.419
      not intractable G40.409
        with status epilepticus G40.401
        without status epilepticus G40.409
  impulsive petit mal — *see* Epilepsy, juvenile myoclonic
  intractable G40.919
    with status epilepticus G40.911
    without status epilepticus G40.919
  juvenile absence G40.A09 (*following G40.3*)
    intractable G40.A19 (*following G40.3*)
      with status epilepticus G40.A11 (*following G40.3*)
      without status epilepticus G40.A19 (*following G40.3*)
    not intractable G40.A09 (*following G40.3*)
      with status epilepticus G40.A01 (*following G40.3*)
      without status epilepticus G40.A09 (*following G40.3*)
  juvenile myoclonic G40.B09 (*following G40.3*)
    intractable G40.B19 (*following G40.3*)
      with status epilepticus G40.B11 (*following G40.3*)
      without status epilepticus G40.B19 (*following G40.3*)
    not intractable G40.B09 (*following G40.3*)
      with status epilepticus G40.B01 (*following G40.3*)
      without status epilepticus G40.B09 (*following G40.3*)
  localization-related (focal) (partial)
    idiopathic G40.009
      with seizures of localized onset G40.009
        intractable G40.019
          with status epilepticus G40.011
          without status epilepticus G40.019
        not intractable G40.009
          with status epilepticus G40.001
          without status epilepticus G40.009
    symptomatic
      with complex partial seizures G40.209
        intractable G40.219
          with status epilepticus G40.211
          without status epilepticus G40.219
        not intractable G40.209
          with status epilepticus G40.201
          without status epilepticus G40.209
      with simple partial seizures G40.109
        intractable G40.119
          with status epilepticus G40.111
          without status epilepticus G40.119
        not intractable G40.109
          with status epilepticus G40.101
          without status epilepticus G40.109
  myoclonus, myoclonic — *see* Epilepsy, generalized, specified NEC
  progressive — *see* Epilepsy, generalized, idiopathic
  not intractable G40.909
    with status epilepticus G40.901

Epilepsy, epileptic, epilepsia — *continued*
  not intractable — *continued*
    without status epilepticus G40.909
  on awakening — *see* Epilepsy, generalized, specified NEC
  parasitic NOS B71.9 [G94]
  partialis continua (*see also* Kozhevnikof's epilepsy) G40.1- ☑
  peripheral — *see* Epilepsy, specified NEC
  procursiva — *see* Epilepsy, localization-related, symptomatic, with simple partial seizures
  progressive (familial) myoclonic — *see* Epilepsy, generalized, idiopathic
  reflex — *see* Epilepsy, specified NEC
  related to
    alcohol G40.509
      not intractable G40.509
        with status epilepticus G40.501
        without status epliepticus G40.509
    drugs G40.509
      not intractable G40.509
        with status epilepticus G40.501
        without status epliepticus G40.509
    external causes G40.509
      not intractable G40.509
        with status epilepticus G40.501
        without status epliepticus G40.509
    hormonal changes G40.509
      not intractable G40.509
        with status epilepticus G40.501
        without status epliepticus G40.509
    sleep deprivation G40.509
      not intractable G40.509
        with status epilepticus G40.501
        without status epliepticus G40.509
    stress G40.509
      not intractable G40.509
        with status epilepticus G40.501
        without status epliepticus G40.509
  somatomotor — *see* Epilepsy, localization-related, symptomatic, with simple partial seizures
  somatosensory — *see* Epilepsy, localization-related, symptomatic, with simple partial seizures
  spasms G40.822
    intractable G40.824
      with status epilepticus G40.823
      without status epilepticus G40.824
    not intractable G40.822
      with status epilepticus G40.821
      without status epilepticus G40.822
  specified NEC G40.802
    intractable G40.804
      with status epilepticus G40.803
      without status epilepticus G40.804
    not intractable G40.802
      with status epilepticus G40.801
      without status epilepticus G40.802
  syndromes
    generalized
      idiopathic G40.309
        intractable G40.319
          with status epilepticus G40.311
          without status epilepticus G40.319
        not intractable G40.309
          with status epilepticus G40.301
          without status epilepticus G40.309
      specified NEC G40.409
        intractable G40.419
          with status epilepticus G40.411
          without status epilepticus G40.419
        not intractable G40.409
          with status epilepticus G40.401
          without status epilepticus G40.409
    localization-related (focal) (partial)
      idiopathic G40.009
        with seizures of localized onset G40.009
          intractable G40.019
            with status epilepticus G40.011
            without status epilepticus G40.019
          not intractable G40.009
            with status epilepticus G40.001
            without status epilepticus G40.009
      symptomatic
        with complex partial seizures G40.209
          intractable G40.219
            with status epilepticus G40.211
            without status epilepticus G40.219
          not intractable G40.209

Epilepsy, epileptic, epilepsia — *continued*
  syndromes — *continued*
    localization-related — *continued*
      symptomatic — *continued*
        with complex partial seizures — *continued*
          not intractable — *continued*
            with status epilepticus G40.201
            without status epilepticus G40.209
        with simple partial seizures G40.109
          intractable G40.119
            with status epilepticus G40.111
            without status epilepticus G40.119
          not intractable G40.109
            with status epilepticus G40.101
            without status epilepticus G40.109
    specified NEC G40.802
      intractable G40.804
        with status epilepticus G40.803
        without status epilepticus G40.804
      not intractable G40.802
        with status epilepticus G40.801
        without status epilepticus G40.802
  tonic (-clonic) — *see* Epilepsy, generalized, specified NEC
  twilight F05
  uncinate (gyrus) — *see* Epilepsy, localization-related, symptomatic, with complex partial seizures
  Unverricht (-Lundborg) (familial myoclonic) — *see* Epilepsy, generalized, idiopathic
  visceral — *see* Epilepsy, specified NEC
  visual — *see* Epilepsy, specified NEC
Epiloia Q85.1
Epimenorrhea N92.0
Epipharyngitis — *see* Nasopharyngitis
Epiphora H04.20- ☑
  due to
    excess lacrimation H04.21- ☑
    insufficient drainage H04.22- ☑
Epiphyseal arrest — *see* Arrest, epiphyseal
Epiphyseolysis, epiphysiolysis — *see* Osteochondropathy
Epiphysitis (*see also* Osteochondropathy)
  juvenile M92.9
  syphilitic (congenital) A50.02
Epiplocele — *see* Hernia, abdomen
Epiploitis — *see* Peritonitis
Epiplosarcomphalocele — *see* Hernia, umbilicus
Episcleritis (suppurative) H15.10- ☑
  in (due to)
    syphilis A52.71
    tuberculosis A18.51
  nodular H15.12- ☑
  periodica fugax H15.11- ☑
    angioneurotic — *see* Edema, angioneurotic
  syphilitic (late) A52.71
  tuberculous A18.51
Episode
  affective, mixed F39
  depersonalization (in neurotic state) F48.1
  depressive F32.9
    major F32.9
      mild F32.0
      moderate F32.1
      severe (without psychotic symptoms) F32.2
        with psychotic symptoms F32.3
    recurrent F33.9
      brief F33.8
    specified NEC F32.89
  hypomanic F30.8
  manic F30.9
    with
      psychotic symptoms F30.2
      remission (full) F30.4
        partial F30.3
    without psychotic symptoms F30.10
      mild F30.11
      moderate F30.12
      severe (without psychotic symptoms) F30.13
        with psychotic symptoms F30.2
    other specified F30.8
    recurrent F31.89
  psychotic F23
    organic F06.8
  schizophrenic (acute) NEC, brief F23
Epispadias (female) (male) Q64.0
Episplenitis D73.89
Epistaxis (multiple) R04.0

Index

Epistaxis — Esthesioneurocytoma

Epistaxis — continued
- hereditary I78.0
- vicarious menstruation N94.89

Epithelioma (malignant) (see also Neoplasm, malignant, by site)
- adenoides cysticum — see Neoplasm, skin, benign
- basal cell — see Neoplasm, skin, malignant
- benign — see Neoplasm, benign, by site
- Bowen's — see Neoplasm, skin, in situ
- calcifying, of Malherbe — see Neoplasm, skin, benign
- external site — see Neoplasm, skin, malignant
- intraepidermal, Jadassohn — see Neoplasm, skin, benign
- squamous cell — see Neoplasm, malignant, by site

Epitheliomatosis pigmented Q82.1
Epitheliopathy, multifocal placoid pigment H30.14- ☑
Epithelium, epithelial — see condition
Epituberculosis (with atelectasis) (allergic) A15.7
Eponychia Q84.6
Epstein's
- nephrosis or syndrome — see Nephrosis
- pearl K09.8

Epulis (gingiva) (fibrous) (giant cell) K06.8
Equinia A24.0
Equinovarus (congenital) (talipes) Q66.0
- acquired — see Deformity, limb, clubfoot

Equivalent
- convulsive (abdominal) — see Epilepsy, specified NEC
- epileptic (psychic) — see Epilepsy, localization-related, symptomatic, with complex partial seizures

Erb (-Duchenne) **paralysis** (birth injury) (newborn) P14.0
Erb-Goldflam disease or syndrome G70.00
- with exacerbation (acute) G70.01
- in crisis G70.01

Erb's
- disease G71.0
- palsy, paralysis (brachial) (birth) (newborn) P14.0
  - spinal (spastic) syphilitic A52.17
- pseudohypertrophic muscular dystrophy G71.0

Erdheim's syndrome (acromegalic macrospondylitis) E22.0
Erection, painful (persistent) — see Priapism
Ergosterol deficiency (vitamin D) E55.9
- with
  - adult osteomalacia M83.8
  - rickets — see Rickets

Ergotism (see also Poisoning, food, noxious, plant)
- from ergot used as drug (migraine therapy) — see Table of Drugs and Chemicals

Erosio interdigitalis blastomycetica B37.2
Erosion
- artery I77.2
  - without rupture I77.89
- bone — see Disorder, bone, density and structure, specified NEC
- bronchus J98.09
- cartilage (joint) — see Disorder, cartilage, specified type NEC
- cervix (uteri) (acquired) (chronic) (congenital) N86
  - with cervicitis N72
- cornea (nontraumatic) — see Ulcer, cornea
  - recurrent H18.83- ☑
  - traumatic — see Abrasion, cornea
- dental (idiopathic) (occupational) (due to diet, drugs or vomiting) K03.2
- duodenum, postpyloric — see Ulcer, duodenum
- esophagus K22.10
  - with bleeding K22.11
- gastric — see Ulcer, stomach
- gastrojejunal — see Ulcer, gastrojejunal
- implanted mesh — see Complications, mesh
- intestine K63.3
- lymphatic vessel I89.8
- pylorus, pyloric (ulcer) — see Ulcer, stomach
- spine, aneurysmal A52.09
- stomach — see Ulcer, stomach
- subcutaneous device pocket
  - nervous system prosthetic device, implant, or graft T85.890 ☑
  - other internal prosthetic device, implant, or graft T85.898 ☑
- teeth (idiopathic) (occupational) (due to diet, drugs or vomiting) K03.2
- urethra N36.8
- uterus N85.8

Erotomania F52.8

Error
- metabolism, inborn — see Disorder, metabolism
- refractive — see Disorder, refraction

Eructation R14.2
- nervous or psychogenic F45.8

Eruption
- creeping B76.9
- drug (generalized) (taken internally) L27.0
  - fixed L27.1
  - in contact with skin — see Dermatitis, due to drugs
  - localized L27.1
- Hutchinson, summer L56.4
- Kaposi's varicelliform B00.0
- napkin L22
- polymorphous light (sun) L56.4
- recalcitrant pustular L13.8
- ringed R23.8
- skin (nonspecific) R21
  - creeping (meaning hookworm) B76.9
  - due to inoculation/vaccination (generalized) (see also Dermatitis, due to, vaccine) L27.0
    - localized L27.1
  - erysipeloid A26.0
  - feigned L98.1
  - Kaposi's varicelliform B00.0
  - lichenoid L28.0
  - meaning dermatitis — see Dermatitis
  - toxic NEC L53.0
- tooth, teeth, abnormal (incomplete) (late) (premature) (sequence) K00.6
- vesicular R23.8

Erysipelas (gangrenous) (infantile) (newborn) (phlegmonous) (suppurative) A46
- external ear A46 [H62.40]
- puerperal, postpartum O86.89

Erysipeloid A26.9
- cutaneous (Rosenbach's) A26.0
- disseminated A26.8
- sepsis A26.7
- specified NEC A26.8

Erythema, erythematous (infectional) (inflammation) L53.9
- ab igne L59.0
- annulare (centrifugum) (rheumaticum) L53.1
- arthriticum epidemicum A25.1
- brucellum — see Brucellosis
- chronic figurate NEC L53.3
- chronicum migrans (Borrelia burgdorferi) A69.20
- diaper L22
- due to
  - chemical NEC L53.0
    - in contact with skin L24.5
  - drug (internal use) — see Dermatitis, due to, drugs
- elevatum diutinum L95.1
- endemic E52
- epidemic, arthritic A25.1
- figuratum perstans L53.3
- gluteal L22
- heat — code by site under Burn, first degree
- ichthyosiforme congenitum bullous Q80.3
- in diseases classified elsewhere L54
- induratum (nontuberculous) L52
  - tuberculous A18.4
- infectiosum B08.3
- intertrigo L30.4
- iris L51.9
- marginatum L53.2
  - in (due to) acute rheumatic fever I00
- medicamentosum — see Dermatitis, due to, drugs
- migrans A26.0
  - chronicum A69.20
  - tongue K14.1
- multiforme (major) (minor) L51.9
  - bullous, bullosum L51.1
  - conjunctiva L51.1
  - nonbullous L51.0
  - pemphigoides L12.0
  - specified NEC L51.8
- napkin L22
- neonatorum P83.88
  - toxic P83.1
- nodosum L52
  - tuberculous A18.4
- palmar L53.8
- pernio T69.1 ☑
- rash, newborn P83.88
- scarlatiniform (recurrent) (exfoliative) L53.8
- solare L55.0

Erythema, erythematous — continued
- specified NEC L53.8
- toxic, toxicum NEC L53.0
  - newborn P83.1
- tuberculous (primary) A18.4

Erythematous, erythematosus — see condition
Erythermalgia (primary) I73.81
Erythralgia I73.81
Erythrasma L08.1
Erythredema (polyneuropathy) — see Poisoning, mercury
Erythremia (acute) C94.0- ☑
- chronic D45
- secondary D75.1

Erythroblastopenia (see also Aplasia, red cell) D60.9
- congenital D61.01

Erythroblastophthisis D61.09
Erythroblastosis (fetalis) (newborn) P55.9
- due to
  - ABO (antibodies) (incompatibility) (isoimmunization) P55.1
  - Rh (antibodies) (incompatibility) (isoimmunization) P55.0

Erythrocyanosis (crurum) I73.89
Erythrocythemia — see Erythremia
Erythrocytosis (megalosplenic) (secondary) D75.1
- familial D75.0
- oval, hereditary — see Elliptocytosis
- secondary D75.1
- stress D75.1

Erythroderma (secondary) (see also Erythema) L53.9
- bullous ichthyosiform, congenital Q80.3
- desquamativum L21.1
- ichthyosiform, congenital (bullous) Q80.3
- neonatorum P83.88
- psoriaticum L40.8

Erythrodysesthesia, palmar plantar (PPE) L27.1
Erythrogenesis imperfecta D61.09
Erythroleukemia C94.0- ☑
Erythromelalgia I73.81
Erythrophagocytosis D75.89
Erythrophobia F40.298
Erythroplakia, oral epithelium, and tongue K13.29
Erythroplasia (Queyrat) D07.4
- specified site — see Neoplasm, skin, in situ
- unspecified site D07.4

Escherichia coli (E. coli), **as cause of disease classified elsewhere** B96.20
- non-O157 Shiga toxin-producing (with known O group) B96.22
- non-Shiga toxin-producing B96.29
- O157 B96.21
- O157 with confirmation of Shiga toxin when H antigen is unknown, or is not H7 B96.21
- O157:H- (nonmotile) with confirmation of Shiga toxin B96.21
- O157:H7 with or without confirmation of Shiga toxin-production B96.21
- Shiga toxin-producing (with unspecified O group) (STEC) B96.23
- specified NEC B96.29

Esophagismus K22.4
Esophagitis (acute) (alkaline) (chemical) (chronic) (infectional) (necrotic) (peptic) (postoperative) K20.9
- candidal B37.81
- due to gastrointestinal reflux disease K21.0
- eosinophilic K20.0
- reflux K21.0
- specified NEC K20.8
- tuberculous A18.83
- ulcerative K22.10
  - with bleeding K22.11

Esophagocele K22.5
Esophagomalacia K22.8
Esophagospasm K22.4
Esophagostenosis K22.2
Esophagostomiasis B81.8
Esophagotracheal — see condition
Esophagus — see condition
Esophoria H50.51
- convergence, excess H51.12
- divergence, insufficiency H51.8

Esotropia — see Strabismus, convergent concomitant
Espundia B55.2
Essential — see condition
Esthesioneuroblastoma C30.0
Esthesioneurocytoma C30.0

☑ Additional Character Required — Refer to the Tabular List for Character Selection
⬢ Subterms under main terms may continue to next column or page

Esthesioneuroepithelioma C30.0
Esthiomene A55
Estivo-autumnal malaria (fever) B50.9
Estrangement (marital) Z63.5
  parent-child NEC Z62.890
Estriasis — see Myiasis
Ethanolism — see Alcoholism
Etherism — see Dependence, drug, inhalant
Ethmoid, ethmoidal — see condition
Ethmoiditis (chronic) (nonpurulent) (purulent) (see also
  Sinusitis, ethmoidal)
  influenzal — see Influenza, with, respiratory manifes-
    tations NEC
  Woakes' J33.1
Ethylism — see Alcoholism
Eulenburg's disease (congenital paramyotonia) G71.19
Eumycetoma B47.0
Eunuchoidism E29.1
  hypogonadotropic E23.0
European blastomycosis — see Cryptococcosis
Eustachian — see condition
Evaluation (for) (of)
  development state
    adolescent Z00.3
    period of
      delayed growth in childhood Z00.70
        with abnormal findings Z00.71
      rapid growth in childhood Z00.2
      puberty Z00.3
  growth and developmental state (period of rapid
    growth) Z00.2
    delayed growth Z00.70
      with abnormal findings Z00.71
  mental health (status) Z00.8
    requested by authority Z04.6
  period of
    delayed growth in childhood Z00.70
      with abnormal findings Z00.71
    rapid growth in childhood Z00.2
  suspected condition — see Observation
Evans syndrome D69.41
Event
  apparent life threatening in newborn and infant (ALTE)
    R68.13
  brief resolved unexplained event (BRUE) R68.13
Eventration (see also Hernia, ventral)
  colon into chest — see Hernia, diaphragm
  diaphragm (congenital) Q79.1
Eversion
  bladder N32.89
  cervix (uteri) N86
    with cervicitis N72
  foot NEC (see also Deformity, valgus, ankle)
    congenital Q66.6
  punctum lacrimale (postinfectional) (senile) H04.52- ☑
  ureter (meatus) N28.89
  urethra (meatus) N36.8
  uterus N81.4
Evidence
  cytologic
    of malignancy on anal smear R85.614
    of malignancy on cervical smear R87.614
    of malignancy on vaginal smear R87.624
Evisceration
  birth injury P15.8
  traumatic NEC
    eye — see Enucleated eye
Evulsion — see Avulsion
Ewing's sarcoma or tumor — see Neoplasm, bone,
  malignant
Examination (for) (following) (general) (of) (routine)
  Z00.00
  with abnormal findings Z00.01
  abuse, physical (alleged), ruled out
    adult Z04.71
    child Z04.72
  adolescent (development state) Z00.3
  alleged rape or sexual assault (victim), ruled out
    adult Z04.41
    child Z04.42
  allergy Z01.82
  annual (adult) (periodic) (physical) Z00.00
    with abnormal findings Z00.01
    gynecological Z01.419
      with abnormal findings Z01.411
  antibody response Z01.84
  blood — see Examination, laboratory
  blood pressure Z01.30

Examination — continued
  blood pressure — continued
    with abnormal findings Z01.31
  cancer staging — see Neoplasm, malignant, by site
  cervical Papanicolaou smear Z12.4
    as part of routine gynecological examination
      Z01.419
    with abnormal findings Z01.411
  child (over 28 days old) Z00.129
    with abnormal findings Z00.121
    under 28 days old — see Newborn, examination
  clinical research control or normal comparison (con-
    trol) (participant) Z00.6
  contraceptive (drug) maintenance (routine) Z30.8
    device (intrauterine) Z30.431
  dental Z01.20
    with abnormal findings Z01.21
  developmental — see Examination, child
  donor (potential) Z00.5
  ear Z01.10
    with abnormal findings NEC Z01.118
  eye Z01.00
    with abnormal findings Z01.01
  following
    accident NEC Z04.3
      transport Z04.1
      work Z04.2
    assault, alleged, ruled out
      adult Z04.71
      child Z04.72
    motor vehicle accident Z04.1
    treatment (for) Z09
      combined NEC Z09
        fracture Z09
        malignant neoplasm Z08
      malignant neoplasm Z08
      mental disorder Z09
      specified condition NEC Z09
  follow-up (routine) (following) Z09
    chemotherapy NEC Z09
      malignant neoplasm Z08
    fracture Z09
    malignant neoplasm Z08
    postpartum Z39.2
    psychotherapy Z09
    radiotherapy NEC Z09
      malignant neoplasm Z08
    surgery NEC Z09
      malignant neoplasm Z08
  gynecological Z01.419
    with abnormal findings Z01.411
    for contraceptive maintenance Z30.8
  health — see Examination, medical
  hearing Z01.10
    with abnormal findings NEC Z01.118
    following failed hearing screening Z01.110
  immunity status testing Z01.84
  laboratory (as part of a general medical examination)
    Z00.00
    with abnormal findings Z00.01
    preprocedural Z01.812
  lactating mother Z39.1
  medical (adult) (for) (of) Z00.00
    with abnormal findings Z00.01
    administrative purpose only Z02.9
      specified NEC Z02.89
    admission to
      armed forces Z02.3
      old age home Z02.2
      prison Z02.89
      residential institution Z02.2
      school Z02.0
        following illness or medical treatment Z02.0
      summer camp Z02.89
    adoption Z02.82
    blood alcohol or drug level Z02.83
    camp (summer) Z02.89
    clinical research, normal subject (control) (partici-
      pant) Z00.6
    control subject in clinical research (normal compar-
      ison) (participant) Z00.6
    donor (potential) Z00.5
    driving license Z02.4
    general (adult) Z00.00
      with abnormal findings Z00.01
    immigration Z02.89
    insurance purposes Z02.6
    marriage Z02.89
    medicolegal reasons NEC Z04.8

Examination — continued
  medical — continued
    naturalization Z02.89
    participation in sport Z02.5
    paternity testing Z02.81
    population survey Z00.8
    pre-employment Z02.1
    pre-operative — see Examination, pre-procedural
    pre-procedural
      cardiovascular Z01.810
      respiratory Z01.811
      specified NEC Z01.818
    preschool children
      for admission to school Z02.0
    prisoners
      for entrance into prison Z02.89
    recruitment for armed forces Z02.3
    specified NEC Z00.8
    sport competition Z02.5
  medicolegal reason NEC Z04.8
  newborn — see Newborn, examination
  pelvic (annual) (periodic) Z01.419
    with abnormal findings Z01.411
  period of rapid growth in childhood Z00.2
  periodic (adult) (annual) (routine) Z00.00
    with abnormal findings Z00.01
  physical (adult) (see also Examination, medical) Z00.00
    sports Z02.5
  postpartum
    immediately after delivery Z39.0
    routine follow-up Z39.2
  pre-chemotherapy (antineoplastic) Z01.818
  prenatal (normal pregnancy) (see also Pregnancy,
    normal) Z34.9- ☑
  pre-procedural (pre-operative)
    cardiovascular Z01.810
    laboratory Z01.812
    respiratory Z01.811
    specified NEC Z01.818
  prior to chemotherapy (antineoplastic) Z01.818
  psychiatric NEC Z00.8
    follow-up not needing further care Z09
    requested by authority Z04.6
  radiological (as part of a general medical examination)
    Z00.00
    with abnormal findings Z00.01
  repeat cervical smear to confirm findings of recent
    normal smear following initial abnormal smear
    Z01.42
  skin (hypersensitivity) Z01.82
  special (see also Examination, by type) Z01.89
    specified type NEC Z01.89
  specified type or reason NEC Z04.8
  teeth Z01.20
    with abnormal findings Z01.21
  urine — see Examination, laboratory
  vision Z01.00
    with abnormal findings Z01.01
Exanthem, exanthema (see also Rash)
  with enteroviral vesicular stomatitis B08.4
  Boston A88.0
  epidemic with meningitis A88.0 [G02]
  subitum B08.20
    due to human herpesvirus 6 B08.21
    due to human herpesvirus 7 B08.22
  viral, virus B09
    specified type NEC B08.8
Excess, excessive, excessively
  alcohol level in blood R78.0
  androgen (ovarian) E28.1
  attrition, tooth, teeth K03.0
  carotene, carotin (dietary) E67.1
  cold, effects of T69.9 ☑
    specified effect NEC T69.8 ☑
  convergence H51.12
  crying
    in child, adolescent, or adult R45.83
    in infant R68.11
  development, breast N62
  divergence H51.8
  drinking (alcohol) NEC (without dependence) F10.10
    habitual (continual) (without remission) F10.20
  eating R63.2
  estrogen E28.0
  fat (see also Obesity)
    in heart — see Degeneration, myocardial
    localized E65
  foreskin N47.8

Excess, excessive, excessively — continued
  gas R14.0
  glucagon E16.3
  heat — see Heat
  intermaxillary vertical dimension of fully erupted teeth M26.37
  interocclusal distance of fully erupted teeth M26.37
  kalium E87.5
  large
    colon K59.39
      congenital Q43.8
    infant P08.0
    organ or site, congenital NEC — see Anomaly, by site
  long
    organ or site, congenital NEC — see Anomaly, by site
  menstruation (with regular cycle) N92.0
    with irregular cycle N92.1
  napping Z72.821
  natrium E87.0
  number of teeth K00.1
  nutrient (dietary) NEC R63.2
  potassium (K) E87.5
  salivation K11.7
  secretion (see also Hypersecretion)
    milk O92.6
    sputum R09.3
    sweat R61
  sexual drive F52.8
  short
    organ or site, congenital NEC — see Anomaly, by site
    umbilical cord in labor or delivery O69.3 ☑
  skin L98.7
    and subcutaneous tissue L98.7
    eyelid (acquired) — see Blepharochalasis
      congenital Q10.3
  sodium (Na) E87.0
  spacing of fully erupted teeth M26.32
  sputum R09.3
  sweating R61
  thirst R63.1
    due to deprivation of water T73.1 ☑
  tuberosity of jaw M26.07
  vitamin
    A (dietary) E67.0
      administered as drug (prolonged intake) — see Table of Drugs and Chemicals, vitamins, adverse effect
      overdose or wrong substance given or taken — see Table of Drugs and Chemicals, vitamins, poisoning
    D (dietary) E67.3
      administered as drug (prolonged intake) — see Table of Drugs and Chemicals, vitamins, adverse effect
      overdose or wrong substance given or taken — see Table of Drugs and Chemicals, vitamins, poisoning
  weight
    gain R63.5
    loss R63.4
Excitability, abnormal, under minor stress (personality disorder) F60.3
Excitation
  anomalous atrioventricular I45.6
  psychogenic F30.8
  reactive (from emotional stress, psychological trauma) F30.8
Excitement
  hypomanic F30.8
  manic F30.9
  mental, reactive (from emotional stress, psychological trauma) F30.8
  state, reactive (from emotional stress, psychological trauma) F30.8
Excoriation (traumatic) (see also Abrasion)
  neurotic L98.1
  skin picking disorder F42.4
Exfoliation
  due to erythematous conditions according to extent of body surface involved L49.0
    less than 10 percent of body surface L49.0
    10-19 percent of body surface L49.1
    20-29 percent of body surface L49.2
    30-39 percent of body surface L49.3
    40-49 percent of body surface L49.4

Exfoliation — continued
  due to erythematous conditions according to extent of body surface involved — continued
    50-59 percent of body surface L49.5
    60-69 percent of body surface L49.6
    70-79 percent of body surface L49.7
    80-89 percent of body surface L49.8
    90-99 percent of body surface L49.9
  teeth, due to systemic causes K08.0
Exfoliative — see condition
Exhaustion, exhaustive (physical NEC) R53.83
  battle F43.0
  cardiac — see Failure, heart
  delirium F43.0
  due to
    cold T69.8 ☑
    excessive exertion T73.3 ☑
    exposure T73.2 ☑
    neurasthenia F48.8
  heart — see Failure, heart
  heat (see also Heat, exhaustion) T67.5 ☑
    due to
      salt depletion T67.4 ☑
      water depletion T67.3 ☑
  maternal, complicating delivery O75.81
  mental F48.8
  myocardium, myocardial — see Failure, heart
  nervous F48.8
  old age R54
  psychogenic F48.8
  psychosis F43.0
  senile R54
  vital NEC Z73.0
Exhibitionism F65.2
Exocervicitis — see Cervicitis
Exomphalos Q79.2
  meaning hernia — see Hernia, umbilicus
Exophoria H50.52
  convergence, insufficiency H51.11
  divergence, excess H51.8
Exophthalmos H05.2- ☑
  congenital Q15.8
  constant NEC H05.24- ☑
  displacement, globe — see Displacement, globe
  due to thyrotoxicosis (hyperthyroidism) — see Hyperthyroidism, with, goiter (diffuse)
  dysthyroid — see Hyperthyroidism, with, goiter (diffuse)
  goiter — see Hyperthyroidism, with, goiter (diffuse)
  intermittent NEC H05.25- ☑
  malignant — see Hyperthyroidism, with, goiter (diffuse)
  orbital
    edema — see Edema, orbit
    hemorrhage — see Hemorrhage, orbit
  pulsating NEC H05.26- ☑
  thyrotoxic, thyrotropic — see Hyperthyroidism, with, goiter (diffuse)
Exostosis (see also Disorder, bone)
  cartilaginous — see Neoplasm, bone, benign
  congenital (multiple) Q78.6
  external ear canal H61.81- ☑
  gonococcal A54.49
  jaw (bone) M27.8
  multiple, congenital Q78.6
  orbit H05.35- ☑
  osteocartilaginous — see Neoplasm, bone, benign
  syphilitic A52.77
Exotropia — see Strabismus, divergent concomitant
Explanation of
  investigation finding Z71.2
  medication Z71.89
Exposure (to) (see also Contact, with) T75.89 ☑
  acariasis Z20.7
  AIDS virus Z20.6
  air pollution Z77.110
  algae and algae toxins Z77.121
  algae bloom Z77.121
  anthrax Z20.810
  aromatic amines Z77.020
  aromatic (hazardous) compounds NEC Z77.028
  aromatic dyes NOS Z77.028
  arsenic Z77.010
  asbestos Z77.090
  bacterial disease NEC Z20.818
  benzene Z77.021
  blue-green algae bloom Z77.121

Exposure — continued
  body fluids (potentially hazardous) Z77.21
  brown tide Z77.121
  chemicals (chiefly nonmedicinal) (hazardous) NEC Z77.098
  cholera Z20.09
  chromium compounds Z77.018
  cold, effects of T69.9 ☑
    specified effect NEC T69.8 ☑
  communicable disease Z20.9
    bacterial NEC Z20.818
    specified NEC Z20.89
    viral NEC Z20.828
  cyanobacteria bloom Z77.121
  disaster Z65.5
  discrimination Z60.5
  dyes Z77.098
  effects of T73.9 ☑
  environmental tobacco smoke (acute) (chronic) Z77.22
  Escherichia coli (E. coli) Z20.01
  exhaustion due to T73.2 ☑
  fiberglass — see Table of Drugs and Chemicals, fiberglass
  German measles Z20.4
  gonorrhea Z20.2
  hazardous metals NEC Z77.018
  hazardous substances NEC Z77.29
  hazards in the physical environment NEC Z77.128
  hazards to health NEC Z77.9
  human immunodeficiency virus (HIV) Z20.6
  human T-lymphotropic virus type-1 (HTLV-1) Z20.89
  implanted
    mesh — see Complications, mesh
    prosthetic materials NEC — see Complications, prosthetic materials NEC
  infestation (parasitic) NEC Z20.7
  intestinal infectious disease NEC Z20.09
    Escherichia coli (E. coli) Z20.01
  lead Z77.011
  meningococcus Z20.811
  mold (toxic) Z77.120
  nickel dust Z77.018
  noise Z77.122
  occupational
    air contaminants NEC Z57.39
    dust Z57.2
    environmental tobacco smoke Z57.31
    extreme temperature Z57.6
    noise Z57.0
    radiation Z57.1
    risk factors Z57.9
      specified NEC Z57.8
    toxic agents (gases) (liquids) (solids) (vapors) in agriculture Z57.4
    toxic agents (gases) (liquids) (solids) (vapors) in industry NEC Z57.5
    vibration Z57.7
  parasitic disease NEC Z20.7
  pediculosis Z20.7
  persecution Z60.5
  pfiesteria piscicida Z77.121
  poliomyelitis Z20.89
  pollution
    air Z77.110
    environmental NEC Z77.118
    soil Z77.112
    water Z77.111
  polycyclic aromatic hydrocarbons Z77.028
  prenatal (drugs) (toxic chemicals) — see Newborn, affected by, noxious substances transmitted via placenta or breast milk
  rabies Z20.3
  radiation, naturally occurring NEC Z77.123
  radon Z77.123
  red tide (Florida) Z77.121
  rubella Z20.4
  second hand tobacco smoke (acute) (chronic) Z77.22
    in the perinatal period P96.81
  sexually-transmitted disease Z20.2
  smallpox (laboratory) Z20.89
  syphilis Z20.2
  terrorism Z65.4
  torture Z65.4
  tuberculosis Z20.1
  uranium Z77.012
  varicella Z20.820
  venereal disease Z20.2
  viral disease NEC Z20.828

☑ Additional Character Required — Refer to the Tabular List for Character Selection   ⬱ Subterms under main terms may continue to next column or page

Exposure — continued
war Z65.5
water pollution Z77.111
Exsanguination — see Hemorrhage
Exstrophy
abdominal contents Q45.8
bladder Q64.10
cloacal Q64.12
specified type NEC Q64.19
supravesical fissure Q64.11
Extensive — see condition
Extra (see also Accessory)
marker chromosomes (normal individual) Q92.61
in abnormal individual Q92.62
rib Q76.6
cervical Q76.5
Extrasystoles (supraventricular) I49.49
atrial I49.1
auricular I49.1
junctional I49.2
ventricular I49.3
Extrauterine gestation or pregnancy — see Pregnancy, by site
Extravasation
blood R58
chyle into mesentery I89.8
pelvicalyceal N13.8
pyelosinus N13.8
urine (from ureter) R39.0
vesicant agent
antineoplastic chemotherapy T80.810 ☑
other agent NEC T80.818 ☑
Extremity — see condition, limb
Extrophy — see Exstrophy
Extroversion
bladder Q64.19
uterus N81.4
complicating delivery O71.2
postpartal (old) N81.4
Extruded tooth (teeth) M26.34
Extrusion
breast implant (prosthetic) T85.42 ☑
eye implant (globe) (ball) T85.328 ☑
intervertebral disc — see Displacement, intervertebral disc
ocular lens implant (prosthetic) — see Complications, intraocular lens
vitreous — see Prolapse, vitreous
Exudate
pleural — see Effusion, pleura
retina H35.89
Exudative — see condition
Eye, eyeball, eyelid — see condition
Eyestrain — see Disturbance, vision, subjective
Eyeworm disease of Africa B74.3

F

Faber's syndrome (achlorhydric anemia) D50.9
Fabry (-Anderson) **disease** E75.21
Faciocephalalgia, autonomic (see also Neuropathy, peripheral, autonomic) G90.09
Factor(s)
psychic, associated with diseases classified elsewhere F54
psychological
affecting physical conditions F54
or behavioral
affecting general medical condition F54
associated with disorders or diseases classified elsewhere F54
Fahr disease (of brain) G23.8
Fahr Volhard disease (of kidney) I12.- ☑
Failure, failed
abortion — see Abortion, attempted
aortic (valve) I35.8
rheumatic I06.8
attempted abortion — see Abortion, attempted
biventricular I50.82
due to left heart failure I50.814
bone marrow — see Anemia, aplastic
cardiac — see Failure, heart
cardiorenal (chronic) (see also Failure, renal, and Failure, heart) I50.9
hypertensive I13.2
cardiorespiratory (see also Failure, heart) R09.2
cardiovascular (chronic) — see Failure, heart

Failure, failed — continued
cerebrovascular I67.9
cervical dilatation in labor O62.0
circulation, circulatory (peripheral) R57.9
newborn P29.89
compensation — see Disease, heart
compliance with medical treatment or regimen — see Noncompliance
congestive — see Failure, heart, congestive
dental implant (endosseous) M27.69
due to
failure of dental prosthesis M27.63
lack of attached gingiva M27.62
occlusal trauma (poor prosthetic design) M27.62
parafunctional habits M27.62
periodontal infection (peri-implantitis) M27.62
poor oral hygiene M27.62
osseointegration M27.61
due to
complications of systemic disease M27.61
poor bone quality M27.61
iatrogenic M27.61
post-osseointegration
biological M27.62
due to complications of systemic disease M27.62
iatrogenic M27.62
mechanical M27.63
pre-integration M27.61
pre-osseointegration M27.61
specified NEC M27.69
descent of head (at term) of pregnancy (mother) O32.4 ☑
endosseous dental implant — see Failure, dental implant
engagement of head (term of pregnancy) (mother) O32.4 ☑
erection (penile) (see also Dysfunction, sexual, male, erectile) N52.9
nonorganic F52.21
examination(s), anxiety concerning Z55.2
expansion terminal respiratory units (newborn) (primary) P28.0
forceps NOS (with subsequent cesarean delivery) O66.5
gain weight (child over 28 days old) R62.51
adult R62.7
newborn P92.6
genital response (male) F52.21
female F52.22
heart (acute) (senile) (sudden) I50.9
with
acute pulmonary edema — see Failure, ventricular, left
decompensation (see also Failure, heart, by type as diastolic or systolic, acute and chronic) I50.9
dilatation — see Disease, heart
normal ejection fraction — see Failure, heart, diastolic
preserved ejection fraction — see Failure, heart, diastolic
reduced ejection fraction — see Failure, heart, systolic
arteriosclerotic I70.90
biventricular I50.82
due to left heart failure I50.814
combined left-right sided I50.82
due to left heart failure I50.814
compensated (see also Failure, heart, by type as diastolic or systolic, chronic) I50.9
complicating
anesthesia (general) (local) or other sedation in labor and delivery O74.2
in pregnancy O29.12- ☑
postpartum, puerperal O89.1
delivery (cesarean) (instrumental) O75.4
congestive I50.9
with rheumatic fever (conditions in I00)
active I01.8
inactive or quiescent (with chorea) I09.81
newborn P29.0
rheumatic (chronic) (inactive) (with chorea) I09.81
active or acute I01.8
with chorea I02.0
decompensated (see also Failure, heart, by type as diastolic or systolic, acute and chronic) I50.9

Failure, failed — continued
heart — continued
degenerative — see Degeneration, myocardial
diastolic (congestive) (left ventricular) I50.30
acute (congestive) I50.31
and (on) chronic (congestive) I50.33
chronic (congestive) I50.32
and (on) acute (congestive) I50.33
combined with systolic (congestive) I50.40
acute (congestive) I50.41
and (on) chronic (congestive) I50.43
chronic (congestive) I50.42
and (on) acute (congestive) I50.43
due to presence of cardiac prosthesis I97.13- ☑
end stage (see also Failure, heart, by type as diastolic or systolic, chronic) I50.84
following cardiac surgery I97.13- ☑
high output NOS I50.83
hypertensive — see Hypertension, heart
left (ventricular) (see also Failure, ventricular, left)
combined diastolic and systolic — see Failure, heart, diastolic, combined with systolic
diastolic — see Failure, heart, diastolic
systolic — see Failure, heart, systolic
low output (syndrome) NOS I50.9
newborn P29.0
organic — see Disease, heart
peripartum O90.3
postprocedural I97.13- ☑
rheumatic (chronic) (inactive) I09.9
right (isolated) (ventricular) I50.810
acute I50.811
and (on) chronic I50.813
chronic I50.812
and acute I50.813
secondary to left heart failure I50.814
specified NEC I50.89

Note: heart failure stages A, B, C, and D are based on the American College of Cardiology and American Heart Association stages of heart failure, which complement and should not be confused with the New York Heart Association Classification of Heart Failure, into Class I, Class II, Class III, and Class IV

stage A Z91.89
stage B (see also Failure, heart, by type as diastolic or systolic) I50.9
stage C (see also Failure, heart, by type as diastolic or systolic) I50.9
stage D (see also Failure, heart, by type as diastolic or systolic, chronic) I50.84
systolic (congestive) (left ventricular) I50.20
acute (congestive) I50.21
and (on) chronic (congestive) I50.23
chronic (congestive) I50.22
and (on) acute (congestive) I50.23
combined with diastolic (congestive) I50.40
acute (congestive) I50.41
and (on) chronic (congestive) I50.43
chronic (congestive) I50.42
and (on) acute (congestive) I50.43
thyrotoxic (see also Thyrotoxicosis) E05.90 [I43]
with
high output (see also Thyrotoxicosis) I50.83
thyroid storm E05.91 [I43]
high output (see also Thyrotoxicosis) I50.83
valvular — see Endocarditis
hepatic K72.90
with coma K72.91
acute or subacute K72.00
with coma K72.01
due to drugs K71.10
with coma K71.11
alcoholic (acute) (chronic) (subacute) K70.40
with coma K70.41
chronic K72.10
with coma K72.11
due to drugs (acute) (subacute) (chronic) K71.10
with coma K71.11
due to drugs (acute) (subacute) (chronic) K71.10
with coma K71.11
postprocedural K91.82
hepatorenal K76.7
induction (of labor) O61.9
abortion — see Abortion, attempted
by
oxytocic drugs O61.0

Failure, failed — *continued*
  induction — *continued*
    by — *continued*
      prostaglandins O61.0
    instrumental O61.1
    mechanical O61.1
    medical O61.0
    specified NEC O61.8
    surgical O61.1
  intubation during anesthesia T88.4 ☑
    in pregnancy O29.6- ☑
    labor and delivery O74.7
    postpartum, puerperal O89.6
  involution, thymus (gland) E32.0
  kidney (*see also* Disease, kidney, chronic) N19
    acute (*see also* Failure, renal, acute) N17.9
  lactation (complete) O92.3
    partial O92.4
  Leydig's cell, adult E29.1
  liver — *see* Failure, hepatic
  menstruation at puberty N91.0
  mitral I05.8
  myocardial, myocardium (*see also* Failure, heart) I50.9
    chronic (*see also* Failure, heart, congestive) I50.9
    congestive (*see also* Failure, heart, congestive) I50.9
  orgasm (female) (psychogenic) F52.31
    male F52.32
  ovarian (primary) E28.39
    iatrogenic E89.40
      asymptomatic E89.40
      symptomatic E89.41
    postprocedural (postablative) (postirradiation) (postsurgical) E89.40
      asymptomatic E89.40
      symptomatic E89.41
  ovulation causing infertility N97.0
  polyglandular, autoimmune E31.0
  prosthetic joint implant — *see* Complications, joint prosthesis, mechanical, breakdown, by site
  renal N19
    with
      tubular necrosis (acute) N17.0
    acute N17.9
      with
        cortical necrosis N17.1
        medullary necrosis N17.2
        tubular necrosis N17.0
      specified NEC N17.8
    chronic N18.9
    hypertensive — *see* Hypertension, kidney
    congenital P96.0
    end stage (chronic) N18.6
      due to hypertension I12.0
    following
      abortion — *see* Abortion by type complicated by specified condition NEC
      crushing T79.5 ☑
      ectopic or molar pregnancy O08.4
      labor and delivery (acute) O90.4
    hypertensive — *see* Hypertension, kidney
    postprocedural N99.0
  respiration, respiratory J96.90
    with
      hypercapnia J96.92
      hypercarbia J96.02
      hypoxia J96.91
    acute J96.00
      with
        hypercapnia J96.02
        hypercarbia J96.02
        hypoxia J96.01
    acute and (on) chronic J96.20
      with
        hypercapnia J96.22
        hypercarbia J96.22
        hypoxia J96.21
    center G93.89
    chronic J96.10
      with
        hypercapnia J96.12
        hypercarbia J96.12
        hypoxia J96.11
    newborn P28.5
    postprocedural (acute) J95.821
      acute and chronic J95.822
  rotation
    cecum Q43.3
    colon Q43.3

Failure, failed — *continued*
  rotation — *continued*
    intestine Q43.3
    kidney Q63.2
  sedation (conscious) (moderate) during procedure T88.52 ☑
    history of Z92.83
  segmentation (*see also* Fusion)
    fingers — *see* Syndactylism, complex, fingers
    vertebra Q76.49
      with scoliosis Q76.3
  seminiferous tubule, adult E29.1
  senile (general) R54
  sexual arousal (male) F52.21
    female F52.22
  testicular endocrine function E29.1
  to thrive (child over 28 days old) R62.51
    adult R62.7
    newborn P92.6
  transplant T86.92
    bone T86.831
      marrow T86.02
    cornea T86.841
    heart T86.22
      with lung(s) T86.32
    intestine T86.851
    kidney T86.12
    liver T86.42
    lung(s) T86.811
      with heart T86.32
    pancreas T86.891
    skin (allograft) (autograft) T86.821
    specified organ or tissue NEC T86.891
    stem cell (peripheral blood) (umbilical cord) T86.5
  trial of labor (with subsequent cesarean delivery) O66.40
    following previous cesarean delivery O66.41
  tubal ligation N99.89
  urinary — *see* Disease, kidney, chronic
  vacuum extraction NOS (with subsequent cesarean delivery) O66.5
  vasectomy N99.89
  ventouse NOS (with subsequent cesarean delivery) O66.5
  ventricular (*see also* Failure, heart) I50.9
    left (*see also* Failure, heart, left) I50.1
      with rheumatic fever (conditions in I00)
        active I01.8
          with chorea I02.0
        inactive or quiescent (with chorea) I09.81
      rheumatic (chronic) (inactive) (with chorea) I09.81
        active or acute I01.8
          with chorea I02.0
    right — *see* Failure, heart, right
  vital centers, newborn P91.88
Fainting (fit) R55
Fallen arches — *see* Deformity, limb, flat foot
Falling, falls (repeated) R29.6
  any organ or part — *see* Prolapse
Fallopian
  insufflation Z31.41
  tube — *see* condition
Fallot's
  pentalogy Q21.8
  tetrad or tetralogy Q21.3
  triad or trilogy Q22.3
False (*see also* condition)
  croup J38.5
  joint — *see* Nonunion, fracture
  labor (pains) O47.9
    at or after 37 completed weeks of gestation O47.1
    before 37 completed weeks of gestation O47.0- ☑
  passage, urethra (prostatic) N36.5
  pregnancy F45.8
Family, familial (*see also* condition)
  disruption Z63.8
    involving divorce or separation Z63.5
  Li-Fraumeni (syndrome) Z15.01
  planning advice Z30.09
  problem Z63.9
    specified NEC Z63.8
  retinoblastoma C69.2- ☑
Famine (effects of) T73.0 ☑
  edema — *see* Malnutrition, severe
Fanconi (-de Toni)(-Debré) **syndrome** E72.09
  with cystinosis E72.04
Fanconi's anemia (congenital pancytopenia) D61.09

Farber's disease or syndrome E75.29
Farcy A24.0
Farmer's
  lung J67.0
  skin L57.8
Farsightedness — *see* Hypermetropia
Fascia — *see* condition
Fasciculation R25.3
Fasciitis M72.9
  diffuse (eosinophilic) M35.4
  infective M72.8
    necrotizing M72.6
  necrotizing M72.6
  nodular M72.4
  perirenal (with ureteral obstruction) N13.5
    with infection N13.6
  plantar M72.2
  specified NEC M72.8
  traumatic (old) M72.8
    current — *code by* site under Sprain
Fascioliasis B66.3
Fasciolopsis, fasciolopsiasis (intestinal) B66.5
Fascioscapulohumeral myopathy G71.0
Fast pulse R00.0
Fat
  embolism — *see* Embolism, fat
  excessive (*see also* Obesity)
    in heart — *see* Degeneration, myocardial
  in stool R19.5
  localized (pad) E65
    heart — *see* Degeneration, myocardial
    knee M79.4
    retropatellar M79.4
  necrosis
    breast N64.1
    mesentery K65.4
    omentum K65.4
  pad E65
    knee M79.4
Fatigue R53.83
  auditory deafness — *see* Deafness
  chronic R53.82
  combat F43.0
  general R53.83
    psychogenic F48.8
  heat (transient) T67.6 ☑
  muscle M62.89
  myocardium — *see* Failure, heart
  neoplasm-related R53.0
  nervous, neurosis F48.8
  operational F48.8
  psychogenic (general) F48.8
  senile R54
  voice R49.8
Fatness — *see* Obesity
Fatty (*see also* condition)
  apron E65
  degeneration — *see* Degeneration, fatty
  heart (enlarged) — *see* Degeneration, myocardial
  liver NEC K76.0
    alcoholic K70.0
    nonalcoholic K76.0
  necrosis — *see* Degeneration, fatty
Fauces — *see* condition
Fauchard's disease (periodontitis) — *see* Periodontitis
Faucitis J02.9
Favism (anemia) D55.0
Favus — *see* Dermatophytosis
Fazio-Londe disease or syndrome G12.1
Fear complex or reaction F40.9
Fear of — *see* Phobia
Feared complaint unfounded Z71.1
Febris, febrile (*see also* Fever)
  flava (*see also* Fever, yellow) A95.9
  melitensis A23.0
  pestis — *see* Plague
  recurrens — *see* Fever, relapsing
  rubra A38.9
Fecal
  incontinence R15.9
  smearing R15.1
  soiling R15.1
  urgency R15.2
Fecalith (impaction) K56.41
  appendix K38.1
  congenital P76.8
Fede's disease K14.0

Feeble rapid pulse due to shock following injury T79.4 ☑
Feeble-minded F70
Feeding
 difficulties R63.3
 problem R63.3
  newborn P92.9
   specified NEC P92.8
  nonorganic (adult) — see Disorder, eating
Feeling (of)
 foreign body in throat R09.89
Feer's disease — see Poisoning, mercury
Feet — see condition
Feigned illness Z76.5
Feil-Klippel syndrome (brevicollis) Q76.1
Feinmesser's (hidrotic) **ectodermal dysplasia** Q82.4
Felinophobia F40.218
Felon (see also Cellulitis, digit)
 with lymphangitis — see Lymphangitis, acute, digit
Felty's syndrome M05.00
 ankle M05.07- ☑
 elbow M05.02- ☑
 foot joint M05.07- ☑
 hand joint M05.04- ☑
 hip M05.05- ☑
 knee M05.06- ☑
 multiple site M05.09
 shoulder M05.01- ☑
 vertebra — see Spondylitis, ankylosing
 wrist M05.03- ☑
Female genital cutting status — see Female genital mutilation status (FGM)
Female genital mutilation status (FGM) N90.810
 specified NEC N90.818
 type I (clitorectomy status) N90.811
 type II (clitorectomy with excision of labia minora status) N90.812
 type III (infibulation status) N90.813
 type IV N90.818
Femur, femoral — see condition
Fenestration, fenestrated (see also Imperfect, closure)
 aortico-pulmonary Q21.4
 cusps, heart valve NEC Q24.8
  pulmonary Q22.3
 pulmonic cusps Q22.3
Fernell's disease (aortic aneurysm) I71.9
Fertile eunuch syndrome E23.0
Fetid
 breath R19.6
 sweat L75.0
Fetishism F65.0
 transvestic F65.1
Fetus, fetal (see also condition)
 alcohol syndrome (dysmorphic) Q86.0
 compressus O31.0- ☑
 hydantoin syndrome Q86.1
 lung tissue P28.0
 papyraceous O31.0- ☑
Fever (inanition) (of unknown origin) (persistent) (with chills) (with rigor) R50.9
 abortus A23.1
 Aden (dengue) A90
 African tick-borne A68.1
 American
  mountain (tick) A93.2
  spotted A77.0
 aphthous B08.8
 arbovirus, arboviral A94
  hemorrhagic A94
  specified NEC A93.8
 Argentinian hemorrhagic A96.0
 Assam B55.0
 Australian Q A78
 Bangkok hemorrhagic A91
 Barmah forest A92.8
 Bartonella A44.0
 bilious, hemoglobinuric B50.8
 blackwater B50.8
 blister B00.1
 Bolivian hemorrhagic A96.1
 Bonvale dam T73.3 ☑
 boutonneuse A77.1
 brain — see Encephalitis
 Brazilian purpuric A48.4
 breakbone A90
 Bullis A77.0
 Bunyamwera A92.8

Fever — continued
 Burdwan B55.0
 Bwamba A92.8
 Cameroon — see Malaria
 Canton A75.9
 catarrhal (acute) J00
  chronic J31.0
 cat-scratch A28.1
 Central Asian hemorrhagic A98.0
 cerebral — see Encephalitis
 cerebrospinal meningococcal A39.0
 Chagres B50.9
 Chandipura A92.8
 Changuinola A93.1
 Charcot's (biliary) (hepatic) (intermittent) — see Calculus, bile duct
 Chikungunya (viral) (hemorrhagic) A92.0
 Chitral A93.1
 Colombo — see Fever, paratyphoid
 Colorado tick (virus) A93.2
 congestive (remittent) — see Malaria
 Congo virus A98.0
 continued malarial B50.9
 Corsican — see Malaria
 Crimean-Congo hemorrhagic A98.0
 Cyprus — see Brucellosis
 dandy A90
 deer fly — see Tularemia
 dengue (virus) A90
  hemorrhagic A91
  sandfly A93.1
 desert B38.0
 drug induced R50.2
 due to
  conditions classified elsewhere R50.81
  heat T67.0 ☑
 enteric A01.00
 enteroviral exanthematous (Boston exanthem) A88.0
 ephemeral (of unknown origin) R50.9
 epidemic hemorrhagic A98.5
 erysipelatous — see Erysipelas
 estivo-autumnal (malarial) B50.9
 famine A75.0
 five day A79.0
 following delivery O86.4
 Fort Bragg A27.89
 gastroenteric A01.00
 gastromalarial — see Malaria
 Gibraltar — see Brucellosis
 glandular — see Mononucleosis, infectious
 Guama (viral) A92.8
 Haverhill A25.1
 hay (allergic) J30.1
  with asthma (bronchial) J45.909
   with
    exacerbation (acute) J45.901
    status asthmaticus J45.902
   due to
    allergen other than pollen J30.89
    pollen, any plant or tree J30.1
 heat (effects) T67.0 ☑
 hematuric, bilious B50.8
 hemoglobinuric (malarial) (bilious) B50.8
 hemorrhagic (arthropod-borne) NOS A94
  with renal syndrome A98.5
  arenaviral A96.9
   specified NEC A96.8
  Argentinian A96.0
  Bangkok A91
  Bolivian A96.1
  Central Asian A98.0
  Chikungunya A92.0
  Crimean-Congo A98.0
  dengue (virus) A91
  epidemic A98.5
  Junin (virus) A96.0
  Korean A98.5
  Kyasanur forest A98.2
  Machupo (virus) A96.1
  mite-borne A93.8
  mosquito-borne A92.8
  Omsk A98.1
  Philippine A91
  Russian A98.5
  Singapore A91
  Southeast Asia A91
  Thailand A91
  tick-borne NEC A93.8

Fever — continued
 hemorrhagic — continued
  viral A99
   specified NEC A98.8
 hepatic — see Cholecystitis
 herpetic — see Herpes
 icterohemorrhagic A27.0
 Indiana A93.8
 infective B99.9
  specified NEC B99.8
 intermittent (bilious) (see also Malaria)
  of unknown origin R50.9
  pernicious B50.9
 iodide R50.2
 Japanese river A75.3
 jungle (see also Malaria)
  yellow A95.0
 Junin (virus) hemorrhagic A96.0
 Katayama B65.2
 kedani A75.3
 Kenya (tick) A77.1
 Kew Garden A79.1
 Korean hemorrhagic A98.5
 Lassa A96.2
 Lone Star A77.0
 Machupo (virus) hemorrhagic A96.1
 malaria, malarial — see Malaria
 Malta A23.9
 Marseilles A77.1
 marsh — see Malaria
 Mayaro (viral) A92.8
 Mediterranean (see also Brucellosis) A23.9
  familial M04.1
  tick A77.1
 meningeal — see Meningitis
 Meuse A79.0
 Mexican A75.2
 mianeh A68.1
 miasmatic — see Malaria
 mosquito-borne (viral) A92.9
  hemorrhagic A92.8
 mountain (see also Brucellosis)
  meaning Rocky Mountain spotted fever A77.0
  tick (American) (Colorado) (viral) A93.2
 Mucambo (viral) A92.8
 mud A27.9
 Neapolitan — see Brucellosis
 neutropenic D70.9
 newborn P81.9
  environmental P81.0
 Nine-Mile A78
 non-exanthematous tick A93.2
 North Asian tick-borne A77.2
 Omsk hemorrhagic A98.1
 O'nyong-nyong (viral) A92.1
 Oropouche (viral) A93.0
 Oroya A44.0
 paludal — see Malaria
 Panama (malarial) B50.9
 Pappataci A93.1
 paratyphoid A01.4
  A A01.1
  B A01.2
  C A01.3
 parrot A70
 periodic (Mediterranean) M04.1
 persistent (of unknown origin) R50.9
 petechial A39.0
 pharyngoconjunctival B30.2
 Philippine hemorrhagic A91
 phlebotomus A93.1
 Piry (virus) A93.8
 Pixuna (viral) A92.8
 Plasmodium ovale B53.0
 polioviral (nonparalytic) A80.4
 Pontiac A48.2
 postimmunization R50.83
 postoperative R50.82
  due to infection T81.4 ☑
 posttransfusion R50.84
 postvaccination R50.83
 presenting with conditions classified elsewhere R50.81
 pretibial A27.89
 puerperal O86.4
 Q A78
 quadrilateral A78
 quartan (malaria) B52.9
 Queensland (coastal) (tick) A77.3

Fever — *continued*
- quintan A79.0
- rabbit — *see* Tularemia
- rat-bite A25.9
  - due to
    - Spirillum A25.0
    - Streptobacillus moniliformis A25.1
- recurrent — *see* Fever, relapsing
- relapsing (Borrelia) A68.9
  - Carter's (Asiatic) A68.1
  - Dutton's (West African) A68.1
  - Koch's A68.9
  - louse-borne A68.0
  - Novy's
    - louse-borne A68.0
    - tick-borne A68.1
  - Obermeyer's (European) A68.0
  - tick-borne A68.1
- remittent (bilious) (congestive) (gastric) — *see* Malaria
- rheumatic (active) (acute) (chronic) (subacute) I00
  - with central nervous system involvement I02.9
  - active with heart involvement — *see* category I01 ☑
  - inactive or quiescent with
    - cardiac hypertrophy I09.89
    - carditis I09.9
    - endocarditis I09.1
      - aortic (valve) I06.9
        - with mitral (valve) disease I08.0
      - mitral (valve) I05.9
        - with aortic (valve) disease I08.0
      - pulmonary (valve) I09.89
      - tricuspid (valve) I07.8
    - heart disease NEC I09.89
    - heart failure (congestive) (conditions in I50.) I09.81
    - left ventricular failure (conditions in I50.1-I50.4-) I09.81
    - myocarditis, myocardial degeneration (conditions in I51.4) I09.0
    - pancarditis I09.9
    - pericarditis I09.2
- Rift Valley (viral) A92.4
- Rocky Mountain spotted A77.0
- rose J30.1
- Ross River B33.1
- Russian hemorrhagic A98.5
- San Joaquin (Valley) B38.0
- sandfly A93.1
- Sao Paulo A77.0
- scarlet A38.9
- seven day (leptospirosis) (autumnal) (Japanese) A27.89
  - dengue A90
- shin-bone A79.0
- Singapore hemorrhagic A91
- solar A90
- Songo A98.5
- sore B00.1
- South African tick-bite A68.1
- Southeast Asia hemorrhagic A91
- spinal — *see* Meningitis
- spirillary A25.0
- splenic — *see* Anthrax
- spotted A77.9
  - American A77.0
  - Brazilian A77.0
  - cerebrospinal meningitis A39.0
  - Colombian A77.0
  - due to Rickettsia
    - australis A77.3
    - conorii A77.1
    - rickettsii A77.0
    - sibirica A77.2
    - specified type NEC A77.8
  - Ehrlichiosis A77.40
    - due to
      - E. chaffeensis A77.41
      - specified organism NEC A77.49
  - Rocky Mountain A77.0
- steroid R50.2
- streptobacillary A25.1
- subtertian B50.9
- Sumatran mite A75.3
- sun A90
- swamp A27.9
- swine A02.8
- sylvatic, yellow A95.0
- Tahyna B33.8

Fever — *continued*
- tertian — *see* Malaria, tertian
- Thailand hemorrhagic A91
- thermic T67.0 ☑
- three-day A93.1
- tick
  - American mountain A93.2
  - Colorado A93.2
  - Kemerovo A93.8
  - Mediterranean A77.1
  - mountain A93.2
  - nonexanthematous A93.2
  - Quaranfil A93.8
- tick-bite NEC A93.8
- tick-borne (hemorrhagic) NEC A93.8
- trench A79.0
- tsutsugamushi A75.3
- typhogastric A01.00
- typhoid (abortive) (hemorrhagic) (intermittent) (malignant) A01.00
  - complicated by
    - arthritis A01.04
    - heart involvement A01.02
    - meningitis A01.01
    - osteomyelitis A01.05
    - pneumonia A01.03
    - specified NEC A01.09
- typhomalarial — *see* Malaria
- typhus — *see* Typhus (fever)
- undulant — *see* Brucellosis
- unknown origin R50.9
- uveoparotid D86.89
- valley B38.0
- Venezuelan equine A92.2
- vesicular stomatitis A93.8
- viral hemorrhagic — *see* Fever, hemorrhagic, by type of virus
- Volhynian A79.0
- Wesselsbron (viral) A92.8
- West
  - African B50.8
  - Nile (viral) A92.30
    - with
      - complications NEC A92.39
      - cranial nerve disorders A92.32
      - encephalitis A92.31
      - encephalomyelitis A92.31
      - neurologic manifestation NEC A92.32
      - optic neuritis A92.32
      - polyradiculitis A92.32
- Whitmore's — *see* Melioidosis
- Wolhynian A79.0
- worm B83.9
- yellow A95.9
  - jungle A95.0
  - sylvatic A95.0
  - urban A95.1
- Zika virus A92.5

Fibrillation
- atrial or auricular (established) I48.91
  - chronic I48.2
  - paroxysmal I48.0
  - permanent I48.2
  - persistent I48.1
- cardiac I49.8
- heart I49.8
- muscular M62.89
- ventricular I49.01

Fibrin
- ball or bodies, pleural (sac) J94.1
- chamber, anterior (eye) (gelatinous exudate) — *see* Iridocyclitis, acute

Fibrinogenolysis — *see* Fibrinolysis

Fibrinogenopenia D68.8
- acquired D65
- congenital D68.2

Fibrinolysis (hemorrhagic) (acquired) D65
- antepartum hemorrhage — *see* Hemorrhage, antepartum, with coagulation defect
- following
  - abortion — *see* Abortion by type complicated by hemorrhage
  - ectopic or molar pregnancy O08.1
- intrapartum O67.0
- newborn, transient P60
- postpartum O72.3

Fibrinopenia (hereditary) D68.2
- acquired D68.4

Fibrinopurulent — *see* condition

Fibrinous — *see* condition

Fibroadenoma
- cellular intracanalicular D24- ☑
- giant D24- ☑
- intracanalicular
  - cellular D24- ☑
  - giant D24- ☑
  - specified site — *see* Neoplasm, benign, by site
  - unspecified site D24- ☑
- juvenile D24- ☑
- pericanalicular
  - specified site — *see* Neoplasm, benign, by site
  - unspecified site D24- ☑
- phyllodes D24- ☑
- prostate D29.1
- specified site NEC — *see* Neoplasm, benign, by site
- unspecified site D24- ☑

Fibroadenosis, breast (chronic) (cystic) (diffuse) (periodic) (segmental) N60.2- ☑

Fibroangioma (*see also* Neoplasm, benign, by site)
- juvenile
  - specified site — *see* Neoplasm, benign, by site
  - unspecified site D10.6

Fibrochondrosarcoma — *see* Neoplasm, cartilage, malignant

Fibrocystic
- disease (*see also* Fibrosis, cystic)
  - breast — *see* Mastopathy, cystic
  - jaw M27.49
  - kidney (congenital) Q61.8
  - liver Q44.6
  - pancreas E84.9
- kidney (congenital) Q61.8

Fibrodysplasia ossificans progressiva — *see* Myositis, ossificans, progressiva

Fibroelastosis (cordis) (endocardial) (endomyocardial) I42.4

Fibroid (tumor) (*see also* Neoplasm, connective tissue, benign)
- disease, lung (chronic) — *see* Fibrosis, lung
- heart (disease) — *see* Myocarditis
- in pregnancy or childbirth O34.1- ☑
  - causing obstructed labor O65.5
- induration, lung (chronic) — *see* Fibrosis, lung
- lung — *see* Fibrosis, lung
- pneumonia (chronic) — *see* Fibrosis, lung
- uterus (*see also* Leiomyoma, uterus) D25.9

Fibrolipoma — *see* Lipoma

Fibroliposarcoma — *see* Neoplasm, connective tissue, malignant

Fibroma (*see also* Neoplasm, connective tissue, benign)
- ameloblastic — *see* Cyst, calcifying odontogenic
- bone (nonossifying) — *see* Disorder, bone, specified type NEC
  - ossifying — *see* Neoplasm, bone, benign
- cementifying — *see* Neoplasm, bone, benign
- chondromyxoid — *see* Neoplasm, bone, benign
- desmoplastic — *see* Neoplasm, connective tissue, uncertain behavior
- durum — *see* Neoplasm, connective tissue, benign
- fascial — *see* Neoplasm, connective tissue, benign
- invasive — *see* Neoplasm, connective tissue, uncertain behavior
- molle — *see* Lipoma
- myxoid — *see* Neoplasm, connective tissue, benign
- nasopharynx, nasopharyngeal (juvenile) D10.6
- nonosteogenic (nonossifying) — *see* Dysplasia, fibrous
- odontogenic (central) — *see* Cyst, calcifying odontogenic
- ossifying — *see* Neoplasm, bone, benign
- periosteal — *see* Neoplasm, bone, benign
- soft — *see* Lipoma

Fibromatosis M72.9
- abdominal — *see* Neoplasm, connective tissue, uncertain behavior
- aggressive — *see* Neoplasm, connective tissue, uncertain behavior
- congenital generalized — *see* Neoplasm, connective tissue, uncertain behavior
- Dupuytren's M72.0
- gingival K06.1
- palmar (fascial) M72.0
- plantar (fascial) M72.2
- pseudosarcomatous (proliferative) (subcutaneous) M72.4
- retroperitoneal D48.3

☑ Additional Character Required — Refer to the Tabular List for Character Selection   〰 Subterms under main terms may continue to next column or page

Fibromatosis — *continued*
  specified NEC M72.8
Fibromyalgia M79.7
Fibromyoma (*see also* Neoplasm, connective tissue, benign)
  uterus (corpus) (*see also* Leiomyoma, uterus)
    in pregnancy or childbirth — *see* Fibroid, in pregnancy or childbirth
      causing obstructed labor O65.5
Fibromyositis M79.7
Fibromyxolipoma D17.9
Fibromyxoma — *see* Neoplasm, connective tissue, benign
Fibromyxosarcoma — *see* Neoplasm, connective tissue, malignant
Fibro-odontoma, ameloblastic — *see* Cyst, calcifying odontogenic
Fibro-osteoma — *see* Neoplasm, bone, benign
Fibroplasia, retrolental H35.17- ☑
Fibropurulent — *see* condition
Fibrosarcoma (*see also* Neoplasm, connective tissue, malignant)
  ameloblastic C41.1
    upper jaw (bone) C41.0
  congenital — *see* Neoplasm, connective tissue, malignant
  fascial — *see* Neoplasm, connective tissue, malignant
  infantile — *see* Neoplasm, connective tissue, malignant
  odontogenic C41.1
    upper jaw (bone) C41.0
  periosteal — *see* Neoplasm, bone, malignant
Fibrosclerosis
  breast N60.3- ☑
  multifocal M35.5
  penis (corpora cavernosa) N48.6
Fibrosis, fibrotic
  adrenal (gland) E27.8
  amnion O41.8X- ☑
  anal papillae K62.89
  arteriocapillary — *see* Arteriosclerosis
  bladder N32.89
    interstitial — *see* Cystitis, chronic, interstitial
    localized submucosal — *see* Cystitis, chronic, interstitial
    panmural — *see* Cystitis, chronic, interstitial
  breast — *see* Fibrosclerosis, breast
  capillary (*see also* Arteriosclerosis) I70.90
    lung (chronic) — *see* Fibrosis, lung
  cardiac — *see* Myocarditis
  cervix N88.8
  chorion O41.8X- ☑
  corpus cavernosum (sclerosing) N48.6
  cystic (of pancreas) E84.9
    with
      distal intestinal obstruction syndrome E84.19
      fecal impaction E84.19
      intestinal manifestations NEC E84.19
      pulmonary manifestations E84.0
      specified manifestations NEC E84.8
  due to device, implant or graft (*see also* Complications, by site and type, specified NEC) T85.828 ☑
    arterial graft NEC T82.828 ☑
    breast (implant) T85.828 ☑
    catheter NEC T85.828 ☑
      dialysis (renal) T82.828 ☑
        intraperitoneal T85.828 ☑
      infusion NEC T82.828 ☑
        spinal (epidural) (subdural) T85.820 ☑
      urinary (indwelling) T83.82 ☑
    electronic (electrode) (pulse generator) (stimulator)
      bone T84.82 ☑
      cardiac T82.827 ☑
      nervous system (brain) (peripheral nerve) (spinal) T85.820 ☑
      urinary T83.82 ☑
    fixation, internal (orthopedic) NEC T84.82 ☑
    gastrointestinal (bile duct) (esophagus) T85.828 ☑
    genital NEC T83.82 ☑
    heart NEC T82.827 ☑
    joint prosthesis T84.82 ☑
    ocular (corneal graft) (orbital implant) NEC T85.828 ☑
    orthopedic NEC T84.82 ☑
    specified NEC T85.828 ☑
    urinary NEC T83.82 ☑
    vascular NEC T82.828 ☑

Fibrosis, fibrotic — *continued*
  due to device, implant or graft (*see also* Complications, by site and type, specified) — *continued*
    ventricular intracranial shunt T85.820 ☑
  ejaculatory duct N50.89
  endocardium — *see* Endocarditis
  endomyocardial (tropical) I42.3
  epididymis N50.89
  eye muscle — *see* Strabismus, mechanical
  heart — *see* Myocarditis
  hepatic — *see* Fibrosis, liver
  hepatolienal (portal hypertension) K76.6
  hepatosplenic (portal hypertension) K76.6
  infrapatellar fat pad M79.4
  intrascrotal N50.89
  kidney N26.9
  liver K74.0
    with sclerosis K74.2
    alcoholic K70.2
  lung (atrophic) (chronic) (confluent) (massive) (perialveolar) (peribronchial) J84.10
    with
      anthracosilicosis J60
      anthracosis J60
      asbestosis J61
      bagassosis J67.1
      bauxite J63.1
      berylliosis J63.2
      byssinosis J66.0
      calcicosis J62.8
      chalicosis J62.8
      dust reticulation J64
      farmer's lung J67.0
      ganister disease J62.8
      graphite J63.3
      pneumoconiosis NOS J64
      siderosis J63.4
      silicosis J62.8
    capillary J84.10
    congenital P27.8
    diffuse (idiopathic) J84.10
      chemicals, gases, fumes or vapors (inhalation) J68.4
      interstitial J84.10
        acute J84.114
      talc J62.0
    following radiation J70.1
    idiopathic J84.112
    postinflammatory J84.10
    silicotic J62.8
    tuberculous — *see* Tuberculosis, pulmonary
  lymphatic gland I89.8
  median bar — *see* Hyperplasia, prostate
  mediastinum (idiopathic) J98.59
  meninges G96.19
  myocardium, myocardial — *see* Myocarditis
  ovary N83.8
  oviduct N83.8
  pancreas K86.89
  penis NEC N48.6
  pericardium I31.0
  perineum, in pregnancy or childbirth O34.7- ☑
    causing obstructed labor O65.5
  pleura J94.1
  popliteal fat pad M79.4
  prostate (chronic) — *see* Hyperplasia, prostate
  pulmonary (*see also* Fibrosis, lung) J84.10
    congenital P27.8
    idiopathic J84.112
  rectal sphincter K62.89
  retroperitoneal, idiopathic (with ureteral obstruction) N13.5
    with infection N13.6
  sclerosing mesenteric (idiopathic) K65.4
  scrotum N50.89
  seminal vesicle N50.89
  senile R54
  skin L90.5
  spermatic cord N50.89
  spleen D73.89
    in schistosomiasis (bilharziasis) B65.9 [D77]
  subepidermal nodular — *see* Neoplasm, skin, benign
  submucous (oral) (tongue) K13.5
  testis N44.8
    chronic, due to syphilis A52.76
  thymus (gland) E32.8
  tongue, submucous K13.5
  tunica vaginalis N50.89

Fibrosis, fibrotic — *continued*
  uterus (non-neoplastic) N85.8
  vagina N89.8
  valve, heart — *see* Endocarditis
  vas deferens N50.89
  vein I87.8
Fibrositis (periarticular) M79.7
  nodular, chronic (Jaccoud's) (rheumatoid) — *see* Arthropathy, postrheumatic, chronic
Fibrothorax J94.1
Fibrotic — *see* Fibrosis
Fibrous — *see* condition
Fibroxanthoma (*see also* Neoplasm, connective tissue, benign)
  atypical — *see* Neoplasm, connective tissue, uncertain behavior
  malignant — *see* Neoplasm, connective tissue, malignant
Fibroxanthosarcoma — *see* Neoplasm, connective tissue, malignant
Fiedler's
  disease (icterohemorrhagic leptospirosis) A27.0
  myocarditis (acute) I40.1
Fifth disease B08.3
  venereal A55
Filaria, filarial, filariasis — *see* Infestation, filarial
Filatov's disease — *see* Mononucleosis, infectious
File-cutter's disease — *see* Poisoning, lead
Filling defect
  biliary tract R93.2
  bladder R93.41
  duodenum R93.3
  gallbladder R93.2
  gastrointestinal tract R93.3
  intestine R93.3
  kidney R93.42- ☑
  stomach R93.3
  ureter R93.41
  urinary organs, specified NEC R93.49
Fimbrial cyst Q50.4
Financial problem affecting care NOS Z59.9
  bankruptcy Z59.8
  foreclosure on loan Z59.8
Findings, abnormal, inconclusive, without diagnosis (*see also* Abnormal)
  17-ketosteroids, elevated R82.5
  acetonuria R82.4
  alcohol in blood R78.0
  anisocytosis R71.8
  antenatal screening of mother O28.9
    biochemical O28.1
    chromosomal O28.5
    cytological O28.2
    genetic O28.5
    hematological O28.0
    radiological O28.4
    specified NEC O28.8
    ultrasonic O28.3
  antibody titer, elevated R76.0
  anticardiolipin antibody R76.0
  antiphosphatidylglycerol antibody R76.0
  antiphosphatidylinositol antibody R76.0
  antiphosphatidylserine antibody R76.0
  antiphospholipid antibody R76.0
  bacteriuria R82.71
  bicarbonate E87.8
  bile in urine R82.2
  blood sugar R73.09
    high R73.9
    low (transient) E16.2
  body fluid or substance, specified NEC R88.8
  casts, urine R82.99
  catecholamines R82.5
  cells, urine R82.99
  chloride E87.8
  cholesterol E78.9
    high E78.00
      with high triglycerides E78.2
  chyluria R82.0
  cloudy
    dialysis effluent R88.0
    urine R82.90
  creatinine clearance R94.4
  crystals, urine R82.99
  culture
    blood R78.81
    positive — *see* Positive, culture
  echocardiogram R93.1

Findings, abnormal, inconclusive, without diagnosis
— *continued*
electrolyte level, urinary R82.99
function study NEC R94.8
 bladder R94.8
 endocrine NEC R94.7
  thyroid R94.6
 kidney R94.4
 liver R94.5
 pancreas R94.8
 placenta R94.8
 pulmonary R94.2
 spleen R94.8
gallbladder, nonvisualization R93.2
glucose (tolerance test) (non-fasting) R73.09
glycosuria R81
heart
 shadow R93.1
 sounds R01.2
hematinuria R82.3
hematocrit drop (precipitous) R71.0
hemoglobinuria R82.3
human papillomavirus (HPV) DNA test positive
 cervix
  high risk R87.810
  low risk R87.820
 vagina
  high risk R87.811
  low risk R87.821
in blood (of substance not normally found in blood) R78.9
 addictive drug NEC R78.4
 alcohol (excessive level) R78.0
 cocaine R78.2
 hallucinogen R78.3
 heavy metals (abnormal level) R78.79
 lead R78.71
 lithium (abnormal level) R78.89
 opiate drug R78.1
 psychotropic drug R78.5
 specified substance NEC R78.89
 steroid agent R78.6
indoleacetic acid, elevated R82.5
ketonuria R82.4
lactic acid dehydrogenase (LDH) R74.0
liver function test R79.89
mammogram NEC R92.8
 calcification (calculus) R92.1
 inconclusive result (due to dense breasts) R92.2
 microcalcification R92.0
mediastinal shift R93.8
melanin, urine R82.99
myoglobinuria R82.1
neonatal screening P09
nonvisualization of gallbladder R93.2
odor of urine NOS R82.90
Papanicolaou cervix R87.619
 non-atypical endometrial cells R87.618
pneumoencephalogram R93.0
poikilocytosis R71.8
potassium (deficiency) E87.6
 excess E87.5
PPD R76.11
radiologic (X-ray) R93.8
 abdomen R93.5
 biliary tract R93.2
 breast R92.8
 gastrointestinal tract R93.3
 genitourinary organs R93.8
 head R93.0
 inconclusive due to excess body fat of patient R93.9
 intrathoracic organs NEC R93.1
 placenta R93.8
 retroperitoneum R93.5
 skin R93.8
 skull R93.0
 subcutaneous tissue R93.8
red blood cell (count) (morphology) (sickling) (volume) R71.8
scan NEC R94.8
 bladder R94.8
 bone R94.8
 kidney R94.4
 liver R93.2
 lung R94.2
 pancreas R94.8
 placental R94.8
 spleen R94.8
 thyroid R94.6

Findings, abnormal, inconclusive, without diagnosis
— *continued*
sedimentation rate, elevated R70.0
SGOT R74.0
SGPT R74.0
sodium (deficiency) E87.1
 excess E87.0
specified body fluid NEC R88.8
stress test R94.39
thyroid (function) (metabolic rate) (scan) (uptake) R94.6
transaminase (level) R74.0
triglycerides E78.9
 high E78.1
  with high cholesterol E78.2
tuberculin skin test (without active tuberculosis) R76.11
urine R82.90
 acetone R82.4
 bacteria R82.71
 bile R82.2
 casts or cells R82.99
 chyle R82.0
 culture positive R82.79
 glucose R81
 hemoglobin R82.3
 ketone R82.4
 sugar R81
vanillylmandelic acid (VMA), elevated R82.5
vectorcardiogram (VCG) R94.39
ventriculogram R93.0
white blood cell (count) (differential) (morphology) D72.9
xerography R92.8
Finger — *see* condition
Fire, Saint Anthony's — *see* Erysipelas
Fire-setting
pathological (compulsive) F63.1
Fish hook stomach K31.89
Fishmeal-worker's lung J67.8
Fissure, fissured
anus, anal K60.2
 acute K60.0
 chronic K60.1
 congenital Q43.8
ear, lobule, congenital Q17.8
epiglottis (congenital) Q31.8
larynx J38.7
 congenital Q31.8
lip K13.0
 congenital — *see* Cleft, lip
nipple N64.0
 associated with
  lactation O92.13
  pregnancy O92.11- ☑
  puerperium O92.12
nose Q30.2
palate (congenital) — *see* Cleft, palate
skin R23.4
spine (congenital) (*see also* Spina bifida)
 with hydrocephalus — *see* Spina bifida, by site, with hydrocephalus
tongue (acquired) K14.5
 congenital Q38.3
Fistula (cutaneous) L98.8
abdomen (wall) K63.2
 bladder N32.2
 intestine NEC K63.2
 ureter N28.89
 uterus N82.5
abdominorectal K63.2
abdominosigmoidal K63.2
abdominothoracic J86.0
abdominouterine N82.5
 congenital Q51.7
abdominovesical N32.2
accessory sinuses — *see* Sinusitis
actinomycotic — *see* Actinomycosis
alveolar antrum — *see* Sinusitis, maxillary
alveolar process K04.6
anorectal K60.5
antrobuccal — *see* Sinusitis, maxillary
antrum — *see* Sinusitis, maxillary
anus, anal (recurrent) (infectional) K60.3
 congenital Q43.6
  with absence, atresia and stenosis Q42.2
 tuberculous A18.32
aorta-duodenal I77.2

Fistula — *continued*
appendix, appendicular K38.3
arteriovenous (acquired) (nonruptured) I77.0
 brain I67.1
  congenital Q28.2
   ruptured I60.8
  ruptured I60.8
 cerebral — *see* Fistula, arteriovenous, brain
 congenital (peripheral) (*see also* Malformation, arteriovenous)
  brain Q28.2
   ruptured I60.8
  coronary Q24.5
  pulmonary Q25.72
 coronary I25.41
  congenital Q24.5
 pulmonary I28.0
  congenital Q25.72
 surgically created (for dialysis) Z99.2
  complication — *see* Complication, arteriovenous, fistula, surgically created
 traumatic — *see* Injury, blood vessel
artery I77.2
aural (mastoid) — *see* Mastoiditis, chronic
auricle (*see also* Disorder, pinna, specified type NEC)
 congenital Q18.1
Bartholin's gland N82.8
bile duct (common) (hepatic) K83.3
 with calculus, stones — *see* Calculus, bile duct
biliary (tract) — *see* Fistula, bile duct
bladder (sphincter) NEC (*see also* Fistula, vesico-) N32.2
 into seminal vesicle N32.2
bone (*see also* Disorder, bone, specified type NEC)
 with osteomyelitis, chronic — *see* Osteomyelitis, chronic, with draining sinus
brain G93.89
 arteriovenous (acquired) I67.1
  congenital Q28.2
branchial (cleft) Q18.0
branchiogenous Q18.0
breast N61.0
 puerperal, postpartum or gestational, due to mastitis (purulent) — *see* Mastitis, obstetric, purulent
bronchial J86.0
bronchocutaneous, bronchomediastinal, bronchopleural, bronchopleuromediastinal (infective) J86.0
 tuberculous NEC A15.5
bronchoesophageal J86.0
 congenital Q39.2
  with atresia of esophagus Q39.1
bronchovisceral J86.0
buccal cavity (infective) K12.2
cecosigmoidal K63.2
cecum K63.2
cerebrospinal (fluid) G96.0
cervical, lateral Q18.1
cervicoaural Q18.1
cervicosigmoidal N82.4
cervicovesical N82.1
cervix N82.8
chest (wall) J86.0
cholecystenteric — *see* Fistula, gallbladder
cholecystocolic — *see* Fistula, gallbladder
cholecystocolonic — *see* Fistula, gallbladder
cholecystoduodenal — *see* Fistula, gallbladder
cholecystogastric — *see* Fistula, gallbladder
cholecystointestinal — *see* Fistula, gallbladder
choledochoduodenal — *see* Fistula, bile duct
cholocolic K82.3
coccyx — *see* Sinus, pilonidal
colon K63.2
colostomy K94.09
common duct — *see* Fistula, bile duct
congenital, site not listed — *see* Anomaly, by site
coronary, arteriovenous I25.41
 congenital Q24.5
costal region J86.0
cul-de-sac, Douglas' N82.8
cystic duct (*see also* Fistula, gallbladder)
 congenital Q44.5
dental K04.6
diaphragm J86.0
duodenum K31.6
ear (external) (canal) — *see* Disorder, ear, external, specified type NEC
enterocolic K63.2
enterocutaneous K63.2

☑ **Additional Character Required** — Refer to the Tabular List for Character Selection Subterms under main terms may continue to next column or page

Fistula — *continued*
  enterouterine N82.4
    congenital Q51.7
  enterovaginal N82.4
    congenital Q52.2
    large intestine N82.3
    small intestine N82.2
  enterovesical N32.1
  epididymis N50.89
    tuberculous A18.15
  esophagobronchial J86.0
    congenital Q39.2
      with atresia of esophagus Q39.1
  esophagocutaneous K22.8
  esophagopleural-cutaneous J86.0
  esophagotracheal J86.0
    congenital Q39.2
      with atresia of esophagus Q39.1
  esophagus K22.8
    congenital Q39.2
      with atresia of esophagus Q39.1
  ethmoid — *see* Sinusitis, ethmoidal
  eyeball (cornea) (sclera) — *see* Disorder, globe, hypotony
  eyelid H01.8
  fallopian tube, external N82.5
  fecal K63.2
    congenital Q43.6
  from periapical abscess K04.6
  frontal sinus — *see* Sinusitis, frontal
  gallbladder K82.3
    with calculus, cholelithiasis, stones — *see* Calculus, gallbladder
  gastric K31.6
  gastrocolic K31.6
    congenital Q40.2
    tuberculous A18.32
  gastroenterocolic K31.6
  gastroesophageal K31.6
  gastrojejunal K31.6
  gastrojejunocolic K31.6
  genital tract (female) N82.9
    specified NEC N82.8
    to intestine NEC N82.4
    to skin N82.5
  hepatic artery-portal vein, congenital Q26.6
  hepatopleural J86.0
  hepatopulmonary J86.0
  ileorectal or ileosigmoidal K63.2
  ileovaginal N82.2
  ileovesical N32.1
  ileum K63.2
  in ano K60.3
    tuberculous A18.32
  inner ear (labyrinth) — *see* subcategory H83.1 ☑
  intestine NEC K63.2
  intestinocolonic (abdominal) K63.2
  intestinoureteral N28.89
  intestinouterine N82.4
  intestinovaginal N82.4
    large intestine N82.3
    small intestine N82.2
  intestinovesical N32.1
  ischiorectal (fossa) K61.3
  jejunum K63.2
  joint M25.10
    ankle M25.17- ☑
    elbow M25.12- ☑
    foot joint M25.17- ☑
    hand joint M25.14- ☑
    hip M25.15- ☑
    knee M25.16- ☑
    shoulder M25.11- ☑
    specified joint NEC M25.18
    tuberculous — *see* Tuberculosis, joint
    vertebrae M25.18
    wrist M25.13- ☑
  kidney N28.89
  labium (majus) (minus) N82.8
  labyrinth — *see* subcategory H83.1 ☑
  lacrimal (gland) (sac) H04.61- ☑
  lacrimonasal duct — *see* Fistula, lacrimal
  laryngotracheal, congenital Q34.8
  larynx J38.7
  lip K13.0
    congenital Q38.0
  lumbar, tuberculous A18.01
  lung J86.0

Fistula — *continued*
  lymphatic I89.8
  mammary (gland) N61.0
  mastoid (process) (region) — *see* Mastoiditis, chronic
  maxillary J32.0
  medial, face and neck Q18.8
  mediastinal J86.0
  mediastinobronchial J86.0
  mediastinocutaneous J86.0
  middle ear — *see* subcategory H74.8 ☑
  mouth K12.2
  nasal J34.89
    sinus — *see* Sinusitis
  nasopharynx J39.2
  nipple N64.0
  nose J34.89
  oral (cutaneous) K12.2
    maxillary J32.0
    nasal (with cleft palate) — *see* Cleft, palate
  orbit, orbital — *see* Disorder, orbit, specified type NEC
  oroantral J32.0
  oviduct, external N82.5
  palate (hard) M27.8
  pancreatic K86.89
  pancreaticoduodenal K86.89
  parotid (gland) K11.4
    region K12.2
  penis N48.89
  perianal K60.3
  pericardium (pleura) (sac) — *see* Pericarditis
  pericecal K63.2
  perineorectal K60.4
  perineosigmoidal K63.2
  perineum, perineal (with urethral involvement) NEC N36.0
    tuberculous A18.13
    ureter N28.89
  perirectal K60.4
    tuberculous A18.32
  peritoneum K65.9
  pharyngoesophageal J39.2
  pharynx J39.2
    branchial cleft (congenital) Q18.0
  pilonidal (infected) (rectum) — *see* Sinus, pilonidal
  pleura, pleural, pleurocutaneous, pleuroperitoneal J86.0
    tuberculous NEC A15.6
  pleuropericardial I31.8
  portal vein-hepatic artery, congenital Q26.6
  postauricular H70.81- ☑
  postoperative, persistent T81.83 ☑
    specified site — *see* Fistula, by site
  preauricular (congenital) Q18.1
  prostate N42.89
  pulmonary J86.0
    arteriovenous I28.0
      congenital Q25.72
    tuberculous — *see* Tuberculosis, pulmonary
  pulmonoperitoneal J86.0
  rectolabial N82.4
  rectosigmoid (intercommunicating) K63.2
  rectoureteral N28.89
  rectourethral N36.0
    congenital Q64.73
  rectouterine N82.4
    congenital Q51.7
  rectovaginal N82.3
    congenital Q52.2
    tuberculous A18.18
  rectovesical N32.1
    congenital Q64.79
  rectovesicovaginal N82.3
  rectovulval N82.4
    congenital Q52.79
  rectum (to skin) K60.4
    congenital Q43.6
      with absence, atresia and stenosis Q42.0
    tuberculous A18.32
  renal N28.89
  retroauricular — *see* Fistula, postauricular
  salivary duct or gland (any) K11.4
    congenital Q38.4
  scrotum (urinary) N50.89
    tuberculous A18.15
  semicircular canals — *see* subcategory H83.1 ☑
  sigmoid K63.2
    to bladder N32.1
  sinus — *see* Sinusitis

Fistula — *continued*
  skin L98.8
    to genital tract (female) N82.5
  splenocolic D73.89
  stercoral K63.2
  stomach K31.6
  sublingual gland K11.4
  submandibular gland K11.4
  submaxillary (gland) K11.4
    region K12.2
  thoracic J86.0
    duct I89.8
  thoracoabdominal J86.0
  thoracogastric J86.0
  thoracointestinal J86.0
  thorax J86.0
  thyroglossal duct Q89.2
  thyroid E07.89
  trachea, congenital (external) (internal) Q32.1
  tracheoesophageal J86.0
    congenital Q39.2
      with atresia of esophagus Q39.1
    following tracheostomy J95.04
  traumatic arteriovenous — *see* Injury, blood vessel, by site
  tuberculous — *code by* site under Tuberculosis
  typhoid A01.09
  umbilicourinary Q64.8
  urachus, congenital Q64.4
  ureter (persistent) N28.89
  ureteroabdominal N28.89
  ureterorectal N28.89
  ureterosigmoido-abdominal N28.89
  ureterovaginal N82.1
  ureterovesical N32.2
  urethra N36.0
    congenital Q64.79
    tuberculous A18.13
  urethroperineal N36.0
  urethroperineovesical N32.2
  urethrorectal N36.0
    congenital Q64.73
  urethroscrotal N50.89
  urethrovaginal N82.1
  urethrovesical N32.2
  urinary (tract) (persistent) (recurrent) N36.0
  uteroabdominal N82.5
    congenital Q51.7
  uteroenteric, uterointestinal N82.4
    congenital Q51.7
  uterorectal N82.4
    congenital Q51.7
  uteroureteric N82.1
  uterourethral Q51.7
  uterovaginal N82.8
  uterovesical N82.1
    congenital Q51.7
  uterus N82.8
  vagina (postpartal) (wall) N82.8
  vaginocutaneous (postpartal) N82.5
  vaginointestinal NEC N82.4
    large intestine N82.3
    small intestine N82.2
  vaginoperineal N82.5
  vasocutaneous, congenital Q55.7
  vesical NEC N32.2
  vesicoabdominal N32.2
  vesicocervicovaginal N82.1
  vesicocolic N32.1
  vesicocutaneous N32.2
  vesicoenteric N32.1
  vesicointestinal N32.1
  vesicometrorectal N82.4
  vesicoperineal N32.2
  vesicorectal N32.1
    congenital Q64.79
  vesicosigmoidal N32.1
  vesicosigmoidovaginal N82.3
  vesicoureteral N32.2
  vesicoureterovaginal N82.1
  vesicourethral N32.2
  vesicourethrorectal N32.1
  vesicouterine N82.1
    congenital Q51.7
  vesicovaginal N82.0
  vulvorectal N82.4
    congenital Q52.79
Fit R56.9
  epileptic — *see* Epilepsy

🔖 Subterms under main terms may continue to next column or page   ☑ Additional Character Required — Refer to the Tabular List for Character Selection   145

Fistula — Fit

Fit — *continued*
  fainting R55
  hysterical F44.5
  newborn P90
Fitting (and adjustment) (of)
  artificial
    arm — *see* Admission, adjustment, artificial, arm
    breast Z44.3 ☑
    eye Z44.2 ☑
    leg — *see* Admission, adjustment, artificial, leg
  automatic implantable cardiac defibrillator (with synchronous cardiac pacemaker) Z45.02
  brain neuropacemaker Z46.2
    implanted Z45.42
  cardiac defibrillator — *see* Fitting (and adjustment) (of), automatic implantable cardiac defibrillator
  catheter, non-vascular Z46.82
  colostomy belt Z46.89
  contact lenses Z46.0
  CRT-D (resynchronization therapy defibrillator) Z45.02
  CRT-P (cardiac resynchronization therapy pacemaker) Z45.018
    pulse generator Z45.010
  cystostomy device Z46.6
  defibrillator, cardiac — *see* Fitting (and adjustment) (of), automatic implantable cardiac defibrillator
  dentures Z46.3
  device NOS Z46.9
    abdominal Z46.89
    gastrointestinal NEC Z46.59
    implanted NEC Z45.89
    nervous system Z46.2
      implanted — *see* Admission, adjustment, device, implanted, nervous system
    orthodontic Z46.4
    orthoptic Z46.0
    orthotic Z46.89
    prosthetic (external) Z44.9
      breast Z44.3 ☑
      dental Z46.3
      eye Z44.2 ☑
      specified NEC Z44.8
    specified NEC Z46.89
    substitution
      auditory Z46.2
        implanted — *see* Admission, adjustment, device, implanted, hearing device
      nervous system Z46.2
        implanted — *see* Admission, adjustment, device, implanted, nervous system
      visual Z46.2
        implanted Z45.31
    urinary Z46.6
  gastric lap band Z46.51
  gastrointestinal appliance NEC Z46.59
  glasses (reading) Z46.0
  hearing aid Z46.1
  ileostomy device Z46.89
  insulin pump Z46.81
  intestinal appliance NEC Z46.89
  myringotomy device (stent) (tube) Z45.82
  neuropacemaker Z46.2
    implanted Z45.42
  non-vascular catheter Z46.82
  orthodontic device Z46.4
  orthopedic device (brace) (cast) (corset) (shoes) Z46.89
  pacemaker (cardiac) (cardiac resynchronization therapy (CRT-P)) Z45.018
    nervous system (brain) (peripheral nerve) (spinal cord) Z46.2
      implanted Z45.42
    pulse generator Z45.010
  portacath (port-a-cath) Z45.2
  prosthesis (external) Z44.9
    arm — *see* Admission, adjustment, artificial, arm
    breast Z44.3 ☑
    dental Z46.3
    eye Z44.2 ☑
    leg — *see* Admission, adjustment, artificial, leg
    specified NEC Z44.8
  spectacles Z46.0
  wheelchair Z46.89
Fitzhugh-Curtis syndrome
  due to
    Chlamydia trachomatis A74.81
    Neisseria gonorrhorea (gonococcal peritonitis) A54.85

Fitz's syndrome (acute hemorrhagic pancreatitis) (*see also* Pancreatitis, acute) K85.80
Fixation
  joint — *see* Ankylosis
  larynx J38.7
  stapes — *see* Ankylosis, ear ossicles
    deafness — *see* Deafness, conductive
  uterus (acquired) — *see* Malposition, uterus
  vocal cord J38.3
Flabby ridge K06.8
Flaccid (*see also* condition)
  palate, congenital Q38.5
Flail
  chest S22.5 ☑
    newborn (birth injury) P13.8
  joint (paralytic) M25.20
    ankle M25.27- ☑
    elbow M25.22- ☑
    foot joint M25.27- ☑
    hand joint M25.24- ☑
    hip M25.25- ☑
    knee M25.26- ☑
    shoulder M25.21- ☑
    specified joint NEC M25.28
    wrist M25.23- ☑
Flajani's disease — *see* Hyperthyroidism, with, goiter (diffuse)
Flap, liver K71.3
Flashbacks (residual to hallucinogen use) F16.283
Flat
  chamber (eye) — *see* Disorder, globe, hypotony, flat anterior chamber
  chest, congenital Q67.8
  foot (acquired) (fixed type) (painful) (postural) (*see also* Deformity, limb, flat foot)
    congenital (rigid) (spastic (everted)) Q66.5- ☑
    rachitic sequelae (late effect) E64.3
  organ or site, congenital NEC — *see* Anomaly, by site
  pelvis M95.5
    with disproportion (fetopelvic) O33.0
      causing obstructed labor O65.0
    congenital Q74.2
Flatau-Schilder disease G37.0
Flatback syndrome M40.30
  lumbar region M40.36
  lumbosacral region M40.37
  thoracolumbar region M40.35
Flattening
  head, femur M89.8X5
  hip — *see* Coxa, plana
  lip (congenital) Q18.8
  nose (congenital) Q67.4
    acquired M95.0
Flatulence R14.3
  psychogenic F45.8
Flatus R14.3
  vaginalis N89.8
Flax-dresser's disease J66.1
Flea bite — *see* Injury, bite, by site, superficial, insect
Flecks, glaucomatous (subcapsular) — *see* Cataract, complicated
Fleischer (-Kayser) **ring** (cornea) H18.04- ☑
Fleshy mole O02.0
Flexibilitas cerea — *see* Catalepsy
Flexion
  amputation stump (surgical) T87.89
  cervix — *see* Malposition, uterus
  contracture, joint — *see* Contraction, joint
  deformity, joint (*see also* Deformity, limb, flexion) M21.20
    hip, congenital Q65.89
  uterus (*see also* Malposition, uterus)
    lateral — *see* Lateroversion, uterus
Flexner-Boyd dysentery A03.2
Flexner's dysentery A03.1
Flexure — *see* Flexion
Flint murmur (aortic insufficiency) I35.1
Floater, vitreous — *see* Opacity, vitreous
Floating
  cartilage (joint) (*see also* Loose, body, joint)
    knee — *see* Derangement, knee, loose body
  gallbladder, congenital Q44.1
  kidney N28.89
    congenital Q63.8
  spleen D73.89
Flooding N92.0
Floor — *see* condition

Floppy
  baby syndrome (nonspecific) P94.2
  iris syndrome (intraoperative) (IFIS) H21.81
  nonrheumatic mitral valve syndrome I34.1
Flu (*see also* Influenza)
  avian (*see also* Influenza, due to, identified novel influenza A virus) J09.X2
  bird (*see also* Influenza, due to, identified novel influenza A virus) J09.X2
  intestinal A08.4
  swine (viruses that normally cause infections in pigs) (*see also* Influenza, due to, identified novel influenza A virus) J09.X2
Fluctuating blood pressure I99.8
Fluid
  abdomen R18.8
  chest J94.8
  heart — *see* Failure, heart, congestive
  joint — *see* Effusion, joint
  loss (acute) E86.9
  lung — *see* Edema, lung
  overload E87.70
    specified NEC E87.79
  peritoneal cavity R18.8
  pleural cavity J94.8
  retention R60.9
Flukes NEC (*see also* Infestation, fluke)
  blood NEC — *see* Schistosomiasis
  liver B66.3
Fluor (vaginalis) N89.8
  trichomonal or due to Trichomonas (vaginalis) A59.00
Fluorosis
  dental K00.3
  skeletal M85.10
    ankle M85.17- ☑
    foot M85.17- ☑
    forearm M85.13- ☑
    hand M85.14- ☑
    lower leg M85.16- ☑
    multiple site M85.19
    neck M85.18
    rib M85.18
    shoulder M85.11- ☑
    skull M85.18
    specified site NEC M85.18
    thigh M85.15- ☑
    toe M85.17- ☑
    upper arm M85.12- ☑
    vertebra M85.18
Flush syndrome E34.0
Flushing R23.2
  menopausal N95.1
Flutter
  atrial or auricular I48.92
    atypical I48.4
    type I I48.3
    type II I48.4
    typical I48.3
  heart I49.8
    atrial or auricular I48.92
      atypical I48.4
      type I I48.3
      type II I48.4
      typical I48.3
    ventricular I49.02
  ventricular I49.02
FNHTR (febrile nonhemolytic transfusion reaction) R50.84
Fochier's abscess — *code by* site under Abscess
Focus, Assmann's — *see* Tuberculosis, pulmonary
Fogo selvagem L10.3
Foix-Alajouanine syndrome G95.19
Fold, folds (anomalous) (*see also* Anomaly, by site)
  Descemet's membrane — *see* Change, corneal membrane, Descemet's, fold
  epicanthic Q10.3
  heart Q24.8
Folie à deux F24
Follicle
  cervix (nabothian) (ruptured) N88.8
  graafian, ruptured, with hemorrhage N83.0- ☑
  nabothian N88.8
Follicular — *see* condition
Folliculitis (superficial) L73.9
  abscedens et suffodiens L66.3
  cyst N83.0- ☑
  decalvans L66.2
  deep — *see* Furuncle, by site

☑ **Additional Character Required — Refer to the Tabular List for Character Selection**

🔻 **Subterms under main terms may continue to next column or page**

Folliculitis — *continued*
  gonococcal (acute) (chronic) A54.01
  keloid, keloidalis L73.0
  pustular L01.02
  ulerythematosa reticulata L66.4
Folliculome lipidique
  specified site — *see* Neoplasm, benign, by site
  unspecified site
    female D27.9
    male D29.20
Følling's disease E70.0
Follow-up — *see* Examination, follow-up
Fong's syndrome (hereditary osteo-onychodysplasia) Q87.2
Food
  allergy L27.2
  asphyxia (from aspiration or inhalation) — *see* Foreign body, by site
  choked on — *see* Foreign body, by site
  deprivation T73.0 ☑
    specified kind of food NEC E63.8
  intoxication — *see* Poisoning, food
  lack of T73.0 ☑
  poisoning — *see* Poisoning, food
  rejection NEC — *see* Disorder, eating
  strangulation or suffocation — *see* Foreign body, by site
  toxemia — *see* Poisoning, food
Foot — *see* condition
Foramen ovale (nonclosure) (patent) (persistent) Q21.1
Forbes' glycogen storage disease E74.03
Fordyce-Fox disease L75.2
Fordyce's disease (mouth) Q38.6
Forearm — *see* condition
Foreign body
  with
    laceration — *see* Laceration, by site, with foreign body
    puncture wound — *see* Puncture, by site, with foreign body
  accidentally left following a procedure T81.509 ☑
    aspiration T81.506 ☑
      resulting in
        adhesions T81.516 ☑
        obstruction T81.526 ☑
        perforation T81.536 ☑
        specified complication NEC T81.596 ☑
    cardiac catheterization T81.505 ☑
      resulting in
        acute reaction T81.60 ☑
          aseptic peritonitis T81.61 ☑
            specified NEC T81.69 ☑
        adhesions T81.515 ☑
        obstruction T81.525 ☑
        perforation T81.535 ☑
        specified complication NEC T81.595 ☑
      causing
        acute reaction T81.60 ☑
          aseptic peritonitis T81.61 ☑
          specified complication NEC T81.69 ☑
        adhesions T81.519 ☑
        aseptic peritonitis T81.61 ☑
        obstruction T81.529 ☑
        perforation T81.539 ☑
        specified complication NEC T81.599 ☑
    endoscopy T81.504 ☑
      resulting in
        adhesions T81.514 ☑
        obstruction T81.524 ☑
        perforation T81.534 ☑
        specified complication NEC T81.594 ☑
    immunization T81.503 ☑
      resulting in
        adhesions T81.513 ☑
        obstruction T81.523 ☑
        perforation T81.533 ☑
        specified complication NEC T81.593 ☑
    infusion T81.501 ☑
      resulting in
        adhesions T81.511 ☑
        obstruction T81.521 ☑
        perforation T81.531 ☑
        specified complication NEC T81.591 ☑
    injection T81.503 ☑
      resulting in
        adhesions T81.513 ☑

Foreign body — *continued*
  accidentally left following a procedure — *continued*
    injection — *continued*
      resulting in — *continued*
        obstruction T81.523 ☑
        perforation T81.533 ☑
        specified complication NEC T81.593 ☑
    kidney dialysis T81.502 ☑
      resulting in
        adhesions T81.512 ☑
        obstruction T81.522 ☑
        perforation T81.532 ☑
        specified complication NEC T81.592 ☑
    packing removal T81.507 ☑
      resulting in
        acute reaction T81.60 ☑
          aseptic peritonitis T81.61 ☑
            specified NEC T81.69 ☑
        adhesions T81.517 ☑
        obstruction T81.527 ☑
        perforation T81.537 ☑
        specified complication NEC T81.597 ☑
    puncture T81.506 ☑
      resulting in
        adhesions T81.516 ☑
        obstruction T81.526 ☑
        perforation T81.536 ☑
        specified complication NEC T81.596 ☑
    specified procedure NEC T81.508 ☑
      resulting in
        acute reaction T81.60 ☑
          aseptic peritonitis T81.61 ☑
            specified NEC T81.69 ☑
        adhesions T81.518 ☑
        obstruction T81.528 ☑
        perforation T81.538 ☑
        specified complication NEC T81.598 ☑
    surgical operation T81.500 ☑
      resulting in
        acute reaction T81.60 ☑
          aseptic peritonitis T81.61 ☑
            specified NEC T81.69 ☑
        adhesions T81.510 ☑
        obstruction T81.520 ☑
        perforation T81.530 ☑
        specified complication NEC T81.590 ☑
    transfusion T81.501 ☑
      resulting in
        adhesions T81.511 ☑
        obstruction T81.521 ☑
        perforation T81.531 ☑
        specified complication NEC T81.591 ☑
  alimentary tract T18.9 ☑
    anus T18.5 ☑
    colon T18.4 ☑
    esophagus — *see* Foreign body, esophagus
    mouth T18.0 ☑
    multiple sites T18.8 ☑
    rectosigmoid (junction) T18.5 ☑
    rectum T18.5 ☑
    small intestine T18.3 ☑
    specified site NEC T18.8 ☑
    stomach T18.2 ☑
  anterior chamber (eye) S05.5- ☑
  auditory canal — *see* Foreign body, entering through orifice, ear
  bronchus T17.508 ☑
    causing
      asphyxiation T17.500 ☑
        food (bone) (seed) T17.520 ☑
        gastric contents (vomitus) T17.510 ☑
        specified type NEC T17.590 ☑
      injury NEC T17.508 ☑
        food (bone) (seed) T17.528 ☑
        gastric contents (vomitus) T17.518 ☑
        specified type NEC T17.598 ☑
  canthus — *see* Foreign body, conjunctival sac
  ciliary body (eye) S05.5- ☑
  conjunctival sac T15.1- ☑
  cornea T15.0- ☑
  entering through orifice
    accessory sinus T17.0 ☑
    alimentary canal T18.9 ☑
      multiple parts T18.8 ☑
      specified part NEC T18.8 ☑

Foreign body — *continued*
  entering through orifice — *continued*
    alveolar process T18.0 ☑
    antrum (Highmore's) T17.0 ☑
    anus T18.5 ☑
    appendix T18.4 ☑
    auditory canal — *see* Foreign body, entering through orifice, ear
    auricle — *see* Foreign body, entering through orifice, ear
    bladder T19.1 ☑
    bronchioles — *see* Foreign body, respiratory tract, specified site NEC
    bronchus (main) — *see* Foreign body, bronchus
    buccal cavity T18.0 ☑
    canthus (inner) — *see* Foreign body, conjunctival sac
    cecum T18.4 ☑
    cervix (canal) (uteri) T19.3 ☑
    colon T18.4 ☑
    conjunctival sac — *see* Foreign body, conjunctival sac
    cornea — *see* Foreign body, cornea
    digestive organ or tract NOS T18.9 ☑
      multiple parts T18.8 ☑
      specified part NEC T18.8 ☑
    duodenum T18.3 ☑
    ear (external) T16.- ☑
    esophagus — *see* Foreign body, esophagus
    eye (external) NOS T15.9- ☑
      conjunctival sac — *see* Foreign body, conjunctival sac
      cornea — *see* Foreign body, cornea
      specified part NEC T15.8- ☑
    eyeball (*see also* Foreign body, entering through orifice, eye, specified part NEC)
      with penetrating wound — *see* Puncture, eyeball
    eyelid (*see also* Foreign body, conjunctival sac)
      with
        laceration — *see* Laceration, eyelid, with foreign body
        puncture — *see* Puncture, eyelid, with foreign body
        superficial injury — *see* Foreign body, superficial, eyelid
    gastrointestinal tract T18.9 ☑
      multiple parts T18.8 ☑
      specified part NEC T18.8 ☑
    genitourinary tract T19.9 ☑
      multiple parts T19.8 ☑
      specified part NEC T19.8 ☑
    globe — *see* Foreign body, entering through orifice, eyeball
    gum T18.0 ☑
    Highmore's antrum T17.0 ☑
    hypopharynx — *see* Foreign body, pharynx
    ileum T18.3 ☑
    intestine (small) T18.3 ☑
      large T18.4 ☑
    lacrimal apparatus (punctum) — *see* Foreign body, entering through orifice, eye, specified part NEC
    large intestine T18.4 ☑
    larynx — *see* Foreign body, larynx
    lung — *see* Foreign body, respiratory tract, specified site NEC
    maxillary sinus T17.0 ☑
    mouth T18.0 ☑
    nasal sinus T17.0 ☑
    nasopharynx — *see* Foreign body, pharynx
    nose (passage) T17.1 ☑
    nostril T17.1 ☑
    oral cavity T18.0 ☑
    palate T18.0 ☑
    penis T19.4 ☑
    pharynx — *see* Foreign body, pharynx
    piriform sinus — *see* Foreign body, pharynx
    rectosigmoid (junction) T18.5 ☑
    rectum T18.5 ☑
    respiratory tract — *see* Foreign body, respiratory tract
    sinus (accessory) (frontal) (maxillary) (nasal) T17.0 ☑
      piriform — *see* Foreign body, pharynx
    small intestine T18.3 ☑

🐦 Subterms under main terms may continue to next column or page   ☑ Additional Character Required — Refer to the Tabular List for Character Selection   **147**

Folliculitis — Foreign body

Foreign body — *continued*
- superficial, without open wound — *continued*
  - jaw S00.85 ☑
  - knee S80.25- ☑
  - labium (majus) (minus) S30.854 ☑
  - larynx S10.15 ☑
  - leg (lower) S80.85- ☑
    - knee — *see* Foreign body, superficial, knee
    - upper — *see* Foreign body, superficial, thigh
  - lip S00.551 ☑
  - lower back S30.850 ☑
  - lumbar region S30.850 ☑
  - malar region S00.85 ☑
  - mammary — *see* Foreign body, superficial, breast
  - mastoid region S00.85 ☑
  - mouth S00.552 ☑
  - nail
    - finger — *see* Foreign body, superficial, finger
    - toe — *see* Foreign body, superficial, toe
  - nape S10.85 ☑
  - nasal S00.35 ☑
  - neck S10.95 ☑
    - specified site NEC S10.85 ☑
    - throat S10.15 ☑
  - nose S00.35 ☑
  - occipital region S00.05 ☑
  - oral cavity S00.552 ☑
  - orbital region — *see* Foreign body, superficial, eyelid
  - palate S00.552 ☑
  - palm — *see* Foreign body, superficial, hand
  - parietal region S00.05 ☑
  - pelvis S30.850 ☑
  - penis S30.852 ☑
  - perineum
    - female S30.854 ☑
    - male S30.850 ☑
  - periocular area — *see* Foreign body, superficial, eyelid
  - phalanges
    - finger — *see* Foreign body, superficial, finger
    - toe — *see* Foreign body, superficial, toe
  - pharynx S10.15 ☑
  - pinna — *see* Foreign body, superficial, ear
  - popliteal space — *see* Foreign body, superficial, knee
  - prepuce S30.852 ☑
  - pubic region S30.850 ☑
  - pudendum
    - female S30.856 ☑
    - male S30.855 ☑
  - sacral region S30.850 ☑
  - scalp S00.05 ☑
  - scapular region — *see* Foreign body, superficial, shoulder
  - scrotum S30.853 ☑
  - shin — *see* Foreign body, superficial, leg
  - shoulder S40.25- ☑
  - sternal region S20.359 ☑
  - submaxillary region S00.85 ☑
  - submental region S00.85 ☑
  - subungual
    - finger(s) — *see* Foreign body, superficial, finger
    - toe(s) — *see* Foreign body, superficial, toe
  - supraclavicular fossa S10.85 ☑
  - supraorbital S00.85 ☑
  - temple S00.85 ☑
  - temporal region S00.85 ☑
  - testis S30.853 ☑
  - thigh S70.35- ☑
  - thorax, thoracic (wall) S20.95 ☑
    - back S20.45- ☑
    - front S20.35- ☑
  - throat S10.15 ☑
  - thumb S60.35- ☑
  - toe(s) (lesser) S90.456 ☑
    - great S90.45- ☑
  - tongue S00.552 ☑
  - trachea S10.15 ☑
  - tunica vaginalis S30.853 ☑
  - tympanum, tympanic membrane — *see* Foreign body, superficial, ear
  - uvula S00.552 ☑
  - vagina S30.854 ☑
  - vocal cords S10.15 ☑
  - vulva S30.854 ☑

Foreign body — *continued*
- superficial, without open wound — *continued*
  - wrist S60.85- ☑
  - swallowed T18.9 ☑
  - trachea T17.408 ☑
    - causing
      - asphyxiation T17.400 ☑
        - food (bone) (seed) T17.420 ☑
        - gastric contents (vomitus) T17.410 ☑
        - specified type NEC T17.490 ☑
      - injury NEC T17.408 ☑
        - food (bone) (seed) T17.428 ☑
        - gastric contents (vomitus) T17.418 ☑
        - specified type NEC T17.498 ☑
  - type of fragment — *see* Retained, foreign body fragments (type of)
  - vitreous (humor) S05.5- ☑
Forestier's disease (rhizomelic pseudopolyarthritis) M35.3
- meaning ankylosing hyperostosis — *see* Hyperostosis, ankylosing
Formation
- hyalin in cornea — *see* Degeneration, cornea
- sequestrum in bone (due to infection) — *see* Osteomyelitis, chronic
- valve
  - colon, congenital Q43.8
  - ureter (congenital) Q62.39
Formication R20.2
Fort Bragg fever A27.89
Fossa (*see also* condition)
- pyriform — *see* condition
Foster-Kennedy syndrome H47.14- ☑
Fothergill's
- disease (trigeminal neuralgia) (*see also* Neuralgia, trigeminal)
  - scarlatina anginosa A38.9
Foul breath R19.6
Foundling Z76.1
Fournier disease or gangrene N49.3
- female N76.89
Fourth
- cranial nerve — *see* condition
- molar K00.1
Foville's (peduncular) **disease or syndrome** G46.3
Fox (-Fordyce) disease (apocrine miliaria) L75.2
Fracture, burst — *see* Fracture, traumatic, by site
Fracture, chronic — *see* Fracture, pathological, by site
Fracture, insufficiency — *see* Fracture, pathological, by site
Fracture, nontraumatic, NEC
- atypical
  - femur M84.750- ☑
    - complete
      - oblique M84.759 ☑
        - left side M84.758 ☑
        - right side M84.757 ☑
      - transverse M84.756 ☑
        - left side M84.755 ☑
        - right side M84.754 ☑
    - incomplete M84.753 ☑
      - left side M84.752 ☑
      - right side M84.751 ☑
Fracture, pathological (pathologic) (*see also* Fracture, traumatic) M84.40 ☑
- ankle M84.47- ☑
- carpus M84.44- ☑
- clavicle M84.41- ☑
- compression (not due to trauma) (*see also* Collapse, vertebra) M48.50- ☑
- dental implant M27.63
- dental restorative material K08.539
  - with loss of material K08.531
  - without loss of material K08.530
- due to
  - neoplastic disease NEC (*see also* Neoplasm) M84.50 ☑
    - ankle M84.57- ☑
    - carpus M84.54- ☑
    - clavicle M84.51- ☑
    - femur M84.55- ☑
    - fibula M84.56- ☑
    - finger M84.54- ☑
    - hip M84.559 ☑
    - humerus M84.52- ☑
    - ilium M84.550 ☑

Fracture, pathological — *continued*
- due to — *continued*
  - neoplastic disease (*see also* Neoplasm) — *continued*
    - ischium M84.550 ☑
    - metacarpus M84.54- ☑
    - metatarsus M84.57- ☑
    - neck M84.58 ☑
    - pelvis M84.550 ☑
    - radius M84.53- ☑
    - rib M84.58 ☑
    - scapula M84.51- ☑
    - skull M84.58 ☑
    - specified site NEC M84.58 ☑
    - tarsus M84.57- ☑
    - tibia M84.56- ☑
    - toe M84.57- ☑
    - ulna M84.53- ☑
    - vertebra M84.58 ☑
  - osteoporosis M80.00 ☑
    - disuse — *see* Osteoporosis, specified type NEC, with pathological fracture
    - drug-induced — *see* Osteoporosis, drug induced, with pathological fracture
    - idiopathic — *see* Osteoporosis, specified type NEC, with pathological fracture
    - postmenopausal — *see* Osteoporosis, postmenopausal, with pathological fracture
    - postoophorectomy — *see* Osteoporosis, postoophorectomy, with pathological fracture
    - postsurgical malabsorption — *see* Osteoporosis, specified type NEC, with pathological fracture
    - specified cause NEC — *see* Osteoporosis, specified type NEC, with pathological fracture
  - specified disease NEC M84.60 ☑
    - ankle M84.67- ☑
    - carpus M84.64- ☑
    - clavicle M84.61- ☑
    - femur M84.65- ☑
    - fibula M84.66- ☑
    - finger M84.64- ☑
    - hip M84.65- ☑
    - humerus M84.62- ☑
    - ilium M84.650 ☑
    - ischium M84.650 ☑
    - metacarpus M84.64- ☑
    - metatarsus M84.67- ☑
    - neck M84.68 ☑
    - radius M84.63- ☑
    - rib M84.68 ☑
    - scapula M84.61- ☑
    - skull M84.68 ☑
    - tarsus M84.67- ☑
    - tibia M84.66- ☑
    - toe M84.67- ☑
    - ulna M84.63- ☑
    - vertebra M84.68 ☑
- femur M84.45- ☑
- fibula M84.46- ☑
- finger M84.44- ☑
- hip M84.459 ☑
- humerus M84.42- ☑
- ilium M84.454 ☑
- ischium M84.454 ☑
- joint prosthesis — *see* Complications, joint prosthesis, mechanical, breakdown, by site
  - periprosthetic — *see* Fracture, pathological, periprosthetic
- metacarpus M84.44- ☑
- metatarsus M84.47- ☑
- neck M84.48 ☑
- pelvis M84.454 ☑
- periprosthetic M97.9 ☑
  - ankle M97.2- ☑
  - elbow M97.4- ☑
  - finger M97.8 ☑
  - hip M97.0- ☑
  - knee M97.1- ☑
  - other specified joint M97.8 ☑
  - shoulder M97.3- ☑
  - spinal joint M97.8 ☑
  - toe joint M97.8 ☑
  - wrist joint M97.8 ☑
- radius M84.43- ☑

Index

Fracture, pathological — Fracture, traumatic

Fracture, pathological — *continued*
restorative material (dental) K08.539
with loss of material K08.531
without loss of material K08.530
rib M84.48 ☑
scapula M84.41- ☑
skull M84.48 ☑
tarsus M84.47- ☑
tibia M84.46- ☑
toe M84.47- ☑
ulna M84.43- ☑
vertebra M84.48 ☑
Fracture, traumatic (abduction) (adduction) (separation)
(*see also* Fracture, pathological) T14.8 ☑
acetabulum S32.40- ☑
column
anterior (displaced) (iliopubic) S32.43- ☑
nondisplaced S32.436 ☑
posterior (displaced) (ilioischial) S32.443 ☑
nondisplaced S32.44- ☑
dome (displaced) S32.48- ☑
nondisplaced S32.48 ☑
specified NEC S32.49- ☑
transverse (displaced) S32.45- ☑
with associated posterior wall fracture (displaced) S32.46- ☑
nondisplaced S32.46- ☑
nondisplaced S32.45- ☑
wall
anterior (displaced) S32.41- ☑
nondisplaced S32.41- ☑
medial (displaced) S32.47- ☑
nondisplaced S32.47- ☑
posterior (displaced) S32.42- ☑
with associated transverse fracture (displaced) S32.46- ☑
nondisplaced S32.46- ☑
nondisplaced S32.42- ☑
acromion — *see* Fracture, scapula, acromial process
ankle S82.899 ☑
bimalleolar (displaced) S82.84- ☑
nondisplaced S82.84- ☑
lateral malleolus only (displaced) S82.6- ☑
nondisplaced S82.6- ☑
medial malleolus (displaced) S82.5- ☑
associated with Maisonneuve's fracture — *see* Fracture, Maisonneuve's
nondisplaced S82.5- ☑
talus — *see* Fracture, tarsal, talus
trimalleolar (displaced) S82.85- ☑
nondisplaced S82.85- ☑
arm (upper) (*see also* Fracture, humerus, shaft)
humerus — *see* Fracture, humerus
radius — *see* Fracture, radius
ulna — *see* Fracture, ulna
astragalus — *see* Fracture, tarsal, talus
atlas — *see* Fracture, neck, cervical vertebra, first
axis — *see* Fracture, neck, cervical vertebra, second
back — *see* Fracture, vertebra
Barton's — *see* Barton's fracture
base of skull — *see* Fracture, skull, base
basicervical (basal) (femoral) S72.0 ☑
Bennett's — *see* Bennett's fracture
bimalleolar — *see* Fracture, ankle, bimalleolar
blow-out S02.3- ☑
bone NEC T14.8 ☑
birth injury P13.9
following insertion of orthopedic implant, joint prosthesis or bone plate — *see* Fracture, following insertion of orthopedic implant, joint prosthesis or bone plate
in (due to) neoplastic disease NEC — *see* Fracture, pathological, due to, neoplastic disease
pathological (cause unknown) — *see* Fracture, pathological
breast bone — *see* Fracture, sternum
bucket handle (semilunar cartilage) — *see* Tear, meniscus
burst — *see* Fracture, traumatic, by site
calcaneus — *see* Fracture, tarsal, calcaneus
carpal bone(s) S62.10- ☑
capitate (displaced) S62.13- ☑
nondisplaced S62.13- ☑
cuneiform — *see* Fracture, carpal bone, triquetrum
hamate (body) (displaced) S62.143 ☑
hook process (displaced) S62.15- ☑

Fracture, traumatic — *continued*
carpal bone(s) — *continued*
hamate — *continued*
hook process — *continued*
nondisplaced S62.15- ☑
nondisplaced S62.14- ☑
larger multangular — *see* Fracture, carpal bones, trapezium
lunate (displaced) S62.12- ☑
nondisplaced S62.12- ☑
navicular S62.00- ☑
distal pole (displaced) S62.01- ☑
nondisplaced S62.01- ☑
middle third (displaced) S62.02- ☑
nondisplaced S62.02- ☑
proximal third (displaced) S62.03- ☑
nondisplaced S62.03- ☑
volar tuberosity — *see* Fracture, carpal bones, navicular, distal pole
os magnum — *see* Fracture, carpal bones, capitate
pisiform (displaced) S62.16- ☑
nondisplaced S62.16- ☑
semilunar — *see* Fracture, carpal bones, lunate
smaller multangular — *see* Fracture, carpal bones, trapezoid
trapezium (displaced) S62.17- ☑
nondisplaced S62.17- ☑
trapezoid (displaced) S62.18- ☑
nondisplaced S62.18- ☑
triquetrum (displaced) S62.11- ☑
nondisplaced S62.11- ☑
unciform — *see* Fracture, carpal bones, hamate
cervical — *see* Fracture, vertebra, cervical
clavicle S42.00- ☑
acromial end (displaced) S42.03- ☑
nondisplaced S42.03- ☑
birth injury P13.4
lateral end — *see* Fracture, clavicle, acromial end
shaft (displaced) S42.02- ☑
nondisplaced S42.02- ☑
sternal end (anterior) (displaced) S42.01- ☑
nondisplaced S42.01- ☑
posterior S42.01- ☑
coccyx S32.2 ☑
collapsed — *see* Collapse, vertebra
collar bone — *see* Fracture, clavicle
Colles' — *see* Colles' fracture
coronoid process — *see* Fracture, ulna, upper end, coronoid process
corpus cavernosum penis S39.840 ☑
costochondral cartilage S23.41 ☑
costochondral, costosternal junction — *see* Fracture, rib
cranium — *see* Fracture, skull
cricoid cartilage S12.8 ☑
cuboid (ankle) — *see* Fracture, tarsal, cuboid
cuneiform
foot — *see* Fracture, tarsal, cuneiform
wrist — *see* Fracture, carpal, triquetrum
delayed union — *see* Delay, union, fracture
dental restorative material K08.539
with loss of material K08.531
without loss of material K08.530
due to
birth injury — *see* Birth, injury, fracture
osteoporosis — *see* Osteoporosis, with fracture
Dupuytren's — *see* Fracture, ankle, lateral malleolus
elbow S42.40- ☑
ethmoid (bone) (sinus) — *see* Fracture, skull, base
face bone S02.92 ☑
fatigue (*see also* Fracture, stress)
vertebra M48.40 ☑
cervical region M48.42 ☑
cervicothoracic region M48.43 ☑
lumbar region M48.46 ☑
lumbosacral region M48.47 ☑
occipito-atlanto-axial region M48.41 ☑
sacrococcygeal region M48.48 ☑
thoracic region M48.44 ☑
thoracolumbar region M48.45 ☑
femur, femoral S72.9- ☑
basicervical (basal) S72.0 ☑
birth injury P13.2
capital epiphyseal S79.01- ☑
condyles, epicondyles — *see* Fracture, femur, lower end

Fracture, traumatic — *continued*
femur, femoral — *continued*
distal end — *see* Fracture, femur, lower end
epiphysis
head — *see* Fracture, femur, upper end, epiphysis
lower — *see* Fracture, femur, lower end, epiphysis
upper — *see* Fracture, femur, upper end, epiphysis
following insertion of implant, prosthesis or plate M96.66- ☑
head — *see* Fracture, femur, upper end, head
intertrochanteric — *see* Fracture, femur, trochanteric
intratrochanteric — *see* Fracture, femur, trochanteric
lower end S72.40- ☑
condyle (displaced) S72.41- ☑
lateral (displaced) S72.42- ☑
nondisplaced S72.42- ☑
medial (displaced) S72.43- ☑
nondisplaced S72.43- ☑
nondisplaced S72.41- ☑
epiphysis (displaced) S72.44- ☑
nondisplaced S72.44- ☑
physeal S79.10- ☑
Salter-Harris
Type I S79.11- ☑
Type II S79.12- ☑
Type III S79.13- ☑
Type IV S79.14- ☑
specified NEC S79.19- ☑
specified NEC S72.49- ☑
supracondylar (displaced) S72.45- ☑
with intracondylar extension (displaced) S72.46- ☑
nondisplaced S72.46- ☑
nondisplaced S72.45- ☑
torus S72.47- ☑
neck — *see* Fracture, femur, upper end, neck
pertrochanteric — *see* Fracture, femur, trochanteric
shaft (lower third) (middle third) (upper third) S72.30- ☑
comminuted (displaced) S72.35- ☑
nondisplaced S72.35- ☑
oblique (displaced) S72.33- ☑
nondisplaced S72.33- ☑
segmental (displaced) S72.36- ☑
nondisplaced S72.36- ☑
specified NEC S72.39- ☑
spiral (displaced) S72.34- ☑
nondisplaced S72.34- ☑
transverse (displaced) S72.32- ☑
nondisplaced S72.32- ☑
specified site NEC — *see* subcategory S72.8 ☑
subcapital (displaced) S72.01- ☑
subtrochanteric (region) (section) (displaced) S72.2- ☑
nondisplaced S72.2- ☑
transcervical — *see* Fracture, femur, upper end, neck
transtrochanteric — *see* Fracture, femur, trochanteric
trochanteric S72.10- ☑
apophyseal (displaced) S72.13- ☑
nondisplaced S72.13- ☑
greater trochanter (displaced) S72.11- ☑
nondisplaced S72.11- ☑
intertrochanteric (displaced) S72.14- ☑
nondisplaced S72.14- ☑
lesser trochanter (displaced) S72.12- ☑
nondisplaced S72.12- ☑
upper end S72.00- ☑
apophyseal (displaced) S72.13- ☑
nondisplaced S72.13- ☑
cervicotrochanteric — *see* Fracture, femur, upper end, neck, base
epiphysis (displaced) S72.02- ☑
nondisplaced S72.02- ☑
head S72.05- ☑
articular (displaced) S72.06- ☑
nondisplaced S72.06- ☑
specified NEC S72.09- ☑
intertrochanteric (displaced) S72.14- ☑

Fracture, traumatic — *continued*
  femur, femoral — *continued*
    upper end — *continued*
      intertrochanteric — *continued*
        nondisplaced S72.14- ☑
      intracapsular S72.01- ☑
      midcervical (displaced) S72.03- ☑
        nondisplaced S72.03- ☑
      neck S72.00- ☑
        base (displaced) S72.04- ☑
          nondisplaced S72.04- ☑
        specified NEC S72.09- ☑
      pertrochanteric — *see* Fracture, femur, upper
          end, trochanteric
      physeal S79.00- ☑
        Salter-Harris type I S79.01- ☑
        specified NEC S79.09- ☑
      subcapital (displaced) S72.01- ☑
      subtrochanteric (displaced) S72.2- ☑
        nondisplaced S72.2- ☑
      transcervical — *see* Fracture, femur, upper end,
          midcervical
      trochanteric S72.10- ☑
        greater (displaced) S72.11- ☑
          nondisplaced S72.11- ☑
        lesser (displaced) S72.12- ☑
          nondisplaced S72.12- ☑
  fibula (shaft) (styloid) S82.40- ☑
    comminuted (displaced) S82.45- ☑
      nondisplaced S82.45- ☑
    following insertion of implant, prosthesis or plate
        M96.67- ☑
    involving ankle or malleolus — *see* Fracture, fibula,
        lateral malleolus
    lateral malleolus (displaced) S82.6- ☑
      nondisplaced S82.6- ☑
    lower end
      physeal S89.30- ☑
        Salter-Harris
          Type I S89.31- ☑
          Type II S89.32- ☑
        specified NEC S89.39- ☑
      specified NEC S82.83- ☑
      torus S82.82- ☑
    oblique (displaced) S82.43- ☑
      nondisplaced S82.43- ☑
    segmental (displaced) S82.46- ☑
      nondisplaced S82.46- ☑
    specified NEC S82.49- ☑
    spiral (displaced) S82.44- ☑
      nondisplaced S82.44- ☑
    transverse (displaced) S82.42- ☑
      nondisplaced S82.42- ☑
    upper end
      physeal S89.20- ☑
        Salter-Harris
          Type I S89.21- ☑
          Type II S89.22- ☑
        specified NEC S89.29- ☑
      specified NEC S82.83- ☑
      torus S82.81- ☑
  finger (except thumb) S62.60- ☑
    distal phalanx (displaced) S62.63- ☑
      nondisplaced S62.66- ☑
    index S62.60- ☑
      distal phalanx (displaced) S62.63- ☑
        nondisplaced S62.66- ☑
      medial phalanx (displaced) S62.62- ☑
        nondisplaced S62.65- ☑
      proximal phalanx (displaced) S62.61- ☑
        nondisplaced S62.64- ☑
    little S62.60- ☑
      distal phalanx (displaced) S62.63- ☑
        nondisplaced S62.66- ☑
      medial phalanx (displaced) S62.62- ☑
        nondisplaced S62.65- ☑
      proximal phalanx (displaced) S62.61- ☑
        nondisplaced S62.64- ☑
    medial phalanx (displaced) S62.62- ☑
      nondisplaced S62.65- ☑
    middle S62.60- ☑
      distal phalanx (displaced) S62.63- ☑
        nondisplaced S62.66- ☑
      medial phalanx (displaced) S62.62- ☑
        nondisplaced S62.65- ☑
      proximal phalanx (displaced) S62.61- ☑

Fracture, traumatic — *continued*
  finger — *continued*
    middle — *continued*
      proximal phalanx — *continued*
        nondisplaced S62.64- ☑
      proximal phalanx (displaced) S62.61- ☑
        nondisplaced S62.64- ☑
    ring S62.60- ☑
      distal phalanx (displaced) S62.63- ☑
        nondisplaced S62.66- ☑
      medial phalanx (displaced) S62.62- ☑
        nondisplaced S62.65- ☑
      proximal phalanx (displaced) S62.61- ☑
        nondisplaced S62.64- ☑
    thumb — *see* Fracture, thumb
  following insertion (intraoperative) (postoperative) of
      orthopedic implant, joint prosthesis or bone
      plate M96.69
    femur M96.66- ☑
    fibula M96.67- ☑
    humerus M96.62- ☑
    pelvis M96.65
    radius M96.63- ☑
    specified bone NEC M96.69
    tibia M96.67- ☑
    ulna M96.63- ☑
  foot S92.90- ☑
    astragalus — *see* Fracture, tarsal, talus
    calcaneus — *see* Fracture, tarsal, calcaneus
    cuboid — *see* Fracture, tarsal, cuboid
    cuneiform — *see* Fracture, tarsal, cuneiform
    metatarsal — *see* Fracture, metatarsal
    navicular — *see* Fracture, tarsal, navicular
    sesamoid S92.81- ☑
    specified NEC S92.81- ☑
    talus — *see* Fracture, tarsal, talus
    tarsal — *see* Fracture, tarsal
    toe — *see* Fracture, toe
  forearm S52.9- ☑
    radius — *see* Fracture, radius
    ulna — *see* Fracture, ulna
  fossa (anterior) (middle) (posterior) S02.19 ☑
  frontal (bone) (skull) S02.0 ☑
    sinus S02.19 ☑
  glenoid (cavity) (scapula) — *see* Fracture, scapula,
      glenoid cavity
  greenstick — *see* Fracture, by site
  hallux — *see* Fracture, toe, great
  hand S62.9- ☑
    carpal — *see* Fracture, carpal bone
    finger (except thumb) — *see* Fracture, finger
    metacarpal — *see* Fracture, metacarpal
    navicular (scaphoid) (hand) — *see* Fracture, carpal
        bone, navicular
    thumb — *see* Fracture, thumb
  healed or old
    with complications — *code by* Nature of the com-
        plication
  heel bone — *see* Fracture, tarsal, calcaneus
  Hill-Sachs S42.29- ☑
  hip — *see* Fracture, femur, neck
  humerus S42.30- ☑
    anatomical neck — *see* Fracture, humerus, upper
        end
    articular process — *see* Fracture, humerus, lower
        end
    capitellum — *see* Fracture, humerus, lower end,
        condyle, lateral
    distal end — *see* Fracture, humerus, lower end
    epiphysis
      lower — *see* Fracture, humerus, lower end,
          physeal
      upper — *see* Fracture, humerus, upper end,
          physeal
    external condyle — *see* Fracture, humerus, lower
        end, condyle, lateral
    following insertion of implant, prosthesis or plate
        M96.62- ☑
    great tuberosity — *see* Fracture, humerus, upper
        end, greater tuberosity
    intercondylar — *see* Fracture, humerus, lower end
    internal epicondyle — *see* Fracture, humerus,
        lower end, epicondyle, medial
    lesser tuberosity — *see* Fracture, humerus, upper
        end, lesser tuberosity
    lower end S42.40- ☑

Fracture, traumatic — *continued*
  humerus — *continued*
    lower end — *continued*
      condyle
        lateral (displaced) S42.45- ☑
          nondisplaced S42.45- ☑
        medial (displaced) S42.46- ☑
          nondisplaced S42.46- ☑
      epicondyle
        lateral (displaced) S42.43- ☑
          nondisplaced S42.43- ☑
        medial (displaced) S42.44- ☑
          incarcerated S42.44- ☑
          nondisplaced S42.44- ☑
      physeal S49.10- ☑
        Salter-Harris
          Type I S49.11- ☑
          Type II S49.12- ☑
          Type III S49.13- ☑
          Type IV S49.14- ☑
        specified NEC S49.19- ☑
      specified NEC (displaced) S42.49- ☑
        nondisplaced S42.49- ☑
      supracondylar (simple) (displaced) S42.41- ☑
        with intercondylar fracture — *see* Fracture,
            humerus, lower end
        comminuted (displaced) S42.42- ☑
          nondisplaced S42.42- ☑
        nondisplaced S42.41- ☑
      torus S42.48- ☑
      transcondylar (displaced) S42.47- ☑
        nondisplaced S42.47- ☑
    proximal end — *see* Fracture, humerus, upper end
    shaft S42.30- ☑
      comminuted (displaced) S42.35- ☑
        nondisplaced S42.35- ☑
      greenstick S42.31- ☑
      oblique (displaced) S42.33- ☑
        nondisplaced S42.33- ☑
      segmental (displaced) S42.36- ☑
        nondisplaced S42.36- ☑
      specified NEC S42.39- ☑
      spiral (displaced) S42.34- ☑
        nondisplaced S42.34- ☑
      transverse (displaced) S42.32- ☑
        nondisplaced S42.32- ☑
    supracondylar — *see* Fracture, humerus, lower end
    surgical neck — *see* Fracture, humerus, upper end,
        surgical neck
    trochlea — *see* Fracture, humerus, lower end,
        condyle, medial
    tuberosity — *see* Fracture, humerus, upper end
    upper end S42.20- ☑
      anatomical neck — *see* Fracture, humerus, up-
          per end, specified NEC
      articular head — *see* Fracture, humerus, upper
          end, specified NEC
      epiphysis — *see* Fracture, humerus, upper end,
          physeal
      greater tuberosity (displaced) S42.25- ☑
        nondisplaced S42.25- ☑
      lesser tuberosity (displaced) S42.26- ☑
        nondisplaced S42.26- ☑
      physeal S49.00- ☑
        Salter-Harris
          Type I S49.01- ☑
          Type II S49.02- ☑
          Type III S49.03- ☑
          Type IV S49.04- ☑
        specified NEC S49.09- ☑
      specified NEC (displaced) S42.29- ☑
        nondisplaced S42.29- ☑
      surgical neck (displaced) S42.21- ☑
        four-part S42.24- ☑
        nondisplaced S42.21- ☑
        three-part S42.23- ☑
        two-part (displaced) S42.22- ☑
          nondisplaced S42.22- ☑
      torus S42.27- ☑
      transepiphyseal — *see* Fracture, humerus, up-
          per end, physeal
  hyoid bone S12.8 ☑
  ilium S32.30- ☑
    with disruption of pelvic ring — *see* Disruption,
        pelvic ring
    avulsion (displaced) S32.31- ☑

Fracture, traumatic — *continued*
  ilium — *continued*
    avulsion — *continued*
      nondisplaced S32.31- ✓
      specified NEC S32.39- ✓
  impaction, impacted — *code as* Fracture, by site
  innominate bone — *see* Fracture, ilium
  instep — *see* Fracture, foot
  ischium S32.60- ✓
    with disruption of pelvic ring — *see* Disruption, pelvic ring
    avulsion (displaced) S32.61- ✓
      nondisplaced S32.61- ✓
    specified NEC S32.69- ✓
  jaw (bone) (lower) — *see* Fracture, mandible
    upper — *see* Fracture, maxilla
  joint prosthesis — *see* Complications, joint prosthesis, mechanical, breakdown, by site
    periprosthetic — *see* Fracture, traumatic, periprosthetic
  knee cap — *see* Fracture, patella
  larynx S12.8 ✓
  late effects — *see* Sequelae, fracture
  leg (lower) S82.9- ✓
    ankle — *see* Fracture, ankle
    femur — *see* Fracture, femur
    fibula — *see* Fracture, fibula
    malleolus — *see* Fracture, ankle
    patella — *see* Fracture, patella
    specified site NEC S82.89- ✓
    tibia — *see* Fracture, tibia
  lumbar spine — *see* Fracture, vertebra, lumbar
  lumbosacral spine S32.9 ✓
  Maisonneuve's (displaced) S82.86- ✓
    nondisplaced S82.86- ✓
  malar bone (*see also* Fracture, maxilla) S02.40Ø ✓
    left side S02.40B ✓
    right side S02.40A ✓
  malleolus — *see* Fracture, ankle
  malunion — *see* Fracture, by site
  mandible (lower jaw (bone)) S02.609 ✓
    alveolus S02.67- ✓
    angle (of jaw) S02.65- ✓
    body, unspecified S02.600 ✓
      left side S02.602 ✓
      right side S02.601 ✓
    condylar process S02.61- ✓
    coronoid process S02.63- ✓
    ramus, unspecified S02.64- ✓
    specified site NEC S02.69- ✓
    subcondylar process S02.62- ✓
    symphysis S02.66 ✓
  manubrium (sterni) S22.21 ✓
    dissociation from sternum S22.23 ✓
  march — *see* Fracture, traumatic, stress, by site
  maxilla, maxillary (bone) (sinus) (superior) (upper jaw) S02.401 ✓
    alveolus S02.42 ✓
    inferior — *see* Fracture, mandible
    LeFort I S02.411 ✓
    LeFort II S02.412 ✓
    LeFort III S02.413 ✓
    left side S02.40D ✓
    right side S02.40C ✓
  metacarpal S62.309 ✓
    base (displaced) S62.319 ✓
      nondisplaced S62.349 ✓
    fifth S62.30- ✓
      base (displaced) S62.31- ✓
        nondisplaced S62.34- ✓
      neck (displaced) S62.33- ✓
        nondisplaced S62.36- ✓
      shaft (displaced) S62.32- ✓
        nondisplaced S62.35- ✓
      specified NEC S62.398 ✓
    first S62.20- ✓
      base NEC (displaced) S62.23- ✓
        nondisplaced S62.23- ✓
      Bennett's — *see* Bennett's fracture
      neck (displaced) S62.25- ✓
        nondisplaced S62.25- ✓
      shaft (displaced) S62.24- ✓
        nondisplaced S62.24- ✓
      specified NEC S62.29- ✓
    fourth S62.30- ✓
      base (displaced) S62.31- ✓

Fracture, traumatic — *continued*
  metacarpal — *continued*
    fourth — *continued*
      base — *continued*
        nondisplaced S62.34- ✓
      neck (displaced) S62.33- ✓
        nondisplaced S62.36- ✓
      shaft (displaced) S62.32- ✓
        nondisplaced S62.35- ✓
      specified NEC S62.39- ✓
    neck (displaced) S62.33- ✓
      nondisplaced S62.36 ✓
    Rolando's — *see* Rolando's fracture
    second S62.30- ✓
      base (displaced) S62.31- ✓
        nondisplaced S62.34- ✓
      neck (displaced) S62.33- ✓
        nondisplaced S62.36- ✓
      shaft (displaced) S62.32- ✓
        nondisplaced S62.35- ✓
      specified NEC S62.39- ✓
    shaft (displaced) S62.32- ✓
      nondisplaced S62.35- ✓
    specified NEC S62.399 ✓
    third S62.30- ✓
      base (displaced) S62.31- ✓
        nondisplaced S62.34- ✓
      neck (displaced) S62.33- ✓
        nondisplaced S62.36- ✓
      shaft (displaced) S62.32- ✓
        nondisplaced S62.35- ✓
      specified NEC S62.39- ✓
  metastatic — *see* Fracture, pathological, due to, neoplastic disease (*see also* Neoplasm)
  metatarsal bone S92.30- ✓
    fifth (displaced) S92.35- ✓
      nondisplaced S92.35- ✓
    first (displaced) S92.31- ✓
      nondisplaced S92.31- ✓
    fourth (displaced) S92.34- ✓
      nondisplaced S92.34- ✓
    physeal S99.10- ✓
    Salter-Harris
      Type I S99.11- ✓
      Type II S99.12- ✓
      Type III S99.13- ✓
      Type IV S99.14- ✓
      specified NEC S99.19- ✓
    second (displaced) S92.32- ✓
      nondisplaced S92.32- ✓
    third (displaced) S92.33- ✓
      nondisplaced S92.33- ✓
  Monteggia's — *see* Monteggia's fracture
  multiple
    hand (and wrist) NEC — *see* Fracture, by site
    ribs — *see* Fracture, rib, multiple
  nasal (bone(s)) S02.2 ✓
  navicular (scaphoid) (foot) (*see also* Fracture, tarsal, navicular)
    hand — *see* Fracture, carpal, navicular
  neck S12.9 ✓
    cervical vertebra S12.9 ✓
      fifth (displaced) S12.400 ✓
        nondisplaced S12.401 ✓
        specified type NEC (displaced) S12.490 ✓
          nondisplaced S12.491 ✓
      first (displaced) S12.000 ✓
        burst (stable) S12.01 ✓
        unstable S12.02 ✓
        lateral mass (displaced) S12.040 ✓
          nondisplaced S12.041 ✓
        nondisplaced S12.001 ✓
        posterior arch (displaced) S12.030 ✓
          nondisplaced S12.031 ✓
        specified type NEC (displaced) S12.090 ✓
          nondisplaced S12.091 ✓
      fourth (displaced) S12.300 ✓
        nondisplaced S12.301 ✓
        specified type NEC (displaced) S12.390 ✓
          nondisplaced S12.391 ✓
      second (displaced) S12.100 ✓
        dens (anterior) (displaced) (type II) S12.110 ✓
          nondisplaced S12.112 ✓
          posterior S12.111 ✓

Fracture, traumatic — *continued*
  neck — *continued*
    cervical vertebra — *continued*
      second — *continued*
        dens — *continued*
          specified type NEC (displaced) S12.120 ✓
            nondisplaced S12.121 ✓
        nondisplaced S12.101 ✓
        specified type NEC (displaced) S12.190 ✓
          nondisplaced S12.191 ✓
      seventh (displaced) S12.600 ✓
        nondisplaced S12.601 ✓
        specified type NEC (displaced) S12.690 ✓
          nondisplaced S12.691 ✓
      sixth (displaced) S12.500 ✓
        nondisplaced S12.501 ✓
        specified type NEC (displaced) S12.590 ✓
          nondisplaced S12.591 ✓
      third (displaced) S12.200 ✓
        nondisplaced S12.201 ✓
        specified type NEC (displaced) S12.290 ✓
          nondisplaced S12.291 ✓
    hyoid bone S12.8 ✓
    larynx S12.8 ✓
    specified site NEC S12.8 ✓
    thyroid cartilage S12.8 ✓
    trachea S12.8 ✓
  neoplastic NEC — *see* Fracture, pathological, due to, neoplastic disease
  neural arch — *see* Fracture, vertebra
  newborn — *see* Birth, injury, fracture
  nontraumatic — *see* Fracture, pathological
  nonunion — *see* Nonunion, fracture
  nose, nasal (bone) (septum) S02.2
  occiput — *see* Fracture, skull, base, occiput
  odontoid process — *see* Fracture, neck, cervical vertebra, second
  olecranon (process) (ulna) — *see* Fracture, ulna, upper end, olecranon process
  orbit, orbital (bone) (region) S02.8- ✓
    floor (blow-out) S02.3- ✓
    roof S02.19 ✓
  os
    calcis — *see* Fracture, tarsal, calcaneus
    magnum — *see* Fracture, carpal, capitate
    pubis — *see* Fracture, pubis
  palate S02.8- ✓
  parietal bone (skull) S02.0 ✓
  patella S82.00- ✓
    comminuted (displaced) S82.04- ✓
      nondisplaced S82.04- ✓
    longitudinal (displaced) S82.02- ✓
      nondisplaced S82.02- ✓
    osteochondral (displaced) S82.01- ✓
      nondisplaced S82.01- ✓
    specified NEC S82.09- ✓
    transverse (displaced) S82.03- ✓
      nondisplaced S82.03- ✓
  pedicle (of vertebral arch) — *see* Fracture, vertebra
  pelvis, pelvic (bone) S32.9 ✓
    acetabulum — *see* Fracture, acetabulum
    circle — *see* Disruption, pelvic ring
    following insertion of implant, prosthesis or plate M96.65
    ilium — *see* Fracture, ilium
    ischium — *see* Fracture, ischium
    multiple
      with disruption of pelvic ring (circle) — *see* Disruption, pelvic ring
      without disruption of pelvic ring (circle) S32.82 ✓
    pubis — *see* Fracture, pubis
    sacrum — *see* Fracture, sacrum
    specified site NEC S32.89 ✓
  periprosthetic, around internal prosthetic joint M97.9
    ankle M97.2- ✓
    elbow M97.4- ✓
    finger M97.8 ✓
    hip M97.0- ✓
    knee M97.1- ✓
    shoulder M97.3- ✓
    specified joint NEC M97.8 ✓
    spine M97.8 ✓
    toe M97.8 ✓

✓ **Additional Character Required** — Refer to the Tabular List for Character Selection   ⬙ **Subterms under main terms may continue to next column or page**

Fracture, traumatic — *continued*
  periprosthetic, around internal prosthetic joint —
    continued
    wrist M97.8 ☑
  phalanx
    foot — *see* Fracture, toe
    hand — *see* Fracture, finger
  pisiform — *see* Fracture, carpal, pisiform
  pond — *see* Fracture, skull
  prosthetic device, internal — *see* Complications,
    prosthetic device, by site, mechanical
  pubis S32.50- ☑
    with disruption of pelvic ring — *see* Disruption,
      pelvic ring
    specified site NEC S32.59- ☑
    superior rim S32.51- ☑
  radius S52.9- ☑
    distal end — *see* Fracture, radius, lower end
    following insertion of implant, prosthesis or plate
      M96.63- ☑
    head — *see* Fracture, radius, upper end, head
    lower end S52.50- ☑
      Barton's — *see* Barton's fracture
      Colles' — *see* Colles' fracture
      extraarticular NEC S52.55- ☑
      intraarticular NEC S52.57- ☑
      physeal S59.20- ☑
        Salter-Harris
          Type I S59.21- ☑
          Type II S59.22- ☑
          Type III S59.23- ☑
          Type IV S59.24- ☑
        specified NEC S59.29- ☑
      Smith's — *see* Smith's fracture
      specified NEC S52.59- ☑
      styloid process (displaced) S52.51- ☑
        nondisplaced S52.51- ☑
      torus S52.52- ☑
    neck — *see* Fracture, radius, upper end
    proximal end — *see* Fracture, radius, upper end
    shaft S52.30- ☑
      bent bone S52.38- ☑
      comminuted (displaced) S52.35- ☑
        nondisplaced S52.35- ☑
      Galeazzi's — *see* Galeazzi's fracture
      greenstick S52.31- ☑
      oblique (displaced) S52.33- ☑
        nondisplaced S52.33- ☑
      segmental (displaced) S52.36- ☑
        nondisplaced S52.36- ☑
      specified NEC S52.39- ☑
      spiral (displaced) S52.34- ☑
        nondisplaced S52.34- ☑
      transverse (displaced) S52.32- ☑
        nondisplaced S52.32- ☑
    upper end S52.10- ☑
      head (displaced) S52.12- ☑
        nondisplaced S52.12- ☑
      neck (displaced) S52.13- ☑
        nondisplaced S52.13- ☑
      physeal S59.10- ☑
        Salter-Harris
          Type I S59.11- ☑
          Type II S59.12- ☑
          Type III S59.13- ☑
          Type IV S59.14- ☑
        specified NEC S59.19- ☑
      specified NEC S52.18- ☑
      torus S52.11- ☑
  ramus
    inferior or superior, pubis — *see* Fracture, pubis
    mandible — *see* Fracture, mandible
  restorative material (dental) K08.539
    with loss of material K08.531
    without loss of material K08.530
  rib S22.3- ☑
    with flail chest — *see* Flail, chest
    multiple S22.4- ☑
      with flail chest — *see* Flail, chest
  root, tooth — *see* Fracture, tooth
  sacrum S32.10 ☑
    specified NEC S32.19 ☑
    Type
      1 S32.14 ☑
      2 S32.15 ☑
      3 S32.16 ☑

Fracture, traumatic — *continued*
  sacrum — *continued*
    Type — *continued*
      4 S32.17 ☑
    Zone
      I S32.119 ☑
        displaced (minimally) S32.111 ☑
          severely S32.112 ☑
        nondisplaced S32.110 ☑
      II S32.129 ☑
        displaced (minimally) S32.121 ☑
          severely S32.122 ☑
        nondisplaced S32.120 ☑
      III S32.139 ☑
        displaced (minimally) S32.131 ☑
          severely S32.132 ☑
        nondisplaced S32.130 ☑
  scaphoid (hand) (*see also* Fracture, carpal, navicular)
    foot — *see* Fracture, tarsal, navicular
  scapula S42.10- ☑
    acromial process (displaced) S42.12- ☑
      nondisplaced S42.12- ☑
    body (displaced) S42.11- ☑
      nondisplaced S42.11- ☑
    coracoid process (displaced) S42.13- ☑
      nondisplaced S42.13- ☑
    glenoid cavity (displaced) S42.14- ☑
      nondisplaced S42.14- ☑
    neck (displaced) S42.15- ☑
      nondisplaced S42.15- ☑
    specified NEC S42.19- ☑
  semilunar bone, wrist — *see* Fracture, carpal, lunate
  sequelae — *see* Sequelae, fracture
  sesamoid bone
    foot S92.81-
    hand — *see* Fracture, carpal
    other — *see* Fracture, traumatic, by site
  shepherd's — *see* Fracture, tarsal, talus
  shoulder (girdle) S42.9- ☑
    blade — *see* Fracture, scapula
  sinus (ethmoid) (frontal) S02.19 ☑
  skull S02.91 ☑
    base S02.10- ☑
      occiput S02.119 ☑
        condyle S02.113 ☑
          specified NEC S02.118 ☑
            left side S02.11H ☑
            right side S02.11G ☑
          type I S02.110 ☑
            left side S02.11B ☑
            right side S02.11A ☑
          type II S02.111 ☑
            left side S02.11D ☑
            right side S02.11C ☑
          type III S02.112 ☑
            left side S02.11F ☑
            right side S02.11E ☑
      specified NEC S02.19 ☑
    birth injury P13.0
    frontal bone S02.0 ☑
    parietal bone S02.0 ☑
    specified site NEC S02.8- ☑
    temporal bone S02.19 ☑
    vault S02.0 ☑
  Smith's — *see* Smith's fracture
  sphenoid (bone) (sinus) S02.19 ☑
  spine — *see* Fracture, vertebra
  spinous process — *see* Fracture, vertebra
  spontaneous (cause unknown) — *see* Fracture,
    pathological
  stave (of thumb) — *see* Fracture, metacarpal, first
  sternum S22.20 ☑
    with flail chest — *see* Flail, chest
    body S22.22 ☑
    manubrium S22.21 ☑
    xiphoid (process) S22.24 ☑
  stress M84.30 ☑
    ankle M84.37- ☑
    carpus M84.34- ☑
    clavicle M84.31- ☑
    femoral neck M84.359 ☑
    femur M84.35- ☑
    fibula M84.36- ☑
    finger M84.34- ☑
    hip M84.359 ☑
    humerus M84.32- ☑

Fracture, traumatic — *continued*
  stress — *continued*
    ilium M84.350 ☑
    ischium M84.350 ☑
    metacarpus M84.34- ☑
    metatarsus M84.37- ☑
    neck — *see* Fracture, fatigue, vertebra
    pelvis M84.350 ☑
    radius M84.33- ☑
    rib M84.38 ☑
    scapula M84.31- ☑
    skull M84.38 ☑
    tarsus M84.37- ☑
    tibia M84.36- ☑
    toe M84.37- ☑
    ulna M84.33- ☑
    vertebra — *see* Fracture, fatigue, vertebra
  supracondylar, elbow — *see* Fracture, humerus, lower
    end, supracondylar
  symphysis pubis — *see* Fracture, pubis
  talus (ankle bone) — *see* Fracture, tarsal, talus
  tarsal bone(s) S92.20- ☑
    astragalus — *see* Fracture, tarsal, talus
    calcaneus S92.00- ☑
      anterior process (displaced) S92.02- ☑
        nondisplaced S92.02- ☑
      body (displaced) S92.01- ☑
        nondisplaced S92.01- ☑
      extraarticular NEC (displaced) S92.05- ☑
        nondisplaced S92.05- ☑
      intraarticular (displaced) S92.06- ☑
        nondisplaced S92.06- ☑
      physeal S99.00- ☑
        Salter-Harris
          Type I S99.01- ☑
          Type II S99.02- ☑
          Type III S99.03- ☑
          Type IV S99.04- ☑
        specified NEC S99.09- ☑
      tuberosity (displaced) S92.04- ☑
        avulsion (displaced) S92.03- ☑
          nondisplaced S92.03- ☑
        nondisplaced S92.04- ☑
    cuboid (displaced) S92.21- ☑
      nondisplaced S92.21- ☑
    cuneiform
      intermediate (displaced) S92.23- ☑
        nondisplaced S92.23- ☑
      lateral (displaced) S92.22- ☑
        nondisplaced S92.22- ☑
      medial (displaced) S92.24- ☑
        nondisplaced S92.24- ☑
    navicular (displaced) S92.25- ☑
      nondisplaced S92.25- ☑
    scaphoid — *see* Fracture, tarsal, navicular
    talus S92.10- ☑
      avulsion (displaced) S92.15- ☑
        nondisplaced S92.15- ☑
      body (displaced) S92.12- ☑
        nondisplaced S92.12- ☑
      dome (displaced) S92.14- ☑
        nondisplaced S92.14- ☑
      head (displaced) S92.12- ☑
        nondisplaced S92.12- ☑
      lateral process (displaced) S92.14- ☑
        nondisplaced S92.14- ☑
      neck (displaced) S92.11- ☑
        nondisplaced S92.11- ☑
      posterior process (displaced) S92.13- ☑
        nondisplaced S92.13- ☑
      specified NEC S92.19- ☑
  temporal bone (styloid) S02.19 ☑
  thorax (bony) S22.9 ☑
    with flail chest — *see* Flail, chest
    rib S22.3- ☑
      multiple S22.4- ☑
        with flail chest — *see* Flail, chest
    sternum S22.20 ☑
      body S22.22 ☑
      manubrium S22.21 ☑
      xiphoid process S22.24 ☑
    vertebra (displaced) S22.009 ☑
      burst (stable) S22.001 ☑
        unstable S22.002 ☑
      eighth S22.069 ☑
        burst (stable) S22.061 ☑

Index

Fracture, traumatic — Fracture, traumatic

Fracture, traumatic — *continued*
  thorax — *continued*
    vertebra — *continued*
      eighth — *continued*
        burst — *continued*
          unstable S22.062 ☑
        specified type NEC S22.068 ☑
        wedge compression S22.060 ☑
      eleventh S22.089 ☑
        burst (stable) S22.081 ☑
          unstable S22.082 ☑
        specified type NEC S22.088 ☑
        wedge compression S22.080 ☑
      fifth S22.059 ☑
        burst (stable) S22.051 ☑
          unstable S22.052 ☑
        specified type NEC S22.058 ☑
        wedge compression S22.050 ☑
      first S22.019 ☑
        burst (stable) S22.011 ☑
          unstable S22.012 ☑
        specified type NEC S22.018 ☑
        wedge compression S22.010 ☑
      fourth S22.049 ☑
        burst (stable) S22.041 ☑
          unstable S22.042 ☑
        specified type NEC S22.048 ☑
        wedge compression S22.040 ☑
      ninth S22.079 ☑
        burst (stable) S22.071 ☑
          unstable S22.072 ☑
        specified type NEC S22.078 ☑
        wedge compression S22.070 ☑
      nondisplaced S22.001 ☑
      second S22.029 ☑
        burst (stable) S22.021 ☑
          unstable S22.022 ☑
        specified type NEC S22.028 ☑
        wedge compression S22.020 ☑
      seventh S22.069 ☑
        burst (stable) S22.061 ☑
          unstable S22.062 ☑
        specified type NEC S22.068 ☑
        wedge compression S22.060 ☑
      sixth S22.059 ☑
        burst (stable) S22.051 ☑
          unstable S22.052 ☑
        specified type NEC S22.058 ☑
        wedge compression S22.050 ☑
      specified type NEC S22.008 ☑
      tenth S22.079 ☑
        burst (stable) S22.071 ☑
          unstable S22.072 ☑
        specified type NEC S22.078 ☑
        wedge compression S22.070 ☑
      third S22.039 ☑
        burst (stable) S22.031 ☑
          unstable S22.032 ☑
        specified type NEC S22.038 ☑
        wedge compression S22.030 ☑
      twelfth S22.089 ☑
        burst (stable) S22.081 ☑
          unstable S22.082 ☑
        specified type NEC S22.088 ☑
        wedge compression S22.080 ☑
      wedge compression S22.000 ☑
  thumb S62.50- ☑
    distal phalanx (displaced) S62.52- ☑
      nondisplaced S62.52- ☑
    proximal phalanx (displaced) S62.51- ☑
      nondisplaced S62.51- ☑
  thyroid cartilage S12.8 ☑
  tibia (shaft) S82.20- ☑
    comminuted (displaced) S82.25- ☑
      nondisplaced S82.25- ☑
    condyles — *see* Fracture, tibia, upper end
    distal end — *see* Fracture, tibia, lower end
    epiphysis
      lower — *see* Fracture, tibia, lower end
      upper — *see* Fracture, tibia, upper end
    following insertion of implant, prosthesis or plate M96.67- ☑
    head (involving knee joint) — *see* Fracture, tibia, upper end
    intercondyloid eminence — *see* Fracture, tibia, upper end

Fracture, traumatic — *continued*
  tibia — *continued*
    involving ankle or malleolus — *see* Fracture, ankle, medial malleolus
    lower end S82.30- ☑
      physeal S89.10- ☑
        Salter-Harris
          Type I S89.11- ☑
          Type II S89.12- ☑
          Type III S89.13- ☑
          Type IV S89.14- ☑
        specified NEC S89.19- ☑
      pilon (displaced) S82.87- ☑
        nondisplaced S82.87- ☑
      specified NEC S82.39- ☑
      torus S82.31- ☑
    malleolus — *see* Fracture, ankle, medial malleolus
    oblique (displaced) S82.23- ☑
      nondisplaced S82.23- ☑
    pilon — *see* Fracture, tibia, lower end, pilon
    proximal end — *see* Fracture, tibia, upper end
    segmental (displaced) S82.26- ☑
      nondisplaced S82.26- ☑
    specified NEC S82.29- ☑
    spine — *see* Fracture, tibia, upper end, spine
    spiral (displaced) S82.24- ☑
      nondisplaced S82.24- ☑
    transverse (displaced) S82.22- ☑
      nondisplaced S82.22- ☑
    tuberosity — *see* Fracture, tibia, upper end, tuberosity
    upper end S82.10- ☑
      bicondylar (displaced) S82.14- ☑
        nondisplaced S82.14- ☑
      lateral condyle (displaced) S82.12- ☑
        nondisplaced S82.12- ☑
      medial condyle (displaced) S82.13- ☑
        nondisplaced S82.13- ☑
      physeal S89.00- ☑
        Salter-Harris
          Type I S89.01- ☑
          Type II S89.02- ☑
          Type III S89.03- ☑
          Type IV S89.04- ☑
        specified NEC S89.09- ☑
      plateau — *see* Fracture, tibia, upper end, bicondylar
      specified NEC S82.19- ☑
      spine (displaced) S82.11- ☑
        nondisplaced S82.11- ☑
      torus S82.16- ☑
      tuberosity (displaced) S82.15- ☑
        nondisplaced S82.15- ☑
  toe S92.91- ☑
    great (displaced) S92.40- ☑
      distal phalanx (displaced) S92.42- ☑
        nondisplaced S92.42- ☑
      nondisplaced S92.40- ☑
      proximal phalanx (displaced) S92.41- ☑
        nondisplaced S92.41- ☑
      specified NEC S92.49- ☑
    lesser (displaced) S92.50- ☑
      distal phalanx (displaced) S92.53- ☑
        nondisplaced S92.53- ☑
      medial phalanx (displaced) S92.52- ☑
        nondisplaced S92.52- ☑
      nondisplaced S92.50- ☑
      proximal phalanx (displaced) S92.51- ☑
        nondisplaced S92.51- ☑
      specified NEC S92.59- ☑
    physeal
      phalanx S99.20- ☑
        Salter-Harris
          Type I S99.21- ☑
          Type II S99.22- ☑
          Type III S99.23- ☑
          Type IV S99.24- ☑
        specified NEC S99.29- ☑
  tooth (root) S02.5 ☑
  trachea (cartilage) S12.8 ☑
  transverse process — *see* Fracture, vertebra
  trapezium or trapezoid bone — *see* Fracture, carpal
  trimalleolar — *see* Fracture, ankle, trimalleolar
  triquetrum (cuneiform of carpus) — *see* Fracture, carpal, triquetrum
  trochanter — *see* Fracture, femur, trochanteric

Fracture, traumatic — *continued*
  tuberosity (external) — *see* Fracture, traumatic, by site
  ulna (shaft) S52.20- ☑
    bent bone S52.28- ☑
    coronoid process — *see* Fracture, ulna, upper end, coronoid process
    distal end — *see* Fracture, ulna, lower end
    following insertion of implant, prosthesis or plate M96.63- ☑
    head S52.60- ☑
    lower end S52.60- ☑
      physeal S59.00- ☑
        Salter-Harris
          Type I S59.01- ☑
          Type II S59.02- ☑
          Type III S59.03- ☑
          Type IV S59.04- ☑
        specified NEC S59.09- ☑
      specified NEC S52.69- ☑
      styloid process (displaced) S52.61- ☑
        nondisplaced S52.61- ☑
      torus S52.62- ☑
    proximal end — *see* Fracture, ulna, upper end
    shaft S52.20- ☑
      comminuted (displaced) S52.25- ☑
        nondisplaced S52.25- ☑
      greenstick S52.21- ☑
      Monteggia's — *see* Monteggia's fracture
      oblique (displaced) S52.23- ☑
        nondisplaced S52.23- ☑
      segmental (displaced) S52.26- ☑
        nondisplaced S52.26- ☑
      specified NEC S52.29- ☑
      spiral (displaced) S52.24- ☑
        nondisplaced S52.24- ☑
      transverse (displaced) S52.22- ☑
        nondisplaced S52.22- ☑
    upper end S52.00- ☑
      coronoid process (displaced) S52.04- ☑
        nondisplaced S52.04- ☑
      olecranon process (displaced) S52.02- ☑
        with intraarticular extension S52.03- ☑
        nondisplaced S52.02- ☑
          with intraarticular extension S52.03- ☑
      specified NEC S52.09- ☑
      torus S52.01- ☑
  unciform — *see* Fracture, carpal, hamate
  vault of skull S02.0 ☑
  vertebra, vertebral (arch) (body) (column) (neural arch) (pedicle) (spinous process) (transverse process)
    atlas — *see* Fracture, neck, cervical vertebra, first
    axis — *see* Fracture, neck, cervical vertebra, second
    cervical (teardrop) S12.9 ☑
      axis — *see* Fracture, neck, cervical vertebra, second
      first (atlas) — *see* Fracture, neck, cervical vertebra, first
      second (axis) — *see* Fracture, neck, cervical vertebra, second
    chronic M84.48 ☑
    coccyx S32.2 ☑
    dorsal — *see* Fracture, thorax, vertebra
    lumbar S32.009 ☑
      burst (stable) S32.001 ☑
        unstable S32.002 ☑
      fifth S32.059 ☑
        burst (stable) S32.051 ☑
          unstable S32.052 ☑
        specified type NEC S32.058 ☑
        wedge compression S32.050 ☑
      first S32.019 ☑
        burst (stable) S32.011 ☑
          unstable S32.012 ☑
        specified type NEC S32.018 ☑
        wedge compression S32.010 ☑
      fourth S32.049 ☑
        burst (stable) S32.041 ☑
          unstable S32.042 ☑
        specified type NEC S32.048 ☑
        wedge compression S32.040 ☑
      second S32.029 ☑
        burst (stable) S32.021 ☑
          unstable S32.022 ☑
        specified type NEC S32.028 ☑
        wedge compression S32.020 ☑
      specified type NEC S32.008 ☑

☑ **Additional Character Required** — **Refer to the Tabular List for Character Selection**

Subterms under main terms may continue to next column or page

Fracture, traumatic — *continued*
  vertebra, vertebral — *continued*
    lumbar — *continued*
      third S32.039 ☑
        burst (stable) S32.031 ☑
          unstable S32.032 ☑
        specified type NEC S32.038 ☑
        wedge compression S32.030 ☑
      wedge compression S32.000 ☑
    metastatic — *see* Collapse, vertebra, in, specified
      disease NEC (*see also* Neoplasm)
    newborn (birth injury) P11.5
    sacrum S32.10 ☑
      specified NEC S32.19 ☑
      Type
        1 S32.14 ☑
        2 S32.15 ☑
        3 S32.16 ☑
        4 S32.17 ☑
      Zone
        I S32.119 ☑
          displaced (minimally) S32.111 ☑
            severely S32.112 ☑
          nondisplaced S32.110 ☑
        II S32.129 ☑
          displaced (minimally) S32.121 ☑
            severely S32.122 ☑
          nondisplaced S32.120 ☑
        III S32.139 ☑
          displaced (minimally) S32.131 ☑
            severely S32.132 ☑
          nondisplaced S32.130 ☑
    thoracic — *see* Fracture, thorax, vertebra
  vertex S02.0 ☑
  vomer (bone) S02.2 ☑
  wrist S62.10- ☑
    carpal — *see* Fracture, carpal bone
    navicular (scaphoid) (hand) — *see* Fracture, carpal,
      navicular
  xiphisternum, xiphoid (process) S22.24 ☑
  zygoma S02.402 ☑
    left side S02.40F ☑
    right side S02.40E ☑
Fragile, fragility
  autosomal site Q95.5
  bone, congenital (with blue sclera) Q78.0
  capillary (hereditary) D69.8
  hair L67.8
  nails L60.3
  non-sex chromosome site Q95.5
  X chromosome Q99.2
Fragilitas
  crinium L67.8
  ossium (with blue sclerae) (hereditary) Q78.0
  unguium L60.3
    congenital Q84.6
Fragments, cataract (lens), **following cataract surgery**
  H59.02- ☑
  retained foreign body — *see* Retained, foreign body
    fragments (type of)
Frailty (frail) R54
  mental R41.81
Frambesia, frambesial (tropica) (*see also* Yaws)
  initial lesion or ulcer A66.0
  primary A66.0
Frambeside
  gummatous A66.4
  of early yaws A66.2
Frambesioma A66.1
Franceschetti-Klein (-Wildervanck) **disease or syn-**
  drome Q75.4
Francis' disease — *see* Tularemia
Franklin disease C88.2
Frank's essential thrombocytopenia D69.3
Fraser's syndrome Q87.0
Freckle(s) L81.2
  malignant melanoma in — *see* Melanoma
  melanotic (Hutchinson's) — *see* Melanoma, in situ
  retinal D49.81
Frederickson's hyperlipoproteinemia, type
  I and V E78.3
  IIA E78.00
  IIB and III E78.2
  IV E78.1
Freeman Sheldon syndrome Q87.0
Freezing (*see also* Effect, adverse, cold) T69.9 ☑

Freiberg's disease (infraction of metatarsal head or osteochondrosis) — *see* Osteochondrosis, juvenile,
  metatarsus
Frei's disease A55
Fremitus, friction, cardiac R01.2
Frenum, frenulum
  external os Q51.828
  tongue (shortening) (congenital) Q38.1
Frequency micturition (nocturnal) R35.0
  psychogenic F45.8
Frey's syndrome
  auriculotemporal G50.8
  hyperhidrosis L74.52
Friction
  burn — *see* Burn, by site
  fremitus, cardiac R01.2
  precordial R01.2
  sounds, chest R09.89
Friderichsen-Waterhouse syndrome or disease A39.1
Friedländer's B (bacillus) **NEC** (*see also* condition) A49.8
Friedreich's
  ataxia G11.1
  combined systemic disease G11.1
  facial hemihypertrophy Q67.4
  sclerosis (cerebellum) (spinal cord) G11.1
Frigidity F52.22
Fröhlich's syndrome E23.6
Frontal (*see also* condition)
  lobe syndrome F07.0
Frostbite (superficial) T33.90 ☑
  with
    partial thickness skin loss — *see* Frostbite (superfi-
      cial), by site
    tissue necrosis T34.90 ☑
  abdominal wall T33.3 ☑
    with tissue necrosis T34.3 ☑
  ankle T33.81- ☑
    with tissue necrosis T34.81- ☑
  arm T33.4- ☑
    with tissue necrosis T34.4- ☑
    finger(s) — *see* Frostbite, finger
    hand — *see* Frostbite, hand
    wrist — *see* Frostbite, wrist
  ear T33.01- ☑
    with tissue necrosis T34.01- ☑
  face T33.09 ☑
    with tissue necrosis T34.09 ☑
  finger T33.53- ☑
    with tissue necrosis T34.53- ☑
  foot T33.82- ☑
    with tissue necrosis T34.82- ☑
  hand T33.52- ☑
    with tissue necrosis T34.52- ☑
  head T33.09 ☑
    with tissue necrosis T34.09 ☑
    ear — *see* Frostbite, ear
    nose — *see* Frostbite, nose
  hip (and thigh) T33.6- ☑
    with tissue necrosis T34.6- ☑
  knee T33.7- ☑
    with tissue necrosis T34.7- ☑
  leg T33.9- ☑
    with tissue necrosis T34.9- ☑
    ankle — *see* Frostbite, ankle
    foot — *see* Frostbite, foot
    knee — *see* Frostbite, knee
    lower T33.7- ☑
      with tissue necrosis T34.7- ☑
    thigh — *see* Frostbite, hip
    toe — *see* Frostbite, toe
  limb
    lower T33.99 ☑
      with tissue necrosis T34.99 ☑
    upper — *see* Frostbite, arm
  neck T33.1 ☑
    with tissue necrosis T34.1 ☑
  nose T33.02 ☑
    with tissue necrosis T34.02 ☑
  pelvis T33.3 ☑
    with tissue necrosis T34.3 ☑
  specified site NEC T33.99 ☑
    with tissue necrosis T34.99 ☑
  thigh — *see* Frostbite, hip
  thorax T33.2 ☑
    with tissue necrosis T34.2 ☑
  toes T33.83- ☑

Frostbite — *continued*
  toes — *continued*
    with tissue necrosis T34.83- ☑
  trunk T33.99 ☑
    with tissue necrosis T34.99 ☑
  wrist T33.51- ☑
    with tissue necrosis T34.51- ☑
Frotteurism F65.81
Frozen (*see also* Effect, adverse, cold) T69.9 ☑
  pelvis (female) N94.89
    male K66.8
  shoulder — *see* Capsulitis, adhesive
Fructokinase deficiency E74.11
Fructose 1,6 diphosphatase deficiency E74.19
Fructosemia (benign) (essential) E74.12
Fructosuria (benign) (essential) E74.11
Fuchs'
  black spot (myopic) (*see also* Myopia, degenerative)
    H44.2- ☑
  dystrophy (corneal endothelium) H18.51
  heterochromic cyclitis — *see* Cyclitis, Fuchs' hete-
    rochromic
Fucosidosis E77.1
Fugue R68.89
  dissociative F44.1
  hysterical (dissociative) F44.1
  postictal in epilepsy — *see* Epilepsy
  reaction to exceptional stress (transient) F43.0
Fulminant, fulminating — *see* condition
Functional (*see also* condition)
  bleeding (uterus) N93.8
Functioning, intellectual, borderline R41.83
Fundus — *see* condition
Fungemia NOS B49
Fungus, fungous
  cerebral G93.89
  disease NOS B49
  infection — *see* Infection, fungus
Funiculitis (acute) (chronic) (endemic) N49.1
  gonococcal (acute) (chronic) A54.23
  tuberculous A18.15
Funnel
  breast (acquired) M95.4
    congenital Q67.6
    sequelae (late effect) of rickets E64.3
  chest (acquired) M95.4
    congenital Q67.6
    sequelae (late effect) of rickets E64.3
  pelvis (acquired) M95.5
    with disproportion (fetopelvic) O33.3 ☑
      causing obstructed labor O65.3
    congenital Q74.2
FUO (fever of unknown origin) R50.9
Furfur L21.0
  microsporon B36.0
Furrier's lung J67.8
Furrowed K14.5
  nail(s) (transverse) L60.4
    congenital Q84.6
  tongue K14.5
    congenital Q38.3
Furuncle L02.92
  abdominal wall L02.221
  ankle — *see* Furuncle, lower limb
  antecubital space — *see* Furuncle, upper limb
  anus K61.0
  arm — *see* Furuncle, upper limb
  auditory canal, external — *see* Abscess, ear, external
  auricle (ear) — *see* Abscess, ear, external
  axilla (region) L02.42- ☑
  back (any part) L02.222
  breast N61.1
  buttock L02.32
  cheek (external) L02.02
  chest wall L02.223
  chin L02.02
  corpus cavernosum N48.21
  ear, external — *see* Abscess, ear, external
  external auditory canal — *see* Abscess, ear, external
  eyelid — *see* Abscess, eyelid
  face L02.02
  femoral (region) — *see* Furuncle, lower limb
  finger — *see* Furuncle, hand
  flank L02.221
  foot L02.62- ☑
  forehead L02.02
  gluteal (region) L02.32

Furuncle — *continued*
  groin L02.224
  hand L02.52- ☑
  head L02.821
    face L02.02
  hip — *see* Furuncle, lower limb
  kidney — *see* Abscess, kidney
  knee — *see* Furuncle, lower limb
  labium (majus) (minus) N76.4
  lacrimal
    gland — *see* Dacryoadenitis
    passages (duct) (sac) — *see* Inflammation, lacrimal,
      passages, acute
  leg (any part) — *see* Furuncle, lower limb
  lower limb L02.42- ☑
  malignant A22.0
  mouth K12.2
  navel L02.226
  neck L02.12
  nose J34.0
  orbit, orbital — *see* Abscess, orbit
  palmar (space) — *see* Furuncle, hand
  partes posteriores L02.32
  pectoral region L02.223
  penis N48.21
  perineum L02.225
  pinna — *see* Abscess, ear, external
  popliteal — *see* Furuncle, lower limb
  prepatellar — *see* Furuncle, lower limb
  scalp L02.821
  seminal vesicle N49.0
  shoulder — *see* Furuncle, upper limb
  specified site NEC L02.828
  submandibular K12.2
  temple (region) L02.02
  thumb — *see* Furuncle, hand
  toe — *see* Furuncle, foot
  trunk L02.229
    abdominal wall L02.221
    back L02.222

Furuncle — *continued*
  trunk — *continued*
    chest wall L02.223
    groin L02.224
    perineum L02.225
    umbilicus L02.226
  umbilicus L02.226
  upper limb L02.42- ☑
  vulva N76.4
Furunculosis — *see* Furuncle
Fused — *see* Fusion, fused
Fusion, fused (congenital)
  astragaloscaphoid Q74.2
  atria Q21.1
  auditory canal Q16.1
  auricles, heart Q21.1
  binocular with defective stereopsis H53.32
  bone Q79.8
  cervical spine M43.22
  choanal Q30.0
  commissure, mitral valve Q23.2
  cusps, heart valve NEC Q24.8
    mitral Q23.2
    pulmonary Q22.1
    tricuspid Q22.4
  ear ossicles Q16.3
  fingers Q70.0 ☑
  hymen Q52.3
  joint (acquired) (*see also* Ankylosis)
    congenital Q74.8
  kidneys (incomplete) Q63.1
  labium (majus) (minus) Q52.5
  larynx and trachea Q34.8
  limb, congenital Q74.8
    lower Q74.2
    upper Q74.0
  lobes, lung Q33.8
  lumbosacral (acquired) M43.27
    arthrodesis status Z98.1
    congenital Q76.49

Fusion, fused — *continued*
  lumbosacral — *continued*
    postprocedural status Z98.1
  nares, nose, nasal, nostril(s) Q30.0
  organ or site not listed — *see* Anomaly, by site
  ossicles Q79.9
    auditory Q16.3
  pulmonic cusps Q22.1
  ribs Q76.6
  sacroiliac (joint) (acquired) M43.28
    arthrodesis status Z98.1
    congenital Q74.2
    postprocedural status Z98.1
  spine (acquired) NEC M43.20
    arthrodesis status Z98.1
    cervical region M43.22
    cervicothoracic region M43.23
    congenital Q76.49
    lumbar M43.26
    lumbosacral region M43.27
    occipito-atlanto-axial region M43.21
    postoperative status Z98.1
    sacrococcygeal region M43.28
    thoracic region M43.24
    thoracolumbar region M43.25
  sublingual duct with submaxillary duct at opening in
    mouth Q38.4
  testes Q55.1
  toes Q70.2- ☑
  tooth, teeth K00.2
  trachea and esophagus Q39.8
  twins Q89.4
  vagina Q52.4
  ventricles, heart Q21.0
  vertebra (arch) — *see* Fusion, spine
  vulva Q52.5
Fusospirillosis (mouth) (tongue) (tonsil) A69.1
Fussy baby R68.12

G

Gain in weight (abnormal) (excessive) (see also Weight, gain)
Gaisböck's disease (polycythemia hypertonica) D75.1
Gait abnormality R26.9
  ataxic R26.0
  falling R29.6
  hysterical (ataxic) (staggering) F44.4
  paralytic R26.1
  spastic R26.1
  specified type NEC R26.89
  staggering R26.0
  unsteadiness R26.81
  walking difficulty NEC R26.2
Galactocele (breast) N64.89
  puerperal, postpartum O92.79
Galactokinase deficiency E74.29
Galactophoritis N61.0
  gestational, puerperal, postpartum O91.2- ☑
Galactorrhea O92.6
  not associated with childbirth N64.3
Galactosemia (classic) (congenital) E74.21
Galactosuria E74.29
Galacturia R82.0
  schistosomiasis (bilharziasis) B65.0
GALD (gestational alloimmune liver disease) P78.84
Galeazzi's fracture S52.37- ☑
Galen's vein — see condition
Galeophobia F40.218
Gall duct — see condition
Gallbladder (see also condition)
  acute K81.0
Gallop rhythm R00.8
Gallstone (colic) (cystic duct) (gallbladder) (impacted) (multiple) (see also Calculus, gallbladder)
  with
    cholecystitis — see Calculus, gallbladder, with cholecystitis
    bile duct (common) (hepatic) — see Calculus, bile duct
  causing intestinal obstruction K56.3
  specified NEC K80.80
    with obstruction K80.81
Gambling Z72.6
  pathological (compulsive) F63.0
Gammopathy (of undetermined significance [MGUS]) D47.2
  associated with lymphoplasmacytic dyscrasia D47.2
  monoclonal D47.2
  polyclonal D89.0
Gamna's disease (siderotic splenomegaly) D73.1
Gamophobia F40.298
Gampsodactylia (congenital) Q66.7
Gamstorp's disease (adynamia episodica hereditaria) G72.3
Gandy-Nanta disease (siderotic splenomegaly) D73.1
Gang
  membership offenses Z72.810
Gangliocytoma D36.10
Ganglioglioma — see Neoplasm, uncertain behavior, by site
Ganglion (compound) (diffuse) (joint) (tendon (sheath)) M67.40
  ankle M67.47- ☑
  foot M67.47- ☑
  forearm M67.43- ☑
  hand M67.44- ☑
  lower leg M67.46- ☑
  multiple sites M67.49
  of yaws (early) (late) A66.6
  pelvic region M67.45- ☑
  periosteal — see Periostitis
  shoulder region M67.41- ☑
  specified site NEC M67.48
  thigh region M67.45- ☑
  tuberculous A18.09
  upper arm M67.42- ☑
  wrist M67.43- ☑
Ganglioneuroblastoma — see Neoplasm, nerve, malignant
Ganglioneuroma D36.10
  malignant — see Neoplasm, nerve, malignant
Ganglioneuromatosis D36.10
Ganglionitis
  fifth nerve — see Neuralgia, trigeminal
  gasserian (postherpetic) (postzoster) B02.21

Ganglionitis — continued
  geniculate G51.1
    newborn (birth injury) P11.3
    postherpetic, postzoster B02.21
  herpes zoster B02.21
  postherpetic geniculate B02.21
Gangliosidosis E75.10
  GM1 E75.19
  GM2 E75.00
    other specified E75.09
    Sandhoff disease E75.01
    Tay-Sachs disease E75.02
  GM3 E75.19
  mucolipidosis IV E75.11
Gangosa A66.5
Gangrene, gangrenous (connective tissue) (dropsical) (dry) (moist) (skin) (ulcer) (see also Necrosis) I96
  with diabetes (mellitus) — see Diabetes, gangrene
  abdomen (wall) I96
  alveolar M27.3
  appendix K35.80
    with
      perforation or rupture K35.2
      peritoneal abscess K35.3
      peritonitis NEC K35.3
        generalized (with perforation or rupture) K35.2
        localized (with perforation or rupture) K35.3
  arteriosclerotic (general) (senile) — see Arteriosclerosis, extremities, with, gangrene
  auricle I96
  Bacillus welchii A48.0
  bladder (infectious) — see Cystitis, specified type NEC
  bowel, cecum, or colon — see Gangrene, intestine
  Clostridium perfringens or welchii A48.0
  cornea H18.89- ☑
  corpora cavernosa N48.29
    noninfective N48.89
  cutaneous, spreading I96
  decubital — see Ulcer, pressure, by site
  diabetic (any site) — see Diabetes, gangrene
  emphysematous — see Gangrene, gas
  epidemic — see Poisoning, food, noxious, plant
  epididymis (infectional) N45.1
  erysipelas — see Erysipelas
  extremity (lower) (upper) I96
  Fournier N49.3
    female N76.89
  fusospirochetal A69.0
  gallbladder — see Cholecystitis, acute
  gas (bacillus) A48.0
    following
      abortion — see Abortion by type complicated by infection
      ectopic or molar pregnancy O08.0
  glossitis K14.0
  hernia — see Hernia, by site, with gangrene
  intestine, intestinal (hemorrhagic) (massive) (see also Infarct, intestine) K55.069
    with
      mesenteric embolism (see also Infarct, intestine) K55.069
      obstruction — see Obstruction, intestine
  laryngitis J04.0
  limb (lower) (upper) I96
  lung J85.0
    spirochetal A69.8
  lymphangitis I89.1
  Meleney's (synergistic) — see Ulcer, skin
  mesentery (see also Infarct, intestine) K55.069
    with
      embolism (see also Infarct, intestine) K55.069
      intestinal obstruction — see Obstruction, intestine
  mouth A69.0
  ovary — see Oophoritis
  pancreas — see Pancreatitis, acute
  penis N48.29
    noninfective N48.89
  perineum I96
  pharynx (see also Pharyngitis)
    Vincent's A69.1
  presenile I73.1
  progressive synergistic — see Ulcer, skin
  pulmonary J85.0
  pulpal (dental) K04.1
  quinsy J36
  Raynaud's (symmetric gangrene) I73.01

Gangrene, gangrenous — continued
  retropharyngeal J39.2
  scrotum N49.3
    noninfective N50.89
  senile (atherosclerotic) — see Arteriosclerosis, extremities, with, gangrene
  spermatic cord N49.1
    noninfective N50.89
  spine I96
  spirochetal NEC A69.8
  spreading cutaneous I96
  stomatitis A69.0
  symmetrical I73.01
  testis (infectional) N45.2
    noninfective N44.8
  throat (see also Pharyngitis)
    diphtheritic A36.0
    Vincent's A69.1
  thyroid (gland) E07.89
  tooth (pulp) K04.1
  tuberculous NEC — see Tuberculosis
  tunica vaginalis N49.1
    noninfective N50.89
  umbilicus I96
  uterus — see Endometritis
  uvulitis K12.2
  vas deferens N49.1
    noninfective N50.89
  vulva N76.89
Ganister disease J62.8
Ganser's syndrome (hysterical) F44.89
Gardner-Diamond syndrome (autoerythrocyte sensitization) D69.2
Gargoylism E76.01
Garré's disease, osteitis (sclerosing), osteomyelitis — see Osteomyelitis, specified type NEC
Garrod's pad, knuckle M72.1
Gartner's duct
  cyst Q52.4
  persistent Q50.6
Gas R14.3
  asphyxiation, inhalation, poisoning, suffocation NEC — see Table of Drugs and Chemicals
  excessive R14.0
  gangrene A48.0
    following
      abortion — see Abortion by type complicated by infection
      ectopic or molar pregnancy O08.0
  on stomach R14.0
  pains R14.1
Gastralgia (see also Pain, abdominal)
Gastrectasis K31.0
  psychogenic F45.8
Gastric — see condition
Gastrinoma
  malignant
    pancreas C25.4
    specified site NEC — see Neoplasm, malignant, by site
    unspecified site C25.4
  specified site — see Neoplasm, uncertain behavior
  unspecified site D37.9
Gastritis (simple) K29.70
  with bleeding K29.71
  acute (erosive) K29.00
    with bleeding K29.01
  alcoholic K29.20
    with bleeding K29.21
  allergic K29.60
    with bleeding K29.61
  atrophic (chronic) K29.40
    with bleeding K29.41
  chronic (antral) (fundal) K29.50
    with bleeding K29.51
    atrophic K29.40
      with bleeding K29.41
    superficial K29.30
      with bleeding K29.31
  dietary counseling and surveillance Z71.3
  due to diet deficiency E63.9
  eosinophilic K52.81
  giant hypertrophic K29.60
    with bleeding K29.61
  granulomatous K29.60
    with bleeding K29.61
  hypertrophic (mucosa) K29.60
    with bleeding K29.61

🐦 Subterms under main terms may continue to next column or page   ☑ Additional Character Required — Refer to the Tabular List for Character Selection   **157**

Gain in weight — Gastritis

Gastritis — continued
- nervous F54
- spastic K29.60
  - with bleeding K29.61
  - specified NEC K29.60
    - with bleeding K29.61
- superficial chronic K29.30
  - with bleeding K29.31
- tuberculous A18.83
- viral NEC A08.4

Gastrocarcinoma — see Neoplasm, malignant, stomach
Gastrocolic — see condition
Gastrodisciasis, gastrodiscoidiasis B66.8
Gastroduodenitis K29.90
- with bleeding K29.91
- virus, viral A08.4
  - specified type NEC A08.39

Gastrodynia — see Pain, abdominal
Gastroenteritis (acute) (chronic) (noninfectious) (see also Enteritis) K52.9
- allergic K52.29
  - with
    - eosinophilic gastritis or gastroenteritis K52.81
    - food protein-induced enterocolitis syndrome K52.21
    - food protein-induced enteropathy K52.22
- dietetic (see also Gastroenteritis, allergic) K52.29
- drug-induced K52.1
- due to
  - Cryptosporidium A07.2
  - drugs K52.1
  - food poisoning — see Intoxication, foodborne
  - radiation K52.0
- eosinophilic K52.81
- epidemic (infectious) A09
- food hypersensitivity (see also Gastroenteritis, allergic) K52.29
- infectious — see Enteritis, infectious
- influenzal — see Influenza, with gastroenteritis
- noninfectious K52.9
  - specified NEC K52.89
- rotaviral A08.0
- Salmonella A02.0
- toxic K52.1
- viral NEC A08.4
  - acute infectious A08.39
    - type Norwalk A08.11
  - infantile (acute) A08.39
  - Norwalk agent A08.11
  - rotaviral A08.0
  - severe of infants A08.39
  - specified type NEC A08.39

Gastroenteropathy (see also Gastroenteritis) K52.9
- acute, due to Norovirus A08.11
- acute, due to Norwalk agent A08.11
- infectious A09

Gastroenteroptosis K63.4
Gastroesophageal laceration- hemorrhage syndrome K22.6
Gastrointestinal — see condition
Gastrojejunal — see condition
Gastrojejunitis (see also Enteritis) K52.9
Gastrojejunocolic — see condition
Gastroliths K31.89
Gastromalacia K31.89
Gastroparalysis K31.84
- diabetic — see Diabetes, gastroparalysis

Gastroparesis K31.84
- diabetic — see Diabetes, by type, with gastroparesis

Gastropathy K31.9
- congestive portal K31.89
- erythematous K29.70
- exudative K90.89
- portal hypertensive K31.89

Gastroptosis K31.89
Gastrorrhagia K92.2
- psychogenic F45.8

Gastroschisis (congenital) Q79.3
Gastrospasm (neurogenic) (reflex) K31.89
- neurotic F45.8
- psychogenic F45.8

Gastrostaxis — see Gastritis, with bleeding
Gastrostenosis K31.89
Gastrostomy
- attention to Z43.1
- status Z93.1

Gastrosuccorrhea (continuous) (intermittent) K31.89
- neurotic F45.8

Gastrosuccorrhea — continued
- psychogenic F45.8

Gatophobia F40.218
Gaucher's disease or splenomegaly (adult) (infantile) E75.22
Gee (-Herter)(-Thaysen) **disease** (nontropical sprue) K90.0
Gélineau's syndrome G47.419
- with cataplexy G47.411

Gemination, tooth, teeth K00.2
Gemistocytoma
- specified site — see Neoplasm, malignant, by site
- unspecified site C71.9

General, generalized — see condition
Genetic
- carrier (status)
  - cystic fibrosis Z14.1
  - hemophilia A (asymptomatic) Z14.01
    - symptomatic Z14.02
  - specified NEC Z14.8
- susceptibility to disease NEC Z15.89
  - malignant neoplasm Z15.09
    - breast Z15.01
    - endometrium Z15.04
    - ovary Z15.02
    - prostate Z15.03
    - specified NEC Z15.09
  - multiple endocrine neoplasia Z15.81

Genital — see condition
Genito-anorectal syndrome A55
Genitourinary system — see condition
Genu
- congenital Q74.1
- extrorsum (acquired) (see also Deformity, varus, knee)
  - congenital Q74.1
  - sequelae (late effect) of rickets E64.3
- introrsum (acquired) (see also Deformity, valgus, knee)
  - congenital Q74.1
  - sequelae (late effect) of rickets E64.3
- rachitic (old) E64.3
- recurvatum (acquired) (see also Deformity, limb, specified type NEC, lower leg)
  - congenital Q68.2
  - sequelae (late effect) of rickets E64.3
- valgum (acquired) (knock-knee) M21.06- ☑
  - congenital Q74.1
  - sequelae (late effect) of rickets E64.3
- varum (acquired) (bowleg) M21.16- ☑
  - congenital Q74.1
  - sequelae (late effect) of rickets E64.3

Geographic tongue K14.1
Geophagia — see Pica
Geotrichosis B48.3
- stomatitis B48.3

Gephyrophobia F40.242
Gerbode defect Q21.0
GERD (gastroesophageal reflux disease) K21.9
Gerhardt's
- disease (erythromelalgia) I73.81
- syndrome (vocal cord paralysis) J38.00
  - bilateral J38.02
  - unilateral J38.01

German measles (see also Rubella)
- exposure to Z20.4

Germinoblastoma (diffuse) C85.9- ☑
- follicular C82.9- ☑

Germinoma — see Neoplasm, malignant, by site
Gerontoxon — see Degeneration, cornea, senile
Gerstmann's syndrome R48.8
- developmental F81.2

Gerstmann-Sträussler-Scheinker syndrome (GSS) A81.82
Gestation (period) (see also Pregnancy)
- ectopic — see Pregnancy, by site
- multiple O30.9- ☑
  - greater than quadruplets — see Pregnancy, multiple (gestation), specified NEC
  - specified NEC — see Pregnancy, multiple (gestation), specified NEC

Gestational
- mammary abscess O91.11- ☑
- purulent mastitis O91.11- ☑
- subareolar abscess O91.11- ☑

Ghon tubercle, primary infection A15.7
Ghost
- teeth K00.4
- vessels (cornea) H16.41- ☑

Ghoul hand A66.3

Gianotti-Crosti disease L44.4
Giant
- cell
  - epulis K06.8
  - peripheral granuloma K06.8
- esophagus, congenital Q39.5
- kidney, congenital Q63.3
- urticaria T78.3 ☑
  - hereditary D84.1

Giardiasis A07.1
Gibert's disease or pityriasis L42
Giddiness R42
- hysterical F44.89
- psychogenic F45.8

Gierke's disease (glycogenosis I) E74.01
Gigantism (cerebral) (hypophyseal) (pituitary) E22.0
- constitutional E34.4

Gilbert's disease or syndrome E80.4
Gilchrist's disease B40.9
Gilford-Hutchinson disease E34.8
Gilles de la Tourette's disease or syndrome (motor-verbal tic) F95.2
Gingivitis K05.10
- acute (catarrhal) K05.00
  - necrotizing A69.1
  - nonplaque induced K05.01
  - plaque induced K05.00
- chronic (desquamative) (hyperplastic) (simple marginal) (pregnancy associated) (ulcerative) K05.10
  - nonplaque induced K05.11
  - plaque induced K05.10
- expulsiva — see Periodontitis
- necrotizing ulcerative (acute) A69.1
- pellagrous E52
  - acute necrotizing A69.1
- Vincent's A69.1

Gingivoglossitis K14.0
Gingivopericementitis — see Periodontitis
Gingivosis — see Gingivitis, chronic
Gingivostomatitis K05.10
- herpesviral B00.2
- necrotizing ulcerative (acute) A69.1

Gland, glandular — see condition
Glanders A24.0
Glanzmann (-Naegeli) **disease or thrombasthenia** D69.1
Glasgow coma scale
- total score
  - 3-8 R40.243 ☑
  - 9-12 R40.242 ☑
  - 13-15 R40.241 ☑

Glass-blower's disease (cataract) — see Cataract, specified NEC
Glaucoma H40.9
- with
  - increased episcleral venous pressure H40.81- ☑
  - pseudoexfoliation of lens — see Glaucoma, open angle, primary, capsular
- absolute H44.51- ☑
- angle-closure (primary) H40.20- ☑
  - acute (attack) (crisis) H40.21- ☑
  - chronic H40.22- ☑
  - intermittent H40.23- ☑
  - residual stage H40.24- ☑
- borderline H40.00- ☑
- capsular (with pseudoexfoliation of lens) — see Glaucoma, open angle, primary, capsular
- childhood Q15.0
- closed angle — see Glaucoma, angle-closure
- congenital Q15.0
- corticosteroid-induced — see Glaucoma, secondary, drugs
- hypersecretion H40.82- ☑
- in (due to)
  - amyloidosis E85.4 [H42]
  - aniridia Q13.1 [H42]
  - concussion of globe — see Glaucoma, secondary, trauma
  - dislocation of lens — see Glaucoma, secondary
  - disorder of lens NEC — see Glaucoma, secondary
  - drugs — see Glaucoma, secondary, drugs
  - endocrine disease NOS E34.9 [H42]
  - eye
    - inflammation — see Glaucoma, secondary, inflammation
    - trauma — see Glaucoma, secondary, trauma

Glaucoma — *continued*
  in — *continued*
    hypermature cataract — *see* Glaucoma, secondary
    iridocyclitis — *see* Glaucoma, secondary, inflammation
    lens disorder — *see* Glaucoma, secondary
    Lowe's syndrome E72.03 [H42]
    metabolic disease NOS E88.9 [H42]
    ocular disorders NEC — *see* Glaucoma, secondary
    onchocerciasis B73.02
    pupillary block — *see* Glaucoma, secondary
    retinal vein occlusion — *see* Glaucoma, secondary
    Rieger's anomaly Q13.81 [H42]
    rubeosis of iris — *see* Glaucoma, secondary
    tumor of globe — *see* Glaucoma, secondary
  infantile Q15.0
  low tension — *see* Glaucoma, open angle, primary, low-tension
  malignant H40.83- ☑
  narrow angle — *see* Glaucoma, angle-closure
  newborn Q15.0
  noncongestive (chronic) — *see* Glaucoma, open angle
  nonobstructive — *see* Glaucoma, open angle
  obstructive (*see also* Glaucoma, angle-closure)
    due to lens changes — *see* Glaucoma, secondary
  open angle H40.10- ☑
    primary H40.11- ☑
      capsular (with pseudoexfoliation of lens) H40.14- ☑
      low-tension H40.12- ☑
      pigmentary H40.13- ☑
      residual stage H40.15- ☑
  phacolytic — *see* Glaucoma, secondary
  pigmentary — *see* Glaucoma, open angle, primary, pigmentary
  postinfectious — *see* Glaucoma, secondary, inflammation
  secondary (to) H40.5- ☑
    drugs H40.6- ☑
    inflammation H40.4- ☑
    trauma H40.3- ☑
  simple (chronic) H40.11- ☑
  simplex H40.11- ☑
  specified type NEC H40.89
  suspect H40.00- ☑
  syphilitic A52.71
  traumatic (*see also* Glaucoma, secondary, trauma)
    newborn (birth injury) P15.3
  tuberculous A18.59
Glaucomatous flecks (subcapsular) — *see* Cataract, complicated
Glazed tongue K14.4
Gleet (gonococcal) A54.01
Glénard's disease K63.4
Glioblastoma (multiforme)
  with sarcomatous component
    specified site — *see* Neoplasm, malignant, by site
    unspecified site C71.9
  giant cell
    specified site — *see* Neoplasm, malignant, by site
    unspecified site C71.9
  specified site — *see* Neoplasm, malignant, by site
  unspecified site C71.9
Glioma (malignant)
  astrocytic
    specified site — *see* Neoplasm, malignant, by site
    unspecified site C71.9
  mixed
    specified site — *see* Neoplasm, malignant, by site
    unspecified site C71.9
  nose Q30.8
  specified site NEC — *see* Neoplasm, malignant, by site
  subependymal D43.2
    specified site — *see* Neoplasm, uncertain behavior, by site
    unspecified site D43.2
  unspecified site C71.9
Gliomatosis cerebri C71.0
Glioneuroma — *see* Neoplasm, uncertain behavior, by site
Gliosarcoma
  specified site — *see* Neoplasm, malignant, by site
  unspecified site C71.9
Gliosis (cerebral) G93.89
  spinal G95.89
Glisson's disease — *see* Rickets
Globinuria R82.3

Globus (hystericus) F45.8
Glomangioma D18.00
  intra-abdominal D18.03
  intracranial D18.02
  skin D18.01
  specified site NEC D18.09
Glomangiomyoma D18.00
  intra-abdominal D18.03
  intracranial D18.02
  skin D18.01
  specified site NEC D18.09
Glomangiosarcoma — *see* Neoplasm, connective tissue, malignant
Glomerular
  disease in syphilis A52.75
  nephritis — *see* Glomerulonephritis
Glomerulitis — *see* Glomerulonephritis
Glomerulonephritis (*see also* Nephritis) N05.9
  with
    edema — *see* Nephrosis
    minimal change N05.0
    minor glomerular abnormality N05.0
  acute N00.9
  chronic N03.9
  crescentic (diffuse) NEC (*see also* N00-N07 with fourth character .7) N05.7
  dense deposit (*see also* N00-N07 with fourth character .6) N05.6
  diffuse
    crescentic (*see also* N00-N07 with fourth character .7) N05.7
    endocapillary proliferative (*see also* N00-N07 with fourth character .4) N05.4
    membranous (*see also* N00-N07 with fourth character .2) N05.2
    mesangial proliferative (*see also* N00-N07 with fourth character .3) N05.3
    mesangiocapillary (*see also* N00-N07 with fourth character .5) N05.5
    sclerosing N18.9
  endocapillary proliferative (diffuse) NEC (*see also* N00-N07 with fourth character .4) N05.4
  extracapillary NEC (*see also* N00-N07 with fourth character .7) N05.7
  focal (and segmental) (*see also* N00-N07 with fourth character .1) N05.1
  hypocomplementemic — *see* Glomerulonephritis, membranoproliferative
  IgA — *see* Nephropathy, IgA
  immune complex (circulating) NEC N05.8
  in (due to)
    amyloidosis E85.4 [N08]
    bilharziasis B65.9 [N08]
    cryoglobulinemia D89.1 [N08]
    defibrination syndrome D65 [N08]
    diabetes mellitus — *see* Diabetes, glomerulosclerosis
    disseminated intravascular coagulation D65 [N08]
    Fabry (-Anderson) disease E75.21 [N08]
    Goodpasture's syndrome M31.0
    hemolytic-uremic syndrome D59.3
    Henoch (-Schönlein) purpura D69.0 [N08]
    lecithin cholesterol acyltransferase deficiency E78.6 [N08]
    microscopic polyangiitis M31.7 [N08]
    multiple myeloma C90.0- ☑ [N08]
    Plasmodium malariae B52.0
    schistosomiasis B65.9 [N08]
    sepsis A41.9 [N08]
      streptococcal A40- ☑ [N08]
    sickle-cell disorders D57.- ☑ [N08]
    strongyloidiasis B78.9 [N08]
    subacute bacterial endocarditis I33.0 [N08]
    syphilis (late) congenital A50.59 [N08]
    systemic lupus erythematosus M32.14
    thrombotic thrombocytopenic purpura M31.1 [N08]
    typhoid fever A01.09
    Waldenström macroglobulinemia C88.0 [N08]
    Wegener's granulomatosis M31.31
  latent or quiescent N03.9
  lobular, lobulonodular — *see* Glomerulonephritis, membranoproliferative
  membranoproliferative (diffuse)(type 1 or 3) (*see also* N00-N07 with fourth character .5) N05.5
    dense deposit (type 2) NEC (*see also* N00-N07 with fourth character .6) N05.6

Glomerulonephritis — *continued*
  membranous (diffuse) NEC (*see also* N00-N07 with fourth character .2) N05.2
  mesangial
    IgA/IgG — *see* Nephropathy, IgA
    proliferative (diffuse) NEC (*see also* N00-N07 with fourth character .3) N05.3
  mesangiocapillary (diffuse) NEC (*see also* N00-N07 with fourth character .5) N05.5
  necrotic, necrotizing NEC (*see also* N00-N07 with fourth character .8) N05.8
  nodular — *see* Glomerulonephritis, membranoproliferative
  poststreptococcal NEC N05.9
    acute N00.9
    chronic N03.9
    rapidly progressive N01.9
  proliferative NEC (*see also* N00-N07 with fourth character .8) N05.8
    diffuse (lupus) M32.14
  rapidly progressive N01.9
  sclerosing, diffuse N18.9
  specified pathology NEC (*see also* N00-N07 with fourth character .8) N05.8
  subacute N01.9
Glomerulopathy — *see* Glomerulonephritis
Glomerulosclerosis (*see also* Sclerosis, renal)
  intercapillary (nodular) (with diabetes) — *see* Diabetes, glomerulosclerosis
  intracapillary — *see* Diabetes, glomerulosclerosis
Glossagra K14.6
Glossalgia K14.6
Glossitis (chronic superficial) (gangrenous) (Moeller's) K14.0
  areata exfoliativa K14.1
  atrophic K14.4
  benign migratory K14.1
  cortical superficial, sclerotic K14.0
  Hunter's D51.0
  interstitial, sclerous K14.0
  median rhomboid K14.2
  pellagrous E52
  superficial, chronic K14.0
Glossocele K14.8
Glossodynia K14.6
  exfoliativa K14.4
Glossoncus K14.8
Glossopathy K14.9
Glossophytia K14.3
Glossoplegia K14.8
Glossoptosis K14.8
Glossopyrosis K14.6
Glossotrichia K14.3
Glossy skin L90.8
Glottis — *see* condition
Glottitis (*see also* Laryngitis) J04.0
Glucagonoma
  pancreas
    benign D13.7
    malignant C25.4
    uncertain behavior D37.8
  specified site NEC
    benign — *see* Neoplasm, benign, by site
    malignant — *see* Neoplasm, malignant, by site
    uncertain behavior — *see* Neoplasm, uncertain behavior, by site
  unspecified site
    benign D13.7
    malignant C25.4
    uncertain behavior D37.8
Glucoglycinuria E72.51
Glucose-galactose malabsorption E74.39
Glue
  ear — *see* Otitis, media, nonsuppurative, chronic, mucoid
  sniffing (airplane) — *see* Abuse, drug, inhalant
    dependence — *see* Dependence, drug, inhalant
Glutaric aciduria E72.3
Glycinemia E72.51
Glycinuria (renal) (with ketosis) E72.09
Glycogen
  infiltration — *see* Disease, glycogen storage
  storage disease — *see* Disease, glycogen storage
Glycogenosis (diffuse) (generalized) (*see also* Disease, glycogen storage)
  cardiac E74.02 [I43]

Glycogenosis — continued
  diabetic, secondary — see Diabetes, glycogenosis, secondary
  pulmonary interstitial J84.842
Glycopenia E16.2
Glycosuria R81
  renal E74.8
Gnathostoma spinigerum (infection) (infestation), **gnathostomiasis** (wandering swelling) B83.1
Goiter (plunging) (substernal) E04.9
  with
    hyperthyroidism (recurrent) — see Hyperthyroidism, with, goiter
    thyrotoxicosis — see Hyperthyroidism, with, goiter
  adenomatous — see Goiter, nodular
  cancerous C73
  congenital (nontoxic) E03.0
    diffuse E03.0
    parenchymatous E03.0
    transitory, with normal functioning P72.0
  cystic E04.2
    due to iodine-deficiency E01.1
  due to
    enzyme defect in synthesis of thyroid hormone E07.1
    iodine-deficiency (endemic) E01.2
  dyshormonogenetic (familial) E07.1
  endemic (iodine-deficiency) E01.2
    diffuse E01.0
    multinodular E01.1
  exophthalmic — see Hyperthyroidism, with, goiter
  iodine-deficiency (endemic) E01.2
    diffuse E01.0
    multinodular E01.1
    nodular E01.1
  lingual Q89.2
  lymphadenoid E06.3
  malignant C73
  multinodular (cystic) (nontoxic) E04.2
    toxic or with hyperthyroidism E05.20
      with thyroid storm E05.21
  neonatal NEC P72.0
  nodular (nontoxic) (due to) E04.9
    with
      hyperthyroidism E05.20
        with thyroid storm E05.21
      thyrotoxicosis E05.20
        with thyroid storm E05.21
    endemic E01.1
    iodine-deficiency E01.1
    sporadic E04.9
    toxic E05.20
      with thyroid storm E05.21
  nontoxic E04.9
    diffuse (colloid) E04.0
    multinodular E04.2
    simple E04.0
    specified NEC E04.8
    uninodular E04.1
  simple E04.0
  toxic — see Hyperthyroidism, with, goiter
  uninodular (nontoxic) E04.1
    toxic or with hyperthyroidism E05.10
      with thyroid storm E05.11
Goiter-deafness syndrome E07.1
Goldberg syndrome Q89.8
Goldberg-Maxwell syndrome E34.51
Goldblatt's hypertension or kidney I70.1
Goldenhar (-Gorlin) **syndrome** Q87.0
Goldflam-Erb disease or syndrome G70.00
  with exacerbation (acute) G70.01
  in crisis G70.01
Goldscheider's disease Q81.8
Goldstein's disease (familial hemorrhagic telangiectasia) I78.0
Golfer's elbow — see Epicondylitis, medial
Gonadoblastoma
  specified site — see Neoplasm, uncertain behavior, by site
  unspecified site
    female D39.10
    male D40.10
Gonecystitis — see Vesiculitis
Gongylonemiasis B83.8
Goniosynechiae — see Adhesions, iris, goniosynechiae
Gonococcemia A54.86
Gonococcus, gonococcal (disease) (infection) (see also condition) A54.9

Gonococcus, gonococcal — continued
  anus A54.6
  bursa, bursitis A54.49
  conjunctiva, conjunctivitis (neonatorum) A54.31
  endocardium A54.83
  eye A54.30
    conjunctivitis A54.31
    iridocyclitis A54.32
    keratitis A54.33
    newborn A54.31
    other specified A54.39
  fallopian tubes (acute) (chronic) A54.24
  genitourinary (organ) (system) (tract) (acute)
    lower A54.00
      with abscess (accessory gland) (periurethral) A54.1
    upper (see also condition) A54.29
  heart A54.83
  iridocyclitis A54.32
  joint A54.42
  lymphatic (gland) (node) A54.89
  meninges, meningitis A54.81
  musculoskeletal A54.40
    arthritis A54.42
    osteomyelitis A54.43
    other specified A54.49
    spondylopathy A54.41
  pelviperitonitis A54.24
  pelvis (acute) (chronic) A54.24
  pharynx A54.5
  proctitis A54.6
  pyosalpinx (acute) (chronic) A54.24
  rectum A54.6
  skin A54.89
  specified site NEC A54.89
  tendon sheath A54.49
  throat A54.5
  urethra (acute) (chronic) A54.01
    with abscess (accessory gland) (periurethral) A54.1
  vulva (acute) (chronic) A54.02
Gonocytoma
  specified site — see Neoplasm, uncertain behavior, by site
  unspecified site
    female D39.10
    male D40.10
Gonorrhea (acute) (chronic) A54.9
  Bartholin's gland (acute) (chronic) (purulent) A54.02
    with abscess (accessory gland) (periurethral) A54.1
  bladder A54.01
  cervix A54.03
  conjunctiva, conjunctivitis (neonatorum) A54.31
  contact Z20.2
  Cowper's gland (with abscess) A54.1
  exposure to Z20.2
  fallopian tube (acute) (chronic) A54.24
  kidney (acute) (chronic) A54.21
  lower genitourinary tract A54.00
    with abscess (accessory gland) (periurethral) A54.1
  ovary (acute) (chronic) A54.24
  pelvis (acute) (chronic) A54.24
    female pelvic inflammatory disease A54.24
  penis A54.09
  prostate (acute) (chronic) A54.22
  seminal vesicle (acute) (chronic) A54.23
  specified site not listed (see also Gonococcus) A54.89
  spermatic cord (acute) (chronic) A54.23
  urethra A54.01
    with abscess (accessory gland) (periurethral) A54.1
  vagina A54.02
  vas deferens (acute) (chronic) A54.23
  vulva A54.02
Goodall's disease A08.19
Goodpasture's syndrome M31.0
Gopalan's syndrome (burning feet) E53.0
Gorlin-Chaudry-Moss syndrome Q87.0
Gottron's papules L94.4
Gougerot-Blum syndrome (pigmented purpuric lichenoid dermatitis) L81.7
Gougerot-Carteaud disease or syndrome (confluent reticulate papillomatosis) L83
Gougerot's syndrome (trisymptomatic) L81.7
Gouley's syndrome (constrictive pericarditis) I31.1
Goundou A66.6
Gout, chronic (see also Gout, gouty) M1A.9 ☑ (following M08)
  drug-induced M1A.20 ☑ (following M08)
    ankle M1A.27- ☑ (following M08)

Gout, chronic — continued
  drug-induced — continued
    elbow M1A.22- ☑ (following M08)
    foot joint M1A.27- ☑ (following M08)
    hand joint M1A.24- ☑ (following M08)
    hip M1A.25- ☑ (following M08)
    knee M1A.26- ☑ (following M08)
    multiple site M1A.29- ☑ (following M08)
    shoulder M1A.21- ☑ (following M08)
    vertebrae M1A.28 ☑ (following M08)
    wrist M1A.23- ☑ (following M08)
  idiopathic M1A.00 ☑ (following M08)
    ankle M1A.07- ☑ (following M08)
    elbow M1A.02- ☑ (following M08)
    foot joint M1A.07- ☑ (following M08)
    hand joint M1A.04- ☑ (following M08)
    hip M1A.05- ☑ (following M08)
    knee M1A.06- ☑ (following M08)
    multiple site M1A.09 ☑ (following M08)
    shoulder M1A.01- ☑ (following M08)
    vertebrae M1A.08 ☑ (following M08)
    wrist M1A.03- ☑ (following M08)
  in (due to) renal impairment M1A.30 ☑ (following M08)
    ankle M1A.37- ☑ (following M08)
    elbow M1A.32- ☑ (following M08)
    foot joint M1A.37- ☑ (following M08)
    hand joint M1A.34- ☑ (following M08)
    hip M1A.35- ☑ (following M08)
    knee M1A.36- ☑ (following M08)
    multiple site M1A.39 ☑ (following M08)
    shoulder M1A.31- ☑ (following M08)
    vertebrae M1A.38 ☑ (following M08)
    wrist M1A.33- ☑ (following M08)
  lead-induced M1A.10 ☑ (following M08)
    ankle M1A.17- ☑ (following M08)
    elbow M1A.12- ☑ (following M08)
    foot joint M1A.17- ☑ (following M08)
    hand joint M1A.14- ☑ (following M08)
    hip M1A.15- ☑ (following M08)
    knee M1A.16- ☑ (following M08)
    multiple site M1A.19 ☑ (following M08)
    shoulder M1A.11- ☑ (following M08)
    vertebrae M1A.18 ☑ (following M08)
    wrist M1A.13- ☑ (following M08)
  primary — see Gout, chronic, idiopathic
  saturnine — see Gout, chronic, lead-induced
  secondary NEC M1A.40 ☑ (following M08)
    ankle M1A.47- ☑ (following M08)
    elbow M1A.42- ☑ (following M08)
    foot joint M1A.47- ☑ (following M08)
    hand joint M1A.44- ☑ (following M08)
    hip M1A.45- ☑ (following M08)
    knee M1A.46- ☑ (following M08)
    multiple site M1A.49 ☑ (following M08)
    shoulder M1A.41- ☑ (following M08)
    vertebrae M1A.48 ☑ (following M08)
    wrist M1A.43- ☑ (following M08)
  syphilitic (see also subcategory M14.8-) A52.77
  tophi M1A.9 ☑ (following M08)
Gout, gouty (acute) (attack) (flare) (see also Gout, chronic) M10.9
  drug-induced M10.20
    ankle M10.27- ☑
    elbow M10.22- ☑
    foot joint M10.27- ☑
    hand joint M10.24- ☑
    hip M10.25- ☑
    knee M10.26- ☑
    multiple site M10.29
    shoulder M10.21- ☑
    vertebrae M10.28
    wrist M10.23- ☑
  idiopathic M10.00
    ankle M10.07- ☑
    elbow M10.02- ☑
    foot joint M10.07- ☑
    hand joint M10.04- ☑
    hip M10.05- ☑
    knee M10.06- ☑
    multiple site M10.09
    shoulder M10.01- ☑
    vertebrae M10.08
    wrist M10.03- ☑
  in (due to) renal impairment M10.30
    ankle M10.37- ☑

☑ **Additional Character Required** — Refer to the Tabular List for Character Selection

▽ Subterms under main terms may continue to next column or page

Gout, gouty — *continued*
  in renal impairment — *continued*
    elbow M10.32- ☑
    foot joint M10.37- ☑
    hand joint M10.34- ☑
    hip M10.35- ☑
    knee M10.36- ☑
    multiple site M10.39
    shoulder M10.31- ☑
    vertebrae M10.38
    wrist M10.33- ☑
  lead-induced M10.10
    ankle M10.17- ☑
    elbow M10.12- ☑
    foot joint M10.17- ☑
    hand joint M10.14- ☑
    hip M10.15- ☑
    knee M10.16- ☑
    multiple site M10.19
    shoulder M10.11- ☑
    vertebrae M10.18
    wrist M10.13- ☑
  primary — *see* Gout, idiopathic
  saturnine — *see* Gout, lead-induced
  secondary NEC M10.40
    ankle M10.47- ☑
    elbow M10.42- ☑
    foot joint M10.47- ☑
    hand joint M10.44- ☑
    hip M10.45- ☑
    knee M10.46- ☑
    multiple site M10.49
    shoulder M10.41- ☑
    vertebrae M10.48
    wrist M10.43- ☑
  syphilitic (*see also* subcategory M14.8-) A52.77
  tophi — *see* Gout, chronic
Gower's
  muscular dystrophy G71.0
  syndrome (vasovagal attack) R55
Gradenigo's syndrome — *see* Otitis, media, suppurative, acute
Graefe's disease — *see* Strabismus, paralytic, ophthalmoplegia, progressive
Graft-versus-host disease D89.813
  acute D89.810
  acute on chronic D89.812
  chronic D89.811
Grain mite (itch) B88.0
Grainhandler's disease or lung J67.8
Grand mal — *see* Epilepsy, generalized, specified NEC
Grand multipara status only (not pregnant) Z64.1
  pregnant — *see* Pregnancy, complicated by, grand multiparity
Granite worker's lung J62.8
Granular (*see also* condition)
  inflammation, pharynx J31.2
  kidney (contracting) — *see* Sclerosis, renal
  liver K74.69
Granulation tissue (abnormal) (excessive) L92.9
  postmastoidectomy cavity — *see* Complications, postmastoidectomy, granulation
Granulocytopenia (primary) (malignant) — *see* Agranulocytosis
Granuloma L92.9
  abdomen K66.8
    from residual foreign body L92.3
    pyogenicum L98.0
  actinic L57.5
  annulare (perforating) L92.0
  apical K04.5
  aural — *see* Otitis, externa, specified NEC
  beryllium (skin) L92.3
  bone
    eosinophilic C96.6
    from residual foreign body — *see* Osteomyelitis, specified type NEC
    lung C96.6
  brain (any site) G06.0
    schistosomiasis B65.9 [G07]
  canaliculus lacrimalis — *see* Granuloma, lacrimal
  candidal (cutaneous) B37.2
  cerebral (any site) G06.0
  coccidioidal (primary) (progressive) B38.7
    lung B38.1
    meninges B38.4
  colon K63.89

Granuloma — *continued*
  conjunctiva H11.22- ☑
  dental K04.5
  ear, middle — *see* Cholesteatoma
  eosinophilic C96.6
    bone C96.6
    lung C96.6
    oral mucosa K13.4
    skin L92.2
  eyelid H01.8
  facial (e) L92.2
  foreign body (in soft tissue) NEC M60.20
    ankle M60.27- ☑
    foot M60.27- ☑
    forearm M60.23- ☑
    hand M60.24- ☑
    in operation wound — *see* Foreign body, accidentally left during a procedure
    lower leg M60.26- ☑
    pelvic region M60.25- ☑
    shoulder region M60.21- ☑
    skin L92.3
    specified site NEC M60.28
    subcutaneous tissue L92.3
    thigh M60.25- ☑
    upper arm M60.22- ☑
  gangraenescens M31.2
  genito-inguinale A58
  giant cell (central) (reparative) (jaw) M27.1
    gingiva (peripheral) K06.8
  gland (lymph) I88.8
  hepatic NEC K75.3
    in (due to)
      berylliosis J63.2 [K77]
      sarcoidosis D86.89
  Hodgkin C81.9 ☑
  ileum K63.89
  infectious B99.9
    specified NEC B99.8
  inguinale (Donovan) (venereal) A58
  intestine NEC K63.89
  intracranial (any site) G06.0
  intraspinal (any part) G06.1
  iridocyclitis — *see* Iridocyclitis, chronic
  jaw (bone) (central) M27.1
    reparative giant cell M27.1
  kidney (*see also* Infection, kidney) N15.8
  lacrimal H04.81- ☑
  larynx J38.7
  lethal midline (faciale(e)) M31.2
  liver NEC — *see* Granuloma, hepatic
  lung (infectious) (*see also* Fibrosis, lung)
    coccidioidal B38.1
    eosinophilic C96.6
  Majocchi's B35.8
  malignant (facial(e)) M31.2
  mandible (central) M27.1
  midline (lethal) M31.2
  monilial (cutaneous) B37.2
  nasal sinus — *see* Sinusitis
  operation wound T81.89 ☑
    foreign body — *see* Foreign body, accidentally left during a procedure
    stitch T81.89 ☑
    talc — *see* Foreign body, accidentally left during a procedure
  oral mucosa K13.4
  orbit, orbital H05.11- ☑
  paracoccidioidal B41.8
  penis, venereal A58
  periapical K04.5
  peritoneum K66.8
    due to ova of helminths NOS (*see also* Helminthiasis) B83.9 [K67]
  postmastoidectomy cavity — *see* Complications, postmastoidectomy, recurrent cholesteatoma
  prostate N42.89
  pudendi (ulcerating) A58
  pulp, internal (tooth) K03.3
  pyogenic, pyogenicum (of) (skin) L98.0
    gingiva K06.8
    maxillary alveolar ridge K04.5
    oral mucosa K13.4
  rectum K62.89
  reticulohistiocytic D76.3
  rubrum nasi L74.8
  Schistosoma — *see* Schistosomiasis
  septic (skin) L98.0

Granuloma — *continued*
  silica (skin) L92.3
  sinus (accessory) (infective) (nasal) — *see* Sinusitis
  skin L92.9
    from residual foreign body L92.3
    pyogenicum L98.0
  spine
    syphilitic (epidural) A52.19
    tuberculous A18.01
  stitch (postoperative) T81.89 ☑
  suppurative (skin) L98.0
  swimming pool A31.1
  talc (*see also* Granuloma, foreign body)
    in operation wound — *see* Foreign body, accidentally left during a procedure
  telangiectaticum (skin) L98.0
  tracheostomy J95.09
  trichophyticum B35.8
  tropicum A66.4
  umbilical P83.81
  umbilicus P83.81
  urethra N36.8
  uveitis — *see* Iridocyclitis, chronic
  vagina A58
  venereum A58
  vocal cord J38.3
Granulomatosis L92.9
  lymphoid C83.8- ☑
  miliary (listerial) A32.89
  necrotizing, respiratory M31.30
  progressive septic D71
  specified NEC L92.8
  Wegener's M31.30
    with renal involvement M31.31
Granulomatous tissue (abnormal) (excessive) L92.9
Granulosis rubra nasi L74.8
Graphite fibrosis (of lung) J63.3
Graphospasm F48.8
  organic G25.89
Grating scapula M89.8X1
Gravel (urinary) — *see* Calculus, urinary
Graves' disease — *see* Hyperthyroidism, with, goiter
Gravis — *see* condition
Grawitz tumor C64.- ☑
Gray syndrome (newborn) P93.0
Grayness, hair (premature) L67.1
  congenital Q84.2
Green sickness D50.8
Greenfield's disease
  meaning
    concentric sclerosis (encephalitis periaxialis concentrica) G37.5
    metachromatic leukodystrophy E75.25
Greenstick fracture — *code as* Fracture, by site
Grey syndrome (newborn) P93.0
Grief F43.21
  prolonged F43.29
  reaction (*see also* Disorder, adjustment) F43.20
Griesinger's disease B76.9
Grinder's lung or pneumoconiosis J62.8
Grinding, teeth
  psychogenic F45.8
  sleep related G47.63
Grip
  Dabney's B33.0
  devil's B33.0
Grippe, grippal (*see also* Influenza)
  Balkan A78
  summer, of Italy A93.1
Grisel's disease M43.6
Groin — *see* condition
Grooved tongue K14.5
Ground itch B76.9
Grover's disease or syndrome L11.1
Growing pains, children R29.898
Growth (fungoid) (neoplastic) (new) (*see also* Neoplasm)
  adenoid (vegetative) J35.8
  benign — *see* Neoplasm, benign, by site
  malignant — *see* Neoplasm, malignant, by site
  rapid, childhood Z00.2
  secondary — *see* Neoplasm, secondary, by site
Gruby's disease B35.0
Gubler-Millard paralysis or syndrome G46.3
Guerin-Stern syndrome Q74.3
Guidance, insufficient anterior (occlusal) M26.54
Guillain-Barré disease or syndrome G61.0
  sequelae G65.0

Guinea worms (infection) (infestation) B72
Guinon's disease (motor-verbal tic) F95.2
Gull's disease E03.4
Gum — see condition
Gumboil K04.7
  with sinus K04.6
Gumma (syphilitic) A52.79
  artery A52.09
    cerebral A52.04
  bone A52.77
    of yaws (late) A66.6
  brain A52.19
  cauda equina A52.19
  central nervous system A52.3
  ciliary body A52.71
  congenital A50.59
  eyelid A52.71
  heart A52.06
  intracranial A52.19
  iris A52.71
  kidney A52.75
  larynx A52.73
  leptomeninges A52.19
  liver A52.74
  meninges A52.19
  myocardium A52.06
  nasopharynx A52.73
  neurosyphilitic A52.3
  nose A52.73
  orbit A52.71
  palate (soft) A52.79
  penis A52.76
  pericardium A52.06
  pharynx A52.73
  pituitary A52.79
  scrofulous (tuberculous) A18.4
  skin A52.79
  specified site NEC A52.79
  spinal cord A52.19
  tongue A52.79
  tonsil A52.73
  trachea A52.73
  tuberculous A18.4
  ulcerative due to yaws A66.4
  ureter A52.75
  yaws A66.4
    bone A66.6
Gunn's syndrome Q07.8
Gunshot wound (see also Wound, open)
  fracture — code as Fracture, by site
  internal organs — see Injury, by site
Gynandrism Q56.0
Gynandroblastoma
  specified site — see Neoplasm, uncertain behavior, by site
  unspecified site
    female D39.10
    male D40.10
Gynecological examination (periodic) (routine) Z01.419
  with abnormal findings Z01.411
Gynecomastia N62
Gynephobia F40.291
Gyrate scalp Q82.8

H

H (Hartnup's) **disease** E72.02
Haas' disease or osteochondrosis (juvenile) (head of humerus) — see Osteochondrosis, juvenile, humerus
Habit, habituation
  bad sleep Z72.821
  chorea F95.8
  disturbance, child F98.9
  drug — see Dependence, drug
  irregular sleep Z72.821
  laxative F55.2
  spasm — see Tic
  tic — see Tic
Haemophilus (H.) **influenzae, as cause of disease classified elsewhere** B96.3
Haff disease — see Poisoning, mercury
Hageman's factor defect, deficiency or disease D68.2
Haglund's disease or osteochondrosis (juvenile) (os tibiale externum) — see Osteochondrosis, juvenile, tarsus
Hailey-Hailey disease Q82.8

Hair (see also condition)
  plucking F63.3
    in stereotyped movement disorder F98.4
  tourniquet syndrome (see also Constriction, external, by site)
    finger S60.44- ☑
    penis S30.842 ☑
    thumb S60.34- ☑
    toe S90.44- ☑
Hairball in stomach T18.2 ☑
Hair-pulling, pathological (compulsive) F63.3
Hairy black tongue K14.3
Half vertebra Q76.49
Halitosis R19.6
Hallerman-Streiff syndrome Q87.0
Hallervorden-Spatz disease G23.0
Hallopeau's acrodermatitis or disease L40.2
Hallucination R44.3
  auditory R44.0
  gustatory R44.2
  olfactory R44.2
  specified NEC R44.2
  tactile R44.2
  visual R44.1
Hallucinosis (chronic) F28
  alcoholic (acute) F10.951
    in
      abuse F10.151
      dependence F10.251
  drug-induced F19.951
    cannabis F12.951
    cocaine F14.951
    hallucinogen F16.151
    in
      abuse F19.151
        cannabis F12.151
        cocaine F14.151
        hallucinogen F16.151
        inhalant F18.151
        opioid F11.151
        sedative, anxiolytic or hypnotic F13.151
        stimulant NEC F15.151
      dependence F19.251
        cannabis F12.251
        cocaine F14.251
        hallucinogen F16.251
        inhalant F18.251
        opioid F11.251
        sedative, anxiolytic or hypnotic F13.251
        stimulant NEC F15.251
    inhalant F18.951
    opioid F11.951
    sedative, anxiolytic or hypnotic F13.951
    stimulant NEC F15.951
  organic F06.0
Hallux
  deformity (acquired) NEC M20.5X- ☑
  limitus M20.5X- ☑
  malleus (acquired) NEC M20.3- ☑
  rigidus (acquired) M20.2- ☑
    congenital Q74.2
    sequelae (late effect) of rickets E64.3
  valgus (acquired) M20.1- ☑
    congenital Q66.6
  varus (acquired) M20.3- ☑
    congenital Q66.3
Halo, visual H53.19
Hamartoma, hamartoblastoma Q85.9
  epithelial (gingival), odontogenic, central or peripheral — see Cyst, calcifying odontogenic
Hamartosis Q85.9
Hamman-Rich syndrome J84.114
Hammer toe (acquired) NEC (see also Deformity, toe, hammer toe)
  congenital Q66.89
  sequelae (late effect) of rickets E64.3
Hand — see condition
Hand-foot syndrome L27.1
Handicap, handicapped
  educational Z55.9
  specified NEC Z55.8
Hand-Schüller-Christian disease or syndrome C96.5
Hanging (asphyxia) (strangulation) (suffocation) — see Asphyxia, traumatic, due to mechanical threat
Hangnail (see also Cellulitis, digit)
  with lymphangitis — see Lymphangitis, acute, digit
Hangover (alcohol) F10.129

Hanhart's syndrome Q87.0
Hanot-Chauffard (-Troisier) **syndrome** E83.19
Hanot's cirrhosis or disease K74.3
Hansen's disease — see Leprosy
Hantaan virus disease (Korean hemorrhagic fever) A98.5
Hantavirus disease (with renal manifestations) (Dobrava) (Puumala) (Seoul) A98.5
  with pulmonary manifestations (Andes) (Bayou) (Bermejo) (Black Creek Canal) (Choclo) (Juquitiba) (Laguna negra) (Lechiguanas) (New York) (Oran) (Sin nombre) B33.4
Happy puppet syndrome Q93.5
Harada's disease or syndrome H30.81- ☑
Hardening
  artery — see Arteriosclerosis
  brain G93.89
Harelip (complete) (incomplete) — see Cleft, lip
Harlequin (newborn) Q80.4
Harley's disease D59.6
Harmful use (of)
  alcohol F10.10
  anxiolytics — see Abuse, drug, sedative
  cannabinoids — see Abuse, drug, cannabis
  cocaine — see Abuse, drug, cocaine
  drug — see Abuse, drug
  hallucinogens — see Abuse, drug, hallucinogen
  hypnotics — see Abuse, drug, sedative
  opioids — see Abuse, drug, opioid
  PCP (phencyclidine) — see Abuse, drug, hallucinogen
  sedatives — see Abuse, drug, sedative
  stimulants NEC — see Abuse, drug, stimulant
Harris' lines — see Arrest, epiphyseal
Hartnup's disease E72.02
Harvester's lung J67.0
Harvesting ovum for in vitro fertilization Z31.83
Hashimoto's disease or thyroiditis E06.3
Hashitoxicosis (transient) E06.3
Hassal-Henle bodies or warts (cornea) H18.49
Haut mal — see Epilepsy, generalized, specified NEC
Haverhill fever A25.1
Hay fever (see also Fever, hay) J30.1
Hayem-Widal syndrome D59.8
Haygarth's nodes M15.8
Haymaker's lung J67.0
Hb (abnormal)
  Bart's disease D56.0
  disease — see Disease, hemoglobin
  trait — see Trait
Head — see condition
Headache R51
  allergic NEC G44.89
  associated with sexual activity G44.82
  chronic daily R51
  cluster G44.009
    chronic G44.029
      intractable G44.021
      not intractable G44.029
    episodic G44.019
      intractable G44.011
      not intractable G44.019
    intractable G44.001
    not intractable G44.009
  cough (primary) G44.83
  daily chronic R51
  drug-induced NEC G44.40
    intractable G44.41
    not intractable G44.40
  exertional (primary) G44.84
  histamine G44.009
    intractable G44.001
    not intractable G44.009
  hypnic G44.81
  lumbar puncture G97.1
  medication overuse G44.40
    intractable G44.41
    not intractable G44.40
  menstrual — see Migraine, menstrual
  migraine (type) (see also Migraine) G43.909
  nasal septum R51
  neuralgiform, short lasting unilateral, with conjunctival injection and tearing (SUNCT) G44.059
    intractable G44.051
    not intractable G44.059
  new daily persistent (NDPH) G44.52
  orgasmic G44.82
  periodic syndromes in adults and children G43.C0 (following G43.7)

☑ **Additional Character Required** — Refer to the Tabular List for Character Selection   Subterms under main terms may continue to next column or page

Headache — *continued*
  periodic syndromes in adults and children — *continued*
    with refractory migraine G43.C1 (*following* G43.7)
    without refractory migraine G43.C0 (*following* G43.7)
    intractable G43.C1 (*following* G43.7)
    not intractable G43.C0 (*following* G43.7)
  postspinal puncture G97.1
  post-traumatic G44.309
    acute G44.319
      intractable G44.311
      not intractable G44.319
    chronic G44.329
      intractable G44.321
      not intractable G44.329
    intractable G44.301
    not intractable G44.309
  pre-menstrual — *see* Migraine, menstrual
  preorgasmic G44.82
  primary
    cough G44.83
    exertional G44.84
    stabbing G44.85
    thunderclap G44.53
  rebound G44.40
    intractable G44.41
    not intractable G44.40
  short lasting unilateral neuralgiform, with conjunctival injection and tearing (SUNCT) G44.059
    intractable G44.051
    not intractable G44.059
  specified syndrome NEC G44.89
  spinal and epidural anesthesia - induced T88.59 ☑
    in labor and delivery O74.5
    in pregnancy O29.4- ☑
    postpartum, puerperal O89.4
  spinal fluid loss (from puncture) G97.1
  stabbing (primary) G44.85
  tension (-type) G44.209
    chronic G44.229
      intractable G44.221
      not intractable G44.229
    episodic G44.219
      intractable G44.211
      not intractable G44.219
    intractable G44.201
    not intractable G44.209
  thunderclap (primary) G44.53
  vascular NEC G44.1
Healthy
  infant
    accompanying sick mother Z76.3
    receiving care Z76.2
  person accompanying sick person Z76.3
Hearing examination Z01.10
  with abnormal findings NEC Z01.118
  following failed hearing screening Z01.110
  for hearing conservation and treatment Z01.12
Heart — *see* condition
Heart beat
  abnormality R00.9
    specified NEC R00.8
  awareness R00.2
  rapid R00.0
  slow R00.1
Heartburn R12
  psychogenic F45.8
Heartland virus disease A93.8
Heat (effects) T67.9 ☑
  apoplexy T67.0 ☑
  burn (*see also* Burn) L55.9
  collapse T67.1 ☑
  cramps T67.2 ☑
  dermatitis or eczema L59.0
  edema T67.7 ☑
  erythema — *code by site under* Burn, first degree
  excessive T67.9 ☑
    specified effect NEC T67.8 ☑
  exhaustion T67.5 ☑
    anhydrotic T67.3 ☑
    due to
      salt (and water) depletion T67.4 ☑
      water depletion T67.3 ☑
        with salt depletion T67.4 ☑
  fatigue (transient) T67.6 ☑
  fever T67.0 ☑
  hyperpyrexia T67.0 ☑

Heat — *continued*
  prickly L74.0
  prostration — *see* Heat, exhaustion
  pyrexia T67.0 ☑
  rash L74.0
  specified effect NEC T67.8 ☑
  stroke T67.0 ☑
  sunburn — *see* Sunburn
  syncope T67.1 ☑
Heavy-for-dates NEC (infant) (4000g to 4499g) P08.1
  exceptionally (4500g or more) P08.0
Hebephrenia, hebephrenic (schizophrenia) F20.1
Heberden's disease or nodes (with arthropathy) M15.1
Hebra's
  pityriasis L26
  prurigo L28.2
Heel — *see* condition
Heerfordt's disease D86.89
Hegglin's anomaly or syndrome D72.0
Heilmeyer-Schoner disease D45
Heine-Medin disease A80.9
Heinz body anemia, congenital D58.2
Heliophobia F40.228
Heller's disease or syndrome F84.3
HELLP syndrome (hemolysis, elevated liver enzymes and low platelet count) O14.2- ☑
  complicating
    childbirth O14.24
    puerperium O14.25
Helminthiasis (*see also* Infestation, helminth)
  Ancylostoma B76.0
  intestinal B82.0
    mixed types (types classifiable to more than one of the titles B65.0-B81.3 and B81.8) B81.4
    specified type NEC B81.8
  mixed types (intestinal) (types classifiable to more than one of the titles B65.0-B81.3 and B81.8) B81.4
  Necator (americanus) B76.1
  specified type NEC B83.8
Heloma L84
Hemangioblastoma — *see* Neoplasm, connective tissue, uncertain behavior
  malignant — *see* Neoplasm, connective tissue, malignant
Hemangioendothelioma (*see also* Neoplasm, uncertain behavior, by site)
  benign D18.00
    intra-abdominal D18.03
    intracranial D18.02
    skin D18.01
    specified site NEC D18.09
  bone (diffuse) — *see* Neoplasm, bone, malignant
  epithelioid (*see also* Neoplasm, uncertain behavior, by site)
    malignant — *see* Neoplasm, malignant, by site
  malignant — *see* Neoplasm, connective tissue, malignant
Hemangiofibroma — *see* Neoplasm, benign, by site
Hemangiolipoma — *see* Lipoma
Hemangioma D18.00
  arteriovenous D18.00
    intra-abdominal D18.03
    intracranial D18.02
    skin D18.01
    specified site NEC D18.09
  capillary D18.00
    intra-abdominal D18.03
    intracranial D18.02
    skin D18.01
    specified site NEC D18.09
  cavernous D18.00
    intra-abdominal D18.03
    intracranial D18.02
    skin D18.01
    specified site NEC D18.09
  epithelioid D18.00
    intra-abdominal D18.03
    intracranial D18.02
    skin D18.01
    specified site NEC D18.09
  histiocytoid D18.00
    intra-abdominal D18.03
    intracranial D18.02
    skin D18.01
    specified site NEC D18.09
  infantile D18.00
    intra-abdominal D18.03

Hemangioma — *continued*
  infantile — *continued*
    intracranial D18.02
    skin D18.01
    specified site NEC D18.09
  intra-abdominal D18.03
  intracranial D18.02
  intramuscular D18.00
    intra-abdominal D18.03
    intracranial D18.02
    skin D18.01
    specified site NEC D18.09
  intrathoracic structures D18.09
  juvenile D18.00
  malignant — *see* Neoplasm, connective tissue, malignant
  plexiform D18.00
    intra-abdominal D18.03
    intracranial D18.02
    skin D18.01
    specified site NEC D18.09
  racemose D18.00
    intra-abdominal D18.03
    intracranial D18.02
    skin D18.01
    specified site NEC D18.09
  sclerosing — *see* Neoplasm, skin, benign
  simplex D18.00
    intra-abdominal D18.03
    intracranial D18.02
    skin D18.01
    specified site NEC D18.09
  skin D18.01
  specified site NEC D18.09
  venous D18.00
    intra-abdominal D18.03
    intracranial D18.02
    skin D18.01
    specified site NEC D18.09
  verrucous keratotic D18.00
    intra-abdominal D18.03
    intracranial D18.02
    skin D18.01
    specified site NEC D18.09
Hemangiomatosis (systemic) I78.8
  involving single site — *see* Hemangioma
Hemangiopericytoma (*see also* Neoplasm, connective tissue, uncertain behavior)
  benign — *see* Neoplasm, connective tissue, benign
  malignant — *see* Neoplasm, connective tissue, malignant
Hemangiosarcoma — *see* Neoplasm, connective tissue, malignant
Hemarthrosis (nontraumatic) M25.00
  ankle M25.07- ☑
  elbow M25.02- ☑
  foot joint M25.07- ☑
  hand joint M25.04- ☑
  hip M25.05- ☑
  in hemophilic arthropathy — *see* Arthropathy, hemophilic
  knee M25.06- ☑
  shoulder M25.01- ☑
  specified joint NEC M25.08
  traumatic — *see* Sprain, by site
  vertebrae M25.08
  wrist M25.03- ☑
Hematemesis K92.0
  with ulcer — *code by site under* Ulcer, with hemorrhage K27.4
  newborn, neonatal P54.0
    due to swallowed maternal blood P78.2
Hematidrosis L74.8
Hematinuria (*see also* Hemoglobinuria)
  malarial B50.8
Hematobilia K83.8
Hematocele
  female NEC N94.89
    with ectopic pregnancy O00.90
      with intrauterine pregnancy O00.91
    ovary N83.8
  male N50.1
Hematochezia (*see also* Melena) K92.1
Hematochyluria (*see also* Infestation, filarial)
  schistosomiasis (bilharziasis) B65.0
Hematocolpos (with hematometra or hematosalpinx) N89.7
Hematocornea — *see* Pigmentation, cornea, stromal

Index

Hematogenous — Hemiplegia

Hematogenous — *see* condition
Hematoma (traumatic) (skin surface intact) (*see also* Contusion)
  with
    injury of internal organs — *see* Injury, by site
    open wound — *see* Wound, open
  amputation stump (surgical) (late) T87.89
  aorta, dissecting I71.00
    abdominal I71.02
    thoracic I71.01
    thoracoabdominal I71.03
  aortic intramural — *see* Dissection, aorta
  arterial (complicating trauma) — *see* Injury, blood vessel, by site
  auricle — *see* Contusion, ear
    nontraumatic — *see* Disorder, pinna, hematoma
  birth injury NEC P15.8
  brain (traumatic)
    with
      cerebral laceration or contusion (diffuse) — *see* Injury, intracranial, diffuse
        focal — *see* Injury, intracranial, focal
    cerebellar, traumatic S06.37- ☑
    intracerebral, traumatic — *see* Injury, intracranial, intracerebral hemorrhage
    newborn NEC P52.4
      birth injury P10.1
    nontraumatic — *see* Hemorrhage, intracranial
    subarachnoid, arachnoid, traumatic — *see* Injury, intracranial, subarachnoid hemorrhage
    subdural, traumatic — *see* Injury, intracranial, subdural hemorrhage
  breast (nontraumatic) N64.89
  broad ligament (nontraumatic) N83.7
    traumatic S37.892 ☑
  cerebellar, traumatic S06.37- ☑
  cerebral — *see* Hematoma, brain
  cerebrum S06.36- ☑
    left S06.35- ☑
    right S06.34- ☑
  cesarean delivery wound O90.2
  complicating delivery (perineal) (pelvic) (vagina) (vulva) O71.7
  corpus cavernosum (nontraumatic) N48.89
  epididymis (nontraumatic) N50.1
  epidural (traumatic) — *see* Injury, intracranial, epidural hemorrhage
    spinal — *see* Injury, spinal cord, by region
  episiotomy O90.2
  face, birth injury P15.4
  genital organ NEC (nontraumatic)
    female (nonobstetric) N94.89
      traumatic S30.202 ☑
    male N50.1
      traumatic S30.201 ☑
  internal organs — *see* Injury, by site
  intracerebral, traumatic — *see* Injury, intracranial, intracerebral hemorrhage
  intraoperative — *see* Complications, intraoperative, hemorrhage
  labia (nontraumatic) (nonobstetric) N90.89
  liver (subcapsular) (nontraumatic) K76.89
    birth injury P15.0
  mediastinum — *see* Injury, intrathoracic
  mesosalpinx (nontraumatic) N83.7
    traumatic S37.898 ☑
  muscle — code by site under Contusion
  nontraumatic
    muscle M79.81
    soft tissue M79.81
  obstetrical surgical wound O90.2
  orbit, orbital (nontraumatic) (*see also* Hemorrhage, orbit)
    traumatic — *see* Contusion, orbit
  pelvis (female) (nontraumatic) (nonobstetric) N94.89
    obstetric O71.7
    traumatic — *see* Injury, by site
  penis (nontraumatic) N48.89
    birth injury P15.5
  perianal (nontraumatic) K64.5
  perineal S30.23 ☑
    complicating delivery O71.7
  perirenal — *see* Injury, kidney
  pinna — *see* Contusion, ear
    nontraumatic — *see* Disorder, pinna, hematoma
  placenta O43.89- ☑

Hematoma — *continued*
  postoperative (postprocedural) — *see* Complication, postprocedural, hematoma
  retroperitoneal (nontraumatic) K66.1
    traumatic S36.892 ☑
  scrotum, superficial S30.22 ☑
    birth injury P15.5
  seminal vesicle (nontraumatic) N50.1
    traumatic S37.892 ☑
  spermatic cord (traumatic) S37.892 ☑
    nontraumatic N50.1
  spinal (cord) (meninges) (*see also* Injury, spinal cord, by region)
    newborn (birth injury) P11.5
  spleen D73.5
    intraoperative — *see* Complications, intraoperative, hemorrhage, spleen
    postprocedural (postoperative) — *see* Complications, postprocedural, hemorrhage, spleen
  sternocleidomastoid, birth injury P15.2
  sternomastoid, birth injury P15.2
  subarachnoid (traumatic) — *see* Injury, intracranial, subarachnoid hemorrhage
    newborn (nontraumatic) P52.5
      due to birth injury P10.3
    nontraumatic — *see* Hemorrhage, intracranial, subarachnoid
  subdural (traumatic) — *see* Injury, intracranial, subdural hemorrhage
    newborn (localized) P52.8
      birth injury P10.0
    nontraumatic — *see* Hemorrhage, intracranial, subdural
  superficial, newborn P54.5
  testis (nontraumatic) N50.1
    birth injury P15.5
  tunica vaginalis (nontraumatic) N50.1
  umbilical cord, complicating delivery O69.5 ☑
  uterine ligament (broad) (nontraumatic) N83.7
    traumatic S37.892 ☑
  vagina (ruptured) (nontraumatic) N89.8
    complicating delivery O71.7
  vas deferens (nontraumatic) N50.1
    traumatic S37.892 ☑
  vitreous — *see* Hemorrhage, vitreous
  vulva (nontraumatic) (nonobstetric) N90.89
    complicating delivery O71.7
    newborn (birth injury) P15.5
Hematometra N85.7
  with hematocolpos N89.7
Hematomyelia (central) G95.19
  newborn (birth injury) P11.5
  traumatic T14.8 ☑
Hematomyelitis G04.90
Hematoperitoneum — *see* Hemoperitoneum
Hematophobia F40.230
Hematopneumothorax (see Hemothorax)
Hematopoiesis, cyclic D70.4
Hematoporphyria — *see* Porphyria
Hematorachis, hematorrhachis G95.19
  newborn (birth injury) P11.5
Hematosalpinx N83.6
  with
    hematocolpos N89.7
    hematometra N85.7
      with hematocolpos N89.7
  infectional — *see* Salpingitis
Hematospermia R36.1
Hematothorax (see Hemothorax)
Hematuria R31.9
  benign (familial) (of childhood) (*see also* Hematuria, idiopathic)
    essential microscopic R31.1
  due to sulphonamide, sulfonamide — *see* Table of Drugs and Chemicals, by drug
  endemic (*see also* Schistosomiasis) B65.0
  gross R31.0
  idiopathic N02.9
    with glomerular lesion
      crescentic (diffuse) glomerulonephritis N02.7
      dense deposit disease N02.6
      endocapillary proliferative glomerulonephritis N02.4
      focal and segmental hyalinosis or sclerosis N02.1
      membranoproliferative (diffuse) N02.5
      membranous (diffuse) N02.2
      mesangial proliferative (diffuse) N02.3

Hematuria — *continued*
  idiopathic — *continued*
    with glomerular lesion — *continued*
      mesangiocapillary (diffuse) N02.5
      minor abnormality N02.0
      proliferative NEC N02.8
      specified pathology NEC N02.8
  intermittent — *see* Hematuria, idiopathic
  malarial B50.8
  microscopic NEC (with symptoms) R31.29
    asymptomatic R31.21
    benign essential R31.1
  paroxysmal (*see also* Hematuria, idiopathic)
    nocturnal D59.5
  persistent — *see* Hematuria, idiopathic
  recurrent — *see* Hematuria, idiopathic
  tropical (*see also* Schistosomiasis) B65.0
  tuberculous A18.13
Hemeralopia (day blindness) H53.11
  vitamin A deficiency E50.5
Hemi-akinesia R41.4
Hemianalgesia R20.0
Hemianencephaly Q00.0
Hemianesthesia R20.0
Hemianopia, hemianopsia (heteronymous) H53.47
  homonymous H53.46- ☑
  syphilitic A52.71
Hemiathetosis R25.8
Hemiatrophy R68.89
  cerebellar G31.9
  face, facial, progressive (Romberg) G51.8
  tongue K14.8
Hemiballism (us) G25.5
Hemicardia Q24.8
Hemicephalus, hemicephaly Q00.0
Hemichorea G25.5
Hemicolitis, left — *see* Colitis, left sided
Hemicrania
  congenital
    malformation Q00.0
  continua G44.51
  meaning migraine (*see also* Migraine) G43.909
  paroxysmal G44.039
    chronic G44.049
      intractable G44.041
      not intractable G44.049
    episodic G44.039
      intractable G44.031
      not intractable G44.039
    intractable G44.031
    not intractable G44.039
Hemidystrophy — *see* Hemiatrophy
Hemiectromelia Q73.8
Hemihypalgesia R20.8
Hemihypesthesia R20.1
Hemi-inattention R41.4
Hemimelia Q73.8
  lower limb — *see* Defect, reduction, lower limb, specified type NEC
  upper limb — *see* Defect, reduction, upper limb, specified type NEC
Hemiparalysis — *see* Hemiplegia
Hemiparesis — *see* Hemiplegia
Hemiparesthesia R20.2
Hemiparkinsonism G20
Hemiplegia G81.9- ☑
  alternans facialis G83.89
  ascending NEC G81.90
    spinal G95.89
  congenital (cerebral) G80.8
    spastic G80.2
  embolic (current episode) I63.4- ☑
  flaccid G81.0- ☑
  following
    cerebrovascular disease I69.959
      cerebral infarction I69.35- ☑
      intracerebral hemorrhage I69.15- ☑
      nontraumatic intracranial hemorrhage NEC I69.25- ☑
      specified disease NEC I69.85- ☑
      stroke NOS I69.35- ☑
      subarachnoid hemorrhage I69.05- ☑
  hysterical F44.4
  newborn NEC P91.88
    birth injury P11.9
  spastic G81.1- ☑
    congenital G80.2
  thrombotic (current episode) I63.3- ☑

Hemisection, spinal cord — see Injury, spinal cord, by
   region
Hemispasm (facial) R25.2
Hemisporosis B48.8
Hemitremor R25.1
Hemivertebra Q76.49
   failure of segmentation with scoliosis Q76.3
   fusion with scoliosis Q76.3
Hemochromatosis E83.119
   with refractory anemia D46.1
   due to repeated red blood cell transfusion E83.111
   hereditary (primary) E83.110
   neonatal P78.84
   primary E83.110
   specified NEC E83.118
Hemoglobin (see also condition)
   abnormal (disease) — see Disease, hemoglobin
   AS genotype D57.3
   Constant Spring D58.2
   E-beta thalassemia D56.5
   fetal, hereditary persistence (HPFH) D56.4
   H Constant Spring D56.0
   low NOS D64.9
   S (Hb S), heterozygous D57.3
Hemoglobinemia D59.9
   due to blood transfusion T80.89 ☑
   paroxysmal D59.6
      nocturnal D59.5
Hemoglobinopathy (mixed) D58.2
   with thalassemia D56.8
   sickle-cell D57.1
      with thalassemia D57.40
         with crisis (vasoocclusive pain) D57.419
            with
               acute chest syndrome D57.411
               splenic sequestration D57.412
         without crisis D57.40
Hemoglobinuria R82.3
   with anemia, hemolytic, acquired (chronic) NEC D59.6
   cold (agglutinin) (paroxysmal) (with Raynaud's syn-
      drome) D59.6
   due to exertion or hemolysis NEC D59.6
   intermittent D59.6
   malarial B50.8
   march D59.6
   nocturnal (paroxysmal) D59.5
   paroxysmal (cold) D59.6
      nocturnal D59.5
Hemolymphangioma D18.1
Hemolysis
   intravascular
      with
         abortion — see Abortion, by type, complicated
            by, hemorrhage
         ectopic or molar pregnancy O08.1
         hemorrhage
            antepartum — see Hemorrhage, antepar-
               tum, with coagulation defect
            intrapartum (see also Hemorrhage, compli-
               cating, delivery) O67.0
         postpartum O72.3
   neonatal (excessive) P58.9
      specified NEC P58.8
Hemolytic — see condition
Hemopericardium I31.2
   following acute myocardial infarction (current compli-
      cation) I23.0
   newborn P54.8
   traumatic — see Injury, heart, with hemopericardium
Hemoperitoneum K66.1
   infectional K65.9
   traumatic S36.899 ☑
      with open wound — see Wound, open, with pene-
         tration into peritoneal cavity
Hemophilia (classical) (familial) (hereditary) D66
   A D66
   acquired D68.311
   autoimmune D68.311
   B D67
   C D68.1
   calcipriva (see also Defect, coagulation) D68.4
   nonfamilial (see also Defect, coagulation) D68.4
   secondary D68.311
   vascular D68.0
Hemophthalmos H44.81- ☑
Hemopneumothorax (see also Hemothorax)
   traumatic S27.2 ☑
Hemoptysis R04.2

Hemoptysis — continued
   newborn P26.9
   tuberculous — see Tuberculosis, pulmonary
Hemorrhage, hemorrhagic (concealed) R58
   abdomen R58
   accidental antepartum — see Hemorrhage, antepar-
      tum
   acute idiopathic pulmonary, in infants R04.81
   adenoid J35.8
   adrenal (capsule) (gland) E27.49
      medulla E27.8
      newborn P54.4
   after delivery — see Hemorrhage, postpartum
   alveolar
      lung, newborn P26.8
      process K08.89
   alveolus K08.89
   amputation stump (surgical) T87.89
   anemia (chronic) D50.0
      acute D62
   antepartum (with) O46.90
      with coagulation defect O46.00- ☑
         afibrinogenemia O46.01- ☑
         disseminated intravascular coagulation
            O46.02- ☑
         hypofibrinogenemia O46.01- ☑
         specified defect NEC O46.09- ☑
      before 20 weeks gestation O20.9
         specified type NEC O20.8
         threatened abortion O20.0
      due to
         abruptio placenta (see also Abruptio placentae)
            O45.9- ☑
         leiomyoma, uterus — see Hemorrhage, antepar-
            tum, specified cause NEC
         placenta previa O44.1- ☑
         specified cause NEC — see subcategory O46.8X- ☑
   anus (sphincter) K62.5
   apoplexy (stroke) — see Hemorrhage, intracranial, in-
      tracerebral
   arachnoid — see Hemorrhage, intracranial, subarach-
      noid
   artery R58
      brain — see Hemorrhage, intracranial, intracerebral
   basilar (ganglion) I61.0
   bladder N32.89
   bowel K92.2
      newborn P54.3
   brain (miliary) (nontraumatic) — see Hemorrhage, in-
      tracranial, intracerebral
      due to
         birth injury P10.1
         syphilis A52.05
      epidural or extradural (traumatic) — see Injury,
         intracranial, epidural hemorrhage
      newborn P52.4
         birth injury P10.1
      subarachnoid — see Hemorrhage, intracranial,
         subarachnoid
      subdural — see Hemorrhage, intracranial, subdural
   brainstem (nontraumatic) I61.3
      traumatic S06.38- ☑
   breast N64.59
   bronchial tube — see Hemorrhage, lung
   bronchopulmonary — see Hemorrhage, lung
   bronchus — see Hemorrhage, lung
   bulbar I61.5
   capillary I78.8
      primary D69.8
   cecum K92.2
   cerebellar, cerebellum (nontraumatic) I61.4
      newborn P52.6
      traumatic S06.37- ☑
   cerebral, cerebrum (see also Hemorrhage, intracranial,
      intracerebral)
      lobe I61.1
      newborn (anoxic) P52.4
         birth injury P10.1
   cerebromeningeal I61.8
   cerebrospinal — see Hemorrhage, intracranial, intrac-
      erebral
   cervix (uteri) (stump) NEC N88.8
   chamber, anterior (eye) — see Hyphema
   childbirth — see Hemorrhage, complicating, delivery
   choroid H31.30- ☑
      expulsive H31.31- ☑
   ciliary body — see Hyphema
   cochlea — see subcategory H83.8 ☑

Hemorrhage, hemorrhagic — continued
   colon K92.2
   complicating
      abortion — see Abortion, by type, complicated by,
         hemorrhage
      delivery O67.9
         associated with coagulation defect (afibrinogen-
            emia) (DIC) (hyperfibrinolysis) O67.0
         specified cause NEC O67.8
      surgical procedure — see Hemorrhage, intraoper-
         ative
   conjunctiva H11.3- ☑
      newborn P54.8
   cord, newborn (stump) P51.9
   corpus luteum (ruptured) cyst N83.1- ☑
   cortical (brain) I61.1
   cranial — see Hemorrhage, intracranial
   cutaneous R23.3
      due to autosensitivity, erythrocyte D69.2
      newborn P54.5
   delayed
      following ectopic or molar pregnancy O08.1
      postpartum O72.2
   diathesis (familial) D69.9
   disease D69.9
      newborn P53
      specified type NEC D69.8
   due to or associated with
      afibrinogenemia or other coagulation defect
         (conditions in categories D65- D69)
         antepartum — see Hemorrhage, antepartum,
            with coagulation defect
         intrapartum O67.0
      dental implant M27.61
      device, implant or graft (see also Complications,
         by site and type, specified NEC) T85.838 ☑
         arterial graft NEC T82.838 ☑
         breast T85.838 ☑
         catheter NEC T85.838 ☑
            dialysis (renal) T82.838 ☑
               intraperitoneal T85.838 ☑
            infusion NEC T82.838 ☑
               spinal (epidural) (subdural) T85.830 ☑
            urinary (indwelling) T83.83 ☑
         electronic (electrode) (pulse generator) (stimu-
            lator)
            bone T84.83 ☑
            cardiac T82.837 ☑
            nervous system (brain) (peripheral nerve)
               (spinal) T85.830 ☑
            urinary T83.83 ☑
         fixation, internal (orthopedic) NEC T84.83 ☑
         gastrointestinal (bile duct) (esophagus)
            T85.838 ☑
         genital NEC T83.83 ☑
         heart NEC T82.837 ☑
         joint prosthesis T84.83 ☑
         ocular (corneal graft) (orbital implant) NEC
            T85.838 ☑
         orthopedic NEC T84.83 ☑
            bone graft T86.838 ☑
         specified NEC T85.838 ☑
         urinary NEC T83.83 ☑
         vascular NEC T82.838 ☑
         ventricular intracranial shunt T85.830 ☑
   duodenum, duodenal K92.2
      ulcer — see Ulcer, duodenum, with hemorrhage
   dura mater — see Hemorrhage, intracranial, subdural
   endotracheal — see Hemorrhage, lung
   epicranial subaponeurotic (massive), birth injury P12.2
   epidural (traumatic) (see also Injury, intracranial,
      epidural hemorrhage)
      nontraumatic I62.1
   esophagus K22.8
      varix I85.01
         secondary I85.11
   excessive, following ectopic gestation (subsequent
      episode) O08.1
   extradural (traumatic) — see Injury, intracranial,
      epidural hemorrhage
      birth injury P10.8
      newborn (anoxic) (nontraumatic) P52.8
      nontraumatic I62.1
   eye NEC H57.8
      fundus — see Hemorrhage, retina
      lid — see Disorder, eyelid, specified type NEC
   fallopian tube N83.6

Hemorrhage, hemorrhagic — *continued*
fibrinogenolysis — *see* Fibrinolysis
fibrinolytic (acquired) — *see* Fibrinolysis
from
  ear (nontraumatic) — *see* Otorrhagia
  tracheostomy stoma J95.01
fundus, eye — *see* Hemorrhage, retina
funis — *see* Hemorrhage, umbilicus, cord
gastric — *see* Hemorrhage, stomach
gastroenteric K92.2
  newborn P54.3
gastrointestinal (tract) K92.2
  newborn P54.3
genital organ, male N50.1
genitourinary (tract) NOS R31.9
gingiva K06.8
globe (eye) — *see* Hemophthalmos
graafian follicle cyst (ruptured) N83.0- ☑
gum K06.8
heart I51.89
hypopharyngeal (throat) R04.1
intermenstrual (regular) N92.3
  irregular N92.1
internal (organs) NEC R58
  capsule I61.0
  ear — *see* subcategory H83.8 ☑
    newborn P54.8
intestine K92.2
  newborn P54.3
intra-abdominal R58
intra-alveolar (lung), newborn P26.8
intracerebral (nontraumatic) — *see* Hemorrhage, intracranial, intracerebral
intracranial (nontraumatic) I62.9
  birth injury P10.9
  epidural, nontraumatic I62.1
  extradural, nontraumatic I62.1
  intracerebral (nontraumatic) (in) I61.9
    brain stem I61.3
    cerebellum I61.4
    hemisphere I61.2
      cortical (superficial) I61.1
      subcortical (deep) I61.0
    intraoperative
      during a nervous system procedure G97.31
      during other procedure G97.32
    intraventricular I61.5
    multiple localized I61.6
    newborn P52.4
      birth injury P10.1
    postprocedural
      following a nervous system procedure G97.51
      following other procedure G97.52
    specified NEC I61.8
    superficial I61.1
    traumatic (diffuse) — *see* Injury, intracranial, diffuse
      focal — *see* Injury, intracranial, focal
  newborn P52.9
    specified NEC P52.8
  subarachnoid (nontraumatic) (from) I60.9
    intracranial (cerebral) artery I60.7
      anterior communicating I60.2
      basilar I60.4
      carotid siphon and bifurcation I60.0- ☑
      communicating I60.7
        anterior I60.2
        posterior I60.3- ☑
      middle cerebral I60.1- ☑
      posterior communicating I60.3- ☑
      specified artery NEC I60.6
      vertebral I60.5- ☑
    newborn P52.5
      birth injury P10.3
    specified NEC I60.8
    traumatic S06.6X- ☑
  subdural (nontraumatic) I62.00
    acute I62.01
    birth injury P10.0
    chronic I62.03
    newborn (anoxic) (hypoxic) P52.8
      birth injury P10.0
    spinal G95.19
    subacute I62.02
    traumatic — *see* Injury, intracranial, subdural hemorrhage

Hemorrhage, hemorrhagic — *continued*
intracranial — *continued*
  traumatic — *see* Injury, intracranial, focal brain injury
intramedullary NEC G95.19
intraocular — *see* Hemophthalmos
intraoperative, intraprocedural — *see* Complication, hemorrhage (hematoma), intraoperative (intraprocedural), by site
intrapartum — *see* Hemorrhage, complicating, delivery
intrapelvic
  female N94.89
  male K66.1
intraperitoneal K66.1
intrapontine I61.3
intraprocedural — *see* Complication, hemorrhage (hematoma), intraoperative (intraprocedural), by site
intrauterine N85.7
  complicating delivery (*see also* Hemorrhage, complicating, delivery) O67.9
  postpartum — *see* Hemorrhage, postpartum
intraventricular I61.5
  newborn (nontraumatic) (*see also* Newborn, affected by, hemorrhage) P52.3
    due to birth injury P10.2
    grade
      1 P52.0
      2 P52.1
      3 P52.21
      4 P52.22
intravesical N32.89
iris (postinfectional) (postinflammatory) (toxic) — *see* Hyphema
joint (nontraumatic) — *see* Hemarthrosis
kidney N28.89
knee (joint) (nontraumatic) — *see* Hemarthrosis, knee
labyrinth — *see* subcategory H83.8 ☑
lenticular striate artery I61.0
ligature, vessel — *see* Hemorrhage, postoperative
liver K76.89
lung R04.89
  newborn P26.9
    massive P26.1
    specified NEC P26.8
  tuberculous — *see* Tuberculosis, pulmonary
massive umbilical, newborn P51.0
mediastinum — *see* Hemorrhage, lung
medulla I61.3
membrane (brain) I60.8
  spinal cord — *see* Hemorrhage, spinal cord
meninges, meningeal (brain) (middle) I60.8
  spinal cord — *see* Hemorrhage, spinal cord
mesentery K66.1
metritis — *see* Endometritis
mouth K13.79
mucous membrane NEC R58
  newborn P54.8
muscle M62.89
nail (subungual) L60.8
nasal turbinate R04.0
  newborn P54.8
navel, newborn P51.9
newborn P54.9
  specified NEC P54.8
nipple N64.59
nose R04.0
  newborn P54.8
omentum K66.1
optic nerve (sheath) H47.02- ☑
orbit, orbital H05.23- ☑
ovary NEC N83.8
oviduct N83.6
pancreas K86.89
parathyroid (gland) (spontaneous) E21.4
parturition — *see* Hemorrhage, complicating, delivery
penis N48.89
pericardium, pericarditis I31.2
peritoneum, peritoneal K66.1
peritonsillar tissue J35.8
  due to infection J36
petechial R23.3
  due to autosensitivity, erythrocyte D69.2
pituitary (gland) E23.6
pleura — *see* Hemorrhage, lung
polioencephalitis, superior E51.2
polymyositis — *see* Polymyositis

Hemorrhage, hemorrhagic — *continued*
pons, pontine I61.3
posterior fossa (nontraumatic) I61.8
  newborn P52.6
postmenopausal N95.0
postnasal R04.0
postoperative — *see* Complications, postprocedural, hemorrhage, by site
postpartum NEC (following delivery of placenta) O72.1
  delayed or secondary O72.2
  retained placenta O72.0
  third stage O72.0
pregnancy — *see* Hemorrhage, antepartum
preretinal — *see* Hemorrhage, retina
prostate N42.1
puerperal — *see* Hemorrhage, postpartum
  delayed or secondary O72.2
pulmonary R04.89
  newborn P26.9
    massive P26.1
    specified NEC P26.8
  tuberculous — *see* Tuberculosis, pulmonary
purpura (primary) D69.3
rectum (sphincter) K62.5
  newborn P54.2
recurring, following initial hemorrhage at time of injury T79.2 ☑
renal N28.89
respiratory passage or tract R04.9
  specified NEC R04.89
retina, retinal (vessels) H35.6- ☑
  diabetic — *see* Diabetes, retinal, hemorrhage
retroperitoneal R58
scalp R58
scrotum N50.1
secondary (nontraumatic) R58
  following initial hemorrhage at time of injury T79.2 ☑
seminal vesicle N50.1
skin R23.3
  newborn P54.5
slipped umbilical ligature P51.8
spermatic cord N50.1
spinal (cord) G95.19
  newborn (birth injury) P11.5
spleen D73.5
  intraoperative — *see* Complications, intraoperative, hemorrhage, spleen
  postprocedural — *see* Complications, postprocedural, hemorrhage, spleen
stomach K92.2
  newborn P54.3
  ulcer — *see* Ulcer, stomach, with hemorrhage
subarachnoid (nontraumatic) — *see* Hemorrhage, intracranial, subarachnoid
subconjunctival (*see also* Hemorrhage, conjunctiva)
  birth injury P15.3
subcortical (brain) I61.0
subcutaneous R23.3
subdiaphragmatic R58
subdural (acute) (nontraumatic) — *see* Hemorrhage, intracranial, subdural
subependymal
  newborn P52.0
    with intraventricular extension P52.1
      and intracerebral extension P52.22
subgaleal P12.2
subhyaloid — *see* Hemorrhage, retina
subperiosteal — *see* Disorder, bone, specified type NEC
subretinal — *see* Hemorrhage, retina
subtentorial — *see* Hemorrhage, intracranial, subdural
subungual L60.8
suprarenal (capsule) (gland) E27.49
  newborn P54.4
tentorium (traumatic) NEC — *see* Hemorrhage, brain
  newborn (birth injury) P10.4
testis N50.1
third stage (postpartum) O72.0
thorax — *see* Hemorrhage, lung
throat R04.1
thymus (gland) E32.8
thyroid (cyst) (gland) E07.89
tongue K14.8
tonsil J35.8
trachea — *see* Hemorrhage, lung
tracheobronchial R04.89
  newborn P26.0

☑ Additional Character Required — Refer to the Tabular List for Character Selection   ▽ Subterms under main terms may continue to next column or page

Index

Hemorrhage, hemorrhagic — *continued*
  traumatic — *code to* specific injury
    cerebellar — *see* Hemorrhage, brain
    intracranial — *see* Hemorrhage, brain
    recurring or secondary (following initial hemor-
      rhage at time of injury) T79.2 ☑
  tuberculous NEC (*see also* Tuberculosis, pulmonary)
    A15.0
  tunica vaginalis N50.1
  ulcer — *code by* site under Ulcer, with hemorrhage
    K27.4
  umbilicus, umbilical
    cord
      after birth, newborn P51.9
      complicating delivery O69.5 ☑
    newborn P51.9
      massive P51.0
      slipped ligature P51.8
    stump P51.9
  urethra (idiopathic) N36.8
  uterus, uterine (abnormal) N93.9
    climacteric N92.4
    complicating delivery — *see* Hemorrhage, compli-
      cating, delivery
    dysfunctional or functional N93.8
    intermenstrual (regular) N92.3
      irregular N92.1
    postmenopausal N95.0
    postpartum — *see* Hemorrhage, postpartum
    preclimacteric or premenopausal N92.4
    prepubertal N93.8
    pubertal N92.2
  vagina (abnormal) N93.9
    newborn P54.6
  vas deferens N50.1
  vasa previa O69.4 ☑
  ventricular I61.5
  vesical N32.89
  viscera NEC R58
    newborn P54.8
  vitreous (humor) (intraocular) H43.1- ☑
  vulva N90.89
Hemorrhoids (bleeding) (without mention of degree)
  K64.9
  1st degree (grade/stage I) (without prolapse outside
    of anal canal) K64.0
  2nd degree (grade/stage II) (that prolapse with
    straining but retract spontaneously) K64.1
  3rd degree (grade/stage III) (that prolapse with
    straining and require manual replacement back
    inside anal canal) K64.2
  4th degree (grade/stage IV) (with prolapsed tissue that
    cannot be manually replaced) K64.3
  complicating
    pregnancy O22.4 ☑
    puerperium O87.2
  external K64.4
    with
      thrombosis K64.5
  internal (without mention of degree) K64.8
  prolapsed K64.8
  skin tags
    anus K64.4
    residual K64.4
  specified NEC K64.8
  strangulated (*see also* Hemorrhoids, by degree) K64.8
  thrombosed (*see also* Hemorrhoids, by degree) K64.5
  ulcerated (*see also* Hemorrhoids, by degree) K64.8
Hemosalpinx N83.6
  with
    hematocolpos N89.7
    hematometra N85.7
      with hematocolpos N89.7
Hemosiderosis (dietary) E83.19
  pulmonary, idiopathic E83.1- ☑ [J84.03]
  transfusion T80.89 ☑
Hemothorax (bacterial) (nontuberculous) J94.2
  newborn P54.8
  traumatic S27.1 ☑
    with pneumothorax S27.2 ☑
  tuberculous NEC A15.6
Henoch (-Schönlein) **disease or syndrome** (purpura)
  D69.0
Henpue, henpuye A66.6
Hepar lobatum (syphilitic) A52.74
Hepatalgia K76.89
Hepatitis K75.9
  acute B17.9

Hepatitis — *continued*
  acute — *continued*
    with coma K72.01
    with hepatic failure — *see* Failure, hepatic
    alcoholic — *see* Hepatitis, alcoholic
    infectious B17.9
    non-viral K72.0 ☑
    viral B17.9
  alcoholic (acute) (chronic) K70.10
    with ascites K70.11
  amebic — *see* Abscess, liver, amebic
  anicteric, (viral) — *see* Hepatitis, viral
  antigen-associated (HAA) — *see* Hepatitis, B
  Australia-antigen (positive) — *see* Hepatitis, B
  autoimmune K75.4
  B B19.10
    with hepatic coma B19.11
    acute B16.9
      with
        delta-agent (coinfection) (without hepatic
          coma) B16.1
          with hepatic coma B16.0
        hepatic coma (without delta-agent coinfec-
          tion) B16.2
    chronic B18.1
      with delta-agent B18.0
  bacterial NEC K75.89
  C (viral) B19.20
    with hepatic coma B19.21
    acute B17.10
      with hepatic coma B17.11
    chronic B18.2
  catarrhal (acute) B15.9
    with hepatic coma B15.0
  cholangiolitic K75.89
  cholestatic K75.89
  chronic K73.9
    active NEC K73.2
    lobular NEC K73.1
    persistent NEC K73.0
    specified NEC K73.8
  cytomegaloviral B25.1
  due to ethanol (acute) (chronic) — *see* Hepatitis, alco-
    holic
  epidemic B15.9
    with hepatic coma B15.0
  fulminant NEC (viral) — *see* Hepatitis, viral
  granulomatous NEC K75.3
  herpesviral B00.81
  history of
    B Z86.19
    C Z86.19
  homologous serum — *see* Hepatitis, viral, type B
  in (due to)
    mumps B26.81
    toxoplasmosis (acquired) B58.1
      congenital (active) P37.1 [K77]
  infectious, infective B15.9
    acute (subacute) B17.9
    chronic B18.9
  inoculation — *see* Hepatitis, viral, type B
  interstitial (chronic) K74.69
  lupoid NEC K75.4
  malignant NEC (with hepatic failure) K72.90
    with coma K72.91
  neonatal (idiopathic) (toxic) P59.29
  neonatal giant cell P59.29
  newborn P59.29
  non-viral K72.0 ☑
  postimmunization — *see* Hepatitis, viral, type B
  post-transfusion — *see* Hepatitis, viral, type B
  reactive, nonspecific K75.2
  serum — *see* Hepatitis, viral, type B
  specified type NEC
    with hepatic failure — *see* Failure, hepatic
  syphilitic (late) A52.74
    congenital (early) A50.08 [K77]
      late A50.59 [K77]
    secondary A51.45
  toxic (*see also* Disease, liver, toxic) K71.6
  tuberculous A18.83
  viral, virus B19.9
    with hepatic coma B19.0
    acute B17.9
    chronic B18.9
      specified NEC B18.8
      type
        B B18.1

Hepatitis — *continued*
  viral, virus — *continued*
    chronic — *continued*
      type — *continued*
        B — *continued*
          with delta-agent B18.0
        C B18.2
    congenital P35.3
    coxsackie B33.8 [K77]
    cytomegalic inclusion B25.1
    in remission, any type — *code to* Hepatitis, chronic,
      by type
    non-A, non-B B17.8
    specified type NEC (with or without coma) B17.8
    type
      A B15.9
        with hepatic coma B15.0
      B B19.10
        with hepatic coma B19.11
        acute B16.9
          with
            delta-agent (coinfection) (without
              hepatic coma) B16.1
              with hepatic coma B16.0
            hepatic coma (without delta-agent
              coinfection) B16.2
        chronic B18.1
          with delta-agent B18.0
      C B19.20
        with hepatic coma B19.21
        acute B17.10
          with hepatic coma B17.11
        chronic B18.2
      E B17.2
      non-A, non-B B17.8
Hepatization lung (acute) — *see* Pneumonia, lobar
Hepatoblastoma C22.2
Hepatocarcinoma C22.0
Hepatocholangiocarcinoma C22.0
Hepatocholangioma, benign D13.4
Hepatocholangitis K75.89
Hepatolenticular degeneration E83.01
Hepatoma (malignant) C22.0
  benign D13.4
  embryonal C22.0
Hepatomegaly (*see also* Hypertrophy, liver)
  with splenomegaly R16.2
  congenital Q44.7
  in mononucleosis
    gammaherpesviral B27.09
    infectious specified NEC B27.89
Hepatoptosis K76.89
Hepatorenal syndrome following labor and delivery
  O90.4
Hepatosis K76.89
Hepatosplenomegaly R16.2
  hyperlipemic (Bürger-Grütz type) E78.3 [K77]
Hereditary — *see* condition
Heredodegeneration, macular — *see* Dystrophy, retina
Heredopathia atactica polyneuritiformis G60.1
Heredosyphilis — *see* Syphilis, congenital
Herlitz' syndrome Q81.1
Hermansky-Pudlak syndrome E70.331
Hermaphrodite, hermaphroditism (true) Q56.0
  46,XX with streak gonads Q99.1
  46,XX/46,XY Q99.1
  46,XY with streak gonads Q99.1
  chimera 46,XX/46,XY Q99.0
Hernia, hernial (acquired) (recurrent) K46.9
  with
    gangrene — *see* Hernia, by site, with, gangrene
    incarceration — *see* Hernia, by site, with, obstruc-
      tion
    irreducible — *see* Hernia, by site, with, obstruction
    obstruction — *see* Hernia, by site, with, obstruction
    strangulation — *see* Hernia, by site, with, obstruc-
      tion
  abdomen, abdominal K46.9
    with
      gangrene (and obstruction) K46.1
      obstruction K46.0
    femoral — *see* Hernia, femoral
    incisional — *see* Hernia, incisional
    inguinal — *see* Hernia, inguinal
    specified site NEC K45.8
      with
        gangrene (and obstruction) K45.1
        obstruction K45.0

Hemorrhage, hemorrhagic — Hernia, hernial

Index

Hernia, hernial — Herpes, herpesvirus, herpetic

Hernia, hernial — *continued*
  abdomen, abdominal — *continued*
    umbilical — *see* Hernia, umbilical
    wall — *see* Hernia, ventral
  appendix — *see* Hernia, abdomen
  bladder (mucosa) (sphincter)
    congenital (female) (male) Q79.51
    female — *see* Cystocele
    male N32.89
  brain, congenital — *see* Encephalocele
  cartilage, vertebra — *see* Displacement, intervertebral
      disc
  cerebral, congenital (*see also* Encephalocele)
    endaural Q01.8
  ciliary body (traumatic) S05.2- ☑
  colon — *see* Hernia, abdomen
  Cooper's — *see* Hernia, abdomen, specified site NEC
  crural — *see* Hernia, femoral
  diaphragm, diaphragmatic K44.9
    with
      gangrene (and obstruction) K44.1
      obstruction K44.0
    congenital Q79.0
  direct (inguinal) — *see* Hernia, inguinal
  diverticulum, intestine — *see* Hernia, abdomen
  double (inguinal) — *see* Hernia, inguinal, bilateral
  due to adhesions (with obstruction) K56.50
  epigastric (*see also* Hernia, ventral) K43.9
  esophageal hiatus — *see* Hernia, hiatal
  external (inguinal) — *see* Hernia, inguinal
  fallopian tube N83.4- ☑
  fascia M62.89
  femoral K41.90
    with
      gangrene (and obstruction) K41.40
        not specified as recurrent K41.40
        recurrent K41.41
      obstruction K41.30
        not specified as recurrent K41.30
        recurrent K41.31
    bilateral K41.20
      with
        gangrene (and obstruction) K41.10
          not specified as recurrent K41.10
          recurrent K41.11
        obstruction K41.00
          not specified as recurrent K41.00
          recurrent K41.01
      not specified as recurrent K41.20
      recurrent K41.21
    not specified as recurrent K41.90
    recurrent K41.91
    unilateral K41.90
      with
        gangrene (and obstruction) K41.40
          not specified as recurrent K41.40
          recurrent K41.41
        obstruction K41.30
          not specified as recurrent K41.30
          recurrent K41.31
      not specified as recurrent K41.90
      recurrent K41.91
  foramen magnum G93.5
    congenital Q01.8
  funicular (umbilical) (*see also* Hernia, umbilicus)
    spermatic (cord) — *see* Hernia, inguinal
  gastrointestinal tract — *see* Hernia, abdomen
  Hesselbach's — *see* Hernia, femoral, specified site NEC
  hiatal (esophageal) (sliding) K44.9
    with
      gangrene (and obstruction) K44.1
      obstruction K44.0
    congenital Q40.1
  hypogastric — *see* Hernia, ventral
  incarcerated (*see also* Hernia, by site, with obstruction)
    with gangrene — *see* Hernia, by site, with gangrene
  incisional K43.2
    with
      gangrene (and obstruction) K43.1
      obstruction K43.0
  indirect (inguinal) — *see* Hernia, inguinal
  inguinal (direct) (external) (funicular) (indirect) (internal) (oblique) (scrotal) (sliding) K40.90
    with
      gangrene (and obstruction) K40.40
        not specified as recurrent K40.40
        recurrent K40.41

Hernia, hernial — *continued*
  inguinal — *continued*
    with — *continued*
      obstruction K40.30
        not specified as recurrent K40.30
        recurrent K40.31
    bilateral K40.20
      with
        gangrene (and obstruction) K40.10
          not specified as recurrent K40.10
          recurrent K40.11
        obstruction K40.00
          not specified as recurrent K40.00
          recurrent K40.01
      not specified as recurrent K40.20
      recurrent K40.21
    not specified as recurrent K40.90
    recurrent K40.91
    unilateral K40.90
      with
        gangrene (and obstruction) K40.40
          not specified as recurrent K40.40
          recurrent K40.41
        obstruction K40.30
          not specified as recurrent K40.30
          recurrent K40.31
      not specified as recurrent K40.90
      recurrent K40.91
  internal (*see also* Hernia, abdomen)
    inguinal — *see* Hernia, inguinal
  interstitial — *see* Hernia, abdomen
  intervertebral cartilage or disc — *see* Displacement,
      intervertebral disc
  intestine, intestinal — *see* Hernia, by site
  intra-abdominal — *see* Hernia, abdomen
  iris (traumatic) S05.2- ☑
  irreducible (*see also* Hernia, by site, with obstruction)
    with gangrene — *see* Hernia, by site, with gangrene
  ischiatic — *see* Hernia, abdomen, specified site NEC
  ischiorectal — *see* Hernia, abdomen, specified site
      NEC
  lens (traumatic) S05.2- ☑
  linea (alba) (semilunaris) — *see* Hernia, ventral
  Littre's — *see* Hernia, abdomen
  lumbar — *see* Hernia, abdomen, specified site NEC
  lung (subcutaneous) J98.4
  mediastinum J98.59
  mesenteric (internal) — *see* Hernia, abdomen
  midline — *see* Hernia, ventral
  muscle (sheath) M62.89
  nucleus pulposus — *see* Displacement, intervertebral
      disc
  oblique (inguinal) — *see* Hernia, inguinal
  obstructive (*see also* Hernia, by site, with obstruction)
    with gangrene — *see* Hernia, by site, with gangrene
  obturator — *see* Hernia, abdomen, specified site NEC
  omental — *see* Hernia, abdomen
  ovary N83.4- ☑
  oviduct N83.4- ☑
  paraesophageal (*see also* Hernia, diaphragm)
    congenital Q40.1
  parastomal K43.5
    with
      gangrene (and obstruction) K43.4
      obstruction K43.3
  paraumbilical — *see* Hernia, umbilicus
  perineal — *see* Hernia, abdomen, specified site NEC
  Petit's — *see* Hernia, abdomen, specified site NEC
  postoperative — *see* Hernia, incisional
  pregnant uterus — *see* Abnormal, uterus in pregnancy
      or childbirth
  prevesical N32.89
  properitoneal — *see* Hernia, abdomen, specified site
      NEC
  pudendal — *see* Hernia, abdomen, specified site NEC
  rectovaginal N81.6
  retroperitoneal — *see* Hernia, abdomen, specified site
      NEC
  Richter's — *see* Hernia, abdomen, with obstruction
  Rieux's, Rieux's — *see* Hernia, abdomen, specified site
      NEC
  sac condition (adhesion) (dropsy) (inflammation)
      (laceration) (suppuration) — *code by site under*
      Hernia
  sciatic — *see* Hernia, abdomen, specified site NEC

Hernia, hernial — *continued*
  scrotum, scrotal — *see* Hernia, inguinal
  sliding (inguinal) (*see also* Hernia, inguinal)
    hiatus — *see* Hernia, hiatal
  spigelian — *see* Hernia, ventral
  spinal — *see* Spina bifida
  strangulated (*see also* Hernia, by site, with obstruction)
    with gangrene — *see* Hernia, by site; with gangrene
  subxiphoid — *see* Hernia, ventral
  supra-umbilicus — *see* Hernia, ventral
  tendon — *see* Disorder, tendon, specified type NEC
  Treitz's (fossa) — *see* Hernia, abdomen, specified site
      NEC
  tunica vaginalis Q55.29
  umbilicus, umbilical K42.9
    with
      gangrene (and obstruction) K42.1
      obstruction K42.0
  ureter N28.89
  urethra, congenital Q64.79
  urinary meatus, congenital Q64.79
  uterus N81.4
    pregnant — *see* Abnormal, uterus in pregnancy or
        childbirth
  vaginal (anterior) (wall) — *see* Cystocele
  Velpeau's — *see* Hernia, femoral
  ventral K43.9
    with
      gangrene (and obstruction) K43.7
      obstruction K43.6
    incisional K43.2
      with
        gangrene (and obstruction) K43.1
        obstruction K43.0
      recurrent — *see* Hernia, incisional
    specified NEC K43.9
      with
        gangrene (and obstruction) K43.7
        obstruction K43.6
  vesical
    congenital (female) (male) Q79.51
    female — *see* Cystocele
    male N32.89
  vitreous (into wound) S05.2- ☑
    into anterior chamber — *see* Prolapse, vitreous
Herniation (*see also* Hernia)
  brain (stem) G93.5
  cerebral G93.5
  mediastinum J98.59
  nucleus pulposus — *see* Displacement, intervertebral
      disc
Herpangina B08.5
Herpes, herpesvirus, herpetic B00.9
  anogenital A60.9
    perianal skin A60.1
    rectum A60.1
    urogenital tract A60.00
      cervix A60.03
      male genital organ NEC A60.02
      penis A60.01
      specified site NEC A60.09
      vagina A60.04
      vulva A60.04
  blepharitis (zoster) B02.39
    simplex B00.59
  circinatus B35.4
    bullosus L12.0
  conjunctivitis (simplex) B00.53
    zoster B02.31
  cornea B02.33
  encephalitis B00.4
    due to herpesvirus 6 B10.01
    due to herpesvirus 7 B10.09
    specified NEC B10.09
  eye (zoster) B02.30
    simplex B00.50
  eyelid (zoster) B02.39
    simplex B00.59
  facialis B00.1
  febrilis B00.1
  geniculate ganglionitis B02.21
  genital, genitalis A60.00
    female A60.09
    male A60.02
  gestational, gestationis O26.4- ☑
  gingivostomatitis B00.2
  human B00.9

Index

Herpes, herpesvirus, herpetic — *continued*
  human — *continued*
    1 — *see* Herpes, simplex
    2 — *see* Herpes, simplex
    3 — *see* Varicella
    4 — *see* Mononucleosis, Epstein-Barr (virus)
    5 — *see* Disease, cytomegalic inclusion (generalized)
    6
      encephalitis B10.01
      specified NEC B10.81
    7
      encephalitis B10.09
      specified NEC B10.82
    8 B10.89
  infection NEC B10.89
    Kaposi's sarcoma associated B10.89
  iridocyclitis (simplex) B00.51
    zoster B02.32
  iris (vesicular erythema multiforme) L51.9
  iritis (simplex) B00.51
  Kaposi's sarcoma associated B10.89
  keratitis (simplex) (dendritic) (disciform) (interstitial) B00.52
    zoster (interstitial) B02.33
  keratoconjunctivitis (simplex) B00.52
    zoster B02.33
  labialis B00.1
  lip B00.1
  meningitis (simplex) B00.3
    zoster B02.1
  ophthalmicus (zoster) NEC B02.30
    simplex B00.50
  penis A60.01
  perianal skin A60.1
  pharyngitis, pharyngotonsillitis B00.2
  rectum A60.1
  scrotum A60.02
  sepsis B00.7
  simplex B00.9
    complicated NEC B00.89
    congenital P35.2
    conjunctivitis B00.53
    external ear B00.1
    eyelid B00.59
    hepatitis B00.81
    keratitis (interstitial) B00.52
    myleitis B00.82
    specified complication NEC B00.89
    visceral B00.89
  stomatitis B00.2
  tonsurans B35.0
  visceral B00.89
  vulva A60.04
  whitlow B00.89
  zoster (*see also* condition) B02.9
    auricularis B02.21
    complicated NEC B02.8
    conjunctivitis B02.31
    disseminated B02.7
    encephalitis B02.0
    eye (lid) B02.39
    geniculate ganglionitis B02.21
    keratitis (interstitial) B02.33
    meningitis B02.1
    myelitis B02.24
    neuritis, neuralgia B02.29
    ophthalmicus NEC B02.30
    oticus B02.21
    polyneuropathy B02.23
    specified complication NEC B02.8
    trigeminal neuralgia B02.22
Herpesvirus (human) — *see* Herpes
Herpetophobia F40.218
Herrick's anemia — *see* Disease, sickle-cell
Hers' disease E74.09
Herter-Gee syndrome K90.0
Herxheimer's reaction R68.89
Hesitancy
  of micturition R39.11
  urinary R39.11
Hesselbach's hernia — *see* Hernia, femoral, specified site NEC
Heterochromia (congenital) Q13.2
  cataract — *see* Cataract, complicated
  cyclitis (Fuchs) — *see* Cyclitis, Fuchs' heterochromic
  hair L67.1
  iritis — *see* Cyclitis, Fuchs' heterochromic

Heterochromia — *continued*
  retained metallic foreign body (nonmagnetic) — *see* Foreign body, intraocular, old, retained
    magnetic — *see* Foreign body, intraocular, old, retained, magnetic
  uveitis — *see* Cyclitis, Fuchs' heterochromic
Heterophoria — *see* Strabismus, heterophoria
Heterophyes, heterophyiasis (small intestine) B66.8
Heterotopia, heterotopic (*see also* Malposition, congenital)
  cerebralis Q04.8
Heterotropia — *see* Strabismus
Heubner-Herter disease K90.0
Hexadactylism Q69.9
HGSIL (cytology finding) (high grade squamous intraepithelial lesion on cytologic smear) (Pap smear finding)
  anus R85.613
  cervix R87.613
    biopsy (histology) finding — *see* Neoplasia, intraepithelial, cervix, grade II or grade III
  vagina R87.623
    biopsy (histology) finding — *see* Neoplasia, intraepithelial, cervix, grade II or grade III
Hibernoma — *see* Lipoma
Hiccup, hiccough R06.6
  epidemic B33.0
  psychogenic F45.8
Hidden penis (congenital) Q55.64
  acquired N48.83
Hidradenitis (axillaris) (suppurative) L73.2
Hidradenoma (nodular) (*see also* Neoplasm, skin, benign)
  clear cell — *see* Neoplasm, skin, benign
  papillary — *see* Neoplasm, skin, benign
Hidrocystoma — *see* Neoplasm, skin, benign
High
  altitude effects T70.20 ☑
    anoxia T70.29 ☑
    on
      ears T70.0 ☑
      sinuses T70.1 ☑
    polycythemia D75.1
  arch
    foot Q66.7
    palate, congenital Q38.5
  arterial tension — *see* Hypertension
  basal metabolic rate R94.8
  blood pressure (*see also* Hypertension)
    borderline R03.0
    reading (incidental) (isolated) (nonspecific), without diagnosis of hypertension R03.0
  cholesterol E78.00
    with high triglycerides E78.2
  diaphragm (congenital) Q79.1
  expressed emotional level within family Z63.8
  head at term O32.4 ☑
  palate, congenital Q38.5
  risk
    infant NEC Z76.2
    sexual behavior (heterosexual) Z72.51
      bisexual Z72.53
      homosexual Z72.52
  scrotal testis, testes
    bilateral Q53.23
    unilateral Q53.13
  temperature (of unknown origin) R50.9
  thoracic rib Q76.6
  triglycerides E78.1
    with high cholesterol E78.2
Hildenbrand's disease A75.0
Hilum — *see* condition
Hip — *see* condition
Hippel's disease Q85.8
Hippophobia F40.218
Hippus H57.09
Hirschsprung's disease or megacolon Q43.1
Hirsutism, hirsuties L68.0
Hirudiniasis
  external B88.3
  internal B83.4
Hiss-Russell dysentery A03.1
Histidinemia, histidinuria E70.41
Histiocytoma (*see also* Neoplasm, skin, benign)
  fibrous (*see also* Neoplasm, skin, benign)
    atypical — *see* Neoplasm, connective tissue, uncertain behavior

Histiocytoma — *continued*
  fibrous (*see also* Neoplasm, skin, benign) — *continued*
    malignant — *see* Neoplasm, connective tissue, malignant
Histiocytosis D76.3
  acute differentiated progressive C96.0
  Langerhans' cell NEC C96.6
    multifocal X
      multisystemic (disseminated) C96.0
      unisystemic C96.5
    pulmonary, adult (adult PLCH) J84.82
    unifocal (X) C96.6
  lipid, lipoid D76.3
    essential E75.29
  malignant C96.A (*following* C96.6)
  mononuclear phagocytes NEC D76.1
    Langerhans' cells C96.6
  non-Langerhans cell D76.3
  polyostotic sclerosing D76.3
  sinus, with massive lymphadenopathy D76.3
  syndrome NEC D76.3
  X NEC C96.6
    acute (progressive) C96.0
    chronic C96.6
    multifocal C96.5
    multisystemic C96.0
    unifocal C96.6
Histoplasmosis B39.9
  with pneumonia NEC B39.2
  African B39.5
  American — *see* Histoplasmosis, capsulati
  capsulati B39.4
    disseminated B39.3
    generalized B39.3
    pulmonary B39.2
      acute B39.0
      chronic B39.1
  Darling's B39.4
  duboisii B39.5
  lung NEC B39.2
History
  family (of) (*see also* History, personal (of))
    alcohol abuse Z81.1
    allergy NEC Z84.89
    anemia Z83.2
    arthritis Z82.61
    asthma Z82.5
    blindness Z82.1
    cardiac death (sudden) Z82.41
    carrier of genetic disease Z84.81
    chromosomal anomaly Z82.79
    chronic
      disabling disease NEC Z82.8
      lower respiratory disease Z82.5
    colonic polyps Z83.71
    congenital malformations and deformations Z82.79
      polycystic kidney Z82.71
    consanguinity Z84.3
    deafness Z82.2
    diabetes mellitus Z83.3
    disability NEC Z82.8
    disease or disorder (of)
      allergic NEC Z84.89
      behavioral NEC Z81.8
      blood and blood-forming organs Z83.2
      cardiovascular NEC Z82.49
      chronic disabling NEC Z82.8
      digestive Z83.79
      ear NEC Z83.52
      endocrine NEC Z83.49
      eye NEC Z83.518
        glaucoma Z83.511
      familial hypercholesterolemia Z83.42
      genitourinary NEC Z84.2
      glaucoma Z83.511
      hematological Z83.2
      immune mechanism Z83.2
      infectious NEC Z83.1
      ischemic heart Z82.49
      kidney Z84.1
      mental NEC Z81.8
      metabolic Z83.49
      musculoskeletal NEC Z82.69
      neurological NEC Z82.0
      nutritional Z83.49
      parasitic NEC Z83.1
      psychiatric NEC Z81.8
      respiratory NEC Z83.6

Herpes, herpesvirus, herpetic — History

Index

History — History

History — continued
  family (see also History, personal) — continued
    disease or disorder — continued
      skin and subcutaneous tissue NEC Z84.0
      specified NEC Z84.89
    drug abuse NEC Z81.3
    epilepsy Z82.0
    familial hypercholesterolemia Z83.42
    genetic disease carrier Z84.81
    glaucoma Z83.511
    hearing loss Z82.2
    human immunodeficiency virus (HIV) infection
        Z83.0
    Huntington's chorea Z82.0
    intellectual disability Z81.0
    leukemia Z80.6
    malignant neoplasm (of) NOS Z80.9
      bladder Z80.52
      breast Z80.3
      bronchus Z80.1
      digestive organ Z80.0
      gastrointestinal tract Z80.0
      genital organ Z80.49
        ovary Z80.41
        prostate Z80.42
        specified organ NEC Z80.49
        testis Z80.43
      hematopoietic NEC Z80.7
      intrathoracic organ NEC Z80.2
      kidney Z80.51
      lung Z80.1
      lymphatic NEC Z80.7
      ovary Z80.41
      prostate Z80.42
      respiratory organ NEC Z80.2
      specified site NEC Z80.8
      testis Z80.43
      trachea Z80.1
      urinary organ or tract Z80.59
        bladder Z80.52
        kidney Z80.51
    mental
      disorder NEC Z81.8
    multiple endocrine neoplasia (MEN) syndrome
        Z83.41
    osteoporosis Z82.62
    polycystic kidney Z82.71
    polyps (colon) Z83.71
    psychiatric disorder Z81.8
    psychoactive substance abuse NEC Z81.3
    respiratory condition NEC Z83.6
      asthma and other lower respiratory conditions
          Z82.5
    self-harmful behavior Z81.8
    SIDS (sudden infant death syndrome) Z84.82
    skin condition Z84.0
    specified condition NEC Z84.89
    stroke (cerebrovascular) Z82.3
    substance abuse NEC Z81.4
      alcohol Z81.1
      drug NEC Z81.3
      psychoactive NEC Z81.3
      tobacco Z81.2
    sudden
      cardiac death Z82.41
      infant death syndrome (SIDS) Z84.82
    tobacco abuse Z81.2
    violence, violent behavior Z81.8
    visual loss Z82.1
  personal (of) (see also History, family (of))
    abuse
      adult Z91.419
        physical and sexual Z91.410
        psychological Z91.411
      childhood Z62.819
        physical Z62.810
        psychological Z62.811
        sexual Z62.810
    alcohol dependence F10.21
    allergy (to) Z88.9
      analgesic agent NEC Z88.6
      anesthetic Z88.4
      antibiotic agent NEC Z88.1
      anti-infective agent NEC Z88.3
      contrast media Z91.041
      drugs, medicaments and biological substances
          Z88.9
        specified NEC Z88.8
      food Z91.018

History — continued
  personal (see also History, family) — continued
    allergy — continued
      food — continued
        additives Z91.02
        eggs Z91.012
        milk products Z91.011
        peanuts Z91.010
        seafood Z91.013
        specified food NEC Z91.018
      insect Z91.038
        bee Z91.030
      latex Z91.040
      medicinal agents Z88.9
        specified NEC Z88.8
      narcotic agent Z88.5
      nonmedicinal agents Z91.048
      penicillin Z88.0
      serum Z88.7
      specified NEC Z91.09
      sulfonamides Z88.2
      vaccine Z88.7
    anaphylactic shock Z87.892
    anaphylaxis Z87.892
    behavioral disorders Z86.59
    benign carcinoid tumor Z86.012
    benign neoplasm Z86.018
      brain Z86.011
      carcinoid Z86.012
      colonic polyps Z86.010
    brain injury (traumatic) Z87.820
    breast implant removal Z98.86
    calculi, renal Z87.442
    cancer — see History, personal (of), malignant
        neoplasm (of)
    cardiac arrest (death), successfully resuscitated
        Z86.74
    cerebral infarction without residual deficit Z86.73
    cervical dysplasia Z87.410
    chemotherapy for neoplastic condition Z92.21
    childhood abuse — see History, personal (of),
        abuse
    cleft lip (corrected) Z87.730
    cleft palate (corrected) Z87.730
    collapsed vertebra (healed) Z87.311
      due to osteoporosis Z87.310
    combat and operational stress reaction Z86.51
    congenital malformation (corrected) Z87.798
      circulatory system (corrected) Z87.74
      digestive system (corrected) NEC Z87.738
      ear (corrected) Z87.721
      eye (corrected) Z87.720
      face and neck (corrected) Z87.790
      genitourinary system (corrected) NEC Z87.718
      heart (corrected) Z87.74
      integument (corrected) Z87.76
      limb(s) (corrected) Z87.76
      musculoskeletal system (corrected) Z87.76
      neck (corrected) Z87.790
      nervous system (corrected) NEC Z87.728
      respiratory system (corrected) Z87.75
      sense organs (corrected) NEC Z87.728
      specified NEC Z87.798
    contraception Z92.0
    deployment (military) Z91.82
    diabetic foot ulcer Z86.31
    disease or disorder (of) Z87.898
      anaphylaxis Z87.892
      blood and blood-forming organs Z86.2
      circulatory system Z86.79
        specified condition NEC Z86.79
      connective tissue Z87.39
      digestive system Z87.19
        colonic polyp Z86.010
        peptic ulcer disease Z87.11
        specified condition NEC Z87.19
      ear Z86.69
      endocrine Z86.39
        diabetic foot ulcer Z86.31
        gestational diabetes Z86.32
        specified type NEC Z86.39
      eye Z86.69
      genital (track) system NEC
        female Z87.42
        male Z87.438
      hematological Z86.2
      Hodgkin Z85.71
      immune mechanism Z86.2
      infectious Z86.19

History — continued
  personal (see also History, family) — continued
    disease or disorder — continued
      infectious — continued
        malaria Z86.13
        Methicillin resistant Staphylococcus aureus
            (MRSA) Z86.14
        poliomyelitis Z86.12
        specified NEC Z86.19
        tuberculosis Z86.11
      mental NEC Z86.59
      metabolic Z86.39
        diabetic foot ulcer Z86.31
        gestational diabetes Z86.32
        specified type NEC Z86.39
      musculoskeletal NEC Z87.39
      nervous system Z86.69
      nutritional Z86.39
      parasitic Z86.19
      respiratory system NEC Z87.09
      sense organs Z86.69
      skin Z87.2
      specified site or type NEC Z87.898
      subcutaneous tissue Z87.2
      trophoblastic Z87.59
      urinary system NEC Z87.448
    drug dependence — see Dependence, drug, by
        type, in remission
    drug therapy
      antineoplastic chemotherapy Z92.21
      estrogen Z92.23
      immunosupression Z92.25
      inhaled steroids Z92.240
      monoclonal drug Z92.22
      specified NEC Z92.29
      steroid Z92.241
      systemic steroids Z92.241
    dysplasia
      cervical (mild) (moderate) Z87.410
        severe (grade III) Z86.001
      prostatic Z87.430
      vaginal (mild) (moderate) Z87.411
        severe (grade III) Z86.008
      vulvar (mild) (moderate) Z87.412
        severe (grade III) Z86.008
    embolism (venous) Z86.718
      pulmonary Z86.711
    encephalitis Z86.61
    estrogen therapy Z92.23
    extracorporeal membrane oxygenation (ECMO)
        Z92.81
    failed conscious sedation Z92.83
    failed moderate sedation Z92.83
    fall, falling Z91.81
    fracture (healed)
      fatigue Z87.312
      fragility Z87.310
      osteoporosis Z87.310
      pathological NEC Z87.311
      stress Z87.312
      traumatic Z87.81
    gestational diabetes Z86.32
    hepatitis
      B Z86.19
      C Z86.19
    Hodgkin disease Z85.71
    hyperthermia, malignant Z88.4
    hypospadias (corrected) Z87.710
    hysterectomy Z90.710
    immunosupression therapy Z92.25
    in situ neoplasm
      breast Z86.000
      cervix uteri Z86.001
      specified NEC Z86.008
    in utero procedure during pregnancy Z98.870
    in utero procedure while a fetus Z98.871
    infection NEC Z86.19
      central nervous system Z86.61
      Methicillin resistant Staphylococcus aureus
          (MRSA) Z86.14
      urinary (recurrent) (tract) Z87.440
    injury NEC Z87.828
    irradiation Z92.3
    kidney stones Z87.442
    leukemia Z85.6
    lymphoma (non-Hodgkin) Z85.72
    malignant melanoma (skin) Z85.820
    malignant neoplasm (of) Z85.9
      accessory sinuses Z85.22

☑ **Additional Character Required — Refer to the Tabular List for Character Selection**   ▽ **Subterms under main terms may continue to next column or page**

History — *continued*
  personal (*see also* History, family) — *continued*
    malignant neoplasm — *continued*
      anus NEC Z85.048
        carcinoid Z85.040
      bladder Z85.51
      bone Z85.830
      brain Z85.841
      breast Z85.3
      bronchus NEC Z85.118
        carcinoid Z85.110
      carcinoid — *see* History, personal (of), malignant neoplasm, by site, carcinioid
      cervix Z85.41
      colon NEC Z85.038
        carcinoid Z85.030
      digestive organ Z85.00
        specified NEC Z85.09
      endocrine gland NEC Z85.858
      epididymis Z85.48
      esophagus Z85.01
      eye Z85.840
      gastrointestinal tract — *see* History, malignant neoplasm, digestive organ
      genital organ
        female Z85.40
          specified NEC Z85.44
        male Z85.45
          specified NEC Z85.49
      hematopoietic NEC Z85.79
      intrathoracic organ Z85.20
      kidney NEC Z85.528
        carcinoid Z85.520
      large intestine NEC Z85.038
        carcinoid Z85.030
      larynx Z85.21
      liver Z85.05
      lung NEC Z85.118
        carcinoid Z85.110
      mediastinum Z85.29
      Merkel cell Z85.821
      middle ear Z85.22
      nasal cavities Z85.22
      nervous system NEC Z85.848
      oral cavity Z85.819
        specified site NEC Z85.818
      ovary Z85.43
      pancreas Z85.07
      pelvis Z85.53
      pharynx Z85.819
        specified site NEC Z85.818
      pleura Z85.29
      prostate Z85.46
      rectosigmoid junction NEC Z85.048
        carcinoid Z85.040
      rectum NEC Z85.048
        carcinoid Z85.040
      respiratory organ Z85.20
      sinuses, accessory Z85.22
      skin NEC Z85.828
        melanoma Z85.820
        Merkel cell Z85.821
      small intestine NEC Z85.068
        carcinoid Z85.060
      soft tissue Z85.831
      specified site NEC Z85.89
      stomach NEC Z85.028
        carcinoid Z85.020
      testis Z85.47
      thymus NEC Z85.238
        carcinoid Z85.230
      thyroid Z85.850
      tongue Z85.810
      trachea Z85.12
      urinary organ or tract Z85.50
        specified NEC Z85.59
      uterus Z85.42
    maltreatment Z91.89
    medical treatment NEC Z92.89
    melanoma (malignant) (skin) Z85.820
    meningitis Z86.61
    mental disorder Z86.59
    Merkel cell carcinoma (skin) Z85.821
    Methicillin resistant Staphylococcus aureus (MRSA) Z86.14
    military deployment Z91.82
    military war, peacekeeping and humanitarian deployment (current or past conflict) Z91.82
    myocardial infarction (old) I25.2

History — *continued*
  personal (*see also* History, family) — *continued*
    neglect (in)
      adult Z91.412
      childhood Z62.812
    neoplasm
      benign Z86.018
        brain Z86.011
        colon polyp Z86.010
      in situ
        breast Z86.000
        cervix uteri Z86.001
        specified NEC Z86.008
      malignant — *see* History of, malignant neoplasm
      uncertain behavior Z86.03
    nephrotic syndrome Z87.441
    nicotine dependence Z87.891
    noncompliance with medical treatment or regimen — *see* Noncompliance
    nutritional deficiency Z86.39
    obstetric complications Z87.59
      childbirth Z87.59
      pregnancy Z87.59
      pre-term labor Z87.51
      puerperium Z87.59
    osteoporosis fractures Z87.31 ☑
    parasuicide (attempt) Z91.5
    physical trauma NEC Z87.828
      self-harm or suicide attempt Z91.5
    pneumonia (recurrent) Z87.01
    poisoning NEC Z91.89
      self-harm or suicide attempt Z91.5
    poor personal hygiene Z91.89
    preterm labor Z87.51
    procedure during pregnancy Z98.870
    procedure while a fetus Z98.871
    prolonged reversible ischemic neurologic deficit (PRIND) Z86.73
    prostatic dysplasia Z87.430
    psychological
      abuse
        adult Z91.411
        child Z62.811
      trauma, specified NEC Z91.49
    radiation therapy Z92.3
    removal
      implant
        breast Z98.86
    renal calculi Z87.442
    respiratory condition NEC Z87.09
    retained foreign body fully removed Z87.821
    risk factors NEC Z91.89
    self-harm Z91.5
    self-poisoning attempt Z91.5
    sex reassignment Z87.890
    sleep-wake cycle problem Z72.821
    specified NEC Z87.898
    steroid therapy (systemic) Z92.241
      inhaled Z92.240
    stroke without residual deficits Z86.73
    substance abuse NEC F10-F19
    sudden cardiac arrest Z86.74
    sudden cardiac death successfully resuscitated Z86.74
    suicide attempt Z91.5
    surgery NEC Z98.890
      with uterine scar Z98.891
      sex reassignment Z87.890
      transplant — *see* Transplant
    thrombophlebitis Z86.72
    thrombosis (venous) Z86.718
      pulmonary Z86.711
    tobacco dependence Z87.891
    transient ischemic attack (TIA) without residual deficits Z86.73
    trauma (physical) NEC Z87.828
      psychological NEC Z91.49
      self-harm Z91.5
    traumatic brain injury Z87.820
    unhealthy sleep-wake cycle Z72.821
    unintended awareness under general anesthesia Z92.84
    urinary calculi Z87.442
    urinary (recurrent) (tract) infection(s) Z87.440
    uterine scar from previous surgery Z98.891
    vaginal dysplasia Z87.411
    venous thrombosis or embolism Z86.718
      pulmonary Z86.711

History — *continued*
  personal (*see also* History, family) — *continued*
    vulvar dysplasia Z87.412
His-Werner disease A79.0
HIV (*see also* Human, immunodeficiency virus) B20
  laboratory evidence (nonconclusive) R75
  nonconclusive test (in infants) R75
  positive, seropositive Z21
Hives (bold) — *see* Urticaria
Hoarseness R49.0
Hobo Z59.0
Hodgkin disease — *see* Lymphoma, Hodgkin
Hodgson's disease I71.2
  ruptured I71.1
Hoffa-Kastert disease E88.89
Hoffa's disease E88.89
Hoffmann-Bouveret syndrome I47.9
Hoffmann's syndrome E03.9 [G73.7]
Hole (round)
  macula H35.34- ☑
  retina (without detachment) — *see* Break, retina, round hole
    with detachment — *see* Detachment, retina, with retinal, break
Holiday relief care Z75.5
Hollenhorst's plaque — *see* Occlusion, artery, retina
Hollow foot (congenital) Q66.7
  acquired — *see* Deformity, limb, foot, specified NEC
Holoprosencephaly Q04.2
Holt-Oram syndrome Q87.2
Homelessness Z59.0
Homesickness — *see* Disorder, adjustment
Homocystinemia, homocystinuria E72.11
Homogentisate 1,2-dioxygenase deficiency E70.29
Homologous serum hepatitis (prophylactic) (therapeutic) — *see* Hepatitis, viral, type B
Honeycomb lung J98.4
  congenital Q33.0
Hooded
  clitoris Q52.6
  penis Q55.69
Hookworm (anemia) (disease) (infection) (infestation) B76.9
  specified NEC B76.8
Hordeolum (eyelid) (externum) (recurrent) H00.019
  internum H00.029
    left H00.026
      lower H00.025
      upper H00.024
    right H00.023
      lower H00.022
      upper H00.021
  left H00.016
    lower H00.015
    upper H00.014
  right H00.013
    lower H00.012
    upper H00.011
Horn
  cutaneous L85.8
  nail L60.2
    congenital Q84.6
Horner (-Claude Bernard) **syndrome** G90.2
  traumatic — *see* Injury, nerve, cervical sympathetic
Horseshoe kidney (congenital) Q63.1
Horton's headache or neuralgia G44.099
  intractable G44.091
  not intractable G44.099
Hospital hopper syndrome — *see* Disorder, factitious
Hospitalism in children — *see* Disorder, adjustment
Hostility R45.5
  towards child Z62.3
Hot flashes
  menopausal N95.1
Hourglass (contracture) (*see also* Contraction, hourglass)
  stomach K31.89
    congenital Q40.2
    stricture K31.2
Household, housing circumstance affecting care Z59.9
  specified NEC Z59.8
Housemaid's knee — *see* Bursitis, prepatellar
Hudson (-Stähli) **line** (cornea) — *see* Pigmentation, cornea, anterior
Human
  bite (open wound) (*see also* Bite)
    intact skin surface — *see* Bite, superficial

Human — continued
  herpesvirus — see Herpes
  immunodeficiency virus (HIV) disease (infection) B20
    asymptomatic status Z21
    contact Z20.6
    counseling Z71.7
    dementia B20 [F02.80]
      with behavioral disturbance B20 [F02.81]
    exposure to Z20.6
    laboratory evidence R75
    type-2 (HIV 2) as cause of disease classified else-
      where B97.35
  papillomavirus (HPV)
    DNA test positive
      high risk
        cervix R87.810
        vagina R87.811
      low risk
        cervix R87.820
        vagina R87.821
    screening for Z11.51
  T-cell lymphotropic virus
    type-1 (HTLV-I) infection B33.3
      as cause of disease classified elsewhere B97.33
      carrier Z22.6
    type-2 (HTLV-II) as cause of disease classified else-
      where B97.34
Humidifier lung or pneumonitis J67.7
Humiliation (experience) **in childhood** Z62.898
Humpback (acquired) — see Kyphosis
Hunchback (acquired) — see Kyphosis
Hunger T73.0 ☑
  air, psychogenic F45.8
Hungry bone syndrome E83.81
Hunner's ulcer — see Cystitis, chronic, interstitial
Hunter's
  glossitis D51.0
  syndrome E76.1
Huntington's disease or chorea G10
  with dementia G10 [F02.80]
    with behavioral disturbance G10 [F02.81]
Hunt's
  disease or syndrome (herpetic geniculate ganglionitis)
    B02.21
    dyssynergia cerebellaris myoclonica G11.1
  neuralgia B02.21
Hurler (-Scheie) **disease or syndrome** E76.02
Hurst's disease G36.1
Hurthle cell
  adenocarcinoma C73
  adenoma D34
  carcinoma C73
  tumor D34
Hutchinson-Boeck disease or syndrome — see Sarcoidosis
Hutchinson-Gilford disease or syndrome E34.8
Hutchinson's
  disease, meaning
    angioma serpiginosum L81.7
    pompholyx (cheiropompholyx) L30.1
    prurigo estivalis L56.4
    summer eruption or summer prurigo L56.4
  melanotic freckle — see Melanoma, in situ
    malignant melanoma in — see Melanoma
  teeth or incisors (congenital syphilis) A50.52
  triad (congenital syphilis) A50.53
Hyalin plaque, sclera, senile H15.89
Hyaline membrane (disease) (lung) (pulmonary) (newborn) P22.0
Hyalinosis
  cutis (et mucosae) E78.89
  focal and segmental (glomerular) (see also N00-N07
    with fourth character .1) N05.1
Hyalitis, hyalosis, asteroid (see also Deposit, crystalline)
  syphilitic (late) A52.71
Hydatid
  cyst or tumor — see Echinococcus
  mole — see Hydatidiform mole
  Morgagni
    female Q50.5
    male (epididymal) Q55.4
      testicular Q55.29
Hydatidiform mole (benign) (complicating pregnancy)
  (delivered) (undelivered) O01.9
  classical O01.0
  complete O01.0
  incomplete O01.1
  invasive D39.2

Hydatidiform mole — continued
  malignant D39.2
  partial O01.1
Hydatidosis — see Echinococcus
Hydradenitis (axillaris) (suppurative) L73.2
Hydradenoma — see Hidradenoma
Hydramnios O40.-
Hydrancephaly, hydranencephaly Q04.3
  with spina bifida — see Spina bifida, with hydro-
    cephalus
Hydrargyrism NEC — see Poisoning, mercury
Hydrarthrosis (see also Effusion, joint)
  gonococcal A54.42
  intermittent M12.40
    ankle M12.47- ☑
    elbow M12.42- ☑
    foot joint M12.47- ☑
    hand joint M12.44- ☑
    hip M12.45- ☑
    knee M12.46- ☑
    multiple site M12.49
    shoulder M12.41- ☑
    specified joint NEC M12.48
    wrist M12.43- ☑
  of yaws (early) (late) (see also subcategory M14.8-)
    A66.6
  syphilitic (late) A52.77
    congenital A50.55 [M12.80]
Hydremia D64.89
Hydrencephalocele (congenital) — see Encephalocele
Hydrencephalomeningocele (congenital) — see Encephalocele
Hydroa R23.8
  aestivale L56.4
  vacciniforme L56.4
Hydroadenitis (axillaris) (suppurative) L73.2
Hydrocalycosis — see Hydronephrosis
Hydrocele (spermatic cord) (testis) (tunica vaginalis)
  N43.3
  canal of Nuck N94.89
  communicating N43.2
    congenital P83.5
  congenital P83.5
  encysted N43.0
  female NEC N94.89
  infected N43.1
  newborn P83.5
  round ligament N94.89
  specified NEC N43.2
  spinalis — see Spina bifida
  vulva N90.89
Hydrocephalus (acquired) (external) (internal) (malignant) (recurrent) G91.9
  aqueduct Sylvius stricture Q03.0
  causing disproportion O33.6 ☑
    with obstructed labor O66.3
  communicating G91.0
  congenital (external) (internal) Q03.9
    with spina bifida Q05.4
      cervical Q05.0
      dorsal Q05.1
      lumbar Q05.2
      lumbosacral Q05.2
      sacral Q05.3
      thoracic Q05.1
      thoracolumbar Q05.1
    specified NEC Q03.8
  due to toxoplasmosis (congenital) P37.1
  foramen Magendie block (acquired) G91.1
    congenital (see also Hydrocephalus, congenital)
      Q03.1
  in (due to)
    infectious disease NEC B89 [G91.4]
    neoplastic disease NEC (see also Neoplasm) G91.4
    parasitic disease B89 [G91.4]
  newborn Q03.9
    with spina bifida — see Spina bifida, with hydro-
      cephalus
  noncommunicating G91.1
  normal pressure G91.2
    secondary G91.0
  obstructive G91.1
  otitic G93.2
  post-traumatic NEC G91.3
  secondary G91.4
    post-traumatic G91.3
  specified NEC G91.8
  syphilitic, congenital A50.49

Hydrocolpos (congenital) N89.8
Hydrocystoma — see Neoplasm, skin, benign
Hydroencephalocele (congenital) — see Encephalocele
Hydroencephalomeningocele (congenital) — see En-
  cephalocele
Hydrohematopneumothorax — see Hemothorax
Hydromeningitis — see Meningitis
Hydromeningocele (spinal) (see also Spina bifida)
  cranial — see Encephalocele
Hydrometra N85.8
Hydrometrocolpos N89.8
Hydromicrocephaly Q02
Hydromphalos (since birth) Q45.8
Hydromyelia Q06.4
Hydromyelocele — see Spina bifida
Hydronephrosis (atrophic) (early) (functionless) (inter-
  mittent) (primary) (secondary) NEC N13.30
  with
    infection N13.6
    obstruction (by) (of)
      renal calculus N13.2
        with infection N13.6
      ureteral NEC N13.1
        with infection N13.6
        calculus N13.2
          with infection N13.6
      ureteropelvic junction (congenital) Q62.11
        acquired N13.0
          with infection N13.6
    ureteral stricture NEC N13.1
      with infection N13.6
  congenital Q62.0
  due to acquired occlusion of ureteropelvic junction
    N13.0
  specified type NEC N13.39
  tuberculous A18.11
Hydropericarditis — see Pericarditis
Hydropericardium — see Pericarditis
Hydroperitoneum R18.8
Hydrophobia — see Rabies
Hydrophthalmos Q15.0
Hydropneumohemothorax — see Hemothorax
Hydropneumopericarditis — see Pericarditis
Hydropneumopericardium — see Pericarditis
Hydropneumothorax J94.8
  traumatic — see Injury, intrathoracic, lung
  tuberculous NEC A15.6
Hydrops R60.9
  abdominis R18.8
  articulorum intermittens — see Hydrarthrosis, inter-
    mittent
  cardiac — see Failure, heart, congestive
  causing obstructed labor (mother) O66.3
  endolymphatic H81.0- ☑
  fetal — see Pregnancy, complicated by, hydrops, fetalis
  fetalis P83.2
    due to
      ABO isoimmunization P56.0
      alpha thalassemia D56.0
      hemolytic disease P56.90
        specified NEC P56.99
      isoimmunization (ABO) (Rh) P56.0
      other specified nonhemolytic disease NEC P83.2
      Rh incompatibility P56.0
    during pregnancy — see Pregnancy, complicated
      by, hydrops, fetalis
  gallbladder K82.1
  joint — see Effusion, joint
  labyrinth H81.0- ☑
  newborn (idiopathic) P83.2
    due to
      ABO isoimmunization P56.0
      alpha thalassemia D56.0
      hemolytic disease P56.90
        specified NEC P56.99
      isoimmunization (ABO) (Rh) P56.0
      Rh incompatibility P56.0
  nutritional — see Malnutrition, severe
  pericardium — see Pericarditis
  pleura — see Hydrothorax
  spermatic cord — see Hydrocele
Hydropyonephrosis N13.6
Hydrorachis Q06.4
Hydrorrhea (nasal) J34.89
  pregnancy — see Rupture, membranes, premature
Hydrosadenitis (axillaris) (suppurative) L73.2
Hydrosalpinx (fallopian tube) (follicularis) N70.11

Hydrothorax (double) (pleura) J94.8
  chylous (nonfilarial) I89.8
    filarial (*see also* Infestation, filarial) B74.9 [J91.8]
  traumatic — *see* Injury, intrathoracic
  tuberculous NEC (non primary) A15.6
Hydroureter (*see also* Hydronephrosis) N13.4
  with infection N13.6
  congenital Q62.39
Hydroureteronephrosis — *see* Hydronephrosis
Hydrourethra N36.8
Hydroxykynureninuria E70.8
Hydroxylysinemia E72.3
Hydroxyprolinemia E72.59
Hygiene, sleep
  abuse Z72.821
  inadequate Z72.821
  poor Z72.821
Hygroma (congenital) (cystic) D18.1
  praepatellare, prepatellar — *see* Bursitis, prepatellar
  subdural I62.03
Hymen — *see* condition
Hymenolepis, hymenolepiasis (diminuta) (infection) (infestation) (nana) B71.0
Hypalgesia R20.8
Hyperacidity (gastric) K31.89
  psychogenic F45.8
Hyperactive, hyperactivity F90.9
  basal cell, uterine cervix — *see* Dysplasia, cervix
  bowel sounds R19.12
  cervix epithelial (basal) — *see* Dysplasia, cervix
  child F90.9
    attention deficit — *see* Disorder, attention-deficit hyperactivity
  detrusor muscle N32.81
  gastrointestinal K31.89
    psychogenic F45.8
  nasal mucous membrane J34.3
  stomach K31.89
  thyroid (gland) — *see* Hyperthyroidism
Hyperacusis H93.23- ☑
Hyperadrenalism E27.5
Hyperadrenocorticism E24.9
  congenital E25.0
  iatrogenic E24.2
    correct substance properly administered — *see* Table of Drugs and Chemicals, by drug, adverse effect
    overdose or wrong substance given or taken — *see* Table of Drugs and Chemicals, by drug, poisoning
  not associated with Cushing's syndrome E27.0
  pituitary-dependent E24.0
Hyperaldosteronism E26.9
  familial (type I) E26.02
  glucocorticoid-remediable E26.02
  primary (due to (bilateral) adrenal hyperplasia) E26.09
  primary NEC E26.09
  secondary E26.1
  specified NEC E26.89
Hyperalgesia R20.8
Hyperalimentation R63.2
  carotene, carotin E67.1
  specified NEC E67.8
  vitamin
    A E67.0
    D E67.3
Hyperaminoaciduria
  arginine E72.21
  cystine E72.01
  lysine E72.3
  ornithine E72.4
Hyperammonemia (congenital) E72.20
Hyperazotemia — *see* Uremia
Hyperbetalipoproteinemia (familial) E78.00
  with prebetalipoproteinemia E78.2
Hyperbilirubinemia
  constitutional E80.6
  familial conjugated E80.6
  neonatal (transient) — *see* Jaundice, newborn
Hypercalcemia, hypocalciuric, familial E83.52
Hypercalciuria, idiopathic E83.52
Hypercapnia R06.89
  newborn P84
Hypercarotenemia, hypercarotinemia (dietary) E67.1
Hypercementosis K03.4
Hyperchloremia E87.8
Hyperchlorhydria K31.89

Hyperchlorhydria — *continued*
  neurotic F45.8
  psychogenic F45.8
Hypercholesterinemia — *see* Hypercholesterolemia
Hypercholesterolemia (essential) (primary) (pure) E78.00
  with hyperglyceridemia, endogenous E78.2
  dietary counseling and surveillance Z71.3
  familial E78.01
  hereditary E78.01
Hyperchylia gastrica, psychogenic F45.8
Hyperchylomicronemia (familial) (primary) E78.3
  with hyperbetalipoproteinemia E78.3
Hypercoagulable (state) D68.59
  activated protein C resistance D68.51
  antithrombin III deficiency D68.59
  factor V Leiden mutation D68.51
  primary NEC D68.59
  protein C deficiency D68.59
  protein S deficiency D68.59
  prothrombin gene mutation D68.52
  secondary D68.69
  specified NEC D68.69
Hypercoagulation (state) D68.59
Hypercorticalism, pituitary-dependent E24.0
Hypercorticosolism — *see* Cushing's, syndrome
Hypercorticosteronism E24.2
  correct substance properly administered — *see* Table of Drugs and Chemicals, by drug, adverse effect
  overdose or wrong substance given or taken — *see* Table of Drugs and Chemicals, by drug, poisoning
Hypercortisonism E24.2
  correct substance properly administered — *see* Table of Drugs and Chemicals, by drug, adverse effect
  overdose or wrong substance given or taken — *see* Table of Drugs and Chemicals, by drug, poisoning
Hyperekplexia Q89.8
Hyperelectrolytemia E87.8
Hyperemesis R11.10
  with nausea R11.2
  gravidarum (mild) O21.0
    with
      carbohydrate depletion O21.1
      dehydration O21.1
      electrolyte imbalance O21.1
      metabolic disturbance O21.1
    severe (with metabolic disturbance) O21.1
  projectile R11.12
  psychogenic F45.8
Hyperemia (acute) (passive) R68.89
  anal mucosa K62.89
  bladder N32.89
  cerebral I67.89
  conjunctiva H11.43- ☑
  ear internal, acute — *see* subcategory H83.0 ☑
  enteric K59.8
  eye — *see* Hyperemia, conjunctiva
  eyelid (active) (passive) — *see* Disorder, eyelid, specified type NEC
  intestine K59.8
  iris — *see* Disorder, iris, vascular
  kidney N28.89
  labyrinth — *see* subcategory H83.0 ☑
  liver (active) K76.89
  lung (passive) — *see* Edema, lung
  pulmonary (passive) — *see* Edema, lung
  renal N28.89
  retina H35.89
  stomach K31.89
Hyperesthesia (body surface) R20.3
  larynx (reflex) J38.7
    hysterical F44.89
  pharynx (reflex) J39.2
    hysterical F44.89
Hyperestrogenism (drug-induced) (iatrogenic) E28.0
Hyperexplexia Q89.8
Hyperfibrinolysis — *see* Fibrinolysis
Hyperfructosemia E74.19
Hyperfunction
  adrenal cortex, not associated with Cushing's syndrome E27.0
  medulla E27.5
    adrenomedullary E27.5
  virilism E25.9
    congenital E25.0
  ovarian E28.8

Hyperfunction — *continued*
  pancreas K86.89
  parathyroid (gland) E21.3
  pituitary (gland) (anterior) E22.9
    specified NEC E22.8
  polyglandular E31.1
  testicular E29.0
Hypergammaglobulinemia D89.2
  polyclonal D89.0
  Waldenström D89.0
Hypergastrinemia E16.4
Hyperglobulinemia R77.1
Hyperglycemia, hyperglycemic (transient) R73.9
  coma — *see* Diabetes, by type, with coma
  postpancreatectomy E89.1
Hyperglyceridemia (endogenous) (essential) (familial) (hereditary) (pure) E78.1
  mixed E78.3
Hyperglycinemia (non-ketotic) E72.51
Hypergonadism
  ovarian E28.8
  testicular (primary) (infantile) E29.0
Hyperheparinemia D68.32
Hyperhidrosis, hyperidrosis R61
  focal
    primary L74.519
      axilla L74.510
      face L74.511
      palms L74.512
      soles L74.513
    secondary L74.52
  generalized R61
  localized
    primary L74.519
      axilla L74.510
      face L74.511
      palms L74.512
      soles L74.513
    secondary L74.52
  psychogenic F45.8
  secondary R61
    focal L74.52
Hyperhistidinemia E70.41
Hyperhomocysteinemia E72.11
Hyperhydroxyprolinemia E72.59
Hyperinsulinism (functional) E16.1
  with
    coma (hypoglycemic) E15
    encephalopathy E16.1 [G94]
  ectopic E16.1
  therapeutic misadventure (from administration of insulin) — *see* subcategory T38.3 ☑
Hyperkalemia E87.5
Hyperkeratosis (*see also* Keratosis) L85.9
  cervix N88.0
  due to yaws (early) (late) (palmar or plantar) A66.3
  follicularis Q82.8
    penetrans (in cutem) L87.0
  palmoplantaris climacterica L85.1
  pinta A67.1
  senile (with pruritus) L57.0
  universalis congenita Q80.8
  vocal cord J38.3
  vulva N90.4
Hyperkinesia, hyperkinetic (disease) (reaction) (syndrome) (childhood) (adolescence) (*see also* Disorder, attention-deficit hyperactivity)
  heart I51.89
Hyperleucine-isoleucinemia E71.19
Hyperlipemia, hyperlipidemia E78.5
  combined E78.2
    familial E78.4
  group
    A E78.00
    B E78.1
    C E78.2
    D E78.3
  mixed E78.2
  specified NEC E78.4
Hyperlipidosis E75.6
  hereditary NEC E75.5
Hyperlipoproteinemia E78.5
  Fredrickson's type
    I E78.3
    IIa E78.00
    IIb E78.2
    III E78.2
    IV E78.1

Hyperlipoproteinemia — continued
   Fredrickson's type — continued
     V E78.3
   low-density-lipoprotein-type (LDL) E78.00
   very-low-density-lipoprotein-type (VLDL) E78.1
Hyperlucent lung, unilateral J43.0
Hyperlysinemia E72.3
Hypermagnesemia E83.41
   neonatal P71.8
Hypermenorrhea N92.0
Hypermethioninemia E72.19
Hypermetropia (congenital) H52.0- ☑
Hypermobility, hypermotility
   cecum — see Syndrome, irritable bowel
   coccyx — see subcategory M53.2 ☑
   colon — see Syndrome, irritable bowel
     psychogenic F45.8
   ileum K58.9
   intestine (see also Syndrome, irritable bowel) K58.9
     psychogenic F45.8
   meniscus (knee) — see Derangement, knee, meniscus
   scapula — see Instability, joint, shoulder
   stomach K31.89
     psychogenic F45.8
   syndrome M35.7
   urethra N36.41
     with intrinsic sphincter deficiency N36.43
Hypernasality R49.21
Hypernatremia E87.0
Hypernephroma C64.- ☑
Hyperopia — see Hypermetropia
Hyperorexia nervosa F50.2
Hyperornithinemia E72.4
Hyperosmia R43.1
Hyperosmolality E87.0
Hyperostosis (monomelic) (see also Disorder, bone, density and structure, specified NEC)
   ankylosing (spine) M48.10
     cervical region M48.12
     cervicothoracic region M48.13
     lumbar region M48.16
     lumbosacral region M48.17
     multiple sites M48.19
     occipito-atlanto-axial region M48.11
     sacrococcygeal region M48.18
     thoracic region M48.14
     thoracolumbar region M48.15
   cortical (skull) M85.2
     infantile M89.8X- ☑
   frontal, internal of skull M85.2
   interna frontalis M85.2
   skeletal, diffuse idiopathic — see Hyperostosis, ankylosing
   skull M85.2
     congenital Q75.8
   vertebral, ankylosing — see Hyperostosis, ankylosing
Hyperovarism E28.8
Hyperoxaluria (primary) E72.53
Hyperparathyroidism E21.3
   primary E21.0
   secondary (renal) N25.81
     non-renal E21.1
   specified NEC E21.2
   tertiary E21.2
Hyperpathia R20.8
Hyperperistalsis R19.2
   psychogenic F45.8
Hyperpermeability, capillary I78.8
Hyperphagia R63.2
Hyperphenylalaninemia NEC E70.1
Hyperphoria (alternating) H50.53
Hyperphosphatemia E83.39
Hyperpiesis, hyperpiesia — see Hypertension
Hyperpigmentation (see also Pigmentation)
   melanin NEC L81.4
   postinflammatory L81.0
Hyperpinealism E34.8
Hyperpituitarism E22.9
Hyperplasia, hyperplastic
   adenoids J35.2
   adrenal (capsule) (cortex) (gland) E27.8
     with
       sexual precocity (male) E25.9
         congenital E25.0
       virilism, adrenal E25.9
         congenital E25.0
       virilization (female) E25.9

Hyperplasia, hyperplastic — continued
   adrenal — continued
     with — continued
       virilization — continued
         congenital E25.0
     congenital E25.0
     salt-losing E25.0
   adrenomedullary E27.5
   angiolymphoid, eosinophilia (ALHE) D18.01
   appendix (lymphoid) K38.0
   artery, fibromuscular I77.3
   bone (see also Hypertrophy, bone)
     marrow D75.89
   breast (see also Hypertrophy, breast)
     ductal (atypical) N60.9- ☑
   C-cell, thyroid E07.0
   cementation (tooth) (teeth) K03.4
   cervical gland R59.0
   cervix (uteri) (basal cell) (endometrium) (polypoid) (see also Dysplasia, cervix)
     congenital Q51.828
   clitoris, congenital Q52.6
   denture K06.2
   endocervicitis N72
   endometrium, endometrial (adenomatous) (benign) (cystic) (glandular) (glandular-cystic) (polypoid) N85.00
     with atypia N85.02
     cervix — see Dysplasia, cervix
     complex (without atypia) N85.01
     simple (without atypia) N85.01
   epithelial L85.9
     focal, oral, including tongue K13.29
     nipple N62
     skin L85.9
     tongue K13.29
     vaginal wall N89.3
   erythroid D75.89
   fibromuscular of artery (carotid) (renal) I77.3
   genital
     female NEC N94.89
     male N50.89
   gingiva K06.1
   glandularis cystica uteri (interstitialis) (see also Hyperplasia, endometrial) N85.00
   gum K06.1
   hymen, congenital Q52.4
   irritative, edentulous (alveolar) K06.2
   jaw M26.09
     alveolar M26.79
     lower M26.03
       alveolar M26.72
     upper M26.01
       alveolar M26.71
   kidney (congenital) Q63.3
   labia N90.69
     epithelial N90.3
   liver (congenital) Q44.7
     nodular, focal K76.89
   lymph gland or node R59.9
   mandible, mandibular M26.03
     alveolar M26.72
     unilateral condylar M27.8
   maxilla, maxillary M26.01
     alveolar M26.71
   myometrium, myometrial N85.2
   neuroendocrine cell, of infancy J84.841
   nose
     lymphoid J34.89
     polypoid J33.9
   oral mucosa (irritative) K13.6
   organ or site, congenital NEC — see Anomaly, by site
   ovary N83.8
   palate, papillary (irritative) K13.6
   pancreatic islet cells E16.9
     alpha E16.8
       with excess
         gastrin E16.4
         glucagon E16.3
     beta E16.1
   parathyroid (gland) E21.0
   pharynx (lymphoid) J39.2
   prostate (adenofibromatous) (nodular) N40.0
     with lower urinary tract symptoms (LUTS) N40.1
     without lower urinary tract symtpoms (LUTS) N40.0
   renal artery I77.89
   reticulo-endothelial (cell) D75.89
   salivary gland (any) K11.1

Hyperplasia, hyperplastic — continued
   Schimmelbusch's — see Mastopathy, cystic
   suprarenal capsule (gland) E27.8
   thymus (gland) (persistent) E32.0
   thyroid (gland) — see Goiter
   tonsils (faucial) (infective) (lingual) (lymphoid) J35.1
     with adenoids J35.3
   unilateral condylar M27.8
   uterus, uterine N85.2
     endometrium (glandular) (see also Hyperplasia, endometrial) N85.00
   vulva N90.69
     epithelial N90.3
Hyperpnea — see Hyperventilation
Hyperpotassemia E87.5
Hyperprebetalipoproteinemia (familial) E78.1
Hyperprolactinemia E22.1
Hyperprolinemia (type I) (type II) E72.59
Hyperproteinemia E88.09
Hyperprothrombinemia, causing coagulation factor deficiency D68.4
Hyperpyrexia R50.9
   heat (effects) T67.0 ☑
   malignant, due to anesthetic T88.3 ☑
   rheumatic — see Fever, rheumatic
   unknown origin R50.9
Hyper-reflexia R29.2
Hypersalivation K11.7
Hypersecretion
   ACTH (not associated with Cushing's syndrome) E27.0
     pituitary E24.0
   adrenaline E27.5
   adrenomedullary E27.5
   androgen (testicular) E29.0
     ovarian (drug-induced) (iatrogenic) E28.1
   calcitonin E07.0
   catecholamine E27.5
   corticoadrenal E24.9
   cortisol E24.9
   epinephrine E27.5
   estrogen E28.0
   gastric K31.89
     psychogenic F45.8
   gastrin E16.4
   glucagon E16.3
   hormone(s)
     ACTH (not associated with Cushing's syndrome) E27.0
       pituitary E24.0
     antidiuretic E22.2
     growth E22.0
     intestinal NEC E34.1
     ovarian androgen E28.1
     pituitary E22.9
     testicular E29.0
     thyroid stimulating E05.80
       with thyroid storm E05.81
   insulin — see Hyperinsulinism
   lacrimal glands — see Epiphora
   medulloadrenal E27.5
   milk O92.6
   ovarian androgens E28.1
   salivary gland (any) K11.7
   thyrocalcitonin E07.0
   upper respiratory J39.8
Hypersegmentation, leukocytic, hereditary D72.0
Hypersensitive, hypersensitiveness, hypersensitivity (see also Allergy)
   carotid sinus G90.01
   colon — see Irritable, colon
   drug T88.7 ☑
   gastrointestinal K52.29
     immediate K52.29
     psychogenic F45.8
   labyrinth — see subcategory H83.2 ☑
   pain R20.8
   pneumonitis — see Pneumonitis, allergic
   reaction T78.40 ☑
     upper respiratory tract NEC J39.3
Hypersomnia (organic) G47.10
   due to
     alcohol
       abuse F10.182
       dependence F10.282
       use F10.982
     amphetamines
       abuse F15.182
       dependence F15.282

☑ **Additional Character Required** — Refer to the Tabular List for Character Selection

▽ **Subterms under main terms may continue to next column or page**

Hypersomnia — *continued*
- due to — *continued*
  - amphetamines — *continued*
    - use F15.982
  - caffeine
    - abuse F15.182
    - dependence F15.282
    - use F15.982
  - cocaine
    - abuse F14.182
    - dependence F14.282
    - use F14.982
  - drug NEC
    - abuse F19.182
    - dependence F19.282
    - use F19.982
  - medical condition G47.14
  - mental disorder F51.13
  - opioid
    - abuse F11.182
    - dependence F11.282
    - use F11.982
  - psychoactive substance NEC
    - abuse F19.182
    - dependence F19.282
    - use F19.982
  - sedative, hypnotic, or anxiolytic
    - abuse F13.182
    - dependence F13.282
    - use F13.982
  - stimulant NEC
    - abuse F15.182
    - dependence F15.282
    - use F15.982
- idiopathic G47.11
  - with long sleep time G47.11
  - without long sleep time G47.12
- menstrual related G47.13
- nonorganic origin F51.11
  - specified NEC F51.19
- not due to a substance or known physiological condition F51.11
  - specified NEC F51.19
- primary F51.11
- recurrent G47.13
- specified NEC G47.19

Hypersplenia, hypersplenism D73.1
Hyperstimulation, ovaries (associated with induced ovulation) N98.1
Hypersusceptibility — *see* Allergy
Hypertelorism (ocular) (orbital) Q75.2
Hypertension, hypertensive (accelerated) (benign) (essential) (idiopathic) (malignant) (systemic) I10
- with
  - heart failure (congestive) I11.0
  - heart involvement (conditions in I50.-, I51.4- I51.9 due to hypertension) — *see* Hypertension, heart
  - kidney involvement — *see* Hypertension, kidney
- benign, intracranial G93.2
- borderline R03.0
- cardiorenal (disease) I13.10
  - with heart failure I13.0
    - with stage 1 through stage 4 chronic kidney disease I13.0
    - with stage 5 or end stage renal disease I13.2
  - without heart failure I13.10
    - with stage 1 through stage 4 chronic kidney disease I13.10
    - with stage 5 or end stage renal disease I13.11
- cardiovascular
  - disease (arteriosclerotic) (sclerotic) — *see* Hypertension, heart
  - renal (disease) — *see* Hypertension, cardiorenal
- chronic venous — *see* Hypertension, venous (chronic)
- complicating
  - childbirth (labor) O16.4
    - pre-existing O10.92
      - with
        - heart disease O10.12
          - with renal disease O10.32
        - pre-eclampsia O11.4
        - renal disease O10.22
          - with heart disease O10.32
        - essential O10.02
        - secondary O10.42
  - pregnancy O16.- ☑
    - with edema (*see also* Pre-eclampsia) O14.9- ☑

Hypertension, hypertensive — *continued*
- complicating — *continued*
  - pregnancy — *continued*
    - gestational (pregnancy induced) (without proteinuria) O13.- ☑
      - with proteinuria O14.9- ☑
        - mild pre-eclampsia O14.0- ☑
        - moderate pre-eclampsia O14.0- ☑
        - severe pre-eclampsia O14.1- ☑
          - with hemolysis, elevated liver enzymes and low platelet count (HELLP) O14.2- ☑
    - pre-existing O10.91- ☑
      - with
        - heart disease O10.11- ☑
          - with renal disease O10.31- ☑
        - pre-eclampsia — *see* category O11
        - renal disease O10.21- ☑
          - with heart disease O10.31- ☑
        - essential O10.01- ☑
        - secondary O10.41- ☑
    - transient O13- ☑
  - puerperium, pre-existing O16.5
    - pre-existing
      - with
        - heart disease O10.13
          - with renal disease O10.33
        - pre-eclampsia O11.5
        - renal disease O10.23
          - with heart disease O10.33
        - essential O10.03
      - pregnancy-induced O13.9
      - secondary O10.43
- crisis I16.9
- due to
  - endocrine disorders I15.2
  - pheochromocytoma I15.2
  - renal disorders NEC I15.1
    - arterial I15.0
  - renovascular disorders I15.0
  - specified disease NEC I15.8
- emergency I16.1
- encephalopathy I67.4
- gestational (without significant proteinuria) (pregnancy-induced) (transient) O13.- ☑
  - with significant proteinuria — *see* Pre-eclampsia
  - complicating
    - delivery O13.4
    - puerperium O13.5
- Goldblatt's I70.1
- heart (disease) (conditions in I51.4-I51.9 due to hypertension) I11.9
  - with
    - heart failure (congestive) I11.0
    - kidney disease (chronic) — *see* Hypertension, cardiorenal
- intracranial (benign) G93.2
- kidney I12.9
  - with
    - heart disease — *see* Hypertension, cardiorenal
    - stage 1 through stage 4 chronic kidney disease I12.9
    - stage 5 chronic kidney disease (CKD) or end stage renal disease (ESRD) I12.0
- lesser circulation I27.0
- maternal O16- ☑
- newborn P29.2
  - pulmonary (persistent) P29.30
- ocular H40.05- ☑
- pancreatic duct — *code to* underlying condition
  - with chronic pancreatitis K86.1
- portal (due to chronic liver disease) (idiopathic) K76.6
  - gastropathy K31.89
  - in (due to) schistosomiasis (bilharziasis) B65.9 [K77]
- postoperative I97.3
- psychogenic F45.8
- pulmonary I27.20
  - with
    - cor pulmonale (chronic) I27.29
      - acute I26.09
    - right heart ventricular strain/failure I27.29
      - acute I26.09
    - right to left shunt related to congenital heart disease I27.83
    - unclear multifactorial mechanisms I27.29
  - arterial (associated) (drug-induced) (toxin-induced) I27.21
  - chronic thromboembolic I27.24

Hypertension, hypertensive — *continued*
- pulmonary — *continued*
  - due to
    - hematologic disorders I27.29
    - left heart disease I27.22
    - lung diseases and hypoxia I27.23
    - metabolic disorders I27.29
    - specified systemic disorders I27.29
  - group 1 (associated) (drug-induced) (toxin-induced) I27.21
  - group 2 I27.22
  - group 3 I27.23
  - group 4 I27.24
  - group 5 I27.29
  - of newborn (persistent) P29.30
  - primary (idiopathic) I27.0
  - secondary
    - arterial I27.21
    - specified NEC I27.29
- renal — *see* Hypertension, kidney
- renovascular I15.0
- secondary NEC I15.9
  - due to
    - endocrine disorders I15.2
    - pheochromocytoma I15.2
    - renal disorders NEC I15.1
      - arterial I15.0
    - renovascular disorders I15.0
  - specified NEC I15.8
- transient, of pregnancy O13- ☑
- urgency I16.0
- venous (chronic)
  - due to
    - deep vein thrombosis — *see* Syndrome, post-thrombotic
  - idiopathic I87.309
    - with
      - inflammation I87.32- ☑
        - with ulcer I87.33- ☑
      - specified complication NEC I87.39- ☑
      - ulcer I87.31- ☑
        - with inflammation I87.33- ☑
      - asymptomatic I87.30- ☑

Hypertensive urgency — *see* Hypertension
Hyperthecosis ovary E28.8
Hyperthermia (of unknown origin) (*see also* Hyperpyrexia)
- malignant, due to anesthesia T88.3 ☑
- newborn P81.9
  - environmental P81.0

Hyperthyroid (recurrent) — *see* Hyperthyroidism
Hyperthyroidism (latent) (pre-adult) (recurrent) E05.90
- with
  - goiter (diffuse) E05.00
    - with thyroid storm E05.01
    - nodular (multinodular) E05.20
      - with thyroid storm E05.21
      - uninodular E05.10
        - with thyroid storm E05.11
  - storm E05.91
- due to ectopic thyroid tissue E05.30
  - with thyroid storm E05.31
- neonatal, transitory P72.1
- specified NEC E05.80
  - with thyroid storm E05.81

Hypertony, hypertonia, hypertonicity
- bladder N31.8
- congenital P94.1
- stomach K31.89
  - psychogenic F45.8
- uterus, uterine (contractions) (complicating delivery) O62.4

Hypertrichosis L68.9
- congenital Q84.2
- eyelid H02.869
  - left H02.866
    - lower H02.865
    - upper H02.864
  - right H02.863
    - lower H02.862
    - upper H02.861
- lanuginosa Q84.2
  - acquired L68.1
- localized L68.2
- specified NEC L68.8

Hypertriglyceridemia, essential E78.1

Hypertrophy, hypertrophic
adenofibromatous, prostate — see Enlargement, enlarged, prostate
adenoids (infective) J35.2
  with tonsils J35.3
adrenal cortex E27.8
alveolar process or ridge — see Anomaly, alveolar
anal papillae K62.89
artery I77.89
  congenital NEC Q27.8
    digestive system Q27.8
    lower limb Q27.8
    specified site NEC Q27.8
    upper limb Q27.8
auricular — see Hypertrophy, cardiac
Bartholin's gland N75.8
bile duct (common) (hepatic) K83.8
bladder (sphincter) (trigone) N32.89
bone M89.30
  carpus M89.34- ☑
  clavicle M89.31- ☑
  femur M89.35- ☑
  fibula M89.36- ☑
  finger M89.34- ☑
  humerus M89.32- ☑
  ilium M89.359
  ischium M89.359
  metacarpus M89.34- ☑
  metatarsus M89.37- ☑
  multiple sites M89.39
  neck M89.38
  radius M89.33- ☑
  rib M89.38
  scapula M89.31- ☑
  skull M89.38
  tarsus M89.37- ☑
  tibia M89.36- ☑
  toe M89.37- ☑
  ulna M89.33- ☑
  vertebra M89.38
brain G93.89
breast N62
  cystic — see Mastopathy, cystic
  newborn P83.4
  pubertal, massive N62
  puerperal, postpartum — see Disorder, breast, specified type NEC
  senile (parenchymatous) N62
cardiac (chronic) (idiopathic) I51.7
  with rheumatic fever (conditions in I00)
    active I01.8
    inactive or quiescent (with chorea) I09.89
  congenital NEC Q24.8
  fatty — see Degeneration, myocardial
  hypertensive — see Hypertension, heart
  rheumatic (with chorea) I09.89
    active or acute I01.8
      with chorea I02.0
  valve — see Endocarditis
cartilage — see Disorder, cartilage, specified type NEC
cecum — see Megacolon
cervix (uteri) N88.8
  congenital Q51.828
  elongation N88.4
clitoris (cirrhotic) N90.89
  congenital Q52.6
colon (see also Megacolon)
  congenital Q43.2
conjunctiva, lymphoid H11.89
corpora cavernosa N48.89
cystic duct K82.8
duodenum K31.89
endometrium (glandular) (see also Hyperplasia, endometrial) N85.00
  cervix N88.8
epididymis N50.89
esophageal hiatus (congenital) Q79.1
  with hernia — see Hernia, hiatal
eyelid — see Disorder, eyelid, specified type NEC
fat pad E65
  knee (infrapatellar) (popliteal) (prepatellar) (retropatellar) M79.4
foot (congenital) Q74.2
frenulum, frenum (tongue) K14.8
  lip K13.0
gallbladder K82.8
gastric mucosa K29.60
  with bleeding K29.61

Hypertrophy, hypertrophic — continued
gland, glandular R59.9
  generalized R59.1
  localized R59.0
gum (mucous membrane) K06.1
heart (idiopathic) (see also Hypertrophy, cardiac)
  valve (see also Endocarditis) I38
hemifacial Q67.4
hepatic — see Hypertrophy, liver
hiatus (esophageal) Q79.1
hilus gland R59.0
hymen, congenital Q52.4
ileum K63.89
intestine NEC K63.89
jejunum K63.89
kidney (compensatory) N28.81
  congenital Q63.3
labium (majus) (minus) N90.60
ligament — see Disorder, ligament
lingual tonsil (infective) J35.1
  with adenoids J35.3
lip K13.0
  congenital Q18.6
liver R16.0
  acute K76.89
  cirrhotic — see Cirrhosis, liver
  congenital Q44.7
  fatty — see Fatty, liver
lymph, lymphatic gland R59.9
  generalized R59.1
  localized R59.0
  tuberculous — see Tuberculosis, lymph gland
mammary gland — see Hypertrophy, breast
Meckel's diverticulum (congenital) Q43.0
  malignant — see Table of Neoplasms, small intestine, malignant
median bar — see Hyperplasia, prostate
meibomian gland — see Chalazion
meniscus, knee, congenital Q74.1
metatarsal head — see Hypertrophy, bone, metatarsus
metatarsus — see Hypertrophy, bone, metatarsus
mucous membrane
  alveolar ridge K06.2
  gum K06.1
  nose (turbinate) J34.3
muscle M62.89
muscular coat, artery I77.89
myocardium (see also Hypertrophy, cardiac)
  idiopathic I42.2
myometrium N85.2
nail L60.2
  congenital Q84.5
nasal J34.89
  alae J34.89
  bone J34.89
  cartilage J34.89
  mucous membrane (septum) J34.3
  sinus J34.89
  turbinate J34.3
nasopharynx, lymphoid (infectional) (tissue) (wall) J35.2
nipple N62
organ or site, congenital NEC — see Anomaly, by site
ovary N83.8
palate (hard) M27.8
  soft K13.79
pancreas, congenital Q45.3
parathyroid (gland) E21.0
parotid gland K11.1
penis N48.89
pharyngeal tonsil J35.2
pharynx J39.2
  lymphoid (infectional) (tissue) (wall) J35.2
pituitary (anterior) (fossa) (gland) E23.6
prepuce (congenital) N47.8
  female N90.89
prostate — see Enlargement, enlarged, prostate
  congenital Q55.4
pseudomuscular G71.0
pylorus (adult) (muscle) (sphincter) K31.1
  congenital or infantile Q40.0
rectal, rectum (sphincter) K62.89
rhinitis (turbinate) J31.0
salivary gland (any) K11.1
  congenital Q38.4
scaphoid (tarsal) — see Hypertrophy, bone, tarsus
scar L91.0
scrotum N50.89

Hypertrophy, hypertrophic — continued
seminal vesicle N50.89
sigmoid — see Megacolon
skin L91.9
  specified NEC L91.8
spermatic cord N50.89
spleen — see Splenomegaly
spondylitis — see Spondylosis
stomach K31.89
sublingual gland K11.1
submandibular gland K11.1
suprarenal cortex (gland) E27.8
synovial NEC M67.20
  acromioclavicular M67.21- ☑
  ankle M67.27- ☑
  elbow M67.22- ☑
  foot M67.27- ☑
  hand M67.24- ☑
  hip M67.25- ☑
  knee M67.26- ☑
  multiple sites M67.29
  specified site NEC M67.28
  wrist M67.23- ☑
tendon — see Disorder, tendon, specified type NEC
testis N44.8
  congenital Q55.29
thymic, thymus (gland) (congenital) E32.0
thyroid (gland) — see Goiter
toe (congenital) Q74.2
  acquired (see also Deformity, toe, specified NEC)
tongue K14.8
  congenital Q38.2
  papillae (foliate) K14.3
tonsils (faucial) (infective) (lingual) (lymphoid) J35.1
  with adenoids J35.3
tunica vaginalis N50.89
ureter N28.89
urethra N36.8
uterus N85.2
  neck (with elongation) N88.4
  puerperal O90.89
uvula K13.79
vagina N89.8
vas deferens N50.89
vein I87.8
ventricle, ventricular (heart) (see also Hypertrophy, cardiac)
  congenital Q24.8
  in tetralogy of Fallot Q21.3
verumontanum N36.8
vocal cord J38.3
vulva N90.60
  stasis (nonfilarial) N90.69
Hypertropia H50.2- ☑
Hypertyrosinemia E70.21
Hyperuricemia (asymptomatic) E79.0
Hypervalinemia E71.19
Hyperventilation (tetany) R06.4
  hysterical F45.8
  psychogenic F45.8
  syndrome F45.8
Hypervitaminosis (dietary) NEC E67.8
  A E67.0
    administered as drug (prolonged intake) — see Table of Drugs and Chemicals, vitamins, adverse effect
    overdose or wrong substance given or taken — see Table of Drugs and Chemicals, vitamins, poisoning
  B6 E67.2
  D E67.3
    administered as drug (prolonged intake) — see Table of Drugs and Chemicals, vitamins, adverse effect
    overdose or wrong substance given or taken — see Table of Drugs and Chemicals, vitamins, poisoning
  K E67.8
    administered as drug (prolonged intake) — see Table of Drugs and Chemicals, vitamins, adverse effect
    overdose or wrong substance given or taken — see Table of Drugs and Chemicals, vitamins, poisoning
Hypervolemia E87.70
  specified NEC E87.79
Hypesthesia R20.1
  cornea — see Anesthesia, cornea

☑ **Additional Character Required** — Refer to the Tabular List for Character Selection   ⬇ **Subterms under main terms may continue to next column or page**

Hyphema H21.0- ☑
  traumatic S05.1- ☑
Hypoacidity, gastric K31.89
  psychogenic F45.8
Hypoadrenalism, hypoadrenia E27.40
  primary E27.1
  tuberculous A18.7
Hypoadrenocorticism E27.40
  pituitary E23.0
  primary E27.1
Hypoalbuminemia E88.09
Hypoaldosteronism E27.40
Hypoalphalipoproteinemia E78.6
Hypobarism T70.29 ☑
Hypobaropathy T70.29 ☑
Hypobetalipoproteinemia (familial) E78.6
Hypocalcemia E83.51
  dietary E58
  neonatal P71.1
    due to cow's milk P71.0
  phosphate-loading (newborn) P71.1
Hypochloremia E87.8
Hypochlorhydria K31.89
  neurotic F45.8
  psychogenic F45.8
Hypochondria, hypochondriac, hypochondriasis
  (reaction) F45.21
  sleep F51.03
Hypochondrogenesis Q77.0
Hypochondroplasia Q77.4
Hypochromasia, blood cells D50.8
Hypodontia — see Anodontia
Hypoeeosinophilia D72.89
Hypoesthesia R20.1
Hypofibrinogenemia D68.8
  acquired D65
  congenital (hereditary) D68.2
Hypofunction
  adrenocortical E27.40
    drug-induced E27.3
    postprocedural E89.6
    primary E27.1
  adrenomedullary, postprocedural E89.6
  cerebral R29.818
  corticoadrenal NEC E27.40
  intestinal K59.8
  labyrinth — see subcategory H83.2 ☑
  ovary E28.39
  pituitary (gland) (anterior) E23.0
  testicular E29.1
    postprocedural (postsurgical) (postirradiation) (ia-
      trogenic) E89.5
Hypogalactia O92.4
Hypogammaglobulinemia (see also Agammaglobulinemia) D80.1
  hereditary D80.0
  nonfamilial D80.1
  transient, of infancy D80.7
Hypogenitalism (congenital) — see Hypogonadism
Hypoglossia Q38.3
Hypoglycemia (spontaneous) E16.2
  coma E15
    diabetic — see Diabetes, by type, with hypo-
      glycemia, with coma
  diabetic — see Diabetes, hypoglycemia
  dietary counseling and surveillance Z71.3
  drug-induced E16.0
    with coma (nondiabetic) E15
  due to insulin E16.0
    with coma (nondiabetic) E15
    therapeutic misadventure — see subcategory
      T38.3 ☑
  functional, nonhyperinsulinemic E16.1
  iatrogenic E16.0
    with coma (nondiabetic) E15
  in infant of diabetic mother P70.1
    gestational diabetes P70.0
  infantile E16.1
  leucine-induced E71.19
  neonatal (transitory) P70.4
    iatrogenic P70.3
  reactive (not drug-induced) E16.1
  transitory neonatal P70.4
Hypogonadism
  female E28.39
  hypogonadotropic E23.0
  male E29.1
  ovarian (primary) E28.39

Hypogonadism — continued
  pituitary E23.0
  testicular (primary) E29.1
Hypohidrosis, hypoidrosis L74.4
Hypoinsulinemia, postprocedural E89.1
Hypokalemia E87.6
Hypoleukocytosis — see Agranulocytosis
Hypolipoproteinemia (alpha) (beta) E78.6
Hypomagnesemia E83.42
  neonatal P71.2
Hypomania, hypomanic reaction F30.8
Hypomenorrhea — see Oligomenorrhea
Hypometabolism R63.8
Hypomotility
  gastrointestinal (tract) K31.89
    psychogenic F45.8
  intestine K59.8
    psychogenic F45.8
  stomach K31.89
    psychogenic F45.8
Hyponasality R49.22
Hyponatremia E87.1
Hypo-osmolality E87.1
Hypo-ovarianism, hypo-ovarism E28.39
Hypoparathyroidism E20.9
  familial E20.8
  idiopathic E20.0
  neonatal, transitory P71.4
  postprocedural E89.2
  specified NEC E20.8
Hypoperfusion (in)
  newborn P96.89
Hypopharyngitis — see Laryngopharyngitis
Hypophoria H50.53
Hypophosphatemia, hypophosphatasia (acquired)
  (congenital) (renal) E83.39
  familial E83.31
Hypophyseal, hypophysis (see also condition)
  dwarfism E23.0
  gigantism E22.0
Hypopiesis — see Hypotension
Hypopinealism E34.8
Hypopituitarism (juvenile) E23.0
  drug-induced E23.1
  due to
    hypophysectomy E89.3
    radiotherapy E89.3
  iatrogenic NEC E23.1
  postirradiation E89.3
  postpartum O99.285
  postprocedural E89.3
Hypoplasia, hypoplastic
  adrenal (gland), congenital Q89.1
  alimentary tract, congenital Q45.8
    upper Q40.8
  anus, anal (canal) Q42.3
    with fistula Q42.2
  aorta, aortic Q25.42
    ascending, in hypoplastic left heart syndrome
      Q23.4
    valve Q23.1
      in hypoplastic left heart syndrome Q23.4
  areola, congenital Q83.8
  arm (congenital) — see Defect, reduction, upper limb
  artery (peripheral) Q27.8
    brain (congenital) Q28.3
    coronary Q24.5
    digestive system Q27.8
    lower limb Q27.8
    pulmonary Q25.79
      functional, unilateral J43.0
    retinal (congenital) Q14.1
    specified site NEC Q27.8
    umbilical Q27.0
    upper limb Q27.8
  auditory canal Q17.8
    causing impairment of hearing Q16.9
  biliary duct or passage Q44.5
  bone NOS Q79.9
    face Q75.8
    marrow D61.9
      megakaryocytic D69.49
    skull — see Hypoplasia, skull
  brain Q02
    gyri Q04.3
    part of Q04.3
  breast (areola) N64.82
  bronchus Q32.4

Hypoplasia, hypoplastic — continued
  cardiac Q24.8
  carpus — see Defect, reduction, upper limb, specified
    type NEC
  cartilage hair Q78.8
  cecum Q42.8
  cementum K00.4
  cephalic Q02
  cerebellum Q04.3
  cervix (uteri), congenital Q51.821
  clavicle (congenital) Q74.0
  coccyx Q76.49
  colon Q42.9
    specified NEC Q42.8
  corpus callosum Q04.0
  cricoid cartilage Q31.2
  digestive organ(s) or tract NEC Q45.8
    upper (congenital) Q40.8
  ear (auricle) (lobe) Q17.2
    middle Q16.4
  enamel of teeth (neonatal) (postnatal) (prenatal) K00.4
  endocrine (gland) NEC Q89.2
  endometrium N85.8
  epididymis (congenital) Q55.4
  epiglottis Q31.2
  erythroid, congenital D61.01
  esophagus (congenital) Q39.8
  eustachian tube Q17.8
  eye Q11.2
  eyelid (congenital) Q10.3
  face Q18.8
    bone(s) Q75.8
  femur (congenital) — see Defect, reduction, lower
    limb, specified type NEC
  fibula (congenital) — see Defect, reduction, lower
    limb, specified type NEC
  finger (congenital) — see Defect, reduction, upper
    limb, specified type NEC
  focal dermal Q82.8
  foot — see Defect, reduction, lower limb, specified
    type NEC
  gallbladder Q44.0
  genitalia, genital organ(s)
    female, congenital Q52.8
      external Q52.79
      internal NEC Q52.8
    in adiposogenital dystrophy E23.6
  glottis Q31.2
  hair Q84.2
  hand (congenital) — see Defect, reduction, upper limb,
    specified type NEC
  heart Q24.8
  humerus (congenital) — see Defect, reduction, upper
    limb, specified type NEC
  intestine (small) Q41.9
    large Q42.9
      specified NEC Q42.8
  jaw M26.09
    alveolar M26.79
      lower M26.04
        alveolar M26.74
      upper M26.02
        alveolar M26.73
  kidney(s) Q60.5
    bilateral Q60.4
    unilateral Q60.3
  labium (majus) (minus), congenital Q52.79
  larynx Q31.2
  left heart syndrome Q23.4
  leg (congenital) — see Defect, reduction, lower limb
  limb Q73.8
    lower (congenital) — see Defect, reduction, lower
      limb
    upper (congenital) — see Defect, reduction, upper
      limb
  liver Q44.7
  lung (lobe) (not associated with short gestation) Q33.6
    associated with immaturity, low birth weight, pre-
      maturity, or short gestation P28.0
  mammary (areola), congenital Q83.8
  mandible, mandibular M26.04
    alveolar M26.74
    unilateral condylar M27.8
  maxillary M26.02
    alveolar M26.73
  medullary D61.9
  megakaryocytic D69.49

Hypoplasia, hypoplastic — *continued*
  metacarpus — *see* Defect, reduction, upper limb, specified type NEC
  metatarsus — *see* Defect, reduction, lower limb, specified type NEC
  muscle Q79.8
  nail(s) Q84.6
  nose, nasal Q30.1
  optic nerve H47.03- ☑
  osseous meatus (ear) Q17.8
  ovary, congenital Q50.39
  pancreas Q45.0
  parathyroid (gland) Q89.2
  parotid gland Q38.4
  patella Q74.1
  pelvis, pelvic girdle Q74.2
  penis (congenital) Q55.62
  peripheral vascular system Q27.8
    digestive system Q27.8
    lower limb Q27.8
    specified site NEC Q27.8
    upper limb Q27.8
  pituitary (gland) (congenital) Q89.2
  pulmonary (not associated with short gestation) Q33.6
    artery, functional J43.0
    associated with short gestation P28.0
  radioulnar — *see* Defect, reduction, upper limb, specified type NEC
  radius — *see* Defect, reduction, upper limb
  rectum Q42.1
    with fistula Q42.0
  respiratory system NEC Q34.8
  rib Q76.6
  right heart syndrome Q22.6
  sacrum Q76.49
  scapula Q74.0
  scrotum Q55.1
  shoulder girdle Q74.0
  skin Q82.8
  skull (bone) Q75.8
    with
      anencephaly Q00.0
      encephalocele — *see* Encephalocele
      hydrocephalus Q03.9
        with spina bifida — *see* Spina bifida, by site, with hydrocephalus
      microcephaly Q02
  spinal (cord) (ventral horn cell) Q06.1
  spine Q76.49
  sternum Q76.7
  tarsus — *see* Defect, reduction, lower limb, specified type NEC
  testis Q55.1
  thymic, with immunodeficiency D82.1
  thymus (gland) Q89.2
    with immunodeficiency D82.1
  thyroid (gland) E03.1
    cartilage Q31.2
  tibiofibular (congenital) — *see* Defect, reduction, lower limb, specified type NEC
  toe — *see* Defect, reduction, lower limb, specified type NEC
  tongue Q38.3
  Turner's K00.4
  ulna (congenital) — *see* Defect, reduction, upper limb
  umbilical artery Q27.0
  unilateral condylar M27.8
  ureter Q62.8
  uterus, congenital Q51.811
  vagina Q52.4
  vascular NEC peripheral Q27.8
    brain Q28.3
    digestive system Q27.8
    lower limb Q27.8
    specified site NEC Q27.8
    upper limb Q27.8
  vein(s) (peripheral) Q27.8
    brain Q28.3
    digestive system Q27.8
    great Q26.8
    lower limb Q27.8
    specified site NEC Q27.8
    upper limb Q27.8
  vena cava (inferior) (superior) Q26.8
  vertebra Q76.49
  vulva, congenital Q52.79
  zonule (ciliary) Q12.8
Hypopnea, obstructive sleep apnea G47.33

Hypopotassemia E87.6
Hypoproconvertinemia, congenital (hereditary) D68.2
Hypoproteinemia E77.8
Hypoprothrombinemia (congenital) (hereditary) (idiopathic) D68.2
  acquired D68.4
  newborn, transient P61.6
Hypoptyalism K11.7
Hypopyon (eye) (anterior chamber) — *see* Iridocyclitis, acute, hypopyon
Hypopyrexia R68.0
Hyporeflexia R29.2
Hyposecretion
  ACTH E23.0
  antidiuretic hormone E23.2
  ovary E28.39
  salivary gland (any) K11.7
  vasopressin E23.2
Hyposegmentation, leukocytic, hereditary D72.0
Hyposiderinemia D50.9
Hypospadias Q54.9
  balanic Q54.0
  coronal Q54.0
  glandular Q54.0
  penile Q54.1
  penoscrotal Q54.2
  perineal Q54.3
  specified NEC Q54.8
Hypospermatogenesis — *see* Oligospermia
Hyposplenism D73.0
Hypostasis pulmonary, passive — *see* Edema, lung
Hypostatic — *see* condition
Hyposthenuria N28.89
Hypotension (arterial) (constitutional) I95.9
  chronic I95.89
  drug-induced I95.2
  due to (of) hemodialysis I95.3
  iatrogenic I95.89
  idiopathic (permanent) I95.0
  intracranial, following ventricular shunting (ventriculostomy) G97.2
  intra-dialytic I95.3
  maternal, syndrome (following labor and delivery) O26.5- ☑
  neurogenic, orthostatic G90.3
  orthostatic (chronic) I95.1
    due to drugs I95.2
    neurogenic G90.3
  postoperative I95.81
  postural I95.1
  specified NEC I95.89
Hypothermia (accidental) T68 ☑
  due to anesthesia, anesthetic T88.51 ☑
  low environmental temperature T68 ☑
  neonatal P80.9
    environmental (mild) NEC P80.8
    mild P80.8
    severe (chronic) (cold injury syndrome) P80.0
    specified NEC P80.8
  not associated with low environmental temperature R68.0
Hypothyroidism (acquired) E03.9
  autoimmune — *see* Thyroiditis, autoimmune
  congenital (without goiter) E03.1
    with goiter (diffuse) E03.0
  due to
    exogenous substance NEC E03.2
    iodine-deficiency, acquired E01.8
      subclinical E02
    irradiation therapy E89.0
    medicament NEC E03.2
    P-aminosalicylic acid (PAS) E03.2
    phenylbutazone E03.2
    resorcinol E03.2
    sulfonamide E03.2
    surgery E89.0
    thiourea group drugs E03.2
  iatrogenic NEC E03.2
  iodine-deficiency (acquired) E01.8
    congenital — *see* Syndrome, iodine- deficiency, congenital
    subclinical E02
  neonatal, transitory P72.2
  postinfectious E03.3
  postirradiation E89.0
  postprocedural E89.0
  postsurgical E89.0
  specified NEC E03.8

Hypothyroidism — *continued*
  subclinical, iodine-deficiency related E02
Hypotonia, hypotonicity, hypotony
  bladder N31.2
  congenital (benign) P94.2
  eye — *see* Disorder, globe, hypotony
Hypotrichosis — *see* Alopecia
Hypotropia H50.2- ☑
Hypoventilation R06.89
  congenital central alveolar G47.35
  sleep related
    idiopathic nonobstructive alveolar G47.34
    in conditions classified elsewhere G47.36
Hypovitaminosis — *see* Deficiency, vitamin
Hypovolemia E86.1
  surgical shock T81.19 ☑
  traumatic (shock) T79.4 ☑
Hypoxemia R09.02
  newborn P84
  sleep related, in conditions classified elsewhere G47.36
Hypoxia (*see also* Anoxia) R09.02
  cerebral, during a procedure NEC G97.81
    postprocedural NEC G97.82
  intrauterine P84
  myocardial — *see* Insufficiency, coronary
  newborn P84
  sleep-related G47.34
Hypsarhythmia — *see* Epilepsy, generalized, specified NEC
Hysteralgia, pregnant uterus O26.89- ☑
Hysteria, hysterical (conversion) (dissociative state) F44.9
  anxiety F41.8
  convulsions F44.5
  psychosis, acute F44.9
Hysteroepilepsy F44.5

I

IBDU (colonic inflammatory bowel dissease unclassified) K52.3
Ichthyoparasitism due to Vandellia cirrhosa B88.8
Ichthyosis (congenital) Q80.9
  acquired L85.0
  fetalis Q80.4
  hystrix Q80.8
  lamellar Q80.2
  lingual K13.29
  palmaris and plantaris Q82.8
  simplex Q80.0
  vera Q80.8
  vulgaris Q80.0
  X-linked Q80.1
Ichthyotoxism — *see* Poisoning, fish
  bacterial — *see* Intoxication, foodborne
Icteroanemia, hemolytic (acquired) D59.9
  congenital — *see* Spherocytosis
Icterus (*see also* Jaundice)
  conjunctiva R17
  gravis, newborn P55.0
  hematogenous (acquired) D59.9
  hemolytic (acquired) D59.9
    congenital — *see* Spherocytosis
  hemorrhagic (acute) (leptospiral) (spirochetal) A27.0
    newborn P53
  infectious B15.9
    with hepatic coma B15.0
    leptospiral A27.0
    spirochetal A27.0
  neonatorum — *see* Jaundice, newborn
  newborn P59.9
  spirochetal A27.0
Ictus solaris, solis T67.0 ☑
Id reaction (due to bacteria) L30.2
Ideation
  homicidal R45.850
  suicidal R45.851
Identity disorder (child) F64.9
  gender role F64.2
  psychosexual F64.2
Idioglossia F80.0
Idiopathic — *see* condition
Idiot, idiocy (congenital) F73
  amaurotic (Bielschowsky(-Jansky)) (family) (infantile (late)) (juvenile (late)) (Vogt-Spielmeyer) E75.4
  microcephalic Q02
IgE asthma J45.909

☑ Additional Character Required — Refer to the Tabular List for Character Selection   ☜ Subterms under main terms may continue to next column or page

IIAC (idiopathic infantile arterial calcification) Q28.8
Ileitis (chronic) (noninfectious) (see also Enteritis) K52.9
 backwash — see Pancolitis, ulcerative (chronic)
 infectious A09
 regional (ulcerative) — see Enteritis, regional, small
  intestine
 segmental — see Enteritis, regional
 terminal (ulcerative) — see Enteritis, regional, small
  intestine
Ileocolitis (see also Enteritis) K52.9
 infectious A09
 regional — see Enteritis, regional
 ulcerative K51.0- ☑
Ileostomy
 attention to Z43.2
 malfunctioning K94.13
 status Z93.2
  with complication — see Complications, enterostomy
Ileotyphus — see Typhoid
Ileum — see condition
Ileus (bowel) (colon) (inhibitory) (intestine) K56.7
 adynamic K56.0
 due to gallstone (in intestine) K56.3
 duodenal (chronic) K31.5
 gallstone K56.3
 mechanical NEC (see also Obstruction, intestine, specified NEC) K56.699
 meconium P76.0
  in cystic fibrosis E84.11
  meaning meconium plug (without cystic fibrosis) P76.0
 myxedema K59.8
 neurogenic K56.0
  Hirschsprung's disease or megacolon Q43.1
 newborn
  due to meconium P76.0
   in cystic fibrosis E84.11
   meaning meconium plug (without cystic fibrosis) P76.0
  transitory P76.1
 obstructive (see also Obstruction, intestine, specified NEC) K56.699
 paralytic K56.0
 postoperative K91.89
Iliac — see condition
Iliotibial band syndrome M76.3- ☑
Illiteracy Z55.0
Illness (see also Disease) R69
 manic-depressive — see Disorder, bipolar
Imbalance R26.89
 autonomic G90.8
 constituents of food intake E63.1
 electrolyte E87.8
  with
   abortion — see Abortion by type, complicated by, electrolyte imbalance
   molar pregnancy O08.5
  due to hyperemesis gravidarum O21.1
  following ectopic or molar pregnancy O08.5
  neonatal, transitory NEC P74.4
   potassium P74.3
   sodium P74.2
 endocrine E34.9
 eye muscle NOS H50.9
 hormone E34.9
 hysterical F44.4
 labyrinth — see subcategory H83.2 ☑
 posture R29.3
 protein-energy — see Malnutrition
 sympathetic G90.8
Imbecile, imbecility (I.Q. 35-49) F71
Imbedding, intrauterine device T83.39 ☑
Imbibition, cholesterol (gallbladder) K82.4
Imbrication, teeth,, fully erupted M26.30
Imerslund (-Gräsbeck) **syndrome** D51.1
Immature (see also Immaturity)
 birth (less than 37 completed weeks) — see Preterm, newborn
  extremely (less than 28 completed weeks) — see Immaturity, extreme
 personality F60.89
Immaturity (less than 37 completed weeks) (see also Preterm, newborn)
 extreme of newborn (less than 28 completed weeks of gestation) (less than 196 completed days of gestation) (unspecified weeks of gestation) P07.20

Immaturity — continued
 extreme of newborn — continued
  gestational age
   less than 23 completed weeks P07.21
   23 completed weeks (23 weeks, 0 days through 23 weeks, 6 days) P07.22
   24 completed weeks (24 weeks, 0 days through 24 weeks, 6 days) P07.23
   25 completed weeks (25 weeks, 0 days through 25 weeks, 6 days) P07.24
   26 completed weeks (26 weeks, 0 days through 26 weeks, 6 days) P07.25
   27 completed weeks (27 weeks, 0 days through 27 weeks, 6 days) P07.26
 fetus or infant light-for-dates — see Light-for-dates
 lung, newborn P28.0
 organ or site NEC — see Hypoplasia
 pulmonary, newborn P28.0
 reaction F60.89
 sexual (female) (male), after puberty E30.0
Immersion T75.1 ☑
 foot T69.02- ☑
 hand T69.01- ☑
Immobile, immobility
 complete, due to severe physical disability or frailty R53.2
 intestine K59.8
 syndrome (paraplegic) M62.3
Immune reconstitution (inflammatory) syndrome [IRIS] D89.3
Immunization (see also Vaccination)
 ABO — see Incompatibility, ABO
  in newborn P55.1
 complication — see Complications, vaccination
 encounter for Z23
 not done (not carried out) Z28.9
  because of (of)
   acute illness of patient Z28.01
   allergy to vaccine (or component) Z28.04
   caregiver refusal Z28.82
   chronic illness of patient Z28.02
   contraindication NEC Z28.09
   group pressure Z28.1
   guardian refusal Z28.82
   immune compromised state of patient Z28.03
   parent refusal Z28.82
   patient had disease being vaccinated against Z28.81
   patient refusal Z28.21
   patient's belief Z28.1
   religious beliefs of patient Z28.1
   specified reason NEC Z28.89
    of patient Z28.29
   unspecified patient reason Z28.20
 Rh factor
  affecting management of pregnancy NEC O36.09- ☑
   anti-D antibody O36.01- ☑
  from transfusion — see Complication(s), transfusion, incompatibility reaction, Rh (factor)
Immunocytoma C83.0- ☑
Immunodeficiency D84.9
 with
  adenosine-deaminase deficiency D81.3
  antibody defects D80.9
   specified type NEC D80.8
  hyperimmunoglobulinemia D80.6
  increased immunoglobulin M (IgM) D80.5
  major defect D82.9
   specified type NEC D82.8
  partial albinism D82.8
  short-limbed stature D82.2
  thrombocytopenia and eczema D82.0
 antibody with
  hyperimmunoglobulinemia D80.6
  near-normal immunoglobulins D80.6
 autosomal recessive, Swiss type D80.0
 combined D81.9
  biotin-dependent carboxylase D81.819
   biotinidase D81.810
   holocarboxylase synthetase D81.818
   specified type NEC D81.818
  severe (SCID) D81.9
   with
    low or normal B-cell numbers D81.2
    low T- and B-cell numbers D81.1
    reticular dysgenesis D81.0
  specified type NEC D81.89

Immunodeficiency — continued
 common variable D83.9
  with
   abnormalities of B-cell numbers and function D83.0
   autoantibodies to B- or T-cells D83.2
   immunoregulatory T-cell disorders D83.1
   specified type NEC D83.8
 following hereditary defective response to Epstein-Barr virus (EBV) D82.3
 selective, immunoglobulin
  A (IgA) D80.2
  G (IgG) (subclasses) D80.3
  M (IgM) D80.4
 severe combined (SCID) D81.9
 specified type NEC D84.8
 X-linked, with increased IgM D80.5
Immunotherapy (encounter for)
 antineoplastic Z51.12
Impaction, impacted
 bowel, colon, rectum (see also Impaction, fecal) K56.49
  by gallstone K56.3
 calculus — see Calculus
 cerumen (ear) (external) H61.2- ☑
 cuspid — see Impaction, tooth
 dental (same or adjacent tooth) K01.1
 fecal, feces K56.41
 fracture — see Fracture, by site
 gallbladder — see Calculus, gallbladder
 gallstone(s) — see Calculus, gallbladder
  bile duct (common) (hepatic) — see Calculus, bile duct
  cystic duct — see Calculus, gallbladder
  in intestine, with obstruction (any part) K56.3
 intestine (calculous) NEC (see also Impaction, fecal) K56.49
  gallstone, with ileus K56.3
 intrauterine device (IUD) T83.39 ☑
 molar — see Impaction, tooth
 shoulder, causing obstructed labor O66.0
 tooth, teeth K01.1
 turbinate J34.89
Impaired, impairment (function)
 auditory discrimination — see Abnormal, auditory perception
 cognitive, mild, so stated G31.84
 dual sensory Z73.82
 fasting glucose R73.01
 glucose tolerance (oral) R73.02
 hearing — see Deafness
 heart — see Disease, heart
 kidney N28.9
  disorder resulting from N25.9
   specified NEC N25.89
 liver K72.90
  with coma K72.91
 mastication K08.89
 mild cognitive, so stated G31.84
 mobility
  ear ossicles — see Ankylosis, ear ossicles
  requiring care provider Z74.09
 myocardium, myocardial — see Insufficiency, myocardial
 rectal sphincter R19.8
 renal (acute) (chronic) N28.9
  disorder resulting from N25.9
   specified NEC N25.89
 vision NEC H54.7
  both eyes H54.3
Impediment, speech R47.9
 psychogenic (childhood) F98.8
 slurring R47.81
 specified NEC R47.89
Impending
 coronary syndrome I20.0
 delirium tremens F10.239
 myocardial infarction I20.0
Imperception auditory (acquired) (see also Deafness)
 congenital H93.25
Imperfect
 aeration, lung (newborn) NEC — see Atelectasis
 closure (congenital)
  alimentary tract NEC Q45.8
   lower Q43.8
   upper Q40.8
  atrioventricular ostium Q21.2
  atrium (secundum) Q21.1
  branchial cleft NOS Q18.2

Index

Imperfect — Inclusion

Imperfect — continued
  closure — continued
    branchial cleft — continued
        cyst Q18.0
        fistula Q18.0
        sinus Q18.0
      choroid Q14.3
      cricoid cartilage Q31.8
      cusps, heart valve NEC Q24.8
        pulmonary Q22.3
      ductus
        arteriosus Q25.0
        Botalli Q25.0
      ear drum (causing impairment of hearing) Q16.4
      esophagus with communication to bronchus or
          trachea Q39.1
      eyelid Q10.3
      foramen
        botalli Q21.1
        ovale Q21.1
      genitalia, genital organ(s) or system
        female Q52.8
          external Q52.79
          internal NEC Q52.8
        male Q55.8
      glottis Q31.8
      interatrial ostium or septum Q21.1
      interauricular ostium or septum Q21.1
      interventricular ostium or septum Q21.0
      larynx Q31.8
      lip — see Cleft, lip
      nasal septum Q30.3
      nose Q30.2
      omphalomesenteric duct Q43.0
      optic nerve entry Q14.2
      organ or site not listed — see Anomaly, by site
      ostium
        interatrial Q21.1
        interauricular Q21.1
        interventricular Q21.0
      palate — see Cleft, palate
      preauricular sinus Q18.1
      retina Q14.1
      roof of orbit Q75.8
      sclera Q13.5
      septum
        aorticopulmonary Q21.4
        atrial (secundum) Q21.1
        between aorta and pulmonary artery Q21.4
        heart Q21.9
        interatrial (secundum) Q21.1
        interauricular (secundum) Q21.1
        interventricular Q21.0
          in tetralogy of Fallot Q21.3
        nasal Q30.3
        ventricular Q21.0
          with pulmonary stenosis or atresia, dextra-
              position of aorta, and hypertrophy of
              right ventricle Q21.3
          in tetralogy of Fallot Q21.3
      skull Q75.0
        with
          anencephaly Q00.0
          encephalocele — see Encephalocele
          hydrocephalus Q03.9
            with spina bifida — see Spina bifida, by
                site, with hydrocephalus
          microcephaly Q02
      spine (with meningocele) — see Spina bifida
      trachea Q32.1
      tympanic membrane (causing impairment of
          hearing) Q16.4
      uterus Q51.818
      vitelline duct Q43.0
    erection — see Dysfunction, sexual, male, erectile
    fusion — see Imperfect, closure
    inflation, lung (newborn) — see Atelectasis
    posture R29.3
    rotation, intestine Q43.3
    septum, ventricular Q21.0
Imperfectly descended testis — see Cryptorchid
Imperforate (congenital) (see also Atresia)
  anus Q42.3
    with fistula Q42.2
  cervix (uteri) Q51.828
  esophagus Q39.0
    with tracheoesophageal fistula Q39.1
  hymen Q52.3

Imperforate — continued
  jejunum Q41.1
  pharynx Q38.8
  rectum Q42.1
    with fistula Q42.0
  urethra Q64.39
  vagina Q52.4
Impervious (congenital) (see also Atresia)
  anus Q42.3
    with fistula Q42.2
  bile duct Q44.2
  esophagus Q39.0
    with tracheoesophageal fistula Q39.1
  intestine (small) Q41.9
    large Q42.9
      specified NEC Q42.8
  rectum Q42.1
    with fistula Q42.0
  ureter — see Atresia, ureter
  urethra Q64.39
Impetiginization of dermatoses L01.1
Impetigo (any organism) (any site) (circinate) (conta-
    giosa) (simplex) (vulgaris) L01.00
  Bockhart's L01.02
  bullous, bullosa L01.03
  external ear L01.00 [H62.40]
  follicularis L01.02
  furfuracea L30.5
  herpetiformis L40.1
    nonobstetrical L40.1
  neonatorum L01.03
  nonbullous L01.01
  specified type NEC L01.09
  ulcerative L01.09
Impingement (on teeth)
  soft tissue
    anterior M26.81
    posterior M26.82
Implant, endometrial N80.9
Implantation
  anomalous — see Anomaly, by site
    ureter Q62.63
  cyst
    external area or site (skin) NEC L72.0
    iris — see Cyst, iris, implantation
    vagina N89.8
    vulva N90.7
  dermoid (cyst) — see Implantation, cyst
Impotence (sexual) N52.9
  counseling Z70.1
  organic origin (see also Dysfunction, sexual, male,
    erectile) N52.9
  psychogenic F52.21
Impression, basilar Q75.8
Imprisonment, anxiety concerning Z65.1
Improper care (child) (newborn) — see Maltreatment
Improperly tied umbilical cord (causing hemorrhage)
  P51.8
Impulsiveness (impulsive) R45.87
Inability to swallow — see Aphagia
Inaccessible, inaccessibility
  health care NEC Z75.3
    due to
      waiting period Z75.2
        for admission to facility elsewhere Z75.1
  other helping agencies Z75.4
Inactive — see condition
Inadequate, inadequacy
  aesthetics of dental restoration K08.56
  biologic, constitutional, functional, or social F60.7
  development
    child R62.50
    genitalia
      after puberty NEC E30.0
      congenital
        female Q52.8
          external Q52.79
          internal Q52.8
        male Q55.8
    lungs Q33.6
      associated with short gestation P28.0
    organ or site not listed — see Anomaly, by site
  diet (causing nutritional deficiency) E63.9
  eating habits Z72.4
  environment, household Z59.1
  family support Z63.8
  food (supply) NEC Z59.4
    hunger effects T73.0 ☑

Inadequate, inadequacy — continued
  functional F60.7
  household care, due to
    family member
      handicapped or ill Z74.2
        on vacation Z75.5
      temporarily away from home Z74.2
    technical defects in home Z59.1
    temporary absence from home of person rendering
        care Z74.2
  housing (heating) (space) Z59.1
  income (financial) Z59.6
  intrafamilial communication Z63.8
  material resources Z59.9
  mental — see Disability, intellectual
  parental supervision or control of child Z62.0
  personality F60.7
  pulmonary
    function R06.89
      newborn P28.5
    ventilation, newborn P28.5
  sample of cytologic smear
    anus R85.615
    cervix R87.615
    vagina R87.625
  social F60.7
    insurance Z59.7
    skills NEC Z73.4
  supervision of child by parent Z62.0
  teaching affecting education Z55.8
  welfare support Z59.7
Inanition R64
  with edema — see Malnutrition, severe
  due to
    deprivation of food T73.0 ☑
    malnutrition — see Malnutrition
  fever R50.9
Inappropriate
  change in quantitative human chorionic gonadotropin
      (hCG) in early pregnancy O02.81
  diet or eating habits Z72.4
  level of quantitative human chorionic gonadotropin
      (hCG) for gestational age in early pregnancy
      O02.81
  secretion
    antidiuretic hormone (ADH) (excessive) E22.2
      deficiency E23.2
    pituitary (posterior) E22.2
Inattention at or after birth — see Neglect
Incarceration, incarcerated
  enterocele K46.0
    gangrenous K46.1
  epiplocele K46.0
    gangrenous K46.1
  exomphalos K42.0
    gangrenous K42.1
  hernia (see also Hernia, by site, with obstruction)
    with gangrene — see Hernia, by site, with gan-
        grene
  iris, in wound — see Injury, eye, laceration, with pro-
      lapse
  lens, in wound — see Injury, eye, laceration, with
      prolapse
  omphalocele K42.0
  prison, anxiety concerning Z65.1
  rupture — see Hernia, by site
  sarcoepiplocele K46.0
    gangrenous K46.1
  sarcoepiplomphalocele K42.0
    with gangrene K42.1
  uterus N85.8
    gravid O34.51- ☑
      causing obstructed labor O65.5
Incised wound
  external — see Laceration
  internal organs — see Injury, by site
Incision, incisional
  hernia K43.2
    with
      gangrene (and obstruction) K43.1
      obstruction K43.0
  surgical, complication — see Complications, surgical
      procedure
  traumatic
    external — see Laceration
    internal organs — see Injury, by site
Inclusion
  azurophilic leukocytic D72.0

☑ Additional Character Required — Refer to the Tabular List for Character Selection   Subterms under main terms may continue to next column or page

Inclusion — *continued*
  blennorrhea (neonatal) (newborn) P39.1
  gallbladder in liver (congenital) Q44.1
Incompatibility
  ABO
    affecting management of pregnancy O36.11- ☑
      anti-A sensitization O36.11- ☑
      anti-B sensitization O36.19- ☑
      specified NEC O36.19- ☑
    infusion or transfusion reaction — *see* Complica-
        tion(s), transfusion, incompatibility reaction,
        ABO
    newborn P55.1
  blood (group) (Duffy) (K(ell)) (Kidd) (Lewis) (M) (S) NEC
    affecting management of pregnancy O36.11- ☑
      anti-A sensitization O36.11- ☑
      anti-B sensitization O36.19- ☑
    infusion or transfusion reaction T80.89 ☑
    newborn P55.8
  divorce or estrangement Z63.5
  Rh (blood group) (factor) Z31.82
    affecting management of pregnancy NEC
      O36.09- ☑
      anti-D antibody O36.01- ☑
    infusion or transfusion reaction — *see* Complica-
        tion(s), transfusion, incompatibility reaction,
        Rh (factor)
    newborn P55.0
  rhesus — *see* Incompatibility, Rh
Incompetency, incompetent, incompetence
  annular
    aortic (valve) — *see* Insufficiency, aortic
    mitral (valve) I34.0
    pulmonary valve (heart) I37.1
  aortic (valve) — *see* Insufficiency, aortic
  cardiac valve — *see* Endocarditis
  cervix, cervical (os) N88.3
    in pregnancy O34.3- ☑
  chronotropic I45.89
    with
      autonomic dysfunction G90.8
      ischemic heart disease I25.89
      left ventricular dysfunction I51.89
      sinus node dysfunction I49.8
  esophagogastric (junction) (sphincter) K22.0
  mitral (valve) — *see* Insufficiency, mitral
  pelvic fundus N81.89
  pubocervical tissue N81.82
  pulmonary valve (heart) I37.1
    congenital Q22.3
  rectovaginal tissue N81.83
  tricuspid (annular) (valve) — *see* Insufficiency, tricuspid
  valvular — *see* Endocarditis
    congenital Q24.8
  vein, venous (saphenous) (varicose) — *see* Varix, leg
Incomplete (*see also* condition)
  bladder, emptying R33.9
  defecation R15.0
  expansion lungs (newborn) NEC — *see* Atelectasis
  rotation, intestine Q43.3
Inconclusive
  diagnostic imaging due to excess body fat of patient
    R93.9
  findings on diagnostic imaging of breast NEC R92.8
  mammogram (due to dense breasts) R92.2
Incontinence R32
  anal sphincter R15.9
  coital N39.491
  feces R15.9
    nonorganic origin F98.1
  insensible (urinary) N39.42
  overflow N39.490
  postural (urinary) N39.492
  psychogenic F45.8
  rectal R15.9
  reflex N39.498
  stress (female) (male) N39.3
    and urge N39.46
  urethral sphincter R32
  urge N39.41
    and stress (female) (male) N39.46
  urine (urinary) R32
    continuous N39.45
    due to cognitive impairment, or severe physical
      disability or immobility R39.81
    functional R39.81
    insensible N39.42
    mixed (stress and urge) N39.46

Incontinence — *continued*
  urine — *continued*
    nocturnal N39.44
    nonorganic origin F98.0
    overflow N39.490
    post dribbling N39.43
    postural N39.492
    reflex N39.498
    specified NEC N39.498
    stress (female) (male) N39.3
      and urge N39.46
    total N39.498
    unaware N39.42
    urge N39.41
      and stress (female) (male) N39.46
Incontinentia pigmenti Q82.3
Incoordinate, incoordination
  esophageal-pharyngeal (newborn) — *see* Dysphagia
  muscular R27.8
  uterus (action) (contractions) (complicating delivery)
    O62.4
Increase, increased
  abnormal, in development R63.8
  androgens (ovarian) E28.1
  anticoagulants (antithrombin) (anti-VIIIa) (anti-IXa)
    (anti-Xa) (anti-XIa) — *see* Circulating anticoagu-
    lants
  cold sense R20.8
  estrogen E28.0
  function
    adrenal
      cortex — *see* Cushing's, syndrome
      medulla E27.5
    pituitary (gland) (anterior) (lobe) E22.9
      posterior E22.2
  heat sense R20.8
  intracranial pressure (benign) G93.2
  permeability, capillaries I78.8
  pressure, intracranial G93.2
  secretion
    gastrin E16.4
    glucagon E16.3
    pancreas, endocrine E16.9
      growth hormone-releasing hormone E16.8
      pancreatic polypeptide E16.8
      somatostatin E16.8
      vasoactive-intestinal polypeptide E16.8
  sphericity, lens Q12.4
  splenic activity D73.1
  venous pressure I87.8
    portal K76.6
Increta placenta O43.22- ☑
Incrustation, cornea, foreign body (lead)(zinc) — *see*
  Foreign body, cornea
Incyclophoria H50.54
Incyclotropia — *see* Cyclotropia
Indeterminate sex Q56.4
India rubber skin Q82.8
Indigestion (acid) (bilious) (functional) K30
  catarrhal K31.89
  due to decomposed food NOS A05.9
  nervous F45.8
  psychogenic F45.8
Indirect — *see* condition
Induratio penis plastica N48.6
Induration, indurated
  brain G93.89
  breast (fibrous) N64.51
    puerperal, postpartum O92.29
  broad ligament N83.8
  chancre
    anus A51.1
    congenital A50.07
    extragenital NEC A51.2
  corpora cavernosa (penis) (plastic) N48.6
  liver (chronic) K76.89
  lung (black) (chronic) (fibroid) (*see also* Fibrosis, lung)
    J84.10
    essential brown J84.03
  penile (plastic) N48.6
  phlebitic — *see* Phlebitis
  skin R23.4
Inebriety (without dependence) — *see* Alcohol, intoxication
Inefficiency, kidney N28.9
Inelasticity, skin R23.4
Inequality, leg (length) (acquired) (*see also* Deformity,
  limb, unequal length)
  congenital — *see* Defect, reduction, lower limb

Inequality, leg — *continued*
  lower leg — *see* Deformity, limb, unequal
    length
Inertia
  bladder (neurogenic) N31.2
  stomach K31.89
    psychogenic F45.8
  uterus, uterine during labor O62.2
    during latent phase of labor O62.0
    primary O62.0
    secondary O62.1
  vesical (neurogenic) N31.2
Infancy, infantile, infantilism (*see also* condition)
  celiac K90.0
  genitalia, genitals (after puberty) E30.0
  Herter's (nontropical sprue) K90.0
  intestinal K90.0
  Lorain E23.0
  pancreatic K86.89
  pelvis M95.5
    with disproportion (fetopelvic) O33.1
      causing obstructed labor O65.1
  pituitary E23.0
  renal N25.0
  uterus — *see* Infantile, genitalia
Infant(s) (*see also* Infancy)
  excessive crying R68.11
  irritable child R68.12
  lack of care — *see* Neglect
  liveborn (singleton) Z38.2
    born in hospital Z38.00
      by cesarean Z38.01
    born outside hospital Z38.1
    multiple NEC Z38.8
      born in hospital Z38.68
        by cesarean Z38.69
      born outside hospital Z38.7
    quadruplet Z38.8
      born in hospital Z38.63
        by cesarean Z38.64
      born outside hospital Z38.7
    quintuplet Z38.8
      born in hospital Z38.65
        by cesarean Z38.66
      born outside hospital Z38.7
    triplet Z38.8
      born in hospital Z38.61
        by cesarean Z38.62
      born outside hospital Z38.7
    twin Z38.5
      born in hospital Z38.30
        by cesarean Z38.31
      born outside hospital Z38.4
  of diabetic mother (syndrome of) P70.1
    gestational diabetes P70.0
Infantile (*see also* condition)
  genitalia, genitals E30.0
  os, uterine E30.0
  penis E30.0
  testis E29.1
  uterus E30.0
Infantilism — *see* Infancy
Infarct, infarction
  adrenal (capsule) (gland) E27.49
  appendices epiploicae (*see also* Infarct, intestine)
    K55.069
  bowel (*see also* Infarct, intestine) K55.069
  brain (stem) — *see* Infarct, cerebral
  breast N64.89
  brewer's (kidney) N28.0
  cardiac — *see* Infarct, myocardium
  cerebellar — *see* Infarct, cerebral
  cerebral (*see also* Occlusion, artery cerebral or precere-
    bral, with infarction) I63.9
    aborted I63.9
    cortical I63.9
    due to
      cerebral venous thrombosis, nonpyogenic I63.6
      embolism
        cerebral arteries I63.4- ☑
        precerebral arteries I63.1- ☑
      occlusion NEC
        cerebral arteries I63.5- ☑
        precerebral arteries I63.2- ☑
      stenosis NEC
        cerebral arteries I63.5- ☑
        precerebral arteries I63.2- ☑

Index *(side tab)*

Infarct, infarction — Index — Infection, infected, infective *(side tab)*

Infarct, infarction — *continued*
  cerebral (*see also* Occlusion, artery cerebral or precerebral, with infarction) — *continued*
    due to — *continued*
      thrombosis
        cerebral artery I63.3- ☑
        precerebral artery I63.0- ☑
      intraoperative
        during cardiac surgery I97.810
        during other surgery I97.811
      postprocedural
        following cardiac surgery I97.820
        following other surgery I97.821
      specified NEC I63.8
  colon (acute) (agnogenic) (embolic) (hemorrhagic) (nonocclusive) (nonthrombotic) (occlusive) (segmental) (thrombotic) (with gangrene) (*see also* Infarct, intestine) K55.049
  coronary artery — *see* Infarct, myocardium
  embolic — *see* Embolism
  fallopian tube N83.8
  gallbladder K82.8
  heart — *see* Infarct, myocardium
  hepatic K76.3
  hypophysis (anterior lobe) E23.6
  impending (myocardium) I20.0
  intestine (acute) (agnogenic) (embolic) (hemorrhagic) (nonocclusive) (nonthrombotic) (occlusive) (thrombotic) (with gangrene) K55.069
    diffuse K55.062
    focal K55.061
    large K55.049
      diffuse K55.042
      focal K55.041
    small K55.029
      diffuse K55.022
      focal K55.021
  kidney N28.0
  liver K76.3
  lung (embolic) (thrombotic) — *see* Embolism, pulmonary
  lymph node I89.8
  mesentery, mesenteric (embolic) (thrombotic) (with gangrene) (*see also* Infarct, intestine) K55.069
  muscle (ischemic) M62.20
    ankle M62.27- ☑
    foot M62.27- ☑
    forearm M62.23- ☑
    hand M62.24- ☑
    lower leg M62.26- ☑
    pelvic region M62.25- ☑
    shoulder region M62.21- ☑
    specified site NEC M62.28
    thigh M62.25- ☑
    upper arm M62.22- ☑
  myocardium, myocardial (acute) (with stated duration of 4 weeks or less) I21.9
    associated with revascularization procedure I21.A9
    diagnosed on ECG, but presenting no symptoms I25.2
    due to
      demand ischemia I21.A1
      ischemic imbalance I21.A1
    healed or old I25.2
    intraoperative (*see also* Infarct, myocardium, associated with revascularization procedure)
      during cardiac surgery I97.790
      during other surgery I97.791
    non-Q wave I21.4
    non-ST elevation (NSTEMI) I21.4
      subsequent I22.2
    nontransmural I21.4
    past (diagnosed on ECG or other investigation, but currently presenting no symptoms) I25.2
    postprocedural (*see also* Infarct, myocardium, associated with revascularization procedure)
      following cardiac surgery (*see also* Infarct, myocardium, type 4 or type 5) I97.190
      following other surgery I97.191
    Q wave (see also, Infarct, myocardium, by site) I21.3
    secondary to
      demand ischemia I21.A1
      ischemic imbalance I21.A1
    ST elevation (STEMI) I21.3
      anterior (anteroapical) (anterolateral) (anteroseptal) (Q wave) (wall) I21.09
        subsequent I22.0

Infarct, infarction — *continued*
  myocardium, myocardial — *continued*
    ST elevation — *continued*
      inferior (diaphragmatic) (inferolateral) (inferoposterior) (wall) NEC I21.19
        subsequent I22.1
      inferoposterior transmural (Q wave) I21.11
      involving
        coronary artery of anterior wall NEC I21.09
        coronary artery of inferior wall NEC I21.19
        diagonal coronary artery I21.02
        left anterior descending coronary artery I21.02
        left circumflex coronary artery I21.21
        left main coronary artery I21.01
        oblique marginal coronary artery I21.21
        right coronary artery I21.11
      lateral (apical-lateral) (basal-lateral) (high) I21.29
        subsequent I22.8
      posterior (posterobasal) (posterolateral) (posteroseptal) (true) I21.29
        subsequent I22.8
      septal I21.29
        subsequent I22.8
      specified NEC I21.29
        subsequent I22.8
      subsequent I22.9
    subsequent (recurrent) (reinfarction) I22.9
      anterior (anteroapical) (anterolateral) (anteroseptal) (wall) I22.0
      diaphragmatic (wall) I22.1
      inferior (diaphragmatic) (inferolateral) (inferoposterior) (wall) I22.1
      lateral (apical-lateral) (basal-lateral) (high) I22.8
      non-ST elevation (NSTEMI) I22.2
      posterior (posterobasal) (posterolateral) (posteroseptal) (true) I22.8
      septal I22.8
      specified NEC I22.8
      ST elevation I22.9
        anterior (anteroapical) (anterolateral) (anteroseptal) (wall) I22.0
        inferior (diaphragmatic) (inferolateral) (inferoposterior) (wall) I22.1
        specified NEC I22.8
      subendocardial I22.2
      transmural I22.9
        anterior (anteroapical) (anterolateral) (anteroseptal) (wall) I22.0
        diaphragmatic (wall) I22.1
        inferior (diaphragmatic) (inferolateral) (inferoposterior) (wall) I22.1
        lateral (apical-lateral) (basal-lateral) (high) I22.8
        posterior (posterobasal) (posterolateral) (posteroseptal) (true) I22.8
        specified NEC I22.8
      type 1 (*see also* Infarction, myocardial, subsequent, by site, or by ST elevation or non-ST elevation) I22.9
      type 2 I21.A1
      type 3 I21.A9
      type 4 I21.A9
      type 5 I21.A9
    syphilitic A52.06
    transmural I21.9
      anterior (anteroapical) (anterolateral) (anteroseptal) (Q wave) (wall) NEC I21.09
      inferior (diaphragmatic) (inferolateral) (inferoposterior) (Q wave) (wall) NEC I21.19
      inferoposterior (Q wave) I21.11
      lateral (apical-lateral) (basal-lateral) (high) NEC I21.29
      posterior (posterobasal) (posterolateral) (posteroseptal) (true) NEC I21.29
      septal NEC I21.29
      specified NEC I21.29
    type 1 (*see also* Infarction, myocardial, by site, or by ST elevation or non-ST elevation) I21.9
    type 2 I21.A1
    type 3 I21.A9
    type 4 (a) (b) (c) I21.A9
    type 5 I21.A9
  nontransmural I21.4
  omentum (*see also* Infarct, intestine) K55.069
  ovary N83.8
  pancreas K86.89
  papillary muscle — *see* Infarct, myocardium

Infarct, infarction — *continued*
  parathyroid gland E21.4
  pituitary (gland) E23.6
  placenta O43.81- ☑
  prostate N42.89
  pulmonary (artery) (vein) (hemorrhagic) — *see* Embolism, pulmonary
  renal (embolic) (thrombotic) N28.0
  retina, retinal (artery) — *see* Occlusion, artery, retina
  spinal (cord) (acute) (embolic) (nonembolic) G95.11
  spleen D73.5
    embolic or thrombotic I74.8
  subendocardial (acute) (nontransmural) I21.4
  suprarenal (capsule) (gland) E27.49
  testis N50.1
  thrombotic (*see also* Thrombosis)
    artery, arterial — *see* Embolism
  thyroid (gland) E07.89
  ventricle (heart) — *see* Infarct, myocardium
Infecting — *see* condition
Infection, infected, infective (opportunistic) B99.9
  with
    drug resistant organism — *see* Resistance (to), drug (*see also* specific organism)
    lymphangitis — *see* Lymphangitis
    organ dysfunction (acute) R65.20
      with septic shock R65.21
  abscess (skin) — *code by* site under Abscess
  Absidia — *see* Mucormycosis
  Acanthamoeba — *see* Acanthamebiasis
  Acanthocheilonema (perstans) (streptocerca) B74.4
  accessory sinus (chronic) — *see* Sinusitis
  achorion — *see* Dermatophytosis
  Acremonium falciforme B47.0
  acromioclavicular M00.9
  Actinobacillus (actinomycetem-comitans) A28.8
    mallei A24.0
    muris A25.1
  Actinomadura B47.1
  Actinomyces (israelii) (*see also* Actinomycosis) A42.9
  Actinomycetales — *see* Actinomycosis
  actinomycotic NOS — *see* Actinomycosis
  adenoid (and tonsil) J03.90
    chronic J35.02
  adenovirus NEC
    as cause of disease classified elsewhere B97.0
    unspecified nature or site B34.0
  aerogenes capsulatus A48.0
  aertrycke — *see* Infection, salmonella
  alimentary canal NOS — *see* Enteritis, infectious
  Allescheria boydii B48.2
  Alternaria B48.8
  alveolus, alveolar (process) K04.7
  Ameba, amebic (histolytica) — *see* Amebiasis
  amniotic fluid, sac or cavity O41.10- ☑
    chorioamnionitis O41.12- ☑
    placentitis O41.14- ☑
  amputation stump (surgical) — *see* Complication, amputation stump, infection
  Ancylostoma (duodenalis) B76.0
  Anisakiasis, Anisakis larvae B81.0
  anthrax — *see* Anthrax
  antrum (chronic) — *see* Sinusitis, maxillary
  anus, anal (papillae) (sphincter) K62.89
  arbovirus (arbor virus) A94
    specified type NEC A93.8
  artificial insemination N98.0
  Ascaris lumbricoides — *see* Ascariasis
  Ascomycetes B47.0
  Aspergillus (flavus) (fumigatus) (terreus) — *see* Aspergillosis
  atypical
    acid-fast (bacilli) — *see* Mycobacterium, atypical
    mycobacteria — *see* Mycobacterium, atypical
    virus A81.9
      specified type NEC A81.89
  auditory meatus (external) — *see* Otitis, externa, infective
  auricle (ear) — *see* Otitis, externa, infective
  axillary gland (lymph) L04.2
  Bacillus A49.9
    abortus A23.1
    anthracis — *see* Anthrax
    Ducrey's (any location) A57
    Flexner's A03.1
    Friedländer's NEC A49.8
    gas (gangrene) A48.0
    mallei A24.0

☑ Additional Character Required — Refer to the Tabular List for Character Selection   ▽ Subterms under main terms may continue to next column or page

Infection, infected, infective — *continued*
  Bacillus — *continued*
    melitensis A23.0
    paratyphoid, paratyphosus A01.4
      A A01.1
      B A01.2
      C A01.3
    Shiga (-Kruse) A03.0
    suipestifer — *see* Infection, salmonella
    swimming pool A31.1
    typhosa A01.00
    welchii — *see* Gangrene, gas
  bacterial NOS A49.9
    as cause of disease classified elsewhere B96.89
      Bacteroides fragilis [B. fragilis] B96.6
      Clostridium perfringens [C. perfringens] B96.7
      Enterobacter sakazakii B96.89
      Enterococcus B95.2
      Escherichia coli [E. coli] (*see also* Escherichia coli) B96.20
      Helicobacter pylori [H.pylori] B96.81
      Hemophilus influenzae [H. influenzae] B96.3
      Klebsiella pneumoniae [K. pneumoniae] B96.1
      Mycoplasma pneumoniae [M. pneumoniae] B96.0
      Proteus (mirabilis) (morganii) B96.4
      Pseudomonas (aeruginosa) (mallei) (pseudomallei) B96.5
      Staphylococcus B95.8
        aureus (methicillin susceptible) (MSSA) B95.61
          methicillin resistant (MRSA) B95.62
        specified NEC B95.7
      Streptococcus B95.5
        group A B95.0
        group B B95.1
        pneumoniae B95.3
        specified NEC B95.4
      Vibrio vulnificus B96.82
    specified NEC A48.8
  Bacterium
    paratyphosum A01.4
      A A01.1
      B A01.2
      C A01.3
    typhosum A01.00
  Bacteroides NEC A49.8
    fragilis, as cause of disease classified elsewhere B96.6
  Balantidium coli A07.0
  Bartholin's gland N75.8
  Basidiobolus B46.8
  bile duct (common) (hepatic) — *see* Cholangitis
  bladder — *see* Cystitis
  Blastomyces, blastomycotic (*see also* Blastomycosis)
    brasiliensis — *see* Paracoccidioidomycosis
    dermatitidis — *see* Blastomycosis
    European — *see* Cryptococcosis
    Loboi B48.0
    North American B40.9
    South American — *see* Paracoccidioidomycosis
  bleb, postprocedure — *see* Blebitis
  bone — *see* Osteomyelitis
  Bordetella — *see* Whooping cough
  Borrelia bergdorfi A69.20
  brain (*see also* Encephalitis) G04.90
    membranes — *see* Meningitis
    septic G06.0
      meninges — *see* Meningitis, bacterial
  branchial cyst Q18.0
  breast — *see* Mastitis
  bronchus — *see* Bronchitis
  Brucella A23.9
    abortus A23.1
    canis A23.3
    melitensis A23.0
    mixed A23.8
    specified NEC A23.8
    suis A23.2
  Brugia (malayi) B74.1
    timori B74.2
  bursa — *see* Bursitis, infective
  buttocks (skin) L08.9
  Campylobacter, intestinal A04.5
    as cause of disease classified elsewhere B96.81
  Candida (albicans) (tropicalis) — *see* Candidiasis
  candiru B88.8
  Capillaria (intestinal) B81.1

Infection, infected, infective — *continued*
  Capillaria — *continued*
    hepatica B83.8
    philippinensis B81.1
  cartilage — *see* Disorder, cartilage, specified type NEC
  cat liver fluke B66.0
  catheter-related bloodstream (CRBSI) T80.211 ☑
  cellulitis — *code by* site under Cellulitis
  central line-associated T80.219 ☑
    bloodstream (CLABSI) T80.211 ☑
    specified NEC T80.218 ☑
  Cephalosporium falciforme B47.0
  cerebrospinal — *see* Meningitis
  cervical gland (lymph) L04.0
  cervix — *see* Cervicitis
  cesarean delivery wound (puerperal) O86.0
  cestodes — *see* Infestation, cestodes
  chest J22
  Chilomastix (intestinal) A07.8
  Chlamydia, chlamydial A74.9
    anus A56.3
    genitourinary tract A56.2
      lower A56.00
      specified NEC A56.19
    lymphogranuloma A55
    pharynx A56.4
    psittaci A70
    rectum A56.3
    sexually transmitted NEC A56.8
  cholera — *see* Cholera
  Cladosporium
    bantianum (brain abscess) B43.1
    carrionii B43.0
    castellanii B36.1
    trichoides (brain abscess) B43.1
    werneckii B36.1
  Clonorchis (sinensis) (liver) B66.1
  Clostridium NEC
    bifermentans A48.0
    botulinum (food poisoning) A05.1
      infant A48.51
      wound A48.52
    difficile
      as cause of disease classified elsewhere B96.89
      foodborne (disease)
        not specified as recurrent A04.72
        recurrent A04.71
      gas gangrene A48.0
      necrotizing enterocolitis
        not specified as recurrent A04.72
        recurrent A04.71
      sepsis A41.4
    gas-forming NEC A48.0
    histolyticum A48.0
    novyi, causing gas gangrene A48.0
    oedematiens A48.0
    perfringens
      as cause of disease classified elsewhere B96.7
      due to food A05.2
      foodborne (disease) A05.2
      gas gangrene A48.0
      sepsis A41.4
    septicum, causing gas gangrene A48.0
    sordellii, causing gas gangrene A48.0
    welchii
      as cause of disease classified elsewhere B96.7
      foodborne (disease) A05.2
      gas gangrene A48.0
      necrotizing enteritis A05.2
      sepsis A41.4
  Coccidioides (immitis) — *see* Coccidioidomycosis
  colon — *see* Enteritis, infectious
  colostomy K94.02
  common duct — *see* Cholangitis
  congenital P39.9
    Candida (albicans) P37.5
    cytomegalovirus P35.1
    hepatitis, viral P35.3
    herpes simplex P35.2
    infectious or parasitic disease P37.9
      specified NEC P37.8
    listeriosis (disseminated) P37.2
    malaria NEC P37.4
      falciparum P37.3
    Plasmodium falciparum P37.3
    poliomyelitis P35.8
    rubella P35.0
    skin P39.4

Infection, infected, infective — *continued*
  congenital — *continued*
    toxoplasmosis (acute) (subacute) (chronic) P37.1
    tuberculosis P37.0
    urinary (tract) P39.3
    vaccinia P35.8
    virus P35.9
      specified type NEC P35.8
  Conidiobolus B46.8
  coronavirus NEC B34.2
    as cause of disease classified elsewhere B97.29
    severe acute respiratory syndrome (SARS associated) B97.21
  corpus luteum — *see* Salpingo-oophoritis
  Corynebacterium diphtheriae — *see* Diphtheria
  cotia virus B08.8
  Coxiella burnetii A78
  coxsackie — *see* Coxsackie
  Cryptococcus neoformans — *see* Cryptococcosis
  Cryptosporidium A07.2
  Cunninghamella — *see* Mucormycosis
  cyst — *see* Cyst
  cystic duct (*see also* Cholecystitis) K81.9
  Cysticercus cellulosae — *see* Cysticercosis
  cytomegalovirus, cytomegaloviral B25.9
    congenital P35.1
    maternal, maternal care for (suspected) damage to fetus O35.3 ☑
    mononucleosis B27.10
      with
        complication NEC B27.19
        meningitis B27.12
        polyneuropathy B27.11
  delta-agent (acute), in hepatitis B carrier B17.0
  dental (pulpal origin) K04.7
  Deuteromycetes B47.0
  Dicrocoelium dendriticum B66.2
  Dipetalonema (perstans) (streptocerca) B74.4
  diphtherial — *see* Diphtheria
  Diphyllobothrium (adult) (latum) (pacificum) B70.0
    larval B70.1
  Diplogonoporus (grandis) B71.8
  Dipylidium caninum B67.4
  Dirofilaria B74.8
  Dracunculus medinensis B72
  Drechslera (hawaiiensis) B43.8
  Ducrey Haemophilus (any location) A57
  due to or resulting from
    artificial insemination N98.0
    central venous catheter T80.219 ☑
      bloodstream T80.211 ☑
      exit or insertion site T80.212 ☑
      localized T80.212 ☑
      port or reservoir T80.212 ☑
      specified NEC T80.218 ☑
      tunnel T80.212 ☑
    device, implant or graft (*see also* Complications, by site and type, infection or inflammation) T85.79 ☑
      arterial graft NEC T82.7 ☑
      breast (implant) T85.79 ☑
      catheter NEC T85.79 ☑
        dialysis (renal) T82.7 ☑
          intraperitoneal T85.71 ☑
        infusion NEC T82.7 ☑
          cranial T85.735 ☑
          intrathecal T85.735 ☑
          spinal (epidural) (subdural) T85.735 ☑
          subarachnoid T85.735 ☑
        urinary T83.518 ☑
          cystostomy T83.510 ☑
          Hopkins T83.518 ☑
          ileostomy T83.518 ☑
          nephrostomy T83.512 ☑
          specified NEC T83.518 ☑
          urethral indwelling T83.511 ☑
          urostomy T83.518 ☑
      electronic (electrode) (pulse generator) (stimulator)
        bone T84.7 ☑
        cardiac T82.7 ☑
        nervous system T85.738 ☑
          brain T85.738 ☑
          cranial nerve T85.732 ☑
          gastric nerve T85.732 ☑
          generator pocket T85.734 ☑
          neurostimulator generator T85.734 ☑

⬛ Subterms under main terms may continue to next column or page   ☑ Additional Character Required — Refer to the Tabular List for Character Selection   183

Infection, infected, infective — Infection, infected, infective

Infection, infected, infective — *continued*
- due to or resulting from — *continued*
  - device, implant or graft (*see also* Complications, by site, infection or inflammation) — *continued*
    - electronic — *continued*
      - nervous system — *continued*
        - peripheral nerve T85.732 ☑
        - sacral nerve T85.732 ☑
        - spinal cord T85.733 ☑
        - vagal nerve T85.732 ☑
      - urinary (indwelling) T83.51 ☑
    - fixation, internal (orthopedic) NEC — *see* Complication, fixation device, infection
    - gastrointestinal (bile duct) (esophagus) T85.79 ☑
      - neurostimulator electrode (lead) T85.732 ☑
    - genital NEC T83.69 ☑
    - heart NEC T82.7 ☑
      - valve (prosthesis) T82.6 ☑
        - graft T82.7 ☑
    - joint prosthesis — *see* Complication, joint prosthesis, infection
    - ocular (corneal graft) (orbital implant) NEC T85.79 ☑
    - orthopedic NEC T84.7 ☑
    - penile (cylinder) (pump) (resevoir) T83.61 ☑
    - specified NEC T85.79 ☑
    - testicular T83.62 ☑
    - urinary NEC T83.598 ☑
      - ileal conduit stent T83.593 ☑
      - implanted neurostimulation T83.590 ☑
      - implanted sphincter T83.591 ☑
      - indwelling ureteral stent T83.592 ☑
      - nephroureteral stent T83.593 ☑
      - specified stent NEC T83.593 ☑
    - vascular NEC T82.7 ☑
    - ventricular intracranial (communicating) shunt T85.730 ☑
  - Hickman catheter T80.219 ☑
    - bloodstream T80.211 ☑
    - localized T80.212 ☑
    - specified NEC T80.218 ☑
  - immunization or vaccination T88.0 ☑
  - infusion, injection or transfusion NEC T80.29 ☑
  - injury NEC — *code by* site under Wound, open
  - peripherally inserted central catheter (PICC) T80.219 ☑
    - bloodstream T80.211 ☑
    - localized T80.212 ☑
    - specified NEC T80.218 ☑
  - portacath (port-a-cath) T80.219 ☑
    - bloodstream T80.211 ☑
    - localized T80.212 ☑
    - specified NEC T80.218 ☑
  - pulmonary artery catheter — *see* Infection, due to or resulting from, central venous catheter
  - surgery T81.4 ☑
  - Swan Ganz catheter — *see* Infection, due to or resulting from, central venous catheter
  - triple lumen catheter T80.219 ☑
    - bloodstream T80.211 ☑
    - localized T80.212 ☑
    - specified NEC T80.218 ☑
  - umbilical venous catheter T80.219 ☑
    - bloodstream T80.211 ☑
    - localized T80.212 ☑
    - specified NEC T80.218 ☑
- during labor NEC O75.3
- ear (middle) (*see also* Otitis media)
  - external — *see* Otitis, externa, infective
  - inner — *see* subcategory H83.0 ☑
- Eberthella typhosa A01.00
- Echinococcus — *see* Echinococcus
- echovirus
  - as cause of disease classified elsewhere B97.12
  - unspecified nature or site B34.1
- endocardium I33.0
- endocervix — *see* Cervicitis
- Entamoeba — *see* Amebiasis
- enteric — *see* Enteritis, infectious
- Enterobacter sakazakii B96.89
- Enterobius vermicularis B80
- enterostomy K94.12
- enterovirus B34.1
  - as cause of disease classified elsewhere B97.10

enterovirus — *continued*
- as cause of disease classified elsewhere — *continued*
  - coxsackievirus B97.11
  - echovirus B97.12
  - specified NEC B97.19
- Entomophthora B46.8
- Epidermophyton — *see* Dermatophytosis
- epididymis — *see* Epididymitis
- episiotomy (puerperal) O86.0
- Erysipelothrix (insidiosa) (rhusiopathiae) — *see* Erysipeloid
- erythema infectiosum B08.3
- Escherichia (E.) coli NEC A49.8
  - as cause of disease classified elsewhere (*see also* Escherichia coli) B96.20
  - congenital P39.8
    - sepsis P36.4
  - generalized A41.51
  - intestinal — *see* Enteritis, infectious, due to, Escherichia coli
- ethmoidal (chronic) (sinus) — *see* Sinusitis, ethmoidal
- eustachian tube (ear) — *see* Salpingitis, eustachian
- external auditory canal (meatus) NEC — *see* Otitis, externa, infective
- eye (purulent) — *see* Endophthalmitis, purulent
- eyelid — *see* Inflammation, eyelid
- fallopian tube — *see* Salpingo-oophoritis
- Fasciola (gigantica) (hepatica) (indica) B66.3
- Fasciolopsis (buski) B66.5
- filarial — *see* Infestation, filarial
- finger (skin) L08.9
  - nail L03.01- ☑
    - fungus B35.1
- fish tapeworm B70.0
  - larval B70.1
- flagellate, intestinal A07.9
- fluke — *see* Infestation, fluke
- focal
  - teeth (pulpal origin) K04.7
  - tonsils J35.01
- Fonsecaea (compactum) (pedrosoi) B43.0
- food — *see* Intoxication, foodborne
- foot (skin) L08.9
  - dermatophytic fungus B35.3
- Francisella tularensis — *see* Tularemia
- frontal (sinus) (chronic) — *see* Sinusitis, frontal
- fungus NOS B49
  - beard B35.0
  - dermatophytic — *see* Dermatophytosis
  - foot B35.3
  - groin B35.6
  - hand B35.2
  - nail B35.1
  - pathogenic to compromised host only B48.8
  - perianal (area) B35.6
  - scalp B35.0
  - skin B36.9
    - foot B35.3
    - hand B35.2
    - toenails B35.1
- Fusarium B48.8
- gallbladder — *see* Cholecystitis
- gas bacillus — *see* Gangrene, gas
- gastrointestinal — *see* Enteritis, infectious
- generalized NEC — *see* Sepsis
- generator pocket, implanted electronic neurostimulator T85.734 ☑
- genital organ or tract
  - female — *see* Disease, pelvis, inflammatory
  - male N49.9
    - multiple sites N49.8
    - specified NEC N49.8
- Ghon tubercle, primary A15.7
- Giardia lamblia A07.1
- gingiva (chronic) K05.10
  - acute K05.00
    - nonplaque induced K05.01
    - plaque induced K05.00
  - nonplaque induced K05.11
  - plaque induced K05.10
- glanders A24.0
- glenosporopsis B48.0
- Gnathostoma (spinigerum) B83.1
- Gongylonema B83.8
- gonococcal — *see* Gonococcus
- gram-negative bacilli NOS A49.9

Infection, infected, infective — *continued*
- guinea worm B72
- gum (chronic) K05.10
  - acute K05.00
    - nonplaque induced K05.01
    - plaque induced K05.00
  - nonplaque induced K05.11
  - plaque induced K05.10
- Haemophilus — *see* Infection, Hemophilus
- heart — *see* Carditis
- Helicobacter pylori A04.8
  - as cause of disease classified elsewhere B96.81
- helminths B83.9
  - intestinal B82.0
    - mixed (types classifiable to more than one of the titles B65.0-B81.3 and B81.8) B81.4
    - specified type NEC B81.8
  - specified type NEC B83.8
- Hemophilus
  - aegyptius, systemic A48.4
  - ducreyi (any location) A57
  - generalized A41.3
  - influenzae NEC A49.2
    - as cause of disease classified elsewhere B96.3
- herpes (simplex) (*see also* Herpes)
  - congenital P35.2
  - disseminated B00.7
  - zoster B02.9
- herpesvirus, herpesviral — *see* Herpes
- Heterophyes (heterophyes) B66.8
- hip (joint) NEC M00.9
  - due to internal joint prosthesis
    - left T84.52 ☑
    - right T84.51 ☑
  - skin NEC L08.9
- Histoplasma — *see* Histoplasmosis
  - American B39.4
  - capsulatum B39.4
- hookworm B76.9
- human
  - papilloma virus A63.0
  - T-cell lymphotropic virus type-1 (HTLV-1) B33.3
- hydrocele N43.0
- Hymenolepis B71.0
- hypopharynx — *see* Pharyngitis
- inguinal (lymph) glands L04.1
  - due to soft chancre A57
- intervertebral disc, pyogenic M46.30
  - cervical region M46.32
  - cervicothoracic region M46.33
  - lumbar region M46.36
  - lumbosacral region M46.37
  - multiple sites M46.39
  - occipito-atlanto-axial region M46.31
  - sacrococcygeal region M46.38
  - thoracic region M46.34
  - thoracolumbar region M46.35
- intestine, intestinal — *see* Enteritis, infectious
  - specified NEC A08.8
- intra-amniotic affecting newborn NEC P39.2
- Isospora belli or hominis A07.3
- Japanese B encephalitis A83.0
- jaw (bone) (lower) (upper) M27.2
- joint NEC M00.9
  - due to internal joint prosthesis T84.50 ☑
- kidney (cortex) (hematogenous) N15.9
  - with calculus N20.0
    - with hydronephrosis N13.6
  - following ectopic gestation O08.83
  - pelvis and ureter (cystic) N28.85
  - puerperal (postpartum) O86.21
  - specified NEC N15.8
- Klebsiella (K.) pneumoniae NEC A49.8
  - as cause of disease classified elsewhere B96.1
- knee (joint) NEC M00.9
  - due to internal joint prosthesis
    - left T84.54 ☑
    - right T84.53 ☑
  - joint M00.9
  - skin L08.9
- Koch's — *see* Tuberculosis
- labia (majora) (minora) (acute) — *see* Vulvitis
- lacrimal
  - gland — *see* Dacryoadenitis
  - passages (duct) (sac) — *see* Inflammation, lacrimal, passages
- lancet fluke B66.2
- larynx NEC J38.7

Infection, infected, infective — continued
leg (skin) NOS L08.9
Legionella pneumophila A48.1
  nonpneumonic A48.2
Leishmania (see also Leishmaniasis)
  aethiopica B55.1
  braziliensis B55.2
  chagasi B55.0
  donovani B55.0
  infantum B55.0
  major B55.1
  mexicana B55.1
  tropica B55.1
lentivirus, as cause of disease classified elsewhere
  B97.31
Leptosphaeria senegalensis B47.0
Leptospira interrogans A27.9
  autumnalis A27.89
  canicola A27.89
  hebdomadis A27.89
  icterohaemorrhagiae A27.0
  pomona A27.89
  specified type NEC A27.89
leptospirochetal NEC — see Leptospirosis
Listeria monocytogenes (see also Listeriosis)
  congenital P37.2
Loa loa B74.3
  with conjunctival infestation B74.3
  eyelid B74.3
Loboa loboi B48.0
local, skin (staphylococcal) (streptococcal) L08.9
  abscess — code by site under Abscess
  cellulitis — code by site under Cellulitis
  specified NEC L08.89
  ulcer — see Ulcer, skin
Loefflerella mallei A24.0
lung (see also Pneumonia) J18.9
  atypical Mycobacterium A31.0
  spirochetal A69.8
  tuberculous — see Tuberculosis, pulmonary
  virus — see Pneumonia, viral
lymph gland (see also Lymphadenitis, acute)
  mesenteric I88.0
lymphoid tissue, base of tongue or posterior pharynx,
  NEC (chronic) J35.03
Madurella (grisea) (mycetomii) B47.0
major
  following ectopic or molar pregnancy O08.0
  puerperal, postpartum, childbirth O85
Malassezia furfur B36.0
Malleomyces
  mallei A24.0
  pseudomallei (whitmori) — see Melioidosis
mammary gland N61.0
Mansonella (ozzardi) (perstans) (streptocerca) B74.4
mastoid — see Mastoiditis
maxilla, maxillary M27.2
  sinus (chronic) — see Sinusitis, maxillary
mediastinum J98.51
Medina (worm) B72
meibomian cyst or gland — see Hordeolum
meninges — see Meningitis, bacterial
meningococcal (see also condition) A39.9
  adrenals A39.1
  brain A39.81
  cerebrospinal A39.0
  conjunctiva A39.89
  endocardium A39.51
  heart A39.50
    endocardium A39.51
    myocardium A39.52
    pericardium A39.53
  joint A39.83
  meninges A39.0
  meningococcemia A39.4
    acute A39.2
    chronic A39.3
  myocardium A39.52
  pericardium A39.53
  retrobulbar neuritis A39.82
  specified site NEC A39.89
mesenteric lymph nodes or glands NEC I88.0
Metagonimus B66.8
metatarsophalangeal M00.9
methicillin
  resistant Staphylococcus aureus (MRSA) A49.02
  susceptible Staphylococcus aureus (MSSA) A49.01
Microsporum, microsporic — see Dermatophytosis

Infection, infected, infective — continued
mixed flora (bacterial) NEC A49.8
Monilia — see Candidiasis
Monosporium apiospermum B48.2
mouth, parasitic B37.0
Mucor — see Mucormycosis
muscle NEC — see Myositis, infective
mycelium NOS B49
mycetoma B47.9
  actinomycotic NEC B47.1
  mycotic NEC B47.0
Mycobacterium, mycobacterial — see Mycobacterium
Mycoplasma NEC A49.3
  pneumoniae, as cause of disease classified else-
    where B96.0
mycotic NOS B49
  pathogenic to compromised host only B48.8
  skin NOS B36.9
myocardium NEC I40.0
nail (chronic)
  with lymphangitis — see Lymphangitis, acute,
    digit
  finger L03.01- ☑
    fungus B35.1
  ingrowing L60.0
  toe L03.03- ☑
    fungus B35.1
nasal sinus (chronic) — see Sinusitis
nasopharynx — see Nasopharyngitis
navel L08.82
Necator americanus B76.1
Neisseria — see Gonococcus
Neotestudina rosatii B47.0
newborn P39.9
  intra-amniotic NEC P39.2
  skin P39.4
  specified type NEC P39.8
nipple N61.0
  associated with
    lactation O91.03
    pregnancy O91.01- ☑
    puerperium O91.02
Nocardia — see Nocardiosis
obstetrical surgical wound (puerperal) O86.0
Oesophagostomum (apiostomum) B81.8
Oestrus ovis — see Myiasis
Oidium albicans B37.9
Onchocerca (volvulus) — see Onchocerciasis
oncovirus, as cause of disease classified elsewhere
  B97.32
operation wound T81.4 ☑
Opisthorchis (felineus) (viverrini) B66.0
orbit, orbital — see Inflammation, orbit
orthopoxvirus NEC B08.09
ovary — see Salpingo-oophoritis
Oxyuris vermicularis B80
pancreas (acute) — see Pancreatitis, acute
  abscess — see Pancreatitis, acute
  specified NEC (see also Pancreatitis, acute) K85.80
papillomavirus, as cause of disease classified elsewhere
  B97.7
papovavirus NEC B34.4
Paracoccidioides brasiliensis — see Paracoccidioidomycosis
Paragonimus (westermani) B66.4
parainfluenza virus B34.8
parameningococcus NOS A39.9
parapoxvirus B08.60
  specified NEC B08.69
parasitic B89
Parastrongylus
  cantonensis B83.2
  costaricensis B81.3
  paratyphoid A01.4
    Type A A01.1
    Type B A01.2
    Type C A01.3
paraurethral ducts N34.2
parotid gland — see Sialoadenitis
parvovirus NEC B34.3
  as cause of disease classified elsewhere B97.6
Pasteurella NEC A28.0
  multocida A28.0
  pestis — see Plague
  pseudotuberculosis A28.0
  septica (cat bite) (dog bite) A28.0
  tularensis — see Tularemia
pelvic, female — see Disease, pelvis, inflammatory

Infection, infected, infective — continued
Penicillium (marneffei) B48.4
penis (glans) (retention) NEC N48.29
periapical K04.5
peridental, periodontal K05.20
  generalized — see Peridontitis, aggressive, gener-
    alized
  localized — see Peridontitis, aggressive, localized
perinatal period P39.9
  specified type NEC P39.8
perineal repair (puerperal) O86.0
periorbital — see Inflammation, orbit
perirectal K62.89
perirenal — see Infection, kidney
peritoneal — see Peritonitis
periureteral N28.89
Petriellidium boydii B48.2
pharynx (see also Pharyngitis)
  coxsackievirus B08.5
  posterior, lymphoid (chronic) J35.03
Phialophora
  gougerotii (subcutaneous abscess or cyst) B43.2
  jeanselmei (subcutaneous abscess or cyst) B43.2
  verrucosa (skin) B43.0
Piedraia hortae B36.3
pinta A67.9
  intermediate A67.1
  late A67.2
  mixed A67.3
  primary A67.0
pinworm B80
pityrosporum furfur B36.0
pleuro-pneumonia-like organism (PPLO) NEC A49.3
  as cause of disease classified elsewhere B96.0
pneumococcus, pneumococcal NEC A49.1
  as cause of disease classified elsewhere B95.3
  generalized (purulent) A40.3
    with pneumonia J13
Pneumocystis carinii (pneumonia) B59
Pneumocystis jiroveci (pneumonia) B59
port or reservoir T80.212 ☑
postoperative T81.4 ☑
postoperative wound T81.4 ☑
postprocedural T81.4 ☑
postvaccinal T88.0 ☑
prepuce NEC N47.7
  with penile inflammation N47.6
prion — see Disease, prion, central nervous system
prostate (capsule) — see Prostatitis
Proteus (mirabilis) (morganii) (vulgaris) NEC A49.8
  as cause of disease classified elsewhere B96.4
protozoal NEC B64
  intestinal A07.9
    specified NEC A07.8
  specified NEC B60.8
Pseudoallescheria boydii B48.2
Pseudomonas NEC A49.8
  as cause of disease classified elsewhere B96.5
  mallei A24.0
  pneumonia J15.1
  pseudomallei — see Melioidosis
puerperal O86.4
  genitourinary tract NEC O86.89
  major or generalized O85
  minor O86.4
  specified NEC O86.89
pulmonary — see Infection, lung
purulent — see Abscess
Pyrenochaeta romeroi B47.0
Q fever A78
rectum (sphincter) K62.89
renal (see also Infection, kidney)
  pelvis and ureter (cystic) N28.85
reovirus, as cause of disease classified elsewhere B97.5
respiratory (tract) NEC J98.8
  acute J22
  chronic J98.8
  influenzal (upper) (acute) — see Influenza, with,
    respiratory manifestations NEC
  lower (acute) J22
    chronic — see Bronchitis, chronic
  rhinovirus J00
  syncytial virus, as cause of disease classified else-
    where B97.4
  upper (acute) NOS J06.9
    chronic J39.8
    streptococcal J06.9
    viral NOS J06.9

Infection, infected, infective — *continued*
resulting from
  presence of internal prosthesis, implant, graft —
      see Complications, by site and type, infection
retortamoniasis A07.8
retroperitoneal NEC K68.9
retrovirus B33.3
  as cause of disease classified elsewhere B97.30
    human
      immunodeficiency, type 2 (HIV 2) B97.35
      T-cell lymphotropic
        type I (HTLV-I) B97.33
        type II (HTLV-II) B97.34
    lentivirus B97.31
    oncovirus B97.32
    specified NEC B97.39
Rhinosporidium (seeberi) B48.1
rhinovirus
  as cause of disease classified elsewhere B97.89
  unspecified nature or site B34.8
Rhizopus — *see* Mucormycosis
rickettsial NOS A79.9
roundworm (large) NEC B82.0
  Ascariasis (*see also* Ascariasis) B77.9
rubella — *see* Rubella
Saccharomyces — *see* Candidiasis
salivary duct or gland (any) — *see* Sialoadenitis
Salmonella (aertrycke) (arizonae) (callinarum)
  (cholerae-suis) (enteritidis) (suipestifer) (typhimurium) A02.9
  with
    (gastro)enteritis A02.0
    sepsis A02.1
    specified manifestation NEC A02.8
  due to food (poisoning) A02.9
  hirschfeldii A01.3
  localized A02.20
    arthritis A02.23
    meningitis A02.21
    osteomyelitis A02.24
    pneumonia A02.22
    pyelonephritis A02.25
    specified NEC A02.29
  paratyphi A01.4
    A A01.1
    B A01.2
    C A01.3
  schottmuelleri A01.2
  typhi, typhosa — *see* Typhoid
Sarcocystis A07.8
scabies B86
Schistosoma — *see* Infestation, Schistosoma
scrotum (acute) NEC N49.2
seminal vesicle — *see* Vesiculitis
septic
  localized, skin — *see* Abscess
sheep liver fluke B66.3
Shigella A03.9
  boydii A03.2
  dysenteriae A03.0
  flexneri A03.1
  group
    A A03.0
    B A03.1
    C A03.2
    D A03.3
  Schmitz (-Stutzer) A03.0
  schmitzii A03.0
  shigae A03.0
  sonnei A03.3
  specified NEC A03.8
shoulder (joint) NEC M00.9
  due to internal joint prosthesis T84.59 ☑
  skin NEC L08.9
sinus (accessory) (chronic) (nasal) (*see also* Sinusitis)
  pilonidal — *see* Sinus, pilonidal
  skin NEC L08.89
Skene's duct or gland — *see* Urethritis
skin (local) (staphylococcal) (streptococcal) L08.9
  abscess — *code by* site under Abscess
  cellulitis — *code by* site under Cellulitis
  due to fungus B36.9
    specified type NEC B36.8
  mycotic B36.9
    specified type NEC B36.8
  newborn P39.4
  ulcer — *see* Ulcer, skin
slow virus A81.9

Infection, infected, infective — *continued*
slow virus — *continued*
  specified NEC A81.89
Sparganum (mansoni) (proliferum) (baxteri) B70.1
specific (*see also* Syphilis)
  to perinatal period — *see* Infection, congenital
specified NEC B99.8
spermatic cord NEC N49.1
sphenoidal (sinus) — *see* Sinusitis, sphenoidal
spinal cord NOS (*see also* Myelitis) G04.91
  abscess G06.1
  meninges — *see* Meningitis
  streptococcal G04.89
Spirillum A25.0
spirochetal NOS A69.9
  lung A69.8
  specified NEC A69.8
Spirometra larvae B70.1
spleen D73.89
Sporotrichum, Sporothrix (schenckii) — *see* Sporotrichosis
staphylococcal, unspecified site
  as cause of disease classified elsewhere B95.8
    aureus (methicillin susceptible) (MSSA) B95.61
      methicillin resistant (MRSA) B95.62
    specified NEC B95.7
  aureus (methicillin susceptible) (MSSA) A49.01
    methicillin resistant (MRSA) A49.02
  food poisoning A05.0
  generalized (purulent) A41.2
  pneumonia — *see* Pneumonia, staphylococcal
Stellantchasmus falcatus B66.8
streptobacillus moniliformis A25.1
streptococcal NEC A49.1
  as cause of disease classified elsewhere B95.5
  B genitourinary complicating
    childbirth O98.82
    pregnancy O98.81- ☑
    puerperium O98.83
  congenital
    sepsis P36.10
      group B P36.0
      specified NEC P36.19
  generalized (purulent) A40.9
Streptomyces B47.1
Strongyloides (stercoralis) — *see* Strongyloidiasis
stump (amputation) (surgical) — *see* Complication,
  amputation stump, infection
subcutaneous tissue, local L08.9
suipestifer — *see* Infection, salmonella
swimming pool bacillus A31.1
Taenia — *see* Infestation, Taenia
Taeniarhynchus saginatus B68.1
tapeworm — *see* Infestation, tapeworm
tendon (sheath) — *see* Tenosynovitis, infective NEC
Ternidens diminutus B81.8
testis — *see* Orchitis
threadworm B80
throat — *see* Pharyngitis
thyroglossal duct K14.8
toe (skin) L08.9
  cellulitis L03.03- ☑
    fungus B35.1
  nail L03.03- ☑
    fungus B35.1
tongue NEC K14.0
  parasitic B37.0
tonsil (and adenoid) (faucial) (lingual) (pharyngeal) —
  see Tonsillitis
tooth, teeth K04.7
  periapical K04.7
  peridental, periodontal K05.20
    generalized — *see* Peridontitis, aggressive,
      generalized
    localized — *see* Peridontitis, aggressive, local-
      ized
  pulp K04.01
    irreversible K04.02
    reversible K04.01
  socket M27.3
TORCH — *see* Infection, congenital
  without active infection P00.2
Torula histolytica — *see* Cryptococcosis
Toxocara (canis) (cati) (felis) B83.0
Toxoplasma gondii — *see* Toxoplasma
trachea, chronic J42
trematode NEC — *see* Infestation, fluke
trench fever A79.0

Infection, infected, infective — *continued*
Treponema pallidum — *see* Syphilis
Trichinella (spiralis) B75
Trichomonas A59.9
  cervix A59.09
  intestine A07.8
  prostate A59.02
  specified site NEC A59.8
  urethra A59.03
  urogenitalis A59.00
  vagina A59.01
  vulva A59.01
Trichophyton, trichophytic — *see* Dermatophytosis
Trichosporon (beigelii) cutaneum B36.2
Trichostrongylus B81.2
Trichuris (trichiura) B79
Trombicula (irritans) B88.0
Trypanosoma
  brucei
    gambiense B56.0
    rhodesiense B56.1
  cruzi — *see* Chagas' disease
tubal — *see* Salpingo-oophoritis
tuberculous NEC — *see* Tuberculosis
tubo-ovarian — *see* Salpingo-oophoritis
tunica vaginalis N49.1
tunnel T80.212 ☑
tympanic membrane NEC — *see* Myringitis
typhoid (abortive) (ambulant) (bacillus) — *see* Typhoid
typhus A75.9
  flea-borne A75.2
  mite-borne A75.3
  recrudescent A75.1
  tick-borne A77.9
    African A77.1
    North Asian A77.2
umbilicus L08.82
ureter N28.86
urethra — *see* Urethritis
urinary (tract) N39.0
  bladder — *see* Cystitis
  complicating
    pregnancy O23.4- ☑
      specified type NEC O23.3- ☑
  kidney — *see* Infection, kidney
  newborn P39.3
  puerperal (postpartum) O86.20
  tuberculous A18.13
  urethra — *see* Urethritis
uterus, uterine — *see* Endometritis
vaccination T88.0 ☑
vaccinia not from vaccination B08.011
vagina (acute) — *see* Vaginitis
varicella B01.9
varicose veins — *see* Varix
vas deferens NEC N49.1
vesical — *see* Cystitis
Vibrio
  cholerae A00.0
    El Tor A00.1
  parahaemolyticus (food poisoning) A05.3
  vulnificus
    as cause of disease classified elsewhere B96.82
    foodborne intoxication A05.5
Vincent's (gum) (mouth) (tonsil) A69.1
virus, viral NOS B34.9
  adenovirus
    as cause of disease classified elsewhere B97.0
    unspecified nature or site B34.0
  arborvirus, arbovirus arthropod-borne A94
  as cause of disease classified elsewhere B97.89
    adenovirus B97.0
    coronavirus B97.29
      SARS-associated B97.21
    coxsackievirus B97.11
    echovirus B97.12
    enterovirus B97.10
      coxsackievirus B97.11
      echovirus B97.12
      specified NEC B97.19
    human
      immunodeficiency, type 2 (HIV 2) B97.35
      metapneumovirus B97.81
      T-cell lymphotropic,
        type I (HTLV-I) B97.33
        type II (HTLV-II) B97.34
    papillomavirus B97.7
    parvovirus B97.6

Infection, infected, infective — *continued*
  virus, viral — *continued*
    as cause of disease classified elsewhere — *continued*
      reovirus B97.5
      respiratory syncytial B97.4
      retrovirus B97.30
        human
          immunodeficiency, type 2 (HIV 2) B97.35
          T-cell lymphotropic,
            type I (HTLV-I) B97.33
            type II (HTLV-II) B97.34
        lentivirus B97.31
        oncovirus B97.32
        specified NEC B97.39
      specified NEC B97.89
    central nervous system A89
      atypical A81.9
        specified NEC A81.89
      enterovirus NEC A88.8
        meningitis A87.0
      slow virus A81.9
        specified NEC A81.89
      specified NEC A88.8
    chest J98.8
    cotia B08.8
    coxsackie (*see also* Infection, coxsackie) B34.1
      as cause of disease classified elsewhere B97.11
    ECHO
      as cause of disease classified elsewhere B97.12
      unspecified nature or site B34.1
    encephalitis, tick-borne A84.9
    enterovirus, as cause of disease classified elsewhere
        B97.10
      coxsackievirus B97.11
      echovirus B97.12
      specified NEC B97.19
    exanthem NOS B09
    human metapneumovirus as cause of disease
        classified elsewhere B97.81
    human papilloma as cause of disease classified
        elsewhere B97.7
    intestine — *see* Enteritis, viral
    respiratory syncytial
      as cause of disease classified elsewhere B97.4
      bronchopneumonia J12.1
      common cold syndrome J00
      nasopharyngitis (acute) J00
    rhinovirus
      as cause of disease classified elsewhere B97.89
      unspecified nature or site B34.8
    slow A81.9
      specified NEC A81.89
    specified type NEC B33.8
      as cause of disease classified elsewhere B97.89
      unspecified nature or site B34.8
    West Nile — *see* Virus, West Nile
  vulva (acute) — *see* Vulvitis
  West Nile — *see* Virus, West Nile
  whipworm B79
  worms B83.9
    specified type NEC B83.8
  Wuchereria (bancrofti) B74.0
    malayi B74.1
  yatapoxvirus B08.70
    specified NEC B08.79
  yeast (*see also* Candidiasis) B37.9
  yellow fever — *see* Fever, yellow
  Yersinia
    enterocolitica (intestinal) A04.6
    pestis — *see* Plague
    pseudotuberculosis A28.2
  Zeis' gland — *see* Hordeolum
  Zika virus A92.5
  zoonotic bacterial NOS A28.9
  Zopfia senegalensis B47.0
Infective, infectious — *see* condition
Infertility
  female N97.9
    age-related N97.8
    associated with
      anovulation N97.0
      cervical (mucus) disease or anomaly N88.3
      congenital anomaly
        cervix N88.3
        fallopian tube N97.1
        uterus N97.2

Infertility — *continued*
  female — *continued*
    associated with — *continued*
      congenital anomaly — *continued*
        vagina N97.8
      dysmucorrhea N88.3
      fallopian tube disease or anomaly N97.1
      pituitary-hypothalamic origin E23.0
      specified origin NEC N97.8
      Stein-Leventhal syndrome E28.2
      uterine disease or anomaly N97.2
      vaginal disease or anomaly N97.8
    due to
      cervical anomaly N88.3
      fallopian tube anomaly N97.1
      ovarian failure E28.39
      Stein-Leventhal syndrome E28.2
      uterine anomaly N97.2
      vaginal anomaly N97.8
    nonimplantation N97.2
    origin
      cervical N88.3
      tubal (block) (occlusion) (stenosis) N97.1
      uterine N97.2
      vaginal N97.8
  male N46.9
    azoospermia N46.01
      extratesticular cause N46.029
        drug therapy N46.021
        efferent duct obstruction N46.023
        infection N46.022
        radiation N46.024
        specified cause NEC N46.029
        systemic disease N46.025
    oligospermia N46.11
      extratesticular cause N46.129
        drug therapy N46.121
        efferent duct obstruction N46.123
        infection N46.122
        radiation N46.124
        specified cause NEC N46.129
        systemic disease N46.125
    specified type NEC N46.8
Infestation B88.9
  Acanthocheilonema (perstans) (streptocerca) B74.4
  Acariasis B88.0
    demodex folliculorum B88.0
    sarcoptes scabiei B86
    trombiculae B88.0
  Agamofilaria streptocerca B74.4
  Ancylostoma, ankylostoma (braziliense) (caninum)
    (ceylanicum) (duodenale) B76.0
    americanum B76.1
    new world B76.1
  Anisakis larvae, anisakiasis B81.0
  arthropod NEC B88.2
  Ascaris lumbricoides — *see* Ascariasis
  Balantidium coli A07.0
  beef tapeworm B68.1
  Bothriocephalus (latus) B70.0
    larval B70.1
  broad tapeworm B70.0
    larval B70.1
  Brugia (malayi) B74.1
    timori B74.2
  candiru B88.8
  Capillaria
    hepatica B83.8
    philippinensis B81.1
  cat liver fluke B66.0
  cestodes B71.9
    diphyllobothrium — *see* Infestation, diphyllobothrium
    dipylidiasis B71.1
    hymenolepiasis B71.0
    specified type NEC B71.8
  chigger B88.0
  chigo, chigoe B88.1
  Clonorchis (sinensis) (liver) B66.1
  coccidial A07.3
  crab-lice B85.3
  Cysticercus cellulosae — *see* Cysticercosis
  Demodex (folliculorum) B88.0
  Dermanyssus gallinae B88.0
  Dermatobia (hominis) — *see* Myiasis
  Dibothriocephalus (latus) B70.0
    larval B70.1
  Dicrocoelium dendriticum B66.2

Infestation — *continued*
  Diphyllobothrium (adult) (latum) (intestinal) (pacificum) B70.0
    larval B70.1
  Diplogonoporus (grandis) B71.8
  Dipylidium caninum B67.4
  Distoma hepaticum B66.3
  dog tapeworm B67.4
  Dracunculus medinensis B72
  dragon worm B72
  dwarf tapeworm B71.0
  Echinococcus — *see* Echinococcus
  Echinostomum ilocanum B66.8
  Entamoeba (histolytica) — *see* Infection, Ameba
  Enterobius vermicularis B80
  eyelid
    in (due to)
      leishmaniasis B55.1
      loiasis B74.3
      onchocerciasis B73.09
      phthiriasis B85.3
      parasitic NOS B89
  eyeworm B74.3
  Fasciola (gigantica) (hepatica) (indica) B66.3
  Fasciolopsis (buski) (intestine) B66.5
  filarial B74.9
    bancroftian B74.0
    conjunctiva B74.9
    due to
      Acanthocheilonema (perstans) (streptocerca)
        B74.4
      Brugia (malayi) B74.1
        timori B74.2
      Dracunculus medinensis B72
      guinea worm B72
      loa loa B74.3
      Mansonella (ozzardi) (perstans) (streptocerca)
        B74.4
      Onchocerca volvulus B73.00
        eye B73.00
        eyelid B73.09
      Wuchereria (bancrofti) B74.0
    Malayan B74.1
    ozzardi B74.4
    specified type NEC B74.8
  fish tapeworm B70.0
    larval B70.1
  fluke B66.9
    blood NOS — *see* Schistosomiasis
    cat liver B66.0
    intestinal B66.5
    lancet B66.2
    liver (sheep) B66.3
      cat B66.0
      Chinese B66.1
      due to clonorchiasis B66.1
      oriental B66.1
    lung (oriental) B66.4
    sheep liver B66.3
    specified type NEC B66.8
  fly larvae — *see* Myiasis
  Gasterophilus (intestinalis) — *see* Myiasis
  Gastrodiscoides hominis B66.8
  Giardia lamblia A07.1
  Gnathostoma (spinigerum) B83.1
  Gongylonema B83.8
  guinea worm B72
  helminth B83.9
    angiostrongyliasis B83.2
      intestinal B81.3
    gnathostomiasis B83.1
    hirudiniasis, internal B83.4
    intestinal B82.0
      angiostrongyliasis B81.3
      anisakiasis B81.0
      ascariasis — *see* Ascariasis
      capillariasis B81.1
      cysticercosis — *see* Cysticercosis
      diphyllobothriasis — *see* Infestation, diphyllobothriasis
      dracunculiasis B72
      echinococcus — *see* Echinococcosis
      enterobiasis B80
      filariasis — *see* Infestation, filarial
      fluke — *see* Infestation, fluke
      hookworm — *see* Infestation, hookworm
      mixed (types classifiable to more than one of
        the titles B65.0-B81.3 and B81.8) B81.4

Infestation — *continued*
- helminth — *continued*
  - intestinal — *continued*
    - onchocerciasis — *see* Onchocerciasis
    - schistosomiasis — *see* Infestation, schistosoma
    - specified
      - cestode NEC — *see* Infestation, cestode
        - type NEC B81.8
      - strongyloidiasis — *see* Strongyloidiasis
      - taenia — *see* Infestation, taenia
      - trichinellosis B75
      - trichostrongyliasis B81.2
      - trichuriasis B79
    - specified type NEC B83.8
    - syngamiasis B83.3
    - visceral larva migrans B83.0
  - Heterophyes (heterophyes) B66.8
  - hookworm B76.9
    - ancylostomiasis B76.0
    - necatoriasis B76.1
    - specified type NEC B76.8
  - Hymenolepis (diminuta) (nana) B71.0
  - intestinal NEC B82.9
  - leeches (aquatic) (land) — *see* Hirudiniasis
  - Leishmania — *see* Leishmaniasis
  - lice, louse — *see* Infestation, Pediculus
  - Linguatula B88.8
  - Liponyssoides sanguineus B88.0
  - Loa loa B74.3
    - conjunctival B74.3
    - eyelid B74.3
  - louse — *see* Infestation, Pediculus
  - maggots — *see* Myiasis
  - Mansonella (ozzardi) (perstans) (streptocerca) B74.4
  - Medina (worm) B72
  - Metagonimus (yokogawai) B66.8
  - microfilaria streptocerca — *see* Onchocerciasis
    - eye B73.00
    - eyelid B73.09
  - mites B88.9
    - scabic B86
  - Monilia (albicans) — *see* Candidiasis
  - mouth B37.0
  - Necator americanus B76.1
  - nematode NEC (intestinal) B82.0
    - Ancylostoma B76.0
    - conjunctiva NEC B83.9
    - Enterobius vermicularis B80
    - Gnathostoma spinigerum B83.1
    - physaloptera B80
    - specified NEC B81.8
    - trichostrongylus B81.2
    - trichuris (trichuria) B79
  - Oesophagostomum (apiostomum) B81.8
  - Oestrus ovis (see also Myiasis) B87.9
  - Onchocerca (volvulus) — *see* Onchocerciasis
  - Opisthorchis (felineus) (viverrini) B66.0
  - orbit, parasitic NOS B89
  - Oxyuris vermicularis B80
  - Paragonimus (westermani) B66.4
  - parasite, parasitic B89
    - eyelid B89
    - intestinal NOS B82.9
    - mouth B37.0
    - skin B88.9
    - tongue B37.0
  - Parastrongylus
    - cantonensis B83.2
    - costaricensis B81.3
  - Pediculus B85.2
    - body B85.1
    - capitis (humanus) (any site) B85.0
    - corporis (humanus) (any site) B85.1
    - head B85.0
    - mixed (classifiable to more than one of the titles B85.0 - B85.3) B85.4
    - pubis (any site) B85.3
  - Pentastoma B88.8
  - Phthirus (pubis) (any site) B85.3
    - with any infestation classifiable to B85.0 - B85.2 B85.4
  - pinworm B80
  - pork tapeworm (adult) B68.0
  - protozoal NEC B64
    - intestinal A07.9
      - specified NEC A07.8
    - specified NEC B60.8
  - pubic, louse B85.3

Infestation — *continued*
- rat tapeworm B71.0
- red bug B88.0
- roundworm (large) NEC B82.0
  - Ascariasis (see also Ascariasis) B77.9
- sandflea B88.1
- Sarcoptes scabiei B86
- scabies B86
- Schistosoma B65.9
  - bovis B65.8
  - cercariae B65.3
  - haematobium B65.0
  - intercalatum B65.8
  - japonicum B65.2
  - mansoni B65.1
  - mattheei B65.8
  - mekongi B65.8
  - specified type NEC B65.8
  - spindale B65.8
- screw worms — *see* Myiasis
- skin NOS B88.9
- Sparganum (mansoni) (proliferum) (baxteri) B70.1
  - larval B70.1
- specified type NEC B88.8
- Spirometra larvae B70.1
- Stellantchasmus falcatus B66.8
- Strongyloides stercoralis — *see* Strongyloidiasis
- Taenia B68.9
  - diminuta B71.0
  - echinococcus — *see* Echinococcus
  - mediocanellata B68.1
  - nana B71.0
  - saginata B68.1
  - solium (intestinal form) B68.0
    - larval form — *see* Cysticercosis
- Taeniarhynchus saginatus B68.1
- tapeworm B71.9
  - beef B68.1
  - broad B70.0
    - larval B70.1
  - dog B67.4
  - dwarf B71.0
  - fish B70.0
    - larval B70.1
  - pork B68.0
  - rat B71.0
- Ternidens diminutus B81.8
- Tetranychus molestissimus B88.0
- threadworm B80
- tongue B37.0
- Toxocara (canis) (cati) (felis) B83.0
- trematode(s) NEC — *see* Infestation, fluke
- Trichinella (spiralis) B75
- Trichocephalus B79
- Trichomonas — *see* Trichomoniasis
- Trichostrongylus B81.2
- Trichuris (trichiura) B79
- Trombicula (irritans) B88.0
- Tunga penetrans B88.1
- Uncinaria americana B76.1
- Vandellia cirrhosa B88.8
- whipworm B79
- worms B83.9
  - intestinal B82.0
- Wuchereria (bancrofti) B74.0

Infiltrate, infiltration
- amyloid (generalized) (localized) — *see* Amyloidosis
- calcareous NEC R89.7
  - localized — *see* Degeneration, by site
- calcium salt R89.7
- cardiac
  - fatty — *see* Degeneration, myocardial
  - glycogenic E74.02 [I43]
- corneal — *see* Edema, cornea
- eyelid — *see* Inflammation, eyelid
- glycogen, glycogenic — *see* Disease, glycogen storage
- heart, cardiac
  - fatty — *see* Degeneration, myocardial
  - glycogenic E74.02 [I43]
- inflammatory in vitreous H43.89
- kidney N28.89
- leukemic — *see* Leukemia
- liver K76.89
  - fatty — *see* Fatty, liver NEC
  - glycogen (see also Disease, glycogen storage) E74.03 [K77]
- lung R91.8
  - eosinophilic J82

Infiltrate, infiltration — *continued*
- lymphatic (see also Leukemia, lymphatic) C91.9- ☑
  - gland I88.9
- muscle, fatty M62.89
- myocardium, myocardial
  - fatty — *see* Degeneration, myocardial
  - glycogenic E74.02 [I43]
- on chest x-ray R91.8
- pulmonary R91.8
  - with eosinophilia J82
- skin (lymphocytic) L98.6
- thymus (gland) (fatty) E32.8
- urine R39.0
- vesicant agent
  - antineoplastic chemotherapy T80.810 ☑
  - other agent NEC T80.818 ☑
- vitreous body H43.89

Infirmity R68.89
- senile R54

Inflammation, inflamed, inflammatory (with exudation)
- abducent (nerve) — *see* Strabismus, paralytic, sixth nerve
- accessory sinus (chronic) — *see* Sinusitis
- adrenal (gland) E27.8
- alveoli, teeth M27.3
  - scorbutic E54
- anal canal, anus K62.89
- antrum (chronic) — *see* Sinusitis, maxillary
- appendix — *see* Appendicitis
- arachnoid — *see* Meningitis
- areola N61.0
  - puerperal, postpartum or gestational — *see* Infection, nipple
- areolar tissue NOS L08.9
- artery — *see* Arteritis
- auditory meatus (external) — *see* Otitis, externa
- Bartholin's gland N75.8
- bile duct (common) (hepatic) or passage — *see* Cholangitis
- bladder — *see* Cystitis
- bone — *see* Osteomyelitis
- brain (see also Encephalitis)
  - membrane — *see* Meningitis
- breast N61.0
  - puerperal, postpartum, gestational — *see* Mastitis, obstetric
- broad ligament — *see* Disease, pelvis, inflammatory
- bronchi — *see* Bronchitis
- catarrhal J00
- cecum — *see* Appendicitis
- cerebral (see also Encephalitis)
  - membrane — *see* Meningitis
- cerebrospinal
  - meningococcal A39.0
- cervix (uteri) — *see* Cervicitis
- chest J98.8
- chorioretinal H30.9- ☑
  - cyclitis — *see* Cyclitis
  - disseminated H30.10- ☑
    - generalized H30.13- ☑
    - peripheral H30.12- ☑
    - posterior pole H30.11- ☑
  - epitheliopathy — *see* Epitheliopathy
  - focal H30.00- ☑
    - juxtapapillary H30.01- ☑
    - macular H30.04- ☑
    - paramacular — *see* Inflammation, chorioretinal, focal, macular
    - peripheral H30.03- ☑
    - posterior pole H30.02- ☑
  - specified type NEC H30.89- ☑
- choroid — *see* Inflammation, chorioretinal
- chronic, postmastoidectomy cavity — *see* Complications, postmastoidectomy, inflammation
- colon — *see* Enteritis
- connective tissue (diffuse) NEC — *see* Disorder, soft tissue, specified type NEC
- cornea — *see* Keratitis
- corpora cavernosa N48.29
- cranial nerve — *see* Disorder, nerve, cranial
- Douglas' cul-de-sac or pouch (chronic) N73.0
- due to device, implant or graft (see also Complications, by site and type, infection or inflammation)
  - arterial graft T82.7 ☑
  - breast (implant) T85.79 ☑
  - catheter T85.79 ☑

☑ **Additional Character Required** — Refer to the Tabular List for Character Selection   ⬙ Subterms under main terms may continue to next column or page

Inflammation, inflamed, inflammatory —
continued
- due to device, implant or graft (*see also* Complications, by site and type, infection or inflammation) — *continued*
  - catheter — *continued*
    - dialysis (renal) T82.7 ☑
      - intraperitoneal T85.71 ☑
    - infusion T82.7 ☑
      - cranial T85.735 ☑
      - intrathecal T85.735 ☑
      - spinal (epidural) (subdural) T85.735 ☑
      - subarachnoid T85.735 ☑
    - urinary T83.518 ☑
      - cystostomy T83.510 ☑
      - Hopkins T83.518 ☑
      - ileostomy T83.518 ☑
      - nephrostomy T83.512 ☑
      - specified NEC T83.518 ☑
      - urethral indwelling T83.511 ☑
      - urostomy T83.518 ☑
  - electronic (electrode) (pulse generator) (stimulator)
    - bone T84.7 ☑
    - cardiac T82.7 ☑
    - nervous system T85.738 ☑
      - brain T85.731 ☑
      - cranial nerve T85.732 ☑
      - gastric nerve T85.732 ☑
      - neurostimulator generator T85.734 ☑
      - peripheral nerve T85.732 ☑
      - sacral nerve T85.732 ☑
      - spinal cord T85.733 ☑
      - vagal nerve T85.732 ☑
    - urinary T83.590 ☑
  - fixation, internal (orthopedic) NEC — *see* Complication, fixation device, infection
  - gastrointestinal (bile duct) (esophagus) T85.79 ☑
    - neurostimulator electrode (lead) T85.732 ☑
  - genital NEC T83.69 ☑
  - heart NEC T82.7 ☑
    - valve (prosthesis) T82.6 ☑
      - graft T82.7 ☑
  - joint prosthesis — *see* Complication, joint prosthesis, infection
  - ocular (corneal graft) (orbital implant) NEC T85.79 ☑
  - orthopedic NEC T84.7 ☑
  - penile (cylinder) (pump) (resevoir) T83.61 ☑
  - specified NEC T85.79 ☑
  - testicular T83.62 ☑
  - urinary NEC T83.598 ☑
    - ileal conduit stent T83.593 ☑
    - implanted neurostimulation T83.590 ☑
    - implanted sphincter T83.591 ☑
    - indwelling ureteral stent T83.592 ☑
    - nephroureteral stent T83.593 ☑
    - specified stent NEC T83.593 ☑
  - vascular NEC T82.7 ☑
  - ventricular intracranial (communicating) shunt T85.730 ☑
- duodenum K29.80
  - with bleeding K29.81
- dura mater — *see* Meningitis
- ear (middle) (*see also* Otitis, media)
  - external — *see* Otitis, externa
  - inner — *see* subcategory H83.0 ☑
- epididymis — *see* Epididymitis
- esophagus K20.9
- ethmoidal (sinus) (chronic) — *see* Sinusitis, ethmoidal
- eustachian tube (catarrhal) — *see* Salpingitis, eustachian
- eyelid H01.9
  - abscess — *see* Abscess, eyelid
  - blepharitis — *see* Blepharitis
  - chalazion — *see* Chalazion
  - dermatosis (noninfectious) — *see* Dermatosis, eyelid
  - hordeolum — *see* Hordeolum
  - specified NEC H01.8
- fallopian tube — *see* Salpingo-oophoritis
- fascia — *see* Myositis
- follicular, pharynx J31.2
- frontal (sinus) (chronic) — *see* Sinusitis, frontal
- gallbladder — *see* Cholecystitis
- gastric — *see* Gastritis
- gastrointestinal — *see* Enteritis

Inflammation, inflamed, inflammatory —
continued
- genital organ (internal) (diffuse)
  - female — *see* Disease, pelvis, inflammatory
  - male N49.9
    - multiple sites N49.8
    - specified NEC N49.8
- gland (lymph) — *see* Lymphadenitis
- glottis — *see* Laryngitis
- granular, pharynx J31.2
- gum K05.10
  - nonplaque induced K05.11
  - plaque induced K05.10
- heart — *see* Carditis
- hepatic duct — *see* Cholangitis
- ileoanal (internal) pouch K91.850
- ileum (*see also* Enteritis)
  - regional or terminal — *see* Enteritis, regional
- intestinal pouch K91.850
- intestine (any part) — *see* Enteritis
- jaw (acute) (bone) (chronic) (lower) (suppurative) (upper) M27.2
- joint NEC — *see* Arthritis
  - sacroiliac M46.1
- kidney — *see* Nephritis
- knee (joint) M13.169
  - tuberculous A18.02
- labium (majus) (minus) — *see* Vulvitis
- lacrimal
  - gland — *see* Dacryoadenitis
  - passages (duct) (sac) (*see also* Dacryocystitis)
    - canaliculitis — *see* Canaliculitis, lacrimal
- larynx — *see* Laryngitis
- leg NOS L08.9
- lip K13.0
- liver (capsule) (*see also* Hepatitis)
  - chronic K73.9
  - suppurative K75.0
- lung (acute) (*see also* Pneumonia)
  - chronic J98.4
- lymph gland or node — *see* Lymphadenitis
- lymphatic vessel — *see* Lymphangitis
- maxilla, maxillary M27.2
  - sinus (chronic) — *see* Sinusitis, maxillary
- membranes of brain or spinal cord — *see* Meningitis
- meninges — *see* Meningitis
- mouth K12.1
- muscle — *see* Myositis
- myocardium — *see* Myocarditis
- nasal sinus (chronic) — *see* Sinusitis
- nasopharynx — *see* Nasopharyngitis
- navel L08.82
- nerve NEC — *see* Neuralgia
- nipple N61.0
  - puerperal, postpartum or gestational — *see* Infection, nipple
- nose — *see* Rhinitis
- oculomotor (nerve) — *see* Strabismus, paralytic, third nerve
- optic nerve — *see* Neuritis, optic
- orbit (chronic) H05.10
  - acute H05.00
    - abscess — *see* Abscess, orbit
    - cellulitis — *see* Cellulitis, orbit
    - osteomyelitis — *see* Osteomyelitis, orbit
    - periostitis — *see* Periostitis, orbital
    - tenonitis — *see* Tenonitis, eye
  - granuloma — *see* Granuloma, orbit
  - myositis — *see* Myositis, orbital
- ovary — *see* Salpingo-oophoritis
- oviduct — *see* Salpingo-oophoritis
- pancreas (acute) — *see* Pancreatitis
- parametrium N73.0
- parotid region L08.9
- pelvis, female — *see* Disease, pelvis, inflammatory
- penis (corpora cavernosa) N48.29
- perianal K62.89
- pericardium — *see* Pericarditis
- perineum (female) (male) L08.9
- perirectal K62.89
- peritoneum — *see* Peritonitis
- periuterine — *see* Disease, pelvis, inflammatory
- perivesical — *see* Cystitis
- petrous bone (acute) (chronic) — *see* Petrositis
- pharynx (acute) — *see* Pharyngitis
- pia mater — *see* Meningitis
- pleura — *see* Pleurisy

Inflammation, inflamed, inflammatory —
continued
- polyp, colon (*see also* Polyp, colon, inflammatory) K51.40
- prostate (*see also* Prostatitis)
  - specified type NEC N41.8
- rectosigmoid — *see* Rectosigmoiditis
- rectum (*see also* Proctitis) K62.89
- respiratory, upper (*see also* Infection, respiratory, upper) J06.9
  - acute, due to radiation J70.0
  - chronic, due to external agent — *see* condition, respiratory, chronic, due to
  - due to
    - chemicals, gases, fumes or vapors (inhalation) J68.2
    - radiation J70.1
- retina — *see* Chorioretinitis
- retrocecal — *see* Appendicitis
- retroperitoneal — *see* Peritonitis
- salivary duct or gland (any) (suppurative) — *see* Sialoadenitis
- scorbutic, alveoli, teeth E54
- scrotum N49.2
- seminal vesicle — *see* Vesiculitis
- sigmoid — *see* Enteritis
- sinus — *see* Sinusitis
- Skene's duct or gland — *see* Urethritis
- skin L08.9
- spermatic cord N49.1
- sphenoidal (sinus) — *see* Sinusitis, sphenoidal
- spinal
  - cord — *see* Encephalitis
  - membrane — *see* Meningitis
  - nerve — *see* Disorder, nerve
- spine — *see* Spondylopathy, inflammatory
- spleen (capsule) D73.89
- stomach — *see* Gastritis
- subcutaneous tissue L08.9
- suprarenal (gland) E27.8
- synovial — *see* Tenosynovitis
- tendon (sheath) NEC — *see* Tenosynovitis
- testis — *see* Orchitis
- throat (acute) — *see* Pharyngitis
- thymus (gland) E32.8
- thyroid (gland) — *see* Thyroiditis
- tongue K14.0
- tonsil — *see* Tonsillitis
- trachea — *see* Tracheitis
- trochlear (nerve) — *see* Strabismus, paralytic, fourth nerve
- tubal — *see* Salpingo-oophoritis
- tuberculous NEC — *see* Tuberculosis
- tubo-ovarian — *see* Salpingo-oophoritis
- tunica vaginalis N49.1
- tympanic membrane — *see* Tympanitis
- umbilicus, umbilical L08.82
- uterine ligament — *see* Disease, pelvis, inflammatory
- uterus (catarrhal) — *see* Endometritis
- uveal tract (anterior) NOS (*see also* Iridocyclitis)
  - posterior — *see* Chorioretinitis
- vagina — *see* Vaginitis
- vas deferens N49.1
- vein (*see also* Phlebitis)
  - intracranial or intraspinal (septic) G08
  - thrombotic I80.9
    - leg — *see* Phlebitis, leg
    - lower extremity — *see* Phlebitis, leg
- vocal cord J38.3
- vulva — *see* Vulvitis
- Wharton's duct (suppurative) — *see* Sialoadenitis

Inflation, lung, imperfect (newborn) — *see* Atelectasis

Influenza (bronchial) (epidemic) (respiratory (upper)) (unidentified influenza virus) J11.1
- with
  - digestive manifestations J11.2
  - encephalopathy J11.81
  - enteritis J11.2
  - gastroenteritis J11.2
  - gastrointestinal manifestations J11.2
  - laryngitis J11.1
  - myocarditis J11.82
  - otitis media J11.83
  - pharyngitis J11.1
  - pneumonia J11.00
    - specified type J11.08
  - respiratory manifestations NEC J11.1

Index

Influenza — Injury

Influenza — continued
with — continued
specified manifestation NEC J11.89
A/H5N1 (see also Influenza, due to, identified novel
influenza A virus) J09.X2
avian (see also Influenza, due to, identified novel influenza A virus) J09.X2
bird (see also Influenza, due to, identified novel influenza A virus) J09.X2
due to
avian (see also Influenza, due to, identified novel
influenza A virus) J09.X2
identified influenza virus NEC J10.1
with
digestive manifestations J10.2
encephalopathy J10.81
enteritis J10.2
gastroenteritis J10.2
gastrointestinal manifestations J10.2
laryngitis J10.1
myocarditis J10.82
otitis media J10.83
pharyngitis J10.1
pneumonia (unspecified type) J10.00
with same identified influenza virus
J10.01
specified type NEC J10.08
respiratory manifestations NEC J10.1
specified manifestation NEC J10.89
identified novel influenza A virus J09.X2
with
digestive manifestations J09.X3
encephalopathy J09.X9
enteritis J09.X3
gastroenteritis J09.X3
gastrointestinal manifestations J09.X3
laryngitis J09.X2
myocarditis J09.X9
otitis media J09.X9
pharyngitis J09.X2
pneumonia J09.X1
respiratory manifestations NEC J09.X2
specified manifestation NEC J09.X9
upper respiratory symptoms J09.X2
novel (2009) H1N1 influenza (see also Influenza, due
to, identified influenza virus NEC) J10.1
novel influenza A/H1N1 (see also Influenza, due to,
identified influenza virus NEC) J10.1
of other animal origin, not bird or swine (see also Influenza, due to, identified novel influenza A
virus) J09.X2
swine (viruses that normally cause infections in pigs)
(see also Influenza, due to, identified novel influenza A virus) J09.X2
Influenzal — see Influenza
Influenza-like disease — see Influenza
Infraction, Freiberg's (metatarsal head) — see Osteochondrosis, juvenile, metatarsus
Infraeruption of tooth (teeth) M26.34
Infusion complication, misadventure, or reaction
— see Complications, infusion
Ingestion
chemical — see Table of Drugs and Chemicals, by
substance, poisoning
drug or medicament
correct substance properly administered — see
Table of Drugs and Chemicals, by drug, adverse effect
overdose or wrong substance given or taken —
see Table of Drugs and Chemicals, by drug,
poisoning
foreign body — see Foreign body, alimentary tract
tularemia A21.3
Ingrowing
hair (beard) L73.1
nail (finger) (toe) L60.0
Inguinal (see also condition)
testicle Q53.9
bilateral Q53.212
unilateral Q53.112
Inhalant-induced
anxiety disorder F18.980
depressive disorder F18.94
major neurocognitive disorder F18.97
mild neurocognitive disorder F18.988
psychotic disorder F18.959
Inhalation
anthrax A22.1

Inhalation — continued
flame T27.3 ☑
food or foreign body — see Foreign body, by site
gases, fumes, or vapors NEC T59.9- ☑
specified agent — see Table of Drugs and Chemicals, by substance
liquid or vomitus — see Asphyxia
meconium (newborn) P24.00
with
with respiratory symptoms P24.01
pneumonia (pneumonitis) P24.01
mucus — see Asphyxia, mucus
oil or gasoline (causing suffocation) — see Foreign
body, by site
smoke J70.5
due to chemicals, gases, fumes and vapors J68.9
steam — see Toxicity, vapors
stomach contents or secretions — see Foreign body,
by site
due to anesthesia (general) (local) or other sedation
T88.59 ☑
in labor and delivery O74.0
in pregnancy O29.01- ☑
postpartum, puerperal O89.01
Inhibition, orgasm
female F52.31
male F52.32
Inhibitor, systemic lupus erythematosus (presence
of) D68.62
Iniencephalus, iniencephaly Q00.2
Injection, traumatic jet (air) (industrial) (water) (paint
or dye) T70.4 ☑
Injury (see also specified injury type) T14.90 ☑
abdomen, abdominal S39.91 ☑
blood vessel — see Injury, blood vessel, abdomen
cavity — see Injury, intra-abdominal
contusion S30.1 ☑
internal — see Injury, intra-abdominal
intra-abdominal organ — see Injury, intra-abdominal
nerve — see Injury, nerve, abdomen
open — see Wound, open, abdomen
specified NEC S39.81 ☑
superficial — see Injury, superficial, abdomen
Achilles tendon S86.00- ☑
laceration S86.02- ☑
specified type NEC S86.09- ☑
strain S86.01- ☑
acoustic, resulting in deafness — see Injury, nerve,
acoustic
adrenal (gland) S37.819 ☑
contusion S37.812 ☑
laceration S37.813 ☑
specified type NEC S37.818 ☑
alveolar (process) S09.93 ☑
ankle S99.91- ☑
contusion — see Contusion, ankle
dislocation — see Dislocation, ankle
fracture — see Fracture, ankle
nerve — see Injury, nerve, ankle
open — see Wound, open, ankle
specified type NEC S99.81- ☑
sprain — see Sprain, ankle
superficial — see Injury, superficial, ankle
anterior chamber, eye — see Injury, eye, specified site
NEC
anus — see Injury, abdomen
aorta (thoracic) S25.00 ☑
abdominal S35.00 ☑
laceration (minor) (superficial) S35.01 ☑
major S35.02 ☑
specified type NEC S35.09 ☑
laceration (minor) (superficial) S25.01 ☑
major S25.02 ☑
specified type NEC S25.09 ☑
arm (upper) S49.9- ☑
blood vessel — see Injury, blood vessel, arm
contusion — see Contusion, arm, upper
fracture — see Fracture, humerus
lower — see Injury, forearm
muscle — see Injury, muscle, shoulder
nerve — see Injury, nerve, arm
open — see Wound, open, arm
specified type NEC S49.8- ☑
superficial — see Injury, superficial, arm

Injury — continued
artery (complicating trauma) (see also Injury, blood
vessel, by site)
cerebral or meningeal — see Injury, intracranial
auditory canal (external) (meatus) S09.91 ☑
auricle, auris, ear S09.91 ☑
axilla — see Injury, shoulder
back — see Injury, back, lower
bile duct S36.13 ☑
birth (see also Birth, injury) P15.9
bladder (sphincter) S37.20 ☑
at delivery O71.5
contusion S37.22 ☑
laceration S37.23 ☑
obstetrical trauma O71.5
specified type NEC S37.29 ☑
blast (air) (hydraulic) (immersion) (underwater) NEC
T14.8 ☑
acoustic nerve trauma — see Injury, nerve, acoustic
bladder — see Injury, bladder
brain — see Concussion
colon — see Injury, intestine, large
ear (primary) S09.31- ☑
secondary S09.39- ☑
generalized T70.8 ☑
lung — see Injury, intrathoracic, lung
multiple body organs T70.8 ☑
peritoneum S36.81 ☑
rectum S36.61 ☑
retroperitoneum S36.898 ☑
small intestine S36.419 ☑
duodenum S36.410 ☑
specified site NEC S36.418 ☑
specified
intra-abdominal organ NEC S36.898 ☑
pelvic organ NEC S37.899 ☑
blood vessel NEC T14.8 ☑
abdomen S35.9 ☑
aorta — see Injury, aorta, abdominal
celiac artery — see Injury, blood vessel, celiac
artery
iliac vessel — see Injury, blood vessel, iliac
laceration S35.91 ☑
mesenteric vessel — see Injury, mesenteric
portal vein — see Injury, blood vessel, portal
vein
renal vessel — see Injury, blood vessel, renal
specified vessel NEC S35.8X- ☑
splenic vessel — see Injury, blood vessel,
splenic
vena cava — see Injury, vena cava, inferior
ankle — see Injury, blood vessel, foot
aorta (abdominal) (thoracic) — see Injury, aorta
arm (upper) NEC S45.90- ☑
forearm — see Injury, blood vessel, forearm
laceration S45.91- ☑
specified
site NEC S45.80- ☑
laceration S45.81- ☑
specified type NEC S45.89- ☑
type NEC S45.99- ☑
superficial vein S45.30- ☑
laceration S45.31- ☑
specified type NEC S45.39- ☑
axillary
artery S45.00- ☑
laceration S45.01- ☑
specified type NEC S45.09- ☑
vein S45.20- ☑
laceration S45.21- ☑
specified type NEC S45.29- ☑
azygos vein — see Injury, blood vessel, thoracic,
specified site NEC
brachial
artery S45.10- ☑
laceration S45.11- ☑
specified type NEC S45.19- ☑
vein S45.20- ☑
laceration S45.219 ☑
specified type NEC S45.29- ☑
carotid artery (common) (external) (internal, extracranial) S15.00- ☑
internal, intracranial S06.8- ☑
laceration (minor) (superficial) S15.01- ☑
major S15.02- ☑
specified type NEC S15.09- ☑

☑ Additional Character Required — Refer to the Tabular List for Character Selection   ▽ Subterms under main terms may continue to next column or page

Injury — *continued*
  blood vessel — *continued*
    celiac artery S35.219 ☑
      branch S35.299 ☑
        laceration (minor) (superficial) S35.291 ☑
          major S35.292 ☑
        specified NEC S35.298 ☑
      laceration (minor) (superficial) S35.211 ☑
        major S35.212 ☑
      specified type NEC S35.218 ☑
    cerebral — *see* Injury, intracranial
    deep plantar — *see* Injury, blood vessel, plantar artery
    digital (hand) — *see* Injury, blood vessel, finger
    dorsal
      artery (foot) S95.00- ☑
        laceration S95.01- ☑
        specified type NEC S95.09- ☑
      vein (foot) S95.20- ☑
        laceration S95.21- ☑
        specified type NEC S95.29- ☑
    due to accidental laceration during procedure — *see* Laceration, accidental complicating surgery
    extremity — *see* Injury, blood vessel, limb
    femoral
      artery (common) (superficial) S75.00- ☑
        laceration (minor) (superficial) S75.01- ☑
          major S75.02- ☑
        specified type NEC S75.09- ☑
      vein (hip level) (thigh level) S75.10- ☑
        laceration (minor) (superficial) S75.11- ☑
          major S75.12- ☑
        specified type NEC S75.19- ☑
    finger S65.50- ☑
      index S65.50- ☑
        laceration S65.51- ☑
        specified type NEC S65.59- ☑
      laceration S65.51- ☑
      little S65.50- ☑
        laceration S65.51- ☑
        specified type NEC S65.59- ☑
      middle S65.50- ☑
        laceration S65.51- ☑
        specified type NEC S65.59- ☑
      specified type NEC S65.59- ☑
      thumb — *see* Injury, blood vessel, thumb
    foot S95.90- ☑
      dorsal
        artery — *see* Injury, blood vessel, dorsal, artery
        vein — *see* Injury, blood vessel, dorsal, vein
      laceration S95.91- ☑
      plantar artery — *see* Injury, blood vessel, plantar artery
      specified
        site NEC S95.80- ☑
          laceration S95.81- ☑
          specified type NEC S95.89- ☑
        specified type NEC S95.99- ☑
    forearm S55.90- ☑
      laceration S55.91- ☑
      radial artery — *see* Injury, blood vessel, radial artery
      specified
        site NEC S55.80- ☑
          laceration S55.81- ☑
          specified type NEC S55.89- ☑
        type NEC S55.99- ☑
      ulnar artery — *see* Injury, blood vessel, ulnar artery
      vein S55.20- ☑
        laceration S55.21- ☑
        specified type NEC S55.29- ☑
    gastric
      artery — *see* Injury, mesenteric, artery, branch
      vein — *see* Injury, blood vessel, abdomen
    gastroduodenal artery — *see* Injury, mesenteric, artery, branch
    greater saphenous vein (lower leg level) S85.30- ☑
      hip (and thigh) level S75.20- ☑
        laceration (minor) (superficial) S75.21- ☑
          major S75.22- ☑
        specified type NEC S75.29- ☑
      laceration S85.31- ☑
      specified type NEC S85.39- ☑

Injury — *continued*
  blood vessel — *continued*
    hand (level) S65.90- ☑
      finger — *see* Injury, blood vessel, finger
      laceration S65.91- ☑
      palmar arch — *see* Injury, blood vessel, palmar arch
      radial artery — *see* Injury, blood vessel, radial artery, hand
      specified
        site NEC S65.80- ☑
          laceration S65.81- ☑
          specified type NEC S65.89- ☑
        type NEC S65.99- ☑
      thumb — *see* Injury, blood vessel, thumb
      ulnar artery — *see* Injury, blood vessel, ulnar artery, hand
    head S09.0 ☑
      intracranial — *see* Injury, intracranial
      multiple S09.0 ☑
    hepatic
      artery — *see* Injury, mesenteric, artery
      vein — *see* Injury, vena cava, inferior
    hip S75.90- ☑
      femoral artery — *see* Injury, blood vessel, femoral, artery
      femoral vein — *see* Injury, blood vessel, femoral, vein
      greater saphenous vein — *see* Injury, blood vessel, greater saphenous, hip level
      laceration S75.91- ☑
      specified
        site NEC S75.80- ☑
          laceration S75.81- ☑
          specified type NEC S75.89- ☑
        type NEC S75.99- ☑
    hypogastric (artery) (vein) — *see* Injury, blood vessel, iliac
    iliac S35.5-
      artery S35.51- ☑
      specified vessel NEC S35.5-
      uterine vessel — *see* Injury, blood vessel, uterine
      vein S35.51- ☑
    innominate — *see* Injury, blood vessel, thoracic, innominate
    intercostal (artery) (vein) — *see* Injury, blood vessel, thoracic, intercostal
    jugular vein (external) S15.20- ☑
      internal S15.30- ☑
        laceration (minor) (superficial) S15.31- ☑
          major S15.32- ☑
        specified type NEC S15.39- ☑
      laceration (minor) (superficial) S15.21- ☑
        major S15.22- ☑
      specified type NEC S15.29- ☑
    leg (level) (lower) S85.90- ☑
      greater saphenous — *see* Injury, blood vessel, greater saphenous
      laceration S85.91- ☑
      lesser saphenous — *see* Injury, blood vessel, lesser saphenous
      peroneal artery — *see* Injury, blood vessel, peroneal artery
      popliteal
        artery — *see* Injury, blood vessel, popliteal, artery
        vein — *see* Injury, blood vessel, popliteal, vein
      specified
        site NEC S85.80- ☑
          laceration S85.81- ☑
          specified type NEC S85.89- ☑
        type NEC S85.99- ☑
      thigh — *see* Injury, blood vessel, hip
      tibial artery — *see* Injury, blood vessel, tibial artery
    lesser saphenous vein (lower leg level) S85.40- ☑
      laceration S85.41- ☑
      specified type NEC S85.49- ☑
    limb
      lower — *see* Injury, blood vessel, leg
      upper — *see* Injury, blood vessel, arm
    lower back — *see* Injury, blood vessel, abdomen
      specified NEC — *see* Injury, blood vessel, abdomen, specified, site NEC

Injury — *continued*
  blood vessel — *continued*
    mammary (artery) (vein) — *see* Injury, blood vessel, thoracic, specified site NEC
    mesenteric (inferior) (superior)
      artery — *see* Injury, mesenteric, artery
      vein — *see* Injury, blood vessel, mesenteric, vein
    neck S15.9 ☑
      specified site NEC S15.8 ☑
    ovarian (artery) (vein) — *see* subcategory S35.8 ☑
    palmar arch (superficial) S65.20- ☑
      deep S65.30- ☑
        laceration S65.31- ☑
        specified type NEC S65.39- ☑
      laceration S65.21- ☑
      specified type NEC S65.29- ☑
    pelvis — *see* Injury, blood vessel, abdomen
      specified NEC — *see* Injury, blood vessel, abdomen, specified, site NEC
    peroneal artery S85.20- ☑
      laceration S85.21- ☑
      specified type NEC S85.29- ☑
    plantar artery (deep) (foot) S95.10- ☑
      laceration S95.11- ☑
      specified type NEC S95.19- ☑
    popliteal
      artery S85.00- ☑
        laceration S85.01- ☑
        specified type NEC S85.09- ☑
      vein S85.50- ☑
        laceration S85.51- ☑
        specified type NEC S85.59- ☑
    portal vein S35.319 ☑
      laceration S35.311 ☑
      specified type NEC S35.318 ☑
    precerebral — *see* Injury, blood vessel, neck
    pulmonary (artery) (vein) — *see* Injury, blood vessel, thoracic, pulmonary
    radial artery (forearm level) S55.10- ☑
      hand and wrist (level) S65.10- ☑
        laceration S65.11- ☑
        specified type NEC S65.19- ☑
      laceration S55.11- ☑
      specified type NEC S55.19- ☑
    renal
      artery S35.40- ☑
        laceration S35.41- ☑
        specified NEC S35.49- ☑
      vein S35.40- ☑
        laceration S35.41- ☑
        specified NEC S35.49- ☑
    saphenous vein (greater) (lower leg level) — *see* Injury, blood vessel, greater saphenous
      hip and thigh level — *see* Injury, blood vessel, greater saphenous, hip level
      lesser — *see* Injury, blood vessel, lesser saphenous
    shoulder
      specified NEC — *see* Injury, blood vessel, arm, specified site NEC
      superficial vein — *see* Injury, blood vessel, arm, superficial vein
    specified NEC T14.8 ☑
    splenic
      artery — *see* Injury, blood vessel, celiac artery, branch
      vein S35.329 ☑
        laceration S35.321 ☑
        specified NEC S35.328 ☑
    subclavian — *see* Injury, blood vessel, thoracic, innominate
    thigh — *see* Injury, blood vessel, hip
    thoracic S25.90 ☑
      aorta S25.00 ☑
        laceration (minor) (superficial) S25.01 ☑
          major S25.02 ☑
        specified type NEC S25.09 ☑
      azygos vein — *see* Injury, blood vessel, thoracic, specified, site NEC
      innominate
        artery S25.10- ☑
          laceration (minor) (superficial) S25.11- ☑
            major S25.12- ☑
          specified type NEC S25.19- ☑

Injury — continued
  blood vessel — continued
    thoracic — continued
      innominate — continued
        vein S25.30- ☑
          laceration (minor) (superficial)
            S25.31- ☑
          major S25.32- ☑
          specified type NEC S25.39- ☑
      intercostal S25.50- ☑
        laceration S25.51- ☑
        specified type NEC S25.59- ☑
      laceration S25.91 ☑
      mammary vessel — see Injury, blood vessel, thoracic, specified, site NEC
      pulmonary S25.40- ☑
        laceration (minor) (superficial) S25.41- ☑
          major S25.42- ☑
        specified type NEC S25.49- ☑
      specified
        site NEC S25.80- ☑
          laceration S25.81 ☑
          specified type NEC S25.89 ☑
        type NEC S25.99 ☑
      subclavian — see Injury, blood vessel, thoracic, innominate
      vena cava (superior) S25.20 ☑
        laceration (minor) (superficial) S25.21 ☑
          major S25.22 ☑
        specified type NEC S25.29 ☑
    thumb S65.40- ☑
      laceration S65.41- ☑
      specified type NEC S65.49- ☑
    tibial artery S85.10- ☑
      anterior S85.13- ☑
        laceration S85.14- ☑
        specified injury NEC S85.15- ☑
      laceration S85.11- ☑
      posterior S85.16- ☑
        laceration S85.17- ☑
        specified injury NEC S85.18- ☑
      specified injury NEC S85.12- ☑
    ulnar artery (forearm level) S55.00- ☑
      hand and wrist (level) S65.00- ☑
        laceration S65.01- ☑
        specified type NEC S65.09- ☑
      laceration S55.01- ☑
      specified type NEC S55.09- ☑
    upper arm (level) — see Injury, blood vessel, arm
      superficial vein — see Injury, blood vessel, arm, superficial vein
    uterine S35.5- ☑
      artery S35.53- ☑
      vein S35.53- ☑
    vena cava — see Injury, vena cava
    vertebral artery S15.10- ☑
      laceration (minor) (superficial) S15.11- ☑
        major S15.12- ☑
      specified type NEC S15.19- ☑
    wrist (level) — see Injury, blood vessel, hand
  brachial plexus S14.3 ☑
    newborn P14.3
  brain (traumatic) S06.9- ☑
    diffuse (axonal) S06.2X- ☑
    focal S06.30- ☑
  brainstem S06.38- ☑
  breast NOS S29.9
  broad ligament — see Injury, pelvic organ, specified site NEC
  bronchus, bronchi — see Injury, intrathoracic, bronchus
  brow S09.90 ☑
  buttock S39.92 ☑
  canthus, eye S05.90 ☑
  cardiac plexus — see Injury, nerve, thorax, sympathetic
  cauda equina S34.3 ☑
  cavernous sinus — see Injury, intracranial
  cecum — see Injury, colon
  celiac ganglion or plexus — see Injury, nerve, lumbosacral, sympathetic
  cerebellum — see Injury, intracranial
  cerebral — see Injury, intracranial
  cervix (uteri) — see Injury, uterus
  cheek (wall) S09.93 ☑
  chest — see Injury, thorax

  childbirth (newborn) (see also Birth, injury)
    maternal NEC O71.9
  chin S09.93 ☑
  choroid (eye) — see Injury, eye, specified site NEC
  clitoris S39.94 ☑
  coccyx (see also Injury, back, lower)
    complicating delivery O71.6
  colon — see Injury, intestine, large
  common bile duct — see Injury, liver
  conjunctiva (superficial) — see Injury, eye, conjunctiva
  conus medullaris — see Injury, spinal, sacral
  cord
    spermatic (pelvic region) S37.898 ☑
      scrotal region S39.848 ☑
    spinal — see Injury, spinal cord, by region
  cornea — see Injury, eye, specified site NEC
    abrasion — see Injury, eye, cornea, abrasion
  cortex (cerebral) (see also Injury, intracranial)
    visual — see Injury, nerve, optic
  costal region NEC S29.9 ☑
  costochondral NEC S29.9 ☑
  cranial
    cavity — see Injury, intracranial
    nerve — see Injury, nerve, cranial
  crushing — see Crush
  cutaneous sensory nerve
  cystic duct — see Injury, liver
  deep tissue — see Contusion, by site
    meaning pressure ulcer — see Ulcer, pressure, unstageable, by site
  delivery (newborn) P15.9
    maternal NEC O71.9
  Descemet's membrane — see Injury, eyeball, penetrating
  diaphragm — see Injury, intrathoracic, diaphragm
  duodenum — see Injury, intestine, small, duodenum
  ear (auricle) (external) (canal) S09.91 ☑
    abrasion — see Abrasion, ear
    bite — see Bite, ear
    blister — see Blister, ear
    bruise — see Contusion, ear
    contusion — see Contusion, ear
    external constriction — see Constriction, external, ear
    hematoma — see Hematoma, ear
    inner — see Injury, ear, middle
    laceration — see Laceration, ear
    middle S09.30- ☑
      blast — see Injury, blast, ear
      specified NEC S09.39- ☑
    puncture — see Puncture, ear
    superficial — see Injury, superficial, ear
  eighth cranial nerve (acoustic or auditory) — see Injury, nerve, acoustic
  elbow S59.90- ☑
    contusion — see Contusion, elbow
    dislocation — see Dislocation, elbow
    fracture — see Fracture, ulna, upper end
    open — see Wound, open, elbow
    specified NEC S59.80- ☑
    sprain — see Sprain, elbow
    superficial — see Injury, superficial, elbow
  eleventh cranial nerve (accessory) — see Injury, nerve, accessory
  epididymis S39.94 ☑
  epigastric region S39.91 ☑
  epiglottis NEC S19.89 ☑
  esophageal plexus — see Injury, nerve, thorax, sympathetic
  esophagus (thoracic part) (see also Injury, intrathoracic, esophagus)
    cervical NEC S19.85 ☑
  eustachian tube S09.30 ☑
  eye S05.9- ☑
    avulsion S05.7- ☑
    ball — see Injury, eyeball
    conjunctiva S05.0- ☑
    cornea
      abrasion S05.0- ☑
    laceration S05.3- ☑
      with prolapse S05.2- ☑
    lacrimal apparatus S05.8X- ☑
    orbit penetration S05.4- ☑
    specified site NEC S05.8X- ☑
  eyeball S05.8X- ☑

  eyeball — continued
    contusion S05.1- ☑
    penetrating S05.6- ☑
      with
        foreign body S05.5- ☑
        prolapse or loss of intraocular tissue S05.2- ☑
        without prolapse or loss of intraocular tissue S05.3- ☑
    specified type NEC S05.8- ☑
  eyebrow S09.93 ☑
  eyelid S09.93 ☑
    abrasion — see Abrasion, eyelid
    contusion — see Contusion, eyelid
    open — see Wound, open, eyelid
  face S09.93 ☑
  fallopian tube S37.509 ☑
    bilateral S37.502 ☑
      blast injury S37.512 ☑
      contusion S37.522 ☑
      laceration S37.532 ☑
      specified type NEC S37.592 ☑
    blast injury (primary) S37.519 ☑
      bilateral S37.512 ☑
      secondary — see Injury, fallopian tube, specified type NEC
      unilateral S37.511 ☑
    contusion S37.529 ☑
      bilateral S37.522 ☑
      unilateral S37.521 ☑
    laceration S37.539 ☑
      bilateral S37.532 ☑
      unilateral S37.531 ☑
    specified type NEC S37.599 ☑
      bilateral S37.592 ☑
      unilateral S37.591 ☑
    unilateral S37.501 ☑
      blast injury S37.511 ☑
      contusion S37.521 ☑
      laceration S37.531 ☑
      specified type NEC S37.591 ☑
  fascia — see Injury, muscle
  fifth cranial nerve (trigeminal) — see Injury, nerve, trigeminal
  finger (nail) S69.9- ☑
    blood vessel — see Injury, blood vessel, finger
    contusion — see Contusion, finger
    dislocation — see Dislocation, finger
    fracture — see Fracture, finger
    muscle — see Injury, muscle, finger
    nerve — see Injury, nerve, digital, finger
    open — see Wound, open, finger
    specified NEC S69.8- ☑
    sprain — see Sprain, finger
    superficial — see Injury, superficial, finger
  first cranial nerve (olfactory) — see Injury, nerve, olfactory
  flank — see Injury, abdomen
  foot S99.92- ☑
    blood vessel — see Injury, blood vessel, foot
    contusion — see Contusion, foot
    dislocation — see Dislocation, foot
    fracture — see Fracture, foot
    muscle — see Injury, muscle, foot
    open — see Wound, open, foot
    specified type NEC S99.82- ☑
    sprain — see Sprain, foot
    superficial — see Injury, superficial, foot
  forceps NOS P15.9
  forearm S59.91- ☑
    blood vessel — see Injury, blood vessel, forearm
    contusion — see Contusion, forearm
    fracture — see Fracture, forearm
    muscle — see Injury, muscle, forearm
    nerve — see Injury, nerve, forearm
    open — see Wound, open, forearm
    specified NEC S59.81- ☑
    superficial — see Injury, superficial, forearm
  forehead S09.90 ☑
  fourth cranial nerve (trochlear) — see Injury, nerve, trochlear
  gallbladder S36.129 ☑
    contusion S36.122 ☑
    laceration S36.123 ☑
    specified NEC S36.128 ☑

☑ Additional Character Required — Refer to the Tabular List for Character Selection   Subterms under main terms may continue to next column or page

Injury — continued
  ganglion
    celiac, coeliac — see Injury, nerve, lumbosacral,
      sympathetic
    gasserian — see Injury, nerve, trigeminal
    stellate — see Injury, nerve, thorax, sympathetic
    thoracic sympathetic — see Injury, nerve, thorax,
      sympathetic
  gasserian ganglion — see Injury, nerve, trigeminal
  gastric artery — see Injury, blood vessel, celiac artery,
    branch
  gastroduodenal artery — see Injury, blood vessel,
    celiac artery, branch
  gastrointestinal tract — see Injury, intra-abdominal
    with open wound into abdominal cavity — see
      Wound, open, with penetration into peri-
      toneal cavity
    colon — see Injury, intestine, large
    rectum — see Injury, intestine, large, rectum
      with open wound into abdominal cavity
        S36.61
    small intestine — see Injury, intestine, small
    specified site NEC — see Injury, intra-abdominal,
      specified, site NEC
    stomach — see Injury, stomach
  genital organ(s)
    external S39.94 ☑
      specified NEC S39.848 ☑
    internal S37.90 ☑
      fallopian tube — see Injury, fallopian tube
      ovary — see Injury, ovary
      prostate — see Injury, prostate
      seminal vesicle — see Injury, pelvis, organ,
        specified site NEC
      uterus — see Injury, uterus
      vas deferens — see Injury, pelvis, organ, speci-
        fied site NEC
    obstetrical trauma O71.9
  gland
    lacrimal laceration — see Injury, eye, specified site
      NEC
    salivary S09.93 ☑
    thyroid NEC S19.84 ☑
  globe (eye) S05.90 ☑
    specified NEC S05.8X- ☑
  groin — see Injury, abdomen
  gum S09.90 ☑
  hand S69.9- ☑
    blood vessel — see Injury, blood vessel, hand
    contusion — see Contusion, hand
    fracture — see Fracture, hand
    muscle — see Injury, muscle, hand
    nerve — see Injury, nerve, hand
    open — see Wound, open, hand
    specified NEC S69.8- ☑
    sprain — see Sprain, hand
    superficial — see Injury, superficial, hand
  head S09.90 ☑
    with loss of consciousness S06.9- ☑
    specified NEC S09.8 ☑
  heart S26.90 ☑
    with hemopericardium S26.00 ☑
      contusion S26.01 ☑
      laceration (mild) S26.020 ☑
        major S26.022 ☑
        moderate S26.021 ☑
      specified type NEC S26.09 ☑
    without hemopericardium S26.10 ☑
      contusion S26.11 ☑
      laceration S26.12 ☑
      specified type NEC S26.19 ☑
    contusion S26.91 ☑
    laceration S26.92 ☑
    specified type NEC S26.99 ☑
  heel — see Injury, foot
  hepatic
    artery — see Injury, blood vessel, celiac artery,
      branch
    duct — see Injury, liver
    vein — see Injury, vena cava, inferior
  hip S79.91- ☑
    blood vessel — see Injury, blood vessel, hip
    contusion — see Contusion, hip
    dislocation — see Dislocation, hip
    fracture — see Fracture, femur, neck
    muscle — see Injury, muscle, hip

Injury — continued
  hip — continued
    nerve — see Injury, nerve, hip
    open — see Wound, open, hip
    specified NEC S79.81- ☑
    sprain — see Sprain, hip
    superficial — see Injury, superficial, hip
  hymen S39.94 ☑
  hypogastric
    blood vessel — see Injury, blood vessel, iliac
    plexus — see Injury, nerve, lumbosacral, sympa-
      thetic
  ileum — see Injury, intestine, small
  iliac region S39.91 ☑
  instrumental (during surgery) — see Laceration, acci-
    dental complicating surgery
    birth injury — see Birth, injury
    nonsurgical — see Injury, by site
    obstetrical O71.9
      bladder O71.5
      cervix O71.3
      high vaginal O71.4
      perineal NOS O70.9
      urethra O71.5
      uterus O71.5
        with rupture or perforation O71.1
  internal T14.8 ☑
    aorta — see Injury, aorta
    bladder (sphincter) — see Injury, bladder
      with
        ectopic or molar pregnancy O08.6
      following ectopic or molar pregnancy O08.6
      obstetrical trauma O71.5
    bronchus, bronchi — see Injury, intrathoracic,
      bronchus
    cecum — see Injury, intestine, large
    cervix (uteri) (see also Injury, uterus)
      with ectopic or molar pregnancy O08.6
      following ectopic or molar pregnancy O08.6
      obstetrical trauma O71.3
    chest — see Injury, intrathoracic
    gastrointestinal tract — see Injury, intra-abdominal
    heart — see Injury, heart
    intestine NEC — see Injury, intestine
    intrauterine — see Injury, uterus
    mesentery — see Injury, intra-abdominal, specified,
      site NEC
    pelvis, pelvic (organ) S37.90 ☑
      following ectopic or molar pregnancy (subse-
        quent episode) O08.6
      obstetrical trauma NEC O71.5
        rupture or perforation O71.1
      specified NEC S39.83 ☑
    rectum — see Injury, intestine, large, rectum
    stomach — see Injury, stomach
    ureter — see Injury, ureter
    urethra (sphincter) following ectopic or molar
      pregnancy O08.6
    uterus — see Injury, uterus
  interscapular area — see Injury, thorax
  intestine
    large S36.509 ☑
      ascending (right) S36.500 ☑
        blast injury (primary) S36.510 ☑
          secondary S36.590 ☑
        contusion S36.520 ☑
        laceration S36.530 ☑
        specified type NEC S36.590 ☑
      blast injury (primary) S36.519 ☑
        ascending (right) S36.510 ☑
        descending (left) S36.512 ☑
        rectum S36.61 ☑
        sigmoid S36.513 ☑
        specified site NEC S36.518 ☑
        transverse S36.511 ☑
      contusion S36.529 ☑
        ascending (right) S36.520 ☑
        descending (left) S36.522 ☑
        rectum S36.62 ☑
        sigmoid S36.523 ☑
        specified site NEC S36.528 ☑
        transverse S36.521 ☑
      descending (left) S36.502 ☑
        blast injury (primary) S36.512 ☑
          secondary S36.592 ☑
        contusion S36.522 ☑
        laceration S36.532 ☑

Injury — continued
  intestine — continued
    large — continued
      descending — continued
        specified type NEC S36.592 ☑
      laceration S36.539 ☑
        ascending (right) S36.530 ☑
        descending (left) S36.532 ☑
        rectum S36.63 ☑
        sigmoid S36.533 ☑
        specified site NEC S36.538 ☑
        transverse S36.531 ☑
      rectum S36.60 ☑
        blast injury (primary) S36.61 ☑
          secondary S36.69 ☑
        contusion S36.62 ☑
        laceration S36.63 ☑
        specified type NEC S36.69 ☑
      sigmoid S36.503 ☑
        blast injury (primary) S36.513 ☑
          secondary S36.593 ☑
        contusion S36.523 ☑
        laceration S36.533 ☑
        specified type NEC S36.593 ☑
      specified
        site NEC S36.508 ☑
          blast injury (primary) S36.518 ☑
            secondary S36.598 ☑
          contusion S36.528 ☑
          laceration S36.538 ☑
          specified type NEC S36.598 ☑
        type NEC S36.599 ☑
          ascending (right) S36.590 ☑
          descending (left) S36.592 ☑
          rectum S36.69 ☑
          sigmoid S36.593 ☑
          specified site NEC S36.598 ☑
          transverse S36.591 ☑
      transverse S36.501 ☑
        blast injury (primary) S36.511 ☑
          secondary S36.591 ☑
        contusion S36.521 ☑
        laceration S36.531 ☑
        specified type NEC S36.591 ☑
    small S36.409 ☑
      blast injury (primary) S36.419 ☑
        duodenum S36.410 ☑
        secondary S36.499 ☑
          duodenum S36.490 ☑
          specified site NEC S36.498 ☑
        specified site NEC S36.418 ☑
      contusion S36.429 ☑
        duodenum S36.420 ☑
        specified site NEC S36.428 ☑
      duodenum S36.400 ☑
        blast injury (primary) S36.410 ☑
          secondary S36.490 ☑
        contusion S36.420 ☑
        laceration S36.430 ☑
        specified NEC S36.490 ☑
      laceration S36.439 ☑
        duodenum S36.430 ☑
        specified site NEC S36.438 ☑
      specified
        site NEC S36.408 ☑
        type NEC S36.499 ☑
          duodenum S36.490 ☑
          specified site NEC S36.498 ☑
  intra-abdominal S36.90 ☑
    adrenal gland — see Injury, adrenal gland
    bladder — see Injury, bladder
    colon — see Injury, intestine, large
    contusion S36.92 ☑
    fallopian tube — see Injury, fallopian tube
    gallbladder — see Injury, gallbladder
    intestine — see Injury, intestine
    kidney — see Injury, kidney
    laceration S36.93 ☑
    liver — see Injury, liver
    ovary — see Injury, ovary
    pancreas — see Injury, pancreas
    pelvic NOS S37.90 ☑
    peritoneum — see Injury, intra-abdominal, speci-
      fied, site NEC
    prostate — see Injury, prostate
    rectum — see Injury, intestine, large, rectum

⛛ Subterms under main terms may continue to next column or page   ☑ Additional Character Required — Refer to the Tabular List for Character Selection   193

Injury — Injury

Injury — *continued*
  intra-abdominal — *continued*
    retroperitoneum — *see* Injury, intra-abdominal, specified, site NEC
    seminal vesicle — *see* Injury, pelvis, organ, specified site NEC
    small intestine — *see* Injury, intestine, small
    specified
      pelvic S37.90 ☑
        specified
          site NEC S37.899 ☑
            specified type NEC S37.898 ☑
          type NEC S37.99 ☑
      site NEC S36.899 ☑
        contusion S36.892 ☑
        laceration S36.893 ☑
        specified type NEC S36.898 ☑
      type NEC S36.99 ☑
    spleen — *see* Injury, spleen
    stomach — *see* Injury, stomach
    ureter — *see* Injury, ureter
    urethra — *see* Injury, urethra
    uterus — *see* Injury, uterus
    vas deferens — *see* Injury, pelvis, organ, specified site NEC
  intracranial (traumatic) S06.9- ☑
    cerebellar hemorrhage, traumatic — *see* Injury, intracranial, focal
    cerebral edema, traumatic S06.1X- ☑
      diffuse S06.1X- ☑
      focal S06.1X- ☑
    diffuse (axonal) S06.2X- ☑
    epidural hemorrhage (traumatic) S06.4X- ☑
    focal brain injury S06.30- ☑
      contusion — *see* Contusion, cerebral
      laceration — *see* Laceration, cerebral
      intracerebral hemorrhage, traumatic S06.36- ☑
        left side S06.35- ☑
        right side S06.34- ☑
    subarachnoid hemorrhage, traumatic S06.6X- ☑
    subdural hemorrhage, traumatic S06.5X- ☑
  intraocular — *see* Injury, eyeball, penetrating
  intrathoracic S27.9
    bronchus S27.409 ☑
      bilateral S27.402 ☑
      blast injury (primary) S27.419 ☑
        bilateral S27.412 ☑
        secondary — *see* Injury, intrathoracic, bronchus, specified type NEC
        unilateral S27.411 ☑
      contusion S27.429 ☑
        bilateral S27.422 ☑
        unilateral S27.421 ☑
      laceration S27.439 ☑
        bilateral S27.432 ☑
        unilateral S27.431 ☑
      specified type NEC S27.499 ☑
        bilateral S27.492 ☑
        unilateral S27.491 ☑
      unilateral S27.401 ☑
    diaphragm S27.809 ☑
      contusion S27.802 ☑
      laceration S27.803 ☑
      specified type NEC S27.808 ☑
    esophagus (thoracic) S27.819 ☑
      contusion S27.812 ☑
      laceration S27.813 ☑
      specified type NEC S27.818 ☑
    heart — *see* Injury, heart
    hemopneumothorax S27.2 ☑
    hemothorax S27.1 ☑
    lung S27.309 ☑
      aspiration J69.0
      bilateral S27.302 ☑
      blast injury (primary) S27.319 ☑
        bilateral S27.312 ☑
        secondary — *see* Injury, intrathoracic, lung, specified type NEC
        unilateral S27.311 ☑
      contusion S27.329 ☑
        bilateral S27.322 ☑
        unilateral S27.321 ☑
      laceration S27.339 ☑
        bilateral S27.332 ☑
        unilateral S27.331 ☑
      specified type NEC S27.399 ☑

Injury — *continued*
  intrathoracic — *continued*
    lung — *continued*
      specified type — *continued*
        bilateral S27.392 ☑
        unilateral S27.391 ☑
        unilateral S27.301 ☑
      pleura S27.60 ☑
        laceration S27.63 ☑
        specified type NEC S27.69 ☑
      pneumothorax S27.0 ☑
      specified organ NEC S27.899 ☑
        contusion S27.892 ☑
        laceration S27.893 ☑
        specified type NEC S27.898 ☑
      thoracic duct — *see* Injury, intrathoracic, specified organ NEC
      thymus gland — *see* Injury, intrathoracic, specified organ NEC
      trachea, thoracic S27.50 ☑
        blast (primary) S27.51 ☑
        contusion S27.52 ☑
        laceration S27.53 ☑
        specified type NEC S27.59 ☑
  iris — *see* Injury, eye, specified site NEC
    penetrating — *see* Injury, eyeball, penetrating
  jaw S09.93 ☑
  jejunum — *see* Injury, intestine, small
  joint NOS T14.8 ☑
    old or residual — *see* Disorder, joint, specified type NEC
  kidney S37.00- ☑
    acute (nontraumatic) N17.9
    contusion — *see* Contusion, kidney
    laceration — *see* Laceration, kidney
    specified NEC S37.09- ☑
  knee S89.9- ☑
    contusion — *see* Contusion, knee
    dislocation — *see* Dislocation, knee
    meniscus (lateral) (medial) — *see* Sprain, knee, specified site NEC
      old injury or tear — *see* Derangement, knee, meniscus, due to old injury
    open — *see* Wound, open, knee
    specified NEC S89.8- ☑
    sprain — *see* Sprain, knee
    superficial — *see* Injury, superficial, knee
  labium (majus) (minus) S39.94 ☑
  labyrinth, ear S09.30- ☑
  lacrimal apparatus, duct, gland, or sac — *see* Injury, eye, specified site NEC
  larynx NEC S19.81 ☑
  leg (lower) S89.9- ☑
    blood vessel — *see* Injury, blood vessel, leg
    contusion — *see* Contusion, leg
    fracture — *see* Fracture, leg
    muscle — *see* Injury, muscle, leg
    nerve — *see* Injury, nerve, leg
    open — *see* Wound, open, leg
    specified NEC S89.8- ☑
    superficial — *see* Injury, superficial, leg
  lens, eye — *see* Injury, eye, specified site NEC
    penetrating — *see* Injury, eyeball, penetrating
  limb NEC T14.8 ☑
  lip S09.93 ☑
  liver S36.119 ☑
    contusion S36.112 ☑
    laceration S36.113 ☑
      major (stellate) S36.116 ☑
      minor S36.114 ☑
      moderate S36.115 ☑
    specified NEC S36.118 ☑
  lower back S39.92 ☑
    specified NEC S39.82 ☑
  lumbar, lumbosacral (region) S39.92 ☑
    plexus — *see* Injury, lumbosacral plexus
  lumbosacral plexus S34.4 ☑
  lung (*see also* Injury, intrathoracic, lung)
    aspiration J69.0
    transfusion-related (TRALI) J95.84
  lymphatic thoracic duct — *see* Injury, intrathoracic, specified organ NEC
  malar region S09.93 ☑
  mastoid region S09.90 ☑
  maxilla S09.93 ☑

Injury — *continued*
  mediastinum — *see* Injury, intrathoracic, specified organ NEC
  membrane, brain — *see* Injury, intracranial
  meningeal artery — *see* Injury, intracranial, subdural hemorrhage
  meninges (cerebral) — *see* Injury, intracranial
  mesenteric
    artery
      branch S35.299 ☑
        laceration (minor) (superficial) S35.291 ☑
          major S35.292 ☑
        specified NEC S35.298 ☑
      inferior S35.239 ☑
        laceration (minor) (superficial) S35.231 ☑
          major S35.232 ☑
        specified NEC S35.238 ☑
      superior S35.229 ☑
        laceration (minor) (superficial) S35.221 ☑
          major S35.222 ☑
        specified NEC S35.228 ☑
    plexus (inferior) (superior) — *see* Injury, nerve, lumbosacral, sympathetic
    vein
      inferior S35.349 ☑
        laceration S35.341 ☑
        specified NEC S35.348 ☑
      superior S35.339 ☑
        laceration S35.331 ☑
        specified NEC S35.338 ☑
  mesentery — *see* Injury, intra-abdominal, specified site NEC
  mesosalpinx — *see* Injury, pelvic organ, specified site NEC
  middle ear S09.30- ☑
  midthoracic region NOS S29.9 ☑
  mouth S09.93 ☑
  multiple NOS T07 ☑
  muscle (and fascia) (and tendon)
    abdomen S39.001 ☑
      laceration S39.021 ☑
      specified type NEC S39.091 ☑
      strain S39.011 ☑
    abductor
      thumb, forearm level — *see* Injury, muscle, thumb, abductor
    adductor
      thigh S76.20- ☑
        laceration S76.22- ☑
        specified type NEC S76.29- ☑
        strain S76.21- ☑
    ankle — *see* Injury, muscle, foot
    anterior muscle group, at leg level (lower) S86.20- ☑
      laceration S86.22- ☑
      specified type NEC S86.29- ☑
      strain S86.21- ☑
    arm (upper) — *see* Injury, muscle, shoulder
    biceps (parts NEC) S46.20- ☑
      laceration S46.22- ☑
      long head S46.10- ☑
        laceration S46.12- ☑
        specified type NEC S46.19- ☑
        strain S46.11- ☑
      specified type NEC S46.29- ☑
      strain S46.21- ☑
    extensor
      finger(s) (other than thumb) — *see* Injury, muscle, finger by site, extensor
      forearm level, specified NEC — *see* Injury, muscle, forearm, extensor
      thumb — *see* Injury, muscle, thumb, extensor
      toe (large) (ankle level) (foot level) — *see* Injury, muscle, toe, extensor
    finger
      extensor (forearm level) S56.40- ☑
        hand level S66.309 ☑
          laceration S66.329 ☑
          specified type NEC S66.399 ☑
          strain S66.319 ☑
        laceration S56.429 ☑
        specified type NEC S56.499 ☑
        strain S56.419 ☑
      flexor (forearm level) S56.10- ☑
        hand level S66.109 ☑
          laceration S66.129 ☑

☑ **Additional Character Required** — **Refer to the Tabular List for Character Selection**   ▽ **Subterms under main terms may continue to next column or page**

Injury — continued
muscle — continued
finger — continued
flexor — continued
hand level — continued
specified type NEC S66.199 ☑
strain S66.119 ☑
laceration S56.129 ☑
specified type NEC S56.199 ☑
strain S56.119 ☑
index
extensor (forearm level)
hand level S66.308 ☑
laceration S66.32- ☑
specified type NEC S66.39- ☑
strain S66.31- ☑
specified type NEC S56.492- ☑
flexor (forearm level)
hand level S66.108 ☑
laceration S66.12- ☑
specified type NEC S66.19- ☑
strain S66.11- ☑
specified type NEC S56.19- ☑
strain S56.11- ☑
intrinsic S66.50- ☑
laceration S66.52- ☑
specified type NEC S66.59- ☑
strain S66.51- ☑
intrinsic S66.509 ☑
laceration S66.529 ☑
specified type NEC S66.599 ☑
strain S66.519 ☑
little
extensor (forearm level)
hand level S66.30- ☑
laceration S66.32- ☑
specified type NEC S66.39- ☑
strain S66.31- ☑
laceration S56.42- ☑
specified type NEC S56.49- ☑
strain S56.41- ☑
flexor (forearm level)
hand level S66.10- ☑
laceration S66.12- ☑
specified type NEC S66.19- ☑
strain S66.11- ☑
laceration S56.12- ☑
specified type NEC S56.19- ☑
strain S56.11- ☑
intrinsic S66.50- ☑
laceration S66.52- ☑
specified type NEC S66.59- ☑
strain S66.51- ☑
middle
extensor (forearm level)
hand level S66.30- ☑
laceration S66.32- ☑
specified type NEC S66.39- ☑
strain S66.31- ☑
laceration S56.42- ☑
specified type NEC S56.49- ☑
strain S56.41- ☑
flexor (forearm level)
hand level S66.10- ☑
laceration S66.12- ☑
specified type NEC S66.19- ☑
strain S66.11- ☑
laceration S56.12- ☑
specified type NEC S56.19- ☑
strain S56.11- ☑
intrinsic S66.50- ☑
laceration S66.52- ☑
specified type NEC S66.59- ☑
strain S66.51- ☑
ring
extensor (forearm level)
hand level S66.30- ☑
laceration S66.32- ☑
specified type NEC S66.39- ☑
strain S66.31- ☑
laceration S56.42- ☑
specified type NEC S56.49- ☑
strain S56.41- ☑
flexor (forearm level)
hand level S66.10- ☑
laceration S66.12- ☑

Injury — continued
muscle — continued
finger — continued
ring — continued
flexor — continued
hand level — continued
specified type NEC S66.19- ☑
strain S66.11- ☑
laceration S56.12- ☑
specified type NEC S56.19- ☑
strain S56.11- ☑
intrinsic S66.50- ☑
laceration S66.52- ☑
specified type NEC S66.59- ☑
strain S66.51- ☑
flexor
finger(s) (other than thumb) — see Injury,
muscle, finger
forearm level, specified NEC — see Injury,
muscle, forearm, flexor
thumb — see Injury, muscle, thumb, flexor
toe (long) (ankle level) (foot level) — see Injury,
muscle, toe, flexor
foot S96.90- ☑
intrinsic S96.20- ☑
laceration S96.22- ☑
specified type NEC S96.29- ☑
strain S96.21- ☑
laceration S96.92- ☑
long extensor, toe — see Injury, muscle, toe,
extensor
long flexor, toe — see Injury, muscle, toe, flexor
specified
site NEC S96.80- ☑
laceration S96.82- ☑
specified type NEC S96.89- ☑
strain S96.81- ☑
type S96.99- ☑
strain S96.91- ☑
forearm (level) S56.90- ☑
extensor S56.50- ☑
laceration S56.52- ☑
specified type NEC S56.59- ☑
strain S56.51- ☑
flexor S56.20- ☑
laceration S56.22- ☑
specified type NEC S56.29- ☑
strain S56.21- ☑
laceration S56.92- ☑
specified S56.99- ☑
site NEC S56.80- ☑
laceration S56.82- ☑
strain S56.81- ☑
type NEC S56.89- ☑
strain S56.91- ☑
hand (level) S66.90- ☑
laceration S66.92- ☑
specified
site NEC S66.80- ☑
laceration S66.82- ☑
specified type NEC S66.89- ☑
strain S66.81- ☑
type NEC S66.99- ☑
strain S66.91- ☑
head S09.10 ☑
laceration S09.12 ☑
specified type NEC S09.19 ☑
strain S09.11 ☑
hip NEC S76.00- ☑
laceration S76.02- ☑
specified type NEC S76.09- ☑
strain S76.01- ☑
intrinsic
ankle and foot level — see Injury, muscle, foot,
intrinsic
finger (other than thumb) — see Injury, muscle,
finger by site, intrinsic
foot (level) — see Injury, muscle, foot, intrinsic
thumb — see Injury, muscle, thumb, intrinsic
leg (level) (lower) S86.90- ☑
Achilles tendon — see Injury, Achilles tendon
anterior muscle group — see Injury, muscle,
anterior muscle group
laceration S86.92- ☑
peroneal muscle group — see Injury, muscle,
peroneal muscle group

Injury — continued
muscle — continued
leg — continued
posterior muscle group — see Injury, muscle,
posterior muscle group, leg level
specified
site NEC S86.80- ☑
laceration S86.82- ☑
specified type NEC S86.89- ☑
strain S86.81- ☑
type NEC S86.99- ☑
strain S86.91- ☑
long
extensor toe, at ankle and foot level — see Injury, muscle, toe, extensor
flexor, toe, at ankle and foot level — see Injury,
muscle, toe, flexor
head, biceps — see Injury, muscle, biceps, long
head
lower back S39.002 ☑
laceration S39.022 ☑
specified type NEC S39.092 ☑
strain S39.012 ☑
neck (level) S16.9 ☑
laceration S16.2 ☑
specified type NEC S16.8 ☑
strain S16.1 ☑
pelvis S39.003 ☑
laceration S39.023 ☑
specified type NEC S39.093 ☑
strain S39.013 ☑
peroneal muscle group, at leg level (lower)
S86.30- ☑
laceration S86.32- ☑
specified type NEC S86.39- ☑
strain S86.31- ☑
posterior muscle (group)
leg level (lower) S86.10- ☑
laceration S86.12- ☑
specified type NEC S86.19- ☑
strain S86.11- ☑
thigh level S76.30- ☑
laceration S76.32- ☑
specified type NEC S76.39- ☑
strain S76.31- ☑
quadriceps (thigh) S76.10- ☑
laceration S76.12- ☑
specified type NEC S76.19- ☑
strain S76.11- ☑
shoulder S46.90- ☑
laceration S46.92- ☑
rotator cuff — see Injury, rotator cuff
specified site NEC S46.80- ☑
laceration S46.82- ☑
specified type NEC S46.89- ☑
strain S46.81- ☑
specified type NEC S46.99- ☑
strain S46.91- ☑
thigh NEC (level) S76.90- ☑
adductor — see Injury, muscle, adductor, thigh
laceration S76.92- ☑
posterior muscle (group) — see Injury, muscle,
posterior muscle, thigh level
quadriceps — see Injury, muscle, quadriceps
specified
site NEC S76.80- ☑
laceration S76.82- ☑
specified type NEC S76.89- ☑
strain S76.81- ☑
type NEC S76.99- ☑
strain S76.91- ☑
thorax (level) S29.009 ☑
back wall S29.002 ☑
front wall S29.001 ☑
laceration S29.029 ☑
back wall S29.022 ☑
front wall S29.021 ☑
specified type NEC S29.099 ☑
back wall S29.092 ☑
front wall S29.091 ☑
strain S29.019 ☑
back wall S29.012 ☑
front wall S29.011 ☑
thumb
abductor (forearm level) S56.30- ☑
laceration S56.32- ☑

⚐ Subterms under main terms may continue to next column or page   ☑ Additional Character Required — Refer to the Tabular List for Character Selection   195

Injury — Injury

Injury — *continued*
  muscle — *continued*
    thumb — *continued*
      abductor — *continued*
        specified type NEC S56.39- ☑
        strain S56.31- ☑
      extensor (forearm level) S56.30- ☑
        hand level S66.20- ☑
          laceration S66.22- ☑
          specified type NEC S66.29- ☑
          strain S66.21- ☑
        laceration S56.32- ☑
        specified type NEC S56.39- ☑
        strain S56.31- ☑
      flexor (forearm level) S56.00- ☑
        hand level S66.00- ☑
          laceration S66.02- ☑
          specified type NEC S66.09- ☑
          strain S66.01- ☑
        laceration S56.02- ☑
        specified type NEC S56.09- ☑
        strain S56.01- ☑
        wrist level — *see* Injury, muscle, thumb, flexor, hand level
      intrinsic S66.40- ☑
        laceration S66.42- ☑
        specified type NEC S66.49- ☑
        strain S66.41- ☑
    toe (*see also* Injury, muscle, foot)
      extensor, long S96.10- ☑
        laceration S96.12- ☑
        specified type NEC S96.19- ☑
        strain S96.11- ☑
      flexor, long S96.00- ☑
        laceration S96.02- ☑
        specified type NEC S96.09- ☑
        strain S96.01- ☑
    triceps S46.30- ☑
      laceration S46.32- ☑
      specified type NEC S46.39- ☑
      strain S46.31- ☑
    wrist (and hand) level — *see* Injury, muscle, hand
  musculocutaneous nerve — *see* Injury, nerve, musculocutaneous
  myocardium — *see* Injury, heart
  nape — *see* Injury, neck
  nasal (septum) (sinus) S09.92 ☑
  nasopharynx S09.92 ☑
  neck S19.9 ☑
    specified NEC S19.80 ☑
      specified site NEC S19.89 ☑
  nerve NEC T14.8 ☑
    abdomen S34.9 ☑
      peripheral S34.6 ☑
      specified site NEC S34.8 ☑
    abducens S04.4- ☑
      contusion S04.4- ☑
      laceration S04.4- ☑
      specified type NEC S04.4- ☑
    abducent — *see* Injury, nerve, abducens
    accessory S04.7- ☑
      contusion S04.7- ☑
      laceration S04.7- ☑
      specified type NEC S04.7- ☑
    acoustic S04.6- ☑
      contusion S04.6- ☑
      laceration S04.6- ☑
      specified type NEC S04.6- ☑
    ankle S94.9- ☑
      cutaneous sensory S94.3- ☑
      specified site NEC — *see* subcategory S94.8 ☑
    anterior crural, femoral — *see* Injury, nerve, femoral
    arm (upper) S44.9- ☑
      axillary — *see* Injury, nerve, axillary
      cutaneous — *see* Injury, nerve, cutaneous, arm
      median — *see* Injury, nerve, median, upper arm
      musculocutaneous — *see* Injury, nerve, musculocutaneous
      radial — *see* Injury, nerve, radial, upper arm
      specified site NEC — *see* subcategory S44.8 ☑
      ulnar — *see* Injury, nerve, ulnar, arm
    auditory — *see* Injury, nerve, acoustic
    axillary S44.3- ☑
    brachial plexus — *see* Injury, brachial plexus
    cervical sympathetic S14.5 ☑
    cranial S04.9 ☑

Injury — *continued*
  nerve — *continued*
    cranial — *continued*
      contusion S04.9 ☑
      eighth (acoustic or auditory) — *see* Injury, nerve, acoustic
      eleventh (accessory) — *see* Injury, nerve, accessory
      fifth (trigeminal) — *see* Injury, nerve, trigeminal
      first (olfactory) — *see* Injury, nerve, olfactory
      fourth (trochlear) — *see* Injury, nerve, trochlear
      laceration S04.9 ☑
      ninth (glossopharyngeal) — *see* Injury, nerve, glossopharyngeal
      second (optic) — *see* Injury, nerve, optic
      seventh (facial) — *see* Injury, nerve, facial
      sixth (abducent) — *see* Injury, nerve, abducens
      specified
        nerve NEC S04.89- ☑
          contusion S04.89- ☑
          laceration S04.89- ☑
          specified type NEC S04.89- ☑
        type NEC S04.9 ☑
      tenth (pneumogastric or vagus) — *see* Injury, nerve, vagus
      third (oculomotor) — *see* Injury, nerve, oculomotor
      twelfth (hypoglossal) — *see* Injury, nerve, hypoglossal
    cutaneous sensory
      ankle (level) S94.3- ☑
      arm (upper) (level) S44.5- ☑
      foot (level) — *see* Injury, nerve, cutaneous sensory, ankle
      forearm (level) S54.3- ☑
      hip (level) S74.2- ☑
      leg (lower level) S84.2- ☑
      shoulder (level) — *see* Injury, nerve, cutaneous sensory, arm
      thigh (level) — *see* Injury, nerve, cutaneous sensory, hip
    deep peroneal — *see* Injury, nerve, peroneal, foot
    digital
      finger S64.4- ☑
        index S64.49- ☑
        little S64.49- ☑
        middle S64.49- ☑
        ring S64.49- ☑
      thumb S64.3- ☑
      toe — *see* Injury, nerve, ankle, specified site NEC
    eighth cranial (acoustic or auditory) — *see* Injury, nerve, acoustic
    eleventh cranial (accessory) — *see* Injury, nerve, accessory
    facial S04.5- ☑
      contusion S04.5- ☑
      laceration S04.5- ☑
      newborn P11.3
      specified type NEC S04.5- ☑
    femoral (hip level) (thigh level) S74.1- ☑
    fifth cranial (trigeminal) — *see* Injury, nerve, trigeminal
    finger (digital) — *see* Injury, nerve, digital, finger
    first cranial (olfactory) — *see* Injury, nerve, olfactory
    foot S94.9- ☑
      cutaneous sensory S94.3- ☑
      deep peroneal S94.2- ☑
      lateral plantar S94.0- ☑
      medial plantar S94.1- ☑
      specified site NEC — *see* subcategory S94.8 ☑
    forearm (level) S54.9- ☑
      cutaneous sensory — *see* Injury, nerve, cutaneous sensory, forearm
      median — *see* Injury, nerve, median
      radial — *see* Injury, nerve, radial
      specified site NEC — *see* subcategory S54.8 ☑
      ulnar — *see* Injury, nerve, ulnar
    fourth cranial (trochlear) — *see* Injury, nerve, trochlear
    glossopharyngeal S04.89- ☑
      specified type NEC S04.89- ☑
    hand S64.9- ☑
      median — *see* Injury, nerve, median, hand
      radial — *see* Injury, nerve, radial, hand
      specified NEC — *see* subcategory S64.8 ☑

Injury — *continued*
  nerve — *continued*
    hand — *continued*
      ulnar — *see* Injury, nerve, ulnar, hand
    hip (level) S74.9- ☑
      cutaneous sensory — *see* Injury, nerve, cutaneous sensory, hip
      femoral — *see* Injury, nerve, femoral
      sciatic — *see* Injury, nerve, sciatic
      specified site NEC — *see* subcategory S74.8 ☑
    hypoglossal S04.89- ☑
      specified type NEC S04.89- ☑
    lateral plantar S94.0- ☑
    leg (lower) S84.9- ☑
      cutaneous sensory — *see* Injury, nerve, cutaneous sensory, leg
      peroneal — *see* Injury, nerve, peroneal
      specified site NEC — *see* subcategory S84.8 ☑
      tibial — *see* Injury, nerve, tibial
      upper — *see* Injury, nerve, thigh
    lower
      back — *see* Injury, nerve, abdomen, specified site NEC
        peripheral — *see* Injury, nerve, abdomen, peripheral
      limb — *see* Injury, nerve, leg
    lumbar plexus — *see* Injury, nerve, lumbosacral, sympathetic
    lumbar spinal — *see* Injury, nerve, spinal, lumbar
    lumbosacral
      plexus — *see* Injury, nerve, lumbosacral, sympathetic
      sympathetic S34.5 ☑
    medial plantar S94.1- ☑
    median (forearm level) S54.1- ☑
      hand (level) S64.1- ☑
      upper arm (level) S44.1- ☑
      wrist (level) — *see* Injury, nerve, median, hand
    musculocutaneous S44.4- ☑
    musculospiral (upper arm level) — *see* Injury, nerve, radial, upper arm
    neck S14.9 ☑
      peripheral S14.4 ☑
      specified site NEC S14.8 ☑
      sympathetic S14.5 ☑
    ninth cranial (glossopharyngeal) — *see* Injury, nerve, glossopharyngeal
    oculomotor S04.1- ☑
      contusion S04.1- ☑
      laceration S04.1- ☑
      specified type NEC S04.1- ☑
    olfactory S04.81- ☑
      specified type NEC S04.81- ☑
    optic S04.01- ☑
      contusion S04.01- ☑
      laceration S04.01- ☑
      specified type NEC S04.01- ☑
    pelvic girdle — *see* Injury, nerve, hip
    pelvis — *see* Injury, nerve, abdomen, specified site NEC
      peripheral — *see* Injury, nerve, abdomen, peripheral
    peripheral NEC T14.8 ☑
      abdomen — *see* Injury, nerve, abdomen, peripheral
      lower back — *see* Injury, nerve, abdomen, peripheral
      neck — *see* Injury, nerve, neck, peripheral
      pelvis — *see* Injury, nerve, abdomen, peripheral
      specified NEC T14.8 ☑
    peroneal (lower leg level) S84.1- ☑
      foot S94.2- ☑
    plexus
      brachial — *see* Injury, brachial plexus
      celiac, coeliac — *see* Injury, nerve, lumbosacral, sympathetic
      mesenteric, inferior — *see* Injury, nerve, lumbosacral, sympathetic
      sacral — *see* Injury, lumbosacral plexus
      spinal
        brachial — *see* Injury, brachial plexus
        lumbosacral — *see* Injury, lumbosacral plexus
    pneumogastric — *see* Injury, nerve, vagus
    radial (forearm level) S54.2- ☑
      hand (level) S64.2- ☑

☑ **Additional Character Required — Refer to the Tabular List for Character Selection**   ▽ **Subterms under main terms may continue to next column or page**

Injury — continued
  nerve — continued
    radial — continued
      upper arm (level) S44.2- ☑
      wrist (level) — see Injury, nerve, radial, hand
    root — see Injury, nerve, spinal, root
    sacral plexus — see Injury, lumbosacral plexus
    sacral spinal — see Injury, nerve, spinal, sacral
    sciatic (hip level) (thigh level) S74.0- ☑
    second cranial (optic) — see Injury, nerve, optic
    seventh cranial (facial) — see Injury, nerve, facial
    shoulder — see Injury, nerve, arm
    sixth cranial (abducent) — see Injury, nerve, abducens
    spinal
      plexus — see Injury, nerve, plexus, spinal
      root
        cervical S14.2 ☑
        dorsal S24.2 ☑
        lumbar S34.21 ☑
        sacral S34.22 ☑
        thoracic — see Injury, nerve, spinal, root, dorsal
    splanchnic — see Injury, nerve, lumbosacral, sympathetic
    sympathetic NEC — see Injury, nerve, lumbosacral, sympathetic
      cervical — see Injury, nerve, cervical sympathetic
    tenth cranial (pneumogastric or vagus) — see Injury, nerve, vagus
    thigh (level) — see Injury, nerve, hip
      cutaneous sensory — see Injury, nerve, cutaneous sensory, hip
      femoral — see Injury, nerve, femoral
      sciatic — see Injury, nerve, sciatic
      specified NEC — see Injury, nerve, hip
    third cranial (oculomotor) — see Injury, nerve, oculomotor
    thorax S24.9 ☑
      peripheral S24.3 ☑
      specified site NEC S24.8 ☑
      sympathetic S24.4 ☑
    thumb, digital — see Injury, nerve, digital, thumb
    tibial (lower leg level) (posterior) S84.0- ☑
    toe — see Injury, nerve, ankle
    trigeminal S04.3- ☑
      contusion S04.3- ☑
      laceration S04.3- ☑
      specified type NEC S04.3- ☑
    trochlear S04.2- ☑
      contusion S04.2- ☑
      laceration S04.2- ☑
      specified type NEC S04.2- ☑
    twelfth cranial (hypoglossal) — see Injury, nerve, hypoglossal
    ulnar (forearm level) S54.0- ☑
      arm (upper) (level) S44.0- ☑
      hand (level) S64.0- ☑
      wrist (level) — see Injury, nerve, ulnar, hand
    vagus S04.89- ☑
      specified type NEC S04.89- ☑
    wrist (level) — see Injury, nerve, hand
  ninth cranial nerve (glossopharyngeal) — see Injury, nerve, glossopharyngeal
  nose (septum) S09.92 ☑
  obstetrical O71.9
    specified NEC O71.89
  occipital (region) (scalp) S09.90 ☑
    lobe — see Injury, intracranial
  optic chiasm S04.02 ☑
  optic radiation S04.03- ☑
  optic tract and pathways S04.03- ☑
  orbit, orbital (region) — see Injury, eye
    penetrating (with foreign body) — see Injury, eye, orbit, penetrating
    specified NEC — see Injury, eye, specified site NEC
  ovary, ovarian S37.409 ☑
    bilateral S37.402 ☑
      contusion S37.422 ☑
      laceration S37.432 ☑
      specified type NEC S37.492 ☑
    blood vessel — see Injury, blood vessel, ovarian
    contusion S37.429 ☑
      bilateral S37.422 ☑
      unilateral S37.421 ☑

Injury — continued
  ovary, ovarian — continued
    laceration S37.439 ☑
      bilateral S37.432 ☑
      unilateral S37.431 ☑
    specified type NEC S37.499 ☑
      bilateral S37.492 ☑
      unilateral S37.491 ☑
    unilateral S37.401 ☑
      contusion S37.421 ☑
      laceration S37.431 ☑
      specified type NEC S37.491 ☑
  palate (hard) (soft) S09.93 ☑
  pancreas S36.209 ☑
    body S36.201 ☑
      contusion S36.221 ☑
      laceration S36.231 ☑
        major S36.261 ☑
        minor S36.241 ☑
        moderate S36.251 ☑
      specified type NEC S36.291 ☑
    contusion S36.229 ☑
    head S36.200 ☑
      contusion S36.220 ☑
      laceration S36.230 ☑
        major S36.260 ☑
        minor S36.240 ☑
        moderate S36.250 ☑
      specified type NEC S36.290 ☑
    laceration S36.239 ☑
      major S36.269 ☑
      minor S36.249 ☑
      moderate S36.259 ☑
    specified type NEC S36.299 ☑
    tail S36.202 ☑
      contusion S36.222 ☑
      laceration S36.232 ☑
        major S36.262 ☑
        minor S36.242 ☑
        moderate S36.252 ☑
      specified type NEC S36.292 ☑
  parietal (region) (scalp) S09.90 ☑
    lobe — see Injury, intracranial
  patellar ligament (tendon) S76.10- ☑
    laceration S76.12- ☑
    specified NEC S76.19- ☑
    strain S76.11- ☑
  pelvis, pelvic (floor) S39.93 ☑
    complicating delivery O70.1
    joint or ligament, complicating delivery O71.6
    organ S37.90 ☑
      with ectopic or molar pregnancy O08.6
      complication of abortion — see Abortion
      contusion S37.92 ☑
      following ectopic or molar pregnancy O08.6
      laceration S37.93 ☑
      obstetrical trauma NEC O71.5
      specified
        site NEC S37.899 ☑
          contusion S37.892 ☑
          laceration S37.893 ☑
          specified type NEC S37.898 ☑
        type NEC S37.99 ☑
    specified NEC S39.83 ☑
  penis S39.94 ☑
  perineum S39.94 ☑
  peritoneum S36.81 ☑
    laceration S36.893 ☑
  periurethral tissue — see Injury, urethra
    complicating delivery O71.82
  phalanges
    foot — see Injury, foot
    hand — see Injury, hand
  pharynx NEC S19.85 ☑
  pleura — see Injury, intrathoracic, pleura
  plexus
    brachial — see Injury, brachial plexus
    cardiac — see Injury, nerve, thorax, sympathetic
    celiac, coeliac — see Injury, nerve, lumbosacral, sympathetic
    esophageal — see Injury, nerve, thorax, sympathetic
    hypogastric — see Injury, nerve, lumbosacral, sympathetic
    lumbar, lumbosacral — see Injury, lumbosacral plexus

Injury — continued
  plexus — continued
    mesenteric — see Injury, nerve, lumbosacral, sympathetic
    pulmonary — see Injury, nerve, thorax, sympathetic
  postcardiac surgery (syndrome) I97.0
  prepuce S39.94 ☑
  prostate S37.829 ☑
    contusion S37.822 ☑
    laceration S37.823 ☑
    specified type NEC S37.828 ☑
  pubic region S39.94 ☑
  pudendum S39.94 ☑
  pulmonary plexus — see Injury, nerve, thorax, sympathetic
  rectovaginal septum NEC S39.83 ☑
  rectum — see Injury, intestine, large, rectum
  retina — see Injury, eye, specified site NEC
    penetrating — see Injury, eyeball, penetrating
  retroperitoneal — see Injury, intra-abdominal, specified site NEC
  rotator cuff (muscle(s)) (tendon(s)) S46.00- ☑
    laceration S46.02- ☑
    specified type NEC S46.09- ☑
    strain S46.01- ☑
  round ligament — see Injury, pelvic organ, specified site NEC
  sacral plexus — see Injury, lumbosacral plexus
  salivary duct or gland S09.93 ☑
  scalp S09.90 ☑
    newborn (birth injury) P12.9
      due to monitoring (electrode) (sampling incision) P12.4
      specified NEC P12.89
        caput succedaneum P12.81
  scapular region — see Injury, shoulder
  sclera — see Injury, eye, specified site NEC
    penetrating — see Injury, eyeball, penetrating
  scrotum S39.94 ☑
  second cranial nerve (optic) — see Injury, nerve, optic
  seminal vesicle — see Injury, pelvic organ, specified site NEC
  seventh cranial nerve (facial) — see Injury, nerve, facial
  shoulder S49.9- ☑
    blood vessel — see Injury, blood vessel, arm
    contusion — see Contusion, shoulder
    dislocation — see Dislocation, shoulder
    fracture — see Fracture, shoulder
    muscle — see Injury, muscle, shoulder
    nerve — see Injury, nerve, shoulder
    open — see Wound, open, shoulder
    specified type NEC S49.8- ☑
    sprain — see Sprain, shoulder girdle
    superficial — see Injury, superficial, shoulder
  sinus
    cavernous — see Injury, intracranial
    nasal S09.92 ☑
  sixth cranial nerve (abducent) — see Injury, nerve, abducens
  skeleton, birth injury P13.9
    specified part NEC P13.8
  skin NEC T14.8 ☑
    surface intact — see Injury, superficial
  skull NEC S09.90 ☑
  specified NEC T14.8 ☑
  spermatic cord (pelvic region) S37.898 ☑
    scrotal region S39.848 ☑
  spinal (cord)
    cervical (neck) S14.109 ☑
      anterior cord syndrome S14.139 ☑
        C1 level S14.131 ☑
        C2 level S14.132 ☑
        C3 level S14.133 ☑
        C4 level S14.134 ☑
        C5 level S14.135 ☑
        C6 level S14.136 ☑
        C7 level S14.137 ☑
        C8 level S14.138 ☑
      Brown-Séquard syndrome S14.149 ☑
        C1 level S14.141 ☑
        C2 level S14.142 ☑
        C3 level S14.143 ☑
        C4 level S14.144 ☑
        C5 level S14.145 ☑
        C6 level S14.146 ☑

Index

Injury — Injury

Injury — continued
 spinal — continued
  cervical — continued
   Brown-Séquard syndrome — continued
    C7 level S14.147 ☑
    C8 level S14.148 ☑
   C1 level S14.101 ☑
   C2 level S14.102 ☑
   C3 level S14.103 ☑
   C4 level S14.104 ☑
   C5 level S14.105 ☑
   C6 level S14.106 ☑
   C7 level S14.107 ☑
   C8 level S14.108 ☑
   central cord syndrome S14.129 ☑
    C1 level S14.121 ☑
    C2 level S14.122 ☑
    C3 level S14.123 ☑
    C4 level S14.124 ☑
    C5 level S14.125 ☑
    C6 level S14.126 ☑
    C7 level S14.127 ☑
    C8 level S14.128 ☑
   complete lesion S14.119 ☑
    C1 level S14.111 ☑
    C2 level S14.112 ☑
    C3 level S14.113 ☑
    C4 level S14.114 ☑
    C5 level S14.115 ☑
    C6 level S14.116 ☑
    C7 level S14.117 ☑
    C8 level S14.118 ☑
   concussion S14.0 ☑
   edema S14.0 ☑
   incomplete lesion specified NEC S14.159 ☑
    C1 level S14.151 ☑
    C2 level S14.152 ☑
    C3 level S14.153 ☑
    C4 level S14.154 ☑
    C5 level S14.155 ☑
    C6 level S14.156 ☑
    C7 level S14.157 ☑
    C8 level S14.158 ☑
   posterior cord syndrome S14.159 ☑
    C1 level S14.151 ☑
    C2 level S14.152 ☑
    C3 level S14.153 ☑
    C4 level S14.154 ☑
    C5 level S14.155 ☑
    C6 level S14.156 ☑
    C7 level S14.157 ☑
    C8 level S14.158 ☑
  dorsal — see Injury, spinal, thoracic
  lumbar S34.109 ☑
   complete lesion S34.119 ☑
    L1 level S34.111 ☑
    L2 level S34.112 ☑
    L3 level S34.113 ☑
    L4 level S34.114 ☑
    L5 level S34.115 ☑
   concussion S34.01 ☑
   edema S34.01 ☑
   incomplete lesion S34.129 ☑
    L1 level S34.121 ☑
    L2 level S34.122 ☑
    L3 level S34.123 ☑
    L4 level S34.124 ☑
    L5 level S34.125 ☑
   L1 level S34.101 ☑
   L2 level S34.102 ☑
   L3 level S34.103 ☑
   L4 level S34.104 ☑
   L5 level S34.105 ☑
  nerve root NEC
   cervical — see Injury, nerve, spinal, root, cervical
   dorsal — see Injury, nerve, spinal, root, dorsal
   lumbar S34.21 ☑
   sacral S34.22 ☑
   thoracic — see Injury, nerve, spinal, root, dorsal
  plexus
   brachial — see Injury, brachial plexus
   lumbosacral — see Injury, lumbosacral plexus
  sacral S34.139 ☑
   complete lesion S34.131 ☑
   incomplete lesion S34.132 ☑

Injury — continued
 spinal — continued
  thoracic S24.109 ☑
   anterior cord syndrome S24.139 ☑
    T1 level S24.131 ☑
    T2-T6 level S24.132 ☑
    T7-T10 level S24.133 ☑
    T11-T12 level S24.134 ☑
   Brown-Séquard syndrome S24.149 ☑
    T1 level S24.141 ☑
    T2-T6 level S24.142 ☑
    T7-T10 level S24.143 ☑
    T11-T12 level S24.144 ☑
   complete lesion S24.119 ☑
    T1 level S24.111 ☑
    T2-T6 level S24.112 ☑
    T7-T10 level S24.113 ☑
    T11-T12 level S24.114 ☑
   concussion S24.0 ☑
   edema S24.0 ☑
   incomplete lesion specified NEC S24.159 ☑
    T1 level S24.151 ☑
    T2-T6 level S24.152 ☑
    T7-T10 level S24.153 ☑
    T11-T12 level S24.154 ☑
   posterior cord syndrome S24.159 ☑
    T1 level S24.151 ☑
    T2-T6 level S24.152 ☑
    T7-T10 level S24.153 ☑
    T11-T12 level S24.154 ☑
   T1 level S24.101 ☑
   T2-T6 level S24.102 ☑
   T7-T10 level S24.103 ☑
   T11-T12 level S24.104 ☑
  splanchnic nerve — see Injury, nerve, lumbosacral, sympathetic
  spleen S36.00 ☑
   contusion S36.029 ☑
    major S36.021 ☑
    minor S36.020 ☑
   laceration S36.039 ☑
    major (massive) (stellate) S36.032 ☑
    moderate S36.031 ☑
    superficial (capsular) (minor) S36.030 ☑
   specified type NEC S36.09 ☑
  splenic artery — see Injury, blood vessel, celiac artery, branch
  stellate ganglion — see Injury, nerve, thorax, sympathetic
  sternal region S29.9 ☑
  stomach S36.30 ☑
   contusion S36.32 ☑
   laceration S36.33 ☑
   specified type NEC S36.39 ☑
  subconjunctival — see Injury, eye, conjunctiva
  subcutaneous NEC T14.8 ☑
  submaxillary region S09.93 ☑
  submental region S09.93 ☑
  subungual
   fingers — see Injury, hand
   toes — see Injury, foot
  superficial NEC T14.8 ☑
   abdomen, abdominal (wall) S30.92 ☑
    abrasion S30.811 ☑
    bite S30.871 ☑
     insect S30.861 ☑
    contusion S30.1 ☑
    external constriction S30.841 ☑
    foreign body S30.851 ☑
   abrasion — see Abrasion, by site
   adnexa, eye NEC — see Injury, eye, specified site NEC
   alveolar process — see Injury, superficial, oral cavity
   ankle S90.91- ☑
    abrasion — see Abrasion, ankle
    bite — see Bite, ankle
    blister — see Blister, ankle
    contusion — see Contusion, ankle
    external constriction — see Constriction, external, ankle
    foreign body — see Foreign body, superficial, ankle
   anus S30.98 ☑
   arm (upper) S40.92- ☑
    abrasion — see Abrasion, arm

Injury — continued
 superficial — continued
  arm — continued
   bite — see Bite, superficial, arm
   blister — see Blister, arm (upper)
   contusion — see Contusion, arm
   external constriction — see Constriction, external, arm
   foreign body — see Foreign body, superficial, arm
  auditory canal (external) (meatus) — see Injury, superficial, ear
  auricle — see Injury, superficial, ear
  axilla — see Injury, superficial, arm
  back (see also Injury, superficial, thorax, back)
   lower S30.91 ☑
    abrasion S30.810 ☑
    contusion S30.0 ☑
    external constriction S30.840 ☑
    superficial
     bite NEC S30.870 ☑
      insect S30.860 ☑
     foreign body S30.850 ☑
  bite NEC — see Bite, superficial NEC, by site
  blister — see Blister, by site
  breast S20.10- ☑
   abrasion — see Abrasion, breast
   bite — see Bite, superficial, breast
   contusion — see Contusion, breast
   external constriction — see Constriction, external, breast
   foreign body — see Foreign body, superficial, breast
  brow — see Injury, superficial, head, specified NEC
  buttock S30.91 ☑
  calf — see Injury, superficial, leg
  canthus, eye — see Injury, superficial, periocular area
  cheek (external) — see Injury, superficial, head, specified NEC
   internal — see Injury, superficial, oral cavity
  chest wall — see Injury, superficial, thorax
  chin — see Injury, superficial, head NEC
  clitoris S30.95 ☑
  conjunctiva — see Injury, eye, conjunctiva
   with foreign body (in conjunctival sac) — see Foreign body, conjunctival sac
  contusion — see Contusion, by site
  costal region — see Injury, superficial, thorax
  digit(s)
   hand — see Injury, superficial, finger
  ear (auricle) (canal) (external) S00.40- ☑
   abrasion — see Abrasion, ear
   bite — see Bite, superficial, ear
   contusion — see Contusion, ear
   external constriction — see Constriction, external, ear
   foreign body — see Foreign body, superficial, ear
  elbow S50.90- ☑
   abrasion — see Abrasion, elbow
   bite — see Bite, superficial, elbow
   blister — see Blister, elbow
   contusion — see Contusion, elbow
   external constriction — see Constriction, external, elbow
   foreign body — see Foreign body, superficial, elbow
  epididymis S30.94 ☑
  epigastric region S30.92 ☑
  epiglottis — see Injury, superficial, throat
  esophagus
   cervical — see Injury, superficial, throat
  external constriction — see Constriction, external, by site
  extremity NEC T14.8 ☑
  eyeball NEC — see Injury, eye, specified site NEC
  eyebrow — see Injury, superficial, periocular area
  eyelid S00.20- ☑
   abrasion — see Abrasion, eyelid
   bite — see Bite, superficial, eyelid
   contusion — see Contusion, eyelid
   external constriction — see Constriction, external, eyelid
   foreign body — see Foreign body, superficial, eyelid

☑ Additional Character Required — Refer to the Tabular List for Character Selection   ⬝ Subterms under main terms may continue to next column or page

Injury — *continued*
  superficial — *continued*
    face NEC — *see* Injury, superficial, head, specified NEC
    finger(s) S60.949 ☑
      abrasion — *see* Abrasion, finger
      bite — *see* Bite, superficial, finger
      blister — *see* Blister, finger
      contusion — *see* Contusion, finger
      external constriction — *see* Constriction, external, finger
      foreign body — *see* Foreign body, superficial, finger
      index S60.94- ☑
      insect bite — *see* Bite, by site, superficial, insect
      little S60.94- ☑
      middle S60.94- ☑
      ring S60.94- ☑
    flank S30.92 ☑
    foot S90.92- ☑
      abrasion — *see* Abrasion, foot
      bite — *see* Bite, foot
      blister — *see* Blister, foot
      contusion — *see* Contusion, foot
      external constriction — *see* Constriction, external, foot
      foreign body — *see* Foreign body, superficial, foot
    forearm S50.91- ☑
      abrasion — *see* Abrasion, forearm
      bite — *see* Bite, forearm, superficial
      blister — *see* Blister, forearm
      contusion — *see* Contusion, forearm
      elbow only — *see* Injury, superficial, elbow
      external constriction — *see* Constriction, external, forearm
      foreign body — *see* Foreign body, superficial, forearm
    forehead — *see* Injury, superficial, head NEC
    foreign body — *see* Foreign body, superficial
    genital organs, external
      female S30.97 ☑
      male S30.96 ☑
    globe (eye) — *see* Injury, eye, specified site NEC
    groin S30.92 ☑
    gum — *see* Injury, superficial, oral cavity
    hand S60.92- ☑
      abrasion — *see* Abrasion, hand
      bite — *see* Bite, superficial, hand
      contusion — *see* Contusion, hand
      external constriction — *see* Constriction, external, hand
      foreign body — *see* Foreign body, superficial, hand
    head S00.90 ☑
      ear — *see* Injury, superficial, ear
      eyelid — *see* Injury, superficial, eyelid
      nose S00.30 ☑
      oral cavity S00.502 ☑
      scalp S00.00 ☑
      specified site NEC S00.80 ☑
    heel — *see* Injury, superficial, foot
    hip S70.91- ☑
      abrasion — *see* Abrasion, hip
      bite — *see* Bite, superficial, hip
      blister — *see* Blister, hip
      contusion — *see* Contusion, hip
      external constriction — *see* Constriction, external, hip
      foreign body — *see* Foreign body, superficial, hip
    iliac region — *see* Injury, superficial, abdomen
    inguinal region — *see* Injury, superficial, abdomen
    insect bite — *see* Bite, by site, superficial, insect
    interscapular region — *see* Injury, superficial, thorax, back
    jaw — *see* Injury, superficial, head, specified NEC
    knee S80.91- ☑
      abrasion — *see* Abrasion, knee
      bite — *see* Bite, superficial, knee
      blister — *see* Blister, knee
      contusion — *see* Contusion, knee
      external constriction — *see* Constriction, external, knee
      foreign body — *see* Foreign body, superficial, knee

Injury — *continued*
  superficial — *continued*
    labium (majus) (minus) S30.95 ☑
    lacrimal (apparatus) (gland) (sac) — *see* Injury, eye, specified site NEC
    larynx — *see* Injury, superficial, throat
    leg (lower) S80.92- ☑
      abrasion — *see* Abrasion, leg
      bite — *see* Bite, superficial, leg
      contusion — *see* Contusion, leg
      external constriction — *see* Constriction, external, leg
      foreign body — *see* Foreign body, superficial, leg
      knee — *see* Injury, superficial, knee
    limb NEC T14.8 ☑
    lip S00.501 ☑
    lower back S30.91 ☑
    lumbar region S30.91 ☑
    malar region — *see* Injury, superficial, head, specified NEC
    mammary — *see* Injury, superficial, breast
    mastoid region — *see* Injury, superficial, head, specified NEC
    mouth — *see* Injury, superficial, oral cavity
    muscle NEC T14.8 ☑
    nail NEC T14.8 ☑
      finger — *see* Injury, superficial, finger
      toe — *see* Injury, superficial, toe
    nasal (septum) — *see* Injury, superficial, nose
    neck S10.90 ☑
      specified site NEC S10.80 ☑
    nose (septum) S00.30 ☑
    occipital region — *see* Injury, superficial, scalp
    oral cavity S00.502 ☑
    orbital region — *see* Injury, superficial, periocular area
    palate — *see* Injury, superficial, oral cavity
    palm — *see* Injury, superficial, hand
    parietal region — *see* Injury, superficial, scalp
    pelvis S30.91 ☑
      girdle — *see* Injury, superficial, hip
    penis S30.93 ☑
    perineum
      female S30.95 ☑
      male S30.91 ☑
    periocular area S00.20- ☑
      abrasion — *see* Abrasion, eyelid
      bite — *see* Bite, superficial, eyelid
      contusion — *see* Contusion, eyelid
      external constriction — *see* Constriction, external, eyelid
      foreign body — *see* Foreign body, superficial, eyelid
    phalanges
      finger — *see* Injury, superficial, finger
      toe — *see* Injury, superficial, toe
    pharynx — *see* Injury, superficial, throat
    pinna — *see* Injury, superficial, ear
    popliteal space — *see* Injury, superficial, knee
    prepuce S30.93 ☑
    pubic region S30.91 ☑
    pudendum
      female S30.97 ☑
      male S30.96 ☑
    sacral region S30.91 ☑
    scalp S00.00 ☑
    scapular region — *see* Injury, superficial, shoulder
    sclera — *see* Injury, eye, specified site NEC
    scrotum S30.94 ☑
    shin — *see* Injury, superficial, leg
    shoulder S40.91- ☑
      abrasion — *see* Abrasion, shoulder
      bite — *see* Bite, superficial, shoulder
      blister — *see* Blister, shoulder
      contusion — *see* Contusion, shoulder
      external constriction — *see* Constriction, external, shoulder
      foreign body — *see* Foreign body, superficial, shoulder
    skin NEC T14.8 ☑
    sternal region — *see* Injury, superficial, thorax, front
    subconjunctival — *see* Injury, eye, specified site NEC
    subcutaneous NEC T14.8 ☑

Injury — *continued*
  superficial — *continued*
    submaxillary region — *see* Injury, superficial, head, specified NEC
    submental region — *see* Injury, superficial, head, specified NEC
    subungual
      finger(s) — *see* Injury, superficial, finger
      toe(s) — *see* Injury, superficial, toe
    supraclavicular fossa — *see* Injury, superficial, neck
    supraorbital — *see* Injury, superficial, head, specified NEC
    temple — *see* Injury, superficial, head, specified NEC
    temporal region — *see* Injury, superficial, head, specified NEC
    testis S30.94 ☑
    thigh S70.92- ☑
      abrasion — *see* Abrasion, thigh
      bite — *see* Bite, superficial, thigh
      blister — *see* Blister, thigh
      contusion — *see* Contusion, thigh
      external constriction — *see* Constriction, external, thigh
      foreign body — *see* Foreign body, superficial, thigh
    thorax, thoracic (wall) S20.90 ☑
      abrasion — *see* Abrasion, thorax
      back S20.40- ☑
      bite — *see* Bite, thorax, superficial
      blister — *see* Blister, thorax
      contusion — *see* Contusion, thorax
      external constriction — *see* Constriction, external, thorax
      foreign body — *see* Foreign body, superficial, thorax
      front S20.30- ☑
    throat S10.10 ☑
      abrasion S10.11 ☑
      bite S10.17 ☑
        insect S10.16 ☑
      blister S10.12 ☑
      contusion S10.0 ☑
      external constriction S10.14 ☑
      foreign body S10.15 ☑
    thumb S60.93- ☑
      abrasion — *see* Abrasion, thumb
      bite — *see* Bite, superficial, thumb
      blister — *see* Blister, thumb
      contusion — *see* Contusion, thumb
      external constriction — *see* Constriction, external, thumb
      foreign body — *see* Foreign body, superficial, thumb
      insect bite — *see* Bite, by site, superficial, insect
      specified type NEC S60.39 ☑
    toe(s) S90.93- ☑
      abrasion — *see* Abrasion, toe
      bite — *see* Bite, toe
      blister — *see* Blister, toe
      contusion — *see* Contusion, toe
      external constriction — *see* Constriction, external, toe
      foreign body — *see* Foreign body, superficial, toe
      great S90.93- ☑
    tongue — *see* Injury, superficial, oral cavity
    tooth, teeth — *see* Injury, superficial, oral cavity
    trachea S10.10 ☑
    tunica vaginalis S30.94 ☑
    tympanum, tympanic membrane — *see* Injury, superficial, ear
    uvula — *see* Injury, superficial, oral cavity
    vagina S30.95 ☑
    vocal cords — *see* Injury, superficial, throat
    vulva S30.95 ☑
    wrist S60.91- ☑
  supraclavicular region — *see* Injury, neck
  supraorbital S09.93 ☑
  suprarenal gland (multiple) — *see* Injury, adrenal
  surgical complication (external or internal site) — *see* Laceration, accidental complicating surgery
  temple S09.90 ☑
  temporal region S09.90 ☑
  tendon (*see also* Injury, muscle, by site)
    abdomen — *see* Injury, muscle, abdomen

⟁ **Subterms under main terms may continue to next column or page**   ☑ **Additional Character Required — Refer to the Tabular List for Character Selection**   **199**

Injury — Injury

Injury — *continued*
  tendon (*see also* Injury, muscle, by site) — *continued*
    Achilles — *see* Injury, Achilles tendon
    lower back — *see* Injury, muscle, lower back
    pelvic organs — *see* Injury, muscle, pelvis
  tenth cranial nerve (pneumogastric or vagus) — *see* Injury, nerve, vagus
  testis S39.94 ☑
  thigh S79.92- ☑
    blood vessel — *see* Injury, blood vessel, hip
    contusion — *see* Contusion, thigh
    fracture — *see* Fracture, femur
    muscle — *see* Injury, muscle, thigh
    nerve — *see* Injury, nerve, thigh
    open — *see* Wound, open, thigh
    specified NEC S79.82- ☑
    superficial — *see* Injury, superficial, thigh
  third cranial nerve (oculomotor) — *see* Injury, nerve, oculomotor
  thorax, thoracic S29.9 ☑
    blood vessel — *see* Injury, blood vessel, thorax
    cavity — *see* Injury, intrathoracic
    dislocation — *see* Dislocation, thorax
    external (wall) S29.9 ☑
      contusion — *see* Contusion, thorax
      nerve — *see* Injury, nerve, thorax
      open — *see* Wound, open, thorax
      specified NEC S29.8 ☑
      sprain — *see* Sprain, thorax
      superficial — *see* Injury, superficial, thorax
    fracture — *see* Fracture, thorax
    internal — *see* Injury, intrathoracic
    intrathoracic organ — *see* Injury, intrathoracic
    sympathetic ganglion — *see* Injury, nerve, thorax, sympathetic
  throat (*see also* Injury, neck) S19.9 ☑
  thumb S69.9- ☑
    blood vessel — *see* Injury, blood vessel, thumb
    contusion — *see* Contusion, thumb
    dislocation — *see* Dislocation, thumb
    fracture — *see* Fracture, thumb
    muscle — *see* Injury, muscle, thumb
    nerve — *see* Injury, nerve, digital, thumb
    open — *see* Wound, open, thumb
    specified NEC S69.8- ☑
    sprain — *see* Sprain, thumb
    superficial — *see* Injury, superficial, thumb
  thymus (gland) — *see* Injury, intrathoracic, specified organ NEC
  thyroid (gland) NEC S19.84 ☑
  toe S99.92- ☑
    contusion — *see* Contusion, toe
    dislocation — *see* Dislocation, toe
    fracture — *see* Fracture, toe
    muscle — *see* Injury, muscle, toe
    open — *see* Wound, open, toe
    specified type NEC S99.82- ☑
    sprain — *see* Sprain, toe
    superficial — *see* Injury, superficial, toe
  tongue S09.93 ☑
  tonsil S09.93 ☑
  tooth S09.93 ☑
  trachea (cervical) NEC S19.82 ☑
    thoracic — *see* Injury, intrathoracic, trachea, thoracic
  transfusion-related acute lung (TRALI) J95.84
  tunica vaginalis S39.94 ☑
  twelfth cranial nerve (hypoglossal) — *see* Injury, nerve, hypoglossal
  ureter S37.10 ☑
    contusion S37.12 ☑
    laceration S37.13 ☑
    specified type NEC S37.19 ☑
  urethra (sphincter) S37.30 ☑
    at delivery O71.5
    contusion S37.32 ☑
    laceration S37.33 ☑
    specified type NEC S37.39 ☑
  urinary organ S37.90 ☑
    contusion S37.92 ☑
    laceration S37.93 ☑
    specified
      site NEC S37.899 ☑
        contusion S37.892 ☑
        laceration S37.893 ☑

Injury — *continued*
  urinary organ — *continued*
    specified — *continued*
      site — *continued*
        specified type NEC S37.898 ☑
      type NEC S37.99 ☑
  uterus, uterine S37.60 ☑
    with ectopic or molar pregnancy O08.6
    blood vessel — *see* Injury, blood vessel, iliac
    contusion S37.62 ☑
    laceration S37.63 ☑
      cervix at delivery O71.3
    rupture associated with obstetrics — *see* Rupture, uterus
    specified type NEC S37.69 ☑
  uvula S09.93 ☑
  vagina S39.93 ☑
    abrasion S30.814 ☑
    bite S31.45 ☑
      insect S30.864 ☑
      superficial NEC S30.874 ☑
    contusion S30.23 ☑
    crush S38.03 ☑
    during delivery — *see* Laceration, vagina, during delivery
    external constriction S30.844 ☑
    insect bite S30.864 ☑
    laceration S31.41 ☑
      with foreign body S31.42 ☑
    open wound S31.40 ☑
    puncture S31.43 ☑
      with foreign body S31.44 ☑
    superficial S30.95 ☑
      foreign body S30.854 ☑
  vas deferens — *see* Injury, pelvic organ, specified site NEC
  vascular NEC T14.8 ☑
  vein — *see* Injury, blood vessel
  vena cava (superior) S25.20 ☑
    inferior S35.10 ☑
      laceration (minor) (superficial) S35.11 ☑
        major S35.12 ☑
      specified type NEC S35.19 ☑
    laceration (minor) (superficial) S25.21 ☑
      major S25.22 ☑
    specified type NEC S25.29 ☑
  vesical (sphincter) — *see* Injury, bladder
  visual cortex S04.04- ☑
  vitreous (humor) S05.90 ☑
    specified NEC S05.8X- ☑
  vocal cord NEC S19.83 ☑
  vulva S39.94 ☑
    abrasion S30.814 ☑
    bite S31.45 ☑
      insect S30.864 ☑
      superficial NEC S30.874 ☑
    contusion S30.23 ☑
    crush S38.03 ☑
    during delivery — *see* Laceration, perineum, female, during delivery
    external constriction S30.844 ☑
    insect bite S30.864 ☑
    laceration S31.41 ☑
      with foreign body S31.42 ☑
    open wound S31.40 ☑
    puncture S31.43 ☑
      with foreign body S31.44 ☑
    superficial S30.95 ☑
      foreign body S30.854 ☑
  whiplash (cervical spine) S13.4 ☑
  wrist S69.9- ☑
    blood vessel — *see* Injury, blood vessel, hand
    contusion — *see* Contusion, wrist
    dislocation — *see* Dislocation, wrist
    fracture — *see* Fracture, wrist
    muscle — *see* Injury, muscle, hand
    nerve — *see* Injury, nerve, hand
    open — *see* Wound, open, wrist
    specified NEC S69.8- ☑
    sprain — *see* Sprain, wrist
    superficial — *see* Injury, superficial, wrist
Inoculation (*see also* Vaccination)
  complication or reaction — *see* Complications, vaccination
Insanity, insane (*see also* Psychosis)
  adolescent — *see* Schizophrenia

Insanity, insane — *continued*
  confusional F28
    acute or subacute F05
  delusional F22
  senile F03 ☑
Insect
  bite — *see* Bite, by site, superficial, insect
  venomous, poisoning NEC (by) — *see* Venom, arthropod
Insensitivity
  adrenocorticotropin hormone (ACTH) E27.49
  androgen E34.50
    complete E34.51
    partial E34.52
Insertion
  cord (umbilical) lateral or velamentous O43.12- ☑
  intrauterine contraceptive device (encounter for) — *see* Intrauterine contraceptive device
Insolation (sunstroke) T67.0 ☑
Insomnia (organic) G47.00
  without objective findings F51.02
  adjustment F51.02
  adjustment disorder F51.02
  behavioral, of childhood Z73.819
    combined type Z73.812
    limit setting type Z73.811
    sleep-onset association type Z73.810
  childhood Z73.819
  chronic F51.04
    somatized tension F51.04
  conditioned F51.04
  due to
    alcohol
      abuse F10.182
      dependence F10.282
      use F10.982
    amphetamines
      abuse F15.182
      dependence F15.282
      use F15.982
    anxiety disorder F51.05
    caffeine
      abuse F15.182
      dependence F15.282
      use F15.982
    cocaine
      abuse F14.182
      dependence F14.282
      use F14.982
    depression F51.05
    drug NEC
      abuse F19.182
      dependence F19.282
      use F19.982
    medical condition G47.01
    mental disorder NEC F51.05
    opioid
      abuse F11.182
      dependence F11.282
      use F11.982
    psychoactive substance NEC
      abuse F19.182
      dependence F19.182
      use F19.982
    sedative, hypnotic, or anxiolytic
      abuse F13.182
      dependence F13.282
      use F13.982
    stimulant NEC
      abuse F15.182
      dependence F15.282
      use F15.982
  fatal familial (FFI) A81.83
  idiopathic F51.01
  learned F51.3
  nonorganic origin F51.01
  not due to a substance or known physiological condition F51.01
    specified NEC F51.09
  paradoxical F51.03
  primary F51.01
  psychiatric F51.05
  psychophysiologic F51.04
  related to psychopathology F51.05
  short-term F51.02
  specified NEC G47.09
  stress-related F51.02
  transient F51.02

☑ **Additional Character Required** — Refer to the Tabular List for Character Selection   ▽ Subterms under main terms may continue to next column or page

Inspiration
  food or foreign body — *see* Foreign body, by site
  mucus — *see* Asphyxia, mucus
Inspissated bile syndrome (newborn) P59.1
Instability
  emotional (excessive) F60.3
  joint (post-traumatic) M25.30
    ankle M25.37- ☑
    due to old ligament injury — *see* Disorder, liga-
      ment
    elbow M25.32- ☑
    flail — *see* Flail, joint
    foot M25.37- ☑
    hand M25.34- ☑
    hip M25.35- ☑
    knee M25.36- ☑
    lumbosacral — *see* subcategory M53.2 ☑
    prosthesis — *see* Complications, joint prosthesis,
      mechanical, displacement, by site
    sacroiliac — *see* subcategory M53.2 ☑
    secondary to
      old ligament injury — *see* Disorder, ligament
      removal of joint prosthesis M96.89
    shoulder (region) M25.31- ☑
    spine — *see* subcategory M53.2 ☑
    wrist M25.33- ☑
  knee (chronic) M23.5- ☑
  lumbosacral — *see* subcategory M53.2 ☑
  nervous F48.8
  personality (emotional) F60.3
  spine — *see* Instability, joint, spine
  vasomotor R55
Institutional syndrome (childhood) F94.2
Institutionalization, affecting child Z62.22
  disinhibited attachment F94.2
Insufficiency, insufficient
  accommodation, old age H52.4
  adrenal (gland) E27.40
    primary E27.1
  adrenocortical E27.40
    drug-induced E27.3
    iatrogenic E27.3
    primary E27.1
  anatomic crown height K08.89
  anterior (occlusal) guidance M26.54
  anus K62.89
  aortic (valve) I35.1
    with
      mitral (valve) disease I08.0
        with tricuspid (valve) disease I08.3
      stenosis I35.2
      tricuspid (valve) disease I08.2
        with mitral (valve) disease I08.3
    congenital Q23.1
    rheumatic I06.1
      with
        mitral (valve) disease I08.0
          with tricuspid (valve) disease I08.3
        stenosis I06.2
          with mitral (valve) disease I08.0
            with tricuspid (valve) disease I08.3
        tricuspid (valve) disease I08.2
          with mitral (valve) disease I08.3
    specified cause NEC I35.1
    syphilitic A52.03
  arterial I77.1
    basilar G45.0
    carotid (hemispheric) G45.1
    cerebral I67.81
    coronary (acute or subacute) I24.8
    mesenteric K55.1
    peripheral I73.9
    precerebral (multiple) (bilateral) G45.2
    vertebral G45.0
  arteriovenous I99.8
  biliary K83.8
  cardiac (*see also* Insufficiency, myocardial)
    due to presence of (cardiac) prosthesis I97.11- ☑
      postprocedural I97.11- ☑
  cardiorenal, hypertensive I13.2
  cardiovascular — *see* Disease, cardiovascular
  cerebrovascular (acute) I67.81
    with transient focal neurological signs and symp-
      toms G45.8
  circulatory NEC I99.8
    newborn P29.89
  clinical crown length K08.89
  convergence H51.11

Insufficiency, insufficient — *continued*
  coronary (acute or subacute) I24.8
    chronic or with a stated duration of over 4 weeks
      I25.89
  corticoadrenal E27.40
    primary E27.1
  dietary E63.9
  divergence H51.8
  food T73.0 ☑
  gastroesophageal K22.8
  gonadal
    ovary E28.39
    testis E29.1
  heart (*see also* Insufficiency, myocardial)
    newborn P29.0
    valve — *see* Endocarditis
  hepatic — *see* Failure, hepatic
  idiopathic autonomic G90.09
  interocclusal distance of fully erupted teeth (ridge)
    M26.36
  kidney N28.9
    acute N28.9
    chronic N18.9
  lacrimal (secretion) H04.12- ☑
    passages — *see* Stenosis, lacrimal
  liver — *see* Failure, hepatic
  lung — *see* Insufficiency, pulmonary
  mental (congenital) — *see* Disability, intellectual
  mesenteric K55.1
  mitral (valve) I34.0
    with
      aortic valve disease I08.0
        with tricuspid (valve) disease I08.3
      obstruction or stenosis I05.2
        with aortic valve disease I08.0
      tricuspid (valve) disease I08.1
        with aortic (valve) disease I08.3
    congenital Q23.3
    rheumatic I05.1
      with
        aortic valve disease I08.0
          with tricuspid (valve) disease I08.3
        obstruction or stenosis I05.2
          with aortic valve disease I08.0
            with tricuspid (valve) disease I08.3
        tricuspid (valve) disease I08.1
          with aortic (valve) disease I08.3
    active or acute I01.1
      with chorea, rheumatic (Sydenham's) I02.0
    specified cause, except rheumatic I34.0
  muscle (*see also* Disease, muscle)
    heart — *see* Insufficiency, myocardial
    ocular NEC H50.9
  myocardial, myocardium (with arteriosclerosis) (*see*
    also Failure, heart) I50.9
    with
      rheumatic fever (conditions in I00) I09.0
        active, acute or subacute I01.2
          with chorea I02.0
        inactive or quiescent (with chorea) I09.0
    congenital Q24.8
    hypertensive — *see* Hypertension, heart
    newborn P29.0
    rheumatic I09.0
      active, acute, or subacute I01.2
    syphilitic A52.06
  nourishment T73.0 ☑
  pancreatic K86.89
    exocrine K86.81
  parathyroid (gland) E20.9
  peripheral vascular (arterial) I73.9
  pituitary E23.0
  placental (mother) O36.51- ☑
  platelets D69.6
  prenatal care affecting management of pregnancy
    O09.3- ☑
  progressive pluriglandular E31.0
  pulmonary J98.4
    acute, following surgery (nonthoracic) J95.2
      thoracic J95.1
    chronic, following surgery J95.3
    following
      shock J98.4
      trauma J98.4
    newborn P28.5
    valve I37.1
      with stenosis I37.2
      congenital Q22.2

Insufficiency, insufficient — *continued*
  pulmonary — *continued*
    valve — *continued*
      rheumatic I09.89
        with aortic, mitral or tricuspid (valve) disease
          I08.8
  pyloric K31.89
  renal (acute) N28.9
    chronic N18.9
  respiratory R06.89
    newborn P28.5
  rotation — *see* Malrotation
  sleep syndrome F51.12
  social insurance Z59.7
  suprarenal E27.40
    primary E27.1
  tarso-orbital fascia, congenital Q10.3
  testis E29.1
  thyroid (gland) (acquired) E03.9
    congenital E03.1
  tricuspid (valve) (rheumatic) I07.1
    with
      aortic (valve) disease I08.2
        with mitral (valve) disease I08.3
      mitral (valve) disease I08.1
        with aortic (valve) disease I08.3
      obstruction or stenosis I07.2
        with aortic (valve) disease I08.2
          with mitral (valve) disease I08.3
    congenital Q22.8
    nonrheumatic I36.1
      with stenosis I36.2
  urethral sphincter R32
  valve, valvular (heart) I38
    aortic — *see* Insufficiency, aortic (valve)
    congenital Q24.8
    mitral — *see* Insufficiency, mitral (valve)
    pulmonary — *see* Insufficiency, pulmonary, valve
    tricuspid — *see* Insufficiency, tricuspid (valve)
  vascular I99.8
    intestine K55.9
      acute (*see also* Ischemia, intestine, acute)
        K55.059
    mesenteric K55.1
    peripheral I73.9
    renal — *see* Hypertension, kidney
  velopharyngeal
    acquired K13.79
    congenital Q38.8
  venous (chronic) (peripheral) I87.2
  ventricular — *see* Insufficiency, myocardial
  welfare support Z59.7
Insufflation, fallopian Z31.41
Insular — *see* condition
Insulinoma
  pancreas
    benign D13.7
    malignant C25.4
    uncertain behavior D37.8
  specified site
    benign — *see* Neoplasm, by site, benign
    malignant — *see* Neoplasm, by site, malignant
    uncertain behavior — *see* Neoplasm, by site, uncer-
      tain behavior
  unspecified site
    benign D13.7
    malignant C25.4
    uncertain behavior D37.8
Insuloma — *see* Insulinoma
Interference
  balancing side M26.56
  non-working side M26.56
Intermenstrual — *see* condition
Intermittent — *see* condition
Internal — *see* condition
Interrogation
  cardiac defibrillator (automatic) (implantable) Z45.02
  cardiac pacemaker Z45.018
  cardiac (event) (loop) recorder Z45.09
  infusion pump (implanted) (intrathecal) Z45.1
  neurostimulator Z46.2
Interruption
  aortic arch Q25.21
  bundle of His I44.30
  phase-shift, sleep cycle — *see* Disorder, sleep, circadian
    rhythm
  sleep phase-shift, or 24 hour sleep-wake cycle — *see*
    Disorder, sleep, circadian rhythm

Index

Interstitial — *see* condition
Intertrigo L30.4
  labialis K13.0
Intervertebral disc — *see* condition
Intestine, intestinal — *see* condition
Intolerance
  carbohydrate K90.49
  disaccharide, hereditary E73.0
  fat NEC K90.49
    pancreatic K90.3
  food K90.49
    dietary counseling and surveillance Z71.3
  fructose E74.10
    hereditary E74.12
  glucose (-galactose) E74.39
  gluten K90.41
  lactose E73.9
    specified NEC E73.8
  lysine E72.3
  milk NEC K90.49
    lactose E73.9
  protein K90.49
  starch NEC K90.49
  sucrose (-isomaltose) E74.31
Intoxicated NEC (without dependence) — *see* Alcohol, intoxication
Intoxication
  acid E87.2
  alcoholic (acute) (without dependence) — *see* Alcohol, intoxication
  alimentary canal K52.1
  amphetamine (without dependence) — *see* Abuse, drug, stimulant, with intoxication
    with dependence — *see* Dependence, drug, stimulant, with intoxication
  anxiolytic (acute) (without dependence) — *see* Abuse, drug, sedative, with intoxication
    with dependence — *see* Dependence, drug, sedative, with intoxication
  caffeine F15.929
    with dependence — *see* Dependence, drug, stimulant, with intoxication
  cannabinoids (acute) (without dependence) — *see* Use, cannabis, with intoxication
    with
      abuse — *see* Abuse, drug, cannabis, with intoxication
      dependence — *see* Dependence, drug, cannabis, with intoxication
  chemical — *see* Table of Drugs and Chemicals
    via placenta or breast milk — *see* - Absorption, chemical, through placenta
  cocaine (acute) (without dependence) — *see* Abuse, drug, cocaine, with intoxication
    with dependence — *see* Dependence, drug, cocaine, with intoxication
  drug
    acute (without dependence) — *see* Abuse, drug, by type with intoxication
      with dependence — *see* Dependence, drug, by type with intoxication
    addictive
      via placenta or breast milk — *see* Absorption, drug, addictive, through placenta
    newborn P93.8
      gray baby syndrome P93.0
    overdose or wrong substance given or taken — *see* Table of Drugs and Chemicals, by drug, poisoning
  enteric K52.1
  foodborne A05.9
    bacterial A05.9
    classical (Clostridium botulinum) A05.1
    due to
      Bacillus cereus A05.4
      bacterium A05.9
        specified NEC A05.8
      Clostridium
        botulinum A05.1
        perfringens A05.2
        welchii A05.2
      Salmonella A02.9
        with
          (gastro)enteritis A02.0
          localized infection(s) A02.20
            arthritis A02.23
            meningitis A02.21
            osteomyelitis A02.24

Intoxication — *continued*
  foodborne — *continued*
    due to — *continued*
      Salmonella — *continued*
        with — *continued*
          localized infection(s) — *continued*
            pneumonia A02.22
            pyelonephritis A02.25
            specified NEC A02.29
          sepsis A02.1
          specified manifestation NEC A02.8
      Staphylococcus A05.0
      Vibrio
        parahaemolyticus A05.3
        vulnificus A05.5
    enterotoxin, staphylococcal A05.0
    noxious — *see* Poisoning, food, noxious
  gastrointestinal K52.1
  hallucinogenic (without dependence) — *see* Abuse, drug, hallucinogen, with intoxication
    with dependence — *see* Dependence, drug, hallucinogen, with intoxication
  hypnotic (acute) (without dependence) — *see* Abuse, drug, sedative, with intoxication
    with dependence — *see* Dependence, drug, sedative, with intoxication
  inhalant (acute) (without dependence) — *see* Abuse, drug, inhalant, with intoxication
    with dependence — *see* Dependence, drug, inhalant, with intoxication
  meaning
    inebriation — *see* category F10 ☑
    poisoning — *see* Table of Drugs and Chemicals
  methyl alcohol (acute) (without dependence) — *see* Alcohol, intoxication
  opioid (acute) (without dependence) — *see* Abuse, drug, opioid, with intoxication
    with dependence — *see* Dependence, drug, opioid, with intoxication
  pathologic NEC (without dependence) — *see* Alcohol, intoxication
  phencyclidine (without dependence) — *see* Abuse, drug, hallucinogen, with intoxication
    with dependence — *see* Dependence, drug, hallucinogen, with intoxication
  potassium (K) E87.5
  psychoactive substance NEC (without dependence) — *see* Abuse, drug, psychoactive NEC, with intoxication
    with dependence — *see* Dependence, drug, psychoactive NEC, with intoxication
  sedative (acute) (without dependence) — *see* Abuse, drug, sedative, with intoxication
    with dependence — *see* Dependence, drug, sedative, with intoxication
  serum (*see also* Reaction, serum) T80.69 ☑
  uremic — *see* Uremia
  volatile solvents (acute) (without dependence) — *see* Abuse, drug, inhalant, with intoxication
    with dependence — *see* Dependence, drug, inhalant, with intoxication
  water E87.79
Intraabdominal testis, testes
  bilateral Q53.211
  unilateral Q53.111
Intracranial — *see* condition
Intrahepatic gallbladder Q44.1
Intraligamentous — *see* condition
Intrathoracic (*see also* condition)
  kidney Q63.2
Intrauterine contraceptive device
  checking Z30.431
  in situ Z97.5
  insertion Z30.430
    immediately following removal Z30.433
  management Z30.431
  reinsertion Z30.433
  removal Z30.432
  replacement Z30.433
  retention in pregnancy O26.3- ☑
Intraventricular — *see* condition
Intrinsic deformity — *see* Deformity
Intubation, difficult or failed T88.4 ☑
Intumescence, lens (eye) (cataract) — *see* Cataract
Intussusception (bowel) (colon) (enteric) (ileocecal) (ileocolic) (intestine) (rectum) K56.1
  appendix K38.8
  congenital Q43.8

Intussusception — *continued*
  ureter (with obstruction) N13.5
Invagination (bowel, colon, intestine or rectum) K56.1
Inversion
  albumin-globulin (A-G) ratio E88.09
  bladder N32.89
  cecum — *see* Intussusception
  cervix N88.8
  chromosome in normal individual Q95.1
  circadian rhythm — *see* Disorder, sleep, circadian rhythm
  nipple N64.59
    congenital Q83.8
    gestational — *see* Retraction, nipple
    puerperal, postpartum — *see* Retraction, nipple
  nyctohemeral rhythm — *see* Disorder, sleep, circadian rhythm
  optic papilla Q14.2
  organ or site, congenital NEC — *see* Anomaly, by site
  sleep rhythm — *see* Disorder, sleep, circadian rhythm
  testis (congenital) Q55.29
  uterus (chronic) (postinfectional) (postpartal, old) N85.5
    postpartum O71.2
  vagina (posthysterectomy) N99.3
  ventricular Q20.5
Investigation (*see also* Examination) Z04.9
  clinical research subject (control) (normal comparison) (participant) Z00.6
Involuntary movement, abnormal R25.9
Involution, involutional (*see also* condition)
  breast, cystic — *see* Dysplasia, mammary, specified type NEC
  depression (single episode) F32.89
    recurrent episode F33.9
  melancholia (single episode) F32.89
    recurrent episode F33.8
  ovary, senile — *see* Atrophy, ovary
  thymus failure E32.8
I.Q.
  under 20 F73
  20-34 F72
  35-49 F71
  50-69 F70
IRDS (type I) P22.0
  type II P22.1
Irideremia Q13.1
Iridis rubeosis — *see* Disorder, iris, vascular
Iridochoroiditis (panuveitis) — *see* Panuveitis
Iridocyclitis H20.9
  acute H20.0- ☑
    hypopyon H20.05- ☑
    primary H20.01- ☑
    recurrent H20.02- ☑
    secondary (noninfectious) H20.04- ☑
      infectious H20.03- ☑
  chronic H20.1- ☑
  due to allergy — *see* Iridocyclitis, acute, secondary
  endogenous — *see* Iridocyclitis, acute, primary
  Fuchs' — *see* Cyclitis, Fuchs' heterochromic
  gonococcal A54.32
  granulomatous — *see* Iridocyclitis, chronic
  herpes, herpetic (simplex) B00.51
    zoster B02.32
  hypopyon — *see* Iridocyclitis, acute, hypopyon
  in (due to)
    ankylosing spondylitis M45.9
    gonococcal infection A54.32
    herpes (simplex) virus B00.51
      zoster B02.32
    infectious disease NOS B99 ☑
    parasitic disease NOS B89 [H22]
    sarcoidosis D86.83
    syphilis A51.43
    tuberculosis A18.54
    zoster B02.32
  lens-induced H20.2- ☑
  nongranulomatous — *see* Iridocyclitis, acute
  recurrent — *see* Iridocyclitis, acute, recurrent
  rheumatic — *see* Iridocyclitis, chronic
  subacute — *see* Iridocyclitis, acute
  sympathetic — *see* Uveitis, sympathetic
  syphilitic (secondary) A51.43
  tuberculous (chronic) A18.54
  Vogt-Koyanagi H20.82- ☑
Iridocyclochoroiditis (panuveitis) — *see* Panuveitis
Iridodialysis H21.53- ☑

☑ **Additional Character Required** — **Refer to the Tabular List for Character Selection**   ▽ **Subterms under main terms may continue to next column or page**

Iridodonesis H21.89
Iridoplegia (complete) (partial) (reflex) H57.09
Iridoschisis H21.25- ✓
Iris (see also condition)
  bombé — see Membrane, pupillary
Iritis (see also Iridocyclitis)
  chronic — see Iridocyclitis, chronic
  diabetic — see E08-E13 with .39
  due to
    herpes simplex B00.51
    leprosy A30.9 [H22]
  gonococcal A54.32
  gouty (see also Gout, by type) M10.9 [H22]
  granulomatous — see Iridocyclitis, chronic
  lens induced — see Iridocyclitis, lens-induced
  papulosa (syphilitic) A52.71
  rheumatic — see Iridocyclitis, chronic
  syphilitic (secondary) A51.43
    congenital (early) A50.01
    late A52.71
  tuberculous A18.54
Iron — see condition
Iron-miner's lung J63.4
Irradiated enamel (tooth, teeth) K03.89
Irradiation effects, adverse T66 ✓
Irreducible, irreducibility — see condition
Irregular, irregularity
  action, heart I49.9
  alveolar process K08.89
  bleeding N92.6
  breathing R06.89
  contour of cornea (acquired) — see Deformity, cornea
    congenital Q13.4
  contour, reconstructed breast N65.0
  dentin (in pulp) K04.3
  eye movements H55.89
    nystagmus — see Nystagmus
    saccadic H55.81
  labor O62.2
  menstruation (cause unknown) N92.6
  periods N92.6
  prostate N42.9
  pupil — see Abnormality, pupillary
  reconstructed breast N65.0
  respiratory R06.89
  septum (nasal) J34.2
  shape, organ or site, congenital NEC — see Distortion
  sleep-wake pattern (rhythm) G47.23
Irritable, irritability R45.4
  bladder N32.89
  bowel (syndrome) K58.9
    with
      constipation K58.1
      diarrhea K58.0
    mixed K58.2
    psychogenic F45.8
    specified NEC K58.8
  bronchial — see Bronchitis
  cerebral, in newborn P91.3
  colon (see also Irritable, bowel) K58.9
    with diarrhea K58.0
    psychogenic F45.8
  duodenum K59.8
  heart (psychogenic) F45.8
  hip — see Derangement, joint, specified type NEC, hip
  ileum K59.8
  infant R68.12
  jejunum K59.8
  rectum K59.8
  stomach K31.89
    psychogenic F45.8
  sympathetic G90.8
  urethra N36.8
Irritation
  anus K62.89
  axillary nerve G54.0
  bladder N32.89
  brachial plexus G54.0
  bronchial — see Bronchitis
  cervical plexus G54.2
  cervix — see Cervicitis
  choroid, sympathetic — see Endophthalmitis
  cranial nerve — see Disorder, nerve, cranial
  gastric K31.89
    psychogenic F45.8
  globe, sympathetic — see Uveitis, sympathetic
  labyrinth — see subcategory H83.2 ✓
  lumbosacral plexus G54.1

Irritation — continued
  meninges (traumatic) — see Injury, intracranial
    nontraumatic — see Meningismus
  nerve — see Disorder, nerve
  nervous R45.0
  penis N48.89
  perineum NEC L29.3
  peripheral autonomic nervous system G90.8
  peritoneum — see Peritonitis
  pharynx J39.2
  plantar nerve — see Lesion, nerve, plantar
  spinal (cord) (traumatic) (see also Injury, spinal cord, by region)
    nerve G58.9
      root NEC — see Radiculopathy
    nontraumatic — see Myelopathy
  stomach K31.89
    psychogenic F45.8
  sympathetic nerve NEC G90.8
  ulnar nerve — see Lesion, nerve, ulnar
  vagina N89.8
Ischemia, ischemic I99.8
  bowel (transient)
    acute (see also Ischemia, intestine, acute) K55.059
    chronic K55.1
    due to mesenteric artery insufficiency K55.1
  brain — see Ischemia, cerebral
  cardiac (see Disease, heart, ischemic)
  cardiomyopathy I25.5
  cerebral (chronic) (generalized) I67.82
    arteriosclerotic I67.2
    intermittent G45.9
    newborn P91.0
    recurrent focal G45.8
    transient G45.9
  colon chronic (due to mesenteric artery insufficiency) K55.1
  coronary — see Disease, heart, ischemic
  demand (coronary) (see also Angina) I24.8
    with myocardial infarction I21.A1
    resulting in myocardial infarction I21.A1
  heart (chronic or with a stated duration of over 4 weeks) I25.9
    acute or with a stated duration of 4 weeks or less I24.9
    subacute I24.9
  infarction, muscle — see Infarct, muscle
  intestine (large) (small) (transient) K55.9
    acute K55.059
      diffuse K55.052
      focal K55.051
      large K55.039
        diffuse K55.032
        focal K55.031
      small K55.019
        diffuse K55.012
        focal K55.011
    chronic K55.1
    due to mesenteric artery insufficiency K55.1
  kidney N28.0
  mesenteric, acute (see also Ischemia, intestine, acute) K55.059
  muscle, traumatic T79.6 ✓
  myocardium, myocardial (chronic or with a stated duration of over 4 weeks) I25.9
    acute, without myocardial infarction I51.3
    silent (asymptomatic) I25.6
    transient of newborn P29.4
  renal N28.0
  retina, retinal — see Occlusion, artery, retina
  small bowel
    acute K55.019
      diffuse K55.012
      focal K55.011
    chronic K55.1
    due to mesenteric artery insufficiency K55.1
  spinal cord G95.11
  subendocardial — see Insufficiency, coronary
  supply (coronary) (see also Angina) I25.9
    due to vasospasm I20.1
Ischial spine — see condition
Ischialgia — see Sciatica
Ischiopagus Q89.4
Ischium, ischial — see condition
Ischuria R34
Iselin's disease or osteochondrosis — see Osteochondrosis, juvenile, metatarsus

Islands of
  parotid tissue in
    lymph nodes Q38.6
    neck structures Q38.6
  submaxillary glands in
    fascia Q38.6
    lymph nodes Q38.6
    neck muscles Q38.6
Islet cell tumor, pancreas D13.7
Isoimmunization NEC (see also Incompatibility)
  affecting management of pregnancy (ABO) (with hydrops fetalis) O36.11- ✓
    anti-A sensitization O36.11- ✓
    anti-B sensitization O36.19- ✓
    anti-c sensitization O36.09- ✓
    anti-C sensitization O36.09- ✓
    anti-e sensitization O36.09- ✓
    anti-E sensitization O36.09- ✓
    Rh NEC O36.09- ✓
      anti-D antibody O36.01- ✓
    specified NEC O36.19- ✓
  newborn P55.9
    with
      hydrops fetalis P56.0
      kernicterus P57.0
    ABO (blood groups) P55.1
    Rhesus (Rh) factor P55.0
    specified type NEC P55.8
Isolation, isolated
  dwelling Z59.8
  family Z63.79
  social Z60.4
Isoleucinosis E71.19
Isomerism atrial appendages (with asplenia or polysplenia) Q20.6
Isosporiasis, isosporosis A07.3
Isovaleric acidemia E71.110
Issue of
  medical certificate Z02.79
    for disability determination Z02.71
  repeat prescription (appliance) (glasses) (medicinal substance, medicament, medicine) Z76.0
    contraception — see Contraception
Itch, itching (see also Pruritus)
  baker's L23.6
  barber's B35.0
  bricklayer's L24.5
  cheese B88.0
  clam digger's B65.3
  coolie B76.9
  copra B88.0
  dew B76.9
  dhobi B35.6
  filarial — see Infestation, filarial
  grain B88.0
  grocer's B88.0
  ground B76.9
  harvest B88.0
  jock B35.6
  Malabar B35.5
    beard B35.0
    foot B35.3
    scalp B35.0
  meaning scabies B86
  Norwegian B86
  perianal L29.0
  poultrymen's B88.0
  sarcoptic B86
  scabies B86
  scrub B88.0
  straw B88.0
  swimmer's B65.3
  water B76.9
  winter L29.8
Ivemark's syndrome (asplenia with congenital heart disease) Q89.01
Ivory bones Q78.2
Ixodiasis NEC B88.8

J

Jaccoud's syndrome — see Arthropathy, postrheumatic, chronic
Jackson's
  membrane Q43.3
  paralysis or syndrome G83.89
  veil Q43.3
Jacquet's dermatitis (diaper dermatitis) L22

Subterms under main terms may continue to next column or page | ✓ Additional Character Required — Refer to the Tabular List for Character Selection | 203

Iridodonesis — Jacquet's dermatitis

Jadassohn-Pellizari's disease or anetoderma L90.2
Jadassohn's
 blue nevus — *see* Nevus
 intraepidermal epithelioma — *see* Neoplasm, skin, benign
Jaffe-Lichtenstein (-Uehlinger) **syndrome** — *see* Dysplasia, fibrous, bone NEC
Jakob-Creutzfeldt disease or syndrome — *see* Creutzfeldt-Jakob disease or syndrome
Jaksch-Luzet disease D64.89
Jamaican
 neuropathy G92
 paraplegic tropical ataxic-spastic syndrome G92
Janet's disease F48.8
Janiceps Q89.4
Jansky-Bielschowsky amaurotic idiocy E75.4
Japanese
 B-type encephalitis A83.0
 river fever A75.3
Jaundice (yellow) R17
 acholuric (familial) (splenomegalic) (*see also* Spherocytosis)
  acquired D59.8
 breast-milk (inhibitor) P59.3
 catarrhal (acute) B15.9
  with hepatic coma B15.0
 cholestatic (benign) R17
 due to or associated with
  delayed conjugation P59.8
   associated with (due to) preterm delivery P59.0
  preterm delivery P59.0
 epidemic (catarrhal) B15.9
  with hepatic coma B15.0
  leptospiral A27.0
  spirochetal A27.0
 familial nonhemolytic (congenital) (Gilbert) E80.4
  Crigler-Najjar E80.5
 febrile (acute) B15.9
  with hepatic coma B15.0
  leptospiral A27.0
  spirochetal A27.0
 hematogenous D59.9
 hemolytic (acquired) D59.9
  congenital — *see* Spherocytosis
 hemorrhagic (acute) (leptospiral) (spirochetal) A27.0
 infectious (acute) (subacute) B15.9
  with hepatic coma B15.0
  leptospiral A27.0
  spirochetal A27.0
 leptospiral (hemorrhagic) A27.0
 malignant (without coma) K72.90
  with coma K72.91
 neonatal — *see* Jaundice, newborn
 newborn P59.9
  due to or associated with
   ABO
    antibodies P55.1
    incompatibility, maternal/fetal P55.1
    isoimmunization P55.1
   absence or deficiency of enzyme system for bilirubin conjugation (congenital) P59.8
   bleeding P58.1
   breast milk inhibitors to conjugation P59.3
    associated with preterm delivery P59.0
   bruising P58.0
   Crigler-Najjar syndrome E80.5
   delayed conjugation P59.8
    associated with preterm delivery P59.0
   drugs or toxins
    given to newborn P58.42
    transmitted from mother P58.41
   excessive hemolysis P58.9
    due to
     bleeding P58.1
     bruising P58.0
     drugs or toxins
      given to newborn P58.42
      transmitted from mother P58.41
     infection P58.2
     polycythemia P58.3
     swallowed maternal blood P58.5
    specified type NEC P58.8
   galactosemia E74.21
   Gilbert syndrome E80.4
   hemolytic disease P55.9
    ABO isoimmunization P55.1
    Rh isoimmunization P55.0
    specified NEC P55.8

Jaundice — *continued*
 newborn — *continued*
  due to or associated with — *continued*
   hepatocellular damage P59.20
    specified NEC P59.29
   hereditary hemolytic anemia P58.8
   hypothyroidism, congenital E03.1
   incompatibility, maternal/fetal NOS P55.9
   infection P58.2
   inspissated bile syndrome P59.1
   isoimmunization NOS P55.9
   mucoviscidosis E84.9
   polycythemia P58.3
   preterm delivery P59.0
   Rh
    antibodies P55.0
    incompatibility, maternal/fetal P55.0
    isoimmunization P55.0
   specified cause NEC P59.8
   swallowed maternal blood P58.5
  spherocytosis (congenital) D58.0
 nonhemolytic congenital familial (Gilbert) E80.4
 nuclear, newborn (*see also* Kernicterus of newborn) P57.9
 obstructive (*see also* Obstruction, bile duct) K83.1
 post-immunization — *see* Hepatitis, viral, type, B
 post-transfusion — *see* Hepatitis, viral, type, B
 regurgitation (*see also* Obstruction, bile duct) K83.1
 serum (homologous) (prophylactic) (therapeutic) — *see* Hepatitis, viral, type, B
 spirochetal (hemorrhagic) A27.0
 symptomatic R17
  newborn P59.9
Jaw — *see* condition
Jaw-winking phenomenon or syndrome Q07.8
Jealousy
 alcoholic F10.988
 childhood F93.8
 sibling F93.8
Jejunitis — *see* Enteritis
Jejunostomy status Z93.4
Jejunum, jejunal — *see* condition
Jensen's disease — *see* Inflammation, chorioretinal, focal, juxtapapillary
Jerks, myoclonic G25.3
Jervell-Lange-Nielsen syndrome I45.81
Jeune's disease Q77.2
Jigger disease B88.1
Job's syndrome (chronic granulomatous disease) D71
Joint (*see also* condition)
 mice — *see* Loose, body, joint
  knee M23.4- ☑
Jordan's anomaly or syndrome D72.0
Joseph-Diamond-Blackfan anemia (congenital hypoplastic) D61.01
Jungle yellow fever A95.0
Jüngling's disease — *see* Sarcoidosis
Juvenile — *see* condition

K

Kahler's disease C90.0- ☑
Kakke E51.11
Kala-azar B55.0
Kallmann's syndrome E23.0
Kanner's syndrome (autism) — *see* Psychosis, childhood
Kaposi's
 dermatosis (xeroderma pigmentosum) Q82.1
 lichen ruber L44.0
  acuminatus L44.0
 sarcoma
  colon C46.4
  connective tissue C46.1
  gastrointestinal organ C46.4
  lung C46.5- ☑
  lymph node (multiple) C46.3
  palate (hard) (soft) C46.2
  rectum C46.4
  skin (multiple sites) C46.0
  specified site NEC C46.7
  stomach C46.4
  unspecified site C46.9
 varicelliform eruption B00.0
  vaccinia T88.1 ☑
Kartagener's syndrome or triad (sinusitis, bronchiectasis, situs inversus) Q89.3

Karyotype
 with abnormality except iso (Xq) Q96.2
 45,X Q96.0
 46,X
  iso (Xq) Q96.1
 46,XX Q98.3
  with streak gonads Q50.32
  hermaphrodite (true) Q99.1
  male Q98.3
 46,XY
  with streak gonads Q56.1
  female Q97.3
  hermaphrodite (true) Q99.1
 47,XXX Q97.0
 47,XXY Q98.0
 47,XYY Q98.5
Kaschin-Beck disease — *see* Disease, Kaschin-Beck
Katayama's disease or fever B65.2
Kawasaki's syndrome M30.3
Kayser-Fleischer ring (cornea) (pseudosclerosis) H18.04- ☑
Kaznelson's syndrome (congenital hypoplastic anemia) D61.01
Kearns-Sayre syndrome H49.81- ☑
Kedani fever A75.3
Kelis L91.0
Kelly (-Patterson) **syndrome** (sideropenic dysphagia) D50.1
Keloid, cheloid L91.0
 acne L73.0
 Addison's L94.0
 cornea — *see* Opacity, cornea
 Hawkin's L91.0
 scar L91.0
Keloma L91.0
Kenya fever A77.1
Keratectasia (*see also* Ectasia, cornea)
 congenital Q13.4
Keratinization of alveolar ridge mucosa
 excessive K13.23
 minimal K13.22
Keratinized residual ridge mucosa
 excessive K13.23
 minimal K13.22
Keratitis (nodular) (nonulcerative) (simple) (zonular) H16.9
 with ulceration (central) (marginal) (perforated) (ring) — *see* Ulcer, cornea
 actinic — *see* Photokeratitis
 arborescens (herpes simplex) B00.52
 areolar H16.11- ☑
 bullosa H16.8
 deep H16.309
  specified type NEC H16.399
 dendritic (a) (herpes simplex) B00.52
 disciform (is) (herpes simplex) B00.52
  varicella B01.81
 filamentary H16.12- ☑
 gonococcal (congenital or prenatal) A54.33
 herpes, herpetic (simplex) B00.52
  zoster B02.33
 in (due to)
  acanthamebiasis B60.13
  adenovirus B30.0
  exanthema (*see also* Exanthem) B09
  herpes (simplex) virus B00.52
  measles B05.81
  syphilis A50.31
  tuberculosis A18.52
  zoster B02.33
 interstitial (nonsyphilitic) H16.30- ☑
  diffuse H16.32- ☑
  herpes, herpetic (simplex) B00.52
   zoster B02.33
  sclerosing H16.33- ☑
  specified type NEC H16.39- ☑
  syphilitic (congenital) (late) A50.31
  tuberculous A18.52
 macular H16.11- ☑
 nummular H16.11- ☑
 oyster shuckers' H16.8
 parenchymatous — *see* Keratitis, interstitial
 petrificans H16.8
 postmeasles B05.81
 punctata
  leprosa A30.9 [H16.14-]
  syphilitic (profunda) A50.31
 punctate H16.14- ☑

Keratitis — *continued*
purulent H16.8
rosacea L71.8
sclerosing H16.33- ☑
specified type NEC H16.8
stellate H16.11- ☑
striate H16.11- ☑
superficial H16.10- ☑
with conjunctivitis — *see* Keratoconjunctivitis
due to light — *see* Photokeratitis
suppurative H16.8
syphilitic (congenital) (prenatal) A50.31
trachomatous A71.1
sequelae B94.0
tuberculous A18.52
vesicular H16.8
xerotic (*see also* Keratomalacia) H16.8
vitamin A deficiency E50.4
Keratoacanthoma L85.8
Keratocele — *see* Descemetocele
Keratoconjunctivitis H16.20- ☑
Acanthamoeba B60.13
adenoviral B30.0
epidemic B30.0
exposure H16.21- ☑
herpes, herpetic (simplex) B00.52
zoster B02.33
in exanthema (*see also* Exanthem) B09
infectious B30.0
lagophthalmic — *see* Keratoconjunctivitis, specified type NEC
neurotrophic H16.23- ☑
phlyctenular H16.25- ☑
postmeasles B05.81
shipyard B30.0
sicca (Sjogren's) M35.0- ☑
not Sjogren's H16.22- ☑
specified type NEC H16.29- ☑
tuberculous (phlyctenular) A18.52
vernal H16.26- ☑
Keratoconus H18.60- ☑
congenital Q13.4
stable H18.61- ☑
unstable H18.62- ☑
Keratocyst (dental) (odontogenic) — *see* Cyst, calcifying odontogenic
Keratoderma, keratodermia (congenital) (palmaris et plantaris) (symmetrical) Q82.8
acquired L85.1
in diseases classified elsewhere L86
climactericum L85.1
gonococcal A54.89
gonorrheal A54.89
punctata L85.2
Reiter's — *see* Reiter's disease
Keratodermatocele — *see* Descemetocele
Keratoglobus H18.79 ☑
congenital Q15.8
with glaucoma Q15.0
Keratohemia — *see* Pigmentation, cornea, stromal
Keratoiritis (*see also* Iridocyclitis)
syphilitic A50.39
tuberculous A18.54
Keratoma L57.0
palmaris and plantaris hereditarium Q82.8
senile L57.0
Keratomalacia H18.44- ☑
vitamin A deficiency E50.4
Keratomegaly Q13.4
Keratomycosis B49
nigrans, nigricans (palmaris) B36.1
Keratopathy H18.9
band H18.42- ☑
bullous (aphakic), following cataract surgery H59.01- ☑
bullous H18.1- ☑
Keratoscleritis, tuberculous A18.52
Keratosis L57.0
actinic L57.0
arsenical L85.8
congenital, specified NEC Q80.8
female genital NEC N94.89
follicularis Q82.8
acquired L11.0
congenita Q82.8
et parafollicularis in cutem penetrans L87.0
spinulosa (decalvans) Q82.8

Keratosis — *continued*
follicularis — *continued*
vitamin A deficiency E50.8
gonococcal A54.89
male genital (external) N50.89
nigricans L83
obturans, external ear (canal) — *see* Cholesteatoma, external ear
palmaris et plantaris (inherited) (symmetrical) Q82.8
acquired L85.1
penile N48.89
pharynx J39.2
pilaris, acquired L85.8
punctata (palmaris et plantaris) L85.2
scrotal N50.89
seborrheic L82.1
inflamed L82.0
senile L57.0
solar L57.0
tonsillaris J35.8
vagina N89.4
vegetans Q82.8
vitamin A deficiency E50.8
vocal cord J38.3
Kerato-uveitis — *see* Iridocyclitis
Kerion (celsi) B35.0
Kernicterus of newborn (not due to isoimmunization) P57.9
due to isoimmunization (conditions in P55.0-P55.9) P57.0
specified type NEC P57.8
Kerunoparalysis T75.09 ☑
Keshan disease E59
Ketoacidosis E87.2
diabetic — *see* Diabetes, by type, with ketoacidosis
Ketonuria R82.4
Ketosis NEC E88.89
diabetic — *see* Diabetes, by type, with with ketoacidosis
Kew Garden fever A79.1
Kidney — *see* condition
Kienböck's disease (*see also* Osteochondrosis, juvenile, hand, carpal lunate)
adult M93.1
Kimmelstiel (-Wilson) **disease** — *see* Diabetes, Kimmelstiel (-Wilson) disease
Kink, kinking
artery I77.1
hair (acquired) L67.8
ileum or intestine — *see* Obstruction, intestine
Lane's — *see* Obstruction, intestine
organ or site, congenital NEC — *see* Anomaly, by site
ureter (pelvic junction) N13.5
with
hydronephrosis N13.1
with infection N13.6
pyelonephritis (chronic) N11.1
congenital Q62.39
vein(s) I87.8
caval I87.1
peripheral I87.1
Kinnier Wilson's disease (hepatolenticular degeneration) E83.01
Kissing spine M48.20
cervical region M48.22
cervicothoracic region M48.23
lumbar region M48.26
lumbosacral region M48.27
occipito-atlanto-axial region M48.21
thoracic region M48.24
thoracolumbar region M48.25
Klatskin's tumor C22.1
Klauder's disease A26.8
Klebs' disease (*see also* Glomerulonephritis) N05- ☑
Klebsiella (K.) **pneumoniae, as cause of disease classified elsewhere** B96.1
Klein (e)-**Levin syndrome** G47.13
Kleptomania F63.2
Klinefelter's syndrome Q98.4
karyotype 47,XXY Q98.0
male with more than two X chromosomes Q98.1
Klippel-Feil deficiency, disease, or syndrome (brevicollis) Q76.1
Klippel's disease I67.2
Klippel-Trenaunay (-Weber) **syndrome** Q87.2
Klumpke (-Déjerine) **palsy, paralysis** (birth) (newborn) P14.1
Knee — *see* condition

Knock knee (acquired) M21.06- ☑
congenital Q74.1
Knot(s)
intestinal, syndrome (volvulus) K56.2
surfer S89.8- ☑
umbilical cord (true) O69.2 ☑
Knotting (of)
hair L67.8
intestine K56.2
Knuckle pad (Garrod's) M72.1
Koch's
infection — *see* Tuberculosis
relapsing fever A68.9
Koch-Weeks' conjunctivitis — *see* Conjunctivitis, acute, mucopurulent
Köebner's syndrome Q81.8
Köenig's disease (osteochondritis dissecans) — *see* Osteochondritis, dissecans
Köhler-Pellegrini-Steida disease or syndrome (calcification, knee joint) — *see* Bursitis, tibial collateral
Köhler's disease
patellar — *see* Osteochondrosis, juvenile, patella
tarsal navicular — *see* Osteochondrosis, juvenile, tarsus
Koilonychia L60.3
congenital Q84.6
Kojevnikov's, epilepsy — *see* Kozhevnikof's epilepsy
Koplik's spots B05.9
Kopp's asthma E32.8
Korsakoff's (Wernicke) **disease, psychosis or syndrome** (alcoholic) F10.96
with dependence F10.26
drug-induced
due to drug abuse — *see* Abuse, drug, by type, with amnestic disorder
due to drug dependence — *see* Dependence, drug, by type, with amnestic disorder
nonalcoholic F04
Korsakov's disease, psychosis or syndrome — *see* Korsakoff's disease
Korsakow's disease, psychosis or syndrome — *see* Korsakoff's disease
Kostmann's disease or syndrome (infantile genetic agranulocytosis) — *see* Agranulocytosis
Kozhevnikof's epilepsy G40.109
intractable G40.119
with status epilepticus G40.111
without status epilepticus G40.119
not intractable G40.109
with status epilepticus G40.101
without status epilepticus G40.109
Krabbe's
disease E75.23
syndrome, congenital muscle hypoplasia Q79.8
Kraepelin-Morel disease — *see* Schizophrenia
Kraft-Weber-Dimitri disease Q85.8
Kraurosis
ani K62.89
penis N48.0
vagina N89.8
vulva N90.4
Kreotoxism A05.9
Krukenberg's
spindle — *see* Pigmentation, cornea, posterior
tumor C79.6- ☑
Kufs' disease E75.4
Kugelberg-Welander disease G12.1
Kuhnt-Junius degeneration (*see also* Degeneration, macula) H35.32- ☑
Kümmell's disease or spondylitis — *see* Spondylopathy, traumatic
Kupffer cell sarcoma C22.3
Kuru A81.81
Kussmaul's
disease M30.0
respiration E87.2
in diabetic acidosis — *see* Diabetes, by type, with ketoacidosis
Kwashiorkor E40
marasmic, marasmus type E42
Kyasanur Forest disease A98.2
Kyphoscoliosis, kyphoscoliotic (acquired) (*see also* Scoliosis) M41.9
congenital Q67.5
heart (disease) I27.1
sequelae of rickets E64.3
tuberculous A18.01
Kyphosis, kyphotic (acquired) M40.209

☞ **Subterms under main terms may continue to next column or page**   ☑ **Additional Character Required — Refer to the Tabular List for Character Selection**   205

Keratitis — Kyphosis, kyphotic

Kyphosis, kyphotic — *continued*
  cervical region M40.202
  cervicothoracic region M40.203
  congenital Q76.419
    cervical region Q76.412
    cervicothoracic region Q76.413
    occipito-atlanto-axial region Q76.411
    thoracic region Q76.414
    thoracolumbar region Q76.415
  Morquio-Brailsford type (spinal) (*see also* subcategory M49.8) E76.219
  postlaminectomy M96.3
  postradiation therapy M96.2
  postural (adolescent) M40.00
    cervicothoracic region M40.03
    thoracic region M40.04
    thoracolumbar region M40.05
  secondary NEC M40.10
    cervical region M40.12
    cervicothoracic region M40.13
    thoracic region M40.14
    thoracolumbar region M40.15
  sequelae of rickets E64.3
  specified type NEC M40.299
    cervical region M40.292
    cervicothoracic region M40.293
    thoracic region M40.294
    thoracolumbar region M40.295
  syphilitic, congenital A50.56
  thoracic region M40.204
  thoracolumbar region M40.205
  tuberculous A18.01
Kyrle disease L87.0

L

Labia, labium — *see* condition
Labile
  blood pressure R09.89
  vasomotor system I73.9
Labioglossal paralysis G12.29
Labium leporinum — *see* Cleft, lip
Labor — *see* Delivery
Labored breathing — *see* Hyperventilation
Labyrinthitis (circumscribed) (destructive) (diffuse) (inner ear) (latent) (purulent) (suppurative) (*see also* subcategory) H83.0 ☑
  syphilitic A52.79
Laceration
  with abortion — *see* Abortion, by type, complicated by laceration of pelvic organs
  abdomen, abdominal
    wall S31.119 ☑
      with
        foreign body S31.129 ☑
        penetration into peritoneal cavity S31.619 ☑
          with foreign body S31.629 ☑
      epigastric region S31.112 ☑
        with
          foreign body S31.122 ☑
          penetration into peritoneal cavity S31.612 ☑
            with foreign body S31.622 ☑
      left
        lower quadrant S31.114 ☑
          with
            foreign body S31.124 ☑
            penetration into peritoneal cavity S31.614 ☑
              with foreign body S31.624 ☑
        upper quadrant S31.111 ☑
          with
            foreign body S31.121 ☑
            penetration into peritoneal cavity S31.611 ☑
              with foreign body S31.621 ☑
      periumbilic region S31.115 ☑
        with
          foreign body S31.125 ☑
          penetration into peritoneal cavity S31.615 ☑
            with foreign body S31.625 ☑
      right
        lower quadrant S31.113 ☑
          with
            foreign body S31.123 ☑

Laceration — *continued*
  abdomen, abdominal — *continued*
    wall — *continued*
      right — *continued*
        lower quadrant — *continued*
          with — *continued*
            penetration into peritoneal cavity S31.613 ☑
              with foreign body S31.623 ☑
        upper quadrant S31.110 ☑
          with
            foreign body S31.120 ☑
            penetration into peritoneal cavity S31.610 ☑
              with foreign body S31.620 ☑
    accidental, complicating surgery — *see* Complications, surgical, accidental puncture or laceration
  Achilles tendon S86.02- ☑
  adrenal gland S37.813 ☑
  alveolar (process) — *see* Laceration, oral cavity
  ankle S91.01- ☑
    with
      foreign body S91.02- ☑
  antecubital space — *see* Laceration, elbow
  anus (sphincter) S31.831 ☑
    with
      ectopic or molar pregnancy O08.6
      foreign body S31.832 ☑
    complicating delivery — *see* Delivery, complicated, by, laceration, anus (sphincter)
    following ectopic or molar pregnancy O08.6
    nontraumatic, nonpuerperal — *see* Fissure, anus
  arm (upper) S41.11- ☑
    with foreign body S41.12- ☑
    lower — *see* Laceration, forearm
  auditory canal (external) (meatus) — *see* Laceration, ear
  auricle, ear — *see* Laceration, ear
  axilla — *see* Laceration, arm
  back (*see also* Laceration, thorax, back)
    lower S31.010 ☑
      with
        foreign body S31.020 ☑
          with penetration into retroperitoneal space S31.021 ☑
        penetration into retroperitoneal space S31.011 ☑
  bile duct S36.13 ☑
  bladder S37.23 ☑
    with ectopic or molar pregnancy O08.6
    following ectopic or molar pregnancy O08.6
    obstetrical trauma O71.5
  blood vessel — *see* Injury, blood vessel
  bowel (*see also* Laceration, intestine)
    with ectopic or molar pregnancy O08.6
    complicating abortion — *see* Abortion, by type, complicated by, specified condition NEC
    following ectopic or molar pregnancy O08.6
    obstetrical trauma O71.5
  brain (any part) (cortex) (diffuse) (membrane) (*see also* Injury, intracranial, diffuse)
    during birth P10.8
      with hemorrhage P10.1
    focal — *see* Injury, intracranial, focal brain injury
  brainstem S06.38- ☑
  breast S21.01- ☑
    with foreign body S21.02- ☑
  broad ligament S37.893 ☑
    with ectopic or molar pregnancy O08.6
    following ectopic or molar pregnancy O08.6
    laceration syndrome N83.8
    obstetrical trauma O71.6
    syndrome (laceration) N83.8
  buttock S31.801 ☑
    with foreign body S31.802 ☑
    left S31.821 ☑
      with foreign body S31.822 ☑
    right S31.811 ☑
      with foreign body S31.812 ☑
  calf — *see* Laceration, leg
  canaliculus lacrimalis — *see* Laceration, eyelid
  canthus, eye — *see* Laceration, eyelid
  capsule, joint — *see* Sprain
  causing eversion of cervix uteri (old) N86
  central (perineal), complicating delivery O70.9
  cerebellum, traumatic S06.37- ☑
  cerebral S06.33- ☑

Laceration — *continued*
  cerebral — *continued*
    during birth P10.8
      with hemorrhage P10.1
    left side S06.32- ☑
    right side S06.31- ☑
  cervix (uteri)
    with ectopic or molar pregnancy O08.6
    following ectopic or molar pregnancy O08.6
    nonpuerperal, nontraumatic N88.1
    obstetrical trauma (current) O71.3
    old (postpartal) N88.1
    traumatic S37.63 ☑
  cheek (external) S01.41- ☑
    with foreign body S01.42- ☑
    internal — *see* Laceration, oral cavity
  chest wall — *see* Laceration, thorax
  chin — *see* Laceration, head, specified site NEC
  chordae tendinae NEC I51.1
    concurrent with acute myocardial infarction — *see* Infarct, myocardium
    following acute myocardial infarction (current complication) I23.4
  clitoris — *see* Laceration, vulva
  colon — *see* Laceration, intestine, large, colon
  common bile duct S36.13 ☑
  cortex (cerebral) — *see* Injury, intracranial, diffuse
  costal region — *see* Laceration, thorax
  cystic duct S36.13 ☑
  diaphragm S27.803 ☑
  digit(s)
    foot — *see* Laceration, toe
    hand — *see* Laceration, finger
  duodenum S36.430 ☑
  ear (canal) (external) S01.31- ☑
    with foreign body S01.32- ☑
    drum S09.2- ☑
  elbow S51.01- ☑
    with
      foreign body S51.02- ☑
  epididymis — *see* Laceration, testis
  epigastric region — *see* Laceration, abdomen, wall, epigastric region
  esophagus K22.8
    traumatic
      cervical S11.21 ☑
        with foreign body S11.22 ☑
      thoracic S27.813 ☑
  eye (ball) S05.3- ☑
    with prolapse or loss of intraocular tissue S05.2- ☑
    penetrating S05.6- ☑
  eyebrow — *see* Laceration, eyelid
  eyelid S01.11- ☑
    with foreign body S01.12- ☑
  face NEC — *see* Laceration, head, specified site NEC
  fallopian tube S37.539 ☑
    bilateral S37.532 ☑
    unilateral S37.531 ☑
  finger(s) S61.219 ☑
    with
      damage to nail S61.319 ☑
        with
          foreign body S61.329 ☑
      foreign body S61.229 ☑
    index S61.218 ☑
      with
        damage to nail S61.318 ☑
          with
            foreign body S61.328 ☑
        foreign body S61.228 ☑
      left S61.211 ☑
        with
          damage to nail S61.311 ☑
            with
              foreign body S61.321 ☑
          foreign body S61.221 ☑
      right S61.210 ☑
        with
          damage to nail S61.310 ☑
            with
              foreign body S61.320 ☑
          foreign body S61.220 ☑
    little S61.218 ☑
      with
        damage to nail S61.318 ☑
          with
            foreign body S61.328 ☑

☑ Additional Character Required — Refer to the Tabular List for Character Selection   Subterms under main terms may continue to next column or page

Laceration — *continued*
  finger(s) — *continued*
    little — *continued*
      with — *continued*
        foreign body S61.228 ☑
      left S61.217 ☑
        with
          damage to nail S61.317 ☑
            with
              foreign body S61.327 ☑
          foreign body S61.227 ☑
      right S61.216 ☑
        with
          damage to nail S61.316 ☑
            with
              foreign body S61.326 ☑
          foreign body S61.226 ☑
    middle S61.218 ☑
      with
        damage to nail S61.318 ☑
          with
            foreign body S61.328 ☑
        foreign body S61.228 ☑
      left S61.213 ☑
        with
          damage to nail S61.313 ☑
            with
              foreign body S61.323 ☑
          foreign body S61.223 ☑
      right S61.212 ☑
        with
          damage to nail S61.312 ☑
            with
              foreign body S61.322 ☑
          foreign body S61.222 ☑
    ring S61.218 ☑
      with
        damage to nail S61.318 ☑
          with
            foreign body S61.328 ☑
        foreign body S61.228 ☑
      left S61.215 ☑
        with
          damage to nail S61.315 ☑
            with
              foreign body S61.325 ☑
          foreign body S61.225 ☑
      right S61.214 ☑
        with
          damage to nail S61.314 ☑
            with
              foreign body S61.324 ☑
          foreign body S61.224 ☑
  flank S31.119 ☑
    with foreign body S31.129 ☑
  foot (except toe(s) alone) S91.319 ☑
    with foreign body S91.329 ☑
    left S91.312 ☑
      with foreign body S91.322 ☑
    right S91.311 ☑
      with foreign body S91.321 ☑
    toe — *see* Laceration, toe
  forearm S51.819 ☑
    with
      foreign body S51.829 ☑
    elbow only — *see* Laceration, elbow
    left S51.812 ☑
      with
        foreign body S51.822 ☑
    right S51.811 ☑
      with
        foreign body S51.821 ☑
  forehead S01.81 ☑
    with foreign body S01.82 ☑
  fourchette O70.0
    with ectopic or molar pregnancy O08.6
    complicating delivery O70.0
    following ectopic or molar pregnancy O08.6
  gallbladder S36.123 ☑
  genital organs, external
    female S31.512 ☑
      with foreign body S31.522 ☑
      vagina — *see* Laceration, vagina
      vulva — *see* Laceration, vulva
    male S31.511 ☑
      with foreign body S31.521 ☑

Laceration — *continued*
  genital organs, external — *continued*
    male — *continued*
      penis — *see* Laceration, penis
      scrotum — *see* Laceration, scrotum
      testis — *see* Laceration, testis
  groin — *see* Laceration, abdomen, wall
  gum — *see* Laceration, oral cavity
  hand S61.419 ☑
    with
      foreign body S61.429 ☑
    finger — *see* Laceration, finger
    left S61.412 ☑
      with
        foreign body S61.422 ☑
    right S61.411 ☑
      with
        foreign body S61.421 ☑
    thumb — *see* Laceration, thumb
  head S01.91 ☑
    with foreign body S01.92 ☑
    cheek — *see* Laceration, cheek
    ear — *see* Laceration, ear
    eyelid — *see* Laceration, eyelid
    lip — *see* Laceration, lip
    nose — *see* Laceration, nose
    oral cavity — *see* Laceration, oral cavity
    scalp S01.01 ☑
      with foreign body S01.02 ☑
    specified site NEC S01.81 ☑
      with foreign body S01.82 ☑
    temporomandibular area — *see* Laceration, cheek
  heart — *see* Injury, heart, laceration
  heel — *see* Laceration, foot
  hepatic duct S36.13 ☑
  hip S71.019 ☑
    with foreign body S71.029 ☑
    left S71.012 ☑
      with foreign body S71.022 ☑
    right S71.011 ☑
      with foreign body S71.021 ☑
  hymen — *see* Laceration, vagina
  hypochondrium — *see* Laceration, abdomen, wall
  hypogastric region — *see* Laceration, abdomen, wall
  ileum S36.438 ☑
  inguinal region — *see* Laceration, abdomen, wall
  instep — *see* Laceration, foot
  internal organ — *see* Injury, by site
  interscapular region — *see* Laceration, thorax, back
  intestine
    large
      colon S36.539 ☑
        ascending S36.530 ☑
        descending S36.532 ☑
        sigmoid S36.533 ☑
        specified site NEC S36.538 ☑
      rectum S36.63 ☑
        transverse S36.531 ☑
    small S36.439 ☑
      duodenum S36.430 ☑
      specified site NEC S36.438 ☑
  intra-abdominal organ S36.93 ☑
    intestine — *see* Laceration, intestine
    liver — *see* Laceration, liver
    pancreas — *see* Laceration, pancreas
    peritoneum S36.81 ☑
    specified site NEC S36.893 ☑
    spleen — *see* Laceration, spleen
    stomach — *see* Laceration, stomach
  intracranial NEC (*see also* Injury, intracranial, diffuse)
    birth injury P10.9
  jaw — *see* Laceration, head, specified site NEC
  jejunum S36.438 ☑
  joint capsule — *see* Sprain, by site
  kidney S37.03- ☑
    major (greater than 3 cm) (massive) (stellate) S37.06- ☑
    minor (less than 1 cm) S37.04- ☑
    moderate (1 to 3 cm) S37.05- ☑
      multiple S37.06- ☑
  knee S81.01- ☑
    with foreign body S81.02- ☑
  labium (majus) (minus) — *see* Laceration, vulva
  lacrimal duct — *see* Laceration, eyelid
  large intestine — *see* Laceration, intestine, large
  larynx S11.011 ☑

Laceration — *continued*
  larynx — *continued*
    with foreign body S11.012 ☑
  leg (lower) S81.819 ☑
    with foreign body S81.829 ☑
    foot — *see* Laceration, foot
    knee — *see* Laceration, knee
    left S81.812 ☑
      with foreign body S81.822 ☑
    right S81.811 ☑
      with foreign body S81.821 ☑
    upper — *see* Laceration, thigh
  ligament — *see* Sprain
  lip S01.511 ☑
    with foreign body S01.521 ☑
  liver S36.113 ☑
    major (stellate) S36.116 ☑
    minor S36.114 ☑
    moderate S36.115 ☑
  loin — *see* Laceration, abdomen, wall
  lower back — *see* Laceration, back, lower
  lumbar region — *see* Laceration, back, lower
  lung S27.339 ☑
    bilateral S27.332 ☑
    unilateral S27.331 ☑
  malar region — *see* Laceration, head, specified site NEC
  mammary — *see* Laceration, breast
  mastoid region — *see* Laceration, head, specified site NEC
  meninges — *see* Injury, intracranial, diffuse
  meniscus — *see* Tear, meniscus
  mesentery S36.893 ☑
  mesosalpinx S37.893 ☑
  mouth — *see* Laceration, oral cavity
  muscle — *see* Injury, muscle, by site, laceration
  nail
    finger — *see* Laceration, finger, with damage to nail
    toe — *see* Laceration, toe, with damage to nail
  nasal (septum) (sinus) — *see* Laceration, nose
  nasopharynx — *see* Laceration, head, specified site NEC
  neck S11.91 ☑
    with foreign body S11.92 ☑
    involving
      cervical esophagus S11.21 ☑
        with foreign body S11.22 ☑
      larynx — *see* Laceration, larynx
      pharynx — *see* Laceration, pharynx
      thyroid gland — *see* Laceration, thyroid gland
      trachea — *see* Laceration, trachea
    specified site NEC S11.81 ☑
      with foreign body S11.82 ☑
  nerve — *see* Injury, nerve
  nose (septum) (sinus) S01.21 ☑
    with foreign body S01.22 ☑
  ocular NOS S05.3-
    adnexa NOS S01.11-
  oral cavity S01.512 ☑
    with foreign body S01.522 ☑
  orbit (eye) — *see* Wound, open, ocular, orbit
  ovary S37.439 ☑
    bilateral S37.432 ☑
    unilateral S37.431 ☑
  palate — *see* Laceration, oral cavity
  palm — *see* Laceration, hand
  pancreas S36.239 ☑
  pelvic S31.010 ☑
    with
      foreign body S31.020 ☑
        penetration into retroperitoneal cavity S31.021 ☑
      penetration into retroperitoneal cavity S31.011 ☑
    floor (*see also* Laceration, back, lower)
      with ectopic or molar pregnancy O08.6
      complicating delivery O70.1
      following ectopic or molar pregnancy O08.6
      old (postpartal) N81.89
    organ S37.93 ☑
  penis S31.21 ☑
    with foreign body S31.22 ☑
  perineum
    female S31.41 ☑

Subterms under main terms may continue to next column or page   ☑ Additional Character Required — Refer to the Tabular List for Character Selection   207

Laceration — Laceration

Laceration — *continued*
  perineum — *continued*
    female — *continued*
      with
        ectopic or molar pregnancy O08.6
        foreign body S31.42 ☑
      during delivery O70.9
        first degree O70.0
        fourth degree O70.3
        second degree O70.1
        third degree (*see also* Delivery, complicated, by, laceration, perineum, third degree) O70.20
      old (postpartal) N81.89
      postpartal N81.89
      secondary (postpartal) O90.1
    male S31.119 ☑
      with foreign body S31.129 ☑
  periocular area (with or without lacrimal passages) — *see* Laceration, eyelid
  peritoneum S36.893 ☑
  periumbilic region — *see* Laceration, abdomen, wall, periumbilic
  periurethral tissue — *see* Laceration, urethra
  phalanges
    finger — *see* Laceration, finger
    toe — *see* Laceration, toe
  pharynx S11.21 ☑
    with foreign body S11.22 ☑
  pinna — *see* Laceration, ear
  popliteal space — *see* Laceration, knee
  prepuce — *see* Laceration, penis
  prostate S37.823 ☑
  pubic region S31.119 ☑
    with foreign body S31.129 ☑
  pudendum — *see* Laceration, genital organs, external
  rectovaginal septum — *see* Laceration, vagina
  rectum S36.63 ☑
  retroperitoneum S36.893 ☑
  round ligament S37.893 ☑
  sacral region — *see* Laceration, back, lower
  sacroiliac region — *see* Laceration, back, lower
  salivary gland — *see* Laceration, oral cavity
  scalp S01.01 ☑
    with foreign body S01.02 ☑
  scapular region — *see* Laceration, shoulder
  scrotum S31.31 ☑
    with foreign body S31.32 ☑
  seminal vesicle S37.893 ☑
  shin — *see* Laceration, leg
  shoulder S41.019 ☑
    with foreign body S41.029 ☑
    left S41.012 ☑
      with foreign body S41.022 ☑
    right S41.011 ☑
      with foreign body S41.021 ☑
  small intestine — *see* Laceration, intestine, small
  spermatic cord — *see* Laceration, testis
  spinal cord (meninges) (*see also* Injury, spinal cord, by region)
    due to injury at birth P11.5
    newborn (birth injury) P11.5
  spleen S36.039 ☑
    major (massive) (stellate) S36.032 ☑
    moderate S36.031 ☑
    superficial (minor) S36.030 ☑
  sternal region — *see* Laceration, thorax, front
  stomach S36.33 ☑
  submaxillary region — *see* Laceration, head, specified site NEC
  submental region — *see* Laceration, head, specified site NEC
  subungual
    finger(s) — *see* Laceration, finger, with damage to nail
    toe(s) — *see* Laceration, toe, with damage to nail
  suprarenal gland — *see* Laceration, adrenal gland
  temple, temporal region — *see* Laceration, head, specified site NEC
  temporomandibular area — *see* Laceration, cheek
  tendon — *see* Injury, muscle, by site, laceration
    Achilles S86.02- ☑
  tentorium cerebelli — *see* Injury, intracranial, diffuse
  testis S31.31 ☑
    with foreign body S31.32 ☑
  thigh S71.11- ☑
    with foreign body S71.12- ☑

Laceration — *continued*
  thorax, thoracic (wall) S21.91 ☑
    with foreign body S21.92 ☑
    back S21.22- ☑
      with penetration into thoracic cavity S21.42- ☑
    front S21.12- ☑
      with penetration into thoracic cavity S21.32- ☑
    back S21.21- ☑
      with
        foreign body S21.22- ☑
          with penetration into thoracic cavity S21.42- ☑
        penetration into thoracic cavity S21.41- ☑
    breast — *see* Laceration, breast
    front S21.11- ☑
      with
        foreign body S21.12- ☑
          with penetration into thoracic cavity S21.32- ☑
        penetration into thoracic cavity S21.31- ☑
  thumb S61.019 ☑
    with
      damage to nail S61.119 ☑
        with
          foreign body S61.129 ☑
      foreign body S61.029 ☑
    left S61.012 ☑
      with
        damage to nail S61.112 ☑
          with
            foreign body S61.122 ☑
        foreign body S61.022 ☑
    right S61.011 ☑
      with
        damage to nail S61.111 ☑
          with
            foreign body S61.121 ☑
        foreign body S61.021 ☑
  thyroid gland S11.11 ☑
    with foreign body S11.12 ☑
  toe(s) S91.119 ☑
    with
      damage to nail S91.219 ☑
        with
          foreign body S91.229 ☑
      foreign body S91.129 ☑
    great S91.113 ☑
      with
        damage to nail S91.213 ☑
          with
            foreign body S91.223 ☑
        foreign body S91.123 ☑
      left S91.112 ☑
        with
          damage to nail S91.212 ☑
            with
              foreign body S91.222 ☑
          foreign body S91.122 ☑
      right S91.111 ☑
        with
          damage to nail S91.211 ☑
            with
              foreign body S91.221 ☑
          foreign body S91.121 ☑
    lesser S91.116 ☑
      with
        damage to nail S91.216 ☑
          with
            foreign body S91.226 ☑
        foreign body S91.126 ☑
      left S91.115 ☑
        with
          damage to nail S91.215 ☑
            with
              foreign body S91.225 ☑
          foreign body S91.125 ☑
      right S91.114 ☑
        with
          damage to nail S91.214 ☑
            with
              foreign body S91.224 ☑
          foreign body S91.124 ☑
  tongue — *see* Laceration, oral cavity
  trachea S11.021 ☑

Laceration — *continued*
  trachea — *continued*
    with foreign body S11.022 ☑
  tunica vaginalis — *see* Laceration, testis
  tympanum, tympanic membrane — *see* Laceration, ear, drum
  umbilical region S31.115 ☑
    with foreign body S31.125 ☑
  ureter S37.13 ☑
  urethra S37.33 ☑
    with or following ectopic or molar pregnancy O08.6
    obstetrical trauma O71.5
  urinary organ NEC S37.893 ☑
  uterus S37.63 ☑
    with ectopic or molar pregnancy O08.6
    following ectopic or molar pregnancy O08.6
    nonpuerperal, nontraumatic N85.8
    obstetrical trauma NEC O71.81
    old (postpartal) N85.8
  uvula — *see* Laceration, oral cavity
  vagina S31.41 ☑
    with
      ectopic or molar pregnancy O08.6
      foreign body S31.42 ☑
    during delivery O71.4
      with perineal laceration — *see* Laceration, perineum, female, during delivery
    following ectopic or molar pregnancy O08.6
    nonpuerperal, nontraumatic N89.8
    old (postpartal) N89.8
  vas deferens S37.893 ☑
  vesical — *see* Laceration, bladder
  vocal cords S11.031 ☑
    with foreign body S11.032 ☑
  vulva S31.41 ☑
    with
      ectopic or molar pregnancy O08.6
      foreign body S31.42 ☑
    complicating delivery O70.0
    following ectopic or molar pregnancy O08.6
    nonpuerperal, nontraumatic N90.89
    old (postpartal) N90.89
  wrist S61.519 ☑
    with
      foreign body S61.529 ☑
    left S61.512 ☑
      with
        foreign body S61.522 ☑
    right S61.511 ☑
      with
        foreign body S61.521 ☑

Lack of
  achievement in school Z55.3
  adequate
    food Z59.4
    intermaxillary vertical dimension of fully erupted teeth M26.36
    sleep Z72.820
  appetite (see Anorexia) R63.0
  awareness R41.9
  care
    in home Z74.2
    of infant (at or after birth) T76.02 ☑
      confirmed T74.02 ☑
  cognitive functions R41.9
  coordination R27.9
    ataxia R27.0
    specified type NEC R27.8
  development (physiological) R62.50
    failure to thrive (child over 28 days old) R62.51
      adult R62.7
      newborn P92.6
    short stature R62.52
    specified type NEC R62.59
  energy R53.83
  financial resources Z59.6
  food T73.0
  growth R62.52
  heating Z59.1
  housing (permanent) (temporary) Z59.0
    adequate Z59.1
  learning experiences in childhood Z62.898
  leisure time (affecting life-style) Z73.2
  material resources Z59.9
  memory (*see also* Amnesia)
    mild, following organic brain damage F06.8
  ovulation N97.0
  parental supervision or control of child Z62.0

☑ **Additional Character Required** — Refer to the Tabular List for Character Selection
🔄 **Subterms under main terms may continue to next column or page**

Lack of — *continued*
  person able to render necessary care Z74.2
  physical exercise Z72.3
  play experience in childhood Z62.898
  posterior occlusal support M26.57
  relaxation (affecting life-style) Z73.2
  sexual
    desire F52.0
    enjoyment F52.1
  shelter Z59.0
  sleep (adequate) Z72.820
  supervision of child by parent Z62.0
  support, posterior occlusal M26.57
  water T73.1 ☑
Lacrimal — *see* condition
Lacrimation, abnormal — *see* Epiphora
Lacrimonasal duct — *see* condition
Lactation, lactating (breast) (puerperal, postpartum)
  associated
    cracked nipple O92.13
    retracted nipple O92.03
  defective O92.4
  disorder NEC O92.79
  excessive O92.6
  failed (complete) O92.3
    partial O92.4
  mastitis NEC — *see* Mastitis, obstetric
  mother (care and/or examination) Z39.1
  nonpuerperal N64.3
Lacticemia, excessive E87.2
Lacunar skull Q75.8
Laennec's cirrhosis K70.30
  with ascites K70.31
  nonalcoholic K74.69
Lafora's disease — *see* Epilepsy, generalized, idiopathic
Lag, lid (nervous) — *see* Retraction, lid
Lagophthalmos (eyelid) (nervous) H02.209
  cicatricial H02.219
    left H02.216
      lower H02.215
      upper H02.214
    right H02.213
      lower H02.212
      upper H02.211
  keratoconjunctivitis — *see* Keratoconjunctivitis
  left H02.206
    lower H02.205
    upper H02.204
  mechanical H02.229
    left H02.226
      lower H02.225
      upper H02.224
    right H02.223
      lower H02.222
      upper H02.221
  paralytic H02.239
    left H02.236
      lower H02.235
      upper H02.234
    right H02.233
      lower H02.232
      upper H02.231
  right H02.203
    lower H02.202
    upper H02.201
Laki-Lorand factor deficiency — *see* Defect, coagulation, specified type NEC
Lalling F80.0
Lambert-Eaton syndrome — *see* Syndrome, Lambert-Eaton
Lambliasis, lambliosis A07.1
Landau-Kleffner syndrome — *see* Epilepsy, specified NEC
Landouzy-Déjérine dystrophy or facioscapulohumeral atrophy G71.0
Landouzy's disease (icterohemorrhagic leptospirosis) A27.0
Landry-Guillain-Barré, syndrome or paralysis G61.0
Landry's disease or paralysis G61.0
Lane's
  band Q43.3
  kink — *see* Obstruction, intestine
  syndrome K90.2
Langdon Down syndrome — *see* Trisomy, 21
Lapsed immunization schedule status Z28.3
Large
  baby (regardless of gestational age) (4000g to 4499g) P08.1

Large — *continued*
  ear, congenital Q17.1
  physiological cup Q14.2
  stature R68.89
Large-for-dates NEC (infant) (4000g to 4499g) P08.1
  affecting management of pregnancy O36.6- ☑
  exceptionally (4500g or more) P08.0
Larsen-Johansson disease orosteochondrosis — *see* Osteochondrosis, juvenile, patella
Larsen's syndrome (flattened facies and multiple congenital dislocations) Q74.8
Larva migrans
  cutaneous B76.9
    Ancylostoma B76.0
  visceral B83.0
Laryngeal — *see* condition
Laryngismus (stridulus) J38.5
  congenital P28.89
  diphtheritic A36.2
Laryngitis (acute) (edematous) (fibrinous) (infective) (infiltrative) (malignant) (membranous) (phlegmonous) (pneumococcal) (pseudomembranous) (septic) (subglottic) (suppurative) (ulcerative) J04.0
  with
    influenza, flu, or grippe — *see* Influenza, with, laryngitis
    tracheitis (acute) — *see* Laryngotracheitis
  atrophic J37.0
  catarrhal J37.0
  chronic J37.0
    with tracheitis (chronic) J37.1
  diphtheritic A36.2
  due to external agent — *see* Inflammation, respiratory, upper, due to
  H. influenzae J04.0
  Hemophilus influenzae J04.0
  hypertrophic J37.0
  influenzal — *see* Influenza, with, respiratory manifestations NEC
  obstructive J05.0
  sicca J37.0
  spasmodic J05.0
    acute J04.0
  streptococcal J04.0
  stridulous J05.0
  syphilitic (late) A52.73
    congenital A50.59 [J99]
      early A50.03 [J99]
  tuberculous A15.5
  Vincent's A69.1
Laryngocele (congenital) (ventricular) Q31.3
Laryngofissure J38.7
  congenital Q31.8
Laryngomalacia (congenital) Q31.5
Laryngopharyngitis (acute) J06.0
  chronic J37.0
  due to external agent — *see* Inflammation, respiratory, upper, due to
Laryngoplegia J38.00
  bilateral J38.02
  unilateral J38.01
Laryngoptosis J38.7
Laryngospasm J38.5
Laryngostenosis J38.6
Laryngotracheitis (acute) (Infectional) (infective) (viral) J04.2
  atrophic J37.1
  catarrhal J37.1
  chronic J37.1
  diphtheritic A36.2
  due to external agent — *see* Inflammation, respiratory, upper, due to
  Hemophilus influenzae J04.2
  hypertrophic J37.1
  influenzal — *see* Influenza, with, respiratory manifestations NEC
  pachydermic J38.7
  sicca J37.1
  spasmodic J38.5
    acute J05.0
  streptococcal J04.2
  stridulous J38.5
  syphilitic (late) A52.73
    congenital A50.59 [J99]
      early A50.03 [J99]
  tuberculous A15.5
  Vincent's A69.1
Laryngotracheobronchitis — *see* Bronchitis

Larynx, laryngeal — *see* condition
Lassa fever A96.2
Lassitude — *see* Weakness
Late
  talker R62.0
  walker R62.0
Late effect(s) — *see* Sequelae
Latent — *see* condition
Laterocession — *see* Lateroversion
Lateroflexion — *see* Lateroversion
Lateroversion
  cervix — *see* Lateroversion, uterus
  uterus, uterine (cervix) (postinfectional) (postpartal, old) N85.4
    congenital Q51.818
    in pregnancy or childbirth O34.59- ☑
Lathyrism — *see* Poisoning, food, noxious, plant
Launois' syndrome (pituitary gigantism) E22.0
Launois-Bensaude adenolipomatosis E88.89
Laurence-Moon (-Bardet)-**Biedl syndrome** Q87.89
Lax, laxity (*see also* Relaxation)
  ligament (ous) (*see also* Disorder, ligament)
    familial M35.7
    knee — *see* Derangement, knee
  skin (acquired) L57.4
    congenital Q82.8
Laxative habit F55.2
Lazy leukocyte syndrome D70.8
Lead miner's lung J63.6
Leak, leakage
  air NEC J93.82
    postprocedural J95.812
  amniotic fluid — *see* Rupture, membranes, premature
  blood (microscopic), fetal, into maternal circulation
    affecting management of pregnancy — *see* Pregnancy, complicated by
  cerebrospinal fluid G96.0
    from spinal (lumbar) puncture G97.0
  device, implant or graft (*see also* Complications, by site and type, mechanical)
    arterial graft NEC — *see* Complication, cardiovascular device, mechanical, vascular
    breast (implant) T85.43 ☑
    catheter NEC T85.638 ☑
      dialysis (renal) T82.43 ☑
        intraperitoneal T85.631 ☑
      infusion NEC T82.534 ☑
        spinal (epidural) (subdural) T85.630 ☑
      urinary T83.038 ☑
        cystostomy T83.030 ☑
        Hopkins T83.038 ☑
        ileostomy T83.038 ☑
        indwelling T83.031 ☑
        nephrostomy T83.032 ☑
        specified T83.038 ☑
        urostomy T83.038 ☑
    gastrointestinal — *see* Complications, prosthetic device, mechanical, gastrointestinal device
    genital NEC T83.498 ☑
      penile prosthesis (cylinder) (implanted) (pump) (reservoir) T83.490 ☑
      testicular prosthesis T83.491 ☑
    heart NEC — *see* Complication, cardiovascular device, mechanical
    joint prosthesis — *see* Complications, joint prosthesis, mechanical, specified NEC, by site
    ocular NEC — *see* Complications, prosthetic device, mechanical, ocular device
    orthopedic NEC — *see* Complication, orthopedic, device, mechanical
    persistent air J93.82
    specified NEC T85.638 ☑
    urinary NEC (*see also* Complication, genitourinary, device, urinary, mechanical)
      graft T83.23 ☑
    vascular NEC — *see* Complication, cardiovascular device, mechanical
    ventricular intracranial shunt T85.03 ☑
  urine — *see* Incontinence
Leaky heart — *see* Endocarditis
Learning defect (specific) F81.9
Leather bottle stomach C16.9
Leber's
  congenital amaurosis H35.50
  optic atrophy (hereditary) H47.22
Lederer's anemia D59.1
Leeches (external) — *see* Hirudiniasis

Index

Leg — *see* condition
Legg (-Calvé)-**Perthes disease, syndrome or osteo-
    chondrosis** M91.1- ☑
Legionellosis A48.1
  nonpneumonic A48.2
Legionnaires'
  disease A48.1
    nonpneumonic A48.2
  pneumonia A48.1
Leigh's disease G31.82
Leiner's disease L21.1
Leiofibromyoma — *see* Leiomyoma
Leiomyoblastoma — *see* Neoplasm, connective tissue,
  benign
Leiomyofibroma (*see also* Neoplasm, connective tissue,
  benign)
  uterus (cervix) (corpus) D25.9
Leiomyoma (*see also* Neoplasm, connective tissue, benign)
  bizarre — *see* Neoplasm, connective tissue, benign
  cellular — *see* Neoplasm, connective tissue, benign
  epithelioid — *see* Neoplasm, connective tissue, benign
  uterus (cervix) (corpus) D25.9
    intramural D25.1
    submucous D25.0
    subserosal D25.2
  vascular — *see* Neoplasm, connective tissue, benign
Leiomyoma, leiomyomatosis (intravascular) — *see*
  Neoplasm, connective tissue, uncertain behavior
Leiomyosarcoma (*see also* Neoplasm, connective tissue,
  malignant)
  epithelioid — *see* Neoplasm, connective tissue, malig-
    nant
  myxoid — *see* Neoplasm, connective tissue, malignant
Leishmaniasis B55.9
  American (mucocutaneous) B55.2
    cutaneous B55.1
  Asian Desert B55.1
  Brazilian B55.2
  cutaneous (any type) B55.1
  dermal (*see also* Leishmaniasis, cutaneous)
    post-kala-azar B55.0
  eyelid B55.1
  infantile B55.0
  Mediterranean B55.0
  mucocutaneous (American) (New World) B55.2
  naso-oral B55.2
  nasopharyngeal B55.2
  old world B55.1
  tegumentaria diffusa B55.1
  visceral B55.0
Leishmanoid, dermal (*see also* Leishmaniasis, cutaneous)
  post-kala-azar B55.0
Lenegre's disease I44.2
Lengthening, leg — *see* Deformity, limb, unequal length
Lennert's lymphoma — *see* Lymphoma, Lennert's
Lennox-Gastaut syndrome G40.812
  intractable G40.814
    with status epilepticus G40.813
    without status epilepticus G40.814
  not intractable G40.812
    with status epilepticus G40.811
    without status epilepticus G40.812
Lens — *see* condition
Lenticonus (anterior) (posterior) (congenital) Q12.8
Lenticular degeneration, progressive E83.01
Lentiglobus (posterior) (congenital) Q12.8
Lentigo (congenital) L81.4
  maligna (*see also* Melanoma, in situ)
    melanoma — *see* Melanoma
Lentivirus, as cause of disease classified elsewhere
  B97.31
Leontiasis
  ossium M85.2
  syphilitic (late) A52.78
    congenital A50.59
Lepothrix A48.8
Lepra — *see* Leprosy
Leprechaunism E34.8
Leprosy A30.- ☑
  with muscle disorder A30.9 [M63.80]
    ankle A30.9 [M63.87-] ☑
    foot A30.9 [M63.87-] ☑
    forearm A30.9 [M63.83-] ☑
    hand A30.9 [M63.84-] ☑
    lower leg A30.9 [M63.86-] ☑

Leprosy — *continued*
  with muscle disorder — *continued*
    multiple sites A30.9 [M63.89]
    pelvic region A30.9 [M63.85-] ☑
    shoulder region A30.9 [M63.81-] ☑
    specified site NEC A30.9 [M63.88]
    thigh A30.9 [M63.85-] ☑
    upper arm A30.9 [M63.82-] ☑
  anesthetic A30.9
  BB A30.3
  BL A30.4
  borderline (infiltrated) (neuritic) A30.3
    lepromatous A30.4
    tuberculoid A30.2
  BT A30.2
  dimorphous (infiltrated) (neuritic) A30.3
  I A30.0
  indeterminate (macular) (neuritic) A30.0
  lepromatous (diffuse) (infiltrated) (macular) (neuritic)
    (nodular) A30.5
  LL A30.5
  macular (early) (neuritic) (simple) A30.9
  maculoanesthetic A30.9
  mixed A30.3
  neural A30.9
  nodular A30.5
  primary neuritic A30.3
  specified type NEC A30.8
  TT A30.1
  tuberculoid (major) (minor) A30.1
Leptocytosis, hereditary D56.9
Leptomeningitis (chronic) (circumscribed) (hemorrhagic)
  (nonsuppurative) — *see* Meningitis
Leptomeningopathy G96.19
Leptospiral — *see* condition
Leptospirochetal — *see* condition
Leptospirosis A27.9
  canicola A27.89
  due to Leptospira interrogans serovar icterohaemor-
    rhagiae A27.0
  icterohemorrhagica A27.0
  pomona A27.89
  Weil's disease A27.0
Leptus dermatitis B88.0
Leriche's syndrome (aortic bifurcation occlusion) I74.09
Leri's pleonosteosis Q78.8
Leri-Weill syndrome Q77.8
Lermoyez' syndrome — *see* Vertigo, peripheral NEC
Lesch-Nyhan syndrome E79.1
Leser-Trélat disease L82.1
  inflamed L82.0
Lesion(s) (nontraumatic)
  abducens nerve — *see* Strabismus, paralytic, sixth
    nerve
  alveolar process K08.9
  angiocentric immunoproliferative D47.Z9 (*following*
    D47.4)
  anorectal K62.9
  aortic (valve) I35.9
  auditory nerve — *see* subcategory H93.3 ☑
  basal ganglion G25.9
  bile duct — *see* Disease, bile duct
  biomechanical M99.9
    specified type NEC M99.89
      abdomen M99.89
      acromioclavicular M99.87
      cervical region M99.81
      cervicothoracic M99.81
      costochondral M99.88
      costovertebral M99.88
      head region M99.80
      hip M99.85
      lower extremity M99.86
      lumbar region M99.83
      lumbosacral M99.83
      occipitocervical M99.80
      pelvic region M99.85
      pubic M99.85
      rib cage M99.88
      sacral region M99.84
      sacrococcygeal M99.84
      sacroiliac M99.84
      specified NEC M99.89
      sternochondral M99.88
      sternoclavicular M99.87
      thoracic region M99.82
      thoracolumbar M99.82
      upper extremity M99.87

Lesion(s) — *continued*
  bladder N32.9
  bone — *see* Disorder, bone
  brachial plexus G54.0
  brain G93.9
    congenital Q04.9
    vascular I67.9
      degenerative I67.9
      hypertensive I67.4
  buccal cavity K13.79
  calcified — *see* Calcification
  canthus — *see* Disorder, eyelid
  carate — *see* Pinta, lesions
  cardia K31.9
  cardiac (*see also* Disease, heart) I51.9
    congenital Q24.9
    valvular — *see* Endocarditis
  cauda equina G83.4
  cecum K63.9
  cerebral — *see* Lesion, brain
  cerebrovascular I67.9
    degenerative I67.9
    hypertensive I67.4
  cervical (nerve) root NEC G54.2
  chiasmal — *see* Disorder, optic, chiasm
  chorda tympani G51.8
  coin, lung R91.1
  colon K63.9
  combined periodontic - endodontic K05.5
  congenital — *see* Anomaly, by site
  conjunctiva H11.9
  conus medullaris — *see* Injury, conus medullaris
  coronary artery — *see* Ischemia, heart
  cranial nerve G52.9
    eighth — *see* Disorder, ear
    eleventh G52.9
    fifth G50.9
    first G52.0
    fourth — *see* Strabismus, paralytic, fourth nerve
    seventh G51.9
    sixth — *see* Strabismus, paralytic, sixth nerve
    tenth G52.2
    twelfth G52.3
  cystic — *see* Cyst
  degenerative — *see* Degeneration
  duodenum K31.9
  edentulous (alveolar) ridge, associated with trauma,
    due to traumatic occlusion K06.2
  en coup de sabre L94.1
  eyelid — *see* Disorder, eyelid
  gasserian ganglion G50.8
  gastric K31.9
  gastroduodenal K31.9
  gastrointestinal K63.9
  gingiva, associated with trauma K06.2
  glomerular
    focal and segmental (*see also* N00-N07 with fourth
      character .1) N05.1
    minimal change (*see also* N00-N07 with fourth
      character .0) N05.0
  heart (organic) — *see* Disease, heart
  hyperchromic, due to pinta (carate) A67.1
  hyperkeratotic — *see* Hyperkeratosis
  hypothalamic E23.7
  ileocecal K63.9
  ileum K63.9
  iliohypogastric nerve G57.8- ☑
  inflammatory — *see* Inflammation
  intestine K63.9
  intracerebral — *see* Lesion, brain
  intrachiasmal (optic) — *see* Disorder, optic, chiasm
  intracranial, space-occupying R90.0
  joint — *see* Disorder, joint
    sacroiliac (old) M53.3
  keratotic — *see* Keratosis
  kidney — *see* Disease, renal
  laryngeal nerve (recurrent) G52.2
  lip K13.0
  liver K76.9
  lumbosacral
    plexus G54.1
    root (nerve) NEC G54.4
  lung (coin) R91.1
  maxillary sinus J32.0
  mitral I05.9
  Morel-Lavallée — *see* Hematoma, by site
  motor cortex NEC G93.89
  mouth K13.79

Lesion(s) — *continued*
  nerve G58.9
    femoral G57.2- ☑
    median G56.1- ☑
      carpal tunnel syndrome — *see* Syndrome, carpal tunnel
    plantar G57.6- ☑
    popliteal (lateral) G57.3- ☑
      medial G57.4- ☑
    radial G56.3- ☑
    sciatic G57.0- ☑
    spinal — *see* Injury, nerve, spinal
    ulnar G56.2- ☑
  nervous system, congenital Q07.9
  nonallopathic — *see* Lesion, biomechanical
  nose (internal) J34.89
  obstructive — *see* Obstruction
  obturator nerve G57.8- ☑
  oral mucosa K13.70
  organ or site NEC — *see* Disease, by site
  osteolytic — *see* Osteolysis
  peptic K27.9
  periodontal, due to traumatic occlusion K05.5
  pharynx J39.2
  pigment, pigmented (skin) L81.9
  pinta — *see* Pinta, lesions
  polypoid — *see* Polyp
  prechiasmal (optic) — *see* Disorder, optic, chiasm
  primary (*see also* Syphilis, primary) A51.0
    carate A67.0
    pinta A67.0
    yaws A66.0
  pulmonary J98.4
    valve I37.9
  pylorus K31.9
  rectosigmoid K63.9
  retina, retinal H35.9
  sacroiliac (joint) (old) M53.3
  salivary gland K11.9
    benign lymphoepithelial K11.8
  saphenous nerve G57.8- ☑
  sciatic nerve G57.0- ☑
  secondary — *see* Syphilis, secondary
  shoulder (region) M75.9- ☑
    specified NEC M75.8- ☑
  sigmoid K63.9
  sinus (accessory) (nasal) J34.89
  skin L98.9
    suppurative L08.0
  SLAP S43.43- ☑
  spinal cord G95.9
    congenital Q06.9
  spleen D73.89
  stomach K31.9
  superior glenoid labrum S43.43- ☑
  syphilitic — *see* Syphilis
  tertiary — *see* Syphilis, tertiary
  thoracic root (nerve) NEC G54.3
  tonsillar fossa J35.9
  tooth, teeth K08.9
    white spot
      chewing surface K02.51
      pit and fissure surface K02.51
      smooth surface K02.61
  traumatic — *see* specific type of injury by site
  tricuspid (valve) I07.9
    nonrheumatic I36.9
  trigeminal nerve G50.9
  ulcerated or ulcerative — *see* Ulcer, skin
  uterus N85.9
  vagus nerve G52.2
  valvular — *see* Endocarditis
  vascular I99.9
    affecting central nervous system I67.9
    following trauma NEC T14.8 ☑
    umbilical cord, complicating delivery O69.5 ☑
  warty — *see* Verruca
  white spot (tooth)
    chewing surface K02.51
    pit and fissure surface K02.51
    smooth surface K02.61
Lethargic — *see* condition
Lethargy R53.83
Letterer-Siwe's disease C96.0
Leukemia, leukemic C95.9- ☑
  acute basophilic C94.8- ☑
  acute bilineal C95.0- ☑

Leukemia, leukemic — *continued*
  acute erythroid C94.0- ☑
  acute lymphoblastic C91.0- ☑
  acute megakaryoblastic C94.2- ☑
  acute megakaryocytic C94.2- ☑
  acute mixed lineage C95.0- ☑
  acute monoblastic (monoblastic/monocytic) C93.0- ☑
  acute monocytic (monoblastic/monocytic) C93.0- ☑
  acute myeloblastic (minimal differentiation) (with maturation) C92.0- ☑
  acute myeloid
    with
      11q23-abnormality C92.6- ☑
      dysplasia of remaining hematopoesis and/or myelodysplastic disease in its history C92.A- ☑ (*following* C92.6)
      multilineage dysplasia C92.A- ☑ (*following* C92.6)
      variation of MLL-gene C92.6- ☑
    M6 (a)(b) C94.0- ☑
    M7 C94.2- ☑
  acute myelomonocytic C92.5- ☑
  acute promyelocytic C92.4- ☑
  adult T-cell (HTLV-1-associated) (acute variant) (chronic variant) (lymphomatoid variant) (smouldering variant) C91.5- ☑
  aggressive NK-cell C94.8- ☑
  AML (1/ETO) (M0) (M1) (M2) (without a FAB classification) C92.0- ☑
  AML M3 C92.4- ☑
  AML M4 (Eo with inv(16) or t(16;16)) C92.5- ☑
  AML M5 C93.0- ☑
  AML M5a C93.0- ☑
  AML M5b C93.0- ☑
  AML Me with t (15;17) and variants C92.4- ☑
  atypical chronic myeloid, BCR/ABL-negative C92.2- ☑
  biphenotypic acute C95.0- ☑
  blast cell C95.0- ☑
  Burkitt-type, mature B-cell C91.A- ☑ (*following* C91.6)
  chronic lymphocytic, of B-cell type C91.1- ☑
  chronic monocytic C93.1- ☑
  chronic myelogenous (Philadelphia chromosome (Ph1) positive) (t(9;22)) (q34;q11) (with crisis of blast cells) C92.1- ☑
  chronic myeloid, BCR/ABL-positive C92.1- ☑
    atypical, BCR/ABL-negative C92.2- ☑
  chronic myelomonocytic C93.1- ☑
  chronic neutrophilic D47.1
  CMML (-1) (-2) (with eosinophilia) C93.1- ☑
  granulocytic (*see also* Category C92) C92.9- ☑
  hairy cell C91.4- ☑
  juvenile myelomonocytic C93.3- ☑
  lymphoid C91.9- ☑
    specified NEC C91.Z- ☑ (*following* C91.6)
  mast cell C94.3- ☑
  mature B-cell, Burkitt-type C91.A- ☑ (*following* C91.6)
  monocytic (subacute) C93.9- ☑
    specified NEC C93.Z- ☑ (*following* C93.3)
  myelogenous (*see also* Category C92) C92.9- ☑
  myeloid C92.9- ☑
    specified NEC C92.Z- ☑ (*following* C92.6)
  plasma cell C90.1- ☑
  plasmacytic C90.1- ☑
  prolymphocytic
    of B-cell type C91.3- ☑
    of T-cell type C91.6- ☑
  specified NEC C94.8- ☑
  stem cell, of unclear lineage C95.0- ☑
  subacute lymphocytic C91.9- ☑
  T-cell large granular lymphocytic C91.Z- ☑ (*following* C91.6)
  unspecified cell type C95.9- ☑
    acute C95.0- ☑
    chronic C95.1- ☑
Leukemoid reaction (*see also* Reaction, leukemoid) D72.823
Leukoaraiosis (hypertensive) I67.81
Leukoariosis — *see* Leukoaraiosis
Leukocoria — *see* Disorder, globe, degenerated condition, leucocoria
Leukocytopenia D72.819
Leukocytosis D72.829
  eosinophilic D72.1
Leukoderma, leukodermia NEC L81.5
  syphilitic A51.39
    late A52.79

Leukodystrophy E75.29
Leukoedema, oral epithelium K13.29
Leukoencephalitis G04.81
  acute (subacute) hemorrhagic G36.1
    postimmunization or postvaccinal G04.02
  postinfectious G04.01
  subacute sclerosing A81.1
  van Bogaert's (sclerosing) A81.1
Leukoencephalopathy (*see also* Encephalopathy) G93.49
  Binswanger's I67.3
  heroin vapor G92
  metachromatic E75.25
  multifocal (progressive) A81.2
  postimmunization and postvaccinal G04.02
  progressive multifocal A81.2
  reversible, posterior G93.6
  van Bogaert's (sclerosing) A81.1
  vascular, progressive I67.3
Leukoerythroblastosis D75.9
Leukokeratosis (*see also* Leukoplakia)
  mouth K13.21
  nicotina palati K13.24
  oral mucosa K13.21
  tongue K13.21
  vocal cord J38.3
Leukokraurosis vulva (e) N90.4
Leukoma (cornea) (*see also* Opacity, cornea)
  adherent H17.0-
  interfering with central vision — *see* Opacity, cornea, central
Leukomalacia, cerebral, newborn P91.2
  periventricular P91.2
Leukomelanopathy, hereditary D72.0
Leukonychia (punctata) (striata) L60.8
  congenital Q84.4
Leukopathia unguium L60.8
  congenital Q84.4
Leukopenia D72.819
  basophilic D72.818
  chemotherapy (cancer) induced D70.1
  congenital D70.0
  cyclic D70.0
  drug induced NEC D70.2
    due to cytoreductive cancer chemotherapy D70.1
  eosinophilic D72.818
  familial D70.0
  infantile genetic D70.0
  malignant D70.9
  periodic D70.0
  transitory neonatal P61.5
Leukopenic — *see* condition
Leukoplakia
  anus K62.89
  bladder (postinfectional) N32.89
  buccal K13.21
  cervix (uteri) N88.0
  esophagus K22.8
  gingiva K13.21
  hairy (oral mucosa) (tongue) K13.3
  kidney (pelvis) N28.89
  larynx J38.7
  lip K13.21
  mouth K13.21
  oral epithelium, including tongue (mucosa) K13.21
  palate K13.21
  pelvis (kidney) N28.89
  penis (infectional) N48.0
  rectum K62.89
  syphilitic (late) A52.79
  tongue K13.21
  ureter (postinfectional) N28.89
  urethra (postinfectional) N36.8
  uterus N85.8
  vagina N89.4
  vocal cord J38.3
  vulva N90.4
Leukorrhea N89.8
  due to Trichomonas (vaginalis) A59.00
  trichomonal A59.00
Leukosarcoma C85.9- ☑
Levocardia (isolated) Q24.1
  with situs inversus Q89.3
Levotransposition Q20.5
Lev's disease or syndrome (acquired complete heart block) I44.2
Levulosuria — *see* Fructosuria
Levurid L30.2

⬇ Subterms under main terms may continue to next column or page   ☑ Additional Character Required — Refer to the Tabular List for Character Selection   211

Lesion — Levurid

Lewy body (ies) (dementia) (disease) G31.83
Leyden-Moebius dystrophy G71.Ø
Leydig cell
　carcinoma
　　specified site — *see* Neoplasm, malignant, by site
　　unspecified site
　　　female C56.9
　　　male C62.9- ☑
　tumor
　　benign
　　　specified site — *see* Neoplasm, benign, by site
　　　unspecified site
　　　　female D27.- ☑
　　　　male D29.2- ☑
　　malignant
　　　specified site — *see* Neoplasm, malignant, by
　　　　site
　　　unspecified site
　　　　female C56.- ☑
　　　　male C62.9- ☑
　　specified site — *see* Neoplasm, uncertain behavior,
　　　by site
　　unspecified site
　　　female D39.1- ☑
　　　male D4Ø.1- ☑
Leydig-Sertoli cell tumor
　specified site — *see* Neoplasm, benign, by site
　unspecified site
　　female D27.- ☑
　　male D29.2- ☑
LGSIL (Low grade squamous intraepithelial lesion on cy-
　tologic smear of)
　anus R85.612
　cervix R87.612
　vagina R87.622
Liar, pathologic F6Ø.2
Libido
　decreased R68.82
Libman-Sacks disease M32.11
Lice (infestation) B85.2
　body (Pediculus corporis) B85.1
　crab B85.3
　head (Pediculus capitis) B85.Ø
　mixed (classifiable to more than one of the titles B85.Ø-
　　B85.3) B85.4
　pubic (Phthirus pubis) B85.3
Lichen L28.Ø
　albus L9Ø.Ø
　　penis N48.Ø
　　vulva N9Ø.4
　amyloidosis E85.4 [L99]
　atrophicus L9Ø.Ø
　　penis N48.Ø
　　vulva N9Ø.4
　congenital Q82.8
　myxedematosus L98.5
　nitidus L44.1
　pilaris Q82.8
　　acquired L85.8
　planopilaris L66.1
　planus (chronicus) L43.9
　　annularis L43.8
　　bullous L43.1
　　follicular L66.1
　　hypertrophic L43.Ø
　　moniliformis L44.3
　　of Wilson L43.9
　　specified NEC L43.8
　　subacute (active) L43.3
　　tropicus L43.3
　ruber
　　acuminatus L44.Ø
　　moniliformis L44.3
　　planus L43.9
　sclerosus (et atrophicus) L9Ø.Ø
　　penis N48.Ø
　　vulva N9Ø.4
　scrofulosus (primary) (tuberculous) A18.4
　simplex (chronicus) (circumscriptus) L28.Ø
　striatus L44.2
　urticatus L28.2
Lichenification L28.Ø
Lichenoides tuberculosis (primary) A18.4
Lichtheim's disease or syndrome — *see* Degeneration,
　combined
Lien migrans D73.89
Ligament — *see* condition

Light
　for gestational age — *see* Light for dates
　headedness R42
Light-for-dates (infant) PØ5.ØØ
　with weight of
　　1ØØØ-1249 grams PØ5.Ø4
　　125Ø-1499 grams PØ5.Ø5
　　15ØØ-1749 grams PØ5.Ø6
　　175Ø-1999 grams PØ5.Ø7
　　2ØØØ-2499 grams PØ5.Ø8
　　25ØØ grams and over PØ5.Ø9
　　499 grams or less PØ5.Ø1
　　5ØØ-749 grams PØ5.Ø2
　　75Ø-999 grams PØ5.Ø3
　affecting management of pregnancy O36.59- ☑
　and small-for-dates — *see* Small for dates
　specified NEC PØ5.Ø9
Lightning (effects) (stroke) (struck by) T75.ØØ ☑
　burn — *see* Burn
　foot E53.8
　shock T75.Ø1 ☑
　specified effect NEC T75.Ø9 ☑
Lightwood-Albright syndrome N25.89
Lightwood's disease or syndrome (renal tubular acido-
　sis) N25.89
Lignac (-de Toni) (-Fanconi) (-Debré) **disease or syn-
　drome** E72.Ø9
　with cystinosis E72.Ø4
Ligneous thyroiditis EØ6.5
Likoff's syndrome I2Ø.8
Limb — *see* condition
Limbic epilepsy personality syndrome FØ7.Ø
Limitation, limited
　activities due to disability Z73.6
　cardiac reserve — *see* Disease, heart
　eye muscle duction, traumatic — *see* Strabismus,
　　mechanical
　mandibular range of motion M26.52
Lindau (-von Hippel) **disease** Q85.8
Line(s)
　Beau's L6Ø.4
　Harris' — *see* Arrest, epiphyseal
　Hudson's (cornea) — *see* Pigmentation, cornea, ante-
　　rior
　Stähli's (cornea) — *see* Pigmentation, cornea, anterior
Linea corneae senilis — *see* Change, cornea, senile
Lingua
　geographica K14.1
　nigra (villosa) K14.3
　plicata K14.5
　tylosis K13.29
Lingual — *see* condition
Linguatulosis B88.8
Linitis (gastric) **plastica** C16.9
Lip — *see* condition
Lipedema — *see* Edema
Lipemia (*see also* Hyperlipidemia)
　retina, retinalis E78.3
Lipidosis E75.6
　cerebral (infantile) (juvenile) (late) E75.4
　cerebroretinal E75.4
　cerebroside E75.22
　cholesterol (cerebral) E75.5
　glycolipid E75.21
　hepatosplenomegalic E78.3
　sphingomyelin — *see* Niemann-Pick disease or syn-
　　drome
　sulfatide E75.29
Lipoadenoma — *see* Neoplasm, benign, by site
Lipoblastoma — *see* Lipoma
Lipoblastomatosis — *see* Lipoma
Lipochondrodystrophy E76.Ø1
Lipochrome histiocytosis (familial) D71
Lipodermatosclerosis — *see* Varix, leg, with, inflamma-
　tion
　ulcerated — *see* Varix, leg, with, ulcer, with inflamma-
　　tion by site
Lipodystrophia progressiva E88.1
Lipodystrophy (progressive) E88.1
　insulin E88.1
　intestinal K9Ø.81
　mesenteric K65.4
Lipofibroma — *see* Lipoma
Lipofuscinosis, neuronal (with ceroidosis) E75.4
Lipogranuloma, sclerosing L92.8
Lipogranulomatosis E78.89
Lipoid (*see also* condition)

Lipoid — *continued*
　histiocytosis D76.3
　　essential E75.29
　nephrosis NØ4.9
　proteinosis of Urbach E78.89
Lipoidemia — *see* Hyperlipidemia
Lipoidosis — *see* Lipidosis
Lipoma D17.9
　fetal D17.9
　　fat cell D17.9
　infiltrating D17.9
　intramuscular D17.9
　pleomorphic D17.9
　site classification
　　arms (skin) (subcutaneous) D17.2- ☑
　　connective tissue D17.3Ø
　　　intra-abdominal D17.5
　　　intrathoracic D17.4
　　　peritoneum D17.79
　　　retroperitoneum D17.79
　　　specified site NEC D17.39
　　　spermatic cord D17.6
　　face (skin) (subcutaneous) D17.Ø
　　genitourinary organ NEC D17.72
　　head (skin) (subcutaneous) D17.Ø
　　intra-abdominal D17.5
　　intrathoracic D17.4
　　kidney D17.71
　　legs (skin) (subcutaneous) D17.2- ☑
　　neck (skin) (subcutaneous) D17.Ø
　　peritoneum D17.79
　　retroperitoneum D17.79
　　skin D17.3Ø
　　　specified site NEC D17.39
　　specified site NEC D17.79
　　spermatic cord D17.6
　　subcutaneous D17.3Ø
　　　specified site NEC D17.39
　　trunk (skin) (subcutaneous) D17.1
　　unspecified D17.9
　spindle cell D17.9
Lipomatosis E88.2
　dolorosa (Dercum) E88.2
　fetal — *see* Lipoma
　Launois-Bensaude E88.89
Lipomyoma — *see* Lipoma
Lipomyxoma — *see* Lipoma
Lipomyxosarcoma — *see* Neoplasm, connective tissue,
　malignant
Lipoprotein metabolism disorder E78.9
Lipoproteinemia E78.5
　broad-beta E78.2
　floating-beta E78.2
　hyper-pre-beta E78.1
Liposarcoma (*see also* Neoplasm, connective tissue,
　malignant)
　dedifferentiated — *see* Neoplasm, connective tissue,
　　malignant
　differentiated type — *see* Neoplasm, connective tissue,
　　malignant
　embryonal — *see* Neoplasm, connective tissue, malig-
　　nant
　mixed type — *see* Neoplasm, connective tissue, malig-
　　nant
　myxoid — *see* Neoplasm, connective tissue, malignant
　pleomorphic — *see* Neoplasm, connective tissue,
　　malignant
　round cell — *see* Neoplasm, connective tissue, malig-
　　nant
　well differentiated type — *see* Neoplasm, connective
　　tissue, malignant
Liposynovitis prepatellaris E88.89
Lipping, cervix N86
Lipschütz disease or ulcer N76.6
Lipuria R82.Ø
　schistosomiasis (bilharziasis) B65.9
Lisping F8Ø.Ø
Lissauer's paralysis A52.17
Lissencephalia, lissencephaly QØ4.3
Listeriosis, listerellosis A32.9
　congenital (disseminated) P37.2
　cutaneous A32.Ø
　neonatal, newborn (disseminated) P37.2
　oculoglandular A32.81
　specified NEC A32.89
Lithemia E79.Ø
Lithiasis — *see* Calculus
Lithosis J62.8

☑ Additional Character Required — Refer to the Tabular List for Character Selection　　　　🔻 Subterms under main terms may continue to next column or page

Lithuria R82.99
Litigation, anxiety concerning Z65.3
Little leaguer's elbow — *see* Epicondylitis, medial
Little's disease G80.9
Littre's
  gland — *see* condition
  hernia — *see* Hernia, abdomen
Littritis — *see* Urethritis
Livedo (annularis) (racemosa) (reticularis) R23.1
Liver — *see* condition
Living alone (problems with) Z60.2
  with handicapped person Z74.2
Lloyd's syndrome — *see* Adenomatosis, endocrine
Loa loa, loaiasis, loasis B74.3
Lobar — *see* condition
Lobomycosis B48.0
Lobo's disease B48.0
Lobotomy syndrome F07.0
Lobstein (-Ekman) **disease or syndrome** Q78.0
Lobster-claw hand Q71.6- ☑
Lobulation (congenital) (*see also* Anomaly, by site)
  kidney, Q63.1
  liver, abnormal Q44.7
  spleen Q89.09
Lobule, lobular — *see* condition
Local, localized — *see* condition
Locked twins causing obstructed labor O66.1
Locked-in state G83.5
Locking
  joint — *see* Derangement, joint, specified type NEC
    knee — *see* Derangement, knee
Lockjaw — *see* Tetanus
Löffler's
  endocarditis I42.3
  eosinophilia J82
  pneumonia J82
  syndrome (eosinophilic pneumonitis) J82
Loiasis (with conjunctival infestation) (eyelid) B74.3
Lone Star fever A77.0
Long
  labor O63.9
    first stage O63.0
    second stage O63.1
  QT syndrome I45.81
Longitudinal stripes or grooves, nails L60.8
  congenital Q84.6
Long-term (current) (prophylactic) **drug therapy** (use of)
  agents affecting estrogen receptors and estrogen levels NEC Z79.818
  anastrozole (Arimidex) Z79.811
  antibiotics Z79.2
    short-term use — *omit code*
  anticoagulants Z79.01
  anti-inflammatory, non-steroidal (NSAID) Z79.1
  antiplatelet Z79.02
  antithrombotics Z79.02
  aromatase inhibitors Z79.811
  aspirin Z79.82
  birth control pill or patch Z79.3
  bisphosphonates Z79.83
  contraceptive, oral Z79.3
  drug, specified NEC Z79.899
  estrogen receptor downregulators Z79.818
  Evista Z79.810
  exemestane (Aromasin) Z79.811
  Fareston Z79.810
  fulvestrant (Faslodex) Z79.818
  gonadotropin-releasing hormone (GnRH) agonist Z79.818
  goserelin acetate (Zoladex) Z79.818
  hormone replacement Z79.890
  insulin Z79.4
  letrozole (Femara) Z79.811
  leuprolide acetate (leuprorelin) (Lupron) Z79.818
  megestrol acetate (Megace) Z79.818
  methadone for pain management Z79.891
  Nolvadex Z79.810
  non-steroidal anti-inflammatories (NSAID) Z79.1
  opiate analgesic Z79.891
  oral
    antidiabetic Z79.84
    contraceptive Z79.3
    hypoglycemic Z79.84
  raloxifene (Evista) Z79.810
  selective estrogen receptor modulators (SERMs) Z79.810

Long-term (current) (prophylactic) **drug therapy** — *continued*
  steroids
    inhaled Z79.51
    systemic Z79.52
  tamoxifen (Nolvadex) Z79.810
  toremifene (Fareston) Z79.810
Loop
  intestine — *see* Volvulus
  vascular on papilla (optic) Q14.2
Loose (*see also* condition)
  body
    joint M24.00
      ankle M24.07- ☑
      elbow M24.02- ☑
      hand M24.04- ☑
      hip M24.05- ☑
      knee M23.4- ☑
      shoulder (region) M24.01- ☑
      specified site NEC M24.08
      toe M24.07- ☑
      vertebra M24.08
      wrist M24.03- ☑
    knee M23.4- ☑
    sheath, tendon — *see* Disorder, tendon, specified type NEC
  cartilage — *see* Loose, body, joint
  skin and subcutaneous tissue (following bariatric surgery weight loss) (following dietary weight loss) L98.7
  tooth, teeth K08.89
Loosening
  aseptic
    joint prosthesis — *see* Complications, joint prosthesis, mechanical, loosening, by site
    epiphysis — *see* Osteochondropathy
  mechanical
    joint prosthesis — *see* Complications, joint prosthesis, mechanical, loosening, by site
Looser-Milkman (-Debray) **syndrome** M83.8
Lop ear (deformity) Q17.3
Lorain (-Levi) **short stature syndrome** E23.0
Lordosis M40.50
  acquired — *see* Lordosis, specified type NEC
  congenital Q76.429
    lumbar region Q76.426
    lumbosacral region Q76.427
    sacral region Q76.428
    sacrococcygeal region Q76.428
    thoracolumbar region Q76.425
  lumbar region M40.56
  lumbosacral region M40.57
  postsurgical M96.4
  postural — *see* Lordosis, specified type NEC
  rachitic (late effect) (sequelae) E64.3
  sequelae of rickets E64.3
  specified type NEC M40.40
    lumbar region M40.46
    lumbosacral region M40.47
    thoracolumbar region M40.45
  thoracolumbar region M40.55
  tuberculous A18.01
Loss (of)
  appetite (*see also* Anorexia) R63.0
    hysterical F50.89
    nonorganic origin F50.89
    psychogenic F50.89
  blood — *see* Hemorrhage
  bone — *see* Loss, substance of, bone
  consciousness, transient R55
    traumatic — *see* Injury, intracranial
  control, sphincter, rectum R15.9
    nonorganic origin F98.1
  elasticity, skin R23.4
  family (member) in childhood Z62.898
  fluid (acute) E86.9
  function of labyrinth — *see* subcategory H83.2 ☑
  hair, nonscarring — *see* Alopecia
  hearing (*see also* Deafness)
    central NOS H90.5
    conductive H90.2
      bilateral H90.0
      unilateral
        with
          restricted hearing on the contralateral side H90.A1- ☑
          unrestricted hearing on the contralateral side H90.1- ☑

Loss — *continued*
  hearing (*see also* Deafness) — *continued*
    mixed conductive and sensorineural hearing loss H90.8
      bilateral H90.6
      unilateral
        with
          restricted hearing on the contralateral side H90.A3- ☑
          unrestricted hearing on the contralateral side H90.7- ☑
    neural NOS H90.5
    perceptive NOS H90.5
    sensorineural NOS H90.5
      bilateral H90.3
      unilateral
        with
          restricted hearing onthe contralateral side H90.A2- ☑
          unrestricted hearing on the contralateral side H90.4- ☑
    sensory NOS H90.5
  height R29.890
  limb or member, traumatic, current — *see* Amputation, traumatic
  love relationship in childhood Z62.898
  memory (*see also* Amnesia)
    mild, following organic brain damage F06.8
  mind — *see* Psychosis
  occlusal vertical dimension of fully erupted teeth M26.37
  organ or part — *see* Absence, by site, acquired
  ossicles, ear (partial) H74.32- ☑
  parent in childhood Z63.4
  pregnancy, recurrent N96
    without current pregnancy N96
    care in current pregnancy O26.2- ☑
  recurrent pregnancy — *see* Loss, pregnancy, recurrent
  self-esteem, in childhood Z62.898
  sense of
    smell — *see* Disturbance, sensation, smell
    taste — *see* Disturbance, sensation, taste
    touch R20.8
  sensory R44.9
    dissociative F44.6
  sexual desire F52.0
  sight (acquired) (complete) (congenital) — *see* Blindness
  substance of
    bone — *see* Disorder, bone, density and structure, specified NEC
      horizontal alveolar K06.3
    cartilage — *see* Disorder, cartilage, specified type NEC
    auricle (ear) — *see* Disorder, pinna, specified type NEC
    vitreous (humor) H15.89
  tooth, teeth — *see* Absence, teeth, acquired
  vision, visual H54.7
    both eyes H54.3
    one eye H54.60
      left (normal vision on right) H54.62
      right (normal vision on left) H54.61
    specified as blindness — *see* Blindness
    subjective
      sudden H53.13- ☑
      transient H53.12- ☑
  vitreous — *see* Prolapse, vitreous
  voice — *see* Aphonia
  weight (abnormal) (cause unknown) R63.4
Louis-Bar syndrome (ataxia-telangiectasia) G11.3
Louping ill (encephalitis) A84.8
Louse, lousiness — *see* Lice
Low
  achiever, school Z55.3
  back syndrome M54.5
  basal metabolic rate R94.8
  birthweight (2499 grams or less) P07.10
    with weight of
      1000-1249 grams P07.14
      1250-1499 grams P07.15
      1500-1749 grams P07.16
      1750-1999 grams P07.17
      2000-2499 grams P07.18
    extreme (999 grams or less) P07.00
      with weight of
        499 grams or less P07.01
        500-749 grams P07.02

Low — *continued*
  birthweight — *continued*
    extreme — *continued*
      with weight of — *continued*
        750-999 grams P07.03
    for gestational age — *see* Light for dates
  blood pressure (*see also* Hypotension)
    reading (incidental) (isolated) (nonspecific) R03.1
  cardiac reserve — *see* Disease, heart
  function (*see also* Hypofunction)
    kidney N28.9
  hematocrit D64.9
  hemoglobin D64.9
  income Z59.6
  level of literacy Z55.0
  lying
    kidney N28.89
    organ or site, congenital — *see* Malposition, congenital
  output syndrome (cardiac) — *see* Failure, heart
  platelets (blood) — *see* Thrombocytopenia
  reserve, kidney N28.89
  salt syndrome E87.1
  self esteem R45.81
  set ears Q17.4
  vision H54.2X- ☑
    one eye (other eye normal) H54.50
      left (normal vision on right) H54.52A- ☑
        other eye blind — *see* Blindness
      right (normal vision on left) H54.511- ☑
Low-density-lipoprotein-type (LDL) **hyperlipoproteinemia** E78.00
Lowe's syndrome E72.03
Lown-Ganong-Levine syndrome I45.6
LSD reaction (acute) (without dependence) F16.90
  with dependence F16.20
L-shaped kidney Q63.8
Ludwig's angina or disease K12.2
Lues (venerea), **luetic** — *see* Syphilis
Luetscher's syndrome (dehydration) E86.0
Lumbago, lumbalgia M54.5
  with sciatica M54.4- ☑
    due to intervertebral disc disorder M51.17
  due to displacement, intervertebral disc M51.27
    with sciatica M51.17
Lumbar — *see* condition
Lumbarization, vertebra, congenital Q76.49
Lumbermen's itch B88.0
Lump (*see also* Mass)
  breast N63.0
    axillary tail
      left N63.32
      right N63.31
    left
      lower inner quadrant N63.24
      lower outer quadrant N63.23
      unspecified quadrant N63.20
      upper inner quadrant N63.22
      upper outer quadrant N63.21
    right
      lower inner quadrant N63.14
      lower outer quadrant N63.13
      unspecified quadrant N63.10
      upper inner quadrant N63.12
      upper outer quadrant N63.11
    subareolar
      left N63.42
      right N63.41
Lunacy — *see* Psychosis
Lung — *see* condition
Lupoid (miliary) **of Boeck** D86.3
Lupus
  anticoagulant D68.62
    with
      hemorrhagic disorder D68.312
      hypercoagulable state D68.62
      finding without diagnosis R76.0
  discoid (local) L93.0
  erythematosus (discoid) (local) L93.0
    disseminated — *see* Lupus, erythematosus, systemic
    eyelid H01.129
      left H01.126
        lower H01.125
        upper H01.124
      right H01.123
        lower H01.122
        upper H01.121

Lupus — *continued*
  erythematosus — *continued*
    profundus L93.2
    specified NEC L93.2
    subacute cutaneous L93.1
    systemic M32.9
      with organ or system involvement M32.10
        endocarditis M32.11
        lung M32.13
        pericarditis M32.12
        renal (glomerular) M32.14
          tubulo-interstitial M32.15
        specified organ or system NEC M32.19
      drug-induced M32.0
      inhibitor (presence of) D68.62
        with
          hemorrhagic disorder D68.312
          hypercoagulable state D68.62
          finding without diagnosis R76.0
      specified NEC M32.8
    exedens A18.4
    hydralazine M32.0
      correct substance properly administered — *see* Table of Drugs and Chemicals, by drug, adverse effect
      overdose or wrong substance given or taken — *see* Table of Drugs and Chemicals, by drug, poisoning
    nephritis (chronic) M32.14
    nontuberculous, not disseminated L93.0
    panniculitis L93.2
    pernio (Besnier) D86.3
    systemic — *see* Lupus, erythematosus, systemic
    tuberculous A18.4
      eyelid A18.4
    vulgaris A18.4
      eyelid A18.4
Luteinoma D27.- ☑
Lutembacher's disease or syndrome (atrial septal defect with mitral stenosis) Q21.1
Luteoma D27.- ☑
Lutz (-Splendore-de Almeida) **disease** — *see* Paracoccidioidomycosis
Luxation (*see also* Dislocation)
  eyeball (nontraumatic) — *see* Luxation, globe
    birth injury P15.3
  globe, nontraumatic H44.82- ☑
  lacrimal gland — *see* Dislocation, lacrimal gland
  lens (old) (partial) (spontaneous)
    congenital Q12.1
    syphilitic A50.39
Lycanthropy F22
Lyell's syndrome L51.2
  due to drug L51.2
    correct substance properly administered — *see* Table of Drugs and Chemicals, by drug, adverse effect
    overdose or wrong substance given or taken — *see* Table of Drugs and Chemicals, by drug, poisoning
Lyme disease A69.20
Lymph
  gland or node — *see* condition
  scrotum — *see* Infestation, filarial
Lymphadenitis I88.9
  with ectopic or molar pregnancy O08.0
  acute L04.9
    axilla L04.2
    face L04.0
    head L04.0
    hip L04.3
    limb
      lower L04.3
      upper L04.2
    neck L04.0
    shoulder L04.2
    specified site NEC L04.8
    trunk L04.1
  anthracosis (occupational) J60
  any site, except mesenteric I88.9
    chronic I88.1
    subacute I88.1
  breast
    gestational — *see* Mastitis, obstetric
    puerperal, postpartum (nonpurulent) O91.22
  chancroidal (congenital) A57
  chronic I88.1
    mesenteric I88.0

Lymphadenitis — *continued*
  due to
    Brugia (malayi) B74.1
      timori B74.2
    chlamydial lymphogranuloma A55
    diphtheria (toxin) A36.89
    lymphogranuloma venereum A55
    Wuchereria bancrofti B74.0
  following ectopic or molar pregnancy O08.0
  gonorrheal A54.89
  infective — *see* Lymphadenitis, acute
  mesenteric (acute) (chronic) (nonspecific) (subacute) I88.0
    due to Salmonella typhi A01.09
    tuberculous A18.39
  mycobacterial A31.8
  purulent — *see* Lymphadenitis, acute
  pyogenic — *see* Lymphadenitis, acute
  regional, nonbacterial I88.8
  septic — *see* Lymphadenitis, acute
  subacute, unspecified site I88.1
  suppurative — *see* Lymphadenitis, acute
  syphilitic (early) (secondary) A51.49
    late A52.79
  tuberculous — *see* Tuberculosis, lymph gland
  venereal (chlamydial) A55
Lymphadenoid goiter E06.3
Lymphadenopathy (generalized) R59.1
  angioimmunoblastic, with dysproteinemia (AILD) C86.5
  due to toxoplasmosis (acquired) B58.89
    congenital (acute) (subacute) (chronic) P37.1
  localized R59.0
  syphilitic (early) (secondary) A51.49
Lymphadenosis R59.1
Lymphangiectasis I89.0
  conjunctiva H11.89
  postinfectional I89.0
  scrotum I89.0
Lymphangiectatic elephantiasis, nonfilarial I89.0
Lymphangioendothelioma D18.1
  malignant — *see* Neoplasm, connective tissue, malignant
Lymphangioleiomyomatosis J84.81
Lymphangioma D18.1
  capillary D18.1
  cavernous D18.1
  cystic D18.1
  malignant — *see* Neoplasm, connective tissue, malignant
Lymphangiomyoma D18.1
Lymphangiomyomatosis J84.81
Lymphangiosarcoma — *see* Neoplasm, connective tissue, malignant
Lymphangitis I89.1
  with
    abscess — *code by* site under Abscess
    cellulitis — *code by* site under Cellulitis
    ectopic or molar pregnancy O08.0
  acute L03.91
    abdominal wall L03.321
    ankle — *see* Lymphangitis, acute, lower limb
    arm — *see* Lymphangitis, acute, upper limb
    auricle (ear) — *see* Lymphangitis, acute, ear
    axilla L03.12- ☑
    back (any part) L03.322
    buttock L03.327
    cervical (meaning neck) L03.222
    cheek (external) L03.212
    chest wall L03.323
    digit
      finger — *see* Lymphangitis, acute, finger
      toe — *see* Lymphangitis, acute, toe
    ear (external) H60.1- ☑
    external auditory canal — *see* Lymphangitis, acute, ear
    eyelid — *see* Abscess, eyelid
    face NEC L03.212
    finger (intrathecal) (periosteal) (subcutaneous) (subcuticular) L03.02- ☑
    foot — *see* Lymphangitis, acute, lower limb
    gluteal (region) L03.327
    groin L03.324
    hand — *see* Lymphangitis, acute, upper limb
    head NEC L03.891
      face (any part, except ear, eye and nose) L03.212
    heel — *see* Lymphangitis, acute, lower limb

Lymphangitis — *continued*
  acute — *continued*
    hip — *see* Lymphangitis, acute, lower limb
    jaw (region) LØ3.212
    knee — *see* Lymphangitis, acute, lower limb
    leg — *see* Lymphangitis, acute, lower limb
    lower limb LØ3.12- ☑
      toe — *see* Lymphangitis, acute, toe
    navel LØ3.326
    neck (region) LØ3.222
    orbit, orbital — *see* Cellulitis, orbit
    pectoral (region) LØ3.323
    perineal, perineum LØ3.325
    scalp (any part) LØ3.891
    shoulder — *see* Lymphangitis, acute, upper limb
    specified site NEC LØ3.898
    thigh — *see* Lymphangitis, acute, lower limb
    thumb (intrathecal) (periosteal) (subcutaneous)
        (subcuticular) — *see* Lymphangitis, acute,
        finger
    toe (intrathecal) (periosteal) (subcutaneous) (sub-
        cuticular) LØ3.Ø4- ☑
    trunk LØ3.329
      abdominal wall LØ3.321
      back (any part) LØ3.322
      buttock LØ3.327
      chest wall LØ3.323
      groin LØ3.324
      perineal, perineum LØ3.325
      umbilicus LØ3.326
    upper limb LØ3.12- ☑
      axilla — *see* Lymphangitis, acute, axilla
      finger — *see* Lymphangitis, acute, finger
      thumb — *see* Lymphangitis, acute, finger
    wrist — *see* Lymphangitis, acute, upper limb
  breast
    gestational — *see* Mastitis, obstetric
  chancroidal A57
  chronic (any site) I89.1
  due to
    Brugia (malayi) B74.1
      timori B74.2
    Wuchereria bancrofti B74.Ø
  following ectopic or molar pregnancy OØ8.89
  penis
    acute N48.29
    gonococcal (acute) (chronic) A54.Ø9
  puerperal, postpartum, childbirth O86.89
  strumous, tuberculous A18.2
  subacute (any site) I89.1
  tuberculous — *see* Tuberculosis, lymph gland
Lymphatic (vessel) — *see* condition
Lymphatism E32.8
Lymphectasia I89.Ø
Lymphedema (acquired) (*see also* Elephantiasis)
  congenital Q82.Ø
  hereditary (chronic) (idiopathic) Q82.Ø
  postmastectomy I97.2
  praecox I89.Ø
  secondary I89.Ø
  surgical NEC I97.89
    postmastectomy (syndrome) I97.2
Lymphoblastic — *see* condition
Lymphoblastoma (diffuse) — *see* Lymphoma, lym-
      phoblastic (diffuse)
  giant follicular — *see* Lymphoma, lymphoblastic (dif-
      fuse)
  macrofollicular — *see* Lymphoma, lymphoblastic
      (diffuse)
Lymphocele I89.8
Lymphocytic
  chorioencephalitis (acute) (serous) A87.2
  choriomeningitis (acute) (serous) A87.2
  meningoencephalitis A87.2
Lymphocytoma, benign cutis L98.8
Lymphocytopenia D72.81Ø
Lymphocytosis (symptomatic) D72.82Ø
  infectious (acute) B33.9
Lymphoepithelioma — *see* Neoplasm, malignant, by
      site
Lymphogranuloma (malignant) (*see also* Lymphoma,
      Hodgkin)
  chlamydial A55
  inguinale A55
  venereum (any site) (chlamydial) (with stricture of
      rectum) A55

Lymphogranulomatosis (malignant) (*see also* Lym-
    phoma, Hodgkin)
  benign (Boeck's sarcoid) (Schaumann's) D86.1
Lymphohistiocytosis, hemophagocytic (familial) D76.1
Lymphoid — *see* condition
Lymphoma (of) (malignant) C85.9Ø
  adult T-cell (HTLV-1-associated) (acute variant)
      (chronic variant) (lymphomatoid variant)
      (smouldering variant) C91.5- ☑
  anaplastic large cell
    ALK-negative C84.7- ☑
    ALK-positive C84.6- ☑
    CD3Ø-positive C84.6- ☑
    primary cutaneous C86.6
  angioimmunoblastic T-cell C86.5
  BALT C88.4
  B-cell C85.1- ☑
  blastic NK-cell C86.4
  blastic plasmacytoid dendritic cell neoplasm (BPDCN)
      C86.4
  B-precursor C83.5- ☑
  bronchial-associated lymphoid tissue [BALT-lym-
      phoma] C88.4
  Burkitt (atypical) C83.7- ☑
  Burkitt-like C83.7- ☑
  centrocytic C83.1- ☑
  cutaneous follicle center C82.6- ☑
  cutaneous T-cell C84.A- ☑ (*following* C84.7)
  diffuse follicle center C82.5- ☑
  diffuse large cell C83.3- ☑
    anaplastic C83.3- ☑
    B-cell C83.3- ☑
    CD3Ø-positive C83.3- ☑
    centroblastic C83.3- ☑
    immunoblastic C83.3- ☑
    plasmablastic C83.3- ☑
    subtype not specified C83.3- ☑
    T-cell rich C83.3- ☑
  enteropathy-type (associated) (intestinal) T-cell C86.2
  extranodal marginal zone B-cell lymphoma of mucosa-
      associated lymphoid tissue [MALT-lymphoma]
      C88.4
  extranodal NK/T-cell, nasal type C86.Ø
  follicular C82.9- ☑
    grade
      I C82.Ø- ☑
      II C82.1- ☑
      III C82.2- ☑
      IIIa C82.3- ☑
      IIIb C82.4- ☑
    specified NEC C82.8- ☑
  hepatosplenic T-cell (alpha-beta) (gamma-delta) C86.1
  histiocytic C85.9- ☑
    true C96.A (*following* C96.6)
  Hodgkin C81.9 ☑
    lymphocyte depleted (classical) C81.3- ☑
    lymphocyte-rich (classical) C81.4- ☑
    mixed cellularity (classical) C81.2- ☑
    nodular
      lymphocyte predominant C81.Ø- ☑
      sclerosis (classical) C81.1- ☑
    nodular sclerosis (classical) C81.1- ☑
    specified NEC (classical) C81.7- ☑
  intravascular large B-cell C83.8- ☑
  Lennert's C84.4- ☑
  lymphoblastic (diffuse) C83.5- ☑
  lymphoblastic B-cell C83.5- ☑
  lymphoblastic T-cell C83.5- ☑
  lymphoepithelioid C84.4- ☑
  lymphoplasmacytic C83.Ø- ☑
    with IgM-production C88.Ø
  MALT C88.4
  mantle cell C83.1- ☑
  mature T-cell NEC C84.4- ☑
  mature T/NK-cell C84.9- ☑
    specified NEC C84.Z- ☑ (*following* C84.7)
  mediastinal (thymic) large B-cell C85.2- ☑
  Mediterranean C86.3
  mucosa-associated lymphoid tissue [MALT-lymphoma]
      C88.4
  NK/T cell C84.9- ☑
  nodal marginal zone C83.Ø- ☑
  non-follicular (diffuse) C83.9- ☑
    specified NEC C83.8- ☑
  non-Hodgkin (*see also* Lymphoma, by type) C85.9- ☑
    specified NEC C85.8- ☑

Lymphoma — *continued*
  non-leukemic variant of B-CLL C83.Ø- ☑
  peripheral T-cell, not classified C84.4- ☑
  primary cutaneous
    anaplastic large cell C86.6
    CD3Ø-positive large T-cell C86.6
  primary effusion B-cell C83.8- ☑
  SALT C88.4
  skin-associated lymphoid tissue [SALT-lymphoma]
      C88.4
  small cell B-cell C83.Ø- ☑
  splenic marginal zone C83.Ø- ☑
  subcutaneous panniculitis-like T-cell C86.3
  T-precursor C83.5- ☑
  true histiocytic C96.A (*following* C96.6)
Lymphomatosis — *see* Lymphoma
Lymphopathia venereum, veneris A55
Lymphopenia D72.81Ø
Lymphoplasmacytic leukemia — *see* Leukemia,
    chronic lymphocytic, B-cell type
Lymphoproliferation, X-linked disease D82.3
Lymphoreticulosis, benign (of inoculation) A28.1
Lymphorrhea I89.8
Lymphosarcoma (diffuse) (*see also* Lymphoma)
    C85.9- ☑
Lymphostasis I89.8
Lypemania — *see* Melancholia
Lysine and hydroxylysine metabolism disorder E72.3
Lyssa — *see* Rabies

M

Macacus ear Q17.3
Maceration, wet feet, tropical (syndrome) T69.Ø2- ☑
MacLeod's syndrome J43.Ø
Macrocephalia, macrocephaly Q75.3
Macrocheilia, macrochilia (congenital) Q18.6
Macrocolon (*see also* Megacolon) Q43.1
Macrocornea Q15.8
  with glaucoma Q15.Ø
Macrocytic — *see* condition
Macrocytosis D75.89
Macrodactylia, macrodactylism (fingers) (thumbs)
    Q74.Ø
  toes Q74.2
Macrodontia KØØ.2
Macrogenia M26.Ø5
Macrogenitosomia (adrenal) (male) (praecox) E25.9
  congenital E25.Ø
Macroglobulinemia (idiopathic) (primary) C88.Ø
  monoclonal (essential) D47.2
  Waldenström C88.Ø
Macroglossia (congenital) Q38.2
  acquired K14.8
Macrognathia, macrognathism (congenital)
    (mandibular) (maxillary) M26.Ø9
Macrogyria (congenital) QØ4.8
Macrohydrocephalus — *see* Hydrocephalus
Macromastia — *see* Hypertrophy, breast
Macrophthalmos Q11.3
  in congenital glaucoma Q15.Ø
Macropsia H53.15
Macrosigmoid K59.39
  congenital Q43.2
Macrospondylitis , acromegalic E22.Ø
Macrostomia (congenital) Q18.4
Macrotia (external ear) (congenital) Q17.1
Macula
  cornea, corneal — *see* Opacity, cornea
  degeneration (atrophic) (exudative) (senile) (*see also*
      Degeneration, macula)
  hereditary — *see* Dystrophy, retina
Maculae ceruleae B85.1
Maculopathy, toxic — *see* Degeneration, macula, toxic
Madarosis (eyelid) HØ2.729
  left HØ2.726
    lower HØ2.725
    upper HØ2.724
  right HØ2.723
    lower HØ2.722
    upper HØ2.721
Madelung's
  deformity (radius) Q74.Ø
  disease
    radial deformity Q74.Ø
    symmetrical lipomas, neck E88.89
Madness — *see* Psychosis

Madura
   foot B47.9
      actinomycotic B47.1
      mycotic B47.0
Maduromycosis B47.0
Maffucci's syndrome Q78.4
Magnesium metabolism disorder — *see* Disorder, metabolism, magnesium
Main en griffe (acquired) (*see also* Deformity, limb, clawhand)
   congenital Q74.0
Maintenance (encounter for)
   antineoplastic chemotherapy Z51.11
   antineoplastic radiation therapy Z51.0
   methadone F11.20
Majocchi's
   disease L81.7
   granuloma B35.8
Major — *see* condition
Mal de los pintos — *see* Pinta
Mal de mer T75.3 ☑
Malabar itch (any site) B35.5
Malabsorption K90.9
   calcium K90.89
   carbohydrate K90.49
   disaccharide E73.9
   fat K90.49
   galactose E74.20
   glucose (-galactose) E74.39
   intestinal K90.9
      specified NEC K90.89
   isomaltose E74.31
   lactose E73.9
   methionine E72.19
   monosaccharide E74.39
   postgastrectomy K91.2
   postsurgical K91.2
   protein K90.49
   starch K90.49
   sucrose E74.39
   syndrome K90.9
      postsurgical K91.2
Malacia, bone (adult) M83.9
   juvenile — *see* Rickets
Malacoplakia
   bladder N32.89
   pelvis (kidney) N28.89
   ureter N28.89
   urethra N36.8
Malacosteon, juvenile — *see* Rickets
Maladaptation — *see* Maladjustment
Maladie de Roger Q21.0
Maladjustment
   conjugal Z63.0
      involving divorce or estrangement Z63.5
   educational Z55.4
   family Z63.9
   marital Z63.0
      involving divorce or estrangement Z63.5
   occupational NEC Z56.89
   simple, adult — *see* Disorder, adjustment
   situational — *see* Disorder, adjustment
   social Z60.9
      due to
         acculturation difficulty Z60.3
         discrimination and persecution (perceived) Z60.5
         exclusion and isolation Z60.4
         life-cycle (phase of life) transition Z60.0
         rejection Z60.4
         specified reason NEC Z60.8
Malaise R53.81
Malakoplakia — *see* Malacoplakia
Malaria, malarial (fever) B54
   with
      blackwater fever B50.8
         hemoglobinuric (bilious) B50.8
      hemoglobinuria B50.8
   accidentally induced (therapeutically) — *code by* type under Malaria
   algid B50.9
   cerebral B50.0 [G94]
   clinically diagnosed (without parasitological confirmation) B54
   congenital NEC P37.4
      falciparum P37.3
   congestion, congestive B54
   continued (fever) B50.9

Malaria, malarial — *continued*
   estivo-autumnal B50.9
   falciparum B50.9
      with complications NEC B50.8
         cerebral B50.0 [G94]
      severe B50.8
   hemorrhagic B54
   malariae B52.9
      with
         complications NEC B52.8
         glomerular disorder B52.0
   malignant (tertian) — *see* Malaria, falciparum
   mixed infections — *code to* first listed type in B50-B53
   ovale B53.0
   parasitologically confirmed NEC B53.8
   pernicious, acute — *see* Malaria, falciparum
   Plasmodium (P.)
      falciparum NEC — *see* Malaria, falciparum
      malariae NEC B52.9
         with Plasmodium
            falciparum (and or vivax) — *see* Malaria, falciparum
            vivax (*see also* Malaria, vivax)
               and falciparum — *see* Malaria, falciparum
      ovale B53.0
         with Plasmodium malariae (*see also* Malaria, malariae)
            and vivax (*see also* Malaria, vivax)
               and falciparum — *see* Malaria, falciparum
      simian B53.1
         with Plasmodium malariae (*see also* Malaria, malariae)
            and vivax (*see also* Malaria, vivax)
               and falciparum — *see* Malaria, falciparum
      vivax NEC B51.9
         with Plasmodium falciparum — *see* Malaria, falciparum
   quartan — *see* Malaria, malariae
   quotidian — *see* Malaria, falciparum
   recurrent B54
   remittent B54
   specified type NEC (parasitologically confirmed) B53.8
   spleen B54
   subtertian (fever) — *see* Malaria, falciparum
   tertian (benign) (*see also* Malaria, vivax)
      malignant B50.9
   tropical B50.9
   typhoid B54
   vivax B51.9
      with
         complications NEC B51.8
         ruptured spleen B51.0
Malassez's disease (cystic) N50.89
Malassimilation K90.9
Maldescent, testis Q53.9
   bilateral Q53.20
      abdominal Q53.211
      perineal Q53.22
   unilateral Q53.10
      abdominal Q53.111
      perineal Q53.12
Maldevelopment (*see also* Anomaly)
   brain Q07.9
   colon Q43.9
   hip Q74.2
      congenital dislocation Q65.2
         bilateral Q65.1
         unilateral Q65.0- ☑
   mastoid process Q75.8
   middle ear Q16.4
      except ossicles Q16.4
      ossicles Q16.3
   ossicles Q16.3
   spine Q76.49
   toe Q74.2
Male type pelvis Q74.2
   with disproportion (fetopelvic) O33.3 ☑
      causing obstructed labor O65.3
Malformation (congenital) (*see also* Anomaly)
   adrenal gland Q89.1
   affecting multiple systems with skeletal changes NEC Q87.5
   alimentary tract Q45.9
      specified type NEC Q45.8
      upper Q40.9

Malformation — *continued*
   alimentary tract — *continued*
      upper — *continued*
         specified type NEC Q40.8
   aorta Q25.40
      absence Q25.41
      aneurysm, congenital Q25.43
      aplasia Q25.41
      atresia Q25.29
         aortic arch Q25.21
      coarctation (preductal) (postductal) Q25.1
      dilatation, congenital Q25.44
      hypoplasia Q25.42
      patent ductus arteriosus Q25.0
      specified type NEC Q25.49
      stenosis Q25.1
         supravalvular Q25.3
   aortic valve Q23.9
      specified NEC Q23.8
   arteriovenous, aneurysmatic (congenital) Q27.30
      brain Q28.2
      cerebral Q28.2
      peripheral Q27.30
         digestive system Q27.33
         lower limb Q27.32
         other specified site Q27.39
         renal vessel Q27.34
         upper limb Q27.31
      precerebral vessels (nonruptured) Q28.0
   auricle
      ear (congenital) Q17.3
         acquired H61.119
            left H61.112
               with right H61.113
            right H61.111
               with left H61.113
   bile duct Q44.5
   bladder Q64.79
      aplasia Q64.5
      diverticulum Q64.6
      exstrophy — *see* Exstrophy, bladder
      neck obstruction Q64.31
   bone Q79.9
      face Q75.9
         specified type NEC Q75.8
      skull Q75.9
         specified type NEC Q75.8
   brain (multiple) Q04.9
      arteriovenous Q28.2
      specified type NEC Q04.8
   branchial cleft Q18.2
   breast Q83.9
      specified type NEC Q83.8
   broad ligament Q50.6
   bronchus Q32.4
   bursa Q79.9
   cardiac
      chambers Q20.9
         specified type NEC Q20.8
      septum Q21.9
         specified type NEC Q21.8
   cerebral Q04.9
      vessels Q28.3
   cervix uteri Q51.9
      specified type NEC Q51.828
   Chiari
      Type I G93.5
      Type II Q07.01
   choroid (congenital) Q14.3
      plexus Q07.8
   circulatory system Q28.9
   cochlea Q16.5
   cornea Q13.4
   coronary vessels Q24.5
   corpus callosum (congenital) Q04.0
   diaphragm Q79.1
   digestive system NEC, specified type NEC Q45.8
   dura Q07.9
      brain Q04.9
      spinal Q06.9
   ear Q17.9
      causing impairment of hearing Q16.9
      external Q17.9
         accessory auricle Q17.0
         causing impairment of hearing Q16.9
         absence of
            auditory canal Q16.1
            auricle Q16.0
         macrotia Q17.1

☑ **Additional Character Required** — **Refer to the Tabular List for Character Selection**   ▽ **Subterms under main terms may continue to next column or page**

Malformation — *continued*
 ear — *continued*
  external — *continued*
   microtia Q17.2
   misplacement Q17.4
   misshapen NEC Q17.3
   prominence Q17.5
   specified type NEC Q17.8
  inner Q16.5
  middle Q16.4
   absence of eustachian tube Q16.2
   ossicles (fusion) Q16.3
  ossicles Q16.3
  specified type NEC Q17.8
 epididymis Q55.4
 esophagus Q39.9
  specified type NEC Q39.8
 eye Q15.9
  lid Q10.3
  specified NEC Q15.8
 fallopian tube Q50.6
 genital organ — *see* Anomaly, genitalia
 great
  artery Q25.9
   aorta — *see* Malformation, aorta
   pulmonary artery — *see* Malformation, pulmonary, artery
   specified type NEC Q25.8
  vein Q26.9
   anomalous
    portal venous connection Q26.5
    pulmonary venous connection Q26.4
     partial Q26.3
     total Q26.2
   persistent left superior vena cava Q26.1
   portal vein-hepatic artery fistula Q26.6
   specified type NEC Q26.8
   vena cava stenosis, congenital Q26.0
 gum Q38.6
 hair Q84.2
 heart Q24.9
  specified type NEC Q24.8
 integument Q84.9
  specified type NEC Q84.8
 internal ear Q16.5
 intestine Q43.9
  specified type NEC Q43.8
 iris Q13.2
 joint Q74.9
  ankle Q74.2
  lumbosacral Q76.49
  sacroiliac Q74.2
  specified type NEC Q74.8
 kidney Q63.9
  accessory Q63.0
  giant Q63.3
  horseshoe Q63.1
  hydronephrosis Q62.0
  malposition Q63.2
  specified type NEC Q63.8
 lacrimal apparatus Q10.6
 lingual Q38.3
 lip Q38.0
 liver Q44.7
 lung Q33.9
 meninges or membrane (congenital) Q07.9
  cerebral Q04.8
  spinal (cord) Q06.9
 middle ear Q16.4
  ossicles Q16.3
 mitral valve Q23.9
  specified NEC Q23.8
 Mondini's (congenital) (malformation, cochlea) Q16.5
 mouth (congenital) Q38.6
 multiple types NEC Q89.7
 musculoskeletal system Q79.9
 myocardium Q24.8
 nail Q84.6
 nervous system (central) Q07.9
 nose Q30.9
  specified type NEC Q30.8
 optic disc Q14.2
 orbit Q10.7
 ovary Q50.39
 palate Q38.5
 parathyroid gland Q89.2
 pelvic organs or tissues NEC
  in pregnancy or childbirth O34.8- ☑
   causing obstructed labor O65.5

Malformation — *continued*
 penis Q55.69
  aplasia Q55.5
  curvature (lateral) Q55.61
  hypoplasia Q55.62
 pericardium Q24.8
 peripheral vascular system Q27.9
  specified type NEC Q27.8
 pharynx Q38.8
 precerebral vessels Q28.1
 prostate Q55.4
 pulmonary
  arteriovenous Q25.72
  artery Q25.9
   atresia Q25.5
   specified type NEC Q25.79
   stenosis Q25.6
  valve Q22.3
 renal artery Q27.2
 respiratory system Q34.9
 retina Q14.1
 scrotum — *see* Malformation, testis and scrotum
 seminal vesicles Q55.4
 sense organs NEC Q07.9
 skin Q82.9
 specified NEC Q89.8
 spinal
  cord Q06.9
  nerve root Q07.8
 spine Q76.49
  kyphosis — *see* Kyphosis, congenital
  lordosis — *see* Lordosis, congenital
 spleen Q89.09
 stomach Q40.3
  specified type NEC Q40.2
 teeth, tooth K00.9
 tendon Q79.9
 testis and scrotum Q55.20
  aplasia Q55.0
  hypoplasia Q55.1
  polyorchism Q55.21
  retractile testis Q55.22
  scrotal transposition Q55.23
  specified NEC Q55.29
 thorax, bony Q76.9
 throat Q38.8
 thyroid gland Q89.2
 tongue (congenital) Q38.3
  hypertrophy Q38.2
  tie Q38.1
 trachea Q32.1
 tricuspid valve Q22.9
  specified type NEC Q22.8
 umbilical cord NEC (complicating delivery) O69.89 ☑
 umbilicus Q89.9
 ureter Q62.8
  agenesis Q62.4
  duplication Q62.5
  malposition — *see* Malposition, congenital, ureter
  obstructive defect — *see* Defect, obstructive, ureter
  vesico-uretero-renal reflux Q62.7
 urethra Q64.79
  aplasia Q64.5
  duplication Q64.74
  posterior valves Q64.2
  prolapse Q64.71
  stricture Q64.32
 urinary system Q64.9
 uterus Q51.9
  specified type NEC Q51.818
 vagina Q52.4
 vas deferens Q55.4
  atresia Q55.3
 vascular system, peripheral Q27.9
 venous — *see* Anomaly, vein(s)
 vulva Q52.70
Malfunction (*see also* Dysfunction)
 cardiac electronic device T82.119 ☑
  electrode T82.110 ☑
  pulse generator T82.111 ☑
  specified type NEC T82.118 ☑
 catheter device NEC T85.618 ☑
  cystostomy T83.010 ☑
  dialysis (renal) (vascular) T82.41 ☑
   intraperitoneal T85.611 ☑
  infusion NEC T82.514 ☑
   cranial T85.610 ☑
   epidural T85.610 ☑

Malfunction — *continued*
 catheter device — *continued*
  infusion — *continued*
   intrathecal T85.610 ☑
   spinal T85.610 ☑
   subarachnoid T85.610 ☑
   subdural T85.610 ☑
  urinary (*see also* Breakdown, device, catheter) T83.018 ☑
 colostomy K94.03
  valve K94.03
 cystostomy (stoma) N99.512
  catheter T83.010 ☑
 enteric stoma K94.13
 enterostomy K94.13
 esophagostomy K94.33
 gastroenteric K31.89
 gastrostomy K94.23
 ileostomy K94.13
  valve K94.13
 intrathecal infusion pump T85.615 ☑
 jejunostomy K94.13
 nervous system device, implant or graft, specified NEC T85.615 ☑
 pacemaker — *see* Malfunction, cardiac electronic device
 prosthetic device, internal — *see* Complications, prosthetic device, by site, mechanical
 tracheostomy J95.03
 urinary device NEC — *see* Complication, genitourinary, device, urinary, mechanical
 valve
  colostomy K94.03
  heart T82.09 ☑
  ileostomy K94.13
 vascular graft or shunt NEC — *see* Complication, cardiovascular device, mechanical, vascular
 ventricular (communicating shunt) T85.01 ☑
Malherbe's tumor — *see* Neoplasm, skin, benign
Malibu disease L98.8
Malignancy (*see also* Neoplasm, malignant, by site)
 unspecified site (primary) C80.1
Malignant — *see* condition
Malingerer, malingering Z76.5
Mallet finger (acquired) — *see* Deformity, finger, mallet finger
 congenital Q74.0
 sequelae of rickets E64.3
Malleus A24.0
Mallory's bodies R89.7
Mallory-Weiss syndrome K22.6
Malnutrition E46
 degree
  first E44.1
  mild (protein) E44.1
  moderate (protein) E44.0
  second E44.0
  severe (protein-energy) E43
   intermediate form E42
    with
     kwashiorkor (and marasmus) E42
     marasmus E41
  third E43
 following gastrointestinal surgery K91.2
 intrauterine
  light-for-dates — *see* Light for dates
  small-for-dates — *see* Small for dates
 lack of care, or neglect (child) (infant) T76.02 ☑
  confirmed T74.02 ☑
 malignant E40
 protein E46
  calorie E46
   mild E44.1
   moderate E44.0
   severe E43
    intermediate form E42
     with
      kwashiorkor (and marasmus) E42
      marasmus E41
  energy E46
   mild E44.1
   moderate E44.0
   severe E43
    intermediate form E42
     with
      kwashiorkor (and marasmus) E42
      marasmus E41
 severe (protein-energy) E43

Malnutrition — continued
  severe — continued
    with
      kwashiorkor (and marasmus) E42
      marasmus E41
Malocclusion (teeth) M26.4
  Angle's M26.219
    class I M26.211
    class II M26.212
    class III M26.213
  due to
    abnormal swallowing M26.59
    mouth breathing M26.59
    tongue, lip or finger habits M26.59
  temporomandibular (joint) M26.69
Malposition
  cervix — see Malposition, uterus
  congenital
    adrenal (gland) Q89.1
    alimentary tract Q45.8
      lower Q43.8
      upper Q40.8
    aorta Q25.49
    appendix Q43.8
    arterial trunk Q20.0
    artery (peripheral) Q27.8
      coronary Q24.5
      digestive system Q27.8
      lower limb Q27.8
      pulmonary Q25.79
      specified site NEC Q27.8
      upper limb Q27.8
    auditory canal Q17.8
      causing impairment of hearing Q16.9
    auricle (ear) Q17.4
      causing impairment of hearing Q16.9
      cervical Q18.2
    biliary duct or passage Q44.5
    bladder (mucosa) — see Exstrophy, bladder
    brachial plexus Q07.8
    brain tissue Q04.8
    breast Q83.8
    bronchus Q32.4
    cecum Q43.8
    clavicle Q74.0
    colon Q43.8
    digestive organ or tract NEC Q45.8
      lower Q43.8
      upper Q40.8
    ear (auricle) (external) Q17.4
      ossicles Q16.3
    endocrine (gland) NEC Q89.2
    epiglottis Q31.8
    eustachian tube Q17.8
    eye Q15.8
    facial features Q18.8
    fallopian tube Q50.6
    finger(s) Q68.1
      supernumerary Q69.0
    foot Q66.9
    gallbladder Q44.1
    gastrointestinal tract Q45.8
    genitalia, genital organ(s) or tract
      female Q52.8
        external Q52.79
        internal NEC Q52.8
      male Q55.8
    glottis Q31.8
    hand Q68.1
    heart Q24.8
      dextrocardia Q24.0
        with complete transposition of viscera Q89.3
    hepatic duct Q44.5
    hip (joint) Q65.89
    intestine (large) (small) Q43.8
      with anomalous adhesions, fixation or malrotation Q43.3
    joint NEC Q68.8
    kidney Q63.2
    larynx Q31.8
    limb Q68.8
      lower Q68.8
      upper Q68.8
    liver Q44.7
    lung (lobe) Q33.8
    nail(s) Q84.6
    nerve Q07.8
    nervous system NEC Q07.8
    nose, nasal (septum) Q30.8

Malposition — continued
  congenital — continued
    organ or site not listed — see Anomaly, by site
    ovary Q50.39
    pancreas Q45.3
    parathyroid (gland) Q89.2
    patella Q74.1
    peripheral vascular system Q27.8
    pituitary (gland) Q89.2
    respiratory organ or system NEC Q34.8
    rib (cage) Q76.6
      supernumerary in cervical region Q76.5
    scapula Q74.0
    shoulder Q74.0
    spinal cord Q06.8
    spleen Q89.09
    sternum NEC Q76.7
    stomach Q40.2
    symphysis pubis Q74.2
    thymus (gland) Q89.2
    thyroid (gland) (tissue) Q89.2
      cartilage Q31.8
    toe(s) Q66.9
      supernumerary Q69.2
    tongue Q38.3
    trachea Q32.1
    ureter Q62.60
      deviation Q62.61
      displacement Q62.62
      ectopia Q62.63
      specified type NEC Q62.69
    uterus Q51.818
    vein(s) (peripheral) Q27.8
      great Q26.8
    vena cava (inferior) (superior) Q26.8
  device, implant or graft (see also Complications, by site and type, mechanical) T85.628 ☑
    arterial graft NEC — see Complication, cardiovascular device, mechanical, vascular
    breast (implant) T85.42 ☑
    catheter NEC T85.628 ☑
      cystostomy T83.020 ☑
      dialysis (renal) T82.42 ☑
        intraperitoneal T85.621 ☑
      infusion NEC T82.524 ☑
        spinal (epidural) (subdural) T85.620 ☑
      urinary (see also Displacement, device, catheter, urinary) T83.028 ☑
    electronic (electrode) (pulse generator) (stimulator)
      bone T84.320 ☑
      cardiac T82.129 ☑
        electrode T82.120 ☑
        pulse generator T82.121 ☑
        specified type NEC T82.128 ☑
      nervous system — see Complication, prosthetic device, mechanical, electronic nervous system stimulator
      urinary — see Complication, genitourinary, device, urinary, mechanical
    fixation, internal (orthopedic) NEC — see Complication, fixation device, mechanical
    gastrointestinal — see Complications, prosthetic device, mechanical, gastrointestinal device
    genital NEC T83.428 ☑
      intrauterine contraceptive device (string) T83.32 ☑
      penile prosthesis (cylinder) (implanted) (pump) (reservoir) T83.420 ☑
      testicular prosthesis T83.421 ☑
    heart NEC — see Complication, cardiovascular device, mechanical
    joint prosthesis — see Complication, joint prosthesis, mechanical
    ocular NEC — see Complications, prosthetic device, mechanical, ocular device
    orthopedic NEC — see Complication, orthopedic, device, mechanical
    specified NEC T85.628 ☑
    urinary NEC (see also Complication, genitourinary, device, urinary, mechanical)
      graft T83.22 ☑
    vascular NEC — see Complication, cardiovascular device, mechanical
    ventricular intracranial shunt T85.02 ☑
  fetus — see Pregnancy, complicated by (management affected by), presentation, fetal
  gallbladder K82.8

Malposition — continued
  gastrointestinal tract, congenital Q45.8
  heart, congenital NEC Q24.8
  joint prosthesis — see Complications, joint prosthesis, mechanical, displacement, by site
  stomach K31.89
    congenital Q40.2
  tooth, teeth, fully erupted M26.30
  uterus (acute) (acquired) (adherent) (asymptomatic) (postinfectional) (postpartal, old) N85.4
    anteflexion or anteversion N85.4
      congenital Q51.818
    flexion N85.4
      lateral — see Lateroversion, uterus
    inversion N85.5
    lateral (flexion) (version) — see Lateroversion, uterus
      in pregnancy or childbirth — see subcategory O34.5 ☑
    retroflexion or retroversion — see Retroversion, uterus
Malposture R29.3
Malrotation
  cecum Q43.3
  colon Q43.3
  intestine Q43.3
  kidney Q63.2
Malta fever — see Brucellosis
Maltreatment
  adult
    abandonment
      confirmed T74.01 ☑
      suspected T76.01 ☑
    confirmed T74.91 ☑
    history of Z91.419
    neglect
      confirmed T74.01 ☑
      suspected T76.01 ☑
    physical abuse
      confirmed T74.11 ☑
      suspected T76.11 ☑
    psychological abuse
      confirmed T74.31 ☑
      history of Z91.411
      suspected T76.31 ☑
    sexual abuse
      confirmed T74.21 ☑
      suspected T76.21 ☑
    suspected T76.91 ☑
  child
    abandonment
      confirmed T74.02 ☑
      suspected T76.02 ☑
    confirmed T74.92 ☑
    history of — see History, personal (of), abuse
    neglect
      confirmed T74.02 ☑
      history of — see History, personal (of), abuse
      suspected T76.02 ☑
    physical abuse
      confirmed T74.12 ☑
      history of — see History, personal (of), abuse
      suspected T76.12 ☑
    psychological abuse
      confirmed T74.32 ☑
      history of — see History, personal (of), abuse
      suspected T76.32 ☑
    sexual abuse
      confirmed T74.22 ☑
      history of — see History, personal (of), abuse
      suspected T76.22 ☑
    suspected T76.92 ☑
  personal history of Z91.89
Maltworker's lung J67.4
Malunion, fracture — see Fracture, by site
Mammillitis N61.0
  puerperal, postpartum O91.02
Mammitis — see Mastitis
Mammogram (examination) Z12.39
  routine Z12.31
Mammoplasia N62
Management (of)
  bone conduction hearing device (implanted) Z45.320
  cardiac pacemaker NEC Z45.018
  cerebrospinal fluid drainage device Z45.41
  cochlear device (implanted) Z45.321
  contraceptive Z30.9

☑ Additional Character Required — Refer to the Tabular List for Character Selection   ▽ Subterms under main terms may continue to next column or page

Management — continued
  contraceptive — continued
    specified NEC Z30.8
    implanted device Z45.9
      specified NEC Z45.89
  infusion pump Z45.1
  procreative Z31.9
    male factor infertility in female Z31.81
    specified NEC Z31.89
  prosthesis (external) (see also Fitting) Z44.9
    implanted Z45.9
      specified NEC Z45.89
  renal dialysis catheter Z49.01
  vascular access device Z45.2
Mangled — see specified injury by site
Mania (monopolar) (see also Disorder, mood, manic
    episode)
  with psychotic symptoms F30.2
  without psychotic symptoms F30.10
    mild F30.11
    moderate F30.12
    severe F30.13
  Bell's F30.8
  chronic (recurrent) F31.89
  hysterical F44.89
  puerperal F30.8
  recurrent F31.89
Manic depression F31.9
Manic-depressive insanity, psychosis, or syndrome
    — see Disorder, bipolar
Mannosidosis E77.1
Mansonelliasis, mansonellosis B74.4
Manson's
  disease B65.1
  schistosomiasis B65.1
Manual — see condition
Maple-bark-stripper's lung (disease) J67.6
Maple-syrup-urine disease E71.0
Marable's syndrome (celiac artery compression) I77.4
Marasmus E41
  due to malnutrition E41
  intestinal E41
  nutritional E41
  senile R54
  tuberculous NEC — see Tuberculosis
Marble
  bones Q78.2
  skin R23.8
Marburg virus disease A98.3
March
  fracture — see Fracture, traumatic, stress, by site
  hemoglobinuria D59.6
Marchesani (-Weill) **syndrome** Q87.0
Marchiafava (-Bignami) **syndrome or disease** G37.1
Marchiafava-Micheli syndrome D59.5
Marcus Gunn's syndrome Q07.8
Marfan's syndrome — see Syndrome, Marfan's
Marie-Bamberger disease — see Osteoarthropathy,
    hypertrophic, specified NEC
Marie-Charcot-Tooth neuropathic muscular atrophy
    G60.0
Marie's
  cerebellar ataxia (late-onset) G11.2
  disease or syndrome (acromegaly) E22.0
Marie-Strümpell arthritis, disease or spondylitis —
    see Spondylitis, ankylosing
Marion's disease (bladder neck obstruction) N32.0
Marital conflict Z63.0
Mark
  port wine Q82.5
  raspberry Q82.5
  strawberry Q82.5
  stretch L90.6
  tattoo L81.8
Marker heterochromatin — see Extra, marker chromo-
    somes
Maroteaux-Lamy syndrome (mild) (severe) E76.29
Marrow (bone)
  arrest D61.9
  poor function D75.89
Marseilles fever A77.1
Marsh fever — see Malaria
Marshall's (hidrotic) **ectodermal dysplasia** Q82.4
Marsh's disease (exophthalmic goiter) E05.00
  with storm E05.01
Masculinization (female) **with adrenal hyperplasia**
    E25.9

Masculinization (female) **with adrenal hyperplasia**
    — continued
  congenital E25.0
Masculinovoblastoma D27.- ☑
Masochism (sexual) F65.51
Mason's lung J62.8
Mass
  abdominal R19.00
    epigastric R19.06
    generalized R19.07
    left lower quadrant R19.04
    left upper quadrant R19.02
    periumbilic R19.05
    right lower quadrant R19.03
    right upper quadrant R19.01
    specified site NEC R19.09
  breast (see also Lump, breast) N63.0
  chest R22.2
  cystic — see Cyst
  ear H93.8- ☑
  head R22.0
  intra-abdominal (diffuse) (generalized) — see Mass,
    abdominal
  kidney N28.89
  liver R16.0
  localized (skin) R22.9
    chest R22.2
    head R22.0
    limb
      lower R22.4- ☑
      upper R22.3- ☑
    neck R22.1
    trunk R22.2
  lung R91.8
  malignant — see Neoplasm, malignant, by site
  neck R22.1
  pelvic (diffuse) (generalized) — see Mass, abdominal
  specified organ NEC — see Disease, by site
  splenic R16.1
  substernal thyroid — see Goiter
  superficial (localized) R22.9
  umbilical (diffuse) (generalized) R19.09
Massive — see condition
Mast cell
  disease, systemic tissue D47.02
  leukemia C94.3- ☑
  neoplasm
    malignant C96.20
      specified type NEC C96.29
    of uncertain behavior NEC D47.09
  sarcoma C96.22
  tumor D47.09
Mastalgia N64.4
Masters-Allen syndrome N83.8
Mastitis (acute) (diffuse) (nonpuerperal) (subacute) N61.0
  with abscess N61.1
  without abscess N61.0
  chronic (cystic) — see Mastopathy, cystic
  cystic (Schimmelbusch's type) — see Mastopathy,
    cystic
  fibrocystic — see Mastopathy, cystic
  infective N61.0
    newborn P39.0
  interstitial, gestational or puerperal — see Mastitis,
    obstetric
  neonatal (noninfective) P83.4
    infective P39.0
  obstetric (interstitial) (nonpurulent)
    associated with
      lactation O91.23
      pregnancy O91.21- ☑
      puerperium O91.22
    purulent
      associated with
        lactation O91.13
        pregnancy O91.11- ☑
        puerperium O91.12
  periductal — see Ectasia, mammary duct
  phlegmonous — see Mastopathy, cystic
  plasma cell — see Ectasia, mammary duct
Mastocytoma (extracutaneous) D47.09
  malignant C96.29
  solitary D47.01
Mastocytosis D47.09
  aggressive systemic C96.21
  cutaneous (diffuse) (maculopapular) D47.01
    congenital Q82.2
    of neonatal onset Q82.2

Mastocytosis — continued
  cutaneous — continued
    of newborn onset Q82.2
  indolent systemic D47.02
  isolated bone marrow D47.02
  malignant C96.29
  systemic (indolent) (smoldering)
    with an associated hematological non-mast cell
        lineage disease (SM-AHNMD) D47.02
Mastodynia N64.4
Mastoid — see condition
Mastoidalgia — see subcategory H92.0 ☑
Mastoiditis (coalescent) (hemorrhagic) (suppurative)
    H70.9- ☑
  acute, subacute H70.00- ☑
    complicated NEC H70.09- ☑
    subperiosteal H70.01- ☑
  chronic (necrotic) (recurrent) H70.1- ☑
  in (due to)
    infectious disease NEC B99 ☑ [H75.0-] ☑
    parasitic disease NEC B89 [H75.0-] ☑
    tuberculosis A18.03
  petrositis — see Petrositis
  postauricular fistula — see Fistula, postauricular
  specified NEC H70.89- ☑
  tuberculous A18.03
Mastopathy, mastopathia N64.9
  chronica cystica — see Mastopathy, cystic
  cystic (chronic) (diffuse) N60.1- ☑
    with epithelial proliferation N60.3- ☑
  diffuse cystic — see Mastopathy, cystic
  estrogenic, oestrogenica N64.89
  ovarian origin N64.89
Mastoplasia, mastoplastia N62
Masturbation (excessive) F98.8
Maternal care (for) — see Pregnancy (complicated by)
    (management affected by)
Matheiu's disease (leptospiral jaundice) A27.0
Mauclaire's disease or osteochondrosis — see Osteo-
    chondrosis, juvenile, hand, metacarpal
Maxcy's disease A75.2
Maxilla, maxillary — see condition
May (-Hegglin) **anomaly or syndrome** D72.0
McArdle (-Schmid)(-Pearson) **disease** (glycogen storage)
    E74.04
McCune-Albright syndrome Q78.1
McQuarrie's syndrome (idiopathic familial hypo-
    glycemia) E16.2
Meadow's syndrome Q86.1
Measles (black) (hemorrhagic) (suppressed) B05.9
  with
    complications NEC B05.89
    encephalitis B05.0
    intestinal complications B05.4
    keratitis (keratoconjunctivitis) B05.81
    meningitis B05.1
    otitis media B05.3
    pneumonia B05.2
  French — see Rubella
  German — see Rubella
  Liberty — see Rubella
Meatitis, urethral — see Urethritis
Meatus, meatal — see condition
Meat-wrappers' asthma J68.9
Meckel-Gruber syndrome Q61.9
Meckel's diverticulitis, diverticulum (displaced) (hy-
    pertrophic) Q43.0
  malignant — see Table of Neoplasms, small intestine,
    malignant
Meconium
  ileus, newborn P76.0
    in cystic fibrosis E84.11
    meaning meconium plug (without cystic fibrosis)
        P76.0
  obstruction, newborn P76.0
    due to fecaliths P76.0
    in mucoviscidosis E84.11
  peritonitis P78.0
  plug syndrome (newborn) NEC P76.0
Median (see also condition)
  arcuate ligament syndrome I77.4
  bar (prostate) (vesical orifice) — see Hyperplasia,
    prostate
  rhomboid glossitis K14.2
Mediastinal shift R93.8
Mediastinitis (acute) (chronic) J98.51
  syphilitic A52.73

Mediastinitis — continued
  tuberculous A15.8
Mediastinopericarditis (see also Pericarditis)
  acute I30.9
  adhesive I31.0
  chronic I31.8
  rheumatic I09.2
Mediastinum, mediastinal — see condition
Medicine poisoning — see Table of Drugs and Chemicals, by drug, poisoning
Mediterranean
  fever — see Brucellosis
    familial M04.1
    tick A77.1
  kala-azar B55.0
  leishmaniasis B55.0
  tick fever A77.1
Medulla — see condition
Medullary cystic kidney Q61.5
Medullated fibers
  optic (nerve) Q14.8
  retina Q14.1
Medulloblastoma
  desmoplastic C71.6
  specified site — see Neoplasm, malignant, by site
  unspecified site C71.6
Medulloepithelioma (see also Neoplasm, malignant, by site)
  teratoid — see Neoplasm, malignant, by site
Medullomyoblastoma
  specified site — see Neoplasm, malignant, by site
  unspecified site C71.6
Meekeren-Ehlers-Danlos syndrome Q79.6
Megacolon (acquired) (functional) (not Hirschsprung's disease) (in) K59.39
  Chagas' disease B57.32
  congenital, congenitum (aganglionic) Q43.1
  Hirschsprung's (disease) Q43.1
  toxic NEC K59.31
    due to Clostridium difficile
      not specified as recurrent A04.72
      recurrent A04.71
Megaesophagus (functional) K22.0
  congenital Q39.5
  in (due to) Chagas' disease B57.31
Megalencephaly Q04.5
Megalerythema (epidemic) B08.3
Megaloappendix Q43.8
Megalocephalus, megalocephaly NEC Q75.3
Megalocornea Q15.8
  with glaucoma Q15.0
Megalocytic anemia D53.1
Megalodactylia (fingers) (thumbs) (congenital) Q74.0
  toes Q74.2
Megaloduodenum Q43.8
Megaloesophagus (functional) K22.0
  congenital Q39.5
Megalogastria (acquired) K31.89
  congenital Q40.2
Megalophthalmos Q11.3
Megalopsia H53.15
Megalosplenia — see Splenomegaly
Megaloureter N28.82
  congenital Q62.2
Megarectum K62.89
Megasigmoid K59.39
  congenital Q43.2
Megaureter N28.82
  congenital Q62.2
Megavitamin-B6 syndrome E67.2
Megrim — see Migraine
Meibomian
  cyst, infected — see Hordeolum
  gland — see condition
  sty, stye — see Hordeolum
Meibomitis — see Hordeolum
Meige-Milroy disease (chronic hereditary edema) Q82.0
Meige's syndrome Q82.0
Melalgia, nutritional E53.8
Melancholia F32.9
  climacteric (single episode) F32.89
    recurrent episode F33.8
  hypochondriac F45.29
  intermittent (single episode) F32.89
    recurrent episode F33.8
  involutional (single episode) F32.89
    recurrent episode F33.8

Melancholia — continued
  menopausal (single episode) F32.89
    recurrent episode F33.8
  puerperal F32.89
  reactive (emotional stress or trauma) F32.3
  recurrent F33.9
  senile F03 ☑
  stuporous (single episode) F32.89
    recurrent episode F33.8
Melanemia R79.89
Melanoameloblastoma — see Neoplasm, bone, benign
Melanoblastoma — see Melanoma
Melanocarcinoma — see Melanoma
Melanocytoma, eyeball D31.9- ☑
Melanocytosis, neurocutaneous Q82.8
Melanoderma, melanodermia L81.4
Melanodontia, infantile K03.89
Melanodontoclasia K03.89
Melanoepithelioma — see Melanoma
Melanoma (malignant) C43.9
  acral lentiginous, malignant — see Melanoma, skin, by site
  amelanotic — see Melanoma, skin, by site
  balloon cell — see Melanoma, skin, by site
  benign — see Nevus
  desmoplastic, malignant — see Melanoma, skin, by site
  epithelioid cell — see Melanoma, skin, by site
    with spindle cell, mixed — see Melanoma, skin, by site
  in
    giant pigmented nevus — see Melanoma, skin, by site
    Hutchinson's melanotic freckle — see Melanoma, skin, by site
    junctional nevus — see Melanoma, skin, by site
    precancerous melanosis — see Melanoma, skin, by site
  in situ D03.9
    abdominal wall D03.59
    ala nasi D03.39
    ankle D03.7- ☑
    anus, anal (margin) (skin) D03.51
    arm D03.6- ☑
    auditory canal D03.2- ☑
    auricle (ear) D03.2- ☑
    auricular canal (external) D03.2- ☑
    axilla, axillary fold D03.59
    back D03.59
    breast D03.52
    brow D03.39
    buttock D03.59
    canthus (eye) D03.1- ☑
    cheek (external) D03.39
    chest wall D03.59
    chin D03.39
    choroid D03.8
    conjunctiva D03.8
    ear (external) D03.2- ☑
    external meatus (ear) D03.2- ☑
    eye D03.8
    eyebrow D03.39
    eyelid (lower) (upper) D03.1- ☑
    face D03.30
      specified NEC D03.39
    female genital organ (external) NEC D03.8
    finger D03.6- ☑
    flank D03.59
    foot D03.7- ☑
    forearm D03.6- ☑
    forehead D03.39
    foreskin D03.8
    gluteal region D03.59
    groin D03.59
    hand D03.6- ☑
    heel D03.7- ☑
    helix D03.2- ☑
    hip D03.7- ☑
    interscapular region D03.59
    iris D03.8
    jaw D03.39
    knee D03.7- ☑
    labium (majus) (minus) D03.8
    lacrimal gland D03.8
    leg D03.7- ☑
    lip (lower) (upper) D03.0
    lower limb NEC D03.7- ☑

Melanoma — continued
  in situ — continued
    male genital organ (external) NEC D03.8
    nail D03.9
      finger D03.6- ☑
      toe D03.7- ☑
    neck D03.4
    nose (external) D03.39
    orbit D03.8
    penis D03.8
    perianal skin D03.51
    perineum D03.51
    pinna D03.2- ☑
    popliteal fossa or space D03.7- ☑
    prepuce D03.8
    pudendum D03.8
    retina D03.8
    retrobulbar D03.8
    scalp D03.4
    scrotum D03.8
    shoulder D03.6- ☑
    specified site NEC D03.8
    submammary fold D03.52
    temple D03.39
    thigh D03.7- ☑
    toe D03.7- ☑
    trunk NEC D03.59
    umbilicus D03.59
    upper limb NEC D03.6- ☑
    vulva D03.8
  juvenile — see Nevus
  malignant, of soft parts except skin — see Neoplasm, connective tissue, malignant
  metastatic
    breast C79.81
    genital organ C79.82
    specified site NEC C79.89
  neurotropic, malignant — see Melanoma, skin, by site
  nodular — see Melanoma, skin, by site
  regressing, malignant — see Melanoma, skin, by site
  skin C43.9
    abdominal wall C43.59
    ala nasi C43.31
    ankle C43.7- ☑
    anus, anal (skin) C43.51
    arm C43.6- ☑
    auditory canal (external) C43.2- ☑
    auricle (ear) C43.2- ☑
    auricular canal (external) C43.2- ☑
    axilla, axillary fold C43.59
    back C43.59
    breast (female) (male) C43.52
    brow C43.39
    buttock C43.59
    canthus (eye) C43.1- ☑
    cheek (external) C43.39
    chest wall C43.59
    chin C43.39
    ear (external) C43.2- ☑
    elbow C43.6- ☑
    external meatus (ear) C43.2- ☑
    eyebrow C43.39
    eyelid (lower) (upper) C43.1- ☑
    face C43.30
      specified NEC C43.39
    female genital organ (external) NEC C51.9
    finger C43.6- ☑
    flank C43.59
    foot C43.7- ☑
    forearm C43.6- ☑
    forehead C43.39
    foreskin C60.0
    glabella C43.39
    gluteal region C43.59
    groin C43.59
    hand C43.6- ☑
    heel C43.7- ☑
    helix C43.2- ☑
    hip C43.7- ☑
    interscapular region C43.59
    jaw (external) C43.39
    knee C43.7- ☑
    labium C51.9
      majus C51.0
      minus C51.1
    leg C43.7- ☑
    lip (lower) (upper) C43.0

  ☑ **Additional Character Required** — Refer to the Tabular List for Character Selection   ⚐ Subterms under main terms may continue to next column or page

Melanoma — *continued*
  skin — *continued*
    lower limb NEC C43.7- ☑
    male genital organ (external) NEC C63.9
    nail
        finger C43.6- ☑
        toe C43.7- ☑
    nasolabial groove C43.39
    nates C43.59
    neck C43.4
    nose (external) C43.31
    overlapping site C43.8
    palpebra C43.1- ☑
    penis C60.9
    perianal skin C43.51
    perineum C43.51
    pinna C43.2- ☑
    popliteal fossa or space C43.7- ☑
    prepuce C60.0
    pudendum C51.9
    scalp C43.4
    scrotum C63.2
    shoulder C43.6- ☑
    skin NEC C43.9
    submammary fold C43.52
    temple C43.39
    thigh C43.7- ☑
    toe C43.7- ☑
    trunk NEC C43.59
    umbilicus C43.59
    upper limb NEC C43.6- ☑
    vulva C51.9
        overlapping sites C51.8
  spindle cell
    with epithelioid, mixed — *see* Melanoma, skin, by site
    type A C69.4- ☑
    type B C69.4- ☑
  superficial spreading — *see* Melanoma, skin, by site
Melanosarcoma (*see also* Melanoma)
  epithelioid cell — *see* Melanoma
Melanosis L81.4
  addisonian E27.1
    tuberculous A18.7
  adrenal E27.1
  colon K63.89
  conjunctiva — *see* Pigmentation, conjunctiva
    congenital Q13.89
  cornea (presenile) (senile) (*see also* Pigmentation, cornea)
    congenital Q13.4
  eye NEC H57.8
    congenital Q15.8
  lenticularis progressiva Q82.1
  liver K76.89
  precancerous (*see also* Melanoma, in situ)
    malignant melanoma in — *see* Melanoma
  Riehl's L81.4
  sclera H15.89
    congenital Q13.89
  suprarenal E27.1
  tar L81.4
  toxic L81.4
Melanuria R82.99
MELAS syndrome E88.41
Melasma L81.1
  adrenal (gland) E27.1
  suprarenal (gland) E27.1
Melena K92.1
  with ulcer — *code by* site under Ulcer, with hemorrhage K27.4
  due to swallowed maternal blood P78.2
  newborn, neonatal P54.1
    due to swallowed maternal blood P78.2
Meleney's
  gangrene (cutaneous) — *see* Ulcer, skin
  ulcer (chronic undermining) — *see* Ulcer, skin
Melioidosis A24.9
  acute A24.1
  chronic A24.2
  fulminating A24.1
  pneumonia A24.1
  pulmonary (chronic) A24.2
    acute A24.1
    subacute A24.2
  sepsis A24.1
  specified NEC A24.3
  subacute A24.2

Melitensis, febris A23.0
Melkersson (-Rosenthal) **syndrome** G51.2
Mellitus, diabetes — *see* Diabetes
Melorheostosis (bone) — *see* Disorder, bone, density and structure, specified NEC
Meloschisis Q18.4
Melotia Q17.4
Membrana
  capsularis lentis posterior Q13.89
  epipapillaris Q14.2
Membranacea placenta O43.19- ☑
Membranaceous uterus N85.8
Membrane(s), membranous (*see also* condition)
  cyclitic — *see* Membrane, pupillary
  folds, congenital — *see* Web
  Jackson's Q43.3
  over face of newborn P28.9
  premature rupture — *see* Rupture, membranes, premature
  pupillary H21.4- ☑
    persistent Q13.89
  retained (with hemorrhage) (complicating delivery) O72.2
    without hemorrhage O73.1
  secondary cataract — *see* Cataract, secondary
  unruptured (causing asphyxia) — *see* Asphyxia, newborn
  vitreous — *see* Opacity, vitreous, membranes and strands
Membranitis — *see* Chorioamnionitis
Memory disturbance, lack or loss (*see also* Amnesia)
  mild, following organic brain damage F06.8
Menadione deficiency E56.1
Menarche
  delayed E30.0
  precocious E30.1
Mendacity, pathologic F60.2
Mendelson's syndrome (due to anesthesia) J95.4
  in labor and delivery O74.0
  in pregnancy O29.01- ☑
  obstetric O74.0
  postpartum, puerperal O89.01
Ménétrier's disease or syndrome K29.60
  with bleeding K29.61
Ménière's disease, syndrome or vertigo H81.0- ☑
Meninges, meningeal — *see* condition
Meningioma (*see also* Neoplasm, meninges, benign)
  angioblastic — *see* Neoplasm, meninges, benign
  angiomatous — *see* Neoplasm, meninges, benign
  endotheliomatous — *see* Neoplasm, meninges, benign
  fibroblastic — *see* Neoplasm, meninges, benign
  fibrous — *see* Neoplasm, meninges, benign
  hemangioblastic — *see* Neoplasm, meninges, benign
  hemangiopericytic — *see* Neoplasm, meninges, benign
  malignant — *see* Neoplasm, meninges, malignant
  meningiothelial — *see* Neoplasm, meninges, benign
  meningotheliomatous — *see* Neoplasm, meninges, benign
  mixed — *see* Neoplasm, meninges, benign
  multiple — *see* Neoplasm, meninges, uncertain behavior
  papillary — *see* Neoplasm, meninges, uncertain behavior
  psammomatous — *see* Neoplasm, meninges, benign
  syncytial — *see* Neoplasm, meninges, benign
  transitional — *see* Neoplasm, meninges, benign
Meningiomatosis (diffuse) — *see* Neoplasm, meninges, uncertain behavior
Meningism — *see* Meningismus
Meningismus (infectional) (pneumococcal) R29.1
  due to serum or vaccine R29.1
  influenzal — *see* Influenza, with, manifestations NEC
Meningitis (basal) (basic) (brain) (cerebral) (cervical) (congestive) (diffuse) (hemorrhagic) (infantile) (membranous) (metastatic) (nonspecific) (pontine) (progressive) (simple) (spinal) (subacute) (sympathetic) (toxic) G03.9
  abacterial G03.0
  actinomycotic A42.81
  adenoviral A87.1
  arbovirus A87.8
  aseptic (acute) G03.0
  bacterial G00.9
    Escherichia coli (E. coli) G00.8
    Friedländer (bacillus) G00.8
    gram-negative G00.9

Meningitis — *continued*
  bacterial — *continued*
    H. influenzae G00.0
    Klebsiella G00.8
    pneumococcal G00.1
    specified organism NEC G00.8
    staphylococcal G00.3
    streptococcal (acute) G00.2
  benign recurrent (Mollaret) G03.2
  candidal B37.5
  caseous (tuberculous) A17.0
  cerebrospinal A39.0
  chronic NEC G03.1
  clear cerebrospinal fluid NEC G03.0
  coxsackievirus A87.0
  cryptococcal B45.1
  diplococcal (gram positive) A39.0
  echovirus A87.0
  enteroviral A87.0
  eosinophilic B83.2
  epidemic NEC A39.0
  Escherichia coli (E. coli) G00.8
  fibrinopurulent G00.9
    specified organism NEC G00.8
  Friedländer (bacillus) G00.8
  gonococcal A54.81
  gram-negative cocci G00.9
  gram-positive cocci G00.9
  H. influenzae G00.0
  Haemophilus (influenzae) G00.0
  in (due to)
    adenovirus A87.1
    African trypanosomiasis B56.9 [G02]
    anthrax A22.8
    bacterial disease NEC A48.8 [G01]
    Chagas' disease (chronic) B57.41
    chickenpox B01.0
    coccidioidomycosis B38.4
    Diplococcus pneumoniae G00.1
    enterovirus A87.0
    herpes (simplex) virus B00.3
        zoster B02.1
    infectious mononucleosis B27.92
    leptospirosis A27.81
    Listeria monocytogenes A32.11
    Lyme disease A69.21
    measles B05.1
    mumps (virus) B26.1
    neurosyphilis (late) A52.13
    parasitic disease NEC B89 [G02]
    poliovirus A80.9 [G02]
    preventive immunization, inoculation or vaccination G03.8
    rubella B06.02
    Salmonella infection A02.21
    specified cause NEC G03.8
    Streptococcal pneumoniae G00.1
    typhoid fever A01.01
    varicella B01.0
    viral disease NEC A87.8
    whooping cough A37.90
    zoster B02.1
  infectious G00.9
  influenzal (H. influenzae) G00.0
  Klebsiella G00.8
  leptospiral (aseptic) A27.81
  lymphocytic (acute) (benign) (serous) A87.2
  meningococcal A39.0
  Mima polymorpha G00.8
  Mollaret (benign recurrent) G03.2
  monilial B37.5
  mycotic NEC B49 [G02]
  Neisseria A39.0
  nonbacterial G03.0
  nonpyogenic NEC G03.0
  ossificans G96.19
  pneumococcal streptococcus pneumoniae G00.1
  poliovirus A80.9 [G02]
  postmeasles B05.1
  purulent G00.9
    specified organism NEC G00.8
  pyogenic G00.9
    specified organism NEC G00.8
  Salmonella (arizonae) (Cholerae-Suis) (enteritidis) (typhimurium) A02.21
  septic G00.9
    specified organism NEC G00.8
  serosa circumscripta NEC G03.0
  serous NEC G93.2

Meningitis — *continued*
specified organism NEC G00.8
sporotrichosis B42.81
staphylococcal G00.3
sterile G03.0
Streptococcal (acute) G00.2
pneumoniae G00.1
suppurative G00.9
specified organism NEC G00.8
syphilitic (late) (tertiary) A52.13
acute A51.41
congenital A50.41
secondary A51.41
Torula histolytica (cryptococcal) B45.1
traumatic (complication of injury) T79.8 ☑
tuberculous A17.0
typhoid A01.01
viral NEC A87.9
Yersinia pestis A20.3
Meningocele (spinal) (*see also* Spina bifida)
with hydrocephalus — *see* Spina bifida, by site, with
hydrocephalus
acquired (traumatic) G96.19
cerebral — *see* Encephalocele
Meningocerebritis — *see* Meningoencephalitis
Meningococcemia A39.4
acute A39.2
chronic A39.3
Meningococcus, meningococcal (*see also* condition)
A39.9
adrenalitis, hemorrhagic A39.1
carrier (suspected) of Z22.31
meningitis (cerebrospinal) A39.0
Meningoencephalitis (*see also* Encephalitis) G04.90
acute NEC (*see also* Encephalitis, viral) A86
bacterial NEC G04.2
California A83.5
diphasic A84.1
eosinophilic B83.2
epidemic A39.81
herpesviral, herpetic B00.4
due to herpesvirus 6 B10.01
due to herpesvirus 7 B10.09
specified NEC B10.09
in (due to)
blastomycosis NEC B40.81
diseases classified elsewhere G05.3
free-living amebae B60.2
H. influenzae G00.0
Hemophilus influenzae (H .influenzae) G00.0
herpes B00.4
due to herpesvirus 6 B10.01
due to herpesvirus 7 B10.09
specified NEC B10.09
Lyme disease A69.22
mercury — *see* subcategory T56.1 ☑
mumps B26.2
Naegleria (amebae) (organisms) (fowleri) B60.2
Parastrongylus cantonensis B83.2
toxoplasmosis (acquired) B58.2
congenital P37.1
infectious (acute) (viral) A86
influenzal (H. influenzae) G00.0
Listeria monocytogenes A32.12
lymphocytic (serous) A87.2
mumps B26.2
parasitic NEC B89 [G05.3]
pneumococcal G04.2
primary amebic B60.2
specific (syphilitic) A52.14
specified organism NEC G04.81
staphylococcal G04.2
streptococcal G04.2
syphilitic A52.14
toxic NEC G92
due to mercury — *see* subcategory T56.1 ☑
tuberculous A17.82
virus NEC A86
Meningoencephalocele (*see also* Encephalocele)
syphilitic A52.19
congenital A50.49
Meningoencephalomyelitis (*see also* Meningoencephalitis)
acute NEC (viral) A86
disseminated G04.00
postimmunization or postvaccination G04.02
postinfectious G04.01

Meningoencephalomyelitis — *continued*
due to
actinomycosis A42.82
Torula B45.1
Toxoplasma or toxoplasmosis (acquired) B58.2
congenital P37.1
postimmunization or postvaccination G04.02
Meningoencephalomyelopathy G96.9
Meningoencephalopathy G96.9
Meningomyelitis (*see also* Meningoencephalitis)
bacterial NEC G04.2
blastomycotic NEC B40.81
cryptococcal B45.1
in diseases classified elsewhere G05.4
meningococcal A39.81
syphilitic A52.19
tuberculous A17.82
Meningomyelocele (*see also* Spina bifida)
syphilitic A52.19
Meningomyeloneuritis — *see* Meningoencephalitis
Meningoradiculitis — *see* Meningitis
Meningovascular — *see* condition
Menkes' disease or syndrome E83.09
meaning maple-syrup-urine disease E71.0
Menometrorrhagia N92.1
Menopause, menopausal (asymptomatic) (state) Z78.0
arthritis (any site) NEC — *see* Arthritis, specified form
NEC
bleeding N92.4
depression (single episode) F32.89
agitated (single episode) F32.2
recurrent episode F33.9
psychotic (single episode) F32.89
recurrent episode F33.9
recurrent episode F33.8
melancholia (single episode) F32.89
recurrent episode F33.8
paranoid state F22
premature E28.319
asymptomatic E28.319
postirradiation E89.40
postsurgical E89.40
symptomatic E28.310
postirradiation E89.41
postsurgical E89.41
psychosis NEC F28
symptomatic N95.1
toxic polyarthritis NEC — *see* Arthritis, specified form
NEC
Menorrhagia (primary) N92.0
climacteric N92.4
menopausal N92.4
menopausal N92.4
postclimacteric N95.0
postmenopausal N95.0
preclimacteric or premenopausal N92.4
pubertal (menses retained) N92.2
Menostaxis N92.0
Menses, retention N94.89
Menstrual — *see* Menstruation
Menstruation
absent — *see* Amenorrhea
anovulatory N97.0
cycle, irregular N92.6
delayed N91.0
disorder N93.9
psychogenic F45.8
during pregnancy O20.8
excessive (with regular cycle) N92.0
with irregular cycle N92.1
at puberty N92.2
frequent N92.0
infrequent — *see* Oligomenorrhea
irregular N92.6
specified NEC N92.5
latent N92.5
membranous N92.5
painful (*see also* Dysmenorrhea) N94.6
primary N94.4
psychogenic F45.8
secondary N94.5
passage of clots N92.0
precocious E30.1
protracted N92.5
rare — *see* Oligomenorrhea
retained N94.89
retrograde N92.5
scanty — *see* Oligomenorrhea

Menstruation — *continued*
suppression N94.89
vicarious (nasal) N94.89
Mental (*see also* condition)
deficiency — *see* Disability, intellectual
deterioration — *see* Psychosis
disorder — *see* Disorder, mental
exhaustion F48.8
insufficiency (congenital) — *see* Disability, intellectual
observation without need for further medical care
Z03.89
retardation — *see* Disability, intellectual
subnormality — *see* Disability, intellectuall
upset — *see* Disorder, mental
Meralgia paresthetica G57.1- ☑
Mercurial — *see* condition
Mercurialism — *see* subcategory T56.1 ☑
Merkel cell tumor — *see* Carcinoma, Merkel cell
Merocele — *see* Hernia, femoral
Meromelia
lower limb — *see* Defect, reduction, lower limb
intercalary
femur — *see* Defect, reduction, lower limb,
specified type NEC
tibiofibular (complete) (incomplete) — *see*
Defect, reduction, lower limb
upper limb — *see* Defect, reduction, upper limb
intercalary, humeral, radioulnar — *see* Agenesis,
arm, with hand present
MERRF syndrome (myoclonic epilepsy associated with
ragged-red fiber) E88.42
Merzbacher-Pelizaeus disease E75.29
Mesaortitis — *see* Aortitis
Mesarteritis — *see* Arteritis
Mesencephalitis — *see* Encephalitis
Mesenchymoma (*see also* Neoplasm, connective tissue,
uncertain behavior)
benign — *see* Neoplasm, connective tissue, benign
malignant — *see* Neoplasm, connective tissue, malignant
Mesenteritis
retractile K65.4
sclerosing K65.4
Mesentery, mesenteric — *see* condition
Mesiodens, mesiodentes K00.1
Mesio-occlusion M26.213
Mesocolon — *see* condition
Mesonephroma (malignant) — *see* Neoplasm, malignant, by site
benign — *see* Neoplasm, benign, by site
Mesophlebitis — *see* Phlebitis
Mesostromal dysgenesia Q13.89
Mesothelioma (malignant) C45.9
benign
mesentery D19.1
mesocolon D19.1
omentum D19.1
peritoneum D19.1
pleura D19.0
specified site NEC D19.7
unspecified site D19.9
biphasic C45.9
benign
mesentery D19.1
mesocolon D19.1
omentum D19.1
peritoneum D19.1
pleura D19.0
specified site NEC D19.7
unspecified site D19.9
cystic D48.4
epithelioid C45.9
benign
mesentery D19.1
mesocolon D19.1
omentum D19.1
peritoneum D19.1
pleura D19.0
specified site NEC D19.7
unspecified site D19.9
fibrous C45.9
benign
mesentery D19.1
mesocolon D19.1
omentum D19.1
peritoneum D19.1
pleura D19.0
specified site NEC D19.7

Mesothelioma — *continued*
  fibrous — *continued*
    benign — *continued*
      unspecified site D19.9
    site classification
      liver C45.7
      lung C45.7
      mediastinum C45.7
      mesentery C45.1
      mesocolon C45.1
      omentum C45.1
      pericardium C45.2
      peritoneum C45.1
      pleura C45.0
        parietal C45.0
      retroperitoneum C45.7
      specified site NEC C45.7
      unspecified C45.9
Metabolic syndrome E88.81
Metagonimiasis B66.8
Metagonimus infestation (intestine) B66.8
Metal
  pigmentation L81.8
  polisher's disease J62.8
Metamorphopsia H53.15
Metaplasia
  apocrine (breast) — *see* Dysplasia, mammary, specified type NEC
  cervix (squamous) — *see* Dysplasia, cervix
  endometrium (squamous) (uterus) N85.8
  esophagus K22.7- ☑
  kidney (pelvis) (squamous) N28.89
  myelogenous D73.1
  myeloid (agnogenic) (megakaryocytic) D73.1
  spleen D73.1
  squamous cell, bladder N32.89
Metastasis, metastatic
  abscess — *see* Abscess
  calcification E83.59
  cancer
    from specified site — *see* Neoplasm, malignant, by site
    to specified site — *see* Neoplasm, secondary, by site
  deposits (in) — *see* Neoplasm, secondary, by site
  disease (*see also* Neoplasm, secondary, by site) C79.9
  spread (to) — *see* Neoplasm, secondary, by site
Metastrongyliasis B83.8
Metatarsalgia M77.4- ☑
  anterior G57.6- ☑
  Morton's G57.6- ☑
Metatarsus, metatarsal (*see also* condition)
  adductus, congenital Q66.22
  valgus (abductus), congenital Q66.6
  varus (congenital) Q66.22
    primus Q66.21
Methadone use — *see* Use, opioid
Methemoglobinemia D74.9
  acquired (with sulfhemoglobinemia) D74.8
  congenital D74.0
  enzymatic (congenital) D74.0
  Hb M disease D74.0
  hereditary D74.0
  toxic D74.8
Methemoglobinuria — *see* Hemoglobinuria
Methioninemia E72.19
Methylmalonic acidemia E71.120
Metritis (catarrhal) (hemorrhagic) (septic) (suppurative) (*see also* Endometritis)
  cervical — *see* Cervicitis
Metropathia hemorrhagica N93.8
Metroperitonitis — *see* Peritonitis, pelvic, female
Metrorrhagia N92.1
  climacteric N92.4
  menopausal N92.4
  postpartum NEC (atonic) (following delivery of placenta) O72.1
    delayed or secondary O72.2
  preclimacteric or premenopausal N92.4
  psychogenic F45.8
Metrorrhexis — *see* Rupture, uterus
Metrosalpingitis N70.91
Metrostaxis N93.8
Metrovaginitis — *see* Endometritis
Meyer-Schwickerath and Weyers syndrome Q87.0
Meynert's amentia (nonalcoholic) F04
  alcoholic F10.96

Meynert's amentia — *continued*
  alcoholic — *continued*
    with dependence F10.26
Mibelli's disease (porokeratosis) Q82.8
Mice, joint — *see* Loose, body, joint
  knee M23.4- ☑
Micrencephalon, micrencephaly Q02
Microalbuminuria R80.9
Microaneurysm, retinal (*see also* Disorder, retina, microaneurysms)
  diabetic — *see* E08-E13 with .31
Microangiopathy (peripheral) I73.9
  thrombotic M31.1
Microcalcifications, breast R92.0
Microcephalus, microcephalic, microcephaly Q02
  due to toxoplasmosis (congenital) P37.1
Microcheilia Q18.7
Microcolon (congenital) Q43.8
Microcornea (congenital) Q13.4
Microcytic — *see* condition
Microdeletions NEC Q93.88
Microdontia K00.2
Microdrepanocytosis D57.40
  with crisis (vasoocclusive pain) D57.419
    with
      acute chest syndrome D57.411
      splenic sequestration D57.412
Microembolism
  atherothrombotic — *see* Atheroembolism
  retinal — *see* Occlusion, artery, retina
Microencephalon Q02
Microfilaria streptocerca infestation — *see* Onchocerciasis
Microgastria (congenital) Q40.2
Microgenia M26.06
Microgenitalia, congenital
  female Q52.8
  male Q55.8
Microglioma — *see* Lymphoma, non-Hodgkin, specified NEC
Microglossia (congenital) Q38.3
Micrognathia, micrognathism (congenital) (mandibular) (maxillary) M26.09
Microgyria (congenital) Q04.3
Microinfarct of heart — *see* Insufficiency, coronary
Microlentia (congenital) Q12.8
Microlithiasis, alveolar, pulmonary J84.02
Micromastia N64.82
Micromyelia (congenital) Q06.8
Micropenis Q55.62
Microphakia (congenital) Q12.8
Microphthalmos, microphthalmia (congenital) Q11.2
  due to toxoplasmosis P37.1
Micropsia H53.15
Microscopic polyangiitis (polyarteritis) M31.7
Microsporidiosis B60.8
  intestinal A07.8
Microsporon furfur infestation B36.0
Microsporosis (*see also* Dermatophytosis)
  nigra B36.1
Microstomia (congenital) Q18.5
Microtia (congenital) (external ear) Q17.2
Microtropia H50.40
Microvillus inclusion disease (MVD) (MVID) Q43.8
Micturition
  disorder NEC (*see also* Difficulty, micturition) R39.198
    psychogenic F45.8
  frequency R35.0
    psychogenic F45.8
  hesitancy R39.11
  incomplete emptying R39.14
  nocturnal R35.1
  painful R30.9
    dysuria R30.0
    psychogenic F45.8
    tenesmus R30.1
  poor stream R39.12
  position dependent R39.192
  split stream R39.13
  straining R39.16
  urgency R39.15
Mid plane — *see* condition
Middle
  ear — *see* condition
  lobe (right) syndrome J98.19
Miescher's elastoma L87.2
Mietens' syndrome Q87.2

Migraine (idiopathic) G43.909
  with aura (acute-onset) (prolonged) (typical) (without headache) G43.109
    with refractory migraine G43.119
      with status migrainosus G43.111
      without status migrainosus G43.119
    without mention of refractory migraine G43.109
      with status migrainosus G43.101
      without status migrainosus G43.109
    intractable G43.119
      with status migrainosus G43.111
      without status migrainosus G43.119
    not intractable G43.109
      with status migrainosus G43.101
      without status migrainosus G43.109
    persistent G43.509
      with cerebral infarction G43.609
        with refractory migraine G43.619
          with status migrainosus G43.611
          without status migrainosus G43.619
        without refractory migraine G43.609
          with status migrainosus G43.601
          without status migrainosus G43.609
        intractable G43.619
          with status migrainosus G43.611
          without status migrainosus G43.619
        not intractable G43.609
          with status migrainosus G43.601
          without status migrainosus G43.609
      without cerebral infarction G43.509
        with refractory migraine G43.519
          with status migrainosus G43.511
          without status migrainosus G43.519
        without refractory migraine G43.509
          with status migrainosus G43.501
          without status migrainosus G43.509
        intractable G43.519
          with status migrainosus G43.511
          without status migrainosus G43.519
        not intractable G43.509
          with status migrainosus G43.501
          without status migrainosus G43.509
  with refractory migraine G43.919
    with status migrainosus G43.911
    without status migrainosus G43.919
  without aura G43.009
    with refractory migraine G43.019
      with status migrainosus G43.011
      without status migrainosus G43.019
    without mention of refractory migraine G43.009
      with status migrainosus G43.001
      without status migrainosus G43.009
  chronic G43.709
    with refractory migraine G43.719
      with status migrainosus G43.711
      without status migrainosus G43.719
    without refractory migraine G43.709
      with status migrainosus G43.701
      without status migrainosus G43.709
    intractable
      with status migrainosus G43.711
      without status migrainosus G43.719
    not intractable
      with status migrainosus G43.701
      without status migrainosus G43.709
  intractable
    with status migrainosus G43.011
    without status migrainosus G43.019
  not intractable
    with status migrainosus G43.001
    without status migrainosus G43.009
  without refractory migraine G43.909
    with status migrainosus G43.901
    without status migrainosus G43.919
  abdominal G43.D0 (*following* G43.7)
    with refractory migraine G43.D1 (*following* G43.7)
    without refractory migraine G43.D0 (*following* G43.7)
    intractable G43.D1 (*following* G43.7)
    not intractable G43.D0 (*following* G43.7)
  basilar — *see* Migraine, with aura
  classical — *see* Migraine, with aura
  common — *see* Migraine, without aura
  complicated G43.109
  equivalents — *see* Migraine, with aura
  familiar — *see* Migraine, hemiplegic
  hemiplegic G43.409
    with refractory migraine G43.419
      with status migrainosus G43.411

☑ Subterms under main terms may continue to next column or page   ☑ Additional Character Required — Refer to the Tabular List for Character Selection   223

Mesothelioma — Migraine

Migraine — *continued*
  hemiplegic — *continued*
    with refractory migraine — *continued*
      without status migrainosus G43.419
    without refractory migraine G43.409
      with status migrainosus G43.401
      without status migrainosus G43.409
    intractable G43.419
      with status migrainosus G43.411
      without status migrainosus G43.419
    not intractable G43.409
      with status migrainosus G43.401
      without status migrainosus G43.409
  intractable G43.919
    with status migrainosus G43.911
    without status migrainosus G43.919
  menstrual G43.829
    with refractory migraine G43.839
      with status migrainosus G43.831
      without status migrainosus G43.839
    without refractory migraine G43.829
      with status migrainosus G43.821
      without status migrainosus G43.829
    intractable G43.839
      with status migrainosus G43.831
      without status migrainosus G43.839
    not intractable 4G43.829
      with status migrainosus G43.821
      without status migrainosus G43.829
  menstrually related — *see* Migraine, menstrual
  not intractable G43.909
    with status migrainosus G43.901
    without status migrainosus G43.919
  ophthalmoplegic G43.B0 (*following* G43.7)
    with refractory migraine G43.B1 (*following* G43.7)
    without refractory migraine G43.B0 (*following* G43.7)
    intractable G43.B1 (*following* G43.7)
    not intractable G43.B0 (*following* G43.7)
  persistent aura (with, without) cerebral infarction — *see* Migraine, with aura, persistent
  preceded or accompanied by transient focal neurological phenomena — *see* Migraine, with aura
  pre-menstrual — *see* Migraine, menstrual
  pure menstrual — *see* Migraine, menstrual
  retinal — *see* Migraine, with aura
  specified NEC G43.809
    intractable G43.819
      with status migrainosus G43.811
      without status migrainosus G43.819
    not intractable G43.809
      with status migrainosus G43.801
      without status migrainosus G43.809
  sporadic — *see* Migraine, hemiplegic
  transformed — *see* Migraine, without aura, chronic
  triggered seizures — *see* Migraine, with aura
Migrant, social Z59.0
Migration, anxiety concerning Z60.3
Migratory, migrating (*see also* condition)
  person Z59.0
  testis Q55.29
Mikity-Wilson disease or syndrome P27.0
Mikulicz' disease or syndrome K11.8
Miliaria L74.3
  alba L74.1
  apocrine L75.2
  crystallina L74.1
  profunda L74.2
  rubra L74.0
  tropicalis L74.2
Miliary — *see* condition
Milium L72.0
  colloid L57.8
Milk
  crust L21.0
  excessive secretion O92.6
  poisoning — *see* Poisoning, food, noxious
  retention O92.79
  sickness — *see* Poisoning, food, noxious
  spots I31.0
Milk-alkali disease or syndrome E83.52
Milk-leg (deep vessels) (nonpuerperal) — *see* Embolism, vein, lower extremity
  complicating pregnancy O22.3- ☑
  puerperal, postpartum, childbirth O87.1
Milkman's disease or syndrome M83.8
Milky urine — *see* Chyluria
Millard-Gubler (-Foville) **paralysis or syndrome** G46.3

Millar's asthma J38.5
Miller Fisher syndrome G61.0
Mills' disease — *see* Hemiplegia
Millstone maker's pneumoconiosis J62.8
Milroy's disease (chronic hereditary edema) Q82.0
Minamata disease T56.1 ☑
Miners' asthma or lung J60
Minkowski-Chauffard syndrome — *see* Spherocytosis
Minor — *see* condition
Minor's disease (hematomyelia) G95.19
Minot's disease (hemorrhagic disease), newborn P53
Minot-von Willebrand-Jurgens disease or syndrome (angiohemophilia) D68.0
Minus (and plus) **hand** (intrinsic) — *see* Deformity, limb, specified type NEC, forearm
Miosis (pupil) H57.03
Mirizzi's syndrome (hepatic duct stenosis) K83.1
Mirror writing F81.0
Misadventure (of) (prophylactic) (therapeutic) (*see also* Complications) T88.9 ☑
  administration of insulin (by accident) — *see* subcategory T38.3 ☑
  infusion — *see* Complications, infusion
  local applications (of fomentations, plasters, etc.) T88.9 ☑
    burn or scald — *see* Burn
    specified NEC T88.8 ☑
  medical care (early) (late) T88.9 ☑
    adverse effect of drugs or chemicals — *see* Table of Drugs and Chemicals
    burn or scald — *see* Burn
    specified NEC T88.8 ☑
  specified NEC T88.8 ☑
  surgical procedure (early) (late) — *see* Complications, surgical procedure
  transfusion — *see* Complications, transfusion
  vaccination or other immunological procedure — *see* Complications, vaccination
Miscarriage O03.9
Misdirection, aqueous H40.83- ☑
Misperception, sleep state F51.02
Misplaced, misplacement
  ear Q17.4
  kidney (acquired) N28.89
    congenital Q63.2
  organ or site, congenital NEC — *see* Malposition, congenital
Missed
  abortion O02.1
  delivery O36.4 ☑
Missing (*see also* Absence)
  string of intrauterine contraceptive device T83.32- ☑
Misuse of drugs F19.99
Mitchell's disease (erythromelalgia) I73.81
Mite(s) (infestation) B88.9
  diarrhea B88.0
  grain (itch) B88.0
  hair follicle (itch) B88.0
  in sputum B88.0
Mitral — *see* condition
Mittelschmerz N94.0
Mixed — *see* condition
MMN (multifocal motor neuropathy) G61.82
MNGIE (Mitochondrial Neurogastrointestinal Encephalopathy) **syndrome** E88.49
Mobile, mobility
  cecum Q43.3
  excessive — *see* Hypermobility
  gallbladder, congenital Q44.1
  kidney N28.89
  organ or site, congenital NEC — *see* Malposition, congenital
Mobitz heart block (atrioventricular) I44.1
Moebius, Möbius
  disease (ophthalmoplegic migraine) — *see* Migraine, ophthalmoplegic
  syndrome Q87.0
    congenital oculofacial paralysis (with other anomalies) Q87.0
    ophthalmoplegic migraine — *see* Migraine, ophthalmoplegic
Moeller's glossitis K14.0
Mohr's syndrome (Types I and II) Q87.0
Mola destruens D39.2
Molar pregnancy O02.0
Molarization of premolars K00.2

Molding, head (during birth) — *omit code*
Mole (pigmented) (*see also* Nevus)
  blood O02.0
  Breus' O02.0
  cancerous — *see* Melanoma
  carneous O02.0
  destructive D39.2
  fleshy O02.0
  hydatid, hydatidiform (benign) (complicating pregnancy) (delivered) (undelivered) O01.9
    classical O01.0
    complete O01.0
    incomplete O01.1
    invasive D39.2
    malignant D39.2
    partial O01.1
  intrauterine O02.0
  invasive (hydatidiform) D39.2
  malignant
    meaning
      malignant hydatidiform mole D39.2
      melanoma — *see* Melanoma
  nonhydatidiform O02.0
  nonpigmented — *see* Nevus
  pregnancy NEC O02.0
  skin — *see* Nevus
  tubal O00.10- ☑
    with intrauterine pregnancy O00.11- ☑
  vesicular — *see* Mole, hydatidiform
Molimen, molimina (menstrual) N94.3
Molluscum contagiosum (epitheliale) B08.1
Mönckeberg's arteriosclerosis, disease, or sclerosis — *see* Arteriosclerosis, extremities
Mondini's malformation (cochlea) Q16.5
Mondor's disease I80.8
Monge's disease T70.29 ☑
Monilethrix (congenital) Q84.1
Moniliasis (*see also* Candidiasis) B37.9
  neonatal P37.5
Monitoring (encounter for)
  therapeutic drug level Z51.81
Monkey malaria B53.1
Monkeypox B04
Monoarthritis M13.10
  ankle M13.17- ☑
  elbow M13.12- ☑
  foot joint M13.17- ☑
  hand joint M13.14- ☑
  hip M13.15- ☑
  knee M13.16- ☑
  shoulder M13.11- ☑
  wrist M13.13- ☑
Monoblastic — *see* condition
Monochromat (ism), monochromatopsia (acquired) (congenital) H53.51
Monocytic — *see* condition
Monocytopenia D72.818
Monocytosis (symptomatic) D72.821
Monomania — *see* Psychosis
Mononeuritis G58.9
  cranial nerve — *see* Disorder, nerve, cranial
  femoral nerve G57.2- ☑
  lateral
    cutaneous nerve of thigh G57.1- ☑
    popliteal nerve G57.3- ☑
  lower limb G57.9- ☑
    specified nerve NEC G57.8- ☑
  medial popliteal nerve G57.4- ☑
  median nerve G56.1- ☑
  multiplex G58.7
  plantar nerve G57.6- ☑
  posterior tibial nerve G57.5- ☑
  radial nerve G56.3- ☑
  sciatic nerve G57.0- ☑
  specified NEC G58.8
  tibial nerve G57.4- ☑
  ulnar nerve G56.2- ☑
  upper limb G56.9- ☑
    specified nerve NEC G56.8- ☑
  vestibular — *see* subcategory H93.3 ☑
Mononeuropathy G58.9
  carpal tunnel syndrome — *see* Syndrome, carpal tunnel
  diabetic NEC — *see* E08-E13 with .41
  femoral nerve — *see* Lesion, nerve, femoral
  ilioinguinal nerve G57.8- ☑
  in diseases classified elsewhere — *see* category G59

☑ **Additional Character Required** — **Refer to the Tabular List for Character Selection**
⩗ **Subterms under main terms may continue to next column or page**

Mononeuropathy — *continued*
  intercostal G58.0
  lower limb G57.9- ☑
    causalgia — *see* Causalgia, lower limb
    femoral nerve — *see* Lesion, nerve, femoral
    meralgia paresthetica G57.1- ☑
    plantar nerve — *see* Lesion, nerve, plantar
    popliteal nerve — *see* Lesion, nerve, popliteal
    sciatic nerve — *see* Lesion, nerve, sciatic
    specified NEC G57.8- ☑
    tarsal tunnel syndrome — *see* Syndrome, tarsal
        tunnel
  median nerve — *see* Lesion, nerve, median
  multiplex G58.7
  obturator nerve G57.8- ☑
  popliteal nerve — *see* Lesion, nerve, popliteal
  radial nerve — *see* Lesion, nerve, radial
  saphenous nerve G57.8- ☑
  specified NEC G58.8
  tarsal tunnel syndrome — *see* Syndrome, tarsal tunnel
  tuberculous A17.83
  ulnar nerve — *see* Lesion, nerve, ulnar
  upper limb G56.9- ☑
    carpal tunnel syndrome — *see* Syndrome, carpal
        tunnel
    causalgia — *see* Causalgia
    median nerve — *see* Lesion, nerve, median
    radial nerve — *see* Lesion, nerve, radial
    specified site NEC G56.8- ☑
    ulnar nerve — *see* Lesion, nerve, ulnar
Mononucleosis, infectious B27.90
  with
    complication NEC B27.99
    meningitis B27.92
    polyneuropathy B27.91
  cytomegaloviral B27.10
    with
      complication NEC B27.19
      meningitis B27.12
      polyneuropathy B27.11
  Epstein-Barr (virus) B27.00
    with
      complication NEC B27.09
      meningitis B27.02
      polyneuropathy B27.01
  gammaherpesviral B27.00
    with
      complication NEC B27.09
      meningitis B27.02
      polyneuropathy B27.01
  specified NEC B27.80
    with
      complication NEC B27.89
      meningitis B27.82
      polyneuropathy B27.81
Monoplegia G83.3- ☑
  congenital (cerebral) G80.8
    spastic G80.1
  embolic (current episode) I63.4- ☑
  following
    cerebrovascular disease
      cerebral infarction
        lower limb I69.34- ☑
        upper limb I69.33- ☑
      intracerebral hemorrhage
        lower limb I69.14- ☑
        upper limb I69.13- ☑
      lower limb I69.94- ☑
      nontraumatic intracranial hemorrhage NEC
        lower limb I69.24- ☑
        upper limb I69.23- ☑
      specified disease NEC
        lower limb I69.84- ☑
        upper limb I69.83- ☑
      stroke NOS
        lower limb I69.34- ☑
        upper limb I69.33- ☑
      subarachnoid hemorrhage
        lower limb I69.04- ☑
        upper limb I69.03- ☑
      upper limb I69.93- ☑
  hysterical (transient) F44.4
  lower limb G83.1- ☑
  psychogenic (conversion reaction) F44.4
  thrombotic (current episode) I63.3- ☑
  transient R29.818
  upper limb G83.2- ☑

Monorchism, monorchidism Q55.0
Monosomy (*see also* Deletion, chromosome) Q93.9
  specified NEC Q93.89
  whole chromosome
    meiotic nondisjunction Q93.0
    mitotic nondisjunction Q93.1
    mosaicism Q93.1
  X Q96.9
Monster, monstrosity (single) Q89.7
  acephalic Q00.0
  twin Q89.4
Monteggia's fracture (-dislocation) S52.27- ☑
Mooren's ulcer (cornea) — *see* Ulcer, cornea, Mooren's
Moore's syndrome — *see* Epilepsy, specified NEC
Mooser-Neill reaction A75.2
Mooser's bodies A75.2
Morbidity not stated or unknown R69
Morbilli — *see* Measles
Morbus (*see also* Disease)
  angelicus, anglorum E55.0
  Beigel B36.2
  caducus — *see* Epilepsy
  celiacus K90.0
  comitialis — *see* Epilepsy
  cordis (*see also* Disease, heart) I51.9
    valvulorum — *see* Endocarditis
  coxae senilis M16.9
    tuberculous A18.02
  hemorrhagicus neonatorum P53
  maculosus neonatorum P54.5
Morel (-Stewart)(-Morgagni) **syndrome** M85.2
Morel-Kraepelin disease — *see* Schizophrenia
Morel-Moore syndrome M85.2
Morgagni's
  cyst, organ, hydatid, or appendage
    female Q50.5
    male (epididymal) Q55.4
      testicular Q55.29
  syndrome M85.2
Morgagni-Stewart-Morel syndrome M85.2
Morgagni-Stokes-Adams syndrome I45.9
Morgagni-Turner (-Albright) **syndrome** Q96.9
Moria F07.0
Moron (I.Q. 50-69) F70
Morphea L94.0
Morphinism (without remission) F11.20
  with remission F11.21
Morphinomania (without remission) F11.20
  with remission F11.21
Morquio (-Ullrich)(-Brailsford) **disease or syndrome** —
    see Mucopolysaccharidosis
Mortification (dry) (moist) — *see* Gangrene
Morton's metatarsalgia (neuralgia)(neuroma) (syndrome) G57.6- ☑
Morvan's disease or syndrome G60.8
Mosaicism, mosaic (autosomal) (chromosomal)
  45,X/46,XX Q96.3
  45,X/other cell lines NEC with abnormal sex chromosome Q96.4
  sex chromosome
    female Q97.8
    lines with various numbers of X chromosomes Q97.2
    male Q98.7
  XY Q96.3
Moschowitz' disease M31.1
Mother yaw A66.0
Motion sickness (from travel, any vehicle) (from roundabouts or swings) T75.3 ☑
Mottled, mottling, teeth (enamel) (endemic) (nonendemic) K00.3
Mounier-Kuhn syndrome Q32.4
  with bronchiectasis J47.9
    exacerbation (acute) J47.1
    lower respiratory infection J47.0
  acquired J98.09
    with bronchiectasis J47.9
      with
        exacerbation (acute) J47.1
        lower respiratory infection J47.0
Mountain
  sickness T70.29 ☑
    with polycythemia , acquired (acute) D75.1
  tick fever A93.2
Mouse, joint — *see* Loose, body, joint
  knee M23.4- ☑
Mouth — *see* condition

Movable
  coccyx — *see* subcategory M53.2 ☑
  kidney N28.89
    congenital Q63.8
  spleen D73.89
Movements, dystonic R25.8
Moyamoya disease I67.5
MRSA (Methicillin resistant Staphylococcus aureus)
  infection A49.02
    as the cause of diseases classified elsewhere B95.62
  sepsis A41.02
MSSA (Methicillin susceptible Staphylococcus aureus)
  infection A49.01
    as the cause of diseases classified elsewhere B95.61
  sepsis A41.01
Mucha-Habermann disease L41.0
Mucinosis (cutaneous) (focal) (papular) (skin) L98.5
  oral K13.79
Mucocele
  appendix K38.8
  buccal cavity K13.79
  gallbladder K82.1
  lacrimal sac, chronic H04.43- ☑
  nasal sinus J34.1
  nose J34.1
  salivary gland (any) K11.6
  sinus (accessory) (nasal) J34.1
  turbinate (bone) (middle) (nasal) J34.1
  uterus N85.8
Mucolipidosis
  I E77.1
  II, III E77.0
  IV E75.11
Mucopolysaccharidosis E76.3
  beta-gluduronidase deficiency E76.29
  cardiopathy E76.3 [I52]
  Hunter's syndrome E76.1
  Hurler's syndrome E76.01
  Hurler-Scheie syndrome E76.02
  Maroteaux-Lamy syndrome E76.29
  Morquio syndrome E76.219
    A E76.210
    B E76.211
    classic E76.210
  Sanfilippo syndrome E76.22
  Scheie's syndrome E76.03
  specified NEC E76.29
  type
    I
      Hurler's syndrome E76.01
      Hurler-Scheie syndrome E76.02
      Scheie's syndrome E76.03
    II E76.1
    III E76.22
    IV E76.219
    IVA E76.210
    IVB E76.211
    VI E76.29
    VII E76.29
Mucormycosis B46.5
  cutaneous B46.3
  disseminated B46.4
  gastrointestinal B46.2
  generalized B46.4
  pulmonary B46.0
  rhinocerebral B46.1
  skin B46.3
  subcutaneous B46.3
Mucositis (ulcerative) K12.30
  due to drugs NEC K12.32
  gastrointestinal K92.81
  mouth (oral) (oropharyngeal) K12.30
    due to antineoplastic therapy K12.31
    due to drugs NEC K12.32
    due to radiation K12.33
    specified NEC K12.39
    viral K12.39
  nasal J34.81
  oral cavity — *see* Mucositis, mouth
  oral soft tissues — *see* Mucositis, mouth
  vagina and vulva N76.81
Mucositis necroticans agranulocytica — *see* Agranulocytosis
Mucous (*see also* condition)
  patches (syphilitic) A51.39
    congenital A50.07
Mucoviscidosis E84.9
  with meconium obstruction E84.11

☑ Subterms under main terms may continue to next column or page   ☑ Additional Character Required — Refer to the Tabular List for Character Selection   225

Mononeuropathy — Mucoviscidosis

Mucus
asphyxia or suffocation — *see* Asphyxia, mucus
in stool R19.5
plug — *see* Asphyxia, mucus
Muguet B37.0
Mulberry molars (congenital syphilis) A50.52
Müllerian mixed tumor
specified site — *see* Neoplasm, malignant, by site
unspecified site C54.9
Multicystic kidney (development) Q61.4
Multiparity (grand) Z64.1
affecting management of pregnancy, labor and delivery (supervision only) O09.4- ☑
requiring contraceptive management — *see* Contraception
Multipartita placenta O43.19- ☑
Multiple, multiplex (*see also* condition)
digits (congenital) Q69.9
endocrine neoplasia — *see* Neoplasia, endocrine, multiple (MEN)
personality F44.81
Mumps B26.9
arthritis B26.85
complication NEC B26.89
encephalitis B26.2
hepatitis B26.81
meningitis (aseptic) B26.1
meningoencephalitis B26.2
myocarditis B26.82
oophoritis B26.89
orchitis B26.0
pancreatitis B26.3
polyneuropathy B26.84
Mumu (*see also* Infestation, filarial) B74.9 [N51]
Münchhausen's syndrome — *see* Disorder, factitious
Münchmeyer's syndrome — *see* Myositis, ossificans, progressiva
Mural — *see* condition
Murmur (cardiac) (heart) (organic) R01.1
abdominal R19.15
aortic (valve) — *see* Endocarditis, aortic
benign R01.0
diastolic — *see* Endocarditis
Flint I35.1
functional R01.0
Graham Steell I37.1
innocent R01.0
mitral (valve) — *see* Insufficiency, mitral
nonorganic R01.0
presystolic, mitral — *see* Insufficiency, mitral
pulmonic (valve) I37.8
systolic R01.1
tricuspid (valve) I07.9
valvular — *see* Endocarditis
Murri's disease (intermittent hemoglobinuria) D59.6
Muscle, muscular (*see also* condition)
carnitine (palmityltransferase) deficiency E71.314
Musculoneuralgia — *see* Neuralgia
Mushrooming hip — *see* Derangement, joint, specified NEC, hip
Mushroom-workers' (pickers') **disease or lung** J67.5
Mutation(s)
factor V Leiden D68.51
prothrombin gene D68.52
surfactant, of lung J84.83
Mutism (*see also* Aphasia)
deaf (acquired) (congenital) NEC H91.3
elective (adjustment reaction) (childhood) F94.0
hysterical F44.4
selective (childhood) F94.0
MVD (microvillus inclusion disease) Q43.8
MVID (microvillus inclusion disease) Q43.8
Myalgia M79.1
epidemic (cervical) B33.0
traumatic NEC T14.8 ☑
Myasthenia G70.9
congenital G70.2
cordis — *see* Failure, heart
developmental G70.2
gravis G70.00
with exacerbation (acute) G70.01
in crisis G70.01
neonatal, transient P94.0
pseudoparalytica G70.00
with exacerbation (acute) G70.01
in crisis G70.01
stomach, psychogenic F45.8

Myasthenia — *continued*
syndrome
in
diabetes mellitus — *see* E08-E13 with .44
neoplastic disease (*see also* Neoplasm)
D49.9 [G73.3]
pernicious anemia D51.0 [G73.3]
thyrotoxicosis E05.90 [G73.3]
with thyroid storm E05.91 [G73.3]
Myasthenic M62.81
Mycelium infection B49
Mycetismus — *see* Poisoning, food, noxious, mushroom
Mycetoma B47.9
actinomycotic B47.1
bone (mycotic) B47.9 [M90.80]
eumycotic B47.0
foot B47.9
actinomycotic B47.1
mycotic B47.0
madurae NEC B47.9
mycotic B47.0
maduromycotic B47.0
mycotic B47.0
nocardial B47.1
Mycobacteriosis — *see* Mycobacterium
Mycobacterium, mycobacterial (infection) A31.9
anonymous A31.9
atypical A31.9
cutaneous A31.1
pulmonary A31.0
tuberculous — *see* Tuberculosis, pulmonary
specified site NEC A31.8
avium (intracellulare complex) A31.0
balnei A31.1
Battey A31.0
chelonei A31.8
cutaneous A31.1
extrapulmonary systemic A31.8
fortuitum A31.8
intracellulare (Battey bacillus) A31.0
kakaferifu A31.8
kansasii (yellow bacillus) A31.0
kasongo A31.8
leprae (*see also* Leprosy) A30.9
luciflavum A31.1
marinum (M. balnei) A31.1
nonspecific — *see* Mycobacterium, atypical
pulmonary (atypical) A31.0
tuberculous — *see* Tuberculosis, pulmonary
scrofulaceum A31.8
simiae A31.8
systemic, extrapulmonary A31.8
szulgai A31.8
terrae A31.8
triviale A31.8
tuberculosis (human, bovine) — *see* Tuberculosis
ulcerans A31.1
xenopi A31.8
Mycoplasma (M.) **pneumoniae, as cause of disease classified elsewhere** B96.0
Mycosis, mycotic B49
cutaneous NEC B36.9
ear B36.9
in
aspergillosis B44.89
candidiasis B37.84
moniliasis B37.84
fungoides (extranodal) (solid organ) C84.0- ☑
mouth B37.0
nails B35.1
opportunistic B48.8
skin NEC B36.9
specified NEC B48.8
stomatitis B37.0
vagina, vaginitis (candidal) B37.3
Mydriasis (pupil) H57.04
Myelatelia Q06.1
Myelinolysis, pontine, central G37.2
Myelitis (acute) (ascending) (childhood) (chronic) (descending) (diffuse) (disseminated) (idiopathic) (pressure) (progressive) (spinal cord) (subacute) (*see also* Encephalitis) G04.91
herpes simplex B00.82
herpes zoster B02.24
in diseases classified elsewhere G05.4
necrotizing, subacute G37.4
optic neuritis in G36.0
postchickenpox B01.12

Myelitis — *continued*
postherpetic B02.24
postimmunization G04.02
postinfectious NEC G04.89
postvaccinal G04.02
specified NEC G04.89
syphilitic (transverse) A52.14
toxic G92
transverse (in demyelinating diseases of central nervous system) G37.3
tuberculous A17.82
varicella B01.12
Myeloblastic — *see* condition
Myeloblastoma
granular cell (*see also* Neoplasm, connective tissue)
malignant — *see* Neoplasm, connective tissue, malignant
tongue D10.1
Myelocele — *see* Spina bifida
Myelocystocele — *see* Spina bifida
Myelocytic — *see* condition
Myelodysplasia D46.9
specified NEC D46.Z (*following* D46.4)
spinal cord (congenital) Q06.1
Myelodysplastic syndrome D46.9
with
5q deletion D46.C (*following* D46.2)
isolated del (5q) chromosomal abnormality D46.C (*following* D46.2)
specified NEC D46.Z (*following* D46.4)
Myeloencephalitis — *see* Encephalitis
Myelofibrosis D75.81
with myeloid metaplasia D47.4
acute C94.4- ☑
idiopathic (chronic) D47.4
primary D47.1
secondary D75.81
in myeloproliferative disease D47.4
Myelogenous — *see* condition
Myeloid — *see* condition
Myelokathexis D70.9
Myeloleukodystrophy E75.29
Myelolipoma — *see* Lipoma
Myeloma (multiple) C90.0- ☑
monostotic C90.3 ☑
plasma cell C90.0- ☑
plasma cell C90.0- ☑
solitary (*see also* Plasmacytoma, solitary) C90.3- ☑
Myelomalacia G95.89
Myelomatosis C90.0- ☑
Myelomeningitis — *see* Meningoencephalitis
Myelomeningocele (spinal cord) — *see* Spina bifida
Myelo-osteo-musculodysplasia hereditaria Q79.8
Myelopathic
anemia D64.89
muscle atrophy — *see* Atrophy, muscle, spinal
pain syndrome G89.0
Myelopathy (spinal cord) G95.9
drug-induced G95.89
in (due to)
degeneration or displacement, intervertebral disc NEC — *see* Disorder, disc, with, myelopathy
infection — *see* Encephalitis
intervertebral disc disorder (*see also* Disorder, disc, with, myelopathy)
mercury — *see* subcategory T56.1 ☑
neoplastic disease (*see also* Neoplasm)
D49.9 [G99.2]
pernicious anemia D51.0 [G99.2]
spondylosis — *see* Spondylosis, with myelopathy NEC
necrotic (subacute) (vascular) G95.19
radiation-induced G95.89
spondylogenic NEC — *see* Spondylosis, with myelopathy NEC
toxic G95.89
transverse, acute G37.3
vascular G95.19
vitamin B12 E53.8 [G32.0]
Myelophthisis D61.82
Myeloradiculitis G04.91
Myeloradiculodysplasia (spinal) Q06.1
Myelosarcoma C92.3- ☑
Myelosclerosis D75.89
with myeloid metaplasia D47.4
disseminated, of nervous system G35
megakaryocytic D47.4

☑ Additional Character Required — Refer to the Tabular List for Character Selection   ▽ Subterms under main terms may continue to next column or page

Myelosclerosis — *continued*
  megakaryocytic — *continued*
    with myeloid metaplasia D47.4
Myelosis
  acute C92.0- ☑
  aleukemic C92.9- ☑
  chronic D47.1
  erythremic (acute) C94.0- ☑
  megakaryocytic C94.2- ☑
  nonleukemic D72.828
  subacute C92.9- ☑
Myiasis (cavernous) B87.9
  aural B87.4
  creeping B87.0
  cutaneous B87.0
  dermal B87.0
  ear (external) (middle) B87.4
  eye B87.2
  genitourinary B87.81
  intestinal B87.82
  laryngeal B87.3
  nasopharyngeal B87.3
  ocular B87.2
  orbit B87.2
  skin B87.0
  specified site NEC B87.89
  traumatic B87.1
  wound B87.1
Myoadenoma, prostate — *see* Hyperplasia, prostate
Myoblastoma
  granular cell (*see also* Neoplasm, connective tissue, benign)
    malignant — *see* Neoplasm, connective tissue, malignant
  tongue D10.1
Myocardial — *see* condition
Myocardiopathy (congestive) (constrictive) (familial) (hypertrophic nonobstructive) (idiopathic) (infiltrative) (obstructive) (primary) (restrictive) (sporadic) (*see also* Cardiomyopathy) I42.9
  alcoholic I42.6
  cobalt-beer I42.6
  glycogen storage E74.02 [I43]
  hypertrophic obstructive I42.1
  in (due to)
    beriberi E51.12
    cardiac glycogenosis E74.02 [I43]
    Friedreich's ataxia G11.1 [I43]
    myotonia atrophica G71.11 [I43]
    progressive muscular dystrophy G71.0 [I43]
  obscure (African) I42.8
  secondary I42.9
  thyrotoxic E05.90 [I43]
    with storm E05.91 [I43]
  toxic NEC I42.7
Myocarditis (with arteriosclerosis)(chronic)(fibroid) (interstitial) (old) (progressive) (senile) I51.4
  with
    rheumatic fever (conditions in I00) I09.0
      active — *see* Myocarditis, acute, rheumatic
      inactive or quiescent (with chorea) I09.0
  active I40.9
    rheumatic I01.2
      with chorea (acute) (rheumatic) (Sydenham's) I02.0
  acute or subacute (interstitial) I40.9
    due to
      streptococcus (beta-hemolytic) I01.2
    idiopathic I40.1
    rheumatic I01.2
      with chorea (acute) (rheumatic) (Sydenham's) I02.0
    specified NEC I40.8
  aseptic of newborn B33.22
  bacterial (acute) I40.0
  Coxsackie (virus) B33.22
  diphtheritic A36.81
  eosinophilic I40.1
  epidemic of newborn (Coxsackie) B33.22
  Fiedler's (acute) (isolated) I40.1
  giant cell (acute) (subacute) I40.1
  gonococcal A54.83
  granulomatous (idiopathic) (isolated) (nonspecific) I40.1
  hypertensive — *see* Hypertension, heart
  idiopathic (granulomatous) I40.1
  in (due to)
    diphtheria A36.81

Myocarditis — *continued*
  in — *continued*
    epidemic louse-borne typhus A75.0 [I41]
    Lyme disease A69.29
    sarcoidosis D86.85
    scarlet fever A38.1
    toxoplasmosis (acquired) B58.81
    typhoid A01.02
    typhus NEC A75.9 [I41]
  infective I40.0
  influenzal — *see* Influenza, with, myocarditis
  isolated (acute) I40.1
  meningococcal A39.52
  mumps B26.82
  nonrheumatic, active I40.9
  parenchymatous I40.9
  pneumococcal I40.0
  rheumatic (chronic) (inactive) (with chorea) I09.0
    active or acute I01.2
      with chorea (acute) (rheumatic) (Sydenham's) I02.0
  rheumatoid — *see* Rheumatoid, carditis
  septic I40.0
  staphylococcal I40.0
  suppurative I40.0
  syphilitic (chronic) A52.06
  toxic I40.8
    rheumatic — *see* Myocarditis, acute, rheumatic
  tuberculous A18.84
  typhoid A01.02
  valvular — *see* Endocarditis
  virus, viral I40.0
    of newborn (Coxsackie) B33.22
Myocardium, myocardial — *see* condition
Myocardosis — *see* Cardiomyopathy
Myoclonus, myoclonic, myoclonia (familial) (essential) (multifocal) (simplex) G25.3
  drug-induced G25.3
  epilepsy (*see also* Epilepsy, generalized, specified NEC) G40.4- ☑
    familial (progressive) G25.3
  epileptica G40.409
    with status epilepticus G40.401
  facial G51.3
  familial progressive G25.3
  Friedreich's G25.3
  jerks G25.3
  massive G25.3
  palatal G25.3
  pharyngeal G25.3
Myocytolysis I51.5
Myodiastasis — *see* Diastasis, muscle
Myoendocarditis — *see* Endocarditis
Myoepithelioma — *see* Neoplasm, benign, by site
Myofasciitis (acute) — *see* Myositis
Myofibroma (*see also* Neoplasm, connective tissue, benign)
  uterus (cervix) (corpus) — *see* Leiomyoma
Myofibromatosis D48.1
  infantile Q89.8
Myofibrosis M62.89
  heart — *see* Myocarditis
  scapulohumeral — *see* Lesion, shoulder, specified NEC
Myofibrositis M79.7
  scapulohumeral — *see* Lesion, shoulder, specified NEC
Myoglobulinuria, myoglobinuria (primary) R82.1
Myokymia, facial G51.4
Myolipoma — *see* Lipoma
Myoma (*see also* Neoplasm, connective tissue, benign)
  malignant — *see* Neoplasm, connective tissue, malignant
  prostate D29.1
  uterus (cervix) (corpus) — *see* Leiomyoma
Myomalacia M62.89
Myometritis — *see* Endometritis
Myometrium — *see* condition
Myonecrosis, clostridial A48.0
Myopathy G72.9
  acute
    necrotizing G72.81
    quadriplegic G72.81
  alcoholic G72.1
  benign congenital G71.2
  central core G71.2
  centronuclear G71.2
  congenital (benign) G71.2
  critical illness G72.81
  distal G71.0

Myopathy — *continued*
  drug-induced G72.0
  endocrine NEC E34.9 [G73.7]
  extraocular muscles H05.82- ☑
  facioscapulohumeral G71.0
  hereditary G71.9
    specified NEC G71.8
  immune NEC G72.49
  in (due to)
    Addison's disease E27.1 [G73.7]
    alcohol G72.1
    amyloidosis E85.0 [G73.7]
    cretinism E00.9 [G73.7]
    Cushing's syndrome E24.9 [G73.7]
    drugs G72.0
    endocrine disease NEC E34.9 [G73.7]
    giant cell arteritis M31.6 [G73.7]
    glycogen storage disease E74.00 [G73.7]
    hyperadrenocorticism E24.9 [G73.7]
    hyperparathyroidism NEC E21.3 [G73.7]
    hypoparathyroidism E20.9 [G73.7]
    hypopituitarism E23.0 [G73.7]
    hypothyroidism E03.9 [G73.7]
    infectious disease NEC B99 ☑ [G73.7]
    lipid storage disease E75.6 [G73.7]
    metabolic disease NEC E88.9 [G73.7]
    myxedema E03.9 [G73.7]
    parasitic disease NEC B89 [G73.7]
    polyarteritis nodosa M30.0 [G73.7]
    rheumatoid arthritis — *see* Rheumatoid, myopathy
    sarcoidosis D86.87
    scleroderma M34.82
    sicca syndrome M35.03
    Sjögren's syndrome M35.03
    systemic lupus erythematosus M32.19
    thyrotoxicosis (hyperthyroidism) E05.90 [G73.7]
      with thyroid storm E05.91 [G73.7]
    toxic agent NEC G72.2
  inflammatory NEC G72.49
  intensive care (ICU) G72.81
  limb-girdle G71.0
  mitochondrial NEC G71.3
  myotubular G71.2
  myotonic, proximal (PROMM) G71.11
  nemaline G71.2
  ocular G71.0
  oculopharyngeal G71.0
  of critical illness G72.81
  primary G71.9
    specified NEC G71.8
  progressive NEC G72.89
  proximal myotonic (PROMM) G71.11
  rod G71.2
  scapulohumeral G71.0
  specified NEC G72.89
  toxic G72.2
Myopericarditis (*see also* Pericarditis)
  chronic rheumatic I09.2
Myopia (axial) (congenital) H52.1- ☑
  degenerative (malignant) H44.20
    with
      choroidal neovascularization H44.2A- ☑
      foveoschisis H44.2D- ☑
      macular hole H44.2B- ☑
      retinal detachment H44.2C- ☑
      specified maculopathy NEC H44.2E- ☑
    bilateral H44.23
    left eye H44.22
    right eye H44.21
  malignant (*see also* Myopia, degenerative) H44.2- ☑
  pernicious (*see also* Myopia, degenerative) H44.2- ☑
  progressive high (degenerative) (*see also* Myopia, degenerative) H44.2- ☑
Myosarcoma — *see* Neoplasm, connective tissue, malignant
Myosis (pupil) H57.03
  stromal (endolymphatic) D39.0
Myositis M60.9
  clostridial A48.0
  due to posture — *see* Myositis, specified type NEC
  epidemic B33.0
  fibrosa or fibrous (chronic), Volkmann's T79.6 ☑
  foreign body granuloma — *see* Granuloma, foreign body
  in (due to)
    bilharziasis B65.9 [M63.8-] ☑
    cysticercosis B69.81
    leprosy A30.9 [M63.8-] ☑

Myositis — *continued*
- in — *continued*
  - mycosis B49 [M63.8-] ☑
  - sarcoidosis D86.87
  - schistosomiasis B65.9 [M63.8-] ☑
  - syphilis
    - late A52.78
    - secondary A51.49
  - toxoplasmosis (acquired) B58.82
  - trichinellosis B75 [M63.8-] ☑
  - tuberculosis A18.09
- inclusion body [IBM] G72.41
- infective M60.009
  - arm M60.002
    - left M60.001
    - right M60.000
  - leg M60.005
    - left M60.004
    - right M60.003
  - lower limb M60.005
    - ankle M60.07- ☑
    - foot M60.07- ☑
    - lower leg M60.06- ☑
    - thigh M60.05- ☑
    - toe M60.07- ☑
  - multiple sites M60.09
  - specified site NEC M60.08
  - upper limb M60.002
    - finger M60.04- ☑
    - forearm M60.03- ☑
    - hand M60.04- ☑
    - shoulder region M60.01- ☑
    - upper arm M60.02- ☑
- interstitial M60.10
  - ankle M60.17- ☑
  - foot M60.17- ☑
  - forearm M60.13- ☑
  - hand M60.14- ☑
  - lower leg M60.16- ☑
  - multiple sites M60.19
  - shoulder region M60.11- ☑
  - specified site NEC M60.18
  - thigh M60.15- ☑
  - upper arm M60.12- ☑
- mycotic B49 [M63.8-] ☑
- orbital, chronic H05.12-
- ossificans or ossifying (circumscripta) (*see also* Ossification, muscle, specified NEC)
  - in (due to)
    - burns M61.30
      - ankle M61.37- ☑
      - foot M61.37- ☑
      - forearm M61.33- ☑
      - hand M61.34- ☑
      - lower leg M61.36- ☑
      - multiple sites M61.39
      - pelvic region M61.35- ☑

Myositis — *continued*
- ossificans or ossifying (*see also* Ossification, muscle, specified) — *continued*
  - in — *continued*
    - burns — *continued*
      - shoulder region M61.31- ☑
      - specified site NEC M61.38
      - thigh M61.35- ☑
      - upper arm M61.32- ☑
    - quadriplegia or paraplegia M61.20
      - ankle M61.27- ☑
      - foot M61.27- ☑
      - forearm M61.23- ☑
      - hand M61.24- ☑
      - lower leg M61.26- ☑
      - multiple sites M61.29
      - pelvic region M61.25- ☑
      - shoulder region M61.21- ☑
      - specified site NEC M61.28
      - thigh M61.25- ☑
      - upper arm M61.22- ☑
  - progressiva M61.10
    - ankle M61.17- ☑
    - finger M61.14- ☑
    - foot M61.17- ☑
    - forearm M61.13- ☑
    - hand M61.14- ☑
    - lower leg M61.16- ☑
    - multiple sites M61.19
    - pelvic region M61.15- ☑
    - shoulder region M61.11- ☑
    - specified site NEC M61.18
    - thigh M61.15- ☑
    - toe M61.17- ☑
    - upper arm M61.12- ☑
  - traumatica M61.00
    - ankle M61.07- ☑
    - foot M61.07- ☑
    - forearm M61.03- ☑
    - hand M61.04- ☑
    - lower leg M61.06- ☑
    - multiple sites M61.09
    - pelvic region M61.05- ☑
    - shoulder region M61.01- ☑
    - specified site NEC M61.08
    - thigh M61.05- ☑
    - upper arm M61.02- ☑
- purulent — *see* Myositis, infective
- specified type NEC M60.80
  - ankle M60.87- ☑
  - foot M60.87- ☑
  - forearm M60.83- ☑
  - hand M60.84- ☑
  - lower leg M60.86- ☑
  - multiple sites M60.89
  - pelvic region M60.85- ☑
  - shoulder region M60.81- ☑

Myositis — *continued*
- specified type — *continued*
  - specified site NEC M60.88
  - thigh M60.85- ☑
  - upper arm M60.82- ☑
- suppurative — *see* Myositis, infective
- traumatic (old) — *see* Myositis, specified type NEC

Myospasia impulsiva F95.2

Myotonia (acquisita) (intermittens) M62.89
- atrophica G71.11
- chondrodystrophic G71.13
- congenita (acetazolamide responsive) (dominant) (recessive) G71.12
- drug-induced G71.14
- dystrophica G71.11
- fluctuans G71.19
- levior G71.12
- permanens G71.19
- symptomatic G71.19

Myotonic pupil — *see* Anomaly, pupil, function, tonic pupil

Myriapodiasis B88.2

Myringitis H73.2- ☑
- with otitis media — *see* Otitis, media
- acute H73.00- ☑
  - bullous H73.01- ☑
  - specified NEC H73.09- ☑
- bullous — *see* Myringitis, acute, bullous
- chronic H73.1- ☑

Mysophobia F40.228

Mytilotoxism — *see* Poisoning, fish

Myxadenitis labialis K13.0

Myxedema (adult) (idiocy) (infantile) (juvenile) (*see also* Hypothyroidism) E03.9
- circumscribed E05.90
  - with storm E05.91
- coma E03.5
- congenital E00.1
- cutis L98.5
- localized (pretibial) E05.90
  - with storm E05.91
- papular L98.5

Myxochondrosarcoma — *see* Neoplasm, cartilage, malignant

Myxofibroma — *see* Neoplasm, connective tissue, benign
- odontogenic — *see* Cyst, calcifying odontogenic

Myxofibrosarcoma — *see* Neoplasm, connective tissue, malignant

Myxolipoma D17.9

Myxoliposarcoma — *see* Neoplasm, connective tissue, malignant

Myxoma (*see also* Neoplasm, connective tissue, benign)
- nerve sheath — *see* Neoplasm, nerve, benign
- odontogenic — *see* Cyst, calcifying odontogenic

Myxosarcoma — *see* Neoplasm, connective tissue, malignant

Myositis — Myxosarcoma

228   ☑ **Additional Character Required — Refer to the Tabular List for Character Selection**   ☜ **Subterms under main terms may continue to next column or page**

N

Naegeli's
- disease Q82.8
- leukemia, monocytic C93.1- ☑

Naegleriasis (with meningoencephalitis) B60.2
Naffziger's syndrome G54.0
Naga sore — *see* Ulcer, skin
Nägele's pelvis M95.5
- with disproportion (fetopelvic) O33.0
  - causing obstructed labor O65.0

Nail (*see also* condition)
- biting F98.8
- patella syndrome Q87.2

Nanism, nanosomia — *see* Dwarfism
Nanophyetiasis B66.8
Nanukayami A27.89
Napkin rash L22
Narcolepsy G47.419
- with cataplexy G47.411
- in conditions classified elsewhere G47.429
  - with cataplexy G47.421

Narcosis R06.89
Narcotism — *see* Dependence
NARP (Neuropathy, Ataxia and Retinitis pigmentosa) syndrome E88.49
Narrow
- anterior chamber angle H40.03- ☑
- gingival width (of periodontal soft tissue) K05.5
- pelvis — *see* Contraction, pelvis

Narrowing (*see also* Stenosis)
- artery I77.1
  - auditory, internal I65.8
    - basilar — *see* Occlusion, artery, basilar
    - carotid — *see* Occlusion, artery, carotid
    - cerebellar — *see* Occlusion, artery, cerebellar
    - cerebral — *see* Occlusion artery, cerebral
    - choroidal — *see* Occlusion, artery, cerebral, specified NEC
    - communicating posterior — *see* Occlusion, artery, cerebral, specified NEC
    - coronary (*see also* Disease, heart, ischemic, atherosclerotic)
      - congenital Q24.5
        - syphilitic A50.54 [I52]
      - due to syphilis NEC A52.06
    - hypophyseal — *see* Occlusion, artery, cerebral, specified NEC
    - pontine — *see* Occlusion, artery, cerebral, specified NEC
    - precerebral — *see* Occlusion, artery, precerebral
    - vertebral — *see* Occlusion, artery, vertebral
- auditory canal (external) — *see* Stenosis, external ear canal
- eustachian tube — *see* Obstruction, eustachian tube
- eyelid — *see* Disorder, eyelid function
- larynx J38.6
- mesenteric artery (*see also* Ischemia, intestine, acute) K55.059
- palate M26.89
- palpebral fissure — *see* Disorder, eyelid function
- ureter N13.5
  - with infection N13.6
- urethra — *see* Stricture, urethra

Narrowness, abnormal, eyelid Q10.3
Nasal — *see* condition
Nasolachrymal, nasolacrimal — *see* condition
Nasopharyngeal (*see also* condition)
- pituitary gland Q89.2
- torticollis M43.6

Nasopharyngitis (acute) (infective) (streptococcal) (subacute) J00
- chronic (suppurative) (ulcerative) J31.1

Nasopharynx, nasopharyngeal — *see* condition
Natal tooth, teeth K00.6
Nausea (without vomiting) R11.0
- with vomiting R11.2
- gravidarum — *see* Hyperemesis, gravidarum
- marina T75.3 ☑
- navalis T75.3 ☑

Navel — *see* condition
Neapolitan fever — *see* Brucellosis
Near drowning T75.1 ☑
Nearsightedness — *see* Myopia
Near-syncope R55
Nebula, cornea — *see* Opacity, cornea

Necator americanus infestation B76.1
Necatoriasis B76.1
Neck — *see* condition
Necrobiosis R68.89
- lipoidica NEC L92.1
  - with diabetes — *see* E08-E13 with .620

Necrolysis, toxic epidermal L51.2
- due to drug
  - correct substance properly administered — *see* Table of Drugs and Chemicals, by drug, adverse effect
  - overdose or wrong substance given or taken — *see* Table of Drugs and Chemicals, by drug, poisoning

Necrophilia F65.89
Necrosis, necrotic (ischemic) (*see also* Gangrene)
- adrenal (capsule) (gland) E27.49
- amputation stump (surgical) (late) T87.50
  - arm T87.5- ☑
  - leg T87.5- ☑
- antrum J32.0
- aorta (hyaline) (*see also* Aneurysm, aorta)
  - cystic medial — *see* Dissection, aorta
- artery I77.5
- bladder (aseptic) (sphincter) N32.89
- bone (*see also* Osteonecrosis) M87.9
  - aseptic or avascular — *see* Osteonecrosis
    - idiopathic M87.00
  - ethmoid J32.2
  - jaw M27.2
  - tuberculous — *see* Tuberculosis, bone
- brain I67.89
- breast (aseptic) (fat) (segmental) N64.1
- bronchus J98.09
- central nervous system NEC I67.89
- cerebellar I67.89
- cerebral I67.89
- colon (*see also* Infarct, intestine) K55.049
- cornea H18.89- ☑
- cortical (acute) (renal) N17.1
- cystic medial (aorta) — *see* Dissection, aorta
- dental pulp K04.1
- esophagus K22.8
- ethmoid (bone) J32.2
- eyelid — *see* Disorder, eyelid, degenerative
- fat, fatty (generalized) (*see also* Disorder, soft tissue, specified type NEC)
  - abdominal wall K65.4
  - breast (aseptic) (segmental) N64.1
  - localized — *see* Degeneration, by site, fatty
  - mesentery K65.4
  - omentum K65.4
  - pancreas K86.89
  - peritoneum K65.4
  - skin (subcutaneous), newborn P83.0
  - subcutaneous, due to birth injury P15.6
- gallbladder — *see* Cholecystitis, acute
- heart — *see* Infarct, myocardium
- hip, aseptic or avascular — *see* Osteonecrosis, by type, femur
- intestine (acute) (hemorrhagic) (massive) (*see also* Infarct, intestine) K55.069
- jaw M27.2
- kidney (bilateral) N28.0
  - acute N17.9
  - cortical (acute) (bilateral) N17.1
    - with ectopic or molar pregnancy O08.4
  - medullary (bilateral) (in acute renal failure) (papillary) N17.2
  - papillary (bilateral) (in acute renal failure) N17.2
  - tubular N17.0
    - with ectopic or molar pregnancy O08.4
    - complicating
      - abortion — *see* Abortion, by type, complicated by, tubular necrosis
      - ectopic or molar pregnancy O08.4
      - pregnancy — *see* Pregnancy, complicated by, diseases of, specified type or system NEC
    - following ectopic or molar pregnancy O08.4
    - traumatic T79.5 ☑
- larynx J38.7
- liver (with hepatic failure) (cell) — *see* Failure, hepatic
  - hemorrhagic, central K76.2
- lung J85.0
- lymphatic gland — *see* Lymphadenitis, acute
- mammary gland (fat) (segmental) N64.1
- mastoid (chronic) — *see* Mastoiditis, chronic

Necrosis, necrotic — *continued*
- medullary (acute) (renal) N17.2
- mesentery (*see also* Infarct, intestine) K55.069
  - fat K65.4
- mitral valve — *see* Insufficiency, mitral
- myocardium, myocardial — *see* Infarct, myocardium
- nose J34.0
- omentum (with mesenteric infarction) (*see also* Infarct, intestine) K55.069
  - fat K65.4
- orbit, orbital — *see* Osteomyelitis, orbit
- ossicles, ear — *see* Abnormal, ear ossicles
- ovary N70.92
- pancreas (aseptic) (duct) (fat) K86.89
  - acute (infective) — *see* Pancreatitis, acute
  - infective — *see* Pancreatitis, acute
- papillary (acute) (renal) N17.2
- perineum N90.89
- peritoneum (with mesenteric infarction) (*see also* Infarct, intestine) K55.069
  - fat K65.4
- pharynx J02.9
  - in granulocytopenia — *see* Neutropenia
  - Vincent's A69.1
- phosphorus — *see* subcategory T54.2 ☑
- pituitary (gland) E23.0
  - postpartum O99.285
  - Sheehan O99.285
- pressure — *see* Ulcer, pressure, by site
- pulmonary J85.0
- pulp (dental) K04.1
- radiation — *see* Necrosis, by site
- radium — *see* Necrosis, by site
- renal — *see* Necrosis, kidney
- sclera H15.89
- scrotum N50.89
- skin or subcutaneous tissue NEC I96
- spine, spinal (column) (*see also* Osteonecrosis, by type, vertebra)
  - cord G95.19
- spleen D73.5
- stomach K31.89
- stomatitis (ulcerative) A69.0
- subcutaneous fat, newborn P83.88
- subendocardial (acute) I21.4
  - chronic I25.89
- suprarenal (capsule) (gland) E27.49
- testis N50.89
- thymus (gland) E32.8
- tonsil J35.8
- trachea J39.8
- tuberculous NEC — *see* Tuberculosis
- tubular (acute) (anoxic) (renal) (toxic) N17.0
  - postprocedural N99.0
- vagina N89.8
- vertebra (*see also* Osteonecrosis, by type, vertebra)
  - tuberculous A18.01
- vulva N90.89
- X-ray — *see* Necrosis, by site

Necrospermia — *see* Infertility, male
Need (for)
- care provider because (of)
  - assistance with personal care Z74.1
  - continuous supervision required Z74.3
  - impaired mobility Z74.09
  - no other household member able to render care Z74.2
  - specified reason NEC Z74.8
- immunization — *see* Vaccination
- vaccination — *see* Vaccination

Neglect
- adult
  - confirmed T74.01 ☑
  - history of Z91.412
  - suspected T76.01 ☑
- child (childhood)
  - confirmed T74.02 ☑
  - history of Z62.812
  - suspected T76.02 ☑
- emotional, in childhood Z62.898
- hemispatial R41.4
- left-sided R41.4
- sensory R41.4
- visuospatial R41.4

Neisserian infection NEC — *see* Gonococcus
Nelaton's syndrome G60.8
Nelson's syndrome E24.1
Nematodiasis (intestinal) B82.0

🖑 Subterms under main terms may continue to next column or page   ☑ Additional Character Required — Refer to the Tabular List for Character Selection   **229**

Naegeli's — Nematodiasis

Nematodiasis — *continued*
  Ancylostoma B76.0
Neonatal (*see also* Newborn)
  acne L70.4
  bradycardia P29.12
  screening, abnormal findings on P09
  tachycardia P29.11
  tooth, teeth K00.6
Neonatorum — *see* condition
Neoplasia
  endocrine, multiple (MEN) E31.20
    type I E31.21
    type IIA E31.22
    type IIB E31.23
  intraepithelial (histologically confirmed)
    anal (AIN) (histologically confirmed) K62.82
      grade I K62.82
      grade II K62.82
      severe D01.3
    cervical glandular (histologically confirmed) D06.9
    cervix (uteri) (CIN) (histologically confirmed) N87.9
      glandular D06.9
      grade I N87.0
      grade II N87.1
      grade III (severe dysplasia) (*see also* Carcinoma, cervix uteri, in situ) D06.9
    prostate (histologically confirmed) (PIN) N42.31
      grade I N42.31
      grade II N42.31
      grade III (severe dysplasia) D07.5
    vagina (histologically confirmed) (VAIN) N89.3
      grade I N89.0
      grade II N89.1
      grade III (severe dysplasia) D07.2
    vulva (histologically confirmed) (VIN) N90.3
      grade I N90.0
      grade II N90.1
      grade III (severe dysplasia) D07.1
Neoplasm, neoplastic (*see also* Table of Neoplasms)
  lipomatous, benign — *see* Lipoma
  malignant mast cell C96.20
    specified type NEC C96.29
  mast cell, of uncertain behavior NEC D47.09
Neovascularization
  ciliary body — *see* Disorder, iris, vascular
  cornea H16.40- ☑
    deep H16.44- ☑
    ghost vessels — *see* Ghost, vessels
    localized H16.43- ☑
    pannus — *see* Pannus
  iris — *see* Disorder, iris, vascular
  retina H35.05- ☑
Nephralgia N23
Nephritis, nephritic (albuminuric) (azotemic) (congenital) (disseminated) (epithelial) (familial) (focal) (granulomatous) (hemorrhagic) (infantile) (nonsuppurative, excretory) (uremic) N05.9
  with
    dense deposit disease N05.6
    diffuse
      crescentic glomerulonephritis N05.7
      endocapillary proliferative glomerulonephritis N05.4
      membranous glomerulonephritis N05.2
      mesangial proliferative glomerulonephritis N05.3
      mesangiocapillary glomerulonephritis N05.5
    edema — *see* Nephrosis
    focal and segmental glomerular lesions N05.1
    foot process disease N04.9
    glomerular lesion
      diffuse sclerosing N05.8
      hypocomplementemic — *see* Nephritis, membranoproliferative
      IgA — *see* Nephropathy, IgA
      lobular, lobulonodular — *see* Nephritis, membranoproliferative
      nodular — *see* Nephritis, membranoproliferative
    lesion of
      glomerulonephritis, proliferative N05.8
      renal necrosis N05.9
    minor glomerular abnormality N05.0
    specified morphological changes NEC N05.8
  acute N00.9
    with
      dense deposit disease N00.6

Nephritis, nephritic — *continued*
  acute — *continued*
    with — *continued*
      diffuse
        crescentic glomerulonephritis N00.7
        endocapillary proliferative glomerulonephritis N00.4
        membranous glomerulonephritis N00.2
        mesangial proliferative glomerulonephritis N00.3
        mesangiocapillary glomerulonephritis N00.5
      focal and segmental glomerular lesions N00.1
      minor glomerular abnormality N00.0
      specified morphological changes NEC N00.8
  amyloid E85.4 [N08]
  antiglomerular basement membrane (anti-GBM) antibody NEC
    in Goodpasture's syndrome M31.0
  antitubular basement membrane (tubulo-interstitial) NEC N12
    toxic — *see* Nephropathy, toxic
  arteriolar — *see* Hypertension, kidney
  arteriosclerotic — *see* Hypertension, kidney
  ascending — *see* Nephritis, tubulo-interstitial
  atrophic N03.9
  Balkan (endemic) N15.0
  calculous, calculus — *see* Calculus, kidney
  cardiac — *see* Hypertension, kidney
  cardiovascular — *see* Hypertension, kidney
  chronic N03.9
    with
      dense deposit disease N03.6
      diffuse
        crescentic glomerulonephritis N03.7
        endocapillary proliferative glomerulonephritis N03.4
        membranous glomerulonephritis N03.2
        mesangial proliferative glomerulonephritis N03.3
        mesangiocapillary glomerulonephritis N03.5
      focal and segmental glomerular lesions N03.1
      minor glomerular abnormality N03.0
      specified morphological changes NEC N03.8
    arteriosclerotic — *see* Hypertension, kidney
  cirrhotic N26.9
  complicating pregnancy O26.83- ☑
  croupous N00.9
  degenerative — *see* Nephrosis
  diffuse sclerosing N05.8
  due to
    diabetes mellitus — *see* E08-E13 with .21
    subacute bacterial endocarditis I33.0
    systemic lupus erythematosus (chronic) M32.14
    typhoid fever A01.09
  gonococcal (acute) (chronic) A54.21
  hypocomplementemic — *see* Nephritis, membranoproliferative
  IgA — *see* Nephropathy, IgA
  immune complex (circulating) NEC N05.8
  infective — *see* Nephritis, tubulo-interstitial
  interstitial — *see* Nephritis, tubulo-interstitial
  lead N14.3
  membranoproliferative (diffuse) (type 1 or 3) (*see also* N00-N07 with fourth character .5) N05.5
    type 2 (*see also* N00-N07 with fourth character .6) N05.6
  minimal change N05.0
  necrotic, necrotizing NEC (*see also* N00-N07 with fourth character .8) N05.8
  nephrotic — *see* Nephrosis
  nodular — *see* Nephritis, membranoproliferative
  polycystic Q61.3
    adult type Q61.2
    autosomal
      dominant Q61.2
      recessive NEC Q61.19
    childhood type NEC Q61.19
    infantile type NEC Q61.19
  poststreptococcal N05.9
    acute N00.9
    chronic N03.9
    rapidly progressive N01.9
  proliferative NEC (*see also* N00-N07 with fourth character .8) N05.8
  purulent — *see* Nephritis, tubulo-interstitial
  rapidly progressive N01.9
    with
      dense deposit disease N01.6

Nephritis, nephritic — *continued*
  rapidly progressive — *continued*
    with — *continued*
      diffuse
        crescentic glomerulonephritis N01.7
        endocapillary proliferative glomerulonephritis N01.4
        membranous glomerulonephritis N01.2
        mesangial proliferative glomerulonephritis N01.3
        mesangiocapillary glomerulonephritis N01.5
      focal and segmental glomerular lesions N01.1
      minor glomerular abnormality N01.0
      specified morphological changes NEC N01.8
  salt losing or wasting NEC N28.89
  saturnine N14.3
  sclerosing, diffuse N05.8
  septic — *see* Nephritis, tubulo-interstitial
  specified pathology NEC (*see also* N00-N07 with fourth character .8) N05.8
  subacute N01.9
  suppurative — *see* Nephritis, tubulo-interstitial
  syphilitic (late) A52.75
    congenital A50.59 [N08]
    early (secondary) A51.44
  toxic — *see* Nephropathy, toxic
  tubal, tubular — *see* Nephritis, tubulo-interstitial
  tuberculous A18.11
  tubulo-interstitial (in) N12
    acute (infectious) N10
    chronic (infectious) N11.9
      nonobstructive N11.8
        reflux-associated N11.0
      obstructive N11.1
      specified NEC N11.8
    due to
      brucellosis A23.9 [N16]
      cryoglobulinemia D89.1 [N16]
      glycogen storage disease E74.00 [N16]
      Sjögren's syndrome M35.04
  vascular — *see* Hypertension, kidney
  war N00.9
Nephroblastoma (epithelial) (mesenchymal) C64- ☑
Nephrocalcinosis E83.59 [N29]
Nephrocystitis, pustular — *see* Nephritis, tubulo-interstitial
Nephrolithiasis (congenital) (pelvis) (recurrent) (*see also* Calculus, kidney)
Nephroma C64- ☑
  mesoblastic D41.0- ☑
Nephronephritis — *see* Nephrosis
Nephronophthisis Q61.5
Nephropathia epidemica A98.5
Nephropathy (*see also* Nephritis) N28.9
  with
    edema — *see* Nephrosis
    glomerular lesion — *see* Glomerulonephritis
  amyloid, hereditary E85.0
  analgesic N14.0
    with medullary necrosis, acute N17.2
  Balkan (endemic) N15.0
  chemical — *see* Nephropathy, toxic
  diabetic — *see* E08-E13 with .21
  drug-induced N14.2
    specified NEC N14.1
  focal and segmental hyalinosis or sclerosis N02.1
  heavy metal-induced N14.3
  hereditary NEC N07.9
    with
      dense deposit disease N07.6
      diffuse
        crescentic glomerulonephritis N07.7
        endocapillary proliferative glomerulonephritis N07.4
        membranous glomerulonephritis N07.2
        mesangial proliferative glomerulonephritis N07.3
        mesangiocapillary glomerulonephritis N07.5
      focal and segmental glomerular lesions N07.1
      minor glomerular abnormality N07.0
      specified morphological changes NEC N07.8
  hypercalcemic N25.89
  hypertensive — *see* Hypertension, kidney
  hypokalemic (vacuolar) N25.89
  IgA N02.8
    with glomerular lesion N02.9
      focal and segmental hyalinosis or sclerosis N02.1

Nephropathy — continued
  IgA — continued
    with glomerular lesion — continued
      membranoproliferative (diffuse) N02.5
      membranous (diffuse) N02.2
      mesangial proliferative (diffuse) N02.3
      mesangiocapillary (diffuse) N02.5
      proliferative NEC N02.8
      specified pathology NEC N02.8
  lead N14.3
  membranoproliferative (diffuse) N02.5
  membranous (diffuse) N02.2
  mesangial (IgA/IgG) — see Nephropathy, IgA
    proliferative (diffuse) N02.3
  mesangiocapillary (diffuse) N02.5
  obstructive N13.8
  phenacetin N17.2
  phosphate-losing N25.0
  potassium depletion N25.89
  pregnancy-related O26.83- ☑
  proliferative NEC (see also N00-N07 with fourth character .8) N05.8
  protein-losing N25.89
  saturnine N14.3
  sickle-cell D57.- ☑ [N08]
  toxic NEC N14.4
    due to
      drugs N14.2
        analgesic N14.0
        specified NEC N14.1
      heavy metals N14.3
  vasomotor N17.0
  water-losing N25.89
Nephroptosis N28.83
Nephropyosis — see Abscess, kidney
Nephrorrhagia N28.89
Nephrosclerosis (arteriolar)(arteriosclerotic) (chronic) (hyaline) (see also Hypertension, kidney)
  hyperplastic — see Hypertension, kidney
  senile N26.9
Nephrosis, nephrotic (Epstein's) (syndrome) (congenital) N04.9
  with
    foot process disease N04.9
    glomerular lesion N04.1
    hypocomplementemic N04.5
  acute N04.9
  anoxic — see Nephrosis, tubular
  chemical — see Nephrosis, tubular
  cholemic K76.7
  diabetic — see E08-E13 with .21
  Finnish type (congenital) Q89.8
  hemoglobin N10
  hemoglobinuric — see Nephrosis, tubular
  in
    amyloidosis E85.4 [N08]
    diabetes mellitus — see E08-E13 with .21
    epidemic hemorrhagic fever A98.5
    malaria (malariae) B52.0
  ischemic — see Nephrosis, tubular
  lipoid N04.9
  lower nephron — see Nephrosis, tubular
  malarial (malariae) B52.0
  minimal change N04.0
  myoglobin N10
  necrotizing — see Nephrosis, tubular
  osmotic (sucrose) N25.89
  radiation N04.9
  syphilitic (late) A52.75
  toxic — see Nephrosis, tubular
  tubular (acute) N17.0
    postprocedural N99.0
    radiation N04.9
Nephrosonephritis, hemorrhagic (endemic) A98.5
Nephrostomy
  attention to Z43.6
  status Z93.6
Nerve (see also condition)
  injury — see Injury, nerve, by body site
Nerves R45.0
Nervous (see also condition) R45.0
  heart F45.8
  stomach F45.8
  tension R45.0
Nervousness R45.0
Nesidioblastoma
  pancreas D13.7
  specified site NEC — see Neoplasm, benign, by site

Nesidioblastoma — continued
  unspecified site D13.7
Nettleship's syndrome — see Urticaria pigmentosa
Neumann's disease or syndrome L10.1
Neuralgia, neuralgic (acute) M79.2
  accessory (nerve) G52.8
  acoustic (nerve) — see subcategory H93.3 ☑
  auditory (nerve) — see subcategory H93.3 ☑
  ciliary G44.009
    intractable G44.001
    not intractable G44.009
  cranial
    nerve (see also Disorder, nerve, cranial)
      fifth or trigeminal — see Neuralgia, trigeminal
      postherpetic, postzoster B02.29
  ear — see subcategory H92.0 ☑
  facialis vera G51.1
  Fothergill's — see Neuralgia, trigeminal
  glossopharyngeal (nerve) G52.1
  Horton's G44.099
    intractable G44.091
    not intractable G44.099
  Hunt's B02.21
  hypoglossal (nerve) G52.3
  infraorbital — see Neuralgia, trigeminal
  malarial — see Malaria
  migrainous G44.009
    intractable G44.001
    not intractable G44.009
  Morton's G57.6- ☑
  nerve, cranial — see Disorder, nerve, cranial
  nose G52.0
  occipital M54.81
  olfactory G52.0
  penis N48.9
  perineum R10.2
  postherpetic NEC B02.29
    trigeminal B02.22
  pubic region R10.2
  scrotum R10.2
  Sluder's G44.89
  specified nerve NEC G58.8
  spermatic cord R10.2
  sphenopalatine (ganglion) G90.09
  trifacial — see Neuralgia, trigeminal
  trigeminal G50.0
    postherpetic, postzoster B02.22
  vagus (nerve) G52.2
  writer's F48.8
    organic G25.89
Neurapraxia — see Injury, nerve
Neurasthenia F48.8
  cardiac F45.8
  gastric F45.8
  heart F45.8
Neurilemmoma (see also Neoplasm, nerve, benign)
  acoustic (nerve) D33.3
  malignant (see also Neoplasm, nerve, malignant)
    acoustic (nerve) C72.4- ☑
Neurilemmosarcoma — see Neoplasm, nerve, malignant
Neurinoma — see Neoplasm, nerve, benign
Neurinomatosis — see Neoplasm, nerve, uncertain behavior
Neuritis (rheumatoid) M79.2
  abducens (nerve) — see Strabismus, paralytic, sixth nerve
  accessory (nerve) G52.8
  acoustic (nerve) (see also subcategory) H93.3 ☑
    in (due to)
      infectious disease NEC B99 ☑ [H94.0-] ☑
      parasitic disease NEC B89 [H94.0-] ☑
    syphilitic A52.15
  alcoholic G62.1
    with psychosis — see Psychosis, alcoholic
  amyloid, any site E85.4 [G63]
  auditory (nerve) — see subcategory H93.3 ☑
  brachial — see Radiculopathy
    due to displacement, intervertebral disc — see Disorder, disc, cervical, with neuritis
  cranial nerve
    due to Lyme disease A69.22
    eighth or acoustic or auditory — see subcategory H93.3 ☑
    eleventh or accessory G52.8
    fifth or trigeminal G51.0
    first or olfactory G52.0

Neuritis — continued
  cranial nerve — continued
    fourth or trochlear — see Strabismus, paralytic, fourth nerve
    second or optic — see Neuritis, optic
    seventh or facial G51.8
      newborn (birth injury) P11.3
    sixth or abducent — see Strabismus, paralytic, sixth nerve
    tenth or vagus G52.2
    third or oculomotor — see Strabismus, paralytic, third nerve
    twelfth or hypoglossal G52.3
  Déjérine-Sottas G60.0
  diabetic (mononeuropathy) — see E08-E13 with .41
    polyneuropathy — see E08-E13 with .42
  due to
    beriberi E51.11
    displacement, prolapse or rupture, intervertebral disc — see Disorder, disc, with, radiculopathy
    herniation, nucleus pulposus M51.9 [G55]
  endemic E51.11
  facial G51.8
    newborn (birth injury) P11.3
  general — see Polyneuropathy
  geniculate ganglion G51.1
    due to herpes (zoster) B02.21
  gouty (see also Gout, by type) M10.9 [G63]
  hypoglossal (nerve) G52.3
  ilioinguinal (nerve) G57.9- ☑
  infectious (multiple) NEC G61.0
  interstitial hypertrophic progressive G60.0
  lumbar M54.16
  lumbosacral M54.17
  multiple (see also Polyneuropathy)
    endemic E51.11
    infective, acute G61.0
  multiplex endemica E51.11
  nerve root — see Radiculopathy
  oculomotor (nerve) — see Strabismus, paralytic, third nerve
  olfactory nerve G52.0
  optic (nerve) (hereditary) (sympathetic) H46.9
    with demyelination G36.0
    in myelitis G36.0
    nutritional H46.2
    papillitis — see Papillitis, optic
    retrobulbar H46.1- ☑
    specified type NEC H46.8
    toxic H46.3
  peripheral (nerve) G62.9
    multiple — see Polyneuropathy
    single — see Mononeuritis
  pneumogastric (nerve) G52.2
  postherpetic, postzoster B02.29
  progressive hypertrophic interstitial G60.0
  retrobulbar (see also Neuritis, optic, retrobulbar)
    in (due to)
      late syphilis A52.15
      meningococcal infection A39.82
    meningococcal A39.82
    syphilitic A52.15
  sciatic (nerve) (see also Sciatica)
    due to displacement of intervertebral disc — see Disorder, disc, with, radiculopathy
  serum (see also Reaction, serum) T80.69 ☑
  shoulder-girdle G54.5
  specified nerve NEC G58.8
  spinal (nerve) root — see Radiculopathy
  syphilitic A52.15
  thenar (median) G56.1- ☑
  thoracic M54.14
  toxic NEC G62.2
  trochlear (nerve) — see Strabismus, paralytic, fourth nerve
  vagus (nerve) G52.2
Neuroastrocytoma — see Neoplasm, uncertain behavior, by site
Neuroavitaminosis E56.9 [G99.8]
Neuroblastoma
  olfactory C30.0
  specified site — see Neoplasm, malignant, by site
  unspecified site C74.90
Neurochorioretinitis — see Chorioretinitis
Neurocirculatory asthenia F45.8
Neurocysticercosis B69.0
Neurocytoma — see Neoplasm, benign, by site

Index

Neurodermatitis (circumscribed) (circumscripta) (local) L28.0
  atopic L20.81
  diffuse (Brocq) L20.81
  disseminated L20.81
Neuroencephalomyelopathy, optic G36.0
Neuroepithelioma (see also Neoplasm, malignant, by site)
  olfactory C30.0
Neurofibroma (see also Neoplasm, nerve, benign)
  melanotic — see Neoplasm, nerve, benign
  multiple — see Neurofibromatosis
  plexiform — see Neoplasm, nerve, benign
Neurofibromatosis (multiple) (nonmalignant) Q85.00
  acoustic Q85.02
  malignant — see Neoplasm, nerve, malignant
  specified NEC Q85.09
  type 1 (von Recklinghausen) Q85.01
  type 2 Q85.02
Neurofibrosarcoma — see Neoplasm, nerve, malignant
Neurogenic (see also condition)
  bladder (see also Dysfunction, bladder, neuromuscular) N31.9
    cauda equina syndrome G83.4
  bowel NEC K59.2
  heart F45.8
Neuroglioma — see Neoplasm, uncertain behavior, by site
Neurolabyrinthitis (of Dix and Hallpike) — see Neuronitis, vestibular
Neurolathyrism — see Poisoning, food, noxious, plant
Neuroleprosy A30.9
Neuroma (see also Neoplasm, nerve, benign)
  acoustic (nerve) D33.3
  amputation (stump) (traumatic) (surgical complication) (late) T87.3- ☑
    arm T87.3- ☑
    leg T87.3- ☑
  digital (toe) G57.6- ☑
  interdigital G58.8
    lower limb (toe) G57.8- ☑
    upper limb G56.8- ☑
  intermetatarsal G57.8- ☑
  Morton's G57.6- ☑
  nonneoplastic
    arm G56.9- ☑
    leg G57.9- ☑
    lower extremity G57.9- ☑
    upper extremity G56.9- ☑
  optic (nerve) D33.3
  plantar G57.6- ☑
  plexiform — see Neoplasm, nerve, benign
  surgical (nonneoplastic)
    arm G56.9- ☑
    leg G57.9- ☑
    lower extremity G57.9- ☑
    upper extremity G56.9- ☑
Neuromyalgia — see Neuralgia
Neuromyasthenia (epidemic) (postinfectious) G93.3
Neuromyelitis G36.9
  ascending G61.0
  optica G36.0
Neuromyopathy G70.9
  paraneoplastic D49.9 [G13.0]
Neuromyotonia (Isaacs) G71.19
Neuronevus — see Nevus
Neuronitis G58.9
  ascending (acute) G57.2- ☑
  vestibular H81.2- ☑
Neuroparalytic — see condition
Neuropathy, neuropathic G62.9
  acute motor G62.81
  alcoholic G62.1
    with psychosis — see Psychosis, alcoholic
  arm G56.9- ☑
  autonomic, peripheral — see Neuropathy, peripheral, autonomic
  axillary G56.9- ☑
  bladder N31.9
    atonic (motor) (sensory) N31.2
    autonomous N31.2
    flaccid N31.2
    nonreflex N31.2
    reflex N31.1
    uninhibited N31.0
  brachial plexus G54.0
  cervical plexus G54.2

Neuropathy, neuropathic — continued
  chronic
    progressive segmentally demyelinating G62.89
    relapsing demyelinating G62.89
  Déjérine-Sottas G60.0
  diabetic — see E08-E13 with .40
    mononeuropathy — see E08-E13 with .41
    polyneuropathy — see E08-E13 with .42
  entrapment G58.9
    iliohypogastric nerve G57.8- ☑
    ilioinguinal nerve G57.8- ☑
    lateral cutaneous nerve of thigh G57.1- ☑
    median nerve G56.0- ☑
    obturator nerve G57.8- ☑
    peroneal nerve G57.3- ☑
    posterior tibial nerve G57.5- ☑
    saphenous nerve G57.8- ☑
    ulnar nerve G56.2- ☑
  facial nerve G51.9
  hereditary G60.9
    motor and sensory (types I-IV) G60.0
    sensory G60.8
    specified NEC G60.8
  hypertrophic G60.0
    Charcot-Marie-Tooth G60.0
    Déjérine-Sottas G60.0
    interstitial progressive G60.0
    of infancy G60.0
    Refsum G60.1
  idiopathic G60.9
    progressive G60.3
    specified NEC G60.8
  in association with hereditary ataxia G60.2
  intercostal G58.0
  ischemic — see Disorder, nerve
  Jamaica (ginger) G62.2
  leg NEC G57.9- ☑
  lower extremity G57.9- ☑
  lumbar plexus G54.1
  median nerve G56.1- ☑
  motor and sensory (see also Polyneuropathy)
    hereditary (types I-IV) G60.0
  multifocal motor (MMN) G61.82
  multiple (acute) (chronic) — see Polyneuropathy
  optic (nerve) (see also Neuritis, optic)
    ischemic H47.01- ☑
  paraneoplastic (sensorial) (Denny Brown) D49.9 [G13.0]
  peripheral (nerve) (see also Polyneuropathy) G62.9
    autonomic G90.9
      idiopathic G90.09
      in (due to)
        amyloidosis E85.4 [G99.0]
        diabetes mellitus — see E08-E13 with .43
        endocrine disease NEC E34.9 [G99.0]
        gout M10.00 [G99.0]
        hyperthyroidism E05.90 [G99.0]
          with thyroid storm E05.91 [G99.0]
        metabolic disease NEC E88.9 [G99.0]
    idiopathic G60.9
      progressive G60.3
    in (due to)
      antitetanus serum G62.0
      arsenic G62.2
      drugs NEC G62.0
      lead G62.2
      organophosphate compounds G62.2
      toxic agent NEC G62.2
  plantar nerves G57.6- ☑
  progressive
    hypertrophic interstitial G60.0
    inflammatory G62.81
  radicular NEC — see Radiculopathy
  sacral plexus G54.1
  sciatic G57.0- ☑
  serum G61.1
  toxic NEC G62.2
  trigeminal sensory G50.8
  ulnar nerve G56.2- ☑
  uremic N18.9 [G63]
  vitamin B12 E53.8 [G63]
    with anemia (pernicious) D51.0 [G63]
    due to dietary deficiency D51.3 [G63]
Neurophthisis (see also Disorder, nerve)
  peripheral, diabetic — see E08-E13 with .42
Neuroretinitis — see Chorioretinitis
Neuroretinopathy, hereditary optic H47.22
Neurosarcoma — see Neoplasm, nerve, malignant
Neurosclerosis — see Disorder, nerve

Neurosis, neurotic F48.9
  anankastic F42.8
  anxiety (state) F41.1
    panic type F41.0
  asthenic F48.8
  bladder F45.8
  cardiac (reflex) F45.8
  cardiovascular F45.8
  character F60.9
  colon F45.8
  compensation F68.1 ☑
  compulsive, compulsion F42.8
  conversion F44.9
  craft F48.8
  cutaneous F45.8
  depersonalization F48.1
  depressive (reaction) (type) F34.1
  environmental F48.8
  excoriation L98.1
  fatigue F48.8
  functional — see Disorder, somatoform
  gastric F45.8
  gastrointestinal F45.8
  heart F45.8
  hypochondriacal F45.21
  hysterical F44.9
  incoordination F45.8
    larynx F45.8
    vocal cord F45.8
  intestine F45.8
  larynx (sensory) F45.8
    hysterical F44.4
  mixed NEC F48.8
  musculoskeletal F45.8
  obsessional F42.8
  obsessive-compulsive F42.8
  occupational F48.8
  ocular NEC F45.8
  organ — see Disorder, somatoform
  pharynx F45.8
  phobic F40.9
  posttraumatic (situational) F43.10
    acute F43.11
    chronic F43.12
  psychasthenic (type) F48.8
  railroad F48.8
  rectum F45.8
  respiratory F45.8
  rumination F45.8
  sexual F65.9
  situational F48.8
  social F40.10
    generalized F40.11
  specified type NEC F48.8
  state F48.9
    with depersonalization episode F48.1
  stomach F45.8
  traumatic F43.10
    acute F43.11
    chronic F43.12
  vasomotor F45.8
  visceral F45.8
  war F48.8
Neurospongioblastosis diffusa Q85.1
Neurosyphilis (arrested) (early) (gumma) (late) (latent) (recurrent) (relapse) A52.3
  with ataxia (cerebellar) (locomotor) (spastic) (spinal) A52.19
  aneurysm (cerebral) A52.05
  arachnoid (adhesive) A52.13
  arteritis (any artery) (cerebral) A52.04
  asymptomatic A52.2
  congenital A50.40
  dura (mater) A52.13
  general paresis A52.17
  hemorrhagic A52.05
  juvenile (asymptomatic) (meningeal) A50.40
  leptomeninges (aseptic) A52.13
  meningeal, meninges (adhesive) A52.13
  meningitis A52.13
  meningovascular (diffuse) A52.13
  optic atrophy A52.15
  parenchymatous (degenerative) A52.19
  paresis, paretic A52.17
    juvenile A50.45
  remission in (sustained) A52.3
  serological (without symptoms) A52.2
  specified nature or site NEC A52.19
  tabes, tabetic (dorsalis) A52.11

Neurodermatitis — Neurosyphilis

☑ **Additional Character Required** — Refer to the Tabular List for Character Selection   ▽ Subterms under main terms may continue to next column or page

Neurosyphilis — *continued*
  tabes, tabetic — *continued*
    juvenile A50.45
   taboparesis A52.17
    juvenile A50.45
   thrombosis (cerebral) A52.05
   vascular (cerebral) NEC A52.05
Neurothekeoma — *see* Neoplasm, nerve, benign
Neurotic — *see* Neurosis
Neurotoxemia — *see* Toxemia
Neutroclusion M26.211
Neutropenia, neutropenic (chronic) (genetic) (idiopathic) (immune) (infantile) (malignant) (pernicious) (splenic) D70.9
  congenital (primary) D70.0
  cyclic D70.4
  cytoreductive cancer chemotherapy sequela D70.1
  drug-induced D70.2
   due to cytoreductive cancer chemotherapy D70.1
  due to infection D70.3
  fever D70.9
  neonatal, transitory (isoimmune) (maternal transfer) P61.5
  periodic D70.4
  secondary (cyclic) (periodic) (splenic) D70.4
   drug-induced D70.2
    due to cytoreductive cancer chemotherapy D70.1
  toxic D70.8
Neutrophilia, hereditary giant D72.0
Nevocarcinoma — *see* Melanoma
Nevus D22.9
  achromic — *see* Neoplasm, skin, benign
  amelanotic — *see* Neoplasm, skin, benign
  angiomatous D18.00
   intra-abdominal D18.03
   intracranial D18.02
   skin D18.01
   specified site NEC D18.09
  araneus I78.1
  balloon cell — *see* Neoplasm, skin, benign
  bathing trunk D48.5
  blue — *see* Neoplasm, skin, benign
   cellular — *see* Neoplasm, skin, benign
   giant — *see* Neoplasm, skin, benign
   Jadassohn's — *see* Neoplasm, skin, benign
   malignant — *see* Melanoma
  capillary D18.00
   intra-abdominal D18.03
   intracranial D18.02
   skin D18.01
   specified site NEC D18.09
  cavernous D18.00
   intra-abdominal D18.03
   intracranial D18.02
   skin D18.01
   specified site NEC D18.09
  cellular — *see* Neoplasm, skin, benign
   blue — *see* Neoplasm, skin, benign
  choroid D31.3- ☑
  comedonicus Q82.5
  conjunctiva D31.0- ☑
  dermal — *see* Neoplasm, skin, benign
   with epidermal nevus — *see* Neoplasm, skin, benign
  dysplastic — *see* Neoplasm, skin, benign
  eye D31.9- ☑
  flammeus Q82.5
  hemangiomatous D18.00
   intra-abdominal D18.03
   intracranial D18.02
   skin D18.01
   specified site NEC D18.09
  iris D31.4- ☑
  lacrimal gland D31.5- ☑
  lymphatic D18.1
  magnocellular
   specified site — *see* Neoplasm, benign, by site
   unspecified site D31.40
  malignant — *see* Melanoma
  meaning hemangioma D18.00
   intra-abdominal D18.03
   intracranial D18.02
   skin D18.01
   specified site NEC D18.09
  mouth (mucosa) D10.30
   specified site NEC D10.39
   white sponge Q38.6

Nevus — *continued*
  multiplex Q85.1
  non-neoplastic I78.1
  oral mucosa D10.30
   specified site NEC D10.39
   white sponge Q38.6
  orbit D31.6- ☑
  pigmented
   giant (*see also* Neoplasm, skin, uncertain behavior) D48.5
    malignant melanoma in — *see* Melanoma
  portwine Q82.5
  retina D31.2- ☑
  retrobulbar D31.6- ☑
  sanguineous Q82.5
  senile I78.1
  skin D22.9
   abdominal wall D22.5
   ala nasi D22.39
   ankle D22.7- ☑
   anus, anal D22.5
   arm D22.6- ☑
   auditory canal (external) D22.2- ☑
   auricle (ear) D22.2- ☑
   auricular canal (external) D22.2- ☑
   axilla, axillary fold D22.5
   back D22.5
   breast D22.5
   brow D22.39
   buttock D22.5
   canthus (eye) D22.1- ☑
   cheek (external) D22.39
   chest wall D22.5
   chin D22.39
   ear (external) D22.2- ☑
   external meatus (ear) D22.2- ☑
   eyebrow D22.39
   eyelid (lower) (upper) D22.1- ☑
   face D22.30
    specified NEC D22.39
   female genital organ (external) NEC D28.0
   finger D22.6- ☑
   flank D22.5
   foot D22.7- ☑
   forearm D22.6- ☑
   forehead D22.39
   foreskin D29.0
   genital organ (external) NEC
    female D28.0
    male D29.9
   gluteal region D22.5
   groin D22.5
   hand D22.6- ☑
   heel D22.7- ☑
   helix D22.2- ☑
   hip D22.7- ☑
   interscapular region D22.5
   jaw D22.39
   knee D22.7- ☑
   labium (majus) (minus) D28.0
   leg D22.7- ☑
   lip (lower) (upper) D22.0
   lower limb D22.7- ☑
   male genital organ (external) D29.9
   nail D22.9
    finger D22.6- ☑
    toe D22.7- ☑
   nasolabial groove D22.39
   nates D22.5
   neck D22.4
   nose (external) D22.39
   palpebra D22.1- ☑
   penis D29.0
   perianal skin D22.5
   perineum D22.5
   pinna D22.2- ☑
   popliteal fossa or space D22.7- ☑
   prepuce D29.0
   pudendum D28.0
   scalp D22.4
   scrotum D29.4
   shoulder D22.6- ☑
   submammary fold D22.5
   temple D22.39
   thigh D22.7- ☑
   toe D22.7- ☑
   trunk NEC D22.5

Nevus — *continued*
  skin — *continued*
   umbilicus D22.5
    upper limb D22.6- ☑
   vulva D28.0
  specified site NEC — *see* Neoplasm, by site, benign
  spider I78.1
  stellar I78.1
  strawberry Q82.5
  Sutton's benign D22.9
  unius lateris Q82.5
  Unna's Q82.5
  vascular Q82.5
  verrucous Q82.5
Newborn (infant) (liveborn) (singleton) Z38.2
  abstinence syndrome P96.1
  acne L70.4
  affected by
   abnormalities of membranes P02.9
    specified NEC P02.8
   abruptio placenta P02.1
   amino-acid metabolic disorder, transitory P74.8
   amniocentesis (while in utero) P00.6
   amnionitis P02.7
   apparent life threatening event (ALTE) R68.13
   bleeding (into)
    cerebral cortex P52.22
    germinal matrix P52.0
    ventricles P52.1
   breech delivery P03.0
   cardiac arrest P29.81
   cardiomyopathy I42.8
    congenital I42.4
   cerebral ischemia P91.0
   Cesarean delivery P03.4
   chemotherapy agents P04.1
   chorioamnionitis P02.7
   cocaine (crack) P04.41
   complications of labor and delivery P03.9
    specified NEC P03.89
   compression of umbilical cord NEC P02.5
   contracted pelvis P03.1
   delivery P03.9
    Cesarean P03.4
    forceps P03.2
    vacuum extractor P03.3
   entanglement (knot) in umbilical cord P02.5
   environmental chemicals P04.6
   fetal (intrauterine)
    growth retardation P05.9
    malnutrition not light or small for gestational age P05.2
   forceps delivery P03.2
   heart rate abnormalities
    bradycardia P29.12
    intrauterine P03.819
     before onset of labor P03.810
     during labor P03.811
    tachycardia P29.11
   hemorrhage (antepartum) P02.1
    cerebellar (nontraumatic) P52.6
    intracerebral (nontraumatic) P52.4
    intracranial (nontraumatic) P52.9
     specified NEC P52.8
    intraventricular (nontraumatic) P52.3
     grade 1 P52.0
     grade 2 P52.1
     grade 3 P52.21
     grade 4 P52.22
    posterior fossa (nontraumatic) P52.6
    subarachnoid (nontraumatic) P52.5
    subependymal P52.0
     with intracerebral extension P52.22
     with intraventricular extension P52.1
      with enlargment of ventricles P52.21
     without intraventricular extension P52.0
   hypoxic ischemic encephalopathy [HIE] P91.60
    mild P91.61
    moderate P91.62
    severe P91.63
   induction of labor P03.89
   intestinal perforation P78.0
   intrauterine (fetal) blood loss P50.9
    due to (from)
     cut end of co-twin cord P50.5
     hemorrhage into
      co-twin P50.3
      maternal circulation P50.4
     placenta P50.2

Newborn — continued
  affected by — continued
    intrauterine blood loss — continued
      due to — continued
        ruptured cord blood P50.1
        vasa previa P50.0
      specified NEC P50.8
    intrauterine (fetal) hemorrhage P50.9
    intrauterine (in utero) procedure P96.5
    malpresentation (malposition) NEC P03.1
    maternal (complication of) (use of)
      alcohol P04.3
      analgesia (maternal) P04.0
      anesthesia (maternal) P04.0
      blood loss P02.1
      circulatory disease P00.3
      condition P00.9
        specified NEC P00.89
      delivery P03.9
        Cesarean P03.4
        forceps P03.2
        vacuum extractor P03.3
      diabetes mellitus (pre-existing) P70.1
      disorder P00.9
        specified NEC P00.89
      drugs (addictive) (illegal) NEC P04.49
      ectopic pregnancy P01.4
      gestational diabetes P70.0
      hemorrhage P02.1
      hypertensive disorder P00.0
      incompetent cervix P01.0
      infectious disease P00.2
      injury P00.5
      labor and delivery P03.9
      malpresentation before labor P01.7
      maternal death P01.6
      medical procedure P00.7
      medication P04.1
      multiple pregnancy P01.5
      nutritional disorder P00.4
      oligohydramnios P01.2
      parasitic disease P00.2
      periodontal disease P00.81
      placenta previa P02.0
      polyhydramnios P01.3
      precipitate delivery P03.5
      pregnancy P01.9
        specified NEC P01.8
      premature rupture of membranes P01.1
      renal disease P00.1
      respiratory disease P00.3
      surgical procedure P00.6
      urinary tract disease P00.1
      uterine contraction (abnormal) P03.6
    meconium peritonitis P78.0
    medication (legal) (maternal use) (prescribed) P04.1
    membrane abnormalities P02.9
      specified NEC P02.8
    membranitis P02.7
    methamphetamine(s) P04.49
    mixed metabolic and respiratory acidosis P84
    neonatal abstinence syndrome P96.1
    noxious substances transmitted via placenta or
        breast milk P04.9
      specified NEC P04.8
    nutritional supplements P04.5
    placenta previa P02.0
    placental
      abnormality (functional) (morphological)
          P02.20
        specified NEC P02.29
      dysfunction P02.29
      infarction P02.29
      insufficiency P02.29
      separation NEC P02.1
      transfusion syndromes P02.3
    placentitis P02.7
    precipitate delivery P03.5
    prolapsed cord P02.4
    respiratory arrest P28.81
    slow intrauterine growth P05.9
    tobacco P04.2
    twin to twin transplacental transfusion P02.3
    umbilical cord (tightly) around neck P02.5
    umbilical cord condition P02.60
      short cord P02.69
      specified NEC P02.69
    uterine contractions (abnormal) P03.6
    vasa previa P02.69

Newborn — continued
  affected by — continued
    vasa previa — continued
      from intrauterine blood loss P50.0
  apnea P28.4
    obstructive P28.4
    primary P28.3
    sleep (central) (obstructive) (primary) P28.3
  born in hospital Z38.00
    by cesarean Z38.01
  born outside hospital Z38.1
  breast buds P96.89
  breast engorgement P83.4
  check-up — see Newborn, examination
  convulsion P90
  dehydration P74.1
  examination
    8 to 28 days old Z00.111
    under 8 days old Z00.110
  fever P81.9
    environmentally-induced P81.0
  hyperbilirubinemia P59.9
    of prematurity P59.0
  hypernatremia P74.2
  hyponatremia P74.2
  infection P39.9
    candidal P37.5
    specified NEC P39.8
    urinary tract P39.3
  jaundice P59.9
    due to
      breast milk inhibitor P59.3
      hepatocellular damage P59.20
        specified NEC P59.29
      preterm delivery P59.0
    of prematurity P59.0
    specified NEC P59.8
  late metabolic acidosis P74.0
  mastitis P39.0
    infective P39.0
    noninfective P83.4
  multiple born NEC Z38.8
    born in hospital Z38.68
      by cesarean Z38.69
    born outside hospital Z38.7
  omphalitis P38.9
    with mild hemorrhage P38.1
    without hemorrhage P38.9
  post-term P08.21
  prolonged gestation (over 42 completed weeks)
      P08.22
  quadruplet Z38.8
    born in hospital Z38.63
      by cesarean Z38.64
    born outside hospital Z38.7
  quintuplet Z38.8
    born in hospital Z38.65
      by cesarean Z38.66
    born outside hospital Z38.7
  seizure P90
  sepsis (congenital) P36.9
    due to
      anaerobes NEC P36.5
      Escherichia coli P36.4
      Staphylococcus P36.30
        aureus P36.2
        specified NEC P36.39
      Streptococcus P36.10
        group B P36.0
        specified NEC P36.19
    specified NEC P36.8
  triplet Z38.8
    born in hospital Z38.61
      by cesarean Z38.62
    born outside hospital Z38.7
  twin Z38.5
    born in hospital Z38.30
      by cesarean Z38.31
    born outside hospital Z38.4
  vomiting P92.09
    bilious P92.01
  weight check Z00.111
Newcastle conjunctivitis or disease B30.8
Nezelof's syndrome (pure alymphocytosis) D81.4
Niacin (amide) **deficiency** E52
Nicolas (-Durand)-**Favre disease** A55
Nicotine — see Tobacco
Nicotinic acid deficiency E52

Niemann-Pick disease or syndrome E75.249
  specified NEC E75.248
  type
    A E75.240
    B E75.241
    C E75.242
    D E75.243
Night
  blindness — see Blindness, night
  sweats R61
  terrors (child) F51.4
Nightmares (REM sleep type) F51.5
NIHSS (National Institutes of Health Stroke Scale) **score**
  R29.7- ☑
Nipple — see condition
Nisbet's chancre A57
Nishimoto (-Takeuchi) **disease** I67.5
Nitritoid crisis or reaction — see Crisis, nitritoid
Nitrosohemoglobinemia D74.8
Njovera A65
Nocardiosis, nocardiasis A43.9
  cutaneous A43.1
  lung A43.0
  pneumonia A43.0
  pulmonary A43.0
  specified site NEC A43.8
Nocturia R35.1
  psychogenic F45.8
Nocturnal — see condition
Nodal rhythm I49.8
Node(s) (see also Nodule)
  Bouchard's (with arthropathy) M15.2
  Haygarth's M15.8
  Heberden's (with arthropathy) M15.1
  larynx J38.7
  lymph — see condition
  milker's B08.03
  Osler's I33.0
  Schmorl's — see Schmorl's disease
  singer's J38.2
  teacher's J38.2
  tuberculous — see Tuberculosis, lymph gland
  vocal cord J38.2
Nodule(s), **nodular**
  actinomycotic — see Actinomycosis
  breast NEC (see also Lump, breast) N63.0
  colloid (cystic), thyroid E04.1
  cutaneous — see Swelling, localized
  endometrial (stromal) D26.1
  Haygarth's M15.8
  inflammatory — see Inflammation
  juxta-articular
    syphilitic A52.77
    yaws A66.7
  larynx J38.7
  lung, solitary (subsegmental branch of the bronchial
      tree) R91.1
    multiple R91.8
  milker's B08.03
  prostate N40.2
    with lower urinary tract symptoms (LUTS) N40.3
    without lower urinary tract symtpoms (LUTS) N40.2
  pulmonary, solitary (subsegmental branch of the
      bronchial tree) R91.1
  retrocardiac R09.89
  rheumatoid M06.30
    ankle M06.37- ☑
    elbow M06.32- ☑
    foot joint M06.37- ☑
    hand joint M06.34- ☑
    hip M06.35- ☑
    knee M06.36- ☑
    multiple site M06.39
    shoulder M06.31- ☑
    vertebra M06.38
    wrist M06.33- ☑
  scrotum (inflammatory) N49.2
  singer's J38.2
  solitary, lung (subsegmental branch of the bronchial
      tree) R91.1
    multiple R91.8
  subcutaneous — see Swelling, localized
  teacher's J38.2
  thyroid (cold) (gland) (nontoxic) E04.1
    with thyrotoxicosis E05.20
      with thyroid storm E05.21
    toxic or with hyperthyroidism E05.20
      with thyroid storm E05.21

Nodule(s), **nodular** — *continued*
  vocal cord J38.2
Noma (gangrenous) (hospital) (infective) A69.0
  auricle I96
  mouth A69.0
  pudendi N76.89
  vulvae N76.89
Nomad, nomadism Z59.0
NOMID (neonatal onset multisystemic inflammatory disorder) M04.2
Nonadherence to medical treatment Z91.19
Nonautoimmune hemolytic anemia D59.4
  drug-induced D59.2
Nonclosure (*see also* Imperfect, closure)
  ductus arteriosus (Botallo's) Q25.0
  foramen
    botalli Q21.1
    ovale Q21.1
Noncompliance Z91.19
  with
    dialysis Z91.15
    dietary regimen Z91.11
    medical treatment Z91.19
    medication regimen NEC Z91.14
      underdosing (*see also* Table of Drugs and Chemicals, categories T36-T50, with final character 6) Z91.14
        intentional NEC Z91.128
          due to financial hardship of patient Z91.120
        unintentional NEC Z91.138
          due to patient's age related debility Z91.130
    renal dialysis Z91.15
Nondescent (congenital) (*see also* Malposition, congenital)
  cecum Q43.3
  colon Q43.3
  testicle Q53.9
    bilateral Q53.20
      abdominal Q53.211
      perineal Q53.22
    unilateral Q53.10
      abdominal Q53.111
      perineal Q53.12
Nondevelopment
  brain Q02
    part of Q04.3
  heart Q24.8
  organ or site, congenital NEC — *see* Hypoplasia
Nonengagement
  head NEC O32.4 ☑
    in labor, causing obstructed labor O64.8 ☑
Nonexanthematous tick fever A93.2
Nonexpansion, lung (newborn) P28.0
Nonfunctioning
  cystic duct (*see also* Disease, gallbladder) K82.8
  gallbladder (*see also* Disease, gallbladder) K82.8
  kidney N28.9
  labyrinth — *see* subcategory H83.2 ☑
Non-Hodgkin lymphoma NEC — *see* Lymphoma, non-Hodgkin
Nonimplantation, ovum N97.2
Noninsufflation, fallopian tube N97.1
Non-ketotic hyperglycinemia E72.51
Nonne-Milroy syndrome Q82.0
Nonovulation N97.0
Non-palpable testicle(s)
  bilateral R39.84
  unilateral R39.83
Nonpatent fallopian tube N97.1
Nonpneumatization, lung NEC P28.0
Nonrotation — *see* Malrotation
Nonsecretion, urine — *see* Anuria
Nonunion
  fracture — *see* Fracture, by site
  joint, following fusion or arthrodesis M96.0
  organ or site, congenital NEC — *see* Imperfect, closure
  symphysis pubis, congenital Q74.2
Nonvisualization, gallbladder R93.2
Nonvital, nonvitalized tooth K04.99
Non-working side interference M26.56
Noonan's syndrome Q87.1
Normocytic anemia (infectional) due to blood loss (chronic) D50.0
  acute D62
Norrie's disease (congenital) Q15.8

North American blastomycosis B40.9
Norwegian itch B86
Nose, nasal — *see* condition
Nosebleed R04.0
Nose-picking F98.8
Nosomania F45.21
Nosophobia F45.22
Nostalgia F43.20
Notch of iris Q13.2
Notching nose, congenital (tip) Q30.2
Nothnagel's
  syndrome — *see* Strabismus, paralytic, third nerve
  vasomotor acroparesthesia I73.89
Novy's relapsing fever A68.9
  louse-borne A68.0
  tick-borne A68.1
Noxious
  foodstuffs, poisoning by — *see* Poisoning, food, noxious, plant
  substances transmitted through placenta or breast milk P04.9
Nucleus pulposus — *see* condition
Numbness R20.0
Nuns' knee — *see* Bursitis, prepatellar
Nursemaid's elbow S53.03- ☑
Nutcracker esophagus K22.4
Nutmeg liver K76.1
Nutrient element deficiency E61.9
  specified NEC E61.8
Nutrition deficient or insufficient (*see also* Malnutrition) E46
  due to
    insufficient food T73.0 ☑
    lack of
      care (child) T76.02 ☑
        adult T76.01 ☑
      food T73.0 ☑
Nutritional stunting E45
Nyctalopia (night blindness) — *see* Blindness, night
Nycturia R35.1
  psychogenic F45.8
Nymphomania F52.8
Nystagmus H55.00
  benign paroxysmal — *see* Vertigo, benign paroxysmal
  central positional H81.4- ☑
  congenital H55.01
  dissociated H55.04
  latent H55.02
  miners' H55.09
  positional
    benign paroxysmal H81.4- ☑
    central H81.4- ☑
  specified form NEC H55.09
  visual deprivation H55.03

O

Obermeyer's relapsing fever (European) A68.0
Obesity E66.9
  with alveolar hypoventilation E66.2
  adrenal E27.8
  complicating
    childbirth O99.214
    pregnancy O99.21- ☑
    puerperium O99.215
  constitutional E66.8
  dietary counseling and surveillance Z71.3
  drug-induced E66.1
  due to
    drug E66.1
    excess calories E66.09
      morbid E66.01
      severe E66.01
  endocrine E66.8
  endogenous E66.8
  exogenous E66.09
  familial E66.8
  glandular E66.8
  hypothyroid — *see* Hypothyroidism
  hypoventilation syndrome (OHS) E66.2
  morbid E66.01
    with
      alveolar hypoventilation E66.2
      obesity hypoventilation syndrome (OHS) E66.2
    due to excess calories E66.01
  nutritional E66.09
  pituitary E23.6

Obesity — *continued*
  severe E66.01
  specified type NEC E66.8
Oblique — *see* condition
Obliteration
  appendix (lumen) K38.8
  artery I77.1
  bile duct (noncalculous) K83.1
  common duct (noncalculous) K83.1
  cystic duct — *see* Obstruction, gallbladder
  disease, arteriolar I77.1
  endometrium N85.8
  eye, anterior chamber — *see* Disorder, globe, hypotony
  fallopian tube N97.1
  lymphatic vessel I89.0
    due to mastectomy I97.2
  organ or site, congenital NEC — *see* Atresia, by site
  ureter N13.5
    with infection N13.6
  urethra — *see* Stricture, urethra
  vein I87.8
  vestibule (oral) K08.89
Observation (following) (for) (without need for further medical care) Z04.9
  accident NEC Z04.3
    at work Z04.2
    transport Z04.1
  adverse effect of drug Z03.6
  alleged rape or sexual assault (victim), ruled out
    adult Z04.41
    child Z04.42
  criminal assault Z04.8
  development state
    adolescent Z00.3
    period of rapid growth in childhood Z00.2
    puberty Z00.3
  disease, specified NEC Z03.89
  following work accident Z04.2
  growth and development state — *see* Observation, development state
  injuries (accidental) NEC (*see also* Observation, accident)
  newborn (for)
    suspected condition, related to exposure from the mother or birth process — *see* Newborn, affected by, maternal
    ruled out Z05.9
      cardiac Z05.0
      connective tissue Z05.73
      gastrointestinal Z05.5
      genetic Z05.41
      genitourinary Z05.6
      immunologic Z05.43
      infectious Z05.1
      metabolic Z05.42
      musculoskeletal Z05.72
      neurological Z05.2
      respiratory Z05.3
      skin and subcutaneous tissue Z05.71
      specified condition NEC Z05.8
  postpartum
    immediately after delivery Z39.0
    routine follow-up Z39.2
  pregnancy (normal) (without complication) Z34.9- ☑
    high risk O09.9- ☑
  suicide attempt, alleged NEC Z03.89
    self-poisoning Z03.6
  suspected, ruled out (*see also* Suspected condition, ruled out)
    abuse, physical
      adult Z04.71
      child Z04.72
    accident at work Z04.2
    adult battering victim Z04.71
    child battering victim Z04.72
    condition NEC Z03.89
      newborn (*see also* Observation, newborn (for), suspected condition, ruled out) Z05.9
    drug poisoning or adverse effect Z03.6
    exposure (to)
      anthrax Z03.810
      biological agent NEC Z03.818
    inflicted injury NEC Z04.8
    suicide attempt, alleged Z03.89
      self-poisoning Z03.6
    toxic effects from ingested substance (drug) (poison) Z03.6

⚕ Subterms under main terms may continue to next column or page   ☑ Additional Character Required — Refer to the Tabular List for Character Selection   235

Nodule — Observation

Observation — *continued*
  toxic effects from ingested substance (drug) (poison) Z03.6
Obsession, obsessional state F42.8
  mixed thoughts and acts F42.2
Obsessive-compulsive neurosis or reaction F42.8
Obstetric embolism, septic — *see* Embolism, obstetric, septic
Obstetrical trauma (complicating delivery) O71.9
  with or following ectopic or molar pregnancy O08.6
  specified type NEC O71.89
Obstipation — *see* Constipation
Obstruction, obstructed, obstructive
  airway J98.8
    with
      allergic alveolitis J67.9
      asthma J45.909
        with
          exacerbation (acute) J45.901
          status asthmaticus J45.902
      bronchiectasis J47.9
        with
          exacerbation (acute) J47.1
          lower respiratory infection J47.0
      bronchitis (chronic) J44.9
      emphysema J43.9
    chronic J44.9
      with
        allergic alveolitis — *see* Pneumonitis, hypersensitivity
        bronchiectasis J47.9
          with
            exacerbation (acute) J47.1
            lower respiratory infection J47.0
    due to
      foreign body — *see* Foreign body, by site, causing asphyxia
      inhalation of fumes or vapors J68.9
      laryngospasm J38.5
  ampulla of Vater K83.1
  aortic (heart) (valve) — *see* Stenosis, aortic
  aortoiliac I74.09
  aqueduct of Sylvius G91.1
    congenital Q03.0
      with spina bifida — *see* Spina bifida, by site, with hydrocephalus
  Arnold-Chiari — *see* Arnold-Chiari disease
  artery (*see also* Atherosclerosis, artery) I70.9 ☑
    basilar (complete) (partial) — *see* Occlusion, artery, basilar
    carotid (complete) (partial) — *see* Occlusion, artery, carotid
    cerebellar — *see* Occlusion, artery, cerebellar
    cerebral (anterior) (middle) (posterior) — *see* Occlusion, artery, cerebral
    precerebral — *see* Occlusion, artery, precerebral
    renal N28.0
    retinal NEC — *see* Occlusion, artery, retina
    stent — *see* Restenosis, stent
    vertebral (complete) (partial) — *see* Occlusion, artery, vertebral
  band (intestinal) (*see also* Obstruction, intestine, specified NEC) K56.699
  bile duct or passage (common) (hepatic) (noncalculous) K83.1
    with calculus K80.51
    congenital (causing jaundice) Q44.3
  biliary (duct) (tract) K83.1
    gallbladder K82.0
  bladder-neck (acquired) N32.0
    congenital Q64.31
    due to hyperplasia (hypertrophy) of prostate — *see* Hyperplasia, prostate
  bowel — *see* Obstruction, intestine
  bronchus J98.09
  canal, ear — *see* Stenosis, external ear canal
  cardia K22.2
  caval veins (inferior) (superior) I87.1
  cecum — *see* Obstruction, intestine
  circulatory I99.8
  colon — *see* Obstruction, intestine
  common duct (noncalculous) K83.1
  coronary (artery) — *see* Occlusion, coronary
  cystic duct (*see also* Obstruction, gallbladder)
    with calculus K80.21
  device, implant or graft (*see also* Complications, by site and type, mechanical) T85.698 ☑

Obstruction, obstructed, obstructive — *continued*
  device, implant or graft (*see also* Complications, by site and type, mechanical) — *continued*
    arterial graft NEC — *see* Complication, cardiovascular device, mechanical, vascular
    catheter NEC T85.628 ☑
      cystostomy T83.090 ☑
      dialysis (renal) T82.49 ☑
        intraperitoneal T85.691 ☑
      Hopkins T83.098 ☑
      ileostomy T83.098 ☑
      infusion NEC T82.594 ☑
        spinal (epidural) (subdural) T85.690 ☑
      nephrostomy T83.092 ☑
      urethral indwelling T83.091 ☑
      urinary T83.098 ☑
      urostomy T83.098 ☑
    due to infection T85.79 ☑
    gastrointestinal — *see* Complications, prosthetic device, mechanical, gastrointestinal device
    genital NEC T83.498 ☑
      intrauterine contraceptive device T83.39 ☑
      penile prosthesis (cylinder) (implanted) (pump) (resevoir) T83.490 ☑
      testicular prosthesis T83.491 ☑
    heart NEC — *see* Complication, cardiovascular device, mechanical
    joint prosthesis — *see* Complications, joint prosthesis, mechanical, specified NEC, by site
    orthopedic NEC — *see* Complication, orthopedic, device, mechanical
    specified NEC T85.628 ☑
    urinary NEC (*see also* Complication, genitourinary, device, urinary, mechanical)
      graft T83.29 ☑
    vascular NEC — *see* Complication, cardiovascular device, mechanical
    ventricular intracranial shunt T85.09 ☑
  due to foreign body accidentally left in operative wound T81.529 ☑
  duodenum K31.5
  ejaculatory duct N50.89
  esophagus K22.2
  eustachian tube (complete) (partial) H68.10- ☑
    cartilagenous (extrinsic) H68.13- ☑
      intrinsic H68.12- ☑
    osseous H68.11- ☑
  fallopian tube (bilateral) N97.1
  fecal K56.41
    with hernia — *see* Hernia, by site, with obstruction
  foramen of Monro (congenital) Q03.8
    with spina bifida — *see* Spina bifida, by site, with hydrocephalus
  foreign body — *see* Foreign body
  gallbladder K82.0
    with calculus, stones K80.21
    congenital Q44.1
  gastric outlet K31.1
  gastrointestinal — *see* Obstruction, intestine
  hepatic K76.89
    duct (noncalculous) K83.1
  ileum — *see* Obstruction, intestine
  iliofemoral (artery) I74.5
  intestine K56.609
    with
      adhesions (intestinal) (peritoneal) K56.50
        complete K56.52
        incomplete K56.51
        partial K56.51
    adynamic K56.0
    by gallstone K56.3
    complete K56.601
    congenital (small) Q41.9
      large Q42.9
        specified part NEC Q42.8
    incomplete K56.600
    neurogenic K56.0
      Hirschsprung's disease or megacolon Q43.1
    newborn P76.9
      due to
        fecaliths P76.8
        inspissated milk P76.2
        meconium (plug) P76.0
          in mucoviscidosis E84.11
      specified NEC P76.8
    partial K56.600
    postoperative K91.30

Obstruction, obstructed, obstructive — *continued*
  intestine — *continued*
    postoperative — *continued*
      complete K91.32
      incomplete K91.31
      partial K91.31
    reflex K56.0
    specified NEC K56.699
      complete K56.691
      incomplete K56.690
      partial K56.690
    volvulus K56.2
  intracardiac ball valve prosthesis T82.09 ☑
  jejunum — *see* Obstruction, intestine
  joint prosthesis — *see* Complications, joint prosthesis, mechanical, specified NEC, by site
  kidney (calices) N28.89
  labor — *see* Delivery
  lacrimal (passages) (duct)
    by
      dacryolith — *see* Dacryolith
      stenosis — *see* Stenosis, lacrimal
    congenital Q10.5
    neonatal H04.53- ☑
  lacrimonasal duct — *see* Obstruction, lacrimal
  lacteal, with steatorrhea K90.2
  laryngitis — *see* Laryngitis
  larynx NEC J38.6
    congenital Q31.8
  lung J98.4
    disease, chronic J44.9
  lymphatic I89.0
  meconium (plug)
    newborn P76.0
      due to fecaliths P76.0
      in mucoviscidosis E84.11
  mitral — *see* Stenosis, mitral
  nasal J34.89
  nasolacrimal duct (*see also* Obstruction, lacrimal)
    congenital Q10.5
  nasopharynx J39.2
  nose J34.89
  organ or site, congenital NEC — *see* Atresia, by site
  pancreatic duct K86.89
  parotid duct or gland K11.8
  pelviureteral junction N13.5
    with hydronephrosis N13.0
    congenital Q62.39
  pharynx J39.2
  portal (circulation) (vein) I81
  prostate (*see also* Hyperplasia, prostate)
    valve (urinary) N32.0
  pulmonary valve (heart) I37.0
  pyelonephritis (chronic) N11.1
  pylorus
    adult K31.1
    congenital or infantile Q40.0
  rectosigmoid — *see* Obstruction, intestine
  rectum K62.4
  renal N28.89
    outflow N13.8
    pelvis, congenital Q62.39
  respiratory J98.8
    chronic J44.9
  retinal (vessels) H34.9
  salivary duct (any) K11.8
    with calculus K11.5
  sigmoid — *see* Obstruction, intestine
  sinus (accessory) (nasal) J34.89
  Stensen's duct K11.8
  stomach NEC K31.89
    acute K31.0
    congenital Q40.2
    due to pylorospasm K31.3
  submandibular duct K11.8
  submaxillary gland K11.8
    with calculus K11.5
  thoracic duct I89.0
  thrombotic — *see* Thrombosis
  trachea J39.8
  tracheostomy airway J95.03
  tricuspid (valve) — *see* Stenosis, tricuspid
  upper respiratory, congenital Q34.8
  ureter (functional) (pelvic junction) NEC N13.5
    with
      hydronephrosis N13.1
        with infection N13.6
      pyelonephritis (chronic) N11.1

Obstruction, obstructed, obstructive — *continued*
  ureter — *continued*
    congenital Q62.39
    due to calculus — *see* Calculus, ureter
  urethra NEC N36.8
    congenital Q64.39
  urinary (moderate) N13.9
    due to hyperplasia (hypertrophy) of prostate —
      see Hyperplasia, prostate
    organ or tract (lower) N13.9
    prostatic valve N32.0
    specified NEC N13.8
  uropathy N13.9
  uterus N85.8
  vagina N89.5
  valvular — *see* Endocarditis
  vein, venous I87.1
    caval (inferior) (superior) I87.1
    thrombotic — *see* Thrombosis
    vena cava (inferior) (superior) I87.1
  vesical NEC N32.0
  vesicourethral orifice N32.0
    congenital Q64.31
  vessel NEC I99.8
    stent — *see* Restenosis, stent
Obturator — *see* condition
Occlusal wear, teeth K03.0
Occlusio pupillae — *see* Membrane, pupillary
Occlusion, occluded
  anus K62.4
    congenital Q42.3
      with fistula Q42.2
  aortoiliac (chronic) I74.09
  aqueduct of Sylvius G91.1
    congenital Q03.0
      with spina bifida — *see* Spina bifida, by site,
        with hydrocephalus
  artery (*see also* Atherosclerosis, artery) I70.9 ☑
    auditory, internal I65.8
    basilar I65.1
      with
        infarction I63.22
          due to
            embolism I63.12
            thrombosis I63.02
    brain or cerebral I66.9
      with infarction (due to) I63.5- ☑
        embolism I63.4- ☑
        thrombosis I63.3- ☑
    carotid I65.2- ☑
      with
        infarction I63.23- ☑
          due to
            embolism I63.13- ☑
            thrombosis I63.03- ☑
    cerebellar (anterior inferior) (posterior inferior)
      (superior) I66.3
      with infarction I63.54- ☑
        due to
          embolism I63.44- ☑
          thrombosis I63.34- ☑
    cerebral I66.9
      with infarction I63.50
        due to
          embolism I63.40
            specified NEC I63.49
          thrombosis I63.30
            specified NEC I63.39
      anterior I66.1-
        with infarction I63.52- ☑
          due to
            embolism I63.42- ☑
            thrombosis I63.32- ☑
      middle I66.0- ☑
        with infarction I63.51- ☑
          due to
            embolism I63.41- ☑
            thrombosis I63.31- ☑
      posterior I66.2- ☑
        with infarction I63.53- ☑
          due to
            embolism I63.43- ☑
            thrombosis I63.33- ☑
      specified NEC I66.8
        with infarction I63.59
          due to
            embolism I63.4- ☑

Occlusion, occluded — *continued*
  artery (*see also* Atherosclerosis, artery) — *contin-
    ued*
    cerebral — *continued*
      specified — *continued*
        with infarction — *continued*
          due to — *continued*
            thrombosis I63.3- ☑
    choroidal (anterior) — *see* Occlusion, artery, pre-
      cerebral, specified NEC
    communicating posterior — *see* Occlusion, artery,
      precerebral, specified NEC
    complete
      coronary I25.82
      extremities I70.92
    coronary (acute) (thrombotic) (without myocardial
      infarction) I24.0
      with myocardial infarction — *see* Infarction,
        myocardium
      chronic total I25.82
      complete I25.82
      healed or old I25.2
      total (chronic) I25.82
    hypophyseal — *see* Occlusion, artery, precerebral,
      specified NEC
    iliac I74.5
    lower extremities due to stenosis or stricture I77.1
    mesenteric (embolic) (thrombotic) (*see also* Infarct,
      intestine) K55.069
    perforating — *see* Occlusion, artery, cerebral,
      specified NEC
    peripheral I77.9
      thrombotic or embolic I74.4
    pontine — *see* Occlusion, artery, precerebral,
      specified NEC
    precerebral I65.9
      with infarction I63.20
        due to
          embolism I63.10
            specified NEC I63.19
          thrombosis I63.00
            specified NEC I63.09
        specified NEC I63.29
      basilar — *see* Occlusion, artery, basilar
      carotid — *see* Occlusion, artery, carotid
      puerperal O88.23
      specified NEC I65.8
        with infarction I63.29
          due to
            embolism I63.19
            thrombosis I63.09
      vertebral — *see* Occlusion, artery, vertebral
    renal N28.0
    retinal
      branch H34.23- ☑
      central H34.1- ☑
      partial H34.21- ☑
      transient H34.0- ☑
    spinal — *see* Occlusion, artery, precerebral, verte-
      bral
    total (chronic)
      coronary I25.82
      extremities I70.92
    vertebral I65.0- ☑
      with
        infarction I63.21- ☑
          due to
            embolism I63.11- ☑
            thrombosis I63.01- ☑
  basilar artery — *see* Occlusion, artery, basilar
  bile duct (common) (hepatic) (noncalculous) K83.1
  bowel — *see* Obstruction, intestine
  carotid (artery) (common) (internal) — *see* Occlusion,
    artery, carotid
  centric (of teeth) M26.59
    maximum intercuspation discrepancy M26.55
  cerebellar (artery) — *see* Occlusion, artery, cerebellar
  cerebral (artery) — *see* Occlusion, artery, cerebral
  cerebrovascular (*see also* Occlusion, artery, cerebral)
    with infarction I63.5- ☑
  cervical canal — *see* Stricture, cervix
  cervix (uteri) — *see* Stricture, cervix
  choanal Q30.0
  choroidal (artery) — *see* Occlusion, artery, precerebral,
    specified NEC
  colon — *see* Obstruction, intestine
  communicating posterior artery — *see* Occlusion,
    artery, precerebral, specified NEC

Occlusion, occluded — *continued*
  coronary (artery) (vein) (thrombotic) (*see also* Infarct,
    myocardium)
    chronic total I25.82
    healed or old I25.2
    not resulting in infarction I24.0
    total (chronic) I25.82
  cystic duct — *see* Obstruction, gallbladder
  embolic — *see* Embolism
  fallopian tube N97.1
    congenital Q50.6
  gallbladder (*see also* Obstruction, gallbladder)
    congenital (causing jaundice) Q44.1
  gingiva, traumatic K06.2
  hymen N89.6
    congenital Q52.3
  hypophyseal (artery) — *see* Occlusion, artery, precere-
    bral, specified NEC
  iliac artery I74.5
  intestine — *see* Obstruction, intestine
  lacrimal passages — *see* Obstruction, lacrimal
  lung J98.4
  lymph or lymphatic channel I89.0
  mammary duct N64.89
  mesenteric artery (embolic) (thrombotic) (*see also* In-
    farct, intestine) K55.069
  nose J34.89
    congenital Q30.0
  organ or site, congenital NEC — *see* Atresia, by site
  oviduct N97.1
    congenital Q50.6
  peripheral arteries
    due to stricture or stenosis I77.1
    upper extremity I74.2
  pontine (artery) — *see* Occlusion, artery, precerebral,
    specified NEC
  posterior lingual, of mandibular teeth M26.29
  precerebral artery — *see* Occlusion, artery, precerebral
  punctum lacrimale — *see* Obstruction, lacrimal
  pupil — *see* Membrane, pupillary
  pylorus, adult (*see also* Stricture, pylorus) K31.1
  renal artery N28.0
  retina, retinal
    artery — *see* Occlusion, artery, retinal
    vein (central) H34.81- ☑
      engorgement H34.82- ☑
      tributary H34.83- ☑
    vessels H34.9
  spinal artery — *see* Occlusion, artery, precerebral,
    vertebral
  teeth (mandibular) (posterior lingual) M26.29
  thoracic duct I89.0
  thrombotic — *see* Thrombosis, artery
  traumatic
    edentulous (alveolar) ridge K06.2
    gingiva K06.2
    periodontal K05.5
  tubal N97.1
  ureter (complete) (partial) N13.5
    congenital Q62.10
  ureteropelvic junction N13.5
    congenital Q62.11
  ureterovesical orifice N13.5
    congenital Q62.12
  urethra — *see* Stricture, urethra
  uterus N85.8
  vagina N89.5
  vascular NEC I99.8
  vein — *see* Thrombosis
    retinal — *see* Occlusion, retinal, vein
  vena cava (inferior) (superior) — *see* Embolism, vena
    cava
  ventricle (brain) NEC G91.1
  vertebral (artery) — *see* Occlusion, artery, vertebral
  vessel (blood) I99.8
  vulva N90.5
Occult
  blood in feces (stools) R19.5
Occupational
  problems NEC Z56.89
Ochlophobia — *see* Agoraphobia
Ochronosis (endogenous) E70.29
Ocular muscle — *see* condition
Oculogyric crisis or disturbance H51.8
  psychogenic F45.8
Oculomotor syndrome H51.9
Oculopathy
  syphilitic NEC A52.71

Oculopathy — *continued*
  syphilitic — *continued*
    congenital
      early A50.01
      late A50.30
    early (secondary) A51.43
    late A52.71
Oddi's sphincter spasm K83.4
Odontalgia K08.89
Odontoameloblastoma — *see* Cyst, calcifying odontogenic
Odontoclasia K03.89
Odontodysplasia, regional K00.4
Odontogenesis imperfecta K00.5
Odontoma (ameloblastic) (complex) (compound) (fibroameloblastic) — *see* Cyst, calcifying odontogenic
Odontomyelitis (closed) (open) K04.01
  irreversible K04.02
  reversible K04.01
Odontorrhagia K08.89
Odontosarcoma, ameloblastic C41.1
  upper jaw (bone) C41.0
Oestriasis — *see* Myiasis
Oguchi's disease H53.63
Ohara's disease — *see* Tularemia
OHS (obesity hypoventilation syndrome) E66.2
Oidiomycosis — *see* Candidiasis
Oidium albicans infection — *see* Candidiasis
Old age (without mention of debility) R54
  dementia F03 ☑
Old (previous) **myocardial infarction** I25.2
Olfactory — *see* condition
Oligemia — *see* Anemia
Oligoastrocytoma
  specified site — *see* Neoplasm, malignant, by site
  unspecified site C71.9
Oligocythemia D64.9
Oligodendroblastoma
  specified site — *see* Neoplasm, malignant
  unspecified site C71.9
Oligodendroglioma
  anaplastic type
    specified site — *see* Neoplasm, malignant, by site
    unspecified site C71.9
  specified site — *see* Neoplasm, malignant, by site
  unspecified site C71.9
Oligodontia — *see* Anodontia
Oligoencephalon Q02
Oligohidrosis L74.4
Oligohydramnios O41.0- ☑
Oligohydrosis L74.4
Oligomenorrhea N91.5
  primary N91.3
  secondary N91.4
Oligophrenia (*see also* Disability, intellectual)
  phenylpyruvic E70.0
Oligospermia N46.11
  due to
    drug therapy N46.121
    efferent duct obstruction N46.123
    infection N46.122
    radiation N46.124
    specified cause NEC N46.129
    systemic disease N46.125
Oligotrichia — *see* Alopecia
Oliguria R34
  postprocedural N99.0
  with, complicating or following ectopic or molar
    pregnancy O08.4
Ollier's disease Q78.4
Omenotocele — *see* Hernia, abdomen, specified site
  NEC
Omentitis — *see* Peritonitis
Omentum, omental — *see* condition
Omphalitis (congenital) (newborn) P38.9
  with mild hemorrhage P38.1
  without hemorrhage P38.9
  not of newborn L08.82
  tetanus A33
Omphalocele Q79.2
Omphalomesenteric duct, persistent Q43.0
Omphalorrhagia, newborn P51.9
Omsk hemorrhagic fever A98.1
Onanism (excessive) F98.8
Onchocerciasis, onchocercosis B73.1
  with
    eye disease B73.00

Onchocerciasis, onchocercosis — *continued*
  with — *continued*
    eye disease — *continued*
      endophthalmitis B73.01
      eyelid B73.09
      glaucoma B73.02
      specified NEC B73.09
  eyelid B73.09
  eye NEC B73.00
Oncocytoma — *see* Neoplasm, benign, by site
Oncovirus, as cause of disease classified elsewhere B97.32
Ondine's curse — *see* Apnea, sleep
Oneirophrenia F23
Onychauxis L60.2
  congenital Q84.5
Onychia (*see also* Cellulitis, digit)
  with lymphangitis — *see* Lymphangitis, acute, digit
  candidal B37.2
  dermatophytic B35.1
Onychitis (*see also* Cellulitis, digit)
  with lymphangitis — *see* Lymphangitis, acute, digit
Onychocryptosis L60.0
Onychodystrophy L60.3
  congenital Q84.6
Onychogryphosis, onychogryposis L60.2
Onycholysis L60.1
Onychomadesis L60.8
Onychomalacia L60.3
Onychomycosis (finger) (toe) B35.1
Onycho-osteodysplasia Q87.2
Onychophagia F98.8
Onychophosis L60.8
Onychoptosis L60.8
Onychorrhexis L60.3
  congenital Q84.6
Onychoschizia L60.3
Onyxis (finger) (toe) L60.0
Onyxitis (*see also* Cellulitis, digit)
  with lymphangitis — *see* Lymphangitis, acute, digit
Oophoritis (cystic) (infectional) (interstitial) N70.92
  with salpingitis N70.93
  acute N70.02
    with salpingitis N70.03
  chronic N70.12
    with salpingitis N70.13
  complicating abortion — *see* Abortion, by type, complicated by, oophoritis
Oophorocele N83.4- ☑
Opacity, opacities
  cornea H17.-
    central H17.1- ☑
    congenital Q13.3
    degenerative — *see* Degeneration, cornea
    hereditary — *see* Dystrophy, cornea
    inflammatory — *see* Keratitis
    minor H17.81- ☑
    peripheral H17.82- ☑
    sequelae of trachoma (healed) B94.0
    specified NEC H17.89
  enamel (teeth) (fluoride) (nonfluoride) K00.3
  lens — *see* Cataract
  snowball — *see* Deposit, crystalline
  vitreous (humor) NEC H43.39- ☑
    congenital Q14.0
    membranes and strands H43.31- ☑
Opalescent dentin (hereditary) K00.5
Open, opening
  abnormal, organ or site, congenital — *see* Imperfect,
    closure
  angle with
    borderline
      findings
        high risk H40.02- ☑
        low risk H40.01- ☑
      intraocular pressure H40.00- ☑
    cupping of discs H40.01- ☑
    glaucoma (primary) — *see* Glaucoma, open angle
  bite
    anterior M26.220
    posterior M26.221
  false — *see* Imperfect, closure
  margin on tooth restoration K08.51
  restoration margins of tooth K08.51
  wound — *see* Wound, open
Operational fatigue F48.8
Operative — *see* condition

Operculitis — *see* Periodontitis
Operculum — *see* Break, retina
Ophiasis L63.2
Ophthalmia (*see also* Conjunctivitis) H10.9
  actinic rays — *see* Photokeratitis
  allergic (acute) — *see* Conjunctivitis, acute, atopic
  blennorrhagic (gonococcal) (neonatorum) A54.31
  diphtheritic A36.86
  Egyptian A71.1
  electrica — *see* Photokeratitis
  gonococcal (neonatorum) A54.31
  metastatic — *see* Endophthalmitis, purulent
  migraine — *see* Migraine, ophthalmoplegic
  neonatorum, newborn P39.1
    gonococcal A54.31
  nodosa H16.24- ☑
  purulent — *see* Conjunctivitis, acute, mucopurulent
  spring — *see* Conjunctivitis, acute, atopic
  sympathetic — *see* Uveitis, sympathetic
Ophthalmitis — *see* Ophthalmia
Ophthalmocele (congenital) Q15.8
Ophthalmoneuromyelitis G36.0
Ophthalmoplegia (*see also* Strabismus, paralytic)
  anterior internuclear — *see* Ophthalmoplegia, internuclear
  ataxia-areflexia G61.0
  diabetic — *see* E08-E13 with .39
  exophthalmic E05.00
    with thyroid storm E05.01
  external H49.88- ☑
    progressive H49.4- ☑
      with pigmentary retinopathy — *see* Kearns-Sayre syndrome
    total H49.3- ☑
  internal (complete) (total) H52.51- ☑
  internuclear H51.2- ☑
  migraine — *see* Migraine, ophthalmoplegic
  Parinaud's H49.88- ☑
  progressive external — *see* Ophthalmoplegia, external, progressive
  supranuclear, progressive G23.1
  total (external) — *see* Ophthalmoplegia, external, total
Opioid(s)
  abuse — *see* Abuse, drug, opioids
  dependence — *see* Dependence, drug, opioids
  induced, without use disorder
    anxiety disorder F11.988
    delirium F11.921
    depressive disorder F11.94
    sexual dysfunction F11.981
    sleep disorder F11.982
Opisthognathism M26.09
Opisthorchiasis (felineus) (viverrini) B66.0
Opitz' disease D73.2
Opiumism — *see* Dependence, drug, opioid
Oppenheim's disease G70.2
Oppenheim-Urbach disease (necrobiosis lipoidica diabeticorum) — *see* E08-E13 with .620
Optic nerve — *see* condition
Orbit — *see* condition
Orchioblastoma C62.9- ☑
Orchitis (gangrenous) (nonspecific) (septic) (suppurative) N45.2
  blennorrhagic (gonococcal) (acute) (chronic) A54.23
  chlamydial A56.19
  filarial (*see also* Infestation, filarial) B74.9 [N51]
  gonococcal (acute) (chronic) A54.23
  mumps B26.0
  syphilitic A52.76
  tuberculous A18.15
Orf (virus disease) B08.02
Organic (*see also* condition)
  brain syndrome F09
  heart — *see* Disease, heart
  mental disorder F09
  psychosis F09
Orgasm
  anejaculatory N53.13
Oriental
  bilharziasis B65.2
  schistosomiasis B65.2
Orifice — *see* condition
Origin of both great vessels from right ventricle Q20.1
Ormond's disease (with ureteral obstruction) N13.5
  with infection N13.6
Ornithine metabolism disorder E72.4

Ornithinemia (Type I) (Type II) E72.4
Ornithosis A70
Orotaciduria, oroticaciduria (congenital) (hereditary) (pyrimidine deficiency) E79.8
  anemia D53.0
Orthodontics
  adjustment Z46.4
  fitting Z46.4
Orthopnea R06.01
Orthopoxvirus B08.09
  specified NEC B08.09
Os, uterus — see condition
Osgood-Schlatter disease or osteochondrosis — see Osteochondrosis, juvenile, tibia
Osler (-Weber)-**Rendu disease** I78.0
Osler's nodes I33.0
Osmidrosis L75.0
Osseous — see condition
Ossification
  artery — see Arteriosclerosis
  auricle (ear) — see Disorder, pinna, specified type NEC
  bronchial J98.09
  cardiac — see Degeneration, myocardial
  cartilage (senile) — see Disorder, cartilage, specified type NEC
  coronary (artery) — see Disease, heart, ischemic, atherosclerotic
  diaphragm J98.6
  ear, middle — see Otosclerosis
  falx cerebri G96.19
  fontanel, premature Q75.0
  heart (see also Degeneration, myocardial)
    valve — see Endocarditis
  larynx J38.7
  ligament — see Disorder, tendon, specified type NEC
    posterior longitudinal — see Spondylopathy, specified NEC
  meninges (cerebral) (spinal) G96.19
  multiple, eccentric centers — see Disorder, bone, development or growth
  muscle (see also Calcification, muscle)
    due to burns — see Myositis, ossificans, in, burns
    paralytic — see Myositis, ossificans, in, quadriplegia
    progressive — see Myositis, ossificans, progressiva
    specified NEC M61.50
      ankle M61.57- ☑
      foot M61.57- ☑
      forearm M61.53- ☑
      hand M61.54- ☑
      lower leg M61.56- ☑
      multiple sites M61.59
      pelvic region M61.55- ☑
      shoulder region M61.51- ☑
      specified site NEC M61.58
      thigh M61.55- ☑
      upper arm M61.52- ☑
    traumatic — see Myositis, ossificans, traumatica
  myocardium, myocardial — see Degeneration, myocardial
  penis N48.89
  periarticular — see Disorder, joint, specified type NEC
  pinna — see Disorder, pinna, specified type NEC
  rider's bone — see Ossification, muscle, specified NEC
  sclera H15.89
  subperiosteal, post-traumatic M89.8X- ☑
  tendon — see Disorder, tendon, specified type NEC
  trachea J39.8
  tympanic membrane — see Disorder, tympanic membrane, specified NEC
  vitreous (humor) — see Deposit, crystalline
Osteitis (see also Osteomyelitis)
  alveolar M27.3
  condensans M85.30
    ankle M85.37- ☑
    foot M85.37- ☑
    forearm M85.33- ☑
    hand M85.34- ☑
    lower leg M85.36- ☑
    multiple site M85.39
    neck M85.38
    rib M85.38
    shoulder M85.31- ☑
    skull M85.38
    specified site NEC M85.38
    thigh M85.35- ☑
    toe M85.37- ☑
    upper arm M85.32- ☑

Osteitis — continued
  condensans — continued
    vertebra M85.38
  deformans M88.9
    in (due to)
      malignant neoplasm of bone C41.9 [M90.60]
      neoplastic disease (see also Neoplasm) D49.9 [M90.60]
        carpus D49.9 [M90.64-] ☑
        clavicle D49.9 [M90.61-] ☑
        femur D49.9 [M90.65-] ☑
        fibula D49.9 [M90.66-] ☑
        finger D49.9 [M90.64-] ☑
        humerus D49.9 [M90.62-] ☑
        ilium D49.9 [M90.65-] ☑
        ischium D49.9 [M90.65-] ☑
        metacarpus D49.9 [M90.64-] ☑
        metatarsus D49.9 [M90.67-] ☑
        multiple sites D49.9 [M90.69]
        neck D49.9 [M90.68]
        radius D49.9 [M90.63-] ☑
        rib D49.9 [M90.68]
        scapula D49.9 [M90.61-] ☑
        skull D49.9 [M90.68]
        tarsus D49.9 [M90.67-] ☑
        tibia D49.9 [M90.66-] ☑
        toe D49.9 [M90.67-] ☑
        ulna D49.9 [M90.63-] ☑
        vertebra D49.9 [M90.68]
    skull M88.0
    specified NEC — see Paget's disease, bone, by site
    vertebra M88.1
  due to yaws A66.6
  fibrosa NEC — see Cyst, bone, by site
    circumscripta — see Dysplasia, fibrous, bone NEC
    cystica (generalisata) E21.0
    disseminata Q78.1
    osteoplastica E21.0
  fragilitans Q78.0
  Garr's (sclerosing) — see Osteomyelitis, specified type NEC
  jaw (acute) (chronic) (lower) (suppurative) (upper) M27.2
  parathyroid E21.0
  petrous bone (acute) (chronic) — see Petrositis
  sclerotic, nonsuppurative — see Osteomyelitis, specified type NEC
  tuberculosa A18.09
    cystica D86.89
    multiplex cystoides D86.89
Osteoarthritis M19.90
  ankle M19.07- ☑
  elbow M19.02- ☑
  foot joint M19.07- ☑
  generalized M15.9
    erosive M15.4
    primary M15.0
    specified NEC M15.8
  hand joint M19.04- ☑
    first carpometacarpal joint M18.9
  hip M16.1- ☑
    bilateral M16.0
    due to hip dysplasia (unilateral) M16.3- ☑
      bilateral M16.2
  interphalangeal
    distal (Heberden) M15.1
    proximal (Bouchard) M15.2
  knee M17.1- ☑
    bilateral M17.0
  post-traumatic NEC M19.92
    ankle M19.17- ☑
    elbow M19.12- ☑
    foot joint M19.17- ☑
    hand joint M19.14- ☑
      first carpometacarpal joint M18.3- ☑
        bilateral M18.2
    hip M16.5- ☑
      bilateral M16.4
    knee M17.3- ☑
      bilateral M17.2
    shoulder M19.11- ☑
    wrist M19.13- ☑
  primary M19.91
    ankle M19.07- ☑
    elbow M19.02- ☑
    foot joint M19.07- ☑
    hand joint M19.04- ☑

Osteoarthritis — continued
  primary — continued
    hand joint — continued
      first carpometacarpal joint M18.1- ☑
        bilateral M18.0
    hip M16.1- ☑
      bilateral M16.0
    knee M17.1- ☑
      bilateral M17.0
    shoulder M19.01- ☑
    spine — see Spondylosis
    wrist M19.03- ☑
  secondary M19.93
    ankle M19.27- ☑
    elbow M19.22- ☑
    foot joint M19.27- ☑
    hand joint M19.24- ☑
      first carpometacarpal joint M18.5- ☑
        bilateral M18.4
    hip M16.7
      bilateral M16.6
    knee M17.5
      bilateral M17.4
    multiple M15.3
    shoulder M19.21- ☑
    spine — see Spondylosis
    wrist M19.23- ☑
  shoulder M19.01- ☑
  spine — see Spondylosis
  wrist M19.03- ☑
Osteoarthropathy (hypertrophic) M19.90
  ankle — see Osteoarthritis, primary, ankle
  elbow — see Osteoarthritis, primary, elbow
  foot joint — see Osteoarthritis, primary, foot
  hand joint — see Osteoarthritis, primary, hand joint
  knee joint — see Osteoarthritis, primary, knee
  multiple site — see Osteoarthritis, primary, multiple joint
  pulmonary (see also Osteoarthropathy, specified type NEC)
    hypertrophic — see Osteoarthropathy, hypertrophic, specified type NEC
  secondary — see Osteoarthropathy, specified type NEC
  secondary hypertrophic — see Osteoarthropathy, specified type NEC
  shoulder — see Osteoarthritis, primary, shoulder
  specified joint NEC — see Osteoarthritis, primary, specified joint NEC
  specified type NEC M89.40
    carpus M89.44- ☑
    clavicle M89.41- ☑
    femur M89.45- ☑
    fibula M89.46- ☑
    finger M89.44- ☑
    humerus M89.42- ☑
    ilium M89.459
    ischium M89.459
    metacarpus M89.44- ☑
    metatarsus M89.47- ☑
    multiple sites M89.49
    neck M89.48
    radius M89.43- ☑
    rib M89.48
    scapula M89.41- ☑
    skull M89.48
    tarsus M89.47- ☑
    tibia M89.46- ☑
    toe M89.47- ☑
    ulna M89.43- ☑
    vertebra M89.48
  spine — see Spondylosis
  wrist — see Osteoarthritis, primary, wrist
Osteoarthrosis (degenerative) (hypertrophic) (joint) (see also Osteoarthritis)
  deformans alkaptonurica E70.29 [M36.8]
  erosive M15.4
  generalized M15.9
    primary M15.0
  polyarticular M15.9
  spine — see Spondylosis
Osteoblastoma — see Neoplasm, bone, benign
  aggressive — see Neoplasm, bone, uncertain behavior
Osteochondritis (see also Osteochondropathy, by site)
  Brailsford's — see Osteochondrosis, juvenile, radius
  dissecans M93.20
    ankle M93.27- ☑

Osteochondritis — *continued*
  dissecans — *continued*
    elbow M93.22- ☑
    foot M93.27- ☑
    hand M93.24- ☑
    hip M93.25-
    knee M93.26- ☑
    multiple sites M93.29
    shoulder joint M93.21- ☑
    specified site NEC M93.28
    wrist M93.23- ☑
  juvenile M92.9
    patellar — *see* Osteochondrosis, juvenile, patella
  syphilitic (congenital) (early) A50.02 [M90.80]
    ankle A50.02 [M90.87-] ☑
    elbow A50.02 [M90.82-] ☑
    foot A50.02 [M90.87-] ☑
    forearm A50.02 [M90.83-] ☑
    hand A50.02 [M90.84-] ☑
    hip A50.02 [M90.85-] ☑
    knee A50.02 [M90.86-] ☑
    multiple sites A50.02 [M90.89]
    shoulder joint A50.02 [M90.81-] ☑
    specified site NEC A50.02 [M90.88]
Osteochondroarthrosis deformans endemica — *see* Disease, Kaschin-Beck
Osteochondrodysplasia Q78.9
  with defects of growth of tubular bones and spine Q77.9
    specified NEC Q77.8
  specified NEC Q78.8
Osteochondrodystrophy E78.9
Osteochondrolysis — *see* Osteochondritis, dissecans
Osteochondroma — *see* Neoplasm, bone, benign
Osteochondromatosis D48.0
  syndrome Q78.4
Osteochondromyxosarcoma — *see* Neoplasm, bone, malignant
Osteochondropathy M93.90
  ankle M93.97- ☑
  elbow M93.92- ☑
  foot M93.97- ☑
  hand M93.94- ☑
  hip M93.95- ☑
  Kienböck's disease of adults M93.1
  knee M93.96- ☑
  multiple joints M93.99
  osteochondritis dissecans — *see* Osteochondritis, dissecans
  osteochondrosis — *see* Osteochondrosis
  shoulder region M93.91- ☑
  slipped upper femoral epiphysis — *see* Slipped, epiphysis, upper femoral
  specified joint NEC M93.98
  specified type NEC M93.80
    ankle M93.87- ☑
    elbow M93.82- ☑
    foot M93.87- ☑
    hand M93.84- ☑
    hip M93.85- ☑
    knee M93.86- ☑
    multiple joints M93.89
    shoulder region M93.81- ☑
    specified joint NEC M93.88
    wrist M93.83- ☑
  syphilitic, congenital
    early A50.02 [M90.80]
    late A50.56 [M90.80]
  wrist M93.93- ☑
Osteochondrosarcoma — *see* Neoplasm, bone, malignant
Osteochondrosis (see also Osteochondropathy, by site)
  acetabulum (juvenile) M91.0
  adult — *see* Osteochondropathy, specified type NEC, by site
  astragalus (juvenile) — *see* Osteochondrosis, juvenile, tarsus
  Blount's — *see* Osteochondrosis, juvenile, tibia
  Buchanan's M91.0
  Burns' — *see* Osteochondrosis, juvenile, ulna
  calcaneus (juvenile) — *see* Osteochondrosis, juvenile, tarsus
  capitular epiphysis (femur) (juvenile) — *see* Legg-Calvé-Perthes disease
  carpal (juvenile) (lunate) (scaphoid) — *see* Osteochondrosis, juvenile, hand, carpal lunate
    adult M93.1

Osteochondrosis — *continued*
  coxae juvenilis — *see* Legg-Calvé-Perthes disease
  deformans juvenilis, coxae — *see* Legg-Calvé-Perthes disease
  Diaz's — *see* Osteochondrosis, juvenile, tarsus
  dissecans (knee) (shoulder) — *see* Osteochondritis, dissecans
  femoral capital epiphysis (juvenile) — *see* Legg-Calvé-Perthes disease
  femur (head), juvenile — *see* Legg-Calvé-Perthes disease
  fibula (juvenile) — *see* Osteochondrosis, juvenile, fibula
  foot NEC (juvenile) M92.8
  Freiberg's — *see* Osteochondrosis, juvenile, metatarsus
  Haas' (juvenile) — *see* Osteochondrosis, juvenile, humerus
  Haglund's — *see* Osteochondrosis, juvenile, tarsus
  hip (juvenile) — *see* Legg-Calvé-Perthes disease
  humerus (capitulum) (head) (juvenile) — *see* Osteochondrosis, juvenile, humerus
  ilium, iliac crest (juvenile) M91.0
  ischiopubic synchondrosis M91.0
  Iselin's — *see* Osteochondrosis, juvenile, metatarsus
  juvenile, juvenilis M92.9
    after congenital dislocation of hip reduction — *see* Osteochondrosis, juvenile, hip, specified NEC
    arm — *see* Osteochondrosis, juvenile, upper limb NEC
    capitular epiphysis (femur) — *see* Legg-Calvé-Perthes disease
    clavicle, sternal epiphysis — *see* Osteochondrosis, juvenile, upper limb NEC
    coxae — *see* Legg-Calvé-Perthes disease
    deformans M92.9
    fibula M92.5- ☑
    foot NEC M92.8
    hand M92.20- ☑
      carpal lunate M92.21- ☑
      metacarpal head M92.22- ☑
      specified site NEC M92.29- ☑
    head of femur — *see* Legg-Calvé-Perthes disease
    hip and pelvis M91.9- ☑
      coxa plana — *see* Coxa, plana
      femoral head — *see* Legg-Calvé-Perthes disease
      pelvis M91.0
      pseudocoxalgia — *see* Pseudocoxalgia
      specified NEC M91.8- ☑
    humerus M92.0- ☑
    limb
      lower NEC M92.8
      upper NEC — *see* Osteochondrosis, juvenile, upper limb NEC
    medial cuneiform bone — *see* Osteochondrosis, juvenile, tarsus
    metatarsus M92.7- ☑
    patella M92.4- ☑
    radius M92.1- ☑
    specified site NEC M92.8
    spine M42.00
      cervical region M42.02
      cervicothoracic region M42.03
      lumbar region M42.06
      lumbosacral region M42.07
      multiple sites M42.09
      occipito-atlanto-axial region M42.01
      sacrococcygeal region M42.08
      thoracic region M42.04
      thoracolumbar region M42.05
    tarsus M92.6- ☑
    tibia M92.5- ☑
    ulna M92.1- ☑
    upper limb NEC M92.3- ☑
    vertebra (body) (epiphyseal plates) (Calvé's) (Scheuermann's) — *see* Osteochondrosis, juvenile, spine
  Kienböck's — *see* Osteochondrosis, juvenile, hand, carpal lunate
    adult M93.1
  Köhler's
    patellar — *see* Osteochondrosis, juvenile, patella
    tarsal navicular — *see* Osteochondrosis, juvenile, tarsus
  Legg-Perthes (-Calvé)(-Waldenström) — *see* Legg-Calvé-Perthes disease
  limb
    lower NEC (juvenile) M92.8

Osteochondrosis — *continued*
  limb — *continued*
    upper NEC (juvenile) — *see* Osteochondrosis, juvenile, upper limb NEC
  lunate bone (carpal) (juvenile) (see also Osteochondrosis, juvenile, hand, carpal lunate)
    adult M93.1
  Mauclaire's — *see* Osteochondrosis, juvenile, hand, metacarpal
  metacarpal (head) (juvenile) — *see* Osteochondrosis, juvenile, hand, metacarpal
  metatarsus (fifth) (head) (juvenile) (second) — *see* Osteochondrosis, juvenile, metatarsus
  navicular (juvenile) — *see* Osteochondrosis, juvenile, tarsus
  os
    calcis (juvenile) — *see* Osteochondrosis, juvenile, tarsus
    tibiale externum (juvenile) — *see* Osteochondrosis, juvenile, tarsus
  Osgood-Schlatter — *see* Osteochondrosis, juvenile, tibia
  Panner's — *see* Osteochondrosis, juvenile, humerus
  patellar center (juvenile) (primary) (secondary) — *see* Osteochondrosis, juvenile, patella
  pelvis (juvenile) M91.0
  Pierson's M91.0
  radius (head) (juvenile) — *see* Osteochondrosis, juvenile, radius
  Scheuermann's — *see* Osteochondrosis, juvenile, spine
  Sever's — *see* Osteochondrosis, juvenile, tarsus
  Sinding-Larsen — *see* Osteochondrosis, juvenile, patella
  spine M42.9
    adult M42.10
      cervical region M42.12
      cervicothoracic region M42.13
      lumbar region M42.16
      lumbosacral region M42.17
      multiple sites M42.19
      occipito-atlanto-axial region M42.11
      sacrococcygeal region M42.18
      thoracic region M42.14
      thoracolumbar region M42.15
    juvenile — *see* Osteochondrosis, juvenile, spine
  symphysis pubis (juvenile) M91.0
  syphilitic (congenital) A50.02
  talus (juvenile) — *see* Osteochondrosis, juvenile, tarsus
  tarsus (navicular) (juvenile) — *see* Osteochondrosis, juvenile, tarsus
  tibia (proximal) (tubercle) (juvenile) — *see* Osteochondrosis, juvenile, tibia
  tuberculous — *see* Tuberculosis, bone
  ulna (lower) (juvenile) — *see* Osteochondrosis, juvenile, ulna
  van Neck's M91.0
  vertebral — *see* Osteochondrosis, spine
Osteoclastoma D48.0
  malignant — *see* Neoplasm, bone, malignant
Osteodynia — *see* Disorder, bone, specified type NEC
Osteodystrophy Q78.9
  azotemic N25.0
  congenital Q78.9
  parathyroid, secondary E21.1
  renal N25.0
Osteofibroma — *see* Neoplasm, bone, benign
Osteofibrosarcoma — *see* Neoplasm, bone, malignant
Osteogenesis imperfecta Q78.0
Osteogenic — *see* condition
Osteolysis M89.50
  carpus M89.54- ☑
  clavicle M89.51- ☑
  femur M89.55- ☑
  fibula M89.56- ☑
  finger M89.54- ☑
  humerus M89.52- ☑
  ilium M89.559
  ischium M89.559
  joint prosthesis (periprosthetic) — *see* Complications, joint prosthesis, mechanical, periprosthetic, osteolysis, by site
  metacarpus M89.54- ☑
  metatarsus M89.57- ☑
  multiple sites M89.59
  neck M89.58
  periprosthetic — *see* Complications, joint prosthesis, mechanical, periprosthetic, osteolysis, by site

Osteolysis — *continued*
  radius M89.53- ☑
  rib M89.58
  scapula M89.51- ☑
  skull M89.58
  tarsus M89.57- ☑
  tibia M89.56- ☑
  toe M89.57- ☑
  ulna M89.53- ☑
  vertebra M89.58
Osteoma (*see also* Neoplasm, bone, benign)
  osteoid (*see also* Neoplasm, bone, benign)
    giant — *see* Neoplasm, bone, benign
Osteomalacia M83.9
  adult M83.9
    drug-induced NEC M83.5
    due to
      malabsorption (postsurgical) M83.2
      malnutrition M83.3
    specified NEC M83.8
  aluminium-induced M83.4
  infantile — *see* Rickets
  juvenile — *see* Rickets
  oncogenic E83.89
  pelvis M83.8
  puerperal M83.0
  senile M83.1
  vitamin-D-resistant in adults E83.31 [M90.8-] ☑
    carpus E83.31 [M90.84-] ☑
    clavicle E83.31 [M90.81-] ☑
    femur E83.31 [M90.85-] ☑
    fibula E83.31 [M90.86-] ☑
    finger E83.31 [M90.84-] ☑
    humerus E83.31 [M90.82-] ☑
    ilium E83.31 [M90.859]
    ischium E83.31 [M90.859]
    metacarpus E83.31 [M90.84-] ☑
    metatarsus E83.31 [M90.87-] ☑
    multiple sites E83.31 [M90.89]
    neck E83.31 [M90.88]
    radius E83.31 [M90.83-] ☑
    rib E83.31 [M90.88]
    scapula E83.31 [M90.819]
    skull E83.31 [M90.88]
    tarsus E83.31 [M90.879]
    tibia E83.31 [M90.869]
    toe E83.31 [M90.879]
    ulna E83.31 [M90.839]
    vertebra E83.31 [M90.88]
Osteomyelitis (general) (infective) (localized) (neonatal) (purulent) (septic) (staphylococcal) (streptococcal) (suppurative) (with periostitis) M86.9
  acute M86.10
    carpus M86.14- ☑
    clavicle M86.11- ☑
    femur M86.15- ☑
    fibula M86.16- ☑
    finger M86.14- ☑
    hematogenous M86.00
      carpus M86.04- ☑
      clavicle M86.01- ☑
      femur M86.05- ☑
      fibula M86.06- ☑
      finger M86.04- ☑
      humerus M86.02- ☑
      ilium M86.059
      ischium M86.059
      mandible M27.2
      metacarpus M86.04- ☑
      metatarsus M86.07- ☑
      multiple sites M86.09
      neck M86.08
      orbit H05.02- ☑
      petrous bone — *see* Petrositis
      radius M86.03- ☑
      rib M86.08
      scapula M86.01- ☑
      skull M86.08
      tarsus M86.07- ☑
      tibia M86.06- ☑
      toe M86.07- ☑
      ulna M86.03- ☑
      vertebra — *see* Osteomyelitis, vertebra
    humerus M86.12- ☑
    ilium M86.159
    ischium M86.159
    mandible M27.2

Osteomyelitis — *continued*
  acute — *continued*
    metacarpus M86.14- ☑
    metatarsus M86.17- ☑
    multiple sites M86.19
    neck M86.18
    orbit H05.02- ☑
    petrous bone — *see* Petrositis
    radius M86.13- ☑
    rib M86.18
    scapula M86.11- ☑
    skull M86.18
    tarsus M86.17- ☑
    tibia M86.16- ☑
    toe M86.17- ☑
    ulna M86.13- ☑
    vertebra — *see* Osteomyelitis, vertebra
  chronic (or old) M86.60
    with draining sinus M86.40
      carpus M86.44- ☑
      clavicle M86.41- ☑
      femur M86.45- ☑
      fibula M86.46- ☑
      finger M86.44- ☑
      humerus M86.42- ☑
      ilium M86.459
      ischium M86.459
      mandible M27.2
      metacarpus M86.44- ☑
      metatarsus M86.47- ☑
      multiple sites M86.49
      neck M86.48
      orbit H05.02- ☑
      petrous bone — *see* Petrositis
      radius M86.43- ☑
      rib M86.48
      scapula M86.41- ☑
      skull M86.48
      tarsus M86.47- ☑
      tibia M86.46- ☑
      toe M86.47- ☑
      ulna M86.43- ☑
      vertebra — *see* Osteomyelitis, vertebra
    carpus M86.64- ☑
    clavicle M86.61- ☑
    femur M86.65- ☑
    fibula M86.66- ☑
    finger M86.64- ☑
    hematogenous NEC M86.50
      carpus M86.54- ☑
      clavicle M86.51- ☑
      femur M86.55- ☑
      fibula M86.56- ☑
      finger M86.54- ☑
      humerus M86.52- ☑
      ilium M86.559
      ischium M86.559
      mandible M27.2
      metacarpus M86.54- ☑
      metatarsus M86.57- ☑
      multifocal M86.30
        carpus M86.34- ☑
        clavicle M86.31- ☑
        femur M86.35- ☑
        fibula M86.36- ☑
        finger M86.34- ☑
        humerus M86.32- ☑
        ilium M86.359
        ischium M86.359
        metacarpus M86.34- ☑
        metatarsus M86.37- ☑
        multiple sites M86.39
        neck M86.38
        radius M86.33- ☑
        rib M86.38
        scapula M86.31- ☑
        skull M86.38
        tarsus M86.37- ☑
        tibia M86.36- ☑
        toe M86.37- ☑
        ulna M86.33- ☑
        vertebra — *see* Osteomyelitis, vertebra
      multiple sites M86.59
      neck M86.58
      orbit H05.02- ☑
      petrous bone — *see* Petrositis

Osteomyelitis — *continued*
  chronic — *continued*
    hematogenous — *continued*
      radius M86.53- ☑
      rib M86.58
      scapula M86.51- ☑
      skull M86.58
      tarsus M86.57- ☑
      tibia M86.56- ☑
      toe M86.57- ☑
      ulna M86.53- ☑
      vertebra — *see* Osteomyelitis, vertebra
    humerus M86.62- ☑
    ilium M86.659
    ischium M86.659
    mandible M27.2
    metacarpus M86.64- ☑
    metatarsus M86.67- ☑
    multifocal — *see* Osteomyelitis, chronic, hematogenous, multifocal
    multiple sites M86.69
    neck M86.68
    orbit H05.02- ☑
    petrous bone — *see* Petrositis
    radius M86.63- ☑
    rib M86.68
    scapula M86.61- ☑
    skull M86.68
    tarsus M86.67- ☑
    tibia M86.66- ☑
    toe M86.67- ☑
    ulna M86.63- ☑
    vertebra — *see* Osteomyelitis, vertebra
  echinococcal B67.2
  Garr's — *see* Osteomyelitis, specified type NEC
  in diabetes mellitus — *see* E08-E13 with .69
  jaw (acute) (chronic) (lower) (neonatal) (suppurative) (upper) M27.2
  nonsuppurating — *see* Osteomyelitis, specified type NEC
  orbit H05.02- ☑
  petrous bone — *see* Petrositis
  Salmonella (arizonae) (cholerae-suis) (enteritidis) (typhimurium) A02.24
  sclerosing, nonsuppurative — *see* Osteomyelitis, specified type NEC
  specified type NEC (*see also* subcategory) M86.8X- ☑
    mandible M27.2
    orbit H05.02- ☑
    petrous bone — *see* Petrositis
    vertebra — *see* Osteomyelitis, vertebra
  subacute M86.20
    carpus M86.24- ☑
    clavicle M86.21- ☑
    femur M86.25- ☑
    fibula M86.26- ☑
    finger M86.24- ☑
    humerus M86.22- ☑
    mandible M27.2
    metacarpus M86.24- ☑
    metatarsus M86.27- ☑
    multiple sites M86.29
    neck M86.28
    orbit H05.02- ☑
    petrous bone — *see* Petrositis
    radius M86.23- ☑
    rib M86.28
    scapula M86.21- ☑
    skull M86.28
    tarsus M86.27- ☑
    tibia M86.26- ☑
    toe M86.27- ☑
    ulna M86.23- ☑
    vertebra — *see* Osteomyelitis, vertebra
  syphilitic A52.77
    congenital (early) A50.02 [M90.80]
  tuberculous — *see* Tuberculosis, bone
  typhoid A01.05
  vertebra M46.20
    cervical region M46.22
    cervicothoracic region M46.23
    lumbar region M46.26
    lumbosacral region M46.27
    occipito-atlanto-axial region M46.21
    sacrococcygeal region M46.28
    thoracic region M46.24
    thoracolumbar region M46.25

Osteomyelofibrosis D47.4
Osteomyelosclerosis D75.89
Osteonecrosis M87.9
  due to
    drugs — *see* Osteonecrosis, secondary, due to,
      drugs
    trauma — *see* Osteonecrosis, secondary, due to,
      trauma
  idiopathic aseptic M87.00
    ankle M87.07- ☑
    carpus M87.03- ☑
    clavicle M87.01- ☑
    femur M87.05- ☑
    fibula M87.06- ☑
    finger M87.04- ☑
    humerus M87.02- ☑
    ilium M87.050
    ischium M87.050
    metacarpus M87.04- ☑
    metatarsus M87.07- ☑
    multiple sites M87.09
    neck M87.08
    pelvis M87.050
    radius M87.03- ☑
    rib M87.08
    scapula M87.01- ☑
    skull M87.08
    tarsus M87.07- ☑
    tibia M87.06- ☑
    toe M87.07- ☑
    ulna M87.03- ☑
    vertebra M87.08
  secondary NEC M87.30
    carpus M87.33- ☑
    clavicle M87.31- ☑
    due to
      drugs M87.10
        carpus M87.13- ☑
        clavicle M87.11- ☑
        femur M87.15- ☑
        fibula M87.16- ☑
        finger M87.14- ☑
        humerus M87.12- ☑
        ilium M87.159
        ischium M87.159
        jaw M87.180
        metacarpus M87.14- ☑
        metatarsus M87.17- ☑
        multiple sites M87.19
        neck M87.18 ☑
        radius M87.13- ☑
        rib M87.18 ☑
        scapula M87.11- ☑
        skull M87.18 ☑
        tarsus M87.17- ☑
        tibia M87.16- ☑
        toe M87.17- ☑
        ulna M87.13- ☑
        vertebra M87.18 ☑
      hemoglobinopathy NEC D58.2 [M90.50]
        carpus D58.2 [M90.54-] ☑
        clavicle D58.2 [M90.51-] ☑
        femur D58.2 [M90.55-] ☑
        fibula D58.2 [M90.56-] ☑
        finger D58.2 [M90.54-] ☑
        humerus D58.2 [M90.52-] ☑
        ilium D58.2 [M90.55-] ☑
        ischium D58.2 [M90.55-] ☑
        metacarpus D58.2 [M90.54-] ☑
        metatarsus D58.2 [M90.57-] ☑
        multiple sites D58.2 [M90.58]
        neck D58.2 [M90.58]
        radius D58.2 [M90.53-] ☑
        rib D58.2 [M90.58]
        scapula D58.2 [M90.51-] ☑
        skull D58.2 [M90.58]
        tarsus D58.2 [M90.57-] ☑
        tibia D58.2 [M90.56-] ☑
        toe D58.2 [M90.57-] ☑
        ulna D58.2 [M90.53-] ☑
        vertebra D58.2 [M90.58]
      trauma (previous) M87.20
        carpus M87.23- ☑
        clavicle M87.21- ☑
        femur M87.25- ☑
        fibula M87.26- ☑

Osteonecrosis — *continued*
  secondary — *continued*
    due to — *continued*
      trauma — *continued*
        finger M87.24- ☑
        humerus M87.22- ☑
        ilium M87.25- ☑
        ischium M87.25- ☑
        metacarpus M87.24- ☑
        metatarsus M87.27- ☑
        multiple sites M87.29
        neck M87.28
        radius M87.23- ☑
        rib M87.28
        scapula M87.21- ☑
        skull M87.28
        tarsus M87.27- ☑
        tibia M87.26- ☑
        toe M87.27- ☑
        ulna M87.23- ☑
        vertebra M87.28
    femur M87.35- ☑
    fibula M87.36- ☑
    finger M87.34- ☑
    humerus M87.32- ☑
    ilium M87.350
    in
      caisson disease T70.3 ☑ [M90.50]
        carpus T70.3 ☑ [M90.54-] ☑
        clavicle T70.3 ☑ [M90.51-] ☑
        femur T70.3 ☑ [M90.55-] ☑
        fibula T70.3 ☑ [M90.56-] ☑
        finger T70.3 ☑ [M90.54-] ☑
        humerus T70.3 ☑ [M90.52-] ☑
        ilium T70.3 ☑ [M90.55-] ☑
        ischium T70.3 ☑ [M90.55-] ☑
        metacarpus T70.3 ☑ [M90.54-] ☑
        metatarsus T70.3 ☑ [M90.57-] ☑
        multiple sites T70.3 ☑ [M90.59]
        neck T70.3 ☑ [M90.58]
        radius T70.3 ☑ [M90.53-] ☑
        rib T70.3 ☑ [M90.58]
        scapula T70.3 ☑ [M90.51-] ☑
        skull T70.3 ☑ [M90.58]
        tarsus T70.3 ☑ [M90.57-] ☑
        tibia T70.3 ☑ [M90.56-] ☑
        toe T70.3 ☑ [M90.57-] ☑
        ulna T70.3 ☑ [M90.53-] ☑
        vertebra T70.3 ☑ [M90.58]
    ischium M87.350
    metacarpus M87.34- ☑
    metatarsus M87.37- ☑
    multiple site M87.39
    neck M87.38
    radius M87.33- ☑
    rib M87.38
    scapula M87.319
    skull M87.38
    tarsus M87.379
    tibia M87.366
    toe M87.379
    ulna M87.33- ☑
    vertebra M87.38
  specified type NEC M87.80
    carpus M87.83- ☑
    clavicle M87.81- ☑
    femur M87.85- ☑
    fibula M87.86- ☑
    finger M87.84- ☑
    humerus M87.82- ☑
    ilium M87.85- ☑
    ischium M87.85- ☑
    metacarpus M87.84- ☑
    metatarsus M87.87- ☑
    multiple sites M87.89
    neck M87.88
    radius M87.83- ☑
    rib M87.88
    scapula M87.81- ☑
    skull M87.88
    tarsus M87.87- ☑
    tibia M87.86- ☑
    toe M87.87- ☑
    ulna M87.83- ☑
    vertebra M87.88
Osteo-onycho-arthro-dysplasia Q87.2

Osteo-onychodysplasia, hereditary Q87.2
Osteopathia condensans disseminata Q78.8
Osteopathy (*see also* Osteomyelitis, Osteonecrosis, Osteoporosis)
  after poliomyelitis M89.60
    carpus M89.64- ☑
    clavicle M89.61- ☑
    femur M89.65- ☑
    fibula M89.66- ☑
    finger M89.64- ☑
    humerus M89.62- ☑
    ilium M89.659
    ischium M89.659
    metacarpus M89.64- ☑
    metatarsus M89.67- ☑
    multiple sites M89.69
    neck M89.68
    radius M89.63- ☑
    rib M89.68
    scapula M89.61- ☑
    skull M89.68
    tarsus M89.67- ☑
    tibia M89.66- ☑
    toe M89.67- ☑
    ulna M89.63- ☑
    vertebra M89.68
  in (due to)
    renal osteodystrophy N25.0
    specified diseases classified elsewhere — *see* subcategory M90.8 ☑
Osteopenia M85.8- ☑
  borderline M85.8- ☑
Osteoperiostitis — *see* Osteomyelitis, specified type NEC
Osteopetrosis (familial) Q78.2
Osteophyte M25.70
  ankle M25.77- ☑
  elbow M25.72- ☑
  foot joint M25.77- ☑
  hand joint M25.74- ☑
  hip M25.75- ☑
  knee M25.76- ☑
  shoulder M25.71- ☑
  spine M25.78
  vertebrae M25.78
  wrist M25.73- ☑
Osteopoikilosis Q78.8
Osteoporosis (female) (male) M81.0
  with current pathological fracture M80.00 ☑
  age-related M81.0
    with current pathologic fracture M80.00 ☑
      carpus M80.04- ☑
      clavicle M80.01- ☑
      fibula M80.06- ☑
      finger M80.04- ☑
      humerus M80.02- ☑
      ilium M80.05- ☑
      ischium M80.05- ☑
      metacarpus M80.04- ☑
      metatarsus M80.07- ☑
      pelvis M80.05- ☑
      radius M80.03- ☑
      scapula M80.01- ☑
      tarsus M80.07- ☑
      tibia M80.06- ☑
      toe M80.07- ☑
      ulna M80.03- ☑
      vertebra M80.08 ☑
  disuse M81.8
    with current pathological fracture M80.80 ☑
      carpus M80.84- ☑
      clavicle M80.81- ☑
      fibula M80.86- ☑
      finger M80.84- ☑
      humerus M80.82- ☑
      ilium M80.85- ☑
      ischium M80.85- ☑
      metacarpus M80.84- ☑
      metatarsus M80.87- ☑
      pelvis M80.85- ☑
      radius M80.83- ☑
      scapula M80.81- ☑
      tarsus M80.87- ☑
      tibia M80.86- ☑
      toe M80.87- ☑
      ulna M80.83- ☑

☑ **Additional Character Required — Refer to the Tabular List for Character Selection**
🔻 **Subterms under main terms may continue to next column or page**

Osteoporosis — continued
  disuse — continued
    with current pathological fracture — continued
      vertebra M80.88 ☑
  drug-induced — see Osteoporosis, specified type NEC
  idiopathic — see Osteoporosis, specified type NEC
  involutional — see Osteoporosis, age-related
  Lequesne M81.6
  localized M81.6
  postmenopausal M81.0
    with pathological fracture M80.00 ☑
      carpus M80.04- ☑
      clavicle M80.01- ☑
      fibula M80.06- ☑
      finger M80.04- ☑
      humerus M80.02- ☑
      ilium M80.05- ☑
      ischium M80.05- ☑
      metacarpus M80.04- ☑
      metatarsus M80.07- ☑
      pelvis M80.05- ☑
      radius M80.03- ☑
      scapula M80.01- ☑
      tarsus M80.07- ☑
      tibia M80.06- ☑
      toe M80.07- ☑
      ulna M80.03- ☑
      vertebra M80.08 ☑
  postoophorectomy — see Osteoporosis, specified type NEC
  postsurgical malabsorption — see Osteoporosis, specified type NEC
  post-traumatic — see Osteoporosis, specified type NEC
  senile — see Osteoporosis, age-related
  specified type NEC M81.8
    with pathological fracture M80.80 ☑
      carpus M80.84- ☑
      clavicle M80.81- ☑
      fibula M80.86- ☑
      finger M80.84- ☑
      humerus M80.82- ☑
      ilium M80.85- ☑
      ischium M80.85- ☑
      metacarpus M80.84- ☑
      metatarsus M80.87- ☑
      pelvis M80.85- ☑
      radius M80.83- ☑
      scapula M80.81- ☑
      tarsus M80.87- ☑
      tibia M80.86- ☑
      toe M80.87- ☑
      ulna M80.83- ☑
      vertebra M80.88 ☑
Osteopsathyrosis (idiopathica) Q78.0
Osteoradionecrosis, jaw (acute) (chronic) (lower) (suppurative) (upper) M27.2
Osteosarcoma (any form) — see Neoplasm, bone, malignant
Osteosclerosis Q78.2
  acquired M85.8- ☑
  congenita Q77.4
  fragilitas (generalisata) Q78.2
  myelofibrosis D75.81
Osteosclerotic anemia D64.89
Osteosis
  cutis L94.2
  renal fibrocystic N25.0
Österreicher-Turner syndrome Q87.2
Ostium
  atrioventriculare commune Q21.2
  primum (arteriosum) (defect) (persistent) Q21.2
  secundum (arteriosum) (defect) (patent) (persistent) Q21.1
Ostrum-Furst syndrome Q75.8
Otalgia H92.0 ☑
Otitis (acute) H66.90
  with effusion (see also Otitis, media, nonsuppurative)
    purulent — see Otitis, media, suppurative
  adhesive — see subcategory H74.1
  chronic (see also Otitis, media, chronic)
    with effusion (see also Otitis, media, nonsuppurative, chronic)
  externa H60.9- ☑
    abscess — see Abscess, ear, external
    acute (noninfective) H60.50- ☑

Otitis — continued
  externa — continued
    acute — continued
      actinic H60.51- ☑
      chemical H60.52- ☑
      contact H60.53- ☑
      eczematoid H60.54- ☑
      infective — see Otitis, externa, infective
      reactive H60.55- ☑
      specified NEC H60.59- ☑
    cellulitis — see Cellulitis, ear
    chronic H60.6- ☑
    diffuse — see Otitis, externa, infective, diffuse
    hemorrhagic — see Otitis, externa, infective, hemorrhagic
    in (due to)
      aspergillosis B44.89
      candidiasis B37.84
      erysipelas A46 [H62.40]
      herpes (simplex) virus infection B00.1
        zoster B02.8
      impetigo L01.00 [H62.40]
      infectious disease NEC B99 ☑ [H62.4-] ☑
      mycosis NEC B36.9 [H62.40]
      parasitic disease NEC B89 [H62.40]
      viral disease NEC B34.9 [H62.40]
      zoster B02.8
    infective NEC H60.39- ☑
      abscess — see Abscess, ear, external
      cellulitis — see Cellulitis, ear
      diffuse H60.31- ☑
      hemorrhagic H60.32- ☑
      swimmer's ear — see Swimmer's, ear
    malignant H60.2- ☑
    mycotic NEC B36.9 [H62.40]
      in
        aspergillosis B44.89
        candidiasis B37.84
        moniliasis B37.84
    necrotizing — see Otitis, externa, malignant
    Pseudomonas aeruginosa — see Otitis, externa, malignant
    reactive — see Otitis, externa, acute, reactive
    specified NEC — see subcategory H60.8 ☑
    tropical NEC B36.9 [H62.40]
      in
        aspergillosis B44.89
        candidiasis B37.84
        moniliasis B37.84
  insidiosa — see Otosclerosis
  interna H83.0 ☑
  media (hemorrhagic) (staphylococcal) (streptococcal) H66.9- ☑
    with effusion (nonpurulent) — see Otitis, media, nonsuppurative
    acute, subacute H66.90
      allergic — see Otitis, media, nonsuppurative, acute, allergic
      exudative — see Otitis, media, suppurative, acute
      mucoid — see Otitis, media, nonsuppurative, acute
      necrotizing (see also Otitis, media, suppurative, acute)
        in
          measles B05.3
          scarlet fever A38.0
      nonsuppurative NEC — see Otitis, media, nonsuppurative, acute
      purulent — see Otitis, media, suppurative, acute
      sanguinous — see Otitis, media, nonsuppurative, acute
      secretory — see Otitis, media, nonsuppurative, acute, serous
      seromucinous — see Otitis, media, nonsuppurative, acute
      serous — see Otitis, media, nonsuppurative, acute, serous
      suppurative — see Otitis, media, suppurative, acute
    allergic — see Otitis, media, nonsuppurative
    catarrhal — see Otitis, media, nonsuppurative
    chronic H66.90
      with effusion (nonpurulent) — see Otitis, media, nonsuppurative, chronic

Otitis — continued
  media — continued
    chronic — continued
      allergic — see Otitis, media, nonsuppurative, chronic, allergic
      benign suppurative — see Otitis, media, suppurative, chronic, tubotympanic
      catarrhal — see Otitis, media, nonsuppurative, chronic, serous
      exudative — see Otitis, media, nonsuppurative, chronic
      mucinous — see Otitis, media, nonsuppurative, chronic, mucoid
      mucoid — see Otitis, media, nonsuppurative, chronic, mucoid
      nonsuppurative NEC — see Otitis, media, nonsuppurative, chronic
      purulent — see Otitis, media, suppurative, chronic
      secretory — see Otitis, media, nonsuppurative, chronic, mucoid
      seromucinous — see Otitis, media, nonsuppurative, chronic
      serous — see Otitis, media, nonsuppurative, chronic, serous
      suppurative — see Otitis, media, suppurative, chronic
      transudative — see Otitis, media, nonsuppurative, chronic, mucoid
    exudative — see Otitis, media, suppurative
    in (due to) (with)
      influenza — see Influenza, with, otitis media
      measles B05.3
      scarlet fever A38.0
      tuberculosis A18.6
      viral disease NEC B34.- ☑ [H67.-] ☑
    mucoid — see Otitis, media, nonsuppurative
    nonsuppurative H65.9- ☑
      acute or subacute NEC H65.19- ☑
        allergic H65.11- ☑
          recurrent H65.11- ☑
        recurrent H65.19- ☑
        secretory — see Otitis, media, nonsuppurative, serous
        serous H65.0- ☑
          recurrent H65.0- ☑
      chronic H65.49- ☑
        allergic H65.41- ☑
        mucoid H65.3- ☑
        serous H65.2- ☑
    postmeasles B05.3
    purulent — see Otitis, media, suppurative
    secretory — see Otitis, media, nonsuppurative
    seromucinous — see Otitis, media, nonsuppurative
    serous — see Otitis, media, nonsuppurative
    suppurative H66.4- ☑
      acute H66.00- ☑
        with rupture of ear drum H66.01- ☑
        recurrent H66.00- ☑
          with rupture of ear drum H66.01- ☑
      chronic (see also subcategory) H66.3 ☑
        atticoantral H66.2- ☑
        benign — see Otitis, media, suppurative, chronic, tubotympanic
        tubotympanic H66.1- ☑
    transudative — see Otitis, media, nonsuppurative
    tuberculous A18.6
Otocephaly Q18.2
Otolith syndrome — see subcategory H81.8 ☑
Otomycosis (diffuse) NEC B36.9 [H62.40]
  in
    aspergillosis B44.89
    candidiasis B37.84
    moniliasis B37.84
Otoporosis — see Otosclerosis
Otorrhagia (nontraumatic) H92.2- ☑
  traumatic — code by Type of injury
Otorrhea H92.1- ☑
  cerebrospinal G96.0
Otosclerosis (general) H80.9- ☑
  cochlear (endosteal) H80.2- ☑
  involving
    otic capsule — see Otosclerosis, cochlear
    oval window
      nonobliterative H80.0- ☑
      obliterative H80.1- ☑
    round window — see Otosclerosis, cochlear

Subterms under main terms may continue to next column or page   ☑ Additional Character Required — Refer to the Tabular List for Character Selection   243

Osteoporosis — Otosclerosis

Otosclerosis — *continued*
  nonobliterative — *see* Otosclerosis, involving, oval window, nonobliterative
  obliterative — *see* Otosclerosis, involving, oval window, obliterative
  specified NEC H80.8- ☑
Otospongiosis — *see* Otosclerosis
Otto's disease or pelvis M24.7
Outcome of delivery Z37.9
  multiple births Z37.9
    all liveborn Z37.50
      quadruplets Z37.52
      quintuplets Z37.53
      sextuplets Z37.54
      specified number NEC Z37.59
      triplets Z37.51
    all stillborn Z37.7
    some liveborn Z37.60
      quadruplets Z37.62
      quintuplets Z37.63
      sextuplets Z37.64
      specified number NEC Z37.69
      triplets Z37.61
  single NEC Z37.9
    liveborn Z37.0
    stillborn Z37.1
  twins NEC Z37.9
    both liveborn Z37.2
    both stillborn Z37.4
    one liveborn, one stillborn Z37.3
Outlet — *see* condition
Ovalocytosis (congenital) (hereditary) — *see* Elliptocytosis
Ovarian — *see* Condition
Ovariocele N83.4- ☑
Ovaritis (cystic) — *see* Oophoritis
Ovary, ovarian (*see also* condition)
  resistant syndrome E28.39
  vein syndrome N13.8
Overactive (*see also* Hyperfunction)
  adrenal cortex NEC E27.0
  bladder N32.81
  hypothalamus E23.3
  thyroid — *see* Hyperthyroidism
Overactivity R46.3
  child — *see* Disorder, attention-deficit hyperactivity
Overbite (deep) (excessive) (horizontal) (vertical) M26.29
Overbreathing — *see* Hyperventilation
Overconscientious personality F60.5
Overdevelopment — *see* Hypertrophy
Overdistension — *see* Distension
Overdose, overdosage (drug) — *see* Table of Drugs and Chemicals, by drug, poisoning
Overeating R63.2
  nonorganic origin F50.89
  psychogenic F50.89
Overexertion (effects) (exhaustion) T73.3 ☑
Overexposure (effects) T73.9 ☑
  exhaustion T73.2 ☑
Overfeeding — *see* Overeating
  newborn P92.4
Overfill, endodontic M27.52
Overgrowth, bone — *see* Hypertrophy, bone
Overhanging of dental restorative material (unrepairable) K08.52
Overheated (places) (effects) — *see* Heat
Overjet (excessive horizontal) M26.23
Overlaid, overlying (suffocation) — *see* Asphyxia, traumatic, due to mechanical threat
Overlap, excessive horizontal (teeth) M26.23
Overlapping toe (acquired) (*see also* Deformity, toe, specified NEC)
  congenital (fifth toe) Q66.89
Overload
  circulatory, due to transfusion (blood) (blood components) (TACO) E87.71
  fluid E87.70
    due to transfusion (blood) (blood components) E87.71
    specified NEC E87.79
  iron, due to repeated red blood cell transfusions E83.111
  potassium (K) E87.5
  sodium (Na) E87.0
Overnutrition — *see* Hyperalimentation
Overproduction (*see also* Hypersecretion)
  ACTH E27.0

Overproduction — *continued*
  catecholamine E27.5
  growth hormone E22.0
Overprotection, child by parent Z62.1
Overriding
  aorta Q25.49
  finger (acquired) — *see* Deformity, finger
    congenital Q68.1
  toe (acquired) (*see also* Deformity, toe, specified NEC)
    congenital Q66.89
Overstrained R53.83
  heart — *see* Hypertrophy, cardiac
Overuse, muscle NEC M70.8- ☑
Overweight E66.3
Overworked R53.83
Oviduct — *see* condition
Ovotestis Q56.0
Ovulation (cycle)
  failure or lack of N97.0
  pain N94.0
Ovum — *see* condition
Owren's disease or syndrome (parahemophilia) D68.2
Ox heart — *see* Hypertrophy, cardiac
Oxalosis E72.53
Oxaluria E72.53
Oxycephaly, oxycephalic Q75.0
  syphilitic, congenital A50.02
Oxyuriasis B80
Oxyuris vermicularis (infestation) B80
Ozena J31.0

P

Pachyderma, pachydermia L85.9
  larynx (verrucosa) J38.7
Pachydermatocele (congenital) Q82.8
Pachydermoperiostosis (*see also* Osteoarthropathy, hypertrophic, specified type NEC)
  clubbed nail M89.40 [L62]
Pachygyria Q04.3
Pachymeningitis (adhesive) (basal) (brain) (cervical) (chronic)(circumscribed) (external) (fibrous) (hemorrhagic) (hypertrophic) (internal) (purulent) (spinal) (suppurative) — *see* Meningitis
Pachyonychia (congenital) Q84.5
Pacinian tumor — *see* Neoplasm, skin, benign
Pad, knuckle or Garrod's M72.1
Paget's disease
  with infiltrating duct carcinoma — *see* Neoplasm, breast, malignant
  bone M88.9
    carpus M88.84- ☑
    clavicle M88.81- ☑
    femur M88.85- ☑
    fibula M88.86- ☑
    finger M88.84- ☑
    humerus M88.82- ☑
    ilium M88.85- ☑
    in neoplastic disease — *see* Osteitis, deformans, in neoplastic disease
    ischium M88.85- ☑
    metacarpus M88.84- ☑
    metatarsus M88.87- ☑
    multiple sites M88.89
    neck M88.88
    radius M88.83- ☑
    rib M88.88
    scapula M88.81- ☑
    skull M88.0
    tarsus M88.87- ☑
    tibia M88.86- ☑
    toe M88.87- ☑
    ulna M88.83- ☑
    vertebra M88.88
  breast (female) C50.01- ☑
    male C50.02- ☑
  extramammary (*see also* Neoplasm, skin, malignant)
    anus C21.0
      margin C44.590
      skin C44.590
    intraductal carcinoma — *see* Neoplasm, breast, malignant
    malignant — *see* Neoplasm, skin, malignant
      breast (female) C50.01- ☑
        male C50.02- ☑
      unspecified site (female) C50.01- ☑
        male C50.02- ☑

Paget's disease — *continued*
  mammary — *see* Paget's disease, breast
  nipple — *see* Paget's disease, breast
  osteitis deformans — *see* Paget's disease, bone
Paget-Schroetter syndrome I82.890
Pain(s) (*see also* Painful) R52
  abdominal R10.9
    colic R10.83
    generalized R10.84
      with acute abdomen R10.0
    lower R10.30
      left quadrant R10.32
      pelvic or perineal R10.2
      periumbilical R10.33
      right quadrant R10.31
    rebound — *see* Tenderness, abdominal, rebound
    severe with abdominal rigidity R10.0
    tenderness — *see* Tenderness, abdominal
    upper R10.10
      epigastric R10.13
      left quadrant R10.12
      right quadrant R10.11
  acute R52
    due to trauma G89.11
    neoplasm related G89.3
    postprocedural NEC G89.18
    post-thoracotomy G89.12
    specified by site — *code to* Pain, by site
  adnexa (uteri) R10.2
  anginoid — *see* Pain, precordial
  anus K62.89
  arm — *see* Pain, limb, upper
  axillary (axilla) M79.62- ☑
  back (postural) M54.9
  bladder R39.89
    associated with micturition — *see* Micturition, painful
    chronic R39.82
  bone — *see* Disorder, bone, specified type NEC
  breast N64.4
  broad ligament R10.2
  cancer associated (acute) (chronic) G89.3
  cecum — *see* Pain, abdominal
  cervicobrachial M53.1
  chest (central) R07.9
    anterior wall R07.89
    atypical R07.89
    ischemic I20.9
    musculoskeletal R07.89
    non-cardiac R07.89
    on breathing R07.1
    pleurodynia R07.81
    precordial R07.2
    wall (anterior) R07.89
  chronic G89.29
    associated with significant psychosocial dysfunction G89.4
    due to trauma G89.21
    neoplasm related G89.3
    postoperative NEC G89.28
    postprocedural NEC G89.28
    post-thoracotomy G89.22
    specified NEC G89.29
  coccyx M53.3
  colon — *see* Pain, abdominal
  coronary — *see* Angina
  costochondral R07.89
  diaphragm R07.1
  due to cancer G89.3
  due to device, implant or graft (*see also* Complications, by site and type, specified NEC) T85.848 ☑
    arterial graft NEC T82.848 ☑
    breast (implant) T85.848 ☑
    catheter NEC T85.848 ☑
      dialysis (renal) T82.848 ☑
        intraperitoneal T85.848 ☑
      infusion NEC T82.848 ☑
        spinal (epidural) (subdural) T85.840 ☑
      urinary (indwelling) T83.84 ☑
    electronic (electrode) (pulse generator) (stimulator)
      bone T85.840 ☑
      cardiac T82.847 ☑
      nervous system (brain) (peripheral nerve) (spinal) T85.84 ☑
      urinary T83.84 ☑
    fixation, internal (orthopedic) NEC T84.84 ☑
    gastrointestinal (bile duct) (esophagus) T85.848 ☑
    genital NEC T83.84 ☑

Pain(s) — *continued*
  due to device, implant or graft (*see also* Complications, by site and type, specified) — *continued*
    heart NEC T82.847 ☑
    infusion NEC T85.848 ☑
    joint prosthesis T84.84 ☑
    ocular (corneal graft) (orbital implant) NEC T85.848 ☑
    orthopedic NEC T84.84 ☑
    specified NEC T85.848 ☑
    urinary NEC T83.84 ☑
    vascular NEC T82.848 ☑
    ventricular intracranial shunt T85.840 ☑
  due to malignancy (primary) (secondary) G89.3
  ear — *see* subcategory H92.0 ☑
  epigastric, epigastrium R10.13
  eye — *see* Pain, ocular
  face, facial R51
    atypical G50.1
  female genital organs NEC N94.89
  finger — *see* Pain, limb, upper
  flank — *see* Pain, abdominal
  foot — *see* Pain, limb, lower
  gallbladder K82.9
  gas (intestinal) R14.1
  gastric — *see* Pain, abdominal
  generalized NOS R52
  genital organ
    female N94.89
    male N50.89
  groin — *see* Pain, abdominal, lower
  hand — *see* Pain, limb, upper
  head — *see* Headache
  heart — *see* Pain, precordial
  infra-orbital — *see* Neuralgia, trigeminal
  intercostal R07.82
  intermenstrual N94.0
  jaw R68.84
  joint M25.50
    ankle M25.57- ☑
    elbow M25.52- ☑
    finger M25.54- ☑
    foot M25.57- ☑
    hand M25.54- ☑
    hip M25.55- ☑
    knee M25.56- ☑
    shoulder M25.51- ☑
    toe M25.57- ☑
    wrist M25.53- ☑
  kidney N23
  laryngeal R07.0
  leg — *see* Pain, limb, lower
  limb M79.609
    lower M79.60- ☑
      foot M79.67- ☑
      lower leg M79.66- ☑
      thigh M79.65- ☑
      toe M79.67- ☑
    upper M79.60- ☑
      axilla M79.62- ☑
      finger M79.64- ☑
      forearm M79.63- ☑
      hand M79.64- ☑
      upper arm M79.62- ☑
  loin M54.5
  low back M54.5
  lumbar region M54.5
  mandibular R68.84
  mastoid — *see* subcategory H92.0 ☑
  maxilla R68.84
  menstrual (*see also* Dysmenorrhea) N94.6
  metacarpophalangeal (joint) — *see* Pain, joint, hand
  metatarsophalangeal (joint) — *see* Pain, joint, foot
  mouth K13.79
  muscle — *see* Myalgia
  musculoskeletal (*see also* Pain, by site) M79.1
  myofascial M79.1
  nasal J34.89
  nasopharynx J39.2
  neck NEC M54.2
  nerve NEC — *see* Neuralgia
  neuromuscular — *see* Neuralgia
  nose J34.89
  ocular H57.1- ☑
  ophthalmic — *see* Pain, ocular
  orbital region — *see* Pain, ocular
  ovary N94.89

Pain(s) — *continued*
  over heart — *see* Pain, precordial
  ovulation N94.0
  pelvic (female) R10.2
  penis N48.89
  pericardial — *see* Pain, precordial
  perineal, perineum R10.2
  pharynx J39.2
  pleura, pleural, pleuritic R07.81
  postoperative NOS G89.18
  postprocedural NOS G89.18
  post-thoracotomy G89.12
  precordial (region) R07.2
  premenstrual N94.3
  psychogenic (persistent) (any site) F45.41
  radicular (spinal) — *see* Radiculopathy
  rectum K62.89
  respiration R07.1
  retrosternal R07.2
  rheumatoid, muscular — *see* Myalgia
  rib R07.81
  root (spinal) — *see* Radiculopathy
  round ligament (stretch) R10.2
  sacroiliac M53.3
  sciatic — *see* Sciatica
  scrotum N50.82
  seminal vesicle N50.89
  shoulder M25.51- ☑
  spermatic cord N50.89
  spinal root — *see* Radiculopathy
  spine M54.9
    cervical M54.2
    low back M54.5
      with sciatica M54.4- ☑
    thoracic M54.6
  stomach — *see* Pain, abdominal
  substernal R07.2
  temporomandibular (joint) M26.62- ☑
  testis N50.81- ☑
  thoracic spine M54.6
    with radicular and visceral pain M54.14
  throat R07.0
  tibia — *see* Pain, limb, lower
  toe — *see* Pain, limb, lower
  tongue K14.6
  tooth K08.89
  trigeminal — *see* Neuralgia, trigeminal
  tumor associated G89.3
  ureter N23
  urinary (organ) (system) N23
  uterus NEC N94.89
  vagina R10.2
  vertebrogenic (syndrome) M54.89
  vesical R39.89
    associated with micturition — *see* Micturition, painful
  vulva R10.2

Painful (*see also* Pain)
  coitus
    female N94.10
    male N53.12
    psychogenic F52.6
  ejaculation (semen) N53.12
    psychogenic F52.6
  erection — *see* Priapism
  feet syndrome E53.8
  joint replacement (hip) (knee) T84.84 ☑
  menstruation — *see* Dysmenorrhea
    psychogenic F45.8
  micturition — *see* Micturition, painful
  respiration R07.1
  scar NEC L90.5
  wire sutures T81.89 ☑

Painter's colic — *see* subcategory T56.0 ☑
Palate — *see* condition
Palatoplegia K13.79
Palatoschisis — *see* Cleft, palate
Palilalia R48.8
Palliative care Z51.5
Pallor R23.1
  optic disc, temporal — *see* Atrophy, optic
Palmar (*see also* condition)
  fascia — *see* condition
Palpable
  cecum K63.89
  kidney N28.89
  ovary N83.8
  prostate N42.9

Palpable — *continued*
  spleen — *see* Splenomegaly
Palpitations (heart) R00.2
  psychogenic F45.8
Palsy (*see also* Paralysis) G83.9
  atrophic diffuse (progressive) G12.22
  Bell's (*see also* Palsy, facial)
    newborn P11.3
  brachial plexus NEC G54.0
    newborn (birth injury) P14.3
  brain — *see* Palsy, cerebral
  bulbar (progressive) (chronic) G12.22
    of childhood (Fazio-Londe) G12.1
    pseudo NEC G12.29
    supranuclear (progressive) G23.1
  cerebral (congenital) G80.9
    ataxic G80.4
    athetoid G80.3
    choreathetoid G80.3
    diplegic G80.8
      spastic G80.1
    dyskinetic G80.3
      athetoid G80.3
      choreathetoid G80.3
      distonic G80.3
    dystonic G80.3
    hemiplegic G80.8
      spastic G80.2
    mixed G80.8
    monoplegic G80.8
      spastic G80.1
    paraplegic G80.8
      spastic G80.1
    quadriplegic G80.8
      spastic G80.0
    spastic G80.1
      diplegic G80.1
      hemiplegic G80.2
      monoplegic G80.1
      quadriplegic G80.0
      specified NEC G80.1
      tetrapelgic G80.0
    specified NEC G80.8
    syphilitic A52.12
      congenital A50.49
    tetraplegic G80.8
      spastic G80.0
  cranial nerve (*see also* Disorder, nerve, cranial)
    multiple G52.7
      in
        infectious disease B99 ☑ [G53]
        neoplastic disease (*see also* Neoplasm) D49.9 [G53]
        parasitic disease B89 [G53]
        sarcoidosis D86.82
  creeping G12.22
  diver's T70.3 ☑
  Erb's P14.0
  facial G51.0
    newborn (birth injury) P11.3
  glossopharyngeal G52.1
  Klumpke (-Déjérine) P14.1
  lead — *see* subcategory T56.0 ☑
  median nerve (tardy) G56.1- ☑
  nerve G58.9
    specified NEC G58.8
  peroneal nerve (acute) (tardy) G57.3- ☑
  progressive supranuclear G23.1
  pseudobulbar NEC G12.29
  radial nerve (acute) G56.3- ☑
  seventh nerve (*see also* Palsy, facial)
    newborn P11.3
  shaking — *see* Parkinsonism
  spastic (cerebral) (spinal) G80.1
  ulnar nerve (tardy) G56.2- ☑
  wasting G12.29
Paludism — *see* Malaria
Panangiitis M30.0
Panaris, panaritium (*see also* Cellulitis, digit)
  with lymphangitis — *see* Lymphangitis, acute, digit
Panarteritis nodosa M30.0
  brain or cerebral I67.7
Pancake heart R93.1
  with cor pulmonale (chronic) I27.81
Pancarditis (acute) (chronic) I51.89
  rheumatic I09.89
    active or acute I01.8
Pancoast's syndrome or tumor C34.1- ☑

☞ **Subterms under main terms may continue to next column or page**   ☑ **Additional Character Required — Refer to the Tabular List for Character Selection**   **245**

Pain — Pancoast's syndrome or tumor

Pancolitis, ulcerative (chronic) K51.00
  with
    abscess K51.014
    complication K51.019
    fistula K51.013
    obstruction K51.012
    rectal bleeding K51.011
    specified complication NEC K51.018
Pancreas, pancreatic — *see* condition
Pancreatitis (annular) (apoplectic) (calcareous) (edematous) (hemorrhagic) (malignant) (recurrent) (subacute) (suppurative) K85.90
  with necrosis (uninfected) K85.91
    infected K85.92
  acute (without necrosis or infection) K85.90
    with necrosis (uninfected) K85.91
      infected K85.92
    alcohol induced (without necrosis or infection) K85.20
      with necrosis (uninfected) K85.21
        infected K85.22
    biliary (without necrosis or infection) K85.10
      with necrosis (uninfected) K85.11
        infected K85.12
    drug induced (without necrosis or infection) K85.30
      with necrosis (uninfected) K85.31
        infected K85.32
    gallstone (without necrosis or infection) K85.10
      with necrosis (uninfected) K85.11
        infected K85.12
    idiopathic (without necrosis or infection) K85.00
      with necrosis (uninfected) K85.01
        infected K85.02
    specified NEC (without necrosis or infection) K85.80
      with necrosis (uninfected) K85.81
        infected K85.82
  chronic (infectious) K86.1
    alcohol-induced K86.0
    recurrent K86.1
    relapsing K86.1
  cystic (chronic) K86.1
  cytomegaloviral B25.2
  fibrous (chronic) K86.1
  gallstone (without necrosis or infection) K85.10
    with necrosis (uninfected) K85.11
      infected K85.12
  gangrenous — *see* Pancreatitis, acute
  interstitial (chronic) K86.1
    acute (*see also* Pancreatitis, acute) K85.80
  mumps B26.3
  recurrent (chronic) K86.1
  relapsing, chronic K86.1
  syphilitic A52.74
Pancreatoblastoma — *see* Neoplasm, pancreas, malignant
Pancreolithiasis K86.89
Pancytolysis D75.89
Pancytopenia (acquired) D61.818
  with
    malformations D61.09
    myelodysplastic syndrome — *see* Syndrome, myelodysplastic
  antineoplastic chemotherapy induced D61.810
  congenital D61.09
  drug-induced NEC D61.811
PANDAS (pediatric autoimmune neuropsychiatric disorders associated with streptococcal infections syndrome) D89.89
Panencephalitis, subacute, sclerosing A81.1
Panhematopenia D61.9
  congenital D61.09
  constitutional D61.09
  splenic, primary D73.1
Panhemocytopenia D61.9
  congenital D61.09
  constitutional D61.09
Panhypogonadism E29.1
Panhypopituitarism E23.0
  prepubertal E23.0
Panic (attack) (state) F41.0
  reaction to exceptional stress (transient) F43.0
Panmyelopathy, familial, constitutional D61.09
Panmyelophthisis D61.82
  congenital D61.09
Panmyelosis (acute) (with myelofibrosis) C94.4- ☑
Panner's disease — *see* Osteochondrosis, juvenile, humerus
Panneuritis endemica E51.11

Panniculitis (nodular) (nonsuppurative) M79.3
  back M54.00
    cervical region M54.02
    cervicothoracic region M54.03
    lumbar region M54.06
    lumbosacral region M54.07
    multiple sites M54.09
    occipito-atlanto-axial region M54.01
    sacrococcygeal region M54.08
    thoracic region M54.04
    thoracolumbar region M54.05
  lupus L93.2
  mesenteric K65.4
  neck M54.02
    cervicothoracic region M54.03
    occipito-atlanto-axial region M54.01
  relapsing M35.6
Panniculus adiposus (abdominal) E65
Pannus (allergic) (cornea) (degenerativus) (keratic) H16.42- ☑
  abdominal (symptomatic) E65
  trachomatosus, trachomatous (active) A71.1
Panophthalmitis H44.01- ☑
Pansinusitis (chronic) (hyperplastic) (nonpurulent) (purulent) J32.4
  acute J01.40
    recurrent J01.41
  tuberculous A15.8
Panuveitis (sympathetic) H44.11- ☑
Panvalvular disease I08.9
  specified NEC I08.8
PAPA (pyogenic arthritis, pyoderma gangrenosum, and acne syndrome) M04.8
Papanicolaou smear, cervix Z12.4
  as part of routine gynecological examination Z01.419
    with abnormal findings Z01.411
  for suspected neoplasm Z12.4
  nonspecific abnormal finding R87.619
  routine Z01.419
    with abnormal findings Z01.411
Papilledema (choked disc) H47.10
  associated with
    decreased ocular pressure H47.12
    increased intracranial pressure H47.11
    retinal disorder H47.13
  Foster-Kennedy syndrome H47.14- ☑
Papillitis H46.00
  anus K62.89
  chronic lingual K14.4
  necrotizing, kidney N17.2
  optic H46.0- ☑
  rectum K62.89
  renal, necrotizing N17.2
  tongue K14.0
Papilloma (*see also* Neoplasm, benign, by site)
  acuminatum (female) (male) (anogenital) A63.0
  basal cell L82.1
    inflamed L82.0
  benign pinta (primary) A67.0
  bladder (urinary) (transitional cell) D41.4
  choroid plexus (lateral ventricle) (third ventricle) D33.0
    anaplastic C71.5
    fourth ventricle D33.1
    malignant C71.5
  renal pelvis (transitional cell) D41.1- ☑
    benign D30.1- ☑
  Schneiderian
    specified site — *see* Neoplasm, benign, by site
    unspecified site D14.0
  serous surface
    borderline malignancy
      specified site — *see* Neoplasm, uncertain behavior, by site
      unspecified site D39.10
    specified site — *see* Neoplasm, benign, by site
    unspecified site D27.9
  transitional (cell)
    bladder (urinary) D41.4
    inverted type — *see* Neoplasm, uncertain behavior, by site
    renal pelvis D41.1- ☑
    ureter D41.2- ☑
  ureter (transitional cell) D41.2- ☑
    benign D30.2- ☑
  urothelial — *see* Neoplasm, uncertain behavior, by site
  villous — *see* Neoplasm, uncertain behavior, by site

Papilloma — *continued*
  villous — *see* Neoplasm, uncertain behavior, by site — *continued*
    adenocarcinoma in — *see* Neoplasm, malignant, by site
    in situ — *see* Neoplasm, in situ
  yaws, plantar or palmar A66.1
Papillomata, multiple, of yaws A66.1
Papillomatosis (*see also* Neoplasm, benign, by site)
  confluent and reticulated L83
  cystic, breast — *see* Mastopathy, cystic
  ductal, breast — *see* Mastopathy, cystic
  intraductal (diffuse) — *see* Neoplasm, benign, by site
  subareolar duct D24- ☑
Papillomavirus, as cause of disease classified elsewhere B97.7
Papillon-Léage and Psaume syndrome Q87.0
Papule(s) R23.8
  carate (primary) A67.0
  fibrous, of nose D22.39
  Gottron's L94.4
  pinta (primary) A67.0
Papulosis
  lymphomatoid C86.6
  malignant I77.89
Papyraceous fetus O31.0- ☑
Para-albuminemia E88.09
Paracephalus Q89.7
Parachute mitral valve Q23.2
Paracoccidioidomycosis B41.9
  disseminated B41.7
  generalized B41.7
  mucocutaneous-lymphangitic B41.8
  pulmonary B41.0
  specified NEC B41.8
  visceral B41.8
Paradentosis K05.4
Paraffinoma T88.8 ☑
Paraganglioma D44.7
  adrenal D35.0- ☑
    malignant C74.1- ☑
  aortic body D44.7
    malignant C75.5
  carotid body D44.6
    malignant C75.4
  chromaffin (*see also* Neoplasm, benign, by site)
    malignant — *see* Neoplasm, malignant, by site
  extra-adrenal D44.7
    malignant C75.5
      specified site — *see* Neoplasm, malignant, by site
      unspecified site C75.5
    specified site — *see* Neoplasm, uncertain behavior, by site
    unspecified site D44.7
  gangliocytic D13.2
    specified site — *see* Neoplasm, benign, by site
    unspecified site D13.2
  glomus jugulare D44.7
    malignant C75.5
  jugular D44.7
  malignant C75.5
    specified site — *see* Neoplasm, malignant, by site
    unspecified site C75.5
  nonchromaffin D44.7
    malignant C75.5
      specified site — *see* Neoplasm, malignant, by site
      unspecified site C75.5
    specified site — *see* Neoplasm, uncertain behavior, by site
    unspecified site D44.7
  parasympathetic D44.7
    specified site — *see* Neoplasm, uncertain behavior, by site
    unspecified site D44.7
  specified site — *see* Neoplasm, uncertain behavior, by site
  sympathetic D44.7
    specified site — *see* Neoplasm, uncertain behavior, by site
    unspecified site D44.7
  unspecified site D44.7
Parageusia R43.2
  psychogenic F45.8
Paragonimiasis B66.4

☑ **Additional Character Required** — Refer to the Tabular List for Character Selection   ▽ Subterms under main terms may continue to next column or page

Paragranuloma, Hodgkin — *see* Lymphoma, Hodgkin, specified NEC
Parahemophilia (*see also* Defect, coagulation) D68.2
Parakeratosis R23.4
  variegata L41.0
Paralysis, paralytic (complete) (incomplete) G83.9
  with
    syphilis A52.17
  abducens, abducent (nerve) — *see* Strabismus, paralytic, sixth nerve
  abductor, lower extremity G57.9- ☑
  accessory nerve G52.8
  accommodation (*see also* Paresis, of accommodation)
    hysterical F44.89
  acoustic nerve (except Deafness) H93.3 ☑
  agitans (*see also* Parkinsonism) G20
    arteriosclerotic G21.4
  alternating (oculomotor) G83.89
  amyotrophic G12.21
  ankle G57.9- ☑
  anus (sphincter) K62.89
  arm — *see* Monoplegia, upper limb
  ascending (spinal), acute G61.0
  association G12.29
  asthenic bulbar G70.00
    with exacerbation (acute) G70.01
    in crisis G70.01
  ataxic (hereditary) G11.9
    general (syphilitic) A52.17
  atrophic G58.9
    infantile, acute — *see* Poliomyelitis, paralytic
    progressive G12.22
    spinal (acute) — *see* Poliomyelitis, paralytic
  axillary G54.0
  Babinski-Nageotte's G83.89
  Bell's G51.0
    newborn P11.3
  Benedikt's G46.3
  birth injury P14.9
    spinal cord P11.5
  bladder (neurogenic) (sphincter) N31.2
  bowel, colon or intestine K56.0
  brachial plexus G54.0
    birth injury P14.3
    newborn (birth injury) P14.3
  brain G83.9
    diplegia G83.0
    triplegia G83.89
  bronchial J98.09
  Brown-Séquard G83.81
  bulbar (chronic) (progressive) G12.22
    infantile — *see* Poliomyelitis, paralytic
    poliomyelitic — *see* Poliomyelitis, paralytic
    pseudo G12.29
  bulbospinal G70.00
    with exacerbation (acute) G70.01
    in crisis G70.01
  cardiac (*see also* Failure, heart) I50.9
  cerebrocerebellar, diplegic G80.1
  cervical
    plexus G54.2
    sympathetic G90.09
  Céstan-Chenais G46.3
  Charcot-Marie-Tooth type G60.0
  Clark's G80.9
  colon K56.0
  compressed air T70.3 ☑
  compression
    arm G56.9- ☑
    leg G57.9- ☑
    lower extremity G57.9- ☑
    upper extremity G56.9- ☑
  congenital (cerebral) — *see* Palsy, cerebral
  conjugate movement (gaze) (of eye) H51.0
    cortical (nuclear) (supranuclear) H51.0
  cordis — *see* Failure, heart
  cranial or cerebral nerve G52.9
  creeping G12.22
  crossed leg G83.89
  crutch — *see* Injury, brachial plexus
  deglutition R13.0
    hysterical F44.4
  dementia A52.17
  descending (spinal) NEC G12.29
  diaphragm (flaccid) J98.6
    due to accidental dissection of phrenic nerve during procedure — *see* Puncture, accidental complicating surgery

Paralysis, paralytic — *continued*
  digestive organs NEC K59.8
  diplegic — *see* Diplegia
  divergence (nuclear) H51.8
  diver's T70.3 ☑
  Duchenne's
    birth injury P14.0
    due to or associated with
      motor neuron disease G12.22
      muscular dystrophy G71.0
  due to intracranial or spinal birth injury — *see* Palsy, cerebral
  embolic (current episode) I63.4- ☑
  Erb (-Duchenne) (birth) (newborn) P14.0
  Erb's syphilitic spastic spinal A52.17
  esophagus K22.8
  eye muscle (extrinsic) H49.9
    intrinsic (*see also* Paresis, of accommodation)
  facial (nerve) G51.0
    birth injury P11.3
    congenital P11.3
    following operation NEC — *see* Puncture, accidental complicating surgery
    newborn (birth injury) P11.3
  familial (recurrent) (periodic) G72.3
    spastic G11.4
  fauces J39.2
  finger G56.9- ☑
  gait R26.1
  gastric nerve (nondiabetic) G52.2
  gaze, conjugate H51.0
  general (progressive) (syphilitic) A52.17
    juvenile A50.45
  glottis J38.00
    bilateral J38.02
    unilateral J38.01
  gluteal G54.1
  Gubler (-Millard) G46.3
  hand — *see* Monoplegia, upper limb
  heart — *see* Arrest, cardiac
  hemiplegic — *see* Hemiplegia
  hyperkalemic periodic (familial) G72.3
  hypoglossal (nerve) G52.3
  hypokalemic periodic G72.3
  hysterical F44.4
  ileus K56.0
  infantile (*see also* Poliomyelitis, paralytic) A80.30
    bulbar — *see* Poliomyelitis, paralytic
    cerebral — *see* Palsy, cerebral
    spastic — *see* Palsy, cerebral, spastic
  infective — *see* Poliomyelitis, paralytic
  inferior nuclear G83.9
  internuclear — *see* Ophthalmoplegia, internuclear
  intestine K56.0
  iris H57.09
    due to diphtheria (toxin) A36.89
  ischemic, Volkmann's (complicating trauma) T79.6 ☑
  Jackson's G83.89
  jake — *see* Poisoning, food, noxious, plant
  Jamaica ginger (jake) G62.2
  juvenile general A50.45
  Klumpke (-Déjérine) (birth) (newborn) P14.1
  labioglossal (laryngeal) (pharyngeal) G12.29
  Landry's G61.0
  laryngeal nerve (recurrent) (superior) (unilateral) J38.00
    bilateral J38.02
    unilateral J38.01
  larynx J38.00
    bilateral J38.02
    due to diphtheria (toxin) A36.2
    unilateral J38.01
  lateral G12.23
  lead T56.0 ☑
  left side — *see* Hemiplegia
  leg G83.1- ☑
    both — *see* Paraplegia
    crossed G83.89
    hysterical F44.4
    psychogenic F44.4
    transient or transitory R29.818
      traumatic NEC — *see* Injury, nerve, leg
  levator palpebrae superioris — *see* Blepharoptosis, paralytic
  limb — *see* Monoplegia
  lip K13.0
  Lissauer's A52.17
  lower limb — *see* Monoplegia, lower limb
    both — *see* Paraplegia

Paralysis, paralytic — *continued*
  lung J98.4
  median nerve G56.1- ☑
  medullary (tegmental) G83.89
  mesencephalic NEC G83.89
    tegmental G83.89
  middle alternating G83.89
  Millard-Gubler-Foville G46.3
  monoplegic — *see* Monoplegia
  motor G83.9
  muscle, muscular NEC G72.89
    due to nerve lesion G58.9
    eye (extrinsic) H49.9
      intrinsic — *see* Paresis, of accommodation
      oblique — *see* Strabismus, paralytic, fourth nerve
    iris sphincter H21.9
    ischemic (Volkmann's) (complicating trauma) T79.6 ☑
    progressive G12.21
    pseudohypertrophic G71.0
  musculocutaneous nerve G56.9- ☑
  musculospiral G56.9- ☑
  nerve (*see also* Disorder, nerve)
    abducent — *see* Strabismus, paralytic, sixth nerve
    accessory G52.8
    auditory (except Deafness) H93.3 ☑
    birth injury P14.9
    cranial or cerebral G52.9
    facial G51.0
      birth injury P11.3
      congenital P11.3
      newborn (birth injury) P11.3
    fourth or trochlear — *see* Strabismus, paralytic, fourth nerve
    newborn (birth injury) P14.9
    oculomotor — *see* Strabismus, paralytic, third nerve
    phrenic (birth injury) P14.2
    radial G56.3- ☑
    seventh or facial G51.0
      newborn (birth injury) P11.3
    sixth or abducent — *see* Strabismus, paralytic, sixth nerve
    syphilitic A52.15
    third or oculomotor — *see* Strabismus, paralytic, third nerve
    trigeminal G50.9
    trochlear — *see* Strabismus, paralytic, fourth nerve
    ulnar G56.2- ☑
  normokalemic periodic G72.3
  ocular H49.9
    alternating G83.89
  oculofacial, congenital (Moebius) Q87.0
  oculomotor (external bilateral) (nerve) — *see* Strabismus, paralytic, third nerve
  palate (soft) K13.79
  paratrigeminal G50.9
  periodic (familial) (hyperkalemic) (hypokalemic) (myotonic) (normokalemic) (potassium sensitive) (secondary) G72.3
  peripheral autonomic nervous system — *see* Neuropathy, peripheral, autonomic
  peroneal (nerve) G57.3- ☑
  pharynx J39.2
  phrenic nerve G56.8- ☑
  plantar nerve(s) G57.6- ☑
  pneumogastric nerve G52.2
  poliomyelitis (current) — *see* Poliomyelitis, paralytic
  popliteal nerve G57.3- ☑
  postepileptic transitory G83.84
  progressive (atrophic) (bulbar) (spinal) G12.22
    general A52.17
    infantile acute — *see* Poliomyelitis, paralytic
    supranuclear G23.1
  pseudobulbar G12.29
  pseudohypertrophic (muscle) G71.0
  psychogenic F44.4
  quadriceps G57.9- ☑
  quadriplegic — *see* Tetraplegia
  radial nerve G56.3- ☑
  rectus muscle (eye) H49.9
  recurrent isolated sleep G47.53
  respiratory (muscle) (system) (tract) R06.81
    center NEC G93.89
    congenital P28.89
    newborn P28.89
  right side — *see* Hemiplegia

Index

Paralysis, paralytic — Parkinsonism

Paralysis, paralytic — continued
  saturnine T56.0 ☑
  sciatic nerve G57.0- ☑
  senile G83.9
  shaking — see Parkinsonism
  shoulder G56.9- ☑
  sleep, recurrent isolated G47.53
  spastic G83.9
    cerebral — see Palsy, cerebral, spastic
    congenital (cerebral) — see Palsy, cerebral, spastic
    familial G11.4
    hereditary G11.4
    quadriplegic G80.0
    syphilitic (spinal) A52.17
  sphincter, bladder — see Paralysis, bladder
  spinal (cord) G83.9
    accessory nerve G52.8
    acute — see Poliomyelitis, paralytic
    ascending acute G61.0
    atrophic (acute) (see also Poliomyelitis, paralytic)
      spastic, syphilitic A52.17
    congenital NEC — see Palsy, cerebral
    hereditary G95.89
    infantile — see Poliomyelitis, paralytic
    progressive G12.21
    sequelae NEC G83.89
  sternomastoid G52.8
  stomach K31.84
    diabetic — see Diabetes, by type, with gastroparesis
    nerve G52.2
      diabetic — see Diabetes, by type, with gastroparesis
  stroke — see Infarct, brain
  subcapsularis G56.8- ☑
  supranuclear (progressive) G23.1
  sympathetic G90.8
    cervical G90.09
    nervous system — see Neuropathy, peripheral, autonomic
  syndrome G83.9
    specified NEC G83.89
  syphilitic spastic spinal (Erb's) A52.17
  thigh G57.9- ☑
  throat J39.2
    diphtheritic A36.0
    muscle J39.2
  thrombotic (current episode) I63.3- ☑
  thumb G56.9- ☑
  tick — see Toxicity, venom, arthropod, specified NEC
  Todd's (postepileptic transitory paralysis) G83.84
  toe G57.6- ☑
  tongue K14.8
  transient R29.5
    arm or leg NEC R29.818
    traumatic NEC — see Injury, nerve
  trapezius G52.8
  traumatic, transient NEC — see Injury, nerve
  trembling — see Parkinsonism
  triceps brachii G56.9- ☑
  trigeminal nerve G50.9
  trochlear (nerve) — see Strabismus, paralytic, fourth nerve
  ulnar nerve G56.2- ☑
  upper limb — see Monoplegia, upper limb
  uremic N18.9 [G99.8]
  uveoparotitic D86.89
  uvula K13.79
    postdiphtheritic A36.0
  vagus nerve G52.2
  vasomotor NEC G90.8
  velum palati K13.79
  vesical — see Paralysis, bladder
  vestibular nerve (except Vertigo) H93.3 ☑
  vocal cords J38.00
    bilateral J38.02
    unilateral J38.01
  Volkmann's (complicating trauma) T79.6 ☑
  wasting G12.29
  Weber's G46.3
  wrist G56.9- ☑
Paramedial urethrovesical orifice Q64.79
Paramenia N92.6
Parametritis (see also Disease, pelvis, inflammatory) N73.2
  acute N73.0

Parametritis — continued
  complicating abortion — see Abortion, by type, complicated by, parametritis
Parametrium, parametric — see condition
Paramnesia — see Amnesia
Paramolar K00.1
Paramyloidosis E85.89
Paramyoclonus multiplex G25.3
Paramyotonia (congenita) G71.19
Parangi — see Yaws
Paranoia (querulans) F22
  senile F03 ☑
Paranoid
  dementia (senile) F03 ☑
    praecox — see Schizophrenia
  personality F60.0
  psychosis (climacteric) (involutional) (menopausal) F22
    psychogenic (acute) F23
    senile F03 ☑
  reaction (acute) F23
    chronic F22
  schizophrenia F20.0
  state (climacteric) (involutional) (menopausal) (simple) F22
    senile F03 ☑
  tendencies F60.0
  traits F60.0
  trends F60.0
  type, psychopathic personality F60.0
Paraparesis — see Paraplegia
Paraphasia R47.02
Paraphilia F65.9
Paraphimosis (congenital) N47.2
  chancroidal A57
Paraphrenia, paraphrenic (late) F22
  schizophrenia F20.0
Paraplegia (lower) G82.20
  ataxic — see Degeneration, combined, spinal cord
  complete G82.21
  congenital (cerebral) G80.8
    spastic G80.1
  familial spastic G11.4
  functional (hysterical) F44.4
  hereditary, spastic G11.4
  hysterical F44.4
  incomplete G82.22
  Pott's A18.01
  psychogenic F44.4
  spastic
    Erb's spinal, syphilitic A52.17
    hereditary G11.4
    tropical G04.1
  syphilitic (spastic) A52.17
  tropical spastic G04.1
Parapoxvirus B08.60
  specified NEC B08.69
Paraproteinemia D89.2
  benign (familial) D89.2
  monoclonal D47.2
  secondary to malignant disease D47.2
Parapsoriasis L41.9
  en plaques L41.4
  guttata L41.1
  large plaque L41.4
  retiform, retiformis L41.5
  small plaque L41.3
  specified NEC L41.8
  varioliformis (acuta) L41.0
Parasitic (see also condition)
  disease NEC B89
  stomatitis B37.0
  sycosis (beard) (scalp) B35.0
  twin Q89.4
Parasitism B89
  intestinal B82.9
  skin B88.9
  specified — see Infestation
Parasitophobia F40.218
Parasomnia G47.50
  due to
    alcohol
      abuse F10.182
      dependence F10.282
      use F10.982
    amphetamines
      abuse F15.182
      dependence F15.282

Parasomnia — continued
  due to — continued
    amphetamines — continued
      use F15.982
    caffeine
      abuse F15.182
      dependence F15.282
      use F15.982
    cocaine
      abuse F14.182
      dependence F14.282
      use F14.982
    drug NEC
      abuse F19.182
      dependence F19.282
      use F19.982
    opioid
      abuse F11.182
      dependence F11.282
      use F11.982
    psychoactive substance NEC
      abuse F19.182
      dependence F19.282
      use F19.982
    sedative, hypnotic, or anxiolytic
      abuse F13.182
      dependence F13.282
      use F13.982
    stimulant NEC
      abuse F15.182
      dependence F15.282
      use F15.982
  in conditions classified elsewhere G47.54
  nonorganic origin F51.8
  organic G47.50
  specified NEC G47.59
Paraspadias Q54.9
Paraspasmus facialis G51.8
Parasuicide (attempt)
  history of (personal) Z91.5
    in family Z81.8
Parathyroid gland — see condition
Parathyroid tetany E20.9
Paratrachoma A74.0
Paratyphilitis — see Appendicitis
Paratyphoid (fever) — see Fever, paratyphoid
Paratyphus — see Fever, paratyphoid
Paraurethral duct Q64.79
  nonorganic origin F51.5
Paraurethritis (see also Urethritis)
  gonococcal (acute) (chronic) (with abscess) A54.1
Paravaccinia NEC B08.04
Paravaginitis — see Vaginitis
Parencephalitis (see also Encephalitis)
  sequelae G09
Parent-child conflict — see Conflict, parent-child
  estrangement NEC Z62.890
Paresis (see also Paralysis)
  accommodation — see Paresis, of accommodation
  Bernhardt's G57.1- ☑
  bladder (sphincter) (see also Paralysis, bladder)
    tabetic A52.17
  bowel, colon or intestine K56.0
  extrinsic muscle, eye H49.9
  general (progressive) (syphilitic) A52.17
    juvenile A50.45
  heart — see Failure, heart
  insane (syphilitic) A52.17
  juvenile (general) A50.45
  of accommodation H52.52- ☑
  peripheral progressive (idiopathic) G60.3
  pseudohypertrophic G71.0
  senile G83.9
  syphilitic (general) A52.17
    congenital A50.45
  vesical NEC N31.2
Paresthesia (see also Disturbance, sensation, skin) R20.2
  Bernhardt G57.1- ☑
Paretic — see condition
Parinaud's
  conjunctivitis H10.89
  oculoglandular syndrome H10.89
  ophthalmoplegia H49.88- ☑
Parkinsonism (idiopathic) (primary) G20
  with neurogenic orthostatic hypotension (symptomatic) G90.3
  arteriosclerotic G21.4
  dementia G31.83 [F02.80]

☑ Additional Character Required — Refer to the Tabular List for Character Selection   ▽ Subterms under main terms may continue to next column or page

Parkinsonism — *continued*
  dementia — *continued*
    with behavioral disturbance G31.83 [F02.81]
  due to
    drugs NEC G21.19
      neuroleptic G21.11
    medication-induced NEC G21.19
  neuroleptic induced G21.11
  postencephalitic G21.3
  secondary G21.9
    due to
      arteriosclerosis G21.4
      drugs NEC G21.19
        neuroleptic G21.11
      encephalitis G21.3
      external agents NEC G21.2
      syphilis A52.19
    specified NEC G21.8
  syphilitic A52.19
  treatment-induced NEC G21.19
  vascular G21.4
Parkinson's disease, syndrome or tremor — *see* Parkinsonism
Parodontitis — *see* Periodontitis
Parodontosis K05.4
Paronychia (*see also* Cellulitis, digit)
  with lymphangitis — *see* Lymphangitis, acute, digit
  candidal (chronic) B37.2
  tuberculous (primary) A18.4
Parorexia (psychogenic) F50.89
Parosmia R43.1
  psychogenic F45.8
Parotid gland — *see* condition
Parotitis, parotiditis (allergic)(nonspecific toxic) (purulent) (septic) (suppurative) (*see also* Sialoadenitis)
  epidemic — *see* Mumps
  infectious — *see* Mumps
  postoperative K91.89
  surgical K91.89
Parrot fever A70
Parrot's disease (early congenital syphilitic pseudoparalysis) A50.02
Parry-Romberg syndrome G51.8
Parry's disease or syndrome E05.00
  with thyroid storm E05.01
Pars planitis — *see* Cyclitis
Parsonage (-Aldren)-**Turner syndrome** G54.5
Parson's disease (exophthalmic goiter) E05.00
  with thyroid storm E05.01
Particolored infant Q82.8
Parturition — *see* Delivery
Parulis K04.7
  with sinus K04.6
Parvovirus, as cause of disease classified elsewhere B97.6
Pasini and Pierini's atrophoderma L90.3
Passage
  false, urethra N36.5
  meconium (newborn) during delivery P03.82
  of sounds or bougies — *see* Attention to, artificial, opening
Passive — *see* condition
  smoking Z77.22
Pasteurella septica A28.0
Pasteurellosis — *see* Infection, Pasteurella
PAT (paroxysmal atrial tachycardia) I47.1
Patau's syndrome — *see* Trisomy, 13
Patches
  mucous (syphilitic) A51.39
    congenital A50.07
  smokers' (mouth) K13.24
Patellar — *see* condition
Patent (*see also* Imperfect, closure)
  canal of Nuck Q52.4
  cervix N88.3
  ductus arteriosus or Botallo's Q25.0
  foramen
    botalli Q21.1
    ovale Q21.1
  interauricular septum Q21.1
  interventricular septum Q21.0
  omphalomesenteric duct Q43.0
  os (uteri) — *see* Patent, cervix
  ostium secundum Q21.1
  urachus Q64.4
  vitelline duct Q43.0
Paterson (-Brown)(-Kelly) **syndrome or web** D50.1

Pathologic, pathological (*see also* condition)
  asphyxia R09.01
  fire-setting F63.1
  gambling F63.0
  ovum O02.0
  resorption, tooth K03.3
  stealing F63.2
Pathology (of) — *see* Disease
  periradicular, associated with previous endodontic treatment NEC M27.59
Pattern, sleep-wake, irregular G47.23
Patulous (*see also* Imperfect, closure (congenital))
  alimentary tract Q45.8
    lower Q43.8
    upper Q40.8
  eustachian tube H69.0- ☑
Pause, sinoatrial I49.5
Paxton's disease B36.2
Pearl(s)
  enamel K00.2
  Epstein's K09.8
Pearl-worker's disease — *see* Osteomyelitis, specified type NEC
Pectenosis K62.4
Pectoral — *see* condition
Pectus
  carinatum (congenital) Q67.7
    acquired M95.4
      rachitic sequelae (late effect) E64.3
  excavatum (congenital) Q67.6
    acquired M95.4
      rachitic sequelae (late effect) E64.3
  recurvatum (congenital) Q67.6
Pedatrophia E41
Pederosis F65.4
Pediculosis (infestation) B85.2
  capitis (head-louse) (any site) B85.0
  corporis (body-louse) (any site) B85.1
  eyelid B85.0
  mixed (classifiable to more than one of the titles B85.0-B85.3) B85.4
  pubis (pubic louse) (any site) B85.3
  vestimenti B85.1
  vulvae B85.3
Pediculus (infestation) — *see* Pediculosis
Pedophilia F65.4
Peg-shaped teeth K00.2
Pelade — *see* Alopecia, areata
Pelger-Huët anomaly or syndrome D72.0
Peliosis (rheumatica) D69.0
  hepatis K76.4
    with toxic liver disease K71.8
Pelizaeus-Merzbacher disease E75.29
Pellagra (alcoholic) (with polyneuropathy) E52
Pellagra-cerebellar-ataxia-renal aminoaciduria syndrome E72.02
Pellegrini (-Stieda) **disease or syndrome** — *see* Bursitis, tibial collateral
Pellizzi's syndrome E34.8
Pel's crisis A52.11
Pelvic (*see also* condition)
  examination (periodic) (routine) Z01.419
    with abnormal findings Z01.411
  kidney, congenital Q63.2
Pelviolithiasis — *see* Calculus, kidney
Pelviperitonitis (*see also* Peritonitis, pelvic)
  gonococcal A54.24
  puerperal O85
Pelvis — *see* condition or type
Pemphigoid L12.9
  benign, mucous membrane L12.1
  bullous L12.0
  cicatricial L12.1
  juvenile L12.2
  ocular L12.1
  specified NEC L12.8
Pemphigus L10.9
  benign familial (chronic) Q82.8
  Brazilian L10.3
  circinatus L13.0
  conjunctiva L12.1
  drug-induced L10.5
  erythematosus L10.4
  foliaceous L10.2
  gangrenous — *see* Gangrene
  neonatorum L01.03
  ocular L12.1
  paraneoplastic L10.81

Pemphigus — *continued*
  specified NEC L10.89
  syphilitic (congenital) A50.06
  vegetans L10.1
  vulgaris L10.0
  wildfire L10.3
Pendred's syndrome E07.1
Pendulous
  abdomen, in pregnancy — *see* Pregnancy, complicated by, abnormal, pelvic organs or tissues NEC
  breast N64.89
Penetrating wound (*see also* Puncture)
  with internal injury — *see* Injury, by site
  eyeball — *see* Puncture, eyeball
  orbit (with or without foreign body) — *see* Puncture, orbit
  uterus by instrument with or following ectopic or molar pregnancy O08.6
Penicillosis B48.4
Penis — *see* condition
Penitis N48.29
Pentalogy of Fallot Q21.8
Pentasomy X syndrome Q97.1
Pentosuria (essential) E74.8
Percreta placenta - O43.23 ☑
Peregrinating patient — *see* Disorder, factitious
Perforation, perforated (nontraumatic) (of)
  accidental during procedure (blood vessel) (nerve) (organ) — *see* Complication, accidental puncture or laceration
  antrum — *see* Sinusitis, maxillary
  appendix K35.2
    with localized peritonitis K35.3
  atrial septum, multiple Q21.1
  attic, ear — *see* Perforation, tympanum, attic
  bile duct (common) (hepatic) K83.2
    cystic K82.2
  bladder (urinary)
    with or following ectopic or molar pregnancy O08.6
    obstetrical trauma O71.5
    traumatic S37.29 ☑
      at delivery O71.5
  bowel K63.1
    with or following ectopic or molar pregnancy O08.6
    newborn P78.0
    obstetrical trauma O71.5
    traumatic — *see* Laceration, intestine
  broad ligament N83.8
    with or following ectopic or molar pregnancy O08.6
    obstetrical trauma O71.6
  by
    device, implant or graft (*see also* Complications, by site and type, mechanical) T85.628 ☑
      arterial graft NEC — *see* Complication, cardiovascular device, mechanical, vascular
      breast (implant) T85.49 ☑
      catheter NEC T85.698 ☑
        cystostomy T83.090 ☑
        dialysis (renal) T82.49 ☑
          intraperitoneal T85.691 ☑
        infusion NEC T82.594 ☑
          spinal (epidural) (subdural) T85.690 ☑
        urinary (*see also* Complications, catheter, urinary T83.098 ☑
      electronic (electrode) (pulse generator) (stimulator)
        bone T84.390 ☑
        cardiac T82.199 ☑
          electrode T82.190 ☑
          pulse generator T82.191 ☑
          specified type NEC T82.198 ☑
        nervous system — *see* Complication, prosthetic device, mechanical, electronic nervous system stimulator
        urinary — *see* Complication, genitourinary, device, urinary, mechanical
      fixation, internal (orthopedic) NEC — *see* Complication, fixation device, mechanical
      gastrointestinal — *see* Complications, prosthetic device, mechanical, gastrointestinal device
      genital NEC T83.498 ☑
        intrauterine contraceptive device T83.39 ☑
        penile prosthesis T83.490 ☑
      heart NEC — *see* Complication, cardiovascular device, mechanical

Perforation, perforated — *continued*
  by — *continued*
    device, implant or graft (*see also* Complications, by site and type, mechanical) — *continued*
      joint prosthesis — *see* Complications, joint prosthesis, mechanical, specified NEC, by site
      ocular NEC — *see* Complications, prosthetic device, mechanical, ocular device
      orthopedic NEC — *see* Complication, orthopedic, device, mechanical
      specified NEC T85.628 ☑
      urinary NEC (*see also* Complication, genitourinary, device, urinary, mechanical)
        graft T83.29 ☑
      vascular NEC — *see* Complication, cardiovascular device, mechanical
      ventricular intracranial shunt T85.09 ☑
      foreign body left accidentally in operative wound T81.539 ☑
      instrument (any) during a procedure, accidental — *see* Puncture, accidental complicating surgery
    cecum K35.2
      with localized peritonitis K35.3
    cervix (uteri) N88.8
      with or following ectopic or molar pregnancy O08.6
      obstetrical trauma O71.3
    colon K63.1
      newborn P78.0
      obstetrical trauma O71.5
      traumatic — *see* Laceration, intestine, large
    common duct (bile) K83.2
    cornea (due to ulceration) — *see* Ulcer, cornea, perforated
    cystic duct K82.2
    diverticulum (intestine) K57.80
      with bleeding K57.81
      large intestine K57.20
        with
          bleeding K57.21
          small intestine K57.40
            with bleeding K57.41
      small intestine K57.00
        with
          bleeding K57.01
          large intestine K57.40
            with bleeding K57.41
    ear drum — *see* Perforation, tympanum
    esophagus K22.3
    ethmoidal sinus — *see* Sinusitis, ethmoidal
    frontal sinus — *see* Sinusitis, frontal
    gallbladder K82.2
    heart valve — *see* Endocarditis
    ileum K63.1
      newborn P78.0
      obstetrical trauma O71.5
      traumatic — *see* Laceration, intestine, small
    instrumental, surgical (accidental) (blood vessel) (nerve) (organ) — *see* Puncture, accidental complicating surgery
    intestine NEC K63.1
      with ectopic or molar pregnancy O08.6
      newborn P78.0
      obstetrical trauma O71.5
      traumatic — *see* Laceration, intestine
      ulcerative NEC K63.1
        newborn P78.0
    jejunum, jejunal K63.1
      obstetrical trauma O71.5
      traumatic — *see* Laceration, intestine, small
      ulcer — *see* Ulcer, gastrojejunal, with perforation
    joint prosthesis — *see* Complications, joint prosthesis, mechanical, specified NEC, by site
    mastoid (antrum) (cell) — *see* Disorder, mastoid, specified NEC
    maxillary sinus — *see* Sinusitis, maxillary
    membrana tympani — *see* Perforation, tympanum
    nasal
      septum J34.89
        congenital Q30.3
        syphilitic A52.73
      sinus J34.89
        congenital Q30.8
        due to sinusitis — *see* Sinusitis
    palate (*see also* Cleft, palate) Q35.9
      syphilitic A52.79
    palatine vault (*see also* Cleft, palate, hard) Q35.1

Perforation, perforated — *continued*
  palatine vault (*see also* Cleft, palate, hard) — *continued*
    syphilitic A52.79
    congenital A50.59
  pars flaccida (ear drum) — *see* Perforation, tympanum, attic
  pelvic
    floor S31.030 ☑
      with
        ectopic or molar pregnancy O08.6
        penetration into retroperitoneal space S31.031 ☑
        retained foreign body S31.040 ☑
          with penetration into retroperitoneal space S31.041 ☑
      following ectopic or molar pregnancy O08.6
      obstetrical trauma O70.1
    organ S37.99 ☑
      adrenal gland S37.818 ☑
      bladder — *see* Perforation, bladder
      fallopian tube S37.599 ☑
        bilateral S37.592 ☑
        unilateral S37.591 ☑
      kidney S37.09-
      obstetrical trauma O71.5
      ovary S37.499 ☑
        bilateral S37.492 ☑
        unilateral S37.491 ☑
      prostate S37.828 ☑
      specified organ NEC S37.898 ☑
      ureter — *see* Perforation, ureter
      urethra — *see* Perforation, urethra
      uterus — *see* Perforation, uterus
  perineum — *see* Laceration, perineum
  pharynx J39.2
  rectum K63.1
    newborn P78.0
    obstetrical trauma O71.5
    traumatic S36.63 ☑
  root canal space due to endodontic treatment M27.51
  sigmoid K63.1
    newborn P78.0
    obstetrical trauma O71.5
    traumatic S36.533 ☑
  sinus (accessory) (chronic) (nasal) J34.89
  sphenoidal sinus — *see* Sinusitis, sphenoidal
  surgical (accidental) (by instrument) (blood vessel) (nerve) (organ) — *see* Puncture, accidental complicating surgery
  traumatic
    external — *see* Puncture
    eye — *see* Puncture, eyeball
    internal organ — *see* Injury, by site
  tympanum, tympanic (membrane) (persistent post-traumatic) (postinflammatory) H72.9- ☑
    attic H72.1- ☑
      multiple — *see* Perforation, tympanum, multiple
      total — *see* Perforation, tympanum, total
    central H72.0- ☑
      multiple — *see* Perforation, tympanum, multiple
      total — *see* Perforation, tympanum, total
    marginal NEC — *see* subcategory H72.2 ☑
    multiple H72.81- ☑
    pars flaccida — *see* Perforation, tympanum, attic
    total H72.82- ☑
    traumatic, current episode S09.2- ☑
  typhoid, gastrointestinal — *see* Typhoid
  ulcer — *see* Ulcer, by site, with perforation
  ureter N28.89
    traumatic S37.19 ☑
  urethra N36.8
    with ectopic or molar pregnancy O08.6
    following ectopic or molar pregnancy O08.6
    obstetrical trauma O71.5
    traumatic S37.39 ☑
      at delivery O71.5
  uterus
    with ectopic or molar pregnancy O08.6
    by intrauterine contraceptive device T83.39 ☑
    following ectopic or molar pregnancy O08.6
    obstetrical trauma O71.1
    traumatic S37.69 ☑
      obstetric O71.1
  uvula K13.79

Perforation, perforated — *continued*
  uvula — *continued*
    syphilitic A52.79
  vagina O71.4
    obstetrical trauma O71.4
    other trauma — *see* Puncture, vagina
Periadenitis mucosa necrotica recurrens K12.0
Periappendicitis (acute) — *see* Appendicitis
Periarteritis nodosa (disseminated) (infectious) (necrotizing) M30.0
Periarthritis (joint) (*see also* Enthesopathy)
  Duplay's M75.0 ☑
  gonococcal A54.42
  humeroscapularis — *see* Capsulitis, adhesive
  scapulohumeral — *see* Capsulitis, adhesive
  shoulder — *see* Capsulitis, adhesive
  wrist M77.2-
Periarthrosis (angioneural) — *see* Enthesopathy
Pericapsulitis, adhesive (shoulder) — *see* Capsulitis, adhesive
Pericarditis (with decompensation) (with effusion) I31.9
  with rheumatic fever (conditions in I00)
    active — *see* Pericarditis, rheumatic
    inactive or quiescent I09.2
  acute (hemorrhagic) (nonrheumatic) (Sicca) I30.9
    with chorea (acute) (rheumatic) (Sydenham's) I02.0
    benign I30.8
    nonspecific I30.0
    rheumatic I01.0
      with chorea (acute) (Sydenham's) I02.0
  adhesive or adherent (chronic) (external) (internal) I31.0
    acute — *see* Pericarditis, acute
    rheumatic I09.2
  bacterial (acute) (subacute) (with serous or seropurulent effusion) I30.1
  calcareous I31.1
  cholesterol (chronic) I31.8
    acute I30.9
  chronic (nonrheumatic) I31.9
    rheumatic I09.2
  constrictive (chronic) I31.1
  coxsackie B33.23
  fibrinocaseous (tuberculous) A18.84
  fibrinopurulent I30.1
  fibrinous I30.8
  fibrous I31.0
  gonococcal A54.83
  idiopathic I30.0
  in systemic lupus erythematosus M32.12
  infective I30.1
  meningococcal A39.53
  neoplastic (chronic) I31.8
    acute I30.9
  obliterans, obliterating I31.0
  plastic I31.0
  pneumococcal I30.1
  postinfarction I24.1
  purulent I30.1
  rheumatic (active) (acute) (with effusion) (with pneumonia) I01.0
    with chorea (acute) (rheumatic) (Sydenham's) I02.0
    chronic or inactive (with chorea) I09.2
  rheumatoid — *see* Rheumatoid, carditis
  septic I30.1
  serofibrinous I30.8
  staphylococcal I30.1
  streptococcal I30.1
  suppurative I30.1
  syphilitic A52.06
  tuberculous A18.84
  uremic N18.9 [I32]
  viral I30.1
Pericardium, pericardial — *see* condition
Pericellulitis — *see* Cellulitis
Pericementitis (chronic) (suppurative) (*see also* Periodontitis)
  acute K05.20
    generalized — *see* Peridontitis, aggressive, generalized
    localized — *see* Peridontitis, aggressive, localized
Perichondritis
  auricle — *see* Perichondritis, ear
  bronchus J98.09
  ear (external) H61.00- ☑
    acute H61.01- ☑
    chronic H61.02- ☑
  external auditory canal — *see* Perichondritis, ear

Perichondritis — continued
　larynx J38.7
　　syphilitic A52.73
　　typhoid A01.09
　nose J34.89
　pinna — see Perichondritis, ear
　trachea J39.8
Periclasia K05.4
Pericoronitis — see Periodontitis
Pericystitis N30.90
　with hematuria N30.91
Peridiverticulitis (intestine) K57.92
　cecum — see Diverticulitis, intestine, large
　colon — see Diverticulitis, intestine, large
　duodenum — see Diverticulitis, intestine, small
　intestine — see Diverticulitis, intestine
　jejunum — see Diverticulitis, intestine, small
　rectosigmoid — see Diverticulitis, intestine, large
　rectum — see Diverticulitis, intestine, large
　sigmoid — see Diverticulitis, intestine, large
Periendocarditis — see Endocarditis
Periepididymitis N45.1
Perifolliculitis L01.02
　abscedens, caput, scalp L66.3
　capitis, abscedens (et suffodiens) L66.3
　superficial pustular L01.02
Perihepatitis K65.8
Perilabyrinthitis (acute) — see subcategory H83.0 ☑
Perimeningitis — see Meningitis
Perimetritis — see Endometritis
Perimetrosalpingitis — see Salpingo-oophoritis
Perineocele N81.81
Perinephric, perinephritic — see condition
Perinephritis (see also Infection, kidney)
　purulent — see Abscess, kidney
Perineum, perineal — see condition
Perineuritis NEC — see Neuralgia
Periodic — see condition
Periodontitis (chronic) (complex) (compound) (local)
　　(simplex) K05.30
　acute K05.20
　　generalized K05.229
　　　moderate K05.222
　　　severe K05.223
　　　slight K05.221
　　localized K05.219
　　　moderate K05.212
　　　severe K05.213
　　　slight K05.211
　apical K04.5
　　acute (pulpal origin) K04.4
　generalized K05.329
　　moderate K05.322
　　severe K05.323
　　slight K05.321
　localized K05.319
　　moderate K05.312
　　severe K05.313
　　slight K05.311
Periodontoclasia K05.4
Periodontosis (juvenile) K05.4
Periods (see also Menstruation)
　heavy N92.0
　irregular N92.6
　shortened intervals (irregular) N92.1
Perionychia (see also Cellulitis, digit)
　with lymphangitis — see Lymphangitis, acute, digit
Perioophoritis — see Salpingo-oophoritis
Periorchitis N45.2
Periosteum, periosteal — see condition
Periostitis (albuminosa) (circumscribed) (diffuse) (infective) (monomelic) (see also Osteomyelitis)
　alveolar M27.3
　alveolodental M27.3
　dental M27.3
　gonorrheal A54.43
　jaw (lower) (upper) M27.2
　orbit H05.03- ☑
　syphilitic A52.77
　　congenital (early) A50.02 [M90.80]
　　secondary A51.46
　tuberculous — see Tuberculosis, bone
　yaws (hypertrophic) (early) (late) A66.6 [M90.80]
Periostosis (hyperplastic) (see also Disorder, bone, specified type NEC)
　with osteomyelitis — see Osteomyelitis, specified type
　　NEC

Peripartum
　cardiomyopathy O90.3
Periphlebitis — see Phlebitis
Periproctitis K62.89
Periprostatitis — see Prostatitis
Perirectal — see condition
Perirenal — see condition
Perisalpingitis — see Salpingo-oophoritis
Perisplenitis (infectional) D73.89
Peristalsis, visible or reversed R19.2
Peritendinitis — see Enthesopathy
Peritoneum, peritoneal — see condition
Peritonitis (adhesive) (bacterial) (fibrinous) (hemorrhagic) (idiopathic) (localized) (perforative) (primary)
　　(with adhesions) (with effusion) K65.9
　with or following
　　abscess K65.1
　　appendicitis K35.3
　　　with perforation or rupture K35.2
　　　generalized K35.2
　　　localized K35.3
　　diverticular disease (intestine) K57.80
　　　with bleeding K57.81
　　　ectopic or molar pregnancy O08.0
　　　large intestine K57.20
　　　　with
　　　　　bleeding K57.21
　　　　　small intestine K57.40
　　　　　　with bleeding K57.41
　　　small intestine K57.00
　　　　with
　　　　　bleeding K57.01
　　　　　large intestine K57.40
　　　　　　with bleeding K57.41
　acute (generalized) K65.0
　aseptic T81.61 ☑
　bile, biliary K65.3
　chemical T81.61 ☑
　chlamydial A74.81
　chronic proliferative K65.8
　complicating abortion — see Abortion, by type, complicated by, pelvic peritonitis
　congenital P78.1
　diaphragmatic K65.0
　diffuse K65.0
　diphtheritic A36.89
　disseminated K65.0
　due to
　　bile K65.3
　　foreign
　　　body or object accidentally left during a procedure (instrument) (sponge) (swab)
　　　　T81.599 ☑
　　　substance accidentally left during a procedure
　　　　(chemical) (powder) (talc) T81.61 ☑
　　talc T81.61 ☑
　　urine K65.8
　eosinophilic K65.8
　　acute K65.0
　fibrocaseous (tuberculous) A18.31
　fibropurulent K65.0
　following ectopic or molar pregnancy O08.0
　general (ized) K65.0
　gonococcal A54.85
　meconium (newborn) P78.0
　neonatal P78.1
　　meconium P78.0
　pancreatic K65.0
　paroxysmal, familial E85.0
　　benign E85.0
　pelvic
　　female N73.5
　　　acute N73.3
　　　chronic N73.4
　　　　with adhesions N73.6
　　male K65.0
　periodic, familial E85.0
　proliferative, chronic K65.8
　puerperal, postpartum, childbirth O85
　purulent K65.0
　septic K65.0
　specified NEC K65.8
　spontaneous bacterial K65.2
　subdiaphragmatic K65.0
　subphrenic K65.0
　suppurative K65.0
　syphilitic A52.74
　　congenital (early) A50.08 [K67]

Peritonitis — continued
　talc T81.61 ☑
　tuberculous A18.31
　urine K65.8
Peritonsillar — see condition
Peritonsillitis J36
Perityphlitis K37
Periureteritis N28.89
Periurethral — see condition
Periurethritis (gangrenous) — see Urethritis
Periuterine — see condition
Perivaginitis — see Vaginitis
Perivasculitis, retinal H35.06- ☑
Perivasitis (chronic) N49.1
Perivesiculitis (seminal) — see Vesiculitis
Perlèche NEC K13.0
　due to
　　candidiasis B37.83
　　moniliasis B37.83
　　riboflavin deficiency E53.0
　　vitamin B2 (riboflavin) deficiency E53.0
Pernicious — see condition
Pernio, perniosis T69.1 ☑
Perpetrator (of abuse) — see Index to External Causes
　of Injury, Perpetrator
Persecution
　delusion F22
　social Z60.5
Perseveration (tonic) R48.8
Persistence, persistent (congenital)
　anal membrane Q42.3
　　with fistula Q42.2
　arteria stapedia Q16.3
　atrioventricular canal Q21.2
　branchial cleft NOS Q18.2
　　cyst Q18.0
　　fistula Q18.0
　　sinus Q18.0
　bulbus cordis in left ventricle Q21.8
　canal of Cloquet Q14.0
　capsule (opaque) Q12.8
　cilioretinal artery or vein Q14.8
　cloaca Q43.7
　communication — see Fistula, congenital
　convolutions
　　aortic arch Q25.46
　　fallopian tube Q50.6
　　oviduct Q50.6
　　uterine tube Q50.6
　double aortic arch Q25.45
　ductus arteriosus (Botalli) Q25.0
　fetal
　　circulation P29.38
　　form of cervix (uteri) Q51.828
　　hemoglobin, hereditary (HPFH) D56.4
　foramen
　　Botalli Q21.1
　　ovale Q21.1
　Gartner's duct Q52.4
　hemoglobin, fetal (hereditary) (HPFH) D56.4
　hyaloid
　　artery (generally incomplete) Q14.0
　　system Q14.8
　hymen, in pregnancy or childbirth — see Pregnancy,
　　complicated by, abnormal, vulva
　lanugo Q84.2
　left
　　posterior cardinal vein Q26.8
　　root with right arch of aorta Q25.49
　　superior vena cava Q26.1
　Meckel's diverticulum Q43.0
　　malignant — see Table of Neoplasms, small intestine, malignant
　mucosal disease (middle ear) — see Otitis, media,
　　suppurative, chronic, tubotympanic
　nail(s), anomalous Q84.6
　omphalomesenteric duct Q43.0
　organ or site not listed — see Anomaly, by site
　ostium
　　atrioventriculare commune Q21.2
　　primum Q21.2
　　secundum Q21.1
　ovarian rests in fallopian tube Q50.6
　pancreatic tissue in intestinal tract Q43.8
　primary (deciduous)
　　teeth K00.6
　　vitreous hyperplasia Q14.0
　pupillary membrane Q13.89

☑ **Additional Character Required — Refer to the Tabular List for Character Selection**   ▽ **Subterms under main terms may continue to next column or page**

Persistence, persistent — Phlebitis

Phlebitis — *continued*
  leg — *continued*
      femoral vein (superficial) I80.1- ☑
      superficial (vessels) I80.0- ☑
  longitudinal sinus — *see* Phlebitis, intracranial (venous) sinus
  lower limb — *see* Phlebitis, leg
  migrans, migrating (superficial) I82.1
  pelvic
      with ectopic or molar pregnancy O08.0
      following ectopic or molar pregnancy O08.0
      puerperal, postpartum O87.1
  popliteal vein — *see* Phlebitis, leg, deep, popliteal
  portal (vein) K75.1
  postoperative T81.72 ☑
  pregnancy — *see* Thrombophlebitis, antepartum
  puerperal, postpartum, childbirth O87.0
      deep O87.1
      pelvic O87.1
      superficial O87.0
  retina — *see* Vasculitis, retina
  saphenous (accessory) (great) (long) (small) — *see* Phlebitis, leg, superficial
  sinus (meninges) — *see* Phlebitis, intracranial (venous) sinus
  specified site NEC I80.8
  syphilitic A52.09
  tibial vein — *see* Phlebitis, leg, deep, tibial
  ulcerative I80.9
      leg — *see* Phlebitis, leg
  umbilicus I80.8
  uterus (septic) — *see* Endometritis
  varicose (leg) (lower limb) — *see* Varix, leg, with, inflammation
Phlebofibrosis I87.8
Phleboliths I87.8
Phlebopathy,
  gestational O22.9- ☑
  puerperal O87.9
Phlebosclerosis I87.8
Phlebothrombosis (*see also* Thrombosis)
  antepartum — *see* Thrombophlebitis, antepartum
  pregnancy — *see* Thrombophlebitis, antepartum
  puerperal — *see* Thrombophlebitis, puerperal
Phlebotomus fever A93.1
Phlegmasia
  alba dolens O87.1
      nonpuerperal — *see* Phlebitis, femoral vein
  cerulea dolens — *see* Phlebitis, leg, deep
Phlegmon — *see* Abscess
Phlegmonous — *see* condition
Phlyctenulosis (allergic) (keratoconjunctivitis) (nontuberculous) (*see also* Keratoconjunctivitis)
  cornea — *see* Keratoconjunctivitis
  tuberculous A18.52
Phobia, phobic F40.9
  animal F40.218
      spiders F40.210
  examination F40.298
  reaction F40.9
  simple F40.298
  social F40.10
      generalized F40.11
  specific (isolated) F40.298
      animal F40.218
         spiders F40.210
      blood F40.230
      injection F40.231
      injury F40.233
      men F40.290
      natural environment F40.228
         thunderstorms F40.220
      situational F40.248
         bridges F40.242
         closed in spaces F40.240
         flying F40.243
         heights F40.241
      specified focus NEC F40.298
      transfusion F40.231
      women F40.291
  specified NEC F40.8
      medical care NEC F40.232
  state F40.9
Phocas' disease — *see* Mastopathy, cystic
Phocomelia Q73.1
  lower limb — *see* Agenesis, leg, with foot present
  upper limb — *see* Agenesis, arm, with hand present

Phoria H50.50
Phosphate-losing tubular disorder N25.0
Phosphatemia E83.39
Phosphaturia E83.39
Photodermatitis (sun) L56.8
  chronic L57.8
  due to drug L56.8
  light other than sun L59.8
Photokeratitis H16.13- ☑
Photophobia H53.14- ☑
Photophthalmia — *see* Photokeratitis
Photopsia H53.19
Photoretinitis — *see* Retinopathy, solar
Photosensitivity, photosensitization (sun) skin L56.8
  light other than sun L59.8
Phrenitis — *see* Encephalitis
Phrynoderma (vitamin A deficiency) E50.8
Phthiriasis (pubis) B85.3
  with any infestation classifiable to B85.0-B85.2 B85.4
Phthirus infestation — *see* Phthiriasis
Phthisis (*see also* Tuberculosis)
  bulbi (infectional) — *see* Disorder, globe, degenerated condition, atrophy
  eyeball (due to infection) — *see* Disorder, globe, degenerated condition, atrophy
Phycomycosis — *see* Zygomycosis
Physalopteriasis B81.8
Physical restraint status Z78.1
Phytobezoar T18.9 ☑
  intestine T18.3 ☑
  stomach T18.2 ☑
Pian — *see* Yaws
Pianoma A66.1
Pica F50.89
  in adults F50.89
  infant or child F98.3
Picking, nose F98.8
Pick-Niemann disease — *see* Niemann-Pick disease or syndrome
Pick's
  cerebral atrophy G31.01 [F02.80]
      with behavioral disturbance G31.01 [F02.81]
  disease or syndrome (brain) G31.01 [F02.80]
      with behavioral disturbance G31.01 [F02.81]
      brain G31.01 [F02.80]
         with behavioral disturbance G31.01 [F02.81]
         pericardium (pericardial pseudocirrhosis of liver) I31.1
      syndrome
         brain G31.01 [F02.80]
            with behavioral disturbance G31.01 [F02.81]
         of heart (pericardial pseudocirrhosis of liver) I31.1
Pickwickian syndrome E66.2
Piebaldism E70.39
Piedra (beard) (scalp) B36.8
  black B36.3
  white B36.2
Pierre Robin deformity or syndrome Q87.0
Pierson's disease or osteochondrosis M91.0
Pig-bel A05.2
Pigeon
  breast or chest (acquired) M95.4
      congenital Q67.7
      rachitic sequelae (late effect) E64.3
  breeder's disease or lung J67.2
  fancier's disease or lung J67.2
  toe — *see* Deformity, toe, specified NEC
Pigmentation (abnormal) (anomaly) L81.9
  conjunctiva H11.13- ☑
  cornea (anterior) H18.01- ☑
      posterior H18.05- ☑
      stromal H18.06- ☑
  diminished melanin formation NEC L81.6
  iron L81.8
  lids, congenital Q82.8
  limbus corneae — *see* Pigmentation, cornea
  metals L81.8
  optic papilla, congenital Q14.2
  retina, congenital (grouped) (nevoid) Q14.1
  scrotum, congenital Q82.8
  tattoo L81.8
Piles (*see also* Hemorrhoids) K64.9
Pili
  annulati or torti (congenital) Q84.1
  incarnati L73.1
Pill roller hand (intrinsic) — *see* Parkinsonism
Pilomatrixoma — *see* Neoplasm, skin, benign

Pilomatrixoma — *continued*
  malignant — *see* Neoplasm, skin, malignant
Pilonidal — *see* condition
Pimple R23.8
PIN — *see* Neoplasia, intraepithelial, prostate
Pinched nerve — *see* Neuropathy, entrapment
Pindborg tumor — *see* Cyst, calcifying odontogenic
Pineal body or gland — *see* condition
Pinealoblastoma C75.3
Pinealoma D44.5
  malignant C75.3
Pineoblastoma C75.3
Pineocytoma D44.5
Pinguecula H11.15- ☑
Pingueculitis H10.81- ☑
Pinhole meatus (*see also* Stricture, urethra) N35.9
Pink
  disease — *see* subcategory T56.1 ☑
  eye — *see* Conjunctivitis, acute, mucopurulent
Pinkus' disease (lichen nitidus) L44.1
Pinpoint
  meatus — *see* Stricture, urethra
  os (uteri) — *see* Stricture, cervix
Pins and needles R20.2
Pinta A67.9
  cardiovascular lesions A67.2
  chancre (primary) A67.0
  erythematous plaques A67.1
  hyperchromic lesions A67.1
  hyperkeratosis A67.1
  lesions A67.9
      cardiovascular A67.2
      hyperchromic A67.1
      intermediate A67.1
      late A67.2
      mixed A67.3
      primary A67.0
      skin (achromic) (cicatricial) (dyschromic) A67.2
         hyperchromic A67.1
         mixed (achromic and hyperchromic) A67.3
  papule (primary) A67.0
  skin lesions (achromic) (cicatricial) (dyschromic) A67.2
      hyperchromic A67.1
      mixed (achromic and hyperchromic) A67.3
  vitiligo A67.2
Pintids A67.1
Pinworm (disease) (infection) (infestation) B80
Piroplasmosis B60.0
Pistol wound — *see* Gunshot wound
Pitchers' elbow — *see* Derangement, joint, specified type NEC, elbow
Pithecoid pelvis Q74.2
  with disproportion (fetopelvic) O33.0
      causing obstructed labor O65.0
Pithiatism F48.8
Pitted — *see* Pitting
Pitting (*see also* Edema) R60.9
  lip R60.0
  nail L60.8
  teeth K00.4
Pituitary gland — *see* condition
Pituitary-snuff-taker's disease J67.8
Pityriasis (capitis) L21.0
  alba L30.5
  circinata (et maculata) L42
  furfuracea L21.0
  Hebra's L26
  lichenoides L41.0
      chronica L41.1
      et varioliformis (acuta) L41.0
  maculata (et circinata) L30.5
  nigra B36.1
  pilaris, Hebra's L44.0
  rosea L42
  rotunda L44.8
  rubra (Hebra) pilaris L44.0
  simplex L30.5
  specified type NEC L30.5
  streptogenes L30.5
  versicolor (scrotal) B36.0
Placenta, placental — *see* Pregnancy, complicated by (care of) (management affected by), specified condition
Placentitis O41.14- ☑
Plagiocephaly Q67.3
Plague A20.9
  abortive A20.8

▽ Subterms under main terms may continue to next column or page   ☑ Additional Character Required — Refer to the Tabular List for Character Selection   253

Phlebitis — Plague

Pneumonia — *continued*
  congenital — *continued*
    due to
      bacterium NEC P23.6
      Chlamydia P23.1
      Escherichia coli P23.4
      Haemophilus influenzae P23.6
      infective organism NEC P23.8
      Klebsiella pneumoniae P23.6
      Mycoplasma P23.6
      Pseudomonas P23.5
      Staphylococcus P23.2
      Streptococcus (except group B) P23.6
        group B P23.3
      viral agent P23.0
    specified NEC P23.8
  croupous — *see* Pneumonia, lobar
  cryptogenic organizing J84.116
  cytomegalic inclusion B25.0
  cytomegaloviral B25.0
  deglutition — *see* Pneumonia, aspiration
  desquamative interstitial J84.117
  diffuse — *see* Pneumonia, broncho
  diplococcal, diplococcus (broncho-) (lobar) J13
  disseminated (focal) — *see* Pneumonia, broncho
  Eaton's agent J15.7
  embolic, embolism — *see* Embolism, pulmonary
  Enterobacter J15.6
  eosinophilic J82
  Escherichia coli (E. coli) J15.5
  Eubacterium J15.8
  fibrinous — *see* Pneumonia, lobar
  fibroid, fibrous (chronic) — *see* Fibrosis, lung
  Friedländer's bacillus J15.0
  Fusobacterium (nucleatum) J15.8
  gangrenous J85.0
  giant cell (measles) B05.2
  gonococcal A54.84
  gram-negative bacteria NEC J15.6
    anaerobic J15.8
  Hemophilus influenzae (broncho) (lobar) J14
  human metapneumovirus J12.3
  hypostatic (broncho) (lobar) J18.2
  in (due to)
    actinomycosis A42.0
    adenovirus J12.0
    anthrax A22.1
    ascariasis B77.81
    aspergillosis B44.9
    Bacillus anthracis A22.1
    Bacterium anitratum J15.6
    candidiasis B37.1
    chickenpox B01.2
    Chlamydia J16.0
      neonatal P23.1
    coccidioidomycosis B38.2
      acute B38.0
      chronic B38.1
    cytomegalovirus disease B25.0
    Diplococcus (pneumoniae) J13
    Eaton's agent J15.7
    Enterobacter J15.6
    Escherichia coli (E. coli) J15.5
    Friedländer's bacillus J15.0
    fumes and vapors (chemical) (inhalation) J68.0
    gonorrhea A54.84
    Hemophilus influenzae (H. influenzae) J14
    Herellea J15.6
    histoplasmosis B39.2
      acute B39.0
      chronic B39.1
    human metapneumovirus J12.3
    Klebsiella (pneumoniae) J15.0
    measles B05.2
    Mycoplasma (pneumoniae) J15.7
    nocardiosis, nocardiasis A43.0
    ornithosis A70
    parainfluenza virus J12.2
    pleuro-pneumonia-like-organism (PPLO) J15.7
    pneumococcus J13
    pneumocystosis (Pneumocystis carinii) (Pneumo-
      cystis jiroveci) B59
    Proteus J15.6
    Pseudomonas NEC J15.1
      pseudomallei A24.1
    psittacosis A70
    Q fever A78
    respiratory syncytial virus J12.1

Pneumonia — *continued*
  in — *continued*
    rheumatic fever I00 [J17]
    rubella B06.81
    Salmonella (infection) A02.22
      typhi A01.03
    schistosomiasis B65.9 [J17]
    Serratia marcescens J15.6
    specified
      bacterium NEC J15.8
      organism NEC J16.8
    spirochetal NEC A69.8
    Staphylococcus J15.20
      aureus (methicillin susceptible) (MSSA) J15.211
        methicillin resistant (MRSA) J15.212
      specified NEC J15.29
    Streptococcus J15.4
      group B J15.3
      pneumoniae J13
      specified NEC J15.4
    toxoplasmosis B58.3
    tularemia A21.2
    typhoid (fever) A01.03
    varicella B01.2
    virus — *see* Pneumonia, viral
    whooping cough A37.91
      due to
        Bordetella parapertussis A37.11
        Bordetella pertussis A37.01
        specified NEC A37.81
    Yersinia pestis A20.2
  inhalation of food or vomit — *see* Pneumonia, aspira-
    tion
  interstitial J84.9
    chronic J84.111
    desquamative J84.117
    due to
      collagen vascular disease J84.17
      known underlying cause J84.17
    idiopathic NOS J84.111
    in disease classified elsewhere J84.17
    lymphocytic (due to collagen vascular disease) (in
      diseases classified elsewhere) J84.17
    lymphoid J84.2
    non-specific J84.89
      due to
        collagen vascular disease J84.17
        known underlying cause J84.17
      idiopathic J84.113
      in diseases classified elsewhere J84.17
    plasma cell B59
    pseudomonas J15.1
    usual J84.112
      due to collagen vascular disease J84.17
      idiopathic J84.112
      in diseases classified elsewhere J84.17
  Klebsiella (pneumoniae) J15.0
  lipid, lipoid (exogenous) J69.1
    endogenous J84.89
  lobar (disseminated) (double) (interstitial) J18.1
    bacterial J15.9
      specified NEC J15.8
    chronic — *see* Fibrosis, lung
    Escherichia coli (E. coli) J15.5
    Friedländer's bacillus J15.0
    Hemophilus influenzae J14
    hypostatic J18.2
    Klebsiella (pneumoniae) J15.0
    pneumococcal J13
    Proteus J15.6
    Pseudomonas J15.1
    specified organism NEC J16.8
    staphylococcal — *see* Pneumonia, staphylococcal
    streptococcal NEC J15.4
    Streptococcus pneumoniae J13
    viral, virus — *see* Pneumonia, viral
  lobular — *see* Pneumonia, broncho
  Löffler's J82
  lymphoid interstitial J84.2
  massive — *see* Pneumonia, lobar
  meconium P24.01
  MRSA (methicillin resistant Staphylococcus aureus)
    J15.212
  MSSA (methicillin susceptible Staphylococcus aureus)
    J15.211
  multilobar — *see* Pneumonia, by type
  Mycoplasma (pneumoniae) J15.7
  necrotic J85.0

Pneumonia — *continued*
  neonatal P23.9
    aspiration — *see* Aspiration, by substance, with
      pneumonia
  nitrogen dioxide J68.0
  organizing J84.89
    due to
      collagen vascular disease J84.17
      known underlying cause J84.17
    in diseases classified elsewhere J84.17
  orthostatic J18.2
  parainfluenza virus J12.2
  parenchymatous — *see* Fibrosis, lung
  passive J18.2
  patchy — *see* Pneumonia, broncho
  Peptococcus J15.8
  Peptostreptococcus J15.8
  plasma cell (of infants) B59
  pleurolobar — *see* Pneumonia, lobar
  pleuro-pneumonia-like organism (PPLO) J15.7
  pneumococcal (broncho) (lobar) J13
  Pneumocystis (carinii) (jiroveci) B59
  postinfectional NEC B99 ☑ [J17]
  postmeasles B05.2
  Proteus J15.6
  Pseudomonas J15.1
  psittacosis A70
  radiation J70.0
  respiratory syncytial virus J12.1
  resulting from a procedure J95.89
  rheumatic I00 [J17]
  Salmonella (arizonae) (cholerae-suis) (enteritidis) (ty-
    phimurium) A02.22
    typhi A01.03
    typhoid fever A01.03
  SARS-associated coronavirus J12.81
  segmented, segmental — *see* Pneumonia, broncho-
  Serratia marcescens J15.6
  specified NEC J18.8
    bacterium NEC J15.8
    organism NEC J16.8
    virus NEC J12.89
  spirochetal NEC A69.8
  staphylococcal (broncho) (lobar) J15.20
    aureus (methicillin susceptible) (MSSA) J15.211
      methicillin resistant (MRSA) J15.212
    specified NEC J15.29
  static, stasis J18.2
  streptococcal NEC (broncho) (lobar) J15.4
    group
      A J15.4
      B J15.3
    specified NEC J15.4
  Streptococcus pneumoniae J13
  syphilitic, congenital (early) A50.04
  traumatic (complication) (early) (secondary) T79.8 ☑
  tuberculous (any) — *see* Tuberculosis, pulmonary
  tularemic A21.2
  varicella B01.2
  Veillonella J15.8
  ventilator associated J95.851
  viral, virus (broncho) (interstitial) (lobar) J12.9
    adenoviral J12.0
    congenital P23.0
    human metapneumovirus J12.3
    parainfluenza J12.2
    respiratory syncytial J12.1
    SARS-associated coronavirus J12.81
    specified NEC J12.89
  white (congenital) A50.04
Pneumonic — *see* condition
Pneumonitis (acute) (primary) (*see also* Pneumonia)
  air-conditioner J67.7
  allergic (due to) J67.9
    organic dust NEC J67.8
    red cedar dust J67.8
    sequoiosis J67.8
    wood dust J67.8
  aspiration J69.0
    due to
      anesthesia J95.4
        during
          labor and delivery O74.0
          pregnancy O29.01- ☑
          puerperium O89.01
      fumes or gases J68.0
    obstetric O74.0

Pneumonitis — *continued*
  chemical (due to gases, fumes or vapors) (inhalation) J68.0
    due to anesthesia J95.4
  cholesterol J84.89
  chronic — *see* Fibrosis, lung
  congenital rubella P35.0
  crack (cocaine) J68.0
  due to
    beryllium J68.0
    cadmium J68.0
    crack (cocaine) J68.0
    detergent J69.8
    fluorocarbon-polymer J68.0
    food, vomit (aspiration) J69.0
    fumes or vapors J68.0
    gases, fumes or vapors (inhalation) J68.0
    inhalation
      blood J69.8
      essences J69.1
      food (regurgitated), milk, vomit J69.0
      oils, essences J69.1
      saliva J69.0
      solids, liquids NEC J69.8
    manganese J68.0
    nitrogen dioxide J68.0
    oils, essences J69.1
    solids, liquids NEC J69.8
    toxoplasmosis (acquired) B58.3
      congenital P37.1
    vanadium J68.0
    ventilator J95.851
  eosinophilic J82
  hypersensitivity J67.9
    air conditioner lung J67.7
    bagassosis J67.1
    bird fancier's lung J67.2
    farmer's lung J67.0
    maltworker's lung J67.4
    maple bark-stripper's lung J67.6
    mushroom worker's lung J67.5
    specified organic dust NEC J67.8
    suberosis J67.3
  interstitial (chronic) J84.89
    acute J84.114
    lymphoid J84.2
    non-specific J84.89
      idiopathic J84.113
  lymphoid, interstitial J84.2
  meconium P24.01
  postanesthetic J95.4
    correct substance properly administered — *see* Table of Drugs and Chemicals, by drug, adverse effect
    in labor and delivery O74.0
    in pregnancy O29.01- ☑
    obstetric O74.0
    overdose or wrong substance given or taken (by accident) — *see* Table of Drugs and Chemicals, by drug, poisoning
    postpartum, puerperal O89.01
  postoperative J95.4
    obstetric O74.0
  radiation J70.0
  rubella, congenital P35.0
  ventilation (air-conditioning) J67.7
  ventilator associated J95.851
  wood-dust J67.8
Pneumonoconiosis — *see* Pneumoconiosis
Pneumoparotid K11.8
Pneumopathy NEC J98.4
  alveolar J84.09
  due to organic dust NEC J66.8
  parietoalveolar J84.09
Pneumopericarditis (*see also* Pericarditis)
  acute I30.9
Pneumopericardium (*see also* Pericarditis)
  congenital P25.3
  newborn P25.3
  traumatic (post) — *see* Injury, heart
Pneumophagia (psychogenic) F45.8
Pneumopleurisy, pneumopleuritis (*see also* Pneumonia) J18.8
Pneumopyopericardium I30.1
Pneumopyothorax — *see* Pyopneumothorax
  with fistula J86.0
Pneumorrhagia (*see also* Hemorrhage, lung)
  tuberculous — *see* Tuberculosis, pulmonary

Pneumothorax NOS J93.9
  acute J93.83
  chronic J93.81
  congenital P25.1
  perinatal period P25.1
  postprocedural J95.811
  specified NEC J93.83
  spontaneous NOS J93.83
    newborn P25.1
    primary J93.11
    secondary J93.12
    tension J93.0
  tense valvular, infectional J93.0
  tension (spontaneous) J93.0
  traumatic S27.0 ☑
    with hemothorax S27.2 ☑
  tuberculous — *see* Tuberculosis, pulmonary
Podagra (*see also* Gout) M10.9
Podencephalus Q01.9
Poikilocytosis R71.8
Poikiloderma L81.6
  Civatte's L57.3
  congenital Q82.8
  vasculare atrophicans L94.5
Poikilodermatomyositis M33.10
  with
    myopathy M33.12
    respiratory involvement M33.11
    specified organ involvement NEC M33.19
Pointed ear (congenital) Q17.3
Poison ivy, oak, sumac or other plant dermatitis (allergic) (contact) L23.7
Poisoning (acute) (*see also* Table of Drugs and Chemicals)
  algae and toxins T65.82- ☑
  Bacillus B (aertrycke (cholerae (suis)) (paratyphosus) (suipestifer) A02.9
  botulinus A05.1
  bacterial toxins A05.9
  berries, noxious — *see* Poisoning, food, noxious, berries
  botulism A05.1
  ciguatera fish T61.0- ☑
  Clostridium botulinum A05.1
  death-cap (Amanita phalloides) (Amanita verna) — *see* Poisoning, food, noxious, mushrooms
  drug — *see* Table of Drugs and Chemicals, by drug, poisoning
  epidemic, fish (noxious) — *see* Poisoning, seafood
    bacterial A05.9
  fava bean D55.0
  fish (noxious) T61.9- ☑
    bacterial — *see* Intoxication, foodborne, by agent
    ciguatera fish — *see* Poisoning, ciguatera fish
    scombroid fish — *see* Poisoning, scombroid fish
    specified type NEC T61.77- ☑
  food (acute) (diseased) (infected) (noxious) NEC T62.9- ☑
    bacterial — *see* Intoxication, foodborne, by agent
    due to
      Bacillus (aertrycke) (choleraesuis) (paratyphosus) (suipestifer) A02.9
        botulinus A05.1
      Clostridium (perfringens) (Welchii) A05.2
      salmonella (aertrycke) (callinarum) (choleraesuis) (enteritidis) (paratyphi) (suipestifer) A02.9
        with
          gastroenteritis A02.0
          sepsis A02.1
      staphylococcus A05.0
      Vibrio
        parahaemolyticus A05.3
        vulnificus A05.5
    noxious or naturally toxic T62.9- ☑
      berries — *see* subcategory T62.1 ☑
      fish — *see* Poisoning, seafood
      mushrooms — *see* subcategory T62.0X ☑
      plants NEC — *see* subcategory T62.2X ☑
      seafood — *see* Poisoning, seafood
      specified NEC — *see* subcategory T62.8X ☑
  ichthyotoxism — *see* Poisoning, seafood
  kreotoxism, food A05.9
  latex T65.81- ☑
  lead T56.0- ☑
  mushroom — *see* Poisoning, food, noxious, mushroom
  mussels (*see also* Poisoning, shellfish)
    bacterial — *see* Intoxication, foodborne, by agent

Poisoning — *continued*
  nicotine (tobacco) T65.2- ☑
  noxious foodstuffs — *see* Poisoning, food, noxious
  plants, noxious — *see* Poisoning, food, noxious, plants NEC
  ptomaine — *see* Poisoning, food
  radiation J70.0
  Salmonella (arizonae) (cholerae-suis) (enteritidis) (typhimurium) A02.9
  scombroid fish T61.1- ☑
  seafood (noxious) T61.9- ☑
    bacterial — *see* Intoxication, foodborne, by agent
    fish — *see* Poisoning, fish
    shellfish — *see* Poisoning, shellfish
    specified NEC — *see* subcategory T61.8X ☑
  shellfish (amnesic) (azaspiracid) (diarrheic) (neurotoxic) (noxious) (paralytic) T61.78- ☑
    bacterial — *see* Intoxication, foodborne, by agent
    ciguatera mollusk — *see* Poisoning, ciguatera fish
  specified substance NEC T65.891 ☑
  Staphylococcus, food A05.0
  tobacco (nicotine) T65.2- ☑
  water E87.79
Poker spine — *see* Spondylitis, ankylosing
Poland syndrome Q79.8
Polioencephalitis (acute) (bulbar) A80.9
  inferior G12.22
  influenzal — *see* Influenza, with, encephalopathy
  superior hemorrhagic (acute) (Wernicke's) E51.2
  Wernicke's E51.2
Polioencephalomyelitis (acute) (anterior) A80.9
  with beriberi E51.2
Polioencephalopathy, superior hemorrhagic E51.2
  with
    beriberi E51.11
    pellagra E52
Poliomeningoencephalitis — *see* Meningoencephalitis
Poliomyelitis (acute) (anterior) (epidemic) A80.9
  with paralysis (bulbar) — *see* Poliomyelitis, paralytic
  abortive A80.4
  ascending (progressive) — *see* Poliomyelitis, paralytic
  bulbar (paralytic) — *see* Poliomyelitis, paralytic
  congenital P35.8
  nonepidemic A80.9
  nonparalytic A80.4
  paralytic A80.30
    specified NEC A80.39
    vaccine-associated A80.0
    wild virus
      imported A80.1
      indigenous A80.2
  spinal, acute A80.9
Poliosis (eyebrow) (eyelashes) L67.1
  circumscripta, acquired L67.1
Pollakiuria R35.0
  psychogenic F45.8
Pollinosis J30.1
Pollitzer's disease L73.2
Polyadenitis (*see also* Lymphadenitis)
  malignant A20.0
Polyalgia M79.89
Polyangiitis M30.0
  microscopic M31.7
  overlap syndrome M30.8
Polyarteritis
  microscopic M31.7
  nodosa M30.0
    with lung involvement M30.1
    juvenile M30.2
    related condition NEC M30.8
Polyarthralgia — *see* Pain, joint
Polyarthritis, polyarthropathy (*see also* Arthritis) M13.0
  due to or associated with other specified conditions — *see* Arthritis
  epidemic (Australian) (with exanthema) B33.1
  infective — *see* Arthritis, pyogenic or pyemic
  inflammatory M06.4
  juvenile (chronic) (seronegative) M08.3
  migratory — *see* Fever, rheumatic
  rheumatic, acute — *see* Fever, rheumatic
Polyarthrosis M15.9
  post-traumatic M15.3
  primary M15.0
  specified NEC M15.8
Polycarential syndrome of infancy E40
Polychondritis (atrophic) (chronic) (*see also* Disorder, cartilage, specified type NEC)
  relapsing M94.1

Polycoria Q13.2
Polycystic (disease)
  degeneration, kidney Q61.3
    autosomal dominant (adult type) Q61.2
    autosomal recessive (infantile type)
      NEC Q61.19
  kidney Q61.3
    autosomal
      dominant Q61.2
      recessive NEC Q61.19
    autosomal dominant (adult type) Q61.2
    autosomal recessive (childhood type) NEC Q61.19
    infantile type NEC Q61.19
  liver Q44.6
  lung J98.4
    congenital Q33.0
  ovary, ovaries E28.2
  spleen Q89.09
Polycythemia (secondary) D75.1
  acquired D75.1
  benign (familial) D75.0
  due to
    donor twin P61.1
    erythropoietin D75.1
    fall in plasma volume D75.1
    high altitude D75.1
    maternal-fetal transfusion P61.1
    stress D75.1
  emotional D75.1
  erythropoietin D75.1
  familial (benign) D75.0
  Gaisböck's (hypertonica) D75.1
  high altitude D75.1
  hypertonica D75.1
  hypoxemic D75.1
  neonatorum P61.1
  nephrogenous D75.1
  relative D75.1
  secondary D75.1
  spurious D75.1
  stress D75.1
  vera D45
Polycytosis cryptogenica D75.1
Polydactylism, polydactyly Q69.9
  toes Q69.2
Polydipsia R63.1
Polydystrophy, pseudo-Hurler E77.0
Polyembryoma — see Neoplasm, malignant, by site
Polyglandular
  deficiency E31.0
  dyscrasia E31.9
  dysfunction E31.9
  syndrome E31.8
Polyhydramnios O40.- ☑
Polymastia Q83.1
Polymenorrhea N92.0
Polymyalgia M35.3
  arteritica, giant cell M31.5
  rheumatica M35.3
    with giant cell arteritis M31.5
Polymyositis (acute) (chronic) (hemorrhagic) M33.20
  with
    myopathy M33.22
    respiratory involvement M33.21
    skin involvement — see Dermatopolymyositis
    specified organ involvement NEC M33.29
  ossificans (generalisata) (progressiva) — see Myositis,
    ossificans, progressiva
Polyneuritis, polyneuritic (see also Polyneuropathy)
  acute (post-)infective G61.0
  alcoholic G62.1
  cranialis G52.7
  demyelinating, chronic inflammatory (CIDP) G61.81
  diabetic — see Diabetes, polyneuropathy
  diphtheritic A36.83
  due to lack of vitamin NEC E56.9 [G63]
  endemic E51.11
  erythredema — see subcategory T56.1 ☑
  febrile, acute G61.0
  hereditary ataxic G60.1
  idiopathic, acute G61.0
  infective (acute) G61.0
  inflammatory, chronic demyelinating (CIDP) G61.81
  nutritional E63.9 [G63]
  postinfective (acute) G61.0
  specified NEC G62.89
Polyneuropathy (peripheral) G62.9

Polyneuropathy — continued
  alcoholic G62.1
  amyloid (Portuguese) E85.1 [G63]
    transthyretin-related (ATTR) familial E85.1
  arsenical G62.2
  critical illness G62.81
  demyelinating, chronic inflammatory (CIDP) G61.81
  diabetic — see Diabetes, polyneuropathy
  drug-induced G62.0
  hereditary G60.9
    specified NEC G60.8
  idiopathic G60.9
    progressive G60.3
  in (due to)
    alcohol G62.1
      sequelae G65.2
    amyloidosis, familial (Portuguese) E85.1 [G63]
    antitetanus serum G61.1
    arsenic G62.2
      sequelae G65.2
    avitaminosis NEC E56.9 [G63]
    beriberi E51.11
    collagen vascular disease NEC M35.9 [G63]
    deficiency (of)
      B (-complex) vitamins E53.9 [G63]
      vitamin B6 E53.1 [G63]
    diabetes — see Diabetes, polyneuropathy
    diphtheria A36.83
    drug or medicament G62.0
      correct substance properly administered — see
        Table of Drugs and Chemicals, by drug,
        adverse effect
      overdose or wrong substance given or taken
        — see Table of Drugs and Chemicals, by
        drug, poisoning
    endocrine disease NEC E34.9 [G63]
    herpes zoster B02.23
    hypoglycemia E16.2 [G63]
    infectious
      disease NEC B99 ☑ [G63]
      mononucleosis B27.91
    lack of vitamin NEC E56.9 [G63]
    lead G62.2
      sequelae G65.2
    leprosy A30.9 [G63]
    Lyme disease A69.22
    metabolic disease NEC E88.9 [G63]
    microscopic polyangiitis M31.7 [G63]
    mumps B26.84
    neoplastic disease (see also Neoplasm) D49.9 [G63]
    nutritional deficiency NEC E63.9 [G63]
    organophosphate compounds G62.2
      sequelae G65.2
    parasitic disease NEC B89 [G63]
    pellagra E52 [G63]
    polyarteritis nodosa M30.0
    porphyria E80.20 [G63]
    radiation G62.82
    rheumatoid arthritis — see Rheumatoid, polyneu-
      ropathy
    sarcoidosis D86.89
    serum G61.1
    syphilis (late) A52.15
      congenital A50.43
    systemic
      connective tissue disorder M35.9 [G63]
      lupus erythematosus M32.19
    toxic agent NEC G62.2
      sequelae G65.2
  inflammatory G61.9
    chronic demyelinating (CIDP) G61.81
    sequelae G65.1
    specified NEC G61.89
  lead G62.2
    sequelae G65.2
  nutritional NEC E63.9 [G63]
  postherpetic (zoster) B02.23
  progressive G60.3
  radiation-induced G62.82
  sensory (hereditary) (idiopathic) G60.8
  specified NEC G62.89
  syphilitic (late) A52.15
    congenital A50.43
  transthyretin-related (ATTR) familial amyloid E85.1
    triorthocresyl phosphate G62.2
      sequelae G65.2
    tuberculosis A17.89
    uremia N18.9 [G63]

Polyneuropathy — continued
  transthyretin-related familial amyloid — continued
    vitamin B12 deficiency E53.8 [G63]
      with anemia (pernicious) D51.0 [G63]
        due to dietary deficiency D51.3 [G63]
    zoster B02.23
Polyopia H53.8
Polyorchism, polyorchidism Q55.21
Polyosteoarthritis (see also Osteoarthritis, generalized)
  M15.9
  post-traumatic M15.3
  specified NEC M15.8
Polyostotic fibrous dysplasia Q78.1
Polyotia Q17.0
Polyp, polypus
  accessory sinus J33.8
  adenocarcinoma in — see Neoplasm, malignant, by
    site
  adenocarcinoma in situ in — see Neoplasm, in situ, by
    site
  adenoid tissue J33.0
  adenomatous (see also Neoplasm, benign, by site)
    adenocarcinoma in — see Neoplasm, malignant,
      by site
    adenocarcinoma in situ in — see Neoplasm, in situ,
      by site
    carcinoma in — see Neoplasm, malignant, by site
    carcinoma in situ in — see Neoplasm, in situ, by
      site
    multiple — see Neoplasm, benign
      adenocarcinoma in — see Neoplasm, malig-
        nant, by site
      adenocarcinoma in situ in — see Neoplasm, in
        situ, by site
  antrum J33.8
  anus, anal (canal) K62.0
  Bartholin's gland N84.3
  bladder D41.4
  carcinoma in — see Neoplasm, malignant, by site
  carcinoma in situ in — see Neoplasm, in situ, by site
  cecum D12.0
  cervix (uteri) N84.1
    in pregnancy or childbirth — see Pregnancy,
      complicated by, abnormal, cervix
    mucous N84.1
    nonneoplastic N84.1
  choanal J33.0
  cholesterol K82.4
  clitoris N84.3
  colon K63.5
    adenomatous D12.6
    ascending D12.2
    cecum D12.0
    descending D12.4
    inflammatory K51.40
      with
        abscess K51.414
        complication K51.419
          specified NEC K51.418
        fistula K51.413
        intestinal obstruction K51.412
        rectal bleeding K51.411
    sigmoid D12.5
    transverse D12.3
  corpus uteri N84.0
  dental K04.01
    irreversible K04.02
    reversible K04.01
  duodenum K31.7
  ear (middle) H74.4- ☑
  endometrium N84.0
  ethmoidal (sinus) J33.8
  fallopian tube N84.8
  female genital tract N84.9
    specified NEC N84.8
  frontal (sinus) J33.8
  gallbladder K82.4
  gingiva, gum K06.8
  labia, labium (majus) (minus) N84.3
  larynx (mucous) J38.1
    adenomatous D14.1
  malignant — see Neoplasm, malignant, by site
  maxillary (sinus) J33.8
  middle ear — see Polyp, ear (middle)
  myometrium N84.0
  nares
    anterior J33.9
    posterior J33.0

Polyp, polypus — *continued*
- nasal (mucous) J33.9
  - cavity J33.0
  - septum J33.0
- nasopharyngeal J33.0
- nose (mucous) J33.9
- oviduct N84.8
- pharynx J39.2
- placenta O90.89
- prostate — *see* Enlargement, enlarged, prostate
- pudenda, pudendum N84.3
- pulpal (dental) K04.01
  - irreversible K04.02
  - reversible K04.01
- rectum (nonadenomatous) K62.1
  - adenomatous — *see* Polyp, adenomatous
- septum (nasal) J33.0
- sinus (accessory) (ethmoidal) (frontal) (maxillary) (sphenoidal) J33.8
- sphenoidal (sinus) J33.8
- stomach K31.7
  - adenomatous D13.1
- tube, fallopian N84.8
- turbinate, mucous membrane J33.8
- umbilical, newborn P83.6
- ureter N28.89
- urethra N36.2
- uterus (body) (corpus) (mucous) N84.0
  - cervix N84.1
  - in pregnancy or childbirth — *see* Pregnancy, complicated by, tumor, uterus
- vagina N84.2
- vocal cord (mucous) J38.1
- vulva N84.3

Polyphagia R63.2
Polyploidy Q92.7
Polypoid — *see* condition
Polyposis (*see also* Polyp)
- coli (adenomatous) D12.6
  - adenocarcinoma in C18.9
  - adenocarcinoma in situ in — *see* Neoplasm, in situ, by site
  - carcinoma in C18.9
- colon (adenomatous) D12.6
- familial D12.6
  - adenocarcinoma in situ in — *see* Neoplasm, in situ, by site
- intestinal (adenomatous) D12.6
- malignant lymphomatous C83.1- ☑
- multiple, adenomatous (*see also* Neoplasm, benign) D36.9

Polyradiculitis — *see* Polyneuropathy
Polyradiculoneuropathy (acute) (postinfective) (segmentally demyelinating) G61.0
Polyserositis
- due to pericarditis I31.1
- pericardial I31.1
- periodic, familial E85.0
- tuberculous A19.9
  - acute A19.1
  - chronic A19.8

Polysplenia syndrome Q89.09
Polysyndactyly (*see also* Syndactylism, syndactyly) Q70.4
Polytrichia L68.3
Polyunguia Q84.6
Polyuria R35.8
- nocturnal R35.1
- psychogenic F45.8

Pompe's disease (glycogen storage) E74.02
Pompholyx L30.1
Poncet's disease (tuberculous rheumatism) A18.09
Pond fracture — *see* Fracture, skull
Ponos B55.0
Pons, pontine — *see* condition
Poor
- aesthetic of existing restoration of tooth K08.56
- contractions, labor O62.2
- gingival margin to tooth restoration K08.51
- personal hygiene R46.0
- prenatal care, affecting management of pregnancy — *see* Pregnancy, complicated by, insufficient, prenatal care
- sucking reflex (newborn) R29.2
- urinary stream R39.12
- vision NEC H54.7

Poradenitis, nostras inguinalis or venerea A55
Porencephaly (congenital) (developmental) (true) Q04.6
- acquired G93.0

Porencephaly — *continued*
- nondevelopmental G93.0
- traumatic (post) F07.89
Porocephaliasis B88.8
Porokeratosis Q82.8
Poroma, eccrine — *see* Neoplasm, skin, benign
Porphyria (South African) E80.20
- acquired E80.20
- acute intermittent (hepatic) (Swedish) E80.21
- cutanea tarda (hereditary) (symptomatic) E80.1
- due to drugs E80.20
  - correct substance properly administered — *see* Table of Drugs and Chemicals, by drug, adverse effect
  - overdose or wrong substance given or taken — *see* Table of Drugs and Chemicals, by drug, poisoning
- erythropoietic (congenital) (hereditary) E80.0
- hepatocutaneous type E80.1
- secondary E80.20
- toxic NEC E80.20
- variegata E80.20
Porphyrinuria — *see* Porphyria
Porphyruria — *see* Porphyria
Port wine nevus, mark, or stain Q82.5
Portal — *see* condition
Posadas-Wernicke disease B38.9
Positive
- culture (nonspecific)
  - blood R78.81
  - bronchial washings R84.5
  - cerebrospinal fluid R83.5
  - cervix uteri R87.5
  - nasal secretions R84.5
  - nipple discharge R89.5
  - nose R84.5
    - staphylococcus (Methicillin susceptible) Z22.321
      - Methicillin resistant Z22.322
  - peritoneal fluid R85.5
  - pleural fluid R84.5
  - prostatic secretions R86.5
  - saliva R85.5
  - seminal fluid R86.5
  - sputum R84.5
  - synovial fluid R89.5
  - throat scrapings R84.5
  - urine R82.79
  - vagina R87.5
  - vulva R87.5
  - wound secretions R89.5
- PPD (skin test) R76.11
- serology for syphilis A53.0
  - with signs or symptoms — *code as* Syphilis, by site and stage
  - false R76.8
- skin test, tuberculin (without active tuberculosis) R76.11
- test, human immunodeficiency virus (HIV) R75
- VDRL A53.0
  - with signs or symptoms — *code by* site and stage under Syphilis A53.9
- Wassermann reaction A53.0
Postcardiotomy syndrome I97.0
Postcaval ureter Q62.62
Postcholecystectomy syndrome K91.5
Postclimacteric bleeding N95.0
Postcommissurotomy syndrome I97.0
Postconcussional syndrome F07.81
Postcontusional syndrome F07.81
Postcricoid region — *see* condition
Post-dates (40-42 weeks) (pregnancy) (mother) O48.0
- more than 42 weeks gestation O48.1
Postencephalitic syndrome F07.89
Posterior — *see* condition
Posterolateral sclerosis (spinal cord) — *see* Degeneration, combined
Postexanthematous — *see* condition
Postfebrile — *see* condition
Postgastrectomy dumping syndrome K91.1
Posthemiplegic chorea — *see* Monoplegia
Posthemorrhagic anemia (chronic) D50.0
- acute D62
- newborn P61.3
Postherpetic neuralgia (zoster) B02.29
- trigeminal B02.22
Posthitis N47.7
Postimmunization complication or reaction — *see* Complications, vaccination

Postinfectious — *see* condition
Postlaminectomy syndrome NEC M96.1
Postleukotomy syndrome F07.0
Postmastectomy lymphedema (syndrome) I97.2
Postmaturity, postmature (over 42 weeks)
- maternal (over 42 weeks gestation) O48.1
- newborn P08.22
Postmeasles complication NEC (*see also* condition) B05.89
Postmenopausal
- endometrium (atrophic) N95.8
  - suppurative (*see also* Endometritis) N71.9
- osteoporosis — *see* Osteoporosis, postmenopausal
Postnasal drip R09.82
- due to
  - allergic rhinitis — *see* Rhinitis, allergic
  - common cold J00
  - gastroesophageal reflux — *see* Reflux, gastroesophageal
  - nasopharyngitis — *see* Nasopharyngitis
  - other known condition — *code to* condition
  - sinusitis — *see* Sinusitis
Postnatal — *see* condition
Postoperative (postprocedural) — *see* Complication, postoperative
- pneumothorax, therapeutic Z98.3
- state NEC Z98.890
Postpancreatectomy hyperglycemia E89.1
Postpartum — *see* Puerperal
Postphlebitic syndrome — *see* Syndrome, postthrombotic
Postpolio (myelitic) **syndrome** G14
Postpoliomyelitic (*see also* condition)
- osteopathy — *see* Osteopathy, after poliomyelitis
Postprocedural (*see also* Postoperative)
- hypoinsulinemia E89.1
Postschizophrenic depression F32.89
Postsurgery status (*see also* Status (post))
- pneumothorax, therapeutic Z98.3
Post-term (40-42 weeks) (pregnancy) (mother) O48.0
- infant P08.21
- more than 42 weeks gestation (mother) O48.1
Post-traumatic brain syndrome, nonpsychotic F07.81
Post-typhoid abscess A01.09
Postures, hysterical F44.2
Postvaccinal reaction or complication — *see* Complications, vaccination
Postvalvulotomy syndrome I97.0
Potain's
- disease (pulmonary edema) — *see* Edema, lung
- syndrome (gastrectasis with dyspepsia) K31.0
Potter's
- asthma J62.8
- facies Q60.6
- lung J62.8
- syndrome (with renal agenesis) Q60.6
Pott's
- curvature (spinal) A18.01
- disease or paraplegia A18.01
- spinal curvature A18.01
- tumor, puffy — *see* Osteomyelitis, specified type NEC
Pouch
- bronchus Q32.4
- Douglas' — *see* condition
- esophagus, esophageal, congenital Q39.6
  - acquired K22.5
- gastric K31.4
- Hartmann's K82.8
- pharynx, pharyngeal (congenital) Q38.7
Pouchitis K91.850
Poultrymen's itch B88.0
Poverty NEC Z59.6
- extreme Z59.5
Poxvirus NEC B08.8
Prader-Willi syndrome Q87.1
Preauricular appendage or tag Q17.0
Prebetalipoproteinemia (acquired) (essential) (familial) (hereditary) (primary) (secondary) E78.1
- with chylomicronemia E78.3
Precipitate labor or delivery O62.3
Preclimacteric bleeding (menorrhagia) N92.4
Precocious
- adrenarche E30.1
- menarche E30.1
- menstruation E30.1
- pubarche E30.1
- puberty E30.1

Precocious — *continued*
  puberty — *continued*
    central E22.8
    sexual development NEC E30.1
    thelarche E30.8
Precocity, sexual (constitutional) (cryptogenic) (female) (idiopathic) (male) E30.1
  with adrenal hyperplasia E25.9
    congenital E25.0
Precordial pain R07.2
Predeciduous teeth K00.2
Prediabetes, prediabetic R73.03
  complicating
    pregnancy — *see* Pregnancy, complicated by, diseases of, specified type or system NEC
    puerperium O99.89
Predislocation status of hip at birth Q65.6
Pre-eclampsia O14.9- ☑
  with pre-existing hypertension — *see* Hypertension, complicating pregnancy, pre-existing, with, pre-eclampsia
  complicating
    childbirth O14.94
    puerperium O14.95
  mild O14.0- ☑
    complicating
      childbirth O14.04
      puerperium O14.05
  moderate O14.0- ☑
    complicating
      childbirth O14.04
      puerperium O14.05
  severe O14.1- ☑
    with hemolysis, elevated liver enzymes and low platelet count (HELLP) O14.2- ☑
    complicating
      childbirth O14.24
      puerperium O14.25
    complicating
      childbirth O14.14
      puerperium O14.15
Pre-eruptive color change, teeth, tooth K00.8
Pre-excitation atrioventricular conduction I45.6
Preglaucoma H40.00- ☑
Pregnancy (single) (uterine) (*see also* Delivery and Puerperal)

Note: The Tabular must be reviewed for assignment of appropriate seventh character for multiple gestation codes in Chapter 15

Note: The Tabular must be reviewed for assignment of the appropriate character indicating the trimester of the pregnancy

  abdominal (ectopic) O00.00
    with intrauterine pregnancy O00.01
    with viable fetus O36.7- ☑
  ampullar O00.10- ☑
    with intrauterine pregnancy O00.11- ☑
  biochemical O02.81
  broad ligament O00.80
    with intrauterine pregnancy O00.81
  cervical O00.8
    with intrauterine pregnancy O00.81
  chemical O02.81
  complicated by (care of) (management affected by)
    abnormal, abnormality
      cervix O34.4- ☑
        causing obstructed labor O65.5
      cord (umbilical) O69.9 ☑
      fetal heart rate or rhythm O36.83- ☑
      findings on antenatal screening of mother O28.9
        biochemical O28.1
        chromosomal O28.5
        cytological O28.2
        genetic O28.5
        hematological O28.0
        radiological O28.4
        specified NEC O28.8
        ultrasonic O28.3
      glucose (tolerance) NEC O99.810
      pelvic organs O34.9- ☑
        specified NEC O34.8- ☑
          causing obstructed labor O65.5
      pelvis (bony) (major) NEC O33.0
      perineum O34.7- ☑

Pregnancy — *continued*
  complicated by — *continued*
    abnormal, abnormality — *continued*
      position
        placenta O44.0- ☑
          with hemorrhage O44.1- ☑
        uterus O34.59- ☑
      uterus O34.59- ☑
        causing obstructed labor O65.5
        congenital O34.0- ☑
      vagina O34.6- ☑
        causing obstructed labor O65.5
      vulva O34.7- ☑
        causing obstructed labor O65.5
    abruptio placentae — *see* Abruptio placentae
    abscess or cellulitis
      bladder O23.1- ☑
      breast O91.11- ☑
      genital organ or tract O23.9- ☑
    abuse
      physical O9A.31 ☑ (*following* O99)
      psychological O9A.51 ☑ (*following* O99)
      sexual O9A.41 ☑ (*following* O99)
    adverse effect anesthesia O29.9- ☑
      aspiration pneumonitis O29.01- ☑
      cardiac arrest O29.11- ☑
      cardiac complication NEC O29.19- ☑
      cardiac failure O29.12- ☑
      central nervous system complication NEC O29.29- ☑
      cerebral anoxia O29.21- ☑
      failed or difficult intubation O29.6- ☑
      inhalation of stomach contents or secretions NOS O29.01- ☑
      local, toxic reaction O29.3X ☑
      Mendelson's syndrome O29.01- ☑
      pressure collapse of lung O29.02- ☑
      pulmonary complications NEC O29.09- ☑
      specified NEC O29.8X- ☑
      spinal and epidural type NEC O29.5X ☑
        induced headache O29.4- ☑
    albuminuria (*see also* Proteinuria, gestational) O12.1- ☑
    alcohol use O99.31- ☑
    amnionitis O41.12- ☑
    anaphylactoid syndrome of pregnancy O88.01- ☑
    anemia (conditions in D50-D64) (pre-existing) O99.01- ☑
      complicating the puerperium O99.03
    antepartum hemorrhage O46.9- ☑
      with coagulation defect — *see* Hemorrhage, antepartum, with coagulation defect
      specified NEC O46.8X- ☑
    appendicitis O99.61- ☑
    atrophy (yellow) (acute) liver (subacute) O26.61- ☑
    bariatric surgery status O99.84- ☑
    bicornis or bicornuate uterus O34.0- ☑
    biliary tract problems O26.61- ☑
    breech presentation O32.1 ☑
    cardiovascular diseases (conditions in I00-I09, I20-I52, I70-I99) O99.41- ☑
    cerebrovascular disorders (conditions in I60-I69) O99.41- ☑
    cervical shortening O26.87- ☑
    cervicitis O23.51- ☑
    chloasma (gravidarum) O26.89- ☑
    cholecystitis O99.61- ☑
    cholestasis (intrahepatic) O26.61- ☑
    chorioamnionitis O41.12- ☑
    circulatory system disorder (conditions in I00-I09, I20-I99, O99.41-)
    compound presentation O32.6 ☑
    conjoined twins O30.02- ☑
    connective system disorders (conditions in M00-M99) O99.89
    contracted pelvis (general) O33.1
      inlet O33.2
      outlet O33.3 ☑
    convulsions (eclamptic) (uremic) (*see also* Eclampsia) O15.9
    cracked nipple O92.11- ☑
    cystitis O23.1- ☑
    cystocele O34.8- ☑
    death of fetus (near term) O36.4 ☑
      early pregnancy O02.1

Pregnancy — *continued*
  complicated by — *continued*
    death of fetus — *continued*
      of one fetus or more in multiple gestation O31.2- ☑
    deciduitis O41.14- ☑
    decreased fetal movement O36.81- ☑
    dental problems O99.61- ☑
    diabetes (mellitus) O24.91- ☑
      gestational (pregnancy induced) — *see* Diabetes, gestational
      pre-existing O24.31- ☑
        specified NEC O24.81- ☑
        type 1 O24.01- ☑
        type 2 O24.11- ☑
    digestive system disorders (conditions in K00-K93) O99.61- ☑
    diseases of — *see* Pregnancy, complicated by, specified body system disease
      biliary tract O26.61- ☑
      blood NEC (conditions in D65-D77) O99.11- ☑
      liver O26.61- ☑
      specified NEC O99.89
    disorders of — *see* Pregnancy, complicated by, specified body system disorder
      amniotic fluid and membranes O41.9- ☑
        specified NEC O41.8X- ☑
      biliary tract O26.61- ☑
      ear and mastoid process (conditions in H60-H95) O99.89
      eye and adnexa (conditions in H00-H59) O99.89
      liver O26.61- ☑
      skin (conditions in L00-L99) O99.71- ☑
      specified NEC O99.89
    displacement, uterus NEC O34.59- ☑
      causing obstructed labor O65.5
    disproportion (due to) O33.9
      fetal (ascites) (hydrops) (meningomyelocele) (sacral teratoma) (tumor) deformities NEC O33.7 ☑
      generally contracted pelvis O33.1
      hydrocephalic fetus O33.6 ☑
      inlet contraction of pelvis O33.2
      mixed maternal and fetal origin O33.4 ☑
      specified NEC O33.8
    double uterus O34.0- ☑
      causing obstructed labor O65.5
    drug use (conditions in F11-F19) O99.32- ☑
    eclampsia, eclamptic (coma) (convulsions) (delirium) (nephritis) (uremia) (*see also* Eclampsia) O15.- ☑
    ectopic pregnancy — *see* Pregnancy, ectopic
    edema O12.0- ☑
      with
        gestational hypertension, mild (*see also* Pre-eclampsia) O14.0- ☑
        proteinuria O12.2- ☑
    effusion, amniotic fluid — *see* Pregnancy, complicated by, premature rupture of membranes
    elderly
      multigravida O09.52- ☑
      primigravida O09.51- ☑
    embolism (*see also* Embolism, obstetric, pregnancy) O88.- ☑
    endocrine diseases NEC O99.28- ☑
    endometritis O86.12
    excessive weight gain O26.0- ☑
    exhaustion O26.81- ☑
      during labor and delivery O75.81
    face presentation O32.3 ☑
    failed induction of labor O61.9
      instrumental O61.1
      mechanical O61.1
      medical O61.0
      specified NEC O61.8
      surgical O61.1
    failed or difficult intubation for anesthesia O29.6- ☑
    false labor (pains) O47.9
      at or after 37 completed weeks of pregnancy O47.1
      before 37 completed weeks of pregnancy O47.0- ☑
    fatigue O26.81- ☑
      during labor and delivery O75.81
    fatty metamorphosis of liver O26.61- ☑
    female genital mutilation O34.8- ☑ [N90.81-] ☑

▽ Subterms under main terms may continue to next column or page   ☑ Additional Character Required — Refer to the Tabular List for Character Selection   259

Precocious — Pregnancy

Index

Pregnancy — Pregnancy

Pregnancy — continued
  complicated by — continued
    placental transfusion syndromes
      fetomaternal O43.01- ☑
      fetus to fetus O43.02- ☑
      maternofetal O43.01- ☑
    placentitis O41.14- ☑
    pneumonia O99.51- ☑
    poisoning (see also Table of Drugs and Chemicals)
      O9A.21 ☑ (following O99)
    polyhydramnios O40- ☑
    polymorphic eruption of pregnancy O26.86
    poor obstetric history NEC O09.29- ☑
    postmaturity (post-term) (40 to 42 weeks) O48.0
      more than 42 completed weeks gestation
        (prolonged) O48.1
    pre-eclampsia O14.9- ☑
      mild O14.0- ☑
      moderate O14.0- ☑
      severe O14.1- ☑
        with hemolysis, elevated liver enzymes and
          low platelet count (HELLP) O14.2- ☑
    premature labor — see Pregnancy, complicated
      by, preterm labor
    premature rupture of membranes O42.90
      with onset of labor
        after 24 hours O42.10
          at or after 37 weeks gestation, onset of
            labor more than 24 hours follow-
            ing rupture O42.12
          pre-term (before 37 completed weeks
            of gestation) O42.11- ☑
        within 24 hours O42.00
          at or after 37 weeks gestation, onset of
            labor within 24 hours of rupture
            O42.02
          pre-term (before 37 completed weeks
            of gestation) O42.01- ☑
      at or after 37 weeks gestation, unspecified as
        to length of time between rupture and
        onset of labor O42.92
      full-term, unspecified as to length of time be-
        tween rupture and onset of labor O42.92
      pre-term (before 37 completed weeks of gesta-
        tion) O42.91- ☑
    premature separation of placenta (see also Abrup-
      tio placentae) O45.9- ☑
    presentation, fetal — see Delivery, complicated
      by, malposition
    preterm delivery O60.10 ☑
    preterm labor
      with delivery O60.10 ☑
        preterm O60.10 ☑
        term O60.20 ☑
      without delivery O60.00
        second trimester O60.02
        third trimester O60.03
      second trimester
        with preterm delivery
          second trimester O60.12 ☑
          third trimester O60.13 ☑
        with term delivery O60.22 ☑
        without delivery O60.02
      third trimester
        with term delivery O60.23 ☑
        with third trimester preterm delivery
          O60.14 ☑
        without delivery O60.03
    previous history of — see Pregnancy, supervision
      of, high-risk
    prolapse, uterus O34.52- ☑
    proteinuria (gestational) (see also Proteinuria,
      gestational) O12.1- ☑
      with edema O12.2- ☑
    pruritic urticarial papules and plaques of pregnancy
      (PUPPP) O26.86
    pruritus (neurogenic) O26.89- ☑
    psychosis or psychoneurosis (puerperal) F53
    ptyalism O26.89- ☑
    PUPPP (pruritic urticarial papules and plaques of
      pregnancy) O26.86
    pyelitis O23.0- ☑
    recurrent pregnancy loss O26.2- ☑
    renal disease or failure NEC O26.83- ☑
      with secondary hypertension, pre-existing —
        see Hypertension, complicating, pregnan-
        cy, pre-existing, secondary

Pregnancy — continued
  complicated by — continued
    renal disease or failure — continued
      hypertensive, pre-existing — see Hypertension,
        complicating, pregnancy, pre-existing,
        with, renal disease
    respiratory condition (conditions in J00-J99)
      O99.51- ☑
    retained, retention
      dead ovum O02.0
      intrauterine contraceptive device O26.3- ☑
    retroversion, uterus O34.53- ☑
    Rh immunization, incompatibility or sensitization
      NEC O36.09- ☑
      anti-D antibody O36.01- ☑
    rupture
      amnion (premature) (see also Pregnancy, com-
        plicated by, premature rupture of mem-
        branes) O42- ☑
      membranes (premature) (see also Pregnancy,
        complicated by, premature rupture of
        membranes) O42- ☑
      uterus (during labor) O71.1
        before onset of labor O71.0- ☑
    salivation (excessive) O26.89- ☑
    salpingitis O23.52- ☑
    salpingo-oophoritis O23.52- ☑
    sepsis (conditions in A40, A41) O98.81- ☑
    size date discrepancy (uterine) O26.84- ☑
    skin condition (conditions in L00-L99) O99.71- ☑
    smoking (tobacco) O99.33- ☑
    social problem O09.7- ☑
    specified condition NEC O26.89- ☑
    spotting O26.85- ☑
    streptococcus group B (GBS) carrier state O99.820
    subluxation of symphysis (pubis) O26.71- ☑
    syphilis (conditions in A50-A53) O98.11- ☑
    threatened
      abortion O20.0
      labor O47.9
        at or after 37 completed weeks of gestation
          O47.1
        before 37 completed weeks of gestation
          O47.0- ☑
    thrombophlebitis (superficial) O22.2- ☑
    thrombosis O22.9- ☑
      cerebral venous O22.5- ☑
      cerebrovenous sinus O22.5- ☑
      deep O22.3- ☑
    tobacco use disorder (smoking) O99.33- ☑
    torsion of uterus O34.59- ☑
    toxemia O14.9- ☑
    transverse lie or presentation O32.2 ☑
    tuberculosis (conditions in A15-A19) O98.01- ☑
    tumor (benign)
      cervix O34.4- ☑
      malignant O9A.11- ☑ (following O99)
      uterus O34.1- ☑
    unstable lie O32.0 ☑
    upper respiratory infection O99.51- ☑
    urethritis O23.2- ☑
    uterine size date discrepancy O26.84- ☑
    vaginitis or vulvitis O23.59- ☑
    varicose veins (lower extremities) O22.0- ☑
      genitals O22.1- ☑
      legs O22.0- ☑
      perineal O22.1- ☑
      vaginal or vulval O22.1- ☑
    venereal disease NEC (conditions in A63.8)
      O98.31- ☑
    venous disorders O22.9- ☑
      specified NEC O22.8X- ☑
    very young mother — see Pregnancy, complicated
      by, young mother
    viral diseases (conditions in A80-B09, B25-B34)
      O98.51- ☑
    vomiting O21.9
      due to diseases classified elsewhere O21.8
      hyperemesis gravidarum (mild) (see also Hyper-
        emesis, gravidarum) O21.0
      late (occurring after 20 weeks of gestation)
        O21.2
    young mother
      multigravida O09.62- ☑
      primigravida O09.61- ☑
  complicated NOS O26.9- ☑
  concealed O09.3- ☑

Pregnancy — continued
  continuing following
    elective fetal reduction of one or more fetus
      O31.3- ☑
    intrauterine death of one or more fetus O31.2- ☑
    spontaneous abortion of one or more fetus
      O31.1- ☑
  cornual O00.80
    with intrauterine pregnancy O00.81
  ectopic (ruptured) O00.90
    with intrauterine pregnancy O00.91
    abdominal O00.00
      with
        intrauterine pregnancy O00.01
        viable fetus O36.7- ☑
    cervical O00.80
      with intrauterine pregnancy O00.81
    complicated (by) O08.9
      afibrinogenemia O08.1
      cardiac arrest O08.81
      chemical damage of pelvic organ(s) O08.6
      circulatory collapse O08.3
      defibrination syndrome O08.1
      electrolyte imbalance O08.5
      embolism (amniotic fluid) (blood clot) (pul-
        monary) (septic) O08.2
      endometritis O08.0
      genital tract and pelvic infection O08.0
      hemorrhage (delayed) (excessive) O08.1
      infection
        genital tract or pelvic O08.0
        kidney O08.83
        urinary tract O08.3
      intravascular coagulation O08.1
      laceration of pelvic organ(s) O08.6
      metabolic disorder O08.5
      oliguria O08.4
      oophoritis O08.0
      parametritis O08.0
      pelvic peritonitis O08.0
      perforation of pelvic organ(s) O08.6
      renal failure or shutdown O08.4
      salpingitis or salpingo-oophoritis O08.0
      sepsis O08.82
      shock O08.83
        septic O08.82
      specified condition NEC O08.89
      tubular necrosis (renal) O08.4
      uremia O08.4
      urinary infection O08.83
      venous complication NEC O08.7
        embolism O08.2
    cornual O00.80
      with intrauterine pregnancy O00.81
    intraligamentous O00.80
      with intrauterine pregnancy O00.81
    mural O00.80
      with intrauterine pregnancy O00.81
    ovarian O00.20- ☑
      with intrauterine pregnancy O00.21- ☑
    specified site NEC O00.80
      with intrauterine pregnancy O00.81
    tubal (ruptured) O00.10- ☑
      with intrauterine pregnancy O00.11- ☑
  examination (normal) Z34.9- ☑
    first Z34.0- ☑
    high-risk — see Pregnancy, supervision of, high-
      risk
    specified Z34.8- ☑
  extrauterine — see Pregnancy, ectopic
  fallopian O00.10- ☑
    with intrauterine pregnancy O00.11- ☑
  false F45.8
  gestational carrier Z33.3
  hidden O09.3- ☑
  high-risk — see Pregnancy, supervision of, high-risk
  incidental finding Z33.1
  interstitial O00.80
    with intrauterine pregnancy O00.81
  intraligamentous O00.80
    with intrauterine pregnancy O00.81
  intramural O00.80
    with intrauterine pregnancy O00.81
  intraperitoneal O00.00
    with intrauterine pregnancy O00.01
  isthmian O00.10- ☑
    with intrauterine pregnancy O00.11- ☑
  mesometric (mural) O00.80

Prescription of contraceptives — *continued*
  barrier Z30.018
  diaphragm Z30.018
  emergency (postcoital) Z30.012
  implantable subdermal Z30.017
  injectable Z30.013
  intrauterine contraceptive device Z30.014
  pills Z30.011
  postcoital (emergency) Z30.012
  repeat Z30.40
    barrier Z30.49
    diaphragm Z30.49
    implantable subdermal Z30.46
    injectable Z30.42
    pills Z30.41
    specified type NEC Z30.49
    transdermal patch hormonal Z30.45
    vaginal ring hormonal Z30.44
  specified type NEC Z30.018
    transdermal patch hormonal Z30.016
    vaginal ring hormonal Z30.015
Presence (of)
  ankle-joint implant (functional) (prosthesis) Z96.66- ☑
  aortocoronary (bypass) graft Z95.1
  arterial-venous shunt (dialysis) Z99.2
  artificial
    eye (globe) Z97.0
    heart (fully implantable) (mechanical) Z95.812
      valve Z95.2
    larynx Z96.3
    lens (intraocular) Z96.1
    limb (complete) (partial) Z97.1- ☑
      arm Z97.1-
        bilateral Z97.15
      leg Z97.1- ☑
        bilateral Z97.16
  audiological implant (functional) Z96.29
  bladder implant (functional) Z96.0
  bone
    conduction hearing device Z96.29
    implant (functional) NEC Z96.7
    joint (prosthesis) — *see* Presence, joint implant
  cardiac
    defibrillator (functional) (with synchronous cardiac
      pacemaker) Z95.810
    implant or graft Z95.9
      specified type NEC Z95.818
    pacemaker Z95.0
    resynchronization therapy
      defibrillator Z95.810
      pacemaker Z95.0
  cardioverter-defibrillator (ICD) Z95.810
  cerebrospinal fluid drainage device Z98.2
  cochlear implant (functional) Z96.21
  contact lens (es) Z97.3
  coronary artery graft or prosthesis Z95.5
  CRT-D (cardiac resynchronization therapy defibrillator)
    Z95.810
  CRT-P (cardiac resynchronization therapy pacemaker)
    Z95.0
  CSF shunt Z98.2
  dental prosthesis device Z97.2
  dentures Z97.2
  device (external) NEC Z97.8
    cardiac NEC Z95.818
    heart assist Z95.811
    implanted (functional) Z96.9
      specified NEC Z96.89
    prosthetic Z97.8
  ear implant Z96.20
    cochlear implant Z96.21
    myringotomy tube Z96.22
    specified type NEC Z96.29
  elbow-joint implant (functional) (prosthesis)
    Z96.62- ☑
  endocrine implant (functional) NEC Z96.49
  eustachian tube stent or device (functional) Z96.29
  external hearing-aid or device Z97.4
  finger-joint implant (functional) (prosthetic) Z96.69- ☑
  functional implant Z96.9
    specified NEC Z96.89
  graft
    cardiac NEC Z95.818
    vascular NEC Z95.828
  hearing-aid or device (external) Z97.4
    implant (bone) (cochlear) (functional) Z96.21
  heart assist device Z95.811
  heart valve implant (functional) Z95.2

Presence — *continued*
  heart valve implant — *continued*
    prosthetic Z95.2
    specified type NEC Z95.4
    xenogenic Z95.3
  hip-joint implant (functional) (prosthesis) Z96.64- ☑
  ICD (cardioverter-defibrillator) Z95.810
  implanted device (artificial) (functional) (prosthetic)
    Z96.9
    automatic cardiac defibrillator (with synchronous
      cardiac pacemaker) Z95.810
    cardiac pacemaker Z95.0
    cochlear Z96.21
    dental Z96.5
    heart Z95.812
    heart valve Z95.2
      prosthetic Z95.2
      specified NEC Z95.4
      xenogenic Z95.3
    insulin pump Z96.41
    intraocular lens Z96.1
    joint Z96.60
      ankle Z96.66- ☑
      elbow Z96.62- ☑
      finger Z96.69- ☑
      hip Z96.64- ☑
      knee Z96.65- ☑
      shoulder Z96.61- ☑
      specified NEC Z96.698
      wrist Z96.63- ☑
    larynx Z96.3
    myringotomy tube Z96.22
    otological Z96.20
      cochlear Z96.21
      eustachian stent Z96.29
      myringotomy Z96.22
      specified NEC Z96.29
      stapes Z96.29
    skin Z96.81
    skull plate Z96.7
    specified NEC Z96.89
    urogenital Z96.0
  insulin pump (functional) Z96.41
  intestinal bypass or anastomosis Z98.0
  intraocular lens (functional) Z96.1
  intrauterine contraceptive device (IUD) Z97.5
  intravascular implant (functional) (prosthetic) NEC
    Z95.9
    coronary artery Z95.5
    defibrillator (with synchronous cardiac pacemaker)
      Z95.810
    peripheral vessel (with angioplasty) Z95.820
  joint implant (prosthetic) (any) Z96.60
    ankle — *see* Presence, ankle joint implant
    elbow — *see* Presence, elbow joint implant
    finger — *see* Presence, finger joint implant
    hip — *see* Presence, hip joint implant
    knee — *see* Presence, knee joint implant
    shoulder — *see* Presence, shoulder joint implant
    specified joint NEC Z96.698
    wrist — *see* Presence, wrist joint implant
  knee-joint implant (functional) (prosthesis) Z96.65- ☑
  laryngeal implant (functional) Z96.3
  mandibular implant (dental) Z96.5
  myringotomy tube(s) Z96.22
  orthopedic-joint implant (prosthetic) (any) — *see*
    Presence, joint implant
  otological implant (functional) Z96.29
  shoulder-joint implant (functional) (prosthesis)
    Z96.61- ☑
  skull-plate implant Z96.7
  spectacles Z97.3
  stapes implant (functional) Z96.29
  systemic lupus erythematosus [SLE] inhibitor D68.62
  tendon implant (functional) (graft) Z96.7
  tooth root(s) implant Z96.5
  ureteral stent Z96.0
  urethral stent Z96.0
  urogenital implant (functional) Z96.0
  vascular implant or device Z95.9
    access port device Z95.828
    specified type NEC Z95.828
  wrist-joint implant (functional) (prosthesis) Z96.63- ☑
Presenile (*see also* condition)
  dementia F03 ☑
  premature aging E34.8
Presentation, fetal — *see* Delivery, complicated by,
  malposition

Prespondylolisthesis (congenital) Q76.2
Pressure
  area, skin — *see* Ulcer, pressure, by site
  brachial plexus G54.0
  brain G93.5
    injury at birth NEC P11.1
  cerebral — *see* Pressure, brain
  chest R07.89
  cone, tentorial G93.5
  hyposystolic (*see also* Hypotension)
    incidental reading, without diagnosis of hypoten-
      sion R03.1
  increased
    intracranial (benign) G93.2
      injury at birth P11.0
    intraocular H40.05- ☑
  lumbosacral plexus G54.1
  mediastinum J98.59
  necrosis (chronic) — *see* Ulcer, pressure, by site
  parental, inappropriate (excessive) Z62.6
  sore (chronic) — *see* Ulcer, pressure, by site
  spinal cord G95.20
  ulcer (chronic) — *see* Ulcer, pressure, by site
  venous, increased I87.8
Pre-syncope R55
Preterm
  delivery (*see also* Pregnancy, complicated by, preterm
    labor) O60.10 ☑
  labor — *see* Pregnancy, complicated by, preterm labor
  newborn (infant) P07.30
    gestational age
      28 completed weeks (28 weeks, 0 days through
        28 weeks, 6 days) P07.31
      29 completed weeks (29 weeks, 0 days through
        29 weeks, 6 days) P07.32
      30 completed weeks (30 weeks, 0 days through
        30 weeks, 6 days) P07.33
      31 completed weeks (31 weeks, 0 days through
        31 weeks, 6 days) P07.34
      32 completed weeks (32 weeks, 0 days through
        32 weeks, 6 days) P07.35
      33 completed weeks (33 weeks, 0 days through
        33 weeks, 6 days) P07.36
      34 completed weeks (34 weeks, 0 days through
        34 weeks, 6 days) P07.37
      35 completed weeks (35 weeks, 0 days through
        35 weeks, 6 days) P07.38
      36 completed weeks (36 weeks, 0 days through
        36 weeks, 6 days) P07.39
Previa
  placenta (total) (without hemorrhage) O44.0- ☑
    with hemorrhage O44.1- ☑
    complete O44.0- ☑
      with hemorrhage O44.1- ☑
    low (*see also* Delivery, complicated, by, placenta,
      low) O44.4- ☑
      with hemorrhage O44.5- ☑
    marginal O44.2- ☑
      with hemorrhage O44.3- ☑
    partial O44.2- ☑
      with hemorrhage O44.3- ☑
  vasa O69.4 ☑
Priapism N48.30
  due to
    disease classified elsewhere N48.32
    drug N48.33
    specified cause NEC N48.39
    trauma N48.31
Prickling sensation (skin) R20.2
Prickly heat L74.0
Primary — *see* condition
Primigravida
  elderly, affecting management of pregnancy, labor
    and delivery (supervision only) — *see* Pregnan-
    cy, complicated by, elderly, primigravida
  older, affecting management of pregnancy, labor and
    delivery (supervision only) — *see* Pregnancy,
    complicated by, elderly, primigravida
  very young, affecting management of pregnancy, labor
    and delivery (supervision only) — *see* Pregnan-
    cy, complicated by, young mother, primigravida
Primipara
  elderly, affecting management of pregnancy, labor
    and delivery (supervision only) — *see* Pregnan-
    cy, complicated by, elderly, primigravida

Primipara — *continued*
  older, affecting management of pregnancy, labor and delivery (supervision only) — *see* Pregnancy, complicated by, elderly, primigravida
  very young, affecting management of pregnancy, labor and delivery (supervision only) — *see* Pregnancy, complicated by, young mother, primigravida
Primus varus (bilateral) Q66.2 ☑
PRIND (Prolonged reversible ischemic neurologic deficit) I63.9
Pringle's disease (tuberous sclerosis) Q85.1
Prinzmetal angina I20.1
Prizefighter ear — *see* Cauliflower ear
Problem (with) (related to)
  academic Z55.8
  acculturation Z60.3
  adjustment (to)
    change of job Z56.1
    life-cycle transition Z60.0
    pension Z60.0
    retirement Z60.0
  adopted child Z62.821
  alcoholism in family Z63.72
  atypical parenting situation Z62.9
  bankruptcy Z59.8
  behavioral (adult) F69
    drug seeking Z76.5
  birth of sibling affecting child Z62.898
  care (of)
    provider dependency Z74.9
      specified NEC Z74.8
    sick or handicapped person in family or household Z63.6
  child
    abuse (affecting the child) — *see* Maltreatment, child
    custody or support proceedings Z65.3
    in care of non-parental family member Z62.21
    in foster care Z62.21
    in welfare custody Z62.21
    living in orphanage or group home Z62.22
  child-rearing Z62.9
    specified NEC Z62.898
  communication (developmental) F80.9
  conflict or discord (with)
    boss Z56.4
    classmates Z55.4
    counselor Z64.4
    employer Z56.4
    family Z63.9
      specified NEC Z63.8
    probation officer Z64.4
    social worker Z64.4
    teachers Z55.4
    workmates Z56.4
  conviction in legal proceedings Z65.0
    with imprisonment Z65.1
  counselor Z64.4
  creditors Z59.8
  digestive K92.9
  drug addict in family Z63.72
  ear — *see* Disorder, ear
  economic Z59.9
    affecting care Z59.9
    specified NEC Z59.8
  education Z55.9
    specified NEC Z55.8
  employment Z56.9
    change of job Z56.1
    discord Z56.4
    environment Z56.5
    sexual harassment Z56.81
    specified NEC Z56.89
    stressful schedule Z56.3
    stress NEC Z56.6
    threat of job loss Z56.2
    unemployment Z56.0
  enuresis, child F98.0
  eye H57.9
  failed examinations (school) Z55.2
  falling Z91.81
  family (*see also* Disruption, family) Z63.9
    specified NEC Z63.8
  feeding (elderly) (infant) R63.3
    newborn P92.9
      breast P92.5
      overfeeding P92.4
      slow P92.2

Problem — *continued*
  feeding — *continued*
    newborn — *continued*
      specified NEC P92.8
      underfeeding P92.3
    nonorganic F50.89
  finance Z59.9
    specified NEC Z59.8
  foreclosure on loan Z59.8
  foster child Z62.822
  frightening experience(s) in childhood Z62.898
  genital NEC
    female N94.9
    male N50.9
  health care Z75.9
    specified NEC Z75.8
  hearing — *see* Deafness
  homelessness Z59.0
  housing Z59.9
    inadequate Z59.1
    isolated Z59.8
    specified NEC Z59.8
  identity (of childhood) F93.8
  illegitimate pregnancy (unwanted) Z64.0
  illiteracy Z55.0
  impaired mobility Z74.09
  imprisonment or incarceration Z65.1
  inadequate teaching affecting education Z55.8
  inappropriate (excessive) parental pressure Z62.6
  influencing health status NEC Z78.9
  in-law Z63.1
  institutionalization, affecting child Z62.22
  intrafamilial communication Z63.8
  jealousy, child F93.8
  landlord Z59.2
  language (developmental) F80.9
  learning (developmental) F81.9
  legal Z65.3
    conviction without imprisonment Z65.0
    imprisonment Z65.1
    release from prison Z65.2
  life-management Z73.9
    specified NEC Z73.89
  life-style Z72.9
    gambling Z72.6
    high-risk sexual behavior (heterosexual) Z72.51
      bisexual Z72.53
      homosexual Z72.52
    inappropriate eating habits Z72.4
    self-damaging behavior NEC Z72.89
    specified NEC Z72.89
    tobacco use Z72.0
  literacy Z55.9
    low level Z55.0
    specified NEC Z55.8
  living alone Z60.2
  lodgers Z59.2
  loss of love relationship in childhood Z62.898
  marital Z63.0
    involving
      divorce Z63.5
      estrangement Z63.5
      gender identity F66
  mastication K08.89
  medical
    care, within family Z63.6
    facilities Z75.9
      specified NEC Z75.8
  mental F48.9
  multiparity Z64.1
  negative life events in childhood Z62.9
    altered pattern of family relationships Z62.898
    frightening experience Z62.898
    loss of
      love relationship Z62.898
      self-esteem Z62.898
    physical abuse (alleged) — *see* Maltreatment, child
    removal from home Z62.29
    specified event NEC Z62.898
  neighbor Z59.2
  neurological NEC R29.818
  new step-parent affecting child Z62.898
  none (feared complaint unfounded) Z71.1
  occupational NEC Z56.89
  parent-child — *see* Conflict, parent-child
  personal hygiene Z91.89
  personality F69
  phase-of-life transition, adjustment Z60.0

Problem — *continued*
  presence of sick or disabled person in family or household Z63.79
    needing care Z63.6
  primary support group (family) Z63.9
    specified NEC Z63.8
  probation officer Z64.4
  psychiatric F99
  psychosexual (development) F66
  psychosocial Z65.9
    religious or spiritual Z65.8
    specified NEC Z65.8
  relationship Z63.9
    childhood F93.8
  release from prison Z65.2
    religious or spiritual Z65.8
  removal from home affecting child Z62.29
  seeking and accepting known hazardous and harmful behavioral or psychological interventions Z65.8
    chemical, nutritional or physical interventions Z65.8
  sexual function (nonorganic) F52.9
  sight H54.7
  sleep disorder, child F51.9
  smell — *see* Disturbance, sensation, smell
  social
    environment Z60.9
      specified NEC Z60.8
    exclusion and rejection Z60.4
    worker Z64.4
  speech R47.9
    developmental F80.9
    specified NEC R47.89
  swallowing — *see* Dysphagia
  taste — *see* Disturbance, sensation, taste
  tic, child F95.0
  underachievement in school Z55.3
  unemployment Z56.0
    threatened Z56.2
  unwanted pregnancy Z64.0
  upbringing Z62.9
    specified NEC Z62.898
  urinary N39.9
  voice production R47.89
  work schedule (stressful) Z56.3
Procedure (surgical)
  converted
    arthroscopic to open Z53.33
    laparoscopic to open Z53.31
    specified procedure NEC to open Z53.39
    thoracoscopic to open Z53.32
  for purpose other than remedying health state Z41.9
    specified NEC Z41.8
  not done Z53.9
    because of
      administrative reasons Z53.8
      contraindication Z53.09
        smoking Z53.01
      patient's decision Z53.20
        for reasons of belief or group pressure Z53.1
        left against medical advice (AMA) Z53.21
        specified reason NEC Z53.29
      specified reason NEC Z53.8
Procidentia (uteri) N81.3
Proctalgia K62.89
  fugax K59.4
  spasmodic K59.4
Proctitis K62.89
  amebic (acute) A06.0
  chlamydial A56.3
  gonococcal A54.6
  granulomatous — *see* Enteritis, regional, large intestine
  herpetic A60.1
  radiation K62.7
  tuberculous A18.32
  ulcerative (chronic) K51.20
    with
      complication K51.219
        abscess K51.214
        fistula K51.213
        obstruction K51.212
        rectal bleeding K51.211
        specified NEC K51.218
Proctocele
  female (without uterine prolapse) N81.6
    with uterine prolapse N81.2
      complete N81.3
  male K62.3

☑ **Additional Character Required — Refer to the Tabular List for Character Selection**   ▽ Subterms under main terms may continue to next column or page

Proctocolitis
  food protein-induced K52.82
  food-induced eosinophilic K52.82
  milk protein-induced K52.82
  mucosal — see Rectosigmoiditis, ulcerative
Proctoptosis K62.3
Proctorrhagia K62.5
Proctosigmoiditis K63.89
  ulcerative (chronic) — see Rectosigmoiditis, ulcerative
Proctospasm K59.4
  psychogenic F45.8
Profichet's disease — see Disorder, soft tissue, specified
    type NEC
Progeria E34.8
Prognathism (mandibular) (maxillary) M26.19
Progonoma (melanotic) — see Neoplasm, benign, by
    site
Progressive — see condition
Prolactinoma
  specified site — see Neoplasm, benign, by site
  unspecified site D35.2
Prolapse, prolapsed
  anus, anal (canal) (sphincter) K62.2
  arm or hand O32.2 ☑
    causing obstructed labor O64.4 ☑
  bladder (mucosa) (sphincter) (acquired)
    congenital Q79.4
    female — see Cystocele
    male N32.89
  breast implant (prosthetic) T85.49 ☑
  cecostomy K94.09
  cecum K63.4
  cervix, cervical (hypertrophied) N81.2
    anterior lip, obstructing labor O65.5
    congenital Q51.828
    postpartal, old N81.2
    stump N81.85
  ciliary body (traumatic) — see Laceration, eye(ball),
    with prolapse or loss of interocular tissue
  colon (pedunculated) K63.4
  colostomy K94.09
  disc (intervertebral) — see Displacement, interverte-
    bral disc
  eye implant (orbital) T85.398 ☑
    lens (ocular) — see Complications, intraocular lens
  fallopian tube N83.4- ☑
  gastric (mucosa) K31.89
  genital, female N81.9
    specified NEC N81.89
  globe, nontraumatic — see Luxation, globe
  ileostomy bud K94.19
  intervertebral disc — see Displacement, intervertebral
    disc
  intestine (small) K63.4
  iris (traumatic) — see Laceration, eye(ball), with pro-
    lapse or loss of interocular tissue
    nontraumatic H21.89
  kidney N28.83
    congenital Q63.2
  laryngeal muscles or ventricle J38.7
  liver K76.89
  meatus urinarius N36.8
  mitral (valve) I34.1
  ocular lens implant — see Complications, intraocular
    lens
  organ or site, congenital NEC — see Malposition,
    congenital
  ovary N83.4- ☑
  pelvic floor, female N81.89
  perineum, female N81.89
  rectum (mucosa) (sphincter) K62.3
    due to trichuris trichuria B79
  spleen D73.89
  stomach K31.89
  umbilical cord
    complicating delivery O69.0 ☑
  urachus, congenital Q64.4
  ureter N28.89
    with obstruction N13.5
      with infection N13.6
  ureterovesical orifice N28.89
  urethra (acquired) (infected) (mucosa) N36.8
    congenital Q64.71
  urinary meatus N36.8
    congenital Q64.72
  uterovaginal N81.4
    complete N81.3
    incomplete N81.2

Prolapse, prolapsed — continued
  uterus (with prolapse of vagina) N81.4
    complete N81.3
    congenital Q51.818
    first degree N81.2
    in pregnancy or childbirth — see Pregnancy,
      complicated by, abnormal, uterus
    incomplete N81.2
    postpartal (old) N81.4
    second degree N81.2
    third degree N81.3
  uveal (traumatic) — see Laceration, eye(ball), with
    prolapse or loss of interocular tissue
  vagina (anterior) (wall) — see Cystocele
    with prolapse of uterus N81.4
      complete N81.3
      incomplete N81.2
    posterior wall N81.6
    posthysterectomy N99.3
  vitreous (humor) H43.0- ☑
    in wound — see Laceration, eye(ball), with pro-
      lapse or loss of interocular tissue
  womb — see Prolapse, uterus
Prolapsus, female N81.9
  specified NEC N81.89
Proliferation(s)
  primary cutaneous CD30-positive large T-cell C86.6
  prostate, atypical small acinar N42.32
Proliferative — see condition
Prolonged, prolongation (of)
  bleeding (time) (idiopathic) R79.1
  coagulation (time) R79.1
  gestation (over 42 completed weeks)
    mother O48.1
    newborn P08.22
  interval I44.0
  labor O63.9
    first stage O63.0
    second stage O63.1
  partial thromboplastin time (PTT) R79.1
  pregnancy (more than 42 weeks gestation) O48.1
  prothrombin time R79.1
  QT interval I45.81
  uterine contractions in labor O62.4
Prominence, prominent
  auricle (congenital) (ear) Q17.5
  ischial spine or sacral promontory
    with disproportion (fetopelvic) O33.0
      causing obstructed labor O65.0
  nose (congenital) acquired M95.0
Promiscuity — see High, risk, sexual behavior
Pronation
  ankle — see Deformity, limb, foot, specified NEC
  foot (see also Deformity, limb, foot, specified NEC)
    congenital Q74.2
Prophylactic
  administration of
    antibiotics, long-term Z79.2
      short-term use — omit code
    drug (see also Long-term (current) drug therapy
      (use of)) Z79.899
  medication Z79.899
  organ removal (for neoplasia management) Z40.00
    breast Z40.01
    fallopian tube(s) Z40.03
      with ovary(s) Z40.02
    ovary(s) Z40.02
    specified site NEC Z40.09
  surgery Z40.9
    for risk factors related to malignant neoplasm —
      see Prophylactic, organ removal
    specified NEC Z40.8
  vaccination Z23
Propionic acidemia E71.121
Proptosis (ocular) (see also Exophthalmos)
  thyroid — see Hyperthyroidism, with goiter
Prosecution, anxiety concerning Z65.3
Prosopagnosia R48.3
Prostadynia N42.81
Prostate, prostatic — see condition
Prostatism — see Hyperplasia, prostate
Prostatitis (congestive) (suppurative) (with cystitis) N41.9
  acute N41.0
  cavitary N41.8
  chronic N41.1
  diverticular N41.8
  due to Trichomonas (vaginalis) A59.02
  fibrous N41.1

Prostatitis — continued
  gonococcal (acute) (chronic) A54.22
  granulomatous N41.4
  hypertrophic N41.1
  subacute N41.1
  trichomonal A59.02
  tuberculous A18.14
Prostatocystitis N41.3
Prostatorrhea N42.89
Prostatosis N42.82
Prostration R53.83
  heat (see also Heat, exhaustion)
    anhydrotic T67.3 ☑
    due to
      salt (and water) depletion T67.4 ☑
      water depletion T67.3 ☑
  nervous F48.8
  senile R54
Protanomaly (anomalous trichromat) H53.54
Protanopia (complete) (incomplete) H53.54
Protection (against) (from) — see Prophylactic
Protein
  deficiency NEC — see Malnutrition
  malnutrition — see Malnutrition
  sickness (see also Reaction, serum) T80.69 ☑
Proteinemia R77.9
Proteinosis
  alveolar (pulmonary) J84.01
  lipid or lipoid (of Urbach) E78.89
Proteinuria R80.9
  Bence Jones R80.3
  complicating pregnancy — see Proteinuria, gestational
  gestational
    complicating
      childbirth O12.14
      pregnancy O12.1- ☑
        with edema O12.2- ☑
      puerperium O12.15
  idiopathic R80.0
  isolated R80.0
    with glomerular lesion N06.9
      dense deposit disease N06.6
      diffuse
        crescentic glomerulonephritis N06.7
        endocapillary proliferative glomerulonephri-
          tis N06.4
        mesangiocapillary glomerulonephritis N06.5
        focal and segmental hyalinosis or sclerosis
          N06.1
        membranous (diffuse) N06.2
        mesangial proliferative (diffuse) N06.3
        minimal change N06.0
        specified pathology NEC N06.8
  orthostatic R80.2
    with glomerular lesion — see Proteinuria, isolated,
      with glomerular lesion
  persistent R80.1
    with glomerular lesion — see Proteinuria, isolated,
      with glomerular lesion
  postural R80.2
    with glomerular lesion — see Proteinuria, isolated,
      with glomerular lesion
  pre-eclamptic — see Pre-eclampsia
  puerperal O12.15
  specified type NEC R80.8
Proteolysis, pathologic D65
Proteus (mirabilis) (morganii), **as cause of disease
  classified elsewhere** B96.4
Prothrombin gene mutation D68.52
Protoporphyria, erythropoietic E80.0
Protozoal (see also condition)
  disease B64
    specified NEC B60.8
Protrusion, protrusio
  acetabuli M24.7
  acetabulum (into pelvis) M24.7
  device, implant or graft (see also Complications, by
    site and type, mechanical) T85.698 ☑
    arterial graft NEC — see Complication, cardiovas-
      cular device, mechanical, vascular
    breast (implant) T85.49 ☑
    catheter NEC T85.698 ☑
      cystostomy T83.090 ☑
      dialysis (renal) T82.49 ☑
        intraperitoneal T85.691 ☑
      infusion NEC T82.594 ☑
        spinal (epidural) (subdural) T85.690 ☑

Protrusion, protrusio — *continued*
  device, implant or graft (*see also* Complications, by site and type, mechanical) — *continued*
    catheter — *continued*
      urinary (*see also* Complications, catheter, urinary) T83.098 ☑
      electronic (electrode) (pulse generator) (stimulator)
        bone T84.390 ☑
        nervous system — *see* Complication, prosthetic device, mechanical, electronic nervous system stimulator
    fixation, internal (orthopedic) NEC — *see* Complication, fixation device, mechanical
    gastrointestinal — *see* Complications, prosthetic device, mechanical, gastrointestinal device
    genital NEC T83.498 ☑
      intrauterine contraceptive device T83.39 ☑
      penile prosthesis (cylinder) (implanted) (pump) (resevoir) T83.490 ☑
      testicular prosthesis T83.491 ☑
    heart NEC — *see* Complication, cardiovascular device, mechanical
    joint prosthesis — *see* Complications, joint prosthesis, mechanical, specified NEC, by site
    ocular NEC — *see* Complications, prosthetic device, mechanical, ocular device
    orthopedic NEC — *see* Complication, orthopedic, device, mechanical
    specified NEC T85.628 ☑
    urinary NEC (*see also* Complication, genitourinary, device, urinary, mechanical)
      graft T83.29 ☑
    vascular NEC — *see* Complication, cardiovascular device, mechanical
    ventricular intracranial shunt T85.09 ☑
  intervertebral disc — *see* Displacement, intervertebral disc
  joint prosthesis — *see* Complications, joint prosthesis, mechanical, specified NEC, by site
  nucleus pulposus — *see* Displacement, intervertebral disc
Prune belly (syndrome) Q79.4
Prurigo (ferox) (gravis) (Hebrae) (Hebra's) (mitis) (simplex) L28.2
  Besnier's L20.0
  estivalis L56.4
  nodularis L28.1
  psychogenic F45.8
Pruritus, pruritic (essential) L29.9
  ani, anus L29.0
    psychogenic F45.8
  anogenital L29.3
    psychogenic F45.8
  due to onchocerca volvulus B73.1
  gravidarum — *see* Pregnancy, complicated by, specified pregnancy-related condition NEC
  hiemalis L29.8
  neurogenic (any site) F45.8
  perianal L29.0
  psychogenic (any site) F45.8
  scroti, scrotum L29.1
    psychogenic F45.8
  senile, senilis L29.8
  specified NEC L29.8
    psychogenic F45.8
  Trichomonas A59.9
  vulva, vulvae L29.2
    psychogenic F45.8
Pseudarthrosis, pseudoarthrosis (bone) — *see* Nonunion, fracture
  clavicle, congenital Q74.0
  joint, following fusion or arthrodesis M96.0
Pseudoaneurysm — *see* Aneurysm
Pseudoangina (pectoris) — *see* Angina
Pseudoangioma I81
Pseudoarteriosus Q28.8
Pseudoarthrosis — *see* Pseudarthrosis
Pseudobulbar affect (PBA) F48.2
Pseudochromhidrosis L67.8
Pseudocirrhosis, liver, pericardial I31.1
Pseudocowpox B08.03
Pseudocoxalgia M91.3- ☑
Pseudocroup J38.5
Pseudo-Cushing's syndrome, alcohol-induced E24.4
Pseudocyesis F45.8
Pseudocyst
  lung J98.4

Pseudocyst — *continued*
  pancreas K86.3
  retina — *see* Cyst, retina
Pseudoelephantiasis neuroarthritica Q82.0
Pseudoexfoliation, capsule (lens) — *see* Cataract, specified NEC
Pseudofolliculitis barbae L73.1
Pseudoglioma H44.89
Pseudohemophilia (Bernuth's) (hereditary) (type B) D68.0
  Type A D69.8
  vascular D69.8
Pseudohermaphroditism Q56.3
  adrenal E25.8
  female Q56.2
    with adrenocortical disorder E25.8
    without adrenocortical disorder Q56.2
    adrenal (congenital) E25.0
    unspecified E25.9
  male Q56.1
    with
      5-alpha-reductase deficiency E29.1
      adrenocortical disorder E25.8
      androgen resistance E34.51
      cleft scrotum Q56.1
      feminizing testis E34.51
    without gonadal disorder Q56.1
  adrenal E25.8
  unspecified E25.9
Pseudo-Hurler's polydystrophy E77.0
Pseudohydrocephalus G93.2
Pseudohypertrophic muscular dystrophy (Erb's) G71.0
Pseudohypertrophy, muscle G71.0
Pseudohypoparathyroidism E20.1
Pseudoinsomnia F51.03
Pseudoleukemia, infantile D64.89
Pseudomembranous — *see* condition
Pseudomeningocele (cerebral) (infective) (post-traumatic) G96.19
  postprocedural (spinal) G97.82
Pseudomenses (newborn) P54.6
Pseudomenstruation (newborn) P54.6
Pseudomonas
  aeruginosa, as cause of disease classified elsewhere B96.5
  mallei infection A24.0
    as cause of disease classified elsewhere B96.5
  pseudomallei, as cause of disease classified elsewhere B96.5
Pseudomyotonia G71.19
Pseudomyxoma peritonei C78.6
Pseudoneuritis, optic (nerve) (disc) (papilla), **congenital** Q14.2
Pseudo-obstruction intestine (acute) (chronic) (idiopathic) (intermittent secondary) (primary) K59.8
Pseudopapilledema H47.33- ☑
  congenital Q14.2
Pseudoparalysis
  arm or leg R29.818
  atonic, congenital P94.2
Pseudopelade L66.0
Pseudophakia Z96.1
Pseudopolyarthritis, rhizomelic M35.3
Pseudopolycythemia D75.1
Pseudopseudohypoparathyroidism E20.1
Pseudopterygium H11.81- ☑
Pseudoptosis (eyelid) — *see* Blepharochalasis
Pseudopuberty, precocious
  female heterosexual E25.8
  male isosexual E25.8
Pseudorickets (renal) N25.0
Pseudorubella B08.20
Pseudosclerema, newborn P83.88
Pseudosclerosis (brain)
  Jakob's — *see* Creutzfeldt-Jakob disease or syndrome of Westphal (Strümpell) E83.01
  spastic — *see* Creutzfeldt-Jakob disease or syndrome
Pseudotetanus — *see* Convulsions
Pseudotetany R29.0
  hysterical F44.5
Pseudotruncus arteriosus Q25.49
Pseudotuberculosis A28.2
  enterocolitis A04.8
  pasteurella (infection) A28.0
Pseudotumor
  cerebri G93.2
  orbital H05.11 ☑

Pseudoxanthoma elasticum Q82.8
Psilosis (sprue) (tropical) K90.1
  nontropical K90.0
Psittacosis A70
Psoitis M60.88
Psoriasis L40.9
  arthropathic L40.50
    arthritis mutilans L40.52
    distal interphalangeal L40.51
    juvenile L40.54
    other specified L40.59
    spondylitis L40.53
  buccal K13.29
  flexural L40.8
  guttate L40.4
  mouth K13.29
  nummular L40.0
  plaque L40.0
  psychogenic F54
  pustular (generalized) L40.1
    palmaris et plantaris L40.3
  specified NEC L40.8
  vulgaris L40.0
Psychasthenia F48.8
Psychiatric disorder or problem F99
Psychogenic (*see also* condition)
  factors associated with physical conditions F54
Psychological and behavioral factors affecting medical condition F59
Psychoneurosis, psychoneurotic (*see also* Neurosis)
  anxiety (state) F41.1
  depersonalization F48.1
  hypochondriacal F45.21
  hysteria F44.9
  neurasthenic F48.8
  personality NEC F60.89
Psychopathy, psychopathic
  affectionless F94.2
  autistic F84.5
  constitution, post-traumatic F07.81
  personality — *see* Disorder, personality
  sexual — *see* Deviation, sexual
  state F60.2
Psychosexual identity disorder of childhood F64.2
Psychosis, psychotic F29
  acute (transient) F23
    hysterical F44.9
  affective — *see* Disorder, mood
  alcoholic F10.959
    with
      abuse F10.159
      anxiety disorder F10.980
        with
          abuse F10.180
          dependence F10.280
      delirium tremens F10.231
      delusions F10.950
        with
          abuse F10.150
          dependence F10.250
      dementia F10.97
        with dependence F10.27
      dependence F10.259
      hallucinosis F10.951
        with
          abuse F10.151
          dependence F10.251
      mood disorder F10.94
        with
          abuse F10.14
          dependence F10.24
      paranoia F10.950
        with
          abuse F10.150
          dependence F10.250
      persisting amnesia F10.96
        with dependence F10.26
    amnestic confabulatory F10.96
      with dependence F10.26
    delirium tremens F10.231
    Korsakoff's, Korsakov's, Korsakow's F10.26
    paranoid type F10.950
      with
        abuse F10.150
        dependence F10.250
  anergastic — *see* Psychosis, organic
  arteriosclerotic (simple type) (uncomplicated) F01.50
    with behavioral disturbance F01.51

☑ **Additional Character Required** — Refer to the Tabular List for Character Selection   ᵂᴮ **Subterms under main terms may continue to next column or page**

Psychosis, psychotic — continued
  childhood F84.0
    atypical F84.8
  climacteric — see Psychosis, involutional
  confusional F29
    acute or subacute F05
    reactive F23
  cycloid F23
  depressive — see Disorder, depressive
  disintegrative (childhood) F84.3
  drug-induced — see F11-F19 with .X59
    paranoid and hallucinatory states — see F11-F19
      with .X50 or .X51
  due to or associated with
    addiction, drug — see F11-F19 with .X59
    dependence
      alcohol F10.259
      drug — see F11-F19 with .X59
    epilepsy F06.8
    Huntington's chorea F06.8
    ischemia, cerebrovascular (generalized) F06.8
    multiple sclerosis F06.8
    physical disease F06.8
    presenile dementia F03 ☑
    senile dementia F03 ☑
    vascular disease (arteriosclerotic) (cerebral) F01.50
      with behavioral disturbance F01.51
  epileptic F06.8
  episode F23
    due to or associated with physical condition F06.8
  exhaustive F43.0
  hallucinatory, chronic F28
  hypomanic F30.8
  hysterical (acute) F44.9
  induced F24
  infantile F84.0
    atypical F84.8
  infective (acute) (subacute) F05
  involutional F28
    depressive — see Disorder, depressive
    melancholic — see Disorder, depressive
    paranoid (state) F22
  Korsakoff's, Korsakov's, Korsakow's (nonalcoholic) F04
    alcoholic F10.96
      in dependence F10.26
    induced by other psychoactive substance — see
      categories F11-F19 with .X5X
  mania, manic (single episode) F30.2
    recurrent type F31.89
  manic-depressive — see Disorder, bipolar
  menopausal — see Psychosis, involutional
  mixed schizophrenic and affective F25.8
  multi-infarct (cerebrovascular) F01.50
    with behavioral disturbance F01.51
  nonorganic F29
    specified NEC F28
  organic F09
    due to or associated with
      arteriosclerosis (cerebral) — see Psychosis, ar-
        teriosclerotic
      cerebrovascular disease, arteriosclerotic — see
        Psychosis, arteriosclerotic
      childbirth — see Psychosis, puerperal
      Creutzfeldt-Jakob disease or syndrome — see
        Creutzfeldt-Jakob disease or syndrome
      dependence, alcohol F10.259
      disease
        alcoholic liver F10.259
        brain, arteriosclerotic — see Psychosis, arte-
          riosclerotic
        cerebrovascular F01.50
          with behavioral disturbance F01.51
        Creutzfeldt-Jakob — see Creutzfeldt-Jakob
          disease or syndrome
        endocrine or metabolic F06.8
          acute or subacute F05
        liver, alcoholic F10.259
      epilepsy transient (acute) F05
      infection
        brain (intracranial) F06.8
          acute or subacute F05
      intoxication
        alcoholic (acute) F10.259
        drug F11-F19 with .X59
      ischemia, cerebrovascular (generalized) — see
        Psychosis, arteriosclerotic
      puerperium — see Psychosis, puerperal

Psychosis, psychotic — continued
  organic — continued
    due to or associated with — continued
      trauma, brain (birth) (from electric current)
        (surgical) F06.8
        acute or subacute F05
      infective F06.8
        acute or subacute F05
      post-traumatic F06.8
        acute or subacute F05
  paranoiac F22
  paranoid (climacteric) (involutional) (menopausal) F22
    psychogenic (acute) F23
    schizophrenic F20.0
    senile F03 ☑
  postpartum F53
  presbyophrenic (type) F03 ☑
  presenile F03 ☑
  psychogenic (paranoid) F23
    depressive F32.3
  puerperal F53
    specified type — see Psychosis, by type
  reactive (brief) (transient) (emotional stress) (psycho-
    logical trauma) F23
    depressive F32.3
      recurrent F33.3
    excitative type F30.8
  schizoaffective F25.9
    depressive type F25.1
    manic type F25.0
  schizophrenia, schizophrenic — see Schizophrenia
  schizophrenia-like, in epilepsy F06.2
  schizophreniform F20.81
    affective type F25.9
    brief F23
    confusional type F23
    mixed type F25.0
  senile NEC F03 ☑
    depressed or paranoid type F03 ☑
    simple deterioration F03 ☑
    specified type — code to condition
  shared F24
  situational (reactive) F23
  symbiotic (childhood) F84.3
  symptomatic F09
Psychosomatic — see Disorder, psychosomatic
Psychosyndrome, organic F07.9
Psychotic episode due to or associated with physical condition F06.8
Pterygium (eye) H11.00- ☑
  amyloid H11.01- ☑
  central H11.02- ☑
  colli Q18.3
  double H11.03- ☑
  peripheral
    progressive H11.05- ☑
    stationary H11.04- ☑
  recurrent H11.06- ☑
Ptilosis (eyelid) — see Madarosis
Ptomaine (poisoning) — see Poisoning, food
Ptosis (see also Blepharoptosis)
  adiposa (false) — see Blepharoptosis
  breast N64.81
  cecum K63.4
  colon K63.4
  congenital (eyelid) Q10.0
    specified site NEC — see Anomaly, by site
  eyelid — see Blepharoptosis
    congenital Q10.0
  gastric K31.89
  intestine K63.4
  kidney N28.83
  liver K76.89
  renal N28.83
  splanchnic K63.4
  spleen D73.89
  stomach K31.89
  viscera K63.4
PTP D69.51
Ptyalism (periodic) K11.7
  hysterical F45.8
  pregnancy — see Pregnancy, complicated by, specified
    pregnancy-related condition NEC
  psychogenic F45.8
Ptyalolithiasis K11.5
Pubarche, precocious E30.1
Pubertas praecox E30.1
Puberty (development state) Z00.3

Puberty — continued
  bleeding (excessive) N92.2
  delayed E30.0
  precocious (constitutional) (cryptogenic) (idiopathic)
    E30.1
    central E22.8
    due to
      ovarian hyperfunction E28.1
        estrogen E28.0
      testicular hyperfunction E29.0
  premature E30.1
    due to
      adrenal cortical hyperfunction E25.8
      pineal tumor E34.8
      pituitary (anterior) hyperfunction E22.8
Puckering, macula — see Degeneration, macula, puckering
Pudenda, pudendum — see condition
Puente's disease (simple glandular cheilitis) K13.0
Puerperal, puerperium (complicated by, complications)
  abnormal glucose (tolerance test) O99.815
  abscess
    areola O91.02
      associated with lactation O91.03
    Bartholin's gland O86.19
    breast O91.12
      associated with lactation O91.13
    cervix (uteri) O86.11
    genital organ NEC O86.19
    kidney O86.21
    mammary O91.12
      associated with lactation O91.13
    nipple O91.02
      associated with lactation O91.03
    peritoneum O85
    subareolar O91.12
      associated with lactation O91.13
    urinary tract — see Puerperal, infection, urinary
    uterus O86.12
    vagina (wall) O86.13
    vaginorectal O86.13
    vulvovaginal gland O86.13
  adnexitis O86.19
  afibrinogenemia, or other coagulation defect O72.3
  albuminuria (acute) (subacute) — see Proteinuria,
    gestational
  alcohol use O99.315
  anemia O90.81
    pre-existing (pre-pregnancy) O99.03
  anesthetic death O89.8
  apoplexy O99.43
  bariatric surgery status O99.845
  blood disorder NEC O99.13
  blood dyscrasia O72.3
  cardiomyopathy O90.3
  cerebrovascular disorder (conditions in I60-I69) O99.43
  cervicitis O86.11
  circulatory system disorder O99.43
  coagulopathy (any) O99.13
    with hemorrhage O72.3
  complications O90.9
    specified NEC O90.89
  convulsions — see Eclampsia
  cystitis O86.22
  cystopyelitis O86.29
  delirium NEC F05
  diabetes O24.93
    gestational — see Puerperal, gestational diabetes
    pre-existing O24.33
      specified NEC O24.83
      type 1 O24.03
      type 2 O24.13
  digestive system disorder O99.63
  disease O90.9
    breast NEC O92.29
    cerebrovascular (acute) O99.43
    nonobstetric NEC O99.89
    tubo-ovarian O86.19
    Valsuani's O99.03
  disorder O90.9
    biliary tract O26.63
    lactation O92.70
    liver O26.63
    nonobstetric NEC O99.89
  disruption
    cesarean wound O90.0
    episiotomy wound O90.1
    perineal laceration wound O90.1

Puerperal, puerperium — *continued*
drug use O99.325
eclampsia (with pre-existing hypertension) O15.2
embolism (pulmonary) (blood clot) — *see* Embolism, obstetric, puerperal
endocrine, nutritional or metabolic disease NEC O99.285
endophlebitis — *see* Puerperal, phlebitis
endotrachelitis O86.11
failure
  lactation (complete) O92.3
    partial O92.4
  renal, acute O90.4
fever (of unknown origin) O86.4
  septic O85
fissure, nipple O92.12
  associated with lactation O92.13
fistula
  breast (due to mastitis) O91.12
    associated with lactation O91.13
  nipple O91.02
    associated with lactation O91.03
galactophoritis O91.22
  associated with lactation O91.23
galactorrhea O92.6
gastric banding status O99.845
gastric bypass status O99.845
gastrointestinal disease NEC O99.63
gestational
  diabetes O24.439
    diet controlled O24.430
    insulin (and diet) controlled O24.434
    oral drug controlled (antidiabetic) (hypoglycemic) O24.435
  edema O12.05
    with proteinuria O12.25
  proteinuria O12.15
gonorrhea O98.23
hematoma, subdural O99.43
hemiplegia, cerebral O99.355
  due to cerbrovascular disorder O99.43
hemorrhage O72.1
  brain O99.43
  bulbar O99.43
  cerebellar O99.43
  cerebral O99.43
  cortical O99.43
  delayed or secondary O72.2
  extradural O99.43
  internal capsule O99.43
  intracranial O99.43
  intrapontine O99.43
  meningeal O99.43
  pontine O99.43
  retained placenta O72.0
  subarachnoid O99.43
  subcortical O99.43
  subdural O99.43
  third stage O72.0
  uterine, delayed O72.2
  ventricular O99.43
hemorrhoids O87.2
hepatorenal syndrome O90.4
hypertension — *see* Hypertension, complicating, puerperium
hypertrophy, breast O92.29
induration breast (fibrous) O92.29
infection O86.4
  cervix O86.11
  generalized O85
  genital tract NEC O86.19
    obstetric surgical wound O86.0
  kidney (bacillus coli) O86.21
  maternal O98.93
    carrier state NEC O99.835
    gonorrhea O98.23
    human immunodeficiency virus (HIV) O98.73
    protozoal O98.63
    sexually transmitted NEC O98.33
    specified NEC O98.83
    streptococcus group B (GBS) carrier state O99.825
    syphilis O98.13
    tuberculosis O98.03
    viral hepatitis O98.43
    viral NEC O98.53
  nipple O91.02
    associated with lactation O91.03
  peritoneum O85

Puerperal, puerperium — *continued*
infection — *continued*
  renal O86.21
  specified NEC O86.89
  urinary (asymptomatic) (tract) NEC O86.20
    bladder O86.22
    kidney O86.21
    specified site NEC O86.29
    urethra O86.22
  vagina O86.13
  vein — *see* Puerperal, phlebitis
ischemia, cerebral O99.43
lymphangitis O86.89
  breast O91.22
    associated with lactation O91.23
malignancy O9A.13 (*following* O99)
malnutrition O25.3
mammillitis O91.02
  associated with lactation O91.03
mammitis O91.22
  associated with lactation O91.23
mania F30.8
mastitis O91.22
  associated with lactation O91.23
  purulent O91.12
    associated with lactation O91.13
melancholia — *see* Disorder, depressive
mental disorder NEC O99.345
metroperitonitis O85
metrorrhagia — *see* Hemorrhage, postpartum
metrosalpingitis O86.19
metrovaginitis O86.13
milk leg O87.1
monoplegia, cerebral O99.43
mood disturbance O90.6
necrosis, liver (acute) (subacute) (conditions in subcategory K72.0) O26.63
  with renal failure O90.4
nervous system disorder O99.355
obesity (pre-existing prior to pregnancy) O99.215
obesity surgery status O99.845
occlusion, precerebral artery O99.43
paralysis
  bladder (sphincter) O90.89
  cerebral O99.43
paralytic stroke O99.43
parametritis O85
paravaginitis O86.13
pelviperitonitis O85
perimetritis O86.12
perimetrosalpingitis O86.19
perinephritis O86.21
periphlebitis — *see* Puerperal phlebitis
peritoneal infection O85
peritonitis (pelvic) O85
perivaginitis O86.13
phlebitis O87.0
  deep O87.1
  pelvic O87.1
  superficial O87.0
phlebothrombosis, deep O87.1
phlegmasia alba dolens O87.1
placental polyp O90.89
pneumonia, embolic — *see* Embolism, obstetric, puerperium
pre-eclampsia — *see* Pre-eclampsia
psychosis F53
pyelitis O86.21
pyelocystitis O86.29
pyelonephritis O86.21
pyelonephrosis O86.21
pyemia O85
pyocystitis O86.29
pyohemia O85
pyometra O86.12
pyonephritis O86.21
pyosalpingitis O86.19
pyrexia (of unknown origin) O86.4
renal
  disease NEC O90.89
  failure O90.4
respiratory disease NEC O99.53
retention
  decidua — *see* Retention, decidua
  placenta O72.0
  secundines — *see* Retention, secundines
retrated nipple O92.02
salpingo-ovaritis O86.19

Puerperal, puerperium — *continued*
salpingoperitonitis O85
secondary perineal tear O90.1
sepsis (pelvic) O85
sepsis O85
septic thrombophlebitis O86.81
skin disorder NEC O99.73
specified condition NEC O99.89
stroke O99.43
subinvolution (uterus) O90.89
subluxation of symphysis (pubis) O26.73
suppuration — *see* Puerperal, abscess
tetanus A34
thelitis O91.02
  associated with lactation O91.03
thrombocytopenia O72.3
thrombophlebitis (superficial) O87.0
  deep O87.1
  pelvic O87.1
  septic O86.81
thrombosis (venous) — *see* Thrombosis, puerperal
thyroiditis O90.5
toxemia (eclamptic) (pre-eclamptic) (with convulsions) O15.2
trauma, non-obstetric O9A.23 (*following* O99)
  caused by abuse (physical) (suspected) O9A.33 (*following* O99)
    confirmed O9A.33 (*following* O99)
    psychological (suspected) O9A.53 (*following* O99)
      confirmed O9A.53 (*following* O99)
    sexual (suspected) O9A.43 (*following* O99)
      confirmed O9A.43 (*following* O99)
uremia (due to renal failure) O90.4
urethritis O86.22
vaginitis O86.13
varicose veins (legs) O87.4
  vulva or perineum O87.8
venous O87.9
vulvitis O86.19
vulvovaginitis O86.13
white leg O87.1
Puerperium — *see* Puerperal
Pulmolithiasis J98.4
Pulmonary — *see* condition
Pulpitis (acute) (anachoretic) (chronic) (hyperplastic) (putrescent) (suppurative) (ulcerative) K04.01
irreversible K04.02
reversible K04.01
Pulpless tooth K04.99
Pulse
alternating R00.8
bigeminal R00.8
fast R00.0
feeble, rapid due to shock following injury T79.4 ☑
rapid R00.0
weak R09.89
Pulsus alternans or trigeminus R00.8
Punch drunk F07.81
Punctum lacrimale occlusion — *see* Obstruction, lacrimal
Puncture
abdomen, abdominal
  wall S31.139 ☑
    with
      foreign body S31.149 ☑
      penetration into peritoneal cavity S31.639 ☑
        with foreign body S31.649 ☑
    epigastric region S31.132 ☑
      with
        foreign body S31.142 ☑
        penetration into peritoneal cavity S31.632 ☑
          with foreign body S31.642 ☑
    left
      lower quadrant S31.134 ☑
        with
          foreign body S31.144 ☑
          penetration into peritoneal cavity S31.634 ☑
            with foreign body S31.644 ☑
      upper quadrant S31.131 ☑
        with
          foreign body S31.141 ☑
          penetration into peritoneal cavity S31.631 ☑
            with foreign body S31.641 ☑

Puncture — *continued*
  abdomen, abdominal — *continued*
    wall — *continued*
      periumbilic region S31.135 ☑
        with
          foreign body S31.145 ☑
          penetration into peritoneal cavity S31.635 ☑
            with foreign body S31.645 ☑
      right
        lower quadrant S31.133 ☑
          with
            foreign body S31.143 ☑
            penetration into peritoneal cavity S31.633 ☑
              with foreign body S31.643 ☑
        upper quadrant S31.130 ☑
          with
            foreign body S31.140 ☑
            penetration into peritoneal cavity S31.630 ☑
              with foreign body S31.640 ☑
  accidental, complicating surgery — *see* Complication, accidental puncture or laceration
  alveolar (process) — *see* Puncture, oral cavity
  ankle S91.039 ☑
    with
      foreign body S91.049 ☑
    left S91.032 ☑
      with
        foreign body S91.042 ☑
    right S91.031 ☑
      with
        foreign body S91.041 ☑
  anus S31.833 ☑
    with foreign body S31.834 ☑
  arm (upper) S41.139 ☑
    with foreign body S41.149 ☑
    left S41.132 ☑
      with foreign body S41.142 ☑
    lower — *see* Puncture, forearm
    right S41.131 ☑
      with foreign body S41.141 ☑
  auditory canal (external) (meatus) — *see* Puncture, ear
  auricle, ear — *see* Puncture, ear
  axilla — *see* Puncture, arm
  back (*see also* Puncture, thorax, back)
    lower S31.030 ☑
      with
        foreign body S31.040 ☑
          with penetration into retroperitoneal space S31.041 ☑
        penetration into retroperitoneal space S31.031 ☑
  bladder (traumatic) S37.29 ☑
    nontraumatic N32.89
  breast S21.039 ☑
    with foreign body S21.049 ☑
    left S21.032 ☑
      with foreign body S21.042 ☑
    right S21.031 ☑
      with foreign body S21.041 ☑
  buttock S31.803 ☑
    with foreign body S31.804 ☑
    left S31.823 ☑
      with foreign body S31.824 ☑
    right S31.813 ☑
      with foreign body S31.814 ☑
  by
    device, implant or graft — *see* Complications, by site and type, mechanical
    foreign body left accidentally in operative wound T81.539 ☑
    instrument (any) during a procedure, accidental — *see* Puncture, accidental complicating surgery
  calf — *see* Puncture, leg
  canaliculus lacrimalis — *see* Puncture, eyelid
  canthus, eye — *see* Puncture, eyelid
  cervical esophagus S11.23 ☑
    with foreign body S11.24 ☑
  cheek (external) S01.439 ☑
    with foreign body S01.449 ☑
    internal — *see* Puncture, oral cavity
    left S01.432 ☑

Puncture — *continued*
  cheek — *continued*
    left — *continued*
      with foreign body S01.442 ☑
    right S01.431 ☑
      with foreign body S01.441 ☑
  chest wall — *see* Puncture, thorax
  chin — *see* Puncture, head, specified site NEC
  clitoris — *see* Puncture, vulva
  costal region — *see* Puncture, thorax
  digit(s)
    foot — *see* Puncture, toe
    hand — *see* Puncture, finger
  ear (canal) (external) S01.339 ☑
    with foreign body S01.349 ☑
    drum S09.2-
    left S01.332 ☑
      with foreign body S01.342 ☑
    right S01.331 ☑
      with foreign body S01.341 ☑
  elbow S51.039 ☑
    with
      foreign body S51.049 ☑
    left S51.032 ☑
      with
        foreign body S51.042 ☑
    right S51.031 ☑
      with
        foreign body S51.041 ☑
  epididymis — *see* Puncture, testis
  epigastric region — *see* Puncture, abdomen, wall, epigastric
  epiglottis S11.83 ☑
    with foreign body S11.84 ☑
  esophagus
    cervical S11.23 ☑
      with foreign body S11.24 ☑
    thoracic S27.818 ☑
  eyeball S05.6-
    with foreign body S05.5-
  eyebrow — *see* Puncture, eyelid
  eyelid S01.13-
    with foreign body S01.14-
    left S01.132 ☑
      with foreign body S01.142 ☑
    right S01.131 ☑
      with foreign body S01.141 ☑
  face NEC — *see* Puncture, head, specified site NEC
  finger(s) S61.239 ☑
    with
      damage to nail S61.339 ☑
        with
          foreign body S61.349 ☑
      foreign body S61.249 ☑
    index S61.238 ☑
      with
        damage to nail S61.338 ☑
          with
            foreign body S61.348 ☑
        foreign body S61.248 ☑
      left S61.231 ☑
        with
          damage to nail S61.331 ☑
            with
              foreign body S61.341 ☑
          foreign body S61.241 ☑
      right S61.230 ☑
        with
          damage to nail S61.330 ☑
            with
              foreign body S61.340 ☑
          foreign body S61.240 ☑
    little S61.238 ☑
      with
        damage to nail S61.338 ☑
          with
            foreign body S61.348 ☑
        foreign body S61.248 ☑
      left S61.237 ☑
        with
          damage to nail S61.337 ☑
            with
              foreign body S61.347 ☑
          foreign body S61.247 ☑
      right S61.236 ☑

Puncture — *continued*
  finger(s) — *continued*
    little — *continued*
      right — *continued*
        with
          damage to nail S61.336 ☑
            with
              foreign body S61.346 ☑
          foreign body S61.246 ☑
    middle S61.238 ☑
      with
        damage to nail S61.338 ☑
          with
            foreign body S61.348 ☑
        foreign body S61.248 ☑
      left S61.233 ☑
        with
          damage to nail S61.333 ☑
            with
              foreign body S61.343 ☑
          foreign body S61.243 ☑
      right S61.232 ☑
        with
          damage to nail S61.332 ☑
            with
              foreign body S61.342 ☑
          foreign body S61.242 ☑
    ring S61.238 ☑
      with
        damage to nail S61.338 ☑
          with
            foreign body S61.348 ☑
        foreign body S61.248 ☑
      left S61.235 ☑
        with
          damage to nail S61.335 ☑
            with
              foreign body S61.345 ☑
          foreign body S61.245 ☑
      right S61.234 ☑
        with
          damage to nail S61.334 ☑
            with
              foreign body S61.344 ☑
          foreign body S61.244 ☑
  flank S31.139 ☑
    with foreign body S31.149 ☑
  foot (except toe(s) alone) S91.339 ☑
    with foreign body S91.349 ☑
    left S91.332 ☑
      with foreign body S91.342 ☑
    right S91.331 ☑
      with foreign body S91.341 ☑
    toe — *see* Puncture, toe
  forearm S51.839 ☑
    with
      foreign body S51.849 ☑
    elbow only — *see* Puncture, elbow
    left S51.832 ☑
      with
        foreign body S51.842 ☑
    right S51.831 ☑
      with
        foreign body S51.841 ☑
  forehead — *see* Puncture, head, specified site NEC
  genital organs, external
    female S31.532 ☑
      with foreign body S31.542 ☑
      vagina — *see* Puncture, vagina
      vulva — *see* Puncture, vulva
    male S31.531 ☑
      with foreign body S31.541 ☑
      penis — *see* Puncture, penis
      scrotum — *see* Puncture, scrotum
      testis — *see* Puncture, testis
  groin — *see* Puncture, abdomen, wall
  gum — *see* Puncture, oral cavity
  hand S61.439 ☑
    with
      foreign body S61.449 ☑
    finger — *see* Puncture, finger
    left S61.432 ☑
      with
        foreign body S61.442 ☑
    right S61.431 ☑

Puncture — *continued*
 hand — *continued*
  right — *continued*
   with
    foreign body S61.441 ☑
  thumb — *see* Puncture, thumb
 head S01.93 ☑
  with foreign body S01.94 ☑
  cheek — *see* Puncture, cheek
  ear — *see* Puncture, ear
  eyelid — *see* Puncture, eyelid
  lip — *see* Puncture, oral cavity
  nose — *see* Puncture, nose
  oral cavity — *see* Puncture, oral cavity
  scalp S01.03 ☑
   with foreign body S01.04 ☑
  specified site NEC S01.83 ☑
   with foreign body S01.84 ☑
  temporomandibular area — *see* Puncture, cheek
 heart S26.99 ☑
  with hemopericardium S26.09 ☑
  without hemopericardium S26.19 ☑
 heel — *see* Puncture, foot
 hip S71.039 ☑
  with foreign body S71.049 ☑
  left S71.032 ☑
   with foreign body S71.042 ☑
  right S71.031 ☑
   with foreign body S71.041 ☑
 hymen — *see* Puncture, vagina
 hypochondrium — *see* Puncture, abdomen, wall
 hypogastric region — *see* Puncture, abdomen, wall
 inguinal region — *see* Puncture, abdomen, wall
 instep — *see* Puncture, foot
 internal organs — *see* Injury, by site
 interscapular region — *see* Puncture, thorax, back
 intestine
  large
   colon S36.599 ☑
    ascending S36.590 ☑
    descending S36.592 ☑
    sigmoid S36.593 ☑
    specified site NEC S36.598 ☑
    transverse S36.591 ☑
   rectum S36.69 ☑
  small S36.499 ☑
   duodenum S36.490 ☑
   specified site NEC S36.498 ☑
 intra-abdominal organ S36.99 ☑
  gallbladder S36.128 ☑
  intestine — *see* Puncture, intestine
  liver S36.118 ☑
  pancreas — *see* Puncture, pancreas
  peritoneum S36.81 ☑
  specified site NEC S36.898 ☑
  spleen S36.09 ☑
  stomach S36.39 ☑
 jaw — *see* Puncture, head, specified site NEC
 knee S81.039 ☑
  with foreign body S81.049 ☑
  left S81.032 ☑
   with foreign body S81.042 ☑
  right S81.031 ☑
   with foreign body S81.041 ☑
 labium (majus) (minus) — *see* Puncture, vulva
 lacrimal duct — *see* Puncture, eyelid
 larynx S11.013 ☑
  with foreign body S11.014 ☑
 leg (lower) S81.839 ☑
  with foreign body S81.849 ☑
  foot — *see* Puncture, foot
  knee — *see* Puncture, knee
  left S81.832 ☑
   with foreign body S81.842 ☑
  right S81.831 ☑
   with foreign body S81.841 ☑
  upper — *see* Puncture, thigh
 lip S01.531 ☑
  with foreign body S01.541 ☑
 loin — *see* Puncture, abdomen, wall
 lower back — *see* Puncture, back, lower
 lumbar region — *see* Puncture, back, lower
 malar region — *see* Puncture, head, specified site NEC
 mammary — *see* Puncture, breast
 mastoid region — *see* Puncture, head, specified site NEC

Puncture — *continued*
 mouth — *see* Puncture, oral cavity
 nail
  finger — *see* Puncture, finger, with damage to nail
  toe — *see* Puncture, toe, with damage to nail
 nasal (septum) (sinus) — *see* Puncture, nose
 nasopharynx — *see* Puncture, head, specified site NEC
 neck S11.93 ☑
  with foreign body S11.94 ☑
  involving
   cervical esophagus — *see* Puncture, cervical esophagus
   larynx — *see* Puncture, larynx
   pharynx — *see* Puncture, pharynx
   thyroid gland — *see* Puncture, thyroid gland
   trachea — *see* Puncture, trachea
  specified site NEC S11.83 ☑
   with foreign body S11.84 ☑
 nose (septum) (sinus) S01.23 ☑
  with foreign body S01.24 ☑
 ocular — *see* Puncture, eyeball
 oral cavity S01.532 ☑
  with foreign body S01.542 ☑
 orbit S05.4- ☑
 palate — *see* Puncture, oral cavity
 palm — *see* Puncture, hand
 pancreas S36.299 ☑
  body S36.291 ☑
  head S36.290 ☑
  tail S36.292 ☑
 pelvis — *see* Puncture, back, lower
 penis S31.23 ☑
  with foreign body S31.24 ☑
 perineum
  female S31.43 ☑
   with foreign body S31.44 ☑
  male S31.139 ☑
   with foreign body S31.149 ☑
 periocular area (with or without lacrimal passages) — *see* Puncture, eyelid
 phalanges
  finger — *see* Puncture, finger
  toe — *see* Puncture, toe
 pharynx S11.23 ☑
  with foreign body S11.24 ☑
 pinna — *see* Puncture, ear
 popliteal space — *see* Puncture, knee
 prepuce — *see* Puncture, penis
 pubic region S31.139 ☑
  with foreign body S31.149 ☑
 pudendum — *see* Puncture, genital organs, external
 rectovaginal septum — *see* Puncture, vagina
 sacral region — *see* Puncture, back, lower
 sacroiliac region — *see* Puncture, back, lower
 salivary gland — *see* Puncture, oral cavity
 scalp S01.03 ☑
  with foreign body S01.04 ☑
 scapular region — *see* Puncture, shoulder
 scrotum S31.33 ☑
  with foreign body S31.34 ☑
 shin — *see* Puncture, leg
 shoulder S41.039 ☑
  with foreign body S41.049 ☑
  left S41.032 ☑
   with foreign body S41.042 ☑
  right S41.031 ☑
   with foreign body S41.041 ☑
 spermatic cord — *see* Puncture, testis
 sternal region — *see* Puncture, thorax, front
 submaxillary region — *see* Puncture, head, specified site NEC
 submental region — *see* Puncture, head, specified site NEC
 subungual
  finger(s) — *see* Puncture, finger, with damage to nail
  toe — *see* Puncture, toe, with damage to nail
 supraclavicular fossa — *see* Puncture, neck, specified site NEC
 temple, temporal region — *see* Puncture, head, specified site NEC
 temporomandibular area — *see* Puncture, cheek
 testis S31.33 ☑
  with foreign body S31.34 ☑
 thigh S71.139 ☑
  with foreign body S71.149 ☑

Puncture — *continued*
 thigh — *continued*
  left S71.132 ☑
   with foreign body S71.142 ☑
  right S71.131 ☑
   with foreign body S71.141 ☑
 thorax, thoracic (wall) S21.93 ☑
  with foreign body S21.94 ☑
  back S21.23- ☑
   with
    foreign body S21.24- ☑
     with penetration S21.44 ☑
    penetration S21.43 ☑
  breast — *see* Puncture, breast
  front S21.13- ☑
   with
    foreign body S21.14- ☑
     with penetration S21.34 ☑
    penetration S21.33 ☑
 throat — *see* Puncture, neck
 thumb S61.039 ☑
  with
   damage to nail S61.139 ☑
    with
     foreign body S61.149 ☑
   foreign body S61.049 ☑
  left S61.032 ☑
   with
    damage to nail S61.132 ☑
     with
      foreign body S61.142 ☑
    foreign body S61.042 ☑
  right S61.031 ☑
   with
    damage to nail S61.131 ☑
     with
      foreign body S61.141 ☑
    foreign body S61.041 ☑
 thyroid gland S11.13 ☑
  with foreign body S11.14 ☑
 toe(s) S91.139 ☑
  with
   damage to nail S91.239 ☑
    with
     foreign body S91.249 ☑
   foreign body S91.149 ☑
  great S91.133 ☑
   with
    damage to nail S91.233 ☑
     with
      foreign body S91.243 ☑
    foreign body S91.143 ☑
   left S91.132 ☑
    with
     damage to nail S91.232 ☑
      with
       foreign body S91.242 ☑
     foreign body S91.142 ☑
   right S91.131 ☑
    with
     damage to nail S91.231 ☑
      with
       foreign body S91.241 ☑
     foreign body S91.141 ☑
  lesser S91.136 ☑
   with
    damage to nail S91.236 ☑
     with
      foreign body S91.246 ☑
    foreign body S91.146 ☑
   left S91.135 ☑
    with
     damage to nail S91.235 ☑
      with
       foreign body S91.245 ☑
     foreign body S91.145 ☑
   right S91.134 ☑
    with
     damage to nail S91.234 ☑
      with
       foreign body S91.244 ☑
     foreign body S91.144 ☑
 tongue — *see* Puncture, oral cavity
 trachea S11.023 ☑
  with foreign body S11.024 ☑
 tunica vaginalis — *see* Puncture, testis

☑ **Additional Character Required** — Refer to the Tabular List for Character Selection ▽ **Subterms under main terms may continue to next column or page**

Puncture — *continued*
  tympanum, tympanic membrane S09.2- ☑
  umbilical region S31.135 ☑
    with foreign body S31.145 ☑
  uvula — *see* Puncture, oral cavity
  vagina S31.43 ☑
    with foreign body S31.44 ☑
  vocal cords S11.033 ☑
    with foreign body S11.034 ☑
  vulva S31.43 ☑
    with foreign body S31.44 ☑
  wrist S61.539 ☑
    with
      foreign body S61.549 ☑
    left S61.532 ☑
      with
        foreign body S61.542 ☑
    right S61.531 ☑
      with
        foreign body S61.541 ☑
PUO (pyrexia of unknown origin) R50.9
Pupillary membrane (persistent) Q13.89
Pupillotonia — *see* Anomaly, pupil, function, tonic pupil
Purpura D69.2
  abdominal D69.0
  allergic D69.0
  anaphylactoid D69.0
  annularis telangiectodes L81.7
  arthritic D69.0
  autoerythrocyte sensitization D69.2
  autoimmune D69.0
  bacterial D69.0
  Bateman's (senile) D69.2
  capillary fragility (hereditary) (idiopathic) D69.8
  cryoglobulinemic D89.1
  Devil's pinches D69.2
  fibrinolytic — *see* Fibrinolysis
  fulminans, fulminous D65
  gangrenous D65
  hemorrhagic, hemorrhagica D69.3
    not due to thrombocytopenia D69.0
  Henoch (-Schönlein) (allergic) D69.0
  hypergammaglobulinemic (benign) (Waldenström)
    D89.0
  idiopathic (thrombocytopenic) D69.3
    nonthrombocytopenic D69.0
  immune thrombocytopenic D69.3
  infectious D69.0
  malignant D69.0
  neonatorum P54.5
  nervosa D69.0
  newborn P54.5
  nonthrombocytopenic D69.2
    hemorrhagic D69.0
    idiopathic D69.0
  nonthrombopenic D69.2
  peliosis rheumatica D69.0
  posttransfusion (post-transfusion) (from (fresh) whole
    blood or blood products) D69.51
  primary D69.49
  red cell membrane sensitivity D69.2
  rheumatica D69.0
  Schönlein (-Henoch) (allergic) D69.0
  scorbutic E54 [D77]
  senile D69.2
  simplex D69.2
  symptomatica D69.0
  telangiectasia annularis L81.7
  thrombocytopenic D69.49
    congenital D69.42
    hemorrhagic D69.3
    hereditary D69.42
    idiopathic D69.3
    immune D69.3
    neonatal, transitory P61.0
    thrombotic M31.1
  thrombohemolytic — *see* Fibrinolysis
  thrombolytic — *see* Fibrinolysis
  thrombopenic D69.49
  thrombotic, thrombocytopenic M31.1
  toxic D69.0
  vascular D69.0
  visceral symptoms D69.0
Purpuric spots R23.3
Purulent — *see* condition
Pus
  in
    stool R19.5

Pus — *continued*
  in — *continued*
    urine N39.0
  tube (rupture) — *see* Salpingo-oophoritis
Pustular rash L08.0
Pustule (nonmalignant) L08.9
  malignant A22.0
Pustulosis palmaris et plantaris L40.3
Putnam (-Dana) **disease or syndrome** — *see* Degeneration, combined
Putrescent pulp (dental) K04.1
Pyarthritis, pyarthrosis — *see* Arthritis, pyogenic or pyemic
  tuberculous — *see* Tuberculosis, joint
Pyelectasis — *see* Hydronephrosis
Pyelitis (congenital) (uremic) (*see also* Pyelonephritis)
  with
    calculus — *see* category N20 ☑
      with hydronephrosis N13.2
    contracted kidney N11.9
  acute N10
  chronic N11.9
    with calculus — *see* category N20 ☑
      with hydronephrosis N13.2
  cystica N28.84
  puerperal (postpartum) O86.21
  tuberculous A18.11
Pyelocystitis — *see* Pyelonephritis
Pyelonephritis (*see also* Nephritis, tubulo-interstitial)
  with
    calculus — *see* category N20 ☑
      with hydronephrosis N13.2
    contracted kidney N11.9
  acute N10
  calculous — *see* category N20 ☑
    with hydronephrosis N13.2
  chronic N11.9
    with calculus — *see* category N20 ☑
      with hydronephrosis N13.2
    associated with ureteral obstruction or stricture
      N11.1
    nonobstructive N11.8
      with reflux (vesicoureteral) N11.0
    obstructive N11.1
    specified NEC N11.8
  in (due to)
    brucellosis A23.9 [N16]
    cryoglobulinemia (mixed) D89.1 [N16]
    cystinosis E72.04
    diphtheria A36.84
    glycogen storage disease E74.09 [N16]
    leukemia NEC C95.9- ☑ [N16]
    lymphoma NEC C85.90 [N16]
    multiple myeloma C90.0- ☑ [N16]
    obstruction N11.1
    Salmonella infection A02.25
    sarcoidosis D86.84
    sepsis A41.9 [N16]
    Sjögren's disease M35.04
    toxoplasmosis B58.83
    transplant rejection T86.91 [N16]
    Wilson's disease E83.01 [N16]
  nonobstructive N12
    with reflux (vesicoureteral) N11.0
    chronic N11.8
  syphilitic A52.75
Pyelonephrosis (obstructive) N11.1
  chronic N11.9
Pyelophlebitis I80.8
Pyeloureteritis cystica N28.85
Pyemia, pyemic (fever) (infection) (purulent) (*see also* Sepsis)
  joint — *see* Arthritis, pyogenic or pyemic
  liver K75.1
  pneumococcal A40.3
  portal K75.1
  postvaccinal T88.0 ☑
  puerperal, postpartum, childbirth O85
  specified organism NEC A41.89
  tuberculous — *see* Tuberculosis, miliary
Pygopagus Q89.4
Pyknoepilepsy (idiopathic) — *see* Pyknolepsy
Pyknolepsy G40.A09 (*following* G40.3)
  intractable G40.A19 (*following* G40.3)
    with status epilepticus G40.A11 (*following* G40.3)
    without status epilepticus G40.A19 (*following* G40.3)
  not intractable G40.A09 (*following* G40.3)

Pyknolepsy — *continued*
  not intractable — *continued*
    with status epilepticus G40.A01 (*following* G40.3)
    without status epilepticus G40.A09 (*following* G40.3)
Pylephlebitis K75.1
Pyle's syndrome Q78.5
Pylethrombophlebitis K75.1
Pylethrombosis K75.1
Pyloritis K29.90
  with bleeding K29.91
Pylorospasm (reflex) **NEC** K31.3
  congenital or infantile Q40.0
  neurotic F45.8
  newborn Q40.0
  psychogenic F45.8
Pylorus, pyloric — *see* condition
Pyoarthrosis — *see* Arthritis, pyogenic or pyemic
Pyocele
  mastoid — *see* Mastoiditis, acute
  sinus (accessory) — *see* Sinusitis
  turbinate (bone) J32.9
  urethra (*see also* Urethritis) N34.0
Pyocolpos — *see* Vaginitis
Pyocystitis N30.80
  with hematuria N30.81
Pyoderma, pyodermia L08.0
  gangrenosum L88
  newborn P39.4
  phagedenic L88
  vegetans L08.81
Pyodermatitis L08.0
  vegetans L08.81
Pyogenic — *see* condition
Pyohydronephrosis N13.6
Pyometra, pyometrium, pyometritis — *see* Endometritis
Pyomyositis (tropical) — *see* Myositis, infective
Pyonephritis N12
Pyonephrosis N13.6
  tuberculous A18.11
Pyo-oophoritis — *see* Salpingo-oophoritis
Pyo-ovarium — *see* Salpingo-oophoritis
Pyopericarditis, pyopericardium I30.1
Pyophlebitis — *see* Phlebitis
Pyopneumopericardium I30.1
Pyopneumothorax (infective) J86.9
  with fistula J86.0
  tuberculous NEC A15.6
Pyosalpinx, pyosalpingitis (*see also* Salpingo-oophoritis)
Pyothorax J86.9
  with fistula J86.0
  tuberculous NEC A15.6
Pyoureter N28.89
  tuberculous A18.11
Pyramidopallidonigral syndrome G20
Pyrexia (of unknown origin) R50.9
  atmospheric T67.0 ☑
  during labor NEC O75.2
  heat T67.0 ☑
  newborn P81.9
    environmentally-induced P81.0
  persistent R50.9
  puerperal O86.4
Pyroglobulinemia NEC E88.09
Pyromania F63.1
Pyrosis R12
Pyuria (bacterial) N39.0

Q

Q fever A78
  with pneumonia A78
Quadricuspid aortic valve Q23.8
Quadrilateral fever A78
Quadriparesis — *see* Quadriplegia
  meaning muscle weakness M62.81
Quadriplegia G82.50
  complete
    C1-C4 level G82.51
    C5-C7 level G82.53
  congenital (cerebral) (spinal) G80.8
    spastic G80.0
  embolic (current episode) I63.4- ☑
  functional R53.2

Quadriplegia — continued
  incomplete
    C1-C4 level G82.52
    C5-C7 level G82.54
  thrombotic (current episode) I63.3- ☑
  traumatic — code to injury with seventh character S
    current episode — see Injury, spinal (cord), cervical
Quadruplet, pregnancy — see Pregnancy, quadruplet
Quarrelsomeness F60.3
Queensland fever A77.3
Quervain's disease M65.4
  thyroid E06.1
Queyrat's erythroplasia D07.4
  penis D07.4
  specified site — see Neoplasm, skin, in situ
  unspecified site D07.4
Quincke's disease or edema T78.3 ☑
  hereditary D84.1
Quinsy (gangrenous) J36
Quintan fever A79.0
Quintuplet, pregnancy — see Pregnancy, quintuplet

R

Rabbit fever — see Tularemia
Rabies A82.9
  contact Z20.3
  exposure to Z20.3
  inoculation reaction — see Complications, vaccination
  sylvatic A82.0
  urban A82.1
Rachischisis — see Spina bifida
Rachitic (see also condition)
  deformities of spine (late effect) (sequelae) E64.3
  pelvis (late effect) (sequelae) E64.3
    with disproportion (fetopelvic) O33.0
      causing obstructed labor O65.0
Rachitis, rachitism (acute) (tarda) (see also Rickets)
  renalis N25.0
  sequelae E64.3
Radial nerve — see condition
Radiation
  burn — see Burn
  effects NOS T66 ☑
  sickness NOS T66 ☑
  therapy, encounter for Z51.0
Radiculitis (pressure) (vertebrogenic) — see Radiculopathy
Radiculomyelitis (see also Encephalitis)
  toxic, due to
    Clostridium tetani A35
    Corynebacterium diphtheriae A36.82
Radiculopathy M54.10
  cervical region M54.12
  cervicothoracic region M54.13
  due to
    disc disorder
      C3 M50.11
      C4 M50.11
      C5 M50.121
      C6 M50.122
      C7 M50.123
    displacement of intervertebral disc — see Disorder, disc, with, radiculopathy
  leg M54.1- ☑
  lumbar region M54.16
  lumbosacral region M54.17
  occipito-atlanto-axial region M54.11
  postherpetic B02.29
  sacrococcygeal region M54.18
  syphilitic A52.11
  thoracic region (with visceral pain) M54.14
  thoracolumbar region M54.15
Radiodermal burns (acute, chronic, or occupational) — see Burn
Radiodermatitis L58.9
  acute L58.0
  chronic L58.1
Radiotherapy session Z51.0
RAEB (refractory anemia with excess blasts) D46.2- ☑
Rage, meaning rabies — see Rabies
Ragpicker's disease A22.1
Ragsorter's disease A22.1
Raillietiniasis B71.8
Railroad neurosis F48.8
Railway spine F48.8

Raised (see also Elevated)
  antibody titer R76.0
Rake teeth, tooth M26.39
Rales R09.89
Ramifying renal pelvis Q63.8
Ramsay-Hunt disease or syndrome (see also Hunt's disease) B02.21
  meaning dyssynergia cerebellaris myoclonica G11.1
Ranula K11.6
  congenital Q38.4
Rape
  adult
    confirmed T74.21 ☑
    suspected T76.21 ☑
  alleged, observation or examination, ruled out
    adult Z04.41
    child Z04.42
  child
    confirmed T74.22 ☑
    suspected T76.22 ☑
Rapid
  feeble pulse, due to shock, following injury T79.4 ☑
  heart (beat) R00.0
    psychogenic F45.8
  second stage (delivery) O62.3
  time-zone change syndrome — see Disorder, sleep, circadian rhythm, psychogenic
Rarefaction, bone — see Disorder, bone, density and structure, specified NEC
Rash (toxic) R21
  canker A38.9
  diaper L22
  drug (internal use) L27.0
    contact (see also Dermatitis, due to, drugs, external) L25.1
  following immunization T88.1 ☑
  food — see Dermatitis, due to, food
  heat L74.0
  napkin (psoriasiform) L22
  nettle — see Urticaria
  pustular L08.0
  rose R21
    epidemic B06.9
  scarlet A38.9
  serum (see also Reaction, serum) T80.69 ☑
  wandering tongue K14.1
Rasmussen aneurysm — see Tuberculosis, pulmonary
Rasmussen encephalitis G04.81
Rat-bite fever A25.9
  due to Streptobacillus moniliformis A25.1
  spirochetal (morsus muris) A25.0
Rathke's pouch tumor D44.3
Raymond (-Céstan) **syndrome** I65.8
Raynaud's disease, phenomenon or syndrome (secondary) I73.00
  with gangrene (symmetric) I73.01
RDS (newborn) (type I) P22.0
  type II P22.1
Reaction (see also Disorder)
  adaptation — see Disorder, adjustment
  adjustment (anxiety) (conduct disorder) (depressiveness) (distress) — see Disorder, adjustment
    with
      mutism, elective (child) (adolescent) F94.0
  adverse
    food (any) (ingested) NEC T78.1 ☑
      anaphylactic — see Shock, anaphylactic, due to food
  affective — see Disorder, mood
  allergic — see Allergy
  anaphylactic — see Shock, anaphylactic
  anaphylactoid — see Shock, anaphylactic
  anesthesia — see Anesthesia, complication
  antitoxin (prophylactic) (therapeutic) — see Complications, vaccination
  anxiety F41.1
  Arthus — see Arthus' phenomenon
  asthenic F48.8
  combat and operational stress F43.0
  compulsive F42.8
  conversion F44.9
  crisis, acute F43.0
  deoxyribonuclease (DNA) (DNase) hypersensitivity D69.2
  depressive (single episode) F32.9
    affective (single episode) F31.4
      recurrent episode F33.9

Reaction — continued
  depressive — continued
    neurotic F34.1
    psychoneurotic F34.1
    psychotic F32.3
    recurrent — see Disorder, depressive, recurrent
  dissociative F44.9
  drug NEC T88.7 ☑
    addictive — see Dependence, drug
      transmitted via placenta or breast milk — see Absorption, drug, addictive, through placenta
    allergic — see Allergy, drug
    lichenoid L43.2
    newborn P93.8
      gray baby syndrome P93.0
    overdose or poisoning (by accident) — see Table of Drugs and Chemicals, by drug, poisoning
    photoallergic L56.1
    phototoxic L56.0
    withdrawal — see Dependence, by drug, with, withdrawal
      infant of dependent mother P96.1
      newborn P96.1
    wrong substance given or taken (by accident) — see Table of Drugs and Chemicals, by drug, poisoning
  fear F40.9
    child (abnormal) F93.8
  febrile nonhemolytic transfusion (FNHTR) R50.84
  fluid loss, cerebrospinal G97.1
  foreign
    body NEC — see Granuloma, foreign body
      in operative wound (inadvertently left) — see Foreign body, accidentally left during a procedure
    substance accidentally left during a procedure (chemical) (powder) (talc) T81.60 ☑
      aseptic peritonitis T81.61 ☑
      body or object (instrument) (sponge) (swab) — see Foreign body, accidentally left during a procedure
      specified reaction NEC T81.69 ☑
  grief — see Disorder, adjustment
  Herxheimer's R68.89
  hyperkinetic — see Hyperkinesia
  hypochondriacal F45.20
  hypoglycemic, due to insulin E16.0
    with coma (diabetic) — see Diabetes, coma
    nondiabetic E15
    therapeutic misadventure — see subcategory T38.3 ☑
  hypomanic F30.8
  hysterical F44.9
  immunization — see Complications, vaccination
  incompatibility
    ABO blood group (infusion) (transfusion) — see Complication(s), transfusion, incompatibility reaction, ABO
    delayed serologic T80.39 ☑
    minor blood group (Duffy) (E) (K(ell)) (Kidd) (Lewis) (M) (N) (P) (S) T80.89 ☑
    Rh (factor) (infusion) (transfusion) — see Complication(s), transfusion, incompatibility reaction, Rh (factor)
  inflammatory — see Infection
  infusion — see Complications, infusion
  inoculation (immune serum) — see Complications, vaccination
  insulin T38.3- ☑
  involutional psychotic — see Disorder, depressive
  leukemoid D72.823
    basophilic D72.823
    lymphocytic D72.823
    monocytic D72.823
    myelocytic D72.823
    neutrophilic D72.823
  LSD (acute)
    due to drug abuse — see Abuse, drug, hallucinogen
    due to drug dependence — see Dependence, drug, hallucinogen
  lumbar puncture G97.1
  manic-depressive — see Disorder, bipolar
  neurasthenic F48.8
  neurogenic — see Neurosis
  neurotic F48.9
  neurotic-depressive F34.1

Reaction — *continued*
  nitritoid — *see* Crisis, nitritoid
  nonspecific
    to
      cell mediated immunity measurement of gamma interferon antigen response measurement without active tuberculosis R76.12
      QuantiFERON-TB test (QFT) without active tuberculosis R76.12
      tuberculin test (*see also* Reaction, tuberculin skin test) R76.11
  obsessive-compulsive F42.8
  organic, acute or subacute — *see* Delirium
  paranoid (acute) F23
    chronic F22
    senile F03 ☑
  passive dependency F60.7
  phobic F40.9
  post-traumatic stress, uncomplicated Z73.3
  psychogenic F99
  psychoneurotic (*see also* Neurosis)
    compulsive F42.8
    depersonalization F48.1
    depressive F34.1
    hypochondriacal F45.20
    neurasthenic F48.8
    obsessive F42.8
  psychophysiologic — *see* Disorder, somatoform
  psychosomatic — *see* Disorder, somatoform
  psychotic — *see* Psychosis
  scarlet fever toxin — *see* Complications, vaccination
  schizophrenic F23
    acute (brief) (undifferentiated) F23
    latent F21
    undifferentiated (acute) (brief) F23
  serological for syphilis — *see* Serology for syphilis
  serum T80.69 ☑
    anaphylactic (immediate) (*see also* Shock, anaphylactic) T80.59 ☑
    specified reaction NEC
      due to
        administration of blood and blood products T80.61 ☑
        immunization T80.62 ☑
        serum specified NEC T80.69 ☑
        vaccination T80.62 ☑
  situational — *see* Disorder, adjustment
  somatization — *see* Disorder, somatoform
  spinal puncture G97.1
  stress (severe) F43.9
    acute (agitation) ("daze") (disorientation) (disturbance of consciousness) (flight reaction) (fugue) F43.0
    specified NEC F43.8
  surgical procedure — *see* Complications, surgical procedure
  tetanus antitoxin — *see* Complications, vaccination
  toxic, to local anesthesia T88.59 ☑
    in labor and delivery O74.4
    in pregnancy O29.3X- ☑
    postpartum, puerperal O89.3
  toxin-antitoxin — *see* Complications, vaccination
  transfusion (blood) (bone marrow) (lymphocytes) (allergic) — *see* Complications, transfusion
  tuberculin skin test, abnormal R76.11
  vaccination (any) — *see* Complications, vaccination
  withdrawing, child or adolescent F93.8
Reactive airway disease — *see* Asthma
Reactive depression — *see* Reaction, depressive
Rearrangement
  chromosomal
    balanced (in) Q95.9
      abnormal individual (autosomal) Q95.2
        non-sex (autosomal) chromosomes Q95.2
        sex/non-sex chromosomes Q95.3
      specified NEC Q95.8
Recalcitrant patient — *see* Noncompliance
Recanalization, thrombus — *see* Thrombosis
Recession, receding
  chamber angle (eye) H21.55- ☑
  chin M26.09
  gingival (postinfective) (postoperative)
    generalized K06.020
      minimal K06.021
      moderate K06.022
      severe K06.023
    localized K06.010
      minimal K06.011

Recession, receding — *continued*
  gingival — *continued*
    localized — *continued*
      moderate K06.012
      severe K06.013
Recklinghausen disease Q85.01
  bones E21.0
Reclus' disease (cystic) — *see* Mastopathy, cystic
Recrudescent typhus (fever) A75.1
Recruitment, auditory H93.21- ☑
Rectalgia K62.89
Rectitis K62.89
Rectocele
  female (without uterine prolapse) N81.6
    with uterine prolapse N81.4
      incomplete N81.2
  in pregnancy — *see* Pregnancy, complicated by, abnormal, pelvic organs or tissues NEC
  male K62.3
Rectosigmoid junction — *see* condition
Rectosigmoiditis K63.89
  ulcerative (chronic) K51.30
    with
      complication K51.319
        abscess K51.314
        fistula K51.313
        obstruction K51.312
        rectal bleeding K51.311
        specified NEC K51.318
Rectourethral — *see* condition
Rectovaginal — *see* condition
Rectovesical — *see* condition
Rectum, rectal — *see* condition
Recurrent — *see* condition
  pregnancy loss — *see* Loss (of), pregnancy, recurrent
Red bugs B88.0
Red tide (*see also* Table of Drugs and Chemicals) T65.82- ☑
Red-cedar lung or pneumonitis J67.8
Reduced
  mobility Z74.09
  ventilatory or vital capacity R94.2
Redundant, redundancy
  anus (congenital) Q43.8
  clitoris N90.89
  colon (congenital) Q43.8
  foreskin (congenital) N47.8
  intestine (congenital) Q43.8
  labia N90.69
  organ or site, congenital NEC — *see* Accessory
  panniculus (abdominal) E65
  prepuce (congenital) N47.8
  pylorus K31.89
  rectum (congenital) Q43.8
  scrotum N50.89
  sigmoid (congenital) Q43.8
  skin L98.7
    and subcutaneous tissue L98.7
    of face L57.4
      eyelids — *see* Blepharochalasis
  stomach K31.89
Reduplication — *see* Duplication
Reflex R29.2
  hyperactive gag J39.2
  pupillary, abnormal — *see* Anomaly, pupil, function
  vasoconstriction I73.9
  vasovagal R55
Reflux K21.9
  acid K21.9
  esophageal K21.9
    with esophagitis K21.0
    newborn P78.83
  gastroesophageal K21.9
    with esophagitis K21.0
  mitral — *see* Insufficiency, mitral
  ureteral — *see* Reflux, vesicoureteral
  vesicoureteral (with scarring) N13.70
    with
      nephropathy N13.729
        with hydroureter N13.739
          bilateral N13.732
          unilateral N13.731
        without hydroureter N13.729
          bilateral N13.722
          unilateral N13.721
        bilateral N13.722
        unilateral N13.721
      pyelonephritis (chronic) N11.0

Reflux — *continued*
  vesicoureteral — *continued*
    without nephropathy N13.71
      congenital Q62.7
Reforming, artificial openings — *see* Attention to, artificial, opening
Refractive error — *see* Disorder, refraction
Refsum's disease or syndrome G60.1
Refusal of
  food, psychogenic F50.89
  treatment (because of) Z53.20
    left against medical advice (AMA) Z53.21
    patient's decision NEC Z53.29
    reasons of belief or group pressure Z53.1
Regional — *see* condition
Regurgitation R11.10
  aortic (valve) — *see* Insufficiency, aortic
  food (*see also* Vomiting)
    with reswallowing — *see* Rumination
    newborn P92.1
  gastric contents — *see* Vomiting
  heart — *see* Endocarditis
  mitral (valve) — *see* Insufficiency, mitral
    congenital Q23.3
  myocardial — *see* Endocarditis
  pulmonary (valve) (heart) I37.1
    congenital Q22.2
    syphilitic A52.03
  tricuspid — *see* Insufficiency, tricuspid
  valve, valvular — *see* Endocarditis
    congenital Q24.8
  vesicoureteral — *see* Reflux, vesicoureteral
Reichmann's disease or syndrome K31.89
Reifenstein syndrome E34.52
Reinsertion
  implantable subdermal contraceptive Z30.46
  intrauterine contraceptive device Z30.433
Reiter's disease, syndrome, or urethritis M02.30
  ankle M02.37- ☑
  elbow M02.32- ☑
  foot joint M02.37- ☑
  hand joint M02.34- ☑
  hip M02.35- ☑
  knee M02.36- ☑
  multiple site M02.39
  shoulder M02.31- ☑
  vertebra M02.38
  wrist M02.33- ☑
Rejection
  food, psychogenic F50.89
  transplant T86.91
    bone T86.830
      marrow T86.01
    cornea T86.840
    heart T86.21
      with lung(s) T86.31
    intestine T86.850
    kidney T86.11
    liver T86.41
    lung(s) T86.810
      with heart T86.31
    organ (immune or nonimmune cause) T86.91
    pancreas T86.890
    skin (allograft) (autograft) T86.820
    specified NEC T86.890
    stem cell (peripheral blood) (umbilical cord) T86.5
Relapsing fever A68.9
  Carter's (Asiatic) A68.1
  Dutton's (West African) A68.1
  Koch's A68.9
  louse-borne (epidemic) A68.0
  Novy's (American) A68.1
  Obermeyers's (European) A68.0
  Spirillum A68.9
  tick-borne (endemic) A68.1
Relationship
  occlusal
    open anterior M26.220
    open posterior M26.221
Relaxation
  anus (sphincter) K62.89
    psychogenic F45.8
  arch (foot) (*see also* Deformity, limb, flat foot)
  back ligaments — *see* Instability, joint, spine
  bladder (sphincter) N31.2
  cardioesophageal K21.9
  cervix — *see* Incompetency, cervix
  diaphragm J98.6

Relaxation — *continued*
  joint (capsule) (ligament) (paralytic) — *see* Flail, joint
    congenital NEC Q74.8
  lumbosacral (joint) — *see* subcategory M53.2 ☑
  pelvic floor N81.89
  perineum N81.89
  posture R29.3
  rectum (sphincter) K62.89
  sacroiliac (joint) — *see* subcategory M53.2 ☑
  scrotum N50.89
  urethra (sphincter) N36.44
  vesical N31.2
Release from prison, anxiety concerning Z65.2
Remains
  canal of Cloquet Q14.0
  capsule (opaque) Q14.8
Remittent fever (malarial) B54
Remnant
  canal of Cloquet Q14.0
  capsule (opaque) Q14.8
  cervix, cervical stump (acquired) (postoperative) N88.8
  cystic duct, postcholecystectomy K91.5
  fingernail L60.8
    congenital Q84.6
  meniscus, knee — *see* Derangement, knee, meniscus,
    specified NEC
  thyroglossal duct Q89.2
  tonsil J35.8
    infected (chronic) J35.01
  urachus Q64.4
Removal (from) (of)
  artificial
    arm Z44.00- ☑
      complete Z44.01- ☑
      partial Z44.02- ☑
    eye Z44.2- ☑
    leg Z44.10- ☑
      complete Z44.11- ☑
      partial Z44.12- ☑
  breast implant Z45.81 ☑
  cardiac pulse generator (battery) (end-of-life) Z45.010
  catheter (urinary) (indwelling) Z46.6
    from artificial opening — *see* Attention to, artificial,
      opening
    non-vascular Z46.82
    vascular NEC Z45.2
  device Z46.9
    contraceptive Z30.432
      implantable subdermal Z30.46
    implanted NEC Z45.89
    specified NEC Z46.89
  drains Z48.03
  dressing (nonsurgical) Z48.00
    surgical Z48.01
  external
    fixation device — *code to* fracture with seventh
      character D
    prosthesis, prosthetic device Z44.9
      breast Z44.3- ☑
      specified NEC Z44.8
  home in childhood (to foster home or institution)
    Z62.29
  ileostomy Z43.2
  insulin pump Z46.81
  myringotomy device (stent) (tube) Z45.82
  nervous system device NEC Z46.2
    brain neuropacemaker Z46.2
    visual substitution device Z46.2
      implanted Z45.31
  non-vascular catheter Z46.82
  organ, prophylactic (for neoplasia management) —
    see Prophylactic, organ removal
  orthodontic device Z46.4
  staples Z48.02
  stent
    ureteral Z46.6
  suture Z48.02
  urinary device Z46.6
  vascular access device or catheter Z45.2
Ren
  arcuatus Q63.1
  mobile, mobilis N28.89
    congenital Q63.8
  unguliformis Q63.1
Renal — *see* condition
Rendu-Osler-Weber disease or syndrome I78.0
Reninoma D41.0- ☑
Renon-Delille syndrome E23.3

Reovirus, as cause of disease classified elsewhere
  B97.5
Repeated falls NEC R29.6
Replaced chromosome by dicentric ring Q93.2
Replacement by artificial or mechanical device or
  prosthesis of
  bladder Z96.0
  blood vessel NEC Z95.828
  bone NEC Z96.7
  cochlea Z96.21
  coronary artery Z95.5
  eustachian tube Z96.29
  eye globe Z97.0
  heart Z95.812
    valve Z95.2
      prosthetic Z95.2
      specified NEC Z95.4
      xenogenic Z95.3
  intestine Z96.89
  joint Z96.60
    hip — *see* Presence, hip joint implant
    knee — *see* Presence, knee joint implant
    specified site NEC Z96.698
  larynx Z96.3
  lens Z96.1
  limb(s) — *see* Presence, artificial, limb
  mandible NEC (for tooth root implant(s)) Z96.5
  organ NEC Z96.89
  peripheral vessel NEC Z95.828
  stapes Z96.29
  teeth Z97.2
  tendon Z96.7
  tissue NEC Z96.89
  tooth root(s) Z96.5
  vessel NEC Z95.828
    coronary (artery) Z95.5
Request for expert evidence Z04.8
Reserve, decreased or low
  cardiac — *see* Disease, heart
  kidney N28.89
Residual (*see also* condition)
  ovary syndrome N99.83
  state, schizophrenic F20.5
  urine R39.198
Resistance, resistant (to)
  activated protein C D68.51
  complicating pregnancy O26.89 ☑
  insulin E88.81
  organism(s)
    to
      drug Z16.30
        aminoglycosides Z16.29
        amoxicillin Z16.11
        ampicillin Z16.11
        antibiotic(s) Z16.20
          multiple Z16.24
          specified NEC Z16.29
        antifungal Z16.32
        antimicrobial (single) Z16.30
          multiple Z16.35
          specified NEC Z16.39
        antimycobacterial (single) Z16.341
          multiple Z16.342
        antiparasitic Z16.31
        antiviral Z16.33
        beta lactam antibiotics Z16.10
          specified NEC Z16.19
        cephalosporins Z16.19
        extended beta lactamase (ESBL) Z16.12
        fluoroquinolones Z16.23
        macrolides Z16.29
        methicillin — *see* MRSA
        multiple drugs (MDRO)
          antibiotics Z16.24
          antimicrobial Z16.35
          antimycobacterials Z16.342
        penicillins Z16.11
        quinine (and related compounds) Z16.31
        quinolones Z16.23
        sulfonamides Z16.29
        tetracyclines Z16.29
        tuberculostatics (single) Z16.341
          multiple Z16.342
        vancomycin Z16.21
          related antibiotics Z16.22
    thyroid hormone E07.89
Resorption
  dental (roots) K03.3

Resorption — *continued*
  dental — *continued*
    alveoli M26.79
    teeth (external) (internal) (pathological) (roots) K03.3
Respiration
  Cheyne-Stokes R06.3
  decreased due to shock, following injury T79.4 ☑
  disorder of, psychogenic F45.8
  insufficient, or poor R06.89
    newborn P28.5
  painful R07.1
  sighing, psychogenic F45.8
Respiratory (*see also* condition)
  distress syndrome (newborn) (type I) P22.0
    type II P22.1
  syncytial virus, as cause of disease classified elsewhere
    B97.4
Respite care Z75.5
Response (drug)
  photoallergic L56.1
  phototoxic L56.0
Restenosis
  stent
    vascular
      end stent
        adjacent to stent — *see* Arteriosclerosis
        within the stent
          coronary T82.855 ☑
          peripheral T82.856 ☑
      in stent
        coronary vessel T82.855 ☑
        peripheral vessel T82.856 ☑
Restless legs (syndrome) G25.81
Restlessness R45.1
Restoration (of)
  dental
    aesthetically inadequate or displeasing K08.56
    defective K08.50
      specified NEC K08.59
    failure of marginal integrity K08.51
    failure of periodontal anatomical intergrity K08.54
  organ continuity from previous sterilization (tuboplas-
    ty) (vasoplasty) Z31.0
    aftercare Z31.42
  tooth (existing)
    contours biologically incompatible with oral health
      K08.54
    open margins K08.51
    overhanging K08.52
    poor aesthetic K08.56
    poor gingival margins K08.51
    unsatisfactory, of tooth K08.50
      specified NEC K08.59
Restorative material (dental)
  allergy to K08.55
  fractured K08.539
    with loss of material K08.531
    without loss of material K08.530
  unrepairable overhanging of K08.52
Restriction of housing space Z59.1
Rests, ovarian, in fallopian tube Q50.6
Restzustand (schizophrenic) F20.5
Retained (*see also* Retention)
  cholelithiasis following cholecystectomy K91.86
  foreign body fragments (type of) Z18.9
    acrylics Z18.2
    animal quill(s) or spines Z18.31
    cement Z18.83
    concrete Z18.83
    crystalline Z18.83
    depleted isotope Z18.09
    depleted uranium Z18.01
    diethylhexylphthalates Z18.2
    glass Z18.81
    isocyanate Z18.2
    magnetic metal Z18.11
    metal Z18.10
    nonmagnectic metal Z18.12
    nontherapeutic radioactive Z18.09
    organic NEC Z18.39
    plastic Z18.2
    quill(s) (animal) Z18.31
    radioactive (nontherapeutic) NEC Z18.09
    specified NEC Z18.89
    spine(s) (animal) Z18.31
    stone Z18.83
    tooth (teeth) Z18.32
    wood Z18.33

Retained — continued
  fragments (type of) Z18.9
    acrylics Z18.2
    animal quill(s) or spines Z18.31
    cement Z18.83
    concrete Z18.83
    crystalline Z18.83
    depleted isotope Z18.09
    depleted uranium Z18.01
    diethylhexylphthalates Z18.2
    glass Z18.81
    isocyanate Z18.2
    magnetic metal Z18.11
    metal Z18.10
    nonmagnectic metal Z18.12
    nontherapeutic radioactive Z18.09
    organic NEC Z18.39
    plastic Z18.2
    quill(s) (animal) Z18.31
    radioactive (nontherapeutic) NEC Z18.09
    specified NEC Z18.89
    spine(s) (animal) Z18.31
    stone Z18.83
    tooth (teeth) Z18.32
    wood Z18.33
  gallstones, following cholecystectomy K91.86
Retardation
  development, developmental, specific — see Disorder, developmental
  endochondral bone growth — see Disorder, bone, development or growth
  growth R62.50
    due to malnutrition E45
  mental — see Disability, intellectual
  motor function, specific F82
  physical (child) R62.52
    due to malnutrition E45
  reading (specific) F81.0
  spelling (specific) (without reading disorder) F81.81
Retching — see Vomiting
Retention (see also Retained)
  bladder — see Retention, urine
  carbon dioxide E87.2
  cholelithiasis following cholecystectomy K91.86
  cyst — see Cyst
  dead
    fetus (at or near term) (mother) O36.4 ☑
      early fetal death O02.1
      ovum O02.0
  decidua (fragments) (following delivery) (with hemorrhage) O72.2
    without hemorrhage O73.1
  deciduous tooth K00.6
  dental root K08.3
  fecal — see Constipation
  fetus
    dead O36.4 ☑
      early O02.1
  fluid R60.9
  foreign body (see also Foreign body, retained)
    current trauma — code as Foreign body, by site or type
  gallstones, following cholecystectomy K91.86
  gastric K31.89
  intrauterine contraceptive device, in pregnancy — see Pregnancy, complicated by, retention, intrauterine device
  membranes (complicating delivery) (with hemorrhage) O72.2
    with abortion — see Abortion, by type
    without hemorrhage O73.1
  meniscus — see Derangement, meniscus
  menses N94.89
  milk (puerperal, postpartum) O92.79
  nitrogen, extrarenal R39.2
  ovary syndrome N99.83
  placenta (total) (with hemorrhage) O72.0
    without hemorrhage O73.0
    portions or fragments (with hemorrhage) O72.2
      without hemorrhage O73.1
  products of conception
    early pregnancy (dead fetus) O02.1
    following
      delivery (with hemorrhage) O72.2
        without hemorrhage O73.1
  secundines (following delivery) (with hemorrhage) O72.0
    without hemorrhage O73.0

Retention — continued
  secundines — continued
    complicating puerperium (delayed hemorrhage) O72.2
    partial O72.2
      without hemorrhage O73.1
  smegma, clitoris N90.89
  urine R33.9
    drug-induced R33.0
    due to hyperplasia (hypertrophy) of prostate — see Hyperplasia, prostate
    organic R33.8
      drug-induced R33.0
    psychogenic F45.8
    specified NEC R33.8
  water (in tissues) — see Edema
Reticulation, dust — see Pneumoconiosis
Reticulocytosis R70.1
Reticuloendotheliosis
  acute infantile C96.0
  leukemic C91.4- ☑
  nonlipid C96.0
Reticulohistiocytoma (giant-cell) D76.3
Reticuloid, actinic L57.1
Reticulosis (skin)
  acute of infancy C96.0
  hemophagocytic, familial D76.1
  histiocytic medullary C96.A (following C96.6)
  lipomelanotic I89.8
  malignant (midline) C86.0
  polymorphic C83.8- ☑
  Sézary — see Sézary disease
Retina, retinal (see also condition)
  dark area D49.81
Retinitis (see also Inflammation, chorioretinal)
  albuminurica N18.9 [H32]
  diabetic — see Diabetes, retinitis
  disciformis — see Degeneration, macula
  focal — see Inflammation, chorioretinal, focal
  gravidarum — see Pregnancy, complicated by, specified pregnancy-related condition NEC
  juxtapapillaris — see Inflammation, chorioretinal, focal, juxtapapillary
  luetic — see Retinitis, syphilitic
  pigmentosa H35.52
  proliferans — see Disorder, globe, degenerative, specified type NEC
  proliferating — see Disorder, globe, degenerative, specified type NEC
  renal N18.9 [H32]
  syphilitic (early) (secondary) A51.43
    central, recurrent A52.71
    congenital (early) A50.01 [H32]
    late A52.71
  tuberculous A18.53
Retinoblastoma C69.2- ☑
  differentiated C69.2- ☑
  undifferentiated C69.2- ☑
Retinochoroiditis (see also Inflammation, chorioretinal)
  disseminated — see Inflammation, chorioretinal, disseminated
    syphilitic A52.71
  focal — see Inflammation, chorioretinal
  juxtapapillaris — see Inflammation, chorioretinal, focal, juxtapapillary
Retinopathy (background) H35.00
  arteriosclerotic I70.8 [H35.0-] ☑
  atherosclerotic I70.8 [H35.0-] ☑
  central serous — see Chorioretinopathy, central serous
  Coats H35.02- ☑
  diabetic — see Diabetes, retinopathy
  exudative H35.02- ☑
  hypertensive H35.03- ☑
  in (due to)
    diabetes — see Diabetes, retinopathy
    sickle-cell disorders D57.- ☑ [H36]
  of prematurity H35.10- ☑
    stage 0 H35.11- ☑
    stage 1 H35.12- ☑
    stage 2 H35.13- ☑
    stage 3 H35.14- ☑
    stage 4 H35.15- ☑
    stage 5 H35.16- ☑
  pigmentary, congenital — see Dystrophy, retina
  proliferative NEC H35.2- ☑
    diabetic — see Diabetes, retinopathy, proliferative
    sickle-cell D57.- ☑ [H36]

Retinopathy — continued
  solar H31.02- ☑
Retinoschisis H33.10- ☑
  congenital Q14.1
  specified type NEC H33.19- ☑
Retortamoniasis A07.8
Retractile testis Q55.22
Retraction
  cervix — see Retroversion, uterus
  drum (membrane) — see Disorder, tympanic membrane, specified NEC
  finger — see Deformity, finger
  lid H02.539
    left H02.536
      lower H02.535
      upper H02.534
    right H02.533
      lower H02.532
      upper H02.531
  lung J98.4
  mediastinum J98.59
  nipple N64.53
    associated with
      lactation O92.03
      pregnancy O92.01- ☑
      puerperium O92.02
    congenital Q83.8
  palmar fascia M72.0
  pleura — see Pleurisy
  ring, uterus (Bandl's) (pathological) O62.4
  sternum (congenital) Q76.7
    acquired M95.4
  uterus — see Retroversion, uterus
  valve (heart) — see Endocarditis
Retrobulbar — see condition
Retrocecal — see condition
Retrocession — see Retroversion
Retrodisplacement — see Retroversion
Retroflection, retroflexion — see Retroversion
Retrognathia, retrognathism (mandibular) (maxillary) M26.19
Retrograde menstruation N92.5
Retroperineal — see condition
Retroperitoneal — see condition
Retroperitonitis K68.9
Retropharyngeal — see condition
Retroplacental — see condition
Retroposition — see Retroversion
Retroprosthetic membrane T85.398 ☑
Retrosternal thyroid (congenital) Q89.2
Retroversion, retroverted
  cervix — see Retroversion, uterus
  female NEC — see Retroversion, uterus
  iris H21.89
  testis (congenital) Q55.29
  uterus (acquired) (acute) (any degree) (asymptomatic) (cervix) (postinfectional) (postpartal, old) N85.4
    congenital Q51.818
    in pregnancy O34.53- ☑
Retrovirus, as cause of disease classified elsewhere B97.30
  human
    immunodeficiency, type 2 (HIV 2) B97.35
    T-cell lymphotropic
      type I (HTLV-I) B97.33
      type II (HTLV-II) B97.34
  lentivirus B97.31
  oncovirus B97.32
  specified NEC B97.39
Retrusion, premaxilla (developmental) M26.09
Rett's disease or syndrome F84.2
Reverse peristalsis R19.2
Reye's syndrome G93.7
Rh (factor)
  hemolytic disease (newborn) P55.0
  incompatibility, immunization or sensitization
    affecting management of pregnancy NEC O36.09- ☑
      anti-D antibody O36.01- ☑
    newborn P55.0
    transfusion reaction — see Complication(s), transfusion, incompatibility reaction, Rh (factor)
  negative mother affecting newborn P55.0
  titer elevated — see Complication(s), transfusion, incompatibility reaction, Rh (factor)
  transfusion reaction — see Complication(s), transfusion, incompatibility reaction, Rh (factor)

Rhabdomyolysis (idiopathic) NEC M62.82
  traumatic T79.6 ☑
Rhabdomyoma (see also Neoplasm, connective tissue, benign)
  adult — see Neoplasm, connective tissue, benign
  fetal — see Neoplasm, connective tissue, benign
  glycogenic — see Neoplasm, connective tissue, benign
Rhabdomyosarcoma (any type) — see Neoplasm, connective tissue, malignant
Rhabdosarcoma — see Rhabdomyosarcoma
Rhesus (factor) **incompatibility** — see Rh, incompatibility
Rheumatic (acute) (subacute) (chronic)
  adherent pericardium I09.2
  coronary arteritis I01.9
  degeneration, myocardium I09.0
  fever (acute) — see Fever, rheumatic
  heart — see Disease, heart, rheumatic
  myocardial degeneration — see Degeneration, myocardium
  myocarditis (chronic) (inactive) (with chorea) I09.0
    with chorea (acute) (rheumatic) (Sydenham's) I02.0
    active or acute I01.2
  pancarditis, acute I01.8
    with chorea (rheumatic) Sydenham's) I02.0
  pericarditis (active) (acute) (with effusion) (with pneumonia) I01.0
    with chorea (acute) (rheumatic) (Sydenham's) I02.0
    chronic or inactive I09.2
  pneumonia I00 [J17]
  torticollis M43.6
  typhoid fever A01.09
Rheumatism (articular) (neuralgic) (nonarticular) M79.0
  gout — see Arthritis, rheumatoid
  intercostal, meaning Tietze's disease M94.0
  palindromic (any site) M12.30
    ankle M12.37- ☑
    elbow M12.32- ☑
    foot joint M12.37- ☑
    hand joint M12.34- ☑
    hip M12.35- ☑
    knee M12.36- ☑
    multiple site M12.39
    shoulder M12.31- ☑
    specified joint NEC M12.38
    vertebrae M12.38
    wrist M12.33- ☑
  sciatic M54.4- ☑
Rheumatoid (see also condition)
  arthritis (see also Arthritis, rheumatoid)
    with involvement of organs NEC M05.60
      ankle M05.67- ☑
      elbow M05.62- ☑
      foot joint M05.67- ☑
      hand joint M05.64- ☑
      hip M05.65- ☑
      knee M05.66- ☑
      multiple site M05.69
      shoulder M05.61- ☑
      vertebra — see Spondylitis, ankylosing
      wrist M05.63- ☑
    seronegative — see Arthritis, rheumatoid, seronegative
    seropositive — see Arthritis, rheumatoid, seropositive
  carditis M05.30
    ankle M05.37- ☑
    elbow M05.32- ☑
    foot joint M05.37- ☑
    hand joint M05.34- ☑
    hip M05.35- ☑
    knee M05.36- ☑
    multiple site M05.39
    shoulder M05.31- ☑
    vertebra — see Spondylitis, ankylosing
    wrist M05.33- ☑
  endocarditis — see Rheumatoid, carditis
  lung (disease) M05.10
    ankle M05.17- ☑
    elbow M05.12- ☑
    foot joint M05.17- ☑
    hand joint M05.14- ☑
    hip M05.15- ☑
    knee M05.16- ☑
    multiple site M05.19
    shoulder M05.11- ☑
    vertebra — see Spondylitis, ankylosing

Rheumatoid — continued
  lung — continued
    wrist M05.13- ☑
  myocarditis — see Rheumatoid, carditis
  myopathy M05.40
    ankle M05.47- ☑
    elbow M05.42- ☑
    foot joint M05.47- ☑
    hand joint M05.44- ☑
    hip M05.45- ☑
    knee M05.46- ☑
    multiple site M05.49
    shoulder M05.41- ☑
    vertebra — see Spondylitis, ankylosing
    wrist M05.43- ☑
  pericarditis — see Rheumatoid, carditis
  polyarthritis — see Arthritis, rheumatoid
  polyneuropathy M05.50
    ankle M05.57- ☑
    elbow M05.52- ☑
    foot joint M05.57- ☑
    hand joint M05.54- ☑
    hip M05.55- ☑
    knee M05.56- ☑
    multiple site M05.59
    shoulder M05.51- ☑
    vertebra — see Spondylitis, ankylosing
    wrist M05.53- ☑
  vasculitis M05.20
    ankle M05.27- ☑
    elbow M05.22- ☑
    foot joint M05.27- ☑
    hand joint M05.24- ☑
    hip M05.25- ☑
    knee M05.26- ☑
    multiple site M05.29
    shoulder M05.21- ☑
    vertebra — see Spondylitis, ankylosing
    wrist M05.23- ☑
Rhinitis (atrophic) (catarrhal) (chronic) (croupous) (fibrinous) (granulomatous) (hyperplastic) (hypertrophic) (membranous) (obstructive) (purulent) (suppurative) (ulcerative) J31.0
  with
    sore throat — see Nasopharyngitis
  acute J00
  allergic J30.9
    with asthma J45.909
      with
        exacerbation (acute) J45.901
        status asthmaticus J45.902
    due to
      food J30.5
      pollen J30.1
    nonseasonal J30.89
    perennial J30.89
    seasonal NEC J30.2
    specified NEC J30.89
  infective J00
  pneumococcal J00
  syphilitic A52.73
    congenital A50.05 [J99]
  tuberculous A15.8
  vasomotor J30.0
Rhinoantritis (chronic) — see Sinusitis, maxillary
Rhinodacryolith — see Dacryolith
Rhinolith (nasal sinus) J34.89
Rhinomegaly J34.89
Rhinopharyngitis (acute) (subacute) (see also Nasopharyngitis)
  chronic J31.1
  destructive ulcerating A66.5
  mutilans A66.5
Rhinophyma L71.1
Rhinorrhea J34.89
  cerebrospinal (fluid) G96.0
  paroxysmal — see Rhinitis, allergic
  spasmodic — see Rhinitis, allergic
Rhinosalpingitis — see Salpingitis, eustachian
Rhinoscleroma A48.8
Rhinosporidiosis B48.1
Rhinovirus infection NEC B34.8
Rhizomelic chondrodysplasia punctata E71.540
Rhythm
  atrioventricular nodal I49.8
  disorder I49.9
    coronary sinus I49.8

Rhythm — continued
  disorder — continued
    ectopic I49.8
    nodal I49.8
  escape I49.9
  heart, abnormal I49.9
  idioventricular I44.2
  nodal I49.8
  sleep, inversion G47.2- ☑
    nonorganic origin — see Disorder, sleep, circadian rhythm, psychogenic
Rhytidosis facialis L98.8
Rib (see also condition)
  cervical Q76.5
Riboflavin deficiency E53.0
Rice bodies (see also Loose, body, joint)
  knee M23.4- ☑
Richter syndrome — see Leukemia, chronic lymphocytic, B-cell type
Richter's hernia — see Hernia, abdomen, with obstruction
Ricinism — see Poisoning, food, noxious, plant
Rickets (active) (acute) (adolescent) (chest wall) (congenital) (current) (infantile) (intestinal) E55.0
  adult — see Osteomalacia
  celiac K90.0
  hypophosphatemic with nephrotic-glycosuric dwarfism E72.09
  inactive E64.3
  kidney N25.0
  renal N25.0
  sequelae, any E64.3
  vitamin-D-resistant E83.31 [M90.80]
Rickettsial disease A79.9
  specified type NEC A79.89
Rickettsialpox (Rickettsia akari) A79.1
Rickettsiosis A79.9
  due to
    Ehrlichia sennetsu A79.81
    Rickettsia akari (rickettsialpox) A79.1
  specified type NEC A79.89
  tick-borne A77.9
  vesicular A79.1
Rider's bone — see Ossification, muscle, specified NEC
Ridge, alveolus (see also condition)
  flabby K06.8
Ridged ear, congenital Q17.3
Riedel's
  lobe, liver Q44.7
  struma, thyroiditis or disease E06.5
Rieger's anomaly or syndrome Q13.81
Riehl's melanosis L81.4
Rietti-Greppi-Micheli anemia D56.9
Rieux's hernia — see Hernia, abdomen, specified site NEC
Riga (-Fede) **disease** K14.0
Riggs' disease — see Periodontitis
Right aortic arch Q25.47
Right middle lobe syndrome J98.11
Rigid, rigidity (see also condition)
  abdominal R19.30
    with severe abdominal pain R10.0
    epigastric R19.36
    generalized R19.37
    left lower quadrant R19.34
    left upper quadrant R19.32
    periumbilic R19.35
    right lower quadrant R19.33
    right upper quadrant R19.31
  articular, multiple, congenital Q68.8
  cervix (uteri) in pregnancy — see Pregnancy, complicated by, abnormal, cervix
  hymen (acquired) (congenital) N89.6
  nuchal R29.1
  pelvic floor in pregnancy — see Pregnancy, complicated by, abnormal, pelvic organs or tissues NEC
  perineum or vulva in pregnancy — see Pregnancy, complicated by, abnormal, vulva
  spine — see Dorsopathy, specified NEC
  vagina in pregnancy — see Pregnancy, complicated by, abnormal, vagina
Rigors R68.89
  with fever R50.9
Riley-Day syndrome G90.1
RIND (reversible ischemic neurologic deficit) I63.9
Ring(s)
  aorta (vascular) Q25.45
  Bandl's O62.4

Ring(s) — *continued*
contraction, complicating delivery O62.4
esophageal, lower (muscular) K22.2
Fleischer's (cornea) H18.04- ☑
hymenal, tight (acquired) (congenital) N89.6
Kayser-Fleischer (cornea) H18.04- ☑
retraction, uterus, pathological O62.4
Schatzki's (esophagus) (lower) K22.2
congenital Q39.3
Soemmerring's — *see* Cataract, secondary
vascular (congenital) Q25.8
aorta Q25.45
Ringed hair (congenital) Q84.1
Ringworm B35.9
beard B35.0
black dot B35.0
body B35.4
Burmese B35.5
corporeal B35.4
foot B35.3
groin B35.6
hand B35.2
honeycomb B35.0
nails B35.1
perianal (area) B35.6
scalp B35.0
specified NEC B35.8
Tokelau B35.5
Rise, venous pressure I87.8
**Rising, PSA following treatment for malignant
    neoplasm of prostate** R97.21
Risk
for
dental caries Z91.849
high Z91.843
low Z91.841
moderate Z91.842
suicidal
meaning personal history of attempted suicide
Z91.5
meaning suicidal ideation — *see* Ideation, suicidal
Ritter's disease L00
Rivalry, sibling Z62.891
Rivalta's disease A42.2
River blindness B73.01
Robert's pelvis Q74.2
with disproportion (fetopelvic) O33.0
causing obstructed labor O65.0
Robin (-Pierre) **syndrome** Q87.0
Robinow-Silvermann-Smith syndrome Q87.1
Robinson's (hidrotic) **ectodermal dysplasia or syn-
    drome** Q82.4
Robles' disease B73.01
Rocky Mountain (spotted) **fever** A77.0
Roetheln — *see* Rubella
Roger's disease Q21.0
Rokitansky-Aschoff sinuses (gallbladder) K82.8
Rolando's fracture (displaced) S62.22- ☑
nondisplaced S62.22- ☑
Romano-Ward (prolonged QT interval) **syndrome** I45.81
Romberg's disease or syndrome G51.8
Roof, mouth — *see* condition
Rosacea L71.9
acne L71.0
keratitis L71.8
specified NEC L71.8
Rosary, rachitic E55.0
Rose
cold J30.1
fever J30.1
rash R21
epidemic B06.9
Rosenbach's erysipeloid A26.0
Rosenthal's disease or syndrome D68.1
Roseola B09
infantum B08.20
due to human herpesvirus 6 B08.21
due to human herpesvirus 7 B08.22
Ross River disease or fever B33.1
Rossbach's disease K31.89
psychogenic F45.8
Rostan's asthma (cardiac) — *see* Failure, ventricular, left
Rotation
anomalous, incomplete or insufficient, intestine Q43.3
cecum (congenital) Q43.3
colon (congenital) Q43.3

Rotation — *continued*
spine, incomplete or insufficient — *see* Dorsopathy,
deforming, specified NEC
tooth, teeth, fully erupted M26.35
vertebra, incomplete or insufficient — *see* Dorsopathy,
deforming, specified NEC
Rotes Quérol disease or syndrome — *see* Hyperostosis,
ankylosing
Roth (-Bernhardt) **disease or syndrome** — *see* Meralgia
paraesthetica
Rothmund (-Thomson) **syndrome** Q82.8
Rotor's disease or syndrome E80.6
Round
back (with wedging of vertebrae) — *see* Kyphosis
sequelae (late effect) of rickets E64.3
worms (large) (infestation) NEC B82.0
Ascariasis (*see also* Ascariasis) B77.9
Roussy-Lévy syndrome G60.0
Rubella (German measles) B06.9
complication NEC B06.09
neurological B06.00
congenital P35.0
contact Z20.4
exposure to Z20.4
maternal
care for (suspected) damage to fetus O35.3 ☑
manifest rubella in infant P35.0
suspected damage to fetus affecting management
of pregnancy O35.3 ☑
specified complications NEC B06.89
Rubeola (meaning measles) — *see* Measles
meaning rubella — *see* Rubella
Rubeosis, iris — *see* Disorder, iris, vascular
Rubinstein-Taybi syndrome Q87.2
Rudimentary (congenital) (*see also* Agenesis)
arm — *see* Defect, reduction, upper limb
bone Q79.9
cervix uteri Q51.828
eye Q11.2
lobule of ear Q17.3
patella Q74.1
respiratory organs in thoracopagus Q89.4
tracheal bronchus Q32.4
uterus Q51.818
in male Q56.1
vagina Q52.0
Ruled out condition — *see* Observation, suspected
Rumination R11.10
with nausea R11.2
disorder of infancy F98.21
neurotic F42.8
newborn P92.1
obsessional F42.8
psychogenic F42.8
Runeberg's disease D51.0
Runny nose R09.89
Rupia (syphilitic) A51.39
congenital A50.06
tertiary A52.79
Rupture, ruptured
abscess (spontaneous) — *code by* site under Abscess
aneurysm — *see* Aneurysm
anus (sphincter) — *see* Laceration, anus
aorta, aortic I71.8
abdominal I71.3
arch I71.1
ascending I71.1
descending I71.8
abdominal I71.3
thoracic I71.1
syphilitic A52.01
thoracoabdominal I71.5
thorax, thoracic I71.1
transverse I71.1
traumatic — *see* Injury, aorta, laceration, major
valve or cusp (*see also* Endocarditis, aortic) I35.8
appendix (with peritonitis) K35.2
with localized peritonitis K35.3
arteriovenous fistula, brain I60.8
artery I77.2
brain — *see* Hemorrhage, intracranial, intracerebral
coronary — *see* Infarct, myocardium
heart — *see* Infarct, myocardium
pulmonary I28.8
traumatic (complication) — *see* Injury, blood vessel
bile duct (common) (hepatic) K83.2
cystic K82.2

Rupture, ruptured — *continued*
bladder (sphincter) (nontraumatic) (spontaneous)
N32.89
following ectopic or molar pregnancy O08.6
obstetrical trauma O71.5
traumatic S37.29 ☑
blood vessel (*see also* Hemorrhage)
brain — *see* Hemorrhage, intracranial, intracerebral
heart — *see* Infarct, myocardium
traumatic (complication) — *see* Injury, blood vessel, laceration, major, by site
bone — *see* Fracture
bowel (nontraumatic) K63.1
brain
aneurysm (congenital) (*see also* Hemorrhage, intracranial, subarachnoid)
syphilitic A52.05
hemorrhagic — *see* Hemorrhage, intracranial, intracerebral
capillaries I78.8
cardiac (auricle) (ventricle) (wall) I23.3
with hemopericardium I23.0
infectional I40.9
traumatic — *see* Injury, heart
cartilage (articular) (current) (*see also* Sprain)
knee S83.3- ☑
semilunar — *see* Tear, meniscus
cecum (with peritonitis) K65.0
with peritoneal abscess K35.3
traumatic S36.598 ☑
celiac artery, traumatic — *see* Injury, blood vessel,
celiac artery, laceration, major
cerebral aneurysm (congenital) (see Hemorrhage, intracranial, subarachnoid)
cervix (uteri)
with ectopic or molar pregnancy O08.6
following ectopic or molar pregnancy O08.6
obstetrical trauma O71.3
traumatic S37.69 ☑
chordae tendineae NEC I51.1
concurrent with acute myocardial infarction — *see*
Infarct, myocardium
following acute myocardial infarction (current
complication) I23.4
choroid (direct) (indirect) (traumatic) H31.32- ☑
circle of Willis I60.6
colon (nontraumatic) K63.1
traumatic — *see* Injury, intestine, large
cornea (traumatic) — *see* Injury, eye, laceration
coronary (artery) (thrombotic) — *see* Infarct, myocardium
corpus luteum (infected) (ovary) N83.1- ☑
cyst — *see* Cyst
cystic duct K82.2
Descemet's membrane — *see* Change, corneal membrane, Descemet's, rupture
traumatic — *see* Injury, eye, laceration
diaphragm, traumatic — *see* Injury, intrathoracic, diaphragm
disc — *see* Rupture, intervertebral disc
diverticulum (intestine) K57.80
with bleeding K57.81
bladder N32.3
large intestine K57.20
with
bleeding K57.21
small intestine K57.40
with bleeding K57.41
small intestine K57.00
with
bleeding K57.01
large intestine K57.40
with bleeding K57.41
duodenal stump K31.89
ear drum (nontraumatic) (*see also* Perforation, tympanum)
traumatic S09.2- ☑
due to blast injury — *see* Injury, blast, ear
esophagus K22.3
eye (without prolapse or loss of intraocular tissue) —
see Injury, eye, laceration
fallopian tube NEC (nonobstetric) (nontraumatic) N83.8
due to pregnancy O00.10- ☑
with intrauterine pregnancy O00.11- ☑
fontanel P13.1
gallbladder K82.2
traumatic S36.128 ☑

Index

Rupture, ruptured — Rupture, ruptured

Rupture, ruptured — *continued*
- gastric (*see also* Rupture, stomach)
  - vessel K92.2
- globe (eye) (traumatic) — *see* Injury, eye, laceration
- graafian follicle (hematoma) N83.0- ☑
- heart — *see* Rupture, cardiac
- hymen (nontraumatic) (nonintentional) N89.8
- internal organ, traumatic — *see* Injury, by site
- intervertebral disc — *see* Displacement, intervertebral disc
  - traumatic — *see* Rupture, traumatic, intervertebral disc
- intestine NEC (nontraumatic) K63.1
  - traumatic — *see* Injury, intestine
- iris (*see also* Abnormality, pupillary)
  - traumatic — *see* Injury, eye, laceration
- joint capsule, traumatic — *see* Sprain
- kidney (traumatic) S37.06- ☑
  - birth injury P15.8
  - nontraumatic N28.89
- lacrimal duct (traumatic) — *see* Injury, eye, specified site NEC
- lens (cataract) (traumatic) — *see* Cataract, traumatic
- ligament, traumatic — *see* Rupture, traumatic, ligament, by site
- liver S36.116 ☑
  - birth injury P15.0
- lymphatic vessel I89.8
- marginal sinus (placental) (with hemorrhage) — *see* Hemorrhage, antepartum, specified cause NEC
- membrana tympani (nontraumatic) — *see* Perforation, tympanum
- membranes (spontaneous)
  - artificial
    - delayed delivery following O75.5
  - delayed delivery following — *see* Pregnancy, complicated by, premature rupture of membranes
- meningeal artery I60.8
- meniscus (knee) (*see also* Tear, meniscus)
  - old — *see* Derangement, meniscus
  - site other than knee — *code as* Sprain
- mesenteric artery, traumatic — *see* Injury, mesenteric, artery, laceration, major
- mesentery (nontraumatic) K66.8
  - traumatic — *see* Injury, intra-abdominal, specified, site NEC
- mitral (valve) I34.8
- muscle (traumatic) (*see also* Strain)
  - diastasis — *see* Diastasis, muscle
  - nontraumatic M62.10
    - ankle M62.17- ☑
    - foot M62.17- ☑
    - forearm M62.13- ☑
    - hand M62.14- ☑
    - lower leg M62.16- ☑
    - pelvic region M62.15- ☑
    - shoulder region M62.11- ☑
    - specified site NEC M62.18
    - thigh M62.15- ☑
    - upper arm M62.12- ☑
  - traumatic — *see* Strain, by site
- musculotendinous junction NEC, nontraumatic — *see* Rupture, tendon, spontaneous
- mycotic aneurysm causing cerebral hemorrhage — *see* Hemorrhage, intracranial, subarachnoid
- myocardium, myocardial — *see* Rupture, cardiac
  - traumatic — *see* Injury, heart
- nontraumatic, meaning hernia — *see* Hernia
  - obstructed — *see* Hernia, by site, obstructed
- operation wound — *see* Disruption, wound, operation
- ovary, ovarian N83.8
  - corpus luteum cyst N83.1- ☑
  - follicle (graafian) N83.0- ☑
- oviduct (nonobstetric) (nontraumatic) N83.8
  - due to pregnancy O00.10- ☑
    - with intrauterine pregnancy O00.11- ☑
- pancreas (nontraumatic) K86.89
  - traumatic S36.299 ☑
- papillary muscle NEC I51.2
  - following acute myocardial infarction (current complication) I23.5
- pelvic
  - floor, complicating delivery O70.1
  - organ NEC, obstetrical trauma O71.5
- perineum (nonobstetric) (nontraumatic) N90.89

Rupture, ruptured — *continued*
- perineum — *continued*
  - complicating delivery — *see* Delivery, complicated, by, laceration, anus (sphincter)
- postoperative wound — *see* Disruption, wound, operation
- prostate (traumatic) S37.828 ☑
- pulmonary
  - artery I28.8
  - valve (heart) I37.8
  - vein I28.8
  - vessel I28.8
- pus tube — *see* Salpingitis
- pyosalpinx — *see* Salpingitis
- rectum (nontraumatic) K63.1
  - traumatic S36.69
- retina, retinal (traumatic) (without detachment) (*see also* Break, retina)
  - with detachment — *see* Detachment, retina, with retinal, break
- rotator cuff (nontraumatic) M75.10- ☑
  - complete M75.12- ☑
  - incomplete M75.11- ☑
- sclera — *see* Injury, eye, laceration
- sigmoid (nontraumatic) K63.1
  - traumatic S36.593
- spinal cord (*see also* Injury, spinal cord, by region)
  - due to injury at birth P11.5
  - newborn (birth injury) P11.5
- spleen (traumatic) S36.09 ☑
  - birth injury P15.1
  - congenital (birth injury) P15.1
  - due to P. vivax malaria B51.0
  - nontraumatic D73.5
  - spontaneous D73.5
- splenic vein R58
  - traumatic — *see* Injury, blood vessel, splenic vein
- stomach (nontraumatic) (spontaneous) K31.89
  - traumatic S36.39
- supraspinatus (complete) (incomplete) (nontraumatic) — *see* Tear, rotator cuff
- symphysis pubis
  - obstetric O71.6
  - traumatic S33.4 ☑
- synovium (cyst) M66.10
  - ankle M66.17- ☑
  - elbow M66.12- ☑
  - finger M66.14- ☑
  - foot M66.17- ☑
  - forearm M66.13- ☑
  - hand M66.14- ☑
  - pelvic region M66.15- ☑
  - shoulder region M66.11- ☑
  - specified site NEC M66.18
  - thigh M66.15- ☑
  - toe M66.17- ☑
  - upper arm M66.12- ☑
  - wrist M66.13- ☑
- tendon (traumatic) — *see* Strain
  - nontraumatic (spontaneous) M66.9
    - ankle M66.87- ☑
    - extensor M66.20
      - ankle M66.27- ☑
      - foot M66.27- ☑
      - forearm M66.23- ☑
      - hand M66.24- ☑
      - lower leg M66.26- ☑
      - multiple sites M66.29
      - pelvic region M66.25- ☑
      - shoulder region M66.21- ☑
      - specified site NEC M66.28
      - thigh M66.25- ☑
      - upper arm M66.22- ☑
    - flexor M66.30
      - ankle M66.37- ☑
      - foot M66.37- ☑
      - forearm M66.33- ☑
      - hand M66.34- ☑
      - lower leg M66.36- ☑
      - multiple sites M66.39
      - pelvic region M66.35- ☑
      - shoulder region M66.31- ☑
      - specified site NEC M66.38
      - thigh M66.35- ☑
      - upper arm M66.32- ☑
    - foot M66.87- ☑
    - forearm M66.83- ☑

Rupture, ruptured — *continued*
- tendon — *see* Strain — *continued*
  - nontraumatic — *continued*
    - hand M66.84- ☑
    - lower leg M66.86- ☑
    - multiple sites M66.89
    - pelvic region M66.85- ☑
    - shoulder region M66.81- ☑
    - specified
      - site NEC M66.88
      - tendon M66.80
    - thigh M66.85- ☑
    - upper arm M66.82- ☑
- thoracic duct I89.8
- tonsil J35.8
- traumatic
  - aorta — *see* Injury, aorta, laceration, major
  - diaphragm — *see* Injury, intrathoracic, diaphragm
  - external site — *see* Wound, open, by site
  - eye — *see* Injury, eye, laceration
  - internal organ — *see* Injury, by site
  - intervertebral disc
    - cervical S13.0 ☑
    - lumbar S33.0 ☑
    - thoracic S23.0 ☑
  - kidney S37.06- ☑
  - ligament (*see also* Sprain)
    - ankle — *see* Sprain, ankle
    - carpus — *see* Rupture, traumatic, ligament, wrist
    - collateral (hand) — *see* Rupture, traumatic, ligament, finger, collateral
    - finger (metacarpophalangeal) (interphalangeal) S63.40- ☑
      - collateral S63.41- ☑
        - index S63.41- ☑
        - little S63.41- ☑
        - middle S63.41- ☑
        - ring S63.41- ☑
      - index S63.40- ☑
      - little S63.40- ☑
      - middle S63.40- ☑
      - palmar S63.42- ☑
        - index S63.42- ☑
        - little S63.42- ☑
        - middle S63.42- ☑
        - ring S63.42- ☑
      - ring S63.40- ☑
      - specified site NEC S63.499 ☑
        - index S63.49- ☑
        - little S63.49- ☑
        - middle S63.49- ☑
        - ring S63.49- ☑
      - volar plate S63.43- ☑
        - index S63.43- ☑
        - little S63.43- ☑
        - middle S63.43- ☑
        - ring S63.43- ☑
    - foot — *see* Sprain, foot
    - radial collateral S53.2- ☑
    - radiocarpal — *see* Rupture, traumatic, ligament, wrist, radiocarpal
    - ulnar collateral S53.3- ☑
    - ulnocarpal — *see* Rupture, traumatic, ligament, wrist, ulnocarpal
    - wrist S63.30- ☑
      - collateral S63.31- ☑
      - radiocarpal S63.32- ☑
      - specified site NEC S63.39- ☑
      - ulnocarpal (palmar) S63.33- ☑
  - liver S36.116 ☑
  - membrana tympani — *see* Rupture, ear drum, traumatic
  - muscle or tendon — *see* Strain
  - myocardium — *see* Injury, heart
  - pancreas S36.299 ☑
  - rectum S36.69 ☑
  - sigmoid S36.593 ☑
  - spleen S36.09 ☑
  - stomach S36.39 ☑
  - symphysis pubis S33.4 ☑
  - tympanum, tympanic (membrane) — *see* Rupture, ear drum, traumatic
  - ureter S37.19 ☑
  - uterus S37.69 ☑
  - vagina — *see* Injury, vagina

☑ Additional Character Required — Refer to the Tabular List for Character Selection   Subterms under main terms may continue to next column or page

Rupture, ruptured — continued
  traumatic — continued
    vena cava — see Injury, vena cava, laceration, major
    tricuspid (heart) (valve) I07.8
    tube, tubal (nonobstetric) (nontraumatic) N83.8
      abscess — see Salpingitis
      due to pregnancy O00.10- ☑
        with intrauterine pregnancy O00.11- ☑
    tympanum, tympanic (membrane) (nontraumatic) (see also Perforation, tympanic membrane) H72.9- ☑
      traumatic — see Rupture, ear drum, traumatic
    umbilical cord, complicating delivery O69.89 ☑
    ureter (traumatic) S37.19 ☑
      nontraumatic N28.89
    urethra (nontraumatic) N36.8
      with ectopic or molar pregnancy O08.6
      following ectopic or molar pregnancy O08.6
      obstetrical trauma O71.5
      traumatic S37.39 ☑
    uterosacral ligament (nonobstetric) (nontraumatic) N83.8
    uterus (traumatic) S37.69 ☑
      before labor O71.0- ☑
      during or after labor O71.1
      nonpuerperal, nontraumatic N85.8
      pregnant (during labor) O71.1
        before labor O71.0- ☑
    vagina — see Injury, vagina
    valve, valvular (heart) — see Endocarditis
    varicose vein — see Varix
    varix — see Varix
    vena cava R58
      traumatic — see Injury, vena cava, laceration, major
    vesical (urinary) N32.89
    vessel (blood) R58
      pulmonary I28.8
      traumatic — see Injury, blood vessel
    viscus R19.8
    vulva complicating delivery O70.0
Russell-Silver syndrome Q87.1
Russian spring-summer type encephalitis A84.0
Rust's disease (tuberculous cervical spondylitis) A18.01
Ruvalcaba-Myhre-Smith syndrome E71.440
Rytand-Lipsitch syndrome I44.2

S

Saber, sabre shin or tibia (syphilitic) A50.56 [M90.8-] ☑
Sac lacrimal — see condition
Saccharomyces infection B37.9
Saccharopinuria E72.3
Saccular — see condition
Sacculation
  aorta (nonsyphilitic) — see Aneurysm, aorta
  bladder N32.3
  intralaryngeal (congenital) (ventricular) Q31.3
  larynx (congenital) (ventricular) Q31.3
  organ or site, congenital — see Distortion
  pregnant uterus — see Pregnancy, complicated by, abnormal, uterus
  ureter N28.89
  urethra N36.1
  vesical N32.3
Sachs' amaurotic familial idiocy or disease E75.02
Sachs-Tay disease E75.02
Sacks-Libman disease M32.11
Sacralgia M53.3
Sacralization Q76.49
Sacrodynia M53.3
Sacroiliac joint — see condition
Sacroiliitis NEC M46.1
Sacrum — see condition
Saddle
  back — see Lordosis
  embolus
    abdominal aorta I74.01
    pulmonary artery I26.92
      with acute cor pulmonale I26.02
  injury — code to condition
  nose M95.0
    due to syphilis A50.57
Sadism (sexual) F65.52
Sadness, postpartal O90.6
Sadomasochism F65.50
Saemisch's ulcer (cornea) — see Ulcer, cornea, central

Sagging
  skin and subcutaneous tissue (following bariatric surgery weight loss) (following dietary weight loss) L98.7
Sahib disease B55.0
Sailors' skin L57.8
Saint
  Anthony's fire — see Erysipelas
  triad — see Hernia, diaphragm
  Vitus' dance — see Chorea, Sydenham's
Salaam
  attack(s) — see Epilepsy, spasms
  tic R25.8
Salicylism
  abuse F55.8
  overdose or wrong substance given — see Table of Drugs and Chemicals, by drug, poisoning
Salivary duct or gland — see condition
Salivation, excessive K11.7
Salmonella — see Infection, Salmonella
Salmonellosis A02.0
Salpingitis (catarrhal) (fallopian tube) (nodular) (pseudofollicular) (purulent) (septic) N70.91
  with oophoritis N70.93
  acute N70.01
    with oophoritis N70.03
  chlamydial A56.11
  chronic N70.11
    with oophoritis N70.13
  complicating abortion — see Abortion, by type, complicated by, salpingitis
  ear — see Salpingitis, eustachian
  eustachian (tube) H68.00- ☑
    acute H68.01- ☑
    chronic H68.02- ☑
  follicularis N70.11
    with oophoritis N70.13
  gonococcal (acute) (chronic) A54.24
  interstitial, chronic N70.11
    with oophoritis N70.13
  isthmica nodosa N70.11
    with oophoritis N70.13
  specific (gonococcal) (acute) (chronic) A54.24
  tuberculous (acute) (chronic) A18.17
  venereal (gonococcal) (acute) (chronic) A54.24
Salpingocele N83.4- ☑
Salpingo-oophoritis (catarrhal) (purulent) (ruptured) (septic) (suppurative) N70.93
  acute N70.03
    with ectopic or molar pregnancy O08.0
    following ectopic or molar pregnancy O08.0
      gonococcal A54.24
  chronic N70.13
  following ectopic or molar pregnancy O08.0
  gonococcal (acute) (chronic) A54.24
  puerperal O86.19
  specific (gonococcal) (acute) (chronic) A54.24
  subacute N70.03
  tuberculous (acute) (chronic) A18.17
  venereal (gonococcal) (acute) (chronic) A54.24
Salpingo-ovaritis — see Salpingo-oophoritis
Salpingoperitonitis — see Salpingo-oophoritis
Salzmann's nodular dystrophy — see Degeneration, cornea, nodular
Sampson's cyst or tumor N80.1
San Joaquin (Valley) **fever** B38.0
Sandblaster's asthma, lung or pneumoconiosis J62.8
Sander's disease (paranoia) F22
Sandfly fever A93.1
Sandhoff's disease E75.01
Sanfilippo (Type B) (Type C) (Type D) **syndrome** E76.22
Sanger-Brown ataxia G11.2
Sao Paulo fever or typhus A77.0
Saponification, mesenteric K65.8
Sarcocele (benign)
  syphilitic A52.76
    congenital A50.59
Sarcocystosis A07.8
Sarcoepiplocele — see Hernia
Sarcoepiplomphalocele Q79.2
Sarcoid (see also Sarcoidosis)
  arthropathy D86.86
  Boeck's D86.9
  Darier-Roussy D86.3
  iridocyclitis D86.83
  meningitis D86.81
  myocarditis D86.85

Sarcoid — continued
  myositis D86.87
  pyelonephritis D86.84
  Spiegler-Fendt L08.89
Sarcoidosis D86.9
  with
    cranial nerve palsies D86.82
    hepatic granuloma D86.89
    polyarthritis D86.86
    tubulo-interstitial nephropathy D86.84
  combined sites NEC D86.89
  lung D86.0
    and lymph nodes D86.2
  lymph nodes D86.1
    and lung D86.2
  meninges D86.81
  skin D86.3
  specified type NEC D86.89
Sarcoma (of) (see also Neoplasm, connective tissue, malignant)
  alveolar soft part — see Neoplasm, connective tissue, malignant
  ameloblastic C41.1
    upper jaw (bone) C41.0
  botryoid — see Neoplasm, connective tissue, malignant
  botryoides — see Neoplasm, connective tissue, malignant
  cerebellar C71.6
    circumscribed (arachnoidal) C71.6
  circumscribed (arachnoidal) cerebellar C71.6
  clear cell (see also Neoplasm, connective tissue, malignant)
    kidney C64.- ☑
  dendritic cells (accessory cells) C96.4
  embryonal — see Neoplasm, connective tissue, malignant
  endometrial (stromal) C54.1
    isthmus C54.0
  epithelioid (cell) — see Neoplasm, connective tissue, malignant
  Ewing's — see Neoplasm, bone, malignant
  follicular dendritic cell C96.4
  germinoblastic (diffuse) — see Lymphoma, diffuse large cell
    follicular — see Lymphoma, follicular, specified NEC
  giant cell (except of bone) (see also Neoplasm, connective tissue, malignant)
    bone — see Neoplasm, bone, malignant
  glomoid — see Neoplasm, connective tissue, malignant
  granulocytic C92.3- ☑
  hemangioendothelial — see Neoplasm, connective tissue, malignant
  hemorrhagic, multiple — see Sarcoma, Kaposi's
  histiocytic C96.A (following C96.6)
  Hodgkin — see Lymphoma, Hodgkin
  immunoblastic (diffuse) — see Lymphoma, diffuse large cell
  interdigitating dendritic cell C96.4
  Kaposi's
    colon C46.4
    connective tissue C46.1
    gastrointestinal organ C46.4
    lung C46.5- ☑
    lymph node(s) C46.3
    palate (hard) (soft) C46.2
    rectum C46.4
    skin C46.0
    specified site NEC C46.7
    stomach C46.4
    unspecified site C46.9
  Kupffer cell C22.3
  Langerhans cell C96.4
  leptomeningeal — see Neoplasm, meninges, malignant
  liver NEC C22.4
  lymphangioendothelial — see Neoplasm, connective tissue, malignant
  lymphoblastic — see Lymphoma, lymphoblastic (diffuse)
  lymphocytic — see Lymphoma, small cell B-cell
  mast cell C96.22
  melanotic — see Melanoma
  meningeal — see Neoplasm, meninges, malignant
  meningothelial — see Neoplasm, meninges, malignant

Sarcoma — continued
  mesenchymal (see also Neoplasm, connective tissue, malignant)
    mixed — see Neoplasm, connective tissue, malignant
  mesothelial — see Mesothelioma
  monstrocellular
    specified site — see Neoplasm, malignant, by site
    unspecified site C71.9
  myeloid C92.3- ☑
  neurogenic — see Neoplasm, nerve, malignant
  odontogenic C41.1
    upper jaw (bone) C41.0
  osteoblastic — see Neoplasm, bone, malignant
  osteogenic (see also Neoplasm, bone, malignant)
    juxtacortical — see Neoplasm, bone, malignant
    periosteal — see Neoplasm, bone, malignant
  periosteal (see also Neoplasm, bone, malignant)
    osteogenic — see Neoplasm, bone, malignant
  pleomorphic cell — see Neoplasm, connective tissue, malignant
  reticulum cell (diffuse) — see Lymphoma, diffuse large cell
    nodular — see Lymphoma, follicular
    pleomorphic cell type — see Lymphoma, diffuse large cell
  rhabdoid — see Neoplasm, malignant, by site
  round cell — see Neoplasm, connective tissue, malignant
  small cell — see Neoplasm, connective tissue, malignant
  soft tissue — see Neoplasm, connective tissue, malignant
  spindle cell — see Neoplasm, connective tissue, malignant
  stromal (endometrial) C54.1
    isthmus C54.0
  synovial (see also Neoplasm, connective tissue, malignant)
    biphasic — see Neoplasm, connective tissue, malignant
    epithelioid cell — see Neoplasm, connective tissue, malignant
    spindle cell — see Neoplasm, connective tissue, malignant
Sarcomatosis
  meningeal — see Neoplasm, meninges, malignant
  specified site NEC — see Neoplasm, connective tissue, malignant
  unspecified site C80.1
Sarcopenia (age-related) M62.84
Sarcosinemia E72.59
Sarcosporidiosis (intestinal) A07.8
Satiety, early R68.81
Saturnine — see condition
Saturnism
  overdose or wrong substance given or taken — see Table of Drugs and Chemicals, by drug, poisoning
Satyriasis F52.8
Sauriasis — see Ichthyosis
SBE (subacute bacterial endocarditis) I33.0
Scabies (any site) B86
Scabs R23.4
Scaglietti-Dagnini syndrome E22.0
Scald — see Burn
Scalenus anticus (anterior) **syndrome** G54.0
Scales R23.4
Scaling, skin R23.4
Scalp — see condition
Scapegoating affecting child Z62.3
Scaphocephaly Q75.0
Scapulalgia M89.8X1
Scapulohumeral myopathy G71.0
Scar, scarring (see also Cicatrix) L90.5
  adherent L90.5
  atrophic L90.5
  cervix
    in pregnancy or childbirth — see Pregnancy, complicated by, abnormal cervix
  cheloid L91.0
  chorioretinal H31.00- ☑
    posterior pole macula H31.01- ☑
    postsurgical H59.81- ☑
    solar retinopathy H31.02- ☑
    specified type NEC H31.09- ☑
  choroid — see Scar, chorioretinal

Scar, scarring — continued
  conjunctiva H11.24- ☑
  cornea H17.9
    xerophthalmic (see also Opacity, cornea)
      vitamin A deficiency E50.6
  duodenum, obstructive K31.5
  hypertrophic L91.0
  keloid L91.0
  labia N90.89
  lung (base) J98.4
  macula — see Scar, chorioretinal, posterior pole
  muscle M62.89
  myocardium, myocardial I25.2
  painful L90.5
  posterior pole (eye) — see Scar, chorioretinal, posterior pole
  retina — see Scar, chorioretinal
  trachea J39.8
  transmural uterine, in pregnancy O34.29
  uterus N85.8
    in pregnancy O34.29
  vagina N89.8
    postoperative N99.2
  vulva N90.89
Scarabiasis B88.2
Scarlatina (anginosa) (maligna) A38.9
  myocarditis (acute) A38.1
    old — see Myocarditis
  otitis media A38.0
  ulcerosa A38.8
Scarlet fever (albuminuria) (angina) A38.9
Schamberg's disease (progressive pigmentary dermatosis) L81.7
Schatzki's ring (acquired) (esophagus) (lower) K22.2
  congenital Q39.3
Schaufenster krankheit I20.8
Schaumann's
  benign lymphogranulomatosis D86.1
  disease or syndrome — see Sarcoidosis
Scheie's syndrome E76.03
Schenck's disease B42.1
Scheuermann's disease or osteochondrosis — see Osteochondrosis, juvenile, spine
Schilder (-Flatau) **disease** G37.0
Schilling-type monocytic leukemia C93.0- ☑
Schimmelbusch's disease, cystic mastitis, or hyperplasia — see Mastopathy, cystic
Schistosoma infestation — see Infestation, Schistosoma
Schistosomiasis B65.9
  with muscle disorder B65.9 [M63.80]
    ankle B65.9 [M63.87-] ☑
    foot B65.9 [M63.87-] ☑
    forearm B65.9 [M63.83-] ☑
    hand B65.9 [M63.84-] ☑
    lower leg B65.9 [M63.86-] ☑
    multiple sites B65.9 [M63.89]
    pelvic region B65.9 [M63.85-] ☑
    shoulder region B65.9 [M63.81-] ☑
    specified site NEC B65.9 [M63.88]
    thigh B65.9 [M63.85-] ☑
    upper arm B65.9 [M63.82-] ☑
  Asiatic B65.2
  bladder B65.0
  chestermani B65.8
  colon B65.1
  cutaneous B65.3
  due to
    S. haematobium B65.0
    S. japonicum B65.2
    S. mansoni B65.1
    S. mattheii B65.8
  Eastern B65.2
  genitourinary tract B65.0
  intestinal B65.1
  lung NEC B65.9 [J99]
    pneumonia B65.9 [J17]
  Manson's (intestinal) B65.1
  oriental B65.2
  pulmonary NEC B65.9 [J99]
    pneumonia B65.9
  Schistosoma
    haematobium B65.0
    japonicum B65.2
    mansoni B65.1
  specified type NEC B65.8
  urinary B65.0
  vesical B65.0
Schizencephaly Q04.6

Schizoaffective psychosis F25.9
Schizodontia K00.2
Schizoid personality F60.1
Schizophrenia, schizophrenic F20.9
  acute (brief) (undifferentiated) F23
  atypical (form) F20.3
  borderline F21
  catalepsy F20.2
  catatonic (type) (excited) (withdrawn) F20.2
  cenesthopathic, cenesthesiopathic F20.89
  childhood type F84.5
  chronic undifferentiated F20.5
  cyclic F25.0
  disorganized (type) F20.1
  flexibilitas cerea F20.2
  hebephrenic (type) F20.1
  incipient F21
  latent F21
  negative type F20.5
  paranoid (type) F20.0
  paraphrenic F20.0
  post-psychotic depression F32.89
  prepsychotic F21
  prodromal F21
  pseudoneurotic F21
  pseudopsychopathic F21
  reaction F23
  residual (state) (type) F20.5
  restzustand F20.5
  schizoaffective (type) — see Psychosis, schizoaffective
  simple (type) F20.89
  simplex F20.89
  specified type NEC F20.89
  spectrum and other psychotic disorder F29
    specified NEC F28
  stupor F20.2
  syndrome of childhood F84.5
  undifferentiated (type) F20.3
    chronic F20.5
Schizothymia (persistent) F60.1
Schlatter-Osgood disease or osteochondrosis — see Osteochondrosis, juvenile, tibia
Schlatter's tibia — see Osteochondrosis, juvenile, tibia
Schmidt's syndrome (polyglandular, autoimmune) E31.0
Schmincke's carcinoma or tumor — see Neoplasm, nasopharynx, malignant
Schmitz (-Stutzer) **dysentery** A03.0
Schmorl's disease or nodes
  lumbar region M51.46
  lumbosacral region M51.47
  sacrococcygeal region M53.3
  thoracic region M51.44
  thoracolumbar region M51.45
Schneiderian
  papilloma — see Neoplasm, nasopharynx, benign
    specified site — see Neoplasm, benign, by site
    unspecified site D14.0
  specified site — see Neoplasm, malignant, by site
    unspecified site C30.0
Scholte's syndrome (malignant carcinoid) E34.0
Scholz (-Bielchowsky-Henneberg) **disease or syndrome** E75.25
Schönlein (-Henoch) disease or purpura (primary) (rheumatic) D69.0
Schottmuller's disease A01.4
Schroeder's syndrome (endocrine hypertensive) E27.0
Schüller-Christian disease or syndrome C96.5
Schultze's type acroparesthesia, simple I73.89
Schultz's disease or syndrome — see Agranulocytosis
Schwalbe-Ziehen-Oppenheim disease G24.1
Schwannoma (see also Neoplasm, nerve, benign)
  malignant (see also Neoplasm, nerve, malignant)
    with rhabdomyoblastic differentiation — see Neoplasm, nerve, malignant
  melanocytic — see Neoplasm, nerve, benign
  pigmented — see Neoplasm, nerve, benign
Schwannomatosis Q85.03
Schwartz (-Jampel) **syndrome** G71.13
Schwartz-Bartter syndrome E22.2
Schweniger-Buzzi anetoderma L90.1
Sciatic — see condition
Sciatica (infective)
  with lumbago M54.4- ☑
    due to intervertebral disc disorder — see Disorder, disc, with, radiculopathy
  due to displacement of intervertebral disc (with lumbago) — see Disorder, disc, with, radiculopathy

Sciatica — *continued*
  wallet M54.3- ☑
Scimitar syndrome Q26.8
Sclera — *see* condition
Sclerectasia H15.84- ☑
Scleredema
  adultorum — *see* Sclerosis, systemic
  Buschke's — *see* Sclerosis, systemic
  newborn P83.Ø
Sclerema (adiposum) (edematosum) (neonatorum)
  (newborn) P83.Ø
  adultorum — *see* Sclerosis, systemic
Scleriasis — *see* Scleroderma
Scleritis H15.ØØ- ☑
  with corneal involvement H15.Ø4- ☑
  anterior H15.Ø1- ☑
  brawny H15.Ø2- ☑
  in (due to) zoster BØ2.34
  posterior H15.Ø3- ☑
  specified type NEC H15.Ø9- ☑
  syphilitic A52.71
  tuberculous (nodular) A18.51
Sclerochoroiditis H31.8
Scleroconjunctivitis — *see* Scleritis
Sclerocystic ovary syndrome E28.2
Sclerodactyly, sclerodactylia L94.3
Scleroderma, sclerodermia (acrosclerotic) (diffuse)
  (generalized) (progressive) (pulmonary) (*see also*
  Sclerosis, systemic) M34.9
  circumscribed L94.Ø
  linear L94.1
  localized L94.Ø
  newborn P83.88
  systemic M34.9
Sclerokeratitis H16.8
  tuberculous A18.52
Scleroma nasi A48.8
Scleromalacia (perforans) H15.Ø5- ☑
Scleromyxedema L98.5
Sclérose en plaques G35
Sclerosis, sclerotic
  adrenal (gland) E27.8
  Alzheimer's — *see* Disease, Alzheimer's
  amyotrophic (lateral) G12.21
  aorta, aortic I7Ø.Ø
    valve — *see* Endocarditis, aortic
  artery, arterial, arteriolar, arteriovascular — *see* Arteriosclerosis
  ascending multiple G35
  brain (generalized) (lobular) G37.9
    artery, arterial I67.2
    diffuse G37.Ø
    disseminated G35
    insular G35
    Krabbe's E75.23
    miliary G35
    multiple G35
    presenile (Alzheimer's) — *see* Disease, Alzheimer's,
      early onset
    senile (arteriosclerotic) I67.2
    stem, multiple G35
    tuberous Q85.1
  bulbar, multiple G35
  bundle of His I44.39
  cardiac — *see* Disease, heart, ischemic, atherosclerotic
  cardiorenal — *see* Hypertension, cardiorenal
  cardiovascular (*see also* Disease, cardiovascular)
    renal — *see* Hypertension, cardiorenal
  cerebellar — *see* Sclerosis, brain
  cerebral — *see* Sclerosis, brain
  cerebrospinal (disseminated) (multiple) G35
  cerebrovascular I67.2
  choroid — *see* Degeneration, choroid
  combined (spinal cord) (*see also* Degeneration, combined)
    multiple G35
  concentric (Balo) G37.5
  cornea — *see* Opacity, cornea
  coronary (artery) I25.1Ø
    with angina pectoris — *see* Arteriosclerosis, coronary (artery),
  corpus cavernosum
    female N9Ø.89
    male N48.6
  diffuse (brain) (spinal cord) G37.Ø
  disseminated G35
  dorsal G35

Sclerosis, sclerotic — *continued*
  dorsolateral (spinal cord) — *see* Degeneration, combined
  endometrium N85.5
  extrapyramidal G25.9
  eye, nuclear (senile) — *see* Cataract, senile, nuclear
  focal and segmental (glomerular) (*see also* NØØ-NØ7
    with fourth character .1) NØ5.1
  Friedreich's (spinal cord) G11.1
  funicular (spermatic cord) N5Ø.89
  general (vascular) — *see* Arteriosclerosis
  gland (lymphatic) I89.8
  hepatic K74.1
    alcoholic K7Ø.2
  hereditary
    cerebellar G11.9
    spinal (Friedreich's ataxia) G11.1
  hippocampal G93.81
  insular G35
  kidney — *see* Sclerosis, renal
  larynx J38.7
  lateral (amyotrophic) (descending) (spinal) G12.21
    primary G12.23
  lens, senile nuclear — *see* Cataract, senile, nuclear
  liver K74.1
    with fibrosis K74.2
      alcoholic K7Ø.2
    alcoholic K7Ø.2
    cardiac K76.1
  lung — *see* Fibrosis, lung
  mastoid — *see* Mastoiditis, chronic
  mesial temporal G93.81
  mitral IØ5.8
  Mönckeberg's (medial) — *see* Arteriosclerosis, extremities
  multiple (brain stem) (cerebral) (generalized) (spinal cord) G35
  myocardium, myocardial — *see* Disease, heart, ischemic, atherosclerotic
  nuclear (senile), eye — *see* Cataract, senile, nuclear
  ovary N83.8
  pancreas K86.89
  penis N48.6
  peripheral arteries — *see* Arteriosclerosis, extremities
  plaques G35
  pluriglandular E31.8
  polyglandular E31.8
  posterolateral (spinal cord) — *see* Degeneration, combined
  presenile (Alzheimer's) — *see* Disease, Alzheimer's, early onset
  primary, lateral G12.23
  progressive, systemic M34.Ø
  pulmonary — *see* Fibrosis, lung
    artery I27.Ø
    valve (heart) — *see* Endocarditis, pulmonary
  renal N26.9
    with
      cystine storage disease E72.Ø9
      hypertensive heart disease (conditions in I11) — *see* Hypertension, cardiorenal
      arteriolar (hyaline) (hyperplastic) — *see* Hypertension, kidney
  retina (senile) (vascular) H35.ØØ
  senile (vascular) — *see* Arteriosclerosis
  spinal (cord) (progressive) G95.89
    ascending G61.Ø
    combined (*see also* Degeneration, combined)
      multiple G35
      syphilitic A52.11
    disseminated G35
    dorsolateral — *see* Degeneration, combined
    hereditary (Friedreich's) (mixed form) G11.1
    lateral (amyotrophic) G12.23
    multiple G35
    posterior (syphilitic) A52.11
  stomach K31.89
  subendocardial, congenital I42.4
  systemic M34.9
    with
      lung involvement M34.81
      myopathy M34.82
      polyneuropathy M34.83
    drug-induced M34.2
    due to chemicals NEC M34.2
    progressive M34.Ø
    specified NEC M34.89
  temporal (mesial) G93.81

Sclerosis, sclerotic — *continued*
  tricuspid (heart) (valve) IØ7.8
  tuberous (brain) Q85.1
  tympanic membrane — *see* Disorder, tympanic membrane, specified NEC
  valve, valvular (heart) — *see* Endocarditis
  vascular — *see* Arteriosclerosis
  vein I87.8
Scoliosis (acquired) (postural) M41.9
  adolescent (idiopathic) — *see* Scoliosis, idiopathic, adolescent
  congenital Q67.5
    due to bony malformation Q76.3
    failure of segmentation (hemivertebra) Q76.3
    hemivertebra fusion Q76.3
    postural Q67.5
  idiopathic M41.2Ø
    adolescent M41.129
      cervical region M41.122
      cervicothoracic region M41.123
      lumbar region M41.126
      lumbosacral region M41.127
      thoracic region M41.124
      thoracolumbar region M41.125
    cervical region M41.22
    cervicothoracic region M41.23
    infantile M41.ØØ
      cervical region M41.Ø2
      cervicothoracic region M41.Ø3
      lumbar region M41.Ø6
      lumbosacral region M41.Ø7
      sacrococcygeal region M41.Ø8
      thoracic region M41.Ø4
      thoracolumbar region M41.Ø5
    juvenile M41.119
      cervical region M41.112
      cervicothoracic region M41.113
      lumbar region M41.116
      lumbosacral region M41.117
      thoracic region M41.114
      thoracolumbar region M41.115
    lumbar region M41.26
    lumbosacral region M41.27
    thoracic region M41.24
    thoracolumbar region M41.25
  infantile — *see* Scoliosis, idiopathic, infantile
  neuromuscular M41.4Ø
    cervical region M41.42
    cervicothoracic region M41.43
    lumbar region M41.46
    lumbosacral region M41.47
    occipito-atlanto-axial region M41.41
    thoracic region M41.44
    thoracolumbar region M41.45
  paralytic — *see* Scoliosis, neuromuscular
  postradiation therapy M96.5
  rachitic (late effect or sequelae) E64.3 [M49.8Ø]
    cervical region E64.3 [M49.82]
    cervicothoracic region E64.3 [M49.83]
    lumbar region E64.3 [M49.86]
    lumbosacral region E64.3 [M49.87]
    multiple sites E64.3 [M49.89]
    occipito-atlanto-axial region E64.3 [M49.81]
    sacrococcygeal region E64.3 [M49.88]
    thoracic region E64.3 [M49.84]
    thoracolumbar region E64.3 [M49.85]
  sciatic M54.4- ☑
  secondary (to) NEC M41.5Ø
    cerebral palsy, Friedreich's ataxia, poliomyelitis, neuromuscular disorders — *see* Scoliosis, neuromuscular
    cervical region M41.52
    cervicothoracic region M41.53
    lumbar region M41.56
    lumbosacral region M41.57
    thoracic region M41.54
    thoracolumbar region M41.55
  specified form NEC M41.8Ø
    cervical region M41.82
    cervicothoracic region M41.83
    lumbar region M41.86
    lumbosacral region M41.87
    thoracic region M41.84
    thoracolumbar region M41.85
  thoracogenic M41.3Ø
    thoracic region M41.34
    thoracolumbar region M41.35
  tuberculous A18.Ø1

Index

Scoliotic pelvis — Secondary

Scoliotic pelvis
  with disproportion (fetopelvic) O33.0
    causing obstructed labor O65.0
Scorbutus, scorbutic (*see also* Scurvy)
  anemia D53.2
Score, NIHSS (National Institutes of Health Stroke Scale) R29.7- ☑
Scotoma (arcuate) (Bjerrum) (central) (ring) (*see also* Defect, visual field, localized, scotoma)
  scintillating H53.19
Scratch — *see* Abrasion
Scratchy throat R09.89
Screening (for) Z13.9
  alcoholism Z13.89
  anemia Z13.0
  anomaly, congenital Z13.89
  antenatal, of mother (*see also* Encounter, antenatal screening) Z36.9
  arterial hypertension Z13.6
  arthropod-borne viral disease NEC Z11.59
  bacteriuria, asymptomatic Z13.89
  behavioral disorder Z13.89
  brain injury, traumatic Z13.850
  bronchitis, chronic Z13.83
  brucellosis Z11.2
  cardiovascular disorder Z13.6
  cataract Z13.5
  chlamydial diseases Z11.8
  cholera Z11.0
  chromosomal abnormalities (nonprocreative) NEC Z13.79
  colonoscopy Z12.11
  congenital
    dislocation of hip Z13.89
    eye disorder Z13.5
    malformation or deformation Z13.89
  contamination NEC Z13.88
  cystic fibrosis Z13.228
  dengue fever Z11.59
  dental disorder Z13.84
  depression Z13.89
  developmental handicap Z13.4
    in early childhood Z13.4
    infant Z13.4
  diabetes mellitus Z13.1
  diphtheria Z11.2
  disability, intellectual Z13.4
    infant Z13.4
  disease or disorder Z13.9
    bacterial NEC Z11.2
      intestinal infectious Z11.0
      respiratory tuberculosis Z11.1
    blood or blood-forming organ Z13.0
    cardiovascular Z13.6
    Chagas' Z11.6
    chlamydial Z11.8
    dental Z13.89
    developmental Z13.4
      in child Z13.4
      infant Z13.4
    digestive tract NEC Z13.818
      lower GI Z13.811
      upper GI Z13.810
    ear Z13.5
    endocrine Z13.29
    eye Z13.5
    genitourinary Z13.89
    heart Z13.6
    human immunodeficiency virus (HIV) infection Z11.4
    immunity Z13.0
    infection
      intestinal Z11.0
        specified NEC Z11.6
      infectious Z11.9
    mental Z13.89
    metabolic Z13.228
    neurological Z13.89
    nutritional Z13.21
      metabolic Z13.228
        lipoid disorders Z13.220
    protozoal Z11.6
      intestinal Z11.0
    respiratory Z13.83
    rheumatic Z13.828
    rickettsial Z11.8
    sexually-transmitted NEC Z11.3
      human immunodeficiency virus (HIV) Z11.4

Screening — *continued*
  disease or disorder — *continued*
    sickle-cell (trait) Z13.0
    skin Z13.89
    specified NEC Z13.89
    spirochetal Z11.8
    thyroid Z13.29
    vascular Z13.6
    venereal Z11.3
    viral NEC Z11.59
      human immunodeficiency virus (HIV) Z11.4
      intestinal Z11.0
  elevated titer Z13.89
  emphysema Z13.83
  encephalitis, viral (mosquito- or tick-borne) Z11.59
  exposure to contaminants (toxic) Z13.88
  fever
    dengue Z11.59
    hemorrhagic Z11.59
    yellow Z11.59
  filariasis Z11.6
  galactosemia Z13.228
  gastrointestinal condition Z13.818
  genetic (nonprocreative) - for procreative management — *see* Testing, genetic, for procreative management
    disease carrier status (nonprocreative) Z13.71
    specified NEC (nonprocreative) Z13.79
  genitourinary condition Z13.89
  glaucoma Z13.5
  gonorrhea Z11.3
  gout Z13.89
  helminthiasis (intestinal) Z11.6
  hematopoietic malignancy Z12.89
  hemoglobinopathies NEC Z13.0
  hemorrhagic fever Z11.59
  Hodgkin disease Z12.89
  human immunodeficiency virus (HIV) Z11.4
  human papillomavirus Z11.51
  hypertension Z13.6
  immunity disorders Z13.0
  infection
    mycotic Z11.8
    parasitic Z11.8
  ingestion of radioactive substance Z13.88
  intellectual disability Z13.4
    infant Z13.4
  intestinal
    helminthiasis Z11.6
    infectious disease Z11.0
  leishmaniasis Z11.6
  leprosy Z11.2
  leptospirosis Z11.8
  leukemia Z12.89
  lymphoma Z12.89
  malaria Z11.6
  malnutrition Z13.29
    metabolic Z13.228
    nutritional Z13.21
  measles Z11.59
  mental disorder Z13.89
  metabolic errors, inborn Z13.228
  multiphasic Z13.89
  musculoskeletal disorder Z13.828
    osteoporosis Z13.820
  mycoses Z11.8
  myocardial infarction (acute) Z13.6
  neoplasm (malignant) (of) Z12.9
    bladder Z12.6
    blood Z12.89
    breast Z12.39
      routine mammogram Z12.31
    cervix Z12.4
    colon Z12.11
    genitourinary organs NEC Z12.79
      bladder Z12.6
      cervix Z12.4
      ovary Z12.73
      prostate Z12.5
      testis Z12.71
      vagina Z12.72
    hematopoietic system Z12.89
    intestinal tract Z12.10
      colon Z12.11
      rectum Z12.12
      small intestine Z12.13
    lung Z12.2
    lymph (glands) Z12.89
    nervous system Z12.82

Screening — *continued*
  neoplasm — *continued*
    oral cavity Z12.81
    prostate Z12.5
    rectum Z12.12
    respiratory organs Z12.2
    skin Z12.83
    small intestine Z12.13
    specified site NEC Z12.89
    stomach Z12.0
  nephropathy Z13.89
  nervous system disorders NEC Z13.858
  neurological condition Z13.89
  osteoporosis Z13.820
  parasitic infestation Z11.9
    specified NEC Z11.8
  phenylketonuria Z13.228
  plague Z11.2
  poisoning (chemical) (heavy metal) Z13.88
  poliomyelitis Z11.59
  postnatal, chromosomal abnormalities Z13.89
  prenatal, of mother (*see also* Encounter, antenatal screening) Z36.9
  protozoal disease Z11.6
    intestinal Z11.0
  pulmonary tuberculosis Z11.1
  radiation exposure Z13.88
  respiratory condition Z13.83
  respiratory tuberculosis Z11.1
  rheumatoid arthritis Z13.828
  rubella Z11.59
  schistosomiasis Z11.6
  sexually-transmitted disease NEC Z11.3
    human immunodeficiency virus (HIV) Z11.4
  sickle-cell disease or trait Z13.0
  skin condition Z13.89
  sleeping sickness Z11.6
  special Z13.9
    specified NEC Z13.89
  syphilis Z11.3
  tetanus Z11.2
  trachoma Z11.8
  traumatic brain injury Z13.850
  trypanosomiasis Z11.6
  tuberculosis, respiratory Z11.1
  venereal disease Z11.3
  viral encephalitis (mosquito- or tick-borne) Z11.59
  whooping cough Z11.2
  worms, intestinal Z11.6
  yaws Z11.8
  yellow fever Z11.59
Scrofula, scrofulosis (tuberculosis of cervical lymph glands) A18.2
Scrofulide (primary) (tuberculous) A18.4
Scrofuloderma, scrofulodermia (any site) (primary) A18.4
Scrofulosus lichen (primary) (tuberculous) A18.4
Scrofulous — *see* condition
Scrotal tongue K14.5
Scrotum — *see* condition
Scurvy, scorbutic E54
  anemia D53.2
  gum E54
  infantile E54
  rickets E55.0 [M90.80]
Sealpox B08.62
Seasickness T75.3 ☑
Seatworm (infection) (infestation) B80
Sebaceous (*see also* condition)
  cyst — *see* Cyst, sebaceous
Seborrhea, seborrheic L21.9
  capillitii R23.8
  capitis L21.0
  dermatitis L21.9
    infantile L21.1
  eczema L21.9
    infantile L21.1
  sicca L21.0
Seckel's syndrome Q87.1
Seclusion, pupil — *see* Membrane, pupillary
Second hand tobacco smoke exposure (acute) (chronic) Z77.22
  in the perinatal period P96.81
Secondary
  dentin (in pulp) K04.3
  neoplasm, secondaries — *see* Table of Neoplasms, secondary

☑ Additional Character Required — Refer to the Tabular List for Character Selection   Subterms under main terms may continue to next column or page

Secretion
- antidiuretic hormone, inappropriate E22.2
- catecholamine, by pheochromocytoma E27.5
- hormone
  - antidiuretic, inappropriate (syndrome) E22.2
  - by
    - carcinoid tumor E34.0
    - pheochromocytoma E27.5
  - ectopic NEC E34.2
- urinary
  - excessive R35.8
  - suppression R34

Section
- nerve, traumatic — *see* Injury, nerve

Sedative, hypnotic, or anxiolytic-induced
- anxiety disorder F13.980
- bipolar and related disorder F13.94
- delirium F13.921
- depressive disorder F13.94
- major neurocognitive disorder F13.97
- mild neurocognitive disorder F13.988
- psychotic disorder F13.959
- sexual dysfunction F13.981
- sleep disorder F13.982

Segmentation, incomplete (congenital) (*see also* Fusion)
- bone NEC Q78.8
- lumbosacral (joint) (vertebra) Q76.49

Seitelberger's syndrome (infantile neuraxonal dystrophy) G31.89

Seizure(s) (*see also* Convulsions) R56.9
- akinetic — *see* Epilepsy, generalized, specified NEC
- atonic — *see* Epilepsy, generalized, specified NEC
- autonomic (hysterical) F44.5
- convulsive — *see* Convulsions
- cortical (focal) (motor) — *see* Epilepsy, localization-related, symptomatic, with simple partial seizures
- disorder (*see also* Epilepsy) G40.909
- due to stroke — *see* Sequelae (of), disease, cerebrovascular, by type, specified NEC
- epileptic — *see* Epilepsy
- febrile (simple) R56.00
  - with status epilepticus G40.901
  - complex (atypical) (complicated) R56.01
    - with status epilepticus G40.901
- grand mal G40.409
  - intractable G40.419
    - with status epilepticus G40.411
    - without status epilepticus G40.419
  - not intractable G40.409
    - with status epilepticus G40.401
    - without status epilepticus G40.409
- heart — *see* Disease, heart
- hysterical F44.5
- intractable G40.919
  - with status epilepticus G40.911
- Jacksonian (focal) (motor type) (sensory type) — *see* Epilepsy, localization-related, symptomatic, with simple partial seizures
- newborn P90
- nonspecific epileptic
  - atonic — *see* Epilepsy, generalized, specified NEC
  - clonic — *see* Epilepsy, generalized, specified NEC
  - myoclonic — *see* Epilepsy, generalized, specified NEC
  - tonic — *see* Epilepsy, generalized, specified NEC
  - tonic-clonic — *see* Epilepsy, generalized, specified NEC
- partial, developing into secondarily generalized seizures
  - complex — *see* Epilepsy, localization-related, symptomatic, with complex partial seizures
  - simple — *see* Epilepsy, localization-related, symptomatic, with simple partial seizures
- petit mal G40.409
  - intractable G40.419
    - with status epilepticus G40.411
    - without status epilepticus G40.419
  - not intractable G40.409
    - with status epilepticus G40.401
    - without status epilepticus G40.409
- post traumatic R56.1
- recurrent G40.909
- specified NEC G40.89
- uncinate — *see* Epilepsy, localization-related, symptomatic, with complex partial seizures

Selenium deficiency, dietary E59

Self-damaging behavior (life-style) Z72.89
Self-harm (attempted)
- history (personal) Z91.5
  - in family Z81.8
Self-mutilation (attempted)
- history (personal) Z91.5
  - in family Z81.8
Self-poisoning
- history (personal) Z91.5
  - in family Z81.8
- observation following (alleged) attempt Z03.6
Semicoma R40.1
Seminal vesiculitis N49.0
Seminoma C62.9- ☑
- specified site — *see* Neoplasm, malignant, by site
Senear-Usher disease or syndrome L10.4
Senectus R54
Senescence (without mention of psychosis) R54
Senile, senility (*see also* condition) R41.81
- with
  - acute confusional state F05
    - mental changes NOS F03 ☑
  - psychosis NEC — *see* Psychosis, senile
- asthenia R54
- cervix (atrophic) N88.8
- debility R54
- endometrium (atrophic) N85.8
- fallopian tube (atrophic) — *see* Atrophy, fallopian tube
- heart (failure) R54
- ovary (atrophic) — *see* Atrophy, ovary
- premature E34.8
- vagina, vaginitis (atrophic) N95.2
- wart L82.1
Sensation
- burning (skin) R20.8
  - tongue K14.6
- loss of R20.8
- prickling (skin) R20.2
- tingling (skin) R20.2
Sense loss
- smell — *see* Disturbance, sensation, smell
- taste — *see* Disturbance, sensation, taste
- touch R20.8
Sensibility disturbance (cortical) (deep) (vibratory) R20.9
Sensitive, sensitivity (*see also* Allergy)
- carotid sinus G90.01
- child (excessive) F93.8
- cold, autoimmune D59.1
- dentin K03.89
- gluten (non-celiac) K90.41
- latex Z91.040
- methemoglobin D74.8
- tuberculin, without clinical or radiological symptoms R76.11
- visual
  - glare H53.71
  - impaired contrast H53.72
Sensitiver Beziehungswahn F22
Sensitization, auto-erythrocytic D69.2
Separation
- anxiety, abnormal (of childhood) F93.0
- apophysis, traumatic — *code as* Fracture, by site
- choroid — *see* Detachment, choroid
- epiphysis, epiphyseal
  - nontraumatic (*see also* Osteochondropathy, specified type NEC)
    - upper femoral — *see* Slipped, epiphysis, upper femoral
  - traumatic — *code as* Fracture, by site
- fracture — *see* Fracture
- infundibulum cardiac from right ventricle by a partition Q24.3
- joint (traumatic) (current) — *code by* site under Dislocation
- pubic bone, obstetrical trauma O71.6
- retina, retinal — *see* Detachment, retina
- symphysis pubis, obstetrical trauma O71.6
- tracheal ring, incomplete, congenital Q32.1
Sepsis (generalized) (unspecified organism) A41.9
- with
  - organ dysfunction (acute) (multiple) R65.20
    - with septic shock R65.21
  - actinomycotic A42.7
  - adrenal hemorrhage syndrome (meningococcal) A39.1
  - anaerobic A41.4
  - Bacillus anthracis A22.7
  - Brucella (*see also* Brucellosis) A23.9

Sepsis — *continued*
- candidal B37.7
- cryptogenic A41.9
- due to device, implant or graft T85.79 ☑
  - arterial graft NEC T82.7 ☑
  - breast (implant) T85.79 ☑
  - catheter NEC T85.79 ☑
    - dialysis (renal) T82.7 ☑
      - intraperitoneal T85.71 ☑
    - infusion NEC T82.7 ☑
      - spinal (cranial) (epidural) (intrathecal) (spinal) (subarachnoid) (subdural) T85.735 ☑
    - urethral indwelling T83.511 ☑
    - urinary T83.518 ☑
  - ectopic or molar pregnancy O08.82
  - electronic (electrode) (pulse generator) (stimulator)
    - bone T84.7 ☑
    - cardiac T82.7 ☑
    - nervous system T85.738 ☑
      - brain T85.731 ☑
      - neurostimulator generator T85.734 ☑
      - peripheral nerve T85.732 ☑
      - spinal cord T85.733 ☑
    - urinary T83.590 ☑
  - fixation, internal (orthopedic) — *see* Complication, fixation device, infection
  - gastrointestinal (bile duct) (esophagus) T85.79 ☑
    - neurostimulator electrode (lead) T85.732 ☑
  - genital T83.69 ☑
  - heart NEC T82.7 ☑
    - valve (prosthesis) T82.6 ☑
      - graft T82.7 ☑
  - joint prosthesis — *see* Complication, joint prosthesis, infection
  - ocular (corneal graft) (orbital implant) T85.79 ☑
  - orthopedic NEC T84.7 ☑
    - fixation device, internal — *see* Complication, fixation device, infection
  - specified NEC T85.79 ☑
  - vascular T82.7 ☑
  - ventricular intracranial (communicating) shunt T85.730 ☑
- during labor O75.3
- Enterococcus A41.81
- Erysipelothrix (rhusiopathiae) (erysipeloid) A26.7
- Escherichia coli (E. coli) A41.5 ☑
- extraintestinal yersiniosis A28.2
- following
  - abortion (subsequent episode) O08.0
    - current episode — *see* Abortion
  - ectopic or molar pregnancy O08.82
  - immunization T88.0 ☑
  - infusion, therapeutic injection or transfusion NEC T80.29 ☑
- gangrenous A41.9
- gonococcal A54.86
- Gram-negative (organism) A41.5 ☑
  - anaerobic A41.4
- Haemophilus influenzae A41.3
- herpesviral B00.7
- intra-abdominal K65.1
- intraocular — *see* Endophthalmitis, purulent
- Listeria monocytogenes A32.7
- localized — *code to* specific localized infection
  - in operation wound T81.4 ☑
  - skin — *see* Abscess
- malleus A24.0
- melioidosis A24.1
- meningeal — *see* Meningitis
- meningococcal A39.4
  - acute A39.2
  - chronic A39.3
- MSSA (Methicillin susceptible Staphylococcus aureus) A41.01
- newborn P36.9
  - due to
    - anaerobes NEC P36.5
    - Escherichia coli P36.4
    - Staphylococcus P36.30
      - aureus P36.2
      - specified NEC P36.39
    - Streptococcus P36.10
      - group B P36.0
      - specified NEC P36.19
  - specified NEC P36.8
- Pasteurella multocida A28.0

▽ Subterms under main terms may continue to next column or page   ☑ Additional Character Required — Refer to the Tabular List for Character Selection   283

Secretion — Sepsis

Sepsis — *continued*
  pelvic, puerperal, postpartum, childbirth O85
  pneumococcal A40.3
  postprocedural T81.4 ☑
  puerperal, postpartum, childbirth (pelvic) O85
  Salmonella (arizonae) (cholerae-suis) (enteritidis) (ty-
      phimurium) A02.1
  severe R65.20
      with septic shock R65.21
  Shigella (*see also* Dysentery, bacillary) A03.9
  skin, localized — *see* Abscess
  specified organism NEC A41.89
  Staphylococcus, staphylococcal A41.2
      aureus (methicillin susceptible) (MSSA) A41.01
          methicillin resistant (MRSA) A41.02
      coagulase-negative A41.1
      specified NEC A41.1
  Streptococcus, streptococcal A40.9
      agalactiae A40.1
      group
          A A40.0
          B A40.1
          D A41.81
      neonatal P36.10
          group B P36.0
          specified NEC P36.19
      pneumoniae A40.3
      pyogenes A40.0
      specified NEC A40.8
  tracheostomy stoma J95.02
  tularemic A21.7
  umbilical, umbilical cord (newborn) — *see* Sepsis,
      newborn
  Yersinia pestis A20.7
Septate — *see* Septum
Septic — *see* condition
  arm — *see* Cellulitis, upper limb
      with lymphangitis — *see* Lymphangitis, acute,
          upper limb
  embolus — *see* Embolism
  finger — *see* Cellulitis, digit
      with lymphangitis — *see* Lymphangitis, acute,
          digit
  foot — *see* Cellulitis, lower limb
      with lymphangitis — *see* Lymphangitis, acute,
          lower limb
  gallbladder (acute) K81.0
  hand — *see* Cellulitis, upper limb
      with lymphangitis — *see* Lymphangitis, acute,
          upper limb
  joint — *see* Arthritis, pyogenic or pyemic
  leg — *see* Cellulitis, lower limb
      with lymphangitis — *see* Lymphangitis, acute,
          lower limb
  nail (*see also* Cellulitis, digit)
      with lymphangitis — *see* Lymphangitis, acute,
          digit
  sore (*see also* Abscess)
      throat J02.0
          streptococcal J02.0
  spleen (acute) D73.89
  teeth, tooth (pulpal origin) K04.4
  throat — *see* Pharyngitis
  thrombus — *see* Thrombosis
  toe — *see* Cellulitis, digit
      with lymphangitis — *see* Lymphangitis, acute,
          digit
  tonsils, chronic J35.01
      with adenoiditis J35.03
  uterus — *see* Endometritis
Septicemia A41.9
  meaning sepsis — *see* Sepsis
Septum, septate (congenital) (*see also* Anomaly, by site)
  anal Q42.3
      with fistula Q42.2
  aqueduct of Sylvius Q03.0
      with spina bifida — *see* Spina bifida, by site, with
          hydrocephalus
  uterus (complete) (partial) Q51.2
  vagina Q52.10
      in pregnancy — *see* Pregnancy, complicated by,
          abnormal vagina
          causing obstructed labor O65.5
      longitudinal Q52.129
          microperforate
              left side Q52.124
              right side Q52.123
          nonobstruction Q52.120

Septum, septate — *continued*
  vagina — *continued*
      longitudinal — *continued*
          obstructing Q52.129
              left side Q52.122
              right side Q52.121
      transverse Q52.11
Sequelae (of) (*see also* condition)
  abscess, intracranial or intraspinal (conditions in G06)
      G09
  amputation — *code to* injury with seventh character
      S
  burn and corrosion — *code to* injury with seventh
      character S
  calcium deficiency E64.8
  cerebrovascular disease — *see* Sequelae, disease,
      cerebrovascular
  childbirth O94
  contusion — *code to* injury with seventh character S
  corrosion — *see* Sequelae, burn and corrosion
  crushing injury — *code to* injury with seventh charac-
      ter S
  disease
      cerebrovascular I69.90
          alteration of sensation I69.998
          aphasia I69.920
          apraxia I69.990
          ataxia I69.993
          cognitive deficits I69.91 ☑
          disturbance of vision I69.998
          dysarthria I69.922
          dysphagia I69.991
          dysphasia I69.921
          facial droop I69.992
          facial weakness I69.992
          fluency disorder I69.923
          hemiplegia I69.95- ☑
          hemorrhage
              intracerebral — *see* Sequelae, hemorrhage,
                  intracerebral
              intracranial, nontraumatic NEC — *see* Seque-
                  lae, hemorrhage, intracranial, nontrau-
                  matic
              subarachnoid — *see* Sequelae, hemorrhage,
                  subarachnoid
          language deficit I69.928
          monoplegia
              lower limb I69.94- ☑
              upper limb I69.93- ☑
          paralytic syndrome I69.96- ☑
          specified effect NEC I69.998
          specified type NEC I69.80
              alteration of sensation I69.898
              aphasia I69.820
              apraxia I69.890
              ataxia I69.893
              cognitive deficits I69.81 ☑
              disturbance of vision I69.898
              dysarthria I69.822
              dysphagia I69.891
              dysphasia I69.821
              facial droop I69.892
              facial weakness I69.892
              fluency disorder I69.823
              hemiplegia I69.85- ☑
              language deficit I69.828
              monoplegia
                  lower limb I69.84- ☑
                  upper limb I69.83- ☑
              paralytic syndrome I69.86- ☑
              specified effect NEC I69.898
          speech deficit I69.928
              speech deficit I69.828
          stroke NOS — *see* Sequelae, stroke NOS
  dislocation — *code to* injury with seventh character S
  encephalitis or encephalomyelitis (conditions in G04)
      G09
      in infectious disease NEC B94.8
      viral B94.1
  external cause — *code to* injury with seventh character
      S
  foreign body entering natural orifice — *code to* injury
      with seventh character S
  fracture — *code to* injury with seventh character S
  frostbite — *code to* injury with seventh character S
  Hansen's disease B92
  hemorrhage
      intracerebral I69.10

Sequelae — *continued*
  hemorrhage — *continued*
      intracerebral — *continued*
          alteration of sensation I69.198
          aphasia I69.120
          apraxia I69.190
          ataxia I69.193
          cognitive deficits I69.11 ☑
          disturbance of vision I69.198
          dysarthria I69.122
          dysphagia I69.191
          dysphasia I69.121
          facial droop I69.192
          facial weakness I69.192
          fluency disorder I69.123
          hemiplegia I69.15- ☑
          language deficit NEC I69.128
          monoplegia
              lower limb I69.14- ☑
              upper limb I69.13- ☑
          paralytic syndrome I69.16- ☑
          specified effect NEC I69.198
          speech deficit NEC I69.128
      intracranial, nontraumatic NEC I69.20
          alteration of sensation I69.298
          aphasia I69.220
          apraxia I69.290
          ataxia I69.293
          cognitive deficits I69.21 ☑
          disturbance of vision I69.298
          dysarthria I69.222
          dysphagia I69.291
          dysphasia I69.221
          facial droop I69.292
          facial weakness I69.292
          fluency disorder I69.223
          hemiplegia I69.25- ☑
          language deficit NEC I69.228
          monoplegia
              lower limb I69.24- ☑
              upper limb I69.23- ☑
          paralytic syndrome I69.26- ☑
          specified effect NEC I69.298
          speech deficit NEC I69.228
      subarachnoid I69.00
          alteration of sensation I69.098
          aphasia I69.020
          apraxia I69.090
          ataxia I69.093
          cognitive deficits — *see* subcategory I69.01- ☑
          disturbance of vision I69.098
          dysarthria I69.022
          dysphagia I69.091
          dysphasia I69.021
          facial droop I69.092
          facial weakness I69.092
          fluency disorder I69.023
          hemiplegia I69.05- ☑
          language deficit NEC I69.028
          monoplegia
              lower limb I69.04- ☑
              upper limb I69.03- ☑
          paralytic syndrome I69.06- ☑
          specified effect NEC I69.098
          speech deficit NEC I69.028
  hepatitis, viral B94.2
  hyperalimentation E68
  infarction
      cerebral I69.30
          alteration of sensation I69.398
          aphasia I69.320
          apraxia I69.390
          ataxia I69.393
          cognitive deficits I69.31 ☑
          disturbance of vision I69.398
          dysarthria I69.322
          dysphagia I69.391
          dysphasia I69.321
          facial droop I69.392
          facial weakness I69.392
          fluency disorder I69.323
          hemiplegia I69.35- ☑
          language deficit NEC I69.328
          monoplegia
              lower limb I69.34- ☑
              upper limb I69.33- ☑
          paralytic syndrome I69.36- ☑
          specified effect NEC I69.398

☑ **Additional Character Required — Refer to the Tabular List for Character Selection**   ⏮ **Subterms under main terms may continue to next column or page**

Sequelae — *continued*
  infarction — *continued*
    cerebral — *continued*
      speech deficit NEC I69.328
  infection, pyogenic, intracranial or intraspinal G09
  infectious disease B94.9
    specified NEC B94.8
  injury — *code to* injury with seventh character S
  leprosy B92
  meningitis
    bacterial (conditions in G00) G09
    other or unspecified cause (conditions in G03) G09
  muscle (and tendon) injury — *code to* injury with seventh character S
  myelitis — *see* Sequelae, encephalitis
  niacin deficiency E64.8
  nutritional deficiency E64.9
    specified NEC E64.8
  obstetrical condition O94
  parasitic disease B94.9
  phlebitis or thrombophlebitis of intracranial or intraspinal venous sinuses and veins (conditions in G08) G09
  poisoning — *code to* poisoning with seventh character S
    nonmedicinal substance — *see* Sequelae, toxic effect, nonmedicinal substance
  poliomyelitis (acute) B91
  pregnancy O94
  protein-energy malnutrition E64.0
  puerperium O94
  rickets E64.3
  selenium deficiency E64.8
  sprain and strain — *code to* injury with seventh character S
  stroke NOS I69.30
    alteration in sensation I69.398
    aphasia I69.320
    apraxia I69.390
    ataxia I69.393
    cognitive deficits I69.31 ☑
    disturbance of vision I69.398
    dysarthria I69.322
    dysphagia I69.391
    dysphasia I69.321
    facial droop I69.392
    facial weakness I69.392
    hemiplegia I69.35- ☑
    language deficit NEC I69.328
    monoplegia
      lower limb I69.34- ☑
      upper limb I69.33- ☑
    paralytic syndrome I69.36- ☑
    specified effect NEC I69.398
    speech deficit NEC I69.328
  tendon and muscle injury — *code to* injury with seventh character S
  thiamine deficiency E64.8
  trachoma B94.0
  tuberculosis B90.9
    bones and joints B90.2
    central nervous system B90.0
    genitourinary B90.1
    pulmonary (respiratory) B90.9
    specified organs NEC B90.8
  viral
    encephalitis B94.1
    hepatitis B94.2
  vitamin deficiency NEC E64.8
    A E64.1
    B E64.8
    C E64.2
  wound, open — *code to* injury with seventh character S
Sequestration (*see also* Sequestrum)
  disk — *see* Displacement, intervertebral disk
  lung, congenital Q33.2
Sequestrum
  bone — *see* Osteomyelitis, chronic
  dental M27.2
  jaw bone M27.2
  orbit — *see* Osteomyelitis, orbit
  sinus (accessory) (nasal) — *see* Sinusitis
Sequoiosis lung or pneumonitis J67.8

Serology for syphilis
  doubtful
    with signs or symptoms — *code by* site and stage under Syphilis
    follow-up of latent syphilis — *see* Syphilis, latent
  negative, with signs or symptoms — *code by* site and stage under Syphilis
  positive A53.0
    with signs or symptoms — *code by* site and stage under Syphilis
  reactivated A53.0
Seroma (*see also* Hematoma)
  postprocedural — *see* Complication, postprocedural, seroma
  traumatic, secondary and recurrent T79.2 ☑
Seropurulent — *see* condition
Serositis, multiple K65.8
  pericardial I31.1
  peritoneal K65.8
Serous — *see* condition
Sertoli cell
  adenoma
    specified site — *see* Neoplasm, benign, by site
    unspecified site
      female D27.9
      male D29.20
  carcinoma
    specified site — *see* Neoplasm, malignant, by site
    unspecified site (male) C62.9- ☑
      female C56.9
  tumor
    with lipid storage
      specified site — *see* Neoplasm, benign, by site
      unspecified site
        female D27.9
        male D29.20
    specified site — *see* Neoplasm, benign, by site
    unspecified site
      female D27.9
      male D29.20
Sertoli-Leydig cell tumor — *see* Neoplasm, benign, by site
  specified site — *see* Neoplasm, benign, by site
  unspecified site
    female D27.9
    male D29.20
Serum
  allergy, allergic reaction (*see also* Reaction, serum) T80.69 ☑
    shock (*see also* Shock, anaphylactic) T80.59 ☑
  arthritis (*see also* Reaction, serum) T80.69 ☑
  complication or reaction NEC (*see also* Reaction, serum) T80.69 ☑
  disease NEC (*see also* Reaction, serum) T80.69 ☑
  hepatitis (*see also* Hepatitis, viral, type B)
    carrier (suspected) of B18.1
  intoxication (*see also* Reaction, serum) T80.69 ☑
  neuritis (*see also* Reaction, serum) T80.69 ☑
  neuropathy G61.1
  poisoning NEC (*see also* Reaction, serum) T80.69 ☑
  rash NEC (*see also* Reaction, serum) T80.69 ☑
  reaction NEC (*see also* Reaction, serum) T80.69 ☑
  sickness NEC (*see also* Reaction, serum) T80.69 ☑
  urticaria (*see also* Reaction, serum) T80.69 ☑
Sesamoiditis M25.8- ☑
Severe sepsis R65.20
  with septic shock R65.21
Sever's disease or osteochondrosis — *see* Osteochondrosis, juvenile, tarsus
Sex
  chromosome mosaics Q97.8
    lines with various numbers of X chromosomes Q97.2
  education Z70.8
  reassignment surgery status Z87.890
Sextuplet pregnancy — *see* Pregnancy, sextuplet
Sexual
  function, disorder of (psychogenic) F52.9
  immaturity (female) (male) E30.0
  impotence (psychogenic) organic origin NEC — *see* Dysfunction, sexual, male
  precocity (constitutional) (cryptogenic)(female) (idiopathic) (male) E30.1
Sexuality, pathologic — *see* Deviation, sexual
Sézary disease C84.1- ☑
Shadow, lung R91.8
Shaking palsy or paralysis — *see* Parkinsonism

Shallowness, acetabulum — *see* Derangement, joint, specified type NEC, hip
Shaver's disease J63.1
Sheath (tendon) — *see* condition
Sheathing, retinal vessels H35.01- ☑
Shedding
  nail L60.8
  premature, primary (deciduous) teeth K00.6
Sheehan's disease or syndrome E23.0
Shelf, rectal K62.89
Shell teeth K00.5
Shellshock (current) F43.0
  lasting state — *see* Disorder, post-traumatic stress
Shield kidney Q63.1
Shift
  auditory threshold (temporary) H93.24- ☑
  mediastinal R93.8
Shifting sleep-work schedule (affecting sleep) G47.26
Shiga (-Kruse) **dysentery** A03.0
Shiga's bacillus A03.0
Shigella (dysentery) — *see* Dysentery, bacillary
Shigellosis A03.9
  Group A A03.0
  Group B A03.1
  Group C A03.2
  Group D A03.3
Shin splints S86.89- ☑
Shingles — *see* Herpes, zoster
Shipyard disease or eye B30.0
Shirodkar suture, in pregnancy — *see* Pregnancy, complicated by, incompetent cervix
Shock R57.9
  with ectopic or molar pregnancy O08.3
  adrenal (cortical) (Addisonian) E27.2
  adverse food reaction (anaphylactic) — *see* Shock, anaphylactic, due to food
  allergic — *see* Shock, anaphylactic
  anaphylactic T78.2 ☑
    chemical — *see* Table of Drugs and Chemicals
    due to drug or medicinal substance
      correct substance properly administered T88.6 ☑
      overdose or wrong substance given or taken (by accident) — *see* Table of Drugs and Chemicals, by drug, poisoning
    due to food (nonpoisonous) T78.00 ☑
      additives T78.06 ☑
      dairy products T78.07 ☑
      eggs T78.08 ☑
      fish T78.03 ☑
        shellfish T78.02 ☑
      fruit T78.04 ☑
      milk T78.07 ☑
      nuts T78.05 ☑
        multiple types T78.05 ☑
        peanuts T78.01 ☑
      peanuts T78.01 ☑
      seeds T78.05 ☑
      specified type NEC T78.09 ☑
      vegetable T78.04 ☑
    following sting(s) — *see* Venom
    immunization T80.52 ☑
    serum T80.59 ☑
      blood and blood products T80.51 ☑
      immunization T80.52 ☑
      specified NEC T80.59 ☑
      vaccination T80.52 ☑
  anaphylactoid — *see* Shock, anaphylactic
  anesthetic
    correct substance properly administered T88.2 ☑
    overdose or wrong substance given or taken — *see* Table of Drugs and Chemicals, by drug, poisoning
      specified anesthetic — *see* Table of Drugs and Chemicals, by drug, poisoning
  cardiogenic R57.0
  chemical substance — *see* Table of Drugs and Chemicals
  complicating ectopic or molar pregnancy O08.3
  culture — *see* Disorder, adjustment
  drug
    due to correct substance properly administered T88.6 ☑
    overdose or wrong substance given or taken (by accident) — *see* Table of Drugs and Chemicals, by drug, poisoning
  during or after labor and delivery O75.1

Subterms under main terms may continue to next column or page   ☑ Additional Character Required — Refer to the Tabular List for Character Selection   285

Sequelae — Shock

Shock — *continued*
  electric T75.4 ☑
    (taser) T75.4 ☑
  endotoxic R65.21
    postprocedural (resulting from a procedure, not elsewhere classified) T81.12 ☑
  following
    ectopic or molar pregnancy O08.3
    injury (immediate) (delayed) T79.4 ☑
    labor and delivery O75.1
  food (anaphylactic) — *see* Shock, anaphylactic, due to food
  from electroshock gun (taser) T75.4 ☑
  gram-negative R65.21
    postprocedural (resulting from a procedure, not elsewhere classified) T81.12 ☑
  hematologic R57.8
  hemorrhagic R57.8
    surgery (intraoperative) (postoperative) T81.19 ☑
    trauma T79.4 ☑
  hypovolemic R57.1
    surgical T81.19 ☑
    traumatic T79.4 ☑
  insulin E15
    therapeutic misadventure — *see* subcategory T38.3 ☑
  kidney N17.0
    traumatic (following crushing) T79.5 ☑
  lightning T75.01 ☑
  liver K72.00
  lung J80
  obstetric O75.1
    with ectopic or molar pregnancy O08.3
    following ectopic or molar pregnancy O08.3
  pleural (surgical) T81.19 ☑
    due to trauma T79.4 ☑
  postprocedural (postoperative) T81.10 ☑
    with ectopic or molar pregnancy O08.3
    cardiogenic T81.11 ☑
    endotoxic T81.12 ☑
    following ectopic or molar pregnancy O08.3
    gram-negative T81.12 ☑
    hypovolemic T81.19 ☑
    septic T81.12 ☑
    specified type NEC T81.19 ☑
  psychic F43.0
  septic (due to severe sepsis) R65.21
  specified NEC R57.8
  surgical T81.10 ☑
  taser gun (taser) T75.4 ☑
  therapeutic misadventure NEC T81.10 ☑
  thyroxin
    overdose or wrong substance given or taken — *see* Table of Drugs and Chemicals, by drug, poisoning
  toxic, syndrome A48.3
  transfusion — *see* Complications, transfusion
  traumatic (immediate) (delayed) T79.4 ☑
Shoemaker's chest M95.4
Short, shortening, shortness
  arm (acquired) (*see also* Deformity, limb, unequal length)
    congenital Q71.81- ☑
    forearm — *see* Deformity, limb, unequal length
  bowel syndrome K91.2
  breath R06.02
  cervical (complicating pregnancy) O26.87- ☑
    non-gravid uterus N88.3
  common bile duct, congenital Q44.5
  cord (umbilical), complicating delivery O69.3 ☑
  cystic duct, congenital Q44.5
  esophagus (congenital) Q39.8
  femur (acquired) — *see* Deformity, limb, unequal length, femur
    congenital — *see* Defect, reduction, lower limb, longitudinal, femur
  frenum, frenulum, linguae (congenital) Q38.1
  hip (acquired) (*see also* Deformity, limb, unequal length)
    congenital Q65.89
  leg (acquired) (*see also* Deformity, limb, unequal length)
    congenital Q72.81- ☑
    lower leg (*see also* Deformity, limb, unequal length)
  limbed stature, with immunodeficiency D82.2
  lower limb (acquired) (*see also* Deformity, limb, unequal length)

Short, shortening, shortness — *continued*
  lower limb (*see also* Deformity, limb, unequal length) — *continued*
    congenital Q72.81- ☑
  organ or site, congenital NEC — *see* Distortion
  palate, congenital Q38.5
  radius (acquired) (*see also* Deformity, limb, unequal length)
    congenital — *see* Defect, reduction, upper limb, longitudinal, radius
  rib syndrome Q77.2
  stature (child) (hereditary) (idiopathic) NEC R62.52
    constitutional E34.3
    due to endocrine disorder E34.3
    Laron-type E34.3
  tendon (*see also* Contraction, tendon)
    with contracture of joint — *see* Contraction, joint
    Achilles (acquired) M67.0- ☑
      congenital Q66.89
    congenital Q79.8
  thigh (acquired) (*see also* Deformity, limb, unequal length, femur)
    congenital — *see* Defect, reduction, lower limb, longitudinal, femur
  tibialis anterior (tendon) — *see* Contraction, tendon
  umbilical cord
    complicating delivery O69.3 ☑
  upper limb, congenital — *see* Defect, reduction, upper limb, specified type NEC
  urethra N36.8
  uvula, congenital Q38.5
  vagina (congenital) Q52.4
Shortsightedness — *see* Myopia
Shoshin (acute fulminating beriberi) E51.11
Shoulder — *see* condition
Shovel-shaped incisors K00.2
Shower, thromboembolic — *see* Embolism
Shunt
  arterial-venous (dialysis) Z99.2
  arteriovenous, pulmonary (acquired) I28.0
    congenital Q25.72
  cerebral ventricle (communicating) in situ Z98.2
  surgical, prosthetic, with complications — *see* Complications, cardiovascular, device or implant
Shutdown, renal N28.9
Shy-Drager syndrome G90.3
Sialadenitis, sialadenosis (any gland) (chronic) (periodic) (suppurative) — *see* Sialoadenitis
Sialectasia K11.8
Sialidosis E77.1
Sialitis, silitis (any gland) (chronic) (suppurative) — *see* Sialoadenitis
Sialoadenitis (any gland) (periodic) (suppurative) K11.20
  acute K11.21
    recurrent K11.22
  chronic K11.23
Sialoadenopathy K11.9
Sialoangitis — *see* Sialoadenitis
Sialodochitis (fibrinosa) — *see* Sialoadenitis
Sialodocholithiasis K11.5
Sialolithiasis K11.5
Sialometaplasia, necrotizing K11.8
Sialorrhea (*see also* Ptyalism)
  periodic — *see* Sialoadenitis
Sialosis K11.7
Siamese twin Q89.4
Sibling rivalry Z62.891
Sicard's syndrome G52.7
Sicca syndrome M35.00
  with
    keratoconjunctivitis M35.01
    lung involvement M35.02
    myopathy M35.03
    renal tubulo-interstitial disorders M35.04
  specified organ involvement NEC M35.09
Sick R69
  or handicapped person in family Z63.79
    needing care at home Z63.6
  sinus (syndrome) I49.5
Sick-euthyroid syndrome E07.81
Sickle-cell
  anemia — *see* Disease, sickle-cell
  trait D57.3
Sicklemia (*see also* Disease, sickle-cell)
  trait D57.3
Sickness
  air (travel) T75.3 ☑

Sickness — *continued*
  airplane T75.3 ☑
  alpine T70.29 ☑
  altitude T70.20 ☑
  Andes T70.29 ☑
  aviator's T70.29 ☑
  balloon T70.29 ☑
  car T75.3 ☑
  compressed air T70.3 ☑
  decompression T70.3 ☑
  green D50.8
  milk — *see* Poisoning, food, noxious
  motion T75.3 ☑
  mountain T70.29 ☑
    acute D75.1
  protein (*see also* Reaction, serum) T80.69 ☑
  radiation T66 ☑
  roundabout (motion) T75.3 ☑
  sea T75.3 ☑
  serum NEC (*see also* Reaction, serum) T80.69 ☑
  sleeping (African) B56.9
    by Trypanosoma B56.9
      brucei
        gambiense B56.0
        rhodesiense B56.1
      East African B56.1
      Gambian B56.0
      Rhodesian B56.1
      West African B56.0
  swing (motion) T75.3 ☑
  train (railway) (travel) T75.3 ☑
  travel (any vehicle) T75.3 ☑
Sideropenia — *see* Anemia, iron deficiency
Siderosilicosis J62.8
Siderosis (lung) J63.4
  eye (globe) — *see* Disorder, globe, degenerative, siderosis
Siemens' syndrome (ectodermal dysplasia) Q82.8
Sighing R06.89
  psychogenic F45.8
Sigmoid (*see also* condition)
  flexure — *see* condition
  kidney Q63.1
Sigmoiditis (*see also* Enteritis) K52.9
  infectious A09
  noninfectious K52.9
Silfverskjöld's syndrome Q78.9
Silicosiderosis J62.8
Silicosis, silicotic (simple) (complicated) J62.8
  with tuberculosis J65
Silicotuberculosis J65
Silo-fillers' disease J68.8
  bronchitis J68.0
  pneumonitis J68.0
  pulmonary edema J68.1
Silver's syndrome Q87.1
Simian malaria B53.1
Simmonds' cachexia or disease E23.0
Simons' disease or syndrome (progressive lipodystrophy) E88.1
Simple, simplex — *see* condition
Simulation, conscious (of illness) Z76.5
Simultanagnosia (asimultagnosia) R48.3
Sin Nombre virus disease (Hantavirus) (cardio)-pulmonary syndrome) B33.4
Sinding-Larsen disease or osteochondrosis — *see* Osteochondrosis, juvenile, patella
Singapore hemorrhagic fever A91
Singer's node or nodule J38.2
Single
  atrium Q21.2
  coronary artery Q24.5
  umbilical artery Q27.0
  ventricle Q20.4
Singultus R06.6
  epidemicus B33.0
Sinus (*see also* Fistula)
  abdominal K63.89
  arrest I45.5
  arrhythmia I49.8
  bradycardia R00.1
  branchial cleft (internal) (external) Q18.0
  coccygeal — *see* Sinus, pilonidal
  dental K04.6
  dermal (congenital) Q06.8
    with abscess Q06.8
    coccygeal, pilonidal — *see* Sinus, coccygeal

☑ **Additional Character Required — Refer to the Tabular List for Character Selection**   **Subterms under main terms may continue to next column or page**

Sinus — *continued*
 infected, skin NEC L08.89
 marginal, ruptured or bleeding — *see* Hemorrhage, antepartum, specified cause NEC
 medial, face and neck Q18.8
 pause I45.5
 pericranii Q01.9
 pilonidal (infected) (rectum) L05.92
  with abscess L05.02
 preauricular Q18.1
 rectovaginal N82.3
 Rokitansky-Aschoff (gallbladder) K82.8
 sacrococcygeal (dermoid) (infected) — *see* Sinus, pilonidal
 tachycardia R00.0
  paroxysmal I47.1
 tarsi syndrome M25.57- ☑
 testis N50.89
 tract (postinfective) — *see* Fistula
 urachus Q64.4
Sinusitis (accessory) (chronic) (hyperplastic) (nasal) (nonpurulent) (purulent) J32.9
 acute J01.90
  ethmoidal J01.20
   recurrent J01.21
  frontal J01.10
   recurrent J01.11
  involving more than one sinus, other than pansinusitis J01.80
   recurrent J01.81
  maxillary J01.00
   recurrent J01.01
  pansinusitis J01.40
   recurrent J01.41
  recurrent J01.91
  specified NEC J01.80
   recurrent J01.81
  sphenoidal J01.30
   recurrent J01.31
 allergic — *see* Rhinitis, allergic
 due to high altitude T70.1 ☑
 ethmoidal J32.2
  acute J01.20
   recurrent J01.21
 frontal J32.1
  acute J01.10
   recurrent J01.11
 influenzal — *see* Influenza, with, respiratory manifestations NEC
 involving more than one sinus but not pansinusitis J32.8
  acute J01.80
   recurrent J01.81
 maxillary J32.0
  acute J01.00
   recurrent J01.01
 sphenoidal J32.3
  acute J01.30
   recurrent J01.31
 tuberculous, any sinus A15.8
Sinusitis-bronchiectasis-situs inversus (syndrome) (triad) Q89.3
Sipple's syndrome E31.22
Sirenomelia (syndrome) Q87.2
Siriasis T67.0 ☑
Sirkari's disease B55.0
Siti A65
Situation, psychiatric F99
Situational
 disturbance (transient) — *see* Disorder, adjustment
  acute F43.0
 maladjustment — *see* Disorder, adjustment
 reaction — *see* Disorder, adjustment
  acute F43.0
Situs inversus or transversus (abdominalis) (thoracis) Q89.3
Sixth disease B08.20
 due to human herpesvirus 6 B08.21
 due to human herpesvirus 7 B08.22
Sjögren-Larsson syndrome Q87.1
Sjögren's syndrome or disease — *see* Sicca syndrome
Skeletal — *see* condition
Skene's gland — *see* condition
Skenitis — *see* Urethritis
Skerljevo A65
Skevas-Zerfus disease — *see* Toxicity, venom, marine animal, sea anemone
Skin (*see also* condition)

Skin — *continued*
 clammy R23.1
 donor — *see* Donor, skin
 hidebound M35.9
Slate-dressers' or slate-miners' lung J62.8
Sleep
 apnea — *see* Apnea, sleep
 deprivation Z72.820
 disorder or disturbance G47.9
  child F51.9
  nonorganic origin F51.9
  specified NEC G47.8
 disturbance G47.9
  nonorganic origin F51.9
 drunkenness F51.9
 rhythm inversion G47.2- ☑
 terrors F51.4
 walking F51.3
  hysterical F44.89
Sleep hygiene
 abuse Z72.821
 inadequate Z72.821
 poor Z72.821
Sleeping sickness — *see* Sickness, sleeping
Sleeplessness — *see* Insomnia
 menopausal N95.1
Sleep-wake schedule disorder G47.20
Slim disease (in HIV infection) B20
Slipped, slipping
 epiphysis (traumatic) (*see also* Osteochondropathy, specified type NEC)
  capital femoral (traumatic)
   acute (on chronic) S79.01- ☑
  current traumatic — *code as* Fracture, by site
  upper femoral (nontraumatic) M93.00- ☑
   acute M93.01- ☑
    on chronic M93.03- ☑
   chronic M93.02- ☑
 intervertebral disc — *see* Displacement, intervertebral disc
 ligature, umbilical P51.8
 patella — *see* Disorder, patella, derangement NEC
 rib M89.8X8
 sacroiliac joint — *see* subcategory M53.2 ☑
 tendon — *see* Disorder, tendon
 ulnar nerve, nontraumatic — *see* Lesion, nerve, ulnar
 vertebra NEC — *see* Spondylolisthesis
Slocumb's syndrome E27.0
Sloughing (multiple) (phagedena) (skin) (*see also* Gangrene)
 abscess — *see* Abscess
 appendix K38.8
 fascia — *see* Disorder, soft tissue, specified type NEC
 scrotum N50.89
 tendon — *see* Disorder, tendon
 transplanted organ — *see* Rejection, transplant
 ulcer — *see* Ulcer, skin
Slow
 feeding, newborn P92.2
 flow syndrome, coronary I20.8
 heart (beat) R00.1
Slowing, urinary stream R39.198
Sluder's neuralgia (syndrome) G44.89
Slurred, slurring speech R47.81
Small (ness)
 for gestational age — *see* Small for dates
 introitus, vagina N89.6
 kidney (unknown cause) N27.9
  bilateral N27.1
  unilateral N27.0
 ovary (congenital) Q50.39
 pelvis
  with disproportion (fetopelvic) O33.1
   causing obstructed labor O65.1
 uterus N85.8
 white kidney N03.9
Small-and-light-for-dates — *see* Small for dates
Small-for-dates (infant) P05.10
 with weight of
  499 grams or less P05.11
  500-749 grams P05.12
  750-999 grams P05.13
  1000-1249 grams P05.14
  1250-1499 grams P05.15
  1500-1749 grams P05.16
  1750-1999 grams P05.17
  2000-2499 grams P05.18

Small-for-dates — *continued*
 with weight of — *continued*
  2500 grams and over P05.19
 specified NEC P05.19
Smallpox B03
Smearing, fecal R15.1
Smith-Lemli-Opitz syndrome E78.72
Smith's fracture S52.54- ☑
Smoker — *see* Dependence, drug, nicotine
Smoker's
 bronchitis J41.0
 cough J41.0
 palate K13.24
 throat J31.2
 tongue K13.24
Smoking
 passive Z77.22
Smothering spells R06.81
Snaggle teeth, tooth M26.39
Snapping
 finger — *see* Trigger finger
 hip — *see* Derangement, joint, specified type NEC, hip
  involving the iliotiblial band M76.3- ☑
 knee — *see* Derangement, knee
  involving the iliotiblial band M76.3- ☑
Sneddon-Wilkinson disease or syndrome (sub-corneal pustular dermatosis) L13.1
Sneezing (intractable) R06.7
Sniffing
 cocaine
  abuse — *see* Abuse, drug, cocaine
  dependence — *see* Dependence, drug, cocaine
 gasoline
  abuse — *see* Abuse, drug, inhalant
  dependence — *see* Dependence, drug, inhalant
 glue (airplane)
  abuse — *see* Abuse, drug, inhalant
  drug dependence — *see* Dependence, drug, inhalant
Sniffles
 newborn P28.89
Snoring R06.83
Snow blindness — *see* Photokeratitis
Snuffles (non-syphilitic) R06.5
 newborn P28.89
 syphilitic (infant) A50.05 [J99]
Social
 exclusion Z60.4
  due to discrimination or persecution (perceived) Z60.5
 migrant Z59.0
  acculturation difficulty Z60.3
 rejection Z60.4
  due to discrimination or persecution Z60.5
 role conflict NEC Z73.5
 skills inadequacy NEC Z73.4
 transplantation Z60.3
Sodoku A25.0
Soemmerring's ring — *see* Cataract, secondary
Soft (*see also* condition)
 nails L60.3
Softening
 bone — *see* Osteomalacia
 brain (necrotic) (progressive) G93.89
  congenital Q04.8
  embolic I63.4- ☑
  hemorrhagic — *see* Hemorrhage, intracranial, intracerebral
  occlusive I63.5- ☑
  thrombotic I63.3- ☑
 cartilage M94.2- ☑
  patella M22.4- ☑
 cerebellar — *see* Softening, brain
 cerebral — *see* Softening, brain
 cerebrospinal — *see* Softening, brain
 myocardial, heart — *see* Degeneration, myocardial
 spinal cord G95.89
 stomach K31.89
Soldier's
 heart F45.8
 patches I31.0
Solitary
 cyst, kidney N28.1
 kidney, congenital Q60.0
Solvent abuse — *see* Abuse, drug, inhalant
 dependence — *see* Dependence, drug, inhalant

☑ *Subterms under main terms may continue to next column or page*   ☑ **Additional Character Required** — Refer to the Tabular List for Character Selection   287

Sinus — Solvent abuse

Index

Somatization reaction, somatic reaction — Splenopathy

Somatization reaction, somatic reaction — *see* Disorder, somatoform
Somnambulism F51.3
  hysterical F44.89
Somnolence R40.0
  nonorganic origin F51.11
Sonne dysentery A03.3
Soor B37.0
Sore
  bed — *see* Ulcer, pressure, by site
  chiclero B55.1
  Delhi B55.1
  desert — *see* Ulcer, skin
  eye H57.1- ☑
  Lahore B55.1
  mouth K13.79
    canker K12.0
  muscle M79.1
  Naga — *see* Ulcer, skin
  of skin — *see* Ulcer, skin
  oriental B55.1
  pressure — *see* Ulcer, pressure, by site
  skin L98.9
  soft A57
  throat (acute) (*see also* Pharyngitis)
    with influenza, flu, or grippe — *see* Influenza, with, respiratory manifestations NEC
    chronic J31.2
    coxsackie (virus) B08.5
    diphtheritic A36.0
    herpesviral B00.2
    influenzal — *see* Influenza, with, respiratory manifestations NEC
    septic J02.0
    streptococcal (ulcerative) J02.0
    viral NEC J02.8
      coxsackie B08.5
  tropical — *see* Ulcer, skin
  veldt — *see* Ulcer, skin
Soto's syndrome (cerebral gigantism) Q87.3
South African cardiomyopathy syndrome I42.8
Southeast Asian hemorrhagic fever A91
Spacing
  abnormal, tooth, teeth, fully erupted M26.30
  excessive, tooth, fully erupted M26.32
Spade-like hand (congenital) Q68.1
Spading nail L60.8
  congenital Q84.6
Spanish collar N47.1
Sparganosis B70.1
Spasm(s), **spastic, spasticity** (*see also* condition) R25.2
  accommodation — *see* Spasm, of accommodation
  ampulla of Vater K83.4
  anus, ani (sphincter) (reflex) K59.4
    psychogenic F45.8
  artery I73.9
    cerebral G45.9
  Bell's G51.3
  bladder (sphincter, external or internal) N32.89
    psychogenic F45.8
  bronchus, bronchiole J98.01
  cardia K22.0
  cardiac I20.1
  carpopedal — *see* Tetany
  cerebral (arteries) (vascular) G45.9
  cervix, complicating delivery O62.4
  ciliary body (of accommodation) — *see* Spasm, of accommodation
  colon (*see also* Irritable, bowel) K58.9
    with diarrhea K58.0
    psychogenic F45.8
  common duct K83.8
  compulsive — *see* Tic
  conjugate H51.8
  coronary (artery) I20.1
  diaphragm (reflex) R06.6
    epidemic B33.0
    psychogenic F45.8
  duodenum K59.8
  epidemic diaphragmatic (transient) B33.0
  esophagus (diffuse) K22.4
    psychogenic F45.8
  facial G51.3
  fallopian tube N83.8
  gastrointestinal (tract) K31.89
    psychogenic F45.8
  glottis J38.5
    hysterical F44.4

Spasm(s), **spastic, spasticity** — *continued*
  glottis — *continued*
    psychogenic F45.8
      conversion reaction F44.4
    reflex through recurrent laryngeal nerve J38.5
  habit — *see* Tic
  heart I20.1
  hemifacial (clonic) G51.3
  hourglass — *see* Contraction, hourglass
  hysterical F44.4
  infantile — *see* Epilepsy, spasms
  inferior oblique, eye H51.8
  intestinal (*see also* Syndrome, irritable bowel) K58.9
    psychogenic F45.8
  larynx, laryngeal J38.5
    hysterical F44.4
    psychogenic F45.8
      conversion reaction F44.4
  levator palpebrae superioris — *see* Disorder, eyelid function
  muscle NEC M62.838
    back M62.830
  nerve, trigeminal G51.0
  nervous F45.8
  nodding F98.4
  occupational F48.8
  oculogyric H51.8
    psychogenic F45.8
  of accommodation H52.53- ☑
  ophthalmic artery — *see* Occlusion, artery, retina
  perineal, female N94.89
  peroneo-extensor (*see also* Deformity, limb, flat foot)
  pharynx (reflex) J39.2
    hysterical F45.8
    psychogenic F45.8
    psychogenic F45.8
  pylorus NEC K31.3
    adult hypertrophic K31.89
    congenital or infantile Q40.0
    psychogenic F45.8
  rectum (sphincter) K59.4
    psychogenic F45.8
  retinal (artery) — *see* Occlusion, artery, retina
  sigmoid (*see also* Syndrome, irritable bowel) K58.9
    psychogenic F45.8
  sphincter of Oddi K83.4
  stomach K31.89
    neurotic F45.8
  throat J39.2
    hysterical F45.8
    psychogenic F45.8
  tic F95.9
    chronic F95.1
    transient of childhood F95.0
  tongue K14.8
  torsion (progressive) G24.1
  trigeminal nerve — *see* Neuralgia, trigeminal
  ureter N13.5
  urethra (sphincter) N35.9
  uterus N85.8
    complicating labor O62.4
  vagina N94.2
    psychogenic F52.5
  vascular I73.9
  vasomotor I73.9
  vein NEC I87.8
  viscera — *see* Pain, abdominal
Spasmodic — *see* condition
Spasmophilia — *see* Tetany
Spasmus nutans F98.4
Spastic, spasticity (*see also* Spasm)
  child (cerebral) (congenital) (paralysis) G80.1
Speaker's throat R49.8
Specific, specified — *see* condition
Speech
  defect, disorder, disturbance, impediment R47.9
    psychogenic, in childhood and adolescence F98.8
    slurring R47.81
    specified NEC R47.89
Spencer's disease A08.19
Spens' syndrome (syncope with heart block) I45.9
Sperm counts (fertility testing) Z31.41
  postvasectomy Z30.8
    reversal Z31.42
Spermatic cord — *see* condition
Spermatocele N43.40
  congenital Q55.4
  multiple N43.42

Spermatocele — *continued*
  single N43.41
Spermatocystitis N49.0
Spermatocytoma C62.9- ☑
  specified site — *see* Neoplasm, malignant, by site
Spermatorrhea N50.89
Sphacelus — *see* Gangrene
Sphenoidal — *see* condition
Sphenoiditis (chronic) — *see* Sinusitis, sphenoidal
Sphenopalatine ganglion neuralgia G90.09
Sphericity, increased, lens (congenital) Q12.4
Spherocytosis (congenital) (familial) (hereditary) D58.0
  hemoglobin disease D58.0
  sickle-cell (disease) D57.8- ☑
Spherophakia Q12.4
Sphincter — *see* condition
Sphincteritis, sphincter of Oddi — *see* Cholangitis
Sphingolipidosis E75.3
  specified NEC E75.29
Sphingomyelinosis E75.3
Spicule tooth K00.2
Spider
  bite — *see* Toxicity, venom, spider
  fingers — *see* Syndrome, Marfan's
  nevus I78.1
  toes — *see* Syndrome, Marfan's
  vascular I78.1
Spiegler-Fendt
  benign lymphocytoma L98.8
  sarcoid L08.89
Spielmeyer-Vogt disease E75.4
Spina bifida (aperta) Q05.9
  with hydrocephalus NEC Q05.4
  cervical Q05.5
    with hydrocephalus Q05.0
  dorsal Q05.6
    with hydrocephalus Q05.1
  lumbar Q05.7
    with hydrocephalus Q05.2
  lumbosacral Q05.7
    with hydrocephalus Q05.2
  occulta Q76.0
  sacral Q05.8
    with hydrocephalus Q05.3
  thoracic Q05.6
    with hydrocephalus Q05.1
  thoracolumbar Q05.6
    with hydrocephalus Q05.1
Spindle, Krukenberg's — *see* Pigmentation, cornea, posterior
Spine, spinal — *see* condition
Spiradenoma (eccrine) — *see* Neoplasm, skin, benign
Spirillosis A25.0
Spirillum
  minus A25.0
  obermeieri infection A68.0
Spirochetal — *see* condition
Spirochetosis A69.9
  arthritic, arthritica A69.9
  bronchopulmonary A69.8
  icterohemorrhagic A27.0
  lung A69.8
Spirometrosis B70.1
Spitting blood — *see* Hemoptysis
Splanchnoptosis K63.4
Spleen, splenic — *see* condition
Splenectasis — *see* Splenomegaly
Splenitis (interstitial) (malignant) (nonspecific) D73.89
  malarial (*see also* Malaria) B54 [D77]
  tuberculous A18.85
Splenocele D73.89
Splenomegaly, splenomegalia (Bengal) (cryptogenic) (idiopathic) (tropical) R16.1
  with hepatomegaly R16.2
  cirrhotic D73.2
  congenital Q89.09
  congestive, chronic D73.2
  Egyptian B65.1
  Gaucher's E75.22
  malarial (*see also* Malaria) B54 [D77]
  neutropenic D73.81
  Niemann-Pick — *see* Niemann-Pick disease or syndrome
  siderotic D73.2
  syphilitic A52.79
    congenital (early) A50.08 [D77]
Splenopathy D73.9

  ☑ **Additional Character Required** — Refer to the Tabular List for Character Selection   🔺 Subterms under main terms may continue to next column or page

Splenoptosis D73.89
Splenosis D73.89
Splinter — *see* Foreign body, superficial, by site
Split, splitting
  foot Q72.7- ☑
  hand Q71.6 ☑
  heart sounds R01.2
  lip, congenital — *see* Cleft, lip
  nails L60.3
  urinary stream R39.13
Spondylarthrosis — *see* Spondylosis
Spondylitis (chronic) (*see also* Spondylopathy, inflammatory)
  ankylopoietica — *see* Spondylitis, ankylosing
  ankylosing (chronic) M45.9
    with lung involvement M45.9 [J99]
    cervical region M45.2
    cervicothoracic region M45.3
    juvenile M08.1
    lumbar region M45.6
    lumbosacral region M45.7
    multiple sites M45.0
    occipito-atlanto-axial region M45.1
    sacrococcygeal region M45.8
    thoracic region M45.4
    thoracolumbar region M45.5
  atrophic (ligamentous) — *see* Spondylitis, ankylosing
  deformans (chronic) — *see* Spondylosis
  gonococcal A54.41
  gouty (*see also* Gout, by type, vertebrae) M10.08
  in (due to)
    brucellosis A23.9 [M49.80]
      cervical region A23.9 [M49.82]
      cervicothoracic region A23.9 [M49.83]
      lumbar region A23.9 [M49.86]
      lumbosacral region A23.9 [M49.87]
      multiple sites A23.9 [M49.89]
      occipito-atlanto-axial region A23.9 [M49.81]
      sacrococcygeal region A23.9 [M49.88]
      thoracic region A23.9 [M49.84]
      thoracolumbar region A23.9 [M49.85]
    enterobacteria (*see also* subcategory M49.8) A04.9
    tuberculosis A18.01
  infectious NEC — *see* Spondylopathy, infective
  juvenile ankylosing (chronic) M08.1
  Kümmell's — *see* Spondylopathy, traumatic
  Marie-Strümpell — *see* Spondylitis, ankylosing
  muscularis — *see* Spondylopathy, specified NEC
  psoriatic L40.53
  rheumatoid — *see* Spondylitis, ankylosing
  rhizomelica — *see* Spondylitis, ankylosing
  sacroiliac NEC M46.1
  senescent, senile — *see* Spondylosis
  traumatic (chronic) or post-traumatic — *see* Spondylopathy, traumatic
  tuberculous A18.01
  typhosa A01.05
Spondylolisthesis (acquired) (degenerative) M43.10
  with disproportion (fetopelvic) O33.0
    causing obstructed labor O65.0
  cervical region M43.12
  cervicothoracic region M43.13
  congenital Q76.2
  lumbar region M43.16
  lumbosacral region M43.17
  multiple sites M43.19
  occipito-atlanto-axial region M43.11
  sacrococcygeal region M43.18
  thoracic region M43.14
  thoracolumbar region M43.15
  traumatic (old) M43.10
    acute
      fifth cervical (displaced) S12.430 ☑
        nondisplaced S12.431 ☑
        specified type NEC (displaced) S12.450 ☑
          nondisplaced S12.451 ☑
        type III S12.44 ☑
      fourth cervical (displaced) S12.330 ☑
        nondisplaced S12.331 ☑
        specified type NEC (displaced) S12.350 ☑
          nondisplaced S12.351 ☑
        type III S12.34 ☑
      second cervical (displaced) S12.130 ☑
        nondisplaced S12.131 ☑
        specified type NEC (displaced) S12.150 ☑
          nondisplaced S12.151 ☑
        type III S12.14 ☑

Spondylolisthesis — *continued*
  traumatic — *continued*
    acute — *continued*
      seventh cervical (displaced) S12.630 ☑
        nondisplaced S12.631 ☑
        specified type NEC (displaced) S12.650 ☑
          nondisplaced S12.651 ☑
        type III S12.64 ☑
      sixth cervical (displaced) S12.530 ☑
        nondisplaced S12.531 ☑
        specified type NEC (displaced) S12.550 ☑
          nondisplaced S12.551 ☑
        type III S12.54 ☑
      third cervical (displaced) S12.230 ☑
        nondisplaced S12.231 ☑
        specified type NEC (displaced) S12.250 ☑
          nondisplaced S12.251 ☑
        type III S12.24 ☑
Spondylolysis (acquired) M43.00
  cervical region M43.02
  cervicothoracic region M43.03
  congenital Q76.2
  lumbar region M43.06
  lumbosacral region M43.07
    with disproportion (fetopelvic) O33.0
      causing obstructed labor O65.8
  multiple sites M43.09
  occipito-atlanto-axial region M43.01
  sacrococcygeal region M43.08
  thoracic region M43.04
  thoracolumbar region M43.05
Spondylopathy M48.9
  infective NEC M46.50
    cervical region M46.52
    cervicothoracic region M46.53
    lumbar region M46.56
    lumbosacral region M46.57
    multiple sites M46.59
    occipito-atlanto-axial region M46.51
    sacrococcygeal region M46.58
    thoracic region M46.54
    thoracolumbar region M46.55
  inflammatory M46.90
    cervical region M46.92
    cervicothoracic region M46.93
    lumbar region M46.96
    lumbosacral region M46.97
    multiple sites M46.99
    occipito-atlanto-axial region M46.91
    sacrococcygeal region M46.98
    specified type NEC M46.80
      cervical region M46.82
      cervicothoracic region M46.83
      lumbar region M46.86
      lumbosacral region M46.87
      multiple sites M46.89
      occipito-atlanto-axial region M46.81
      sacrococcygeal region M46.88
      thoracic region M46.84
      thoracolumbar region M46.85
    thoracic region M46.94
    thoracolumbar region M46.95
  neuropathic, in
    syringomyelia and syringobulbia G95.0
    tabes dorsalis A52.11
  specified NEC — *see* subcategory M48.8 ☑
  traumatic M48.30
    cervical region M48.32
    cervicothoracic region M48.33
    lumbar region M48.36
    lumbosacral region M48.37
    occipito-atlanto-axial region M48.31
    sacrococcygeal region M48.38
    thoracic region M48.34
    thoracolumbar region M48.35
Spondylosis M47.9
  with
    disproportion (fetopelvic) O33.0
      causing obstructed labor O65.0
    myelopathy NEC M47.10
      cervical region M47.12
      cervicothoracic region M47.13
      lumbar region M47.16
      occipito-atlanto-axial region M47.11
      thoracic region M47.14
      thoracolumbar region M47.15
    radiculopathy M47.20
      cervical region M47.22

Spondylosis — *continued*
  with — *continued*
    radiculopathy — *continued*
      cervicothoracic region M47.23
      lumbar region M47.26
      lumbosacral region M47.27
      occipito-atlanto-axial region M47.21
      sacrococcygeal region M47.28
      thoracic region M47.24
      thoracolumbar region M47.25
  without myelopathy or radiculopathy M47.819
    cervical region M47.812
    cervicothoracic region M47.813
    lumbar region M47.816
    lumbosacral region M47.817
    occipito-atlanto-axial region M47.811
    sacrococcygeal region M47.818
    thoracic region M47.814
    thoracolumbar region M47.815
  specified NEC M47.899
    cervical region M47.892
    cervicothoracic region M47.893
    lumbar region M47.896
    lumbosacral region M47.897
    occipito-atlanto-axial region M47.891
    sacrococcygeal region M47.898
    thoracic region M47.894
    thoracolumbar region M47.895
  traumatic — *see* Spondylopathy, traumatic
Sponge
  inadvertently left in operation wound — *see* Foreign body, accidentally left during a procedure
  kidney (medullary) Q61.5
Sponge-diver's disease — *see* Toxicity, venom, marine animal, sea anemone
Spongioblastoma (any type) — *see* Neoplasm, malignant, by site
  specified site — *see* Neoplasm, malignant, by site
  unspecified site C71.9
Spongioneuroblastoma — *see* Neoplasm, malignant, by site
Spontaneous (*see also* condition)
  fracture (cause unknown) — *see* Fracture, pathological
Spoon nail L60.3
  congenital Q84.6
Sporadic — *see* condition
Sporothrix schenckii infection — *see* Sporotrichosis
Sporotrichosis B42.9
  arthritis B42.82
  disseminated B42.7
  generalized B42.7
  lymphocutaneous (fixed) (progressive) B42.1
  pulmonary B42.0
  specified NEC B42.89
Spots, spotting (in) (of)
  Bitot's (*see also* Pigmentation, conjunctiva)
    in the young child E50.1
    vitamin A deficiency E50.1
  café, au lait L81.3
  Cayenne pepper I78.1
  cotton wool, retina — *see* Occlusion, artery, retina
  de Morgan's (senile angiomas) I78.1
  Fuchs' black (myopic) (*see also* Myopia, degenerative) H44.2- ☑
  intermenstrual (regular) N92.0
    irregular N92.1
  Koplik's B05.9
  liver L81.4
  pregnancy O26.85- ☑
  purpuric R23.3
  ruby I78.1
Spotted fever — *see* Fever, spotted N92.3
Sprain (joint) (ligament)
  acromioclavicular joint or ligament S43.5- ☑
  ankle S93.40- ☑
    calcaneofibular ligament S93.41- ☑
    deltoid ligament S93.42- ☑
    internal collateral ligament — *see* Sprain, ankle, specified ligament NEC
    specified ligament NEC S93.49- ☑
    talofibular ligament — *see* Sprain, ankle, specified ligament NEC
    tibiofibular ligament S93.43- ☑
  anterior longitudinal, cervical S13.4 ☑
  atlas, atlanto-axial, atlanto-occipital S13.4 ☑
  breast bone — *see* Sprain, sternum
  calcaneofibular — *see* Sprain, ankle
  carpal — *see* Sprain, wrist

▽ Subterms under main terms may continue to next column or page   ☑ Additional Character Required — Refer to the Tabular List for Character Selection   289

Splenoptosis — Sprain

Index

Sprain — Stähli's line

Sprain — *continued*
- carpometacarpal — *see* Sprain, hand, specified site NEC
- cartilage
  - costal S23.41 ☑
  - semilunar (knee) — *see* Sprain, knee, specified site NEC
    - with current tear — *see* Tear, meniscus
  - thyroid region S13.5 ☑
  - xiphoid — *see* Sprain, sternum
- cervical, cervicodorsal, cervicothoracic S13.4 ☑
- chondrosternal S23.421 ☑
- coracoclavicular S43.8- ☑
- coracohumeral S43.41- ☑
- coronary, knee — *see* Sprain, knee, specified site NEC
- costal cartilage S23.41 ☑
- cricoarytenoid articulation or ligament S13.5 ☑
- cricothyroid articulation S13.5 ☑
- cruciate, knee — *see* Sprain, knee, cruciate
- deltoid, ankle — *see* Sprain, ankle
- dorsal (spine) S23.3 ☑
- elbow S53.40- ☑
  - radial collateral ligament S53.43- ☑
  - radiohumeral S53.41- ☑
  - rupture
    - radial collateral ligament — *see* Rupture, traumatic, ligament, radial collateral
    - ulnar collateral ligament — *see* Rupture, traumatic, ligament, ulnar collateral
  - specified type NEC S53.49- ☑
  - ulnar collateral ligament S53.44- ☑
  - ulnohumeral S53.42- ☑
- femur, head — *see* Sprain, hip
- fibular collateral, knee — *see* Sprain, knee, collateral
- fibulocalcaneal — *see* Sprain, ankle
- finger(s) S63.61- ☑
  - index S63.61- ☑
  - interphalangeal (joint) S63.63- ☑
    - index S63.63- ☑
    - little S63.63- ☑
    - middle S63.63- ☑
    - ring S63.63- ☑
  - little S63.61- ☑
  - metacarpophalangeal (joint) S63.65- ☑
  - middle S63.61- ☑
  - ring S63.61- ☑
  - specified site NEC S63.69- ☑
    - index S63.69- ☑
    - little S63.69- ☑
    - middle S63.69- ☑
    - ring S63.69- ☑
- foot S93.60- ☑
  - specified ligament NEC S93.69- ☑
  - tarsal ligament S93.61- ☑
  - tarsometatarsal ligament S93.62- ☑
  - toe — *see* Sprain, toe
- hand S63.9- ☑
  - finger — *see* Sprain, finger
  - specified site NEC — *see* subcategory S63.8 ☑
  - thumb — *see* Sprain, thumb
- head S03.9 ☑
- hip S73.10- ☑
  - iliofemoral ligament S73.11- ☑
  - ischiocapsular (ligament) S73.12- ☑
  - specified NEC S73.19- ☑
- iliofemoral — *see* Sprain, hip
- innominate
  - acetabulum — *see* Sprain, hip
  - sacral junction S33.6 ☑
- internal
  - collateral, ankle — *see* Sprain, ankle
  - semilunar cartilage — *see* Sprain, knee, specified site NEC
- interphalangeal
  - finger — *see* Sprain, finger, interphalangeal (joint)
  - toe — *see* Sprain, toe, interphalangeal joint
- ischiocapsular — *see* Sprain, hip
- ischiofemoral — *see* Sprain, hip
- jaw (articular disc) (cartilage) (meniscus) S03.4- ☑
  - old M26.69
- knee S83.9- ☑
  - collateral ligament S83.40- ☑
    - lateral (fibular) S83.42- ☑
    - medial (tibial) S83.41- ☑
  - cruciate ligament S83.50- ☑
    - anterior S83.51- ☑

Sprain — *continued*
- knee — *continued*
  - cruciate ligament — *continued*
    - posterior S83.52- ☑
  - lateral (fibular) collateral ligament S83.42- ☑
  - medial (tibial) collateral ligament S83.41- ☑
  - patellar ligament S76.11- ☑
  - specified site NEC S83.8X- ☑
  - superior tibiofibular joint (ligament) S83.6- ☑
- lateral collateral, knee — *see* Sprain, knee, collateral
- lumbar (spine) S33.5 ☑
- lumbosacral S33.9 ☑
- mandible (articular disc) S03.4- ☑
  - old M26.69
- medial collateral, knee — *see* Sprain, knee, collateral
- meniscus
  - jaw S03.4- ☑
    - old M26.69
  - knee — *see* Sprain, knee, specified site NEC
    - with current tear — *see* Tear, meniscus
      - old — *see* Derangement, knee, meniscus, due to old tear
  - mandible S03.4- ☑
    - old M26.69
- metacarpal (distal) (proximal) — *see* Sprain, hand, specified site NEC
- metacarpophalangeal — *see* Sprain, finger, metacarpophalangeal (joint)
- metatarsophalangeal — *see* Sprain, toe, metatarsophalangeal joint
- midcarpal — *see* Sprain, hand, specified site NEC
- midtarsal — *see* Sprain, foot, specified site NEC
- neck S13.9 ☑
  - anterior longitudinal cervical ligament S13.4 ☑
  - atlanto-axial joint S13.4 ☑
  - atlanto-occipital joint S13.4 ☑
  - cervical spine S13.4 ☑
  - cricoarytenoid ligament S13.5 ☑
  - cricothyroid ligament S13.5 ☑
  - specified site NEC S13.8 ☑
  - thyroid region (cartilage) S13.5 ☑
- nose S03.8 ☑
- orbicular, hip — *see* Sprain, hip
- patella — *see* Sprain, knee, specified site NEC
- patellar ligament S76.11- ☑
- pelvis NEC S33.8 ☑
- phalanx
  - finger — *see* Sprain, finger
  - toe — *see* Sprain, toe
- pubofemoral — *see* Sprain, hip
- radiocarpal — *see* Sprain, wrist
- radiohumeral — *see* Sprain, elbow
- radius, collateral — *see* Rupture, traumatic, ligament, radial collateral
- rib (cage) S23.41 ☑
- rotator cuff (capsule) S43.42- ☑
- sacroiliac (region)
  - chronic or old — *see* subcategory M53.2 ☑
  - joint S33.6 ☑
- scaphoid (hand) — *see* Sprain, hand, specified site NEC
- scapula (r) — *see* Sprain, shoulder girdle, specified site NEC
- semilunar cartilage (knee) — *see* Sprain, knee, specified site NEC
  - with current tear — *see* Tear, meniscus
    - old — *see* Derangement, knee, meniscus, due to old tear
- shoulder joint S43.40- ☑
  - acromioclavicular joint (ligament) — *see* Sprain, acromioclavicular joint
  - blade — *see* Sprain, shoulder, girdle, specified site NEC
  - coracoclavicular joint (ligament) — *see* Sprain, coracoclavicular joint
  - coracohumeral ligament — *see* Sprain, coracohumeral joint
  - girdle S43.9- ☑
    - specified site NEC S43.8- ☑
  - rotator cuff — *see* Sprain, rotator cuff
  - specified site NEC S43.49- ☑
  - sternoclavicular joint (ligament) — *see* Sprain, sternoclavicular joint
- spine
  - cervical S13.4 ☑
  - lumbar S33.5 ☑

Sprain — *continued*
- spine — *continued*
  - thoracic S23.3 ☑
- sternoclavicular joint S43.6- ☑
- sternum S23.429 ☑
  - chondrosternal joint S23.421 ☑
  - specified site NEC S23.428 ☑
  - sternoclavicular (joint) (ligament) S23.420 ☑
- symphysis
  - jaw S03.4- ☑
    - old M26.69
  - mandibular S03.4- ☑
    - old M26.69
- talofibular — *see* Sprain, ankle
- tarsal — *see* Sprain, foot, specified site NEC
- tarsometatarsal — *see* Sprain, foot, specified site NEC
- temporomandibular S03.4- ☑
  - old M26.69
- thorax S23.9 ☑
  - ribs S23.41 ☑
  - specified site NEC S23.8 ☑
  - spine S23.3 ☑
  - sternum — *see* Sprain, sternum
- thumb S63.60- ☑
  - interphalangeal (joint) S63.62- ☑
  - metacarpophalangeal (joint) S63.64- ☑
  - specified site NEC S63.68- ☑
- thyroid cartilage or region S13.5 ☑
- tibia (proximal end) — *see* Sprain, knee, specified site NEC
- tibial collateral, knee — *see* Sprain, knee, collateral
- tibiofibular
  - distal — *see* Sprain, ankle
  - superior — *see* Sprain, knee, specified site NEC
- toe(s) S93.50- ☑
  - great S93.50- ☑
  - interphalangeal joint S93.51- ☑
    - great S93.51- ☑
    - lesser S93.51- ☑
  - lesser S93.50- ☑
  - metatarsophalangeal joint S93.52- ☑
    - great S93.52- ☑
    - lesser S93.52- ☑
- ulna, collateral — *see* Rupture, traumatic, ligament, ulnar collateral
- ulnohumeral — *see* Sprain, elbow
- wrist S63.50- ☑
  - carpal S63.51- ☑
  - radiocarpal S63.52- ☑
  - specified site NEC S63.59- ☑
- xiphoid cartilage — *see* Sprain, sternum

Sprengel's deformity (congenital) Q74.0
Sprue (tropical) K90.1
- celiac K90.0
- idiopathic K90.49
- meaning thrush B37.0
- nontropical K90.0
Spur, bone (*see also* Enthesopathy)
- calcaneal M77.3- ☑
- iliac crest M76.2- ☑
- nose (septum) J34.89
Spurway's syndrome Q78.0
Sputum
- abnormal (amount) (color) (odor) (purulent) R09.3
- blood-stained R04.2
- excessive (cause unknown) R09.3
Squamous (*see also* condition)
- epithelium in
  - cervical canal (congenital) Q51.828
  - uterine mucosa (congenital) Q51.818
Squashed nose M95.0
- congenital Q67.4
Squeeze, diver's T70.3 ☑
Squint (*see also* Strabismus)
- accommodative — *see* Strabismus, convergent concomitant
St. Hubert's disease A82.9
Stab (*see also* Laceration)
- internal organs — *see* Injury, by site
Stafne's cyst or cavity M27.0
Staggering gait R26.0
- hysterical F44.4
Staghorn calculus — *see* Calculus, kidney
Stähli's line (cornea) (pigment) — *see* Pigmentation, cornea, anterior

☑ Additional Character Required — Refer to the Tabular List for Character Selection   Subterms under main terms may continue to next column or page

Stain, staining
  meconium (newborn) P96.83
  port wine Q82.5
  tooth, teeth (hard tissues) (extrinsic) K03.6
    due to
      accretions K03.6
      deposits (betel) (black) (green) (materia alba)
        (orange) (soft) (tobacco) K03.6
      metals (copper) (silver) K03.7
      nicotine K03.6
      pulpal bleeding K03.7
      tobacco K03.6
    intrinsic K00.8
Stammering (see also Disorder, fluency) F80.81
Standstill
  auricular I45.5
  cardiac — see Arrest, cardiac
  sinoatrial I45.5
  ventricular — see Arrest, cardiac
Stannosis J63.5
Stanton's disease — see Melioidosis
Staphylitis (acute) (catarrhal) (chronic) (gangrenous)
  (membranous) (suppurative) (ulcerative) K12.2
Staphylococcal scalded skin syndrome L00
Staphylococcemia A41.2
Staphylococcus, staphylococcal (see also condition)
  as cause of disease classified elsewhere B95.8
    aureus (methicillin susceptible) B95.61
      methicillin resistant (MRSA) B95.62
  specified NEC, as cause of disease classified elsewhere
    B95.7
Staphyloma (sclera)
  cornea H18.72- ☑
  equatorial H15.81- ☑
  localized (anterior) H15.82- ☑
  posticum H15.83- ☑
  ring H15.85- ☑
Stargardt's disease — see Dystrophy, retina
Starvation (inanition) (due to lack of food) T73.0 ☑
  edema — see Malnutrition, severe
Stasis
  bile (noncalculous) K83.1
  bronchus J98.09
    with infection — see Bronchitis
  cardiac — see Failure, heart, congestive
  cecum K59.8
  colon K59.8
  dermatitis I87.2
    with
      varicose ulcer — see Varix, leg, with ulcer, with
        inflammation
      varicose veins — see Varix, leg, with, inflamma-
        tion
      due to postthrombotic syndrome — see Syndrome,
        postthrombotic
  duodenal K31.5
  eczema — see Varix, leg, with, inflammation
  edema — see Hypertension, venous (chronic), idiopath-
    ic
  foot T69.0- ☑
  ileocecal coil K59.8
  ileum K59.8
  intestinal K59.8
  jejunum K59.8
  kidney N19
  liver (cirrhotic) K76.1
  lymphatic I89.8
  pneumonia J18.2
  pulmonary — see Edema, lung
  rectal K59.8
  renal N19
    tubular N17.0
  ulcer — see Varix, leg, with, ulcer
    without varicose veins I87.2
  urine — see Retention, urine
  venous I87.8
State (of)
  affective and paranoid, mixed, organic psychotic F06.8
  agitated R45.1
    acute reaction to stress F43.0
  anxiety (neurotic) F41.1
  apprehension F41.1
  burn-out Z73.0
  climacteric, female Z78.0
    symptomatic N95.1
  compulsive F42.8
    mixed with obsessional thoughts F42.2
  confusional (psychogenic) F44.89

State — continued
  confusional — continued
    acute (see also Delirium)
      with
        arteriosclerotic dementia F01.50
          with behavioral disturbance F01.51
        senility or dementia F05
      alcoholic F10.231
    epileptic F05
    reactive (from emotional stress, psychological
      trauma) F44.89
    subacute — see Delirium
  convulsive — see Convulsions
  crisis F43.0
  depressive F32.9
    neurotic F34.1
  dissociative F44.9
  emotional shock (stress) R45.7
  hypercoagulation — see Hypercoagulable
  locked-in G83.5
  menopausal Z78.0
    symptomatic N95.1
  neurotic F48.9
    with depersonalization F48.1
  obsessional F42.8
  oneiroid (schizophrenia-like) F23
  organic
    hallucinatory (nonalcoholic) F06.0
    paranoid (-hallucinatory) F06.2
  panic F41.0
  paranoid F22
    climacteric F22
    involutional F22
    menopausal F22
    organic F06.2
    senile F03 ☑
    simple F22
  persistent vegetative R40.3
  phobic F40.9
  postleukotomy F07.0
  pregnant
    gestational carrier Z33.3
    incidental Z33.1
  psychogenic, twilight F44.89
  psychopathic (constitutional) F60.2
  psychotic, organic (see also Psychosis, organic)
    mixed paranoid and affective F06.8
    senile or presenile F03 ☑
    transient NEC F06.8
      with
        depression F06.31
        hallucinations F06.0
  residual schizophrenic F20.5
  restlessness R45.1
  stress (emotional) R45.7
  tension (mental) F48.9
    specified NEC F48.8
  transient organic psychotic NEC F06.8
    depressive type F06.31
    hallucinatory type F06.0
  twilight
    epileptic F05
    psychogenic F44.89
  vegetative, persistent R40.3
  vital exhaustion Z73.0
  withdrawal, — see Withdrawal, state
Status (post) (see also Presence (of))
  absence, epileptic — see Epilepsy, by type, with status
    epilepticus
  administration of tPA (rtPA) in a different facility
    within the last 24 hours prior to admission to
    current facility Z92.82
  adrenalectomy (unilateral) (bilateral) E89.6
  anastomosis Z98.0
  anginosus I20.9
  angioplasty (peripheral) Z98.62
    with implant Z95.820
    coronary artery Z98.61
      with implant Z95.5
  aortocoronary bypass Z95.1
  arthrodesis Z98.1
  artificial opening (of) Z93.9
    gastrointestinal tract Z93.4
    specified NEC Z93.8
    urinary tract Z93.6
    vagina Z93.8
  asthmaticus — see Asthma, by type, with status asth-
    maticus

Status — continued
  awaiting organ transplant Z76.82
  bariatric surgery Z98.84
  bed confinement Z74.01
  bleb, filtering (vitreous), after glaucoma surgery Z98.83
  breast implant Z98.82
    removal Z98.86
  cataract extraction Z98.4- ☑
  cholecystectomy Z90.49
  clitorectomy N90.811
    with excision of labia minora N90.812
  colectomy (complete) (partial) Z90.49
  colonization — see Carrier (suspected) of
  colostomy Z93.3
  convulsivus idiopathicus — see Epilepsy, by type, with
    status epilepticus
  coronary artery angioplasty — see Status, angioplasty,
    coronary artery
  coronary artery bypass graft Z95.1
  cystectomy (urinary bladder) Z90.6
  cystostomy Z93.50
    appendico-vesicostomy Z93.52
    cutaneous Z93.51
    specified NEC Z93.59
  delinquent immunization Z28.3
  dental Z98.818
    crown Z98.811
    fillings Z98.811
    restoration Z98.811
    sealant Z98.810
    specified NEC Z98.818
  deployment (current) (military) Z56.82
  dialysis (hemodialysis) (peritoneal) Z99.2
  do not resuscitate (DNR) Z66
  donor — see Donor
  embedded fragments — see Retained, foreign body
    fragments (type of)
  embedded splinter — see Retained, foreign body
    fragments (type of)
  enterostomy Z93.4
  epileptic, epilepticus (see also Epilepsy, by type, with
    status epilepticus) G40.901
  estrogen receptor
    negative Z17.1
    positive Z17.0
  female genital cutting — see Female genital mutilation
    status
  female genital mutilation — see Female genital muti-
    lation status
  filtering (vitreous) bleb after glaucoma surgery Z98.83
  gastrectomy (complete) (partial) Z90.3
  gastric banding Z98.84
  gastric bypass for obesity Z98.84
  gastrostomy Z93.1
  human immunodeficiency virus (HIV) infection,
    asymptomatic Z21
  hysterectomy (complete) (total) Z90.710
    partial (with remaining cervial stump) Z90.711
  ileostomy Z93.2
  implant
    breast Z98.82
  infibulation N90.813
  intestinal bypass Z98.0
  jejunostomy Z93.4
  lapsed immunization schedule Z28.3
  laryngectomy Z90.02
  lymphaticus E32.8
  malignancy
    castrate resistant prostate Z19.2
    hormone resistant Z19.2
    hormone sensitive Z19.1
  marmoratus G80.3
  mastectomy (unilateral) (bilateral) Z90.1- ☑
  military deployment status (current) Z56.82
    in theater or in support of military war, peacekeep-
      ing and humanitarian operations Z56.82
  nephrectomy (unilateral) (bilateral) Z90.5
  nephrostomy Z93.6
  obesity surgery Z98.84
  oophorectomy
    bilateral Z90.722
    unilateral Z90.721
  organ replacement
    by artificial or mechanical device or prosthesis of
      artery Z95.828
      bladder Z96.0
      blood vessel Z95.828
      breast Z97.8

▽ **Subterms under main terms may continue to next column or page**   ☑ **Additional Character Required — Refer to the Tabular List for Character Selection**   **291**

Stain, staining — Status

Index

Status — Stenosis, stenotic

Status — continued
  organ replacement — continued
    by artificial or mechanical device or prosthesis of
        — continued
      eye globe Z97.0
      heart Z95.812
        valve Z95.2
      intestine Z97.8
      joint Z96.60
        hip — see Presence, hip joint implant
        knee — see Presence, knee joint implant
        specified site NEC Z96.698
      kidney Z97.8
      larynx Z96.3
      lens Z96.1
      limbs — see Presence, artificial, limb
      liver Z97.8
      lung Z97.8
      pancreas Z97.8
    by organ transplant (heterologous)(homologous)
        — see Transplant
  pacemaker
    brain Z96.89
    cardiac Z95.0
    specified NEC Z96.89
  pancreatectomy Z90.410
    complete Z90.410
    partial Z90.411
    total Z90.410
  physical restraint Z78.1
  pneumonectomy (complete) (partial) Z90.2
  pneumothorax, therapeutic Z98.3
  postcommotio cerebri F07.81
  postoperative (postprocedural) NEC Z98.890
    breast implant Z98.82
    dental Z98.818
      crown Z98.811
      fillings Z98.811
      restoration Z98.811
      sealant Z98.810
      specified NEC Z98.818
    pneumothorax, therapeutic Z98.3
    uterine scar Z98.891
  postpartum (routine follow-up) Z39.2
    care immediately after delivery Z39.0
  postsurgical (postprocedural) NEC Z98.890
    pneumothorax, therapeutic Z98.3
  pregnancy, incidental Z33.1
  prosthesis coronary angioplasty Z95.5
  pseudophakia Z96.1
  renal dialysis (hemodialysis) (peritoneal) Z99.2
  retained foreign body — see Retained, foreign body
      fragments (type of)
  reversed jejunal transposition (for bypass) Z98.0
  salpingo-oophorectomy
    bilateral Z90.722
    unilateral Z90.721
  sex reassignment surgery status Z87.890
  shunt
    arteriovenous (for dialysis) Z99.2
    cerebrospinal fluid Z98.2
    ventricular (communicating) (for drainage) Z98.2
  splenectomy Z90.81
  thymicolymphaticus E32.8
  thymicus E32.8
  thymolymphaticus E32.8
  thyroidectomy (hypothyroidism) E89.0
  tooth (teeth) extraction (see also Absence, teeth, ac-
      quired) K08.409
  tPA (rtPA) administration in a different facility within
      the last 24 hours prior to admission to current
      facility Z92.82
  tracheostomy Z93.0
  transplant — see Transplant
    organ removed Z98.85
  tubal ligation Z98.51
  underimmunization Z28.3
  ureterostomy Z93.6
  urethrostomy Z93.6
  vagina, artificial Z93.8
  vasectomy Z98.52
  wheelchair confinement Z99.3
Stealing
  child problem F91.8
    in company with others Z72.810
  pathological (compulsive) F63.2
Steam burn — see Burn
Steatocystoma multiplex L72.2

Steatohepatitis (nonalcoholic) (NASH) K75.81
Steatoma L72.3
  eyelid (cystic) — see Dermatosis, eyelid
    infected — see Hordeolum
Steatorrhea (chronic) K90.9
  with lacteal obstruction K90.2
  idiopathic (adult) (infantile) K90.9
  pancreatic K90.3
  primary K90.0
  tropical K90.1
Steatosis E88.89
  heart — see Degeneration, myocardial
  kidney N28.89
  liver NEC K76.0
Steele-Richardson-Olszewski disease or syndrome
    G23.1
Steinbrocker's syndrome G90.8
Steinert's disease G71.11
Stein-Leventhal syndrome E28.2
Stein's syndrome E28.2
STEMI (see also Infarct, myocardium, ST elevation) I21.3
Stenocardia I20.8
Stenocephaly Q75.8
Stenosis, stenotic (cicatricial) (see also Stricture)
  ampulla of Vater K83.1
  anus, anal (canal) (sphincter) K62.4
    and rectum K62.4
      congenital Q42.3
        with fistula Q42.2
  aorta (ascending) (supraventricular) (congenital) Q25.1
    arteriosclerotic I70.0
    calcified I70.0
    supravalvular Q25.3
  aortic (valve) I35.0
    with insufficiency I35.2
    congenital Q23.0
    rheumatic I06.0
      with
        incompetency, insufficiency or regurgitation
            I06.2
          with mitral (valve) disease I08.0
            with tricuspid (valve) disease I08.3
        mitral (valve) disease I08.0
          with tricuspid (valve) disease I08.3
        tricuspid (valve) disease I08.2
          with mitral (valve) disease I08.3
    specified cause NEC I35.0
    syphilitic A52.03
  aqueduct of Sylvius (congenital) Q03.0
    with spina bifida — see Spina bifida, by site, with
        hydrocephalus
    acquired G91.1
  artery NEC (see also Arteriosclerosis) I77.1
    celiac I77.4
    cerebral — see Occlusion, artery, cerebral
    extremities — see Arteriosclerosis, extremities
    precerebral — see Occlusion, artery, precerebral
    pulmonary (congenital) Q25.6
      acquired I28.8
    renal I70.1
    stent
      coronary T82.855 ☑
      peripheral T82.856 ☑
  bile duct (common) (hepatic) K83.1
    congenital Q44.3
  bladder-neck (acquired) N32.0
    congenital Q64.31
  brain G93.89
  bronchus J98.09
    congenital Q32.3
    syphilitic A52.72
  cardia (stomach) K22.2
    congenital Q39.3
  cardiovascular — see Disease, cardiovascular
  caudal M48.08
  cervix, cervical (canal) N88.2
    congenital Q51.828
    in pregnancy or childbirth — see Pregnancy,
        complicated by, abnormal cervix
  colon (see also Obstruction, intestine)
    congenital Q42.9
      specified NEC Q42.8
  colostomy K94.03
  common (bile) duct K83.1
    congenital Q44.3
  coronary (artery) — see Disease, heart, ischemic,
      atherosclerotic
  cystic duct — see Obstruction, gallbladder

Stenosis, stenotic — continued
  due to presence of device, implant or graft (see also
      Complications, by site and type, specified NEC)
      T85.858 ☑
    arterial graft NEC T82.858 ☑
    breast (implant) T85.858 ☑
    catheter T85.858 ☑
      dialysis (renal) T82.858 ☑
        intraperitoneal T85.858 ☑
      infusion NEC T82.858 ☑
        spinal (epidural) (subdural) T85.850 ☑
      urinary (indwelling) T83.85 ☑
    fixation, internal (orthopedic) NEC T84.85 ☑
    gastrointestinal (bile duct) (esophagus) T85.858 ☑
    genital NEC T83.85 ☑
    heart NEC T82.857 ☑
    joint prosthesis T84.85 ☑
    ocular (corneal graft) (orbital implant) NEC
        T85.858 ☑
    orthopedic NEC T84.85 ☑
    specified NEC T85.858 ☑
    urinary NEC T83.85 ☑
    vascular NEC T82.858 ☑
    ventricular intracranial shunt T85.850 ☑
  duodenum K31.5
    congenital Q41.0
  ejaculatory duct NEC N50.89
    stent
      vascular
        end stent
          adjacent to stent — see Arteriosclerosis
          within the stent
            coronary T82.855 ☑
            peripheral T82.856 ☑
        in stent
          coronary vessel T82.855 ☑
          peripheral vessel T82.856 ☑
  endocervical os — see Stenosis, cervix
  enterostomy K94.13
  esophagus K22.2
    congenital Q39.3
    syphilitic A52.79
      congenital A50.59 [K23]
  eustachian tube — see Obstruction, eustachian tube
  external ear canal (acquired) H61.30- ☑
    congenital Q16.1
    due to
      inflammation H61.32- ☑
      trauma H61.31- ☑
    postprocedural H95.81- ☑
    specified cause NEC H61.39- ☑
  gallbladder — see Obstruction, gallbladder
  glottis J38.6
  heart valve (congenital) Q24.8
    aortic Q23.0
    mitral Q23.2
    pulmonary Q22.1
    tricuspid Q22.4
  hepatic duct K83.1
  hymen N89.6
  hypertrophic subaortic (idiopathic) I42.1
  ileum (see also Obstruction, intestine, specified NEC)
      K56.699
    congenital Q41.2
  infundibulum cardia Q24.3
  intervertebral foramina (see also Lesion, biomechani-
      cal, specified NEC)
    connective tissue M99.79
      abdomen M99.79
      cervical region M99.71
      cervicothoracic M99.71
      head region M99.70
      lumbar region M99.73
      lumbosacral M99.73
      occipitocervical M99.70
      sacral region M99.74
      sacrococcygeal M99.74
      sacroiliac M99.74
      specified NEC M99.79
      thoracic region M99.72
      thoracolumbar M99.72
    disc M99.79
      abdomen M99.79
      cervical region M99.71
      cervicothoracic M99.71
      head region M99.70
      lower extremity M99.76

☑ Additional Character Required — Refer to the Tabular List for Character Selection   ᵀᴿᵁ Subterms under main terms may continue to next column or page

Stenosis, stenotic — *continued*
  intervertebral foramina (*see also* Lesion, biomechanical,
      specified) — *continued*
    disc — *continued*
      lumbar region M99.73
      lumbosacral M99.73
      occipitocervical M99.70
      pelvic M99.75
      rib cage M99.78
      sacral region M99.74
      sacrococcygeal M99.74
      sacroiliac M99.74
      specified NEC M99.79
      thoracic region M99.72
      thoracolumbar M99.72
      upper extremity M99.77
    osseous M99.69
      abdomen M99.69
      cervical region M99.61
      cervicothoracic M99.61
      head region M99.60
      lower extremity M99.66
      lumbar region M99.63
      lumbosacral M99.63
      occipitocervical M99.60
      pelvic M99.65
      rib cage M99.68
      sacral region M99.64
      sacrococcygeal M99.64
      sacroiliac M99.64
      specified NEC M99.69
      thoracic region M99.62
      thoracolumbar M99.62
      upper extremity M99.67
    subluxation — *see* Stenosis, intervertebral forami-
        na, osseous
  intestine (*see also* Obstruction, intestine)
    congenital (small) Q41.9
      large Q42.9
        specified NEC Q42.8
      specified NEC Q41.8
  jejunum (*see also* Obstruction, intestine, specified NEC)
      K56.699
    congenital Q41.1
  lacrimal (passage)
    canaliculi H04.54- ☑
    congenital Q10.5
    duct H04.55- ☑
    punctum H04.56- ☑
    sac H04.57- ☑
  lacrimonasal duct — *see* Stenosis, lacrimal, duct
    congenital Q10.5
  larynx J38.6
    congenital NEC Q31.8
      subglottic Q31.1
    syphilitic A52.73
      congenital A50.59 [J99]
  mitral (chronic) (inactive) (valve) I05.0
    with
      aortic valve disease I08.0
      incompetency, insufficiency or regurgitation
          I05.2
    active or acute I01.1
      with rheumatic or Sydenham's chorea I02.0
    congenital Q23.2
    specified cause, except rheumatic I34.2
    syphilitic A52.03
  myocardium, myocardial (*see also* Degeneration, my-
      ocardial)
    hypertrophic subaortic (idiopathic) I42.1
  nares (anterior) (posterior) J34.89
    congenital Q30.0
  nasal duct (*see also* Stenosis, lacrimal, duct)
    congenital Q10.5
  nasolacrimal duct (*see also* Stenosis, lacrimal, duct)
    congenital Q10.5
  neural canal (*see also* Lesion, biomechanical, specified
      NEC)
    connective tissue M99.49
      abdomen M99.49
      cervical region M99.41
      cervicothoracic M99.41
      head region M99.40
      lower extremity M99.46
      lumbar region M99.43
      lumbosacral M99.43
      occipitocervical M99.40
      pelvic M99.45

Stenosis, stenotic — *continued*
  neural canal (*see also* Lesion, biomechanical, specified)
      — *continued*
    connective tissue — *continued*
      rib cage M99.48
      sacral region M99.44
      sacrococcygeal M99.44
      sacroiliac M99.44
      specified NEC M99.49
      thoracic region M99.42
      thoracolumbar M99.42
      upper extremity M99.47
    intervertebral disc M99.59
      abdomen M99.59
      cervical region M99.51
      cervicothoracic M99.51
      head region M99.50
      lower extremity M99.56
      lumbar region M99.53
      lumbosacral M99.53
      occipitocervical M99.50
      pelvic M99.55
      rib cage M99.58
      sacral region M99.54
      sacrococcygeal M99.54
      sacroiliac M99.54
      specified NEC M99.59
      thoracic region M99.52
      thoracolumbar M99.52
      upper extremity M99.57
    osseous M99.39
      abdomen M99.39
      cervical region M99.31
      cervicothoracic M99.31
      head region M99.30
      lower extremity M99.36
      lumbar region M99.33
      lumbosacral M99.33
      occipitocervical M99.30
      pelvic M99.35
      rib cage M99.38
      sacral region M99.34
      sacrococcygeal M99.34
      sacroiliac M99.34
      specified NEC M99.39
      thoracic region M99.32
      thoracolumbar M99.32
      upper extremity M99.37
    subluxation M99.29
      cervical region M99.21
      cervicothoracic M99.21
      head region M99.20
      lower extremity M99.26
      lumbar region M99.23
      lumbosacral M99.23
      occipitocervical M99.20
      pelvic M99.25
      rib cage M99.28
      sacral region M99.24
      sacrococcygeal M99.24
      sacroiliac M99.24
      specified NEC M99.29
      thoracic region M99.22
      thoracolumbar M99.22
      upper extremity M99.27
  organ or site, congenital NEC — *see* Atresia, by site
  papilla of Vater K83.1
  pulmonary (artery) (congenital) Q25.6
    with ventricular septal defect, transposition of
        aorta, and hypertrophy of right ventricle
        Q21.3
    acquired I28.8
    in tetralogy of Fallot Q21.3
    infundibular Q24.3
    subvalvular Q24.3
    supravalvular Q25.6
    valve I37.0
      with insufficiency I37.2
      congenital Q22.1
      rheumatic I09.89
        with aortic, mitral or tricuspid (valve) disease
            I08.8
    vein, acquired I28.8
    vessel NEC I28.8
  pulmonic (congenital) Q22.1
    infundibular Q24.3
    subvalvular Q24.3
  pylorus (hypertrophic) (acquired) K31.1
    adult K31.1

Stenosis, stenotic — *continued*
  pylorus — *continued*
    congenital Q40.0
    infantile Q40.0
  rectum (sphincter) — *see* Stricture, rectum
  renal artery I70.1
    congenital Q27.1
  salivary duct (any) K11.8
  sphincter of Oddi K83.1
  spinal M48.00
    cervical region M48.02
    cervicothoracic region M48.03
    lumbar region (NOS) (without neurogenic claudi-
        cation) M48.061
      with neurogenic claudication M48.062
    lumbosacral region M48.07
    occipito-atlanto-axial region M48.01
    sacrococcygeal region M48.08
    thoracic region M48.04
    thoracolumbar region M48.05
  stomach, hourglass K31.2
  subaortic (congenital) Q24.4
    hypertrophic (idiopathic) I42.1
  subglottic J38.6
    congenital Q31.1
    postprocedural J95.5
  trachea J39.8
    congenital Q32.1
    syphilitic A52.73
    tuberculous NEC A15.5
  tracheostomy J95.03
  tricuspid (valve) I07.0
    with
      aortic (valve) disease I08.2
      incompetency, insufficiency or regurgitation
          I07.2
        with aortic (valve) disease I08.2
          with mitral (valve) disease I08.3
      mitral (valve) disease I08.1
        with aortic (valve) disease I08.3
    congenital Q22.4
    nonrheumatic I36.0
      with insufficiency I36.2
  tubal N97.1
  ureter — *see* Atresia, ureter
  ureteropelvic junction, congenital Q62.11
  ureterovesical orifice, congenital Q62.12
  urethra (valve) (*see also* Stricture, urethra)
    congenital Q64.32
  urinary meatus, congenital Q64.33
  vagina N89.5
    congenital Q52.4
    in pregnancy — *see* Pregnancy, complicated by,
        abnormal vagina
      causing obstructed labor O65.5
  valve (cardiac) (heart) (*see also* Endocarditis) I38
    congenital Q24.8
      aortic Q23.0
      mitral Q23.2
      pulmonary Q22.1
      tricuspid Q22.4
  vena cava (inferior) (superior) I87.1
    congenital Q26.0
  vesicourethral orifice Q64.31
  vulva N90.5
Stent jail T82.897 ☑
Stercolith (impaction) K56.41
  appendix K38.1
Stercoraceous, stercoral ulcer K63.3
  anus or rectum K62.6
Stereotypies NEC F98.4
Sterility — *see* Infertility
Sterilization — *see* Encounter (for), sterilization
Sternalgia — *see* Angina
Sternopagus Q89.4
Sternum bifidum Q76.7
Steroid
  effects (adverse) (adrenocortical) (iatrogenic)
    cushingoid E24.2
    correct substance properly administered — *see*
        Table of Drugs and Chemicals, by drug,
        adverse effect
    overdose or wrong substance given or taken
        — *see* Table of Drugs and Chemicals, by
        drug, poisoning
  diabetes — *see* subcategory E09 ☑

Steroid — *continued*
  effects — *continued*
    diabetes — *see* subcategory — *continued*
      correct substance properly administered — *see* Table of Drugs and Chemicals, by drug, adverse effect
      overdose or wrong substance given or taken — *see* Table of Drugs and Chemicals, by drug, poisoning
    fever R50.2
    insufficiency E27.3
      correct substance properly administered — *see* Table of Drugs and Chemicals, by drug, adverse effect
      overdose or wrong substance given or taken — *see* Table of Drugs and Chemicals, by drug, poisoning
    responder H40.04- ☑
Stevens-Johnson disease or syndrome L51.1
  toxic epidermal necrolysis overlap L51.3
Stewart-Morel syndrome M85.2
Sticker's disease B08.3
Sticky eye — *see* Conjunctivitis, acute, mucopurulent
Stieda's disease — *see* Bursitis, tibial collateral
Stiff neck — *see* Torticollis
Stiff-man syndrome G25.82
Stiffness, joint NEC M25.60
  ankle M25.67- ☑
  ankylosis — *see* Ankylosis, joint
  contracture — *see* Contraction, joint
  elbow M25.62- ☑
  foot M25.67- ☑
  hand M25.64- ☑
  hip M25.65- ☑
  knee M25.66- ☑
  shoulder M25.61- ☑
  wrist M25.63- ☑
Stigmata congenital syphilis A50.59
Stillbirth P95
Still-Felty syndrome — *see* Felty's syndrome
Still's disease or syndrome (juvenile) M08.20
  adult-onset M06.1
  ankle M08.27- ☑
  elbow M08.22- ☑
  foot joint M08.27- ☑
  hand joint M08.24- ☑
  hip M08.25- ☑
  knee M08.26- ☑
  multiple site M08.29
  shoulder M08.21- ☑
  vertebra M08.28
  wrist M08.23- ☑
Stimulation, ovary E28.1
Sting (venomous) (with allergic or anaphylactic shock) — *see* Table of Drugs and Chemicals, by animal or substance, poisoning
Stippled epiphyses Q78.8
Stitch
  abscess T81.4 ☑
  burst (in operation wound) — *see* Disruption, wound, operation
Stokes' disease E05.00
  with thyroid storm E05.01
Stokes-Adams disease or syndrome I45.9
Stokvis (-Talma) **disease** D74.8
Stoma malfunction
  colostomy K94.03
  enterostomy K94.13
  gastrostomy K94.23
  ileostomy K94.13
  tracheostomy J95.03
Stomach — *see* condition
Stomatitis (denture) (ulcerative) K12.1
  angular K13.0
    due to dietary or vitamin deficiency E53.0
  aphthous K12.0
  bovine B08.61
  candidal B37.0
  catarrhal K12.1
  diphtheritic A36.89
  due to
    dietary deficiency E53.0
    thrush B37.0
    vitamin deficiency
      B group NEC E53.9
      B2 (riboflavin) E53.0
  epidemic B08.8

Stomatitis — *continued*
  epizootic B08.8
  follicular K12.1
  gangrenous A69.0
  Geotrichum B48.3
  herpesviral, herpetic B00.2
  herpetiformis K12.0
  malignant K12.1
  membranous acute K12.1
  monilial B37.0
  mycotic B37.0
  necrotizing ulcerative A69.0
  parasitic B37.0
  septic K12.1
  spirochetal A69.1
  suppurative (acute) K12.2
  ulceromembranous A69.1
  vesicular K12.1
    with exanthem (enteroviral) B08.4
    virus disease A93.8
  Vincent's A69.1
Stomatocytosis D58.8
Stomatomycosis B37.0
Stomatorrhagia K13.79
Stone(s) (*see also* Calculus)
  bladder (diverticulum) N21.0
  cystine E72.09
  heart syndrome I50.1
  kidney N20.0
  prostate N42.0
  pulpal (dental) K04.2
  renal N20.0
  salivary gland or duct (any) K11.5
  urethra (impacted) N21.1
  urinary (duct) (impacted) (passage) N20.9
    bladder (diverticulum) N21.0
    lower tract N21.9
    specified NEC N21.8
  xanthine E79.8 [N22]
Stonecutter's lung J62.8
Stonemason's asthma, disease, lung or pneumoconiosis J62.8
Stoppage
  heart — *see* Arrest, cardiac
  urine — *see* Retention, urine
Storm, thyroid — *see* Thyrotoxicosis
Strabismus (congenital) (nonparalytic) H50.9
  concomitant H50.40
    convergent — *see* Strabismus, convergent concomitant
    divergent — *see* Strabismus, divergent concomitant
  convergent concomitant H50.00
    accommodative component H50.43
    alternating H50.05
      with
        A pattern H50.06
        specified nonconcomitances NEC H50.08
        V pattern H50.07
    monocular H50.01- ☑
      with
        A pattern H50.02- ☑
        specified nonconcomitances NEC H50.04- ☑
        V pattern H50.03- ☑
      intermittent H50.31- ☑
        alternating H50.32
  cyclotropia H50.41 ☑
  divergent concomitant H50.10
    alternating H50.15
      with
        A pattern H50.16
        specified nonconcomitances NEC H50.18
        V pattern H50.17
    monocular H50.11- ☑
      with
        A pattern H50.12- ☑
        specified nonconcomitances NEC H50.14- ☑
        V pattern H50.13- ☑
      intermittent H50.33 ☑
        alternating H50.34
  Duane's syndrome H50.81- ☑
  due to adhesions, scars H50.69
  heterophoria H50.50
    alternating H50.55
    cyclophoria H50.54
    esophoria H50.51
    exophoria H50.52
    vertical H50.53

Strabismus — *continued*
  heterotropia H50.40
    intermittent H50.30
  hypertropia H50.2- ☑
  hypotropia — *see* Hypertropia
  latent H50.50
  mechanical H50.60
    Brown's sheath syndrome H50.61- ☑
    specified type NEC H50.69
  monofixation syndrome H50.42
  paralytic H49.9
    abducens nerve H49.2- ☑
    fourth nerve H49.1- ☑
    Kearns-Sayre syndrome H49.81- ☑
    ophthalmoplegia (external)
      progressive H49.4- ☑
        with pigmentary retinopathy H49.81- ☑
      total H49.3- ☑
    sixth nerve H49.2- ☑
    specified type NEC H49.88- ☑
    third nerve H49.0- ☑
    trochlear nerve H49.1- ☑
  specified type NEC H50.89
  vertical H50.2- ☑
Strain
  back S39.012 ☑
  cervical S16.1 ☑
  eye NEC — *see* Disturbance, vision, subjective
  heart — *see* Disease, heart
  low back S39.012 ☑
  mental NOS Z73.3
    work-related Z56.6
  muscle (tendon) — *see* Injury, muscle, by site, strain
  neck S16.1 ☑
  physical NOS Z73.3
    work-related Z56.6
  postural (*see also* Disorder, soft tissue, due to use)
  psychological NEC Z73.3
  tendon — *see* Injury, muscle, by site, strain
Straining, on urination R39.16
Strand, vitreous — *see* Opacity, vitreous, membranes and strands
Strangulation, strangulated (*see also* Asphyxia, traumatic)
  appendix K38.8
  bladder-neck N32.0
  bowel or colon K56.2
  food or foreign body — *see* Foreign body, by site
  hemorrhoids — *see* Hemorrhoids, with complication
  hernia (*see also* Hernia, by site, with obstruction)
    with gangrene — *see* Hernia, by site, with gangrene
  intestine (large) (small) K56.2
    with hernia (*see also* Hernia, by site, with obstruction)
      with gangrene — *see* Hernia, by site, with gangrene
  mesentery K56.2
  mucus — *see* Asphyxia, mucus
  omentum K56.2
  organ or site, congenital NEC — *see* Atresia, by site
  ovary — *see* Torsion, ovary
  penis N48.89
    foreign body T19.4 ☑
  rupture — *see* Hernia, by site, with obstruction
  stomach due to hernia (*see also* Hernia, by site, with obstruction)
    with gangrene — *see* Hernia, by site, with gangrene
  vesicourethral orifice N32.0
Strangury R30.0
Straw itch B88.0
Strawberry
  gallbladder K82.4
  mark Q82.5
  tongue (red) (white) K14.3
Streak(s)
  macula, angioid H35.33
  ovarian Q50.32
Strephosymbolia F81.0
  secondary to organic lesion R48.8
Streptobacillary fever A25.1
Streptobacillosis A25.1
Streptobacillus moniliformis A25.1
Streptococcus, streptococcal (*see also* condition)
  as cause of disease classified elsewhere B95.5

Streptococcus, streptococcal — *continued*
  group
    A, as cause of disease classified elsewhere B95.0
    B, as cause of disease classified elsewhere B95.1
    D, as cause of disease classified elsewhere B95.2
    pneumoniae, as cause of disease classified elsewhere
      B95.3
    specified NEC, as cause of disease classified elsewhere
      B95.4
Streptomycosis B47.1
Streptotrichosis A48.8
Stress F43.9
  family — *see* Disruption, family
  fetal P84
    complicating pregnancy O77.9
      due to drug administration O77.1
  mental NEC Z73.3
    work-related Z56.6
  physical NEC Z73.3
    work-related Z56.6
  polycythemia D75.1
  reaction (*see also* Reaction, stress) F43.9
  work schedule Z56.3
Stretching, nerve — *see* Injury, nerve
Striae albicantes, atrophicae or distensae (cutis) L90.6
Stricture (*see also* Stenosis)
  ampulla of Vater K83.1
  anus (sphincter) K62.4
    congenital Q42.3
      with fistula Q42.2
      infantile Q42.3
        with fistula Q42.2
  aorta (ascending) (congenital) Q25.1
    arteriosclerotic I70.0
    calcified I70.0
    supravalvular, congenital Q25.3
  aortic (valve) — *see* Stenosis, aortic
  aqueduct of Sylvius (congenital) Q03.0
    with spina bifida — *see* Spina bifida, by site, with
      hydrocephalus
    acquired G91.1
  artery I77.1
    basilar — *see* Occlusion, artery, basilar
    carotid — *see* Occlusion, artery, carotid
    celiac I77.4
    congenital (peripheral) Q27.8
      cerebral Q28.3
      coronary Q24.5
      digestive system Q27.8
      lower limb Q27.8
      retinal Q14.1
      specified site NEC Q27.8
      umbilical Q27.0
      upper limb Q27.8
    coronary — *see* Disease, heart, ischemic,
      atherosclerotic
      congenital Q24.5
    precerebral — *see* Occlusion, artery, precerebral
    pulmonary (congenital) Q25.6
      acquired I28.8
    renal I70.1
    vertebral — *see* Occlusion, artery, vertebral
  auditory canal (external) (congenital)
    acquired — *see* Stenosis, external ear canal
  bile duct (common) (hepatic) K83.1
    congenital Q44.3
    postoperative K91.89
  bladder N32.89
    neck N32.0
  bowel — *see* Obstruction, intestine
  brain G93.89
  bronchus J98.09
    congenital Q32.3
    syphilitic A52.72
  cardia (stomach) K22.2
    congenital Q39.3
  cardiac (*see also* Disease, heart)
    orifice (stomach) K22.2
  cecum — *see* Obstruction, intestine
  cervix, cervical (canal) N88.2
    congenital Q51.828
    in pregnancy — *see* Pregnancy, complicated by,
      abnormal cervix
      causing obstructed labor O65.5
  colon (*see also* Obstruction, intestine)
    congenital Q42.9
      specified NEC Q42.8
  colostomy K94.03

Stricture — *continued*
  common (bile) duct K83.1
  coronary (artery) — *see* Disease, heart, ischemic,
    atherosclerotic
  cystic duct — *see* Obstruction, gallbladder
  digestive organs NEC, congenital Q45.8
  duodenum K31.5
    congenital Q41.0
  ear canal (external) (congenital) Q16.1
    acquired — *see* Stricture, auditory canal, acquired
  ejaculatory duct N50.89
  enterostomy K94.13
  esophagus K22.2
    congenital Q39.3
    syphilitic A52.79
      congenital A50.59 [K23]
  eustachian tube (*see also* Obstruction, eustachian tube)
    congenital Q17.8
  fallopian tube N97.1
    gonococcal A54.24
    tuberculous A18.17
  gallbladder — *see* Obstruction, gallbladder
  glottis J38.6
  heart (*see also* Disease, heart)
    valve (*see also* Endocarditis) I38
      aortic Q23.0
      mitral Q23.2
      pulmonary Q22.1
      tricuspid Q22.4
  hepatic duct K83.1
  hourglass, of stomach K31.2
  hymen N89.6
  hypopharynx J39.2
  ileum (*see also* Obstruction, intestine, specified NEC)
    K56.699
    congenital Q41.2
  intestine (*see also* Obstruction, intestine)
    congenital (small) Q41.9
      large Q42.9
        specified NEC Q42.8
      specified NEC Q41.8
    ischemic K55.1
  jejunum (*see also* Obstruction, intestine, specified NEC)
    K56.699
    congenital Q41.1
  lacrimal passages (*see also* Stenosis, lacrimal)
    congenital Q10.5
  larynx J38.6
    congenital NEC Q31.8
      subglottic Q31.1
    syphilitic A52.73
      congenital A50.59 [J99]
  meatus
    ear (congenital) Q16.1
      acquired — *see* Stricture, auditory canal, ac-
        quired
      osseous (ear) (congenital) Q16.1
        acquired — *see* Stricture, auditory canal, ac-
          quired
    urinarius (*see also* Stricture, urethra)
      congenital Q64.33
  mitral (valve) — *see* Stenosis, mitral
  myocardium, myocardial I51.5
    hypertrophic subaortic (idiopathic) I42.1
  nares (anterior) (posterior) J34.89
    congenital Q30.0
  nasal duct (*see also* Stenosis, lacrimal, duct)
    congenital Q10.5
  nasolacrimal duct (*see also* Stenosis, lacrimal, duct)
    congenital Q10.5
  nasopharynx J39.2
    syphilitic A52.73
  nose J34.89
    congenital Q30.0
  nostril (anterior) (posterior) J34.89
    congenital Q30.0
    syphilitic A52.73
      congenital A50.59 [J99]
  organ or site, congenital NEC — *see* Atresia, by site
  os uteri — *see* Stricture, cervix
  osseous meatus (ear) (congenital) Q16.1
    acquired — *see* Stricture, auditory canal, acquired
  oviduct — *see* Stricture, fallopian tube
  pelviureteric junction (congenital) Q62.11
    acquired, with hydronephrosis N13.0
  penis, by foreign body T19.4 ☑
  pharynx J39.2
  prostate N42.89

Stricture — *continued*
  pulmonary, pulmonic
    artery (congenital) Q25.6
      acquired I28.8
      noncongenital I28.8
    infundibulum (congenital) Q24.3
    valve I37.0
      congenital Q22.1
    vein, acquired I28.8
    vessel NEC I28.8
  punctum lacrimale (*see also* Stenosis, lacrimal, punc-
    tum)
    congenital Q10.5
  pylorus (hypertrophic) K31.1
    adult K31.1
    congenital Q40.0
    infantile Q40.0
  rectosigmoid (*see also* Obstruction, intestine, specified
    NEC) K56.699
  rectum (sphincter) K62.4
    congenital Q42.1
      with fistula Q42.0
    due to
      chlamydial lymphogranuloma A55
      irradiation K91.89
      lymphogranuloma venereum A55
    gonococcal A54.6
    inflammatory (chlamydial) A55
    syphilitic A52.74
    tuberculous A18.32
  renal artery I70.1
    congenital Q27.1
  salivary duct or gland (any) K11.8
  sigmoid (flexure) — *see* Obstruction, intestine
  spermatic cord N50.89
  stoma (following) (of)
    colostomy K94.03
    enterostomy K94.13
    gastrostomy K94.23
    ileostomy K94.13
    tracheostomy J95.03
  stomach K31.89
    congenital Q40.2
    hourglass K31.2
  subaortic Q24.4
    hypertrophic (acquired) (idiopathic) I42.1
  subglottic J38.6
  syphilitic NEC A52.79
  trachea J39.8
    congenital Q32.1
    syphilitic A52.73
    tuberculous NEC A15.5
  tracheostomy J95.03
  tricuspid (valve) — *see* Stenosis, tricuspid
  tunica vaginalis N50.89
  ureter (postoperative) N13.5
    with
      hydronephrosis N13.1
        with infection N13.6
      pyelonephritis (chronic) N11.1
    congenital — *see* Atresia, ureter
    tuberculous A18.11
  ureteropelvic junction (congenital) Q62.11
    acquired, with hydronephrosis N13.0
  ureterovesical orifice N13.5
    with infection N13.6
  urethra (organic) (spasmodic) N35.9
    associated with schistosomiasis B65.0 [N37]
    congenital Q64.39
      valvular (posterior) Q64.2
    due to
      infection — *see* Stricture, urethra, postinfective
      trauma — *see* Stricture, urethra, post-traumatic
    gonococcal, gonorrheal A54.01
    infective NEC — *see* Stricture, urethra, postinfective
    late effect (sequelae) of injury — *see* Stricture,
      urethra, post-traumatic
    postcatheterization — *see* Stricture, urethra, post-
      procedural
    postinfective NEC
      female N35.12
      male N35.119
        anterior urethra N35.114
        bulbous urethra N35.112
        meatal N35.111
        membranous urethra N35.113
    postobstetric N35.021

Index

Stricture—Subluxation

Stricture — *continued*
  urethra — *continued*
    postoperative — *see* Stricture, urethra, postprocedural
    postprocedural
      female N99.12
      male N99.114
        anterior bulbous urethra N99.113
        bulbous urethra N99.111
        fossa navicularis N99.115
        meatal N99.110
        membranous urethra N99.112
    post-traumatic
      female N35.028
        due to childbirth N35.021
      male N35.014
        anterior urethra N35.013
        bulbous urethra N35.011
        meatal N35.010
        membranous urethra N35.012
    sequela (late effect) of
      childbirth N35.021
      injury — *see* Stricture, urethra, post-traumatic
    specified cause NEC N35.8
    syphilitic A52.76
    traumatic — *see* Stricture, urethra, post-traumatic
    valvular (posterior), congenital Q64.2
  urinary meatus — *see* Stricture, urethra
  uterus, uterine (synechiae) N85.6
    os (external) (internal) — *see* Stricture, cervix
  vagina (outlet) — *see* Stenosis, vagina
  valve (cardiac) (heart) (*see also* Endocarditis)
    congenital
      aortic Q23.0
      mitral Q23.2
      pulmonary Q22.1
      tricuspid Q22.4
  vas deferens N50.89
    congenital Q55.4
  vein I87.1
  vena cava (inferior) (superior) NEC I87.1
    congenital Q26.0
  vesicourethral orifice N32.0
    congenital Q64.31
  vulva (acquired) N90.5
Stridor R06.1
  congenital (larynx) P28.89
Stridulous — *see* condition
Stroke (apoplectic) (brain) (embolic) (ischemic) (paralytic) (thrombotic) I63.9
  cryptogenic (*see also* infarction, cerebral) I63.9
  epileptic — *see* Epilepsy
  heat T67.0 ☑
  in evolution I63.9
  intraoperative
    during cardiac surgery I97.810
    during other surgery I97.811
  lightning — *see* Lightning
  meaning
    cerebral hemorrhage — *code to* Hemorrhage, intracranial
    cerebral infarction — *code to* Infarction, cerebral
  postprocedural
    following cardiac surgery I97.820
    following other surgery I97.821
  unspecified (NOS) I63.9
Stromatosis, endometrial D39.0
Strongyloidiasis, strongyloidosis B78.9
  cutaneous B78.1
  disseminated B78.7
  intestinal B78.0
Strophulus pruriginosus L28.2
Struck by lightning — *see* Lightning
Struma (*see also* Goiter)
  Hashimoto E06.3
  lymphomatosa E06.3
  nodosa (simplex) E04.9
    endemic E01.2
      multinodular E01.1
    multinodular E04.2
      iodine-deficiency related E01.1
    toxic or with hyperthyroidism E05.20
      with thyroid storm E05.21
      multinodular E05.20
        with thyroid storm E05.21
      uninodular E05.10
        with thyroid storm E05.11
    toxicosa E05.20

Struma — *continued*
  nodosa — *continued*
    toxicosa — *continued*
      with thyroid storm E05.21
      multinodular E05.20
        with thyroid storm E05.21
      uninodular E05.10
        with thyroid storm E05.11
    uninodular E04.1
  ovarii D27.- ☑
  Riedel's E06.5
Strumipriva cachexia E03.4
Strümpell-Marie spine — *see* Spondylitis, ankylosing
Strümpell-Westphal pseudosclerosis E83.01
Stuart deficiency disease (factor X) D68.2
Stuart-Prower factor deficiency (factor X) D68.2
Student's elbow — *see* Bursitis, elbow, olecranon
Stump — *see* Amputation
Stunting, nutritional E45
Stupor (catatonic) R40.1
  depressive (single episode) F32.89
    recurrent episode F33.8
  dissociative F44.2
  manic F30.2
  manic-depressive F31.89
  psychogenic (anergic) F44.2
  reaction to exceptional stress (transient) F43.0
Sturge (-Weber) (-Dimitri) (-Kalischer) **disease or syndrome** Q85.8
Stuttering F80.81
  adult onset F98.5
  childhood onset F80.81
  following cerebrovascular disease — *see* Disorder, fluency. following cerebrovascular disease
  in conditions classified elsewhere R47.82
Sty, stye (external) (internal) (meibomian) (zeisian) — *see* Hordeolum
Subacidity, gastric K31.89
  psychogenic F45.8
Subacute — *see* condition
Subarachnoid — *see* condition
Subcortical — *see* condition
Subcostal syndrome, nerve compression — *see* Mononeuropathy, upper limb, specified site NEC
Subcutaneous, subcuticular — *see* condition
Subdural — *see* condition
Subendocardium — *see* condition
Subependymoma
  specified site — *see* Neoplasm, uncertain behavior, by site
  unspecified site D43.2
Suberosis J67.3
Subglossitis — *see* Glossitis
Subhemophilia D66
Subinvolution
  breast (postlactational) (postpuerperal) N64.89
  puerperal O90.89
  uterus (chronic) (nonpuerperal) N85.3
    puerperal O90.89
Sublingual — *see* condition
Sublinguitis — *see* Sialoadenitis
Subluxatable hip Q65.6
Subluxation (*see also* Dislocation)
  acromioclavicular S43.11- ☑
  ankle S93.0- ☑
  atlantoaxial, recurrent M43.4
    with myelopathy M43.3
  carpometacarpal (joint) NEC S63.05- ☑
    thumb S63.04- ☑
  complex, vertebral — *see* Complex, subluxation
  congenital (*see also* Malposition, congenital)
    hip — *see* Dislocation, hip, congenital, partial
    joint (excluding hip)
      lower limb Q68.8
      shoulder Q68.8
      upper limb Q68.8
  elbow (traumatic) S53.10- ☑
    anterior S53.11- ☑
    lateral S53.14- ☑
    medial S53.13- ☑
    posterior S53.12- ☑
    specified type NEC S53.19- ☑
  finger S63.20- ☑
    index S63.20- ☑
    interphalangeal S63.22- ☑
      distal S63.24- ☑
        index S63.24-

Subluxation — *continued*
  finger — *continued*
    interphalangeal — *continued*
      distal — *continued*
        little S63.24- ☑
        middle S63.24- ☑
        ring S63.24- ☑
      index S63.22- ☑
      little S63.22- ☑
      middle S63.22- ☑
      proximal S63.23- ☑
        index S63.23- ☑
        little S63.23- ☑
        middle S63.23- ☑
        ring S63.23- ☑
      ring S63.22- ☑
    little S63.20- ☑
    metacarpophalangeal S63.21- ☑
      index S63.21- ☑
      little S63.21- ☑
      middle S63.21- ☑
      ring S63.21- ☑
    middle S63.20- ☑
    ring S63.20- ☑
  foot S93.30- ☑
    specified site NEC S93.33- ☑
    tarsal joint S93.31- ☑
    tarsometatarsal joint S93.32- ☑
    toe — *see* Subluxation, toe
  hip S73.00- ☑
    anterior S73.03- ☑
      obturator S73.02- ☑
    central S73.04- ☑
    posterior S73.01- ☑
  interphalangeal (joint)
    finger S63.22- ☑
      distal joint S63.24- ☑
        index S63.24- ☑
        little S63.24- ☑
        middle S63.24- ☑
        ring S63.24- ☑
      index S63.22- ☑
      little S63.22- ☑
      middle S63.22- ☑
      proximal joint S63.23- ☑
        index S63.23- ☑
        little S63.23- ☑
        middle S63.23- ☑
        ring S63.23- ☑
      ring S63.22- ☑
    thumb S63.12- ☑
      distal joint S63.14- ☑
      proximal joint S63.13- ☑
    toe S93.13- ☑
      great S93.13- ☑
      lesser S93.13- ☑
  joint prosthesis — *see* Complications, joint prosthesis, mechanical, displacement, by site
  knee S83.10- ☑
    cap — *see* Subluxation, patella
    patella — *see* Subluxation, patella
    proximal tibia
      anteriorly S83.11- ☑
      laterally S83.14- ☑
      medially S83.13- ☑
      posteriorly S83.12- ☑
    specified type NEC S83.19- ☑
  lens — *see* Dislocation, lens, partial
  ligament, traumatic — *see* Sprain, by site
  metacarpal (bone)
    proximal end S63.06- ☑
  metacarpophalangeal (joint)
    finger S63.21- ☑
      index S63.21- ☑
      little S63.21- ☑
      middle S63.21- ☑
      ring S63.21- ☑
    thumb S63.11- ☑
  metatarsophalangeal joint S93.14- ☑
    great toe S93.14- ☑
    lesser toe S93.14- ☑
  midcarpal (joint) S63.03- ☑
  patella S83.00- ☑
    lateral S83.01- ☑
    recurrent (nontraumatic) — *see* Dislocation, patella, recurrent, incomplete

☑ **Additional Character Required** — Refer to the Tabular List for Character Selection   Subterms under main terms may continue to next column or page

Subluxation — *continued*
  patella — *continued*
    specified type NEC S83.09- ☑
  pathological — *see* Dislocation, pathological
  radial head S53.00- ☑
    anterior S53.01- ☑
    nursemaid's elbow S53.03- ☑
    posterior S53.02- ☑
    specified type NEC S53.09- ☑
  radiocarpal (joint) S63.02- ☑
  radioulnar (joint)
    distal S63.01- ☑
    proximal — *see* Subluxation, elbow
  shoulder
    congenital Q68.8
    girdle S43.30- ☑
      scapula S43.31- ☑
      specified site NEC S43.39- ☑
    traumatic S43.00- ☑
      anterior S43.01- ☑
      inferior S43.03- ☑
      posterior S43.02- ☑
      specified type NEC S43.08- ☑
  sternoclavicular (joint) S43.20- ☑
    anterior S43.21- ☑
    posterior S43.22- ☑
  symphysis (pubis)
  thumb S63.103 ☑
    interphalangeal joint — *see* Subluxation, interpha-
      langeal (joint), thumb
    metacarpophalangeal joint — *see* Subluxation,
      metacarpophalangeal (joint), thumb
  toe(s) S93.10- ☑
    great S93.10- ☑
      interphalangeal joint S93.13- ☑
      metatarsophalangeal joint S93.14- ☑
    interphalangeal joint S93.13- ☑
    lesser S93.10- ☑
      interphalangeal joint S93.13- ☑
      metatarsophalangeal joint S93.14- ☑
    metatarsophalangeal joint S93.149 ☑
  ulna
    distal end S63.07- ☑
    proximal end — *see* Subluxation, elbow
  ulnohumeral joint — *see* Subluxation, elbow
  vertebral
    recurrent NEC — *see* subcategory M43.5 ☑
    traumatic
      cervical S13.100 ☑
        atlantoaxial joint S13.120 ☑
        atlantooccipital joint S13.110 ☑
        atloidooccipital joint S13.110 ☑
        joint between
          C0 and C1 S13.110 ☑
          C1 and C2 S13.120 ☑
          C2 and C3 S13.130 ☑
          C3 and C4 S13.140 ☑
          C4 and C5 S13.150 ☑
          C5 and C6 S13.160 ☑
          C6 and C7 S13.170 ☑
          C7 and T1 S13.180 ☑
        occipitoatloid joint S13.110 ☑
      lumbar S33.100 ☑
        joint between
          L1 and L2 S33.110 ☑
          L2 and L3 S33.120 ☑
          L3 and L4 S33.130 ☑
          L4 and L5 S33.140 ☑
      thoracic S23.100 ☑
        joint between
          T1 and T2 S23.110 ☑
          T2 and T3 S23.120 ☑
          T3 and T4 S23.122 ☑
          T4 and T5 S23.130 ☑
          T5 and T6 S23.132 ☑
          T6 and T7 S23.140 ☑
          T7 and T8 S23.142 ☑
          T8 and T9 S23.150 ☑
          T9 and T10 S23.152 ☑
          T10 and T11 S23.160 ☑
          T11 and T12 S23.162 ☑
          T12 and L1 S23.170 ☑
  wrist (carpal bone) S63.00- ☑
    carpometacarpal joint — *see* Subluxation, car-
      pometacarpal (joint)

Subluxation — *continued*
  wrist — *continued*
    distal radioulnar joint — *see* Subluxation, radioul-
      nar (joint), distal
    metacarpal bone, proximal — *see* Subluxation,
      metacarpal (bone), proximal end
    midcarpal — *see* Subluxation, midcarpal (joint)
    radiocarpal joint — *see* Subluxation, radiocarpal
      (joint)
    recurrent — *see* Dislocation, recurrent, wrist
    specified site NEC S63.09- ☑
    ulna — *see* Subluxation, ulna, distal end
Submaxillary — *see* condition
Submersion (fatal) (nonfatal) T75.1 ☑
Submucous — *see* condition
Subnormal, subnormality
  accommodation (old age) H52.4
  mental — *see* Disability, intellectual
  temperature (accidental) T68 ☑
Subphrenic — *see* condition
Subscapular nerve — *see* condition
Subseptus uterus Q51.2
Subsiding appendicitis K36
Substance (other psychoactive) **-induced**
  anxiety disorder F19.980
  bipolar and related disorder F19.94
  delirium F19.921
  depressive disorder F19.94
  major neurocognitive disorder F19.97
  mild neurocognitive disorder F19.988
  obsessive-compulsive and related disorder F19.988
  psychotic disorder F19.959
  sexual dysfunction F19.981
  sleep disorder F19.982
Substernal thyroid E04.9
  congenital Q89.2
Substitution disorder F44.9
Subtentorial — *see* condition
Subthyroidism (acquired) (*see also* Hypothyroidism)
  congenital E03.1
Succenturiate placenta O43.19- ☑
Sucking thumb, child (excessive) F98.8
Sudamen, sudamina L74.1
Sudanese kala-azar B55.0
Sudden
  hearing loss — *see* Deafness, sudden
  heart failure — *see* Failure, heart
Sudeck's atrophy, disease, or syndrome — *see* Algoneurodystrophy
Suffocation — *see* Asphyxia, traumatic
Sugar
  blood
    high (transient) R73.9
    low (transient) E16.2
  in urine R81
Suicide, suicidal (attempted) T14.91 ☑
  by poisoning — *see* Table of Drugs and Chemicals
  history of (personal) Z91.5
    in family Z81.8
  ideation — *see* Ideation, suicidal
  risk
    meaning personal history of attempted suicide
      Z91.5
    meaning suicidal ideation — *see* Ideation, suicidal
  tendencies
    meaning personal history of attempted suicide
      Z91.5
    meaning suicidal ideation — *see* Ideation, suicidal
  trauma — *see* nature of injury by site
Suipestifer infection — *see* Infection, salmonella
Sulfhemoglobinemia, sulphemoglobinemia (acquired) (with methemoglobinemia) D74.8
Sumatran mite fever A75.3
Summer — *see* condition
Sunburn L55.9
  due to
    tanning bed (acute) L56.8
      chronic L57.8
    ultraviolet radiation (acute) L56.8
      chronic L57.8
  first degree L55.0
  second degree L55.1
  third degree L55.2
SUNCT (short lasting unilateral neuralgiform headache
  with conjunctival injection and tearing) G44.059
  intractable G44.051
  not intractable G44.059

Sundowning F05
Sunken acetabulum — *see* Derangement, joint, specified type NEC, hip
Sunstroke T67.0 ☑
Superfecundation — *see* Pregnancy, multiple
Superfetation — *see* Pregnancy, multiple
Superinvolution (uterus) N85.8
Supernumerary (congenital)
  aortic cusps Q23.8
  auditory ossicles Q16.3
  bone Q79.8
  breast Q83.1
  carpal bones Q74.0
  cusps, heart valve NEC Q24.8
    aortic Q23.8
    mitral Q23.2
    pulmonary Q22.3
  digit(s) Q69.9
  ear (lobule) Q17.0
  fallopian tube Q50.6
  finger Q69.0
  hymen Q52.4
  kidney Q63.0
  lacrimonasal duct Q10.6
  lobule (ear) Q17.0
  mitral cusps Q23.2
  muscle Q79.8
  nipple(s) Q83.3
  organ or site not listed — *see* Accessory
  ossicles, auditory Q16.3
  ovary Q50.31
  oviduct Q50.6
  pulmonary, pulmonic cusps Q22.3
  rib Q76.6
    cervical or first (syndrome) Q76.5
  roots (of teeth) K00.2
  spleen Q89.09
  tarsal bones Q74.2
  teeth K00.1
  testis Q55.29
  thumb Q69.1
  toe Q69.2
  uterus Q51.2
  vagina Q52.1 ☑
  vertebra Q76.49
Supervision (of)
  contraceptive — *see* Prescription, contraceptives
  dietary (for) Z71.3
    allergy (food) Z71.3
    colitis Z71.3
    diabetes mellitus Z71.3
    food allergy or intolerance Z71.3
    gastritis Z71.3
    hypercholesterolemia Z71.3
    hypoglycemia Z71.3
    intolerance (food) Z71.3
    obesity Z71.3
    specified NEC Z71.3
  healthy infant or child Z76.2
    foundling Z76.1
  high-risk pregnancy — *see* Pregnancy, complicated
    by, high, risk
  lactation Z39.1
  pregnancy — *see* Pregnancy, supervision of
Supplemental teeth K00.1
Suppression
  binocular vision H53.34
  lactation O92.5
  menstruation N94.89
  ovarian secretion E28.39
  renal N28.9
  urine, urinary secretion R34
Suppuration, suppurative (*see also* condition)
  accessory sinus (chronic) — *see* Sinusitis
  adrenal gland
  antrum (chronic) — *see* Sinusitis, maxillary
  bladder — *see* Cystitis
  brain G06.0
    sequelae G09
  breast N61.1
    puerperal, postpartum or gestational — *see* Masti-
      tis, obstetric, purulent
  dental periosteum M27.3
  ear (middle) (*see also* Otitis, media)
    external NEC — *see* Otitis, externa, infective
    internal — *see* subcategory H83.0 ☑
  ethmoidal (chronic) (sinus) — *see* Sinusitis, ethmoidal
  fallopian tube — *see* Salpingo-oophoritis

Suppuration, suppurative — *continued*
  frontal (chronic) (sinus) — *see* Sinusitis, frontal
  gallbladder (acute) K81.0
  gum K05.20
    generalized — *see* Peridontitis, aggressive, generalized
    localized — *see* Peridontitis, aggressive, localized
  intracranial G06.0
  joint — *see* Arthritis, pyogenic or pyemic
  labyrinthine — *see* subcategory H83.0 ☑
  lung — *see* Abscess, lung
  mammary gland N61.1
    puerperal, postpartum O91.12
      associated with lactation O91.13
  maxilla, maxillary M27.2
    sinus (chronic) — *see* Sinusitis, maxillary
  muscle — *see* Myositis, infective
  nasal sinus (chronic) — *see* Sinusitis
  pancreas, acute (*see also* Pancreatitis, acute) K85.80
  parotid gland — *see* Sialoadenitis
  pelvis, pelvic
    female — *see* Disease, pelvis, inflammatory
    male K65.0
  pericranial — *see* Osteomyelitis
  salivary duct or gland (any) — *see* Sialoadenitis
  sinus (accessory) (chronic) (nasal) — *see* Sinusitis
  sphenoidal sinus (chronic) — *see* Sinusitis, sphenoidal
  thymus (gland) E32.1
  thyroid (gland) E06.0
  tonsil — *see* Tonsillitis
  uterus — *see* Endometritis
Supraeruption of tooth (teeth) M26.34
Supraglottitis J04.30
  with obstruction J04.31
Suprarenal (gland) — *see* condition
Suprascapular nerve — *see* condition
Suprasellar — *see* condition
Surfer's knots or nodules S89.8- ☑
Surgical
  emphysema T81.82 ☑
  procedures, complication or misadventure — *see* Complications, surgical procedures
  shock T81.10 ☑
Surveillance (of) (for) (*see also* Observation)
  alcohol abuse Z71.41
  contraceptive — *see* Prescription, contraceptives
  dietary Z71.3
  drug abuse Z71.51
Susceptibility to disease, genetic Z15.89
  malignant neoplasm Z15.09
    breast Z15.01
    endometrium Z15.04
    ovary Z15.02
    prostate Z15.03
    specified NEC Z15.09
  multiple endocrine neoplasia Z15.81
Suspected condition, ruled out (*see also* Observation, suspected)
  amniotic cavity and membrane Z03.71
  cervical shortening Z03.75
  fetal anomaly Z03.73
  fetal growth Z03.74
  maternal and fetal conditions NEC Z03.79
  newborn (*see also* Observation, newborn, suspected condition ruled out) Z05.9
  oligohydramnios Z03.71
  placental problem Z03.72
  polyhydramnios Z03.71
Suspended uterus
  in pregnancy or childbirth — *see* Pregnancy, complicated by, abnormal uterus
Sutton's nevus D22.9
Suture
  burst (in operation wound) T81.31 ☑
    external operation wound T81.31 ☑
    internal operation wound T81.32 ☑
  inadvertently left in operation wound — *see* Foreign body, accidentally left during a procedure
  removal Z48.02
Swab inadvertently left in operation wound — *see* Foreign body, accidentally left during a procedure
Swallowed, swallowing
  difficulty — *see* Dysphagia
  foreign body — *see* Foreign body, alimentary tract
Swan-neck deformity (finger) — *see* Deformity, finger, swan-neck
Swearing, compulsive F42.8

Swearing, compulsive — *continued*
  in Gilles de la Tourette's syndrome F95.2
Sweat, sweats
  fetid L75.0
  night R61
Sweating, excessive R61
Sweeley-Klionsky disease E75.21
Sweet's disease or dermatosis L98.2
Swelling (of) R60.9
  abdomen, abdominal (not referable to any particular organ) — *see* Mass, abdominal
  ankle — *see* Effusion, joint, ankle
  arm M79.89
    forearm M79.89
  breast (*see also* Lump, breast) N63.0
  Calabar B74.3
  cervical gland R59.0
  chest, localized R22.2
  ear H93.8- ☑
  extremity (lower) (upper) — *see* Disorder, soft tissue, specified type NEC
  finger M79.89
  foot M79.89
  glands R59.9
    generalized R59.1
    localized R59.0
  hand M79.89
  head (localized) R22.0
  inflammatory — *see* Inflammation
  intra-abdominal — *see* Mass, abdominal
  joint — *see* Effusion, joint
  leg M79.89
    lower M79.89
  limb — *see* Disorder, soft tissue, specified type NEC
  localized (skin) R22.9
    chest R22.2
    head R22.0
    limb
      lower — *see* Mass, localized, limb, lower
      upper — *see* Mass, localized, limb, upper
    neck R22.1
    trunk R22.2
  neck (localized) R22.1
  pelvic — *see* Mass, abdominal
  scrotum N50.89
  splenic — *see* Splenomegaly
  testis N50.89
  toe M79.89
  umbilical R19.09
  wandering, due to Gnathostoma (spinigerum) B83.1
  white — *see* Tuberculosis, arthritis
Swift (-Feer) **disease**
  overdose or wrong substance given or taken — *see* Table of Drugs and Chemicals, by drug, poisoning
Swimmer's
  cramp T75.1 ☑
  ear H60.33- ☑
  itch B65.3
Swimming in the head R42
Swollen — *see* Swelling
Swyer syndrome Q99.1
Sycosis L73.8
  barbae (not parasitic) L73.8
  contagiosa (mycotic) B35.0
  lupoides L73.8
  mycotic B35.0
  parasitic B35.0
  vulgaris L73.8
Sydenham's chorea — *see* Chorea, Sydenham's
Sylvatic yellow fever A95.0
Sylvest's disease B33.0
Symblepharon H11.23- ☑
  congenital Q10.3
Symond's syndrome G93.2
Sympathetic — *see* condition
Sympatheticotonia G90.8
Sympathicoblastoma
  specified site — *see* Neoplasm, malignant, by site
  unspecified site C74.90
Sympathogonioma — *see* Sympathicoblastoma
Symphalangy (fingers) (toes) Q70.9
Symptoms NEC R68.89
  breast NEC N64.59
  cold J00
  development NEC R63.8
  factitious, self-induced — *see* Disorder, factitious

Symptoms — *continued*
  genital organs, female R10.2
  involving
    abdomen NEC R19.8
    appearance NEC R46.89
    awareness R41.9
      altered mental status R41.82
      amnesia — *see* Amnesia
      borderline intellectual functioning R41.83
      coma — *see* Coma
      disorientation R41.0
      neurologic neglect syndrome R41.4
      senile cognitive decline R41.81
      specified symptom NEC R41.89
    behavior NEC R46.89
    cardiovascular system NEC R09.89
    chest NEC R09.89
    circulatory system NEC R09.89
    cognitive functions R41.9
      altered mental status R41.82
      amnesia — *see* Amnesia
      borderline intellectual functioning R41.83
      coma — *see* Coma
      disorientation R41.0
      neurologic neglect syndrome R41.4
      senile cognitive decline R41.81
      specified symptom NEC R41.89
    development NEC R62.50
    digestive system NEC R19.8
    emotional state NEC R45.89
      emotional lability R45.86
    food and fluid intake R63.8
    general perceptions and sensations R44.9
      specified NEC R44.8
    musculoskeletal system R29.91
      specified NEC R29.898
    nervous system R29.90
      specified NEC R29.818
    pelvis NEC R19.8
    respiratory system NEC R09.89
    skin and integument R23.9
    urinary system R39.9
  menopausal N95.1
  metabolism NEC R63.8
  neurotic F48.8
  of infancy R68.19
  pelvis NEC, female R10.2
  skin and integument NEC R23.9
  subcutaneous tissue NEC R23.9
  viral cold J00
Sympus Q74.2
Syncephalus Q89.4
Synchondrosis
  abnormal (congenital) Q78.8
  ischiopubic M91.0
Synchysis (scintillans) (senile) (vitreous body) H43.89
Syncope (near) (pre-) R55
  anginosa I20.8
  bradycardia R00.1
  cardiac R55
  carotid sinus G90.01
  due to spinal (lumbar) puncture G97.1
  heart R55
  heat T67.1 ☑
  laryngeal R05
  psychogenic F48.8
  tussive R05
  vasoconstriction R55
  vasodepressor R55
  vasomotor R55
  vasovagal R55
Syndactylism, syndactyly Q70.9
  complex (with synostosis)
    fingers Q70.0- ☑
    toes Q70.2- ☑
  simple (without synostosis)
    fingers Q70.1- ☑
    toes Q70.3- ☑
Syndrome (*see also* Disease)
  48,XXXX Q97.1
  49,XXXXX Q97.1
  5q minus NOS D46.C (*following* D46.2)
  abdominal
    acute R10.0
    muscle deficiency Q79.4
  abnormal innervation H02.519
    left H02.516
      lower H02.515

Syndrome — *continued*
- abnormal innervation — *continued*
  - left — *continued*
    - upper H02.514
  - right H02.513
    - lower H02.512
    - upper H02.511
- abstinence, neonatal P96.1
- acid pulmonary aspiration, obstetric O74.0
- acquired immunodeficiency — *see* Human, immunodeficiency virus (HIV) disease
- acute abdominal R10.0
- acute respiratory distress (adult) (child) J80
  - idiopathic J84.114
- Adair-Dighton Q78.0
- Adams-Stokes (-Morgagni) I45.9
- adiposogenital E23.6
- adrenal
  - hemorrhage (meningococcal) A39.1
  - meningococcic A39.1
- adrenocortical — *see* Cushing's, syndrome
- adrenogenital E25.9
  - congenital, associated with enzyme deficiency E25.0
- afferent loop NEC K91.89
- Alagille's Q44.7
- alcohol withdrawal (without convulsions) — *see* Dependence, alcohol, with, withdrawal
- Alder's D72.0
- Aldrich (-Wiskott) D82.0
- alien hand R41.4
- Alport Q87.81
- alveolar hypoventilation E66.2
- alveolocapillary block J84.10
- amnesic, amnestic (confabulatory) (due to) — *see* Disorder, amnesic
- amyostatic (Wilson's disease) E83.01
- androgen insensitivity E34.50
  - complete E34.51
  - partial E34.52
- androgen resistance (*see also* Syndrome, androgen insensitivity) E34.50
- Angelman Q93.5
- anginal — *see* Angina
- ankyloglossia superior Q38.1
- anterior
  - chest wall R07.89
  - cord G83.82
  - spinal artery G95.19
    - compression M47.019
      - cervical region M47.012
      - cervicothoracic region M47.013
      - lumbar region M47.016
      - occipito-atlanto-axial region M47.011
      - thoracic region M47.014
      - thoracolumbar region M47.015
  - tibial M76.81- ☑
- antibody deficiency D80.9
  - agammaglobulinemic D80.1
    - hereditary D80.0
  - congenital D80.0
  - hypogammaglobulinemic D80.1
    - hereditary D80.0
- anticardiolipin (-antibody) D68.61
- antidepressant discontinuation T43.205 ☑
- antiphospholipid (-antibody) D68.61
- aortic
  - arch M31.4
  - bifurcation I74.09
- aortomesenteric duodenum occlusion K31.5
- apical ballooning (transient left ventricular) I51.81
- arcuate ligament I77.4
- argentaffin, argintaffinoma E34.0
- Arnold-Chiari — *see* Arnold-Chiari disease
- Arrillaga-Ayerza I27.0
- arterial tortuosity Q87.82
- arteriovenous steal T82.898- ☑
- Asherman's N85.6
- aspiration, of newborn — *see* Aspiration, by substance, with pneumonia
  - meconium P24.01
- ataxia-telangiectasia G11.3
- auriculotemporal G50.8
- autoerythrocyte sensitization (Gardner-Diamond) D69.2
- autoimmune lymphoproliferative [ALPS] D89.82
- autoimmune polyglandular E31.0
- autoinflammatory M04.9

Syndrome — *continued*
- autoinflammatory — *continued*
  - specified type NEC M04.8
- autosomal — *see* Abnormal, autosomes
- Avellis' G46.8
- Ayerza (-Arrillaga) I27.0
- Babinski-Nageotte G83.89
- Bakwin-Krida Q78.5
- bare lymphocyte D81.6
- Barré-Guillain G61.0
- Barré-Liéou M53.0
- Barrett's — *see* Barrett's, esophagus
- Barsony-Polgar K22.4
- Bársony-Teschendorf K22.4
- Barth E78.71
- Bartter's E26.81
- basal cell nevus Q87.89
- Basedow's E05.00
  - with thyroid storm E05.01
- basilar artery G45.0
- Batten-Steinert G71.11
- battered
  - baby or child — *see* Maltreatment, child, physical abuse
  - spouse — *see* Maltreatment, adult, physical abuse
- Beals Q87.40
- Beau's I51.5
- Beck's I65.8
- Benedikt's G46.3
- Béquez César (-Steinbrinck-Chédiak-Higashi) E70.330
- Bernhardt-Roth — *see* Meralgia paresthetica
- Bernheim's — *see* Failure, heart, right
- big spleen D73.1
- bilateral polycystic ovarian E28.2
- Bing-Horton's — *see* Horton's headache
- Birt-Hogg-Dube syndrome Q87.89
- Björck (-Thorsen) E34.0
- black
  - lung J60
  - widow spider bite — *see* Toxicity, venom, spider, black widow
- Blackfan-Diamond D61.01
- Blau M04.8
- blind loop K90.2
  - congenital Q43.8
  - postsurgical K91.2
- blue sclera Q78.0
- blue toe I75.02- ☑
- Boder-Sedgewick G11.3
- Boerhaave's K22.3
- Borjeson Forssman Lehmann Q89.8
- Bouillaud's I01.9
- Bourneville (-Pringle) Q85.1
- Bouveret (-Hoffman) I47.9
- brachial plexus G54.0
- bradycardia-tachycardia I49.5
- brain (nonpsychotic) F09
  - with psychosis, psychotic reaction F09
  - acute or subacute — *see* Delirium
  - congenital — *see* Disability, intellectual
  - organic F09
    - post-traumatic (nonpsychotic) F07.81
      - psychotic F09
    - personality change F07.0
    - postcontusional F07.81
    - post-traumatic, nonpsychotic F07.81
    - psycho-organic F09
    - psychotic F06.8
- brain stem stroke G46.3
- Brandt's (acrodermatitis enteropathica) E83.2
- broad ligament laceration N83.8
- Brock's J98.11
- bronze baby P83.88
- Brown-Sequard G83.81
- Brugada I49.8
- bubbly lung P27.0
- Buchem's M85.2
- Budd-Chiari I82.0
- bulbar (progressive) G12.22
- Bürger-Grütz E78.3
- Burke's K86.89
- Burnett's (milk-alkali) E83.52
- burning feet E53.9
- Bywaters' T79.5 ☑
- Call-Fleming I67.841
- carbohydrate-deficient glycoprotein (CDGS) E77.8
- carcinogenic thrombophlebitis I82.1
- carcinoid E34.0

Syndrome — *continued*
- cardiac asthma I50.1
- cardiacos negros I27.0
- cardiofaciocutaneous Q87.89
- cardiopulmonary-obesity E66.2
- cardiorenal — *see* Hypertension, cardiorenal
- cardiorespiratory distress (idiopathic), newborn P22.0
- cardiovascular renal — *see* Hypertension, cardiorenal
- carotid
  - artery (hemispheric) (internal) G45.1
  - body G90.01
  - sinus G90.01
- carpal tunnel G56.0- ☑
- Cassidy (-Scholte) E34.0
- cat cry Q93.4
- cat eye Q92.8
- cauda equina G83.4
- causalgia — *see* Causalgia
- celiac K90.0
  - artery compression I77.4
  - axis I77.4
- central pain G89.0
- cerebellar
  - hereditary G11.9
  - stroke G46.4
- cerebellomedullary malformation — *see* Spina bifida
- cerebral
  - artery
    - anterior G46.1
    - middle G46.0
    - posterior G46.2
  - gigantism E22.0
- cervical (root) M53.1
  - disc — *see* Disorder, disc, cervical, with neuritis
  - fusion Q76.1
  - posterior, sympathicus M53.0
  - rib Q76.5
  - sympathetic paralysis G90.2
- cervicobrachial (diffuse) M53.1
- cervicocranial M53.0
- cervicodorsal outlet G54.2
- cervicothoracic outlet G54.0
- Céstan (-Raymond) I65.8
- Charcot's (angina cruris) (intermittent claudication) I73.9
- Charcot-Weiss-Baker G90.09
- CHARGE Q89.8
- Chédiak-Higashi (-Steinbrinck) E70.330
- chest wall R07.1
- Chiari's (hepatic vein thrombosis) I82.0
- Chilaiditi's Q43.3
- child maltreatment — *see* Maltreatment, child
- chondrocostal junction M94.0
- chondroectodermal dysplasia Q77.6
- chromosome 4 short arm deletion Q93.3
- chromosome 5 short arm deletion Q93.4
- chronic
  - infantile neurological, cutaneous and articular (CINCA) M04.2
  - pain G89.4
  - personality F68.8
- Clarke-Hadfield K86.89
- Clerambault's automatism G93.89
- Clouston's (hidrotic ectodermal dysplasia) Q82.4
- clumsiness, clumsy child F82
- cluster headache G44.009
  - intractable G44.001
  - not intractable G44.009
- Coffin-Lowry Q89.8
- cold injury (newborn) P80.0
- combined immunity deficiency D81.9
- compartment (deep) (posterior) (traumatic) T79.A0 ☑ (*following* T79.7)
  - abdomen T79.A3 ☑ (*following* T79.7)
  - lower extremity (hip, buttock, thigh, leg, foot, toes) T79.A2 ☑ (*following* T79.7)
  - nontraumatic
    - abdomen M79.A3 (*following* M79.7)
    - lower extremity (hip, buttock, thigh, leg, foot, toes) M79.A2- ☑ (*following* M79.7)
    - specified site NEC M79.A9 (*following* M79.7)
    - upper extremity (shoulder, arm, forearm, wrist, hand, fingers) M79.A1- ☑ (*following* M79.7)
  - postprocedural — *see* Syndrome, compartment, nontraumatic
  - specified site NEC T79.A9 ☑ (*following* T79.7)

⚐ **Subterms under main terms may continue to next column or page**   ☑ **Additional Character Required — Refer to the Tabular List for Character Selection**   **299**

Syndrome — Syndrome

Syndrome — *continued*
  compartment — *continued*
    upper extremity (shoulder, arm, forearm, wrist, hand, fingers) T79.A1 ☑ (*following* T79.7)
  complex regional pain — *see* Syndrome, pain, complex regional
  compression T79.5 ☑
    anterior spinal — *see* Syndrome, anterior, spinal artery, compression
    cauda equina G83.4
    celiac artery I77.4
    vertebral artery M47.029
      cervical region M47.022
      occipito-atlanto-axial region M47.021
  concussion F07.81
  congenital
    affecting multiple systems NEC Q87.89
    central alveolar hypoventilation G47.35
    facial diplegia Q87.0
    muscular hypertrophy-cerebral Q87.89
    oculo-auriculovertebral Q87.0
    oculofacial diplegia (Moebius) Q87.0
    rubella (manifest) P35.0
  congestion-fibrosis (pelvic), female N94.89
  congestive dysmenorrhea N94.6
  connective tissue M35.9
    overlap NEC M35.1
  Conn's E26.01
  conus medullaris G95.81
  cord
    anterior G83.82
    posterior G83.83
  coronary
    acute NEC I24.9
    insufficiency or intermediate I20.0
    slow flow I20.8
  Costen's (complex) M26.69
  costochondral junction M94.0
  costoclavicular G54.0
  costovertebral E22.0
  Cowden Q85.8
  craniovertebral M53.0
  Creutzfeldt-Jakob — *see* Creutzfeldt-Jakob disease or syndrome
  crib death R99
  cricopharyngeal — *see* Dysphagia
  cri-du-chat Q93.4
  croup J05.0
  CRPS I — *see* Syndrome, pain, complex regional I
  crush T79.5 ☑
  cryopyrin-associated perodic M04.2
  cryptophthalmos Q87.0
  cubital tunnel — *see* Lesion, nerve, ulnar
  Curschmann (-Batten) (-Steinert) G71.11
  Cushing's E24.9
    alcohol-induced E24.4
    drug-induced E24.2
    due to
      alcohol
      drugs E24.2
      ectopic ACTH E24.3
      overproduction of pituitary ACTH E24.0
    overdose or wrong substance given or taken — *see* Table of Drugs and Chemicals, by drug, poisoning
    pituitary-dependent E24.0
    specified type NEC E24.8
  cystic duct stump K91.5
  Dana-Putnam D51.0
  Danbolt (-Cross) (acrodermatitis enteropathica) E83.2
  Dandy-Walker Q03.1
    with spina bifida Q07.01
  Danlos' Q79.6
  De Quervain E34.51
  de Toni-Fanconi (-Debré) E72.09
    with cystinosis E72.04
  defibrination (*see also* Fibrinolysis)
    with
      antepartum hemorrhage — *see* Hemorrhage, antepartum, with coagulation defect
      intrapartum hemorrhage — *see* Hemorrhage, complicating, delivery
    newborn P60
    postpartum O72.3
  Degos' I77.89
  Déjérine-Roussy G89.0
  delayed sleep phase G47.21
  demyelinating G37.9

Syndrome — *continued*
  dependence — *see* F10-F19 with fourth character .2
  depersonalization (-derealization) F48.1
  di George's D82.1
  diabetes mellitus in newborn infant P70.2
  diabetes mellitus-hypertension-nephrosis — *see* Diabetes, nephrosis
  diabetes-nephrosis — *see* Diabetes, nephrosis
  diabetic amyotrophy — *see* Diabetes, amyotrophy
  dialysis associated steal T82.898- ☑
  Diamond-Blackfan D61.01
  Diamond-Gardener D69.2
  DIC (diffuse or disseminated intravascular coagulopathy) D65
  Dighton's Q78.0
  disequilibrium E87.8
  Döhle body-panmyelopathic D72.0
  dorsolateral medullary G46.4
  double athetosis G80.3
  Down (*see also* Down syndrome) Q90.9
  Dresbach's (elliptocytosis) D58.1
  Dressler's (postmyocardial infarction) I24.1
    postcardiotomy I97.0
  drug withdrawal, infant of dependent mother P96.1
  dry eye H04.12- ☑
  due to abnormality
    chromosomal Q99.9
      sex
        female phenotype Q97.9
        male phenotype Q98.9
        specified NEC Q99.8
  dumping (postgastrectomy) K91.1
    nonsurgical K31.89
  Dupré's (meningism) R29.1
  dysmetabolic X E88.81
  dyspraxia, developmental F82
  Eagle-Barrett Q79.4
  Eaton-Lambert — *see* Syndrome, Lambert-Eaton
  Ebstein's Q22.5
  ectopic ACTH E24.3
  eczema-thrombocytopenia D82.0
  Eddowes' Q78.0
  effort (psychogenic) F45.8
  Ehlers-Danlos Q79.6
  Eisenmenger's I27.83
  Ekman's Q78.0
  electric feet E53.8
  Ellis-van Creveld Q77.6
  empty nest Z60.0
  endocrine-hypertensive E27.0
  entrapment — *see* Neuropathy, entrapment
  eosinophilia-myalgia M35.8
  epileptic (*see also* Epilepsy, by type)
    absence G40.A09 (*following* G40.3)
      intractable G40.A19 (*following* G40.3)
        with status epilepticus G40.A11 (*following* G40.3)
        without status epilepticus G40.A19 (*following* G40.3)
      not intractable G40.A09 (*following* G40.3)
        with status epilepticus G40.A01 (*following* G40.3)
        without status epilepticus G40.A09 (*following* G40.3)
  Erdheim-Chester (ECD) E88.89
  Erdheim's E22.0
  erythrocyte fragmentation D59.4
  Evans D69.41
  exhaustion F48.8
  extrapyramidal G25.9
    specified NEC G25.89
  eye retraction — *see* Strabismus
  eyelid-malar-mandible Q87.0
  Faber's D50.9
  facial pain, paroxysmal G50.0
  Fallot's Q21.3
  familial cold autoinflammatory M04.2
  familial eczema-thrombocytopenia (Wiskott-Aldrich) D82.0
  Fanconi (-de Toni) (-Debré) E72.09
    with cystinosis E72.04
  Fanconi's (anemia) (congenital pancytopenia) D61.09
  fatigue
    chronic R53.82
    psychogenic F48.8
  faulty bowel habit K59.39
  Feil-Klippel (brevicollis) Q76.1
  Felty's — *see* Felty's syndrome

Syndrome — *continued*
  fertile eunuch E23.0
  fetal
    alcohol (dysmorphic) Q86.0
    hydantoin Q86.1
  Fiedler's I40.1
  first arch Q87.0
  fish odor E72.8
  Fisher's G61.0
  Fitzhugh-Curtis
    due to
      Chlamydia trachomatis A74.81
      Neisseria gonorrhorea (gonococcal peritonitis) A54.85
  Fitz's (*see also* Pancreatitis, acute) K85.80
  Flajani (-Basedow) E05.00
    with thyroid storm E05.01
  flatback — *see* Flatback syndrome
  floppy
    baby P94.2
    iris (intraoeprative) (IFIS) H21.81
    mitral valve I34.1
  flush E34.0
  Foix-Alajouanine G95.19
  Fong's Q87.2
  food protein-induced enterocolitis K52.21
  foramen magnum G93.5
  Foster-Kennedy H47.14- ☑
  Foville's (peduncular) G46.3
  fragile X Q99.2
  Franceschetti Q75.4
  Frey's
    auriculotemporal G50.8
    hyperhidrosis L74.52
  Friderichsen-Waterhouse A39.1
  Froin's G95.89
  frontal lobe F07.0
  Fukuhara E88.49
  functional
    bowel K59.9
    prepubertal castrate E29.1
  Gaisböck's D75.1
  ganglion (basal ganglia brain) G25.9
    geniculi G51.1
  Gardner-Diamond D69.2
  gastroesophageal
    junction K22.0
    laceration-hemorrhage K22.6
  gastrojejunal loop obstruction K91.89
  Gee-Herter-Heubner K90.0
  Gelineau's G47.419
    with cataplexy G47.411
  genito-anorectal A55
  Gerstmann-Sträussler-Scheinker (GSS) A81.82
  Gianotti-Crosti L44.4
  giant platelet (Bernard-Soulier) D69.1
  Gilles de la Tourette's F95.2
  goiter-deafness E07.1
  Goldberg Q89.8
  Goldberg-Maxwell E34.51
  Good's D83.8
  Gopalan' (burning feet) E53.8
  Gorlin's Q87.89
  Gougerot-Blum L81.7
  Gouley's I31.1
  Gower's R55
  gray or grey (newborn) P93.0
    platelet D69.1
  Gubler-Millard G46.3
  Guillain-Barré (-Strohl) G61.0
  gustatory sweating G50.8
  Hadfield-Clarke K86.89
  hair tourniquet — *see* Constriction, external, by site
  Hamman's J98.19
  hand-foot L27.1
  hand-shoulder G90.8
  hantavirus (cardio)-pulmonary (HPS) (HCPS) B33.4
  happy puppet Q93.5
  Harada's H30.81- ☑
  Hayem-Faber D50.9
  headache NEC G44.89
    complicated NEC G44.59
  Heberden's I20.8
  Hedinger's E34.0
  Hegglin's D72.0
  HELLP (hemolysis, elevated liver enzymes and low platelet count) O14.2- ☑
    complicating
      childbirth O14.24

Syndrome — *continued*
  HELLP — *continued*
    complicating — *continued*
      puerperium O14.25
  hemolytic-uremic D59.3
  hemophagocytic, infection-associated D76.2
  Henoch-Schönlein D69.0
  hepatic flexure K59.8
  hepatopulmonary K76.81
  hepatorenal K76.7
    following delivery O90.4
    postoperative or postprocedural K91.83
    postpartum, puerperal O90.4
  hepatourologic K76.7
  Herter (-Gee) (nontropical sprue) K90.0
  Heubner-Herter K90.0
  Heyd's K76.7
  Hilger's G90.09
  histamine-like (fish poisoning) — *see* Poisoning, fish
  histiocytic D76.3
  histiocytosis NEC D76.3
  HIV infection, acute B20
  Hoffmann-Werdnig G12.0
  Hollander-Simons E88.1
  Hoppe-Goldflam G70.00
    with exacerbation (acute) G70.01
    in crisis G70.01
  Horner's G90.2
  hungry bone E83.81
  hunterian glossitis D51.0
  Hutchinson's triad A50.53
  hyperabduction G54.0
  hyperammonemia-hyperornithinemia-homocitrulline-
    mia E72.4
  hypereosinophilic (idiopathic) D72.1
  hyperimmunoglobulin D M04.1
  hyperimmunoglobulin E (IgE) D82.4
  hyperkalemic E87.5
  hyperkinetic — *see* Hyperkinesia
  hypermobility M35.7
  hypernatremia E87.0
  hyperosmolarity E87.0
  hyperperfusion G97.82
  hypersplenic D73.1
  hypertransfusion, newborn P61.1
  hyperventilation F45.8
  hyperviscosity (of serum)
    polycythemic D75.1
    sclerothymic D58.8
  hypoglycemic (familial) (neonatal) E16.2
  hypokalemic E87.6
  hyponatremic E87.1
  hypopituitarism E23.0
  hypoplastic left-heart Q23.4
  hypopotassemia E87.6
  hyposmolality E87.1
  hypotension, maternal O26.5- ☑
  hypothenar hammer I73.89
  hypoventilation, obesity (OHS) E66.2
  ICF (intravascular coagulation-fibrinolysis) D65
  idiopathic
    cardiorespiratory distress, newborn P22.0
    nephrotic (infantile) N04.9
  iliotibial band M76.3- ☑
  immobility, immobilization (paraplegic) M62.3
  immune reconstitution D89.3
  immune reconstitution inflammatory [IRIS] D89.3
  immunity deficiency, combined D81.9
  immunodeficiency
    acquired — *see* Human, immunodeficiency virus
      (HIV) disease
    combined D81.9
  impending coronary I20.0
  impingement, shoulder M75.4- ☑
  inappropriate secretion of antidiuretic hormone E22.2
  infant
    gestational diabetes P70.0
    of diabetic mother P70.1
  infantilism (pituitary) E23.0
  inferior vena cava I87.1
  inspissated bile (newborn) P59.1
  institutional (childhood) F94.2
  insufficient sleep F51.12
  intermediate coronary (artery) I20.0
  interspinous ligament — *see* Spondylopathy, specified
    NEC
  intestinal
    carcinoid E34.0

Syndrome — *continued*
  intestinal — *continued*
    knot K56.2
  intravascular coagulation-fibrinolysis (ICF) D65
  iodine-deficiency, congenital E00.9
    type
      mixed E00.2
      myxedematous E00.1
      neurological E00.0
  IRDS (idiopathic respiratory distress, newborn) P22.0
  irritable
    bowel K58.9
      with
        constipation K58.1
        diarrhea K58.0
      mixed K58.2
      psychogenic F45.8
      specified NEC K58.8
    heart (psychogenic) F45.8
    weakness F48.8
  ischemic
    bowel (transient) K55.9
      chronic K55.1
      due to mesenteric artery insufficiency K55.1
    steal T82.898 ☑
  IVC (intravascular coagulopathy) D65
  Ivemark's Q89.01
  Jaccoud's — *see* Arthropathy, postrheumatic, chronic
  Jackson's G83.89
  Jakob-Creutzfeldt — *see* Creutzfeldt-Jakob disease or
    syndrome
  jaw-winking Q07.8
  Jervell-Lange-Nielsen I45.81
  jet lag G47.25
  Job's D71
  Joseph-Diamond-Blackfan D61.01
  jugular foramen G52.7
  Kabuki Q89.8
  Kanner's (autism) F84.0
  Kartagener's Q89.3
  Kelly's D50.1
  Kimmelstiel-Wilson — *see* Diabetes, specified type,
    with Kimmelstiel-Wilson disease
  Klein (e)-Levine G47.13
  Klippel-Feil (brevicollis) Q76.1
  Köhler-Pellegrini-Steida — *see* Bursitis, tibial collateral
  König's K59.8
  Korsakoff (-Wernicke) (nonalcoholic) F04
    alcoholic F10.26
  Kostmann's D70.0
  Krabbe's congenital muscle hypoplasia Q79.8
  labyrinthine — *see* subcategory H83.2 ☑
  lacunar NEC G46.7
  Lambert-Eaton G70.80
    in
      neoplastic disease G73.1
      specified disease NEC G70.81
  Landau-Kleffner — *see* Epilepsy, specified NEC
  Larsen's Q74.8
  lateral
    cutaneous nerve of thigh G57.1- ☑
    medullary G46.4
  Launois' E22.0
  lazy
    leukocyte D70.8
    posture M62.3
  Lemiere I80.8
  Lennox-Gastaut G40.812
    intractable G40.814
      with status epilepticus G40.813
      without status epilepticus G40.814
    not intractable G40.812
      with status epilepticus G40.811
      without status epilepticus G40.812
  lenticular, progressive E83.01
  Leopold-Levi's E05.90
  Lev's I44.2
  Lichtheim's D51.0
  Li-Fraumeni Z15.01
  Lightwood's N25.89
  Lignac (de Toni) (-Fanconi) (-Debré) E72.09
    with cystinosis E72.04
  Likoff's I20.8
  limbic epilepsy personality F07.0
  liver-kidney K76.7
  lobotomy F07.0
  Loffler's J82
  long arm 18 or 21 deletion Q93.89

Syndrome — *continued*
  long QT I45.81
  Louis-Barré G11.3
  low
    atmospheric pressure T70.29 ☑
    back M54.5
    output (cardiac) I50.9
  lower radicular, newborn (birth injury) P14.8
  Luetscher's (dehydration) E86.0
  Lupus anticoagulant D68.62
  Lutembacher's Q21.1
  macrophage activation D76.1
    due to infection D76.2
  magnesium-deficiency R29.0
  Majeed M04.8
  Mal de Debarquement R42
  malabsorption K90.9
    postsurgical K91.2
  malformation, congenital, due to
    alcohol Q86.0
    exogenous cause NEC Q86.8
    hydantoin Q86.1
    warfarin Q86.2
  malignant
    carcinoid E34.0
    neuroleptic G21.0
  Mallory-Weiss K22.6
  mandibulofacial dysostosis Q75.4
  manic-depressive — *see* Disorder, bipolar
  maple-syrup-urine E71.0
  Marable's I77.4
  Marfan's Q87.40
    with
      cardiovascular manifestations Q87.418
        aortic dilation Q87.410
      ocular manifestations Q87.42
      skeletal manifestations Q87.43
  Marie's (acromegaly) E22.0
  mast cell activation — *see* Activation, mast cell
  maternal hypotension — *see* Syndrome, hypotension,
    maternal
  May (-Hegglin) D72.0
  McArdle (-Schmidt) (-Pearson) E74.04
  McQuarrie's E16.2
  meconium plug (newborn) P76.0
  median arcuate ligament I77.4
  Meekeren-Ehlers-Danlos Q79.6
  megavitamin-B6 E67.2
  Meige G24.4
  MELAS E88.41
  Mendelson's O74.0
  MERRF (myoclonic epilepsy associated with ragged-
    red fibers) E88.42
  mesenteric
    artery (superior) K55.1
    vascular insufficiency K55.1
  metabolic E88.81
  metastatic carcinoid E34.0
  micrognathia-glossoptosis Q87.0
  midbrain NEC G93.89
  middle lobe (lung) J98.19
  middle radicular G54.0
  migraine (*see also* Migraine) G43.909
  Mikulicz' K11.8
  milk-alkali E83.52
  Millard-Gubler G46.3
  Miller-Dieker Q93.88
  Miller-Fisher G61.0
  Minkowski-Chauffard D58.0
  Mirizzi's K83.1
  MNGIE (Mitochondrial Neurogastrointestinal En-
    cephalopathy) E88.49
  Möbius, ophthalmoplegic migraine — *see* Migraine,
    ophthalmoplegic
  monofixation H50.42
  Morel-Moore M85.2
  Morel-Morgagni M85.2
  Morgagni (-Morel) (-Stewart) M85.2
  Morgagni-Adams-Stokes I45.9
  Mounier-Kuhn Q32.4
    with bronchiectasis J47.9
      with
        exacerbation (acute) J47.1
        lower respiratory infection J47.0
    acquired J98.09
      with bronchiectasis J47.9
        with
          exacerbation (acute) J47.1
          lower respiratory infection J47.0

Index

Syndrome — Syndrome

Syndrome — *continued*
Muckle-Wells M04.2
mucocutaneous lymph node (acute febrile) (MCLS) M30.3
multiple endocrine neoplasia (MEN) — *see* Neoplasia, endocrine, multiple (MEN)
multiple operations — *see* Disorder, factitious
myasthenic G70.9
  in
    diabetes mellitus — *see* Diabetes, amyotrophy
    endocrine disease NEC E34.9 [G73.3]
    neoplastic disease (*see also* Neoplasm) D49.9 [G73.3]
    thyrotoxicosis (hyperthyroidism) E05.90 [G73.3]
      with thyroid storm E05.91 [G73.3]
myelodysplastic D46.9
  with
    5q deletion D46.C (*following* D46.2)
    isolated del (5q) chromosomal abnormality D46.C (*following* D46.2)
    lesions, low grade D46.20
    specified NEC D46.Z (*following* D46.4)
myelopathic pain G89.0
myeloproliferative (chronic) D47.1
myofascial pain M79.1
Naffziger's G54.0
nail patella Q87.2
NARP (Neuropathy, Ataxia and Retinitis pigmentosa) E88.49
neonatal abstinence P96.1
nephritic (*see also* Nephritis)
  with edema — *see* Nephrosis
  acute N00.9
  chronic N03.9
  rapidly progressive N01.9
nephrotic (congenital) (*see also* Nephrosis) N04.9
  with
    dense deposit disease N04.6
    diffuse
      crescentic glomerulonephritis N04.7
      endocapillary proliferative glomerulonephritis N04.4
      membranous glomerulonephritis N04.2
      mesangial proliferative glomerulonephritis N04.3
      mesangiocapillary glomerulonephritis N04.5
    focal and segmental glomerular lesions N04.1
    minor glomerular abnormality N04.0
    specified morphological changes NEC N04.8
  diabetic — *see* Diabetes, nephrosis
neurologic neglect R41.4
Nezelof's D81.4
Nonne-Milroy-Meige Q82.0
Nothnagel's vasomotor acroparesthesia I73.89
obesity hypoventilation (OHS) E66.2
oculomotor H51.9
ophthalmoplegia-cerebellar ataxia — *see* Strabismus, paralytic, third nerve
oral allergy T78.1 ☑
oral-facial-digital Q87.0
organic
  affective F06.30
  amnesic (not alcohol- or drug-induced) F04
  brain F09
  depressive F06.31
  hallucinosis F06.0
  personality F07.0
Ormond's N13.5
oro-facial-digital Q87.0
os trigonum Q68.8
Osler-Weber-Rendu I78.0
osteoporosis-osteomalacia M83.8
Osterreicher-Turner Q87.2
otolith — *see* subcategory H81.8 ☑
oto-palatal-digital Q87.0
outlet (thoracic) G54.0
ovary
  polycystic E28.2
  resistant E28.39
  sclerocystic E28.2
Owren's D68.2
Paget-Schroetter I82.890
pain (*see also* Pain)
  complex regional I G90.50
    lower limb G90.52- ☑
    specified site NEC G90.59
    upper limb G90.51- ☑
  complex regional II — *see* Causalgia

Syndrome — *continued*
painful
  bruising D69.2
    feet E53.8
    prostate N42.81
  paralysis agitans — *see* Parkinsonism
paralytic G83.9
  specified NEC G83.89
Parinaud's H51.0
parkinsonian — *see* Parkinsonism
Parkinson's — *see* Parkinsonism
paroxysmal facial pain G50.0
Parry's E05.00
  with thyroid storm E05.01
Parsonage (-Aldren)-Turner G54.5
patella clunk M25.86- ☑
Paterson (-Brown) (-Kelly) D50.1
pectoral girdle I77.89
pectoralis minor I77.89
pediatric autoimmune neuropsychiatric disorders associated with streptococcal infections (PANDAS) D89.89
Pelger-Huet D72.0
pellagra-cerebellar ataxia-renal aminoaciduria E72.02
pellagroid E52
Pellegrini-Stieda — *see* Bursitis, tibial collateral
pelvic congestion-fibrosis, female N94.89
penta X Q97.1
peptic ulcer — *see* Ulcer, peptic
perabduction I77.89
periodic fever M04.1
periodic fever, aphthous stomatitis, pharyngitis, and adenopathy [PFAPA] M04.8
periodic headache, in adults and children — *see* Headache, periodic syndromes in adults and children
periurethral fibrosis N13.5
phantom limb (without pain) G54.7
  with pain G54.6
pharyngeal pouch D82.1
Pick's — *see* Disease, Pick's
Pickwickian E66.2
PIE (pulmonary infiltration with eosinophilia) J82
pigmentary pallidal degeneration (progressive) G23.0
pineal E34.8
pituitary E22.0
placental transfusion — *see* Pregnancy, complicated by, placental transfusion syndromes
plantar fascia M72.2
plateau iris (post-iridectomy) (postprocedural) H21.82
Plummer-Vinson D50.1
pluricarential of infancy E40
plurideficiency E40
pluriglandular (compensatory) E31.8
  autoimmune E31.0
pneumatic hammer T75.21 ☑
polyangiitis overlap M30.8
polycarential of infancy E40
polyglandular E31.8
  autoimmune E31.0
polysplenia Q89.09
pontine NEC G93.89
popliteal
  artery entrapment I77.89
  web Q87.89
post chemoembolization — *code to* associated conditions
postcardiac injury
  postcardiotomy I97.0
  postmyocardial infarction I24.1
postcardiotomy I97.0
postcholecystectomy K91.5
postcommissurotomy I97.0
postconcussional F07.81
postcontusional F07.81
postencephalitic F07.89
posterior
  cervical sympathetic M53.0
  cord G83.83
  fossa compression G93.5
  reversible encephalopathy (PRES) I67.83
postgastrectomy (dumping) K91.1
postgastric surgery K91.1
postinfarction I24.1
postlaminectomy NEC M96.1
postleukotomy F07.0
postmastectomy lymphedema I97.2
postmyocardial infarction I24.1

Syndrome — *continued*
postoperative NEC T81.9 ☑
  blind loop K90.2
postpartum panhypopituitary (Sheehan) E23.0
postpolio (myelitic) G14
postthrombotic I87.009
  with
    inflammation I87.02- ☑
      with ulcer I87.03- ☑
    specified complication NEC I87.09- ☑
    ulcer I87.01- ☑
      with inflammation I87.03- ☑
    asymptomatic I87.00- ☑
postvagotomy K91.1
postvalvulotomy I97.0
postviral NEC G93.3
  fatigue G93.3
Potain's K31.0
potassium intoxication E87.5
precerebral artery (multiple) (bilateral) G45.2
preinfarction I20.0
preleukemic D46.9
premature senility E34.8
premenstrual dysphoric F32.89
premenstrual tension N94.3
Prinzmetal-Massumi R07.1
prune belly Q79.4
pseudo -Turner's Q87.1
pseudocarpal tunnel (sublimis) — *see* Syndrome, carpal tunnel
pseudoparalytica G70.00
  with exacerbation (acute) G70.01
  in crisis G70.01
psycho-organic (nonpsychotic severity) F07.9
  acute or subacute F05
  depressive type F06.31
  hallucinatory type F06.0
  nonpsychotic severity F07.0
  specified NEC F07.89
pulmonary
  arteriosclerosis I27.0
  dysmaturity (Wilson-Mikity) P27.0
  hypoperfusion (idiopathic) P22.0
  renal (hemorrhagic) (Goodpasture's) M31.0
pure
  motor lacunar G46.5
  sensory lacunar G46.6
Putnam-Dana D51.0
pyogenic arthritis, pyoderma gangrenosum, and acne [PAPA] M04.8
pyramidopallidonigral G20
pyriformis — *see* Lesion, nerve, sciatic
QT interval prolongation I45.81
radicular NEC — *see* Radiculopathy
  upper limbs, newborn (birth injury) P14.3
rapid time-zone change G47.25
Rasmussen G04.81
Raymond (-Céstan) I65.8
Raynaud's I73.00
  with gangrene I73.01
RDS (respiratory distress syndrome, newborn) P22.0
reactive airways dysfunction J68.3
Refsum's G60.1
Reifenstein E34.52
renal glomerulohyalinosis-diabetic — *see* Diabetes, nephrosis
Rendu-Osler-Weber I78.0
residual ovary N99.83
resistant ovary E28.39
respiratory
  distress
    acute J80
      adult J80
      child J80
      idiopathic J84.114
    newborn (idiopathic) (type I) P22.0
      type II P22.1
restless legs G25.81
retinoblastoma (familial) C69.2 ☑
retroperitoneal fibrosis N13.5
retroviral seroconversion (acute) Z21
Reye's G93.7
Richter — *see* Leukemia, chronic lymphocytic, B-cell type
Ridley's I50.1
right
  heart, hypoplastic Q22.6

☑ **Additional Character Required — Refer to the Tabular List for Character Selection**   ▿ **Subterms under main terms may continue to next column or page**

Syndrome — *continued*
  right — *continued*
    ventricular obstruction — *see* Failure, heart, congestive
  Romano-Ward (prolonged QT interval) I45.81
  rotator cuff, shoulder (*see also* Tear, rotator cuff) M75.10- ☑
  Rotes Quérol — *see* Hyperostosis, ankylosing
  Roth — *see* Meralgia paresthetica
  rubella (congenital) P35.0
  Ruvalcaba-Myhre-Smith E71.440
  Rytand-Lipsitch I44.2
  salt
    depletion E87.1
      due to heat NEC T67.8 ☑
        causing heat exhaustion or prostration T67.4 ☑
    low E87.1
  salt-losing N28.89
  Scaglietti-Dagnini E22.0
  scalenus anticus (anterior) G54.0
  scapulocostal — *see* Mononeuropathy, upper limb, specified site NEC
  scapuloperoneal G71.0
  schizophrenic, of childhood NEC F84.5
  Schnitzler D47.2
  Scholte's E34.0
  Schroeder's E27.0
  Schüller-Christian C96.5
  Schwachman's — *see* Syndrome, Shwachman's
  Schwartz (-Jampel) G71.13
  Schwartz-Bartter E22.2
  scimitar Q26.8
  sclerocystic ovary E28.2
  Seitelberger's G31.89
  septicemic adrenal hemorrhage A39.1
  seroconversion, retroviral (acute) Z21
  serous meningitis G93.2
  severe acute respiratory (SARS) J12.81
  shaken infant T74.4 ☑
  shock (traumatic) T79.4 ☑
    kidney N17.0
      following crush injury T79.5 ☑
    toxic A48.3
  shock-lung J80
  Shone's — *code to* specific anomalies
  short
    bowel K91.2
    rib Q77.2
  shoulder-hand — *see* Algoneurodystrophy
  Shwachman's D70.4
  sicca — *see* Sicca syndrome
  sick
    cell E87.1
    sinus I49.5
  sick-euthyroid E07.81
  sideropenic D50.1
  Siemens' ectodermal dysplasia Q82.4
  Silfversköld's Q78.9
  Simons' E88.1
  sinus tarsi M25.57- ☑
  sinusitis-bronchiectasis-situs inversus Q89.3
  Sipple's E31.22
  sirenomelia Q87.2
  Slocumb's E27.0
  slow flow, coronary I20.8
  Sluder's G44.89
  Smith-Magenis Q93.88
  Sneddon-Wilkinson L13.1
  Sotos' Q87.3
  South African cardiomyopathy I42.8
  spasmodic
    upward movement, eyes H51.8
    winking F95.8
  Spen's I45.9
  splenic
    agenesis Q89.01
    flexure K59.8
    neutropenia D73.81
  Spurway's Q78.0
  staphylococcal scalded skin L00
  steal
    arteriovenous T82.898- ☑
    ischemic T82.898- ☑
    subclavian G45.8
  Stein-Leventhal E28.2
  Stein's E28.2
  Stevens-Johnson syndrome L51.1

Syndrome — *continued*
  Stevens-Johnson syndrome — *continued*
    toxic epidermal necrolysis overlap L51.3
  Stewart-Morel M85.2
  Stickler Q89.8
  stiff baby Q89.8
  stiff man G25.82
  Still-Felty — *see* Felty's syndrome
  Stokes (-Adams) I45.9
  stone heart I50.1
  straight back, congenital Q76.49
  subclavian steal G45.8
  subcoracoid-pectoralis minor G54.0
  subcostal nerve compression I77.89
  subphrenic interposition Q43.3
  superior
    cerebellar artery I63.8
    mesenteric artery K55.1
    semi-circular canal dehiscence H83.8X- ☑
    vena cava I87.1
  supine hypotensive (maternal) — *see* Syndrome, hypotension, maternal
  suprarenal cortical E27.0
  supraspinatus (*see also* Tear, rotator cuff) M75.10- ☑
  Susac G93.49
  swallowed blood P78.2
  sweat retention L74.0
  Swyer Q99.1
  Symond's G93.2
  sympathetic
    cervical paralysis G90.2
    pelvic, female N94.89
  systemic inflammatory response (SIRS), of non-infectious origin (without organ dysfunction) R65.10
    with acute organ dysfunction R65.11
  tachycardia-bradycardia I49.5
  takotsubo I51.81
  TAR (thrombocytopenia with absent radius) Q87.2
  tarsal tunnel G57.5- ☑
  teething K00.7
  tegmental G93.89
  telangiectasic-pigmentation-cataract Q82.8
  temporal pyramidal apex — *see* Otitis, media, suppurative, acute
  temporomandibular joint-pain-dysfunction M26.62- ☑
  Terry's (*see also* Myopia, degenerative) H44.2- ☑
  testicular feminization (*see also* Syndrome, androgen insensitivity) E34.51
  thalamic pain (hyperesthetic) G89.0
  thoracic outlet (compression) G54.0
  Thorson-Björck E34.0
  thrombocytopenia with absent radius (TAR) Q87.2
  thyroid-adrenocortical insufficiency E31.0
  tibial
    anterior M76.81- ☑
    posterior M76.82- ☑
  Tietze's M94.0
  time-zone (rapid) G47.25
  Toni-Fanconi E72.09
    with cystinosis E72.04
  Touraine's Q79.8
  tourniquet — *see* Constriction, external, by site
  toxic shock A48.3
  transient left ventricular apical ballooning I51.81
  traumatic vasospastic T75.22 ☑
  Treacher Collins Q75.4
  triple X, female Q97.0
  trisomy Q92.9
    13 Q91.7
      meiotic nondisjunction Q91.4
      mitotic nondisjunction Q91.5
      mosaicism Q91.5
      translocation Q91.6
    18 Q91.3
      meiotic nondisjunction Q91.0
      mitotic nondisjunction Q91.1
      mosaicism Q91.1
      translocation Q91.2
    20 (q)(p) Q92.8
    21 Q90.9
      meiotic nondisjunction Q90.0
      mitotic nondisjunction Q90.1
      mosaicism Q90.1
      translocation Q90.2
    22 Q92.8
  tropical wet feet T69.0- ☑
  Trousseau's I82.1

Syndrome — *continued*
  tumor lysis (following antineoplastic chemotherapy) (spontaneous) NEC E88.3
  tumor necrosis factor receptor associated periodic (TRAPS) M04.1
  Twiddler's (due to)
    automatic implantable defibrillator T82.198 ☑
    cardiac pacemaker T82.198 ☑
  Unverricht (-Lundborg) — *see* Epilepsy, generalized, idiopathic
  upward gaze H51.8
  uremia, chronic (*see also* Disease, kidney, chronic) N18.9
  urethral N34.3
  urethro-oculo-articular — *see* Reiter's disease
  urohepatic K76.7
  vago-hypoglossal G52.7
  van Buchem's M85.2
  van der Hoeve's Q78.0
  vascular NEC in cerebrovascular disease G46.8
  vasoconstriction, reversible cerebrovascular I67.841
  vasomotor I73.9
  vasospastic (traumatic) T75.22 ☑
  vasovagal R55
  VATER Q87.2
  velo-cardio-facial Q93.81
  vena cava (inferior) (superior) (obstruction) I87.1
  vertebral
    artery G45.0
      compression — *see* Syndrome, anterior, spinal artery, compression
    steal G45.0
  vertebro-basilar artery G45.0
  vertebrogenic (pain) M54.89
  vertiginous — *see* Disorder, vestibular function
  Vinson-Plummer D50.1
  virus B34.9
  visceral larva migrans B83.0
  visual disorientation H53.8
  vitamin B6 deficiency E53.1
  vitreal corneal H59.01- ☑
  vitreous (touch) H59.01- ☑
  Vogt-Koyanagi H20.82- ☑
  Volkmann's T79.6 ☑
  von Schroetter's I82.890
  von Willebrand (-Jürgen) D68.0
  Waldenström-Kjellberg D50.1
  Wallenberg's G46.3
  water retention E87.79
  Waterhouse (-Friderichsen) A39.1
  Weber-Gubler G46.3
  Weber-Leyden G46.3
  Weber's G46.3
  Wegener's M31.30
    with
      kidney involvement M31.31
      lung involvement M31.30
        with kidney involvement M31.31
  Weingarten's (tropical eosinophilia) J82
  Weiss-Baker G90.09
  Werdnig-Hoffman G12.0
  Wermer's E31.21
  Werner's E34.8
  Wernicke-Korsakoff (nonalcoholic) F04
    alcoholic F10.26
  Westphal-Strümpell E83.01
  West's — *see* Epilepsy, spasms
  wet
    feet (maceration) (tropical) T69.0- ☑
    lung, newborn P22.1
  whiplash S13.4 ☑
  whistling face Q87.0
  Wilkie's K55.1
  Wilkinson-Sneddon L13.1
  Willebrand (-Jürgens) D68.0
  Wilson's (hepatolenticular degeneration) E83.01
  Wiskott-Aldrich D82.0
  withdrawal — *see* Withdrawal, state
    drug
      infant of dependent mother P96.1
      therapeutic use, newborn P96.2
  Woakes' (ethmoiditis) J33.1
  Wright's (hyperabduction) G54.0
  X I20.9
  XXXX Q97.1
  XXXXX Q97.1
  XXXXY Q98.1
  XXY Q98.0

Syndrome — *continued*
  yellow nail L60.5
  Zahorsky's B08.5
  Zellweger syndrome E71.510
  Zellweger-like syndrome E71.541
Synechia (anterior) (iris) (posterior) (pupil) (*see also* Adhesions, iris)
  intra-uterine (traumatic) N85.6
Synesthesia R20.8
Syngamiasis, syngamosis B83.3
Synodontia K00.2
Synorchidism, synorchism Q55.1
Synostosis (congenital) Q78.8
  astragalo-scaphoid Q74.2
  radioulnar Q74.0
Synovial sarcoma — *see* Neoplasm, connective tissue, malignant
Synovioma (malignant) (*see also* Neoplasm, connective tissue, malignant)
  benign — *see* Neoplasm, connective tissue, benign
Synoviosarcoma — *see* Neoplasm, connective tissue, malignant
Synovitis (*see also* Tenosynovitis) M65.9
  crepitant
    hand M70.0- ☑
    wrist M70.03- ☑
  gonococcal A54.49
  gouty — *see* Gout
  in (due to)
    crystals M65.8- ☑
    gonorrhea A54.49
    syphilis (late) A52.78
    use, overuse, pressure — *see* Disorder, soft tissue, due to use
  infective NEC — *see* Tenosynovitis, infective NEC
  specified NEC — *see* Tenosynovitis, specified type NEC
  syphilitic A52.78
    congenital (early) A50.02
  toxic — *see* Synovitis, transient
  transient M67.3- ☑
    ankle M67.37- ☑
    elbow M67.32- ☑
    foot joint M67.37- ☑
    hand joint M67.34- ☑
    hip M67.35- ☑
    knee M67.36- ☑
    multiple site M67.39
    pelvic region M67.35- ☑
    shoulder M67.31- ☑
    specified joint NEC M67.38
    wrist M67.33- ☑
  traumatic, current — *see* Sprain
  tuberculous — *see* Tuberculosis, synovitis
  villonodular (pigmented) M12.2- ☑
    ankle M12.27- ☑
    elbow M12.22- ☑
    foot joint M12.27- ☑
    hand joint M12.24- ☑
    hip M12.25- ☑
    knee M12.26- ☑
    multiple site M12.29
    pelvic region M12.25- ☑
    shoulder M12.21- ☑
    specified joint NEC M12.28
    vertebrae M12.28
    wrist M12.23- ☑
Syphilid A51.39
  congenital A50.06
  newborn A50.06
  tubercular (late) A52.79
Syphilis, syphilitic (acquired) A53.9
  abdomen (late) A52.79
  acoustic nerve A52.15
  adenopathy (secondary) A51.49
  adrenal (gland) (with cortical hypofunction) A52.79
  age under 2 years NOS (*see also* Syphilis, congenital, early)
    acquired A51.9
  alopecia (secondary) A51.32
  anemia (late) A52.79 [D63.8]
  aneurysm (aorta) (ruptured) A52.01
    central nervous system A52.05
    congenital A50.54 [I79.0]
  anus (late) A52.74
    primary A51.1
    secondary A51.39
  aorta (arch) (abdominal) (thoracic) A52.02

Syphilis, syphilitic — *continued*
  aorta — *continued*
    aneurysm A52.01
  aortic (insufficiency) (regurgitation) (stenosis) A52.03
    aneurysm A52.01
  arachnoid (adhesive) (cerebral) (spinal) A52.13
  asymptomatic — *see* Syphilis, latent
  ataxia (locomotor) A52.11
  atrophoderma maculatum A51.39
  auricular fibrillation A52.06
  bladder (late) A52.76
  bone A52.77
    secondary A51.46
  brain A52.17
  breast (late) A52.79
  bronchus (late) A52.72
  bubo (primary) A51.0
  bulbar palsy A52.19
  bursa (late) A52.78
  cardiac decompensation A52.06
  cardiovascular A52.00
  central nervous system (late) (recurrent) (relapse) (tertiary) A52.3
    with
      ataxia A52.11
      general paralysis A52.17
        juvenile A50.45
      paresis (general) A52.17
        juvenile A50.45
      tabes (dorsalis) A52.11
        juvenile A50.45
      taboparesis A52.17
        juvenile A50.45
    aneurysm A52.05
    congenital A50.40
    juvenile A50.40
    remission in (sustained) A52.3
    serology doubtful, negative, or positive A52.3
    specified nature or site NEC A52.19
    vascular A52.05
  cerebral A52.17
    meningovascular A52.13
    nerves (multiple palsies) A52.15
    sclerosis A52.17
    thrombosis A52.05
  cerebrospinal (tabetic type) A52.12
  cerebrovascular A52.05
  cervix (late) A52.76
  chancre (multiple) A51.0
    extragenital A51.2
    Rollet's A51.0
  Charcot's joint A52.16
  chorioretinitis A51.43
    congenital A50.01
    late A52.71
    prenatal A50.01
  choroiditis — *see* Syphilitic chorioretinitis
  choroidoretinitis — *see* Syphilitic chorioretinitis
  ciliary body (secondary) A51.43
    late A52.71
  colon (late) A52.74
  combined spinal sclerosis A52.11
  condyloma (latum) A51.31
  congenital A50.9
    with
      paresis (general) A50.45
      tabes (dorsalis) A50.45
      taboparesis A50.45
    early, or less than 2 years after birth NEC A50.2
      with manifestations — *see* Syphilis, congenital, early, symptomatic
      latent (without manifestations) A50.1
        negative spinal fluid test A50.1
        serology positive A50.1
      symptomatic A50.09
        cutaneous A50.06
        mucocutaneous A50.07
        oculopathy A50.01
        osteochondropathy A50.02
        pharyngitis A50.03
        pneumonia A50.04
        rhinitis A50.05
        visceral A50.08
    chorioretinitis, choroiditis A50.01 [H32]
    interstitial keratitis A50.31
    juvenile neurosyphilis A50.45
    late, or 2 years or more after birth NEC A50.7
      chorioretinitis, choroiditis A50.32
      interstitial keratitis A50.31

Syphilis, syphilitic — *continued*
  congenital — *continued*
    late, or 2 years or more after birth — *continued*
      juvenile neurosyphilis A50.45
      latent (without manifestations) A50.6
        negative spinal fluid test A50.6
        serology positive A50.6
      symptomatic or with manifestations NEC A50.59
        arthropathy A50.55
        cardiovascular A50.54
        Clutton's joints A50.51
        Hutchinson's teeth A50.52
        Hutchinson's triad A50.53
        osteochondropathy A50.56
        saddle nose A50.57
  conjugal A53.9
    tabes A52.11
  conjunctiva (late) A52.71
  contact Z20.2
  cord bladder A52.19
  cornea, late A52.71
  coronary (artery) (sclerosis) A52.06
  coryza, congenital A50.05
  cranial nerve A52.15
    multiple palsies A52.15
  cutaneous — *see* Syphilis, skin
  dacryocystitis (late) A52.71
  degeneration, spinal cord A52.12
  dementia paralytica A52.17
    juvenilis A50.45
  destruction of bone A52.77
  dilatation, aorta A52.01
  due to blood transfusion A53.9
  dura mater A52.13
  ear A52.79
    inner A52.79
      nerve (eighth) A52.15
      neurorecurrence A52.15
  early A51.9
    cardiovascular A52.00
    central nervous system A52.3
    latent (without manifestations) (less than 2 years after infection) A51.5
      negative spinal fluid test A51.5
      serological relapse after treatment A51.5
      serology positive A51.5
    relapse (treated, untreated) A51.9
    skin A51.39
    symptomatic A51.9
      extragenital chancre A51.2
      primary, except extragenital chancre A51.0
      secondary (*see also* Syphilis, secondary) A51.39
        relapse (treated, untreated) A51.49
    ulcer A51.39
  eighth nerve (neuritis) A52.15
  endemic A65
  endocarditis A52.03
    aortic A52.03
    pulmonary A52.03
  epididymis (late) A52.76
  epiglottis (late) A52.73
  epiphysitis (congenital) (early) A50.02
  episcleritis (late) A52.71
  esophagus A52.79
  eustachian tube A52.73
  exposure to Z20.2
  eye A52.71
  eyelid (late) (with gumma) A52.71
  fallopian tube (late) A52.76
  fracture A52.77
  gallbladder (late) A52.74
  gastric (polyposis) (late) A52.74
  general A53.9
    paralysis A52.17
      juvenile A50.45
  genital (primary) A51.0
  glaucoma A52.71
  gumma NEC A52.79
    cardiovascular system A52.00
    central nervous system A52.3
    congenital A50.59
  heart (block) (decompensation) (disease) (failure) A52.06 [I52]
    valve NEC A52.03
  hemianesthesia A52.19
  hemianopsia A52.71
  hemiparesis A52.17
  hemiplegia A52.17

☑ **Additional Character Required** — Refer to the Tabular List for Character Selection   🖫 **Subterms under main terms may continue to next column or page**

Syphilis, syphilitic — *continued*
- hepatic artery A52.09
- hepatis A52.74
- hepatomegaly, congenital A50.08
- hereditaria tarda — *see* Syphilis, congenital, late
- hereditary — *see* Syphilis, congenital
- Hutchinson's teeth A50.52
- hyalitis A52.71
- inactive — *see* Syphilis, latent
- infantum — *see* Syphilis, congenital
- inherited — *see* Syphilis, congenital
- internal ear A52.79
- intestine (late) A52.74
- iris, iritis (secondary) A51.43
  - late A52.71
- joint (late) A52.77
- keratitis (congenital) (interstitial) (late) A50.31
- kidney (late) A52.75
- lacrimal passages (late) A52.71
- larynx (late) A52.73
- late A52.9
  - cardiovascular A52.00
  - central nervous system A52.3
  - kidney A52.75
  - latent or 2 years or more after infection (without manifestations) A52.8
    - negative spinal fluid test A52.8
    - serology positive A52.8
  - paresis A52.17
  - specified site NEC A52.79
  - symptomatic or with manifestations A52.79
  - tabes A52.11
- latent A53.0
  - with signs or symptoms — *code by* site and stage under Syphilis
  - early, or less than 2 years after infection A51.5
    - central nervous system A52.2
    - date of infection unspecified A53.0
    - follow-up of latent syphilis A53.0
      - date of infection unspecified A53.0
      - late, or 2 years or more after infection A52.8
    - late, or 2 years or more after infection A52.8
    - positive serology (only finding) A53.0
      - early, or less than 2 years after infection A51.5
      - date of infection unspecified A53.0
      - late, or 2 years or more after infection A52.8
- lens (late) A52.71
- leukoderma A51.39
  - late A52.79
- lienitis A52.79
- lip A51.39
  - chancre (primary) A51.2
  - late A52.79
- Lissauer's paralysis A52.17
- liver A52.74
- locomotor ataxia A52.11
- lung A52.72
- lymph gland (early) (secondary) A51.49
  - late A52.79
- lymphadenitis (secondary) A51.49
- macular atrophy of skin A51.39
  - striated A52.79
- mediastinum (late) A52.73
- meninges (adhesive) (brain) (spinal cord) A52.13
- meningitis A52.13
  - acute (secondary) A51.41
  - congenital A50.41
- meningoencephalitis A52.14
- meningovascular A52.13
  - congenital A50.41
- mesarteritis A52.09
  - brain A52.04
- middle ear A52.77
- mitral stenosis A52.03
- monoplegia A52.17
- mouth (secondary) A51.39
  - late A52.79
- mucocutaneous (secondary) A51.39
  - late A52.79
- mucous
  - membrane (secondary) A51.39
    - late A52.79
  - patches A51.39
    - congenital A50.07
- mulberry molars A50.52
- muscle A52.78
- myocardium A52.06
- nasal sinus (late) A52.73

Syphilis, syphilitic — *continued*
- neonatorum — *see* Syphilis, congenital
- nephrotic syndrome (secondary) A51.44
- nerve palsy (any cranial nerve) A52.15
  - multiple A52.15
- nervous system, central A52.3
- neuritis A52.15
  - acoustic A52.15
- neurorecidive of retina A52.19
- neuroretinitis A52.19
- newborn — *see* Syphilis, congenital
- nodular superficial (late) A52.79
- nonvenereal A65
- nose (late) A52.73
  - saddle back deformity A50.57
- occlusive arterial disease A52.09
- oculopathy A52.71
- ophthalmic (late) A52.71
- optic nerve (atrophy) (neuritis) (papilla) A52.15
- orbit (late) A52.71
- organic A53.9
- osseous (late) A52.77
- osteochondritis (congenital) (early) A50.02 [M90.80]
- osteoporosis A52.77
- ovary (late) A52.76
- oviduct (late) A52.76
- palate (late) A52.79
- pancreas (late) A52.74
- paralysis A52.17
  - general A52.17
    - juvenile A50.45
- paresis (general) A52.17
  - juvenile A50.45
- paresthesia A52.19
- Parkinson's disease or syndrome A52.19
- paroxysmal tachycardia A52.06
- pemphigus (congenital) A50.06
- penis (chancre) A51.0
  - late A52.76
- pericardium A52.06
- perichondritis, larynx (late) A52.73
- periosteum (late) A52.77
  - congenital (early) A50.02 [M90.80]
  - early (secondary) A51.46
- peripheral nerve A52.79
- petrous bone (late) A52.77
- pharynx (late) A52.73
  - secondary A51.39
- pituitary (gland) A52.79
- pleura (late) A52.73
- pneumonia, white A50.04
- pontine lesion A52.17
- portal vein A52.09
- primary A51.0
  - anal A51.1
  - and secondary — *see* Syphilis, secondary
  - central nervous system A52.3
  - extragenital chancre NEC A51.2
  - fingers A51.2
  - genital A51.0
  - lip A51.2
  - specified site NEC A51.2
  - tonsils A51.2
- prostate (late) A52.76
- ptosis (eyelid) A52.71
- pulmonary (late) A52.72
  - artery A52.09
- pyelonephritis (late) A52.75
- recently acquired, symptomatic A51.9
- rectum (late) A52.74
- respiratory tract (late) A52.73
- retina, late A52.71
- retrobulbar neuritis A52.15
- salpingitis A52.76
- sclera (late) A52.71
- sclerosis
  - cerebral A52.17
  - coronary A52.06
  - multiple A52.11
- scotoma (central) A52.71
- scrotum (late) A52.76
- secondary (and primary) A51.49
  - adenopathy A51.49
  - anus A51.39
  - bone A51.46
  - chorioretinitis, choroiditis A51.43
  - hepatitis A51.45
  - liver A51.45
  - lymphadenitis A51.49

Syphilis, syphilitic — *continued*
- secondary — *continued*
  - meningitis (acute) A51.41
  - mouth A51.39
  - mucous membranes A51.39
  - periosteum, periostitis A51.46
  - pharynx A51.39
  - relapse (treated, untreated) A51.49
  - skin A51.39
  - specified form NEC A51.49
  - tonsil A51.39
  - ulcer A51.39
  - viscera NEC A51.49
  - vulva A51.39
- seminal vesicle (late) A52.76
- seronegative with signs or symptoms — *code by* site and stage under Syphilis
- seropositive
  - with signs or symptoms — *code by* site and stage under Syphilis
  - follow-up of latent syphilis — *see* Syphilis, latent
  - only finding — *see* Syphilis, latent
- seventh nerve (paralysis) A52.15
- sinus, sinusitis (late) A52.73
- skeletal system A52.77
- skin (with ulceration) (early) (secondary) A51.39
  - late or tertiary A52.79
- small intestine (late) A52.74
- spastic spinal paralysis A52.17
- spermatic cord (late) A52.76
- spinal (cord) A52.12
- spleen A52.79
- splenomegaly A52.79
- spondylitis A52.77
- staphyloma A52.71
- stigmata (congenital) A50.59
- stomach A52.74
- synovium A52.78
- tabes dorsalis (late) A52.11
  - juvenile A50.45
- tabetic type A52.11
  - juvenile A50.45
- taboparesis A52.17
  - juvenile A50.45
- tachycardia A52.06
- tendon (late) A52.78
- tertiary A52.9
  - with symptoms NEC A52.79
  - cardiovascular A52.00
  - central nervous system A52.3
  - multiple NEC A52.79
  - specified site NEC A52.79
- testis A52.76
- thorax A52.73
- throat A52.73
- thymus (gland) (late) A52.79
- thyroid (late) A52.79
- tongue (late) A52.79
- tonsil (lingual) (late) A52.73
  - primary A51.2
  - secondary A51.39
- trachea (late) A52.73
- tunica vaginalis (late) A52.76
- ulcer (any site) (early) (secondary) A51.39
  - late A52.79
  - perforating A52.79
    - foot A52.11
- urethra (late) A52.76
- urogenital (late) A52.76
- uterus (late) A52.76
- uveal tract (secondary) A51.43
  - late A52.71
- uveitis (secondary) A51.43
  - late A52.71
- uvula (late) (perforated) A52.79
- vagina A51.0
  - late A52.76
- valvulitis NEC A52.03
- vascular A52.00
  - brain (cerebral) A52.05
- ventriculi A52.74
- vesicae urinariae (late) A52.76
- viscera (abdominal) (late) A52.74
  - secondary A51.49
- vitreous (opacities) (late) A52.71
  - hemorrhage A52.71
- vulva A51.0
  - late A52.76
  - secondary A51.39

Syphiloma A52.79
  cardiovascular system A52.00
  central nervous system A52.3
  circulatory system A52.00
  congenital A50.59
Syphilophobia F45.29
Syringadenoma (*see also* Neoplasm, skin, benign)
  papillary — *see* Neoplasm, skin, benign

Syringobulbia G95.0
Syringocystadenoma — *see* Neoplasm, skin, benign
  papillary — *see* Neoplasm, skin, benign
Syringoma (*see also* Neoplasm, skin, benign)
  chondroid — *see* Neoplasm, skin, benign
Syringomyelia G95.0
Syringomyelitis — *see* Encephalitis
Syringomyelocele — *see* Spina bifida

Syringopontia G95.0
System, systemic (*see also* condition)
  disease, combined — *see* Degeneration, combined
  inflammatory response syndrome (SIRS) of non-infectious origin (without organ dysfunction) R65.10
    with acute organ dysfunction R65.11
  lupus erythematosus M32.9
    inhibitor present D68.62

☑ **Additional Character Required — Refer to the Tabular List for Character Selection**   ▽ **Subterms under main terms may continue to next column or page**

T

Tabacism, tabacosis, tabagism (see also Poisoning, tobacco)
  meaning dependence (without remission) F17.200
    with
      disorder F17.299
        in remission F17.211
        specified disorder NEC F17.298
        withdrawal F17.203
Tabardillo A75.9
  flea-borne A75.2
  louse-borne A75.0
Tabes, tabetic A52.10
  with
    central nervous system syphilis A52.10
    Charcot's joint A52.16
    cord bladder A52.19
    crisis, viscera (any) A52.19
    paralysis, general A52.17
    paresis (general) A52.17
    perforating ulcer (foot) A52.19
  arthropathy (Charcot) A52.16
  bladder A52.19
  bone A52.11
  cerebrospinal A52.12
  congenital A50.45
  conjugal A52.10
  dorsalis A52.11
    juvenile A50.49
  juvenile A50.49
  latent A52.19
  mesenterica A18.39
  paralysis, insane, general A52.17
  spasmodic A52.17
  syphilis (cerebrospinal) A52.12
Taboparalysis A52.17
Taboparesis (remission) A52.17
  juvenile A50.45
TAC (trigeminal autonomic cephalgia) **NEC** G44.099
  intractable G44.091
  not intractable G44.099
Tache noir S60.22- ☑
Tachyalimentation K91.2
Tachyarrhythmia, tachyrhythmia — see Tachycardia
Tachycardia R00.0
  atrial (paroxysmal) I47.1
  auricular I47.1
  AV nodal re-entry (re-entrant) I47.1
  junctional (paroxysmal) I47.1
  newborn P29.11
  nodal (paroxysmal) I47.1
  non-paroxysmal AV nodal I45.89
  paroxysmal (sustained) (nonsustained) I47.9
    with sinus bradycardia I49.5
    atrial (PAT) I47.1
    atrioventricular (AV) (re-entrant) I47.1
      psychogenic F54
    junctional I47.1
      ectopic I47.1
    nodal I47.1
    psychogenic (atrial) (supraventricular) (ventricular) F54
    supraventricular (sustained) I47.1
      psychogenic F54
    ventricular I47.2
      psychogenic F54
  psychogenic F45.8
  sick sinus I49.5
  sinoauricular NOS R00.0
    paroxysmal I47.1
  sinus [sinusal] NOS R00.0
    paroxysmal I47.1
  supraventricular I47.1
  ventricular (paroxysmal) (sustained) I47.2
    psychogenic F54
Tachygastria K31.89
Tachypnea R06.82
  hysterical F45.8
  newborn (idiopathic) (transitory) P22.1
  psychogenic F45.8
  transitory, of newborn P22.1
TACO (transfusion associated circulatory overload) E87.71
Taenia (infection) (infestation) B68.9
  diminuta B71.0
  echinococcal infestation B67.90
  mediocanellata B68.1

Taenia — continued
  nana B71.0
  saginata B68.1
  solium (intestinal form) B68.0
    larval form — see Cysticercosis
Taeniasis (intestine) — see Taenia
Tag (hypertrophied skin) (infected) L91.8
  adenoid J35.8
  anus K64.4
  hemorrhoidal K64.4
  hymen N89.8
  perineal N90.89
  preauricular Q17.0
  sentinel K64.4
  skin L91.8
    accessory (congenital) Q82.8
    anus K64.4
    congenital Q82.8
    preauricular Q17.0
  tonsil J35.8
  urethra, urethral N36.8
  vulva N90.89
Tahyna fever B33.8
Takahara's disease E80.3
Takayasu's disease or syndrome M31.4
Talcosis (pulmonary) J62.0
Talipes (congenital) Q66.89
  acquired, planus — see Deformity, limb, flat foot
  asymmetric Q66.89
  calcaneovalgus Q66.4
  calcaneovarus Q66.1
  calcaneus Q66.89
  cavus Q66.7
  equinovalgus Q66.6
  equinovarus Q66.0
  equinus Q66.89
  percavus Q66.7
  planovalgus Q66.6
  planus (acquired) (any degree) (see also Deformity, limb, flat foot)
    congenital Q66.5- ☑
    due to rickets (sequelae) E64.3
  valgus Q66.6
  varus Q66.3
Tall stature, constitutional E34.4
Talma's disease M62.89
Talon noir S90.3- ☑
  hand S60.22- ☑
  heel S90.3- ☑
  toe S90.1- ☑
Tamponade, heart I31.4
Tanapox (virus disease) B08.71
Tangier disease E78.6
Tantrum, child problem F91.8
Tapeworm (infection) (infestation) — see Infestation, tapeworm
Tapia's syndrome G52.7
TAR (thrombocytopenia with absent radius) **syndrome** Q87.2
Tarral-Besnier disease L44.0
Tarsal tunnel syndrome — see Syndrome, tarsal tunnel
Tarsalgia — see Pain, limb, lower
Tarsitis (eyelid) H01.8
  syphilitic A52.71
  tuberculous A18.4
Tartar (teeth) (dental calculus) K03.6
Tattoo (mark) L81.8
Tauri's disease E74.09
Taurodontism K00.2
Taussig-Bing syndrome Q20.1
Taybi's syndrome Q87.2
Tay-Sachs amaurotic familial idiocy or disease E75.02
TBI (traumatic brain injury) S06.9 ☑
Teacher's node or nodule J38.2
Tear, torn (traumatic) (see also Laceration)
  with abortion — see Abortion
  annular fibrosis M51.35
  anus, anal (sphincter) S31.831 ☑
    complicating delivery
      with third degree perineal laceration (see also Delivery, complicated, by, laceration, perineum, third degree) O70.20
        with mucosa O70.3
      without third degree perineal laceration O70.4
    nontraumatic (healed) (old) K62.81
  articular cartilage, old — see Derangement, joint, articular cartilage, by site

Tear, torn — continued
  bladder
    with ectopic or molar pregnancy O08.6
    following ectopic or molar pregnancy O08.6
    obstetrical O71.5
    traumatic — see Injury, bladder
  bowel
    with ectopic or molar pregnancy O08.6
    following ectopic or molar pregnancy O08.6
    obstetrical trauma O71.5
  broad ligament
    with ectopic or molar pregnancy O08.6
    following ectopic or molar pregnancy O08.6
    obstetrical trauma O71.6
  bucket handle (knee) (meniscus) — see Tear, meniscus
  capsule, joint — see Sprain
  cartilage (see also Sprain)
    articular, old — see Derangement, joint, articular cartilage, by site
  cervix
    with ectopic or molar pregnancy O08.6
    following ectopic or molar pregnancy O08.6
    obstetrical trauma (current) O71.3
    old N88.1
    traumatic — see Injury, uterus
  dural G97.41
    nontraumatic G96.11
  internal organ — see Injury, by site
  knee cartilage
    articular (current) S83.3- ☑
    old — see Derangement, knee, meniscus, due to old tear
  ligament — see Sprain
  meniscus (knee) (current injury) S83.209 ☑
    bucket-handle S83.20- ☑
    lateral
      bucket-handle S83.25- ☑
      complex S83.27- ☑
      peripheral S83.26- ☑
      specified type NEC S83.28- ☑
    medial
      bucket-handle S83.21- ☑
      complex S83.23- ☑
      peripheral S83.22- ☑
      specified type NEC S83.24- ☑
    old — see Derangement, knee, meniscus, due to old tear
    site other than knee — code as Sprain
    specified type NEC S83.20- ☑
  muscle — see Strain
  pelvic
    floor, complicating delivery O70.1
    organ NEC, obstetrical trauma O71.5
      with ectopic or molar pregnancy O08.6
      following ectopic or molar pregnancy O08.6
  perineal, secondary O90.1
  periurethral tissue, obstetrical trauma O71.82
    with ectopic or molar pregnancy O08.6
    following ectopic or molar pregnancy O08.6
  rectovaginal septum — see Laceration, vagina
  retina, retinal (without detachment) (horseshoe) (see also Break, retina, horseshoe)
    with detachment — see Detachment, retina, with retinal, break
  rotator cuff (nontraumatic) M75.10- ☑
    complete M75.12- ☑
    incomplete M75.11- ☑
    traumatic S46.01- ☑
      capsule S43.42- ☑
  semilunar cartilage, knee — see Tear, meniscus
  supraspinatus (complete) (incomplete) (nontraumatic) (see also Tear, rotator cuff) M75.10- ☑
  tendon — see Strain
  tentorial, at birth P10.4
  umbilical cord
    complicating delivery O69.89 ☑
  urethra
    with ectopic or molar pregnancy O08.6
    following ectopic or molar pregnancy O08.6
    obstetrical trauma O71.5
  uterus — see Injury, uterus
  vagina — see Laceration, vagina
  vessel, from catheter — see Puncture, accidental complicating surgery
  vulva, complicating delivery O70.0
Tear-stone — see Dacryolith

Index

Teeth — Test, tests, testing

Teeth (*see also* condition)
  grinding
    psychogenic F45.8
    sleep related G47.63
Teething (syndrome) K00.7
Telangiectasia, telangiectasis (verrucous) I78.1
  ataxic (cerebellar) (Louis-Bar) G11.3
  familial I78.0
  hemorrhagic, hereditary (congenital) (senile) I78.0
  hereditary, hemorrhagic (congenital) (senile) I78.0
  juxtafoveal H35.07- ☑
  macular H35.07- ☑
  macularis eruptiva perstans D47.01
  parafoveal H35.07- ☑
  retinal (idiopathic) (juxtafoveal) (macular) (parafoveal) H35.07- ☑
  spider I78.1
Telephone scatologia F65.89
Telescoped bowel or intestine K56.1
  congenital Q43.8
Temperature
  body, high (of unknown origin) R50.9
  cold, trauma from T69.9 ☑
    newborn P80.0
    specified effect NEC T69.8 ☑
Temple — *see* condition
Temporal — *see* condition
Temporomandibular joint pain-dysfunction syndrome M26.62- ☑
Temporosphenoidal — *see* condition
Tendency
  bleeding — *see* Defect, coagulation
  suicide
    meaning personal history of attempted suicide Z91.5
    meaning suicidal ideation — *see* Ideation, suicidal
  to fall R29.6
Tenderness, abdominal R10.819
  epigastric R10.816
  generalized R10.817
  left lower quadrant R10.814
  left upper quadrant R10.812
  periumbilic R10.815
  rebound R10.829
    epigastric R10.826
    generalized R10.827
    left lower quadrant R10.824
    left upper quadrant R10.822
    periumbilic R10.825
    right lower quadrant R10.823
    right upper quadrant R10.821
  right lower quadrant R10.813
  right upper quadrant R10.811
Tendinitis, tendonitis (*see also* Enthesopathy)
  Achilles M76.6- ☑
  adhesive — *see* Tenosynovitis, specified type NEC
    shoulder — *see* Capsulitis, adhesive
  bicipital M75.2- ☑
  calcific M65.2- ☑
    ankle M65.27- ☑
    foot M65.27- ☑
    forearm M65.23- ☑
    hand M65.24- ☑
    lower leg M65.26- ☑
    multiple sites M65.29
    pelvic region M65.25- ☑
    shoulder M75.3- ☑
    specified site NEC M65.28
    thigh M65.25- ☑
    upper arm M65.22- ☑
  due to use, overuse, pressure (*see also* Disorder, soft tissue, due to use)
    specified NEC — *see* Disorder, soft tissue, due to use, specified NEC
  gluteal M76.0- ☑
  patellar M76.5- ☑
  peroneal M76.7- ☑
  psoas M76.1- ☑
  tibial (posterior) M76.82- ☑
    anterior M76.81- ☑
  trochanteric — *see* Bursitis, hip, trochanteric
Tendon — *see* condition
Tendosynovitis — *see* Tenosynovitis
Tenesmus (rectal) R19.8
  vesical R30.1
Tennis elbow — *see* Epicondylitis, lateral

Tenonitis (*see also* Tenosynovitis)
  eye (capsule) H05.04- ☑
Tenontosynovitis — *see* Tenosynovitis
Tenontothecitis — *see* Tenosynovitis
Tenophyte — *see* Disorder, synovium, specified type NEC
Tenosynovitis (*see also* Synovitis) M65.9
  adhesive — *see* Tenosynovitis, specified type NEC
    shoulder — *see* Capsulitis, adhesive
  bicipital (calcifying) — *see* Tendinitis, bicipital
  gonococcal A54.49
  in (due to)
    crystals M65.8- ☑
    gonorrhea A54.49
    syphilis (late) A52.78
    use, overuse, pressure (*see also* Disorder, soft tissue, due to use)
      specified NEC — *see* Disorder, soft tissue, due to use, specified NEC
  infective NEC M65.1- ☑
    ankle M65.17- ☑
    foot M65.17- ☑
    forearm M65.13- ☑
    hand M65.14- ☑
    lower leg M65.16- ☑
    multiple sites M65.19
    pelvic region M65.15- ☑
    shoulder region M65.11- ☑
    specified site NEC M65.18
    thigh M65.15- ☑
    upper arm M65.12- ☑
  radial styloid M65.4
  shoulder region M65.81- ☑
    adhesive — *see* Capsulitis, adhesive
  specified type NEC M65.88
    ankle M65.87- ☑
    foot M65.87- ☑
    forearm M65.83- ☑
    hand M65.84- ☑
    lower leg M65.86- ☑
    multiple sites M65.89
    pelvic region M65.85- ☑
    shoulder region M65.81- ☑
    specified site NEC M65.88
    thigh M65.85- ☑
    upper arm M65.82- ☑
  tuberculous — *see* Tuberculosis, tenosynovitis
Tenovaginitis — *see* Tenosynovitis
Tension
  arterial, high (*see also* Hypertension)
    without diagnosis of hypertension R03.0
  headache G44.209
    intractable G44.201
    not intractable G44.209
  nervous R45.0
  pneumothorax J93.0
  premenstrual N94.3
  state (mental) F48.9
Tentorium — *see* condition
Teratencephalus Q89.8
Teratism Q89.7
Teratoblastoma (malignant) — *see* Neoplasm, malignant, by site
Teratocarcinoma (*see also* Neoplasm, malignant, by site)
  liver C22.7
Teratoma (solid) (*see also* Neoplasm, uncertain behavior, by site)
  with embryonal carcinoma, mixed — *see* Neoplasm, malignant, by site
  with malignant transformation — *see* Neoplasm, malignant, by site
  adult (cystic) — *see* Neoplasm, benign, by site
  benign — *see* Neoplasm, benign, by site
  combined with choriocarcinoma — *see* Neoplasm, malignant, by site
  cystic (adult) — *see* Neoplasm, benign, by site
  differentiated — *see* Neoplasm, benign, by site
  embryonal (*see also* Neoplasm, malignant, by site)
    liver C22.7
  immature — *see* Neoplasm, malignant, by site
  liver C22.7
    adult, benign, cystic, differentiated type or mature D13.4
  malignant (*see also* Neoplasm, malignant, by site)
    anaplastic — *see* Neoplasm, malignant, by site
    intermediate — *see* Neoplasm, malignant, by site

Teratoma — *continued*
  malignant (*see also* Neoplasm, malignant, by site) — *continued*
    intermediate — *see* Neoplasm, malignant, by site — *continued*
      specified site — *see* Neoplasm, malignant, by site
      unspecified site C62.90
    undifferentiated — *see* Neoplasm, malignant, by site
  mature — *see* Neoplasm, uncertain behavior, by site
    malignant — *see* Neoplasm, by site, malignant, by site
  ovary D27.- ☑
    embryonal, immature or malignant C56- ☑
  solid — *see* Neoplasm, uncertain behavior, by site
  testis C62.9- ☑
    adult, benign, cystic, differentiated type or mature D29.2- ☑
    scrotal C62.1- ☑
    undescended C62.0- ☑
Termination
  anomalous (*see also* Malposition, congenital)
    right pulmonary vein Q26.3
  pregnancy, elective Z33.2
Ternidens diminutus infestation B81.8
Ternidensiasis B81.8
Terror(s) night (child) F51.4
Terrorism, victim of Z65.4
Terry's syndrome (*see also* Myopia, degenerative) H44.2- ☑
Tertiary — *see* condition
Test, tests, testing (for)
  adequacy (for dialysis)
    hemodialysis Z49.31
    peritoneal Z49.32
  blood pressure Z01.30
    abnormal reading — *see* Blood, pressure
  blood typing Z01.83
    Rh typing Z01.83
  blood-alcohol Z04.8
    positive — *see* Findings, abnormal, in blood
  blood-drug Z04.8
    positive — *see* Findings, abnormal, in blood
  cardiac pulse generator (battery) Z45.010
  fertility Z31.41
  genetic
    disease carrier status for procreative management
      female Z31.430
      male Z31.440
    male partner of patient with recurrent pregnancy loss Z31.441
    procreative management NEC
      female Z31.438
      male Z31.448
  hearing Z01.10
    with abnormal findings NEC Z01.118
  HIV (human immunodeficiency virus)
    nonconclusive (in infants) R75
    positive Z21
    seropositive Z21
  immunity status Z01.84
  intelligence NEC Z01.89
  laboratory (as part of a general medical examination) Z00.00
    with abnormal finding Z00.01
    for medicolegal reason NEC Z04.8
  male partner of patient with recurrent pregnancy loss Z31.441
  Mantoux (for tuberculosis) Z11.1
    abnormal result R76.11
  pregnancy, positive first pregnancy — *see* Pregnancy, normal, first
  procreative Z31.49
    fertility Z31.41
  skin, diagnostic
    allergy Z01.82
      special screening examination — *see* Screening, by name of disease
    Mantoux Z11.1
    tuberculin Z11.1
  specified NEC Z01.89
  tuberculin Z11.1
    abnormal result R76.11
  vision Z01.00
    with abnormal findings Z01.01
  Wassermann Z11.3
    positive — *see* Serology for syphilis, positive

Testicle, testicular, testis (*see also* condition)
  feminization syndrome (*see also* Syndrome, androgen insensitivity) E34.51
  migrans Q55.29
Tetanus, tetanic (cephalic) (convulsions) A35
  with
    abortion A34
    ectopic or molar pregnancy O08.0
  following ectopic or molar pregnancy O08.0
  inoculation reaction (due to serum) — *see* Complications, vaccination
  neonatorum A33
  obstetrical A34
  puerperal, postpartum, childbirth A34
Tetany (due to) R29.0
  alkalosis E87.3
  associated with rickets E55.0
  convulsions R29.0
    hysterical F44.5
  functional (hysterical) F44.5
  hyperkinetic R29.0
    hysterical F44.5
  hyperpnea R06.4
    hysterical F44.5
    psychogenic F45.8
  hyperventilation (*see also* Hyperventilation) R06.4
    hysterical F44.5
  neonatal (without calcium or magnesium deficiency) P71.3
  parathyroid (gland) E20.9
  parathyroprival E89.2
  post- (para)thyroidectomy E89.2
  postoperative E89.2
  pseudotetany R29.0
  psychogenic (conversion reaction) F44.5
Tetralogy of Fallot Q21.3
Tetraplegia (chronic) (*see also* Quadriplegia) G82.50
Thailand hemorrhagic fever A91
Thalassanemia — *see* Thalassemia
Thalassemia (anemia) (disease) D56.9
  with other hemoglobinopathy D56.8
  alpha (major) (severe) (triple gene defect) D56.0
    minor D56.3
    silent carrier D56.3
    trait D56.3
  beta (severe) D56.1
    homozygous D56.1
    major D56.1
    minor D56.3
    trait D56.3
  delta-beta (homozygous) D56.2
    minor D56.3
    trait D56.3
  dominant D56.8
  hemoglobin
    C D56.8
    E-beta D56.5
  intermedia D56.1
  major D56.1
  minor D56.3
  mixed D56.8
  sickle-cell — *see* Disease, sickle-cell, thalassemia
  specified type NEC D56.8
  trait D56.3
  variants D56.8
Thanatophoric dwarfism or short stature Q77.1
Thaysen-Gee disease (nontropical sprue) K90.0
Thaysen's disease K90.0
Thecoma D27- ☑
  luteinized D27- ☑
  malignant C56- ☑
Thelarche, premature E30.8
Thelaziasis B83.8
Thelitis N61.0
  puerperal, postpartum or gestational — *see* Infection, nipple
Therapeutic — *see* condition
Therapy
  drug, long-term (current) (prophylactic)
    agents affecting estrogen receptors and estrogen levels NEC Z79.818
    anastrozole (Arimidex) Z79.811
    antibiotics Z79.2
      short-term use — *omit code*
    anticoagulants Z79.01
    anti-inflammatory Z79.1
    antiplatelet Z79.02
    antithrombotics Z79.02

Therapy — *continued*
  drug, long-term — *continued*
    aromatase inhibitors Z79.811
    aspirin Z79.82
    birth control pill or patch Z79.3
    bisphosphonates Z79.83
    contraceptive, oral Z79.3
    drug, specified NEC Z79.899
    estrogen receptor downregulators Z79.818
    Evista Z79.810
    exemestane (Aromasin) Z79.811
    Fareston Z79.810
    fulvestrant (Faslodex) Z79.818
    gonadotropin-releasing hormone (GnRH) agonist Z79.818
    goserelin acetate (Zoladex) Z79.818
    hormone replacement Z79.890
    insulin Z79.4
    letrozole (Femara) Z79.811
    leuprolide acetate (leuprorelin) (Lupron) Z79.818
    megestrol acetate (Megace) Z79.818
    methadone
      for pain management Z79.891
      maintenance therapy F11.20
    Nolvadex Z79.810
    opiate analgesic Z79.891
    oral contraceptive Z79.3
    raloxifene (Evista) Z79.810
    selective estrogen receptor modulators (SERMs) Z79.810
    short term — *omit code*
    steroids
      inhaled Z79.51
      systemic Z79.52
    tamoxifen (Nolvadex) Z79.810
    toremifene (Fareston) Z79.810
Thermic — *see* condition
Thermography (abnormal) (*see also* Abnormal, diagnostic imaging) R93.8
  breast R92.8
Thermoplegia T67.0 ☑
Thesaurismosis, glycogen — *see* Disease, glycogen storage
Thiamin deficiency E51.9
  specified NEC E51.8
Thiaminic deficiency with beriberi E51.11
Thibierge-Weissenbach syndrome — *see* Sclerosis, systemic
Thickening
  bone — *see* Hypertrophy, bone
  breast N64.59
  endometrium R93.8
  epidermal L85.9
    specified NEC L85.8
  hymen N89.6
  larynx J38.7
  nail L60.2
    congenital Q84.5
  periosteal — *see* Hypertrophy, bone
  pleura J92.9
    with asbestos J92.0
  skin R23.4
  subepiglottic J38.7
  tongue K14.8
  valve, heart — *see* Endocarditis
Thigh — *see* condition
Thinning vertebra — *see* Spondylopathy, specified NEC
Thirst, excessive R63.1
  due to deprivation of water T73.1 ☑
Thomsen disease G71.12
Thoracic (*see also* condition)
  kidney Q63.2
  outlet syndrome G54.0
Thoracogastroschisis (congenital) Q79.8
Thoracopagus Q89.4
Thorax — *see* condition
Thorn's syndrome N28.89
Thorson-Björck syndrome E34.0
Threadworm (infection) (infestation) B80
Threatened
  abortion O20.0
    with subsequent abortion O03.9
  job loss, anxiety concerning Z56.2
  labor (without delivery) O47.9
    at or after 37 completed weeks of gestation O47.1
    before 37 completed weeks of gestation O47.0- ☑
  loss of job, anxiety concerning Z56.2
  miscarriage O20.0

Threatened — *continued*
  unemployment, anxiety concerning Z56.2
Three-day fever A93.1
Threshers' lung J67.0
Thrix annulata (congenital) Q84.1
Throat — *see* condition
Thrombasthenia (Glanzmann) (hemorrhagic) (hereditary) D69.1
Thromboangiitis I73.1
  obliterans (general) I73.1
    cerebral I67.89
    vessels
      brain I67.89
      spinal cord I67.89
Thromboarteritis — *see* Arteritis
Thromboasthenia (Glanzmann) (hemorrhagic) (hereditary) D69.1
Thrombocytasthenia (Glanzmann) D69.1
Thrombocythemia (essential) (hemorrhagic) (idiopathic) (primary) D47.3
Thrombocytopathy (dystrophic) (granulopenic) D69.1
Thrombocytopenia, thrombocytopenic D69.6
  with absent radius (TAR) Q87.2
  congenital D69.42
  dilutional D69.59
  due to
    (massive) blood transfusion D69.59
    drugs D69.59
    extracorporeal circulation of blood D69.59
    platelet alloimmunization D69.59
  essential D69.3
  heparin induced (HIT) D75.82
  hereditary D69.42
  idiopathic D69.3
  neonatal, transitory P61.0
    due to
      exchange transfusion P61.0
      idiopathic maternal thrombocytopenia P61.0
      isoimmunization P61.0
  primary NEC D69.49
    idiopathic D69.3
  puerperal, postpartum O72.3
  secondary D69.59
  transient neonatal P61.0
Thrombocytosis, essential D47.3
  primary D47.3
Thromboembolism — *see* Embolism
Thrombopathy (Bernard-Soulier) D69.1
  constitutional D68.0
  Willebrand-Jurgens D68.0
Thrombopenia — *see* Thrombocytopenia
Thrombophilia D68.59
  primary NEC D68.59
  secondary NEC D68.69
  specified NEC D68.69
Thrombophlebitis I80.9
  antepartum O22.2- ☑
    deep O22.3- ☑
    superficial O22.2- ☑
  cavernous (venous) sinus G08
    complicating pregnancy O22.5- ☑
    nonpyogenic I67.6
  cerebral (sinus) (vein) G08
    nonpyogenic I67.6
    sequelae G09
  due to implanted device — *see* Complications, by site and type, specified NEC
  during or resulting from a procedure NEC T81.72 ☑
  femoral vein (superficial) I80.1- ☑
  femoropopliteal vein I80.0- ☑
  hepatic (vein) I80.8
  idiopathic, recurrent I82.1
  iliofemoral I80.1- ☑
  intracranial venous sinus (any) G08
    nonpyogenic I67.6
    sequelae G09
  intraspinal venous sinuses and veins G08
    nonpyogenic G95.19
  lateral (venous) sinus G08
    nonpyogenic I67.6
  leg I80.3
    superficial I80.0- ☑
  longitudinal (venous) sinus G08
    nonpyogenic I67.6
  lower extremity I80.299
  migrans, migrating I82.1
  pelvic
    with ectopic or molar pregnancy O08.0

Thrombophlebitis — *continued*
pelvic — *continued*
following ectopic or molar pregnancy O08.0
puerperal O87.1
popliteal vein — *see* Phlebitis, leg, deep, popliteal
portal (vein) K75.1
postoperative T81.72 ☑
pregnancy — *see* Thrombophlebitis, antepartum
puerperal, postpartum, childbirth O87.0
deep O87.1
pelvic O87.1
septic O86.81
superficial O87.0
saphenous (greater) (lesser) I80.0- ☑
sinus (intracranial) G08
nonpyogenic I67.6
specified site NEC I80.8
tibial vein I80.23- ☑

Thrombosis, thrombotic (bland) (multiple) (progressive)
(silent) (vessel) I82.90
anal K64.5
antepartum — *see* Thrombophlebitis, antepartum
aorta, aortic I74.10
abdominal I74.09
saddle I74.01
bifurcation I74.09
saddle I74.01
specified site NEC I74.19
terminal I74.09
thoracic I74.11
valve — *see* Endocarditis, aortic
apoplexy I63.3- ☑
artery, arteries (postinfectional) I74.9
auditory, internal — *see* Occlusion, artery, precerebral, specified NEC
basilar — *see* Occlusion, artery, basilar
carotid (common) (internal) — *see* Occlusion,
artery, carotid
cerebellar (anterior inferior) (posterior inferior)
(superior) — *see* Occlusion, artery, cerebellar
cerebral — *see* Occlusion, artery, cerebral
choroidal (anterior) — *see* Occlusion, artery, precerebral, specified NEC
communicating, posterior — *see* Occlusion, artery,
precerebral, specified NEC
coronary (*see also* Infarct, myocardium)
not resulting in infarction I24.0
hepatic I74.8
hypophyseal — *see* Occlusion, artery, precerebral,
specified NEC
iliac I74.5
limb I74.4
lower I74.3
upper I74.2
meningeal, anterior or posterior — *see* Occlusion,
artery, cerebral, specified NEC
mesenteric (with gangrene) (*see also* Infarct, intestine) K55.069
ophthalmic — *see* Occlusion, artery, retina
pontine — *see* Occlusion, artery, precerebral,
specified NEC
precerebral — *see* Occlusion, artery, precerebral
pulmonary (iatrogenic) — *see* Embolism, pulmonary
renal N28.0
retinal — *see* Occlusion, artery, retina
spinal, anterior or posterior G95.11
traumatic NEC T14.8 ☑
vertebral — *see* Occlusion, artery, vertebral
atrium, auricular (*see also* Infarct, myocardium)
following acute myocardial infarction (current
complication) I23.6
not resulting in infarction I51.3
old I51.3
basilar (artery) — *see* Occlusion, artery, basilar
brain (artery) (stem) (*see also* Occlusion, artery, cerebral)
due to syphilis A52.05
puerperal O99.43
sinus — *see* Thrombosis, intracranial venous sinus
capillary I78.8
cardiac (*see also* Infarct, myocardium)
not resulting in infarction I51.3
old I51.3
valve — *see* Endocarditis
carotid (artery) (common) (internal) — *see* Occlusion,
artery, carotid

Thrombosis, thrombotic — *continued*
cavernous (venous) sinus — *see* Thrombosis, intracranial venous sinus
cerebellar artery (anterior inferior) (posterior inferior)
(superior) I66.3
cerebral (artery) — *see* Occlusion, artery, cerebral
cerebrovenous sinus (*see also* Thrombosis, intracranial
venous sinus)
puerperium O87.3
chronic I82.91
coronary (artery) (vein) (*see also* Infarct, myocardium)
not resulting in infarction I24.0
corpus cavernosum N48.89
cortical I66.9
deep — *see* Embolism, vein, lower extremity
due to device, implant or graft (*see also* Complications,
by site and type, specified NEC) T85.868 ☑
arterial graft NEC T82.868 ☑
breast (implant) T85.868 ☑
catheter NEC T85.868 ☑
dialysis (renal) T82.868 ☑
intraperitoneal T85.868 ☑
infusion NEC T82.868 ☑
spinal (epidural) (subdural) T85.860 ☑
urinary (indwelling) T83.86 ☑
electronic (electrode) (pulse generator) (stimulator)
bone T84.86 ☑
cardiac T82.867 ☑
nervous system (brain) (peripheral nerve)
(spinal) T85.860 ☑
urinary T83.86 ☑
fixation, internal (orthopedic) NEC T84.86 ☑
gastrointestinal (bile duct) (esophagus) T85.868 ☑
genital NEC T83.86 ☑
heart T82.867 ☑
joint prosthesis T84.86 ☑
ocular (corneal graft) (orbital implant) NEC
T85.868 ☑
orthopedic NEC T84.86 ☑
specified NEC T85.868 ☑
urinary NEC T83.86 ☑
vascular NEC T82.868 ☑
ventricular intracranial shunt T85.860 ☑
during the puerperium — *see* Thrombosis, puerperal
endocardial (*see also* Infarct, myocardium)
not resulting in infarction I51.3
eye — *see* Occlusion, retina
genital organ
female NEC N94.89
pregnancy — *see* Thrombophlebitis, antepartum
male N50.1
gestational — *see* Phlebopathy, gestational
heart (chamber) (*see also* Infarct, myocardium)
not resulting in infarction I51.3
old I51.3
hepatic (vein) I82.0
artery I74.8
history (of) Z86.718
intestine (with gangrene) (*see also* Infarct, intestine)
K55.069
intracardiac NEC (apical) (atrial) (auricular) (ventricular)
(old) I51.3
intracranial (arterial) I66.9
venous sinus (any) G08
nonpyogenic origin I67.6
puerperium O87.3
intramural (*see also* Infarct, myocardium)
not resulting in infarction I51.3
old I51.3
intraspinal venous sinuses and veins G08
nonpyogenic G95.19
kidney (artery) N28.0
lateral (venous) sinus — *see* Thrombosis, intracranial
venous sinus
leg — *see* Thrombosis, vein, lower extremity
arterial I74.3
liver (venous) I82.0
artery I74.8
portal vein I81
longitudinal (venous) sinus — *see* Thrombosis, intracranial venous sinus
lower limb — *see* Thrombosis, vein, lower extremity
lung (iatrogenic) (postoperative) — *see* Embolism,
pulmonary
meninges (brain) (arterial) I66.8

Thrombosis, thrombotic — *continued*
mesenteric (artery) (with gangrene) (*see also* Infarct,
intestine) K55.069
vein (inferior) (superior) I81
mitral I34.8
mural (*see also* Infarct, myocardium)
due to syphilis A52.06
not resulting in infarction I51.3
old I51.3
omentum (with gangrene) (*see also* Infarct, intestine)
K55.069
ophthalmic — *see* Occlusion, retina
pampiniform plexus (male) N50.1
parietal (*see also* Infarct, myocardium)
not resulting in infarction I24.0
penis, superficial vein N48.81
perianal venous K64.5
peripheral arteries I74.4
upper I74.2
personal history (of) Z86.718
portal I81
due to syphilis A52.09
precerebral artery — *see* Occlusion, artery, precerebral
puerperal, postpartum O87.0
brain (artery) O99.43
venous (sinus) O87.3
cardiac O99.43
cerebral (artery) O99.43
venous (sinus) O87.3
superficial O87.0
pulmonary (artery) (iatrogenic) (postoperative) (vein)
— *see* Embolism, pulmonary
renal (artery) N28.0
vein I82.3
resulting from presence of device, implant or graft —
see Complications, by site and type, specified
NEC
retina, retinal — *see* Occlusion, retina
scrotum N50.1
seminal vesicle N50.1
sigmoid (venous) sinus — *see* Thrombosis, intracranial
venous sinus
sinus, intracranial (any) — *see* Thrombosis, intracranial
venous sinus
specified site NEC I82.890
chronic I82.891
spermatic cord N50.1
spinal cord (arterial) G95.11
due to syphilis A52.09
pyogenic origin G06.1
spleen, splenic D73.5
artery I74.8
testis N50.1
traumatic NEC T14.8 ☑
tricuspid I07.8
tumor — *see* Neoplasm, unspecified behavior, by site
tunica vaginalis N50.1
umbilical cord (vessels), complicating delivery O69.5 ☑
vas deferens N50.1
vein (acute) I82.90
antecubital I82.61- ☑
chronic I82.71- ☑
axillary I82.A1- ☑ (*following* I82.7)
chronic I82.A2- ☑ (*following* I82.7)
basilic I82.61- ☑
chronic I82.71- ☑
brachial I82.62- ☑
chronic I82.72- ☑
brachiocephalic (innominate) I82.290
chronic I82.291
cephalic I82.61- ☑
chronic I82.71- ☑
cerebral, nonpyogenic I67.6
chronic I82.91
deep (DVT) I82.40- ☑
calf I82.4Z- ☑
chronic I82.5Z- ☑
lower leg I82.4Z- ☑
chronic I82.5Z- ☑
thigh I82.4Y- ☑
chronic I82.5Y- ☑
upper leg I82.4Y- ☑
chronic I82.5Y- ☑
femoral I82.41- ☑
chronic I82.51- ☑
iliac (iliofemoral) I82.42- ☑
chronic I82.52- ☑

Thrombosis, thrombotic — *continued*
  vein — *continued*
    innominate I82.290
      chronic I82.291
    internal jugular I82.C1- ☑ (*following* I82.7)
      chronic I82.C2- ☑ (*following* I82.7)
    lower extremity
      deep I82.40- ☑
        chronic I82.50- ☑
        specified NEC I82.49- ☑
          chronic NEC I82.59- ☑
      distal
        deep I82.4Z- ☑
      proximal
        deep I82.4Y- ☑
          chronic I82.5Y- ☑
      superficial I82.81- ☑
    perianal K64.5
    popliteal I82.43- ☑
      chronic I82.53- ☑
    radial I82.62- ☑
      chronic I82.72- ☑
    renal I82.3
    saphenous (greater) (lesser) I82.81- ☑
    specified NEC I82.890
      chronic NEC I82.891
    subclavian I82.B1- ☑ (*following* I82.7)
      chronic I82.B2- ☑ (*following* I82.7)
    thoracic NEC I82.290
      chronic I82.291
    tibial I82.44- ☑
      chronic I82.54- ☑
    ulnar I82.62- ☑
      chronic I82.72- ☑
    upper extremity I82.60- ☑
      chronic I82.70- ☑
      deep I82.62- ☑
        chronic I82.72- ☑
      superficial I82.61- ☑
        chronic I82.71- ☑
  vena cava
    inferior I82.220
      chronic I82.221
    superior I82.210
      chronic I82.211
  venous, perianal K64.5
  ventricle (*see also* Infarct, myocardium)
    following acute myocardial infarction (current complication) I23.6
    not resulting in infarction I24.0
    old I51.3
Thrombus — *see* Thrombosis
Thrush (*see also* Candidiasis)
  newborn P37.5
  oral B37.0
  vaginal B37.3
Thumb (*see also* condition)
  sucking (child problem) F98.8
Thymitis E32.8
Thymoma (benign) D15.0
  malignant C37
Thymus, thymic (gland) — *see* condition
Thyrocele — *see* Goiter
Thyroglossal (*see also* condition)
  cyst Q89.2
  duct, persistent Q89.2
Thyroid (gland) (body) (*see also* condition)
  hormone resistance E07.89
  lingual Q89.2
  nodule (cystic) (nontoxic) (single) E04.1
Thyroiditis E06.9
  acute (nonsuppurative) (pyogenic) (suppurative) E06.0
  autoimmune E06.3
  chronic (nonspecific) (sclerosing) E06.5
    with thyrotoxicosis, transient E06.2
    fibrous E06.5
    lymphadenoid E06.3
    lymphocytic E06.3
    lymphoid E06.3
  de Quervain's E06.1
  drug-induced E06.4
  fibrous (chronic) E06.5
  giant-cell (follicular) E06.1
  granulomatous (de Quervain) (subacute) E06.1
  Hashimoto's (struma lymphomatosa) E06.3
  iatrogenic E06.4
  ligneous E06.5

Thyroiditis — *continued*
  lymphocytic (chronic) E06.3
  lymphoid E06.3
  lymphomatous E06.3
  nonsuppurative E06.1
  postpartum, puerperal O90.5
  pseudotuberculous E06.1
  pyogenic E06.0
  radiation E06.4
  Riedel's E06.5
  subacute (granulomatous) E06.1
  suppurative E06.0
  tuberculous A18.81
  viral E06.1
  woody E06.5
Thyrolingual duct, persistent Q89.2
Thyromegaly E01.0
Thyrotoxic
  crisis — *see* Thyrotoxicosis
  heart disease or failure (*see also* Thyrotoxicosis) E05.90 [I43]
    with thyroid storm E05.91 [I43]
  storm — *see* Thyrotoxicosis
Thyrotoxicosis (recurrent) E05.90
  with
    goiter (diffuse) E05.00
      with thyroid storm E05.01
      adenomatous uninodular E05.10
        with thyroid storm E05.11
      multinodular E05.20
        with thyroid storm E05.21
      nodular E05.20
        with thyroid storm E05.21
      uninodular E05.10
        with thyroid storm E05.11
    infiltrative
      dermopathy E05.00
        with thyroid storm E05.01
      ophthalmopathy E05.00
        with thyroid storm E05.01
    single thyroid nodule E05.10
      with thyroid storm E05.11
    thyroid storm E05.91
  due to
    ectopic thyroid nodule or tissue E05.30
      with thyroid storm E05.31
    ingestion of (excessive) thyroid material E05.40
      with thyroid storm E05.41
    overproduction of thyroid-stimulating hormone E05.80
      with thyroid storm E05.81
    specified cause NEC E05.80
      with thyroid storm E05.81
  factitia E05.40
    with thyroid storm E05.41
  heart (*see also* Failure, heart, high-output) E05.90 [I43]
    with thyroid storm (*see also* Failure, heart, high-output) E05.91 [I43]
  failure (*see also* Failure, heart, high-output) E05.90 [I43]
  neonatal (transient) P72.1
  transient with chronic thyroiditis E06.2
Tibia vara — *see* Osteochondrosis, juvenile, tibia
Tic (disorder) F95.9
  breathing F95.8
  child problem F95.0
  compulsive F95.1
  de la Tourette F95.2
  degenerative (generalized) (localized) G25.69
    facial G25.69
  disorder
    chronic
      motor F95.1
      vocal F95.1
    combined vocal and multiple motor F95.2
    transient F95.0
  douloureux G50.0
    atypical G50.1
    postherpetic, postzoster B02.22
  drug-induced G25.61
  eyelid F95.8
  habit F95.9
    chronic F95.1
    transient of childhood F95.0
  lid, transient of childhood F95.0
  motor-verbal F95.2
  occupational F48.8
  orbicularis F95.8

Tic — *continued*
  orbicularis — *continued*
    transient of childhood F95.0
  organic origin G25.69
  postchoreic G25.69
  provisional F95.0
  psychogenic, compulsive F95.1
  salaam R25.8
  spasm (motor or vocal) F95.9
    chronic F95.1
    transient of childhood F95.0
  specified NEC F95.8
Tick-borne — *see* condition
Tietze's disease or syndrome M94.0
Tight, tightness
  anus K62.89
  chest R07.89
  fascia (lata) M62.89
  foreskin (congenital) N47.1
  hymen, hymenal ring N89.6
  introitus (acquired) (congenital) N89.6
  rectal sphincter K62.89
  tendon — *see* Short, tendon
  urethral sphincter N35.9
Tilting vertebra — *see* Dorsopathy, deforming, specified NEC
Timidity, child F93.8
Tinea (intersecta) (tarsi) B35.9
  amiantacea L44.8
  asbestina B35.0
  barbae B35.0
  beard B35.0
  black dot B35.0
  blanca B36.2
  capitis B35.0
  corporis B35.4
  cruris B35.6
  flava B36.0
  foot B35.3
  furfuracea B36.0
  imbricata (Tokelau) B35.5
  kerion B35.0
  manuum B35.2
  microsporic — *see* Dermatophytosis
  nigra B36.1
  nodosa — *see* Piedra
  pedis B35.3
  scalp B35.0
  specified NEC B35.8
  sycosis B35.0
  tonsurans B35.0
  trichophytic — *see* Dermatophytosis
  unguium B35.1
  versicolor B36.0
Tingling sensation (skin) R20.2
Tin-miner's lung J63.5
Tinnitus NOS H93.1- ☑
  audible H93.1- ☑
  aurium H93.1- ☑
  pulsatile H93.A- ☑
  subjective H93.1- ☑
Tipped tooth (teeth) M26.33
Tipping
  pelvis M95.5
    with disproportion (fetopelvic) O33.0
      causing obstructed labor O65.0
  tooth (teeth), fully erupted M26.33
Tiredness R53.83
Tissue — *see* condition
Tobacco (nicotine)
  abuse — *see* Tobacco, use
  dependence — *see* Dependence, drug, nicotine
  harmful use Z72.0
  heart — *see* Tobacco, toxic effect
  maternal use, affecting newborn P04.2
  toxic effect — *see* Table of Drugs and Chemicals, by substance, poisoning
    chewing tobacco — *see* Table of Drugs and Chemicals, by substance, poisoning
    cigarettes — *see* Table of Drugs and Chemicals, by substance, poisoning
  use Z72.0
    complicating
      childbirth O99.334 ☑
      pregnancy O99.33- ☑
      puerperium O99.335
    counseling and surveillance Z71.6
    history Z87.891

Index

Tobacco — Trance

Tobacco — *continued*
withdrawal state (*see also* Dependence, drug, nicotine) F17.203
Tocopherol deficiency E56.0
Todd's
cirrhosis K74.3
paralysis (postepileptic) (transitory) G83.84
Toe — *see* condition
Toilet, artificial opening — *see* Attention to, artificial, opening
Tokelau (ringworm) B35.5
Tollwut — *see* Rabies
Tommaselli's disease R31.9
correct substance properly administered — *see* Table of Drugs and Chemicals, by drug, adverse effect
overdose or wrong substance given or taken — *see* Table of Drugs and Chemicals, by drug, poisoning
Tongue (*see also* condition)
tie Q38.1
Tonic pupil — *see* Anomaly, pupil, function, tonic pupil
Toni-Fanconi syndrome (cystinosis) E72.09
with cystinosis E72.04
Tonsil — *see* condition
Tonsillitis (acute) (catarrhal) (croupous) (follicular) (gangrenous) (infective) (lacunar) (lingual) (malignant) (membranous) (parenchymatous) (phlegmonous) (pseudomembranous) (purulent) (septic) (subacute) (suppurative) (toxic) (ulcerative) (vesicular) (viral) J03.90
chronic J35.01
with adenoiditis J35.03
diphtheritic A36.0
hypertrophic J35.01
with adenoiditis J35.03
recurrent J03.91
specified organism NEC J03.80
recurrent J03.81
staphylococcal J03.80
recurrent J03.81
streptococcal J03.00
recurrent J03.01
tuberculous A15.8
Vincent's A69.1
Tooth, teeth — *see* condition
Toothache K08.89
Topagnosis R20.8
Tophi — *see* Gout, chronic
TORCH infection — *see* Infection, congenital
without active infection P00.2
Torn — *see* Tear
Tornwaldt's cyst or disease J39.2
Torsion
accessory tube — *see* Torsion, fallopian tube
adnexa (female) — *see* Torsion, fallopian tube
aorta, acquired I77.1
appendix epididymis N44.04
appendix testis N44.03
bile duct (common) (hepatic) K83.8
congenital Q44.5
bowel, colon or intestine K56.2
cervix — *see* Malposition, uterus
cystic duct K82.8
dystonia — *see* Dystonia, torsion
epididymis (appendix) N44.04
fallopian tube N83.52- ☑
with ovary N83.53
gallbladder K82.8
congenital Q44.1
hydatid of Morgagni
female N83.52- ☑
male N44.03
kidney (pedicle) (leading to infarction) N28.0
Meckel's diverticulum (congenital) Q43.0
malignant — *see* Table of Neoplasms, small intestine, malignant
mesentery K56.2
omentum K56.2
organ or site, congenital NEC — *see* Anomaly, by site
ovary (pedicle) N83.51- ☑
with fallopian tube N83.53
congenital Q50.2
oviduct — *see* Torsion, fallopian tube
penis (acquired) N48.82
congenital Q55.63
spasm — *see* Dystonia, torsion
spermatic cord N44.02
extravaginal N44.01

Torsion — *continued*
spermatic cord — *continued*
intravaginal N44.02
spleen D73.5
testis, testicle N44.00
appendix N44.03
tibia — *see* Deformity, limb, specified type NEC, lower leg
uterus — *see* Malposition, uterus
Torticollis (intermittent) (spastic) M43.6
congenital (sternomastoid) Q68.0
due to birth injury P15.8
hysterical F44.4
ocular R29.891
psychogenic F45.8
conversion reaction F44.4
rheumatic M43.6
rheumatoid M06.88
spasmodic G24.3
traumatic, current S13.4 ☑
Tortipelvis G24.1
Tortuous
aortic arch Q25.46
artery I77.1
organ or site, congenital NEC — *see* Distortion
retinal vessel, congenital Q14.1
ureter N13.8
urethra N36.8
vein — *see* Varix
Torture, victim of Z65.4
Torula, torular (histolytica) (infection) — *see* Cryptococcosis
Torulosis — *see* Cryptococcosis
Torus (mandibularis) (palatinus) M27.0
fracture — *see* Fracture, by site, torus
Touraine's syndrome Q79.8
Tourette's syndrome F95.2
Tourniquet syndrome — *see* Constriction, external, by site
Tower skull Q75.0
with exophthalmos Q87.0
Toxemia R68.89
bacterial — *see* Sepsis
burn — *see* Burn
eclamptic (with pre-existing hypertension) — *see* Eclampsia
erysipelatous — *see* Erysipelas
fatigue R68.89
food — *see* Poisoning, food
gastrointestinal K52.1
intestinal K52.1
kidney — *see* Uremia
malarial — *see* Malaria
myocardial — *see* Myocarditis, toxic
of pregnancy — *see* Pre-eclampsia
pre-eclamptic — *see* Pre-eclampsia
small intestine K52.1
staphylococcal, due to food A05.0
stasis R68.89
uremic — *see* Uremia
urinary — *see* Uremia
Toxemica cerebropathia psychica (nonalcoholic) F04
alcoholic — *see* Alcohol, amnestic disorder
Toxic (poisoning) (*see also* condition) T65.91 ☑
effect — *see* Table of Drugs and Chemicals, by substance, poisoning
shock syndrome A48.3
thyroid (gland) — *see* Thyrotoxicosis
Toxicemia — *see* Toxemia
Toxicity — *see* Table of Drugs and Chemicals, by substance, poisoning
fava bean D55.0
food, noxious — *see* Poisoning, food
from drug or nonmedicinal substance — *see* Table of Drugs and Chemicals, by drug
Toxicosis (*see also* Toxemia)
capillary, hemorrhagic D69.0
Toxinfection, gastrointestinal K52.1
Toxocariasis B83.0
Toxoplasma, toxoplasmosis (acquired) B58.9
with
hepatitis B58.1
meningoencephalitis B58.2
ocular involvement B58.00
other organ involvement B58.89
pneumonia, pneumonitis B58.3
congenital (acute) (subacute) (chronic) P37.1

Toxoplasma, toxoplasmosis — *continued*
maternal, manifest toxoplasmosis in infant (acute) (subacute) (chronic) P37.1
tPA (rtPA) administration in a different facility within the last 24 hours prior to admission to current facility Z92.82
Trabeculation, bladder N32.89
Trachea — *see* condition
Tracheitis (catarrhal) (infantile) (membranous) (plastic) (septal) (suppurative) (viral) J04.10
with
bronchitis (15 years of age and above) J40
acute or subacute — *see* Bronchitis, acute
chronic J42
tuberculous NEC A15.5
under 15 years of age J20.9
laryngitis (acute) J04.2
chronic J37.1
tuberculous NEC A15.5
acute J04.10
with obstruction J04.11
chronic J42
with
bronchitis (chronic) J42
laryngitis (chronic) J37.1
diphtheritic (membranous) A36.89
due to external agent — *see* Inflammation, respiratory, upper, due to
syphilitic A52.73
tuberculous A15.5
Trachelitis (nonvenereal) — *see* Cervicitis
Tracheobronchial — *see* condition
Tracheobronchitis (15 years of age and above) (*see also* Bronchitis)
due to
Bordetella bronchiseptica A37.80
with pneumonia A37.81
Francisella tularensis A21.8
Tracheobronchomegaly Q32.4
with bronchiectasis J47.9
with
exacerbation (acute) J47.1
lower respiratory infection J47.0
acquired J98.09
with bronchiectasis J47.9
with
exacerbation (acute) J47.1
lower respiratory infection J47.0
Tracheobronchopneumonitis — *see* Pneumonia, broncho-
Tracheocele (external) (internal) J39.8
congenital Q32.1
Tracheomalacia J39.8
congenital Q32.0
Tracheopharyngitis (acute) J06.9
chronic J42
due to external agent — *see* Inflammation, respiratory, upper, due to
Tracheostenosis J39.8
Tracheostomy
complication — *see* Complication, tracheostomy
status Z93.0
attention to Z43.0
malfunctioning J95.03
Trachoma, trachomatous A71.9
active (stage) A71.1
contraction of conjunctiva A71.1
dubium A71.0
healed or sequelae B94.0
initial (stage) A71.0
pannus A71.1
Türck's J37.0
Traction, vitreomacular H43.82- ☑
Train sickness T75.3 ☑
Trait(s)
Hb-S D57.3
hemoglobin
abnormal NEC D58.2
with thalassemia D56.3
C — *see* Disease, hemoglobin C
S (Hb-S) D57.3
Lepore D56.3
personality, accentuated Z73.1
sickle-cell D57.3
with elliptocytosis or spherocytosis D57.3
type A personality Z73.1
Tramp Z59.0
Trance R41.89

Trance — *continued*
  hysterical F44.89
Transaminasemia R74.0
Transection
  abdomen (partial) S38.3 ☑
  aorta (incomplete) (*see also* Injury, aorta)
    complete — *see* Injury, aorta, laceration, major
  carotid artery (incomplete) (*see also* Injury, blood
      vessel, carotid, laceration)
    complete — *see* Injury, blood vessel, carotid, lacer-
      ation, major
  celiac artery (incomplete) S35.211 ☑
    branch (incomplete) S35.291 ☑
      complete S35.292 ☑
    complete S35.212 ☑
  innominate
    artery (incomplete) (*see also* Injury, blood vessel,
        thoracic, innominate, artery, laceration)
      complete — *see* Injury, blood vessel, thoracic,
        innominate, artery, laceration, major
    vein (incomplete) (*see also* Injury, blood vessel,
        thoracic, innominate, vein, laceration)
      complete — *see* Injury, blood vessel, thoracic,
        innominate, vein, laceration, major
  jugular vein (external) (incomplete) (*see also* Injury,
      blood vessel, jugular vein, laceration)
    complete — *see* Injury, blood vessel, jugular vein,
      laceration, major
  internal (incomplete) (*see also* Injury, blood vessel,
      jugular vein, internal, laceration)
    complete — *see* Injury, blood vessel, jugular
      vein, internal, laceration, major
  mesenteric artery (incomplete) (*see also* Injury,
      mesenteric, artery, laceration)
    complete — *see* Injury, mesenteric artery, lacera-
      tion, major
  pulmonary vessel (incomplete) (*see also* Injury, blood
      vessel, thoracic, pulmonary, laceration)
    complete — *see* Injury, blood vessel, thoracic,
      pulmonary, laceration, major
  subclavian — *see* Transection, innominate
  vena cava (incomplete) (*see also* Injury, vena cava)
    complete — *see* Injury, vena cava, laceration, major
  vertebral artery (incomplete) (*see also* Injury, blood
      vessel, vertebral, laceration)
    complete — *see* Injury, blood vessel, vertebral,
      laceration, major
Transfusion
  associated (red blood cell) hemochromatosis E83.111
  blood
    ABO incompatible — *see* Complication(s), transfu-
      sion, incompatibility reaction, ABO
    minor blood group (Duffy) (E) (K(ell)) (Kidd) (Lewis)
      (M) (N) (P) (S) T80.89 ☑
    reaction or complication — *see* Complications,
      transfusion
  fetomaternal (mother) — *see* Pregnancy, complicated
    by, placenta, transfusion syndrome
  maternofetal (mother) — *see* Pregnancy, complicated
    by, placenta, transfusion syndrome
  placental (syndrome) (mother) — *see* Pregnancy,
    complicated by, placenta, transfusion syndrome
  reaction (adverse) — *see* Complications, transfusion
  related acute lung injury (TRALI) J95.84
  twin-to-twin — *see* Pregnancy, complicated by, pla-
    centa, transfusion syndrome, fetus to fetus
Transient (meaning homeless) (*see also* condition) Z59.0
Translocation
  balanced autosomal Q95.9
    in normal individual Q95.0
  chromosomes NEC Q99.8
    balanced and insertion in normal individual Q95.0
  Down syndrome Q90.2
  trisomy
    13 Q91.6
    18 Q91.2
    21 Q90.2
Translucency, iris — *see* Degeneration, iris
**Transmission of chemical substances through the
    placenta** — *see* Absorption, chemical, through
    placenta
Transparency, lung, unilateral J43.0
Transplant (ed) (status) Z94.9
  awaiting organ Z76.82
  bone Z94.6
    marrow Z94.81
  candidate Z76.82

Transplant — *continued*
  complication — *see* Complication, transplant
  cornea Z94.7
  heart Z94.1
    and lung(s) Z94.3
    valve Z95.2
      prosthetic Z95.2
      specified NEC Z95.4
      xenogenic Z95.3
  intestine Z94.82
  kidney Z94.0
  liver Z94.4
  lung(s) Z94.2
    and heart Z94.3
  organ (failure) (infection) (rejection) Z94.9
    removal status Z98.85
  pancreas Z94.83
  skin Z94.5
  social Z60.3
  specified organ or tissue NEC Z94.89
  stem cells Z94.84
  tissue Z94.9
Transplants, ovarian, endometrial N80.1
Transposed — *see* Transposition
Transposition (congenital) (*see also* Malposition, con-
      genital)
  abdominal viscera Q89.3
  aorta (dextra) Q20.3
  appendix Q43.8
  colon Q43.8
  corrected Q20.5
  great vessels (complete) (partial) Q20.3
  heart Q24.0
    with complete transposition of viscera Q89.3
  intestine (large) (small) Q43.8
  reversed jejunal (for bypass) (status) Z98.0
  scrotum Q55.23
  stomach Q40.2
    with general transposition of viscera Q89.3
  tooth, teeth, fully erupted M26.30
  vessels, great (complete) (partial) Q20.3
  viscera (abdominal) (thoracic) Q89.3
Transsexualism F64.0
Transverse (*see also* condition)
  arrest (deep), in labor O64.0 ☑
  lie (mother) O32.2 ☑
    causing obstructed labor O64.8 ☑
Transvestism, transvestitism (dual-role) F64.1
  fetishistic F65.1
Trapped placenta (with hemorrhage) O72.0
  without hemorrhage O73.0
TRAPS (tumor necrosis factor receptor associated periodic
      syndrome) M04.1
Trauma, traumatism (*see also* Injury)
  acoustic — *see* subcategory H83.3 ☑
  birth — *see* Birth, injury
  complicating ectopic or molar pregnancy O08.6
  during delivery O71.9
  following ectopic or molar pregnancy O08.6
  obstetric O71.9
    specified NEC O71.89
  occlusal
    primary K08.81
    secondary K08.82
Traumatic (*see also* condition)
  brain injury S06.9 ☑
Treacher Collins syndrome Q75.4
Treitz's hernia — *see* Hernia, abdomen, specified site
    NEC
Trematode infestation — *see* Infestation, fluke
Trematodiasis — *see* Infestation, fluke
Trembling paralysis — *see* Parkinsonism
Tremor(s) R25.1
  drug induced G25.1
  essential (benign) G25.0
  familial G25.0
  hereditary G25.0
  hysterical F44.4
  intention G25.2
  medication induced postural G25.1
  mercurial — *see* subcategory T56.1 ☑
  Parkinson's — *see* Parkinsonism
  psychogenic (conversion reaction) F44.4
  senilis R54
  specified type NEC G25.2
Trench
  fever A79.0
  foot — *see* Immersion, foot

Trench — *continued*
  mouth A69.1
Treponema pallidum infection — *see* Syphilis
Treponematosis
  due to
    T. pallidum — *see* Syphilis
    T. pertenue — *see* Yaws
Triad
  Hutchinson's (congenital syphilis) A50.53
  Kartagener's Q89.3
  Saint's — *see* Hernia, diaphragm
Trichiasis (eyelid) H02.059
  with entropion — *see* Entropion
  left H02.056
    lower H02.055
    upper H02.054
  right H02.053
    lower H02.052
    upper H02.051
Trichinella spiralis (infection) (infestation) B75
Trichinellosis, trichiniasis, trichinelliasis, trichinosis
    B75
  with muscle disorder B75 [M63.80]
    ankle B75 [M63.87-] ☑
    foot B75 [M63.87-] ☑
    forearm B75 [M63.83-] ☑
    hand B75 [M63.84-] ☑
    lower leg B75 [M63.86-] ☑
    multiple sites B75 [M63.89]
    pelvic region B75 [M63.85-] ☑
    shoulder region B75 [M63.81-] ☑
    specified site NEC B75 [M63.88]
    thigh B75 [M63.85-] ☑
    upper arm B75 [M63.82-] ☑
Trichobezoar T18.9 ☑
  intestine T18.3 ☑
  stomach T18.2 ☑
Trichocephaliasis, trichocephalosis B79
Trichocephalus infestation B79
Trichoclasis L67.8
Trichoepithelioma (*see also* Neoplasm, skin, benign)
  malignant — *see* Neoplasm, skin, malignant
Trichofolliculoma — *see* Neoplasm, skin, benign
Tricholemmoma — *see* Neoplasm, skin, benign
Trichomoniasis A59.9
  bladder A59.03
  cervix A59.09
  intestinal A07.8
  prostate A59.02
  seminal vesicles A59.09
  specified site NEC A59.8
  urethra A59.03
  urogenitalis A59.00
  vagina A59.01
  vulva A59.01
Trichomycosis
  axillaris A48.8
  nodosa, nodularis B36.8
Trichonodosis L67.8
Trichophytid, trichophyton infection — *see* Dermato-
    phytosis
Trichophytobezoar T18.9 ☑
  intestine T18.3 ☑
  stomach T18.2 ☑
Trichophytosis — *see* Dermatophytosis
Trichoptilosis L67.8
Trichorrhexis (nodosa) (invaginata) L67.0
Trichosis axillaris A48.8
Trichosporosis nodosa B36.2
Trichostasis spinulosa (congenital) Q84.1
Trichostrongyliasis, trichostrongylosis (small intes-
    tine) B81.2
Trichostrongylus infection B81.2
Trichotillomania F63.3
Trichromat, trichromatopsia, anomalous (congenital)
    H53.55
Trichuriasis B79
Trichuris trichiura (infection) (infestation) (any site) B79
Tricuspid (valve) — *see* condition
Trifid (*see also* Accessory)
  kidney (pelvis) Q63.8
  tongue Q38.3
Trigeminal neuralgia — *see* Neuralgia, trigeminal
Trigeminy R00.8
Trigger finger (acquired) M65.30
  congenital Q74.0
  index finger M65.32- ☑

314

☑ **Additional Character Required** — Refer to the Tabular List for Character Selection   ▽ **Subterms under main terms may continue to next column or page**

Tuberculosis, tubercular, tuberculous — *continued*
cystitis A18.12
dactylitis A18.03
diarrhea A18.32
diffuse — *see* Tuberculosis, miliary
digestive tract A18.32
disseminated — *see* Tuberculosis, miliary
duodenum A18.32
dura (mater) (cerebral) (spinal) A17.0
   abscess (cerebral) (spinal) A17.81
dysentery A18.32
ear (inner) (middle) A18.6
   bone A18.03
   external (primary) A18.4
   skin (primary) A18.4
elbow A18.02
emphysema — *see* Tuberculosis, pulmonary
empyema A15.6
encephalitis A17.82
endarteritis A18.89
endocarditis A18.84
   aortic A18.84
   mitral A18.84
   pulmonary A18.84
   tricuspid A18.84
endocrine glands NEC A18.82
endometrium A18.17
enteric, enterica, enteritis A18.32
enterocolitis A18.32
epididymis, epididymitis A18.15
epidural abscess (cerebral) (spinal) A17.81
epiglottis A15.5
episcleritis A18.51
erythema (induratum) (nodosum) (primary) A18.4
esophagus A18.83
eustachian tube A18.6
exposure (to) Z20.1
exudative — *see* Tuberculosis, pulmonary
eye A18.50
eyelid (primary) (lupus) A18.4
fallopian tube (acute) (chronic) A18.17
fascia A18.09
fauces A15.8
female pelvic inflammatory disease A18.17
finger A18.03
first infection A15.7
gallbladder A18.83
ganglion A18.09
gastritis A18.83
gastrocolic fistula A18.32
gastroenteritis A18.32
gastrointestinal tract A18.32
general, generalized — *see* Tuberculosis, miliary
genital organs A18.10
genitourinary A18.10
genu A18.02
glandula suprarenalis A18.7
glandular, general A18.2
glottis A15.5
grinder's J65
gum A18.83
hand A18.03
heart A18.84
hematogenous — *see* Tuberculosis, miliary
hemoptysis — *see* Tuberculosis, pulmonary
hemorrhage NEC — *see* Tuberculosis, pulmonary
hemothorax A15.6
hepatitis A18.83
hilar lymph nodes A15.4
   primary (progressive) A15.7
hip (joint) (disease) (bone) A18.02
hydropneumothorax A15.6
hydrothorax A15.6
hypoadrenalism A18.7
hypopharynx A15.8
ileocecal (hyperplastic) A18.32
ileocolitis A18.32
ileum A18.32
iliac spine (superior) A18.03
immunological findings only A15.7
indurativa (primary) A18.4
infantile A15.7
infection A15.9
   without clinical manifestations A15.7
infraclavicular gland A18.2
inguinal gland A18.2
inguinalis A18.2
intestine (any part) A18.32

Tuberculosis, tubercular, tuberculous — *continued*
iridocyclitis A18.54
iris, iritis A18.54
ischiorectal A18.32
jaw A18.03
jejunum A18.32
joint A18.02
   vertebral A18.01
keratitis (interstitial) A18.52
keratoconjunctivitis A18.52
kidney A18.11
knee (joint) A18.02
kyphosis, kyphoscoliosis A18.01
laryngitis A15.5
larynx A15.5
latent R76.11
leptomeninges, leptomeningitis (cerebral) (spinal) A17.0
lichenoides (primary) A18.4
linguae A18.83
lip A18.83
liver A18.83
lordosis A18.01
lung — *see* Tuberculosis, pulmonary
lupus vulgaris A18.4
lymph gland or node (peripheral) A18.2
   abdomen A18.39
   bronchial A15.4
     primary (progressive) A15.7
   cervical A18.2
   hilar A15.4
     primary (progressive) A15.7
   intrathoracic A15.4
     primary (progressive) A15.7
   mediastinal A15.4
     primary (progressive) A15.7
   mesenteric A18.39
   retroperitoneal A18.39
   tracheobronchial A15.4
     primary (progressive) A15.7
lymphadenitis — *see* Tuberculosis, lymph gland
lymphangitis — *see* Tuberculosis, lymph gland
lymphatic (gland) (vessel) — *see* Tuberculosis, lymph gland
mammary gland A18.89
marasmus A15.9
mastoiditis A18.03
mediastinal lymph gland or node A15.4
   primary (progressive) A15.7
mediastinitis A15.8
   primary (progressive) A15.7
mediastinum A15.8
   primary (progressive) A15.7
medulla A17.81
melanosis, Addisonian A18.7
meninges, meningitis (basilar) (cerebral) (cerebrospinal) (spinal) A17.0
meningoencephalitis A17.82
mesentery, mesenteric (gland or node) A18.39
miliary A19.9
   acute A19.2
     multiple sites A19.1
     single specified site A19.0
   chronic A19.8
   specified NEC A19.8
millstone makers' J65
miner's J65
molder's J65
mouth A18.83
multiple A19.9
   acute A19.1
   chronic A19.8
muscle A18.09
myelitis A17.82
myocardium, myocarditis A18.84
nasal (passage) (sinus) A15.8
nasopharynx A15.8
neck gland A18.2
nephritis A18.11
nerve (mononeuropathy) A17.83
nervous system A17.9
nose (septum) A15.8
ocular A18.50
omentum A18.31
oophoritis (acute) (chronic) A18.17
optic (nerve trunk) (papilla) A18.59
orbit A18.59
orchitis A18.15
organ, specified NEC A18.89

Tuberculosis, tubercular, tuberculous — *continued*
osseous — *see* Tuberculosis, bone
osteitis — *see* Tuberculosis, bone
osteomyelitis — *see* Tuberculosis, bone
otitis media A18.6
ovary, ovaritis (acute) (chronic) A18.17
oviduct (acute) (chronic) A18.17
pachymeningitis A17.0
palate (soft) A18.83
pancreas A18.83
papulonecrotic (a) (primary) A18.4
parathyroid glands A18.82
paronychia (primary) A18.4
parotid gland or region A18.83
pelvis (bony) A18.03
penis A18.15
peribronchitis A15.5
pericardium, pericarditis A18.84
perichondritis, larynx A15.5
periostitis — *see* Tuberculosis, bone
perirectal fistula A18.32
peritoneum NEC A18.31
peritonitis A18.31
pharynx, pharyngitis A15.8
phlyctenulosis (keratoconjunctivitis) A18.52
phthisis NEC — *see* Tuberculosis, pulmonary
pituitary gland A18.82
pleura, pleural, pleurisy, pleuritis (fibrinous) (obliterative) (purulent) (simple plastic) (with effusion) A15.6
   primary (progressive) A15.7
pneumonia, pneumonic — *see* Tuberculosis, pulmonary
pneumothorax (spontaneous) (tense valvular) — *see* Tuberculosis, pulmonary
polyneuropathy A17.89
polyserositis A19.9
   acute A19.1
   chronic A19.8
potter's J65
prepuce A18.15
primary (complex) A15.7
proctitis A18.32
prostate, prostatitis A18.14
pulmonalis — *see* Tuberculosis, pulmonary
pulmonary (cavitated) (fibrotic) (infiltrative) (nodular) A15.0
   childhood type or first infection A15.7
   primary (complex) A15.7
pyelitis A18.11
pyelonephritis A18.11
pyemia — *see* Tuberculosis, miliary
pyonephrosis A18.11
pyopneumothorax A15.6
pyothorax A15.6
rectum (fistula) (with abscess) A18.32
reinfection stage — *see* Tuberculosis, pulmonary
renal A18.11
renis A18.11
respiratory A15.9
   primary A15.7
   specified site NEC A15.8
retina, retinitis A18.53
retroperitoneal (lymph gland or node) A18.39
rheumatism NEC A18.09
rhinitis A15.8
sacroiliac (joint) A18.01
sacrum A18.01
salivary gland A18.83
salpingitis (acute) (chronic) A18.17
sandblaster's J65
sclera A18.51
scoliosis A18.01
scrofulous A18.2
scrotum A18.15
seminal tract or vesicle A18.15
senile A15.9
septic — *see* Tuberculosis, miliary
shoulder (joint) A18.02
   blade A18.03
sigmoid A18.32
sinus (any nasal) A15.8
   bone A18.03
   epididymis A18.15
skeletal NEC A18.03
skin (any site) (primary) A18.4
small intestine A18.32
soft palate A18.83

Tuberculosis, tubercular, tuberculous — *continued*
  spermatic cord A18.15
  spine, spinal (column) A18.01
    cord A17.81
    medulla A17.81
    membrane A17.0
    meninges A17.0
  spleen, splenitis A18.85
  spondylitis A18.01
  sternoclavicular joint A18.02
  stomach A18.83
  stonemason's J65
  subcutaneous tissue (cellular) (primary) A18.4
  subcutis (primary) A18.4
  subdeltoid bursa A18.83
  submaxillary (region) A18.83
  supraclavicular gland A18.2
  suprarenal (capsule) (gland) A18.7
  swelling, joint (*see also* category M01) (*see also* Tuberculosis, joint) A18.02
  symphysis pubis A18.02
  synovitis A18.09
    articular A18.02
    spine or vertebra A18.01
  systemic — *see* Tuberculosis, miliary
  tarsitis A18.4
  tendon (sheath) — *see* Tuberculosis, tenosynovitis
  tenosynovitis A18.09
    spine or vertebra A18.01
  testis A18.15
  throat A15.8
  thymus gland A18.82
  thyroid gland A18.81
  tongue A18.83
  tonsil, tonsillitis A15.8
  trachea, tracheal A15.5
    lymph gland or node A15.4
      primary (progressive) A15.7
  tracheobronchial A15.5
    lymph gland or node A15.4
      primary (progressive) A15.7
  tubal (acute) (chronic) A18.17
  tunica vaginalis A18.15
  ulcer (skin) (primary) A18.4
    bowel or intestine A18.32
    specified NEC — *see* Tuberculosis, by site
  unspecified site A15.9
  ureter A18.11
  urethra, urethral (gland) A18.13
  urinary organ or tract A18.13
  uterus A18.17
  uveal tract A18.54
  uvula A18.83
  vagina A18.18
  vas deferens A18.15
  verruca, verrucosa (cutis) (primary) A18.4
  vertebra (column) A18.01
  vesiculitis A18.15
  vulva A18.18
  wrist (joint) A18.02
Tuberculum
  Carabelli — *see* Excludes Note at K00.2
  occlusal — *see* Excludes Note at K00.2
  paramolare K00.2
Tuberosity, enitre maxillary M26.07
Tuberous sclerosis (brain) Q85.1
Tubo-ovarian — *see* condition
Tuboplasty, after previous sterilization Z31.0
  aftercare Z31.42
Tubotympanitis, catarrhal (chronic) — *see* Otitis, media, nonsuppurative, chronic, serous
Tularemia A21.9
  with
    conjunctivitis A21.1
    pneumonia A21.2
  abdominal A21.3
  bronchopneumonic A21.2
  conjunctivitis A21.1
  cryptogenic A21.3
  enteric A21.3
  gastrointestinal A21.3
  generalized A21.7
  ingestion A21.3
  intestinal A21.3
  oculoglandular A21.1
  ophthalmic A21.1
  pneumonia (any), pneumonic A21.2
  pulmonary A21.2

Tularemia — *continued*
  sepsis A21.7
  specified NEC A21.8
  typhoidal A21.7
  ulceroglandular A21.0
Tularensis conjunctivitis A21.1
Tumefaction (*see also* Swelling)
  liver — *see* Hypertrophy, liver
Tumor (*see also* Neoplasm, unspecified behavior, by site)
  acinar cell — *see* Neoplasm, uncertain behavior, by site
  acinic cell — *see* Neoplasm, uncertain behavior, by site
  adenocarcinoid — *see* Neoplasm, malignant, by site
  adenomatoid (*see also* Neoplasm, benign, by site)
    odontogenic — *see* Cyst, calcifying odontogenic
  adnexal (skin) — *see* Neoplasm, skin, benign, by site
  adrenal
    cortical (benign) D35.0- ☑
      malignant C74.0- ☑
    rest — *see* Neoplasm, benign, by site
  alpha-cell
    malignant
      pancreas C25.4
      specified site NEC — *see* Neoplasm, malignant, by site
      unspecified site C25.4
    pancreas D13.7
    specified site NEC — *see* Neoplasm, benign, by site
    unspecified site D13.7
  aneurysmal — *see* Aneurysm
  aortic body D44.7
    malignant C75.5
  Askin's — *see* Neoplasm, connective tissue, malignant
  basal cell (*see also* Neoplasm, skin, uncertain behavior) D48.5
  Bednar — *see* Neoplasm, skin, malignant
  benign (unclassified) — *see* Neoplasm, benign, by site
  beta-cell
    malignant
      pancreas C25.4
      specified site NEC — *see* Neoplasm, malignant, by site
      unspecified site C25.4
    pancreas D13.7
    specified site NEC — *see* Neoplasm, benign, by site
    unspecified site D13.7
  Brenner D27.9
    borderline malignancy D39.1- ☑
    malignant C56- ☑
    proliferating D39.1- ☑
  bronchial alveolar, intravascular D38.1
  Brooke's — *see* Neoplasm, skin, benign
  brown fat — *see* Lipoma
  Burkitt — *see* Lymphoma, Burkitt
  calcifying epithelial odontogenic — *see* Cyst, calcifying odontogenic
  carcinoid
    benign D3A.00 (*following* D36)
      appendix D3A.020 (*following* D36)
      ascending colon D3A.022 (*following* D36)
      bronchus (lung) D3A.090 (*following* D36)
      cecum D3A.021 (*following* D36)
      colon D3A.029 (*following* D36)
      descending colon D3A.024 (*following* D36)
      duodenum D3A.010 (*following* D36)
      foregut NOS D3A.094 (*following* D36)
      hindgut NOS D3A.096 (*following* D36)
      ileum D3A.012 (*following* D36)
      jejunum D3A.011 (*following* D36)
      kidney D3A.093 (*following* D36)
      large intestine D3A.029 (*following* D36)
      lung (bronchus) D3A.090 (*following* D36)
      midgut NOS D3A.095 (*following* D36)
      rectum D3A.026 (*following* D36)
      sigmoid colon D3A.025 (*following* D36)
      small intestine D3A.019 (*following* D36)
      specified NEC D3A.098 (*following* D36)
      stomach D3A.092 (*following* D36)
      thymus D3A.091 (*following* D36)
      transverse colon D3A.023 (*following* D36)
    malignant C7A.00 (*following* C75)
      appendix C7A.020 (*following* C75)
      ascending colon C7A.022 (*following* C75)
      bronchus (lung) C7A.090 (*following* C75)
      cecum C7A.021 (*following* C75)
      colon C7A.029 (*following* C75)
      descending colon C7A.024 (*following* C75)

Tumor — *continued*
  carcinoid — *continued*
    malignant — *continued*
      duodenum C7A.010 (*following* C75)
      foregut NOS C7A.094 (*following* C75)
      hindgut NOS C7A.096 (*following* C75)
      ileum C7A.012 (*following* C75)
      jejunum C7A.011 (*following* C75)
      kidney C7A.093 (*following* C75)
      large intestine C7A.029 (*following* C75)
      lung (bronchus) C7A.090 (*following* C75)
      midgut NOS C7A.095 (*following* C75)
      rectum C7A.026 (*following* C75)
      sigmoid colon C7A.025 (*following* C75)
      small intestine C7A.019 (*following* C75)
      specified NEC C7A.098 (*following* C75)
      stomach C7A.092 (*following* C75)
      thymus C7A.091 (*following* C75)
      transverse colon C7A.023 (*following* C75)
      mesentary metastasis C7B.04 (*following* C75)
      secondary C7B.00 (*following* C75)
        bone C7B.03 (*following* C75)
        distant lymph nodes C7B.01 (*following* C75)
        liver C7B.02 (*following* C75)
        peritoneum C7B.04 (*following* C75)
        specified NEC C7B.09 (*following* C75)
  carotid body D44.6
    malignant C75.4
  cells (*see also* Neoplasm, unspecified behavior, by site)
    benign — *see* Neoplasm, benign, by site
    malignant — *see* Neoplasm, malignant, by site
    uncertain whether benign or malignant — *see* Neoplasm, uncertain behavior, by site
  cervix, in pregnancy or childbirth — *see* Pregnancy, complicated by, tumor, cervix
  chondromatous giant cell — *see* Neoplasm, bone, benign
  chromaffin (*see also* Neoplasm, benign, by site)
    malignant — *see* Neoplasm, malignant, by site
  Cock's peculiar L72.3
  Codman's — *see* Neoplasm, bone, benign
  dentigerous, mixed — *see* Cyst, calcifying odontogenic
  dermoid — *see* Neoplasm, benign, by site
    with malignant transformation C56- ☑
  desmoid (extra-abdominal) (*see also* Neoplasm, connective tissue, uncertain behavior)
    abdominal — *see* Neoplasm, connective tissue, uncertain behavior
  embolus — *see* Neoplasm, secondary, by site
  embryonal (mixed) (*see also* Neoplasm, uncertain behavior, by site)
    liver C22.7
  endodermal sinus
    specified site — *see* Neoplasm, malignant, by site
    unspecified site
      female C56.- ☑
      male C62.90
  epithelial
    benign — *see* Neoplasm, benign, by site
    malignant — *see* Neoplasm, malignant, by site
  Ewing's — *see* Neoplasm, bone, malignant, by site
  fatty — *see* Lipoma
  fibroid — *see* Leiomyoma
  G cell
    malignant
      pancreas C25.4
      specified site NEC — *see* Neoplasm, malignant, by site
      unspecified site C25.4
    specified site — *see* Neoplasm, uncertain behavior, by site
    unspecified site D37.8
  germ cell (*see also* Neoplasm, malignant, by site)
    mixed — *see* Neoplasm, malignant, by site
  ghost cell, odontogenic — *see* Cyst, calcifying odontogenic
  giant cell (*see also* Neoplasm, uncertain behavior, by site)
    bone D48.0
      malignant — *see* Neoplasm, bone, malignant
    chondromatous — *see* Neoplasm, bone, benign
    malignant — *see* Neoplasm, malignant, by site
    soft parts — *see* Neoplasm, connective tissue, uncertain behavior
      malignant — *see* Neoplasm, connective tissue, malignant
  glomus D18.00
    intra-abdominal D18.03

Tumor — *continued*
  glomus — *continued*
    intracranial D18.02
    jugulare D44.7
      malignant C75.5
    skin D18.01
    specified site NEC D18.09
  gonadal stromal — *see* Neoplasm, uncertain behavior, by site
  granular cell (*see also* Neoplasm, connective tissue, benign)
    malignant — *see* Neoplasm, connective tissue, malignant
  granulosa cell D39.1- ☑
    juvenile D39.1- ☑
    malignant C56- ☑
  granulosa cell-theca cell D39.1- ☑
    malignant C56- ☑
  Grawitz's C64- ☑
  hemorrhoidal — *see* Hemorrhoids
  hilar cell D27- ☑
  hilus cell D27- ☑
  Hurthle cell (benign) D34
    malignant C73
  hydatid — *see* Echinococcus
  hypernephroid (*see also* Neoplasm, uncertain behavior, by site)
  interstitial cell (*see also* Neoplasm, uncertain behavior, by site)
    benign — *see* Neoplasm, benign, by site
    malignant — *see* Neoplasm, malignant, by site
  intravascular bronchial alveolar D38.1
  islet cell — *see* Neoplasm, benign, by site
    malignant — *see* Neoplasm, malignant, by site
      pancreas C25.4
      specified site NEC — *see* Neoplasm, malignant, by site
      unspecified site C25.4
    pancreas D13.7
    specified site NEC — *see* Neoplasm, benign, by site
    unspecified site D13.7
  juxtaglomerular D41.0- ☑
  Klatskin's C22.1
  Krukenberg's C79.6- ☑
  Leydig cell — *see* Neoplasm, uncertain behavior, by site
    benign — *see* Neoplasm, benign, by site
      specified site — *see* Neoplasm, benign, by site
      unspecified site
        female D27.9
        male D29.20
    malignant — *see* Neoplasm, malignant, by site
      specified site — *see* Neoplasm, malignant, by site
      unspecified site
        female C56.9
        male C62.90
    specified site — *see* Neoplasm, uncertain behavior, by site
    unspecified site
      female D39.10
      male D40.10
  lipid cell, ovary D27- ☑
  lipoid cell, ovary D27- ☑
  malignant (*see also* Neoplasm, malignant, by site) C80.1
    fusiform cell (type) C80.1
    giant cell (type) C80.1
    localized, plasma cell — *see* Plasmacytoma, solitary
    mixed NEC C80.1
    small cell (type) C80.1
    spindle cell (type) C80.1
    unclassified C80.1
  mast cell D47.09
  melanotic, neuroectodermal — *see* Neoplasm, benign, by site
  Merkel cell — *see* Carcinoma, Merkel cell
  mesenchymal
    malignant — *see* Neoplasm, connective tissue, malignant
    mixed — *see* Neoplasm, connective tissue, uncertain behavior
  mesodermal, mixed (*see also* Neoplasm, malignant, by site)
    liver C22.4

Tumor — *continued*
  mesonephric (*see also* Neoplasm, uncertain behavior, by site)
    malignant — *see* Neoplasm, malignant, by site
  metastatic
    from specified site — *see* Neoplasm, malignant, by site
    of specified site — *see* Neoplasm, malignant, by site
    to specified site — *see* Neoplasm, secondary, by site
  mixed NEC (*see also* Neoplasm, benign, by site)
    malignant — *see* Neoplasm, malignant, by site
  mucinous of low malignant potential
    specified site — *see* Neoplasm, malignant, by site
    unspecified site C56.9
  mucocarcinoid
    specified site — *see* Neoplasm, malignant, by site
    unspecified site C18.1
  mucoepidermoid — *see* Neoplasm, uncertain behavior, by site
  Müllerian, mixed
    specified site — *see* Neoplasm, malignant, by site
    unspecified site C54.9
  myoepithelial — *see* Neoplasm, benign, by site
  neuroectodermal (peripheral) — *see* Neoplasm, malignant, by site
    primitive
      specified site — *see* Neoplasm, malignant, by site
      unspecified site C71.9
  neuroendocrine D3A.8 (*following* D36)
    malignant poorly differentiated C7A.1 (*following* C75)
    secondary NEC C7B.8 (*following* C75)
    specified NEC C7A.8 (*following* C75)
  neurogenic olfactory C30.0
  nonencapsulated sclerosing C73
  odontogenic (adenomatoid) (benign) (calcifying epithelial) (keratocystic) (squamous) — *see* Cyst, calcifying odontogenic
    malignant C41.1
      upper jaw (bone) C41.0
  ovarian stromal D39.1- ☑
  ovary, in pregnancy — *see* Pregnancy, complicated by
  pacinian — *see* Neoplasm, skin, benign
  Pancoast's — *see* Pancoast's syndrome
  papillary (*see also* Papilloma)
    cystic D37.9
    mucinous of low malignant potential C56- ☑
      specified site — *see* Neoplasm, malignant, by site
      unspecified site C56.9
    serous of low malignant potential
      specified site — *see* Neoplasm, malignant, by site
      unspecified site C56.9
  pelvic, in pregnancy or childbirth — *see* Pregnancy, complicated by
  phantom F45.8
  phyllodes D48.6- ☑
    benign D24- ☑
    malignant — *see* Neoplasm, breast, malignant
  Pindborg — *see* Cyst, calcifying odontogenic
  placental site trophoblastic D39.2
  plasma cell (malignant) (localized) — *see* Plasmacytoma, solitary
  polyvesicular vitelline
    specified site — *see* Neoplasm, malignant, by site
    unspecified site
      female C56.9
      male C62.90
  Pott's puffy — *see* Osteomyelitis, specified NEC
  Rathke's pouch D44.3
  retinal anlage — *see* Neoplasm, benign, by site
  salivary gland type, mixed — *see* Neoplasm, salivary gland, benign
    malignant — *see* Neoplasm, salivary gland, malignant
  Sampson's N80.1
  Schmincke's — *see* Neoplasm, nasopharynx, malignant
  sclerosing stromal D27- ☑
  sebaceous — *see* Cyst, sebaceous
  secondary — *see* Neoplasm, secondary, by site
    carcinoid C7B.00 (*following* C75)
      bone C7B.03 (*following* C75)
      distant lymph nodes C7B.01 (*following* C75)

Tumor — *continued*
  secondary — *see* Neoplasm, secondary, by site — *continued*
    carcinoid — *continued*
      liver C7B.02 (*following* C75)
      peritoneum C7B.04 (*following* C75)
      specified NEC C7B.09 (*following* C75)
    neuroendocrine NEC C7B.8 (*following* C75)
  serous of low malignant potential
    specified site — *see* Neoplasm, malignant, by site
    unspecified site C56.9
  Sertoli cell — *see* Neoplasm, benign, by site
    with lipid storage
      specified site — *see* Neoplasm, benign, by site
      unspecified site
        female D27.9
        male D29.20
    specified site — *see* Neoplasm, benign, by site
    unspecified site
      female D27.9
      male D29.20
  Sertoli-Leydig cell — *see* Neoplasm, benign, by site
    specified site — *see* Neoplasm, benign, by site
    unspecified site
      female D27.9
      male D29.20
  sex cord (-stromal) — *see* Neoplasm, uncertain behavior, by site
    with annular tubules D39.1- ☑
  skin appendage — *see* Neoplasm, skin, benign
  smooth muscle — *see* Neoplasm, connective tissue, uncertain behavior
  soft tissue
    benign — *see* Neoplasm, connective tissue, benign
    malignant — *see* Neoplasm, connective tissue, malignant
  sternomastoid (congenital) Q68.0
  stromal
    endometrial D39.0
    gastric D48.1
      benign D21.4
      malignant C16.9
      uncertain behavior D48.1
    gastrointestinal C49.A- ☑
      benign D21.4
      esophagus C49.A1
      malignant C49.A0
        colon C49.A4
        duodenum C49.A3
        esophagus C49.A1
        ileum C49.A3
        jejunum C49.A3
        large intestine C49.A4
        Meckel diverticulum C49.A3
        omentum C49.A9
        peritoneum C49.A9
        rectum C49.A5
        small intestine C49.A3
        specified site NEC C49.A9
        stomach C49.A2
      rectum C49.A5
      small intestine C49.A3
      specified site NEC C49.A9
      stomach C49.A2
      uncertain behavior D48.1
    intestine
      benign D21.4
      malignant
        large C49.A4
        small C49.A3
      uncertain behavior D48.1
    ovarian D39.1- ☑
    stomach C49.A2
      benign D21.4
      malignant C49.A2
      uncertain behavior D48.1
  sweat gland (*see also* Neoplasm, skin, uncertain behavior)
    benign — *see* Neoplasm, skin, benign
    malignant — *see* Neoplasm, skin, malignant
  syphilitic, brain A52.17
  testicular D40.10
  testicular stromal D40.1- ☑
  theca cell D27- ☑
  theca cell-granulosa cell D39.1- ☑
  Triton, malignant — *see* Neoplasm, nerve, malignant
  trophoblastic, placental site D39.2
  turban D23.4

Tumor — Tumor

Tumor — *continued*
- uterus (body), in pregnancy or childbirth — *see* Pregnancy, complicated by tumor, uterus
- vagina, in pregnancy or childbirth — *see* Pregnancy, complicated by
- varicose — *see* Varix
- von Recklinghausen's — *see* Neurofibromatosis
- vulva or perineum, in pregnancy or childbirth — *see* Pregnancy, complicated by
  - causing obstructed labor O65.5
- Warthin's — *see* Neoplasm, salivary gland, benign
- Wilms' C64- ☑
- yolk sac — *see* Neoplasm, malignant, by site
  - specified site — *see* Neoplasm, malignant, by site
  - unspecified site
    - female C56.9
    - male C62.90

Tumor lysis syndrome (following antineoplastic chemotherapy) (spontaneous) NEC E88.3
Tumorlet — *see* Neoplasm, uncertain behavior, by site
Tungiasis B88.1
Tunica vasculosa lentis Q12.2
Turban tumor D23.4
Türck's trachoma J37.0
Turner-Kieser syndrome Q87.2
Turner-like syndrome Q87.1
Turner's
- hypoplasia (tooth) K00.4
- syndrome Q96.9
  - specified NEC Q96.8
- tooth K00.4
Turner-Ullrich syndrome Q96.9
Tussis convulsiva — *see* Whooping cough
Twiddler's syndrome (due to)
- automatic implantable defibrillator T82.198
- cardiac pacemaker T82.198 ☑
Twilight state
- epileptic F05
- psychogenic F44.89
Twin (newborn) (*see also* Newborn, twin)
- conjoined Q89.4
- pregnancy — *see* Pregnancy, twin
Twinning, teeth K00.2
Twist, twisted
- bowel, colon or intestine K56.2
- hair (congenital) Q84.1
- mesentery K56.2
- omentum K56.2
- organ or site, congenital NEC — *see* Anomaly, by site
- ovarian pedicle — *see* Torsion, ovary
Twitching R25.3
Tylosis (acquired) L84
- buccalis K13.29
- linguae K13.29
- palmaris et plantaris (congenital) (inherited) Q82.8
  - acquired L85.1
Tympanism R14.0
Tympanites (abdominal) (intestinal) R14.0
Tympanitis — *see* Myringitis
Tympanosclerosis H74.0 ☑
Tympanum — *see* condition
Tympany
- abdomen R14.0
- chest R09.89
Type A behavior pattern Z73.1
Typhlitis — *see* Appendicitis
Typhoenteritis — *see* Typhoid
Typhoid (abortive) (ambulant) (any site) (clinical) (fever) (hemorrhagic) (infection) (intermittent) (malignant) (rheumatic) (Widal negative) A01.00
- with pneumonia A01.03
- abdominal A01.09
- arthritis A01.04
- carrier (suspected) of Z22.0
- cholecystitis (current) A01.09
- endocarditis A01.02
- heart involvement A01.02
- inoculation reaction — *see* Complications, vaccination
- meningitis A01.01
- mesenteric lymph nodes A01.09
- myocarditis A01.02
- osteomyelitis A01.05
- perichondritis, larynx A01.09
- pneumonia A01.03
- specified NEC A01.09
- spine A01.05
- ulcer (perforating) A01.09

Typhomalaria (fever) — *see* Malaria
Typhomania A01.00
Typhoperitonitis A01.09
Typhus (fever) A75.9
- abdominal, abdominalis — *see* Typhoid
- African tick A77.1
- amarillic A95.9
- brain A75.9 [G94]
- cerebral A75.9 [G94]
- classical A75.0
- due to Rickettsia
  - prowazekii A75.0
    - recrudescent A75.1
  - tsutsugamushi A75.3
  - typhi A75.2
- endemic (flea-borne) A75.2
- epidemic (louse-borne) A75.0
- exanthematicus SAI A75.0
  - brillii SAI A75.1
  - mexicanus SAI A75.2
  - typhus murinus A75.2
- exanthematic NEC A75.0
- flea-borne A75.2
- India tick A77.1
- Kenya (tick) A77.1
- louse-borne A75.0
- Mexican A75.2
- mite-borne A75.3
- murine A75.2
- North Asian tick-borne A77.2
- petechial A75.9
- Queensland tick A77.3
- rat A75.2
- recrudescent A75.1
- recurrens — *see* Fever, relapsing
- Sao Paulo A77.0
- scrub (China) (India) (Malaysia) (New Guinea) A75.3
- shop (of Malaysia) A75.2
- Siberian tick A77.2
- tick-borne A77.9
- tropical (mite-borne) A75.3
Tyrosinemia E70.21
- newborn, transitory P74.5
Tyrosinosis E70.21
Tyrosinuria E70.29

U

Uhl's anomaly or disease Q24.8
Ulcer, ulcerated, ulcerating, ulceration, ulcerative
- alveolar process M27.3
- amebic (intestine) A06.1
  - skin A06.7
- anastomotic — *see* Ulcer, gastrojejunal
- anorectal K62.6
- antral — *see* Ulcer, stomach
- anus (sphincter) (solitary) K62.6
- aorta — *see* Aneurysm
- aphthous (oral) (recurrent) K12.0
  - genital organ(s)
    - female N76.6
    - male N50.89
- artery I77.2
- atrophic — *see* Ulcer, skin
  - decubitus — *see* Ulcer, pressure, by site
- back L98.429
  - with
    - bone involvement without evidence of necrosis L98.426
    - bone necrosis L98.424
    - exposed fat layer L98.422
    - muscle involvement without evidence of necrosis L98.425
    - muscle necrosis L98.423
    - skin breakdown only L98.421
    - specified severity NEC L98.428
- Barrett's (esophagus) K22.10
  - with bleeding K22.11
- bile duct (common) (hepatic) K83.8
- bladder (solitary) (sphincter) NEC N32.89
  - bilharzial B65.9 [N33]
    - in schistosomiasis (bilharzial) B65.9 [N33]
  - submucosal — *see* Cystitis, interstitial
  - tuberculous A18.12
  - bleeding K27.4
- bone — *see* Osteomyelitis, specified type NEC
- bowel — *see* Ulcer, intestine
- breast N61.1

Ulcer, ulcerated, ulcerating, ulceration, ulcerative — *continued*
- bronchus J98.09
- buccal (cavity) (traumatic) K12.1
- Buruli A31.1
- buttock L98.419
  - with
    - bone involvement without evidence of necrosis L98.416
    - bone necrosis L98.414
    - exposed fat layer L98.412
    - muscle involvement without evidence of necrosis L98.415
    - muscle necrosis L98.413
    - skin breakdown only L98.411
    - specified severity NEC L98.418
- cancerous — *see* Neoplasm, malignant, by site
- cardia K22.10
  - with bleeding K22.11
- cardioesophageal (peptic) K22.10
  - with bleeding K22.11
- cecum — *see* Ulcer, intestine
- cervix (uteri) (decubitus) (trophic) N86
  - with cervicitis N72
- chancroidal A57
- chiclero B55.1
- chronic (cause unknown) — *see* Ulcer, skin
- Cochin-China B55.1
- colon — *see* Ulcer, intestine
- conjunctiva H10.89
- cornea H16.00- ☑
  - with hypopyon H16.03- ☑
  - central H16.01- ☑
  - dendritic (herpes simplex) B00.52
  - marginal H16.04- ☑
  - Mooren's H16.05- ☑
  - mycotic H16.06- ☑
  - perforated H16.07- ☑
  - ring H16.02- ☑
  - tuberculous (phlyctenular) A18.52
- corpus cavernosum (chronic) N48.5
- crural — *see* Ulcer, lower limb
- Curling's — *see* Ulcer, peptic, acute
- Cushing's — *see* Ulcer, peptic, acute
- cystic duct K82.8
- cystitis (interstitial) — *see* Cystitis, interstitial
- decubitus — *see* Ulcer, pressure, by site
- dendritic, cornea (herpes simplex) B00.52
- diabetes, diabetic — *see* Diabetes, ulcer
- Dieulafoy's K25.0
- due to
  - infection NEC — *see* Ulcer, skin
  - radiation NEC L59.8
  - trophic disturbance (any region) — *see* Ulcer, skin
  - X-ray L58.1
- duodenum, duodenal (eroded) (peptic) K26.9
  - with
    - hemorrhage K26.4
      - and perforation K26.6
    - perforation K26.5
  - acute K26.3
    - with
      - hemorrhage K26.0
        - and perforation K26.2
      - perforation K26.1
  - chronic K26.7
    - with
      - hemorrhage K26.4
        - and perforation K26.6
      - perforation K26.5
- dysenteric A09
- elusive — *see* Cystitis, interstitial
- endocarditis (acute) (chronic) (subacute) I28.8
- epiglottis J38.7
- esophagus (peptic) K22.10
  - with bleeding K22.11
  - due to
    - aspirin K22.10
      - with bleeding K22.11
    - gastrointestinal reflux disease K21.0
    - ingestion of chemical or medicament K22.10
      - with bleeding K22.11
  - fungal K22.10
    - with bleeding K22.11
  - infective K22.10
    - with bleeding K22.11
  - varicose — *see* Varix, esophagus
- eyelid (region) H01.8

☑ **Additional Character Required** — Refer to the Tabular List for Character Selection ▽ **Subterms under main terms may continue to next column or page**

Ulcer, ulcerated, ulcerating, ulceration, ulcerative
— *continued*
fauces J39.2
Fenwick (-Hunner) (solitary) — *see* Cystitis, interstitial
fistulous — *see* Ulcer, skin
foot (indolent) (trophic) — *see* Ulcer, lower limb
frambesial, initial A66.0
frenum (tongue) K14.0
gallbladder or duct K82.8
gangrenous — *see* Gangrene
gastric — *see* Ulcer, stomach
gastrocolic — *see* Ulcer, gastrojejunal
gastroduodenal — *see* Ulcer, peptic
gastroesophageal — *see* Ulcer, stomach
gastrointestinal — *see* Ulcer, gastrojejunal
gastrojejunal (peptic) K28.9
 with
  hemorrhage K28.4
   and perforation K28.6
  perforation K28.5
 acute K28.3
  with
   hemorrhage K28.0
    and perforation K28.2
   perforation K28.1
 chronic K28.7
  with
   hemorrhage K28.4
    and perforation K28.6
   perforation K28.5
gastrojejunocolic — *see* Ulcer, gastrojejunal
gingiva K06.8
gingivitis K05.10
 nonplaque induced K05.11
 plaque induced K05.10
glottis J38.7
granuloma of pudenda A58
gum K06.8
gumma, due to yaws A66.4
heel — *see* Ulcer, lower limb
hemorrhoid (*see also* Hemorrhoids, by degree) K64.8
Hunner's — *see* Cystitis, interstitial
hypopharynx J39.2
hypopyon (chronic) (subacute) — *see* Ulcer, cornea, with hypopyon
hypostaticum — *see* Ulcer, varicose
ileum — *see* Ulcer, intestine
intestine, intestinal K63.3
 with perforation K63.1
 amebic A06.1
 duodenal — *see* Ulcer, duodenum
 granulocytopenic (with hemorrhage) — *see* Neutropenia
 marginal — *see* Ulcer, gastrojejunal
 perforating K63.1
  newborn P78.0
 primary, small intestine K63.3
 rectum K62.6
 stercoraceous, stercoral K63.3
 tuberculous A18.32
 typhoid (fever) — *see* Typhoid
 varicose I86.8
jejunum, jejunal — *see* Ulcer, gastrojejunal
keratitis — *see* Ulcer, cornea
knee — *see* Ulcer, lower limb
labium (majus) (minus) N76.6
laryngitis — *see* Laryngitis
larynx (aphthous) (contact) J38.7
 diphtheritic A36.2
leg — *see* Ulcer, lower limb
lip K13.0
Lipschütz's N76.6
lower limb (atrophic) (chronic) (neurogenic) (perforating) (pyogenic) (trophic) (tropical) L97.909
 with
  bone involvement without evidence of necrosis L97.906
  bone necrosis L97.904
  exposed fat layer L97.902
  muscle involvement without evidence of necrosis L97.905
  muscle necrosis L97.903
  skin breakdown only L97.901
  specified severity NEC L97.908
 ankle L97.309
  with
   bone involvement without evidence of necrosis L97.306

Ulcer, ulcerated, ulcerating, ulceration, ulcerative
— *continued*
lower limb — *continued*
 ankle — *continued*
  with — *continued*
   bone necrosis L97.304
   exposed fat layer L97.302
   muscle involvement without evidence of necrosis L97.305
   muscle necrosis L97.303
   skin breakdown only L97.301
   specified severity NEC L97.308
  left L97.329
   with
    bone involvement without evidence of necrosis L97.326
    bone necrosis L97.324
    exposed fat layer L97.322
    muscle involvement without evidence of necrosis L97.325
    muscle necrosis L97.323
    skin breakdown only L97.321
    specified severity NEC L97.328
  right L97.319
   with
    bone involvement without evidence of necrosis L97.316
    bone necrosis L97.314
    exposed fat layer L97.312
    muscle involvement without evidence of necrosis L97.315
    muscle necrosis L97.313
    skin breakdown only L97.311
    specified severity NEC L97.318
 calf L97.209
  with
   bone involvement without evidence of necrosis L97.206
   bone necrosis L97.204
   exposed fat layer L97.202
   muscle involvement without evidence of necrosis L97.205
   muscle necrosis L97.203
   skin breakdown only L97.201
   specified severity NEC L97.208
  left L97.229
   with
    bone involvement without evidence of necrosis L97.226
    bone necrosis L97.224
    exposed fat layer L97.222
    muscle involvement without evidence of necrosis L97.225
    muscle necrosis L97.223
    skin breakdown only L97.221
    specified severity NEC L97.228
  right L97.219
   with
    bone involvement without evidence of necrosis L97.216
    bone necrosis L97.214
    exposed fat layer L97.212
    muscle involvement without evidence of necrosis L97.215
    muscle necrosis L97.213
    skin breakdown only L97.211
    specified severity NEC L97.218
 decubitus — *see* Ulcer, pressure, by site
 foot specified NEC L97.509
  with
   bone involvement without evidence of necrosis L97.506
   bone necrosis L97.504
   exposed fat layer L97.502
   muscle involvement without evidence of necrosis L97.505
   muscle necrosis L97.503
   skin breakdown only L97.501
   specified severity NEC L97.508
  left L97.529
   with
    bone involvement without evidence of necrosis L97.526
    bone necrosis L97.524
    exposed fat layer L97.522
    muscle involvement without evidence of necrosis L97.525
    muscle necrosis L97.523
    skin breakdown only L97.521

Ulcer, ulcerated, ulcerating, ulceration, ulcerative
— *continued*
lower limb — *continued*
 foot specified — *continued*
  left — *continued*
   with — *continued*
    specified severity NEC L97.528
   right L97.519
    with
     bone involvement without evidence of necrosis L97.516
     bone necrosis L97.514
     exposed fat layer L97.512
     muscle involvement without evidence of necrosis L97.515
     muscle necrosis L97.513
     skin breakdown only L97.511
     specified severity NEC L97.518
  heel L97.409
   with
    bone involvement without evidence of necrosis L97.406
    bone necrosis L97.404
    exposed fat layer L97.402
    muscle involvement without evidence of necrosis L97.405
    muscle necrosis L97.403
    skin breakdown only L97.401
    specified severity NEC L97.408
   left L97.429
    with
     bone involvement without evidence of necrosis L97.426
     bone necrosis L97.424
     exposed fat layer L97.422
     muscle involvement without evidence of necrosis L97.425
     muscle necrosis L97.423
     skin breakdown only L97.421
     specified severity NEC L97.428
   right L97.419
    with
     bone involvement without evidence of necrosis L97.416
     bone necrosis L97.414
     exposed fat layer L97.412
     muscle involvement without evidence of necrosis L97.415
     muscle necrosis L97.413
     skin breakdown only L97.411
     specified severity NEC L97.418
  left L97.929
   with
    bone involvement without evidence of necrosis L97.926
    bone necrosis L97.924
    exposed fat layer L97.922
    muscle involvement without evidence of necrosis L97.925
    muscle necrosis L97.923
    skin breakdown only L97.921
    specified severity NEC L97.928
  leprous A30.1
  lower leg NOS L97.909
   with
    bone involvement without evidence of necrosis L97.906
    bone necrosis L97.904
    exposed fat layer L97.902
    muscle involvement without evidence of necrosis L97.905
    muscle necrosis L97.903
    skin breakdown only L97.901
    specified severity NEC L97.908
   left L97.929
    with
     bone involvement without evidence of necrosis L97.926
     bone necrosis L97.924
     exposed fat layer L97.922
     muscle involvement without evidence of necrosis L97.925
     muscle necrosis L97.923
     skin breakdown only L97.921
     specified severity NEC L97.928
   right L97.919
    with
     bone involvement without evidence of necrosis L97.916

Ulcer, ulcerated, ulcerating, ulceration, ulcerative
— continued
 lower limb — continued
  lower leg — continued
   right — continued
    with — continued
     bone necrosis L97.914
     exposed fat layer L97.912
     muscle involvement without evidence
      of necrosis L97.915
     muscle necrosis L97.913
     skin breakdown only L97.911
     specified severity NEC L97.918
    specified site NEC L97.809
     with
      bone involvement without evidence of
       necrosis L97.806
      bone necrosis L97.804
      exposed fat layer L97.802
      muscle involvement without evidence
       of necrosis L97.805
      muscle necrosis L97.803
      skin breakdown only L97.801
      specified severity NEC L97.808
    left L97.829
     with
      bone involvement without evidence
       of necrosis L97.826
      bone necrosis L97.824
      exposed fat layer L97.822
      muscle involvement without evi-
       dence of necrosis L97.825
      muscle necrosis L97.823
      skin breakdown only L97.821
      specified severity NEC L97.828
    right L97.819
     with
      bone involvement without evidence
       of necrosis L97.816
      bone necrosis L97.814
      exposed fat layer L97.812
      muscle involvement without evi-
       dence of necrosis L97.815
      muscle necrosis L97.813
      skin breakdown only L97.811
      specified severity NEC L97.818
 midfoot L97.409
  with
   bone involvement without evidence of
    necrosis L97.406
   bone necrosis L97.404
   exposed fat layer L97.402
   muscle involvement without evidence of
    necrosis L97.405
   muscle necrosis L97.403
   skin breakdown only L97.401
   specified severity NEC L97.408
  left L97.429
   with
    bone involvement without evidence of
     necrosis L97.426
    bone necrosis L97.424
    exposed fat layer L97.422
    muscle involvement without evidence
     of necrosis L97.425
    muscle necrosis L97.423
    skin breakdown only L97.421
    specified severity NEC L97.428
  right L97.419
   with
    bone involvement without evidence of
     necrosis L97.416
    bone necrosis L97.414
    exposed fat layer L97.412
    muscle involvement without evidence
     of necrosis L97.415
    muscle necrosis L97.413
    skin breakdown only L97.411
    specified severity NEC L97.418
 right L97.919
  with
   bone involvement without evidence of
    necrosis L97.916
   bone necrosis L97.914
   exposed fat layer L97.912
   muscle involvement without evidence of
    necrosis L97.915
   muscle necrosis L97.913
   skin breakdown only L97.911

Ulcer, ulcerated, ulcerating, ulceration, ulcerative
— continued
 lower limb — continued
  right — continued
   with — continued
    specified severity NEC L97.918
   syphilitic A52.19
   thigh L97.109
    with
     bone involvement without evidence of
      necrosis L97.106
     bone necrosis L97.104
     exposed fat layer L97.102
     muscle involvement without evidence of
      necrosis L97.105
     muscle necrosis L97.103
     skin breakdown only L97.101
     specified severity NEC L97.108
    left L97.129
     with
      bone involvement without evidence of
       necrosis L97.126
      bone necrosis L97.124
      exposed fat layer L97.122
      muscle involvement without evidence
       of necrosis L97.125
      muscle necrosis L97.123
      skin breakdown only L97.121
      specified severity NEC L97.128
    right L97.119
     with
      bone involvement without evidence of
       necrosis L97.116
      bone necrosis L97.114
      exposed fat layer L97.112
      muscle involvement without evidence
       of necrosis L97.115
      muscle necrosis L97.113
      skin breakdown only L97.111
      specified severity NEC L97.118
   toe L97.509
    with
     bone involvement without evidence of
      necrosis L97.506
     bone necrosis L97.504
     exposed fat layer L97.502
     muscle involvement without evidence of
      necrosis L97.505
     muscle necrosis L97.503
     skin breakdown only L97.501
     specified severity NEC L97.508
    left L97.529
     with
      bone involvement without evidence of
       necrosis L97.526
      bone necrosis L97.524
      exposed fat layer L97.522
      muscle involvement without evidence
       of necrosis L97.525
      muscle necrosis L97.523
      skin breakdown only L97.521
      specified severity NEC L97.528
    right L97.519
     with
      bone involvement without evidence of
       necrosis L97.516
      bone necrosis L97.514
      exposed fat layer L97.512
      muscle involvement without evidence
       of necrosis L97.515
      muscle necrosis L97.513
      skin breakdown only L97.511
      specified severity NEC L97.518
   varicose — see Varix, leg, with, ulcer
  luetic — see Ulcer, syphilitic
  lung J98.4
   tuberculous — see Tuberculosis, pulmonary
 malignant — see Neoplasm, malignant, by site
 marginal NEC — see Ulcer, gastrojejunal
 meatus (urinarius) N34.2
 Meckel's diverticulum Q43.0
  malignant — see Table of Neoplasms, small intestine, malignant
 Meleney's (chronic undermining) — see Ulcer, skin
 Mooren's (cornea) — see Ulcer, cornea, Mooren's
 mycobacterial (skin) A31.1
 nasopharynx J39.2
 neck, uterus N86

Ulcer, ulcerated, ulcerating, ulceration, ulcerative
— continued
 neurogenic NEC — see Ulcer, skin
 nose, nasal (passage) (infective) (septum) J34.0
  skin — see Ulcer, skin
  spirochetal A69.8
  varicose (bleeding) I86.8
 oral mucosa (traumatic) K12.1
 palate (soft) K12.1
 penis (chronic) N48.5
 peptic (site unspecified) K27.9
  with
   hemorrhage K27.4
    and perforation K27.6
   perforation K27.5
  acute K27.3
   with
    hemorrhage K27.0
     and perforation K27.2
    perforation K27.1
  chronic K27.7
   with
    hemorrhage K27.4
     and perforation K27.6
    perforation K27.5
  esophagus K22.10
   with bleeding K22.11
  newborn P78.82
 perforating K27.5
  skin — see Ulcer, skin
 peritonsillar J35.8
 phagedenic (tropical) — see Ulcer, skin
 pharynx J39.2
 phlebitis — see Phlebitis
 plaster — see Ulcer, pressure, by site
 popliteal space — see Ulcer, lower limb
 postpyloric — see Ulcer, duodenum
 prepuce N47.7
 prepyloric — see Ulcer, stomach
 pressure (pressure area) L89.9- ☑
  ankle L89.5- ☑
  back L89.1- ☑
  buttock L89.3- ☑
  coccyx L89.15- ☑
  contiguous site of back, buttock, hip L89.4- ☑
  elbow L89.0- ☑
  face L89.81- ☑
  head L89.81- ☑
  heel L89.6- ☑
  hip L89.2- ☑
  sacral region (tailbone) L89.15- ☑
  specified site NEC L89.89- ☑
  stage 1 (healing) (pre-ulcer skin changes limited
   to persistent focal edema)
   ankle L89.5- ☑
   back L89.1- ☑
   buttock L89.3- ☑
   coccyx L89.15- ☑
   contiguous site of back, buttock, hip L89.4- ☑
   elbow L89.0- ☑
   face L89.81- ☑
   head L89.81- ☑
   heel L89.6- ☑
   hip L89.2- ☑
   sacral region (tailbone) L89.15- ☑
   specified site NEC L89.89- ☑
  stage 2 (healing) (abrasion, blister, partial thickness
   skin loss involving epidermis and/or dermis)
   ankle L89.5- ☑
   back L89.1- ☑
   buttock L89.3- ☑
   coccyx L89.15- ☑
   contiguous site of back, buttock, hip L89.4- ☑
   elbow L89.0- ☑
   face L89.81- ☑
   head L89.81- ☑
   heel L89.6- ☑
   hip L89.2- ☑
   sacral region (tailbone) L89.15- ☑
   specified site NEC L89.89- ☑
  stage 3 (healing) (full thickness skin loss involving
   damage or necrosis of subcutaneous tissue)
   ankle L89.5- ☑
   back L89.1- ☑
   buttock L89.3- ☑
   coccyx L89.15- ☑
   contiguous site of back, buttock, hip L89.4- ☑

☑ Additional Character Required — Refer to the Tabular List for Character Selection   ⮥ Subterms under main terms may continue to next column or page

Index

Ulcer, ulcerated, ulcerating, ulceration, ulcerative
  — *continued*
  pressure — *continued*
    stage 3 — *continued*
      elbow L89.0- ☑
      face L89.81- ☑
      head L89.81- ☑
      heel L89.6- ☑
      hip L89.2- ☑
      sacral region (tailbone) L89.15- ☑
      specified site NEC L89.89- ☑
    stage 4 (healing) (necrosis of soft tissues through
        to underlying muscle, tendon, or bone)
      ankle L89.5- ☑
      back L89.1- ☑
      buttock L89.3- ☑
      coccyx L89.15- ☑
      contiguous site of back, buttock, hip L89.4- ☑
      elbow L89.0- ☑
      face L89.81- ☑
      head L89.81- ☑
      heel L89.6- ☑
      hip L89.2- ☑
      sacral region (tailbone) L89.15- ☑
      specified site NEC L89.89- ☑
    unspecified stage
      ankle L89.5- ☑
      back L89.1- ☑
      buttock L89.3- ☑
      coccyx L89.15- ☑
      contiguous site of back, buttock, hip L89.4- ☑
      elbow L89.0- ☑
      face L89.81- ☑
      head L89.81- ☑
      heel L89.6- ☑
      hip L89.2- ☑
      sacral region (tailbone) L89.15- ☑
      specified site NEC L89.89- ☑
    unstageable
      ankle L89.5- ☑
      back L89.1- ☑
      buttock L89.3- ☑
      coccyx L89.15- ☑
      contiguous site of back, buttock, hip L89.4- ☑
      elbow L89.0- ☑
      face L89.81- ☑
      head L89.81- ☑
      heel L89.6- ☑
      hip L89.2- ☑
      sacral region (tailbone) L89.15- ☑
      specified site NEC L89.89- ☑
  primary of intestine K63.3
    with perforation K63.1
  prostate N41.9
  pyloric — *see* Ulcer, stomach
  rectosigmoid K63.3
    with perforation K63.1
  rectum (sphincter) (solitary) K62.6
    stercoraceous, stercoral K62.6
  retina — *see* Inflammation, chorioretinal
  rodent (*see also* Neoplasm, skin, malignant)
  sclera — *see* Scleritis
  scrofulous (tuberculous) A18.2
  scrotum N50.89
    tuberculous A18.15
    varicose I86.1
  seminal vesicle N50.89
  sigmoid — *see* Ulcer, intestine
  skin (atrophic) (chronic) (neurogenic) (non-healing)
    (perforating) (pyogenic) (trophic) (tropical)
    L98.499
    with gangrene — *see* Gangrene
    amebic A06.7
    back — *see* Ulcer, back
    buttock — *see* Ulcer, buttock
    decubitus — *see* Ulcer, pressure
    lower limb — *see* Ulcer, lower limb
    mycobacterial A31.1
    specified site NEC L98.499
      with
        bone involvement without evidence of
          necrosis L98.496
        bone necrosis L98.494
        exposed fat layer L98.492
        muscle involvement without evidence of
          necrosis L98.495
        muscle necrosis L98.493

Ulcer, ulcerated, ulcerating, ulceration, ulcerative
  — *continued*
  skin — *continued*
    specified site — *continued*
      with — *continued*
        skin breakdown only L98.491
        specified severity NEC L98.498
    tuberculous (primary) A18.4
    varicose — *see* Ulcer, varicose
  sloughing — *see* Ulcer, skin
  solitary, anus or rectum (sphincter) K62.6
  sore throat J02.9
    streptococcal J02.0
  spermatic cord N50.89
  spine (tuberculous) A18.01
  stasis (venous) — *see* Varix, leg, with, ulcer
    without varicose veins I87.2
  stercoraceous, stercoral K63.3
    with perforation K63.1
    anus or rectum K62.6
  stoma, stomal — *see* Ulcer, gastrojejunal
  stomach (eroded) (peptic) (round) K25.9
    with
      hemorrhage K25.4
        and perforation K25.6
      perforation K25.5
    acute K25.3
      with
        hemorrhage K25.0
          and perforation K25.2
        perforation K25.1
    chronic K25.7
      with
        hemorrhage K25.4
          and perforation K25.6
        perforation K25.5
  stomal — *see* Ulcer, gastrojejunal
  stomatitis K12.1
  stress — *see* Ulcer, peptic
  strumous (tuberculous) A18.2
  submucosal, bladder — *see* Cystitis, interstitial
  syphilitic (any site) (early) (secondary) A51.39
    late A52.79
    perforating A52.79
      foot A52.11
  testis N50.89
  thigh — *see* Ulcer, lower limb
  throat J39.2
    diphtheritic A36.0
  toe — *see* Ulcer, lower limb
  tongue (traumatic) K14.0
  tonsil J35.8
    diphtheritic A36.0
  trachea J39.8
  trophic — *see* Ulcer, skin
  tropical — *see* Ulcer, skin
  tuberculous — *see* Tuberculosis, ulcer
  tunica vaginalis N50.89
  turbinate J34.89
  typhoid (perforating) — *see* Typhoid
  unspecified site — *see* Ulcer, skin
  urethra (meatus) — *see* Urethritis
  uterus N85.8
    cervix N86
      with cervicitis N72
    neck N86
      with cervicitis N72
  vagina N76.5
    in Behçet's disease M35.2 [N77.0]
    pessary N89.8
  valve, heart I33.0
  varicose (lower limb, any part) (*see also* Varix, leg, with,
    ulcer)
    broad ligament I86.2
    esophagus — *see* Varix, esophagus
    inflamed or infected — *see* Varix, leg, with ulcer,
      with inflammation
    nasal septum I86.8
    perineum I86.3
    scrotum I86.1
    specified site NEC I86.8
    sublingual I86.0
    vulva I86.3
  vas deferens N50.89
  vulva (acute) (infectional) N76.6
    in (due to)
      Behçet's disease M35.2 [N77.0]
      herpesviral (herpes simplex) infection A60.04

Ulcer, ulcerated, ulcerating, ulceration, ulcerative
  — *continued*
  vulva — *continued*
    in — *continued*
      tuberculosis A18.18
  vulvobuccal, recurring N76.6
  X-ray L58.1
  yaws A66.4
Ulcerosa scarlatina A38.8
Ulcus (*see also* Ulcer)
  cutis tuberculosum A18.4
  duodeni — *see* Ulcer, duodenum
  durum (syphilitic) A51.0
    extragenital A51.2
  gastrojejunale — *see* Ulcer, gastrojejunal
  hypostaticum — *see* Ulcer, varicose
  molle (cutis) (skin) A57
  serpens corneae — *see* Ulcer, cornea, central
  ventriculi — *see* Ulcer, stomach
Ulegyria Q04.8
Ulerythema
  ophryogenes, congenital Q84.2
  sycosiforme L73.8
Ullrich (-Bonnevie)(-Turner) **syndrome** (*see also* Turner's
  syndrome) Q87.1
Ullrich-Feichtiger syndrome Q87.0
Ulnar — *see* condition
Ulorrhagia, ulorrhea K06.8
Umbilicus, umbilical — *see* condition
Unacceptable
  contours of tooth K08.54
  morphology of tooth K08.54
Unavailability (of)
  bed at medical facility Z75.1
  health service-related agencies Z75.4
  medical facilities (at) Z75.3
    due to
      investigation by social service agency Z75.2
      lack of services at home Z75.0
      remoteness from facility Z75.3
      waiting list Z75.1
    home Z75.0
    outpatient clinic Z75.3
  schooling Z55.1
  social service agencies Z75.4
Uncinaria americana infestation B76.1
Uncinariasis B76.9
Uncongenial work Z56.5
Unconscious (ness) — *see* Coma
Under observation — *see* Observation
Underachievement in school Z55.3
Underdevelopment (*see also* Undeveloped)
  nose Q30.1
  sexual E30.0
Underdosing (*see also* Table of Drugs and Chemicals,
  categories T36-T50, with final character 6) Z91.14
  intentional NEC Z91.128
    due to financial hardship of patient Z91.120
  unintentional NEC Z91.138
    due to patient's age related debility Z91.130
Underfeeding, newborn P92.3
Underfill, endodontic M27.53
Underimmunization status Z28.3
Undernourishment — *see* Malnutrition
Undernutrition — *see* Malnutrition
Underweight R63.6
  for gestational age — *see* Light for dates
Underwood's disease P83.0
Undescended (*see also* Malposition, congenital)
  cecum Q43.3
  colon Q43.3
  testicle — *see* Cryptorchid
Undeveloped, undevelopment (*see also* Hypoplasia)
  brain (congenital) Q02
  cerebral (congenital) Q02
  heart Q24.8
  lung Q33.6
  testis E29.1
  uterus E30.0
Undiagnosed (disease) R69
Undulant fever — *see* Brucellosis
Unemployment, anxiety concerning Z56.0
  threatened Z56.2
Unequal length (acquired) (limb) (*see also* Deformity,
  limb, unequal length)
  leg (*see also* Deformity, limb, unequal length)
    congenital Q72.9- ☑

Ulcer, ulcerated, ulcerating, ulceration, ulcerative — Unequal length

Index

Unextracted dental root — Use

Unextracted dental root K08.3
Unguis incarnatus L60.0
Unhappiness R45.2
Unicornate uterus Q51.4
  in pregnancy or childbirth O34.00
Unilateral (*see also* condition)
  development, breast N64.89
  organ or site, congenital NEC — *see* Agenesis, by site
Unilocular heart Q20.8
Union, abnormal (*see also* Fusion)
  larynx and trachea Q34.8
Universal mesentery Q43.3
Unrepairable overhanging of dental restorative
    materials K08.52
Unsatisfactory
  restoration of tooth K08.50
    specified NEC K08.59
  sample of cytologic smear
    anus R85.615
    cervix R87.615
    vagina R87.625
  surroundings Z59.1
  work Z56.5
Unsoundness of mind — *see* Psychosis
Unstable
  back NEC — *see* Instability, joint, spine
  hip (congenital) Q65.6
    acquired — *see* Derangement, joint, specified type
      NEC, hip
  joint — *see* Instability, joint
    secondary to removal of joint prosthesis M96.89
  lie (mother) O32.0 ☑
  lumbosacral joint (congenital)
    acquired — *see* subcategory M53.2 ☑
  sacroiliac — *see* subcategory M53.2 ☑
  spine NEC — *see* Instability, joint, spine
Unsteadiness on feet R26.81
Untruthfulness, child problem F91.8
Unverricht (-Lundborg) **disease or epilepsy** — *see*
    Epilepsy, generalized, idiopathic
Unwanted pregnancy Z64.0
Upbringing, institutional Z62.22
  away from parents NEC Z62.29
  in care of non-parental family member Z62.21
  in foster care Z62.21
  in orphanage or group home Z62.22
  in welfare custody Z62.21
Upper respiratory — *see* condition
Upset
  gastric K30
  gastrointestinal K30
    psychogenic F45.8
  intestinal (large) (small) K59.9
    psychogenic F45.8
  menstruation N93.9
  mental F48.9
  stomach K30
    psychogenic F45.8
Urachus (*see also* condition)
  patent or persistent Q64.4
Urbach-Oppenheim disease (necrobiosis lipoidica dia-
    beticorum) — *see* E08-E13 with .620
Urbach's lipoid proteinosis E78.89
Urbach-Wiethe disease E78.89
Urban yellow fever A95.1
Urea
  blood, high — *see* Uremia
  cycle metabolism disorder — *see* Disorder, urea cycle
    metabolism
Uremia, uremic N19
  with
    ectopic or molar pregnancy O08.4
    polyneuropathy N18.9 [G63]
  chronic NOS (*see also* Disease, kidney, chronic) N18.9
    due to hypertension — *see* Hypertensive, kidney
  complicating
    ectopic or molar pregnancy O08.4
  congenital P96.0
  extrarenal R39.2
  following ectopic or molar pregnancy O08.4
  newborn P96.0
  prerenal R39.2
Ureter, ureteral — *see* condition
Ureteralgia N23
Ureterectasis — *see* Hydroureter
Ureteritis N28.89
  cystica N28.86

Ureteritis — *continued*
  due to calculus N20.1
    with calculus, kidney N20.2
      with hydronephrosis N13.2
  gonococcal (acute) (chronic) A54.21
  nonspecific N28.89
Ureterocele N28.89
  congenital (orthotopic) Q62.31
    ectopic Q62.32
Ureterolith, ureterolithiasis — *see* Calculus, ureter
Ureterostomy
  attention to Z43.6
  status Z93.6
Urethra, urethral — *see* condition
Urethralgia R39.89
Urethritis (anterior) (posterior) N34.2
  calculous N21.1
  candidal B37.41
  chlamydial A56.01
  diplococcal (gonococcal) A54.01
    with abscess (accessory gland) (periurethral) A54.1
  gonococcal A54.01
    with abscess (accessory gland) (periurethral) A54.1
  nongonococcal N34.1
    Reiter's — *see* Reiter's disease
  nonspecific N34.1
  nonvenereal N34.1
  postmenopausal N34.2
  puerperal O86.22
  Reiter's — *see* Reiter's disease
  specified NEC N34.2
  trichomonal or due to Trichomonas (vaginalis) A59.03
Urethrocele N81.0
  with
    cystocele — *see* Cystocele
    prolapse of uterus — *see* Prolapse, uterus
Urethrolithiasis (with colic or infection) N21.1
Urethrorectal — *see* condition
Urethrorrhagia N36.8
Urethrorrhea R36.9
Urethrostomy
  attention to Z43.6
  status Z93.6
Urethrotrigonitis — *see* Trigonitis
Urethrovaginal — *see* condition
Urgency
  fecal R15.2
  hypertensive — *see* Hypertension
  urinary R39.15
Urhidrosis, uridrosis L74.8
Uric acid in blood (increased) E79.0
Uricacidemia (asymptomatic) E79.0
Uricemia (asymptomatic) E79.0
Uricosuria R82.99
Urinary — *see* condition
Urination
  frequent R35.0
  painful R30.9
Urine
  blood in — *see* Hematuria
  discharge, excessive R35.8
  enuresis, nonorganic origin F98.0
  extravasation R39.0
  frequency R35.0
  incontinence R32
    nonorganic origin F98.0
  intermittent stream R39.198
  pus in N39.0
  retention or stasis R33.9
    organic R33.8
      drug-induced R33.0
    psychogenic F45.8
  secretion
    deficient R34
    excessive R35.8
    frequency R35.0
  stream
    intermittent R39.198
    slowing R39.198
    splitting R39.13
    weak R39.12
Urinemia — *see* Uremia
Urinoma, urethra N36.8
Uroarthritis, infectious (Reiter's) — *see* Reiter's disease
Urodialysis R34
Urolithiasis — *see* Calculus, urinary
Uronephrosis — *see* Hydronephrosis
Uropathy N39.9

Uropathy — *continued*
  obstructive N13.9
    specified NEC N13.8
  reflux N13.9
    specified NEC N13.8
  vesicoureteral reflux-associated — *see* Reflux, vesi-
    coureteral
Urosepsis — *code to* condition
Urticaria L50.9
  with angioneurotic edema T78.3 ☑
    hereditary D84.1
  allergic L50.0
  cholinergic L50.5
  chronic L50.8
  cold, familial L50.2
  contact L50.6
  dermatographic L50.3
  due to
    cold or heat L50.2
    drugs L50.0
    food L50.0
    inhalants L50.0
    plants L50.6
    serum (*see also* Reaction, serum) T80.69 ☑
  factitial L50.3
  familial cold M04.2
  giant T78.3 ☑
    hereditary D84.1
  gigantea T78.3 ☑
  idiopathic L50.1
  larynx T78.3 ☑
    hereditary D84.1
  neonatorum P83.88
  nonallergic L50.1
  papulosa (Hebra) L28.2
  pigmentosa D47.01
    congenital Q82.2
    of neonatal onset Q82.2
    of newborn onset Q82.2
  recurrent periodic L50.8
  serum (*see also* Reaction, serum) T80.69 ☑
  solar L56.3
  specified type NEC L50.8
  thermal (cold) (heat) L50.2
  vibratory L50.4
  xanthelasmoidea — *see* Urticaria pigmentosa
Use (of)
  alcohol Z72.89
    with
      intoxication F10.929
      sleep disorder F10.982
    harmful — *see* Abuse, alcohol
  amphetamines — *see* Use, stimulant NEC
  caffeine — *see* Use, stimulant NEC
  cannabis F12.90
    with
      anxiety disorder F12.980
      intoxication F12.929
        with
          delirium F12.921
          perceptual disturbance F12.922
        uncomplicated F12.920
      other specified disorder F12.988
      psychosis F12.959
        delusions F12.950
        hallucinations F12.951
      unspecified disorder F12.99
  cocaine F14.90
    with
      anxiety disorder F14.980
      intoxication F14.929
        with
          delirium F14.921
          perceptual disturbance F14.922
        uncomplicated F14.920
      other specified disorder F14.988
      psychosis F14.959
        delusions F14.950
        hallucinations F14.951
      sexual dysfunction F14.981
      sleep disorder F14.982
      unspecified disorder F14.99
    harmful — *see* Abuse, drug, cocaine
  drug(s) NEC F19.90
    with sleep disorder F19.982
    harmful — *see* Abuse, drug, by type
  hallucinogen NEC F16.90

☑ Additional Character Required — Refer to the Tabular List for Character Selection   ▽ Subterms under main terms may continue to next column or page

Use — *continued*
  hallucinogen — *continued*
    with
      anxiety disorder F16.980
      intoxication F16.929
        with
          delirium F16.921
        uncomplicated F16.920
      mood disorder F16.94
      other specified disorder F16.988
      perception disorder (flashbacks) F16.983
      psychosis F16.959
        delusions F16.950
        hallucinations F16.951
      unspecified disorder F16.99
    harmful — *see* Abuse, drug, hallucinogen NEC
  inhalants F18.90
    with
      anxiety disorder F18.980
      intoxication F18.929
        with delirium F18.921
        uncomplicated F18.920
      mood disorder F18.94
      other specified disorder F18.988
      persisting dementia F18.97
      psychosis F18.959
        delusions F18.950
        hallucinations F18.951
      unspecified disorder F18.99
    harmful — *see* Abuse, drug, inhalant
  methadone — *see* Use, opioid
  nonprescribed drugs F19.90
    harmful — *see* Abuse, non-psychoactive substance
  opioid F11.90
    with
      disorder F11.99
        mood F11.94
        sleep F11.982
        specified type NEC F11.988
      intoxication F11.929
        with
          delirium F11.921
          perceptual disturbance F11.922
        uncomplicated F11.920
      withdrawal F11.93
    harmful — *see* Abuse, drug, opioid
  patent medicines F19.90
    harmful — *see* Abuse, non-psychoactive substance
  psychoactive drug NEC F19.90
    with
      anxiety disorder F19.980
      intoxication F19.929
        with
          delirium F19.921
          perceptual disturbance F19.922
        uncomplicated F19.920
      mood disorder F19.94
      other specified disorder F19.988
      persisting
        amnestic disorder F19.96
        dementia F19.97
      psychosis F19.959
        delusions F19.950
        hallucinations F19.951
      sexual dysfunction F19.981
      sleep disorder F19.982
      unspecified disorder F19.99
      withdrawal F19.939
        with
          delirium F19.931
          perceptual disturbance F19.932
        uncomplicated F19.930
    harmful — *see* Abuse, drug NEC, psychoactive NEC
  sedative, hypnotic, or anxiolytic F13.90
    with
      anxiety disorder F13.980
      intoxication F13.929
        with
          delirium F13.921
        uncomplicated F13.920
      other specified disorder F13.988
      persisting
        amnestic disorder F13.96
        dementia F13.97
      psychosis F13.959
        delusions F13.950
        hallucinations F13.951
      sexual dysfunction F13.981

Use — *continued*
  sedative, hypnotic, or anxiolytic — *continued*
    with — *continued*
      sleep disorder F13.982
      unspecified disorder F13.99
    harmful — *see* Abuse, drug, sedative, hypnotic, or anxiolytic
  stimulant NEC F15.90
    with
      anxiety disorder F15.980
      intoxication F15.929
        with
          delirium F15.921
          perceptual disturbance F15.922
        uncomplicated F15.920
      mood disorder F15.94
      other specified disorder F15.988
      psychosis F15.959
        delusions F15.950
        hallucinations F15.951
      sexual dysfunction F15.981
      sleep disorder F15.982
      unspecified disorder F15.99
      withdrawal F15.93
    harmful — *see* Abuse, drug, stimulant NEC
  tobacco Z72.0
    with dependence — *see* Dependence, drug, nicotine
  volatile solvents (*see also* Use, inhalant) F18.90
    harmful — *see* Abuse, drug, inhalant

Usher-Senear disease or syndrome L10.4
Uta B55.1
Uteromegaly N85.2
Uterovaginal — *see* condition
Uterovesical — *see* condition
Uveal — *see* condition
Uveitis (anterior) (*see also* Iridocyclitis)
  acute — *see* Iridocyclitis, acute
  chronic — *see* Iridocyclitis, chronic
  due to toxoplasmosis (acquired) B58.09
    congenital P37.1
  granulomatous — *see* Iridocyclitis, chronic
  heterochromic — *see* Cyclitis, Fuchs' heterochromic
  lens-induced — *see* Iridocyclitis, lens-induced
  posterior — *see* Chorioretinitis
  sympathetic H44.13- ☑
  syphilitic (secondary) A51.43
    congenital (early) A50.01
    late A52.71
  tuberculous A18.54
Uveoencephalitis — *see* Inflammation, chorioretinal
Uveokeratitis — *see* Iridocyclitis
Uveoparotitis D86.89
Uvula — *see* condition
Uvulitis (acute) (catarrhal) (chronic) (membranous) (suppurative) (ulcerative) K12.2

V

Vaccination (prophylactic)
  complication or reaction — *see* Complications, vaccination
  delayed Z28.9
  encounter for Z23
  not done — *see* Immunization, not done, because (of)
Vaccinia (generalized) (localized) T88.1 ☑
  without vaccination B08.011
  congenital P35.8
Vacuum, in sinus (accessory) (nasal) J34.89
Vagabond, vagabondage Z59.0
Vagabond's disease B85.1
Vagina, vaginal — *see* condition
Vaginalitis (tunica) (testis) N49.1
Vaginismus (reflex) N94.2
  functional F52.5
  nonorganic F52.5
  psychogenic F52.5
  secondary N94.2
Vaginitis (acute) (circumscribed) (diffuse) (emphysematous) (nonvenereal) (ulcerative) N76.0
  with ectopic or molar pregnancy O08.0
  amebic A06.82
  atrophic, postmenopausal N95.2
  bacterial N76.0
  blennorrhagic (gonococcal) A54.02
  candidal B37.3
  chlamydial A56.02

Vaginitis — *continued*
  chronic N76.1
  due to Trichomonas (vaginalis) A59.01
  following ectopic or molar pregnancy O08.0
  gonococcal A54.02
    with abscess (accessory gland) (periurethral) A54.1
  granuloma A58
  in (due to)
    candidiasis B37.3
    herpesviral (herpes simplex) infection A60.04
    pinworm infection B80 [N77.1]
  monilial B37.3
  mycotic (candidal) B37.3
  postmenopausal atrophic N95.2
  puerperal (postpartum) O86.13
  senile (atrophic) N95.2
  subacute or chronic N76.1
  syphilitic (early) A51.0
    late A52.76
  trichomonal A59.01
  tuberculous A18.18
Vaginosis — *see* Vaginitis
Vagotonia G52.2
Vagrancy Z59.0
VAIN — *see* Neoplasia, intraepithelial, vagina
Vallecula — *see* condition
Valley fever B38.0
Valsuani's disease — *see* Anemia, obstetric
Valve, valvular (formation) (*see also* condition)
  cerebral ventricle (communicating) in situ Z98.2
  cervix, internal os Q51.828
  congenital NEC — *see* Atresia, by site
  ureter (pelvic junction) (vesical orifice) Q62.39
  urethra (congenital) (posterior) Q64.2
Valvulitis (chronic) — *see* Endocarditis
Valvulopathy — *see* Endocarditis
Van Bogaert's leukoencephalopathy (sclerosing) (subacute) A81.1
Van Bogaert-Scherer-Epstein disease or syndrome E75.5
Van Buchem's syndrome M85.2
Van Creveld-von Gierke disease E74.01
Van der Hoeve (-de Kleyn) **syndrome** Q78.0
Van der Woude's syndrome Q38.0
Van Neck's disease or osteochondrosis M91.0
Vanishing lung J44.9
Vapor asphyxia or suffocation T59.9 ☑
  specified agent — *see* Table of Drugs and Chemicals
Variance, lethal ball, prosthetic heart valve T82.09 ☑
Variants, thalassemic D56.8
Variations in hair color L67.1
Varicella B01.9
  with
    complications NEC B01.89
    encephalitis B01.11
    encephalomyelitis B01.11
    meningitis B01.0
    myelitis B01.12
    pneumonia B01.2
  congenital P35.8
Varices — *see* Varix
Varicocele (scrotum) (thrombosed) I86.1
  ovary I86.2
  perineum I86.3
  spermatic cord (ulcerated) I86.1
Varicose
  aneurysm (ruptured) I77.0
  dermatitis — *see* Varix, leg, with, inflammation
  eczema — *see* Varix, leg, with, inflammation
  phlebitis — *see* Varix, with, inflammation
  tumor — *see* Varix
  ulcer (lower limb, any part) (*see also* Varix, leg, with, ulcer)
    anus (*see also* Hemorrhoids) K64.8
    esophagus — *see* Varix, esophagus
    inflamed or infected — *see* Varix, leg, with ulcer, with inflammation
    nasal septum I86.8
    perineum I86.3
    scrotum I86.1
    specified site NEC I86.8
    vein — *see* Varix
    vessel — *see* Varix, leg
Varicosis, varicosities, varicosity — *see* Varix
Variola (major) (minor) B03
Varioloid B03
Varix (lower limb) (ruptured) I83.90

▽ Subterms under main terms may continue to next column or page   ☑ Additional Character Required — Refer to the Tabular List for Character Selection   **323**

Use — Varix

Varix — *continued*
  with
    edema I83.899
    inflammation I83.10
      with ulcer (venous) I83.209
    pain I83.819
    specified complication NEC I83.899
    stasis dermatitis I83.10
      with ulcer (venous) I83.209
    swelling I83.899
    ulcer I83.009
      with inflammation I83.209
  aneurysmal I77.0
  asymptomatic I83.9- ☑
  bladder I86.2
  broad ligament I86.2
  complicating
    childbirth (lower extremity) O87.4
      anus or rectum O87.2
      genital (vagina, vulva or perineum) O87.8
    pregnancy (lower extremity) O22.0- ☑
      anus or rectum O22.4- ☑
      genital (vagina, vulva or perineum) O22.1- ☑
    puerperium (lower extremity) O87.4
      anus or rectum O87.2
      genital (vagina, vulva, perineum) O87.8
  congenital (any site) Q27.8
  esophagus (idiopathic) (primary) (ulcerated) I85.00
    bleeding I85.01
    congenital Q27.8
    in (due to)
      alcoholic liver disease I85.10
        bleeding I85.11
      cirrhosis of liver I85.10
        bleeding I85.11
      portal hypertension I85.10
        bleeding I85.11
      schistosomiasis I85.10
        bleeding I85.11
      toxic liver disease I85.10
        bleeding I85.11
    secondary I85.10
      bleeding I85.11
  gastric I86.4
  inflamed or infected I83.10
    ulcerated I83.209
  labia (majora) I86.3
  leg (asymptomatic) I83.90
    with
      edema I83.899
      inflammation I83.10
        with ulcer — *see* Varix, leg, with, ulcer, with inflammation by site
      pain I83.819
      specified complication NEC I83.899
      swelling I83.899
      ulcer I83.009
        with inflammation I83.209
        ankle I83.003
          with inflammation I83.203
        calf I83.002
          with inflammation I83.202
        foot NEC I83.005
          with inflammation I83.205
        heel I83.004
          with inflammation I83.204
        lower leg NEC I83.008
          with inflammation I83.208
        midfoot I83.004
          with inflammation I83.204
        thigh I83.001
          with inflammation I83.201
      bilateral (asymptomatic) I83.93
        with
          edema I83.893
          pain I83.813
          specified complication NEC I83.893
          swelling I83.893
          ulcer I83.0- ☑
            with inflammation I83.209
      left (asymptomatic) I83.92
        with
          edema I83.892
          inflammation I83.12
            with ulcer — *see* Varix, leg, with, ulcer, with inflammation by site
          pain I83.812
          specified complication NEC I83.892

Varix — *continued*
  leg — *continued*
    left — *continued*
      with — *continued*
        swelling I83.892
        ulcer I83.029
          with inflammation I83.229
          ankle I83.023
            with inflammation I83.223
          calf I83.022
            with inflammation I83.222
          foot NEC I83.025
            with inflammation I83.225
          heel I83.024
            with inflammation I83.224
          lower leg NEC I83.028
            with inflammation I83.228
          midfoot I83.024
            with inflammation I83.224
          thigh I83.021
            with inflammation I83.221
      right (asymptomatic) I83.91
        with
          edema I83.891
          inflammation I83.11
            with ulcer — *see* Varix, leg, with, ulcer, with inflammation by site
          pain I83.811
          specified complication NEC I83.891
          swelling I83.891
          ulcer I83.019
            with inflammation I83.219
            ankle I83.013
              with inflammation I83.213
            calf I83.012
              with inflammation I83.212
            foot NEC I83.015
              with inflammation I83.215
            heel I83.014
              with inflammation I83.214
            lower leg NEC I83.018
              with inflammation I83.218
            midfoot I83.014
              with inflammation I83.214
            thigh I83.011
              with inflammation I83.211
  nasal septum I86.8
  orbit I86.8
    congenital Q27.8
  ovary I86.2
  papillary I78.1
  pelvis I86.2
  perineum I86.3
  pharynx I86.8
  placenta O43.89- ☑
  renal papilla I86.8
  retina H35.09
  scrotum (ulcerated) I86.1
  sigmoid colon I86.8
  specified site NEC I86.8
  spinal (cord) (vessels) I86.8
  spleen, splenic (vein) (with phlebolith) I86.8
  stomach I86.4
  sublingual I86.0
  ulcerated I83.009
    inflamed or infected I83.209
  uterine ligament I86.2
  vagina I86.8
  vocal cord I86.8
  vulva I86.3
Vas deferens — *see* condition
Vas deferentitis N49.1
Vasa previa O69.4 ☑
  hemorrhage from, affecting newborn P50.0
Vascular (*see also* condition)
  loop on optic papilla Q14.2
  spasm I73.9
  spider I78.1
Vascularization, cornea — *see* Neovascularization, cornea
Vasculitis I77.6
  allergic D69.0
  cryoglobulinemic D89.1
  disseminated I77.6
  hypocomplementemic M31.8
  kidney I77.89
  livedoid L95.0
  nodular L95.8

Vasculitis — *continued*
  retina H35.06- ☑
  rheumatic — *see* Fever, rheumatic
  rheumatoid — *see* Rheumatoid, vasculitis
  skin (limited to) L95.9
    specified NEC L95.8
  systemic M31.8
Vasculopathy, necrotizing M31.9
  cardiac allograft T86.290
  specified NEC M31.8
Vasitis (nodosa) N49.1
  tuberculous A18.15
Vasodilation I73.9
Vasomotor — *see* condition
Vasoplasty, after previous sterilization Z31.0
  aftercare Z31.42
Vasospasm (vasoconstriction) I73.9
  cerebral (cerebrovascular) (artery) I67.848
    reversible I67.841
  coronary I20.1
  nerve
    arm — *see* Mononeuropathy, upper limb
    brachial plexus G54.0
    cervical plexus G54.2
    leg — *see* Mononeuropathy, lower limb
  peripheral NOS I73.9
  retina (artery) — *see* Occlusion, artery, retina
Vasospastic — *see* condition
Vasovagal attack (paroxysmal) R55
  psychogenic F45.8
VATER syndrome Q87.2
Vater's ampulla — *see* condition
Vegetation, vegetative
  adenoid (nasal fossa) J35.8
  endocarditis (acute) (any valve) (subacute) I33.0
  heart (mycotic) (valve) I33.0
Veil
  Jackson's Q43.3
Vein, venous — *see* condition
Veldt sore — *see* Ulcer, skin
Velpeau's hernia — *see* Hernia, femoral
Venereal
  bubo A55
  disease A64
  granuloma inguinale A58
  lymphogranuloma (Durand-Nicolas-Favre) A55
Venofibrosis I87.8
Venom, venomous — *see* Table of Drugs and Chemicals, by animal or substance, poisoning
Venous — *see* condition
Ventilator lung, newborn P27.8
Ventral — *see* condition
Ventricle, ventricular (*see also* condition)
  escape I49.3
  inversion Q20.5
Ventriculitis (cerebral) (*see also* Encephalitis) G04.90
Ventriculostomy status Z98.2
Vernet's syndrome G52.7
Verneuil's disease (syphilitic bursitis) A52.78
Verruca (due to HPV) (filiformis) (simplex) (viral) (vulgaris) B07.9
  acuminata A63.0
  necrogenica (primary) (tuberculosa) A18.4
  plana B07.8
  plantaris B07.0
  seborrheica L82.1
    inflamed L82.0
  senile (seborrheic) L82.1
    inflamed L82.0
  tuberculosa (primary) A18.4
  venereal A63.0
Verrucosities — *see* Verruca
Verruga peruana, peruviana A44.1
Version
  with extraction
  cervix — *see* Malposition, uterus
  uterus (postinfectional) (postpartal, old) — *see* Malposition, uterus
Vertebra, vertebral — *see* condition
Vertical talus (congenital) Q66.80
  left foot Q66.82
  right foot Q66.81
Vertigo R42
  auditory — *see* Vertigo, aural
  aural H81.31- ☑
  benign paroxysmal (positional) H81.1- ☑
  central (origin) H81.4- ☑

☑ **Additional Character Required — Refer to the Tabular List for Character Selection**   ▽ **Subterms under main terms may continue to next column or page**

Vertigo — *continued*
cerebral H81.4- ☑
Dix and Hallpike (epidemic) — *see* Neuronitis,
   vestibular
due to infrasound T75.23 ☑
epidemic A88.1
   Dix and Hallpike — *see* Neuronitis, vestibular
   Pedersen's — *see* Neuronitis, vestibular
   vestibular neuronitis — *see* Neuronitis, vestibular
hysterical F44.89
infrasound T75.23 ☑
labyrinthine — *see* subcategory H81.0 ☑
laryngeal R05
malignant positional H81.4- ☑
Ménière's — *see* subcategory H81.0 ☑
menopausal N95.1
otogenic — *see* Vertigo, aural
paroxysmal positional, benign — *see* Vertigo, benign
   paroxysmal
Pedersen's (epidemic) — *see* Neuronitis, vestibular
peripheral NEC H81.39- ☑
positional
   benign paroxysmal — *see* Vertigo, benign parox-
     ysmal
   malignant H81.4- ☑
Very-low-density-lipoprotein-type (VLDL) **hyper-**
   lipoproteinemia E78.1
Vesania — *see* Psychosis
Vesical — *see* condition
Vesicle
cutaneous R23.8
seminal — *see* condition
skin R23.8
Vesicocolic — *see* condition
Vesicoperineal — *see* condition
Vesicorectal — *see* condition
Vesicourethrorectal — *see* condition
Vesicovaginal — *see* condition
Vesicular — *see* condition
Vesiculitis (seminal) N49.0
amebic A06.82
gonorrheal (acute) (chronic) A54.23
trichomonal A59.09
tuberculous A18.15
Vestibulitis (ear) (*see also* subcategory) H83.0 ☑
nose (external) J34.89
vulvar N94.810
Vestibulopathy , acute peripheral (recurrent) — *see*
   Neuronitis, vestibular
Vestige, vestigial (*see also* Persistence)
branchial Q18.0
structures in vitreous Q14.0
Vibration
adverse effects T75.20 ☑
   pneumatic hammer syndrome T75.21 ☑
   specified effect NEC T75.29 ☑
   vasospastic syndrome T75.22 ☑
   vertigo from infrasound T75.23 ☑
exposure (occupational) Z57.7
vertigo T75.23 ☑
Vibriosis A28.9
Victim (of)
crime Z65.4
disaster Z65.5
terrorism Z65.4
torture Z65.4
war Z65.5
Vidal's disease L28.0
Villaret's syndrome G52.7
Villous — *see* condition
VIN — *see* Neoplasia, intraepithelial, vulva
Vincent's infection (angina) (gingivitis) A69.1
stomatitis NEC A69.1
Vinson-Plummer syndrome D50.1
Violence, physical R45.6
Viosterol deficiency — *see* Deficiency, calciferol
Vipoma — *see* Neoplasm, malignant, by site
Viremia B34.9
Virilism (adrenal) E25.9
congenital E25.0
Virilization (female) (suprarenal) E25.9
congenital E25.0
isosexual E28.2
Virulent bubo A57
Virus, viral (*see also* condition)
as cause of disease classified elsewhere B97.89
cytomegalovirus B25.9

Virus, viral — *continued*
human immunodeficiency (HIV) — *see* Human, immunodeficiency virus (HIV) disease
infection — *see* Infection, virus
specified NEC B34.8
swine influenza (viruses that normally cause infections
   in pigs) (*see also* Influenza, due to, identified
   novel influenza A virus) J09.X2
West Nile (fever) A92.30
   with
     complications NEC A92.39
     cranial nerve disorders A92.32
     encephalitis A92.31
     encephalomyelitis A92.31
     neurologic manifestation NEC A92.32
     optic neuritis A92.32
     polyradiculitis A92.32
Viscera, visceral — *see* condition
Visceroptosis K63.4
Visible peristalsis R19.2
Vision, visual
binocular, suppression H53.34
blurred, blurring H53.8
   hysterical F44.6
defect, defective NEC H54.7
disorientation (syndrome) H53.8
disturbance H53.9
   hysterical F44.6
double H53.2
examination Z01.00
   with abnormal findings Z01.01
field, limitation (defect) — *see* Defect, visual field
hallucinations R44.1
halos H53.19
loss — *see* Loss, vision
   sudden — *see* Disturbance, vision, subjective, loss,
     sudden
low (both eyes) — *see* Low, vision
perception, simultaneous without fusion H53.33
Vitality, lack or want of R53.83
newborn P96.89
Vitamin deficiency — *see* Deficiency, vitamin
Vitelline duct, persistent Q43.0
Vitiligo L80
eyelid H02.739
   left H02.736
     lower H02.735
     upper H02.734
   right H02.733
     lower H02.732
     upper H02.731
pinta A67.2
vulva N90.89
Vitreal corneal syndrome H59.01- ☑
Vitreoretinopathy, proliferative (*see also* Retinopathy,
   proliferative)
with retinal detachment — *see* Detachment, retina,
   traction
Vitreous (*see also* condition)
touch syndrome — *see* Complication, postprocedural,
   following cataract surgery
Vocal cord — *see* condition
Vogt-Koyanagi syndrome H20.82- ☑
Vogt's disease or syndrome G80.3
Vogt-Spielmeyer amaurotic idiocy or disease E75.4
Voice
change R49.9
   specified NEC R49.8
loss — *see* Aphonia
Volhynian fever A79.0
Volkmann's ischemic contracture or paralysis (complicating trauma) T79.6 ☑
Volvulus (bowel) (colon) (intestine) K56.2
with perforation K56.2
congenital Q43.8
duodenum K31.5
fallopian tube — *see* Torsion, fallopian tube
oviduct — *see* Torsion, fallopian tube
stomach (due to absence of gastrocolic ligament)
   K31.89
Vomiting R11.10
with nausea R11.2
without nausea R11.11
asphyxia — *see* Foreign body, by site, causing asphyxia, gastric contents
bilious (cause unknown) R11.14
   following gastro-intestinal surgery K91.0
   in newborn P92.01

Vomiting — *continued*
blood — *see* Hematemesis
causing asphyxia, choking, or suffocation — *see* Foreign body, by site
cyclical G43.A0 (*following* G43.7)
   with refractory migraine G43.A1 (*following* G43.7)
   without refractory migraine G43.A0 (*following*
     G43.7)
   intractable G43.A1 (*following* G43.7)
   not intractable G43.A0 (*following* G43.7)
   psychogenic F50.89
fecal mater R11.13
following gastrointestinal surgery K91.0
   psychogenic F50.89
functional K31.89
hysterical F50.89
nervous F50.89
neurotic F50.89
newborn NEC P92.09
   bilious P92.01
periodic R11.10
   psychogenic F50.89
projectile R11.12
psychogenic F50.89
uremic — *see* Uremia
Vomito negro — *see* Fever, yellow
Von Bezold's abscess — *see* Mastoiditis, acute
Von Economo-Cruchet disease A85.8
Von Eulenburg's disease G71.19
Von Gierke's disease E74.01
Von Hippel (-Lindau) **disease or syndrome** Q85.8
Von Jaksch's anemia or disease D64.89
Von Recklinghausen
disease (neurofibromatosis) Q85.01
   bones E21.0
Von Schroetter's syndrome I82.890
Von Willebrand (-Jurgens)(-Minot) **disease or syn-**
   drome D68.0
Von Zumbusch's disease L40.1
Voyeurism F65.3
Vrolik's disease Q78.0
Vulva — *see* condition
Vulvismus N94.2
Vulvitis (acute) (allergic) (atrophic) (hypertrophic) (intertriginous) (senile) N76.2
with ectopic or molar pregnancy O08.0
adhesive, congenital Q52.79
blennorrhagic (gonococcal) A54.02
candidal B37.3
chlamydial A56.02
due to Haemophilus ducreyi A57
following ectopic or molar pregnancy O08.0
gonococcal A54.02
   with abscess (accessory gland) (periurethral) A54.1
herpesviral A60.04
leukoplakic N90.4
monilial B37.3
puerperal (postpartum) O86.19
subacute or chronic N76.3
syphilitic (early) A51.0
   late A52.76
trichomonal A59.01
tuberculous A18.18
Vulvodynia N94.819
specified NEC N94.818
Vulvorectal — *see* condition
Vulvovaginitis (acute) — *see* Vaginitis

W

Waiting list, person on Z75.1
for organ transplant Z76.82
undergoing social agency investigation Z75.2
Waldenström
hypergammaglobulinemia D89.0
syndrome or macroglobulinemia C88.0
Waldenström-Kjellberg syndrome D50.1
Walking
difficulty R26.2
   psychogenic F44.4
sleep F51.3
   hysterical F44.89
Wall, abdominal — *see* condition
Wallenberg's disease or syndrome G46.3
Wallgren's disease I87.8
Wandering
gallbladder, congenital Q44.1
in diseases classified elsewhere Z91.83

Index (left margin)

Wandering — Worries (left margin)

Wandering — *continued*
kidney, congenital Q63.8
organ or site, congenital NEC — *see* Malposition, congenital, by site
pacemaker (heart) I49.8
spleen D73.89
War neurosis F48.8
Wart (due to HPV) (filiform) (infectious) (viral) B07.9
anogenital region (venereal) A63.0
common B07.8
external genital organs (venereal) A63.0
flat B07.8
Hassal-Henle's (of cornea) H18.49
Peruvian A44.1
plantar B07.0
prosector (tuberculous) A18.4
seborrheic L82.1
inflamed L82.0
senile (seborrheic) L82.1
inflamed L82.0
tuberculous A18.4
venereal A63.0
Warthin's tumor — *see* Neoplasm, salivary gland, benign
Wassilieff's disease A27.0
Wasting
disease R64
due to malnutrition E41
extreme (due to malnutrition) E41
muscle NEC — *see* Atrophy, muscle
Water
clefts (senile cataract) — *see* Cataract, senile, incipient
deprivation of T73.1 ☑
intoxication E87.79
itch B76.9
lack of T73.1 ☑
loading E87.70
on
brain — *see* Hydrocephalus
chest J94.8
poisoning E87.79
Waterbrash R12
Waterhouse (-Friderichsen) **syndrome or disease** (meningococcal) A39.1
Water-losing nephritis N25.89
Watermelon stomach K31.819
with hemorrhage K31.811
without hemorrhage K31.819
Watsoniasis B66.8
Wax in ear — *see* Impaction, cerumen
Weak, weakening, weakness (generalized) R53.1
arches (acquired) (*see also* Deformity, limb, flat foot)
bladder (sphincter) R32
facial R29.810
following
cerebrovascular disease I69.992
cerebral infarction I69.392
intracerebral hemorrhage I69.192
nontraumatic intracranial hemorrhage NEC I69.292
specified disease NEC I69.892
stroke I69.392
subarachnoid hemorrhage I69.092
foot (double) — *see* Weak, arches
heart, cardiac — *see* Failure, heart
mind F70
muscle M62.81
myocardium — *see* Failure, heart
newborn P96.89
pelvic fundus N81.89
pubocervical tissue N81.82
rectovaginal tissue N81.83
senile R54
urinary stream R39.12
valvular — *see* Endocarditis
Wear, worn (with normal or routine use)
articular bearing surface of internal joint prosthesis — *see* Complications, joint prosthesis, mechanical, wear of articular bearing surfaces, by site
device, implant or graft — *see* Complications, by site, mechanical complication
tooth, teeth (approximal) (hard tissues) (interproximal) (occlusal) K03.0
Weather, weathered
effects of
cold T69.9 ☑
specified effect NEC T69.8 ☑
hot — *see* Heat
skin L57.8

Weaver's syndrome Q87.3
Web, webbed (congenital)
duodenal Q43.8
esophagus Q39.4
fingers Q70.1- ☑
larynx (glottic) (subglottic) Q31.0
neck (pterygium colli) Q18.3
Paterson-Kelly D50.1
popliteal syndrome Q87.89
toes Q70.3- ☑
Weber-Christian disease M35.6
Weber-Cockayne syndrome (epidermolysis bullosa) Q81.8
Weber-Gubler syndrome G46.3
Weber-Leyden syndrome G46.3
Weber-Osler syndrome I78.0
Weber's paralysis or syndrome G46.3
Wedge-shaped or wedging vertebra — *see* Collapse, vertebra NEC
Wegener's granulomatosis or syndrome M31.30
with
kidney involvement M31.31
lung involvement M31.30
with kidney involvement M31.31
Wegner's disease A50.02
Weight
1000-2499 grams at birth (low) — *see* Low, birthweight
999 grams or less at birth (extremely low) — *see* Low, birthweight, extreme
and length below 10th percentile for gestational age P05.1- ☑
below but length above 10th percentile for gestational age P05.0- ☑
gain (abnormal) (excessive) R63.5
in pregnancy — *see* Pregnancy, complicated by, excessive weight gain
low — *see* Pregnancy, complicated by, insufficient, weight gain
loss (abnormal) (cause unknown) R63.4
Weightlessness (effect of) T75.82 ☑
Weil (l)-**Marchesani syndrome** Q87.1
Weil's disease A27.0
Weingarten's syndrome J82
Weir Mitchell's disease I73.81
Weiss-Baker syndrome G90.09
Wells' disease L98.3
Wen — *see* Cyst, sebaceous
Wenckebach's block or phenomenon I44.1
Werdnig-Hoffmann syndrome (muscular atrophy) G12.0
Werlhof's disease D69.3
Wermer's disease or syndrome E31.21
Werner-His disease A79.0
Werner's disease or syndrome E34.8
Wernicke-Korsakoff's syndrome or psychosis (alcoholic) F10.96
with dependence F10.26
drug-induced
due to drug abuse — *see* Abuse, drug, by type, with amnestic disorder
due to drug dependence — *see* Dependence, drug, by type, with amnestic disorder
nonalcoholic F04
Wernicke-Posadas disease B38.9
Wernicke's
developmental aphasia F80.2
disease or syndrome E51.2
encephalopathy E51.2
polioencephalitis, superior E51.2
West African fever B50.8
Westphal-Strümpell syndrome E83.01
West's syndrome — *see* Epilepsy, spasms
Wet
feet, tropical (maceration) (syndrome) — *see* Immersion, foot
lung (syndrome), newborn P22.1
Wharton's duct — *see* condition
Wheal — *see* Urticaria
Wheezing R06.2
Whiplash injury S13.4 ☑
Whipple's disease (*see also* subcategory M14.8-) K90.81
Whipworm (disease) (infection) (infestation) B79
Whistling face Q87.0
White (*see also* condition)
kidney, small N03.9
leg, puerperal, postpartum, childbirth O87.1

White — *continued*
mouth B37.0
patches of mouth K13.29
spot lesions, teeth
chewing surface K02.51
pit and fissure surface K02.51
smooth surface K02.61
Whitehead L70.0
Whitlow (*see also* Cellulitis, digit)
with lymphangitis — *see* Lymphangitis, acute, digit
herpesviral B00.89
Whitmore's disease or fever — *see* Melioidosis
Whooping cough A37.90
with pneumonia A37.91
due to Bordetella
bronchiseptica A37.81
parapertussis A37.11
pertussis A37.01
specified organism NEC A37.81
due to
Bordetella
bronchiseptica A37.80
with pneumonia A37.81
parapertussis A37.10
with pneumonia A37.11
pertussis A37.00
with pneumonia A37.01
specified NEC A37.80
with pneumonia A37.81
Wichman's asthma J38.5
Wide cranial sutures, newborn P96.3
Widening aorta — *see* Ectasia, aorta
with aneurysm — *see* Aneurysm, aorta
Wilkie's disease or syndrome K55.1
Wilkinson-Sneddon disease or syndrome L13.1
Willebrand (-Jürgens) **thrombopathy** D68.0
Willige-Hunt disease or syndrome G23.1
Wilms' tumor C64- ☑
Wilson-Mikity syndrome P27.0
Wilson's
disease or syndrome E83.01
hepatolenticular degeneration E83.01
lichen ruber L43.9
Window (*see also* Imperfect, closure)
aorticopulmonary Q21.4
Winter — *see* condition
Wiskott-Aldrich syndrome D82.0
Withdrawal state (*see also* Dependence, drug by type, with withdrawal)
alcohol
with perceptual disturbances F10.232
without perceptual disturbances F10.239
caffeine F15.93
cannabis F12.288
newborn
correct therapeutic substance properly administered P96.2
infant of dependent mother P96.1
therapeutic substance, neonatal P96.2
Witts' anemia D50.8
Witzelsucht F07.0
Woakes' ethmoiditis or syndrome J33.1
Wolff-Hirschhorn syndrome Q93.3
Wolff-Parkinson-White syndrome I45.6
Wolhynian fever A79.0
Wolman's disease E75.5
Wood lung or pneumonitis J67.8
Woolly, wooly hair (congenital) (nevus) Q84.1
Woolsorter's disease A22.1
Word
blindness (congenital) (developmental) F81.0
deafness (congenital) (developmental) H93.25
Worm(s) (infection) (infestation) (*see also* Infestation, helminth)
guinea B72
in intestine NEC B82.0
Worm-eaten soles A66.3
Worn out — *see* Exhaustion
cardiac
defibrillator (with synchronous cardiace pacemaker) Z45.02
pacemaker
battery Z45.010
lead Z45.018
device, implant or graft — *see* Complications, by site, mechanical
Worried well Z71.1
Worries R45.82

Wound check Z48.0- ☑
    due to injury — *code to* Injury, by site, using appropriate seventh character for subsequent encounter
Wound, open T14.8- ☑
    abdomen, abdominal
        wall S31.109 ☑
            with penetration into peritoneal cavity S31.609 ☑
            bite — *see* Bite, abdomen, wall
            epigastric region S31.102 ☑
                with penetration into peritoneal cavity S31.602 ☑
                bite — *see* Bite, abdomen, wall, epigastric region
                laceration — *see* Laceration, abdomen, wall, epigastric region
                puncture — *see* Puncture, abdomen, wall, epigastric region
            laceration — *see* Laceration, abdomen, wall
            left
                lower quadrant S31.104 ☑
                    with penetration into peritoneal cavity S31.604 ☑
                    bite — *see* Bite, abdomen, wall, left, lower quadrant
                    laceration — *see* Laceration, abdomen, wall, left, lower quadrant
                    puncture — *see* Puncture, abdomen, wall, left, lower quadrant
                upper quadrant S31.101 ☑
                    with penetration into peritoneal cavity S31.601 ☑
                    bite — *see* Bite, abdomen, wall, left, upper quadrant
                    laceration — *see* Laceration, abdomen, wall, left, upper quadrant
                    puncture — *see* Puncture, abdomen, wall, left, upper quadrant
            periumbilic region S31.105 ☑
                with penetration into peritoneal cavity S31.605 ☑
                bite — *see* Bite, abdomen, wall, periumbilic region
                laceration — *see* Laceration, abdomen, wall, periumbilic region
                puncture — *see* Puncture, abdomen, wall, periumbilic region
            puncture — *see* Puncture, abdomen, wall
            right
                lower quadrant S31.103 ☑
                    with penetration into peritoneal cavity S31.603 ☑
                    bite — *see* Bite, abdomen, wall, right, lower quadrant
                    laceration — *see* Laceration, abdomen, wall, right, lower quadrant
                    puncture — *see* Puncture, abdomen, wall, right, lower quadrant
                upper quadrant S31.100 ☑
                    with penetration into peritoneal cavity S31.600 ☑
                    bite — *see* Bite, abdomen, wall, right, upper quadrant
                    laceration — *see* Laceration, abdomen, wall, right, upper quadrant
                    puncture — *see* Puncture, abdomen, wall, right, upper quadrant
    alveolar (process) — *see* Wound, open, oral cavity
    ankle S91.00- ☑
        bite — *see* Bite, ankle
        laceration — *see* Laceration, ankle
        puncture — *see* Puncture, ankle
    antecubital space — *see* Wound, open, elbow
    anterior chamber, eye — *see* Wound, open, ocular
    anus S31.839 ☑
        bite S31.835 ☑
        laceration — *see* Laceration, anus
        puncture — *see* Puncture, anus
    arm (upper) S41.10- ☑
        with amputation — *see* Amputation, traumatic, arm
        bite — *see* Bite, arm
        forearm — *see* Wound, open, forearm
        laceration — *see* Laceration, arm
        puncture — *see* Puncture, arm
    auditory canal (external) (meatus) — *see* Wound, open, ear

Wound, open — *continued*
    auricle, ear — *see* Wound, open, ear
    axilla — *see* Wound, open, arm
    back (*see also* Wound, open, thorax, back)
        lower S31.000 ☑
            with penetration into retroperitoneal space S31.001 ☑
            bite — *see* Bite, back, lower
            laceration — *see* Laceration, back, lower
            puncture — *see* Puncture, back, lower
    bite — *see* Bite
    blood vessel — *see* Injury, blood vessel
    breast S21.00- ☑
        with amputation — *see* Amputation, traumatic, breast
        bite — *see* Bite, breast
        laceration — *see* Laceration, breast
        puncture — *see* Puncture, breast
    buttock S31.809 ☑
        bite — *see* Bite, buttock
        laceration — *see* Laceration, buttock
        left S31.829 ☑
        puncture — *see* Puncture, buttock
        right S31.819 ☑
    calf — *see* Wound, open, leg
    canaliculus lacrimalis — *see* Wound, open, eyelid
    canthus, eye — *see* Wound, open, eyelid
    cervical esophagus S11.20 ☑
        bite S11.25 ☑
        laceration — *see* Laceration, esophagus, traumatic, cervical
        puncture — *see* Puncture, cervical esophagus
    cheek (external) S01.40- ☑
        bite — *see* Bite, cheek
        internal — *see* Wound, open, oral cavity
        laceration — *see* Laceration, cheek
        puncture — *see* Puncture, cheek
    chest wall — *see* Wound, open, thorax
    chin — *see* Wound, open, head, specified site NEC
    choroid — *see* Wound, open, ocular
    ciliary body (eye) — *see* Wound, open, ocular
    clitoris S31.40 ☑
        with amputation — *see* Amputation, traumatic, clitoris
        bite S31.45 ☑
        laceration — *see* Laceration, vulva
        puncture — *see* Puncture, vulva
    conjunctiva — *see* Wound, open, ocular
    cornea — *see* Wound, open, ocular
    costal region — *see* Wound, open, thorax
    Descemet's membrane — *see* Wound, open, ocular
    digit(s)
        foot — *see* Wound, open, toe
        hand — *see* Wound, open, finger
    ear (canal) (external) S01.30- ☑
        with amputation — *see* Amputation, traumatic, ear
        bite — *see* Bite, ear
        drum S09.2- ☑
        laceration — *see* Laceration, ear
        puncture — *see* Puncture, ear
    elbow S51.00- ☑
        bite — *see* Bite, elbow
        laceration — *see* Laceration, elbow
        puncture — *see* Puncture, elbow
    epididymis — *see* Wound, open, testis
    epigastric region S31.102 ☑
        with penetration into peritoneal cavity S31.602 ☑
        bite — *see* Bite, abdomen, wall, epigastric region
        laceration — *see* Laceration, abdomen, wall, epigastric region
        puncture — *see* Puncture, abdomen, wall, epigastric region
    epiglottis — *see* Wound, open, neck, specified site NEC
    esophagus (thoracic) S27.819 ☑
        cervical — *see* Wound, open, cervical esophagus
        laceration S27.813 ☑
        specified type NEC S27.818 ☑
    eye — *see* Wound, open, ocular
    eyeball — *see* Wound, open, ocular
    eyebrow — *see* Wound, open, eyelid
    eyelid S01.10- ☑
        bite — *see* Bite, eyelid
        laceration — *see* Laceration, eyelid
        puncture — *see* Puncture, eyelid

Wound, open — *continued*
    face NEC — *see* Wound, open, head, specified site NEC
    finger(s) S61.209 ☑
        with
            amputation — *see* Amputation, traumatic, finger
            damage to nail S61.309 ☑
        bite — *see* Bite, finger
        index S61.208 ☑
            with
                damage to nail S61.308 ☑
            left S61.201 ☑
                with
                    damage to nail S61.301 ☑
            right S61.200 ☑
                with
                    damage to nail S61.300 ☑
        laceration — *see* Laceration, finger
        little S61.208 ☑
            with
                damage to nail S61.308 ☑
            left S61.207 ☑
                with damage to nail S61.307 ☑
            right S61.206 ☑
                with damage to nail S61.306 ☑
        middle S61.208 ☑
            with
                damage to nail S61.308 ☑
            left S61.203 ☑
                with damage to nail S61.303 ☑
            right S61.202 ☑
                with damage to nail S61.302 ☑
        puncture — *see* Puncture, finger
        ring S61.208 ☑
            with
                damage to nail S61.308 ☑
            left S61.205 ☑
                with damage to nail S61.305 ☑
            right S61.204 ☑
                with damage to nail S61.304 ☑
    flank — *see* Wound, open, abdomen, wall
    foot (except toe(s) alone) S91.30- ☑
        with amputation — *see* Amputation, traumatic, foot
        bite — *see* Bite, foot
        laceration — *see* Laceration, foot
        puncture — *see* Puncture, foot
        toe — *see* Wound, open, toe
    forearm S51.80- ☑
        with
            amputation — *see* Amputation, traumatic, forearm
        bite — *see* Bite, forearm
        elbow only — *see* Wound, open, elbow
        laceration — *see* Laceration, forearm
        puncture — *see* Puncture, forearm
    forehead — *see* Wound, open, head, specified site NEC
    genital organs, external
        with amputation — *see* Amputation, traumatic, genital organs
        bite — *see* Bite, genital organ
        female S31.502 ☑
            vagina S31.40 ☑
            vulva S31.40 ☑
        laceration — *see* Laceration, genital organ
        male S31.501 ☑
            penis S31.20 ☑
            scrotum S31.30 ☑
            testes S31.30 ☑
        puncture — *see* Puncture, genital organ
    globe (eye) — *see* Wound, open, ocular
    groin — *see* Wound, open, abdomen, wall
    gum — *see* Wound, open, oral cavity
    hand S61.40- ☑
        with
            amputation — *see* Amputation, traumatic, hand
        bite — *see* Bite, hand
        finger(s) — *see* Wound, open, finger
        laceration — *see* Laceration, hand
        puncture — *see* Puncture, hand
        thumb — *see* Wound, open, thumb
    head S01.90 ☑
        bite — *see* Bite, head
        cheek — *see* Wound, open, cheek
        ear — *see* Wound, open, ear

☑ **Additional Character Required — Refer to the Tabular List for Character Selection**   ⁿᵉʷ **Subterms under main terms may continue to next column or page**

Index

Wound, open — *continued*
  thorax, thoracic — *continued*
    back — *continued*
      with penetration S21.40 ☑
    bite — *see* Bite, thorax
    breast — *see* Wound, open, breast
    front S21.10- ☑
      with penetration S21.30 ☑
    laceration — *see* Laceration, thorax
    puncture — *see* Puncture, thorax
  throat — *see* Wound, open, neck
  thumb S61.009 ☑
    with
      amputation — *see* Amputation, traumatic, thumb
      damage to nail S61.109 ☑
    bite — *see* Bite, thumb
    laceration — *see* Laceration, thumb
    left S61.002 ☑
      with
        damage to nail S61.102 ☑
    puncture — *see* Puncture, thumb
    right S61.001 ☑
      with
        damage to nail S61.101 ☑
  thyroid (gland) — *see* Wound, open, neck, thyroid
  toe(s) S91.109 ☑
    with
      amputation — *see* Amputation, traumatic, toe
      damage to nail S91.209 ☑
    bite — *see* Bite, toe
    great S91.103 ☑
      with
        damage to nail S91.203 ☑
      left S91.102 ☑
        with
          damage to nail S91.202 ☑
      right S91.101 ☑
        with
          damage to nail S91.201 ☑
    laceration — *see* Laceration, toe
    lesser S91.106 ☑
      with
        damage to nail S91.206 ☑
      left S91.105 ☑
        with
          damage to nail S91.205 ☑
      right S91.104 ☑
        with
          damage to nail S91.204 ☑
    puncture — *see* Puncture, toe
  tongue — *see* Wound, open, oral cavity
  trachea (cervical region) — *see* Wound, open, neck, trachea
  tunica vaginalis — *see* Wound, open, testis
  tympanum, tympanic membrane S09.2- ☑
    laceration — *see* Laceration, ear, drum
    puncture — *see* Puncture, tympanum
  umbilical region — *see* Wound, open, abdomen, wall, periumbilic region
  uvula — *see* Wound, open, oral cavity
  vagina S31.40 ☑
    bite S31.45 ☑
    laceration — *see* Laceration, vagina
    puncture — *see* Puncture, vagina
  vitreous (humor) — *see* Wound, open, ocular
  vocal cord S11.039 ☑
    bite — *see* Bite, vocal cord
    laceration S11.031 ☑
      with foreign body S11.032 ☑
    puncture S11.033 ☑
      with foreign body S11.034 ☑
  vulva S31.40 ☑
    with amputation — *see* Amputation, traumatic, vulva
    bite S31.45 ☑
    laceration — *see* Laceration, vulva
    puncture — *see* Puncture, vulva
  wrist S61.50- ☑
    bite — *see* Bite, wrist
    laceration — *see* Laceration, wrist
    puncture — *see* Puncture, wrist
Wound, superficial — *see* Injury (*see also* specified injury type)

Wright's syndrome G54.0
Wrist — *see* condition
Wrong drug (by accident) (given in error) — *see* Table of Drugs and Chemicals, by drug, poisoning
Wry neck — *see* Torticollis
Wuchereria (bancrofti) **infestation** B74.0
Wuchereriasis B74.0
Wuchernde Struma Langhans C73

X

Xanthelasma (eyelid) (palpebrarum) H02.60
  left H02.66
    lower H02.65
    upper H02.64
  right H02.63
    lower H02.62
    upper H02.61
Xanthelasmatosis (essential) E78.2
Xanthinuria, hereditary E79.8
Xanthoastrocytoma
  specified site — *see* Neoplasm, malignant, by site
  unspecified site C71.9
Xanthofibroma — *see* Neoplasm, connective tissue, benign
Xanthogranuloma D76.3
Xanthoma(s), xanthomatosis (primary) (familial) (hereditary) E75.5
  with
    hyperlipoproteinemia
      Type I E78.3
      Type III E78.2
      Type IV E78.1
      Type V E78.3
  bone (generalisata) C96.5
  cerebrotendinous E75.5
  cutaneotendinous E75.5
  disseminatum (skin) E78.2
  eruptive E78.2
  hypercholesterinemic E78.00
  hypercholesterolemic E78.00
  hyperlipidemic E78.5
  joint E75.5
  multiple (skin) E78.2
  tendon (sheath) E75.5
  tuberosum E78.2
  tuberous E78.2
  tubo-eruptive E78.2
  verrucous, oral mucosa K13.4
Xanthosis R23.8
Xenophobia F40.10
Xeroderma (*see also* Ichthyosis)
  acquired L85.0
  eyelid H01.149
    left H01.146
      lower H01.145
      upper H01.144
    right H01.143
      lower H01.142
      upper H01.141
  pigmentosum Q82.1
  vitamin A deficiency E50.8
Xerophthalmia (vitamin A deficiency) E50.7
  unrelated to vitamin A deficiency — *see* Keratoconjunctivitis
Xerosis
  conjunctiva H11.14- ☑
    with Bitot's spots (*see also* Pigmentation, conjunctiva)
      vitamin A deficiency E50.1
    vitamin A deficiency E50.0
  cornea H18.89- ☑
    with ulceration — *see* Ulcer, cornea
      vitamin A deficiency E50.3
    vitamin A deficiency E50.2
  cutis L85.3
  skin L85.3
Xerostomia K11.7
Xiphopagus Q89.4
XO syndrome Q96.9
X-ray (of)
  abnormal findings — *see* Abnormal, diagnostic imaging
  breast (mammogram) (routine) Z12.31

X-ray — *continued*
  chest
    routine (as part of a general medical examination) Z00.00
      with abnormal findings Z00.01
  routine (as part of a general medical examination) Z00.00
    with abnormal findings Z00.01
XXXXY syndrome Q98.1
XXY syndrome Q98.0

Y

Yaba pox (virus disease) B08.72
Yatapoxvirus B08.70
  specified NEC B08.79
Yawning R06.89
  psychogenic F45.8
Yaws A66.9
  cutaneous, less than five years after infection A66.2
  bone lesions A66.6
  butter A66.1
  chancre A66.0
  early (cutaneous) (macular) (maculopapular) (micropapular) (papular) A66.2
    frambeside A66.2
    skin lesions NEC A66.2
  eyelid A66.2
  ganglion A66.6
  gangosis, gangosa A66.5
  gumma, gummata A66.4
    bone A66.6
  gummatous
    frambeside A66.4
    osteitis A66.6
    periostitis A66.6
  hydrarthrosis (*see also* subcategory M14.8-) A66.6
  hyperkeratosis (early) (late) A66.3
  initial lesions A66.0
  joint lesions (*see also* subcategory M14.8-) A66.6
  juxta-articular nodules A66.7
  late nodular (ulcerated) A66.4
  latent (without clinical manifestations) (with positive serology) A66.8
  mother A66.0
  mucosal A66.7
  multiple papillomata A66.1
  nodular, late (ulcerated) A66.4
  osteitis A66.6
  papilloma, plantar or palmar A66.1
  periostitis (hypertrophic) A66.6
  specified NEC A66.7
  ulcers A66.4
  wet crab A66.1
Yeast infection (*see also* Candidiasis) B37.9
Yellow
  atrophy (liver) — *see* Failure, hepatic
  fever — *see* Fever, yellow
  jack — *see* Fever, yellow
  jaundice — *see* Jaundice
  nail syndrome L60.5
Yersiniosis (*see also* Infection, Yersinia)
  extraintestinal A28.2
  intestinal A04.6

Z

Zahorsky's syndrome (herpangina) B08.5
Zellweger's syndrome Q87.89
Zenker's diverticulum (esophagus) K22.5
Ziehen-Oppenheim disease G24.1
Zieve's syndrome K70.0
Zika NOS A92.5
Zinc
  deficiency, dietary E60
  metabolism disorder E83.2
Zollinger-Ellison syndrome E16.4
Zona — *see* Herpes, zoster
Zoophobia F40.218
Zoster (herpes) — *see* Herpes, zoster
Zygomycosis B46.9
  specified NEC B46.8
Zymotic — *see* condition

Wound, open — Zymotic

Note: The list below gives the code number for neoplasms by anatomical site. For each site there are six possible code numbers according to whether the neoplasm in question is malignant, benign, in situ, of uncertain behavior, or of unspecified nature. The description of the neoplasm will often indicate which of the six columns is appropriate; e.g., malignant melanoma of skin, benign fibroadenoma of breast, carcinoma in situ of cervix uteri. Where such descriptors are not present, the remainder of the Index should be consulted where guidance is given to the appropriate column for each morphological (histological) variety listed; e.g., Mesonephroma – see Neoplasm, malignant; Embryoma (see also Neoplasm, uncertain behavior); Disease, Bowen's – see Neoplasm, skin, in situ. However, the guidance in the Index can be overridden if one of the descriptors mentioned above is present; e.g., malignant adenoma of colon is coded to C18.9 and not to D12.6 as the adjective "malignant" overrides the Index entry "Adenoma (see also Neoplasm, benign, by site)." Codes listed with a dash -, following the code have a required additional character for laterality. The tabular list must be reviewed for the complete code.

	Malignant Primary	Malignant Secondary	Ca in situ	Benign	Uncertain	Unspecified Behavior
Neoplasm, neoplastic	C80.1	C79.9	D09.9	D36.9	D48.9	D49.9
abdomen,						
abdominal	C76.2	C79.8-☑	D09.8	D36.7	D48.7	D49.89
cavity	C76.2	C79.8-☑	D09.8	D36.7	D48.7	D49.89
organ	C76.2	C79.8-☑	D09.8	D36.7	D48.7	D49.89
viscera	C76.2	C79.8-☑	D09.8	D36.7	D48.7	D49.89
wall — see also Neoplasm, abdomen, wall,						
skin	C44.509	C79.2	D04.5	D23.5	D48.5	D49.2
connective tissue	C49.4	C79.8-☑	—	D21.4	D48.1	D49.2
skin	C44.509	—	—	—	—	—
basal cell carcinoma	C44.519	—	—	—	—	—
specified type NEC	C44.599	—	—	—	—	—
squamous cell carcinoma	C44.529	—	—	—	—	—
abdominopelvic	C76.8	C79.8-☑	—	D36.7	D48.7	D49.89
accessory sinus — see Neoplasm, sinus						
acoustic nerve	C72.4-☑	C79.49	—	D33.3	D43.3	D49.7
adenoid (pharynx) (tissue)	C11.1	C79.89	D00.08	D10.6	D37.05	D49.0
adipose tissue — see also Neoplasm, connective						
tissue	C49.4	C79.89	—	D21.9	D48.1	D49.2
adnexa (uterine)	C57.4	C79.89	D07.39	D28.7	D39.8	D49.59
adrenal	C74.9-☑	C79.7-☑	D09.3	D35.0-☑	D44.1-☑	D49.7
capsule	C74.9-☑	C79.7-☑	D09.3	D35.0-☑	D44.1-☑	D49.7
cortex	C74.0-☑	C79.7-☑	D09.3	D35.0-☑	D44.1-☑	D49.7
gland	C74.9-☑	C79.7-☑	D09.3	D35.0-☑	D44.1-☑	D49.7
medulla	C74.1-☑	C79.7-☑	D09.3	D35.0-☑	D44.1-☑	D49.7
ala nasi (external) — see also Neoplasm, skin,						
nose	C44.301	C79.2	D04.39	D23.39	D48.5	D49.2
alimentary canal or tract NEC	C26.9	C78.80	D01.9	D13.9	D37.9	D49.0
alveolar	C03.9	C79.89	D00.03	D10.39	D37.09	D49.0
mucosa	C03.9	C79.89	D00.03	D10.39	D37.09	D49.0
lower	C03.1	C79.89	D00.03	D10.39	D37.09	D49.0
upper	C03.0	C79.89	D00.03	D10.39	D37.09	D49.0
ridge or process	C41.1	C79.51	—	D16.5	D48.0	D49.2
carcinoma	C03.9	C79.8-☑	—	—	—	—
lower	C03.1	C79.8-☑	—	—	—	—
upper	C03.0	C79.8-☑	—	—	—	—
lower	C41.1	C79.51	—	D16.5	D48.0	D49.2
mucosa	C03.9	C79.89	D00.03	D10.39	D37.09	D49.0
lower	C03.1	C79.89	D00.03	D10.39	D37.09	D49.0
upper	C03.0	C79.89	D00.03	D10.39	D37.09	D49.0
upper	C41.0	C79.51	—	D16.4	D48.0	D49.2
sulcus	C06.1	C79.89	D00.02	D10.39	D37.09	D49.0
alveolus	C03.9	C79.89	D00.03	D10.39	D37.09	D49.0
lower	C03.1	C79.89	D00.03	D10.39	D37.09	D49.0
upper	C03.0	C79.89	D00.03	D10.39	D37.09	D49.0
ampulla of Vater	C24.1	C78.89	D01.5	D13.5	D37.6	D49.0
ankle NEC	C76.5-☑	C79.89	D04.7-☑	D36.7	D48.7	D49.89
anorectum, anorectal (junction)	C21.8	C78.5	D01.3	D12.9	D37.8	D49.0
antecubital fossa or space	C76.4-☑	C79.89	D04.6-☑	D36.7	D48.7	D49.89
Neoplasm, neoplastic — continued						
antrum (Highmore) (maxillary)	C31.0	C78.39	D02.3	D14.0	D38.5	D49.1
pyloric	C16.3	C78.89	D00.2	D13.1	D37.1	D49.0
tympanicum	C30.1	C78.39	D02.3	D14.0	D38.5	D49.1
anus, anal	C21.0	C78.5	D01.3	D12.9	D37.8	D49.0
canal	C21.1	C78.5	D01.3	D12.9	D37.8	D49.0
cloacogenic zone	C21.2	C78.5	D01.3	D12.9	D37.8	D49.0
margin — see also Neoplasm, anus, skin	C44.500	C79.2	D04.5	D23.5	D48.5	D49.2
overlapping lesion with rectosigmoid junction or rectum	C21.8	—	—	—	—	—
skin	C44.500	C79.2	D04.5	D23.5	D48.5	D49.2
basal cell carcinoma	C44.510	—	—	—	—	—
specified type NEC	C44.590	—	—	—	—	—
squamous cell carcinoma	C44.520	—	—	—	—	—
sphincter	C21.1	C78.5	D01.3	D12.9	D37.8	D49.0
aorta (thoracic)	C49.3	C79.89	—	D21.3	D48.1	D49.2
abdominal	C49.4	C79.89	—	D21.4	D48.1	D49.2
aortic body	C75.5	C79.89	—	D35.6	D44.7	D49.7
aponeurosis	C49.9	C79.89	—	D21.9	D48.1	D49.2
palmar	C49.1-☑	C79.89	—	D21.1-☑	D48.1	D49.2
plantar	C49.2-☑	C79.89	—	D21.2-☑	D48.1	D49.2
appendix	C18.1	C78.5	D01.0	D12.1	D37.3	D49.0
arachnoid	C70.9	C79.49	—	D32.9	D42.9	D49.7
cerebral	C70.0	C79.32	—	D32.0	D42.0	D49.7
spinal	C70.1	C79.49	—	D32.1	D42.1	D49.7
areola	C50.0-☑	C79.81	D05-☑	D24-☑	D48.6-☑	D49.3
arm NEC	C76.4-☑	C79.89	D04.6-☑	D36.7	D48.7	D49.89
artery — see Neoplasm, connective tissue						
aryepiglottic fold	C13.1	C79.89	D00.08	D10.7	D37.05	D49.0
hypopharyngeal aspect	C13.1	C79.89	D00.08	D10.7	D37.05	D49.0
laryngeal aspect	C32.1	C78.39	D02.0	D14.1	D38.0	D49.1
marginal zone	C13.1	C79.89	D00.08	D10.7	D37.05	D49.0
arytenoid (cartilage)	C32.3	C78.39	D02.0	D14.1	D38.0	D49.1
fold — see Neoplasm, aryepiglottic						
associated with transplanted organ	C80.2	—	—	—	—	—
atlas	C41.2	C79.51	—	D16.6	D48.0	D49.2
atrium, cardiac	C38.0	C79.89	—	D15.1	D48.7	D49.89
auditory						
canal (external) (skin)	C44.20-☑	C79.2	D04.2-☑	D23.2-☑	D48.5	D49.2
internal	C30.1	C78.39	D02.3	D14.0	D38.5	D49.1
nerve	C72.4-☑	C79.49	—	D33.3	D43.3	D49.7
tube	C30.1	C78.39	D02.3	D14.0	D38.5	D49.1
opening	C11.2	C79.89	D00.08	D10.6	D37.05	D49.0
auricle, ear — see also Neoplasm, skin,						
ear	C44.20-☑	C79.2	D04.2-☑	D23.2-☑	D48.5	D49.2
auricular canal (external) — see also Neoplasm, skin, ear	C44.20-☑	C79.2	D04.2-☑	D23.2-☑	D48.5	D49.2
internal	C30.1	C78.39	D02.3	D14.0	D38.5	D49.2
autonomic nerve or nervous system NEC (see Neoplasm, nerve, peripheral)						
axilla, axillary	C76.1	C79.89	D09.8	D36.7	D48.7	D49.89
fold — see also Neoplasm, skin,						
trunk	C44.509	C79.2	D04.5	D23.5	D48.5	D49.2
back NEC	C76.8	C79.89	D04.5	D36.7	D48.7	D49.89
Bartholin's gland	C51.0	C79.82	D07.1	D28.0	D39.8	D49.59
basal ganglia	C71.0	C79.31	—	D33.0	D43.0	D49.6
basis pedunculi	C71.7	C79.31	—	D33.1	D43.1	D49.6
bile or biliary (tract)	C24.9	C78.89	D01.5	D13.5	D37.6	D49.0
canaliculi (biliferi) (intrahepatic)	C22.1	C78.7	D01.5	D13.4	D37.6	D49.0
canals, interlobular	C22.1	C78.89	D01.5	D13.4	D37.6	D49.0

Neoplasm Table

Neoplasm, neoplastic — continued
bile or biliary — continued

	Malignant Primary	Malignant Secondary	Ca in situ	Benign	Uncertain	Unspecified Behavior
duct or passage (common) (cystic) (extrahepatic)	C24.0	C78.89	D01.5	D13.5	D37.6	D49.0
interlobular	C22.1	C78.89	D01.5	D13.4	D37.6	D49.0
intrahepatic	C22.1	C78.7	D01.5	D13.4	D37.6	D49.0
and extrahepatic	C24.8	C78.89	D01.5	D13.5	D37.6	D49.0
bladder (urinary)	C67.9	C79.11	D09.0	D30.3	D41.4	D49.4
dome	C67.1	C79.11	D09.0	D30.3	D41.4	D49.4
neck	C67.5	C79.11	D09.0	D30.3	D41.4	D49.4
orifice	C67.9	C79.11	D09.0	D30.3	D41.4	D49.4
ureteric	C67.6	C79.11	D09.0	D30.3	D41.4	D49.4
urethral	C67.5	C79.11	D09.0	D30.3	D41.4	D49.4
overlapping lesion	C67.8	—	—	—	—	—
sphincter	C67.8	C79.11	D09.0	D30.3	D41.4	D49.4
trigone	C67.0	C79.11	D09.0	D30.3	D41.4	D49.4
urachus	C67.7	C79.11	D09.0	D30.3	D41.4	D49.4
wall	C67.9	C79.11	D09.0	D30.3	D41.4	D49.4
anterior	C67.3	C79.11	D09.0	D30.3	D41.4	D49.4
lateral	C67.2	C79.11	D09.0	D30.3	D41.4	D49.4
posterior	C67.4	C79.11	D09.0	D30.3	D41.4	D49.4
blood vessel — *see* Neoplasm, connective tissue						
bone (periosteum)	C41.9	C79.51	—	D16.9	D48.0	D49.2
acetabulum	C41.4	C79.51	—	D16.8	D48.0	D49.2
ankle	C40.3-☑	C79.51	—	D16.3-☑	—	—
arm NEC	C40.0-☑	C79.51	—	D16.0-☑	—	—
astragalus	C40.3-☑	C79.51	—	D16.3-☑	—	—
atlas	C41.2	C79.51	—	D16.6	D48.0	D49.2
axis	C41.2	C79.51	—	D16.6	D48.0	D49.2
back NEC	C41.2	C79.51	—	D16.6	D48.0	D49.2
calcaneus	C40.3-☑	C79.51	—	D16.3-☑	—	—
calvarium	C41.0	C79.51	—	D16.4	D48.0	D49.2
carpus (any)	C40.1-☑	C79.51	—	D16.1-☑	—	—
cartilage NEC	C41.9	C79.51	—	D16.9	D48.0	D49.2
clavicle	C41.3	C79.51	—	D16.7	D48.0	D49.2
clivus	C41.0	C79.51	—	D16.4	D48.0	D49.2
coccygeal vertebra	C41.4	C79.51	—	D16.8	D48.0	D49.2
coccyx	C41.4	C79.51	—	D16.8	D48.0	D49.2
costal cartilage	C41.3	C79.51	—	D16.7	D48.0	D49.2
costovertebral joint	C41.3	C79.51	—	D16.7	D48.0	D49.2
cranial	C41.0	C79.51	—	D16.4	D48.0	D49.2
cuboid	C40.3-☑	C79.51	—	D16.3-☑	—	—
cuneiform	C41.9	C79.51	—	D16.9	D48.0	D49.2
elbow	C40.0-☑	C79.51	—	D16.0-☑	—	—
ethmoid (labyrinth)	C41.0	C79.51	—	D16.4	D48.0	D49.2
face	C41.0	C79.51	—	D16.4	D48.0	D49.2
femur (any part)	C40.2-☑	C79.51	—	D16.2-☑	—	—
fibula (any part)	C40.2-☑	C79.51	—	D16.2-☑	—	—
finger (any)	C40.1-☑	C79.51	—	D16.1-☑	—	—
foot	C40.3-☑	C79.51	—	D16.3-☑	—	—
forearm	C40.0-☑	C79.51	—	D16.0-☑	—	—
frontal	C41.0	C79.51	—	D16.4	D48.0	D49.2
hand	C40.1-☑	C79.51	—	D16.1-☑	—	—
heel	C40.3-☑	C79.51	—	D16.3-☑	—	—
hip	C41.4	C79.51	—	D16.8	D48.0	D49.2
humerus (any part)	C40.0-☑	C79.51	—	D16.0-☑	—	—
hyoid	C41.0	C79.51	—	D16.4	D48.0	D49.2
ilium	C41.4	C79.51	—	D16.8	D48.0	D49.2
innominate	C41.4	C79.51	—	D16.8	D48.0	D49.2
intervertebral cartilage or disc	C41.2	C79.51	—	D16.6	D48.0	D49.2
ischium	C41.4	C79.51	—	D16.8	D48.0	D49.2
jaw (lower)	C41.1	C79.51	—	D16.5	D48.0	D49.2
knee	C40.2-☑	C79.51	—	D16.2-☑	—	—
leg NEC	C40.2-☑	C79.51	—	D16.2-☑	—	—
limb NEC	C40.9-☑	C79.51	—	D16.9		
lower (long bones)	C40.2-☑	C79.51	—	D16.2-☑	—	—
short bones	C40.3-☑	C79.51	—	D16.3-☑	—	—
upper (long bones)	C40.0-☑	C79.51	—	D16.0-☑	—	—
short bones	C40.1-☑	C79.51	—	D16.1-☑	—	—
malar	C41.0	C79.51	—	D16.4	D48.0	D49.2

Neoplasm, neoplastic — continued
bone — continued

	Malignant Primary	Malignant Secondary	Ca in situ	Benign	Uncertain	Unspecified Behavior
mandible	C41.1	C79.51	—	D16.5	D48.0	D49.2
marrow NEC (any bone)	C96.9	C79.52	—	—	D47.9	D49.89
mastoid	C41.0	C79.51	—	D16.4	D48.0	D49.2
maxilla, maxillary (superior)	C41.0	C79.51	—	D16.4	D48.0	D49.2
inferior	C41.1	C79.51	—	D16.5	D48.0	D49.2
metacarpus (any)	C40.1-☑	C79.51	—	D16.1-☑	—	—
metatarsus (any)	C40.3-☑	C79.51	—	D16.3-☑	—	—
navicular						
ankle	C40.3-☑	C79.51	—			
hand	C40.1-☑	C79.51	—			
nose, nasal	C41.0	C79.51	—	D16.4	D48.0	D49.2
occipital	C41.0	C79.51	—	D16.4	D48.0	D49.2
orbit	C41.0	C79.51	—	D16.4	D48.0	D49.2
overlapping sites	C40.8-☑	—	—	—	—	—
parietal	C41.0	C79.51	—	D16.4	D48.0	D49.2
patella	C40.2-☑	C79.51	—	—	—	—
pelvic	C41.4	C79.51	—	D16.8	D48.0	D49.2
phalanges						
foot	C40.3-☑	C79.51	—	—	—	—
hand	C40.1-☑	C79.51	—	—	—	—
pubic	C41.4	C79.51	—	D16.8	D48.0	D49.2
radius (any part)	C40.0-☑	C79.51	—	D16.0-☑	—	—
rib	C41.3	C79.51	—	D16.7	D48.0	D49.2
sacral vertebra	C41.4	C79.51	—	D16.8	D48.0	D49.2
sacrum	C41.4	C79.51	—	D16.8	D48.0	D49.2
scaphoid						
of ankle	C40.3-☑	C79.51	—	—	—	—
of hand	C40.1-☑	C79.51	—	—	—	—
scapula (any part)	C40.0-☑	C79.51	—	D16.0-☑	—	—
sella turcica	C41.0	C79.51	—	D16.4	D48.0	D49.2
shoulder	C40.0-☑	C79.51	—	D16.0-☑	—	—
skull	C41.0	C79.51	—	D16.4	D48.0	D49.2
sphenoid	C41.0	C79.51	—	D16.4	D48.0	D49.2
spine, spinal (column)	C41.2	C79.51	—	D16.6	D48.0	D49.2
coccyx	C41.4	C79.51	—	D16.8	D48.0	D49.2
sacrum	C41.4	C79.51	—	D16.8	D48.0	D49.2
sternum	C41.3	C79.51	—	D16.7	D48.0	D49.2
tarsus (any)	C40.3-☑	C79.51	—	—	—	—
temporal	C41.0	C79.51	—	D16.4	D48.0	D49.2
thumb	C40.1-☑	C79.51	—	—	—	—
tibia (any part)	C40.2-☑	C79.51	—	—	—	—
toe (any)	C40.3-☑	C79.51	—	—	—	—
trapezium	C40.1-☑	C79.51	—	—	—	—
trapezoid	C40.1-☑	C79.51	—	—	—	—
turbinate	C41.0	C79.51	—	D16.4	D48.0	D49.2
ulna (any part)	C40.0-☑	C79.51	—	D16.0-☑	—	—
unciform	C40.1-☑	C79.51	—	—	—	—
vertebra (column)	C41.2	C79.51	—	D16.6	D48.0	D49.2
coccyx	C41.4	C79.51	—	D16.8	D48.0	D49.2
sacrum	C41.4	C79.51	—	D16.8	D48.0	D49.2
vomer	C41.0	C79.51	—	D16.4	D48.0	D49.2
wrist	C40.1-☑	C79.51	—	—	—	—
xiphoid process	C41.3	C79.51	—	D16.7	D48.0	D49.2
zygomatic	C41.0	C79.51	—	D16.4	D48.0	D49.2
book-leaf (mouth) — *ventral surface of tongue and floor of mouth*	C06.89	C79.89	D00.00	D10.39	D37.09	D49.0
bowel — *see* Neoplasm, intestine						
brachial plexus	C47.1-☑	C79.89	—	D36.12	D48.2	D49.2
brain NEC	C71.9	C79.31	—	D33.2	D43.2	D49.6
basal ganglia	C71.0	C79.31	—	D33.0	D43.0	D49.6
cerebellopontine angle	C71.6	C79.31	—	D33.1	D43.1	D49.6
cerebellum NOS	C71.6	C79.31	—	D33.1	D43.1	D49.6
cerebrum	C71.0	C79.31	—	D33.0	D43.0	D49.6
choroid plexus	C71.7	C79.31	—	D33.1	D43.1	D49.6
corpus callosum	C71.8	C79.31	—	D33.2	D43.2	D49.6
corpus striatum	C71.0	C79.31	—	D33.0	D43.0	D49.6
cortex (cerebral)	C71.0	C79.31	—	D33.0	D43.0	D49.6
frontal lobe	C71.1	C79.31	—	D33.0	D43.0	D49.6
globus pallidus	C71.0	C79.31	—	D33.0	D43.0	D49.6
hippocampus	C71.2	C79.31	—	D33.0	D43.0	D49.6
hypothalamus	C71.0	C79.31	—	D33.0	D43.0	D49.6
internal capsule	C71.0	C79.31	—	D33.0	D43.0	D49.6

☑ Additional Character Required — Refer to the Tabular List for Character Selection   Subterms under main terms may continue to next column or page

Neoplasm, bile or biliary — Neoplasm, brain NEC

Neoplasm, neoplastic — *continued*
brain — *continued*

	Malignant Primary	Malignant Secondary	Ca in situ	Benign	Uncertain	Unspecified Behavior
medulla oblongata	C71.7	C79.31	—	D33.1	D43.1	D49.6
meninges	C70.0	C79.32	—	D32.0	D42.0	D49.7
midbrain	C71.7	C79.31	—	D33.1	D43.1	D49.6
occipital lobe	C71.4	C79.31	—	D33.0	D43.0	D49.6
overlapping lesion	C71.8	C79.31	—	—	—	—
parietal lobe	C71.3	C79.31	—	D33.0	D43.0	D49.6
peduncle	C71.7	C79.31	—	D33.1	D43.1	D49.6
pons	C71.7	C79.31	—	D33.1	D43.1	D49.6
stem	C71.7	C79.31	—	D33.1	D43.1	D49.6
tapetum	C71.8	C79.31	—	D33.2	D43.2	D49.6
temporal lobe	C71.2	C79.31	—	D33.0	D43.0	D49.6
thalamus	C71.0	C79.31	—	D33.0	D43.0	D49.6
uncus	C71.2	C79.31	—	D33.0	D43.0	D49.6
ventricle (floor)	C71.5	C79.31	—	D33.0	D43.0	D49.6
fourth	C71.7	C79.31	—	D33.1	D43.1	D49.6
branchial (cleft) (cyst) (vestiges)	C10.4	C79.89	D00.08	D10.5	D37.05	D49.0
breast (connective tissue) (glandular tissue) (soft parts)	C50.9-✓	C79.81	D05.-✓	D24.-✓	D48.6-✓	D49.3
areola	C50.0-✓	C79.81	D05.-✓	D24.-✓	D48.6-✓	D49.3
axillary tail	C50.6-✓	C79.81	D05.-✓	D24.-✓	D48.6-✓	D49.3
central portion	C50.1-✓	C79.81	D05.-✓	D24.-✓	D48.6-✓	D49.3
inner	C50.8-✓	C79.81	D05.-✓	D24.-✓	D48.6-✓	D49.3
lower	C50.8-✓	C79.81	D05.-✓	D24.-✓	D48.6-✓	D49.3
lower-inner quadrant	C50.3-✓	C79.81	D05.-✓	D24.-✓	D48.6-✓	D49.3
lower-outer quadrant	C50.5-✓	C79.81	D05.-✓	D24.-✓	D48.6-✓	D49.3
mastectomy site (skin) — *see also* Neoplasm, breast, skin	C44.501	C79.2	—	—	—	—
specified as breast tissue	C50.8-✓	C79.81	—	—	—	—
midline	C50.8-✓	C79.81	D05.-✓	D24.-✓	D48.6-✓	D49.3
nipple	C50.0-✓	C79.81	D05.-✓	D24.-✓	D48.6-✓	D49.3
outer	C50.8-✓	C79.81	D05.-✓	D24.-✓	D48.6-✓	D49.3
overlapping lesion	C50.8-✓	—	—	—	—	—
skin	C44.501	C79.2	D04.5	D23.5	D48.5	D49.2
basal cell carcinoma	C44.511	—	—	—	—	—
specified type NEC	C44.591	—	—	—	—	—
squamous cell carcinoma	C44.521	—	—	—	—	—
tail (axillary)	C50.6-✓	C79.81	D05.-✓	D24.-✓	D48.6-✓	D49.3
upper	C50.8-✓	C79.81	D05.-✓	D24.-✓	D48.6-✓	D49.3
upper-inner quadrant	C50.2-✓	C79.81	D05.-✓	D24.-✓	D48.6-✓	D49.3
upper-outer quadrant	C50.4-✓	C79.81	D05.-✓	D24.-✓	D48.6-✓	D49.3
broad ligament	C57.1-✓	C79.82	D07.39	D28.2	D39.8	D49.59
bronchiogenic, bronchogenic (lung)	C34.9-✓	C78.0-✓	D02.2-✓	D14.3-✓	D38.1	D49.1
bronchiole	C34.9-✓	C78.0-✓	D02.2-✓	D14.3-✓	D38.1	D49.1
bronchus	C34.9-✓	C78.0-✓	D02.2-✓	D14.3-✓	D38.1	D49.1
carina	C34.0-✓	C78.0-✓	D02.2-✓	D14.3-✓	D38.1	D49.1
lower lobe of lung	C34.3-✓	C78.0-✓	D02.2-✓	D14.3-✓	D38.1	D49.1
main	C34.0-✓	C78.0-✓	D02.2-✓	D14.3-✓	D38.1	D49.1
middle lobe of lung	C34.2	C78.0-✓	D02.21	D14.31	D38.1	D49.1
overlapping lesion	C34.8-✓	—	—	—	—	—
upper lobe of lung	C34.1-✓	C78.0-✓	D02.2-✓	D14.3-✓	D38.1	D49.1
brow	C44.309	C79.2	D04.39	D23.39	D48.5	D49.2
basal cell carcinoma	C44.319	—	—	—	—	—
specified type NEC	C44.399	—	—	—	—	—
squamous cell carcinoma	C44.329	—	—	—	—	—
buccal (cavity)	C06.9	C79.89	D00.00	D10.39	D37.09	D49.0
commissure	C06.0	C79.89	D00.02	D10.39	D37.09	D49.0
groove (lower) (upper)	C06.1	C79.89	D00.02	D10.39	D37.09	D49.0
mucosa	C06.0	C79.89	D00.02	D10.39	D37.09	D49.0
sulcus (lower) (upper)	C06.1	C79.89	D00.02	D10.39	D37.09	D49.0

Neoplasm, neoplastic — *continued*

	Malignant Primary	Malignant Secondary	Ca in situ	Benign	Uncertain	Unspecified Behavior
bulbourethral gland	C68.0	C79.19	D09.19	D30.4	D41.3	D49.59
bursa — *see* Neoplasm, connective tissue						
buttock NEC	C76.3	C79.89	D04.5	D36.7	D48.7	D49.89
calf	C76.5-✓	C79.89	D04.7-✓	D36.7	D48.7	D49.89
calvarium	C41.0	C79.51	—	D16.4	D48.0	D49.2
calyx, renal	C65.-✓	C79.0-✓	D09.19	D30.1-✓	D41.1-✓	D49.51-✓
canal						
anal	C21.1	C78.5	D01.3	D12.9	D37.8	D49.0
auditory (external) — *see also* Neoplasm, skin, ear	C44.20-✓	C79.2	D04.2-✓	D23.2-✓	D48.5	D49.2
auricular (external) — *see also* Neoplasm, skin, ear	C44.20-✓	C79.2	D04.2-✓	D23.2-✓	D48.5	D49.2
canaliculi, biliary (biliferi) (intrahepatic)	C22.1	C78.7	D01.5	D13.4	D37.6	D49.0
canthus (eye) (inner) (outer)	C44.10-✓	C79.2	D04.1-✓	D23.1-✓	D48.5	D49.2
basal cell carcinoma	C44.11-✓	—	—	—	—	—
specified type NEC	C44.19-✓	—	—	—	—	—
squamous cell carcinoma	C44.12-✓	—	—	—	—	—
capillary — *see* Neoplasm, connective tissue						
caput coli	C18.0	C78.5	D01.0	D12.0	D37.4	D49.0
carcinoid — *see* Tumor, carcinoid						
cardia (gastric)	C16.0	C78.89	D00.2	D13.1	D37.1	D49.0
cardiac orifice (stomach)	C16.0	C78.89	D00.2	D13.1	D37.1	D49.0
cardio-esophageal junction	C16.0	C78.89	D00.2	D13.1	D37.1	D49.0
cardio-esophagus	C16.0	C78.89	D00.2	D13.1	D37.1	D49.0
carina (bronchus)	C34.0-✓	C78.0-✓	D02.2-✓	D14.3-✓	D38.1	D49.1
carotid (artery)	C49.0	C79.89	—	D21.0	D48.1	D49.2
body	C75.4	C79.89	—	D35.5	D44.6	D49.7
carpus (any bone)	C40.1-✓	C79.51	—	D16.1-✓	—	—
cartilage (articular) (joint) NEC — *see also* Neoplasm, bone	C41.9	C79.51	—	D16.9	D48.0	D49.2
arytenoid	C32.3	C78.39	D02.0	D14.1	D38.0	D49.1
auricular	C49.0	C79.89	—	D21.0	D48.1	D49.2
bronchi	C34.0-✓	C78.39	—	D14.3-✓	D38.1	D49.1
costal	C41.3	C79.51	—	D16.7	D48.0	D49.2
cricoid	C32.3	C78.39	D02.0	D14.1	D38.0	D49.1
cuneiform	C32.3	C78.39	D02.0	D14.1	D38.0	D49.1
ear (external)	C49.0	C79.89	—	D21.0	D48.1	D49.2
ensiform	C41.3	C79.51	—	D16.7	D48.0	D49.2
epiglottis	C32.1	C78.39	D02.0	D14.1	D38.0	D49.1
anterior surface	C10.1	C79.89	D00.08	D10.5	D37.05	D49.0
eyelid	C49.0	C79.89	—	D21.0	D48.1	D49.2
intervertebral	C41.2	C79.51	—	D16.6	D48.0	D49.2
larynx, laryngeal	C32.3	C78.39	D02.0	D14.1	D38.0	D49.1
nose, nasal	C30.0	C78.39	D02.3	D14.0	D38.5	D49.1
pinna	C49.0	C79.89	—	D21.0	D48.1	D49.2
rib	C41.3	C79.51	—	D16.7	D48.0	D49.2
semilunar (knee)	C40.2-✓	C79.51	—	D16.2-✓	D48.0	D49.2
thyroid	C32.3	C78.39	D02.0	D14.1	D38.0	D49.1
trachea	C33	C78.39	D02.1	D14.2	D38.1	D49.1
cauda equina	C72.1	C79.49	—	D33.4	D43.4	D49.7
cavity						
buccal	C06.9	C79.89	D00.00	D10.30	D37.09	D49.0
nasal	C30.0	C78.39	D02.3	D14.0	D38.5	D49.1
oral	C06.9	C79.89	D00.00	D10.30	D37.09	D49.0
peritoneal	C48.2	C78.6	—	D20.1	D48.4	D49.0
tympanic	C30.1	C78.39	D02.3	D14.0	D38.5	D49.1
cecum	C18.0	C78.5	D01.0	D12.0	D37.4	D49.0
central nervous system	C72.9	C79.40	—	—	—	—
cerebellopontine (angle)	C71.6	C79.31	—	D33.1	D43.1	D49.6
cerebellum, cerebellar	C71.6	C79.31	—	D33.1	D43.1	D49.6
cerebrum, cerebral (cortex) (hemisphere) (white matter)	C71.0	C79.31	—	D33.0	D43.0	D49.6
meninges	C70.0	C79.32	—	D32.0	D42.0	D49.7
peduncle	C71.7	C79.31	—	D33.1	D43.1	D49.6

Side tab: Neoplasm Table — Neoplasm, brain NEC — Neoplasm, cerebrum, cerebral

Neoplasm Table

Neoplasm, neoplastic — *continued*	Malignant Primary	Malignant Secondary	Ca in situ	Benign	Uncertain	Unspecified Behavior
cerebrum, cerebral — *continued*						
ventricle	C71.5	C79.31	—	D33.0	D43.0	D49.6
fourth	C71.7	C79.31	—	D33.1	D43.1	D49.6
cervical region	C76.0	C79.89	D09.8	D36.7	D48.7	D49.89
cervix (cervical) (uteri) (uterus)	C53.9	C79.82	D06.9	D26.0	D39.0	D49.59
canal	C53.0	C79.82	D06.0	D26.0	D39.0	D49.59
endocervix (canal) (gland)	C53.0	C79.82	D06.0	D26.0	D39.0	D49.59
exocervix	C53.1	C79.82	D06.1	D26.0	D39.0	D49.59
external os	C53.1	C79.82	D06.1	D26.0	D39.0	D49.59
internal os	C53.0	C79.82	D06.0	D26.0	D39.0	D49.59
nabothian gland	C53.0	C79.82	D06.0	D26.0	D39.0	D49.59
overlapping lesion	C53.8	—	—	—	—	—
squamocolumnar junction	C53.8	C79.82	D06.7	D26.0	D39.0	D49.59
stump	C53.8	C79.82	D06.7	D26.0	D39.0	D49.59
cheek	C76.0	C79.89	D09.8	D36.7	D48.7	D49.89
external	C44.309	C79.2	D04.39	D23.39	D48.5	D49.2
basal cell carcinoma	C44.319					
specified type NEC	C44.399	—	—	—	—	—
squamous cell carcinoma	C44.329	—	—	—	—	—
inner aspect	C06.0	C79.89	D00.02	D10.39	D37.09	D49.0
internal	C06.0	C79.89	D00.02	D10.39	D37.09	D49.0
mucosa	C06.0	C79.89	D00.02	D10.39	D37.09	D49.0
chest (wall) NEC	C76.1	C79.89	D09.8	D36.7	D48.7	D49.89
chiasma opticum	C72.3-☑	C79.49	—	D33.3	D43.3	D49.7
chin	C44.309	C79.2	D04.39	D23.39	D48.5	D49.2
basal cell carcinoma	C44.319	—	—	—	—	—
specified type NEC	C44.399	—	—	—	—	—
squamous cell carcinoma	C44.329	—	—	—	—	—
choana	C11.3	C79.89	D00.08	D10.6	D37.05	D49.0
cholangiole	C22.1	C78.89	D01.5	D13.4	D37.6	D49.0
choledochal duct	C24.0	C78.89	D01.5	D13.5	D37.6	D49.0
choroid	C69.3-☑	C79.49	D09.2-☑	D31.3-☑	D48.7	D49.81
plexus	C71.5	C79.31	—	D33.0	D43.0	D49.6
ciliary body	C69.4-☑	C79.49	D09.2-☑	D31.4-☑	D48.7	D49.89
clavicle	C41.3	C79.51	—	D16.7	D48.0	D49.2
clitoris	C51.2	C79.82	D07.1	D28.0	D39.8	D49.59
clivus	C41.0	C79.51	—	D16.4	D48.0	D49.2
cloacogenic zone	C21.2	C78.5	D01.3	D12.9	D37.8	D49.0
coccygeal						
body or glomus	C49.5	C79.89	—	D21.5	D48.1	D49.2
vertebra	C41.4	C79.51	—	D16.8	D48.0	D49.2
coccyx	C41.4	C79.51	—	D16.8	D48.0	D49.2
colon — *see also* Neoplasm, intestine, large	C18.9	C78.5	—	—	—	—
with rectum	C19	C78.5	D01.1	D12.7	D37.5	D49.0
columnella — *see also* Neoplasm, skin, face	C44.390	C79.2	D04.39	D23.39	D48.5	D49.2
column, spinal — *see* Neoplasm, spine						
commissure						
labial, lip	C00.6	C79.89	D00.01	D10.39	D37.01	D49.0
laryngeal	C32.0	C78.39	D02.0	D14.1	D38.0	D49.1
common (bile) duct	C24.0	C78.89	D01.5	D13.5	D37.6	D49.0
concha — *see also* Neoplasm, skin, ear	C44.20-☑	C79.2	D04.2-☑	D23.2-☑	D48.5	D49.2
nose	C30.0	C78.39	D02.3	D14.0	D38.5	D49.1
conjunctiva	C69.0-☑	C79.49	D09.2-☑	D31.0-☑	D48.7	D49.89

Neoplasm, neoplastic — *continued*	Malignant Primary	Malignant Secondary	Ca in situ	Benign	Uncertain	Unspecified Behavior
connective tissue NEC	C49.9	C79.89	—	D21.9	D48.1	D49.2

Note: For neoplasms of connective tissue (blood vessel, bursa, fascia, ligament, muscle, peripheral nerves, sympathetic and parasympathetic nerves and ganglia, synovia, tendon, etc.) or of morphological types that indicate connective tissue, code according to the list under "Neoplasm, connective tissue". For sites that do not appear in this list, code to neoplasm of that site; e.g., fibrosarcoma, pancreas (C25.9)

Note: Morphological types that indicate connective tissue appear in their proper place in the alphabetic index with the instruction "see Neoplasm, connective tissue ...."

	Malignant Primary	Malignant Secondary	Ca in situ	Benign	Uncertain	Unspecified Behavior
abdomen	C49.4	C79.89	—	D21.4	D48.1	D49.2
abdominal wall	C49.4	C79.89	—	D21.4	D48.1	D49.2
ankle	C49.2-☑	C79.89	—	D21.2-☑	D48.1	D49.2
antecubital fossa or space	C49.1-☑	C79.89	—	D21.1-☑	D48.1	D49.2
arm	C49.1-☑	C79.89	—	D21.1-☑	D48.1	D49.2
auricle (ear)	C49.0	C79.89	—	D21.0	D48.1	D49.2
axilla	C49.3	C79.89	—	D21.3	D48.1	D49.2
back	C49.6	C79.89	—	D21.6	D48.1	D49.2
breast — *see* Neoplasm, breast						
buttock	C49.5	C79.89	—	D21.5	D48.1	D49.2
calf	C49.2-☑	C79.89	—	D21.2-☑	D48.1	D49.2
cervical region	C49.0	C79.89	—	D21.0	D48.1	D49.2
cheek	C49.0	C79.89	—	D21.0	D48.1	D49.2
chest (wall)	C49.3	C79.89	—	D21.3	D48.1	D49.2
chin	C49.0	C79.89	—	D21.0	D48.1	D49.2
diaphragm	C49.3	C79.89	—	D21.3	D48.1	D49.2
ear (external)	C49.0	C79.89	—	D21.0	D48.1	D49.2
elbow	C49.1-☑	C79.89	—	D21.1-☑	D48.1	D49.2
extrarectal	C49.5	C79.89	—	D21.5	D48.1	D49.2
extremity	C49.9	C79.89	—	D21.9	D48.1	D49.2
lower	C49.2-☑	C79.89	—	D21.2-☑	D48.1	D49.2
upper	C49.1-☑	C79.89	—	D21.1-☑	D48.1	D49.2
eyelid	C49.0	C79.89	—	D21.0	D48.1	D49.2
face	C49.0	C79.89	—	D21.0	D48.1	D49.2
finger	C49.1-☑	C79.89	—	D21.1-☑	D48.1	D49.2
flank	C49.6	C79.89	—	D21.6	D48.1	D49.2
foot	C49.2-☑	C79.89	—	D21.2-☑	D48.1	D49.2
forearm	C49.1-☑	C79.89	—	D21.1-☑	D48.1	D49.2
forehead	C49.0	C79.89	—	D21.0	D48.1	D49.2
gastric	C49.4	C79.89	—	D21.4	D48.1	D49.2
gastrointestinal	C49.4	C79.89	—	D21.4	D48.1	D49.2
gluteal region	C49.5	C79.89	—	D21.5	D48.1	D49.2
great vessels NEC	C49.3	C79.89	—	D21.3	D48.1	D49.2
groin	C49.5	C79.89	—	D21.5	D48.1	D49.2
hand	C49.1-☑	C79.89	—	D21.1-☑	D48.1	D49.2
head	C49.0	C79.89	—	D21.0	D48.1	D49.2
heel	C49.2-☑	C79.89	—	D21.2-☑	D48.1	D49.2
hip	C49.2-☑	C79.89	—	D21.2-☑	D48.1	D49.2
hypochondrium	C49.4	C79.89	—	D21.4	D48.1	D49.2
iliopsoas muscle	C49.5	C79.89	—	D21.5	D48.1	D49.2
infraclavicular region	C49.3	C79.89	—	D21.3	D48.1	D49.2
inguinal (canal) (region)	C49.5	C79.89	—	D21.5	D48.1	D49.2
intestinal	C49.4	C79.89	—	D21.4	D48.1	D49.2
intrathoracic	C49.3	C79.89	—	D21.3	D48.1	D49.2
ischiorectal fossa	C49.5	C79.89	—	D21.5	D48.1	D49.2
jaw	C03.9	C79.89	D00.03	D10.39	D48.1	D49.0
knee	C49.2-☑	C79.89	—	D21.2-☑	D48.1	D49.2
leg	C49.2-☑	C79.89	—	D21.2-☑	D48.1	D49.2
limb NEC	C49.9	C79.89	—	D21.9	D48.1	D49.2
lower	C49.2-☑	C79.89	—	D21.2-☑	D48.1	D49.2
upper	C49.1-☑	C79.89	—	D21.1-☑	D48.1	D49.2
nates	C49.5	C79.89	—	D21.5	D48.1	D49.2
neck	C49.0	C79.89	—	D21.0	D48.1	D49.2
orbit	C69.6-☑	C79.49	D09.2-☑	D31.6-☑	D48.1	D49.89
overlapping lesion	C49.8	—	—	—	—	—
pararectal	C49.5	C79.89	—	D21.5	D48.1	D49.2
para-urethral	C49.5	C79.89	—	D21.5	D48.1	D49.2
paravaginal	C49.5	C79.89	—	D21.5	D48.1	D49.2
pelvis (floor)	C49.5	C79.89	—	D21.5	D48.1	D49.2
pelvo-abdominal	C49.8	C79.89	—	D21.6	D48.1	D49.2
perineum	C49.5	C79.89	—	D21.5	D48.1	D49.2
perirectal (tissue)	C49.5	C79.89	—	D21.5	D48.1	D49.2

☑ Additional Character Required — Refer to the Tabular List for Character Selection   ⱅ Subterms under main terms may continue to next column or page

Neoplasm, cerebrum, cerebral — Neoplasm, connective tissue NEC

Neoplasm, neoplastic — continued	Malignant Primary	Malignant Secondary	Ca in situ	Benign	Uncertain	Unspecified Behavior
connective tissue — continued						
periurethral (tissue)	C49.5	C79.89	—	D21.5	D48.1	D49.2
popliteal fossa or space	C49.2-✓	C79.89	—	D21.2-✓	D48.1	D49.2
presacral	C49.5	C79.89	—	D21.5	D48.1	D49.2
psoas muscle	C49.4	C79.89	—	D21.4	D48.1	D49.2
pterygoid fossa	C49.0	C79.89	—	D21.0	D48.1	D49.2
rectovaginal septum or wall	C49.5	C79.89	—	D21.5	D48.1	D49.2
rectovesical	C49.5	C79.89	—	D21.5	D48.1	D49.2
retroperitoneum	C48.0	C78.6	—	D20.0	D48.3	D49.0
sacrococcygeal region	C49.5	C79.89	—	D21.5	D48.1	D49.2
scalp	C49.0	C79.89	—	D21.0	D48.1	D49.2
scapular region	C49.3	C79.89	—	D21.3	D48.1	D49.2
shoulder	C49.1-✓	C79.89	—	D21.1-✓	D48.1	D49.2
skin (dermis) NEC — see also Neoplasm, skin, by site	C44.90	C79.2	D04.9	D23.9	D48.5	D49.2
stomach	C49.4	C79.89	—	D21.4	D48.1	D49.2
submental	C49.0	C79.89	—	D21.0	D48.1	D49.2
supraclavicular region	C49.0	C79.89	—	D21.0	D48.1	D49.2
temple	C49.0	C79.89	—	D21.0	D48.1	D49.2
temporal region	C49.0	C79.89	—	D21.0	D48.1	D49.2
thigh	C49.2-✓	C79.89	—	D21.2-✓	D48.1	D49.2
thoracic (duct) (wall)	C49.3	C79.89	—	D21.3	D48.1	D49.2
thorax	C49.3	C79.89	—	D21.3	D48.1	D49.2
thumb	C49.1-✓	C79.89	—	D21.1-✓	D48.1	D49.2
toe	C49.2-✓	C79.89	—	D21.2-✓	D48.1	D49.2
trunk	C49.6	C79.89	—	D21.6	D48.1	D49.2
umbilicus	C49.4	C79.89	—	D21.4	D48.1	D49.2
vesicorectal	C49.5	C79.89	—	D21.5	D48.1	D49.2
wrist	C49.1-✓	C79.89	—	D21.1-✓	D48.1	D49.2
conus medullaris	C72.0	C79.49	—	D33.4	D43.4	D49.7
cord (true) (vocal)	C32.0	C78.39	D02.0	D14.1	D38.0	D49.1
false	C32.1	C78.39	D02.0	D14.1	D38.0	D49.1
spermatic	C63.1-✓	C79.82	D07.69	D29.8	D40.8	D49.59
spinal (cervical) (lumbar) (thoracic)	C72.0	C79.49	—	D33.4	D43.4	D49.7
cornea (limbus)	C69.1-✓	C79.49	D09.2-✓	D31.1-✓	D48.7	D49.89
corpus						
albicans	C56.-✓	C79.6-✓	D07.39	D27.-✓	D39.1-✓	D49.59
callosum, brain	C71.0	C79.31	—	D33.2	D43.2	D49.6
cavernosum	C60.2	C79.82	D07.4	D29.0	D40.8	D49.59
gastric	C16.2	C78.89	D00.2	D13.1	D37.1	D49.0
overlapping sites	C54.8	—	—	—	—	—
penis	C60.2	C79.82	D07.4	D29.0	D40.8	D49.59
striatum, cerebrum	C71.0	C79.31	—	D33.0	D43.0	D49.6
uteri	C54.9	C79.82	D07.0	D26.1	D39.0	D49.59
isthmus	C54.0	C79.82	D07.0	D26.1	D39.0	D49.59
cortex						
adrenal	C74.0-✓	C79.7-✓	D09.3	D35.0-✓	D44.1-✓	D49.7
cerebral	C71.0	C79.31	—	D33.0	D43.0	D49.6
costal cartilage	C41.3	C79.51	—	D16.7	D48.0	D49.2
costovertebral joint	C41.3	C79.51	—	D16.7	D48.0	D49.2
Cowper's gland	C68.0	C79.19	D09.19	D30.4	D41.3	D49.59
cranial (fossa, any)	C71.9	C79.31	—	D33.2	D43.2	D49.6
meninges	C70.0	C79.32	—	D32.0	D42.0	D49.7
nerve	C72.50	C79.49	—	D33.3	D43.3	D49.7
specified NEC	C72.59	C79.49	—	D33.3	D43.3	D49.7
craniobuccal pouch	C75.2	C79.89	D09.3	D35.2	D44.3	D49.7
craniopharyngeal (duct) (pouch)	C75.2	C79.89	D09.3	D35.3	D44.4	D49.7
cricoid	C13.0	C79.89	D00.08	D10.7	D37.05	D49.0
cartilage	C32.3	C78.39	D02.0	D14.1	D38.0	D49.1
cricopharynx	C13.0	C79.89	D00.08	D10.7	D37.05	D49.0
crypt of Morgagni	C21.8	C78.5	D01.3	D12.9	D37.8	D49.0
crystalline lens	C69.4-✓	C79.49	D09.2-✓	D31.4-✓	D48.7	D49.89
cul-de-sac (Douglas')	C48.1	C78.6	—	D20.1	D48.4	D49.0
cuneiform cartilage	C32.3	C78.39	D02.0	D14.1	D38.0	D49.1
cutaneous — see Neoplasm, skin						
cutis — see Neoplasm, skin						

Neoplasm, neoplastic — continued	Malignant Primary	Malignant Secondary	Ca in situ	Benign	Uncertain	Unspecified Behavior
cystic (bile) duct (common)	C24.0	C78.89	D01.5	D13.5	D37.6	D49.0
dermis — see Neoplasm, skin						
diaphragm	C49.3	C79.89	—	D21.3	D48.1	D49.2
digestive organs, system, tube, or tract						
NEC	C26.9	C78.89	D01.9	D13.9	D37.9	D49.0
disc, intervertebral	C41.2	C79.51	—	D16.6	D48.0	D49.2
disease, generalized	C80.0	—	—	—	—	—
disseminated	C80.0	—	—	—	—	—
Douglas' cul-de-sac or pouch	C48.1	C78.6	—	D20.1	D48.4	D49.0
duodenojejunal junction	C17.8	C78.4	D01.49	D13.39	D37.2	D49.0
duodenum	C17.0	C78.4	D01.49	D13.2	D37.2	D49.0
dura (cranial) (mater)	C70.9	C79.49	—	D32.9	D42.9	D49.7
cerebral	C70.0	C79.32	—	D32.0	D42.0	D49.7
spinal	C70.1	C79.49	—	D32.1	D42.1	D49.7
ear (external) — see also Neoplasm, skin, ear	C44.20-✓	C79.2	D04.2-✓	D23.2-✓	D48.5	D49.2
auricle or auris — see also Neoplasm, skin, ear	C44.20-✓	C79.2	D04.2-✓	D23.2-✓	D48.5	D49.2
canal, external — see also Neoplasm, skin, ear	C44.20-✓	C79.2	D04.2-✓	D23.2-✓	D48.5	D49.2
cartilage	C49.0	C79.89	—	D21.0	D48.1	D49.2
external meatus — see also Neoplasm, skin, ear	C44.20-✓	C79.2	D04.2-✓	D23.2-✓	D48.5	D49.2
inner	C30.1	C78.39	D02.3	D14.0	D38.5	D49.1
lobule — see also Neoplasm, skin, ear	C44.20-✓	C79.2	D04.2-✓	D23.2-✓	D48.5	D49.2
middle	C30.1	C78.39	D02.3	D14.0	D38.5	D49.1
overlapping lesion with accessory sinuses	C31.8	—	—	—	—	—
skin	C44.20-✓	C79.2	D04.2-✓	D23.2-✓	D48.5	D49.2
basal cell carcinoma	C44.21-✓	—	—	—	—	—
specified type NEC	C44.29-✓	—	—	—	—	—
squamous cell carcinoma	C44.22-✓	—	—	—	—	—
earlobe	C44.20-✓	C79.2	D04.2-✓	D23.2-✓	D48.5	D49.2
basal cell carcinoma	C44.21-✓	—	—	—	—	—
specified type NEC	C44.29-✓	—	—	—	—	—
squamous cell carcinoma	C44.22-✓	—	—	—	—	—
ejaculatory duct	C63.7	C79.82	D07.69	D29.8	D40.8	D49.59
elbow NEC	C76.4-✓	C79.89	D04.6-✓	D36.7	D48.7	D49.89
endocardium	C38.0	C79.89	—	D15.1	D48.7	D49.89
endocervix (canal) (gland)	C53.0	C79.82	D06.0	D26.0	D39.0	D49.59
endocrine gland						
NEC	C75.9	C79.89	D09.3	D35.9	D44.9	D49.7
pluriglandular	C75.8	C79.89	D09.3	D35.7	D44.9	D49.7
endometrium (gland) (stroma)	C54.1	C79.82	D07.0	D26.1	D39.0	D49.59
ensiform cartilage	C41.3	C79.51	—	D16.7	D48.0	D49.2
enteric — see Neoplasm, intestine						
ependyma (brain)	C71.5	C79.31	—	D33.0	D43.0	D49.6
fourth ventricle	C71.7	C79.31	—	D33.1	D43.1	D49.6
epicardium	C38.0	C79.89	—	D15.1	D48.7	D49.89
epididymis	C63.0-✓	C79.82	D07.69	D29.3-✓	D40.8	D49.59
epidural	C72.9	C79.49	—	D33.9	D43.9	D49.7
epiglottis	C32.1	C78.39	D02.0	D14.1	D38.0	D49.1
anterior aspect or surface	C10.1	C79.89	D00.08	D10.5	D37.05	D49.0
cartilage	C32.3	C78.39	D02.0	D14.1	D38.0	D49.1
free border (margin)	C10.1	C79.89	D00.08	D10.5	D37.05	D49.0
junctional region	C10.8	C79.89	D00.08	D10.5	D37.05	D49.0
posterior (laryngeal) surface	C32.1	C78.39	D02.0	D14.1	D38.0	D49.1

Neoplasm Table

Neoplasm, epiglottis — Neoplasm, gland, glandular

Neoplasm, neoplastic — continued	Malignant Primary	Malignant Secondary	Ca in situ	Benign	Uncertain	Unspecified Behavior
epiglottis — *continued*						
suprahyoid portion	C32.1	C78.39	D02.0	D14.1	D38.0	D49.1
esophagogastric junction	C16.0	C78.89	D00.2	D13.1	D37.1	D49.0
esophagus	C15.9	C78.89	D00.1	D13.0	D37.8	D49.0
abdominal	C15.5	C78.89	D00.1	D13.0	D37.8	D49.0
cervical	C15.3	C78.89	D00.1	D13.0	D37.8	D49.0
distal (third)	C15.5	C78.89	D00.1	D13.0	D37.8	D49.0
lower (third)	C15.5	C78.89	D00.1	D13.0	D37.8	D49.0
middle (third)	C15.4	C78.89	D00.1	D13.0	D37.8	D49.0
overlapping lesion	C15.8	—	—	—	—	—
proximal (third)	C15.3	C78.89	D00.1	D13.0	D37.8	D49.0
thoracic	C15.4	C78.89	D00.1	D13.0	D37.8	D49.0
upper (third)	C15.3	C78.89	D00.1	D13.0	D37.8	D49.0
ethmoid (sinus)	C31.1	C78.39	D02.3	D14.0	D38.5	D49.1
bone or labyrinth	C41.0	C79.51	—	D16.4	D48.0	D49.2
eustachian tube	C30.1	C78.39	D02.3	D14.0	D38.5	D49.1
exocervix	C53.1	C79.82	D06.1	D26.0	D39.0	D49.59
external						
meatus (ear) — *see also* Neoplasm, skin, ear	C44.20-☑	C79.2	D04.2-☑	D23.2-☑	D48.5	D49.2
os, cervix uteri	C53.1	C79.82	D06.1	D26.0	D39.0	D49.59
extradural	C72.9	C79.49	—	D33.9	D43.9	D49.7
extrahepatic (bile) duct	C24.0	C78.89	D01.5	D13.5	D37.6	D49.0
overlapping lesion with gallbladder	C24.8	—	—	—	—	—
extraocular muscle	C69.6-☑	C79.49	D09.2-☑	D31.6-☑	D48.7	D49.89
extrarectal	C76.3	C79.89	D09.8	D36.7	D48.7	D49.89
extremity	C76.8	C79.89	D04.8	D36.7	D48.7	D49.89
lower	C76.5-☑	C79.89	D04.7-☑	D36.7	D48.7	D49.89
upper	C76.4-☑	C79.89	D04.6-☑	D36.7	D48.7	D49.89
eyeball	C69.9-☑	C79.49	D09.2-☑	D31.9-☑	D48.7	D49.89
eyebrow	C44.309	C79.2	D04.39	D23.39	D48.5	D49.2
basal cell carcinoma	C44.319	—	—	—	—	—
specified type NEC	C44.399	—	—	—	—	—
squamous cell carcinoma	C44.329	—	—	—	—	—
eyelid (lower) (skin) (upper)	C44.10-☑	—	—	—	—	—
basal cell carcinoma	C44.11-☑	—	—	—	—	—
cartilage	C49.0	C79.89	—	D21.0	D48.1	D49.2
specified type NEC	C44.19-☑	—	—	—	—	—
squamous cell carcinoma	C44.12-☑	—	—	—	—	—
eye NEC	C69.9-☑	C79.49	D09.2-☑	D31.9-☑	D48.7	D49.89
overlapping sites	C69.8-☑	—	—	—	—	—
face NEC	C76.0	C79.89	D04.39	D36.7	D48.7	D49.89
fallopian tube (accessory)	C57.0-☑	C79.82	D07.39	D28.2	D39.8	D49.59
falx (cerebella) (cerebri)	C70.0	C79.32	—	D32.0	D42.0	D49.7
fascia — *see also* Neoplasm, connective tissue						
palmar	C49.1-☑	C79.89	—	D21.1-☑	D48.1	D49.2
plantar	C49.2-☑	C79.89	—	D21.2-☑	D48.1	D49.2
fatty tissue — *see* Neoplasm, connective tissue						
fauces, faucial NEC	C10.9	C79.89	D00.08	D10.5	D37.05	D49.0
pillars	C09.1	C79.89	D00.08	D10.5	D37.05	D49.0
tonsil	C09.9	C79.89	D00.08	D10.4	D37.05	D49.0
femur (any part)	C40.2-☑	—	—	D16.2-☑	—	—
fetal membrane	C58	C79.82	D07.0	D26.7	D39.2	D49.59
fibrous tissue — *see* Neoplasm, connective tissue						
fibula (any part)	C40.2-☑	C79.51	—	D16.2-☑	—	—
filum terminale	C72.0	C79.49	—	D33.4	D43.4	D49.7
finger NEC	C76.4-☑	C79.89	D04.6-☑	D36.7	D48.7	D49.89
flank NEC	C76.8	C79.89	D04.5	D36.7	D48.7	D49.89
follicle, nabothian	C53.0	C79.82	D06.0	D26.0	D39.0	D49.59
foot NEC	C76.5-☑	C79.89	D04.7-☑	D36.7	D48.7	D49.89
forearm NEC	C76.4-☑	C79.89	D04.6-☑	D36.7	D48.7	D49.89
forehead (skin)	C44.309	C79.2	D04.39	D23.39	D48.5	D49.2

Neoplasm, neoplastic — continued	Malignant Primary	Malignant Secondary	Ca in situ	Benign	Uncertain	Unspecified Behavior
forehead — *continued*						
basal cell carcinoma	C44.319	—	—	—	—	—
specified type NEC	C44.399	—	—	—	—	—
squamous cell carcinoma	C44.329	—	—	—	—	—
foreskin	C60.0	C79.82	D07.4	D29.0	D40.8	D49.59
fornix						
pharyngeal	C11.3	C79.89	D00.08	D10.6	D37.05	D49.0
vagina	C52	C79.82	D07.2	D28.1	D39.8	D49.59
fossa (of)						
anterior (cranial)	C71.9	C79.31	—	D33.2	D43.2	D49.6
cranial	C71.9	C79.31	—	D33.2	D43.2	D49.6
ischiorectal	C76.3	C79.89	D09.8	D36.7	D48.7	D49.89
middle (cranial)	C71.9	C79.31	—	D33.2	D43.2	D49.6
piriform	C12	C79.89	D00.08	D10.7	D37.05	D49.0
pituitary	C75.1	C79.89	D09.3	D35.2	D44.3	D49.7
posterior (cranial)	C71.9	C79.31	—	D33.2	D43.2	D49.6
pterygoid	C49.0	C79.89	—	D21.0	D48.1	D49.2
pyriform	C12	C79.89	D00.08	D10.7	D37.05	D49.0
Rosenmuller	C11.2	C79.89	D00.08	D10.6	D37.05	D49.0
tonsillar	C09.0	C79.89	D00.08	D10.5	D37.05	D49.0
fourchette	C51.9	C79.82	D07.1	D28.0	D39.8	D49.59
frenulum						
labii — *see* Neoplasm, lip, internal						
linguae	C02.2	C79.89	D00.07	D10.1	D37.02	D49.0
frontal						
bone	C41.0	C79.51	—	D16.4	D48.0	D49.2
lobe, brain	C71.1	C79.31	—	D33.0	D43.0	D49.6
pole	C71.1	C79.31	—	D33.0	D43.0	D49.6
sinus	C31.2	C78.39	D02.3	D14.0	D38.5	D49.1
fundus						
stomach	C16.1	C78.89	D00.2	D13.1	D37.1	D49.0
uterus	C54.3	C79.82	D07.0	D26.1	D39.0	D49.59
gallbladder	C23	C78.89	D01.5	D13.5	D37.6	D49.0
overlapping lesion with extrahepatic bile ducts	C24.8	—	—	—	—	—
gall duct (extrahepatic)	C24.0	C78.89	D01.5	D13.5	D37.6	D49.0
intrahepatic	C22.1	C78.7	D01.5	D13.4	D37.6	D49.0
ganglia — *see also* Neoplasm, nerve, peripheral	C47.9	C79.89	—	D36.10	D48.2	D49.2
basal	C71.0	C79.31	—	D33.0	D43.0	D49.6
cranial nerve	C72.50	C79.49	—	D33.3	D43.3	D49.7
Gartner's duct	C52	C79.82	D07.2	D28.1	D39.8	D49.59
gastric — *see* Neoplasm, stomach						
gastrocolic	C26.9	C78.89	D01.9	D13.9	D37.9	D49.0
gastroesophageal junction	C16.0	C78.89	D00.2	D13.1	D37.1	D49.0
gastrointestinal (tract) NEC	C26.9	C78.89	D01.9	D13.9	D37.9	D49.0
generalized	C80.0	—	—	—	—	—
genital organ or tract						
female NEC	C57.9	C79.82	D07.30	D28.9	D39.9	D49.59
overlapping lesion	C57.8	—	—	—	—	—
specified site NEC	C57.7	C79.82	D07.39	D28.7	D39.8	D49.59
male NEC	C63.9	C79.82	D07.60	D29.9	D40.9	D49.59
overlapping lesion	C63.8	—	—	—	—	—
specified site NEC	C63.7	C79.82	D07.69	D29.8	D40.8	D49.59
genitourinary tract						
female	C57.9	C79.82	D07.30	D28.9	D39.9	D49.59
male	C63.9	C79.82	D07.60	D29.9	D40.9	D49.59
gingiva (alveolar) (marginal)	C03.9	C79.89	D00.03	D10.39	D37.09	D49.0
lower	C03.1	C79.89	D00.03	D10.39	D37.09	D49.0
mandibular	C03.1	C79.89	D00.03	D10.39	D37.09	D49.0
maxillary	C03.0	C79.89	D00.03	D10.39	D37.09	D49.0
upper	C03.0	C79.89	D00.03	D10.39	D37.09	D49.0
gland, glandular (lymphatic) (system) — *see also* Neoplasm, lymph gland						
endocrine NEC	C75.9	C79.89	D09.3	D35.9	D44.9	D49.7

☑ Additional Character Required — Refer to the Tabular List for Character Selection   🔻 Subterms under main terms may continue to next column or page

Neoplasm, neoplastic — continued

gland, glandular — *see also* Neoplasm, lymph gland — *continued*
  salivary — *see* Neoplasm, salivary gland

	Malignant Primary	Malignant Secondary	Ca in situ	Benign	Uncertain	Unspecified Behavior
glans penis	C60.1	C79.82	D07.4	D29.0	D40.8	D49.59
globus pallidus	C71.0	C79.31	—	D33.0	D43.0	D49.6
glomus						
coccygeal	C49.5	C79.89	—	D21.5	D48.1	D49.2
jugularis	C75.5	C79.89	—	D35.6	D44.7	D49.7
glosso-epiglottic fold(s)	C10.1	C79.89	D00.08	D10.5	D37.05	D49.0
glossopalatine fold	C09.1	C79.89	D00.08	D10.5	D37.05	D49.0
glossopharyngeal sulcus	C09.0	C79.89	D00.08	D10.5	D37.05	D49.0
glottis	C32.0	C78.39	D02.0	D14.1	D38.0	D49.1
gluteal region	C76.3	C79.89	D04.5	D36.7	D48.7	D49.89
great vessels NEC	C49.3	C79.89	—	D21.3	D48.1	D49.2
groin NEC	C76.3	C79.89	D04.5	D36.7	D48.7	D49.89
gum	C03.9	C79.89	D00.03	D10.39	D37.09	D49.0
lower	C03.1	C79.89	D00.03	D10.39	D37.09	D49.0
upper	C03.0	C79.89	D00.03	D10.39	D37.09	D49.0
hand NEC	C76.4-☑	C79.89	D04.6-☑	D36.7	D48.7	D49.89
head NEC	C76.0	C79.89	D04.4	D36.7	D48.7	D49.89
heart	C38.0	C79.89	—	D15.1	D48.7	D49.89
heel NEC	C76.5-☑	C79.89	D04.7-☑	D36.7	D48.7	D49.89
helix — *see also* Neoplasm, skin, ear	C44.20-☑	C79.2	D04.2-☑	D23.2-☑	D48.5	D49.2
hematopoietic, hemopoietic tissue NEC	C96.9	—	—	—	—	—
specified NEC	C96.Z	—	—	—	—	—
hemisphere, cerebral	C71.0	C79.31	—	D33.0	D43.0	D49.6
hemorrhoidal zone	C21.1	C78.5	D01.3	D12.9	D37.8	D49.0
hepatic — *see also* Index to disease, by histology	C22.9	C78.7	D01.5	D13.4	D37.6	D49.0
duct (bile)	C24.0	C78.89	D01.5	D13.5	D37.6	D49.0
flexure (colon)	C18.3	C78.5	D01.0	D12.3	D37.4	D49.0
primary	C22.8	C78.7	D01.5	D13.4	D37.6	D49.0
hepatobiliary	C24.9	C78.89	D01.5	D13.5	D37.6	D49.0
hepatoblastoma	C22.2	C78.7	D01.5	D13.4	D37.6	D49.0
hepatoma	C22.0	C78.7	D01.5	D13.4	D37.6	D49.0
hilus of lung	C34.0-☑	C78.0-☑	D02.2-☑	D14.3-☑	D38.1	D49.1
hippocampus, brain	C71.2	C79.31	—	D33.0	D43.0	D49.6
hip NEC	C76.5-☑	C79.89	D04.7-☑	D36.7	D48.7	D49.89
humerus (any part)	C40.0-☑	C79.51	—	D16.0-☑	—	—
hymen	C52	C79.82	D07.2	D28.1	D39.8	D49.59
hypopharynx, hypopharyngeal NEC	C13.9	C79.89	D00.08	D10.7	D37.05	D49.0
overlapping lesion	C13.8	—	—	—	—	—
postcricoid region	C13.0	C79.89	D00.08	D10.7	D37.05	D49.0
posterior wall	C13.2	C79.89	D00.08	D10.7	D37.05	D49.0
pyriform fossa (sinus)	C12	C79.89	D00.08	D10.7	D37.05	D49.0
hypophysis	C75.1	C79.89	D09.3	D35.2	D44.3	D49.7
hypothalamus	C71.0	C79.31	—	D33.0	D43.0	D49.6
ileocecum, ileocecal (coil) (junction) (valve)	C18.0	C78.5	D01.0	D12.0	D37.4	D49.0
ileum	C17.2	C78.4	D01.49	D13.39	D37.2	D49.0
ilium	C41.4	C79.51	—	D16.8	D48.0	D49.2
immunoproliferative NEC	C88.9	—	—	—	—	—
infraclavicular (region)	C76.1	C79.89	D04.5	D36.7	D48.7	D49.89
inguinal (region)	C76.3	C79.89	D04.5	D36.7	D48.7	D49.89
insula	C71.0	C79.31	—	D33.0	D43.0	D49.6
insular tissue (pancreas)	C25.4	C78.89	D01.7	D13.7	D37.8	D49.0
brain	C71.0	C79.31	—	D33.0	D43.0	D49.6
interarytenoid fold	C13.1	C78.39	D00.08	D10.7	D37.05	D49.0
hypopharyngeal aspect	C13.1	C79.89	D00.08	D10.7	D37.05	D49.0
laryngeal aspect	C32.1	C78.39	D02.0	D14.1	D38.0	D49.1
marginal zone	C13.1	C79.89	D00.08	D10.7	D37.05	D49.0
interdental papillae	C03.9	C79.89	D00.03	D10.39	D37.09	D49.0

Neoplasm, neoplastic — continued

interdental papillae — *continued*

	Malignant Primary	Malignant Secondary	Ca in situ	Benign	Uncertain	Unspecified Behavior
lower	C03.1	C79.89	D00.03	D10.39	D37.09	D49.0
upper	C03.0	C79.89	D00.03	D10.39	D37.09	D49.0
internal						
capsule	C71.0	C79.31	—	D33.0	D43.0	D49.6
os (cervix)	C53.0	C79.82	D06.0	D26.0	D39.0	D49.59
intervertebral cartilage or disc	C41.2	C79.51	—	D16.6	D48.0	D49.2
intestine, intestinal	C26.0	C78.80	D01.40	D13.9	D37.8	D49.0
large	C18.9	C78.5	D01.0	D12.6	D37.4	D49.0
appendix	C18.1	C78.5	D01.0	D12.1	D37.3	D49.0
caput coli	C18.0	C78.5	D01.0	D12.0	D37.4	D49.0
cecum	C18.0	C78.5	D01.0	D12.0	D37.4	D49.0
colon	C18.9	C78.5	D01.0	D12.6	D37.4	D49.0
and rectum	C19	C78.5	D01.1	D12.7	D37.5	D49.0
ascending	C18.2	C78.5	D01.0	D12.2	D37.4	D49.0
caput	C18.0	C78.5	D01.0	D12.0	D37.4	D49.0
descending	C18.6	C78.5	D01.0	D12.4	D37.4	D49.0
distal	C18.6	C78.5	D01.0	D12.4	D37.4	D49.0
left	C18.6	C78.5	D01.0	D12.4	D37.4	D49.0
overlapping lesion	C18.8	—	—	—	—	—
pelvic	C18.7	C78.5	D01.0	D12.5	D37.4	D49.0
right	C18.2	C78.5	D01.0	D12.2	D37.4	D49.0
sigmoid (flexure)	C18.7	C78.5	D01.0	D12.5	D37.4	D49.0
transverse	C18.4	C78.5	D01.0	D12.3	D37.4	D49.0
hepatic flexure	C18.3	C78.5	D01.0	D12.3	D37.4	D49.0
ileocecum, ileocecal (coil) (valve)	C18.0	C78.5	D01.0	D12.0	D37.4	D49.0
overlapping lesion	C18.8	—	—	—	—	—
sigmoid flexure (lower) (upper)	C18.7	C78.5	D01.0	D12.5	D37.4	D49.0
splenic flexure	C18.5	C78.5	D01.0	D12.3	D37.4	D49.0
small	C17.9	C78.4	D01.40	D13.30	D37.2	D49.0
duodenum	C17.0	C78.4	D01.49	D13.2	D37.2	D49.0
ileum	C17.2	C78.4	D01.49	D13.39	D37.2	D49.0
jejunum	C17.1	C78.4	D01.49	D13.39	D37.2	D49.0
overlapping lesion	C17.8	—	—	—	—	—
tract NEC	C26.0	C78.89	D01.40	D13.9	D37.8	D49.0
intra-abdominal	C76.2	C79.89	D09.8	D36.7	D48.7	D49.89
intracranial NEC	C71.9	C79.31	—	D33.2	D43.2	D49.6
intrahepatic (bile) duct	C22.1	C78.7	D01.5	D13.4	D37.6	D49.0
intraocular	C69.9-☑	C79.49	D09.2-☑	D31.9-☑	D48.7	D49.89
intraorbital	C69.6-☑	C79.49	D09.2-☑	D31.6-☑	D48.7	D49.89
intrasellar	C75.1	C79.89	D09.3	D35.2	D44.3	D49.7
intrathoracic (cavity) (organs)	C76.1	C79.89	D09.8	D15.9	D48.7	D49.89
specified NEC	C76.1	C79.89	D09.8	D15.7	—	—
iris	C69.4-☑	C79.49	D09.2-☑	D31.4-☑	D48.7	D49.89
ischiorectal (fossa)	C76.3	C79.89	D09.8	D36.7	D48.7	D49.89
ischium	C41.4	C79.51	—	D16.8	D48.0	D49.2
island of Reil	C71.0	C79.31	—	D33.0	D43.0	D49.6
islands or islets of Langerhans	C25.4	C78.89	D01.7	D13.7	D37.8	D49.0
isthmus uteri	C54.0	C79.82	D07.0	D26.1	D39.0	D49.59
jaw	C76.0	C79.89	D09.8	D36.7	D48.7	D49.89
bone	C41.1	C79.51	—	D16.5	D48.0	D49.2
lower	C41.1	C79.51	—	D16.5	—	—
upper	C41.0	C79.51	—	D16.4	—	—
carcinoma (any type) (lower) (upper)	C76.0	C79.89		—	—	—
skin — *see also* Neoplasm, skin, face	C44.309	C79.2	D04.39	D23.39	D48.5	D49.2
soft tissues	C03.9	C79.89	D00.03	D10.39	D37.09	D49.0
lower	C03.1	C79.89	D00.03	D10.39	D37.09	D49.0
upper	C03.0	C79.89	D00.03	D10.39	D37.09	D49.0
jejunum	C17.1	C78.4	D01.49	D13.39	D37.2	D49.0
joint NEC — *see also* Neoplasm, bone	C41.9	C79.51		D16.9	D48.0	D49.2
acromioclavicular	C40.0-☑	C79.51	—	D16.0-☑		

Neoplasm Table

	Malignant Primary	Malignant Secondary	Ca in situ	Benign	Uncertain	Unspecified Behavior
Neoplasm, neoplastic — *continued*						
joint — *see also* Neoplasm, bone — *continued*						
bursa or synovial membrane — *see* Neoplasm, connective tissue						
costovertebral	C41.3	C79.51	—	D16.7	D48.Ø	D49.2
sternocostal	C41.3	C79.51	—	D16.7	D48.Ø	D49.2
temporomandibular	C41.1	C79.51	—	D16.5	D48.Ø	D49.2
junction						
anorectal	C21.8	C78.5	DØ1.3	D12.9	D37.8	D49.Ø
cardioesophageal	C16.Ø	C78.89	DØØ.2	D13.1	D37.1	D49.Ø
esophagogastric	C16.Ø	C78.89	DØØ.2	D13.1	D37.1	D49.Ø
gastroesophageal	C16.Ø	C78.89	DØØ.2	D13.1	D37.1	D49.Ø
hard and soft palate	CØ5.9	C79.89	DØØ.ØØ	D1Ø.39	D37.Ø9	D49.Ø
ileocecal	C18.Ø	C78.5	DØ1.Ø	D12.Ø	D37.4	D49.Ø
pelvirectal	C19	C78.5	DØ1.1	D12.7	D37.5	D49.Ø
pelviureteric	C65.-☑	C79.Ø-☑	DØ9.19	D3Ø.1-☑	D41.1-☑	D49.59
rectosigmoid	C19	C78.5	DØ1.1	D12.7	D37.5	D49.Ø
squamocolumnar, of cervix	C53.8	C79.82	DØ6.7	D26.Ø	D39.Ø	D49.59
Kaposi's sarcoma — *see* Kaposi's, sarcoma						
kidney						
(parenchymal)	C64.-☑	C79.Ø-☑	DØ9.19	D3Ø.Ø-☑	D41.Ø-☑	D49.51-☑
calyx	C65.-☑	C79.Ø-☑	DØ9.19	D3Ø.1-☑	D41.1-☑	D49.51-☑
hilus	C65.-☑	C79.Ø-☑	DØ9.19	D3Ø.1-☑	D41.1-☑	D49.51-☑
pelvis	C65.-☑	C79.Ø-☑	DØ9.19	D3Ø.1-☑	D41.1-☑	D49.51-☑
knee NEC	C76.5-☑	C79.89	DØ4.7-☑	D36.7	D48.7	D49.89
labia (skin)	C51.9	C79.82	DØ7.1	D28.Ø	D39.8	D49.59
majora	C51.Ø	C79.82	DØ7.1	D28.Ø	D39.8	D49.59
minora	C51.1	C79.82	DØ7.1	D28.Ø	D39.8	D49.59
labial — *see also* Neoplasm, lip	CØØ.9	C79.89	DØØ.Ø1	D1Ø.Ø	D37.Ø1	D49.Ø
sulcus (lower) (upper)	CØ6.1	C79.89	DØØ.Ø2	D1Ø.39	D37.Ø9	D49.Ø
labium (skin)	C51.9	C79.82	DØ7.1	D28.Ø	D39.8	D49.59
majus	C51.Ø	C79.82	DØ7.1	D28.Ø	D39.8	D49.59
minus	C51.1	C79.82	DØ7.1	D28.Ø	D39.8	D49.59
lacrimal						
canaliculi	C69.5-☑	C79.49	DØ9.2-☑	D31.5-☑	D48.7	D49.89
duct (nasal)	C69.5-☑	C79.49	DØ9.2-☑	D31.5-☑	D48.7	D49.89
gland	C69.5-☑	C79.49	DØ9.2-☑	D31.5-☑	D48.7	D49.89
punctum	C69.5-☑	C79.49	DØ9.2-☑	D31.5-☑	D48.7	D49.89
sac	C69.5-☑	C79.49	DØ9.2-☑	D31.5-☑	D48.7	D49.89
Langerhans, islands or islets	C25.4	C78.89	DØ1.7	D13.7	D37.8	D49.Ø
laryngopharynx	C13.9	C79.89	DØØ.Ø8	D1Ø.7	D37.Ø5	D49.Ø
larynx, laryngeal NEC	C32.9	C78.39	DØ2.Ø	D14.1	D38.Ø	D49.1
aryepiglottic fold	C32.1	C78.39	DØ2.Ø	D14.1	D38.Ø	D49.1
cartilage (arytenoid) (cricoid) (cuneiform) (thyroid)	C32.3	C78.39	DØ2.Ø	D14.1	D38.Ø	D49.1
commissure (anterior) (posterior)	C32.Ø	C78.39	DØ2.Ø	D14.1	D38.Ø	D49.1
extrinsic NEC	C32.1	C78.39	DØ2.Ø	D14.1	D38.Ø	D49.1
meaning hypopharynx	C13.9	C79.89	DØØ.Ø8	D1Ø.7	D37.Ø5	D49.Ø
interarytenoid fold	C32.1	C78.39	DØ2.Ø	D14.1	D38.Ø	D49.1
intrinsic	C32.Ø	C78.39	DØ2.Ø	D14.1	D38.Ø	D49.1
overlapping lesion	C32.8	—	—	—	—	—
ventricular band	C32.1	C78.39	DØ2.Ø	D14.1	D38.Ø	D49.1
leg NEC	C76.5-☑	C79.89	DØ4.7-☑	D36.7	D48.7	D49.89
lens, crystalline	C69.4-☑	C79.49	DØ9.2-☑	D31.4-☑	D48.7	D49.89
lid (lower) (upper)	C44.1Ø-☑	C79.2	DØ4.1-☑	D23.1-☑	D48.5	D49.2
basal cell carcinoma	C44.11-☑	—	—	—	—	—
specified type NEC	C44.19-☑	—	—	—	—	—
squamous cell carcinoma	C44.12-☑	—	—	—	—	—

	Malignant Primary	Malignant Secondary	Ca in situ	Benign	Uncertain	Unspecified Behavior
Neoplasm, neoplastic — *continued*						
ligament — *see also* Neoplasm, connective tissue						
broad	C57.1-☑	C79.82	DØ7.39	D28.2	D39.8	D49.59
Mackenrodt's	C57.7	C79.82	DØ7.39	D28.7	D39.8	D49.59
non-uterine — *see* Neoplasm, connective tissue						
round	C57.2-☑	C79.82	—	D28.2	D39.8	D49.59
sacro-uterine	C57.3	C79.82	—	D28.2	D39.8	D49.59
uterine	C57.3	C79.82	—	D28.2	D39.8	D49.59
utero-ovarian	C57.7	C79.82	DØ7.39	D28.2	D39.8	D49.59
uterosacral	C57.3	C79.82	—	D28.2	D39.8	D49.59
limb	C76.8	C79.89	DØ4.8	D36.7	D48.7	D49.89
lower	C76.5-☑	C79.89	DØ4.7-☑	D36.7	D48.7	D49.89
upper	C76.4-☑	C79.89	DØ4.6-☑	D36.7	D48.7	D49.89
limbus of cornea	C69.1-☑	C79.49	DØ9.2-☑	D31.1-☑	D48.7	D49.89
lingual NEC — *see also* Neoplasm, tongue	CØ2.9	C79.89	DØØ.Ø7	D1Ø.1	D37.Ø2	D49.Ø
lingula, lung	C34.1-☑	C78.Ø-☑	DØ2.2-☑	D14.3-☑	D38.1	D49.1
lip	CØØ.9	C79.89	DØØ.Ø1	D1Ø.Ø	D37.Ø1	D49.Ø
buccal aspect — *see* Neoplasm, lip, internal						
commissure	CØØ.6	C79.89	DØØ.Ø1	D1Ø.Ø	D37.Ø1	D49.Ø
external	CØØ.2	C79.89	DØØ.Ø1	D1Ø.Ø	D37.Ø1	D49.Ø
lower	CØØ.1	C79.89	DØØ.Ø1	D1Ø.Ø	D37.Ø1	D49.Ø
upper	CØØ.Ø	C79.89	DØØ.Ø1	D1Ø.Ø	D37.Ø1	D49.Ø
frenulum — *see* Neoplasm, lip, internal						
inner aspect — *see* Neoplasm, lip, internal						
internal	CØØ.5	C79.89	DØØ.Ø1	D1Ø.Ø	D37.Ø1	D49.Ø
lower	CØØ.4	C79.89	DØØ.Ø1	D1Ø.Ø	D37.Ø1	D49.Ø
upper	CØØ.3	C79.89	DØØ.Ø1	D1Ø.Ø	D37.Ø1	D49.Ø
lipstick area	CØØ.2	C79.89	DØØ.Ø1	D1Ø.Ø	D37.Ø1	D49.Ø
lower	CØØ.1	C79.89	DØØ.Ø1	D1Ø.Ø	D37.Ø1	D49.Ø
upper	CØØ.Ø	C79.89	DØØ.Ø1	D1Ø.Ø	D37.Ø1	D49.Ø
lower	CØØ.1	C79.89	DØØ.Ø1	D1Ø.Ø	D37.Ø1	D49.Ø
internal	CØØ.4	C79.89	DØØ.Ø1	D1Ø.Ø	D37.Ø1	D49.Ø
mucosa — *see* Neoplasm, lip, internal						
oral aspect — *see* Neoplasm, lip, internal						
overlapping lesion with oral cavity or pharynx	CØØ.8 C14.8	— —	— —	— —	— —	— —
skin (commissure) (ligament) (lower) (upper)	C44.ØØ	C79.2	DØ4.Ø	D23.Ø	D48.5	D49.2
basal cell carcinoma	C44.Ø1	—	—	—	—	—
specified type NEC	C44.Ø9	—	—	—	—	—
squamous cell carcinoma	C44.Ø2	—	—	—	—	—
upper	CØØ.Ø	C79.89	DØØ.Ø1	D1Ø.Ø	D37.Ø1	D49.Ø
internal	CØØ.3	C79.89	DØØ.Ø1	D1Ø.Ø	D37.Ø1	D49.Ø
vermilion border	CØØ.2	C79.89	DØØ.Ø1	D1Ø.Ø	D37.Ø1	D49.Ø
lower	CØØ.1	C79.89	DØØ.Ø1	D1Ø.Ø	D37.Ø1	D49.Ø
upper	CØØ.Ø	C79.89	DØØ.Ø1	D1Ø.Ø	D37.Ø1	D49.Ø
lipomatous — *see* Lipoma, by site						
liver — *see also* Index to disease, by histology	C22.9	C78.7	DØ1.5	D13.4	D37.6	D49.Ø
primary	C22.8	C78.7	DØ1.5	D13.4	D37.6	D49.Ø
lumbosacral plexus	C47.5	C79.89	—	D36.16	D48.2	D49.2
lung	C34.9-☑	C78.Ø-☑	DØ2.2-☑	D14.3-☑	D38.1	D49.1
azygos lobe	C34.1-☑	C78.Ø-☑	DØ2.2-☑	D14.3-☑	D38.1	D49.1
carina	C34.Ø-☑	C78.Ø-☑	DØ2.2-☑	D14.3-☑	D38.1	D49.1
hilus	C34.Ø-☑	C78.Ø-☑	DØ2.2-☑	D14.3-☑	D38.1	D49.1
lingula	C34.1-☑	C78.Ø-☑	DØ2.2-☑	D14.3-☑	D38.1	D49.1
lobe NEC	C34.9-☑	C78.Ø-☑	DØ2.2-☑	D14.3-☑	D38.1	D49.1
lower lobe	C34.3-☑	C78.Ø-☑	DØ2.2-☑	D14.3-☑	D38.1	D49.1

   ☑ Additional Character Required — Refer to the Tabular List for Character Selection   ▽ Subterms under main terms may continue to next column or page

Neoplasm, joint NEC — Neoplasm, lung

Neoplasm Table

	Malignant Primary	Malignant Secondary	Ca in situ	Benign	Uncertain	Unspecified Behavior
Neoplasm, neoplastic — *continued*						
lung — *continued*						
main bronchus	C34.0-✓	C78.0-✓	D02.2-✓	D14.3-✓	D38.1	D49.1
mesothelioma — *see* Mesothelioma						
middle lobe	C34.2	C78.0-✓	D02.21	D14.31	D38.1	D49.1
overlapping lesion	C34.8-✓	—				—
upper lobe	C34.1-✓	C78.0-✓	D02.2-✓	D14.3-✓	D38.1	D49.1
lymph, lymphatic channel						
NEC	C49.9	C79.89		D21.9	D48.1	D49.2
gland (secondary)	—	C77.9	—	D36.0	D48.7	D49.89
abdominal	—	C77.2	—	D36.0	D48.7	D49.89
aortic	—	C77.2	—	D36.0	D48.7	D49.89
arm	—	C77.3	—	D36.0	D48.7	D49.89
auricular (anterior) (posterior)	—	C77.0	—	D36.0	D48.7	D49.89
axilla, axillary	—	C77.3	—	D36.0	D48.7	D49.89
brachial	—	C77.3	—	D36.0	D48.7	D49.89
bronchial	—	C77.1	—	D36.0	D48.7	D49.89
bronchopulmonary	—	C77.1	—	D36.0	D48.7	D49.89
celiac	—	C77.2	—	D36.0	D48.7	D49.89
cervical	—	C77.0	—	D36.0	D48.7	D49.89
cervicofacial	—	C77.0	—	D36.0	D48.7	D49.89
Cloquet	—	C77.4	—	D36.0	D48.7	D49.89
colic	—	C77.2	—	D36.0	D48.7	D49.89
common duct	—	C77.2	—	D36.0	D48.7	D49.89
cubital	—	C77.3	—	D36.0	D48.7	D49.89
diaphragmatic	—	C77.1	—	D36.0	D48.7	D49.89
epigastric, inferior	—	C77.1	—	D36.0	D48.7	D49.89
epitrochlear	—	C77.3	—	D36.0	D48.7	D49.89
esophageal	—	C77.1	—	D36.0	D48.7	D49.89
face	—	C77.0	—	D36.0	D48.7	D49.89
femoral	—	C77.4	—	D36.0	D48.7	D49.89
gastric	—	C77.2	—	D36.0	D48.7	D49.89
groin	—	C77.4	—	D36.0	D48.7	D49.89
head	—	C77.0	—	D36.0	D48.7	D49.89
hepatic	—	C77.2	—	D36.0	D48.7	D49.89
hilar (pulmonary)	—	C77.1	—	D36.0	D48.7	D49.89
splenic	—	C77.2	—	D36.0	D48.7	D49.89
hypogastric	—	C77.5	—	D36.0	D48.7	D49.89
ileocolic	—	C77.2	—	D36.0	D48.7	D49.89
iliac	—	C77.5	—	D36.0	D48.7	D49.89
infraclavicular	—	C77.3	—	D36.0	D48.7	D49.89
inguina, inguinal	—	C77.4	—	D36.0	D48.7	D49.89
innominate	—	C77.1	—	D36.0	D48.7	D49.89
intercostal	—	C77.1	—	D36.0	D48.7	D49.89
intestinal	—	C77.2	—	D36.0	D48.7	D49.89
intrabdominal	—	C77.2	—	D36.0	D48.7	D49.89
intrapelvic	—	C77.5	—	D36.0	D48.7	D49.89
intrathoracic	—	C77.1	—	D36.0	D48.7	D49.89
jugular	—	C77.0	—	D36.0	D48.7	D49.89
leg	—	C77.4	—	D36.0	D48.7	D49.89
limb						
lower	—	C77.4	—	D36.0	D48.7	D49.89
upper	—	C77.3	—	D36.0	D48.7	D49.89
lower limb	—	C77.4	—	D36.0	D48.7	D49.89
lumbar	—	C77.2	—	D36.0	D48.7	D49.89
mandibular	—	C77.0	—	D36.0	D48.7	D49.89
mediastinal	—	C77.1	—	D36.0	D48.7	D49.89
mesenteric (inferior) (superior)	—	C77.2	—	D36.0	D48.7	D49.89
midcolic	—	C77.2	—	D36.0	D48.7	D49.89
multiple sites in categories C77.0-C77.5	—	C77.8	—	D36.0	D48.7	D49.89
neck	—	C77.0	—	D36.0	D48.7	D49.89
obturator	—	C77.5	—	D36.0	D48.7	D49.89
occipital	—	C77.0	—	D36.0	D48.7	D49.89
pancreatic	—	C77.2	—	D36.0	D48.7	D49.89
para-aortic	—	C77.2	—	D36.0	D48.7	D49.89
paracervical	—	C77.5	—	D36.0	D48.7	D49.89
parametrial	—	C77.5	—	D36.0	D48.7	D49.89
parasternal	—	C77.1	—	D36.0	D48.7	D49.89
parotid	—	C77.0	—	D36.0	D48.7	D49.89
pectoral	—	C77.3	—	D36.0	D48.7	D49.89
pelvic	—	C77.5	—	D36.0	D48.7	D49.89
peri-aortic	—	C77.2	—	D36.0	D48.7	D49.89
peripancreatic	—	C77.2	—	D36.0	D48.7	D49.89
popliteal	—	C77.4	—	D36.0	D48.7	D49.89
porta hepatis	—	C77.2	—	D36.0	D48.7	D49.89
Neoplasm, neoplastic — *continued*						
lymph, lymphatic channel — *continued*						
gland — *continued*						
portal	—	C77.2	—	D36.0	D48.7	D49.89
preauricular	—	C77.0	—	D36.0	D48.7	D49.89
prelaryngeal	—	C77.0	—	D36.0	D48.7	D49.89
presymphysial	—	C77.5	—	D36.0	D48.7	D49.89
pretracheal	—	C77.0	—	D36.0	D48.7	D49.89
primary (any site) NEC	C96.9	—	—	—	—	—
pulmonary (hiler)	—	C77.1	—	D36.0	D48.7	D49.89
pyloric	—	C77.2	—	D36.0	D48.7	D49.89
retroperitoneal	—	C77.2	—	D36.0	D48.7	D49.89
retropharyngeal	—	C77.0	—	D36.0	D48.7	D49.89
Rosenmuller's	—	C77.4	—	D36.0	D48.7	D49.89
sacral	—	C77.5	—	D36.0	D48.7	D49.89
scalene	—	C77.0	—	D36.0	D48.7	D49.89
site NEC	—	C77.9	—	D36.0	D48.7	D49.89
splenic (hilar)	—	C77.2	—	D36.0	D48.7	D49.89
subclavicular	—	C77.3	—	D36.0	D48.7	D49.89
subinguinal	—	C77.4	—	D36.0	D48.7	D49.89
sublingual	—	C77.0	—	D36.0	D48.7	D49.89
submandibular	—	C77.0	—	D36.0	D48.7	D49.89
submaxillary	—	C77.0	—	D36.0	D48.7	D49.89
submental	—	C77.0	—	D36.0	D48.7	D49.89
subscapular	—	C77.3	—	D36.0	D48.7	D49.89
supraclavicular	—	C77.0	—	D36.0	D48.7	D49.89
thoracic	—	C77.1	—	D36.0	D48.7	D49.89
tibial	—	C77.4	—	D36.0	D48.7	D49.89
tracheal	—	C77.1	—	D36.0	D48.7	D49.89
tracheobronchial	—	C77.1	—	D36.0	D48.7	D49.89
upper limb	—	C77.3	—	D36.0	D48.7	D49.89
Virchow's	—	C77.0	—	D36.0	D48.7	D49.89
node — *see also* Neoplasm, lymph gland						
primary NEC	C96.9	—	—	—	—	—
vessel — *see also* Neoplasm, connective tissue	C49.9	C79.89	—	D21.9	D48.1	D49.2
Mackenrodt's ligament	C57.7	C79.82	D07.39	D28.7	D39.8	D49.59
malar	C41.0	C79.51	—	D16.4	D48.0	D49.2
region — *see* Neoplasm, cheek						
mammary gland — *see* Neoplasm, breast						
mandible	C41.1	C79.51	—	D16.5	D48.0	D49.2
alveolar						
mucosa (carcinoma)	C03.1	C79.89	D00.03	D10.39	D37.09	D49.0
ridge or process	C41.1	C79.51	—	D16.5	D48.0	D49.2
marrow (bone) NEC	C96.9	C79.52	—	—	D47.9	D49.89
mastectomy site (skin) — *see also* Neoplasm, breast, skin	C44.501	C79.2	—	—	—	—
specified as breast tissue	C50.8-✓	C79.81	—	—	—	—
mastoid (air cells) (antrum) (cavity)	C30.1	C78.39	D02.3	D14.0	D38.5	D49.1
bone or process	C41.0	C79.51	—	D16.4	D48.0	D49.2
maxilla, maxillary (superior)	C41.0	C79.51	—	D16.4	D48.0	D49.2
alveolar						
mucosa	C03.0	C79.89	D00.03	D10.39	D37.09	D49.0
ridge or process (carcinoma)	C41.0	C79.51	—	D16.4	D48.0	D49.2
antrum	C31.0	C78.39	D02.3	D14.0	D38.5	D49.1
carcinoma	C03.0	C79.51	—	—	—	—
inferior — *see* Neoplasm, mandible						
sinus	C31.0	C78.39	D02.3	D14.0	D38.5	D49.1
meatus external (ear) — *see also* Neoplasm, skin, ear	C44.20-✓	C79.2	D04.2-✓	D23.2-✓	D48.5	D49.2
Meckel diverticulum, malignant	C17.3	C78.4	D01.49	D13.39	D37.2	D49.0
mediastinum, mediastinal	C38.3	C78.1	—	D15.2	D38.3	D49.89

Neoplasm, lung — Neoplasm, mediastinum, mediastinal

Neoplasm Table

Neoplasm, neoplastic — continued	Malignant Primary	Malignant Secondary	Ca in situ	Benign	Uncertain	Unspecified Behavior
mediastinum, mediastinal — continued						
anterior	C38.1	C78.1	—	D15.2	D38.3	D49.89
posterior	C38.2	C78.1	—	D15.2	D38.3	D49.89
medulla						
adrenal	C74.1-☑	C79.7-☑	D09.3	D35.0-☑	D44.1-☑	D49.7
oblongata	C71.7	C79.31	—	D33.1	D43.1	D49.6
meibomian gland	C44.10-☑	C79.2	D04.1-☑	D23.1-☑	D48.5	D49.2
basal cell carcinoma	C44.11-☑	—	—	—	—	—
specified type NEC	C44.19-☑	—	—	—	—	—
squamous cell carcinoma	C44.12-☑	—	—	—	—	—
melanoma — see Melanoma						
meninges	C70.9	C79.49	—	D32.9	D42.9	D49.7
brain	C70.0	C79.32	—	D32.0	D42.0	D49.7
cerebral	C70.0	C79.32	—	D32.0	D42.0	D49.7
crainial	C70.0	C79.32	—	D32.0	D42.0	D49.7
intracranial	C70.0	C79.32	—	D32.0	D42.0	D49.7
spinal (cord)	C70.1	C79.49	—	D32.1	D42.1	D49.7
meniscus, knee joint (lateral) (medial)	C40.2-☑	C79.51	—	D16.2-☑	D48.0	D49.2
Merkel cell — see Carcinoma, Merkel cell						
mesentery, mesenteric	C48.1	C78.6	—	D20.1	D48.4	D49.0
mesoappendix	C48.1	C78.6	—	D20.1	D48.4	D49.0
mesocolon	C48.1	C78.6	—	D20.1	D48.4	D49.0
mesopharynx — see Neoplasm, oropharynx						
mesosalpinx	C57.1-☑	C79.82	D07.39	D28.2	D39.8	D49.59
mesothelial tissue — see Mesothelioma						
mesothelioma — see Mesothelioma						
mesovarium	C57.1-☑	C79.82	D07.39	D28.2	D39.8	D49.59
metacarpus (any bone)	C40.1-☑	C79.51	—	D16.1-☑	—	—
metastatic NEC — see also Neoplasm, by site, secondary	—	C79.9				
metatarsus (any bone)	C40.3-☑	C79.51	—	D16.3-☑	—	—
midbrain	C71.7	C79.31	—	D33.1	D43.1	D49.6
milk duct — see Neoplasm, breast						
mons						
pubis	C51.9	C79.82	D07.1	D28.0	D39.8	D49.59
veneris	C51.9	C79.82	D07.1	D28.0	D39.8	D49.59
motor tract	C72.9	C79.49	—	D33.9	D43.9	D49.7
brain	C71.9	C79.31	—	D33.2	D43.2	D49.6
cauda equina	C72.1	C79.49	—	D33.4	D43.4	D49.7
spinal	C72.0	C79.49	—	D33.4	D43.4	D49.7
mouth	C06.9	C79.89	D00.00	D10.30	D37.09	D49.0
book-leaf	C06.89	C79.89	—	—	—	—
floor	C04.9	C79.89	D00.06	D10.2	D37.09	D49.0
anterior portion	C04.0	C79.89	D00.06	D10.2	D37.09	D49.0
lateral portion	C04.1	C79.89	D00.06	D10.2	D37.09	D49.0
overlapping lesion	C04.8	—	—	—	—	—
overlapping NEC	C06.80	—	—	—	—	—
roof	C05.9	C79.89	D00.00	D10.39	D37.09	D49.0
specified part NEC	C06.89	C79.89	D00.00	D10.39	D37.09	D49.0
vestibule	C06.1	C79.89	D00.00	D10.39	D37.09	D49.0
mucosa						
alveolar (ridge or process)	C03.9	C79.89	D00.03	D10.39	D37.09	D49.0
lower	C03.1	C79.89	D00.03	D10.39	D37.09	D49.0
upper	C03.0	C79.89	D00.03	D10.39	D37.09	D49.0
buccal	C06.0	C79.89	D00.02	D10.39	D37.09	D49.0
cheek	C06.0	C79.89	D00.02	D10.39	D37.09	D49.0
lip — see Neoplasm, lip, internal						
nasal	C30.0	C78.39	D02.3	D14.0	D38.5	D49.1
oral	C06.0	C79.89	D00.02	D10.39	D37.09	D49.0
Mullerian duct						
female	C57.7	C79.82	D07.39	D28.7	D39.8	D49.59
male	C63.7	C79.82	D07.69	D29.8	D40.8	D49.59

Neoplasm, neoplastic — continued	Malignant Primary	Malignant Secondary	Ca in situ	Benign	Uncertain	Unspecified Behavior
muscle — see also Neoplasm, connective tissue						
extraocular	C69.6-☑	C79.49	D09.2-☑	D31.6-☑	D48.7	D49.89
myocardium	C38.0	C79.89	—	D15.1	D48.7	D49.89
myometrium	C54.2	C79.82	D07.0	D26.1	D39.0	D49.59
myopericardium	C38.0	C79.89	—	D15.1	D48.7	D49.89
nabothian gland (follicle)	C53.0	C79.82	D06.0	D26.0	D39.0	D49.59
nail — see also Neoplasm, skin, limb	C44.90	C79.2	D04.9	D23.9	D48.5	D49.2
finger — see also Neoplasm, skin, limb, upper	C44.60-☑	C79.2	D04.6-☑	D23.6-☑	D48.5	D49.2
toe — see also Neoplasm, skin, limb, lower	C44.70-☑	C79.2	D04.7-☑	D23.7-☑	D48.5	D49.2
nares, naris (anterior) (posterior)	C30.0	C78.39	D02.3	D14.0	D38.5	D49.1
nasal — see Neoplasm, nose						
nasolabial groove — see also Neoplasm, skin, face	C44.309	C79.2	D04.39	D23.39	D48.5	D49.2
nasolacrimal duct	C69.5-☑	C79.49	D09.2-☑	D31.5-☑	D48.7	D49.89
nasopharynx, nasopharyngeal	C11.9	C79.89	D00.08	D10.6	D37.05	D49.0
floor	C11.3	C79.89	D00.08	D10.6	D37.05	D49.0
overlapping lesion	C11.8	—	—	—	—	—
roof	C11.0	C79.89	D00.08	D10.6	D37.05	D49.0
wall	C11.9	C79.89	D00.08	D10.6	D37.05	D49.0
anterior	C11.3	C79.89	D00.08	D10.6	D37.05	D49.0
lateral	C11.2	C79.89	D00.08	D10.6	D37.05	D49.0
posterior	C11.1	C79.89	D00.08	D10.6	D37.05	D49.0
superior	C11.0	C79.89	D00.08	D10.6	D37.05	D49.0
nates — see also Neoplasm, skin, trunk	C44.509	C79.2	D04.5	D23.5	D48.5	D49.2
neck NEC	C76.0	C79.89	D09.8	D36.7	D48.7	D49.89
skin	C44.40	—	—	—	—	—
basal cell carcinoma	C44.41	—	—	—	—	—
specified type NEC	C44.49	—	—	—	—	—
squamous cell carcinoma	C44.42	—	—	—	—	—
nerve (ganglion)	C47.9	C79.89	—	D36.10	D48.2	D49.2
abducens	C72.59	C79.49	—	D33.3	D43.3	D49.7
accessory (spinal)	C72.59	C79.49	—	D33.3	D43.3	D49.7
acoustic	C72.4-☑	C79.49	—	D33.3	D43.3	D49.7
auditory	C72.4-☑	C79.49	—	D33.3	D43.3	D49.7
autonomic NEC — see also Neoplasm, nerve, peripheral	C47.9	C79.89	—	D36.10	D48.2	D49.2
brachial	C47.1-☑	C79.89	—	D36.12	D48.2	D49.2
cranial	C72.50	C79.49	—	D33.3	D43.3	D49.7
specified NEC	C72.59	C79.49	—	D33.3	D43.3	D49.7
facial	C72.59	C79.49	—	D33.3	D43.3	D49.7
femoral	C47.2-☑	C79.89	—	D36.13	D48.2	D49.2
ganglion NEC — see also Neoplasm, nerve, peripheral	C47.9	C79.89	—	D36.10	D48.2	D49.2
glossopharyngeal	C72.59	C79.49	—	D33.3	D43.3	D49.7
hypoglossal	C72.59	C79.49	—	D33.3	D43.3	D49.7
intercostal	C47.3	C79.89	—	D36.14	D48.2	D49.2
lumbar	C47.6	C79.89	—	D36.17	D48.2	D49.2
median	C47.1-☑	C79.89	—	D36.12	D48.2	D49.2
obturator	C47.2-☑	C79.89	—	D36.13	D48.2	D49.2
oculomotor	C72.59	C79.49	—	D33.3	D43.3	D49.7
olfactory	C47.2-☑	C79.49	—	D33.3	D43.3	D49.7
optic	C72.3-☑	C79.49	—	D33.3	D43.3	D49.7
parasympathetic NEC	C47.9	C79.89	—	D36.10	D48.2	D49.2
peripheral NEC	C47.9	C79.89	—	D36.10	D48.2	D49.2
abdomen	C47.4	C79.89	—	D36.15	D48.2	D49.2
abdominal wall	C47.4	C79.89	—	D36.15	D48.2	D49.2
ankle	C47.2-☑	C79.89	—	D36.13	D48.2	D49.2
antecubital fossa or space	C47.1-☑	C79.89	—	D36.12	D48.2	D49.2

☑ Additional Character Required — Refer to the Tabular List for Character Selection   Subterms under main terms may continue to next column or page

Neoplasm Table (right margin)

Neoplasm, neoplastic —	Malignant Primary	Malignant Secondary	Ca in situ	Benign	Uncertain	Unspecified Behavior
continued						
nerve — *continued*						
peripheral — *continued*						
arm	C47.1-☑	C79.89	—	D36.12	D48.2	D49.2
auricle (ear)	C47.0	C79.89	—	D36.11	D48.2	D49.2
axilla	C47.3	C79.89	—	D36.12	D48.2	D49.2
back	C47.6	C79.89	—	D36.17	D48.2	D49.2
buttock	C47.5	C79.89	—	D36.16	D48.2	D49.2
calf	C47.2-☑	C79.89	—	D36.13	D48.2	D49.2
cervical region	C47.0	C79.89	—	D36.11	D48.2	D49.2
cheek	C47.0	C79.89	—	D36.11	D48.2	D49.2
chest (wall)	C47.3	C79.89	—	D36.14	D48.2	D49.2
chin	C47.0	C79.89	—	D36.11	D48.2	D49.2
ear (external)	C47.0	C79.89	—	D36.11	D48.2	D49.2
elbow	C47.1-☑	C79.89	—	D36.12	D48.2	D49.2
extrarectal	C47.5	C79.89	—	D36.16	D48.2	D49.2
extremity	C47.9	C79.89	—	D36.10	D48.2	D49.2
lower	C47.2-☑	C79.89	—	D36.13	D48.2	D49.2
upper	C47.1-☑	C79.89	—	D36.12	D48.2	D49.2
eyelid	C47.0	C79.89	—	D36.11	D48.2	D49.2
face	C47.0	C79.89	—	D36.11	D48.2	D49.2
finger	C47.1-☑	C79.89	—	D36.12	D48.2	D49.2
flank	C47.6	C79.89	—	D36.17	D48.2	D49.2
foot	C47.2-☑	C79.89	—	D36.13	D48.2	D49.2
forearm	C47.1-☑	C79.89	—	D36.12	D48.2	D49.2
forehead	C47.0	C79.89	—	D36.11	D48.2	D49.2
gluteal region	C47.5	C79.89	—	D36.16	D48.2	D49.2
groin	C47.5	C79.89	—	D36.16	D48.2	D49.2
hand	C47.1-☑	C79.89	—	D36.12	D48.2	D49.2
head	C47.0	C79.89	—	D36.11	D48.2	D49.2
heel	C47.2-☑	C79.89	—	D36.13	D48.2	D49.2
hip	C47.2-☑	C79.89	—	D36.13	D48.2	D49.2
infraclavicular region	C47.3	C79.89	—	D36.14	D48.2	D49.2
inguinal (canal) (region)	C47.5	C79.89	—	D36.16	D48.2	D49.2
intrathoracic	C47.3	C79.89	—	D36.14	D48.2	D49.2
ischiorectal fossa	C47.5	C79.89	—	D36.16	D48.2	D49.2
knee	C47.2-☑	C79.89	—	D36.13	D48.2	D49.2
leg	C47.2-☑	C79.89	—	D36.13	D48.2	D49.2
limb NEC	C47.9	C79.89	—	D36.10	D48.2	D49.2
lower	C47.2-☑	C79.89	—	D36.13	D48.2	D49.2
upper	C47.1-☑	C79.89	—	D36.12	D48.2	D49.2
nates	C47.5	C79.89	—	D36.16	D48.2	D49.2
neck	C47.0	C79.89	—	D36.11	D48.2	D49.2
orbit	C69.6-☑	C79.49	—	D31.6-☑	D48.7	D49.2
pararectal	C47.5	C79.89	—	D36.16	D48.2	D49.2
paraurethral	C47.5	C79.89	—	D36.16	D48.2	D49.2
paravaginal	C47.5	C79.89	—	D36.16	D48.2	D49.2
pelvis (floor)	C47.5	C79.89	—	D36.16	D48.2	D49.2
pelvoabdominal	C47.8	C79.89	—	D36.17	D48.2	D49.2
perineum	C47.5	C79.89	—	D36.16	D48.2	D49.2
perirectal (tissue)	C47.5	C79.89	—	D36.16	D48.2	D49.2
periurethral (tissue)	C47.5	C79.89	—	D36.16	D48.2	D49.2
popliteal fossa or space	C47.2-☑	C79.89	—	D36.13	D48.2	D49.2
presacral	C47.5	C79.89	—	D36.16	D48.2	D49.2
pterygoid fossa	C47.0	C79.89	—	D36.11	D48.2	D49.2
rectovaginal septum or wall	C47.5	C79.89	—	D36.16	D48.2	D49.2
rectovesical	C47.5	C79.89	—	D36.16	D48.2	D49.2
sacrococcygeal region	C47.5	C79.89	—	D36.16	D48.2	D49.2
scalp	C47.0	C79.89	—	D36.11	D48.2	D49.2
scapular region	C47.3	C79.89	—	D36.14	D48.2	D49.2
shoulder	C47.1-☑	C79.89	—	D36.12	D48.2	D49.2
submental	C47.0	C79.89	—	D36.11	D48.2	D49.2
supraclavicular region	C47.0	C79.89	—	D36.11	D48.2	D49.2
temple	C47.0	C79.89	—	D36.11	D48.2	D49.2
temporal region	C47.0	C79.89	—	D36.11	D48.2	D49.2
thigh	C47.2-☑	C79.89	—	D36.13	D48.2	D49.2
thoracic (duct) (wall)	C47.3	C79.89	—	D36.14	D48.2	D49.2
thorax	C47.3	C79.89	—	D36.14	D48.2	D49.2
thumb	C47.1-☑	C79.89	—	D36.12	D48.2	D49.2
toe	C47.2-☑	C79.89	—	D36.13	D48.2	D49.2
trunk	C47.6	C79.89	—	D36.17	D48.2	D49.2

Neoplasm, neoplastic —	Malignant Primary	Malignant Secondary	Ca in situ	Benign	Uncertain	Unspecified Behavior
continued						
nerve — *continued*						
peripheral — *continued*						
umbilicus	C47.4	C79.89	—	D36.15	D48.2	D49.2
vesicorectal	C47.5	C79.89	—	D36.16	D48.2	D49.2
wrist	C47.1-☑	C79.89	—	D36.12	D48.2	D49.2
radial	C47.1-☑	C79.89	—	D36.12	D48.2	D49.2
sacral	C47.5	C79.89	—	D36.16	D48.2	D49.2
sciatic	C47.2-☑	C79.89	—	D36.13	D48.2	D49.2
spinal NEC	C47.9	C79.89	—	D36.10	D48.2	D49.2
accessory	C72.59	C79.49		D33.3	D43.3	D49.7
sympathetic NEC — *see also* Neoplasm, nerve, peripheral	C47.9	C79.89	—	D36.10	D48.2	D49.2
trigeminal	C72.59	C79.49		D33.3	D43.3	D49.7
trochlear	C72.59	C79.49		D33.3	D43.3	D49.7
ulnar	C47.1-☑	C79.89	—	D36.12	D48.2	D49.2
vagus	C72.59	C79.49		D33.3	D43.3	D49.7
nervous system (central)	C72.9	C79.40		D33.9	D43.9	D49.7
autonomic — *see* Neoplasm, nerve, peripheral						
parasympathetic — *see* Neoplasm, nerve, peripheral						
specified site NEC	—	C79.49		D33.7	D43.8	—
sympathetic — *see* Neoplasm, nerve, peripheral						
nevus — *see* Nevus						
nipple	C50.0-☑	C79.81	D05.-☑	D24.-☑	—	—
nose, nasal	C76.0	C79.89	D09.8	D36.7	D48.7	D49.89
ala (external) (nasi) — *see also* Neoplasm, nose, skin						
bone	C41.0	C79.51	—	D16.4	D48.0	D49.2
cartilage	C30.0	C78.39	D02.3	D14.0	D38.5	D49.1
cavity	C30.0	C78.39	D02.3	D14.0	D38.5	D49.1
choana	C11.3	C79.89	D00.08	D10.6	D37.05	D49.0
external (skin) — *see also* Neoplasm, nose, skin	C44.301	C79.2	D04.39	D23.39	D48.5	D49.2
fossa	C30.0	C78.39	D02.3	D14.0	D38.5	D49.1
internal	C30.0	C78.39	D02.3	D14.0	D38.5	D49.1
mucosa	C30.0	C78.39	D02.3	D14.0	D38.5	D49.1
septum	C30.0	C78.39	D02.3	D14.0	D38.5	D49.1
posterior margin	C11.3	C79.89	D00.08	D10.6	D37.05	D49.0
sinus — *see* Neoplasm, sinus						
skin	C44.301	C79.2	D04.39	D23.39	D48.5	D49.2
basal cell carcinoma	C44.311	—	—	—	—	—
specified type NEC	C44.391	—	—	—	—	—
squamous cell carcinoma	C44.321	—	—	—	—	—
turbinate (mucosa)	C30.0	C78.39	D02.3	D14.0	D38.5	D49.1
bone	C41.0	C79.51	—	D16.4	D48.0	D49.2
vestibule	C30.0	C78.39	D02.3	D14.0	D38.5	D49.1
nostril	C30.0	C78.39	D02.3	D14.0	D38.5	D49.1
nucleus pulposus	C41.2	C79.51	—	D16.6	D48.0	D49.2
occipital bone	C41.0	C79.51	—	D16.4	D48.0	D49.2
lobe or pole, brain	C71.4	C79.31	—	D33.0	D43.0	D49.6
odontogenic — *see* Neoplasm, jaw bone						
olfactory nerve or bulb	C72.2-☑	C79.49	—	D33.3	D43.3	D49.7
olive (brain)	C71.7	C79.31	—	D33.1	D43.1	D49.6
omentum	C48.1	C78.6	—	D20.1	D48.4	D49.0
operculum (brain)	C71.0	C79.31	—	D33.0	D43.0	D49.6
optic nerve, chiasm, or tract	C72.3-☑	C79.49	—	D33.3	D43.3	D49.7
oral (cavity)	C06.9	C79.89	D00.00	D10.30	D37.09	D49.0
ill-defined	C14.8	C79.89	D00.00	D10.30	D37.09	D49.0
mucosa	C06.0	C79.89	D00.02	D10.30	D37.09	D49.0
orbit	C69.6-☑	C79.49	D09.2-☑	D31.6-☑	D48.7	D49.89
autonomic nerve	C69.6-☑	C79.49	—	D31.6-☑	D48.7	D49.2
bone	C41.0	C79.51	—	D16.4	D48.0	D49.2

	Malignant Primary	Malignant Secondary	Ca in situ	Benign	Uncertain	Unspecified Behavior
Neoplasm, neoplastic — continued						
orbit — continued						
eye	C69.6-✓	C79.49	D09.2-✓	D31.6-✓	D48.7	D49.89
peripheral nerves	C69.6-✓	C79.49	—	D31.6-✓	D48.7	D49.2
soft parts	C69.6-✓	C79.49	D09.2-✓	D31.6-✓	D48.7	D49.89
organ of Zuckerkandl	C75.5	C79.89	—	D35.6	D44.7	D49.7
oropharynx	C10.9	C79.89	D00.08	D10.5	D37.05	D49.0
branchial cleft (vestige)	C10.4	C79.89	D00.08	D10.5	D37.05	D49.0
junctional region	C10.8	C79.89	D00.08	D10.5	D37.05	D49.0
lateral wall	C10.2	C79.89	D00.08	D10.5	D37.05	D49.0
overlapping lesion	C10.8	—	—	—	—	—
pillars or fauces	C09.1	C79.89	D00.08	D10.5	D37.05	D49.0
posterior wall	C10.3	C79.89	D00.08	D10.5	D37.05	D49.0
vallecula	C10.0	C79.89	D00.08	D10.5	D37.05	D49.0
os						
external	C53.1	C79.82	D06.1	D26.0	D39.0	D49.59
internal	C53.0	C79.82	D06.0	D26.0	D39.0	D49.59
ovary	C56.-✓	C79.6-✓	D07.39	D27.-✓	D39.1-✓	D49.59
oviduct	C57.0-✓	C79.82	D07.39	D28.2	D39.8	D49.59
palate	C05.9	C79.89	D00.00	D10.39	D37.09	D49.0
hard	C05.0	C79.89	D00.05	D10.39	D37.09	D49.0
junction of hard and soft palate	C05.9	C79.89	D00.00	D10.39	D37.09	D49.0
overlapping lesions	C05.8	—	—	—	—	—
soft	C05.1	C79.89	D00.04	D10.39	D37.09	D49.0
nasopharyngeal surface	C11.3	C79.89	D00.08	D10.6	D37.05	D49.0
posterior surface	C11.3	C79.89	D00.08	D10.6	D37.05	D49.0
superior surface	C11.3	C79.89	D00.08	D10.6	D37.05	D49.0
palatoglossal arch	C09.1	C79.89	D00.00	D10.5	D37.09	D49.0
palatopharyngeal arch	C09.1	C79.89	D00.00	D10.5	D37.09	D49.0
pallium	C71.9	C79.31		D33.0	D43.0	D49.6
palpebra	C44.10-✓	C79.2	D04.1-✓	D23.1-✓	D48.5	D49.2
basal cell carcinoma	C44.11-✓	—	—	—	—	—
specified type NEC	C44.19-✓	—	—	—	—	—
squamous cell carcinoma	C44.12-✓	—	—	—	—	—
pancreas	C25.9	C78.89	D01.7	D13.6	D37.8	D49.0
body	C25.1	C78.89	D01.7	D13.6	D37.8	D49.0
duct (of Santorini) (of Wirsung)	C25.3	C78.89	D01.7	D13.6	D37.8	D49.0
ectopic tissue	C25.7	C78.89	—	D13.6	D37.8	D49.0
head	C25.0	C78.89	D01.7	D13.6	D37.8	D49.0
islet cells	C25.4	C78.89	D01.7	D13.7	D37.8	D49.0
neck	C25.7	C78.89	D01.7	D13.6	D37.8	D49.0
overlapping lesion	C25.8	—	—	—	—	—
tail	C25.2	C78.89	D01.7	D13.6	D37.8	D49.0
para-aortic body	C75.5	C79.89	—	D35.6	D44.7	D49.7
paraganglion NEC	C75.5	C79.89	—	D35.6	D44.7	D49.7
parametrium	C57.3	C79.82	—	D28.2	D39.8	D49.59
paranephric	C48.0	C78.6	—	D20.0	D48.3	D49.0
pararectal	C76.3	C79.89	—	D36.7	D48.7	D49.89
parasagittal (region)	C76.0	C79.89	D09.8	D36.7	D48.7	D49.89
parasellar	C72.9	C79.49	—	D33.9	D43.8	D49.7
parathyroid (gland)	C75.0	C79.89	D09.3	D35.1	D44.2	D49.7
paraurethral	C76.3	C79.89	—	D36.7	D48.7	D49.89
gland	C68.1	C79.19	D09.19	D30.8	D41.8	D49.59
paravaginal	C76.3	C79.89	—	D36.7	D48.7	D49.89
parenchyma, kidney	C64.-✓	C79.0-✓	D09.19	D30.0-✓	D41.0-✓	D49.51-✓
parietal						
bone	C41.0	C79.51		D16.4	D48.0	D49.2
lobe, brain	C71.3	C79.31	—	D33.0	D43.0	D49.6
paroophoron	C57.1-✓	C79.82	D07.39	D28.2	D39.8	D49.59
parotid (duct) (gland)	C07	C79.89	D00.00	D11.0	D37.030	D49.0
parovarium	C57.1-✓	C79.82	D07.39	D28.2	D39.8	D49.59
patella	C40.20	C79.51				
peduncle, cerebral	C71.7	C79.31	—	D33.1	D43.1	D49.6
pelvirectal junction	C19	C78.5	D01.1	D12.7	D37.5	D49.0
pelvis, pelvic	C76.3	C79.89	D09.8	D36.7	D48.7	D49.89
bone	C41.4	C79.51	—	D16.8	D48.0	D49.2
floor	C76.3	C79.89	D09.8	D36.7	D48.7	D49.89
renal	C65.-✓	C79.0-✓	D09.19	D30.1-✓	D41.1-✓	D49.51-✓
viscera	C76.3	C79.89	D09.8	D36.7	D48.7	D49.89
wall	C76.3	C79.89	D09.8	D36.7	D48.7	D49.89
pelvo-abdominal	C76.8	C79.89	D09.8	D36.7	D48.7	D49.89
penis	C60.9	C79.82	D07.4	D29.0	D40.8	D49.59

	Malignant Primary	Malignant Secondary	Ca in situ	Benign	Uncertain	Unspecified Behavior
Neoplasm, neoplastic — continued						
penis — continued						
body	C60.2	C79.82	D07.4	D29.0	D40.8	D49.59
corpus (cavernosum)	C60.2	C79.82	D07.4	D29.0	D40.8	D49.59
glans	C60.1	C79.82	D07.4	D29.0	D40.8	D49.59
overlapping sites	C60.8	—	—	—	—	—
skin NEC	C60.9	C79.82	D07.4	D29.0	D40.8	D49.59
periadrenal (tissue)	C48.0	C78.6	—	D20.0	D48.3	D49.0
perianal (skin) — see also Neoplasm, anus, skin	C44.500	C79.2	D04.5	D23.5	D48.5	D49.2
pericardium	C38.0	C79.89	—	D15.1	D48.7	D49.89
perinephric	C48.0	C78.6	—	D20.0	D48.3	D49.0
perineum	C76.3	C79.89	D09.8	D36.7	D48.7	D49.89
periodontal tissue NEC	C03.9	C79.89	D00.03	D10.39	D37.09	D49.0
periosteum — see Neoplasm, bone						
peripancreatic	C48.0	C78.6	—	D20.0	D48.3	D49.0
peripheral nerve NEC	C47.9	C79.89	—	D36.10	D48.2	D49.2
perirectal (tissue)	C76.3	C79.89	—	D36.7	D48.7	D49.89
perirenal (tissue)	C48.0	C78.6	—	D20.0	D48.3	D49.0
peritoneum, peritoneal (cavity)	C48.2	C78.6	—	D20.1	D48.4	D49.0
benign mesothelial tissue — see Mesothelioma, benign						
overlapping lesion with digestive organs	C26.9	—	—	—	—	—
parietal	C48.1	C78.6	—	D20.1	D48.4	D49.0
pelvic	C48.1	C78.6	—	D20.1	D48.4	D49.0
specified part NEC	C48.1	C78.6	—	D20.1	D48.4	D49.0
peritonsillar (tissue)	C76.0	C79.89	D09.8	D36.7	D48.7	D49.89
periurethral tissue	C76.3	C79.89	—	D36.7	D48.7	D49.89
phalanges						
foot	C40.3-✓	C79.51	—	D16.3-✓	—	—
hand	C40.1-✓	C79.51	—	D16.1-✓	—	—
pharynx, pharyngeal	C14.0	C79.89	D00.08	D10.9	D37.05	D49.0
bursa	C11.1	C79.89	D00.08	D10.6	D37.05	D49.0
fornix	C11.3	C79.89	D00.08	D10.6	D37.05	D49.0
recess	C11.2	C79.89	D00.08	D10.6	D37.05	D49.0
region	C14.0	C79.89	D00.08	D10.9	D37.05	D49.0
tonsil	C11.1	C79.89	D00.08	D10.6	D37.05	D49.0
wall (lateral) (posterior)	C14.0	C79.89	D00.08	D10.9	D37.05	D49.0
pia mater	C70.9	C79.40	—	D32.9	D42.9	D49.7
cerebral	C70.0	C79.32	—	D32.0	D42.0	D49.7
cranial	C70.0	C79.32	—	D32.0	D42.0	D49.7
spinal	C70.1	C79.49	—	D32.1	D42.1	D49.7
pillars of fauces	C09.1	C79.89	D00.08	D10.5	D37.05	D49.0
pineal (body) (gland)	C75.3	C79.89	D09.3	D35.4	D44.5	D49.7
pinna (ear) NEC — see also Neoplasm, skin, ear	C44.20-✓	C79.2	D04.2-✓	D23.2-✓	D48.5	D49.2
piriform fossa or sinus	C12	C79.89	D00.08	D10.7	D37.05	D49.0
pituitary (body) (fossa) (gland) (lobe)	C75.1	C79.89	D09.3	D35.2	D44.3	D49.7
placenta	C58	C79.82	D07.0	D26.7	D39.2	D49.59
pleura, pleural (cavity)	C38.4	C78.2	—	D19.0	D38.2	D49.1
overlapping lesion with heart or mediastinum	C38.8	—	—	—	—	—
parietal	C38.4	C78.2	—	D19.0	D38.2	D49.1
visceral	C38.4	C78.2	—	D19.0	D38.2	D49.1
plexus						
brachial	C47.1-✓	C79.89	—	D36.12	D48.2	D49.2
cervical	C47.0	C79.89	—	D36.11	D48.2	D49.2
choroid	C71.5	C79.31	—	D33.0	D43.0	D49.6
lumbosacral	C47.5	C79.89	—	D36.16	D48.2	D49.2
sacral	C47.5	C79.89	—	D36.16	D48.2	D49.2
pluriendocrine	C75.8	C79.89	D09.3	D35.7	D44.9	D49.7
pole						
frontal	C71.1	C79.31	—	D33.0	D43.0	D49.6
occipital	C71.4	C79.31	—	D33.0	D43.0	D49.6
pons (varolii)	C71.7	C79.31	—	D33.1	D43.1	D49.6

Neoplasm Table

Neoplasm, orbit — Neoplasm, pons

Neoplasm, neoplastic — continued	Malignant Primary	Malignant Secondary	Ca in situ	Benign	Uncertain	Unspecified Behavior
popliteal fossa or space	C76.5-☑	C79.89	D04.7-☑	D36.7	D48.7	D49.89
postcricoid (region)	C13.0	C79.89	D00.08	D10.7	D37.05	D49.0
posterior fossa (cranial)	C71.9	C79.31	—	D33.2	D43.2	D49.6
postnasal space	C11.9	C79.89	D00.08	D10.6	D37.05	D49.0
prepuce	C60.0	C79.82	D07.4	D29.0	D40.8	D49.59
prepylorus	C16.4	C78.89	D00.2	D13.1	D37.1	D49.0
presacral (region)	C76.3	C79.89	—	D36.7	D48.7	D49.89
prostate (gland)	C61	C79.82	D07.5	D29.1	D40.0	D49.59
utricle	C68.0	C79.19	D09.19	D30.4	D41.3	D49.59
pterygoid fossa	C49.0	C79.89	—	D21.0	D48.1	D49.2
pubic bone	C41.4	C79.51	—	D16.8	D48.0	D49.2
pudenda, pudendum (femaie)	C51.9	C79.82	D07.1	D28.0	D39.8	D49.59
pulmonary — see also Neoplasm, lung	C34.9-☑	C78.0-☑	D02.2-☑	D14.3-☑	D38.1	D49.1
putamen	C71.0	C79.31	—	D33.0	D43.0	D49.6
pyloric						
antrum	C16.3	C78.89	D00.2	D13.1	D37.1	D49.0
canal	C16.4	C78.89	D00.2	D13.1	D37.1	D49.0
pylorus	C16.4	C78.89	D00.2	D13.1	D37.1	D49.0
pyramid (brain)	C71.7	C79.31	—	D33.1	D43.1	D49.6
pyriform fossa or sinus	C12	C79.89	D00.08	D10.7	D37.05	D49.0
radius (any part)	C40.0-☑	C79.51	—	D16.0-☑	—	—
Rathke's pouch	C75.1	C79.89	D09.3	D35.2	D44.3	D49.7
rectosigmoid (junction)	C19	C78.5	D01.1	D12.7	D37.5	D49.0
overlapping lesion with anus or rectum	C21.8	—	—	—	—	—
rectouterine pouch	C48.1	C78.6	—	D20.1	D48.4	D49.0
rectovaginal septum or wall	C76.3	C79.89	D09.8	D36.7	D48.7	D49.89
rectovesical septum	C76.3	C79.89	D09.8	D36.7	D48.7	D49.89
rectum (ampulla)	C20	C78.5	D01.2	D12.8	D37.5	D49.0
and colon	C19	C78.5	D01.1	D12.7	D37.5	D49.0
overlapping lesion with anus or rectosigmoid junction	C21.8	—	—	—	—	—
renal	C64.-☑	C79.0-☑	D09.19	D30.0-☑	D41.0-☑	D49.51-☑
calyx	C65.-☑	C79.0-☑	D09.19	D30.1-☑	D41.1-☑	D49.51-☑
hilus	C65.-☑	C79.0-☑	D09.19	D30.1-☑	D41.1-☑	D49.51-☑
parenchyma	C64.-☑	C79.0-☑	D09.19	D30.0-☑	D41.0-☑	D49.51-☑
pelvis	C65.-☑	C79.0-☑	D09.19	D30.1-☑	D41.1-☑	D49.51-☑
respiratory						
organs or system NEC	C39.9	C78.30	D02.4	D14.4	D38.6	D49.1
tract NEC	C39.9	C78.30	D02.4	D14.4	D38.5	D49.1
upper	C39.0	C78.30	D02.4	D14.4	D38.5	D49.1
retina	C69.2-☑	C79.49	D09.2-☑	D31.2-☑	D48.7	D49.81
retrobulbar	C69.6-☑	C79.49	—	D31.6-☑	D48.7	D49.89
retrocecal	C48.0	C78.6	—	D20.0	D48.3	D49.0
retromolar (area) (triangle) (trigone)	C06.2	C79.89	D00.00	D10.39	D37.09	D49.0
retro-orbital	C76.0	C79.89	D09.8	D36.7	D48.7	D49.89
retroperitoneal (space) (tissue)	C48.0	C78.6	—	D20.0	D48.3	D49.0
retroperitoneum	C48.0	C78.6	—	D20.0	D48.3	D49.0
retropharyngeal	C14.0	C79.89	D00.08	D10.9	D37.05	D49.0
retrovesical (septum)	C76.3	C79.89	D09.8	D36.7	D48.7	D49.89
rhinencephalon	C71.0	C79.31	—	D33.0	D43.0	D49.6
rib	C41.3	C79.51	—	D16.7	D48.0	D49.2
Rosenmuller's fossa	C11.2	C79.89	D00.08	D10.6	D37.05	D49.0
round ligament	C57.2-☑	C79.82	—	D28.2	D39.8	D49.59
sacrococcyx, sacrococcygeal	C41.4	C79.51	—	D16.8	D48.0	D49.2
region	C76.3	C79.89	D09.8	D36.7	D48.7	D49.89
sacrouterine ligament	C57.3	C79.82	—	D28.2	D39.8	D49.59
sacrum, sacral (vertebra)	C41.4	C79.51	—	D16.8	D48.0	D49.2
salivary gland or duct (major)	C08.9	C79.89	D00.00	D11.9	D37.039	D49.0
minor NEC	C06.9	C79.89	D00.00	D10.39	D37.04	D49.0
overlapping lesion	C08.9	—	—	—	—	—
parotid	C07	C79.89	D00.00	D11.0	D37.030	D49.0

Neoplasm, neoplastic — continued	Malignant Primary	Malignant Secondary	Ca in situ	Benign	Uncertain	Unspecified Behavior
salivary gland or duct — continued						
pluriglandular	C08.9	C79.89	D00.00	D11.9	D37.039	D49.0
sublingual	C08.1	C79.89	D00.00	D11.7	D37.031	D49.0
submandibular	C08.0	C79.89	D00.00	D11.7	D37.032	D49.0
submaxillary	C08.0	C79.89	D00.00	D11.7	D37.032	D49.0
salpinx (uterine)	C57.0-☑	C79.82	D07.39	D28.2	D39.8	D49.59
Santorini's duct	C25.3	C78.89	D01.7	D13.6	D37.8	D49.0
scalp	C44.40	C79.2	D04.4	D23.4	D48.5	D49.2
basal cell carcinoma	C44.41	—	—	—	—	—
specified type NEC	C44.49	—	—	—	—	—
squamous cell carcinoma	C44.42	—	—	—	—	—
scapula (any part)	C40.0-☑	C79.51	—	D16.0-☑	—	—
scapular region	C76.1	C79.89	D09.8	D36.7	D48.7	D49.89
scar NEC — see also Neoplasm, skin, by site	C44.90	C79.2	D04.9	D23.9	D48.5	D49.2
sciatic nerve	C47.2-☑	C79.89	—	D36.13	D48.2	D49.2
sclera	C69.4-☑	C79.49	D09.2-☑	D31.4-☑	D48.7	D49.89
scrotum (skin)	C63.2	C79.82	D07.61	D29.4	D40.8	D49.59
sebaceous gland — see Neoplasm, skin						
sella turcica	C75.1	C79.89	D09.3	D35.2	D44.3	D49.7
bone	C41.0	C79.51	—	D16.4	D48.0	D49.2
semilunar cartilage (knee)	C40.2-☑	C79.51	—	D16.2-☑	D48.0	D49.2
seminal vesicle	C63.7	C79.82	D07.69	D29.8	D40.8	D49.59
septum						
nasal	C30.0	C78.39	D02.3	D14.0	D38.5	D49.1
posterior margin	C11.3	C79.89	D00.08	D10.6	D37.05	D49.0
rectovaginal	C76.3	C79.89	D09.8	D36.7	D48.7	D49.89
rectovesical	C76.3	C79.89	D09.8	D36.7	D48.7	D49.89
urethrovaginal	C57.9	C79.82	D07.30	D28.9	D39.9	D49.59
vesicovaginal	C57.9	C79.82	D07.30	D28.9	D39.9	D49.59
shoulder NEC	C76.4-☑	C79.89	D04.6-☑	D36.7	D48.7	D49.89
sigmoid flexure (lower) (upper)	C18.7	C78.5	D01.0	D12.5	D37.4	D49.0
sinus (accessory)	C31.9	C78.39	D02.3	D14.0	D38.5	D49.1
bone (any)	C41.0	C79.51	—	D16.4	D48.0	D49.2
ethmoidal	C31.1	C78.39	D02.3	D14.0	D38.5	D49.1
frontal	C31.2	C78.39	D02.3	D14.0	D38.5	D49.1
maxillary	C31.0	C78.39	D02.3	D14.0	D38.5	D49.1
nasal, paranasal NEC	C31.9	C78.39	D02.3	D14.0	D38.5	D49.1
overlapping lesion	C31.8	—	—	—	—	—
pyriform	C12	C79.89	D00.08	D10.7	D37.05	D49.0
sphenoid	C31.3	C78.39	D02.3	D14.0	D38.5	D49.1
skeleton, skeletal NEC	C41.9	C79.51	—	D16.9	D48.0	D49.2
Skene's gland	C68.1	C79.19	D09.19	D30.8	D41.8	D49.59
skin NOS	C44.90	C79.2	D04.9	D23.9	D48.5	D49.2
abdominal wall	C44.509	C79.2	D04.5	D23.5	D48.5	D49.2
basal cell carcinoma	C44.519	—	—	—	—	—
specified type NEC	C44.599	—	—	—	—	—
squamous cell carcinoma	C44.529	—	—	—	—	—
ala nasi — see also Neoplasm, nose, skin	C44.301	C79.2	D04.39	D23.39	D48.5	D49.2
ankle — see also Neoplasm, skin, limb, lower	C44.70-☑	C79.2	D04.7-☑	D23.7-☑	D48.5	D49.2
antecubital space — see also Neoplasm, skin, limb, upper	C44.60-☑	C79.2	D04.6-☑	D23.6-☑	D48.5	D49.2
anus	C44.500	C79.2	D04.5	D23.5	D48.5	D49.2
basal cell carcinoma	C44.510	—	—	—	—	—
specified type NEC	C44.590	—	—	—	—	—
squamous cell carcinoma	C44.520	—	—	—	—	—
arm — see also Neoplasm, skin, limb, upper	C44.60-☑	C79.2	D04.6-☑	D23.6-☑	D48.5	D49.2

Neoplasm Table

Neoplasm, neoplastic —	Malignant Primary	Malignant Secondary	Ca in situ	Benign	Uncertain	Unspecified Behavior
continued						
skin — *continued*						
auditory canal (external) — *see also* Neoplasm, skin, ear	C44.20-☑	C79.2	D04.2-☑	D23.2-☑	D48.5	D49.2
auricle (ear) — *see also* Neoplasm, skin, ear	C44.20-☑	C79.2	D04.2-☑	D23.2-☑	D48.5	D49.2
auricular canal (external) — *see also* Neoplasm, skin, ear	C44.20-☑	C79.2	D04.2-☑	D23.2-☑	D48.5	D49.2
axilla, axillary fold — *see also* Neoplasm, skin, trunk	C44.509	C79.2	D04.5	D23.5	D48.5	D49.2
back — *see also* Neoplasm, skin, trunk	C44.509	C79.2	D04.5	D23.5	D48.5	D49.2
basal cell carcinoma	C44.91	—	—	—	—	—
breast	C44.501	C79.2	D04.5	D23.5	D48.5	D49.2
basal cell carcinoma	C44.511	—	—	—	—	—
specified type NEC	C44.591	—	—	—	—	—
squamous cell carcinoma	C44.521	—	—	—	—	—
brow — *see also* Neoplasm, skin, face	C44.309	C79.2	D04.39	D23.39	D48.5	D49.2
buttock — *see also* Neoplasm, skin, trunk	C44.509	C79.2	D04.5	D23.5	D48.5	D49.2
calf — *see also* Neoplasm, skin, limb, lower	C44.70-☑	C79.2	D04.7-☑	D23.7-☑	D48.5	D49.2
canthus (eye) (inner) (outer)	C44.10-☑	C79.2	D04.1-☑	D23.1-☑	D48.5	D49.2
basal cell carcinoma	C44.11-☑	—	—	—	—	—
specified type NEC	C44.19-☑	—	—	—	—	—
squamous cell carcinoma	C44.12-☑	—	—	—	—	—
cervical region — *see also* Neoplasm, skin, neck	C44.40	C79.2	D04.4	D23.4	D48.5	D49.2
cheek (external) — *see also* Neoplasm, skin, face	C44.309	C79.2	D04.39	D23.39	D48.5	D49.2
chest (wall) — *see also* Neoplasm, skin, trunk	C44.509	C79.2	D04.5	D23.5	D48.5	D49.2
chin — *see also* Neoplasm, skin, face	C44.309	C79.2	D04.39	D23.39	D48.5	D49.2
clavicular area — *see also* Neoplasm, skin, trunk	C44.509	C79.2	D04.5	D23.5	D48.5	D49.2
clitoris	C51.2	C79.82	D07.1	D28.0	D39.8	D49.59
columnella — *see also* Neoplasm, skin, face	C44.309	C79.2	D04.39	D23.39	D48.5	D49.2
concha — *see also* Neoplasm, skin, ear	C44.20-☑	C79.2	D04.2-☑	D23.2-☑	D48.5	D49.2
ear (external)	C44.20-☑	C79.2	D04.2-☑	D23.2-☑	D48.5	D49.2
basal cell carcinoma	C44.21-☑	—	—	—	—	—
specified type NEC	C44.29-☑	—	—	—	—	—
squamous cell carcinoma	C44.22-☑	—	—	—	—	—
elbow — *see also* Neoplasm, skin, limb, upper	C44.60-☑	C79.2	D04.6-☑	D23.6-☑	D48.5	D49.2
eyebrow — *see also* Neoplasm, skin, face	C44.309	C79.2	D04.39	D23.39	D48.5	D49.2
eyelid	C44.10-☑	C79.2	D04.1-☑	D23.1-☑	D48.5	D49.2

Neoplasm, neoplastic —	Malignant Primary	Malignant Secondary	Ca in situ	Benign	Uncertain	Unspecified Behavior
continued						
skin — *continued*						
eyelid — *continued*						
basal cell carcinoma	C44.11-☑	—	—	—	—	—
specified type NEC	C44.19-☑	—	—	—	—	—
squamous cell carcinoma	C44.12-☑	—	—	—	—	—
face NOS	C44.300	C79.2	D04.30	D23.30	D48.5	D49.2
basal cell carcinoma	C44.310	—	—	—	—	—
specified type NEC	C44.390	—	—	—	—	—
squamous cell carcinoma	C44.320	—	—	—	—	—
female genital organs (external)	C51.9	C79.82	D07.1	D28.0	D39.8	D49.59
clitoris	C51.2	C79.82	D07.1	D28.0	D39.8	D49.59
labium NEC	C51.9	C79.82	D07.1	D28.0	D39.8	D49.59
majus	C51.0	C79.82	D07.1	D28.0	D39.8	D49.59
minus	C51.1	C79.82	D07.1	D28.0	D39.8	D49.59
pudendum	C51.9	C79.82	D07.1	D28.0	D39.8	D49.59
vulva	C51.9	C79.82	D07.1	D28.0	D39.8	D49.59
finger — *see also* Neoplasm, skin, limb, upper	C44.60-☑	C79.2	D04.6-☑	D23.6-☑	D48.5	D49.2
flank — *see also* Neoplasm, skin, trunk	C44.509	C79.2	D04.5	D23.5	D48.5	D49.2
foot — *see also* Neoplasm, skin, limb, lower	C44.70-☑	C79.2	D04.7-☑	D23.7-☑	D48.5	D49.2
forearm — *see also* Neoplasm, skin, limb, upper	C44.60-☑	C79.2	D04.6-☑	D23.6-☑	D48.5	D49.2
forehead — *see also* Neoplasm, skin, face	C44.309	C79.2	D04.39	D23.39	D48.5	D49.2
glabella — *see also* Neoplasm, skin, face	C44.309	C79.2	D04.39	D23.39	D48.5	D49.2
gluteal region — *see also* Neoplasm, skin, trunk	C44.509	C79.2	D04.5	D23.5	D48.5	D49.2
groin — *see also* Neoplasm, skin, trunk	C44.509	C79.2	D04.5	D23.5	D48.5	D49.2
hand — *see also* Neoplasm, skin, limb, upper	C44.60-☑	C79.2	D04.6-☑	D23.6-☑	D48.5	D49.2
head NEC — *see also* Neoplasm, skin, scalp	C44.40	C79.2	D04.4	D23.4	D48.5	D49.2
heel — *see also* Neoplasm, skin, limb, lower	C44.70-☑	C79.2	D04.7-☑	D23.7-☑	D48.5	D49.2
helix — *see also* Neoplasm, skin, ear	C44.20-☑	C79.2	D04.2-☑	D23.2-☑	D48.5	D49.2
hip — *see also* Neoplasm, skin, limb, lower	C44.70-☑	C79.2	D04.7-☑	D23.7-☑	D48.5	D49.2
infraclavicular region — *see also* Neoplasm, skin, trunk	C44.509	C79.2	D04.5	D23.5	D48.5	D49.2
inguinal region — *see also* Neoplasm, skin, trunk	C44.509	C79.2	D04.5	D23.5	D48.5	D49.2
jaw — *see also* Neoplasm, skin, face	C44.309	C79.2	D04.39	D23.39	D48.5	D49.2
Kaposi's sarcoma — *see* Kaposi's, sarcoma, skin						
knee — *see also* Neoplasm, skin, limb, lower	C44.70-☑	C79.2	D04.7-☑	D23.7-☑	D48.5	D49.2
labia						
majora	C51.0	C79.82	D07.1	D28.0	D39.8	D49.59
minora	C51.1	C79.82	D07.1	D28.0	D39.8	D49.59

☑ Additional Character Required — Refer to the Tabular List for Character Selection   ▽ Subterms under main terms may continue to next column or page

	Malignant Primary	Malignant Secondary	Ca in situ	Benign	Uncertain	Unspecified Behavior
Neoplasm, neoplastic —						
continued						
skin — *continued*						
leg — *see also*						
Neoplasm, skin,						
limb, lower	C44.70-☑	C79.2	D04.7-☑	D23.7-☑	D48.5	D49.2
lid (lower) (upper)	C44.10-☑	C79.2	D04.1-☑	D23.1-☑	D48.5	D49.2
basal cell						
carcinoma	C44.11-☑	—	—	—	—	—
specified type						
NEC	C44.19-☑	—	—	—	—	—
squamous cell						
carcinoma	C44.12-☑	—	—	—	—	—
limb NEC	C44.90	C79.2	D04.9	D23.9	D48.5	D49.2
basal cell						
carcinoma	C44.91	—	—	—	—	—
lower	C44.70-☑	C79.2	D04.7-☑	D23.7-☑	D48.5	D49.2
basal cell						
carcinoma	C44.71-☑	—	—	—	—	—
specified type						
NEC	C44.79-☑	—	—	—	—	—
squamous cell						
carcinoma	C44.72-☑	—	—	—	—	—
upper	C44.60-☑	C79.2	D04.6-☑	D23.6-☑	D48.5	D49.2
basal cell						
carcinoma	C44.61-☑	—	—	—	—	—
specified type						
NEC	C44.69-☑	—	—	—	—	—
squamous cell						
carcinoma	C44.62-☑	—	—	—	—	—
lip (lower) (upper)	C44.00	C79.2	D04.0	D23.0	D48.5	D49.2
basal cell						
carcinoma	C44.01					
specified type						
NEC	C44.09	—	—	—	—	—
squamous cell						
carcinoma	C44.02	—	—	—	—	—
male genital						
organs	C63.9	C79.82	D07.60	D29.9	D40.8	D49.59
penis	C60.9	C79.82	D07.4	D29.0	D40.8	D49.59
prepuce	C60.0	C79.82	D07.4	D29.0	D40.8	D49.59
scrotum	C63.2	C79.82	D07.61	D29.4	D40.8	D49.59
mastectomy site (skin)						
— *see also*						
Neoplasm, skin,						
breast	C44.501	C79.2	—	—	—	—
specified as breast						
tissue	C50.8-☑	C79.81	—	—	—	—
meatus, acoustic						
(external) — *see*						
also Neoplasm, skin,						
ear	C44.20-☑	C79.2	D04.2-☑	D23.2-☑	D48.5	D49.2
melanotic — *see*						
Melanoma						
Merkel cell — *see*						
Carcinoma, Merkel						
cell						
nates — *see also*						
Neoplasm, skin,						
trunk	C44.509	C79.2	D04.5	D23.5	D48.5	D49.2
neck	C44.40	C79.2	D04.4	D23.4	D48.5	D49.2
basal cell						
carcinoma	C44.41	—	—	—	—	—
specified type						
NEC	C44.49	—	—	—	—	—
squamous cell						
carcinoma	C44.42	—	—	—	—	—
nevus — *see* Nevus,						
skin						
nose (external) — *see*						
also Neoplasm,						
nose, skin	C44.301	C79.2	D04.39	D23.39	D48.5	D49.2
overlapping lesion	C44.80	—	—	—	—	—
basal cell						
carcinoma	C44.81	—	—	—	—	—
specified type						
NEC	C44.89	—	—	—	—	—
squamous cell						
carcinoma	C44.82	—	—	—	—	—
palm — *see also*						
Neoplasm, skin,						
limb, upper	C44.60-☑	C79.2	D04.6-☑	D23.6-☑	D48.5	D49.2
palpebra	C44.10-☑	C79.2	D04.1-☑	D23.1-☑	D48.5	D49.2

	Malignant Primary	Malignant Secondary	Ca in situ	Benign	Uncertain	Unspecified Behavior
Neoplasm, neoplastic —						
continued						
skin — *continued*						
palpebra — *continued*						
basal cell						
carcinoma	C44.11-☑	—	—	—	—	—
specified type						
NEC	C44.19-☑	—	—	—	—	—
squamous cell						
carcinoma	C44.12-☑	—	—	—	—	—
penis NEC	C60.9	C79.82	D07.4	D29.0	D40.8	D49.59
perianal — *see also*						
Neoplasm, skin,						
anus	C44.500	C79.2	D04.5	D23.5	D48.5	D49.2
perineum — *see also*						
Neoplasm, skin,						
anus	C44.500	C79.2	D04.5	D23.5	D48.5	D49.2
pinna — *see also*						
Neoplasm, skin,						
ear	C44.20-☑	C79.2	D04.2-☑	D23.2-☑	D48.5	D49.2
plantar — *see also*						
Neoplasm, skin,						
limb, lower	C44.70-☑	C79.2	D04.7-☑	D23.7-☑	D48.5	D49.2
popliteal fossa or space						
— *see also*						
Neoplasm, skin,						
limb, lower	C44.70-☑	C79.2	D04.7-☑	D23.7-☑	D48.5	D49.2
prepuce	C60.0	C79.82	D07.4	D29.0	D40.8	D49.59
pubes — *see also*						
Neoplasm, skin,						
trunk	C44.509	C79.2	D04.5	D23.5	D48.5	D49.2
sacrococcygeal region						
— *see also*						
Neoplasm, skin,						
trunk	C44.509	C79.2	D04.5	D23.5	D48.5	D49.2
scalp	C44.40	C79.2	D04.4	D23.4	D48.5	D49.2
basal cell						
carcinoma	C44.41	—	—	—	—	—
specified type						
NEC	C44.49	—	—	—	—	—
squamous cell						
carcinoma	C44.42	—	—	—	—	—
scapular region — *see*						
also Neoplasm, skin,						
trunk	C44.509	C79.2	D04.5	D23.5	D48.5	D49.2
scrotum	C63.2	C79.82	D07.61	D29.4	D40.8	D49.59
shoulder — *see also*						
Neoplasm, skin,						
limb, upper	C44.60-☑	C79.2	D04.6-☑	D23.6-☑	D48.5	D49.2
sole (foot) — *see also*						
Neoplasm, skin,						
limb, lower	C44.70-☑	C79.2	D04.7-☑	D23.7-☑	D48.5	D49.2
specified sites NEC	C44.80	C79.2	D04.8	D23.9	D48.5	D49.2
basal cell						
carcinoma	C44.81	—	—	—	—	—
specified type						
NEC	C44.89	—	—	—	—	—
squamous cell						
carcinoma	C44.82	—	—	—	—	—
specified type NEC	C44.99	—	—	—	—	—
squamous cell						
carcinoma	C44.92	—	—	—	—	—
submammary fold —						
see also Neoplasm,						
skin, trunk	C44.509	C79.2	D04.5	D23.5	D48.5	D49.2
supraclavicular region						
— *see also*						
Neoplasm, skin,						
neck	C44.40	C79.2	D04.4	D23.4	D48.5	D49.2
temple — *see also*						
Neoplasm, skin,						
face	C44.309	C79.2	D04.39	D23.39	D48.5	D49.2
thigh — *see also*						
Neoplasm, skin,						
limb, lower	C44.70-☑	C79.2	D04.7-☑	D23.7-☑	D48.5	D49.2
thoracic wall — *see also*						
Neoplasm, skin,						
trunk	C44.509	C79.2	D04.5	D23.5	D48.5	D49.2
thumb — *see also*						
Neoplasm, skin,						
limb, upper	C44.60-☑	C79.2	D04.6-☑	D23.6-☑	D48.5	D49.2
toe — *see also*						
Neoplasm, skin,						
limb, lower	C44.70-☑	C79.2	D04.7-☑	D23.7-☑	D48.5	D49.2

	Malignant Primary	Malignant Secondary	Ca in situ	Benign	Uncertain	Unspecified Behavior
Neoplasm, neoplastic — *continued*						
skin — *continued*						
tragus — *see also* Neoplasm, skin, ear	C44.20-☑	C79.2	D04.2-☑	D23.2-☑	D48.5	D49.2
trunk	C44.509	C79.2	D04.5	D23.5	D48.5	D49.2
basal cell carcinoma	C44.519	—	—	—	—	—
specified type NEC	C44.599	—	—	—	—	—
squamous cell carcinoma	C44.529	—	—	—	—	—
umbilicus — *see also* Neoplasm, skin, trunk	C44.509	C79.2	D04.5	D23.5	D48.5	D49.2
vulva	C51.9	C79.82	D07.1	D28.0	D39.8	D49.59
overlapping lesion	C51.8	—	—	—	—	—
wrist — *see also* Neoplasm, skin, limb, upper	C44.60-☑	C79.2	D04.6-☑	D23.6-☑	D48.5	D49.2
skull	C41.0	C79.51	—	D16.4	D48.0	D49.2
soft parts or tissues — *see* Neoplasm, connective tissue						
specified site NEC	C76.8	C79.89	D09.8	D36.7	D48.7	D49.89
spermatic cord	C63.1-☑	C79.82	D07.69	D29.8	D40.8	D49.59
sphenoid	C31.3	C78.39	D02.3	D14.0	D38.5	D49.1
bone	C41.0	C79.51	—	D16.4	D48.0	D49.2
sinus	C31.3	C78.39	D02.3	D14.0	D38.5	D49.1
sphincter						
anal	C21.1	C78.5	D01.3	D12.9	D37.8	D49.0
of Oddi	C24.0	C78.89	D01.5	D13.5	D37.6	D49.0
spine, spinal (column)	C41.2	C79.51	—	D16.6	D48.0	D49.2
bulb	C71.7	C79.31	—	D33.1	D43.1	D49.6
coccyx	C41.4	C79.51	—	D16.8	D48.0	D49.2
cord (cervical) (lumbar) (sacral) (thoracic)	C72.0	C79.49	—	D33.4	D43.4	D49.7
dura mater	C70.1	C79.49	—	D32.1	D42.1	D49.7
lumbosacral	C41.2	C79.51	—	D16.6	D48.0	D49.2
marrow NEC	C96.9	C79.52	—	—	D47.9	D49.89
membrane	C70.1	C79.49	—	D32.1	D42.1	D49.7
meninges	C70.1	C79.49	—	D32.1	D42.1	D49.7
nerve (root)	C47.9	C79.89	—	D36.10	D48.2	D49.2
pia mater	C70.1	C79.49	—	D32.1	D42.1	D49.7
root	C47.9	C79.89	—	D36.10	D48.2	D49.2
sacrum	C41.4	C79.51	—	D16.8	D48.0	D49.2
spleen, splenic NEC	C26.1	C78.89	D01.7	D13.9	D37.8	D49.0
flexure (colon)	C18.5	C78.5	D01.0	D12.3	D37.4	D49.0
stem, brain	C71.7	C79.31	—	D33.1	D43.1	D49.6
Stensen's duct	C07	C79.89	D00.00	D11.0	D37.030	D49.0
sternum	C41.3	C79.51	—	D16.7	D48.0	D49.2
stomach	C16.9	C78.89	D00.2	D13.1	D37.1	D49.0
antrum (pyloric)	C16.3	C78.89	D00.2	D13.1	D37.1	D49.0
body	C16.2	C78.89	D00.2	D13.1	D37.1	D49.0
cardia	C16.0	C78.89	D00.2	D13.1	D37.1	D49.0
cardiac orifice	C16.0	C78.89	D00.2	D13.1	D37.1	D49.0
corpus	C16.2	C78.89	D00.2	D13.1	D37.1	D49.0
fundus	C16.1	C78.89	D00.2	D13.1	D37.1	D49.0
greater curvature NEC	C16.6	C78.89	D00.2	D13.1	D37.1	D49.0
lesser curvature NEC	C16.5	C78.89	D00.2	D13.1	D37.1	D49.0
overlapping lesion	C16.8	—	—	—	—	—
prepylorus	C16.4	C78.89	D00.2	D13.1	D37.1	D49.0
pylorus	C16.4	C78.89	D00.2	D13.1	D37.1	D49.0
wall NEC	C16.9	C78.89	D00.2	D13.1	D37.1	D49.0
anterior NEC	C16.8	C78.89	D00.2	D13.1	D37.1	D49.0
posterior NEC	C16.8	C78.89	D00.2	D13.1	D37.1	D49.0
stroma, endometrial	C54.1	C79.82	D07.0	D26.1	D39.0	D49.59
stump, cervical	C53.8	C79.82	D06.7	D26.0	D39.0	D49.59
subcutaneous (nodule) (tissue) NEC — *see* Neoplasm, connective tissue						
subdural	C70.9	C79.32	—	D32.9	D42.9	D49.7
subglottis, subglottic	C32.2	C78.39	D02.0	D14.1	D38.0	D49.1
sublingual	C04.9	C79.89	D00.06	D10.2	D37.09	D49.0
gland or duct	C08.1	C79.89	D00.00	D11.7	D37.031	D49.0

	Malignant Primary	Malignant Secondary	Ca in situ	Benign	Uncertain	Unspecified Behavior
Neoplasm, neoplastic — *continued*						
submandibular gland	C08.0	C79.89	D00.00	D11.7	D37.032	D49.0
submaxillary gland or duct	C08.0	C79.89	D00.00	D11.7	D37.032	D49.0
submental	C76.0	C79.89	D09.8	D36.7	D48.7	D49.89
subpleural	C34.9-☑	C78.0-☑	D02.2-☑	D14.3-☑	D38.1	D49.1
substernal	C38.1	C78.1	—	D15.2	D38.3	D49.89
sudoriferous, sudoriparous gland, site unspecified	C44.90	C79.2	D04.9	D23.9	D48.5	D49.2
specified site — *see* Neoplasm, skin						
supraclavicular region	C76.0	C79.89	D09.8	D36.7	D48.7	D49.89
supraglottis	C32.1	C78.39	D02.0	D14.1	D38.0	D49.1
suprarenal	C74.9-☑	C79.7-☑	D09.3	D35.0-☑	D44.1-☑	D49.7
capsule	C74.9-☑	C79.7-☑	D09.3	D35.0-☑	D44.1-☑	D49.7
cortex	C74.0-☑	C79.7-☑	D09.3	D35.0-☑	D44.1-☑	D49.7
gland	C74.9-☑	C79.7-☑	D09.3	D35.0-☑	D44.1-☑	D49.7
medulla	C74.1-☑	C79.7-☑	D09.3	D35.0-☑	D44.1-☑	D49.7
suprasellar (region)	C71.9	C79.31	—	D33.2	D43.2	D49.6
supratentorial (brain) NEC	C71.0	C79.31	—	D33.0	D43.0	D49.6
sweat gland (apocrine) (eccrine), site unspecified	C44.90	C79.2	D04.9	D23.9	D48.5	D49.2
specified site — *see* Neoplasm, skin						
sympathetic nerve or nervous system NEC	C47.9	C79.89	—	D36.10	D48.2	D49.2
symphysis pubis	C41.4	C79.51	—	D16.8	D48.0	D49.2
synovial membrane — *see* Neoplasm, connective tissue						
tapetum, brain	C71.8	C79.31	—	D33.2	D43.2	D49.6
tarsus (any bone)	C40.3-☑	C79.51	—	D16.3-☑	—	—
temple (skin) — *see also* Neoplasm, skin, face	C44.309	C79.2	D04.39	D23.39	D48.5	D49.2
temporal						
bone	C41.0	C79.51	—	D16.4	D48.0	D49.2
lobe or pole	C71.2	C79.31	—	D33.0	D43.0	D49.6
region	C76.0	C79.89	D09.8	D36.7	D48.7	D49.89
skin — *see also* Neoplasm, skin, face	C44.309	C79.2	D04.39	D23.39	D48.5	D49.2
tendon (sheath) — *see* Neoplasm, connective tissue						
tentorium (cerebelli)	C70.0	C79.32	—	D32.0	D42.0	D49.7
testis, testes	C62.9-☑	C79.82	D07.69	D29.2-☑	D40.1-☑	D49.59
descended	C62.1-☑	C79.82	D07.69	D29.2-☑	D40.1-☑	D49.59
ectopic	C62.0-☑	C79.82	D07.69	D29.2-☑	D40.1-☑	D49.59
retained	C62.0-☑	C79.82	D07.69	D29.2-☑	D40.1-☑	D49.59
scrotal	C62.1-☑	C79.82	D07.69	D29.2-☑	D40.1-☑	D49.59
undescended	C62.0-☑	C79.82	D07.69	D29.2-☑	D40.1-☑	D49.59
unspecified whether descended or undescended	C62.9-☑	C79.82	D07.69	D29.2-☑	D40.1-☑	D49.59
thalamus	C71.0	C79.31	—	D33.0	D43.0	D49.6
thigh NEC	C76.5-☑	C79.89	D04.7-☑	D36.7	D48.7	D49.89
thorax, thoracic (cavity) (organs NEC)	C76.1	C79.89	D09.8	D36.7	D48.7	D49.89
duct	C49.3	C79.89	—	D21.3	D48.1	D49.2
wall NEC	C76.1	C79.89	D09.8	D36.7	D48.7	D49.89
throat	C14.0	C79.89	D00.08	D10.9	D37.05	D49.0
thumb NEC	C76.4-☑	C79.89	D04.6-☑	D36.7	D48.7	D49.89
thymus (gland)	C37	C79.89	D09.3	D15.0	D38.4	D49.89
thyroglossal duct	C73	C79.89	D09.3	D34	D44.0	D49.7
thyroid (gland)	C73	C79.89	D09.3	D34	D44.0	D49.7
cartilage	C32.3	C78.39	D02.0	D14.1	D38.0	D49.1
tibia (any part)	C40.2-☑	C79.51	—	D16.2-☑	—	—
toe NEC	C76.5-☑	C79.89	D04.7-☑	D36.7	D48.7	D49.89
tongue	C02.9	C79.89	D00.07	D10.1	D37.02	D49.0
anterior (two-thirds) NEC	C02.3	C79.89	D00.07	D10.1	D37.02	D49.0
dorsal surface	C02.0	C79.89	D00.07	D10.1	D37.02	D49.0
ventral surface	C02.2	C79.89	D00.07	D10.1	D37.02	D49.0

Neoplasm, neoplastic — continued

	Malignant Primary	Malignant Secondary	Ca in situ	Benign	Uncertain	Unspecified Behavior
tongue — *continued*						
base (dorsal surface)	C01	C79.89	D00.07	D10.1	D37.02	D49.0
border (lateral)	C02.1	C79.89	D00.07	D10.1	D37.02	D49.0
dorsal surface NEC	C02.0	C79.89	D00.07	D10.1	D37.02	D49.0
fixed part NEC	C01	C79.89	D00.07	D10.1	D37.02	D49.0
foreamen cecum	C02.0	C79.89	D00.07	D10.1	D37.02	D49.0
frenulum linguae	C02.2	C79.89	D00.07	D10.1	D37.02	D49.0
junctional zone	C02.8	C79.89	D00.07	D10.1	D37.02	D49.0
margin (lateral)	C02.1	C79.89	D00.07	D10.1	D37.02	D49.0
midline NEC	C02.0	C79.89	D00.07	D10.1	D37.02	D49.0
mobile part NEC	C02.3	C79.89	D00.07	D10.1	D37.02	D49.0
overlapping lesion	C02.8	—	—	—	—	—
posterior (third)	C01	C79.89	D00.07	D10.1	D37.02	D49.0
root	C01	C79.89	D00.07	D10.1	D37.02	D49.0
surface (dorsal)	C02.0	C79.89	D00.07	D10.1	D37.02	D49.0
base	C01	C79.89	D00.07	D10.1	D37.02	D49.0
ventral	C02.2	C79.89	D00.07	D10.1	D37.02	D49.0
tip	C02.1	C79.89	D00.07	D10.1	D37.02	D49.0
tonsil	C02.4	C79.89	D00.07	D10.1	D37.02	D49.0
tonsil	C09.9	C79.89	D00.08	D10.4	D37.05	D49.0
fauces, faucial	C09.9	C79.89	D00.08	D10.4	D37.05	D49.0
lingual	C02.4	C79.89	D00.07	D10.1	D37.02	D49.0
overlapping sites	C09.8	—	—	—	—	—
palatine	C09.9	C79.89	D00.08	D10.4	D37.05	D49.0
pharyngeal	C11.1	C79.89	D00.08	D10.6	D37.05	D49.0
pillar (anterior) (posterior)	C09.1	C79.89	D00.08	D10.5	D37.05	D49.0
tonsillar fossa	C09.0	C79.89	D00.08	D10.5	D37.05	D49.0
tooth socket NEC	C03.9	C79.89	D00.03	D10.39	D37.09	D49.0
trachea (cartilage) (mucosa)	C33	C78.39	D02.1	D14.2	D38.1	D49.1
overlapping lesion with bronchus or lung	C34.8-☑	—	—	—	—	—
tracheobronchial	C34.8-☑	C78.39	D02.1	D14.2	D38.1	D49.1
overlapping lesion with lung	C34.8-☑	—	—	—	—	—
tragus — *see also* Neoplasm, skin, ear	C44.20-☑	C79.2	D04.2-☑	D23.2-☑	D48.5	D49.2
trunk NEC	C76.8	C79.89	D04.5	D36.7	D48.7	D49.89
tubo-ovarian	C57.8	C79.82	D07.39	D28.7	D39.8	D49.59
tunica vaginalis	C63.7	C79.82	D07.69	D29.8	D40.8	D49.59
turbinate (bone)	C41.0	C79.51	—	D16.4	D48.0	D49.2
nasal	C30.0	C78.39	D02.3	D14.0	D38.5	D49.1
tympanic cavity	C30.1	C78.39	D02.3	D14.0	D38.5	D49.1
ulna (any part)	C40.0-☑	C79.51	—	D16.0-☑	—	—
umbilicus, umbilical — *see also* Neoplasm, skin, trunk	C44.509	C79.2	D04.5	D23.5	D48.5	D49.2
uncus, brain	C71.2	C79.31	—	D33.0	D43.0	D49.6
unknown site or unspecified	C80.1	C79.9	D09.9	D36.9	D48.9	D49.9
urachus	C67.7	C79.11	D09.0	D30.3	D41.4	D49.4
ureter-bladder (junction)	C67.6	C79.11	D09.0	D30.3	D41.4	D49.4
ureter, ureteral	C66.-☑	C79.19	D09.19	D30.2-☑	D41.2-☑	D49.59
orifice (bladder)	C67.6	C79.11	D09.0	D30.3	D41.4	D49.4
urethra, urethral (gland)	C68.0	C79.19	D09.19	D30.4	D41.3	D49.59
orifice, internal	C67.5	C79.11	D09.0	D30.3	D41.4	D49.4
urethrovaginal (septum)	C57.9	C79.82	D07.30	D28.9	D39.8	D49.59
urinary organ or system	C68.9	C79.10	D09.10	D30.9	D41.9	D49.59
bladder — *see* Neoplasm, bladder						
overlapping lesion	C68.8	—	—	—	—	—
specified sites NEC	C68.8	C79.19	D09.19	D30.8	D41.8	D49.59
utero-ovarian	C57.8	C79.82	D07.39	D28.7	D39.8	D49.59
ligament	C57.1-☑	C79.82	D07.39	D28.2	D39.8	D49.59
uterosacral ligament	C57.3	C79.82	—	D28.2	D39.8	D49.59
uterus, uteri, uterine	C55	C79.82	D07.0	D26.9	D39.0	D49.59
adnexa NEC	C57.4	C79.82	D07.39	D28.7	D39.8	D49.59
body	C54.9	C79.82	D07.0	D26.1	D39.0	D49.59
cervix	C53.9	C79.82	D06.9	D26.0	D39.0	D49.59
cornu	C54.9	C79.82	D07.0	D26.1	D39.0	D49.59
corpus	C54.9	C79.82	D07.0	D26.1	D39.0	D49.59
endocervix (canal) (gland)	C53.0	C79.82	D06.0	D26.0	D39.0	D49.59

Neoplasm, neoplastic — continued

	Malignant Primary	Malignant Secondary	Ca in situ	Benign	Uncertain	Unspecified Behavior
uterus, uteri, uterine — *continued*						
endometrium	C54.1	C79.82	D07.0	D26.1	D39.0	D49.59
exocervix	C53.1	C79.82	D06.1	D26.0	D39.0	D49.59
external os	C53.1	C79.82	D06.1	D26.0	D39.0	D49.59
fundus	C54.3	C79.82	D07.0	D26.1	D39.0	D49.59
internal os	C53.0	C79.82	D06.0	D26.0	D39.0	D49.59
isthmus	C54.0	C79.82	D07.0	D26.1	D39.0	D49.59
ligament	C57.3	C79.82	—	D28.2	D39.8	D49.59
broad	C57.1-☑	C79.82	D07.39	D28.2	D39.8	D49.59
round	C57.2-☑	C79.82	—	D28.2	D39.8	D49.59
lower segment	C54.0	C79.82	D07.0	D26.1	D39.0	D49.59
myometrium	C54.2	C79.82	D07.0	D26.1	D39.0	D49.59
overlapping sites	C54.8	—	—	—	—	—
squamocolumnar junction	C53.8	C79.82	D06.7	D26.0	D39.0	D49.59
tube	C57.0-☑	C79.82	D07.39	D28.2	D39.8	D49.59
utricle, prostatic	C68.0	C79.19	D09.19	D30.4	D41.3	D49.59
uveal tract	C69.4-☑	C79.49	D09.2-☑	D31.4-☑	D48.7	D49.89
uvula	C05.2	C79.89	D00.04	D10.39	D37.09	D49.0
vagina, vaginal (fornix) (vault) (wall)	C52	C79.82	D07.2	D28.1	D39.8	D49.59
vaginovesical	C57.9	C79.82	D07.30	D28.9	D39.9	D49.59
septum	C57.9	C79.82	D07.30	D28.9	D39.9	D49.59
vallecula (epiglottis)	C10.0	C79.89	D00.08	D10.5	D37.05	D49.0
vascular — *see* Neoplasm, connective tissue						
vas deferens	C63.1-☑	C79.82	D07.69	D29.8	D40.8	D49.59
Vater's ampulla	C24.1	C78.89	D01.5	D13.5	D37.6	D49.0
vein, venous — *see* Neoplasm, connective tissue						
vena cava (abdominal) (inferior)	C49.4	C79.89	—	D21.4	D48.1	D49.2
superior	C49.3	C79.89	—	D21.3	D48.1	D49.2
ventricle (cerebral) (floor) (lateral) (third)	C71.5	C79.31	—	D33.0	D43.0	D49.6
cardiac (left) (right)	C38.0	C79.89	—	D15.1	D48.7	D49.89
fourth	C71.7	C79.31	—	D33.1	D43.1	D49.6
ventricular band of larynx	C32.1	C78.39	D02.0	D14.1	D38.0	D49.1
ventriculus — *see* Neoplasm, stomach						
vermillion border — *see* Neoplasm, lip						
vermis, cerebellum	C71.6	C79.31	—	D33.1	D43.1	D49.6
vertebra (column)	C41.2	C79.51	—	D16.6	D48.0	D49.2
coccyx	C41.4	C79.51	—	D16.8	D48.0	D49.2
marrow NEC	C96.9	C79.52	—		D47.9	D49.89
sacrum	C41.4	C79.51	—	D16.8	D48.0	D49.2
vesical — *see* Neoplasm, bladder						
vesicle, seminal	C63.7	C79.82	D07.69	D29.8	D40.8	D49.59
vesicocervical tissue	C57.9	C79.82	D07.30	D28.9	D39.9	D49.59
vesicorectal	C76.3	C79.82	D09.8	D36.7	D48.7	D49.89
vesicovaginal	C57.9	C79.82	D07.30	D28.9	D39.9	D49.59
septum	C57.9	C79.82	D07.30	D28.9	D39.8	D49.59
vessel (blood) — *see* Neoplasm, connective tissue						
vestibular gland, greater	C51.0	C79.82	D07.1	D28.0	D39.8	D49.59
vestibule						
mouth	C06.1	C79.89	D00.00	D10.39	D37.09	D49.0
nose	C30.0	C78.39	D02.3	D14.0	D38.5	D49.1
Virchow's gland	C77.0	C77.0	—	D36.0	D48.7	D49.89
viscera NEC	C76.8	C79.89	D09.8	D36.7	D48.7	D49.89
vocal cords (true)	C32.0	C78.39	D02.0	D14.1	D38.0	D49.1
false	C32.1	C78.39	D02.0	D14.1	D38.0	D49.1
vomer	C41.0	C79.51	—	D16.4	D48.0	D49.2
vulva	C51.9	C79.82	D07.1	D28.0	D39.8	D49.59
vulvovaginal gland	C51.0	C79.82	D07.1	D28.0	D39.8	D49.59
Waldeyer's ring	C14.2	C79.89	D00.08	D10.9	D37.05	D49.0
Wharton's duct	C08.0	C79.89	D00.00	D11.7	D37.032	D49.0
white matter (central) (cerebral)	C71.0	C79.31	—	D33.0	D43.0	D49.6
windpipe	C33	C78.39	D02.1	D14.2	D38.1	D49.1
Wirsung's duct	C25.3	C78.89	D01.7	D13.6	D37.8	D49.0
wolffian (body) (duct)						
female	C57.7	C79.82	D07.39	D28.7	D39.8	D49.59

	Malignant Primary	Malignant Secondary	Ca in situ	Benign	Uncertain	Unspecified Behavior
Neoplasm, neoplastic — *continued*						
wolffian — *continued*						
male	C63.7	C79.82	D07.69	D29.8	D40.8	D49.59
womb — *see* Neoplasm, uterus						
wrist NEC	C76.4-☑	C79.89	D04.6-☑	D36.7	D48.7	D49.89
xiphoid process	C41.3	C79.51	—	D16.7	D48.0	D49.2
Zuckerkandl organ	C75.5	C79.89	—	D35.6	D44.7	D49.7

☑ **Additional Character Required — Refer to the Tabular List for Character Selection**   ▽ **Subterms under main terms may continue to next column or page**

Substance	Poisoning, Accidental (unintentional)	Poisoning, Intentional Self-harm	Poisoning, Assault	Poisoning, Undetermined	Adverse Effect	Under-dosing
14-Hydroxydihydromorphinone	T40.2X1	T40.2X2	T40.2X3	T40.2X4	T40.2X5	T40.2X6
1-Propanol	T51.3X1	T51.3X2	T51.3X3	T51.3X4	—	—
2,3,7,8-Tetrachlorodibenzo-p-dioxin	T53.7X1	T53.7X2	T53.7X3	T53.7X4	—	—
2,4,5-T (trichlorophenoxyacetic acid)	T60.1X1	T60.1X2	T60.1X3	T60.1X4	—	—
2,4,5-Trichlorophenoxyacetic acid	T60.3X1	T60.3X2	T60.3X3	T60.3X4	—	—
2,4-D (dichlorophenoxyacetic acid)	T60.3X1	T60.3X2	T60.3X3	T60.3X4	—	—
2,4-Toluene diisocyanate	T65.0X1	T65.0X2	T65.0X3	T65.0X4	—	—
2-Deoxy-5-fluorouridine	T45.1X1	T45.1X2	T45.1X3	T45.1X4	T45.1X5	T45.1X6
2-Ethoxyethanol	T52.3X1	T52.3X2	T52.3X3	T52.3X4	—	—
2-Methoxyethanol	T52.3X1	T52.3X2	T52.3X3	T52.3X4	—	—
2-Propanol	T51.2X1	T51.2X2	T51.2X3	T51.2X4	—	—
4-Aminobutyric acid	T43.8X1	T43.8X2	T43.8X3	T43.8X4	T43.8X5	T43.8X6
4-Aminophenol derivatives	T39.1X1	T39.1X2	T39.1X3	T39.1X4	T39.1X5	T39.1X6
5-Deoxy-5-fluorouridine	T45.1X1	T45.1X2	T45.1X3	T45.1X4	T45.1X5	T45.1X6
5-Methoxypsoralen (5-MOP)	T50.991	T50.992	T50.993	T50.994	T50.995	T50.996
8-Aminoquinoline drugs	T37.2X1	T37.2X2	T37.2X3	T37.2X4	T37.2X5	T37.2X6
8-Methoxypsoralen (8-MOP)	T50.991	T50.992	T50.993	T50.994	T50.995	T50.996
ABOB	T37.5X1	T37.5X2	T37.5X3	T37.5X4	T37.5X5	T37.5X6
Abrine	T62.2X1	T62.2X2	T62.2X3	T62.2X4	—	—
Abrus (seed)	T62.2X1	T62.2X2	T62.2X3	T62.2X4	—	—
Absinthe	T51.0X1	T51.0X2	T51.0X3	T51.0X4	—	—
beverage	T51.0X1	T51.0X2	T51.0X3	T51.0X4	—	—
Acaricide	T60.8X1	T60.8X2	T60.8X3	T60.8X4	—	—
Acebutolol	T44.7X1	T44.7X2	T44.7X3	T44.7X4	T44.7X5	T44.7X6
Acecarbromal	T42.6X1	T42.6X2	T42.6X3	T42.6X4	T42.6X5	T42.6X6
Aceclidine	T44.1X1	T44.1X2	T44.1X3	T44.1X4	T44.1X5	T44.1X6
Acedapsone	T37.0X1	T37.0X2	T37.0X3	T37.0X4	T37.0X5	T37.0X6
Acefylline piperazine	T48.6X1	T48.6X2	T48.6X3	T48.6X4	T48.6X5	T48.6X6
Acemorphan	T40.2X1	T40.2X2	T40.2X3	T40.2X4	T40.2X5	T40.2X6
Acenocoumarin	T45.511	T45.512	T45.513	T45.514	T45.515	T45.516
Acenocoumarol	T45.511	T45.512	T45.513	T45.514	T45.515	T45.516
Acepifylline	T48.6X1	T48.6X2	T48.6X3	T48.6X4	T48.6X5	T48.6X6
Acepromazine	T43.3X1	T43.3X2	T43.3X3	T43.3X4	T43.3X5	T43.3X6
Acesulfamethoxypyridazine	T37.0X1	T37.0X2	T37.0X3	T37.0X4	T37.0X5	T37.0X6
Acetal	T52.8X1	T52.8X2	T52.8X3	T52.8X4	—	—
Acetaldehyde (vapor)	T52.8X1	T52.8X2	T52.8X3	T52.8X4	—	—
liquid	T65.891	T65.892	T65.893	T65.894	—	—
Acetaminophen	T39.1X1	T39.1X2	T39.1X3	T39.1X4	T39.1X5	T39.1X6
Acetaminosalol	T39.1X1	T39.1X2	T39.1X3	T39.1X4	T39.1X5	T39.1X6
Acetanilide	T39.1X1	T39.1X2	T39.1X3	T39.1X4	T39.1X5	T39.1X6
Acetarsol	T37.3X1	T37.3X2	T37.3X3	T37.3X4	T37.3X5	T37.3X6
Acetazolamide	T50.2X1	T50.2X2	T50.2X3	T50.2X4	T50.2X5	T50.2X6
Acetiamine	T45.2X1	T45.2X2	T45.2X3	T45.2X4	T45.2X5	T45.2X6
Acetic						
acid	T54.2X1	T54.2X2	T54.2X3	T54.2X4	—	—
with sodium acetate (ointment)	T49.3X1	T49.3X2	T49.3X3	T49.3X4	T49.3X5	T49.3X6
ester (solvent)(vapor)	T52.8X1	T52.8X2	T52.8X3	T52.8X4	—	—
irrigating solution	T50.3X1	T50.3X2	T50.3X3	T50.3X4	T50.3X5	T50.3X6
medicinal (lotion)	T49.2X1	T49.2X2	T49.2X3	T49.2X4	T49.2X5	T49.2X6
anhydride	T65.891	T65.892	T65.893	T65.894	—	—
ether (vapor)	T52.8X1	T52.8X2	T52.8X3	T52.8X4	—	—
Acetohexamide	T38.3X1	T38.3X2	T38.3X3	T38.3X4	T38.3X5	T38.3X6
Acetohydroxamic acid	T50.991	T50.992	T50.993	T50.994	T50.995	T50.996
Acetomenaphthone	T45.7X1	T45.7X2	T45.7X3	T45.7X4	T45.7X5	T45.7X6
Acetomorphine	T40.1X1	T40.1X2	T40.1X3	T40.1X4	—	—
Acetone (oils)	T52.4X1	T52.4X2	T52.4X3	T52.4X4	—	—
chlorinated	T52.4X1	T52.4X2	T52.4X3	T52.4X4	—	—
vapor	T52.4X1	T52.4X2	T52.4X3	T52.4X4	—	—
Acetonitrile	T52.8X1	T52.8X2	T52.8X3	T52.8X4	—	—
Acetophenazine	T43.3X1	T43.3X2	T43.3X3	T43.3X4	T43.3X5	T43.3X6
Acetophenetedin	T39.1X1	T39.1X2	T39.1X3	T39.1X4	T39.1X5	T39.1X6
Acetophenone	T52.4X1	T52.4X2	T52.4X3	T52.4X4	—	—
Acetorphine	T40.2X1	T40.2X2	T40.2X3	T40.2X4	—	—
Acetosulfone (sodium)	T37.1X1	T37.1X2	T37.1X3	T37.1X4	T37.1X5	T37.1X6
Acetrizoate (sodium)	T50.8X1	T50.8X2	T50.8X3	T50.8X4	T50.8X5	T50.8X6
Acetrizoic acid	T50.8X1	T50.8X2	T50.8X3	T50.8X4	T50.8X5	T50.8X6
Acetyl						
bromide	T53.6X1	T53.6X2	T53.6X3	T53.6X4	—	—
chloride	T53.6X1	T53.6X2	T53.6X3	T53.6X4	—	—
Acetylcarbromal	T42.6X1	T42.6X2	T42.6X3	T42.6X4	T42.6X5	T42.6X6
Acetylcholine						
chloride	T44.1X1	T44.1X2	T44.1X3	T44.1X4	T44.1X5	T44.1X6
derivative	T44.1X1	T44.1X2	T44.1X3	T44.1X4	T44.1X5	T44.1X6
Acetylcysteine	T48.4X1	T48.4X2	T48.4X3	T48.4X4	T48.4X5	T48.4X6
Acetyldigitoxin	T46.0X1	T46.0X2	T46.0X3	T46.0X4	T46.0X5	T46.0X6
Acetyldigoxin	T46.0X1	T46.0X2	T46.0X3	T46.0X4	T46.0X5	T46.0X6

Substance	Poisoning, Accidental (unintentional)	Poisoning, Intentional Self-harm	Poisoning, Assault	Poisoning, Undetermined	Adverse Effect	Under-dosing
Acetyldihydrocodeine	T40.2X1	T40.2X2	T40.2X3	T40.2X4	—	—
Acetyldihydrocodeinone	T40.2X1	T40.2X2	T40.2X3	T40.2X4	—	—
Acetylene (gas)	T59.891	T59.892	T59.893	T59.894	—	—
dichloride	T53.6X1	T53.6X2	T53.6X3	T53.6X4	—	—
incomplete combustion of	T58.11	T58.12	T58.13	T58.14	—	—
industrial	T59.891	T59.892	T59.893	T59.894	—	—
tetrachloride	T53.6X1	T53.6X2	T53.6X3	T53.6X4	—	—
vapor	T53.6X1	T53.6X2	T53.6X3	T53.6X4	—	—
Acetylpheneturide	T42.6X1	T42.6X2	T42.6X3	T42.6X4	T42.6X5	T42.6X6
Acetylphenylhydrazine	T39.8X1	T39.8X2	T39.8X3	T39.8X4	T39.8X5	T39.8X6
Acetylsalicylic acid (salts)	T39.011	T39.012	T39.013	T39.014	T39.015	T39.016
enteric coated	T39.011	T39.012	T39.013	T39.014	T39.015	T39.016
Acetylsulfamethoxypyridazine	T37.0X1	T37.0X2	T37.0X3	T37.0X4	T37.0X5	T37.0X6
Achromycin	T36.4X1	T36.4X2	T36.4X3	T36.4X4	T36.4X5	T36.4X6
ophthalmic preparation	T49.5X1	T49.5X2	T49.5X3	T49.5X4	T49.5X5	T49.5X6
topical NEC	T49.0X1	T49.0X2	T49.0X3	T49.0X4	T49.0X5	T49.0X6
Aciclovir	T37.5X1	T37.5X2	T37.5X3	T37.5X4	T37.5X5	T37.5X6
Acidifying agent NEC	T50.901	T50.902	T50.903	T50.904	T50.905	T50.906
Acid (corrosive) NEC	T54.2X1	T54.2X2	T54.2X3	T54.2X4	—	—
Acipimox	T46.6X1	T46.6X2	T46.6X3	T46.6X4	T46.6X5	T46.6X6
Acitretin	T50.991	T50.992	T50.993	T50.994	T50.995	T50.996
Aclarubicin	T45.1X1	T45.1X2	T45.1X3	T45.1X4	T45.1X5	T45.1X6
Aclatonium napadisilate	T48.1X1	T48.1X2	T48.1X3	T48.1X4	T48.1X5	T48.1X6
Aconite (wild)	T46.991	T46.992	T46.993	T46.994	T46.995	T46.996
Aconitine	T46.991	T46.992	T46.993	T46.994	T46.995	T46.996
Aconitum ferox	T46.991	T46.992	T46.993	T46.994	T46.995	T46.996
Acridine	T65.6X1	T65.6X2	T65.6X3	T65.6X4	—	—
vapor	T59.891	T59.892	T59.893	T59.894	—	—
Acriflavine	T37.91	T37.92	T37.93	T37.94	T37.95	T37.96
Acriflavinium chloride	T49.0X1	T49.0X2	T49.0X3	T49.0X4	T49.0X5	T49.0X6
Acrinol	T49.0X1	T49.0X2	T49.0X3	T49.0X4	T49.0X5	T49.0X6
Acrisorcin	T49.0X1	T49.0X2	T49.0X3	T49.0X4	T49.0X5	T49.0X6
Acrivastine	T45.0X1	T45.0X2	T45.0X3	T45.0X4	T45.0X5	T45.0X6
Acrolein (gas)	T59.891	T59.892	T59.893	T59.894	—	—
liquid	T54.1X1	T54.1X2	T54.1X3	T54.1X4	—	—
Acrylamide	T65.891	T65.892	T65.893	T65.894	—	—
Acrylic resin	T49.3X1	T49.3X2	T49.3X3	T49.3X4	T49.3X5	T49.3X6
Acrylonitrile	T65.891	T65.892	T65.893	T65.894	—	—
Actaea spicata	T62.2X1	T62.2X2	T62.2X3	T62.2X4	—	—
berry	T62.1X1	T62.1X2	T62.1X3	T62.1X4	—	—
Acterol	T37.3X1	T37.3X2	T37.3X3	T37.3X4	T37.3X5	T37.3X6
ACTH	T38.811	T38.812	T38.813	T38.814	T38.815	T38.816
Actinomycin C	T45.1X1	T45.1X2	T45.1X3	T45.1X4	T45.1X5	T45.1X6
Actinomycin D	T45.1X1	T45.1X2	T45.1X3	T45.1X4	T45.1X5	T45.1X6
Activated charcoal — *see also* Charcoal, medicinal	T47.6X1	T47.6X2	T47.6X3	T47.6X4	T47.6X5	T47.6X6
Acyclovir	T37.5X1	T37.5X2	T37.5X3	T37.5X4	T37.5X5	T37.5X6
Adenine	T45.2X1	T45.2X2	T45.2X3	T45.2X4	T45.2X5	T45.2X6
arabinoside	T37.5X1	T37.5X2	T37.5X3	T37.5X4	T37.5X5	T37.5X6
Adenosine (phosphate)	T46.2X1	T46.2X2	T46.2X3	T46.2X4	T46.2X5	T46.2X6
ADH	T38.891	T38.892	T38.893	T38.894	T38.895	T38.896
Adhesive NEC	T65.891	T65.892	T65.893	T65.894	—	—
Adicillin	T36.0X1	T36.0X2	T36.0X3	T36.0X4	T36.0X5	T36.0X6
Adiphenine	T44.3X1	T44.3X2	T44.3X3	T44.3X4	T44.3X5	T44.3X6
Adipiodone	T50.8X1	T50.8X2	T50.8X3	T50.8X4	T50.8X5	T50.8X6
Adjunct, pharmaceutical	T50.901	T50.902	T50.903	T50.904	T50.905	T50.906
Adrenal (extract, cortex or medulla) (glucocorticoids) (hormones) (mineralocorticoids)	T38.0X1	T38.0X2	T38.0X3	T38.0X4	T38.0X5	T38.0X6
ENT agent	T49.6X1	T49.6X2	T49.6X3	T49.6X4	T49.6X5	T49.6X6
ophthalmic preparation	T49.5X1	T49.5X2	T49.5X3	T49.5X4	T49.5X5	T49.5X6
topical NEC	T49.0X1	T49.0X2	T49.0X3	T49.0X4	T49.0X5	T49.0X6
Adrenalin — *see* Adrenaline						
Adrenaline	T44.5X1	T44.5X2	T44.5X3	T44.5X4	T44.5X5	T44.5X6
Adrenergic NEC	T44.901	T44.902	T44.903	T44.904	T44.905	T44.906
blocking agent NEC	T44.8X1	T44.8X2	T44.8X3	T44.8X4	T44.8X5	T44.8X6
beta, heart	T44.7X1	T44.7X2	T44.7X3	T44.7X4	T44.7X5	T44.7X6
specified NEC	T44.991	T44.992	T44.993	T44.994	T44.995	T44.996
Adrenochrome						
derivative	T46.991	T46.992	T46.993	T46.994	T46.995	T46.996
(mono) semicarbazone	T46.991	T46.992	T46.993	T46.994	T46.995	T46.996
Adrenocorticotrophic hormone	T38.811	T38.812	T38.813	T38.814	T38.815	T38.816
Adrenocorticotrophin	T38.811	T38.812	T38.813	T38.814	T38.815	T38.816
Adriamycin	T45.1X1	T45.1X2	T45.1X3	T45.1X4	T45.1X5	T45.1X6
Aerosol spray NEC	T65.91	T65.92	T65.93	T65.94	—	—
Aerosporin	T36.8X1	T36.8X2	T36.8X3	T36.8X4	T36.8X5	T36.8X6
ENT agent	T49.6X1	T49.6X2	T49.6X3	T49.6X4	T49.6X5	T49.6X6
ophthalmic preparation	T49.5X1	T49.5X2	T49.5X3	T49.5X4	T49.5X5	T49.5X6
topical NEC	T49.0X1	T49.0X2	T49.0X3	T49.0X4	T49.0X5	T49.0X6
Aethusa cynapium	T62.2X1	T62.2X2	T62.2X3	T62.2X4	—	—
Afghanistan black	T40.7X1	T40.7X2	T40.7X3	T40.7X4	T40.7X5	T40.7X6

Substance	Poisoning, Accidental (unintentional)	Poisoning, Intentional Self-harm	Poisoning, Assault	Poisoning, Undetermined	Adverse Effect	Underdosing
Aflatoxin	T64.01	T64.02	T64.03	T64.04	—	—
Afloqualone	T42.8X1	T42.8X2	T42.8X3	T42.8X4	T42.8X5	T42.8X6
African boxwood	T62.2X1	T62.2X2	T62.2X3	T62.2X4		
Agar	T47.4X1	T47.4X2	T47.4X3	T47.4X4	T47.4X5	T47.4X6
Agonist						
predominantly						
alpha-adrenoreceptor	T44.4X1	T44.4X2	T44.4X3	T44.4X4	T44.4X5	T44.4X6
beta-adrenoreceptor	T44.5X1	T44.5X2	T44.5X3	T44.5X4	T44.5X5	T44.5X6
Agricultural agent NEC	T65.91	T65.92	T65.93	T65.94		
Agrypnal	T42.3X1	T42.3X2	T42.3X3	T42.3X4	T42.3X5	T42.3X6
AHLG	T50.Z11	T50.Z12	T50.Z13	T50.Z14	T50.Z15	T50.Z16
Air contaminant(s), source/type NOS	T65.91	T65.92	T65.93	T65.94		
Ajmaline	T46.2X1	T46.2X2	T46.2X3	T46.2X4	T46.2X5	T46.2X6
Akee	T62.1X1	T62.1X2	T62.1X3	T62.1X4		
Akrinol	T49.0X1	T49.0X2	T49.0X3	T49.0X4	T49.0X5	T49.0X6
Akritoin	T37.8X1	T37.8X2	T37.8X3	T37.8X4	T37.8X5	T37.8X6
Alacepril	T46.4X1	T46.4X2	T46.4X3	T46.4X4	T46.4X5	T46.4X6
Alantolactone	T37.4X1	T37.4X2	T37.4X3	T37.4X4	T37.4X5	T37.4X6
Albamycin	T36.8X1	T36.8X2	T36.8X3	T36.8X4	T36.8X5	T36.8X6
Albendazole	T37.4X1	T37.4X2	T37.4X3	T37.4X4	T37.4X5	T37.4X6
Albumin						
bovine	T45.8X1	T45.8X2	T45.8X3	T45.8X4	T45.8X5	T45.8X6
human serum	T45.8X1	T45.8X2	T45.8X3	T45.8X4	T45.8X5	T45.8X6
salt-poor	T45.8X1	T45.8X2	T45.8X3	T45.8X4	T45.8X5	T45.8X6
normal human serum	T45.8X1	T45.8X2	T45.8X3	T45.8X4	T45.8X5	T45.8X6
Albuterol	T48.6X1	T48.6X2	T48.6X3	T48.6X4	T48.6X5	T48.6X6
Albutoin	T42.0X1	T42.0X2	T42.0X3	T42.0X4	T42.0X5	T42.0X6
Alclometasone	T49.0X1	T49.0X2	T49.0X3	T49.0X4	T49.0X5	T49.0X6
Alcohol	T51.91	T51.92	T51.93	T51.94	—	—
absolute	T51.0X1	T51.0X2	T51.0X3	T51.0X4		
beverage	T51.0X1	T51.0X2	T51.0X3	T51.0X4		
allyl	T51.8X1	T51.8X2	T51.8X3	T51.8X4		
amyl	T51.3X1	T51.3X2	T51.3X3	T51.3X4		
antifreeze	T51.1X1	T51.1X2	T51.1X3	T51.1X4		
beverage	T51.0X1	T51.0X2	T51.0X3	T51.0X4		
butyl	T51.3X1	T51.3X2	T51.3X3	T51.3X4		
dehydrated	T51.0X1	T51.0X2	T51.0X3	T51.0X4		
beverage	T51.0X1	T51.0X2	T51.0X3	T51.0X4		
denatured	T51.0X1	T51.0X2	T51.0X3	T51.0X4		
deterrent NEC	T50.6X1	T50.6X2	T50.6X3	T50.6X4	T50.6X5	T50.6X6
diagnostic (gastric function)	T50.8X1	T50.8X2	T50.8X3	T50.8X4	T50.8X5	T50.8X6
ethyl	T51.0X1	T51.0X2	T51.0X3	T51.0X4		
beverage	T51.0X1	T51.0X2	T51.0X3	T51.0X4		
grain	T51.0X1	T51.0X2	T51.0X3	T51.0X4		
beverage	T51.0X1	T51.0X2	T51.0X3	T51.0X4		
industrial	T51.0X1	T51.0X2	T51.0X3	T51.0X4		
isopropyl	T51.2X1	T51.2X2	T51.2X3	T51.2X4		
methyl	T51.1X1	T51.1X2	T51.1X3	T51.1X4		
preparation for consumption	T51.0X1	T51.0X2	T51.0X3	T51.0X4		
propyl	T51.3X1	T51.3X2	T51.3X3	T51.3X4		
secondary	T51.2X1	T51.2X2	T51.2X3	T51.2X4		
radiator	T51.1X1	T51.1X2	T51.1X3	T51.1X4		
rubbing	T51.2X1	T51.2X2	T51.2X3	T51.2X4		
specified type NEC	T51.8X1	T51.8X2	T51.8X3	T51.8X4		
surgical	T51.0X1	T51.0X2	T51.0X3	T51.0X4		
vapor (from any type of Alcohol)	T59.891	T59.892	T59.893	T59.894		
wood	T51.1X1	T51.1X2	T51.1X3	T51.1X4		
Alcuronium (chloride)	T48.1X1	T48.1X2	T48.1X3	T48.1X4	T48.1X5	T48.1X6
Aldactone	T50.0X1	T50.0X2	T50.0X3	T50.0X4	T50.0X5	T50.0X6
Aldesulfone sodium	T37.1X1	T37.1X2	T37.1X3	T37.1X4	T37.1X5	T37.1X6
Aldicarb	T60.0X1	T60.0X2	T60.0X3	T60.0X4		
Aldomet	T46.5X1	T46.5X2	T46.5X3	T46.5X4	T46.5X5	T46.5X6
Aldosterone	T50.0X1	T50.0X2	T50.0X3	T50.0X4	T50.0X5	T50.0X6
Aldrin (dust)	T60.1X1	T60.1X2	T60.1X3	T60.1X4		
Aleve — see Naproxen						
Alexitol sodium	T47.1X1	T47.1X2	T47.1X3	T47.1X4	T47.1X5	T47.1X6
Alfacalcidol	T45.2X1	T45.2X2	T45.2X3	T45.2X4	T45.2X5	T45.2X6
Alfadolone	T41.1X1	T41.1X2	T41.1X3	T41.1X4	T41.1X5	T41.1X6
Alfaxalone	T41.1X1	T41.1X2	T41.1X3	T41.1X4	T41.1X5	T41.1X6
Alfentanil	T40.4X1	T40.4X2	T40.4X3	T40.4X4	T40.4X5	T40.4X6
Alfuzosin (hydrochloride)	T44.8X1	T44.8X2	T44.8X3	T44.8X4	T44.8X5	T44.8X6
Algae (harmful) (toxin)	T65.821	T65.822	T65.823	T65.824	—	—
Algeldrate	T47.1X1	T47.1X2	T47.1X3	T47.1X4	T47.1X5	T47.1X6
Algin	T47.8X1	T47.8X2	T47.8X3	T47.8X4	T47.8X5	T47.8X6
Alglucerase	T45.3X1	T45.3X2	T45.3X3	T45.3X4	T45.3X5	T45.3X6
Alidase	T45.3X1	T45.3X2	T45.3X3	T45.3X4	T45.3X5	T45.3X6
Alimemazine	T43.3X1	T43.3X2	T43.3X3	T43.3X4	T43.3X5	T43.3X6
Aliphatic thiocyanates	T65.0X1	T65.0X2	T65.0X3	T65.0X4		
Alizapride	T45.0X1	T45.0X2	T45.0X3	T45.0X4	T45.0X5	T45.0X6

Substance	Poisoning, Accidental (unintentional)	Poisoning, Intentional Self-harm	Poisoning, Assault	Poisoning, Undetermined	Adverse Effect	Underdosing
Alkali (caustic)	T54.3X1	T54.3X2	T54.3X3	T54.3X4		
Alkaline antiseptic solution (aromatic)	T49.6X1	T49.6X2	T49.6X3	T49.6X4	T49.6X5	T49.6X6
Alkalinizing agents (medicinal)	T50.901	T50.902	T50.903	T50.904	T50.905	T50.906
Alkalizing agent NEC	T50.901	T50.902	T50.903	T50.904	T50.905	T50.906
Alka-seltzer	T39.011	T39.012	T39.013	T39.014	T39.015	T39.016
Alkavervir	T46.5X1	T46.5X2	T46.5X3	T46.5X4	T46.5X5	T46.5X6
Alkonium (bromide)	T49.0X1	T49.0X2	T49.0X3	T49.0X4	T49.0X5	T49.0X6
Alkylating drug NEC	T45.1X1	T45.1X2	T45.1X3	T45.1X4	T45.1X5	T45.1X6
antimyeloproliferative	T45.1X1	T45.1X2	T45.1X3	T45.1X4	T45.1X5	T45.1X6
lymphatic	T45.1X1	T45.1X2	T45.1X3	T45.1X4	T45.1X5	T45.1X6
Alkylisocyanate	T65.0X1	T65.0X2	T65.0X3	T65.0X4	—	—
Allantoin	T49.4X1	T49.4X2	T49.4X3	T49.4X4	T49.4X5	T49.4X6
Allegron	T43.011	T43.012	T43.013	T43.014	T43.015	T43.016
Allethrin	T49.0X1	T49.0X2	T49.0X3	T49.0X4	T49.0X5	T49.0X6
Allobarbital	T42.3X1	T42.3X2	T42.3X3	T42.3X4	T42.3X5	T42.3X6
Allopurinol	T50.4X1	T50.4X2	T50.4X3	T50.4X4	T50.4X5	T50.4X6
Allyl						
alcohol	T51.8X1	T51.8X2	T51.8X3	T51.8X4	—	—
disulfide	T46.6X1	T46.6X2	T46.6X3	T46.6X4	T46.6X5	T46.6X6
Allylestrenol	T38.5X1	T38.5X2	T38.5X3	T38.5X4	T38.5X5	T38.5X6
Allylisopropylacetylurea	T42.6X1	T42.6X2	T42.6X3	T42.6X4	T42.6X5	T42.6X6
Allylisopropylmalonylurea	T42.3X1	T42.3X2	T42.3X3	T42.3X4	T42.3X5	T42.3X6
Allylthiourea	T49.3X1	T49.3X2	T49.3X3	T49.3X4	T49.3X5	T49.3X6
Allyltribromide	T42.6X1	T42.6X2	T42.6X3	T42.6X4	T42.6X5	T42.6X6
Allypropymal	T42.3X1	T42.3X2	T42.3X3	T42.3X4	T42.3X5	T42.3X6
Almagate	T47.1X1	T47.1X2	T47.1X3	T47.1X4	T47.1X5	T47.1X6
Almasilate	T47.1X1	T47.1X2	T47.1X3	T47.1X4	T47.1X5	T47.1X6
Almitrine	T50.7X1	T50.7X2	T50.7X3	T50.7X4	T50.7X5	T50.7X6
Aloes	T47.2X1	T47.2X2	T47.2X3	T47.2X4	T47.2X5	T47.2X6
Aloglutamol	T47.1X1	T47.1X2	T47.1X3	T47.1X4	T47.1X5	T47.1X6
Aloin	T47.2X1	T47.2X2	T47.2X3	T47.2X4	T47.2X5	T47.2X6
Aloxidone	T42.2X1	T42.2X2	T42.2X3	T42.2X4	T42.2X5	T42.2X6
Alpha						
acetyldigoxin	T46.0X1	T46.0X2	T46.0X3	T46.0X4	T46.0X5	T46.0X6
adrenergic blocking drug	T44.6X1	T44.6X2	T44.6X3	T44.6X4	T44.6X5	T44.6X6
amylase	T45.3X1	T45.3X2	T45.3X3	T45.3X4	T45.3X5	T45.3X6
tocoferol (acetate)	T45.2X1	T45.2X2	T45.2X3	T45.2X4	T45.2X5	T45.2X6
tocopherol	T45.2X1	T45.2X2	T45.2X3	T45.2X4	T45.2X5	T45.2X6
Alphadolone	T41.1X1	T41.1X2	T41.1X3	T41.1X4	T41.1X5	T41.1X6
Alphaprodine	T40.4X1	T40.4X2	T40.4X3	T40.4X4	T40.4X5	T40.4X6
Alphaxalone	T41.1X1	T41.1X2	T41.1X3	T41.1X4	T41.1X5	T41.1X6
Alprazolam	T42.4X1	T42.4X2	T42.4X3	T42.4X4	T42.4X5	T42.4X6
Alprenolol	T44.7X1	T44.7X2	T44.7X3	T44.7X4	T44.7X5	T44.7X6
Alprostadil	T46.7X1	T46.7X2	T46.7X3	T46.7X4	T46.7X5	T46.7X6
Alsactide	T38.811	T38.812	T38.813	T38.814	T38.815	T38.816
Alseroxylon	T46.5X1	T46.5X2	T46.5X3	T46.5X4	T46.5X5	T46.5X6
Alteplase	T45.611	T45.612	T45.613	T45.614	T45.615	T45.616
Altizide	T50.2X1	T50.2X2	T50.2X3	T50.2X4	T50.2X5	T50.2X6
Altretamine	T45.1X1	T45.1X2	T45.1X3	T45.1X4	T45.1X5	T45.1X6
Alum (medicinal)	T49.4X1	T49.4X2	T49.4X3	T49.4X4	T49.4X5	T49.4X6
nonmedicinal (ammonium) (potassium)	T56.891	T56.892	T56.893	T56.894		
Aluminium, aluminum						
acetate	T49.2X1	T49.2X2	T49.2X3	T49.2X4	T49.2X5	T49.2X6
solution	T49.0X1	T49.0X2	T49.0X3	T49.0X4	T49.0X5	T49.0X6
aspirin	T39.011	T39.012	T39.013	T39.014	T39.015	T39.016
bis (acetylsalicylate)	T39.011	T39.012	T39.013	T39.014	T39.015	T39.016
carbonate (gel, basic)	T47.1X1	T47.1X2	T47.1X3	T47.1X4	T47.1X5	T47.1X6
chlorhydroxide-complex	T47.1X1	T47.1X2	T47.1X3	T47.1X4	T47.1X5	T47.1X6
chloride	T49.2X1	T49.2X2	T49.2X3	T49.2X4	T49.2X5	T49.2X6
clofibrate	T46.6X1	T46.6X2	T46.6X3	T46.6X4	T46.6X5	T46.6X6
diacetate	T49.2X1	T49.2X2	T49.2X3	T49.2X4	T49.2X5	T49.2X6
glycinate	T47.1X1	T47.1X2	T47.1X3	T47.1X4	T47.1X5	T47.1X6
hydroxide (gel)	T47.1X1	T47.1X2	T47.1X3	T47.1X4	T47.1X5	T47.1X6
hydroxide-magnesium carb. gel	T47.1X1	T47.1X2	T47.1X3	T47.1X4	T47.1X5	T47.1X6
magnesium silicate	T47.1X1	T47.1X2	T47.1X3	T47.1X4	T47.1X5	T47.1X6
nicotinate	T46.7X1	T46.7X2	T46.7X3	T46.7X4	T46.7X5	T46.7X6
ointment (surgical) (topical)	T49.3X1	T49.3X2	T49.3X3	T49.3X4	T49.3X5	T49.3X6
phosphate	T47.1X1	T47.1X2	T47.1X3	T47.1X4	T47.1X5	T47.1X6
salicylate	T39.091	T39.092	T39.093	T39.094	T39.095	T39.096
silicate	T47.1X1	T47.1X2	T47.1X3	T47.1X4	T47.1X5	T47.1X6
sodium silicate	T47.1X1	T47.1X2	T47.1X3	T47.1X4	T47.1X5	T47.1X6
subacetate	T49.2X1	T49.2X2	T49.2X3	T49.2X4	T49.2X5	T49.2X6
sulfate	T49.0X1	T49.0X2	T49.0X3	T49.0X4	T49.0X5	T49.0X6
tannate	T47.6X1	T47.6X2	T47.6X3	T47.6X4	T47.6X5	T47.6X6
topical NEC	T49.3X1	T49.3X2	T49.3X3	T49.3X4	T49.3X5	T49.3X6
Alurate	T42.3X1	T42.3X2	T42.3X3	T42.3X4	T42.3X5	T42.3X6
Alverine	T44.3X1	T44.3X2	T44.3X3	T44.3X4	T44.3X5	T44.3X6
Alvodine	T40.2X1	T40.2X2	T40.2X3	T40.2X4	T40.2X5	T40.2X6
Amanita phalloides	T62.0X1	T62.0X2	T62.0X3	T62.0X4		

Substance	Poisoning, Accidental (unintentional)	Poisoning, Intentional Self-harm	Poisoning, Assault	Poisoning, Undetermined	Adverse Effect	Under-dosing
Amanitine	T62.0X1	T62.0X2	T62.0X3	T62.0X4	—	—
Amantadine	T42.8X1	T42.8X2	T42.8X3	T42.8X4	T42.8X5	T42.8X6
Ambazone	T49.6X1	T49.6X2	T49.6X3	T49.6X4	T49.6X5	T49.6X6
Ambenonium (chloride)	T44.0X1	T44.0X2	T44.0X3	T44.0X4	T44.0X5	T44.0X6
Ambroxol	T48.4X1	T48.4X2	T48.4X3	T48.4X4	T48.4X5	T48.4X6
Ambuphylline	T48.6X1	T48.6X2	T48.6X3	T48.6X4	T48.6X5	T48.6X6
Ambutonium bromide	T44.3X1	T44.3X2	T44.3X3	T44.3X4	T44.3X5	T44.3X6
Amcinonide	T49.0X1	T49.0X2	T49.0X3	T49.0X4	T49.0X5	T49.0X6
Amdinocilline	T36.0X1	T36.0X2	T36.0X3	T36.0X4	T36.0X5	T36.0X6
Ametazole	T50.8X1	T50.8X2	T50.8X3	T50.8X4	T50.8X5	T50.8X6
Amethocaine	T41.3X1	T41.3X2	T41.3X3	T41.3X4	T41.3X5	T41.3X6
regional	T41.3X1	T41.3X2	T41.3X3	T41.3X4	T41.3X5	T41.3X6
spinal	T41.3X1	T41.3X2	T41.3X3	T41.3X4	T41.3X5	T41.3X6
Amethopterin	T45.1X1	T45.1X2	T45.1X3	T45.1X4	T45.1X5	T45.1X6
Amezinium metilsulfate	T44.991	T44.992	T44.993	T44.994	T44.995	T44.996
Amfebutamone	T43.291	T43.292	T43.293	T43.294	T43.295	T43.296
Amfepramone	T50.5X1	T50.5X2	T50.5X3	T50.5X4	T50.5X5	T50.5X6
Amfetamine	T43.621	T43.622	T43.623	T43.624	T43.625	T43.626
Amfetaminil	T43.621	T43.622	T43.623	T43.624	T43.625	T43.626
Amfomycin	T36.8X1	T36.8X2	T36.8X3	T36.8X4	T36.8X5	T36.8X6
Amidefrine mesilate	T48.5X1	T48.5X2	T48.5X3	T48.5X4	T48.5X5	T48.5X6
Amidone	T40.3X1	T40.3X2	T40.3X3	T40.3X4	T40.3X5	T40.3X6
Amidopyrine	T39.2X1	T39.2X2	T39.2X3	T39.2X4	T39.2X5	T39.2X6
Amidotrizoate	T50.8X1	T50.8X2	T50.8X3	T50.8X4	T50.8X5	T50.8X6
Amiflamine	T43.1X1	T43.1X2	T43.1X3	T43.1X4	T43.1X5	T43.1X6
Amikacin	T36.5X1	T36.5X2	T36.5X3	T36.5X4	T36.5X5	T36.5X6
Amikhelline	T46.3X1	T46.3X2	T46.3X3	T46.3X4	T46.3X5	T46.3X6
Amiloride	T50.2X1	T50.2X2	T50.2X3	T50.2X4	T50.2X5	T50.2X6
Aminacrine	T49.0X1	T49.0X2	T49.0X3	T49.0X4	T49.0X5	T49.0X6
Amineptine	T43.011	T43.012	T43.013	T43.014	T43.015	T43.016
Aminitrozole	T37.3X1	T37.3X2	T37.3X3	T37.3X4	T37.3X5	T37.3X6
Aminoacetic acid (derivatives)	T50.3X1	T50.3X2	T50.3X3	T50.3X4	T50.3X5	T50.3X6
Amino acids	T50.3X1	T50.3X2	T50.3X3	T50.3X4	T50.3X5	T50.3X6
Aminoacridine	T49.0X1	T49.0X2	T49.0X3	T49.0X4	T49.0X5	T49.0X6
Aminobenzoic acid (-p)	T49.3X1	T49.3X2	T49.3X3	T49.3X4	T49.3X5	T49.3X6
Aminocaproic acid	T45.621	T45.622	T45.623	T45.624	T45.625	T45.626
Aminoethylisothiourium	T45.8X1	T45.8X2	T45.8X3	T45.8X4	T45.8X5	T45.8X6
Aminofenazone	T39.2X1	T39.2X2	T39.2X3	T39.2X4	T39.2X5	T39.2X6
Aminoglutethimide	T45.1X1	T45.1X2	T45.1X3	T45.1X4	T45.1X5	T45.1X6
Aminohippuric acid	T50.8X1	T50.8X2	T50.8X3	T50.8X4	T50.8X5	T50.8X6
Aminomethylbenzoic acid	T45.691	T45.692	T45.693	T45.694	T45.695	T45.696
Aminometradine	T50.2X1	T50.2X2	T50.2X3	T50.2X4	T50.2X5	T50.2X6
Aminopentamide	T44.3X1	T44.3X2	T44.3X3	T44.3X4	T44.3X5	T44.3X6
Aminophenazone	T39.2X1	T39.2X2	T39.2X3	T39.2X4	T39.2X5	T39.2X6
Aminophenol	T54.0X1	T54.0X2	T54.0X3	T54.0X4	—	—
Aminophenylpyridone	T43.591	T43.592	T43.593	T43.594	T43.595	T43.596
Aminophylline	T48.6X1	T48.6X2	T48.6X3	T48.6X4	T48.6X5	T48.6X6
Aminopterin sodium	T45.1X1	T45.1X2	T45.1X3	T45.1X4	T45.1X5	T45.1X6
Aminopyrine	T39.2X1	T39.2X2	T39.2X3	T39.2X4	T39.2X5	T39.2X6
Aminorex	T50.5X1	T50.5X2	T50.5X3	T50.5X4	T50.5X5	T50.5X6
Aminosalicylic acid	T37.1X1	T37.1X2	T37.1X3	T37.1X4	T37.1X5	T37.1X6
Aminosalylum	T37.1X1	T37.1X2	T37.1X3	T37.1X4	T37.1X5	T37.1X6
Amiodarone	T46.2X1	T46.2X2	T46.2X3	T46.2X4	T46.2X5	T46.2X6
Amiphenazole	T50.7X1	T50.7X2	T50.7X3	T50.7X4	T50.7X5	T50.7X6
Amiquinsin	T46.5X1	T46.5X2	T46.5X3	T46.5X4	T46.5X5	T46.5X6
Amisometradine	T50.2X1	T50.2X2	T50.2X3	T50.2X4	T50.2X5	T50.2X6
Amisulpride	T43.591	T43.592	T43.593	T43.594	T43.595	T43.596
Amitriptyline	T43.011	T43.012	T43.013	T43.014	T43.015	T43.016
Amitriptylinoxide	T43.011	T43.012	T43.013	T43.014	T43.015	T43.016
Amlexanox	T48.6X1	T48.6X2	T48.6X3	T48.6X4	T48.6X5	T48.6X6
Ammonia (fumes) (gas) (vapor)	T59.891	T59.892	T59.893	T59.894	—	—
aromatic spirit	T48.991	T48.992	T48.993	T48.994	T48.995	T48.996
liquid (household)	T54.3X1	T54.3X2	T54.3X3	T54.3X4	—	—
Ammoniated mercury	T49.0X1	T49.0X2	T49.0X3	T49.0X4	T49.0X5	T49.0X6
Ammonium						
acid tartrate	T49.5X1	T49.5X2	T49.5X3	T49.5X4	T49.5X5	T49.5X6
bromide	T42.6X1	T42.6X2	T42.6X3	T42.6X4	T42.6X5	T42.6X6
carbonate	T54.3X1	T54.3X2	T54.3X3	T54.3X4	—	—
chloride	T50.991	T50.992	T50.993	T50.994	T50.995	T50.996
expectorant	T48.4X1	T48.4X2	T48.4X3	T48.4X4	T48.4X5	T48.4X6
compounds (household) NEC	T54.3X1	T54.3X2	T54.3X3	T54.3X4	—	—
fumes (any usage)	T59.891	T59.892	T59.893	T59.894	—	—
industrial	T54.3X1	T54.3X2	T54.3X3	T54.3X4	—	—
ichthyosulronate	T49.4X1	T49.4X2	T49.4X3	T49.4X4	T49.4X5	T49.4X6
mandelate	T37.91	T37.92	T37.93	T37.94	T37.95	T37.96
sulfamate	T60.3X1	T60.3X2	T60.3X3	T60.3X4	—	—
sulfonate resin	T47.8X1	T47.8X2	T47.8X3	T47.8X4	T47.8X5	T47.8X6
Amobarbital (sodium)	T42.3X1	T42.3X2	T42.3X3	T42.3X4	T42.3X5	T42.3X6
Amodiaquine	T37.2X1	T37.2X2	T37.2X3	T37.2X4	T37.2X5	T37.2X6
Amopyroquin (e)	T37.2X1	T37.2X2	T37.2X3	T37.2X4	T37.2X5	T37.2X6

Substance	Poisoning, Accidental (unintentional)	Poisoning, Intentional Self-harm	Poisoning, Assault	Poisoning, Undetermined	Adverse Effect	Under-dosing
Amoxapine	T43.011	T43.012	T43.013	T43.014	T43.015	T43.016
Amoxicillin	T36.0X1	T36.0X2	T36.0X3	T36.0X4	T36.0X5	T36.0X6
Amperozide	T43.591	T43.592	T43.593	T43.594	T43.595	T43.596
Amphenidone	T43.591	T43.592	T43.593	T43.594	T43.595	T43.596
Amphetamine NEC	T43.621	T43.622	T43.623	T43.624	T43.625	T43.626
Amphomycin	T36.8X1	T36.8X2	T36.8X3	T36.8X4	T36.8X5	T36.8X6
Amphotalide	T37.4X1	T37.4X2	T37.4X3	T37.4X4	T37.4X5	T37.4X6
Amphotericin B	T36.7X1	T36.7X2	T36.7X3	T36.7X4	T36.7X5	T36.7X6
topical	T49.0X1	T49.0X2	T49.0X3	T49.0X4	T49.0X5	T49.0X6
Ampicillin	T36.0X1	T36.0X2	T36.0X3	T36.0X4	T36.0X5	T36.0X6
Amprotropine	T44.3X1	T44.3X2	T44.3X3	T44.3X4	T44.3X5	T44.3X6
Amsacrine	T45.1X1	T45.1X2	T45.1X3	T45.1X4	T45.1X5	T45.1X6
Amygdaline	T62.2X1	T62.2X2	T62.2X3	T62.2X4	—	—
Amyl						
acetate	T52.8X1	T52.8X2	T52.8X3	T52.8X4	—	—
vapor	T59.891	T59.892	T59.893	T59.894	—	—
alcohol	T51.3X1	T51.3X2	T51.3X3	T51.3X4	—	—
chloride	T53.6X1	T53.6X2	T53.6X3	T53.6X4	—	—
formate	T52.8X1	T52.8X2	T52.8X3	T52.8X4	—	—
nitrite	T46.3X1	T46.3X2	T46.3X3	T46.3X4	T46.3X5	T46.3X6
propionate	T65.891	T65.892	T65.893	T65.894	—	—
Amylase	T47.5X1	T47.5X2	T47.5X3	T47.5X4	T47.5X5	T47.5X6
Amyleine, regional	T41.3X1	T41.3X2	T41.3X3	T41.3X4	T41.3X5	T41.3X6
Amylene						
dichloride	T53.6X1	T53.6X2	T53.6X3	T53.6X4	—	—
hydrate	T51.3X1	T51.3X2	T51.3X3	T51.3X4	—	—
Amylmetacresol	T49.6X1	T49.6X2	T49.6X3	T49.6X4	T49.6X5	T49.6X6
Amylobarbitone	T42.3X1	T42.3X2	T42.3X3	T42.3X4	T42.3X5	T42.3X6
Amylocaine, regional	T41.3X1	T41.3X2	T41.3X3	T41.3X4	T41.3X5	T41.3X6
infiltration (subcutaneous)	T41.3X1	T41.3X2	T41.3X3	T41.3X4	T41.3X5	T41.3X6
nerve block (peripheral) (plexus)	T41.3X1	T41.3X2	T41.3X3	T41.3X4	T41.3X5	T41.3X6
spinal	T41.3X1	T41.3X2	T41.3X3	T41.3X4	T41.3X5	T41.3X6
topical (surface)	T41.3X1	T41.3X2	T41.3X3	T41.3X4	T41.3X5	T41.3X6
Amylopectin	T47.6X1	T47.6X2	T47.6X3	T47.6X4	T47.6X5	T47.6X6
Amytal (sodium)	T42.3X1	T42.3X2	T42.3X3	T42.3X4	T42.3X5	T42.3X6
Anabolic steroid	T38.7X1	T38.7X2	T38.7X3	T38.7X4	T38.7X5	T38.7X6
Analeptic NEC	T50.7X1	T50.7X2	T50.7X3	T50.7X4	T50.7X5	T50.7X6
Analgesic	T39.91	T39.92	T39.93	T39.94	T39.95	T39.96
anti-inflammatory NEC	T39.91	T39.92	T39.93	T39.94	T39.95	T39.96
propionic acid derivative	T39.311	T39.312	T39.313	T39.314	T39.315	T39.316
antirheumatic NEC	T39.4X1	T39.4X2	T39.4X3	T39.4X4	T39.4X5	T39.4X6
aromatic NEC	T39.1X1	T39.1X2	T39.1X3	T39.1X4	T39.1X5	T39.1X6
narcotic NEC	T40.601	T40.602	T40.603	T40.604	T40.605	T40.606
combination	T40.601	T40.602	T40.603	T40.604	T40.605	T40.606
obstetric	T40.601	T40.602	T40.603	T40.604	T40.605	T40.606
non-narcotic NEC	T39.91	T39.92	T39.93	T39.94	T39.95	T39.96
combination	T39.91	T39.92	T39.93	T39.94	T39.95	T39.96
pyrazole	T39.2X1	T39.2X2	T39.2X3	T39.2X4	T39.2X5	T39.2X6
specified NEC	T39.8X1	T39.8X2	T39.8X3	T39.8X4	T39.8X5	T39.8X6
Analgin	T39.2X1	T39.2X2	T39.2X3	T39.2X4	T39.2X5	T39.2X6
Anamirta cocculus	T62.1X1	T62.1X2	T62.1X3	T62.1X4	—	—
Ancillin	T36.0X1	T36.0X2	T36.0X3	T36.0X4	T36.0X5	T36.0X6
Ancrod	T45.691	T45.692	T45.693	T45.694	T45.695	T45.696
Androgen	T38.7X1	T38.7X2	T38.7X3	T38.7X4	T38.7X5	T38.7X6
Androgen-estrogen mixture	T38.7X1	T38.7X2	T38.7X3	T38.7X4	T38.7X5	T38.7X6
Androstalone	T38.7X1	T38.7X2	T38.7X3	T38.7X4	T38.7X5	T38.7X6
Androstanolone	T38.7X1	T38.7X2	T38.7X3	T38.7X4	T38.7X5	T38.7X6
Androsterone	T38.7X1	T38.7X2	T38.7X3	T38.7X4	T38.7X5	T38.7X6
Anemone pulsatilla	T62.2X1	T62.2X2	T62.2X3	T62.2X4	—	—
Anesthesia						
caudal	T41.3X1	T41.3X2	T41.3X3	T41.3X4	T41.3X5	T41.3X6
endotracheal	T41.0X1	T41.0X2	T41.0X3	T41.0X4	T41.0X5	T41.0X6
epidural	T41.3X1	T41.3X2	T41.3X3	T41.3X4	T41.3X5	T41.3X6
inhalation	T41.0X1	T41.0X2	T41.0X3	T41.0X4	T41.0X5	T41.0X6
local	T41.3X1	T41.3X2	T41.3X3	T41.3X4	T41.3X5	T41.3X6
mucosal	T41.3X1	T41.3X2	T41.3X3	T41.3X4	T41.3X5	T41.3X6
muscle relaxation	T48.1X1	T48.1X2	T48.1X3	T48.1X4	T48.1X5	T48.1X6
nerve blocking	T41.3X1	T41.3X2	T41.3X3	T41.3X4	T41.3X5	T41.3X6
plexus blocking	T41.3X1	T41.3X2	T41.3X3	T41.3X4	T41.3X5	T41.3X6
potentiated	T41.201	T41.202	T41.203	T41.204	T41.205	T41.206
rectal	T41.201	T41.202	T41.203	T41.204	T41.205	T41.206
general	T41.201	T41.202	T41.203	T41.204	T41.205	T41.206
local	T41.3X1	T41.3X2	T41.3X3	T41.3X4	T41.3X5	T41.3X6
regional	T41.3X1	T41.3X2	T41.3X3	T41.3X4	T41.3X5	T41.3X6
surface	T41.3X1	T41.3X2	T41.3X3	T41.3X4	T41.3X5	T41.3X6
Anesthetic NEC — see also Anesthesia	T41.41	T41.42	T41.43	T41.44	T41.45	T41.46
with muscle relaxant	T41.201	T41.202	T41.203	T41.204	T41.205	T41.206
general	T41.201	T41.202	T41.203	T41.204	T41.205	T41.206
local	T41.3X1	T41.3X2	T41.3X3	T41.3X4	T41.3X5	T41.3X6
gaseous NEC	T41.0X1	T41.0X2	T41.0X3	T41.0X4	T41.0X5	T41.0X6

Table of Drugs and Chemicals

Anesthetic NEC — Antihemophilic

Substance	Poisoning, Accidental (unintentional)	Poisoning, Intentional Self-harm	Poisoning, Assault	Poisoning, Undetermined	Adverse Effect	Under-dosing
Anesthetic — *see also* Anesthesia — *continued*						
general NEC	T41.2Ø1	T41.2Ø2	T41.2Ø3	T41.2Ø4	T41.2Ø5	T41.2Ø6
halogenated hydrocarbon derivatives NEC	T41.ØX1	T41.ØX2	T41.ØX3	T41.ØX4	T41.ØX5	T41.ØX6
infiltration NEC	T41.3X1	T41.3X2	T41.3X3	T41.3X4	T41.3X5	T41.3X6
intravenous NEC	T41.1X1	T41.1X2	T41.1X3	T41.1X4	T41.1X5	T41.1X6
local NEC	T41.3X1	T41.3X2	T41.3X3	T41.3X4	T41.3X5	T41.3X6
rectal	T41.2Ø1	T41.2Ø2	T41.2Ø3	T41.2Ø4	T41.2Ø5	T41.2Ø6
general	T41.2Ø1	T41.2Ø2	T41.2Ø3	T41.2Ø4	T41.2Ø5	T41.2Ø6
local	T41.3X1	T41.3X2	T41.3X3	T41.3X4	T41.3X5	T41.3X6
regional NEC	T41.3X1	T41.3X2	T41.3X3	T41.3X4	T41.3X5	T41.3X6
spinal NEC	T41.3X1	T41.3X2	T41.3X3	T41.3X4	T41.3X5	T41.3X6
thiobarbiturate	T41.1X1	T41.1X2	T41.1X3	T41.1X4	T41.1X5	T41.1X6
topical	T41.3X1	T41.3X2	T41.3X3	T41.3X4	T41.3X5	T41.3X6
Aneurine	T45.2X1	T45.2X2	T45.2X3	T45.2X4	T45.2X5	T45.2X6
Angio-Conray	T50.8X1	T50.8X2	T50.8X3	T50.8X4	T50.8X5	T50.8X6
Angiotensin	T44.5X1	T44.5X2	T44.5X3	T44.5X4	T44.5X5	T44.5X6
Angiotensinamide	T44.991	T44.992	T44.993	T44.994	T44.995	T44.996
Anhydrohydroxy-progesterone	T38.5X1	T38.5X2	T38.5X3	T38.5X4	T38.5X5	T38.5X6
Anhydron	T50.2X1	T50.2X2	T50.2X3	T50.2X4	T50.2X5	T50.2X6
Anileridine	T40.4X1	T40.4X2	T40.4X3	T40.4X4	T40.4X5	T40.4X6
Aniline (dye) (liquid)	T65.3X1	T65.3X2	T65.3X3	T65.3X4	—	—
analgesic	T39.1X1	T39.1X2	T39.1X3	T39.1X4	T39.1X5	T39.1X6
derivatives, therapeutic NEC	T39.1X1	T39.1X2	T39.1X3	T39.1X4	T39.1X5	T39.1X6
vapor	T65.3X1	T65.3X2	T65.3X3	T65.3X4	—	—
Aniscoropine	T44.3X1	T44.3X2	T44.3X3	T44.3X4	T44.3X5	T44.3X6
Anise oil	T47.5X1	T47.5X2	T47.5X3	T47.5X4	T47.5X5	T47.5X6
Anisidine	T65.3X1	T65.3X2	T65.3X3	T65.3X4	—	—
Anisindione	T45.511	T45.512	T45.513	T45.514	T45.515	T45.516
Anisotropine methyl-bromide	T44.3X1	T44.3X2	T44.3X3	T44.3X4	T44.3X5	T44.3X6
Anistreplase	T45.611	T45.612	T45.613	T45.614	T45.615	T45.616
Anorexiant (central)	T50.5X1	T50.5X2	T50.5X3	T50.5X4	T50.5X5	T50.5X6
Anorexic agents	T50.5X1	T50.5X2	T50.5X3	T50.5X4	T50.5X5	T50.5X6
Ansamycin	T36.6X1	T36.6X2	T36.6X3	T36.6X4	T36.6X5	T36.6X6
Ant (bite) (sting)	T63.421	T63.422	T63.423	T63.424	—	—
Antabuse	T50.6X1	T50.6X2	T50.6X3	T50.6X4	T50.6X5	T50.6X6
Antacid NEC	T47.1X1	T47.1X2	T47.1X3	T47.1X4	T47.1X5	T47.1X6
Antagonist						
Aldosterone	T50.ØX1	T50.ØX2	T50.ØX3	T50.ØX4	T50.ØX5	T50.ØX6
alpha-adrenoreceptor	T44.6X1	T44.6X2	T44.6X3	T44.6X4	T44.6X5	T44.6X6
anticoagulant	T45.7X1	T45.7X2	T45.7X3	T45.7X4	T45.7X5	T45.7X6
beta-adrenoreceptor	T44.7X1	T44.7X2	T44.7X3	T44.7X4	T44.7X5	T44.7X6
extrapyramidal NEC	T44.3X1	T44.3X2	T44.3X3	T44.3X4	T44.3X5	T44.3X6
folic acid	T45.1X1	T45.1X2	T45.1X3	T45.1X4	T45.1X5	T45.1X6
H2 receptor	T47.ØX1	T47.ØX2	T47.ØX3	T47.ØX4	T47.ØX5	T47.ØX6
heavy metal	T45.8X1	T45.8X2	T45.8X3	T45.8X4	T45.8X5	T45.8X6
narcotic analgesic	T50.7X1	T50.7X2	T50.7X3	T50.7X4	T50.7X5	T50.7X6
opiate	T50.7X1	T50.7X2	T50.7X3	T50.7X4	T50.7X5	T50.7X6
pyrimidine	T45.1X1	T45.1X2	T45.1X3	T45.1X4	T45.1X5	T45.1X6
serotonin	T46.5X1	T46.5X2	T46.5X3	T46.5X4	T46.5X5	T46.5X6
Antazolin(e)	T45.ØX1	T45.ØX2	T45.ØX3	T45.ØX4	T45.ØX5	T45.ØX6
Anterior pituitary hormone NEC	T38.811	T38.812	T38.813	T38.814	T38.815	T38.816
Anthelmintic NEC	T37.4X1	T37.4X2	T37.4X3	T37.4X4	T37.4X5	T37.4X6
Anthiolimine	T37.4X1	T37.4X2	T37.4X3	T37.4X4	T37.4X5	T37.4X6
Anthralin	T49.4X1	T49.4X2	T49.4X3	T49.4X4	T49.4X5	T49.4X6
Anthramycin	T45.1X1	T45.1X2	T45.1X3	T45.1X4	T45.1X5	T45.1X6
Antiadrenergic NEC	T44.8X1	T44.8X2	T44.8X3	T44.8X4	T44.8X5	T44.8X6
Antiallergic NEC	T45.ØX1	T45.ØX2	T45.ØX3	T45.ØX4	T45.ØX5	T45.ØX6
Antiandrogen NEC	T38.6X1	T38.6X2	T38.6X3	T38.6X4	T38.6X5	T38.6X6
Anti-anemic (drug) (preparation)	T45.8X1	T45.8X2	T45.8X3	T45.8X4	T45.8X5	T45.8X6
Antianxiety drug NEC	T43.5Ø1	T43.5Ø2	T43.5Ø3	T43.5Ø4	T43.5Ø5	T43.5Ø6
Antiaris toxicaria	T65.891	T65.892	T65.893	T65.894	—	—
Antiarteriosclerotic drug	T46.6X1	T46.6X2	T46.6X3	T46.6X4	T46.6X5	T46.6X6
Antiasthmatic drug NEC	T48.6X1	T48.6X2	T48.6X3	T48.6X4	T48.6X5	T48.6X6
Antibiotic NEC	T36.91	T36.92	T36.93	T36.94	T36.95	T36.96
aminoglycoside	T36.5X1	T36.5X2	T36.5X3	T36.5X4	T36.5X5	T36.5X6
anticancer	T45.1X1	T45.1X2	T45.1X3	T45.1X4	T45.1X5	T45.1X6
antifungal	T36.7X1	T36.7X2	T36.7X3	T36.7X4	T36.7X5	T36.7X6
antimycobacterial	T36.5X1	T36.5X2	T36.5X3	T36.5X4	T36.5X5	T36.5X6
antineoplastic	T45.1X1	T45.1X2	T45.1X3	T45.1X4	T45.1X5	T45.1X6
b-lactam NEC	T36.1X1	T36.1X2	T36.1X3	T36.1X4	T36.1X5	T36.1X6
cephalosporin (group)	T36.1X1	T36.1X2	T36.1X3	T36.1X4	T36.1X5	T36.1X6
chloramphenicol (group)	T36.2X1	T36.2X2	T36.2X3	T36.2X4	T36.2X5	T36.2X6
ENT	T49.6X1	T49.6X2	T49.6X3	T49.6X4	T49.6X5	T49.6X6
eye	T49.5X1	T49.5X2	T49.5X3	T49.5X4	T49.5X5	T49.5X6
fungicidal (local)	T49.ØX1	T49.ØX2	T49.ØX3	T49.ØX4	T49.ØX5	T49.ØX6
intestinal	T36.8X1	T36.8X2	T36.8X3	T36.8X4	T36.8X5	T36.8X6
local	T49.ØX1	T49.ØX2	T49.ØX3	T49.ØX4	T49.ØX5	T49.ØX6

Substance	Poisoning, Accidental (unintentional)	Poisoning, Intentional Self-harm	Poisoning, Assault	Poisoning, Undetermined	Adverse Effect	Under-dosing
Antibiotic — *continued*						
macrolides	T36.3X1	T36.3X2	T36.3X3	T36.3X4	T36.3X5	T36.3X6
polypeptide	T36.8X1	T36.8X2	T36.8X3	T36.8X4	T36.8X5	T36.8X6
specified NEC	T36.8X1	T36.8X2	T36.8X3	T36.8X4	T36.8X5	T36.8X6
tetracycline (group)	T36.4X1	T36.4X2	T36.4X3	T36.4X4	T36.4X5	T36.4X6
throat	T49.6X1	T49.6X2	T49.6X3	T49.6X4	T49.6X5	T49.6X6
Anticancer agents NEC	T45.1X1	T45.1X2	T45.1X3	T45.1X4	T45.1X5	T45.1X6
Anticholesterolemic drug NEC	T46.6X1	T46.6X2	T46.6X3	T46.6X4	T46.6X5	T46.6X6
Anticholinergic NEC	T44.3X1	T44.3X2	T44.3X3	T44.3X4	T44.3X5	T44.3X6
Anticholinesterase	T44.ØX1	T44.ØX2	T44.ØX3	T44.ØX4	T44.ØX5	T44.ØX6
organophosphorus	T44.ØX1	T44.ØX2	T44.ØX3	T44.ØX4	T44.ØX5	T44.ØX6
insecticide	T60.ØX1	T60.ØX2	T60.ØX3	T60.ØX4	—	—
nerve gas	T59.891	T59.892	T59.893	T59.894	—	—
reversible	T44.ØX1	T44.ØX2	T44.ØX3	T44.ØX4	T44.ØX5	T44.ØX6
ophthalmological	T49.5X1	T49.5X2	T49.5X3	T49.5X4	T49.5X5	T49.5X6
Anticoagulant NEC	T45.511	T45.512	T45.513	T45.514	T45.515	T45.516
Antagonist	T45.7X1	T45.7X2	T45.7X3	T45.7X4	T45.7X5	T45.7X6
Anti-common-cold drug NEC	T48.5X1	T48.5X2	T48.5X3	T48.5X4	T48.5X5	T48.5X6
Anticonvulsant	T42.71	T42.72	T42.73	T42.74	T42.75	T42.76
barbiturate	T42.3X1	T42.3X2	T42.3X3	T42.3X4	T42.3X5	T42.3X6
combination (with barbiturate)	T42.3X1	T42.3X2	T42.3X3	T42.3X4	T42.3X5	T42.3X6
hydantoin	T42.ØX1	T42.ØX2	T42.ØX3	T42.ØX4	T42.ØX5	T42.ØX6
hypnotic NEC	T42.6X1	T42.6X2	T42.6X3	T42.6X4	T42.6X5	T42.6X6
oxazolidinedione	T42.2X1	T42.2X2	T42.2X3	T42.2X4	T42.2X5	T42.2X6
pyrimidinedione	T42.6X1	T42.6X2	T42.6X3	T42.6X4	T42.6X5	T42.6X6
specified NEC	T42.6X1	T42.6X2	T42.6X3	T42.6X4	T42.6X5	T42.6X6
succinimide	T42.2X1	T42.2X2	T42.2X3	T42.2X4	T42.2X5	T42.2X6
Antidepressant	T43.2Ø1	T43.2Ø2	T43.2Ø3	T43.2Ø4	T43.2Ø5	T43.2Ø6
monoamine oxidase inhibitor	T43.1X1	T43.1X2	T43.1X3	T43.1X4	T43.1X5	T43.1X6
selective serotonin norepinephrine reuptake inhibitor	T43.211	T43.212	T43.213	T43.214	T43.215	T43.216
selective serotonin reuptake inhibitor	T43.221	T43.222	T43.223	T43.224	T43.225	T43.226
specified NEC	T43.291	T43.292	T43.293	T43.294	T43.295	T43.296
tetracyclic	T43.Ø21	T43.Ø22	T43.Ø23	T43.Ø24	T43.Ø25	T43.Ø26
triazolopyridine	T43.211	T43.212	T43.213	T43.214	T43.215	T43.216
tricyclic	T43.Ø11	T43.Ø12	T43.Ø13	T43.Ø14	T43.Ø15	T43.Ø16
Antidiabetic NEC	T38.3X1	T38.3X2	T38.3X3	T38.3X4	T38.3X5	T38.3X6
biguanide	T38.3X1	T38.3X2	T38.3X3	T38.3X4	T38.3X5	T38.3X6
and sulfonyl combined	T38.3X1	T38.3X2	T38.3X3	T38.3X4	T38.3X5	T38.3X6
combined	T38.3X1	T38.3X2	T38.3X3	T38.3X4	T38.3X5	T38.3X6
sulfonylurea	T38.3X1	T38.3X2	T38.3X3	T38.3X4	T38.3X5	T38.3X6
Antidiarrheal drug NEC	T47.6X1	T47.6X2	T47.6X3	T47.6X4	T47.6X5	T47.6X6
absorbent	T47.6X1	T47.6X2	T47.6X3	T47.6X4	T47.6X5	T47.6X6
Anti-D immunoglobulin (human)	T50.Z11	T50.Z12	T50.Z13	T50.Z14	T50.Z15	T50.Z16
Antidiphtheria serum	T50.Z11	T50.Z12	T50.Z13	T50.Z14	T50.Z15	T50.Z16
Antidiuretic hormone	T38.891	T38.892	T38.893	T38.894	T38.895	T38.896
Antidote NEC	T50.6X1	T50.6X2	T50.6X3	T50.6X4	T50.6X5	T50.6X6
heavy metal	T45.8X1	T45.8X2	T45.8X3	T45.8X4	T45.8X5	T45.8X6
Antidysrhythmic NEC	T46.2X1	T46.2X2	T46.2X3	T46.2X4	T46.2X5	T46.2X6
Antiemetic drug	T45.ØX1	T45.ØX2	T45.ØX3	T45.ØX4	T45.ØX5	T45.ØX6
Antiepilepsy agent	T42.71	T42.72	T42.73	T42.74	T42.75	T42.76
combination	T42.5X1	T42.5X2	T42.5X3	T42.5X4	T42.5X5	T42.5X6
mixed	T42.5X1	T42.5X2	T42.5X3	T42.5X4	T42.5X5	T42.5X6
specified, NEC	T42.6X1	T42.6X2	T42.6X3	T42.6X4	T42.6X5	T42.6X6
Antiestrogen NEC	T38.6X1	T38.6X2	T38.6X3	T38.6X4	T38.6X5	T38.6X6
Antifertility pill	T38.4X1	T38.4X2	T38.4X3	T38.4X4	T38.4X5	T38.4X6
Antifibrinolytic drug	T45.621	T45.622	T45.623	T45.624	T45.625	T45.626
Antifilarial drug	T37.4X1	T37.4X2	T37.4X3	T37.4X4	T37.4X5	T37.4X6
Antiflatulent	T47.5X1	T47.5X2	T47.5X3	T47.5X4	T47.5X5	T47.5X6
Antifreeze	T65.91	T65.92	T65.93	T65.94	—	—
alcohol	T51.1X1	T51.1X2	T51.1X3	T51.1X4	—	—
ethylene glycol	T51.8X1	T51.8X2	T51.8X3	T51.8X4	—	—
Antifungal						
antibiotic (systemic)	T36.7X1	T36.7X2	T36.7X3	T36.7X4	T36.7X5	T36.7X6
anti-infective NEC	T37.91	T37.92	T37.93	T37.94	T37.95	T37.96
disinfectant, local	T49.ØX1	T49.ØX2	T49.ØX3	T49.ØX4	T49.ØX5	T49.ØX6
nonmedicinal (spray)	T60.3X1	T60.3X2	T60.3X3	T60.3X4	—	—
topical	T49.ØX1	T49.ØX2	T49.ØX3	T49.ØX4	T49.ØX5	T49.ØX6
Anti-gastric-secretion drug NEC	T47.1X1	T47.1X2	T47.1X3	T47.1X4	T47.1X5	T47.1X6
Antigonadotrophin NEC	T38.6X1	T38.6X2	T38.6X3	T38.6X4	T38.6X5	T38.6X6
Antihallucinogen	T43.5Ø1	T43.5Ø2	T43.5Ø3	T43.5Ø4	T43.5Ø5	T43.5Ø6
Antihelmintics	T37.4X1	T37.4X2	T37.4X3	T37.4X4	T37.4X5	T37.4X6
Antihemophilic						
factor	T45.8X1	T45.8X2	T45.8X3	T45.8X4	T45.8X5	T45.8X6
fraction	T45.8X1	T45.8X2	T45.8X3	T45.8X4	T45.8X5	T45.8X6

Substance	Poisoning, Accidental (unintentional)	Poisoning, Intentional Self-harm	Poisoning, Assault	Poisoning, Undetermined	Adverse Effect	Under-dosing
Antihemophilic — *continued*						
globulin concentrate	T45.7X1	T45.7X2	T45.7X3	T45.7X4	T45.7X5	T45.7X6
human plasma	T45.8X1	T45.8X2	T45.8X3	T45.8X4	T45.8X5	T45.8X6
plasma, dried	T45.7X1	T45.7X2	T45.7X3	T45.7X4	T45.7X5	T45.7X6
Antihemorrhoidal preparation	T49.2X1	T49.2X2	T49.2X3	T49.2X4	T49.2X5	T49.2X6
Antiheparin drug	T45.7X1	T45.7X2	T45.7X3	T45.7X4	T45.7X5	T45.7X6
Antihistamine	T45.0X1	T45.0X2	T45.0X3	T45.0X4	T45.0X5	T45.0X6
Antihookworm drug	T37.4X1	T37.4X2	T37.4X3	T37.4X4	T37.4X5	T37.4X6
Anti-human lymphocytic globulin	T50.Z11	T50.Z12	T50.Z13	T50.Z14	T50.Z15	T50.Z16
Antihyperlipidemic drug	T46.6X1	T46.6X2	T46.6X3	T46.6X4	T46.6X5	T46.6X6
Antihypertensive drug NEC	T46.5X1	T46.5X2	T46.5X3	T46.5X4	T46.5X5	T46.5X6
Anti-infective NEC	T37.91	T37.92	T37.93	T37.94	T37.95	T37.96
anthelmintic	T37.4X1	T37.4X2	T37.4X3	T37.4X4	T37.4X5	T37.4X6
antibiotics	T36.91	T36.92	T36.93	T36.94	T36.95	T36.96
specified NEC	T36.8X1	T36.8X2	T36.8X3	T36.8X4	T36.8X5	T36.8X6
antimalarial	T37.2X1	T37.2X2	T37.2X3	T37.2X4	T37.2X5	T37.2X6
antimycobacterial NEC	T37.1X1	T37.1X2	T37.1X3	T37.1X4	T37.1X5	T37.1X6
antibiotics	T36.5X1	T36.5X2	T36.5X3	T36.5X4	T36.5X5	T36.5X6
antiprotozoal NEC	T37.3X1	T37.3X2	T37.3X3	T37.3X4	T37.3X5	T37.3X6
blood	T37.2X1	T37.2X2	T37.2X3	T37.2X4	T37.2X5	T37.2X6
antiviral	T37.5X1	T37.5X2	T37.5X3	T37.5X4	T37.5X5	T37.5X6
arsenical	T37.8X1	T37.8X2	T37.8X3	T37.8X4	T37.8X5	T37.8X6
bismuth, local	T49.0X1	T49.0X2	T49.0X3	T49.0X4	T49.0X5	T49.0X6
ENT	T49.6X1	T49.6X2	T49.6X3	T49.6X4	T49.6X5	T49.6X6
eye NEC	T49.5X1	T49.5X2	T49.5X3	T49.5X4	T49.5X5	T49.5X6
heavy metals NEC	T37.8X1	T37.8X2	T37.8X3	T37.8X4	T37.8X5	T37.8X6
local NEC	T49.0X1	T49.0X2	T49.0X3	T49.0X4	T49.0X5	T49.0X6
specified NEC	T49.0X1	T49.0X2	T49.0X3	T49.0X4	T49.0X5	T49.0X6
mixed	T37.91	T37.92	T37.93	T37.94	T37.95	T37.96
ophthalmic preparation	T49.5X1	T49.5X2	T49.5X3	T49.5X4	T49.5X5	T49.5X6
topical NEC	T49.0X1	T49.0X2	T49.0X3	T49.0X4	T49.0X5	T49.0X6
Anti-inflammatory drug NEC	T39.391	T39.392	T39.393	T39.394	T39.395	T39.396
local	T49.0X1	T49.0X2	T49.0X3	T49.0X4	T49.0X5	T49.0X6
nonsteroidal NEC	T39.391	T39.392	T39.393	T39.394	T39.395	T39.396
propionic acid derivative	T39.311	T39.312	T39.313	T39.314	T39.315	T39.316
specified NEC	T39.391	T39.392	T39.393	T39.394	T39.395	T39.396
Antikaluretic	T50.3X1	T50.3X2	T50.3X3	T50.3X4	T50.3X5	T50.3X6
Antiknock (tetraethyl lead)	T56.0X1	T56.0X2	T56.0X3	T56.0X4	—	—
Antilipemic drug NEC	T46.6X1	T46.6X2	T46.6X3	T46.6X4	T46.6X5	T46.6X6
Antimalarial	T37.2X1	T37.2X2	T37.2X3	T37.2X4	T37.2X5	T37.2X6
prophylactic NEC	T37.2X1	T37.2X2	T37.2X3	T37.2X4	T37.2X5	T37.2X6
pyrimidine derivative	T37.2X1	T37.2X2	T37.2X3	T37.2X4	T37.2X5	T37.2X6
Antimetabolite	T45.1X1	T45.1X2	T45.1X3	T45.1X4	T45.1X5	T45.1X6
Antimitotic agent	T45.1X1	T45.1X2	T45.1X3	T45.1X4	T45.1X5	T45.1X6
Antimony (compounds) (vapor) NEC	T56.891	T56.892	T56.893	T56.894	—	—
anti-infectives	T37.8X1	T37.8X2	T37.8X3	T37.8X4	T37.8X5	T37.8X6
dimercaptosuccinate	T37.3X1	T37.3X2	T37.3X3	T37.3X4	T37.3X5	T37.3X6
hydride	T56.891	T56.892	T56.893	T56.894	—	—
pesticide (vapor)	T60.8X1	T60.8X2	T60.8X3	T60.8X4	—	—
potassium (sodium) tartrate	T37.8X1	T37.8X2	T37.8X3	T37.8X4	T37.8X5	T37.8X6
sodium	T37.3X1	T37.3X2	T37.3X3	T37.3X4	T37.3X5	T37.3X6
dimercaptosuccinate						
tartrated	T37.8X1	T37.8X2	T37.8X3	T37.8X4	T37.8X5	T37.8X6
Antimuscarinic NEC	T44.3X1	T44.3X2	T44.3X3	T44.3X4	T44.3X5	T44.3X6
Antimycobacterial drug NEC	T37.1X1	T37.1X2	T37.1X3	T37.1X4	T37.1X5	T37.1X6
antibiotics	T36.5X1	T36.5X2	T36.5X3	T36.5X4	T36.5X5	T36.5X6
combination	T37.1X1	T37.1X2	T37.1X3	T37.1X4	T37.1X5	T37.1X6
Antinausea drug	T45.0X1	T45.0X2	T45.0X3	T45.0X4	T45.0X5	T45.0X6
Antinematode drug	T37.4X1	T37.4X2	T37.4X3	T37.4X4	T37.4X5	T37.4X6
Antineoplastic NEC	T45.1X1	T45.1X2	T45.1X3	T45.1X4	T45.1X5	T45.1X6
alkaloidal	T45.1X1	T45.1X2	T45.1X3	T45.1X4	T45.1X5	T45.1X6
antibiotics	T45.1X1	T45.1X2	T45.1X3	T45.1X4	T45.1X5	T45.1X6
combination	T45.1X1	T45.1X2	T45.1X3	T45.1X4	T45.1X5	T45.1X6
estrogen	T38.5X1	T38.5X2	T38.5X3	T38.5X4	T38.5X5	T38.5X6
steroid	T38.7X1	T38.7X2	T38.7X3	T38.7X4	T38.7X5	T38.7X6
Antiparasitic drug (systemic)	T37.91	T37.92	T37.93	T37.94	T37.95	T37.96
local	T49.0X1	T49.0X2	T49.0X3	T49.0X4	T49.0X5	T49.0X6
specified NEC	T37.8X1	T37.8X2	T37.8X3	T37.8X4	T37.8X5	T37.8X6
Antiparkinsonism drug NEC	T42.8X1	T42.8X2	T42.8X3	T42.8X4	T42.8X5	T42.8X6
Antiperspirant NEC	T49.2X1	T49.2X2	T49.2X3	T49.2X4	T49.2X5	T49.2X6
Antiphlogistic NEC	T39.4X1	T39.4X2	T39.4X3	T39.4X4	T39.4X5	T39.4X6
Antiplatyhelmintic drug	T37.4X1	T37.4X2	T37.4X3	T37.4X4	T37.4X5	T37.4X6
Antiprotozoal drug NEC	T37.3X1	T37.3X2	T37.3X3	T37.3X4	T37.3X5	T37.3X6
blood	T37.2X1	T37.2X2	T37.2X3	T37.2X4	T37.2X5	T37.2X6
local	T49.0X1	T49.0X2	T49.0X3	T49.0X4	T49.0X5	T49.0X6
Antipruritic drug NEC	T49.1X1	T49.1X2	T49.1X3	T49.1X4	T49.1X5	T49.1X6
Antipsychotic drug	T43.501	T43.502	T43.503	T43.504	T43.505	T43.506
specified NEC	T43.591	T43.592	T43.593	T43.594	T43.595	T43.596
Antipyretic	T39.91	T39.92	T39.93	T39.94	T39.95	T39.96
specified NEC	T39.8X1	T39.8X2	T39.8X3	T39.8X4	T39.8X5	T39.8X6
Antipyrine	T39.2X1	T39.2X2	T39.2X3	T39.2X4	T39.2X5	T39.2X6
Antirabies hyperimmune serum	T50.Z11	T50.Z12	T50.Z13	T50.Z14	T50.Z15	T50.Z16
Antirheumatic NEC	T39.4X1	T39.4X2	T39.4X3	T39.4X4	T39.4X5	T39.4X6
Antirigidity drug NEC	T42.8X1	T42.8X2	T42.8X3	T42.8X4	T42.8X5	T42.8X6
Antischistosomal drug	T37.4X1	T37.4X2	T37.4X3	T37.4X4	T37.4X5	T37.4X6
Antiscorpion sera	T50.Z11	T50.Z12	T50.Z13	T50.Z14	T50.Z15	T50.Z16
Antiseborrheics	T49.4X1	T49.4X2	T49.4X3	T49.4X4	T49.4X5	T49.4X6
Antiseptics (external) (medicinal)	T49.0X1	T49.0X2	T49.0X3	T49.0X4	T49.0X5	T49.0X6
Antistine	T45.0X1	T45.0X2	T45.0X3	T45.0X4	T45.0X5	T45.0X6
Antitapeworm drug	T37.4X1	T37.4X2	T37.4X3	T37.4X4	T37.4X5	T37.4X6
Antitetanus immunoglobulin	T50.Z11	T50.Z12	T50.Z13	T50.Z14	T50.Z15	T50.Z16
Antithrombotic	T45.521	T45.522	T45.523	T45.524	T45.525	T45.526
Antithyroid drug NEC	T38.2X1	T38.2X2	T38.2X3	T38.2X4	T38.2X5	T38.2X6
Antitoxin	T50.Z11	T50.Z12	T50.Z13	T50.Z14	T50.Z15	T50.Z16
diphtheria	T50.Z11	T50.Z12	T50.Z13	T50.Z14	T50.Z15	T50.Z16
gas gangrene	T50.Z11	T50.Z12	T50.Z13	T50.Z14	T50.Z15	T50.Z16
tetanus	T50.Z11	T50.Z12	T50.Z13	T50.Z14	T50.Z15	T50.Z16
Antitrichomonal drug	T37.3X1	T37.3X2	T37.3X3	T37.3X4	T37.3X5	T37.3X6
Antituberculars	T37.1X1	T37.1X2	T37.1X3	T37.1X4	T37.1X5	T37.1X6
antibiotics	T36.5X1	T36.5X2	T36.5X3	T36.5X4	T36.5X5	T36.5X6
Antitussive NEC	T48.3X1	T48.3X2	T48.3X3	T48.3X4	T48.3X5	T48.3X6
codeine mixture	T40.2X1	T40.2X2	T40.2X3	T40.2X4	T40.2X5	T40.2X6
opiate	T40.2X1	T40.2X2	T40.2X3	T40.2X4	T40.2X5	T40.2X6
Antivaricose drug	T46.8X1	T46.8X2	T46.8X3	T46.8X4	T46.8X5	T46.8X6
Antivenin, antivenom (sera)	T50.Z11	T50.Z12	T50.Z13	T50.Z14	T50.Z15	T50.Z16
crotaline	T50.Z11	T50.Z12	T50.Z13	T50.Z14	T50.Z15	T50.Z16
spider bite	T50.Z11	T50.Z12	T50.Z13	T50.Z14	T50.Z15	T50.Z16
Antivertigo drug	T45.0X1	T45.0X2	T45.0X3	T45.0X4	T45.0X5	T45.0X6
Antiviral drug NEC	T37.5X1	T37.5X2	T37.5X3	T37.5X4	T37.5X5	T37.5X6
eye	T49.5X1	T49.5X2	T49.5X3	T49.5X4	T49.5X5	T49.5X6
Antiwhipworm drug	T37.4X1	T37.4X2	T37.4X3	T37.4X4	T37.4X5	T37.4X6
Ant poison — *see* Insecticide						
Antrol — *see also* by specific chemical substance	T60.91	T60.92	T60.93	T60.94	—	—
fungicide	T60.91	T60.92	T60.93	T60.94	—	—
ANTU (alpha naphthylthiourea)	T60.4X1	T60.4X2	T60.4X3	T60.4X4	—	—
Apalcillin	T36.0X1	T36.0X2	T36.0X3	T36.0X4	T36.0X5	T36.0X6
APC	T48.5X1	T48.5X2	T48.5X3	T48.5X4	T48.5X5	T48.5X6
Aplonidine	T44.4X1	T44.4X2	T44.4X3	T44.4X4	T44.4X5	T44.4X6
Apomorphine	T47.7X1	T47.7X2	T47.7X3	T47.7X4	T47.7X5	T47.7X6
Appetite depressants, central	T50.5X1	T50.5X2	T50.5X3	T50.5X4	T50.5X5	T50.5X6
Apraclonidine (hydrochloride)	T44.4X1	T44.4X2	T44.4X3	T44.4X4	T44.4X5	T44.4X6
Apresoline	T46.5X1	T46.5X2	T46.5X3	T46.5X4	T46.5X5	T46.5X6
Aprindine	T46.2X1	T46.2X2	T46.2X3	T46.2X4	T46.2X5	T46.2X6
Aprobarbital	T42.3X1	T42.3X2	T42.3X3	T42.3X4	T42.3X5	T42.3X6
Apronalide	T42.6X1	T42.6X2	T42.6X3	T42.6X4	T42.6X5	T42.6X6
Aprotinin	T45.621	T45.622	T45.623	T45.624	T45.625	T45.626
Aptocaine	T41.3X1	T41.3X2	T41.3X3	T41.3X4	T41.3X5	T41.3X6
Aqua fortis	T54.2X1	T54.2X2	T54.2X3	T54.2X4	—	—
Ara-A	T37.5X1	T37.5X2	T37.5X3	T37.5X4	T37.5X5	T37.5X6
Ara-C	T45.1X1	T45.1X2	T45.1X3	T45.1X4	T45.1X5	T45.1X6
Arachis oil	T49.3X1	T49.3X2	T49.3X3	T49.3X4	T49.3X5	T49.3X6
cathartic	T47.4X1	T47.4X2	T47.4X3	T47.4X4	T47.4X5	T47.4X6
Aralen	T37.2X1	T37.2X2	T37.2X3	T37.2X4	T37.2X5	T37.2X6
Arecoline	T44.1X1	T44.1X2	T44.1X3	T44.1X4	T44.1X5	T44.1X6
Arginine	T50.991	T50.992	T50.993	T50.994	T50.995	T50.996
glutamate	T50.991	T50.992	T50.993	T50.994	T50.995	T50.996
Argyrol	T49.0X1	T49.0X2	T49.0X3	T49.0X4	T49.0X5	T49.0X6
ENT agent	T49.6X1	T49.6X2	T49.6X3	T49.6X4	T49.6X5	T49.6X6
ophthalmic preparation	T49.5X1	T49.5X2	T49.5X3	T49.5X4	T49.5X5	T49.5X6
Aristocort	T38.0X1	T38.0X2	T38.0X3	T38.0X4	T38.0X5	T38.0X6
ENT agent	T49.6X1	T49.6X2	T49.6X3	T49.6X4	T49.6X5	T49.6X6
ophthalmic preparation	T49.5X1	T49.5X2	T49.5X3	T49.5X4	T49.5X5	T49.5X6
topical NEC	T49.0X1	T49.0X2	T49.0X3	T49.0X4	T49.0X5	T49.0X6
Aromatics, corrosive	T54.1X1	T54.1X2	T54.1X3	T54.1X4	—	—
disinfectants	T54.1X1	T54.1X2	T54.1X3	T54.1X4	—	—
Arsenate of lead	T57.0X1	T57.0X2	T57.0X3	T57.0X4	—	—
herbicide	T57.0X1	T57.0X2	T57.0X3	T57.0X4	—	—
Arsenic, arsenicals (compounds) (dust) (vapor) **NEC**	T57.0X1	T57.0X2	T57.0X3	T57.0X4	—	—
anti-infectives	T37.8X1	T37.8X2	T37.8X3	T37.8X4	T37.8X5	T37.8X6
pesticide (dust) (fumes)	T57.0X1	T57.0X2	T57.0X3	T57.0X4	—	—

Table of Drugs and Chemicals

Substance	Poisoning, Accidental (unintentional)	Poisoning, Intentional Self-harm	Poisoning, Assault	Poisoning, Undetermined	Adverse Effect	Under-dosing
Arsine (gas)	T57.0X1	T57.0X2	T57.0X3	T57.0X4	—	—
Arsphenamine (silver)	T37.8X1	T37.8X2	T37.8X3	T37.8X4	T37.8X5	T37.8X6
Arsthinol	T37.3X1	T37.3X2	T37.3X3	T37.3X4	T37.3X5	T37.3X6
Artane	T44.3X1	T44.3X2	T44.3X3	T44.3X4	T44.3X5	T44.3X6
Arthropod (venomous) **NEC**	T63.481	T63.482	T63.483	T63.484	—	—
Articaine	T41.3X1	T41.3X2	T41.3X3	T41.3X4	T41.3X5	T41.3X6
Asbestos	T57.8X1	T57.8X2	T57.8X3	T57.8X4	—	—
Ascaridole	T37.4X1	T37.4X2	T37.4X3	T37.4X4	T37.4X5	T37.4X6
Ascorbic acid	T45.2X1	T45.2X2	T45.2X3	T45.2X4	T45.2X5	T45.2X6
Asiaticoside	T49.0X1	T49.0X2	T49.0X3	T49.0X4	T49.0X5	T49.0X6
Asparaginase	T45.1X1	T45.1X2	T45.1X3	T45.1X4	T45.1X5	T45.1X6
Aspidium (oleoresin)	T37.4X1	T37.4X2	T37.4X3	T37.4X4	T37.4X5	T37.4X6
Aspirin (aluminum) (soluble)	T39.011	T39.012	T39.013	T39.014	T39.015	T39.016
Aspoxicillin	T36.0X1	T36.0X2	T36.0X3	T36.0X4	T36.0X5	T36.0X6
Astemizole	T45.0X1	T45.0X2	T45.0X3	T45.0X4	T45.0X5	T45.0X6
Astringent (local)	T49.2X1	T49.2X2	T49.2X3	T49.2X4	T49.2X5	T49.2X6
specified NEC	T49.2X1	T49.2X2	T49.2X3	T49.2X4	T49.2X5	T49.2X6
Astromicin	T36.5X1	T36.5X2	T36.5X3	T36.5X4	T36.5X5	T36.5X6
Ataractic drug NEC	T43.501	T43.502	T43.503	T43.504	T43.505	T43.506
Atenolol	T44.7X1	T44.7X2	T44.7X3	T44.7X4	T44.7X5	T44.7X6
Atonia drug, intestinal	T47.4X1	T47.4X2	T47.4X3	T47.4X4	T47.4X5	T47.4X6
Atophan	T50.4X1	T50.4X2	T50.4X3	T50.4X4	T50.4X5	T50.4X6
Atracurium besilate	T48.1X1	T48.1X2	T48.1X3	T48.1X4	T48.1X5	T48.1X6
Atropine	T44.3X1	T44.3X2	T44.3X3	T44.3X4	T44.3X5	T44.3X6
derivative	T44.3X1	T44.3X2	T44.3X3	T44.3X4	T44.3X5	T44.3X6
methonitrate	T44.3X1	T44.3X2	T44.3X3	T44.3X4	T44.3X5	T44.3X6
Attapulgite	T47.6X1	T47.6X2	T47.6X3	T47.6X4	T47.6X5	T47.6X6
Auramine	T65.891	T65.892	T65.893	T65.894	—	—
dye	T65.6X1	T65.6X2	T65.6X3	T65.6X4	—	—
fungicide	T60.3X1	T60.3X2	T60.3X3	T60.3X4	—	—
Auranofin	T39.4X1	T39.4X2	T39.4X3	T39.4X4	T39.4X5	T39.4X6
Aurantiin	T46.991	T46.992	T46.993	T46.994	T46.995	T46.996
Aureomycin	T36.4X1	T36.4X2	T36.4X3	T36.4X4	T36.4X5	T36.4X6
ophthalmic preparation	T49.5X1	T49.5X2	T49.5X3	T49.5X4	T49.5X5	T49.5X6
topical NEC	T49.0X1	T49.0X2	T49.0X3	T49.0X4	T49.0X5	T49.0X6
Aurothioglucose	T39.4X1	T39.4X2	T39.4X3	T39.4X4	T39.4X5	T39.4X6
Aurothioglycanide	T39.4X1	T39.4X2	T39.4X3	T39.4X4	T39.4X5	T39.4X6
Aurothiomalate sodium	T39.4X1	T39.4X2	T39.4X3	T39.4X4	T39.4X5	T39.4X6
Aurotioprol	T39.4X1	T39.4X2	T39.4X3	T39.4X4	T39.4X5	T39.4X6
Automobile fuel	T52.0X1	T52.0X2	T52.0X3	T52.0X4	—	—
Autonomic nervous system agent NEC	T44.901	T44.902	T44.903	T44.904	T44.905	T44.906
Avlosulfon	T37.1X1	T37.1X2	T37.1X3	T37.1X4	T37.1X5	T37.1X6
Avomine	T42.6X1	T42.6X2	T42.6X3	T42.6X4	T42.6X5	T42.6X6
Axerophthol	T45.2X1	T45.2X2	T45.2X3	T45.2X4	T45.2X5	T45.2X6
Azacitidine	T45.1X1	T45.1X2	T45.1X3	T45.1X4	T45.1X5	T45.1X6
Azacyclonol	T43.591	T43.592	T43.593	T43.594	T43.595	T43.596
Azadirachta	T60.2X1	T60.2X2	T60.2X3	T60.2X4	—	—
Azanidazole	T37.3X1	T37.3X2	T37.3X3	T37.3X4	T37.3X5	T37.3X6
Azapetine	T46.7X1	T46.7X2	T46.7X3	T46.7X4	T46.7X5	T46.7X6
Azapropazone	T39.2X1	T39.2X2	T39.2X3	T39.2X4	T39.2X5	T39.2X6
Azaribine	T45.1X1	T45.1X2	T45.1X3	T45.1X4	T45.1X5	T45.1X6
Azaserine	T45.1X1	T45.1X2	T45.1X3	T45.1X4	T45.1X5	T45.1X6
Azatadine	T45.0X1	T45.0X2	T45.0X3	T45.0X4	T45.0X5	T45.0X6
Azatepa	T45.1X1	T45.1X2	T45.1X3	T45.1X4	T45.1X5	T45.1X6
Azathioprine	T45.1X1	T45.1X2	T45.1X3	T45.1X4	T45.1X5	T45.1X6
Azelaic acid	T49.0X1	T49.0X2	T49.0X3	T49.0X4	T49.0X5	T49.0X6
Azelastine	T45.0X1	T45.0X2	T45.0X3	T45.0X4	T45.0X5	T45.0X6
Azidocillin	T36.0X1	T36.0X2	T36.0X3	T36.0X4	T36.0X5	T36.0X6
Azidothymidine	T37.5X1	T37.5X2	T37.5X3	T37.5X4	T37.5X5	T37.5X6
Azinphos (ethyl) (methyl)	T60.0X1	T60.0X2	T60.0X3	T60.0X4	—	—
Aziridine (chelating)	T54.1X1	T54.1X2	T54.1X3	T54.1X4	—	—
Azithromycin	T36.3X1	T36.3X2	T36.3X3	T36.3X4	T36.3X5	T36.3X6
Azlocillin	T36.0X1	T36.0X2	T36.0X3	T36.0X4	T36.0X5	T36.0X6
Azobenzene smoke	T65.3X1	T65.3X2	T65.3X3	T65.3X4	—	—
acaricide	T60.8X1	T60.8X2	T60.8X3	T60.8X4	—	—
Azosulfamide	T37.0X1	T37.0X2	T37.0X3	T37.0X4	T37.0X5	T37.0X6
AZT	T37.5X1	T37.5X2	T37.5X3	T37.5X4	T37.5X5	T37.5X6
Aztreonam	T36.1X1	T36.1X2	T36.1X3	T36.1X4	T36.1X5	T36.1X6
Azulfidine	T37.0X1	T37.0X2	T37.0X3	T37.0X4	T37.0X5	T37.0X6
Azuresin	T50.8X1	T50.8X2	T50.8X3	T50.8X4	T50.8X5	T50.8X6
b-acetyldigoxin	T46.0X1	T46.0X2	T46.0X3	T46.0X4	T46.0X5	T46.0X6
P-Acetamidophenol	T39.1X1	T39.1X2	T39.1X3	T39.1X4	T39.1X5	T39.1X6
Bacampicillin	T36.0X1	T36.0X2	T36.0X3	T36.0X4	T36.0X5	T36.0X6
Bacillus						
lactobacillus	T47.8X1	T47.8X2	T47.8X3	T47.8X4	T47.8X5	T47.8X6
subtilis	T47.6X1	T47.6X2	T47.6X3	T47.6X4	T47.6X5	T47.6X6
Bacimycin	T49.0X1	T49.0X2	T49.0X3	T49.0X4	T49.0X5	T49.0X6
ophthalmic preparation	T49.5X1	T49.5X2	T49.5X3	T49.5X4	T49.5X5	T49.5X6
Bacitracin zinc	T49.0X1	T49.0X2	T49.0X3	T49.0X4	T49.0X5	T49.0X6
with neomycin	T49.0X1	T49.0X2	T49.0X3	T49.0X4	T49.0X5	T49.0X6
ENT agent	T49.6X1	T49.6X2	T49.6X3	T49.6X4	T49.6X5	T49.6X6
ophthalmic preparation	T49.5X1	T49.5X2	T49.5X3	T49.5X4	T49.5X5	T49.5X6

Substance	Poisoning, Accidental (unintentional)	Poisoning, Intentional Self-harm	Poisoning, Assault	Poisoning, Undetermined	Adverse Effect	Under-dosing
Bacitracin zinc — *continued*						
topical NEC	T49.0X1	T49.0X2	T49.0X3	T49.0X4	T49.0X5	T49.0X6
Baclofen	T42.8X1	T42.8X2	T42.8X3	T42.8X4	T42.8X5	T42.8X6
Baking soda	T50.991	T50.992	T50.993	T50.994	T50.995	T50.996
BAL	T45.8X1	T45.8X2	T45.8X3	T45.8X4	T45.8X5	T45.8X6
Bambuterol	T48.6X1	T48.6X2	T48.6X3	T48.6X4	T48.6X5	T48.6X6
Bamethan (sulfate)	T46.7X1	T46.7X2	T46.7X3	T46.7X4	T46.7X5	T46.7X6
Bamifylline	T48.6X1	T48.6X2	T48.6X3	T48.6X4	T48.6X5	T48.6X6
Bamipine	T45.0X1	T45.0X2	T45.0X3	T45.0X4	T45.0X5	T45.0X6
Baneberry — *see* Actaea spicata						
Banewort — *see* Belladonna						
Barbenyl	T42.3X1	T42.3X2	T42.3X3	T42.3X4	T42.3X5	T42.3X6
Barbexaclone	T42.6X1	T42.6X2	T42.6X3	T42.6X4	T42.6X5	T42.6X6
Barbital	T42.3X1	T42.3X2	T42.3X3	T42.3X4	T42.3X5	T42.3X6
sodium	T42.3X1	T42.3X2	T42.3X3	T42.3X4	T42.3X5	T42.3X6
Barbitone	T42.3X1	T42.3X2	T42.3X3	T42.3X4	T42.3X5	T42.3X6
Barbiturate NEC	T42.3X1	T42.3X2	T42.3X3	T42.3X4	T42.3X5	T42.3X6
with tranquilizer	T42.3X1	T42.3X2	T42.3X3	T42.3X4	T42.3X5	T42.3X6
anesthetic (intravenous)	T41.1X1	T41.1X2	T41.1X3	T41.1X4	T41.1X5	T41.1X6
Barium (carbonate) (chloride) (sulfate)	T57.8X1	T57.8X2	T57.8X3	T57.8X4	—	—
diagnostic agent	T50.8X1	T50.8X2	T50.8X3	T50.8X4	T50.8X5	T50.8X6
pesticide	T60.4X1	T60.4X2	T60.4X3	T60.4X4	—	—
rodenticide	T60.4X1	T60.4X2	T60.4X3	T60.4X4	—	—
sulfate (medicinal)	T50.8X1	T50.8X2	T50.8X3	T50.8X4	T50.8X5	T50.8X6
Barrier cream	T49.3X1	T49.3X2	T49.3X3	T49.3X4	T49.3X5	T49.3X6
Basic fuchsin	T49.0X1	T49.0X2	T49.0X3	T49.0X4	T49.0X5	T49.0X6
Battery acid or fluid	T54.2X1	T54.2X2	T54.2X3	T54.2X4	—	—
Bay rum	T51.8X1	T51.8X2	T51.8X3	T51.8X4	—	—
b-benzalbutyramide	T46.6X1	T46.6X2	T46.6X3	T46.6X4	T46.6X5	T46.6X6
BCG (vaccine)	T50.A91	T50.A92	T50.A93	T50.A94	T50.A95	T50.A96
BCNU	T45.1X1	T45.1X2	T45.1X3	T45.1X4	T45.1X5	T45.1X6
Bearsfoot	T62.2X1	T62.2X2	T62.2X3	T62.2X4	—	—
Beclamide	T42.6X1	T42.6X2	T42.6X3	T42.6X4	T42.6X5	T42.6X6
Beclomethasone	T44.5X1	T44.5X2	T44.5X3	T44.5X4	T44.5X5	T44.5X6
Bee (sting) (venom)	T63.441	T63.442	T63.443	T63.444	—	—
Befunolol	T49.5X1	T49.5X2	T49.5X3	T49.5X4	T49.5X5	T49.5X6
Bekanamycin	T36.5X1	T36.5X2	T36.5X3	T36.5X4	T36.5X5	T36.5X6
Belladonna — *see also* Nightshade						
alkaloids	T44.3X1	T44.3X2	T44.3X3	T44.3X4	T44.3X5	T44.3X6
extract	T44.3X1	T44.3X2	T44.3X3	T44.3X4	T44.3X5	T44.3X6
herb	T44.3X1	T44.3X2	T44.3X3	T44.3X4	T44.3X5	T44.3X6
Bemegride	T50.7X1	T50.7X2	T50.7X3	T50.7X4	T50.7X5	T50.7X6
Benactyzine	T44.3X1	T44.3X2	T44.3X3	T44.3X4	T44.3X5	T44.3X6
Benadryl	T45.0X1	T45.0X2	T45.0X3	T45.0X4	T45.0X5	T45.0X6
Benaprizine	T44.3X1	T44.3X2	T44.3X3	T44.3X4	T44.3X5	T44.3X6
Benazepril	T46.4X1	T46.4X2	T46.4X3	T46.4X4	T46.4X5	T46.4X6
Bencyclane	T46.7X1	T46.7X2	T46.7X3	T46.7X4	T46.7X5	T46.7X6
Bendazol	T46.3X1	T46.3X2	T46.3X3	T46.3X4	T46.3X5	T46.3X6
Bendrofluazide	T50.2X1	T50.2X2	T50.2X3	T50.2X4	T50.2X5	T50.2X6
Bendroflumethiazide	T50.2X1	T50.2X2	T50.2X3	T50.2X4	T50.2X5	T50.2X6
Benemid	T50.4X1	T50.4X2	T50.4X3	T50.4X4	T50.4X5	T50.4X6
Benethamine penicillin	T36.0X1	T36.0X2	T36.0X3	T36.0X4	T36.0X5	T36.0X6
Benexate	T47.1X1	T47.1X2	T47.1X3	T47.1X4	T47.1X5	T47.1X6
Benfluorex	T46.6X1	T46.6X2	T46.6X3	T46.6X4	T46.6X5	T46.6X6
Benfotiamine	T45.2X1	T45.2X2	T45.2X3	T45.2X4	T45.2X5	T45.2X6
Benisone	T49.0X1	T49.0X2	T49.0X3	T49.0X4	T49.0X5	T49.0X6
Benomyl	T60.0X1	T60.0X2	T60.0X3	T60.0X4	—	—
Benoquin	T49.8X1	T49.8X2	T49.8X3	T49.8X4	T49.8X5	T49.8X6
Benoxinate	T41.3X1	T41.3X2	T41.3X3	T41.3X4	T41.3X5	T41.3X6
Benperidol	T43.4X1	T43.4X2	T43.4X3	T43.4X4	T43.4X5	T43.4X6
Benproperine	T48.3X1	T48.3X2	T48.3X3	T48.3X4	T48.3X5	T48.3X6
Benserazide	T42.8X1	T42.8X2	T42.8X3	T42.8X4	T42.8X5	T42.8X6
Bentazepam	T42.4X1	T42.4X2	T42.4X3	T42.4X4	T42.4X5	T42.4X6
Bentiromide	T50.8X1	T50.8X2	T50.8X3	T50.8X4	T50.8X5	T50.8X6
Bentonite	T49.3X1	T49.3X2	T49.3X3	T49.3X4	T49.3X5	T49.3X6
Benzalbutyramide	T46.6X1	T46.6X2	T46.6X3	T46.6X4	T46.6X5	T46.6X6
Benzalkonium (chloride)	T49.0X1	T49.0X2	T49.0X3	T49.0X4	T49.0X5	T49.0X6
ophthalmic preparation	T49.5X1	T49.5X2	T49.5X3	T49.5X4	T49.5X5	T49.5X6
Benzamidosalicylate (calcium)	T37.1X1	T37.1X2	T37.1X3	T37.1X4	T37.1X5	T37.1X6
Benzamine	T41.3X1	T41.3X2	T41.3X3	T41.3X4	T41.3X5	T41.3X6
lactate	T49.1X1	T49.1X2	T49.1X3	T49.1X4	T49.1X5	T49.1X6
Benzamphetamine	T50.5X1	T50.5X2	T50.5X3	T50.5X4	T50.5X5	T50.5X6
Benzapril hydrochloride	T46.5X1	T46.5X2	T46.5X3	T46.5X4	T46.5X5	T46.5X6
Benzathine	T36.0X1	T36.0X2	T36.0X3	T36.0X4	T36.0X5	T36.0X6
benzylpenicillin						
Benzathine penicillin	T36.0X1	T36.0X2	T36.0X3	T36.0X4	T36.0X5	T36.0X6
Benzatropine	T42.8X1	T42.8X2	T42.8X3	T42.8X4	T42.8X5	T42.8X6
Benzbromarone	T50.4X1	T50.4X2	T50.4X3	T50.4X4	T50.4X5	T50.4X6
Benzcarbimine	T45.1X1	T45.1X2	T45.1X3	T45.1X4	T45.1X5	T45.1X6
Benzedrex	T44.991	T44.992	T44.993	T44.994	T44.995	T44.996

Additional Character May Be Required — Refer to the Tabular List for Character Selection   ▽ Subterms under main terms may continue to next column or page

Substance	Poisoning, Accidental (unintentional)	Poisoning, Intentional Self-harm	Poisoning, Assault	Poisoning, Undetermined	Adverse Effect	Under-dosing
Benzedrine (amphetamine)	T43.621	T43.622	T43.623	T43.624	T43.625	T43.626
Benzenamine	T65.3X1	T65.3X2	T65.3X3	T65.3X4	—	—
Benzene	T52.1X1	T52.1X2	T52.1X3	T52.1X4	—	—
homologues (acetyl) (dimethyl) (methyl) (solvent)	T52.2X1	T52.2X2	T52.2X3	T52.2X4	—	—
Benzethonium (chloride)	T49.0X1	T49.0X2	T49.0X3	T49.0X4	T49.0X5	T49.0X6
Benzfetamine	T50.5X1	T50.5X2	T50.5X3	T50.5X4	T50.5X5	T50.5X6
Benzhexol	T44.3X1	T44.3X2	T44.3X3	T44.3X4	T44.3X5	T44.3X6
Benzhydramine (chloride)	T45.0X1	T45.0X2	T45.0X3	T45.0X4	T45.0X5	T45.0X6
Benzidine	T65.891	T65.892	T65.893	T65.894	—	—
Benzilonium bromide	T44.3X1	T44.3X2	T44.3X3	T44.3X4	T44.3X5	T44.3X6
Benzimidazole	T60.3X1	T60.3X2	T60.3X3	T60.3X4	—	—
Benzin (e) — see Ligroin						
Benziodarone	T46.3X1	T46.3X2	T46.3X3	T46.3X4	T46.3X5	T46.3X6
Benznidazole	T37.3X1	T37.3X2	T37.3X3	T37.3X4	T37.3X5	T37.3X6
Benzocaine	T41.3X1	T41.3X2	T41.3X3	T41.3X4	T41.3X5	T41.3X6
Benzodiapin	T42.4X1	T42.4X2	T42.4X3	T42.4X4	T42.4X5	T42.4X6
Benzodiazepine NEC	T42.4X1	T42.4X2	T42.4X3	T42.4X4	T42.4X5	T42.4X6
Benzoic acid	T49.0X1	T49.0X2	T49.0X3	T49.0X4	T49.0X5	T49.0X6
with salicylic acid	T49.0X1	T49.0X2	T49.0X3	T49.0X4	T49.0X5	T49.0X6
Benzoin (tincture)	T48.5X1	T48.5X2	T48.5X3	T48.5X4	T48.5X5	T48.5X6
Benzol (benzene)	T52.1X1	T52.1X2	T52.1X3	T52.1X4	—	—
vapor	T52.0X1	T52.0X2	T52.0X3	T52.0X4	—	—
Benzomorphan	T40.2X1	T40.2X2	T40.2X3	T40.2X4	T40.2X5	T40.2X6
Benzonatate	T48.3X1	T48.3X2	T48.3X3	T48.3X4	T48.3X5	T48.3X6
Benzophenones	T49.3X1	T49.3X2	T49.3X3	T49.3X4	T49.3X5	T49.3X6
Benzopyrone	T46.991	T46.992	T46.993	T46.994	T46.995	T46.996
Benzothiadiazides	T50.2X1	T50.2X2	T50.2X3	T50.2X4	T50.2X5	T50.2X6
Benzoxonium chloride	T49.0X1	T49.0X2	T49.0X3	T49.0X4	T49.0X5	T49.0X6
Benzoylpas calcium	T37.1X1	T37.1X2	T37.1X3	T37.1X4	T37.1X5	T37.1X6
Benzoyl peroxide	T49.0X1	T49.0X2	T49.0X3	T49.0X4	T49.0X5	T49.0X6
Benzperidin	T43.591	T43.592	T43.593	T43.594	T43.595	T43.596
Benzperidol	T43.591	T43.592	T43.593	T43.594	T43.595	T43.596
Benzphetamine	T50.5X1	T50.5X2	T50.5X3	T50.5X4	T50.5X5	T50.5X6
Benzpyrinium bromide	T44.1X1	T44.1X2	T44.1X3	T44.1X4	T44.1X5	T44.1X6
Benzquinamide	T45.0X1	T45.0X2	T45.0X3	T45.0X4	T45.0X5	T45.0X6
Benzthiazide	T50.2X1	T50.2X2	T50.2X3	T50.2X4	T50.2X5	T50.2X6
Benztropine						
anticholinergic	T44.3X1	T44.3X2	T44.3X3	T44.3X4	T44.3X5	T44.3X6
antiparkinson	T42.8X1	T42.8X2	T42.8X3	T42.8X4	T42.8X5	T42.8X6
Benzydamine	T49.0X1	T49.0X2	T49.0X3	T49.0X4	T49.0X5	T49.0X6
Benzyl						
acetate	T52.8X1	T52.8X2	T52.8X3	T52.8X4	—	—
alcohol	T49.0X1	T49.0X2	T49.0X3	T49.0X4	T49.0X5	T49.0X6
benzoate	T49.0X1	T49.0X2	T49.0X3	T49.0X4	T49.0X5	T49.0X6
Benzoic acid	T49.0X1	T49.0X2	T49.0X3	T49.0X4	T49.0X5	T49.0X6
morphine	T40.2X1	T40.2X2	T40.2X3	T40.2X4	—	—
nicotinate	T46.6X1	T46.6X2	T46.6X3	T46.6X4	T46.6X5	T46.6X6
penicillin	T36.0X1	T36.0X2	T36.0X3	T36.0X4	T36.0X5	T36.0X6
Benzylhydrochlorthiazide	T50.2X1	T50.2X2	T50.2X3	T50.2X4	T50.2X5	T50.2X6
Benzylpenicillin	T36.0X1	T36.0X2	T36.0X3	T36.0X4	T36.0X5	T36.0X6
Benzylthiouracil	T38.2X1	T38.2X2	T38.2X3	T38.2X4	T38.2X5	T38.2X6
Bephenium	T37.4X1	T37.4X2	T37.4X3	T37.4X4	T37.4X5	T37.4X6
hydroxynaphthoate						
Bepridil	T46.1X1	T46.1X2	T46.1X3	T46.1X4	T46.1X5	T46.1X6
Bergamot oil	T65.891	T65.892	T65.893	T65.894	—	—
Bergapten	T50.991	T50.992	T50.993	T50.994	T50.995	T50.996
Berries, poisonous	T62.1X1	T62.1X2	T62.1X3	T62.1X4	—	—
Beryllium (compounds)	T56.7X1	T56.7X2	T56.7X3	T56.7X4	—	—
beta adrenergic blocking agent, heart	T44.7X1	T44.7X2	T44.7X3	T44.7X4	T44.7X5	T44.7X6
Betacarotene	T45.2X1	T45.2X2	T45.2X3	T45.2X4	T45.2X5	T45.2X6
Beta-Chlor	T42.6X1	T42.6X2	T42.6X3	T42.6X4	T42.6X5	T42.6X6
Betahistine	T46.7X1	T46.7X2	T46.7X3	T46.7X4	T46.7X5	T46.7X6
Betaine	T47.5X1	T47.5X2	T47.5X3	T47.5X4	T47.5X5	T47.5X6
Betamethasone	T49.0X1	T49.0X2	T49.0X3	T49.0X4	T49.0X5	T49.0X6
topical	T49.0X1	T49.0X2	T49.0X3	T49.0X4	T49.0X5	T49.0X6
Betamicin	T36.8X1	T36.8X2	T36.8X3	T36.8X4	T36.8X5	T36.8X6
Betanidine	T46.5X1	T46.5X2	T46.5X3	T46.5X4	T46.5X5	T46.5X6
Betaxolol	T44.7X1	T44.7X2	T44.7X3	T44.7X4	T44.7X5	T44.7X6
Betazole	T50.8X1	T50.8X2	T50.8X3	T50.8X4	T50.8X5	T50.8X6
Bethanechol	T44.1X1	T44.1X2	T44.1X3	T44.1X4	T44.1X5	T44.1X6
chloride	T44.1X1	T44.1X2	T44.1X3	T44.1X4	T44.1X5	T44.1X6
Bethanidine	T46.5X1	T46.5X2	T46.5X3	T46.5X4	T46.5X5	T46.5X6
Betoxycaine	T41.3X1	T41.3X2	T41.3X3	T41.3X4	T41.3X5	T41.3X6
Betula oil	T49.3X1	T49.3X2	T49.3X3	T49.3X4	T49.3X5	T49.3X6
Bevantolol	T44.7X1	T44.7X2	T44.7X3	T44.7X4	T44.7X5	T44.7X6
Bevonium metilsulfate	T44.3X1	T44.3X2	T44.3X3	T44.3X4	T44.3X5	T44.3X6
Bezafibrate	T46.6X1	T46.6X2	T46.6X3	T46.6X4	T46.6X5	T46.6X6
Bezitramide	T40.4X1	T40.4X2	T40.4X3	T40.4X4	T40.4X5	T40.4X6
BHA	T50.991	T50.992	T50.993	T50.994	T50.995	T50.996
Bhang	T40.7X1	T40.7X2	T40.7X3	T40.7X4	T40.7X5	T40.7X6
BHC (medicinal)	T49.0X1	T49.0X2	T49.0X3	T49.0X4	T49.0X5	T49.0X6

Substance	Poisoning, Accidental (unintentional)	Poisoning, Intentional Self-harm	Poisoning, Assault	Poisoning, Undetermined	Adverse Effect	Under-dosing
BHC — continued						
nonmedicinal (vapor)	T53.6X1	T53.6X2	T53.6X3	T53.6X4	—	—
Bialamicol	T37.3X1	T37.3X2	T37.3X3	T37.3X4	T37.3X5	T37.3X6
Bibenzonium bromide	T48.3X1	T48.3X2	T48.3X3	T48.3X4	T48.3X5	T48.3X6
Bibrocathol	T49.5X1	T49.5X2	T49.5X3	T49.5X4	T49.5X5	T49.5X6
Bichloride of mercury — see Mercury, chloride						
Bichromates (calcium) (potassium)(sodium) (crystals)	T57.8X1	T57.8X2	T57.8X3	T57.8X4	—	—
fumes	T56.2X1	T56.2X2	T56.2X3	T56.2X4	—	—
Biclotymol	T49.6X1	T49.6X2	T49.6X3	T49.6X4	T49.6X5	T49.6X6
Bicucculine	T50.7X1	T50.7X2	T50.7X3	T50.7X4	T50.7X5	T50.7X6
Bifemelane	T43.291	T43.292	T43.293	T43.294	T43.295	T43.296
Biguanide derivatives, oral	T38.3X1	T38.3X2	T38.3X3	T38.3X4	T38.3X5	T38.3X6
Bile salts	T47.5X1	T47.5X2	T47.5X3	T47.5X4	T47.5X5	T47.5X6
Biligrafin	T50.8X1	T50.8X2	T50.8X3	T50.8X4	T50.8X5	T50.8X6
Bilopaque	T50.8X1	T50.8X2	T50.8X3	T50.8X4	T50.8X5	T50.8X6
Binifibrate	T46.6X1	T46.6X2	T46.6X3	T46.6X4	T46.6X5	T46.6X6
Binitrobenzol	T65.3X1	T65.3X2	T65.3X3	T65.3X4	—	—
Bioflavonoid(s)	T46.991	T46.992	T46.993	T46.994	T46.995	T46.996
Biological substance NEC	T50.901	T50.902	T50.903	T50.904	T50.905	T50.906
Biotin	T45.2X1	T45.2X2	T45.2X3	T45.2X4	T45.2X5	T45.2X6
Biperiden	T44.3X1	T44.3X2	T44.3X3	T44.3X4	T44.3X5	T44.3X6
Bisacodyl	T47.2X1	T47.2X2	T47.2X3	T47.2X4	T47.2X5	T47.2X6
Bisbentiamine	T45.2X1	T45.2X2	T45.2X3	T45.2X4	T45.2X5	T45.2X6
Bisbutiamine	T45.2X1	T45.2X2	T45.2X3	T45.2X4	T45.2X5	T45.2X6
Bisdequalinium (salts) (diacetate)	T49.6X1	T49.6X2	T49.6X3	T49.6X4	T49.6X5	T49.6X6
Bishydroxycoumarin	T45.511	T45.512	T45.513	T45.514	T45.515	T45.516
Bismarsen	T37.8X1	T37.8X2	T37.8X3	T37.8X4	T37.8X5	T37.8X6
Bismuth salts	T47.6X1	T47.6X2	T47.6X3	T47.6X4	T47.6X5	T47.6X6
aluminate	T47.1X1	T47.1X2	T47.1X3	T47.1X4	T47.1X5	T47.1X6
anti-infectives	T37.8X1	T37.8X2	T37.8X3	T37.8X4	T37.8X5	T37.8X6
formic iodide	T49.0X1	T49.0X2	T49.0X3	T49.0X4	T49.0X5	T49.0X6
glycolylarsenate	T49.0X1	T49.0X2	T49.0X3	T49.0X4	T49.0X5	T49.0X6
nonmedicinal (compounds) NEC	T65.91	T65.92	T65.93	T65.94	—	—
subcarbonate	T47.6X1	T47.6X2	T47.6X3	T47.6X4	T47.6X5	T47.6X6
subsalicylate	T37.8X1	T37.8X2	T37.8X3	T37.8X4	T37.8X5	T37.8X6
sulfarsphenamine	T37.8X1	T37.8X2	T37.8X3	T37.8X4	T37.8X5	T37.8X6
Bisoprolol	T44.7X1	T44.7X2	T44.7X3	T44.7X4	T44.7X5	T44.7X6
Bisoxatin	T47.2X1	T47.2X2	T47.2X3	T47.2X4	T47.2X5	T47.2X6
Bisulepin (hydrochloride)	T45.0X1	T45.0X2	T45.0X3	T45.0X4	T45.0X5	T45.0X6
Bithionol	T37.8X1	T37.8X2	T37.8X3	T37.8X4	T37.8X5	T37.8X6
anthelminthic	T37.4X1	T37.4X2	T37.4X3	T37.4X4	T37.4X5	T37.4X6
Bitolterol	T48.6X1	T48.6X2	T48.6X3	T48.6X4	T48.6X5	T48.6X6
Bitoscanate	T37.4X1	T37.4X2	T37.4X3	T37.4X4	T37.4X5	T37.4X6
Bitter almond oil	T62.8X1	T62.8X2	T62.8X3	T62.8X4	—	—
Bittersweet	T62.2X1	T62.2X2	T62.2X3	T62.2X4	—	—
Black						
flag	T60.91	T60.92	T60.93	T60.94	—	—
henbane	T62.2X1	T62.2X2	T62.2X3	T62.2X4	—	—
leaf (40)	T60.91	T60.92	T60.93	T60.94	—	—
widow spider (bite)	T63.311	T63.312	T63.313	T63.314	—	—
antivenin	T50.Z11	T50.Z12	T50.Z13	T50.Z14	T50.Z15	T50.Z16
Blast furnace gas (carbon monoxide from)	T58.8X1	T58.8X2	T58.8X3	T58.8X4	—	—
Bleach	T54.91	T54.92	T54.93	T54.94	—	—
Bleaching agent (medicinal)	T49.4X1	T49.4X2	T49.4X3	T49.4X4	T49.4X5	T49.4X6
Bleomycin	T45.1X1	T45.1X2	T45.1X3	T45.1X4	T45.1X5	T45.1X6
Blockain	T41.3X1	T41.3X2	T41.3X3	T41.3X4	T41.3X5	T41.3X6
infiltration (subcutaneous)	T41.3X1	T41.3X2	T41.3X3	T41.3X4	T41.3X5	T41.3X6
nerve block (peripheral) (plexus)	T41.3X1	T41.3X2	T41.3X3	T41.3X4	T41.3X5	T41.3X6
topical (surface)	T41.3X1	T41.3X2	T41.3X3	T41.3X4	T41.3X5	T41.3X6
Blockers, calcium channel	T46.1X1	T46.1X2	T46.1X3	T46.1X4	T46.1X5	T46.1X6
Blood (derivatives) (natural) (plasma) (whole)	T45.8X1	T45.8X2	T45.8X3	T45.8X4	T45.8X5	T45.8X6
dried	T45.8X1	T45.8X2	T45.8X3	T45.8X4	T45.8X5	T45.8X6
drug affecting NEC	T45.91	T45.92	T45.93	T45.94	T45.95	T45.96
expander NEC	T45.8X1	T45.8X2	T45.8X3	T45.8X4	T45.8X5	T45.8X6
fraction NEC	T45.8X1	T45.8X2	T45.8X3	T45.8X4	T45.8X5	T45.8X6
substitute (macromolecular)	T45.8X1	T45.8X2	T45.8X3	T45.8X4	T45.8X5	T45.8X6
Blue velvet	T40.2X1	T40.2X2	T40.2X3	T40.2X4	—	—
Bone meal	T62.8X1	T62.8X2	T62.8X3	T62.8X4	—	—
Bonine	T45.0X1	T45.0X2	T45.0X3	T45.0X4	T45.0X5	T45.0X6
Bopindolol	T44.7X1	T44.7X2	T44.7X3	T44.7X4	T44.7X5	T44.7X6
Boracic acid	T49.0X1	T49.0X2	T49.0X3	T49.0X4	T49.0X5	T49.0X6
ENT agent	T49.6X1	T49.6X2	T49.6X3	T49.6X4	T49.6X5	T49.6X6
ophthalmic preparation	T49.5X1	T49.5X2	T49.5X3	T49.5X4	T49.5X5	T49.5X6
Borane complex	T57.8X1	T57.8X2	T57.8X3	T57.8X4	—	—

Table of Drugs and Chemicals

Borate — Cadmium

Substance	Poisoning, Accidental (unintentional)	Poisoning, Intentional Self-harm	Poisoning, Assault	Poisoning, Undetermined	Adverse Effect	Under-dosing
Borate(s)	T57.8X1	T57.8X2	T57.8X3	T57.8X4	—	—
buffer	T50.991	T50.992	T50.993	T50.994	T50.995	T50.996
cleanser	T54.91	T54.92	T54.93	T54.94	—	—
sodium	T57.8X1	T57.8X2	T57.8X3	T57.8X4	—	—
Borax (cleanser)	T54.91	T54.92	T54.93	T54.94	—	—
Bordeaux mixture	T60.3X1	T60.3X2	T60.3X3	T60.3X4	—	—
Boric acid	T49.0X1	T49.0X2	T49.0X3	T49.0X4	T49.0X5	T49.0X6
ENT agent	T49.6X1	T49.6X2	T49.6X3	T49.6X4	T49.6X5	T49.6X6
ophthalmic preparation	T49.5X1	T49.5X2	T49.5X3	T49.5X4	T49.5X5	T49.5X6
Bornaprine	T44.3X1	T44.3X2	T44.3X3	T44.3X4	T44.3X5	T44.3X6
Boron	T57.8X1	T57.8X2	T57.8X3	T57.8X4	—	—
hydride NEC	T57.8X1	T57.8X2	T57.8X3	T57.8X4	—	—
fumes or gas	T57.8X1	T57.8X2	T57.8X3	T57.8X4	—	—
trifluoride	T59.891	T59.892	T59.893	T59.894	—	—
Botox	T48.291	T48.292	T48.293	T48.294	T48.295	T48.296
Botulinus anti-toxin (type A, B)	T50.Z11	T50.Z12	T50.Z13	T50.Z14	T50.Z15	T50.Z16
Brake fluid vapor	T59.891	T59.892	T59.893	T59.894	—	—
Brallobarbital	T42.3X1	T42.3X2	T42.3X3	T42.3X4	T42.3X5	T42.3X6
Bran (wheat)	T47.4X1	T47.4X2	T47.4X3	T47.4X4	T47.4X5	T47.4X6
Brass (fumes)	T56.891	T56.892	T56.893	T56.894	—	—
Brasso	T52.0X1	T52.0X2	T52.0X3	T52.0X4	—	—
Bretylium tosilate	T46.2X1	T46.2X2	T46.2X3	T46.2X4	T46.2X5	T46.2X6
Brevital (sodium)	T41.1X1	T41.1X2	T41.1X3	T41.1X4	T41.1X5	T41.1X6
Brinase	T45.3X1	T45.3X2	T45.3X3	T45.3X4	T45.3X5	T45.3X6
British antilewisite	T45.8X1	T45.8X2	T45.8X3	T45.8X4	T45.8X5	T45.8X6
Brodifacoum	T60.4X1	T60.4X2	T60.4X3	T60.4X4	—	—
Bromal (hydrate)	T42.6X1	T42.6X2	T42.6X3	T42.6X4	T42.6X5	T42.6X6
Bromazepam	T42.4X1	T42.4X2	T42.4X3	T42.4X4	T42.4X5	T42.4X6
Bromazine	T45.0X1	T45.0X2	T45.0X3	T45.0X4	T45.0X5	T45.0X6
Brombenzylcyanide	T59.3X1	T59.3X2	T59.3X3	T59.3X4	—	—
Bromelains	T45.3X1	T45.3X2	T45.3X3	T45.3X4	T45.3X5	T45.3X6
Bromethalin	T60.4X1	T60.4X2	T60.4X3	T60.4X4	—	—
Bromhexine	T48.4X1	T48.4X2	T48.4X3	T48.4X4	T48.4X5	T48.4X6
Bromide salts	T42.6X1	T42.6X2	T42.6X3	T42.6X4	T42.6X5	T42.6X6
Bromindione	T45.511	T45.512	T45.513	T45.514	T45.515	T45.516
Bromine						
compounds (medicinal)	T42.6X1	T42.6X2	T42.6X3	T42.6X4	T42.6X5	T42.6X6
sedative	T42.6X1	T42.6X2	T42.6X3	T42.6X4	T42.6X5	T42.6X6
vapor	T59.891	T59.892	T59.893	T59.894	—	—
Bromisoval	T42.6X1	T42.6X2	T42.6X3	T42.6X4	T42.6X5	T42.6X6
Bromisovalum	T42.6X1	T42.6X2	T42.6X3	T42.6X4	T42.6X5	T42.6X6
Bromobenzylcyanide	T59.3X1	T59.3X2	T59.3X3	T59.3X4	—	—
Bromochlorosalicylani-lide	T49.0X1	T49.0X2	T49.0X3	T49.0X4	T49.0X5	T49.0X6
Bromocriptine	T42.8X1	T42.8X2	T42.8X3	T42.8X4	T42.8X5	T42.8X6
Bromodiphenhydramine	T45.0X1	T45.0X2	T45.0X3	T45.0X4	T45.0X5	T45.0X6
Bromoform	T42.6X1	T42.6X2	T42.6X3	T42.6X4	T42.6X5	T42.6X6
Bromophenol blue reagent	T50.991	T50.992	T50.993	T50.994	T50.995	T50.996
Bromopride	T47.8X1	T47.8X2	T47.8X3	T47.8X4	T47.8X5	T47.8X6
Bromosalicylchloranitide	T49.0X1	T49.0X2	T49.0X3	T49.0X4	T49.0X5	T49.0X6
Bromosalicylhydroxamic acid	T37.1X1	T37.1X2	T37.1X3	T37.1X4	T37.1X5	T37.1X6
Bromo-seltzer	T39.1X1	T39.1X2	T39.1X3	T39.1X4	T39.1X5	T39.1X6
Bromoxynil	T60.3X1	T60.3X2	T60.3X3	T60.3X4	—	—
Bromperidol	T43.4X1	T43.4X2	T43.4X3	T43.4X4	T43.4X5	T43.4X6
Brompheniramine	T45.0X1	T45.0X2	T45.0X3	T45.0X4	T45.0X5	T45.0X6
Bromsulfophthalein	T50.8X1	T50.8X2	T50.8X3	T50.8X4	T50.8X5	T50.8X6
Bromural	T42.6X1	T42.6X2	T42.6X3	T42.6X4	T42.6X5	T42.6X6
Bromvaletone	T42.6X1	T42.6X2	T42.6X3	T42.6X4	T42.6X5	T42.6X6
Bronchodilator NEC	T48.6X1	T48.6X2	T48.6X3	T48.6X4	T48.6X5	T48.6X6
Brotizolam	T42.4X1	T42.4X2	T42.4X3	T42.4X4	T42.4X5	T42.4X6
Brovincamine	T46.7X1	T46.7X2	T46.7X3	T46.7X4	T46.7X5	T46.7X6
Brown recluse spider (bite) (venom)	T63.331	T63.332	T63.333	T63.334	—	—
Brown spider (bite) (venom)	T63.391	T63.392	T63.393	T63.394	—	—
Broxaterol	T48.6X1	T48.6X2	T48.6X3	T48.6X4	T48.6X5	T48.6X6
Broxuridine	T45.1X1	T45.1X2	T45.1X3	T45.1X4	T45.1X5	T45.1X6
Broxyquinoline	T37.8X1	T37.8X2	T37.8X3	T37.8X4	T37.8X5	T37.8X6
Bruceine	T48.291	T48.292	T48.293	T48.294	T48.295	T48.296
Brucia	T62.2X1	T62.2X2	T62.2X3	T62.2X4	—	—
Brucine	T65.1X1	T65.1X2	T65.1X3	T65.1X4	—	—
Brunswick green — *see* Copper						
Bruten — *see* Ibuprofen						
Bryonia	T47.2X1	T47.2X2	T47.2X3	T47.2X4	T47.2X5	T47.2X6
Buclizine	T45.0X1	T45.0X2	T45.0X3	T45.0X4	T45.0X5	T45.0X6
Buclosamide	T49.0X1	T49.0X2	T49.0X3	T49.0X4	T49.0X5	T49.0X6
Budesonide	T44.5X1	T44.5X2	T44.5X3	T44.5X4	T44.5X5	T44.5X6
Budralazine	T46.5X1	T46.5X2	T46.5X3	T46.5X4	T46.5X5	T46.5X6
Bufferin	T39.011	T39.012	T39.013	T39.014	T39.015	T39.016
Buflomedil	T46.7X1	T46.7X2	T46.7X3	T46.7X4	T46.7X5	T46.7X6
Buformin	T38.3X1	T38.3X2	T38.3X3	T38.3X4	T38.3X5	T38.3X6
Bufotenine	T40.991	T40.992	T40.993	T40.994	—	—
Bufrolin	T48.6X1	T48.6X2	T48.6X3	T48.6X4	T48.6X5	T48.6X6

Substance	Poisoning, Accidental (unintentional)	Poisoning, Intentional Self-harm	Poisoning, Assault	Poisoning, Undetermined	Adverse Effect	Under-dosing
Bufylline	T48.6X1	T48.6X2	T48.6X3	T48.6X4	T48.6X5	T48.6X6
Bulk filler	T50.5X1	T50.5X2	T50.5X3	T50.5X4	T50.5X5	T50.5X6
cathartic	T47.4X1	T47.4X2	T47.4X3	T47.4X4	T47.4X5	T47.4X6
Bumetanide	T50.1X1	T50.1X2	T50.1X3	T50.1X4	T50.1X5	T50.1X6
Bunaftine	T46.2X1	T46.2X2	T46.2X3	T46.2X4	T46.2X5	T46.2X6
Bunamiodyl	T50.8X1	T50.8X2	T50.8X3	T50.8X4	T50.8X5	T50.8X6
Bunazosin	T44.6X1	T44.6X2	T44.6X3	T44.6X4	T44.6X5	T44.6X6
Bunitrolol	T44.7X1	T44.7X2	T44.7X3	T44.7X4	T44.7X5	T44.7X6
Buphenine	T46.7X1	T46.7X2	T46.7X3	T46.7X4	T46.7X5	T46.7X6
Bupivacaine	T41.3X1	T41.3X2	T41.3X3	T41.3X4	T41.3X5	T41.3X6
infiltration (subcutaneous)	T41.3X1	T41.3X2	T41.3X3	T41.3X4	T41.3X5	T41.3X6
nerve block (peripheral) (plexus)	T41.3X1	T41.3X2	T41.3X3	T41.3X4	T41.3X5	T41.3X6
spinal	T41.3X1	T41.3X2	T41.3X3	T41.3X4	T41.3X5	T41.3X6
Bupranolol	T44.7X1	T44.7X2	T44.7X3	T44.7X4	T44.7X5	T44.7X6
Buprenorphine	T40.4X1	T40.4X2	T40.4X3	T40.4X4	T40.4X5	T40.4X6
Bupropion	T43.291	T43.292	T43.293	T43.294	T43.295	T43.296
Burimamide	T47.1X1	T47.1X2	T47.1X3	T47.1X4	T47.1X5	T47.1X6
Buserelin	T38.891	T38.892	T38.893	T38.894	T38.895	T38.896
Buspirone	T43.591	T43.592	T43.593	T43.594	T43.595	T43.596
Busulfan, busulphan	T45.1X1	T45.1X2	T45.1X3	T45.1X4	T45.1X5	T45.1X6
Butabarbital (sodium)	T42.3X1	T42.3X2	T42.3X3	T42.3X4	T42.3X5	T42.3X6
Butabarbitone	T42.3X1	T42.3X2	T42.3X3	T42.3X4	T42.3X5	T42.3X6
Butabarpal	T42.3X1	T42.3X2	T42.3X3	T42.3X4	T42.3X5	T42.3X6
Butacaine	T41.3X1	T41.3X2	T41.3X3	T41.3X4	T41.3X5	T41.3X6
Butalamine	T46.7X1	T46.7X2	T46.7X3	T46.7X4	T46.7X5	T46.7X6
Butalbital	T42.3X1	T42.3X2	T42.3X3	T42.3X4	T42.3X5	T42.3X6
Butallylonal	T42.3X1	T42.3X2	T42.3X3	T42.3X4	T42.3X5	T42.3X6
Butamben	T41.3X1	T41.3X2	T41.3X3	T41.3X4	T41.3X5	T41.3X6
Butamirate	T48.3X1	T48.3X2	T48.3X3	T48.3X4	T48.3X5	T48.3X6
Butane (distributed in mobile container)	T59.891	T59.892	T59.893	T59.894	—	—
distributed through pipes	T59.891	T59.892	T59.893	T59.894	—	—
incomplete combustion	T58.11	T58.12	T58.13	T58.14	—	—
Butanilicaine	T41.3X1	T41.3X2	T41.3X3	T41.3X4	T41.3X5	T41.3X6
Butanol	T51.3X1	T51.3X2	T51.3X3	T51.3X4	—	—
Butanone, 2-butanone	T52.4X1	T52.4X2	T52.4X3	T52.4X4	—	—
Butantrone	T49.4X1	T49.4X2	T49.4X3	T49.4X4	T49.4X5	T49.4X6
Butaperazine	T43.3X1	T43.3X2	T43.3X3	T43.3X4	T43.3X5	T43.3X6
Butazolidin	T39.2X1	T39.2X2	T39.2X3	T39.2X4	T39.2X5	T39.2X6
Butetamate	T48.6X1	T48.6X2	T48.6X3	T48.6X4	T48.6X5	T48.6X6
Butethal	T42.3X1	T42.3X2	T42.3X3	T42.3X4	T42.3X5	T42.3X6
Butethamate	T44.3X1	T44.3X2	T44.3X3	T44.3X4	T44.3X5	T44.3X6
Buthalitone (sodium)	T41.1X1	T41.1X2	T41.1X3	T41.1X4	T41.1X5	T41.1X6
Butisol (sodium)	T42.3X1	T42.3X2	T42.3X3	T42.3X4	T42.3X5	T42.3X6
Butizide	T50.2X1	T50.2X2	T50.2X3	T50.2X4	T50.2X5	T50.2X6
Butobarbital	T42.3X1	T42.3X2	T42.3X3	T42.3X4	T42.3X5	T42.3X6
sodium	T42.3X1	T42.3X2	T42.3X3	T42.3X4	T42.3X5	T42.3X6
Butobarbitone	T42.3X1	T42.3X2	T42.3X3	T42.3X4	T42.3X5	T42.3X6
Butoconazole (nitrate)	T49.0X1	T49.0X2	T49.0X3	T49.0X4	T49.0X5	T49.0X6
Butorphanol	T40.4X1	T40.4X2	T40.4X3	T40.4X4	T40.4X5	T40.4X6
Butriptyline	T43.011	T43.012	T43.013	T43.014	T43.015	T43.016
Butropium bromide	T44.3X1	T44.3X2	T44.3X3	T44.3X4	T44.3X5	T44.3X6
Buttercups	T62.2X1	T62.2X2	T62.2X3	T62.2X4	—	—
Butter of antimony — *see* Antimony						
Butyl						
acetate (secondary)	T52.8X1	T52.8X2	T52.8X3	T52.8X4	—	—
alcohol	T51.3X1	T51.3X2	T51.3X3	T51.3X4	—	—
aminobenzoate	T41.3X1	T41.3X2	T41.3X3	T41.3X4	T41.3X5	T41.3X6
butyrate	T52.8X1	T52.8X2	T52.8X3	T52.8X4	—	—
carbinol	T51.3X1	T51.3X2	T51.3X3	T51.3X4	—	—
carbitol	T52.3X1	T52.3X2	T52.3X3	T52.3X4	—	—
cellosolve	T52.3X1	T52.3X2	T52.3X3	T52.3X4	—	—
chloral (hydrate)	T42.6X1	T42.6X2	T42.6X3	T42.6X4	T42.6X5	T42.6X6
formate	T52.8X1	T52.8X2	T52.8X3	T52.8X4	—	—
lactate	T52.8X1	T52.8X2	T52.8X3	T52.8X4	—	—
propionate	T52.8X1	T52.8X2	T52.8X3	T52.8X4	—	—
scopolamine bromide	T44.3X1	T44.3X2	T44.3X3	T44.3X4	T44.3X5	T44.3X6
thiobarbital sodium	T41.1X1	T41.1X2	T41.1X3	T41.1X4	T41.1X5	T41.1X6
Butylated hydroxyanisole	T50.991	T50.992	T50.993	T50.994	T50.995	T50.996
Butylchloral hydrate	T42.6X1	T42.6X2	T42.6X3	T42.6X4	T42.6X5	T42.6X6
Butyltoluene	T52.2X1	T52.2X2	T52.2X3	T52.2X4	—	—
Butyn	T41.3X1	T41.3X2	T41.3X3	T41.3X4	T41.3X5	T41.3X6
Butyrophenone (-based tranquilizers)	T43.4X1	T43.4X2	T43.4X3	T43.4X4	T43.4X5	T43.4X6
Cabergoline	T42.8X1	T42.8X2	T42.8X3	T42.8X4	T42.8X5	T42.8X6
Cacodyl, cacodylic acid	T57.0X1	T57.0X2	T57.0X3	T57.0X4	—	—
Cactinomycin	T45.1X1	T45.1X2	T45.1X3	T45.1X4	T45.1X5	T45.1X6
Cade oil	T49.4X1	T49.4X2	T49.4X3	T49.4X4	T49.4X5	T49.4X6
Cadexomer iodine	T49.0X1	T49.0X2	T49.0X3	T49.0X4	T49.0X5	T49.0X6
Cadmium (chloride) (fumes) (oxide)	T56.3X1	T56.3X2	T56.3X3	T56.3X4	—	—

Substance	Poisoning, Accidental (unintentional)	Poisoning, Intentional Self-harm	Poisoning, Assault	Poisoning, Undetermined	Adverse Effect	Under-dosing
Cadmium — *continued*						
sulfide (medicinal) NEC	T49.4X1	T49.4X2	T49.4X3	T49.4X4	T49.4X5	T49.4X6
Cadralazine	T46.5X1	T46.5X2	T46.5X3	T46.5X4	T46.5X5	T46.5X6
Caffeine	T43.611	T43.612	T43.613	T43.614	T43.615	T43.616
Calabar bean	T62.2X1	T62.2X2	T62.2X3	T62.2X4	—	—
Caladium seguinum	T62.2X1	T62.2X2	T62.2X3	T62.2X4	—	—
Calamine (lotion)	T49.3X1	T49.3X2	T49.3X3	T49.3X4	T49.3X5	T49.3X6
Calcifediol	T45.2X1	T45.2X2	T45.2X3	T45.2X4	T45.2X5	T45.2X6
Calciferol	T45.2X1	T45.2X2	T45.2X3	T45.2X4	T45.2X5	T45.2X6
Calcitonin	T50.991	T50.992	T50.993	T50.994	T50.995	T50.996
Calcitriol	T45.2X1	T45.2X2	T45.2X3	T45.2X4	T45.2X5	T45.2X6
Calcium	T50.3X1	T50.3X2	T50.3X3	T50.3X4	T50.3X5	T50.3X6
actylsalicylate	T39.011	T39.012	T39.013	T39.014	T39.015	T39.016
benzamidosalicylate	T37.1X1	T37.1X2	T37.1X3	T37.1X4	T37.1X5	T37.1X6
bromide	T42.6X1	T42.6X2	T42.6X3	T42.6X4	T42.6X5	T42.6X6
bromolactobionate	T42.6X1	T42.6X2	T42.6X3	T42.6X4	T42.6X5	T42.6X6
carbaspirin	T39.011	T39.012	T39.013	T39.014	T39.015	T39.016
carbimide	T50.6X1	T50.6X2	T50.6X3	T50.6X4	T50.6X5	T50.6X6
carbonate	T47.1X1	T47.1X2	T47.1X3	T47.1X4	T47.1X5	T47.1X6
chloride	T50.991	T50.992	T50.993	T50.994	T50.995	T50.996
anhydrous	T50.991	T50.992	T50.993	T50.994	T50.995	T50.996
cyanide	T57.8X1	T57.8X2	T57.8X3	T57.8X4	—	—
dioctyl sulfosuccinate	T47.4X1	T47.4X2	T47.4X3	T47.4X4	T47.4X5	T47.4X6
disodium edathamil	T45.8X1	T45.8X2	T45.8X3	T45.8X4	T45.8X5	T45.8X6
disodium edetate	T45.8X1	T45.8X2	T45.8X3	T45.8X4	T45.8X5	T45.8X6
dobesilate	T46.991	T46.992	T46.993	T46.994	T46.995	T46.996
EDTA	T45.8X1	T45.8X2	T45.8X3	T45.8X4	T45.8X5	T45.8X6
ferrous citrate	T45.4X1	T45.4X2	T45.4X3	T45.4X4	T45.4X5	T45.4X6
folinate	T45.8X1	T45.8X2	T45.8X3	T45.8X4	T45.8X5	T45.8X6
glubionate	T50.3X1	T50.3X2	T50.3X3	T50.3X4	T50.3X5	T50.3X6
gluconate	T50.3X1	T50.3X2	T50.3X3	T50.3X4	T50.3X5	T50.3X6
gluconogalactogluconate	T50.3X1	T50.3X2	T50.3X3	T50.3X4	T50.3X5	T50.3X6
hydrate, hydroxide	T54.3X1	T54.3X2	T54.3X3	T54.3X4	—	—
hypochlorite	T54.3X1	T54.3X2	T54.3X3	T54.3X4	—	—
iodide	T48.4X1	T48.4X2	T48.4X3	T48.4X4	T48.4X5	T48.4X6
ipodate	T50.8X1	T50.8X2	T50.8X3	T50.8X4	T50.8X5	T50.8X6
lactate	T50.3X1	T50.3X2	T50.3X3	T50.3X4	T50.3X5	T50.3X6
leucovorin	T45.8X1	T45.8X2	T45.8X3	T45.8X4	T45.8X5	T45.8X6
mandelate	T37.91	T37.92	T37.93	T37.94	T37.95	T37.96
oxide	T54.3X1	T54.3X2	T54.3X3	T54.3X4	—	—
pantothenate	T45.2X1	T45.2X2	T45.2X3	T45.2X4	T45.2X5	T45.2X6
phosphate	T50.3X1	T50.3X2	T50.3X3	T50.3X4	T50.3X5	T50.3X6
salicylate	T39.091	T39.092	T39.093	T39.094	T39.095	T39.096
salts	T50.3X1	T50.3X2	T50.3X3	T50.3X4	T50.3X5	T50.3X6
Calculus-dissolving drug	T50.991	T50.992	T50.993	T50.994	T50.995	T50.996
Calomel	T49.0X1	T49.0X2	T49.0X3	T49.0X4	T49.0X5	T49.0X6
Caloric agent	T50.3X1	T50.3X2	T50.3X3	T50.3X4	T50.3X5	T50.3X6
Calusterone	T38.7X1	T38.7X2	T38.7X3	T38.7X4	T38.7X5	T38.7X6
Camazepam	T42.4X1	T42.4X2	T42.4X3	T42.4X4	T42.4X5	T42.4X6
Camomile	T49.0X1	T49.0X2	T49.0X3	T49.0X4	T49.0X5	T49.0X6
Camoquin	T37.2X1	T37.2X2	T37.2X3	T37.2X4	T37.2X5	T37.2X6
Camphor						
insecticide	T60.2X1	T60.2X2	T60.2X3	T60.2X4	—	—
medicinal	T49.8X1	T49.8X2	T49.8X3	T49.8X4	T49.8X5	T49.8X6
Camylofin	T44.3X1	T44.3X2	T44.3X3	T44.3X4	T44.3X5	T44.3X6
Cancer chemotherapy drug regimen	T45.1X1	T45.1X2	T45.1X3	T45.1X4	T45.1X5	T45.1X6
Candeptin	T49.0X1	T49.0X2	T49.0X3	T49.0X4	T49.0X5	T49.0X6
Candicidin	T49.0X1	T49.0X2	T49.0X3	T49.0X4	T49.0X5	T49.0X6
Cannabinol	T40.7X1	T40.7X2	T40.7X3	T40.7X4	T40.7X5	T40.7X6
Cannabis (derivatives)	T40.7X1	T40.7X2	T40.7X3	T40.7X4	T40.7X5	T40.7X6
Canned heat	T51.1X1	T51.1X2	T51.1X3	T51.1X4	—	—
Canrenoic acid	T50.0X1	T50.0X2	T50.0X3	T50.0X4	T50.0X5	T50.0X6
Canrenone	T50.0X1	T50.0X2	T50.0X3	T50.0X4	T50.0X5	T50.0X6
Cantharides, cantharidin, cantharis	T49.8X1	T49.8X2	T49.8X3	T49.8X4	T49.8X5	T49.8X6
Canthaxanthin	T50.991	T50.992	T50.993	T50.994	T50.995	T50.996
Capillary-active drug NEC	T46.901	T46.902	T46.903	T46.904	T46.905	T46.906
Capreomycin	T36.8X1	T36.8X2	T36.8X3	T36.8X4	T36.8X5	T36.8X6
Capsicum	T49.4X1	T49.4X2	T49.4X3	T49.4X4	T49.4X5	T49.4X6
Captafol	T60.3X1	T60.3X2	T60.3X3	T60.3X4	—	—
Captan	T60.3X1	T60.3X2	T60.3X3	T60.3X4	—	—
Captodiame, captodiamine	T43.591	T43.592	T43.593	T43.594	T43.595	T43.596
Captopril	T46.4X1	T46.4X2	T46.4X3	T46.4X4	T46.4X5	T46.4X6
Caramiphen	T44.3X1	T44.3X2	T44.3X3	T44.3X4	T44.3X5	T44.3X6
Carazolol	T44.7X1	T44.7X2	T44.7X3	T44.7X4	T44.7X5	T44.7X6
Carbachol	T44.1X1	T44.1X2	T44.1X3	T44.1X4	T44.1X5	T44.1X6
Carbacrylamine (resin)	T50.3X1	T50.3X2	T50.3X3	T50.3X4	T50.3X5	T50.3X6
Carbamate (insecticide)	T60.0X1	T60.0X2	T60.0X3	T60.0X4	—	—
Carbamate (sedative)	T42.6X1	T42.6X2	T42.6X3	T42.6X4	T42.6X5	T42.6X6
herbicide	T60.0X1	T60.0X2	T60.0X3	T60.0X4	—	—
insecticide	T60.0X1	T60.0X2	T60.0X3	T60.0X4	—	—
Carbamazepine	T42.1X1	T42.1X2	T42.1X3	T42.1X4	T42.1X5	T42.1X6
Carbamide	T47.3X1	T47.3X2	T47.3X3	T47.3X4	T47.3X5	T47.3X6
peroxide	T49.0X1	T49.0X2	T49.0X3	T49.0X4	T49.0X5	T49.0X6
topical	T49.8X1	T49.8X2	T49.8X3	T49.8X4	T49.8X5	T49.8X6
Carbamylcholine chloride	T44.1X1	T44.1X2	T44.1X3	T44.1X4	T44.1X5	T44.1X6
Carbaril	T60.0X1	T60.0X2	T60.0X3	T60.0X4	—	—
Carbarsone	T37.3X1	T37.3X2	T37.3X3	T37.3X4	T37.3X5	T37.3X6
Carbaryl	T60.0X1	T60.0X2	T60.0X3	T60.0X4	—	—
Carbaspirin	T39.011	T39.012	T39.013	T39.014	T39.015	T39.016
Carbazochrome (salicylate) (sodium sulfonate)	T49.4X1	T49.4X2	T49.4X3	T49.4X4	T49.4X5	T49.4X6
Carbenicillin	T36.0X1	T36.0X2	T36.0X3	T36.0X4	T36.0X5	T36.0X6
Carbenoxolone	T47.1X1	T47.1X2	T47.1X3	T47.1X4	T47.1X5	T47.1X6
Carbetapentane	T48.3X1	T48.3X2	T48.3X3	T48.3X4	T48.3X5	T48.3X6
Carbethyl salicylate	T39.091	T39.092	T39.093	T39.094	T39.095	T39.096
Carbidopa (with levodopa)	T42.8X1	T42.8X2	T42.8X3	T42.8X4	T42.8X5	T42.8X6
Carbimazole	T38.2X1	T38.2X2	T38.2X3	T38.2X4	T38.2X5	T38.2X6
Carbinol	T51.1X1	T51.1X2	T51.1X3	T51.1X4	—	—
Carbinoxamine	T45.0X1	T45.0X2	T45.0X3	T45.0X4	T45.0X5	T45.0X6
Carbiphene	T39.8X1	T39.8X2	T39.8X3	T39.8X4	T39.8X5	T39.8X6
Carbitol	T52.3X1	T52.3X2	T52.3X3	T52.3X4	—	—
Carbocaine	T41.3X1	T41.3X2	T41.3X3	T41.3X4	T41.3X5	T41.3X6
infiltration (subcutaneous)	T41.3X1	T41.3X2	T41.3X3	T41.3X4	T41.3X5	T41.3X6
nerve block (peripheral) (plexus)	T41.3X1	T41.3X2	T41.3X3	T41.3X4	T41.3X5	T41.3X6
topical (surface)	T41.3X1	T41.3X2	T41.3X3	T41.3X4	T41.3X5	T41.3X6
Carbocisteine	T48.4X1	T48.4X2	T48.4X3	T48.4X4	T48.4X5	T48.4X6
Carbocromen	T46.3X1	T46.3X2	T46.3X3	T46.3X4	T46.3X5	T46.3X6
Carbol fuchsin	T49.0X1	T49.0X2	T49.0X3	T49.0X4	T49.0X5	T49.0X6
Carbolic acid — *see also* Phenol	T54.0X1	T54.0X2	T54.0X3	T54.0X4	—	—
Carbolonium (bromide)	T48.1X1	T48.1X2	T48.1X3	T48.1X4	T48.1X5	T48.1X6
Carbo medicinalis	T47.6X1	T47.6X2	T47.6X3	T47.6X4	T47.6X5	T47.6X6
Carbomycin	T36.8X1	T36.8X2	T36.8X3	T36.8X4	T36.8X5	T36.8X6
Carbon						
bisulfide (liquid)	T65.4X1	T65.4X2	T65.4X3	T65.4X4	—	—
vapor	T65.4X1	T65.4X2	T65.4X3	T65.4X4	—	—
dioxide (gas)	T59.7X1	T59.7X2	T59.7X3	T59.7X4	—	—
medicinal	T41.5X1	T41.5X2	T41.5X3	T41.5X4	T41.5X5	T41.5X6
nonmedicinal	T59.7X1	T59.7X2	T59.7X3	T59.7X4	—	—
snow	T49.4X1	T49.4X2	T49.4X3	T49.4X4	T49.4X5	T49.4X6
disulfide (liquid)	T65.4X1	T65.4X2	T65.4X3	T65.4X4	—	—
vapor	T65.4X1	T65.4X2	T65.4X3	T65.4X4	—	—
monoxide (from incomplete combustion)	T58.91	T58.92	T58.93	T58.94	—	—
blast furnace gas	T58.8X1	T58.8X2	T58.8X3	T58.8X4	—	—
butane (distributed in mobile container)	T58.11	T58.12	T58.13	T58.14	—	—
distributed through pipes	T58.11	T58.12		T58.14	—	—
charcoal fumes	T58.2X1	T58.2X2	T58.2X3	T58.2X4	—	—
coal	T58.2X1	T58.2X2	T58.2X3	T58.2X4	—	—
coke (in domestic stoves, fireplaces)	T58.2X1	T58.2X2	T58.2X3	T58.2X4	—	—
exhaust gas (motor) not in transit	T58.01	T58.02	T58.03	T58.04	—	—
combustion engine, any not in watercraft	T58.01	T58.02	T58.03	T58.04	—	—
farm tractor, not in transit	T58.01	T58.02	T58.03	T58.04	—	—
gas engine	T58.01	T58.02	T58.03	T58.04	—	—
motor pump	T58.01	T58.02	T58.03	T58.04	—	—
motor vehicle, not in transit	T58.01	T58.02	T58.03	T58.04	—	—
fuel (in domestic use)	T58.2X1	T58.2X2	T58.2X3	T58.2X4	—	—
gas (piped)	T58.11	T58.12	T58.13	T58.14	—	—
in mobile container	T58.11	T58.12	T58.13	T58.14	—	—
piped (natural)	T58.11	T58.12	T58.13	T58.14	—	—
utility	T58.11	T58.12	T58.13	T58.14	—	—
in mobile container	T58.11	T58.12	T58.13	T58.14	—	—
gas (piped)	T58.11	T58.12	T58.13	T58.14	—	—
illuminating gas	T58.11	T58.12	T58.13	T58.14	—	—
industrial fuels or gases, any	T58.8X1	T58.8X2	T58.8X3	T58.8X4	—	—
kerosene (in domestic stoves, fireplaces)	T58.2X1	T58.2X2	T58.2X3	T58.2X4	—	—
kiln gas or vapor	T58.8X1	T58.8X2	T58.8X3	T58.8X4	—	—
motor exhaust gas, not in transit	T58.01	T58.02	T58.03	T58.04	—	—
piped gas (manufactured) (natural)	T58.11	T58.12	T58.13	T58.14	—	—
producer gas	T58.8X1	T58.8X2	T58.8X3	T58.8X4	—	—
propane (distributed in mobile container)	T58.11	T58.12	T58.13	T58.14	—	—

Substance	Poisoning, Accidental (unintentional)	Poisoning, Intentional Self-harm	Poisoning, Assault	Poisoning, Undetermined	Adverse Effect	Under-dosing
Carbon — *continued*						
monoxide — *continued*						
propane — *continued*						
distributed through pipes	T58.11	T58.12	T58.13	T58.14	—	—
solid (in domestic stoves, fireplaces)	T58.2X1	T58.2X2	T58.2X3	T58.2X4	—	—
specified source NEC	T58.8X1	T58.8X2	T58.8X3	T58.8X4	—	—
stove gas	T58.11	T58.12	T58.13	T58.14	—	—
piped	T58.11	T58.12	T58.13	T58.14	—	—
utility gas	T58.11	T58.12	T58.13	T58.14	—	—
piped	T58.11	T58.12	T58.13	T58.14	—	—
water gas	T58.11	T58.12	T58.13	T58.14	—	—
wood (in domestic stoves, fireplaces)	T58.2X1	T58.2X2	T58.2X3	T58.2X4	—	—
tetrachloride (vapor) NEC	T53.0X1	T53.0X2	T53.0X3	T53.0X4	—	—
liquid (cleansing agent) NEC	T53.0X1	T53.0X2	T53.0X3	T53.0X4	—	—
solvent	T53.0X1	T53.0X2	T53.0X3	T53.0X4	—	—
Carbonic acid gas	T59.7X1	T59.7X2	T59.7X3	T59.7X4	—	—
anhydrase inhibitor NEC	T50.2X1	T50.2X2	T50.2X3	T50.2X4	T50.2X5	T50.2X6
Carbophenothion	T60.0X1	T60.0X2	T60.0X3	T60.0X4	—	—
Carboplatin	T45.1X1	T45.1X2	T45.1X3	T45.1X4	T45.1X5	T45.1X6
Carboprost	T48.0X1	T48.0X2	T48.0X3	T48.0X4	T48.0X5	T48.0X6
Carboquone	T45.1X1	T45.1X2	T45.1X3	T45.1X4	T45.1X5	T45.1X6
Carbowax	T49.3X1	T49.3X2	T49.3X3	T49.3X4	T49.3X5	T49.3X6
Carboxymethylcellulose	T47.4X1	T47.4X2	T47.4X3	T47.4X4	T47.4X5	T47.4X6
Carbrital	T42.3X1	T42.3X2	T42.3X3	T42.3X4	T42.3X5	T42.3X6
Carbromal	T42.6X1	T42.6X2	T42.6X3	T42.6X4	T42.6X5	T42.6X6
Carbutamide	T38.3X1	T38.3X2	T38.3X3	T38.3X4	T38.3X5	T38.3X6
Carbuterol	T48.6X1	T48.6X2	T48.6X3	T48.6X4	T48.6X5	T48.6X6
Cardiac						
depressants	T46.2X1	T46.2X2	T46.2X3	T46.2X4	T46.2X5	T46.2X6
rhythm regulator	T46.2X1	T46.2X2	T46.2X3	T46.2X4	T46.2X5	T46.2X6
specified NEC	T46.2X1	T46.2X2	T46.2X3	T46.2X4	T46.2X5	T46.2X6
Cardiografin	T50.8X1	T50.8X2	T50.8X3	T50.8X4	T50.8X5	T50.8X6
Cardiogreen	T50.8X1	T50.8X2	T50.8X3	T50.8X4	T50.8X5	T50.8X6
Cardiotonic (glycoside) **NEC**	T46.0X1	T46.0X2	T46.0X3	T46.0X4	T46.0X5	T46.0X6
Cardiovascular drug NEC	T46.901	T46.902	T46.903	T46.904	T46.905	T46.906
Cardrase	T50.2X1	T50.2X2	T50.2X3	T50.2X4	T50.2X5	T50.2X6
Carfecillin	T36.0X1	T36.0X2	T36.0X3	T36.0X4	T36.0X5	T36.0X6
Carfenazine	T43.3X1	T43.3X2	T43.3X3	T43.3X4	T43.3X5	T43.3X6
Carfusin	T49.0X1	T49.0X2	T49.0X3	T49.0X4	T49.0X5	T49.0X6
Carindacillin	T36.0X1	T36.0X2	T36.0X3	T36.0X4	T36.0X5	T36.0X6
Carisoprodol	T42.8X1	T42.8X2	T42.8X3	T42.8X4	T42.8X5	T42.8X6
Carmellose	T47.4X1	T47.4X2	T47.4X3	T47.4X4	T47.4X5	T47.4X6
Carminative	T47.5X1	T47.5X2	T47.5X3	T47.5X4	T47.5X5	T47.5X6
Carmofur	T45.1X1	T45.1X2	T45.1X3	T45.1X4	T45.1X5	T45.1X6
Carmustine	T45.1X1	T45.1X2	T45.1X3	T45.1X4	T45.1X5	T45.1X6
Carotene	T45.2X1	T45.2X2	T45.2X3	T45.2X4	T45.2X5	T45.2X6
Carphenazine	T43.3X1	T43.3X2	T43.3X3	T43.3X4	T43.3X5	T43.3X6
Carpipramine	T42.4X1	T42.4X2	T42.4X3	T42.4X4	T42.4X5	T42.4X6
Carprofen	T39.311	T39.312	T39.313	T39.314	T39.315	T39.316
Carpronium chloride	T44.3X1	T44.3X2	T44.3X3	T44.3X4	T44.3X5	T44.3X6
Carrageenan	T47.8X1	T47.8X2	T47.8X3	T47.8X4	T47.8X5	T47.8X6
Carteolol	T44.7X1	T44.7X2	T44.7X3	T44.7X4	T44.7X5	T44.7X6
Carter's Little Pills	T47.2X1	T47.2X2	T47.2X3	T47.2X4	T47.2X5	T47.2X6
Cascara (sagrada)	T47.2X1	T47.2X2	T47.2X3	T47.2X4	T47.2X5	T47.2X6
Cassava	T62.2X1	T62.2X2	T62.2X3	T62.2X4	—	—
Castellani's paint	T49.0X1	T49.0X2	T49.0X3	T49.0X4	T49.0X5	T49.0X6
Castor						
bean	T62.2X1	T62.2X2	T62.2X3	T62.2X4	—	—
oil	T47.2X1	T47.2X2	T47.2X3	T47.2X4	T47.2X5	T47.2X6
Catalase	T45.3X1	T45.3X2	T45.3X3	T45.3X4	T45.3X5	T45.3X6
Caterpillar (sting)	T63.431	T63.432	T63.433	T63.434	—	—
Catha (edulis) (tea)	T43.691	T43.692	T43.693	T43.694	—	—
Cathartic NEC	T47.4X1	T47.4X2	T47.4X3	T47.4X4	T47.4X5	T47.4X6
anthacene derivative	T47.2X1	T47.2X2	T47.2X3	T47.2X4	T47.2X5	T47.2X6
bulk	T47.4X1	T47.4X2	T47.4X3	T47.4X4	T47.4X5	T47.4X6
contact	T47.2X1	T47.2X2	T47.2X3	T47.2X4	T47.2X5	T47.2X6
emollient NEC	T47.4X1	T47.4X2	T47.4X3	T47.4X4	T47.4X5	T47.4X6
irritant NEC	T47.2X1	T47.2X2	T47.2X3	T47.2X4	T47.2X5	T47.2X6
mucilage	T47.4X1	T47.4X2	T47.4X3	T47.4X4	T47.4X5	T47.4X6
saline	T47.3X1	T47.3X2	T47.3X3	T47.3X4	T47.3X5	T47.3X6
vegetable	T47.2X1	T47.2X2	T47.2X3	T47.2X4	T47.2X5	T47.2X6
Cathine	T50.5X1	T50.5X2	T50.5X3	T50.5X4	T50.5X5	T50.5X6
Cathomycin	T36.8X1	T36.8X2	T36.8X3	T36.8X4	T36.8X5	T36.8X6
Cation exchange resin	T50.3X1	T50.3X2	T50.3X3	T50.3X4	T50.3X5	T50.3X6
Caustic(s) NEC	T54.91	T54.92	T54.93	T54.94	—	—
alkali	T54.3X1	T54.3X2	T54.3X3	T54.3X4	—	—
hydroxide	T54.3X1	T54.3X2	T54.3X3	T54.3X4	—	—
potash	T54.3X1	T54.3X2	T54.3X3	T54.3X4	—	—
soda	T54.3X1	T54.3X2	T54.3X3	T54.3X4	—	—

Substance	Poisoning, Accidental (unintentional)	Poisoning, Intentional Self-harm	Poisoning, Assault	Poisoning, Undetermined	Adverse Effect	Under-dosing
Caustic(s) NEC — *continued*						
specified NEC	T54.91	T54.92	T54.93	T54.94	—	—
Ceepryn	T49.0X1	T49.0X2	T49.0X3	T49.0X4	T49.0X5	T49.0X6
ENT agent	T49.6X1	T49.6X2	T49.6X3	T49.6X4	T49.6X5	T49.6X6
lozenges	T49.6X1	T49.6X2	T49.6X3	T49.6X4	T49.6X5	T49.6X6
Cefacetrile	T36.1X1	T36.1X2	T36.1X3	T36.1X4	T36.1X5	T36.1X6
Cefaclor	T36.1X1	T36.1X2	T36.1X3	T36.1X4	T36.1X5	T36.1X6
Cefadroxil	T36.1X1	T36.1X2	T36.1X3	T36.1X4	T36.1X5	T36.1X6
Cefalexin	T36.1X1	T36.1X2	T36.1X3	T36.1X4	T36.1X5	T36.1X6
Cefaloglycin	T36.1X1	T36.1X2	T36.1X3	T36.1X4	T36.1X5	T36.1X6
Cefaloridine	T36.1X1	T36.1X2	T36.1X3	T36.1X4	T36.1X5	T36.1X6
Cefalosporins	T36.1X1	T36.1X2	T36.1X3	T36.1X4	T36.1X5	T36.1X6
Cefalotin	T36.1X1	T36.1X2	T36.1X3	T36.1X4	T36.1X5	T36.1X6
Cefamandole	T36.1X1	T36.1X2	T36.1X3	T36.1X4	T36.1X5	T36.1X6
Cefamycin antibiotic	T36.1X1	T36.1X2	T36.1X3	T36.1X4	T36.1X5	T36.1X6
Cefapirin	T36.1X1	T36.1X2	T36.1X3	T36.1X4	T36.1X5	T36.1X6
Cefatrizine	T36.1X1	T36.1X2	T36.1X3	T36.1X4	T36.1X5	T36.1X6
Cefazedone	T36.1X1	T36.1X2	T36.1X3	T36.1X4		T36.1X6
Cefazolin	T36.1X1	T36.1X2	T36.1X3	T36.1X4	T36.1X5	T36.1X6
Cefbuperazone	T36.1X1	T36.1X2	T36.1X3	T36.1X4	T36.1X5	T36.1X6
Cefetamet	T36.1X1	T36.1X2	T36.1X3	T36.1X4	T36.1X5	T36.1X6
Cefixime	T36.1X1	T36.1X2	T36.1X3	T36.1X4	T36.1X5	T36.1X6
Cefmenoxime	T36.1X1	T36.1X2	T36.1X3	T36.1X4	T36.1X5	T36.1X6
Cefmetazole	T36.1X1	T36.1X2	T36.1X3	T36.1X4	T36.1X5	T36.1X6
Cefminox	T36.1X1	T36.1X2	T36.1X3	T36.1X4	T36.1X5	T36.1X6
Cefonicid	T36.1X1	T36.1X2	T36.1X3	T36.1X4	T36.1X5	T36.1X6
Cefoperazone	T36.1X1	T36.1X2	T36.1X3	T36.1X4	T36.1X5	T36.1X6
Ceforanide	T36.1X1	T36.1X2	T36.1X3	T36.1X4	T36.1X5	T36.1X6
Cefotaxime	T36.1X1	T36.1X2	T36.1X3	T36.1X4	T36.1X5	T36.1X6
Cefotetan	T36.1X1	T36.1X2	T36.1X3	T36.1X4	T36.1X5	T36.1X6
Cefotiam	T36.1X1	T36.1X2	T36.1X3	T36.1X4	T36.1X5	T36.1X6
Cefoxitin	T36.1X1	T36.1X2	T36.1X3	T36.1X4	T36.1X5	T36.1X6
Cefpimizole	T36.1X1	T36.1X2	T36.1X3	T36.1X4	T36.1X5	T36.1X6
Cefpiramide	T36.1X1	T36.1X2	T36.1X3	T36.1X4	T36.1X5	T36.1X6
Cefradine	T36.1X1	T36.1X2	T36.1X3	T36.1X4	T36.1X5	T36.1X6
Cefroxadine	T36.1X1	T36.1X2	T36.1X3	T36.1X4	T36.1X5	T36.1X6
Cefsulodin	T36.1X1	T36.1X2	T36.1X3	T36.1X4	T36.1X5	T36.1X6
Ceftazidime	T36.1X1	T36.1X2	T36.1X3	T36.1X4	T36.1X5	T36.1X6
Cefteram	T36.1X1	T36.1X2	T36.1X3	T36.1X4	T36.1X5	T36.1X6
Ceftezole	T36.1X1	T36.1X2	T36.1X3	T36.1X4	T36.1X5	T36.1X6
Ceftizoxime	T36.1X1	T36.1X2	T36.1X3	T36.1X4	T36.1X5	T36.1X6
Ceftriaxone	T36.1X1	T36.1X2	T36.1X3	T36.1X4	T36.1X5	T36.1X6
Cefuroxime	T36.1X1	T36.1X2	T36.1X3	T36.1X4	T36.1X5	T36.1X6
Cefuzonam	T36.1X1	T36.1X2	T36.1X3	T36.1X4	T36.1X5	T36.1X6
Celestone	T38.0X1	T38.0X2	T38.0X3	T38.0X4	T38.0X5	T38.0X6
topical	T49.0X1	T49.0X2	T49.0X3	T49.0X4	T49.0X5	T49.0X6
Celiprolol	T44.7X1	T44.7X2	T44.7X3	T44.7X4	T44.7X5	T44.7X6
Cellosolve	T52.91	T52.92	T52.93	T52.94	—	—
Cell stimulants and proliferants	T49.8X1	T49.8X2	T49.8X3	T49.8X4	T49.8X5	T49.8X6
Cellulose						
cathartic	T47.4X1	T47.4X2	T47.4X3	T47.4X4	T47.4X5	T47.4X6
hydroxyethyl	T47.4X1	T47.4X2	T47.4X3	T47.4X4	T47.4X5	T47.4X6
nitrates (topical)	T49.3X1	T49.3X2	T49.3X3	T49.3X4	T49.3X5	T49.3X6
oxidized	T49.4X1	T49.4X2	T49.4X3	T49.4X4	T49.4X5	T49.4X6
Centipede (bite)	T63.411	T63.412	T63.413	T63.414	—	—
Central nervous system						
depressants	T42.71	T42.72	T42.73	T42.74	T42.75	T42.76
anesthetic (general) NEC	T41.201	T41.202	T41.203	T41.204	T41.205	T41.206
gases NEC	T41.0X1	T41.0X2	T41.0X3	T41.0X4	T41.0X5	T41.0X6
intravenous	T41.1X1	T41.1X2	T41.1X3	T41.1X4	T41.1X5	T41.1X6
barbiturates	T42.3X1	T42.3X2	T42.3X3	T42.3X4	T42.3X5	T42.3X6
benzodiazepines	T42.4X1	T42.4X2	T42.4X3	T42.4X4	T42.4X5	T42.4X6
bromides	T42.6X1	T42.6X2	T42.6X3	T42.6X4	T42.6X5	T42.6X6
cannabis sativa	T40.7X1	T40.7X2	T40.7X3	T40.7X4	T40.7X5	T40.7X6
chloral hydrate	T42.6X1	T42.6X2	T42.6X3	T42.6X4	T42.6X5	T42.6X6
ethanol	T51.0X1	T51.0X2	T51.0X3	T51.0X4	—	—
hallucinogenics	T40.901	T40.902	T40.903	T40.904	T40.905	T40.906
hypnotics	T42.71	T42.72	T42.73	T42.74	T42.75	T42.76
specified NEC	T42.6X1	T42.6X2	T42.6X3	T42.6X4	T42.6X5	T42.6X6
muscle relaxants	T42.8X1	T42.8X2	T42.8X3	T42.8X4	T42.8X5	T42.8X6
paraldehyde	T42.6X1	T42.6X2	T42.6X3	T42.6X4	T42.6X5	T42.6X6
sedatives; sedative-hypnotics	T42.71	T42.72	T42.73	T42.74	T42.75	T42.76
mixed NEC	T42.6X1	T42.6X2	T42.6X3	T42.6X4	T42.6X5	T42.6X6
specified NEC	T42.6X1	T42.6X2	T42.6X3	T42.6X4	T42.6X5	T42.6X6
muscle-tone depressants	T42.8X1	T42.8X2	T42.8X3	T42.8X4	T42.8X5	T42.8X6
stimulants	T43.601	T43.602	T43.603	T43.604	T43.605	T43.606
amphetamines	T43.621	T43.622	T43.623	T43.624	T43.625	T43.626
analeptics	T50.7X1	T50.7X2	T50.7X3	T50.7X4	T50.7X5	T50.7X6
antidepressants	T43.201	T43.202	T43.203	T43.204	T43.205	T43.206
opiate antagonists	T50.7X1	T50.7X2	T50.7X3	T50.7X4	T50.7X5	T50.7X6
specified NEC	T43.691	T43.692	T43.693	T43.694	T43.695	T43.696

Substance	Poisoning, Accidental (unintentional)	Poisoning, Intentional Self-harm	Poisoning, Assault	Poisoning, Undetermined	Adverse Effect	Under-dosing
Cephalexin	T36.1X1	T36.1X2	T36.1X3	T36.1X4	T36.1X5	T36.1X6
Cephaloglycin	T36.1X1	T36.1X2	T36.1X3	T36.1X4	T36.1X5	T36.1X6
Cephaloridine	T36.1X1	T36.1X2	T36.1X3	T36.1X4	T36.1X5	T36.1X6
Cephalosporins	T36.1X1	T36.1X2	T36.1X3	T36.1X4	T36.1X5	T36.1X6
N (adicillin)	T36.0X1	T36.0X2	T36.0X3	T36.0X4	T36.0X5	T36.0X6
Cephalothin	T36.1X1	T36.1X2	T36.1X3	T36.1X4	T36.1X5	T36.1X6
Cephalotin	T36.1X1	T36.1X2	T36.1X3	T36.1X4	T36.1X5	T36.1X6
Cephradine	T36.1X1	T36.1X2	T36.1X3	T36.1X4	T36.1X5	T36.1X6
Cerbera (odallam)	T62.2X1	T62.2X2	T62.2X3	T62.2X4	—	—
Cerberin	T46.0X1	T46.0X2	T46.0X3	T46.0X4	T46.0X5	T46.0X6
Cerebral stimulants	T43.601	T43.602	T43.603	T43.604	T43.605	T43.606
psychotherapeutic	T43.601	T43.602	T43.603	T43.604	T43.605	T43.606
specified NEC	T43.691	T43.692	T43.693	T43.694	T43.695	T43.696
Cerium oxalate	T45.0X1	T45.0X2	T45.0X3	T45.0X4	T45.0X5	T45.0X6
Cerous oxalate	T45.0X1	T45.0X2	T45.0X3	T45.0X4	T45.0X5	T45.0X6
Ceruletide	T50.8X1	T50.8X2	T50.8X3	T50.8X4	T50.8X5	T50.8X6
Cetalkonium (chloride)	T49.0X1	T49.0X2	T49.0X3	T49.0X4	T49.0X5	T49.0X6
Cethexonium chloride	T49.0X1	T49.0X2	T49.0X3	T49.0X4	T49.0X5	T49.0X6
Cetiedil	T46.7X1	T46.7X2	T46.7X3	T46.7X4	T46.7X5	T46.7X6
Cetirizine	T45.0X1	T45.0X2	T45.0X3	T45.0X4	T45.0X5	T45.0X6
Cetomacrogol	T50.991	T50.992	T50.993	T50.994	T50.995	T50.996
Cetotiamine	T45.2X1	T45.2X2	T45.2X3	T45.2X4	T45.2X5	T45.2X6
Cetoxime	T45.0X1	T45.0X2	T45.0X3	T45.0X4	T45.0X5	T45.0X6
Cetraxate	T47.1X1	T47.1X2	T47.1X3	T47.1X4	T47.1X5	T47.1X6
Cetrimide	T49.0X1	T49.0X2	T49.0X3	T49.0X4	T49.0X5	T49.0X6
Cetrimonium (bromide)	T49.0X1	T49.0X2	T49.0X3	T49.0X4	T49.0X5	T49.0X6
Cetylpyridinium chloride	T49.0X1	T49.0X2	T49.0X3	T49.0X4	T49.0X5	T49.0X6
ENT agent	T49.6X1	T49.6X2	T49.6X3	T49.6X4	T49.6X5	T49.6X6
lozenges	T49.6X1	T49.6X2	T49.6X3	T49.6X4	T49.6X5	T49.6X6
Cevadilla — see Sabadilla						
Cevitamic acid	T45.2X1	T45.2X2	T45.2X3	T45.2X4	T45.2X5	T45.2X6
Chalk, precipitated	T47.1X1	T47.1X2	T47.1X3	T47.1X4	T47.1X5	T47.1X6
Chamomile	T49.0X1	T49.0X2	T49.0X3	T49.0X4	T49.0X5	T49.0X6
Ch'an su	T46.0X1	T46.0X2	T46.0X3	T46.0X4	T46.0X5	T46.0X6
Charcoal	T47.6X1	T47.6X2	T47.6X3	T47.6X4	T47.6X5	T47.6X6
activated — see also Charcoal, medicinal						
fumes (Carbon monoxide)	T58.2X1	T58.2X2	T58.2X3	T58.2X4	—	—
industrial	T58.8X1	T58.8X2	T58.8X3	T58.8X4	—	—
medicinal (activated)	T47.6X1	T47.6X2	T47.6X3	T47.6X4	T47.6X5	T47.6X6
antidiarrheal	T47.6X1	T47.6X2	T47.6X3	T47.6X4	T47.6X5	T47.6X6
poison control	T47.8X1	T47.8X2	T47.8X3	T47.8X4	T47.8X5	T47.8X6
specified use other than for diarrhea	T47.8X1	T47.8X2	T47.8X3	T47.8X4	T47.8X5	T47.8X6
topical	T49.8X1	T49.8X2	T49.8X3	T49.8X4	T49.8X5	T49.8X6
Chaulmosulfone	T37.1X1	T37.1X2	T37.1X3	T37.1X4	T37.1X5	T37.1X6
Chelating agent NEC	T50.6X1	T50.6X2	T50.6X3	T50.6X4	T50.6X5	T50.6X6
Chelidonium majus	T62.2X1	T62.2X2	T62.2X3	T62.2X4	—	—
Chemical substance NEC	T65.91	T65.92	T65.93	T65.94	—	—
Chenodeoxycholic acid	T47.5X1	T47.5X2	T47.5X3	T47.5X4	T47.5X5	T47.5X6
Chenodiol	T47.5X1	T47.5X2	T47.5X3	T47.5X4	T47.5X5	T47.5X6
Chenopodium	T37.4X1	T37.4X2	T37.4X3	T37.4X4	T37.4X5	T37.4X6
Cherry laurel	T62.2X1	T62.2X2	T62.2X3	T62.2X4	—	—
Chinidin (e)	T46.2X1	T46.2X2	T46.2X3	T46.2X4	T46.2X5	T46.2X6
Chiniofon	T37.8X1	T37.8X2	T37.8X3	T37.8X4	T37.8X5	T37.8X6
Chlophedianol	T48.3X1	T48.3X2	T48.3X3	T48.3X4	T48.3X5	T48.3X6
Chloral	T42.6X1	T42.6X2	T42.6X3	T42.6X4	T42.6X5	T42.6X6
derivative	T42.6X1	T42.6X2	T42.6X3	T42.6X4	T42.6X5	T42.6X6
hydrate	T42.6X1	T42.6X2	T42.6X3	T42.6X4	T42.6X5	T42.6X6
Chloralamide	T42.6X1	T42.6X2	T42.6X3	T42.6X4	T42.6X5	T42.6X6
Chloralodol	T42.6X1	T42.6X2	T42.6X3	T42.6X4	T42.6X5	T42.6X6
Chloralose	T60.4X1	T60.4X2	T60.4X3	T60.4X4	—	—
Chlorambucil	T45.1X1	T45.1X2	T45.1X3	T45.1X4	T45.1X5	T45.1X6
Chloramine	T57.8X1	T57.8X2	T57.8X3	T57.8X4	—	—
T	T49.0X1	T49.0X2	T49.0X3	T49.0X4	T49.0X5	T49.0X6
topical	T49.0X1	T49.0X2	T49.0X3	T49.0X4	T49.0X5	T49.0X6
Chloramphenicol	T36.2X1	T36.2X2	T36.2X3	T36.2X4	T36.2X5	T36.2X6
ENT agent	T49.6X1	T49.6X2	T49.6X3	T49.6X4	T49.6X5	T49.6X6
ophthalmic preparation	T49.5X1	T49.5X2	T49.5X3	T49.5X4	T49.5X5	T49.5X6
topical NEC	T49.0X1	T49.0X2	T49.0X3	T49.0X4	T49.0X5	T49.0X6
Chlorate (potassium) (sodium) NEC	T60.3X1	T60.3X2	T60.3X3	T60.3X4	—	—
herbicide	T60.3X1	T60.3X2	T60.3X3	T60.3X4	—	—
Chlorazanil	T50.2X1	T50.2X2	T50.2X3	T50.2X4	T50.2X5	T50.2X6
Chlorbenzene, chlorbenzol	T53.7X1	T53.7X2	T53.7X3	T53.7X4	—	—
Chlorbenzoxamine	T44.3X1	T44.3X2	T44.3X3	T44.3X4	T44.3X5	T44.3X6
Chlorbutol	T42.6X1	T42.6X2	T42.6X3	T42.6X4	T42.6X5	T42.6X6
Chlorcyclizine	T45.0X1	T45.0X2	T45.0X3	T45.0X4	T45.0X5	T45.0X6
Chlordan (e) (dust)	T60.1X1	T60.1X2	T60.1X3	T60.1X4	—	—
Chlordantoin	T49.0X1	T49.0X2	T49.0X3	T49.0X4	T49.0X5	T49.0X6
Chlordiazepoxide	T42.4X1	T42.4X2	T42.4X3	T42.4X4	T42.4X5	T42.4X6
Chlordiethyl benzamide	T49.3X1	T49.3X2	T49.3X3	T49.3X4	T49.3X5	T49.3X6
Chloresium	T49.8X1	T49.8X2	T49.8X3	T49.8X4	T49.8X5	T49.8X6
Chlorethiazol	T42.6X1	T42.6X2	T42.6X3	T42.6X4	T42.6X5	T42.6X6
Chlorethyl — see Ethyl chloride						
Chloretone	T42.6X1	T42.6X2	T42.6X3	T42.6X4	T42.6X5	T42.6X6
Chlorex	T53.6X1	T53.6X2	T53.6X3	T53.6X4	—	—
insecticide	T60.1X1	T60.1X2	T60.1X3	T60.1X4	—	—
Chlorfenvinphos	T60.0X1	T60.0X2	T60.0X3	T60.0X4	—	—
Chlorhexadol	T42.6X1	T42.6X2	T42.6X3	T42.6X4	T42.6X5	T42.6X6
Chlorhexamide	T45.1X1	T45.1X2	T45.1X3	T45.1X4	T45.1X5	T45.1X6
Chlorhexidine	T49.0X1	T49.0X2	T49.0X3	T49.0X4	T49.0X5	T49.0X6
Chlorhydroxyquinolin	T49.0X1	T49.0X2	T49.0X3	T49.0X4	T49.0X5	T49.0X6
Chloride of lime (bleach)	T54.3X1	T54.3X2	T54.3X3	T54.3X4	—	—
Chlorimipramine	T43.011	T43.012	T43.013	T43.014	T43.015	T43.016
Chlorinated						
camphene	T53.6X1	T53.6X2	T53.6X3	T53.6X4	—	—
diphenyl	T53.7X1	T53.7X2	T53.7X3	T53.7X4	—	—
hydrocarbons NEC	T53.91	T53.92	T53.93	T53.94	—	—
solvents	T53.91	T53.92	T53.93	T53.94	—	—
lime (bleach)	T54.3X1	T54.3X2	T54.3X3	T54.3X4	—	—
and boric acid solution	T49.0X1	T49.0X2	T49.0X3	T49.0X4	T49.0X5	T49.0X6
naphthalene (insecticide)	T60.1X1	T60.1X2	T60.1X3	T60.1X4	—	—
industrial (non-pesticide)	T53.7X1	T53.7X2	T53.7X3	T53.7X4	—	—
pesticide NEC	T60.8X1	T60.8X2	T60.8X3	T60.8X4	—	—
soda — see also sodium hypochlorite						
solution	T49.0X1	T49.0X2	T49.0X3	T49.0X4	▼T49.0X5	T49.0X6
Chlorine (fumes) (gas)	T59.4X1	T59.4X2	T59.4X3	T59.4X4	—	—
bleach	T54.3X1	T54.3X2	T54.3X3	T54.3X4	—	—
compound gas NEC	T59.4X1	T59.4X2	T59.4X3	T59.4X4	—	—
disinfectant	T59.4X1	T59.4X2	T59.4X3	T59.4X4	—	—
releasing agents NEC	T59.4X1	T59.4X2	T59.4X3	T59.4X4	—	—
Chlorisondamine chloride	T46.991	T46.992	T46.993	T46.994	T46.995	T46.996
Chlormadinone	T38.5X1	T38.5X2	T38.5X3	T38.5X4	T38.5X5	T38.5X6
Chlormephos	T60.0X1	T60.0X2	T60.0X3	T60.0X4	—	—
Chlormerodrin	T50.2X1	T50.2X2	T50.2X3	T50.2X4	T50.2X5	T50.2X6
Chlormethiazole	T42.6X1	T42.6X2	T42.6X3	T42.6X4	T42.6X5	T42.6X6
Chlormethine	T45.1X1	T45.1X2	T45.1X3	T45.1X4	T45.1X5	T45.1X6
Chlormethylenecycline	T36.4X1	T36.4X2	T36.4X3	T36.4X4	T36.4X5	T36.4X6
Chlormezanone	T42.6X1	T42.6X2	T42.6X3	T42.6X4	T42.6X5	T42.6X6
Chloroacetic acid	T60.3X1	T60.3X2	T60.3X3	T60.3X4	—	—
Chloroacetone	T59.3X1	T59.3X2	T59.3X3	T59.3X4	—	—
Chloroacetophenone	T59.3X1	T59.3X2	T59.3X3	T59.3X4	—	—
Chloroaniline	T53.7X1	T53.7X2	T53.7X3	T53.7X4	—	—
Chlorobenzene, chlorobenzol	T53.7X1	T53.7X2	T53.7X3	T53.7X4	—	—
Chlorobromomethane (fire extinguisher)	T53.6X1	T53.6X2	T53.6X3	T53.6X4	—	—
Chlorobutanol	T49.0X1	T49.0X2	T49.0X3	T49.0X4	T49.0X5	T49.0X6
Chlorocresol	T49.0X1	T49.0X2	T49.0X3	T49.0X4	T49.0X5	T49.0X6
Chlorodehydromethyltestosterone	T38.7X1	T38.7X2	T38.7X3	T38.7X4	T38.7X5	T38.7X6
Chlorodinitrobenzene	T53.7X1	T53.7X2	T53.7X3	T53.7X4	—	—
dust or vapor	T53.7X1	T53.7X2	T53.7X3	T53.7X4	—	—
Chlorodiphenyl	T53.7X1	T53.7X2	T53.7X3	T53.7X4	—	—
Chloroethane — see Ethyl chloride						
Chloroethylene	T53.6X1	T53.6X2	T53.6X3	T53.6X4	—	—
Chlorofluorocarbons	T53.5X1	T53.5X2	T53.5X3	T53.5X4	—	—
Chloroform (fumes) (vapor)	T53.1X1	T53.1X2	T53.1X3	T53.1X4	—	—
anesthetic	T41.0X1	T41.0X2	T41.0X3	T41.0X4	T41.0X5	T41.0X6
solvent	T53.1X1	T53.1X2	T53.1X3	T53.1X4	—	—
water, concentrated	T41.0X1	T41.0X2	T41.0X3	T41.0X4	T41.0X5	T41.0X6
Chloroguanide	T37.2X1	T37.2X2	T37.2X3	T37.2X4	T37.2X5	T37.2X6
Chloromycetin	T36.2X1	T36.2X2	T36.2X3	T36.2X4	T36.2X5	T36.2X6
ENT agent	T49.6X1	T49.6X2	T49.6X3	T49.6X4	T49.6X5	T49.6X6
ophthalmic preparation	T49.5X1	T49.5X2	T49.5X3	T49.5X4	T49.5X5	T49.5X6
otic solution	T49.6X1	T49.6X2	T49.6X3	T49.6X4	T49.6X5	T49.6X6
topical NEC	T49.0X1	T49.0X2	T49.0X3	T49.0X4	T49.0X5	T49.0X6
Chloronitrobenzene	T53.7X1	T53.7X2	T53.7X3	T53.7X4	—	—
dust or vapor	T53.7X1	T53.7X2	T53.7X3	T53.7X4	—	—
Chlorophacinone	T60.4X1	T60.4X2	T60.4X3	T60.4X4	—	—
Chlorophenol	T53.7X1	T53.7X2	T53.7X3	T53.7X4	—	—
Chlorophenothane	T60.1X1	T60.1X2	T60.1X3	T60.1X4	—	—
Chlorophyll	T50.991	T50.992	T50.993	T50.994	T50.995	T50.996
Chloropicrin (fumes)	T53.6X1	T53.6X2	T53.6X3	T53.6X4	—	—
fumigant	T60.8X1	T60.8X2	T60.8X3	T60.8X4	—	—
fungicide	T60.3X1	T60.3X2	T60.3X3	T60.3X4	—	—
pesticide	T60.8X1	T60.8X2	T60.8X3	T60.8X4	—	—
Chloroprocaine	T41.3X1	T41.3X2	T41.3X3	T41.3X4	T41.3X5	T41.3X6
infiltration (subcutaneous)	T41.3X1	T41.3X2	T41.3X3	T41.3X4	T41.3X5	T41.3X6
nerve block (peripheral) (plexus)	T41.3X1	T41.3X2	T41.3X3	T41.3X4	T41.3X5	T41.3X6
spinal	T41.3X1	T41.3X2	T41.3X3	T41.3X4	T41.3X5	T41.3X6
Chloroptic	T49.5X1	T49.5X2	T49.5X3	T49.5X4	T49.5X5	T49.5X6
Chloropurine	T45.1X1	T45.1X2	T45.1X3	T45.1X4	T45.1X5	T45.1X6

Table of Drugs and Chemicals

Chloropyramine — Cloponone

Substance	Poisoning, Accidental (unintentional)	Poisoning, Intentional Self-harm	Poisoning, Assault	Poisoning, Undetermined	Adverse Effect	Under-dosing
Chloropyramine	T45.0X1	T45.0X2	T45.0X3	T45.0X4	T45.0X5	T45.0X6
Chloropyrifos	T60.0X1	T60.0X2	T60.0X3	T60.0X4	—	—
Chloropyrilene	T45.0X1	T45.0X2	T45.0X3	T45.0X4	T45.0X5	T45.0X6
Chloroquine	T37.2X1	T37.2X2	T37.2X3	T37.2X4	T37.2X5	T37.2X6
Chlorothalonil	T60.3X1	T60.3X2	T60.3X3	T60.3X4	—	—
Chlorothen	T45.0X1	T45.0X2	T45.0X3	T45.0X4	T45.0X5	T45.0X6
Chlorothiazide	T50.2X1	T50.2X2	T50.2X3	T50.2X4	T50.2X5	T50.2X6
Chlorothymol	T49.4X1	T49.4X2	T49.4X3	T49.4X4	T49.4X5	T49.4X6
Chlorotrianisene	T38.5X1	T38.5X2	T38.5X3	T38.5X4	T38.5X5	T38.5X6
Chlorovinyldichloroarsine, not in war	T57.0X1	T57.0X2	T57.0X3	T57.0X4	—	—
Chloroxine	T49.4X1	T49.4X2	T49.4X3	T49.4X4	T49.4X5	T49.4X6
Chloroxylenol	T49.0X1	T49.0X2	T49.0X3	T49.0X4	T49.0X5	T49.0X6
Chlorphenamine	T45.0X1	T45.0X2	T45.0X3	T45.0X4	T45.0X5	T45.0X6
Chlorphenesin	T42.8X1	T42.8X2	T42.8X3	T42.8X4	T42.8X5	T42.8X6
topical (antifungal)	T49.0X1	T49.0X2	T49.0X3	T49.0X4	T49.0X5	T49.0X6
Chlorpheniramine	T45.0X1	T45.0X2	T45.0X3	T45.0X4	T45.0X5	T45.0X6
Chlorphenoxamine	T45.0X1	T45.0X2	T45.0X3	T45.0X4	T45.0X5	T45.0X6
Chlorphentermine	T50.5X1	T50.5X2	T50.5X3	T50.5X4	T50.5X5	T50.5X6
Chlorprocaine — see Chloroprocaine						
Chlorproguanil	T37.2X1	T37.2X2	T37.2X3	T37.2X4	T37.2X5	T37.2X6
Chlorpromazine	T43.3X1	T43.3X2	T43.3X3	T43.3X4	T43.3X5	T43.3X6
Chlorpropamide	T38.3X1	T38.3X2	T38.3X3	T38.3X4	T38.3X5	T38.3X6
Chlorprothixene	T43.4X1	T43.4X2	T43.4X3	T43.4X4	T43.4X5	T43.4X6
Chlorquinaldol	T49.0X1	T49.0X2	T49.0X3	T49.0X4	T49.0X5	T49.0X6
Chlorquinol	T49.0X1	T49.0X2	T49.0X3	T49.0X4	T49.0X5	T49.0X6
Chlortalidone	T50.2X1	T50.2X2	T50.2X3	T50.2X4	T50.2X5	T50.2X6
Chlortetracycline	T36.4X1	T36.4X2	T36.4X3	T36.4X4	T36.4X5	T36.4X6
Chlorthalidone	T50.2X1	T50.2X2	T50.2X3	T50.2X4	T50.2X5	T50.2X6
Chlorthion	T60.0X1	T60.0X2	T60.0X3	T60.0X4	—	—
Chlorthiophos	T60.0X1	T60.0X2	T60.0X3	T60.0X4	—	—
Chlortrianisene	T38.5X1	T38.5X2	T38.5X3	T38.5X4	T38.5X5	T38.5X6
Chlor-Trimeton	T45.0X1	T45.0X2	T45.0X3	T45.0X4	T45.0X5	T45.0X6
Chlorzoxazone	T42.8X1	T42.8X2	T42.8X3	T42.8X4	T42.8X5	T42.8X6
Choke damp	T59.7X1	T59.7X2	T59.7X3	T59.7X4	—	—
Cholagogues	T47.5X1	T47.5X2	T47.5X3	T47.5X4	T47.5X5	T47.5X6
Cholebrine	T50.8X1	T50.8X2	T50.8X3	T50.8X4	T50.8X5	T50.8X6
Cholecalciferol	T45.2X1	T45.2X2	T45.2X3	T45.2X4	T45.2X5	T45.2X6
Cholecystokinin	T50.8X1	T50.8X2	T50.8X3	T50.8X4	T50.8X5	T50.8X6
Cholera vaccine	T50.A91	T50.A92	T50.A93	T50.A94	T50.A95	T50.A96
Choleretic	T47.5X1	T47.5X2	T47.5X3	T47.5X4	T47.5X5	T47.5X6
Cholesterol-lowering agents	T46.6X1	T46.6X2	T46.6X3	T46.6X4	T46.6X5	T46.6X6
Cholestyramine (resin)	T46.6X1	T46.6X2	T46.6X3	T46.6X4	T46.6X5	T46.6X6
Cholic acid	T47.5X1	T47.5X2	T47.5X3	T47.5X4	T47.5X5	T47.5X6
Choline	T48.6X1	T48.6X2	T48.6X3	T48.6X4	T48.6X5	T48.6X6
chloride	T50.991	T50.992	T50.993	T50.994	T50.995	T50.996
dihydrogen citrate	T50.991	T50.992	T50.993	T50.994	T50.995	T50.996
salicylate	T39.091	T39.092	T39.093	T39.094	T39.095	T39.096
theophyllinate	T48.6X1	T48.6X2	T48.6X3	T48.6X4	T48.6X5	T48.6X6
Cholinergic (drug) NEC	T44.1X1	T44.1X2	T44.1X3	T44.1X4	T44.1X5	T44.1X6
muscle tone enhancer	T44.1X1	T44.1X2	T44.1X3	T44.1X4	T44.1X5	T44.1X6
organophosphorus	T44.0X1	T44.0X2	T44.0X3	T44.0X4	T44.0X5	T44.0X6
insecticide	T60.0X1	T60.0X2	T60.0X3	T60.0X4	—	—
nerve gas	T59.891	T59.892	T59.893	T59.894	—	—
trimethyl ammonium propanediol	T44.1X1	T44.1X2	T44.1X3	T44.1X4	T44.1X5	T44.1X6
Cholinesterase reactivator	T50.6X1	T50.6X2	T50.6X3	T50.6X4	T50.6X5	T50.6X6
Cholografin	T50.8X1	T50.8X2	T50.8X3	T50.8X4	T50.8X5	T50.8X6
Chorionic gonadotropin	T38.891	T38.892	T38.893	T38.894	T38.895	T38.896
Chromate	T56.2X1	T56.2X2	T56.2X3	T56.2X4	—	—
dust or mist	T56.2X1	T56.2X2	T56.2X3	T56.2X4	—	—
lead — see also lead	T56.0X1	T56.0X2	T56.0X3	T56.0X4	—	—
paint	T56.0X1	T56.0X2	T56.0X3	T56.0X4	—	—
Chromic						
acid	T56.2X1	T56.2X2	T56.2X3	T56.2X4	—	—
dust or mist	T56.2X1	T56.2X2	T56.2X3	T56.2X4	—	—
phosphate 32P	T45.1X1	T45.1X2	T45.1X3	T45.1X4	T45.1X5	T45.1X6
Chromium	T56.2X1	T56.2X2	T56.2X3	T56.2X4	—	—
compounds — see Chromate						
sesquioxide	T50.8X1	T50.8X2	T50.8X3	T50.8X4	T50.8X5	T50.8X6
Chromomycin A3	T45.1X1	T45.1X2	T45.1X3	T45.1X4	T45.1X5	T45.1X6
Chromonar	T46.3X1	T46.3X2	T46.3X3	T46.3X4	T46.3X5	T46.3X6
Chromyl chloride	T56.2X1	T56.2X2	T56.2X3	T56.2X4	—	—
Chrysarobin	T49.4X1	T49.4X2	T49.4X3	T49.4X4	T49.4X5	T49.4X6
Chrysazin	T47.2X1	T47.2X2	T47.2X3	T47.2X4	T47.2X5	T47.2X6
Chymar	T45.3X1	T45.3X2	T45.3X3	T45.3X4	T45.3X5	T45.3X6
ophthalmic preparation	T49.5X1	T49.5X2	T49.5X3	T49.5X4	T49.5X5	T49.5X6
Chymopapain	T45.3X1	T45.3X2	T45.3X3	T45.3X4	T45.3X5	T45.3X6
Chymotrypsin	T45.3X1	T45.3X2	T45.3X3	T45.3X4	T45.3X5	T45.3X6
ophthalmic preparation	T49.5X1	T49.5X2	T49.5X3	T49.5X4	T49.5X5	T49.5X6
Cianidanol	T50.991	T50.992	T50.993	T50.994	T50.995	T50.996
Cianopramine	T43.011	T43.012	T43.013	T43.014	T43.015	T43.016
Cibenzoline	T46.2X1	T46.2X2	T46.2X3	T46.2X4	T46.2X5	T46.2X6
Ciclacillin	T36.0X1	T36.0X2	T36.0X3	T36.0X4	T36.0X5	T36.0X6
Ciclobarbital — see Hexobarbital						
Ciclonicate	T46.7X1	T46.7X2	T46.7X3	T46.7X4	T46.7X5	T46.7X6
Ciclopirox (olamine)	T49.0X1	T49.0X2	T49.0X3	T49.0X4	T49.0X5	T49.0X6
Ciclosporin	T45.1X1	T45.1X2	T45.1X3	T45.1X4	T45.1X5	T45.1X6
Cicuta maculata or virosa	T62.2X1	T62.2X2	T62.2X3	T62.2X4	—	—
Cicutoxin	T62.2X1	T62.2X2	T62.2X3	T62.2X4	—	—
Cigarette lighter fluid	T52.0X1	T52.0X2	T52.0X3	T52.0X4	—	—
Cigarettes (tobacco)	T65.221	T65.222	T65.223	T65.224	—	—
Ciguatoxin	T61.01	T61.02	T61.03	T61.04	—	—
Cilazapril	T46.4X1	T46.4X2	T46.4X3	T46.4X4	T46.4X5	T46.4X6
Cimetidine	T47.0X1	T47.0X2	T47.0X3	T47.0X4	T47.0X5	T47.0X6
Cimetropium bromide	T44.3X1	T44.3X2	T44.3X3	T44.3X4	T44.3X5	T44.3X6
Cinchocaine	T41.3X1	T41.3X2	T41.3X3	T41.3X4	T41.3X5	T41.3X6
topical (surface)	T41.3X1	T41.3X2	T41.3X3	T41.3X4	T41.3X5	T41.3X6
Cinchona	T37.2X1	T37.2X2	T37.2X3	T37.2X4	T37.2X5	T37.2X6
Cinchonine alkaloids	T37.2X1	T37.2X2	T37.2X3	T37.2X4	T37.2X5	T37.2X6
Cinchophen	T50.4X1	T50.4X2	T50.4X3	T50.4X4	T50.4X5	T50.4X6
Cinepazide	T46.7X1	T46.7X2	T46.7X3	T46.7X4	T46.7X5	T46.7X6
Cinnamedrine	T48.5X1	T48.5X2	T48.5X3	T48.5X4	T48.5X5	T48.5X6
Cinnarizine	T45.0X1	T45.0X2	T45.0X3	T45.0X4	T45.0X5	T45.0X6
Cinoxacin	T37.8X1	T37.8X2	T37.8X3	T37.8X4	T37.8X5	T37.8X6
Ciprofibrate	T46.6X1	T46.6X2	T46.6X3	T46.6X4	T46.6X5	T46.6X6
Ciprofloxacin	T36.8X1	T36.8X2	T36.8X3	T36.8X4	T36.8X5	T36.8X6
Cisapride	T47.8X1	T47.8X2	T47.8X3	T47.8X4	T47.8X5	T47.8X6
Cisplatin	T45.1X1	T45.1X2	T45.1X3	T45.1X4	T45.1X5	T45.1X6
Citalopram	T43.221	T43.222	T43.223	T43.224	T43.225	T43.226
Citanest	T41.3X1	T41.3X2	T41.3X3	T41.3X4	T41.3X5	T41.3X6
infiltration (subcutaneous)	T41.3X1	T41.3X2	T41.3X3	T41.3X4	T41.3X5	T41.3X6
nerve block (peripheral) (plexus)	T41.3X1	T41.3X2	T41.3X3	T41.3X4	T41.3X5	T41.3X6
Citric acid	T47.5X1	T47.5X2	T47.5X3	T47.5X4	T47.5X5	T47.5X6
Citrovorum (factor)	T45.8X1	T45.8X2	T45.8X3	T45.8X4	T45.8X5	T45.8X6
Claviceps purpurea	T62.2X1	T62.2X2	T62.2X3	T62.2X4	—	—
Clavulanic acid	T36.1X1	T36.1X2	T36.1X3	T36.1X4	T36.1X5	T36.1X6
Cleaner, cleansing agent, type not specified	T65.891	T65.892	T65.893	T65.894	—	—
of paint or varnish	T52.91	T52.92	T52.93	T52.94	—	—
specified type NEC	T65.891	T65.892	T65.893	T65.894	—	—
Clebopride	T47.8X1	T47.8X2	T47.8X3	T47.8X4	T47.8X5	T47.8X6
Clefamide	T37.3X1	T37.3X2	T37.3X3	T37.3X4	T37.3X5	T37.3X6
Clemastine	T45.0X1	T45.0X2	T45.0X3	T45.0X4	T45.0X5	T45.0X6
Clematis vitalba	T62.2X1	T62.2X2	T62.2X3	T62.2X4	—	—
Clemizole	T45.0X1	T45.0X2	T45.0X3	T45.0X4	T45.0X5	T45.0X6
penicillin	T36.0X1	T36.0X2	T36.0X3	T36.0X4	T36.0X5	T36.0X6
Clenbuterol	T48.6X1	T48.6X2	T48.6X3	T48.6X4	T48.6X5	T48.6X6
Clidinium bromide	T44.3X1	T44.3X2	T44.3X3	T44.3X4	T44.3X5	T44.3X6
Clindamycin	T36.8X1	T36.8X2	T36.8X3	T36.8X4	T36.8X5	T36.8X6
Clinofibrate	T46.6X1	T46.6X2	T46.6X3	T46.6X4	T46.6X5	T46.6X6
Clioquinol	T37.8X1	T37.8X2	T37.8X3	T37.8X4	T37.8X5	T37.8X6
Cliradon	T40.2X1	T40.2X2	T40.2X3	T40.2X4	—	—
Clobazam	T42.4X1	T42.4X2	T42.4X3	T42.4X4	T42.4X5	T42.4X6
Clobenzorex	T50.5X1	T50.5X2	T50.5X3	T50.5X4	T50.5X5	T50.5X6
Clobetasol	T49.0X1	T49.0X2	T49.0X3	T49.0X4	T49.0X5	T49.0X6
Clobetasone	T49.0X1	T49.0X2	T49.0X3	T49.0X4	T49.0X5	T49.0X6
Clobutinol	T48.3X1	T48.3X2	T48.3X3	T48.3X4	T48.3X5	T48.3X6
Clocortolone	T38.0X1	T38.0X2	T38.0X3	T38.0X4	T38.0X5	T38.0X6
Clodantoin	T49.0X1	T49.0X2	T49.0X3	T49.0X4	T49.0X5	T49.0X6
Clodronic acid	T50.991	T50.992	T50.993	T50.994	T50.995	T50.996
Clofazimine	T37.1X1	T37.1X2	T37.1X3	T37.1X4	T37.1X5	T37.1X6
Clofedanol	T48.3X1	T48.3X2	T48.3X3	T48.3X4	T48.3X5	T48.3X6
Clofenamide	T50.2X1	T50.2X2	T50.2X3	T50.2X4	T50.2X5	T50.2X6
Clofenotane	T49.0X1	T49.0X2	T49.0X3	T49.0X4	T49.0X5	T49.0X6
Clofezone	T39.2X1	T39.2X2	T39.2X3	T39.2X4	T39.2X5	T39.2X6
Clofibrate	T46.6X1	T46.6X2	T46.6X3	T46.6X4	T46.6X5	T46.6X6
Clofibride	T46.6X1	T46.6X2	T46.6X3	T46.6X4	T46.6X5	T46.6X6
Cloforex	T50.5X1	T50.5X2	T50.5X3	T50.5X4	T50.5X5	T50.5X6
Clomethiazole	T42.6X1	T42.6X2	T42.6X3	T42.6X4	T42.6X5	T42.6X6
Clometocillin	T36.0X1	T36.0X2	T36.0X3	T36.0X4	T36.0X5	T36.0X6
Clomifene	T38.5X1	T38.5X2	T38.5X3	T38.5X4	T38.5X5	T38.5X6
Clomiphene	T38.5X1	T38.5X2	T38.5X3	T38.5X4	T38.5X5	T38.5X6
Clomipramine	T43.011	T43.012	T43.013	T43.014	T43.015	T43.016
Clomocycline	T36.4X1	T36.4X2	T36.4X3	T36.4X4	T36.4X5	T36.4X6
Clonazepam	T42.4X1	T42.4X2	T42.4X3	T42.4X4	T42.4X5	T42.4X6
Clonidine	T46.5X1	T46.5X2	T46.5X3	T46.5X4	T46.5X5	T46.5X6
Clonixin	T39.8X1	T39.8X2	T39.8X3	T39.8X4	T39.8X5	T39.8X6
Clopamide	T50.2X1	T50.2X2	T50.2X3	T50.2X4	T50.2X5	T50.2X6
Clopenthixol	T43.4X1	T43.4X2	T43.4X3	T43.4X4	T43.4X5	T43.4X6
Cloperastine	T48.3X1	T48.3X2	T48.3X3	T48.3X4	T48.3X5	T48.3X6
Clophedianol	T48.3X1	T48.3X2	T48.3X3	T48.3X4	T48.3X5	T48.3X6
Cloponone	T36.2X1	T36.2X2	T36.2X3	T36.2X4	T36.2X5	T36.2X6

Additional Character May Be Required — Refer to the Tabular List for Character Selection ▽ Subterms under main terms may continue to next column or page

Substance	Poisoning, Accidental (unintentional)	Poisoning, Intentional Self-harm	Poisoning, Assault	Poisoning, Undetermined	Adverse Effect	Under-dosing
Cloprednol	T38.0X1	T38.0X2	T38.0X3	T38.0X4	T38.0X5	T38.0X6
Cloral betaine	T42.6X1	T42.6X2	T42.6X3	T42.6X4	T42.6X5	T42.6X6
Cloramfenicol	T36.2X1	T36.2X2	T36.2X3	T36.2X4	T36.2X5	T36.2X6
Clorazepate (dipotassium)	T42.4X1	T42.4X2	T42.4X3	T42.4X4	T42.4X5	T42.4X6
Clorexolone	T50.2X1	T50.2X2	T50.2X3	T50.2X4	T50.2X5	T50.2X6
Clorfenamine	T45.0X1	T45.0X2	T45.0X3	T45.0X4	T45.0X5	T45.0X6
Clorgiline	T43.1X1	T43.1X2	T43.1X3	T43.1X4	T43.1X5	T43.1X6
Clorotepine	T44.3X1	T44.3X2	T44.3X3	T44.3X4	T44.3X5	T44.3X6
Clorox (bleach)	T54.91	T54.92	T54.93	T54.94	—	—
Clorprenaline	T48.6X1	T48.6X2	T48.6X3	T48.6X4	T48.6X5	T48.6X6
Clortermine	T50.5X1	T50.5X2	T50.5X3	T50.5X4	T50.5X5	T50.5X6
Clotiapine	T43.591	T43.592	T43.593	T43.594	T43.595	T43.596
Clotiazepam	T42.4X1	T42.4X2	T42.4X3	T42.4X4	T42.4X5	T42.4X6
Clotibric acid	T46.6X1	T46.6X2	T46.6X3	T46.6X4	T46.6X5	T46.6X6
Clotrimazole	T49.0X1	T49.0X2	T49.0X3	T49.0X4	T49.0X5	T49.0X6
Cloxacillin	T36.0X1	T36.0X2	T36.0X3	T36.0X4	T36.0X5	T36.0X6
Cloxazolam	T42.4X1	T42.4X2	T42.4X3	T42.4X4	T42.4X5	T42.4X6
Cloxiquine	T49.0X1	T49.0X2	T49.0X3	T49.0X4	T49.0X5	T49.0X6
Clozapine	T42.4X1	T42.4X2	T42.4X3	T42.4X4	T42.4X5	T42.4X6
Coagulant NEC	T45.7X1	T45.7X2	T45.7X3	T45.7X4	T45.7X5	T45.7X6
Coal (carbon monoxide from) — see also Carbon, monoxide, coal	T58.2X1	T58.2X2	T58.2X3	T58.2X4	—	—
oil — see Kerosene						
tar	T49.1X1	T49.1X2	T49.1X3	T49.1X4	T49.1X5	T49.1X6
fumes	T59.891	T59.892	T59.893	T59.894	—	—
medicinal (ointment)	T49.4X1	T49.4X2	T49.4X3	T49.4X4	T49.4X5	T49.4X6
analgesics NEC	T39.2X1	T39.2X2	T39.2X3	T39.2X4	T39.2X5	T39.2X6
naphtha (solvent)	T52.0X1	T52.0X2	T52.0X3	T52.0X4	—	—
Cobalamine	T45.2X1	T45.2X2	T45.2X3	T45.2X4	T45.2X5	T45.2X6
Cobalt (nonmedicinal) (fumes) (industrial)	T56.891	T56.892	T56.893	T56.894	—	—
medicinal (trace) (chloride)	T45.8X1	T45.8X2	T45.8X3	T45.8X4	T45.8X5	T45.8X6
Cobra (venom)	T63.041	T63.042	T63.043	T63.044	—	—
Coca (leaf)	T40.5X1	T40.5X2	T40.5X3	T40.5X4	T40.5X5	T40.5X6
Cocaine	T40.5X1	T40.5X2	T40.5X3	T40.5X4	T40.5X5	T40.5X6
topical anesthetic	T41.3X1	T41.3X2	T41.3X3	T41.3X4	T41.3X5	T41.3X6
Cocarboxylase	T45.3X1	T45.3X2	T45.3X3	T45.3X4	T45.3X5	T45.3X6
Coccidioidin	T50.8X1	T50.8X2	T50.8X3	T50.8X4	T50.8X5	T50.8X6
Cocculus indicus	T62.1X1	T62.1X2	T62.1X3	T62.1X4	—	—
Cochineal	T65.6X1	T65.6X2	T65.6X3	T65.6X4	—	—
medicinal products	T50.991	T50.992	T50.993	T50.994	T50.995	T50.996
Codeine	T40.2X1	T40.2X2	T40.2X3	T40.2X4	T40.2X5	T40.2X6
Cod-liver oil	T45.2X1	T45.2X2	T45.2X3	T45.2X4	T45.2X5	T45.2X6
Coenzyme A	T50.991	T50.992	T50.993	T50.994	T50.995	T50.996
Coffee	T62.8X1	T62.8X2	T62.8X3	T62.8X4	—	—
Cogalactoisomerase	T50.991	T50.992	T50.993	T50.994	T50.995	T50.996
Cogentin	T44.3X1	T44.3X2	T44.3X3	T44.3X4	T44.3X5	T44.3X6
Coke fumes or gas (carbon monoxide)	T58.2X1	T58.2X2	T58.2X3	T58.2X4	—	—
industrial use	T58.8X1	T58.8X2	T58.8X3	T58.8X4	—	—
Colace	T47.4X1	T47.4X2	T47.4X3	T47.4X4	T47.4X5	T47.4X6
Colaspase	T45.1X1	T45.1X2	T45.1X3	T45.1X4	T45.1X5	T45.1X6
Colchicine	T50.4X1	T50.4X2	T50.4X3	T50.4X4	T50.4X5	T50.4X6
Colchicum	T62.2X1	T62.2X2	T62.2X3	T62.2X4	—	—
Cold cream	T49.3X1	T49.3X2	T49.3X3	T49.3X4	T49.3X5	T49.3X6
Colecalciferol	T45.2X1	T45.2X2	T45.2X3	T45.2X4	T45.2X5	T45.2X6
Colestipol	T46.6X1	T46.6X2	T46.6X3	T46.6X4	T46.6X5	T46.6X6
Colestyramine	T46.6X1	T46.6X2	T46.6X3	T46.6X4	T46.6X5	T46.6X6
Colimycin	T36.8X1	T36.8X2	T36.8X3	T36.8X4	T36.8X5	T36.8X6
Colistimethate	T36.8X1	T36.8X2	T36.8X3	T36.8X4	T36.8X5	T36.8X6
Colistin	T36.8X1	T36.8X2	T36.8X3	T36.8X4	T36.8X5	T36.8X6
sulfate (eye preparation)	T49.5X1	T49.5X2	T49.5X3	T49.5X4	T49.5X5	T49.5X6
Collagen	T50.991	T50.992	T50.993	T50.994	T50.995	T50.996
Collagenase	T49.4X1	T49.4X2	T49.4X3	T49.4X4	T49.4X5	T49.4X6
Collodion	T49.3X1	T49.3X2	T49.3X3	T49.3X4	T49.3X5	T49.3X6
Colocynth	T47.2X1	T47.2X2	T47.2X3	T47.2X4	T47.2X5	T47.2X6
Colophony adhesive	T49.3X1	T49.3X2	T49.3X3	T49.3X4	T49.3X5	T49.3X6
Colorant — see also Dye	T50.991	T50.992	T50.993	T50.994	T50.995	T50.996
Coloring matter — see Dye(s)						
Combustion gas (after combustion) — see Carbon, monoxide						
prior to combustion	T59.891	T59.892	T59.893	T59.894	—	—
Compazine	T43.3X1	T43.3X2	T43.3X3	T43.3X4	T43.3X5	T43.3X6
Compound						
42 (warfarin)	T60.4X1	T60.4X2	T60.4X3	T60.4X4	—	—
269 (endrin)	T60.1X1	T60.1X2	T60.1X3	T60.1X4	—	—
497 (dieldrin)	T60.1X1	T60.1X2	T60.1X3	T60.1X4	—	—
1080 (sodium fluoroacetate)	T60.4X1	T60.4X2	T60.4X3	T60.4X4	—	—
3422 (parathion)	T60.0X1	T60.0X2	T60.0X3	T60.0X4	—	—
3911 (phorate)	T60.0X1	T60.0X2	T60.0X3	T60.0X4	—	—
Compound — continued						
3956 (toxaphene)	T60.1X1	T60.1X2	T60.1X3	T60.1X4	—	—
4049 (malathion)	T60.0X1	T60.0X2	T60.0X3	T60.0X4	—	—
4069 (malathion)	T60.0X1	T60.0X2	T60.0X3	T60.0X4	—	—
4124 (dicapthon)	T60.0X1	T60.0X2	T60.0X3	T60.0X4	—	—
E (cortisone)	T38.0X1	T38.0X2	T38.0X3	T38.0X4	T38.0X5	T38.0X6
F (hydrocortisone)	T38.0X1	T38.0X2	T38.0X3	T38.0X4	T38.0X5	T38.0X6
Congener, anabolic	T38.7X1	T38.7X2	T38.7X3	T38.7X4	T38.7X5	T38.7X6
Congo red	T50.8X1	T50.8X2	T50.8X3	T50.8X4	T50.8X5	T50.8X6
Coniine, conine	T62.2X1	T62.2X2	T62.2X3	T62.2X4	—	—
Conium (maculatum)	T62.2X1	T62.2X2	T62.2X3	T62.2X4	—	—
Conjugated estrogenic substances	T38.5X1	T38.5X2	T38.5X3	T38.5X4	T38.5X5	T38.5X6
Contac	T48.5X1	T48.5X2	T48.5X3	T48.5X4	T48.5X5	T48.5X6
Contact lens solution	T49.5X1	T49.5X2	T49.5X3	T49.5X4	T49.5X5	T49.5X6
Contraceptive (oral)	T38.4X1	T38.4X2	T38.4X3	T38.4X4	T38.4X5	T38.4X6
vaginal	T49.8X1	T49.8X2	T49.8X3	T49.8X4	T49.8X5	T49.8X6
Contrast medium, radiography	T50.8X1	T50.8X2	T50.8X3	T50.8X4	T50.8X5	T50.8X6
Convallaria glycosides	T46.0X1	T46.0X2	T46.0X3	T46.0X4	T46.0X5	T46.0X6
Convallaria majalis	T62.2X1	T62.2X2	T62.2X3	T62.2X4	—	—
berry	T62.1X1	T62.1X2	T62.1X3	T62.1X4	—	—
Copperhead snake (bite) (venom)	T63.061	T63.062	T63.063	T63.064	—	—
Copper (dust) (fumes) (nonmedicinal) NEC	T56.4X1	T56.4X2	T56.4X3	T56.4X4	—	—
arsenate, arsenite	T57.0X1	T57.0X2	T57.0X3	T57.0X4	—	—
insecticide	T60.2X1	T60.2X2	T60.2X3	T60.2X4	—	—
emetic	T47.7X1	T47.7X2	T47.7X3	T47.7X4	T47.7X5	T47.7X6
fungicide	T60.3X1	T60.3X2	T60.3X3	T60.3X4	—	—
gluconate	T49.0X1	T49.0X2	T49.0X3	T49.0X4	T49.0X5	T49.0X6
insecticide	T60.2X1	T60.2X2	T60.2X3	T60.2X4	—	—
medicinal (trace)	T45.8X1	T45.8X2	T45.8X3	T45.8X4	T45.8X5	T45.8X6
oleate	T49.0X1	T49.0X2	T49.0X3	T49.0X4	T49.0X5	T49.0X6
sulfate	T56.4X1	T56.4X2	T56.4X3	T56.4X4	—	—
cupric	T56.4X1	T56.4X2	T56.4X3	T56.4X4	—	—
fungicide	T60.3X1	T60.3X2	T60.3X3	T60.3X4	—	—
medicinal						
ear	T49.6X1	T49.6X2	T49.6X3	T49.6X4	T49.6X5	T49.6X6
emetic	T47.7X1	T47.7X2	T47.7X3	T47.7X4	T47.7X5	T47.7X6
eye	T49.5X1	T49.5X2	T49.5X3	T49.5X4	T49.5X5	T49.5X6
cuprous	T56.4X1	T56.4X2	T56.4X3	T56.4X4	—	—
fungicide	T60.3X1	T60.3X2	T60.3X3	T60.3X4	—	—
medicinal						
ear	T49.6X1	T49.6X2	T49.6X3	T49.6X4	T49.6X5	T49.6X6
emetic	T47.7X1	T47.7X2	T47.7X3	T47.7X4	T47.7X5	T47.7X6
eye	T49.5X1	T49.5X2	T49.5X3	T49.5X4	T49.5X5	T49.5X6
Coral (sting)	T63.691	T63.692	T63.693	T63.694	—	—
snake (bite) (venom)	T63.021	T63.022	T63.023	T63.024	—	—
Corbadrine	T49.6X1	T49.6X2	T49.6X3	T49.6X4	T49.6X5	T49.6X6
Cordite	T65.891	T65.892	T65.893	T65.894	—	—
vapor	T59.891	T59.892	T59.893	T59.894	—	—
Cordran	T49.0X1	T49.0X2	T49.0X3	T49.0X4	T49.0X5	T49.0X6
Corn cures	T49.4X1	T49.4X2	T49.4X3	T49.4X4	T49.4X5	T49.4X6
Cornhusker's lotion	T49.3X1	T49.3X2	T49.3X3	T49.3X4	T49.3X5	T49.3X6
Corn starch	T49.3X1	T49.3X2	T49.3X3	T49.3X4	T49.3X5	T49.3X6
Coronary vasodilator NEC	T46.3X1	T46.3X2	T46.3X3	T46.3X4	T46.3X5	T46.3X6
Corrosive NEC	T54.91	T54.92	T54.93	T54.94	—	—
acid NEC	T54.2X1	T54.2X2	T54.2X3	T54.2X4	—	—
aromatics	T54.1X1	T54.1X2	T54.1X3	T54.1X4	—	—
disinfectant	T54.1X1	T54.1X2	T54.1X3	T54.1X4	—	—
fumes NEC	T54.91	T54.92	T54.93	T54.94	—	—
specified NEC	T54.91	T54.92	T54.93	T54.94	—	—
sublimate	T56.1X1	T56.1X2	T56.1X3	T56.1X4	—	—
Cortate	T38.0X1	T38.0X2	T38.0X3	T38.0X4	T38.0X5	T38.0X6
Cort-Dome	T38.0X1	T38.0X2	T38.0X3	T38.0X4	T38.0X5	T38.0X6
ENT agent	T49.6X1	T49.6X2	T49.6X3	T49.6X4	T49.6X5	T49.6X6
ophthalmic preparation	T49.5X1	T49.5X2	T49.5X3	T49.5X4	T49.5X5	T49.5X6
topical NEC	T49.0X1	T49.0X2	T49.0X3	T49.0X4	T49.0X5	T49.0X6
Cortef	T38.0X1	T38.0X2	T38.0X3	T38.0X4	T38.0X5	T38.0X6
ENT agent	T49.6X1	T49.6X2	T49.6X3	T49.6X4	T49.6X5	T49.6X6
ophthalmic preparation	T49.5X1	T49.5X2	T49.5X3	T49.5X4	T49.5X5	T49.5X6
topical NEC	T49.0X1	T49.0X2	T49.0X3	T49.0X4	T49.0X5	T49.0X6
Corticosteroid	T38.0X1	T38.0X2	T38.0X3	T38.0X4	T38.0X5	T38.0X6
ENT agent	T49.6X1	T49.6X2	T49.6X3	T49.6X4	T49.6X5	T49.6X6
mineral	T50.0X1	T50.0X2	T50.0X3	T50.0X4	T50.0X5	T50.0X6
ophthalmic	T49.5X1	T49.5X2	T49.5X3	T49.5X4	T49.5X5	T49.5X6
topical NEC	T49.0X1	T49.0X2	T49.0X3	T49.0X4	T49.0X5	T49.0X6
Corticotropin	T38.811	T38.812	T38.813	T38.814	T38.815	T38.816
Cortisol	T38.0X1	T38.0X2	T38.0X3	T38.0X4	T38.0X5	T38.0X6
ENT agent	T49.6X1	T49.6X2	T49.6X3	T49.6X4	T49.6X5	T49.6X6
ophthalmic preparation	T49.5X1	T49.5X2	T49.5X3	T49.5X4	T49.5X5	T49.5X6
topical NEC	T49.0X1	T49.0X2	T49.0X3	T49.0X4	T49.0X5	T49.0X6

Cloprednol — Cortisol

Subterms under main terms may continue to next column or page   Additional Character May Be Required — Refer to the Tabular List for Character Selection   361

Substance	Poisoning, Accidental (unintentional)	Poisoning, Intentional Self-harm	Poisoning, Assault	Poisoning, Undetermined	Adverse Effect	Under-dosing
Cortisone (acetate)	T38.0X1	T38.0X2	T38.0X3	T38.0X4	T38.0X5	T38.0X6
ENT agent	T49.6X1	T49.6X2	T49.6X3	T49.6X4	T49.6X5	T49.6X6
ophthalmic preparation	T49.5X1	T49.5X2	T49.5X3	T49.5X4	T49.5X5	T49.5X6
topical NEC	T49.0X1	T49.0X2	T49.0X3	T49.0X4	T49.0X5	T49.0X6
Cortivazol	T38.0X1	T38.0X2	T38.0X3	T38.0X4	T38.0X5	T38.0X6
Cortogen	T38.0X1	T38.0X2	T38.0X3	T38.0X4	T38.0X5	T38.0X6
ENT agent	T49.6X1	T49.6X2	T49.6X3	T49.6X4	T49.6X5	T49.6X6
ophthalmic preparation	T49.5X1	T49.5X2	T49.5X3	T49.5X4	T49.5X5	T49.5X6
Cortone	T38.0X1	T38.0X2	T38.0X3	T38.0X4	T38.0X5	T38.0X6
ENT agent	T49.6X1	T49.6X2	T49.6X3	T49.6X4	T49.6X5	T49.6X6
ophthalmic preparation	T49.5X1	T49.5X2	T49.5X3	T49.5X4	T49.5X5	T49.5X6
Cortril	T38.0X1	T38.0X2	T38.0X3	T38.0X4	T38.0X5	T38.0X6
ENT agent	T49.6X1	T49.6X2	T49.6X3	T49.6X4	T49.6X5	T49.6X6
ophthalmic preparation	T49.5X1	T49.5X2	T49.5X3	T49.5X4	T49.5X5	T49.5X6
topical NEC	T49.0X1	T49.0X2	T49.0X3	T49.0X4	T49.0X5	T49.0X6
Corynebacterium parvum	T45.1X1	T45.1X2	T45.1X3	T45.1X4	T45.1X5	T45.1X6
Cosmetic preparation	T49.8X1	T49.8X2	T49.8X3	T49.8X4	T49.8X5	T49.8X6
Cosmetics	T49.8X1	T49.8X2	T49.8X3	T49.8X4	T49.8X5	T49.8X6
Cosyntropin	T38.811	T38.812	T38.813	T38.814	T38.815	T38.816
Cotarnine	T45.7X1	T45.7X2	T45.7X3	T45.7X4	T45.7X5	T45.7X6
Co-trimoxazole	T36.8X1	T36.8X2	T36.8X3	T36.8X4	T36.8X5	T36.8X6
Cottonseed oil	T49.3X1	T49.3X2	T49.3X3	T49.3X4	T49.3X5	T49.3X6
Cough mixture (syrup)	T48.4X1	T48.4X2	T48.4X3	T48.4X4	T48.4X5	T48.4X6
containing opiates	T40.2X1	T40.2X2	T40.2X3	T40.2X4	T40.2X5	T40.2X6
expectorants	T48.4X1	T48.4X2	T48.4X3	T48.4X4	T48.4X5	T48.4X6
Coumadin	T45.511	T45.512	T45.513	T45.514	T45.515	T45.516
rodenticide	T60.4X1	T60.4X2	T60.4X3	T60.4X4	—	—
Coumaphos	T60.0X1	T60.0X2	T60.0X3	T60.0X4	—	—
Coumarin	T45.511	T45.512	T45.513	T45.514	T45.515	T45.516
Coumetarol	T45.511	T45.512	T45.513	T45.514	T45.515	T45.516
Cowbane	T62.2X1	T62.2X2	T62.2X3	T62.2X4	—	—
Cozyme	T45.2X1	T45.2X2	T45.2X3	T45.2X4	T45.2X5	T45.2X6
Crack	T40.5X1	T40.5X2	T40.5X3	T40.5X4	—	—
Crataegus extract	T46.0X1	T46.0X2	T46.0X3	T46.0X4	T46.0X5	T46.0X6
Creolin	T54.1X1	T54.1X2	T54.1X3	T54.1X4	—	—
disinfectant	T54.1X1	T54.1X2	T54.1X3	T54.1X4	—	—
Creosol (compound)	T49.0X1	T49.0X2	T49.0X3	T49.0X4	T49.0X5	T49.0X6
Creosote (coal tar)	T49.0X1	T49.0X2	T49.0X3	T49.0X4	T49.0X5	T49.0X6
(beechwood)						
medicinal (expectorant)	T48.4X1	T48.4X2	T48.4X3	T48.4X4	T48.4X5	T48.4X6
syrup	T48.4X1	T48.4X2	T48.4X3	T48.4X4	T48.4X5	T48.4X6
Cresol(s)	T49.0X1	T49.0X2	T49.0X3	T49.0X4	T49.0X5	T49.0X6
and soap solution	T49.0X1	T49.0X2	T49.0X3	T49.0X4	T49.0X5	T49.0X6
Cresyl acetate	T49.0X1	T49.0X2	T49.0X3	T49.0X4	T49.0X5	T49.0X6
Cresylic acid	T49.0X1	T49.0X2	T49.0X3	T49.0X4	T49.0X5	T49.0X6
Crimidine	T60.4X1	T60.4X2	T60.4X3	T60.4X4	—	—
Croconazole	T37.8X1	T37.8X2	T37.8X3	T37.8X4	T37.8X5	T37.8X6
Cromoglicic acid	T48.6X1	T48.6X2	T48.6X3	T48.6X4	T48.6X5	T48.6X6
Cromolyn	T48.6X1	T48.6X2	T48.6X3	T48.6X4	T48.6X5	T48.6X6
Cromonar	T46.3X1	T46.3X2	T46.3X3	T46.3X4	T46.3X5	T46.3X6
Cropropamide	T39.8X1	T39.8X2	T39.8X3	T39.8X4	T39.8X5	T39.8X6
with crotethamide	T50.7X1	T50.7X2	T50.7X3	T50.7X4	T50.7X5	T50.7X6
Crotamiton	T49.0X1	T49.0X2	T49.0X3	T49.0X4	T49.0X5	T49.0X6
Crotethamide	T39.8X1	T39.8X2	T39.8X3	T39.8X4	T39.8X5	T39.8X6
with cropropamide	T50.7X1	T50.7X2	T50.7X3	T50.7X4	T50.7X5	T50.7X6
Croton (oil)	T47.2X1	T47.2X2	T47.2X3	T47.2X4	T47.2X5	T47.2X6
chloral	T42.6X1	T42.6X2	T42.6X3	T42.6X4	T42.6X5	T42.6X6
Crude oil	T52.0X1	T52.0X2	T52.0X3	T52.0X4	—	—
Cryogenine	T39.8X1	T39.8X2	T39.8X3	T39.8X4	T39.8X5	T39.8X6
Cryolite (vapor)	T60.1X1	T60.1X2	T60.1X3	T60.1X4	—	—
insecticide	T60.1X1	T60.1X2	T60.1X3	T60.1X4	—	—
Cryptenamine (tannates)	T46.5X1	T46.5X2	T46.5X3	T46.5X4	T46.5X5	T46.5X6
Crystal violet	T49.0X1	T49.0X2	T49.0X3	T49.0X4	T49.0X5	T49.0X6
Cuckoopint	T62.2X1	T62.2X2	T62.2X3	T62.2X4	—	—
Cumetharol	T45.511	T45.512	T45.513	T45.514	T45.515	T45.516
Cupric						
acetate	T60.3X1	T60.3X2	T60.3X3	T60.3X4	—	—
acetoarsenite	T57.0X1	T57.0X2	T57.0X3	T57.0X4	—	—
arsenate	T57.0X1	T57.0X2	T57.0X3	T57.0X4	—	—
gluconate	T49.0X1	T49.0X2	T49.0X3	T49.0X4	T49.0X5	T49.0X6
oleate	T49.0X1	T49.0X2	T49.0X3	T49.0X4	T49.0X5	T49.0X6
sulfate	T56.4X1	T56.4X2	T56.4X3	T56.4X4	—	—
Cuprous sulfate — see also Copper sulfate	T56.4X1	T56.4X2	T56.4X3	T56.4X4	—	—
Curare, curarine	T48.1X1	T48.1X2	T48.1X3	T48.1X4	T48.1X5	T48.1X6
Cyamemazine	T43.3X1	T43.3X2	T43.3X3	T43.3X4	T43.3X5	T43.3X6
Cyamopsis tetragonoloba	T46.6X1	T46.6X2	T46.6X3	T46.6X4	T46.6X5	T46.6X6
Cyanacetyl hydrazide	T37.1X1	T37.1X2	T37.1X3	T37.1X4	T37.1X5	T37.1X6
Cyanic acid (gas)	T59.891	T59.892	T59.893	T59.894	—	—
Cyanide(s) (compounds)	T65.0X1	T65.0X2	T65.0X3	T65.0X4	—	—
(potassium) (sodium)						
NEC						
dust or gas (inhalation) NEC	T57.3X1	T57.3X2	T57.3X3	T57.3X4	—	—
Cyanide(s) (compounds) (potassium) (sodium) NEC — continued						
fumigant	T65.0X1	T65.0X2	T65.0X3	T65.0X4	—	—
hydrogen	T57.3X1	T57.3X2	T57.3X3	T57.3X4	—	—
mercuric see Mercury						
pesticide (dust) (fumes)	T65.0X1	T65.0X2	T65.0X3	T65.0X4	—	—
Cyanoacrylate adhesive	T49.3X1	T49.3X2	T49.3X3	T49.3X4	T49.3X5	T49.3X6
Cyanocobalamin	T45.8X1	T45.8X2	T45.8X3	T45.8X4	T45.8X5	T45.8X6
Cyanogen (chloride) (gas)	T59.891	T59.892	T59.893	T59.894	—	—
NEC						
Cyclacillin	T36.0X1	T36.0X2	T36.0X3	T36.0X4	T36.0X5	T36.0X6
Cyclaine	T41.3X1	T41.3X2	T41.3X3	T41.3X4	T41.3X5	T41.3X6
Cyclamate	T50.991	T50.992	T50.993	T50.994	T50.995	T50.996
Cyclamen europaeum	T62.2X1	T62.2X2	T62.2X3	T62.2X4	—	—
Cyclandelate	T46.7X1	T46.7X2	T46.7X3	T46.7X4	T46.7X5	T46.7X6
Cyclazocine	T50.7X1	T50.7X2	T50.7X3	T50.7X4	T50.7X5	T50.7X6
Cyclizine	T45.0X1	T45.0X2	T45.0X3	T45.0X4	T45.0X5	T45.0X6
Cyclobarbital	T42.3X1	T42.3X2	T42.3X3	T42.3X4	T42.3X5	T42.3X6
Cyclobarbitone	T42.3X1	T42.3X2	T42.3X3	T42.3X4	T42.3X5	T42.3X6
Cyclobenzaprine	T48.1X1	T48.1X2	T48.1X3	T48.1X4	T48.1X5	T48.1X6
Cyclodrine	T44.3X1	T44.3X2	T44.3X3	T44.3X4	T44.3X5	T44.3X6
Cycloguanil embonate	T37.2X1	T37.2X2	T37.2X3	T37.2X4	T37.2X5	T37.2X6
Cyclohexane	T52.8X1	T52.8X2	T52.8X3	T52.8X4	—	—
Cyclohexanol	T51.8X1	T51.8X2	T51.8X3	T51.8X4	—	—
Cyclohexanone	T52.4X1	T52.4X2	T52.4X3	T52.4X4	—	—
Cycloheximide	T60.3X1	T60.3X2	T60.3X3	T60.3X4	—	—
Cyclohexyl acetate	T52.8X1	T52.8X2	T52.8X3	T52.8X4	—	—
Cycloleucin	T45.1X1	T45.1X2	T45.1X3	T45.1X4	T45.1X5	T45.1X6
Cyclomethycaine	T41.3X1	T41.3X2	T41.3X3	T41.3X4	T41.3X5	T41.3X6
Cyclopentamine	T44.4X1	T44.4X2	T44.4X3	T44.4X4	T44.4X5	T44.4X6
Cyclopenthiazide	T50.2X1	T50.2X2	T50.2X3	T50.2X4	T50.2X5	T50.2X6
Cyclopentolate	T44.3X1	T44.3X2	T44.3X3	T44.3X4	T44.3X5	T44.3X6
Cyclophosphamide	T45.1X1	T45.1X2	T45.1X3	T45.1X4	T45.1X5	T45.1X6
Cycloplegic drug	T49.5X1	T49.5X2	T49.5X3	T49.5X4	T49.5X5	T49.5X6
Cyclopropane	T41.291	T41.292	T41.293	T41.294	T41.295	T41.296
Cyclopyrabital	T39.8X1	T39.8X2	T39.8X3	T39.8X4	T39.8X5	T39.8X6
Cycloserine	T37.1X1	T37.1X2	T37.1X3	T37.1X4	T37.1X5	T37.1X6
Cyclosporin	T45.1X1	T45.1X2	T45.1X3	T45.1X4	T45.1X5	T45.1X6
Cyclothiazide	T50.2X1	T50.2X2	T50.2X3	T50.2X4	T50.2X5	T50.2X6
Cycrimine	T44.3X1	T44.3X2	T44.3X3	T44.3X4	T44.3X5	T44.3X6
Cyhalothrin	T60.1X1	T60.1X2	T60.1X3	T60.1X4	—	—
Cymarin	T46.0X1	T46.0X2	T46.0X3	T46.0X4	T46.0X5	T46.0X6
Cypermethrin	T60.1X1	T60.1X2	T60.1X3	T60.1X4	—	—
Cyphenothrin	T60.2X1	T60.2X2	T60.2X3	T60.2X4	—	—
Cyproheptadine	T45.0X1	T45.0X2	T45.0X3	T45.0X4	T45.0X5	T45.0X6
Cyproterone	T38.6X1	T38.6X2	T38.6X3	T38.6X4	T38.6X5	T38.6X6
Cysteamine	T50.6X1	T50.6X2	T50.6X3	T50.6X4	T50.6X5	T50.6X6
Cytarabine	T45.1X1	T45.1X2	T45.1X3	T45.1X4	T45.1X5	T45.1X6
Cytisus						
laburnum	T62.2X1	T62.2X2	T62.2X3	T62.2X4	—	—
scoparius	T62.2X1	T62.2X2	T62.2X3	T62.2X4	—	—
Cytochrome C	T47.5X1	T47.5X2	T47.5X3	T47.5X4	T47.5X5	T47.5X6
Cytomel	T38.1X1	T38.1X2	T38.1X3	T38.1X4	T38.1X5	T38.1X6
Cytosine arabinoside	T45.1X1	T45.1X2	T45.1X3	T45.1X4	T45.1X5	T45.1X6
Cytoxan	T45.1X1	T45.1X2	T45.1X3	T45.1X4	T45.1X5	T45.1X6
Cytozyme	T45.7X1	T45.7X2	T45.7X3	T45.7X4	T45.7X5	T45.7X6
S-Carboxymethylcysteine	T48.4X1	T48.4X2	T48.4X3	T48.4X4	T48.4X5	T48.4X6
Dacarbazine	T45.1X1	T45.1X2	T45.1X3	T45.1X4	T45.1X5	T45.1X6
Dactinomycin	T45.1X1	T45.1X2	T45.1X3	T45.1X4	T45.1X5	T45.1X6
DADPS	T37.1X1	T37.1X2	T37.1X3	T37.1X4	T37.1X5	T37.1X6
Dakin's solution	T49.0X1	T49.0X2	T49.0X3	T49.0X4	T49.0X5	T49.0X6
Dalapon (sodium)	T60.3X1	T60.3X2	T60.3X3	T60.3X4	—	—
Dalmane	T42.4X1	T42.4X2	T42.4X3	T42.4X4	T42.4X5	T42.4X6
Danazol	T38.6X1	T38.6X2	T38.6X3	T38.6X4	T38.6X5	T38.6X6
Danilone	T45.511	T45.512	T45.513	T45.514	T45.515	T45.516
Danthron	T47.2X1	T47.2X2	T47.2X3	T47.2X4	T47.2X5	T47.2X6
Dantrolene	T42.8X1	T42.8X2	T42.8X3	T42.8X4	T42.8X5	T42.8X6
Dantron	T47.2X1	T47.2X2	T47.2X3	T47.2X4	T47.2X5	T47.2X6
Daphne (gnidium) (mezereum)	T62.2X1	T62.2X2	T62.2X3	T62.2X4	—	—
berry	T62.1X1	T62.1X2	T62.1X3	T62.1X4	—	—
Dapsone	T37.1X1	T37.1X2	T37.1X3	T37.1X4	T37.1X5	T37.1X6
Daraprim	T37.2X1	T37.2X2	T37.2X3	T37.2X4	T37.2X5	T37.2X6
Darnel	T62.2X1	T62.2X2	T62.2X3	T62.2X4	—	—
Darvon	T39.8X1	T39.8X2	T39.8X3	T39.8X4	T39.8X5	T39.8X6
Daunomycin	T45.1X1	T45.1X2	T45.1X3	T45.1X4	T45.1X5	T45.1X6
Daunorubicin	T45.1X1	T45.1X2	T45.1X3	T45.1X4	T45.1X5	T45.1X6
DBI	T38.3X1	T38.3X2	T38.3X3	T38.3X4	T38.3X5	T38.3X6
D-Con	T60.91	T60.92	T60.93	T60.94	—	—
insecticide	T60.2X1	T60.2X2	T60.2X3	T60.2X4	—	—
rodenticide	T60.4X1	T60.4X2	T60.4X3	T60.4X4	—	—
DDAVP	T38.891	T38.892	T38.893	T38.894	T38.895	T38.896

Additional Character May Be Required — Refer to the Tabular List for Character Selection ▽ Subterms under main terms may continue to next column or page

Substance	Poisoning, Accidental (unintentional)	Poisoning, Intentional Self-harm	Poisoning, Assault	Poisoning, Undetermined	Adverse Effect	Under-dosing
DDE (bis(chlorophenyl)-dichloroethylene)	T60.2X1	T60.2X2	T60.2X3	T60.2X4	—	—
DDS	T37.1X1	T37.1X2	T37.1X3	T37.1X4	T37.1X5	T37.1X6
DDT (dust)	T60.1X1	T60.1X2	T60.1X3	T60.1X4	—	—
Deadly nightshade — see also Belladonna	T62.2X1	T62.2X2	T62.2X3	T62.2X4	—	—
berry	T62.1X1	T62.1X2	T62.1X3	T62.1X4	—	—
Deamino-D-arginine vasopressin	T38.891	T38.892	T38.893	T38.894	T38.895	T38.896
Deanol (aceglumate)	T50.991	T50.992	T50.993	T50.994	T50.995	T50.996
Debrisoquine	T46.5X1	T46.5X2	T46.5X3	T46.5X4	T46.5X5	T46.5X6
Decaborane	T57.8X1	T57.8X2	T57.8X3	T57.8X4	—	—
fumes	T59.891	T59.892	T59.893	T59.894		
Decadron	T38.0X1	T38.0X2	T38.0X3	T38.0X4	T38.0X5	T38.0X6
ENT agent	T49.6X1	T49.6X2	T49.6X3	T49.6X4	T49.6X5	T49.6X6
ophthalmic preparation	T49.5X1	T49.5X2	T49.5X3	T49.5X4	T49.5X5	T49.5X6
topical NEC	T49.0X1	T49.0X2	T49.0X3	T49.0X4	T49.0X5	T49.0X6
Decahydronaphthalene	T52.8X1	T52.8X2	T52.8X3	T52.8X4	—	—
Decalin	T52.8X1	T52.8X2	T52.8X3	T52.8X4	—	—
Decamethonium (bromide)	T48.1X1	T48.1X2	T48.1X3	T48.1X4	T48.1X5	T48.1X6
Decholin	T47.5X1	T47.5X2	T47.5X3	T47.5X4	T47.5X5	T47.5X6
Declomycin	T36.4X1	T36.4X2	T36.4X3	T36.4X4	T36.4X5	T36.4X6
Decongestant, nasal (mucosa)	T48.5X1	T48.5X2	T48.5X3	T48.5X4	T48.5X5	T48.5X6
combination	T48.5X1	T48.5X2	T48.5X3	T48.5X4	T48.5X5	T48.5X6
Deet	T60.8X1	T60.8X2	T60.8X3	T60.8X4	—	—
Deferoxamine	T45.8X1	T45.8X2	T45.8X3	T45.8X4	T45.8X5	T45.8X6
Deflazacort	T38.0X1	T38.0X2	T38.0X3	T38.0X4	T38.0X5	T38.0X6
Deglycyrrhizinized extract of licorice	T48.4X1	T48.4X2	T48.4X3	T48.4X4	T48.4X5	T48.4X6
Dehydrocholic acid	T47.5X1	T47.5X2	T47.5X3	T47.5X4	T47.5X5	T47.5X6
Dehydroemetine	T37.3X1	T37.3X2	T37.3X3	T37.3X4	T37.3X5	T37.3X6
Dekalin	T52.8X1	T52.8X2	T52.8X3	T52.8X4	—	—
Delalutin	T38.5X1	T38.5X2	T38.5X3	T38.5X4	T38.5X5	T38.5X6
Delorazepam	T42.4X1	T42.4X2	T42.4X3	T42.4X4	T42.4X5	T42.4X6
Delphinium	T62.2X1	T62.2X2	T62.2X3	T62.2X4	—	—
Deltamethrin	T60.1X1	T60.1X2	T60.1X3	T60.1X4	—	—
Deltasone	T38.0X1	T38.0X2	T38.0X3	T38.0X4	T38.0X5	T38.0X6
Deltra	T38.0X1	T38.0X2	T38.0X3	T38.0X4	T38.0X5	T38.0X6
Delvinal	T42.3X1	T42.3X2	T42.3X3	T42.3X4	T42.3X5	T42.3X6
Demecarium (bromide)	T49.5X1	T49.5X2	T49.5X3	T49.5X4	T49.5X5	T49.5X6
Demeclocycline	T36.4X1	T36.4X2	T36.4X3	T36.4X4	T36.4X5	T36.4X6
Demecolcine	T45.1X1	T45.1X2	T45.1X3	T45.1X4	T45.1X5	T45.1X6
Demegestone	T38.5X1	T38.5X2	T38.5X3	T38.5X4	T38.5X5	T38.5X6
Demelanizing agents	T49.8X1	T49.8X2	T49.8X3	T49.8X4	T49.8X5	T49.8X6
Demephion -O and -S	T60.0X1	T60.0X2	T60.0X3	T60.0X4	—	—
Demerol	T40.2X1	T40.2X2	T40.2X3	T40.2X4	T40.2X5	T40.2X6
Demethylchlortetracycline	T36.4X1	T36.4X2	T36.4X3	T36.4X4	T36.4X5	T36.4X6
Demethyltetracycline	T36.4X1	T36.4X2	T36.4X3	T36.4X4	T36.4X5	T36.4X6
Demeton -O and -S	T60.0X1	T60.0X2	T60.0X3	T60.0X4	—	—
Demulcent (external)	T49.3X1	T49.3X2	T49.3X3	T49.3X4	T49.3X5	T49.3X6
specified NEC	T49.3X1	T49.3X2	T49.3X3	T49.3X4	T49.3X5	T49.3X6
Demulen	T38.4X1	T38.4X2	T38.4X3	T38.4X4	T38.4X5	T38.4X6
Denatured alcohol	T51.0X1	T51.0X2	T51.0X3	T51.0X4	—	—
Dendrid	T49.5X1	T49.5X2	T49.5X3	T49.5X4	T49.5X5	T49.5X6
Dental drug, topical application NEC	T49.7X1	T49.7X2	T49.7X3	T49.7X4	T49.7X5	T49.7X6
Dentifrice	T49.7X1	T49.7X2	T49.7X3	T49.7X4	T49.7X5	T49.7X6
Deodorant spray (feminine hygiene)	T49.8X1	T49.8X2	T49.8X3	T49.8X4	T49.8X5	T49.8X6
Deoxycortone	T50.0X1	T50.0X2	T50.0X3	T50.0X4	T50.0X5	T50.0X6
Deoxyribonuclease (pancreatic)	T45.3X1	T45.3X2	T45.3X3	T45.3X4	T45.3X5	T45.3X6
Depilatory	T49.4X1	T49.4X2	T49.4X3	T49.4X4	T49.4X5	T49.4X6
Deprenalin	T42.8X1	T42.8X2	T42.8X3	T42.8X4	T42.8X5	T42.8X6
Deprenyl	T42.8X1	T42.8X2	T42.8X3	T42.8X4	T42.8X5	T42.8X6
Depressant						
appetite (central)	T50.5X1	T50.5X2	T50.5X3	T50.5X4	T50.5X5	T50.5X6
cardiac	T46.2X1	T46.2X2	T46.2X3	T46.2X4	T46.2X5	T46.2X6
central nervous system (anesthetic) — see also Central nervous system, depressants	T42.71	T42.72	T42.73	T42.74	T42.75	T42.76
general anesthetic	T41.201	T41.202	T41.203	T41.204	T41.205	T41.206
muscle tone	T42.8X1	T42.8X2	T42.8X3	T42.8X4	T42.8X5	T42.8X6
muscle tone, central	T42.8X1	T42.8X2	T42.8X3	T42.8X4	T42.8X5	T42.8X6
psychotherapeutic	T43.501	T43.502	T43.503	T43.504	T43.505	T43.506
Depressant, appetite	T50.5X1	T50.5X2	T50.5X3	T50.5X4	T50.5X5	T50.5X6
Deptropine	T45.0X1	T45.0X2	T45.0X3	T45.0X4	T45.0X5	T45.0X6
Dequalinium (chloride)	T49.0X1	T49.0X2	T49.0X3	T49.0X4	T49.0X5	T49.0X6
Derris root	T60.2X1	T60.2X2	T60.2X3	T60.2X4	—	—
Deserpidine	T46.5X1	T46.5X2	T46.5X3	T46.5X4	T46.5X5	T46.5X6
Desferrioxamine	T45.8X1	T45.8X2	T45.8X3	T45.8X4	T45.8X5	T45.8X6
Desipramine	T43.011	T43.012	T43.013	T43.014	T43.015	T43.016
Deslanoside	T46.0X1	T46.0X2	T46.0X3	T46.0X4	T46.0X5	T46.0X6
Desloughing agent	T49.4X1	T49.4X2	T49.4X3	T49.4X4	T49.4X5	T49.4X6
Desmethylimipramine	T43.011	T43.012	T43.013	T43.014	T43.015	T43.016
Desmopressin	T38.891	T38.892	T38.893	T38.894	T38.895	T38.896
Desocodeine	T40.2X1	T40.2X2	T40.2X3	T40.2X4	T40.2X5	T40.2X6
Desogestrel	T38.5X1	T38.5X2	T38.5X3	T38.5X4	T38.5X5	T38.5X6
Desomorphine	T40.2X1	T40.2X2	T40.2X3	T40.2X4	—	—
Desonide	T49.0X1	T49.0X2	T49.0X3	T49.0X4	T49.0X5	T49.0X6
Desoximetasone	T49.0X1	T49.0X2	T49.0X3	T49.0X4	T49.0X5	T49.0X6
Desoxycorticosteroid	T50.0X1	T50.0X2	T50.0X3	T50.0X4	T50.0X5	T50.0X6
Desoxycortone	T50.0X1	T50.0X2	T50.0X3	T50.0X4	T50.0X5	T50.0X6
Desoxyephedrine	T43.621	T43.622	T43.623	T43.624	T43.625	T43.626
Detaxtran	T46.6X1	T46.6X2	T46.6X3	T46.6X4	T46.6X5	T46.6X6
Detergent	T49.2X1	T49.2X2	T49.2X3	T49.2X4	T49.2X5	T49.2X6
external medication	T49.2X1	T49.2X2	T49.2X3	T49.2X4	T49.2X5	T49.2X6
local	T49.2X1	T49.2X2	T49.2X3	T49.2X4	T49.2X5	T49.2X6
medicinal	T49.2X1	T49.2X2	T49.2X3	T49.2X4	T49.2X5	T49.2X6
nonmedicinal	T55.1X1	T55.1X2	T55.1X3	T55.1X4	—	—
specified NEC	T55.1X1	T55.1X2	T55.1X3	T55.1X4	—	—
Deterrent, alcohol	T50.6X1	T50.6X2	T50.6X3	T50.6X4	T50.6X5	T50.6X6
Detoxifying agent	T50.6X1	T50.6X2	T50.6X3	T50.6X4	T50.6X5	T50.6X6
Detrothyronine	T38.1X1	T38.1X2	T38.1X3	T38.1X4	T38.1X5	T38.1X6
Dettol (external medication)	T49.0X1	T49.0X2	T49.0X3	T49.0X4	T49.0X5	T49.0X6
Dexamethasone	T38.0X1	T38.0X2	T38.0X3	T38.0X4	T38.0X5	T38.0X6
ENT agent	T49.6X1	T49.6X2	T49.6X3	T49.6X4	T49.6X5	T49.6X6
ophthalmic preparation	T49.5X1	T49.5X2	T49.5X3	T49.5X4	T49.5X5	T49.5X6
topical NEC	T49.0X1	T49.0X2	T49.0X3	T49.0X4	T49.0X5	T49.0X6
Dexamfetamine	T43.621	T43.622	T43.623	T43.624	T43.625	T43.626
Dexamphetamine	T43.621	T43.622	T43.623	T43.624	T43.625	T43.626
Dexbrompheniramine	T45.0X1	T45.0X2	T45.0X3	T45.0X4	T45.0X5	T45.0X6
Dexchlorpheniramine	T45.0X1	T45.0X2	T45.0X3	T45.0X4	T45.0X5	T45.0X6
Dexedrine	T43.621	T43.622	T43.623	T43.624	T43.625	T43.626
Dexetimide	T44.3X1	T44.3X2	T44.3X3	T44.3X4	T44.3X5	T44.3X6
Dexfenfluramine	T50.5X1	T50.5X2	T50.5X3	T50.5X4	T50.5X5	T50.5X6
Dexpanthenol	T45.2X1	T45.2X2	T45.2X3	T45.2X4	T45.2X5	T45.2X6
Dextran (40) (70) (150)	T45.8X1	T45.8X2	T45.8X3	T45.8X4	T45.8X5	T45.8X6
Dextriferron	T45.4X1	T45.4X2	T45.4X3	T45.4X4	T45.4X5	T45.4X6
Dextroamphetamine	T43.621	T43.622	T43.623	T43.624	T43.625	T43.626
Dextro calcium pantothenate	T45.2X1	T45.2X2	T45.2X3	T45.2X4	T45.2X5	T45.2X6
Dextromethorphan	T48.3X1	T48.3X2	T48.3X3	T48.3X4	T48.3X5	T48.3X6
Dextromoramide	T40.4X1	T40.4X2	T40.4X3	T40.4X4	—	—
topical	T49.8X1	T49.8X2	T49.8X3	T49.8X4	T49.8X5	T49.8X6
Dextro pantothenyl alcohol	T45.2X1	T45.2X2	T45.2X3	T45.2X4	T45.2X5	T45.2X6
Dextropropoxyphene	T40.4X1	T40.4X2	T40.4X3	T40.4X4	T40.4X5	T40.4X6
Dextrorphan	T40.2X1	T40.2X2	T40.2X3	T40.2X4	T40.2X5	T40.2X6
Dextrose	T50.3X1	T50.3X2	T50.3X3	T50.3X4	T50.3X5	T50.3X6
concentrated solution, intravenous	T46.8X1	T46.8X2	T46.8X3	T46.8X4	T46.8X5	T46.8X6
Dextrothyroxin	T38.1X1	T38.1X2	T38.1X3	T38.1X4	T38.1X5	T38.1X6
Dextrothyroxine sodium	T38.1X1	T38.1X2	T38.1X3	T38.1X4	T38.1X5	T38.1X6
DFP	T44.0X1	T44.0X2	T44.0X3	T44.0X4	T44.0X5	T44.0X6
DHE	T37.3X1	T37.3X2	T37.3X3	T37.3X4	T37.3X5	T37.3X6
45	T46.5X1	T46.5X2	T46.5X3	T46.5X4	T46.5X5	T46.5X6
Diabinese	T38.3X1	T38.3X2	T38.3X3	T38.3X4	T38.3X5	T38.3X6
Diacetone alcohol	T52.4X1	T52.4X2	T52.4X3	T52.4X4	—	—
Diacetyl monoxime	T50.991	T50.992	T50.993	T50.994	—	—
Diacetylmorphine	T40.1X1	T40.1X2	T40.1X3	T40.1X4	—	—
Diachylon plaster	T49.4X1	T49.4X2	T49.4X3	T49.4X4	T49.4X5	T49.4X6
Diaethylstilboestrolum	T38.5X1	T38.5X2	T38.5X3	T38.5X4	T38.5X5	T38.5X6
Diagnostic agent NEC	T50.8X1	T50.8X2	T50.8X3	T50.8X4	T50.8X5	T50.8X6
Dial (soap)	T49.2X1	T49.2X2	T49.2X3	T49.2X4	T49.2X5	T49.2X6
sedative	T42.3X1	T42.3X2	T42.3X3	T42.3X4	T42.3X5	T42.3X6
Dialkyl carbonate	T52.91	T52.92	T52.93	T52.94	—	—
Diallylbarbituric acid	T42.3X1	T42.3X2	T42.3X3	T42.3X4	T42.3X5	T42.3X6
Diallymal	T42.3X1	T42.3X2	T42.3X3	T42.3X4	T42.3X5	T42.3X6
Dialysis solution (intraperitoneal)	T50.3X1	T50.3X2	T50.3X3	T50.3X4	T50.3X5	T50.3X6
Diaminodiphenylsulfone	T37.1X1	T37.1X2	T37.1X3	T37.1X4	T37.1X5	T37.1X6
Diamorphine	T40.1X1	T40.1X2	T40.1X3	T40.1X4	—	—
Diamox	T50.2X1	T50.2X2	T50.2X3	T50.2X4	T50.2X5	T50.2X6
Diamthazole	T49.0X1	T49.0X2	T49.0X3	T49.0X4	T49.0X5	T49.0X6
Dianthone	T47.2X1	T47.2X2	T47.2X3	T47.2X4	T47.2X5	T47.2X6
Diaphenylsulfone	T37.0X1	T37.0X2	T37.0X3	T37.0X4	T37.0X5	T37.0X6
Diasone (sodium)	T37.1X1	T37.1X2	T37.1X3	T37.1X4	T37.1X5	T37.1X6
Diastase	T47.5X1	T47.5X2	T47.5X3	T47.5X4	T47.5X5	T47.5X6
Diatrizoate	T50.8X1	T50.8X2	T50.8X3	T50.8X4	T50.8X5	T50.8X6
Diazepam	T42.4X1	T42.4X2	T42.4X3	T42.4X4	T42.4X5	T42.4X6
Diazinon	T60.0X1	T60.0X2	T60.0X3	T60.0X4	—	—
Diazomethane (gas)	T59.891	T59.892	T59.893	T59.894		
Diazoxide	T46.5X1	T46.5X2	T46.5X3	T46.5X4	T46.5X5	T46.5X6
Dibekacin	T36.5X1	T36.5X2	T36.5X3	T36.5X4	T36.5X5	T36.5X6

Table of Drugs and Chemicals

Substance	Poisoning, Accidental (unintentional)	Poisoning, Intentional Self-harm	Poisoning, Assault	Poisoning, Undetermined	Adverse Effect	Under-dosing
Dibenamine	T44.6X1	T44.6X2	T44.6X3	T44.6X4	T44.6X5	T44.6X6
Dibenzepin	T43.011	T43.012	T43.013	T43.014	T43.015	T43.016
Dibenzheptropine	T45.0X1	T45.0X2	T45.0X3	T45.0X4	T45.0X5	T45.0X6
Dibenzyline	T44.6X1	T44.6X2	T44.6X3	T44.6X4	T44.6X5	T44.6X6
Diborane (gas)	T59.891	T59.892	T59.893	T59.894	—	—
Dibromochloropropane	T60.8X1	T60.8X2	T60.8X3	T60.8X4	—	—
Dibromodulcitol	T45.1X1	T45.1X2	T45.1X3	T45.1X4	T45.1X5	T45.1X6
Dibromoethane	T53.6X1	T53.6X2	T53.6X3	T53.6X4	—	—
Dibromomannitol	T45.1X1	T45.1X2	T45.1X3	T45.1X4	T45.1X5	T45.1X6
Dibromopropamidine isethionate	T49.0X1	T49.0X2	T49.0X3	T49.0X4	T49.0X5	T49.0X6
Dibrompropamidine	T49.0X1	T49.0X2	T49.0X3	T49.0X4	T49.0X5	T49.0X6
Dibucaine	T41.3X1	T41.3X2	T41.3X3	T41.3X4	T41.3X5	T41.3X6
topical (surface)	T41.3X1	T41.3X2	T41.3X3	T41.3X4	T41.3X5	T41.3X6
Dibunate sodium	T48.3X1	T48.3X2	T48.3X3	T48.3X4	T48.3X5	T48.3X6
Dibutoline sulfate	T44.3X1	T44.3X2	T44.3X3	T44.3X4	T44.3X5	T44.3X6
Dicamba	T60.3X1	T60.3X2	T60.3X3	T60.3X4	—	—
Dicapthon	T60.0X1	T60.0X2	T60.0X3	T60.0X4	—	—
Dichlobenil	T60.3X1	T60.3X2	T60.3X3	T60.3X4	—	—
Dichlone	T60.3X1	T60.3X2	T60.3X3	T60.3X4	—	—
Dichloralphenozone	T42.6X1	T42.6X2	T42.6X3	T42.6X4	T42.6X5	T42.6X6
Dichlorbenzidine	T65.3X1	T65.3X2	T65.3X3	T65.3X4	—	—
Dichlorhydrin	T52.8X1	T52.8X2	T52.8X3	T52.8X4	—	—
Dichlorhydroxyquinoline	T37.8X1	T37.8X2	T37.8X3	T37.8X4	T37.8X5	T37.8X6
Dichlorobenzene	T53.7X1	T53.7X2	T53.7X3	T53.7X4	—	—
Dichlorobenzyl alcohol	T49.6X1	T49.6X2	T49.6X3	T49.6X4	T49.6X5	T49.6X6
Dichlorodifluoromethane	T53.5X1	T53.5X2	T53.5X3	T53.5X4	—	—
Dichloroethane	T52.8X1	T52.8X2	T52.8X3	T52.8X4	—	—
Dichloroethylene	T53.6X1	T53.6X2	T53.6X3	T53.6X4	—	—
Dichloroethyl sulfide, not in war	T59.891	T59.892	T59.893	T59.894	—	—
Dichloroformoxine, not in war	T59.891	T59.892	T59.893	T59.894	—	—
Dichlorohydrin, alpha-dichlorohydrin	T52.8X1	T52.8X2	T52.8X3	T52.8X4	—	—
Dichloromethane (solvent)	T53.4X1	T53.4X2	T53.4X3	T53.4X4	—	—
vapor	T53.4X1	T53.4X2	T53.4X3	T53.4X4	—	—
Dichloronaphthoquinone	T60.3X1	T60.3X2	T60.3X3	T60.3X4	—	—
Dichlorophen	T37.4X1	T37.4X2	T37.4X3	T37.4X4	T37.4X5	T37.4X6
Dichloropropene	T60.3X1	T60.3X2	T60.3X3	T60.3X4	—	—
Dichloropropionic acid	T60.3X1	T60.3X2	T60.3X3	T60.3X4	—	—
Dichlorphenamide	T50.2X1	T50.2X2	T50.2X3	T50.2X4	T50.2X5	T50.2X6
Dichlorvos	T60.0X1	T60.0X2	T60.0X3	T60.0X4	—	—
Diclofenac	T39.391	T39.392	T39.393	T39.394	T39.395	T39.396
Diclofenamide	T50.2X1	T50.2X2	T50.2X3	T50.2X4	T50.2X5	T50.2X6
Diclofensine	T43.291	T43.292	T43.293	T43.294	T43.295	T43.296
Diclonixine	T39.8X1	T39.8X2	T39.8X3	T39.8X4	T39.8X5	T39.8X6
Dicloxacillin	T36.0X1	T36.0X2	T36.0X3	T36.0X4	T36.0X5	T36.0X6
Dicophane	T49.0X1	T49.0X2	T49.0X3	T49.0X4	T49.0X5	T49.0X6
Dicoumarol, dicoumarin, dicumarol	T45.511	T45.512	T45.513	T45.514	T45.515	T45.516
Dicrotophos	T60.0X1	T60.0X2	T60.0X3	T60.0X4	—	—
Dicyanogen (gas)	T65.0X1	T65.0X2	T65.0X3	T65.0X4	—	—
Dicyclomine	T44.3X1	T44.3X2	T44.3X3	T44.3X4	T44.3X5	T44.3X6
Dicycloverine	T44.3X1	T44.3X2	T44.3X3	T44.3X4	T44.3X5	T44.3X6
Dideoxycytidine	T37.5X1	T37.5X2	T37.5X3	T37.5X4	T37.5X5	T37.5X6
Dideoxyinosine	T37.5X1	T37.5X2	T37.5X3	T37.5X4	T37.5X5	T37.5X6
Dieldrin (vapor)	T60.1X1	T60.1X2	T60.1X3	T60.1X4	—	—
Diemal	T42.3X1	T42.3X2	T42.3X3	T42.3X4	T42.3X5	T42.3X6
Dienestrol	T38.5X1	T38.5X2	T38.5X3	T38.5X4	T38.5X5	T38.5X6
Dienoestrol	T38.5X1	T38.5X2	T38.5X3	T38.5X4	T38.5X5	T38.5X6
Dietetic drug NEC	T50.901	T50.902	T50.903	T50.904	T50.905	T50.906
Diethazine	T42.8X1	T42.8X2	T42.8X3	T42.8X4	T42.8X5	T42.8X6
Diethyl						
barbituric acid	T42.3X1	T42.3X2	T42.3X3	T42.3X4	T42.3X5	T42.3X6
carbamazine	T37.4X1	T37.4X2	T37.4X3	T37.4X4	T37.4X5	T37.4X6
carbinol	T51.3X1	T51.3X2	T51.3X3	T51.3X4	—	—
carbonate	T52.8X1	T52.8X2	T52.8X3	T52.8X4	—	—
ether (vapor) — see also ether	T41.0X1	T41.0X2	T41.0X3	T41.0X4	T41.0X5	T41.0X6
oxide	T52.8X1	T52.8X2	T52.8X3	T52.8X4	—	—
propion	T50.5X1	T50.5X2	T50.5X3	T50.5X4	T50.5X5	T50.5X6
stilbestrol	T38.5X1	T38.5X2	T38.5X3	T38.5X4	T38.5X5	T38.5X6
toluamide (nonmedicinal)	T60.8X1	T60.8X2	T60.8X3	T60.8X4	—	—
medicinal	T49.3X1	T49.3X2	T49.3X3	T49.3X4	T49.3X5	T49.3X6
Diethylcarbamazine	T37.4X1	T37.4X2	T37.4X3	T37.4X4	T37.4X5	T37.4X6
Diethylene						
dioxide	T52.8X1	T52.8X2	T52.8X3	T52.8X4	—	—
glycol (monoacetate) (monobutyl ether) (monoethyl ether)	T52.3X1	T52.3X2	T52.3X3	T52.3X4	—	—
Diethylhexylphthalate	T65.891	T65.892	T65.893	T65.894	—	—
Diethylpropion	T50.5X1	T50.5X2	T50.5X3	T50.5X4	T50.5X5	T50.5X6

Substance	Poisoning, Accidental (unintentional)	Poisoning, Intentional Self-harm	Poisoning, Assault	Poisoning, Undetermined	Adverse Effect	Under-dosing
Diethylstilbestrol	T38.5X1	T38.5X2	T38.5X3	T38.5X4	T38.5X5	T38.5X6
Diethylstilboestrol	T38.5X1	T38.5X2	T38.5X3	T38.5X4	T38.5X5	T38.5X6
Diethylsulfone-diethylmethane	T42.6X1	T42.6X2	T42.6X3	T42.6X4	T42.6X5	T42.6X6
Diethyltoluamide	T49.0X1	T49.0X2	T49.0X3	T49.0X4	T49.0X5	T49.0X6
Diethyltryptamine (DET)	T40.991	T40.992	T40.993	T40.994	—	—
Difebarbamate	T42.3X1	T42.3X2	T42.3X3	T42.3X4	T42.3X5	T42.3X6
Difencloxazine	T40.2X1	T40.2X2	T40.2X3	T40.2X4	T40.2X5	T40.2X6
Difenidol	T45.0X1	T45.0X2	T45.0X3	T45.0X4	T45.0X5	T45.0X6
Difenoxin	T47.6X1	T47.6X2	T47.6X3	T47.6X4	T47.6X5	T47.6X6
Difetarsone	T37.3X1	T37.3X2	T37.3X3	T37.3X4	T37.3X5	T37.3X6
Diffusin	T45.3X1	T45.3X2	T45.3X3	T45.3X4	T45.3X5	T45.3X6
Diflorasone	T49.0X1	T49.0X2	T49.0X3	T49.0X4	T49.0X5	T49.0X6
Diflos	T44.0X1	T44.0X2	T44.0X3	T44.0X4	T44.0X5	T44.0X6
Diflubenzuron	T60.1X1	T60.1X2	T60.1X3	T60.1X4	—	—
Diflucortolone	T49.0X1	T49.0X2	T49.0X3	T49.0X4	T49.0X5	T49.0X6
Diflunisal	T39.091	T39.092	T39.093	T39.094	T39.095	T39.096
Difluoromethyldopa	T42.8X1	T42.8X2	T42.8X3	T42.8X4	T42.8X5	T42.8X6
Difluorophate	T44.0X1	T44.0X2	T44.0X3	T44.0X4	T44.0X5	T44.0X6
Digestant NEC	T47.5X1	T47.5X2	T47.5X3	T47.5X4	T47.5X5	T47.5X6
Digitalin (e)	T46.0X1	T46.0X2	T46.0X3	T46.0X4	T46.0X5	T46.0X6
Digitalis (leaf)(glycoside)	T46.0X1	T46.0X2	T46.0X3	T46.0X4	T46.0X5	T46.0X6
lanata	T46.0X1	T46.0X2	T46.0X3	T46.0X4	T46.0X5	T46.0X6
purpurea	T46.0X1	T46.0X2	T46.0X3	T46.0X4	T46.0X5	T46.0X6
Digitoxin	T46.0X1	T46.0X2	T46.0X3	T46.0X4	T46.0X5	T46.0X6
Digitoxose	T46.0X1	T46.0X2	T46.0X3	T46.0X4	T46.0X5	T46.0X6
Digoxin	T46.0X1	T46.0X2	T46.0X3	T46.0X4	T46.0X5	T46.0X6
Digoxine	T46.0X1	T46.0X2	T46.0X3	T46.0X4	T46.0X5	T46.0X6
Dihydralazine	T46.5X1	T46.5X2	T46.5X3	T46.5X4	T46.5X5	T46.5X6
Dihydrazine	T46.5X1	T46.5X2	T46.5X3	T46.5X4	T46.5X5	T46.5X6
Dihydrocodeine	T40.2X1	T40.2X2	T40.2X3	T40.2X4	T40.2X5	T40.2X6
Dihydrocodeinone	T40.2X1	T40.2X2	T40.2X3	T40.2X4	T40.2X5	T40.2X6
Dihydroergocornine	T46.7X1	T46.7X2	T46.7X3	T46.7X4	T46.7X5	T46.7X6
Dihydroergocristine (mesilate)	T46.7X1	T46.7X2	T46.7X3	T46.7X4	T46.7X5	T46.7X6
Dihydroergokryptine	T46.7X1	T46.7X2	T46.7X3	T46.7X4	T46.7X5	T46.7X6
Dihydroergotamine	T46.5X1	T46.5X2	T46.5X3	T46.5X4	T46.5X5	T46.5X6
Dihydroergotoxine	T46.7X1	T46.7X2	T46.7X3	T46.7X4	T46.7X5	T46.7X6
mesilate	T46.7X1	T46.7X2	T46.7X3	T46.7X4	T46.7X5	T46.7X6
Dihydrohydroxycodeinone	T40.2X1	T40.2X2	T40.2X3	T40.2X4	T40.2X5	T40.2X6
Dihydrohydroxymorphinone	T40.2X1	T40.2X2	T40.2X3	T40.2X4	T40.2X5	T40.2X6
Dihydroisocodeine	T40.2X1	T40.2X2	T40.2X3	T40.2X4	T40.2X5	T40.2X6
Dihydromorphine	T40.2X1	T40.2X2	T40.2X3	T40.2X4	—	—
Dihydromorphinone	T40.2X1	T40.2X2	T40.2X3	T40.2X4	T40.2X5	T40.2X6
Dihydrostreptomycin	T36.5X1	T36.5X2	T36.5X3	T36.5X4	T36.5X5	T36.5X6
Dihydrotachysterol	T45.2X1	T45.2X2	T45.2X3	T45.2X4	T45.2X5	T45.2X6
Dihydroxyaluminum aminoacetate	T47.1X1	T47.1X2	T47.1X3	T47.1X4	T47.1X5	T47.1X6
Dihydroxyaluminum sodium carbonate	T47.1X1	T47.1X2	T47.1X3	T47.1X4	T47.1X5	T47.1X6
Dihydroxyanthraquinone	T47.2X1	T47.2X2	T47.2X3	T47.2X4	T47.2X5	T47.2X6
Dihydroxycodeinone	T40.2X1	T40.2X2	T40.2X3	T40.2X4	T40.2X5	T40.2X6
Dihydroxypropyl theophylline	T50.2X1	T50.2X2	T50.2X3	T50.2X4	T50.2X5	T50.2X6
Diiodohydroxyquin	T37.8X1	T37.8X2	T37.8X3	T37.8X4	T37.8X5	T37.8X6
topical	T49.0X1	T49.0X2	T49.0X3	T49.0X4	T49.0X5	T49.0X6
Diiodohydroxyquinoline	T37.8X1	T37.8X2	T37.8X3	T37.8X4	T37.8X5	T37.8X6
Diiodotyrosine	T38.2X1	T38.2X2	T38.2X3	T38.2X4	T38.2X5	T38.2X6
Diisopromine	T44.3X1	T44.3X2	T44.3X3	T44.3X4	T44.3X5	T44.3X6
Diisopropylamine	T46.3X1	T46.3X2	T46.3X3	T46.3X4	T46.3X5	T46.3X6
Diisopropylfluorophosphonate	T44.0X1	T44.0X2	T44.0X3	T44.0X4	T44.0X5	T44.0X6
Dilantin	T42.0X1	T42.0X2	T42.0X3	T42.0X4	T42.0X5	T42.0X6
Dilaudid	T40.2X1	T40.2X2	T40.2X3	T40.2X4	T40.2X5	T40.2X6
Dilazep	T46.3X1	T46.3X2	T46.3X3	T46.3X4	T46.3X5	T46.3X6
Dill	T47.5X1	T47.5X2	T47.5X3	T47.5X4	T47.5X5	T47.5X6
Diloxanide	T37.3X1	T37.3X2	T37.3X3	T37.3X4	T37.3X5	T37.3X6
Diltiazem	T46.1X1	T46.1X2	T46.1X3	T46.1X4	T46.1X5	T46.1X6
Dimazole	T49.0X1	T49.0X2	T49.0X3	T49.0X4	T49.0X5	T49.0X6
Dimefline	T50.7X1	T50.7X2	T50.7X3	T50.7X4	T50.7X5	T50.7X6
Dimefox	T60.0X1	T60.0X2	T60.0X3	T60.0X4	—	—
Dimemorfan	T48.3X1	T48.3X2	T48.3X3	T48.3X4	T48.3X5	T48.3X6
Dimenhydrinate	T45.0X1	T45.0X2	T45.0X3	T45.0X4	T45.0X5	T45.0X6
Dimercaprol (British anti-lewisite)	T45.8X1	T45.8X2	T45.8X3	T45.8X4	T45.8X5	T45.8X6
Dimercaptopropanol	T45.8X1	T45.8X2	T45.8X3	T45.8X4	T45.8X5	T45.8X6
Dimestrol	T38.5X1	T38.5X2	T38.5X3	T38.5X4	T38.5X5	T38.5X6
Dimetane	T45.0X1	T45.0X2	T45.0X3	T45.0X4	T45.0X5	T45.0X6
Dimethicone	T47.1X1	T47.1X2	T47.1X3	T47.1X4	T47.1X5	T47.1X6
Dimethindene	T45.0X1	T45.0X2	T45.0X3	T45.0X4	T45.0X5	T45.0X6
Dimethisoquin	T49.1X1	T49.1X2	T49.1X3	T49.1X4	T49.1X5	T49.1X6
Dimethisterone	T38.5X1	T38.5X2	T38.5X3	T38.5X4	T38.5X5	T38.5X6
Dimethoate	T60.0X1	T60.0X2	T60.0X3	T60.0X4	—	—
Dimethocaine	T41.3X1	T41.3X2	T41.3X3	T41.3X4	T41.3X5	T41.3X6
Dimethoxanate	T48.3X1	T48.3X2	T48.3X3	T48.3X4	T48.3X5	T48.3X6

Substance	Poisoning, Accidental (unintentional)	Poisoning, Intentional Self-harm	Poisoning, Assault	Poisoning, Undetermined	Adverse Effect	Under-dosing
Dimethyl						
arsine, arsinic acid	T57.0X1	T57.0X2	T57.0X3	T57.0X4	—	—
carbinol	T51.2X1	T51.2X2	T51.2X3	T51.2X4	—	—
carbonate	T52.8X1	T52.8X2	T52.8X3	T52.8X4	—	—
diguanide	T38.3X1	T38.3X2	T38.3X3	T38.3X4	T38.3X5	T38.3X6
ketone	T52.4X1	T52.4X2	T52.4X3	T52.4X4	—	—
vapor	T52.4X1	T52.4X2	T52.4X3	T52.4X4	—	—
meperidine	T40.2X1	T40.2X2	T40.2X3	T40.2X4	T40.2X5	T40.2X6
parathion	T60.0X1	T60.0X2	T60.0X3	T60.0X4	—	—
phthlate	T49.3X1	T49.3X2	T49.3X3	T49.3X4	T49.3X5	T49.3X6
polysiloxane	T47.8X1	T47.8X2	T47.8X3	T47.8X4	T47.8X5	T47.8X6
sulfate (fumes)	T59.891	T59.892	T59.893	T59.894		
liquid	T65.891	T65.892	T65.893	T65.894	—	—
sulfoxide (nonmedicinal)	T52.8X1	T52.8X2	T52.8X3	T52.8X4	—	—
medicinal	T49.4X1	T49.4X2	T49.4X3	T49.4X4	T49.4X5	T49.4X6
tryptamine	T40.991	T40.992	T40.993	T40.994	—	—
tubocurarine	T48.1X1	T48.1X2	T48.1X3	T48.1X4	T48.1X5	T48.1X6
Dimethylamine sulfate	T49.4X1	T49.4X2	T49.4X3	T49.4X4	T49.4X5	T49.4X6
Dimethylformamide	T52.8X1	T52.8X2	T52.8X3	T52.8X4	—	—
Dimethyltubocurarinium chloride	T48.1X1	T48.1X2	T48.1X3	T48.1X4	T48.1X5	T48.1X6
Dimeticone	T47.1X1	T47.1X2	T47.1X3	T47.1X4	T47.1X5	T47.1X6
Dimetilan	T60.0X1	T60.0X2	T60.0X3	T60.0X4	—	—
Dimetindene	T45.0X1	T45.0X2	T45.0X3	T45.0X4	T45.0X5	T45.0X6
Dimetotiazine	T43.3X1	T43.3X2	T43.3X3	T43.3X4	T43.3X5	T43.3X6
Dimorpholamine	T50.7X1	T50.7X2	T50.7X3	T50.7X4	T50.7X5	T50.7X6
Dimoxyline	T46.3X1	T46.3X2	T46.3X3	T46.3X4	T46.3X5	T46.3X6
Dinitrobenzene	T65.3X1	T65.3X2	T65.3X3	T65.3X4	—	—
vapor	T59.891	T59.892	T59.893	T59.894	—	—
Dinitrobenzol	T65.3X1	T65.3X2	T65.3X3	T65.3X4	—	—
vapor	T59.891	T59.892	T59.893	T59.894	—	—
Dinitrobutylphenol	T65.3X1	T65.3X2	T65.3X3	T65.3X4	—	—
Dinitro (-ortho-)cresol (pesticide) (spray)	T65.3X1	T65.3X2	T65.3X3	T65.3X4	—	—
Dinitrocyclohexylphenol	T65.3X1	T65.3X2	T65.3X3	T65.3X4	—	—
Dinitrophenol	T65.3X1	T65.3X2	T65.3X3	T65.3X4	—	—
Dinoprost	T48.0X1	T48.0X2	T48.0X3	T48.0X4	T48.0X5	T48.0X6
Dinoprostone	T48.0X1	T48.0X2	T48.0X3	T48.0X4	T48.0X5	T48.0X6
Dinoseb	T60.3X1	T60.3X2	T60.3X3	T60.3X4	—	—
Dioctyl sulfosuccinate (calcium) (sodium)	T47.4X1	T47.4X2	T47.4X3	T47.4X4	T47.4X5	T47.4X6
Diodone	T50.8X1	T50.8X2	T50.8X3	T50.8X4	T50.8X5	T50.8X6
Diodoquin	T37.8X1	T37.8X2	T37.8X3	T37.8X4	T37.8X5	T37.8X6
Dionin	T40.2X1	T40.2X2	T40.2X3	T40.2X4	T40.2X5	T40.2X6
Diosmin	T46.991	T46.992	T46.993	T46.994	T46.995	T46.996
Dioxane	T52.8X1	T52.8X2	T52.8X3	T52.8X4	—	—
Dioxathion	T60.0X1	T60.0X2	T60.0X3	T60.0X4	—	—
Dioxin	T53.7X1	T53.7X2	T53.7X3	T53.7X4	—	—
Dioxopromethazine	T43.3X1	T43.3X2	T43.3X3	T43.3X4	T43.3X5	T43.3X6
Dioxyline	T46.3X1	T46.3X2	T46.3X3	T46.3X4	T46.3X5	T46.3X6
Dipentene	T52.8X1	T52.8X2	T52.8X3	T52.8X4	—	—
Diperodon	T41.3X1	T41.3X2	T41.3X3	T41.3X4	T41.3X5	T41.3X6
Diphacinone	T60.4X1	T60.4X2	T60.4X3	T60.4X4	—	—
Diphemanil	T44.3X1	T44.3X2	T44.3X3	T44.3X4	T44.3X5	T44.3X6
metilsulfate	T44.3X1	T44.3X2	T44.3X3	T44.3X4	T44.3X5	T44.3X6
Diphenadione	T45.511	T45.512	T45.513	T45.514	T45.515	T45.516
rodenticide	T60.4X1	T60.4X2	T60.4X3	T60.4X4	—	—
Diphenhydramine	T45.0X1	T45.0X2	T45.0X3	T45.0X4	T45.0X5	T45.0X6
Diphenidol	T45.0X1	T45.0X2	T45.0X3	T45.0X4	T45.0X5	T45.0X6
Diphenoxylate	T47.6X1	T47.6X2	T47.6X3	T47.6X4	T47.6X5	T47.6X6
Diphenylamine	T65.3X1	T65.3X2	T65.3X3	T65.3X4	—	—
Diphenylbutazone	T39.2X1	T39.2X2	T39.2X3	T39.2X4	T39.2X5	T39.2X6
Diphenylchloroarsine, not in war	T57.0X1	T57.0X2	T57.0X3	T57.0X4	—	—
Diphenylhydantoin	T42.0X1	T42.0X2	T42.0X3	T42.0X4	T42.0X5	T42.0X6
Diphenylmethane dye	T52.1X1	T52.1X2	T52.1X3	T52.1X4	—	—
Diphenylpyraline	T45.0X1	T45.0X2	T45.0X3	T45.0X4	T45.0X5	T45.0X6
Diphtheria						
antitoxin	T50.Z11	T50.Z12	T50.Z13	T50.Z14	T50.Z15	T50.Z16
toxoid	T50.A91	T50.A92	T50.A93	T50.A94	T50.A95	T50.A96
with tetanus toxoid	T50.A21	T50.A22	T50.A23	T50.A24	T50.A25	T50.A26
with pertussis component	T50.A11	T50.A12	T50.A13	T50.A14	T50.A15	T50.A16
vaccine	T50.A91	T50.A92	T50.A93	T50.A94	T50.A95	T50.A96
combination						
without pertussis	T50.A21	T50.A22	T50.A23	T50.A24	T50.A25	T50.A26
including pertussis	T50.A11	T50.A12	T50.A13	T50.A14	T50.A15	T50.A16
Diphylline	T50.2X1	T50.2X2	T50.2X3	T50.2X4	T50.2X5	T50.2X6
Dipipanone	T40.4X1	T40.4X2	T40.4X3	T40.4X4	—	—
Dipivefrine	T49.5X1	T49.5X2	T49.5X3	T49.5X4	T49.5X5	T49.5X6
Diplovax	T50.B91	T50.B92	T50.B93	T50.B94	T50.B95	T50.B96
Diprophylline	T50.2X1	T50.2X2	T50.2X3	T50.2X4	T50.2X5	T50.2X6
Dipropyline	T48.291	T48.292	T48.293	T48.294	T48.295	T48.296
Dipyridamole	T46.3X1	T46.3X2	T46.3X3	T46.3X4	T46.3X5	T46.3X6
Dipyrone	T39.2X1	T39.2X2	T39.2X3	T39.2X4	T39.2X5	T39.2X6
Diquat (dibromide)	T60.3X1	T60.3X2	T60.3X3	T60.3X4	—	—
Disinfectant	T65.891	T65.892	T65.893	T65.894	—	—
alkaline	T54.3X1	T54.3X2	T54.3X3	T54.3X4	—	—
aromatic	T54.1X1	T54.1X2	T54.1X3	T54.1X4	—	—
intestinal	T37.8X1	T37.8X2	T37.8X3	T37.8X4	T37.8X5	T37.8X6
Disipal	T42.8X1	T42.8X2	T42.8X3	T42.8X4	T42.8X5	T42.8X6
Disodium edetate	T50.6X1	T50.6X2	T50.6X3	T50.6X4	T50.6X5	T50.6X6
Disoprofol	T41.291	T41.292	T41.293	T41.294	T41.295	T41.296
Disopyramide	T46.2X1	T46.2X2	T46.2X3	T46.2X4	T46.2X5	T46.2X6
Distigmine (bromide)	T44.0X1	T44.0X2	T44.0X3	T44.0X4	T44.0X5	T44.0X6
Disulfamide	T50.2X1	T50.2X2	T50.2X3	T50.2X4	T50.2X5	T50.2X6
Disulfanilamide	T37.0X1	T37.0X2	T37.0X3	T37.0X4	T37.0X5	T37.0X6
Disulfiram	T50.6X1	T50.6X2	T50.6X3	T50.6X4	T50.6X5	T50.6X6
Disulfoton	T60.0X1	T60.0X2	T60.0X3	T60.0X4	—	—
Dithiazanine iodide	T37.4X1	T37.4X2	T37.4X3	T37.4X4	T37.4X5	T37.4X6
Dithiocarbamate	T60.0X1	T60.0X2	T60.0X3	T60.0X4	—	—
Dithranol	T49.4X1	T49.4X2	T49.4X3	T49.4X4	T49.4X5	T49.4X6
Diucardin	T50.2X1	T50.2X2	T50.2X3	T50.2X4	T50.2X5	T50.2X6
Diupres	T50.2X1	T50.2X2	T50.2X3	T50.2X4	T50.2X5	T50.2X6
Diuretic NEC	T50.2X1	T50.2X2	T50.2X3	T50.2X4	T50.2X5	T50.2X6
benzothiadiazine	T50.2X1	T50.2X2	T50.2X3	T50.2X4	T50.2X5	T50.2X6
carbonic acid anhydrase inhibitors	T50.2X1	T50.2X2	T50.2X3	T50.2X4	T50.2X5	T50.2X6
furfuryl NEC	T50.2X1	T50.2X2	T50.2X3	T50.2X4	T50.2X5	T50.2X6
loop (high-ceiling)	T50.1X1	T50.1X2	T50.1X3	T50.1X4	T50.1X5	T50.1X6
mercurial NEC	T50.2X1	T50.2X2	T50.2X3	T50.2X4	T50.2X5	T50.2X6
osmotic	T50.2X1	T50.2X2	T50.2X3	T50.2X4	T50.2X5	T50.2X6
purine NEC	T50.2X1	T50.2X2	T50.2X3	T50.2X4	T50.2X5	T50.2X6
saluretic NEC	T50.2X1	T50.2X2	T50.2X3	T50.2X4	T50.2X5	T50.2X6
sulfonamide	T50.2X1	T50.2X2	T50.2X3	T50.2X4	T50.2X5	T50.2X6
thiazide NEC	T50.2X1	T50.2X2	T50.2X3	T50.2X4	T50.2X5	T50.2X6
xanthine	T50.2X1	T50.2X2	T50.2X3	T50.2X4	T50.2X5	T50.2X6
Diurgin	T50.2X1	T50.2X2	T50.2X3	T50.2X4	T50.2X5	T50.2X6
Diuril	T50.2X1	T50.2X2	T50.2X3	T50.2X4	T50.2X5	T50.2X6
Diuron	T60.3X1	T60.3X2	T60.3X3	T60.3X4	—	—
Divalproex	T42.6X1	T42.6X2	T42.6X3	T42.6X4	T42.6X5	T42.6X6
Divinyl ether	T41.0X1	T41.0X2	T41.0X3	T41.0X4	T41.0X5	T41.0X6
Dixanthogen	T49.0X1	T49.0X2	T49.0X3	T49.0X4	T49.0X5	T49.0X6
Dixyrazine	T43.3X1	T43.3X2	T43.3X3	T43.3X4	T43.3X5	T43.3X6
D-lysergic acid diethylamide	T40.8X1	T40.8X2	T40.8X3	T40.8X4	—	—
DMCT	T36.4X1	T36.4X2	T36.4X3	T36.4X4	T36.4X5	T36.4X6
DMSO — see Dimethyl sulfoxide						
DNBP	T60.3X1	T60.3X2	T60.3X3	T60.3X4	—	—
DNOC	T65.3X1	T65.3X2	T65.3X3	T65.3X4	—	—
Dobutamine	T44.5X1	T44.5X2	T44.5X3	T44.5X4	T44.5X5	T44.5X6
DOCA	T38.0X1	T38.0X2	T38.0X3	T38.0X4	T38.0X5	T38.0X6
Docusate sodium	T47.4X1	T47.4X2	T47.4X3	T47.4X4	T47.4X5	T47.4X6
Dodicin	T49.0X1	T49.0X2	T49.0X3	T49.0X4	T49.0X5	T49.0X6
Dofamium chloride	T49.0X1	T49.0X2	T49.0X3	T49.0X4	T49.0X5	T49.0X6
Dolophine	T40.3X1	T40.3X2	T40.3X3	T40.3X4	T40.3X5	T40.3X6
Doloxene	T39.8X1	T39.8X2	T39.8X3	T39.8X4	T39.8X5	T39.8X6
Domestic gas (after combustion) — see Gas, utility						
prior to combustion	T59.891	T59.892	T59.893	T59.894	—	—
Domiodol	T48.4X1	T48.4X2	T48.4X3	T48.4X4	T48.4X5	T48.4X6
Domiphen (bromide)	T49.0X1	T49.0X2	T49.0X3	T49.0X4	T49.0X5	T49.0X6
Domperidone	T45.0X1	T45.0X2	T45.0X3	T45.0X4	T45.0X5	T45.0X6
Dopa	T42.8X1	T42.8X2	T42.8X3	T42.8X4	T42.8X5	T42.8X6
Dopamine	T44.991	T44.992	T44.993	T44.994	T44.995	T44.996
Doriden	T42.6X1	T42.6X2	T42.6X3	T42.6X4	T42.6X5	T42.6X6
Dormiral	T42.3X1	T42.3X2	T42.3X3	T42.3X4	T42.3X5	T42.3X6
Dormison	T42.6X1	T42.6X2	T42.6X3	T42.6X4	T42.6X5	T42.6X6
Dornase	T48.4X1	T48.4X2	T48.4X3	T48.4X4	T48.4X5	T48.4X6
Dorsacaine	T41.3X1	T41.3X2	T41.3X3	T41.3X4	T41.3X5	T41.3X6
Dosulepin	T43.011	T43.012	T43.013	T43.014	T43.015	T43.016
Dothiepin	T43.011	T43.012	T43.013	T43.014	T43.015	T43.016
Doxantrazole	T48.6X1	T48.6X2	T48.6X3	T48.6X4	T48.6X5	T48.6X6
Doxapram	T50.7X1	T50.7X2	T50.7X3	T50.7X4	T50.7X5	T50.7X6
Doxazosin	T44.6X1	T44.6X2	T44.6X3	T44.6X4	T44.6X5	T44.6X6
Doxepin	T43.011	T43.012	T43.013	T43.014	T43.015	T43.016
Doxifluridine	T45.1X1	T45.1X2	T45.1X3	T45.1X4	T45.1X5	T45.1X6
Doxorubicin	T45.1X1	T45.1X2	T45.1X3	T45.1X4	T45.1X5	T45.1X6
Doxycycline	T36.4X1	T36.4X2	T36.4X3	T36.4X4	T36.4X5	T36.4X6
Doxylamine	T45.0X1	T45.0X2	T45.0X3	T45.0X4	T45.0X5	T45.0X6
Dramamine	T45.0X1	T45.0X2	T45.0X3	T45.0X4	T45.0X5	T45.0X6
Drano (drain cleaner)	T54.3X1	T54.3X2	T54.3X3	T54.3X4	—	—
Dressing, live pulp	T49.7X1	T49.7X2	T49.7X3	T49.7X4	T49.7X5	T49.7X6
Drocode	T40.2X1	T40.2X2	T40.2X3	T40.2X4	T40.2X5	T40.2X6
Dromoran	T40.2X1	T40.2X2	T40.2X3	T40.2X4	T40.2X5	T40.2X6
Dromostanolone	T38.7X1	T38.7X2	T38.7X3	T38.7X4	T38.7X5	T38.7X6

Table of Drugs and Chemicals

Substance	Poisoning, Accidental (unintentional)	Poisoning, Intentional Self-harm	Poisoning, Assault	Poisoning, Undetermined	Adverse Effect	Under-dosing
Dronabinol	T40.7X1	T40.7X2	T40.7X3	T40.7X4	T40.7X5	T40.7X6
Droperidol	T43.591	T43.592	T43.593	T43.594	T43.595	T43.596
Dropropizine	T48.3X1	T48.3X2	T48.3X3	T48.3X4	T48.3X5	T48.3X6
Drostanolone	T38.7X1	T38.7X2	T38.7X3	T38.7X4	T38.7X5	T38.7X6
Drotaverine	T44.3X1	T44.3X2	T44.3X3	T44.3X4	T44.3X5	T44.3X6
Drotrecogin alfa	T45.511	T45.512	T45.513	T45.514	T45.515	T45.516
Drug NEC	T50.901	T50.902	T50.903	T50.904	T50.905	T50.906
specified NEC	T50.991	T50.992	T50.993	T50.994	T50.995	T50.996
DTIC	T45.1X1	T45.1X2	T45.1X3	T45.1X4	T45.1X5	T45.1X6
Duboisine	T44.3X1	T44.3X2	T44.3X3	T44.3X4	T44.3X5	T44.3X6
Dulcolax	T47.2X1	T47.2X2	T47.2X3	T47.2X4	T47.2X5	T47.2X6
Duponol (C) (EP)	T49.2X1	T49.2X2	T49.2X3	T49.2X4	T49.2X5	T49.2X6
Durabolin	T38.7X1	T38.7X2	T38.7X3	T38.7X4	T38.7X5	T38.7X6
Dyclone	T41.3X1	T41.3X2	T41.3X3	T41.3X4	T41.3X5	T41.3X6
Dyclonine	T41.3X1	T41.3X2	T41.3X3	T41.3X4	T41.3X5	T41.3X6
Dydrogesterone	T38.5X1	T38.5X2	T38.5X3	T38.5X4	T38.5X5	T38.5X6
Dye NEC	T65.6X1	T65.6X2	T65.6X3	T65.6X4	—	—
antiseptic	T49.0X1	T49.0X2	T49.0X3	T49.0X4	T49.0X5	T49.0X6
diagnostic agents	T50.8X1	T50.8X2	T50.8X3	T50.8X4	T50.8X5	T50.8X6
pharmaceutical NEC	T50.901	T50.902	T50.903	T50.904	T50.905	T50.906
Dyflos	T44.0X1	T44.0X2	T44.0X3	T44.0X4	T44.0X5	T44.0X6
Dymelor	T38.3X1	T38.3X2	T38.3X3	T38.3X4	T38.3X5	T38.3X6
Dynamite	T65.3X1	T65.3X2	T65.3X3	T65.3X4	—	—
fumes	T59.891	T59.892	T59.893	T59.894	—	—
Dyphylline	T44.3X1	T44.3X2	T44.3X3	T44.3X4	T44.3X5	T44.3X6
b-eucaine	T49.1X1	T49.1X2	T49.1X3	T49.1X4	T49.1X5	T49.1X6
Ear drug NEC	T49.6X1	T49.6X2	T49.6X3	T49.6X4	T49.6X5	T49.6X6
Ear preparations	T49.6X1	T49.6X2	T49.6X3	T49.6X4	T49.6X5	T49.6X6
Echothiophate, echothiopate, ecothiopate	T49.5X1	T49.5X2	T49.5X3	T49.5X4	T49.5X5	T49.5X6
Econazole	T49.0X1	T49.0X2	T49.0X3	T49.0X4	T49.0X5	T49.0X6
Ecothiopate iodide	T49.5X1	T49.5X2	T49.5X3	T49.5X4	T49.5X5	T49.5X6
Ecstasy	T43.621	T43.622	T43.623	T43.624	T43.625	T43.626
Ectylurea	T42.6X1	T42.6X2	T42.6X3	T42.6X4	T42.6X5	T42.6X6
Edathamil disodium	T45.8X1	T45.8X2	T45.8X3	T45.8X4	T45.8X5	T45.8X6
Edecrin	T50.1X1	T50.1X2	T50.1X3	T50.1X4	T50.1X5	T50.1X6
Edetate, disodium (calcium)	T45.8X1	T45.8X2	T45.8X3	T45.8X4	T45.8X5	T45.8X6
Edoxudine	T49.5X1	T49.5X2	T49.5X3	T49.5X4	T49.5X5	T49.5X6
Edrophonium	T44.0X1	T44.0X2	T44.0X3	T44.0X4	T44.0X5	T44.0X6
chloride	T44.0X1	T44.0X2	T44.0X3	T44.0X4	T44.0X5	T44.0X6
EDTA	T50.6X1	T50.6X2	T50.6X3	T50.6X4	T50.6X5	T50.6X6
Eflornithine	T37.2X1	T37.2X2	T37.2X3	T37.2X4	T37.2X5	T37.2X6
Efloxate	T46.3X1	T46.3X2	T46.3X3	T46.3X4	T46.3X5	T46.3X6
Elase	T49.8X1	T49.8X2	T49.8X3	T49.8X4	T49.8X5	T49.8X6
Elastase	T47.5X1	T47.5X2	T47.5X3	T47.5X4	T47.5X5	T47.5X6
Elaterium	T47.2X1	T47.2X2	T47.2X3	T47.2X4	T47.2X5	T47.2X6
Elcatonin	T50.991	T50.992	T50.993	T50.994	T50.995	T50.996
Elder	T62.2X1	T62.2X2	T62.2X3	T62.2X4	—	—
berry, (unripe)	T62.1X1	T62.1X2	T62.1X3	T62.1X4	—	—
Electrolyte balance drug	T50.3X1	T50.3X2	T50.3X3	T50.3X4	T50.3X5	T50.3X6
Electrolytes NEC	T50.3X1	T50.3X2	T50.3X3	T50.3X4	T50.3X5	T50.3X6
Electrolytic agent NEC	T50.3X1	T50.3X2	T50.3X3	T50.3X4	T50.3X5	T50.3X6
Elemental diet	T50.901	T50.902	T50.903	T50.904	T50.905	T50.906
Elliptinium acetate	T45.1X1	T45.1X2	T45.1X3	T45.1X4	T45.1X5	T45.1X6
Embramine	T45.0X1	T45.0X2	T45.0X3	T45.0X4	T45.0X5	T45.0X6
Emepronium (salts)	T44.3X1	T44.3X2	T44.3X3	T44.3X4	T44.3X5	T44.3X6
bromide	T44.3X1	T44.3X2	T44.3X3	T44.3X4	T44.3X5	T44.3X6
Emetic NEC	T47.7X1	T47.7X2	T47.7X3	T47.7X4	T47.7X5	T47.7X6
Emetine	T37.3X1	T37.3X2	T37.3X3	T37.3X4	T37.3X5	T37.3X6
Emollient NEC	T49.3X1	T49.3X2	T49.3X3	T49.3X4	T49.3X5	T49.3X6
Emorfazone	T39.8X1	T39.8X2	T39.8X3	T39.8X4	T39.8X5	T39.8X6
Emylcamate	T43.591	T43.592	T43.593	T43.594	T43.595	T43.596
Enalapril	T46.4X1	T46.4X2	T46.4X3	T46.4X4	T46.4X5	T46.4X6
Enalaprilat	T46.4X1	T46.4X2	T46.4X3	T46.4X4	T46.4X5	T46.4X6
Encainide	T46.2X1	T46.2X2	T46.2X3	T46.2X4	T46.2X5	T46.2X6
Endocaine	T41.3X1	T41.3X2	T41.3X3	T41.3X4	T41.3X5	T41.3X6
Endosulfan	T60.2X1	T60.2X2	T60.2X3	T60.2X4	—	—
Endothall	T60.3X1	T60.3X2	T60.3X3	T60.3X4	—	—
Endralazine	T46.5X1	T46.5X2	T46.5X3	T46.5X4	T46.5X5	T46.5X6
Endrin	T60.1X1	T60.1X2	T60.1X3	T60.1X4	—	—
Enflurane	T41.0X1	T41.0X2	T41.0X3	T41.0X4	T41.0X5	T41.0X6
Enhexymal	T42.3X1	T42.3X2	T42.3X3	T42.3X4	T42.3X5	T42.3X6
Enocitabine	T45.1X1	T45.1X2	T45.1X3	T45.1X4	T45.1X5	T45.1X6
Enovid	T38.4X1	T38.4X2	T38.4X3	T38.4X4	T38.4X5	T38.4X6
Enoxacin	T36.8X1	T36.8X2	T36.8X3	T36.8X4	T36.8X5	T36.8X6
Enoxaparin (sodium)	T45.511	T45.512	T45.513	T45.514	T45.515	T45.516
Enpiprazole	T43.591	T43.592	T43.593	T43.594	T43.595	T43.596
Enprofylline	T48.6X1	T48.6X2	T48.6X3	T48.6X4	T48.6X5	T48.6X6
Enprostil	T47.1X1	T47.1X2	T47.1X3	T47.1X4	T47.1X5	T47.1X6
Enterogastrone	T38.891	T38.892	T38.893	T38.894	T38.895	T38.896
ENT preparations (anti-infectives)	T49.6X1	T49.6X2	T49.6X3	T49.6X4	T49.6X5	T49.6X6
Enviomycin	T36.8X1	T36.8X2	T36.8X3	T36.8X4	T36.8X5	T36.8X6
Enzodase	T45.3X1	T45.3X2	T45.3X3	T45.3X4	T45.3X5	T45.3X6
Enzyme NEC	T45.3X1	T45.3X2	T45.3X3	T45.3X4	T45.3X5	T45.3X6
depolymerizing	T49.8X1	T49.8X2	T49.8X3	T49.8X4	T49.8X5	T49.8X6
fibrolytic	T45.3X1	T45.3X2	T45.3X3	T45.3X4	T45.3X5	T45.3X6
gastric	T47.5X1	T47.5X2	T47.5X3	T47.5X4	T47.5X5	T47.5X6
intestinal	T47.5X1	T47.5X2	T47.5X3	T47.5X4	T47.5X5	T47.5X6
local action	T49.4X1	T49.4X2	T49.4X3	T49.4X4	T49.4X5	T49.4X6
proteolytic	T49.4X1	T49.4X2	T49.4X3	T49.4X4	T49.4X5	T49.4X6
thrombolytic	T45.3X1	T45.3X2	T45.3X3	T45.3X4	T45.3X5	T45.3X6
EPAB	T41.3X1	T41.3X2	T41.3X3	T41.3X4	T41.3X5	T41.3X6
Epanutin	T42.0X1	T42.0X2	T42.0X3	T42.0X4	T42.0X5	T42.0X6
Ephedra	T44.991	T44.992	T44.993	T44.994	T44.995	T44.996
Ephedrine	T44.991	T44.992	T44.993	T44.994	T44.995	T44.996
Epichlorhydrin, epichlorohydrin	T52.8X1	T52.8X2	T52.8X3	T52.8X4	—	—
Epicillin	T36.0X1	T36.0X2	T36.0X3	T36.0X4	T36.0X5	T36.0X6
Epiestriol	T38.5X1	T38.5X2	T38.5X3	T38.5X4	T38.5X5	T38.5X6
Epilim — *see* Sodium valproate						
Epimestrol	T38.5X1	T38.5X2	T38.5X3	T38.5X4	T38.5X5	T38.5X6
Epinephrine	T44.5X1	T44.5X2	T44.5X3	T44.5X4	T44.5X5	T44.5X6
Epirubicin	T45.1X1	T45.1X2	T45.1X3	T45.1X4	T45.1X5	T45.1X6
Epitiostanol	T38.7X1	T38.7X2	T38.7X3	T38.7X4	T38.7X5	T38.7X6
Epitizide	T50.2X1	T50.2X2	T50.2X3	T50.2X4	T50.2X5	T50.2X6
EPN	T60.0X1	T60.0X2	T60.0X3	T60.0X4	—	—
EPO	T45.8X1	T45.8X2	T45.8X3	T45.8X4	T45.8X5	T45.8X6
Epoetin alpha	T45.8X1	T45.8X2	T45.8X3	T45.8X4	T45.8X5	T45.8X6
Epomediol	T50.991	T50.992	T50.993	T50.994	T50.995	T50.996
Epoprostenol	T45.521	T45.522	T45.523	T45.524	T45.525	T45.526
Epoxy resin	T65.891	T65.892	T65.893	T65.894	—	—
Eprazinone	T48.4X1	T48.4X2	T48.4X3	T48.4X4	T48.4X5	T48.4X6
Epsilon aminocaproic acid	T45.621	T45.622	T45.623	T45.624	T45.625	T45.626
Epsom salt	T47.3X1	T47.3X2	T47.3X3	T47.3X4	T47.3X5	T47.3X6
Eptazocine	T40.4X1	T40.4X2	T40.4X3	T40.4X4	T40.4X5	T40.4X6
Equanil	T43.591	T43.592	T43.593	T43.594	T43.595	T43.596
Equisetum	T62.2X1	T62.2X2	T62.2X3	T62.2X4	—	—
diuretic	T50.2X1	T50.2X2	T50.2X3	T50.2X4	T50.2X5	T50.2X6
Ergobasine	T48.0X1	T48.0X2	T48.0X3	T48.0X4	T48.0X5	T48.0X6
Ergocalciferol	T45.2X1	T45.2X2	T45.2X3	T45.2X4	T45.2X5	T45.2X6
Ergoloid mesylates	T46.7X1	T46.7X2	T46.7X3	T46.7X4	T46.7X5	T46.7X6
Ergometrine	T48.0X1	T48.0X2	T48.0X3	T48.0X4	T48.0X5	T48.0X6
Ergonovine	T48.0X1	T48.0X2	T48.0X3	T48.0X4	T48.0X5	T48.0X6
Ergotamine	T46.5X1	T46.5X2	T46.5X3	T46.5X4	T46.5X5	T46.5X6
Ergotocine	T48.0X1	T48.0X2	T48.0X3	T48.0X4	T48.0X5	T48.0X6
Ergotrate	T48.0X1	T48.0X2	T48.0X3	T48.0X4	T48.0X5	T48.0X6
Ergot NEC	T64.81	T64.82	T64.83	T64.84	—	—
derivative	T48.0X1	T48.0X2	T48.0X3	T48.0X4	T48.0X5	T48.0X6
medicinal (alkaloids)	T48.0X1	T48.0X2	T48.0X3	T48.0X4	T48.0X5	T48.0X6
prepared	T48.0X1	T48.0X2	T48.0X3	T48.0X4	T48.0X5	T48.0X6
Eritrityl tetranitrate	T46.3X1	T46.3X2	T46.3X3	T46.3X4	T46.3X5	T46.3X6
Erythrityl tetranitrate	T46.3X1	T46.3X2	T46.3X3	T46.3X4	T46.3X5	T46.3X6
Erythrol tetranitrate	T46.3X1	T46.3X2	T46.3X3	T46.3X4	T46.3X5	T46.3X6
Erythromycin (salts)	T36.3X1	T36.3X2	T36.3X3	T36.3X4	T36.3X5	T36.3X6
ophthalmic preparation	T49.5X1	T49.5X2	T49.5X3	T49.5X4	T49.5X5	T49.5X6
topical NEC	T49.0X1	T49.0X2	T49.0X3	T49.0X4	T49.0X5	T49.0X6
Erythropoietin	T45.8X1	T45.8X2	T45.8X3	T45.8X4	T45.8X5	T45.8X6
human	T45.8X1	T45.8X2	T45.8X3	T45.8X4	T45.8X5	T45.8X6
Escin	T46.991	T46.992	T46.993	T46.994	T46.995	T46.996
Esculin	T45.2X1	T45.2X2	T45.2X3	T45.2X4	T45.2X5	T45.2X6
Esculoside	T45.2X1	T45.2X2	T45.2X3	T45.2X4	T45.2X5	T45.2X6
ESDT (ether-soluble tar distillate)	T49.1X1	T49.1X2	T49.1X3	T49.1X4	T49.1X5	T49.1X6
Eserine	T49.5X1	T49.5X2	T49.5X3	T49.5X4	T49.5X5	T49.5X6
Esflurbiprofen	T39.311	T39.312	T39.313	T39.314	T39.315	T39.316
Eskabarb	T42.3X1	T42.3X2	T42.3X3	T42.3X4	T42.3X5	T42.3X6
Eskalith	T43.8X1	T43.8X2	T43.8X3	T43.8X4	T43.8X5	T43.8X6
Esmolol	T44.7X1	T44.7X2	T44.7X3	T44.7X4	T44.7X5	T44.7X6
Estanozolol	T38.7X1	T38.7X2	T38.7X3	T38.7X4	T38.7X5	T38.7X6
Estazolam	T42.4X1	T42.4X2	T42.4X3	T42.4X4	T42.4X5	T42.4X6
Estradiol	T38.5X1	T38.5X2	T38.5X3	T38.5X4	T38.5X5	T38.5X6
with testosterone	T38.7X1	T38.7X2	T38.7X3	T38.7X4	T38.7X5	T38.7X6
benzoate	T38.5X1	T38.5X2	T38.5X3	T38.5X4	T38.5X5	T38.5X6
Estramustine	T45.1X1	T45.1X2	T45.1X3	T45.1X4	T45.1X5	T45.1X6
Estriol	T38.5X1	T38.5X2	T38.5X3	T38.5X4	T38.5X5	T38.5X6
Estrogen	T38.5X1	T38.5X2	T38.5X3	T38.5X4	T38.5X5	T38.5X6
with progesterone	T38.5X1	T38.5X2	T38.5X3	T38.5X4	T38.5X5	T38.5X6
conjugated	T38.5X1	T38.5X2	T38.5X3	T38.5X4	T38.5X5	T38.5X6
Estrone	T38.5X1	T38.5X2	T38.5X3	T38.5X4	T38.5X5	T38.5X6
Estropipate	T38.5X1	T38.5X2	T38.5X3	T38.5X4	T38.5X5	T38.5X6
Etacrynate sodium	T50.1X1	T50.1X2	T50.1X3	T50.1X4	T50.1X5	T50.1X6
Etacrynic acid	T50.1X1	T50.1X2	T50.1X3	T50.1X4	T50.1X5	T50.1X6
Etafedrine	T48.6X1	T48.6X2	T48.6X3	T48.6X4	T48.6X5	T48.6X6
Etafenone	T46.3X1	T46.3X2	T46.3X3	T46.3X4	T46.3X5	T46.3X6
Etambutol	T37.1X1	T37.1X2	T37.1X3	T37.1X4	T37.1X5	T37.1X6

Dronabinol — Etambutol

Substance	Poisoning, Accidental (unintentional)	Poisoning, Intentional Self-harm	Poisoning, Assault	Poisoning, Undetermined	Adverse Effect	Under-dosing
Etamiphyllin	T48.6X1	T48.6X2	T48.6X3	T48.6X4	T48.6X5	T48.6X6
Etamivan	T50.7X1	T50.7X2	T50.7X3	T50.7X4	T50.7X5	T50.7X6
Etamsylate	T45.7X1	T45.7X2	T45.7X3	T45.7X4	T45.7X5	T45.7X6
Etebenecid	T50.4X1	T50.4X2	T50.4X3	T50.4X4	T50.4X5	T50.4X6
Ethacridine	T49.0X1	T49.0X2	T49.0X3	T49.0X4	T49.0X5	T49.0X6
Ethacrynic acid	T50.1X1	T50.1X2	T50.1X3	T50.1X4	T50.1X5	T50.1X6
Ethadione	T42.2X1	T42.2X2	T42.2X3	T42.2X4	T42.2X5	T42.2X6
Ethambutol	T37.1X1	T37.1X2	T37.1X3	T37.1X4	T37.1X5	T37.1X6
Ethamide	T50.2X1	T50.2X2	T50.2X3	T50.2X4	T50.2X5	T50.2X6
Ethamivan	T50.7X1	T50.7X2	T50.7X3	T50.7X4	T50.7X5	T50.7X6
Ethamsylate	T45.7X1	T45.7X2	T45.7X3	T45.7X4	T45.7X5	T45.7X6
Ethanol	T51.0X1	T51.0X2	T51.0X3	T51.0X4	—	—
beverage	T51.0X1	T51.0X2	T51.0X3	T51.0X4	—	—
Ethanolamine oleate	T46.8X1	T46.8X2	T46.8X3	T46.8X4	T46.8X5	T46.8X6
Ethaverine	T44.3X1	T44.3X2	T44.3X3	T44.3X4	T44.3X5	T44.3X6
Ethchlorvynol	T42.6X1	T42.6X2	T42.6X3	T42.6X4	T42.6X5	T42.6X6
Ethebenecid	T50.4X1	T50.4X2	T50.4X3	T50.4X4	T50.4X5	T50.4X6
Ether (vapor)	T41.0X1	T41.0X2	T41.0X3	T41.0X4	T41.0X5	T41.0X6
anesthetic	T41.0X1	T41.0X2	T41.0X3	T41.0X4	T41.0X5	T41.0X6
divinyl	T41.0X1	T41.0X2	T41.0X3	T41.0X4	T41.0X5	T41.0X6
ethyl (medicinal)	T41.0X1	T41.0X2	T41.0X3	T41.0X4	T41.0X5	T41.0X6
nonmedicinal	T52.8X1	T52.8X2	T52.8X3	T52.8X4	—	—
petroleum — see Ligroin						
solvent	T52.8X1	T52.8X2	T52.8X3	T52.8X4	—	—
Ethiazide	T50.2X1	T50.2X2	T50.2X3	T50.2X4	T50.2X5	T50.2X6
Ethidium chloride (vapor)	T59.891	T59.892	T59.893	T59.894		
Ethinamate	T42.6X1	T42.6X2	T42.6X3	T42.6X4	T42.6X5	T42.6X6
Ethinylestradiol, ethinyloestradiol	T38.5X1	T38.5X2	T38.5X3	T38.5X4	T38.5X5	T38.5X6
with						
levonorgestrel	T38.4X1	T38.4X2	T38.4X3	T38.4X4	T38.4X5	T38.4X6
norethisterone	T38.4X1	T38.4X2	T38.4X3	T38.4X4	T38.4X5	T38.4X6
Ethiodized oil (131 I)	T50.8X1	T50.8X2	T50.8X3	T50.8X4	T50.8X5	T50.8X6
Ethion	T60.0X1	T60.0X2	T60.0X3	T60.0X4	—	—
Ethionamide	T37.1X1	T37.1X2	T37.1X3	T37.1X4	T37.1X5	T37.1X6
Ethioniamide	T37.1X1	T37.1X2	T37.1X3	T37.1X4	T37.1X5	T37.1X6
Ethisterone	T38.5X1	T38.5X2	T38.5X3	T38.5X4	T38.5X5	T38.5X6
Ethobral	T42.3X1	T42.3X2	T42.3X3	T42.3X4	T42.3X5	T42.3X6
Ethocaine (infiltration)	T41.3X1	T41.3X2	T41.3X3	T41.3X4	T41.3X5	T41.3X6
(topical)						
nerve block (peripheral) (plexus)	T41.3X1	T41.3X2	T41.3X3	T41.3X4	T41.3X5	T41.3X6
spinal	T41.3X1	T41.3X2	T41.3X3	T41.3X4	T41.3X5	T41.3X6
Ethoheptazine	T40.4X1	T40.4X2	T40.4X3	T40.4X4	T40.4X5	T40.4X6
Ethopropazine	T44.3X1	T44.3X2	T44.3X3	T44.3X4	T44.3X5	T44.3X6
Ethosuximide	T42.2X1	T42.2X2	T42.2X3	T42.2X4	T42.2X5	T42.2X6
Ethotoin	T42.0X1	T42.0X2	T42.0X3	T42.0X4	T42.0X5	T42.0X6
Ethoxazene	T37.91	T37.92	T37.93	T37.94	T37.95	T37.96
Ethoxazorutoside	T46.991	T46.992	T46.993	T46.994	T46.995	T46.996
Ethoxzolamide	T50.2X1	T50.2X2	T50.2X3	T50.2X4	T50.2X5	T50.2X6
Ethyl						
acetate	T52.8X1	T52.8X2	T52.8X3	T52.8X4	—	—
alcohol	T51.0X1	T51.0X2	T51.0X3	T51.0X4	—	—
beverage	T51.0X1	T51.0X2	T51.0X3	T51.0X4	—	—
aldehyde (vapor)	T59.891	T59.892	T59.893	T59.894	—	—
liquid	T52.8X1	T52.8X2	T52.8X3	T52.8X4	—	—
aminobenzoate	T41.3X1	T41.3X2	T41.3X3	T41.3X4	T41.3X5	T41.3X6
aminophenothiazine	T43.3X1	T43.3X2	T43.3X3	T43.3X4	T43.3X5	T43.3X6
benzoate	T52.8X1	T52.8X2	T52.8X3	T52.8X4	—	—
biscoumacetate	T45.511	T45.512	T45.513	T45.514	T45.515	T45.516
bromide (anesthetic)	T41.0X1	T41.0X2	T41.0X3	T41.0X4	T41.0X5	T41.0X6
carbamate	T45.1X1	T45.1X2	T45.1X3	T45.1X4	T45.1X5	T45.1X6
carbinol	T51.3X1	T51.3X2	T51.3X3	T51.3X4	—	—
carbonate	T52.8X1	T52.8X2	T52.8X3	T52.8X4	—	—
chaulmoograte	T37.1X1	T37.1X2	T37.1X3	T37.1X4	T37.1X5	T37.1X6
chloride (anesthetic)	T41.0X1	T41.0X2	T41.0X3	T41.0X4	T41.0X5	T41.0X6
anesthetic (local)	T41.3X1	T41.3X2	T41.3X3	T41.3X4	T41.3X5	T41.3X6
inhaled	T41.0X1	T41.0X2	T41.0X3	T41.0X4	T41.0X5	T41.0X6
local	T49.4X1	T49.4X2	T49.4X3	T49.4X4	T49.4X5	T49.4X6
solvent	T53.6X1	T53.6X2	T53.6X3	T53.6X4	—	—
dibunate	T48.3X1	T48.3X2	T48.3X3	T48.3X4	T48.3X5	T48.3X6
dichloroarsine (vapor)	T57.0X1	T57.0X2	T57.0X3	T57.0X4	—	—
estranol	T38.7X1	T38.7X2	T38.7X3	T38.7X4	T38.7X5	T38.7X6
ether — see also ether	T52.8X1	T52.8X2	T52.8X3	T52.8X4	—	—
formate NEC (solvent)	T52.0X1	T52.0X2	T52.0X3	T52.0X4	—	—
fumarate	T49.4X1	T49.4X2	T49.4X3	T49.4X4	T49.4X5	T49.4X6
hydroxyisobutyrate NEC (solvent)	T52.8X1	T52.8X2	T52.8X3	T52.8X4	—	—
iodoacetate	T59.3X1	T59.3X2	T59.3X3	T59.3X4	—	—
lactate NEC (solvent)	T52.8X1	T52.8X2	T52.8X3	T52.8X4	—	—
loflazepate	T42.4X1	T42.4X2	T42.4X3	T42.4X4	T42.4X5	T42.4X6
mercuric chloride	T56.1X1	T56.1X2	T56.1X3	T56.1X4	—	—
methylcarbinol	T51.8X1	T51.8X2	T51.8X3	T51.8X4	—	—

Substance	Poisoning, Accidental (unintentional)	Poisoning, Intentional Self-harm	Poisoning, Assault	Poisoning, Undetermined	Adverse Effect	Under-dosing
Ethyl — continued						
morphine	T40.2X1	T40.2X2	T40.2X3	T40.2X4	T40.2X5	T40.2X6
noradrenaline	T48.6X1	T48.6X2	T48.6X3	T48.6X4	T48.6X5	T48.6X6
oxybutyrate NEC (solvent)	T52.8X1	T52.8X2	T52.8X3	T52.8X4	—	—
Ethylene (gas)	T59.891	T59.892	T59.893	T59.894		
anesthetic (general)	T41.0X1	T41.0X2	T41.0X3	T41.0X4	T41.0X5	T41.0X6
chlorohydrin	T52.8X1	T52.8X2	T52.8X3	T52.8X4	—	—
vapor	T53.6X1	T53.6X2	T53.6X3	T53.6X4		
dichloride	T52.8X1	T52.8X2	T52.8X3	T52.8X4		
vapor	T53.6X1	T53.6X2	T53.6X3	T53.6X4		
dinitrate	T52.3X1	T52.3X2	T52.3X3	T52.3X4		
glycol(s)	T52.8X1	T52.8X2	T52.8X3	T52.8X4		
dinitrate	T52.3X1	T52.3X2	T52.3X3	T52.3X4		
monobutyl ether	T52.3X1	T52.3X2	T52.3X3	T52.3X4		
imine	T54.1X1	T54.1X2	T54.1X3	T54.1X4		
oxide (fumigant)	T59.891	T59.892	T59.893	T59.894		
(nonmedicinal)						
medicinal	T49.0X1	T49.0X2	T49.0X3	T49.0X4	T49.0X5	T49.0X6
Ethylenediaminetetra-acetic acid	T50.6X1	T50.6X2	T50.6X3	T50.6X4	T50.6X5	T50.6X6
Ethylenediamine theophylline	T48.6X1	T48.6X2	T48.6X3	T48.6X4	T48.6X5	T48.6X6
Ethylenedinitrilotetra-acetate	T50.6X1	T50.6X2	T50.6X3	T50.6X4	T50.6X5	T50.6X6
Ethylestrenol	T38.7X1	T38.7X2	T38.7X3	T38.7X4	T38.7X5	T38.7X6
Ethylhydroxycellulose	T47.4X1	T47.4X2	T47.4X3	T47.4X4	T47.4X5	T47.4X6
Ethylidene						
chloride NEC	T53.6X1	T53.6X2	T53.6X3	T53.6X4		
diacetate	T60.3X1	T60.3X2	T60.3X3	T60.3X4		
dicoumarin	T45.511	T45.512	T45.513	T45.514	T45.515	T45.516
dicoumarol	T45.511	T45.512	T45.513	T45.514	T45.515	T45.516
diethyl ether	T52.0X1	T52.0X2	T52.0X3	T52.0X4		
Ethylmorphine	T40.2X1	T40.2X2	T40.2X3	T40.2X4	T40.2X5	T40.2X6
Ethylnorepinephrine	T48.6X1	T48.6X2	T48.6X3	T48.6X4	T48.6X5	T48.6X6
Ethylparachlorophen-oxyisobutyrate	T46.6X1	T46.6X2	T46.6X3	T46.6X4	T46.6X5	T46.6X6
Ethynodiol	T38.4X1	T38.4X2	T38.4X3	T38.4X4	T38.4X5	T38.4X6
with mestranol diacetate	T38.4X1	T38.4X2	T38.4X3	T38.4X4	T38.4X5	T38.4X6
Etidocaine	T41.3X1	T41.3X2	T41.3X3	T41.3X4	T41.3X5	T41.3X6
infiltration (subcutaneous)	T41.3X1	T41.3X2	T41.3X3	T41.3X4	T41.3X5	T41.3X6
nerve (peripheral) (plexus)	T41.3X1	T41.3X2	T41.3X3	T41.3X4	T41.3X5	T41.3X6
Etidronate	T50.991	T50.992	T50.993	T50.994	T50.995	T50.996
Etidronic acid (disodium salt)	T50.991	T50.992	T50.993	T50.994	T50.995	T50.996
Etifoxine	T42.6X1	T42.6X2	T42.6X3	T42.6X4	T42.6X5	T42.6X6
Etilefrine	T44.4X1	T44.4X2	T44.4X3	T44.4X4	T44.4X5	T44.4X6
Etilfen	T42.3X1	T42.3X2	T42.3X3	T42.3X4	T42.3X5	T42.3X6
Etinodiol	T38.4X1	T38.4X2	T38.4X3	T38.4X4	T38.4X5	T38.4X6
Etiroxate	T46.6X1	T46.6X2	T46.6X3	T46.6X4	T46.6X5	T46.6X6
Etizolam	T42.4X1	T42.4X2	T42.4X3	T42.4X4	T42.4X5	T42.4X6
Etodolac	T39.391	T39.392	T39.393	T39.394	T39.395	T39.396
Etofamide	T37.3X1	T37.3X2	T37.3X3	T37.3X4	T37.3X5	T37.3X6
Etofibrate	T46.6X1	T46.6X2	T46.6X3	T46.6X4	T46.6X5	T46.6X6
Etofylline	T46.7X1	T46.7X2	T46.7X3	T46.7X4	T46.7X5	T46.7X6
clofibrate	T46.6X1	T46.6X2	T46.6X3	T46.6X4	T46.6X5	T46.6X6
Etoglucid	T45.1X1	T45.1X2	T45.1X3	T45.1X4	T45.1X5	T45.1X6
Etomidate	T41.1X1	T41.1X2	T41.1X3	T41.1X4	T41.1X5	T41.1X6
Etomide	T39.8X1	T39.8X2	T39.8X3	T39.8X4	T39.8X5	T39.8X6
Etomidoline	T44.3X1	T44.3X2	T44.3X3	T44.3X4	T44.3X5	T44.3X6
Etoposide	T45.1X1	T45.1X2	T45.1X3	T45.1X4	T45.1X5	T45.1X6
Etorphine	T40.2X1	T40.2X2	T40.2X3	T40.2X4	T40.2X5	T40.2X6
Etoval	T42.3X1	T42.3X2	T42.3X3	T42.3X4	T42.3X5	T42.3X6
Etozolin	T50.1X1	T50.1X2	T50.1X3	T50.1X4	T50.1X5	T50.1X6
Etretinate	T50.991	T50.992	T50.993	T50.994	T50.995	T50.996
Etryptamine	T43.691	T43.692	T43.693	T43.694	T43.695	T43.696
Etybenzatropine	T44.3X1	T44.3X2	T44.3X3	T44.3X4	T44.3X5	T44.3X6
Etynodiol	T38.4X1	T38.4X2	T38.4X3	T38.4X4	T38.4X5	T38.4X6
Eucaine	T41.3X1	T41.3X2	T41.3X3	T41.3X4	T41.3X5	T41.3X6
Eucalyptus oil	T49.7X1	T49.7X2	T49.7X3	T49.7X4	T49.7X5	T49.7X6
Eucatropine	T49.5X1	T49.5X2	T49.5X3	T49.5X4	T49.5X5	T49.5X6
Eucodal	T40.2X1	T40.2X2	T40.2X3	T40.2X4	T40.2X5	T40.2X6
Euneryl	T42.3X1	T42.3X2	T42.3X3	T42.3X4	T42.3X5	T42.3X6
Euphthalmine	T44.3X1	T44.3X2	T44.3X3	T44.3X4	T44.3X5	T44.3X6
Eurax	T49.0X1	T49.0X2	T49.0X3	T49.0X4	T49.0X5	T49.0X6
Euresol	T49.4X1	T49.4X2	T49.4X3	T49.4X4	T49.4X5	T49.4X6
Euthroid	T38.1X1	T38.1X2	T38.1X3	T38.1X4	T38.1X5	T38.1X6
Evans blue	T50.8X1	T50.8X2	T50.8X3	T50.8X4	T50.8X5	T50.8X6
Evipal	T42.3X1	T42.3X2	T42.3X3	T42.3X4	T42.3X5	T42.3X6
sodium	T41.1X1	T41.1X2	T41.1X3	T41.1X4	T41.1X5	T41.1X6
Evipan	T42.3X1	T42.3X2	T42.3X3	T42.3X4	T42.3X5	T42.3X6
sodium	T41.1X1	T41.1X2	T41.1X3	T41.1X4	T41.1X5	T41.1X6
Exalamide	T49.0X1	T49.0X2	T49.0X3	T49.0X4	T49.0X5	T49.0X6
Exalgin	T39.1X1	T39.1X2	T39.1X3	T39.1X4	T39.1X5	T39.1X6
Excipients, pharmaceutical	T50.901	T50.902	T50.903	T50.904	T50.905	T50.906

Table of Drugs and Chemicals

Etamiphyllin — Excipients, pharmaceutical

Table of Drugs and Chemicals

Exhaust gas — Fluorinated corticosteroids

Substance	Poisoning, Accidental (unintentional)	Poisoning, Intentional Self-harm	Poisoning, Assault	Poisoning, Undetermined	Adverse Effect	Under-dosing
Exhaust gas (engine) (motor vehicle)	T58.01	T58.02	T58.03	T58.04	—	—
Ex-Lax (phenolphthalein)	T47.2X1	T47.2X2	T47.2X3	T47.2X4	T47.2X5	T47.2X6
Expectorant NEC	T48.4X1	T48.4X2	T48.4X3	T48.4X4	T48.4X5	T48.4X6
Extended insulin zinc suspension	T38.3X1	T38.3X2	T38.3X3	T38.3X4	T38.3X5	T38.3X6
External medications (skin) (mucous membrane)	T49.91	T49.92	T49.93	T49.94	T49.95	T49.96
dental agent	T49.7X1	T49.7X2	T49.7X3	T49.7X4	T49.7X5	T49.7X6
ENT agent	T49.6X1	T49.6X2	T49.6X3	T49.6X4	T49.6X5	T49.6X6
ophthalmic preparation	T49.5X1	T49.5X2	T49.5X3	T49.5X4	T49.5X5	T49.5X6
specified NEC	T49.8X1	T49.8X2	T49.8X3	T49.8X4	T49.8X5	T49.8X6
Extrapyramidal antagonist NEC	T44.3X1	T44.3X2	T44.3X3	T44.3X4	T44.3X5	T44.3X6
Eye agents (anti-infective)	T49.5X1	T49.5X2	T49.5X3	T49.5X4	T49.5X5	T49.5X6
Eye drug NEC	T49.5X1	T49.5X2	T49.5X3	T49.5X4	T49.5X5	T49.5X6
FAC (fluorouracil + doxorubicin + cyclophosphamide)	T45.1X1	T45.1X2	T45.1X3	T45.1X4	T45.1X5	T45.1X6
Factor						
I (fibrinogen)	T45.8X1	T45.8X2	T45.8X3	T45.8X4	T45.8X5	T45.8X6
III (thromboplastin)	T45.8X1	T45.8X2	T45.8X3	T45.8X4	T45.8X5	T45.8X6
VIII (antihemophilic Factor) (concentrate)	T45.8X1	T45.8X2	T45.8X3	T45.8X4	T45.8X5	T45.8X6
IX complex	T45.7X1	T45.7X2	T45.7X3	T45.7X4	T45.7X5	T45.7X6
human	T45.8X1	T45.8X2	T45.8X3	T45.8X4	T45.8X5	T45.8X6
Famotidine	T47.0X1	T47.0X2	T47.0X3	T47.0X4	T47.0X5	T47.0X6
Fat suspension, intravenous	T50.991	T50.992	T50.993	T50.994	T50.995	T50.996
Fazadinium bromide	T48.1X1	T48.1X2	T48.1X3	T48.1X4	T48.1X5	T48.1X6
Febarbamate	T42.3X1	T42.3X2	T42.3X3	T42.3X4	T42.3X5	T42.3X6
Fecal softener	T47.4X1	T47.4X2	T47.4X3	T47.4X4	T47.4X5	T47.4X6
Fedrilate	T48.3X1	T48.3X2	T48.3X3	T48.3X4	T48.3X5	T48.3X6
Felodipine	T46.1X1	T46.1X2	T46.1X3	T46.1X4	T46.1X5	T46.1X6
Felypressin	T38.891	T38.892	T38.893	T38.894	T38.895	T38.896
Femoxetine	T43.221	T43.222	T43.223	T43.224	T43.225	T43.226
Fenalcomine	T46.3X1	T46.3X2	T46.3X3	T46.3X4	T46.3X5	T46.3X6
Fenamisal	T37.1X1	T37.1X2	T37.1X3	T37.1X4	T37.1X5	T37.1X6
Fenazone	T39.2X1	T39.2X2	T39.2X3	T39.2X4	T39.2X5	T39.2X6
Fenbendazole	T37.4X1	T37.4X2	T37.4X3	T37.4X4	T37.4X5	T37.4X6
Fenbutrazate	T50.5X1	T50.5X2	T50.5X3	T50.5X4	T50.5X5	T50.5X6
Fencamfamine	T43.691	T43.692	T43.693	T43.694	T43.695	T43.696
Fendiline	T46.1X1	T46.1X2	T46.1X3	T46.1X4	T46.1X5	T46.1X6
Fenetylline	T43.691	T43.692	T43.693	T43.694	T43.695	T43.696
Fenflumizole	T39.391	T39.392	T39.393	T39.394	T39.395	T39.396
Fenfluramine	T50.5X1	T50.5X2	T50.5X3	T50.5X4	T50.5X5	T50.5X6
Fenobarbital	T42.3X1	T42.3X2	T42.3X3	T42.3X4	T42.3X5	T42.3X6
Fenofibrate	T46.6X1	T46.6X2	T46.6X3	T46.6X4	T46.6X5	T46.6X6
Fenoprofen	T39.311	T39.312	T39.313	T39.314	T39.315	T39.316
Fenoterol	T48.6X1	T48.6X2	T48.6X3	T48.6X4	T48.6X5	T48.6X6
Fenoverine	T44.3X1	T44.3X2	T44.3X3	T44.3X4	T44.3X5	T44.3X6
Fenoxazoline	T48.5X1	T48.5X2	T48.5X3	T48.5X4	T48.5X5	T48.5X6
Fenproporex	T50.5X1	T50.5X2	T50.5X3	T50.5X4	T50.5X5	T50.5X6
Fenquizone	T50.2X1	T50.2X2	T50.2X3	T50.2X4	T50.2X5	T50.2X6
Fentanyl	T40.4X1	T40.4X2	T40.4X3	T40.4X4	T40.4X5	T40.4X6
Fentazin	T43.3X1	T43.3X2	T43.3X3	T43.3X4	T43.3X5	T43.3X6
Fenthion	T60.0X1	T60.0X2	T60.0X3	T60.0X4	—	—
Fenticlor	T49.0X1	T49.0X2	T49.0X3	T49.0X4	T49.0X5	T49.0X6
Fenylbutazone	T39.2X1	T39.2X2	T39.2X3	T39.2X4	T39.2X5	T39.2X6
Feprazone	T39.2X1	T39.2X2	T39.2X3	T39.2X4	T39.2X5	T39.2X6
Fer de lance (bite) (venom)	T63.061	T63.062	T63.063	T63.064	—	—
Ferric — see also Iron						
chloride	T45.4X1	T45.4X2	T45.4X3	T45.4X4	T45.4X5	T45.4X6
citrate	T45.4X1	T45.4X2	T45.4X3	T45.4X4	T45.4X5	T45.4X6
hydroxide						
colloidal	T45.4X1	T45.4X2	T45.4X3	T45.4X4	T45.4X5	T45.4X6
polymaltose	T45.4X1	T45.4X2	T45.4X3	T45.4X4	T45.4X5	T45.4X6
pyrophosphate	T45.4X1	T45.4X2	T45.4X3	T45.4X4	T45.4X5	T45.4X6
Ferritin	T45.4X1	T45.4X2	T45.4X3	T45.4X4	T45.4X5	T45.4X6
Ferrocholinate	T45.4X1	T45.4X2	T45.4X3	T45.4X4	T45.4X5	T45.4X6
Ferrodextrane	T45.4X1	T45.4X2	T45.4X3	T45.4X4	T45.4X5	T45.4X6
Ferropolimaler	T45.4X1	T45.4X2	T45.4X3	T45.4X4	T45.4X5	T45.4X6
Ferrous — see also Iron						
phosphate	T45.4X1	T45.4X2	T45.4X3	T45.4X4	T45.4X5	T45.4X6
salt	T45.4X1	T45.4X2	T45.4X3	T45.4X4	T45.4X5	T45.4X6
with folic acid	T45.4X1	T45.4X2	T45.4X3	T45.4X4	T45.4X5	T45.4X6
Ferrous fumarate, gluconate, lactate, salt NEC, sulfate (medicinal)	T45.4X1	T45.4X2	T45.4X3	T45.4X4	T45.4X5	T45.4X6
Ferrovanadium (fumes)	T59.891	T59.892	T59.893	T59.894	—	—
Ferrum — see Iron						
Fertilizers NEC	T65.891	T65.892	T65.893	T65.894	—	—
with herbicide mixture	T60.3X1	T60.3X2	T60.3X3	T60.3X4	—	—
Fetoxilate	T47.6X1	T47.6X2	T47.6X3	T47.6X4	T47.6X5	T47.6X6
Fiber, dietary	T47.4X1	T47.4X2	T47.4X3	T47.4X4	T47.4X5	T47.4X6
Fiberglass	T65.831	T65.832	T65.833	T65.834	—	—
Fibrinogen (human)	T45.8X1	T45.8X2	T45.8X3	T45.8X4	T45.8X5	T45.8X6
Fibrinolysin (human)	T45.691	T45.692	T45.693	T45.694	T45.695	T45.696
Fibrinolysis						
affecting drug	T45.601	T45.602	T45.603	T45.604	T45.605	T45.606
inhibitor NEC	T45.621	T45.622	T45.623	T45.624	T45.625	T45.626
Fibrinolytic drug	T45.611	T45.612	T45.613	T45.614	T45.615	T45.616
Filix mas	T37.4X1	T37.4X2	T37.4X3	T37.4X4	T37.4X5	T37.4X6
Filtering cream	T49.3X1	T49.3X2	T49.3X3	T49.3X4	T49.3X5	T49.3X6
Fiorinal	T39.011	T39.012	T39.013	T39.014	T39.015	T39.016
Firedamp	T59.891	T59.892	T59.893	T59.894	—	—
Fish, noxious, nonbacterial	T61.91	T61.92	T61.93	T61.94	—	—
ciguatera	T61.01	T61.02	T61.03	T61.04	—	—
scombroid	T61.11	T61.12	T61.13	T61.14	—	—
shell	T61.781	T61.782	T61.783	T61.784	—	—
specified NEC	T61.771	T61.772	T61.773	T61.774	—	—
Flagyl	T37.3X1	T37.3X2	T37.3X3	T37.3X4	T37.3X5	T37.3X6
Flavine adenine dinucleotide	T45.2X1	T45.2X2	T45.2X3	T45.2X4	T45.2X5	T45.2X6
Flavodic acid	T46.991	T46.992	T46.993	T46.994	T46.995	T46.996
Flavoxate	T44.3X1	T44.3X2	T44.3X3	T44.3X4	T44.3X5	T44.3X6
Flaxedil	T48.1X1	T48.1X2	T48.1X3	T48.1X4	T48.1X5	T48.1X6
Flaxseed (medicinal)	T49.3X1	T49.3X2	T49.3X3	T49.3X4	T49.3X5	T49.3X6
Flecainide	T46.2X1	T46.2X2	T46.2X3	T46.2X4	T46.2X5	T46.2X6
Fleroxacin	T36.8X1	T36.8X2	T36.8X3	T36.8X4	T36.8X5	T36.8X6
Floctafenine	T39.8X1	T39.8X2	T39.8X3	T39.8X4	T39.8X5	T39.8X6
Flomax	T44.6X1	T44.6X2	T44.6X3	T44.6X4	T44.6X5	T44.6X6
Flomoxef	T36.1X1	T36.1X2	T36.1X3	T36.1X4	T36.1X5	T36.1X6
Flopropione	T44.3X1	T44.3X2	T44.3X3	T44.3X4	T44.3X5	T44.3X6
Florantyrone	T47.5X1	T47.5X2	T47.5X3	T47.5X4	T47.5X5	T47.5X6
Floraquin	T37.8X1	T37.8X2	T37.8X3	T37.8X4	T37.8X5	T37.8X6
Florinef	T38.0X1	T38.0X2	T38.0X3	T38.0X4	T38.0X5	T38.0X6
ENT agent	T49.6X1	T49.6X2	T49.6X3	T49.6X4	T49.6X5	T49.6X6
ophthalmic preparation	T49.5X1	T49.5X2	T49.5X3	T49.5X4	T49.5X5	T49.5X6
topical NEC	T49.0X1	T49.0X2	T49.0X3	T49.0X4	T49.0X5	T49.0X6
Flowers of sulfur	T49.4X1	T49.4X2	T49.4X3	T49.4X4	T49.4X5	T49.4X6
Floxuridine	T45.1X1	T45.1X2	T45.1X3	T45.1X4	T45.1X5	T45.1X6
Fluanisone	T43.4X1	T43.4X2	T43.4X3	T43.4X4	T43.4X5	T43.4X6
Flubendazole	T37.4X1	T37.4X2	T37.4X3	T37.4X4	T37.4X5	T37.4X6
Fluclorolone acetonide	T49.0X1	T49.0X2	T49.0X3	T49.0X4	T49.0X5	T49.0X6
Flucloxacillin	T36.0X1	T36.0X2	T36.0X3	T36.0X4	T36.0X5	T36.0X6
Fluconazole	T37.8X1	T37.8X2	T37.8X3	T37.8X4	T37.8X5	T37.8X6
Flucytosine	T37.8X1	T37.8X2	T37.8X3	T37.8X4	T37.8X5	T37.8X6
Fludeoxyglucose (18F)	T50.8X1	T50.8X2	T50.8X3	T50.8X4	T50.8X5	T50.8X6
Fludiazepam	T42.4X1	T42.4X2	T42.4X3	T42.4X4	T42.4X5	T42.4X6
Fludrocortisone	T50.0X1	T50.0X2	T50.0X3	T50.0X4	T50.0X5	T50.0X6
ENT agent	T49.6X1	T49.6X2	T49.6X3	T49.6X4	T49.6X5	T49.6X6
ophthalmic preparation	T49.5X1	T49.5X2	T49.5X3	T49.5X4	T49.5X5	T49.5X6
topical NEC	T49.0X1	T49.0X2	T49.0X3	T49.0X4	T49.0X5	T49.0X6
Fludroxycortide	T49.0X1	T49.0X2	T49.0X3	T49.0X4	T49.0X5	T49.0X6
Flufenamic acid	T39.391	T39.392	T39.393	T39.394	T39.395	T39.396
Fluindione	T45.511	T45.512	T45.513	T45.514	T45.515	T45.516
Flumequine	T37.8X1	T37.8X2	T37.8X3	T37.8X4	T37.8X5	T37.8X6
Flumethasone	T49.0X1	T49.0X2	T49.0X3	T49.0X4	T49.0X5	T49.0X6
Flumethiazide	T50.2X1	T50.2X2	T50.2X3	T50.2X4	T50.2X5	T50.2X6
Flumidin	T37.5X1	T37.5X2	T37.5X3	T37.5X4	T37.5X5	T37.5X6
Flunarizine	T46.7X1	T46.7X2	T46.7X3	T46.7X4	T46.7X5	T46.7X6
Flunidazole	T37.8X1	T37.8X2	T37.8X3	T37.8X4	T37.8X5	T37.8X6
Flunisolide	T48.6X1	T48.6X2	T48.6X3	T48.6X4	T48.6X5	T48.6X6
Flunitrazepam	T42.4X1	T42.4X2	T42.4X3	T42.4X4	T42.4X5	T42.4X6
Fluocinolone (acetonide)	T49.0X1	T49.0X2	T49.0X3	T49.0X4	T49.0X5	T49.0X6
Fluocinonide	T49.0X1	T49.0X2	T49.0X3	T49.0X4	T49.0X5	T49.0X6
Fluocortin (butyl)	T49.0X1	T49.0X2	T49.0X3	T49.0X4	T49.0X5	T49.0X6
Fluocortolone	T49.0X1	T49.0X2	T49.0X3	T49.0X4	T49.0X5	T49.0X6
Fluohydrocortisone	T38.0X1	T38.0X2	T38.0X3	T38.0X4	T38.0X5	T38.0X6
ENT agent	T49.6X1	T49.6X2	T49.6X3	T49.6X4	T49.6X5	T49.6X6
ophthalmic preparation	T49.5X1	T49.5X2	T49.5X3	T49.5X4	T49.5X5	T49.5X6
topical NEC	T49.0X1	T49.0X2	T49.0X3	T49.0X4	T49.0X5	T49.0X6
Fluonid	T49.0X1	T49.0X2	T49.0X3	T49.0X4	T49.0X5	T49.0X6
Fluopromazine	T43.3X1	T43.3X2	T43.3X3	T43.3X4	T43.3X5	T43.3X6
Fluoracetate	T60.8X1	T60.8X2	T60.8X3	T60.8X4	—	—
Fluorescein	T50.8X1	T50.8X2	T50.8X3	T50.8X4	T50.8X5	T50.8X6
Fluorhydrocortisone	T50.0X1	T50.0X2	T50.0X3	T50.0X4	T50.0X5	T50.0X6
Fluoride (nonmedicinal) (pesticide) (sodium) NEC	T60.8X1	T60.8X2	T60.8X3	T60.8X4	—	—
hydrogen — see Hydrofluoric acid						
medicinal NEC	T50.991	T50.992	T50.993	T50.994	T50.995	T50.996
dental use	T49.7X1	T49.7X2	T49.7X3	T49.7X4	T49.7X5	T49.7X6
not pesticide NEC	T54.91	T54.92	T54.93	T54.94	—	—
stannous	T49.7X1	T49.7X2	T49.7X3	T49.7X4	T49.7X5	T49.7X6
Fluorinated corticosteroids	T38.0X1	T38.0X2	T38.0X3	T38.0X4	T38.0X5	T38.0X6

Substance	Poisoning, Accidental (unintentional)	Poisoning, Intentional Self-harm	Poisoning, Assault	Poisoning, Undetermined	Adverse Effect	Under-dosing
Fluorine (gas)	T59.5X1	T59.5X2	T59.5X3	T59.5X4	—	—
salt — see Fluoride(s)						
Fluoristan	T49.7X1	T49.7X2	T49.7X3	T49.7X4	T49.7X5	T49.7X6
Fluormetholone	T49.0X1	T49.0X2	T49.0X3	T49.0X4	T49.0X5	T49.0X6
Fluoroacetate	T60.8X1	T60.8X2	T60.8X3	T60.8X4	—	—
Fluorocarbon monomer	T53.6X1	T53.6X2	T53.6X3	T53.6X4	—	—
Fluorocytosine	T37.8X1	T37.8X2	T37.8X3	T37.8X4	T37.8X5	T37.8X6
Fluorodeoxyuridine	T45.1X1	T45.1X2	T45.1X3	T45.1X4	T45.1X5	T45.1X6
Fluorometholone	T49.0X1	T49.0X2	T49.0X3	T49.0X4	T49.0X5	T49.0X6
ophthalmic preparation	T49.5X1	T49.5X2	T49.5X3	T49.5X4	T49.5X5	T49.5X6
Fluorophosphate insecticide	T60.0X1	T60.0X2	T60.0X3	T60.0X4	—	—
Fluorosol	T46.3X1	T46.3X2	T46.3X3	T46.3X4	T46.3X5	T46.3X6
Fluorouracil	T45.1X1	T45.1X2	T45.1X3	T45.1X4	T45.1X5	T45.1X6
Fluorphenylalanine	T49.5X1	T49.5X2	T49.5X3	T49.5X4	T49.5X5	T49.5X6
Fluothane	T41.0X1	T41.0X2	T41.0X3	T41.0X4	T41.0X5	T41.0X6
Fluoxetine	T43.221	T43.222	T43.223	T43.224	T43.225	T43.226
Fluoxymesterone	T38.7X1	T38.7X2	T38.7X3	T38.7X4	T38.7X5	T38.7X6
Flupenthixol	T43.4X1	T43.4X2	T43.4X3	T43.4X4	T43.4X5	T43.4X6
Flupentixol	T43.4X1	T43.4X2	T43.4X3	T43.4X4	T43.4X5	T43.4X6
Fluphenazine	T43.3X1	T43.3X2	T43.3X3	T43.3X4	T43.3X5	T43.3X6
Fluprednidene	T49.0X1	T49.0X2	T49.0X3	T49.0X4	T49.0X5	T49.0X6
Fluprednisolone	T38.0X1	T38.0X2	T38.0X3	T38.0X4	T38.0X5	T38.0X6
Fluradoline	T39.8X1	T39.8X2	T39.8X3	T39.8X4	T39.8X5	T39.8X6
Flurandrenolide	T49.0X1	T49.0X2	T49.0X3	T49.0X4	T49.0X5	T49.0X6
Flurandrenolone	T49.0X1	T49.0X2	T49.0X3	T49.0X4	T49.0X5	T49.0X6
Flurazepam	T42.4X1	T42.4X2	T42.4X3	T42.4X4	T42.4X5	T42.4X6
Flurbiprofen	T39.311	T39.312	T39.313	T39.314	T39.315	T39.316
Flurobate	T49.0X1	T49.0X2	T49.0X3	T49.0X4	T49.0X5	T49.0X6
Fluroxene	T41.0X1	T41.0X2	T41.0X3	T41.0X4	T41.0X5	T41.0X6
Fluspirilene	T43.591	T43.592	T43.593	T43.594	T43.595	T43.596
Flutamide	T38.6X1	T38.6X2	T38.6X3	T38.6X4	T38.6X5	T38.6X6
Flutazolam	T38.0X1	T38.0X2	T38.0X3	T38.0X4	T38.0X5	T38.0X6
Fluticasone propionate	T38.0X1	T38.0X2	T38.0X3	T38.0X4	T38.0X5	T38.0X6
Flutoprazepam	T42.4X1	T42.4X2	T42.4X3	T42.4X4	T42.4X5	T42.4X6
Flutropium bromide	T48.6X1	T48.6X2	T48.6X3	T48.6X4	T48.6X5	T48.6X6
Fluvoxamine	T43.221	T43.222	T43.223	T43.224	T43.225	T43.226
Folacin	T45.8X1	T45.8X2	T45.8X3	T45.8X4	T45.8X5	T45.8X6
Folic acid	T45.8X1	T45.8X2	T45.8X3	T45.8X4	T45.8X5	T45.8X6
with ferrous salt	T45.2X1	T45.2X2	T45.2X3	T45.2X4	T45.2X5	T45.2X6
antagonist	T45.1X1	T45.1X2	T45.1X3	T45.1X4	T45.1X5	T45.1X6
Folinic acid	T45.8X1	T45.8X2	T45.8X3	T45.8X4	T45.8X5	T45.8X6
Folium stramoniae	T48.6X1	T48.6X2	T48.6X3	T48.6X4	T48.6X5	T48.6X6
Follicle-stimulating hormone, human	T38.811	T38.812	T38.813	T38.814	T38.815	T38.816
Folpet	T60.3X1	T60.3X2	T60.3X3	T60.3X4	—	—
Fominoben	T48.3X1	T48.3X2	T48.3X3	T48.3X4	T48.3X5	T48.3X6
Food, foodstuffs, noxious, nonbacterial, NEC	T62.91	T62.92	T62.93	T62.94	—	—
berries	T62.1X1	T62.1X2	T62.1X3	T62.1X4	—	—
fish — see also Fish	T61.91	T61.92	T61.93	T61.94	—	—
mushrooms	T62.0X1	T62.0X2	T62.0X3	T62.0X4	—	—
plants	T62.2X1	T62.2X2	T62.2X3	T62.2X4	—	—
seafood	T61.91	T61.92	T61.93	T61.94	—	—
specified NEC	T61.8X1	T61.8X2	T61.8X3	T61.8X4	—	—
seeds	T62.2X1	T62.2X2	T62.2X3	T62.2X4	—	—
shellfish	T61.781	T61.782	T61.783	T61.784	—	—
specified NEC	T62.8X1	T62.8X2	T62.8X3	T62.8X4	—	—
Fool's parsley	T62.2X1	T62.2X2	T62.2X3	T62.2X4	—	—
Formaldehyde (solution), gas or vapor	T59.2X1	T59.2X2	T59.2X3	T59.2X4	—	—
fungicide	T60.3X1	T60.3X2	T60.3X3	T60.3X4	—	—
Formalin	T59.2X1	T59.2X2	T59.2X3	T59.2X4	—	—
fungicide	T60.3X1	T60.3X2	T60.3X3	T60.3X4	—	—
vapor	T59.2X1	T59.2X2	T59.2X3	T59.2X4	—	—
Formic acid	T54.2X1	T54.2X2	T54.2X3	T54.2X4	—	—
vapor	T59.891	T59.892	T59.893	T59.894	—	—
Foscarnet sodium	T37.5X1	T37.5X2	T37.5X3	T37.5X4	T37.5X5	T37.5X6
Fosfestrol	T38.5X1	T38.5X2	T38.5X3	T38.5X4	T38.5X5	T38.5X6
Fosfomycin	T36.8X1	T36.8X2	T36.8X3	T36.8X4	T36.8X5	T36.8X6
Fosfonet sodium	T37.5X1	T37.5X2	T37.5X3	T37.5X4	T37.5X5	T37.5X6
Fosinopril	T46.4X1	T46.4X2	T46.4X3	T46.4X4	T46.4X5	T46.4X6
sodium	T46.4X1	T46.4X2	T46.4X3	T46.4X4	T46.4X5	T46.4X6
Fowler's solution	T57.0X1	T57.0X2	T57.0X3	T57.0X4	—	—
Foxglove	T62.2X1	T62.2X2	T62.2X3	T62.2X4	—	—
Framycetin	T36.5X1	T36.5X2	T36.5X3	T36.5X4	T36.5X5	T36.5X6
Frangula	T47.2X1	T47.2X2	T47.2X3	T47.2X4	T47.2X5	T47.2X6
extract	T47.2X1	T47.2X2	T47.2X3	T47.2X4	T47.2X5	T47.2X6
Frei antigen	T50.8X1	T50.8X2	T50.8X3	T50.8X4	T50.8X5	T50.8X6
Freon	T53.5X1	T53.5X2	T53.5X3	T53.5X4	—	—
Fructose	T50.3X1	T50.3X2	T50.3X3	T50.3X4	T50.3X5	T50.3X6
Frusemide	T50.1X1	T50.1X2	T50.1X3	T50.1X4	T50.1X5	T50.1X6
FSH	T38.811	T38.812	T38.813	T38.814	T38.815	T38.816

Substance	Poisoning, Accidental (unintentional)	Poisoning, Intentional Self-harm	Poisoning, Assault	Poisoning, Undetermined	Adverse Effect	Under-dosing
Ftorafur	T45.1X1	T45.1X2	T45.1X3	T45.1X4	T45.1X5	T45.1X6
Fuel						
automobile	T52.0X1	T52.0X2	T52.0X3	T52.0X4	—	—
exhaust gas, not in transit	T58.01	T58.02	T58.03	T58.04	—	—
vapor NEC	T52.0X1	T52.0X2	T52.0X3	T52.0X4	—	—
gas (domestic use) — see also Carbon, monoxide, fuel, utility	T59.891	T59.892	T59.893	T59.894	—	—
utility	T59.891	T59.892	T59.893	T59.894	—	—
incomplete combustion of — see Carbon, monoxide, fuel, utility						
in mobile container	T59.891	T59.892	T59.893	T59.894	—	—
piped (natural)	T59.891	T59.892	T59.893	T59.894	—	—
industrial, incomplete combustion	T58.8X1	T58.8X2	T58.8X3	T58.8X4	—	—
Fugillin	T36.8X1	T36.8X2	T36.8X3	T36.8X4	T36.8X5	T36.8X6
Fulminate of mercury	T56.1X1	T56.1X2	T56.1X3	T56.1X4	—	—
Fulvicin	T36.7X1	T36.7X2	T36.7X3	T36.7X4	T36.7X5	T36.7X6
Fumadil	T36.8X1	T36.8X2	T36.8X3	T36.8X4	T36.8X5	T36.8X6
Fumagillin	T36.8X1	T36.8X2	T36.8X3	T36.8X4	T36.8X5	T36.8X6
Fumaric acid	T49.4X1	T49.4X2	T49.4X3	T49.4X4	T49.4X5	T49.4X6
Fumes (from)	T59.91	T59.92	T59.93	T59.94	—	—
carbon monoxide — see Carbon, monoxide						
charcoal (domestic use) — see Charcoal, fumes						
chloroform — see Chloroform						
coke (in domestic stoves, fireplaces) — see Coke fumes						
corrosive NEC	T54.91	T54.92	T54.93	T54.94	—	—
ether — see ether						
freons	T53.5X1	T53.5X2	T53.5X3	T53.5X4	—	—
hydrocarbons	T59.891	T59.892	T59.893	T59.894	—	—
petroleum (liquefied)	T59.891	T59.892	T59.893	T59.894	—	—
distributed through pipes (pure or mixed with air)	T59.891	T59.892	T59.893	T59.894	—	—
lead — see lead						
metal — see Metals, or the specified metal						
nitrogen dioxide	T59.0X1	T59.0X2	T59.0X3	T59.0X4	—	—
pesticides — see Pesticides						
petroleum (liquefied)	T59.891	T59.892	T59.893	T59.894	—	—
distributed through pipes (pure or mixed with air)	T59.891	T59.892	T59.893	T59.894	—	—
polyester	T59.891	T59.892	T59.893	T59.894	—	—
specified source NEC — see also substance specified	T59.891	T59.892	T59.893	T59.894	—	—
sulfur dioxide	T59.1X1	T59.1X2	T59.1X3	T59.1X4	—	—
Fumigant NEC	T60.91	T60.92	T60.93	T60.94	—	—
Fungicide NEC (nonmedicinal)	T60.3X1	T60.3X2	T60.3X3	T60.3X4	—	—
Fungi, noxious, used as food	T62.0X1	T62.0X2	T62.0X3	T62.0X4	—	—
Fungizone	T36.7X1	T36.7X2	T36.7X3	T36.7X4	T36.7X5	T36.7X6
topical	T49.0X1	T49.0X2	T49.0X3	T49.0X4	T49.0X5	T49.0X6
Furacin	T49.0X1	T49.0X2	T49.0X3	T49.0X4	T49.0X5	T49.0X6
Furadantin	T37.91	T37.92	T37.93	T37.94	T37.95	T37.96
Furazolidone	T37.8X1	T37.8X2	T37.8X3	T37.8X4	T37.8X5	T37.8X6
Furazolium chloride	T49.0X1	T49.0X2	T49.0X3	T49.0X4	T49.0X5	T49.0X6
Furfural	T52.8X1	T52.8X2	T52.8X3	T52.8X4	—	—
Furnace (coal burning) (domestic), gas from	T58.2X1	T58.2X2	T58.2X3	T58.2X4	—	—
industrial	T58.8X1	T58.8X2	T58.8X3	T58.8X4	—	—
Furniture polish	T65.891	T65.892	T65.893	T65.894	—	—
Furosemide	T50.1X1	T50.1X2	T50.1X3	T50.1X4	T50.1X5	T50.1X6
Furoxone	T37.91	T37.92	T37.93	T37.94	T37.95	T37.96
Fursultiamine	T45.2X1	T45.2X2	T45.2X3	T45.2X4	T45.2X5	T45.2X6
Fusafungine	T36.8X1	T36.8X2	T36.8X3	T36.8X4	T36.8X5	T36.8X6
Fusel oil (any) (amyl) (butyl) (propyl), vapor	T51.3X1	T51.3X2	T51.3X3	T51.3X4	—	—
Fusidate (ethanolamine) (sodium)	T36.8X1	T36.8X2	T36.8X3	T36.8X4	T36.8X5	T36.8X6
Fusidic acid	T36.8X1	T36.8X2	T36.8X3	T36.8X4	T36.8X5	T36.8X6
Fytic acid, nonasodium	T50.6X1	T50.6X2	T50.6X3	T50.6X4	T50.6X5	T50.6X6
b-Galactosidase	T47.5X1	T47.5X2	T47.5X3	T47.5X4	T47.5X5	T47.5X6
GABA	T43.8X1	T43.8X2	T43.8X3	T43.8X4	T43.8X5	T43.8X6
Gadopentetic acid	T50.8X1	T50.8X2	T50.8X3	T50.8X4	T50.8X5	T50.8X6
Galactose	T50.3X1	T50.3X2	T50.3X3	T50.3X4	T50.3X5	T50.3X6
Galantamine	T44.0X1	T44.0X2	T44.0X3	T44.0X4	T44.0X5	T44.0X6

▽ Subterms under main terms may continue to next column or page   Additional Character May Be Required — Refer to the Tabular List for Character Selection

Table of Drugs and Chemicals

Substance	Poisoning, Accidental (unintentional)	Poisoning, Intentional Self-harm	Poisoning, Assault	Poisoning, Undetermined	Adverse Effect	Under-dosing
Gallamine (triethiodide)	T48.1X1	T48.1X2	T48.1X3	T48.1X4	T48.1X5	T48.1X6
Gallium citrate	T50.991	T50.992	T50.993	T50.994	T50.995	T50.996
Gallopamil	T46.1X1	T46.1X2	T46.1X3	T46.1X4	T46.1X5	T46.1X6
Gamboge	T47.2X1	T47.2X2	T47.2X3	T47.2X4	T47.2X5	T47.2X6
Gamimune	T50.Z11	T50.Z12	T50.Z13	T50.Z14	T50.Z15	T50.Z16
Gamma-aminobutyric acid	T43.8X1	T43.8X2	T43.8X3	T43.8X4	T43.8X5	T43.8X6
Gamma-benzene hexachloride (medicinal)	T49.0X1	T49.0X2	T49.0X3	T49.0X4	T49.0X5	T49.0X6
nonmedicinal, vapor	T53.6X1	T53.6X2	T53.6X3	T53.6X4	—	—
Gamma-BHC (medicinal) — *see also* Gamma-benzene hexachloride	T49.0X1	T49.0X2	T49.0X3	T49.0X4	T49.0X5	T49.0X6
Gamma globulin	T50.Z11	T50.Z12	T50.Z13	T50.Z14	T50.Z15	T50.Z16
Gamulin	T50.Z11	T50.Z12	T50.Z13	T50.Z14	T50.Z15	T50.Z16
Ganciclovir (sodium)	T37.5X1	T37.5X2	T37.5X3	T37.5X4	T37.5X5	T37.5X6
Ganglionic blocking drug NEC	T44.2X1	T44.2X2	T44.2X3	T44.2X4	T44.2X5	T44.2X6
specified NEC	T44.2X1	T44.2X2	T44.2X3	T44.2X4	T44.2X5	T44.2X6
Ganja	T40.7X1	T40.7X2	T40.7X3	T40.7X4	T40.7X5	T40.7X6
Garamycin	T36.5X1	T36.5X2	T36.5X3	T36.5X4	T36.5X5	T36.5X6
ophthalmic preparation	T49.5X1	T49.5X2	T49.5X3	T49.5X4	T49.5X5	T49.5X6
topical NEC	T49.0X1	T49.0X2	T49.0X3	T49.0X4	T49.0X5	T49.0X6
Gardenal	T42.3X1	T42.3X2	T42.3X3	T42.3X4	T42.3X5	T42.3X6
Gardepanyl	T42.3X1	T42.3X2	T42.3X3	T42.3X4	T42.3X5	T42.3X6
Gaseous substance — *see* Gas						
Gasoline	T52.0X1	T52.0X2	T52.0X3	T52.0X4	—	—
vapor	T52.0X1	T52.0X2	T52.0X3	T52.0X4	—	—
Gastric enzymes	T47.5X1	T47.5X2	T47.5X3	T47.5X4	T47.5X5	T47.5X6
Gastrografin	T50.8X1	T50.8X2	T50.8X3	T50.8X4	T50.8X5	T50.8X6
Gastrointestinal drug	T47.91	T47.92	T47.93	T47.94	T47.95	T47.96
biological	T47.8X1	T47.8X2	T47.8X3	T47.8X4	T47.8X5	T47.8X6
specified NEC	T47.8X1	T47.8X2	T47.8X3	T47.8X4	T47.8X5	T47.8X6
Gas NEC	T59.91	T59.92	T59.93	T59.94	—	—
acetylene	T59.891	T59.892	T59.893	T59.894	—	—
incomplete combustion of	T58.11	T58.12	T58.13	T58.14	—	—
air contaminants, source or type not specified	T59.91	T59.92	T59.93	T59.94	—	—
anesthetic	T41.0X1	T41.0X2	T41.0X3	T41.0X4	T41.0X5	T41.0X6
blast furnace	T58.8X1	T58.8X2	T58.8X3	T58.8X4	—	—
butane — *see* butane						
carbon monoxide — *see* Carbon, monoxide						
chlorine	T59.4X1	T59.4X2	T59.4X3	T59.4X4	—	—
coal	T58.2X1	T58.2X2	T58.2X3	T58.2X4	—	—
cyanide	T57.3X1	T57.3X2	T57.3X3	T57.3X4	—	—
dicyanogen	T65.0X1	T65.0X2	T65.0X3	T65.0X4	—	—
domestic — *see* Domestic gas						
exhaust	T58.01	T58.02	T58.03	T58.04	—	—
from utility (for cooking, heating, or lighting) (after combustion) — *see* Carbon, monoxide, fuel, utility						
prior to combustion	T59.891	T59.892	T59.893	T59.894	—	—
from wood- or coal-burning stove or fireplace	T58.2X1	T58.2X2	T58.2X3	T58.2X4	—	—
fuel (domestic use) (after combustion) — *see also* Carbon, monoxide, fuel						
industrial use	T58.8X1	T58.8X2	T58.8X3	T58.8X4	—	—
prior to combustion	T59.891	T59.892	T59.893	T59.894	—	—
utility	T59.891	T59.892	T59.893	T59.894	—	—
incomplete combustion of — *see* Carbon, monoxide, fuel, utility						
in mobile container	T59.891	T59.892	T59.893	T59.894	—	—
piped (natural)	T59.891	T59.892	T59.893	T59.894	—	—
garage	T58.01	T58.02	T58.03	T58.04	—	—
hydrocarbon NEC	T59.891	T59.892	T59.893	T59.894	—	—
incomplete combustion of — *see* Carbon, monoxide, fuel, utility						
liquefied — *see* butane						
piped	T59.891	T59.892	T59.893	T59.894	—	—
hydrocyanic acid	T65.0X1	T65.0X2	T65.0X3	T65.0X4	—	—
illuminating (after combustion)	T58.11	T58.12	T58.13	T58.14	—	—
prior to combustion	T59.891	T59.892	T59.893	T59.894	—	—
incomplete combustion, any — *see* Carbon, monoxide						
kiln	T58.8X1	T58.8X2	T58.8X3	T58.8X4	—	—
lacrimogenic	T59.3X1	T59.3X2	T59.3X3	T59.3X4	—	—

Substance	Poisoning, Accidental (unintentional)	Poisoning, Intentional Self-harm	Poisoning, Assault	Poisoning, Undetermined	Adverse Effect	Under-dosing
Gas — *continued*						
liquefied petroleum — *see* butane						
marsh	T59.891	T59.892	T59.893	T59.894	—	—
motor exhaust, not in transit	T58.01	T58.02	T58.03	T58.04	—	—
mustard, not in war	T59.891	T59.892	T59.893	T59.894	—	—
natural	T59.891	T59.892	T59.893	T59.894	—	—
nerve, not in war	T59.91	T59.92	T59.93	T59.94	—	—
oil	T52.0X1	T52.0X2	T52.0X3	T52.0X4	—	—
petroleum (liquefied) (distributed in mobile containers)	T59.891	T59.892	T59.893	T59.894	—	—
piped (pure or mixed with air)	T59.891	T59.892	T59.893	T59.894	—	—
piped (manufactured) (natural) NEC	T59.891	T59.892	T59.893	T59.894	—	—
producer	T58.8X1	T58.8X2	T58.8X3	T58.8X4	—	—
propane — *see* propane						
refrigerant (chlorofluoro-carbon)	T53.5X1	T53.5X2	T53.5X3	T53.5X4	—	—
not chlorofluoro-carbon	T59.891	T59.892	T59.893	T59.894	—	—
sewer	T59.91	T59.92	T59.93	T59.94	—	—
specified source NEC	T59.91	T59.92	T59.93	T59.94	—	—
stove (after combustion)	T58.11	T58.12	T58.13	T58.14	—	—
prior to combustion	T59.891	T59.892	T59.893	T59.894	—	—
tear	T59.3X1	T59.3X2	T59.3X3	T59.3X4	—	—
therapeutic	T41.5X1	T41.5X2	T41.5X3	T41.5X4	T41.5X5	T41.5X6
utility (for cooking, heating, or lighting) (piped) NEC	T59.891	T59.892	T59.893	T59.894	—	—
incomplete combustion of — *see* Carbon, monoxide, fuel, utilty						
in mobile container	T59.891	T59.892	T59.893	T59.894	—	—
piped (natural)	T59.891	T59.892	T59.893	T59.894	—	—
water	T58.11	T58.12	T58.13	T58.14	—	—
incomplete combustion of — *see* Carbon, monoxide, fuel, utility						
Gaultheria procumbens	T62.2X1	T62.2X2	T62.2X3	T62.2X4	—	—
Gefarnate	T44.3X1	T44.3X2	T44.3X3	T44.3X4	T44.3X5	T44.3X6
Gelatin (intravenous)	T45.8X1	T45.8X2	T45.8X3	T45.8X4	T45.8X5	T45.8X6
absorbable (sponge)	T45.7X1	T45.7X2	T45.7X3	T45.7X4	T45.7X5	T45.7X6
Gelfilm	T49.8X1	T49.8X2	T49.8X3	T49.8X4	T49.8X5	T49.8X6
Gelfoam	T45.7X1	T45.7X2	T45.7X3	T45.7X4	T45.7X5	T45.7X6
Gelsemine	T50.991	T50.992	T50.993	T50.994	T50.995	T50.996
Gelsemium (sempervirens)	T62.2X1	T62.2X2	T62.2X3	T62.2X4	—	—
Gemeprost	T48.0X1	T48.0X2	T48.0X3	T48.0X4	T48.0X5	T48.0X6
Gemfibrozil	T46.6X1	T46.6X2	T46.6X3	T46.6X4	T46.6X5	T46.6X6
Gemonil	T42.3X1	T42.3X2	T42.3X3	T42.3X4	T42.3X5	T42.3X6
Gentamicin	T36.5X1	T36.5X2	T36.5X3	T36.5X4	T36.5X5	T36.5X6
ophthalmic preparation	T49.5X1	T49.5X2	T49.5X3	T49.5X4	T49.5X5	T49.5X6
topical NEC	T49.0X1	T49.0X2	T49.0X3	T49.0X4	T49.0X5	T49.0X6
Gentian	T47.5X1	T47.5X2	T47.5X3	T47.5X4	T47.5X5	T47.5X6
violet	T49.0X1	T49.0X2	T49.0X3	T49.0X4	T49.0X5	T49.0X6
Gepefrine	T44.4X1	T44.4X2	T44.4X3	T44.4X4	T44.4X5	T44.4X6
Gestonorone caproate	T38.5X1	T38.5X2	T38.5X3	T38.5X4	T38.5X5	T38.5X6
Gexane	T49.0X1	T49.0X2	T49.0X3	T49.0X4	T49.0X5	T49.0X6
Gila monster (venom)	T63.111	T63.112	T63.113	T63.114	—	—
Ginger	T47.5X1	T47.5X2	T47.5X3	T47.5X4	T47.5X5	T47.5X6
Jamaica — *see* Jamaica, ginger						
Gitalin	T46.0X1	T46.0X2	T46.0X3	T46.0X4	T46.0X5	T46.0X6
amorphous	T46.0X1	T46.0X2	T46.0X3	T46.0X4	T46.0X5	T46.0X6
Gitaloxin	T46.0X1	T46.0X2	T46.0X3	T46.0X4	T46.0X5	T46.0X6
Gitoxin	T46.0X1	T46.0X2	T46.0X3	T46.0X4	T46.0X5	T46.0X6
Glafenine	T39.8X1	T39.8X2	T39.8X3	T39.8X4	T39.8X5	T39.8X6
Glandular extract (medicinal) **NEC**	T50.Z91	T50.Z92	T50.Z93	T50.Z94	T50.Z95	T50.Z96
Glaucarubin	T37.3X1	T37.3X2	T37.3X3	T37.3X4	T37.3X5	T37.3X6
Glibenclamide	T38.3X1	T38.3X2	T38.3X3	T38.3X4	T38.3X5	T38.3X6
Glibornuride	T38.3X1	T38.3X2	T38.3X3	T38.3X4	T38.3X5	T38.3X6
Gliclazide	T38.3X1	T38.3X2	T38.3X3	T38.3X4	T38.3X5	T38.3X6
Glimidine	T38.3X1	T38.3X2	T38.3X3	T38.3X4	T38.3X5	T38.3X6
Glipizide	T38.3X1	T38.3X2	T38.3X3	T38.3X4	T38.3X5	T38.3X6
Gliquidone	T38.3X1	T38.3X2	T38.3X3	T38.3X4	T38.3X5	T38.3X6
Glisolamide	T38.3X1	T38.3X2	T38.3X3	T38.3X4	T38.3X5	T38.3X6
Glisoxepide	T38.3X1	T38.3X2	T38.3X3	T38.3X4	T38.3X5	T38.3X6
Globin zinc insulin	T38.3X1	T38.3X2	T38.3X3	T38.3X4	T38.3X5	T38.3X6
Globulin						
antilymphocytic	T50.Z11	T50.Z12	T50.Z13	T50.Z14	T50.Z15	T50.Z16
antirhesus	T50.Z11	T50.Z12	T50.Z13	T50.Z14	T50.Z15	T50.Z16
antivenin	T50.Z11	T50.Z12	T50.Z13	T50.Z14	T50.Z15	T50.Z16
antiviral	T50.Z11	T50.Z12	T50.Z13	T50.Z14	T50.Z15	T50.Z16

Gallamine — Globulin

Substance	Poisoning, Accidental (unintentional)	Poisoning, Intentional Self-harm	Poisoning, Assault	Poisoning, Undetermined	Adverse Effect	Under-dosing
Glucagon	T38.3X1	T38.3X2	T38.3X3	T38.3X4	T38.3X5	T38.3X6
Glucocorticoids	T38.0X1	T38.0X2	T38.0X3	T38.0X4	T38.0X5	T38.0X6
Glucocorticosteroid	T38.0X1	T38.0X2	T38.0X3	T38.0X4	T38.0X5	T38.0X6
Gluconic acid	T50.991	T50.992	T50.993	T50.994	T50.995	T50.996
Glucosamine sulfate	T39.4X1	T39.4X2	T39.4X3	T39.4X4	T39.4X5	T39.4X6
Glucose	T50.3X1	T50.3X2	T50.3X3	T50.3X4	T50.3X5	T50.3X6
with sodium chloride	T50.3X1	T50.3X2	T50.3X3	T50.3X4	T50.3X5	T50.3X6
Glucosulfone sodium	T37.1X1	T37.1X2	T37.1X3	T37.1X4	T37.1X5	T37.1X6
Glucurolactone	T47.8X1	T47.8X2	T47.8X3	T47.8X4	T47.8X5	T47.8X6
Glue NEC	T52.8X1	T52.8X2	T52.8X3	T52.8X4	—	—
Glutamic acid	T47.5X1	T47.5X2	T47.5X3	T47.5X4	T47.5X5	T47.5X6
Glutaral (medicinal)	T49.0X1	T49.0X2	T49.0X3	T49.0X4	T49.0X5	T49.0X6
nonmedicinal	T65.891	T65.892	T65.893	T65.894	—	—
Glutaraldehyde (nonmedicinal)	T65.891	T65.892	T65.893	T65.894	—	—
medicinal	T49.0X1	T49.0X2	T49.0X3	T49.0X4	T49.0X5	T49.0X6
Glutathione	T50.6X1	T50.6X2	T50.6X3	T50.6X4	T50.6X5	T50.6X6
Glutethimide	T42.6X1	T42.6X2	T42.6X3	T42.6X4	T42.6X5	T42.6X6
Glyburide	T38.3X1	T38.3X2	T38.3X3	T38.3X4	T38.3X5	T38.3X6
Glycerin	T47.4X1	T47.4X2	T47.4X3	T47.4X4	T47.4X5	T47.4X6
Glycerol	T47.4X1	T47.4X2	T47.4X3	T47.4X4	T47.4X5	T47.4X6
borax	T49.6X1	T49.6X2	T49.6X3	T49.6X4	T49.6X5	T49.6X6
intravenous	T50.3X1	T50.3X2	T50.3X3	T50.3X4	T50.3X5	T50.3X6
iodinated	T48.4X1	T48.4X2	T48.4X3	T48.4X4	T48.4X5	T48.4X6
Glycerophosphate	T50.991	T50.992	T50.993	T50.994	T50.995	T50.996
Glyceryl						
gualacolate	T48.4X1	T48.4X2	T48.4X3	T48.4X4	T48.4X5	T48.4X6
nitrate	T46.3X1	T46.3X2	T46.3X3	T46.3X4	T46.3X5	T46.3X6
triacetate (topical)	T49.0X1	T49.0X2	T49.0X3	T49.0X4	T49.0X5	T49.0X6
trinitrate	T46.3X1	T46.3X2	T46.3X3	T46.3X4	T46.3X5	T46.3X6
Glycine	T50.3X1	T50.3X2	T50.3X3	T50.3X4	T50.3X5	T50.3X6
Glyclopyramide	T38.3X1	T38.3X2	T38.3X3	T38.3X4	T38.3X5	T38.3X6
Glycobiarsol	T37.3X1	T37.3X2	T37.3X3	T37.3X4	T37.3X5	T37.3X6
Glycols (ether)	T52.3X1	T52.3X2	T52.3X3	T52.3X4	—	—
Glyconiazide	T37.1X1	T37.1X2	T37.1X3	T37.1X4	T37.1X5	T37.1X6
Glycopyrrolate	T44.3X1	T44.3X2	T44.3X3	T44.3X4	T44.3X5	T44.3X6
Glycopyrronium	T44.3X1	T44.3X2	T44.3X3	T44.3X4	T44.3X5	T44.3X6
bromide	T44.3X1	T44.3X2	T44.3X3	T44.3X4	T44.3X5	T44.3X6
Glycoside, cardiac (stimulant)	T46.0X1	T46.0X2	T46.0X3	T46.0X4	T46.0X5	T46.0X6
Glycyclamide	T38.3X1	T38.3X2	T38.3X3	T38.3X4	T38.3X5	T38.3X6
Glycyrrhiza extract	T48.4X1	T48.4X2	T48.4X3	T48.4X4	T48.4X5	T48.4X6
Glycyrrhizic acid	T48.4X1	T48.4X2	T48.4X3	T48.4X4	T48.4X5	T48.4X6
Glycyrrhizinate potassium	T48.4X1	T48.4X2	T48.4X3	T48.4X4	T48.4X5	T48.4X6
Glymidine sodium	T38.3X1	T38.3X2	T38.3X3	T38.3X4	T38.3X5	T38.3X6
Glyphosate	T60.3X1	T60.3X2	T60.3X3	T60.3X4	—	—
Glyphylline	T48.6X1	T48.6X2	T48.6X3	T48.6X4	T48.6X5	T48.6X6
Gold						
colloidal (l98Au)	T45.1X1	T45.1X2	T45.1X3	T45.1X4	T45.1X5	T45.1X6
salts	T39.4X1	T39.4X2	T39.4X3	T39.4X4	T39.4X5	T39.4X6
Golden sulfide of antimony	T56.891	T56.892	T56.893	T56.894	—	—
Goldylocks	T62.2X1	T62.2X2	T62.2X3	T62.2X4	—	—
Gonadal tissue extract	T38.901	T38.902	T38.903	T38.904	T38.905	T38.906
female	T38.5X1	T38.5X2	T38.5X3	T38.5X4	T38.5X5	T38.5X6
male	T38.7X1	T38.7X2	T38.7X3	T38.7X4	T38.7X5	T38.7X6
Gonadorelin	T38.891	T38.892	T38.893	T38.894	T38.895	T38.896
Gonadotropin	T38.891	T38.892	T38.893	T38.894	T38.895	T38.896
chorionic	T38.891	T38.892	T38.893	T38.894	T38.895	T38.896
pituitary	T38.811	T38.812	T38.813	T38.814	T38.815	T38.816
Goserelin	T45.1X1	T45.1X2	T45.1X3	T45.1X4	T45.1X5	T45.1X6
Grain alcohol	T51.0X1	T51.0X2	T51.0X3	T51.0X4	—	—
Gramicidin	T49.0X1	T49.0X2	T49.0X3	T49.0X4	T49.0X5	T49.0X6
Granisetron	T45.0X1	T45.0X2	T45.0X3	T45.0X4	T45.0X5	T45.0X6
Gratiola officinalis	T62.2X1	T62.2X2	T62.2X3	T62.2X4	—	—
Grease	T65.891	T65.892	T65.893	T65.894	—	—
Green hellebore	T62.2X1	T62.2X2	T62.2X3	T62.2X4	—	—
Green soap	T49.2X1	T49.2X2	T49.2X3	T49.2X4	T49.2X5	T49.2X6
Grifulvin	T36.7X1	T36.7X2	T36.7X3	T36.7X4	T36.7X5	T36.7X6
Griseofulvin	T36.7X1	T36.7X2	T36.7X3	T36.7X4	T36.7X5	T36.7X6
Growth hormone	T38.811	T38.812	T38.813	T38.814	T38.815	T38.816
Guaiacol derivatives	T48.4X1	T48.4X2	T48.4X3	T48.4X4	T48.4X5	T48.4X6
Guaiac reagent	T50.991	T50.992	T50.993	T50.994	T50.995	T50.996
Guaifenesin	T48.4X1	T48.4X2	T48.4X3	T48.4X4	T48.4X5	T48.4X6
Guaimesal	T48.4X1	T48.4X2	T48.4X3	T48.4X4	T48.4X5	T48.4X6
Guaiphenesin	T48.4X1	T48.4X2	T48.4X3	T48.4X4	T48.4X5	T48.4X6
Guamecycline	T36.4X1	T36.4X2	T36.4X3	T36.4X4	T36.4X5	T36.4X6
Guanabenz	T46.5X1	T46.5X2	T46.5X3	T46.5X4	T46.5X5	T46.5X6
Guanacline	T46.5X1	T46.5X2	T46.5X3	T46.5X4	T46.5X5	T46.5X6
Guanadrel	T46.5X1	T46.5X2	T46.5X3	T46.5X4	T46.5X5	T46.5X6
Guanatol	T37.2X1	T37.2X2	T37.2X3	T37.2X4	T37.2X5	T37.2X6
Guanethidine	T46.5X1	T46.5X2	T46.5X3	T46.5X4	T46.5X5	T46.5X6
Guanfacine	T46.5X1	T46.5X2	T46.5X3	T46.5X4	T46.5X5	T46.5X6
Guano	T65.891	T65.892	T65.893	T65.894	—	—

Substance	Poisoning, Accidental (unintentional)	Poisoning, Intentional Self-harm	Poisoning, Assault	Poisoning, Undetermined	Adverse Effect	Under-dosing
Guanochlor	T46.5X1	T46.5X2	T46.5X3	T46.5X4	T46.5X5	T46.5X6
Guanoclor	T46.5X1	T46.5X2	T46.5X3	T46.5X4	T46.5X5	T46.5X6
Guanoctine	T46.5X1	T46.5X2	T46.5X3	T46.5X4	T46.5X5	T46.5X6
Guanoxabenz	T46.5X1	T46.5X2	T46.5X3	T46.5X4	T46.5X5	T46.5X6
Guanoxan	T46.5X1	T46.5X2	T46.5X3	T46.5X4	T46.5X5	T46.5X6
Guar gum (medicinal)	T46.6X1	T46.6X2	T46.6X3	T46.6X4	T46.6X5	T46.6X6
Hachimycin	T36.7X1	T36.7X2	T36.7X3	T36.7X4	T36.7X5	T36.7X6
Hair						
dye	T49.4X1	T49.4X2	T49.4X3	T49.4X4	T49.4X5	T49.4X6
preparation NEC	T49.4X1	T49.4X2	T49.4X3	T49.4X4	T49.4X5	T49.4X6
Halazepam	T42.4X1	T42.4X2	T42.4X3	T42.4X4	T42.4X5	T42.4X6
Halcinolone	T49.0X1	T49.0X2	T49.0X3	T49.0X4	T49.0X5	T49.0X6
Halcinonide	T49.0X1	T49.0X2	T49.0X3	T49.0X4	T49.0X5	T49.0X6
Halethazole	T49.0X1	T49.0X2	T49.0X3	T49.0X4	T49.0X5	T49.0X6
Hallucinogen NEC	T40.901	T40.902	T40.903	T40.904	T40.905	T40.906
Halofantrine	T37.2X1	T37.2X2	T37.2X3	T37.2X4	T37.2X5	T37.2X6
Halofenate	T46.6X1	T46.6X2	T46.6X3	T46.6X4	T46.6X5	T46.6X6
Halometasone	T49.0X1	T49.0X2	T49.0X3	T49.0X4	T49.0X5	T49.0X6
Haloperidol	T43.4X1	T43.4X2	T43.4X3	T43.4X4	T43.4X5	T43.4X6
Haloprogin	T49.0X1	T49.0X2	T49.0X3	T49.0X4	T49.0X5	T49.0X6
Halotex	T49.0X1	T49.0X2	T49.0X3	T49.0X4	T49.0X5	T49.0X6
Halothane	T41.0X1	T41.0X2	T41.0X3	T41.0X4	T41.0X5	T41.0X6
Haloxazolam	T42.4X1	T42.4X2	T42.4X3	T42.4X4	T42.4X5	T42.4X6
Halquinols	T49.0X1	T49.0X2	T49.0X3	T49.0X4	T49.0X5	T49.0X6
Hamamelis	T49.2X1	T49.2X2	T49.2X3	T49.2X4	T49.2X5	T49.2X6
Haptendextran	T45.8X1	T45.8X2	T45.8X3	T45.8X4	T45.8X5	T45.8X6
Harmonyl	T46.5X1	T46.5X2	T46.5X3	T46.5X4	T46.5X5	T46.5X6
Hartmann's solution	T50.3X1	T50.3X2	T50.3X3	T50.3X4	T50.3X5	T50.3X6
Hashish	T40.7X1	T40.7X2	T40.7X3	T40.7X4	T40.7X5	T40.7X6
Hawaiian Woodrose seeds	T40.991	T40.992	T40.993	T40.994	—	—
HCB	T60.3X1	T60.3X2	T60.3X3	T60.3X4	—	—
HCH	T53.6X1	T53.6X2	T53.6X3	T53.6X4	—	—
medicinal	T49.0X1	T49.0X2	T49.0X3	T49.0X4	T49.0X5	T49.0X6
HCN	T57.3X1	T57.3X2	T57.3X3	T57.3X4	—	—
Headache cures, drugs, powders NEC	T50.901	T50.902	T50.903	T50.904	T50.905	T50.906
Heavenly Blue (morning glory)	T40.991	T40.992	T40.993	T40.994	—	—
Heavy metal antidote	T45.8X1	T45.8X2	T45.8X3	T45.8X4	T45.8X5	T45.8X6
Hedaquinium	T49.0X1	T49.0X2	T49.0X3	T49.0X4	T49.0X5	T49.0X6
Hedge hyssop	T62.2X1	T62.2X2	T62.2X3	T62.2X4	—	—
Heet	T49.8X1	T49.8X2	T49.8X3	T49.8X4	T49.8X5	T49.8X6
Helenin	T37.4X1	T37.4X2	T37.4X3	T37.4X4	T37.4X5	T37.4X6
Helium (nonmedicinal) NEC	T59.891	T59.892	T59.893	T59.894	—	—
medicinal	T48.991	T48.992	T48.993	T48.994	T48.995	T48.996
Hellebore (black) (green) (white)	T62.2X1	T62.2X2	T62.2X3	T62.2X4	—	—
Hematin	T45.8X1	T45.8X2	T45.8X3	T45.8X4	T45.8X5	T45.8X6
Hematinic preparation	T45.8X1	T45.8X2	T45.8X3	T45.8X4	T45.8X5	T45.8X6
Hematological agent	T45.91	T45.92	T45.93	T45.94	T45.95	T45.96
specified NEC	T45.8X1	T45.8X2	T45.8X3	T45.8X4	T45.8X5	T45.8X6
Hemlock	T62.2X1	T62.2X2	T62.2X3	T62.2X4	—	—
Hemostatic	T45.621	T45.622	T45.623	T45.624	T45.625	T45.626
drug, systemic	T45.621	T45.622	T45.623	T45.624	T45.625	T45.626
Hemostyptic	T49.4X1	T49.4X2	T49.4X3	T49.4X4	T49.4X5	T49.4X6
Henbane	T62.2X1	T62.2X2	T62.2X3	T62.2X4	—	—
Heparin (sodium)	T45.511	T45.512	T45.513	T45.514	T45.515	T45.516
action reverser	T45.7X1	T45.7X2	T45.7X3	T45.7X4	T45.7X5	T45.7X6
Heparin-fraction	T45.511	T45.512	T45.513	T45.514	T45.515	T45.516
Heparinoid (systemic)	T45.511	T45.512	T45.513	T45.514	T45.515	T45.516
Hepatic secretion stimulant	T47.8X1	T47.8X2	T47.8X3	T47.8X4	T47.8X5	T47.8X6
Hepatitis B						
immune globulin	T50.Z11	T50.Z12	T50.Z13	T50.Z14	T50.Z15	T50.Z16
vaccine	T50.B91	T50.B92	T50.B93	T50.B94	T50.B95	T50.B96
Hepronicate	T46.7X1	T46.7X2	T46.7X3	T46.7X4	T46.7X5	T46.7X6
Heptabarb	T42.3X1	T42.3X2	T42.3X3	T42.3X4	T42.3X5	T42.3X6
Heptabarbital	T42.3X1	T42.3X2	T42.3X3	T42.3X4	T42.3X5	T42.3X6
Heptabarbitone	T42.3X1	T42.3X2	T42.3X3	T42.3X4	T42.3X5	T42.3X6
Heptachlor	T60.1X1	T60.1X2	T60.1X3	T60.1X4	—	—
Heptalgin	T40.2X1	T40.2X2	T40.2X3	T40.2X4	T40.2X5	T40.2X6
Heptaminol	T46.3X1	T46.3X2	T46.3X3	T46.3X4	T46.3X5	T46.3X6
Herbicide NEC	T60.3X1	T60.3X2	T60.3X3	T60.3X4	—	—
Heroin	T40.1X1	T40.1X2	T40.1X3	T40.1X4	—	—
Herplex	T49.5X1	T49.5X2	T49.5X3	T49.5X4	T49.5X5	T49.5X6
HES	T45.8X1	T45.8X2	T45.8X3	T45.8X4	T45.8X5	T45.8X6
Hesperidin	T46.991	T46.992	T46.993	T46.994	T46.995	T46.996
Hetacillin	T36.0X1	T36.0X2	T36.0X3	T36.0X4	T36.0X5	T36.0X6
Hetastarch	T45.8X1	T45.8X2	T45.8X3	T45.8X4	T45.8X5	T45.8X6
HETP	T60.0X1	T60.0X2	T60.0X3	T60.0X4	—	—
Hexachlorobenzene (vapor)	T60.3X1	T60.3X2	T60.3X3	T60.3X4	—	—
Hexachlorocyclohexane	T53.6X1	T53.6X2	T53.6X3	T53.6X4	—	—
Hexachlorophene	T49.0X1	T49.0X2	T49.0X3	T49.0X4	T49.0X5	T49.0X6

Substance	Poisoning, Accidental (unintentional)	Poisoning, Intentional Self-harm	Poisoning, Assault	Poisoning, Undetermined	Adverse Effect	Under-dosing
Hexadiline	T46.3X1	T46.3X2	T46.3X3	T46.3X4	T46.3X5	T46.3X6
Hexadimethrine (bromide)	T45.7X1	T45.7X2	T45.7X3	T45.7X4	T45.7X5	T45.7X6
Hexadylamine	T46.3X1	T46.3X2	T46.3X3	T46.3X4	T46.3X5	T46.3X6
Hexaethyl tetraphosphate	T60.0X1	T60.0X2	T60.0X3	T60.0X4	—	—
Hexafluorenium bromide	T48.1X1	T48.1X2	T48.1X3	T48.1X4	T48.1X5	T48.1X6
Hexafluronium (bromide)	T48.1X1	T48.1X2	T48.1X3	T48.1X4	T48.1X5	T48.1X6
Hexa-germ	T49.2X1	T49.2X2	T49.2X3	T49.2X4	T49.2X5	T49.2X6
Hexahydrobenzol	T52.8X1	T52.8X2	T52.8X3	T52.8X4	—	—
Hexahydrocresol(s)	T51.8X1	T51.8X2	T51.8X3	T51.8X4	—	—
arsenide	T57.0X1	T57.0X2	T57.0X3	T57.0X4	—	—
arseniurated	T57.0X1	T57.0X2	T57.0X3	T57.0X4	—	—
cyanide	T57.3X1	T57.3X2	T57.3X3	T57.3X4	—	—
gas	T59.891	T59.892	T59.893	T59.894	—	—
Fluoride (liquid)	T57.8X1	T57.8X2	T57.8X3	T57.8X4	—	—
vapor	T59.891	T59.892	T59.893	T59.894	—	—
phophorated	T60.0X1	T60.0X2	T60.0X3	T60.0X4	—	—
sulfate	T57.8X1	T57.8X2	T57.8X3	T57.8X4	—	—
sulfide (gas)	T59.6X1	T59.6X2	T59.6X3	T59.6X4	—	—
arseniurated	T57.0X1	T57.0X2	T57.0X3	T57.0X4	—	—
sulfurated	T57.8X1	T57.8X2	T57.8X3	T57.8X4	—	—
Hexahydrophenol	T51.8X1	T51.8X2	T51.8X3	T51.8X4	—	—
Hexalen	T51.8X1	T51.8X2	T51.8X3	T51.8X4	—	—
Hexamethonium bromide	T44.2X1	T44.2X2	T44.2X3	T44.2X4	T44.2X5	T44.2X6
Hexamethylene	T52.8X1	T52.8X2	T52.8X3	T52.8X4	—	—
Hexamethylmelamine	T45.1X1	T45.1X2	T45.1X3	T45.1X4	T45.1X5	T45.1X6
Hexamidine	T49.0X1	T49.0X2	T49.0X3	T49.0X4	T49.0X5	T49.0X6
Hexamine (mandelate)	T37.8X1	T37.8X2	T37.8X3	T37.8X4	T37.8X5	T37.8X6
Hexanone, 2-hexanone	T52.4X1	T52.4X2	T52.4X3	T52.4X4	—	—
Hexanuorenium	T48.1X1	T48.1X2	T48.1X3	T48.1X4	T48.1X5	T48.1X6
Hexapropymate	T42.6X1	T42.6X2	T42.6X3	T42.6X4	T42.6X5	T42.6X6
Hexasonium iodide	T44.3X1	T44.3X2	T44.3X3	T44.3X4	T44.3X5	T44.3X6
Hexcarbacholine bromide	T48.1X1	T48.1X2	T48.1X3	T48.1X4	T48.1X5	T48.1X6
Hexemal	T42.3X1	T42.3X2	T42.3X3	T42.3X4	T42.3X5	T42.3X6
Hexestrol	T38.5X1	T38.5X2	T38.5X3	T38.5X4	T38.5X5	T38.5X6
Hexethal (sodium)	T42.3X1	T42.3X2	T42.3X3	T42.3X4	T42.3X5	T42.3X6
Hexetidine	T37.8X1	T37.8X2	T37.8X3	T37.8X4	T37.8X5	T37.8X6
Hexobarbital	T42.3X1	T42.3X2	T42.3X3	T42.3X4	T42.3X5	T42.3X6
rectal	T41.291	T41.292	T41.293	T41.294	T41.295	T41.296
sodium	T41.1X1	T41.1X2	T41.1X3	T41.1X4	T41.1X5	T41.1X6
Hexobendine	T46.3X1	T46.3X2	T46.3X3	T46.3X4	T46.3X5	T46.3X6
Hexocyclium	T44.3X1	T44.3X2	T44.3X3	T44.3X4	T44.3X5	T44.3X6
metilsulfate	T44.3X1	T44.3X2	T44.3X3	T44.3X4	T44.3X5	T44.3X6
Hexoestrol	T38.5X1	T38.5X2	T38.5X3	T38.5X4	T38.5X5	T38.5X6
Hexone	T52.4X1	T52.4X2	T52.4X3	T52.4X4	—	—
Hexoprenaline	T48.6X1	T48.6X2	T48.6X3	T48.6X4	T48.6X5	T48.6X6
Hexylcaine	T41.3X1	T41.3X2	T41.3X3	T41.3X4	T41.3X5	T41.3X6
Hexylresorcinol	T52.2X1	T52.2X2	T52.2X3	T52.2X4	—	—
HGH (human growth hormone)	T38.811	T38.812		T38.814	T38.815	T38.816
Hinkle's pills	T47.2X1	T47.2X2	T47.2X3	T47.2X4	T47.2X5	T47.2X6
Histalog	T50.8X1	T50.8X2	T50.8X3	T50.8X4	T50.8X5	T50.8X6
Histamine (phosphate)	T50.8X1	T50.8X2	T50.8X3	T50.8X4	T50.8X5	T50.8X6
Histoplasmin	T50.8X1	T50.8X2	T50.8X3	T50.8X4	T50.8X5	T50.8X6
Holly berries	T62.2X1	T62.2X2	T62.2X3	T62.2X4	—	—
Homatropine	T44.3X1	T44.3X2	T44.3X3	T44.3X4	T44.3X5	T44.3X6
methylbromide	T44.3X1	T44.3X2	T44.3X3	T44.3X4	T44.3X5	T44.3X6
Homochlorcyclizine	T45.0X1	T45.0X2	T45.0X3	T45.0X4	T45.0X5	T45.0X6
Homosalate	T49.3X1	T49.3X2	T49.3X3	T49.3X4	T49.3X5	T49.3X6
Homo-tet	T50.Z11	T50.Z12	T50.Z13	T50.Z14	T50.Z15	T50.Z16
Hormone	T38.801	T38.802	T38.803	T38.804	T38.805	T38.806
adrenal cortical steroids	T38.0X1	T38.0X2	T38.0X3	T38.0X4	T38.0X5	T38.0X6
androgenic	T38.7X1	T38.7X2	T38.7X3	T38.7X4	T38.7X5	T38.7X6
anterior pituitary NEC	T38.811	T38.812	T38.813	T38.814	T38.815	T38.816
antidiabetic agents	T38.3X1	T38.3X2	T38.3X3	T38.3X4	T38.3X5	T38.3X6
antidiuretic	T38.891	T38.892	T38.893	T38.894	T38.895	T38.896
cancer therapy	T45.1X1	T45.1X2	T45.1X3	T45.1X4	T45.1X5	T45.1X6
follicle stimulating	T38.811	T38.812	T38.813	T38.814	T38.815	T38.816
gonadotropic	T38.891	T38.892	T38.893	T38.894	T38.895	T38.896
pituitary	T38.811	T38.812	T38.813	T38.814	T38.815	T38.816
growth	T38.811	T38.812	T38.813	T38.814	T38.815	T38.816
luteinizing	T38.811	T38.812	T38.813	T38.814	T38.815	T38.816
ovarian	T38.5X1	T38.5X2	T38.5X3	T38.5X4	T38.5X5	T38.5X6
oxytocic	T48.0X1	T48.0X2	T48.0X3	T48.0X4	T48.0X5	T48.0X6
parathyroid (derivatives)	T50.991	T50.992	T50.993	T50.994	T50.995	T50.996
pituitary (posterior) NEC	T38.891	T38.892	T38.893	T38.894	T38.895	T38.896
anterior	T38.811	T38.812	T38.813	T38.814	T38.815	T38.816
specified, NEC	T38.891	T38.892	T38.893	T38.894	T38.895	T38.896
thyroid	T38.1X1	T38.1X2	T38.1X3	T38.1X4	T38.1X5	T38.1X6
Hornet (sting)	T63.451	T63.452	T63.453	T63.454	—	—
Horse anti-human lymphocytic serum	T50.Z11	T50.Z12	T50.Z13	T50.Z14	T50.Z15	T50.Z16
Horticulture agent NEC	T65.91	T65.92	T65.93	T65.94	—	—
with pesticide	T60.91	T60.92	T60.93	T60.94	—	—
Human						
albumin	T45.8X1	T45.8X2	T45.8X3	T45.8X4	T45.8X5	T45.8X6
growth hormone (HGH)	T38.811	T38.812	T38.813	T38.814	T38.815	T38.816
immune serum	T50.Z11	T50.Z12	T50.Z13	T50.Z14	T50.Z15	T50.Z16
Hyaluronidase	T45.3X1	T45.3X2	T45.3X3	T45.3X4	T45.3X5	T45.3X6
Hyazyme	T45.3X1	T45.3X2	T45.3X3	T45.3X4	T45.3X5	T45.3X6
Hycodan	T40.2X1	T40.2X2	T40.2X3	T40.2X4	T40.2X5	T40.2X6
Hydantoin derivative NEC	T42.0X1	T42.0X2	T42.0X3	T42.0X4	T42.0X5	T42.0X6
Hydeltra	T38.0X1	T38.0X2	T38.0X3	T38.0X4	T38.0X5	T38.0X6
Hydergine	T44.6X1	T44.6X2	T44.6X3	T44.6X4	T44.6X5	T44.6X6
Hydrabamine penicillin	T36.0X1	T36.0X2	T36.0X3	T36.0X4	T36.0X5	T36.0X6
Hydralazine	T46.5X1	T46.5X2	T46.5X3	T46.5X4	T46.5X5	T46.5X6
Hydrargaphen	T49.0X1	T49.0X2	T49.0X3	T49.0X4	T49.0X5	T49.0X6
Hydrargyri aminochloridum	T49.0X1	T49.0X2	T49.0X3	T49.0X4	T49.0X5	T49.0X6
Hydrastine	T48.291	T48.292	T48.293	T48.294	T48.295	T48.296
Hydrazine	T54.1X1	T54.1X2	T54.1X3	T54.1X4	—	—
monoamine oxidase inhibitors	T43.1X1	T43.1X2	T43.1X3	T43.1X4	T43.1X5	T43.1X6
Hydrazoic acid, azides	T54.2X1	T54.2X2	T54.2X3	T54.2X4	—	—
Hydriodic acid	T48.4X1	T48.4X2	T48.4X3	T48.4X4	T48.4X5	T48.4X6
Hydrocarbon gas	T59.891	T59.892	T59.893	T59.894		
incomplete combustion of — see Carbon, monoxide, fuel, utility						
liquefied (mobile container)	T59.891	T59.892	T59.893	T59.894	—	—
piped (natural)	T59.891	T59.892	T59.893	T59.894	—	—
Hydrochloric acid (liquid)	T54.2X1	T54.2X2	T54.2X3	T54.2X4	—	—
medicinal (digestant)	T47.5X1	T47.5X2	T47.5X3	T47.5X4	T47.5X5	T47.5X6
vapor	T59.891	T59.892	T59.893	T59.894	—	—
Hydrochlorothiazide	T50.2X1	T50.2X2	T50.2X3	T50.2X4	T50.2X5	T50.2X6
Hydrocodone	T40.2X1	T40.2X2	T40.2X3	T40.2X4	T40.2X5	T40.2X6
Hydrocortisone (derivatives)	T38.0X1	T38.0X2	T38.0X3	T38.0X4	T38.0X5	T38.0X6
aceponate	T49.0X1	T49.0X2	T49.0X3	T49.0X4	T49.0X5	T49.0X6
ENT agent	T49.6X1	T49.6X2	T49.6X3	T49.6X4	T49.6X5	T49.6X6
ophthalmic preparation	T49.5X1	T49.5X2	T49.5X3	T49.5X4	T49.5X5	T49.5X6
topical NEC	T49.0X1	T49.0X2	T49.0X3	T49.0X4	T49.0X5	T49.0X6
Hydrocortone	T38.0X1	T38.0X2	T38.0X3	T38.0X4	T38.0X5	T38.0X6
ENT agent	T49.6X1	T49.6X2	T49.6X3	T49.6X4	T49.6X5	T49.6X6
ophthalmic preparation	T49.5X1	T49.5X2	T49.5X3	T49.5X4	T49.5X5	T49.5X6
topical NEC	T49.0X1	T49.0X2	T49.0X3	T49.0X4	T49.0X5	T49.0X6
Hydrocyanic acid (liquid)	T57.3X1	T57.3X2	T57.3X3	T57.3X4	—	—
gas	T65.0X1	T65.0X2	T65.0X3	T65.0X4	—	—
Hydroflumethiazide	T50.2X1	T50.2X2	T50.2X3	T50.2X4	T50.2X5	T50.2X6
Hydrofluoric acid (liquid)	T54.2X1	T54.2X2	T54.2X3	T54.2X4	—	—
vapor	T59.891	T59.892	T59.893	T59.894	—	—
Hydrogen	T59.891	T59.892	T59.893	T59.894	—	—
arsenide	T57.0X1	T57.0X2	T57.0X3	T57.0X4	—	—
arseniureted	T57.0X1	T57.0X2	T57.0X3	T57.0X4	—	—
chloride	T57.8X1	T57.8X2	T57.8X3	T57.8X4	—	—
cyanide (salts)	T57.3X1	T57.3X2	T57.3X3	T57.3X4	—	—
gas	T57.3X1	T57.3X2	T57.3X3	T57.3X4	—	—
Fluoride	T59.5X1	T59.5X2	T59.5X3	T59.5X4	—	—
vapor	T59.5X1	T59.5X2	T59.5X3	T59.5X4	—	—
peroxide	T49.0X1	T49.0X2	T49.0X3	T49.0X4	T49.0X5	T49.0X6
phosphureted	T57.1X1	T57.1X2	T57.1X3	T57.1X4	—	—
sulfide	T59.6X1	T59.6X2	T59.6X3	T59.6X4	—	—
arseniureted	T57.0X1	T57.0X2	T57.0X3	T57.0X4	—	—
sulfureted	T59.6X1	T59.6X2	T59.6X3	T59.6X4	—	—
Hydromethylpyridine	T46.7X1	T46.7X2	T46.7X3	T46.7X4	T46.7X5	T46.7X6
Hydromorphinol	T40.2X1	T40.2X2	T40.2X3	T40.2X4		
Hydromorphinone	T40.2X1	T40.2X2	T40.2X3	T40.2X4	T40.2X5	T40.2X6
Hydromorphone	T40.2X1	T40.2X2	T40.2X3	T40.2X4	T40.2X5	T40.2X6
Hydromox	T50.2X1	T50.2X2	T50.2X3	T50.2X4	T50.2X5	T50.2X6
Hydrophilic lotion	T49.3X1	T49.3X2	T49.3X3	T49.3X4	T49.3X5	T49.3X6
Hydroquinidine	T46.2X1	T46.2X2	T46.2X3	T46.2X4	T46.2X5	T46.2X6
Hydroquinone	T52.2X1	T52.2X2	T52.2X3	T52.2X4	—	—
vapor	T59.891	T59.892	T59.893	T59.894	—	—
Hydrosulfuric acid (gas)	T59.6X1	T59.6X2	T59.6X3	T59.6X4	—	—
Hydrotalcite	T47.1X1	T47.1X2	T47.1X3	T47.1X4	T47.1X5	T47.1X6
Hydrous wool fat	T49.3X1	T49.3X2	T49.3X3	T49.3X4	T49.3X5	T49.3X6
Hydroxide, caustic	T54.3X1	T54.3X2	T54.3X3	T54.3X4	—	—
Hydroxocobalamin	T45.8X1	T45.8X2	T45.8X3	T45.8X4	T45.8X5	T45.8X6
Hydroxyamphetamine	T49.5X1	T49.5X2	T49.5X3	T49.5X4	T49.5X5	T49.5X6
Hydroxycarbamide	T45.1X1	T45.1X2	T45.1X3	T45.1X4	T45.1X5	T45.1X6
Hydroxychloroquine	T37.8X1	T37.8X2	T37.8X3	T37.8X4	T37.8X5	T37.8X6
Hydroxydihydrocodeinone	T40.2X1	T40.2X2	T40.2X3	T40.2X4	T40.2X5	T40.2X6
Hydroxyestrone	T38.5X1	T38.5X2	T38.5X3	T38.5X4	T38.5X5	T38.5X6
Hydroxyethyl starch	T45.8X1	T45.8X2	T45.8X3	T45.8X4	T45.8X5	T45.8X6
Hydroxymethylpentanone	T52.4X1	T52.4X2	T52.4X3	T52.4X4	—	—
Hydroxyphenamate	T43.591	T43.592	T43.593	T43.594	T43.595	T43.596
Hydroxyphenylbutazone	T39.2X1	T39.2X2	T39.2X3	T39.2X4	T39.2X5	T39.2X6
Hydroxyprogesterone	T38.5X1	T38.5X2	T38.5X3	T38.5X4	T38.5X5	T38.5X6

Additional Character May Be Required — Refer to the Tabular List for Character Selection ▽ **Subterms under main terms may continue to next column or page**

Substance	Poisoning, Accidental (unintentional)	Poisoning, Intentional Self-harm	Poisoning, Assault	Poisoning, Undetermined	Adverse Effect	Under-dosing
Hydroxyprogesterone — *continued*						
caproate	T38.5X1	T38.5X2	T38.5X3	T38.5X4	T38.5X5	T38.5X6
Hydroxyquinoline (derivatives) **NEC**	T37.8X1	T37.8X2	T37.8X3	T37.8X4	T37.8X5	T37.8X6
Hydroxystilbamidine	T37.3X1	T37.3X2	T37.3X3	T37.3X4	T37.3X5	T37.3X6
Hydroxytoluene (nonmedicinal)	T54.0X1	T54.0X2	T54.0X3	T54.0X4	—	—
medicinal	T49.0X1	T49.0X2	T49.0X3	T49.0X4	T49.0X5	T49.0X6
Hydroxyurea	T45.1X1	T45.1X2	T45.1X3	T45.1X4	T45.1X5	T45.1X6
Hydroxyzine	T43.591	T43.592	T43.593	T43.594	T43.595	T43.596
Hyoscine	T44.3X1	T44.3X2	T44.3X3	T44.3X4	T44.3X5	T44.3X6
Hyoscyamine	T44.3X1	T44.3X2	T44.3X3	T44.3X4	T44.3X5	T44.3X6
Hyoscyamus	T44.3X1	T44.3X2	T44.3X3	T44.3X4	T44.3X5	T44.3X6
dry extract	T44.3X1	T44.3X2	T44.3X3	T44.3X4	T44.3X5	T44.3X6
Hypaque	T50.8X1	T50.8X2	T50.8X3	T50.8X4	T50.8X5	T50.8X6
Hypertussis	T50.Z11	T50.Z12	T50.Z13	T50.Z14	T50.Z15	T50.Z16
Hypnotic	T42.71	T42.72	T42.73	T42.74	T42.75	T42.76
anticonvulsant	T42.71	T42.72	T42.73	T42.74	T42.75	T42.76
specified NEC	T42.6X1	T42.6X2	T42.6X3	T42.6X4	T42.6X5	T42.6X6
Hypochlorite	T49.0X1	T49.0X2	T49.0X3	T49.0X4	T49.0X5	T49.0X6
Hypophysis, posterior	T38.891	T38.892	T38.893	T38.894	T38.895	T38.896
Hypotensive NEC	T46.5X1	T46.5X2	T46.5X3	T46.5X4	T46.5X5	T46.5X6
Hypromellose	T49.5X1	T49.5X2	T49.5X3	T49.5X4	T49.5X5	T49.5X6
Ibacitabine	T37.5X1	T37.5X2	T37.5X3	T37.5X4	T37.5X5	T37.5X6
Ibopamine	T44.991	T44.992	T44.993	T44.994	T44.995	T44.996
Ibufenac	T39.311	T39.312	T39.313	T39.314	T39.315	T39.316
Ibuprofen	T39.311	T39.312	T39.313	T39.314	T39.315	T39.316
Ibuproxam	T39.311	T39.312	T39.313	T39.314	T39.315	T39.316
Ibuterol	T48.6X1	T48.6X2	T48.6X3	T48.6X4	T48.6X5	T48.6X6
Ichthammol	T49.0X1	T49.0X2	T49.0X3	T49.0X4	T49.0X5	T49.0X6
Ichthyol	T49.4X1	T49.4X2	T49.4X3	T49.4X4	T49.4X5	T49.4X6
Idarubicin	T45.1X1	T45.1X2	T45.1X3	T45.1X4	T45.1X5	T45.1X6
Idrocilamide	T42.8X1	T42.8X2	T42.8X3	T42.8X4	T42.8X5	T42.8X6
Ifenprodil	T46.7X1	T46.7X2	T46.7X3	T46.7X4	T46.7X5	T46.7X6
Ifosfamide	T45.1X1	T45.1X2	T45.1X3	T45.1X4	T45.1X5	T45.1X6
Iletin	T38.3X1	T38.3X2	T38.3X3	T38.3X4	T38.3X5	T38.3X6
Ilex	T62.2X1	T62.2X2	T62.2X3	T62.2X4	—	—
Illuminating gas (after combustion)	T58.11	T58.12	T58.13	T58.14	—	—
prior to combustion	T59.891	T59.892	T59.893	T59.894	—	—
Ilopan	T45.2X1	T45.2X2	T45.2X3	T45.2X4	T45.2X5	T45.2X6
Iloprost	T46.7X1	T46.7X2	T46.7X3	T46.7X4	T46.7X5	T46.7X6
Ilotycin	T36.3X1	T36.3X2	T36.3X3	T36.3X4	T36.3X5	T36.3X6
ophthalmic preparation	T49.5X1	T49.5X2	T49.5X3	T49.5X4	T49.5X5	T49.5X6
topical NEC	T49.0X1	T49.0X2	T49.0X3	T49.0X4	T49.0X5	T49.0X6
Imidazole-4-carboxamide	T45.1X1	T45.1X2	T45.1X3	T45.1X4	T45.1X5	T45.1X6
Iminostilbene	T42.1X1	T42.1X2	T42.1X3	T42.1X4	T42.1X5	T42.1X6
Imipenem	T36.0X1	T36.0X2	T36.0X3	T36.0X4	T36.0X5	T36.0X6
Imipramine	T43.011	T43.012	T43.013	T43.014	T43.015	T43.016
Immu-G	T50.Z11	T50.Z12	T50.Z13	T50.Z14	T50.Z15	T50.Z16
Immuglobin	T50.Z11	T50.Z12	T50.Z13	T50.Z14	T50.Z15	T50.Z16
Immune						
globulin	T50.Z11	T50.Z12	T50.Z13	T50.Z14	T50.Z15	T50.Z16
serum globulin	T50.Z11	T50.Z12	T50.Z13	T50.Z14	T50.Z15	T50.Z16
Immunoglobin human (intravenous) (normal)	T50.Z11	T50.Z12	T50.Z13	T50.Z14	T50.Z15	T50.Z16
unmodified	T50.Z11	T50.Z12	T50.Z13	T50.Z14	T50.Z15	T50.Z16
Immunosuppressive drug	T45.1X1	T45.1X2	T45.1X3	T45.1X4	T45.1X5	T45.1X6
Immu-tetanus	T50.Z11	T50.Z12	T50.Z13	T50.Z14	T50.Z15	T50.Z16
Indalpine	T43.221	T43.222	T43.223	T43.224	T43.225	T43.226
Indanazoline	T48.5X1	T48.5X2	T48.5X3	T48.5X4	T48.5X5	T48.5X6
Indandione (derivatives)	T45.511	T45.512	T45.513	T45.514	T45.515	T45.516
Indapamide	T46.5X1	T46.5X2	T46.5X3	T46.5X4	T46.5X5	T46.5X6
Indendione (derivatives)	T45.511	T45.512	T45.513	T45.514	T45.515	T45.516
Indenolol	T44.7X1	T44.7X2	T44.7X3	T44.7X4	T44.7X5	T44.7X6
Inderal	T44.7X1	T44.7X2	T44.7X3	T44.7X4	T44.7X5	T44.7X6
Indian						
hemp	T40.7X1	T40.7X2	T40.7X3	T40.7X4	T40.7X5	T40.7X6
tobacco	T62.2X1	T62.2X2	T62.2X3	T62.2X4	—	—
Indigo carmine	T50.8X1	T50.8X2	T50.8X3	T50.8X4	T50.8X5	T50.8X6
Indobufen	T45.521	T45.522	T45.523	T45.524	T45.525	T45.526
Indocin	T39.2X1	T39.2X2	T39.2X3	T39.2X4	T39.2X5	T39.2X6
Indocyanine green	T50.8X1	T50.8X2	T50.8X3	T50.8X4	T50.8X5	T50.8X6
Indometacin	T39.391	T39.392	T39.393	T39.394	T39.395	T39.396
Indomethacin	T39.391	T39.392	T39.393	T39.394	T39.395	T39.396
farnesil	T39.4X1	T39.4X2	T39.4X3	T39.4X4	T39.4X5	T39.4X6
Indoramin	T44.6X1	T44.6X2	T44.6X3	T44.6X4	T44.6X5	T44.6X6
Industrial						
alcohol	T51.0X1	T51.0X2	T51.0X3	T51.0X4	—	—
fumes	T59.891	T59.892	T59.893	T59.894	—	—
solvents (fumes) (vapors)	T52.91	T52.92	T52.93	T52.94	—	—
Influenza vaccine	T50.B91	T50.B92	T50.B93	T50.B94	T50.B95	T50.B96
Ingested substance NEC	T65.91	T65.92	T65.93	T65.94	—	—
INH	T37.1X1	T37.1X2	T37.1X3	T37.1X4	T37.1X5	T37.1X6
Inhalation, gas (noxious) — *see* Gas						
Inhibitor						
angiotensin-converting enzyme	T46.4X1	T46.4X2	T46.4X3	T46.4X4	T46.4X5	T46.4X6
carbonic anhydrase	T50.2X1	T50.2X2	T50.2X3	T50.2X4	T50.2X5	T50.2X6
fibrinolysis	T45.621	T45.622	T45.623	T45.624	T45.625	T45.626
monoamine oxidase NEC	T43.1X1	T43.1X2	T43.1X3	T43.1X4	T43.1X5	T43.1X6
hydrazine	T43.1X1	T43.1X2	T43.1X3	T43.1X4	T43.1X5	T43.1X6
postsynaptic	T43.8X1	T43.8X2	T43.8X3	T43.8X4	T43.8X5	T43.8X6
prothrombin synthesis	T45.511	T45.512	T45.513	T45.514	T45.515	T45.516
Ink	T65.891	T65.892	T65.893	T65.894	—	—
Inorganic substance NEC	T57.91	T57.92	T57.93	T57.94	—	—
Inosine pranobex	T37.5X1	T37.5X2	T37.5X3	T37.5X4	T37.5X5	T37.5X6
Inositol	T50.991	T50.992	T50.993	T50.994	T50.995	T50.996
nicotinate	T46.7X1	T46.7X2	T46.7X3	T46.7X4	T46.7X5	T46.7X6
Inproquone	T45.1X1	T45.1X2	T45.1X3	T45.1X4	T45.1X5	T45.1X6
Insecticide NEC	T60.91	T60.92	T60.93	T60.94	—	—
carbamate	T60.0X1	T60.0X2	T60.0X3	T60.0X4	—	—
chlorinated	T60.1X1	T60.1X2	T60.1X3	T60.1X4	—	—
mixed	T60.91	T60.92	T60.93	T60.94	—	—
organochlorine	T60.1X1	T60.1X2	T60.1X3	T60.1X4	—	—
organophosphorus	T60.0X1	T60.0X2	T60.0X3	T60.0X4	—	—
Insect (sting), venomous	T63.481	T63.482	T63.483	T63.484	—	—
ant	T63.421	T63.422	T63.423	T63.424	—	—
bee	T63.441	T63.442	T63.443	T63.444	—	—
caterpillar	T63.431	T63.432	T63.433	T63.434	—	—
hornet	T63.451	T63.452	T63.453	T63.454	—	—
wasp	T63.461	T63.462	T63.463	T63.464	—	—
Insular tissue extract	T38.3X1	T38.3X2	T38.3X3	T38.3X4	T38.3X5	T38.3X6
Insulin (amorphous) (globin) (isophane) (Lente) (NPH) (Semilente) (Ultralente)	T38.3X1	T38.3X2	T38.3X3	T38.3X4	T38.3X5	T38.3X6
defalan	T38.3X1	T38.3X2	T38.3X3	T38.3X4	T38.3X5	T38.3X6
human	T38.3X1	T38.3X2	T38.3X3	T38.3X4	T38.3X5	T38.3X6
injection, soluble	T38.3X1	T38.3X2	T38.3X3	T38.3X4	T38.3X5	T38.3X6
biphasic	T38.3X1	T38.3X2	T38.3X3	T38.3X4	T38.3X5	T38.3X6
intermediate acting	T38.3X1	T38.3X2	T38.3X3	T38.3X4	T38.3X5	T38.3X6
protamine zinc	T38.3X1	T38.3X2	T38.3X3	T38.3X4	T38.3X5	T38.3X6
slow acting	T38.3X1	T38.3X2	T38.3X3	T38.3X4	T38.3X5	T38.3X6
zinc						
protamine injection	T38.3X1	T38.3X2	T38.3X3	T38.3X4	T38.3X5	T38.3X6
suspension (amorphous) (crystalline)	T38.3X1	T38.3X2	T38.3X3	T38.3X4	T38.3X5	T38.3X6
Interferon (alpha) (beta) (gamma)	T37.5X1	T37.5X2	T37.5X3	T37.5X4	T37.5X5	T37.5X6
Intestinal motility control drug	T47.6X1	T47.6X2	T47.6X3	T47.6X4	T47.6X5	T47.6X6
biological	T47.8X1	T47.8X2	T47.8X3	T47.8X4	T47.8X5	T47.8X6
Intranarcon	T41.1X1	T41.1X2	T41.1X3	T41.1X4	T41.1X5	T41.1X6
Intravenous						
amino acids	T50.991	T50.992	T50.993	T50.994	T50.995	T50.996
fat suspension	T50.991	T50.992	T50.993	T50.994	T50.995	T50.996
Inulin	T50.8X1	T50.8X2	T50.8X3	T50.8X4	T50.8X5	T50.8X6
Invert sugar	T50.3X1	T50.3X2	T50.3X3	T50.3X4	T50.3X5	T50.3X6
Inza — *see* Naproxen						
Iobenzamic acid	T50.8X1	T50.8X2	T50.8X3	T50.8X4	T50.8X5	T50.8X6
Iocarmic acid	T50.8X1	T50.8X2	T50.8X3	T50.8X4	T50.8X5	T50.8X6
Iocetamic acid	T50.8X1	T50.8X2	T50.8X3	T50.8X4	T50.8X5	T50.8X6
Iodamide	T50.8X1	T50.8X2	T50.8X3	T50.8X4	T50.8X5	T50.8X6
Iodide NEC — *see also* Iodine	T49.0X1	T49.0X2	T49.0X3	T49.0X4	T49.0X5	T49.0X6
mercury (ointment)	T49.0X1	T49.0X2	T49.0X3	T49.0X4	T49.0X5	T49.0X6
methylate	T49.0X1	T49.0X2	T49.0X3	T49.0X4	T49.0X5	T49.0X6
potassium (expectorant) NEC	T48.4X1	T48.4X2	T48.4X3	T48.4X4	T48.4X5	T48.4X6
Iodinated						
contrast medium	T50.8X1	T50.8X2	T50.8X3	T50.8X4	T50.8X5	T50.8X6
glycerol	T48.4X1	T48.4X2	T48.4X3	T48.4X4	T48.4X5	T48.4X6
human serum albumin (131I)	T50.8X1	T50.8X2	T50.8X3	T50.8X4	T50.8X5	T50.8X6
Iodine (antiseptic, external) (tincture) **NEC**	T49.0X1	T49.0X2	T49.0X3	T49.0X4	T49.0X5	T49.0X6
125 — *see also* Radiation sickness, and Exposure to radioactivce isotopes	T50.8X1	T50.8X2	T50.8X3	T50.8X4	T50.8X5	T50.8X6
therapeutic	T50.991	T50.992	T50.993	T50.994	T50.995	T50.996
131 — *see also* Radiation sickness, and Exposure to radioactivce isotopes	T50.8X1	T50.8X2	T50.8X3	T50.8X4	T50.8X5	T50.8X6
therapeutic	T38.2X1	T38.2X2	T38.2X3	T38.2X4	T38.2X5	T38.2X6
diagnostic	T50.8X1	T50.8X2	T50.8X3	T50.8X4	T50.8X5	T50.8X6

Table of Drugs and Chemicals

Iodine — Khat

Substance	Poisoning, Accidental (unintentional)	Poisoning, Intentional Self-harm	Poisoning, Assault	Poisoning, Undetermined	Adverse Effect	Under-dosing
Iodine (antiseptic, external) (tincture) **NEC** — *continued*						
for thyroid conditions (antithyroid)	T38.2X1	T38.2X2	T38.2X3	T38.2X4	T38.2X5	T38.2X6
solution	T49.0X1	T49.0X2	T49.0X3	T49.0X4	T49.0X5	T49.0X6
vapor	T59.891	T59.892	T59.893	T59.894	—	—
Iodipamide	T50.8X1	T50.8X2	T50.8X3	T50.8X4	T50.8X5	T50.8X6
Iodized (poppy seed) oil	T50.8X1	T50.8X2	T50.8X3	T50.8X4	T50.8X5	T50.8X6
Iodobismitol	T37.8X1	T37.8X2	T37.8X3	T37.8X4	T37.8X5	T37.8X6
Iodochlorhydroxyquin	T37.8X1	T37.8X2	T37.8X3	T37.8X4	T37.8X5	T37.8X6
topical	T49.0X1	T49.0X2	T49.0X3	T49.0X4	T49.0X5	T49.0X6
Iodochlorhydroxyquinoline	T37.8X1	T37.8X2	T37.8X3	T37.8X4	T37.8X5	T37.8X6
Iodocholesterol (131I)	T50.8X1	T50.8X2	T50.8X3	T50.8X4	T50.8X5	T50.8X6
Iodoform	T49.0X1	T49.0X2	T49.0X3	T49.0X4	T49.0X5	T49.0X6
Iodohippuric acid	T50.8X1	T50.8X2	T50.8X3	T50.8X4	T50.8X5	T50.8X6
Iodopanoic acid	T50.8X1	T50.8X2	T50.8X3	T50.8X4	T50.8X5	T50.8X6
Iodophthalein (sodium)	T50.8X1	T50.8X2	T50.8X3	T50.8X4	T50.8X5	T50.8X6
Iodopyracet	T50.8X1	T50.8X2	T50.8X3	T50.8X4	T50.8X5	T50.8X6
Iodoquinol	T37.8X1	T37.8X2	T37.8X3	T37.8X4	T37.8X5	T37.8X6
Iodoxamic acid	T50.8X1	T50.8X2	T50.8X3	T50.8X4	T50.8X5	T50.8X6
Iofendylate	T50.8X1	T50.8X2	T50.8X3	T50.8X4	T50.8X5	T50.8X6
Ioglycamic acid	T50.8X1	T50.8X2	T50.8X3	T50.8X4	T50.8X5	T50.8X6
Iohexol	T50.8X1	T50.8X2	T50.8X3	T50.8X4	T50.8X5	T50.8X6
Ion exchange resin						
anion	T47.8X1	T47.8X2	T47.8X3	T47.8X4	T47.8X5	T47.8X6
cation	T50.3X1	T50.3X2	T50.3X3	T50.3X4	T50.3X5	T50.3X6
cholestyramine	T46.6X1	T46.6X2	T46.6X3	T46.6X4	T46.6X5	T46.6X6
intestinal	T47.8X1	T47.8X2	T47.8X3	T47.8X4	T47.8X5	T47.8X6
Iopamidol	T50.8X1	T50.8X2	T50.8X3	T50.8X4	T50.8X5	T50.8X6
Iopanoic acid	T50.8X1	T50.8X2	T50.8X3	T50.8X4	T50.8X5	T50.8X6
Iophenoic acid	T50.8X1	T50.8X2	T50.8X3	T50.8X4	T50.8X5	T50.8X6
Iopodate, sodium	T50.8X1	T50.8X2	T50.8X3	T50.8X4	T50.8X5	T50.8X6
Iopodic acid	T50.8X1	T50.8X2	T50.8X3	T50.8X4	T50.8X5	T50.8X6
Iopromide	T50.8X1	T50.8X2	T50.8X3	T50.8X4	T50.8X5	T50.8X6
Iopydol	T50.8X1	T50.8X2	T50.8X3	T50.8X4	T50.8X5	T50.8X6
Iotalamic acid	T50.8X1	T50.8X2	T50.8X3	T50.8X4	T50.8X5	T50.8X6
Iothalamate	T50.8X1	T50.8X2	T50.8X3	T50.8X4	T50.8X5	T50.8X6
Iothiouracil	T38.2X1	T38.2X2	T38.2X3	T38.2X4	T38.2X5	T38.2X6
Iotrol	T50.8X1	T50.8X2	T50.8X3	T50.8X4	T50.8X5	T50.8X6
Iotrolan	T50.8X1	T50.8X2	T50.8X3	T50.8X4	T50.8X5	T50.8X6
Iotroxate	T50.8X1	T50.8X2	T50.8X3	T50.8X4	T50.8X5	T50.8X6
Iotroxic acid	T50.8X1	T50.8X2	T50.8X3	T50.8X4	T50.8X5	T50.8X6
Ioversol	T50.8X1	T50.8X2	T50.8X3	T50.8X4	T50.8X5	T50.8X6
Ioxaglate	T50.8X1	T50.8X2	T50.8X3	T50.8X4	T50.8X5	T50.8X6
Ioxaglic acid	T50.8X1	T50.8X2	T50.8X3	T50.8X4	T50.8X5	T50.8X6
Ioxitalamic acid	T50.8X1	T50.8X2	T50.8X3	T50.8X4	T50.8X5	T50.8X6
Ipecac	T47.7X1	T47.7X2	T47.7X3	T47.7X4	T47.7X5	T47.7X6
Ipecacuanha	T48.4X1	T48.4X2	T48.4X3	T48.4X4	T48.4X5	T48.4X6
Ipodate, calcium	T50.8X1	T50.8X2	T50.8X3	T50.8X4	T50.8X5	T50.8X6
Ipral	T42.3X1	T42.3X2	T42.3X3	T42.3X4	T42.3X5	T42.3X6
Ipratropium (bromide)	T48.6X1	T48.6X2	T48.6X3	T48.6X4	T48.6X5	T48.6X6
Ipriflavone	T46.3X1	T46.3X2	T46.3X3	T46.3X4	T46.3X5	T46.3X6
Iprindole	T43.011	T43.012	T43.013	T43.014	T43.015	T43.016
Iproclozide	T43.1X1	T43.1X2	T43.1X3	T43.1X4	T43.1X5	T43.1X6
Iprofenin	T50.8X1	T50.8X2	T50.8X3	T50.8X4	T50.8X5	T50.8X6
Iproheptine	T49.2X1	T49.2X2	T49.2X3	T49.2X4	T49.2X5	T49.2X6
Iproniazid	T43.1X1	T43.1X2	T43.1X3	T43.1X4	T43.1X5	T43.1X6
Iproplatin	T45.1X1	T45.1X2	T45.1X3	T45.1X4	T45.1X5	T45.1X6
Iproveratril	T46.1X1	T46.1X2	T46.1X3	T46.1X4	T46.1X5	T46.1X6
Iron (compounds) (medicinal) **NEC**	T45.4X1	T45.4X2	T45.4X3	T45.4X4	T45.4X5	T45.4X6
ammonium	T45.4X1	T45.4X2	T45.4X3	T45.4X4	T45.4X5	T45.4X6
dextran injection	T45.4X1	T45.4X2	T45.4X3	T45.4X4	T45.4X5	T45.4X6
nonmedicinal	T56.891	T56.892	T56.893	T56.894	—	—
salts	T45.4X1	T45.4X2	T45.4X3	T45.4X4	T45.4X5	T45.4X6
sorbitex	T45.4X1	T45.4X2	T45.4X3	T45.4X4	T45.4X5	T45.4X6
sorbitol citric acid complex	T45.4X1	T45.4X2	T45.4X3	T45.4X4	T45.4X5	T45.4X6
Irrigating fluid (vaginal)	T49.8X1	T49.8X2	T49.8X3	T49.8X4	T49.8X5	T49.8X6
eye	T49.5X1	T49.5X2	T49.5X3	T49.5X4	T49.5X5	T49.5X6
Isepamicin	T36.5X1	T36.5X2	T36.5X3	T36.5X4	T36.5X5	T36.5X6
Isoaminile (citrate)	T48.3X1	T48.3X2	T48.3X3	T48.3X4	T48.3X5	T48.3X6
Isoamyl nitrite	T46.3X1	T46.3X2	T46.3X3	T46.3X4	T46.3X5	T46.3X6
Isobenzan	T60.1X1	T60.1X2	T60.1X3	T60.1X4	—	—
Isobutyl acetate	T52.8X1	T52.8X2	T52.8X3	T52.8X4	—	—
Isocarboxazid	T43.1X1	T43.1X2	T43.1X3	T43.1X4	T43.1X5	T43.1X6
Isoconazole	T49.0X1	T49.0X2	T49.0X3	T49.0X4	T49.0X5	T49.0X6
Isocyanate	T65.0X1	T65.0X2	T65.0X3	T65.0X4	—	—
Isoephedrine	T44.991	T44.992	T44.993	T44.994	T44.995	T44.996
Isoetarine	T48.6X1	T48.6X2	T48.6X3	T48.6X4	T48.6X5	T48.6X6
Isoethadione	T42.2X1	T42.2X2	T42.2X3	T42.2X4	T42.2X5	T42.2X6
Isoetharine	T44.5X1	T44.5X2	T44.5X3	T44.5X4	T44.5X5	T44.5X6
Isoflurane	T41.0X1	T41.0X2	T41.0X3	T41.0X4	T41.0X5	T41.0X6
Isoflurophate	T44.0X1	T44.0X2	T44.0X3	T44.0X4	T44.0X5	T44.0X6
Isomaltose, ferric complex	T45.4X1	T45.4X2	T45.4X3	T45.4X4	T45.4X5	T45.4X6
Isometheptene	T44.3X1	T44.3X2	T44.3X3	T44.3X4	T44.3X5	T44.3X6
Isoniazid	T37.1X1	T37.1X2	T37.1X3	T37.1X4	T37.1X5	T37.1X6
with rifampicin	T36.6X1	T36.6X2	T36.6X3	T36.6X4	T36.6X5	T36.6X6
thioacetazone	T37.1X1	T37.1X2	T37.1X3	T37.1X4	T37.1X5	T37.1X6
Isonicotinic acid hydrazide	T37.1X1	T37.1X2	T37.1X3	T37.1X4	T37.1X5	T37.1X6
Isonipecaine	T40.4X1	T40.4X2	T40.4X3	T40.4X4	T40.4X5	T40.4X6
Isopentaquine	T37.2X1	T37.2X2	T37.2X3	T37.2X4	T37.2X5	T37.2X6
Isophane insulin	T38.3X1	T38.3X2	T38.3X3	T38.3X4	T38.3X5	T38.3X6
Isophorone	T65.891	T65.892	T65.893	T65.894	—	—
Isophosphamide	T45.1X1	T45.1X2	T45.1X3	T45.1X4	T45.1X5	T45.1X6
Isopregnenone	T38.5X1	T38.5X2	T38.5X3	T38.5X4	T38.5X5	T38.5X6
Isoprenaline	T48.6X1	T48.6X2	T48.6X3	T48.6X4	T48.6X5	T48.6X6
Isopromethazine	T43.3X1	T43.3X2	T43.3X3	T43.3X4	T43.3X5	T43.3X6
Isopropamide	T44.3X1	T44.3X2	T44.3X3	T44.3X4	T44.3X5	T44.3X6
iodide	T44.3X1	T44.3X2	T44.3X3	T44.3X4	T44.3X5	T44.3X6
Isopropanol	T51.2X1	T51.2X2	T51.2X3	T51.2X4	—	—
Isopropyl						
acetate	T52.8X1	T52.8X2	T52.8X3	T52.8X4	—	—
alcohol	T51.2X1	T51.2X2	T51.2X3	T51.2X4	—	—
medicinal	T49.4X1	T49.4X2	T49.4X3	T49.4X4	T49.4X5	T49.4X6
ether	T52.8X1	T52.8X2	T52.8X3	T52.8X4	—	—
Isopropylaminophenazone	T39.2X1	T39.2X2	T39.2X3	T39.2X4	T39.2X5	T39.2X6
Isoproterenol	T48.6X1	T48.6X2	T48.6X3	T48.6X4	T48.6X5	T48.6X6
Isosorbide dinitrate	T46.3X1	T46.3X2	T46.3X3	T46.3X4	T46.3X5	T46.3X6
Isothipendyl	T45.0X1	T45.0X2	T45.0X3	T45.0X4	T45.0X5	T45.0X6
Isotretinoin	T50.991	T50.992	T50.993	T50.994	T50.995	T50.996
Isoxazolyl penicillin	T36.0X1	T36.0X2	T36.0X3	T36.0X4	T36.0X5	T36.0X6
Isoxicam	T39.391	T39.392	T39.393	T39.394	T39.395	T39.396
Isoxsuprine	T46.7X1	T46.7X2	T46.7X3	T46.7X4	T46.7X5	T46.7X6
Ispagula	T47.4X1	T47.4X2	T47.4X3	T47.4X4	T47.4X5	T47.4X6
husk	T47.4X1	T47.4X2	T47.4X3	T47.4X4	T47.4X5	T47.4X6
Isradipine	T46.1X1	T46.1X2	T46.1X3	T46.1X4	T46.1X5	T46.1X6
I-thyroxine sodium	T38.1X1	T38.1X2	T38.1X3	T38.1X4	T38.1X5	T38.1X6
Itraconazole	T37.8X1	T37.8X2	T37.8X3	T37.8X4	T37.8X5	T37.8X6
Itramin tosilate	T46.3X1	T46.3X2	T46.3X3	T46.3X4	T46.3X5	T46.3X6
Ivermectin	T37.4X1	T37.4X2	T37.4X3	T37.4X4	T37.4X5	T37.4X6
Izoniazid	T37.1X1	T37.1X2	T37.1X3	T37.1X4	T37.1X5	T37.1X6
with thioacetazone	T37.1X1	T37.1X2	T37.1X3	T37.1X4	T37.1X5	T37.1X6
Jalap	T47.2X1	T47.2X2	T47.2X3	T47.2X4	T47.2X5	T47.2X6
Jamaica						
dogwood (bark)	T39.8X1	T39.8X2	T39.8X3	T39.8X4	T39.8X5	T39.8X6
ginger	T65.891	T65.892	T65.893	T65.894	—	—
root	T62.2X1	T62.2X2	T62.2X3	T62.2X4	—	—
Jatropha	T62.2X1	T62.2X2	T62.2X3	T62.2X4	—	—
curcas	T62.2X1	T62.2X2	T62.2X3	T62.2X4	—	—
Jectofer	T45.4X1	T45.4X2	T45.4X3	T45.4X4	T45.4X5	T45.4X6
Jellyfish (sting)	T63.621	T63.622	T63.623	T63.624		
Jequirity (bean)	T62.2X1	T62.2X2	T62.2X3	T62.2X4		
Jimson weed (stramonium)	T62.2X1	T62.2X2	T62.2X3	T62.2X4		
seeds	T62.2X1	T62.2X2	T62.2X3	T62.2X4		
Josamycin	T36.3X1	T36.3X2	T36.3X3	T36.3X4	T36.3X5	T36.3X6
Juniper tar	T49.1X1	T49.1X2	T49.1X3	T49.1X4	T49.1X5	T49.1X6
Kallidinogenase	T46.7X1	T46.7X2	T46.7X3	T46.7X4	T46.7X5	T46.7X6
Kallikrein	T46.7X1	T46.7X2	T46.7X3	T46.7X4	T46.7X5	T46.7X6
Kanamycin	T36.5X1	T36.5X2	T36.5X3	T36.5X4	T36.5X5	T36.5X6
Kantrex	T36.5X1	T36.5X2	T36.5X3	T36.5X4	T36.5X5	T36.5X6
Kaolin	T47.6X1	T47.6X2	T47.6X3	T47.6X4	T47.6X5	T47.6X6
light	T47.6X1	T47.6X2	T47.6X3	T47.6X4	T47.6X5	T47.6X6
Karaya (gum)	T47.4X1	T47.4X2	T47.4X3	T47.4X4	T47.4X5	T47.4X6
Kebuzone	T39.2X1	T39.2X2	T39.2X3	T39.2X4	T39.2X5	T39.2X6
Kelevan	T60.1X1	T60.1X2	T60.1X3	T60.1X4	—	—
Kemithal	T41.1X1	T41.1X2	T41.1X3	T41.1X4	T41.1X5	T41.1X6
Kenacort	T38.0X1	T38.0X2	T38.0X3	T38.0X4	T38.0X5	T38.0X6
Keratolytic drug NEC	T49.4X1	T49.4X2	T49.4X3	T49.4X4	T49.4X5	T49.4X6
anthracene	T49.4X1	T49.4X2	T49.4X3	T49.4X4	T49.4X5	T49.4X6
Keratoplastic NEC	T49.4X1	T49.4X2	T49.4X3	T49.4X4	T49.4X5	T49.4X6
Kerosene, kerosine (fuel) (solvent) **NEC**	T52.0X1	T52.0X2	T52.0X3	T52.0X4	—	—
insecticide	T52.0X1	T52.0X2	T52.0X3	T52.0X4	—	—
vapor	T52.0X1	T52.0X2	T52.0X3	T52.0X4	—	—
Ketamine	T41.291	T41.292	T41.293	T41.294	T41.295	T41.296
Ketazolam	T42.4X1	T42.4X2	T42.4X3	T42.4X4	T42.4X5	T42.4X6
Ketazon	T39.2X1	T39.2X2	T39.2X3	T39.2X4	T39.2X5	T39.2X6
Ketobemidone	T40.4X1	T40.4X2	T40.4X3	T40.4X4	—	—
Ketoconazole	T49.0X1	T49.0X2	T49.0X3	T49.0X4	T49.0X5	T49.0X6
Ketols	T52.4X1	T52.4X2	T52.4X3	T52.4X4	—	—
Ketone oils	T52.4X1	T52.4X2	T52.4X3	T52.4X4	—	—
Ketoprofen	T39.311	T39.312	T39.313	T39.314	T39.315	T39.316
Ketorolac	T39.8X1	T39.8X2	T39.8X3	T39.8X4	T39.8X5	T39.8X6
Ketotifen	T45.0X1	T45.0X2	T45.0X3	T45.0X4	T45.0X5	T45.0X6
Khat	T43.691	T43.692	T43.693	T43.694	—	—

Table of Drugs and Chemicals

Khellin — Liquid

Substance	Poisoning, Accidental (unintentional)	Poisoning, Intentional Self-harm	Poisoning, Assault	Poisoning, Undetermined	Adverse Effect	Under-dosing
Khellin	T46.3X1	T46.3X2	T46.3X3	T46.3X4	T46.3X5	T46.3X6
Khelloside	T46.3X1	T46.3X2	T46.3X3	T46.3X4	T46.3X5	T46.3X6
Kiln gas or vapor (carbon monoxide)	T58.8X1	T58.8X2	T58.8X3	T58.8X4	—	—
Kitasamycin	T36.3X1	T36.3X2	T36.3X3	T36.3X4	T36.3X5	T36.3X6
Konsyl	T47.4X1	T47.4X2	T47.4X3	T47.4X4	T47.4X5	T47.4X6
Kosam seed	T62.2X1	T62.2X2	T62.2X3	T62.2X4		
Krait (venom)	T63.091	T63.092	T63.093	T63.094	—	—
Kwell (insecticide)	T60.1X1	T60.1X2	T60.1X3	T60.1X4	—	—
anti-infective (topical)	T49.0X1	T49.0X2	T49.0X3	T49.0X4	T49.0X5	T49.0X6
Labetalol	T44.8X1	T44.8X2	T44.8X3	T44.8X4	T44.8X5	T44.8X6
Laburnum (seeds)	T62.2X1	T62.2X2	T62.2X3	T62.2X4		
leaves	T62.2X1	T62.2X2	T62.2X3	T62.2X4		
Lachesine	T49.5X1	T49.5X2	T49.5X3	T49.5X4	T49.5X5	T49.5X6
Lacidipine	T46.5X1	T46.5X2	T46.5X3	T46.5X4	T46.5X5	T46.5X6
Lacquer	T65.6X1	T65.6X2	T65.6X3	T65.6X4	—	—
Lacrimogenic gas	T59.3X1	T59.3X2	T59.3X3	T59.3X4	—	—
Lactated potassic saline	T50.3X1	T50.3X2	T50.3X3	T50.3X4	T50.3X5	T50.3X6
Lactic acid	T49.8X1	T49.8X2	T49.8X3	T49.8X4	T49.8X5	T49.8X6
Lactobacillus						
acidophilus	T47.6X1	T47.6X2	T47.6X3	T47.6X4	T47.6X5	T47.6X6
compound	T47.6X1	T47.6X2	T47.6X3	T47.6X4	T47.6X5	T47.6X6
bifidus, lyophilized	T47.6X1	T47.6X2	T47.6X3	T47.6X4	T47.6X5	T47.6X6
bulgaricus	T47.6X1	T47.6X2	T47.6X3	T47.6X4	T47.6X5	T47.6X6
sporogenes	T47.6X1	T47.6X2	T47.6X3	T47.6X4	T47.6X5	T47.6X6
Lactoflavin	T45.2X1	T45.2X2	T45.2X3	T45.2X4	T45.2X5	T45.2X6
Lactose (as excipient)	T50.901	T50.902	T50.903	T50.904	T50.905	T50.906
Lactuca (virosa) (extract)	T42.6X1	T42.6X2	T42.6X3	T42.6X4	T42.6X5	T42.6X6
Lactucarium	T42.6X1	T42.6X2	T42.6X3	T42.6X4	T42.6X5	T42.6X6
Lactulose	T47.3X1	T47.3X2	T47.3X3	T47.3X4	T47.3X5	T47.3X6
Laevo— see Levo-						
Lanatosides	T46.0X1	T46.0X2	T46.0X3	T46.0X4	T46.0X5	T46.0X6
Lanolin	T49.3X1	T49.3X2	T49.3X3	T49.3X4	T49.3X5	T49.3X6
Largactil	T43.3X1	T43.3X2	T43.3X3	T43.3X4	T43.3X5	T43.3X6
Larkspur	T62.2X1	T62.2X2	T62.2X3	T62.2X4	—	—
Laroxyl	T43.011	T43.012	T43.013	T43.014	T43.015	T43.016
Lasix	T50.1X1	T50.1X2	T50.1X3	T50.1X4	T50.1X5	T50.1X6
Lassar's paste	T49.4X1	T49.4X2	T49.4X3	T49.4X4	T49.4X5	T49.4X6
Latamoxef	T36.1X1	T36.1X2	T36.1X3	T36.1X4	T36.1X5	T36.1X6
Latex	T65.811	T65.812	T65.813	T65.814	—	—
Lathyrus (seed)	T62.2X1	T62.2X2	T62.2X3	T62.2X4	—	—
Laudanum	T40.0X1	T40.0X2	T40.0X3	T40.0X4	T40.0X5	T40.0X6
Laudexium	T48.1X1	T48.1X2	T48.1X3	T48.1X4	T48.1X5	T48.1X6
Laughing gas	T41.0X1	T41.0X2	T41.0X3	T41.0X4	T41.0X5	T41.0X6
Laurel, black or cherry	T62.2X1	T62.2X2	T62.2X3	T62.2X4	—	—
Laurolinium	T49.0X1	T49.0X2	T49.0X3	T49.0X4	T49.0X5	T49.0X6
Lauryl sulfoacetate	T49.2X1	T49.2X2	T49.2X3	T49.2X4	T49.2X5	T49.2X6
Laxative NEC	T47.4X1	T47.4X2	T47.4X3	T47.4X4	T47.4X5	T47.4X6
osmotic	T47.3X1	T47.3X2	T47.3X3	T47.3X4	T47.3X5	T47.3X6
saline	T47.3X1	T47.3X2	T47.3X3	T47.3X4	T47.3X5	T47.3X6
stimulant	T47.2X1	T47.2X2	T47.2X3	T47.2X4	T47.2X5	T47.2X6
L-dopa	T42.8X1	T42.8X2	T42.8X3	T42.8X4	T42.8X5	T42.8X6
Lead (dust) (fumes) (vapor) NEC	T56.0X1	T56.0X2	T56.0X3	T56.0X4		
acetate	T49.2X1	T49.2X2	T49.2X3	T49.2X4	T49.2X5	T49.2X6
alkyl (fuel additive)	T56.0X1	T56.0X2	T56.0X3	T56.0X4	—	—
anti-infectives	T37.8X1	T37.8X2	T37.8X3	T37.8X4	T37.8X5	T37.8X6
antiknock compound (tetraethyl)	T56.0X1	T56.0X2	T56.0X3	T56.0X4	—	—
arsenate, arsenite (dust)(herbicide) (insecticide) (vapor)	T57.0X1	T57.0X2		T57.0X4		
carbonate	T56.0X1	T56.0X2	T56.0X3	T56.0X4	—	—
paint	T56.0X1	T56.0X2	T56.0X3	T56.0X4	—	—
chromate	T56.0X1	T56.0X2	T56.0X3	T56.0X4	—	—
paint	T56.0X1	T56.0X2	T56.0X3	T56.0X4	—	—
dioxide	T56.0X1	T56.0X2	T56.0X3	T56.0X4	—	—
inorganic	T56.0X1	T56.0X2	T56.0X3	T56.0X4	—	—
iodide	T56.0X1	T56.0X2	T56.0X3	T56.0X4	—	—
pigment (paint)	T56.0X1	T56.0X2	T56.0X3	T56.0X4	—	—
monoxide (dust)	T56.0X1	T56.0X2	T56.0X3	T56.0X4	—	—
paint	T56.0X1	T56.0X2	T56.0X3	T56.0X4	—	—
organic	T56.0X1	T56.0X2	T56.0X3	T56.0X4	—	—
oxide	T56.0X1	T56.0X2	T56.0X3	T56.0X4	—	—
paint	T56.0X1	T56.0X2	T56.0X3	T56.0X4	—	—
paint	T56.0X1	T56.0X2	T56.0X3	T56.0X4	—	—
salts	T56.0X1	T56.0X2	T56.0X3	T56.0X4	—	—
specified compound NEC	T56.0X1	T56.0X2	T56.0X3	T56.0X4	—	—
tetra-ethyl	T56.0X1	T56.0X2	T56.0X3	T56.0X4	—	—
Lebanese red	T40.7X1	T40.7X2	T40.7X3	T40.7X4	T40.7X5	T40.7X6
Lefetamine	T39.8X1	T39.8X2	T39.8X3	T39.8X4	T39.8X5	T39.8X6
Lenperone	T43.4X1	T43.4X2	T43.4X3	T43.4X4	T43.4X5	T43.4X6
Lente lietin (insulin)	T38.3X1	T38.3X2	T38.3X3	T38.3X4	T38.3X5	T38.3X6

Substance	Poisoning, Accidental (unintentional)	Poisoning, Intentional Self-harm	Poisoning, Assault	Poisoning, Undetermined	Adverse Effect	Under-dosing
Leptazol	T50.7X1	T50.7X2	T50.7X3	T50.7X4	T50.7X5	T50.7X6
Leptophos	T60.0X1	T60.0X2	T60.0X3	T60.0X4	—	—
Leritine	T40.2X1	T40.2X2	T40.2X3	T40.2X4	T40.2X5	T40.2X6
Letosteine	T48.4X1	T48.4X2	T48.4X3	T48.4X4	T48.4X5	T48.4X6
Letter	T38.1X1	T38.1X2	T38.1X3	T38.1X4	T38.1X5	T38.1X6
Lettuce opium	T42.6X1	T42.6X2	T42.6X3	T42.6X4	T42.6X5	T42.6X6
Leucinocaine	T41.3X1	T41.3X2	T41.3X3	T41.3X4	T41.3X5	T41.3X6
Leucocianidol	T46.991	T46.992	T46.993	T46.994	T46.995	T46.996
Leucovorin (factor)	T45.8X1	T45.8X2	T45.8X3	T45.8X4	T45.8X5	T45.8X6
Leukeran	T45.1X1	T45.1X2	T45.1X3	T45.1X4	T45.1X5	T45.1X6
Leuprolide	T38.891	T38.892	T38.893	T38.894	T38.895	T38.896
Levalbuterol	T48.6X1	T48.6X2	T48.6X3	T48.6X4	T48.6X5	T48.6X6
Levallorphan	T50.7X1	T50.7X2	T50.7X3	T50.7X4	T50.7X5	T50.7X6
Levamisole	T37.4X1	T37.4X2	T37.4X3	T37.4X4	T37.4X5	T37.4X6
Levanil	T42.6X1	T42.6X2	T42.6X3	T42.6X4	T42.6X5	T42.6X6
Levarterenol	T44.4X1	T44.4X2	T44.4X3	T44.4X4	T44.4X5	T44.4X6
Levdropropizine	T48.3X1	T48.3X2	T48.3X3	T48.3X4	T48.3X5	T48.3X6
Levobunolol	T49.5X1	T49.5X2	T49.5X3	T49.5X4	T49.5X5	T49.5X6
Levocabastine (hydrochloride)	T45.0X1	T45.0X2	T45.0X3	T45.0X4	T45.0X5	T45.0X6
Levocarnitine	T50.991	T50.992	T50.993	T50.994	T50.995	T50.996
Levodopa	T42.8X1	T42.8X2	T42.8X3	T42.8X4	T42.8X5	T42.8X6
with carbidopa	T42.8X1	T42.8X2	T42.8X3	T42.8X4	T42.8X5	T42.8X6
Levo-dromoran	T40.2X1	T40.2X2	T40.2X3	T40.2X4	T40.2X5	T40.2X6
Levoglutamide	T50.991	T50.992	T50.993	T50.994	T50.995	T50.996
Levoid	T38.1X1	T38.1X2	T38.1X3	T38.1X4	T38.1X5	T38.1X6
Levo-isomethadone	T40.3X1	T40.3X2	T40.3X3	T40.3X4	T40.3X5	T40.3X6
Levomepromazine	T43.3X1	T43.3X2	T43.3X3	T43.3X4	T43.3X5	T43.3X6
Levonordefrin	T49.6X1	T49.6X2	T49.6X3	T49.6X4	T49.6X5	T49.6X6
Levonorgestrel	T38.4X1	T38.4X2	T38.4X3	T38.4X4	T38.4X5	T38.4X6
with ethinylestradiol	T38.5X1	T38.5X2	T38.5X3	T38.5X4	T38.5X5	T38.5X6
Levopromazine	T43.3X1	T43.3X2	T43.3X3	T43.3X4	T43.3X5	T43.3X6
Levoprome	T42.6X1	T42.6X2	T42.6X3	T42.6X4	T42.6X5	T42.6X6
Levopropoxyphene	T40.4X1	T40.4X2	T40.4X3	T40.4X4	T40.4X5	T40.4X6
Levopropylhexedrine	T50.5X1	T50.5X2	T50.5X3	T50.5X4	T50.5X5	T50.5X6
Levoproxyphylline	T48.6X1	T48.6X2	T48.6X3	T48.6X4	T48.6X5	T48.6X6
Levorphanol	T40.4X1	T40.4X2	T40.4X3	T40.4X4	T40.4X5	T40.4X6
Levothyroxine	T38.1X1	T38.1X2	T38.1X3	T38.1X4	T38.1X5	T38.1X6
sodium	T38.1X1	T38.1X2	T38.1X3	T38.1X4	T38.1X5	T38.1X6
Levsin	T44.3X1	T44.3X2	T44.3X3	T44.3X4	T44.3X5	T44.3X6
Levulose	T50.3X1	T50.3X2	T50.3X3	T50.3X4	T50.3X5	T50.3X6
Lewisite (gas), not in war	T57.0X1	T57.0X2	T57.0X3	T57.0X4	—	—
Librium	T42.4X1	T42.4X2	T42.4X3	T42.4X4	T42.4X5	T42.4X6
Lidex	T49.0X1	T49.0X2	T49.0X3	T49.0X4	T49.0X5	T49.0X6
Lidocaine	T41.3X1	T41.3X2	T41.3X3	T41.3X4	T41.3X5	T41.3X6
regional	T41.3X1	T41.3X2	T41.3X3	T41.3X4	T41.3X5	T41.3X6
spinal	T41.3X1	T41.3X2	T41.3X3	T41.3X4	T41.3X5	T41.3X6
Lidofenin	T50.8X1	T50.8X2	T50.8X3	T50.8X4	T50.8X5	T50.8X6
Lidoflazine	T46.1X1	T46.1X2	T46.1X3	T46.1X4	T46.1X5	T46.1X6
Lighter fluid	T52.0X1	T52.0X2	T52.0X3	T52.0X4	—	—
Lignin hemicellulose	T47.6X1	T47.6X2	T47.6X3	T47.6X4	T47.6X5	T47.6X6
Lignocaine	T41.3X1	T41.3X2	T41.3X3	T41.3X4	T41.3X5	T41.3X6
regional	T41.3X1	T41.3X2	T41.3X3	T41.3X4	T41.3X5	T41.3X6
spinal	T41.3X1	T41.3X2	T41.3X3	T41.3X4	T41.3X5	T41.3X6
Ligroin (e) (solvent)	T52.0X1	T52.0X2	T52.0X3	T52.0X4	—	—
vapor	T59.891	T59.892	T59.893	T59.894	—	—
Ligustrum vulgare	T62.2X1	T62.2X2	T62.2X3	T62.2X4	—	—
Lily of the valley	T62.2X1	T62.2X2	T62.2X3	T62.2X4	—	—
Lime (chloride)	T54.3X1	T54.3X2	T54.3X3	T54.3X4	—	—
Limonene	T52.8X1	T52.8X2	T52.8X3	T52.8X4	—	—
Lincomycin	T36.8X1	T36.8X2	T36.8X3	T36.8X4	T36.8X5	T36.8X6
Lindane (insecticide) (nonmedicinal) (vapor)	T53.6X1	T53.6X2	T53.6X3	T53.6X4	—	—
medicinal	T49.0X1	T49.0X2	T49.0X3	T49.0X4	T49.0X5	T49.0X6
Liniments NEC	T49.91	T49.92	T49.93	T49.94	T49.95	T49.96
Linoleic acid	T46.6X1	T46.6X2	T46.6X3	T46.6X4	T46.6X5	T46.6X6
Linolenic acid	T46.6X1	T46.6X2	T46.6X3	T46.6X4	T46.6X5	T46.6X6
Linseed	T47.4X1	T47.4X2	T47.4X3	T47.4X4	T47.4X5	T47.4X6
Liothyronine	T38.1X1	T38.1X2	T38.1X3	T38.1X4	T38.1X5	T38.1X6
Liotrix	T38.1X1	T38.1X2	T38.1X3	T38.1X4	T38.1X5	T38.1X6
Lipancreatin	T47.5X1	T47.5X2	T47.5X3	T47.5X4	T47.5X5	T47.5X6
Lipo-alprostadil	T46.7X1	T46.7X2	T46.7X3	T46.7X4	T46.7X5	T46.7X6
Lipo-Lutin	T38.5X1	T38.5X2	T38.5X3	T38.5X4	T38.5X5	T38.5X6
Lipotropic drug NEC	T50.901	T50.902	T50.903	T50.904	T50.905	T50.906
Liquefied petroleum gases	T59.891	T59.892	T59.893	T59.894	—	—
piped (pure or mixed with air)	T59.891	T59.892	T59.893	T59.894	—	—
Liquid						
paraffin	T47.4X1	T47.4X2	T47.4X3	T47.4X4	T47.4X5	T47.4X6
petrolatum	T47.4X1	T47.4X2	T47.4X3	T47.4X4	T47.4X5	T47.4X6
topical	T49.3X1	T49.3X2	T49.3X3	T49.3X4	T49.3X5	T49.3X6
specified NEC	T65.891	T65.892	T65.893	T65.894	—	—
substance	T65.91	T65.92	T65.93	T65.94	—	—

Table of Drugs and Chemicals

Liquor creosolis compositus — Meladrazine

Substance	Poisoning, Accidental (unintentional)	Poisoning, Intentional Self-harm	Poisoning, Assault	Poisoning, Undetermined	Adverse Effect	Under-dosing
Liquor creosolis compositus	T65.891	T65.892	T65.893	T65.894	—	—
Liquorice	T48.4X1	T48.4X2	T48.4X3	T48.4X4	T48.4X5	T48.4X6
extract	T47.8X1	T47.8X2	T47.8X3	T47.8X4	T47.8X5	T47.8X6
Lisinopril	T46.4X1	T46.4X2	T46.4X3	T46.4X4	T46.4X5	T46.4X6
Lisuride	T42.8X1	T42.8X2	T42.8X3	T42.8X4	T42.8X5	T42.8X6
Lithane	T43.8X1	T43.8X2	T43.8X3	T43.8X4	T43.8X5	T43.8X6
Lithium	T56.891	T56.892	T56.893	T56.894	—	—
gluconate	T43.591	T43.592	T43.593	T43.594	T43.595	T43.596
salts (carbonate)	T43.591	T43.592	T43.593	T43.594	T43.595	T43.596
Lithonate	T43.8X1	T43.8X2	T43.8X3	T43.8X4	T43.8X5	T43.8X6
Liver						
extract	T45.8X1	T45.8X2	T45.8X3	T45.8X4	T45.8X5	T45.8X6
for parenteral use	T45.8X1	T45.8X2	T45.8X3	T45.8X4	T45.8X5	T45.8X6
fraction 1	T45.8X1	T45.8X2	T45.8X3	T45.8X4	T45.8X5	T45.8X6
hydrolysate	T45.8X1	T45.8X2	T45.8X3	T45.8X4	T45.8X5	T45.8X6
Lizard (bite) (venom)	T63.121	T63.122	T63.123	T63.124	—	—
LMD	T45.8X1	T45.8X2	T45.8X3	T45.8X4	T45.8X5	T45.8X6
Lobelia	T62.2X1	T62.2X2	T62.2X3	T62.2X4	—	—
Lobeline	T50.7X1	T50.7X2	T50.7X3	T50.7X4	T50.7X5	T50.7X6
Local action drug NEC	T49.8X1	T49.8X2	T49.8X3	T49.8X4	T49.8X5	T49.8X6
Locorten	T49.0X1	T49.0X2	T49.0X3	T49.0X4	T49.0X5	T49.0X6
Lofepramine	T43.011	T43.012	T43.013	T43.014	T43.015	T43.016
Lolium temulentum	T62.2X1	T62.2X2	T62.2X3	T62.2X4	—	—
Lomotil	T47.6X1	T47.6X2	T47.6X3	T47.6X4	T47.6X5	T47.6X6
Lomustine	T45.1X1	T45.1X2	T45.1X3	T45.1X4	T45.1X5	T45.1X6
Lonidamine	T45.1X1	T45.1X2	T45.1X3	T45.1X4	T45.1X5	T45.1X6
Loperamide	T47.6X1	T47.6X2	T47.6X3	T47.6X4	T47.6X5	T47.6X6
Loprazolam	T42.4X1	T42.4X2	T42.4X3	T42.4X4	T42.4X5	T42.4X6
Lorajmine	T46.2X1	T46.2X2	T46.2X3	T46.2X4	T46.2X5	T46.2X6
Loratidine	T45.0X1	T45.0X2	T45.0X3	T45.0X4	T45.0X5	T45.0X6
Lorazepam	T42.4X1	T42.4X2	T42.4X3	T42.4X4	T42.4X5	T42.4X6
Lorcainide	T46.2X1	T46.2X2	T46.2X3	T46.2X4	T46.2X5	T46.2X6
Lormetazepam	T42.4X1	T42.4X2	T42.4X3	T42.4X4	T42.4X5	T42.4X6
Lotions NEC	T49.91	T49.92	T49.93	T49.94	T49.95	T49.96
Lotusate	T42.3X1	T42.3X2	T42.3X3	T42.3X4	T42.3X5	T42.3X6
Lovastatin	T46.6X1	T46.6X2	T46.6X3	T46.6X4	T46.6X5	T46.6X6
Lowila	T49.2X1	T49.2X2	T49.2X3	T49.2X4	T49.2X5	T49.2X6
Loxapine	T43.591	T43.592	T43.593	T43.594	T43.595	T43.596
Lozenges (throat)	T49.6X1	T49.6X2	T49.6X3	T49.6X4	T49.6X5	T49.6X6
LSD	T40.8X1	T40.8X2	T40.8X3	T40.8X4	—	—
L-Tryptophan — see amino acid						
Lubricant, eye	T49.5X1	T49.5X2	T49.5X3	T49.5X4	T49.5X5	T49.5X6
Lubricating oil NEC	T52.0X1	T52.0X2	T52.0X3	T52.0X4		
Lucanthone	T37.4X1	T37.4X2	T37.4X3	T37.4X4	T37.4X5	T37.4X6
Luminal	T42.3X1	T42.3X2	T42.3X3	T42.3X4	T42.3X5	T42.3X6
Lung irritant (gas) NEC	T59.91	T59.92	T59.93	T59.94		
Luteinizing hormone	T38.811	T38.812	T38.813	T38.814	T38.815	T38.816
Lutocylol	T38.5X1	T38.5X2	T38.5X3	T38.5X4	T38.5X5	T38.5X6
Lutromone	T38.5X1	T38.5X2	T38.5X3	T38.5X4	T38.5X5	T38.5X6
Lututrin	T48.291	T48.292	T48.293	T48.294	T48.295	T48.296
Lye (concentrated)	T54.3X1	T54.3X2	T54.3X3	T54.3X4		
Lygranum (skin test)	T50.8X1	T50.8X2	T50.8X3	T50.8X4	T50.8X5	T50.8X6
Lymecycline	T36.4X1	T36.4X2	T36.4X3	T36.4X4	T36.4X5	T36.4X6
Lymphogranuloma venereum antigen	T50.8X1	T50.8X2	T50.8X3	T50.8X4	T50.8X5	T50.8X6
Lynestrenol	T38.4X1	T38.4X2	T38.4X3	T38.4X4	T38.4X5	T38.4X6
Lyovac Sodium Edecrin	T50.1X1	T50.1X2	T50.1X3	T50.1X4	T50.1X5	T50.1X6
Lypressin	T38.891	T38.892	T38.893	T38.894	T38.895	T38.896
Lysergic acid diethylamide	T40.8X1	T40.8X2	T40.8X3	T40.8X4	—	—
Lysergide	T40.8X1	T40.8X2	T40.8X3	T40.8X4	—	—
Lysine vasopressin	T38.891	T38.892	T38.893	T38.894	T38.895	T38.896
Lysol	T54.1X1	T54.1X2	T54.1X3	T54.1X4	—	—
Lysozyme	T49.0X1	T49.0X2	T49.0X3	T49.0X4	T49.0X5	T49.0X6
Lytta (vitatta)	T49.8X1	T49.8X2	T49.8X3	T49.8X4	T49.8X5	T49.8X6
Mace	T59.3X1	T59.3X2	T59.3X3	T59.3X4	—	—
Macrogol	T50.991	T50.992	T50.993	T50.994	T50.995	T50.996
Macrolide						
anabolic drug	T38.7X1	T38.7X2	T38.7X3	T38.7X4	T38.7X5	T38.7X6
antibiotic	T36.3X1	T36.3X2	T36.3X3	T36.3X4	T36.3X5	T36.3X6
Mafenide	T49.0X1	T49.0X2	T49.0X3	T49.0X4	T49.0X5	T49.0X6
Magaldrate	T47.1X1	T47.1X2	T47.1X3	T47.1X4	T47.1X5	T47.1X6
Magic mushroom	T40.991	T40.992	T40.993	T40.994	—	—
Magnamycin	T36.8X1	T36.8X2	T36.8X3	T36.8X4	T36.8X5	T36.8X6
Magnesia magma	T47.1X1	T47.1X2	T47.1X3	T47.1X4	T47.1X5	T47.1X6
Magnesium NEC	T56.891	T56.892	T56.893	T56.894		
carbonate	T47.1X1	T47.1X2	T47.1X3	T47.1X4	T47.1X5	T47.1X6
citrate	T47.4X1	T47.4X2	T47.4X3	T47.4X4	T47.4X5	T47.4X6
hydroxide	T47.1X1	T47.1X2	T47.1X3	T47.1X4	T47.1X5	T47.1X6
oxide	T47.1X1	T47.1X2	T47.1X3	T47.1X4	T47.1X5	T47.1X6
peroxide	T49.0X1	T49.0X2	T49.0X3	T49.0X4	T49.0X5	T49.0X6
salicylate	T39.091	T39.092	T39.093	T39.094	T39.095	T39.096
silicofluoride	T50.3X1	T50.3X2	T50.3X3	T50.3X4	T50.3X5	T50.3X6

Substance	Poisoning, Accidental (unintentional)	Poisoning, Intentional Self-harm	Poisoning, Assault	Poisoning, Undetermined	Adverse Effect	Under-dosing
Magnesium — continued						
sulfate	T47.4X1	T47.4X2	T47.4X3	T47.4X4	T47.4X5	T47.4X6
thiosulfate	T45.0X1	T45.0X2	T45.0X3	T45.0X4	T45.0X5	T45.0X6
trisilicate	T47.1X1	T47.1X2	T47.1X3	T47.1X4	T47.1X5	T47.1X6
Malathion (medicinal)	T49.0X1	T49.0X2	T49.0X3	T49.0X4	T49.0X5	T49.0X6
insecticide	T60.0X1	T60.0X2	T60.0X3	T60.0X4		
Male fern extract	T37.4X1	T37.4X2	T37.4X3	T37.4X4	T37.4X5	T37.4X6
M-AMSA	T45.1X1	T45.1X2	T45.1X3	T45.1X4	T45.1X5	T45.1X6
Mandelic acid	T37.8X1	T37.8X2	T37.8X3	T37.8X4	T37.8X5	T37.8X6
Manganese (dioxide) (salts)	T57.2X1	T57.2X2	T57.2X3	T57.2X4		
medicinal	T50.991	T50.992	T50.993	T50.994	T50.995	T50.996
Mannitol	T47.3X1	T47.3X2	T47.3X3	T47.3X4	T47.3X5	T47.3X6
hexanitrate	T46.3X1	T46.3X2	T46.3X3	T46.3X4	T46.3X5	T46.3X6
Mannomustine	T45.1X1	T45.1X2	T45.1X3	T45.1X4	T45.1X5	T45.1X6
MAO inhibitors	T43.1X1	T43.1X2	T43.1X3	T43.1X4	T43.1X5	T43.1X6
Mapharsen	T37.8X1	T37.8X2	T37.8X3	T37.8X4	T37.8X5	T37.8X6
Maphenide	T49.0X1	T49.0X2	T49.0X3	T49.0X4	T49.0X5	T49.0X6
Maprotiline	T43.021	T43.022	T43.023	T43.024	T43.025	T43.026
Marcaine	T41.3X1	T41.3X2	T41.3X3	T41.3X4	T41.3X5	T41.3X6
infiltration (subcutaneous)	T41.3X1	T41.3X2	T41.3X3	T41.3X4	T41.3X5	T41.3X6
nerve block (peripheral) (plexus)	T41.3X1	T41.3X2	T41.3X3	T41.3X4	T41.3X5	T41.3X6
Marezine	T45.0X1	T45.0X2	T45.0X3	T45.0X4	T45.0X5	T45.0X6
Marihuana	T40.7X1	T40.7X2	T40.7X3	T40.7X4	T40.7X5	T40.7X6
Marijuana	T40.7X1	T40.7X2	T40.7X3	T40.7X4	T40.7X5	T40.7X6
Marine (sting)	T63.691	T63.692	T63.693	T63.694	—	—
animals (sting)	T63.691	T63.692	T63.693	T63.694	—	—
plants (sting)	T63.711	T63.712	T63.713	T63.714	—	—
Marplan	T43.1X1	T43.1X2	T43.1X3	T43.1X4	T43.1X5	T43.1X6
Marsh gas	T59.891	T59.892	T59.893	T59.894	—	—
Marsilid	T43.1X1	T43.1X2	T43.1X3	T43.1X4	T43.1X5	T43.1X6
Matulane	T45.1X1	T45.1X2	T45.1X3	T45.1X4	T45.1X5	T45.1X6
Mazindol	T50.5X1	T50.5X2	T50.5X3	T50.5X4	T50.5X5	T50.5X6
MCPA	T60.3X1	T60.3X2	T60.3X3	T60.3X4		
MDMA	T43.621	T43.622	T43.623	T43.624	T43.625	T43.626
Meadow saffron	T62.2X1	T62.2X2	T62.2X3	T62.2X4	—	—
Measles virus vaccine (attenuated)	T50.B91	T50.B92	T50.B93	T50.B94	T50.B95	T50.B96
Meat, noxious	T62.8X1	T62.8X2	T62.8X3	T62.8X4	—	—
Meballymal	T42.3X1	T42.3X2	T42.3X3	T42.3X4	T42.3X5	T42.3X6
Mebanazine	T43.1X1	T43.1X2	T43.1X3	T43.1X4	T43.1X5	T43.1X6
Mebaral	T42.3X1	T42.3X2	T42.3X3	T42.3X4	T42.3X5	T42.3X6
Mebendazole	T37.4X1	T37.4X2	T37.4X3	T37.4X4	T37.4X5	T37.4X6
Mebeverine	T44.3X1	T44.3X2	T44.3X3	T44.3X4	T44.3X5	T44.3X6
Mebhydrolin	T45.0X1	T45.0X2	T45.0X3	T45.0X4	T45.0X5	T45.0X6
Mebumal	T42.3X1	T42.3X2	T42.3X3	T42.3X4	T42.3X5	T42.3X6
Mebutamate	T43.591	T43.592	T43.593	T43.594	T43.595	T43.596
Mecamylamine	T44.2X1	T44.2X2	T44.2X3	T44.2X4	T44.2X5	T44.2X6
Mechlorethamine	T45.1X1	T45.1X2	T45.1X3	T45.1X4	T45.1X5	T45.1X6
Mecillinam	T36.0X1	T36.0X2	T36.0X3	T36.0X4	T36.0X5	T36.0X6
Meclizine (hydrochloride)	T45.0X1	T45.0X2	T45.0X3	T45.0X4	T45.0X5	T45.0X6
Meclocycline	T36.4X1	T36.4X2	T36.4X3	T36.4X4	T36.4X5	T36.4X6
Meclofenamate	T39.391	T39.392	T39.393	T39.394	T39.395	T39.396
Meclofenamic acid	T39.391	T39.392	T39.393	T39.394	T39.395	T39.396
Meclofenoxate	T43.691	T43.692	T43.693	T43.694	T43.695	T43.696
Meclozine	T45.0X1	T45.0X2	T45.0X3	T45.0X4	T45.0X5	T45.0X6
Mecobalamin	T45.8X1	T45.8X2	T45.8X3	T45.8X4	T45.8X5	T45.8X6
Mecoprop	T60.3X1	T60.3X2	T60.3X3	T60.3X4	—	—
Mecrilate	T49.3X1	T49.3X2	T49.3X3	T49.3X4	T49.3X5	T49.3X6
Mecysteine	T48.4X1	T48.4X2	T48.4X3	T48.4X4	T48.4X5	T48.4X6
Medazepam	T42.4X1	T42.4X2	T42.4X3	T42.4X4	T42.4X5	T42.4X6
Medicament NEC	T50.901	T50.902	T50.903	T50.904	T50.905	T50.906
Medinal	T42.3X1	T42.3X2	T42.3X3	T42.3X4	T42.3X5	T42.3X6
Medomin	T42.3X1	T42.3X2	T42.3X3	T42.3X4	T42.3X5	T42.3X6
Medrogestone	T38.5X1	T38.5X2	T38.5X3	T38.5X4	T38.5X5	T38.5X6
Medroxalol	T44.8X1	T44.8X2	T44.8X3	T44.8X4	T44.8X5	T44.8X6
Medroxyprogesterone acetate (depot)	T38.5X1	T38.5X2	T38.5X3	T38.5X4	T38.5X5	T38.5X6
Medrysone	T49.0X1	T49.0X2	T49.0X3	T49.0X4	T49.0X5	T49.0X6
Mefenamic acid	T39.391	T39.392	T39.393	T39.394	T39.395	T39.396
Mefenorex	T50.5X1	T50.5X2	T50.5X3	T50.5X4	T50.5X5	T50.5X6
Mefloquine	T37.2X1	T37.2X2	T37.2X3	T37.2X4	T37.2X5	T37.2X6
Mefruside	T50.2X1	T50.2X2	T50.2X3	T50.2X4	T50.2X5	T50.2X6
Megahallucinogen	T40.901	T40.902	T40.903	T40.904	T40.905	T40.906
Megestrol	T38.5X1	T38.5X2	T38.5X3	T38.5X4	T38.5X5	T38.5X6
Meglumine						
antimoniate	T37.8X1	T37.8X2	T37.8X3	T37.8X4	T37.8X5	T37.8X6
diatrizoate	T50.8X1	T50.8X2	T50.8X3	T50.8X4	T50.8X5	T50.8X6
iodipamide	T50.8X1	T50.8X2	T50.8X3	T50.8X4	T50.8X5	T50.8X6
iotroxate	T50.8X1	T50.8X2	T50.8X3	T50.8X4	T50.8X5	T50.8X6
MEK (methyl ethyl ketone)	T52.4X1	T52.4X2	T52.4X3	T52.4X4		
Meladinin	T49.3X1	T49.3X2	T49.3X3	T49.3X4	T49.3X5	T49.3X6
Meladrazine	T44.3X1	T44.3X2	T44.3X3	T44.3X4	T44.3X5	T44.3X6

376

Additional Character May Be Required — Refer to the Tabular List for Character Selection   Subterms under main terms may continue to next column or page

Substance	Poisoning, Accidental (unintentional)	Poisoning, Intentional Self-harm	Poisoning, Assault	Poisoning, Undetermined	Adverse Effect	Under-dosing
Melaleuca alternifolia oil	T49.0X1	T49.0X2	T49.0X3	T49.0X4	T49.0X5	T49.0X6
Melanizing agents	T49.3X1	T49.3X2	T49.3X3	T49.3X4	T49.3X5	T49.3X6
Melanocyte-stimulating hormone	T38.891	T38.892	T38.893	T38.894	T38.895	T38.896
Melarsonyl potassium	T37.3X1	T37.3X2	T37.3X3	T37.3X4	T37.3X5	T37.3X6
Melarsoprol	T37.3X1	T37.3X2	T37.3X3	T37.3X4	T37.3X5	T37.3X6
Melia azedarach	T62.2X1	T62.2X2	T62.2X3	T62.2X4	—	—
Melitracen	T43.011	T43.012	T43.013	T43.014	T43.015	T43.016
Mellaril	T43.3X1	T43.3X2	T43.3X3	T43.3X4	T43.3X5	T43.3X6
Meloxine	T49.3X1	T49.3X2	T49.3X3	T49.3X4	T49.3X5	T49.3X6
Melperone	T43.4X1	T43.4X2	T43.4X3	T43.4X4	T43.4X5	T43.4X6
Melphalan	T45.1X1	T45.1X2	T45.1X3	T45.1X4	T45.1X5	T45.1X6
Memantine	T43.8X1	T43.8X2	T43.8X3	T43.8X4	T43.8X5	T43.8X6
Menadiol	T45.7X1	T45.7X2	T45.7X3	T45.7X4	T45.7X5	T45.7X6
sodium sulfate	T45.7X1	T45.7X2	T45.7X3	T45.7X4	T45.7X5	T45.7X6
Menadione	T45.7X1	T45.7X2	T45.7X3	T45.7X4	T45.7X5	T45.7X6
sodium bisulfite	T45.7X1	T45.7X2	T45.7X3	T45.7X4	T45.7X5	T45.7X6
Menaphthone	T45.7X1	T45.7X2	T45.7X3	T45.7X4	T45.7X5	T45.7X6
Menaquinone	T45.7X1	T45.7X2	T45.7X3	T45.7X4	T45.7X5	T45.7X6
Menatetrenone	T45.7X1	T45.7X2	T45.7X3	T45.7X4	T45.7X5	T45.7X6
Meningococcal vaccine	T50.A91	T50.A92	T50.A93	T50.A94	T50.A95	T50.A96
Menningovax (-AC) (-C)	T50.A91	T50.A92	T50.A93	T50.A94	T50.A95	T50.A96
Menotropins	T38.811	T38.812	T38.813	T38.814	T38.815	T38.816
Menthol	T48.5X1	T48.5X2	T48.5X3	T48.5X4	T48.5X5	T48.5X6
Mepacrine	T37.2X1	T37.2X2	T37.2X3	T37.2X4	T37.2X5	T37.2X6
Meparfynol	T42.6X1	T42.6X2	T42.6X3	T42.6X4	T42.6X5	T42.6X6
Mepartricin	T36.7X1	T36.7X2	T36.7X3	T36.7X4	T36.7X5	T36.7X6
Mepazine	T43.3X1	T43.3X2	T43.3X3	T43.3X4	T43.3X5	T43.3X6
Mepenzolate	T44.3X1	T44.3X2	T44.3X3	T44.3X4	T44.3X5	T44.3X6
bromide	T44.3X1	T44.3X2	T44.3X3	T44.3X4	T44.3X5	T44.3X6
Meperidine	T40.4X1	T40.4X2	T40.4X3	T40.4X4	T40.4X5	T40.4X6
Mephebarbital	T42.3X1	T42.3X2	T42.3X3	T42.3X4	T42.3X5	T42.3X6
Mephenamin (e)	T42.8X1	T42.8X2	T42.8X3	T42.8X4	T42.8X5	T42.8X6
Mephenesin	T42.8X1	T42.8X2	T42.8X3	T42.8X4	T42.8X5	T42.8X6
Mephenhydramine	T45.0X1	T45.0X2	T45.0X3	T45.0X4	T45.0X5	T45.0X6
Mephenoxalone	T42.8X1	T42.8X2	T42.8X3	T42.8X4	T42.8X5	T42.8X6
Mephentermine	T44.991	T44.992	T44.993	T44.994	T44.995	T44.996
Mephenytoin	T42.0X1	T42.0X2	T42.0X3	T42.0X4	T42.0X5	T42.0X6
with phenobarbital	T42.3X1	T42.3X2	T42.3X3	T42.3X4	T42.3X5	T42.3X6
Mephobarbital	T42.3X1	T42.3X2	T42.3X3	T42.3X4	T42.3X5	T42.3X6
Mephosfolan	T60.0X1	T60.0X2	T60.0X3	T60.0X4	—	—
Mepindolol	T44.7X1	T44.7X2	T44.7X3	T44.7X4	T44.7X5	T44.7X6
Mepiperphenidol	T44.3X1	T44.3X2	T44.3X3	T44.3X4	T44.3X5	T44.3X6
Mepitiostane	T38.7X1	T38.7X2	T38.7X3	T38.7X4	T38.7X5	T38.7X6
Mepivacaine	T41.3X1	T41.3X2	T41.3X3	T41.3X4	T41.3X5	T41.3X6
epidural	T41.3X1	T41.3X2	T41.3X3	T41.3X4	T41.3X5	T41.3X6
Meprednisone	T38.0X1	T38.0X2	T38.0X3	T38.0X4	T38.0X5	T38.0X6
Meprobam	T43.591	T43.592	T43.593	T43.594	T43.595	T43.596
Meprobamate	T43.591	T43.592	T43.593	T43.594	T43.595	T43.596
Meproscillarin	T46.0X1	T46.0X2	T46.0X3	T46.0X4	T46.0X5	T46.0X6
Meprylcaine	T41.3X1	T41.3X2	T41.3X3	T41.3X4	T41.3X5	T41.3X6
Meptazinol	T39.8X1	T39.8X2	T39.8X3	T39.8X4	T39.8X5	T39.8X6
Mepyramine	T45.0X1	T45.0X2	T45.0X3	T45.0X4	T45.0X5	T45.0X6
Mequitazine	T43.3X1	T43.3X2	T43.3X3	T43.3X4	T43.3X5	T43.3X6
Meralluride	T50.2X1	T50.2X2	T50.2X3	T50.2X4	T50.2X5	T50.2X6
Merbaphen	T50.2X1	T50.2X2	T50.2X3	T50.2X4	T50.2X5	T50.2X6
Merbromin	T49.0X1	T49.0X2	T49.0X3	T49.0X4	T49.0X5	T49.0X6
Mercaptobenzothiazole salts	T49.0X1	T49.0X2	T49.0X3	T49.0X4	T49.0X5	T49.0X6
Mercaptomerin	T50.2X1	T50.2X2	T50.2X3	T50.2X4	T50.2X5	T50.2X6
Mercaptopurine	T45.1X1	T45.1X2	T45.1X3	T45.1X4	T45.1X5	T45.1X6
Mercumatilin	T50.2X1	T50.2X2	T50.2X3	T50.2X4	T50.2X5	T50.2X6
Mercuramide	T50.2X1	T50.2X2	T50.2X3	T50.2X4	T50.2X5	T50.2X6
Mercurochrome	T49.0X1	T49.0X2	T49.0X3	T49.0X4	T49.0X5	T49.0X6
Mercurophylline	T50.2X1	T50.2X2	T50.2X3	T50.2X4	T50.2X5	T50.2X6
Mercury, mercurial, mercuric, mercurous (compounds) (cyanide) (fumes) (nonmedicinal) (vapor) NEC	T56.1X1	T56.1X2	T56.1X3	T56.1X4	—	—
ammoniated	T49.0X1	T49.0X2	T49.0X3	T49.0X4	T49.0X5	T49.0X6
anti-infective						
local	T49.0X1	T49.0X2	T49.0X3	T49.0X4	T49.0X5	T49.0X6
systemic	T37.8X1	T37.8X2	T37.8X3	T37.8X4	T37.8X5	T37.8X6
topical	T49.0X1	T49.0X2	T49.0X3	T49.0X4	T49.0X5	T49.0X6
chloride (ammoniated)	T49.0X1	T49.0X2	T49.0X3	T49.0X4	T49.0X5	T49.0X6
fungicide	T56.1X1	T56.1X2	T56.1X3	T56.1X4	—	—
diuretic NEC	T50.2X1	T50.2X2	T50.2X3	T50.2X4	T50.2X5	T50.2X6
fungicide	T56.1X1	T56.1X2	T56.1X3	T56.1X4	—	—
organic (fungicide)	T56.1X1	T56.1X2	T56.1X3	T56.1X4	—	—
oxide, yellow	T49.0X1	T49.0X2	T49.0X3	T49.0X4	T49.0X5	T49.0X6
Mersalyl	T50.2X1	T50.2X2	T50.2X3	T50.2X4	T50.2X5	T50.2X6
Merthiolate	T49.0X1	T49.0X2	T49.0X3	T49.0X4	T49.0X5	T49.0X6

Substance	Poisoning, Accidental (unintentional)	Poisoning, Intentional Self-harm	Poisoning, Assault	Poisoning, Undetermined	Adverse Effect	Under-dosing
Merthiolate — continued						
ophthalmic preparation	T49.5X1	T49.5X2	T49.5X3	T49.5X4	T49.5X5	T49.5X6
Meruvax	T50.B91	T50.B92	T50.B93	T50.B94	T50.B95	T50.B96
Mesalazine	T47.8X1	T47.8X2	T47.8X3	T47.8X4	T47.8X5	T47.8X6
Mescal buttons	T40.991	T40.992	T40.993	T40.994	—	—
Mescaline	T40.991	T40.992	T40.993	T40.994	—	—
Mesna	T48.4X1	T48.4X2	T48.4X3	T48.4X4	T48.4X5	T48.4X6
Mesoglycan	T46.6X1	T46.6X2	T46.6X3	T46.6X4	T46.6X5	T46.6X6
Mesoridazine	T43.3X1	T43.3X2	T43.3X3	T43.3X4	T43.3X5	T43.3X6
Mestanolone	T38.7X1	T38.7X2	T38.7X3	T38.7X4	T38.7X5	T38.7X6
Mesterolone	T38.7X1	T38.7X2	T38.7X3	T38.7X4	T38.7X5	T38.7X6
Mestranol	T38.5X1	T38.5X2	T38.5X3	T38.5X4	T38.5X5	T38.5X6
Mesulergine	T42.8X1	T42.8X2	T42.8X3	T42.8X4	T42.8X5	T42.8X6
Mesulfen	T49.0X1	T49.0X2	T49.0X3	T49.0X4	T49.0X5	T49.0X6
Mesuximide	T42.2X1	T42.2X2	T42.2X3	T42.2X4	T42.2X5	T42.2X6
Metabutethamine	T41.3X1	T41.3X2	T41.3X3	T41.3X4	T41.3X5	T41.3X6
Metactesylacetate	T49.0X1	T49.0X2	T49.0X3	T49.0X4	T49.0X5	T49.0X6
Metacycline	T36.4X1	T36.4X2	T36.4X3	T36.4X4	T36.4X5	T36.4X6
Metaldehyde (snail killer) NEC	T60.8X1	T60.8X2	T60.8X3	T60.8X4	—	—
Metals (heavy) (nonmedicinal)	T56.91	T56.92	T56.93	T56.94	—	—
dust, fumes, or vapor NEC	T56.91	T56.92	T56.93	T56.94	—	—
light NEC	T56.91	T56.92	T56.93	T56.94	—	—
dust, fumes, or vapor NEC	T56.91	T56.92	T56.93	T56.94	—	—
specified NEC	T56.891	T56.892	T56.893	T56.894	—	—
thallium	T56.811	T56.812	T56.813	T56.814	—	—
Metamfetamine	T43.621	T43.622	T43.623	T43.624	T43.625	T43.626
Metamizole sodium	T39.2X1	T39.2X2	T39.2X3	T39.2X4	T39.2X5	T39.2X6
Metampicillin	T36.0X1	T36.0X2	T36.0X3	T36.0X4	T36.0X5	T36.0X6
Metamucil	T47.4X1	T47.4X2	T47.4X3	T47.4X4	T47.4X5	T47.4X6
Metandienone	T38.7X1	T38.7X2	T38.7X3	T38.7X4	T38.7X5	T38.7X6
Metandrostenolone	T38.7X1	T38.7X2	T38.7X3	T38.7X4	T38.7X5	T38.7X6
Metaphen	T49.0X1	T49.0X2	T49.0X3	T49.0X4	T49.0X5	T49.0X6
Metaphos	T60.0X1	T60.0X2	T60.0X3	T60.0X4	—	—
Metapramine	T43.011	T43.012	T43.013	T43.014	T43.015	T43.016
Metaproterenol	T48.291	T48.292	T48.293	T48.294	T48.295	T48.296
Metaraminol	T44.4X1	T44.4X2	T44.4X3	T44.4X4	T44.4X5	T44.4X6
Metaxalone	T42.8X1	T42.8X2	T42.8X3	T42.8X4	T42.8X5	T42.8X6
Metenolone	T38.7X1	T38.7X2	T38.7X3	T38.7X4	T38.7X5	T38.7X6
Metergoline	T42.8X1	T42.8X2	T42.8X3	T42.8X4	T42.8X5	T42.8X6
Metescufylline	T46.991	T46.992	T46.993	T46.994	T46.995	T46.996
Metetoin	T42.0X1	T42.0X2	T42.0X3	T42.0X4	T42.0X5	T42.0X6
Metformin	T38.3X1	T38.3X2	T38.3X3	T38.3X4	T38.3X5	T38.3X6
Methacholine	T44.1X1	T44.1X2	T44.1X3	T44.1X4	T44.1X5	T44.1X6
Methacycline	T36.4X1	T36.4X2	T36.4X3	T36.4X4	T36.4X5	T36.4X6
Methadone	T40.3X1	T40.3X2	T40.3X3	T40.3X4	T40.3X5	T40.3X6
Methallenestril	T38.5X1	T38.5X2	T38.5X3	T38.5X4	T38.5X5	T38.5X6
Methallenoestril	T38.5X1	T38.5X2	T38.5X3	T38.5X4	T38.5X5	T38.5X6
Methamphetamine	T43.621	T43.622	T43.623	T43.624	T43.625	T43.626
Methampyrone	T39.2X1	T39.2X2	T39.2X3	T39.2X4	T39.2X5	T39.2X6
Methandienone	T38.7X1	T38.7X2	T38.7X3	T38.7X4	T38.7X5	T38.7X6
Methandriol	T38.7X1	T38.7X2	T38.7X3	T38.7X4	T38.7X5	T38.7X6
Methandrostenolone	T38.7X1	T38.7X2	T38.7X3	T38.7X4	T38.7X5	T38.7X6
Methane	T59.891	T59.892	T59.893	T59.894	—	—
Methanethiol	T59.891	T59.892	T59.893	T59.894	—	—
Methaniazide	T37.1X1	T37.1X2	T37.1X3	T37.1X4	T37.1X5	T37.1X6
Methanol (vapor)	T51.1X1	T51.1X2	T51.1X3	T51.1X4	—	—
Methantheline	T44.3X1	T44.3X2	T44.3X3	T44.3X4	T44.3X5	T44.3X6
Methanthelinium bromide	T44.3X1	T44.3X2	T44.3X3	T44.3X4	T44.3X5	T44.3X6
Methaphenilene	T45.0X1	T45.0X2	T45.0X3	T45.0X4	T45.0X5	T45.0X6
Methapyrilene	T45.0X1	T45.0X2	T45.0X3	T45.0X4	T45.0X5	T45.0X6
Methaqualone (compound)	T42.6X1	T42.6X2	T42.6X3	T42.6X4	T42.6X5	T42.6X6
Metharbital	T42.3X1	T42.3X2	T42.3X3	T42.3X4	T42.3X5	T42.3X6
Methazolamide	T50.2X1	T50.2X2	T50.2X3	T50.2X4	T50.2X5	T50.2X6
Methdilazine	T43.3X1	T43.3X2	T43.3X3	T43.3X4	T43.3X5	T43.3X6
Methedrine	T43.621	T43.622	T43.623	T43.624	T43.625	T43.626
Methenamine (mandelate)	T37.8X1	T37.8X2	T37.8X3	T37.8X4	T37.8X5	T37.8X6
Methenolone	T38.7X1	T38.7X2	T38.7X3	T38.7X4	T38.7X5	T38.7X6
Methergine	T48.0X1	T48.0X2	T48.0X3	T48.0X4	T48.0X5	T48.0X6
Methetoin	T42.0X1	T42.0X2	T42.0X3	T42.0X4	T42.0X5	T42.0X6
Methiacil	T38.2X1	T38.2X2	T38.2X3	T38.2X4	T38.2X5	T38.2X6
Methicillin	T36.0X1	T36.0X2	T36.0X3	T36.0X4	T36.0X5	T36.0X6
Methimazole	T38.2X1	T38.2X2	T38.2X3	T38.2X4	T38.2X5	T38.2X6
Methiodal sodium	T50.8X1	T50.8X2	T50.8X3	T50.8X4	T50.8X5	T50.8X6
Methionine	T50.991	T50.992	T50.993	T50.994	T50.995	T50.996
Methisazone	T37.5X1	T37.5X2	T37.5X3	T37.5X4	T37.5X5	T37.5X6
Methisoprinol	T37.5X1	T37.5X2	T37.5X3	T37.5X4	T37.5X5	T37.5X6
Methitural	T42.3X1	T42.3X2	T42.3X3	T42.3X4	T42.3X5	T42.3X6
Methixene	T44.3X1	T44.3X2	T44.3X3	T44.3X4	T44.3X5	T44.3X6
Methobarbital, methobarbitone	T42.3X1	T42.3X2	T42.3X3	T42.3X4	T42.3X5	T42.3X6
Methocarbamol	T42.8X1	T42.8X2	T42.8X3	T42.8X4	T42.8X5	T42.8X6

Table of Drugs and Chemicals

Methocarbamol — Milk of magnesia

Substance	Poisoning, Accidental (unintentional)	Poisoning, Intentional Self-harm	Poisoning, Assault	Poisoning, Undetermined	Adverse Effect	Under-dosing
Methocarbamol — *continued*						
skeletal muscle relaxant	T48.1X1	T48.1X2	T48.1X3	T48.1X4	T48.1X5	T48.1X6
Methohexital	T41.1X1	T41.1X2	T41.1X3	T41.1X4	T41.1X5	T41.1X6
Methohexitone	T41.1X1	T41.1X2	T41.1X3	T41.1X4	T41.1X5	T41.1X6
Methoin	T42.0X1	T42.0X2	T42.0X3	T42.0X4	T42.0X5	T42.0X6
Methopholine	T39.8X1	T39.8X2	T39.8X3	T39.8X4	T39.8X5	T39.8X6
Methopromazine	T43.3X1	T43.3X2	T43.3X3	T43.3X4	T43.3X5	T43.3X6
Methorate	T48.3X1	T48.3X2	T48.3X3	T48.3X4	T48.3X5	T48.3X6
Methoserpidine	T46.5X1	T46.5X2	T46.5X3	T46.5X4	T46.5X5	T46.5X6
Methotrexate	T45.1X1	T45.1X2	T45.1X3	T45.1X4	T45.1X5	T45.1X6
Methotrimeprazine	T43.3X1	T43.3X2	T43.3X3	T43.3X4	T43.3X5	T43.3X6
Methoxa-Dome	T49.3X1	T49.3X2	T49.3X3	T49.3X4	T49.3X5	T49.3X6
Methoxamine	T44.4X1	T44.4X2	T44.4X3	T44.4X4	T44.4X5	T44.4X6
Methoxsalen	T50.991	T50.992	T50.993	T50.994	T50.995	T50.996
Methoxyaniline	T65.3X1	T65.3X2	T65.3X3	T65.3X4	—	—
Methoxybenzyl penicillin	T36.0X1	T36.0X2	T36.0X3	T36.0X4	T36.0X5	T36.0X6
Methoxychlor	T53.7X1	T53.7X2	T53.7X3	T53.7X4	—	—
Methoxy-DDT	T53.7X1	T53.7X2	T53.7X3	T53.7X4	—	—
Methoxyflurane	T41.0X1	T41.0X2	T41.0X3	T41.0X4	T41.0X5	T41.0X6
Methoxyphenamine	T48.6X1	T48.6X2	T48.6X3	T48.6X4	T48.6X5	T48.6X6
Methoxypromazine	T43.3X1	T43.3X2	T43.3X3	T43.3X4	T43.3X5	T43.3X6
Methscopolamine bromide	T44.3X1	T44.3X2	T44.3X3	T44.3X4	T44.3X5	T44.3X6
Methsuximide	T42.2X1	T42.2X2	T42.2X3	T42.2X4	T42.2X5	T42.2X6
Methyclothiazide	T50.2X1	T50.2X2	T50.2X3	T50.2X4	T50.2X5	T50.2X6
Methyl						
acetate	T52.4X1	T52.4X2	T52.4X3	T52.4X4	—	—
acetone	T52.4X1	T52.4X2	T52.4X3	T52.4X4	—	—
acrylate	T65.891	T65.892	T65.893	T65.894	—	—
alcohol	T51.1X1	T51.1X2	T51.1X3	T51.1X4	—	—
aminophenol	T65.3X1	T65.3X2	T65.3X3	T65.3X4	—	—
amphetamine	T43.621	T43.622	T43.623	T43.624	T43.625	T43.626
androstanolone	T38.7X1	T38.7X2	T38.7X3	T38.7X4	T38.7X5	T38.7X6
atropine	T44.3X1	T44.3X2	T44.3X3	T44.3X4	T44.3X5	T44.3X6
benzene	T52.2X1	T52.2X2	T52.2X3	T52.2X4	—	—
benzoate	T52.8X1	T52.8X2	T52.8X3	T52.8X4	—	—
benzol	T52.2X1	T52.2X2	T52.2X3	T52.2X4	—	—
bromide (gas)	T59.891	T59.892	T59.893	T59.894	—	—
fumigant	T60.8X1	T60.8X2	T60.8X3	T60.8X4	—	—
butanol	T51.3X1	T51.3X2	T51.3X3	T51.3X4	—	—
carbinol	T51.1X1	T51.1X2	T51.1X3	T51.1X4	—	—
carbonate	T52.8X1	T52.8X2	T52.8X3	T52.8X4	—	—
CCNU	T45.1X1	T45.1X2	T45.1X3	T45.1X4	T45.1X5	T45.1X6
cellosolve	T52.91	T52.92	T52.93	T52.94	—	—
cellulose	T47.4X1	T47.4X2	T47.4X3	T47.4X4	T47.4X5	T47.4X6
chloride (gas)	T59.891	T59.892	T59.893	T59.894	—	—
chloroformate	T59.3X1	T59.3X2	T59.3X3	T59.3X4	—	—
cyclohexane	T52.8X1	T52.8X2	T52.8X3	T52.8X4	—	—
cyclohexanol	T51.8X1	T51.8X2	T51.8X3	T51.8X4	—	—
cyclohexanone	T52.8X1	T52.8X2	T52.8X3	T52.8X4	—	—
cyclohexyl acetate	T52.8X1	T52.8X2	T52.8X3	T52.8X4	—	—
demeton	T60.0X1	T60.0X2	T60.0X3	T60.0X4	—	—
dihydromorphinone	T40.2X1	T40.2X2	T40.2X3	T40.2X4	T40.2X5	T40.2X6
ergometrine	T48.0X1	T48.0X2	T48.0X3	T48.0X4	T48.0X5	T48.0X6
ergonovine	T48.0X1	T48.0X2	T48.0X3	T48.0X4	T48.0X5	T48.0X6
ethyl ketone	T52.4X1	T52.4X2	T52.4X3	T52.4X4	—	—
glucamine antimonate	T37.8X1	T37.8X2	T37.8X3	T37.8X4	T37.8X5	T37.8X6
hydrazine	T65.891	T65.892	T65.893	T65.894	—	—
iodide	T65.891	T65.892	T65.893	T65.894	—	—
isobutyl ketone	T52.4X1	T52.4X2	T52.4X3	T52.4X4	—	—
isothiocyanate	T60.3X1	T60.3X2	T60.3X3	T60.3X4	—	—
mercaptan	T59.891	T59.892	T59.893	T59.894	—	—
morphine NEC	T40.2X1	T40.2X2	T40.2X3	T40.2X4	T40.2X5	T40.2X6
nicotinate	T49.4X1	T49.4X2	T49.4X3	T49.4X4	T49.4X5	T49.4X6
paraben	T49.0X1	T49.0X2	T49.0X3	T49.0X4	T49.0X5	T49.0X6
parafynol	T42.6X1	T42.6X2	T42.6X3	T42.6X4	T42.6X5	T42.6X6
parathion	T60.0X1	T60.0X2	T60.0X3	T60.0X4	—	—
peridol	T43.4X1	T43.4X2	T43.4X3	T43.4X4	T43.4X5	T43.4X6
phenidate	T43.631	T43.632	T43.633	T43.634	T43.635	T43.636
prednisolone	T38.0X1	T38.0X2	T38.0X3	T38.0X4	T38.0X5	T38.0X6
ENT agent	T49.6X1	T49.6X2	T49.6X3	T49.6X4	T49.6X5	T49.6X6
ophthalmic preparation	T49.5X1	T49.5X2	T49.5X3	T49.5X4	T49.5X5	T49.5X6
topical NEC	T49.0X1	T49.0X2	T49.0X3	T49.0X4	T49.0X5	T49.0X6
propylcarbinol	T51.3X1	T51.3X2	T51.3X3	T51.3X4	—	—
rosaniline NEC	T49.0X1	T49.0X2	T49.0X3	T49.0X4	—	T49.0X6
salicylate	T49.2X1	T49.2X2	T49.2X3	T49.2X4	T49.2X5	T49.2X6
sulfate (fumes)	T59.891	T59.892	T59.893	T59.894	—	—
liquid	T52.8X1	T52.8X2	T52.8X3	T52.8X4	—	—
sulfonal	T42.6X1	T42.6X2	T42.6X3	T42.6X4	T42.6X5	T42.6X6
testosterone	T38.7X1	T38.7X2	T38.7X3	T38.7X4	T38.7X5	T38.7X6
thiouracil	T38.2X1	T38.2X2	T38.2X3	T38.2X4	T38.2X5	T38.2X6
Methylamphetamine	T43.621	T43.622	T43.623	T43.624	T43.625	T43.626
Methylated spirit	T51.1X1	T51.1X2	T51.1X3	T51.1X4	—	—
Methylatropine nitrate	T44.3X1	T44.3X2	T44.3X3	T44.3X4	T44.3X5	T44.3X6

Substance	Poisoning, Accidental (unintentional)	Poisoning, Intentional Self-harm	Poisoning, Assault	Poisoning, Undetermined	Adverse Effect	Under-dosing
Methylbenactyzium bromide	T44.3X1	T44.3X2	T44.3X3	T44.3X4	T44.3X5	T44.3X6
Methylbenzethonium chloride	T49.0X1	T49.0X2	T49.0X3	T49.0X4	T49.0X5	T49.0X6
Methylcellulose	T47.4X1	T47.4X2	T47.4X3	T47.4X4	T47.4X5	T47.4X6
laxative	T47.4X1	T47.4X2	T47.4X3	T47.4X4	T47.4X5	T47.4X6
Methylchlorophenoxyacetic acid	T60.3X1	T60.3X2	T60.3X3	T60.3X4	—	—
Methyldopa	T46.5X1	T46.5X2	T46.5X3	T46.5X4	T46.5X5	T46.5X6
Methyldopate	T46.5X1	T46.5X2	T46.5X3	T46.5X4	T46.5X5	T46.5X6
Methylene						
blue	T50.6X1	T50.6X2	T50.6X3	T50.6X4	T50.6X5	T50.6X6
chloride or dichloride (solvent) NEC	T53.4X1	T53.4X2	T53.4X3	T53.4X4	—	—
Methylenedioxyamphetamine	T43.621	T43.622	T43.623	T43.624	T43.625	T43.626
Methylenedioxymethamphetamine	T43.621	T43.622	T43.623	T43.624	T43.625	T43.626
Methylergometrine	T48.0X1	T48.0X2	T48.0X3	T48.0X4	T48.0X5	T48.0X6
Methylergonovine	T48.0X1	T48.0X2	T48.0X3	T48.0X4	T48.0X5	T48.0X6
Methylestrenolone	T38.5X1	T38.5X2	T38.5X3	T38.5X4	T38.5X5	T38.5X6
Methylethyl cellulose	T50.991	T50.992	T50.993	T50.994	T50.995	T50.996
Methylhexabital	T42.3X1	T42.3X2	T42.3X3	T42.3X4	T42.3X5	T42.3X6
Methylmorphine	T40.2X1	T40.2X2	T40.2X3	T40.2X4	T40.2X5	T40.2X6
Methylparaben (ophthalmic)	T49.5X1	T49.5X2	T49.5X3	T49.5X4	T49.5X5	T49.5X6
Methylparafynol	T42.6X1	T42.6X2	T42.6X3	T42.6X4	T42.6X5	T42.6X6
Methylpentynol, methylpenthynol	T42.6X1	T42.6X2	T42.6X3	T42.6X4	T42.6X5	T42.6X6
Methylphenidate	T43.631	T43.632	T43.633	T43.634	T43.635	T43.636
Methylphenobarbital	T42.3X1	T42.3X2	T42.3X3	T42.3X4	T42.3X5	T42.3X6
Methylpolysiloxane	T47.1X1	T47.1X2	T47.1X3	T47.1X4	T47.1X5	T47.1X6
Methylprednisolone — *see* Methyl, prednisolone						
Methylrosaniline	T49.0X1	T49.0X2	T49.0X3	T49.0X4	T49.0X5	T49.0X6
Methylrosanilinium chloride	T49.0X1	T49.0X2	T49.0X3	T49.0X4	T49.0X5	T49.0X6
Methyltestosterone	T38.7X1	T38.7X2	T38.7X3	T38.7X4	T38.7X5	T38.7X6
Methylthionine chloride	T50.6X1	T50.6X2	T50.6X3	T50.6X4	T50.6X5	T50.6X6
Methylthioninium chloride	T50.6X1	T50.6X2	T50.6X3	T50.6X4	T50.6X5	T50.6X6
Methylthiouracil	T38.2X1	T38.2X2	T38.2X3	T38.2X4	T38.2X5	T38.2X6
Methyprylon	T42.6X1	T42.6X2	T42.6X3	T42.6X4	T42.6X5	T42.6X6
Methysergide	T46.5X1	T46.5X2	T46.5X3	T46.5X4	T46.5X5	T46.5X6
Metiamide	T47.1X1	T47.1X2	T47.1X3	T47.1X4	T47.1X5	T47.1X6
Meticillin	T36.0X1	T36.0X2	T36.0X3	T36.0X4	T36.0X5	T36.0X6
Meticrane	T50.2X1	T50.2X2	T50.2X3	T50.2X4	T50.2X5	T50.2X6
Metildigoxin	T46.0X1	T46.0X2	T46.0X3	T46.0X4	T46.0X5	T46.0X6
Metipranolol	T49.5X1	T49.5X2	T49.5X3	T49.5X4	T49.5X5	T49.5X6
Metirosine	T46.5X1	T46.5X2	T46.5X3	T46.5X4	T46.5X5	T46.5X6
Metisazone	T37.5X1	T37.5X2	T37.5X3	T37.5X4	T37.5X5	T37.5X6
Metixene	T44.3X1	T44.3X2	T44.3X3	T44.3X4	T44.3X5	T44.3X6
Metizoline	T48.5X1	T48.5X2	T48.5X3	T48.5X4	T48.5X5	T48.5X6
Metoclopramide	T45.0X1	T45.0X2	T45.0X3	T45.0X4	T45.0X5	T45.0X6
Metofenazate	T43.3X1	T43.3X2	T43.3X3	T43.3X4	T43.3X5	T43.3X6
Metofoline	T39.8X1	T39.8X2	T39.8X3	T39.8X4	T39.8X5	T39.8X6
Metolazone	T50.2X1	T50.2X2	T50.2X3	T50.2X4	T50.2X5	T50.2X6
Metopon	T40.2X1	T40.2X2	T40.2X3	T40.2X4	T40.2X5	T40.2X6
Metopirine	T45.1X1	T45.1X2	T45.1X3	T45.1X4	T45.1X5	T45.1X6
Metoprolol	T44.7X1	T44.7X2	T44.7X3	T44.7X4	T44.7X5	T44.7X6
Metrifonate	T60.0X1	T60.0X2	T60.0X3	T60.0X4	—	—
Metrizamide	T50.8X1	T50.8X2	T50.8X3	T50.8X4	T50.8X5	T50.8X6
Metrizoic acid	T50.8X1	T50.8X2	T50.8X3	T50.8X4	T50.8X5	T50.8X6
Metronidazole	T37.8X1	T37.8X2	T37.8X3	T37.8X4	T37.8X5	T37.8X6
Metycaine	T41.3X1	T41.3X2	T41.3X3	T41.3X4	T41.3X5	T41.3X6
infiltration (subcutaneous)	T41.3X1	T41.3X2	T41.3X3	T41.3X4	T41.3X5	T41.3X6
nerve block (peripheral) (plexus)	T41.3X1	T41.3X2	T41.3X3	T41.3X4	T41.3X5	T41.3X6
topical (surface)	T41.3X1	T41.3X2	T41.3X3	T41.3X4	T41.3X5	T41.3X6
Metyrapone	T50.8X1	T50.8X2	T50.8X3	T50.8X4	T50.8X5	T50.8X6
Mevinphos	T60.0X1	T60.0X2	T60.0X3	T60.0X4	—	—
Mexazolam	T42.4X1	T42.4X2	T42.4X3	T42.4X4	T42.4X5	T42.4X6
Mexenone	T49.3X1	T49.3X2	T49.3X3	T49.3X4	T49.3X5	T49.3X6
Mexiletine	T46.2X1	T46.2X2	T46.2X3	T46.2X4	T46.2X5	T46.2X6
Mezereon	T62.2X1	T62.2X2	T62.2X3	T62.2X4	—	—
berries	T62.1X1	T62.1X2	T62.1X3	T62.1X4	—	—
Mezlocillin	T36.0X1	T36.0X2	T36.0X3	T36.0X4	T36.0X5	T36.0X6
Mianserin	T43.021	T43.022	T43.023	T43.024	T43.025	T43.026
Micatin	T49.0X1	T49.0X2	T49.0X3	T49.0X4	T49.0X5	T49.0X6
Miconazole	T49.0X1	T49.0X2	T49.0X3	T49.0X4	T49.0X5	T49.0X6
Micronomicin	T36.5X1	T36.5X2	T36.5X3	T36.5X4	T36.5X5	T36.5X6
Midazolam	T42.4X1	T42.4X2	T42.4X3	T42.4X4	T42.4X5	T42.4X6
Midecamycin	T36.3X1	T36.3X2	T36.3X3	T36.3X4	T36.3X5	T36.3X6
Mifepristone	T38.6X1	T38.6X2	T38.6X3	T38.6X4	T38.6X5	T38.6X6
Milk of magnesia	T47.1X1	T47.1X2	T47.1X3	T47.1X4	T47.1X5	T47.1X6

Table of Drugs and Chemicals

Substance	Poisoning, Accidental (unintentional)	Poisoning, Intentional Self-harm	Poisoning, Assault	Poisoning, Undetermined	Adverse Effect	Under-dosing
Millipede (tropical) (venomous)	T63.411	T63.412	T63.413	T63.414	—	—
Miltown	T43.591	T43.592	T43.593	T43.594	T43.595	T43.596
Milverine	T44.3X1	T44.3X2	T44.3X3	T44.3X4	T44.3X5	T44.3X6
Minaprine	T43.291	T43.292	T43.293	T43.294	T43.295	T43.296
Minaxolone	T41.291	T41.292	T41.293	T41.294	T41.295	T41.296
Mineral						
acids	T54.2X1	T54.2X2	T54.2X3	T54.2X4	—	—
oil (laxative)(medicinal)	T47.4X1	T47.4X2	T47.4X3	T47.4X4	T47.4X5	T47.4X6
emulsion	T47.2X1	T47.2X2	T47.2X3	T47.2X4	T47.2X5	T47.2X6
nonmedicinal	T52.0X1	T52.0X2	T52.0X3	T52.0X4	—	—
topical	T49.3X1	T49.3X2	T49.3X3	T49.3X4	T49.3X5	T49.3X6
salt NEC	T50.3X1	T50.3X2	T50.3X3	T50.3X4	T50.3X5	T50.3X6
spirits	T52.0X1	T52.0X2	T52.0X3	T52.0X4	—	—
Mineralocorticosteroid	T50.0X1	T50.0X2	T50.0X3	T50.0X4	T50.0X5	T50.0X6
Minocycline	T36.4X1	T36.4X2	T36.4X3	T36.4X4	T36.4X5	T36.4X6
Minoxidil	T46.7X1	T46.7X2	T46.7X3	T46.7X4	T46.7X5	T46.7X6
Miokamycin	T36.3X1	T36.3X2	T36.3X3	T36.3X4	T36.3X5	T36.3X6
Miotic drug	T49.5X1	T49.5X2	T49.5X3	T49.5X4	T49.5X5	T49.5X6
Mipafox	T60.0X1	T60.0X2	T60.0X3	T60.0X4	—	—
Mirex	T60.1X1	T60.1X2	T60.1X3	T60.1X4	—	—
Mirtazapine	T43.021	T43.022	T43.023	T43.024	T43.025	T43.026
Misonidazole	T37.3X1	T37.3X2	T37.3X3	T37.3X4	T37.3X5	T37.3X6
Misoprostol	T47.1X1	T47.1X2	T47.1X3	T47.1X4	T47.1X5	T47.1X6
Mithramycin	T45.1X1	T45.1X2	T45.1X3	T45.1X4	T45.1X5	T45.1X6
Mitobronitol	T45.1X1	T45.1X2	T45.1X3	T45.1X4	T45.1X5	T45.1X6
Mitoguazone	T45.1X1	T45.1X2	T45.1X3	T45.1X4	T45.1X5	T45.1X6
Mitolactol	T45.1X1	T45.1X2	T45.1X3	T45.1X4	T45.1X5	T45.1X6
Mitomycin	T45.1X1	T45.1X2	T45.1X3	T45.1X4	T45.1X5	T45.1X6
Mitopodozide	T45.1X1	T45.1X2	T45.1X3	T45.1X4	T45.1X5	T45.1X6
Mitotane	T45.1X1	T45.1X2	T45.1X3	T45.1X4	T45.1X5	T45.1X6
Mitoxantrone	T45.1X1	T45.1X2	T45.1X3	T45.1X4	T45.1X5	T45.1X6
Mivacurium chloride	T48.1X1	T48.1X2	T48.1X3	T48.1X4	T48.1X5	T48.1X6
Miyari bacteria	T47.6X1	T47.6X2	T47.6X3	T47.6X4	T47.6X5	T47.6X6
Moclobemide	T43.1X1	T43.1X2	T43.1X3	T43.1X4	T43.1X5	T43.1X6
Moderil	T46.5X1	T46.5X2	T46.5X3	T46.5X4	T46.5X5	T46.5X6
Mofebutazone	T39.2X1	T39.2X2	T39.2X3	T39.2X4	T39.2X5	T39.2X6
Mogadon — see Nitrazepam						
Molindone	T43.591	T43.592	T43.593	T43.594	T43.595	T43.596
Molsidomine	T46.3X1	T46.3X2	T46.3X3	T46.3X4	T46.3X5	T46.3X6
Mometasone	T49.0X1	T49.0X2	T49.0X3	T49.0X4	T49.0X5	T49.0X6
Monistat	T49.0X1	T49.0X2	T49.0X3	T49.0X4	T49.0X5	T49.0X6
Monoamine oxidase inhibitor NEC	T43.1X1	T43.1X2	T43.1X3	T43.1X4	T43.1X5	T43.1X6
hydrazine	T43.1X1	T43.1X2	T43.1X3	T43.1X4	T43.1X5	T43.1X6
Monobenzone	T49.4X1	T49.4X2	T49.4X3	T49.4X4	T49.4X5	T49.4X6
Monochloroacetic acid	T60.3X1	T60.3X2	T60.3X3	T60.3X4	—	—
Monochlorobenzene	T53.7X1	T53.7X2	T53.7X3	T53.7X4	—	—
Monoethanolamine	T46.8X1	T46.8X2	T46.8X3	T46.8X4	T46.8X5	T46.8X6
oleate	T46.8X1	T46.8X2	T46.8X3	T46.8X4	T46.8X5	T46.8X6
Monooctanoin	T50.991	T50.992	T50.993	T50.994	T50.995	T50.996
Monophenylbutazone	T39.2X1	T39.2X2	T39.2X3	T39.2X4	T39.2X5	T39.2X6
Monosodium glutamate	T65.891	T65.892	T65.893	T65.894	—	—
Monosulfiram	T49.0X1	T49.0X2	T49.0X3	T49.0X4	T49.0X5	T49.0X6
Monoxide, carbon — see Carbon, monoxide						
Monoxidine hydrochloride	T46.1X1	T46.1X2	T46.1X3	T46.1X4	T46.1X5	T46.1X6
Monuron	T60.3X1	T60.3X2	T60.3X3	T60.3X4	—	—
Moperone	T43.4X1	T43.4X2	T43.4X3	T43.4X4	T43.4X5	T43.4X6
Mopidamol	T45.1X1	T45.1X2	T45.1X3	T45.1X4	T45.1X5	T45.1X6
MOPP (mechloreth-amine + vincristine + prednisone + procarba-zine)	T45.1X1	T45.1X2	T45.1X3	T45.1X4	T45.1X5	T45.1X6
Morfin	T40.2X1	T40.2X2	T40.2X3	T40.2X4	T40.2X5	T40.2X6
Morinamide	T37.1X1	T37.1X2	T37.1X3	T37.1X4	T37.1X5	T37.1X6
Morning glory seeds	T40.991	T40.992	T40.993	T40.994	—	—
Moroxydine	T37.5X1	T37.5X2	T37.5X3	T37.5X4	T37.5X5	T37.5X6
Morphazinamide	T37.1X1	T37.1X2	T37.1X3	T37.1X4	T37.1X5	T37.1X6
Morphine	T40.2X1	T40.2X2	T40.2X3	T40.2X4	T40.2X5	T40.2X6
antagonist	T50.7X1	T50.7X2	T50.7X3	T50.7X4	T50.7X5	T50.7X6
Morpholinylethylmorphine	T40.2X1	T40.2X2	T40.2X3	T40.2X4	—	—
Morsuximide	T42.2X1	T42.2X2	T42.2X3	T42.2X4	T42.2X5	T42.2X6
Mosapramine	T43.591	T43.592	T43.593	T43.594	T43.595	T43.596
Moth balls — see also Pesticides	T60.2X1	T60.2X2	T60.2X3	T60.2X4	—	—
naphthalene	T60.2X1	T60.2X2	T60.2X3	T60.2X4	—	—
paradichlorobenzene	T60.1X1	T60.1X2	T60.1X3	T60.1X4	—	—
Motor exhaust gas	T58.01	T58.02	T58.03	T58.04	—	—
Mouthwash (antiseptic) (zinc chloride)	T49.6X1	T49.6X2	T49.6X3	T49.6X4	T49.6X5	T49.6X6
Moxastine	T45.0X1	T45.0X2	T45.0X3	T45.0X4	T45.0X5	T45.0X6
Moxaverine	T44.3X1	T44.3X2	T44.3X3	T44.3X4	T44.3X5	T44.3X6
Moxisylyte	T46.7X1	T46.7X2	T46.7X3	T46.7X4	T46.7X5	T46.7X6
Mucilage, plant	T47.4X1	T47.4X2	T47.4X3	T47.4X4	T47.4X5	T47.4X6
Mucolytic drug	T48.4X1	T48.4X2	T48.4X3	T48.4X4	T48.4X5	T48.4X6
Mucomyst	T48.4X1	T48.4X2	T48.4X3	T48.4X4	T48.4X5	T48.4X6
Mucous membrane agents (external)	T49.91	T49.92	T49.93	T49.94	T49.95	T49.96
specified NEC	T49.8X1	T49.8X2	T49.8X3	T49.8X4	T49.8X5	T49.8X6
Mumps						
immune globulin (human)	T50.Z11	T50.Z12	T50.Z13	T50.Z14	T50.Z15	T50.Z16
skin test antigen	T50.8X1	T50.8X2	T50.8X3	T50.8X4	T50.8X5	T50.8X6
vaccine	T50.B91	T50.B92	T50.B93	T50.B94	T50.B95	T50.B96
Mumpsvax	T50.B91	T50.B92	T50.B93	T50.B94	T50.B95	T50.B96
Mupirocin	T49.0X1	T49.0X2	T49.0X3	T49.0X4	T49.0X5	T49.0X6
Muriatic acid — see Hydrochloric acid						
Muromonab-CD3	T45.1X1	T45.1X2	T45.1X3	T45.1X4	T45.1X5	T45.1X6
Muscle-action drug NEC	T48.201	T48.202	T48.203	T48.204	T48.205	T48.206
Muscle affecting agents NEC	T48.201	T48.202	T48.203	T48.204	T48.205	T48.206
oxytocic	T48.0X1	T48.0X2	T48.0X3	T48.0X4	T48.0X5	T48.0X6
relaxants	T48.201	T48.202	T48.203	T48.204	T48.205	T48.206
central nervous system	T42.8X1	T42.8X2	T42.8X3	T42.8X4	T42.8X5	T42.8X6
skeletal	T48.1X1	T48.1X2	T48.1X3	T48.1X4	T48.1X5	T48.1X6
smooth	T44.3X1	T44.3X2	T44.3X3	T44.3X4	T44.3X5	T44.3X6
Muscle relaxant — see Relaxant, muscle						
Muscle-tone depressant, central NEC	T42.8X1	T42.8X2	T42.8X3	T42.8X4	T42.8X5	T42.8X6
specified NEC	T42.8X1	T42.8X2	T42.8X3	T42.8X4	T42.8X5	T42.8X6
Mushroom, noxious	T62.0X1	T62.0X2	T62.0X3	T62.0X4	—	—
Mussel, noxious	T61.781	T61.782	T61.783	T61.784	—	—
Mustard (emetic)	T47.7X1	T47.7X2	T47.7X3	T47.7X4	T47.7X5	T47.7X6
black	T47.7X1	T47.7X2	T47.7X3	T47.7X4	T47.7X5	T47.7X6
gas, not in war	T59.91	T59.92	T59.93	T59.94	—	—
nitrogen	T45.1X1	T45.1X2	T45.1X3	T45.1X4	T45.1X5	T45.1X6
Mustine	T45.1X1	T45.1X2	T45.1X3	T45.1X4	T45.1X5	T45.1X6
M-vac	T45.1X1	T45.1X2	T45.1X3	T45.1X4	T45.1X5	T45.1X6
Mycifradin	T36.5X1	T36.5X2	T36.5X3	T36.5X4	T36.5X5	T36.5X6
topical	T49.0X1	T49.0X2	T49.0X3	T49.0X4	T49.0X5	T49.0X6
Mycitracin	T36.8X1	T36.8X2	T36.8X3	T36.8X4	T36.8X5	T36.8X6
ophthalmic preparation	T49.5X1	T49.5X2	T49.5X3	T49.5X4	T49.5X5	T49.5X6
Mycostatin	T36.7X1	T36.7X2	T36.7X3	T36.7X4	T36.7X5	T36.7X6
topical	T49.0X1	T49.0X2	T49.0X3	T49.0X4	T49.0X5	T49.0X6
Mycotoxins	T64.81	T64.82	T64.83	T64.84	—	—
aflatoxin	T64.01	T64.02	T64.03	T64.04	—	—
specified NEC	T64.81	T64.82	T64.83	T64.84	—	—
Mydriacyl	T44.3X1	T44.3X2	T44.3X3	T44.3X4	T44.3X5	T44.3X6
Mydriatic drug	T49.5X1	T49.5X2	T49.5X3	T49.5X4	T49.5X5	T49.5X6
Myelobromal	T45.1X1	T45.1X2	T45.1X3	T45.1X4	T45.1X5	T45.1X6
Myleran	T45.1X1	T45.1X2	T45.1X3	T45.1X4	T45.1X5	T45.1X6
Myochrysine (e)	T39.2X1	T39.2X2	T39.2X3	T39.2X4	T39.2X5	T39.2X6
Myoneural blocking agents	T48.1X1	T48.1X2	T48.1X3	T48.1X4	T48.1X5	T48.1X6
Myralact	T49.0X1	T49.0X2	T49.0X3	T49.0X4	T49.0X5	T49.0X6
Myristica fragrans	T62.2X1	T62.2X2	T62.2X3	T62.2X4	—	—
Myristicin	T65.891	T65.892	T65.893	T65.894	—	—
Mysoline	T42.3X1	T42.3X2	T42.3X3	T42.3X4	T42.3X5	T42.3X6
Nabilone	T40.7X1	T40.7X2	T40.7X3	T40.7X4	T40.7X5	T40.7X6
Nabumetone	T39.391	T39.392	T39.393	T39.394	T39.395	T39.396
Nadolol	T44.7X1	T44.7X2	T44.7X3	T44.7X4	T44.7X5	T44.7X6
Nafcillin	T36.0X1	T36.0X2	T36.0X3	T36.0X4	T36.0X5	T36.0X6
Nafoxidine	T38.6X1	T38.6X2	T38.6X3	T38.6X4	T38.6X5	T38.6X6
Naftazone	T46.991	T46.992	T46.993	T46.994	T46.995	T46.996
Naftidrofuryl (oxalate)	T46.7X1	T46.7X2	T46.7X3	T46.7X4	T46.7X5	T46.7X6
Naftifine	T49.0X1	T49.0X2	T49.0X3	T49.0X4	T49.0X5	T49.0X6
Nail polish remover	T52.91	T52.92	T52.93	T52.94	—	—
Nalbuphine	T40.4X1	T40.4X2	T40.4X3	T40.4X4	T40.4X5	T40.4X6
Naled	T60.0X1	T60.0X2	T60.0X3	T60.0X4	—	—
Nalidixic acid	T37.8X1	T37.8X2	T37.8X3	T37.8X4	T37.8X5	T37.8X6
Nalorphine	T50.7X1	T50.7X2	T50.7X3	T50.7X4	T50.7X5	T50.7X6
Naloxone	T50.7X1	T50.7X2	T50.7X3	T50.7X4	T50.7X5	T50.7X6
Naltrexone	T50.7X1	T50.7X2	T50.7X3	T50.7X4	T50.7X5	T50.7X6
Namenda	T43.8X1	T43.8X2	T43.8X3	T43.8X4	T43.8X5	T43.8X6
Nandrolone	T38.7X1	T38.7X2	T38.7X3	T38.7X4	T38.7X5	T38.7X6
Naphazoline	T48.5X1	T48.5X2	T48.5X3	T48.5X4	T48.5X5	T48.5X6
Naphtha (painters') (petroleum)	T52.0X1	T52.0X2	T52.0X3	T52.0X4	—	—
solvent	T52.0X1	T52.0X2	T52.0X3	T52.0X4	—	—
vapor	T52.0X1	T52.0X2	T52.0X3	T52.0X4	—	—
Naphthalene (non-chlorinated)	T60.2X1	T60.2X2	T60.2X3	T60.2X4	—	—
chlorinated	T60.1X1	T60.1X2	T60.1X3	T60.1X4	—	—
vapor	T60.1X1	T60.1X2	T60.1X3	T60.1X4	—	—

Table of Drugs and Chemicals

Naphthalene — Nonoxinol

Substance	Poisoning, Accidental (unintentional)	Poisoning, Intentional Self-harm	Poisoning, Assault	Poisoning, Undetermined	Adverse Effect	Under-dosing
Naphthalene — *continued*						
insecticide or moth repellent	T60.2X1	T60.2X2	T60.2X3	T60.2X4	—	—
chlorinated	T60.1X1	T60.1X2	T60.1X3	T60.1X4	—	—
vapor	T60.2X1	T60.2X2	T60.2X3	T60.2X4	—	—
chlorinated	T60.1X1	T60.1X2	T60.1X3	T60.1X4	—	—
Naphthol	T65.891	T65.892	T65.893	T65.894	—	—
Naphthylamine	T65.891	T65.892	T65.893	T65.894	—	—
Naphthylthiourea (ANTU)	T60.4X1	T60.4X2	T60.4X3	T60.4X4	—	—
Naprosyn — *see* Naproxen						
Naproxen	T39.311	T39.312	T39.313	T39.314	T39.315	T39.316
Narcotic (drug)	T40.601	T40.602	T40.603	T40.604	T40.605	T40.606
analgesic NEC	T40.601	T40.602	T40.603	T40.604	T40.605	T40.606
antagonist	T50.7X1	T50.7X2	T50.7X3	T50.7X4	T50.7X5	T50.7X6
specified NEC	T40.691	T40.692	T40.693	T40.694	T40.695	T40.696
synthetic	T40.4X1	T40.4X2	T40.4X3	T40.4X4	T40.4X5	T40.4X6
Narcotine	T48.3X1	T48.3X2	T48.3X3	T48.3X4	T48.3X5	T48.3X6
Nardil	T43.1X1	T43.1X2	T43.1X3	T43.1X4	T43.1X5	T43.1X6
Nasal drug NEC	T49.6X1	T49.6X2	T49.6X3	T49.6X4	T49.6X5	T49.6X6
Natamycin	T49.0X1	T49.0X2	T49.0X3	T49.0X4	T49.0X5	T49.0X6
Natrium cyanide — *see* Cyanide(s)						
Natural						
blood (product)	T45.8X1	T45.8X2	T45.8X3	T45.8X4	T45.8X5	T45.8X6
gas (piped)	T59.891	T59.892	T59.893	T59.894	—	—
incomplete combustion	T58.11	T58.12	T58.13	T58.14	—	—
Nealbarbital	T42.3X1	T42.3X2	T42.3X3	T42.3X4	T42.3X5	T42.3X6
Nectadon	T48.3X1	T48.3X2	T48.3X3	T48.3X4	T48.3X5	T48.3X6
Nedocromil	T48.6X1	T48.6X2	T48.6X3	T48.6X4	T48.6X5	T48.6X6
Nefopam	T39.8X1	T39.8X2	T39.8X3	T39.8X4	T39.8X5	T39.8X6
Nematocyst (sting)	T63.691	T63.692	T63.693	T63.694	—	—
Nembutal	T42.3X1	T42.3X2	T42.3X3	T42.3X4	T42.3X5	T42.3X6
Nemonapride	T43.591	T43.592	T43.593	T43.594	T43.595	T43.596
Neoarsphenamine	T37.8X1	T37.8X2	T37.8X3	T37.8X4	T37.8X5	T37.8X6
Neocinchophen	T50.4X1	T50.4X2	T50.4X3	T50.4X4	T50.4X5	T50.4X6
Neomycin (derivatives)	T36.5X1	T36.5X2	T36.5X3	T36.5X4	T36.5X5	T36.5X6
with						
bacitracin	T49.0X1	T49.0X2	T49.0X3	T49.0X4	T49.0X5	T49.0X6
neostigmine	T44.0X1	T44.0X2	T44.0X3	T44.0X4	T44.0X5	T44.0X6
ENT agent	T49.6X1	T49.6X2	T49.6X3	T49.6X4	T49.6X5	T49.6X6
ophthalmic preparation	T49.5X1	T49.5X2	T49.5X3	T49.5X4	T49.5X5	T49.5X6
topical NEC	T49.0X1	T49.0X2	T49.0X3	T49.0X4	T49.0X5	T49.0X6
Neonal	T42.3X1	T42.3X2	T42.3X3	T42.3X4	T42.3X5	T42.3X6
Neoprontosil	T37.0X1	T37.0X2	T37.0X3	T37.0X4	T37.0X5	T37.0X6
Neosalvarsan	T37.8X1	T37.8X2	T37.8X3	T37.8X4	T37.8X5	T37.8X6
Neosilversalvarsan	T37.8X1	T37.8X2	T37.8X3	T37.8X4	T37.8X5	T37.8X6
Neosporin	T36.8X1	T36.8X2	T36.8X3	T36.8X4	T36.8X5	T36.8X6
ENT agent	T49.6X1	T49.6X2	T49.6X3	T49.6X4	T49.6X5	T49.6X6
opthalmic preparation	T49.5X1	T49.5X2	T49.5X3	T49.5X4	T49.5X5	T49.5X6
topical NEC	T49.0X1	T49.0X2	T49.0X3	T49.0X4	T49.0X5	T49.0X6
Neostigmine bromide	T44.0X1	T44.0X2	T44.0X3	T44.0X4	T44.0X5	T44.0X6
Neraval	T42.3X1	T42.3X2	T42.3X3	T42.3X4	T42.3X5	T42.3X6
Neravan	T42.3X1	T42.3X2	T42.3X3	T42.3X4	T42.3X5	T42.3X6
Nerium oleander	T62.2X1	T62.2X2	T62.2X3	T62.2X4	—	—
Nerve gas, not in war	T59.91	T59.92	T59.93	T59.94	—	—
Nesacaine	T41.3X1	T41.3X2	T41.3X3	T41.3X4	T41.3X5	T41.3X6
infiltration (subcutaneous)	T41.3X1	T41.3X2	T41.3X3	T41.3X4	T41.3X5	T41.3X6
nerve block (peripheral) (plexus)	T41.3X1	T41.3X2	T41.3X3	T41.3X4	T41.3X5	T41.3X6
Netilmicin	T36.5X1	T36.5X2	T36.5X3	T36.5X4	T36.5X5	T36.5X6
Neurobarb	T42.3X1	T42.3X2	T42.3X3	T42.3X4	T42.3X5	T42.3X6
Neuroleptic drug NEC	T43.501	T43.502	T43.503	T43.504	T43.505	T43.506
Neuromuscular blocking drug	T48.1X1	T48.1X2	T48.1X3	T48.1X4	T48.1X5	T48.1X6
Neutral insulin injection	T38.3X1	T38.3X2	T38.3X3	T38.3X4	T38.3X5	T38.3X6
Neutral spirits	T51.0X1	T51.0X2	T51.0X3	T51.0X4	—	—
beverage	T51.0X1	T51.0X2	T51.0X3	T51.0X4	—	—
Niacin	T46.7X1	T46.7X2	T46.7X3	T46.7X4	T46.7X5	T46.7X6
Niacinamide	T45.2X1	T45.2X2	T45.2X3	T45.2X4	T45.2X5	T45.2X6
Nialamide	T43.1X1	T43.1X2	T43.1X3	T43.1X4	T43.1X5	T43.1X6
Niaprazine	T42.6X1	T42.6X2	T42.6X3	T42.6X4	T42.6X5	T42.6X6
Nicametate	T46.7X1	T46.7X2	T46.7X3	T46.7X4	T46.7X5	T46.7X6
Nicardipine	T46.1X1	T46.1X2	T46.1X3	T46.1X4	T46.1X5	T46.1X6
Nicergoline	T46.7X1	T46.7X2	T46.7X3	T46.7X4	T46.7X5	T46.7X6
Nickel (carbonyl) (tetra-carbonyl) (fumes) (vapor)	T56.891	T56.892	T56.893	T56.894	—	—
Nickelocene	T56.891	T56.892	T56.893	T56.894	—	—
Niclosamide	T37.4X1	T37.4X2	T37.4X3	T37.4X4	T37.4X5	T37.4X6
Nicofuranose	T46.7X1	T46.7X2	T46.7X3	T46.7X4	T46.7X5	T46.7X6
Nicomorphine	T40.2X1	T40.2X2	T40.2X3	T40.2X4	—	—
Nicorandil	T46.3X1	T46.3X2	T46.3X3	T46.3X4	T46.3X5	T46.3X6
Nicotiana (plant)	T62.2X1	T62.2X2	T62.2X3	T62.2X4	—	—
Nicotinamide	T45.2X1	T45.2X2	T45.2X3	T45.2X4	T45.2X5	T45.2X6
Nicotine (insecticide) (spray) (sulfate) NEC	T60.2X1	T60.2X2	T60.2X3	T60.2X4	—	—
from tobacco	T65.291	T65.292	T65.293	T65.294	—	—
cigarettes	T65.221	T65.222	T65.223	T65.224	—	—
not insecticide	T65.291	T65.292	T65.293	T65.294	—	—
Nicotinic acid	T46.7X1	T46.7X2	T46.7X3	T46.7X4	T46.7X5	T46.7X6
Nicotinyl alcohol	T46.7X1	T46.7X2	T46.7X3	T46.7X4	T46.7X5	T46.7X6
Nicoumalone	T45.511	T45.512	T45.513	T45.514	T45.515	T45.516
Nifedipine	T46.1X1	T46.1X2	T46.1X3	T46.1X4	T46.1X5	T46.1X6
Nifenazone	T39.2X1	T39.2X2	T39.2X3	T39.2X4	T39.2X5	T39.2X6
Nifuraldezone	T37.91	T37.92	T37.93	T37.94	T37.95	T37.96
Nifuratel	T37.8X1	T37.8X2	T37.8X3	T37.8X4	T37.8X5	T37.8X6
Nifurtimox	T37.3X1	T37.3X2	T37.3X3	T37.3X4	T37.3X5	T37.3X6
Nifurtoinol	T37.8X1	T37.8X2	T37.8X3	T37.8X4	T37.8X5	T37.8X6
Nightshade, deadly (solanum) — *see also* Belladonna	T62.2X1	T62.2X2	T62.2X3	T62.2X4	—	—
berry	T62.1X1	T62.1X2	T62.1X3	T62.1X4	—	—
Nikethamide	T50.7X1	T50.7X2	T50.7X3	T50.7X4	T50.7X5	T50.7X6
Nilstat	T36.7X1	T36.7X2	T36.7X3	T36.7X4	T36.7X5	T36.7X6
topical	T49.0X1	T49.0X2	T49.0X3	T49.0X4	T49.0X5	T49.0X6
Nilutamide	T38.6X1	T38.6X2	T38.6X3	T38.6X4	T38.6X5	T38.6X6
Nimesulide	T39.391	T39.392	T39.393	T39.394	T39.395	T39.396
Nimetazepam	T42.4X1	T42.4X2	T42.4X3	T42.4X4	T42.4X5	T42.4X6
Nimodipine	T46.1X1	T46.1X2	T46.1X3	T46.1X4	T46.1X5	T46.1X6
Nimorazole	T37.3X1	T37.3X2	T37.3X3	T37.3X4	T37.3X5	T37.3X6
Nimustine	T45.1X1	T45.1X2	T45.1X3	T45.1X4	T45.1X5	T45.1X6
Niridazole	T37.4X1	T37.4X2	T37.4X3	T37.4X4	T37.4X5	T37.4X6
Nisentil	T40.2X1	T40.2X2	T40.2X3	T40.2X4	T40.2X5	T40.2X6
Nisoldipine	T46.1X1	T46.1X2	T46.1X3	T46.1X4	T46.1X5	T46.1X6
Nitramine	T65.3X1	T65.3X2	T65.3X3	T65.3X4	—	—
Nitrate, organic	T46.3X1	T46.3X2	T46.3X3	T46.3X4	T46.3X5	T46.3X6
Nitrazepam	T42.4X1	T42.4X2	T42.4X3	T42.4X4	T42.4X5	T42.4X6
Nitrefazole	T50.6X1	T50.6X2	T50.6X3	T50.6X4	T50.6X5	T50.6X6
Nitrendipine	T46.1X1	T46.1X2	T46.1X3	T46.1X4	T46.1X5	T46.1X6
Nitric						
acid (liquid)	T54.2X1	T54.2X2	T54.2X3	T54.2X4	—	—
vapor	T59.891	T59.892	T59.893	T59.894	—	—
oxide (gas)	T59.891	T59.892	T59.893	T59.894	—	—
Nitrimidazine	T37.3X1	T37.3X2	T37.3X3	T37.3X4	T37.3X5	T37.3X6
Nitrite, amyl (medicinal) (vapor)	T46.3X1	T46.3X2	T46.3X3	T46.3X4	T46.3X5	T46.3X6
Nitroaniline	T65.3X1	T65.3X2	T65.3X3	T65.3X4	—	—
vapor	T59.891	T59.892	T59.893	T59.894	—	—
Nitrobenzene, nitrobenzol	T65.3X1	T65.3X2	T65.3X3	T65.3X4	—	—
vapor	T65.3X1	T65.3X2	T65.3X3	T65.3X4	—	—
Nitrocellulose	T65.891	T65.892	T65.893	T65.894	—	—
lacquer	T65.891	T65.892	T65.893	T65.894	—	—
Nitrodiphenyl	T65.3X1	T65.3X2	T65.3X3	T65.3X4	—	—
Nitrofural	T49.0X1	T49.0X2	T49.0X3	T49.0X4	T49.0X5	T49.0X6
Nitrofurantoin	T37.8X1	T37.8X2	T37.8X3	T37.8X4	T37.8X5	T37.8X6
Nitrofurazone	T49.0X1	T49.0X2	T49.0X3	T49.0X4	T49.0X5	T49.0X6
Nitrogen	T59.0X1	T59.0X2	T59.0X3	T59.0X4	—	—
mustard	T45.1X1	T45.1X2	T45.1X3	T45.1X4	T45.1X5	T45.1X6
Nitroglycerin, nitroglycerol (medicinal)	T46.3X1	T46.3X2	T46.3X3	T46.3X4	T46.3X5	T46.3X6
nonmedicinal	T65.5X1	T65.5X2	T65.5X3	T65.5X4	—	—
fumes	T65.5X1	T65.5X2	T65.5X3	T65.5X4	—	—
Nitroglycol	T52.3X1	T52.3X2	T52.3X3	T52.3X4	—	—
Nitrohydrochloric acid	T54.2X1	T54.2X2	T54.2X3	T54.2X4	—	—
Nitromersol	T49.0X1	T49.0X2	T49.0X3	T49.0X4	T49.0X5	T49.0X6
Nitronaphthalene	T65.891	T65.892	T65.893	T65.894	—	—
Nitrophenol	T54.0X1	T54.0X2	T54.0X3	T54.0X4	—	—
Nitropropane	T52.8X1	T52.8X2	T52.8X3	T52.8X4	—	—
Nitroprusside	T46.5X1	T46.5X2	T46.5X3	T46.5X4	T46.5X5	T46.5X6
Nitrosodimethylamine	T65.3X1	T65.3X2	T65.3X3	T65.3X4	—	—
Nitrothiazol	T37.4X1	T37.4X2	T37.4X3	T37.4X4	T37.4X5	T37.4X6
Nitrotoluene, nitrotoluol	T65.3X1	T65.3X2	T65.3X3	T65.3X4	—	—
vapor	T65.3X1	T65.3X2	T65.3X3	T65.3X4	—	—
Nitrous						
acid (liquid)	T54.2X1	T54.2X2	T54.2X3	T54.2X4	—	—
fumes	T59.891	T59.892	T59.893	T59.894	—	—
ether spirit	T46.3X1	T46.3X2	T46.3X3	T46.3X4	T46.3X5	T46.3X6
oxide	T41.0X1	T41.0X2	T41.0X3	T41.0X4	T41.0X5	T41.0X6
Nitroxoline	T37.8X1	T37.8X2	T37.8X3	T37.8X4	T37.8X5	T37.8X6
Nitrozone	T49.0X1	T49.0X2	T49.0X3	T49.0X4	T49.0X5	T49.0X6
Nizatidine	T47.0X1	T47.0X2	T47.0X3	T47.0X4	T47.0X5	T47.0X6
Nizofenone	T43.8X1	T43.8X2	T43.8X3	T43.8X4	T43.8X5	T43.8X6
Noctec	T42.6X1	T42.6X2	T42.6X3	T42.6X4	T42.6X5	T42.6X6
Noludar	T42.6X1	T42.6X2	T42.6X3	T42.6X4	T42.6X5	T42.6X6
Nomegestrol	T38.5X1	T38.5X2	T38.5X3	T38.5X4	T38.5X5	T38.5X6
Nomifensine	T43.291	T43.292	T43.293	T43.294	T43.295	T43.296
Nonoxinol	T49.8X1	T49.8X2	T49.8X3	T49.8X4	T49.8X5	T49.8X6

Substance	Poisoning, Accidental (unintentional)	Poisoning, Intentional Self-harm	Poisoning, Assault	Poisoning, Undetermined	Adverse Effect	Under-dosing
Nonylphenoxy (polyethoxyethanol)	T49.8X1	T49.8X2	T49.8X3	T49.8X4	T49.8X5	T49.8X6
Noptil	T42.3X1	T42.3X2	T42.3X3	T42.3X4	T42.3X5	T42.3X6
Noradrenaline	T44.4X1	T44.4X2	T44.4X3	T44.4X4	T44.4X5	T44.4X6
Noramidopyrine	T39.2X1	T39.2X2	T39.2X3	T39.2X4	T39.2X5	T39.2X6
methanesulfonate sodium	T39.2X1	T39.2X2	T39.2X3	T39.2X4	T39.2X5	T39.2X6
Norbormide	T60.4X1	T60.4X2	T60.4X3	T60.4X4	—	—
Nordazepam	T42.4X1	T42.4X2	T42.4X3	T42.4X4	T42.4X5	T42.4X6
Norepinephrine	T44.4X1	T44.4X2	T44.4X3	T44.4X4	T44.4X5	T44.4X6
Norethandrolone	T38.7X1	T38.7X2	T38.7X3	T38.7X4	T38.7X5	T38.7X6
Norethindrone	T38.4X1	T38.4X2	T38.4X3	T38.4X4	T38.4X5	T38.4X6
Norethisterone (acetate) (enantate)	T38.4X1	T38.4X2	T38.4X3	T38.4X4	T38.4X5	T38.4X6
with ethinylestradiol	T38.5X1	T38.5X2	T38.5X3	T38.5X4	T38.5X5	T38.5X6
Noretynodrel	T38.5X1	T38.5X2	T38.5X3	T38.5X4	T38.5X5	T38.5X6
Norfenefrine	T44.4X1	T44.4X2	T44.4X3	T44.4X4	T44.4X5	T44.4X6
Norfloxacin	T36.8X1	T36.8X2	T36.8X3	T36.8X4	T36.8X5	T36.8X6
Norgestrel	T38.4X1	T38.4X2	T38.4X3	T38.4X4	T38.4X5	T38.4X6
Norgestrienone	T38.4X1	T38.4X2	T38.4X3	T38.4X4	T38.4X5	T38.4X6
Norlestrin	T38.4X1	T38.4X2	T38.4X3	T38.4X4	T38.4X5	T38.4X6
Norlutin	T38.4X1	T38.4X2	T38.4X3	T38.4X4	T38.4X5	T38.4X6
Normal serum albumin (human), salt-poor	T45.8X1	T45.8X2	T45.8X3	T45.8X4	T45.8X5	T45.8X6
Normethandrone	T38.5X1	T38.5X2	T38.5X3	T38.5X4	T38.5X5	T38.5X6
Normison — see Benzodiazepines						
Normorphine	T40.2X1	T40.2X2	T40.2X3	T40.2X4	—	—
Norpseudoephedrine	T50.5X1	T50.5X2	T50.5X3	T50.5X4	T50.5X5	T50.5X6
Nortestosterone (furanpropionate)	T38.7X1	T38.7X2	T38.7X3	T38.7X4	T38.7X5	T38.7X6
Nortriptyline	T43.011	T43.012	T43.013	T43.014	T43.015	T43.016
Noscapine	T48.3X1	T48.3X2	T48.3X3	T48.3X4	T48.3X5	T48.3X6
Nose preparations	T49.6X1	T49.6X2	T49.6X3	T49.6X4	T49.6X5	T49.6X6
Novobiocin	T36.5X1	T36.5X2	T36.5X3	T36.5X4	T36.5X5	T36.5X6
Novocain (infiltration) (topical)	T41.3X1	T41.3X2	T41.3X3	T41.3X4	T41.3X5	T41.3X6
nerve block (peripheral) (plexus)	T41.3X1	T41.3X2	T41.3X3	T41.3X4	T41.3X5	T41.3X6
spinal	T41.3X1	T41.3X2	T41.3X3	T41.3X4	T41.3X5	T41.3X6
Noxious foodstuff	T62.91	T62.92	T62.93	T62.94	—	—
specified NEC	T62.8X1	T62.8X2	T62.8X3	T62.8X4	—	—
Noxiptiline	T43.011	T43.012	T43.013	T43.014	T43.015	T43.016
Noxytiolin	T49.0X1	T49.0X2	T49.0X3	T49.0X4	T49.0X5	T49.0X6
NPH Iletin (insulin)	T38.3X1	T38.3X2	T38.3X3	T38.3X4	T38.3X5	T38.3X6
Numorphan	T40.2X1	T40.2X2	T40.2X3	T40.2X4	T40.2X5	T40.2X6
Nunol	T42.3X1	T42.3X2	T42.3X3	T42.3X4	T42.3X5	T42.3X6
Nupercaine (spinal anesthetic)	T41.3X1	T41.3X2	T41.3X3	T41.3X4	T41.3X5	T41.3X6
topical (surface)	T41.3X1	T41.3X2	T41.3X3	T41.3X4	T41.3X5	T41.3X6
Nutmeg oil (liniment)	T49.3X1	T49.3X2	T49.3X3	T49.3X4	T49.3X5	T49.3X6
Nutritional supplement	T50.901	T50.902	T50.903	T50.904	T50.905	T50.906
Nux vomica	T65.1X1	T65.1X2	T65.1X3	T65.1X4	—	—
Nydrazid	T37.1X1	T37.1X2	T37.1X3	T37.1X4	T37.1X5	T37.1X6
Nylidrin	T46.7X1	T46.7X2	T46.7X3	T46.7X4	T46.7X5	T46.7X6
Nystatin	T36.7X1	T36.7X2	T36.7X3	T36.7X4	T36.7X5	T36.7X6
topical	T49.0X1	T49.0X2	T49.0X3	T49.0X4	T49.0X5	T49.0X6
Nytol	T45.0X1	T45.0X2	T45.0X3	T45.0X4	T45.0X5	T45.0X6
Obidoxime chloride	T50.6X1	T50.6X2	T50.6X3	T50.6X4	T50.6X5	T50.6X6
Octafonium (chloride)	T49.3X1	T49.3X2	T49.3X3	T49.3X4	T49.3X5	T49.3X6
Octamethyl pyrophosphoramide	T60.0X1	T60.0X2	T60.0X3	T60.0X4	—	—
Octanoin	T50.991	T50.992	T50.993	T50.994	T50.995	T50.996
Octatropine methylbromide	T44.3X1	T44.3X2	T44.3X3	T44.3X4	T44.3X5	T44.3X6
Octotiamine	T45.2X1	T45.2X2	T45.2X3	T45.2X4	T45.2X5	T45.2X6
Octoxinol (9)	T49.8X1	T49.8X2	T49.8X3	T49.8X4	T49.8X5	T49.8X6
Octreotide	T38.991	T38.992	T38.993	T38.994	T38.995	T38.996
Octyl nitrite	T46.3X1	T46.3X2	T46.3X3	T46.3X4	T46.3X5	T46.3X6
Oestradiol	T38.5X1	T38.5X2	T38.5X3	T38.5X4	T38.5X5	T38.5X6
Oestriol	T38.5X1	T38.5X2	T38.5X3	T38.5X4	T38.5X5	T38.5X6
Oestrogen	T38.5X1	T38.5X2	T38.5X3	T38.5X4	T38.5X5	T38.5X6
Oestrone	T38.5X1	T38.5X2	T38.5X3	T38.5X4	T38.5X5	T38.5X6
Ofloxacin	T36.8X1	T36.8X2	T36.8X3	T36.8X4	T36.8X5	T36.8X6
Oil (of)	T65.891	T65.892	T65.893	T65.894	—	—
bitter almond	T62.8X1	T62.8X2	T62.8X3	T62.8X4	—	—
cloves	T49.7X1	T49.7X2	T49.7X3	T49.7X4	T49.7X5	T49.7X6
colors	T65.6X1	T65.6X2	T65.6X3	T65.6X4	—	—
fumes	T59.891	T59.892	T59.893	T59.894	—	—
lubricating	T52.0X1	T52.0X2	T52.0X3	T52.0X4	—	—
Niobe	T52.8X1	T52.8X2	T52.8X3	T52.8X4	—	—
vitriol (liquid)	T54.2X1	T54.2X2	T54.2X3	T54.2X4	—	—
fumes	T54.2X1	T54.2X2	T54.2X3	T54.2X4	—	—
wintergreen (bitter) NEC	T49.3X1	T49.3X2	T49.3X3	T49.3X4	T49.3X5	T49.3X6

Substance	Poisoning, Accidental (unintentional)	Poisoning, Intentional Self-harm	Poisoning, Assault	Poisoning, Undetermined	Adverse Effect	Under-dosing
Oily preparation (for skin)	T49.3X1	T49.3X2	T49.3X3	T49.3X4	T49.3X5	T49.3X6
Ointment NEC	T49.3X1	T49.3X2	T49.3X3	T49.3X4	T49.3X5	T49.3X6
Olanzapine	T43.591	T43.592	T43.593	T43.594	T43.595	T43.596
Oleander	T62.2X1	T62.2X2	T62.2X3	T62.2X4	—	—
Oleandomycin	T36.3X1	T36.3X2	T36.3X3	T36.3X4	T36.3X5	T36.3X6
Oleandrin	T46.0X1	T46.0X2	T46.0X3	T46.0X4	T46.0X5	T46.0X6
Oleic acid	T46.6X1	T46.6X2	T46.6X3	T46.6X4	T46.6X5	T46.6X6
Oleovitamin A	T45.2X1	T45.2X2	T45.2X3	T45.2X4	T45.2X5	T45.2X6
Oleum ricini	T47.2X1	T47.2X2	T47.2X3	T47.2X4	T47.2X5	T47.2X6
Olive oil (medicinal) NEC	T47.4X1	T47.4X2	T47.4X3	T47.4X4	T47.4X5	T47.4X6
Olivomycin	T45.1X1	T45.1X2	T45.1X3	T45.1X4	T45.1X5	T45.1X6
Olsalazine	T47.8X1	T47.8X2	T47.8X3	T47.8X4	T47.8X5	T47.8X6
Omeprazole	T47.1X1	T47.1X2	T47.1X3	T47.1X4	T47.1X5	T47.1X6
OMPA	T60.0X1	T60.0X2	T60.0X3	T60.0X4	—	—
Oncovin	T45.1X1	T45.1X2	T45.1X3	T45.1X4	T45.1X5	T45.1X6
Ondansetron	T45.0X1	T45.0X2	T45.0X3	T45.0X4	T45.0X5	T45.0X6
Ophthaine	T41.3X1	T41.3X2	T41.3X3	T41.3X4	T41.3X5	T41.3X6
Ophthetic	T41.3X1	T41.3X2	T41.3X3	T41.3X4	T41.3X5	T41.3X6
Opiate NEC	T40.601	T40.602	T40.603	T40.604	T40.605	T40.606
antagonists	T50.7X1	T50.7X2	T50.7X3	T50.7X4	T50.7X5	T50.7X6
Opioid NEC	T40.2X1	T40.2X2	T40.2X3	T40.2X4	T40.2X5	T40.2X6
Opipramol	T43.011	T43.012	T43.013	T43.014	T43.015	T43.016
Opium alkaloids (total)	T40.0X1	T40.0X2	T40.0X3	T40.0X4	T40.0X5	T40.0X6
standardized powdered	T40.0X1	T40.0X2	T40.0X3	T40.0X4	T40.0X5	T40.0X6
tincture (camphorated)	T40.0X1	T40.0X2	T40.0X3	T40.0X4	T40.0X5	T40.0X6
Oracon	T38.4X1	T38.4X2	T38.4X3	T38.4X4	T38.4X5	T38.4X6
Oragrafin	T50.8X1	T50.8X2	T50.8X3	T50.8X4	T50.8X5	T50.8X6
Oral contraceptives	T38.4X1	T38.4X2	T38.4X3	T38.4X4	T38.4X5	T38.4X6
Oral rehydration salts	T50.3X1	T50.3X2	T50.3X3	T50.3X4	T50.3X5	T50.3X6
Orazamide	T50.991	T50.992	T50.993	T50.994	T50.995	T50.996
Orciprenaline	T48.291	T48.292	T48.293	T48.294	T48.295	T48.296
Organidin	T48.4X1	T48.4X2	T48.4X3	T48.4X4	T48.4X5	T48.4X6
Organonitrate NEC	T46.3X1	T46.3X2	T46.3X3	T46.3X4	T46.3X5	T46.3X6
Organophosphates	T60.0X1	T60.0X2	T60.0X3	T60.0X4	—	—
Orimune	T50.B91	T50.B92	T50.B93	T50.B94	T50.B95	T50.B96
Orinase	T38.3X1	T38.3X2	T38.3X3	T38.3X4	T38.3X5	T38.3X6
Ormeloxifene	T38.6X1	T38.6X2	T38.6X3	T38.6X4	T38.6X5	T38.6X6
Ornidazole	T37.3X1	T37.3X2	T37.3X3	T37.3X4	T37.3X5	T37.3X6
Ornithine aspartate	T50.991	T50.992	T50.993	T50.994	T50.995	T50.996
Ornoprostil	T47.1X1	T47.1X2	T47.1X3	T47.1X4	T47.1X5	T47.1X6
Orphenadrine (hydrochloride)	T42.8X1	T42.8X2	T42.8X3	T42.8X4	T42.8X5	T42.8X6
Ortal (sodium)	T42.3X1	T42.3X2	T42.3X3	T42.3X4	T42.3X5	T42.3X6
Orthoboric acid	T49.0X1	T49.0X2	T49.0X3	T49.0X4	T49.0X5	T49.0X6
ENT agent	T49.6X1	T49.6X2	T49.6X3	T49.6X4	T49.6X5	T49.6X6
ophthalmic preparation	T49.5X1	T49.5X2	T49.5X3	T49.5X4	T49.5X5	T49.5X6
Orthocaine	T41.3X1	T41.3X2	T41.3X3	T41.3X4	T41.3X5	T41.3X6
Orthodichlorobenzene	T53.7X1	T53.7X2	T53.7X3	T53.7X4	—	—
Ortho-Novum	T38.4X1	T38.4X2	T38.4X3	T38.4X4	T38.4X5	T38.4X6
Orthotolidine (reagent)	T54.2X1	T54.2X2	T54.2X3	T54.2X4	—	—
Osmic acid (liquid)	T54.2X1	T54.2X2	T54.2X3	T54.2X4	—	—
fumes	T54.2X1	T54.2X2	T54.2X3	T54.2X4	—	—
Osmotic diuretics	T50.2X1	T50.2X2	T50.2X3	T50.2X4	T50.2X5	T50.2X6
Otilonium bromide	T44.3X1	T44.3X2	T44.3X3	T44.3X4	T44.3X5	T44.3X6
Otorhinolaryngological drug NEC	T49.6X1	T49.6X2	T49.6X3	T49.6X4	T49.6X5	T49.6X6
Ouabain (e)	T46.0X1	T46.0X2	T46.0X3	T46.0X4	T46.0X5	T46.0X6
Ovarian hormone	T38.5X1	T38.5X2	T38.5X3	T38.5X4	T38.5X5	T38.5X6
stimulant	T38.5X1	T38.5X2	T38.5X3	T38.5X4	T38.5X5	T38.5X6
Ovral	T38.4X1	T38.4X2	T38.4X3	T38.4X4	T38.4X5	T38.4X6
Ovulen	T38.4X1	T38.4X2	T38.4X3	T38.4X4	T38.4X5	T38.4X6
Oxacillin	T36.0X1	T36.0X2	T36.0X3	T36.0X4	T36.0X5	T36.0X6
Oxalic acid	T54.2X1	T54.2X2	T54.2X3	T54.2X4	—	—
ammonium salt	T50.991	T50.992	T50.993	T50.994	T50.995	T50.996
Oxamniquine	T37.4X1	T37.4X2	T37.4X3	T37.4X4	T37.4X5	T37.4X6
Oxanamide	T43.591	T43.592	T43.593	T43.594	T43.595	T43.596
Oxandrolone	T38.7X1	T38.7X2	T38.7X3	T38.7X4	T38.7X5	T38.7X6
Oxantel	T37.4X1	T37.4X2	T37.4X3	T37.4X4	T37.4X5	T37.4X6
Oxapium iodide	T44.3X1	T44.3X2	T44.3X3	T44.3X4	T44.3X5	T44.3X6
Oxaprotiline	T43.021	T43.022	T43.023	T43.024	T43.025	T43.026
Oxaprozin	T39.311	T39.312	T39.313	T39.314	T39.315	T39.316
Oxatomide	T45.0X1	T45.0X2	T45.0X3	T45.0X4	T45.0X5	T45.0X6
Oxazepam	T42.4X1	T42.4X2	T42.4X3	T42.4X4	T42.4X5	T42.4X6
Oxazimedrine	T50.5X1	T50.5X2	T50.5X3	T50.5X4	T50.5X5	T50.5X6
Oxazolam	T42.4X1	T42.4X2	T42.4X3	T42.4X4	T42.4X5	T42.4X6
Oxazolidine derivatives	T42.2X1	T42.2X2	T42.2X3	T42.2X4	T42.2X5	T42.2X6
Oxazolidinedione (derivative)	T42.2X1	T42.2X2	T42.2X3	T42.2X4	T42.2X5	T42.2X6
Ox bile extract	T47.5X1	T47.5X2	T47.5X3	T47.5X4	T47.5X5	T47.5X6
Oxcarbazepine	T42.1X1	T42.1X2	T42.1X3	T42.1X4	T42.1X5	T42.1X6
Oxedrine	T44.4X1	T44.4X2	T44.4X3	T44.4X4	T44.4X5	T44.4X6
Oxeladin (citrate)	T48.3X1	T48.3X2	T48.3X3	T48.3X4	T48.3X5	T48.3X6

Subterms under main terms may continue to next column or page   Additional Character May Be Required — Refer to the Tabular List for Character Selection   381

Nonylphenoxy — Oxeladin

Table of Drugs and Chemicals

Substance	Poisoning, Accidental (unintentional)	Poisoning, Intentional Self-harm	Poisoning, Assault	Poisoning, Undetermined	Adverse Effect	Under-dosing
Oxendolone	T38.5X1	T38.5X2	T38.5X3	T38.5X4	T38.5X5	T38.5X6
Oxetacaine	T41.3X1	T41.3X2	T41.3X3	T41.3X4	T41.3X5	T41.3X6
Oxethazine	T41.3X1	T41.3X2	T41.3X3	T41.3X4	T41.3X5	T41.3X6
Oxetorone	T39.8X1	T39.8X2	T39.8X3	T39.8X4	T39.8X5	T39.8X6
Oxiconazole	T49.0X1	T49.0X2	T49.0X3	T49.0X4	T49.0X5	T49.0X6
Oxidizing agent NEC	T54.91	T54.92	T54.93	T54.94	—	—
Oxipurinol	T50.4X1	T50.4X2	T50.4X3	T50.4X4	T50.4X5	T50.4X6
Oxitriptan	T43.291	T43.292	T43.293	T43.294	T43.295	T43.296
Oxitropium bromide	T48.6X1	T48.6X2	T48.6X3	T48.6X4	T48.6X5	T48.6X6
Oxodipine	T46.1X1	T46.1X2	T46.1X3	T46.1X4	T46.1X5	T46.1X6
Oxolamine	T48.3X1	T48.3X2	T48.3X3	T48.3X4	T48.3X5	T48.3X6
Oxolinic acid	T37.8X1	T37.8X2	T37.8X3	T37.8X4	T37.8X5	T37.8X6
Oxomemazine	T43.3X1	T43.3X2	T43.3X3	T43.3X4	T43.3X5	T43.3X6
Oxophenarsine	T37.3X1	T37.3X2	T37.3X3	T37.3X4	T37.3X5	T37.3X6
Oxprenolol	T44.7X1	T44.7X2	T44.7X3	T44.7X4	T44.7X5	T44.7X6
Oxsoralen	T49.3X1	T49.3X2	T49.3X3	T49.3X4	T49.3X5	T49.3X6
Oxtriphylline	T48.6X1	T48.6X2	T48.6X3	T48.6X4	T48.6X5	T48.6X6
Oxybate sodium	T41.291	T41.292	T41.293	T41.294	T41.295	T41.296
Oxybuprocaine	T41.3X1	T41.3X2	T41.3X3	T41.3X4	T41.3X5	T41.3X6
Oxybutynin	T44.3X1	T44.3X2	T44.3X3	T44.3X4	T44.3X5	T44.3X6
Oxychlorosene	T49.0X1	T49.0X2	T49.0X3	T49.0X4	T49.0X5	T49.0X6
Oxycodone	T40.2X1	T40.2X2	T40.2X3	T40.2X4	T40.2X5	T40.2X6
Oxyfedrine	T46.3X1	T46.3X2	T46.3X3	T46.3X4	T46.3X5	T46.3X6
Oxygen	T41.5X1	T41.5X2	T41.5X3	T41.5X4	T41.5X5	T41.5X6
Oxylone	T49.0X1	T49.0X2	T49.0X3	T49.0X4	T49.0X5	T49.0X6
ophthalmic preparation	T49.5X1	T49.5X2	T49.5X3	T49.5X4	T49.5X5	T49.5X6
Oxymesterone	T38.7X1	T38.7X2	T38.7X3	T38.7X4	T38.7X5	T38.7X6
Oxymetazoline	T48.5X1	T48.5X2	T48.5X3	T48.5X4	T48.5X5	T48.5X6
Oxymetholone	T38.7X1	T38.7X2	T38.7X3	T38.7X4	T38.7X5	T38.7X6
Oxymorphone	T40.2X1	T40.2X2	T40.2X3	T40.2X4	T40.2X5	T40.2X6
Oxypertine	T43.591	T43.592	T43.593	T43.594	T43.595	T43.596
Oxyphenbutazone	T39.2X1	T39.2X2	T39.2X3	T39.2X4	T39.2X5	T39.2X6
Oxyphencyclimine	T44.3X1	T44.3X2	T44.3X3	T44.3X4	T44.3X5	T44.3X6
Oxyphenisatine	T47.2X1	T47.2X2	T47.2X3	T47.2X4	T47.2X5	T47.2X6
Oxyphenonium bromide	T44.3X1	T44.3X2	T44.3X3	T44.3X4	T44.3X5	T44.3X6
Oxypolygelatin	T45.8X1	T45.8X2	T45.8X3	T45.8X4	T45.8X5	T45.8X6
Oxyquinoline (derivatives)	T37.8X1	T37.8X2	T37.8X3	T37.8X4	T37.8X5	T37.8X6
Oxytetracycline	T36.4X1	T36.4X2	T36.4X3	T36.4X4	T36.4X5	T36.4X6
Oxytocic drug NEC	T48.0X1	T48.0X2	T48.0X3	T48.0X4	T48.0X5	T48.0X6
Oxytocin (synthetic)	T48.0X1	T48.0X2	T48.0X3	T48.0X4	T48.0X5	T48.0X6
Ozone	T59.891	T59.892	T59.893	T59.894	—	—
PABA	T49.3X1	T49.3X2	T49.3X3	T49.3X4	T49.3X5	T49.3X6
Packed red cells	T45.8X1	T45.8X2	T45.8X3	T45.8X4	T45.8X5	T45.8X6
Padimate	T49.3X1	T49.3X2	T49.3X3	T49.3X4	T49.3X5	T49.3X6
Paint NEC	T65.6X1	T65.6X2	T65.6X3	T65.6X4	—	—
cleaner	T52.91	T52.92	T52.93	T52.94	—	—
fumes NEC	T59.891	T59.892	T59.893	T59.894	—	—
lead (fumes)	T56.0X1	T56.0X2	T56.0X3	T56.0X4	—	—
solvent NEC	T52.8X1	T52.8X2	T52.8X3	T52.8X4	—	—
stripper	T52.8X1	T52.8X2	T52.8X3	T52.8X4	—	—
Palfium	T40.2X1	T40.2X2	T40.2X3	T40.2X4	—	—
Palm kernel oil	T50.991	T50.992	T50.993	T50.994	T50.995	T50.996
Paludrine	T37.2X1	T37.2X2	T37.2X3	T37.2X4	T37.2X5	T37.2X6
PAM (pralidoxime)	T50.6X1	T50.6X2	T50.6X3	T50.6X4	T50.6X5	T50.6X6
Pamaquine (naphthoute)	T37.2X1	T37.2X2	T37.2X3	T37.2X4	T37.2X5	T37.2X6
Panadol	T39.1X1	T39.1X2	T39.1X3	T39.1X4	T39.1X5	T39.1X6
Pancreatic						
digestive secretion stimulant	T47.8X1	T47.8X2	T47.8X3	T47.8X4	T47.8X5	T47.8X6
dornase	T45.3X1	T45.3X2	T45.3X3	T45.3X4	T45.3X5	T45.3X6
Pancreatin	T47.5X1	T47.5X2	T47.5X3	T47.5X4	T47.5X5	T47.5X6
Pancrelipase	T47.5X1	T47.5X2	T47.5X3	T47.5X4	T47.5X5	T47.5X6
Pancuronium (bromide)	T48.1X1	T48.1X2	T48.1X3	T48.1X4	T48.1X5	T48.1X6
Pangamic acid	T45.2X1	T45.2X2	T45.2X3	T45.2X4	T45.2X5	T45.2X6
Panthenol	T45.2X1	T45.2X2	T45.2X3	T45.2X4	T45.2X5	T45.2X6
topical	T49.8X1	T49.8X2	T49.8X3	T49.8X4	T49.8X5	T49.8X6
Pantopon	T40.0X1	T40.0X2	T40.0X3	T40.0X4	T40.0X5	T40.0X6
Pantothenic acid	T45.2X1	T45.2X2	T45.2X3	T45.2X4	T45.2X5	T45.2X6
Panwarfin	T45.511	T45.512	T45.513	T45.514	T45.515	T45.516
Papain	T47.5X1	T47.5X2	T47.5X3	T47.5X4	T47.5X5	T47.5X6
digestant	T47.5X1	T47.5X2	T47.5X3	T47.5X4	T47.5X5	T47.5X6
Papaveretum	T40.0X1	T40.0X2	T40.0X3	T40.0X4	T40.0X5	T40.0X6
Papaverine	T44.3X1	T44.3X2	T44.3X3	T44.3X4	T44.3X5	T44.3X6
Para-acetamidophenol	T39.1X1	T39.1X2	T39.1X3	T39.1X4	T39.1X5	T39.1X6
Para-aminobenzoic acid	T49.3X1	T49.3X2	T49.3X3	T49.3X4	T49.3X5	T49.3X6
Para-aminophenol derivatives	T39.1X1	T39.1X2	T39.1X3	T39.1X4	T39.1X5	T39.1X6
Para-aminosalicylic acid	T37.1X1	T37.1X2	T37.1X3	T37.1X4	T37.1X5	T37.1X6
Paracetaldehyde	T42.6X1	T42.6X2	T42.6X3	T42.6X4	T42.6X5	T42.6X6
Paracetamol	T39.1X1	T39.1X2	T39.1X3	T39.1X4	T39.1X5	T39.1X6
Parachlorophenol (camphorated)	T49.0X1	T49.0X2	T49.0X3	T49.0X4	T49.0X5	T49.0X6
Paracodin	T40.2X1	T40.2X2	T40.2X3	T40.2X4	T40.2X5	T40.2X6
Paradione	T42.2X1	T42.2X2	T42.2X3	T42.2X4	T42.2X5	T42.2X6
Paraffin(s) (wax)	T52.0X1	T52.0X2	T52.0X3	T52.0X4	—	—
liquid (medicinal)	T47.4X1	T47.4X2	T47.4X3	T47.4X4	T47.4X5	T47.4X6
nonmedicinal	T52.0X1	T52.0X2	T52.0X3	T52.0X4	—	—
Paraformaldehyde	T60.3X1	T60.3X2	T60.3X3	T60.3X4	—	—
Paraldehyde	T42.6X1	T42.6X2	T42.6X3	T42.6X4	T42.6X5	T42.6X6
Paramethadione	T42.2X1	T42.2X2	T42.2X3	T42.2X4	T42.2X5	T42.2X6
Paramethasone	T38.0X1	T38.0X2	T38.0X3	T38.0X4	T38.0X5	T38.0X6
acetate	T49.0X1	T49.0X2	T49.0X3	T49.0X4	T49.0X5	T49.0X6
Paraoxon	T60.0X1	T60.0X2	T60.0X3	T60.0X4	—	—
Paraquat	T60.3X1	T60.3X2	T60.3X3	T60.3X4	—	—
Parasympatholytic NEC	T44.3X1	T44.3X2	T44.3X3	T44.3X4	T44.3X5	T44.3X6
Parasympathomimetic drug NEC	T44.1X1	T44.1X2	T44.1X3	T44.1X4	T44.1X5	T44.1X6
Parathion	T60.0X1	T60.0X2	T60.0X3	T60.0X4	—	—
Parathormone	T50.991	T50.992	T50.993	T50.994	T50.995	T50.996
Parathyroid extract	T50.991	T50.992	T50.993	T50.994	T50.995	T50.996
Paratyphoid vaccine	T50.A91	T50.A92	T50.A93	T50.A94	T50.A95	T50.A96
Paredrine	T44.4X1	T44.4X2	T44.4X3	T44.4X4	T44.4X5	T44.4X6
Paregoric	T40.0X1	T40.0X2	T40.0X3	T40.0X4	T40.0X5	T40.0X6
Pargyline	T46.5X1	T46.5X2	T46.5X3	T46.5X4	T46.5X5	T46.5X6
Paris green	T57.0X1	T57.0X2	T57.0X3	T57.0X4	—	—
insecticide	T57.0X1	T57.0X2	T57.0X3	T57.0X4	—	—
Parnate	T43.1X1	T43.1X2	T43.1X3	T43.1X4	T43.1X5	T43.1X6
Paromomycin	T36.5X1	T36.5X2	T36.5X3	T36.5X4	T36.5X5	T36.5X6
Paroxypropione	T45.1X1	T45.1X2	T45.1X3	T45.1X4	T45.1X5	T45.1X6
Parzone	T40.2X1	T40.2X2	T40.2X3	T40.2X4	T40.2X5	T40.2X6
PAS	T37.1X1	T37.1X2	T37.1X3	T37.1X4	T37.1X5	T37.1X6
Pasiniazid	T37.1X1	T37.1X2	T37.1X3	T37.1X4	T37.1X5	T37.1X6
PBB (polybrominated biphenyls)	T65.891	T65.892	T65.893	T65.894	—	—
PCB	T65.891	T65.892	T65.893	T65.894	—	—
PCP						
meaning pentachlorophenol	T60.1X1	T60.1X2	T60.1X3	T60.1X4	—	—
fungicide	T60.3X1	T60.3X2	T60.3X3	T60.3X4	—	—
herbicide	T60.3X1	T60.3X2	T60.3X3	T60.3X4	—	—
insecticide	T60.1X1	T60.1X2	T60.1X3	T60.1X4	—	—
meaning phencyclidine	T40.991	T40.992	T40.993	T40.994	—	—
Peach kernel oil (emulsion)	T47.4X1	T47.4X2	T47.4X3	T47.4X4	T47.4X5	T47.4X6
Peanut oil (emulsion) NEC	T47.4X1	T47.4X2	T47.4X3	T47.4X4	T47.4X5	T47.4X6
topical	T49.3X1	T49.3X2	T49.3X3	T49.3X4	T49.3X5	T49.3X6
Pearly Gates (morning glory seeds)	T40.991	T40.992	T40.993	T40.994	—	—
Pecazine	T43.3X1	T43.3X2	T43.3X3	T43.3X4	T43.3X5	T43.3X6
Pectin	T47.6X1	T47.6X2	T47.6X3	T47.6X4	T47.6X5	T47.6X6
Pefloxacin	T37.8X1	T37.8X2	T37.8X3	T37.8X4	T37.8X5	T37.8X6
Pegademase, bovine	T50.Z91	T50.Z92	T50.Z93	T50.Z94	T50.Z95	T50.Z96
Pelletierine tannate	T37.4X1	T37.4X2	T37.4X3	T37.4X4	T37.4X5	T37.4X6
Pemirolast (potassium)	T48.6X1	T48.6X2	T48.6X3	T48.6X4	T48.6X5	T48.6X6
Pemoline	T50.7X1	T50.7X2	T50.7X3	T50.7X4	T50.7X5	T50.7X6
Pempidine	T44.2X1	T44.2X2	T44.2X3	T44.2X4	T44.2X5	T44.2X6
Penamecillin	T36.0X1	T36.0X2	T36.0X3	T36.0X4	T36.0X5	T36.0X6
Penbutolol	T44.7X1	T44.7X2	T44.7X3	T44.7X4	T44.7X5	T44.7X6
Penethamate	T36.0X1	T36.0X2	T36.0X3	T36.0X4	T36.0X5	T36.0X6
Penfluridol	T43.591	T43.592	T43.593	T43.594	T43.595	T43.596
Penflutizide	T50.2X1	T50.2X2	T50.2X3	T50.2X4	T50.2X5	T50.2X6
Pengitoxin	T46.0X1	T46.0X2	T46.0X3	T46.0X4	T46.0X5	T46.0X6
Penicillamine	T50.6X1	T50.6X2	T50.6X3	T50.6X4	T50.6X5	T50.6X6
Penicillin (any)	T36.0X1	T36.0X2	T36.0X3	T36.0X4	T36.0X5	T36.0X6
Penicillinase	T45.3X1	T45.3X2	T45.3X3	T45.3X4	T45.3X5	T45.3X6
Penicilloyl polylysine	T50.8X1	T50.8X2	T50.8X3	T50.8X4	T50.8X5	T50.8X6
Penimepicycline	T36.4X1	T36.4X2	T36.4X3	T36.4X4	T36.4X5	T36.4X6
Pentachloroethane	T53.6X1	T53.6X2	T53.6X3	T53.6X4	—	—
Pentachloronaphthalene	T53.7X1	T53.7X2	T53.7X3	T53.7X4	—	—
Pentachlorophenol (pesticide)	T60.1X1	T60.1X2	T60.1X3	T60.1X4	—	—
fungicide	T60.3X1	T60.3X2	T60.3X3	T60.3X4	—	—
herbicide	T60.3X1	T60.3X2	T60.3X3	T60.3X4	—	—
insecticide	T60.1X1	T60.1X2	T60.1X3	T60.1X4	—	—
Pentaerythritol	T46.3X1	T46.3X2	T46.3X3	T46.3X4	T46.3X5	T46.3X6
chloral	T42.6X1	T42.6X2	T42.6X3	T42.6X4	T42.6X5	T42.6X6
tetranitrate NEC	T46.3X1	T46.3X2	T46.3X3	T46.3X4	T46.3X5	T46.3X6
Pentaerythrityl tetranitrate	T46.3X1	T46.3X2	T46.3X3	T46.3X4	T46.3X5	T46.3X6
Pentagastrin	T50.8X1	T50.8X2	T50.8X3	T50.8X4		T50.8X6
Pentalin	T53.6X1	T53.6X2	T53.6X3	T53.6X4	—	—
Pentamethonium bromide	T44.2X1	T44.2X2	T44.2X3	T44.2X4	T44.2X5	T44.2X6
Pentamidine	T37.3X1	T37.3X2	T37.3X3	T37.3X4	T37.3X5	T37.3X6
Pentanol	T51.3X1	T51.3X2	T51.3X3	T51.3X4	—	—
Pentapyrrolinium (bitartrate)	T44.2X1	T44.2X2	T44.2X3	T44.2X4	T44.2X5	T44.2X6
Pentaquine	T37.2X1	T37.2X2	T37.2X3	T37.2X4	T37.2X5	T37.2X6

Oxendolone — Pentaquine

Additional Character May Be Required — Refer to the Tabular List for Character Selection   ▽ Subterms under main terms may continue to next column or page

Table of Drugs and Chemicals

Substance	Poisoning, Accidental (unintentional)	Poisoning, Intentional Self-harm	Poisoning, Assault	Poisoning, Undetermined	Adverse Effect	Under-dosing
Pentazocine	T40.4X1	T40.4X2	T40.4X3	T40.4X4	T40.4X5	T40.4X6
Pentetrazole	T50.7X1	T50.7X2	T50.7X3	T50.7X4	T50.7X5	T50.7X6
Penthienate bromide	T44.3X1	T44.3X2	T44.3X3	T44.3X4	T44.3X5	T44.3X6
Pentifylline	T46.7X1	T46.7X2	T46.7X3	T46.7X4	T46.7X5	T46.7X6
Pentobarbital	T42.3X1	T42.3X2	T42.3X3	T42.3X4	T42.3X5	T42.3X6
sodium	T42.3X1	T42.3X2	T42.3X3	T42.3X4	T42.3X5	T42.3X6
Pentobarbitone	T42.3X1	T42.3X2	T42.3X3	T42.3X4	T42.3X5	T42.3X6
Pentolonium tartrate	T44.2X1	T44.2X2	T44.2X3	T44.2X4	T44.2X5	T44.2X6
Pentosan polysulfate	T39.8X1	T39.8X2	T39.8X3	T39.8X4	T39.8X5	T39.8X6
(sodium)						
Pentostatin	T45.1X1	T45.1X2	T45.1X3	T45.1X4	T45.1X5	T45.1X6
Pentothal	T41.1X1	T41.1X2	T41.1X3	T41.1X4	T41.1X5	T41.1X6
Pentoxifylline	T46.7X1	T46.7X2	T46.7X3	T46.7X4	T46.7X5	T46.7X6
Pentoxyverine	T48.3X1	T48.3X2	T48.3X3	T48.3X4	T48.3X5	T48.3X6
Pentrinat	T46.3X1	T46.3X2	T46.3X3	T46.3X4	T46.3X5	T46.3X6
Pentylenetetrazole	T50.7X1	T50.7X2	T50.7X3	T50.7X4	T50.7X5	T50.7X6
Pentylsalicylamide	T37.1X1	T37.1X2	T37.1X3	T37.1X4	T37.1X5	T37.1X6
Pentymal	T42.3X1	T42.3X2	T42.3X3	T42.3X4	T42.3X5	T42.3X6
Peplomycin	T45.1X1	T45.1X2	T45.1X3	T45.1X4	T45.1X5	T45.1X6
Peppermint (oil)	T47.5X1	T47.5X2	T47.5X3	T47.5X4	T47.5X5	T47.5X6
Pepsin	T47.5X1	T47.5X2	T47.5X3	T47.5X4	T47.5X5	T47.5X6
digestant	T47.5X1	T47.5X2	T47.5X3	T47.5X4	T47.5X5	T47.5X6
Pepstatin	T47.1X1	T47.1X2	T47.1X3	T47.1X4	T47.1X5	T47.1X6
Peptavlon	T50.8X1	T50.8X2	T50.8X3	T50.8X4	T50.8X5	T50.8X6
Perazine	T43.3X1	T43.3X2	T43.3X3	T43.3X4	T43.3X5	T43.3X6
Percaine (spinal)	T41.3X1	T41.3X2	T41.3X3	T41.3X4	T41.3X5	T41.3X6
topical (surface)	T41.3X1	T41.3X2	T41.3X3	T41.3X4	T41.3X5	T41.3X6
Perchloroethylene	T53.3X1	T53.3X2	T53.3X3	T53.3X4	—	—
medicinal	T37.4X1	T37.4X2	T37.4X3	T37.4X4	T37.4X5	T37.4X6
vapor	T53.3X1	T53.3X2	T53.3X3	T53.3X4	—	—
Percodan	T40.2X1	T40.2X2	T40.2X3	T40.2X4	T40.2X5	T40.2X6
Percogesic — see also	T45.0X1	T45.0X2	T45.0X3	T45.0X4	T45.0X5	T45.0X6
acetaminophen						
Percorten	T38.0X1	T38.0X2	T38.0X3	T38.0X4	T38.0X5	T38.0X6
Pergolide	T42.8X1	T42.8X2	T42.8X3	T42.8X4	T42.8X5	T42.8X6
Pergonal	T38.811	T38.812	T38.813	T38.814	T38.815	T38.816
Perhexilene	T46.3X1	T46.3X2	T46.3X3	T46.3X4	T46.3X5	T46.3X6
Perhexiline (maleate)	T46.3X1	T46.3X2	T46.3X3	T46.3X4	T46.3X5	T46.3X6
Periactin	T45.0X1	T45.0X2	T45.0X3	T45.0X4	T45.0X5	T45.0X6
Periciazine	T43.3X1	T43.3X2	T43.3X3	T43.3X4	T43.3X5	T43.3X6
Periclor	T42.6X1	T42.6X2	T42.6X3	T42.6X4	T42.6X5	T42.6X6
Perindopril	T46.4X1	T46.4X2	T46.4X3	T46.4X4	T46.4X5	T46.4X6
Perisoxal	T39.8X1	T39.8X2	T39.8X3	T39.8X4	T39.8X5	T39.8X6
Peritoneal dialysis solution	T50.3X1	T50.3X2	T50.3X3	T50.3X4	T50.3X5	T50.3X6
Peritrate	T46.3X1	T46.3X2	T46.3X3	T46.3X4	T46.3X5	T46.3X6
Perlapine	T42.4X1	T42.4X2	T42.4X3	T42.4X4	T42.4X5	T42.4X6
Permanganate	T65.891	T65.892	T65.893	T65.894	—	—
Permethrin	T60.1X1	T60.1X2	T60.1X3	T60.1X4	—	—
Pernocton	T42.3X1	T42.3X2	T42.3X3	T42.3X4	T42.3X5	T42.3X6
Pernoston	T42.3X1	T42.3X2	T42.3X3	T42.3X4	T42.3X5	T42.3X6
Peronine	T40.2X1	T40.2X2	T40.2X3	T40.2X4	—	—
Perphenazine	T43.3X1	T43.3X2	T43.3X3	T43.3X4	T43.3X5	T43.3X6
Pertofrane	T43.011	T43.012	T43.013	T43.014	T43.015	T43.016
Pertussis						
immune serum (human)	T50.Z11	T50.Z12	T50.Z13	T50.Z14	T50.Z15	T50.Z16
vaccine (with diphtheria toxoid)	T50.A11	T50.A12	T50.A13	T50.A14	T50.A15	T50.A16
(with tetanus toxoid)						
Peruvian balsam	T49.0X1	T49.0X2	T49.0X3	T49.0X4	T49.0X5	T49.0X6
Peruvoside	T46.0X1	T46.0X2	T46.0X3	T46.0X4	T46.0X5	T46.0X6
Pesticide (dust) (fumes) (vapor)	T60.91	T60.92	T60.93	T60.94	—	—
NEC						
arsenic	T57.0X1	T57.0X2	T57.0X3	T57.0X4	—	—
chlorinated	T60.1X1	T60.1X2	T60.1X3	T60.1X4	—	—
cyanide	T65.0X1	T65.0X2	T65.0X3	T65.0X4	—	—
kerosene	T52.0X1	T52.0X2	T52.0X3	T52.0X4	—	—
mixture (of compounds)	T60.91	T60.92	T60.93	T60.94	—	—
naphthalene	T60.2X1	T60.2X2	T60.2X3	T60.2X4	—	—
organochlorine	T60.1X1	T60.1X2	T60.1X3	T60.1X4	—	—
(compounds)						
petroleum (distillate) (products)	T60.8X1	T60.8X2	T60.8X3	T60.8X4	—	—
NEC						
specified ingredient NEC	T60.8X1	T60.8X2	T60.8X3	T60.8X4	—	—
strychnine	T65.1X1	T65.1X2	T65.1X3	T65.1X4	—	—
thallium	T60.4X1	T60.4X2	T60.4X3	T60.4X4	—	—
Pethidine	T40.4X1	T40.4X2	T40.4X3	T40.4X4	T40.4X5	T40.4X6
Petrichloral	T42.6X1	T42.6X2	T42.6X3	T42.6X4	T42.6X5	T42.6X6
Petrol	T52.0X1	T52.0X2	T52.0X3	T52.0X4	—	—
vapor	T52.0X1	T52.0X2	T52.0X3	T52.0X4	—	—
Petrolatum	T49.3X1	T49.3X2	T49.3X3	T49.3X4	T49.3X5	T49.3X6
hydrophilic	T49.3X1	T49.3X2	T49.3X3	T49.3X4	T49.3X5	T49.3X6
liquid	T47.4X1	T47.4X2	T47.4X3	T47.4X4	T47.4X5	T47.4X6
topical	T49.3X1	T49.3X2	T49.3X3	T49.3X4	T49.3X5	T49.3X6
nonmedicinal	T52.0X1	T52.0X2	T52.0X3	T52.0X4	—	—

Substance	Poisoning, Accidental (unintentional)	Poisoning, Intentional Self-harm	Poisoning, Assault	Poisoning, Undetermined	Adverse Effect	Under-dosing
Petrolatum — continued						
red veterinary	T49.3X1	T49.3X2	T49.3X3	T49.3X4	T49.3X5	T49.3X6
white	T49.3X1	T49.3X2	T49.3X3	T49.3X4	T49.3X5	T49.3X6
Petroleum (products) NEC	T52.0X1	T52.0X2	T52.0X3	T52.0X4	—	—
benzine(s) — see Ligroin						
ether — see Ligroin						
jelly — see Petrolatum						
naphtha — see Ligroin						
pesticide	T60.8X1	T60.8X2	T60.8X3	T60.8X4	—	—
solids	T52.0X1	T52.0X2	T52.0X3	T52.0X4	—	—
solvents	T52.0X1	T52.0X2	T52.0X3	T52.0X4	—	—
vapor	T52.0X1	T52.0X2	T52.0X3	T52.0X4	—	—
Peyote	T40.991	T40.992	T40.993	T40.994		
Phanodorm, phanodorn	T42.3X1	T42.3X2	T42.3X3	T42.3X4	T42.3X5	T42.3X6
Phanquinone	T37.3X1	T37.3X2	T37.3X3	T37.3X4	T37.3X5	T37.3X6
Phanquone	T37.3X1	T37.3X2	T37.3X3	T37.3X4	T37.3X5	T37.3X6
Pharmaceutical						
adjunct NEC	T50.901	T50.902	T50.903	T50.904	T50.905	T50.906
excipient NEC	T50.901	T50.902	T50.903	T50.904	T50.905	T50.906
sweetener	T50.901	T50.902	T50.903	T50.904	T50.905	T50.906
viscous agent	T50.901	T50.902	T50.903	T50.904	T50.905	T50.906
Phemitone	T42.3X1	T42.3X2	T42.3X3	T42.3X4	T42.3X5	T42.3X6
Phenacaine	T41.3X1	T41.3X2	T41.3X3	T41.3X4	T41.3X5	T41.3X6
Phenacemide	T42.6X1	T42.6X2	T42.6X3	T42.6X4	T42.6X5	T42.6X6
Phenacetin	T39.1X1	T39.1X2	T39.1X3	T39.1X4	T39.1X5	T39.1X6
Phenadoxone	T40.2X1	T40.2X2	T40.2X3	T40.2X4	—	—
Phenaglycodol	T43.591	T43.592	T43.593	T43.594	T43.595	T43.596
Phenantoin	T42.0X1	T42.0X2	T42.0X3	T42.0X4	T42.0X5	T42.0X6
Phenaphthazine reagent	T50.991	T50.992	T50.993	T50.994	T50.995	T50.996
Phenazocine	T40.4X1	T40.4X2	T40.4X3	T40.4X4	T40.4X5	T40.4X6
Phenazone	T39.2X1	T39.2X2	T39.2X3	T39.2X4	T39.2X5	T39.2X6
Phenazopyridine	T39.8X1	T39.8X2	T39.8X3	T39.8X4	T39.8X5	T39.8X6
Phenbenicillin	T36.0X1	T36.0X2	T36.0X3	T36.0X4	T36.0X5	T36.0X6
Phenbutrazate	T50.5X1	T50.5X2	T50.5X3	T50.5X4	T50.5X5	T50.5X6
Phencyclidine	T40.991	T40.992	T40.993	T40.994	T40.995	T40.996
Phendimetrazine	T50.5X1	T50.5X2	T50.5X3	T50.5X4	T50.5X5	T50.5X6
Phenelzine	T43.1X1	T43.1X2	T43.1X3	T43.1X4	T43.1X5	T43.1X6
Phenemal	T42.3X1	T42.3X2	T42.3X3	T42.3X4	T42.3X5	T42.3X6
Phenergan	T42.6X1	T42.6X2	T42.6X3	T42.6X4	T42.6X5	T42.6X6
Pheneticillin	T36.0X1	T36.0X2	T36.0X3	T36.0X4	T36.0X5	T36.0X6
Pheneturide	T42.6X1	T42.6X2	T42.6X3	T42.6X4	T42.6X5	T42.6X6
Phenformin	T38.3X1	T38.3X2	T38.3X3	T38.3X4	T38.3X5	T38.3X6
Phenglutarimide	T44.3X1	T44.3X2	T44.3X3	T44.3X4	T44.3X5	T44.3X6
Phenicarbazide	T39.8X1	T39.8X2	T39.8X3	T39.8X4	T39.8X5	T39.8X6
Phenindamine	T45.0X1	T45.0X2	T45.0X3	T45.0X4	T45.0X5	T45.0X6
Phenindione	T45.511	T45.512	T45.513	T45.514	T45.515	T45.516
Pheniprazine	T43.1X1	T43.1X2	T43.1X3	T43.1X4	T43.1X5	T43.1X6
Pheniramine	T45.0X1	T45.0X2	T45.0X3	T45.0X4	T45.0X5	T45.0X6
Phenisatin	T47.2X1	T47.2X2	T47.2X3	T47.2X4	T47.2X5	T47.2X6
Phenmetrazine	T50.5X1	T50.5X2	T50.5X3	T50.5X4	T50.5X5	T50.5X6
Phenobal	T42.3X1	T42.3X2	T42.3X3	T42.3X4	T42.3X5	T42.3X6
Phenobarbital	T42.3X1	T42.3X2	T42.3X3	T42.3X4	T42.3X5	T42.3X6
with						
mephenytoin	T42.3X1	T42.3X2	T42.3X3	T42.3X4	T42.3X5	T42.3X6
phenytoin	T42.3X1	T42.3X2	T42.3X3	T42.3X4	T42.3X5	T42.3X6
sodium	T42.3X1	T42.3X2	T42.3X3	T42.3X4	T42.3X5	T42.3X6
Phenobarbitone	T42.3X1	T42.3X2	T42.3X3	T42.3X4	T42.3X5	T42.3X6
Phenobutiodil	T50.8X1	T50.8X2	T50.8X3	T50.8X4	T50.8X5	T50.8X6
Phenoctide	T49.0X1	T49.0X2	T49.0X3	T49.0X4	T49.0X5	T49.0X6
Phenol	T49.0X1	T49.0X2	T49.0X3	T49.0X4	T49.0X5	T49.0X6
disinfectant	T54.0X1	T54.0X2	T54.0X3	T54.0X4	—	—
in oil injection	T46.8X1	T46.8X2	T46.8X3	T46.8X4	T46.8X5	T46.8X6
medicinal	T49.1X1	T49.1X2	T49.1X3	T49.1X4	T49.1X5	T49.1X6
nonmedicinal NEC	T54.0X1	T54.0X2	T54.0X3	T54.0X4	—	—
pesticide	T60.8X1	T60.8X2	T60.8X3	T60.8X4	—	—
red	T50.8X1	T50.8X2	T50.8X3	T50.8X4	T50.8X5	T50.8X6
Phenolic preparation	T49.1X1	T49.1X2	T49.1X3	T49.1X4	T49.1X5	T49.1X6
Phenolphthalein	T47.2X1	T47.2X2	T47.2X3	T47.2X4	T47.2X5	T47.2X6
Phenolsulfonphthalein	T50.8X1	T50.8X2	T50.8X3	T50.8X4	T50.8X5	T50.8X6
Phenomorphan	T40.2X1	T40.2X2	T40.2X3	T40.2X4	—	—
Phenonyl	T42.3X1	T42.3X2	T42.3X3	T42.3X4	T42.3X5	T42.3X6
Phenoperidine	T40.4X1	T40.4X2	T40.4X3	T40.4X4	—	—
Phenopyrazone	T46.991	T46.992	T46.993	T46.994	T46.995	T46.996
Phenoquin	T50.4X1	T50.4X2	T50.4X3	T50.4X4	T50.4X5	T50.4X6
Phenothiazine (psychotropic)	T43.3X1	T43.3X2	T43.3X3	T43.3X4	T43.3X5	T43.3X6
NEC						
insecticide	T60.2X1	T60.2X2	T60.2X3	T60.2X4	—	—
Phenothrin	T49.0X1	T49.0X2	T49.0X3	T49.0X4	T49.0X5	T49.0X6
Phenoxybenzamine	T46.7X1	T46.7X2	T46.7X3	T46.7X4	T46.7X5	T46.7X6
Phenoxyethanol	T49.0X1	T49.0X2	T49.0X3	T49.0X4	T49.0X5	T49.0X6
Phenoxymethyl penicillin	T36.0X1	T36.0X2	T36.0X3	T36.0X4	T36.0X5	T36.0X6
Phenprobamate	T42.8X1	T42.8X2	T42.8X3	T42.8X4	T42.8X5	T42.8X6
Phenprocoumon	T45.511	T45.512	T45.513	T45.514	T45.515	T45.516

Pentazocine — Phenprocoumon

Table of Drugs and Chemicals

Phensuximide — Poloxamer

Substance	Poisoning, Accidental (unintentional)	Poisoning, Intentional Self-harm	Poisoning, Assault	Poisoning, Undetermined	Adverse Effect	Under-dosing
Phensuximide	T42.2X1	T42.2X2	T42.2X3	T42.2X4	T42.2X5	T42.2X6
Phentermine	T50.5X1	T50.5X2	T50.5X3	T50.5X4	T50.5X5	T50.5X6
Phenthicillin	T36.0X1	T36.0X2	T36.0X3	T36.0X4	T36.0X5	T36.0X6
Phentolamine	T46.7X1	T46.7X2	T46.7X3	T46.7X4	T46.7X5	T46.7X6
Phenyl						
butazone	T39.2X1	T39.2X2	T39.2X3	T39.2X4	T39.2X5	T39.2X6
enediamine	T65.3X1	T65.3X2	T65.3X3	T65.3X4	—	—
hydrazine	T65.3X1	T65.3X2	T65.3X3	T65.3X4	—	—
antineoplastic	T45.1X1	T45.1X2	T45.1X3	T45.1X4	T45.1X5	T45.1X6
mercuric compounds — see Mercury						
salicylate	T49.3X1	T49.3X2	T49.3X3	T49.3X4	T49.3X5	T49.3X6
Phenylalanine mustard	T45.1X1	T45.1X2	T45.1X3	T45.1X4	T45.1X5	T45.1X6
Phenylbutazone	T39.2X1	T39.2X2	T39.2X3	T39.2X4	T39.2X5	T39.2X6
Phenylenediamine	T65.3X1	T65.3X2	T65.3X3	T65.3X4	—	—
Phenylephrine	T44.4X1	T44.4X2	T44.4X3	T44.4X4	T44.4X5	T44.4X6
Phenylethylbiguanide	T38.3X1	T38.3X2	T38.3X3	T38.3X4	T38.3X5	T38.3X6
Phenylmercuric						
acetate	T49.0X1	T49.0X2	T49.0X3	T49.0X4	T49.0X5	T49.0X6
borate	T49.0X1	T49.0X2	T49.0X3	T49.0X4	T49.0X5	T49.0X6
nitrate	T49.0X1	T49.0X2	T49.0X3	T49.0X4	T49.0X5	T49.0X6
Phenylmethylbarbitone	T42.3X1	T42.3X2	T42.3X3	T42.3X4	T42.3X5	T42.3X6
Phenylpropanol	T47.5X1	T47.5X2	T47.5X3	T47.5X4	T47.5X5	T47.5X6
Phenylpropanolamine	T44.991	T44.992	T44.993	T44.994	T44.995	T44.996
Phenylsulfthion	T60.0X1	T60.0X2	T60.0X3	T60.0X4	—	—
Phenyltoloxamine	T45.0X1	T45.0X2	T45.0X3	T45.0X4	T45.0X5	T45.0X6
Phenyramidol, phenyramidon	T39.8X1	T39.8X2	T39.8X3	T39.8X4	T39.8X5	T39.8X6
Phenytoin	T42.0X1	T42.0X2	T42.0X3	T42.0X4	T42.0X5	T42.0X6
with Phenobarbital	T42.3X1	T42.3X2	T42.3X3	T42.3X4	T42.3X5	T42.3X6
pHisoHex	T49.2X1	T49.2X2	T49.2X3	T49.2X4	T49.2X5	T49.2X6
Pholcodine	T48.3X1	T48.3X2	T48.3X3	T48.3X4	T48.3X5	T48.3X6
Pholedrine	T46.991	T46.992	T46.993	T46.994	T46.995	T46.996
Phorate	T60.0X1	T60.0X2	T60.0X3	T60.0X4	—	—
Phosdrin	T60.0X1	T60.0X2	T60.0X3	T60.0X4	—	—
Phosfolan	T60.0X1	T60.0X2	T60.0X3	T60.0X4	—	—
Phosgene (gas)	T59.891	T59.892	T59.893	T59.894	—	—
Phosphamidon	T60.0X1	T60.0X2	T60.0X3	T60.0X4	—	—
Phosphate	T65.891	T65.892	T65.893	T65.894	—	—
laxative	T47.4X1	T47.4X2	T47.4X3	T47.4X4	T47.4X5	T47.4X6
organic	T60.0X1	T60.0X2	T60.0X3	T60.0X4	—	—
solvent	T52.91	T52.92	T52.93	T52.94	—	—
tricresyl	T65.891	T65.892	T65.893	T65.894	—	—
Phosphine	T57.1X1	T57.1X2	T57.1X3	T57.1X4	—	—
fumigant	T57.1X1	T57.1X2	T57.1X3	T57.1X4	—	—
Phospholine	T49.5X1	T49.5X2	T49.5X3	T49.5X4	T49.5X5	T49.5X6
Phosphoric acid	T54.2X1	T54.2X2	T54.2X3	T54.2X4	—	—
Phosphorus (compound) NEC	T57.1X1	T57.1X2	T57.1X3	T57.1X4	—	—
pesticide	T60.0X1	T60.0X2	T60.0X3	T60.0X4	—	—
Phthalates	T65.891	T65.892	T65.893	T65.894	—	—
Phthalic anhydride	T65.891	T65.892	T65.893	T65.894	—	—
Phthalimidoglutarimide	T42.6X1	T42.6X2	T42.6X3	T42.6X4	T42.6X5	T42.6X6
Phthalylsulfathiazole	T37.0X1	T37.0X2	T37.0X3	T37.0X4	T37.0X5	T37.0X6
Phylloquinone	T45.7X1	T45.7X2	T45.7X3	T45.7X4	T45.7X5	T45.7X6
Physeptone	T40.3X1	T40.3X2	T40.3X3	T40.3X4	T40.3X5	T40.3X6
Physostigma venenosum	T62.2X1	T62.2X2	T62.2X3	T62.2X4	—	—
Physostigmine	T49.5X1	T49.5X2	T49.5X3	T49.5X4	T49.5X5	T49.5X6
Phytolacca decandra	T62.2X1	T62.2X2	T62.2X3	T62.2X4	—	—
berries	T62.1X1	T62.1X2	T62.1X3	T62.1X4	—	—
Phytomenadione	T45.7X1	T45.7X2	T45.7X3	T45.7X4	T45.7X5	T45.7X6
Phytonadione	T45.7X1	T45.7X2	T45.7X3	T45.7X4	T45.7X5	T45.7X6
Picoperine	T48.3X1	T48.3X2	T48.3X3	T48.3X4	T48.3X5	T48.3X6
Picosulfate (sodium)	T47.2X1	T47.2X2	T47.2X3	T47.2X4	T47.2X5	T47.2X6
Picric (acid)	T54.2X1	T54.2X2	T54.2X3	T54.2X4	—	—
Picrotoxin	T50.7X1	T50.7X2	T50.7X3	T50.7X4	T50.7X5	T50.7X6
Piketoprofen	T49.0X1	T49.0X2	T49.0X3	T49.0X4	T49.0X5	T49.0X6
Pilocarpine	T44.1X1	T44.1X2	T44.1X3	T44.1X4	T44.1X5	T44.1X6
Pilocarpus (jaborandi) extract	T44.1X1	T44.1X2	T44.1X3	T44.1X4	T44.1X5	T44.1X6
Pilsicainide (hydrochloride)	T46.2X1	T46.2X2	T46.2X3	T46.2X4	T46.2X5	T46.2X6
Pimaricin	T36.7X1	T36.7X2	T36.7X3	T36.7X4	T36.7X5	T36.7X6
Pimeclone	T50.7X1	T50.7X2	T50.7X3	T50.7X4	T50.7X5	T50.7X6
Pimelic ketone	T52.8X1	T52.8X2	T52.8X3	T52.8X4	—	—
Pimethixene	T45.0X1	T45.0X2	T45.0X3	T45.0X4	T45.0X5	T45.0X6
Piminodine	T40.2X1	T40.2X2	T40.2X3	T40.2X4	T40.2X5	T40.2X6
Pimozide	T43.591	T43.592	T43.593	T43.594	T43.595	T43.596
Pinacidil	T46.5X1	T46.5X2	T46.5X3	T46.5X4	T46.5X5	T46.5X6
Pinaverium bromide	T44.3X1	T44.3X2	T44.3X3	T44.3X4	T44.3X5	T44.3X6
Pinazepam	T42.4X1	T42.4X2	T42.4X3	T42.4X4	T42.4X5	T42.4X6
Pindolol	T44.7X1	T44.7X2	T44.7X3	T44.7X4	T44.7X5	T44.7X6
Pindone	T60.4X1	T60.4X2	T60.4X3	T60.4X4	—	—
Pine oil (disinfectant)	T65.891	T65.892	T65.893	T65.894	—	—

Substance	Poisoning, Accidental (unintentional)	Poisoning, Intentional Self-harm	Poisoning, Assault	Poisoning, Undetermined	Adverse Effect	Under-dosing
Pinkroot	T37.4X1	T37.4X2	T37.4X3	T37.4X4	T37.4X5	T37.4X6
Pipadone	T40.2X1	T40.2X2	T40.2X3	T40.2X4	—	—
Pipamazine	T45.0X1	T45.0X2	T45.0X3	T45.0X4	T45.0X5	T45.0X6
Pipamperone	T43.4X1	T43.4X2	T43.4X3	T43.4X4	T43.4X5	T43.4X6
Pipazetate	T48.3X1	T48.3X2	T48.3X3	T48.3X4	T48.3X5	T48.3X6
Pipemidic acid	T37.8X1	T37.8X2	T37.8X3	T37.8X4	T37.8X5	T37.8X6
Pipenzolate bromide	T44.3X1	T44.3X2	T44.3X3	T44.3X4	T44.3X5	T44.3X6
Piperacetazine	T43.3X1	T43.3X2	T43.3X3	T43.3X4	T43.3X5	T43.3X6
Piperacillin	T36.0X1	T36.0X2	T36.0X3	T36.0X4	T36.0X5	T36.0X6
Piperazine	T37.4X1	T37.4X2	T37.4X3	T37.4X4	T37.4X5	T37.4X6
estrone sulfate	T38.5X1	T38.5X2	T38.5X3	T38.5X4	T38.5X5	T38.5X6
Piper cubeba	T62.2X1	T62.2X2	T62.2X3	T62.2X4	—	—
Piperidione	T48.3X1	T48.3X2	T48.3X3	T48.3X4	T48.3X5	T48.3X6
Piperidolate	T44.3X1	T44.3X2	T44.3X3	T44.3X4	T44.3X5	T44.3X6
Piperocaine	T41.3X1	T41.3X2	T41.3X3	T41.3X4	T41.3X5	T41.3X6
infiltration (subcutaneous)	T41.3X1	T41.3X2	T41.3X3	T41.3X4	T41.3X5	T41.3X6
nerve block (peripheral) (plexus)	T41.3X1	T41.3X2	T41.3X3	T41.3X4	T41.3X5	T41.3X6
topical (surface)	T41.3X1	T41.3X2	T41.3X3	T41.3X4	T41.3X5	T41.3X6
Piperonyl butoxide	T60.8X1	T60.8X2	T60.8X3	T60.8X4	—	—
Pipethanate	T44.3X1	T44.3X2	T44.3X3	T44.3X4	T44.3X5	T44.3X6
Pipobroman	T45.1X1	T45.1X2	T45.1X3	T45.1X4	T45.1X5	T45.1X6
Pipotiazine	T43.3X1	T43.3X2	T43.3X3	T43.3X4	T43.3X5	T43.3X6
Pipoxizine	T45.0X1	T45.0X2	T45.0X3	T45.0X4	T45.0X5	T45.0X6
Pipradrol	T43.691	T43.692	T43.693	T43.694	T43.695	T43.696
Piprinhydrinate	T45.0X1	T45.0X2	T45.0X3	T45.0X4	T45.0X5	T45.0X6
Pirarubicin	T45.1X1	T45.1X2	T45.1X3	T45.1X4	T45.1X5	T45.1X6
Pirazinamide	T37.1X1	T37.1X2	T37.1X3	T37.1X4	T37.1X5	T37.1X6
Pirbuterol	T48.6X1	T48.6X2	T48.6X3	T48.6X4	T48.6X5	T48.6X6
Pirenzepine	T47.1X1	T47.1X2	T47.1X3	T47.1X4	T47.1X5	T47.1X6
Piretanide	T50.1X1	T50.1X2	T50.1X3	T50.1X4	T50.1X5	T50.1X6
Piribedil	T42.8X1	T42.8X2	T42.8X3	T42.8X4	T42.8X5	T42.8X6
Piridoxilate	T46.3X1	T46.3X2	T46.3X3	T46.3X4	T46.3X5	T46.3X6
Piritramide	T40.4X1	T40.4X2	T40.4X3	T40.4X4	—	—
Piromidic acid	T37.8X1	T37.8X2	T37.8X3	T37.8X4	T37.8X5	T37.8X6
Piroxicam	T39.391	T39.392	T39.393	T39.394	T39.395	T39.396
beta-cyclodextrin complex	T39.8X1	T39.8X2	T39.8X3	T39.8X4	T39.8X5	T39.8X6
Pirozadil	T46.6X1	T46.6X2	T46.6X3	T46.6X4	T46.6X5	T46.6X6
Piscidia (bark) (erythrina)	T39.8X1	T39.8X2	T39.8X3	T39.8X4	T39.8X5	T39.8X6
Pitch	T65.891	T65.892	T65.893	T65.894	—	—
Pitkin's solution	T41.3X1	T41.3X2	T41.3X3	T41.3X4	T41.3X5	T41.3X6
Pitocin	T48.0X1	T48.0X2	T48.0X3	T48.0X4	T48.0X5	T48.0X6
Pitressin (tannate)	T38.891	T38.892	T38.893	T38.894	T38.895	T38.896
Pituitary extracts (posterior)	T38.891	T38.892	T38.893	T38.894	T38.895	T38.896
anterior	T38.811	T38.812	T38.813	T38.814	T38.815	T38.816
Pituitrin	T38.891	T38.892	T38.893	T38.894	T38.895	T38.896
Pivampicillin	T36.0X1	T36.0X2	T36.0X3	T36.0X4	T36.0X5	T36.0X6
Pivmecillinam	T36.0X1	T36.0X2	T36.0X3	T36.0X4	T36.0X5	T36.0X6
Placental hormone	T38.891	T38.892	T38.893	T38.894	T38.895	T38.896
Placidyl	T42.6X1	T42.6X2	T42.6X3	T42.6X4	T42.6X5	T42.6X6
Plague vaccine	T50.A91	T50.A92	T50.A93	T50.A94	T50.A95	T50.A96
Plant						
food or fertilizer NEC	T65.891	T65.892	T65.893	T65.894	—	—
containing herbicide	T60.3X1	T60.3X2	T60.3X3	T60.3X4	—	—
noxious, used as food	T62.2X1	T62.2X2	T62.2X3	T62.2X4	—	—
berries	T62.1X1	T62.1X2	T62.1X3	T62.1X4	—	—
seeds	T62.2X1	T62.2X2	T62.2X3	T62.2X4	—	—
specified type NEC	T62.2X1	T62.2X2	T62.2X3	T62.2X4	—	—
Plasma	T45.8X1	T45.8X2	T45.8X3	T45.8X4	T45.8X5	T45.8X6
expander NEC	T45.8X1	T45.8X2	T45.8X3	T45.8X4	T45.8X5	T45.8X6
protein fraction (human)	T45.8X1	T45.8X2	T45.8X3	T45.8X4	T45.8X5	T45.8X6
Plasmanate	T45.8X1	T45.8X2	T45.8X3	T45.8X4	T45.8X5	T45.8X6
Plasminogen (tissue) activator	T45.611	T45.612	T45.613	T45.614	T45.615	T45.616
Plaster dressing	T49.3X1	T49.3X2	T49.3X3	T49.3X4	T49.3X5	T49.3X6
Plastic dressing	T49.3X1	T49.3X2	T49.3X3	T49.3X4	T49.3X5	T49.3X6
Plegicil	T43.3X1	T43.3X2	T43.3X3	T43.3X4	T43.3X5	T43.3X6
Plicamycin	T45.1X1	T45.1X2	T45.1X3	T45.1X4	T45.1X5	T45.1X6
Podophyllotoxin	T49.8X1	T49.8X2	T49.8X3	T49.8X4	T49.8X5	T49.8X6
Podophyllum (resin)	T49.4X1	T49.4X2	T49.4X3	T49.4X4	T49.4X5	T49.4X6
Poisonous berries	T62.1X1	T62.1X2	T62.1X3	T62.1X4	—	—
Poison NEC	T65.91	T65.92	T65.93	T65.94	—	—
Pokeweed (any part)	T62.2X1	T62.2X2	T62.2X3	T62.2X4	—	—
Poldine metilsulfate	T44.3X1	T44.3X2	T44.3X3	T44.3X4	T44.3X5	T44.3X6
Polidexide (sulfate)	T46.6X1	T46.6X2	T46.6X3	T46.6X4	T46.6X5	T46.6X6
Polidocanol	T46.8X1	T46.8X2	T46.8X3	T46.8X4	T46.8X5	T46.8X6
Poliomyelitis vaccine	T50.B91	T50.B92	T50.B93	T50.B94	T50.B95	T50.B96
Polish (car) (floor) (furniture) (metal) (porcelain) (silver)	T65.891	T65.892	T65.893	T65.894	—	—
abrasive	T65.891	T65.892	T65.893	T65.894	—	—
porcelain	T65.891	T65.892	T65.893	T65.894	—	—
Poloxalkol	T47.4X1	T47.4X2	T47.4X3	T47.4X4	T47.4X5	T47.4X6
Poloxamer	T47.4X1	T47.4X2	T47.4X3	T47.4X4	T47.4X5	T47.4X6

Additional Character May Be Required — Refer to the Tabular List for Character Selection

Subterms under main terms may continue to next column or page

Substance	Poisoning, Accidental (unintentional)	Poisoning, Intentional Self-harm	Poisoning, Assault	Poisoning, Undetermined	Adverse Effect	Under-dosing
Polyaminostyrene resins	T50.3X1	T50.3X2	T50.3X3	T50.3X4	T50.3X5	T50.3X6
Polycarbophil	T47.4X1	T47.4X2	T47.4X3	T47.4X4	T47.4X5	T47.4X6
Polychlorinated biphenyl	T65.891	T65.892	T65.893	T65.894	—	—
Polycycline	T36.4X1	T36.4X2	T36.4X3	T36.4X4	T36.4X5	T36.4X6
Polyester fumes	T59.891	T59.892	T59.893	T59.894		
Polyester resin hardener	T52.91	T52.92	T52.93	T52.94	—	—
fumes	T59.891	T59.892	T59.893	T59.894		
Polyestradiol phosphate	T38.5X1	T38.5X2	T38.5X3	T38.5X4	T38.5X5	T38.5X6
Polyethanolamine alkyl sulfate	T49.2X1	T49.2X2	T49.2X3	T49.2X4	T49.2X5	T49.2X6
Polyethylene adhesive	T49.3X1	T49.3X2	T49.3X3	T49.3X4	T49.3X5	T49.3X6
Polyferose	T45.4X1	T45.4X2	T45.4X3	T45.4X4	T45.4X5	T45.4X6
Polygeline	T45.8X1	T45.8X2	T45.8X3	T45.8X4	T45.8X5	T45.8X6
Polymyxin	T36.8X1	T36.8X2	T36.8X3	T36.8X4	T36.8X5	T36.8X6
B	T36.8X1	T36.8X2	T36.8X3	T36.8X4	T36.8X5	T36.8X6
ENT agent	T49.6X1	T49.6X2	T49.6X3	T49.6X4	T49.6X5	T49.6X6
ophthalmic preparation	T49.5X1	T49.5X2	T49.5X3	T49.5X4	T49.5X5	T49.5X6
topical NEC	T49.0X1	T49.0X2	T49.0X3	T49.0X4	T49.0X5	T49.0X6
E sulfate (eye preparation)	T49.5X1	T49.5X2	T49.5X3	T49.5X4	T49.5X5	T49.5X6
Polynoxylin	T49.0X1	T49.0X2	T49.0X3	T49.0X4	T49.0X5	T49.0X6
Polyoestradiol phosphate	T38.5X1	T38.5X2	T38.5X3	T38.5X4	T38.5X5	T38.5X6
Polyoxymethyleneurea	T49.0X1	T49.0X2	T49.0X3	T49.0X4	T49.0X5	T49.0X6
Polysilane	T47.8X1	T47.8X2	T47.8X3	T47.8X4	T47.8X5	T47.8X6
Polytetrafluoroethylene (inhaled)	T59.891	T59.892	T59.893	T59.894	—	—
Polythiazide	T50.2X1	T50.2X2	T50.2X3	T50.2X4	T50.2X5	T50.2X6
Polyvidone	T45.8X1	T45.8X2	T45.8X3	T45.8X4	T45.8X5	T45.8X6
Polyvinylpyrrolidone	T45.8X1	T45.8X2	T45.8X3	T45.8X4	T45.8X5	T45.8X6
Pontocaine (hydrochloride) (infiltration) (topical)	T41.3X1	T41.3X2	T41.3X3	T41.3X4	T41.3X5	T41.3X6
nerve block (peripheral) (plexus)	T41.3X1	T41.3X2	T41.3X3	T41.3X4	T41.3X5	T41.3X6
spinal	T41.3X1	T41.3X2	T41.3X3	T41.3X4	T41.3X5	T41.3X6
Porfiromycin	T45.1X1	T45.1X2	T45.1X3	T45.1X4	T45.1X5	T45.1X6
Posterior pituitary hormone NEC	T38.891	T38.892	T38.893	T38.894	T38.895	T38.896
Pot	T40.7X1	T40.7X2	T40.7X3	T40.7X4	T40.7X5	T40.7X6
Potash (caustic)	T54.3X1	T54.3X2	T54.3X3	T54.3X4	—	—
Potassic saline injection (lactated)	T50.3X1	T50.3X2	T50.3X3	T50.3X4	T50.3X5	T50.3X6
Potassium-removing resin	T50.3X1	T50.3X2	T50.3X3	T50.3X4	T50.3X5	T50.3X6
Potassium-retaining drug	T50.3X1	T50.3X2	T50.3X3	T50.3X4	T50.3X5	T50.3X6
Potassium (salts) NEC	T50.3X1	T50.3X2	T50.3X3	T50.3X4	T50.3X5	T50.3X6
aminobenzoate	T45.8X1	T45.8X2	T45.8X3	T45.8X4	T45.8X5	T45.8X6
aminosalicylate	T37.1X1	T37.1X2	T37.1X3	T37.1X4	T37.1X5	T37.1X6
antimony ' tartrate'	T37.8X1	T37.8X2	T37.8X3	T37.8X4	T37.8X5	T37.8X6
arsenite (solution)	T57.0X1	T57.0X2	T57.0X3	T57.0X4	—	—
bichromate	T56.2X1	T56.2X2	T56.2X3	T56.2X4	—	—
bisulfate	T47.3X1	T47.3X2	T47.3X3	T47.3X4	T47.3X5	T47.3X6
bromide	T42.6X1	T42.6X2	T42.6X3	T42.6X4	T42.6X5	T42.6X6
canrenoate	T50.0X1	T50.0X2	T50.0X3	T50.0X4	T50.0X5	T50.0X6
carbonate	T54.3X1	T54.3X2	T54.3X3	T54.3X4	—	—
chlorate NEC	T65.891	T65.892	T65.893	T65.894	—	—
chloride	T50.3X1	T50.3X2	T50.3X3	T50.3X4	T50.3X5	T50.3X6
citrate	T50.991	T50.992	T50.993	T50.994	T50.995	T50.996
cyanide	T65.0X1	T65.0X2	T65.0X3	T65.0X4	—	—
ferric hexacyanoferrate (medicinal)	T50.6X1	T50.6X2	T50.6X3	T50.6X4	T50.6X5	T50.6X6
nonmedicinal	T65.891	T65.892	T65.893	T65.894	—	—
Fluoride	T57.8X1	T57.8X2	T57.8X3	T57.8X4	—	—
glucaldrate	T47.1X1	T47.1X2	T47.1X3	T47.1X4	T47.1X5	T47.1X6
hydroxide	T54.3X1	T54.3X2	T54.3X3	T54.3X4	—	—
iodate	T49.0X1	T49.0X2	T49.0X3	T49.0X4	T49.0X5	T49.0X6
iodide	T48.4X1	T48.4X2	T48.4X3	T48.4X4	T48.4X5	T48.4X6
nitrate	T57.8X1	T57.8X2	T57.8X3	T57.8X4	—	—
oxalate	T65.891	T65.892	T65.893	T65.894	—	—
perchlorate (nonmedicinal) NEC	T65.891	T65.892	T65.893	T65.894	—	—
antithyroid	T38.2X1	T38.2X2	T38.2X3	T38.2X4	T38.2X5	T38.2X6
medicinal	T38.2X1	T38.2X2	T38.2X3	T38.2X4	T38.2X5	T38.2X6
Permanganate (nonmedicinal)	T65.891	T65.892	T65.893	T65.894	—	—
medicinal	T49.0X1	T49.0X2	T49.0X3	T49.0X4	T49.0X5	T49.0X6
sulfate	T47.2X1	T47.2X2	T47.2X3	T47.2X4	T47.2X5	T47.2X6
Povidone	T45.8X1	T45.8X2	T45.8X3	T45.8X4	T45.8X5	T45.8X6
iodine	T49.0X1	T49.0X2	T49.0X3	T49.0X4	T49.0X5	T49.0X6
Practolol	T44.7X1	T44.7X2	T44.7X3	T44.7X4	T44.7X5	T44.7X6
Prajmalium bitartrate	T46.2X1	T46.2X2	T46.2X3	T46.2X4	T46.2X5	T46.2X6
Pralidoxime (iodide)	T50.6X1	T50.6X2	T50.6X3	T50.6X4	T50.6X5	T50.6X6
chloride	T50.6X1	T50.6X2	T50.6X3	T50.6X4	T50.6X5	T50.6X6
Pramiverine	T44.3X1	T44.3X2	T44.3X3	T44.3X4	T44.3X5	T44.3X6
Pramocaine	T49.1X1	T49.1X2	T49.1X3	T49.1X4	T49.1X5	T49.1X6
Pramoxine	T49.1X1	T49.1X2	T49.1X3	T49.1X4	T49.1X5	T49.1X6
Prasterone	T38.7X1	T38.7X2	T38.7X3	T38.7X4	T38.7X5	T38.7X6
Pravastatin	T46.6X1	T46.6X2	T46.6X3	T46.6X4	T46.6X5	T46.6X6
Prazepam	T42.4X1	T42.4X2	T42.4X3	T42.4X4	T42.4X5	T42.4X6
Praziquantel	T37.4X1	T37.4X2	T37.4X3	T37.4X4	T37.4X5	T37.4X6
Prazitone	T43.291	T43.292	T43.293	T43.294	T43.295	T43.296
Prazosin	T44.6X1	T44.6X2	T44.6X3	T44.6X4	T44.6X5	T44.6X6
Prednicarbate	T49.0X1	T49.0X2	T49.0X3	T49.0X4	T49.0X5	T49.0X6
Prednimustine	T45.1X1	T45.1X2	T45.1X3	T45.1X4	T45.1X5	T45.1X6
Prednisolone	T38.0X1	T38.0X2	T38.0X3	T38.0X4	T38.0X5	T38.0X6
ENT agent	T49.6X1	T49.6X2	T49.6X3	T49.6X4	T49.6X5	T49.6X6
ophthalmic preparation	T49.5X1	T49.5X2	T49.5X3	T49.5X4	T49.5X5	T49.5X6
steaglate	T49.0X1	T49.0X2	T49.0X3	T49.0X4	T49.0X5	T49.0X6
topical NEC	T49.0X1	T49.0X2	T49.0X3	T49.0X4	T49.0X5	T49.0X6
Prednisone	T38.0X1	T38.0X2	T38.0X3	T38.0X4	T38.0X5	T38.0X6
Prednylidene	T38.0X1	T38.0X2	T38.0X3	T38.0X4	T38.0X5	T38.0X6
Pregnandiol	T38.5X1	T38.5X2	T38.5X3	T38.5X4	T38.5X5	T38.5X6
Pregneninolone	T38.5X1	T38.5X2	T38.5X3	T38.5X4	T38.5X5	T38.5X6
Preludin	T43.691	T43.692	T43.693	T43.694	T43.695	T43.696
Premarin	T38.5X1	T38.5X2	T38.5X3	T38.5X4	T38.5X5	T38.5X6
Premedication anesthetic	T41.201	T41.202	T41.203	T41.204	T41.205	T41.206
Prenalterol	T44.5X1	T44.5X2	T44.5X3	T44.5X4	T44.5X5	T44.5X6
Prenoxdiazine	T48.3X1	T48.3X2	T48.3X3	T48.3X4	T48.3X5	T48.3X6
Prenylamine	T46.3X1	T46.3X2	T46.3X3	T46.3X4	T46.3X5	T46.3X6
Preparation H	T49.8X1	T49.8X2	T49.8X3	T49.8X4	T49.8X5	T49.8X6
Preparation, local	T49.4X1	T49.4X2	T49.4X3	T49.4X4	T49.4X5	T49.4X6
Preservative (nonmedicinal)	T65.891	T65.892	T65.893	T65.894	—	—
medicinal	T50.901	T50.902	T50.903	T50.904	T50.905	T50.906
wood	T60.91	T60.92	T60.93	T60.94	—	—
Prethcamide	T50.7X1	T50.7X2	T50.7X3	T50.7X4	T50.7X5	T50.7X6
Pride of China	T62.2X1	T62.2X2	T62.2X3	T62.2X4	—	—
Pridinol	T44.3X1	T44.3X2	T44.3X3	T44.3X4	T44.3X5	T44.3X6
Prifinium bromide	T44.3X1	T44.3X2	T44.3X3	T44.3X4	T44.3X5	T44.3X6
Prilocaine	T41.3X1	T41.3X2	T41.3X3	T41.3X4	T41.3X5	T41.3X6
infiltration (subcutaneous)	T41.3X1	T41.3X2	T41.3X3	T41.3X4	T41.3X5	T41.3X6
nerve block (peripheral) (plexus)	T41.3X1	T41.3X2	T41.3X3	T41.3X4	T41.3X5	T41.3X6
regional	T41.3X1	T41.3X2	T41.3X3	T41.3X4	T41.3X5	T41.3X6
Primaquine	T37.2X1	T37.2X2	T37.2X3	T37.2X4	T37.2X5	T37.2X6
Primidone	T42.6X1	T42.6X2	T42.6X3	T42.6X4	T42.6X5	T42.6X6
Primula (veris)	T62.2X1	T62.2X2	T62.2X3	T62.2X4	—	—
Prinadol	T40.2X1	T40.2X2	T40.2X3	T40.2X4	T40.2X5	T40.2X6
Priscol, Priscoline	T44.6X1	T44.6X2	T44.6X3	T44.6X4	T44.6X5	T44.6X6
Pristinamycin	T36.3X1	T36.3X2	T36.3X3	T36.3X4	T36.3X5	T36.3X6
Privet	T62.2X1	T62.2X2	T62.2X3	T62.2X4	—	—
berries	T62.1X1	T62.1X2	T62.1X3	T62.1X4	—	—
Privine	T44.4X1	T44.4X2	T44.4X3	T44.4X4	T44.4X5	T44.4X6
Pro-Banthine	T44.3X1	T44.3X2	T44.3X3	T44.3X4	T44.3X5	T44.3X6
Probarbital	T42.3X1	T42.3X2	T42.3X3	T42.3X4	T42.3X5	T42.3X6
Probenecid	T50.4X1	T50.4X2	T50.4X3	T50.4X4	T50.4X5	T50.4X6
Probucol	T46.6X1	T46.6X2	T46.6X3	T46.6X4	T46.6X5	T46.6X6
Procainamide	T46.2X1	T46.2X2	T46.2X3	T46.2X4	T46.2X5	T46.2X6
Procaine	T41.3X1	T41.3X2	T41.3X3	T41.3X4	T41.3X5	T41.3X6
benzylpenicillin	T36.0X1	T36.0X2	T36.0X3	T36.0X4	T36.0X5	T36.0X6
nerve block (periphreal) (plexus)	T41.3X1	T41.3X2	T41.3X3	T41.3X4	T41.3X5	T41.3X6
penicillin G	T36.0X1	T36.0X2	T36.0X3	T36.0X4	T36.0X5	T36.0X6
regional	T41.3X1	T41.3X2	T41.3X3	T41.3X4	T41.3X5	T41.3X6
spinal	T41.3X1	T41.3X2	T41.3X3	T41.3X4	T41.3X5	T41.3X6
Procalmidol	T43.591	T43.592	T43.593	T43.594	T43.595	T43.596
Procarbazine	T45.1X1	T45.1X2	T45.1X3	T45.1X4	T45.1X5	T45.1X6
Procaterol	T44.5X1	T44.5X2	T44.5X3	T44.5X4	T44.5X5	T44.5X6
Prochlorperazine	T43.3X1	T43.3X2	T43.3X3	T43.3X4	T43.3X5	T43.3X6
Procyclidine	T44.3X1	T44.3X2	T44.3X3	T44.3X4	T44.3X5	T44.3X6
Producer gas	T58.8X1	T58.8X2	T58.8X3	T58.8X4	—	—
Profadol	T40.4X1	T40.4X2	T40.4X3	T40.4X4	T40.4X5	T40.4X6
Profenamine	T44.3X1	T44.3X2	T44.3X3	T44.3X4	T44.3X5	T44.3X6
Profenil	T44.3X1	T44.3X2	T44.3X3	T44.3X4	T44.3X5	T44.3X6
Proflavine	T49.0X1	T49.0X2	T49.0X3	T49.0X4	T49.0X5	T49.0X6
Progabide	T42.6X1	T42.6X2	T42.6X3	T42.6X4	T42.6X5	T42.6X6
Progesterone	T38.5X1	T38.5X2	T38.5X3	T38.5X4	T38.5X5	T38.5X6
Progestin	T38.5X1	T38.5X2	T38.5X3	T38.5X4	T38.5X5	T38.5X6
oral contraceptive	T38.4X1	T38.4X2	T38.4X3	T38.4X4	T38.4X5	T38.4X6
Progestogen NEC	T38.5X1	T38.5X2	T38.5X3	T38.5X4	T38.5X5	T38.5X6
Progestone	T38.5X1	T38.5X2	T38.5X3	T38.5X4	T38.5X5	T38.5X6
Proglumide	T47.1X1	T47.1X2	T47.1X3	T47.1X4	T47.1X5	T47.1X6
Proguanil	T37.2X1	T37.2X2	T37.2X3	T37.2X4	T37.2X5	T37.2X6
Prolactin	T38.811	T38.812	T38.813	T38.814	T38.815	T38.816
Prolintane	T43.691	T43.692	T43.693	T43.694	T43.695	T43.696
Proloid	T38.1X1	T38.1X2	T38.1X3	T38.1X4	T38.1X5	T38.1X6
Proluton	T38.5X1	T38.5X2	T38.5X3	T38.5X4	T38.5X5	T38.5X6
Promacetin	T37.1X1	T37.1X2	T37.1X3	T37.1X4	T37.1X5	T37.1X6
Promazine	T43.3X1	T43.3X2	T43.3X3	T43.3X4	T43.3X5	T43.3X6
Promedol	T40.2X1	T40.2X2	T40.2X3	T40.2X4		

▼ Subterms under main terms may continue to next column or page   Additional Character May Be Required — Refer to the Tabular List for Character Selection   385

Polyaminostyrene resins — Promedol

Substance	Poisoning, Accidental (unintentional)	Poisoning, Intentional Self-harm	Poisoning, Assault	Poisoning, Undetermined	Adverse Effect	Under-dosing
Promegestone	T38.5X1	T38.5X2	T38.5X3	T38.5X4	T38.5X5	T38.5X6
Promethazine (teoclate)	T43.3X1	T43.3X2	T43.3X3	T43.3X4	T43.3X5	T43.3X6
Promin	T37.1X1	T37.1X2	T37.1X3	T37.1X4	T37.1X5	T37.1X6
Pronase	T45.3X1	T45.3X2	T45.3X3	T45.3X4	T45.3X5	T45.3X6
Pronestyl (hydrochloride)	T46.2X1	T46.2X2	T46.2X3	T46.2X4	T46.2X5	T46.2X6
Pronetalol	T44.7X1	T44.7X2	T44.7X3	T44.7X4	T44.7X5	T44.7X6
Prontosil	T37.0X1	T37.0X2	T37.0X3	T37.0X4	T37.0X5	T37.0X6
Propachlor	T60.3X1	T60.3X2	T60.3X3	T60.3X4	—	—
Propafenone	T46.2X1	T46.2X2	T46.2X3	T46.2X4	T46.2X5	T46.2X6
Propallylonal	T42.3X1	T42.3X2	T42.3X3	T42.3X4	T42.3X5	T42.3X6
Propamidine	T49.0X1	T49.0X2	T49.0X3	T49.0X4	T49.0X5	T49.0X6
Propane (distributed in mobile container)	T59.891	T59.892	T59.893	T59.894	—	—
distributed through pipes	T59.891	T59.892	T59.893	T59.894	—	—
incomplete combustion	T58.11	T58.12	T58.13	T58.14	—	—
Propanidid	T41.291	T41.292	T41.293	T41.294	T41.295	T41.296
Propanil	T60.3X1	T60.3X2	T60.3X3	T60.3X4	—	—
Propantheline	T44.3X1	T44.3X2	T44.3X3	T44.3X4	T44.3X5	T44.3X6
bromide	T44.3X1	T44.3X2	T44.3X3	T44.3X4	T44.3X5	T44.3X6
Proparacaine	T41.3X1	T41.3X2	T41.3X3	T41.3X4	T41.3X5	T41.3X6
Propatylnitrate	T46.3X1	T46.3X2	T46.3X3	T46.3X4	T46.3X5	T46.3X6
Propicillin	T36.0X1	T36.0X2	T36.0X3	T36.0X4	T36.0X5	T36.0X6
Propiolactone	T49.0X1	T49.0X2	T49.0X3	T49.0X4	T49.0X5	T49.0X6
Propiomazine	T45.0X1	T45.0X2	T45.0X3	T45.0X4	T45.0X5	T45.0X6
Propionaldehyde (medicinal)	T42.6X1	T42.6X2	T42.6X3	T42.6X4	T42.6X5	T42.6X6
Propionate (calcium) (sodium)	T49.0X1	T49.0X2	T49.0X3	T49.0X4	T49.0X5	T49.0X6
Propion gel	T49.0X1	T49.0X2	T49.0X3	T49.0X4	T49.0X5	T49.0X6
Propitocaine	T41.3X1	T41.3X2	T41.3X3	T41.3X4	T41.3X5	T41.3X6
infiltration (subcutaneous)	T41.3X1	T41.3X2	T41.3X3	T41.3X4	T41.3X5	T41.3X6
nerve block (peripheral) (plexus)	T41.3X1	T41.3X2	T41.3X3	T41.3X4	T41.3X5	T41.3X6
Propofol	T41.291	T41.292	T41.293	T41.294	T41.295	T41.296
Propoxur	T60.0X1	T60.0X2	T60.0X3	T60.0X4	—	—
Propoxycaine	T41.3X1	T41.3X2	T41.3X3	T41.3X4	T41.3X5	T41.3X6
infiltration (subcutaneous)	T41.3X1	T41.3X2	T41.3X3	T41.3X4	T41.3X5	T41.3X6
nerve block (peripheral) (plexus)	T41.3X1	T41.3X2	T41.3X3	T41.3X4	T41.3X5	T41.3X6
topical (surface)	T41.3X1	T41.3X2	T41.3X3	T41.3X4	T41.3X5	T41.3X6
Propoxyphene	T40.4X1	T40.4X2	T40.4X3	T40.4X4	T40.4X5	T40.4X6
Propranolol	T44.7X1	T44.7X2	T44.7X3	T44.7X4	T44.7X5	T44.7X6
Propyl						
alcohol	T51.3X1	T51.3X2	T51.3X3	T51.3X4	—	—
carbinol	T51.3X1	T51.3X2	T51.3X3	T51.3X4	—	—
hexadrine	T44.4X1	T44.4X2	T44.4X3	T44.4X4	T44.4X5	T44.4X6
iodone	T50.8X1	T50.8X2	T50.8X3	T50.8X4	T50.8X5	T50.8X6
thiouracil	T38.2X1	T38.2X2	T38.2X3	T38.2X4	T38.2X5	T38.2X6
Propylaminophenothiazine	T43.3X1	T43.3X2	T43.3X3	T43.3X4	T43.3X5	T43.3X6
Propylene	T59.891	T59.892	T59.893	T59.894	—	—
Propylhexedrine	T48.5X1	T48.5X2	T48.5X3	T48.5X4	T48.5X5	T48.5X6
Propyliodone	T50.8X1	T50.8X2	T50.8X3	T50.8X4	T50.8X5	T50.8X6
Propylparaben (ophthalmic)	T49.5X1	T49.5X2	T49.5X3	T49.5X4	T49.5X5	T49.5X6
Propylthiouracil	T38.2X1	T38.2X2	T38.2X3	T38.2X4	T38.2X5	T38.2X6
Propyphenazone	T39.2X1	T39.2X2	T39.2X3	T39.2X4	T39.2X5	T39.2X6
Proquazone	T39.391	T39.392	T39.393	T39.394	T39.395	T39.396
Proscillaridin	T46.0X1	T46.0X2	T46.0X3	T46.0X4	T46.0X5	T46.0X6
Prostacyclin	T45.521	T45.522	T45.523	T45.524	T45.525	T45.526
Prostaglandin (I2)	T45.521	T45.522	T45.523	T45.524	T45.525	T45.526
E1	T46.7X1	T46.7X2	T46.7X3	T46.7X4	T46.7X5	T46.7X6
E2	T48.0X1	T48.0X2	T48.0X3	T48.0X4	T48.0X5	T48.0X6
F2 alpha	T48.0X1	T48.0X2	T48.0X3	T48.0X4	T48.0X5	T48.0X6
Prostigmin	T44.0X1	T44.0X2	T44.0X3	T44.0X4	T44.0X5	T44.0X6
Prosultiamine	T45.2X1	T45.2X2	T45.2X3	T45.2X4	T45.2X5	T45.2X6
Protamine sulfate	T45.7X1	T45.7X2	T45.7X3	T45.7X4	T45.7X5	T45.7X6
zinc insulin	T38.3X1	T38.3X2	T38.3X3	T38.3X4	T38.3X5	T38.3X6
Protease	T47.5X1	T47.5X2	T47.5X3	T47.5X4	T47.5X5	T47.5X6
Protectant, skin NEC	T49.3X1	T49.3X2	T49.3X3	T49.3X4	T49.3X5	T49.3X6
Protein hydrolysate	T50.991	T50.992	T50.993	T50.994	T50.995	T50.996
Prothiaden — see Dothiepin hydrochloride						
Prothionamide	T37.1X1	T37.1X2	T37.1X3	T37.1X4	T37.1X5	T37.1X6
Prothipendyl	T43.591	T43.592	T43.593	T43.594	T43.595	T43.596
Prothoate	T60.0X1	T60.0X2	T60.0X3	T60.0X4	—	—
Prothrombin						
activator	T45.7X1	T45.7X2	T45.7X3	T45.7X4	T45.7X5	T45.7X6
synthesis inhibitor	T45.511	T45.512	T45.513	T45.514	T45.515	T45.516
Protionamide	T37.1X1	T37.1X2	T37.1X3	T37.1X4	T37.1X5	T37.1X6
Protirelin	T38.891	T38.892	T38.893	T38.894	T38.895	T38.896
Protokylol	T48.6X1	T48.6X2	T48.6X3	T48.6X4	T48.6X5	T48.6X6
Protopam	T50.6X1	T50.6X2	T50.6X3	T50.6X4	T50.6X5	T50.6X6
Protoveratrine(s) (A) (B)	T46.5X1	T46.5X2	T46.5X3	T46.5X4	T46.5X5	T46.5X6
Protriptyline	T43.011	T43.012	T43.013	T43.014	T43.015	T43.016
Provera	T38.5X1	T38.5X2	T38.5X3	T38.5X4	T38.5X5	T38.5X6
Provitamin A	T45.2X1	T45.2X2	T45.2X3	T45.2X4	T45.2X5	T45.2X6
Proxibarbal	T42.3X1	T42.3X2	T42.3X3	T42.3X4	T42.3X5	T42.3X6
Proxymetacaine	T41.3X1	T41.3X2	T41.3X3	T41.3X4	T41.3X5	T41.3X6
Proxyphylline	T48.6X1	T48.6X2	T48.6X3	T48.6X4	T48.6X5	T48.6X6
Prozac — see Fluoxetine hydrochloride						
Prunus						
laurocerasus	T62.2X1	T62.2X2	T62.2X3	T62.2X4	—	—
virginiana	T62.2X1	T62.2X2	T62.2X3	T62.2X4	—	—
Prussian blue						
commercial	T65.891	T65.892	T65.893	T65.894	—	—
therapeutic	T50.6X1	T50.6X2	T50.6X3	T50.6X4	T50.6X5	T50.6X6
Prussic acid	T65.0X1	T65.0X2	T65.0X3	T65.0X4	—	—
vapor	T57.3X1	T57.3X2	T57.3X3	T57.3X4	—	—
Pseudoephedrine	T44.991	T44.992	T44.993	T44.994	T44.995	T44.996
Psilocin	T40.991	T40.992	T40.993	T40.994	—	—
Psilocybin	T40.991	T40.992	T40.993	T40.994	—	—
Psilocybine	T40.991	T40.992	T40.993	T40.994	—	—
Psoralene (nonmedicinal)	T65.891	T65.892	T65.893	T65.894	—	—
Psoralens (medicinal)	T50.991	T50.992	T50.993	T50.994	T50.995	T50.996
PSP (phenolsulfonphthalein)	T50.8X1	T50.8X2	T50.8X3	T50.8X4	T50.8X5	T50.8X6
Psychodysleptic drug NEC	T40.901	T40.902	T40.903	T40.904	T40.905	T40.906
Psychostimulant	T43.601	T43.602	T43.603	T43.604	T43.605	T43.606
amphetamine	T43.621	T43.622	T43.623	T43.624	T43.625	T43.626
caffeine	T43.611	T43.612	T43.613	T43.614	T43.615	T43.616
methylphenidate	T43.631	T43.632	T43.633	T43.634	T43.635	T43.636
specified NEC	T43.691	T43.692	T43.693	T43.694	T43.695	T43.696
Psychotherapeutic drug NEC	T43.91	T43.92	T43.93	T43.94	T43.95	T43.96
antidepressants — see also Antidepressant	T43.201	T43.202	T43.203	T43.204	T43.205	T43.206
specified NEC	T43.8X1	T43.8X2	T43.8X3	T43.8X4	T43.8X5	T43.8X6
tranquilizers NEC	T43.501	T43.502	T43.503	T43.504	T43.505	T43.506
Psychotomimetic agents	T40.901	T40.902	T40.903	T40.904	T40.905	T40.906
Psychotropic drug NEC	T43.91	T43.92	T43.93	T43.94	T43.95	T43.96
specified NEC	T43.8X1	T43.8X2	T43.8X3	T43.8X4	T43.8X5	T43.8X6
Psyllium hydrophilic mucilloid	T47.4X1	T47.4X2	T47.4X3	T47.4X4	T47.4X5	T47.4X6
Pteroylglutamic acid	T45.8X1	T45.8X2	T45.8X3	T45.8X4	T45.8X5	T45.8X6
Pteroyltriglutamate	T45.1X1	T45.1X2	T45.1X3	T45.1X4	T45.1X5	T45.1X6
PTFE — see Polytetrafluoroethylene						
Pulp						
devitalizing paste	T49.7X1	T49.7X2	T49.7X3	T49.7X4	T49.7X5	T49.7X6
dressing	T49.7X1	T49.7X2	T49.7X3	T49.7X4	T49.7X5	T49.7X6
Pulsatilla	T62.2X1	T62.2X2	T62.2X3	T62.2X4	—	—
Pumpkin seed extract	T37.4X1	T37.4X2	T37.4X3	T37.4X4	T37.4X5	T37.4X6
Purex (bleach)	T54.91	T54.92	T54.93	T54.94	—	—
Purgative NEC — see also Cathartic	T47.4X1	T47.4X2	T47.4X3	T47.4X4	T47.4X5	T47.4X6
Purine analogue (antineoplastic)	T45.1X1	T45.1X2	T45.1X3	T45.1X4	T45.1X5	T45.1X6
Purine diuretics	T50.2X1	T50.2X2	T50.2X3	T50.2X4	T50.2X5	T50.2X6
Purinethol	T45.1X1	T45.1X2	T45.1X3	T45.1X4	T45.1X5	T45.1X6
PVP	T45.8X1	T45.8X2	T45.8X3	T45.8X4	T45.8X5	T45.8X6
Pyrabital	T39.8X1	T39.8X2	T39.8X3	T39.8X4	T39.8X5	T39.8X6
Pyramidon	T39.2X1	T39.2X2	T39.2X3	T39.2X4	T39.2X5	T39.2X6
Pyrantel	T37.4X1	T37.4X2	T37.4X3	T37.4X4	T37.4X5	T37.4X6
Pyrathiazine	T45.0X1	T45.0X2	T45.0X3	T45.0X4	T45.0X5	T45.0X6
Pyrazinamide	T37.1X1	T37.1X2	T37.1X3	T37.1X4	T37.1X5	T37.1X6
Pyrazinoic acid (amide)	T37.1X1	T37.1X2	T37.1X3	T37.1X4	T37.1X5	T37.1X6
Pyrazole (derivatives)	T39.2X1	T39.2X2	T39.2X3	T39.2X4	T39.2X5	T39.2X6
Pyrazolone analgesic NEC	T39.2X1	T39.2X2	T39.2X3	T39.2X4	T39.2X5	T39.2X6
Pyrethrin, pyrethrum (nonmedicinal)	T60.2X1	T60.2X2	T60.2X3	T60.2X4	—	—
Pyrethrum extract	T49.0X1	T49.0X2	T49.0X3	T49.0X4	T49.0X5	T49.0X6
Pyribenzamine	T45.0X1	T45.0X2	T45.0X3	T45.0X4	T45.0X5	T45.0X6
Pyridine	T52.8X1	T52.8X2	T52.8X3	T52.8X4	—	—
aldoxime methiodide	T50.6X1	T50.6X2	T50.6X3	T50.6X4	T50.6X5	T50.6X6
aldoxime methyl chloride	T50.6X1	T50.6X2	T50.6X3	T50.6X4	T50.6X5	T50.6X6
vapor	T59.891	T59.892	T59.893	T59.894	—	—
Pyridium	T39.8X1	T39.8X2	T39.8X3	T39.8X4	T39.8X5	T39.8X6
Pyridostigmine bromide	T44.0X1	T44.0X2	T44.0X3	T44.0X4	T44.0X5	T44.0X6
Pyridoxal phosphate	T45.2X1	T45.2X2	T45.2X3	T45.2X4	T45.2X5	T45.2X6
Pyridoxine	T45.2X1	T45.2X2	T45.2X3	T45.2X4	T45.2X5	T45.2X6
Pyrilamine	T45.0X1	T45.0X2	T45.0X3	T45.0X4	T45.0X5	T45.0X6
Pyrimethamine	T37.2X1	T37.2X2	T37.2X3	T37.2X4	T37.2X5	T37.2X6
with sulfadoxine	T37.2X1	T37.2X2	T37.2X3	T37.2X4	T37.2X5	T37.2X6
Pyrimidine antagonist	T45.1X1	T45.1X2	T45.1X3	T45.1X4	ICD.1X5	T45.1X6
Pyriminil	T60.4X1	T60.4X2	T60.4X3	T60.4X4	—	—
Pyrithione zinc	T49.4X1	T49.4X2	T49.4X3	T49.4X4	T49.4X5	T49.4X6
Pyrithyldione	T42.6X1	T42.6X2	T42.6X3	T42.6X4	T42.6X5	T42.6X6

Substance	Poisoning, Accidental (unintentional)	Poisoning, Intentional Self-harm	Poisoning, Assault	Poisoning, Undetermined	Adverse Effect	Under-dosing
Pyrogallic acid	T49.0X1	T49.0X2	T49.0X3	T49.0X4	T49.0X5	T49.0X6
Pyrogallol	T49.0X1	T49.0X2	T49.0X3	T49.0X4	T49.0X5	T49.0X6
Pyroxylin	T49.3X1	T49.3X2	T49.3X3	T49.3X4	T49.3X5	T49.3X6
Pyrrobutamine	T45.0X1	T45.0X2	T45.0X3	T45.0X4	T45.0X5	T45.0X6
Pyrrolizidine alkaloids	T62.8X1	T62.8X2	T62.8X3	T62.8X4	—	—
Pyrvinium chloride	T37.4X1	T37.4X2	T37.4X3	T37.4X4	T37.4X5	T37.4X6
PZI	T38.3X1	T38.3X2	T38.3X3	T38.3X4	T38.3X5	T38.3X6
Quaalude	T42.6X1	T42.6X2	T42.6X3	T42.6X4	T42.6X5	T42.6X6
Quarternary ammonium						
anti-infective	T49.0X1	T49.0X2	T49.0X3	T49.0X4	T49.0X5	T49.0X6
ganglion blocking	T44.2X1	T44.2X2	T44.2X3	T44.2X4	T44.2X5	T44.2X6
parasympatholytic	T44.3X1	T44.3X2	T44.3X3	T44.3X4	T44.3X5	T44.3X6
Quazepam	T42.4X1	T42.4X2	T42.4X3	T42.4X4	T42.4X5	T42.4X6
Quicklime	T54.3X1	T54.3X2	T54.3X3	T54.3X4	—	—
Quillaja extract	T48.4X1	T48.4X2	T48.4X3	T48.4X4	T48.4X5	T48.4X6
Quinacrine	T37.2X1	T37.2X2	T37.2X3	T37.2X4	T37.2X5	T37.2X6
Quinaglute	T46.2X1	T46.2X2	T46.2X3	T46.2X4	T46.2X5	T46.2X6
Quinalbarbital	T42.3X1	T42.3X2	T42.3X3	T42.3X4	T42.3X5	T42.3X6
Quinalbarbitone sodium	T42.3X1	T42.3X2	T42.3X3	T42.3X4	T42.3X5	T42.3X6
Quinalphos	T60.0X1	T60.0X2	T60.0X3	T60.0X4		
Quinapril	T46.4X1	T46.4X2	T46.4X3	T46.4X4	T46.4X5	T46.4X6
Quinestradiol	T38.5X1	T38.5X2	T38.5X3	T38.5X4	T38.5X5	T38.5X6
Quinestradol	T38.5X1	T38.5X2	T38.5X3	T38.5X4	T38.5X5	T38.5X6
Quinestrol	T38.5X1	T38.5X2	T38.5X3	T38.5X4	T38.5X5	T38.5X6
Quinethazone	T50.2X1	T50.2X2	T50.2X3	T50.2X4	T50.2X5	T50.2X6
Quingestanol	T38.4X1	T38.4X2	T38.4X3	T38.4X4	T38.4X5	T38.4X6
Quinidine	T46.2X1	T46.2X2	T46.2X3	T46.2X4	T46.2X5	T46.2X6
Quinine	T37.2X1	T37.2X2	T37.2X3	T37.2X4	T37.2X5	T37.2X6
Quiniobine	T37.8X1	T37.8X2	T37.8X3	T37.8X4	T37.8X5	T37.8X6
Quinisocaine	T49.1X1	T49.1X2	T49.1X3	T49.1X4	T49.1X5	T49.1X6
Quinocide	T37.2X1	T37.2X2	T37.2X3	T37.2X4	T37.2X5	T37.2X6
Quinoline (derivatives) NEC	T37.8X1	T37.8X2	T37.8X3	T37.8X4	T37.8X5	T37.8X6
Quinupramine	T43.011	T43.012	T43.013	T43.014	T43.015	T43.016
Quotane	T41.3X1	T41.3X2	T41.3X3	T41.3X4	T41.3X5	T41.3X6
Rabies						
immune globulin (human)	T50.Z11	T50.Z12	T50.Z13	T50.Z14	T50.Z15	T50.Z16
vaccine	T50.B91	T50.B92	T50.B93	T50.B94	T50.B95	T50.B96
Racemoramide	T40.2X1	T40.2X2	T40.2X3	T40.2X4		
Racemorphan	T40.2X1	T40.2X2	T40.2X3	T40.2X4	T40.2X5	T40.2X6
Racepinefrin	T44.5X1	T44.5X2	T44.5X3	T44.5X4	T44.5X5	T44.5X6
Raclopride	T43.591	T43.592	T43.593	T43.594	T43.595	T43.596
Radiator alcohol	T51.1X1	T51.1X2	T51.1X3	T51.1X4		
Radioactive drug NEC	T50.8X1	T50.8X2	T50.8X3	T50.8X4	T50.8X5	T50.8X6
Radio-opaque (drugs) (materials)	T50.8X1	T50.8X2	T50.8X3	T50.8X4	T50.8X5	T50.8X6
Ramifenazone	T39.2X1	T39.2X2	T39.2X3	T39.2X4	T39.2X5	T39.2X6
Ramipril	T46.4X1	T46.4X2	T46.4X3	T46.4X4	T46.4X5	T46.4X6
Ranitidine	T47.0X1	T47.0X2	T47.0X3	T47.0X4	T47.0X5	T47.0X6
Ranunculus	T62.2X1	T62.2X2	T62.2X3	T62.2X4	—	—
Rat poison NEC	T60.4X1	T60.4X2	T60.4X3	T60.4X4		
Rattlesnake (venom)	T63.011	T63.012	T63.013	T63.014	—	—
Raubasine	T46.7X1	T46.7X2	T46.7X3	T46.7X4	T46.7X5	T46.7X6
Raudixin	T46.5X1	T46.5X2	T46.5X3	T46.5X4	T46.5X5	T46.5X6
Rautensin	T46.5X1	T46.5X2	T46.5X3	T46.5X4	T46.5X5	T46.5X6
Rautina	T46.5X1	T46.5X2	T46.5X3	T46.5X4	T46.5X5	T46.5X6
Rautotal	T46.5X1	T46.5X2	T46.5X3	T46.5X4	T46.5X5	T46.5X6
Rauwiloid	T46.5X1	T46.5X2	T46.5X3	T46.5X4	T46.5X5	T46.5X6
Rauwoldin	T46.5X1	T46.5X2	T46.5X3	T46.5X4	T46.5X5	T46.5X6
Rauwolfia (alkaloids)	T46.5X1	T46.5X2	T46.5X3	T46.5X4	T46.5X5	T46.5X6
Razoxane	T45.1X1	T45.1X2	T45.1X3	T45.1X4	T45.1X5	T45.1X6
Realgar	T57.0X1	T57.0X2	T57.0X3	T57.0X4	—	—
Recombinant (R) — see specific protein						
Red blood cells, packed	T45.8X1	T45.8X2	T45.8X3	T45.8X4	T45.8X5	T45.8X6
Red squill (scilliroside)	T60.4X1	T60.4X2	T60.4X3	T60.4X4	—	—
Reducing agent, industrial NEC	T65.891	T65.892	T65.893	T65.894	—	—
Refrigerant gas (chlorofluorocarbon)	T53.5X1	T53.5X2	T53.5X3	T53.5X4	—	—
not chlorofluorocarbon	T59.891	T59.892	T59.893	T59.894	—	—
Regroton	T50.2X1	T50.2X2	T50.2X3	T50.2X4	T50.2X5	T50.2X6
Rehydration salts (oral)	T50.3X1	T50.3X2	T50.3X3	T50.3X4	T50.3X5	T50.3X6
Rela	T42.8X1	T42.8X2	T42.8X3	T42.8X4	T42.8X5	T42.8X6
Relaxant, muscle						
anesthetic	T48.1X1	T48.1X2	T48.1X3	T48.1X4	T48.1X5	T48.1X6
central nervous system	T42.8X1	T42.8X2	T42.8X3	T42.8X4	T42.8X5	T42.8X6
skeletal NEC	T48.1X1	T48.1X2	T48.1X3	T48.1X4	T48.1X5	T48.1X6
smooth NEC	T44.3X1	T44.3X2	T44.3X3	T44.3X4	T44.3X5	T44.3X6
Remoxipride	T43.591	T43.592	T43.593	T43.594	T43.595	T43.596
Renese	T50.2X1	T50.2X2	T50.2X3	T50.2X4	T50.2X5	T50.2X6
Renografin	T50.8X1	T50.8X2	T50.8X3	T50.8X4	T50.8X5	T50.8X6
Replacement solution	T50.3X1	T50.3X2	T50.3X3	T50.3X4	T50.3X5	T50.3X6
Reproterol	T48.6X1	T48.6X2	T48.6X3	T48.6X4	T48.6X5	T48.6X6
Rescinnamine	T46.5X1	T46.5X2	T46.5X3	T46.5X4	T46.5X5	T46.5X6
Reserpin (e)	T46.5X1	T46.5X2	T46.5X3	T46.5X4	T46.5X5	T46.5X6
Resorcin, resorcinol (nonmedicinal)	T65.891	T65.892	T65.893	T65.894	—	
medicinal	T49.4X1	T49.4X2	T49.4X3	T49.4X4	T49.4X5	T49.4X6
Respaire	T48.4X1	T48.4X2	T48.4X3	T48.4X4	T48.4X5	T48.4X6
Respiratory drug NEC	T48.901	T48.902	T48.903	T48.904	T48.905	T48.906
antiasthmatic NEC	T48.6X1	T48.6X2	T48.6X3	T48.6X4	T48.6X5	T48.6X6
anti-common-cold NEC	T48.5X1	T48.5X2	T48.5X3	T48.5X4	T48.5X5	T48.5X6
expectorant NEC	T48.4X1	T48.4X2	T48.4X3	T48.4X4	T48.4X5	T48.4X6
stimulant	T48.901	T48.902	T48.903	T48.904	T48.905	T48.906
Retinoic acid	T49.0X1	T49.0X2	T49.0X3	T49.0X4	T49.0X5	T49.0X6
Retinol	T45.2X1	T45.2X2	T45.2X3	T45.2X4	T45.2X5	T45.2X6
Rh (D) immune globulin (human)	T50.Z11	T50.Z12	T50.Z13	T50.Z14	T50.Z15	T50.Z16
Rhodine	T39.011	T39.012	T39.013	T39.014	T39.015	T39.016
RhoGAM	T50.Z11	T50.Z12	T50.Z13	T50.Z14	T50.Z15	T50.Z16
Rhubarb						
dry extract	T47.2X1	T47.2X2	T47.2X3	T47.2X4	T47.2X5	T47.2X6
tincture, compound	T47.2X1	T47.2X2	T47.2X3	T47.2X4	T47.2X5	T47.2X6
Ribavirin	T37.5X1	T37.5X2	T37.5X3	T37.5X4	T37.5X5	T37.5X6
Riboflavin	T45.2X1	T45.2X2	T45.2X3	T45.2X4	T45.2X5	T45.2X6
Ribostamycin	T36.5X1	T36.5X2	T36.5X3	T36.5X4	T36.5X5	T36.5X6
Ricin	T62.2X1	T62.2X2	T62.2X3	T62.2X4		
Ricinus communis	T62.2X1	T62.2X2	T62.2X3	T62.2X4	—	—
Rickettsial vaccine NEC	T50.A91	T50.A92	T50.A93	T50.A94	T50.A95	T50.A96
Rifabutin	T36.6X1	T36.6X2	T36.6X3	T36.6X4	T36.6X5	T36.6X6
Rifamide	T36.6X1	T36.6X2	T36.6X3	T36.6X4	T36.6X5	T36.6X6
Rifampicin	T36.6X1	T36.6X2	T36.6X3	T36.6X4	T36.6X5	T36.6X6
with isoniazid	T37.1X1	T37.1X2	T37.1X3	T37.1X4	T37.1X5	T37.1X6
Rifampin	T36.6X1	T36.6X2	T36.6X3	T36.6X4	T36.6X5	T36.6X6
Rifamycin	T36.6X1	T36.6X2	T36.6X3	T36.6X4	T36.6X5	T36.6X6
Rifaximin	T36.6X1	T36.6X2	T36.6X3	T36.6X4	T36.6X5	T36.6X6
Rimantadine	T37.5X1	T37.5X2	T37.5X3	T37.5X4	T37.5X5	T37.5X6
Rimazolium metilsulfate	T39.8X1	T39.8X2	T39.8X3	T39.8X4	T39.8X5	T39.8X6
Rimifon	T37.1X1	T37.1X2	T37.1X3	T37.1X4	T37.1X5	T37.1X6
Rimiterol	T48.6X1	T48.6X2	T48.6X3	T48.6X4	T48.6X5	T48.6X6
Ringer (lactate) solution	T50.3X1	T50.3X2	T50.3X3	T50.3X4	T50.3X5	T50.3X6
Ristocetin	T36.8X1	T36.8X2	T36.8X3	T36.8X4	T36.8X5	T36.8X6
Ritalin	T43.631	T43.632	T43.633	T43.634	T43.635	T43.636
Ritodrine	T44.5X1	T44.5X2	T44.5X3	T44.5X4	T44.5X5	T44.5X6
Roach killer — see Insecticide						
Rociverine	T44.3X1	T44.3X2	T44.3X3	T44.3X4	T44.3X5	T44.3X6
Rocky Mountain spotted fever vaccine	T50.A91	T50.A92	T50.A93	T50.A94	T50.A95	T50.A96
Rodenticide NEC	T60.4X1	T60.4X2	T60.4X3	T60.4X4	—	—
Rohypnol	T42.4X1	T42.4X2	T42.4X3	T42.4X4	T42.4X5	T42.4X6
Rokitamycin	T36.3X1	T36.3X2	T36.3X3	T36.3X4	T36.3X5	T36.3X6
Rolaids	T47.1X1	T47.1X2	T47.1X3	T47.1X4	T47.1X5	T47.1X6
Rolitetracycline	T36.4X1	T36.4X2	T36.4X3	T36.4X4	T36.4X5	T36.4X6
Romilar	T48.3X1	T48.3X2	T48.3X3	T48.3X4	T48.3X5	T48.3X6
Ronifibrate	T46.6X1	T46.6X2	T46.6X3	T46.6X4	T46.6X5	T46.6X6
Rosaprostol	T47.1X1	T47.1X2	T47.1X3	T47.1X4	T47.1X5	T47.1X6
Rose bengal sodium (131I)	T50.8X1	T50.8X2	T50.8X3	T50.8X4	T50.8X5	T50.8X6
Rose water ointment	T49.3X1	T49.3X2	T49.3X3	T49.3X4	T49.3X5	T49.3X6
Rosoxacin	T37.8X1	T37.8X2	T37.8X3	T37.8X4	T37.8X5	T37.8X6
Rotenone	T60.2X1	T60.2X2	T60.2X3	T60.2X4	—	—
Rotoxamine	T45.0X1	T45.0X2	T45.0X3	T45.0X4	T45.0X5	T45.0X6
Rough-on-rats	T60.4X1	T60.4X2	T60.4X3	T60.4X4	—	—
Roxatidine	T47.0X1	T47.0X2	T47.0X3	T47.0X4	T47.0X5	T47.0X6
Roxithromycin	T36.3X1	T36.3X2	T36.3X3	T36.3X4	T36.3X5	T36.3X6
Rt-PA	T45.611	T45.612	T45.613	T45.614	T45.615	T45.616
Rubbing alcohol	T51.2X1	T51.2X2	T51.2X3	T51.2X4		
Rubefacient	T49.4X1	T49.4X2	T49.4X3	T49.4X4	T49.4X5	T49.4X6
Rubella vaccine	T50.B91	T50.B92	T50.B93	T50.B94	T50.B95	T50.B96
Rubeola vaccine	T50.B91	T50.B92	T50.B93	T50.B94	T50.B95	T50.B96
Rubidium chloride Rb82	T50.8X1	T50.8X2	T50.8X3	T50.8X4	T50.8X5	T50.8X6
Rubidomycin	T45.1X1	T45.1X2	T45.1X3	T45.1X4	T45.1X5	T45.1X6
Rue	T62.2X1	T62.2X2	T62.2X3	T62.2X4	—	—
Rufocromomycin	T45.1X1	T45.1X2	T45.1X3	T45.1X4	T45.1X5	T45.1X6
Russel's viper venin	T45.7X1	T45.7X2	T45.7X3	T45.7X4	T45.7X5	T45.7X6
Ruta (graveolens)	T62.2X1	T62.2X2	T62.2X3	T62.2X4	—	—
Rutinum	T46.991	T46.992	T46.993	T46.994	T46.995	T46.996
Rutoside	T46.991	T46.992	T46.993	T46.994	T46.995	T46.996
b-sitosterol(s)	T46.6X1	T46.6X2	T46.6X3	T46.6X4	T46.6X5	T46.6X6
Sabadilla (plant)	T62.2X1	T62.2X2	T62.2X3	T62.2X4	—	—
pesticide	T60.2X1	T60.2X2	T60.2X3	T60.2X4	—	—
Saccharated iron oxide	T45.8X1	T45.8X2	T45.8X3	T45.8X4	T45.8X5	T45.8X6
Saccharin	T50.901	T50.902	T50.903	T50.904	T50.905	T50.906
Saccharomyces boulardii	T47.6X1	T47.6X2	T47.6X3	T47.6X4	T47.6X5	T47.6X6
Safflower oil	T46.6X1	T46.6X2	T46.6X3	T46.6X4	T46.6X5	T46.6X6
Safrazine	T43.1X1	T43.1X2	T43.1X3	T43.1X4	T43.1X5	T43.1X6
Salazosulfapyridine	T37.0X1	T37.0X2	T37.0X3	T37.0X4	T37.0X5	T37.0X6

Substance	Poisoning, Accidental (unintentional)	Poisoning, Intentional Self-harm	Poisoning, Assault	Poisoning, Undetermined	Adverse Effect	Under-dosing
Salbutamol	T48.6X1	T48.6X2	T48.6X3	T48.6X4	T48.6X5	T48.6X6
Salicylamide	T39.091	T39.092	T39.093	T39.094	T39.095	T39.096
Salicylate NEC	T39.091	T39.092	T39.093	T39.094	T39.095	T39.096
methyl	T49.3X1	T49.3X2	T49.3X3	T49.3X4	T49.3X5	T49.3X6
theobromine calcium	T50.2X1	T50.2X2	T50.2X3	T50.2X4	T50.2X5	T50.2X6
Salicylazosulfapyridine	T37.0X1	T37.0X2	T37.0X3	T37.0X4	T37.0X5	T37.0X6
Salicylhydroxamic acid	T49.0X1	T49.0X2	T49.0X3	T49.0X4	T49.0X5	T49.0X6
Salicylic acid	T49.4X1	T49.4X2	T49.4X3	T49.4X4	T49.4X5	T49.4X6
with benzoic acid	T49.4X1	T49.4X2	T49.4X3	T49.4X4	T49.4X5	T49.4X6
congeners	T39.091	T39.092	T39.093	T39.094	T39.095	T39.096
derivative	T39.091	T39.092	T39.093	T39.094	T39.095	T39.096
salts	T39.091	T39.092	T39.093	T39.094	T39.095	T39.096
Salinazid	T37.1X1	T37.1X2	T37.1X3	T37.1X4	T37.1X5	T37.1X6
Salmeterol	T48.6X1	T48.6X2	T48.6X3	T48.6X4	T48.6X5	T48.6X6
Salol	T49.3X1	T49.3X2	T49.3X3	T49.3X4	T49.3X5	T49.3X6
Salsalate	T39.091	T39.092	T39.093	T39.094	T39.095	T39.096
Salt-replacing drug	T50.901	T50.902	T50.903	T50.904	T50.905	T50.906
Salt-retaining mineralocorticoid	T50.0X1	T50.0X2	T50.0X3	T50.0X4	T50.0X5	T50.0X6
Salt substitute	T50.901	T50.902	T50.903	T50.904	T50.905	T50.906
Saluretic NEC	T50.2X1	T50.2X2	T50.2X3	T50.2X4	T50.2X5	T50.2X6
Saluron	T50.2X1	T50.2X2	T50.2X3	T50.2X4	T50.2X5	T50.2X6
Salvarsan 606 (neosilver) (silver)	T37.8X1	T37.8X2	T37.8X3	T37.8X4	T37.8X5	T37.8X6
Sambucus canadensis	T62.2X1	T62.2X2	T62.2X3	T62.2X4	—	—
berry	T62.1X1	T62.1X2	T62.1X3	T62.1X4	—	—
Sandril	T46.5X1	T46.5X2	T46.5X3	T46.5X4	T46.5X5	T46.5X6
Sanguinaria canadensis	T62.2X1	T62.2X2	T62.2X3	T62.2X4	—	—
Saniflush (cleaner)	T54.2X1	T54.2X2	T54.2X3	T54.2X4	—	—
Santonin	T37.4X1	T37.4X2	T37.4X3	T37.4X4	T37.4X5	T37.4X6
Santyl	T49.8X1	T49.8X2	T49.8X3	T49.8X4	T49.8X5	T49.8X6
Saralasin	T46.5X1	T46.5X2	T46.5X3	T46.5X4	T46.5X5	T46.5X6
Sarcolysin	T45.1X1	T45.1X2	T45.1X3	T45.1X4	T45.1X5	T45.1X6
Sarkomycin	T45.1X1	T45.1X2	T45.1X3	T45.1X4	T45.1X5	T45.1X6
Saroten	T43.011	T43.012	T43.013	T43.014	T43.015	T43.016
Saturnine — see Lead						
Savin (oil)	T49.4X1	T49.4X2	T49.4X3	T49.4X4	T49.4X5	T49.4X6
Scammony	T47.2X1	T47.2X2	T47.2X3	T47.2X4	T47.2X5	T47.2X6
Scarlet red	T49.8X1	T49.8X2	T49.8X3	T49.8X4	T49.8X5	T49.8X6
Scheele's green	T57.0X1	T57.0X2	T57.0X3	T57.0X4	—	—
insecticide	T57.0X1	T57.0X2	T57.0X3	T57.0X4	—	—
Schizontozide (blood) (tissue)	T37.2X1	T37.2X2	T37.2X3	T37.2X4	T37.2X5	T37.2X6
Schradan	T60.0X1	T60.0X2	T60.0X3	T60.0X4	—	—
Schweinfurth green	T57.0X1	T57.0X2	T57.0X3	T57.0X4	—	—
insecticide	T57.0X1	T57.0X2	T57.0X3	T57.0X4	—	—
Scilla, rat poison	T60.4X1	T60.4X2	T60.4X3	T60.4X4	—	—
Scillaren	T60.4X1	T60.4X2	T60.4X3	T60.4X4	—	—
Sclerosing agent	T46.8X1	T46.8X2	T46.8X3	T46.8X4	T46.8X5	T46.8X6
Scombrotoxin	T61.11	T61.12	T61.13	T61.14	—	—
Scopolamine	T44.3X1	T44.3X2	T44.3X3	T44.3X4	T44.3X5	T44.3X6
Scopolia extract	T44.3X1	T44.3X2	T44.3X3	T44.3X4	T44.3X5	T44.3X6
Scouring powder	T65.891	T65.892	T65.893	T65.894	—	—
Sea						
anemone (sting)	T63.631	T63.632	T63.633	T63.634	—	—
cucumber (sting)	T63.691	T63.692	T63.693	T63.694	—	—
snake (bite) (venom)	T63.091	T63.092	T63.093	T63.094	—	—
urchin spine (puncture)	T63.691	T63.692	T63.693	T63.694	—	—
Seafood	T61.91	T61.92	T61.93	T61.94	—	—
specified NEC	T61.8X1	T61.8X2	T61.8X3	T61.8X4	—	—
Secbutabarbital	T42.3X1	T42.3X2	T42.3X3	T42.3X4	T42.3X5	T42.3X6
Secbutabarbitone	T42.3X1	T42.3X2	T42.3X3	T42.3X4	T42.3X5	T42.3X6
Secnidazole	T37.3X1	T37.3X2	T37.3X3	T37.3X4	T37.3X5	T37.3X6
Secobarbital	T42.3X1	T42.3X2	T42.3X3	T42.3X4	T42.3X5	T42.3X6
Seconal	T42.3X1	T42.3X2	T42.3X3	T42.3X4	T42.3X5	T42.3X6
Secretin	T50.8X1	T50.8X2	T50.8X3	T50.8X4	T50.8X5	T50.8X6
Sedative NEC	T42.71	T42.72	T42.73	T42.74	T42.75	T42.76
mixed NEC	T42.6X1	T42.6X2	T42.6X3	T42.6X4	T42.6X5	T42.6X6
Sedormid	T42.6X1	T42.6X2	T42.6X3	T42.6X4	T42.6X5	T42.6X6
Seed disinfectant or dressing	T60.8X1	T60.8X2	T60.8X3	T60.8X4	—	—
Seeds (poisonous)	T62.2X1	T62.2X2	T62.2X3	T62.2X4	—	—
Selegiline	T42.8X1	T42.8X2	T42.8X3	T42.8X4	T42.8X5	T42.8X6
Selenium NEC	T56.891	T56.892	T56.893	T56.894	—	—
disulfide or sulfide	T49.4X1	T49.4X2	T49.4X3	T49.4X4	T49.4X5	T49.4X6
fumes	T59.891	T59.892	T59.893	T59.894	—	—
sulfide	T49.4X1	T49.4X2	T49.4X3	T49.4X4	T49.4X5	T49.4X6
Selenomethionine (75Se)	T50.8X1	T50.8X2	T50.8X3	T50.8X4	T50.8X5	T50.8X6
Selsun	T49.4X1	T49.4X2	T49.4X3	T49.4X4	T49.4X5	T49.4X6
Semustine	T45.1X1	T45.1X2	T45.1X3	T45.1X4	T45.1X5	T45.1X6
Senega syrup	T48.4X1	T48.4X2	T48.4X3	T48.4X4	T48.4X5	T48.4X6
Senna	T47.2X1	T47.2X2	T47.2X3	T47.2X4	T47.2X5	T47.2X6
Sennoside A+B	T47.2X1	T47.2X2	T47.2X3	T47.2X4	T47.2X5	T47.2X6
Septisol	T49.2X1	T49.2X2	T49.2X3	T49.2X4	T49.2X5	T49.2X6
Seractide	T38.811	T38.812	T38.813	T38.814	T38.815	T38.816
Serax	T42.4X1	T42.4X2	T42.4X3	T42.4X4	T42.4X5	T42.4X6
Serenesil	T42.6X1	T42.6X2	T42.6X3	T42.6X4	T42.6X5	T42.6X6
Serenium (hydrochloride)	T37.91	T37.92	T37.93	T37.94	T37.95	T37.96
Serepax — see Oxazepam						
Sermorelin	T38.891	T38.892	T38.893	T38.894	T38.895	T38.896
Sernyl	T41.1X1	T41.1X2	T41.1X3	T41.1X4	T41.1X5	T41.1X6
Serotonin	T50.991	T50.992	T50.993	T50.994	T50.995	T50.996
Serpasil	T46.5X1	T46.5X2	T46.5X3	T46.5X4	T46.5X5	T46.5X6
Serrapeptase	T45.3X1	T45.3X2	T45.3X3	T45.3X4	T45.3X5	T45.3X6
Serum						
antibotulinus	T50.Z11	T50.Z12	T50.Z13	T50.Z14	T50.Z15	T50.Z16
anticytotoxic	T50.Z11	T50.Z12	T50.Z13	T50.Z14	T50.Z15	T50.Z16
antidiphtheria	T50.Z11	T50.Z12	T50.Z13	T50.Z14	T50.Z15	T50.Z16
antimeningococcus	T50.Z11	T50.Z12	T50.Z13	T50.Z14	T50.Z15	T50.Z16
anti-Rh	T50.Z11	T50.Z12	T50.Z13	T50.Z14	T50.Z15	T50.Z16
anti-snake-bite	T50.Z11	T50.Z12	T50.Z13	T50.Z14	T50.Z15	T50.Z16
antitetanic	T50.Z11	T50.Z12	T50.Z13	T50.Z14	T50.Z15	T50.Z16
antitoxic	T50.Z11	T50.Z12	T50.Z13	T50.Z14	T50.Z15	T50.Z16
complement (inhibitor)	T45.8X1	T45.8X2	T45.8X3	T45.8X4	T45.8X5	T45.8X6
convalescent	T50.Z11	T50.Z12	T50.Z13	T50.Z14	T50.Z15	T50.Z16
hemolytic complement	T45.8X1	T45.8X2	T45.8X3	T45.8X4	T45.8X5	T45.8X6
immune (human)	T50.Z11	T50.Z12	T50.Z13	T50.Z14	T50.Z15	T50.Z16
protective NEC	T50.Z11	T50.Z12	T50.Z13	T50.Z14	T50.Z15	T50.Z16
Setastine	T45.0X1	T45.0X2	T45.0X3	T45.0X4	T45.0X5	T45.0X6
Setoperone	T43.591	T43.592	T43.593	T43.594	T43.595	T43.596
Sewer gas	T59.91	T59.92	T59.93	T59.94	—	—
Shampoo	T55.0X1	T55.0X2	T55.0X3	T55.0X4	—	—
Shellfish, noxious, nonbacterial	T61.781	T61.782	T61.783	T61.784	—	—
Sildenafil	T46.7X1	T46.7X2	T46.7X3	T46.7X4	T46.7X5	T46.7X6
Silibinin	T50.991	T50.992	T50.993	T50.994	T50.995	T50.996
Silicone NEC	T65.891	T65.892	T65.893	T65.894	—	—
medicinal	T49.3X1	T49.3X2	T49.3X3	T49.3X4	T49.3X5	T49.3X6
Silvadene	T49.0X1	T49.0X2	T49.0X3	T49.0X4	T49.0X5	T49.0X6
Silver	T49.0X1	T49.0X2	T49.0X3	T49.0X4	T49.0X5	T49.0X6
anti-infectives	T49.0X1	T49.0X2	T49.0X3	T49.0X4	T49.0X5	T49.0X6
arsphenamine	T37.8X1	T37.8X2	T37.8X3	T37.8X4	T37.8X5	T37.8X6
colloidal	T49.0X1	T49.0X2	T49.0X3	T49.0X4	T49.0X5	T49.0X6
nitrate	T49.0X1	T49.0X2	T49.0X3	T49.0X4	T49.0X5	T49.0X6
ophthalmic preparation	T49.5X1	T49.5X2	T49.5X3	T49.5X4	T49.5X5	T49.5X6
toughened (keratolytic)	T49.4X1	T49.4X2	T49.4X3	T49.4X4	T49.4X5	T49.4X6
nonmedicinal (dust)	T56.891	T56.892	T56.893	T56.894	—	—
protein	T49.5X1	T49.5X2	T49.5X3	T49.5X4	T49.5X5	T49.5X6
salvarsan	T37.8X1	T37.8X2	T37.8X3	T37.8X4	T37.8X5	T37.8X6
sulfadiazine	T49.4X1	T49.4X2	T49.4X3	T49.4X4	T49.4X5	T49.4X6
Silymarin	T50.991	T50.992	T50.993	T50.994	T50.995	T50.996
Simaldrate	T47.1X1	T47.1X2	T47.1X3	T47.1X4	T47.1X5	T47.1X6
Simazine	T60.3X1	T60.3X2	T60.3X3	T60.3X4	—	—
Simethicone	T47.1X1	T47.1X2	T47.1X3	T47.1X4	T47.1X5	T47.1X6
Simfibrate	T46.6X1	T46.6X2	T46.6X3	T46.6X4	T46.6X5	T46.6X6
Simvastatin	T46.6X1	T46.6X2	T46.6X3	T46.6X4	T46.6X5	T46.6X6
Sincalide	T50.8X1	T50.8X2	T50.8X3	T50.8X4	T50.8X5	T50.8X6
Sinequan	T43.011	T43.012	T43.013	T43.014	T43.015	T43.016
Singoserp	T46.5X1	T46.5X2	T46.5X3	T46.5X4	T46.5X5	T46.5X6
Sintrom	T45.511	T45.512	T45.513	T45.514	T45.515	T45.516
Sisomicin	T36.5X1	T36.5X2	T36.5X3	T36.5X4	T36.5X5	T36.5X6
Sitosterols	T46.6X1	T46.6X2	T46.6X3	T46.6X4	T46.6X5	T46.6X6
Skeletal muscle relaxants	T48.1X1	T48.1X2	T48.1X3	T48.1X4	T48.1X5	T48.1X6
Skin						
agents (external)	T49.91	T49.92	T49.93	T49.94	T49.95	T49.96
specified NEC	T49.8X1	T49.8X2	T49.8X3	T49.8X4	T49.8X5	T49.8X6
test antigen	T50.8X1	T50.8X2	T50.8X3	T50.8X4	T50.8X5	T50.8X6
Sleep-eze	T45.0X1	T45.0X2	T45.0X3	T45.0X4	T45.0X5	T45.0X6
Sleeping draught, pill	T42.71	T42.72	T42.73	T42.74	T42.75	T42.76
Smallpox vaccine	T50.B11	T50.B12	T50.B13	T50.B14	T50.B15	T50.B16
Smelter fumes NEC	T56.91	T56.92	T56.93	T56.94	—	—
Smog	T59.1X1	T59.1X2	T59.1X3	T59.1X4	—	—
Smoke NEC	T59.811	T59.812	T59.813	T59.814	—	—
Smooth muscle relaxant	T44.3X1	T44.3X2	T44.3X3	T44.3X4	T44.3X5	T44.3X6
Snail killer NEC	T60.8X1	T60.8X2	T60.8X3	T60.8X4	—	—
Snake venom or bite	T63.001	T63.002	T63.003	T63.004	—	—
hemocoagulase	T45.7X1	T45.7X2	T45.7X3	T45.7X4	T45.7X5	T45.7X6
Snuff	T65.211	T65.212	T65.213	T65.214	—	—
Soap (powder) (product)	T55.0X1	T55.0X2	T55.0X3	T55.0X4	—	—
enema	T47.4X1	T47.4X2	T47.4X3	T47.4X4	T47.4X5	T47.4X6
medicinal, soft	T49.2X1	T49.2X2	T49.2X3	T49.2X4	T49.2X5	T49.2X6
superfatted	T49.2X1	T49.2X2	T49.2X3	T49.2X4	T49.2X5	T49.2X6
Sobrerol	T48.4X1	T48.4X2	T48.4X3	T48.4X4	T48.4X5	T48.4X6
Soda (caustic)	T54.3X1	T54.3X2	T54.3X3	T54.3X4	—	—
bicarb	T47.1X1	T47.1X2	T47.1X3	T47.1X4	T47.1X5	T47.1X6

Additional Character May Be Required — Refer to the Tabular List for Character Selection   ▶ **Subterms under main terms may continue to next column or page**

Substance	Poisoning, Accidental (unintentional)	Poisoning, Intentional Self-harm	Poisoning, Assault	Poisoning, Undetermined	Adverse Effect	Under-dosing
Soda — *continued*						
chlorinated — *see* Sodium, hypochlorite						
Sodium						
acetosulfone	T37.1X1	T37.1X2	T37.1X3	T37.1X4	T37.1X5	T37.1X6
acetrizoate	T50.8X1	T50.8X2	T50.8X3	T50.8X4	T50.8X5	T50.8X6
acid phosphate	T50.3X1	T50.3X2	T50.3X3	T50.3X4	T50.3X5	T50.3X6
alginate	T47.8X1	T47.8X2	T47.8X3	T47.8X4	T47.8X5	T47.8X6
amidotrizoate	T50.8X1	T50.8X2	T50.8X3	T50.8X4	T50.8X5	T50.8X6
aminopterin	T45.1X1	T45.1X2	T45.1X3	T45.1X4	T45.1X5	T45.1X6
amylosulfate	T47.8X1	T47.8X2	T47.8X3	T47.8X4	T47.8X5	T47.8X6
amytal	T42.3X1	T42.3X2	T42.3X3	T42.3X4	T42.3X5	T42.3X6
antimony gluconate	T37.3X1	T37.3X2	T37.3X3	T37.3X4	T37.3X5	T37.3X6
arsenate	T57.0X1	T57.0X2	T57.0X3	T57.0X4	—	—
aurothiomalate	T39.4X1	T39.4X2	T39.4X3	T39.4X4	T39.4X5	T39.4X6
aurothiosulfate	T39.4X1	T39.4X2	T39.4X3	T39.4X4	T39.4X5	T39.4X6
barbiturate	T42.3X1	T42.3X2	T42.3X3	T42.3X4	T42.3X5	T42.3X6
basic phosphate	T47.4X1	T47.4X2	T47.4X3	T47.4X4	T47.4X5	T47.4X6
bicarbonate	T47.1X1	T47.1X2	T47.1X3	T47.1X4	T47.1X5	T47.1X6
bichromate	T57.8X1	T57.8X2	T57.8X3	T57.8X4	—	—
biphosphate	T50.3X1	T50.3X2	T50.3X3	T50.3X4	T50.3X5	T50.3X6
bisulfate	T65.891	T65.892	T65.893	T65.894	—	—
borate						
cleanser	T57.8X1	T57.8X2	T57.8X3	T57.8X4	—	—
eye	T49.5X1	T49.5X2	T49.5X3	T49.5X4	T49.5X5	T49.5X6
therapeutic	T49.8X1	T49.8X2	T49.8X3	T49.8X4	T49.8X5	T49.8X6
bromide	T42.6X1	T42.6X2	T42.6X3	T42.6X4	T42.6X5	T42.6X6
cacodylate (nonmedicinal) NEC	T50.8X1	T50.8X2	T50.8X3	T50.8X4	T50.8X5	T50.8X6
anti-infective	T37.8X1	T37.8X2	T37.8X3	T37.8X4	T37.8X5	T37.8X6
herbicide	T60.3X1	T60.3X2	T60.3X3	T60.3X4	—	—
calcium edetate	T45.8X1	T45.8X2	T45.8X3	T45.8X4	T45.8X5	T45.8X6
carbonate NEC	T54.3X1	T54.3X2	T54.3X3	T54.3X4	—	—
chlorate NEC	T65.891	T65.892	T65.893	T65.894	—	—
herbicide	T54.91	T54.92	T54.93	T54.94	—	—
chloride	T50.3X1	T50.3X2	T50.3X3	T50.3X4	T50.3X5	T50.3X6
with glucose	T50.3X1	T50.3X2	T50.3X3	T50.3X4	T50.3X5	T50.3X6
chromate	T65.891	T65.892	T65.893	T65.894	—	—
citrate	T50.991	T50.992	T50.993	T50.994	T50.995	T50.996
cromoglicate	T48.6X1	T48.6X2	T48.6X3	T48.6X4	T48.6X5	T48.6X6
cyanide	T65.0X1	T65.0X2	T65.0X3	T65.0X4	—	—
cyclamate	T50.3X1	T50.3X2	T50.3X3	T50.3X4	T50.3X5	T50.3X6
dehydrocholate	T45.8X1	T45.8X2	T45.8X3	T45.8X4	T45.8X5	T45.8X6
diatrizoate	T50.8X1	T50.8X2	T50.8X3	T50.8X4	T50.8X5	T50.8X6
dibunate	T48.4X1	T48.4X2	T48.4X3	T48.4X4	T48.4X5	T48.4X6
dioctyl sulfosuccinate	T47.4X1	T47.4X2	T47.4X3	T47.4X4	T47.4X5	T47.4X6
dipantoyl ferrate	T45.8X1	T45.8X2	T45.8X3	T45.8X4	T45.8X5	T45.8X6
edetate	T45.8X1	T45.8X2	T45.8X3	T45.8X4	T45.8X5	T45.8X6
ethacrynate	T50.1X1	T50.1X2	T50.1X3	T50.1X4	T50.1X5	T50.1X6
feredetate	T45.8X1	T45.8X2	T45.8X3	T45.8X4	T45.8X5	T45.8X6
Fluoride — *see* Fluoride						
fluoroacetate (dust) (pesticide)	T60.4X1	T60.4X2	T60.4X3	T60.4X4	—	—
free salt	T50.3X1	T50.3X2	T50.3X3	T50.3X4	T50.3X5	T50.3X6
fusidate	T36.8X1	T36.8X2	T36.8X3	T36.8X4	T36.8X5	T36.8X6
glucaldrate	T47.1X1	T47.1X2	T47.1X3	T47.1X4	T47.1X5	T47.1X6
glucosulfone	T37.1X1	T37.1X2	T37.1X3	T37.1X4	T37.1X5	T37.1X6
glutamate	T45.8X1	T45.8X2	T45.8X3	T45.8X4	T45.8X5	T45.8X6
hydrogen carbonate	T50.3X1	T50.3X2	T50.3X3	T50.3X4	T50.3X5	T50.3X6
hydroxide	T54.3X1	T54.3X2	T54.3X3	T54.3X4	—	—
hypochlorite (bleach) NEC	T54.3X1	T54.3X2	T54.3X3	T54.3X4	—	—
disinfectant	T54.3X1	T54.3X2	T54.3X3	T54.3X4	—	—
medicinal (anti-infective) (external)	T49.0X1	T49.0X2	T49.0X3	T49.0X4	T49.0X5	T49.0X6
vapor	T54.3X1	T54.3X2	T54.3X3	T54.3X4	—	—
hyposulfite	T49.0X1	T49.0X2	T49.0X3	T49.0X4	T49.0X5	T49.0X6
indigotin disulfonate	T50.8X1	T50.8X2	T50.8X3	T50.8X4	T50.8X5	T50.8X6
iodide	T50.991	T50.992	T50.993	T50.994	T50.995	T50.996
I-131	T50.8X1	T50.8X2	T50.8X3	T50.8X4	T50.8X5	T50.8X6
therapeutic	T38.2X1	T38.2X2	T38.2X3	T38.2X4	T38.2X5	T38.2X6
iodohippurate (131I)	T50.8X1	T50.8X2	T50.8X3	T50.8X4	T50.8X5	T50.8X6
iopodate	T50.8X1	T50.8X2	T50.8X3	T50.8X4	T50.8X5	T50.8X6
iothalamate	T50.8X1	T50.8X2	T50.8X3	T50.8X4	T50.8X5	T50.8X6
iron edetate	T45.4X1	T45.4X2	T45.4X3	T45.4X4	T45.4X5	T45.4X6
lactate (compound solution)	T45.8X1	T45.8X2	T45.8X3	T45.8X4	T45.8X5	T45.8X6
lauryl (sulfate)	T49.2X1	T49.2X2	T49.2X3	T49.2X4	T49.2X5	T49.2X6
L-triiodothyronine	T38.1X1	T38.1X2	T38.1X3	T38.1X4	T38.1X5	T38.1X6
magnesium citrate	T50.991	T50.992	T50.993	T50.994	T50.995	T50.996
mersalate	T50.2X1	T50.2X2	T50.2X3	T50.2X4	T50.2X5	T50.2X6
metasilicate	T65.891	T65.892	T65.893	T65.894	—	—
metrizoate	T50.8X1	T50.8X2	T50.8X3	T50.8X4	T50.8X5	T50.8X6

Substance	Poisoning, Accidental (unintentional)	Poisoning, Intentional Self-harm	Poisoning, Assault	Poisoning, Undetermined	Adverse Effect	Under-dosing
Sodium — *continued*						
monofluoroacetate (pesticide)	T60.1X1	T60.1X2	T60.1X3	T60.1X4	—	—
morrhuate	T46.8X1	T46.8X2	T46.8X3	T46.8X4	T46.8X5	T46.8X6
nafcillin	T36.0X1	T36.0X2	T36.0X3	T36.0X4	T36.0X5	T36.0X6
nitrate (oxidizing agent)	T65.891	T65.892	T65.893	T65.894	—	—
nitrite	T50.6X1	T50.6X2	T50.6X3	T50.6X4	T50.6X5	T50.6X6
nitroferricyanide	T46.5X1	T46.5X2	T46.5X3	T46.5X4	T46.5X5	T46.5X6
nitroprusside	T46.5X1	T46.5X2	T46.5X3	T46.5X4	T46.5X5	T46.5X6
oxalate	T65.891	T65.892	T65.893	T65.894	—	—
oxide/peroxide	T65.891	T65.892	T65.893	T65.894	—	—
oxybate	T41.291	T41.292	T41.293	T41.294	T41.295	T41.296
para-aminohippurate	T50.8X1	T50.8X2	T50.8X3	T50.8X4	T50.8X5	T50.8X6
perborate (nonmedicinal) NEC	T65.891	T65.892	T65.893	T65.894	—	—
medicinal	T49.0X1	T49.0X2	T49.0X3	T49.0X4	T49.0X5	T49.0X6
soap	T55.0X1	T55.0X2	T55.0X3	T55.0X4	—	—
percarbonate — *see* Sodium, perborate						
pertechnetate Tc99m	T50.8X1	T50.8X2	T50.8X3	T50.8X4	T50.8X5	T50.8X6
phosphate						
cellulose	T45.8X1	T45.8X2	T45.8X3	T45.8X4	T45.8X5	T45.8X6
dibasic	T47.2X1	T47.2X2	T47.2X3	T47.2X4	T47.2X5	T47.2X6
monobasic	T47.2X1	T47.2X2	T47.2X3	T47.2X4	T47.2X5	T47.2X6
phytate	T50.6X1	T50.6X2	T50.6X3	T50.6X4	T50.6X5	T50.6X6
picosulfate	T47.2X1	T47.2X2	T47.2X3	T47.2X4	T47.2X5	T47.2X6
polyhydroxyaluminium monocarbonate	T47.1X1	T47.1X2	T47.1X3	T47.1X4	T47.1X5	T47.1X6
polystyrene sulfonate	T50.3X1	T50.3X2	T50.3X3	T50.3X4	T50.3X5	T50.3X6
propionate	T49.0X1	T49.0X2	T49.0X3	T49.0X4	T49.0X5	T49.0X6
propyl hydroxybenzoate	T50.991	T50.992	T50.993	T50.994	T50.995	T50.996
psylliate	T46.8X1	T46.8X2	T46.8X3	T46.8X4	T46.8X5	T46.8X6
removing resins	T50.3X1	T50.3X2	T50.3X3	T50.3X4	T50.3X5	T50.3X6
salicylate	T39.091	T39.092	T39.093	T39.094	T39.095	T39.096
salt NEC	T50.3X1	T50.3X2	T50.3X3	T50.3X4	T50.3X5	T50.3X6
selenate	T60.2X1	T60.2X2	T60.2X3	T60.2X4	—	—
stibogluconate	T37.3X1	T37.3X2	T37.3X3	T37.3X4	T37.3X5	T37.3X6
sulfate	T47.4X1	T47.4X2	T47.4X3	T47.4X4	T47.4X5	T47.4X6
sulfoxone	T37.1X1	T37.1X2	T37.1X3	T37.1X4	T37.1X5	T37.1X6
tetradecyl sulfate	T46.8X1	T46.8X2	T46.8X3	T46.8X4	T46.8X5	T46.8X6
thiopental	T41.1X1	T41.1X2	T41.1X3	T41.1X4	T41.1X5	T41.1X6
thiosalicylate	T39.091	T39.092	T39.093	T39.094	T39.095	T39.096
thiosulfate	T50.6X1	T50.6X2	T50.6X3	T50.6X4	T50.6X5	T50.6X6
tolbutamide	T38.3X1	T38.3X2	T38.3X3	T38.3X4	T38.3X5	T38.3X6
(L)-triiodothyronine	T38.1X1	T38.1X2	T38.1X3	T38.1X4	T38.1X5	T38.1X6
tyropanoate	T50.8X1	T50.8X2	T50.8X3	T50.8X4	T50.8X5	T50.8X6
valproate	T42.6X1	T42.6X2	T42.6X3	T42.6X4	T42.6X5	T42.6X6
versenate	T50.6X1	T50.6X2	T50.6X3	T50.6X4	T50.6X5	T50.6X6
Sodium-free salt	T50.901	T50.902	T50.903	T50.904	T50.905	T50.906
Sodium-removing resin	T50.3X1	T50.3X2	T50.3X3	T50.3X4	T50.3X5	T50.3X6
Soft soap	T55.0X1	T55.0X2	T55.0X3	T55.0X4	—	—
Solanine	T62.2X1	T62.2X2	T62.2X3	T62.2X4	—	—
berries	T62.1X1	T62.1X2	T62.1X3	T62.1X4	—	—
Solanum dulcamara	T62.2X1	T62.2X2	T62.2X3	T62.2X4	—	—
berries	T62.1X1	T62.1X2	T62.1X3	T62.1X4	—	—
Solapsone	T37.1X1	T37.1X2	T37.1X3	T37.1X4	T37.1X5	T37.1X6
Solar lotion	T49.3X1	T49.3X2	T49.3X3	T49.3X4	T49.3X5	T49.3X6
Solasulfone	T37.1X1	T37.1X2	T37.1X3	T37.1X4	T37.1X5	T37.1X6
Soldering fluid	T65.891	T65.892	T65.893	T65.894	—	—
Solid substance	T65.91	T65.92	T65.93	T65.94	—	—
specified NEC	T65.891	T65.892	T65.893	T65.894	—	—
Solvent, industrial NEC	T52.91	T52.92	T52.93	T52.94	—	—
naphtha	T52.0X1	T52.0X2	T52.0X3	T52.0X4	—	—
petroleum	T52.0X1	T52.0X2	T52.0X3	T52.0X4	—	—
specified NEC	T52.8X1	T52.8X2	T52.8X3	T52.8X4	—	—
Soma	T42.8X1	T42.8X2	T42.8X3	T42.8X4	T42.8X5	T42.8X6
Somatorelin	T38.891	T38.892	T38.893	T38.894	T38.895	T38.896
Somatostatin	T38.991	T38.992	T38.993	T38.994	T38.995	T38.996
Somatotropin	T38.811	T38.812	T38.813	T38.814	T38.815	T38.816
Somatrem	T38.811	T38.812	T38.813	T38.814	T38.815	T38.816
Somatropin	T38.811	T38.812	T38.813	T38.814	T38.815	T38.816
Sominex	T45.0X1	T45.0X2	T45.0X3	T45.0X4	T45.0X5	T45.0X6
Somnos	T42.6X1	T42.6X2	T42.6X3	T42.6X4	T42.6X5	T42.6X6
Somonal	T42.3X1	T42.3X2	T42.3X3	T42.3X4	T42.3X5	T42.3X6
Soneryl	T42.3X1	T42.3X2	T42.3X3	T42.3X4	T42.3X5	T42.3X6
Soothing syrup	T50.901	T50.902	T50.903	T50.904	T50.905	T50.906
Sopor	T42.6X1	T42.6X2	T42.6X3	T42.6X4	T42.6X5	T42.6X6
Soporific	T42.71	T42.72	T42.73	T42.74	T42.75	T42.76
Soporific drug	T42.71	T42.72	T42.73	T42.74	T42.75	T42.76
specified type NEC	T42.6X1	T42.6X2	T42.6X3	T42.6X4	T42.6X5	T42.6X6
Sorbide nitrate	T46.3X1	T46.3X2	T46.3X3	T46.3X4	T46.3X5	T46.3X6
Sorbitol	T47.4X1	T47.4X2	T47.4X3	T47.4X4	T47.4X5	T47.4X6
Sotalol	T44.7X1	T44.7X2	T44.7X3	T44.7X4	T44.7X5	T44.7X6

Table of Drugs and Chemicals

Sotradecol — Sulfanilylguanidine

Substance	Poisoning, Accidental (unintentional)	Poisoning, Intentional Self-harm	Poisoning, Assault	Poisoning, Undetermined	Adverse Effect	Under-dosing
Sotradecol	T46.8X1	T46.8X2	T46.8X3	T46.8X4	T46.8X5	T46.8X6
Soysterol	T46.6X1	T46.6X2	T46.6X3	T46.6X4	T46.6X5	T46.6X6
Spacoline	T44.3X1	T44.3X2	T44.3X3	T44.3X4	T44.3X5	T44.3X6
Spanish fly	T49.8X1	T49.8X2	T49.8X3	T49.8X4	T49.8X5	T49.8X6
Sparine	T43.3X1	T43.3X2	T43.3X3	T43.3X4	T43.3X5	T43.3X6
Sparteine	T48.0X1	T48.0X2	T48.0X3	T48.0X4	T48.0X5	T48.0X6
Spasmolytic						
anticholinergics	T44.3X1	T44.3X2	T44.3X3	T44.3X4	T44.3X5	T44.3X6
autonomic	T44.3X1	T44.3X2	T44.3X3	T44.3X4	T44.3X5	T44.3X6
bronchial NEC	T48.6X1	T48.6X2	T48.6X3	T48.6X4	T48.6X5	T48.6X6
quaternary ammonium	T44.3X1	T44.3X2	T44.3X3	T44.3X4	T44.3X5	T44.3X6
skeletal muscle NEC	T48.1X1	T48.1X2	T48.1X3	T48.1X4	T48.1X5	T48.1X6
Spectinomycin	T36.5X1	T36.5X2	T36.5X3	T36.5X4	T36.5X5	T36.5X6
Speed	T43.621	T43.622	T43.623	T43.624	T43.625	T43.626
Spermicide	T49.8X1	T49.8X2	T49.8X3	T49.8X4	T49.8X5	T49.8X6
Spider (bite) (venom)	T63.391	T63.392	T63.393	T63.394		
antivenin	T50.Z11	T50.Z12	T50.Z13	T50.Z14	T50.Z15	T50.Z16
Spigelia (root)	T37.4X1	T37.4X2	T37.4X3	T37.4X4	T37.4X5	T37.4X6
Spindle inactivator	T50.4X1	T50.4X2	T50.4X3	T50.4X4	T50.4X5	T50.4X6
Spiperone	T43.4X1	T43.4X2	T43.4X3	T43.4X4	T43.4X5	T43.4X6
Spiramycin	T36.3X1	T36.3X2	T36.3X3	T36.3X4	T36.3X5	T36.3X6
Spirapril	T46.4X1	T46.4X2	T46.4X3	T46.4X4	T46.4X5	T46.4X6
Spirilene	T43.591	T43.592	T43.593	T43.594	T43.595	T43.596
Spirit(s) (neutral) NEC	T51.0X1	T51.0X2	T51.0X3	T51.0X4	—	—
beverage	T51.0X1	T51.0X2	T51.0X3	T51.0X4	—	—
industrial	T51.0X1	T51.0X2	T51.0X3	T51.0X4	—	—
mineral	T52.0X1	T52.0X2	T52.0X3	T52.0X4	—	—
of salt — see Hydrochloric acid						
surgical	T51.0X1	T51.0X2	T51.0X3	T51.0X4	—	—
Spironolactone	T50.0X1	T50.0X2	T50.0X3	T50.0X4	T50.0X5	T50.0X6
Spiroperidol	T43.4X1	T43.4X2	T43.4X3	T43.4X4	T43.4X5	T43.4X6
Sponge, absorbable (gelatin)	T45.7X1	T45.7X2	T45.7X3	T45.7X4	T45.7X5	T45.7X6
Sporostacin	T49.0X1	T49.0X2	T49.0X3	T49.0X4	T49.0X5	T49.0X6
Spray (aerosol)	T65.91	T65.92	T65.93	T65.94	—	—
cosmetic	T65.891	T65.892	T65.893	T65.894	—	—
medicinal NEC	T50.901	T50.902	T50.903	T50.904	T50.905	T50.906
pesticides — see Pesticides						
specified content — see specific substance						
Spurge flax	T62.2X1	T62.2X2	T62.2X3	T62.2X4	—	—
Spurges	T62.2X1	T62.2X2	T62.2X3	T62.2X4	—	—
Sputum viscosity-lowering drug	T48.4X1	T48.4X2	T48.4X3	T48.4X4	T48.4X5	T48.4X6
Squill	T46.0X1	T46.0X2	T46.0X3	T46.0X4	T46.0X5	T46.0X6
rat poison	T60.4X1	T60.4X2	T60.4X3	T60.4X4	—	—
Squirting cucumber (cathartic)	T47.2X1	T47.2X2	T47.2X3	T47.2X4	T47.2X5	T47.2X6
Stains	T65.6X1	T65.6X2	T65.6X3	T65.6X4	—	—
Stannous fluoride	T49.7X1	T49.7X2	T49.7X3	T49.7X4	T49.7X5	T49.7X6
Stanolone	T38.7X1	T38.7X2	T38.7X3	T38.7X4	T38.7X5	T38.7X6
Stanozolol	T38.7X1	T38.7X2	T38.7X3	T38.7X4	T38.7X5	T38.7X6
Staphisagria or stavesacre (pediculicide)	T49.0X1	T49.0X2	T49.0X3	T49.0X4	T49.0X5	T49.0X6
Starch	T50.901	T50.902	T50.903	T50.904	T50.905	T50.906
Stelazine	T43.3X1	T43.3X2	T43.3X3	T43.3X4	T43.3X5	T43.3X6
Stemetil	T43.3X1	T43.3X2	T43.3X3	T43.3X4	T43.3X5	T43.3X6
Stepronin	T48.4X1	T48.4X2	T48.4X3	T48.4X4	T48.4X5	T48.4X6
Sterculia	T47.4X1	T47.4X2	T47.4X3	T47.4X4	T47.4X5	T47.4X6
Sternutator gas	T59.891	T59.892	T59.893	T59.894	—	—
Steroid	T38.0X1	T38.0X2	T38.0X3	T38.0X4	T38.0X5	T38.0X6
anabolic	T38.7X1	T38.7X2	T38.7X3	T38.7X4	T38.7X5	T38.7X6
androgenic	T38.7X1	T38.7X2	T38.7X3	T38.7X4	T38.7X5	T38.7X6
antineoplastic, hormone	T38.7X1	T38.7X2	T38.7X3	T38.7X4	T38.7X5	T38.7X6
estrogen	T38.5X1	T38.5X2	T38.5X3	T38.5X4	T38.5X5	T38.5X6
ENT agent	T49.6X1	T49.6X2	T49.6X3	T49.6X4	T49.6X5	T49.6X6
ophthalmic preparation	T49.5X1	T49.5X2	T49.5X3	T49.5X4	T49.5X5	T49.5X6
topical NEC	T49.0X1	T49.0X2	T49.0X3	T49.0X4	T49.0X5	T49.0X6
Stibine	T56.891	T56.892	T56.893	T56.894	—	—
Stibogluconate	T37.3X1	T37.3X2	T37.3X3	T37.3X4	T37.3X5	T37.3X6
Stibophen	T37.4X1	T37.4X2	T37.4X3	T37.4X4	T37.4X5	T37.4X6
Stilbamidine (isetionate)	T37.3X1	T37.3X2	T37.3X3	T37.3X4	T37.3X5	T37.3X6
Stilbestrol	T38.5X1	T38.5X2	T38.5X3	T38.5X4	T38.5X5	T38.5X6
Stilboestrol	T38.5X1	T38.5X2	T38.5X3	T38.5X4	T38.5X5	T38.5X6
Stimulant						
central nervous system — see also Psychostimulant	T43.601	T43.602	T43.603	T43.604	T43.605	T43.606
analeptics	T50.7X1	T50.7X2	T50.7X3	T50.7X4	T50.7X5	T50.7X6
opiate antagonist	T50.7X1	T50.7X2	T50.7X3	T50.7X4	T50.7X5	T50.7X6
psychotherapeutic NEC — see also Psychotherapeutic drug	T43.601	T43.602	T43.603	T43.604	T43.605	T43.606
specified NEC	T43.691	T43.692	T43.693	T43.694	T43.695	T43.696

Substance	Poisoning, Accidental (unintentional)	Poisoning, Intentional Self-harm	Poisoning, Assault	Poisoning, Undetermined	Adverse Effect	Under-dosing
Stimulant — continued						
respiratory	T48.901	T48.902	T48.903	T48.904	T48.905	T48.906
Stone-dissolving drug	T50.901	T50.902	T50.903	T50.904	T50.905	T50.906
Storage battery (cells) (acid)	T54.2X1	T54.2X2	T54.2X3	T54.2X4	—	—
Stovaine	T41.3X1	T41.3X2	T41.3X3	T41.3X4	T41.3X5	T41.3X6
infiltration (subcutaneous)	T41.3X1	T41.3X2	T41.3X3	T41.3X4	T41.3X5	T41.3X6
nerve block (peripheral) (plexus)	T41.3X1	T41.3X2	T41.3X3	T41.3X4	T41.3X5	T41.3X6
spinal	T41.3X1	T41.3X2	T41.3X3	T41.3X4	T41.3X5	T41.3X6
topical (surface)	T41.3X1	T41.3X2	T41.3X3	T41.3X4	T41.3X5	T41.3X6
Stovarsal	T37.8X1	T37.8X2	T37.8X3	T37.8X4	T37.8X5	T37.8X6
Stove gas — see Gas, stove						
Stoxil	T49.5X1	T49.5X2	T49.5X3	T49.5X4	T49.5X5	T49.5X6
Stramonium	T48.6X1	T48.6X2	T48.6X3	T48.6X4	T48.6X5	T48.6X6
natural state	T62.2X1	T62.2X2	T62.2X3	T62.2X4	—	—
Streptodornase	T45.3X1	T45.3X2	T45.3X3	T45.3X4	T45.3X5	T45.3X6
Streptoduocin	T36.5X1	T36.5X2	T36.5X3	T36.5X4	T36.5X5	T36.5X6
Streptokinase	T45.611	T45.612	T45.613	T45.614	T45.615	T45.616
Streptomycin (derivative)	T36.5X1	T36.5X2	T36.5X3	T36.5X4	T36.5X5	T36.5X6
Streptonivicin	T36.5X1	T36.5X2	T36.5X3	T36.5X4	T36.5X5	T36.5X6
Streptovarycin	T36.5X1	T36.5X2	T36.5X3	T36.5X4	T36.5X5	T36.5X6
Streptozocin	T45.1X1	T45.1X2	T45.1X3	T45.1X4	T45.1X5	T45.1X6
Streptozotocin	T45.1X1	T45.1X2	T45.1X3	T45.1X4	T45.1X5	T45.1X6
Stripper (paint) (solvent)	T52.8X1	T52.8X2	T52.8X3	T52.8X4	—	—
Strobane	T60.1X1	T60.1X2	T60.1X3	T60.1X4	—	—
Strofantina	T46.0X1	T46.0X2	T46.0X3	T46.0X4	T46.0X5	T46.0X6
Strophanthin (g) (k)	T46.0X1	T46.0X2	T46.0X3	T46.0X4	T46.0X5	T46.0X6
Strophanthus	T46.0X1	T46.0X2	T46.0X3	T46.0X4	T46.0X5	T46.0X6
Strophantin	T46.0X1	T46.0X2	T46.0X3	T46.0X4	T46.0X5	T46.0X6
Strophantin-g	T46.0X1	T46.0X2	T46.0X3	T46.0X4	T46.0X5	T46.0X6
Strychnine (nonmedicinal) (pesticide) (salts)	T65.1X1	T65.1X2	T65.1X3	T65.1X4	—	—
medicinal	T48.291	T48.292	T48.293	T48.294	T48.295	T48.296
Strychnos (ignatii) — see Strychnine						
Styramate	T42.8X1	T42.8X2	T42.8X3	T42.8X4	T42.8X5	T42.8X6
Styrene	T65.891	T65.892	T65.893	T65.894	—	—
Succinimide, antiepileptic or anticonvulsant	T42.2X1	T42.2X2	T42.2X3	T42.2X4	T42.2X5	T42.2X6
mercuric — see Mercury						
Succinylcholine	T48.1X1	T48.1X2	T48.1X3	T48.1X4	T48.1X5	T48.1X6
Succinylsulfathiazole	T37.0X1	T37.0X2	T37.0X3	T37.0X4	T37.0X5	T37.0X6
Sucralfate	T47.1X1	T47.1X2	T47.1X3	T47.1X4	T47.1X5	T47.1X6
Sucrose	T50.3X1	T50.3X2	T50.3X3	T50.3X4	T50.3X5	T50.3X6
Sufentanil	T40.4X1	T40.4X2	T40.4X3	T40.4X4	T40.4X5	T40.4X6
Sulbactam	T36.0X1	T36.0X2	T36.0X3	T36.0X4	T36.0X5	T36.0X6
Sulbenicillin	T36.0X1	T36.0X2	T36.0X3	T36.0X4	T36.0X5	T36.0X6
Sulbentine	T49.0X1	T49.0X2	T49.0X3	T49.0X4	T49.0X5	T49.0X6
Sulfacetamide	T49.0X1	T49.0X2	T49.0X3	T49.0X4	T49.0X5	T49.0X6
ophthalmic preparation	T49.5X1	T49.5X2	T49.5X3	T49.5X4	T49.5X5	T49.5X6
Sulfachlorpyridazine	T37.0X1	T37.0X2	T37.0X3	T37.0X4	T37.0X5	T37.0X6
Sulfacitine	T37.0X1	T37.0X2	T37.0X3	T37.0X4	T37.0X5	T37.0X6
Sulfadiasulfone sodium	T37.0X1	T37.0X2	T37.0X3	T37.0X4	T37.0X5	T37.0X6
Sulfadiazine	T37.0X1	T37.0X2	T37.0X3	T37.0X4	T37.0X5	T37.0X6
silver (topical)	T49.0X1	T49.0X2	T49.0X3	T49.0X4	T49.0X5	T49.0X6
Sulfadimethoxine	T37.0X1	T37.0X2	T37.0X3	T37.0X4	T37.0X5	T37.0X6
Sulfadimidine	T37.0X1	T37.0X2	T37.0X3	T37.0X4	T37.0X5	T37.0X6
Sulfadoxine	T37.0X1	T37.0X2	T37.0X3	T37.0X4	T37.0X5	T37.0X6
with pyrimethamine	T37.2X1	T37.2X2	T37.2X3	T37.2X4	T37.2X5	T37.2X6
Sulfaethidole	T37.0X1	T37.0X2	T37.0X3	T37.0X4	T37.0X5	T37.0X6
Sulfafurazole	T37.0X1	T37.0X2	T37.0X3	T37.0X4	T37.0X5	T37.0X6
Sulfaguanidine	T37.0X1	T37.0X2	T37.0X3	T37.0X4	T37.0X5	T37.0X6
Sulfalene	T37.0X1	T37.0X2	T37.0X3	T37.0X4	T37.0X5	T37.0X6
Sulfaloxate	T37.0X1	T37.0X2	T37.0X3	T37.0X4	T37.0X5	T37.0X6
Sulfaloxic acid	T37.0X1	T37.0X2	T37.0X3	T37.0X4	T37.0X5	T37.0X6
Sulfamazone	T39.2X1	T39.2X2	T39.2X3	T39.2X4	T39.2X5	T39.2X6
Sulfamerazine	T37.0X1	T37.0X2	T37.0X3	T37.0X4	T37.0X5	T37.0X6
Sulfameter	T37.0X1	T37.0X2	T37.0X3	T37.0X4	T37.0X5	T37.0X6
Sulfamethazine	T37.0X1	T37.0X2	T37.0X3	T37.0X4	T37.0X5	T37.0X6
Sulfamethizole	T37.0X1	T37.0X2	T37.0X3	T37.0X4	T37.0X5	T37.0X6
Sulfamethoxazole	T37.0X1	T37.0X2	T37.0X3	T37.0X4	T37.0X5	T37.0X6
with trimethoprim	T36.8X1	T36.8X2	T36.8X3	T36.8X4	T36.8X5	T36.8X6
Sulfamethoxydiazine	T37.0X1	T37.0X2	T37.0X3	T37.0X4	T37.0X5	T37.0X6
Sulfamethoxypyridazine	T37.0X1	T37.0X2	T37.0X3	T37.0X4	T37.0X5	T37.0X6
Sulfamethylthiazole	T37.0X1	T37.0X2	T37.0X3	T37.0X4	T37.0X5	T37.0X6
Sulfametoxydiazine	T37.0X1	T37.0X2	T37.0X3	T37.0X4	T37.0X5	T37.0X6
Sulfamidopyrine	T39.2X1	T39.2X2	T39.2X3	T39.2X4	T39.2X5	T39.2X6
Sulfamonomethoxine	T37.0X1	T37.0X2	T37.0X3	T37.0X4	T37.0X5	T37.0X6
Sulfamoxole	T37.0X1	T37.0X2	T37.0X3	T37.0X4	T37.0X5	T37.0X6
Sulfamylon	T49.0X1	T49.0X2	T49.0X3	T49.0X4	T49.0X5	T49.0X6
Sulfan blue (diagnostic dye)	T50.8X1	T50.8X2	T50.8X3	T50.8X4	T50.8X5	T50.8X6
Sulfanilamide	T37.0X1	T37.0X2	T37.0X3	T37.0X4	T37.0X5	T37.0X6
Sulfanilylguanidine	T37.0X1	T37.0X2	T37.0X3	T37.0X4	T37.0X5	T37.0X6

Substance	Poisoning, Accidental (unintentional)	Poisoning, Intentional Self-harm	Poisoning, Assault	Poisoning, Undetermined	Adverse Effect	Under-dosing
Sulfaperin	T37.0X1	T37.0X2	T37.0X3	T37.0X4	T37.0X5	T37.0X6
Sulfaphenazole	T37.0X1	T37.0X2	T37.0X3	T37.0X4	T37.0X5	T37.0X6
Sulfaphenylthiazole	T37.0X1	T37.0X2	T37.0X3	T37.0X4	T37.0X5	T37.0X6
Sulfaproxyline	T37.0X1	T37.0X2	T37.0X3	T37.0X4	T37.0X5	T37.0X6
Sulfapyridine	T37.0X1	T37.0X2	T37.0X3	T37.0X4	T37.0X5	T37.0X6
Sulfapyrimidine	T37.0X1	T37.0X2	T37.0X3	T37.0X4	T37.0X5	T37.0X6
Sulfarsphenamine	T37.8X1	T37.8X2	T37.8X3	T37.8X4	T37.8X5	T37.8X6
Sulfasalazine	T37.0X1	T37.0X2	T37.0X3	T37.0X4	T37.0X5	T37.0X6
Sulfasuxidine	T37.0X1	T37.0X2	T37.0X3	T37.0X4	T37.0X5	T37.0X6
Sulfasymazine	T37.0X1	T37.0X2	T37.0X3	T37.0X4	T37.0X5	T37.0X6
Sulfated amylopectin	T47.8X1	T47.8X2	T47.8X3	T47.8X4	T47.8X5	T47.8X6
Sulfathiazole	T37.0X1	T37.0X2	T37.0X3	T37.0X4	T37.0X5	T37.0X6
Sulfatostearate	T49.2X1	T49.2X2	T49.2X3	T49.2X4	T49.2X5	T49.2X6
Sulfinpyrazone	T50.4X1	T50.4X2	T50.4X3	T50.4X4	T50.4X5	T50.4X6
Sulfiram	T49.0X1	T49.0X2	T49.0X3	T49.0X4	T49.0X5	T49.0X6
Sulfisomidine	T37.0X1	T37.0X2	T37.0X3	T37.0X4	T37.0X5	T37.0X6
Sulfisoxazole	T37.0X1	T37.0X2	T37.0X3	T37.0X4	T37.0X5	T37.0X6
ophthalmic preparation	T49.5X1	T49.5X2	T49.5X3	T49.5X4	T49.5X5	T49.5X6
Sulfobromophthalein (sodium)	T50.8X1	T50.8X2	T50.8X3	T50.8X4	T50.8X5	T50.8X6
Sulfobromphthalein	T50.8X1	T50.8X2	T50.8X3	T50.8X4	T50.8X5	T50.8X6
Sulfogaiacol	T48.4X1	T48.4X2	T48.4X3	T48.4X4	T48.4X5	T48.4X6
Sulfomyxin	T36.8X1	T36.8X2	T36.8X3	T36.8X4	T36.8X5	T36.8X6
Sulfonal	T42.6X1	T42.6X2	T42.6X3	T42.6X4	T42.6X5	T42.6X6
Sulfonamide NEC	T37.0X1	T37.0X2	T37.0X3	T37.0X4	T37.0X5	T37.0X6
eye	T49.5X1	T49.5X2	T49.5X3	T49.5X4	T49.5X5	T49.5X6
Sulfonazide	T37.1X1	T37.1X2	T37.1X3	T37.1X4	T37.1X5	T37.1X6
Sulfones	T37.1X1	T37.1X2	T37.1X3	T37.1X4	T37.1X5	T37.1X6
Sulfonethylmethane	T42.6X1	T42.6X2	T42.6X3	T42.6X4	T42.6X5	T42.6X6
Sulfonmethane	T42.6X1	T42.6X2	T42.6X3	T42.6X4	T42.6X5	T42.6X6
Sulfonphthal, sulfonphthol	T50.8X1	T50.8X2	T50.8X3	T50.8X4	T50.8X5	T50.8X6
Sulfonylurea derivatives, oral	T38.3X1	T38.3X2	T38.3X3	T38.3X4	T38.3X5	T38.3X6
Sulforidazine	T43.3X1	T43.3X2	T43.3X3	T43.3X4	T43.3X5	T43.3X6
Sulfoxone	T37.1X1	T37.1X2	T37.1X3	T37.1X4	T37.1X5	T37.1X6
Sulfuric acid	T54.2X1	T54.2X2	T54.2X3	T54.2X4	—	—
Sulfur, sulfurated, sulfuric, sulfurous, sulfuryl (compounds NEC) (medicinal)	T49.4X1	T49.4X2	T49.4X3	T49.4X4	T49.4X5	T49.4X6
acid	T54.2X1	T54.2X2	T54.2X3	T54.2X4	—	—
dioxide (gas)	T59.1X1	T59.1X2	T59.1X3	T59.1X4	—	—
ether — see Ether(s)						
hydrogen	T59.6X1	T59.6X2	T59.6X3	T59.6X4	—	—
medicinal (keratolytic) (ointment) NEC	T49.4X1	T49.4X2	T49.4X3	T49.4X4	T49.4X5	T49.4X6
ointment	T49.0X1	T49.0X2	T49.0X3	T49.0X4	T49.0X5	T49.0X6
pesticide (vapor)	T60.91	T60.92	T60.93	T60.94	—	—
vapor NEC	T59.891	T59.892	T59.893	T59.894	—	—
Sulglicotide	T47.1X1	T47.1X2	T47.1X3	T47.1X4	T47.1X5	T47.1X6
Sulindac	T39.391	T39.392	T39.393	T39.394	T39.395	T39.396
Sulisatin	T47.2X1	T47.2X2	T47.2X3	T47.2X4	T47.2X5	T47.2X6
Sulisobenzone	T49.3X1	T49.3X2	T49.3X3	T49.3X4	T49.3X5	T49.3X6
Sulkowitch's reagent	T50.8X1	T50.8X2	T50.8X3	T50.8X4	T50.8X5	T50.8X6
Sulmetozine	T44.3X1	T44.3X2	T44.3X3	T44.3X4	T44.3X5	T44.3X6
Suloctidil	T46.7X1	T46.7X2	T46.7X3	T46.7X4	T46.7X5	T46.7X6
Sulph- — see also Sulf-						
Sulphadiazine	T37.0X1	T37.0X2	T37.0X3	T37.0X4	T37.0X5	T37.0X6
Sulphadimethoxine	T37.0X1	T37.0X2	T37.0X3	T37.0X4	T37.0X5	T37.0X6
Sulphadimidine	T37.0X1	T37.0X2	T37.0X3	T37.0X4	T37.0X5	T37.0X6
Sulphadione	T37.1X1	T37.1X2	T37.1X3	T37.1X4	T37.1X5	T37.1X6
Sulphafurazole	T37.0X1	T37.0X2	T37.0X3	T37.0X4	T37.0X5	T37.0X6
Sulphamethizole	T37.0X1	T37.0X2	T37.0X3	T37.0X4	T37.0X5	T37.0X6
Sulphamethoxazole	T37.0X1	T37.0X2	T37.0X3	T37.0X4	T37.0X5	T37.0X6
Sulphan blue	T50.8X1	T50.8X2	T50.8X3	T50.8X4	T50.8X5	T50.8X6
Sulphaphenazole	T37.0X1	T37.0X2	T37.0X3	T37.0X4	T37.0X5	T37.0X6
Sulphapyridine	T37.0X1	T37.0X2	T37.0X3	T37.0X4	T37.0X5	T37.0X6
Sulphasalazine	T37.0X1	T37.0X2	T37.0X3	T37.0X4	T37.0X5	T37.0X6
Sulphinpyrazone	T50.4X1	T50.4X2	T50.4X3	T50.4X4	T50.4X5	T50.4X6
Sulpiride	T43.591	T43.592	T43.593	T43.594	T43.595	T43.596
Sulprostone	T48.0X1	T48.0X2	T48.0X3	T48.0X4	T48.0X5	T48.0X6
Sulpyrine	T39.2X1	T39.2X2	T39.2X3	T39.2X4	T39.2X5	T39.2X6
Sultamicillin	T36.0X1	T36.0X2	T36.0X3	T36.0X4	T36.0X5	T36.0X6
Sulthiame	T42.6X1	T42.6X2	T42.6X3	T42.6X4	T42.6X5	T42.6X6
Sultiame	T42.6X1	T42.6X2	T42.6X3	T42.6X4	T42.6X5	T42.6X6
Sultopride	T43.591	T43.592	T43.593	T43.594	T43.595	T43.596
Sumatriptan	T39.8X1	T39.8X2	T39.8X3	T39.8X4	T39.8X5	T39.8X6
Sunflower seed oil	T46.6X1	T46.6X2	T46.6X3	T46.6X4	T46.6X5	T46.6X6
Superinone	T48.4X1	T48.4X2	T48.4X3	T48.4X4	T48.4X5	T48.4X6
Suprofen	T39.311	T39.312	T39.313	T39.314	T39.315	T39.316
Suramin (sodium)	T37.4X1	T37.4X2	T37.4X3	T37.4X4	T37.4X5	T37.4X6
Surfacaine	T41.3X1	T41.3X2	T41.3X3	T41.3X4	T41.3X5	T41.3X6
Surital	T41.1X1	T41.1X2	T41.1X3	T41.1X4	T41.1X5	T41.1X6

Substance	Poisoning, Accidental (unintentional)	Poisoning, Intentional Self-harm	Poisoning, Assault	Poisoning, Undetermined	Adverse Effect	Under-dosing
Sutilains	T45.3X1	T45.3X2	T45.3X3	T45.3X4	T45.3X5	T45.3X6
Suxamethonium (chloride)	T48.1X1	T48.1X2	T48.1X3	T48.1X4	T48.1X5	T48.1X6
Suxethonium (chloride)	T48.1X1	T48.1X2	T48.1X3	T48.1X4	T48.1X5	T48.1X6
Suxibuzone	T39.2X1	T39.2X2	T39.2X3	T39.2X4	T39.2X5	T39.2X6
Sweetener	T50.901	T50.902	T50.903	T50.904	T50.905	T50.906
Sweet niter spirit	T46.3X1	T46.3X2	T46.3X3	T46.3X4	T46.3X5	T46.3X6
Sweet oil (birch)	T49.3X1	T49.3X2	T49.3X3	T49.3X4	T49.3X5	T49.3X6
Sym-dichloroethyl ether	T53.6X1	T53.6X2	T53.6X3	T53.6X4	—	—
Sympatholytic NEC	T44.8X1	T44.8X2	T44.8X3	T44.8X4	T44.8X5	T44.8X6
haloalkylamine	T44.8X1	T44.8X2	T44.8X3	T44.8X4	T44.8X5	T44.8X6
Sympathomimetic NEC	T44.901	T44.902	T44.903	T44.904	T44.905	T44.906
anti-common-cold	T48.5X1	T48.5X2	T48.5X3	T48.5X4	T48.5X5	T48.5X6
bronchodilator	T48.6X1	T48.6X2	T48.6X3	T48.6X4	T48.6X5	T48.6X6
specified NEC	T44.991	T44.992	T44.993	T44.994	T44.995	T44.996
Synagis	T50.B91	T50.B92	T50.B93	T50.B94	T50.B95	T50.B96
Synalar	T49.0X1	T49.0X2	T49.0X3	T49.0X4	T49.0X5	T49.0X6
Synthroid	T38.1X1	T38.1X2	T38.1X3	T38.1X4	T38.1X5	T38.1X6
Syntocinon	T48.0X1	T48.0X2	T48.0X3	T48.0X4	T48.0X5	T48.0X6
Syrosingopine	T46.5X1	T46.5X2	T46.5X3	T46.5X4	T46.5X5	T46.5X6
Systemic drug	T45.91	T45.92	T45.93	T45.94	T45.95	T45.96
specified NEC	T45.8X1	T45.8X2	T45.8X3	T45.8X4	T45.8X5	T45.8X6
Tablets — see also specified substance	T50.901	T50.902	T50.903	T50.904	T50.905	T50.906
Tace	T38.5X1	T38.5X2	T38.5X3	T38.5X4	T38.5X5	T38.5X6
Tacrine	T44.0X1	T44.0X2	T44.0X3	T44.0X4	T44.0X5	T44.0X6
Tadalafil	T46.7X1	T46.7X2	T46.7X3	T46.7X4	T46.7X5	T46.7X6
Talampicillin	T36.0X1	T36.0X2	T36.0X3	T36.0X4	T36.0X5	T36.0X6
Talbutal	T42.3X1	T42.3X2	T42.3X3	T42.3X4	T42.3X5	T42.3X6
Talc powder	T49.3X1	T49.3X2	T49.3X3	T49.3X4	T49.3X5	T49.3X6
Talcum	T49.3X1	T49.3X2	T49.3X3	T49.3X4	T49.3X5	T49.3X6
Taleranol	T38.6X1	T38.6X2	T38.6X3	T38.6X4	T38.6X5	T38.6X6
Tamoxifen	T38.6X1	T38.6X2	T38.6X3	T38.6X4	T38.6X5	T38.6X6
Tamsulosin	T44.6X1	T44.6X2	T44.6X3	T44.6X4	T44.6X5	T44.6X6
Tandearil, tanderil	T39.2X1	T39.2X2	T39.2X3	T39.2X4	T39.2X5	T39.2X6
Tannic acid	T49.2X1	T49.2X2	T49.2X3	T49.2X4	T49.2X5	T49.2X6
medicinal (astringent)	T49.2X1	T49.2X2	T49.2X3	T49.2X4	T49.2X5	T49.2X6
Tannin — see Tannic acid						
Tansy	T62.2X1	T62.2X2	T62.2X3	T62.2X4	—	—
TAO	T36.3X1	T36.3X2	T36.3X3	T36.3X4	T36.3X5	T36.3X6
Tapazole	T38.2X1	T38.2X2	T38.2X3	T38.2X4	T38.2X5	T38.2X6
Taractan	T43.591	T43.592	T43.593	T43.594	T43.595	T43.596
Tarantula (venomous)	T63.321	T63.322	T63.323	T63.324		
Tartar emetic	T37.8X1	T37.8X2	T37.8X3	T37.8X4	T37.8X5	T37.8X6
Tartaric acid	T65.891	T65.892	T65.893	T65.894	—	—
Tartrated antimony (anti-infective)	T37.8X1	T37.8X2	T37.8X3	T37.8X4	T37.8X5	T37.8X6
Tartrate, laxative	T47.4X1	T47.4X2	T47.4X3	T47.4X4	T47.4X5	T47.4X6
Tar NEC	T52.0X1	T52.0X2	T52.0X3	T52.0X4	—	—
camphor	T60.1X1	T60.1X2	T60.1X3	T60.1X4	—	—
distillate	T49.1X1	T49.1X2	T49.1X3	T49.1X4	T49.1X5	T49.1X6
fumes	T59.891	T59.892	T59.893	T59.894	—	—
medicinal	T49.1X1	T49.1X2	T49.1X3	T49.1X4	T49.1X5	T49.1X6
ointment	T49.1X1	T49.1X2	T49.1X3	T49.1X4	T49.1X5	T49.1X6
Tauromustine	T45.1X1	T45.1X2	T45.1X3	T45.1X4	T45.1X5	T45.1X6
TCA — see Trichloroacetic acid						
TCDD	T53.7X1	T53.7X2	T53.7X3	T53.7X4	—	—
TDI (vapor)	T65.0X1	T65.0X2	T65.0X3	T65.0X4	—	—
Tear						
gas	T59.3X1	T59.3X2	T59.3X3	T59.3X4	—	—
solution	T49.5X1	T49.5X2	T49.5X3	T49.5X4	T49.5X5	T49.5X6
Teclothiazide	T50.2X1	T50.2X2	T50.2X3	T50.2X4	T50.2X5	T50.2X6
Teclozan	T37.3X1	T37.3X2	T37.3X3	T37.3X4	T37.3X5	T37.3X6
Tegafur	T45.1X1	T45.1X2	T45.1X3	T45.1X4	T45.1X5	T45.1X6
Tegretol	T42.1X1	T42.1X2	T42.1X3	T42.1X4	T42.1X5	T42.1X6
Teicoplanin	T36.8X1	T36.8X2	T36.8X3	T36.8X4	T36.8X5	T36.8X6
Telepaque	T50.8X1	T50.8X2	T50.8X3	T50.8X4	T50.8X5	T50.8X6
Tellurium	T56.891	T56.892	T56.893	T56.894	—	—
fumes	T56.891	T56.892	T56.893	T56.894	—	—
TEM	T45.1X1	T45.1X2	T45.1X3	T45.1X4	T45.1X5	T45.1X6
Temazepam	T42.4X1	T42.4X2	T42.4X3	T42.4X4	T42.4X5	T42.4X6
Temocillin	T36.0X1	T36.0X2	T36.0X3	T36.0X4	T36.0X5	T36.0X6
Tenamfetamine	T43.621	T43.622	T43.623	T43.624	T43.625	T43.626
Teniposide	T45.1X1	T45.1X2	T45.1X3	T45.1X4	T45.1X5	T45.1X6
Tenitramine	T46.3X1	T46.3X2	T46.3X3	T46.3X4	T46.3X5	T46.3X6
Tenoglicin	T48.4X1	T48.4X2	T48.4X3	T48.4X4	T48.4X5	T48.4X6
Tenonitrozole	T37.3X1	T37.3X2	T37.3X3	T37.3X4	T37.3X5	T37.3X6
Tenoxicam	T39.391	T39.392	T39.393	T39.394	T39.395	T39.396
TEPA	T45.1X1	T45.1X2	T45.1X3	T45.1X4	T45.1X5	T45.1X6
TEPP	T60.0X1	T60.0X2	T60.0X3	T60.0X4	—	—
Teprotide	T46.5X1	T46.5X2	T46.5X3	T46.5X4	T46.5X5	T46.5X6
Terazosin	T44.6X1	T44.6X2	T44.6X3	T44.6X4	T44.6X5	T44.6X6
Terbufos	T60.0X1	T60.0X2	T60.0X3	T60.0X4	—	—
Terbutaline	T48.6X1	T48.6X2	T48.6X3	T48.6X4	T48.6X5	T48.6X6

Substance	Poisoning, Accidental (unintentional)	Poisoning, Intentional Self-harm	Poisoning, Assault	Poisoning, Undetermined	Adverse Effect	Under-dosing
Terconazole	T49.0X1	T49.0X2	T49.0X3	T49.0X4	T49.0X5	T49.0X6
Terfenadine	T45.0X1	T45.0X2	T45.0X3	T45.0X4	T45.0X5	T45.0X6
Teriparatide (acetate)	T50.991	T50.992	T50.993	T50.994	T50.995	T50.996
Terizidone	T37.1X1	T37.1X2	T37.1X3	T37.1X4	T37.1X5	T37.1X6
Terlipressin	T38.891	T38.892	T38.893	T38.894	T38.895	T38.896
Terodiline	T46.3X1	T46.3X2	T46.3X3	T46.3X4	T46.3X5	T46.3X6
Teroxalene	T37.4X1	T37.4X2	T37.4X3	T37.4X4	T37.4X5	T37.4X6
Terpin (cis) hydrate	T48.4X1	T48.4X2	T48.4X3	T48.4X4	T48.4X5	T48.4X6
Terramycin	T36.4X1	T36.4X2	T36.4X3	T36.4X4	T36.4X5	T36.4X6
Tertatolol	T44.7X1	T44.7X2	T44.7X3	T44.7X4	T44.7X5	T44.7X6
Tessalon	T48.3X1	T48.3X2	T48.3X3	T48.3X4	T48.3X5	T48.3X6
Testolactone	T38.7X1	T38.7X2	T38.7X3	T38.7X4	T38.7X5	T38.7X6
Testosterone	T38.7X1	T38.7X2	T38.7X3	T38.7X4	T38.7X5	T38.7X6
Tetanus toxoid or vaccine	T50.A91	T50.A92	T50.A93	T50.A94	T50.A95	T50.A96
antitoxin	T50.Z11	T50.Z12	T50.Z13	T50.Z14	T50.Z15	T50.Z16
immune globulin (human)	T50.Z11	T50.Z12	T50.Z13	T50.Z14	T50.Z15	T50.Z16
toxoid	T50.A91	T50.A92	T50.A93	T50.A94	T50.A95	T50.A96
with diphtheria toxoid	T50.A21	T50.A22	T50.A23	T50.A24	T50.A25	T50.A26
with pertussis	T50.A11	T50.A12	T50.A13	T50.A14	T50.A15	T50.A16
Tetrabenazine	T43.591	T43.592	T43.593	T43.594	T43.595	T43.596
Tetracaine	T41.3X1	T41.3X2	T41.3X3	T41.3X4	T41.3X5	T41.3X6
nerve block (peripheral) (plexus)	T41.3X1	T41.3X2	T41.3X3	T41.3X4	T41.3X5	T41.3X6
regional	T41.3X1	T41.3X2	T41.3X3	T41.3X4	T41.3X5	T41.3X6
spinal	T41.3X1	T41.3X2	T41.3X3	T41.3X4	T41.3X5	T41.3X6
Tetrachlorethylene — see Tetrachloroethylene						
Tetrachlormethiazide	T50.2X1	T50.2X2	T50.2X3	T50.2X4	T50.2X5	T50.2X6
Tetrachloroethane	T53.6X1	T53.6X2	T53.6X3	T53.6X4	—	—
vapor	T53.6X1	T53.6X2	T53.6X3	T53.6X4	—	—
paint or varnish	T53.6X1	T53.6X2	T53.6X3	T53.6X4	—	—
Tetrachloroethylene (liquid)	T53.3X1	T53.3X2	T53.3X3	T53.3X4	—	—
medicinal	T37.4X1	T37.4X2	T37.4X3	T37.4X4	T37.4X5	T37.4X6
vapor	T53.3X1	T53.3X2	T53.3X3	T53.3X4	—	—
Tetrachloromethane — see Carbon tetrachloride						
Tetracosactide	T38.811	T38.812	T38.813	T38.814	T38.815	T38.816
Tetracosactrin	T38.811	T38.812	T38.813	T38.814	T38.815	T38.816
Tetracycline	T36.4X1	T36.4X2	T36.4X3	T36.4X4	T36.4X5	T36.4X6
ophthalmic preparation	T49.5X1	T49.5X2	T49.5X3	T49.5X4	T49.5X5	T49.5X6
topical NEC	T49.0X1	T49.0X2	T49.0X3	T49.0X4	T49.0X5	T49.0X6
Tetradifon	T60.8X1	T60.8X2	T60.8X3	T60.8X4	—	—
Tetradotoxin	T61.771	T61.772	T61.773	T61.774	—	—
Tetraethyl						
lead	T56.0X1	T56.0X2	T56.0X3	T56.0X4	—	—
pyrophosphate	T60.0X1	T60.0X2	T60.0X3	T60.0X4	—	—
Tetraethylammonium chloride	T44.2X1	T44.2X2	T44.2X3	T44.2X4	T44.2X5	T44.2X6
Tetraethylthiuram disulfide	T50.6X1	T50.6X2	T50.6X3	T50.6X4	T50.6X5	T50.6X6
Tetrahydroaminoacridine	T44.0X1	T44.0X2	T44.0X3	T44.0X4	T44.0X5	T44.0X6
Tetrahydrocannabinol	T40.7X1	T40.7X2	T40.7X3	T40.7X4	T40.7X5	T40.7X6
Tetrahydrofuran	T52.8X1	T52.8X2	T52.8X3	T52.8X4	—	—
Tetrahydronaphthalene	T52.8X1	T52.8X2	T52.8X3	T52.8X4	—	—
Tetrahydrozoline	T49.5X1	T49.5X2	T49.5X3	T49.5X4	T49.5X5	T49.5X6
Tetralin	T52.8X1	T52.8X2	T52.8X3	T52.8X4	—	—
Tetramethrin	T60.2X1	T60.2X2	T60.2X3	T60.2X4	—	—
Tetramethylthiuram (disulfide) NEC	T60.3X1	T60.3X2	T60.3X3	T60.3X4	—	—
medicinal	T49.0X1	T49.0X2	T49.0X3	T49.0X4	T49.0X5	T49.0X6
Tetramisole	T37.4X1	T37.4X2	T37.4X3	T37.4X4	T37.4X5	T37.4X6
Tetranicotinoyl fructose	T46.7X1	T46.7X2	T46.7X3	T46.7X4	T46.7X5	T46.7X6
Tetrazepam	T42.4X1	T42.4X2	T42.4X3	T42.4X4	T42.4X5	T42.4X6
Tetronal	T42.6X1	T42.6X2	T42.6X3	T42.6X4	T42.6X5	T42.6X6
Tetryl	T65.3X1	T65.3X2	T65.3X3	T65.3X4	—	—
Tetrylammonium chloride	T44.2X1	T44.2X2	T44.2X3	T44.2X4	T44.2X5	T44.2X6
Tetryzoline	T49.5X1	T49.5X2	T49.5X3	T49.5X4	T49.5X5	T49.5X6
Thalidomide	T45.1X1	T45.1X2	T45.1X3	T45.1X4	T45.1X5	T45.1X6
Thallium (compounds) (dust) NEC	T56.811	T56.812	T56.813	T56.814	—	—
pesticide	T60.4X1	T60.4X2	T60.4X3	T60.4X4	—	—
THC	T40.7X1	T40.7X2	T40.7X3	T40.7X4	T40.7X5	T40.7X6
Thebacon	T48.3X1	T48.3X2	T48.3X3	T48.3X4	T48.3X5	T48.3X6
Thebaine	T40.2X1	T40.2X2	T40.2X3	T40.2X4	T40.2X5	T40.2X6
Thenoic acid	T49.6X1	T49.6X2	T49.6X3	T49.6X4	T49.6X5	T49.6X6
Thenyldiamine	T45.0X1	T45.0X2	T45.0X3	T45.0X4	T45.0X5	T45.0X6
Theobromine (calcium salicylate)	T48.6X1	T48.6X2	T48.6X3	T48.6X4	T48.6X5	T48.6X6
sodium salicylate	T48.6X1	T48.6X2	T48.6X3	T48.6X4	T48.6X5	T48.6X6
Theophyllamine	T48.6X1	T48.6X2	T48.6X3	T48.6X4	T48.6X5	T48.6X6
Theophylline	T48.6X1	T48.6X2	T48.6X3	T48.6X4	T48.6X5	T48.6X6
aminobenzoic acid	T48.6X1	T48.6X2	T48.6X3	T48.6X4	T48.6X5	T48.6X6

Substance	Poisoning, Accidental (unintentional)	Poisoning, Intentional Self-harm	Poisoning, Assault	Poisoning, Undetermined	Adverse Effect	Under-dosing
Theophylline — continued						
ethylenediamine	T48.6X1	T48.6X2	T48.6X3	T48.6X4	T48.6X5	T48.6X6
piperazine	T48.6X1	T48.6X2	T48.6X3	T48.6X4	T48.6X5	T48.6X6
p-amino-benzoate						
Thiabendazole	T37.4X1	T37.4X2	T37.4X3	T37.4X4	T37.4X5	T37.4X6
Thialbarbital	T41.1X1	T41.1X2	T41.1X3	T41.1X4	T41.1X5	T41.1X6
Thiamazole	T38.2X1	T38.2X2	T38.2X3	T38.2X4	T38.2X5	T38.2X6
Thiambutosine	T37.1X1	T37.1X2	T37.1X3	T37.1X4	T37.1X5	T37.1X6
Thiamine	T45.2X1	T45.2X2	T45.2X3	T45.2X4	T45.2X5	T45.2X6
Thiamphenicol	T36.2X1	T36.2X2	T36.2X3	T36.2X4	T36.2X5	T36.2X6
Thiamylal	T41.1X1	T41.1X2	T41.1X3	T41.1X4	T41.1X5	T41.1X6
sodium	T41.1X1	T41.1X2	T41.1X3	T41.1X4	T41.1X5	T41.1X6
Thiazesim	T43.291	T43.292	T43.293	T43.294	T43.295	T43.296
Thiazides (diuretics)	T50.2X1	T50.2X2	T50.2X3	T50.2X4	T50.2X5	T50.2X6
Thiazinamium metilsulfate	T43.3X1	T43.3X2	T43.3X3	T43.3X4	T43.3X5	T43.3X6
Thiethylperazine	T43.3X1	T43.3X2	T43.3X3	T43.3X4	T43.3X5	T43.3X6
Thimerosal	T49.0X1	T49.0X2	T49.0X3	T49.0X4	T49.0X5	T49.0X6
ophthalmic preparation	T49.5X1	T49.5X2	T49.5X3	T49.5X4	T49.5X5	T49.5X6
Thioacetazone	T37.1X1	T37.1X2	T37.1X3	T37.1X4	T37.1X5	T37.1X6
with isoniazid	T37.1X1	T37.1X2	T37.1X3	T37.1X4	T37.1X5	T37.1X6
Thiobarbital sodium	T41.1X1	T41.1X2	T41.1X3	T41.1X4	T41.1X5	T41.1X6
Thiobarbiturate anesthetic	T41.1X1	T41.1X2	T41.1X3	T41.1X4	T41.1X5	T41.1X6
Thiobismol	T37.8X1	T37.8X2	T37.8X3	T37.8X4	T37.8X5	T37.8X6
Thiobutabarbital sodium	T41.1X1	T41.1X2	T41.1X3	T41.1X4	T41.1X5	T41.1X6
Thiocarbamate (insecticide)	T60.0X1	T60.0X2	T60.0X3	T60.0X4	—	—
Thiocarbamide	T38.2X1	T38.2X2	T38.2X3	T38.2X4	T38.2X5	T38.2X6
Thiocarbarsone	T37.8X1	T37.8X2	T37.8X3	T37.8X4	T37.8X5	T37.8X6
Thiocarlide	T37.1X1	T37.1X2	T37.1X3	T37.1X4	T37.1X5	T37.1X6
Thioctamide	T50.991	T50.992	T50.993	T50.994	T50.995	T50.996
Thioctic acid	T50.991	T50.992	T50.993	T50.994	T50.995	T50.996
Thiofos	T60.0X1	T60.0X2	T60.0X3	T60.0X4	—	—
Thioglycolate	T49.4X1	T49.4X2	T49.4X3	T49.4X4	T49.4X5	T49.4X6
Thioglycolic acid	T65.891	T65.892	T65.893	T65.894	—	—
Thioguanine	T45.1X1	T45.1X2	T45.1X3	T45.1X4	T45.1X5	T45.1X6
Thiomercaptomerin	T50.2X1	T50.2X2	T50.2X3	T50.2X4	T50.2X5	T50.2X6
Thiomerin	T50.2X1	T50.2X2	T50.2X3	T50.2X4	T50.2X5	T50.2X6
Thiomersal	T49.0X1	T49.0X2	T49.0X3	T49.0X4	T49.0X5	T49.0X6
Thionazin	T60.0X1	T60.0X2	T60.0X3	T60.0X4	—	—
Thiopental (sodium)	T41.1X1	T41.1X2	T41.1X3	T41.1X4	T41.1X5	T41.1X6
Thiopentone (sodium)	T41.1X1	T41.1X2	T41.1X3	T41.1X4	T41.1X5	T41.1X6
Thiopropazate	T43.3X1	T43.3X2	T43.3X3	T43.3X4	T43.3X5	T43.3X6
Thioproperazine	T43.3X1	T43.3X2	T43.3X3	T43.3X4	T43.3X5	T43.3X6
Thioridazine	T43.3X1	T43.3X2	T43.3X3	T43.3X4	T43.3X5	T43.3X6
Thiosinamine	T49.3X1	T49.3X2	T49.3X3	T49.3X4	T49.3X5	T49.3X6
Thiotepa	T45.1X1	T45.1X2	T45.1X3	T45.1X4	T45.1X5	T45.1X6
Thiothixene	T43.4X1	T43.4X2	T43.4X3	T43.4X4	T43.4X5	T43.4X6
Thiouracil (benzyl) (methyl) (propyl)	T38.2X1	T38.2X2	T38.2X3	T38.2X4	T38.2X5	T38.2X6
Thiourea	T38.2X1	T38.2X2	T38.2X3	T38.2X4	T38.2X5	T38.2X6
Thiphenamil	T44.3X1	T44.3X2	T44.3X3	T44.3X4	T44.3X5	T44.3X6
Thiram	T60.3X1	T60.3X2	T60.3X3	T60.3X4	—	—
medicinal	T49.2X1	T49.2X2	T49.2X3	T49.2X4	T49.2X5	T49.2X6
Thonzylamine (systemic)	T45.0X1	T45.0X2	T45.0X3	T45.0X4	T45.0X5	T45.0X6
mucosal decongestant	T48.5X1	T48.5X2	T48.5X3	T48.5X4	T48.5X5	T48.5X6
Thorazine	T43.3X1	T43.3X2	T43.3X3	T43.3X4	T43.3X5	T43.3X6
Thorium dioxide suspension	T50.8X1	T50.8X2	T50.8X3	T50.8X4	T50.8X5	T50.8X6
Thornapple	T62.2X1	T62.2X2	T62.2X3	T62.2X4	—	—
Throat drug NEC	T49.6X1	T49.6X2	T49.6X3	T49.6X4	T49.6X5	T49.6X6
Thrombin	T45.7X1	T45.7X2	T45.7X3	T45.7X4	T45.7X5	T45.7X6
Thrombolysin	T45.611	T45.612	T45.613	T45.614	T45.615	T45.616
Thromboplastin	T45.7X1	T45.7X2	T45.7X3	T45.7X4	T45.7X5	T45.7X6
Thurfyl nicotinate	T46.7X1	T46.7X2	T46.7X3	T46.7X4	T46.7X5	T46.7X6
Thymol	T49.0X1	T49.0X2	T49.0X3	T49.0X4	T49.0X5	T49.0X6
Thymopentin	T37.5X1	T37.5X2	T37.5X3	T37.5X4	T37.5X5	T37.5X6
Thymoxamine	T46.7X1	T46.7X2	T46.7X3	T46.7X4	T46.7X5	T46.7X6
Thymus extract	T38.891	T38.892	T38.893	T38.894	T38.895	T38.896
Thyreotrophic hormone	T38.811	T38.812	T38.813	T38.814	T38.815	T38.816
Thyroglobulin	T38.1X1	T38.1X2	T38.1X3	T38.1X4	T38.1X5	T38.1X6
Thyroid (hormone)	T38.1X1	T38.1X2	T38.1X3	T38.1X4	T38.1X5	T38.1X6
Thyrolar	T38.1X1	T38.1X2	T38.1X3	T38.1X4	T38.1X5	T38.1X6
Thyrotrophin	T38.811	T38.812	T38.813	T38.814	T38.815	T38.816
Thyrotropic hormone	T38.811	T38.812	T38.813	T38.814	T38.815	T38.816
Thyroxine	T38.1X1	T38.1X2	T38.1X3	T38.1X4	T38.1X5	T38.1X6
Tiabendazole	T37.4X1	T37.4X2	T37.4X3	T37.4X4	T37.4X5	T37.4X6
Tiamizide	T50.2X1	T50.2X2	T50.2X3	T50.2X4	T50.2X5	T50.2X6
Tianeptine	T43.291	T43.292	T43.293	T43.294	T43.295	T43.296
Tiapamil	T46.1X1	T46.1X2	T46.1X3	T46.1X4	T46.1X5	T46.1X6
Tiapride	T43.591	T43.592	T43.593	T43.594	T43.595	T43.596
Tiaprofenic acid	T39.311	T39.312	T39.313	T39.314	ICD39.315	T39.316
Tiaramide	T39.8X1	T39.8X2	T39.8X3	T39.8X4	T39.8X5	T39.8X6
Ticarcillin	T36.0X1	T36.0X2	T36.0X3	T36.0X4	T36.0X5	T36.0X6
Ticlatone	T49.0X1	T49.0X2	T49.0X3	T49.0X4	T49.0X5	T49.0X6

Substance	Poisoning, Accidental (unintentional)	Poisoning, Intentional Self-harm	Poisoning, Assault	Poisoning, Undetermined	Adverse Effect	Under-dosing
Ticlopidine	T45.521	T45.522	T45.523	T45.524	T45.525	T45.526
Ticrynafen	T50.1X1	T50.1X2	T50.1X3	T50.1X4	T50.1X5	T50.1X6
Tidiacic	T50.991	T50.992	T50.993	T50.994	T50.995	T50.996
Tiemonium	T44.3X1	T44.3X2	T44.3X3	T44.3X4	T44.3X5	T44.3X6
iodide	T44.3X1	T44.3X2	T44.3X3	T44.3X4	T44.3X5	T44.3X6
Tienilic acid	T50.1X1	T50.1X2	T50.1X3	T50.1X4	T50.1X5	T50.1X6
Tifenamil	T44.3X1	T44.3X2	T44.3X3	T44.3X4	T44.3X5	T44.3X6
Tigan	T45.0X1	T45.0X2	T45.0X3	T45.0X4	T45.0X5	T45.0X6
Tigloidine	T44.3X1	T44.3X2	T44.3X3	T44.3X4	T44.3X5	T44.3X6
Tilactase	T47.5X1	T47.5X2	T47.5X3	T47.5X4	T47.5X5	T47.5X6
Tiletamine	T41.291	T41.292	T41.293	T41.294	T41.295	T41.296
Tilidine	T40.4X1	T40.4X2	T40.4X3	T40.4X4		
Timepidium bromide	T44.3X1	T44.3X2	T44.3X3	T44.3X4	T44.3X5	T44.3X6
Timiperone	T43.4X1	T43.4X2	T43.4X3	T43.4X4	T43.4X5	T43.4X6
Timolol	T44.7X1	T44.7X2	T44.7X3	T44.7X4	T44.7X5	T44.7X6
Tincture, iodine — see Iodine						
Tindal	T43.3X1	T43.3X2	T43.3X3	T43.3X4	T43.3X5	T43.3X6
Tinidazole	T37.3X1	T37.3X2	T37.3X3	T37.3X4	T37.3X5	T37.3X6
Tinoridine	T39.8X1	T39.8X2	T39.8X3	T39.8X4	T39.8X5	T39.8X6
Tin (chloride) (dust) (oxide) NEC	T56.6X1	T56.6X2	T56.6X3	T56.6X4	—	—
anti-infectives	T37.8X1	T37.8X2	T37.8X3	T37.8X4	T37.8X5	T37.8X6
Tiocarlide	T37.1X1	T37.1X2	T37.1X3	T37.1X4	T37.1X5	T37.1X6
Tioclomarol	T45.511	T45.512	T45.513	T45.514	T45.515	T45.516
Tioconazole	T49.0X1	T49.0X2	T49.0X3	T49.0X4	T49.0X5	T49.0X6
Tioguanine	T45.1X1	T45.1X2	T45.1X3	T45.1X4	T45.1X5	T45.1X6
Tiopronin	T50.991	T50.992	T50.993	T50.994	T50.995	T50.996
Tiotixene	T43.4X1	T43.4X2	T43.4X3	T43.4X4	T43.4X5	T43.4X6
Tioxolone	T49.4X1	T49.4X2	T49.4X3	T49.4X4	T49.4X5	T49.4X6
Tipepidine	T48.3X1	T48.3X2	T48.3X3	T48.3X4	T48.3X5	T48.3X6
Tiquizium bromide	T44.3X1	T44.3X2	T44.3X3	T44.3X4	T44.3X5	T44.3X6
Tiratricol	T38.1X1	T38.1X2	T38.1X3	T38.1X4	T38.1X5	T38.1X6
Tisopurine	T50.4X1	T50.4X2	T50.4X3	T50.4X4	T50.4X5	T50.4X6
Titanium (compounds) (vapor)	T56.891	T56.892	T56.893	T56.894	—	—
dioxide	T49.3X1	T49.3X2	T49.3X3	T49.3X4	T49.3X5	T49.3X6
ointment	T49.3X1	T49.3X2	T49.3X3	T49.3X4	T49.3X5	T49.3X6
oxide	T49.3X1	T49.3X2	T49.3X3	T49.3X4	T49.3X5	T49.3X6
tetrachloride	T56.891	T56.892	T56.893	T56.894	—	—
Titanocene	T56.891	T56.892	T56.893	T56.894	—	—
Titroid	T38.1X1	T38.1X2	T38.1X3	T38.1X4	T38.1X5	T38.1X6
Tizanidine	T42.8X1	T42.8X2	T42.8X3	T42.8X4	T42.8X5	T42.8X6
TMTD	T60.3X1	T60.3X2	T60.3X3	T60.3X4		
TNT (fumes)	T65.3X1	T65.3X2	T65.3X3	T65.3X4		
Toadstool	T62.0X1	T62.0X2	T62.0X3	T62.0X4	—	—
Tobacco NEC	T65.291	T65.292	T65.293	T65.294	—	—
cigarettes	T65.221	T65.222	T65.223	T65.224		
Indian	T62.2X1	T62.2X2	T62.2X3	T62.2X4		
smoke, second-hand	T65.221	T65.222	T65.223	T65.224		
Tobramycin	T36.5X1	T36.5X2	T36.5X3	T36.5X4	T36.5X5	T36.5X6
Tocainide	T46.2X1	T46.2X2	T46.2X3	T46.2X4	T46.2X5	T46.2X6
Tocoferol	T45.2X1	T45.2X2	T45.2X3	T45.2X4	T45.2X5	T45.2X6
Tocopherol	T45.2X1	T45.2X2	T45.2X3	T45.2X4	T45.2X5	T45.2X6
acetate	T45.2X1	T45.2X2	T45.2X3	T45.2X4	T45.2X5	T45.2X6
Tocosamine	T48.0X1	T48.0X2	T48.0X3	T48.0X4	T48.0X5	T48.0X6
Todralazine	T46.5X1	T46.5X2	T46.5X3	T46.5X4	T46.5X5	T46.5X6
Tofisopam	T42.4X1	T42.4X2	T42.4X3	T42.4X4	T42.4X5	T42.4X6
Tofranil	T43.011	T43.012	T43.013	T43.014	T43.015	T43.016
Toilet deodorizer	T65.891	T65.892	T65.893	T65.894	—	—
Tolamolol	T44.7X1	T44.7X2	T44.7X3	T44.7X4	T44.7X5	T44.7X6
Tolazamide	T38.3X1	T38.3X2	T38.3X3	T38.3X4	T38.3X5	T38.3X6
Tolazoline	T46.7X1	T46.7X2	T46.7X3	T46.7X4	T46.7X5	T46.7X6
Tolbutamide (sodium)	T38.3X1	T38.3X2	T38.3X3	T38.3X4	T38.3X5	T38.3X6
Tolciclate	T49.0X1	T49.0X2	T49.0X3	T49.0X4	T49.0X5	T49.0X6
Tolmetin	T39.391	T39.392	T39.393	T39.394	T39.395	T39.396
Tolnaftate	T49.0X1	T49.0X2	T49.0X3	T49.0X4	T49.0X5	T49.0X6
Tolonidine	T46.5X1	T46.5X2	T46.5X3	T46.5X4	T46.5X5	T46.5X6
Toloxatone	T42.6X1	T42.6X2	T42.6X3	T42.6X4	T42.6X5	T42.6X6
Tolperisone	T44.3X1	T44.3X2	T44.3X3	T44.3X4	T44.3X5	T44.3X6
Tolserol	T42.8X1	T42.8X2	T42.8X3	T42.8X4	T42.8X5	T42.8X6
Toluene (liquid)	T52.2X1	T52.2X2	T52.2X3	T52.2X4	—	—
diisocyanate	T65.0X1	T65.0X2	T65.0X3	T65.0X4	—	—
Toluidine	T65.891	T65.892	T65.893	T65.894	—	—
vapor	T59.891	T59.892	T59.893	T59.894	—	—
Toluol (liquid)	T52.2X1	T52.2X2	T52.2X3	T52.2X4	—	—
vapor	T52.2X1	T52.2X2	T52.2X3	T52.2X4	—	—
Toluylenediamine	T65.3X1	T65.3X2	T65.3X3	T65.3X4	—	—
Tolylene-2,4-diisocyanate	T65.0X1	T65.0X2	T65.0X3	T65.0X4	—	—
Tonic NEC	T50.901	T50.902	T50.903	T50.904	T50.905	T50.906
Topical action drug NEC	T49.91	T49.92	T49.93	T49.94	T49.95	T49.96
ear, nose or throat	T49.6X1	T49.6X2	T49.6X3	T49.6X4	T49.6X5	T49.6X6
eye	T49.5X1	T49.5X2	T49.5X3	T49.5X4	T49.5X5	T49.5X6
skin	T49.91	T49.92	T49.93	T49.94	T49.95	T49.96

Substance	Poisoning, Accidental (unintentional)	Poisoning, Intentional Self-harm	Poisoning, Assault	Poisoning, Undetermined	Adverse Effect	Under-dosing
Topical action drug — continued						
specified NEC	T49.8X1	T49.8X2	T49.8X3	T49.8X4	T49.8X5	T49.8X6
Toquizine	T44.3X1	T44.3X2	T44.3X3	T44.3X4	T44.3X5	T44.3X6
Toremifene	T38.6X1	T38.6X2	T38.6X3	T38.6X4	T38.6X5	T38.6X6
Tosylchloramide sodium	T49.8X1	T49.8X2	T49.8X3	T49.8X4	T49.8X5	T49.8X6
Toxaphene (dust) (spray)	T60.1X1	T60.1X2	T60.1X3	T60.1X4	—	—
Toxin, diphtheria (Schick Test)	T50.8X1	T50.8X2	T50.8X3	T50.8X4	T50.8X5	T50.8X6
Toxoid						
combined	T50.A21	T50.A22	T50.A23	T50.A24	T50.A25	T50.A26
diphtheria	T50.A91	T50.A92	T50.A93	T50.A94	T50.A95	T50.A96
tetanus	T50.A91	T50.A92	T50.A93	T50.A94	T50.A95	T50.A96
Trace element NEC	T45.8X1	T45.8X2	T45.8X3	T45.8X4	T45.8X5	T45.8X6
Tractor fuel NEC	T52.0X1	T52.0X2	T52.0X3	T52.0X4	—	—
Tragacanth	T50.991	T50.992	T50.993	T50.994	T50.995	T50.996
Tramadol	T40.4X1	T40.4X2	T40.4X3	T40.4X4	T40.4X5	T40.4X6
Tramazoline	T48.5X1	T48.5X2	T48.5X3	T48.5X4	T48.5X5	T48.5X6
Tranexamic acid	T45.621	T45.622	T45.623	T45.624	T45.625	T45.626
Tranilast	T45.0X1	T45.0X2	T45.0X3	T45.0X4	T45.0X5	T45.0X6
Tranquilizer NEC	T43.501	T43.502	T43.503	T43.504	T43.505	T43.506
with hypnotic or sedative	T42.6X1	T42.6X2	T42.6X3	T42.6X4	T42.6X5	T42.6X6
benzodiazepine NEC	T42.4X1	T42.4X2	T42.4X3	T42.4X4	T42.4X5	T42.4X6
butyrophenone NEC	T43.4X1	T43.4X2	T43.4X3	T43.4X4	T43.4X5	T43.4X6
carbamate	T43.591	T43.592	T43.593	T43.594	T43.595	T43.596
dimethylamine	T43.3X1	T43.3X2	T43.3X3	T43.3X4	T43.3X5	T43.3X6
ethylamine	T43.3X1	T43.3X2	T43.3X3	T43.3X4	T43.3X5	T43.3X6
hydroxyzine	T43.591	T43.592	T43.593	T43.594	T43.595	T43.596
major NEC	T43.501	T43.502	T43.503	T43.504	T43.505	T43.506
penothiazine NEC	T43.3X1	T43.3X2	T43.3X3	T43.3X4	T43.3X5	T43.3X6
phenothiazine-based	T43.3X1	T43.3X2	T43.3X3	T43.3X4	T43.3X5	T43.3X6
piperazine NEC	T43.3X1	T43.3X2	T43.3X3	T43.3X4	T43.3X5	T43.3X6
piperidine	T43.3X1	T43.3X2	T43.3X3	T43.3X4	T43.3X5	T43.3X6
propylamine	T43.3X1	T43.3X2	T43.3X3	T43.3X4	T43.3X5	T43.3X6
specified NEC	T43.591	T43.592	T43.593	T43.594	T43.595	T43.596
thioxanthene NEC	T43.591	T43.592	T43.593	T43.594	T43.595	T43.596
Tranxene	T42.4X1	T42.4X2	T42.4X3	T42.4X4	T42.4X5	T42.4X6
Tranylcypromine	T43.1X1	T43.1X2	T43.1X3	T43.1X4	T43.1X5	T43.1X6
Trapidil	T46.3X1	T46.3X2	T46.3X3	T46.3X4	T46.3X5	T46.3X6
Trasentine	T44.3X1	T44.3X2	T44.3X3	T44.3X4	T44.3X5	T44.3X6
Travert	T50.3X1	T50.3X2	T50.3X3	T50.3X4	T50.3X5	T50.3X6
Trazodone	T43.211	T43.212	T43.213	T43.214	T43.215	T43.216
Trecator	T37.1X1	T37.1X2	T37.1X3	T37.1X4	T37.1X5	T37.1X6
Treosulfan	T45.1X1	T45.1X2	T45.1X3	T45.1X4	T45.1X5	T45.1X6
Tretamine	T45.1X1	T45.1X2	T45.1X3	T45.1X4	T45.1X5	T45.1X6
Tretinoin	T49.0X1	T49.0X2	T49.0X3	T49.0X4	T49.0X5	T49.0X6
Tretoquinol	T48.6X1	T48.6X2	T48.6X3	T48.6X4	T48.6X5	T48.6X6
Triacetin	T49.0X1	T49.0X2	T49.0X3	T49.0X4	T49.0X5	T49.0X6
Triacetoxyanthracene	T49.4X1	T49.4X2	T49.4X3	T49.4X4	T49.4X5	T49.4X6
Triacetyloleandomycin	T36.3X1	T36.3X2	T36.3X3	T36.3X4	T36.3X5	T36.3X6
Triamcinolone	T38.0X1	T38.0X2	T38.0X3	T38.0X4	T38.0X5	T38.0X6
ENT agent	T49.6X1	T49.6X2	T49.6X3	T49.6X4	T49.6X5	T49.6X6
hexacetonide	T49.0X1	T49.0X2	T49.0X3	T49.0X4	T49.0X5	T49.0X6
ophthalmic preparation	T49.5X1	T49.5X2	T49.5X3	T49.5X4	T49.5X5	T49.5X6
topical NEC	T49.0X1	T49.0X2	T49.0X3	T49.0X4	T49.0X5	T49.0X6
Triampyzine	T44.3X1	T44.3X2	T44.3X3	T44.3X4	T44.3X5	T44.3X6
Triamterene	T50.2X1	T50.2X2	T50.2X3	T50.2X4	T50.2X5	T50.2X6
Triazine (herbicide)	T60.3X1	T60.3X2	T60.3X3	T60.3X4		
Triaziquone	T45.1X1	T45.1X2	T45.1X3	T45.1X4	T45.1X5	T45.1X6
Triazolam	T42.4X1	T42.4X2	T42.4X3	T42.4X4	T42.4X5	T42.4X6
Triazole (herbicide)	T60.3X1	T60.3X2	T60.3X3	T60.3X4		
Tribenoside	T46.991	T46.992	T46.993	T46.994	T46.995	T46.996
Tribromacetaldehyde	T42.6X1	T42.6X2	T42.6X3	T42.6X4	T42.6X5	T42.6X6
Tribromoethanol, rectal	T41.291	T41.292	T41.293	T41.294	T41.295	T41.296
Tribromomethane	T42.6X1	T42.6X2	T42.6X3	T42.6X4	T42.6X5	T42.6X6
Trichlorethane	T53.2X1	T53.2X2	T53.2X3	T53.2X4	—	—
Trichlorethylene	T53.2X1	T53.2X2	T53.2X3	T53.2X4	—	—
Trichlorfon	T60.0X1	T60.0X2	T60.0X3	T60.0X4	—	—
Trichlormethiazide	T50.2X1	T50.2X2	T50.2X3	T50.2X4	T50.2X5	T50.2X6
Trichlormethine	T45.1X1	T45.1X2	T45.1X3	T45.1X4	T45.1X5	T45.1X6
Trichloroacetic acid, Trichloracetic acid	T54.2X1	T54.2X2	T54.2X3	T54.2X4		
medicinal	T49.4X1	T49.4X2	T49.4X3	T49.4X4	T49.4X5	T49.4X6
Trichloroethane	T53.2X1	T53.2X2	T53.2X3	T53.2X4	—	—
Trichloroethanol	T42.6X1	T42.6X2	T42.6X3	T42.6X4	T42.6X5	T42.6X6
Trichloroethylene (liquid)	T53.2X1	T53.2X2	T53.2X3	T53.2X4	—	—
(vapor)						
anesthetic (gas)	T41.0X1	T41.0X2	T41.0X3	T41.0X4	T41.0X5	T41.0X6
vapor NEC	T53.2X1	T53.2X2	T53.2X3	T53.2X4	—	—
Trichloroethyl phosphate	T42.6X1	T42.6X2	T42.6X3	T42.6X4	T42.6X5	T42.6X6
Trichlorofluoromethane NEC	T53.5X1	T53.5X2	T53.5X3	T53.5X4	—	—
Trichloronate	T60.0X1	T60.0X2	T60.0X3	T60.0X4	—	—
Trichloropropane	T53.6X1	T53.6X2	T53.6X3	T53.6X4	—	—

Subterms under main terms may continue to next column or page   Additional Character May Be Required — Refer to the Tabular List for Character Selection   393

Ticlopidine — Trichloropropane

Table of Drugs and Chemicals

Substance	Poisoning, Accidental (unintentional)	Poisoning, Intentional Self-harm	Poisoning, Assault	Poisoning, Undetermined	Adverse Effect	Under-dosing
Trichlorotriethylamine	T45.1X1	T45.1X2	T45.1X3	T45.1X4	T45.1X5	T45.1X6
Trichomonacides NEC	T37.3X1	T37.3X2	T37.3X3	T37.3X4	T37.3X5	T37.3X6
Trichomycin	T36.7X1	T36.7X2	T36.7X3	T36.7X4	T36.7X5	T36.7X6
Triclobisonium chloride	T49.0X1	T49.0X2	T49.0X3	T49.0X4	T49.0X5	T49.0X6
Triclocarban	T49.0X1	T49.0X2	T49.0X3	T49.0X4	T49.0X5	T49.0X6
Triclofos	T42.6X1	T42.6X2	T42.6X3	T42.6X4	T42.6X5	T42.6X6
Triclosan	T49.0X1	T49.0X2	T49.0X3	T49.0X4	T49.0X5	T49.0X6
Tricresyl phosphate	T65.891	T65.892	T65.893	T65.894	—	—
solvent	T52.91	T52.92	T52.93	T52.94	—	—
Tricyclamol chloride	T44.3X1	T44.3X2	T44.3X3	T44.3X4	T44.3X5	T44.3X6
Tridesilon	T49.0X1	T49.0X2	T49.0X3	T49.0X4	T49.0X5	T49.0X6
Tridihexethyl iodide	T44.3X1	T44.3X2	T44.3X3	T44.3X4	T44.3X5	T44.3X6
Tridione	T42.2X1	T42.2X2	T42.2X3	T42.2X4	T42.2X5	T42.2X6
Trientine	T45.8X1	T45.8X2	T45.8X3	T45.8X4	T45.8X5	T45.8X6
Triethanolamine NEC	T54.3X1	T54.3X2	T54.3X3	T54.3X4	—	—
detergent	T54.3X1	T54.3X2	T54.3X3	T54.3X4	—	—
trinitrate (biphosphate)	T46.3X1	T46.3X2	T46.3X3	T46.3X4	T46.3X5	T46.3X6
Triethanomelamine	T45.1X1	T45.1X2	T45.1X3	T45.1X4	T45.1X5	T45.1X6
Triethylenemelamine	T45.1X1	T45.1X2	T45.1X3	T45.1X4	T45.1X5	T45.1X6
Triethylenephosphoramide	T45.1X1	T45.1X2	T45.1X3	T45.1X4	T45.1X5	T45.1X6
Triethylenethiophosphoramide	T45.1X1	T45.1X2	T45.1X3	T45.1X4	T45.1X5	T45.1X6
Trifluoperazine	T43.3X1	T43.3X2	T43.3X3	T43.3X4	T43.3X5	T43.3X6
Trifluoroethyl vinyl ether	T41.0X1	T41.0X2	T41.0X3	T41.0X4	T41.0X5	T41.0X6
Trifluperidol	T43.4X1	T43.4X2	T43.4X3	T43.4X4	T43.4X5	T43.4X6
Triflupromazine	T43.3X1	T43.3X2	T43.3X3	T43.3X4	T43.3X5	T43.3X6
Trifluridine	T37.5X1	T37.5X2	T37.5X3	T37.5X4	T37.5X5	T37.5X6
Triflusal	T45.521	T45.522	T45.523	T45.524	T45.525	T45.526
Trihexyphenidyl	T44.3X1	T44.3X2	T44.3X3	T44.3X4	T44.3X5	T44.3X6
Triiodothyronine	T38.1X1	T38.1X2	T38.1X3	T38.1X4	T38.1X5	T38.1X6
Trilene	T41.0X1	T41.0X2	T41.0X3	T41.0X4	T41.0X5	T41.0X6
Trilostane	T38.991	T38.992	T38.993	T38.994	T38.995	T38.996
Trimebutine	T44.3X1	T44.3X2	T44.3X3	T44.3X4	T44.3X5	T44.3X6
Trimecaine	T41.3X1	T41.3X2	T41.3X3	T41.3X4	T41.3X5	T41.3X6
Trimeprazine (tartrate)	T44.3X1	T44.3X2	T44.3X3	T44.3X4	T44.3X5	T44.3X6
Trimetaphan camsilate	T44.2X1	T44.2X2	T44.2X3	T44.2X4	T44.2X5	T44.2X6
Trimetazidine	T46.7X1	T46.7X2	T46.7X3	T46.7X4	T46.7X5	T46.7X6
Trimethadione	T42.2X1	T42.2X2	T42.2X3	T42.2X4	T42.2X5	T42.2X6
Trimethaphan	T44.2X1	T44.2X2	T44.2X3	T44.2X4	T44.2X5	T44.2X6
Trimethidinium	T44.2X1	T44.2X2	T44.2X3	T44.2X4	T44.2X5	T44.2X6
Trimethobenzamide	T45.0X1	T45.0X2	T45.0X3	T45.0X4	T45.0X5	T45.0X6
Trimethoprim	T37.8X1	T37.8X2	T37.8X3	T37.8X4	T37.8X5	T37.8X6
with sulfamethoxazole	T36.8X1	T36.8X2	T36.8X3	T36.8X4	T36.8X5	T36.8X6
Trimethylcarbinol	T51.3X1	T51.3X2	T51.3X3	T51.3X4	—	—
Trimethylpsoralen	T49.3X1	T49.3X2	T49.3X3	T49.3X4	T49.3X5	T49.3X6
Trimeton	T45.0X1	T45.0X2	T45.0X3	T45.0X4	T45.0X5	T45.0X6
Trimetrexate	T45.1X1	T45.1X2	T45.1X3	T45.1X4	T45.1X5	T45.1X6
Trimipramine	T43.011	T43.012	T43.013	T43.014	T43.015	T43.016
Trimustine	T45.1X1	T45.1X2	T45.1X3	T45.1X4	T45.1X5	T45.1X6
Trinitrine	T46.3X1	T46.3X2	T46.3X3	T46.3X4	T46.3X5	T46.3X6
Trinitrobenzol	T65.3X1	T65.3X2	T65.3X3	T65.3X4	—	—
Trinitrophenol	T65.3X1	T65.3X2	T65.3X3	T65.3X4	—	—
Trinitrotoluene (fumes)	T65.3X1	T65.3X2	T65.3X3	T65.3X4	—	—
Trional	T42.6X1	T42.6X2	T42.6X3	T42.6X4	T42.6X5	T42.6X6
Triorthocresyl phosphate	T65.891	T65.892	T65.893	T65.894	—	—
Trioxide of arsenic	T57.0X1	T57.0X2	T57.0X3	T57.0X4	—	—
Trioxysalen	T49.4X1	T49.4X2	T49.4X3	T49.4X4	T49.4X5	T49.4X6
Tripamide	T50.2X1	T50.2X2	T50.2X3	T50.2X4	T50.2X5	T50.2X6
Triparanol	T46.6X1	T46.6X2	T46.6X3	T46.6X4	T46.6X5	T46.6X6
Tripelennamine	T45.0X1	T45.0X2	T45.0X3	T45.0X4	T45.0X5	T45.0X6
Triperiden	T44.3X1	T44.3X2	T44.3X3	T44.3X4	T44.3X5	T44.3X6
Triperidol	T43.4X1	T43.4X2	T43.4X3	T43.4X4	T43.4X5	T43.4X6
Triphenylphosphate	T65.891	T65.892	T65.893	T65.894	—	—
Triple						
bromides	T42.6X1	T42.6X2	T42.6X3	T42.6X4	T42.6X5	T42.6X6
carbonate	T47.1X1	T47.1X2	T47.1X3	T47.1X4	T47.1X5	T47.1X6
vaccine						
DPT	T50.A11	T50.A12	T50.A13	T50.A14	T50.A15	T50.A16
including pertussis	T50.A11	T50.A12	T50.A13	T50.A14	T50.A15	T50.A16
MMR	T50.B91	T50.B92	T50.B93	T50.B94	T50.B95	T50.B96
Triprolidine	T45.0X1	T45.0X2	T45.0X3	T45.0X4	T45.0X5	T45.0X6
Trisodium hydrogen edetate	T50.6X1	T50.6X2	T50.6X3	T50.6X4	T50.6X5	T50.6X6
Trisoralen	T49.3X1	T49.3X2	T49.3X3	T49.3X4	T49.3X5	T49.3X6
Trisulfapyrimidines	T37.0X1	T37.0X2	T37.0X3	T37.0X4	T37.0X5	T37.0X6
Trithiozine	T44.3X1	T44.3X2	T44.3X3	T44.3X4	T44.3X5	T44.3X6
Tritiozine	T44.3X1	T44.3X2	T44.3X3	T44.3X4	T44.3X5	T44.3X6
Tritoqualine	T45.0X1	T45.0X2	T45.0X3	T45.0X4	T45.0X5	T45.0X6
Trofosfamide	T45.1X1	T45.1X2	T45.1X3	T45.1X4	T45.1X5	T45.1X6
Troleandomycin	T36.3X1	T36.3X2	T36.3X3	T36.3X4	T36.3X5	T36.3X6
Trolnitrate (phosphate)	T46.3X1	T46.3X2	T46.3X3	T46.3X4	T46.3X5	T46.3X6
Tromantadine	T37.5X1	T37.5X2	T37.5X3	T37.5X4	T37.5X5	T37.5X6
Trometamol	T50.2X1	T50.2X2	T50.2X3	T50.2X4	T50.2X5	T50.2X6
Tromethamine	T50.2X1	T50.2X2	T50.2X3	T50.2X4	T50.2X5	T50.2X6
Tronothane	T41.3X1	T41.3X2	T41.3X3	T41.3X4	T41.3X5	T41.3X6
Tropacine	T44.3X1	T44.3X2	T44.3X3	T44.3X4	T44.3X5	T44.3X6
Tropatepine	T44.3X1	T44.3X2	T44.3X3	T44.3X4	T44.3X5	T44.3X6
Tropicamide	T44.3X1	T44.3X2	T44.3X3	T44.3X4	T44.3X5	T44.3X6
Trospium chloride	T44.3X1	T44.3X2	T44.3X3	T44.3X4	T44.3X5	T44.3X6
Troxerutin	T46.991	T46.992	T46.993	T46.994	T46.995	T46.996
Troxidone	T42.2X1	T42.2X2	T42.2X3	T42.2X4	T42.2X5	T42.2X6
Tryparsamide	T37.3X1	T37.3X2	T37.3X3	T37.3X4	T37.3X5	T37.3X6
Trypsin	T45.3X1	T45.3X2	T45.3X3	T45.3X4	T45.3X5	T45.3X6
Tryptizol	T43.011	T43.012	T43.013	T43.014	T43.015	T43.016
TSH	T38.811	T38.812	T38.813	T38.814	T38.815	T38.816
Tuaminoheptane	T48.5X1	T48.5X2	T48.5X3	T48.5X4	T48.5X5	T48.5X6
Tuberculin, purified protein derivative (PPD)	T50.8X1	T50.8X2	T50.8X3	T50.8X4	T50.8X5	T50.8X6
Tubocurare	T48.1X1	T48.1X2	T48.1X3	T48.1X4	T48.1X5	T48.1X6
Tubocurarine (chloride)	T48.1X1	T48.1X2	T48.1X3	T48.1X4	T48.1X5	T48.1X6
Tulobuterol	T48.6X1	T48.6X2	T48.6X3	T48.6X4	T48.6X5	T48.6X6
Turpentine (spirits of)	T52.8X1	T52.8X2	T52.8X3	T52.8X4	—	—
vapor	T52.8X1	T52.8X2	T52.8X3	T52.8X4	—	—
Tybamate	T43.591	T43.592	T43.593	T43.594	T43.595	T43.596
Tyloxapol	T48.4X1	T48.4X2	T48.4X3	T48.4X4	T48.4X5	T48.4X6
Tymazoline	T48.5X1	T48.5X2	T48.5X3	T48.5X4	T48.5X5	T48.5X6
Typhoid-paratyphoid vaccine	T50.A91	T50.A92	T50.A93	T50.A94	T50.A95	T50.A96
Typhus vaccine	T50.A91	T50.A92	T50.A93	T50.A94	T50.A95	T50.A96
Tyropanoate	T50.8X1	T50.8X2	T50.8X3	T50.8X4	T50.8X5	T50.8X6
Tyrothricin	T49.6X1	T49.6X2	T49.6X3	T49.6X4	T49.6X5	T49.6X6
ENT agent	T49.6X1	T49.6X2	T49.6X3	T49.6X4	T49.6X5	T49.6X6
ophthalmic preparation	T49.5X1	T49.5X2	T49.5X3	T49.5X4	T49.5X5	T49.5X6
Ufenamate	T39.391	T39.392	T39.393	T39.394	T39.395	T39.396
Ultraviolet light protectant	T49.3X1	T49.3X2	T49.3X3	T49.3X4	T49.3X5	T49.3X6
Undecenoic acid	T49.0X1	T49.0X2	T49.0X3	T49.0X4	T49.0X5	T49.0X6
Undecoylium	T49.0X1	T49.0X2	T49.0X3	T49.0X4	T49.0X5	T49.0X6
Undecylenic acid (derivatives)	T49.0X1	T49.0X2	T49.0X3	T49.0X4	T49.0X5	T49.0X6
Unna's boot	T49.3X1	T49.3X2	T49.3X3	T49.3X4	T49.3X5	T49.3X6
Unsaturated fatty acid	T46.6X1	T46.6X2	T46.6X3	T46.6X4	T46.6X5	T46.6X6
Uracil mustard	T45.1X1	T45.1X2	T45.1X3	T45.1X4	T45.1X5	T45.1X6
Uramustine	T45.1X1	T45.1X2	T45.1X3	T45.1X4	T45.1X5	T45.1X6
Urapidil	T46.5X1	T46.5X2	T46.5X3	T46.5X4	T46.5X5	T46.5X6
Urari	T48.1X1	T48.1X2	T48.1X3	T48.1X4	T48.1X5	T48.1X6
Urate oxidase	T50.4X1	T50.4X2	T50.4X3	T50.4X4	T50.4X5	T50.4X6
Urea	T47.3X1	T47.3X2	T47.3X3	T47.3X4	T47.3X5	T47.3X6
peroxide	T49.0X1	T49.0X2	T49.0X3	T49.0X4	T49.0X5	T49.0X6
stibamine	T37.4X1	T37.4X2	T37.4X3	T37.4X4	T37.4X5	T37.4X6
topical	T49.8X1	T49.8X2	T49.8X3	T49.8X4	T49.8X5	T49.8X6
Urethane	T45.1X1	T45.1X2	T45.1X3	T45.1X4	T45.1X5	T45.1X6
Urginea (maritima) (scilla) — *see* Squill						
Uric acid metabolism drug NEC	T50.4X1	T50.4X2	T50.4X3	T50.4X4	T50.4X5	T50.4X6
Uricosuric agent	T50.4X1	T50.4X2	T50.4X3	T50.4X4	T50.4X5	T50.4X6
Urinary anti-infective	T37.8X1	T37.8X2	T37.8X3	T37.8X4	T37.8X5	T37.8X6
Urofollitropin	T38.811	T38.812	T38.813	T38.814	T38.815	T38.816
Urokinase	T45.611	T45.612	T45.613	T45.614	T45.615	T45.616
Urokon	T50.8X1	T50.8X2	T50.8X3	T50.8X4	T50.8X5	T50.8X6
Ursodeoxycholic acid	T50.991	T50.992	T50.993	T50.994	T50.995	T50.996
Ursodiol	T50.991	T50.992	T50.993	T50.994	T50.995	T50.996
Urtica	T62.2X1	T62.2X2	T62.2X3	T62.2X4	—	—
Utility gas — *see* Gas, utility						
Vaccine NEC	T50.Z91	T50.Z92	T50.Z93	T50.Z94	T50.Z95	T50.Z96
antineoplastic	T50.Z91	T50.Z92	T50.Z93	T50.Z94	T50.Z95	T50.Z96
bacterial NEC	T50.A91	T50.A92	T50.A93	T50.A94	T50.A95	T50.A96
with						
other bacterial component	T50.A21	T50.A22	T50.A23	T50.A24	T50.A25	T50.A26
pertussis component	T50.A11	T50.A12	T50.A13	T50.A14	T50.A15	T50.A16
viral-rickettsial component	T50.A21	T50.A22	T50.A23	T50.A24	T50.A25	T50.A26
mixed NEC	T50.A21	T50.A22	T50.A23	T50.A24	T50.A25	T50.A26
BCG	T50.A91	T50.A92	T50.A93	T50.A94	T50.A95	T50.A96
cholera	T50.A91	T50.A92	T50.A93	T50.A94	T50.A95	T50.A96
diphtheria	T50.A91	T50.A92	T50.A93	T50.A94	T50.A95	T50.A96
with tetanus	T50.A21	T50.A22	T50.A23	T50.A24	T50.A25	T50.A26
and pertussis	T50.A11	T50.A12	T50.A13	T50.A14	T50.A15	T50.A16
influenza	T50.B91	T50.B92	T50.B93	T50.B94	T50.B95	T50.B96
measles	T50.B91	T50.B92	T50.B93	T50.B94	T50.B95	T50.B96
with mumps and rubella	T50.B91	T50.B92	T50.B93	T50.B94	T50.B95	T50.B96
meningococcal	T50.A91	T50.A92	T50.A93	T50.A94	T50.A95	T50.A96
mumps	T50.B91	T50.B92	T50.B93	T50.B94	T50.B95	T50.B96
paratyphoid	T50.A91	T50.A92	T50.A93	T50.A94	T50.A95	T50.A96
pertussis	T50.A11	T50.A12	T50.A13	T50.A14	T50.A15	T50.A16
with diphtheria	T50.A11	T50.A12	T50.A13	T50.A14	T50.A15	T50.A16

Trichlorotriethylamine — Vaccine NEC

Substance	Poisoning, Accidental (unintentional)	Poisoning, Intentional Self-harm	Poisoning, Assault	Poisoning, Undetermined	Adverse Effect	Under-dosing
Vaccine — *continued*						
pertussis — *continued*						
with diphtheria — *continued*						
and tetanus	T50.A11	T50.A12	T50.A13	T50.A14	T50.A15	T50.A16
with other component	T50.A11	T50.A12	T50.A13	T50.A14	T50.A15	T50.A16
plague	T50.A91	T50.A92	T50.A93	T50.A94	T50.A95	T50.A96
poliomyelitis	T50.B91	T50.B92	T50.B93	T50.B94	T50.B95	T50.B96
poliovirus	T50.B91	T50.B92	T50.B93	T50.B94	T50.B95	T50.B96
rabies	T50.B91	T50.B92	T50.B93	T50.B94	T50.B95	T50.B96
respiratory syncytial virus	T50.B91	T50.B92	T50.B93	T50.B94	T50.B95	T50.B96
rickettsial NEC	T50.A91	T50.A92	T50.A93	T50.A94	T50.A95	T50.A96
with						
bacterial component	T50.A21	T50.A22	T50.A23	T50.A24	T50.A25	T50.A26
Rocky Mountain spotted fever	T50.A91	T50.A92	T50.A93	T50.A94	T50.A95	T50.A96
rubella	T50.B91	T50.B92	T50.B93	T50.B94	T50.B95	T50.B96
sabin oral	T50.B91	T50.B92	T50.B93	T50.B94	T50.B95	T50.B96
smallpox	T50.B11	T50.B12	T50.B13	T50.B14	T50.B15	T50.B16
TAB	T50.A91	T50.A92	T50.A93	T50.A94	T50.A95	T50.A96
tetanus	T50.A91	T50.A92	T50.A93	T50.A94	T50.A95	T50.A96
typhoid	T50.A91	T50.A92	T50.A93	T50.A94	T50.A95	T50.A96
typhus	T50.A91	T50.A92	T50.A93	T50.A94	T50.A95	T50.A96
viral NEC	T50.B91	T50.B92	T50.B93	T50.B94	T50.B95	T50.B96
yellow fever	T50.B91	T50.B92	T50.B93	T50.B94	T50.B95	T50.B96
Vaccinia immune globulin	T50.Z11	T50.Z12	T50.Z13	T50.Z14	T50.Z15	T50.Z16
Vaginal contraceptives	T49.8X1	T49.8X2	T49.8X3	T49.8X4	T49.8X5	T49.8X6
Valerian						
root	T42.6X1	T42.6X2	T42.6X3	T42.6X4	T42.6X5	T42.6X6
tincture	T42.6X1	T42.6X2	T42.6X3	T42.6X4	T42.6X5	T42.6X6
Valethamate bromide	T44.3X1	T44.3X2	T44.3X3	T44.3X4	T44.3X5	T44.3X6
Valisone	T49.0X1	T49.0X2	T49.0X3	T49.0X4	T49.0X5	T49.0X6
Valium	T42.4X1	T42.4X2	T42.4X3	T42.4X4	T42.4X5	T42.4X6
Valmid	T42.6X1	T42.6X2	T42.6X3	T42.6X4	T42.6X5	T42.6X6
Valnoctamide	T42.6X1	T42.6X2	T42.6X3	T42.6X4	T42.6X5	T42.6X6
Valproate (sodium)	T42.6X1	T42.6X2	T42.6X3	T42.6X4	T42.6X5	T42.6X6
Valproic acid	T42.6X1	T42.6X2	T42.6X3	T42.6X4	T42.6X5	T42.6X6
Valpromide	T42.6X1	T42.6X2	T42.6X3	T42.6X4	T42.6X5	T42.6X6
Vanadium	T56.891	T56.892	T56.893	T56.894	—	—
Vancomycin	T36.8X1	T36.8X2	T36.8X3	T36.8X4	T36.8X5	T36.8X6
Vapor — *see also* Gas	T59.91	T59.92	T59.93	T59.94	—	—
kiln (carbon monoxide)	T58.8X1	T58.8X2	T58.8X3	T58.8X4	—	—
lead — *see* lead						
specified source NEC	T59.891	T59.892	T59.893	T59.894	—	—
Vardenafil	T46.7X1	T46.7X2	T46.7X3	T46.7X4	T46.7X5	T46.7X6
Varicose reduction drug	T46.8X1	T46.8X2	T46.8X3	T46.8X4	T46.8X5	T46.8X6
Varnish	T65.4X1	T65.4X2	T65.4X3	T65.4X4	—	—
cleaner	T52.91	T52.92	T52.93	T52.94	—	—
Vaseline	T49.3X1	T49.3X2	T49.3X3	T49.3X4	T49.3X5	T49.3X6
Vasodilan	T46.7X1	T46.7X2	T46.7X3	T46.7X4	T46.7X5	T46.7X6
Vasodilator						
coronary NEC	T46.3X1	T46.3X2	T46.3X3	T46.3X4	T46.3X5	T46.3X6
peripheral NEC	T46.7X1	T46.7X2	T46.7X3	T46.7X4	T46.7X5	T46.7X6
Vasopressin	T38.891	T38.892	T38.893	T38.894	T38.895	T38.896
Vasopressor drugs	T38.891	T38.892	T38.893	T38.894	T38.895	T38.896
Vecuronium bromide	T48.1X1	T48.1X2	T48.1X3	T48.1X4	T48.1X5	T48.1X6
Vegetable extract, astringent	T49.2X1	T49.2X2	T49.2X3	T49.2X4	T49.2X5	T49.2X6
Venlafaxine	T43.211	T43.212	T43.213	T43.214	T43.215	T43.216
Venom, venomous (bite) (sting)	T63.91	T63.92	T63.93	T63.94	—	—
amphibian NEC	T63.831	T63.832	T63.833	T63.834	—	—
animal NEC	T63.891	T63.892	T63.893	T63.894	—	—
ant	T63.421	T63.422	T63.423	T63.424	—	—
arthropod NEC	T63.481	T63.482	T63.483	T63.484	—	—
bee	T63.441	T63.442	T63.443	T63.444	—	—
centipede	T63.411	T63.412	T63.413	T63.414	—	—
fish	T63.591	T63.592	T63.593	T63.594	—	—
frog	T63.811	T63.812	T63.813	T63.814	—	—
hornet	T63.451	T63.452	T63.453	T63.454	—	—
insect NEC	T63.481	T63.482	T63.483	T63.484	—	—
lizard	T63.121	T63.122	T63.123	T63.124	—	—
marine						
animals	T63.691	T63.692	T63.693	T63.694	—	—
bluebottle	T63.611	T63.612	T63.613	T63.614	—	—
jellyfish NEC	T63.621	T63.622	T63.623	T63.624	—	—
Portugese Man-o-war	T63.611	T63.612	T63.613	T63.614	—	—
sea anemone	T63.631	T63.632	T63.633	T63.634	—	—
specified NEC	T63.691	T63.692	T63.693	T63.694	—	—
fish	T63.591	T63.592	T63.593	T63.594	—	—
plants	T63.711	T63.712	T63.713	T63.714	—	—
sting ray	T63.511	T63.512	T63.513	T63.514	—	—
millipede (tropical)	T63.411	T63.412	T63.413	T63.414	—	—
plant NEC	T63.791	T63.792	T63.793	T63.794	—	—

Substance	Poisoning, Accidental (unintentional)	Poisoning, Intentional Self-harm	Poisoning, Assault	Poisoning, Undetermined	Adverse Effect	Under-dosing
Venom, venomous — *continued*						
plant — *continued*						
marine	T63.711	T63.712	T63.713	T63.714	—	—
reptile	T63.191	T63.192	T63.193	T63.194	—	—
gila monster	T63.111	T63.112	T63.113	T63.114	—	—
lizard NEC	T63.121	T63.122	T63.123	T63.124	—	—
scorpion	T63.2X1	T63.2X2	T63.2X3	T63.2X4	—	—
snake	T63.001	T63.002	T63.003	T63.004	—	—
African NEC	T63.081	T63.082	T63.083	T63.084	—	—
American (North) (South) NEC	T63.061	T63.062	T63.063	T63.064	—	—
Asian	T63.081	T63.082	T63.083	T63.084	—	—
Australian	T63.071	T63.072	T63.073	T63.074	—	—
cobra	T63.041	T63.042	T63.043	T63.044	—	—
coral snake	T63.021	T63.022	T63.023	T63.024	—	—
rattlesnake	T63.011	T63.012	T63.013	T63.014	—	—
specified NEC	T63.091	T63.092	T63.093	T63.094	—	—
taipan	T63.031	T63.032	T63.033	T63.034	—	—
specified NEC	T63.891	T63.892	T63.893	T63.894	—	—
spider	T63.301	T63.302	T63.303	T63.304	—	—
black widow	T63.311	T63.312	T63.313	T63.314	—	—
brown recluse	T63.331	T63.332	T63.333	T63.334	—	—
specified NEC	T63.391	T63.392	T63.393	T63.394	—	—
tarantula	T63.321	T63.322	T63.323	T63.324	—	—
sting ray	T63.511	T63.512	T63.513	T63.514	—	—
toad	T63.821	T63.822	T63.823	T63.824	—	—
wasp	T63.461	T63.462	T63.463	T63.464	—	—
Venous sclerosing drug NEC	T46.8X1	T46.8X2	T46.8X3	T46.8X4	T46.8X5	T46.8X6
Ventolin — *see* Albuterol						
Veramon	T42.3X1	T42.3X2	T42.3X3	T42.3X4	T42.3X5	T42.3X6
Verapamil	T46.1X1	T46.1X2	T46.1X3	T46.1X4	T46.1X5	T46.1X6
Veratrine	T46.5X1	T46.5X2	T46.5X3	T46.5X4	T46.5X5	T46.5X6
Veratrum						
album	T62.2X1	T62.2X2	T62.2X3	T62.2X4	—	—
alkaloids	T46.5X1	T46.5X2	T46.5X3	T46.5X4	T46.5X5	T46.5X6
viride	T62.2X1	T62.2X2	T62.2X3	T62.2X4	—	—
Verdigris	T60.3X1	T60.3X2	T60.3X3	T60.3X4	—	—
Veronal	T42.3X1	T42.3X2	T42.3X3	T42.3X4	T42.3X5	T42.3X6
Veroxil	T37.4X1	T37.4X2	T37.4X3	T37.4X4	T37.4X5	T37.4X6
Versenate	T50.6X1	T50.6X2	T50.6X3	T50.6X4	T50.6X5	T50.6X6
Versidyne	T39.8X1	T39.8X2	T39.8X3	T39.8X4	T39.8X5	T39.8X6
Vetrabutine	T48.0X1	T48.0X2	T48.0X3	T48.0X4	T48.0X5	T48.0X6
Vidarabine	T37.5X1	T37.5X2	T37.5X3	T37.5X4	T37.5X5	T37.5X6
Vienna						
green	T57.0X1	T57.0X2	T57.0X3	T57.0X4	—	—
insecticide	T60.2X1	T60.2X2	T60.2X3	T60.2X4	—	—
red	T57.0X1	T57.0X2	T57.0X3	T57.0X4	—	—
pharmaceutical dye	T50.991	T50.992	T50.993	T50.994	T50.995	T50.996
Vigabatrin	T42.6X1	T42.6X2	T42.6X3	T42.6X4	T42.6X5	T42.6X6
Viloxazine	T43.291	T43.292	T43.293	T43.294	T43.295	T43.296
Viminol	T39.8X1	T39.8X2	T39.8X3	T39.8X4	T39.8X5	T39.8X6
Vinbarbital, vinbarbitone	T42.3X1	T42.3X2	T42.3X3	T42.3X4	T42.3X5	T42.3X6
Vinblastine	T45.1X1	T45.1X2	T45.1X3	T45.1X4	T45.1X5	T45.1X6
Vinburnine	T46.7X1	T46.7X2	T46.7X3	T46.7X4	T46.7X5	T46.7X6
Vincamine	T45.1X1	T45.1X2	T45.1X3	T45.1X4	T45.1X5	T45.1X6
Vincristine	T45.1X1	T45.1X2	T45.1X3	T45.1X4	T45.1X5	T45.1X6
Vindesine	T45.1X1	T45.1X2	T45.1X3	T45.1X4	T45.1X5	T45.1X6
Vinesthene, vinethene	T41.0X1	T41.0X2	T41.0X3	T41.0X4	T41.0X5	T41.0X6
Vinorelbine tartrate	T45.1X1	T45.1X2	T45.1X3	T45.1X4	T45.1X5	T45.1X6
Vinpocetine	T46.7X1	T46.7X2	T46.7X3	T46.7X4	T46.7X5	T46.7X6
Vinyl						
acetate	T65.891	T65.892	T65.893	T65.894	—	—
bital	T42.3X1	T42.3X2	T42.3X3	T42.3X4	T42.3X5	T42.3X6
bromide	T65.891	T65.892	T65.893	T65.894	—	—
chloride	T59.891	T59.892	T59.893	T59.894	—	—
ether	T41.0X1	T41.0X2	T41.0X3	T41.0X4	T41.0X5	T41.0X6
Vinylbital	T42.3X1	T42.3X2	T42.3X3	T42.3X4	T42.3X5	T42.3X6
Vinylidene chloride	T65.891	T65.892	T65.893	T65.894	—	—
Vioform	T37.8X1	T37.8X2	T37.8X3	T37.8X4	T37.8X5	T37.8X6
topical	T49.0X1	T49.0X2	T49.0X3	T49.0X4	T49.0X5	T49.0X6
Viomycin	T36.8X1	T36.8X2	T36.8X3	T36.8X4	T36.8X5	T36.8X6
Viosterol	T45.2X1	T45.2X2	T45.2X3	T45.2X4	T45.2X5	T45.2X6
Viper (venom)	T63.091	T63.092	T63.093	T63.094	—	—
Viprynium	T37.4X1	T37.4X2	T37.4X3	T37.4X4	T37.4X5	T37.4X6
Viquidil	T46.7X1	T46.7X2	T46.7X3	T46.7X4	T46.7X5	T46.7X6
Viral vaccine NEC	T50.B91	T50.B92	T50.B93	T50.B94	T50.B95	T50.B96
Virginiamycin	T36.8X1	T36.8X2	T36.8X3	T36.8X4	T36.8X5	T36.8X6
Virugon	T37.5X1	T37.5X2	T37.5X3	T37.5X4	T37.5X5	T37.5X6
Viscous agent	T50.901	T50.902	T50.903	T50.904	T50.905	T50.906
Visine	T49.5X1	T49.5X2	T49.5X3	T49.5X4	T49.5X5	T49.5X6
Visnadine	T46.3X1	T46.3X2	T46.3X3	T46.3X4	T46.3X5	T46.3X6
Vitamin NEC	T45.2X1	T45.2X2	T45.2X3	T45.2X4	T45.2X5	T45.2X6

Table of Drugs and Chemicals

Substance	Poisoning, Accidental (unintentional)	Poisoning, Intentional Self-harm	Poisoning, Assault	Poisoning, Undetermined	Adverse Effect	Under-dosing
Vitamin — *continued*						
A	T45.2X1	T45.2X2	T45.2X3	T45.2X4	T45.2X5	T45.2X6
B1	T45.2X1	T45.2X2	T45.2X3	T45.2X4	T45.2X5	T45.2X6
B2	T45.2X1	T45.2X2	T45.2X3	T45.2X4	T45.2X5	T45.2X6
B6	T45.2X1	T45.2X2	T45.2X3	T45.2X4	T45.2X5	T45.2X6
B12	T45.2X1	T45.2X2	T45.2X3	T45.2X4	T45.2X5	T45.2X6
B15	T45.2X1	T45.2X2	T45.2X3	T45.2X4	T45.2X5	T45.2X6
B NEC	T45.2X1	T45.2X2	T45.2X3	T45.2X4	T45.2X5	T45.2X6
nicotinic acid	T46.7X1	T46.7X2	T46.7X3	T46.7X4	T46.7X5	T46.7X6
C	T45.2X1	T45.2X2	T45.2X3	T45.2X4	T45.2X5	T45.2X6
D	T45.2X1	T45.2X2	T45.2X3	T45.2X4	T45.2X5	T45.2X6
D2	T45.2X1	T45.2X2	T45.2X3	T45.2X4	T45.2X5	T45.2X6
D3	T45.2X1	T45.2X2	T45.2X3	T45.2X4	T45.2X5	T45.2X6
E	T45.2X1	T45.2X2	T45.2X3	T45.2X4	T45.2X5	T45.2X6
E acetate	T45.2X1	T45.2X2	T45.2X3	T45.2X4	T45.2X5	T45.2X6
hematopoietic	T45.8X1	T45.8X2	T45.8X3	T45.8X4	T45.8X5	T45.8X6
K1	T45.7X1	T45.7X2	T45.7X3	T45.7X4	T45.7X5	T45.7X6
K2	T45.7X1	T45.7X2	T45.7X3	T45.7X4	T45.7X5	T45.7X6
K NEC	T45.7X1	T45.7X2	T45.7X3	T45.7X4	T45.7X5	T45.7X6
PP	T45.2X1	T45.2X2	T45.2X3	T45.2X4	T45.2X5	T45.2X6
ulceroprotectant	T47.1X1	T47.1X2	T47.1X3	T47.1X4	T47.1X5	T47.1X6
Vleminckx's solution	T49.4X1	T49.4X2	T49.4X3	T49.4X4	T49.4X5	T49.4X6
Voltaren — *see* Diclofenac						
sodium						
Warfarin	T45.511	T45.512	T45.513	T45.514	T45.515	T45.516
rodenticide	T45.511	T45.512	T45.513	T45.514	T45.515	T45.516
sodium	T45.511	T45.512	T45.513	T45.514	T45.515	T45.516
Wasp (sting)	T63.461	T63.462	T63.463	T63.464	—	—
Water						
balance drug	T50.3X1	T50.3X2	T50.3X3	T50.3X4	T50.3X5	T50.3X6
distilled	T50.3X1	T50.3X2	T50.3X3	T50.3X4	T50.3X5	T50.3X6
gas — *see* Gas, water						
incomplete combustion of —						
see Carbon, monoxide,						
fuel, utility						
hemlock	T62.2X1	T62.2X2	T62.2X3	T62.2X4	—	—
moccasin (venom)	T63.061	T63.062	T63.063	T63.064	—	—
purified	T50.3X1	T50.3X2	T50.3X3	T50.3X4	T50.3X5	T50.3X6
Wax (paraffin) (petroleum)	T52.0X1	T52.0X2	T52.0X3	T52.0X4	—	—
automobile	T65.891	T65.892	T65.893	T65.894	—	—
floor	T52.0X1	T52.0X2	T52.0X3	T52.0X4	—	—
Weed killers NEC	T60.3X1	T60.3X2	T60.3X3	T60.3X4	—	—
Welldorm	T42.6X1	T42.6X2	T42.6X3	T42.6X4	T42.6X5	T42.6X6
White						
arsenic	T57.0X1	T57.0X2	T57.0X3	T57.0X4	—	—
helleborne	T62.2X1	T62.2X2	T62.2X3	T62.2X4	—	—
lotion (keratolytic)	T49.4X1	T49.4X2	T49.4X3	T49.4X4	T49.4X5	T49.4X6
spirit	T52.0X1	T52.0X2	T52.0X3	T52.0X4	—	—
Whitewash	T65.891	T65.892	T65.893	T65.894	—	—
Whole blood (human)	T45.8X1	T45.8X2	T45.8X3	T45.8X4	T45.8X5	T45.8X6
Wild						
black cherry	T62.2X1	T62.2X2	T62.2X3	T62.2X4	—	—
poisonous plants NEC	T62.2X1	T62.2X2	T62.2X3	T62.2X4	—	—
Window cleaning fluid	T65.891	T65.892	T65.893	T65.894	—	—
Wintergreen (oil)	T49.3X1	T49.3X2	T49.3X3	T49.3X4	T49.3X5	T49.3X6
Wisterine	T62.2X1	T62.2X2	T62.2X3	T62.2X4	—	—
Witch hazel	T49.2X1	T49.2X2	T49.2X3	T49.2X4	T49.2X5	T49.2X6
Wood alcohol or spirit	T51.1X1	T51.1X2	T51.1X3	T51.1X4	—	—
Wool fat (hydrous)	T49.3X1	T49.3X2	T49.3X3	T49.3X4	T49.3X5	T49.3X6
Woorali	T48.1X1	T48.1X2	T48.1X3	T48.1X4	T48.1X5	T48.1X6
Wormseed, American	T37.4X1	T37.4X2	T37.4X3	T37.4X4	T37.4X5	T37.4X6
Xamoterol	T44.5X1	T44.5X2	T44.5X3	T44.5X4	T44.5X5	T44.5X6
Xanthine diuretics	T50.2X1	T50.2X2	T50.2X3	T50.2X4	T50.2X5	T50.2X6
Xanthinol nicotinate	T46.7X1	T46.7X2	T46.7X3	T46.7X4	T46.7X5	T46.7X6
Xanthotoxin	T49.3X1	T49.3X2	T49.3X3	T49.3X4	T49.3X5	T49.3X6
Xantinol nicotinate	T46.7X1	T46.7X2	T46.7X3	T46.7X4	T46.7X5	T46.7X6
Xantocillin	T36.0X1	T36.0X2	T36.0X3	T36.0X4	T36.0X5	T36.0X6
Xenon (127Xe) (133Xe)	T50.8X1	T50.8X2	T50.8X3	T50.8X4	T50.8X5	T50.8X6
Xenysalate	T49.4X1	T49.4X2	T49.4X3	T49.4X4	T49.4X5	T49.4X6
Xibornol	T37.8X1	T37.8X2	T37.8X3	T37.8X4	T37.8X5	T37.8X6
Xigris	T45.511	T45.512	T45.513	T45.514	T45.515	T45.516
Xipamide	T50.2X1	T50.2X2	T50.2X3	T50.2X4	T50.2X5	T50.2X6
Xylene (vapor)	T52.2X1	T52.2X2	T52.2X3	T52.2X4	—	—
Xylocaine (infiltration) (topical)	T41.3X1	T41.3X2	T41.3X3	T41.3X4	T41.3X5	T41.3X6
nerve block (peripheral) (plexus)	T41.3X1	T41.3X2	T41.3X3	T41.3X4	T41.3X5	T41.3X6
spinal	T41.3X1	T41.3X2	T41.3X3	T41.3X4	T41.3X5	T41.3X6
Xylol (vapor)	T52.2X1	T52.2X2	T52.2X3	T52.2X4	—	—
Xylometazoline	T48.5X1	T48.5X2	T48.5X3	T48.5X4	T48.5X5	T48.5X6
Yeast	T45.2X1	T45.2X2	T45.2X3	T45.2X4	T45.2X5	T45.2X6
dried	T45.2X1	T45.2X2	T45.2X3	T45.2X4	T45.2X5	T45.2X6
Yellow						
fever vaccine	T50.B91	T50.B92	T50.B93	T50.B94	T50.B95	T50.B96
jasmine	T62.2X1	T62.2X2	T62.2X3	T62.2X4	—	—
phenolphthalein	T47.2X1	T47.2X2	T47.2X3	T47.2X4	T47.2X5	T47.2X6
Yew	T62.2X1	T62.2X2	T62.2X3	T62.2X4		
Yohimbic acid	T40.991	T40.992	T40.993	T40.994	T40.995	T40.996
Zactane	T39.8X1	T39.8X2	T39.8X3	T39.8X4	T39.8X5	T39.8X6
Zalcitabine	T37.5X1	T37.5X2	T37.5X3	T37.5X4	T37.5X5	T37.5X6
Zaroxolyn	T50.2X1	T50.2X2	T50.2X3	T50.2X4	T50.2X5	T50.2X6
Zephiran (topical)	T49.0X1	T49.0X2	T49.0X3	T49.0X4	T49.0X5	T49.0X6
ophthalmic preparation	T49.5X1	T49.5X2	T49.5X3	T49.5X4	T49.5X5	T49.5X6
Zeranol	T38.7X1	T38.7X2	T38.7X3	T38.7X4	T38.7X5	T38.7X6
Zerone	T51.1X1	T51.1X2	T51.1X3	T51.1X4		
Zidovudine	T37.5X1	T37.5X2	T37.5X3	T37.5X4	T37.5X5	T37.5X6
Zimeldine	T43.221	T43.222	T43.223	T43.224	T43.225	T43.226
Zinc (compounds) (fumes) (vapor)	T56.5X1	T56.5X2	T56.5X3	T56.5X4	—	—
NEC						
anti-infectives	T49.0X1	T49.0X2	T49.0X3	T49.0X4	T49.0X5	T49.0X6
antivaricose	T46.8X1	T46.8X2	T46.8X3	T46.8X4	T46.8X5	T46.8X6
bacitracin	T49.0X1	T49.0X2	T49.0X3	T49.0X4	T49.0X5	T49.0X6
chloride (mouthwash)	T49.6X1	T49.6X2	T49.6X3	T49.6X4	T49.6X5	T49.6X6
chromate	T56.5X1	T56.5X2	T56.5X3	T56.5X4	—	—
gelatin	T49.3X1	T49.3X2	T49.3X3	T49.3X4	T49.3X5	T49.3X6
oxide	T49.3X1	T49.3X2	T49.3X3	T49.3X4	T49.3X5	T49.3X6
plaster	T49.3X1	T49.3X2	T49.3X3	T49.3X4	T49.3X5	T49.3X6
peroxide	T49.0X1	T49.0X2	T49.0X3	T49.0X4	T49.0X5	T49.0X6
pesticides	T56.5X1	T56.5X2	T56.5X3	T56.5X4	—	—
phosphide	T60.4X1	T60.4X2	T60.4X3	T60.4X4	—	—
pyrithionate	T49.4X1	T49.4X2	T49.4X3	T49.4X4	T49.4X5	T49.4X6
stearate	T49.3X1	T49.3X2	T49.3X3	T49.3X4	T49.3X5	T49.3X6
sulfate	T49.5X1	T49.5X2	T49.5X3	T49.5X4	T49.5X5	T49.5X6
ENT agent	T49.6X1	T49.6X2	T49.6X3	T49.6X4	T49.6X5	T49.6X6
ophthalmic solution	T49.5X1	T49.5X2	T49.5X3	T49.5X4	T49.5X5	T49.5X6
topical NEC	T49.0X1	T49.0X2	T49.0X3	T49.0X4	T49.0X5	T49.0X6
undecylenate	T49.0X1	T49.0X2	T49.0X3	T49.0X4	T49.0X5	T49.0X6
Zineb	T60.0X1	T60.0X2	T60.0X3	T60.0X4	—	—
Zinostatin	T45.1X1	T45.1X2	T45.1X3	T45.1X4	T45.1X5	T45.1X6
Zipeprol	T48.3X1	T48.3X2	T48.3X3	T48.3X4	T48.3X5	T48.3X6
Zofenopril	T46.4X1	T46.4X2	T46.4X3	T46.4X4	T46.4X5	T46.4X6
Zolpidem	T42.6X1	T42.6X2	T42.6X3	T42.6X4	T42.6X5	T42.6X6
Zomepirac	T39.391	T39.392	T39.393	T39.394	T39.395	T39.396
Zopiclone	T42.6X1	T42.6X2	T42.6X3	T42.6X4	T42.6X5	T42.6X6
Zorubicin	T45.1X1	T45.1X2	T45.1X3	T45.1X4	T45.1X5	T45.1X6
Zotepine	T43.591	T43.592	T43.593	T43.594	T43.595	T43.596
Zovant	T45.511	T45.512	T45.513	T45.514	T45.515	T45.516
Zoxazolamine	T42.8X1	T42.8X2	T42.8X3	T42.8X4	T42.8X5	T42.8X6
Zuclopenthixol	T43.4X1	T43.4X2	T43.4X3	T43.4X4	T43.4X5	T43.4X6
Zygadenus (venenosus)	T62.2X1	T62.2X2	T62.2X3	T62.2X4	—	—
Zyprexa	T43.591	T43.592	T43.593	T43.594	T43.595	T43.596

Additional Character May Be Required — Refer to the Tabular List for Character Selection

▽ Subterms under main terms may continue to next column or page

A

Abandonment (causing exposure to weather conditions) (with intent to injure or kill) NEC X58 ☑
Abuse (adult) (child) (mental) (physical) (sexual) X58 ☑
Accident (to) X58 ☑
  aircraft (in transit) (powered) (*see also* Accident, transport, aircraft)
    due to, caused by cataclysm — *see* Forces of nature, by type
  animal-drawn vehicle — *see* Accident, transport, animal-drawn vehicle occupant
  animal-rider — *see* Accident, transport, animal-rider
  automobile — *see* Accident, transport, car occupant
  bare foot water skier V94.4 ☑
  boat, boating (*see also* Accident, watercraft)
    striking swimmer
      powered V94.11 ☑
      unpowered V94.12 ☑
  bus — *see* Accident, transport, bus occupant
  cable car, not on rails V98.0 ☑
    on rails — *see* Accident, transport, streetcar occupant
  car — *see* Accident, transport, car occupant
  caused by, due to
    animal NEC W64 ☑
    chain hoist W24.0 ☑
    cold (excessive) — *see* Exposure, cold
    corrosive liquid, substance — *see* Table of Drugs and Chemicals
    cutting or piercing instrument — *see* Contact, with, by type of instrument
    drive belt W24.0 ☑
    electric
      current — *see* Exposure, electric current
      motor (*see also* Contact, with, by type of machine) W31.3 ☑
      current (of) W86.8 ☑
    environmental factor NEC X58 ☑
    explosive material — *see* Explosion
    fire, flames — *see* Exposure, fire
    firearm missile — *see* Discharge, firearm by type
    heat (excessive) — *see* Heat
    hot — *see* Contact, with, hot
    ignition — *see* Ignition
    lifting device W24.0 ☑
    lightning — *see* subcategory T75.0 ☑
      causing fire — *see* Exposure, fire
    machine, machinery — *see* Contact, with, by type of machine
    natural factor NEC X58 ☑
    pulley (block) W24.0 ☑
    radiation — *see* Radiation
    steam X13.1 ☑
      inhalation X13.0 ☑
      pipe X16 ☑
    thunderbolt — *see* subcategory T75.0 ☑
      causing fire — *see* Exposure, fire
    transmission device W24.1 ☑
  coach — *see* Accident, transport, bus occupant
  coal car — *see* Accident, transport, industrial vehicle occupant
  diving (*see also* Fall, into, water)
    with
      drowning or submersion — *see* Drowning
  forklift — *see* Accident, transport, industrial vehicle occupant
  heavy transport vehicle NOS — *see* Accident, transport, truck occupant
  ice yacht V98.2 ☑
  in
    medical, surgical procedure
      as, or due to misadventure — *see* Misadventure
      causing an abnormal reaction or later complication without mention of misadventure (*see also* Complication of or following, by type of procedure) Y84.9
  land yacht V98.1 ☑
  late effect of — *see* W00-X58 with 7th character S
  logging car — *see* Accident, transport, industrial vehicle occupant
  machine, machinery (*see also* Contact, with, by type of machine)
    on board watercraft V93.69 ☑
      explosion — *see* Explosion, in, watercraft

Accident — *continued*
  machine, machinery (*see also* Contact, with, by type of machine) — *continued*
    on board watercraft — *continued*
      fire — *see* Burn, on board watercraft
      powered craft V93.63 ☑
        ferry boat V93.61 ☑
        fishing boat V93.62 ☑
        jetskis V93.63 ☑
        liner V93.61 ☑
        merchant ship V93.60 ☑
        passenger ship V93.61 ☑
        sailboat V93.64 ☑
  mine tram — *see* Accident, transport, industrial vehicle occupant
  mobility scooter (motorized) — *see* Accident, transport, pedestrian, conveyance, specified type NEC
  motor scooter — *see* Accident, transport, motorcyclist
  motor vehicle NOS (traffic) (*see also* Accident, transport) V89.2 ☑
    nontraffic NEC V89.0 ☑
    three-wheeled NOS — *see* Accident, transport, three-wheeled motor vehicle occupant
  motorcycle NOS — *see* Accident, transport, motorcyclist
  nonmotor vehicle NOS (nontraffic) (*see also* Accident, transport) V89.1 ☑
    traffic NOS V89.3 ☑
  nontraffic (victim's mode of transport NOS) V88.9 ☑
    collision (between) V88.7 ☑
      bus and truck V88.5 ☑
      car and:
        bus V88.3 ☑
        pickup V88.2 ☑
        three-wheeled motor vehicle V88.0 ☑
        train V88.6 ☑
        truck V88.4 ☑
        two-wheeled motor vehicle V88.0 ☑
        van V88.2 ☑
      specified vehicle NEC and:
        three-wheeled motor vehicle V88.1 ☑
        two-wheeled motor vehicle V88.1 ☑
      known mode of transport — *see* Accident, transport, by type of vehicle
    noncollision V88.8 ☑
  on board watercraft V93.89 ☑
    powered craft V93.83 ☑
      ferry boat V93.81 ☑
      fishing boat V93.82 ☑
      jetskis V93.83 ☑
      liner V93.81 ☑
      merchant ship V93.80 ☑
      passenger ship V93.81 ☑
    unpowered craft V93.88 ☑
      canoe V93.85 ☑
      inflatable V93.86 ☑
        in tow
          recreational V94.31 ☑
          specified NEC V94.32 ☑
      kayak V93.85 ☑
      sailboat V93.84 ☑
      surf-board V93.88 ☑
      water skis V93.87 ☑
      windsurfer V93.88 ☑
  parachutist V97.29 ☑
    entangled in object V97.21 ☑
    injured on landing V97.22 ☑
  pedal cycle — *see* Accident, transport, pedal cyclist
  pedestrian (on foot)
    with
      another pedestrian W51 ☑
        with fall W03 ☑
          due to ice or snow W00.0 ☑
      on pedestrian conveyance NEC V00.09 ☑
      roller skater (in-line) V00.01 ☑
      skate boarder V00.02 ☑
      transport vehicle — *see* Accident, transport
    on pedestrian conveyance — *see* Accident, transport, pedestrian, conveyance
  pick-up truck or van — *see* Accident, transport, pickup truck occupant
  quarry truck — *see* Accident, transport, industrial vehicle occupant
  railway vehicle (any) (in motion) — *see* Accident, transport, railway vehicle occupant
    due to cataclysm — *see* Forces of nature, by type

Accident — *continued*
  scooter (non-motorized) — *see* Accident, transport, pedestrian, conveyance, scooter
  sequelae of — *see* categories W00-X58 with 7th character S
  skateboard — *see* Accident, transport, pedestrian, conveyance, skateboard
  ski(ing) — *see* Accident, transport, pedestrian, conveyance
    lift V98.3 ☑
  specified cause NEC X58 ☑
  streetcar — *see* Accident, transport, streetcar occupant
  traffic (victim's mode of transport NOS) V87.9 ☑
    collision (between) V87.7 ☑
      bus and truck V87.5 ☑
      car and:
        bus V87.3 ☑
        pickup V87.2 ☑
        three-wheeled motor vehicle V87.0 ☑
        train V87.6 ☑
        truck V87.4 ☑
        two-wheeled motor vehicle V87.0 ☑
        van V87.2 ☑
      specified vehicle NEC and:
        three-wheeled motor vehicle V87.1 ☑
        two-wheeled motor vehicle V87.1 ☑
    known mode of transport — *see* Accident, transport, by type of vehicle
    noncollision V87.8 ☑
  transport (involving injury to) V99 ☑
    18 wheeler — *see* Accident, transport, truck occupant
    agricultural vehicle occupant (nontraffic) V84.9 ☑
      driver V84.5 ☑
      hanger-on V84.7 ☑
      passenger V84.6 ☑
      traffic V84.3 ☑
        driver V84.0 ☑
        hanger-on V84.2 ☑
        passenger V84.1 ☑
      while boarding or alighting V84.4 ☑
    aircraft NEC V97.89 ☑
      military NEC V97.818 ☑
        with civilian aircraft V97.810 ☑
        civilian injured by V97.811 ☑
      occupant injured (in)
        nonpowered craft accident V96.9 ☑
          balloon V96.00 ☑
            collision V96.03 ☑
            crash V96.01 ☑
            explosion V96.05 ☑
            fire V96.04 ☑
            forced landing V96.02 ☑
            specified type NEC V96.09 ☑
          glider V96.20 ☑
            collision V96.23 ☑
            crash V96.21 ☑
            explosion V96.25 ☑
            fire V96.24 ☑
            forced landing V96.22 ☑
            specified type NEC V96.29 ☑
          hang glider V96.10 ☑
            collision V96.13 ☑
            crash V96.11 ☑
            explosion V96.15 ☑
            fire V96.14 ☑
            forced landing V96.12 ☑
            specified type NEC V96.19 ☑
          specified craft NEC V96.8 ☑
        powered craft accident V95.9 ☑
          fixed wing NEC
            commercial V95.30 ☑
              collision V95.33 ☑
              crash V95.31 ☑
              explosion V95.35 ☑
              fire V95.34 ☑
              forced landing V95.32 ☑
              specified type NEC V95.39 ☑
            private V95.20 ☑
              collision V95.23 ☑
              crash V95.21 ☑
              explosion V95.25 ☑
              fire V95.24 ☑
              forced landing V95.22 ☑
              specified type NEC V95.29 ☑
          glider V95.10 ☑

Accident — *continued*
 transport — *continued*
  aircraft — *continued*
   occupant injured — *continued*
    powered craft accident — *continued*
     glider — *continued*
      collision V95.13 ☑
      crash V95.11 ☑
      explosion V95.15 ☑
      fire V95.14 ☑
      forced landing V95.12 ☑
      specified type NEC V95.19 ☑
     helicopter V95.00 ☑
      collision V95.03 ☑
      crash V95.01 ☑
      explosion V95.05 ☑
      fire V95.04 ☑
      forced landing V95.02 ☑
      specified type NEC V95.09 ☑
     spacecraft V95.40 ☑
      collision V95.43 ☑
      crash V95.41 ☑
      explosion V95.45 ☑
      fire V95.44 ☑
      forced landing V95.42 ☑
      specified type NEC V95.49 ☑
     specified craft NEC V95.8 ☑
     ultralight V95.10 ☑
      collision V95.13 ☑
      crash V95.11 ☑
      explosion V95.15 ☑
      fire V95.14 ☑
      forced landing V95.12 ☑
      specified type NEC V95.19 ☑
    specified accident NEC V97.0 ☑
    while boarding or alighting V97.1 ☑
   person (injured by)
    falling from, in or on aircraft V97.0 ☑
    machinery on aircraft V97.89 ☑
    on ground with aircraft involvement V97.39 ☑
    rotating propeller V97.32 ☑
    struck by object falling from aircraft V97.31 ☑
    sucked into aircraft jet V97.33 ☑
    while boarding or alighting aircraft V97.1 ☑
   airport (battery-powered) passenger vehicle — *see* Accident, transport, industrial vehicle occupant
  all-terrain vehicle occupant (nontraffic) V86.95 ☑
   driver V86.55 ☑
   dune buggy — *see* Accident, transport, dune buggy occupant
   hanger-on V86.75 ☑
   passenger V86.65 ☑
   snowmobile — *see* Accident, transport, snowmobile occupant
   specified type NEC V86.99 ☑
   traffic V86.35 ☑
    driver V86.05 ☑
    hanger-on V86.25 ☑
    passenger V86.15 ☑
   while boarding or alighting V86.45 ☑
  ambulance occupant (traffic) V86.31 ☑
   driver V86.01 ☑
   hanger-on V86.21 ☑
   nontraffic V86.91 ☑
    driver V86.51 ☑
    hanger-on V86.71 ☑
    passenger V86.61 ☑
   passenger V86.11 ☑
   while boarding or alighting V86.41 ☑
  animal-drawn vehicle occupant (in) V80.929 ☑
   collision (with)
    animal V80.12 ☑
     being ridden V80.711 ☑
    animal-drawn vehicle V80.721 ☑
    bus V80.42 ☑
    car V80.42 ☑
    fixed or stationary object V80.82 ☑
    military vehicle V80.920 ☑
    nonmotor vehicle V80.791 ☑
    pedal cycle V80.22 ☑
    pedestrian V80.12 ☑
    pickup V80.42 ☑
    railway train or vehicle V80.62 ☑

Accident — *continued*
 transport — *continued*
  animal-drawn vehicle occupant — *continued*
   collision — *continued*
    specified motor vehicle NEC V80.52 ☑
    streetcar V80.731 ☑
    truck V80.42 ☑
    two- or three-wheeled motor vehicle V80.32 ☑
    van V80.42 ☑
   noncollision V80.02 ☑
   specified circumstance NEC V80.928 ☑
  animal-rider V80.919 ☑
   collision (with)
    animal V80.11 ☑
     being ridden V80.710 ☑
    animal-drawn vehicle V80.720 ☑
    bus V80.41 ☑
    car V80.41 ☑
    fixed or stationary object V80.81 ☑
    military vehicle V80.910 ☑
    nonmotor vehicle V80.790 ☑
    pedal cycle V80.21 ☑
    pedestrian V80.11 ☑
    pickup V80.41 ☑
    railway train or vehicle V80.61 ☑
    specified motor vehicle NEC V80.51 ☑
    streetcar V80.730 ☑
    truck V80.41 ☑
    two- or three-wheeled motor vehicle V80.31 ☑
    van V80.41 ☑
   noncollision V80.018 ☑
    specified as horse rider V80.010 ☑
   specified circumstance NEC V80.918 ☑
  armored car — *see* Accident, transport, truck occupant
  battery-powered truck (baggage) (mail) — *see* Accident, transport, industrial vehicle occupant
  bus occupant V79.9 ☑
   collision (with)
    animal (traffic) V70.9 ☑
     being ridden (traffic) V76.9 ☑
      nontraffic V76.3 ☑
      while boarding or alighting V76.4 ☑
     nontraffic V70.3 ☑
     while boarding or alighting V70.4 ☑
    animal-drawn vehicle (traffic) V76.9 ☑
     nontraffic V76.3 ☑
     while boarding or alighting V76.4 ☑
    bus (traffic) V74.9 ☑
     nontraffic V74.3 ☑
     while boarding or alighting V74.4 ☑
    car (traffic) V73.9 ☑
     nontraffic V73.3 ☑
     while boarding or alighting V73.4 ☑
    motor vehicle NOS (traffic) V79.60 ☑
     nontraffic V79.20 ☑
     specified type NEC (traffic) V79.69 ☑
      nontraffic V79.29 ☑
    pedal cycle (traffic) V71.9 ☑
     nontraffic V71.3 ☑
     while boarding or alighting V71.4 ☑
    pickup truck (traffic) V73.9 ☑
     nontraffic V73.3 ☑
     while boarding or alighting V73.4 ☑
    railway vehicle (traffic) V75.9 ☑
     nontraffic V75.3 ☑
     while boarding or alighting V75.4 ☑
    specified vehicle NEC (traffic) V76.9 ☑
     nontraffic V76.3 ☑
     while boarding or alighting V76.4 ☑
    stationary object (traffic) V77.9 ☑
     nontraffic V77.3 ☑
     while boarding or alighting V77.4 ☑
    streetcar (traffic) V76.9 ☑
     nontraffic V76.3 ☑
     while boarding or alighting V76.4 ☑
    three wheeled motor vehicle (traffic) V72.9 ☑
     nontraffic V72.3 ☑
     while boarding or alighting V72.4 ☑
    truck (traffic) V74.9 ☑
     nontraffic V74.3 ☑
     while boarding or alighting V74.4 ☑

Accident — *continued*
 transport — *continued*
  bus occupant — *continued*
   collision — *continued*
    two wheeled motor vehicle (traffic) V72.9 ☑
     nontraffic V72.3 ☑
     while boarding or alighting V72.4 ☑
    van (traffic) V73.9 ☑
     nontraffic V73.3 ☑
     while boarding or alighting V73.4 ☑
   driver
    collision (with)
     animal (traffic) V70.5 ☑
      being ridden (traffic) V76.5 ☑
       nontraffic V76.0 ☑
      nontraffic V70.0 ☑
     animal-drawn vehicle (traffic) V76.5 ☑
      nontraffic V76.0 ☑
     bus (traffic) V74.5 ☑
      nontraffic V74.0 ☑
     car (traffic) V73.5 ☑
      nontraffic V73.0 ☑
     motor vehicle NOS (traffic) V79.40 ☑
      nontraffic V79.00 ☑
      specified type NEC (traffic) V79.49 ☑
       nontraffic V79.09 ☑
     pedal cycle (traffic) V71.5 ☑
      nontraffic V71.0 ☑
     pickup truck (traffic) V73.5 ☑
      nontraffic V73.0 ☑
     railway vehicle (traffic) V75.5 ☑
      nontraffic V75.0 ☑
     specified vehicle NEC (traffic) V76.5 ☑
      nontraffic V76.0 ☑
     stationary object (traffic) V77.5 ☑
      nontraffic V77.0 ☑
     streetcar (traffic) V76.5 ☑
      nontraffic V76.0 ☑
     three wheeled motor vehicle (traffic) V72.5 ☑
      nontraffic V72.0 ☑
     truck (traffic) V74.5 ☑
      nontraffic V74.0 ☑
     two wheeled motor vehicle (traffic) V72.5 ☑
      nontraffic V72.0 ☑
     van (traffic) V73.5 ☑
      nontraffic V73.0 ☑
    noncollision accident (traffic) V78.5 ☑
     nontraffic V78.0 ☑
   hanger-on
    collision (with)
     animal (traffic) V70.7 ☑
      being ridden (traffic) V76.7 ☑
       nontraffic V76.2 ☑
      nontraffic V70.2 ☑
     animal-drawn vehicle (traffic) V76.7 ☑
      nontraffic V76.2 ☑
     bus (traffic) V74.7 ☑
      nontraffic V74.2 ☑
     car (traffic) V73.7 ☑
      nontraffic V73.2 ☑
     pedal cycle (traffic) V71.7 ☑
      nontraffic V71.2 ☑
     pickup truck (traffic) V73.7 ☑
      nontraffic V73.2 ☑
     railway vehicle (traffic) V75.7 ☑
      nontraffic V75.2 ☑
     specified vehicle NEC (traffic) V76.7 ☑
      nontraffic V76.2 ☑
     stationary object (traffic) V77.7 ☑
      nontraffic V77.2 ☑
     streetcar (traffic) V76.7 ☑
      nontraffic V76.2 ☑
     three wheeled motor vehicle (traffic) V72.7 ☑
      nontraffic V72.2 ☑
     truck (traffic) V74.7 ☑
      nontraffic V74.2 ☑
     two wheeled motor vehicle (traffic) V72.7 ☑
      nontraffic V72.2 ☑
     van (traffic) V73.7 ☑
      nontraffic V73.2 ☑
    noncollision accident (traffic) V78.7 ☑
     nontraffic V78.2 ☑

☑ **Additional Character Required — Refer to the Tabular List for Character Selection**   ▽ **Subterms under main terms may continue to next column or page**

Accident — *continued*
　transport — *continued*
　　bus occupant — *continued*
　　　noncollision accident (traffic) V78.9 ☑
　　　　nontraffic V78.3 ☑
　　　　while boarding or alighting V78.4 ☑
　　　nontraffic V79.3 ☑
　　　passenger
　　　　collision (with)
　　　　　animal (traffic) V70.6 ☑
　　　　　　being ridden (traffic) V76.6 ☑
　　　　　　　nontraffic V76.1 ☑
　　　　　　nontraffic V70.1 ☑
　　　　　animal-drawn vehicle (traffic) V76.6 ☑
　　　　　　nontraffic V76.1 ☑
　　　　　bus (traffic) V74.6 ☑
　　　　　　nontraffic V74.1 ☑
　　　　　car (traffic) V73.6 ☑
　　　　　　nontraffic V73.1 ☑
　　　　　motor vehicle NOS (traffic) V79.50 ☑
　　　　　　nontraffic V79.10 ☑
　　　　　　specified type NEC (traffic) V79.59 ☑
　　　　　　　nontraffic V79.19 ☑
　　　　　pedal cycle (traffic) V71.6 ☑
　　　　　　nontraffic V71.1 ☑
　　　　　pickup truck (traffic) V73.6 ☑
　　　　　　nontraffic V73.1 ☑
　　　　　railway vehicle (traffic) V75.6 ☑
　　　　　　nontraffic V75.1 ☑
　　　　　specified vehicle NEC (traffic) V76.6 ☑
　　　　　　nontraffic V76.1 ☑
　　　　　stationary object (traffic) V77.6 ☑
　　　　　　nontraffic V77.1 ☑
　　　　　streetcar (traffic) V76.6 ☑
　　　　　　nontraffic V76.1 ☑
　　　　　three wheeled motor vehicle (traffic)
　　　　　　V72.6 ☑
　　　　　　nontraffic V72.1 ☑
　　　　　truck (traffic) V74.6 ☑
　　　　　　nontraffic V74.1 ☑
　　　　　two wheeled motor vehicle (traffic)
　　　　　　V72.6 ☑
　　　　　　nontraffic V72.1 ☑
　　　　　van (traffic) V73.6 ☑
　　　　　　nontraffic V73.1 ☑
　　　　noncollision accident (traffic) V78.6 ☑
　　　　　nontraffic V78.1 ☑
　　　specified type NEC V79.88 ☑
　　　military vehicle V79.81 ☑
　　cable car, not on rails V98.0 ☑
　　　on rails — *see* Accident, transport, streetcar
　　　　occupant
　　car occupant V49.9 ☑
　　　ambulance occupant — *see* Accident, transport,
　　　　ambulance occupant
　　　collision (with)
　　　　animal (traffic) V40.9 ☑
　　　　　being ridden (traffic) V46.9 ☑
　　　　　　nontraffic V46.3 ☑
　　　　　　while boarding or alighting V46.4 ☑
　　　　　nontraffic V40.3 ☑
　　　　　while boarding or alighting V40.4 ☑
　　　　animal-drawn vehicle (traffic) V46.9 ☑
　　　　　nontraffic V46.3 ☑
　　　　　while boarding or alighting V46.4 ☑
　　　　bus (traffic) V44.9 ☑
　　　　　nontraffic V44.3 ☑
　　　　　while boarding or alighting V44.4 ☑
　　　　car (traffic) V43.92 ☑
　　　　　nontraffic V43.32 ☑
　　　　　while boarding or alighting V43.42 ☑
　　　　motor vehicle NOS (traffic) V49.60 ☑
　　　　　nontraffic V49.20 ☑
　　　　　specified type NEC (traffic) V49.69 ☑
　　　　　　nontraffic V49.29 ☑
　　　　pedal cycle (traffic) V41.9 ☑
　　　　　nontraffic V41.3 ☑
　　　　　while boarding or alighting V41.4 ☑
　　　　pickup truck (traffic) V43.93 ☑
　　　　　nontraffic V43.33 ☑
　　　　　while boarding or alighting V43.43 ☑
　　　　railway vehicle (traffic) V45.9 ☑
　　　　　nontraffic V45.3 ☑
　　　　　while boarding or alighting V45.4 ☑
　　　　specified vehicle NEC (traffic) V46.9 ☑
　　　　　nontraffic V46.3 ☑

Accident — *continued*
　transport — *continued*
　　car occupant — *continued*
　　　collision — *continued*
　　　　specified vehicle — *continued*
　　　　　while boarding or alighting V46.4 ☑
　　　　sport utility vehicle (traffic) V43.91 ☑
　　　　　nontraffic V43.31 ☑
　　　　　while boarding or alighting V43.41 ☑
　　　　stationary object (traffic) V47.9 ☑
　　　　　nontraffic V47.3 ☑
　　　　　while boarding or alighting V47.4 ☑
　　　　streetcar (traffic) V46.9 ☑
　　　　　nontraffic V46.3 ☑
　　　　　while boarding or alighting V46.4 ☑
　　　　three wheeled motor vehicle (traffic)
　　　　　V42.9 ☑
　　　　　nontraffic V42.3 ☑
　　　　　while boarding or alighting V42.4 ☑
　　　　truck (traffic) V44.9 ☑
　　　　　nontraffic V44.3 ☑
　　　　　while boarding or alighting V44.4 ☑
　　　　two wheeled motor vehicle (traffic) V42.9 ☑
　　　　　nontraffic V42.3 ☑
　　　　　while boarding or alighting V42.4 ☑
　　　　van (traffic) V43.94 ☑
　　　　　nontraffic V43.34 ☑
　　　　　while boarding or alighting V43.44 ☑
　　　driver
　　　　collision (with)
　　　　　animal (traffic) V40.5 ☑
　　　　　　being ridden (traffic) V46.5 ☑
　　　　　　　nontraffic V46.0 ☑
　　　　　　nontraffic V40.0 ☑
　　　　　animal-drawn vehicle (traffic) V46.5 ☑
　　　　　　nontraffic V46.0 ☑
　　　　　bus (traffic) V44.5 ☑
　　　　　　nontraffic V44.0 ☑
　　　　　car (traffic) V43.52 ☑
　　　　　　nontraffic V43.02 ☑
　　　　　motor vehicle NOS (traffic) V49.40 ☑
　　　　　　nontraffic V49.00 ☑
　　　　　　specified type NEC (traffic) V49.49 ☑
　　　　　　　nontraffic V49.09 ☑
　　　　　pedal cycle (traffic) V41.5 ☑
　　　　　　nontraffic V41.0 ☑
　　　　　pickup truck (traffic) V43.53 ☑
　　　　　　nontraffic V43.03 ☑
　　　　　railway vehicle (traffic) V45.5 ☑
　　　　　　nontraffic V45.0 ☑
　　　　　specified vehicle NEC (traffic) V46.5 ☑
　　　　　　nontraffic V46.0 ☑
　　　　　sport utility vehicle (traffic) V43.51 ☑
　　　　　　nontraffic V43.01 ☑
　　　　　stationary object (traffic) V47.5 ☑
　　　　　　nontraffic V47.0 ☑
　　　　　streetcar (traffic) V46.5 ☑
　　　　　　nontraffic V46.0 ☑
　　　　　three wheeled motor vehicle (traffic)
　　　　　　V42.5 ☑
　　　　　　nontraffic V42.0 ☑
　　　　　truck (traffic) V44.5 ☑
　　　　　　nontraffic V44.0 ☑
　　　　　two wheeled motor vehicle (traffic)
　　　　　　V42.5 ☑
　　　　　　nontraffic V42.0 ☑
　　　　　van (traffic) V43.54 ☑
　　　　　　nontraffic V43.04 ☑
　　　　noncollision accident (traffic) V48.5 ☑
　　　　　nontraffic V48.0 ☑
　　　hanger-on
　　　　collision (with)
　　　　　animal (traffic) V40.7 ☑
　　　　　　being ridden (traffic) V46.7 ☑
　　　　　　　nontraffic V46.2 ☑
　　　　　　nontraffic V40.2 ☑
　　　　　animal-drawn vehicle (traffic) V46.7 ☑
　　　　　　nontraffic V46.2 ☑
　　　　　bus (traffic) V44.7 ☑
　　　　　　nontraffic V44.2 ☑
　　　　　car (traffic) V43.72 ☑
　　　　　　nontraffic V43.22 ☑
　　　　　pedal cycle (traffic) V41.7 ☑
　　　　　　nontraffic V41.2 ☑
　　　　　pickup truck (traffic) V43.73 ☑
　　　　　　nontraffic V43.23 ☑

Accident — *continued*
　transport — *continued*
　　car occupant — *continued*
　　　hanger-on — *continued*
　　　　collision — *continued*
　　　　　railway vehicle (traffic) V45.7 ☑
　　　　　　nontraffic V45.2 ☑
　　　　　specified vehicle NEC (traffic) V46.7 ☑
　　　　　　nontraffic V46.2 ☑
　　　　　sport utility vehicle (traffic) V43.71 ☑
　　　　　　nontraffic V43.21 ☑
　　　　　stationary object (traffic) V47.7 ☑
　　　　　　nontraffic V47.2 ☑
　　　　　streetcar (traffic) V46.7 ☑
　　　　　　nontraffic V46.2 ☑
　　　　　three wheeled motor vehicle (traffic)
　　　　　　V42.7 ☑
　　　　　　nontraffic V42.2 ☑
　　　　　truck (traffic) V44.7 ☑
　　　　　　nontraffic V44.2 ☑
　　　　　two wheeled motor vehicle (traffic)
　　　　　　V42.7 ☑
　　　　　　nontraffic V42.2 ☑
　　　　　van (traffic) V43.74 ☑
　　　　　　nontraffic V43.24 ☑
　　　　noncollision accident (traffic) V48.7 ☑
　　　　　nontraffic V48.2 ☑
　　　noncollision accident (traffic) V48.9 ☑
　　　　nontraffic V48.3 ☑
　　　　while boarding or alighting V48.4 ☑
　　　nontraffic V49.3 ☑
　　　passenger
　　　　collision (with)
　　　　　animal (traffic) V40.6 ☑
　　　　　　being ridden (traffic) V46.6 ☑
　　　　　　　nontraffic V46.1 ☑
　　　　　　nontraffic V40.1 ☑
　　　　　animal-drawn vehicle (traffic) V46.6 ☑
　　　　　　nontraffic V46.1 ☑
　　　　　bus (traffic) V44.6 ☑
　　　　　　nontraffic V44.1 ☑
　　　　　car (traffic) V43.62 ☑
　　　　　　nontraffic V43.12 ☑
　　　　　motor vehicle NOS (traffic) V49.50 ☑
　　　　　　nontraffic V49.10 ☑
　　　　　　specified type NEC (traffic) V49.59 ☑
　　　　　　　nontraffic V49.19 ☑
　　　　　pedal cycle (traffic) V41.6 ☑
　　　　　　nontraffic V41.1 ☑
　　　　　pickup truck (traffic) V43.63 ☑
　　　　　　nontraffic V43.13 ☑
　　　　　railway vehicle (traffic) V45.6 ☑
　　　　　　nontraffic V45.1 ☑
　　　　　specified vehicle NEC (traffic) V46.6 ☑
　　　　　　nontraffic V46.1 ☑
　　　　　sport utility vehicle (traffic) V43.61 ☑
　　　　　　nontraffic V43.11 ☑
　　　　　stationary object (traffic) V47.6 ☑
　　　　　　nontraffic V47.1 ☑
　　　　　streetcar (traffic) V46.6 ☑
　　　　　　nontraffic V46.1 ☑
　　　　　three wheeled motor vehicle (traffic)
　　　　　　V42.6 ☑
　　　　　　nontraffic V42.1 ☑
　　　　　truck (traffic) V44.6 ☑
　　　　　　nontraffic V44.1 ☑
　　　　　two wheeled motor vehicle (traffic)
　　　　　　V42.6 ☑
　　　　　　nontraffic V42.1 ☑
　　　　　van (traffic) V43.64 ☑
　　　　　　nontraffic V43.14 ☑
　　　　noncollision accident (traffic) V48.6 ☑
　　　　　nontraffic V48.1 ☑
　　　specified type NEC V49.88 ☑
　　　military vehicle V49.81 ☑
　　coal car — *see* Accident, transport, industrial vehi-
　　　cle occupant
　　construction vehicle occupant (nontraffic) V85.9 ☑
　　　driver V85.5 ☑
　　　hanger-on V85.7 ☑
　　　passenger V85.6 ☑
　　　traffic V85.3 ☑
　　　　driver V85.0 ☑
　　　　hanger-on V85.2 ☑
　　　　passenger V85.1 ☑
　　　while boarding or alighting V85.4 ☑

External Causes Index

Accident — *continued*
  transport — *continued*
    dirt bike rider (nontraffic) V86.96 ☑
      driver V86.56 ☑
      hanger-on V86.76 ☑
      passenger V86.66 ☑
      traffic V86.36 ☑
        driver V86.06 ☑
        hanger-on V86.26 ☑
        passenger V86.16 ☑
      while boarding or alighting V86.46 ☑
    due to cataclysm — *see* Forces of nature, by type
    dune buggy occupant (nontraffic) V86.93 ☑
      driver V86.53 ☑
      hanger-on V86.73 ☑
      passenger V86.63 ☑
      traffic V86.33 ☑
        driver V86.03 ☑
        hanger-on V86.23 ☑
        passenger V86.13 ☑
      while boarding or alighting V86.43 ☑
    forklift — *see* Accident, transport, industrial vehicle occupant
    go cart — *see* Accident, transport, all-terrain vehicle occupant
    golf cart — *see* Accident, transport, all-terrain vehicle occupant
    heavy transport vehicle occupant — *see* Accident, transport, truck occupant
    ice yacht V98.2 ☑
    industrial vehicle occupant (nontraffic) V83.9 ☑
      driver V83.5 ☑
      hanger-on V83.7 ☑
      passenger V83.6 ☑
      traffic V83.3 ☑
        driver V83.0 ☑
        hanger-on V83.2 ☑
        passenger V83.1 ☑
      while boarding or alighting V83.4 ☑
    interurban electric car — *see* Accident, transport, streetcar
    land yacht V98.1 ☑
    logging car — *see* Accident, transport, industrial vehicle occupant
    military vehicle occupant (traffic) V86.34 ☑
      driver V86.04 ☑
      hanger-on V86.24 ☑
      nontraffic V86.94 ☑
        driver V86.54 ☑
        hanger-on V86.74 ☑
        passenger V86.64 ☑
      passenger V86.14 ☑
      while boarding or alighting V86.44 ☑
    mine tram — *see* Accident, transport, industrial vehicle occupant
    motor vehicle NEC occupant (traffic) V89.2 ☑
    motorcoach — *see* Accident, transport, bus occupant
    motor/cross bike rider (*see also* Accident, transport, dirt bike rider) V86.96 ☑
    motorcyclist V29.9 ☑
      collision (with)
        animal (traffic) V20.9 ☑
          being ridden (traffic) V26.9 ☑
            nontraffic V26.2 ☑
            while boarding or alighting V26.3 ☑
          nontraffic V20.2 ☑
          while boarding or alighting V20.3 ☑
        animal-drawn vehicle (traffic) V26.9 ☑
          nontraffic V26.2 ☑
          while boarding or alighting V26.3 ☑
        bus (traffic) V24.9 ☑
          nontraffic V24.2 ☑
          while boarding or alighting V24.3 ☑
        car (traffic) V23.9 ☑
          nontraffic V23.2 ☑
          while boarding or alighting V23.3 ☑
        motor vehicle NOS (traffic) V29.60 ☑
          nontraffic V29.20 ☑
          specified type NEC (traffic) V29.69 ☑
            nontraffic V29.29 ☑
        pedal cycle (traffic) V21.9 ☑
          nontraffic V21.2 ☑
          while boarding or alighting V21.3 ☑
        pickup truck (traffic) V23.9 ☑
          nontraffic V23.2 ☑

Accident — *continued*
  transport — *continued*
    motorcyclist — *continued*
      collision — *continued*
        pickup truck — *continued*
          while boarding or alighting V23.3 ☑
        railway vehicle (traffic) V25.9 ☑
          nontraffic V25.2 ☑
          while boarding or alighting V25.3 ☑
        specified vehicle NEC (traffic) V26.9 ☑
          nontraffic V26.2 ☑
          while boarding or alighting V26.3 ☑
        stationary object (traffic) V27.9 ☑
          nontraffic V27.2 ☑
          while boarding or alighting V27.3 ☑
        streetcar (traffic) V26.9 ☑
          nontraffic V26.2 ☑
          while boarding or alighting V26.3 ☑
        three wheeled motor vehicle (traffic) V22.9 ☑
          nontraffic V22.2 ☑
          while boarding or alighting V22.3 ☑
        truck (traffic) V24.9 ☑
          nontraffic V24.2 ☑
          while boarding or alighting V24.3 ☑
        two wheeled motor vehicle (traffic) V22.9 ☑
          nontraffic V22.2 ☑
          while boarding or alighting V22.3 ☑
        van (traffic) V23.9 ☑
          nontraffic V23.2 ☑
          while boarding or alighting V23.3 ☑
      driver
        collision (with)
          animal (traffic) V20.4 ☑
            being ridden (traffic) V26.4 ☑
              nontraffic V26.0 ☑
            nontraffic V20.0 ☑
          animal-drawn vehicle (traffic) V26.4 ☑
            nontraffic V26.0 ☑
          bus (traffic) V24.4 ☑
            nontraffic V24.0 ☑
          car (traffic) V23.4 ☑
            nontraffic V23.0 ☑
          motor vehicle NOS (traffic) V29.40 ☑
            nontraffic V29.00 ☑
            specified type NEC (traffic) V29.49 ☑
              nontraffic V29.09 ☑
          pedal cycle (traffic) V21.4 ☑
            nontraffic V21.0 ☑
          pickup truck (traffic) V23.4 ☑
            nontraffic V23.0 ☑
          railway vehicle (traffic) V25.4 ☑
            nontraffic V25.0 ☑
          specified vehicle NEC (traffic) V26.4 ☑
            nontraffic V26.0 ☑
          stationary object (traffic) V27.4 ☑
            nontraffic V27.0 ☑
          streetcar (traffic) V26.4 ☑
            nontraffic V26.0 ☑
          three wheeled motor vehicle (traffic) V22.4 ☑
            nontraffic V22.0 ☑
          truck (traffic) V24.4 ☑
            nontraffic V24.0 ☑
          two wheeled motor vehicle (traffic) V22.4 ☑
            nontraffic V22.0 ☑
          van (traffic) V23.4 ☑
            nontraffic V23.0 ☑
          noncollision accident (traffic) V28.4 ☑
            nontraffic V28.0 ☑
      noncollision accident (traffic) V28.9 ☑
        nontraffic V28.2 ☑
        while boarding or alighting V28.3 ☑
      nontraffic V29.3 ☑
      passenger
        collision (with)
          animal (traffic) V20.5 ☑
            being ridden (traffic) V26.5 ☑
              nontraffic V26.1 ☑
            nontraffic V20.1 ☑
          animal-drawn vehicle (traffic) V26.5 ☑
            nontraffic V26.1 ☑
          bus (traffic) V24.5 ☑
            nontraffic V24.1 ☑
          car (traffic) V23.5 ☑

Accident — *continued*
  transport — *continued*
    motorcyclist — *continued*
      passenger — *continued*
        collision — *continued*
          car — *continued*
            nontraffic V23.1 ☑
          motor vehicle NOS (traffic) V29.50 ☑
            nontraffic V29.10 ☑
            specified type NEC (traffic) V29.59 ☑
              nontraffic V29.19 ☑
          pedal cycle (traffic) V21.5 ☑
            nontraffic V21.1 ☑
          pickup truck (traffic) V23.5 ☑
            nontraffic V23.1 ☑
          railway vehicle (traffic) V25.5 ☑
            nontraffic V25.1 ☑
          specified vehicle NEC (traffic) V26.5 ☑
            nontraffic V26.1 ☑
          stationary object (traffic) V27.5 ☑
            nontraffic V27.1 ☑
          streetcar (traffic) V26.5 ☑
            nontraffic V26.1 ☑
          three wheeled motor vehicle (traffic) V22.5 ☑
            nontraffic V22.1 ☑
          truck (traffic) V24.5 ☑
            nontraffic V24.1 ☑
          two wheeled motor vehicle (traffic) V22.5 ☑
            nontraffic V22.1 ☑
          van (traffic) V23.5 ☑
            nontraffic V23.1 ☑
        noncollision accident (traffic) V28.5 ☑
          nontraffic V28.1 ☑
      specified type NEC V29.88 ☑
        military vehicle V29.81 ☑
    occupant (of)
      aircraft (powered) V95.9 ☑
        fixed wing
          commercial — *see* Accident, transport, aircraft, occupant, powered, fixed wing, commercial
          private — *see* Accident, transport, aircraft, occupant, powered, fixed wing, private
        nonpowered V96.9 ☑
        specified NEC V95.8 ☑
      airport battery-powered vehicle — *see* Accident, transport, industrial vehicle occupant
      all-terrain vehicle (ATV) — *see* Accident, transport, all-terrain vehicle occupant
      animal-drawn vehicle — *see* Accident, transport, animal-drawn vehicle occupant
      automobile — *see* Accident, transport, car occupant
      balloon V96.00 ☑
      battery-powered vehicle — *see* Accident, transport, industrial vehicle occupant
      bicycle — *see* Accident, transport, pedal cyclist
        motorized — *see* Accident, transport, motorcycle rider
      boat NEC — *see* Accident, watercraft
      bulldozer — *see* Accident, transport, construction vehicle occupant
      bus — *see* Accident, transport, bus occupant
      cable car (on rails) (*see also* Accident, transport, streetcar occupant)
        not on rails V98.0 ☑
      car (*see also* Accident, transport, car occupant)
        cable (on rails) (*see also* Accident, transport, streetcar occupant)
          not on rails V98.0 ☑
      coach — *see* Accident, transport, bus occupant
      coal-car — *see* Accident, transport, industrial vehicle occupant
      digger — *see* Accident, transport, construction vehicle occupant
      dump truck — *see* Accident, transport, construction vehicle occupant
      earth-leveler — *see* Accident, transport, construction vehicle occupant
      farm machinery (self-propelled) — *see* Accident, transport, agricultural vehicle occupant

   ☑ **Additional Character Required — Refer to the Tabular List for Character Selection**   ▽ **Subterms under main terms may continue to next column or page**

Accident — *continued*
  transport — *continued*
    occupant — *continued*
      forklift — *see* Accident, transport, industrial vehicle occupant
      glider (unpowered) V96.20 ☑
        hang V96.10 ☑
        powered (microlight) (ultralight) — *see* Accident, transport, aircraft, occupant, powered, glider
      glider (unpowered) NEC V96.20 ☑
      hang-glider V96.10 ☑
      harvester — *see* Accident, transport, agricultural vehicle occupant
      heavy (transport) vehicle — *see* Accident, transport, truck occupant
      helicopter — *see* Accident, transport, aircraft, occupant, helicopter
      ice-yacht V98.2 ☑
      kite (carrying person) V96.8 ☑
      land-yacht V98.1 ☑
      logging car — *see* Accident, transport, industrial vehicle occupant
      mechanical shovel — *see* Accident, transport, construction vehicle occupant
      microlight — *see* Accident, transport, aircraft, occupant, powered, glider
      minibus — *see* Accident, transport, pickup truck occupant
      minivan — *see* Accident, transport, pickup truck occupant
      moped — *see* Accident, transport, motorcycle
      motor scooter — *see* Accident, transport, motorcycle
      motorcycle (with sidecar) — *see* Accident, transport, motorcycle
      off-road motor-vehicle (*see also* Accident, transport, all-terrain vehicle occupant) V86.99 ☑
      pedal cycle (*see also* Accident, transport, pedal cyclist)
      pick-up (truck) — *see* Accident, transport, pickup truck occupant
      railway (train) (vehicle) (subterranean) (elevated) — *see* Accident, transport, railway vehicle occupant
      rickshaw — *see* Accident, transport, pedal cycle
        motorized — *see* Accident, transport, three-wheeled motor vehicle
        pedal driven — *see* Accident, transport, pedal cyclist
      road-roller — *see* Accident, transport, construction vehicle occupant
      ship NOS V94.9 ☑
      ski-lift (chair) (gondola) V98.3 ☑
      snowmobile — *see* Accident, transport, snowmobile occupant
      spacecraft, spaceship — *see* Accident, transport, aircraft, occupant, spacecraft
      sport utility vehicle — *see* Accident, transport, pickup truck occupant
      streetcar (interurban) (operating on public street or highway) — *see* Accident, transport, streetcar occupant
      SUV — *see* Accident, transport, pickup truck occupant
      téléférique V98.0 ☑
      three-wheeled vehicle (motorized) (*see also* Accident, transport, three-wheeled motor vehicle occupant)
        nonmotorized — *see* Accident, transport, pedal cycle
      tractor (farm) (and trailer) — *see* Accident, transport, agricultural vehicle occupant
      train — *see* Accident, transport, railway vehicle occupant
      tram — *see* Accident, transport, streetcar occupant
        in mine or quarry — *see* Accident, transport, industrial vehicle occupant
      tricycle — *see* Accident, transport, pedal cycle
        motorized — *see* Accident, transport, three-wheeled motor vehicle
      trolley — *see* Accident, transport, streetcar occupant
        in mine or quarry — *see* Accident, transport, industrial vehicle occupant

Accident — *continued*
  transport — *continued*
    occupant — *continued*
      tub, in mine or quarry — *see* Accident, transport, industrial vehicle occupant
      ultralight — *see* Accident, transport, aircraft, occupant, powered, glider
      van — *see* Accident, transport, van occupant
      vehicle NEC V89.9 ☑
        heavy transport — *see* Accident, transport, truck occupant
        motor (traffic) NEC V89.2 ☑
        nontraffic NEC V89.0 ☑
      watercraft NOS V94.9 ☑
        causing drowning — *see* Drowning, resulting from accident to boat
    off-road motor-vehicle (*see also* Accident, transport, all-terrain vehicle occupant) V86.99 ☑
    parachutist V97.29 ☑
      after accident to aircraft — *see* Accident, transport, aircraft
      entangled in object V97.21 ☑
      injured on landing V97.22 ☑
    pedal cyclist V19.9 ☑
      collision (with)
        animal (traffic) V10.9 ☑
          being ridden (traffic) V16.9 ☑
            nontraffic V16.2 ☑
            while boarding or alighting V16.3 ☑
          nontraffic V10.2 ☑
          while boarding or alighting V10.3 ☑
        animal-drawn vehicle (traffic) V16.9 ☑
          nontraffic V16.2 ☑
          while boarding or alighting V16.3 ☑
        bus (traffic) V14.9 ☑
          nontraffic V14.2 ☑
          while boarding or alighting V14.3 ☑
        car (traffic) V13.9 ☑
          nontraffic V13.2 ☑
          while boarding or alighting V13.3 ☑
        motor vehicle NOS (traffic) V19.60 ☑
          nontraffic V19.20 ☑
          specified type NEC (traffic) V19.69 ☑
            nontraffic V19.29 ☑
        pedal cycle (traffic) V11.9 ☑
          nontraffic V11.2 ☑
          while boarding or alighting V11.3 ☑
        pickup truck (traffic) V13.9 ☑
          nontraffic V13.2 ☑
          while boarding or alighting V13.3 ☑
        railway vehicle (traffic) V15.9 ☑
          nontraffic V15.2 ☑
          while boarding or alighting V15.3 ☑
        specified vehicle NEC (traffic) V16.9 ☑
          nontraffic V16.2 ☑
          while boarding or alighting V16.3 ☑
        stationary object (traffic) V17.9 ☑
          nontraffic V17.2 ☑
          while boarding or alighting V17.3 ☑
        streetcar (traffic) V16.9 ☑
          nontraffic V16.2 ☑
          while boarding or alighting V16.3 ☑
        three wheeled motor vehicle (traffic) V12.9 ☑
          nontraffic V12.2 ☑
          while boarding or alighting V12.3 ☑
        truck (traffic) V14.9 ☑
          nontraffic V14.2 ☑
          while boarding or alighting V14.3 ☑
        two wheeled motor vehicle (traffic) V12.9 ☑
          nontraffic V12.2 ☑
          while boarding or alighting V12.3 ☑
        van (traffic) V13.9 ☑
          nontraffic V13.2 ☑
          while boarding or alighting V13.3 ☑
      driver
        collision (with)
          animal (traffic) V10.4 ☑
            being ridden (traffic) V16.4 ☑
              nontraffic V16.0 ☑
            nontraffic V10.0 ☑
          animal-drawn vehicle (traffic) V16.4 ☑
            nontraffic V16.0 ☑
          bus (traffic) V14.4 ☑
            nontraffic V14.0 ☑
          car (traffic) V13.4 ☑

Accident — *continued*
  transport — *continued*
    pedal cyclist — *continued*
      driver — *continued*
        collision — *continued*
          car — *continued*
            nontraffic V13.0 ☑
          motor vehicle NOS (traffic) V19.40 ☑
            nontraffic V19.00 ☑
            specified type NEC (traffic) V19.49 ☑
              nontraffic V19.09 ☑
          pedal cycle (traffic) V11.4 ☑
            nontraffic V11.0 ☑
          pickup truck (traffic) V13.4 ☑
            nontraffic V13.0 ☑
          railway vehicle (traffic) V15.4 ☑
            nontraffic V15.0 ☑
          specified vehicle NEC (traffic) V16.4 ☑
            nontraffic V16.0 ☑
          stationary object (traffic) V17.4 ☑
            nontraffic V17.0 ☑
          streetcar (traffic) V16.4 ☑
            nontraffic V16.0 ☑
          three wheeled motor vehicle (traffic) V12.4 ☑
            nontraffic V12.0 ☑
          truck (traffic) V14.4 ☑
            nontraffic V14.0 ☑
          two wheeled motor vehicle (traffic) V12.4 ☑
            nontraffic V12.0 ☑
          van (traffic) V13.4 ☑
            nontraffic V13.0 ☑
        noncollision accident (traffic) V18.4 ☑
          nontraffic V18.0 ☑
      noncollision accident (traffic) V18.9 ☑
        nontraffic V18.2 ☑
        while boarding or alighting V18.3 ☑
      nontraffic V19.3 ☑
      passenger
        collision (with)
          animal (traffic) V10.5 ☑
            being ridden (traffic) V16.5 ☑
              nontraffic V16.1 ☑
            nontraffic V10.1 ☑
          animal-drawn vehicle (traffic) V16.5 ☑
            nontraffic V16.1 ☑
          bus (traffic) V14.5 ☑
            nontraffic V14.1 ☑
          car (traffic) V13.5 ☑
            nontraffic V13.1 ☑
          motor vehicle NOS (traffic) V19.50 ☑
            nontraffic V19.10 ☑
            specified type NEC (traffic) V19.59 ☑
              nontraffic V19.19 ☑
          pedal cycle (traffic) V11.5 ☑
            nontraffic V11.1 ☑
          pickup truck (traffic) V13.5 ☑
            nontraffic V13.1 ☑
          railway vehicle (traffic) V15.5 ☑
            nontraffic V15.1 ☑
          specified vehicle NEC (traffic) V16.5 ☑
            nontraffic V16.1 ☑
          stationary object (traffic) V17.5 ☑
            nontraffic V17.1 ☑
          streetcar (traffic) V16.5 ☑
            nontraffic V16.1 ☑
          three wheeled motor vehicle (traffic) V12.5 ☑
            nontraffic V12.1 ☑
          truck (traffic) V14.5 ☑
            nontraffic V14.1 ☑
          two wheeled motor vehicle (traffic) V12.5 ☑
            nontraffic V12.1 ☑
          van (traffic) V13.5 ☑
            nontraffic V13.1 ☑
        noncollision accident (traffic) V18.5 ☑
          nontraffic V18.1 ☑
      specified type NEC V19.88 ☑
        military vehicle V19.81 ☑
    pedestrian
      conveyance (occupant) V09.9 ☑
        babystroller V00.828 ☑
          collision (with) V09.9 ☑

Accident — *continued*
  transport — *continued*
    pedestrian — *continued*
      conveyance — *continued*
        babystroller — *continued*
          collision — *continued*
            animal being ridden or animal drawn vehicle V06.99 ☑
              nontraffic V06.09 ☑
              traffic V06.19 ☑
            bus or heavy transport V04.99 ☑
              nontraffic V04.09 ☑
              traffic V04.19 ☑
            car V03.99 ☑
              nontraffic V03.09 ☑
              traffic V03.19 ☑
            pedal cycle V01.99 ☑
              nontraffic V01.09 ☑
              traffic V01.19 ☑
            pick-up truck or van V03.99 ☑
              nontraffic V03.09 ☑
              traffic V03.19 ☑
            railway (train) (vehicle) V05.99 ☑
              nontraffic V05.09 ☑
              traffic V05.19 ☑
            stationary object V00.822 ☑
            streetcar V06.99 ☑
              nontraffic V06.09 ☑
              traffic V06.19 ☑
            two- or three-wheeled motor vehicle V02.99 ☑
              nontraffic V02.09 ☑
              traffic V02.19 ☑
            vehicle V09.9 ☑
              animal-drawn V06.99 ☑
                nontraffic V06.09 ☑
                traffic V06.19 ☑
              motor
                nontraffic V09.00 ☑
                traffic V09.20 ☑
           fall V00.821 ☑
          nontraffic V09.1 ☑
            involving motor vehicle NEC V09.00 ☑
          traffic V09.3 ☑
            involving motor vehicle NEC V09.20 ☑
        flat-bottomed NEC V00.388 ☑
          collision (with) V09.9 ☑
            animal being ridden or animal drawn vehicle V06.99 ☑
              nontraffic V06.09 ☑
              traffic V06.19 ☑
            bus or heavy transport V04.99 ☑
              nontraffic V04.09 ☑
              traffic V04.19 ☑
            car V03.99 ☑
              nontraffic V03.09 ☑
              traffic V03.19 ☑
            pedal cycle V01.99 ☑
              nontraffic V01.09 ☑
              traffic V01.19 ☑
            pick-up truck or van V03.99 ☑
              nontraffic V03.09 ☑
              traffic V03.19 ☑
            railway (train) (vehicle) V05.99 ☑
              nontraffic V05.09 ☑
              traffic V05.19 ☑
            stationary object V00.382 ☑
            streetcar V06.99 ☑
              nontraffic V06.09 ☑
              traffic V06.19 ☑
            two- or three-wheeled motor vehicle V02.99 ☑
              nontraffic V02.09 ☑
              traffic V02.19 ☑
            vehicle V09.9 ☑
              animal-drawn V06.99 ☑
                nontraffic V06.09 ☑
                traffic V06.19 ☑
              motor
                nontraffic V09.00 ☑
                traffic V09.20 ☑
           fall V00.381 ☑
          nontraffic V09.1 ☑

Accident — *continued*
  transport — *continued*
    pedestrian — *continued*
      conveyance — *continued*
        flat-bottomed — *continued*
          nontraffic — *continued*
            involving motor vehicle NEC V09.00 ☑
          snow
            board — *see* Accident, transport, pedestrian, conveyance, snow board
            ski — *see* Accident, transport, pedestrian, conveyance, skis (snow)
          traffic V09.3 ☑
            involving motor vehicle NEC V09.20 ☑
        gliding type NEC V00.288 ☑
          collision (with) V09.9 ☑
            animal being ridden or animal drawn vehicle V06.99 ☑
              nontraffic V06.09 ☑
              traffic V06.19 ☑
            bus or heavy transport V04.99 ☑
              nontraffic V04.09 ☑
              traffic V04.19 ☑
            car V03.99 ☑
              nontraffic V03.09 ☑
              traffic V03.19 ☑
            pedal cycle V01.99 ☑
              nontraffic V01.09 ☑
              traffic V01.19 ☑
            pick-up truck or van V03.99 ☑
              nontraffic V03.09 ☑
              traffic V03.19 ☑
            railway (train) (vehicle) V05.99 ☑
              nontraffic V05.09 ☑
              traffic V05.19 ☑
            stationary object V00.282 ☑
            streetcar V06.99 ☑
              nontraffic V06.09 ☑
              traffic V02.19 ☑
            two- or three-wheeled motor vehicle V02.99 ☑
              nontraffic V02.09 ☑
              traffic V02.19 ☑
            vehicle V09.9 ☑
              animal-drawn V06.99 ☑
                nontraffic V06.09 ☑
                traffic V06.19 ☑
              motor
                nontraffic V09.00 ☑
                traffic V09.20 ☑
         fall V00.281 ☑
        heelies — *see* Accident, transport, pedestrian, conveyance, heelies
        ice skate — *see* Accident, transport, pedestrian, conveyance, ice skate
        nontraffic V09.1 ☑
          involving motor vehicle NEC V09.00 ☑
        sled — *see* Accident, transport, pedestrian, conveyance, sled
        traffic V09.3 ☑
          involving motor vehicle NEC V09.20 ☑
          wheelies — *see* Accident, transport, pedestrian, conveyance, heelies
        heelies V00.158 ☑
          colliding with stationary object V00.152 ☑
          fall V00.151 ☑
        ice skates V00.218 ☑
          collision (with) V09.9 ☑
            animal being ridden or animal drawn vehicle V06.99 ☑
              nontraffic V06.09 ☑
              traffic V06.19 ☑
            bus or heavy transport V04.99 ☑
              nontraffic V04.09 ☑
              traffic V04.19 ☑
            car V03.99 ☑
              nontraffic V03.09 ☑
              traffic V03.19 ☑

Accident — *continued*
  transport — *continued*
    pedestrian — *continued*
      conveyance — *continued*
        ice skates — *continued*
          collision — *continued*
            pedal cycle V01.99 ☑
              nontraffic V01.09 ☑
              traffic V01.19 ☑
            pick-up truck or van V03.99 ☑
              nontraffic V03.09 ☑
              traffic V03.19 ☑
            railway (train) (vehicle) V05.99 ☑
              nontraffic V05.09 ☑
              traffic V05.19 ☑
            stationary object V00.212 ☑
            streetcar V06.99 ☑
              nontraffic V06.09 ☑
              traffic V06.19 ☑
            two- or three-wheeled motor vehicle V02.99 ☑
              nontraffic V02.09 ☑
              traffic V02.19 ☑
            vehicle V09.9 ☑
              animal-drawn V06.99 ☑
                nontraffic V06.09 ☑
                traffic V06.19 ☑
              motor
                nontraffic V09.00 ☑
                traffic V09.20 ☑
         fall V00.211 ☑
        nontraffic V09.1 ☑
          involving motor vehicle NEC V09.00 ☑
        traffic V09.3 ☑
          involving motor vehicle NEC V09.20 ☑
        motorized mobility scooter V00.838 ☑
          collision with stationary object V00.832 ☑
          fall from V00.831 ☑
        nontraffic V09.1 ☑
          involving motor vehicle V09.00 ☑
            military V09.01 ☑
            specified type NEC V09.09 ☑
        roller skates (non in-line) V00.128 ☑
          collision (with) V09.9 ☑
            animal being ridden or animal drawn vehicle V06.91 ☑
              nontraffic V06.01 ☑
              traffic V06.11 ☑
            bus or heavy transport V04.91 ☑
              nontraffic V04.01 ☑
              traffic V04.11 ☑
            car V03.91 ☑
              nontraffic V03.01 ☑
              traffic V03.11 ☑
            pedal cycle V01.91 ☑
              nontraffic V01.01 ☑
              traffic V01.11 ☑
            pick-up truck or van V03.91 ☑
              nontraffic V03.01 ☑
              traffic V03.11 ☑
            railway (train) (vehicle) V05.91 ☑
              nontraffic V05.01 ☑
              traffic V05.11 ☑
            stationary object V00.122 ☑
            streetcar V06.91 ☑
              nontraffic V06.01 ☑
              traffic V06.11 ☑
            two- or three-wheeled motor vehicle V02.91 ☑
              nontraffic V02.01 ☑
              traffic V02.11 ☑
            vehicle V09.9 ☑
              animal-drawn V06.91 ☑
                nontraffic V06.01 ☑
                traffic V06.11 ☑
              motor
                nontraffic V09.00 ☑
                traffic V09.20 ☑
        fall V00.121 ☑
        in-line V00.118 ☑

☑ **Additional Character Required — Refer to the Tabular List for Character Selection**   ▽ **Subterms under main terms may continue to next column or page**

Accident — *continued*
  transport — *continued*
    pedestrian — *continued*
      conveyance — *continued*
        roller skates — *continued*
          in-line — *continued*
            collision — *see also Accident, transport, pedestrian, conveyance occupant, roller skates, collision*
              with stationary object V00.112 ☑
            fall V00.111 ☑
            nontraffic V09.1 ☑
              involving motor vehicle NEC V09.00 ☑
            traffic V09.3 ☑
              involving motor vehicle NEC V09.20 ☑
        rolling shoes V00.158 ☑
          colliding with stationary object V00.152 ☑
          fall V00.151 ☑
        rolling type NEC V00.188 ☑
          collision (with) V09.9 ☑
            animal being ridden or animal drawn vehicle V06.99 ☑
              nontraffic V06.09 ☑
              traffic V06.19 ☑
            bus or heavy transport V04.99 ☑
              nontraffic V04.09 ☑
              traffic V04.19 ☑
            car V03.99 ☑
              nontraffic V03.09 ☑
              traffic V03.19 ☑
            pedal cycle V01.99 ☑
              nontraffic V01.09 ☑
              traffic V01.19 ☑
            pick-up truck or van V03.99 ☑
              nontraffic V03.09 ☑
              traffic V03.19 ☑
            railway (train) (vehicle) V05.99 ☑
              nontraffic V05.09 ☑
              traffic V05.19 ☑
            stationary object V00.182 ☑
            streetcar V06.99 ☑
              nontraffic V06.09 ☑
              traffic V06.19 ☑
            two- or three-wheeled motor vehicle V02.99 ☑
              nontraffic V02.09 ☑
              traffic V02.19 ☑
            vehicle V09.9 ☑
              animal-drawn V06.99 ☑
                nontraffic V06.09 ☑
                traffic V06.19 ☑
              motor
                nontraffic V09.00 ☑
                traffic V09.20 ☑
        fall V00.181 ☑
        in-line roller skate — *see Accident, transport, pedestrian, conveyance, roller skate, in-line*
        nontraffic V09.1 ☑
          involving motor vehicle NEC V09.00 ☑
        roller skate — *see Accident, transport, pedestrian, conveyance, roller skate*
        scooter (non-motorized) — *see Accident, transport, pedestrian, conveyance, scooter*
        skateboard — *see Accident, transport, pedestrian, conveyance, skateboard*
        traffic V09.3 ☑
          involving motor vehicle NEC V09.20 ☑
        scooter (non-motorized) V00.148 ☑
          collision (with) V09.9 ☑
            animal being ridden or animal drawn vehicle V06.99 ☑
              nontraffic V06.09 ☑
              traffic V06.19 ☑
            bus or heavy transport V04.99 ☑
              nontraffic V04.09 ☑
              traffic V04.19 ☑

scooter — *continued*
  collision — *continued*
    car V03.99 ☑
      nontraffic V03.09 ☑
      traffic V03.19 ☑
    pedal cycle V01.99 ☑
      nontraffic V01.09 ☑
      traffic V01.19 ☑
    pick-up truck or van V03.99 ☑
      nontraffic V03.09 ☑
      traffic V03.19 ☑
    railway (train) (vehicle) V05.99 ☑
      nontraffic V05.09 ☑
      traffic V05.19 ☑
    stationary object V00.142 ☑
    streetcar V06.99 ☑
      nontraffic V06.09 ☑
      traffic V06.19 ☑
    two- or three-wheeled motor vehicle V02.99 ☑
      nontraffic V02.09 ☑
      traffic V02.19 ☑
    vehicle V09.9 ☑
      animal-drawn V06.99 ☑
        nontraffic V06.09 ☑
        traffic V06.19 ☑
      motor
        nontraffic V09.00 ☑
        traffic V09.20 ☑
  fall V00.141 ☑
  nontraffic V09.1 ☑
    involving motor vehicle NEC V09.00 ☑
  traffic V09.3 ☑
    involving motor vehicle NEC V09.20 ☑
skate board V00.138 ☑
  collision (with) V09.9 ☑
    animal being ridden or animal drawn vehicle V06.92 ☑
      nontraffic V06.02 ☑
      traffic V06.12 ☑
    bus or heavy transport V04.92 ☑
      nontraffic V04.02 ☑
      traffic V04.12 ☑
    car V03.92 ☑
      nontraffic V03.02 ☑
      traffic V03.12 ☑
    pedal cycle V01.92 ☑
      nontraffic V01.02 ☑
      traffic V01.12 ☑
    pick-up truck or van V03.92 ☑
      nontraffic V03.02 ☑
      traffic V03.12 ☑
    railway (train) (vehicle) V05.92 ☑
      nontraffic V05.02 ☑
      traffic V05.12 ☑
    stationary object V00.132 ☑
    streetcar V06.92 ☑
      nontraffic V06.02 ☑
      traffic V06.12 ☑
    two- or three-wheeled motor vehicle V02.92 ☑
      nontraffic V02.02 ☑
      traffic V02.12 ☑
    vehicle V09.9 ☑
      animal-drawn V06.92 ☑
        nontraffic V06.02 ☑
        traffic V06.12 ☑
      motor
        nontraffic V09.00 ☑
        traffic V09.20 ☑
  fall V00.131 ☑
  nontraffic V09.1 ☑
    involving motor vehicle NEC V09.00 ☑
  traffic V09.3 ☑
    involving motor vehicle NEC V09.20 ☑
skis (snow) V00.328 ☑
  collision (with) V09.9 ☑

skis — *continued*
  collision — *continued*
    animal being ridden or animal drawn vehicle V06.99 ☑
      nontraffic V06.09 ☑
      traffic V06.19 ☑
    bus or heavy transport V04.99 ☑
      nontraffic V04.09 ☑
      traffic V04.19 ☑
    car V03.99 ☑
      nontraffic V03.09 ☑
      traffic V03.19 ☑
    pedal cycle V01.99 ☑
      nontraffic V01.09 ☑
      traffic V01.19 ☑
    pick-up truck or van V03.99 ☑
      nontraffic V03.09 ☑
      traffic V03.19 ☑
    railway (train) (vehicle) V05.99 ☑
      nontraffic V05.09 ☑
      traffic V05.19 ☑
    stationary object V00.322 ☑
    streetcar V06.99 ☑
      nontraffic V06.09 ☑
      traffic V06.19 ☑
    two- or three-wheeled motor vehicle V02.99 ☑
      nontraffic V02.09 ☑
      traffic V02.19 ☑
    vehicle V09.9 ☑
      animal-drawn V06.99 ☑
        nontraffic V06.09 ☑
        traffic V06.19 ☑
      motor
        nontraffic V09.00 ☑
        traffic V09.20 ☑
  fall V00.321 ☑
  nontraffic V09.1 ☑
    involving motor vehicle NEC V09.00 ☑
  traffic V09.3 ☑
    involving motor vehicle NEC V09.20 ☑
sled V00.228 ☑
  collision (with) V09.9 ☑
    animal being ridden or animal drawn vehicle V06.99 ☑
      nontraffic V06.09 ☑
      traffic V06.19 ☑
    bus or heavy transport V04.99 ☑
      nontraffic V04.09 ☑
      traffic V04.19 ☑
    car V03.99 ☑
      nontraffic V03.09 ☑
      traffic V03.19 ☑
    pedal cycle V01.99 ☑
      nontraffic V01.09 ☑
      traffic V01.19 ☑
    pick-up truck or van V03.99 ☑
      nontraffic V03.09 ☑
      traffic V03.19 ☑
    railway (train) (vehicle) V05.99 ☑
      nontraffic V05.09 ☑
      traffic V05.19 ☑
    stationary object V00.222 ☑
    streetcar V06.99 ☑
      nontraffic V06.09 ☑
      traffic V06.19 ☑
    two- or three-wheeled motor vehicle V02.99 ☑
      nontraffic V02.09 ☑
      traffic V02.19 ☑
    vehicle V09.9 ☑
      animal-drawn V06.99 ☑
        nontraffic V06.09 ☑
        traffic V06.19 ☑
      motor
        nontraffic V09.00 ☑
        traffic V09.20 ☑
  fall V00.221 ☑
  nontraffic V09.1 ☑

Accident — *continued*
  transport — *continued*
    pedestrian — *continued*
      conveyance — *continued*
        sled — *continued*
          nontraffic — *continued*
            involving motor vehicle NEC V09.00 ☑
          traffic V09.3 ☑
            involving motor vehicle NEC V09.20 ☑
        snow board V00.318 ☑
          collision (with) V09.9 ☑
            animal being ridden or animal drawn vehicle V06.99 ☑
              nontraffic V06.09 ☑
              traffic V06.19 ☑
            bus or heavy transport V04.99 ☑
              nontraffic V04.09 ☑
              traffic V04.19 ☑
            car V03.99 ☑
              nontraffic V03.09 ☑
              traffic V03.19 ☑
            pedal cycle V01.99 ☑
              nontraffic V01.09 ☑
              traffic V01.19 ☑
            pick-up truck or van V03.99 ☑
              nontraffic V03.09 ☑
              traffic V03.19 ☑
            railway (train) (vehicle) V05.99 ☑
              nontraffic V05.09 ☑
              traffic V05.19 ☑
            stationary object V00.312 ☑
            streetcar V06.99 ☑
              nontraffic V06.09 ☑
              traffic V06.19 ☑
            two- or three-wheeled motor vehicle V02.99 ☑
              nontraffic V02.09 ☑
              traffic V02.19 ☑
            vehicle V09.9 ☑
              animal-drawn V06.99 ☑
                nontraffic V06.09 ☑
                traffic V06.19 ☑
              motor
                nontraffic V09.00 ☑
                traffic V09.20 ☑
          fall V00.311 ☑
          nontraffic V09.1 ☑
            involving motor vehicle NEC V09.00 ☑
          traffic V09.3 ☑
            involving motor vehicle NEC V09.20 ☑
        specified type NEC V00.898 ☑
          collision (with) V09.9 ☑
            animal being ridden or animal drawn vehicle V06.99 ☑
              nontraffic V06.09 ☑
              traffic V06.19 ☑
            bus or heavy transport V04.99 ☑
              nontraffic V04.09 ☑
              traffic V04.19 ☑
            car V03.99 ☑
              nontraffic V03.09 ☑
              traffic V03.19 ☑
            pedal cycle V01.99 ☑
              nontraffic V01.09 ☑
              traffic V01.19 ☑
            pick-up truck or van V03.99 ☑
              nontraffic V03.09 ☑
              traffic V03.19 ☑
            railway (train) (vehicle) V05.99 ☑
              nontraffic V05.09 ☑
              traffic V05.19 ☑
            stationary object V00.892 ☑
            streetcar V06.99 ☑
              nontraffic V06.09 ☑
              traffic V06.19 ☑
            two- or three-wheeled motor vehicle V02.99 ☑
              nontraffic V02.09 ☑
              traffic V02.19 ☑
            vehicle V09.9 ☑
              animal-drawn V06.99 ☑
                nontraffic V06.09 ☑

Accident — *continued*
  transport — *continued*
    pedestrian — *continued*
      conveyance — *continued*
        specified type — *continued*
          collision — *continued*
            vehicle — *continued*
              animal-drawn — *continued*
                traffic V06.19 ☑
              motor
                nontraffic V09.00 ☑
                traffic V09.20 ☑
          fall V00.891 ☑
          nontraffic V09.1 ☑
            involving motor vehicle NEC V09.00 ☑
          traffic V09.3 ☑
            involving motor vehicle NEC V09.20 ☑
        traffic V09.3 ☑
          involving motor vehicle V09.20 ☑
            military V09.21 ☑
            specified type NEC V09.29 ☑
        wheelchair (powered) V00.818 ☑
          collision (with) V09.9 ☑
            animal being ridden or animal drawn vehicle V06.99 ☑
              nontraffic V06.09 ☑
              traffic V06.19 ☑
            bus or heavy transport V04.99 ☑
              nontraffic V04.09 ☑
              traffic V04.19 ☑
            car V03.99 ☑
              nontraffic V03.09 ☑
              traffic V03.19 ☑
            pedal cycle V01.99 ☑
              nontraffic V01.09 ☑
              traffic V01.19 ☑
            pick-up truck or van V03.99 ☑
              nontraffic V03.09 ☑
              traffic V03.19 ☑
            railway (train) (vehicle) V05.99 ☑
              nontraffic V05.09 ☑
              traffic V05.19 ☑
            stationary object V00.812 ☑
            streetcar V06.99 ☑
              nontraffic V06.09 ☑
              traffic V06.19 ☑
            two- or three-wheeled motor vehicle V02.99 ☑
              nontraffic V02.09 ☑
              traffic V02.19 ☑
            vehicle V09.9 ☑
              animal-drawn V06.99 ☑
                nontraffic V06.09 ☑
                traffic V06.19 ☑
              motor
                nontraffic V09.00 ☑
                traffic V09.20 ☑
          fall V00.811 ☑
          nontraffic V09.1 ☑
            involving motor vehicle NEC V09.00 ☑
          traffic V09.3 ☑
            involving motor vehicle NEC V09.20 ☑
        wheeled shoe V00.158 ☑
          colliding with stationary object V00.152 ☑
          fall V00.151 ☑
      on foot (*see also* Accident, pedestrian)
        collision (with)
          animal being ridden or animal drawn vehicle V06.90 ☑
            nontraffic V06.00 ☑
            traffic V06.10 ☑
          bus or heavy transport V04.90 ☑
            nontraffic V04.00 ☑
            traffic V04.10 ☑
          car V03.90 ☑
            nontraffic V03.00 ☑
            traffic V03.10 ☑
          pedal cycle V01.90 ☑
            nontraffic V01.00 ☑
            traffic V01.10 ☑
          pick-up truck or van V03.90 ☑

Accident — *continued*
  transport — *continued*
    pedestrian — *continued*
      on foot (*see also* Accident, pedestrian) — *continued*
        collision — *continued*
          pick-up truck or van — *continued*
            nontraffic V03.00 ☑
            traffic V03.10 ☑
          railway (train) (vehicle) V05.90 ☑
            nontraffic V05.00 ☑
            traffic V05.10 ☑
          streetcar V06.90 ☑
            nontraffic V06.00 ☑
            traffic V06.10 ☑
          two- or three-wheeled motor vehicle V02.90 ☑
            nontraffic V02.00 ☑
            traffic V02.10 ☑
          vehicle V09.9 ☑
            animal-drawn V06.90 ☑
              nontraffic V06.00 ☑
              traffic V06.10 ☑
            motor
          nontraffic V09.1 ☑
            involving motor vehicle V09.00 ☑
              military V09.01 ☑
              specified type NEC V09.09 ☑
          traffic V09.3 ☑
            involving motor vehicle V09.20 ☑
              military V09.21 ☑
              specified type NEC V09.29 ☑
      person NEC (unknown way or transportation) V99 ☑
      collision (between)
        bus (with)
          heavy transport vehicle (traffic) V87.5 ☑
            nontraffic V88.5 ☑
        car (with)
          bus (traffic) V87.3 ☑
            nontraffic V88.3 ☑
          heavy transport vehicle (traffic) V87.4 ☑
            nontraffic V88.4 ☑
            nontraffic V88.5 ☑
          pick-up truck or van (traffic) V87.2 ☑
            nontraffic V88.2 ☑
          train or railway vehicle (traffic) V87.6 ☑
            nontraffic V88.6 ☑
          two-or three-wheeled motor vehicle (traffic) V87.0 ☑
            nontraffic V88.0 ☑
        motor vehicle (traffic) NEC V87.7 ☑
          nontraffic V88.7 ☑
        two-or three-wheeled vehicle (with) (traffic)
          motor vehicle NEC V87.1 ☑
            nontraffic V88.1 ☑
        nonmotor vehicle (collision) (noncollision) (traffic) V87.9 ☑
          nontraffic V88.9 ☑
      pickup truck occupant V59.9 ☑
        collision (with)
          animal (traffic) V50.9 ☑
            being ridden (traffic) V56.9 ☑
              nontraffic V56.3 ☑
              while boarding or alighting V56.4 ☑
            nontraffic V50.3 ☑
            while boarding or alighting V50.4 ☑
          animal-drawn vehicle (traffic) V56.9 ☑
            nontraffic V56.3 ☑
            while boarding or alighting V56.4 ☑
          bus (traffic) V54.9 ☑
            nontraffic V54.3 ☑
            while boarding or alighting V54.4 ☑
          car (traffic) V53.9 ☑
            nontraffic V53.3 ☑
            while boarding or alighting V53.4 ☑
          motor vehicle NOS (traffic) V59.60 ☑
            nontraffic V59.20 ☑
            specified type NEC (traffic) V59.69 ☑
              nontraffic V59.29 ☑
          pedal cycle (traffic) V51.9 ☑
            nontraffic V51.3 ☑
            while boarding or alighting V51.4 ☑
          pickup truck (traffic) V53.9 ☑
            nontraffic V53.3 ☑
            while boarding or alighting V53.4 ☑

Accident — *continued*
  transport — *continued*
    pickup truck occupant — *continued*
      collision — *continued*
        railway vehicle (traffic) V55.9 ☑
          nontraffic V55.3 ☑
          while boarding or alighting V55.4 ☑
        specified vehicle NEC (traffic) V56.9 ☑
          nontraffic V56.3 ☑
          while boarding or alighting V56.4 ☑
        stationary object (traffic) V57.9 ☑
          nontraffic V57.3 ☑
          while boarding or alighting V57.4 ☑
        streetcar (traffic) V56.9 ☑
          nontraffic V56.3 ☑
          while boarding or alighting V56.4 ☑
        three wheeled motor vehicle (traffic) V52.9 ☑
          nontraffic V52.3 ☑
          while boarding or alighting V52.4 ☑
        truck (traffic) V54.9 ☑
          nontraffic V54.3 ☑
          while boarding or alighting V54.4 ☑
        two wheeled motor vehicle (traffic) V52.9 ☑
          nontraffic V52.3 ☑
          while boarding or alighting V52.4 ☑
        van (traffic) V53.9 ☑
          nontraffic V53.3 ☑
          while boarding or alighting V53.4 ☑
      driver
        collision (with)
          animal (traffic) V50.5 ☑
            being ridden (traffic) V56.5 ☑
              nontraffic V56.0 ☑
            nontraffic V50.0 ☑
          animal-drawn vehicle (traffic) V56.5 ☑
            nontraffic V56.0 ☑
          bus (traffic) V54.5 ☑
            nontraffic V54.0 ☑
          car (traffic) V53.5 ☑
            nontraffic V53.0 ☑
          motor vehicle NOS (traffic) V59.40 ☑
            nontraffic V59.00 ☑
            specified type NEC (traffic) V59.49 ☑
              nontraffic V59.09 ☑
          pedal cycle (traffic) V51.5 ☑
            nontraffic V51.0 ☑
          pickup truck (traffic) V53.5 ☑
            nontraffic V53.0 ☑
          railway vehicle (traffic) V55.5 ☑
            nontraffic V55.0 ☑
          specified vehicle NEC (traffic) V56.5 ☑
            nontraffic V56.0 ☑
          stationary object (traffic) V57.5 ☑
            nontraffic V57.0 ☑
          streetcar (traffic) V56.5 ☑
            nontraffic V56.0 ☑
          three wheeled motor vehicle (traffic) V52.5 ☑
            nontraffic V52.0 ☑
          truck (traffic) V54.5 ☑
            nontraffic V54.0 ☑
          two wheeled motor vehicle (traffic) V52.5 ☑
            nontraffic V52.0 ☑
          van (traffic) V53.5 ☑
            nontraffic V53.0 ☑
        noncollision accident (traffic) V58.5 ☑
          nontraffic V58.0 ☑
      hanger-on
        collision (with)
          animal (traffic) V50.7 ☑
            being ridden (traffic) V56.7 ☑
              nontraffic V56.2 ☑
            nontraffic V50.2 ☑
          animal-drawn vehicle (traffic) V56.7 ☑
            nontraffic V56.2 ☑
          bus (traffic) V54.7 ☑
            nontraffic V54.2 ☑
          car (traffic) V53.7 ☑
            nontraffic V53.2 ☑
          pedal cycle (traffic) V51.7 ☑
            nontraffic V51.2 ☑
          pickup truck (traffic) V53.7 ☑
            nontraffic V53.2 ☑
          railway vehicle (traffic) V55.7 ☑

Accident — *continued*
  transport — *continued*
    pickup truck occupant — *continued*
      hanger-on — *continued*
        collision — *continued*
          railway vehicle — *continued*
            nontraffic V55.2 ☑
          specified vehicle NEC (traffic) V56.7 ☑
            nontraffic V56.2 ☑
          stationary object (traffic) V57.7 ☑
            nontraffic V57.2 ☑
          streetcar (traffic) V56.7 ☑
            nontraffic V56.2 ☑
          three wheeled motor vehicle (traffic) V52.7 ☑
            nontraffic V52.2 ☑
          truck (traffic) V54.7 ☑
            nontraffic V54.2 ☑
          two wheeled motor vehicle (traffic) V52.7 ☑
            nontraffic V52.2 ☑
          van (traffic) V53.7 ☑
            nontraffic V53.2 ☑
        noncollision accident (traffic) V58.7 ☑
          nontraffic V58.2 ☑
      noncollision accident (traffic) V58.9 ☑
        nontraffic V58.3 ☑
        while boarding or alighting V58.4 ☑
      nontraffic V59.3 ☑
      passenger
        collision (with)
          animal (traffic) V50.6 ☑
            being ridden (traffic) V56.6 ☑
              nontraffic V56.1 ☑
            nontraffic V50.1 ☑
          animal-drawn vehicle (traffic) V56.6 ☑
            nontraffic V56.1 ☑
          bus (traffic) V54.6 ☑
            nontraffic V54.1 ☑
          car (traffic) V53.6 ☑
            nontraffic V53.1 ☑
          motor vehicle NOS (traffic) V59.50 ☑
            nontraffic V59.10 ☑
            specified type NEC (traffic) V59.59 ☑
              nontraffic V59.19 ☑
          pedal cycle (traffic) V51.6 ☑
            nontraffic V51.1 ☑
          pickup truck (traffic) V53.6 ☑
            nontraffic V53.1 ☑
          railway vehicle (traffic) V55.6 ☑
            nontraffic V55.1 ☑
          specified vehicle NEC (traffic) V56.6 ☑
            nontraffic V56.1 ☑
          stationary object (traffic) V57.6 ☑
            nontraffic V57.1 ☑
          streetcar (traffic) V56.6 ☑
            nontraffic V56.1 ☑
          three wheeled motor vehicle (traffic) V52.6 ☑
            nontraffic V52.1 ☑
          truck (traffic) V54.6 ☑
            nontraffic V54.1 ☑
          two wheeled motor vehicle (traffic) V52.6 ☑
            nontraffic V52.1 ☑
          van (traffic) V53.6 ☑
            nontraffic V53.1 ☑
        noncollision accident (traffic) V58.6 ☑
          nontraffic V58.1 ☑
      specified type NEC V59.88 ☑
        military vehicle V59.81 ☑
      quarry truck — *see* Accident, transport, industrial vehicle occupant
      race car — *see* Accident, transport, motor vehicle NEC occupant
    railway vehicle occupant V81.9 ☑
      collision (with) V81.3 ☑
        motor vehicle (non-military) (traffic) V81.1 ☑
          military V81.83 ☑
          nontraffic V81.0 ☑
        rolling stock V81.2 ☑
        specified object NEC V81.3 ☑
      during derailment V81.7 ☑

Accident — *continued*
  transport — *continued*
    railway vehicle occupant — *continued*
      during derailment — *continued*
        with antecedent collision — *see* Accident, transport, railway vehicle occupant, collision
      explosion V81.81 ☑
      fall (in railway vehicle) V81.5 ☑
        during derailment V81.7 ☑
          with antecedent collision — *see* Accident, transport, railway vehicle occupant, collision
        from railway vehicle V81.6 ☑
          during derailment V81.7 ☑
            with antecedent collision — *see* Accident, transport, railway vehicle occupant, collision
        while boarding or alighting V81.4 ☑
      fire V81.81 ☑
      object falling onto train V81.82 ☑
      specified type NEC V81.89 ☑
      while boarding or alighting V81.4 ☑
    ski lift V98.3 ☑
    snowmobile occupant (nontraffic) V86.92 ☑
      driver V86.52 ☑
      hanger-on V86.72 ☑
      passenger V86.62 ☑
      traffic V86.32 ☑
        driver V86.02 ☑
        hanger-on V86.22 ☑
        passenger V86.12 ☑
      while boarding or alighting V86.42 ☑
    specified NEC V98.8 ☑
    sport utility vehicle occupant (*see also* Accident, transport, pickup truck occupant)
    streetcar occupant V82.9 ☑
      collision (with) V82.3 ☑
        motor vehicle (traffic) V82.1 ☑
          nontraffic V82.0 ☑
        rolling stock V82.2 ☑
      during derailment V82.7 ☑
        with antecedent collision — *see* Accident, transport, streetcar occupant, collision
      fall (in streetcar) V82.5 ☑
        during derailment V82.7 ☑
          with antecedent collision — *see* Accident, transport, streetcar occupant, collision
        from streetcar V82.6 ☑
          during derailment V82.7 ☑
            with antecedent collision — *see* Accident, transport, streetcar occupant, collision
        while boarding or alighting V82.4 ☑
      while boarding or alighting V82.4 ☑
      specified type NEC V82.8 ☑
      while boarding or alighting V82.4 ☑
    three-wheeled motor vehicle occupant V39.9 ☑
      collision (with)
        animal (traffic) V30.9 ☑
          being ridden (traffic) V36.9 ☑
            nontraffic V36.3 ☑
            while boarding or alighting V36.4 ☑
          nontraffic V30.3 ☑
          while boarding or alighting V30.4 ☑
        animal-drawn vehicle (traffic) V36.9 ☑
          nontraffic V36.3 ☑
          while boarding or alighting V36.4 ☑
        bus (traffic) V34.9 ☑
          nontraffic V34.3 ☑
          while boarding or alighting V34.4 ☑
        car (traffic) V33.9 ☑
          nontraffic V33.3 ☑
          while boarding or alighting V33.4 ☑
        motor vehicle NOS (traffic) V39.60 ☑
          nontraffic V39.20 ☑
          specified type NEC (traffic) V39.69 ☑
            nontraffic V39.29 ☑
        pedal cycle (traffic) V31.9 ☑
          nontraffic V31.3 ☑
          while boarding or alighting V31.4 ☑
        pickup truck (traffic) V33.9 ☑
          nontraffic V33.3 ☑
          while boarding or alighting V33.4 ☑
        railway vehicle (traffic) V35.9 ☑

▽ **Subterms under main terms may continue to next column or page**   ☑ **Additional Character Required — Refer to the Tabular List for Character Selection**   **405**

Accident — Accident

External Causes Index

Accident — Accident

Accident — *continued*
 transport — *continued*
  three-wheeled motor vehicle occupant — *continued*
   collision — *continued*
    railway vehicle — *continued*
     nontraffic V35.3 ☑
     while boarding or alighting V35.4 ☑
    specified vehicle NEC (traffic) V36.9 ☑
     nontraffic V36.3 ☑
     while boarding or alighting V36.4 ☑
    stationary object (traffic) V37.9 ☑
     nontraffic V37.3 ☑
     while boarding or alighting V37.4 ☑
    streetcar (traffic) V36.9 ☑
     nontraffic V36.3 ☑
     while boarding or alighting V36.4 ☑
    three wheeled motor vehicle (traffic) V32.9 ☑
     nontraffic V32.3 ☑
     while boarding or alighting V32.4 ☑
    truck (traffic) V34.9 ☑
     nontraffic V34.3 ☑
     while boarding or alighting V34.4 ☑
    two wheeled motor vehicle (traffic) V32.9 ☑
     nontraffic V32.3 ☑
     while boarding or alighting V32.4 ☑
    van (traffic) V33.9 ☑
     nontraffic V33.3 ☑
     while boarding or alighting V33.4 ☑
   driver
    collision (with)
     animal (traffic) V30.5 ☑
      being ridden (traffic) V36.5 ☑
       nontraffic V36.0 ☑
      nontraffic V30.0 ☑
     animal-drawn vehicle (traffic) V36.5 ☑
      nontraffic V36.0 ☑
     bus (traffic) V34.5 ☑
      nontraffic V34.0 ☑
     car (traffic) V33.5 ☑
      nontraffic V33.0 ☑
     motor vehicle NOS (traffic) V39.40 ☑
      nontraffic V39.00 ☑
      specified type NEC (traffic) V39.49 ☑
       nontraffic V39.09 ☑
     pedal cycle (traffic) V31.5 ☑
      nontraffic V31.0 ☑
     pickup truck (traffic) V33.5 ☑
      nontraffic V33.0 ☑
     railway vehicle (traffic) V35.5 ☑
      nontraffic V35.0 ☑
     specified vehicle NEC (traffic) V36.5 ☑
      nontraffic V36.0 ☑
     stationary object (traffic) V37.5 ☑
      nontraffic V37.0 ☑
     streetcar (traffic) V36.5 ☑
      nontraffic V36.0 ☑
     three wheeled motor vehicle (traffic) V32.5 ☑
      nontraffic V32.0 ☑
     truck (traffic) V34.5 ☑
      nontraffic V34.0 ☑
     two wheeled motor vehicle (traffic) V32.5 ☑
      nontraffic V32.0 ☑
     van (traffic) V33.5 ☑
      nontraffic V33.0 ☑
    noncollision accident (traffic) V38.5 ☑
     nontraffic V38.0 ☑
   hanger-on
    collision (with)
     animal (traffic) V30.7 ☑
      being ridden (traffic) V36.7 ☑
       nontraffic V36.2 ☑
      nontraffic V30.2 ☑
     animal-drawn vehicle (traffic) V36.7 ☑
      nontraffic V36.2 ☑
     bus (traffic) V34.7 ☑
      nontraffic V34.2 ☑
     car (traffic) V33.7 ☑
      nontraffic V33.2 ☑
     pedal cycle (traffic) V31.7 ☑
      nontraffic V31.2 ☑
     pickup truck (traffic) V33.7 ☑
      nontraffic V33.2 ☑

Accident — *continued*
 transport — *continued*
  three-wheeled motor vehicle occupant — *continued*
   hanger-on — *continued*
    collision — *continued*
     railway vehicle (traffic) V35.7 ☑
      nontraffic V35.2 ☑
     specified vehicle NEC (traffic) V36.7 ☑
      nontraffic V36.2 ☑
     stationary object (traffic) V37.7 ☑
      nontraffic V37.2 ☑
     streetcar (traffic) V36.7 ☑
      nontraffic V36.2 ☑
     three wheeled motor vehicle (traffic) V32.7 ☑
      nontraffic V32.2 ☑
     truck (traffic) V34.7 ☑
      nontraffic V34.2 ☑
     two wheeled motor vehicle (traffic) V32.7 ☑
      nontraffic V32.2 ☑
     van (traffic) V33.7 ☑
      nontraffic V33.2 ☑
    noncollision accident (traffic) V38.7 ☑
     nontraffic V38.2 ☑
   noncollision accident (traffic) V38.9 ☑
    nontraffic V38.3 ☑
    while boarding or alighting V38.4 ☑
   nontraffic V39.3 ☑
   passenger
    collision (with)
     animal (traffic) V30.6 ☑
      being ridden (traffic) V36.6 ☑
       nontraffic V36.1 ☑
      nontraffic V30.1 ☑
     animal-drawn vehicle (traffic) V36.6 ☑
      nontraffic V36.1 ☑
     bus (traffic) V34.6 ☑
      nontraffic V34.1 ☑
     car (traffic) V33.6 ☑
      nontraffic V33.1 ☑
     motor vehicle NOS (traffic) V39.50 ☑
      nontraffic V39.10 ☑
      specified type NEC (traffic) V39.59 ☑
       nontraffic V39.19 ☑
     pedal cycle (traffic) V31.6 ☑
      nontraffic V31.1 ☑
     pickup truck (traffic) V33.6 ☑
      nontraffic V33.1 ☑
     railway vehicle (traffic) V35.6 ☑
      nontraffic V35.1 ☑
     specified vehicle NEC (traffic) V36.6 ☑
      nontraffic V36.1 ☑
     stationary object (traffic) V37.6 ☑
      nontraffic V37.1 ☑
     streetcar (traffic) V36.6 ☑
      nontraffic V36.1 ☑
     three wheeled motor vehicle (traffic) V32.6 ☑
      nontraffic V32.1 ☑
     truck (traffic) V34.6 ☑
      nontraffic V34.1 ☑
     two wheeled motor vehicle (traffic) V32.6 ☑
      nontraffic V32.1 ☑
     van (traffic) V33.6 ☑
      nontraffic V33.1 ☑
    noncollision accident (traffic) V38.6 ☑
     nontraffic V38.1 ☑
   specified type NEC V39.89 ☑
    military vehicle V39.81 ☑
  tractor (farm) (and trailer) — *see* Accident, transport, agricultural vehicle occupant
  tram — *see* Accident, transport, streetcar
   in mine or quarry — *see* Accident, transport, industrial vehicle occupant
  trolley — *see* Accident, transport, streetcar
   in mine or quarry — *see* Accident, transport, industrial vehicle occupant
  truck (heavy) occupant V69.9 ☑
   collision (with)
    animal (traffic) V60.9 ☑
     being ridden (traffic) V66.9 ☑
      nontraffic V66.3 ☑
      while boarding or alighting V66.4 ☑

Accident — *continued*
 transport — *continued*
  truck occupant — *continued*
   collision — *continued*
    animal — *continued*
     nontraffic V60.3 ☑
     while boarding or alighting V60.4 ☑
    animal-drawn vehicle (traffic) V66.9 ☑
     nontraffic V66.3 ☑
     while boarding or alighting V66.4 ☑
    bus (traffic) V64.9 ☑
     nontraffic V64.3 ☑
     while boarding or alighting V64.4 ☑
    car (traffic) V63.9 ☑
     nontraffic V63.3 ☑
     while boarding or alighting V63.4 ☑
    motor vehicle NOS (traffic) V69.60 ☑
     nontraffic V69.20 ☑
     specified type NEC (traffic) V69.69 ☑
      nontraffic V69.29 ☑
    pedal cycle (traffic) V61.9 ☑
     nontraffic V61.3 ☑
     while boarding or alighting V61.4 ☑
    pickup truck (traffic) V63.9 ☑
     nontraffic V63.3 ☑
     while boarding or alighting V63.4 ☑
    railway vehicle (traffic) V65.9 ☑
     nontraffic V65.3 ☑
     while boarding or alighting V65.4 ☑
    specified vehicle NEC (traffic) V66.9 ☑
     nontraffic V66.3 ☑
     while boarding or alighting V66.4 ☑
    stationary object (traffic) V67.9 ☑
     nontraffic V67.3 ☑
     while boarding or alighting V67.4 ☑
    streetcar (traffic) V66.9 ☑
     nontraffic V66.3 ☑
     while boarding or alighting V66.4 ☑
    three wheeled motor vehicle (traffic) V62.9 ☑
     nontraffic V62.3 ☑
     while boarding or alighting V62.4 ☑
    truck (traffic) V64.9 ☑
     nontraffic V64.3 ☑
     while boarding or alighting V64.4 ☑
    two wheeled motor vehicle (traffic) V62.9 ☑
     nontraffic V62.3 ☑
     while boarding or alighting V62.4 ☑
    van (traffic) V63.9 ☑
     nontraffic V63.3 ☑
     while boarding or alighting V63.4 ☑
   driver
    collision (with)
     animal (traffic) V60.5 ☑
      being ridden (traffic) V66.5 ☑
       nontraffic V66.0 ☑
      nontraffic V60.0 ☑
     animal-drawn vehicle (traffic) V66.5 ☑
      nontraffic V66.0 ☑
     bus (traffic) V64.5 ☑
      nontraffic V64.0 ☑
     car (traffic) V63.5 ☑
      nontraffic V63.0 ☑
     motor vehicle NOS (traffic) V69.40 ☑
      nontraffic V69.00 ☑
      specified type NEC (traffic) V69.49 ☑
       nontraffic V69.09 ☑
     pedal cycle (traffic) V61.5 ☑
      nontraffic V61.0 ☑
     pickup truck (traffic) V63.5 ☑
      nontraffic V63.0 ☑
     railway vehicle (traffic) V65.5 ☑
      nontraffic V65.0 ☑
     specified vehicle NEC (traffic) V66.5 ☑
      nontraffic V66.0 ☑
     stationary object (traffic) V67.5 ☑
      nontraffic V67.0 ☑
     streetcar (traffic) V66.5 ☑
      nontraffic V66.0 ☑
     three wheeled motor vehicle (traffic) V62.5 ☑
      nontraffic V62.0 ☑
     truck (traffic) V64.5 ☑
      nontraffic V64.0 ☑
     two wheeled motor vehicle (traffic) V62.5 ☑

☑ Additional Character Required — Refer to the Tabular List for Character Selection   🔻 Subterms under main terms may continue to next column or page

Accident — *continued*
  transport — *continued*
    truck occupant — *continued*
      driver — *continued*
        collision — *continued*
          two wheeled motor vehicle — *continued*
            nontraffic V62.0 ☑
            van (traffic) V63.5 ☑
            nontraffic V63.0 ☑
          noncollision accident (traffic) V68.5 ☑
            nontraffic V68.0 ☑
      dump — *see* Accident, transport, construction vehicle occupant
      hanger-on
        collision (with)
          animal (traffic) V60.7 ☑
            being ridden (traffic) V66.7 ☑
              nontraffic V66.2 ☑
            nontraffic V60.2 ☑
          animal-drawn vehicle (traffic) V66.7 ☑
            nontraffic V66.2 ☑
          bus (traffic) V64.7 ☑
            nontraffic V64.2 ☑
          car (traffic) V63.7 ☑
            nontraffic V63.2 ☑
          pedal cycle (traffic) V61.7 ☑
            nontraffic V61.2 ☑
          pickup truck (traffic) V63.7 ☑
            nontraffic V63.2 ☑
          railway vehicle (traffic) V65.7 ☑
            nontraffic V65.2 ☑
          specified vehicle NEC (traffic) V66.7 ☑
            nontraffic V66.2 ☑
          stationary object (traffic) V67.7 ☑
            nontraffic V67.2 ☑
          streetcar (traffic) V66.7 ☑
            nontraffic V66.2 ☑
          three wheeled motor vehicle (traffic) V62.7 ☑
            nontraffic V62.2 ☑
          truck (traffic) V64.7 ☑
            nontraffic V64.2 ☑
          two wheeled motor vehicle (traffic) V62.7 ☑
            nontraffic V62.2 ☑
          van (traffic) V63.7 ☑
            nontraffic V63.2 ☑
        noncollision accident (traffic) V68.7 ☑
          nontraffic V68.2 ☑
      noncollision accident (traffic) V68.9 ☑
        nontraffic V68.3 ☑
        while boarding or alighting V68.4 ☑
      nontraffic V69.3 ☑
      passenger
        collision (with)
          animal (traffic) V60.6 ☑
            being ridden (traffic) V66.6 ☑
              nontraffic V66.1- ☑
            nontraffic V60.1 ☑
          animal-drawn vehicle (traffic) V66.6 ☑
            nontraffic V66.1 ☑
          bus (traffic) V64.6 ☑
            nontraffic V64.1 ☑
          car (traffic) V63.6 ☑
            nontraffic V63.1 ☑
          motor vehicle NOS (traffic) V69.50 ☑
            nontraffic V69.10 ☑
            specified type NEC (traffic) V69.59 ☑
              nontraffic V69.19 ☑
          pedal cycle (traffic) V61.6 ☑
            nontraffic V61.1 ☑
          pickup truck (traffic) V63.6 ☑
            nontraffic V63.1 ☑
          railway vehicle (traffic) V65.6 ☑
            nontraffic V65.1 ☑
          specified vehicle NEC (traffic) V66.6 ☑
            nontraffic V66.1 ☑
          stationary object (traffic) V67.6 ☑
            nontraffic V67.1 ☑
          streetcar (traffic) V66.6 ☑
            nontraffic V66.1 ☑
          three wheeled motor vehicle (traffic) V62.6 ☑
            nontraffic V62.1 ☑
          truck (traffic) V64.6 ☑

Accident — *continued*
  transport — *continued*
    truck occupant — *continued*
      passenger — *continued*
        collision — *continued*
          truck — *continued*
            nontraffic V64.1 ☑
          two wheeled motor vehicle (traffic) V62.6 ☑
            nontraffic V62.1 ☑
          van (traffic) V63.6 ☑
            nontraffic V63.1 ☑
          noncollision accident (traffic) V68.6 ☑
            nontraffic V68.1 ☑
      pickup — *see* Accident, transport, pickup truck occupant
      specified type NEC V69.88 ☑
        military vehicle V69.81 ☑
    van occupant V59.9 ☑
      collision (with)
        animal (traffic) V50.9 ☑
          being ridden (traffic) V56.9 ☑
            nontraffic V56.3 ☑
            while boarding or alighting V56.4 ☑
          nontraffic V50.3 ☑
          while boarding or alighting V50.4 ☑
        animal-drawn vehicle (traffic) V56.9 ☑
          nontraffic V56.3 ☑
          while boarding or alighting V56.4 ☑
        bus (traffic) V54.9 ☑
          nontraffic V54.3 ☑
          while boarding or alighting V54.4 ☑
        car (traffic) V53.9 ☑
          nontraffic V53.3 ☑
          while boarding or alighting V53.4 ☑
        motor vehicle NOS (traffic) V59.60 ☑
          nontraffic V59.20 ☑
          specified type NEC (traffic) V59.69 ☑
            nontraffic V59.29 ☑
        pedal cycle (traffic) V51.9 ☑
          nontraffic V51.3 ☑
          while boarding or alighting V51.4 ☑
        pickup truck (traffic) V53.9 ☑
          nontraffic V53.3 ☑
          while boarding or alighting V53.4 ☑
        railway vehicle (traffic) V55.9 ☑
          nontraffic V55.3 ☑
          while boarding or alighting V55.4 ☑
        specified vehicle NEC (traffic) V56.9 ☑
          nontraffic V56.3 ☑
          while boarding or alighting V56.4 ☑
        stationary object (traffic) V57.9 ☑
          nontraffic V57.3 ☑
          while boarding or alighting V57.4 ☑
        streetcar (traffic) V56.9 ☑
          nontraffic V56.3 ☑
          while boarding or alighting V56.4 ☑
        three wheeled motor vehicle (traffic) V52.9 ☑
          nontraffic V52.3 ☑
          while boarding or alighting V52.4 ☑
        truck (traffic) V54.9 ☑
          nontraffic V54.3 ☑
          while boarding or alighting V54.4 ☑
        two wheeled motor vehicle (traffic) V52.9 ☑
          nontraffic V52.3 ☑
          while boarding or alighting V52.4 ☑
        van (traffic) V53.9 ☑
          nontraffic V53.3 ☑
          while boarding or alighting V53.4 ☑
      driver
        collision (with)
          animal (traffic) V50.5 ☑
            being ridden (traffic) V56.5 ☑
              nontraffic V56.0 ☑
            nontraffic V50.0 ☑
          animal-drawn vehicle (traffic) V56.5 ☑
            nontraffic V56.0 ☑
          bus (traffic) V54.5 ☑
            nontraffic V54.0 ☑
          car (traffic) V53.5 ☑
            nontraffic V53.0 ☑
          motor vehicle NOS (traffic) V59.40 ☑
            nontraffic V59.00 ☑
          specified type NEC (traffic) V59.49 ☑
            nontraffic V59.09 ☑

Accident — *continued*
  transport — *continued*
    van occupant — *continued*
      driver — *continued*
        collision — *continued*
          pedal cycle (traffic) V51.5 ☑
            nontraffic V51.0 ☑
          pickup truck (traffic) V53.5 ☑
            nontraffic V53.0 ☑
          railway vehicle (traffic) V55.5 ☑
            nontraffic V55.0 ☑
          specified vehicle NEC (traffic) V56.5 ☑
            nontraffic V56.0 ☑
          stationary object (traffic) V57.5 ☑
            nontraffic V57.0 ☑
          streetcar (traffic) V56.5 ☑
            nontraffic V56.0 ☑
          three wheeled motor vehicle (traffic) V52.5 ☑
            nontraffic V52.0 ☑
          truck (traffic) V54.5 ☑
            nontraffic V54.0 ☑
          two wheeled motor vehicle (traffic) V52.5 ☑
            nontraffic V52.0 ☑
          van (traffic) V53.5 ☑
            nontraffic V53.0 ☑
        noncollision accident (traffic) V58.5 ☑
          nontraffic V58.0 ☑
      hanger-on
        collision (with)
          animal (traffic) V50.7 ☑
            being ridden (traffic) V56.7 ☑
              nontraffic V56.2 ☑
            nontraffic V50.2 ☑
          animal-drawn vehicle (traffic) V56.7 ☑
            nontraffic V56.2 ☑
          bus (traffic) V54.7 ☑
            nontraffic V54.2 ☑
          car (traffic) V53.7 ☑
            nontraffic V53.2 ☑
          pedal cycle (traffic) V51.7 ☑
            nontraffic V51.2 ☑
          pickup truck (traffic) V53.7 ☑
            nontraffic V53.2 ☑
          railway vehicle (traffic) V55.7 ☑
            nontraffic V55.2 ☑
          specified vehicle NEC (traffic) V56.7 ☑
            nontraffic V56.2 ☑
          stationary object (traffic) V57.7 ☑
            nontraffic V57.2 ☑
          streetcar (traffic) V56.7 ☑
            nontraffic V56.2 ☑
          three wheeled motor vehicle (traffic) V52.7 ☑
            nontraffic V52.2 ☑
          truck (traffic) V54.7 ☑
            nontraffic V54.2 ☑
          two wheeled motor vehicle (traffic) V52.7 ☑
            nontraffic V52.2 ☑
          van (traffic) V53.7 ☑
            nontraffic V53.2 ☑
        noncollision accident (traffic) V58.7 ☑
          nontraffic V58.2 ☑
      noncollision accident (traffic) V58.9 ☑
        nontraffic V58.3 ☑
        while boarding or alighting V58.4 ☑
      nontraffic V59.3 ☑
      passenger
        collision (with)
          animal (traffic) V50.6 ☑
            being ridden (traffic) V56.6 ☑
              nontraffic V56.1 ☑
            nontraffic V50.1 ☑
          animal-drawn vehicle (traffic) V56.6 ☑
            nontraffic V56.1 ☑
          bus (traffic) V54.6 ☑
            nontraffic V54.1 ☑
          car (traffic) V53.6 ☑
            nontraffic V53.1 ☑
          motor vehicle NOS (traffic) V59.50 ☑
            nontraffic V59.10 ☑
          specified type NEC (traffic) V59.59 ☑
            nontraffic V59.19 ☑
          pedal cycle (traffic) V51.6 ☑

External Causes Index

Accident — Activity

Accident — continued
  transport — continued
    van occupant — continued
      passenger — continued
        collision — continued
          pedal cycle — continued
            nontraffic V51.1 ☑
          pickup truck (traffic) V53.6 ☑
            nontraffic V53.1 ☑
          railway vehicle (traffic) V55.6 ☑
            nontraffic V55.1 ☑
          specified vehicle NEC (traffic) V56.6 ☑
            nontraffic V56.1 ☑
          stationary object (traffic) V57.6 ☑
            nontraffic V57.1 ☑
          streetcar (traffic) V56.6 ☑
            nontraffic V56.1 ☑
          three wheeled motor vehicle (traffic) V52.6 ☑
            nontraffic V52.1 ☑
          truck (traffic) V54.6 ☑
            nontraffic V54.1 ☑
          two wheeled motor vehicle (traffic) V52.6 ☑
            nontraffic V52.1 ☑
          van (traffic) V53.6 ☑
            nontraffic V53.1 ☑
          noncollision accident (traffic) V58.6 ☑
            nontraffic V58.1 ☑
        specified type NEC V59.88 ☑
        military vehicle V59.81 ☑
  watercraft occupant — see Accident, watercraft
  vehicle NEC V89.9 ☑
    animal-drawn NEC — see Accident, transport, animal-drawn vehicle occupant
    special
      agricultural — see Accident, transport, agricultural vehicle occupant
      construction — see Accident, transport, construction vehicle occupant
      industrial — see Accident, transport, industrial vehicle occupant
    three-wheeled NEC (motorized) — see Accident, transport, three-wheeled motor vehicle occupant
  watercraft V94.9 ☑
    causing
      drowning — see Drowning, due to, accident to, watercraft
      injury NEC V91.89 ☑
        crushed between craft and object V91.19 ☑
          powered craft V91.13 ☑
            ferry boat V91.11 ☑
            fishing boat V91.12 ☑
            jetskis V91.13 ☑
            liner V91.11 ☑
            merchant ship V91.10 ☑
            passenger ship V91.11 ☑
          unpowered craft V91.18 ☑
            canoe V91.15 ☑
            inflatable V91.16 ☑
            kayak V91.15 ☑
            sailboat V91.14 ☑
            surf-board V91.18 ☑
            windsurfer V91.18 ☑
        fall on board V91.29 ☑
          powered craft V91.23 ☑
            ferry boat V91.21 ☑
            fishing boat V91.22 ☑
            jetskis V91.23 ☑
            liner V91.21 ☑
            merchant ship V91.20 ☑
            passenger ship V91.21 ☑
          unpowered craft
            canoe V91.25 ☑
            inflatable V91.26 ☑
            kayak V91.25 ☑
            sailboat V91.24 ☑
        fire on board causing burn V91.09 ☑
          powered craft V91.03 ☑
            ferry boat V91.01 ☑
            fishing boat V91.02 ☑
            jetskis V91.03 ☑
            liner V91.01 ☑
            merchant ship V91.00 ☑
            passenger ship V91.01 ☑

Accident — continued
  watercraft — continued
    causing — continued
      injury — continued
        fire on board causing burn — continued
          unpowered craft V91.08 ☑
            canoe V91.05 ☑
            inflatable V91.06 ☑
            kayak V91.05 ☑
            sailboat V91.04 ☑
            surf-board V91.08 ☑
            water skis V91.07 ☑
            windsurfer V91.08 ☑
        hit by falling object V91.39 ☑
          powered craft V91.33 ☑
            ferry boat V91.31 ☑
            fishing boat V91.32 ☑
            jetskis V91.33 ☑
            liner V91.31 ☑
            merchant ship V91.30 ☑
            passenger ship V91.31 ☑
          unpowered craft V91.38 ☑
            canoe V91.35 ☑
            inflatable V91.36 ☑
            kayak V91.35 ☑
            sailboat V91.34 ☑
            surf-board V91.38 ☑
            water skis V91.37 ☑
            windsurfer V91.38 ☑
        specified type NEC V91.89 ☑
          powered craft V91.83 ☑
            ferry boat V91.81 ☑
            fishing boat V91.82 ☑
            jetskis V91.83 ☑
            liner V91.81 ☑
            merchant ship V91.80 ☑
            passenger ship V91.81 ☑
          unpowered craft V91.88 ☑
            canoe V91.85 ☑
            inflatable V91.86 ☑
            kayak V91.85 ☑
            sailboat V91.84 ☑
            surf-board V91.88 ☑
            water skis V91.87 ☑
            windsurfer V91.88 ☑
      due to, caused by cataclysm — see Forces of nature, by type
      military NEC V94.818 ☑
        with civilian watercraft V94.810 ☑
        civilian in water injured by V94.811 ☑
      nonpowered, struck by
        nonpowered vessel V94.22 ☑
        powered vessel V94.21 ☑
      specified type NEC V94.89 ☑
      striking swimmer
        powered V94.11 ☑
        unpowered V94.12 ☑

Acid throwing (assault) Y08.89 ☑
Activity (involving) (of victim at time of event) Y93.9
  aerobic and step exercise (class) Y93.A3 (following Y93.7)
  alpine skiing Y93.23
  animal care NEC Y93.K9 (following Y93.7)
  arts and handcrafts NEC Y93.D9 (following Y93.7)
  athletics played as a team or group NEC Y93.69
  athletics played individually NEC Y93.59
  athletics NEC Y93.79
  baking Y93.G3 (following Y93.7)
  ballet Y93.41
  barbells Y93.B3 (following Y93.7)
  BASE (Building, Antenna, Span, Earth) jumping Y93.33
  baseball Y93.64
  basketball Y93.67
  bathing (personal) Y93.E1 (following Y93.7)
  beach volleyball Y93.68
  bike riding Y93.55
  blackout game Y93.85
  boogie boarding Y93.18
  bowling Y93.54
  boxing Y93.71
  brass instrument playing Y93.J4 (following Y93.7)
  building construction Y93.H3 (following Y93.7)
  bungee jumping Y93.34
  calisthenics Y93.A2 (following Y93.7)
  canoeing (in calm and turbulent water) Y93.16
  capture the flag Y93.6A
  cardiorespiratory exercise NEC Y93.A9 (following Y93.7)

Activity — continued
  caregiving (providing) NEC Y93.F9 (following Y93.7)
    bathing Y93.F1 (following Y93.7)
    lifting Y93.F2 (following Y93.7)
  cellular
    communication device Y93.C2 (following Y93.7)
    telephone Y93.C2 (following Y93.7)
  challenge course Y93.A5 (following Y93.7)
  cheerleading Y93.45
  choking game Y93.85
  circuit training Y93.A4 (following Y93.7)
  cleaning
    floor Y93.E5 (following Y93.7)
  climbing NEC Y93.39
    mountain Y93.31
    rock Y93.31
    wall Y93.31
  clothing care and maintenance NEC Y93.E9 (following Y93.7)
  combatives Y93.75
  computer
    keyboarding Y93.C1 (following Y93.7)
    technology NEC Y93.C9 (following Y93.7)
  confidence course Y93.A5 (following Y93.7)
  construction (building) Y93.H3 (following Y93.7)
  cooking and baking Y93.G3 (following Y93.7)
  cool down exercises Y93.A2 (following Y93.7)
  cricket Y93.69
  crocheting Y93.D1 (following Y93.7)
  cross country skiing Y93.24
  dancing (all types) Y93.41
  digging
    dirt Y93.H1 (following Y93.7)
  dirt digging Y93.H1 (following Y93.7)
  dishwashing Y93.G1 (following Y93.7)
  diving (platform) (springboard) Y93.12
    underwater Y93.15
  dodge ball Y93.6A
  downhill skiing Y93.23
  drum playing Y93.J2 (following Y93.7)
  dumbbells Y93.B3 (following Y93.7)
  electronic
    devices NEC Y93.C9 (following Y93.7)
      hand held interactive Y93.C2 (following Y93.7)
    game playing (using) (with)
      interactive device Y93.C2 (following Y93.7)
      keyboard or other stationary device Y93.C1 (following Y93.7)
  elliptical machine Y93.A1 (following Y93.7)
  exercise(s)
    machines ((primarily) for)
      cardiorespiratory conditioning Y93.A1 (following Y93.7)
      muscle strengthening Y93.B1 (following Y93.7)
    muscle strengthening (non-machine) NEC Y93.B9 (following Y93.7)
  external motion NEC Y93.I9 (following Y93.7)
    rollercoaster Y93.I1 (following Y93.7)
  fainting game Y93.85
  field hockey Y93.65
  figure skating (pairs) (singles) Y93.21
  flag football Y93.62
  floor mopping and cleaning Y93.E5 (following Y93.7)
  food preparation and clean up Y93.G1 (following Y93.7)
  football (American) NOS Y93.61
    flag Y93.62
    tackle Y93.61
    touch Y93.62
  four square Y93.6A
  free weights Y93.B3 (following Y93.7)
  frisbee (ultimate) Y93.74
  furniture
    building Y93.D3 (following Y93.7)
    finishing Y93.D3 (following Y93.7)
    repair Y93.D3 (following Y93.7)
  game playing (electronic)
    using interactive device Y93.C2 (following Y93.7)
    using keyboard or other stationary device Y93.C1 (following Y93.7)
  gardening Y93.H2 (following Y93.7)
  golf Y93.53
  grass drills Y93.A6 (following Y93.7)
  grilling and smoking food Y93.G2 (following Y93.7)
  grooming and shearing an animal Y93.K3 (following Y93.7)
  guerilla drills Y93.A6 (following Y93.7)
  gymnastics (rhythmic) Y93.43
  hand held interactive electronic device Y93.C2 (following Y93.7)

Activity — Assault

Assault — *continued*
  burning, burns — *continued*
    cigarette(s) X97 ☑
    hot object X98.9 ☑
      fluid NEC X98.2 ☑
      household appliance X98.3 ☑
      specified NEC X98.8 ☑
      steam X98.0 ☑
      tap water X98.1 ☑
      vapors X98.0 ☑
    scalding — *see* Assault, burning
    steam X98.0 ☑
    vitriol Y08.89 ☑
  caustic, corrosive substance (gas) Y08.89 ☑
  crashing of
    aircraft Y08.81 ☑
    motor vehicle Y03.8 ☑
      pushed in front of Y02.0 ☑
      run over Y03.0 ☑
      specified NEC Y03.8 ☑
  cutting or piercing instrument X99.9 ☑
    dagger X99.2 ☑
    glass X99.0 ☑
    knife X99.1 ☑
    specified NEC X99.8 ☑
    sword X99.2 ☑
  dagger X99.2 ☑
  drowning (in) X92.9 ☑
    bathtub X92.0 ☑
    natural water X92.3 ☑
    specified NEC X92.8 ☑
    swimming pool X92.1 ☑
      following fall X92.2 ☑
  dynamite X96.8 ☑
  explosive(s) (material) X96.9 ☑
  fight (hand) (fists) (foot) (unarmed) Y04.0 ☑
    with weapon — *see* Assault, by type of weapon
  fire X97 ☑
  firearm X95.9 ☑
    airgun X95.01 ☑
    handgun X93 ☑
    hunting rifle X94.1 ☑
    larger X94.9 ☑
      specified NEC X94.8 ☑
    machine gun X94.2 ☑
    shotgun X94.0 ☑
    specified NEC X95.8 ☑
  from high place Y01 ☑
  gunshot (wound) NEC — *see* Assault, firearm, by type
  incendiary device X97 ☑
  injury Y09
    to child due to criminal abortion attempt NEC Y08.89 ☑
  knife X99.1 ☑
  late effect of — *see* categories X92-Y08 with 7th character S
  placing before moving object NEC Y02.8 ☑
    motor vehicle Y02.0 ☑
  poisoning — *see* categories T36-T65 with 7th character S
  puncture, any part of body — *see* Assault, cutting or piercing instrument
  pushing
    before moving object NEC Y02.8 ☑
      motor vehicle Y02.0 ☑
      subway train Y02.1 ☑
      train Y02.1 ☑
    from high place Y01 ☑
  rape T74.2- ☑
  scalding — *see* Assault, burning
  sequelae of — *see* categories X92-Y08 with 7th character S
  sexual (by bodily force) T74.2- ☑
  shooting — *see* Assault, firearm
  specified means NEC Y08.89 ☑
  stab, any part of body — *see* Assault, cutting or piercing instrument
  steam X98.0 ☑
  striking against
    other person Y04.2 ☑
    sports equipment Y08.09 ☑
      baseball bat Y08.02 ☑
      hockey stick Y08.01 ☑
  struck by
    sports equipment Y08.09 ☑
      baseball bat Y08.02 ☑

Assault — *continued*
  struck by — *continued*
    sports equipment — *continued*
      hockey stick Y08.01 ☑
  submersion — *see* Assault, drowning
  violence Y09
  weapon Y09
    blunt Y00 ☑
    cutting or piercing — *see* Assault, cutting or piercing instrument
    firearm — *see* Assault, firearm
  wound Y09
    cutting — *see* Assault, cutting or piercing instrument
    gunshot — *see* Assault, firearm
    knife X99.1 ☑
    piercing — *see* Assault, cutting or piercing instrument
    puncture — *see* Assault, cutting or piercing instrument
    stab — *see* Assault, cutting or piercing instrument
Attack by mammals NEC W55.89 ☑
Avalanche — *see* Landslide
Aviator's disease — *see* Air, pressure

B

Barotitis, barodontalgia, barosinusitis, barotrauma (otitic) (sinus) — *see* Air, pressure
Battered (baby) (child) (person) (syndrome) X58 ☑
Bayonet wound W26.1 ☑
  in
    legal intervention — *see* Legal, intervention, sharp object, bayonet
    war operations — *see* War operations, combat
  stated as undetermined whether accidental or intentional Y28.8 ☑
  suicide (attempt) X78.2 ☑
Bean in nose — *see* categories T17 and T18 ☑
Bed set on fire NEC — *see* Exposure, fire, uncontrolled, building, bed
Beheading (by guillotine)
  homicide X99.9 ☑
  legal execution — *see* Legal, intervention
Bending, injury in (prolonged) (static) X50.1 ☑
Bends — *see* Air, pressure, change
Bite, bitten by
  alligator W58.01 ☑
  arthropod (nonvenomous) NEC W57 ☑
  bull W55.21 ☑
  cat W55.01 ☑
  cow W55.21 ☑
  crocodile W58.11 ☑
  dog W54.0 ☑
  goat W55.31 ☑
  hoof stock NEC W55.31 ☑
  horse W55.11 ☑
  human being (accidentally) W50.3 ☑
    with intent to injure or kill Y04.1 ☑
    as, or caused by, a crowd or human stampede (with fall) W52 ☑
    assault Y04.1 ☑
    homicide (attempt) Y04.1 ☑
    in
      fight Y04.1 ☑
  insect (nonvenomous) W57 ☑
  lizard (nonvenomous) W59.01 ☑
  mammal NEC W55.81 ☑
    marine W56.31 ☑
  marine animal (nonvenomous) W56.81 ☑
  millipede W57 ☑
  moray eel W56.51 ☑
  mouse W53.01 ☑
  person(s) (accidentally) W50.3 ☑
    with intent to injure or kill Y04.1 ☑
    as, or caused by, a crowd or human stampede (with fall) W52 ☑
    assault Y04.1 ☑
    homicide (attempt) Y04.1 ☑
    in
      fight Y04.1 ☑
  pig W55.41 ☑
  raccoon W55.51 ☑
  rat W53.11 ☑
  reptile W59.81 ☑
    lizard W59.01 ☑

Bite, bitten by — *continued*
  reptile — *continued*
    snake W59.11 ☑
    turtle W59.21 ☑
      terrestrial W59.81 ☑
  rodent W53.81 ☑
    mouse W53.01 ☑
    rat W53.11 ☑
    specified NEC W53.81 ☑
    squirrel W53.21 ☑
  shark W56.41 ☑
  sheep W55.31 ☑
  snake (nonvenomous) W59.11 ☑
  spider (nonvenomous) W57 ☑
  squirrel W53.21 ☑
Blast (air) in war operations — *see* War operations, blast
Blizzard X37.2 ☑
Blood alcohol level Y90.9
  less than 20mg/100ml Y90.0
  20-39mg/100ml Y90.1
  40-59mg/100ml Y90.2
  60-79mg/100ml Y90.3
  80-99mg/100ml Y90.4
  100-119mg/100ml Y90.5
  120-199mg/100ml Y90.6
  200-239mg/100ml Y90.7
  presence in blood, level not specified Y90.9
Blow X58 ☑
  by law-enforcing agent, police (on duty) — *see* Legal, intervention, manhandling
    blunt object — *see* Legal, intervention, blunt object
Blowing up — *see* Explosion
Brawl (hand) (fists) (foot) Y04.0 ☑
Breakage (accidental) (part of)
  ladder (causing fall) W11 ☑
  scaffolding (causing fall) W12 ☑
Broken
  glass, contact with — *see* Contact, with, glass
  power line (causing electric shock) W85 ☑
Bumping against, into (accidentally)
  object NEC W22.8 ☑
    with fall — *see* Fall, due to, bumping against, object
    caused by crowd or human stampede (with fall) W52 ☑
    sports equipment W21.9 ☑
  person(s) W51 ☑
    with fall W03 ☑
      due to ice or snow W00.0 ☑
    assault Y04.2 ☑
    caused by, a crowd or human stampede (with fall) W52 ☑
    homicide (attempt) Y04.2 ☑
  sports equipment W21.9 ☑
Burn, burned, burning (accidental) (by) (from) (on)
  acid NEC — *see* Table of Drugs and Chemicals
  bed linen — *see* Exposure, fire, uncontrolled, in building, bed
  blowtorch X08.8 ☑
    with ignition of clothing NEC X06.2 ☑
      nightwear X05 ☑
  bonfire, campfire (controlled) (*see also* Exposure, fire, controlled, not in building)
    uncontrolled — *see* Exposure, fire, uncontrolled, not in building
  candle X08.8 ☑
    with ignition of clothing NEC X06.2 ☑
      nightwear X05 ☑
  caustic liquid, substance (external) (internal) NEC — *see* Table of Drugs and Chemicals
  chemical (external) (internal) (*see also* Table of Drugs and Chemicals)
    in war operations — *see* War operations. fire
  cigar(s) or cigarette(s) X08.8 ☑
    with ignition of clothing NEC X06.2 ☑
      nightwear X05 ☑
  clothes, clothing NEC (from controlled fire) X06.2 ☑
    with conflagration — *see* Exposure, fire, uncontrolled, building
      not in building or structure — *see* Exposure, fire, uncontrolled, not in building
  cooker (hot) X15.8 ☑
    stated as undetermined whether accidental or intentional Y27.3 ☑
    suicide (attempt) X77.3 ☑
  electric blanket X16 ☑

Burn, burned, burning — *continued*
engine (hot) X17 ✓
fire, flames — *see* Exposure, fire
flare, Very pistol — *see* Discharge, firearm NEC
heat
  from appliance (electrical) (household) X15.8 ✓
    cooker X15.8 ✓
    hotplate X15.2 ✓
    kettle X15.8 ✓
    light bulb X15.8 ✓
    saucepan X15.3 ✓
    skillet X15.3 ✓
    stated as undetermined whether accidental or
      intentional Y27.3 ✓
    stove X15.0 ✓
    suicide (attempt) X77.3 ✓
    toaster X15.1 ✓
  in local application or packing during medical or
    surgical procedure Y63.5
heating
  appliance, radiator or pipe X16 ✓
homicide (attempt) — *see* Assault, burning
hot
  air X14.1 ✓
  cooker X15.8 ✓
  drink X10.0 ✓
  engine X17 ✓
  fat X10.2 ✓
  fluid NEC X12 ✓
  food X10.1 ✓
  gases X14.1 ✓
  heating appliance X16 ✓
  household appliance NEC X15.8 ✓
  kettle X15.8 ✓
  liquid NEC X12 ✓
  machinery X17 ✓
  metal (molten) (liquid) NEC X18 ✓
  object (not producing fire or flames) NEC X19 ✓
  oil (cooking) X10.2 ✓
  pipe(s) X16 ✓
  radiator X16 ✓
  saucepan (glass) (metal) X15.3 ✓
  stove (kitchen) X15.0 ✓
  substance NEC X19 ✓
    caustic or corrosive NEC — *see* Table of Drugs
      and Chemicals
  toaster X15.1 ✓
  tool X17 ✓
  vapor X13.1 ✓
  water (tap) — *see* Contact, with, hot, tap water
hotplate X15.2 ✓
  suicide (attempt) X77.3 ✓
ignition — *see* Ignition
in war operations — *see* War operations, fire
inflicted by other person X97 ✓
  by hot objects, hot vapor, and steam — *see* Assault,
    burning, hot object
internal, from swallowed caustic, corrosive liquid,
  substance — *see* Table of Drugs and Chemicals
iron (hot) X15.8 ✓
  stated as undetermined whether accidental or in-
    tentional Y27.3 ✓
  suicide (attempt) X77.3 ✓
kettle (hot) X15.8 ✓
  stated as undetermined whether accidental or in-
    tentional Y27.3 ✓
  suicide (attempt) X77.3 ✓
lamp (flame) X08.8 ✓
  with ignition of clothing NEC X06.2 ✓
    nightwear X05 ✓
lighter (cigar) (cigarette) X08.8 ✓
  with ignition of clothing NEC X06.2 ✓
    nightwear X05 ✓
lightning — *see* subcategory T75.0 ✓
  causing fire — *see* Exposure, fire
liquid (boiling) (hot) NEC X12 ✓
  stated as undetermined whether accidental or in-
    tentional Y27.2 ✓
  suicide (attempt) X77.2 ✓
local application of externally applied substance in
  medical or surgical care Y63.5
machinery (hot) X17 ✓
matches X08.8 ✓
  with ignition of clothing NEC X06.2 ✓
    nightwear X05 ✓

Burn, burned, burning — *continued*
mattress — *see* Exposure, fire, uncontrolled, building,
  bed
medicament, externally applied Y63.5
metal (hot) (liquid) (molten) NEC X18 ✓
nightwear (nightclothes, nightdress, gown, pajamas,
  robe) X05 ✓
object (hot) NEC X19 ✓
on board watercraft
  due to
    accident to watercraft V91.09 ✓
      powered craft V91.03 ✓
        ferry boat V91.01 ✓
        fishing boat V91.02 ✓
        jetskis V91.03 ✓
        liner V91.01 ✓
        merchant ship V91.00 ✓
        passenger ship V91.01 ✓
      unpowered craft V91.08 ✓
        canoe V91.05 ✓
        inflatable V91.06 ✓
        kayak V91.05 ✓
        sailboat V91.04 ✓
        surf-board V91.08 ✓
        water skis V91.07 ✓
        windsurfer V91.08 ✓
    fire on board V93.09 ✓
      ferry boat V93.01 ✓
      fishing boat V93.02 ✓
      jetskis V93.03 ✓
      liner V93.01 ✓
      merchant ship V93.00 ✓
      passenger ship V93.01 ✓
      powered craft NEC V93.03 ✓
      sailboat V93.04 ✓
    specified heat source NEC on board V93.19 ✓
      ferry boat V93.11 ✓
      fishing boat V93.12 ✓
      jetskis V93.13 ✓
      liner V93.11 ✓
      merchant ship V93.10 ✓
      passenger ship V93.11 ✓
      powered craft NEC V93.13 ✓
      sailboat V93.14 ✓
pipe (hot) X16 ✓
  smoking X08.8 ✓
    with ignition of clothing NEC X06.2 ✓
      nightwear X05 ✓
powder — *see* Powder burn
radiator (hot) X16 ✓
saucepan (hot) (glass) (metal) X15.3 ✓
  stated as undetermined whether accidental or in-
    tentional Y27.3 ✓
  suicide (attempt) X77.3 ✓
self-inflicted X76 ✓
  stated as undetermined whether accidental or in-
    tentional Y26 ✓
stated as undetermined whether accidental or intentional Y27.0 ✓
steam X13.1 ✓
  pipe X16 ✓
    stated as undetermined whether accidental or
      intentional Y27.8 ✓
  stated as undetermined whether accidental or in-
    tentional Y27.0 ✓
  suicide (attempt) X77.0 ✓
stove (hot) (kitchen) X15.0 ✓
  stated as undetermined whether accidental or in-
    tentional Y27.3 ✓
  suicide (attempt) X77.3 ✓
substance (hot) NEC X19 ✓
  boiling X12 ✓
    stated as undetermined whether accidental or
      intentional Y27.2 ✓
    suicide (attempt) X77.2 ✓
  molten (metal) X18 ✓
suicide (attempt) NEC X76 ✓
  hot
    household appliance X77.3 ✓
    object X77.9 ✓
therapeutic misadventure
  heat in local application or packing during medical
    or surgical procedure Y63.5
  overdose of radiation Y63.2
toaster (hot) X15.1 ✓

Burn, burned, burning — *continued*
toaster — *continued*
    stated as undetermined whether accidental or in-
      tentional Y27.3 ✓
    suicide (attempt) X77.3 ✓
tool (hot) X17 ✓
torch, welding X08.8 ✓
  with ignition of clothing NEC X06.2 ✓
    nightwear X05 ✓
trash fire (controlled) — *see* Exposure, fire, controlled,
  not in building
  uncontrolled — *see* Exposure, fire, uncontrolled,
    not in building
vapor (hot) X13.1 ✓
  stated as undetermined whether accidental or in-
    tentional Y27.0 ✓
  suicide (attempt) X77.0 ✓
Very pistol — *see* Discharge, firearm NEC
Butted by animal W55.82 ✓
bull W55.22 ✓
cow W55.22 ✓
goat W55.32 ✓
horse W55.12 ✓
pig W55.42 ✓
sheep W55.32 ✓

C

Caisson disease — *see* Air, pressure, change
Campfire (exposure to) (controlled) (*see also* Exposure,
  fire, controlled, not in building)
  uncontrolled — *see* Exposure, fire, uncontrolled, not
    in building
Capital punishment (any means) — *see* Legal, intervention
Car sickness T75.3 ✓
Casualty (not due to war) NEC X58 ✓
war — *see* War operations
Cat
bite W55.01 ✓
scratch W55.03 ✓
Cataclysm, cataclysmic (any injury) NEC — *see* Forces
  of nature
Catching fire — *see* Exposure, fire
Caught
between
  folding object W23.0 ✓
  objects (moving) (stationary and moving) W23.0 ✓
    and machinery — *see* Contact, with, by type of
      machine
    stationary W23.1 ✓
  sliding door and door frame W23.0 ✓
by, in
  machinery (moving parts of) — *see* Contact, with,
    by type of machine
  washing-machine wringer W23.0 ✓
under packing crate (due to losing grip) W23.1 ✓
Cave-in caused by cataclysmic earth surface move-
ment or eruption — *see* Landslide
Change(s) in air pressure — *see* Air, pressure, change
Choked, choking (on) (any object except food or vomitus)
food (bone) (seed) — *see* categories T17 and T18 ✓
vomitus T17.81- ✓
Civil insurrection — *see* War operations
Cloudburst (any injury) X37.8 ✓
Cold, exposure to (accidental) (excessive) (extreme)
  (natural) (place) NEC — *see* Exposure, cold
Collapse
building W20.1 ✓
  burning (uncontrolled fire) X00.2 ✓
dam or man-made structure (causing earth movement)
  X36.0 ✓
machinery — *see* Contact, with, by type of machine
structure W20.1 ✓
  burning (uncontrolled fire) X00.2 ✓
Collision (accidental) NEC (*see also* Accident, transport)
  V89.9 ✓
pedestrian W51 ✓
  with fall W03 ✓
    due to ice or snow W00.0 ✓
    involving pedestrian conveyance — *see* Acci-
      dent, transport, pedestrian, conveyance
  and
    crowd or human stampede (with fall) W52 ✓
    object W22.8 ✓

External Causes Index

Collision — Contact

Collision — *continued*
  pedestrian — *continued*
    and — *continued*
      object — *continued*
        with fall — *see* Fall, due to, bumping
          against, object
    person(s) — *see* Collision, pedestrian
    transport vehicle NEC V89.9 ☑
    and
      avalanche, fallen or not moving — *see* Accident,
        transport
      falling or moving — *see* Landslide
      landslide, fallen or not moving — *see* Accident,
        transport
      falling or moving — *see* Landslide
      due to cataclysm — *see* Forces of nature, by type
      intentional, purposeful suicide (attempt) — *see*
        Suicide, collision
Combustion, spontaneous — *see* Ignition
Complication (delayed) **of or following** (medical or
    surgical procedure) Y84.9
  with misadventure — *see* Misadventure
  amputation of limb(s) Y83.5
  anastomosis (arteriovenous) (blood vessel) (gastroje-
    junal) (tendon) (natural or artificial material)
    Y83.2
  aspiration (of fluid) Y84.4
    tissue Y84.8
  biopsy Y84.8
  blood
    sampling Y84.7
    transfusion
      procedure Y84.8
  bypass Y83.2
  catheterization (urinary) Y84.6
    cardiac Y84.0
  colostomy Y83.3
  cystostomy Y83.3
  dialysis (kidney) Y84.1
  drug — *see* Table of Drugs and Chemicals
  due to misadventure — *see* Misadventure
  duodenostomy Y83.3
  electroshock therapy Y84.3
  external stoma, creation of Y83.3
  formation of external stoma Y83.3
  gastrostomy Y83.3
  graft Y83.2
  hypothermia (medically-induced) Y84.8
  implant, implantation (of)
    artificial
      internal device (cardiac pacemaker) (electrodes
        in brain) (heart valve prosthesis) (ortho-
        pedic) Y83.1
      material or tissue (for anastomosis or bypass)
        Y83.2
        with creation of external stoma Y83.3
      natural tissues (for anastomosis or bypass) Y83.2
        with creation of external stoma Y83.3
  infusion
    procedure Y84.8
  injection — *see* Table of Drugs and Chemicals
    procedure Y84.8
  insertion of gastric or duodenal sound Y84.5
  insulin-shock therapy Y84.3
  paracentesis (abdominal) (thoracic) (aspirative) Y84.4
  procedures other than surgical operation — *see*
    Complication of or following, by type of proce-
    dure
  radiological procedure or therapy Y84.2
  removal of organ (partial) (total) NEC Y83.6
  sampling
    blood Y84.7
    fluid NEC Y84.4
    tissue Y84.8
  shock therapy Y84.3
  surgical operation NEC (*see also* Complication of or
    following, by type of operation) Y83.9
    reconstructive NEC Y83.4
      with
        anastomosis, bypass or graft Y83.2
        formation of external stoma Y83.3
    specified NEC Y83.8
  transfusion (*see also* Table of Drugs and Chemicals)
    procedure Y84.8
  transplant, transplantation (heart) (kidney) (liver)
    (whole organ, any) Y83.0
    partial organ Y83.4
  ureterostomy Y83.3

Complication (delayed) **of or following** —
    continued
  vaccination (*see also* Table of Drugs and Chemicals)
    procedure Y84.8
Compression
  divers' squeeze — *see* Air, pressure, change
  trachea by
    food (lodged in esophagus) — *see* categories T17
      and T18 ☑
    vomitus (lodged in esophagus) T17.81- ☑
Conflagration — *see* Exposure, fire, uncontrolled
Constriction (external)
  hair W49.01 ☑
  jewelry W49.04 ☑
  ring W49.04 ☑
  rubber band W49.03 ☑
  specified item NEC W49.09 ☑
  string W49.02 ☑
  thread W49.02 ☑
Contact (accidental)
  with
    abrasive wheel (metalworking) W31.1 ☑
    alligator W58.09 ☑
      bite W58.01 ☑
      crushing W58.03 ☑
      strike W58.02 ☑
    amphibian W62.9 ☑
      frog W62.0 ☑
      toad W62.1 ☑
    animal (nonvenomous) NEC W64 ☑
      marine W56.89 ☑
        bite W56.81 ☑
        dolphin — *see* Contact, with, dolphin
        fish NEC — *see* Contact, with, fish
        mammal — *see* Contact, with, mammal,
          marine
        orca — *see* Contact, with, orca
        sea lion — *see* Contact, with, sea lion
        shark — *see* Contact, with, shark
        strike W56.82 ☑
    animate mechanical force NEC W64 ☑
    arrow W21.89 ☑
      not thrown, projected or falling W45.8 ☑
    arthropods (nonvenomous) W57 ☑
    axe W27.0 ☑
    band-saw (industrial) W31.2 ☑
    bayonet — *see* Bayonet wound
    bee(s) X58 ☑
    bench-saw (industrial) W31.2 ☑
    bird W61.99 ☑
      bite W61.91 ☑
      chicken — *see* Contact, with, chicken
      duck — *see* Contact, with, duck
      goose — *see* Contact, with, goose
      macaw — *see* Contact, with, macaw
      parrot — *see* Contact, with, parrot
      psittacine — *see* Contact, with, psittacine
      strike W61.92 ☑
      turkey — *see* Contact, with, turkey
    blender W29.0 ☑
    boiling water X12 ☑
      stated as undetermined whether accidental or
        intentional Y27.2 ☑
      suicide (attempt) X77.2 ☑
    bore, earth-drilling or mining (land) (seabed)
      W31.0 ☑
    buffalo — *see* Contact, with, hoof stock NEC
    bull W55.29 ☑
      bite W55.21 ☑
      gored W55.22 ☑
      strike W55.22 ☑
    bumper cars W31.81 ☑
    camel — *see* Contact, with, hoof stock NEC
    can
      lid W26.8 ☑
      opener W27.4 ☑
        powered W29.0 ☑
    cat W55.09 ☑
      bite W55.01 ☑
      scratch W55.03 ☑
    caterpillar (venomous) X58 ☑
    centipede (venomous) X58 ☑
    chain
      hoist W24.0 ☑
        agricultural operations W30.89 ☑
      saw W29.3 ☑

Contact — *continued*
  with — *continued*
    chicken W61.39 ☑
      peck W61.33 ☑
      strike W61.32 ☑
    chisel W27.0 ☑
    circular saw W31.2 ☑
    cobra X58 ☑
    combine (harvester) W30.0 ☑
    conveyer belt W24.1 ☑
    cooker (hot) X15.8 ☑
      stated as undetermined whether accidental or
        intentional Y27.3 ☑
      suicide (attempt) X77.3 ☑
    coral X58 ☑
    cotton gin W31.82 ☑
    cow W55.29 ☑
      bite W55.21 ☑
      strike W55.22 ☑
    crane W24.0 ☑
      agricultural operations W30.89 ☑
    crocodile W58.19 ☑
      bite W58.11 ☑
      crushing W58.13 ☑
      strike W58.12 ☑
    dagger W26.1 ☑
      stated as undetermined whether accidental or
        intentional Y28.2 ☑
      suicide (attempt) X78.2 ☑
    dairy equipment W31.82 ☑
    dart W21.89 ☑
      not thrown, projected or falling W45.8 ☑
    deer — *see* Contact, with, hoof stock NEC
    derrick W24.0 ☑
      agricultural operations W30.89 ☑
        hay W30.2 ☑
    dog W54.8 ☑
      bite W54.0 ☑
      strike W54.1 ☑
    dolphin W56.09 ☑
      bite W56.01 ☑
      strike W56.02 ☑
    donkey — *see* Contact, with, hoof stock NEC
    drill (powered) W29.8 ☑
      earth (land) (seabed) W31.0 ☑
      nonpowered W27.8 ☑
    drive belt W24.0 ☑
      agricultural operations W30.89 ☑
    dry ice — *see* Exposure, cold, man-made
    dryer (clothes) (powered) (spin) W29.2 ☑
    duck W61.69 ☑
      bite W61.61 ☑
      strike W61.62 ☑
    earth (-)
      drilling machine (industrial) W31.0 ☑
      scraping machine in stationary use W31.83 ☑
    edge of stiff paper W26.2 ☑
    electric
      beater W29.0 ☑
      blanket X16 ☑
      fan W29.2 ☑
        commercial W31.82 ☑
      knife W29.1 ☑
      mixer W29.0 ☑
    elevator (building) W24.0 ☑
      agricultural operations W30.89 ☑
        grain W30.3 ☑
    engine(s), hot NEC X17 ☑
    excavating machine W31.0 ☑
    farm machine W30.9 ☑
    feces — *see* Contact, with, by type of animal
    fer de lance X58 ☑
    fish W56.59 ☑
      bite W56.51 ☑
      shark — *see* Contact, with, shark
      strike W56.52 ☑
    flying horses W31.81 ☑
    forging (metalworking) machine W31.1 ☑
    fork W27.4 ☑
    forklift (truck) W24.0 ☑
      agricultural operations W30.89 ☑
    frog W62.0 ☑
    garden
      cultivator (powered) W29.3 ☑
        riding W30.89 ☑
      fork W27.1 ☑

☑ Additional Character Required — Refer to the Tabular List for Character Selection

�快 Subterms under main terms may continue to next column or page

Contact — *continued*
  with — *continued*
    gas turbine W31.3 ☑
    Gila monster X58 ☑
    giraffe — *see* Contact, with, hoof stock NEC
    glass (sharp) (broken) W25 ☑
      with subsequent fall W18.02 ☑
      assault X99.0 ☑
      due to fall — *see* Fall, by type
      stated as undetermined whether accidental or
        intentional Y28.0 ☑
      suicide (attempt) X78.0 ☑
    goat W55.39 ☑
      bite W55.31 ☑
      strike W55.32 ☑
    goose W61.59 ☑
      bite W61.51 ☑
      strike W61.52 ☑
    hand
      saw W27.0 ☑
      tool (not powered) NEC W27.8 ☑
        powered W29.8 ☑
    harvester W30.0 ☑
    hay-derrick W30.2 ☑
    heating
      appliance (hot) X16 ☑
      pad (electric) X16 ☑
    heat NEC X19 ☑
      from appliance (electrical) (household) — *see*
        Contact, with, hot, household appliance
        heating appliance X16 ☑
    hedge-trimmer (powered) W29.3 ☑
    hoe W27.1 ☑
    hoist (chain) (shaft) NEC W24.0 ☑
      agricultural W30.89 ☑
    hoof stock NEC W55.39 ☑
      bite W55.31 ☑
      strike W55.32 ☑
    hornet(s) X58 ☑
    horse W55.19 ☑
      bite W55.11 ☑
      strike W55.12 ☑
    hot
      air X14.1 ☑
        inhalation X14.0 ☑
      cooker X15.8 ☑
      drinks X10.0 ☑
      engine X17 ☑
      fats X10.2 ☑
      fluids NEC X12 ☑
        assault X98.2 ☑
        suicide (attempt) X77.2 ☑
        undetermined whether accidental or inten-
          tional Y27.2 ☑
      food X10.1 ☑
      gases X14.1 ☑
        inhalation X14.0 ☑
      heating appliance X16 ☑
      household appliance X15.8 ☑
        assault X98.3 ☑
        cooker X15.8 ☑
        hotplate X15.2 ☑
        kettle X15.8 ☑
        light bulb X15.8 ☑
        object NEC X19 ☑
          assault X98.8 ☑
          stated as undetermined whether acciden-
            tal or intentional Y27.9 ☑
          suicide (attempt) X77.8 ☑
        saucepan X15.3 ☑
        skillet X15.3 ☑
        stated as undetermined whether accidental
          or intentional Y27.3 ☑
        stove X15.0 ☑
        suicide (attempt) X77.3 ☑
        toaster X15.1 ☑
      kettle X15.8 ☑
      light bulb X15.8 ☑
      liquid NEC (*see also* Burn) X12 ☑
        drinks X10.0 ☑
        stated as undetermined whether accidental
          or intentional Y27.2 ☑
        suicide (attempt) X77.2 ☑
        tap water X11.8 ☑
          stated as undetermined whether acciden-
            tal or intentional Y27.1 ☑

Contact — *continued*
  with — *continued*
    hot — *continued*
      liquid (*see also* Burn) — *continued*
        tap water — *continued*
          suicide (attempt) X77.1 ☑
      machinery X17 ☑
      metal (molten) (liquid) NEC X18 ☑
      object (not producing fire or flames) NEC X19 ☑
      oil (cooking) X10.2 ☑
      pipe X16 ☑
      plate X15.2 ☑
      radiator X16 ☑
      saucepan (glass) (metal) X15.3 ☑
      skillet X15.3 ☑
      stove (kitchen) X15.0 ☑
      substance NEC X19 ☑
      tap-water X11.8 ☑
        assault X98.1 ☑
        heated on stove X12 ☑
          stated as undetermined whether acciden-
            tal or intentional Y27.2 ☑
          suicide (attempt) X77.2 ☑
        in bathtub X11.0 ☑
        running X11.1 ☑
        stated as undetermined whether accidental
          or intentional Y27.1 ☑
        suicide (attempt) X77.1 ☑
      toaster X15.1 ☑
      tool X17 ☑
      vapors X13.1 ☑
        inhalation X13.0 ☑
      water (tap) X11.8 ☑
        boiling X12 ☑
          stated as undetermined whether acciden-
            tal or intentional Y27.2 ☑
          suicide (attempt) X77.2 ☑
        heated on stove X12 ☑
          stated as undetermined whether acciden-
            tal or intentional Y27.2 ☑
          suicide (attempt) X77.2 ☑
        in bathtub X11.0 ☑
        running X11.1 ☑
        stated as undetermined whether accidental
          or intentional Y27.1 ☑
        suicide (attempt) X77.1 ☑
    hotplate X15.2 ☑
    ice-pick W27.4 ☑
    insect (nonvenomous) NEC W57 ☑
    kettle (hot) X15.8 ☑
    knife W26.0 ☑
      assault X99.1 ☑
      electric W29.1 ☑
      stated as undetermined whether accidental or
        intentional Y28.1 ☑
      suicide (attempt) X78.1 ☑
    lathe (metalworking) W31.1 ☑
      turnings W45.8 ☑
      woodworking W31.2 ☑
    lawnmower (powered) (ridden) W28 ☑
      causing electrocution W86.8 ☑
        suicide (attempt) X83.1 ☑
      unpowered W27.1 ☑
    lift, lifting (devices) W24.0 ☑
      agricultural operations W30.89 ☑
      shaft W24.0 ☑
    liquefied gas — *see* Exposure, cold, man-made
    liquid air, hydrogen, nitrogen — *see* Exposure, cold,
      man-made
    lizard (nonvenomous) W59.09 ☑
      bite W59.01 ☑
      strike W59.02 ☑
    llama — *see* Contact, with, hoof stock NEC
    macaw W61.19 ☑
      bite W61.11 ☑
      strike W61.12 ☑
    machine, machinery W31.9 ☑
      abrasive wheel W31.1 ☑
      agricultural including animal-powered
        W30.9 ☑
        combine harvester W30.0 ☑
        grain storage elevator W30.3 ☑
        hay derrick W30.2 ☑
        power take-off device W30.1 ☑
        reaper W30.0 ☑
        specified NEC W30.89 ☑

Contact — *continued*
  with — *continued*
    machine, machinery — *continued*
      agricultural including animal-powered — *con-*
        tinued
        thresher W30.0 ☑
        transport vehicle, stationary W30.81 ☑
      band saw W31.2 ☑
      bench saw W31.2 ☑
      circular saw W31.2 ☑
      commercial NEC W31.82 ☑
      drilling, metal (industrial) W31.1 ☑
      earth-drilling W31.0 ☑
      earthmoving or scraping W31.89 ☑
      excavating W31.89 ☑
      forging machine W31.1 ☑
      gas turbine W31.3 ☑
      hot X17 ☑
      internal combustion engine W31.3 ☑
      land drill W31.0 ☑
      lathe W31.1 ☑
      lifting (devices) W24.0 ☑
      metal drill W31.1 ☑
      metalworking (industrial) W31.1 ☑
      milling, metal W31.1 ☑
      mining W31.0 ☑
      molding W31.2 ☑
      overhead plane W31.2 ☑
      power press, metal W31.1 ☑
      prime mover W31.3 ☑
      printing W31.89 ☑
      radial saw W31.2 ☑
      recreational W31.81 ☑
      roller-coaster W31.81 ☑
      rolling mill, metal W31.1 ☑
      sander W31.2 ☑
      seabed drill W31.0 ☑
      shaft
        hoist W31.0 ☑
        lift W31.0 ☑
      specified NEC W31.89 ☑
      spinning W31.89 ☑
      steam engine W31.3 ☑
      transmission W24.1 ☑
      undercutter W31.0 ☑
      water driven turbine W31.3 ☑
      weaving W31.89 ☑
      woodworking or forming (industrial) W31.2 ☑
    mammal (feces) (urine) W55.89 ☑
      bull — *see* Contact, with, bull
      cat — *see* Contact, with, cat
      cow — *see* Contact, with, cow
      goat — *see* Contact, with, goat
      hoof stock — *see* Contact, with, hoof stock
      horse — *see* Contact, with, horse
      marine W56.39 ☑
        dolphin — *see* Contact, with, dolphin
        orca — *see* Contact, with, orca
        sea lion — *see* Contact, with, sea lion
        specified NEC W56.39 ☑
          bite W56.31 ☑
          strike W56.32 ☑
      pig — *see* Contact, with, pig
      raccoon — *see* Contact, with, raccoon
      rodent — *see* Contact, with, rodent
      sheep — *see* Contact, with, sheep
      specified NEC W55.89 ☑
        bite W55.81 ☑
        strike W55.82 ☑
    marine
      animal W56.89 ☑
        bite W56.81 ☑
        dolphin — *see* Contact, with, dolphin
        fish NEC — *see* Contact, with, fish
        mammal — *see* Contact, with, mammal,
          marine
        orca — *see* Contact, with, orca
        sea lion — *see* Contact, with, sea lion
        shark — *see* Contact, with, shark
        strike W56.82 ☑
    meat
      grinder (domestic) W29.0 ☑
        industrial W31.82 ☑
        nonpowered W27.4 ☑
      slicer (domestic) W29.0 ☑
        industrial W31.82 ☑

▽ Subterms under main terms may continue to next column or page   ☑ Additional Character Required — Refer to the Tabular List for Character Selection   413

Contact — Contact

Contact — *continued*
  with — *continued*
    merry go round W31.81 ☑
    metal, hot (liquid) (molten) NEC X18 ☑
    millipede W57 ☑
    nail W45.0 ☑
      gun W29.4 ☑
    needle (sewing) W27.3 ☑
      hypodermic W46.0 ☑
        contaminated W46.1 ☑
    object (blunt) NEC
      hot NEC X19 ☑
      legal intervention — *see* Legal, intervention, blunt object
      sharp NEC W45.8 ☑
        inflicted by other person NEC W45.8 ☑
          stated as
            intentional homicide (attempt) — *see* Assault, cutting or piercing instrument
        legal intervention — *see* Legal, intervention, sharp object
        self-inflicted X78.9 ☑
    orca W56.29 ☑
      bite W56.21 ☑
      strike W56.22 ☑
    overhead plane W31.2 ☑
    paper (as sharp object) W26.2 ☑
    paper-cutter W27.5 ☑
    parrot W61.09 ☑
      bite W61.01 ☑
      strike W61.02 ☑
    pig W55.49 ☑
      bite W55.41 ☑
      strike W55.42 ☑
    pipe, hot X16 ☑
    pitchfork W27.1 ☑
    plane (metal) (wood) W27.0 ☑
      overhead W31.2 ☑
    plant thorns, spines, sharp leaves or other mechanisms W60 ☑
    powered
      garden cultivator W29.3 ☑
      household appliance, implement, or machine W29.8 ☑
      saw (industrial) W31.2 ☑
        hand W29.8 ☑
    printing machine W31.89 ☑
    psittacine bird W61.29 ☑
      bite W61.21 ☑
      macaw — *see* Contact, with, macaw
      parrot — *see* Contact, with, parrot
      strike W61.22 ☑
    pulley (block) (transmission) W24.0 ☑
      agricultural operations W30.89 ☑
    raccoon W55.59 ☑
      bite W55.51 ☑
      strike W55.52 ☑
    radial-saw (industrial) W31.2 ☑
    radiator (hot) X16 ☑
    rake W27.1 ☑
    rattlesnake X58 ☑
    reaper W30.0 ☑
    reptile W59.89 ☑
      lizard — *see* Contact, with, lizard
      snake — *see* Contact, with, snake
      specified NEC W59.89 ☑
        bite W59.81 ☑
        crushing W59.83 ☑
        strike W59.82 ☑
      turtle — *see* Contact, with, turtle
    rivet gun (powered) W29.4 ☑
    road scraper — *see* Accident, transport, construction vehicle
    rodent (feces) (urine) W53.89 ☑
      bite W53.81 ☑
      mouse W53.09 ☑
        bite W53.01 ☑
      rat W53.19 ☑
        bite W53.11 ☑
      specified NEC W53.89 ☑
        bite W53.81 ☑
      squirrel W53.29 ☑
        bite W53.21 ☑
    roller coaster W31.81 ☑
    rope NEC W24.0 ☑

Contact — *continued*
  with — *continued*
    rope — *continued*
      agricultural operations W30.89 ☑
    saliva — *see* Contact, with, by type of animal
    sander W29.8 ☑
      industrial W31.2 ☑
    saucepan (hot) (glass) (metal) X15.3 ☑
    saw W27.0 ☑
      band (industrial) W31.2 ☑
      bench (industrial) W31.2 ☑
      chain W29.3 ☑
      hand W27.0 ☑
    sawing machine, metal W31.1 ☑
    scissors W27.2 ☑
    scorpion X58 ☑
    screwdriver W27.0 ☑
      powered W29.8 ☑
    sea
      anemone, cucumber or urchin (spine) X58 ☑
      lion W56.19 ☑
        bite W56.11 ☑
        strike W56.12 ☑
    serpent — *see* Contact, with, snake, by type
    sewing-machine (electric) (powered) W29.2 ☑
      not powered W27.8 ☑
    shaft (hoist) (lift) (transmission) NEC W24.0 ☑
      agricultural W30.89 ☑
    shark W56.49 ☑
      bite W56.41 ☑
      strike W56.42 ☑
    sharp object(s) W26.9 ☑
      specified NEC W26.8 ☑
    shears (hand) W27.2 ☑
      powered (industrial) W31.1 ☑
        domestic W29.2 ☑
    sheep W55.39 ☑
      bite W55.31 ☑
      strike W55.32 ☑
    shovel W27.8 ☑
      steam — *see* Accident, transport, construction vehicle
    snake (nonvenomous) W59.19 ☑
      bite W59.11 ☑
      crushing W59.13 ☑
      strike W59.12 ☑
    spade W27.1 ☑
    spider (venomous) X58 ☑
    spin-drier W29.2 ☑
    spinning machine W31.89 ☑
    splinter W45.8 ☑
    sports equipment W21.9 ☑
    staple gun (powered) W29.8 ☑
    steam X13.1 ☑
      engine W31.3 ☑
      inhalation X13.0 ☑
      pipe X16 ☑
      shovel W31.89 ☑
    stove (hot) (kitchen) X15.0 ☑
    substance, hot NEC X19 ☑
      molten (metal) X18 ☑
    sword W26.1 ☑
      assault X99.2 ☑
      stated as undetermined whether accidental or intentional Y28.2 ☑
      suicide (attempt) X78.2 ☑
    tarantula X58 ☑
    thresher W30.0 ☑
    tin can lid W26.8 ☑
    toad W62.1 ☑
    toaster (hot) X15.1 ☑
    tool W27.8 ☑
      hand (not powered) W27.8 ☑
        auger W27.0 ☑
        axe W27.0 ☑
        can opener W27.4 ☑
        chisel W27.0 ☑
        fork W27.4 ☑
        garden W27.1 ☑
        handsaw W27.0 ☑
        hoe W27.1 ☑
        ice-pick W27.4 ☑
        kitchen utensil W27.4 ☑
        manual
          lawn mower W27.1 ☑
          sewing machine W27.8 ☑

Contact — *continued*
  with — *continued*
    tool — *continued*
      hand — *continued*
        meat grinder W27.4 ☑
        needle (sewing) W27.3 ☑
          hypodermic W46.0 ☑
            contaminated W46.1 ☑
        paper cutter W27.5 ☑
        pitchfork W27.1 ☑
        rake W27.1 ☑
        scissors W27.2 ☑
        screwdriver W27.0 ☑
        specified NEC W27.8 ☑
        workbench W27.0 ☑
      hot X17 ☑
      powered W29.8 ☑
        blender W29.0 ☑
          commercial W31.82 ☑
        can opener W29.0 ☑
          commercial W31.82 ☑
        chainsaw W29.3 ☑
        clothes dryer W29.2 ☑
          commercial W31.82 ☑
        dishwasher W29.2 ☑
          commercial W31.82 ☑
        edger W29.3 ☑
        electric fan W29.2 ☑
          commercial W31.82 ☑
        electric knife W29.1 ☑
        food processor W29.0 ☑
          commercial W31.82 ☑
        garbage disposal W29.0 ☑
          commercial W31.82 ☑
        garden tool W29.3 ☑
        hedge trimmer W29.3 ☑
        ice maker W29.0 ☑
          commercial W31.82 ☑
        kitchen appliance W29.0 ☑
          commercial W31.82 ☑
        lawn mower W28 ☑
        meat grinder W29.0 ☑
          commercial W31.82 ☑
        mixer W29.0 ☑
          commercial W31.82 ☑
        rototiller W29.3 ☑
        sewing machine W29.2 ☑
          commercial W31.82 ☑
        washing machine W29.2 ☑
          commercial W31.82 ☑
    transmission device (belt, cable, chain, gear, pinion, shaft) W24.1 ☑
      agricultural operations W30.89 ☑
    turbine (gas) (water-driven) W31.3 ☑
    turkey W61.49 ☑
      peck W61.43 ☑
      strike W61.42 ☑
    turtle (nonvenomous) W59.29 ☑
      bite W59.21 ☑
      strike W59.22 ☑
      terrestrial W59.89 ☑
        bite W59.81 ☑
        crushing W59.83 ☑
        strike W59.82 ☑
    under-cutter W31.0 ☑
    urine — *see* Contact, with, by type of animal
    vehicle
      agricultural use (transport) — *see* Accident, transport, agricultural vehicle
        not on public highway W30.81 ☑
      industrial use (transport) — *see* Accident, transport, industrial vehicle
        not on public highway W31.83 ☑
      off-road use (transport) — *see* Accident, transport, all-terrain or off-road vehicle
        not on public highway W31.83 ☑
      special construction use (transport) — *see* Accident, transport, construction vehicle
        not on public highway W31.83 ☑
    venomous
      animal X58 ☑
      arthropods X58 ☑
      lizard X58 ☑
      marine animal NEC X58 ☑
      marine plant NEC X58 ☑
      millipedes (tropical) X58 ☑

Contact — *continued*
  with — *continued*
    venomous — *continued*
      plant(s) X58 ☑
      snake X58 ☑
      spider X58 ☑
      viper X58 ☑
      washing-machine (powered) W29.2 ☑
      wasp X58 ☑
      weaving-machine W31.89 ☑
      winch W24.0 ☑
        agricultural operations W30.89 ☑
      wire NEC W24.0 ☑
        agricultural operations W30.89 ☑
      wood slivers W45.8 ☑
      yellow jacket X58 ☑
      zebra — *see* Contact, with, hoof stock NEC
    pressure X50.9 ☑
    stress X50.9 ☑
Coup de soleil X32 ☑
Crash
  aircraft (in transit) (powered) V95.9 ☑
    balloon V96.01 ☑
    fixed wing NEC (private) V95.21 ☑
      commercial V95.31 ☑
    glider V96.21 ☑
      hang V96.11 ☑
      powered V95.11 ☑
    helicopter V95.01 ☑
    in war operations — *see* War operations, destruction of aircraft
    microlight V95.11 ☑
    nonpowered V96.9 ☑
      specified NEC V96.8 ☑
    powered NEC V95.8 ☑
    stated as
      homicide (attempt) Y08.81 ☑
      suicide (attempt) X83.0 ☑
    ultralight V95.11 ☑
  spacecraft V95.41 ☑
  transport vehicle NEC (*see also* Accident, transport) V89.9 ☑
    homicide (attempt) Y03.8 ☑
    motor NEC (traffic) V89.2 ☑
      homicide (attempt) Y03.8 ☑
      suicide (attempt) — *see* Suicide, collision
Cruelty (mental) (physical) (sexual) X58 ☑
Crushed (accidentally) X58 ☑
  between objects (moving) (stationary and moving) W23.0 ☑
    stationary W23.1 ☑
  by
    alligator W58.03 ☑
    avalanche NEC — *see* Landslide
    cave-in W20.0 ☑
      caused by cataclysmic earth surface movement — *see* Landslide
    crocodile W58.13 ☑
    crowd or human stampede W52 ☑
    falling
      aircraft V97.39 ☑
        in war operations — *see* War operations, destruction of aircraft
      earth, material W20.0 ☑
        caused by cataclysmic earth surface movement — *see* Landslide
      object NEC W20.8 ☑
    landslide NEC — *see* Landslide
    lizard (nonvenomous) W59.09 ☑
    machinery — *see* Contact, with, by type of machine
    reptile NEC W59.89 ☑
    snake (nonvenomous) W59.13 ☑
  in
    machinery — *see* Contact, with, by type of machine
Cut, cutting (any part of body) (accidental) (*see also* Contact, with, by object or machine)
  during medical or surgical treatment as misadventure — *see* Index to Diseases and Injuries, Complications
  homicide (attempt) — *see* Assault, cutting or piercing instrument
  inflicted by other person — *see* Assault, cutting or piercing instrument
  legal
    execution — *see* Legal, intervention

Cut, cutting — *continued*
  legal — *continued*
    intervention — *see* Legal, intervention, sharp object
  machine NEC (*see also* Contact, with, by type of machine) W31.9 ☑
  self-inflicted — *see* Suicide, cutting or piercing instrument
  suicide (attempt) — *see* Suicide, cutting or piercing instrument
Cyclone (any injury) X37.1 ☑

D

Decapitation (accidental circumstances) NEC X58 ☑
  homicide X99.9 ☑
  legal execution — *see* Legal, intervention
Dehydration from lack of water X58 ☑
Deprivation X58 ☑
Derailment (accidental)
  railway (rolling stock) (train) (vehicle) (without antecedent collision) V81.7 ☑
    with antecedent collision — *see* Accident, transport, railway vehicle occupant
  streetcar (without antecedent collision) V82.7 ☑
    with antecedent collision — *see* Accident, transport, streetcar occupant
Descent
  parachute (voluntary) (without accident to aircraft) V97.29 ☑
    due to accident to aircraft — *see* Accident, transport, aircraft
Desertion X58 ☑
Destitution X58 ☑
Disability, late effect or sequela of injury — *see* Sequelae
Discharge (accidental)
  airgun W34.010 ☑
    assault X95.01 ☑
    homicide (attempt) X95.01 ☑
    stated as undetermined whether accidental or intentional Y24.0 ☑
    suicide (attempt) X74.01 ☑
  BB gun — *see* Discharge, airgun
  firearm (accidental) W34.00 ☑
    assault X95.9 ☑
    handgun (pistol) (revolver) W32.0 ☑
      assault X93 ☑
      homicide (attempt) X93 ☑
      legal intervention — *see* Legal, intervention, firearm, handgun
      stated as undetermined whether accidental or intentional Y22 ☑
      suicide (attempt) X72 ☑
    homicide (attempt) X95.9 ☑
    hunting rifle W33.02 ☑
      assault X94.1 ☑
      homicide (attempt) X94.1 ☑
      legal intervention
        injuring
          bystander Y35.032 ☑
          law enforcement personnel Y35.031 ☑
          suspect Y35.033 ☑
      stated as undetermined whether accidental or intentional Y23.1 ☑
      suicide (attempt) X73.1 ☑
    larger W33.00 ☑
      assault X94.9 ☑
      homicide (attempt) X94.9 ☑
      hunting rifle — *see* Discharge, firearm, hunting rifle
      legal intervention — *see* Legal, intervention, firearm by type of firearm
      machine gun — *see* Discharge, firearm, machine gun
      shotgun — *see* Discharge, firearm, shotgun
      specified NEC W33.09 ☑
        assault X94.8 ☑
        homicide (attempt) X94.8 ☑
        legal intervention
          injuring
            bystander Y35.092 ☑
            law enforcement personnel Y35.091 ☑
            suspect Y35.093 ☑

Discharge — *continued*
  firearm — *continued*
    larger — *continued*
      specified — *continued*
        stated as undetermined whether accidental or intentional Y23.8 ☑
        suicide (attempt) X73.8 ☑
      stated as undetermined whether accidental or intentional Y23.9 ☑
      suicide (attempt) X73.9 ☑
    legal intervention
      injuring
        bystander Y35.002 ☑
        law enforcement personnel Y35.001 ☑
        suspect Y35.03 ☑
      using rubber bullet
        injuring
          bystander Y35.042 ☑
          law enforcement personnel Y35.041 ☑
          suspect Y35.043 ☑
    machine gun W33.03 ☑
      assault X94.2 ☑
      homicide (attempt) X94.2 ☑
      legal intervention — *see* Legal, intervention, firearm, machine gun
      stated as undetermined whether accidental or intentional Y23.3 ☑
      suicide (attempt) X73.2 ☑
    pellet gun — *see* Discharge, airgun
    shotgun W33.01 ☑
      assault X94.0 ☑
      homicide (attempt) X94.0 ☑
      legal intervention — *see* Legal, intervention, firearm, specified NEC
      stated as undetermined whether accidental or intentional Y23.0 ☑
      suicide (attempt) X73.0 ☑
    specified NEC W34.09 ☑
      assault X95.8 ☑
      homicide (attempt) X95.8 ☑
      legal intervention — *see* Legal, intervention, firearm, specified NEC
      stated as undetermined whether accidental or intentional Y24.8 ☑
      suicide (attempt) X74.8 ☑
    stated as undetermined whether accidental or intentional Y24.9 ☑
    suicide (attempt) X74.9 ☑
    Very pistol W34.09 ☑
      assault X95.8 ☑
      homicide (attempt) X95.8 ☑
      stated as undetermined whether accidental or intentional Y24.8 ☑
      suicide (attempt) X74.8 ☑
  firework(s) W39 ☑
    stated as undetermined whether accidental or intentional Y25 ☑
  gas-operated gun NEC W34.018 ☑
    airgun — *see* Discharge, airgun
    assault X95.09 ☑
    homicide (attempt) X95.09 ☑
    paintball gun — *see* Discharge, paintball gun
    stated as undetermined whether accidental or intentional Y24.8 ☑
    suicide (attempt) X74.09 ☑
  gun NEC (*see also* Discharge, firearm NEC)
    air — *see* Discharge, airgun
    BB — *see* Discharge, airgun
    for single hand use — *see* Discharge, firearm, handgun
    hand — *see* Discharge, firearm, handgun
    machine — *see* Discharge, firearm, machine gun
    other specified — *see* Discharge, firearm NEC
    paintball — *see* Discharge, paintball gun
    pellet — *see* Discharge, airgun
  handgun — *see* Discharge, firearm, handgun
  machine gun — *see* Discharge, firearm, machine gun
  paintball gun W34.011 ☑
    assault X95.02 ☑
    homicide (attempt) X95.02 ☑
    stated as undetermined whether accidental or intentional Y24.8 ☑
    suicide (attempt) X74.02 ☑
  pistol — *see* Discharge, firearm, handgun
    flare — *see* Discharge, firearm, Very pistol
    pellet — *see* Discharge, airgun

Discharge — *continued*
pistol — *see* Discharge, firearm, handgun — *continued*
    Very — *see* Discharge, firearm, Very pistol
revolver — *see* Discharge, firearm, handgun
rifle (hunting) — *see* Discharge, firearm, hunting rifle
shotgun — *see* Discharge, firearm, shotgun
spring-operated gun NEC W34.018 ☑
    assault X95.09 ☑
    homicide (attempt) X95.09 ☑
    stated as undetermined whether accidental or intentional Y24.8 ☑
    suicide (attempt) X74.09 ☑

Disease
Andes W94.11 ☑
aviator's — *see* Air, pressure
range W94.11 ☑

Diver's disease, palsy, paralysis, squeeze — *see* Air, pressure

Diving (into water) — *see* Accident, diving

Dog bite W54.0 ☑

Dragged by transport vehicle NEC (*see also* Accident, transport) V09.9 ☑

Drinking poison (accidental) — *see* Table of Drugs and Chemicals

Dropped (accidentally) **while being carried or supported by other person** W04 ☑

Drowning (accidental) W74 ☑
assault X92.9 ☑
due to
  accident (to)
    machinery — *see* Contact, with, by type of machine
    watercraft V90.89 ☑
      burning V90.29 ☑
        powered V90.23 ☑
          fishing boat V90.22 ☑
          jetskis V90.23 ☑
          merchant ship V90.20 ☑
          passenger ship V90.21 ☑
        unpowered V90.28 ☑
          canoe V90.25 ☑
          inflatable V90.26 ☑
          kayak V90.25 ☑
          sailboat V90.24 ☑
          water skis V90.27 ☑
      crushed V90.39 ☑
        powered V90.33 ☑
          fishing boat V90.32 ☑
          jetskis V90.33 ☑
          merchant ship V90.30 ☑
          passenger ship V90.31 ☑
        unpowered V90.38 ☑
          canoe V90.35 ☑
          inflatable V90.36 ☑
          kayak V90.35 ☑
          sailboat V90.34 ☑
          water skis V90.37 ☑
      overturning V90.09 ☑
        powered V90.03 ☑
          fishing boat V90.02 ☑
          jetskis V90.03 ☑
          merchant ship V90.00 ☑
          passenger ship V90.01 ☑
        unpowered V90.08 ☑
          canoe V90.05 ☑
          inflatable V90.06 ☑
          kayak V90.05 ☑
          sailboat V90.04 ☑
      sinking V90.19 ☑
        powered V90.13 ☑
          fishing boat V90.12 ☑
          jetskis V90.13 ☑
          merchant ship V90.10 ☑
          passenger ship V90.11 ☑
        unpowered V90.18 ☑
          canoe V90.15 ☑
          inflatable V90.16 ☑
          kayak V90.15 ☑
          sailboat V90.14 ☑
      specified type NEC V90.89 ☑
        powered V90.83 ☑
          fishing boat V90.82 ☑
          jetskis V90.83 ☑
          merchant ship V90.80 ☑
          passenger ship V90.81 ☑

Drowning — *continued*
due to — *continued*
  accident — *continued*
    watercraft — *continued*
      specified type — *continued*
        unpowered V90.88 ☑
          canoe V90.85 ☑
          inflatable V90.86 ☑
          kayak V90.85 ☑
          sailboat V90.84 ☑
          water skis V90.87 ☑
  avalanche — *see* Landslide
  cataclysmic
    earth surface movement NEC — *see* Forces of nature, earth movement
    storm — *see* Forces of nature, cataclysmic storm
  cloudburst X37.8 ☑
  cyclone X37.1 ☑
  fall overboard (from) V92.09 ☑
    powered craft V92.03 ☑
      ferry boat V92.01 ☑
      fishing boat V92.02 ☑
      jetskis V92.03 ☑
      liner V92.01 ☑
      merchant ship V92.00 ☑
      passenger ship V92.01 ☑
  resulting from
    accident to watercraft — *see* Drowning, due to, accident to, watercraft
    being washed overboard (from) V92.29 ☑
      powered craft V92.23 ☑
        ferry boat V92.21 ☑
        fishing boat V92.22 ☑
        jetskis V92.23 ☑
        liner V92.21 ☑
        merchant ship V92.20 ☑
        passenger ship V92.21 ☑
      unpowered craft V92.28 ☑
        canoe V92.25 ☑
        inflatable V92.26 ☑
        kayak V92.25 ☑
        sailboat V92.24 ☑
        surf-board V92.28 ☑
        water skis V92.27 ☑
        windsurfer V92.28 ☑
    motion of watercraft V92.19 ☑
      powered craft V92.13 ☑
        ferry boat V92.11 ☑
        fishing boat V92.12 ☑
        jetskis V92.13 ☑
        liner V92.11 ☑
        merchant ship V92.10 ☑
        passenger ship V92.11 ☑
      unpowered craft
        canoe V92.15 ☑
        inflatable V92.16 ☑
        kayak V92.15 ☑
        sailboat V92.14 ☑
    unpowered craft V92.08 ☑
      canoe V92.05 ☑
      inflatable V92.06 ☑
      kayak V92.05 ☑
      sailboat V92.04 ☑
      surf-board V92.08 ☑
      water skis V92.07 ☑
      windsurfer V92.08 ☑
  hurricane X37.0 ☑
  jumping into water from watercraft (involved in accident) (*see also* Drowning, due to, accident to, watercraft)
    without accident to or on watercraft W16.711 ☑
  tidal wave NEC — *see* Forces of nature, tidal wave
  torrential rain X37.8 ☑
following
  fall
    into
      bathtub W16.211 ☑
      bucket W16.221 ☑
      fountain — *see* Drowning, following, fall, into, water, specified NEC
      quarry — *see* Drowning, following, fall, into, water, specified NEC
      reservoir — *see* Drowning, following, fall, into, water, specified NEC

Drowning — *continued*
following — *continued*
  fall — *continued*
    into — *continued*
      swimming-pool W16.011 ☑
        stated as undetermined whether accidental or intentional Y21.3 ☑
        striking
          bottom W16.021 ☑
          wall W16.031 ☑
        suicide (attempt) X71.2 ☑
      water NOS W16.41 ☑
        natural (lake) (open sea) (river) (stream) (pond) W16.111 ☑
          striking
            bottom W16.121 ☑
            side W16.131 ☑
        specified NEC W16.311 ☑
          striking
            bottom W16.321 ☑
            wall W16.331 ☑
    overboard NEC — *see* Drowning, due to, fall overboard
  jump or dive
    from boat W16.711 ☑
      striking bottom W16.721 ☑
    into
      fountain — *see* Drowning, following, jump or dive, into, water, specified NEC
      quarry — *see* Drowning, following, jump or dive, into, water, specified NEC
      reservoir — *see* Drowning, following, jump or dive, into, water, specified NEC
      swimming-pool W16.511 ☑
        striking
          bottom W16.521 ☑
          wall W16.531 ☑
        suicide (attempt) X71.2 ☑
      water NOS W16.91 ☑
        natural (lake) (open sea) (river) (stream) (pond) W16.611 ☑
        specified NEC W16.811 ☑
          bottom W16.821 ☑
          striking
            bottom W16.821 ☑
            wall W16.831 ☑
        striking
          bottom W16.821 ☑
          wall W16.831 ☑
        striking bottom W16.621 ☑
homicide (attempt) X92.9 ☑
in
  bathtub (accidental) W65 ☑
    assault X92.0 ☑
    following fall W16.211 ☑
      stated as undetermined whether accidental or intentional Y21.1 ☑
    stated as undetermined whether accidental or intentional Y21.0 ☑
    suicide (attempt) X71.0 ☑
  lake — *see* Drowning, in, natural water
  natural water (lake) (open sea) (river) (stream) (pond) W69 ☑
    assault X92.3 ☑
    following
      dive or jump W16.611 ☑
        striking bottom W16.621 ☑
      fall W16.111 ☑
        striking
          bottom W16.121 ☑
          side W16.131 ☑
    stated as undetermined whether accidental or intentional Y21.4 ☑
    suicide (attempt) X71.3 ☑
  quarry — *see* Drowning, in, specified place NEC
  quenching tank — *see* Drowning, in, specified place NEC
  reservoir — *see* Drowning, in, specified place NEC
  river — *see* Drowning, in, natural water
  sea — *see* Drowning, in, natural water
  specified place NEC W73 ☑
    assault X92.8 ☑
    following
      dive or jump W16.811 ☑
        striking
          bottom W16.821 ☑
          wall W16.831 ☑

☑ **Additional Character Required — Refer to the Tabular List for Character Selection**   ◿ **Subterms under main terms may continue to next column or page**

Drowning — *continued*
  in — *continued*
    specified place — *continued*
      following — *continued*
        fall W16.311 ☑
          striking
            bottom W16.321 ☑
            wall W16.331 ☑
      stated as undetermined whether accidental or
        intentional Y21.8 ☑
      suicide (attempt) X71.8 ☑
    stream — *see* Drowning, in, natural water
    swimming-pool W67 ☑
      assault X92.1 ☑
        following fall X92.2 ☑
      following
        dive or jump W16.511 ☑
          striking
            bottom W16.521 ☑
            wall W16.531 ☑
        fall W16.011 ☑
          striking
            bottom W16.021 ☑
            wall W16.031 ☑
      stated as undetermined whether accidental or
        intentional Y21.2 ☑
        following fall Y21.3 ☑
      suicide (attempt) X71.1 ☑
        following fall X71.2 ☑
    war operations — *see* War operations, restriction
      of airway
  resulting from accident to watercraft — *see* Drowning,
    due to, accident, watercraft
  self-inflicted X71.9 ☑
  stated as undetermined whether accidental or inten-
    tional Y21.9 ☑
  suicide (attempt) X71.9 ☑

E

Earth falling (on) W20.0 ☑
  caused by cataclysmic earth surface movement or
    eruption — *see* Landslide
Earth (surface) **movement NEC** — *see* Forces of nature,
  earth movement
Earthquake (any injury) X34 ☑
Effect(s) (adverse) **of**
  air pressure (any) — *see* Air, pressure
  cold, excessive (exposure to) — *see* Exposure, cold
  heat (excessive) — *see* Heat
  hot place (weather) — *see* Heat
  insolation X30 ☑
  late — *see* Sequelae
  motion — *see* Motion
  nuclear explosion or weapon in war operations — *see*
    War operations, nuclear weapon
  radiation — *see* Radiation
  travel — *see* Travel
Electric shock (accidental) (by) (in) — *see* Exposure,
  electric current
Electrocution (accidental) — *see* Exposure, electric current
**Endotracheal tube wrongly placed during anesthetic
  procedure**
Entanglement
  in
    bed linen, causing suffocation T71 ☑
    wheel of pedal cycle V19.88 ☑
Entry of foreign body or material — *see* Foreign body
Environmental pollution related condition — *see*
  category Z57 ☑
Execution, legal (any method) — *see* Legal, intervention
Exhaustion
  cold — *see* Exposure, cold
  due to excessive exertion (*see also* Overexertion)
    X50.9 ☑
  heat — *see* Heat
Explosion (accidental) (of) (with secondary fire) W40.9 ☑
  acetylene W40.1 ☑
  aerosol can W36.1 ☑
  air tank (compressed) (in machinery) W36.2 ☑
  aircraft (in transit) (powered) NEC V95.9 ☑
    balloon V96.05 ☑
    fixed wing NEC (private) V95.25 ☑
      commercial V95.35 ☑
    glider V96.25 ☑

Explosion — *continued*
  aircraft — *continued*
    glider — *continued*
      hang V96.15 ☑
      powered V95.15 ☑
    helicopter V95.05 ☑
    in war operations — *see* War operations, destruc-
      tion of aircraft
    microlight V95.15 ☑
    nonpowered V96.9 ☑
      specified NEC V96.8 ☑
    powered NEC V95.8 ☑
    stated as
      homicide (attempt) Y03.8 ☑
      suicide (attempt) X83.0 ☑
    ultralight V95.15 ☑
  anesthetic gas in operating room W40.1 ☑
  antipersonnel bomb W40.8 ☑
    assault X96.0 ☑
    homicide (attempt) X96.0 ☑
    suicide (attempt) X75 ☑
  assault X96.9 ☑
  bicycle tire W37.0 ☑
  blasting (cap) (materials) W40.0 ☑
  boiler (machinery), not on transport vehicle W35 ☑
    on watercraft — *see* Explosion, in, watercraft
  butane W40.1 ☑
  caused by other person X96.9 ☑
  coal gas W40.1 ☑
  detonator W40.0 ☑
  dump (munitions) W40.8 ☑
  dynamite W40.0 ☑
    in
      assault X96.8 ☑
      homicide (attempt) X96.8 ☑
      legal intervention
        injuring
          bystander Y35.112 ☑
          law enforcement personnel Y35.111 ☑
          suspect Y35.113 ☑
      suicide (attempt) X75 ☑
  explosive (material) W40.9 ☑
    gas W40.1 ☑
    in blasting operation W40.0 ☑
    specified NEC W40.8 ☑
      in
        assault X96.8 ☑
        homicide (attempt) X96.8 ☑
        legal intervention
          injuring
            bystander Y35.192 ☑
            law enforcement personnel
              Y35.191 ☑
            suspect Y35.193 ☑
        suicide (attempt) X75 ☑
  factory (munitions) W40.8 ☑
  fertilizer bomb W40.8 ☑
    assault X96.3 ☑
    homicide (attempt) X96.3 ☑
    suicide (attempt) X75 ☑
  firearm (parts) NEC W34.19 ☑
    airgun W34.110 ☑
    BB gun W34.110 ☑
    gas, air or spring-operated gun NEC W34.118 ☑
    hangun W32.1 ☑
    hunting rifle W33.12 ☑
    larger firearm W33.10 ☑
      specified NEC W33.19 ☑
    machine gun W33.13 ☑
    paintball gun W34.111 ☑
    pellet gun W34.110 ☑
    shotgun W33.11 ☑
    Very pistol [flare] W34.19 ☑
  fire-damp W40.1 ☑
  fireworks W39 ☑
  gas (coal) (explosive) W40.1 ☑
    cylinder W36.9 ☑
      aerosol can W36.1 ☑
      air tank W36.2 ☑
      pressurized W36.3 ☑
      specified NEC W36.8 ☑
  gasoline (fumes) (tank) not in moving motor vehicle
    W40.1 ☑
    bomb W40.8 ☑
      assault X96.1 ☑
      homicide (attempt) X96.1 ☑

Explosion — *continued*
  gasoline not in moving motor vehicle — *continued*
    bomb — *continued*
      suicide (attempt) X75 ☑
    in motor vehicle — *see* Accident, transport, by type
      of vehicle
  grain store W40.8 ☑
  grenade W40.8 ☑
    in
      assault X96.8 ☑
      homicide (attempt) X96.8 ☑
      legal intervention
        injuring
          bystander Y35.192 ☑
          law enforcement personnel Y35.191 ☑
          suspect Y35.193 ☑
      suicide (attempt) X75 ☑
  handgun (parts) — *see* Explosion, firearm, hangun
    (parts)
  homicide (attempt) X96.9 ☑
    antipersonnel bomb — *see* Explosion, antiperson-
      nel bomb
    fertilizer bomb — *see* Explosion, fertilizer bomb
    gasoline bomb — *see* Explosion, gasoline bomb
    letter bomb — *see* Explosion, letter bomb
    pipe bomb — *see* Explosion, pipe bomb
    specified NEC X96.8 ☑
  hose, pressurized W37.8 ☑
  hot water heater, tank (in machinery) W35 ☑
    on watercraft — *see* Explosion, in, watercraft
  in, on
    dump W40.8 ☑
    factory W40.8 ☑
    mine (of explosive gases) NEC W40.1 ☑
    watercraft V93.59 ☑
      powered craft V93.53 ☑
        ferry boat V93.51 ☑
        fishing boat V93.52 ☑
        jetskis V93.53 ☑
        liner V93.51 ☑
        merchant ship V93.50 ☑
        passenger ship V93.51 ☑
        sailboat V93.54 ☑
  letter bomb W40.8 ☑
    assault X96.2 ☑
    homicide (attempt) X96.2 ☑
    suicide (attempt) X75 ☑
  machinery (*see also* Contact, with, by type of machine)
    on board watercraft — *see* Explosion, in, watercraft
    pressure vessel — *see* Explosion, by type of vessel
  methane W40.1 ☑
  mine W40.1 ☑
  missile NEC W40.8 ☑
  mortar bomb W40.8 ☑
    in
      assault X96.8 ☑
      homicide (attempt) X96.8 ☑
      legal intervention
        injuring
          bystander Y35.192 ☑
          law enforcement personnel Y35.191 ☑
          suspect Y35.193 ☑
      suicide (attempt) X75 ☑
  munitions (dump) (factory) W40.8 ☑
  pipe, pressurized W37.8 ☑
    bomb W40.8 ☑
      assault X96.4 ☑
      homicide (attempt) X96.4 ☑
      suicide (attempt) X75 ☑
  pressure, pressurized
    cooker W38 ☑
    gas tank (in machinery) W36.3 ☑
    hose W37.8 ☑
    pipe W37.8 ☑
    specified device NEC W38 ☑
    tire W37.8 ☑
      bicycle W37.0 ☑
    vessel (in machinery) W38 ☑
  propane W40.1 ☑
  self-inflicted X75 ☑
  shell (artillery) NEC W40.8 ☑
    during war operations — *see* War operations, ex-
      plosion

External Causes Index

Explosion — External cause status

Explosion — *continued*
  shell — *continued*
    in
      legal intervention
        injuring
          bystander Y35.122 ☑
          law enforcement personnel Y35.121 ☑
          suspect Y35.123 ☑
      war — *see* War operations, explosion
  spacecraft V95.45 ☑
  stated as undetermined whether accidental or intentional Y25 ☑
  steam or water lines (in machinery) W37.8 ☑
  stove W40.9 ☑
  suicide (attempt) X75 ☑
  tire, pressurized W37.8 ☑
    bicycle W37.0 ☑
  undetermined whether accidental or intentional Y25 ☑
  vehicle tire NEC W37.8 ☑
    bicycle W37.0 ☑
  war operations — *see* War operations, explosion
Exposure (to) X58 ☑
  air pressure change — *see* Air, pressure
  cold (accidental) (excessive) (extreme) (natural) (place) X31 ☑
    assault Y08.89 ☑
    due to
      man-made conditions W93.8 ☑
        dry ice (contact) W93.01 ☑
          inhalation W93.02 ☑
        liquid air (contact) (hydrogen) (nitrogen) W93.11 ☑
          inhalation W93.12 ☑
        refrigeration unit (deep freeze) W93.2 ☑
        suicide (attempt) X83.2 ☑
      weather (conditions) X31 ☑
    homicide (attempt) Y08.89 ☑
    self-inflicted X83.2 ☑
  due to abandonment or neglect X58 ☑
  electric current W86.8 ☑
    appliance (faulty) W86.8 ☑
      domestic W86.0 ☑
    caused by other person Y08.89 ☑
    conductor (faulty) W86.1 ☑
    control apparatus (faulty) W86.1 ☑
    electric power generating plant, distribution station W86.1 ☑
    electroshock gun — *see* Exposure, electric current, taser
    high-voltage cable W85 ☑
    homicide (attempt) Y08.89 ☑
    legal execution — *see* Legal, intervention, specified means NEC
    lightning — *see* subcategory T75.0 ☑
    live rail W86.8 ☑
    misadventure in medical or surgical procedure in electroshock therapy Y63.4
    motor (electric) (faulty) W86.8 ☑
      domestic W86.0 ☑
    self-inflicted X83.1 ☑
    specified NEC W86.8 ☑
      domestic W86.0 ☑
    stun gun — *see* Exposure, electric current, taser
    suicide (attempt) X83.1 ☑
    taser W86.8 ☑
      assault Y08.89 ☑
      legal intervention — *see* category Y35 ☑
      self-harm (intentional) X83.8 ☑
      undetermined intent Y33 ☑
    third rail W86.8 ☑
    transformer (faulty) W86.1 ☑
    transmission lines W85 ☑
  environmental tobacco smoke X58 ☑
  excessive
    cold — *see* Exposure, cold
    heat (natural) NEC X30 ☑
      man-made W92 ☑
  factor(s) NOS X58 ☑
    environmental NEC X58 ☑
      man-made NEC W99 ☑
      natural NEC — *see* Forces of nature
    specified NEC X58 ☑
  fire, flames (accidental) X08.8 ☑
    assault X97 ☑

Exposure — *continued*
  fire, flames — *continued*
    campfire — *see* Exposure, fire, controlled, not in building
    controlled (in)
      with ignition (of) clothing (*see also* Ignition, clothes) X06.2 ☑
        nightwear X05 ☑
      bonfire — *see* Exposure, fire, controlled, not in building
      brazier (in building or structure) (*see also* Exposure, fire, controlled, building)
        not in building or structure — *see* Exposure, fire, controlled, not in building
      building or structure X02.0 ☑
        with
          fall from building X02.3 ☑
          from building X02.5 ☑
          injury due to building collapse X02.2 ☑
          smoke inhalation X02.1 ☑
        hit by object from building X02.4 ☑
        specified mode of injury NEC X02.8 ☑
      fireplace, furnace or stove — *see* Exposure, fire, controlled, building
      not in building or structure X03.0 ☑
        with
          fall X03.3 ☑
          smoke inhalation X03.1 ☑
        hit by object X03.4 ☑
        specified mode of injury NEC X03.8 ☑
      trash — *see* Exposure, fire, controlled, not in building
    fireplace — *see* Exposure, fire, controlled, building
    fittings or furniture (in building or structure) (uncontrolled) — *see* Exposure, fire, uncontrolled, building
    forest (uncontrolled) — *see* Exposure, fire, uncontrolled, not in building
    grass (uncontrolled) — *see* Exposure, fire, uncontrolled, not in building
    hay (uncontrolled) — *see* Exposure, fire, uncontrolled, not in building
    homicide (attempt) X97 ☑
    ignition of highly flammable material X04 ☑
    in, of, on, starting in
      machinery — *see* Contact, with, by type of machine
      motor vehicle (in motion) (*see also* Accident, transport, occupant by type of vehicle) V87.8 ☑
        with collision — *see* Collision
      railway rolling stock, train, vehicle V81.81 ☑
        with collision — *see* Accident, transport, railway vehicle occupant
      street car (in motion) V82.8 ☑
        with collision — *see* Accident, transport, streetcar occupant
      transport vehicle NEC (*see also* Accident, transport)
        with collision — *see* Collision
      war operations (*see also* War operations, fire)
        from nuclear explosion — *see* War operations, nuclear weapons
      watercraft (in transit) (not in transit) V91.09 ☑
        localized — *see* Burn, on board watercraft, due to, fire on board
        powered craft V91.03 ☑
          ferry boat V91.01 ☑
          fishing boat V91.02 ☑
          jet skis V91.03 ☑
          liner V91.01 ☑
          merchant ship V91.00 ☑
          passenger ship V91.01 ☑
        unpowered craft V91.08 ☑
          canoe V91.05 ☑
          inflatable V91.06 ☑
          kayak V91.05 ☑
          sailboat V91.04 ☑
          surf-board V91.08 ☑
          waterskis V91.07 ☑
          windsurfer V91.08 ☑
    lumber (uncontrolled) — *see* Exposure, fire, uncontrolled, not in building
    mine (uncontrolled) — *see* Exposure, fire, uncontrolled, not in building
    prairie (uncontrolled) — *see* Exposure, fire, uncontrolled, not in building

Exposure — *continued*
  fire, flames — *continued*
    resulting from
      explosion — *see* Explosion
      lightning X08.8 ☑
    self-inflicted X76
    specified NEC X08.8 ☑
    started by other person X97 ☑
    stated as undetermined whether accidental or intentional Y26 ☑
    stove — *see* Exposure, fire, controlled, building
    suicide (attempt) X76 ☑
    tunnel (uncontrolled) — *see* Exposure, fire, uncontrolled, not in building
    uncontrolled
      in building or structure X00.0 ☑
        with
          fall from building X00.3 ☑
          injury due to building collapse X00.2 ☑
          jump from building X00.5 ☑
          smoke inhalation X00.1 ☑
        bed X08.00 ☑
          due to
            cigarette X08.01 ☑
            specified material NEC X08.09 ☑
        furniture NEC X08.20 ☑
          due to
            cigarette X08.21 ☑
            specified material NEC X08.29 ☑
        hit by object from building X00.4 ☑
        sofa X08.10 ☑
          due to
            cigarette X08.11 ☑
            specified material NEC X08.19 ☑
        specified mode of injury NEC X00.8 ☑
      not in building or structure (any) X01.0 ☑
        with
          fall X01.3 ☑
          smoke inhalation X01.1 ☑
        hit by object X01.4 ☑
        specified mode of injury NEC X01.8 ☑
      undetermined whether accidental or intentional Y26 ☑
  forces of nature NEC — *see* Forces of nature
  G-forces (abnormal) W49.9 ☑
  gravitational forces (abnormal) W49.9 ☑
  heat (natural) NEC — *see* Heat
  high-pressure jet (hydraulic) (pneumatic) W49.9 ☑
  hydraulic jet W49.9 ☑
  inanimate mechanical force W49.9 ☑
  jet, high-pressure (hydraulic) (pneumatic) W49.9 ☑
  lightning — *see* subcategory T75.0 ☑
    causing fire — *see* Exposure, fire
  mechanical forces NEC W49.9 ☑
    animate NEC W64
    inanimate NEC W49.9 ☑
  noise W42.9 ☑
    supersonic W42.0 ☑
  noxious substance — *see* Table of Drugs and Chemicals
  pneumatic jet W49.9 ☑
  prolonged in deep-freeze unit or refrigerator W93.2 ☑
  radiation — *see* Radiation
  smoke (*see also* Exposure, fire)
    tobacco, second hand Z77.22
  specified factors NEC X58 ☑
  sunlight X32 ☑
    man-made (sun lamp) W89.8 ☑
      tanning bed W89.1 ☑
  supersonic waves W42.0 ☑
  transmission line(s), electric W85 ☑
  vibration W49.9 ☑
  waves
    infrasound W49.9 ☑
    sound W42.9 ☑
    supersonic W42.0 ☑
  weather NEC — *see* Forces of nature
External cause status Y99.9
  child assisting in compensated work for family Y99.8
  civilian activity done for financial or other compensation Y99.0
  civilian activity done for income or pay Y99.0
  family member assisting in compensated work for other family member Y99.8
  hobby not done for income Y99.8
  leisure activity Y99.8

External cause status — *continued*
> military activity Y99.1
> off-duty activity of military personnel Y99.8
> recreation or sport not for income or while a student
>> Y99.8
> specified NEC Y99.8
> student activity Y99.8
> volunteer activity Y99.2

F

Factors, supplemental
> alcohol
>> blood level
>>> less than 20mg/100ml Y90.0
>>> 20-39mg/100ml Y90.1
>>> 40-59mg/100ml Y90.2
>>> 60-79mg/100ml Y90.3
>>> 80-99mg/100ml Y90.4
>>> 100-119mg/100ml Y90.5
>>> 120-199mg/100ml Y90.6
>>> 200-239mg/100ml Y90.7
>>> 240mg/100ml or more Y90.8
>>> presence in blood, level not specified Y90.9
>> presence in blood, but level not specified Y90.9
> environmental-pollution-related condition- see Z57 ☑
> nosocomial condition Y95
> work-related condition Y99.0

Failure
> in suture or ligature during surgical procedure Y65.2
> mechanical, of instrument or apparatus (any) (during
>> any medical or surgical procedure) Y65.8
> sterile precautions (during medical and surgical care)
>> — *see* Misadventure, failure, sterile precautions,
>> by type of procedure
> to
>> introduce tube or instrument Y65.4
>>> endotracheal tube during anesthesia Y65.3
>> make curve (transport vehicle) NEC — *see* Accident,
>>> transport
>> remove tube or instrument Y65.4

Fall, falling (accidental) W19 ☑
> building W20.1
>> burning (uncontrolled fire) X00.3 ☑
> down
>> embankment W17.81 ☑
>> escalator W10.0 ☑
>> hill W17.81 ☑
>> ladder W11 ☑
>> ramp W10.2 ☑
>> stairs, steps W10.9 ☑
> due to
>> bumping against
>>> object W18.00 ☑
>>>> sharp glass W18.02 ☑
>>>> specified NEC W18.09 ☑
>>>> sports equipment W18.01 ☑
>>> person W03 ☑
>>>> due to ice or snow W00.0 ☑
>>>> on pedestrian conveyance — *see* Accident,
>>>>> transport, pedestrian, conveyance
>> collision with another person W03 ☑
>>> due to ice or snow W00.0 ☑
>>> involving pedestrian conveyance — *see* Acci-
>>>> dent, transport, pedestrian, conveyance
>> grocery cart tipping over W17.82 ☑
>> ice or snow W00.9 ☑
>>> from one level to another W00.2 ☑
>>> on stairs or steps W00.1 ☑
>>> involving pedestrian conveyance — *see* Acci-
>>>> dent, transport, pedestrian, conveyance
>>> on same level W00.0 ☑
>> slipping (on moving sidewalk) W01.0 ☑
>>> with subsequent striking against object
>>>> W01.10 ☑
>>>> furniture W01.190 ☑
>>>> sharp object W01.119 ☑
>>>>> glass W01.110 ☑
>>>>> power tool or machine W01.111 ☑
>>>>> specified NEC W01.118 ☑
>>>> specified NEC W01.198 ☑
>> striking against
>>> object W18.00 ☑
>>>> sharp glass W18.02 ☑
>>>> specified NEC W18.09 ☑
>>>> sports equipment W18.01 ☑
>>> person W03 ☑

Fall, falling — *continued*
> due to — *continued*
>> striking against — *continued*
>>> person — *continued*
>>>> due to ice or snow W00.0 ☑
>>>> on pedestrian conveyance — *see* Accident,
>>>>> transport, pedestrian, conveyance
> earth (with asphyxia or suffocation (by pressure)) —
>> *see* Earth, falling
> from, off, out of
>> aircraft NEC (with accident to aircraft NEC) V97.0 ☑
>>> while boarding or alighting V97.1 ☑
>> balcony W13.0 ☑
>> bed W06 ☑
>> boat, ship, watercraft NEC (with drowning or sub-
>>> mersion) — *see* Drowning, due to, fall over-
>>> board
>>> with hitting bottom or object V94.0 ☑
>> bridge W13.1 ☑
>> building W13.9 ☑
>>> burning (uncontrolled fire) X00.3 ☑
>> cavity W17.2 ☑
>> chair W07 ☑
>> cherry picker W17.89 ☑
>> cliff W15 ☑
>> dock W17.4 ☑
>> embankment W17.81 ☑
>> escalator W10.0 ☑
>> flagpole W13.8 ☑
>> furniture NEC W08 ☑
>> grocery cart W17.82 ☑
>> haystack W17.89 ☑
>> high place NEC W17.89 ☑
>>> stated as undetermined whether accidental or
>>>> intentional Y30 ☑
>> hole W17.2 ☑
>> incline W10.2 ☑
>> ladder W11 ☑
>> lifting device W17.89 ☑
>> machine, machinery (*see also* Contact, with, by
>>> type of machine)
>>> not in operation W17.89 ☑
>> manhole W17.1 ☑
>> mobile elevated work platform [MEWP] W17.89 ☑
>> motorized mobility scooter W05.2 ☑
>> one level to another NEC W17.89 ☑
>>> intentional, purposeful, suicide (attempt)
>>>> X80 ☑
>>> stated as undetermined whether accidental or
>>>> intentional Y30 ☑
>> pit W17.2 ☑
>> playground equipment W09.8 ☑
>>> jungle gym W09.2 ☑
>>> slide W09.0 ☑
>>> swing W09.1 ☑
>> quarry W17.89 ☑
>> railing W13.9 ☑
>> ramp W10.2 ☑
>> roof W13.2 ☑
>> scaffolding W12 ☑
>> scooter (nonmotorized) W05.1 ☑
>>> motorized mobility W05.2 ☑
>> sky lift W17.89 ☑
>> stairs, steps W10.9 ☑
>>> curb W10.1 ☑
>>> due to ice or snow W00.1 ☑
>>> escalator W10.0 ☑
>>> incline W10.2 ☑
>>> ramp W10.2 ☑
>>> sidewalk curb W10.1 ☑
>>> specified NEC W10.8 ☑
>> stepladder W11 ☑
>> storm drain W17.1 ☑
>> streetcar NEC V82.6 ☑
>>> with antecedent collision — *see* Accident,
>>>> transport, streetcar occupant
>>> while boarding or alighting V82.4 ☑
>> structure NEC W13.8 ☑
>>> burning (uncontrolled fire) X00.3 ☑
>> table W08 ☑
>> toilet W18.11 ☑
>>> with subsequent striking against object
>>>> W18.12 ☑
>> train NEC V81.6 ☑
>>> during derailment (without antecedent colli-
>>>> sion) V81.7 ☑

Fall, falling — *continued*
> from, off, out of — *continued*
>> train — *continued*
>>> during derailment — *continued*
>>>> with antecedent collision — *see* Accident,
>>>>> transport, railway vehicle occupant
>>> while boarding or alighting V81.4 ☑
>> transport vehicle after collision — *see* Accident,
>>> transport, by type of vehicle, collision
>> tree W14 ☑
>> vehicle (in motion) NEC (*see also* Accident, trans-
>>> port) V89.9 ☑
>>> motor NEC (*see also* Accident, transport, occu-
>>>> pant, by type of vehicle) V87.8 ☑
>>> stationary W17.89 ☑
>>>> while boarding or alighting — *see* Accident,
>>>>> transport, by type of vehicle, while
>>>>> boarding or alighting
>> viaduct W13.8 ☑
>> wall W13.8 ☑
>> watercraft (*see also* Drowning, due to, fall over-
>>> board)
>>> with hitting bottom or object V94.0 ☑
>> well W17.0 ☑
>> wheelchair, non-moving W05.0 ☑
>>> powered — *see* Accident, transport, pedestrian,
>>>> conveyance occupant, specified type NEC
>> window W13.4 ☑
> in, on
>> aircraft NEC V97.0 ☑
>>> with accident to aircraft V97.0 ☑
>>> while boarding or alighting V97.1 ☑
>> bathtub (empty) W18.2 ☑
>>> filled W16.212 ☑
>>>> causing drowning W16.211 ☑
>> escalator W10.0 ☑
>> incline W10.2 ☑
>> ladder W11 ☑
>> machine, machinery — *see* Contact, with, by type
>>> of machine
>> object, edged, pointed or sharp (with cut) — *see*
>>> Fall, by type
>> playground equipment W09.8 ☑
>>> jungle gym W09.2 ☑
>>> slide W09.0 ☑
>>> swing W09.1 ☑
>> ramp W10.2 ☑
>> scaffolding W12 ☑
>> shower W18.2 ☑
>>> causing drowning W16.211 ☑
>> staircase, stairs, steps W10.9 ☑
>>> curb W10.1 ☑
>>> due to ice or snow W00.1 ☑
>>> escalator W10.0 ☑
>>> incline W10.2 ☑
>>> specified NEC W10.8 ☑
>> streetcar (without antecedent collision) V82.5 ☑
>>> with antecedent collision — *see* Accident,
>>>> transport, streetcar occupant
>>> while boarding or alighting V82.4 ☑
>> train (without antecedent collision) V81.5 ☑
>>> with antecedent collision — *see* Accident,
>>>> transport, railway vehicle occupant
>>> during derailment (without antecedent colli-
>>>> sion) V81.7 ☑
>>>> with antecedent collision — *see* Accident,
>>>>> transport, railway vehicle occupant
>>> while boarding or alighting V81.4 ☑
>> transport vehicle after collision — *see* Accident,
>>> transport, by type of vehicle, collision
>> watercraft V93.39 ☑
>>> due to
>>>> accident to craft V91.29 ☑
>>>>> powered craft V91.23 ☑
>>>>>> ferry boat V91.21 ☑
>>>>>> fishing boat V91.22 ☑
>>>>>> jetskis V91.23 ☑
>>>>>> liner V91.21 ☑
>>>>>> merchant ship V91.20 ☑
>>>>>> passenger ship V91.21 ☑
>>>>> unpowered craft
>>>>>> canoe V91.25 ☑
>>>>>> inflatable V91.26 ☑
>>>>>> kayak V91.25 ☑
>>>>>> sailboat V91.24 ☑
>>>> powered craft V93.33 ☑

Fall, falling — *continued*
  in, on — *continued*
    watercraft — *continued*
      powered craft — *continued*
        ferry boat V93.31 ☑
        fishing boat V93.32 ☑
        jetskis V93.33 ☑
        liner V93.31 ☑
        merchant ship V93.30 ☑
        passenger ship V93.31 ☑
      unpowered craft V93.38 ☑
        canoe V93.35 ☑
        inflatable V93.36 ☑
        kayak V93.35 ☑
        sailboat V93.34 ☑
        surf-board V93.38 ☑
        windsurfer V93.38 ☑
  into
    cavity W17.2 ☑
    dock W17.4 ☑
    fire — *see* Exposure, fire, by type
    haystack W17.89 ☑
    hole W17.2 ☑
    lake — *see* Fall, into, water
    manhole W17.1 ☑
    moving part of machinery — *see* Contact, with, by
      type of machine
    ocean — *see* Fall, into, water
    opening in surface NEC W17.89 ☑
    pit W17.2 ☑
    pond — *see* Fall, into, water
    quarry W17.89 ☑
    river — *see* Fall, into, water
    shaft W17.89 ☑
    storm drain W17.1 ☑
    stream — *see* Fall, into, water
    swimming pool (*see also* Fall, into, water, in,
      swimming pool)
      empty W17.3 ☑
    tank W17.89 ☑
    water W16.42 ☑
      causing drowning W16.41 ☑
      from watercraft — *see* Drowning, due to, fall
        overboard
      hitting diving board W21.4 ☑
      in
        bathtub W16.212 ☑
          causing drowning W16.211 ☑
        bucket W16.222 ☑
          causing drowning W16.221 ☑
        natural body of water W16.112 ☑
          causing drowning W16.111 ☑
          striking
            bottom W16.122 ☑
              causing drowning W16.121 ☑
            side W16.132 ☑
              causing drowning W16.131 ☑
        specified water NEC W16.312 ☑
          causing drowning W16.311 ☑
          striking
            bottom W16.322 ☑
              causing drowning W16.321 ☑
            wall W16.332 ☑
              causing drowning W16.331 ☑
        swimming pool W16.012 ☑
          causing drowning W16.011 ☑
          striking
            bottom W16.022 ☑
              causing drowning W16.031 ☑
            wall W16.032 ☑
              causing drowning W16.021 ☑
        utility bucket W16.222 ☑
          causing drowning W16.221 ☑
    well W17.0 ☑
  involving
    bed W06 ☑
    chair W07 ☑
    furniture NEC W08 ☑
    glass — *see* Fall, by type
    playground equipment W09.8 ☑
      jungle gym W09.2 ☑
      slide W09.0 ☑
      swing W09.1 ☑
    roller blades — *see* Accident, transport, pedestrian,
      conveyance

Fall, falling — *continued*
  involving — *continued*
    skateboard(s) — *see* Accident, transport, pedestri-
      an, conveyance
    skates (ice) (in line) (roller) — *see* Accident, trans-
      port, pedestrian, conveyance
    skis — *see* Accident, transport, pedestrian, con-
      veyance
    table W08 ☑
    wheelchair, non-moving W05.0 ☑
      powered — *see* Accident, transport, pedestrian,
        conveyance, specified type NEC
  object — *see* Struck by, object, falling
  off
    toilet W18.11 ☑
      with subsequent striking against object
        W18.12 ☑
  on same level W18.30 ☑
    due to
      specified NEC W18.39 ☑
      stepping on an object W18.31 ☑
  out of
    bed W06 ☑
    building NEC W13.8 ☑
    chair W07 ☑
    furniture NEC W08 ☑
    wheelchair, non-moving W05.0 ☑
      powered — *see* Accident, transport, pedestrian,
        conveyance, specified type NEC
    window W13.4 ☑
  over
    animal W01.0 ☑
    cliff W15 ☑
    embankment W17.81 ☑
    small object W01.0 ☑
  rock W20.8 ☑
  same level W18.30 ☑
    from
      being crushed, pushed, or stepped on by a
        crowd or human stampede W52 ☑
      collision, pushing, shoving, by or with other
        person W03 ☑
      slipping, stumbling, tripping W01.0 ☑
    involving ice or snow W00.0 ☑
      involving skates (ice) (roller), skateboard, skis
        — *see* Accident, transport, pedestrian,
        conveyance
  snowslide (avalanche) — *see* Landslide
  stone W20.8 ☑
  structure W20.1 ☑
    burning (uncontrolled fire) X00.3 ☑
  through
    bridge W13.1 ☑
    floor W13.3 ☑
    roof W13.2 ☑
    wall W13.8 ☑
    window W13.4 ☑
  timber W20.8 ☑
  tree (caused by lightning) W20.8 ☑
  while being carried or supported by other person(s)
    W04 ☑

Fallen on by
  animal (not being ridden) NEC W55.89 ☑
Felo-de-se — *see* Suicide
Fight (hand) (fists) (foot) — *see* Assault, fight
Fire (accidental) — *see* Exposure, fire
Firearm discharge — *see* Discharge, firearm
Fireball effects from nuclear explosion in war oper-
  ations — *see* War operations, nuclear weapons
Fireworks (explosion) W39 ☑
Flash burns from explosion — *see* Explosion
Flood (any injury) (caused by) X38 ☑
  collapse of man-made structure causing earth move-
    ment X36.0 ☑
  tidal wave — *see* Forces of nature, tidal wave
Food (any type) **in**
  air passages (with asphyxia, obstruction, or suffoca-
    tion) — *see* categories T17 and T18 ☑
  alimentary tract causing asphyxia (due to compression
    of trachea) — *see* categories T17 and T18 ☑
Forces of nature X39.8 ☑
  avalanche X36.1 ☑
    causing transport accident — *see* Accident, trans-
      port, by type of vehicle
  blizzard X37.2 ☑
  cataclysmic storm X37.9 ☑

Forces of nature — *continued*
  cataclysmic storm — *continued*
    with flood X38 ☑
    blizzard X37.2 ☑
    cloudburst X37.8 ☑
    cyclone X37.1 ☑
    dust storm X37.3 ☑
    hurricane X37.0 ☑
    specified storm NEC X37.8 ☑
    storm surge X37.0 ☑
    tornado X37.1 ☑
    twister X37.1 ☑
    typhoon X37.0 ☑
  cloudburst X37.8 ☑
  cold (natural) X31 ☑
  cyclone X37.1 ☑
  dam collapse causing earth movement X36.0 ☑
  dust storm X37.3 ☑
  earth movement X36.1 ☑
    caused by dam or structure collapse X36.0 ☑
    earthquake X34 ☑
  earthquake X34 ☑
  flood (caused by) X38 ☑
    dam collapse X36.0 ☑
    tidal wave — *see* Forces of nature, tidal wave
  heat (natural) X30 ☑
  hurricane X37.0 ☑
  landslide X36.1 ☑
    causing transport accident — *see* Accident, trans-
      port, by type of vehicle
  lightning — *see* subcategory T75.0 ☑
    causing fire — *see* Exposure, fire
  mudslide X36.1 ☑
    causing transport accident — *see* Accident, trans-
      port, by type of vehicle
  radiation (natural) X39.08 ☑
    radon X39.01 ☑
  radon X39.01 ☑
  specified force NEC X39.8 ☑
  storm surge X37.0 ☑
  structure collapse causing earth movement X36.0 ☑
  sunlight X32 ☑
  tidal wave X37.41 ☑
    due to
      earthquake X37.41 ☑
      landslide X37.43 ☑
      storm X37.42 ☑
      volcanic eruption X37.41 ☑
  tornado X37.1 ☑
  tsunami X37.41 ☑
  twister X37.1 ☑
  typhoon X37.0 ☑
  volcanic eruption X35 ☑
Foreign body
  aspiration — *see* Index to Diseases and Injuries, For-
    eign body, respiratory tract
  embedded in skin W45 ☑
  entering through skin W45.8 ☑
    can lid W26.8 ☑
    nail W45.0 ☑
    paper W26.2 ☑
    specified NEC W45.8 ☑
    splinter W45.8 ☑
Forest fire (exposure to) — *see* Exposure, fire, uncontrolled, not in building
Found injured X58 ☑
  from exposure (to) — *see* Exposure
  on
    highway, road(way), street V89.9 ☑
    railway right of way V81.9 ☑
Fracture (circumstances unknown or unspecified) X58 ☑
  due to specified cause NEC X58 ☑
Freezing — *see* Exposure, cold
Frostbite X31 ☑
  due to man-made conditions — *see* Exposure, cold,
    man-made
Frozen — *see* Exposure, cold

G

Gored by bull W55.22 ☑
Gunshot wound W34.00 ☑

H

Hailstones, injured by X39.8 ☑

Hanged herself or himself — *see* Hanging, self-inflicted
Hanging (accidental) (*see also* category) T71 ☑
  legal execution — *see* Legal, intervention, specified
    means NEC
Heat (effects of) (excessive) X30 ☑
  due to
    man-made conditions W92 ☑
      on board watercraft V93.29 ☑
        fishing boat V93.22 ☑
        merchant ship V93.20 ☑
        passenger ship V93.21 ☑
        sailboat V93.24 ☑
        specified powered craft NEC V93.23 ☑
    weather (conditions) X30 ☑
  from
    electric heating apparatus causing burning X16 ☑
    nuclear explosion in war operations — *see* War
      operations, nuclear weapons
  inappropriate in local application or packing in medical
    or surgical procedure Y63.5
Hemorrhage
  delayed following medical or surgical treatment
    without mention of misadventure — *see* Index
    to Diseases and Injuries, Complication(s)
  during medical or surgical treatment as misadventure
    — *see* Index to Diseases and Injuries, Complica-
    tion(s)
High
  altitude (effects) — *see* Air, pressure, low
  level of radioactivity, effects — *see* Radiation
  pressure (effects) — *see* Air, pressure, high
  temperature, effects — *see* Heat
Hit, hitting (accidental) by — *see* Struck by
Hitting against — *see* Striking against
Homicide (attempt) (justifiable) — *see* Assault
Hot
  place, effects (*see also* Heat)
  weather, effects X30 ☑
House fire (uncontrolled) — *see* Exposure, fire, uncon-
    trolled, building
Humidity, causing problem X39.8 ☑
Hunger X58 ☑
Hurricane (any injury) X37.0 ☑
Hypobarism, hypobaropathy — *see* Air, pressure, low

I

Ictus
  caloris (*see also* Heat)
  solaris X30 ☑
Ignition (accidental) (*see also* Exposure, fire) X08.8 ☑
  anesthetic gas in operating room W40.1 ☑
  apparel X06.2 ☑
    from highly flammable material X04 ☑
    nightwear X05 ☑
  bed linen (sheets) (spreads) (pillows) (mattress) — *see*
    Exposure, fire, uncontrolled, building, bed
  benzine X04 ☑
  clothes, clothing NEC (from controlled fire) X06.2 ☑
    from
      highly flammable material X04 ☑
  ether X04 ☑
    in operating room W40.1 ☑
  explosive material — *see* Explosion
  gasoline X04 ☑
  jewelry (plastic) (any) X06.0 ☑
  kerosene X04 ☑
  material
    explosive — *see* Explosion
    highly flammable with secondary explosion X04 ☑
  nightwear X05 ☑
  paraffin X04 ☑
  petrol X04 ☑
Immersion (accidental) (*see also* Drowning)
  hand or foot due to cold (excessive) X31 ☑
Implantation of quills of porcupine W55.89 ☑
Inanition (from) (hunger) X58 ☑
  thirst X58 ☑
Inappropriate operation performed
  correct operation on wrong side or body part (wrong
    side) (wrong site) Y65.53
  operation intended for another patient done on wrong
    patient Y65.52
  wrong operation performed on correct patient Y65.51
Inattention after, at birth (homicidal intent) (infantici-
  dal intent) X58 ☑

Incident, adverse
  device
    anesthesiology Y70.8
      accessory Y70.2
      diagnostic Y70.0
      miscellaneous Y70.8
      monitoring Y70.0
      prosthetic Y70.2
      rehabilitative Y70.1
      surgical Y70.3
      therapeutic Y70.1
    cardiovascular Y71.8
      accessory Y71.2
      diagnostic Y71.0
      miscellaneous Y71.8
      monitoring Y71.0
      prosthetic Y71.2
      rehabilitative Y71.1
      surgical Y71.3
      therapeutic Y71.1
    gastroenterology Y73.8
      accessory Y73.2
      diagnostic Y73.0
      miscellaneous Y73.8
      monitoring Y73.0
      prosthetic Y73.2
      rehabilitative Y73.1
      surgical Y73.3
      therapeutic Y73.1
    general
      hospital Y74.8
        accessory Y74.2
        diagnostic Y74.0
        miscellaneous Y74.8
        monitoring Y74.0
        prosthetic Y74.2
        rehabilitative Y74.1
        surgical Y74.3
        therapeutic Y74.1
      surgical Y81.8
        accessory Y81.2
        diagnostic Y81.0
        miscellaneous Y81.8
        monitoring Y81.0
        prosthetic Y81.2
        rehabilitative Y81.1
        surgical Y81.3
        therapeutic Y81.1
    gynecological Y76.8
      accessory Y76.2
      diagnostic Y76.0
      miscellaneous Y76.8
      monitoring Y76.0
      prosthetic Y76.2
      rehabilitative Y76.1
      surgical Y76.3
      therapeutic Y76.1
    medical Y82.9
      specified type NEC Y82.8
    neurological Y75.8
      accessory Y75.2
      diagnostic Y75.0
      miscellaneous Y75.8
      monitoring Y75.0
      prosthetic Y75.2
      rehabilitative Y75.1
      surgical Y75.3
      therapeutic Y75.1
    obstetrical Y76.8
      accessory Y76.2
      diagnostic Y76.0
      miscellaneous Y76.8
      monitoring Y76.0
      prosthetic Y76.2
      rehabilitative Y76.1
      surgical Y76.3
      therapeutic Y76.1
    ophthalmic Y77.8
      accessory Y77.2
      diagnostic Y77.0
      miscellaneous Y77.8
      monitoring Y77.0
      prosthetic Y77.2
      rehabilitative Y77.1
      surgical Y77.3
      therapeutic Y77.1
    orthopedic Y79.8
      accessory Y79.2
      diagnostic Y79.0

Incident, adverse — *continued*
  device — *continued*
    orthopedic — *continued*
      miscellaneous Y79.8
      monitoring Y79.0
      prosthetic Y79.2
      rehabilitative Y79.1
      surgical Y79.3
      therapeutic Y79.1
    otorhinolaryngological Y72.8
      accessory Y72.2
      diagnostic Y72.0
      miscellaneous Y72.8
      monitoring Y72.0
      prosthetic Y72.2
      rehabilitative Y72.1
      surgical Y72.3
      therapeutic Y72.1
    personal use Y74.8
      accessory Y74.2
      diagnostic Y74.0
      miscellaneous Y74.8
      monitoring Y74.0
      prosthetic Y74.2
      rehabilitative Y74.1
      surgical Y74.3
      therapeutic Y74.1
    physical medicine Y80.8
      accessory Y80.2
      diagnostic Y80.0
      miscellaneous Y80.8
      monitoring Y80.0
      prosthetic Y80.2
      rehabilitative Y80.1
      surgical Y80.3
      therapeutic Y80.1
    plastic surgical Y81.8
      accessory Y81.2
      diagnostic Y81.0
      miscellaneous Y81.8
      monitoring Y81.0
      prosthetic Y81.2
      rehabilitative Y81.1
      surgical Y81.3
      therapeutic Y81.1
    radiological Y78.8
      accessory Y78.2
      diagnostic Y78.0
      miscellaneous Y78.8
      monitoring Y78.0
      prosthetic Y78.2
      rehabilitative Y78.1
      surgical Y78.3
      therapeutic Y78.1
    urology Y73.8
      accessory Y73.2
      diagnostic Y73.0
      miscellaneous Y73.8
      monitoring Y73.0
      prosthetic Y73.2
      rehabilitative Y73.1
      surgical Y73.3
      therapeutic Y73.1
Incineration (accidental) — *see* Exposure, fire
Infanticide — *see* Assault
Infrasound waves (causing injury) W49.9 ☑
Ingestion
  foreign body (causing injury) (with obstruction) — *see*
    Foreign body, alimentary canal
  poisonous
    plant(s) X58 ☑
    substance NEC — *see* Table of Drugs and Chemicals
Inhalation
  excessively cold substance, man-made — *see* Expo-
    sure, cold, man-made
  food (any type) (into respiratory tract) (with asphyxia,
    obstruction respiratory tract, suffocation) — *see*
    categories T17 and T18 ☑
  foreign body — *see* Foreign body, aspiration
  gastric contents (with asphyxia, obstruction respiratory
    passage, suffocation) T17.81- ☑
  hot air or gases X14.0 ☑
  liquid air, hydrogen, nitrogen W93.12 ☑
    suicide (attempt) X83.2 ☑
  steam X13.0 ☑
    assault X98.0 ☑
    stated as undetermined whether accidental or in-
      tentional Y27.0 ☑

Inhalation — *continued*
steam — *continued*
suicide (attempt) X77.0 ☑
toxic gas — *see* Table of Drugs and Chemicals
vomitus (with asphyxia, obstruction respiratory passage, suffocation) T17.81- ☑
Injury, injured (accidental(ly)) NOS X58 ☑
by, caused by, from
assault — *see* Assault
law-enforcing agent, police, in course of legal intervention — *see* Legal intervention
suicide (attempt) X83.8 ☑
due to, in
civil insurrection — *see* War operations
fight (*see also* Assault, fight) Y04.0 ☑
war operations — *see* War operations
homicide (*see also* Assault) Y09
inflicted (by)
in course of arrest (attempted), suppression of disturbance, maintenance of order, by law-enforcing agents — *see* Legal intervention
other person
stated as
accidental X58 ☑
intentional, homicide (attempt) — *see* Assault
undetermined whether accidental or intentional Y33 ☑
purposely (inflicted) by other person(s) — *see* Assault
self-inflicted X83.8 ☑
stated as accidental X58 ☑
specified cause NEC X58 ☑
undetermined whether accidental or intentional Y33 ☑
Insolation, effects X30 ☑
Insufficient nourishment X58 ☑
Interruption of respiration (by)
food (lodged in esophagus) — *see* categories T17 and T18 ☑
vomitus (lodged in esophagus) T17.81- ☑
Intervention, legal — *see* Legal intervention
Intoxication
drug — *see* Table of Drugs and Chemicals
poison — *see* Table of Drugs and Chemicals

J

Jammed (accidentally)
between objects (moving) (stationary and moving) W23.0 ☑
stationary W23.1 ☑
Jumped, jumping
before moving object NEC X81.8 ☑
motor vehicle X81.0 ☑
subway train X81.1 ☑
train X81.1 ☑
undetermined whether accidental or intentional Y31 ☑
from
boat (into water) voluntarily, without accident (to or on boat) W16.712 ☑
with
accident to or on boat — *see* Accident, watercraft
drowning or submersion W16.711 ☑
suicide (attempt) X71.3 ☑
striking bottom W16.722 ☑
causing drowning W16.721 ☑
building (*see also* Jumped, from, high place) W13.9 ☑
burning (uncontrolled fire) X00.5 ☑
high place NEC W17.89 ☑
suicide (attempt) X80 ☑
undetermined whether accidental or intentional Y30 ☑
structure (*see also* Jumped, from, high place) W13.9 ☑
burning (uncontrolled fire) X00.5 ☑
into water W16.92 ☑
causing drowning W16.91 ☑
from, off watercraft — *see* Jumped, from, boat
in
natural body W16.612 ☑
causing drowning W16.611 ☑
striking bottom W16.622 ☑
causing drowning W16.621 ☑

Jumped, jumping — *continued*
into water — *continued*
in — *continued*
specified place NEC W16.812 ☑
causing drowning W16.811 ☑
striking
bottom W16.822 ☑
causing drowning W16.821 ☑
wall W16.832 ☑
causing drowning W16.831 ☑
swimming pool W16.512 ☑
causing drowning W16.511 ☑
striking
bottom W16.522 ☑
causing drowning W16.521 ☑
wall W16.532 ☑
causing drowning W16.531 ☑
suicide (attempt) X71.3 ☑

K

Kicked by
animal NEC W55.82 ☑
person(s) (accidentally) W50.1 ☑
with intent to injure or kill Y04.0 ☑
as, or caused by, a crowd or human stampede (with fall) W52 ☑
assault Y04.0 ☑
homicide (attempt) Y04.0 ☑
in
fight Y04.0 ☑
legal intervention
injuring
bystander Y35.812 ☑
law enforcement personnel Y35.811 ☑
suspect Y35.813 ☑
Kicking
against
object W22.8 ☑
sports equipment W21.9 ☑
stationary W22.09 ☑
sports equipment W21.89 ☑
person — *see* Striking against, person
sports equipment W21.9 ☑
carpet stretcher with knee X50.3 ☑
Killed, killing (accidentally) NOS (*see also* Injury) X58 ☑
in
action — *see* War operations
brawl, fight (hand) (fists) (foot) Y04.0 ☑
by weapon (*see also* Assault)
cutting, piercing — *see* Assault, cutting or piercing instrument
firearm — *see* Discharge, firearm, by type, homicide
self
stated as
accident NOS X58 ☑
suicide — *see* Suicide
undetermined whether accidental or intentional Y33 ☑
Kneeling (prolonged (static) X50.1 ☑
Knocked down (accidentally) (by) NOS X58 ☑
animal (not being ridden) NEC (*see also* Struck by, by type of animal)
crowd or human stampede W52 ☑
person W51 ☑
in brawl, fight Y04.0 ☑
transport vehicle NEC (*see also* Accident, transport) V09.9 ☑

L

Laceration NEC — *see* Injury
Lack of
care (helpless person) (infant) (newborn) X58 ☑
food except as result of abandonment or neglect X58 ☑
due to abandonment or neglect X58 ☑
water except as result of transport accident X58 ☑
due to transport accident — *see* Accident, transport, by type
helpless person, infant, newborn X58 ☑
Landslide (falling on transport vehicle) X36.1 ☑
caused by collapse of man-made structure X36.0 ☑
Late effect — *see* Sequelae

Legal
execution (any method) — *see* Legal, intervention
intervention (by)
baton — *see* Legal, intervention, blunt object, baton
bayonet — *see* Legal, intervention, sharp object, bayonet
blow — *see* Legal, intervention, manhandling
blunt object
baton
injuring
bystander Y35.312 ☑
law enforcement personnel Y35.311 ☑
suspect Y35.313 ☑
injuring
bystander Y35.302 ☑
law enforcement personnel Y35.301 ☑
suspect Y35.303 ☑
specified NEC
injuring
bystander Y35.392 ☑
law enforcement personnel Y35.391 ☑
suspect Y35.393 ☑
stave
injuring
bystander Y35.392 ☑
law enforcement personnel Y35.391 ☑
suspect Y35.393 ☑
bomb — *see* Legal, intervention, explosive
cutting or piercing instrument — *see* Legal, intervention, sharp object
dynamite — *see* Legal, intervention, explosive, dynamite
explosive(s)
dynamite
injuring
bystander Y35.112 ☑
law enforcement personnel Y35.111 ☑
suspect Y35.113 ☑
grenade
injuring
bystander Y35.192 ☑
law enforcement personnel Y35.191 ☑
suspect Y35.193 ☑
injuring
bystander Y35.102 ☑
law enforcement personnel Y35.101 ☑
suspect Y35.103 ☑
mortar bomb
injuring
bystander Y35.192 ☑
law enforcement personnel Y35.191 ☑
suspect Y35.193 ☑
shell
injuring
bystander Y35.122 ☑
law enforcement personnel Y35.121 ☑
suspect Y35.123 ☑
specified NEC
injuring
bystander Y35.192 ☑
law enforcement personnel Y35.191 ☑
suspect Y35.193 ☑
firearm(s) (discharge)
handgun
injuring
bystander Y35.022 ☑
law enforcement personnel Y35.021 ☑
suspect Y35.023 ☑
injuring
bystander Y35.002 ☑
law enforcement personnel Y35.001 ☑
suspect Y35.003 ☑
machine gun
injuring
bystander Y35.012 ☑
law enforcement personnel Y35.011 ☑
suspect Y35.013 ☑
rifle pellet
injuring
bystander Y35.032 ☑
law enforcement personnel Y35.031 ☑
suspect Y35.033 ☑
rubber bullet
injuring
bystander Y35.042 ☑
law enforcement personnel Y35.041 ☑

Legal — *continued*
  intervention — *continued*
    firearm(s) — *continued*
      rubber bullet — *continued*
        injuring — *continued*
          suspect Y35.043 ☑
      shotgun — *see* Legal, intervention, firearm, specified NEC
      specified NEC
        injuring
          bystander Y35.092 ☑
          law enforcement personnel Y35.091 ☑
          suspect Y35.093 ☑
    gas (asphyxiation) (poisoning)
      injuring
        bystander Y35.202 ☑
        law enforcement personnel Y35.201 ☑
        suspect Y35.203 ☑
      specified NEC
        injuring
          bystander Y35.292 ☑
          law enforcement personnel Y35.291 ☑
          suspect Y35.293 ☑
      tear gas
        injuring
          bystander Y35.212 ☑
          law enforcement personnel Y35.211 ☑
          suspect Y35.213 ☑
    grenade — *see* Legal, intervention, explosive, grenade
    injuring
      bystander Y35.92 ☑
      law enforcement personnel Y35.91 ☑
      suspect Y35.93 ☑
    late effect (of) — *see* with 7th character S Y35 ☑
    manhandling
      injuring
        bystander Y35.812 ☑
        law enforcement personnel Y35.811 ☑
        suspect Y35.813 ☑
    sequelae (of) — *see* with 7th character S Y35 ☑
    sharp objects
      bayonet
        injuring
          bystander Y35.412 ☑
          law enforcement personnel Y35.411 ☑
          suspect Y35.413 ☑
      injuring
        bystander Y35.402 ☑
        law enforcement personnel Y35.401 ☑
        suspect Y35.403 ☑
      specified NEC
        injuring
          bystander Y35.492 ☑
          law enforcement personnel Y35.491 ☑
          suspect Y35.493 ☑
    specified means NEC
      injuring
        bystander Y35.892 ☑
        law enforcement personnel Y35.891 ☑
        suspect Y35.893 ☑
    stabbing — *see* Legal, intervention, sharp object
    stave — *see* Legal, intervention, blunt object, stave
    tear gas — *see* Legal, intervention, gas, tear gas
    truncheon — *see* Legal, intervention, blunt object, stave

Lifting — *see also* Overexertion
  heavy objects X50.0 ☑
  weights X50.0 ☑
Lightning (shock) (stroke) (struck by) — *see* subcategory T75.0 ☑
  causing fire — *see* Exposure, fire
Loss of control (transport vehicle) NEC — *see* Accident, transport
Lost at sea NOS — *see* Drowning, due to, fall overboard
Low
  pressure (effects) — *see* Air, pressure, low
  temperature (effects) — *see* Exposure, cold
Lying before train, vehicle or other moving object X81.8 ☑
  subway train X81.1 ☑
  train X81.1 ☑
  undetermined whether accidental or intentional Y31 ☑
Lynching — *see* Assault

M

Malfunction (mechanism or component) (of)
  firearm W34.10 ☑
    airgun W34.110 ☑
    BB gun W34.110 ☑
    gas, air or spring-operated gun NEC W34.118 ☑
    handgun W32.1 ☑
    hunting rifle W33.12 ☑
    larger firearm W33.10 ☑
      specified NEC W33.19 ☑
    machine gun W33.13 ☑
    paintball gun W34.111 ☑
    pellet gun W34.110 ☑
    shotgun W33.11 ☑
    specified NEC W34.19 ☑
    Very pistol [flare] W34.19 ☑
  handgun — *see* Malfunction, firearm, handgun
Maltreatment — *see* Perpetrator
Mangled (accidentally) NOS X58 ☑
Manhandling (in brawl, fight) Y04.0 ☑
  legal intervention — *see* Legal, intervention, manhandling
Manslaughter (nonaccidental) — *see* Assault
Mauled by animal NEC W55.89 ☑
Medical procedure, complication of (delayed or as an abnormal reaction without mention of misadventure) — *see* Complication of or following, by specified type of procedure
  due to or as a result of misadventure — *see* Misadventure
Melting (due to fire) (*see also* Exposure, fire)
  apparel NEC X06.3 ☑
  clothes, clothing NEC X06.3 ☑
    nightwear X05 ☑
  fittings or furniture (burning building) (uncontrolled fire) X00.8 ☑
  nightwear X05 ☑
  plastic jewelry X06.1 ☑
Mental cruelty X58 ☑
Military operations (injuries to military and civilians occuring during peacetime on military property and during routine military exercises and operations) (by) (from) (involving) Y37.90- ☑
  air blast Y37.20- ☑
  aircraft
    destruction — *see* Military operations, destruction of aircraft
    airway restriction — *see* Military operations, restriction of airways
  asphyxiation — *see* Military operations, restriction of airways
  biological weapons Y37.6X- ☑
  blast Y37.20- ☑
  blast fragments Y37.20- ☑
  blast wave Y37.20- ☑
  blast wind Y37.20- ☑
  bomb Y37.20- ☑
    dirty Y37.50- ☑
    gasoline Y37.31- ☑
    incendiary Y37.31- ☑
    petrol Y37.31- ☑
  bullet Y37.43- ☑
    incendiary Y37.32- ☑
    rubber Y37.41- ☑
  chemical weapons Y37.7X- ☑
  combat
    hand to hand (unarmed) combat Y37.44- ☑
    using blunt or piercing object Y37.45- ☑
  conflagration — *see* Military operations, fire
  conventional warfare NEC Y37.49- ☑
  depth-charge Y37.01- ☑
  destruction of aircraft Y37.10- ☑
    due to
      air to air missile Y37.11- ☑
      collision with other aircraft Y37.12- ☑
      detonation (accidental) of onboard munitions and explosives Y37.14- ☑
      enemy fire or explosives Y37.11- ☑
      explosive placed on aircraft Y37.11- ☑
      onboard fire Y37.13- ☑
      rocket propelled grenade [RPG] Y37.11- ☑
      small arms fire Y37.11- ☑
      surface to air missile Y37.11- ☑
    specified NEC Y37.19- ☑

Military operations — *continued*
  detonation (accidental) of
    onboard marine weapons Y37.05- ☑
    own munitions or munitions launch device Y37.24- ☑
  dirty bomb Y37.50- ☑
  explosion (of) Y37.20- ☑
    aerial bomb Y37.21- ☑
    bomb NOS (*see also* Military operations, bomb(s)) Y37.20- ☑
    fragments Y37.20- ☑
    grenade Y37.29- ☑
    guided missile Y37.22- ☑
    improvised explosive device [IED] (person-borne) (roadside) (vehicle-borne) Y37.23- ☑
    land mine Y37.29- ☑
    marine mine (at sea) (in harbor) Y37.02- ☑
    marine weapon Y37.00- ☑
      specified NEC Y37.09- ☑
    own munitions or munitions launch device (accidental) Y37.24- ☑
    sea-based artillery shell Y37.03- ☑
    specified NEC Y37.29- ☑
    torpedo Y37.04- ☑
  fire Y37.30- ☑
    specified NEC Y37.39- ☑
  firearms
    discharge Y37.43- ☑
    pellets Y37.42- ☑
  flamethrower Y37.33- ☑
  fragments (from) (of)
    improvised explosive device [IED] (person-borne) (roadside) (vehicle-borne) Y37.26- ☑
    munitions Y37.25- ☑
    specified NEC Y37.29- ☑
    weapons Y37.27- ☑
  friendly fire Y37.92- ☑
  hand to hand (unarmed) combat Y37.44- ☑
  hot substances — *see* Military operations, fire
  incendiary bullet Y37.32- ☑
  nuclear weapon (effects of) Y37.50- ☑
    acute radiation exposure Y37.54- ☑
    blast pressure Y37.51- ☑
    direct blast Y37.51- ☑
    direct heat Y37.53- ☑
    fallout exposure Y37.54- ☑
    fireball Y37.53- ☑
    indirect blast (struck or crushed by blast debris) (being thrown by blast) Y37.52- ☑
    ionizing radiation (immediate exposure) Y37.54- ☑
    nuclear radiation Y37.54- ☑
    radiation
      ionizing (immediate exposure) Y37.54- ☑
      nuclear Y37.54- ☑
      thermal Y37.53- ☑
    secondary effects Y37.54- ☑
    specified NEC Y37.59- ☑
    thermal radiation Y37.53- ☑
  restriction of air (airway)
    intentional Y37.46- ☑
    unintentional Y37.47- ☑
  rubber bullets Y37.41- ☑
  shrapnel NOS Y37.29- ☑
  suffocation — *see* Military operations, restriction of airways
  unconventional warfare NEC Y37.7X- ☑
  underwater blast NOS Y37.00- ☑
  warfare
    conventional NEC Y37.49- ☑
    unconventional NEC Y37.7X- ☑
  weapon of mass destruction [WMD] Y37.91- ☑
  weapons
    biological weapons Y37.6X- ☑
    chemical Y37.7X- ☑
    nuclear (effects of) Y37.50- ☑
      acute radiation exposure Y37.54- ☑
      blast pressure Y37.51- ☑
      direct blast Y37.51- ☑
      direct heat Y37.53- ☑
      fallout exposure Y37.54- ☑
      fireball Y37.53- ☑
      radiation
        ionizing (immediate exposure) Y37.54- ☑
        nuclear Y37.54- ☑
        thermal Y37.53- ☑
      secondary effects Y37.54- ☑

External Causes Index

Military operations — Place of occurrence

Military operations — *continued*
  weapons — *continued*
    nuclear — *continued*
      specified NEC Y37.59- ☑
    of mass destruction [WMD] Y37.91- ☑
Misadventure(s) to patient(s) during surgical or medical care Y69
  contaminated medical or biological substance (blood, drug, fluid) Y64.9
    administered (by) NEC Y64.9
      immunization Y64.1
      infusion Y64.0
      injection Y64.1
      specified means NEC Y64.8
      transfusion Y64.0
      vaccination Y64.1
  excessive amount of blood or other fluid during transfusion or infusion Y63.0
  failure
    in dosage Y63.9
      electroshock therapy Y63.4
      inappropriate temperature (too hot or too cold) in local application and packing Y63.5
      infusion
        excessive amount of fluid Y63.0
        incorrect dilution of fluid Y63.1
      insulin-shock therapy Y63.4
      nonadministration of necessary drug or biological substance Y63.6
      overdose — *see* Table of Drugs and Chemicals
      radiation, in therapy Y63.2
      radiation
        overdose Y63.2
      specified procedure NEC Y63.8
      transfusion
        excessive amount of blood Y63.0
  mechanical, of instrument or apparatus (any) (during any procedure) Y65.8
    sterile precautions (during procedure) Y62.9
      aspiration of fluid or tissue (by puncture or catheterization, except heart) Y62.6
      biopsy (except needle aspiration) Y62.8
        needle (aspirating) Y62.6
      blood sampling Y62.6
      catheterization Y62.6
        heart Y62.5
      dialysis (kidney) Y62.2
      endoscopic examination Y62.4
      enema Y62.8
      immunization Y62.3
      infusion Y62.1
      injection Y62.3
      needle biopsy Y62.6
      paracentesis (abdominal) (thoracic) Y62.6
      perfusion Y62.2
      puncture (lumbar) Y62.6
      removal of catheter or packing Y62.8
      specified procedure NEC Y62.8
      surgical operation Y62.0
      transfusion Y62.1
      vaccination Y62.3
  suture or ligature during surgical procedure Y65.2
  to introduce or to remove tube or instrument — *see* Failure, to
  hemorrhage — *see* Index to Diseases and Injuries, Complication(s)
  inadvertent exposure of patient to radiation Y63.3
  inappropriate
    operation performed — *see* Inappropriate operation performed
    temperature (too hot or too cold) in local application or packing Y63.5
  infusion (*see also* Misadventure, by type, infusion) Y69
    excessive amount of fluid Y63.0
    incorrect dilution of fluid Y63.1
    wrong fluid Y65.1
  mismatched blood in transfusion Y65.0
  nonadministration of necessary drug or biological substance Y63.6
  overdose — *see* Table of Drugs and Chemicals
    radiation (in therapy) Y63.2
  perforation — *see* Index to Diseases and Injuries, Complication(s)
  performance of inappropriate operation — *see* Inappropriate operation performed
  puncture — *see* Index to Diseases and Injuries, Complication(s)
  specified type NEC Y65.8

Misadventure(s) to patient(s) during surgical or medical care — *continued*
  specified type — *continued*
    failure
      suture or ligature during surgical operation Y65.2
      to introduce or to remove tube or instrument — *see* Failure, to
    infusion of wrong fluid Y65.1
    performance of inappropriate operation — *see* Inappropriate operation performed
    transfusion of mismatched blood Y65.0
    wrong
      fluid in infusion Y65.1
      placement of endotracheal tube during anesthetic procedure Y65.3
  transfusion — *see* Misadventure, by type, transfusion
    excessive amount of blood Y63.0
    mismatched blood Y65.0
  wrong
    drug given in error — *see* Table of Drugs and Chemicals
    fluid in infusion Y65.1
    placement of endotracheal tube during anesthetic procedure Y65.3
Mismatched blood in transfusion Y65.0
Motion sickness T75.3 ☑
Mountain sickness W94.11 ☑
Mudslide (of cataclysmic nature) — *see* Landslide
Murder (attempt) — *see* Assault

N

Nail
  contact with W45.0 ☑
    gun W29.4 ☑
  embedded in skin W45.0 ☑
Neglect (criminal) (homicidal intent) X58 ☑
Noise (causing injury) (pollution) W42.9 ☑
  supersonic W42.0 ☑
Nonadministration (of)
  drug or biological substance (necessary) Y63.6
  surgical and medical care Y66
Nosocomial condition Y95

O

Object
  falling
    from, in, on, hitting
      machinery — *see* Contact, with, by type of machine
  set in motion by
    accidental explosion or rupture of pressure vessel W38 ☑
    firearm — *see* Discharge, firearm, by type
    machine(ry) — *see* Contact, with, by type of machine
Overdose (drug) — *see* Table of Drugs and Chemicals
  radiation Y63.2
Overexertion X50.9 ☑
  from
    prolonged static or awkward postures X50.1 ☑
    repetitive movements X50.3 ☑
    specified strenuous movements or postures NEC X50.9 ☑
    strenuous movement or load X50.0 ☑
Overexposure (accidental) (to)
  cold (*see also* Exposure, cold) X31 ☑
    due to man-made conditions — *see* Exposure, cold, man-made
  heat (*see also* Heat) X30 ☑
  radiation — *see* Radiation
  radioactivity W88.0 ☑
  sun (sunburn) X32 ☑
  weather NEC — *see* Forces of nature
  wind NEC — *see* Forces of nature
Overheated — *see* Heat
Overturning (accidental)
  machinery — *see* Contact, with, by type of machine
  transport vehicle NEC (*see also* Accident, transport) V89.9 ☑
  watercraft (causing drowning, submersion) (*see also* Drowning, due to, accident to, watercraft, overturning)
    causing injury except drowning or submersion — *see* Accident, watercraft, causing, injury NEC

P

Parachute descent (voluntary) (without accident to aircraft) V97.29 ☑
  due to accident to aircraft — *see* Accident, transport, aircraft
Pecked by bird W61.99 ☑
Perforation during medical or surgical treatment as misadventure — *see* Index to Diseases and Injuries, Complication(s)
Perpetrator, perpetration, of assault, maltreatment and neglect (by) Y07.9
  boyfriend Y07.03
  brother Y07.410
    stepbrother Y07.435
  coach Y07.53
  cousin
    female Y07.491
    male Y07.490
  daycare provider Y07.519
    at-home
      adult care Y07.512
      childcare Y07.510
    care center
      adult care Y07.513
      childcare Y07.511
  family member NEC Y07.499
  father Y07.11
    adoptive Y07.13
    foster Y07.420
    stepfather Y07.430
  foster father Y07.420
  foster mother Y07.421
  girl friend Y07.04
  healthcare provider Y07.529
    mental health Y07.521
    specified NEC Y07.528
  husband Y07.01
  instructor Y07.53
  mother Y07.12
    adoptive Y07.14
    foster Y07.421
    stepmother Y07.433
  nonfamily member Y07.50
    specified NEC Y07.59
  nurse Y07.528
  occupational therapist Y07.528
  partner of parent
    female Y07.434
    male Y07.432
  physical therapist Y07.528
  sister Y07.411
  speech therapist Y07.528
  stepbrother Y07.435
  stepfather Y07.430
  stepmother Y07.433
  stepsister Y07.436
  teacher Y07.53
  wife Y07.02
Piercing — *see* Contact, with, by type of object or machine
Pinched
  between objects (moving) (stationary and moving) W23.0 ☑
  stationary W23.1 ☑
Pinned under machine(ry) — *see* Contact, with, by type of machine
Place of occurrence Y92.9
  abandoned house Y92.89
  airplane Y92.813
  airport Y92.520
  ambulatory health services establishment NEC Y92.538
  ambulatory surgery center Y92.530
  amusement park Y92.831
  apartment (co-op) — *see* Place of occurrence, residence, apartment
  assembly hall Y92.29
  bank Y92.510
  barn Y92.71
  baseball field Y92.320
  basketball court Y92.310
  beach Y92.832
  boarding house — *see* Place of occurrence, residence, boarding house
  boat Y92.814
  bowling alley Y92.39
  bridge Y92.89

Place of occurrence — *continued*
building under construction Y92.61
bus Y92.811
    station Y92.521
cafe Y92.511
campsite Y92.833
campus — *see* Place of occurrence, school
canal Y92.89
car Y92.810
casino Y92.59
children's home — *see* Place of occurrence, residence,
    institutional, orphanage
church Y92.22
cinema Y92.26
clubhouse Y92.29
coal pit Y92.64
college (community) Y92.214
condominium — *see* Place of occurrence, residence,
    apartment
construction area — *see* Place of occurrence, industrial
    and construction area
convalescent home — *see* Place of occurrence, resi-
    dence, institutional, nursing home
court-house Y92.240
cricket ground Y92.328
cultural building Y92.258
    art gallery Y92.250
    museum Y92.251
    music hall Y92.252
    opera house Y92.253
    specified NEC Y92.258
    theater Y92.254
dancehall Y92.252
day nursery Y92.210
dentist office Y92.531
derelict house Y92.89
desert Y92.820
dockyard Y92.62
dock NOS Y92.89
doctor's office Y92.531
dormitory — *see* Place of occurrence, residence, insti-
    tutional, school dormitory
dry dock Y92.62
factory (building) (premises) Y92.63
farm (land under cultivation) (outbuildings) Y92.79
    barn Y92.71
    chicken coop Y92.72
    field Y92.73
    hen house Y92.72
    house — *see* Place of occurrence, residence, house
    orchard Y92.74
    specified NEC Y92.79
football field Y92.321
forest Y92.821
freeway Y92.411
gallery Y92.250
garage (commercial) Y92.59
    boarding house Y92.044
    military base Y92.135
    mobile home Y92.025
    nursing home Y92.124
    orphanage Y92.114
    private house Y92.015
    reform school Y92.155
gas station Y92.524
gasworks Y92.69
golf course Y92.39
gravel pit Y92.64
grocery Y92.512
gymnasium Y92.39
handball court Y92.318
harbor Y92.89
harness racing course Y92.39
healthcare provider office Y92.531
highway (interstate) Y92.411
hill Y92.828
hockey rink Y92.330
home — *see* Place of occurrence, residence
hospice — *see* Place of occurrence, residence, institu-
    tional, nursing home
hospital Y92.239
    cafeteria Y92.233
    corridor Y92.232
    operating room Y92.234
    patient
        bathroom Y92.231
        room Y92.230
    specified NEC Y92.238

Place of occurrence — *continued*
hotel Y92.59
house (*see also* Place of occurrence, residence)
    abandoned Y92.89
    under construction Y92.61
industrial and construction area (yard) Y92.69
    building under construction Y92.61
    dock Y92.62
    dry dock Y92.62
    factory Y92.63
    gasworks Y92.69
    mine Y92.64
    oil rig Y92.65
    pit Y92.64
    power station Y92.69
    shipyard Y92.62
    specified NEC Y92.69
    tunnel under construction Y92.69
    workshop Y92.69
kindergarten Y92.211
lacrosse field Y92.328
lake Y92.828
library Y92.241
mall Y92.59
market Y92.512
marsh Y92.828
military
    base — *see* Place of occurrence, residence, institu-
        tional, military base
    training ground Y92.84
mine Y92.64
mosque Y92.22
motel Y92.59
motorway (interstate) Y92.411
mountain Y92.828
movie-house Y92.26
museum Y92.251
music-hall Y92.252
not applicable Y92.9
nuclear power station Y92.69
nursing home — *see* Place of occurrence, residence,
    institutional, nursing home
office building Y92.59
offshore installation Y92.65
oil rig Y92.65
old people's home — *see* Place of occurrence, resi-
    dence, institutional, specified NEC
opera-house Y92.253
orphanage — *see* Place of occurrence, residence, insti-
    tutional, orphanage
outpatient surgery center Y92.530
park (public) Y92.830
    amusement Y92.831
parking garage Y92.89
    lot Y92.481
pavement Y92.480
physician office Y92.531
polo field Y92.328
pond Y92.828
post office Y92.242
power station Y92.69
prairie Y92.828
prison — *see* Place of occurrence, residence, institu-
    tional, prison
public
    administration building Y92.248
        city hall Y92.243
        courthouse Y92.240
        library Y92.241
        post office Y92.242
        specified NEC Y92.248
    building NEC Y92.29
    hall Y92.29
    place NOS Y92.89
race course Y92.39
radio station Y92.59
railway line (bridge) Y92.85
ranch (outbuildings) — *see* Place of occurrence, farm
recreation area Y92.838
    amusement park Y92.831
    beach Y92.832
    campsite Y92.833
    park (public) Y92.830
    seashore Y92.832
    specified NEC Y92.838
reform school - — *see* Place of occurrence, residence,
    institutional, reform school
religious institution Y92.22

Place of occurrence — *continued*
residence (non-institutional) (private) Y92.009
    apartment Y92.039
        bathroom Y92.031
        bedroom Y92.032
        kitchen Y92.030
        specified NEC Y92.038
    bathroom Y92.002
    bedroom Y92.003
    boarding house Y92.049
        bathroom Y92.041
        bedroom Y92.042
        driveway Y92.043
        garage Y92.044
        garden Y92.046
        kitchen Y92.040
        specified NEC Y92.048
        swimming pool Y92.045
        yard Y92.046
    dining room Y92.001
    garden Y92.007
    home Y92.009
    house, single family Y92.019
        bathroom Y92.012
        bedroom Y92.013
        dining room Y92.011
        driveway Y92.014
        garage Y92.015
        garden Y92.017
        kitchen Y92.010
        specified NEC Y92.018
        swimming pool Y92.016
        yard Y92.017
    institutional Y92.10
        children's home — *see* Place of occurrence,
            residence, institutional, orphanage
        hospice — *see* Place of occurrence, residence,
            institutional, nursing home
        military base Y92.139
            barracks Y92.133
            garage Y92.135
            garden Y92.137
            kitchen Y92.130
            mess hall Y92.131
            specified NEC Y92.138
            swimming pool Y92.136
            yard Y92.137
        nursing home Y92.129
            bathroom Y92.121
            bedroom Y92.122
            driveway Y92.123
            garage Y92.124
            garden Y92.126
            kitchen Y92.120
            specified NEC Y92.128
            swimming pool Y92.125
            yard Y92.126
        orphanage Y92.119
            bathroom Y92.111
            bedroom Y92.112
            driveway Y92.113
            garage Y92.114
            garden Y92.116
            kitchen Y92.110
            specified NEC Y92.118
            swimming pool Y92.115
            yard Y92.116
        prison Y92.149
            bathroom Y92.142
            cell Y92.143
            courtyard Y92.147
            dining room Y92.141
            kitchen Y92.140
            specified NEC Y92.148
            swimming pool Y92.146
        reform school Y92.159
            bathroom Y92.152
            bedroom Y92.153
            dining room Y92.151
            driveway Y92.154
            garage Y92.155
            garden Y92.157
            kitchen Y92.150
            specified NEC Y92.158
            swimming pool Y92.156
            yard Y92.157
        school dormitory Y92.169
            bathroom Y92.162
            bedroom Y92.163

⩔ Subterms under main terms may continue to next column or page   ☑ Additional Character Required — Refer to the Tabular List for Character Selection

Place of occurrence — *continued*
  residence — *continued*
    institutional — *continued*
      school dormitory — *continued*
        dining room Y92.161
        kitchen Y92.160
        specified NEC Y92.168
      specified NEC Y92.199
        bathroom Y92.192
        bedroom Y92.193
        dining room Y92.191
        driveway Y92.194
        garage Y92.195
        garden Y92.197
        kitchen Y92.190
        specified NEC Y92.198
        swimming pool Y92.196
        yard Y92.197
    kitchen Y92.000
    mobile home Y92.029
      bathroom Y92.022
      bedroom Y92.023
      dining room Y92.021
      driveway Y92.024
      garage Y92.025
      garden Y92.027
      kitchen Y92.020
      specified NEC Y92.028
      swimming pool Y92.026
      yard Y92.027
    specified place in residence NEC Y92.008
    specified residence type NEC Y92.099
      bathroom Y92.091
      bedroom Y92.092
      driveway Y92.093
      garage Y92.094
      garden Y92.096
      kitchen Y92.090
      specified NEC Y92.098
      swimming pool Y92.095
      yard Y92.096
  restaurant Y92.511
  riding school Y92.39
  river Y92.828
  road Y92.488
  rodeo ring Y92.39
  rugby field Y92.328
  same day surgery center Y92.530
  sand pit Y92.64
  school (private) (public) (state) Y92.219
    college Y92.214
    daycare center Y92.210
    elementary school Y92.211
    high school Y92.213
    kindergarten Y92.211
    middle school Y92.212
    specified NEC Y92.218
    trace school Y92.215
    university Y92.214
    vocational school Y92.215
  sea (shore) Y92.832
  senior citizen center Y92.29
  service area
    airport Y92.520
    bus station Y92.521
    gas station Y92.524
    highway rest stop Y92.523
    railway station Y92.522
  shipyard Y92.62
  shop (commercial) Y92.513
  sidewalk Y92.480
  silo Y92.79
  skating rink (roller) Y92.331
    ice Y92.330
  slaughter house Y92.86
  soccer field Y92.322
  specified place NEC Y92.89
  sports area Y92.39
    athletic
      court Y92.318
        basketball Y92.310
        specified NEC Y92.318
        squash Y92.311
        tennis Y92.312
      field Y92.328
        baseball Y92.320
        cricket ground Y92.328
        football Y92.321
        hockey Y92.328

Place of occurrence — *continued*
  sports area — *continued*
    athletic — *continued*
      field — *continued*
        soccer Y92.322
        specified NEC Y92.328
    golf course Y92.39
    gymnasium Y92.39
    riding school Y92.39
    skating rink (roller) Y92.331
      ice Y92.330
    stadium Y92.39
    swimming pool Y92.34
    squash court Y92.311
  stadium Y92.39
  steeplechasing course Y92.39
  store Y92.512
  stream Y92.828
  street and highway Y92.410
    bike path Y92.482
    freeway Y92.411
    highway ramp Y92.415
    interstate highway Y92.411
    local residential or business street Y92.414
    motorway Y92.411
    parking lot Y92.481
    parkway Y92.412
    sidewalk Y92.480
    specified NEC Y92.488
    state road Y92.413
  subway car Y92.816
  supermarket Y92.512
  swamp Y92.828
  swimming pool (public) Y92.34
    private (at) Y92.095
      boarding house Y92.045
      military base Y92.136
      mobile home Y92.026
      nursing home Y92.125
      orphanage Y92.115
      prison Y92.146
      reform school Y92.156
      single family residence Y92.016
  synagogue Y92.22
  television station Y92.59
  tennis court Y92.312
  theater Y92.254
  trade area Y92.59
    bank Y92.510
    cafe Y92.511
    casino Y92.59
    garage Y92.59
    hotel Y92.59
    market Y92.512
    office building Y92.59
    radio station Y92.59
    restaurant Y92.511
    shop Y92.513
    shopping mall Y92.59
    store Y92.512
    supermarket Y92.512
    television station Y92.59
    warehouse Y92.59
  trailer park, residential — *see* Place of occurrence, residence, mobile home
  trailer site NOS Y92.89
  train Y92.815
    station Y92.522
  truck Y92.812
  tunnel under construction Y92.69
  university Y92.214
  urgent (health) care center Y92.532
  vehicle (transport) Y92.818
    airplane Y92.813
    boat Y92.814
    bus Y92.811
    car Y92.810
    specified NEC Y92.818
    subway car Y92.816
    train Y92.815
    truck Y92.812
  warehouse Y92.59
  water reservoir Y92.89
  wilderness area Y92.828
    desert Y92.820
    forest Y92.821
    marsh Y92.828
    mountain Y92.828
    prairie Y92.828

Place of occurrence — *continued*
  wilderness area — *continued*
    specified NEC Y92.828
    swamp Y92.828
  workshop Y92.69
  yard, private Y92.096
    boarding house Y92.046
    mobile home Y92.027
    single family house Y92.017
  youth center Y92.29
  zoo (zoological garden) Y92.834
Plumbism — *see* Table of Drugs and Chemicals, lead
Poisoning (accidental) (by) (*see also* Table of Drugs and Chemicals)
  by plant, thorns, spines, sharp leaves or other mechanisms NEC X58 ☑
  carbon monoxide
    generated by
      motor vehicle — *see* Accident, transport
      watercraft (in transit) (not in transit) V93.89 ☑
        ferry boat V93.81 ☑
        fishing boat V93.82 ☑
        jet skis V93.83 ☑
        liner V93.81 ☑
        merchant ship V93.80 ☑
        passenger ship V93.81 ☑
        powered craft NEC V93.83 ☑
  caused by injection of poisons into skin by plant thorns, spines, sharp leaves X58 ☑
  marine or sea plants (venomous) X58 ☑
  execution — *see* Legal, intervention, gas
  intervention
    by gas — *see* Legal, intervention, gas
    other specified means — *see* Legal, intervention, specified means NEC
  exhaust gas
    generated by
      motor vehicle — *see* Accident, transport
      watercraft (in transit) (not in transit) V93.89 ☑
        ferry boat V93.81 ☑
        fishing boat V93.82 ☑
        jet skis V93.83 ☑
        liner V93.81 ☑
        merchant ship V93.80 ☑
        passenger ship V93.81 ☑
        powered craft NEC V93.83 ☑
  fumes or smoke due to
    explosion (*see also* Explosion) W40.9 ☑
    fire — *see* Exposure, fire
    ignition — *see* Ignition
  gas
    in legal intervention — *see* Legal, intervention, gas
    legal execution — *see* Legal, intervention, gas
  in war operations — *see* War operations
  legal
Powder burn (by) (from)
  airgun W34.110 ☑
  BB gun W34.110 ☑
  firearm NEC W34.19 ☑
  gas, air or spring-operated gun NEC W34.118 ☑
  handgun W32.1 ☑
  hunting rifle W33.12 ☑
  larger firearm W33.10 ☑
    specified NEC W33.19 ☑
  machine gun W33.13 ☑
  paintball gun W34.111 ☑
  pellet gun W34.110 ☑
  shotgun W33.11 ☑
  Very pistol [flare] W34.19 ☑
Premature cessation (of) **surgical and medical care** Y66
Privation (food) (water) X58 ☑
Procedure (operation)
  correct, on wrong side or body part (wrong side) (wrong site) Y65.53
  intended for another patient done on wrong patient Y65.52
  performed on patient not scheduled for surgery Y65.52
  performed on wrong patient Y65.52
  wrong, performed on correct patient Y65.51
Prolonged
  sitting in transport vehicle — *see* Travel, by type of vehicle
  stay in
    high altitude as cause of anoxia, barodontalgia, barotitis or hypoxia W94.11 ☑
    weightless environment X52 ☑

Pulling, excessive (*see also* Overexertion) X50.9- ☑
Puncture, puncturing (*see also* Contact, with, by type of object or machine)
  by
    plant thorns, spines, sharp leaves or other mechanisms NEC W60 ☑
    during medical or surgical treatment as misadventure — *see* Index to Diseases and Injuries, Complication(s)
Pushed, pushing (accidental) (injury in)
  by other person(s) (accidental) W51 ☑
    with fall W03 ☑
      due to ice or snow W00.0 ☑
    as, or caused by, a crowd or human stampede (with fall) W52 ☑
    before moving object NEC Y02.8 ☑
      motor vehicle Y02.0 ☑
      subway train Y02.1 ☑
      train Y02.1 ☑
    from
      high place NEC
        in accidental circumstances W17.89 ☑
        stated as
          intentional, homicide (attempt) Y01
          undetermined whether accidental or intentional Y30 ☑
      transport vehicle NEC (*see also* Accident, transport) V89.9 ☑
        stated as
          intentional, homicide (attempt) Y08.89 ☑
  overexertion X50.9 ☑

R

Radiation (exposure to)
  arc lamps W89.0 ☑
  atomic power plant (malfunction) NEC W88.1 ☑
  complication of or abnormal reaction to medical radiotherapy Y84.2
  electromagnetic, ionizing W88.0 ☑
  gamma rays W88.1 ☑
  in
    war operations (from or following nuclear explosion) — *see* War operations
  inadvertent exposure of patient (receiving test or therapy) Y63.3
  infrared (heaters and lamps) W90.1 ☑
    excessive heat from W92 ☑
  ionized, ionizing (particles, artificially accelerated)
    radioisotopes W88.1 ☑
    specified NEC W88.8 ☑
    x-rays W88.0 ☑
  isotopes, radioactive — *see* Radiation, radioactive isotopes
  laser(s) W90.2 ☑
    in war operations — *see* War operations
    misadventure in medical care Y63.2
  light sources (man-made visible and ultraviolet) W89.9 ☑
    natural X32 ☑
    specified NEC W89.8 ☑
    tanning bed W89.1 ☑
    welding light W89.0 ☑
  man-made visible light W89.9 ☑
    specified NEC W89.8 ☑
    tanning bed W89.1 ☑
    welding light W89.0 ☑
  microwave W90.8 ☑
  misadventure in medical or surgical procedure Y63.2
  natural NEC X39.08 ☑
    radon X39.01 ☑
  overdose (in medical or surgical procedure) Y63.2
  radar W90.0 ☑
  radioactive isotopes (any) W88.1 ☑
    atomic power plant malfunction W88.1 ☑
    misadventure in medical or surgical treatment Y63.2
  radiofrequency W90.0 ☑
  radium NEC W88.1 ☑
  sun X32 ☑
  ultraviolet (light) (man-made) W89.9 ☑
    natural X32 ☑
    specified NEC W89.8 ☑
    tanning bed W89.1 ☑
    welding light W89.0 ☑

Radiation — *continued*
  welding arc, torch, or light W89.0 ☑
    excessive heat from W92 ☑
  x-rays (hard) (soft) W88.0 ☑
Range disease W94.11 ☑
Rape (attempted) T74.2- ☑
Rat bite W53.11 ☑
Reaching (prolonged) (static) X50.1 ☑
Reaction, abnormal to medical procedure (*see also* Complication of or following, by type of procedure) Y84.9
  with misadventure — *see* Misadventure
  biologicals — *see* Table of Drugs and Chemicals
  drugs — *see* Table of Drugs and Chemicals
  vaccine — *see* Table of Drugs and Chemicals
Recoil
  airgun W34.110 ☑
  BB gun W34.110 ☑
  firearm NEC W34.19 ☑
  gas, air or spring-operated gun NEC W34.118 ☑
  handgun W32.1 ☑
  hunting rifle W33.12 ☑
  larger firearm W33.10 ☑
    specified NEC W33.19 ☑
  machine gun W33.13 ☑
  paintball gun W34.111 ☑
  pellet W34.110 ☑
  shotgun W33.11 ☑
  Very pistol [flare] W34.19 ☑
Reduction in
  atmospheric pressure — *see* Air, pressure, change
Rock falling on or hitting (accidentally) (person) W20.8 ☑
  in cave-in W20.0 ☑
Run over (accidentally) (by)
  animal (not being ridden) NEC W55.89 ☑
  machinery — *see* Contact, with, by specified type of machine
  transport vehicle NEC (*see also* Accident, transport) V09.9 ☑
    intentional homicide (attempt) Y03.0 ☑
    motor NEC V09.20 ☑
      intentional homicide (attempt) Y03.0 ☑
Running
  before moving object X81.8 ☑
    motor vehicle X81.0 ☑
Running off, away
  animal (being ridden) (*see also* Accident, transport) V80.918 ☑
    not being ridden W55.89 ☑
  animal-drawn vehicle NEC (*see also* Accident, transport) V80.928 ☑
  highway, road(way), street
    transport vehicle NEC (*see also* Accident, transport) V89.9 ☑
Rupture pressurized devices — *see* Explosion, by type of device

S

Saturnism — *see* Table of Drugs and Chemicals, lead
Scald, scalding (accidental) (by) (from) (in) X19 ☑
  air (hot) X14.1 ☑
  gases (hot) X14.1 ☑
  homicide (attempt) — *see* Assault, burning, hot object
  inflicted by other person
    stated as intentional, homicide (attempt) — *see* Assault, burning, hot object
  liquid (boiling) (hot) NEC X12 ☑
    stated as undetermined whether accidental or intentional Y27.2 ☑
    suicide (attempt) X77.2 ☑
  local application of externally applied substance in medical or surgical care Y63.5
  metal (molten) (liquid) (hot) NEC X18 ☑
  self-inflicted X77.9 ☑
  stated as undetermined whether accidental or intentional Y27.8 ☑
  steam X13.1 ☑
    assault X98.0 ☑
    stated as undetermined whether accidental or intentional Y27.0 ☑
    suicide (attempt) X77.0 ☑
  suicide (attempt) X77.9 ☑
  vapor (hot) X13.1 ☑
    assault X98.0 ☑

Scald, scalding — *continued*
  vapor — *continued*
    stated as undetermined whether accidental or intentional Y27.0 ☑
    suicide (attempt) X77.0 ☑
Scratched by
  cat W55.03 ☑
  person(s) (accidentally) W50.4 ☑
    with intent to injure or kill Y04.0 ☑
    as, or caused by, a crowd or human stampede (with fall) W52 ☑
    assault Y04.0 ☑
    homicide (attempt) Y04.0 ☑
    in
      fight Y04.0 ☑
      legal intervention
        injuring
          bystander Y35.892 ☑
          law enforcement personnel Y35.891 ☑
          suspect Y35.893 ☑
Seasickness T75.3 ☑
Self-harm NEC (*see also* External cause by type, undetermined whether accidental or intentional)
  intentional — *see* Suicide
  poisoning NEC — *see* Table of Drugs and Chemicals, poisoning, accidental
Self-inflicted (injury) NEC (*see also* External cause by type, undetermined whether accidental or intentional)
  intentional — *see* Suicide
  poisoning NEC — *see* Table of Drugs and Chemicals, poisoning, accidental
Sequelae (of)
  accident NEC — *see* W00-X58 with 7th character S
  assault (homicidal) (any means) — *see* X92-Y08 with 7th character S
  homicide, attempt (any means) — *see* X92-Y08 with 7th character S
  injury undetermined whether accidentally or purposely inflicted — *see* Y21-Y33 with 7th character S
  intentional self-harm (classifiable to X71-X83) — *see* X71-X83 with 7th character S
  legal intervention — *see* with 7th character S Y35 ☑
  motor vehicle accident — *see* V00-V99 with 7th character S
  suicide, attempt (any means) — *see* X71-X83 with 7th character S
  transport accident — *see* V00-V99 with 7th character S
  war operations — *see* War operations
Shock
  electric — *see* Exposure, electric current
  from electric appliance (any) (faulty) W86.8 ☑
    domestic W86.0 ☑
    suicide (attempt) X83.1 ☑
Shooting, shot (accidental(ly)) (*see also* Discharge, firearm, by type)
  herself or himself — *see* Discharge, firearm by type, self-inflicted
  homicide (attempt) — *see* Discharge, firearm by type, homicide
  in war operations — *see* War operations
  inflicted by other person — *see* Discharge, firearm by type, homicide
    accidental — *see* Discharge, firearm, by type of firearm
  legal
    execution — *see* Legal, intervention, firearm
    intervention — *see* Legal, intervention, firearm
  self-inflicted — *see* Discharge, firearm by type, suicide
    accidental — *see* Discharge, firearm, by type of firearm
  suicide (attempt) — *see* Discharge, firearm by type, suicide
Shoving (accidentally) **by other person** — *see* Pushed, by other person
Sickness
  alpine W94.11 ☑
  motion — *see* Motion
  mountain W94.11 ☑
Sinking (accidental)
  watercraft (causing drowning, submersion) (*see also* Drowning, due to, accident to, watercraft, sinking)
    causing injury except drowning or submersion — *see* Accident, watercraft, causing, injury NEC
Siriasis X32 ☑

Sitting (prolonged) (static) X50.1 ☑
Slashed wrists — *see* Cut, self-inflicted
Slipping (accidental) (on same level) (with fall) W01.0 ☑
 without fall W18.40 ☑
  due to
   specified NEC W18.49 ☑
   stepping from one level to another W18.43 ☑
   stepping into hole or opening W18.42 ☑
   stepping on object W18.41 ☑
 on
  ice W00.0 ☑
   with skates — *see* Accident, transport, pedestrian, conveyance
  mud W01.0 ☑
  oil W01.0 ☑
  snow W00.0 ☑
   with skis — *see* Accident, transport, pedestrian, conveyance
  surface (slippery) (wet) NEC W01.0 ☑
Sliver, wood, contact with W45.8 ☑
Smoldering (due to fire) — *see* Exposure, fire
Sodomy (attempted) **by force** T74.2 ☑
Sound waves (causing injury) W42.9 ☑
 supersonic W42.0 ☑
Splinter, contact with W45.8 ☑
Stab, stabbing — *see* Cut
Standing (prolonged) (static) X50.1 ☑
Starvation X58 ☑
Status of external cause Y99.9
 child assisting in compensated work for family Y99.8
 civilian activity done for financial or other compensation Y99.0
 civilian activity done for income or pay Y99.0
 family member assisting in compensated work for other family member Y99.8
 hobby not done for income Y99.8
 leisure activity Y99.8
 military activity Y99.1
 off-duty activity of military personnel Y99.8
 recreation or sport not for income or while a student Y99.8
 specified NEC Y99.8
 student activity Y99.8
 volunteer activity Y99.2
Stepped on
 by
  animal (not being ridden) NEC W55.89 ☑
  crowd or human stampede W52 ☑
  person W50.0 ☑
Stepping on
 object W22.8 ☑
  with fall W18.31 ☑
  sports equipment W21.9 ☑
  stationary W22.09 ☑
   sports equipment W21.89 ☑
 person W51 ☑
  by crowd or human stampede W52 ☑
 sports equipment W21.9 ☑
Sting
 arthropod, nonvenomous W57 ☑
 insect, nonvenomous W57 ☑
Storm (cataclysmic) — *see* Forces of nature, cataclysmic storm
Straining, excessive (*see also* Overexertion) X50.9 ☑
Strangling — *see* Strangulation
Strangulation (accidental) T71 ☑
Strenuous movements (*see also* Overexertion) X50.9 ☑
Striking against
 airbag (automobile) W22.10 ☑
  driver side W22.11 ☑
  front passenger side W22.12 ☑
  specified NEC W22.19 ☑
 bottom when
  diving or jumping into water (in) W16.822 ☑
   causing drowning W16.821 ☑
   from boat W16.722 ☑
    causing drowning W16.721 ☑
   natural body W16.622 ☑
    causing drowning W16.821 ☑
   swimming pool W16.522 ☑
    causing drowning W16.521 ☑
  falling into water (in) W16.322 ☑
   causing drowning W16.321 ☑
   fountain — *see* Striking against, bottom when, falling into water, specified NEC
   natural body W16.122 ☑

Striking against — *continued*
 bottom when — *continued*
  falling into water — *continued*
   natural body — *continued*
    causing drowning W16.121 ☑
   reservoir — *see* Striking against, bottom when, falling into water, specified NEC
   specified NEC W16.322 ☑
    causing drowning W16.321 ☑
   swimming pool W16.022 ☑
    causing drowning W16.021 ☑
 diving board (swimming-pool) W21.4 ☑
 object W22.8 ☑
  with
   drowning or submersion — *see* Drowning
   fall — *see* Fall, due to, bumping against, object
  caused by crowd or human stampede (with fall) W52 ☑
  furniture W22.03 ☑
  lamppost W22.02 ☑
  sports equipment W21.9 ☑
  stationary W22.09 ☑
   sports equipment W21.89 ☑
  wall W22.01 ☑
 person(s) W51 ☑
  with fall W03 ☑
   due to ice or snow W00.0 ☑
  as, or caused by, a crowd or human stampede (with fall) W52 ☑
  assault Y04.2 ☑
  homicide (attempt) Y04.2 ☑
 sports equipment W21.9 ☑
 wall (when) W22.01 ☑
  diving or jumping into water (in) W16.832 ☑
   causing drowning W16.831 ☑
   swimming pool W16.532 ☑
    causing drowning W16.531 ☑
  falling into water (in) W16.332 ☑
   causing drowning W16.331 ☑
   fountain — *see* Striking against, wall when, falling into water, specified NEC
   natural body W16.132 ☑
    causing drowning W16.131 ☑
   reservoir — *see* Striking against, wall when, falling into water, specified NEC
   specified NEC W16.332 ☑
    causing drowning W16.331 ☑
   swimming pool W16.032 ☑
    causing drowning W16.031 ☑
  swimming pool (when) W22.042 ☑
   causing drowning W22.041 ☑
   diving or jumping into water W16.532 ☑
    causing drowning W16.531 ☑
   falling into water W16.032 ☑
    causing drowning W16.031 ☑
Struck (accidentally) **by**
 airbag (automobile) W22.10 ☑
  driver side W22.11 ☑
  front passenger side W22.12 ☑
  specified NEC W22.19 ☑
 alligator W58.02 ☑
 animal (not being ridden) NEC W55.89 ☑
 avalanche — *see* Landslide
 ball (hit) (thrown) W21.00 ☑
  assault Y08.09 ☑
  baseball W21.03 ☑
  basketball W21.05 ☑
  football W21.01 ☑
  golf ball W21.04 ☑
  soccer W21.02 ☑
  softball W21.07 ☑
  specified NEC W21.09 ☑
  volleyball W21.06 ☑
 bat or racquet
  baseball bat W21.11 ☑
   assault Y08.02 ☑
  golf club W21.13 ☑
   assault Y08.09 ☑
  specified NEC W21.19 ☑
   assault Y08.09 ☑
  tennis racquet W21.12 ☑
   assault Y08.09 ☑
 bullet (*see also* Discharge, firearm by type)
  in war operations — *see* War operations
 crocodile W58.12 ☑
 dog W54.1 ☑

Struck (accidentally) **by** — *continued*
 flare, Very pistol — *see* Discharge, firearm NEC
 hailstones X39.8 ☑
 hockey (ice)
  field
   puck W21.221 ☑
   stick W21.211 ☑
  puck W21.220 ☑
  stick W21.210 ☑
   assault Y08.01 ☑
 landslide — *see* Landslide
 law-enforcement agent (on duty) — *see* Legal, intervention, manhandling
  with blunt object — *see* Legal, intervention, blunt object
 lightning T75.0 ☑
  causing fire — *see* Exposure, fire
 machine — *see* Contact, with, by type of machine
 mammal NEC W55.89 ☑
  marine W56.32 ☑
 marine animal W56.82 ☑
 missile
  firearm — *see* Discharge, firearm by type
  in war operations — *see* War operations, missile
 object W22.8 ☑
  blunt W22.8 ☑
   assault Y00 ☑
   suicide (attempt) X79 ☑
   undetermined whether accidental or intentional Y29 ☑
  falling W20.8 ☑
   from, in, on
    building W20.1 ☑
     burning (uncontrolled fire) X00.4 ☑
    cataclysmic
     earth surface movement NEC — *see* Landslide
     storm — *see* Forces of nature, cataclysmic storm
    cave-in W20.0 ☑
    earthquake X34 ☑
    machine (in operation) — *see* Contact, with, by type of machine
    structure W20.1 ☑
     burning X00.4 ☑
    transport vehicle (in motion) — *see* Accident, transport, by type of vehicle
    watercraft V93.49 ☑
     due to
      accident to craft V91.39 ☑
       powered craft V91.33 ☑
        ferry boat V91.31 ☑
        fishing boat V91.32 ☑
        jetskis V91.33 ☑
        liner V91.31 ☑
        merchant ship V91.30 ☑
        passenger ship V91.31 ☑
       unpowered craft V91.38 ☑
        canoe V91.35 ☑
        inflatable V91.36 ☑
        kayak V91.35 ☑
        sailboat V91.34 ☑
        surf-board V91.38 ☑
        windsurfer V91.38 ☑
      powered craft V93.43 ☑
       ferry boat V93.41 ☑
       fishing boat V93.42 ☑
       jetskis V93.43 ☑
       liner V93.41 ☑
       merchant ship V93.40 ☑
       passenger ship V93.41 ☑
      unpowered craft V93.48 ☑
       sailboat V93.44 ☑
       surf-board V93.48 ☑
       windsurfer V93.48 ☑
 moving NEC W20.8 ☑
 projected W20.8 ☑
  assault Y00 ☑
  in sports W21.9 ☑
   assault Y08.09 ☑
   ball W21.00 ☑
    baseball W21.03 ☑
    basketball W21.05 ☑
    football W21.01 ☑
    golf ball W21.04 ☑
    soccer W21.02 ☑

Struck (accidentally) **by** — *continued*
  object — *continued*
    projected — *continued*
      in sports — *continued*
        ball — *continued*
          softball W21.07 ☑
          specified NEC W21.09 ☑
          volleyball W21.06 ☑
        bat or racquet
          baseball bat W21.11 ☑
            assault Y08.02 ☑
          golf club W21.13 ☑
            assault Y08.09 ☑
          specified NEC W21.19 ☑
            assault Y08.09 ☑
          tennis racquet W21.12 ☑
            assault Y08.09 ☑
        hockey (ice)
          field
            puck W21.221 ☑
            stick W21.211 ☑
          puck W21.220 ☑
          stick W21.210 ☑
            assault Y08.01 ☑
        specified NEC W21.89 ☑
    set in motion by explosion — *see* Explosion
    thrown W20.8 ☑
      assault Y00 ☑
      in sports W21.9 ☑
        assault Y08.09 ☑
        ball W21.00 ☑
          baseball W21.03 ☑
          basketball W21.05 ☑
          football W21.01 ☑
          golf ball W21.04 ☑
          soccer W21.02 ☑
          soft ball W21.07 ☑
          specified NEC W21.09 ☑
          volleyball W21.06 ☑
        bat or racquet
          baseball bat W21.11 ☑
            assault Y08.02 ☑
          golf club W21.13 ☑
            assault Y08.09 ☑
          specified NEC W21.19 ☑
            assault Y08.09 ☑
          tennis racquet W21.12 ☑
            assault Y08.09 ☑
        hockey (ice)
          field
            puck W21.221 ☑
            stick W21.211 ☑
          puck W21.220 ☑
          stick W21.210 ☑
            assault Y08.01 ☑
        specified NEC W21.89 ☑
  other person(s) W50.0 ☑
    with
      blunt object W22.8 ☑
        intentional, homicide (attempt) Y00 ☑
        sports equipment W21.9 ☑
        undetermined whether accidental or intentional Y29 ☑
      fall W03 ☑
        due to ice or snow W00.0 ☑
    as, or caused by, a crowd or human stampede (with fall) W52 ☑
    assault Y04.2 ☑
    homicide (attempt) Y04.2 ☑
    in legal intervention
      injuring
        bystander Y35.812 ☑
        law enforcement personnel Y35.811 ☑
        suspect Y35.813 ☑
    sports equipment W21.9 ☑
  police (on duty) — *see* Legal, intervention, manhandling
    with blunt object — *see* Legal, intervention, blunt object
  sports equipment W21.9 ☑
    assault Y08.09 ☑
    ball W21.00 ☑
      baseball W21.03 ☑
      basketball W21.05 ☑
      football W21.01 ☑
      golf ball W21.04 ☑

Struck (accidentally) **by** — *continued*
  sports equipment — *continued*
    ball — *continued*
      soccer W21.02 ☑
      soft ball W21.07 ☑
      specified NEC W21.09 ☑
      volleyball W21.06 ☑
    bat or racquet
      baseball bat W21.11 ☑
        assault Y08.02 ☑
      golf club W21.13 ☑
        assault Y08.09 ☑
      specified NEC W21.19 ☑
      tennis racquet W21.12 ☑
        assault Y08.09 ☑
    cleats (shoe) W21.31 ☑
    foot wear NEC W21.39 ☑
    football helmet W21.81 ☑
    hockey (ice)
      field
        puck W21.221 ☑
        stick W21.211 ☑
      puck W21.220 ☑
      stick W21.210 ☑
        assault Y08.01 ☑
    skate blades W21.32 ☑
    specified NEC W21.89 ☑
      assault Y08.09 ☑
  thunderbolt — *see* subcategory T75.0 ☑
    causing fire — *see* Exposure, fire
  transport vehicle NEC (*see also* Accident, transport) V09.9 ☑
    intentional, homicide (attempt) Y03.0 ☑
    motor NEC (*see also* Accident, transport) V09.20 ☑
      homicide Y03.0 ☑
  vehicle (transport) NEC — *see* Accident, transport, by type of vehicle
    stationary (falling from jack, hydraulic lift, ramp) W20.8 ☑

Stumbling
  without fall W18.40 ☑
    due to
      specified NEC W18.49 ☑
      stepping from one level to another W18.43 ☑
      stepping into hole or opening W18.42 ☑
      stepping on object W18.41 ☑
    over
      animal NEC W01.0 ☑
        with fall W18.09 ☑
      carpet, rug or (small) object W22.8 ☑
        with fall W18.09 ☑
      person W51 ☑
        with fall W03 ☑
          due to ice or snow W00.0 ☑

Submersion (accidental) — *see* Drowning
Suffocation (accidental) (by external means) (by pressure) (mechanical) (*see also* category) T71 ☑
  due to, by
    avalanche — *see* Landslide
    explosion — *see* Explosion
    fire — *see* Exposure, fire
    food, any type (aspiration) (ingestion) (inhalation) — *see* categories T17 and T18
    ignition — *see* Ignition
    landslide — *see* Landslide
    machine(ry) — *see* Contact, with, by type of machine
    vomitus (aspiration) (inhalation) T17.81- ☑
  in
    burning building X00.8 ☑

Suicide, suicidal (attempted) (by) X83.8 ☑
  blunt object X79 ☑
  burning, burns X76 ☑
    hot object X77.9 ☑
      fluid NEC X77.2 ☑
      household appliance X77.3 ☑
      specified NEC X77.8 ☑
      steam X77.0 ☑
      tap water X77.1 ☑
      vapors X77.0 ☑
  caustic substance — *see* Table of Drugs and Chemicals
  cold, extreme X83.2 ☑
  collision of motor vehicle with
    motor vehicle X82.0 ☑
    specified NEC X82.8 ☑
    train X82.1 ☑

Suicide, suicidal — *continued*
  collision of motor vehicle with — *continued*
    tree X82.2 ☑
  crashing of aircraft X83.0 ☑
  cut (any part of body) X78.9 ☑
  cutting or piercing instrument X78.9 ☑
    dagger X78.2 ☑
    glass X78.0 ☑
    knife X78.1 ☑
    specified NEC X78.8 ☑
    sword X78.2 ☑
  drowning (in) X71.9 ☑
    bathtub X71.0 ☑
    natural water X71.3 ☑
    specified NEC X71.8 ☑
    swimming pool X71.1 ☑
      following fall X71.2 ☑
  electrocution X83.1 ☑
  explosive(s) (material) X75 ☑
  fire, flames X76 ☑
  firearm X74.9 ☑
    airgun X74.01 ☑
    handgun X72 ☑
    hunting rifle X73.1 ☑
    larger X73.9 ☑
      specified NEC X73.8 ☑
    machine gun X73.2 ☑
    shotgun X73.0 ☑
    specified NEC X74.8 ☑
  hanging X83.8 ☑
  hot object — *see* Suicide, burning, hot object
  jumping
    before moving object X81.8 ☑
      motor vehicle X81.0 ☑
      subway train X81.1 ☑
      train X81.1 ☑
    from high place X80 ☑
  late effect of attempt — *see* X71-X83 with 7th character S
  lying before moving object, train, vehicle X81.8 ☑
  poisoning — *see* Table of Drugs and Chemicals
  puncture (any part of body) — *see* Suicide, cutting or piercing instrument
  scald — *see* Suicide, burning, hot object
  sequelae of attempt — *see* X71-X83 with 7th character S
  sharp object (any) — *see* Suicide, cutting or piercing instrument
  shooting — *see* Suicide, firearm
  specified means NEC X83.8 ☑
  stab (any part of body) — *see* Suicide, cutting or piercing instrument
  steam, hot vapors X77.0 ☑
  strangulation X83.8 ☑
  submersion — *see* Suicide, drowning
  suffocation X83.8 ☑
  wound NEC X83.8 ☑
Sunstroke X32 ☑
Supersonic waves (causing injury) W42.0 ☑
Surgical procedure, complication of (delayed or as an abnormal reaction without mention of misadventure) (*see also* Complication of or following, by type of procedure)
  due to or as a result of misadventure — *see* Misadventure
Swallowed, swallowing
  foreign body — *see* Foreign body, alimentary canal
  poison — *see* Table of Drugs and Chemicals
  substance
    caustic or corrosive — *see* Table of Drugs and Chemicals
    poisonous — *see* Table of Drugs and Chemicals

T

Tackle in sport W03 ☑
Terrorism (involving) Y38.80 ☑
  biological weapons Y38.6X- ☑
  chemical weapons Y38.7X- ☑
  conflagration Y38.3X- ☑
  drowning and submersion Y38.89- ☑
  explosion Y38.2X- ☑
    destruction of aircraft Y38.1X- ☑
    marine weapons Y38.0X- ☑
  fire Y38.3X- ☑
  firearms Y38.4X- ☑

Terrorism — *continued*
  hot substances Y38.3X- ☑
  lasers Y38.89-
  nuclear weapons Y38.5X- ☑
  piercing or stabbing instruments Y38.89- ☑
  secondary effects Y38.9X- ☑
  specified method NEC Y38.89- ☑
  suicide bomber Y38.81- ☑
Thirst X58 ☑
Threat to breathing
  aspiration — *see* Aspiration
  due to cave-in, falling earth or substance NEC T71 ☑
Thrown (accidentally)
  against part (any) of or object in transport vehicle (in motion) NEC (*see also* Accident, transport)
  from
    high place, homicide (attempt) Y01 ☑
    machinery — *see* Contact, with, by type of machine
    transport vehicle NEC (*see also* Accident, transport) V89.9 ☑
  off — *see* Thrown, from
Thunderbolt — *see* subcategory T75.0 ☑
  causing fire — *see* Exposure, fire
Tidal wave (any injury) **NEC** — *see* Forces of nature, tidal wave
Took
  overdose (drug) — *see* Table of Drugs and Chemicals
  poison — *see* Table of Drugs and Chemicals
Tornado (any injury) X37.1 ☑
Torrential rain (any injury) X37.8 ☑
Torture X58 ☑
Trampled by animal NEC W55.89 ☑
Trapped (accidentally)
  between objects (moving) (stationary and moving) — *see* Caught
  by part (any) of
    motorcycle V29.88 ☑
    pedal cycle V19.88 ☑
    transport vehicle NEC (*see also* Accident, transport) V89.9 ☑
Travel (effects) (sickness) T75.3 ☑
Tree falling on or hitting (accidentally) (person) W20.8 ☑
Tripping
  without fall W18.40 ☑
    due to
      specified NEC W18.49 ☑
      stepping from one level to another W18.43 ☑
      stepping into hole or opening W18.42 ☑
      stepping on object W18.41 ☑
    over
      animal W01.0 ☑
        with fall W01.0 ☑
      carpet, rug or (small) object W22.8 ☑
        with fall W18.09 ☑
      person W51 ☑
        with fall W03 ☑
          due to ice or snow W00.0 ☑
Twisted by person(s) (accidentally) W50.2 ☑
  with intent to injure or kill Y04.0 ☑
  as, or caused by, a crowd or human stampede (with fall) W52 ☑
  assault Y04.0 ☑
  homicide (attempt) Y04.0 ☑
  in
    fight Y04.0 ☑
    legal intervention — *see* Legal, intervention, manhandling
Twisting (prolonged) (static) X50.1- ☑

U

Underdosing of necessary drugs, medicaments or biological substances Y63.6
Undetermined intent (contact) (exposure)
  automobile collision Y32 ☑
  blunt object Y29 ☑
  drowning (submersion) (in) Y21.9 ☑
    bathtub Y21.0 ☑
      after fall Y21.1 ☑
    natural water (lake) (ocean) (pond) (river) (stream) Y21.4 ☑
    specified place NEC Y21.8 ☑
    swimming pool Y21.2 ☑
      after fall Y21.3 ☑
  explosive material Y25 ☑

Undetermined intent — *continued*
  fall, jump or push from high place Y30 ☑
  falling, lying or running before moving object Y31 ☑
  fire Y26 ☑
  firearm discharge Y24.9 ☑
    airgun (BB) (pellet) Y24.0 ☑
    handgun (pistol) (revolver) Y22 ☑
    hunting rifle Y23.1 ☑
    larger Y23.9 ☑
      hunting rifle Y23.1 ☑
      machine gun Y23.3 ☑
      military Y23.2 ☑
      shotgun Y23.0 ☑
      specified type NEC Y23.8 ☑
    machine gun Y23.3 ☑
    military Y23.2 ☑
    shotgun Y23.0 ☑
    specified type NEC Y24.8 ☑
    Very pistol Y24.8 ☑
  hot object Y27.9 ☑
    fluid NEC Y27.2 ☑
    household appliance Y27.3 ☑
    specified object NEC Y27.8 ☑
    steam Y27.0 ☑
    tap water Y27.1 ☑
    vapor Y27.0 ☑
  jump, fall or push from high place Y30 ☑
  lying, falling or running before moving object Y31 ☑
  motor vehicle crash Y32 ☑
  push, fall or jump from high place Y30 ☑
  running, falling or lying before moving object Y31 ☑
  sharp object Y28.9 ☑
    dagger Y28.2 ☑
    glass Y28.0 ☑
    knife Y28.1 ☑
    specified object NEC Y28.8 ☑
    sword Y28.2 ☑
  smoke Y26 ☑
  specified event NEC Y33 ☑
Use of hand as hammer X50.3 ☑

V

Vibration (causing injury) W49.9 ☑
Victim (of)
  avalanche — *see* Landslide
  earth movements NEC — *see* Forces of nature, earth movement
  earthquake X34 ☑
  flood — *see* Flood
  landslide — *see* Landslide
  lightning — *see* subcategory T75.0 ☑
    causing fire — *see* Exposure, fire
  storm (cataclysmic) NEC — *see* Forces of nature, cataclysmic storm
  volcanic eruption X35 ☑
Volcanic eruption (any injury) X35 ☑
Vomitus, gastric contents in air passages (with asphyxia, obstruction or suffocation) T17.81- ☑

W

Walked into stationary object (any) W22.09 ☑
  furniture W22.03 ☑
  lamppost W22.02 ☑
  wall W22.01 ☑
War operations (injuries to military personnel and civilians during war, civil insurrection and peacekeeping missions) (by) (from) (involving) Y36.90 ☑
  after cessation of hostilities Y36.89- ☑
    explosion (of)
      bomb placed during war operations Y36.82- ☑
      mine placed during war operations Y36.81- ☑
      specified NEC Y36.88- ☑
  air blast Y36.20- ☑
  aircraft
    destruction — *see* War operations, destruction of aircraft
    airway restriction — *see* War operations, restriction of airways
  asphyxiation — *see* War operations, restriction of airways
  biological weapons Y36.6X- ☑
  blast Y36.20- ☑
  blast fragments Y36.20- ☑
  blast wave Y36.20- ☑

War operations — *continued*
  blast wind Y36.20- ☑
  bomb Y36.20- ☑
    dirty Y36.50- ☑
    gasoline Y36.31- ☑
    incendiary Y36.31- ☑
    petrol Y36.31- ☑
  bullet Y36.43- ☑
    incendiary Y36.32- ☑
    rubber Y36.41- ☑
  chemical weapons Y36.7X- ☑
  combat
    hand to hand (unarmed) combat Y36.44- ☑
    using blunt or piercing object Y36.45- ☑
  conflagration — *see* War operations, fire
  conventional warfare NEC Y36.49- ☑
  depth-charge Y36.01- ☑
  destruction of aircraft Y36.10- ☑
    due to
      air to air missile Y36.11- ☑
      collision with other aircraft Y36.12- ☑
      detonation (accidental) of onboard munitions and explosives Y36.14- ☑
      enemy fire or explosives Y36.11- ☑
      explosive placed on aircraft Y36.11- ☑
      onboard fire Y36.13- ☑
      rocket propelled grenade [RPG] Y36.11- ☑
      small arms fire Y36.11- ☑
      surface to air missile Y36.11- ☑
    specified NEC Y36.19- ☑
  detonation (accidental) of
    onboard marine weapons Y36.05- ☑
    own munitions or munitions launch device Y36.24- ☑
  dirty bomb Y36.50- ☑
  explosion (of) Y36.20- ☑
    aerial bomb Y36.21- ☑
    after cessation of hostilities
      bomb placed during war operations Y36.82- ☑
      mine placed during war operations Y36.81- ☑
    bomb NOS (*see also* War operations, bomb(s)) Y36.20- ☑
    fragments Y36.20- ☑
    grenade Y36.29- ☑
    guided missile Y36.22- ☑
    improvised explosive device [IED] (person-borne) (roadside) (vehicle-borne) Y36.23- ☑
    land mine Y36.29- ☑
    marine mine (at sea) (in harbor) Y36.02- ☑
    marine weapon Y36.00- ☑
      specified NEC Y36.09- ☑
    own munitions or munitions launch device (accidental) Y36.24- ☑
    sea-based artillery shell Y36.03- ☑
    specified NEC Y36.29- ☑
    torpedo Y36.04- ☑
  fire Y36.30- ☑
    specified NEC Y36.39- ☑
  firearms
    discharge Y36.43- ☑
    pellets Y36.42- ☑
  flamethrower Y36.33- ☑
  fragments (from) (of)
    improvised explosive device [IED] (person-borne) (roadside) (vehicle-borne) Y36.26- ☑
    munitions Y36.25- ☑
    specified NEC Y36.29- ☑
    weapons Y36.27- ☑
  friendly fire Y36.92 ☑
  hand to hand (unarmed) combat Y36.44- ☑
  hot substances — *see* War operations, fire
  incendiary bullet Y36.32- ☑
  nuclear weapon (effects of) Y36.50- ☑
    acute radiation exposure Y36.54- ☑
    blast pressure Y36.51- ☑
    direct blast Y36.51- ☑
    direct heat Y36.53- ☑
    fallout exposure Y36.54- ☑
    fireball Y36.53- ☑
    indirect blast (struck or crushed by blast debris) (being thrown by blast) Y36.52- ☑
    ionizing radiation (immediate exposure) Y36.54- ☑
    nuclear radiation Y36.54- ☑
    radiation
      ionizing (immediate exposure) Y36.54- ☑
      nuclear Y36.54- ☑

War operations — *continued*
  nuclear weapon — *continued*
    radiation — *continued*
      thermal Y36.53- ☑
    secondary effects Y36.54- ☑
    specified NEC Y36.59- ☑
    thermal radiation Y36.53- ☑
  restriction of air (airway)
    intentional Y36.46- ☑
    unintentional Y36.47- ☑
  rubber bullets Y36.41- ☑
  shrapnel NOS Y36.29- ☑
  suffocation — *see* War operations, restriction of airways
  unconventional warfare NEC Y36.7X- ☑
  underwater blast NOS Y36.00- ☑
  warfare
    conventional NEC Y36.49- ☑
    unconventional NEC Y36.7X- ☑

War operations — *continued*
  weapon of mass destruction [WMD] Y36.91 ☑
  weapons
    biological weapons Y36.6X- ☑
    chemical Y36.7X- ☑
    nuclear (effects of) Y36.50- ☑
      acute radiation exposure Y36.54- ☑
      blast pressure Y36.51- ☑
      direct blast Y36.51- ☑
      direct heat Y36.53- ☑
      fallout exposure Y36.54- ☑
      fireball Y36.53- ☑
      radiation
        ionizing (immediate exposure) Y36.54- ☑
        nuclear Y36.54- ☑
        thermal Y36.53- ☑
      secondary effects Y36.54- ☑
      specified NEC Y36.59- ☑
    of mass destruction [WMD] Y36.91 ☑

Washed
  away by flood — *see* Flood
  off road by storm (transport vehicle) — *see* Forces of nature, cataclysmic storm
Weather exposure NEC — *see* Forces of nature
Weightlessness (causing injury) (effects of) (in spacecraft, real or simulated) X52 ☑
Work related condition Y99.0
Wound (accidental) NEC (*see also* Injury) X58 ☑
  battle (*see also* War operations) Y36.90 ☑
  gunshot — *see* Discharge, firearm by type
Wreck transport vehicle NEC (*see also* Accident, transport) V89.9 ☑
Wrong
  device implanted into correct surgical site Y65.51
  fluid in infusion Y65.1
  patient, procedure performed on Y65.52
  procedure (operation) on correct patient Y65.51

Chapter 1. Certain Infectious and Parasitic Diseases (A00–B99)

Chapter Specific Guidelines with Coding Examples

The chapter specific guidelines from the ICD-10-CM Official Guidelines for Coding and Reporting have been provided below. Along with these guidelines are coding examples, contained in the shaded boxes, that have been developed to help illustrate the coding and/or sequencing guidance found in these guidelines.

a. Human immunodeficiency virus (HIV) infections

1) Code only confirmed cases

Code only confirmed cases of HIV infection/illness. This is an exception to the hospital inpatient guideline Section II, H.

In this context, "confirmation" does not require documentation of positive serology or culture for HIV; the provider's diagnostic statement that the patient is HIV positive, or has an HIV-related illness is sufficient.

> Patient admitted with anemia with possible HIV infection
>
> **D64.9**   **Anemia, unspecified**
>
> *Explanation:* Only the anemia is coded in this scenario because it has not been confirmed that an HIV infection is present. This is an exception to the guideline Section II, H for hospital inpatient coding.

2) Selection and sequencing of HIV codes

(a) Patient admitted for HIV-related condition

If a patient is admitted for an HIV-related condition, the principal diagnosis should be B20, Human immunodeficiency virus [HIV] disease followed by additional diagnosis codes for all reported HIV-related conditions.

> HIV with PCP
>
> **B20**   **Human immunodeficiency virus [HIV] disease**
>
> **B59**   **Pneumocystosis**
>
> *Explanation:* Pneumonia due to *Pneumocystis carinii* is an HIV related condition, so the HIV diagnosis code is reported first, followed by the code for the pneumonia.

(b) Patient with HIV disease admitted for unrelated condition

If a patient with HIV disease is admitted for an unrelated condition (such as a traumatic injury), the code for the unrelated condition (e.g., the nature of injury code) should be the principal diagnosis. Other diagnoses would be B20 followed by additional diagnosis codes for all reported HIV-related conditions.

> Unstable angina, native coronary artery atherosclerosis, HIV
>
> **I25.110**   **Atherosclerotic heart disease of native coronary artery with unstable angina pectoris**
>
> **B20**   **Human immunodeficiency virus [HIV] disease**
>
> *Explanation:* The arteriosclerotic coronary artery disease and the unstable angina are not related to HIV, so those conditions are reported first using a combination code, and HIV is reported secondarily.

(c) Whether the patient is newly diagnosed

Whether the patient is newly diagnosed or has had previous admissions/encounters for HIV conditions is irrelevant to the sequencing decision.

> Newly diagnosed multiple cutaneous Kaposi's sarcoma lesions in previously diagnosed HIV disease.
>
> **B20**   **Human immunodeficiency virus [HIV] disease**
>
> **C46.0**   **Kaposi's sarcoma of skin**
>
> *Explanation:* Even though the HIV was diagnosed on a previous encounter, it is still sequenced first when coded with an HIV related condition. Kaposi's sarcoma is an HIV-related condition.

(d) Asymptomatic human immunodeficiency virus

Z21, Asymptomatic human immunodeficiency virus [HIV] infection status, is to be applied when the patient without any documentation of symptoms is listed as being "HIV positive," "known HIV," "HIV test

positive," or similar terminology. Do not use this code if the term "AIDS" is used or if the patient is treated for any HIV-related illness or is described as having any condition(s) resulting from his/her HIV positive status; use B20 in these cases.

> Patient admitted for aftercare and rehabilitation post-appendectomy for acute appendicitis; status post-positive HIV test on Atripla, with no prior or current symptoms
>
> **Z48.815**   **Encounter for surgical aftercare following surgery on the digestive system**
>
> **Z21**   **Asymptomatic human immunodeficiency virus [HIV] infection status**
>
> *Explanation:* Code Z21 is used to document that the patient has had a positive HIV test but has been asymptomatic. Being on medication for HIV does not indicate that the infection is active and B20 Human immunodeficiency virus [HIV] disease, should not be assigned unless there is documentation that the patient has had *current or prior* symptoms or HIV-related complications. The aftercare being provided post-appendectomy is sequenced first.

(e) Patients with inconclusive HIV serology

Patients with inconclusive HIV serology, but no definitive diagnosis or manifestations of the illness, may be assigned code R75, Inconclusive laboratory evidence of human immunodeficiency virus [HIV].

(f) Previously diagnosed HIV-related illness

Patients with any known prior diagnosis of an HIV-related illness should be coded to B20. Once a patient has developed an HIV-related illness, the patient should always be assigned code B20 on every subsequent admission/encounter. Patients previously diagnosed with any HIV illness (B20) should never be assigned to R75 or Z21, Asymptomatic human immunodeficiency virus [HIV] infection status.

(g) HIV infection in pregnancy, childbirth and the puerperium

During pregnancy, childbirth or the puerperium, a patient admitted (or presenting for a health care encounter) because of an HIV-related illness should receive a principal diagnosis code of O98.7-, Human immunodeficiency [HIV] disease complicating pregnancy, childbirth and the puerperium, followed by B20 and the code(s) for the HIV-related illness(es). Codes from Chapter 15 always take sequencing priority.

Patients with asymptomatic HIV infection status admitted (or presenting for a health care encounter) during pregnancy, childbirth, or the puerperium should receive codes of O98.7- and Z21.

(h) Encounters for testing for HIV

If a patient is being seen to determine his/her HIV status, use code Z11.4, Encounter for screening for human immunodeficiency virus [HIV]. Use additional codes for any associated high risk behavior.

If a patient with signs or symptoms is being seen for HIV testing, code the signs and symptoms. An additional counseling code Z71.7, Human immunodeficiency virus [HIV] counseling, may be used if counseling is provided during the encounter for the test.

When a patient returns to be informed of his/her HIV test results and the test result is negative, use code Z71.7, Human immunodeficiency virus [HIV] counseling.

If the results are positive, see previous guidelines and assign codes as appropriate.

b. Infectious agents as the cause of diseases classified to other chapters

Certain infections are classified in chapters other than Chapter 1 and no organism is identified as part of the infection code. In these instances, it is necessary to use an additional code from Chapter 1 to identify the organism. A code from category B95, Streptococcus, Staphylococcus, and Enterococcus as the cause of diseases classified to other chapters, B96, Other bacterial agents as the cause of diseases classified to other chapters, or B97, Viral agents as the cause of diseases classified to other chapters, is to be used as an additional code to identify the organism. An instructional note will be found at the infection code advising that an additional organism code is required.

Chapter 1. Certain Infectious and Parasitic Diseases

E. coli UTI.

N39.Ø	Urinary tract infection, site not specified
B96.2Ø	Unspecified Escherichia coli [E.coli] as the cause of diseases classified elsewhere

Explanation: An instructional note under the code for the urinary tract infection indicates to code also the specific organism.

c. Infections resistant to antibiotics

Many bacterial infections are resistant to current antibiotics. It is necessary to identify all infections documented as antibiotic resistant. Assign a code from category Z16, Resistance to antimicrobial drugs, following the infection code only if the infection code does not identify drug resistance.

Antimycobacterial-resistant primary pulmonary tuberculosis.

A15.Ø	Tuberculosis of lung
Z16.341	Resistance to single antimycobacterial drug

Explanation: Code Z16.341 is assigned as a secondary code to represent the antimycobacterial resistance. This code includes resistance to antimycobacterial drug "NOS"; if multiple drug resistance is not specified, classification defaults to the single drug resistance code.

d. Sepsis, severe sepsis, and septic shock

1) Coding of sepsis and severe sepsis

(a) Sepsis

For a diagnosis of sepsis, assign the appropriate code for the underlying systemic infection. If the type of infection or causal organism is not further specified, assign code A41.9, Sepsis, unspecified organism.

A code from subcategory R65.2, Severe sepsis, should not be assigned unless severe sepsis or an associated acute organ dysfunction is documented.

Gram-negative sepsis.

A41.5Ø	Gram-negative sepsis, unspecified

Staphylococcal sepsis

A41.2	Sepsis due to unspecified staphylococcus

Explanation: In both examples above the organism causing the sepsis is identified, therefore A41.9 Sepsis, unspecified organism, would not be appropriate as this code would not capture the highest degree of specificity found in the documentation. Do not use an additional code for severe sepsis unless an acute organ dysfunction was also documented as "associated with" or "due to" the sepsis or the sepsis was documented as "severe."

(i) Negative or inconclusive blood cultures and sepsis

Negative or inconclusive blood cultures do not preclude a diagnosis of sepsis in patients with clinical evidence of the condition; however, the provider should be queried.

(ii) Urosepsis

The term urosepsis is a nonspecific term. It is not to be considered synonymous with sepsis. It has no default code in the Alphabetic Index. Should a provider use this term, he/she must be queried for clarification.

(iii) Sepsis with organ dysfunction

If a patient has sepsis and associated acute organ dysfunction or multiple organ dysfunction (MOD), follow the instructions for coding severe sepsis.

(iv) Acute organ dysfunction that is not clearly associated with the sepsis

If a patient has sepsis and an acute organ dysfunction, but the medical record documentation indicates that the acute organ dysfunction is related to a medical condition other than the sepsis, do not assign a code from subcategory R65.2, Severe sepsis. An acute organ dysfunction must be associated with the sepsis in order to assign the severe sepsis code. If the documentation is not clear as to whether an acute organ dysfunction is related to the sepsis or another medical condition, query the provider.

Sepsis and acute respiratory failure due to COPD exacerbation.

A41.9	Sepsis, unspecified organism
J44.1	Chronic obstructive pulmonary disease with (acute) exacerbation
J96.ØØ	Acute respiratory failure, unspecified whether with hypoxia or hypercapnia

Explanation: Although acute organ dysfunction is present in the form of acute respiratory failure, severe sepsis (R65.2) is not coded in this example, as the acute respiratory failure is attributed to the COPD exacerbation rather than the sepsis. Sequencing of these codes would be determined by the circumstances of the admission.

(b) Severe sepsis

The coding of severe sepsis requires a minimum of 2 codes: first a code for the underlying systemic infection, followed by a code from subcategory R65.2, Severe sepsis. If the causal organism is not documented, assign code A41.9, Sepsis, unspecified organism, for the infection. Additional code(s) for the associated acute organ dysfunction are also required.

Due to the complex nature of severe sepsis, some cases may require querying the provider prior to assignment of the codes.

2) Septic shock

(a) Septic shock generally refers to circulatory failure associated with severe sepsis, and therefore, it represents a type of acute organ dysfunction.

For cases of septic shock, the code for the systemic infection should be sequenced first, followed by code R65.21, Severe sepsis with septic shock or code T81.12, Postprocedural septic shock. Any additional codes for the other acute organ dysfunctions should also be assigned. As noted in the sequencing instructions in the Tabular List, the code for septic shock cannot be assigned as a principal diagnosis.

Sepsis with septic shock.

A41.9	Sepsis, unspecified organism
R65.21	Severe sepsis with septic shock

Explanation: Documentation of septic shock automatically implies severe sepsis as it is a form of acute organ dysfunction. Septic shock is not coded as the principal diagnosis; it is always preceded by the code for the systemic infection.

3) Sequencing of severe sepsis

If severe sepsis is present on admission, and meets the definition of principal diagnosis, the underlying systemic infection should be assigned as principal diagnosis followed by the appropriate code from subcategory R65.2 as required by the sequencing rules in the Tabular List. A code from subcategory R65.2 can never be assigned as a principal diagnosis.

When severe sepsis develops during an encounter (it was not present on admission), the underlying systemic infection and the appropriate code from subcategory R65.2 should be assigned as secondary diagnoses.

Severe sepsis may be present on admission, but the diagnosis may not be confirmed until sometime after admission. If the documentation is not clear whether severe sepsis was present on admission, the provider should be queried.

4) Sepsis and severe sepsis with a localized infection

If the reason for admission is both sepsis or severe sepsis and a localized infection, such as pneumonia or cellulitis, a code(s) for the underlying systemic infection should be assigned first and the code for the localized infection should be assigned as a secondary diagnosis. If the patient has severe sepsis, a code from subcategory R65.2 should also be assigned as a secondary diagnosis. If the patient is admitted with a localized infection, such as pneumonia, and sepsis/severe sepsis doesn't develop until after admission, the localized infection should be assigned first, followed by the appropriate sepsis/severe sepsis codes.

Patient presents with acute renal failure due to severe sepsis from *Pseudomonas pneumonia*.

A41.9	**Sepsis, unspecified organism**
J15.1	**Pneumonia due to Pseudomonas**
R65.20	**Severe sepsis without septic shock**
N17.9	**Acute kidney failure, unspecified**

Explanation: If all conditions are present on admission, the systemic infection (sepsis) is sequenced first followed by the codes for the localized infection (pneumonia), severe sepsis and any organ dysfunction. If only the pneumonia was present on admission with the sepsis and resulting renal failure developing later in the admission, then the pneumonia would be sequenced first.

5) **Sepsis due to a postprocedural infection**
   (a) **Documentation of causal relationship**

   As with all postprocedural complications, code assignment is based on the provider's documentation of the relationship between the infection and the procedure.

   (b) **Sepsis due to a postprocedural infection**

   For such cases, the postprocedural infection code, such as T80.2, Infections following infusion, transfusion, and therapeutic injection, T81.4, Infection following a procedure, T88.0, Infection following immunization, or O86.0, Infection of obstetric surgical wound, should be coded first, followed by the code for the specific infection. If the patient has severe sepsis, the appropriate code from subcategory R65.2 should also be assigned with the additional code(s) for any acute organ dysfunction.

   (c) **Postprocedural infection and postprocedural septic shock**

   In cases where a postprocedural infection has occurred and has resulted in severe sepsis the code for the precipitating complication such as code T81.4, Infection following a procedure, or O86.0, Infection of obstetrical surgical wound should be coded first followed by code R65.20, Severe sepsis without septic shock. A code for the systemic infection should also be assigned.

   If a postprocedural infection has resulted in postprocedural septic shock, the code for the precipitating complication such as code T81.4, Infection following a procedure, or O86.0, Infection of obstetrical surgical wound should be coded first followed by code T81.12-, Postprocedural septic shock. A code for the systemic infection should also be assigned.

6) **Sepsis and severe sepsis associated with a noninfectious process (condition)**

   In some cases a noninfectious process (condition), such as trauma, may lead to an infection which can result in sepsis or severe sepsis. If sepsis or severe sepsis is documented as associated with a noninfectious condition, such as a burn or serious injury, and this condition meets the definition for principal diagnosis, the code for the noninfectious condition should be sequenced first, followed by the code for the resulting infection. If severe sepsis is present, a code from subcategory R65.2 should also be assigned with any associated organ dysfunction(s) codes. It is not necessary to assign a code from subcategory R65.1, Systemic inflammatory response syndrome (SIRS) of non-infectious origin, for these cases.

   If the infection meets the definition of principal diagnosis, it should be sequenced before the non-infectious condition. When both the associated non-infectious condition and the infection meet the definition of principal diagnosis, either may be assigned as principal diagnosis.

   Only one code from category R65, Symptoms and signs specifically associated with systemic inflammation and infection, should be assigned. Therefore, when a non-infectious condition leads to an infection resulting in severe sepsis, assign the appropriate code from subcategory R65.2, Severe sepsis. Do not additionally assign a code from subcategory R65.1, Systemic inflammatory response syndrome (SIRS) of non-infectious origin.

   See Section I.C.18. SIRS due to non-infectious process

Patient admitted from hospital to home health for management of multiple third-degree burns of the right upper arm extending from the elbow to shoulder. The patient became septic during the hospital admission and will be continued on IV antibiotic treatment for MSSA sepsis until follow-up blood cultures return negative. The patient requires routine dressing changes three times a week to the burned areas, which are healing well with scarring present.

A41.02	**Sepsis due to Methicillin susceptible Staphylococcus aureus**
T22.391D	**Burn of third degree of multiple sites of right shoulder and upper arm limb, except wrist and hand, subsequent encounter**
Z45.2	**Encounter for adjustment and management of vascular access device**

Explanation: Although the burn is a noninfectious condition, it gave rise to a systemic "infection," as opposed to a less critical inflammatory response. The systemic infection (sepsis) code is all that is required, and a code for SIRS due to noninfectious process is not needed. The code for systemic infection is coded first as the wounds are uncomplicated and healing well, while the sepsis still requires active treatment with IV antibiotics. The seventh character D is appropriate when coding the burn with the routine dressing changes with no wound complications.

7) **Sepsis and septic shock complicating abortion, pregnancy, childbirth, and the puerperium**

   See Section I.C.15. Sepsis and septic shock complicating abortion, pregnancy, childbirth and the puerperium

8) **Newborn sepsis**

   See Section I.C.16. f. Bacterial sepsis of Newborn

e. **Methicillin resistant Staphylococcus aureus (MRSA) conditions**

   1) **Selection and sequencing of MRSA codes**
      (a) **Combination codes for MRSA infection**

      When a patient is diagnosed with an infection that is due to methicillin resistant *Staphylococcus aureus* (MRSA), and that infection has a combination code that includes the causal organism (e.g., sepsis, pneumonia) assign the appropriate combination code for the condition (e.g., code A41.02, Sepsis due to Methicillin resistant Staphylococcus aureus or code J15.212, Pneumonia due to Methicillin resistant Staphylococcus aureus). Do not assign code B95.62, Methicillin resistant Staphylococcus aureus infection as the cause of diseases classified elsewhere, as an additional code, because the combination code includes the type of infection and the MRSA organism. Do not assign a code from subcategory Z16.11, Resistance to penicillins, as an additional diagnosis.

      See Section C.1. for instructions on coding and sequencing of sepsis and severe sepsis.

      (b) **Other codes for MRSA infection**

      When there is documentation of a current infection (e.g., wound infection, stitch abscess, urinary tract infection) due to MRSA, and that infection does not have a combination code that includes the causal organism, assign the appropriate code to identify the condition along with code B95.62, Methicillin resistant Staphylococcus aureus infection as the cause of diseases classified elsewhere for the MRSA infection. Do not assign a code from subcategory Z16.11, Resistance to penicillins.

      (c) **Methicillin susceptible Staphylococcus aureus (MSSA) and MRSA colonization**

      The condition or state of being colonized or carrying MSSA or MRSA is called colonization or carriage, while an individual person is described as being colonized or being a carrier. Colonization means that MSSA or MSRA is present on or in the body without necessarily causing illness. A positive MRSA colonization test might be documented by the provider as "MRSA screen positive" or "MRSA nasal swab positive".

      Assign code Z22.322, Carrier or suspected carrier of Methicillin resistant Staphylococcus aureus, for patients documented as having MRSA colonization. Assign code Z22.321, Carrier or suspected carrier of Methicillin susceptible Staphylococcus aureus, for patient documented as having MSSA colonization. Colonization is not necessarily indicative of a disease process or as the cause of a specific condition the patient may have unless documented as such by the provider.

      (d) **MRSA colonization and infection**

      If a patient is documented as having both MRSA colonization and infection during a hospital admission, code Z22.322, Carrier or suspected carrier of Methicillin resistant Staphylococcus aureus, and a code for the MRSA infection may both be assigned.

f. Zika virus infections

1) Code only confirmed cases

Code only a confirmed diagnosis of Zika virus (A92.5, Zika virus disease) as documented by the provider. This is an exception to the hospital inpatient guideline Section II, H. In this context, "confirmation" does not require documentation of the type of test performed; the physician's diagnostic statement that the condition is confirmed is sufficient. This code should be assigned regardless of the stated mode of transmission.

If the provider documents "suspected", "possible" or "probable" Zika, do not assign code A92.5. Assign a code(s) explaining the reason for encounter (such as fever, rash, or joint pain) or Z20.828, Contact with and (suspected) exposure to other viral communicable diseases.

Chapter 1. Certain Infectious and Parasitic Diseases (A00-B99)

INCLUDES diseases generally recognized as communicable or transmissible

Use additional code to identify resistance to antimicrobial drugs (Z16.-)

EXCLUDES 1 *certain localized infections—see body system-related chapters*

EXCLUDES 2 *carrier or suspected carrier of infectious disease (Z22.-)*
infectious and parasitic diseases specific to the perinatal period (P35-P39)
infectious and parasitic diseases complicating pregnancy, childbirth and the puerperium (O98.-)
influenza and other acute respiratory infections (J00-J22)

This chapter contains the following blocks:

A00-A09	Intestinal infectious diseases
A15-A19	Tuberculosis
A20-A28	Certain zoonotic bacterial diseases
A30-A49	Other bacterial diseases
A50-A64	Infections with a predominantly sexual mode of transmission
A65-A69	Other spirochetal diseases
A70-A74	Other diseases caused by chlamydiae
A75-A79	Rickettsioses
A80-A89	Viral infections of the central nervous system
A90-A99	Arthropod-borne viral fevers and viral hemorrhagic fevers
B00-B09	Viral infections characterized by skin and mucous membrane lesions
B10	Other human herpesviruses
B15-B19	Viral hepatitis
B20	Human immunodeficiency virus [HIV] disease
B25-B34	Other viral diseases
B35-B49	Mycoses
B50-B64	Protozoal diseases
B65-B83	Helminthiases
B85-B89	Pediculosis, acariasis and other infestations
B90-B94	Sequelae of infectious and parasitic diseases
B95-B97	Bacterial and viral infectious agents
B99	Other infectious diseases

Intestinal Infectious Diseases (A00-A09)

✓4ᵗʰ A00 Cholera

A00.0 Cholera due to Vibrio cholerae 01, biovar cholerae
Classical cholera

A00.1 Cholera due to Vibrio cholerae 01, biovar eltor
Cholera eltor

A00.9 Cholera, unspecified ▽

✓4ᵗʰ A01 Typhoid and paratyphoid fevers
DEF: Typhoid fever: An acute generalized illness caused by *Salmonella typhi;* clinical features are fever, headache, abdominal pain, cough, toxemia, leukopenia, abnormal pulse, rose spots on the skin, bacteremia, hyperplasia of intestinal lymph nodes, mesenteric lymphadenopathy, and Peyer's patches in the intestines.
DEF: Paratyphoid fever: A prolonged febrile illness, caused by *Salmonella* serotypes other than *S. typhi,* especially *S. enterica* serotypes paratyphi A, B, and C.

✓5ᵗʰ A01.0 Typhoid fever
Infection due to Salmonella typhi

A01.00 Typhoid fever, unspecified ▽

A01.01 Typhoid meningitis

A01.02 Typhoid fever with heart involvement
Typhoid endocarditis
Typhoid myocarditis

A01.03 Typhoid pneumonia

A01.04 Typhoid arthritis

A01.05 Typhoid osteomyelitis

A01.09 Typhoid fever with other complications

A01.1 Paratyphoid fever A

A01.2 Paratyphoid fever B

A01.3 Paratyphoid fever C

A01.4 Paratyphoid fever, unspecified ▽
Infection due to Salmonella paratyphi NOS

✓4ᵗʰ A02 Other salmonella infections
INCLUDES infection or foodborne intoxication due to any Salmonella species other than S. typhi and S. paratyphi

A02.0 Salmonella enteritis
Salmonellosis

A02.1 Salmonella sepsis

✓5ᵗʰ A02.2 Localized salmonella infections

A02.20 Localized salmonella infection, unspecified ▽

A02.21 Salmonella meningitis

A02.22 Salmonella pneumonia

A02.23 Salmonella arthritis

A02.24 Salmonella osteomyelitis

A02.25 Salmonella pyelonephritis
Salmonella tubulo-interstitial nephropathy

A02.29 Salmonella with other localized infection

A02.8 Other specified salmonella infections

A02.9 Salmonella infection, unspecified ▽

✓4ᵗʰ A03 Shigellosis
DEF: Infection caused by the genus *Shigella,* of the family *Enterobacteriaceae;* known to cause an acute dysenteric infection of the bowel with fever, drowsiness, anorexia, nausea, vomiting, bloody diarrhea, abdominal cramps, and distention.

A03.0 Shigellosis due to Shigella dysenteriae
Group A shigellosis [Shiga-Kruse dysentery]

A03.1 Shigellosis due to Shigella flexneri
Group B shigellosis

A03.2 Shigellosis due to Shigella boydii
Group C shigellosis

A03.3 Shigellosis due to Shigella sonnei
Group D shigellosis

A03.8 Other shigellosis

A03.9 Shigellosis, unspecified ▽
Bacillary dysentery NOS

✓4ᵗʰ A04 Other bacterial intestinal infections
EXCLUDES 1 *bacterial foodborne intoxications, NEC (A05.-)*
tuberculous enteritis (A18.32)

A04.0 Enteropathogenic Escherichia coli infection

A04.1 Enterotoxigenic Escherichia coli infection

A04.2 Enteroinvasive Escherichia coli infection

A04.3 Enterohemorrhagic Escherichia coli infection
DEF: *E. coli* infection penetrating the intestinal mucosa, producing microscopic ulceration and bleeding.

A04.4 Other intestinal Escherichia coli infections
Escherichia coli enteritis NOS

A04.5 Campylobacter enteritis

A04.6 Enteritis due to Yersinia enterocolitica
EXCLUDES 1 *extraintestinal yersiniosis (A28.2)*

✓5ᵗʰ A04.7 Enterocolitis due to Clostridium difficile
Foodborne intoxication by Clostridium difficile
Pseudomembraneous colitis

● **A04.71 Enterocolitis due to Clostridium difficile,** recurrent

● **A04.72 Enterocolitis due to Clostridium difficile,** not specified as recurrent

A04.8 Other specified bacterial intestinal infections

A04.9 Bacterial intestinal infection, unspecified ▽
Bacterial enteritis NOS

✓4ᵗʰ A05 Other bacterial foodborne intoxications, not elsewhere classified
EXCLUDES 1 *Clostridium difficile foodborne intoxication and infection* ▶*(A04.7-)*◀
Escherichia coli infection (A04.0-A04.4)
listeriosis (A32.-)
salmonella foodborne intoxication and infection (A02.-)
toxic effect of noxious foodstuffs (T61-T62)

A05.0 Foodborne staphylococcal intoxication

A05.1 Botulism food poisoning
Botulism NOS
Classical foodborne intoxication due to Clostridium botulinum
EXCLUDES 1 *infant botulism (A48.51)*
wound botulism (A48.52)

A05.2 Foodborne Clostridium perfringens [Clostridium welchii] intoxication
Enteritis necroticans
Pig-bel

A05.3 Foodborne Vibrio parahaemolyticus intoxication

A05.4 Foodborne Bacillus cereus intoxication

A05.5 Foodborne Vibrio vulnificus intoxication

A05.8 Other specified bacterial foodborne intoxications

A05.9 Bacterial foodborne intoxication, unspecified ▽

✓ Additional Character Req   **✓x7ᵗʰ** Placeholder Alert   Case-Mix Diagnosis   Manifestation   ▽ Unspecified Dx   **EXCLUDES 1** Not coded here   **EXCLUDES 2** Not included here

Chapter 1. Certain Infectious and Parasitic Diseases

A06–A17.0

✓4ᵗʰ **A06 Amebiasis**

    INCLUDES   infection due to Entamoeba histolytica

    EXCLUDES 1   *other protozoal intestinal diseases (A07.-)*

    EXCLUDES 2   *acanthamebiasis (B60.1-)*

           Naegleriasis (B60.2)

    A06.0 Acute ambebic dysentery

         Acute amebiasis

         Intestinal amebiasis NOS

    A06.1 Chronic intestinal amebiasis

    A06.2 Amebic nondysenteric colitis

    A06.3 Ameboma of intestine

         Ameboma NOS

    A06.4 Amebic liver abscess

         Hepatic amebiasis

    A06.5 Amebic lung abscess

         Amebic abscess of lung (and liver)

    A06.6 Amebic brain abscess

         Amebic abscess of brain (and liver) (and lung)

    A06.7 Cutaneous amebiasis

✓5ᵗʰ **A06.8 Amebic infection of other sites**

        A06.81 Amebic cystitis

        A06.82 Other amebic genitourinary infections

             Amebic balanitis

             Amebic vesiculitis

             Amebic vulvovaginitis

        A06.89 Other amebic infections

             Amebic appendicitis

             Amebic splenic abscess

    A06.9 Amebiasis, unspecified   ▽

✓4ᵗʰ **A07 Other protozoal intestinal diseases**

    A07.0 Balantidiasis

         Balantidial dysentery

    A07.1 Giardiasis [lambliasis]

    A07.2 Cryptosporidiosis

    A07.3 Isosporiasis

         Infection due to Isospora belli and Isospora hominis

         Intestinal coccidiosis

         Isosporosis

    A07.4 Cyclosporiasis

    A07.8 Other specified protozoal intestinal diseases

         Intestinal microsporidiosis

         Intestinal trichomoniasis

         Sarcocystosis

         Sarcosporidiosis

    A07.9 Protozoal intestinal disease, unspecified   ▽

         Flagellate diarrhea   Protozoal diarrhea

         Protozoal colitis   Protozoal dysentery

✓4ᵗʰ **A08 Viral and other specified intestinal infections**

    EXCLUDES 1   *influenza with involvement of gastrointestinal tract (J09.X3, J10.2, J11.2)*

    A08.0 Rotaviral enteritis

✓5ᵗʰ **A08.1 Acute gastroenteropathy due to Norwalk agent and other small round viruses**

        A08.11 Acute gastroenteropathy due to Norwalk agent

             Acute gastroenteropathy due to Norovirus

             Acute gastroenteropathy due to Norwalk-like agent

        A08.19 Acute gastroenteropathy due to other small round viruses

             Acute gastroenteropathy due to small round virus [SRV] NOS

    A08.2 Adenoviral enteritis

✓5ᵗʰ **A08.3 Other viral enteritis**

        A08.31 Calicivirus enteritis

        A08.32 Astrovirus enteritis

        A08.39 Other viral enteritis

             Coxsackie virus enteritis

             Echovirus enteritis

             Enterovirus enteritis NEC

             Torovirus enteritis

    A08.4 Viral intestinal infection, unspecified   ▽

         Viral enteritis NOS

         Viral gastroenteritis NOS

         Viral gastroenteropathy NOS

         AHA: 2016, 3Q, 12

    A08.8 Other specified intestinal infections

A09 Infectious gastroenteritis and colitis, unspecified   ▽

     Infectious colitis NOS

     Infectious enteritis NOS

     Infectious gastroenteritis NOS

    EXCLUDES 1   *colitis NOS (K52.9)*

           diarrhea NOS (R19.7)

           enteritis NOS (K52.9)

           gastroenteritis NOS (K52.9)

           noninfective gastroenteritis and colitis, unspecified (K52.9)

DEF: Colitis: An inflammation of mucous membranes of the colon.

DEF: Enteritis: An inflammation of mucous membranes of the small intestine.

DEF: Gastroenteritis: An inflammation of mucous membranes of stomach and intestines.

Tuberculosis (A15-A19)

    INCLUDES   infections due to Mycobacterium tuberculosis and Mycobacterium bovis

    EXCLUDES 1   *congenital tuberculosis (P37.0)*

           nonspecific reaction to test for tuberculosis without active tuberculosis (R76.1-)

           pneumoconiosis associated with tuberculosis, any type in A15 (J65)

           positive PPD (R76.11)

           positive tuberculin skin test without active tuberculosis (R76.11)

           sequelae of tuberculosis (B90.-)

           silicotuberculosis (J65)

✓4ᵗʰ **A15 Respiratory tuberculosis**

    A15.0 Tuberculosis of lung

         Tuberculous bronchiectasis

         Tuberculous fibrosis of lung

         Tuberculous pneumonia

         Tuberculous pneumothorax

    A15.4 Tuberculosis of intrathoracic lymph nodes

         Tuberculosis of hilar lymph nodes

         Tuberculosis of mediastinal lymph nodes

         Tuberculosis of tracheobronchial lymph nodes

        EXCLUDES 1   *tuberculosis specified as primary (A15.7)*

    A15.5 Tuberculosis of larynx, trachea and bronchus

         Tuberculosis of bronchus

         Tuberculosis of glottis

         Tuberculosis of larynx

         Tuberculosis of trachea

    A15.6 Tuberculous pleurisy

         Tuberculosis of pleura Tuberculous empyema

        EXCLUDES 1   *primary respiratory tuberculosis (A15.7)*

    A15.7 Primary respiratory tuberculosis

    A15.8 Other respiratory tuberculosis

         Mediastinal tuberculosis

         Nasopharyngeal tuberculosis

         Tuberculosis of nose

         Tuberculosis of sinus [any nasal]

    A15.9 Respiratory tuberculosis unspecified   ▽

✓4ᵗʰ **A17 Tuberculosis of nervous system**

    A17.0 Tuberculous meningitis

         Tuberculosis of meninges (cerebral) (spinal)

         Tuberculous leptomeningitis

        EXCLUDES 1   *tuberculous meningoencephalitis (A17.82)*

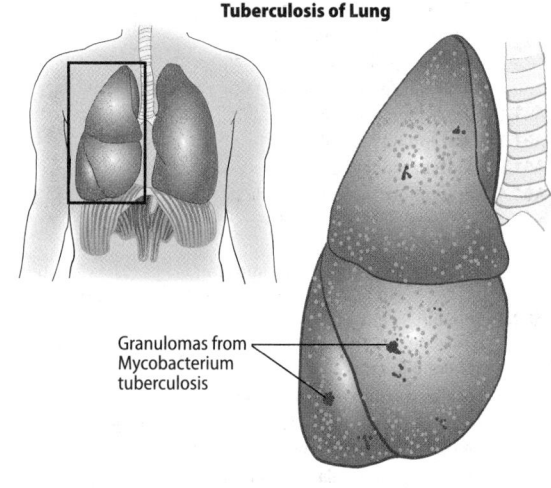

Tuberculosis of Lung

Granulomas from Mycobacterium tuberculosis

N Newborn: 0   P Pediatric: 0-17   M Maternity: 12-55   A Adult: 15-124   NRS Nonroutine supply Dx   NC Dx Noncancer Dx   PDx Primary Dx   ►◄ Revised Text   ● New Code   ▲ Revised Title

438   ICD-10-CM 2018

A17.1   **Meningeal tuberculoma**
Tuberculoma of meninges (cerebral) (spinal)
EXCLUDES 2   *tuberculoma of brain and spinal cord (A17.81)*

✓5ᵗʰ **A17.8**   Other **tuberculosis of nervous system**

     A17.81   **Tuberculoma of** brain and spinal cord
Tuberculous abscess of brain and spinal cord

     A17.82   **Tuberculous** meningoencephalitis
Tuberculous myelitis

     A17.83   **Tuberculous** neuritis
Tuberculous mononeuropathy

     A17.89   **Other tuberculosis of nervous system**
Tuberculous polyneuropathy

A17.9   **Tuberculosis of nervous system, unspecified**   ▽

✓4ᵗʰ **A18**   **Tuberculosis of** other organs

   ✓5ᵗʰ **A18.0**   **Tuberculosis of** bones and joints

     A18.01   **Tuberculosis of** spine
Pott's disease or curvature of spine
Tuberculous arthritis
Tuberculous osteomyelitis of spine
Tuberculous spondylitis

     A18.02   **Tuberculous** arthritis of other joints
Tuberculosis of hip (joint)
Tuberculosis of knee (joint)

     A18.03   **Tuberculosis of** other bones
Tuberculous mastoiditis
Tuberculous osteomyelitis

     A18.09   **Other musculoskeletal** tuberculosis
Tuberculous myositis
Tuberculous synovitis
Tuberculous tenosynovitis

   ✓5ᵗʰ **A18.1**   **Tuberculosis of** genitourinary system

     A18.10   **Tuberculosis of genitourinary system, unspecified**   ▽

     A18.11   **Tuberculosis of** kidney and ureter

     A18.12   **Tuberculosis of** bladder

     A18.13   **Tuberculosis of** other urinary organs
Tuberculous urethritis

     A18.14   **Tuberculosis of** prostate   🅰♂

     A18.15   **Tuberculosis of** other male genital organs   ♂

     A18.16   **Tuberculosis of** cervix   ♀

     A18.17   **Tuberculous female** pelvic inflammatory disease   ♀
Tuberculous endometritis
Tuberculous oophoritis and salpingitis

     A18.18   **Tuberculosis of** other female genital organs   ♀
Tuberculous ulceration of vulva

   A18.2   **Tuberculous** peripheral lymphadenopathy
Tuberculous adenitis
EXCLUDES 2   *tuberculosis of bronchial and mediastinal lymph nodes (A15.4)*
tuberculosis of mesenteric and retroperitoneal lymph nodes (A18.39)
tuberculous tracheobronchial adenopathy (A15.4)

   ✓5ᵗʰ **A18.3**   **Tuberculosis of** intestines, peritoneum and mesenteric glands

     A18.31   **Tuberculous** peritonitis
Tuberculous ascites
DEF: Tuberculous inflammation of the membrane lining the abdomen.

     A18.32   **Tuberculous** enteritis
Tuberculosis of anus and rectum
Tuberculosis of intestine (large) (small)

     A18.39   **Retroperitoneal** tuberculosis
Tuberculosis of mesenteric glands
Tuberculosis of retroperitoneal (lymph glands)

   A18.4   **Tuberculosis of** skin and subcutaneous tissue
Erythema induratum, tuberculous
Lupus excedens
Lupus vulgaris NOS
Lupus vulgaris of eyelid
Scrofuloderma
Tuberculosis of external ear
EXCLUDES 2   *lupus erythematosus (L93.-)*
lupus NOS (M32.9)
systemic (M32.-)

   ✓5ᵗʰ **A18.5**   **Tuberculosis of** eye
EXCLUDES 2   *lupus vulgaris of eyelid (A18.4)*

     A18.50   **Tuberculosis of eye, unspecified**   ▽

     A18.51   **Tuberculous** episcleritis

     A18.52   **Tuberculous** keratitis
Tuberculous interstitial keratitis
Tuberculous keratoconjunctivitis (interstitial) (phlyctenular)

     A18.53   **Tuberculous** chorioretinitis

     A18.54   **Tuberculous** iridocyclitis

     A18.59   **Other tuberculosis of eye**
Tuberculous conjunctivitis

   A18.6   **Tuberculosis of (inner) (middle)** ear
Tuberculous otitis media
EXCLUDES 2   *tuberculosis of external ear (A18.4)*
tuberculous mastoiditis (A18.03)

   A18.7   **Tuberculosis of** adrenal glands
Tuberculous Addison's disease

   ✓5ᵗʰ **A18.8**   **Tuberculosis of** other specified organs

     A18.81   **Tuberculosis of** thyroid gland

     A18.82   **Tuberculosis of** other endocrine glands
Tuberculosis of pituitary gland
Tuberculosis of thymus gland

     A18.83   **Tuberculosis of** digestive tract organs**, not elsewhere classified**
EXCLUDES 1   *tuberculosis of intestine (A18.32)*

     A18.84   **Tuberculosis of** heart
Tuberculous cardiomyopathy
Tuberculous endocarditis
Tuberculous myocarditis
Tuberculous pericarditis

     A18.85   **Tuberculosis of** spleen

     A18.89   **Tuberculosis of other sites**
Tuberculosis of muscle
Tuberculous cerebral arteritis

✓4ᵗʰ **A19**   **Miliary tuberculosis**
INCLUDES   disseminated tuberculosis
generalized tuberculosis
tuberculous polyserositis

   A19.0   **Acute miliary tuberculosis of a** single specified site

   A19.1   **Acute miliary tuberculosis of** multiple sites

   A19.2   **Acute miliary tuberculosis, unspecified**   ▽

   A19.8   **Other miliary tuberculosis**

   A19.9   **Miliary tuberculosis, unspecified**   ▽

Certain zoonotic bacterial diseases (A20-A28)

✓4ᵗʰ **A20**   **Plague**
INCLUDES   infection due to Yersinia pestis

   A20.0   Bubonic **plague**

   A20.1   Cellulocutaneous **plague**

   A20.2   Pneumonic **plague**

   A20.3   **Plague** meningitis

   A20.7   Septicemic **plague**

   A20.8   **Other forms of plague**
Abortive plague
Asymptomatic plague
Pestis minor

   A20.9   **Plague, unspecified**   ▽

✓4ᵗʰ **A21**   **Tularemia**
INCLUDES   deer-fly fever
infection due to Francisella tularensis
rabbit fever
DEF: A febrile disease transmitted to humans by the bites of deer flies, fleas, and ticks; by inhaling aerosolized *F. tularensis*; or by ingesting contaminated food or water. Patients quickly develop fever, chills, weakness, headache, backache, and malaise.

   A21.0   Ulceroglandular **tularemia**

   A21.1   Oculoglandular **tularemia**
Ophthalmic tularemia

   A21.2   Pulmonary **tularemia**

   A21.3   Gastrointestinal **tularemia**
Abdominal tularemia

   A21.7   Generalized **tularemia**

   A21.8   **Other forms of tularemia**

   A21.9   **Tularemia, unspecified**   ▽

✓4ᵗʰ **A22**   **Anthrax**
INCLUDES   infection due to Bacillus anthracis

   A22.0   Cutaneous **anthrax**   NRS
Malignant carbuncle
Malignant pustule

A22.1 Pulmonary anthrax
Inhalation anthrax
Ragpicker's disease
Woolsorter's disease

A22.2 Gastrointestinal anthrax

A22.7 Anthrax sepsis

A22.8 Other forms of anthrax
Anthrax meningitis

A22.9 Anthrax, unspecified ▽

✓4ᵗʰ **A23 Brucellosis**
INCLUDES   Malta fever
Mediterranean fever
undulant fever

A23.0 Brucellosis due to Brucella melitensis

A23.1 Brucellosis due to Brucella abortus

A23.2 Brucellosis due to Brucella suis

A23.3 Brucellosis due to Brucella canis

A23.8 Other brucellosis

A23.9 Brucellosis, unspecified ▽

✓4ᵗʰ **A24 Glanders and melioidosis**

A24.0 Glanders
Infection due to Pseudomonas mallei
Malleus

A24.1 Acute and fulminating melioidosis
Melioidosis pneumonia
Melioidosis sepsis

A24.2 Subacute and chronic melioidosis

A24.3 Other melioidosis

A24.9 Melioidosis, unspecified ▽
Infection due to Pseudomonas pseudomallei NOS
Whitmore's disease

✓4ᵗʰ **A25 Rat-bite fevers**

A25.0 Spirillosis
Sodoku

A25.1 Streptobacillosis
Epidemic arthritic erythema
Haverhill fever
Streptobacillary rat-bite fever

A25.9 Rat-bite fever, unspecified ▽

✓4ᵗʰ **A26 Erysipeloid**

A26.0 Cutaneous erysipeloid NRS
Erythema migrans

A26.7 Erysipelothrix sepsis

A26.8 Other forms of erysipeloid

A26.9 Erysipeloid, unspecified ▽

✓4ᵗʰ **A27 Leptospirosis**

A27.0 Leptospirosis icterohemorrhagica
Leptospiral or spirochetal jaundice (hemorrhagic)
Weil's disease

✓5ᵗʰ **A27.8 Other forms of leptospirosis**

A27.81 Aseptic meningitis in leptospirosis

A27.89 Other forms of leptospirosis

A27.9 Leptospirosis, unspecified ▽

✓4ᵗʰ **A28 Other zoonotic bacterial diseases, not elsewhere classified**

A28.0 Pasteurellosis

A28.1 Cat-scratch disease
Cat-scratch fever

A28.2 Extraintestinal yersiniosis
EXCLUDES 1   enteritis due to Yersinia enterocolitica (A04.6)
plague (A20.-)

A28.8 Other specified zoonotic bacterial diseases, not elsewhere classified

A28.9 Zoonotic bacterial disease, unspecified ▽

Other bacterial diseases (A30-A49)
AHA: 2016, 3Q, 8-14

✓4ᵗʰ **A30 Leprosy [Hansen's disease]**
INCLUDES   infection due to Mycobacterium leprae
EXCLUDES 1   sequelae of leprosy (B92)

A30.0 Indeterminate leprosy
I leprosy

A30.1 Tuberculoid leprosy
TT leprosy

A30.2 Borderline tuberculoid leprosy
BT leprosy

A30.3 Borderline leprosy
BB leprosy

A30.4 Borderline lepromatous leprosy
BL leprosy

A30.5 Lepromatous leprosy
LL leprosy

A30.8 Other forms of leprosy

A30.9 Leprosy, unspecified ▽

✓4ᵗʰ **A31 Infection due to other mycobacteria**
EXCLUDES 2   leprosy (A30.-)
tuberculosis (A15-A19)

A31.0 Pulmonary mycobacterial infection
Infection due to Mycobacterium avium
Infection due to Mycobacterium intracellulare [Battey bacillus]
Infection due to Mycobacterium kansasii

A31.1 Cutaneous mycobacterial infection
Buruli ulcer
Infection due to Mycobacterium marinum
Infection due to Mycobacterium ulcerans

A31.2 Disseminated mycobacterium avium-intracellulare complex (DMAC)
MAC sepsis

A31.8 Other mycobacterial infections

A31.9 Mycobacterial infection, unspecified ▽
Atypical mycobacterial infection NOS
Mycobacteriosis NOS

✓4ᵗʰ **A32 Listeriosis**
INCLUDES   listerial foodborne infection
EXCLUDES 1   neonatal (disseminated) listeriosis (P37.2)

A32.0 Cutaneous listeriosis

✓5ᵗʰ **A32.1 Listerial meningitis and meningoencephalitis**

A32.11 Listerial meningitis

A32.12 Listerial meningoencephalitis

A32.7 Listerial sepsis

✓5ᵗʰ **A32.8 Other forms of listeriosis**

A32.81 Oculoglandular listeriosis

A32.82 Listerial endocarditis

A32.89 Other forms of listeriosis
Listerial cerebral arteritis

A32.9 Listeriosis, unspecified ▽

A33 Tetanus neonatorum Ⓝ
AHA: 2016, 3Q, 8-14

A34 Obstetrical tetanus Ⓜ♀
AHA: 2016, 3Q, 8-14

A35 Other tetanus
Tetanus NOS
EXCLUDES 1   obstetrical tetanus (A34)
tetanus neonatorum (A33)
AHA: 2016, 3Q, 8-14

✓4ᵗʰ **A36 Diphtheria**

A36.0 Pharyngeal diphtheria
Diphtheritic membranous angina
Tonsillar diphtheria

A36.1 Nasopharyngeal diphtheria

A36.2 Laryngeal diphtheria
Diphtheritic laryngotracheitis

A36.3 Cutaneous diphtheria
EXCLUDES 2   erythrasma (L08.1)

✓5ᵗʰ **A36.8 Other diphtheria**

A36.81 Diphtheritic cardiomyopathy
Diphtheritic myocarditis

A36.82 Diphtheritic radiculomyelitis

A36.83 Diphtheritic polyneuritis

A36.84 Diphtheritic tubulo-interstitial nephropathy

A36.85 Diphtheritic cystitis

A36.86 Diphtheritic conjunctivitis

A36.89 Other diphtheritic complications
Diphtheritic peritonitis

A36.9 Diphtheria, unspecified ▽

Ⓝ Newborn: 0   Ⓟ Pediatric: 0-17   Ⓜ Maternity: 12-55   Ⓐ Adult: 15-124   NRS Nonroutine supply Dx   NCDx Noncancer Dx   PDx Primary Dx   ▶◀ Revised Text   ● New Code   ▲ Revised Title

440   ICD-10-CM 2018

✓4ᵗʰ A37 Whooping cough

✓5ᵗʰ A37.0 Whooping cough due to Bordetella pertussis

A37.00 Whooping cough due to Bordetella pertussis without pneumonia

A37.01 Whooping cough due to Bordetella pertussis with pneumonia

✓5ᵗʰ A37.1 Whooping cough due to Bordetella parapertussis

A37.10 Whooping cough due to Bordetella parapertussis without pneumonia

A37.11 Whooping cough due to Bordetella parapertussis with pneumonia

✓5ᵗʰ A37.8 Whooping cough due to other Bordetella species

A37.80 Whooping cough due to other Bordetella species without pneumonia

A37.81 Whooping cough due to other Bordetella species with pneumonia

✓5ᵗʰ A37.9 Whooping cough, unspecified species

A37.90 Whooping cough, unspecified species without pneumonia ▽

A37.91 Whooping cough, unspecified species with pneumonia ▽

✓4ᵗʰ A38 Scarlet fever

INCLUDES scarlatina
EXCLUDES 2 streptococcal sore throat (J02.0)

A38.0 Scarlet fever with otitis media

A38.1 Scarlet fever with myocarditis

A38.8 Scarlet fever with other complications

A38.9 Scarlet fever, uncomplicated ▽
Scarlet fever, NOS

✓4ᵗʰ A39 Meningococcal infection

A39.0 Meningococcal meningitis

A39.1 Waterhouse-Friderichsen syndrome
Meningococcal hemorrhagic adrenalitis
Meningococcic adrenal syndrome

A39.2 Acute meningococcemia

A39.3 Chronic meningococcemia

A39.4 Meningococcemia, unspecified ▽

✓5ᵗʰ A39.5 Meningococcal heart disease

A39.50 Meningococcal carditis, unspecified ▽

A39.51 Meningococcal endocarditis

A39.52 Meningococcal myocarditis

A39.53 Meningococcal pericarditis

✓5ᵗʰ A39.8 Other meningococcal infections

A39.81 Meningococcal encephalitis

A39.82 Meningococcal retrobulbar neuritis

A39.83 Meningococcal arthritis

A39.84 Postmeningococcal arthritis

A39.89 Other meningococcal infections
Meningococcal conjunctivitis

A39.9 Meningococcal infection, unspecified ▽
Meningococcal disease NOS

✓4ᵗʰ A40 Streptococcal sepsis

Code first: postprocedural streptococcal sepsis (T81.4-)
streptococcal sepsis during labor (O75.3)
streptococcal sepsis following abortion or ectopic or molar pregnancy (O03-O07, O08.0)
streptococcal sepsis following immunization (T88.0)
streptococcal sepsis following infusion, transfusion or therapeutic injection (T80.2-)

EXCLUDES 1 neonatal (P36.0-P36.1)
puerperal sepsis (O85)
sepsis due to Streptococcus, group D (A41.81)

AHA: 2016, 1Q, 32
TIP: Sepsis should not be coded after it has been resolved or documented as resolving; code the underlying infection if still under treatment.

A40.0 Sepsis due to streptococcus, group A

A40.1 Sepsis due to streptococcus, group B

A40.3 Sepsis due to Streptococcus pneumoniae
Pneumococcal sepsis

A40.8 Other streptococcal sepsis

A40.9 Streptococcal sepsis, unspecified ▽

✓4ᵗʰ A41 Other sepsis

Code first: postprocedural sepsis (T81.4-)
sepsis during labor (O75.3)
sepsis following abortion, ectopic or molar pregnancy (O03-O07, O08.0)
sepsis following immunization (T88.0)
sepsis following infusion, transfusion or therapeutic injection (T80.2-)

EXCLUDES 1 bacteremia NOS (R78.81)
neonatal (P36.-)
puerperal sepsis (O85)
streptococcal sepsis (A40.-)

EXCLUDES 2 sepsis (due to) (in) actinomycotic (A42.7)
sepsis (due to) (in) anthrax (A22.7)
sepsis (due to) (in) candidal (B37.7)
sepsis (due to) (in) Erysipelothrix (A26.7)
sepsis (due to) (in) extraintestinal yersiniosis (A28.2)
sepsis (due to) (in) gonococcal (A54.86)
sepsis (due to) (in) herpesviral (B00.7)
sepsis (due to) (in) listerial (A32.7)
sepsis (due to) (in) melioidosis (A24.1)
sepsis (due to) (in) meningococcal (A39.2-A39.4)
sepsis (due to) (in) plague (A20.7)
sepsis (due to) (in) tularemia (A21.7)
toxic shock syndrome (A48.3)

AHA: 2016, 1Q, 32; 2014, 2Q, 13
TIP: Sepsis should not be coded after it has been resolved or documented as resolving; code the underlying infection if still under treatment.

✓5ᵗʰ A41.0 Sepsis due to Staphylococcus aureus

A41.01 Sepsis due to Methicillin susceptible Staphylococcus aureus
MSSA sepsis
Staphylococcus aureus sepsis NOS

A41.02 Sepsis due to Methicillin resistant Staphylococcus aureus

A41.1 Sepsis due to other specified staphylococcus
Coagulase negative staphylococcus sepsis

A41.2 Sepsis due to unspecified staphylococcus ▽

A41.3 Sepsis due to Hemophilus influenzae

A41.4 Sepsis due to anaerobes
EXCLUDES 1 gas gangrene (A48.0)

✓5ᵗʰ A41.5 Sepsis due to other Gram-negative organisms

A41.50 Gram-negative sepsis, unspecified ▽
Gram-negative sepsis NOS

A41.51 Sepsis due to Escherichia coli [E. coli]

A41.52 Sepsis due to Pseudomonas
Pseudomonas aeroginosa

A41.53 Sepsis due to Serratia

A41.59 Other Gram-negative sepsis

✓5ᵗʰ A41.8 Other specified sepsis

A41.81 Sepsis due to Enterococcus

A41.89 Other specified sepsis
AHA: 2017, 1Q, 51; 2016, 3Q, 8-14

A41.9 Sepsis, unspecified organism ▽
Septicemia NOS

✓4ᵗʰ A42 Actinomycosis

EXCLUDES 1 actinomycetoma (B47.1)

A42.0 Pulmonary actinomycosis

A42.1 Abdominal actinomycosis

A42.2 Cervicofacial actinomycosis

A42.7 Actinomycotic sepsis

✓5ᵗʰ A42.8 Other forms of actinomycosis

A42.81 Actinomycotic meningitis

A42.82 Actinomycotic encephalitis

A42.89 Other forms of actinomycosis

A42.9 Actinomycosis, unspecified ▽

✓4ᵗʰ A43 Nocardiosis

A43.0 Pulmonary nocardiosis

A43.1 Cutaneous nocardiosis

A43.8 Other forms of nocardiosis

A43.9 Nocardiosis, unspecified ▽

✓4ᵗʰ A44 Bartonellosis

A44.0 Systemic bartonellosis
Oroya fever

A44.1 Cutaneous and mucocutaneous bartonellosis
Verruga peruana

✓ Additional Character Req   ✓x7ᵗʰ Placeholder Alert   Case-Mix Diagnosis   Manifestation   ▽ Unspecified Dx   **EXCLUDES 1** Not coded here   **EXCLUDES 2** Not included here

A44.8   **Other forms of bartonellosis**

A44.9   **Bartonellosis, unspecified** ▽

A46   Erysipelas
> EXCLUDES 1   *postpartum or puerperal erysipelas (O86.89)*
> **DEF:** A skin infection affecting the upper dermis and superficial dermal lymphatics; lesion edges are well-demarcated with distinct raised borders; it is often caused by group A *Streptococci.*

✓4ᵗʰ **A48   Other bacterial diseases, not elsewhere classified**
> EXCLUDES 1   *actinomycetoma (B47.1)*

A48.0   **Gas gangrene**
Clostridial cellulitis
Clostridial myonecrosis

A48.1   **Legionnaires' disease**
> **DEF:** Severe and often fatal infection by *Legionella pneumophila;* symptoms include high fever, gastrointestinal pain, headache, myalgia, dry cough, and pneumonia; usually transmitted through airborne water droplets via air conditioning systems or hot tubs.

A48.2   **Nonpneumonic Legionnaires' disease [Pontiac fever]**

A48.3   **Toxic shock syndrome**
Use additional code to identify the organism (B95, B96)
> EXCLUDES 1   *endotoxic shock NOS (R57.8)*
> *sepsis NOS (A41.9)*

A48.4   **Brazilian purpuric fever**
Systemic Hemophilus aegyptius infection

✓5ᵗʰ A48.5   **Other specified botulism**
Non-foodborne intoxication due to toxins of Clostridium botulinum [C. botulinum]
> EXCLUDES 1   *food poisoning due to toxins of Clostridium botulinum (A05.1)*

A48.51   **Infant botulism** ℗

A48.52   **Wound botulism**
Non-foodborne botulism NOS
Use additional code for associated wound

A48.8   **Other specified bacterial diseases**

✓4ᵗʰ **A49   Bacterial infection of unspecified site**
> EXCLUDES 1   *bacterial agents as the cause of diseases classified elsewhere (B95-B96)*
> *chlamydial infection NOS (A74.9)*
> *meningococcal infection NOS (A39.9)*
> *rickettsial infection NOS (A79.9)*
> *spirochetal infection NOS (A69.9)*

✓5ᵗʰ A49.0   Staphylococcal infection, unspecified site

A49.01   Methicillin susceptible **Staphylococcus aureus infection, unspecified site** ▽
Methicillin susceptible Staphylococcus aureus (MSSA) infection
Staphylococcus aureus infection NOS

A49.02   Methicillin resistant **Staphylococcus aureus infection, unspecified site** ▽
Methicillin resistant Staphylococcus aureus (MRSA) infection

A49.1   Streptococcal **infection, unspecified site** ▽

A49.2   Hemophilus influenzae **infection, unspecified site** ▽

A49.3   Mycoplasma **infection, unspecified site** ▽

A49.8   Other bacterial infections of unspecified site ▽

A49.9   Bacterial infection, unspecified ▽
> EXCLUDES 1   *bacteremia NOS (R78.81)*

Infections with a predominantly sexual mode of transmission (A50-A64)

> EXCLUDES 1   *human immunodeficiency virus [HIV] disease (B20)*
> *nonspecific and nongonococcal urethritis (N34.1)*
> *Reiter's disease (M02.3-)*

✓4ᵗʰ **A50   Congenital syphilis**

✓5ᵗʰ A50.0   Early **congenital syphilis,** symptomatic
Any congenital syphilitic condition specified as early or manifest less than two years after birth.

A50.01   **Early congenital syphilitic** oculopathy

A50.02   **Early congenital syphilitic** osteochondropathy

A50.03   **Early congenital syphilitic** pharyngitis
Early congenital syphilitic laryngitis

A50.04   **Early congenital syphilitic** pneumonia

A50.05   **Early congenital syphilitic** rhinitis

A50.06   **Early** cutaneous **congenital syphilis** NRS

A50.07   **Early** mucocutaneous **congenital syphilis** NRS

A50.08   **Early** visceral **congenital syphilis**

A50.09   **Other early congenital syphilis, symptomatic**

A50.1   Early **congenital syphilis,** latent
Congenital syphilis without clinical manifestations, with positive serological reaction and negative spinal fluid test, less than two years after birth.

A50.2   **Early congenital syphilis, unspecified** ▽
Congenital syphilis NOS less than two years after birth.

✓5ᵗʰ A50.3   Late **congenital syphilitic** oculopathy
> EXCLUDES 1   *Hutchinson's triad (A50.53)*

A50.30   **Late congenital syphilitic oculopathy, unspecified** ▽

A50.31   **Late congenital syphilitic** interstitial keratitis

A50.32   **Late congenital syphilitic** chorioretinitis

A50.39   **Other late congenital syphilitic oculopathy**

✓5ᵗʰ A50.4   Late **congenital** neurosyphilis [juvenile neurosyphilis]
Use additional code to identify any associated mental disorder
> EXCLUDES 1   *Hutchinson's triad (A50.53)*

A50.40   **Late congenital neurosyphilis, unspecified** ▽
Juvenile neurosyphilis NOS

A50.41   **Late congenital syphilitic** meningitis

A50.42   **Late congenital syphilitic** encephalitis

A50.43   **Late congenital syphilitic** polyneuropathy

A50.44   **Late congenital syphilitic** optic nerve atrophy

A50.45   **Juvenile general paresis**
Dementia paralytica juvenilis
Juvenile tabetoparetic neurosyphilis

A50.49   **Other late congenital neurosyphilis**
Juvenile tabes dorsalis

✓5ᵗʰ A50.5   Other late **congenital syphilis,** symptomatic
Any congenital syphilitic condition specified as late or manifest two years or more after birth.

A50.51   **Clutton's joints**

A50.52   **Hutchinson's teeth**

A50.53   **Hutchinson's triad**

A50.54   **Late congenital cardiovascular syphilis**

A50.55   **Late congenital syphilitic arthropathy**

A50.56   **Late congenital syphilitic osteochondropathy**

A50.57   **Syphilitic saddle nose**

A50.59   **Other late congenital syphilis, symptomatic**

A50.6   Late **congenital syphilis,** latent
Congenital syphilis without clinical manifestations, with positive serological reaction and negative spinal fluid test, two years or more after birth.

A50.7   Late **congenital syphilis, unspecified** ▽
Congenital syphilis NOS two years or more after birth.

A50.9   **Congenital syphilis, unspecified** ▽

✓4ᵗʰ **A51   Early syphilis**

A51.0   Primary genital **syphilis**
Syphilitic chancre NOS

A51.1   Primary anal **syphilis**

A51.2   Primary **syphilis of other sites**

✓5ᵗʰ A51.3   Secondary **syphilis of** skin and mucous membranes
> **DEF:** Transitory or chronic cutaneous eruptions that present within two to 10 weeks following initial syphilis infection that may include nontender lymphadenopathy along with alopecia and condylomata lata.

A51.31   **Condyloma latum**

A51.32   **Syphilitic alopecia**

A51.39   **Other secondary syphilis of skin**
Syphilitic leukoderma
Syphilitic mucous patch
> EXCLUDES 1   *late syphilitic leukoderma (A52.79)*

✓5ᵗʰ A51.4   Other secondary **syphilis**

A51.41   **Secondary syphilitic** meningitis

A51.42   **Secondary syphilitic** female pelvic disease ♀

A51.43   **Secondary syphilitic** oculopathy
Secondary syphilitic chorioretinitis
Secondary syphilitic iridocyclitis, iritis
Secondary syphilitic uveitis

A51.44   **Secondary syphilitic** nephritis

A51.45   **Secondary syphilitic** hepatitis

A51.46   **Secondary syphilitic** osteopathy

A51.49   **Other secondary syphilitic conditions**
Secondary syphilitic lymphadenopathy
Secondary syphilitic myositis

A51.5   Early **syphilis,** latent
Syphilis (acquired) without clinical manifestations, with positive serological reaction and negative spinal fluid test, less than two years after infection.

A51.9   Early **syphilis, unspecified** ▽

☑4ᵗʰ **A52**   Late **syphilis**

☑5ᵗʰ **A52.0**   Cardiovascular and cerebrovascular **syphilis**

     A52.00   **Cardiovascular syphilis, unspecified** ▽

     A52.01   **Syphilitic** aneurysm of aorta

     A52.02   **Syphilitic** aortitis

     A52.03   **Syphilitic** endocarditis
         Syphilitic aortic valve incompetence or stenosis
         Syphilitic mitral valve stenosis
         Syphilitic pulmonary valve regurgitation

     A52.04   **Syphilitic cerebral** arteritis

     A52.05   Other cerebrovascular **syphilis**
         Syphilitic cerebral aneurysm (ruptured)
            (non-ruptured)
         Syphilitic cerebral thrombosis

     A52.06   Other **syphilitic heart involvement**
         Syphilitic coronary artery disease
         Syphilitic myocarditis
         Syphilitic pericarditis

     A52.09   Other **cardiovascular syphilis**

☑5ᵗʰ **A52.1**   Symptomatic neurosyphilis

     A52.10   **Symptomatic neurosyphilis, unspecified** ▽

     A52.11   Tabes dorsalis
         Locomotor ataxia (progressive)
         Tabetic neurosyphilis

     A52.12   Other **cerebrospinal syphilis**

     A52.13   **Late syphilitic** meningitis

     A52.14   **Late syphilitic** encephalitis

     A52.15   **Late syphilitic** neuropathy
         Late syphilitic acoustic neuritis
         Late syphilitic optic (nerve) atrophy
         Late syphilitic polyneuropathy
         Late syphilitic retrobulbar neuritis

     A52.16   Charcôt's arthropathy **(tabetic)**

     A52.17   General paresis
         Dementia paralytica

     A52.19   **Other symptomatic neurosyphilis**
         Syphilitic parkinsonism

A52.2   Asymptomatic **neurosyphilis**

A52.3   **Neurosyphilis, unspecified** ▽
     Gumma (syphilitic)
     Syphilis (late)
     Syphiloma

☑5ᵗʰ **A52.7**   Other **symptomatic late syphilis**

     A52.71   **Late syphilitic** oculopathy
         Late syphilitic chorioretinitis
         Late syphilitic episcleritis

     A52.72   **Syphilis of** lung and bronchus

     A52.73   **Symptomatic late syphilis of** other respiratory organs

     A52.74   **Syphilis of** liver and other viscera
         Late syphilitic peritonitis

     A52.75   **Syphilis of** kidney and ureter
         Syphilitic glomerular disease

     A52.76   Other genitourinary **symptomatic late syphilis**
         Late syphilitic female pelvic inflammatory disease

     A52.77   **Syphilis of** bone and joint

     A52.78   **Syphilis of other** musculoskeletal tissue
         Late syphilitic bursitis
         Syphilis [stage unspecified] of bursa
         Syphilis [stage unspecified] of muscle
         Syphilis [stage unspecified] of synovium
         Syphilis [stage unspecified] of tendon

     A52.79   **Other symptomatic late syphilis**
         Late syphilitic leukoderma
         Syphilis of adrenal gland
         Syphilis of pituitary gland
         Syphilis of thyroid gland
         Syphilitic splenomegaly
         EXCLUDES 1   *syphilitic leukoderma (secondary) (A51.39)*

A52.8   Late **syphilis,** latent
     Syphilis (acquired) without clinical manifestations, with positive serological reaction and negative spinal fluid test, two years or more after infection

A52.9   Late syphilis, unspecified ▽

☑4ᵗʰ **A53**   Other and unspecified **syphilis**

A53.0   Latent **syphilis, unspecified as early or late**
     Latent syphilis NOS
     Positive serological reaction for syphilis

A53.9   **Syphilis, unspecified** ▽
     Infection due to Treponema pallidum NOS
     Syphilis (acquired) NOS
     EXCLUDES 1   *syphilis NOS under two years of age (A50.2)*

☑4ᵗʰ **A54**   Gonococcal infection

☑5ᵗʰ **A54.0**   **Gonococcal infection of** lower genitourinary tract without periurethral or accessory gland abscess
     EXCLUDES 1   *gonococcal infection with genitourinary gland abscess (A54.1)*
            gonococcal infection with periurethral abscess (A54.1)

     A54.00   **Gonococcal infection of lower genitourinary tract, unspecified** ▽

     A54.01   **Gonococcal** cystitis and urethritis, unspecified ▽

     A54.02   **Gonococcal** vulvovaginitis, unspecified ♀▽

     A54.03   **Gonococcal** cervicitis, unspecified ♀▽

     A54.09   **Other gonococcal infection of lower genitourinary tract**

A54.1   **Gonococcal infection of lower genitourinary tract** with periurethral and accessory gland abscess
     Gonococcal Bartholin's gland abscess

☑5ᵗʰ **A54.2**   **Gonococcal** pelviperitonitis and other **gonococcal genitourinary infection**

     A54.21   **Gonococcal infection of** kidney and ureter

     A54.22   **Gonococcal** prostatitis ♂

     A54.23   **Gonococcal infection of** other male genital organs ♂
         Gonococcal epididymitis
         Gonococcal orchitis

     A54.24   **Gonococcal** female pelvic inflammatory disease ♀
         Gonococcal pelviperitonitis
         EXCLUDES 1   *gonococcal peritonitis (A54.85)*

     A54.29   **Other gonococcal genitourinary infections**

☑5ᵗʰ **A54.3**   **Gonococcal infection of** eye

     A54.30   **Gonococcal infection of eye, unspecified** ▽

     A54.31   **Gonococcal** conjunctivitis
         Ophthalmia neonatorum due to gonococcus

     A54.32   **Gonococcal** iridocyclitis

     A54.33   **Gonococcal** keratitis

     A54.39   **Other gonococcal eye infection**
         Gonococcal endophthalmia

☑5ᵗʰ **A54.4**   **Gonococcal infection of** musculoskeletal system

     A54.40   **Gonococcal infection of musculoskeletal system, unspecified** ▽

     A54.41   **Gonococcal** spondylopathy

     A54.42   **Gonococcal** arthritis
         EXCLUDES 2   *gonococcal infection of spine (A54.41)*

     A54.43   **Gonococcal** osteomyelitis
         EXCLUDES 2   *gonococcal infection of spine (A54.41)*

     A54.49   **Gonococcal infection of** other **musculoskeletal tissue**
         Gonococcal bursitis
         Gonococcal myositis
         Gonococcal synovitis
         Gonococcal tenosynovitis

A54.5   **Gonococcal** pharyngitis

A54.6   **Gonococcal infection of** anus and rectum

☑5ᵗʰ **A54.8**   Other gonococcal infections

     A54.81   **Gonococcal** meningitis

     A54.82   **Gonococcal** brain abscess

     A54.83   **Gonococcal** heart infection
         Gonococcal endocarditis
         Gonococcal myocarditis
         Gonococcal pericarditis

     A54.84   **Gonococcal** pneumonia

     A54.85   **Gonococcal** peritonitis
         EXCLUDES 1   *gonococcal pelviperitonitis (A54.24)*

     A54.86   **Gonococcal** sepsis

     A54.89   **Other gonococcal infections**
         Gonococcal keratoderma
         Gonococcal lymphadenitis

A54.9   **Gonococcal infection, unspecified** ▽

☑ Additional Character Req   ☑x7ᵗʰ Placeholder Alert   Case-Mix Diagnosis   Manifestation   ▽ Unspecified Dx   **EXCLUDES 1** Not coded here   **EXCLUDES 2** Not included here

Chapter 1. Certain Infectious and Parasitic Diseases

A55–A68.9

A55 Chlamydial lymphogranuloma (venereum)
Climatic or tropical bubo
Durand-Nicolas-Favre disease
Esthiomene
Lymphogranuloma inguinale

✓4ᵗʰ **A56 Other sexually transmitted chlamydial diseases**
INCLUDES sexually transmitted diseases due to Chlamydia trachomatis
EXCLUDES 1 neonatal chlamydial conjunctivitis (P39.1)
neonatal chlamydial pneumonia (P23.1)
EXCLUDES 2 chlamydial lymphogranuloma (A55)
conditions classified to A74-

✓5ᵗʰ **A56.0 Chlamydial infection of lower genitourinary tract**
A56.00 Chlamydial infection of lower genitourinary tract, unspecified ▽
A56.01 Chlamydial cystitis and urethritis
A56.02 Chlamydial vulvovaginitis ♀
A56.09 Other chlamydial infection of lower genitourinary tract
Chlamydial cervicitis

✓5ᵗʰ **A56.1 Chlamydial infection of pelviperitoneum and other genitourinary organs**
A56.11 Chlamydial female pelvic inflammatory disease ♀
A56.19 Other chlamydial genitourinary infection
Chlamydial epididymitis
Chlamydial orchitis

A56.2 Chlamydial infection of genitourinary tract, unspecified ▽
A56.3 Chlamydial infection of anus and rectum
A56.4 Chlamydial infection of pharynx
A56.8 Sexually transmitted chlamydial infection of other sites

A57 Chancroid
Ulcus molle

A58 Granuloma inguinale
Donovanosis

✓4ᵗʰ **A59 Trichomoniasis**
EXCLUDES 2 intestinal trichomoniasis (A07.8)

✓5ᵗʰ **A59.0 Urogenital trichomoniasis**
A59.00 Urogenital trichomoniasis, unspecified ▽
Fluor (vaginalis) due to Trichomonas
Leukorrhea (vaginalis) due to Trichomonas
A59.01 Trichomonal vulvovaginitis ♀
A59.02 Trichomonal prostatitis ♂
A59.03 Trichomonal cystitis and urethritis
A59.09 Other urogenital trichomoniasis
Trichomonas cervicitis

A59.8 Trichomoniasis of other sites
A59.9 Trichomoniasis, unspecified ▽

✓4ᵗʰ **A60 Anogenital herpesviral [herpes simplex] infections**
✓5ᵗʰ **A60.0 Herpesviral infection of genitalia and urogenital tract**
A60.00 Herpesviral infection of urogenital system, unspecified ▽
A60.01 Herpesviral infection of penis ♂
A60.02 Herpesviral infection of other male genital organs ♂
A60.03 Herpesviral cervicitis ♀
A60.04 Herpesviral vulvovaginitis ♀
Herpesviral [herpes simplex] ulceration
Herpesviral [herpes simplex] vaginitis
Herpesviral [herpes simplex] vulvitis
A60.09 Herpesviral infection of other urogenital tract

A60.1 Herpesviral infection of perianal skin and rectum
A60.9 Anogenital herpesviral infection, unspecified ▽

✓4ᵗʰ **A63 Other predominantly sexually transmitted diseases, not elsewhere classified**
EXCLUDES 2 molluscum contagiosum (B08.1)
papilloma of cervix (D26.0)

A63.0 Anogenital (venereal) warts
Anogenital warts due to (human) papillomavirus [HPV]
Condyloma acuminatum
A63.8 Other specified predominantly sexually transmitted diseases

A64 Unspecified sexually transmitted disease ▽

Other spirochetal diseases (A65-A69)
EXCLUDES 2 leptospirosis (A27.-)
syphilis (A50-A53)

A65 Nonvenereal syphilis
Bejel
Endemic syphilis
Njovera

✓4ᵗʰ **A66 Yaws**
INCLUDES bouba
frambesia (tropica)
pian

A66.0 Initial lesions of yaws
Chancre of yaws
Frambesia, initial or primary
Initial frambesial ulcer
Mother yaw

A66.1 Multiple papillomata and wet crab yaws
Frambesioma
Pianoma
Plantar or palmar papilloma of yaws

A66.2 Other early skin lesions of yaws
Cutaneous yaws, less than five years after infection
Early yaws (cutaneous) (macular) (maculopapular) (micropapular) (papular)
Frambeside of early yaws

A66.3 Hyperkeratosis of yaws
Ghoul hand
Hyperkeratosis, palmar or plantar (early) (late) due to yaws
Worm-eaten soles

A66.4 Gummata and ulcers of yaws
Gummatous frambeside
Nodular late yaws (ulcerated)

A66.5 Gangosa
Rhinopharyngitis mutilans

A66.6 Bone and joint lesions of yaws
Yaws ganglion
Yaws goundou
Yaws gumma, bone or periostitis
Yaws hydrarthrosis
Yaws osteitis
Yaws gummatous osteitis
Yaws periostitis (hypertrophic)

A66.7 Other manifestations of yaws
Juxta-articular nodules of yaws
Mucosal yaws

A66.8 Latent yaws
Yaws without clinical manifestations, with positive serology

A66.9 Yaws, unspecified ▽

✓4ᵗʰ **A67 Pinta [carate]**
A67.0 Primary lesions of pinta
Chancre (primary) of pinta
Papule (primary) of pinta

A67.1 Intermediate lesions of pinta
Erythematous plaques of pinta
Hyperchromic lesions of pinta
Hyperkeratosis of pinta
Pintids

A67.2 Late lesions of pinta
Achromic skin lesions of pinta
Cicatricial skin lesions of pinta
Dyschromic skin lesions of pinta

A67.3 Mixed lesions of pinta
Achromic with hyperchromic skin lesions of pinta [carate]

A67.9 Pinta, unspecified ▽

✓4ᵗʰ **A68 Relapsing fevers**
INCLUDES recurrent fever
EXCLUDES 2 Lyme disease (A69.2-)

A68.0 Louse-borne relapsing fever
Relapsing fever due to Borrelia recurrentis

A68.1 Tick-borne relapsing fever
Relapsing fever due to any Borrelia species other than Borrelia recurrentis

A68.9 Relapsing fever, unspecified ▽

Ⓝ Newborn: 0   Ⓟ Pediatric: 0-17   Ⓜ Maternity: 12-55   Ⓐ Adult: 15-124   **NRS** Nonroutine supply Dx   **NC Dx** Noncancer Dx   **PDx** Primary Dx   ►◄ Revised Text   ● New Code   ▲ Revised Title

✓4ᵗʰ A69 Other spirochetal infections

A69.0 Necrotizing ulcerative stomatitis
Cancrum oris
Fusospirochetal gangrene
Noma
Stomatitis gangrenosa

A69.1 Other Vincent's infections
Fusospirochetal pharyngitis
Necrotizing ulcerative (acute) gingivitis
Necrotizing ulcerative (acute) gingivostomatitis
Spirochetal stomatitis
Trench mouth
Vincent's angina
Vincent's gingivitis

✓5ᵗʰ A69.2 Lyme disease
Erythema chronicum migrans due to Borrelia burgdorferi
DEF: A recurrent multisystem disorder through tick bites; begins with lesions of erythema chronicum migrans; followed by arthritis of the large joints, myalgia, malaise, and neurological and cardiac manifestations.

A69.20 Lyme disease, unspecified ▽
A69.21 Meningitis due to Lyme disease
A69.22 Other neurologic disorders in Lyme disease
Cranial neuritis
Meningoencephalitis
Polyneuropathy
A69.23 Arthritis due to Lyme disease
A69.29 Other conditions associated with Lyme disease
Myopericarditis due to Lyme disease
AHA: 2016, 3Q, 12

A69.8 Other specified spirochetal infections
A69.9 Spirochetal infection, unspecified ▽

Other diseases caused by chlamydiae (A70-A74)
EXCLUDES 1 sexually transmitted chlamydial diseases (A55-A56)

A70 Chlamydia psittaci infections
Ornithosis
Parrot fever
Psittacosis

✓4ᵗʰ A71 Trachoma
EXCLUDES 1 sequelae of trachoma (B94.0)

A71.0 Initial stage of trachoma
Trachoma dubium
A71.1 Active stage of trachoma
Granular conjunctivitis (trachomatous)
Trachomatous follicular conjunctivitis
Trachomatous pannus
A71.9 Trachoma, unspecified ▽

✓4ᵗʰ A74 Other diseases caused by chlamydiae
EXCLUDES 1 neonatal chlamydial conjunctivitis (P39.1)
neonatal chlamydial pneumonia (P23.1)
Reiter's disease (M02.3-)
sexually transmitted chlamydial diseases (A55-A56)
EXCLUDES 2 chlamydial pneumonia (J16.0)

A74.0 Chlamydial conjunctivitis
Paratrachoma
✓5ᵗʰ A74.8 Other chlamydial diseases
A74.81 Chlamydial peritonitis
A74.89 Other chlamydial diseases
A74.9 Chlamydial infection, unspecified ▽
Chlamydiosis NOS

Rickettsioses (A75-A79)

✓4ᵗʰ A75 Typhus fever
EXCLUDES 1 rickettsiosis due to Ehrlichia sennetsu (A79.81)

A75.0 Epidemic louse-borne typhus fever due to Rickettsia prowazekii
Classical typhus (fever)
Epidemic (louse-borne) typhus
A75.1 Recrudescent typhus [Brill's disease]
Brill-Zinsser disease
A75.2 Typhus fever due to Rickettsia typhi
Murine (flea-borne) typhus
A75.3 Typhus fever due to Rickettsia tsutsugamushi
Scrub (mite-borne) typhus
Tsutsugamushi fever

A75.9 Typhus fever, unspecified ▽
Typhus (fever) NOS

✓4ᵗʰ A77 Spotted fever [tick-borne rickettsioses]
A77.0 Spotted fever due to Rickettsia rickettsii
Rocky Mountain spotted fever
Sao Paulo fever
A77.1 Spotted fever due to Rickettsia conorii
African tick typhus
Boutonneuse fever
India tick typhus
Kenya tick typhus
Marseilles fever
Mediterranean tick fever
A77.2 Spotted fever due to Rickettsia siberica
North Asian tick fever
Siberian tick typhus
A77.3 Spotted fever due to Rickettsia australis
Queensland tick typhus
✓5ᵗʰ A77.4 Ehrlichiosis
EXCLUDES 1 rickettsiosis due to Ehrlichia sennetsu (A79.81)
A77.40 Ehrlichiosis, unspecified ▽
A77.41 Ehrlichiosis chaffeensis [E. chafeensis]
A77.49 Other ehrlichiosis
A77.8 Other spotted fevers
A77.9 Spotted fever, unspecified ▽
Tick-borne typhus NOS

A78 Q fever
Infection due to Coxiella burnetii
Nine Mile fever
Quadrilateral fever

✓4ᵗʰ A79 Other rickettsioses
A79.0 Trench fever
Quintan fever
Wolhynian fever
A79.1 Rickettsialpox due to Rickettsia akari
Kew Garden fever
Vesicular rickettsiosis
✓5ᵗʰ A79.8 Other specified rickettsioses
A79.81 Rickettsiosis due to Ehrlichia sennetsu
A79.89 Other specified rickettsioses
A79.9 Rickettsiosis, unspecified ▽
Rickettsial infection NOS

Viral and prion infections of the central nervous system (A80-A89)
EXCLUDES 1 postpolio syndrome (G14)
sequelae of poliomyelitis (B91)
sequelae of viral encephalitis (B94.1)

✓4ᵗʰ A80 Acute poliomyelitis
A80.0 Acute paralytic poliomyelitis, vaccine-associated
A80.1 Acute paralytic poliomyelitis, wild virus, imported
A80.2 Acute paralytic poliomyelitis, wild virus, indigenous
✓5ᵗʰ A80.3 Acute paralytic poliomyelitis, other and unspecified
A80.30 Acute paralytic poliomyelitis, unspecified ▽
A80.39 Other acute paralytic poliomyelitis
A80.4 Acute nonparalytic poliomyelitis
A80.9 Acute poliomyelitis, unspecified ▽

✓4ᵗʰ A81 Atypical virus infections of central nervous system
INCLUDES diseases of the central nervous system caused by prions
Use additional code to identify:
dementia with behavioral disturbance (F02.81)
dementia without behavioral disturbance (F02.80)
✓5ᵗʰ A81.0 Creutzfeldt-Jakob disease
A81.00 Creutzfeldt-Jakob disease, unspecified ▽
Jakob-Creutzfeldt disease, unspecified
A81.01 Variant Creutzfeldt-Jakob disease
vCJD
A81.09 Other Creutzfeldt-Jakob disease
CJD
Familial Creutzfeldt-Jakob disease
Iatrogenic Creutzfeldt-Jakob disease
Sporadic Creutzfeldt-Jakob disease
Subacute spongiform encephalopathy (with dementia)

Chapter 1. Certain Infectious and Parasitic Diseases

A81.1   Subacute sclerosing panencephalitis
Dawson's inclusion body encephalitis
Van Bogaert's sclerosing leukoencephalopathy

A81.2   Progressive multifocal leukoencephalopathy
Multifocal leukoencephalopathy NOS

☑5ʰ **A81.8   Other atypical virus infections of central nervous system**

     A81.81   Kuru

     A81.82   Gerstmann-Sträussler-Scheinker syndrome
         GSS syndrome

     A81.83   Fatal familial insomnia
         FFI

     A81.89   Other atypical virus infections of central nervous system

A81.9   Atypical virus infection of central nervous system, unspecified ▽
     Prion diseases of the central nervous system NOS

☑4ʰ **A82   Rabies**

A82.0   Sylvatic rabies

A82.1   Urban rabies

A82.9   Rabies, unspecified ▽

☑4ʰ **A83   Mosquito-borne viral encephalitis**
INCLUDES   mosquito-borne viral meningoencephalitis
EXCLUDES 2   *Venezuelan equine encephalitis (A92.2)*
         West Nile fever (A92.3-)
         West Nile virus (A92.3-)

A83.0   Japanese encephalitis

A83.1   Western equine encephalitis

A83.2   Eastern equine encephalitis

A83.3   St Louis encephalitis

A83.4   Australian encephalitis
Kunjin virus disease

A83.5   California encephalitis
California meningoencephalitis
La Crosse encephalitis

A83.6   Rocio virus disease

A83.8   Other mosquito-borne viral encephalitis

A83.9   Mosquito-borne viral encephalitis, unspecified ▽

☑4ʰ **A84   Tick-borne viral encephalitis**
INCLUDES   tick-borne viral meningoencephalitis

A84.0   Far Eastern tick-borne encephalitis [Russian spring-summer encephalitis]

A84.1   Central European tick-borne encephalitis

A84.8   Other tick-borne viral encephalitis
Louping ill
Powassan virus disease

A84.9   Tick-borne viral encephalitis, unspecified ▽

☑4ʰ **A85   Other viral encephalitis, not elsewhere classified**
INCLUDES   specified viral encephalomyelitis NEC
         specified viral meningoencephalitis NEC
EXCLUDES 1   *benign myalgic encephalomyelitis (G93.3)*
         encephalitis due to cytomegalovirus (B25.8)
         encephalitis due to herpesvirus NEC (B10.0-)
         encephalitis due to herpesvirus [herpes simplex] (B00.4)
         encephalitis due to measles virus (B05.0)
         encephalitis due to mumps virus (B26.2)
         encephalitis due to poliomyelitis virus (A80.-)
         encephalitis due to zoster (B02.0)
         lymphocytic choriomeningitis (A87.2)

A85.0   Enteroviral encephalitis
Enteroviral encephalomyelitis

A85.1   Adenoviral encephalitis
Adenoviral meningoencephalitis

A85.2   Arthropod-borne viral encephalitis, unspecified ▽
EXCLUDES 1   *West nile virus with encephalitis (A92.31)*

A85.8   Other specified viral encephalitis
Encephalitis lethargica
Von Economo-Cruchet disease

A86   Unspecified viral encephalitis ▽
Viral encephalomyelitis NOS
Viral meningoencephalitis NOS

☑4ʰ **A87   Viral meningitis**
EXCLUDES 1   *meningitis due to herpesvirus [herpes simplex] (B00.3)*
         meningitis due to measles virus (B05.1)
         meningitis due to mumps virus (B26.1)
         meningitis due to poliomyelitis virus (A80.-)
         meningitis due to zoster (B02.1)

A87.0   Enteroviral meningitis
Coxsackievirus meningitis
Echovirus meningitis

A87.1   Adenoviral meningitis

A87.2   Lymphocytic choriomeningitis
Lymphocytic meningoencephalitis

A87.8   Other viral meningitis

A87.9   Viral meningitis, unspecified ▽

☑4ʰ **A88   Other viral infections of central nervous system, not elsewhere classified**
EXCLUDES 1   *viral encephalitis NOS (A86)*
         viral meningitis NOS (A87.9)

A88.0   Enteroviral exanthematous fever [Boston exanthem]

A88.1   Epidemic vertigo

A88.8   Other specified viral infections of central nervous system

A89   Unspecified viral infection of central nervous system ▽

Arthropod-borne viral fevers and viral hemorrhagic fevers (A90-A99)

A90   Dengue fever [classical dengue]
EXCLUDES 1   *dengue hemorrhagic fever (A91)*
AHA: 2016, 3Q, 13

A91   Dengue hemorrhagic fever

☑4ʰ **A92   Other mosquito-borne viral fevers**
EXCLUDES 1   *Ross River disease (B33.1)*

A92.0   Chikungunya virus disease
Chikungunya (hemorrhagic) fever

A92.1   O'nyong-nyong fever

A92.2   Venezuelan equine fever
Venezuelan equine encephalitis
Venezuelan equine encephalomyelitis virus disease

☑5ʰ **A92.3   West Nile virus infection**
West Nile fever
AHA: 2016, 3Q, 12

     A92.30   West Nile virus infection, unspecified ▽
         West Nile fever NOS
         West Nile fever without complications
         West Nile virus NOS

     A92.31   West Nile virus infection with encephalitis
         West Nile encephalitis
         West Nile encephalomyelitis

     A92.32   West Nile virus infection with other neurologic manifestation
         Use additional code to specify the neurologic manifestation

     A92.39   West Nile virus infection with other complications
         Use additional code to specify the other conditions

A92.4   Rift Valley fever

A92.5   Zika virus disease
Zika virus fever
Zika virus infection
Zika NOS

A92.8   Other specified mosquito-borne viral fevers

A92.9   Mosquito-borne viral fever, unspecified ▽

☑4ʰ **A93   Other arthropod-borne viral fevers, not elsewhere classified**

A93.0   Oropouche virus disease
Oropouche fever

A93.1   Sandfly fever
Pappataci fever
Phlebotomus fever

A93.2   Colorado tick fever

A93.8   Other specified arthropod-borne viral fevers
Piry virus disease
Vesicular stomatitis virus disease [Indiana fever]

A94   Unspecified arthropod-borne viral fever ▽
Arboviral fever NOS
Arbovirus infection NOS

Ⓝ Newborn: 0   Ⓟ Pediatric: 0-17   Ⓜ Maternity: 12-55   Ⓐ Adult: 15-124   NRS Nonroutine supply Dx   NCDx Noncancer Dx   PDx Primary Dx   ►◄ Revised Text   ● New Code   ▲ Revised Title

446   ICD-10-CM 2018

✓4ᵗʰ A95 Yellow fever

A95.0 **Sylvatic** yellow fever
Jungle yellow fever

A95.1 **Urban** yellow fever

A95.9 Yellow fever, unspecified ▽

✓4ᵗʰ A96 Arenaviral hemorrhagic fever

A96.0 **Junin** hemorrhagic fever
Argentinian hemorrhagic fever

A96.1 **Machupo** hemorrhagic fever
Bolivian hemorrhagic fever

A96.2 **Lassa** fever

A96.8 Other arenaviral hemorrhagic fevers

A96.9 Arenaviral hemorrhagic fever, unspecified ▽

✓4ᵗʰ A98 Other viral hemorrhagic fevers, not elsewhere classified

EXCLUDES 1 *chikungunya hemorrhagic fever (A92.0)*
dengue hemorrhagic fever (A91)

A98.0 Crimean-Congo hemorrhagic fever
Central Asian hemorrhagic fever

A98.1 Omsk hemorrhagic fever

A98.2 Kyasanur Forest disease

A98.3 Marburg virus disease

A98.4 Ebola virus disease

A98.5 Hemorrhagic fever with renal syndrome
Epidemic hemorrhagic fever
Korean hemorrhagic fever
Russian hemorrhagic fever
Hantaan virus disease
Hantavirus disease with renal manifestations
Nephropathia epidemica
Songo fever
EXCLUDES 1 *hantavirus (cardio)-pulmonary syndrome (B33.4)*

A98.8 Other specified viral hemorrhagic fevers

A99 Unspecified viral hemorrhagic fever ▽

Viral infections characterized by skin and mucous membrane lesions (B00-B09)

✓4ᵗʰ B00 Herpesviral [herpes simplex] infections

EXCLUDES 1 *congenital herpesviral infections (P35.2)*
EXCLUDES 2 *anogenital herpesviral infection (A60.-)*
gammaherpesviral mononucleosis (B27.0-)
herpangina (B08.5)

B00.0 **Eczema herpeticum**
Kaposi's varicelliform eruption

B00.1 **Herpesviral** vesicular dermatitis
Herpes simplex facialis
Herpes simplex labialis
Herpes simplex otitis externa
Vesicular dermatitis of ear
Vesicular dermatitis of lip

B00.2 **Herpesviral** gingivostomatitis and pharyngotonsillitis
Herpesviral pharyngitis

B00.3 **Herpesviral** meningitis

B00.4 **Herpesviral** encephalitis
Herpesviral meningoencephalitis
Simian B disease
EXCLUDES 1 *herpesviral encephalitis due to herpesvirus 6 and 7 (B10.01, B10.09)*
non-simplex herpesviral encephalitis (B10.0-)

✓5ᵗʰ B00.5 **Herpesviral** ocular disease

B00.50 **Herpesviral** ocular disease, unspecified ▽

B00.51 **Herpesviral** iridocyclitis
Herpesviral iritis
Herpesviral uveitis, anterior

B00.52 **Herpesviral** keratitis
Herpesviral keratoconjunctivitis

B00.53 **Herpesviral** conjunctivitis

B00.59 **Other herpesviral disease of eye**
Herpesviral dermatitis of eyelid

B00.7 **Disseminated herpesviral disease**
Herpesviral sepsis

✓5ᵗʰ B00.8 **Other** forms of herpesviral infections

B00.81 **Herpesviral** hepatitis

B00.82 **Herpes simplex** myelitis

B00.89 **Other herpesviral infection**
Herpesviral whitlow

B00.9 Herpesviral infection, unspecified ▽
Herpes simplex infection NOS

✓4ᵗʰ B01 Varicella [chickenpox]

B01.0 **Varicella** meningitis

✓5ᵗʰ B01.1 **Varicella** encephalitis, myelitis and encephalomyelitis
Postchickenpox encephalitis, myelitis and encephalomyelitis

B01.11 **Varicella** encephalitis and encephalomyelitis
Postchickenpox encephalitis and encephalomyelitis

B01.12 **Varicella** myelitis
Postchickenpox myelitis

B01.2 **Varicella** pneumonia

✓5ᵗʰ B01.8 **Varicella with** other complications

B01.81 **Varicella** keratitis

B01.89 **Other varicella complications**

B01.9 **Varicella** without complication ▽
Varicella NOS

✓4ᵗʰ B02 Zoster [herpes zoster]

INCLUDES shingles
zona

B02.0 **Zoster** encephalitis
Zoster meningoencephalitis

B02.1 **Zoster** meningitis

✓5ᵗʰ B02.2 **Zoster with** other nervous system involvement

B02.21 **Postherpetic** geniculate ganglionitis

B02.22 **Postherpetic** trigeminal neuralgia

B02.23 **Postherpetic** polyneuropathy

B02.24 **Postherpetic** myelitis
Herpes zoster myelitis

B02.29 **Other postherpetic nervous system involvement**
Postherpetic radiculopathy

✓5ᵗʰ B02.3 **Zoster** ocular disease

B02.30 **Zoster ocular disease, unspecified** ▽

B02.31 **Zoster** conjunctivitis

B02.32 **Zoster** iridocyclitis

B02.33 **Zoster** keratitis
Herpes zoster keratoconjunctivitis

B02.34 **Zoster** scleritis

B02.39 **Other herpes zoster eye disease**
Zoster blepharitis

B02.7 **Disseminated** zoster

B02.8 **Zoster with** other complications
Herpes zoster otitis externa

B02.9 **Zoster** without complications ▽
Zoster NOS

B03 Smallpox

NOTE In 1980 the 33rd World Health Assembly declared that smallpox had been eradicated.
The classification is maintained for surveillance purposes.

B04 Monkeypox

✓4ᵗʰ B05 Measles

INCLUDES morbilli
EXCLUDES 1 *subacute sclerosing panencephalitis (A81.1)*

B05.0 **Measles complicated by** encephalitis
Postmeasles encephalitis

B05.1 **Measles complicated by** meningitis
Postmeasles meningitis

B05.2 **Measles complicated by** pneumonia
Postmeasles pneumonia

B05.3 **Measles complicated by** otitis media
Postmeasles otitis media

B05.4 **Measles with** intestinal complications

✓5ᵗʰ B05.8 **Measles with** other complications

B05.81 **Measles** keratitis and keratoconjunctivitis

B05.89 **Other measles complications**

B05.9 **Measles** without complication ▽
Measles NOS

✓4ᵗʰ B06 Rubella [German measles]

EXCLUDES 1 *congenital rubella (P35.0)*

✓5ᵗʰ B06.0 **Rubella with** neurological complications

B06.00 **Rubella with neurological complication, unspecified** ▽

B06.01 **Rubella** encephalitis
Rubella meningoencephalitis

B06.02   Rubella meningitis

B06.09   Other neurological complications of rubella

✓5ᵗʰ **B06.8**   Rubella with other complications

B06.81   Rubella pneumonia

B06.82   Rubella arthritis

B06.89   Other rubella complications

B06.9   Rubella without complication   ▽
Rubella NOS

✓4ᵗʰ **B07**   **Viral warts**

INCLUDES   verruca simplex
verruca vulgaris
viral warts due to human papillomavirus

EXCLUDES 2   anogenital (venereal) warts (A63.0)
papilloma of bladder (D41.4)
papilloma of cervix (D26.0)
papilloma larynx (D14.1)

B07.0   Plantar wart
Verruca plantaris

B07.8   Other viral warts
Common wart
Flat wart
Verruca plana

B07.9   Viral wart, unspecified   ▽

✓4ᵗʰ **B08**   **Other viral infections characterized by skin and mucous membrane lesions, not elsewhere classified**

EXCLUDES 1   vesicular stomatitis virus disease (A93.8)

✓5ᵗʰ **B08.0**   Other orthopoxvirus infections

EXCLUDES 2   monkeypox (B04)

✓6ᵗʰ **B08.01**   Cowpox and vaccinia not from vaccine

B08.010   Cowpox
DEF: A disease contracted by milking infected cows; vesicles usually appear on the fingers, hands, and adjacent areas and usually disappear without scarring; other symptoms: local edema, lymphangitis, and regional lymphadenitis with or without fever.

B08.011   Vaccinia not from vaccine
EXCLUDES 1   vaccinia (from vaccination) (generalized) (T88.1)

B08.02   Orf virus disease
Contagious pustular dermatitis
Ecthyma contagiosum

B08.03   Pseudocowpox [milker's node]

B08.04   Paravaccinia, unspecified   ▽

B08.09   Other orthopoxvirus infections
Orthopoxvirus infection NOS

B08.1   Molluscum contagiosum
DEF: Benign poxvirus infection causing small bumps on the skin or conjunctiva; transmitted by close contact.

✓5ᵗʰ **B08.2**   Exanthema subitum [sixth disease]
Roseola infantum

B08.20   Exanthema subitum [sixth disease], unspecified   P ▽
Roseola infantum, unspecified

B08.21   Exanthema subitum [sixth disease] due to human herpesvirus 6   P
Roseola infantum due to human herpesvirus 6

B08.22   Exanthema subitum [sixth disease] due to human herpesvirus 7   P
Roseola infantum due to human herpesvirus 7

B08.3   Erythema infectiosum [fifth disease]

B08.4   Enteroviral vesicular stomatitis with exanthem
Hand, foot and mouth disease

B08.5   Enteroviral vesicular pharyngitis
Herpangina
DEF: Acute infectious Coxsackie virus infection causing throat lesions, fever, and vomiting; generally affects children in summer.

✓5ᵗʰ **B08.6**   Parapoxvirus infections

B08.60   Parapoxvirus infection, unspecified   ▽

B08.61   Bovine stomatitis

B08.62   Sealpox

B08.69   Other parapoxvirus infections

✓5ᵗʰ **B08.7**   Yatapoxvirus infections

B08.70   Yatapoxvirus infection, unspecified   ▽

B08.71   Tanapox virus disease

B08.72   Yaba pox virus disease
Yaba monkey tumor disease

B08.79   Other yatapoxvirus infections

B08.8   Other specified viral infections characterized by skin and mucous membrane lesions
Enteroviral lymphonodular pharyngitis
Foot-and-mouth disease
Poxvirus NEC

B09   **Unspecified viral infection characterized by skin and mucous**   ▽
membrane lesions
Viral enanthema NOS
Viral exanthema NOS

Other human herpesviruses (B10)

✓4ᵗʰ **B10**   **Other human herpesviruses**

EXCLUDES 2   cytomegalovirus (B25.9)
Epstein-Barr virus (B27.0-)
herpes NOS (B00.9)
herpes simplex (B00.-)
herpes zoster (B02.-)
human herpesvirus NOS (B00.-)
human herpesvirus 1 and 2 (B00.-)
human herpesvirus 3 (B01.-, B02.-)
human herpesvirus 4 (B27.0-)
human herpesvirus 5 (B25.-)
varicella (B01.-)
zoster (B02.-)

✓5ᵗʰ **B10.0**   Other human herpesvirus encephalitis

EXCLUDES 2   herpes encephalitis NOS (B00.4)
herpes simplex encephalitis (B00.4)
human herpesvirus encephalitis (B00.4)
simian B herpes virus encephalitis (B00.4)

B10.01   Human herpesvirus 6 encephalitis

B10.09   Other human herpesvirus encephalitis
Human herpesvirus 7 encephalitis

✓5ᵗʰ **B10.8**   Other human herpesvirus infection

B10.81   Human herpesvirus 6 infection

B10.82   Human herpesvirus 7 infection

B10.89   Other human herpesvirus infection
Human herpesvirus 8 infection
Kaposi's sarcoma-associated herpesvirus infection

Viral hepatitis (B15-B19)

EXCLUDES 1   sequelae of viral hepatitis (B94.2)
EXCLUDES 2   cytomegaloviral hepatitis (B25.1)
herpesviral [herpes simplex] hepatitis (B00.81)

DEF: Hepatitis A: HAV infection is self-limiting with flulike symptoms; transmission, fecal-oral.
DEF: Hepatitis B: HBV infection can be chronic and systemic; transmission, bodily fluids.
DEF: Hepatitis C: HCV infection can be chronic and systemic; transmission, blood transfusion and unidentified agents.
DEF: Hepatitis D (delta): HDV occurs only in the presence of hepatitis B virus; transmission, contaminated blood in contact with mucous membranes.
DEF: Hepatitis E: HEV is epidemic form; transmission, fecal-oral, most often from contaminated water.

✓4ᵗʰ **B15**   **Acute hepatitis A**

B15.0   Hepatitis A with hepatic coma   NC Dx

B15.9   Hepatitis A without hepatic coma
Hepatitis A (acute)(viral) NOS

✓4ᵗʰ **B16**   **Acute hepatitis B**
AHA: 2016, 3Q, 13

B16.0   Acute hepatitis B with delta-agent with hepatic coma   NC Dx

B16.1   Acute hepatitis B with delta-agent without hepatic coma

B16.2   Acute hepatitis B without delta-agent with hepatic coma   NC Dx

B16.9   Acute hepatitis B without delta-agent and without hepatic coma
Hepatitis B (acute) (viral) NOS

✓4ᵗʰ **B17**   **Other acute viral hepatitis**

B17.0   Acute delta-(super) infection of hepatitis B carrier

✓5ᵗʰ **B17.1**   Acute hepatitis C

B17.10   Acute hepatitis C without hepatic coma
Acute hepatitis C NOS

B17.11   Acute hepatitis C with hepatic coma   NC Dx

B17.2   Acute hepatitis E

B17.8   Other specified acute viral hepatitis
Hepatitis non-A non-B (acute) (viral) NEC

B17.9 Acute viral hepatitis, unspecified ▽
    Acute hepatitis NOS
    Acute infectious hepatitis NOS

✓4ᵗʰ **B18 Chronic viral hepatitis**
    INCLUDES carrier of viral hepatitis
    AHA: 2017, 1Q, 41

    B18.0 Chronic viral hepatitis B with delta-agent NC Dx

    B18.1 Chronic viral hepatitis B without delta-agent NC Dx
        Carrier of viral hepatitis B
        Chronic (viral) hepatitis B

    B18.2 Chronic viral hepatitis C NC Dx
        Carrier of viral hepatitis C

    B18.8 Other chronic viral hepatitis NC Dx
        Carrier of other viral hepatitis

    B18.9 Chronic viral hepatitis, unspecified NC Dx ▽
        Carrier of unspecified viral hepatitis

✓4ᵗʰ **B19 Unspecified viral hepatitis**
    B19.0 Unspecified viral hepatitis with hepatic coma NC Dx ▽

    ✓5ᵗʰ **B19.1 Unspecified viral hepatitis B**
        B19.10 Unspecified viral hepatitis B without hepatic ▽
            coma
            Unspecified viral hepatitis B NOS

        B19.11 Unspecified viral hepatitis B with hepatic NC Dx ▽
            coma

    ✓5ᵗʰ **B19.2 Unspecified viral hepatitis C**
        B19.20 Unspecified viral hepatitis C without hepatic ▽
            coma
            Viral hepatitis C NOS

        B19.21 Unspecified viral hepatitis C with hepatic NC Dx ▽
            coma

    B19.9 Unspecified viral hepatitis without hepatic coma ▽
        Viral hepatitis NOS

Human immunodeficiency virus [HIV] disease (B20)

B20 Human immunodeficiency virus [HIV] disease NC Dx
    INCLUDES acquired immune deficiency syndrome [AIDS]
        AIDS-related complex [ARC]
        HIV infection, symptomatic
    Code first human immunodeficiency virus [HIV] disease complicating
        pregnancy, childbirth and the puerperium, if applicable (O98.7-)
    Use additional code(s) to identify all manifestations of HIV infection
    EXCLUDES 1 asymptomatic human immunodeficiency virus [HIV] infection
            status (Z21)
            exposure to HIV virus (Z20.6)
            inconclusive serologic evidence of HIV (R75)

Other viral diseases (B25-B34)

✓4ᵗʰ **B25 Cytomegaloviral disease**
    EXCLUDES 1 congenital cytomegalovirus infection (P35.1)
            cytomegaloviral mononucleosis (B27.1-)

    B25.0 Cytomegaloviral pneumonitis
    B25.1 Cytomegaloviral hepatitis
    B25.2 Cytomegaloviral pancreatitis
    B25.8 Other cytomegaloviral diseases
        Cytomegaloviral encephalitis
    B25.9 Cytomegaloviral disease, unspecified ▽

✓4ᵗʰ **B26 Mumps**
    INCLUDES epidemic parotitis
        infectious parotitis

    B26.0 Mumps orchitis ♂
    B26.1 Mumps meningitis
    B26.2 Mumps encephalitis
    B26.3 Mumps pancreatitis
    ✓5ᵗʰ **B26.8 Mumps with other complications**
        B26.81 Mumps hepatitis
        B26.82 Mumps myocarditis
        B26.83 Mumps nephritis
        B26.84 Mumps polyneuropathy
        B26.85 Mumps arthritis
        B26.89 Other mumps complications
    B26.9 Mumps without complication ▽
        Mumps NOS
        Mumps parotitis NOS

✓4ᵗʰ **B27 Infectious mononucleosis**
    INCLUDES glandular fever
        monocytic angina
        Pfeiffer's disease

    ✓5ᵗʰ **B27.0 Gammaherpesviral mononucleosis**
        Mononucleosis due to Epstein-Barr virus
        B27.00 Gammaherpesviral mononucleosis without
            complication
        B27.01 Gammaherpesviral mononucleosis with
            polyneuropathy
        B27.02 Gammaherpesviral mononucleosis with meningitis
        B27.09 Gammaherpesviral mononucleosis with other
            complications
            Hepatomegaly in gammaherpesviral mononucleosis

    ✓5ᵗʰ **B27.1 Cytomegaloviral mononucleosis**
        B27.10 Cytomegaloviral mononucleosis without
            complications
        B27.11 Cytomegaloviral mononucleosis with
            polyneuropathy
        B27.12 Cytomegaloviral mononucleosis with meningitis
        B27.19 Cytomegaloviral mononucleosis with other
            complication
            Hepatomegaly in cytomegaloviral mononucleosis

    ✓5ᵗʰ **B27.8 Other infectious mononucleosis**
        B27.80 Other infectious mononucleosis without
            complication
        B27.81 Other infectious mononucleosis with
            polyneuropathy
        B27.82 Other infectious mononucleosis with meningitis
        B27.89 Other infectious mononucleosis with other
            complication
            Hepatomegaly in other infectious mononucleosis

    ✓5ᵗʰ **B27.9 Infectious mononucleosis, unspecified**
        B27.90 Infectious mononucleosis, unspecified without ▽
            complication
        B27.91 Infectious mononucleosis, unspecified with ▽
            polyneuropathy
        B27.92 Infectious mononucleosis, unspecified with ▽
            meningitis
        B27.99 Infectious mononucleosis, unspecified with ▽
            other complication
            Hepatomegaly in unspecified infectious
            mononucleosis

✓4ᵗʰ **B30 Viral conjunctivitis**
    EXCLUDES 1 herpesviral [herpes simplex] ocular disease (B00.5)
            ocular zoster (B02.3)

    B30.0 Keratoconjunctivitis due to adenovirus
        Epidemic keratoconjunctivitis
        Shipyard eye

    B30.1 Conjunctivitis due to adenovirus
        Acute adenoviral follicular conjunctivitis
        Swimming-pool conjunctivitis

    B30.2 Viral pharyngoconjunctivitis

    B30.3 Acute epidemic hemorrhagic conjunctivitis (enteroviral)
        Conjunctivitis due to coxsackievirus 24
        Conjunctivitis due to enterovirus 70
        Hemorrhagic conjunctivitis (acute)(epidemic)

Viral Conjunctivitis

Normal conjunctiva

Inflamed conjunctiva

B30.8 Other viral conjunctivitis
Newcastle conjunctivitis

B30.9 Viral conjunctivitis, unspecified ▽

✓4ᵗʰ B33 Other viral diseases, not elsewhere classified

B33.0 Epidemic myalgia
Bornholm disease

B33.1 Ross River disease
Epidemic polyarthritis and exanthema
Ross River fever

✓5ᵗʰ B33.2 Viral carditis
Coxsackie (virus) carditis

    B33.20 Viral carditis, unspecified ▽
    B33.21 Viral endocarditis
    B33.22 Viral myocarditis
    B33.23 Viral pericarditis
    B33.24 Viral cardiomyopathy

B33.3 Retrovirus infections, not elsewhere classified
Retrovirus infection NOS

B33.4 Hantavirus (cardio)-pulmonary syndrome [HPS] [HCPS]
Hantavirus disease with pulmonary manifestations
Sin nombre virus disease
Use additional code to identify any associated acute kidney failure (N17.9)
   EXCLUDES 1   *hantavirus disease with renal manifestations (A98.5)*
             hemorrhagic fever with renal manifestations (A98.5)

B33.8 Other specified viral diseases
   EXCLUDES 1   *anogenital human papillomavirus infection (A63.0)*
             viral warts due to human papillomavirus infection (B07)

✓4ᵗʰ B34 Viral infection of unspecified site
   EXCLUDES 1   *anogenital human papillomavirus infection (A63.0)*
             cytomegaloviral disease NOS (B25.9)
             herpesvirus [herpes simplex] infection NOS (B00.9)
             retrovirus infection NOS (B33.3)
             viral agents as the cause of diseases classified elsewhere (B97.-)
             viral warts due to human papillomavirus infection (B07)

B34.0 Adenovirus infection, unspecified ▽
B34.1 Enterovirus infection, unspecified ▽
Coxsackievirus infection NOS
Echovirus infection NOS
B34.2 Coronavirus infection, unspecified ▽
   EXCLUDES 1   *pneumonia due to SARS-associated coronavirus (J12.81)*
B34.3 Parvovirus infection, unspecified ▽
B34.4 Papovavirus infection, unspecified ▽
B34.8 Other viral infections of unspecified site ▽
B34.9 Viral infection, unspecified ▽
Viremia NOS
AHA: 2016, 3Q, 10

Mycoses (B35-B49)
EXCLUDES 2   *hypersensitivity pneumonitis due to organic dust (J67.-)*
            mycosis fungoides (C84.0-)

✓4ᵗʰ B35 Dermatophytosis
INCLUDES   favus
         infections due to species of Epidermophyton, Micro-sporum and Trichophyton
         tinea, any type except those in B36-
DEF: Contagious superficial fungal infection of the skin that invades and grows in dead keratin.

B35.0 Tinea barbae and tinea capitis
Beard ringworm
Kerion
Scalp ringworm
Sycosis, mycotic

B35.1 Tinea unguium NRS
Dermatophytic onychia
Dermatophytosis of nail
Onychomycosis
Ringworm of nails

B35.2 Tinea manuum NRS
Dermatophytosis of hand
Hand ringworm

B35.3 Tinea pedis NRS
Athlete's foot
Dermatophytosis of foot
Foot ringworm

B35.4 Tinea corporis NRS
Ringworm of the body

B35.5 Tinea imbricata NRS
Tokelau

B35.6 Tinea cruris NRS
Dhobi itch
Groin ringworm
Jock itch

B35.8 Other dermatophytoses NRS
Disseminated dermatophytosis
Granulomatous dermatophytosis

B35.9 Dermatophytosis, unspecified NRS ▽
Ringworm NOS

✓4ᵗʰ B36 Other superficial mycoses

B36.0 Pityriasis versicolor NRS
Tinea flava
Tinea versicolor

B36.1 Tinea nigra NRS
Keratomycosis nigricans palmaris
Microsporosis nigra
Pityriasis nigra

B36.2 White piedra NRS
Tinea blanca

B36.3 Black piedra NRS

B36.8 Other specified superficial mycoses NRS

B36.9 Superficial mycosis, unspecified NRS ▽

✓4ᵗʰ B37 Candidiasis
INCLUDES   candidosis
         moniliasis
EXCLUDES 1   *neonatal candidiasis (P37.5)*

B37.0 Candidal stomatitis
Oral thrush

B37.1 Pulmonary candidiasis
Candidal bronchitis
Candidal pneumonia

B37.2 Candidiasis of skin and nail NRS
Candidal onychia
Candidal paronychia
   EXCLUDES 2   *diaper dermatitis (L22)*

B37.3 Candidiasis of vulva and vagina ♀
Candidal vulvovaginitis
Monilial vulvovaginitis
Vaginal thrush

✓5ᵗʰ B37.4 Candidiasis of other urogenital sites
    B37.41 Candidal cystitis and urethritis
    B37.42 Candidal balanitis
    B37.49 Other urogenital candidiasis
         Candidal pyelonephritis

B37.5 Candidal meningitis

B37.6 Candidal endocarditis

B37.7 Candidal sepsis
Disseminated candidiasis
Systemic candidiasis
AHA: 2014, 4Q, 46

✓5ᵗʰ B37.8 Candidiasis of other sites
    B37.81 Candidal esophagitis
    B37.82 Candidal enteritis
         Candidal proctitis
    B37.83 Candidal cheilitis
    B37.84 Candidal otitis externa
    B37.89 Other sites of candidiasis
         Candidal osteomyelitis

B37.9 Candidiasis, unspecified ▽
Thrush NOS

✓4ᵗʰ B38 Coccidioidomycosis

B38.0 Acute pulmonary coccidioidomycosis
B38.1 Chronic pulmonary coccidioidomycosis
B38.2 Pulmonary coccidioidomycosis, unspecified ▽
B38.3 Cutaneous coccidioidomycosis NRS
B38.4 Coccidioidomycosis meningitis
   DEF: *Coccidioides immitis* infection of the lining of the brain and/or spinal cord.

N Newborn: 0   P Pediatric: 0-17   M Maternity: 12-55   A Adult: 15-124   NRS Nonroutine supply Dx   NCDx Noncancer Dx   PDx Primary Dx   ▶◀ Revised Text   ● New Code   ▲ Revised Title

450   ICD-10-CM 2018

Histoplasmosis

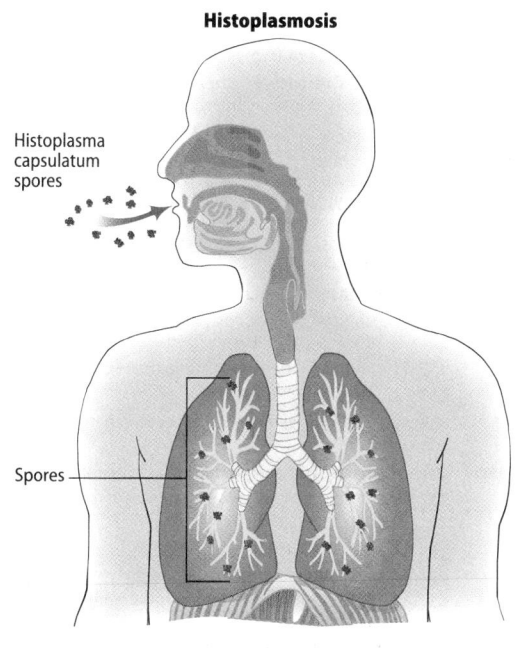

Histoplasma capsulatum spores

Spores

B38.7   Disseminated **coccidioidomycosis**
     Generalized coccidioidomycosis

✓5ᵗʰ **B38.8**   Other **forms of coccidioidomycosis**

     B38.81   Prostatic **coccidioidomycosis**   ♂

     B38.89   Other forms of coccidioidomycosis

B38.9   Coccidioidomycosis, unspecified   ▽

✓4ᵗʰ **B39**   **Histoplasmosis**

     Code first associated AIDS (B20)

     Use additional code for any associated manifestations, such as:
        endocarditis (I39)
        meningitis (G02)
        pericarditis (I32)
        retinitits (H32)
     DEF: Type of lung infection caused by breathing in fungal spores often found in the droppings of bats and birds or soil contaminated by their droppings.

     B39.0   Acute pulmonary **histoplasmosis capsulati**

     B39.1   Chronic pulmonary **histoplasmosis capsulati**

     B39.2   Pulmonary histoplasmosis capsulati, unspecified   ▽

     B39.3   Disseminated **histoplasmosis capsulati**
        Generalized histoplasmosis capsulati

     B39.4   Histoplasmosis **capsulati, unspecified**   ▽
        American histoplasmosis

     B39.5   Histoplasmosis **duboisii**
        African histoplasmosis

     B39.9   Histoplasmosis, unspecified   ▽

✓4ᵗʰ **B40**   **Blastomycosis**

     EXCLUDES 1   Brazilian blastomycosis (B41.-)
               keloidal blastomycosis (B48.0)

     B40.0   Acute pulmonary **blastomycosis**

     B40.1   Chronic pulmonary **blastomycosis**

     B40.2   Pulmonary blastomycosis, unspecified   ▽

     B40.3   Cutaneous **blastomycosis**   NRS

     B40.7   Disseminated **blastomycosis**
        Generalized blastomycosis

✓5ᵗʰ **B40.8**   Other **forms of blastomycosis**

        B40.81   Blastomycotic **meningoencephalitis**
             Meningomyelitis due to blastomycosis

        B40.89   Other forms of blastomycosis

     B40.9   Blastomycosis, unspecified   ▽

✓4ᵗʰ **B41**   **Paracoccidioidomycosis**

     INCLUDES   Brazilian blastomycosis
               Lutz' disease

     B41.0   Pulmonary **paracoccidioidomycosis**

     B41.7   Disseminated **paracoccidioidomycosis**
        Generalized paracoccidioidomycosis

     B41.8   Other forms of paracoccidioidomycosis

     B41.9   Paracoccidioidomycosis, unspecified   ▽

✓4ᵗʰ **B42**   **Sporotrichosis**

     B42.0   Pulmonary **sporotrichosis**

     B42.1   Lymphocutaneous **sporotrichosis**

     B42.7   Disseminated **sporotrichosis**
        Generalized sporotrichosis

✓5ᵗʰ **B42.8**   Other **forms of sporotrichosis**

        B42.81   Cerebral **sporotrichosis**
             Meningitis due to sporotrichosis

        B42.82   Sporotrichosis **arthritis**

        B42.89   Other forms of sporotrichosis

     B42.9   Sporotrichosis, unspecified   ▽

✓4ᵗʰ **B43**   **Chromomycosis and pheomycotic abscess**

     B43.0   Cutaneous **chromomycosis**   NRS
        Dermatitis verrucosa

     B43.1   Pheomycotic **brain abscess**   NRS
        Cerebral chromomycosis

     B43.2   Subcutaneous **pheomycotic abscess and cyst**   NRS

     B43.8   Other forms of chromomycosis   NRS

     B43.9   Chromomycosis, unspecified   NRS ▽

✓4ᵗʰ **B44**   **Aspergillosis**

     INCLUDES   aspergilloma

     B44.0   Invasive pulmonary **aspergillosis**

     B44.1   Other **pulmonary aspergillosis**

     B44.2   Tonsillar **aspergillosis**

     B44.7   Disseminated **aspergillosis**
        Generalized aspergillosis

✓5ᵗʰ **B44.8**   Other **forms of aspergillosis**

        B44.81   Allergic bronchopulmonary **aspergillosis**

        B44.89   Other forms of aspergillosis

     B44.9   Aspergillosis, unspecified   ▽

✓4ᵗʰ **B45**   **Cryptococcosis**

     B45.0   Pulmonary **cryptococcosis**

     B45.1   Cerebral **cryptococcosis**
        Cryptococcal meningitis
        Cryptococcosis meningocerebralis

     B45.2   Cutaneous **cryptococcosis**   NRS

     B45.3   Osseous **cryptococcosis**

     B45.7   Disseminated **cryptococcosis**
        Generalized cryptococcosis

     B45.8   Other forms of cryptococcosis

     B45.9   Cryptococcosis, unspecified   ▽

✓4ᵗʰ **B46**   **Zygomycosis**

     B46.0   Pulmonary **mucormycosis**

     B46.1   Rhinocerebral **mucormycosis**

     B46.2   Gastrointestinal **mucormycosis**

     B46.3   Cutaneous **mucormycosis**   NRS
        Subcutaneous mucormycosis

     B46.4   Disseminated **mucormycosis**
        Generalized mucormycosis

     B46.5   Mucormycosis, unspecified   ▽

     B46.8   Other zygomycoses
        Entomophthoromycosis

     B46.9   Zygomycosis, unspecified   ▽
        Phycomycosis NOS

✓4ᵗʰ **B47**   **Mycetoma**

     B47.0   Eumycetoma   NRS
        Madura foot, mycotic
        Maduromycosis

     B47.1   Actinomycetoma   NRS

     B47.9   Mycetoma, unspecified   NRS ▽
        Madura foot NOS

✓4ᵗʰ **B48**   **Other mycoses, not elsewhere classified**

     B48.0   Lobomycosis   NRS
        Keloidal blastomycosis
        Lobo's disease

     B48.1   Rhinosporidiosis

     B48.2   Allescheriasis
        Infection due to Pseudallescheria boydii
        EXCLUDES 1   eumycetoma (B47.0)

     B48.3   Geotrichosis
        Geotrichum stomatitis

✓ Additional Character Req   ✓x7ᵗʰ Placeholder Alert   Case-Mix Diagnosis   Manifestation   ▽ Unspecified Dx   **EXCLUDES 1** Not coded here   **EXCLUDES 2** Not included here

ICD-10-CM 2018   **451**

B48.4 Penicillosis

B48.8 Other specified mycoses
Adiaspiromycosis
Infection of tissue and organs by Alternaria
Infection of tissue and organs by Drechslera
Infection of tissue and organs by Fusarium
Infection of tissue and organs by saprophytic fungi NEC
AHA: 2014, 4Q, 46; 2014, 2Q, 13

B49 Unspecified mycosis ▽
Fungemia NOS

Protozoal diseases (B50-B64)

EXCLUDES 1 *amebiasis (AØ6.-)*
other protozoal intestinal diseases (AØ7.-)

✓4ᵗʰ **B50 Plasmodium falciparum malaria**
INCLUDES mixed infections of Plasmodium falciparum with any other Plasmodium species

B50.0 Plasmodium falciparum malaria with cerebral complications
Cerebral malaria NOS

B50.8 Other severe and complicated Plasmodium falciparum malaria
Severe or complicated Plasmodium falciparum malaria NOS

B50.9 Plasmodium falciparum malaria, unspecified ▽

✓4ᵗʰ **B51 Plasmodium vivax malaria**
INCLUDES mixed infections of Plasmodium vivax with other Plasmodium species, except Plasmodium falciparum
EXCLUDES 1 *plasmodium vivax with Plasmodium falciparum (B50.-)*

B51.0 Plasmodium vivax malaria with rupture of spleen

B51.8 Plasmodium vivax malaria with other complications

B51.9 Plasmodium vivax malaria without complication ▽
Plasmodium vivax malaria NOS

✓4ᵗʰ **B52 Plasmodium malariae malaria**
INCLUDES mixed infections of Plasmodium malariae with other Plasmodium species, except Plasmodium falciparum and Plasmodium vivax
EXCLUDES 1 *Plasmodium falciparum (B50.-)*
Plasmodium vivax (B51.-)

B52.0 Plasmodium malariae malaria with nephropathy

B52.8 Plasmodium malariae malaria with other complications

B52.9 Plasmodium malariae malaria without complication ▽
Plasmodium malariae malaria NOS

✓4ᵗʰ **B53 Other specified malaria**

B53.0 Plasmodium ovale malaria
EXCLUDES 1 *Plasmodium ovale with Plasmodium falciparum (B50.-)*
Plasmodium ovale with Plasmodium malariae (B52.-)
Plasmodium ovale with Plasmodium vivax (B51.-)

B53.1 Malaria due to simian plasmodia
EXCLUDES 1 *Malaria due to simian plasmodia with Plasmodium falciparum (B50.-)*
Malaria due to simian plasmodia with Plasmodium malariae (B52.-)
Malaria due to simian plasmodia with Plasmodium ovale (B53.0)
Malaria due to simian plasmodia with Plasmodium vivax (B51.-)

B53.8 Other malaria, not elsewhere classified

B54 Unspecified malaria ▽

✓4ᵗʰ **B55 Leishmaniasis**

B55.0 Visceral leishmaniasis
Kala-azar
Post-kala-azar dermal leishmaniasis

B55.1 Cutaneous leishmaniasis

B55.2 Mucocutaneous leishmaniasis

B55.9 Leishmaniasis, unspecified ▽

✓4ᵗʰ **B56 African trypanosomiasis**

B56.0 Gambiense trypanosomiasis
Infection due to Trypanosoma brucei gambiense
West African sleeping sickness

B56.1 Rhodesiense trypanosomiasis
East African sleeping sickness
Infection due to Trypanosoma brucei rhodesiense

B56.9 African trypanosomiasis, unspecified
Sleeping sickness NOS

✓4ᵗʰ **B57 Chagas' disease**
INCLUDES American trypanosomiasis
infection due to Trypanosoma cruzi

B57.0 Acute Chagas' disease with heart involvement
Acute Chagas' disease with myocarditis

B57.1 Acute Chagas' disease without heart involvement
Acute Chagas' disease NOS

B57.2 Chagas' disease (chronic) with heart involvement
American trypanosomiasis NOS
Chagas' disease (chronic) NOS
Chagas' disease (chronic) with myocarditis
Trypanosomiasis NOS

✓5ᵗʰ **B57.3 Chagas' disease (chronic) with digestive system involvement**

B57.30 Chagas' disease with digestive system involvement, unspecified ▽

B57.31 Megaesophagus in Chagas' disease

B57.32 Megacolon in Chagas' disease

B57.39 Other digestive system involvement in Chagas' disease

✓5ᵗʰ **B57.4 Chagas' disease (chronic) with nervous system involvement**

B57.40 Chagas' disease with nervous system involvement, unspecified ▽

B57.41 Meningitis in Chagas' disease

B57.42 Meningoencephalitis in Chagas' disease

B57.49 Other nervous system involvement in Chagas' disease

B57.5 Chagas' disease (chronic) with other organ involvement

✓4ᵗʰ **B58 Toxoplasmosis**
INCLUDES infection due to Toxoplasma gondii
EXCLUDES 1 *congenital toxoplasmosis (P37.1)*

✓5ᵗʰ **B58.0 Toxoplasma oculopathy**

B58.00 Toxoplasma oculopathy, unspecified ▽

B58.01 Toxoplasma chorioretinitis

B58.09 Other toxoplasma oculopathy
Toxoplasma uveitis

B58.1 Toxoplasma hepatitis

B58.2 Toxoplasma meningoencephalitis

B58.3 Pulmonary toxoplasmosis

✓5ᵗʰ **B58.8 Toxoplasmosis with other organ involvement**

B58.81 Toxoplasma myocarditis

B58.82 Toxoplasma myositis

B58.83 Toxoplasma tubulo-interstitial nephropathy
Toxoplasma pyelonephritis

B58.89 Toxoplasmosis with other organ involvement

B58.9 Toxoplasmosis, unspecified ▽

B59 Pneumocystosis
Pneumonia due to Pneumocystis carinii
Pneumonia due to Pneumocystis jiroveci

✓4ᵗʰ **B60 Other protozoal diseases, not elsewhere classified**
EXCLUDES 1 *cryptosporidiosis (AØ7.2)*
intestinal microsporidiosis (AØ7.8)
isosporiasis (AØ7.3)

B60.0 Babesiosis
Piroplasmosis

✓5ᵗʰ **B60.1 Acanthamebiasis**

B60.10 Acanthamebiasis, unspecified ▽

B60.11 Meningoencephalitis due to Acanthamoeba (culbertsoni)

B60.12 Conjunctivitis due to Acanthamoeba

B60.13 Keratoconjunctivitis due to Acanthamoeba

B60.19 Other acanthamebic disease

B60.2 Naegleriasis
Primary amebic meningoencephalitis

B60.8 Other specified protozoal diseases
Microsporidiosis

B64 Unspecified protozoal disease ▽

Helminthiases (B65-B83)

✓4ᵗʰ **B65 Schistosomiasis [bilharziasis]**
INCLUDES snail fever

B65.0 Schistosomiasis due to Schistosoma haematobium [urinary schistosomiasis]

N Newborn: 0 ▪ P Pediatric: 0-17 ▪ M Maternity: 12-55 ▪ A Adult: 15-124 ▪ NRS Nonroutine supply Dx ▪ NC Dx Noncancer Dx ▪ PDx Primary Dx ▪ ►◄ Revised Text ▪ ● New Code ▪ ▲ Revised Title

452 | ICD-10-CM 2018

B65.1 Schistosomiasis due to Schistosoma mansoni [intestinal schistosomiasis]

B65.2 Schistosomiasis due to Schistosoma japonicum
Asiatic schistosomiasis

B65.3 Cercarial dermatitis   NRS
Swimmer's itch

B65.8 Other schistosomiasis
Infection due to Schistosoma intercalatum
Infection due to Schistosoma mattheei
Infection due to Schistosoma mekongi

B65.9 Schistosomiasis, unspecified ▽

☑4th **B66 Other fluke infections**

B66.0 Opisthorchiasis
Infection due to cat liver fluke
Infection due to Opisthorchis (felineus)(viverrini)

B66.1 Clonorchiasis
Chinese liver fluke disease
Infection due to Clonorchis sinensis
Oriental liver fluke disease

B66.2 Dicroceliasis
Infection due to Dicrocoelium dendriticum
Lancet fluke infection

B66.3 Fascioliasis
Infection due to Fasciola gigantica
Infection due to Fasciola hepatica
Infection due to Fasciola indica
Sheep liver fluke disease

B66.4 Paragonimiasis
Infection due to Paragonimus species
Lung fluke disease
Pulmonary distomiasis

B66.5 Fasciolopsiasis
Infection due to Fasciolopsis buski
Intestinal distomiasis

B66.8 Other specified fluke infections
Echinostomiasis   Nanophyetiasis
Heterophyiasis   Watsoniasis
Metagonimiasis

B66.9 Fluke infection, unspecified ▽

☑4th **B67 Echinococcosis**
INCLUDES hydatidosis

B67.0 Echinococcus granulosus infection of liver

B67.1 Echinococcus granulosus infection of lung

B67.2 Echinococcus granulosus infection of bone

☑5th **B67.3 Echinococcus granulosus infection, other and multiple sites**

    B67.31 Echinococcus granulosus infection, thyroid gland

    B67.32 Echinococcus granulosus infection, multiple sites

    B67.39 Echinococcus granulosus infection, other sites

B67.4 Echinococcus granulosus infection, unspecified ▽
Dog tapeworm (infection)

B67.5 Echinococcus multilocularis infection of liver

☑5th **B67.6 Echinococcus multilocularis infection, other and multiple sites**

    B67.61 Echinococcus multilocularis infection, multiple sites

    B67.69 Echinococcus multilocularis infection, other sites

B67.7 Echinococcus multilocularis infection, unspecified ▽

B67.8 Echinococcosis, unspecified, of liver ▽

☑5th **B67.9 Echinococcosis, other and unspecified**

    B67.90 Echinococcosis, unspecified ▽
Echinococcosis NOS

    B67.99 Other echinococcosis

☑4th **B68 Taeniasis**
EXCLUDES 1 cysticercosis (B69.-)

B68.0 Taenia solium taeniasis
Pork tapeworm (infection)

B68.1 Taenia saginata taeniasis
Beef tapeworm (infection)
Infection due to adult tapeworm Taenia saginata

B68.9 Taeniasis, unspecified ▽

☑4th **B69 Cysticercosis**
INCLUDES cysticerciasis infection due to larval form of Taenia solium

B69.0 Cysticercosis of central nervous system

B69.1 Cysticercosis of eye

☑5th **B69.8 Cysticercosis of other sites**

    B69.81 Myositis in cysticercosis

    B69.89 Cysticercosis of other sites

B69.9 Cysticercosis, unspecified ▽

☑4th **B70 Diphyllobothriasis and sparganosis**

B70.0 Diphyllobothriasis
Diphyllobothrium (adult) (latum) (pacificum) infection
Fish tapeworm (infection)
EXCLUDES 2 larval diphyllobothriasis (B70.1)

B70.1 Sparganosis
Infection due to Sparganum (mansoni) (proliferum)
Infection due to Spirometra larva
Larval diphyllobothriasis
Spirometrosis

☑4th **B71 Other cestode infections**

B71.0 Hymenolepiasis
Dwarf tapeworm infection
Rat tapeworm (infection)

B71.1 Dipylidiasis

B71.8 Other specified cestode infections
Coenurosis

B71.9 Cestode infection, unspecified ▽
Tapeworm (infection) NOS

B72 Dracunculiasis
INCLUDES guinea worm infection
infection due to Dracunculus medinensis

☑4th **B73 Onchocerciasis**
INCLUDES onchocerca volvulus infection
onchocercosis
river blindness

☑5th **B73.0 Onchocerciasis with eye disease**

    B73.00 Onchocerciasis with eye involvement, unspecified ▽

    B73.01 Onchocerciasis with endophthalmitis

    B73.02 Onchocerciasis with glaucoma

    B73.09 Onchocerciasis with other eye involvement
Infestation of eyelid due to onchocerciasis

B73.1 Onchocerciasis without eye disease

☑4th **B74 Filariasis**
EXCLUDES 2 onchocerciasis (B73)
tropical (pulmonary) eosinophilia NOS (J82)

B74.0 Filariasis due to Wuchereria bancrofti
Bancroftian elephantiasis
Bancroftian filariasis

B74.1 Filariasis due to Brugia malayi

B74.2 Filariasis due to Brugia timori

B74.3 Loiasis
Calabar swelling
Eyeworm disease of Africa
Loa loa infection

B74.4 Mansonelliasis
Infection due to Mansonella ozzardi
Infection due to Mansonella perstans
Infection due to Mansonella streptocerca

B74.8 Other filariases
Dirofilariasis

B74.9 Filariasis, unspecified ▽

B75 Trichinellosis
INCLUDES infection due to Trichinella species
trichiniasis

☑4th **B76 Hookworm diseases**
INCLUDES uncinariasis

B76.0 Ancylostomiasis
Infection due to Ancylostoma species

B76.1 Necatoriasis
Infection due to Necator americanus

B76.8 Other hookworm diseases

B76.9 Hookworm disease, unspecified ▽
Cutaneous larva migrans NOS

☑4th **B77 Ascariasis**
INCLUDES ascaridiasis
roundworm infection

B77.0 Ascariasis with intestinal complications

☑5th **B77.8 Ascariasis with other complications**

    B77.81 Ascariasis pneumonia

    B77.89 Ascariasis with other complications

B77.9 Ascariasis, unspecified ▽

☑ Additional Character Req   ✓x7th Placeholder Alert   Case-Mix Diagnosis   Manifestation   ▽ Unspecified Dx   EXCLUDES 1 Not coded here   EXCLUDES 2 Not included here

Chapter 1. Certain Infectious and Parasitic Diseases

✓4ᵗʰ **B78 Strongyloidiasis**
    EXCLUDES 1   *trichostrongyliasis (B81.2)*
  B78.0   Intestinal **strongyloidiasis**
  B78.1   Cutaneous **strongyloidiasis**   **NRS**
  B78.7   Disseminated **strongyloidiasis**
  B78.9   **Strongyloidiasis, unspecified**   ▽

B79 Trichuriasis
    INCLUDES   trichocephaliasis
                whipworm (disease)(infection)

B80 Enterobiasis
    INCLUDES   oxyuriasis
                pinworm infection
                threadworm infection

✓4ᵗʰ **B81 Other intestinal helminthiases, not elsewhere classified**
    EXCLUDES 1 ►*angiostrongyliasis due to:*
             angiostrongylus cantonensis (B83.2)
             parastrongylus cantonensis (B83.2) ◄
  B81.0   **Anisakiasis**
          Infection due to Anisakis larva
  B81.1   **Intestinal capillariasis**
          Capillariasis NOS
          Infection due to Capillaria philippinensis
         EXCLUDES 2   *hepatic capillariasis (B83.8)*
  B81.2   **Trichostrongyliasis**
  B81.3   **Intestinal angiostrongyliasis**
          ►Angiostrongyliasis due to:
             angiostrongylus costaricensis
             parastrongylus costaricensis◄
  B81.4   **Mixed intestinal helminthiases**
          Infection due to intestinal helminths classified to more than one
            of the categories B65.0-B81.3 and B81.8
          Mixed helminthiasis NOS
  B81.8   **Other specified intestinal helminthiases**
          Infection due to Oesophagostomum species
            [esophagostomiasis]
          Infection due to Ternidens diminutus [ternidensiasis]

✓4ᵗʰ **B82 Unspecified intestinal parasitism**
  B82.0   Intestinal **helminthiasis, unspecified**   ▽
  B82.9   Intestinal **parasitism, unspecified**   ▽

✓4ᵗʰ **B83 Other helminthiases**
    EXCLUDES 1   *capillariasis NOS (B81.1)*
    EXCLUDES 2   *intestinal capillariasis (B81.1)*
  B83.0   **Visceral larva migrans**
          Toxocariasis
  B83.1   **Gnathostomiasis**
          Wandering swelling
  B83.2   **Angiostrongyliasis due to Parastrongylus cantonensis**
          Eosinophilic meningoencephalitis due to Parastrongylus
            cantonensis
         EXCLUDES 2   *intestinal angiostrongyliasis (B81.3)*
  B83.3   **Syngamiasis**
          Syngamosis
  B83.4   **Internal hirudiniasis**
         EXCLUDES 2   *external hirudiniasis (B88.3)*
  B83.8   **Other specified helminthiases**
          Acanthocephaliasis
          Gongylonemiasis
          Hepatic capillariasis
          Metastrongyliasis
          Thelaziasis
  B83.9   **Helminthiasis, unspecified**   ▽
          Worms NOS
         EXCLUDES 1   *intestinal helminthiasis NOS (B82.0)*

Pediculosis, acariasis and other infestations (B85-B89)

✓4ᵗʰ **B85 Pediculosis and phthiriasis**
  B85.0   **Pediculosis due to** Pediculus humanus capitis
          Head-louse infestation
  B85.1   **Pediculosis due to** Pediculus humanus corporis
          Body-louse infestation
  B85.2   **Pediculosis, unspecified**   ▽
  B85.3   Phthiriasis
          Infestation by crab-louse
          Infestation by Phthirus pubis

  B85.4   Mixed **pediculosis and phthiriasis**
          Infestation classifiable to more than one of the categories B85.0-
            B85.3

B86 Scabies
     Sarcoptic itch

✓4ᵗʰ **B87 Myiasis**
    INCLUDES   infestation by larva of flies
  B87.0   **Cutaneous myiasis**
          Creeping myiasis
  B87.1   **Wound myiasis**
          Traumatic myiasis
  B87.2   **Ocular myiasis**
  B87.3   **Nasopharyngeal myiasis**
          Laryngeal myiasis
  B87.4   **Aural myiasis**
  ✓5ᵗʰ **B87.8**   **Myiasis of** other sites
      B87.81   **Genitourinary myiasis**
      B87.82   **Intestinal myiasis**
      B87.89   **Myiasis of other sites**
  B87.9   **Myiasis, unspecified**   ▽

✓4ᵗʰ **B88 Other infestations**
  B88.0   **Other acariasis**
          Acarine dermatitis
          Dermatitis due to Demodex species
          Dermatitis due to Dermanyssus gallinae
          Dermatitis due to Liponyssoides sanguineus
          Trombiculosis
         EXCLUDES 2   *scabies (B86)*
  B88.1   **Tungiasis [sandflea infestation]**
  B88.2   **Other arthropod infestations**
          Scarabiasis
  B88.3   **External hirudiniasis**
          Leech infestation NOS
         EXCLUDES 2   *internal hirudiniasis (B83.4)*
  B88.8   **Other specified infestations**
          Ichthyoparasitism due to Vandellia cirrhosa
          Linguatulosis
          Porocephaliasis
  B88.9   **Infestation, unspecified**   ▽
          Infestation (skin) NOS
          Infestation by mites NOS
          Skin parasites NOS

B89 Unspecified parasitic disease   ▽

Sequelae of infectious and parasitic diseases (B90-B94)

    NOTE   Categories B90-B94 are to be used to indicate conditions in
           categories A00-B89 as the cause of sequelae, which are themselves
           classified elsewhere. The "sequelae" include conditions specified as
           such; they also include residuals of diseases classifiable to the above
           categories if there is evidence that the disease itself is no longer
           present. Codes from these categories are not to be used for chronic
           infections. Code chronic current infections to active infectious
           disease as appropriate.

  Code first condition resulting from (sequela) the infectious or parasitic disease

✓4ᵗʰ **B90 Sequelae of** tuberculosis
  B90.0   **Sequelae of** central nervous system **tuberculosis**
  B90.1   **Sequelae of** genitourinary **tuberculosis**
  B90.2   **Sequelae of tuberculosis of** bones and joints
  B90.8   **Sequelae of tuberculosis of other organs**
         EXCLUDES 2   *sequelae of respiratory tuberculosis (B90.9)*
  B90.9   **Sequelae of** respiratory **and unspecified tuberculosis**   ▽
          Sequelae of tuberculosis NOS

B91 Sequelae of poliomyelitis
    EXCLUDES 1   *postpolio syndrome (G14)*

B92 Sequelae of leprosy

✓4ᵗʰ **B94 Sequelae of** other and unspecified **infectious and parasitic diseases**
  B94.0   **Sequelae of** trachoma
  B94.1   **Sequelae of** viral encephalitis
  B94.2   **Sequelae of** viral hepatitis
  B94.8   **Sequelae of other specified infectious and parasitic diseases**
  B94.9   **Sequelae of unspecified infectious and parasitic disease**   ▽

N Newborn: 0   **P** Pediatric: 0-17   **M** Maternity: 12-55   **A** Adult: 15-124   **NRS** Nonroutine supply Dx   **NC Dx** Noncancer Dx   **PDx** Primary Dx   ►◄ Revised Text   ● New Code   ▲ Revised Title

454   ICD-10-CM 2018

Bacterial and viral infectious agents (B95-B97)

NOTE　These categories are provided for use as supplementary or additional codes to identify the infectious agent(s) in diseases classified elsewhere.

✓4ᵗʰ **B95** **Streptococcus, Staphylococcus, and Enterococcus as the cause of diseases classified elsewhere**

B95.0 Streptococcus, group A, as the cause of diseases classified elsewhere

B95.1 Streptococcus, group B, as the cause of diseases classified elsewhere

B95.2 Enterococcus as the cause of diseases classified elsewhere

B95.3 Streptococcus pneumoniae as the cause of diseases classified elsewhere

B95.4 Other streptococcus as the cause of diseases classified elsewhere

B95.5 Unspecified streptococcus as the cause of diseases classified elsewhere ▽

✓5ᵗʰ **B95.6** Staphylococcus aureus as the cause of diseases classified elsewhere

B95.61 Methicillin susceptible **Staphylococcus aureus infection as the cause of diseases classified elsewhere**
Methicillin susceptible Staphylococcus aureus (MSSA) infection as the cause of diseases classified elsewhere
Staphylococcus aureus infection NOS as the cause of diseases classified elsewhere

B95.62 Methicillin resistant **Staphylococcus aureus infection as the cause of diseases classified elsewhere**
Methicillin resistant Staphylococcus aureus (MRSA) infection as the cause of diseases classified elsewhere
AHA: 2016, 1Q, 12

B95.7 Other staphylococcus as the cause of diseases classified elsewhere

B95.8 Unspecified staphylococcus as the cause of diseases classified elsewhere ▽

✓4ᵗʰ **B96** **Other bacterial agents as the cause of diseases classified elsewhere**

B96.0 Mycoplasma pneumoniae [M. pneumoniae] as the cause of diseases classified elsewhere
Pleuro-pneumonia-like-organism [PPLO]

B96.1 Klebsiella pneumoniae [K. pneumoniae] as the cause of diseases classified elsewhere

✓5ᵗʰ **B96.2** Escherichia coli [E. coli] as the cause of diseases classified elsewhere

B96.20 Unspecified Escherichia coli [E. coli] as the cause of diseases classified elsewhere ▽
Escherichia coli [E. coli] NOS

B96.21 Shiga toxin-producing **Escherichia coli [E. coli] (STEC) O157 as the cause of diseases classified elsewhere**
E. coli O157:H- (nonmotile) with confirmation of Shiga toxin
E. coli O157 with confirmation of Shiga toxin when H antigen is unknown, or is not H7
O157:H7 Escherichia coli [E.coli] with or without confirmation of Shiga toxin-production
Shiga toxin-producing Escherichia coli [E.coli] O157:H7 with or without confirmation of Shiga toxin-production
STEC O157:H7 with or without confirmation of Shiga toxin-production

B96.22 Other specified Shiga toxin-producing **Escherichia coli [E. coli] (STEC) as the cause of diseases classified elsewhere**
Non-O157 Shiga toxin-producing Escherichia coli [E.coli]
Non-O157 Shiga toxin-producing Escherichia coli [E.coli] with known O group

B96.23 Unspecified Shiga toxin-producing **Escherichia coli [E. coli] (STEC) as the cause of diseases classified elsewhere** ▽
Shiga toxin-producing Escherichia coli [E. coli] with unspecified O group
STEC NOS

B96.29 Other Escherichia coli [E. coli] as the cause of diseases classified elsewhere
Non-Shiga toxin-producing E. coli

B96.3 Hemophilus influenzae [H. influenzae] as the cause of diseases classified elsewhere

B96.4 Proteus (mirabilis) (morganii) as the cause of diseases classified elsewhere

B96.5 Pseudomonas (aeruginosa) (mallei) (pseudomallei) as the cause of diseases classified elsewhere
AHA: 2015, 1Q, 18

B96.6 Bacteroides fragilis [B. fragilis] as the cause of diseases classified elsewhere

B96.7 Clostridium perfringens [C. perfringens] as the cause of diseases classified elsewhere

✓5ᵗʰ **B96.8** Other specified bacterial agents as the cause of diseases classified elsewhere

B96.81 Helicobacter pylori [H. pylori] as the cause of diseases classified elsewhere

B96.82 Vibrio vulnificus as the cause of diseases classified elsewhere

B96.89 Other specified bacterial agents as the cause of diseases classified elsewhere

✓4ᵗʰ **B97** **Viral agents as the cause of diseases classified elsewhere**
AHA: 2016, 3Q, 8-10, 14

B97.0 Adenovirus as the cause of diseases classified elsewhere

✓5ᵗʰ **B97.1** Enterovirus as the cause of diseases classified elsewhere

B97.10 Unspecified enterovirus as the cause of diseases classified elsewhere ▽

B97.11 Coxsackievirus as the cause of diseases classified elsewhere

B97.12 Echovirus as the cause of diseases classified elsewhere

B97.19 Other enterovirus as the cause of diseases classified elsewhere

✓5ᵗʰ **B97.2** Coronavirus as the cause of diseases classified elsewhere

B97.21 SARS-associated **coronavirus as the cause of diseases classified elsewhere**
EXCLUDES 1 pneumonia due to SARS-associated coronavirus (J12.81)

B97.29 Other coronavirus as the cause of diseases classified elsewhere

✓5ᵗʰ **B97.3** Retrovirus as the cause of diseases classified elsewhere
EXCLUDES 1 human immunodeficiency virus [HIV] disease (B20)

B97.30 Unspecified retrovirus as the cause of diseases classified elsewhere ▽

B97.31 Lentivirus as the cause of diseases classified elsewhere

B97.32 Oncovirus as the cause of diseases classified elsewhere

B97.33 Human T-cell lymphotrophic virus, type I [HTLV-I] as the cause of diseases classified elsewhere

B97.34 Human T-cell lymphotrophic virus, type II [HTLV-II] as the cause of diseases classified elsewhere

B97.35 Human immunodeficiency virus, type 2 [HIV 2] as the cause of diseases classified elsewhere

B97.39 Other retrovirus as the cause of diseases classified elsewhere

B97.4 Respiratory syncytial **virus as the cause of diseases classified elsewhere**

B97.5 Reovirus as the cause of diseases classified elsewhere

B97.6 Parvovirus as the cause of diseases classified elsewhere

B97.7 Papillomavirus as the cause of diseases classified elsewhere

✓5ᵗʰ **B97.8** Other viral agents as the cause of diseases classified elsewhere

B97.81 Human metapneumovirus as the cause of diseases classified elsewhere

B97.89 Other viral agents as the cause of diseases classified elsewhere

Other infectious diseases (B99)

✓4ᵗʰ **B99** **Other and unspecified infectious diseases**

B99.8 Other infectious disease

B99.9 Unspecified infectious disease ▽

✓ Additional Character Req　✓x7ᵗʰ Placeholder Alert　Case-Mix Diagnosis　Manifestation　▽ Unspecified Dx　**EXCLUDES 1** Not coded here　**EXCLUDES 2** Not included here

ICD-10-CM 2018　　　　　　　　　　　　　　　　　　　　　　**455**

Chapter 2. Neoplasms (C00–D49)

Chapter Specific Guidelines with Coding Examples

The chapter specific guidelines from the ICD-10-CM Official Guidelines for Coding and Reporting have been provided below. Along with these guidelines are coding examples, contained in the shaded boxes, that have been developed to help illustrate the coding and/or sequencing guidance found in these guidelines.

General guidelines

Chapter 2 of the ICD-10-CM contains the codes for most benign and all malignant neoplasms. Certain benign neoplasms, such as prostatic adenomas, may be found in the specific body system chapters. To properly code a neoplasm it is necessary to determine from the record if the neoplasm is benign, in-situ, malignant, or of uncertain histologic behavior. If malignant, any secondary (metastatic) sites should also be determined.

Primary malignant neoplasms overlapping site boundaries

A primary malignant neoplasm that overlaps two or more contiguous (next to each other) sites should be classified to the subcategory/code .8 ('overlapping lesion'), unless the combination is specifically indexed elsewhere. For multiple neoplasms of the same site that are not contiguous such as tumors in different quadrants of the same breast, codes for each site should be assigned.

> A 73-year-old white female with a large rapidly growing malignant tumor in the left breast extending from the upper outer quadrant into the axillary tail.
>
> **C50.812   Malignant neoplasm of overlapping sites of left female breast**
>
> *Explanation*: Because this is a single large tumor that overlaps two contiguous sites, a single code for overlapping sites is assigned.

> A 52-year old white female with two distinct lesions of the right breast, one (0.5 cm) in the upper outer quadrant and a second (1.5 cm) in the lower outer quadrant; path report indicates both lesions are malignant
>
> **C50.411   Malignant neoplasm of upper-outer quadrant of breast, female**
>
> **C50.511   Malignant neoplasm of lower-outer quadrant of breast, female**
>
> *Explanation*: This patient has two distinct malignant lesions of right breast in adjacent quadrants. Because the lesions are not contiguous, two codes are reported.

Malignant neoplasm of ectopic tissue

Malignant neoplasms of ectopic tissue are to be coded to the site of origin mentioned, e.g., ectopic pancreatic malignant neoplasms involving the stomach are coded to **malignant neoplasm of** pancreas, unspecified (C25.9).

The neoplasm table in the Alphabetic Index should be referenced first. However, if the histological term is documented, that term should be referenced first, rather than going immediately to the Neoplasm Table, in order to determine which column in the Neoplasm Table is appropriate. For example, if the documentation indicates "adenoma," refer to the term in the Alphabetic Index to review the entries under this term and the instructional note to "see also neoplasm, by site, benign." The table provides the proper code based on the type of neoplasm and the site. It is important to select the proper column in the table that corresponds to the type of neoplasm. The Tabular List should then be referenced to verify that the correct code has been selected from the table and that a more specific site code does not exist.

See Section I.C.21. Factors influencing health status and contact with health services, Status, for information regarding Z15.0, codes for genetic susceptibility to cancer.

a. Treatment directed at the malignancy

If the treatment is directed at the malignancy, designate the malignancy as the principal diagnosis.

The only exception to this guideline is if a patient admission/encounter is solely for the administration of chemotherapy, immunotherapy or **external beam** radiation therapy, assign the appropriate Z51.-- code as the first-listed or principal diagnosis, and the diagnosis or problem for which the service is being performed as a secondary diagnosis.

b. Treatment of secondary site

When a patient is admitted because of a primary neoplasm with metastasis and treatment is directed toward the secondary site only, the secondary neoplasm is designated as the principal diagnosis even though the primary malignancy is still present.

> Patient with unresolved primary prostate cancer is admitted for respiratory care and rehabilitation related to new diagnosis of right lung metastasis.
>
> **C78.01   Secondary malignant neoplasm of right lung**
>
> **C61   Malignant neoplasm of prostate**
>
> *Explanation*: The patient was admitted for treatment of the secondary neoplastic disease of the right lung with respiratory care. The code for the secondary lung metastasis is sequenced before the code for primary prostate cancer.

c. Coding and sequencing of complications

Coding and sequencing of complications associated with the malignancies or with the therapy thereof are subject to the following guidelines:

1) Anemia associated with malignancy

When admission/encounter is for management of an anemia associated with the malignancy, and the treatment is only for anemia, the appropriate code for the malignancy is sequenced as the principal or first-listed diagnosis followed by the appropriate code for the anemia (such as code D63.0, Anemia in neoplastic disease).

> Patient is admitted for treatment of anemia in advanced colon cancer.
>
> **C18.9   Malignant neoplasm of colon, unspecified**
>
> **D63.0   Anemia in neoplastic disease**
>
> *Explanation*: Even though the admission was solely to treat the anemia, this guideline indicates that the code for the malignancy is sequenced first.

2) Anemia associated with chemotherapy, immunotherapy and radiation therapy

When the admission/encounter is for management of an anemia associated with an adverse effect of the administration of chemotherapy or immunotherapy and the only treatment is for the anemia, the anemia code is sequenced first followed by the appropriate codes for the neoplasm and the adverse effect (T45.1X5, Adverse effect of antineoplastic and immunosuppressive drugs).

> A 52-year-old male with chronic lymphocytic leukemia noted with Richter transformation following acute mononucleosis infection, now resolved, is admitted for assessment and monitoring of labs. The clinical record notes anemia secondary to chemotherapy and weekly lab orders. The patient continues to receive chemotherapy.
>
> **D64.81   Anemia due to antineoplastic chemotherapy**
>
> **T45.1X5D   Adverse effect of antineoplastic drugs and immunosuppressive drugs, subsequent encounter**
>
> **C91.10   Chronic lymphocytic leukemia of B-Cell type not having achieved remission**
>
> *Explanation*: The code for anemia is sequenced before the code for the neoplasm and the adverse effect of chemotherapy. The seventh character D is applied to code T45.1X5-, as active treatment of the adverse effect, the anemia, is no longer required.

When the admission/encounter is for management of an anemia associated with an adverse effect of radiotherapy, the anemia code should be sequenced first, followed by the appropriate neoplasm code and code Y84.2, Radiological procedure and radiotherapy as the cause of abnormal reaction of the patient, or of later complication, without mention of misadventure at the time of the procedure.

> A 65-year-old female is admitted following hospitalization for multiple blood transfusions to treat anemia secondary to radiation therapy. She has been receiving radiation treatments for right breast cancer.
>
> **D64.89**   **Other specified anemias**
>
> **C50.911**   **Malignant neoplasm of unspecified site of right female breast**
>
> **Y84.2**   **Radiological procedure and radiotherapy as the cause of abnormal reaction of the patient, or of later complication, without mention of misadventure at the time of the procedure**
>
> *Explanation*: The code for the anemia is sequenced first, followed by the code for the malignancy, and last the code for the abnormal reaction due to radiotherapy.

3) Management of dehydration due to the malignancy

When the admission/encounter is for management of dehydration due to the malignancy and only the dehydration is being treated (intravenous rehydration), the dehydration is sequenced first, followed by the code(s) for the malignancy.

4) Treatment of a complication resulting from a surgical procedure

When the admission/encounter is for treatment of a complication resulting from a surgical procedure, designate the complication as the principal or first-listed diagnosis if treatment is directed at resolving the complication.

d. Primary malignancy previously excised

When a primary malignancy has been previously excised or eradicated from its site and there is no further treatment directed to that site and there is no evidence of any existing primary malignancy, a code from category Z85, Personal history of malignant neoplasm, should be used to indicate the former site of the malignancy. Any mention of extension, invasion, or metastasis to another site is coded as a secondary malignant neoplasm to that site. The secondary site may be the principal or first-listed with the Z85 code used as a secondary code.

> History of breast cancer, left radical mastectomy 18 months ago with no current treatment; bronchoscopy with lung biopsy shows metastatic disease in the right lung.
>
> **C78.01**   **Secondary malignant neoplasm of right lung**
>
> **Z85.3**   **Personal history of malignant neoplasm of breast**
>
> *Explanation*: The patient has undergone a diagnostic procedure that revealed metastatic breast cancer in the right lung. The code for the secondary (metastatic) site is sequenced first followed by a personal history code to identify the former site of the primary malignancy.

e. Admissions/Encounters involving chemotherapy, immunotherapy and radiation therapy

1) Episode of care involves surgical removal of neoplasm

When an episode of care involves the surgical removal of a neoplasm, primary or secondary site, followed by adjunct chemotherapy or radiation treatment during the same episode of care, the code for the neoplasm should be assigned as principal or first-listed diagnosis.

2) Patient admission/encounter solely for administration of chemotherapy, immunotherapy and radiation therapy

If a patient admission/encounter is solely for the administration of chemotherapy, immunotherapy or **external beam** radiation therapy assign code Z51.0, Encounter for antineoplastic radiation therapy, or Z51.11, Encounter for antineoplastic chemotherapy, or Z51.12, Encounter for antineoplastic immunotherapy as the first-listed or principal diagnosis. If a patient receives more than one of these therapies during the same admission more than one of these codes may be assigned, in any sequence.

The malignancy for which the therapy is being administered should be assigned as a secondary diagnosis.

If a patient admission/encounter is for the insertion or implantation of radioactive elements (e.g., brachytherapy) the appropriate code for the malignancy is sequenced as the principal or first-listed diagnosis. Code Z51.0 should not be assigned.

3) Patient admitted for radiation therapy, chemotherapy or immunotherapy and develops complications

When a patient is admitted for the purpose of **external beam** radiotherapy, immunotherapy or chemotherapy and develops complications such as uncontrolled nausea and vomiting or dehydration, the principal or first-listed diagnosis is Z51.0, Encounter for antineoplastic radiation therapy, or Z51.11, Encounter for antineoplastic chemotherapy, or Z51.12, Encounter for antineoplastic immunotherapy followed by any codes for the complications.

When a patient is admitted for the purpose of insertion or implantation of radioactive elements (e.g., brachytherapy) and develops complications such as uncontrolled nausea and vomiting or dehydration, the principal or first-listed diagnosis is the appropriate code for the malignancy followed by any codes for the complications.

f. Admission/encounter to determine extent of malignancy

When the reason for admission/encounter is to determine the extent of the malignancy, or for a procedure such as paracentesis or thoracentesis, the primary malignancy or appropriate metastatic site is designated as the principal or first-listed diagnosis, even though chemotherapy or radiotherapy is administered.

g. Symptoms, signs, and abnormal findings listed in Chapter 18 associated with neoplasms

Symptoms, signs, and ill-defined conditions listed in Chapter 18 characteristic of, or associated with, an existing primary or secondary site malignancy cannot be used to replace the malignancy as principal or first-listed diagnosis, regardless of the number of admissions or encounters for treatment and care of the neoplasm.

See Section I.C.21. Factors influencing health status and contact with health services, Encounter for prophylactic organ removal.

> Patient is admitted for respiratory decline with severe shortness of breath and new onset use of continuous oxygen, related to inoperable neoplasm of the right lung.
>
> **C34.91**   **Malignant neoplasm of unspecified part of right bronchus or lung**
>
> **Z99.81**   **Dependence on supplemental oxygen**
>
> *Explanation*: No code is assigned for shortness of breath, as this symptom is an integral part of the neoplastic lung disease and should not take the place of a code for the neoplasm, regardless of encounter.

h. Admission/encounter for pain control/management

See Section I.C.6. for information on coding admission/encounter for pain control/management.

i. Malignancy in two or more noncontiguous sites

A patient may have more than one malignant tumor in the same organ. These tumors may represent different primaries or metastatic disease, depending on the site. Should the documentation be unclear, the provider should be queried as to the status of each tumor so that the correct codes can be assigned.

j. Disseminated malignant neoplasm, unspecified

Code C80.0, Disseminated malignant neoplasm, unspecified, is for use only in those cases where the patient has advanced metastatic disease and no known primary or secondary sites are specified. It should not be used in place of assigning codes for the primary site and all known secondary sites.

> Patient who has had no regular medical care for over 10 years until recent symptoms developed is admitted post-hospital stay with a new diagnosis of carcinomatosis.
>
> **C80.0**   **Disseminated malignant neoplasm, unspecified**
>
> *Explanation*: Carcinomatosis NOS is an "inclusion term" under code C80.0 Disseminated malignant neoplasm, unspecified. This code should seldom be used but is available for use in cases such as this.

k. Malignant neoplasm without specification of site

Code C80.1, Malignant (primary) neoplasm, unspecified, equates to Cancer, unspecified. This code should only be used when no determination can be made as to the primary site of a malignancy. This code should rarely be used in the inpatient setting.

> Evaluation of painful hip leads to diagnosis of a metastatic bone lesion from an unknown primary neoplasm source.
>
> **C79.51**   **Secondary malignant neoplasm of bone**
>
> **C80.1**   **Malignant (primary) neoplasm, unspecified**
>
> *Explanation*: If only the secondary site is known, use code C80.1 for the unknown primary site.

l. Sequencing of neoplasm codes

1) Encounter for treatment of primary malignancy

If the reason for the encounter is for treatment of a primary malignancy, assign the malignancy as the principal/first-listed diagnosis. The primary site is to be sequenced first, followed by any metastatic sites.

2) Encounter for treatment of secondary malignancy

When an encounter is for a primary malignancy with metastasis and treatment is directed toward the metastatic (secondary) site(s) only, the metastatic site(s) is designated as the principal/first-listed diagnosis. The primary malignancy is coded as an additional code.

> Patient is admitted with primary colon cancer with new onset metastasis to the ribs resulting in shortness of breath and pain.
>
> **C79.51**   **Secondary malignant neoplasm of bone**
>
> **C18.9**   **Malignant neoplasm of colon, unspecified**
>
> **G89.3**   **Neoplasm related pain (acute) (chronic)**
>
> *Explanation*: The focus of care for this admission is on the newly diagnosed metastasis to the ribs (bone) rather than the primary colon cancer, indicating a need to code the metastasis to the bone as primary. Provider documentation supports pain due to neoplastic disease, as well.

3) Malignant neoplasm in a pregnant patient

When a pregnant woman has a malignant neoplasm, a code from subcategory O9A.1-, Malignant neoplasm complicating pregnancy, childbirth, and the puerperium, should be sequenced first, followed by the appropriate code from Chapter 2 to indicate the type of neoplasm.

4) Encounter for complication associated with a neoplasm

When an encounter is for management of a complication associated with a neoplasm, such as dehydration, and the treatment is only for the complication, the complication is coded first, followed by the appropriate code(s) for the neoplasm.

The exception to this guideline is anemia. When the admission/encounter is for management of an anemia associated with the malignancy, and the treatment is only for anemia, the appropriate code for the malignancy is sequenced as the principal or first-listed diagnosis followed by code D63.0, Anemia in neoplastic disease.

> Patient with pancreatic cancer is seen for initiation of TPN for cancer-related moderate protein-calorie malnutrition.
>
> **E44.0**   **Moderate protein-calorie malnutrition**
>
> **C25.9**   **Malignant neoplasm of pancreas, unspecified**
>
> *Explanation*: The encounter is to initiate treatment for malnutrition, a common complication of many types of neoplasms, and is sequenced first.

5) Complication from surgical procedure for treatment of a neoplasm

When an encounter is for treatment of a complication resulting from a surgical procedure performed for the treatment of the neoplasm, designate the complication as the principal/first-listed diagnosis. See guideline regarding the coding of a current malignancy versus personal history to determine if the code for the neoplasm should also be assigned.

6) Pathologic fracture due to a neoplasm

When an encounter is for a pathological fracture due to a neoplasm, and the focus of treatment is the fracture, a code from subcategory M84.5, Pathological fracture in neoplastic disease, should be sequenced first, followed by the code for the neoplasm.

If the focus of treatment is the neoplasm with an associated pathological fracture, the neoplasm code should be sequenced first, followed by a code from M84.5 for the pathological fracture.

m. Current malignancy versus personal history of malignancy

When a primary malignancy has been excised but further treatment, such as an additional surgery for the malignancy, radiation therapy or chemotherapy is directed to that site, the primary malignancy code should be used until treatment is completed.

When a primary malignancy has been previously excised or eradicated from its site, there is no further treatment (of the malignancy) directed to that site, and there is no evidence of any existing primary malignancy, a code from category Z85, Personal history of malignant neoplasm, should be used to indicate the former site of the malignancy.

See Section I.C.21. Factors influencing health status and contact with health services, History (of)

> Female patient with ongoing chemotherapy after right mastectomy for breast cancer.
>
> **C50.911**   **Malignant neoplasm of unspecified site of right female breast**
>
> **Z90.11**   **Acquired absence of right breast and nipple**
>
> *Explanation*: Even though the breast has been removed, the breast cancer is still being treated with chemotherapy and therefore is still coded as a current condition rather than personal history.

n. Leukemia, multiple myeloma, and malignant plasma cell neoplasms in remission versus personal history

The categories for leukemia, and category C90, Multiple myeloma and malignant plasma cell neoplasms, have codes indicating whether or not the leukemia has achieved remission. There are also codes Z85.6, Personal history of leukemia, and Z85.79, Personal history of other malignant neoplasms of lymphoid, hematopoietic and related tissues. If the documentation is unclear as to whether the leukemia has achieved remission, the provider should be queried.

See Section I.C.21. Factors influencing health status and contact with health services, History (of)

o. Aftercare following surgery for neoplasm

See Section I.C.21. Factors influencing health status and contact with health services, Aftercare

p. Follow-up care for completed treatment of a malignancy

See Section I.C.21. Factors influencing health status and contact with health services, Follow-up

q. Prophylactic organ removal for prevention of malignancy

See Section I.C. 21, Factors influencing health status and contact with health services, Prophylactic organ removal

r. Malignant neoplasm associated with transplanted organ

A malignant neoplasm of a transplanted organ should be coded as a transplant complication. Assign first the appropriate code from category T86.-, Complications of transplanted organs and tissue, followed by code C80.2, Malignant neoplasm associated with transplanted organ. Use an additional code for the specific malignancy.

Chapter 2. Neoplasms (C00-D49)

NOTE

Functional activity
All neoplasms are classified in this chapter, whether they are functionally active or not. An additional code from Chapter 4 may be used, to identify functional activity associated with any neoplasm.

Morphology [Histology]
Chapter 2 classifies neoplasms primarily by site (topography), with broad groupings for behavior, malignant, in situ, benign, etc. The Table of Neoplasms should be used to identify the correct topography code. In a few cases, such as for malignant melanoma and certain neuroendocrine tumors, the morphology (histologic type) is included in the category and codes.

Primary malignant neoplasms overlapping site boundaries
A primary malignant neoplasm that overlaps two or more contiguous (next to each other) sites should be classified to the subcategory/code .8 ("overlapping lesion"), unless the combination is specifically indexed elsewhere. For multiple neoplasms of the same site that are not contiguous, such as tumors in different quadrants of the same breast, codes for each site should be assigned.

Malignant neoplasm of ectopic tissue
Malignant neoplasms of ectopic tissue are to be coded to the site mentioned, e.g., ectopic pancreatic malignant neoplasms are coded to pancreas, unspecified (C25.9).

AHA: 2017, 1Q, 4, 5-6, 8

This chapter contains the following blocks:

C00-C14	Malignant neoplasms of lip, oral cavity and pharynx
C15-C26	Malignant neoplasms of digestive organs
C30-C39	Malignant neoplasms of respiratory and intrathoracic organs
C40-C41	Malignant neoplasms of bone and articular cartilage
C43-C44	Melanoma and other malignant neoplasms of skin
C45-C49	Malignant neoplasms of mesothelial and soft tissue
C50	Malignant neoplasms of breast
C51-C58	Malignant neoplasms of female genital organs
C60-C63	Malignant neoplasms of male genital organs
C64-C68	Malignant neoplasms of urinary tract
C69-C72	Malignant neoplasms of eye, brain and other parts of central nervous system
C73-C75	Malignant neoplasms of thyroid and other endocrine glands
C7A	Malignant neuroendocrine tumors
C7B	Secondary neuroendocrine tumors
C76-C80	Malignant neoplasms of ill-defined, other secondary and unspecified sites
C81-C96	Malignant neoplasms of lymphoid, hematopoietic and related tissue
D00-D09	In situ neoplasms
D10-D36	Benign neoplasms, except benign neuroendocrine tumors
D3A	Benign neuroendocrine tumors
D37-D48	Neoplasms of uncertain behavior, polycythemia vera and myelodysplastic syndromes
D49	Neoplasms of unspecified behavior

MALIGNANT NEOPLASMS (C00-C96)

Malignant neoplasms, stated or presumed to be primary (of specified sites), and certain specified histologies, except neuroendocrine, and of lymphoid, hematopoietic and related tissue (C00-C75)

Malignant neoplasms of lip, oral cavity and pharynx (C00-C14)

☑4ᵗʰ C00 Malignant neoplasm of lip
    Use additional code to identify:
        alcohol abuse and dependence (F10.-)
        history of tobacco dependence (Z87.891)
        tobacco dependence (F17.-)
        tobacco use (Z72.0)
        EXCLUDES 1 malignant melanoma of lip (C43.0)
                Merkel cell carcinoma of lip (C4A.0)
                other and unspecified malignant neoplasm of skin of lip (C44.0-)

    C00.0 Malignant neoplasm of external upper lip
        Malignant neoplasm of lipstick area of upper lip
        Malignant neoplasm of upper lip NOS
        Malignant neoplasm of vermilion border of upper lip

    C00.1 Malignant neoplasm of external lower lip
        Malignant neoplasm of lower lip NOS
        Malignant neoplasm of lipstick area of lower lip
        Malignant neoplasm of vermilion border of lower lip

    C00.2 Malignant neoplasm of external lip, unspecified ▽
        Malignant neoplasm of vermilion border of lip NO

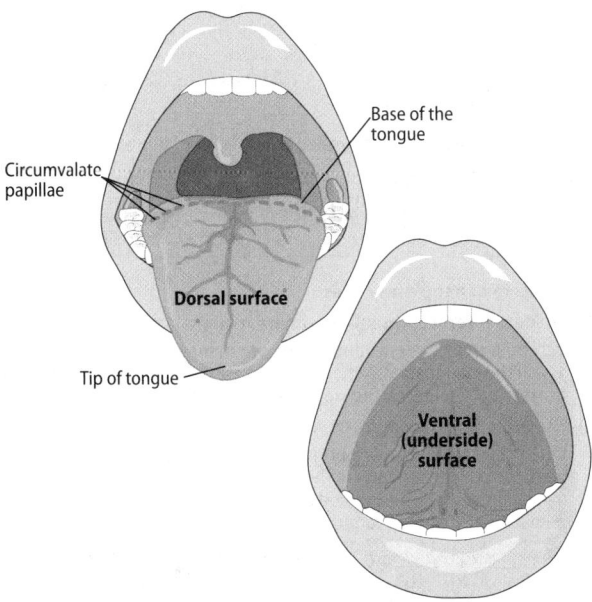

Malignant Neoplasm of Tongue

Base of the tongue
Circumvallate papillae
Dorsal surface
Tip of tongue
Ventral (underside) surface

    C00.3 Malignant neoplasm of upper lip, inner aspect
        Malignant neoplasm of buccal aspect of upper lip
        Malignant neoplasm of frenulum of upper lip
        Malignant neoplasm of mucosa of upper lip
        Malignant neoplasm of oral aspect of upper lip

    C00.4 Malignant neoplasm of lower lip, inner aspect
        Malignant neoplasm of buccal aspect of lower lip
        Malignant neoplasm of frenulum of lower lip
        Malignant neoplasm of mucosa of lower lip
        Malignant neoplasm of oral aspect of lower lip

    C00.5 Malignant neoplasm of lip, unspecified, inner aspect ▽
        Malignant neoplasm of buccal aspect of lip, unspecified
        Malignant neoplasm of frenulum of lip, unspecified
        Malignant neoplasm of mucosa of lip, unspecified
        Malignant neoplasm of oral aspect of lip, unspecified

    C00.6 Malignant neoplasm of commissure of lip, unspecified ▽

    C00.8 Malignant neoplasm of overlapping sites of lip

    C00.9 Malignant neoplasm of lip, unspecified ▽

C01 Malignant neoplasm of base of tongue
    Malignant neoplasm of dorsal surface of base of tongue
    Malignant neoplasm of fixed part of tongue NOS
    Malignant neoplasm of posterior third of tongue
    Use additional code to identify:
        alcohol abuse and dependence (F10.-)
        history of tobacco dependence (Z87.891)
        tobacco dependence (F17.-)
        tobacco use (Z72.0)

☑4ᵗʰ C02 Malignant neoplasm of other and unspecified parts of tongue
    Use additional code to identify:
        alcohol abuse and dependence (F10.-)
        history of tobacco dependence (Z87.891)
        tobacco dependence (F17.-)
        tobacco use (Z72.0)

    C02.0 Malignant neoplasm of dorsal surface of tongue
        Malignant neoplasm of anterior two-thirds of tongue, dorsal surface
        EXCLUDES 2 malignant neoplasm of dorsal surface of base of tongue (C01)

    C02.1 Malignant neoplasm of border of tongue
        Malignant neoplasm of tip of tongue

    C02.2 Malignant neoplasm of ventral surface of tongue
        Malignant neoplasm of anterior two-thirds of tongue, ventral surface
        Malignant neoplasm of frenulum linguae

    C02.3 Malignant neoplasm of anterior two-thirds of tongue, part unspecified
        Malignant neoplasm of middle third of tongue NOS
        Malignant neoplasm of mobile part of tongue NOS

    C02.4 Malignant neoplasm of lingual tonsil
        EXCLUDES 2 malignant neoplasm of tonsil NOS (C09.9)

☑ Newborn: 0   ☑ Pediatric: 0-17   ☑ Maternity: 12-55   ☑ Adult: 15-124   **NRS** Nonroutine supply Dx   **NCDx** Noncancer Dx   **PDx** Primary Dx   ▶◀ Revised Text   ● New Code   ▲ Revised Title

460   ICD-10-CM 2018

C02.8 **Malignant neoplasm of** overlapping sites **of tongue**
    Malignant neoplasm of two or more contiguous sites of tongue

C02.9 **Malignant neoplasm of tongue, unspecified** ▽

✓4ᵗʰ **C03** **Malignant neoplasm of** gum
    INCLUDES malignant neoplasm of alveolar (ridge) mucosa
                malignant neoplasm of gingiva
    Use additional code to identify:
        alcohol abuse and dependence (F10.-)
        history of tobacco dependence (Z87.891)
        tobacco dependence (F17.-)
        tobacco use (Z72.0)
    EXCLUDES 2 *malignant odontogenic neoplasms (C41.0-C41.1)*

C03.0 **Malignant neoplasm of** upper gum

C03.1 **Malignant neoplasm of** lower gum

C03.9 **Malignant neoplasm of gum, unspecified** ▽

✓4ᵗʰ **C04** **Malignant neoplasm of** floor of mouth
    Use additional code to identify:
        alcohol abuse and dependence (F10.-)
        history of tobacco dependence (Z87.891)
        tobacco dependence (F17.-)
        tobacco use (Z72.0)

C04.0 **Malignant neoplasm of** anterior **floor of mouth**
    Malignant neoplasm of anterior to the premolar-canine
    junction

C04.1 **Malignant neoplasm of** lateral **floor of mouth**

C04.8 **Malignant neoplasm of** overlapping sites **of floor of mouth**

C04.9 **Malignant neoplasm of floor of mouth, unspecified** ▽

✓4ᵗʰ **C05** **Malignant neoplasm of** palate
    Use additional code to identify:
        alcohol abuse and dependence (F10.-)
        history of tobacco dependence (Z87.891)
        tobacco dependence (F17.-)
        tobacco use (Z72.0)
    EXCLUDES 1 *Kaposi's sarcoma of palate (C46.2)*

C05.0 **Malignant neoplasm of** hard **palate**

C05.1 **Malignant neoplasm of** soft **palate**
        EXCLUDES 2 *malignant neoplasm of nasopharyngeal surface of soft palate (C11.3)*

C05.2 **Malignant neoplasm of** uvula

C05.8 **Malignant neoplasm of** overlapping sites **of palate**

C05.9 **Malignant neoplasm of palate, unspecified** ▽
    Malignant neoplasm of roof of mouth

✓4ᵗʰ **C06** **Malignant neoplasm of** other and unspecified parts of mouth
    Use additional code to identify:
        alcohol abuse and dependence (F10.-)
        history of tobacco dependence (Z87.891)
        tobacco dependence (F17.-)
        tobacco use (Z72.0)

C06.0 **Malignant neoplasm of** cheek mucosa
    Malignant neoplasm of buccal mucosa NOS
    Malignant neoplasm of internal cheek

C06.1 **Malignant neoplasm of** vestibule **of mouth**
    Malignant neoplasm of buccal sulcus (upper) (lower)
    Malignant neoplasm of labial sulcus (upper) (lower)

C06.2 **Malignant neoplasm of** retromolar area

✓5ᵗʰ **C06.8** **Malignant neoplasm of** overlapping sites of other and unspecified **parts of mouth**

    C06.80 **Malignant neoplasm of overlapping sites of** ▽
        unspecified parts of mouth

    C06.89 **Malignant neoplasm of overlapping sites of other parts of mouth**
        "book leaf" neoplasm [ventral surface of tongue and
        floor of mouth]

C06.9 **Malignant neoplasm of mouth, unspecified** ▽
    Malignant neoplasm of minor salivary gland, unspecified site
    Malignant neoplasm of oral cavity NOS

C07 **Malignant neoplasm of** parotid gland
    Use additional code to identify:
        alcohol abuse and dependence (F10.-)
        exposure to environmental tobacco smoke (Z77.22)
        exposure to tobacco smoke in the perinatal period (P96.81)
        history of tobacco dependence (Z87.891)
        occupational exposure to environmental tobacco smoke (Z57.31)
        tobacco dependence (F17.-)
        tobacco use (Z72.0)

✓4ᵗʰ **C08** **Malignant neoplasm of** other and unspecified major salivary glands
    INCLUDES malignant neoplasm of salivary ducts
    Use additional code to identify:
        alcohol abuse and dependence (F10.-)
        exposure to environmental tobacco smoke (Z77.22)
        exposure to tobacco smoke in the perinatal period (P96.81)
        history of tobacco dependence (Z87.891)
        occupational exposure to environmental tobacco smoke (Z57.31)
        tobacco dependence (F17.-)
        tobacco use (Z72.0)
    EXCLUDES 1 *malignant neoplasms of specified minor salivary glands which are classified according to their anatomical location*
    EXCLUDES 2 *malignant neoplasms of minor salivary glands NOS (C06.9)*
                   malignant neoplasm of parotid gland (C07)

C08.0 **Malignant neoplasm of** submandibular **gland**
    Malignant neoplasm of submaxillary gland

C08.1 **Malignant neoplasm of** sublingual **gland**

C08.9 **Malignant neoplasm of** major salivary gland, unspecified ▽
    Malignant neoplasm of salivary gland (major) NOS

✓4ᵗʰ **C09** **Malignant neoplasm of** tonsil
    Use additional code to identify:
        alcohol abuse and dependence (F10.-)
        exposure to environmental tobacco smoke (Z77.22)
        exposure to tobacco smoke in the perinatal period (P96.81)
        history of tobacco dependence (Z87.891)
        occupational exposure to environmental tobacco smoke (Z57.31)
        tobacco dependence (F17.-)
        tobacco use (Z72.0)
    EXCLUDES 2 *malignant neoplasm of lingual tonsil (C02.4)*
                   malignant neoplasm of pharyngeal tonsil (C11.1)

C09.0 **Malignant neoplasm of** tonsillar fossa

C09.1 **Malignant neoplasm of** tonsillar pillar **(anterior) (posterior)**

C09.8 **Malignant neoplasm of** overlapping sites **of tonsil**

C09.9 **Malignant neoplasm of tonsil, unspecified** ▽
    Malignant neoplasm of tonsil NOS
    Malignant neoplasm of faucial tonsils
    Malignant neoplasm of palatine tonsils

✓4ᵗʰ **C10** **Malignant neoplasm of** oropharynx
    Use additional code to identify:
        alcohol abuse and dependence (F10.-)
        exposure to environmental tobacco smoke (Z77.22)
        exposure to tobacco smoke in the perinatal period (P96.81)
        history of tobacco dependence (Z87.891)
        occupational exposure to environmental tobacco smoke (Z57.31)
        tobacco dependence (F17.-)
        tobacco use (Z72.0)
    EXCLUDES 2 *malignant neoplasm of tonsil (C09.-)*

C10.0 **Malignant neoplasm of** vallecula

C10.1 **Malignant neoplasm of** anterior surface of epiglottis
    Malignant neoplasm of epiglottis, free border [margin]
    Malignant neoplasm of glossoepiglottic fold(s)
        EXCLUDES 2 *malignant neoplasm of epiglottis (suprahyoid portion) NOS (C32.1)*

C10.2 **Malignant neoplasm of** lateral wall **of oropharynx**

C10.3 **Malignant neoplasm of** posterior wall **of oropharynx**

C10.4 **Malignant neoplasm of** branchial cleft
    Malignant neoplasm of branchial cyst [site of neoplasm]

C10.8 **Malignant neoplasm of** overlapping sites **of oropharynx**
    Malignant neoplasm of junctional region of oropharynx

C10.9 **Malignant neoplasm of oropharynx, unspecified** ▽

✓4ᵗʰ **C11** **Malignant neoplasm of** nasopharynx
    Use additional code to identify:
        exposure to environmental tobacco smoke (Z77.22)
        exposure to tobacco smoke in the perinatal period (P96.81)
        history of tobacco dependence (Z87.891)
        occupational exposure to environmental tobacco smoke (Z57.31)
        tobacco dependence (F17.-)
        tobacco use (Z72.0)

C11.0 **Malignant neoplasm of** superior wall **of nasopharynx**
    Malignant neoplasm of roof of nasopharynx

C11.1 **Malignant neoplasm of** posterior wall **of nasopharynx**
    Malignant neoplasm of adenoid
    Malignant neoplasm of pharyngeal tonsil

C11.2 **Malignant neoplasm of** lateral wall **of nasopharynx**
    Malignant neoplasm of fossa of Rosenmüller
    Malignant neoplasm of opening of auditory tube
    Malignant neoplasm of pharyngeal recess

✓ Additional Character Req   ✓7ᵗʰ Placeholder Alert   Case-Mix Diagnosis   Manifestation   ▽ Unspecified Dx   **EXCLUDES 1** Not coded here   **EXCLUDES 2** Not included here

ICD-10-CM 2018   **461**

C02.8–C11.2

C11.3 Malignant neoplasm of anterior wall of nasopharynx
Malignant neoplasm of floor of nasopharynx
Malignant neoplasm of nasopharyngeal (anterior) (posterior)
    surface of soft palate
Malignant neoplasm of posterior margin of nasal choana
Malignant neoplasm of posterior margin of nasal septum

C11.8 Malignant neoplasm of overlapping sites of nasopharynx

C11.9 Malignant neoplasm of nasopharynx, unspecified   ▽
Malignant neoplasm of nasopharyngeal wall NOS

C12 Malignant neoplasm of pyriform sinus
Malignant neoplasm of pyriform fossa
Use additional code to identify:
    exposure to environmental tobacco smoke (Z77.22)
    exposure to tobacco smoke in the perinatal period (P96.81)
    history of tobacco dependence (Z87.891)
    occupational exposure to environmental tobacco smoke (Z57.31)
    tobacco dependence (F17.-)
    tobacco use (Z72.0)

✓4ᵗʰ C13 Malignant neoplasm of hypopharynx
Use additional code to identify:
    exposure to environmental tobacco smoke (Z77.22)
    exposure to tobacco smoke in the perinatal period (P96.81)
    history of tobacco dependence (Z87.891)
    occupational exposure to environmental tobacco smoke (Z57.31)
    tobacco dependence (F17.-)
    tobacco use (Z72.0)
EXCLUDES 2   *malignant neoplasm of pyriform sinus (C12)*

C13.0 Malignant neoplasm of postcricoid region

C13.1 Malignant neoplasm of aryepiglottic fold, hypopharyngeal aspect
Malignant neoplasm of aryepiglottic fold, marginal zone
Malignant neoplasm of aryepiglottic fold NOS
Malignant neoplasm of interarytenoid fold, marginal zone
Malignant neoplasm of interarytenoid fold NOS
EXCLUDES 2   *malignant neoplasm of aryepiglottic fold or interarytenoid fold, laryngeal aspect (C32.1)*

C13.2 Malignant neoplasm of posterior wall of hypopharynx

C13.8 Malignant neoplasm of overlapping sites of hypopharynx

C13.9 Malignant neoplasm of hypopharynx, unspecified   ▽
Malignant neoplasm of hypopharyngeal wall NOS

✓4ᵗʰ C14 Malignant neoplasm of other and ill-defined sites in the lip, oral cavity and pharynx
Use additional code to identify:
    alcohol abuse and dependence (F10.-)
    exposure to environmental tobacco smoke (Z77.22)
    exposure to tobacco smoke in the perinatal period (P96.81)
    history of tobacco dependence (Z87.891)
    occupational exposure to environmental tobacco smoke (Z57.31)
    tobacco dependence (F17.-)
    tobacco use (Z72.0)
EXCLUDES 1   *malignant neoplasm of oral cavity NOS (C06.9)*

C14.0 Malignant neoplasm of pharynx, unspecified   ▽

C14.2 Malignant neoplasm of Waldeyer's ring

C14.8 Malignant neoplasm of overlapping sites of lip, oral cavity and pharynx
Primary malignant neoplasm of two or more contiguous sites of
    lip, oral cavity and pharynx
EXCLUDES 1   *"book leaf" neoplasm [ventral surface of tongue and floor of mouth] (C06.89)*

Malignant neoplasms of digestive organs (C15-C26)

EXCLUDES 1   *Kaposi's sarcoma of gastrointestinal sites (C46.4)*
EXCLUDES 2   *gastrointestinal stromal tumors (C49.A-)*

✓4ᵗʰ C15 Malignant neoplasm of esophagus
Use additional code to identify:
    alcohol abuse and dependence (F10.-)

C15.3 Malignant neoplasm of upper third of esophagus

C15.4 Malignant neoplasm of middle third of esophagus

C15.5 Malignant neoplasm of lower third of esophagus
EXCLUDES 1   *malignant neoplasm of cardio-esophageal junction (C16.0)*

C15.8 Malignant neoplasm of overlapping sites of esophagus

C15.9 Malignant neoplasm of esophagus, unspecified   ▽

✓4ᵗʰ C16 Malignant neoplasm of stomach
Use additional code to identify:
    alcohol abuse and dependence (F10.-)
EXCLUDES 2   *malignant carcinoid tumor of the stomach (C7A.092)*

C16.0 Malignant neoplasm of cardia
Malignant neoplasm of cardiac orifice
Malignant neoplasm of cardio-esophageal junction
Malignant neoplasm of esophagus and stomach
Malignant neoplasm of gastro-esophageal junction

C16.1 Malignant neoplasm of fundus of stomach

C16.2 Malignant neoplasm of body of stomach

C16.3 Malignant neoplasm of pyloric antrum
Malignant neoplasm of gastric antrum

C16.4 Malignant neoplasm of pylorus
Malignant neoplasm of prepylorus
Malignant neoplasm of pyloric canal

C16.5 Malignant neoplasm of lesser curvature of stomach, unspecified   ▽
Malignant neoplasm of lesser curvature of stomach, not
    classifiable to C16.1-C16.4

C16.6 Malignant neoplasm of greater curvature of stomach, unspecified   ▽
Malignant neoplasm of greater curvature of stomach, not
    classifiable to C16.0-C16.4

C16.8 Malignant neoplasm of overlapping sites of stomach

C16.9 Malignant neoplasm of stomach, unspecified   ▽
Gastric cancer NOS

✓4ᵗʰ C17 Malignant neoplasm of small intestine
EXCLUDES 1   *malignant carcinoid tumors of the small intestine (C7A.01)*
AHA: 2016, 1Q, 19

C17.0 Malignant neoplasm of duodenum

C17.1 Malignant neoplasm of jejunum

C17.2 Malignant neoplasm of ileum
EXCLUDES 1   *malignant neoplasm of ileocecal valve (C18.0)*

C17.3 Meckel's diverticulum, malignant
EXCLUDES 1   *Meckel's diverticulum, congenital (Q43.0)*

C17.8 Malignant neoplasm of overlapping sites of small intestine

C17.9 Malignant neoplasm of small intestine, unspecified   ▽

✓4ᵗʰ C18 Malignant neoplasm of colon
EXCLUDES 1   *malignant carcinoid tumors of the colon (C7A.02-)*

C18.0 Malignant neoplasm of cecum
Malignant neoplasm of ileocecal valve

C18.1 Malignant neoplasm of appendix

C18.2 Malignant neoplasm of ascending colon

C18.3 Malignant neoplasm of hepatic flexure

C18.4 Malignant neoplasm of transverse colon

C18.5 Malignant neoplasm of splenic flexure

C18.6 Malignant neoplasm of descending colon

C18.7 Malignant neoplasm of sigmoid colon
Malignant neoplasm of sigmoid (flexure)
EXCLUDES 1   *malignant neoplasm of rectosigmoid junction (C19)*

C18.8 Malignant neoplasm of overlapping sites of colon

C18.9 Malignant neoplasm of colon, unspecified   ▽
Malignant neoplasm of large intestine NOS

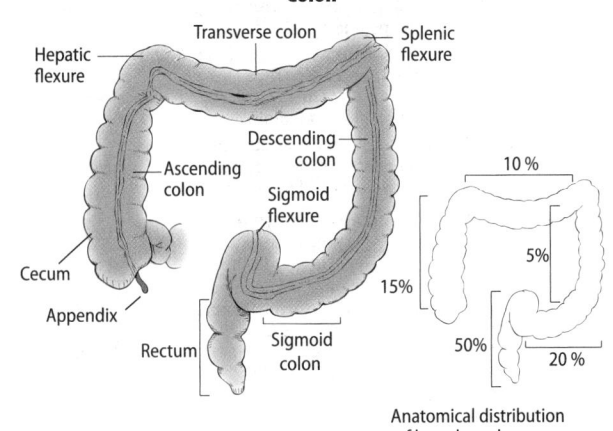

Colon

Anatomical distribution
of large bowel cancers

N Newborn: 0   P Pediatric: 0-17   M Maternity: 12-55   A Adult: 15-124   NRS Nonroutine supply Dx   NCDx Noncancer Dx   PDx Primary Dx   ►◄ Revised Text   ● New Code   ▲ Revised Title

462   ICD-10-CM 2018

C19 Malignant neoplasm of rectosigmoid junction
Malignant neoplasm of colon with rectum
Malignant neoplasm of rectosigmoid (colon)
EXCLUDES 1   *malignant carcinoid tumors of the colon (C7A.02-)*

C20 Malignant neoplasm of rectum
Malignant neoplasm of rectal ampulla
EXCLUDES 1   *malignant carcinoid tumor of the rectum (C7A.026)*

✓4ᵗʰ C21 Malignant neoplasm of anus and anal canal
EXCLUDES 2   *malignant carcinoid tumors of the colon (C7A.02-)*
     malignant melanoma of anal margin (C43.51)
     malignant melanoma of anal skin (C43.51)
     malignant melanoma of perianal skin (C43.51)
     other and unspecified malignant neoplasm of anal margin
       (C44.500, C44.510, C44.520, C44.590)
     other and unspecified malignant neoplasm of anal skin
       (C44.500, C44.510, C44.520, C44.590)
     other and unspecified malignant neoplasm of perianal skin
       (C44.500, C44.510, C44.520, C44.590)

C21.0 Malignant neoplasm of anus, unspecified ▽

C21.1 Malignant neoplasm of anal canal
Malignant neoplasm of anal sphincter

C21.2 Malignant neoplasm of cloacogenic zone

C21.8 Malignant neoplasm of overlapping sites of rectum, anus and anal canal
Malignant neoplasm of anorectal junction
Malignant neoplasm of anorectum
Primary malignant neoplasm of two or more contiguous sites of rectum, anus and anal canal

✓4ᵗʰ C22 Malignant neoplasm of liver and intrahepatic bile ducts
Use additional code to identify:
   alcohol abuse and dependence (F10.-)
   hepatitis B (B16.-, B18.0-B18.1)
   hepatitis C (B17.1-, B18.2)
EXCLUDES 1   *malignant neoplasm of biliary tract NOS (C24.9)*
     secondary malignant neoplasm of liver and intrahepatic bile duct (C78.7)

C22.0 Liver cell carcinoma
Hepatocellular carcinoma
Hepatoma
AHA: 2016, 1Q, 18

C22.1 Intrahepatic bile duct carcinoma
Cholangiocarcinoma
EXCLUDES 1   *malignant neoplasm of hepatic duct (C24.0)*

C22.2 Hepatoblastoma

C22.3 Angiosarcoma of liver
Kupffer cell sarcoma

C22.4 Other sarcomas of liver

C22.7 Other specified carcinomas of liver

C22.8 Malignant neoplasm of liver, primary, unspecified as to type ▽

C22.9 Malignant neoplasm of liver, not specified as primary or secondary ▽

C23 Malignant neoplasm of gallbladder

✓4ᵗʰ C24 Malignant neoplasm of other and unspecified parts of biliary tract
EXCLUDES 1   *malignant neoplasm of intrahepatic bile duct (C22.1)*

C24.0 Malignant neoplasm of extrahepatic bile duct
Malignant neoplasm of biliary duct or passage NOS
Malignant neoplasm of common bile duct
Malignant neoplasm of cystic duct
Malignant neoplasm of hepatic duct

C24.1 Malignant neoplasm of ampulla of Vater
DEF: Malignant neoplasm in the area of dilation at the juncture of the common bile and pancreatic ducts near the opening into the lumen of the duodenum.

C24.8 Malignant neoplasm of overlapping sites of biliary tract
Malignant neoplasm involving both intrahepatic and extrahepatic bile ducts
Primary malignant neoplasm of two or more contiguous sites of biliary tract

C24.9 Malignant neoplasm of biliary tract, unspecified ▽

✓4ᵗʰ C25 Malignant neoplasm of pancreas
Code also exocrine pancreatic insufficiency (K86.81)
Use additional code to identify:
   alcohol abuse and dependence (F10.-)

C25.0 Malignant neoplasm of head of pancreas

C25.1 Malignant neoplasm of body of pancreas

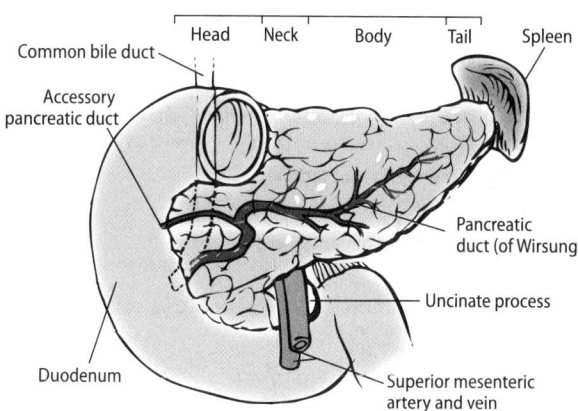

Pancreas

C25.2 Malignant neoplasm of tail of pancreas

C25.3 Malignant neoplasm of pancreatic duct

C25.4 Malignant neoplasm of endocrine pancreas
Malignant neoplasm of islets of Langerhans
Use additional code to identify any functional activity

C25.7 Malignant neoplasm of other parts of pancreas
Malignant neoplasm of neck of pancreas

C25.8 Malignant neoplasm of overlapping sites of pancreas

C25.9 Malignant neoplasm of pancreas, unspecified ▽

✓4ᵗʰ C26 Malignant neoplasm of other and ill-defined digestive organs
EXCLUDES 1   *malignant neoplasm of peritoneum and retroperitoneum (C48.-)*

C26.0 Malignant neoplasm of intestinal tract, part unspecified ▽
Malignant neoplasm of intestine NOS

C26.1 Malignant neoplasm of spleen
EXCLUDES 1   *Hodgkin lymphoma (C81.-)*
     non-Hodgkin lymphoma (C82-C85)

C26.9 Malignant neoplasm of ill-defined sites within the digestive system ▽
Malignant neoplasm of alimentary canal or tract NOS
Malignant neoplasm of gastrointestinal tract NOS
EXCLUDES 1   *malignant neoplasm of abdominal NOS (C76.2)*
     malignant neoplasm of intra-abdominal NOS (C76.2)

Malignant neoplasms of respiratory and intrathoracic organs (C30-C39)

INCLUDES   malignant neoplasm of middle ear
EXCLUDES 1   *mesothelioma (C45.-)*

✓4ᵗʰ C30 Malignant neoplasm of nasal cavity and middle ear

C30.0 Malignant neoplasm of nasal cavity
Malignant neoplasm of cartilage of nose
Malignant neoplasm of nasal concha
Malignant neoplasm of internal nose
Malignant neoplasm of septum of nose
Malignant neoplasm of vestibule of nose
EXCLUDES 1   *malignant melanoma of skin of nose (C43.31)*
     malignant neoplasm of nasal bone (C41.0)
     malignant neoplasm of nose NOS (C76.0)
     malignant neoplasm of olfactory bulb (C72.2-)
     malignant neoplasm of posterior margin of nasal septum and choana (C11.3)
     malignant neoplasm of turbinates (C41.0)
     other and unspecified malignant neoplasm of skin of nose (C44.301, C44.311, C44.321, C44.391)

C30.1 Malignant neoplasm of middle ear
Malignant neoplasm of antrum tympanicum
Malignant neoplasm of auditory tube
Malignant neoplasm of eustachian tube
Malignant neoplasm of inner ear
Malignant neoplasm of mastoid air cells
Malignant neoplasm of tympanic cavity
EXCLUDES 1   *malignant melanoma of skin of (external) ear (C43.2-)*
     malignant neoplasm of auricular canal (external) (C43.2-,C44.2-)
     malignant neoplasm of bone of ear (meatus) (C41.0)
     malignant neoplasm of cartilage of ear (C49.0)
     other and unspecified malignant neoplasm of skin of (external) ear (C44.2-)

✓ Additional Character Req   ✓x7ᵗʰ Placeholder Alert   Case-Mix Diagnosis   Manifestation   ▽ Unspecified Dx   *EXCLUDES 1* Not coded here   *EXCLUDES 2* Not included here

ICD-10-CM 2018   463

Chapter 2. Neoplasms

C19–C30.1

Chapter 2. Neoplasms

✓4th **C31** **Malignant neoplasm of accessory sinuses**

     C31.0 **Malignant neoplasm of maxillary sinus**
         Malignant neoplasm of antrum (Highmore) (maxillary)

     C31.1 **Malignant neoplasm of ethmoidal sinus**

     C31.2 **Malignant neoplasm of frontal sinus**

     C31.3 **Malignant neoplasm of sphenoid sinus**

     C31.8 **Malignant neoplasm of overlapping sites of accessory sinuses**

     C31.9 **Malignant neoplasm of accessory sinus, unspecified** ▽

✓4th **C32** **Malignant neoplasm of larynx**
     Use additional code to identify:
         alcohol abuse and dependence (F10.-)
         exposure to environmental tobacco smoke (Z77.22)
         exposure to tobacco smoke in the perinatal period (P96.81)
         history of tobacco dependence (Z87.891)
         occupational exposure to environmental tobacco smoke (Z57.31)
         tobacco dependence (F17.-)
         tobacco use (Z72.0)

     C32.0 **Malignant neoplasm of glottis**
         Malignant neoplasm of intrinsic larynx
         Malignant neoplasm of laryngeal commissure
           (anterior)(posterior)
         Malignant neoplasm of vocal cord (true) NOS

     C32.1 **Malignant neoplasm of supraglottis**
         Malignant neoplasm of aryepiglottic fold or interarytenoid fold,
           laryngeal aspect
         Malignant neoplasm of epiglottis (suprahyoid portion) NOS
         Malignant neoplasm of extrinsic larynx
         Malignant neoplasm of false vocal cord
         Malignant neoplasm of posterior (laryngeal) surface of epiglottis
         Malignant neoplasm of ventricular bands
         EXCLUDES 2   malignant neoplasm of anterior surface of epiglottis
                  (C10.1)
                   malignant neoplasm of aryepiglottic fold or
                     interarytenoid fold, hypopharyngeal aspect
                     (C13.1)
                   malignant neoplasm of aryepiglottic fold or
                     interarytenoid fold, marginal zone (C13.1)
                   malignant neoplasm of aryepiglottic fold or
                     interarytenoid fold NOS (C13.1)

     C32.2 **Malignant neoplasm of subglottis**

     C32.3 **Malignant neoplasm of laryngeal cartilage**

     C32.8 **Malignant neoplasm of overlapping sites of larynx**

     C32.9 **Malignant neoplasm of larynx, unspecified** ▽

C33 **Malignant neoplasm of trachea**
     Use additional code to identify:
         exposure to environmental tobacco smoke (Z77.22)
         exposure to tobacco smoke in the perinatal period (P96.81)
         history of tobacco dependence (Z87.891)
         occupational exposure to environmental tobacco smoke (Z57.31)
         tobacco dependence (F17.-)
         tobacco use (Z72.0)

✓4th **C34** **Malignant neoplasm of bronchus and lung**
     Use additional code to identify:
         exposure to environmental tobacco smoke (Z77.22)
         exposure to tobacco smoke in the perinatal period (P96.81)
         history of tobacco dependence (Z87.891)
         occupational exposure to environmental tobacco smoke (Z57.31)
         tobacco dependence (F17.-)
         tobacco use (Z72.0)
     EXCLUDES 1   Kaposi's sarcoma of lung (C46.5-)
                  malignant carcinoid tumor of the bronchus and lung (C7A.090)

     ✓5th **C34.0** **Malignant neoplasm of main bronchus**
         Malignant neoplasm of carina
         Malignant neoplasm of hilus (of lung)

         C34.00 **Malignant neoplasm of unspecified main bronchus** ▽

         C34.01 **Malignant neoplasm of right main bronchus**

         C34.02 **Malignant neoplasm of left main bronchus**

     ✓5th **C34.1** **Malignant neoplasm of upper lobe, bronchus or lung**

         C34.10 **Malignant neoplasm of upper lobe, unspecified bronchus or lung** ▽

         C34.11 **Malignant neoplasm of upper lobe, right bronchus or lung**

         C34.12 **Malignant neoplasm of upper lobe, left bronchus or lung**

     C34.2 **Malignant neoplasm of middle lobe, bronchus or lung**

✓5th **C34.3** **Malignant neoplasm of lower lobe, bronchus or lung**

     C34.30 **Malignant neoplasm of lower lobe, unspecified bronchus or lung** ▽

     C34.31 **Malignant neoplasm of lower lobe, right bronchus or lung**

     C34.32 **Malignant neoplasm of lower lobe, left bronchus or lung**

✓5th **C34.8** **Malignant neoplasm of overlapping sites of bronchus and lung**

     C34.80 **Malignant neoplasm of overlapping sites of unspecified bronchus and lung** ▽

     C34.81 **Malignant neoplasm of overlapping sites of right bronchus and lung**

     C34.82 **Malignant neoplasm of overlapping sites of left bronchus and lung**

✓5th **C34.9** **Malignant neoplasm of unspecified part of bronchus or lung**

     C34.90 **Malignant neoplasm of unspecified part of unspecified bronchus or lung** ▽
         Lung cancer NOS

     C34.91 **Malignant neoplasm of unspecified part of right bronchus or lung** ▽

     C34.92 **Malignant neoplasm of unspecified part of left bronchus or lung** ▽

C37 **Malignant neoplasm of thymus**
     EXCLUDES 1   malignant carcinoid tumor of the thymus (C7A.091)

✓4th **C38** **Malignant neoplasm of heart, mediastinum and pleura**
     EXCLUDES 1   mesothelioma (C45.-)

     C38.0 **Malignant neoplasm of heart**
         Malignant neoplasm of pericardium
         EXCLUDES 1   malignant neoplasm of great vessels (C49.3)

     C38.1 **Malignant neoplasm of anterior mediastinum**

     C38.2 **Malignant neoplasm of posterior mediastinum**

     C38.3 **Malignant neoplasm of mediastinum, part unspecified** ▽

     C38.4 **Malignant neoplasm of pleura**

     C38.8 **Malignant neoplasm of overlapping sites of heart, mediastinum and pleura**

✓4th **C39** **Malignant neoplasm of other and ill-defined sites in the respiratory system and intrathoracic organs**
     Use additional code to identify:
         exposure to environmental tobacco smoke (Z77.22)
         exposure to tobacco smoke in the perinatal period (P96.81)
         history of tobacco dependence (Z87.891)
         occupational exposure to environmental tobacco smoke (Z57.31)
         tobacco dependence (F17.-)
         tobacco use (Z72.0)
     EXCLUDES 1   intrathoracic malignant neoplasm NOS (C76.1)
                  thoracic malignant neoplasm NOS (C76.1)

     C39.0 **Malignant neoplasm of upper respiratory tract, part unspecified** ▽

     C39.9 **Malignant neoplasm of lower respiratory tract, part unspecified** ▽
         Malignant neoplasm of respiratory tract NOS

Malignant neoplasms of bone and articular cartilage (C40-C41)

     INCLUDES   malignant neoplasm of cartilage (articular) (joint)
               malignant neoplasm of periosteum
     EXCLUDES 1   malignant neoplasm of bone marrow NOS (C96.9)
                  malignant neoplasm of synovia (C49.-)

✓4th **C40** **Malignant neoplasm of bone and articular cartilage of limbs**
     Use additional code to identify major osseous defect, if applicable
     (M89.7-)

     ✓5th **C40.0** **Malignant neoplasm of scapula and long bones of upper limb**

         C40.00 **Malignant neoplasm of scapula and long bones of unspecified upper limb** ▽

         C40.01 **Malignant neoplasm of scapula and long bones of right upper limb**

         C40.02 **Malignant neoplasm of scapula and long bones of left upper limb**

     ✓5th **C40.1** **Malignant neoplasm of short bones of upper limb**

         C40.10 **Malignant neoplasm of short bones of unspecified upper limb** ▽

         C40.11 **Malignant neoplasm of short bones of right upper limb**

         C40.12 **Malignant neoplasm of short bones of left upper limb**

✓5ᵗʰ C40.2 Malignant neoplasm of long bones of lower limb

C40.20 **Malignant neoplasm of long bones of unspecified lower limb** ▽

C40.21 **Malignant neoplasm of long bones of** right **lower limb**

C40.22 **Malignant neoplasm of long bones of** left **lower limb**

✓5ᵗʰ C40.3 Malignant neoplasm of short bones of lower limb

C40.30 **Malignant neoplasm of short bones of unspecified lower limb** ▽

C40.31 **Malignant neoplasm of short bones of** right **lower limb**

C40.32 **Malignant neoplasm of short bones of** left **lower limb**

✓5ᵗʰ C40.8 Malignant neoplasm of overlapping sites **of bone and articular cartilage of limb**

C40.80 **Malignant neoplasm of overlapping sites of bone and articular cartilage of unspecified limb** ▽

C40.81 **Malignant neoplasm of overlapping sites of bone and articular cartilage of** right **limb**

C40.82 **Malignant neoplasm of overlapping sites of bone and articular cartilage of** left **limb**

✓5ᵗʰ C40.9 Malignant neoplasm of unspecified **bones and articular cartilage of limb**

C40.90 **Malignant neoplasm of unspecified bones and articular cartilage of unspecified limb** ▽

C40.91 **Malignant neoplasm of unspecified bones and articular cartilage of** right **limb** ▽

C40.92 **Malignant neoplasm of unspecified bones and articular cartilage of** left **limb** ▽

✓4ᵗʰ C41 Malignant neoplasm of bone and articular cartilage of other and unspecified sites

EXCLUDES 1   malignant neoplasm of bones of limbs (C40.-)
malignant neoplasm of cartilage of ear (C49.0)
malignant neoplasm of cartilage of eyelid (C49.0)
malignant neoplasm of cartilage of larynx (C32.3)
malignant neoplasm of cartilage of limbs (C40.-)
malignant neoplasm of cartilage of nose (C30.0)

C41.0 **Malignant neoplasm of bones of** skull and face

Malignant neoplasm of maxilla (superior)
Malignant neoplasm of orbital bone

EXCLUDES 2   carcinoma, any type except intraosseous or odontogenic of:
maxillary sinus (C31.0)
upper jaw (C03.0)
malignant neoplasm of jaw bone (lower) (C41.1)

C41.1 **Malignant neoplasm of** mandible

Malignant neoplasm of inferior maxilla
Malignant neoplasm of lower jaw bone

EXCLUDES 2   carcinoma, any type except intraosseous or odontogenic of:
jaw NOS (C03.9)
lower (C03.1)
malignant neoplasm of upper jaw bone (C41.0)

C41.2 **Malignant neoplasm of** vertebral column

EXCLUDES 1   malignant neoplasm of sacrum and coccyx (C41.4)

C41.3 **Malignant neoplasm of** ribs, sternum and clavicle

C41.4 **Malignant neoplasm of** pelvic bones, sacrum and coccyx

C41.9 **Malignant neoplasm of** bone and articular cartilage, **unspecified** ▽

Melanoma and other malignant neoplasms of skin (C43-C44)

✓4ᵗʰ C43 Malignant **melanoma of** skin

EXCLUDES 1   melanoma in situ (D03.-)

EXCLUDES 2   malignant melanoma of skin of genital organs (C51-C52, C60.-, C63.-)
Merkel cell carcinoma (C4A.-)
sites other than skin—code to malignant neoplasm of the site

C43.0 **Malignant melanoma of** lip   NRS

EXCLUDES 1   malignant neoplasm of vermilion border of lip (C00.0-C00.2)

✓5ᵗʰ C43.1 Malignant melanoma of eyelid, including canthus

C43.10 **Malignant melanoma of unspecified eyelid, including canthus** NRS ▽

C43.11 **Malignant melanoma of** right **eyelid, including canthus** NRS

C43.12 **Malignant melanoma of** left **eyelid, including canthus** NRS

✓5ᵗʰ C43.2 Malignant melanoma of ear and external auricular canal

C43.20 **Malignant melanoma of unspecified ear and external auricular canal** NRS ▽

C43.21 **Malignant melanoma of** right **ear and external auricular canal** NRS

C43.22 **Malignant melanoma of** left **ear and external auricular canal** NRS

✓5ᵗʰ C43.3 Malignant melanoma of other and unspecified parts of face

C43.30 **Malignant melanoma of unspecified part of face** NRS ▽

C43.31 **Malignant melanoma of** nose   NRS

C43.39 **Malignant melanoma of other parts of face** NRS

C43.4 **Malignant melanoma of** scalp and neck   NRS

✓5ᵗʰ C43.5 Malignant melanoma of trunk

EXCLUDES 2   malignant neoplasm of anus NOS (C21.0)
malignant neoplasm of scrotum (C63.2)

C43.51 **Malignant melanoma of** anal skin   NRS

Malignant melanoma of anal margin
Malignant melanoma of perianal skin

C43.52 **Malignant melanoma of** skin of breast   NRS

C43.59 **Malignant melanoma of other part of trunk** NRS

✓5ᵗʰ C43.6 Malignant melanoma of upper limb, including shoulder

C43.60 **Malignant melanoma of unspecified upper limb, including shoulder** NRS ▽

C43.61 **Malignant melanoma of** right **upper limb, including shoulder** NRS

C43.62 **Malignant melanoma of** left **upper limb, including shoulder** NRS

✓5ᵗʰ C43.7 Malignant melanoma of lower limb, including hip

C43.70 **Malignant melanoma of unspecified lower limb, including hip** NRS ▽

C43.71 **Malignant melanoma of** right **lower limb, including hip** NRS

C43.72 **Malignant melanoma of** left **lower limb, including hip** NRS

C43.8 **Malignant melanoma of** overlapping sites **of skin** NRS

C43.9 **Malignant melanoma of skin, unspecified** NRS ▽

Malignant melanoma of unspecified site of skin
Melanoma (malignant) NOS

✓4ᵗʰ C4A Merkel cell carcinoma

DEF: Malignant cutaneous cancer predominantly found in elderly patients with sun exposure that usually presents as a flesh-colored or bluish-red lump typically seen on the neck, head and face.

C4A.0 **Merkel cell carcinoma of** lip   NRS

EXCLUDES 1   malignant neoplasm of vermilion border of lip (C00.0-C00.2)

✓5ᵗʰ C4A.1 Merkel cell carcinoma of eyelid, including canthus

C4A.10 **Merkel cell carcinoma of unspecified eyelid, including canthus** NRS ▽

C4A.11 **Merkel cell carcinoma of** right **eyelid, including canthus** NRS

C4A.12 **Merkel cell carcinoma of** left **eyelid, including canthus** NRS

✓5ᵗʰ C4A.2 Merkel cell carcinoma of ear and external auricular canal

C4A.20 **Merkel cell carcinoma of unspecified ear and external auricular canal** NRS ▽

C4A.21 **Merkel cell carcinoma of** right **ear and external auricular canal** NRS

C4A.22 **Merkel cell carcinoma of** left **ear and external auricular canal** NRS

✓5ᵗʰ C4A.3 Merkel cell carcinoma of other and unspecified **parts of face**

C4A.30 **Merkel cell carcinoma of unspecified part of face** NRS ▽

C4A.31 **Merkel cell carcinoma of** nose   NRS

C4A.39 **Merkel cell carcinoma of other parts of face** NRS

C4A.4 **Merkel cell carcinoma of** scalp and neck   NRS

✓5ᵗʰ C4A.5 Merkel cell carcinoma of trunk

EXCLUDES 2   malignant neoplasm of anus NOS (C21.0)
malignant neoplasm of scrotum (C63.2)

C4A.51 **Merkel cell carcinoma of** anal skin   NRS

Merkel cell carcinoma of anal margin
Merkel cell carcinoma of perianal skin

C4A.52 **Merkel cell carcinoma of** skin of breast   NRS

C4A.59 **Merkel cell carcinoma of other part of trunk** NRS

✓ Additional Character Req   ✓x7ᵗʰ Placeholder Alert   Case-Mix Diagnosis   Manifestation   ▽ Unspecified Dx   *EXCLUDES 1* Not coded here   *EXCLUDES 2* Not included here

✓5th **C4A.6** Merkel cell carcinoma of upper limb, including shoulder

  C4A.60 Merkel cell carcinoma of unspecified upper limb, including shoulder `NRS` ▽

  C4A.61 Merkel cell carcinoma of right upper limb, including shoulder `NRS`

  C4A.62 Merkel cell carcinoma of left upper limb, including shoulder `NRS`

✓5th **C4A.7** Merkel cell carcinoma of lower limb, including hip

  C4A.70 Merkel cell carcinoma of unspecified lower limb, including hip `NRS` ▽

  C4A.71 Merkel cell carcinoma of right lower limb, including hip `NRS`

  C4A.72 Merkel cell carcinoma of left lower limb, including hip `NRS`

C4A.8 Merkel cell carcinoma of overlapping sites `NRS`

C4A.9 Merkel cell carcinoma, unspecified `NRS` ▽
    Merkel cell carcinoma of unspecified site
    Merkel cell carcinoma NOS

✓4th **C44** Other and unspecified malignant neoplasm of skin
  INCLUDES malignant neoplasm of sebaceous glands
           malignant neoplasm of sweat glands
  EXCLUDES 1 Kaposi's sarcoma of skin (C46.0)
           malignant melanoma of skin (C43.-)
           malignant neoplasm of skin of genital organs (C51-C52, C60-, C63.2)
           Merkel cell carcinoma (C4A.-)

DEF: Basal cell carcinoma: An abnormal growth of skin cells that arises from the deepest layer of the epidermis and may present as an open sore, red patches, pink growth, or scar. One of the most common forms of skin cancer, typically caused by sun exposure.
DEF: Squamous cell carcinoma: An uncontrolled growth of abnormal skin cells that arises from the skin's outer layers (epidermis) and may present as an open sore; firm, red nodule; elevated growth with a central depression; or flat sore with a scaly crust.

✓5th **C44.0** Other and unspecified malignant neoplasm of skin of lip
  EXCLUDES 1 malignant neoplasm of lip (C00.-)

  C44.00 Unspecified malignant neoplasm of skin of lip `NRS` ▽

  C44.01 Basal cell carcinoma of skin of lip `NRS`

  C44.02 Squamous cell carcinoma of skin of lip `NRS`

  C44.09 Other specified malignant neoplasm of skin of lip `NRS`

✓5th **C44.1** Other and unspecified malignant neoplasm of skin of eyelid, including canthus
  EXCLUDES 1 connective tissue of eyelid (C49.0)

  ✓6th **C44.10** Unspecified malignant neoplasm of skin of eyelid, including canthus

    C44.101 Unspecified malignant neoplasm of skin of unspecified eyelid, including canthus `NRS` ▽

    C44.102 Unspecified malignant neoplasm of skin of right eyelid, including canthus `NRS` ▽

    C44.109 Unspecified malignant neoplasm of skin of left eyelid, including canthus `NRS` ▽

  ✓6th **C44.11** Basal cell carcinoma of skin of eyelid, including canthus

    C44.111 Basal cell carcinoma of skin of unspecified eyelid, including canthus `NRS` ▽

    C44.112 Basal cell carcinoma of skin of right eyelid, including canthus `NRS`

    C44.119 Basal cell carcinoma of skin of left eyelid, including canthus `NRS`

  ✓6th **C44.12** Squamous cell carcinoma of skin of eyelid, including canthus

    C44.121 Squamous cell carcinoma of skin of unspecified eyelid, including canthus `NRS` ▽

    C44.122 Squamous cell carcinoma of skin of right eyelid, including canthus `NRS`

    C44.129 Squamous cell carcinoma of skin of left eyelid, including canthus `NRS`

  ✓6th **C44.19** Other specified malignant neoplasm of skin of eyelid, including canthus

    C44.191 Other specified malignant neoplasm of skin of unspecified eyelid, including canthus `NRS` ▽

    C44.192 Other specified malignant neoplasm of skin of right eyelid, including canthus `NRS`

    C44.199 Other specified malignant neoplasm of skin of left eyelid, including canthus `NRS`

✓5th **C44.2** Other and unspecified malignant neoplasm of skin of ear and external auricular canal
  EXCLUDES 1 connective tissue of ear (C49.0)

  ✓6th **C44.20** Unspecified malignant neoplasm of skin of ear and external auricular canal

    C44.201 Unspecified malignant neoplasm of skin of unspecified ear and external auricular canal `NRS` ▽

    C44.202 Unspecified malignant neoplasm of skin of right ear and external auricular canal `NRS` ▽

    C44.209 Unspecified malignant neoplasm of skin of left ear and external auricular canal `NRS` ▽

  ✓6th **C44.21** Basal cell carcinoma of skin of ear and external auricular canal

    C44.211 Basal cell carcinoma of skin of unspecified ear and external auricular canal `NRS` ▽

    C44.212 Basal cell carcinoma of skin of right ear and external auricular canal `NRS`

    C44.219 Basal cell carcinoma of skin of left ear and external auricular canal `NRS`

  ✓6th **C44.22** Squamous cell carcinoma of skin of ear and external auricular canal

    C44.221 Squamous cell carcinoma of skin of unspecified ear and external auricular canal `NRS` ▽

    C44.222 Squamous cell carcinoma of skin of right ear and external auricular canal `NRS`

    C44.229 Squamous cell carcinoma of skin of left ear and external auricular canal `NRS`

  ✓6th **C44.29** Other specified malignant neoplasm of skin of ear and external auricular canal

    C44.291 Other specified malignant neoplasm of skin of unspecified ear and external auricular canal `NRS` ▽

    C44.292 Other specified malignant neoplasm of skin of right ear and external auricular canal `NRS`

    C44.299 Other specified malignant neoplasm of skin of left ear and external auricular canal `NRS`

✓5th **C44.3** Other and unspecified malignant neoplasm of skin of other and unspecified parts of face

  ✓6th **C44.30** Unspecified malignant neoplasm of skin of other and unspecified parts of face

    C44.300 Unspecified malignant neoplasm of skin of unspecified part of face `NRS` ▽

    C44.301 Unspecified malignant neoplasm of skin of nose `NRS` ▽

    C44.309 Unspecified malignant neoplasm of skin of other parts of face `NRS` ▽

  ✓6th **C44.31** Basal cell carcinoma of skin of other and unspecified parts of face

    C44.310 Basal cell carcinoma of skin of unspecified parts of face `NRS` ▽

    C44.311 Basal cell carcinoma of skin of nose `NRS`

    C44.319 Basal cell carcinoma of skin of other parts of face `NRS`

  ✓6th **C44.32** Squamous cell carcinoma of skin of other and unspecified parts of face

    C44.320 Squamous cell carcinoma of skin of unspecified parts of face `NRS` ▽

    C44.321 Squamous cell carcinoma of skin of nose `NRS`

    C44.329 Squamous cell carcinoma of skin of other parts of face `NRS`

  ✓6th **C44.39** Other specified malignant neoplasm of skin of other and unspecified parts of face

    C44.390 Other specified malignant neoplasm of skin of unspecified parts of face `NRS` ▽

    C44.391 Other specified malignant neoplasm of skin of nose `NRS`

    C44.399 Other specified malignant neoplasm of skin of other parts of face `NRS`

N Newborn: 0   **P** Pediatric: 0-17   **M** Maternity: 12-55   **A** Adult: 15-124   `NRS` Nonroutine supply Dx   `NCDx` Noncancer Dx   `PDx` Primary Dx   ▶◀ Revised Text   ● New Code   ▲ Revised Title

466   ICD-10-CM 2018

✓5th **C44.4 Other and unspecified malignant neoplasm of skin of** scalp and neck

     C44.40 Unspecified malignant neoplasm of skin of NRS ▽
scalp and neck

     C44.41 Basal cell carcinoma **of skin of scalp and neck** NRS

     C44.42 Squamous cell carcinoma **of skin of scalp and neck** NRS

     C44.49 Other specified malignant neoplasm of skin of scalp and neck NRS

✓5th **C44.5 Other and unspecified malignant neoplasm of** skin of trunk

     EXCLUDES 1   anus NOS (C21.0)
                scrotum (C63.2)

   ✓6th **C44.50** Unspecified **malignant neoplasm of skin of trunk**

     C44.500 Unspecified malignant neoplasm of NRS ▽
anal skin

         Unspecified malignant neoplasm of anal
margin
         Unspecified malignant neoplasm of
perianal skin

     C44.501 Unspecified malignant neoplasm of NRS ▽
skin of breast

     C44.509 Unspecified malignant neoplasm of NRS ▽
skin of other part of trunk

   ✓6th **C44.51** Basal cell carcinoma **of skin of trunk**

     C44.510 Basal cell carcinoma of anal skin NRS

         Basal cell carcinoma of anal margin
         Basal cell carcinoma of perianal skin

     C44.511 Basal cell carcinoma of skin of breast NRS

     C44.519 Basal cell carcinoma of skin of other part of trunk NRS

   ✓6th **C44.52** Squamous cell carcinoma **of skin of trunk**

     C44.520 Squamous cell carcinoma of anal skin NRS

         Squamous cell carcinoma of anal margin
         Squamous cell carcinoma of perianal skin

     C44.521 Squamous cell carcinoma of skin of breast NRS

     C44.529 Squamous cell carcinoma of skin of other part of trunk NRS

   ✓6th **C44.59** Other **specified malignant neoplasm of skin of trunk**

     C44.590 Other specified malignant neoplasm of anal skin NRS

         Other specified malignant neoplasm of
anal margin
         Other specified malignant neoplasm of
perianal skin

     C44.591 Other specified malignant neoplasm of skin of breast NRS

     C44.599 Other specified malignant neoplasm of skin of other part of trunk NRS

✓5th **C44.6 Other and unspecified malignant neoplasm of skin of** upper limb, including shoulder

   ✓6th **C44.60 Unspecified malignant neoplasm of skin of upper limb, including shoulder**

     C44.601 Unspecified malignant neoplasm of skin of unspecified upper limb, including shoulder NRS ▽

     C44.602 Unspecified malignant neoplasm of skin of right **upper limb, including shoulder** NRS ▽

     C44.609 Unspecified malignant neoplasm of skin of left **upper limb, including shoulder** NRS ▽

   ✓6th **C44.61** Basal cell carcinoma **of skin of upper limb, including shoulder**

     C44.611 Basal cell carcinoma of skin of unspecified upper limb, including shoulder NRS ▽

     C44.612 Basal cell carcinoma of skin of right **upper limb, including shoulder** NRS

     C44.619 Basal cell carcinoma of skin of left **upper limb, including shoulder** NRS

   ✓6th **C44.62** Squamous cell carcinoma **of skin of upper limb, including shoulder**

     C44.621 Squamous cell carcinoma of skin of unspecified upper limb, including shoulder NRS ▽

     C44.622 Squamous cell carcinoma of skin of right **upper limb, including shoulder** NRS

     C44.629 Squamous cell carcinoma of skin of left **upper limb, including shoulder** NRS

   ✓6th **C44.69** Other **specified malignant neoplasm of skin of upper limb, including shoulder**

     C44.691 Other specified malignant neoplasm of skin of unspecified upper limb, including shoulder NRS ▽

     C44.692 Other specified malignant neoplasm of skin of right **upper limb, including shoulder** NRS

     C44.699 Other specified malignant neoplasm of skin of left **upper limb, including shoulder** NRS

✓5th **C44.7 Other and unspecified malignant neoplasm of skin of** lower limb, including hip

   ✓6th **C44.70** Unspecified **malignant neoplasm of skin of lower limb, including hip**

     C44.701 Unspecified malignant neoplasm of skin of unspecified lower limb, including hip NRS ▽

     C44.702 Unspecified malignant neoplasm of skin of right **lower limb, including hip** NRS ▽

     C44.709 Unspecified malignant neoplasm of skin of left **lower limb, including hip** NRS ▽

   ✓6th **C44.71** Basal cell carcinoma **of skin of lower limb, including hip**

     C44.711 Basal cell carcinoma of skin of unspecified lower limb, including hip NRS ▽

     C44.712 Basal cell carcinoma of skin of right **lower limb, including hip** NRS

     C44.719 Basal cell carcinoma of skin of left **lower limb, including hip** NRS

   ✓6th **C44.72** Squamous cell carcinoma **of skin of lower limb, including hip**

     C44.721 Squamous cell carcinoma of skin of unspecified lower limb, including hip NRS ▽

     C44.722 Squamous cell carcinoma of skin of right **lower limb, including hip** NRS

     C44.729 Squamous cell carcinoma of skin of left **lower limb, including hip** NRS

   ✓6th **C44.79 Other specified malignant neoplasm of skin of lower limb, including hip**

     C44.791 Other specified malignant neoplasm of skin of unspecified lower limb, including hip NRS ▽

     C44.792 Other specified malignant neoplasm of skin of right **lower limb, including hip** NRS

     C44.799 Other specified malignant neoplasm of skin of left **lower limb, including hip** NRS

✓5th **C44.8 Other and unspecified malignant neoplasm of** overlapping sites of skin

     C44.80 Unspecified malignant neoplasm of overlapping sites of skin NRS ▽

     C44.81 Basal cell carcinoma **of overlapping sites of skin** NRS

     C44.82 Squamous cell carcinoma **of overlapping sites of skin** NRS

     C44.89 Other specified malignant neoplasm of overlapping sites of skin NRS

✓5th **C44.9 Other and unspecified malignant neoplasm of skin, unspecified**

     C44.90 Unspecified malignant neoplasm of skin, unspecified NRS ▽

         Malignant neoplasm of unspecified site of skin

     C44.91 Basal cell carcinoma **of skin, unspecified** NRS ▽

     C44.92 Squamous cell carcinoma **of skin, unspecified** NRS ▽

     C44.99 Other specified malignant neoplasm of skin, unspecified NRS ▽

✓ Additional Character Req   ✓x7th Placeholder Alert   Case-Mix Diagnosis   Manifestation   ▽ Unspecified Dx   EXCLUDES 1 Not coded here   EXCLUDES 2 Not included here

ICD-10-CM 2018   467

C44.4–C44.99

Malignant neoplasms of mesothelial and soft tissue (C45-C49)

✓4ᵗʰ C45 Mesothelioma

DEF: Rare type of cancer that forms in the thin layer of protective tissue that covers the majority of internal organs (mesothelium).

C45.0 Mesothelioma of pleura

EXCLUDES 1 *other malignant neoplasm of pleura (C38.4)*

AHA: 2017, 2Q, 11

C45.1 Mesothelioma of peritoneum

Mesothelioma of cul-de-sac
Mesothelioma of mesentery
Mesothelioma of mesocolon
Mesothelioma of omentum
Mesothelioma of peritoneum (parietal) (pelvic)

EXCLUDES 1 *other malignant neoplasm of soft tissue of peritoneum (C48.-)*

C45.2 Mesothelioma of pericardium

EXCLUDES 1 *other malignant neoplasm of pericardium (C38.0)*

C45.7 Mesothelioma of other sites

C45.9 Mesothelioma, unspecified ▽

✓4ᵗʰ C46 Kaposi's sarcoma

Code first any human immunodeficiency virus [HIV] disease (B20)
DEF: Malignant neoplasm that causes patches of abnormal tissue to grow under the skin, in the lining of the mouth, nose, and throat, in lymph nodes, or in other visceral organs. Kaposi's sarcoma is caused by human herpesvirus8 (HHV8).

C46.0 Kaposi's sarcoma of skin NRS

C46.1 Kaposi's sarcoma of soft tissue

Kaposi's sarcoma of blood vessel
Kaposi's sarcoma of connective tissue
Kaposi's sarcoma of fascia
Kaposi's sarcoma of ligament
Kaposi's sarcoma of lymphatic(s) NEC
Kaposi's sarcoma of muscle

EXCLUDES 2 *Kaposi's sarcoma of lymph glands and nodes (C46.3)*

C46.2 Kaposi's sarcoma of palate

C46.3 Kaposi's sarcoma of lymph nodes

C46.4 Kaposi's sarcoma of gastrointestinal sites

✓5ᵗʰ C46.5 Kaposi's sarcoma of lung

C46.50 Kaposi's sarcoma of unspecified lung ▽

C46.51 Kaposi's sarcoma of right lung

C46.52 Kaposi's sarcoma of left lung

C46.7 Kaposi's sarcoma of other sites

C46.9 Kaposi's sarcoma, unspecified ▽

Kaposi's sarcoma of unspecified site

✓4ᵗʰ C47 Malignant neoplasm of peripheral nerves and autonomic nervous system

INCLUDES malignant neoplasm of sympathetic and parasympathetic nerves and ganglia

EXCLUDES 1 *Kaposi's sarcoma of soft tissue (C46.1)*

C47.0 Malignant neoplasm of peripheral nerves of head, face and neck

EXCLUDES 1 *malignant neoplasm of peripheral nerves of orbit (C69.6-)*

✓5ᵗʰ C47.1 Malignant neoplasm of peripheral nerves of upper limb, including shoulder

C47.10 Malignant neoplasm of peripheral nerves of unspecified upper limb, including shoulder ▽

C47.11 Malignant neoplasm of peripheral nerves of right upper limb, including shoulder

C47.12 Malignant neoplasm of peripheral nerves of left upper limb, including shoulder

✓5ᵗʰ C47.2 Malignant neoplasm of peripheral nerves of lower limb, including hip

C47.20 Malignant neoplasm of peripheral nerves of unspecified lower limb, including hip ▽

C47.21 Malignant neoplasm of peripheral nerves of right lower limb, including hip

C47.22 Malignant neoplasm of peripheral nerves of left lower limb, including hip

C47.3 Malignant neoplasm of peripheral nerves of thorax

C47.4 Malignant neoplasm of peripheral nerves of abdomen

C47.5 Malignant neoplasm of peripheral nerves of pelvis

C47.6 Malignant neoplasm of peripheral nerves of trunk, unspecified ▽

Malignant neoplasm of peripheral nerves of unspecified part of trunk

C47.8 Malignant neoplasm of overlapping sites of peripheral nerves and autonomic nervous system

C47.9 Malignant neoplasm of peripheral nerves and autonomic nervous system, unspecified ▽

Malignant neoplasm of unspecified site of peripheral nerves and autonomic nervous system

✓4ᵗʰ C48 Malignant neoplasm of retroperitoneum and peritoneum

EXCLUDES 1 *Kaposi's sarcoma of connective tissue (C46.1)*
mesothelioma (C45.-)

C48.0 Malignant neoplasm of retroperitoneum

C48.1 Malignant neoplasm of specified parts of peritoneum

Malignant neoplasm of cul-de-sac
Malignant neoplasm of mesentery
Malignant neoplasm of mesocolon
Malignant neoplasm of omentum
Malignant neoplasm of parietal peritoneum
Malignant neoplasm of pelvic peritoneum

C48.2 Malignant neoplasm of peritoneum, unspecified ▽

C48.8 Malignant neoplasm of overlapping sites of retroperitoneum and peritoneum

✓4ᵗʰ C49 Malignant neoplasm of other connective and soft tissue

INCLUDES malignant neoplasm of blood vessel
malignant neoplasm of bursa
malignant neoplasm of cartilage
malignant neoplasm of fascia
malignant neoplasm of fat
malignant neoplasm of ligament, except uterine
malignant neoplasm of lymphatic vessel
malignant neoplasm of muscle
malignant neoplasm of synovia
malignant neoplasm of tendon (sheath)

EXCLUDES 1 *malignant neoplasm of cartilage (of):*
articular (C40-C41)
larynx (C32.3)
nose (C30.0)
malignant neoplasm of connective tissue of breast (C50.-)

EXCLUDES 2 *Kaposi's sarcoma of soft tissue (C46.1)*
malignant neoplasm of heart (C38.0)
malignant neoplasm of peripheral nerves and autonomic nervous system (C47.-)
malignant neoplasm of peritoneum (C48.2)
malignant neoplasm of retroperitoneum (C48.0)
malignant neoplasm of uterine ligament (C57.3)
mesothelioma (C45.-)

C49.0 Malignant neoplasm of connective and soft tissue of head, face and neck

Malignant neoplasm of connective tissue of ear
Malignant neoplasm of connective tissue of eyelid

EXCLUDES 1 *connective tissue of orbit (C69.6-)*

✓5ᵗʰ C49.1 Malignant neoplasm of connective and soft tissue of upper limb, including shoulder

C49.10 Malignant neoplasm of connective and soft tissue of unspecified upper limb, including shoulder ▽

C49.11 Malignant neoplasm of connective and soft tissue of right upper limb, including shoulder

C49.12 Malignant neoplasm of connective and soft tissue of left upper limb, including shoulder

✓5ᵗʰ C49.2 Malignant neoplasm of connective and soft tissue of lower limb, including hip

C49.20 Malignant neoplasm of connective and soft tissue of unspecified lower limb, including hip ▽

C49.21 Malignant neoplasm of connective and soft tissue of right lower limb, including hip

C49.22 Malignant neoplasm of connective and soft tissue of left lower limb, including hip

C49.3 Malignant neoplasm of connective and soft tissue of thorax

Malignant neoplasm of axilla
Malignant neoplasm of diaphragm
Malignant neoplasm of great vessels

EXCLUDES 1 *malignant neoplasm of breast (C50.-)*
malignant neoplasm of heart (C38.0)
malignant neoplasm of mediastinum (C38.1-C38.3)
malignant neoplasm of thymus (C37)

AHA: 2015, 3Q, 19

C49.4 Malignant neoplasm of connective and soft tissue of abdomen

Malignant neoplasm of abdominal wall
Malignant neoplasm of hypochondrium

C49.5   **Malignant neoplasm of connective and soft tissue of pelvis**
   Malignant neoplasm of buttock
   Malignant neoplasm of groin
   Malignant neoplasm of perineum

C49.6   **Malignant neoplasm of connective and soft tissue of trunk, unspecified** ▽
   Malignant neoplasm of back NOS

C49.8   **Malignant neoplasm of overlapping sites of connective and soft tissue**
   Primary malignant neoplasm of two or more contiguous sites of connective and soft tissue

C49.9   **Malignant neoplasm of connective and soft tissue, unspecified** ▽

✓5th **C49.A**   **Gastrointestinal stromal tumor**
   C49.A0   Gastrointestinal stromal tumor, unspecified site ▽
   C49.A1   Gastrointestinal stromal tumor of esophagus
   C49.A2   Gastrointestinal stromal tumor of stomach
   C49.A3   Gastrointestinal stromal tumor of small intestine
   C49.A4   Gastrointestinal stromal tumor of large intestine
   C49.A5   Gastrointestinal stromal tumor of rectum
   C49.A9   Gastrointestinal stromal tumor of other sites

Malignant neoplasms of breast (C50)

✓4th **C50**   **Malignant neoplasm of breast**
   INCLUDES   connective tissue of breast
     Paget's disease of breast
     Paget's disease of nipple
   Use additional code to identify estrogen receptor status (Z17.0, Z17.1)
   EXCLUDES 1   *skin of breast (C44.501, C44.511, C44.521, C44.591)*

✓5th **C50.0**   **Malignant neoplasm of nipple and areola**
   ✓6th **C50.01**   Malignant neoplasm of nipple and areola, female
     C50.011   Malignant neoplasm of nipple and areola, right female breast ♀
     C50.012   Malignant neoplasm of nipple and areola, left female breast ♀
     C50.019   Malignant neoplasm of nipple and areola, unspecified female breast ♀▽
   ✓6th **C50.02**   Malignant neoplasm of nipple and areola, male
     C50.021   Malignant neoplasm of nipple and areola, right male breast ♂
     C50.022   Malignant neoplasm of nipple and areola, left male breast ♂
     C50.029   Malignant neoplasm of nipple and areola, unspecified male breast ♂▽

✓5th **C50.1**   **Malignant neoplasm of central portion of breast**
   ✓6th **C50.11**   Malignant neoplasm of central portion of breast, female
     C50.111   Malignant neoplasm of central portion of right female breast ♀
     C50.112   Malignant neoplasm of central portion of left female breast ♀
     C50.119   Malignant neoplasm of central portion of unspecified female breast ♀▽

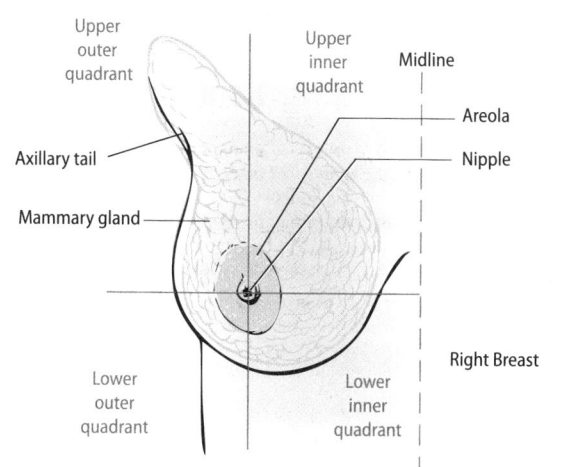

Female Breast

Upper outer quadrant

Upper inner quadrant

Midline

Areola

Nipple

Axillary tail

Mammary gland

Right Breast

Lower outer quadrant

Lower inner quadrant

✓6th **C50.12**   Malignant neoplasm of central portion of breast, male
   C50.121   Malignant neoplasm of central portion of right male breast ♂
   C50.122   Malignant neoplasm of central portion of left male breast ♂
   C50.129   Malignant neoplasm of central portion of unspecified male breast ♂▽

✓5th **C50.2**   **Malignant neoplasm of upper-inner quadrant of breast**
   ✓6th **C50.21**   Malignant neoplasm of upper-inner quadrant of breast, female
     C50.211   Malignant neoplasm of upper-inner quadrant of right female breast ♀
     C50.212   Malignant neoplasm of upper-inner quadrant of left female breast ♀
     C50.219   Malignant neoplasm of upper-inner quadrant of unspecified female breast ♀▽
   ✓6th **C50.22**   Malignant neoplasm of upper-inner quadrant of breast, male
     C50.221   Malignant neoplasm of upper-inner quadrant of right male breast ♂
     C50.222   Malignant neoplasm of upper-inner quadrant of left male breast ♂
     C50.229   Malignant neoplasm of upper-inner quadrant of unspecified male breast ♂▽

✓5th **C50.3**   **Malignant neoplasm of lower-inner quadrant of breast**
   ✓6th **C50.31**   Malignant neoplasm of lower-inner quadrant of breast, female
     C50.311   Malignant neoplasm of lower-inner quadrant of right female breast ♀
     C50.312   Malignant neoplasm of lower-inner quadrant of left female breast ♀
     C50.319   Malignant neoplasm of lower-inner quadrant of unspecified female breast ♀▽
   ✓6th **C50.32**   Malignant neoplasm of lower-inner quadrant of breast, male
     C50.321   Malignant neoplasm of lower-inner quadrant of right male breast ♂
     C50.322   Malignant neoplasm of lower-inner quadrant of left male breast ♂
     C50.329   Malignant neoplasm of lower-inner quadrant of unspecified male breast ♂▽

✓5th **C50.4**   **Malignant neoplasm of upper-outer quadrant of breast**
   ✓6th **C50.41**   Malignant neoplasm of upper-outer quadrant of breast, female
     C50.411   Malignant neoplasm of upper-outer quadrant of right female breast ♀
     C50.412   Malignant neoplasm of upper-outer quadrant of left female breast ♀
     C50.419   Malignant neoplasm of upper-outer quadrant of unspecified female breast ♀▽
   ✓6th **C50.42**   Malignant neoplasm of upper-outer quadrant of breast, male
     C50.421   Malignant neoplasm of upper-outer quadrant of right male breast ♂
     C50.422   Malignant neoplasm of upper-outer quadrant of left male breast ♂
     C50.429   Malignant neoplasm of upper-outer quadrant of unspecified male breast ♂▽

✓5th **C50.5**   **Malignant neoplasm of lower-outer quadrant of breast**
   ✓6th **C50.51**   Malignant neoplasm of lower-outer quadrant of breast, female
     C50.511   Malignant neoplasm of lower-outer quadrant of right female breast ♀
     C50.512   Malignant neoplasm of lower-outer quadrant of left female breast ♀
     C50.519   Malignant neoplasm of lower-outer quadrant of unspecified female breast ♀▽
   ✓6th **C50.52**   Malignant neoplasm of lower-outer quadrant of breast, male
     C50.521   Malignant neoplasm of lower-outer quadrant of right male breast ♂
     C50.522   Malignant neoplasm of lower-outer quadrant of left male breast ♂
     C50.529   Malignant neoplasm of lower-outer quadrant of unspecified male breast ♂▽

✓ Additional Character Req   ✓x7th Placeholder Alert   Case-Mix Diagnosis   Manifestation   ▽ Unspecified Dx   EXCLUDES 1 Not coded here   EXCLUDES 2 Not included here

ICD-10-CM 2018   469

C49.5–C50.529

Chapter 2. Neoplasms

C50.6–C61

✓5ᵗʰ **C50.6 Malignant neoplasm of** axillary tail **of breast**

    ✓6ᵗʰ **C50.61 Malignant neoplasm of axillary tail of breast,** female

        C50.611 Malignant neoplasm of axillary tail of right **female breast** ♀

        C50.612 Malignant neoplasm of axillary tail of left **female breast** ♀

        C50.619 Malignant neoplasm of axillary tail of unspecified female breast ♀▽

    ✓6ᵗʰ **C50.62 Malignant neoplasm of axillary tail of breast,** male

        C50.621 Malignant neoplasm of axillary tail of right **male breast** ♂

        C50.622 Malignant neoplasm of axillary tail of left **male breast** ♂

        C50.629 Malignant neoplasm of axillary tail of unspecified male breast ♂▽

✓5ᵗʰ **C50.8 Malignant neoplasm of** overlapping sites **of breast**

    ✓6ᵗʰ **C50.81 Malignant neoplasm of overlapping sites of breast,** female

        C50.811 Malignant neoplasm of overlapping sites of right **female breast** ♀

        C50.812 Malignant neoplasm of overlapping sites of left **female breast** ♀

        C50.819 Malignant neoplasm of overlapping sites of unspecified female breast ♀▽

    ✓6ᵗʰ **C50.82 Malignant neoplasm of overlapping sites of breast,** male

        C50.821 Malignant neoplasm of overlapping sites of right **male breast** ♂

        C50.822 Malignant neoplasm of overlapping sites of left **male breast** ♂

        C50.829 Malignant neoplasm of overlapping sites of unspecified male breast ♂▽

✓5ᵗʰ **C50.9 Malignant neoplasm of breast of** unspecified site

    ✓6ᵗʰ **C50.91 Malignant neoplasm of breast of unspecified site,** female

        C50.911 Malignant neoplasm of unspecified site of right **female breast** ♀

        C50.912 Malignant neoplasm of unspecified site of left **female breast** ♀

        C50.919 Malignant neoplasm of unspecified site of unspecified female breast ♀▽

    ✓6ᵗʰ **C50.92 Malignant neoplasm of breast of unspecified site,** male

        C50.921 Malignant neoplasm of unspecified site of right **male breast** ♂

        C50.922 Malignant neoplasm of unspecified site of left **male breast** ♂

        C50.929 Malignant neoplasm of unspecified site of unspecified male breast ♂▽

Malignant neoplasms of female genital organs (C51-C58)

INCLUDES   malignant neoplasm of skin of female genital organs

✓4ᵗʰ **C51 Malignant neoplasm of vulva**

    EXCLUDES 1   *carcinoma in situ of vulva (D07.1)*

    C51.0 Malignant neoplasm of labium majus ♀
        Malignant neoplasm of Bartholin's [greater vestibular] gland

    C51.1 Malignant neoplasm of labium minus ♀

    C51.2 Malignant neoplasm of clitoris ♀

    C51.8 Malignant neoplasm of overlapping sites **of vulva** ♀

    C51.9 Malignant neoplasm of vulva, unspecified ♀▽
        Malignant neoplasm of external female genitalia NOS
        Malignant neoplasm of pudendum

  C52 Malignant neoplasm of vagina ♀
    EXCLUDES 1   *carcinoma in situ of vagina (D07.2)*

✓4ᵗʰ **C53 Malignant neoplasm of** cervix uteri
    EXCLUDES 1   *carcinoma in situ of cervix uteri (D06.-)*

    C53.0 Malignant neoplasm of endocervix ♀

    C53.1 Malignant neoplasm of exocervix ♀

    C53.8 Malignant neoplasm of overlapping sites **of cervix uteri** ♀

    C53.9 Malignant neoplasm of cervix uteri, unspecified ♀▽

✓4ᵗʰ **C54 Malignant neoplasm of** corpus uteri

    C54.0 Malignant neoplasm of isthmus **uteri** ♀
        Malignant neoplasm of lower uterine segment

    C54.1 Malignant neoplasm of endometrium ♀

    C54.2 Malignant neoplasm of myometrium ♀

    C54.3 Malignant neoplasm of fundus uteri ♀

    C54.8 Malignant neoplasm of overlapping sites **of corpus uteri** ♀

    C54.9 Malignant neoplasm of corpus uteri, unspecified ♀▽

  C55 Malignant neoplasm of uterus, part unspecified ♀▽

✓4ᵗʰ **C56 Malignant neoplasm of** ovary
    Use additional code to identify any functional activity

    C56.1 Malignant neoplasm of right **ovary** ♀

    C56.2 Malignant neoplasm of left **ovary** ♀

    C56.9 Malignant neoplasm of unspecified ovary ♀▽

✓4ᵗʰ **C57 Malignant neoplasm of** other and unspecified female genital organs

    ✓5ᵗʰ **C57.0 Malignant neoplasm of** fallopian tube
        Malignant neoplasm of oviduct
        Malignant neoplasm of uterine tube

        C57.00 Malignant neoplasm of unspecified fallopian tube ♀▽

        C57.01 Malignant neoplasm of right **fallopian tube** ♀

        C57.02 Malignant neoplasm of left **fallopian tube** ♀

    ✓5ᵗʰ **C57.1 Malignant neoplasm of** broad ligament

        C57.10 Malignant neoplasm of unspecified broad ligament ♀▽

        C57.11 Malignant neoplasm of right **broad ligament** ♀

        C57.12 Malignant neoplasm of left **broad ligament** ♀

    ✓5ᵗʰ **C57.2 Malignant neoplasm of** round ligament

        C57.20 Malignant neoplasm of unspecified round ligament ♀▽

        C57.21 Malignant neoplasm of right **round ligament** ♀

        C57.22 Malignant neoplasm of left **round ligament** ♀

    C57.3 Malignant neoplasm of parametrium ♀
        Malignant neoplasm of uterine ligament NOS

    C57.4 Malignant neoplasm of uterine adnexa, **unspecified** ♀▽

    C57.7 Malignant neoplasm of other specified female genital organs ♀
        Malignant neoplasm of wolffian body or duct

    C57.8 Malignant neoplasm of overlapping sites **of female genital organs** ♀
        Primary malignant neoplasm of two or more contiguous sites of the female genital organs whose point of origin cannot be determined
        Primary tubo-ovarian malignant neoplasm whose point of origin cannot be determined
        Primary utero-ovarian malignant neoplasm whose point of origin cannot be determined

    C57.9 Malignant neoplasm of female genital organ, unspecified ♀▽
        Malignant neoplasm of female genitourinary tract NOS

  C58 Malignant neoplasm of placenta Ⓜ♀
    INCLUDES   choriocarcinoma NOS
         chorionepithelioma NOS
    EXCLUDES 1   *chorioadenoma (destruens) (D39.2)*
         hydatidiform mole NOS (O01.9)
         invasive hydatidiform mole (D39.2)
         male choriocarcinoma NOS (C62.9-)
         malignant hydatidiform mole (D39.2)

Malignant neoplasms of male genital organs (C60-C63)

INCLUDES   malignant neoplasm of skin of male genital organs

✓4ᵗʰ **C60 Malignant neoplasm of** penis

    C60.0 Malignant neoplasm of prepuce ♂
        Malignant neoplasm of foreskin

    C60.1 Malignant neoplasm of glans **penis** ♂

    C60.2 Malignant neoplasm of body **of penis** ♂
        Malignant neoplasm of corpus cavernosum

    C60.8 Malignant neoplasm of overlapping sites **of penis** ♂

    C60.9 Malignant neoplasm of penis, unspecified ♂▽
        Malignant neoplasm of skin of penis NOS

  C61 Malignant neoplasm of prostate ♂
    Use additional code to identify:
        hormone sensitivity status (Z19.1-Z19.2)
        rising PSA following treatment for malignant neoplasm of prostate (R97.21)
    EXCLUDES 1   *malignant neoplasm of seminal vesicle (C63.7)*
    AHA: 2017, 1Q, 17

Ⓝ Newborn: 0   Ⓟ Pediatric: 0-17   Ⓜ Maternity: 12-55   Ⓐ Adult: 15-124   NRS Nonroutine supply Dx   NCDx Noncancer Dx   PDx Primary Dx   ▶◀ Revised Text   ● New Code   ▲ Revised Title

470   ICD-10-CM 2018

✓4th C62 Malignant neoplasm of testis
Use additional code to identify any functional activity

✓5th C62.0 Malignant neoplasm of undescended testis
Malignant neoplasm of ectopic testis
Malignant neoplasm of retained testis

C62.00 Malignant neoplasm of unspecified undescended testis ♂▽

C62.01 Malignant neoplasm of undescended right testis ♂

C62.02 Malignant neoplasm of undescended left testis ♂

✓5th C62.1 Malignant neoplasm of descended testis
Malignant neoplasm of scrotal testis

C62.10 Malignant neoplasm of unspecified descended testis ♂▽

C62.11 Malignant neoplasm of descended right testis ♂

C62.12 Malignant neoplasm of descended left testis ♂

✓5th C62.9 Malignant neoplasm of testis, unspecified whether descended or undescended

C62.90 Malignant neoplasm of unspecified testis, unspecified whether descended or undescended ♂▽
Malignant neoplasm of testis NOS

C62.91 Malignant neoplasm of right testis, unspecified whether descended or undescended ♂▽

C62.92 Malignant neoplasm of left testis, unspecified whether descended or undescended ♂▽

✓4th C63 Malignant neoplasm of other and unspecified male genital organs

✓5th C63.0 Malignant neoplasm of epididymis
C63.00 Malignant neoplasm of unspecified epididymis ♂▽
C63.01 Malignant neoplasm of right epididymis ♂
C63.02 Malignant neoplasm of left epididymis ♂

✓5th C63.1 Malignant neoplasm of spermatic cord
C63.10 Malignant neoplasm of unspecified spermatic cord ♂▽
C63.11 Malignant neoplasm of right spermatic cord ♂
C63.12 Malignant neoplasm of left spermatic cord ♂

C63.2 Malignant neoplasm of scrotum ♂
Malignant neoplasm of skin of scrotum

C63.7 Malignant neoplasm of other specified male genital organs ♂
Malignant neoplasm of seminal vesicle
Malignant neoplasm of tunica vaginalis

C63.8 Malignant neoplasm of overlapping sites of male genital organs ♂
Primary malignant neoplasm of two or more contiguous sites of male genital organs whose point of origin cannot be determined

C63.9 Malignant neoplasm of male genital organ, unspecified ♂▽
Malignant neoplasm of male genitourinary tract NOS

Malignant neoplasms of urinary tract (C64-C68)

✓4th C64 Malignant neoplasm of kidney, except renal pelvis
EXCLUDES 1 malignant carcinoid tumor of the kidney (C7A.093)
malignant neoplasm of renal calyces (C65.-)
malignant neoplasm of renal pelvis (C65.-)

C64.1 Malignant neoplasm of right kidney, except renal pelvis
C64.2 Malignant neoplasm of left kidney, except renal pelvis
C64.9 Malignant neoplasm of unspecified kidney, except renal pelvis ▽

✓4th C65 Malignant neoplasm of renal pelvis
INCLUDES malignant neoplasm of pelviureteric junction
malignant neoplasm of renal calyces

C65.1 Malignant neoplasm of right renal pelvis
C65.2 Malignant neoplasm of left renal pelvis
C65.9 Malignant neoplasm of unspecified renal pelvis ▽

✓4th C66 Malignant neoplasm of ureter
EXCLUDES 1 malignant neoplasm of ureteric orifice of bladder (C67.6)

C66.1 Malignant neoplasm of right ureter
C66.2 Malignant neoplasm of left ureter
C66.9 Malignant neoplasm of unspecified ureter ▽

✓4th C67 Malignant neoplasm of bladder
C67.0 Malignant neoplasm of trigone of bladder
C67.1 Malignant neoplasm of dome of bladder
C67.2 Malignant neoplasm of lateral wall of bladder

C67.3 Malignant neoplasm of anterior wall of bladder
C67.4 Malignant neoplasm of posterior wall of bladder
C67.5 Malignant neoplasm of bladder neck
Malignant neoplasm of internal urethral orifice
C67.6 Malignant neoplasm of ureteric orifice
C67.7 Malignant neoplasm of urachus
C67.8 Malignant neoplasm of overlapping sites of bladder
C67.9 Malignant neoplasm of bladder, unspecified ▽
AHA: 2016, 1Q, 19

✓4th C68 Malignant neoplasm of other and unspecified urinary organs
EXCLUDES 1 malignant neoplasm of female genitourinary tract NOS (C57.9)
malignant neoplasm of male genitourinary tract NOS (C63.9)

C68.0 Malignant neoplasm of urethra
EXCLUDES 1 malignant neoplasm of urethral orifice of bladder (C67.5)

C68.1 Malignant neoplasm of paraurethral glands
C68.8 Malignant neoplasm of overlapping sites of urinary organs
Primary malignant neoplasm of two or more contiguous sites of urinary organs whose point of origin cannot be determined
C68.9 Malignant neoplasm of urinary organ, unspecified ▽
Malignant neoplasm of urinary system NOS

Malignant neoplasms of eye, brain and other parts of central nervous system (C69-C72)

✓4th C69 Malignant neoplasm of eye and adnexa
EXCLUDES 1 malignant neoplasm of connective tissue of eyelid (C49.0)
malignant neoplasm of eyelid (skin) (C43.1-, C44.1-)
malignant neoplasm of optic nerve (C72.3-)

✓5th C69.0 Malignant neoplasm of conjunctiva
C69.00 Malignant neoplasm of unspecified conjunctiva ▽
C69.01 Malignant neoplasm of right conjunctiva
C69.02 Malignant neoplasm of left conjunctiva

✓5th C69.1 Malignant neoplasm of cornea
C69.10 Malignant neoplasm of unspecified cornea ▽
C69.11 Malignant neoplasm of right cornea
C69.12 Malignant neoplasm of left cornea

✓5th C69.2 Malignant neoplasm of retina
EXCLUDES 1 dark area on retina (D49.81)
neoplasm of unspecified behavior of retina and choroid (D49.81)
retinal freckle (D49.81)
C69.20 Malignant neoplasm of unspecified retina ▽
C69.21 Malignant neoplasm of right retina
C69.22 Malignant neoplasm of left retina

✓5th C69.3 Malignant neoplasm of choroid
C69.30 Malignant neoplasm of unspecified choroid ▽
C69.31 Malignant neoplasm of right choroid
C69.32 Malignant neoplasm of left choroid

✓5th C69.4 Malignant neoplasm of ciliary body
C69.40 Malignant neoplasm of unspecified ciliary body ▽
C69.41 Malignant neoplasm of right ciliary body
C69.42 Malignant neoplasm of left ciliary body

✓5th C69.5 Malignant neoplasm of lacrimal gland and duct
Malignant neoplasm of lacrimal sac
Malignant neoplasm of nasolacrimal duct
C69.50 Malignant neoplasm of unspecified lacrimal gland and duct ▽
C69.51 Malignant neoplasm of right lacrimal gland and duct
C69.52 Malignant neoplasm of left lacrimal gland and duct

✓5th C69.6 Malignant neoplasm of orbit
Malignant neoplasm of connective tissue of orbit
Malignant neoplasm of extraocular muscle
Malignant neoplasm of peripheral nerves of orbit
Malignant neoplasm of retrobulbar tissue
Malignant neoplasm of retro-ocular tissue
EXCLUDES 1 malignant neoplasm of orbital bone (C41.0)
C69.60 Malignant neoplasm of unspecified orbit ▽
C69.61 Malignant neoplasm of right orbit
C69.62 Malignant neoplasm of left orbit

✓5th C69.8 Malignant neoplasm of overlapping sites of eye and adnexa
C69.80 Malignant neoplasm of overlapping sites of unspecified eye and adnexa ▽

✓ Additional Character Req   ✓x7th Placeholder Alert   Case-Mix Diagnosis   Manifestation   ▽ Unspecified Dx   EXCLUDES 1 Not coded here   EXCLUDES 2 Not included here

Chapter 2. Neoplasms

    C69.81   **Malignant neoplasm of overlapping sites of right eye and adnexa**

    C69.82   **Malignant neoplasm of overlapping sites of left eye and adnexa**

✓5ᵗʰ C69.9   **Malignant neoplasm of unspecified site of eye**
    Malignant neoplasm of eyeball

    C69.9Ø   **Malignant neoplasm of unspecified site of unspecified eye** ▽

    C69.91   **Malignant neoplasm of unspecified site of right eye** ▽

    C69.92   **Malignant neoplasm of unspecified site of left eye** ▽

✓4ᵗʰ **C7Ø**   **Malignant neoplasm of meninges**

    C7Ø.Ø   **Malignant neoplasm of cerebral meninges**

    C7Ø.1   **Malignant neoplasm of spinal meninges**

    C7Ø.9   **Malignant neoplasm of meninges, unspecified** ▽

✓4ᵗʰ **C71**   **Malignant neoplasm of brain**
    EXCLUDES 1   *malignant neoplasm of cranial nerves (C72.2-C72.5)*
              retrobulbar malignant neoplasm (C69.6-)

    C71.Ø   **Malignant neoplasm of cerebrum, except lobes and ventricles**
           Malignant neoplasm of supratentorial NOS

    C71.1   **Malignant neoplasm of frontal lobe**

    C71.2   **Malignant neoplasm of temporal lobe**

    C71.3   **Malignant neoplasm of parietal lobe**

    C71.4   **Malignant neoplasm of occipital lobe**

    C71.5   **Malignant neoplasm of cerebral ventricle**
        EXCLUDES 1   *malignant neoplasm of fourth cerebral ventricle (C71.7)*

    C71.6   **Malignant neoplasm of cerebellum**

    C71.7   **Malignant neoplasm of brain stem**
           Malignant neoplasm of fourth cerebral ventricle
           Infratentorial malignant neoplasm NOS

    C71.8   **Malignant neoplasm of overlapping sites of brain**

    C71.9   **Malignant neoplasm of brain, unspecified** ▽
           AHA: 2014, 3Q, 3

✓4ᵗʰ **C72**   **Malignant neoplasm of spinal cord, cranial nerves and other parts of central nervous system**
    EXCLUDES 1   *malignant neoplasm of meninges (C7Ø.-)*
              malignant neoplasm of peripheral nerves and autonomic nervous system (C47.-)

    C72.Ø   **Malignant neoplasm of spinal cord**

    C72.1   **Malignant neoplasm of cauda equina**

✓5ᵗʰ C72.2   **Malignant neoplasm of olfactory nerve**
    Malignant neoplasm of olfactory bulb

    C72.2Ø   **Malignant neoplasm of unspecified olfactory nerve** ▽

    C72.21   **Malignant neoplasm of right olfactory nerve**

    C72.22   **Malignant neoplasm of left olfactory nerve**

✓5ᵗʰ C72.3   **Malignant neoplasm of optic nerve**

    C72.3Ø   **Malignant neoplasm of unspecified optic nerve** ▽

    C72.31   **Malignant neoplasm of right optic nerve**

    C72.32   **Malignant neoplasm of left optic nerve**

Lobes of the Brain

✓5ᵗʰ C72.4   **Malignant neoplasm of acoustic nerve**

    C72.4Ø   **Malignant neoplasm of unspecified acoustic nerve** ▽

    C72.41   **Malignant neoplasm of right acoustic nerve**

    C72.42   **Malignant neoplasm of left acoustic nerve**

✓5ᵗʰ C72.5   **Malignant neoplasm of other and unspecified cranial nerves**

    C72.5Ø   **Malignant neoplasm of unspecified cranial nerve** ▽
           Malignant neoplasm of cranial nerve NOS

    C72.59   **Malignant neoplasm of other cranial nerves**

    C72.9   **Malignant neoplasm of central nervous system, unspecified** ▽
           Malignant neoplasm of unspecified site of central nervous system
           Malignant neoplasm of nervous system NOS

Malignant neoplasms of thyroid and other endocrine glands (C73-C75)

C73   **Malignant neoplasm of thyroid gland**
    Use additional code to identify any functional activity

✓4ᵗʰ **C74**   **Malignant neoplasm of adrenal gland**

✓5ᵗʰ C74.Ø   **Malignant neoplasm of cortex of adrenal gland**

    C74.ØØ   **Malignant neoplasm of cortex of unspecified adrenal gland** ▽

    C74.Ø1   **Malignant neoplasm of cortex of right adrenal gland**

    C74.Ø2   **Malignant neoplasm of cortex of left adrenal gland**

✓5ᵗʰ C74.1   **Malignant neoplasm of medulla of adrenal gland**

    C74.1Ø   **Malignant neoplasm of medulla of unspecified adrenal gland** ▽

    C74.11   **Malignant neoplasm of medulla of right adrenal gland**

    C74.12   **Malignant neoplasm of medulla of left adrenal gland**

✓5ᵗʰ C74.9   **Malignant neoplasm of unspecified part of adrenal gland**

    C74.9Ø   **Malignant neoplasm of unspecified part of unspecified adrenal gland** ▽

    C74.91   **Malignant neoplasm of unspecified part of right adrenal gland** ▽

    C74.92   **Malignant neoplasm of unspecified part of left adrenal gland** ▽

✓4ᵗʰ **C75**   **Malignant neoplasm of other endocrine glands and related structures**
    EXCLUDES 1   *malignant carcinoid tumors (C7A.Ø-)*
              malignant neoplasm of adrenal gland (C74.-)
              malignant neoplasm of endocrine pancreas (C25.4)
              malignant neoplasm of islets of Langerhans (C25.4)
              malignant neoplasm of ovary (C56.-)
              malignant neoplasm of testis (C62.-)
              malignant neoplasm of thymus (C37)
              malignant neoplasm of thyroid gland (C73)
              malignant neuroendocrine tumors (C7A.-)

    C75.Ø   **Malignant neoplasm of parathyroid gland**

    C75.1   **Malignant neoplasm of pituitary gland**

    C75.2   **Malignant neoplasm of craniopharyngeal duct**

    C75.3   **Malignant neoplasm of pineal gland**

    C75.4   **Malignant neoplasm of carotid body**

    C75.5   **Malignant neoplasm of aortic body and other paraganglia**

    C75.8   **Malignant neoplasm with pluriglandular involvement, unspecified** ▽

    C75.9   **Malignant neoplasm of endocrine gland, unspecified** ▽

Malignant neuroendocrine tumors (C7A)

✓4ᵗʰ **C7A**   **Malignant neuroendocrine tumors**
    Use additional code to identify any associated endocrine syndrome, such as:
      carcinoid syndrome (E34.Ø)
    Code also any associated multiple endocrine neoplasia [MEN] syndromes (E31.2-)
    EXCLUDES 2   *malignant pancreatic islet cell tumors (C25.4)*
              Merkel cell carcinoma (C4A.-)

✓5ᵗʰ C7A.Ø   **Malignant carcinoid tumors**

    C7A.ØØ   **Malignant carcinoid tumor of unspecified site** ▽

✓6ᵗʰ C7A.Ø1   **Malignant carcinoid tumors of the small intestine**

        C7A.Ø1Ø   **Malignant carcinoid tumor of the duodenum**

        C7A.Ø11   **Malignant carcinoid tumor of the jejunum**

Ⓝ Newborn: 0   Ⓟ Pediatric: 0-17   Ⓜ Maternity: 12-55   Ⓐ Adult: 15-124   **NRS** Nonroutine supply Dx   **NCDx** Noncancer Dx   **PDx** Primary Dx   ▶◀ Revised Text   ● New Code   ▲ Revised Title

472   ICD-10-CM 2018

C7A.Ø12 **Malignant carcinoid tumor of the** ileum

C7A.Ø19 **Malignant carcinoid tumor of the small** ▽
intestine, unspecified portion

✓6th C7A.Ø2 **Malignant carcinoid tumors of the** appendix, large intestine, and rectum

C7A.Ø2Ø **Malignant carcinoid tumor of the** **appendix**

C7A.Ø21 **Malignant carcinoid tumor of the** cecum

C7A.Ø22 **Malignant carcinoid tumor of the** ascending colon

C7A.Ø23 **Malignant carcinoid tumor of the** transverse colon

C7A.Ø24 **Malignant carcinoid tumor of the** descending colon

C7A.Ø25 **Malignant carcinoid tumor of the** sigmoid colon

C7A.Ø26 **Malignant carcinoid tumor of the** rectum

C7A.Ø29 **Malignant carcinoid tumor of the** ▽ **large intestine, unspecified portion**
Malignant carcinoid tumor of the colon NOS

✓6th C7A.Ø9 **Malignant carcinoid tumors of** other sites

C7A.Ø9Ø **Malignant carcinoid tumor of the** bronchus and lung

C7A.Ø91 **Malignant carcinoid tumor of the** thymus

C7A.Ø92 **Malignant carcinoid tumor of the** stomach

C7A.Ø93 **Malignant carcinoid tumor of the** kidney

C7A.Ø94 **Malignant carcinoid tumor of the** ▽ **foregut, unspecified**

C7A.Ø95 **Malignant carcinoid tumor of the** ▽ **midgut, unspecified**

C7A.Ø96 **Malignant carcinoid tumor of the** ▽ **hindgut, unspecified**

C7A.Ø98 **Malignant carcinoid tumors of** other sites

C7A.1 **Malignant** poorly differentiated **neuroendocrine tumors**
High grade neuroendocrine carcinoma, any site
Malignant poorly differentiated neuroendocrine tumor NOS
Malignant poorly differentiated neuroendocrine carcinoma, any site

C7A.8 **Other malignant neuroendocrine tumors**

Secondary neuroendocrine tumors (C7B)

✓4th C7B **Secondary neuroendocrine tumors**
Use additional code to identify any functional activity

✓5th C7B.Ø **Secondary** carcinoid tumors

C7B.ØØ **Secondary carcinoid tumors, unspecified site** ▽

C7B.Ø1 **Secondary carcinoid tumors of** distant lymph nodes

C7B.Ø2 **Secondary carcinoid tumors of** liver

C7B.Ø3 **Secondary carcinoid tumors of** bone

C7B.Ø4 **Secondary carcinoid tumors of** peritoneum
Mesentery metastasis of carcinoid tumor

C7B.Ø9 **Secondary carcinoid tumors of other sites**

C7B.1 **Secondary** Merkel cell carcinoma   NRS
Merkel cell carcinoma nodal presentation
Merkel cell carcinoma visceral metastatic presentation

C7B.8 **Other secondary neuroendocrine tumors**

Malignant neoplasms of ill-defined, other secondary and unspecified sites (C76-C8Ø)

✓4th C76 **Malignant neoplasm of** other and ill-defined sites
EXCLUDES 1   *malignant neoplasm of female genitourinary tract NOS (C57.9)*
malignant neoplasm of male genitourinary tract NOS (C63.9)
malignant neoplasm of lymphoid, hematopoietic and related tissue (C81-C96)
malignant neoplasm of skin (C44.-)
malignant neoplasm of unspecified site NOS (C8Ø.1)

C76.Ø **Malignant neoplasm of** head, face and neck
Malignant neoplasm of cheek NOS
Malignant neoplasm of nose NOS

C76.1 **Malignant neoplasm of** thorax
Intrathoracic malignant neoplasm NOS
Malignant neoplasm of axilla NOS
Thoracic malignant neoplasm NOS

C76.2 **Malignant neoplasm of** abdomen

C76.3 **Malignant neoplasm of** pelvis
Malignant neoplasm of groin NOS
Malignant neoplasm of sites overlapping systems within the pelvis
Rectovaginal (septum) malignant neoplasm
Rectovesical (septum) malignant neoplasm

✓5th C76.4 **Malignant neoplasm of** upper limb

C76.4Ø **Malignant neoplasm of unspecified upper limb** ▽

C76.41 **Malignant neoplasm of** right **upper limb**

C76.42 **Malignant neoplasm of** left **upper limb**

✓5th C76.5 **Malignant neoplasm of** lower limb

C76.5Ø **Malignant neoplasm of unspecified lower limb** ▽

C76.51 **Malignant neoplasm of** right **lower limb**

C76.52 **Malignant neoplasm of** left **lower limb**

C76.8 **Malignant neoplasm of other** specified ill-defined sites
Malignant neoplasm of overlapping ill-defined sites

✓4th C77 **Secondary and unspecified malignant neoplasm of** lymph nodes
EXCLUDES 1   *malignant neoplasm of lymph nodes, specified as primary (C81-C86, C88, C96.-)*
mesentery metastasis of carcinoid tumor (C7B.Ø4)
secondary carcinoid tumors of distant lymph nodes (C7B.Ø1)

C77.Ø **Secondary and unspecified malignant neoplasm of lymph nodes of** head, face and neck
Secondary and unspecified malignant neoplasm of supraclavicular lymph nodes

C77.1 **Secondary and unspecified malignant neoplasm of** intrathoracic **lymph nodes**

C77.2 **Secondary and unspecified malignant neoplasm of** intra-abdominal lymph nodes

C77.3 **Secondary and unspecified malignant neoplasm of** axilla and upper limb **lymph nodes**
Secondary and unspecified malignant neoplasm of pectoral lymph nodes

C77.4 **Secondary and unspecified malignant neoplasm of** inguinal and lower limb **lymph nodes**

C77.5 **Secondary and unspecified malignant neoplasm of** intrapelvic **lymph nodes**

C77.8 **Secondary and unspecified malignant neoplasm of lymph nodes of** multiple regions

C77.9 **Secondary and unspecified malignant neoplasm of** ▽ **lymph node, unspecified**

✓4th C78 **Secondary malignant neoplasm of** respiratory and digestive organs
EXCLUDES 1   *secondary carcinoid tumors of liver (C7B.Ø2)*
secondary carcinoid tumors of peritoneum (C7B.Ø4)
EXCLUDES 2   *lymph node metastases (C77.Ø)*

✓5th C78.Ø **Secondary malignant neoplasm of** lung

C78.ØØ **Secondary malignant neoplasm of unspecified** ▽ **lung**

C78.Ø1 **Secondary malignant neoplasm of** right **lung**

C78.Ø2 **Secondary malignant neoplasm of** left **lung**

C78.1 **Secondary malignant neoplasm of** mediastinum

C78.2 **Secondary malignant neoplasm of** pleura

✓5th C78.3 **Secondary malignant neoplasm of** other and unspecified respiratory organs

C78.3Ø **Secondary malignant neoplasm of unspecified** ▽ **respiratory organ**

C78.39 **Secondary malignant neoplasm of other respiratory organs**

C78.4 **Secondary malignant neoplasm of** small intestine

C78.5 **Secondary malignant neoplasm of** large intestine and rectum

C78.6 **Secondary malignant neoplasm of** retroperitoneum and peritoneum
AHA: 2017, 2Q, 12

C78.7 **Secondary malignant neoplasm of** liver and intrahepatic bile duct

✓5th C78.8 **Secondary malignant neoplasm of** other and unspecified digestive organs

C78.8Ø **Secondary malignant neoplasm of unspecified** ▽ **digestive organ**

C78.89 **Secondary malignant neoplasm of other digestive organs**
Code also exocrine pancreatic insufficiency (K86.81)

Chapter 2. Neoplasms

C79–C81.29

✓4ᵗʰ **C79 Secondary malignant neoplasm of** other and unspecified sites
    EXCLUDES 1   *secondary carcinoid tumors (C7B.-)*
              secondary neuroendocrine tumors (C7B.-)
    EXCLUDES 2   *lymph node metastases (C77.0)*

  ✓5ᵗʰ **C79.0 Secondary malignant neoplasm of** kidney and renal pelvis
      C79.00 Secondary malignant neoplasm of unspecified kidney and renal pelvis ▽
      C79.01 Secondary malignant neoplasm of right **kidney and renal pelvis**
      C79.02 Secondary malignant neoplasm of left **kidney and renal pelvis**

  ✓5ᵗʰ **C79.1 Secondary malignant neoplasm of** bladder and other and unspecified urinary organs
      C79.10 Secondary malignant neoplasm of unspecified urinary organs ▽
      C79.11 Secondary malignant neoplasm of bladder
         EXCLUDES 2 ▶*lymph node metastases (C77.0)*◀
      C79.19 Secondary malignant neoplasm of other urinary organs

  C79.2 Secondary malignant neoplasm of skin
      EXCLUDES 1   *secondary Merkel cell carcinoma (C7B.1)*

  ✓5ᵗʰ **C79.3 Secondary malignant neoplasm of** brain and cerebral meninges
      C79.31 Secondary malignant neoplasm of brain
      C79.32 Secondary malignant neoplasm of cerebral meninges

  ✓5ᵗʰ **C79.4 Secondary malignant neoplasm of** other and unspecified parts of nervous system
      C79.40 Secondary malignant neoplasm of unspecified part of nervous system ▽
      C79.49 Secondary malignant neoplasm of other parts of nervous system

  ✓5ᵗʰ **C79.5 Secondary malignant neoplasm of** bone and bone marrow
      EXCLUDES 1   *secondary carcinoid tumors of bone (C7B.03)*
      C79.51 Secondary malignant neoplasm of bone
      C79.52 Secondary malignant neoplasm of bone marrow

  ✓5ᵗʰ **C79.6 Secondary malignant neoplasm of** ovary
      C79.60 Secondary malignant neoplasm of unspecified ovary ♀▽
      C79.61 Secondary malignant neoplasm of right **ovary** ♀
      C79.62 Secondary malignant neoplasm of left **ovary** ♀

  ✓5ᵗʰ **C79.7 Secondary malignant neoplasm of** adrenal gland
      C79.70 Secondary malignant neoplasm of unspecified adrenal gland ▽
      C79.71 Secondary malignant neoplasm of right **adrenal gland**
      C79.72 Secondary malignant neoplasm of left **adrenal gland**

  ✓5ᵗʰ **C79.8 Secondary malignant neoplasm of** other specified sites
      C79.81 Secondary malignant neoplasm of breast
      C79.82 Secondary malignant neoplasm of genital organs
      C79.89 Secondary malignant neoplasm of other specified sites
         AHA: 2017, 2Q, 11

  C79.9 Secondary malignant neoplasm of unspecified site ▽
      Metastatic cancer NOS
      Metastatic disease NOS
      EXCLUDES 1   *carcinomatosis NOS (C80.0)*
              generalized cancer NOS (C80.0)
              malignant (primary) neoplasm of unspecified site (C80.1)

✓4ᵗʰ **C80 Malignant neoplasm** without specification of site
    EXCLUDES 1   *malignant carcinoid tumor of unspecified site (C7A.00)*
               malignant neoplasm of specified multiple sites—code to each site

  C80.0 Disseminated malignant neoplasm, unspecified ▽
      Carcinomatosis NOS
      Generalized cancer, unspecified site (primary) (secondary)
      Generalized malignancy, unspecified site (primary) (secondary)

  C80.1 Malignant (primary) **neoplasm, unspecified** ▽
      Cancer NOS
      Cancer unspecified site (primary)
      Carcinoma unspecified site (primary)
      Malignancy unspecified site (primary)
      EXCLUDES 1   *secondary malignant neoplasm of unspecified site (C79.9)*

  C80.2 Malignant neoplasm associated with transplanted organ
      Code first complication of transplanted organ (T86.-)
      Use additional code to identify the specific malignancy

Malignant neoplasms of lymphoid, hematopoietic and related tissue (C81-C96)

    EXCLUDES 2   *Kaposi's sarcoma of lymph nodes (C46.3)*
              secondary and unspecified neoplasm of lymph nodes (C77.-)
              secondary neoplasm of bone marrow (C79.52)
              secondary neoplasm of spleen (C78.89)

✓4ᵗʰ **C81 Hodgkin lymphoma**
    EXCLUDES 1   *personal history of Hodgkin lymphoma (Z85.71)*

  ✓5ᵗʰ **C81.0 Nodular lymphocyte predominant Hodgkin lymphoma**
      C81.00 Nodular lymphocyte predominant Hodgkin lymphoma, unspecified site ▽
      C81.01 Nodular lymphocyte predominant Hodgkin lymphoma, lymph nodes of head, face, and neck
      C81.02 Nodular lymphocyte predominant Hodgkin lymphoma, intrathoracic **lymph nodes**
      C81.03 Nodular lymphocyte predominant Hodgkin lymphoma, intra-abdominal **lymph nodes**
      C81.04 Nodular lymphocyte predominant Hodgkin lymphoma, lymph nodes of axilla and upper limb
      C81.05 Nodular lymphocyte predominant Hodgkin lymphoma, lymph nodes of inguinal region and lower limb
      C81.06 Nodular lymphocyte predominant Hodgkin lymphoma, intrapelvic **lymph nodes**
      C81.07 Nodular lymphocyte predominant Hodgkin lymphoma, spleen
      C81.08 Nodular lymphocyte predominant Hodgkin lymphoma, lymph nodes of multiple sites
      C81.09 Nodular lymphocyte predominant Hodgkin lymphoma, extranodal and solid organ sites

  ✓5ᵗʰ **C81.1 Nodular sclerosis Hodgkin lymphoma**
      Nodular sclerosis classical Hodgkin lymphoma
      C81.10 Nodular sclerosis Hodgkin lymphoma, unspecified site ▽
      C81.11 Nodular sclerosis Hodgkin lymphoma, lymph nodes of head, face, and neck
      C81.12 Nodular sclerosis Hodgkin lymphoma, intrathoracic **lymph nodes**
      C81.13 Nodular sclerosis Hodgkin lymphoma, intra-abdominal **lymph nodes**
      C81.14 Nodular sclerosis Hodgkin lymphoma, lymph nodes of axilla and upper limb
      C81.15 Nodular sclerosis Hodgkin lymphoma, lymph nodes of inguinal region and lower limb
      C81.16 Nodular sclerosis Hodgkin lymphoma, intrapelvic **lymph nodes**
      C81.17 Nodular sclerosis Hodgkin lymphoma, spleen
      C81.18 Nodular sclerosis Hodgkin lymphoma, lymph nodes of multiple sites
      C81.19 Nodular sclerosis Hodgkin lymphoma, extranodal and solid organ sites

  ✓5ᵗʰ **C81.2 Mixed cellularity Hodgkin lymphoma**
      Mixed cellularity classical Hodgkin lymphoma
      C81.20 Mixed cellularity Hodgkin lymphoma, unspecified site ▽
      C81.21 Mixed cellularity Hodgkin lymphoma, lymph nodes of head, face, and neck
      C81.22 Mixed cellularity Hodgkin lymphoma, intrathoracic **lymph nodes**
      C81.23 Mixed cellularity Hodgkin lymphoma, intra-abdominal **lymph nodes**
      C81.24 Mixed cellularity Hodgkin lymphoma, lymph nodes of axilla and upper limb
      C81.25 Mixed cellularity Hodgkin lymphoma, lymph nodes of inguinal region and lower limb
      C81.26 Mixed cellularity Hodgkin lymphoma, intrapelvic **lymph nodes**
      C81.27 Mixed cellularity Hodgkin lymphoma, spleen
      C81.28 Mixed cellularity Hodgkin lymphoma, lymph nodes of multiple sites
      C81.29 Mixed cellularity Hodgkin lymphoma, extranodal and solid organ sites

---

Ⓝ Newborn: 0   Ⓟ Pediatric: 0-17   Ⓜ Maternity: 12-55   Ⓐ Adult: 15-124   **NRS** Nonroutine supply Dx   **NC Dx** Noncancer Dx   **PDx** Primary Dx   ▶◀ Revised Text   ● New Code   ▲ Revised Title

✓5th **C81.3 Lymphocyte depleted Hodgkin lymphoma**
Lymphocyte depleted classical Hodgkin lymphoma

C81.30 **Lymphocyte depleted Hodgkin lymphoma, unspecified site** ▽

C81.31 **Lymphocyte depleted Hodgkin lymphoma, lymph nodes of head, face, and neck**

C81.32 **Lymphocyte depleted Hodgkin lymphoma, intrathoracic lymph nodes**

C81.33 **Lymphocyte depleted Hodgkin lymphoma, intra-abdominal lymph nodes**

C81.34 **Lymphocyte depleted Hodgkin lymphoma, lymph nodes of axilla and upper limb**

C81.35 **Lymphocyte depleted Hodgkin lymphoma, lymph nodes of inguinal region and lower limb**

C81.36 **Lymphocyte depleted Hodgkin lymphoma, intrapelvic lymph nodes**

C81.37 **Lymphocyte depleted Hodgkin lymphoma, spleen**

C81.38 **Lymphocyte depleted Hodgkin lymphoma, lymph nodes of multiple sites**

C81.39 **Lymphocyte depleted Hodgkin lymphoma, extranodal and solid organ sites**

✓5th **C81.4 Lymphocyte-rich Hodgkin lymphoma**
Lymphocyte-rich classical Hodgkin lymphoma

EXCLUDES 1 *nodular lymphocyte predominant Hodgkin lymphoma (C81.0-)*

C81.40 **Lymphocyte-rich Hodgkin lymphoma, unspecified site** ▽

C81.41 **Lymphocyte-rich Hodgkin lymphoma, lymph nodes of head, face, and neck**

C81.42 **Lymphocyte-rich Hodgkin lymphoma, intrathoracic lymph nodes**

C81.43 **Lymphocyte-rich Hodgkin lymphoma, intra-abdominal lymph nodes**

C81.44 **Lymphocyte-rich Hodgkin lymphoma, lymph nodes of axilla and upper limb**

C81.45 **Lymphocyte-rich Hodgkin lymphoma, lymph nodes of inguinal region and lower limb**

C81.46 **Lymphocyte-rich Hodgkin lymphoma, intrapelvic lymph nodes**

C81.47 **Lymphocyte-rich Hodgkin lymphoma, spleen**

C81.48 **Lymphocyte-rich Hodgkin lymphoma, lymph nodes of multiple sites**

C81.49 **Lymphocyte-rich Hodgkin lymphoma, extranodal and solid organ sites**

✓5th **C81.7 Other Hodgkin lymphoma**
Classical Hodgkin lymphoma NOS
Other classical Hodgkin lymphoma

C81.70 **Other Hodgkin lymphoma, unspecified site** ▽

C81.71 **Other Hodgkin lymphoma, lymph nodes of head, face, and neck**

C81.72 **Other Hodgkin lymphoma, intrathoracic lymph nodes**

C81.73 **Other Hodgkin lymphoma, intra-abdominal lymph nodes**

C81.74 **Other Hodgkin lymphoma, lymph nodes of axilla and upper limb**

C81.75 **Other Hodgkin lymphoma, lymph nodes of inguinal region and lower limb**

C81.76 **Other Hodgkin lymphoma, intrapelvic lymph nodes**

C81.77 **Other Hodgkin lymphoma, spleen**

C81.78 **Other Hodgkin lymphoma, lymph nodes of multiple sites**

C81.79 **Other Hodgkin lymphoma, extranodal and solid organ sites**

✓5th **C81.9 Hodgkin lymphoma, unspecified**

C81.90 **Hodgkin lymphoma, unspecified, unspecified site** ▽

C81.91 **Hodgkin lymphoma, unspecified, lymph nodes of head, face, and neck** ▽

C81.92 **Hodgkin lymphoma, unspecified, intrathoracic lymph nodes** ▽

C81.93 **Hodgkin lymphoma, unspecified, intra-abdominal lymph nodes** ▽

C81.94 **Hodgkin lymphoma, unspecified, lymph nodes of axilla and upper limb** ▽

C81.95 **Hodgkin lymphoma, unspecified, lymph nodes of inguinal region and lower limb** ▽

C81.96 **Hodgkin lymphoma, unspecified, intrapelvic lymph nodes** ▽

C81.97 **Hodgkin lymphoma, unspecified, spleen** ▽

C81.98 **Hodgkin lymphoma, unspecified, lymph nodes of multiple sites** ▽

C81.99 **Hodgkin lymphoma, unspecified, extranodal and solid organ sites** ▽

✓4th **C82 Follicular lymphoma**
INCLUDES follicular lymphoma with or without diffuse areas
EXCLUDES 1 *mature T/NK-cell lymphomas (C84.-)*
personal history of non-Hodgkin lymphoma (Z85.72)

✓5th **C82.0 Follicular lymphoma grade I**

C82.00 **Follicular lymphoma grade I, unspecified site** ▽

C82.01 **Follicular lymphoma grade I, lymph nodes of head, face, and neck**

C82.02 **Follicular lymphoma grade I, intrathoracic lymph nodes**

C82.03 **Follicular lymphoma grade I, intra-abdominal lymph nodes**

C82.04 **Follicular lymphoma grade I, lymph nodes of axilla and upper limb**

C82.05 **Follicular lymphoma grade I, lymph nodes of inguinal region and lower limb**

C82.06 **Follicular lymphoma grade I, intrapelvic lymph nodes**

C82.07 **Follicular lymphoma grade I, spleen**

C82.08 **Follicular lymphoma grade I, lymph nodes of multiple sites**

C82.09 **Follicular lymphoma grade I, extranodal and solid organ sites**

✓6th **C82.1 Follicular lymphoma grade II**

C82.10 **Follicular lymphoma grade II, unspecified site** ▽

C82.11 **Follicular lymphoma grade II, lymph nodes of head, face, and neck**

C82.12 **Follicular lymphoma grade II, intrathoracic lymph nodes**

C82.13 **Follicular lymphoma grade II, intra-abdominal lymph nodes**

C82.14 **Follicular lymphoma grade II, lymph nodes of axilla and upper limb**

C82.15 **Follicular lymphoma grade II, lymph nodes of inguinal region and lower limb**

C82.16 **Follicular lymphoma grade II, intrapelvic lymph nodes**

C82.17 **Follicular lymphoma grade II, spleen**

C82.18 **Follicular lymphoma grade II, lymph nodes of multiple sites**

C82.19 **Follicular lymphoma grade II, extranodal and solid organ sites**

✓5th **C82.2 Follicular lymphoma grade III, unspecified**

C82.20 **Follicular lymphoma grade III, unspecified, unspecified site** ▽

C82.21 **Follicular lymphoma grade III, unspecified, lymph nodes of head, face, and neck** ▽

C82.22 **Follicular lymphoma grade III, unspecified, intrathoracic lymph nodes** ▽

C82.23 **Follicular lymphoma grade III, unspecified, intra-abdominal lymph nodes** ▽

C82.24 **Follicular lymphoma grade III, unspecified, lymph nodes of axilla and upper limb** ▽

C82.25 **Follicular lymphoma grade III, unspecified, lymph nodes of inguinal region and lower limb** ▽

C82.26 **Follicular lymphoma grade III, unspecified, intrapelvic lymph nodes** ▽

C82.27 **Follicular lymphoma grade III, unspecified, spleen** ▽

C82.28 **Follicular lymphoma grade III, unspecified, lymph nodes of multiple sites** ▽

C82.29 **Follicular lymphoma grade III, unspecified, extranodal and solid organ sites** ▽

✓5th **C82.3 Follicular lymphoma grade IIIa**

C82.30 **Follicular lymphoma grade IIIa, unspecified site** ▽

C82.31 **Follicular lymphoma grade IIIa, lymph nodes of head, face, and neck**

C82.32 **Follicular lymphoma grade IIIa, intrathoracic lymph nodes**

☑ Additional Character Req   v1 7th Placeholder Alert   Case-Mix Diagnosis   Manifestation   ▽ Unspecified Dx   EXCLUDES 1 Not coded here   EXCLUDES 2 Not included here

ICD-10-CM 2018   475

Chapter 2. Neoplasms

C82.33 Follicular lymphoma grade IIIa, intra-abdominal lymph nodes

C82.34 Follicular lymphoma grade IIIa, lymph nodes of axilla and upper limb

C82.35 Follicular lymphoma grade IIIa, lymph nodes of inguinal region and lower limb

C82.36 Follicular lymphoma grade IIIa, intrapelvic lymph nodes

C82.37 Follicular lymphoma grade IIIa, spleen

C82.38 Follicular lymphoma grade IIIa, lymph nodes of multiple sites

C82.39 Follicular lymphoma grade IIIa, extranodal and solid organ sites

✓5ᵗʰ C82.4 Follicular lymphoma grade IIIb

C82.40 Follicular lymphoma grade IIIb, unspecified site ▽

C82.41 Follicular lymphoma grade IIIb, lymph nodes of head, face, and neck

C82.42 Follicular lymphoma grade IIIb, intrathoracic lymph nodes

C82.43 Follicular lymphoma grade IIIb, intra-abdominal lymph nodes

C82.44 Follicular lymphoma grade IIIb, lymph nodes of axilla and upper limb

C82.45 Follicular lymphoma grade IIIb, lymph nodes of inguinal region and lower limb

C82.46 Follicular lymphoma grade IIIb, intrapelvic lymph nodes

C82.47 Follicular lymphoma grade IIIb, spleen

C82.48 Follicular lymphoma grade IIIb, lymph nodes of multiple sites

C82.49 Follicular lymphoma grade IIIb, extranodal and solid organ sites

✓5ᵗʰ C82.5 Diffuse follicle center lymphoma

C82.50 Diffuse follicle center lymphoma, unspecified site ▽

C82.51 Diffuse follicle center lymphoma, lymph nodes of head, face, and neck

C82.52 Diffuse follicle center lymphoma, intrathoracic lymph nodes

C82.53 Diffuse follicle center lymphoma, intra-abdominal lymph nodes

C82.54 Diffuse follicle center lymphoma, lymph nodes of axilla and upper limb

C82.55 Diffuse follicle center lymphoma, lymph nodes of inguinal region and lower limb

C82.56 Diffuse follicle center lymphoma, intrapelvic lymph nodes

C82.57 Diffuse follicle center lymphoma, spleen

C82.58 Diffuse follicle center lymphoma, lymph nodes of multiple sites

C82.59 Diffuse follicle center lymphoma, extranodal and solid organ sites

✓5ᵗʰ C82.6 Cutaneous follicle center lymphoma

C82.60 Cutaneous follicle center lymphoma, unspecified site NRS ▽

C82.61 Cutaneous follicle center lymphoma, lymph nodes of head, face, and neck NRS

C82.62 Cutaneous follicle center lymphoma, intrathoracic lymph nodes NRS

C82.63 Cutaneous follicle center lymphoma, intra-abdominal lymph nodes NRS

C82.64 Cutaneous follicle center lymphoma, lymph nodes of axilla and upper limb NRS

C82.65 Cutaneous follicle center lymphoma, lymph nodes of inguinal region and lower limb NRS

C82.66 Cutaneous follicle center lymphoma, intrapelvic lymph nodes NRS

C82.67 Cutaneous follicle center lymphoma, spleen NRS

C82.68 Cutaneous follicle center lymphoma, lymph nodes of multiple sites NRS

C82.69 Cutaneous follicle center lymphoma, extranodal and solid organ sites NRS

✓5ᵗʰ C82.8 Other types of follicular lymphoma

C82.80 Other types of follicular lymphoma, unspecified site NRS ▽

C82.81 Other types of follicular lymphoma, lymph nodes of head, face, and neck NRS

C82.82 Other types of follicular lymphoma, intrathoracic lymph nodes NRS

C82.83 Other types of follicular lymphoma, intra-abdominal lymph nodes NRS

C82.84 Other types of follicular lymphoma, lymph nodes of axilla and upper limb NRS

C82.85 Other types of follicular lymphoma, lymph nodes of inguinal region and lower limb NRS

C82.86 Other types of follicular lymphoma, intrapelvic lymph nodes NRS

C82.87 Other types of follicular lymphoma, spleen NRS

C82.88 Other types of follicular lymphoma, lymph nodes of multiple sites NRS

C82.89 Other types of follicular lymphoma, extranodal and solid organ sites NRS

✓5ᵗʰ C82.9 Follicular lymphoma, unspecified

C82.90 Follicular lymphoma, unspecified, unspecified site NRS ▽

C82.91 Follicular lymphoma, unspecified, lymph nodes of head, face, and neck NRS ▽

C82.92 Follicular lymphoma, unspecified, intrathoracic lymph nodes NRS ▽

C82.93 Follicular lymphoma, unspecified, intra-abdominal lymph nodes NRS ▽

C82.94 Follicular lymphoma, unspecified, lymph nodes of axilla and upper limb NRS ▽

C82.95 Follicular lymphoma, unspecified, lymph nodes of inguinal region and lower limb NRS ▽

C82.96 Follicular lymphoma, unspecified, intrapelvic lymph nodes NRS ▽

C82.97 Follicular lymphoma, unspecified, spleen NRS ▽

C82.98 Follicular lymphoma, unspecified, lymph nodes of multiple sites NRS ▽

C82.99 Follicular lymphoma, unspecified, extranodal and solid organ sites NRS ▽

✓4ᵗʰ C83 Non-follicular lymphoma

EXCLUDES 1   personal history of non-Hodgkin lymphoma (Z85.72)

✓5ᵗʰ C83.0 Small cell B-cell lymphoma

Lymphoplasmacytic lymphoma
Nodal marginal zone lymphoma
Non-leukemic variant of B-CLL
Splenic marginal zone lymphoma

EXCLUDES 1   chronic lymphocytic leukemia (C91.1)
mature T/NK-cell lymphomas (C84.-)
Waldenström macroglobulinemia (C88.0)

C83.00 Small cell B-cell lymphoma, unspecified site NRS ▽

C83.01 Small cell B-cell lymphoma, lymph nodes of head, face, and neck NRS

C83.02 Small cell B-cell lymphoma, intrathoracic lymph nodes NRS

C83.03 Small cell B-cell lymphoma, intra-abdominal lymph nodes NRS

C83.04 Small cell B-cell lymphoma, lymph nodes of axilla and upper limb NRS

C83.05 Small cell B-cell lymphoma, lymph nodes of inguinal region and lower limb NRS

C83.06 Small cell B-cell lymphoma, intrapelvic lymph nodes

C83.07 Small cell B-cell lymphoma, spleen

C83.08 Small cell B-cell lymphoma, lymph nodes of multiple sites

C83.09 Small cell B-cell lymphoma, extranodal and solid organ sites

✓5ᵗʰ C83.1 Mantle cell lymphoma

Centrocytic lymphoma
Malignant lymphomatous polyposis

DEF: Rare form of B-cell non-Hodgkin lymphoma named for the location of tumor cell production, the mantle zone of the lymph nodes.

C83.10 Mantle cell lymphoma, unspecified site ▽

C83.11 Mantle cell lymphoma, lymph nodes of head, face, and neck

C83.12 Mantle cell lymphoma, intrathoracic lymph nodes

C83.13 Mantle cell lymphoma, intra-abdominal lymph nodes

C83.14 Mantle cell lymphoma, lymph nodes of axilla and upper limb

N Newborn: 0   P Pediatric: 0-17   M Maternity: 12-55   A Adult: 15-124   NRS Nonroutine supply Dx   NCDx Noncancer Dx   PDx Primary Dx   ►◄ Revised Text   ● New Code   ▲ Revised Title

476   ICD-10-CM 2018

C83.15   Mantle cell lymphoma, lymph nodes of inguinal region and lower limb

C83.16   Mantle cell lymphoma, intrapelvic lymph nodes

C83.17   Mantle cell lymphoma, spleen

C83.18   Mantle cell lymphoma, lymph nodes of multiple sites

C83.19   Mantle cell lymphoma, extranodal and solid organ sites

✓5th **C83.3**   Diffuse large B-cell lymphoma
     Anaplastic diffuse large B-cell lymphoma
     CD30-positive diffuse large B-cell lymphoma
     Centroblastic diffuse large B-cell lymphoma
     Diffuse large B-cell lymphoma, subtype not specified
     Immunoblastic diffuse large B-cell lymphoma
     Plasmablastic diffuse large B-cell lymphoma
     T-cell rich diffuse large B-cell lymphoma
     EXCLUDES 1   mature T/NK-cell lymphomas (C84.-)
                mediastinal (thymic) large B-cell lymphoma (C85.2-)

C83.30   Diffuse large B-cell lymphoma, unspecified site   ▽

C83.31   Diffuse large B-cell lymphoma, lymph nodes of head, face, and neck

C83.32   Diffuse large B-cell lymphoma, intrathoracic lymph nodes

C83.33   Diffuse large B-cell lymphoma, intra-abdominal lymph nodes

C83.34   Diffuse large B-cell lymphoma, lymph nodes of axilla and upper limb

C83.35   Diffuse large B-cell lymphoma, lymph nodes of inguinal region and lower limb

C83.36   Diffuse large B-cell lymphoma, intrapelvic lymph nodes

C83.37   Diffuse large B-cell lymphoma, spleen

C83.38   Diffuse large B-cell lymphoma, lymph nodes of multiple sites

C83.39   Diffuse large B-cell lymphoma, extranodal and solid organ sites

✓5th **C83.5**   Lymphoblastic (diffuse) lymphoma
     B-precursor lymphoma
     Lymphoblastic B-cell lymphoma
     Lymphoblastic lymphoma NOS
     Lymphoblastic T-cell lymphoma
     T-precursor lymphoma

C83.50   Lymphoblastic (diffuse) lymphoma, unspecified site   ▽

C83.51   Lymphoblastic (diffuse) lymphoma, lymph nodes of head, face, and neck

C83.52   Lymphoblastic (diffuse) lymphoma, intrathoracic lymph nodes

C83.53   Lymphoblastic (diffuse) lymphoma, intra-abdominal lymph nodes

C83.54   Lymphoblastic (diffuse) lymphoma, lymph nodes of axilla and upper limb

C83.55   Lymphoblastic (diffuse) lymphoma, lymph nodes of inguinal region and lower limb

C83.56   Lymphoblastic (diffuse) lymphoma, intrapelvic lymph nodes

C83.57   Lymphoblastic (diffuse) lymphoma, spleen

C83.58   Lymphoblastic (diffuse) lymphoma, lymph nodes of multiple sites

C83.59   Lymphoblastic (diffuse) lymphoma, extranodal and solid organ sites

✓5th **C83.7**   Burkitt lymphoma
     Atypical Burkitt lymphoma
     Burkitt-like lymphoma
     EXCLUDES 1   mature B-cell leukemia Burkitt type (C91.A-)
     DEF: Malignancy of the lymphatic system, most often seen as a large bone-deteriorating lesion within the jaw or as an abdominal mass. It is a form of non-Hodgkin's lymphoma and is recognized as the fastest growing human tumor.

C83.70   Burkitt lymphoma, unspecified site   ▽

C83.71   Burkitt lymphoma, lymph nodes of head, face, and neck

C83.72   Burkitt lymphoma, intrathoracic lymph nodes

C83.73   Burkitt lymphoma, intra-abdominal lymph nodes

C83.74   Burkitt lymphoma, lymph nodes of axilla and upper limb

C83.75   Burkitt lymphoma, lymph nodes of inguinal region and lower limb

C83.76   Burkitt lymphoma, intrapelvic lymph nodes

C83.77   Burkitt lymphoma, spleen

C83.78   Burkitt lymphoma, lymph nodes of multiple sites

C83.79   Burkitt lymphoma, extranodal and solid organ sites

✓5th **C83.8**   Other non-follicular lymphoma
     Intravascular large B-cell lymphoma
     Lymphoid granulomatosis
     Primary effusion B-cell lymphoma
     EXCLUDES 1   mediastinal (thymic) large B-cell lymphoma (C85.2-)
                T-cell rich B-cell lymphoma (C83.3-)

C83.80   Other non-follicular lymphoma, unspecified site   ▽

C83.81   Other non-follicular lymphoma, lymph nodes of head, face, and neck

C83.82   Other non-follicular lymphoma, intrathoracic lymph nodes

C83.83   Other non-follicular lymphoma, intra-abdominal lymph nodes

C83.84   Other non-follicular lymphoma, lymph nodes of axilla and upper limb

C83.85   Other non-follicular lymphoma, lymph nodes of inguinal region and lower limb

C83.86   Other non-follicular lymphoma, intrapelvic lymph nodes

C83.87   Other non-follicular lymphoma, spleen

C83.88   Other non-follicular lymphoma, lymph nodes of multiple sites

C83.89   Other non-follicular lymphoma, extranodal and solid organ sites

✓5th **C83.9**   Non-follicular (diffuse) lymphoma, unspecified

C83.90   Non-follicular (diffuse) lymphoma, unspecified, unspecified site   ▽

C83.91   Non-follicular (diffuse) lymphoma, unspecified, lymph nodes of head, face, and neck   ▽

C83.92   Non-follicular (diffuse) lymphoma, unspecified, intrathoracic lymph nodes   ▽

C83.93   Non-follicular (diffuse) lymphoma, unspecified, intra-abdominal lymph nodes   ▽

C83.94   Non-follicular (diffuse) lymphoma, unspecified, lymph nodes of axilla and upper limb   ▽

C83.95   Non-follicular (diffuse) lymphoma, unspecified, lymph nodes of inguinal region and lower limb   ▽

C83.96   Non-follicular (diffuse) lymphoma, unspecified, intrapelvic lymph nodes   ▽

C83.97   Non-follicular (diffuse) lymphoma, unspecified, spleen   ▽

C83.98   Non-follicular (diffuse) lymphoma, unspecified, lymph nodes of multiple sites   ▽

C83.99   Non-follicular (diffuse) lymphoma, unspecified, extranodal and solid organ sites   ▽

✓4th **C84**   Mature T/NK-cell lymphomas
     EXCLUDES 1   personal history of non-Hodgkin lymphoma (Z85.72)

✓5th **C84.0**   Mycosis fungoides
     EXCLUDES 1   peripheral T-cell lymphoma, not classified (C84.4-)
     DEF: Most common form of cutaneous T-cell lymphoma, also known as Alibert-Bazin syndrome. A type of non-Hodgkin lymphoma in which white blood cells become cancerous and affect the skin and sometimes internal organs.

C84.00   Mycosis fungoides, unspecified site   NRS ▽

C84.01   Mycosis fungoides, lymph nodes of head, face, and neck   NRS

C84.02   Mycosis fungoides, intrathoracic lymph nodes   NRS

C84.03   Mycosis fungoides, intra-abdominal lymph nodes   NRS

C84.04   Mycosis fungoides, lymph nodes of axilla and upper limb   NRS

C84.05   Mycosis fungoides, lymph nodes of inguinal region and lower limb   NRS

C84.06   Mycosis fungoides, intrapelvic lymph nodes   NRS

C84.07   Mycosis fungoides, spleen   NRS

C84.08   Mycosis fungoides, lymph nodes of multiple sites   NRS

C84.09   Mycosis fungoides, extranodal and solid organ sites   NRS

✓5th **C84.1**   Sézary disease

C84.10   Sézary disease, unspecified site   NRS ▽

Chapter 2. Neoplasms

C83.15–C84.10

Chapter 2. Neoplasms

C84.11   Sézary disease, lymph nodes of head, face, and neck   `NRS`

C84.12   Sézary disease, intrathoracic lymph nodes   `NRS`

C84.13   Sézary disease, intra-abdominal lymph nodes   `NRS`

C84.14   Sézary disease, lymph nodes of axilla and upper limb   `NRS`

C84.15   Sézary disease, lymph nodes of inguinal region and lower limb   `NRS`

C84.16   Sézary disease, intrapelvic lymph nodes   `NRS`

C84.17   Sézary disease, spleen   `NRS`

C84.18   Sézary disease, lymph nodes of multiple sites   `NRS`

C84.19   Sézary disease, extranodal and solid organ sites   `NRS`

✓5ᵗʰ **C84.4**   **Peripheral T-cell lymphoma, not classified**
Lennert's lymphoma
Lymphoepithelioid lymphoma
Mature T-cell lymphoma, not elsewhere classified

C84.40   Peripheral T-cell lymphoma, not classified, unspecified site   ▽

C84.41   Peripheral T-cell lymphoma, not classified, lymph nodes of head, face, and neck

C84.42   Peripheral T-cell lymphoma, not classified, intrathoracic lymph nodes

C84.43   Peripheral T-cell lymphoma, not classified, intra-abdominal lymph nodes

C84.44   Peripheral T-cell lymphoma, not classified, lymph nodes of axilla and upper limb

C84.45   Peripheral T-cell lymphoma, not classified, lymph nodes of inguinal region and lower limb

C84.46   Peripheral T-cell lymphoma, not classified, intrapelvic lymph nodes

C84.47   Peripheral T-cell lymphoma, not classified, spleen

C84.48   Peripheral T-cell lymphoma, not classified, lymph nodes of multiple sites

C84.49   Peripheral T-cell lymphoma, not classified, extranodal and solid organ sites

✓5ᵗʰ **C84.6**   **Anaplastic large cell lymphoma, ALK-positive**
Anaplastic large cell lymphoma, CD3Ø-positive

C84.60   Anaplastic large cell lymphoma, ALK-positive, unspecified site   ▽

C84.61   Anaplastic large cell lymphoma, ALK-positive, lymph nodes of head, face, and neck

C84.62   Anaplastic large cell lymphoma, ALK-positive, intrathoracic lymph nodes

C84.63   Anaplastic large cell lymphoma, ALK-positive, intra-abdominal lymph nodes

C84.64   Anaplastic large cell lymphoma, ALK-positive, lymph nodes of axilla and upper limb

C84.65   Anaplastic large cell lymphoma, ALK-positive, lymph nodes of inguinal region and lower limb

C84.66   Anaplastic large cell lymphoma, ALK-positive, intrapelvic lymph nodes

C84.67   Anaplastic large cell lymphoma, ALK-positive, spleen

C84.68   Anaplastic large cell lymphoma, ALK-positive, lymph nodes of multiple sites

C84.69   Anaplastic large cell lymphoma, ALK-positive, extranodal and solid organ sites

✓5ᵗʰ **C84.7**   **Anaplastic large cell lymphoma, ALK-negative**
   `EXCLUDES 1`   primary cutaneous CD3Ø-positive T-cell proliferations (C86.6-)

C84.70   Anaplastic large cell lymphoma, ALK-negative, unspecified site   ▽

C84.71   Anaplastic large cell lymphoma, ALK-negative, lymph nodes of head, face, and neck

C84.72   Anaplastic large cell lymphoma, ALK-negative, intrathoracic lymph nodes

C84.73   Anaplastic large cell lymphoma, ALK-negative, intra-abdominal lymph nodes

C84.74   Anaplastic large cell lymphoma, ALK-negative, lymph nodes of axilla and upper limb

C84.75   Anaplastic large cell lymphoma, ALK-negative, lymph nodes of inguinal region and lower limb

C84.76   Anaplastic large cell lymphoma, ALK-negative, intrapelvic lymph nodes

C84.77   Anaplastic large cell lymphoma, ALK-negative, spleen

C84.78   Anaplastic large cell lymphoma, ALK-negative, lymph nodes of multiple sites

C84.79   Anaplastic large cell lymphoma, ALK-negative, extranodal and solid organ sites

✓5ᵗʰ **C84.A**   **Cutaneous T-cell lymphoma, unspecified**

C84.AØ   Cutaneous T-cell lymphoma, unspecified, unspecified site   `NRS` ▽

C84.A1   Cutaneous T-cell lymphoma, unspecified, lymph nodes of head, face, and neck   `NRS` ▽

C84.A2   Cutaneous T-cell lymphoma, unspecified, intrathoracic lymph nodes   `NRS` ▽

C84.A3   Cutaneous T-cell lymphoma, unspecified, intra-abdominal lymph nodes   `NRS` ▽

C84.A4   Cutaneous T-cell lymphoma, unspecified, lymph nodes of axilla and upper limb   `NRS` ▽

C84.A5   Cutaneous T-cell lymphoma, unspecified, lymph nodes of inguinal region and lower limb   `NRS` ▽

C84.A6   Cutaneous T-cell lymphoma, unspecified, intrapelvic lymph nodes   `NRS` ▽

C84.A7   Cutaneous T-cell lymphoma, unspecified, spleen   `NRS` ▽

C84.A8   Cutaneous T-cell lymphoma, unspecified, lymph nodes of multiple sites   `NRS` ▽

C84.A9   Cutaneous T-cell lymphoma, unspecified, extranodal and solid organ sites   `NRS` ▽

✓5ᵗʰ **C84.Z**   **Other mature T/NK-cell lymphomas**
   `NOTE`   If T-cell lineage or involvement is mentioned in conjunction with a specific lymphoma, code to the more specific description.
   `EXCLUDES 1`   angioimmunoblastic T-cell lymphoma (C86.5)
      blastic NK-cell lymphoma (C86.4)
      enteropathy-type T-cell lymphoma (C86.2)
      extranodal NK-cell lymphoma, nasal type (C86.Ø)
      hepatosplenic T-cell lymphoma (C86.1)
      primary cutaneous CD3Ø-positive T-cell proliferations (C86.6)
      subcutaneous panniculitis-like T-cell lymphoma (C86.3)
      T-cell leukemia (C91.1-)

C84.ZØ   Other mature T/NK-cell lymphomas, unspecified site   ▽

C84.Z1   Other mature T/NK-cell lymphomas, lymph nodes of head, face, and neck

C84.Z2   Other mature T/NK-cell lymphomas, intrathoracic lymph nodes

C84.Z3   Other mature T/NK-cell lymphomas, intra-abdominal lymph nodes

C84.Z4   Other mature T/NK-cell lymphomas, lymph nodes of axilla and upper limb

C84.Z5   Other mature T/NK-cell lymphomas, lymph nodes of inguinal region and lower limb

C84.Z6   Other mature T/NK-cell lymphomas, intrapelvic lymph nodes

C84.Z7   Other mature T/NK-cell lymphomas, spleen

C84.Z8   Other mature T/NK-cell lymphomas, lymph nodes of multiple sites

C84.Z9   Other mature T/NK-cell lymphomas, extranodal and solid organ sites

✓5ᵗʰ **C84.9**   **Mature T/NK-cell lymphomas, unspecified**
NK/T cell lymphoma NOS
   `EXCLUDES 1`   mature T-cell lymphoma, not elsewhere classified (C84.4-)

C84.9Ø   Mature T/NK-cell lymphomas, unspecified, unspecified site   ▽

C84.91   Mature T/NK-cell lymphomas, unspecified, lymph nodes of head, face, and neck   ▽

C84.92   Mature T/NK-cell lymphomas, unspecified, intrathoracic lymph nodes   ▽

C84.93   Mature T/NK-cell lymphomas, unspecified, intra-abdominal lymph nodes   ▽

C84.94   Mature T/NK-cell lymphomas, unspecified, lymph nodes of axilla and upper limb   ▽

C84.95   Mature T/NK-cell lymphomas, unspecified, lymph nodes of inguinal region and lower limb   ▽

C84.96   Mature T/NK-cell lymphomas, unspecified, intrapelvic lymph nodes   ▽

C84.97   Mature T/NK-cell lymphomas, unspecified, spleen   ▽

N Newborn: 0   P Pediatric: 0-17   M Maternity: 12-55   A Adult: 15-124   `NRS` Nonroutine supply Dx   `NC Dx` Noncancer Dx   `PDx` Primary Dx   ►◄ Revised Text   ● New Code   ▲ Revised Title

478   ICD-10-CM 2018

C84.98　Mature T/NK-cell lymphomas, unspecified, lymph nodes of multiple sites ▽

C84.99　Mature T/NK-cell lymphomas, unspecified, extranodal and solid organ sites ▽

✓4ᵗʰ C85　Other specified and unspecified types of non-Hodgkin lymphoma

EXCLUDES 1　other specified types of T/NK-cell lymphoma (C86.-)
　　　　　　　personal history of non-Hodgkin lymphoma (Z85.72)

✓5ᵗʰ C85.1　Unspecified B-cell lymphoma

NOTE　If B-cell lineage or involvement is mentioned in conjunction with a specific lymphoma, code to the more specific description.

C85.10　Unspecified B-cell lymphoma, unspecified site ▽

C85.11　Unspecified B-cell lymphoma, lymph nodes of head, face, and neck ▽

C85.12　Unspecified B-cell lymphoma, intrathoracic lymph nodes ▽

C85.13　Unspecified B-cell lymphoma, intra-abdominal lymph nodes ▽

C85.14　Unspecified B-cell lymphoma, lymph nodes of axilla and upper limb ▽

C85.15　Unspecified B-cell lymphoma, lymph nodes of inguinal region and lower limb ▽

C85.16　Unspecified B-cell lymphoma, intrapelvic lymph nodes ▽

C85.17　Unspecified B-cell lymphoma, spleen ▽

C85.18　Unspecified B-cell lymphoma, lymph nodes of multiple sites ▽

C85.19　Unspecified B-cell lymphoma, extranodal and solid organ sites ▽

✓5ᵗʰ C85.2　Mediastinal (thymic) large B-cell lymphoma

C85.20　Mediastinal (thymic) large B-cell lymphoma, unspecified site ▽

C85.21　Mediastinal (thymic) large B-cell lymphoma, lymph nodes of head, face, and neck

C85.22　Mediastinal (thymic) large B-cell lymphoma, intrathoracic lymph nodes

C85.23　Mediastinal (thymic) large B-cell lymphoma, intra-abdominal lymph nodes

C85.24　Mediastinal (thymic) large B-cell lymphoma, lymph nodes of axilla and upper limb

C85.25　Mediastinal (thymic) large B-cell lymphoma, lymph nodes of inguinal region and lower limb

C85.26　Mediastinal (thymic) large B-cell lymphoma, intrapelvic lymph nodes

C85.27　Mediastinal (thymic) large B-cell lymphoma, spleen

C85.28　Mediastinal (thymic) large B-cell lymphoma, lymph nodes of multiple sites

C85.29　Mediastinal (thymic) large B-cell lymphoma, extranodal and solid organ sites

✓5ᵗʰ C85.8　Other specified types of non-Hodgkin lymphoma

C85.80　Other specified types of non-Hodgkin lymphoma, unspecified site ▽

C85.81　Other specified types of non-Hodgkin lymphoma, lymph nodes of head, face, and neck

C85.82　Other specified types of non-Hodgkin lymphoma, intrathoracic lymph nodes

C85.83　Other specified types of non-Hodgkin lymphoma, intra-abdominal lymph nodes

C85.84　Other specified types of non-Hodgkin lymphoma, lymph nodes of axilla and upper limb

C85.85　Other specified types of non-Hodgkin lymphoma, lymph nodes of inguinal region and lower limb

C85.86　Other specified types of non-Hodgkin lymphoma, intrapelvic lymph nodes

C85.87　Other specified types of non-Hodgkin lymphoma, spleen

C85.88　Other specified types of non-Hodgkin lymphoma, lymph nodes of multiple sites

C85.89　Other specified types of non-Hodgkin lymphoma, extranodal and solid organ sites

✓5ᵗʰ C85.9　Non-Hodgkin lymphoma, unspecified

Lymphoma NOS
Malignant lymphoma NOS
Non-Hodgkin lymphoma NOS

C85.90　Non-Hodgkin lymphoma, unspecified, unspecified site ▽

C85.91　Non-Hodgkin lymphoma, unspecified, lymph nodes of head, face, and neck ▽

C85.92　Non-Hodgkin lymphoma, unspecified, intrathoracic lymph nodes ▽

C85.93　Non-Hodgkin lymphoma, unspecified, intra-abdominal lymph nodes ▽

C85.94　Non-Hodgkin lymphoma, unspecified, lymph nodes of axilla and upper limb ▽

C85.95　Non-Hodgkin lymphoma, unspecified, lymph nodes of inguinal region and lower limb ▽

C85.96　Non-Hodgkin lymphoma, unspecified, intrapelvic lymph nodes ▽

C85.97　Non-Hodgkin lymphoma, unspecified, spleen ▽

C85.98　Non-Hodgkin lymphoma, unspecified, lymph nodes of multiple sites ▽

C85.99　Non-Hodgkin lymphoma, unspecified, extranodal and solid organ sites ▽

✓4ᵗʰ C86　Other specified types of T/NK-cell lymphoma

EXCLUDES 1　anaplastic large cell lymphoma, ALK negative (C84.7-)
　　　　　　　anaplastic large cell lymphoma, ALK positive (C84.6-)
　　　　　　　mature T/NK-cell lymphomas (C84.-)
　　　　　　　other specified types of non-Hodgkin lymphoma (C85.8-)

C86.0　Extranodal NK/T-cell lymphoma, nasal type

C86.1　Hepatosplenic T-cell lymphoma
Alpha-beta and gamma delta types

C86.2　Enteropathy-type (intestinal) T-cell lymphoma
Enteropathy associated T-cell lymphoma

C86.3　Subcutaneous panniculitis-like T-cell lymphoma

C86.4　Blastic NK-cell lymphoma
▶Blastic plasmacytoid dendritic cell neoplasm (BPDCN)◀

C86.5　Angioimmunoblastic T-cell lymphoma
Angioimmunoblastic lymphadenopathy with dysproteinemia [AILD]

C86.6　Primary cutaneous CD30-positive T-cell proliferations
Lymphomatoid papulosis
Primary cutaneous anaplastic large cell lymphoma
Primary cutaneous CD30-positive large T-cell lymphoma

✓4ᵗʰ C88　Malignant immunoproliferative diseases and certain other B-cell lymphomas

EXCLUDES 1　B-cell lymphoma, unspecified (C85.1-)
　　　　　　　personal history of other malignant neoplasms of lymphoid, hematopoietic and related tissues (Z85.79)

C88.0　Waldenström macroglobulinemia
Lymphoplasmacytic lymphoma with IgM-production
Macroglobulinemia (idiopathic) (primary)
EXCLUDES 1　small cell B-cell lymphoma (C83.0)

C88.2　Heavy chain disease
Franklin disease
Gamma heavy chain disease
Mu heavy chain disease

C88.3　Immunoproliferative small intestinal disease
Alpha heavy chain disease
Mediterranean lymphoma

C88.4　Extranodal marginal zone B-cell lymphoma of mucosa-associated lymphoid tissue [MALT-lymphoma]
Lymphoma of skin-associated lymphoid tissue [SALT-lymphoma]
Lymphoma of bronchial-associated lymphoid tissue [BALT-lymphoma]
EXCLUDES 1　high malignant (diffuse large B-cell) lymphoma (C83.3-)

C88.8　Other malignant immunoproliferative diseases

C88.9　Malignant immunoproliferative disease, unspecified ▽
Immunoproliferative disease NOS

✓ Additional Character Req　　✓7ᵗʰ Placeholder Alert　　Case-Mix Diagnosis　　Manifestation　　▽ Unspecified Dx　　**EXCLUDES 1** Not coded here　　**EXCLUDES 2** Not included here

ICD-10-CM 2018　　　　　　　　　　　　　　　　　　　　　　　　　　　　　　　　　　　　　　　479

✓4th C90 Multiple myeloma and malignant plasma cell neoplasms

> EXCLUDES 1   *personal history of other malignant neoplasms of lymphoid, hematopoietic and related tissues (Z85.79)*

✓5th C90.0 Multiple myeloma
     Kahler's disease
     Medullary plasmacytoma
     Myelomatosis
     Plasma cell myeloma
> EXCLUDES 1   *solitary myeloma (C90.3-)*
>   *solitary plasmactyoma (C90.3-)*

     C90.00 Multiple myeloma not having achieved remission
         Multiple myeloma with failed remission
         Multiple myeloma NOS

     C90.01 Multiple myeloma in remission

     C90.02 Multiple myeloma in relapse

✓5th C90.1 Plasma cell leukemia
     Plasmacytic leukemia

     C90.10 Plasma cell leukemia not having achieved remission
         Plasma cell leukemia with failed remission
         Plasma cell leukemia NOS

     C90.11 Plasma cell leukemia in remission

     C90.12 Plasma cell leukemia in relapse

✓5th C90.2 Extramedullary plasmacytoma

     C90.20 Extramedullary plasmacytoma not having achieved remission
         Extramedullary plasmacytoma with failed remission
         Extramedullary plasmacytoma NOS

     C90.21 Extramedullary plasmacytoma in remission

     C90.22 Extramedullary plasmacytoma in relapse

✓5th C90.3 Solitary plasmacytoma
     Localized malignant plasma cell tumor NOS
     Plasmacytoma NOS
     Solitary myeloma

     C90.30 Solitary plasmacytoma not having achieved remission
         Solitary plasmacytoma with failed remission
         Solitary plasmacytoma NOS

     C90.31 Solitary plasmacytoma in remission

     C90.32 Solitary plasmacytoma in relapse

✓4th C91 Lymphoid leukemia

> EXCLUDES 1   *personal history of leukemia (Z85.6)*

✓5th C91.0 Acute lymphoblastic leukemia [ALL]
> NOTE   Code C91.0 should only be used for T-cell and B-cell precursor leukemia

     C91.00 Acute lymphoblastic leukemia not having achieved remission
         Acute lymphoblastic leukemia with failed remission
         Acute lymphoblastic leukemia NOS

     C91.01 Acute lymphoblastic leukemia, in remission

     C91.02 Acute lymphoblastic leukemia, in relapse

✓5th C91.1 Chronic lymphocytic leukemia of B-cell type
     Lymphoplasmacytic leukemia
     Richter syndrome
> EXCLUDES 1   *lymphoplasmacytic lymphoma (C83.0-)*

     C91.10 Chronic lymphocytic leukemia of B-cell type not having achieved remission
         Chronic lymphocytic leukemia of B-cell type with failed remission
         Chronic lymphocytic leukemia of B-cell type NOS

     C91.11 Chronic lymphocytic leukemia of B-cell type in remission

     C91.12 Chronic lymphocytic leukemia of B-cell type in relapse

✓5th C91.3 Prolymphocytic leukemia of B-cell type

     C91.30 Prolymphocytic leukemia of B-cell type not having achieved remission
         Prolymphocytic leukemia of B-cell type with failed remission
         Prolymphocytic leukemia of B-cell type NOS

     C91.31 Prolymphocytic leukemia of B-cell type, in remission

     C91.32 Prolymphocytic leukemia of B-cell type, in relapse

✓5th C91.4 Hairy cell leukemia
     Leukemic reticuloendotheliosis

     C91.40 Hairy cell leukemia not having achieved remission
         Hairy cell leukemia with failed remission
         Hairy cell leukemia NOS

     C91.41 Hairy cell leukemia, in remission

     C91.42 Hairy cell leukemia, in relapse

✓5th C91.5 Adult T-cell lymphoma/leukemia (HTLV-1-associated)
     Acute variant of adult T-cell lymphoma/leukemia (HTLV-1-associated)
     Chronic variant of adult T-cell lymphoma/leukemia (HTLV-1-associated)
     Lymphomatoid variant of adult T-cell lymphoma/leukemia (HTLV-1-associated)
     Smouldering variant of adult T-cell lymphoma/leukemia (HTLV-1-associated)

     C91.50 Adult T-cell lymphoma/leukemia (HTLV-1-associated) not having achieved remission   A
         Adult T-cell lymphoma/leukemia (HTLV-1-associated) with failed remission
         Adult T-cell lymphoma/leukemia (HTLV-1-associated) NOS

     C91.51 Adult T-cell lymphoma/leukemia (HTLV-1-associated), in remission   A

     C91.52 Adult T-cell lymphoma/leukemia (HTLV-1-associated), in relapse   A

✓5th C91.6 Prolymphocytic leukemia of T-cell type

     C91.60 Prolymphocytic leukemia of T-cell type not having achieved remission
         Prolymphocytic leukemia of T-cell type with failed remission
         Prolymphocytic leukemia of T-cell type NOS

     C91.61 Prolymphocytic leukemia of T-cell type, in remission

     C91.62 Prolymphocytic leukemia of T-cell type, in relapse

✓5th C91.A Mature B-cell leukemia Burkitt-type
> EXCLUDES 1   *Burkitt lymphoma (C83.7-)*

     C91.A0 Mature B-cell leukemia Burkitt-type not having achieved remission
         Mature B-cell leukemia Burkitt-type with failed remission
         Mature B-cell leukemia Burkitt-type NOS

     C91.A1 Mature B-cell leukemia Burkitt-type, in remission

     C91.A2 Mature B-cell leukemia Burkitt-type, in relapse

✓5th C91.Z Other lymphoid leukemia
     T-cell large granular lymphocytic leukemia (associated with rheumatoid arthritis)

     C91.Z0 Other lymphoid leukemia not having achieved remission
         Other lymphoid leukemia with failed remission
         Other lymphoid leukemia NOS

     C91.Z1 Other lymphoid leukemia, in remission

     C91.Z2 Other lymphoid leukemia, in relapse

✓5th C91.9 Lymphoid leukemia, unspecified

     C91.90 Lymphoid leukemia, unspecified not having achieved remission   ▽
         Lymphoid leukemia with failed remission
         Lymphoid leukemia NOS

     C91.91 Lymphoid leukemia, unspecified, in remission   ▽

     C91.92 Lymphoid leukemia, unspecified, in relapse   ▽

✓4th C92 Myeloid leukemia
> INCLUDES   granulocytic leukemia
>   myelogenous leukemia
> EXCLUDES 1   *personal history of leukemia (Z85.6)*

✓5th C92.0 Acute myeloblastic leukemia
     Acute myeloblastic leukemia, minimal differentiation
     Acute myeloblastic leukemia (with maturation)
     Acute myeloblastic leukemia 1/ETO
     Acute myeloblastic leukemia M0
     Acute myeloblastic leukemia M1
     Acute myeloblastic leukemia M2
     Acute myeloblastic leukemia with t(8;21)
     Acute myeloblastic leukemia (without a FAB classification) NOS
     Refractory anemia with excess blasts in transformation [RAEB T]
> EXCLUDES 1   *acute exacerbation of chronic myeloid leukemia (C92.10)*
>   *refractory anemia with excess of blasts not in transformation (D46.2-)*

     C92.00 Acute myeloblastic leukemia, not having achieved remission
         Acute myeloblastic leukemia with failed remission
         Acute myeloblastic leukemia NOS

     C92.01 Acute myeloblastic leukemia, in remission

     C92.02 Acute myeloblastic leukemia, in relapse

✅5ᵗʰ **C92.1** Chronic **myeloid leukemia, BCR/ABL-positive**
Chronic myelogenous leukemia, Philadelphia chromosome (Ph1) positive
Chronic myelogenous leukemia, t(9;22) (q34;q11)
Chronic myelogenous leukemia with crisis of blast cells
> *EXCLUDES 1*   atypical chronic myeloid leukemia BCR/ABL-negative (C92.2-)
> chronic myelomonocytic leukemia (C93.1-)
> chronic myeloproliferative disease (D47.1)

     C92.10 **Chronic myeloid leukemia, BCR/ABL-positive, not having achieved remission**
Chronic myeloid leukemia, BCR/ABL-positive with failed remission
Chronic myeloid leukemia, BCR/ABL-positive NOS

     C92.11 **Chronic myeloid leukemia, BCR/ABL-positive, in remission**

     C92.12 **Chronic myeloid leukemia, BCR/ABL-positive, in relapse**

✅5ᵗʰ **C92.2** Atypical chronic **myeloid leukemia, BCR/ABL-negative**

     C92.20 **Atypical chronic myeloid leukemia, BCR/ABL-negative, not having achieved remission**
Atypical chronic myeloid leukemia, BCR/ABL-negative with failed remission
Atypical chronic myeloid leukemia, BCR/ABL-negative NOS

     C92.21 **Atypical chronic myeloid leukemia, BCR/ABL-negative, in remission**

     C92.22 **Atypical chronic myeloid leukemia, BCR/ABL-negative, in relapse**

✅5ᵗʰ **C92.3** Myeloid **sarcoma**
A malignant tumor of immature myeloid cells
Chloroma
Granulocytic sarcoma

     C92.30 **Myeloid sarcoma, not having achieved remission**
Myeloid sarcoma with failed remission
Myeloid sarcoma NOS

     C92.31 **Myeloid sarcoma, in remission**

     C92.32 **Myeloid sarcoma, in relapse**

✅5ᵗʰ **C92.4** Acute promyelocytic **leukemia**
AML M3   AML Me with t(15;17) and variants

     C92.40 **Acute promyelocytic leukemia, not having achieved remission**
Acute promyelocytic leukemia with failed remission
Acute promyelocytic leukemia NOS

     C92.41 **Acute promyelocytic leukemia, in remission**

     C92.42 **Acute promyelocytic leukemia, in relapse**

✅5ᵗʰ **C92.5** Acute myelomonocytic **leukemia**
AML M4   AML M4 Eo with inv(16) or t(16;16)

     C92.50 **Acute myelomonocytic leukemia, not having achieved remission**
Acute myelomonocytic leukemia with failed remission
Acute myelomonocytic leukemia NOS

     C92.51 **Acute myelomonocytic leukemia, in remission**

     C92.52 **Acute myelomonocytic leukemia, in relapse**

✅5ᵗʰ **C92.6** Acute myeloid **leukemia with 11q23-abnormality**
Acute myeloid leukemia with variation of MLL-gene

     C92.60 **Acute myeloid leukemia with 11q23-abnormality not having achieved remission**
Acute myeloid leukemia with 11q23-abnormality with failed remission
Acute myeloid leukemia with 11q23-abnormality NOS

     C92.61 **Acute myeloid leukemia with 11q23-abnormality in remission**

     C92.62 **Acute myeloid leukemia with 11q23-abnormality in relapse**

✅5ᵗʰ **C92.A** Acute myeloid **leukemia with multilineage dysplasia**
Acute myeloid leukemia with dysplasia of remaining hematopoesis and/or myelodysplastic disease in its history

     C92.A0 **Acute myeloid leukemia with multilineage dysplasia, not having achieved remission**
Acute myeloid leukemia with multilineage dysplasia with failed remission
Acute myeloid leukemia with multilineage dysplasia NOS

     C92.A1 **Acute myeloid leukemia with multilineage dysplasia, in remission**

     C92.A2 **Acute myeloid leukemia with multilineage dysplasia, in relapse**

✅5ᵗʰ **C92.Z** Other **myeloid leukemia**

     C92.Z0 **Other myeloid leukemia not having achieved remission**
Myeloid leukemia NEC with failed remission
Myeloid leukemia NEC

     C92.Z1 **Other myeloid leukemia, in remission**

     C92.Z2 **Other myeloid leukemia, in relapse**

✅5ᵗʰ **C92.9** Myeloid **leukemia, unspecified**

     C92.90 **Myeloid leukemia, unspecified, not having achieved remission** ▽
Myeloid leukemia, unspecified with failed remission
Myeloid leukemia, unspecified NOS

     C92.91 **Myeloid leukemia, unspecified in remission** ▽

     C92.92 **Myeloid leukemia, unspecified in relapse** ▽

✅4ᵗʰ **C93** **Monocytic leukemia**
> *INCLUDES*   monocytoid leukemia
> *EXCLUDES 1*   personal history of leukemia (Z85.6)

✅5ᵗʰ **C93.0** Acute **monoblastic/monocytic leukemia**
AML M5   AML M5b
AML M5a

     C93.00 **Acute monoblastic/monocytic leukemia, not having achieved remission**
Acute monoblastic/monocytic leukemia with failed remission
Acute monoblastic/monocytic leukemia NOS

     C93.01 **Acute monoblastic/monocytic leukemia, in remission**

     C93.02 **Acute monoblastic/monocytic leukemia, in relapse**

✅5ᵗʰ **C93.1** Chronic **myelomonocytic leukemia**
Chronic monocytic leukemia   CMML-2
CMML-1   CMML with eosinophilia

     C93.10 **Chronic myelomonocytic leukemia not having achieved remission**
Chronic myelomonocytic leukemia with failed remission
Chronic myelomonocytic leukemia NOS

     C93.11 **Chronic myelomonocytic leukemia, in remission**

     C93.12 **Chronic myelomonocytic leukemia, in relapse**

✅5ᵗʰ **C93.3** Juvenile **myelomonocytic leukemia**

     C93.30 **Juvenile myelomonocytic leukemia, not having achieved remission** 🄿
Juvenile myelomonocytic leukemia with failed remission
Juvenile myelomonocytic leukemia NOS

     C93.31 **Juvenile myelomonocytic leukemia, in remission** 🄿

     C93.32 **Juvenile myelomonocytic leukemia, in relapse** 🄿

✅5ᵗʰ **C93.Z** Other **monocytic leukemia**

     C93.Z0 **Other monocytic leukemia, not having achieved remission**
Other monocytic leukemia NOS

     C93.Z1 **Other monocytic leukemia, in remission**

     C93.Z2 **Other monocytic leukemia, in relapse**

✅5ᵗʰ **C93.9** Monocytic **leukemia, unspecified**

     C93.90 **Monocytic leukemia, unspecified, not having achieved remission** ▽
Monocytic leukemia, unspecified with failed remission
Monocytic leukemia, unspecified NOS

     C93.91 **Monocytic leukemia, unspecified in remission** ▽

     C93.92 **Monocytic leukemia, unspecified in relapse** ▽

✅4ᵗʰ **C94** Other **leukemias of specified cell type**
> *EXCLUDES 1*   leukemic reticuloendotheliosis (C91.4-)
> myelodysplastic syndromes (D46.-)
> personal history of leukemia (Z85.6)
> plasma cell leukemia (C90.1-)

✅5ᵗʰ **C94.0** Acute **erythroid leukemia**
Acute myeloid leukemia M6(a)(b)
Erythroleukemia
DEF: Erythroleukemia: A malignant blood dyscrasia (a myeloproliferative disorder).

     C94.00 **Acute erythroid leukemia, not having achieved remission**
Acute erythroid leukemia with failed remission
Acute erythroid leukemia NOS

     C94.01 **Acute erythroid leukemia, in remission**

     C94.02 **Acute erythroid leukemia, in relapse**

✅ Additional Character Req   ✅xᵗʰ Placeholder Alert   Case-Mix Diagnosis   Manifestation   ▽ Unspecified Dx   *EXCLUDES 1* Not coded here   *EXCLUDES 2* Not included here

ICD-10-CM 2018   **481**

Chapter 2. Neoplasms

✓5ᵗʰ **C94.2 Acute megakaryoblastic leukemia**
Acute myeloid leukemia M7
Acute megakaryocytic leukemia

    C94.20 Acute megakaryoblastic leukemia not having achieved remission
Acute megakaryoblastic leukemia with failed remission
Acute megakaryoblastic leukemia NOS

    C94.21 Acute megakaryoblastic leukemia, in remission

    C94.22 Acute megakaryoblastic leukemia, in relapse

✓5ᵗʰ **C94.3 Mast cell leukemia**

    C94.30 Mast cell leukemia not having achieved remission
Mast cell leukemia with failed remission
Mast cell leukemia NOS

    C94.31 Mast cell leukemia, in remission

    C94.32 Mast cell leukemia, in relapse

✓5ᵗʰ **C94.4 Acute panmyelosis with myelofibrosis**
Acute myelofibrosis
    EXCLUDES 1   *myelofibrosis NOS (D75.81)*
               secondary myelofibrosis NOS (D75.81)

    C94.40 Acute panmyelosis with myelofibrosis not having achieved remission
Acute myelofibrosis NOS
Acute panmyelosis with myelofibrosis with failed remission
Acute panmyelosis NOS

    C94.41 Acute panmyelosis with myelofibrosis, in remission

    C94.42 Acute panmyelosis with myelofibrosis, in relapse

C94.6 Myelodysplastic disease, not classified
Myeloproliferative disease, not classified

✓5ᵗʰ **C94.8 Other specified leukemias**
Aggressive NK-cell leukemia
Acute basophilic leukemia

    C94.80 Other specified leukemias not having achieved remission
Other specified leukemias with failed remission
Other specified leukemias NOS

    C94.81 Other specified leukemias, in remission

    C94.82 Other specified leukemias, in relapse

✓4ᵗʰ **C95 Leukemia of unspecified cell type**
    EXCLUDES 1   *personal history of leukemia (Z85.6)*

✓5ᵗʰ **C95.0 Acute leukemia of unspecified cell type**
Acute bilineal leukemia
Acute mixed lineage leukemia
Biphenotypic acute leukemia
Stem cell leukemia of unclear lineage
    EXCLUDES 1   *acute exacerbation of unspecified chronic leukemia (C95.10)*

    C95.00 Acute leukemia of unspecified cell type not having achieved remission
Acute leukemia of unspecified cell type with failed remission
Acute leukemia NOS

    C95.01 Acute leukemia of unspecified cell type, in remission

    C95.02 Acute leukemia of unspecified cell type, in relapse

✓5ᵗʰ **C95.1 Chronic leukemia of unspecified cell type**

    C95.10 Chronic leukemia of unspecified cell type not having achieved remission
Chronic leukemia of unspecified cell type with failed remission
Chronic leukemia NOS

    C95.11 Chronic leukemia of unspecified cell type, in remission

    C95.12 Chronic leukemia of unspecified cell type, in relapse

✓5ᵗʰ **C95.9 Leukemia, unspecified**

    C95.90 Leukemia, unspecified not having achieved remission ▽
Leukemia, unspecified with failed remission
Leukemia NOS

    C95.91 Leukemia, unspecified, in remission ▽

    C95.92 Leukemia, unspecified, in relapse ▽

✓4ᵗʰ **C96 Other and unspecified malignant neoplasms of lymphoid, hematopoietic and related tissue**
    EXCLUDES 1   *personal history of other malignant neoplasms of lymphoid, hematopoietic and related tissues (Z85.79)*

C96.0 Multifocal and multisystemic (disseminated) Langerhans-cell histiocytosis
Histiocytosis X, multisystemic
Letterer-Siwe disease
    EXCLUDES 1   *adult pulmonary Langerhans cell histiocytosis (J84.82)*
               multifocal and unisystemic Langerhans-cell histiocytosis (C96.5)
               unifocal Langerhans-cell histiocytosis (C96.6)

▲ ✓5ᵗʰ **C96.2 Malignant mast cell neoplasm**
~~Aggressive systemic mastocytosis~~
~~Mast cell sarcoma~~
    EXCLUDES 1   *indolent mastocytosis ▶(D47.02)◀*
               mast cell leukemia (C94.30)
               mastocytosis (congenital) (cutaneous) (Q82.2)

●   **C96.20 Malignant mast cell neoplasm, unspecified** ▽

●   **C96.21 Aggressive systemic mastocytosis**

●   **C96.22 Mast cell sarcoma**

●   **C96.29 Other malignant mast cell neoplasm**

C96.4 Sarcoma of dendritic cells (accessory cells)
Follicular dendritic cell sarcoma
Interdigitating dendritic cell sarcoma
Langerhans cell sarcoma

C96.5 Multifocal and unisystemic Langerhans-cell histiocytosis
Hand-Schüller-Christian disease
Histiocytosis X, multifocal
    EXCLUDES 1   *multifocal and multisystemic (disseminated) Langerhans-cell histiocytosis (C96.0)*
               unifocal Langerhans-cell histiocytosis (C96.6)

C96.6 Unifocal Langerhans-cell histiocytosis
Eosinophilic granuloma
Histiocytosis X, unifocal
Histiocytosis X NOS
Langerhans-cell histiocytosis NOS
    EXCLUDES 1   *multifocal and multisysemic (disseminated) Langerhans-cell histiocytosis (C96.0)*
               multifocal and unisystemic Langerhans-cell histiocytosis (C96.5)

C96.A Histiocytic sarcoma
Malignant histiocytosis

C96.Z Other specified malignant neoplasms of lymphoid, hematopoietic and related tissue

C96.9 Malignant neoplasm of lymphoid, hematopoietic and related tissue, unspecified ▽

In situ neoplasms (D00-D09)

INCLUDES   Bowen's disease
             erythroplasia
             grade III intraepithelial neoplasia
             Queyrat's erythroplasia

✓4ᵗʰ **D00 Carcinoma in situ of oral cavity, esophagus and stomach**
    EXCLUDES 1   *melanoma in situ (D03.-)*

✓5ᵗʰ **D00.0 Carcinoma in situ of lip, oral cavity and pharynx**
Use additional code to identify:
    exposure to environmental tobacco smoke (Z77.22)
    exposure to tobacco smoke in the perinatal period (P96.81)
    history of tobacco dependence (Z87.891)
    occupational exposure to environmental tobacco smoke (Z57.31)
    tobacco dependence (F17.-)
    tobacco use (Z72.0)
    EXCLUDES 1   *carcinoma in situ of aryepiglottic fold or interarytenoid fold, laryngeal aspect (D02.0)*
               carcinoma in situ of epiglottis NOS (D02.0)
               carcinoma in situ of epiglottis suprahyoid portion (D02.0)
               carcinoma in situ of skin of lip (D03.0, D04.0)

    D00.00 Carcinoma in situ of oral cavity, unspecified site ▽

    D00.01 Carcinoma in situ of labial mucosa and vermilion border

    D00.02 Carcinoma in situ of buccal mucosa

    D00.03 Carcinoma in situ of gingiva and edentulous alveolar ridge

    D00.04 Carcinoma in situ of soft palate

    D00.05 Carcinoma in situ of hard palate

    D00.06 Carcinoma in situ of floor of mouth

Ⓝ Newborn: 0   Ⓟ Pediatric: 0-17   Ⓜ Maternity: 12-55   Ⓐ Adult: 15-124   **NRS** Nonroutine supply Dx   **NC Dx** Noncancer Dx   **PDx** Primary Dx   ▶◀ Revised Text   ● New Code   ▲ Revised Title

482   ICD-10-CM 2018

Chapter 2. Neoplasms (side tab)

D00.07   **Carcinoma in situ of** tongue

D00.08   **Carcinoma in situ of** pharynx
  Carcinoma in situ of aryepiglottic fold NOS
  Carcinoma in situ of hypopharyngeal aspect of
    aryepiglottic fold
  Carcinoma in situ of marginal zone of aryepiglottic
    fold

D00.1   **Carcinoma in situ of** esophagus

D00.2   **Carcinoma in situ of** stomach

✓4ᵗʰ **D01   Carcinoma in situ of** other and unspecified digestive organs
  EXCLUDES 1   melanoma in situ (D03.-)

D01.0   **Carcinoma in situ of** colon
  EXCLUDES 1   carcinoma in situ of rectosigmoid junction (D01.1)

D01.1   **Carcinoma in situ of** rectosigmoid junction

D01.2   **Carcinoma in situ of** rectum

D01.3   **Carcinoma in situ of** anus and anal canal
  Anal intraepithelial neoplasia III [AIN III]
  Severe dysplasia of anus
  EXCLUDES 1   anal intraepithelial neoplasia I and II [AIN I and AIN II]
      (K62.82)
    carcinoma in situ of anal margin (D04.5)
    carcinoma in situ of anal skin (D04.5)
    carcinoma in situ of perianal skin (D04.5)

✓5ᵗʰ D01.4   **Carcinoma in situ of** other and unspecified parts of intestine
  EXCLUDES 1   carcinoma in situ of ampulla of Vater (D01.5)

D01.40   **Carcinoma in situ of unspecified part of intestine** ▽

D01.49   **Carcinoma in situ of other parts of intestine**

D01.5   **Carcinoma in situ of** liver, gallbladder and bile ducts
  Carcinoma in situ of ampulla of Vater

D01.7   **Carcinoma in situ of** other specified digestive organs
  Carcinoma in situ of pancreas

D01.9   **Carcinoma in situ of** digestive organ, unspecified ▽

✓4ᵗʰ **D02   Carcinoma in situ of** middle ear and respiratory system
  Use additional code to identify:
  exposure to environmental tobacco smoke (Z77.22)
  exposure to tobacco smoke in the perinatal period (P96.81)
  history of tobacco dependence (Z87.891)
  occupational exposure to environmental tobacco smoke (Z57.31)
  tobacco dependence (F17.-)
  tobacco use (Z72.0)
  EXCLUDES 1   melanoma in situ (D03.-)

D02.0   **Carcinoma in situ of** larynx
  Carcinoma in situ of aryepiglottic fold or interarytenoid fold,
    laryngeal aspect
  Carcinoma in situ of epiglottis (suprahyoid portion)
  EXCLUDES 1   carcinoma in situ of aryepiglottic fold or interarytenoid
      fold NOS (D00.08)
    carcinoma in situ of hypopharyngeal aspect (D00.08)
    carcinoma in situ of marginal zone (D00.08)

D02.1   **Carcinoma in situ of** trachea

✓5ᵗʰ D02.2   **Carcinoma in situ of** bronchus and lung

D02.20   **Carcinoma in situ of unspecified bronchus and lung** ▽

D02.21   **Carcinoma in situ of** right **bronchus and lung**

D02.22   **Carcinoma in situ of** left **bronchus and lung**

D02.3   **Carcinoma in situ of** other parts of respiratory system
  Carcinoma in situ of accessory sinuses
  Carcinoma in situ of middle ear
  Carcinoma in situ of nasal cavities
  EXCLUDES 1   carcinoma in situ of ear (external) (skin) (D04.2-)
    carcinoma in situ of nose NOS (D09.8)
    carcinoma in situ of skin of nose (D04.3)

D02.4   **Carcinoma in situ of** respiratory system, unspecified ▽

✓4ᵗʰ **D03   Melanoma in situ**

D03.0   **Melanoma in situ of** lip   NRS

✓5ᵗʰ D03.1   **Melanoma in situ of** eyelid, including canthus

D03.10   **Melanoma in situ of unspecified eyelid, including canthus** ▽

D03.11   **Melanoma in situ of** right **eyelid, including canthus**   NRS

D03.12   **Melanoma in situ of** left **eyelid, including canthus**   NRS

✓5ᵗʰ D03.2   **Melanoma in situ of** ear and external auricular canal

D03.20   **Melanoma in situ of unspecified ear and external auricular canal** ▽

D03.21   **Melanoma in situ of** right **ear and external auricular canal**   NRS

D03.22   **Melanoma in situ of** left **ear and external auricular canal**   NRS

✓5ᵗʰ D03.3   **Melanoma in situ of** other and unspecified parts of face

D03.30   **Melanoma in situ of unspecified part of face** ▽

D03.39   **Melanoma in situ of other parts of face**   NRS

D03.4   **Melanoma in situ of** scalp and neck   NRS

✓5ᵗʰ D03.5   **Melanoma in situ of** trunk

D03.51   **Melanoma in situ of** anal skin   NRS
  Melanoma in situ of anal margin
  Melanoma in situ of perianal skin

D03.52   **Melanoma in situ of** breast (skin) (soft tissue)   NRS

D03.59   **Melanoma in situ of** other part of trunk   NRS

✓5ᵗʰ D03.6   **Melanoma in situ of** upper limb, including shoulder

D03.60   **Melanoma in situ of unspecified upper limb, including shoulder** ▽

D03.61   **Melanoma in situ of** right **upper limb, including shoulder**   NRS

D03.62   **Melanoma in situ of** left **upper limb, including shoulder**   NRS

✓5ᵗʰ D03.7   **Melanoma in situ of** lower limb, including hip

D03.70   **Melanoma in situ of unspecified lower limb, including hip** ▽

D03.71   **Melanoma in situ of** right **lower limb, including hip**   NRS

D03.72   **Melanoma in situ of** left **lower limb, including hip**   NRS

D03.8   **Melanoma in situ of** other sites   NRS
  Melanoma in situ of scrotum
  EXCLUDES 1   carcinoma in situ of scrotum (D07.61)

D03.9   **Melanoma in situ, unspecified** ▽

✓4ᵗʰ **D04   Carcinoma in situ of** skin
  EXCLUDES 1   erythroplasia of Queyrat (penis) NOS (D07.4)
    melanoma in situ (D03.-)

D04.0   **Carcinoma in situ of skin of** lip   NRS
  EXCLUDES 1   carcinoma in situ of vermilion border of lip (D00.01)

✓5ᵗʰ D04.1   **Carcinoma in situ of skin of** eyelid, including canthus

D04.10   **Carcinoma in situ of skin of unspecified eyelid, including canthus**   NRS ▽

D04.11   **Carcinoma in situ of skin of** right **eyelid, including canthus**   NRS

D04.12   **Carcinoma in situ of skin of** left **eyelid, including canthus**   NRS

✓5ᵗʰ D04.2   **Carcinoma in situ of skin of** ear and external auricular canal

D04.20   **Carcinoma in situ of skin of unspecified ear and external auricular canal**   NRS ▽

D04.21   **Carcinoma in situ of skin of** right **ear and external auricular canal**   NRS

D04.22   **Carcinoma in situ of skin of** left **ear and external auricular canal**   NRS

✓5ᵗʰ D04.3   **Carcinoma in situ of skin of** other and unspecified parts of face

D04.30   **Carcinoma in situ of skin of unspecified part of face**   NRS ▽

D04.39   **Carcinoma in situ of skin of other parts of face**   NRS

D04.4   **Carcinoma in situ of skin of** scalp and neck   NRS

D04.5   **Carcinoma in situ of skin of** trunk   NRS
  Carcinoma in situ of anal margin
  Carcinoma in situ of anal skin
  Carcinoma in situ of perianal skin
  Carcinoma in situ of skin of breast
  EXCLUDES 1   carcinoma in situ of anus NOS (D01.3)
    carcinoma in situ of scrotum (D07.61)
    carcinoma in situ of skin of genital organs (D07.-)

✓5ᵗʰ D04.6   **Carcinoma in situ of skin of** upper limb, including shoulder

D04.60   **Carcinoma in situ of skin of unspecified upper limb, including shoulder**   NRS ▽

D04.61   **Carcinoma in situ of skin of** right **upper limb, including shoulder**   NRS

D04.62   **Carcinoma in situ of skin of** left **upper limb, including shoulder**   NRS

✓5ᵗʰ D04.7   **Carcinoma in situ of skin of** lower limb, including hip

D04.70   **Carcinoma in situ of skin of unspecified lower limb, including hip**   NRS ▽

✓ Additional Character Req   ✓x7ᵗʰ Placeholder Alert   Case-Mix Diagnosis   Manifestation   ▽ Unspecified Dx   *EXCLUDES 1* Not coded here   *EXCLUDES 2* Not included here

D04.71　Carcinoma in situ of skin of right lower limb, including hip　NRS

D04.72　Carcinoma in situ of skin of left lower limb, including hip　NRS

D04.8　Carcinoma in situ of skin of other sites　NRS

D04.9　Carcinoma in situ of skin, unspecified　NRS ▽

✓4ᵗʰ **D05** Carcinoma in situ of breast
    EXCLUDES 1　carcinoma in situ of skin of breast (D04.5)
          melanoma in situ of breast (skin) (D03.5)
          Paget's disease of breast or nipple (C50.-)

  ✓5ᵗʰ **D05.0** Lobular carcinoma in situ of breast
    D05.00　Lobular carcinoma in situ of unspecified breast　▽
    D05.01　Lobular carcinoma in situ of right breast
    D05.02　Lobular carcinoma in situ of left breast

  ✓5ᵗʰ **D05.1** Intraductal carcinoma in situ of breast
    D05.10　Intraductal carcinoma in situ of unspecified breast　▽
    D05.11　Intraductal carcinoma in situ of right breast
    D05.12　Intraductal carcinoma in situ of left breast

  ✓5ᵗʰ **D05.8** Other specified type of carcinoma in situ of breast
    D05.80　Other specified type of carcinoma in situ of unspecified breast　▽
    D05.81　Other specified type of carcinoma in situ of right breast
    D05.82　Other specified type of carcinoma in situ of left breast

  ✓5ᵗʰ **D05.9** Unspecified type of carcinoma in situ of breast
    D05.90　Unspecified type of carcinoma in situ of unspecified breast　▽
    D05.91　Unspecified type of carcinoma in situ of right breast　▽
    D05.92　Unspecified type of carcinoma in situ of left breast　▽

✓4ᵗʰ **D06** Carcinoma in situ of cervix uteri
    INCLUDES　cervical adenocarcinoma in situ
          cervical intraepithelial glandular neoplasia
          cervical intraepithelial neoplasia III [CIN III]
          severe dysplasia of cervix uteri
    EXCLUDES 1　cervical intraepithelial neoplasia II [CIN II] (N87.1)
          cytologic evidence of malignancy of cervix without histologic confirmation (R87.614)
          high grade squamous intraepithelial lesion (HGSIL) of cervix (R87.613)
          melanoma in situ of cervix (D03.5)
          moderate cervical dysplasia (N87.1)

  D06.0　Carcinoma in situ of endocervix　♀
  D06.1　Carcinoma in situ of exocervix　♀
  D06.7　Carcinoma in situ of other parts of cervix　♀
  D06.9　Carcinoma in situ of cervix, unspecified　♀ ▽

✓4ᵗʰ **D07** Carcinoma in situ of other and unspecified genital organs
    EXCLUDES 1　melanoma in situ of trunk (D03.5)

  D07.0　Carcinoma in situ of endometrium　♀
  D07.1　Carcinoma in situ of vulva　♀
    Severe dysplasia of vulva
    Vulvar intraepithelial neoplasia III [VIN III]
    EXCLUDES 1　moderate dysplasia of vulva (N90.1)
          vulvar intraepithelial neoplasia II [VIN II] (N90.1)

  D07.2　Carcinoma in situ of vagina　♀
    Severe dysplasia of vagina
    Vaginal intraepithelial neoplasia III [VAIN III]
    EXCLUDES 1　moderate dysplasia of vagina (N89.1)
          vaginal intraepithelial neoplasia II [VIN II] (N89.1)

  ✓5ᵗʰ **D07.3** Carcinoma in situ of other and unspecified female genital organs
    D07.30　Carcinoma in situ of unspecified female genital organs　♀ ▽
    D07.39　Carcinoma in situ of other female genital organs　♀

  D07.4　Carcinoma in situ of penis　♂
    Erythroplasia of Queyrat NOS

  D07.5　Carcinoma in situ of prostate　♂
    Prostatic intraepithelial neoplasia III (PIN III)
    Severe dysplasia of prostate
    EXCLUDES 1　dysplasia (mild) (moderate) of prostate (N42.3-)
          prostatic intraepithelial neoplasia II [PIN II] (N42.3-)

  D07.6　Carcinoma in situ of other and unspecified male genital organs
    D07.60　Carcinoma in situ of unspecified male genital organs　♂ ▽
    D07.61　Carcinoma in situ of scrotum　♂
    D07.69　Carcinoma in situ of other male genital organs　♂

✓4ᵗʰ **D09** Carcinoma in situ of other and unspecified sites
    EXCLUDES 1　melanoma in situ (D03.-)

  D09.0　Carcinoma in situ of bladder

  ✓5ᵗʰ **D09.1** Carcinoma in situ of other and unspecified urinary organs
    D09.10　Carcinoma in situ of unspecified urinary organ　▽
    D09.19　Carcinoma in situ of other urinary organs

  ✓5ᵗʰ **D09.2** Carcinoma in situ of eye
    EXCLUDES 1　carcinoma in situ of skin of eyelid (D04.1-)
    D09.20　Carcinoma in situ of unspecified eye　▽
    D09.21　Carcinoma in situ of right eye
    D09.22　Carcinoma in situ of left eye

  D09.3　Carcinoma in situ of thyroid and other endocrine glands
    EXCLUDES 1　carcinoma in situ of endocrine pancreas (D01.7)
          carcinoma in situ of ovary (D07.39)
          carcinoma in situ of testis (D07.69)

  D09.8　Carcinoma in situ of other specified sites
  D09.9　Carcinoma in situ, unspecified　▽

Benign neoplasms, except benign neuroendocrine tumors (D10-D36)

✓4ᵗʰ **D10** Benign neoplasm of mouth and pharynx

  D10.0　Benign neoplasm of lip
    Benign neoplasm of lip (frenulum) (inner aspect) (mucosa) (vermilion border)
    EXCLUDES 1　benign neoplasm of skin of lip (D22.0, D23.0)

  D10.1　Benign neoplasm of tongue
    Benign neoplasm of lingual tonsil

  D10.2　Benign neoplasm of floor of mouth

  ✓5ᵗʰ **D10.3** Benign neoplasm of other and unspecified parts of mouth
    D10.30　Benign neoplasm of unspecified part of mouth　▽
    D10.39　Benign neoplasm of other parts of mouth
       Benign neoplasm of minor salivary gland NOS
       EXCLUDES 1　benign odontogenic neoplasms (D16.4-D16.5)
            benign neoplasm of mucosa of lip (D10.0)
            benign neoplasm of nasopharyngeal surface of soft palate (D10.6)

  D10.4　Benign neoplasm of tonsil
    Benign neoplasm of tonsil (faucial) (palatine)
    EXCLUDES 1　benign neoplasm of lingual tonsil (D10.1)
          benign neoplasm of pharyngeal tonsil (D10.6)
          benign neoplasm of tonsillar fossa (D10.5)
          benign neoplasm of tonsillar pillars (D10.5)

  D10.5　Benign neoplasm of other parts of oropharynx
    Benign neoplasm of epiglottis, anterior aspect
    Benign neoplasm of tonsillar fossa
    Benign neoplasm of tonsillar pillars
    Benign neoplasm of vallecula
    EXCLUDES 1　benign neoplasm of epiglottis NOS (D14.1)
          benign neoplasm of epiglottis, suprahyoid portion (D14.1)

  D10.6　Benign neoplasm of nasopharynx
    Benign neoplasm of pharyngeal tonsil
    Benign neoplasm of posterior margin of septum and choanae

  D10.7　Benign neoplasm of hypopharynx
  D10.9　Benign neoplasm of pharynx, unspecified　▽

✓4ᵗʰ **D11** Benign neoplasm of major salivary glands
    EXCLUDES 1　benign neoplasms of specified minor salivary glands which are classified according to their anatomical location
          benign neoplasms of minor salivary glands NOS (D10.39)

  D11.0　Benign neoplasm of parotid gland
  D11.7　Benign neoplasm of other major salivary glands
    Benign neoplasm of sublingual salivary gland
    Benign neoplasm of submandibular salivary gland

  D11.9　Benign neoplasm of major salivary gland, unspecified　▽

N Newborn: 0　P Pediatric: 0-17　M Maternity: 12-55　A Adult: 15-124　NRS Nonroutine supply Dx　NC Dx Noncancer Dx　PDx Primary Dx　▶◀ Revised Text　● New Code　▲ Revised Title

✓4ᵗʰ **D12**   **Benign neoplasm of colon, rectum, anus and anal canal**
> *EXCLUDES 1*   *benign carcinoid tumors of the large intestine, and rectum (D3A.Ø2-)*
> **AHA:** 2017, 1Q, 15; 2015, 2Q, 14

    D12.Ø   **Benign neoplasm of cecum**
       Benign neoplasm of ileocecal valve

    D12.1   **Benign neoplasm of appendix**
       EXCLUDES 1   *benign carcinoid tumor of the appendix (D3A.Ø2Ø)*

    D12.2   **Benign neoplasm of ascending colon**

    D12.3   **Benign neoplasm of transverse colon**
       Benign neoplasm of hepatic flexure
       Benign neoplasm of splenic flexure
       AHA: 2017, 1Q, 16

    D12.4   **Benign neoplasm of descending colon**

    D12.5   **Benign neoplasm of sigmoid colon**

    D12.6   **Benign neoplasm of colon, unspecified**   ▽
       Adenomatosis of colon
       Benign neoplasm of large intestine NOS
       Polyposis (hereditary) of colon
       EXCLUDES 1   *inflammatory polyp of colon (K51.4-)*
               polyp of colon NOS (K63.5)

    D12.7   **Benign neoplasm of rectosigmoid junction**

    D12.8   **Benign neoplasm of rectum**
       EXCLUDES 1   *benign carcinoid tumor of the rectum (D3A.Ø26)*

    D12.9   **Benign neoplasm of anus and anal canal**
       Benign neoplasm of anus NOS
       EXCLUDES 1   *benign neoplasm of anal margin (D22.5, D23.5)*
               benign neoplasm of anal skin (D22.5, D23.5)
               benign neoplasm of perianal skin (D22.5, D23.5)

✓4ᵗʰ **D13**   **Benign neoplasm of other and ill-defined parts of digestive system**
> *EXCLUDES 1*   *benign stromal tumors of digestive system (D21.4)*

    D13.Ø   **Benign neoplasm of esophagus**

    D13.1   **Benign neoplasm of stomach**
       EXCLUDES 1   *benign carcinoid tumor of the stomach (D3A.Ø92)*

    D13.2   **Benign neoplasm of duodenum**
       EXCLUDES 1   *benign carcinoid tumor of the duodenum (D3A.Ø1Ø)*

✓5ᵗʰ   **D13.3**   **Benign neoplasm of other and unspecified parts of small intestine**
       EXCLUDES 1   *benign carcinoid tumors of the small intestine (D3A.Ø1-)*
               benign neoplasm of ileocecal valve (D12.Ø)

       D13.3Ø   **Benign neoplasm of unspecified part of small intestine**   ▽

       D13.39   **Benign neoplasm of other parts of small intestine**

    D13.4   **Benign neoplasm of liver**
       Benign neoplasm of intrahepatic bile ducts

    D13.5   **Benign neoplasm of extrahepatic bile ducts**

    D13.6   **Benign neoplasm of pancreas**
       EXCLUDES 1   *benign neoplasm of endocrine pancreas (D13.7)*

    D13.7   **Benign neoplasm of endocrine pancreas**
       Islet cell tumor   Benign neoplasm of islets of Langerhans
       Use additional code to identify any functional activity

    D13.9   **Benign neoplasm of ill-defined sites within the digestive system**   ▽
       Benign neoplasm of digestive system NOS
       Benign neoplasm of intestine NOS
       Benign neoplasm of spleen

✓4ᵗʰ **D14**   **Benign neoplasm of middle ear and respiratory system**

    D14.Ø   **Benign neoplasm of middle ear, nasal cavity and accessory sinuses**
       Benign neoplasm of cartilage of nose
       EXCLUDES 1   *benign neoplasm of auricular canal (external) (D22.2-, D23.2-)*
               benign neoplasm of bone of ear (D16.4)
               benign neoplasm of bone of nose (D16.4)
               benign neoplasm of cartilage of ear (D21.Ø)
               benign neoplasm of ear (external)(skin) (D22.2-, D23.2-)
               benign neoplasm of nose NOS (D36.7)
               benign neoplasm of skin of nose (D22.39, D23.39)
               benign neoplasm of olfactory bulb (D33.3)
               benign neoplasm of posterior margin of septum and choanae (D10.6)
               polyp of accessory sinus (J33.8)
               polyp of ear (middle) (H74.4)
               polyp of nasal (cavity) (J33.-)

    D14.1   **Benign neoplasm of larynx**
       Adenomatous polyp of larynx
       Benign neoplasm of epiglottis (suprahyoid portion)
       EXCLUDES 1   *benign neoplasm of epiglottis, anterior aspect (D10.5)*
               polyp (nonadenomatous) of vocal cord or larynx (J38.1)

    D14.2   **Benign neoplasm of trachea**

✓5ᵗʰ   **D14.3**   **Benign neoplasm of bronchus and lung**
       EXCLUDES 1   *benign carcinoid tumor of the bronchus and lung (D3A.Ø9Ø)*

       D14.3Ø   **Benign neoplasm of unspecified bronchus and lung**   ▽

       D14.31   **Benign neoplasm of right bronchus and lung**

       D14.32   **Benign neoplasm of left bronchus and lung**

    D14.4   **Benign neoplasm of respiratory system, unspecified**   ▽

✓4ᵗʰ **D15**   **Benign neoplasm of other and unspecified intrathoracic organs**
> *EXCLUDES 1*   *benign neoplasm of mesothelial tissue (D19.-)*

    D15.Ø   **Benign neoplasm of thymus**
       EXCLUDES 1   *benign carcinoid tumor of the thymus (D3A.Ø91)*

    D15.1   **Benign neoplasm of heart**
       EXCLUDES 1   *benign neoplasm of great vessels (D21.3)*

    D15.2   **Benign neoplasm of mediastinum**

    D15.7   **Benign neoplasm of other specified intrathoracic organs**

    D15.9   **Benign neoplasm of intrathoracic organ, unspecified**   ▽

✓4ᵗʰ **D16**   **Benign neoplasm of bone and articular cartilage**
> *EXCLUDES 1*   *benign neoplasm of connective tissue of ear (D21.Ø)*
>   *benign neoplasm of connective tissue of eyelid (D21.Ø)*
>   *benign neoplasm of connective tissue of larynx (D14.1)*
>   *benign neoplasm of connective tissue of nose (D14.Ø)*
>   *benign neoplasm of synovia (D21.-)*

✓5ᵗʰ   **D16.Ø**   **Benign neoplasm of scapula and long bones of upper limb**

       D16.ØØ   **Benign neoplasm of scapula and long bones of unspecified upper limb**   ▽

       D16.Ø1   **Benign neoplasm of scapula and long bones of right upper limb**

       D16.Ø2   **Benign neoplasm of scapula and long bones of left upper limb**

✓5ᵗʰ   **D16.1**   **Benign neoplasm of short bones of upper limb**

       D16.1Ø   **Benign neoplasm of short bones of unspecified upper limb**   ▽

       D16.11   **Benign neoplasm of short bones of right upper limb**

       D16.12   **Benign neoplasm of short bones of left upper limb**

✓5ᵗʰ   **D16.2**   **Benign neoplasm of long bones of lower limb**

       D16.2Ø   **Benign neoplasm of long bones of unspecified lower limb**   ▽

       D16.21   **Benign neoplasm of long bones of right lower limb**

       D16.22   **Benign neoplasm of long bones of left lower limb**

✓5ᵗʰ   **D16.3**   **Benign neoplasm of short bones of lower limb**

       D16.3Ø   **Benign neoplasm of short bones of unspecified lower limb**   ▽

       D16.31   **Benign neoplasm of short bones of right lower limb**

       D16.32   **Benign neoplasm of short bones of left lower limb**

    D16.4   **Benign neoplasm of bones of skull and face**
       Benign neoplasm of maxilla (superior)
       Benign neoplasm of orbital bone
       Keratocyst of maxilla
       Keratocystic odontogenic tumor of maxilla
       EXCLUDES 2   *benign neoplasm of lower jaw bone (D16.5)*

    D16.5   **Benign neoplasm of lower jaw bone**
       Keratocyst of mandible
       Keratocystic odontogenic tumor of mandible

    D16.6   **Benign neoplasm of vertebral column**
       EXCLUDES 1   *benign neoplasm of sacrum and coccyx (D16.8)*

    D16.7   **Benign neoplasm of ribs, sternum and clavicle**

    D16.8   **Benign neoplasm of pelvic bones, sacrum and coccyx**

    D16.9   **Benign neoplasm of bone and articular cartilage, unspecified**   ▽

✓4ᵗʰ **D17**   **Benign lipomatous neoplasm**

    D17.Ø   **Benign lipomatous neoplasm of skin and subcutaneous tissue of head, face and neck**

    D17.1   **Benign lipomatous neoplasm of skin and subcutaneous tissue of trunk**

✓ Additional Character Req   ✓x7ᵗʰ Placeholder Alert   Case-Mix Diagnosis   Manifestation   ▽ Unspecified Dx   *EXCLUDES 1* Not coded here   *EXCLUDES 2* Not included here

ICD-10-CM 2018   **485**

D12–D17.1

Chapter 2. Neoplasms

D17.2–D22.12

☑5ᵗʰ **D17.2 Benign lipomatous neoplasm of** skin and subcutaneous tissue of limb

    D17.20 Benign lipomatous neoplasm of skin and subcutaneous tissue of unspecified limb ▽

    D17.21 Benign lipomatous neoplasm of skin and subcutaneous tissue of right arm

    D17.22 Benign lipomatous neoplasm of skin and subcutaneous tissue of left arm

    D17.23 Benign lipomatous neoplasm of skin and subcutaneous tissue of right leg

    D17.24 Benign lipomatous neoplasm of skin and subcutaneous tissue of left leg

☑5ᵗʰ **D17.3 Benign lipomatous neoplasm of** skin and subcutaneous tissue of other and unspecified sites

    D17.30 Benign lipomatous neoplasm of skin and subcutaneous tissue of unspecified sites ▽

    D17.39 Benign lipomatous neoplasm of skin and subcutaneous tissue of other sites

D17.4 Benign lipomatous neoplasm of intrathoracic organs

D17.5 Benign lipomatous neoplasm of intra-abdominal organs

    EXCLUDES 1   *benign lipomatous neoplasm of peritoneum and retroperitoneum (D17.79)*

D17.6 Benign lipomatous neoplasm of spermatic cord   ♂

☑5ᵗʰ **D17.7 Benign lipomatous neoplasm of** other sites

    D17.71 Benign lipomatous neoplasm of kidney

    D17.72 Benign lipomatous neoplasm of other genitourinary organ

    D17.79 Benign lipomatous neoplasm of other sites
        Benign lipomatous neoplasm of peritoneum
        Benign lipomatous neoplasm of retroperitoneum

D17.9 Benign lipomatous neoplasm, unspecified ▽
    Lipoma NOS

☑4ᵗʰ **D18 Hemangioma and lymphangioma, any site**

    EXCLUDES 1   *benign neoplasm of glomus jugulare (D35.6)*
         blue or pigmented nevus (D22.-)
         nevus NOS (D22.-)
         vascular nevus (Q82.5)

☑5ᵗʰ **D18.0 Hemangioma**
    Angioma NOS
    Cavernous nevus
    DEF: A common benign tumor usually occurring in infancy; composed of newly formed blood vessels due to malformation of angioblastic tissue.

    D18.00 Hemangioma unspecified site ▽

    D18.01 Hemangioma of skin and subcutaneous tissue

    D18.02 Hemangioma of intracranial structures

    D18.03 Hemangioma of intra-abdominal structures

    D18.09 Hemangioma of other sites

D18.1 Lymphangioma, any site

☑4ᵗʰ **D19 Benign neoplasm of** mesothelial tissue

D19.0 Benign neoplasm of mesothelial tissue of pleura

D19.1 Benign neoplasm of mesothelial tissue of peritoneum

D19.7 Benign neoplasm of mesothelial tissue of other sites

D19.9 Benign neoplasm of mesothelial tissue, unspecified ▽
    Benign mesothelioma NOS

☑4ᵗʰ **D20 Benign neoplasm of soft tissue of** retroperitoneum and peritoneum

    EXCLUDES 1   *benign lipomatous neoplasm of peritoneum and retroperitoneum (D17.79)*
         benign neoplasm of mesothelial tissue (D19.-)

D20.0 Benign neoplasm of soft tissue of retroperitoneum

D20.1 Benign neoplasm of soft tissue of peritoneum

☑4ᵗʰ **D21 Other benign neoplasms of** connective and other soft tissue

    INCLUDES   benign neoplasm of blood vessel
         benign neoplasm of bursa
         benign neoplasm of cartilage
         benign neoplasm of fascia
         benign neoplasm of fat
         benign neoplasm of ligament, except uterine
         benign neoplasm of lymphatic channel
         benign neoplasm of muscle
         benign neoplasm of synovia
         benign neoplasm of tendon (sheath)
         benign stromal tumors

    EXCLUDES 1   *benign neoplasm of articular cartilage (D16.-)*
         benign neoplasm of cartilage of larynx (D14.1)
         benign neoplasm of cartilage of nose (D14.0)
         benign neoplasm of connective tissue of breast (D24.-)
         benign neoplasm of peripheral nerves and autonomic nervous system (D36.1-)
         benign neoplasm of peritoneum (D20.1)
         benign neoplasm of retroperitoneum (D20.0)
         benign neoplasm of uterine ligament, any (D28.2)
         benign neoplasm of vascular tissue (D18.-)
         hemangioma (D18.0-)
         lipomatous neoplasm (D17.-)
         lymphangioma (D18.1)
         uterine leiomyoma (D25.-)

D21.0 Benign neoplasm of connective and other soft tissue of head, face and neck
    Benign neoplasm of connective tissue of ear
    Benign neoplasm of connective tissue of eyelid
    EXCLUDES 1   *benign neoplasm of connective tissue of orbit (D31.6-)*

☑5ᵗʰ **D21.1 Benign neoplasm of connective and other soft tissue of** upper limb, including shoulder

    D21.10 Benign neoplasm of connective and other soft tissue of unspecified upper limb, including shoulder ▽

    D21.11 Benign neoplasm of connective and other soft tissue of right upper limb, including shoulder

    D21.12 Benign neoplasm of connective and other soft tissue of left upper limb, including shoulder

☑5ᵗʰ **D21.2 Benign neoplasm of connective and other soft tissue of** lower limb, including hip

    D21.20 Benign neoplasm of connective and other soft tissue of unspecified lower limb, including hip ▽

    D21.21 Benign neoplasm of connective and other soft tissue of right lower limb, including hip

    D21.22 Benign neoplasm of connective and other soft tissue of left lower limb, including hip

D21.3 Benign neoplasm of connective and other soft tissue of thorax
    Benign neoplasm of axilla
    Benign neoplasm of diaphragm
    Benign neoplasm of great vessels
    EXCLUDES 1   *benign neoplasm of heart (D15.1)*
         benign neoplasm of mediastinum (D15.2)
         benign neoplasm of thymus (D15.0)

D21.4 Benign neoplasm of connective and other soft tissue of abdomen
    Benign stromal tumors of abdomen

D21.5 Benign neoplasm of connective and other soft tissue of pelvis
    EXCLUDES 1   *benign neoplasm of any uterine ligament (D28.2)*
         uterine leiomyoma (D25.-)

D21.6 Benign neoplasm of connective and other soft tissue of trunk, unspecified ▽
    Benign neoplasm of back NOS

D21.9 Benign neoplasm of connective and other soft tissue, unspecified ▽

☑4ᵗʰ **D22 Melanocytic nevi**

    INCLUDES   atypical nevus
         blue hairy pigmented nevus
         nevus NOS

D22.0 Melanocytic nevi of lip

☑5ᵗʰ **D22.1 Melanocytic nevi of** eyelid, including canthus

    D22.10 Melanocytic nevi of unspecified eyelid, including canthus ▽

    D22.11 Melanocytic nevi of right eyelid, including canthus

    D22.12 Melanocytic nevi of left eyelid, including canthus

Ⓝ Newborn: 0   Ⓟ Pediatric: 0-17   Ⓜ Maternity: 12-55   Ⓐ Adult: 15-124   NRS Nonroutine supply Dx   NCDx Noncancer Dx   PDx Primary Dx   ▶◀ Revised Text   ● New Code   ▲ Revised Title

486   ICD-10-CM 2018

Chapter 2. Neoplasms

✓5ᵗʰ **D22.2 Melanocytic nevi of** ear and external auricular canal

    D22.20 Melanocytic nevi of unspecified ear and external ▽
          auricular canal

    D22.21 Melanocytic nevi of right **ear and external auricular canal**

    D22.22 Melanocytic nevi of left **ear and external auricular canal**

✓5ᵗʰ **D22.3 Melanocytic nevi of** other and unspecified parts of face

    D22.30 Melanocytic nevi of unspecified part of face ▽

    D22.39 Melanocytic nevi of other parts of face

D22.4 Melanocytic nevi of scalp and neck

D22.5 Melanocytic nevi of trunk
    Melanocytic nevi of anal margin
    Melanocytic nevi of anal skin
    Melanocytic nevi of perianal skin
    Melanocytic nevi of skin of breast

✓5ᵗʰ **D22.6 Melanocytic nevi of** upper limb, including shoulder

    D22.60 Melanocytic nevi of unspecified upper limb, ▽
          including shoulder

    D22.61 Melanocytic nevi of right **upper limb, including shoulder**

    D22.62 Melanocytic nevi of left **upper limb, including shoulder**

✓5ᵗʰ **D22.7 Melanocytic nevi of** lower limb, including hip

    D22.70 Melanocytic nevi of unspecified lower limb, ▽
          including hip

    D22.71 Melanocytic nevi of right **lower limb, including hip**

    D22.72 Melanocytic nevi of left **lower limb, including hip**

D22.9 Melanocytic nevi, unspecified ▽

✓4ᵗʰ **D23 Other benign neoplasms of** skin
    INCLUDES benign neoplasm of hair follicles
          benign neoplasm of sebaceous glands
          benign neoplasm of sweat glands
    EXCLUDES 1 benign lipomatous neoplasms of skin (D17.0-D17.3)
          melanocytic nevi (D22.-)

D23.0 Other benign neoplasm of skin of lip
    EXCLUDES 1 benign neoplasm of vermilion border of lip (D10.0)

✓5ᵗʰ **D23.1 Other benign neoplasm of skin of** eyelid, including canthus

    D23.10 Other benign neoplasm of skin of unspecified ▽
          eyelid, including canthus

    D23.11 Other benign neoplasm of skin of right **eyelid, including canthus**

    D23.12 Other benign neoplasm of skin of left **eyelid, including canthus**

✓5ᵗʰ **D23.2 Other benign neoplasm of skin of** ear and external auricular canal

    D23.20 Other benign neoplasm of skin of unspecified ▽
          ear and external auricular canal

    D23.21 Other benign neoplasm of skin of right **ear and external auricular canal**

    D23.22 Other benign neoplasm of skin of left **ear and external auricular canal**

✓5ᵗʰ **D23.3 Other benign neoplasm of skin of** other and unspecified parts of face

    D23.30 Other benign neoplasm of skin of unspecified ▽
          part of face

    D23.39 Other benign neoplasm of skin of other parts of face

D23.4 Other benign neoplasm of skin of scalp and neck

D23.5 Other benign neoplasm of skin of trunk
    Other benign neoplasm of anal margin
    Other benign neoplasm of anal skin
    Other benign neoplasm of perianal skin
    Other benign neoplasm of skin of breast
    EXCLUDES 1 benign neoplasm of anus NOS (D12.9)

✓5ᵗʰ **D23.6 Other benign neoplasm of skin of** upper limb, including shoulder

    D23.60 Other benign neoplasm of skin of unspecified ▽
          upper limb, including shoulder

    D23.61 Other benign neoplasm of skin of right **upper limb, including shoulder**

    D23.62 Other benign neoplasm of skin of left **upper limb, including shoulder**

✓5ᵗʰ **D23.7 Other benign neoplasm of skin of** lower limb, including hip

    D23.70 Other benign neoplasm of skin of unspecified ▽
          lower limb, including hip

Uterine Leiomyomas (Fibroids)

    D23.71 Other benign neoplasm of skin of right **lower limb, including hip**

    D23.72 Other benign neoplasm of skin of left **lower limb, including hip**

D23.9 Other benign neoplasm of skin, unspecified ▽

✓4ᵗʰ **D24 Benign neoplasm of** breast
    INCLUDES benign neoplasm of connective tissue of breast
          benign neoplasm of soft parts of breast
          fibroadenoma of breast
    EXCLUDES 2 adenofibrosis of breast (N60.2)
          benign cyst of breast (N60.-)
          benign mammary dysplasia (N60.-)
          benign neoplasm of skin of breast (D22.5, D23.5)
          fibrocystic disease of breast (N60.-)

D24.1 Benign neoplasm of right **breast**

D24.2 Benign neoplasm of left **breast**

D24.9 Benign neoplasm of unspecified breast ▽

✓4ᵗʰ **D25 Leiomyoma of uterus**
    INCLUDES uterine fibroid
          uterine fibromyoma
          uterine myoma

D25.0 Submucous leiomyoma of uterus ♀

D25.1 Intramural leiomyoma of uterus ♀
    Interstitial leiomyoma of uterus

D25.2 Subserosal leiomyoma of uterus ♀
    Subperitoneal leiomyoma of uterus

D25.9 Leiomyoma of uterus, unspecified ♀▽

✓4ᵗʰ **D26 Other benign neoplasms of** uterus

D26.0 Other benign neoplasm of cervix uteri ♀

D26.1 Other benign neoplasm of corpus uteri ♀

D26.7 Other benign neoplasm of other parts of uterus ♀

D26.9 Other benign neoplasm of uterus, unspecified ♀▽

✓4ᵗʰ **D27 Benign neoplasm of** ovary
    Use additional code to identify any functional activity
    EXCLUDES 2 corpus albicans cyst (N83.2-)
          corpus luteum cyst (N83.1-)
          endometrial cyst (N80.1)
          follicular (atretic) cyst (N83.0-)
          graafian follicle cyst (N83.0-)
          ovarian cyst NEC (N83.2-)x
          ovarian retention cyst w(N83.2-)

D27.0 Benign neoplasm of right **ovary** ♀

D27.1 Benign neoplasm of left **ovary** ♀

D27.9 Benign neoplasm of unspecified ovary ♀▽

✓4ᵗʰ **D28 Benign neoplasm of** other and unspecified female genital organs
    INCLUDES adenomatous polyp
          benign neoplasm of skin of female genital organs
          benign teratoma
    EXCLUDES 1 epoophoron cyst (Q50.5)
          fimbrial cyst (Q50.4)
          Gartner's duct cyst (Q52.4)
          parovarian cyst (Q50.5)

D28.0 Benign neoplasm of vulva ♀

D28.1 Benign neoplasm of vagina ♀

☑ Additional Character Req   ✓x7ᵗʰ Placeholder Alert   <u>Case-Mix Diagnosis</u>   Manifestation   ▽ Unspecified Dx   EXCLUDES 1 Not coded here   EXCLUDES 2 Not included here

Chapter 2. Neoplasms *(left margin)*

D28.2 **Benign neoplasm of** uterine tubes and ligaments ♀
Benign neoplasm of fallopian tube
Benign neoplasm of uterine ligament (broad) (round)

D28.7 **Benign neoplasm of other specified female genital organs** ♀

D28.9 **Benign neoplasm of female genital organ, unspecified** ♀▽

✓4ᵗʰ **D29** **Benign neoplasm of** male genital organs
INCLUDES benign neoplasm of skin of male genital organs

D29.0 **Benign neoplasm of** penis ♂

D29.1 **Benign neoplasm of** prostate ♂
EXCLUDES 1 *enlarged prostate (N40.-)*

✓5ᵗʰ **D29.2** **Benign neoplasm of** testis
Use additional code to identify any functional activity

D29.20 **Benign neoplasm of unspecified testis** ♂▽

D29.21 **Benign neoplasm of** right testis ♂

D29.22 **Benign neoplasm of** left testis ♂

✓5ᵗʰ **D29.3** **Benign neoplasm of** epididymis

D29.30 **Benign neoplasm of unspecified epididymis** ♂▽

D29.31 **Benign neoplasm of** right epididymis ♂

D29.32 **Benign neoplasm of** left epididymis ♂

D29.4 **Benign neoplasm of** scrotum ♂
Benign neoplasm of skin of scrotum

D29.8 **Benign neoplasm of other specified male genital organs** ♂
Benign neoplasm of seminal vesicle
Benign neoplasm of spermatic cord
Benign neoplasm of tunica vaginalis

D29.9 **Benign neoplasm of male genital organ, unspecified** ♂▽

✓4ᵗʰ **D30** **Benign neoplasm of** urinary organs

✓5ᵗʰ **D30.0** **Benign neoplasm of** kidney
EXCLUDES 1 *benign carcinoid tumor of the kidney (D3A.093)*
benign neoplasm of renal calyces (D30.1-)
benign neoplasm of renal pelvis (D30.1-)

D30.00 **Benign neoplasm of unspecified kidney** ▽

D30.01 **Benign neoplasm of** right kidney

D30.02 **Benign neoplasm of** left kidney

✓5ᵗʰ **D30.1** **Benign neoplasm of** renal pelvis

D30.10 **Benign neoplasm of unspecified renal pelvis** ▽

D30.11 **Benign neoplasm of** right renal pelvis

D30.12 **Benign neoplasm of** left renal pelvis

✓5ᵗʰ **D30.2** **Benign neoplasm of** ureter
EXCLUDES 1 *benign neoplasm of ureteric orifice of bladder (D30.3)*

D30.20 **Benign neoplasm of unspecified ureter** ▽

D30.21 **Benign neoplasm of** right ureter

D30.22 **Benign neoplasm of** left ureter

D30.3 **Benign neoplasm of** bladder
Benign neoplasm of ureteric orifice of bladder
Benign neoplasm of urethral orifice of bladder

D30.4 **Benign neoplasm of** urethra
EXCLUDES 1 *benign neoplasm of urethral orifice of bladder (D30.3)*

D30.8 **Benign neoplasm of other specified urinary organs**
Benign neoplasm of paraurethral glands

D30.9 **Benign neoplasm of urinary organ, unspecified** ▽
Benign neoplasm of urinary system NOS

✓4ᵗʰ **D31** **Benign neoplasm of** eye and adnexa
EXCLUDES 1 *benign neoplasm of connective tissue of eyelid (D21.0)*
benign neoplasm of optic nerve (D33.3)
benign neoplasm of skin of eyelid (D22.1-, D23.1-)

✓5ᵗʰ **D31.0** **Benign neoplasm of** conjunctiva

D31.00 **Benign neoplasm of unspecified conjunctiva** ▽

D31.01 **Benign neoplasm of** right conjunctiva

D31.02 **Benign neoplasm of** left conjunctiva

✓5ᵗʰ **D31.1** **Benign neoplasm of** cornea

D31.10 **Benign neoplasm of unspecified cornea** ▽

D31.11 **Benign neoplasm of** right cornea

D31.12 **Benign neoplasm of** left cornea

✓5ᵗʰ **D31.2** **Benign neoplasm of** retina
EXCLUDES 1 *dark area on retina (D49.81)*
hemangioma of retina (D49.81)
neoplasm of unspecified behavior of retina and
    choroid (D49.81)
retinal freckle (D49.81)

D31.20 **Benign neoplasm of unspecified retina** ▽

D31.21 **Benign neoplasm of** right retina

D31.22 **Benign neoplasm of** left retina

✓5ᵗʰ **D31.3** **Benign neoplasm of** choroid

D31.30 **Benign neoplasm of unspecified choroid** ▽

D31.31 **Benign neoplasm of** right choroid

D31.32 **Benign neoplasm of** left choroid

✓5ᵗʰ **D31.4** **Benign neoplasm of** ciliary body

D31.40 **Benign neoplasm of unspecified ciliary body** ▽

D31.41 **Benign neoplasm of** right ciliary body

D31.42 **Benign neoplasm of** left ciliary body

✓5ᵗʰ **D31.5** **Benign neoplasm of** lacrimal gland and duct
Benign neoplasm of lacrimal sac
Benign neoplasm of nasolacrimal duct

D31.50 **Benign neoplasm of unspecified lacrimal gland** ▽
and duct

D31.51 **Benign neoplasm of** right lacrimal gland and duct

D31.52 **Benign neoplasm of** left lacrimal gland and duct

✓5ᵗʰ **D31.6** **Benign neoplasm of unspecified site of** orbit
Benign neoplasm of connective tissue of orbit
Benign neoplasm of extraocular muscle
Benign neoplasm of peripheral nerves of orbit
Benign neoplasm of retrobulbar tissue
Benign neoplasm of retro-ocular tissue
EXCLUDES 1 *benign neoplasm of orbital bone (D16.4)*

D31.60 **Benign neoplasm of unspecified site of** ▽
unspecified orbit

D31.61 **Benign neoplasm of unspecified site of** right orbit ▽

D31.62 **Benign neoplasm of unspecified site of** left orbit ▽

✓5ᵗʰ **D31.9** **Benign neoplasm of** unspecified part of eye
Benign neoplasm of eyeball

D31.90 **Benign neoplasm of unspecified part of** ▽
unspecified eye

D31.91 **Benign neoplasm of unspecified part of** right eye ▽

D31.92 **Benign neoplasm of unspecified part of** left eye ▽

✓4ᵗʰ **D32** **Benign neoplasm of** meninges

D32.0 **Benign neoplasm of** cerebral **meninges**

D32.1 **Benign neoplasm of** spinal **meninges**

D32.9 **Benign neoplasm of meninges, unspecified** ▽
Meningioma NOS

✓4ᵗʰ **D33** **Benign neoplasm of** brain and other parts of central nervous
system
EXCLUDES 1 *angioma (D18.0-)*
benign neoplasm of meninges (D32.-)
benign neoplasm of peripheral nerves and autonomic nervous
    system (D36.1-)
hemangioma (D18.0-)
neurofibromatosis (Q85.0-)
retro-ocular benign neoplasm (D31.6-)

D33.0 **Benign neoplasm of** brain, supratentorial
Benign neoplasm of cerebral ventricle
Benign neoplasm of cerebrum
Benign neoplasm of frontal lobe
Benign neoplasm of occipital lobe
Benign neoplasm of parietal lobe
Benign neoplasm of temporal lobe
EXCLUDES 1 *benign neoplasm of fourth ventricle (D33.1)*

D33.1 **Benign neoplasm of** brain, infratentorial
Benign neoplasm of brain stem
Benign neoplasm of cerebellum
Benign neoplasm of fourth ventricle

D33.2 **Benign neoplasm of** brain, unspecified ▽

D33.3 **Benign neoplasm of** cranial nerves
Benign neoplasm of olfactory bulb

D33.4 **Benign neoplasm of** spinal cord

D33.7 **Benign neoplasm of other specified parts of central nervous**
system

D33.9 **Benign neoplasm of central nervous system, unspecified** ▽
Benign neoplasm of nervous system (central) NOS

D34 **Benign neoplasm of** thyroid gland
Use additional code to identify any functional activity

Ⓝ Newborn: 0 Ⓟ Pediatric: 0-17 Ⓜ Maternity: 12-55 Ⓐ Adult: 15-124 NRS Nonroutine supply Dx NCDx Noncancer Dx PDx Primary Dx ▶◀ Revised Text ● New Code ▲ Revised Title

488   ICD-10-CM 2018

✓4ᵗʰ **D35** **Benign neoplasm of** other and unspecified endocrine glands

Use additional code to identify any functional activity

EXCLUDES 1   *benign neoplasm of endocrine pancreas (D13.7)*
benign neoplasm of ovary (D27.-)
benign neoplasm of testis (D29.2-)
benign neoplasm of thymus (D15.0)

✓5ᵗʰ **D35.0** **Benign neoplasm of** adrenal gland

D35.00 **Benign neoplasm of unspecified adrenal gland** ▽

D35.01 **Benign neoplasm of** right **adrenal gland**

D35.02 **Benign neoplasm of** left **adrenal gland**

D35.1 **Benign neoplasm of** parathyroid gland

D35.2 **Benign neoplasm of** pituitary gland
AHA: 2014, 3Q, 22

D35.3 **Benign neoplasm of** craniopharyngeal duct

D35.4 **Benign neoplasm of** pineal gland

D35.5 **Benign neoplasm of** carotid body

D35.6 **Benign neoplasm of** aortic body and other paraganglia
Benign tumor of glomus jugulare

D35.7 **Benign neoplasm of other specified endocrine glands**

D35.9 **Benign neoplasm of endocrine gland, unspecified** ▽
Benign neoplasm of unspecified endocrine gland

✓4ᵗʰ **D36** **Benign neoplasm of** other and unspecified sites

D36.0 **Benign neoplasm of** lymph nodes
EXCLUDES 1 *lymphangioma (D18.1)*

✓5ᵗʰ **D36.1** **Benign neoplasm of** peripheral nerves and autonomic nervous system
EXCLUDES 1   *benign neoplasm of peripheral nerves of orbit (D31.6-)*
neurofibromatosis (Q85.0-)

D36.10 **Benign neoplasm of peripheral nerves and** ▽
autonomic nervous system, unspecified

D36.11 **Benign neoplasm of peripheral nerves and**
autonomic nervous system of face, head, and neck

D36.12 **Benign neoplasm of peripheral nerves and**
autonomic nervous system, upper limb, including shoulder

D36.13 **Benign neoplasm of peripheral nerves and**
autonomic nervous system of lower limb, including hip

D36.14 **Benign neoplasm of peripheral nerves and**
autonomic nervous system of thorax

D36.15 **Benign neoplasm of peripheral nerves and**
autonomic nervous system of abdomen

D36.16 **Benign neoplasm of peripheral nerves and**
autonomic nervous system of pelvis

D36.17 **Benign neoplasm of peripheral nerves and** ▽
autonomic nervous system of trunk, **unspecified**

D36.7 **Benign neoplasm of other specified sites**
Benign neoplasm of nose NOS

D36.9 **Benign neoplasm, unspecified site** ▽

Benign neuroendocrine tumors (D3A)

✓4ᵗʰ **D3A** **Benign neuroendocrine tumors**

Use additional code to identify any associated endocrine syndrome, such as:
carcinoid syndrome (E34.0)
Code also any associated multiple endocrine neoplasia [MEN] syndromes (E31.2-)
EXCLUDES 2 *benign pancreatic islet cell tumors (D13.7)*

✓5ᵗʰ **D3A.0** **Benign** carcinoid tumors

D3A.00 **Benign carcinoid tumor of unspecified site** ▽
Carcinoid tumor NOS

✓6ᵗʰ **D3A.01** **Benign carcinoid tumors of the** small intestine

D3A.010 **Benign carcinoid tumor of the** duodenum

D3A.011 **Benign carcinoid tumor of the** jejunum

D3A.012 **Benign carcinoid tumor of the** ileum

D3A.019 **Benign carcinoid tumor of the small** ▽
intestine, unspecified portion

✓6ᵗʰ **D3A.02** **Benign carcinoid tumors of the** appendix, large intestine, and rectum

D3A.020 **Benign carcinoid tumor of the** appendix

D3A.021 **Benign carcinoid tumor of the** cecum

D3A.022 **Benign carcinoid tumor of the** ascending colon

D3A.023 **Benign carcinoid tumor of the** transverse colon

D3A.024 **Benign carcinoid tumor of the** descending colon

D3A.025 **Benign carcinoid tumor of the** sigmoid colon

D3A.026 **Benign carcinoid tumor of the** rectum

D3A.029 **Benign carcinoid tumor of the large** ▽
intestine, unspecified portion
Benign carcinoid tumor of the colon NOS

✓6ᵗʰ **D3A.09** **Benign carcinoid tumors of** other sites

D3A.090 **Benign carcinoid tumor of the** bronchus and lung

D3A.091 **Benign carcinoid tumor of the** thymus

D3A.092 **Benign carcinoid tumor of the** stomach

D3A.093 **Benign carcinoid tumor of the** kidney

D3A.094 **Benign carcinoid tumor of the** foregut ▽
unspecified

D3A.095 **Benign carcinoid tumor of the** midgut ▽
unspecified

D3A.096 **Benign carcinoid tumor of the** hindgut ▽
unspecified

D3A.098 **Benign carcinoid tumors of** other sites

D3A.8 **Other benign neuroendocrine tumors** ▽
Neuroendocrine tumor NOS

Neoplasms of uncertain behavior, polycythemia vera and myelodysplastic syndromes (D37-D48)

NOTE   Categories D37-D44, and D48 classify by site neoplasms of uncertain behavior, i.e., histologic confirmation whether the neoplasm is malignant or benign cannot be made.

EXCLUDES 1 *neoplasms of unspecified behavior (D49.-)*

✓4ᵗʰ **D37** **Neoplasm of uncertain behavior of** oral cavity and digestive organs
EXCLUDES 1 *stromal tumors of uncertain behavior of digestive system (D48.1)*

✓5ᵗʰ **D37.0** **Neoplasm of uncertain behavior of** lip, oral cavity and pharynx
EXCLUDES 1   *neoplasm of uncertain behavior of aryepiglottic fold or interarytenoid fold, laryngeal aspect (D38.0)*
neoplasm of uncertain behavior of epiglottis NOS (D38.0)
neoplasm of uncertain behavior of skin of lip (D48.5)
neoplasm of uncertain behavior of suprahyoid portion of epiglottis (D38.0)

D37.01 **Neoplasm of uncertain behavior of** lip
Neoplasm of uncertain behavior of vermilion border of lip

D37.02 **Neoplasm of uncertain behavior of** tongue

✓6ᵗʰ **D37.03** **Neoplasm of uncertain behavior of the** major salivary glands

D37.030 **Neoplasm of uncertain behavior of the** parotid **salivary glands**

D37.031 **Neoplasm of uncertain behavior of the** sublingual **salivary glands**

D37.032 **Neoplasm of uncertain behavior of the** submandibular **salivary glands**

D37.039 **Neoplasm of uncertain behavior of** ▽
the major salivary glands, unspecified

D37.04 **Neoplasm of uncertain behavior of the** minor salivary glands
Neoplasm of uncertain behavior of submucosal salivary glands of lip
Neoplasm of uncertain behavior of submucosal salivary glands of cheek
Neoplasm of uncertain behavior of submucosal salivary glands of hard palate
Neoplasm of uncertain behavior of submucosal salivary glands of soft palate

D37.05 **Neoplasm of uncertain behavior of** pharynx
Neoplasm of uncertain behavior of aryepiglottic fold of pharynx NOS
Neoplasm of uncertain behavior of hypopharyngeal aspect of aryepiglottic fold of pharynx
Neoplasm of uncertain behavior of marginal zone of aryepiglottic fold of pharynx

D37.09 **Neoplasm of uncertain behavior of other specified sites of the oral cavity**

D37.1 **Neoplasm of uncertain behavior of** stomach

D37.2 **Neoplasm of uncertain behavior of** small intestine

D37.3 **Neoplasm of uncertain behavior of** appendix

☑ Additional Character Req   ✓x7ᵗʰ Placeholder Alert   Case-Mix Diagnosis   Manifestation   ▽ Unspecified Dx   **EXCLUDES 1** Not coded here   **EXCLUDES 2** Not included here

ICD-10-CM 2018   **489**

Chapter 2. Neoplasms

D37.4–D44.2

D37.4   **Neoplasm of uncertain behavior of** colon

D37.5   **Neoplasm of uncertain behavior of** rectum
Neoplasm of uncertain behavior of rectosigmoid junction

D37.6   **Neoplasm of uncertain behavior of** liver, gallbladder and bile ducts
Neoplasm of uncertain behavior of ampulla of Vater

D37.8   **Neoplasm of uncertain behavior of other specified digestive organs**
Neoplasm of uncertain behavior of anal canal
Neoplasm of uncertain behavior of anal sphincter
Neoplasm of uncertain behavior of anus NOS
Neoplasm of uncertain behavior of esophagus
Neoplasm of uncertain behavior of intestine NOS
Neoplasm of uncertain behavior of pancreas
> **EXCLUDES 1**   neoplasm of uncertain behavior of anal margin (D48.5)
> neoplasm of uncertain behavior of anal skin (D48.5)
> neoplasm of uncertain behavior of perianal skin (D48.5)

D37.9   **Neoplasm of uncertain behavior of digestive organ, unspecified** ▽

✓4ᵗʰ D38   **Neoplasm of uncertain behavior of** middle ear and respiratory and intrathoracic organs
> **EXCLUDES 1**   neoplasm of uncertain behavior of heart (D48.7)

D38.0   **Neoplasm of uncertain behavior of** larynx
Neoplasm of uncertain behavior of aryepiglottic fold or interarytenoid fold, laryngeal aspect
Neoplasm of uncertain behavior of epiglottis (suprahyoid portion)
> **EXCLUDES 1**   neoplasm of uncertain behavior of aryepiglottic fold or interarytenoid fold NOS (D37.05)
> neoplasm of uncertain behavior of hypopharyngeal aspect of aryepiglottic fold (D37.05)
> neoplasm of uncertain behavior of marginal zone of aryepiglottic fold (D37.05)

D38.1   **Neoplasm of uncertain behavior of** trachea, bronchus and lung

D38.2   **Neoplasm of uncertain behavior of** pleura

D38.3   **Neoplasm of uncertain behavior of** mediastinum

D38.4   **Neoplasm of uncertain behavior of** thymus

D38.5   **Neoplasm of uncertain behavior of other respiratory organs**
Neoplasm of uncertain behavior of accessory sinuses
Neoplasm of uncertain behavior of cartilage of nose
Neoplasm of uncertain behavior of middle ear
Neoplasm of uncertain behavior of nasal cavities
> **EXCLUDES 1**   neoplasm of uncertain behavior of ear (external) (skin) (D48.5)
> neoplasm of uncertain behavior of nose NOS (D48.7)
> neoplasm of uncertain behavior of skin of nose (D48.5)

D38.6   **Neoplasm of uncertain behavior of respiratory organ, unspecified** ▽

✓4ᵗʰ D39   **Neoplasm of uncertain behavior of** female genital organs

D39.0   **Neoplasm of uncertain behavior of** uterus   ♀

✓5ᵗʰ D39.1   **Neoplasm of uncertain behavior of** ovary
Use additional code to identify any functional activity

D39.10   **Neoplasm of uncertain behavior of unspecified ovary**   ♀▽

D39.11   **Neoplasm of uncertain behavior of** right ovary   ♀

D39.12   **Neoplasm of uncertain behavior of** left ovary   ♀

D39.2   **Neoplasm of uncertain behavior of** placenta   Ⓜ♀
Chorioadenoma destruens
Invasive hydatidiform mole
Malignant hydatidiform mole
> **EXCLUDES 1**   hydatidiform mole NOS (O01.9)

D39.8   **Neoplasm of uncertain behavior of other specified female genital organs**   ♀
Neoplasm of uncertain behavior of skin of female genital organs

D39.9   **Neoplasm of uncertain behavior of female genital organ, unspecified**   ♀▽

✓4ᵗʰ D40   **Neoplasm of uncertain behavior of** male genital organs

D40.0   **Neoplasm of uncertain behavior of** prostate   ♂

✓5ᵗʰ D40.1   **Neoplasm of uncertain behavior of** testis

D40.10   **Neoplasm of uncertain behavior of unspecified testis**   ♂▽

D40.11   **Neoplasm of uncertain behavior of** right testis   ♂

D40.12   **Neoplasm of uncertain behavior of** left testis   ♂

D40.8   **Neoplasm of uncertain behavior of other specified male genital organs**   ♂
Neoplasm of uncertain behavior of skin of male genital organs

D40.9   **Neoplasm of uncertain behavior of male genital organ, unspecified**   ♂▽

✓4ᵗʰ D41   **Neoplasm of uncertain behavior of** urinary organs

✓5ᵗʰ D41.0   **Neoplasm of uncertain behavior of** kidney
> **EXCLUDES 1**   neoplasm of uncertain behavior of renal pelvis (D41.1-)

D41.00   **Neoplasm of uncertain behavior of unspecified kidney** ▽

D41.01   **Neoplasm of uncertain behavior of** right kidney

D41.02   **Neoplasm of uncertain behavior of** left kidney

✓5ᵗʰ D41.1   **Neoplasm of uncertain behavior of** renal pelvis

D41.10   **Neoplasm of uncertain behavior of unspecified renal pelvis** ▽

D41.11   **Neoplasm of uncertain behavior of** right renal pelvis

D41.12   **Neoplasm of uncertain behavior of** left renal pelvis

✓5ᵗʰ D41.2   **Neoplasm of uncertain behavior of** ureter

D41.20   **Neoplasm of uncertain behavior of unspecified ureter** ▽

D41.21   **Neoplasm of uncertain behavior of** right ureter

D41.22   **Neoplasm of uncertain behavior of** left ureter

D41.3   **Neoplasm of uncertain behavior of** urethra

D41.4   **Neoplasm of uncertain behavior of** bladder

D41.8   **Neoplasm of uncertain behavior of other specified urinary organs**

D41.9   **Neoplasm of uncertain behavior of unspecified urinary organ** ▽

✓4ᵗʰ D42   **Neoplasm of uncertain behavior of** meninges

D42.0   **Neoplasm of uncertain behavior of** cerebral meninges

D42.1   **Neoplasm of uncertain behavior of** spinal meninges

D42.9   **Neoplasm of uncertain behavior of** meninges, unspecified ▽

✓4ᵗʰ D43   **Neoplasm of uncertain behavior of** brain and central nervous system
> **EXCLUDES 1**   neoplasm of uncertain behavior of peripheral nerves and autonomic nervous system (D48.2)

D43.0   **Neoplasm of uncertain behavior of** brain, supratentorial
Neoplasm of uncertain behavior of cerebral ventricle
Neoplasm of uncertain behavior of cerebrum
Neoplasm of uncertain behavior of frontal lobe
Neoplasm of uncertain behavior of occipital lobe
Neoplasm of uncertain behavior of parietal lobe
Neoplasm of uncertain behavior of temporal lobe
> **EXCLUDES 1**   neoplasm of uncertain behavior of fourth ventricle (D43.1)

D43.1   **Neoplasm of uncertain behavior of** brain, infratentorial
Neoplasm of uncertain behavior of brain stem
Neoplasm of uncertain behavior of cerebellum
Neoplasm of uncertain behavior of fourth ventricle

D43.2   **Neoplasm of uncertain behavior of** brain, unspecified ▽

D43.3   **Neoplasm of uncertain behavior of** cranial nerves

D43.4   **Neoplasm of uncertain behavior of** spinal cord

D43.8   **Neoplasm of uncertain behavior of other** specified parts of central nervous system

D43.9   **Neoplasm of uncertain behavior of central nervous system, unspecified** ▽
Neoplasm of uncertain behavior of nervous system (central) NOS

✓4ᵗʰ D44   **Neoplasm of uncertain behavior of** endocrine glands
> **EXCLUDES 1**   multiple endocrine adenomatosis (E31.2-)
> multiple endocrine neoplasia (E31.2-)
> neoplasm of uncertain behavior of endocrine pancreas (D37.8)
> neoplasm of uncertain behavior of ovary (D39.1-)
> neoplasm of uncertain behavior of testis (D40.1-)
> neoplasm of uncertain behavior of thymus (D38.4)

D44.0   **Neoplasm of uncertain behavior of** thyroid gland

✓5ᵗʰ D44.1   **Neoplasm of uncertain behavior of** adrenal gland
Use additional code to identify any functional activity

D44.10   **Neoplasm of uncertain behavior of unspecified adrenal gland** ▽

D44.11   **Neoplasm of uncertain behavior of** right adrenal gland

D44.12   **Neoplasm of uncertain behavior of** left adrenal gland

D44.2   **Neoplasm of uncertain behavior of** parathyroid gland

---

Ⓝ Newborn: 0   Ⓟ Pediatric: 0-17   Ⓜ Maternity: 12-55   Ⓐ Adult: 15-124   **NRS** Nonroutine supply Dx   **NC Dx** Noncancer Dx   **PDx** Primary Dx   ►◄ Revised Text   ● New Code   ▲ Revised Title

490   ICD-10-CM 2018

Chapter 2. Neoplasms

D44.3   **Neoplasm of uncertain behavior of** pituitary gland
Use additional code to identify any functional activity

D44.4   **Neoplasm of uncertain behavior of** craniopharyngeal duct

D44.5   **Neoplasm of uncertain behavior of** pineal gland

D44.6   **Neoplasm of uncertain behavior of** carotid body

D44.7   **Neoplasm of uncertain behavior of** aortic body and other paraganglia

D44.9   **Neoplasm of uncertain behavior of unspecified** ▽
endocrine gland

D45   **Polycythemia vera**
> EXCLUDES 1   *familial polycythemia (D75.0)*
> *secondary polycythemia (D75.1)*
DEF: Abnormal proliferation of all bone marrow elements, increased red cell mass, and total blood volume; unknown etiology, frequently associated with splenomegaly, leukocytosis, and thrombocythemia.

✓4ᵗʰ **D46**   **Myelodysplastic syndromes**
Use additional code for adverse effect, if applicable, to identify drug (T36-T50 with fifth or sixth character 5)
> EXCLUDES 2   *drug-induced aplastic anemia (D61.1)*

D46.0   **Refractory anemia** without ring sideroblasts, **so stated**
Refractory anemia without sideroblasts, without excess of blasts

D46.1   **Refractory anemia** with ring sideroblasts
RARS

✓5ᵗʰ **D46.2**   **Refractory anemia** with excess of blasts [RAEB]

     D46.20   **Refractory anemia with excess of blasts,** ▽
unspecified
RAEB NOS

     D46.21   **Refractory anemia with excess of** blasts 1
RAEB 1

     D46.22   **Refractory anemia with excess of** blasts 2
RAEB 2

D46.A   **Refractory** cytopenia with multilineage dysplasia

D46.B   **Refractory** cytopenia with multilineage dysplasia and ring sideroblasts
RCMD RS

D46.C   **Myelodysplastic syndrome** with isolated del(5q) chromosomal abnormality
Myelodysplastic syndrome with 5q deletion
5q minus syndrome NOS

D46.4   **Refractory anemia, unspecified** ▽

D46.Z   **Other myelodysplastic syndromes**
> EXCLUDES 1   *chronic myelomonocytic leukemia (C93.1-)*

D46.9   **Myelodysplastic syndrome, unspecified** ▽
Myelodysplasia NOS

✓4ᵗʰ **D47**   **Other neoplasms of uncertain behavior of** lymphoid, hematopoietic and related tissue

▲ ✓5ᵗʰ **D47.0**   **Mast cell neoplasms of uncertain behavior**
~~Indolent systemic mastocytosis~~
~~Mast cell tumor NOS~~
~~Mastocytoma NOS~~
> EXCLUDES 1   ▶*congenital cutaneous mastocytosis (Q82.2-)*
> *histiocytic neoplasms of uncertain behavior (D47.Z9)*
> *malignant mast cell neoplasm (C96.2-)*◀
> *mastocytosis (congenital) (cutaneous) (Q82.2)*

     D47.01   **Cutaneous** mastocytosis
Diffuse cutaneous mastocytosis
Maculopapular cutaneous mastocytosis
Solitary mastocytoma
Telangiectasia macularis eruptiva perstans
Urticaria pigmentosa
> EXCLUDES 1   *congenital (diffuse) (maculopapular)*
> *cutaneous mastocytosis (Q82.2)*
> *congenital urticaria pigmentosa (Q82.2)*
> *extracutaneous mastocytoma (D47.09)*

     D47.02   **Systemic** mastocytosis
Indolent systemic mastocytosis
Isolated bone marrow mastocytosis
Smoldering systemic mastocytosis
Systemic mastocytosis, with an associated hematological non-mast cell lineage disease (SM-AHNMD)
Code also, if applicable, any associated hematological non-mast cell lineage disease, such as:
acute myeloid leukemia (C92.6-, C92.A-)
chronic myelomonocytic leukemia (C93.1-)
essential thrombocytosis (D47.3)
hypereosinophilic syndrome (D72.1)
myelodysplastic syndrome (D46.9)
myeloproliferative syndrome (D47.1)
non-Hodgkin lymphoma (C82-C85)
plasma cell myeloma (C90.0-)
polycythemia vera (D45)
> EXCLUDES 1   *aggressive systemic mastocytosis (C96.21)*
> *mast cell leukemia (C94.3-)*

     D47.09   **Other mast cell neoplasms of uncertain behavior**
Extracutaneous mastocytoma
Mast cell tumor NOS
Mastocytoma NOS
Mastocytosis NOS

D47.1   **Chronic myeloproliferative disease**
Chronic neutrophilic leukemia
Myeloproliferative disease, unspecified
> EXCLUDES 1   *atypical chronic myeloid leukemia BCR/ABL-negative (C92.2-)*
> *chronic myeloid leukemia BCR/ABL-positive (C92.1-)*
> *myelofibrosis NOS (D75.81)*
> *myelophthisic anemia (D61.82)*
> *myelophthisis (D61.82)*
> *secondary myelofibrosis NOS (D75.81)*

D47.2   **Monoclonal gammopathy**
Monoclonal gammopathy of undetermined significance [MGUS]

D47.3   **Essential (hemorrhagic) thrombocythemia**
Essential thrombocytosis
Idiopathic hemorrhagic thrombocythemia

D47.4   **Osteomyelofibrosis**
Chronic idiopathic myelofibrosis
Myelofibrosis (idiopathic) (with myeloid metaplasia)
Myelosclerosis (megakaryocytic) with myeloid metaplasia
Secondary myelofibrosis in myeloproliferative disease
> EXCLUDES 1   *acute myelofibrosis (C94.4-)*

✓5ᵗʰ **D47.Z**   **Other** specified neoplasms of uncertain behavior of lymphoid, hematopoietic and related tissue

     D47.Z1   **Post-transplant lymphoproliferative disorder (PTLD)**
Code first complications of transplanted organs and tissue (T86.-)
DEF: Excessive proliferation of B-cell lymphocytes following Epstein-Barr virus infection in organ transplant patients; may progress to non-Hodgkin lymphoma.

     D47.Z2   **Castleman disease**
Code also if applicable human herpesvirus 8 infection (B10.89)
> EXCLUDES 2   *Kaposi's sarcoma (C46-)*

     D47.Z9   **Other specified neoplasms of uncertain behavior of lymphoid, hematopoietic and related tissue**
Histiocytic tumors of uncertain behavior

D47.9   **Neoplasm of uncertain behavior of lymphoid,** ▽
hematopoietic and related tissue, unspecified
Lymphoproliferative disease NOS

✓4ᵗʰ **D48**   **Neoplasm of uncertain behavior of other and unspecified sites**
> EXCLUDES 1   *neurofibromatosis (nonmalignant) (Q85.0-)*

D48.0   **Neoplasm of uncertain behavior of** bone and articular cartilage
> EXCLUDES 1   *neoplasm of uncertain behavior of cartilage of ear (D48.1)*
> *neoplasm of uncertain behavior of cartilage of larynx (D38.0)*
> *neoplasm of uncertain behavior of cartilage of nose (D38.5)*
> *neoplasm of uncertain behavior of connective tissue of eyelid (D48.1)*
> *neoplasm of uncertain behavior of synovia (D48.1)*

D48.1 **Neoplasm of uncertain behavior of** connective and other soft tissue
     Neoplasm of uncertain behavior of connective tissue of ear
     Neoplasm of uncertain behavior of connective tissue of eyelid
     Stromal tumors of uncertain behavior of digestive system
     EXCLUDES 1   *neoplasm of uncertain behavior of articular cartilage (D48.0)*
        neoplasm of uncertain behavior of cartilage of larynx (D38.0)
        neoplasm of uncertain behavior of cartilage of nose (D38.5)
        neoplasm of uncertain behavior of connective tissue of breast (D48.6-)

D48.2 **Neoplasm of uncertain behavior of** peripheral nerves and autonomic nervous system
     EXCLUDES 1   *neoplasm of uncertain behavior of peripheral nerves of orbit (D48.7)*

D48.3 **Neoplasm of uncertain behavior of** retroperitoneum

D48.4 **Neoplasm of uncertain behavior of** peritoneum

D48.5 **Neoplasm of uncertain behavior of** skin
     Neoplasm of uncertain behavior of anal margin
     Neoplasm of uncertain behavior of anal skin
     Neoplasm of uncertain behavior of perianal skin
     Neoplasm of uncertain behavior of skin of breast
     EXCLUDES 1   *neoplasm of uncertain behavior of anus NOS (D37.8)*
        neoplasm of uncertain behavior of skin of genital organs (D39.8, D40.8)
        neoplasm of uncertain behavior of vermilion border of lip (D37.0)

√5ᵗʰ **D48.6** **Neoplasm of uncertain behavior of** breast
     Neoplasm of uncertain behavior of connective tissue of breast
     Cystosarcoma phyllodes
     EXCLUDES 1   *neoplasm of uncertain behavior of skin of breast (D48.5)*

     D48.60 **Neoplasm of uncertain behavior of unspecified breast** ▽

     D48.61 **Neoplasm of uncertain behavior of** right **breast**

     D48.62 **Neoplasm of uncertain behavior of** left **breast**

D48.7 **Neoplasm of uncertain behavior of other specified sites**
     Neoplasm of uncertain behavior of eye
     Neoplasm of uncertain behavior of heart
     Neoplasm of uncertain behavior of peripheral nerves of orbit
     EXCLUDES 1   *neoplasm of uncertain behavior of connective tissue (D48.1)*
        neoplasm of uncertain behavior of skin of eyelid (D48.5)

D48.9 **Neoplasm of uncertain behavior, unspecified** ▽

Neoplasms of unspecified behavior (D49)

√4ᵗʰ **D49** **Neoplasms of unspecified behavior**
     NOTE   Category D49 classifies by site neoplasms of unspecified morphology and behavior. The term "mass", unless otherwise stated, is not to be regarded as a neoplastic growth.
     INCLUDES   "growth" NOS
        neoplasm NOS
        new growth NOS
        tumor NOS
     EXCLUDES 1   *neoplasms of uncertain behavior (D37-D44, D48)*

D49.0 **Neoplasm of unspecified behavior of** digestive system
     EXCLUDES 1   *neoplasm of unspecified behavior of margin of anus (D49.2)*
        neoplasm of unspecified behavior of perianal skin (D49.2)
        neoplasm of unspecified behavior of skin of anus (D49.2)

D49.1 **Neoplasm of unspecified behavior of** respiratory system

D49.2 **Neoplasm of unspecified behavior of** bone, soft tissue, and skin
     EXCLUDES 1   *neoplasm of unspecified behavior of anal canal (D49.0)*
        neoplasm of unspecified behavior of anus NOS (D49.0)
        neoplasm of unspecified behavior of bone marrow (D49.89)
        neoplasm of unspecified behavior of cartilage of larynx (D49.1)
        neoplasm of unspecified behavior of cartilage of nose (D49.1)
        neoplasm of unspecified behavior of connective tissue of breast (D49.3)
        neoplasm of unspecified behavior of skin of genital organs (D49.59)
        neoplasm of unspecified behavior of vermilion border of lip (D49.0)

D49.3 **Neoplasm of unspecified behavior of** breast
     EXCLUDES 1   *neoplasm of unspecified behavior of skin of breast (D49.2)*

D49.4 **Neoplasm of unspecified behavior of** bladder

√5ᵗʰ **D49.5** **Neoplasm of unspecified behavior of** other genitourinary organs

     √6ᵗʰ **D49.51** **Neoplasm of unspecified behavior of** kidney

        D49.511 **Neoplasm of unspecified behavior of** right **kidney**

        D49.512 **Neoplasm of unspecified behavior of** left **kidney**

        D49.519 **Neoplasm of unspecified behavior of** unspecified **kidney** ▽

     D49.59 **Neoplasm of unspecified behavior of other genitourinary organ**

D49.6 **Neoplasm of unspecified behavior of** brain
     EXCLUDES 1   *neoplasm of unspecified behavior of cerebral meninges (D49.7)*
        neoplasm of unspecified behavior of cranial nerves (D49.7)

D49.7 **Neoplasm of unspecified behavior of** endocrine glands and other parts of nervous system
     EXCLUDES 1   *neoplasm of unspecified behavior of peripheral, sympathetic, and parasympathetic nerves and ganglia (D49.2)*

√5ᵗʰ **D49.8** **Neoplasm of unspecified behavior of** other specified sites
     EXCLUDES 1   *neoplasm of unspecified behavior of eyelid (skin) (D49.2)*
        neoplasm of unspecified behavior of eyelid cartilage (D49.2)
        neoplasm of unspecified behavior of great vessels (D49.2)
        neoplasm of unspecified behavior of optic nerve (D49.7)

     D49.81 **Neoplasm of unspecified behavior of** retina and choroid
        Dark area on retina
        Retinal freckle

     D49.89 **Neoplasm of unspecified behavior of other specified sites**

D49.9 **Neoplasm of unspecified behavior of unspecified site** ▽

Chapter 3. Diseases of the Blood and Blood-forming Organs and Certain Disorders Involving the Immune Mechanism (D5Ø–D89)

Chapter Specific Coding Guidelines and Examples
Reserved for future guideline expansion

Chapter 3. Diseases of the Blood and Blood-forming Organs *(left margin, vertical)*

Chapter 3. Diseases of the Blood and Blood-forming Organs and Certain Disorders Involving the Immune Mechanism (D5Ø-D89)

EXCLUDES 2   *autoimmune disease (systemic) NOS (M35.9)*
certain conditions originating in the perinatal period (PØØ-P96)
complications of pregnancy, childbirth and the puerperium (OØØ-O9A)
congenital malformations, deformations and chromosomal abnormalities (QØØ-Q99)
endocrine, nutritional and metabolic diseases (EØØ-E88)
human immunodeficiency virus [HIV] disease (B2Ø)
injury, poisoning and certain other consequences of external causes (SØØ-T88)
neoplasms (CØØ-D49)
symptoms, signs and abnormal clinical and laboratory findings, not elsewhere classified (RØØ-R94)

This chapter contains the following blocks:

D5Ø-D53   Nutritional anemias
D55-D59   Hemolytic anemias
D6Ø-D64   Aplastic and other anemias and other bone marrow failure syndromes
D65-D69   Coagulation defects, purpura and other hemorrhagic conditions
D7Ø-D77   Other disorders of blood and blood-forming organs
D78   Intraoperative and postprocedural complications of the spleen
D8Ø-D89   Certain disorders involving the immune mechanism

Nutritional anemias (D5Ø-D53)

✓4ᵗʰ D5Ø   Iron deficiency anemia
   INCLUDES   asiderotic anemia
       hypochromic anemia

   D5Ø.Ø   Iron deficiency anemia secondary to blood loss (chronic)
     Posthemorrhagic anemia (chronic)
     EXCLUDES 1   *acute posthemorrhagic anemia (D62)*
         congenital anemia from fetal blood loss (P61.3)

   D5Ø.1   Sideropenic dysphagia
     Kelly-Paterson syndrome
     Plummer-Vinson syndrome

   D5Ø.8   Other iron deficiency anemias
     Iron deficiency anemia due to inadequate dietary iron intake

   D5Ø.9   Iron deficiency anemia, unspecified   ▽

✓4ᵗʰ D51   Vitamin B12 deficiency anemia
   EXCLUDES 1   *vitamin B12 deficiency (E53.8)*

   D51.Ø   Vitamin B12 deficiency anemia due to intrinsic factor deficiency
     Addison anemia
     Biermer anemia
     Pernicious (congenital) anemia
     Congenital intrinsic factor deficiency
     DEF: Chronic progressive anemia due to vitamin B12 malabsorption; caused by lack of secretion of intrinsic factor, which is produced by the gastric mucosa of the stomach.

   D51.1   Vitamin B12 deficiency anemia due to selective vitamin B12 malabsorption with proteinuria
     Imerslund (Gräsbeck) syndrome
     Megaloblastic hereditary anemia

   D51.2   Transcobalamin II deficiency

   D51.3   Other dietary vitamin B12 deficiency anemia
     Vegan anemia

   D51.8   Other vitamin B12 deficiency anemias

   D51.9   Vitamin B12 deficiency anemia, unspecified   ▽

✓4ᵗʰ D52   Folate deficiency anemia
   EXCLUDES 1   *folate deficiency without anemia (E53.8)*

   D52.Ø   Dietary folate deficiency anemia
     Nutritional megaloblastic anemia
     DEF: The result of a poor diet with inadequate intake of folate, which is needed to produce healthy red blood cells.

   D52.1   Drug-induced folate deficiency anemia
     Use additional code for adverse effect, if applicable, to identify drug (T36-T5Ø with fifth or sixth character 5)

   D52.8   Other folate deficiency anemias

   D52.9   Folate deficiency anemia, unspecified   ▽
     Folic acid deficiency anemia NOS

✓4ᵗʰ D53   Other nutritional anemias
   INCLUDES   megaloblastic anemia unresponsive to vitamin B12 or folate therapy

   D53.Ø   Protein deficiency anemia
     Amino-acid deficiency anemia
     Orotaciduric anemia
     EXCLUDES 1   *Lesch-Nyhan syndrome (E79.1)*

   D53.1   Other megaloblastic anemias, not elsewhere classified
     Megaloblastic anemia NOS
     EXCLUDES 1   *Di Guglielmo's disease (C94.Ø)*

   D53.2   Scorbutic anemia
     EXCLUDES 1   *scurvy (E54)*

   D53.8   Other specified nutritional anemias
     Anemia associated with deficiency of copper
     Anemia associated with deficiency of molybdenum
     Anemia associated with deficiency of zinc
     EXCLUDES 1   *nutritional deficiencies without anemia, such as:*
         copper deficiency NOS (E61.Ø)
         molybdenum deficiency NOS (E61.5)
         zinc deficiency NOS (E6Ø)

   D53.9   Nutritional anemia, unspecified   ▽
     Simple chronic anemia
     EXCLUDES 1   *anemia NOS (D64.9)*

Hemolytic anemias (D55-D59)

✓4ᵗʰ D55   Anemia due to enzyme disorders
   EXCLUDES 1   *drug-induced enzyme deficiency anemia (D59.2)*

   D55.Ø   Anemia due to glucose-6-phosphate dehydrogenase [G6PD] deficiency
     Favism
     G6PD deficiency anemia

   D55.1   Anemia due to other disorders of glutathione metabolism
     Anemia (due to) enzyme deficiencies, except G6PD, related to the hexose monophosphate [HMP] shunt pathway
     Anemia (due to) hemolytic nonspherocytic (hereditary), type I

   D55.2   Anemia due to disorders of glycolytic enzymes
     Hemolytic nonspherocytic (hereditary) anemia, type II
     Hexokinase deficiency anemia
     Pyruvate kinase [PK] deficiency anemia
     Triose-phosphate isomerase deficiency anemia
     EXCLUDES 1   *disorders of glycolysis not associated with anemia (E74.8)*

   D55.3   Anemia due to disorders of nucleotide metabolism

   D55.8   Other anemias due to enzyme disorders

   D55.9   Anemia due to enzyme disorder, unspecified   ▽

✓4ᵗʰ D56   Thalassemia
   EXCLUDES 1   *sickle-cell thalassemia (D57.4-)*

   D56.Ø   Alpha thalassemia
     Alpha thalassemia major
     Hemoglobin H Constant Spring
     Hemoglobin H disease
     Hydrops fetalis due to alpha thalassemia
     Severe alpha thalassemia
     Triple gene defect alpha thalassemia
     Use additional code, if applicable, for hydrops fetalis due to alpha thalassemia (P56.99)
     EXCLUDES 1   *alpha thalassemia trait or minor (D56.3)*
         asymptomatic alpha thalassemia (D56.3)
         hydrops fetalis due to isoimmunization (P56.Ø)
         hydrops fetalis not due to immune hemolysis (P83.2)
     DEF: HBA1 and HBA2 genetic variant of chromosome 16 prevalent among those of African and Southeast Asian descent; associated with a wide spectrum of anemic presentation; includes hemoglobin H disease subtypes.

   D56.1   Beta thalassemia
     Beta thalassemia major
     Cooley's anemia
     Homozygous beta thalassemia
     Severe beta thalassemia
     Thalassemia intermedia
     Thalassemia major
     EXCLUDES 1   *beta thalassemia minor (D56.3)*
         beta thalassemia trait (D56.3)
         delta-beta thalassemia (D56.2)
         hemoglobin E-beta thalassemia (D56.5)
         sickle-cell beta thalassemia (D57.4-)

N Newborn: 0   P Pediatric: 0-17   M Maternity: 12-55   A Adult: 15-124   NRS Nonroutine supply Dx   NC Dx Noncancer Dx   PDx Primary Dx   ▶◀ Revised Text   ● New Code   ▲ Revised Title

494   ICD-10-CM 2018

Thalassemia

Misshapen RBC

Misshapen RBC

Healthy RBC

Sickle cell

Sickle cells

Normal RBCs

D56.2　Delta-beta thalassemia
　　　Homozygous delta-beta thalassemia
　　　EXCLUDES 1　delta-beta thalassemia minor (D56.3)
　　　　　　　　delta-beta thalassemia trait (D56.3)

D56.3　Thalassemia minor
　　　Alpha thalassemia minor
　　　Alpha thalassemia silent carrier
　　　Alpha thalassemia trait
　　　Beta thalassemia minor
　　　Beta thalassemia trait
　　　Delta-beta thalassemia minor
　　　Delta-beta thalassemia trait
　　　Thalassemia trait NOS
　　　EXCLUDES 1　alpha thalassemia (D56.0)
　　　　　　　　beta thalassemia (D56.1)
　　　　　　　　delta-beta thalassemia (D56.2)
　　　　　　　　hemoglobin E-beta thalassemia (D56.5)
　　　　　　　　sickle-cell trait (D57.3)
　　　DEF: Solitary abnormal gene that identifies a carrier of the disease, yet with an absence of symptoms or a clinically mild anemic presentation.

D56.4　Hereditary persistence of fetal hemoglobin [HPFH]

D56.5　Hemoglobin E-beta thalassemia
　　　EXCLUDES 1　beta thalassemia (D56.1)
　　　　　　　　beta thalassemia minor (D56.3)
　　　　　　　　beta thalassemia trait (D56.3)
　　　　　　　　delta-beta thalassemia (D56.2)
　　　　　　　　delta-beta thalassemia trait (D56.3)
　　　　　　　　hemoglobin E disease (D58.2)
　　　　　　　　other hemoglobinopathies (D58.2)
　　　　　　　　sickle-cell beta thalassemia (D57.4-)

D56.8　Other thalassemias
　　　Dominant thalassemia
　　　Hemoglobin C thalassemia
　　　Mixed thalassemia
　　　Thalassemia with other hemoglobinopathy
　　　EXCLUDES 1　hemoglobin C disease (D58.2)
　　　　　　　　hemoglobin E disease (D58.2)
　　　　　　　　other hemoglobinopathies (D58.2)
　　　　　　　　sickle-cell anemia (D57.-)
　　　　　　　　sickle-cell thalassemia (D57.4)

D56.9　Thalassemia, unspecified　　　　▽
　　　Mediterranean anemia (with other hemoglobinopathy)

☑4ᵗʰ D57　Sickle-cell disorders
　　　Use additional code for any associated fever (R50.81)
　　　EXCLUDES 1　other hemoglobinopathies (D58.-)

☑5ᵗʰ D57.0　Hb-SS disease with crisis
　　　Sickle-cell disease NOS with crisis
　　　Hb-SS disease with vasoocclusive pain
　　　　D57.00　Hb-SS disease with crisis, unspecified　　▽
　　　　D57.01　Hb-SS disease with acute chest syndrome
　　　　D57.02　Hb-SS disease with splenic sequestration

D57.1　Sickle-cell disease without crisis　　　▽
　　　Hb-SS disease without crisis
　　　Sickle-cell anemia NOS
　　　Sickle-cell disease NOS
　　　Sickle-cell disorder NOS

☑5ᵗʰ D57.2　Sickle-cell/Hb-C disease
　　　Hb-SC disease
　　　Hb-S/Hb-C disease
　　　　D57.20　Sickle-cell/Hb-C disease without crisis　　▽
　　　☑6ᵗʰ **D57.21　Sickle-cell/Hb-C disease with crisis**
　　　　　　D57.211　Sickle-cell/Hb-C disease with acute chest syndrome
　　　　　　D57.212　Sickle-cell/Hb-C disease with splenic sequestration
　　　　　　D57.219　Sickle-cell/Hb-C disease with crisis, unspecified　　▽
　　　　　　　　Sickle-cell/Hb-C disease with crisis NOS

D57.3　Sickle-cell trait
　　　Hb-S trait
　　　Heterozygous hemoglobin S
　　　DEF: Heterozygous genetic makeup characterized by one gene for normal hemoglobin and one for sickle-cell hemoglobin; clinical disease rarely present.

☑5ᵗʰ D57.4　Sickle-cell thalassemia
　　　Sickle-cell beta thalassemia
　　　Thalassemia Hb-S disease
　　　　D57.40　Sickle-cell thalassemia without crisis　　▽
　　　　　　Microdrepanocytosis
　　　　　　Sickle-cell thalassemia NOS
　　　☑6ᵗʰ **D57.41　Sickle-cell thalassemia with crisis**
　　　　　　Sickle-cell thalassemia with vasoocclusive pain
　　　　　　D57.411　Sickle-cell thalassemia with acute chest syndrome
　　　　　　D57.412　Sickle-cell thalassemia with splenic sequestration
　　　　　　D57.419　Sickle-cell thalassemia with crisis, unspecified　　▽
　　　　　　　　Sickle-cell thalassemia with crisis NOS

☑5ᵗʰ D57.8　Other sickle-cell disorders
　　　Hb-SD disease
　　　Hb-SE disease
　　　　D57.80　Other sickle-cell disorders without crisis　　▽
　　　☑6ᵗʰ **D57.81　Other sickle-cell disorders with crisis**
　　　　　　D57.811　Other sickle-cell disorders with acute chest syndrome
　　　　　　D57.812　Other sickle-cell disorders with splenic sequestration　　▽
　　　　　　D57.819　Other sickle-cell disorders with crisis, unspecified　　▽
　　　　　　　　Other sickle-cell disorders with crisis NOS

☑4ᵗʰ D58　Other hereditary hemolytic anemias
　　　EXCLUDES 1　hemolytic anemia of the newborn (P55.-)

D58.0　Hereditary spherocytosis
　　　Acholuric (familial) jaundice
　　　Congenital (spherocytic) hemolytic icterus
　　　Minkowski-Chauffard syndrome

D58.1　Hereditary elliptocytosis
　　　Elliptocytosis (congenital)
　　　Ovalocytosis (congenital) (hereditary)

Chapter 3. Diseases of the Blood and Blood-forming Organs

D58.2 **Other hemoglobinopathies**
Abnormal hemoglobin NOS
Congenital Heinz body anemia
Hb-C disease
Hb-D disease
Hb-E disease
Hemoglobinopathy NOS
Unstable hemoglobin hemolytic disease
EXCLUDES 1 *familial polycythemia (D75.0)*
Hb-M disease (D74.0)
hemoglobin E-beta thalassemia (D56.5)
hereditary persistence of fetal hemoglobin [HPFH] (D56.4)
high-altitude polycythemia (D75.1)
methemoglobinemia (D74.-)
other hemoglobinopathies with thalassemia (D56.8)

D58.8 **Other specified hereditary hemolytic anemias**
Stomatocytosis

D58.9 **Hereditary hemolytic anemia, unspecified** ▽

✓4th **D59** **Acquired hemolytic anemia**
DEF: Non-hereditary anemia characterized by premature destruction of red blood cells; caused by infectious organisms, poisons, and physical agents.

D59.0 **Drug-induced autoimmune hemolytic anemia**
Use additional code for adverse effect, if applicable, to identify drug (T36-T50 with fifth or sixth character 5)

D59.1 **Other autoimmune hemolytic anemias**
Autoimmune hemolytic disease (cold type) (warm type)
Chronic cold hemagglutinin disease
Cold agglutinin disease
Cold agglutinin hemoglobinuria
Cold type (secondary) (symptomatic) hemolytic anemia
Warm type (secondary) (symptomatic) hemolytic anemia
EXCLUDES 1 *Evans syndrome (D69.41)*
hemolytic disease of newborn (P55.-)
paroxysmal cold hemoglobinuria (D59.6)

D59.2 **Drug-induced nonautoimmune hemolytic anemia**
Drug-induced enzyme deficiency anemia
Use additional code for adverse effect, if applicable, to identify drug (T36-T50 with fifth or sixth character 5)

D59.3 **Hemolytic-uremic syndrome**
Use additional code to identify associated:
E. coli infection (B96.2-)
Pneumococcal pneumonia (J13)
Shigella dysenteriae (A03.9)

D59.4 **Other nonautoimmune hemolytic anemias**
Mechanical hemolytic anemia
Microangiopathic hemolytic anemia
Toxic hemolytic anemia

D59.5 **Paroxysmal nocturnal hemoglobinuria [Marchiafava-Micheli]**
EXCLUDES 1 *hemoglobinuria NOS (R82.3)*

D59.6 **Hemoglobinuria due to hemolysis from other external causes**
Hemoglobinuria from exertion
March hemoglobinuria
Paroxysmal cold hemoglobinuria
Use additional code (Chapter 20) to identify external cause
EXCLUDES 1 *hemoglobinuria NOS (R82.3)*

D59.8 **Other acquired hemolytic anemias**

D59.9 **Acquired hemolytic anemia, unspecified** ▽
Idiopathic hemolytic anemia, chronic

Aplastic and other anemias and other bone marrow failure syndromes (D60-D64)

✓4th **D60** **Acquired pure red cell aplasia [erythroblastopenia]**
INCLUDES red cell aplasia (acquired) (adult) (with thymoma)
EXCLUDES 1 *congenital red cell aplasia (D61.01)*

D60.0 **Chronic acquired pure red cell aplasia**

D60.1 **Transient acquired pure red cell aplasia**

D60.8 **Other acquired pure red cell aplasias**

D60.9 **Acquired pure red cell aplasia, unspecified** ▽

✓4th **D61** **Other aplastic anemias and other bone marrow failure syndromes**
EXCLUDES 1 *neutropenia (D70.-)*
AHA: 2014, 4Q, 22

✓5th **D61.0** **Constitutional aplastic anemia**

D61.01 **Constitutional (pure) red blood cell aplasia**
Blackfan-Diamond syndrome
Congenital (pure) red cell aplasia
Familial hypoplastic anemia
Primary (pure) red cell aplasia
Red cell (pure) aplasia of infants
EXCLUDES 1 *acquired red cell aplasia (D60.9)*

D61.09 **Other constitutional aplastic anemia**
Fanconi's anemia
Pancytopenia with malformations

D61.1 **Drug-induced aplastic anemia**
Use additional code for adverse effect, if applicable, to identify drug (T36-T50 with fifth or sixth character 5)

D61.2 **Aplastic anemia due to other external agents**
Code first, if applicable, toxic effects of substances chiefly nonmedicinal as to source (T51-T65)

D61.3 **Idiopathic aplastic anemia**

✓5th **D61.8** **Other specified aplastic anemias and other bone marrow failure syndromes**

✓6th **D61.81** **Pancytopenia**
EXCLUDES 1 *pancytopenia (due to) (with) aplastic anemia (D61.9)*
pancytopenia (due to) (with) bone marrow infiltration (D61.82)
pancytopenia (due to) (with) congenital (pure) red cell aplasia (D61.01)
pancytopenia (due to) (with) hairy cell leukemia (C91.4-)
pancytopenia (due to) (with) human immunodeficiency virus disease (B20)
pancytopenia (due to) (with) leukoerythroblastic anemia (D61.82)
pancytopenia (due to) (with) myeloproliferative disease (D47.1)
EXCLUDES 2 *pancytopenia (due to) (with) myelodysplastic syndromes (D46.-)*
DEF: Occurs when a person has a shortage of all three blood cells: white, red, and platelets.

D61.810 **Antineoplastic chemotherapy induced pancytopenia**
EXCLUDES 2 *aplastic anemia due to antineoplastic chemotherapy (D61.1)*

D61.811 **Other drug-induced pancytopenia**
EXCLUDES 2 *aplastic anemia due to drugs (D61.1)*

D61.818 **Other pancytopenia**

D61.82 **Myelophthisis**
Leukoerythroblastic anemia
Myelophthisic anemia
Panmyelophthisis
Code also the underlying disorder, such as:
malignant neoplasm of breast (C50.-)
tuberculosis (A15.-)
EXCLUDES 1 *idiopathic myelofibrosis (D47.1)*
myelofibrosis NOS (D75.81)
myelofibrosis with myeloid metaplasia (D47.4)
primary myelofibrosis (D47.1)
secondary myelofibrosis (D75.81)

D61.89 **Other specified aplastic anemias and other bone marrow failure syndromes**

D61.9 **Aplastic anemia, unspecified** ▽
Hypoplastic anemia NOS
Medullary hypoplasia

D62 **Acute posthemorrhagic anemia**
EXCLUDES 1 *anemia due to chronic blood loss (D50.0)*
blood loss anemia NOS (D50.0)
congenital anemia from fetal blood loss (P61.3)

N Newborn: 0   P Pediatric: 0-17   M Maternity: 12-55   A Adult: 15-124   NRS Nonroutine supply Dx   NCDx Noncancer Dx   PDx Primary Dx   ►◄ Revised Text   ● New Code   ▲ Revised Title

496   ICD-10-CM 2018

D58.2–D62

☑️⁴ᵗʰ **D63 Anemia in chronic diseases classified elsewhere**

D63.0 Anemia in neoplastic disease
Code first neoplasm (C00-D49)
EXCLUDES 1 anemia due to antineoplastic chemotherapy (D64.81)
aplastic anemia due to antineoplastic chemotherapy
(D61.1)
EXCLUDES 2 ▶anemia due to antineoplastic chemotherapy
(D64.81)◀

D63.1 Anemia in chronic kidney disease
Erythropoietin resistant anemia (EPO resistant anemia)
Code first underlying chronic kidney disease (CKD) (N18.-)

D63.8 Anemia in other chronic diseases classified elsewhere
Code first underlying disease, such as:
diphyllobothriasis (B70.0)
hookworm disease (B76.0-B76.9)
hypothyroidism (E00.0-E03.9)
malaria (B50.0-B54)
symptomatic late syphilis (A52.79)
tuberculosis (A18.89)

☑️⁴ᵗʰ **D64 Other anemias**
EXCLUDES 1 refractory anemia (D46.-)
refractory anemia with excess blasts in transformation
[RAEB T] (C92.0-)

D64.0 Hereditary sideroblastic anemia
Sex-linked hypochromic sideroblastic anemia

D64.1 Secondary sideroblastic anemia due to disease
Code first underlying disease

D64.2 Secondary sideroblastic anemia due to drugs and toxins
Code first poisoning due to drug or toxin, if applicable (T36-T65
with fifth or sixth character 1-4 or 6)
Use additional code for adverse effect, if applicable, to identify
drug (T36-T50 with fifth or sixth character 5)

D64.3 Other sideroblastic anemias
Sideroblastic anemia NOS
Pyridoxine-responsive sideroblastic anemia NEC

D64.4 Congenital dyserythropoietic anemia
Dyshematopoietic anemia (congenital)
EXCLUDES 1 Blackfan-Diamond syndrome (D61.01)
Di Guglielmo's disease (C94.0)

☑️⁵ᵗʰ **D64.8 Other specified anemias**

D64.81 Anemia due to antineoplastic chemotherapy
Antineoplastic chemotherapy induced anemia
EXCLUDES 1 aplastic anemia due to antineoplastic
chemotherapy (D61.1)
EXCLUDES 2 anemia in neoplastic disease (D63.0)
AHA: 2014, 4Q, 22
DEF: Reversible adverse effect of chemotherapy,
causing inhibition of bone marrow production; decrease
in red blood cell production prevents adequate
oxygenation of the tissues and organs causing fatigue,
SOB, and exacerbation of other medical conditions.

D64.89 Other specified anemias
Infantile pseudoleukemia

D64.9 Anemia, unspecified   ▽
AHA: 2017, 1Q, 7

Coagulation defects, purpura and other hemorrhagic conditions (D65-D69)

D65 Disseminated intravascular coagulation [defibrination syndrome]
Afibrinogenemia, acquired
Consumption coagulopathy
Diffuse or disseminated intravascular coagulation [DIC]
Fibrinolytic hemorrhage, acquired
Fibrinolytic purpura
Purpura fulminans
EXCLUDES 1 disseminated intravascular coagulation (complicating):
abortion or ectopic or molar pregnancy (O00-O07, O08.1)
in newborn (P60)
pregnancy, childbirth and the puerperium (O45.0, O46.0,
O67.0, O72.3)

D66 Hereditary factor VIII deficiency
Classical hemophilia   Deficiency factor VIII (with functional defect)
Hemophilia A   Hemophilia NOS
EXCLUDES 1 factor VIII deficiency with vascular defect (D68.0)
DEF: Hereditary, sex-linked lack of antihemophilic globulin (AHG) (factor
VIII); causes abnormal coagulation characterized by increased bleeding,
large bruises of skin, bleeding in mouth, nose, gastrointestinal tract;
hemorrhages into joints, resulting in swelling and impaired function.

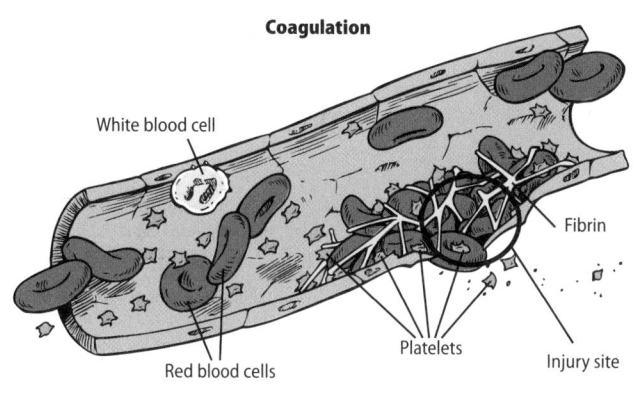

Coagulation

White blood cell
Fibrin
Platelets
Injury site
Red blood cells

D67 Hereditary factor IX deficiency
Christmas disease
Factor IX deficiency (with functional defect)
Hemophilia B
Plasma thromboplastin component [PTC] deficiency

☑️⁴ᵗʰ **D68 Other coagulation defects**
EXCLUDES 1 abnormal coagulation profile (R79.1)
coagulation defects complicating abortion or ectopic or molar
pregnancy (O00-O07, O08.1)
coagulation defects complicating pregnancy, childbirth and the
puerperium (O45.0, O46.0, O67.0, O72.3)
AHA: 2016, 1Q, 14
TIP: Do not assign to identify routine therapeutic anticoagulation effects;
assign only for documented adverse effects.

D68.0 Von Willebrand's disease
Angiohemophilia
Factor VIII deficiency with vascular defect
Vascular hemophilia
EXCLUDES 1 capillary fragility (hereditary) (D69.8)
factor VIII deficiency NOS (D66)
factor VIII deficiency with functional defect (D66)
DEF: Abnormal blood coagulation caused by deficient blood
factor VII; congenital; symptoms include excess or prolonged
bleeding.

D68.1 Hereditary factor XI deficiency
Hemophilia C
Plasma thromboplastin antecedent [PTA] deficiency
Rosenthal's disease

D68.2 Hereditary deficiency of other clotting factors
AC globulin deficiency
Congenital afibrinogenemia
Deficiency of factor I [fibrinogen]
Deficiency of factor II [prothrombin]
Deficiency of factor V [labile]
Deficiency of factor VII [stable]
Deficiency of factor X [Stuart-Prower]
Deficiency of factor XII [Hageman]
Deficiency of factor XIII [fibrin stabilizing]
Dysfibrinogenemia (congenital)
Hypoproconvertinemia
Owren's disease
Proaccelerin deficiency

☑️⁵ᵗʰ **D68.3 Hemorrhagic disorder due to circulating anticoagulants**

☑️⁶ᵗʰ **D68.31 Hemorrhagic disorder due to intrinsic circulating anticoagulants, antibodies, or inhibitors**

D68.311 Acquired hemophilia
Autoimmune hemophilia
Autoimmune inhibitors to clotting factors
Secondary hemophilia

Chapter 3. Diseases of the Blood and Blood-forming Organs

D68.312   Antiphospholipid antibody with hemorrhagic disorder
Lupus anticoagulant (LAC) with hemorrhagic disorder
Systemic lupus erythematosus [SLE] inhibitor with hemorrhagic disorder
> **EXCLUDES 1**   *antiphospholipid antibody, finding without diagnosis (R76.0)*
> *antiphospholipid antibody syndrome (D68.61)*
> *antiphospholipid antibody with hypercoagulable state (D68.61)*
> *lupus anticoagulant (LAC) finding without diagnosis (R76.0)*
> *lupus anticoagulant (LAC) with hypercoagulable state (D68.62)*
> *systemic lupus erythematosus [SLE] inhibitor finding without diagnosis (R76.0)*
> *systemic lupus erythematosus [SLE] inhibitor with hypercoagulable state (D68.62)*

D68.318   Other hemorrhagic disorder due to intrinsic circulating anticoagulants, antibodies, or inhibitors
Antithromboplastinemia
Antithromboplastinogenemia
Hemorrhagic disorder due to intrinsic increase in antithrombin
Hemorrhagic disorder due to intrinsic increase in anti-VIIIa
Hemorrhagic disorder due to intrinsic increase in anti-IXa
Hemorrhagic disorder due to intrinsic increase in anti-XIa

D68.32   Hemorrhagic disorder due to extrinsic circulating anticoagulants
Drug-induced hemorrhagic disorder
Hemorrhagic disorder due to increase in anti-IIa
Hemorrhagic disorder due to increase in anti-Xa
Hyperheparinemia
Use additional code for adverse effect, if applicable, to identify drug (T45.515, T45.525)
AHA: 2016, 1Q, 14-15

D68.4   Acquired coagulation factor deficiency
Deficiency of coagulation factor due to liver disease
Deficiency of coagulation factor due to vitamin K deficiency
> **EXCLUDES 1**   *vitamin K deficiency of newborn (P53)*

☑5ᵗʰ **D68.5**   Primary thrombophilia
Primary hypercoagulable states
> **EXCLUDES 1**   *antiphospholipid syndrome (D68.61)*
> *lupus anticoagulant (D68.62)*
> *secondary activated protein C resistance (D68.69)*
> *secondary antiphospholipid antibody syndrome (D68.69)*
> *secondary lupus anticoagulant with hypercoagulable state (D68.69)*
> *secondary systemic lupus erythematosus [SLE] inhibitor with hypercoagulable state (D68.69)*
> *systemic lupus erythematosus [SLE] inhibitor finding without diagnosis (R76.0)*
> *systemic lupus erythematosus [SLE] inhibitor with hemorrhagic disorder (D68.312)*
> *thrombotic thrombocytopenic purpura (M31.1)*

D68.51   Activated protein C resistance
Factor V Leiden mutation

D68.52   Prothrombin gene mutation

D68.59   Other primary thrombophilia
Antithrombin III deficiency   Protein C deficiency
Hypercoagulable state NOS   Protein S deficiency
Primary hypercoagulable state NEC   Thrombophilia NOS
Primary thrombophilia NEC

☑5ᵗʰ **D68.6**   Other thrombophilia
Other hypercoagulable states
> **EXCLUDES 1**   *diffuse or disseminated intravascular coagulation [DIC] (D65)*
> *heparin induced thrombocytopenia (HIT) (D75.82)*
> *hyperhomocysteinemia (E72.11)*

D68.61   Antiphospholipid syndrome
Anticardiolipin syndrome
Antiphospholipid antibody syndrome
> **EXCLUDES 1**   *antiphospholipid antibody, finding without diagnosis (R76.0)*
> *antiphospholipid antibody with hemorrhagic disorder (D68.312)*
> *lupus anticoagulant syndrome (D68.62)*

D68.62   Lupus anticoagulant syndrome
Lupus anticoagulant
Presence of systemic lupus erythematosus [SLE] inhibitor
> **EXCLUDES 1**   *anticardiolipin syndrome (D68.61)*
> *antiphospholipid syndrome (D68.61)*
> *lupus anticoagulant (LAC) finding without diagnosis (R76.0)*
> *lupus anticoagulant (LAC) with hemorrhagic disorder (D68.312)*

D68.69   Other thrombophilia
Hypercoagulable states NEC
Secondary hypercoagulable state NOS

D68.8   Other specified coagulation defects
> **EXCLUDES 1**   *hemorrhagic disease of newborn (P53)*

D68.9   Coagulation defect, unspecified   ▽

☑4ᵗʰ **D69**   Purpura and other hemorrhagic conditions
> **EXCLUDES 1**   *benign hypergammaglobulinemic purpura (D89.0)*
> *cryoglobulinemic purpura (D89.1)*
> *essential (hemorrhagic) thrombocythemia (D47.3)*
> *hemorrhagic thrombocythemia (D47.3)*
> *purpura fulminans (D65)*
> *thrombotic thrombocytopenic purpura (M31.1)*
> *Waldenström hypergammaglobulinemic purpura (D89.0)*

D69.0   Allergic purpura
Allergic vasculitis
Nonthrombocytopenic hemorrhagic purpura
Nonthrombocytopenic idiopathic purpura
Purpura anaphylactoid
Purpura Henoch(-Schönlein)
Purpura rheumatica
Vascular purpura
> **EXCLUDES 1**   *thrombocytopenic hemorrhagic purpura (D69.3)*
DEF: Any hemorrhagic condition, thrombocytic or nonthrombocytopenic in origin, caused by a presumed allergic reaction.

D69.1   Qualitative platelet defects
Bernard-Soulier [giant platelet] syndrome
Glanzmann's disease
Grey platelet syndrome
Thromboasthenia (hemorrhagic) (hereditary)
Thrombocytopathy
> **EXCLUDES 1**   *von Willebrand's disease (D68.0)*

D69.2   Other nonthrombocytopenic purpura
Purpura NOS   Senile purpura
Purpura simplex

D69.3   Immune thrombocytopenic purpura
Hemorrhagic (thrombocytopenic) purpura
Idiopathic thrombocytopenic purpura
Tidal platelet dysgenesis
DEF: Tidal platelet dysgenesis: Platelet counts fluctuate from normal to very low within periods of 20 to 40 days and may involve autoimmune platelet destruction.

☑5ᵗʰ **D69.4**   Other primary thrombocytopenia
> **EXCLUDES 1**   *transient neonatal thrombocytopenia (P61.0)*
> *Wiskott-Aldrich syndrome (D82.0)*

D69.41   Evans syndrome

D69.42   Congenital and hereditary thrombocytopenia purpura
Congenital thrombocytopenia
Hereditary thrombocytopenia
Code first congenital or hereditary disorder, such as: thrombocytopenia with absent radius (TAR syndrome) (Q87.2)

D69.49   Other primary thrombocytopenia
Megakaryocytic hypoplasia
Primary thrombocytopenia NOS

N Newborn: 0   P Pediatric: 0-17   M Maternity: 12-55   A Adult: 15-124   NRS Nonroutine supply Dx   NCDx Noncancer Dx   PDx Primary Dx   ►◄ Revised Text   ● New Code   ▲ Revised Title

498   ICD-10-CM 2018

✓5ᵗʰ **D69.5 Secondary thrombocytopenia**
     EXCLUDES 1   *heparin induced thrombocytopenia (HIT) (D75.82)*
           transient thrombocytopenia of newborn (P61.0)

     D69.51 Posttransfusion purpura
         Posttransfusion purpura from whole blood (fresh) or
           blood products
         PTP

     D69.59 Other secondary thrombocytopenia
         AHA: 2014, 4Q, 22

D69.6 Thrombocytopenia, unspecified   ▽

D69.8 Other specified hemorrhagic conditions
     Capillary fragility (hereditary)
     Vascular pseudohemophilia

D69.9 Hemorrhagic condition, unspecified   ▽

Other disorders of blood and blood-forming organs (D70-D77)

✓4ᵗʰ **D70 Neutropenia**
     INCLUDES   agranulocytosis
           decreased absolute neurophile count (ANC)
     Use additional code for any associated:
         fever (R50.81)
         mucositis (J34.81, K12.3-, K92.81, N76.81)
     EXCLUDES 1   *neutropenic splenomegaly (D73.81)*
           transient neonatal neutropenia (P61.5)

     D70.0 Congenital agranulocytosis
         Congenital neutropenia
         Infantile genetic agranulocytosis
         Kostmann's disease

     D70.1 Agranulocytosis secondary to cancer chemotherapy
         Use additional code for adverse effect, if applicable, to identify
           drug (T45.1X5)
         Code also underlying neoplasm
         AHA: 2014, 4Q, 22

     D70.2 Other drug-induced agranulocytosis
         Use additional code for adverse effect, if applicable, to identify
           drug (T36-T50 with fifth or sixth character 5)

     D70.3 Neutropenia due to infection

     D70.4 Cyclic neutropenia
         Cyclic hematopoiesis
         Periodic neutropenia

     D70.8 Other neutropenia

     D70.9 Neutropenia, unspecified   ▽

D71 Functional disorders of polymorphonuclear neutrophils
     Cell membrane receptor complex [CR3] defect
     Chronic (childhood) granulomatous disease
     Congenital dysphagocytosis
     Progressive septic granulomatosis

✓4ᵗʰ **D72 Other disorders of white blood cells**
     EXCLUDES 1   *basophilia (D72.824)*
           immunity disorders (D80-D89)
           neutropenia (D70)
           preleukemia (syndrome) (D46.9)

     D72.0 Genetic anomalies of leukocytes
         Alder (granulation) (granulocyte) anomaly
         Alder syndrome
         Hereditary leukocytic hypersegmentation
         Hereditary leukocytic hyposegmentation
         Hereditary leukomelanopathy
         May-Hegglin (granulation) (granulocyte) anomaly
         May-Hegglin syndrome
         Pelger-Huët (granulation) (granulocyte) anomaly
         Pelger-Huët syndrome
         EXCLUDES 1   *Chédiak (-Steinbrinck)-Higashi syndrome (E70.330)*

     D72.1 Eosinophilia
         Allergic eosinophilia
         Hereditary eosinophilia
         EXCLUDES 1   *Löffler's syndrome (J82)*
           pulmonary eosinophilia (J82)

✓5ᵗʰ   **D72.8 Other specified disorders of white blood cells**
     EXCLUDES 1   *leukemia (C91-C95)*

     ✓6ᵗʰ   **D72.81 Decreased white blood cell count**
         EXCLUDES 1   *neutropenia (D70.-)*

         D72.810 Lymphocytopenia
           Decreased lymphocytes

         D72.818 Other decreased white blood cell count
           Basophilic leukopenia
           Eosinophilic leukopenia
           Monocytopenia
           Other decreased leukocytes
           Plasmacytopenia

         D72.819 Decreased white blood cell count, unspecified   ▽
           Decreased leukocytes, unspecified
           Leukocytopenia, unspecified
           Leukopenia
           EXCLUDES 1   *malignant leukopenia (D70.9)*

     ✓6ᵗʰ   **D72.82 Elevated white blood cell count**
         EXCLUDES 1   *eosinophilia (D72.1)*

         D72.820 Lymphocytosis (symptomatic)
           Elevated lymphocytes

         D72.821 Monocytosis (symptomatic)
           EXCLUDES 1   *infectious mononucleosis (B27.-)*

         D72.822 Plasmacytosis

         D72.823 Leukemoid reaction
           Basophilic leukemoid reaction
           Leukemoid reaction NOS
           Lymphocytic leukemoid reaction
           Monocytic leukemoid reaction
           Myelocytic leukemoid reaction
           Neutrophilic leukemoid reaction

         D72.824 Basophilia

         D72.825 Bandemia
           Bandemia without diagnosis of specific
             infection
           EXCLUDES 1   *confirmed infection—code to*
             infection
             leukemia (C91.-, C92.-, C93.-,
               C94.-, C95.-)
           DEF: Increase in early neutrophil cells, called
             band cells; may indicate infection.

         D72.828 Other elevated white blood cell count

         D72.829 Elevated white blood cell count, unspecified   ▽
           Elevated leukocytes, unspecified
           Leukocytosis, unspecified

     D72.89 Other specified disorders of white blood cells
         Abnormality of white blood cells NEC

     D72.9 Disorder of white blood cells, unspecified   ▽
         Abnormal leukocyte differential NOS

✓4ᵗʰ **D73 Diseases of spleen**

     D73.0 Hyposplenism
         Atrophy of spleen
         EXCLUDES 1   *asplenia (congenital) (Q89.01)*
           postsurgical absence of spleen (Z90.81)

     D73.1 Hypersplenism
         EXCLUDES 1   *neutropenic splenomegaly (D73.81)*
           primary splenic neutropenia (D73.81)
           splenitis, splenomegaly in late syphilis (A52.79)
           splenitis, splenomegaly in tuberculosis (A18.85)
           splenomegaly NOS (R16.1)
           splenomegaly congenital (Q89.0)

     D73.2 Chronic congestive splenomegaly

     D73.3 Abscess of spleen

     D73.4 Cyst of spleen

     D73.5 Infarction of spleen
         Splenic rupture, nontraumatic
         Torsion of spleen
         EXCLUDES 1   *rupture of spleen due to Plasmodium vivax malaria*
           (B51.0)
           traumatic rupture of spleen (S36.03-)

✓5ᵗʰ   **D73.8 Other diseases of spleen**

     D73.81 Neutropenic splenomegaly
         Werner-Schultz disease

     D73.89 Other diseases of spleen
         Fibrosis of spleen NOS
         Perisplenitis
         Splenitis NOS

     D73.9 Disease of spleen, unspecified   ▽

✓4ᵗʰ **D74 Methemoglobinemia**

     D74.0 Congenital methemoglobinemia
         Congenital NADH-methemoglobin reductase deficiency
         Hemoglobin-M [Hb-M] disease
         Methemoglobinemia, hereditary

✓ Additional Character Req   ✓x7ᵗʰ Placeholder Alert   Case-Mix Diagnosis   Manifestation   ▽ Unspecified Dx   EXCLUDES 1 Not coded here   EXCLUDES 2 Not included here

ICD-10-CM 2018   499

Chapter 3. Diseases of the Blood and Blood-forming Organs

D74.8   **Other methemoglobinemias**
Acquired methemoglobinemia (with sulfhemoglobinemia)
Toxic methemoglobinemia

D74.9   **Methemoglobinemia, unspecified** ▽

√4ᵗʰ **D75**   **Other and unspecified diseases of blood and blood-forming organs**
   EXCLUDES 2   acute lymphadenitis (L04.-)
       chronic lymphadenitis (I88.1)
       enlarged lymph nodes (R59.-)
       hypergammaglobulinemia NOS (D89.2)
       lymphadenitis NOS (I88.9)
       mesenteric lymphadenitis (acute) (chronic) (I88.0)

D75.0   **Familial erythrocytosis**
Benign polycythemia
Familial polycythemia
  EXCLUDES 1   hereditary ovalocytosis (D58.1)

D75.1   **Secondary polycythemia**
Acquired polycythemia
Emotional polycythemia
Erythrocytosis NOS
Hypoxemic polycythemia
Nephrogenous polycythemia
Polycythemia due to erythropoietin
Polycythemia due to fall in plasma volume
Polycythemia due to high altitude
Polycythemia due to stress
Polycythemia NOS
Relative polycythemia
  EXCLUDES 1   polycythemia neonatorum (P61.1)
       polycythemia vera (D45)
DEF: Elevated number of red blood cells in circulating blood as a result of reduced oxygen supply to the tissues.

√5ᵗʰ **D75.8**   **Other specified diseases of blood and blood-forming organs**

D75.81   **Myelofibrosis**
Myelofibrosis NOS
Secondary myelofibrosis NOS
Code first the underlying disorder, such as: malignant neoplasm of breast (C50.-)
Use additional code, if applicable, for associated therapy-related myelodysplastic syndrome (D46.-)
Use additional code for adverse effect, if applicable, to identify drug (T45.1X5)
  EXCLUDES 1   acute myelofibrosis (C94.4-)
       idiopathic myelofibrosis (D47.1)
       leukoerythroblastic anemia (D61.82)
       myelofibrosis with myeloid metaplasia (D47.4)
       myelophthisic anemia (D61.82)
       myelophthisis (D61.82)
       primary myelofibrosis (D47.1)

D75.82   **Heparin induced thrombocytopenia (HIT)**
DEF: Immune-mediated reaction to heparin therapy causing an abrupt fall in platelet count and serious complications such as pulmonary embolism, stroke, AMI, or DVT.

D75.89   **Other specified diseases of blood and blood-forming organs**

D75.9   **Disease of blood and blood-forming organs, unspecified** ▽

√4ᵗʰ **D76**   **Other specified diseases with participation of lymphoreticular and reticulohistiocytic tissue**
  EXCLUDES 1   (Abt-) Letterer-Siwe disease (C96.0)
       eosinophilic granuloma (C96.6)
       Hand-Schüller-Christian disease (C96.5)
       histiocytic medullary reticulosis (C96.9)x
       histiocytic sarcoma (C96.A)
       histiocytosis X, multifocal (C96.5)
       histiocytosis X, unifocal (C96.6)
       Langerhans-cell histiocytosis, multifocal (C96.5)
       Langerhans-cell histiocytosis NOS (C96.6)
       Langerhans-cell histiocytosis, unifocal (C96.6)
       leukemic reticuloendotheliosis (C91.4-)
       lipomelanotic reticulosis (I89.8)
       malignant histiocytosis (C96.A)
       malignant reticulosis (C86.0)
       nonlipid reticuloendotheliosis (C96.0)

D76.1   **Hemophagocytic lymphohistiocytosis**
Familial hemophagocytic reticulosis
Histiocytoses of mononuclear phagocytes

D76.2   **Hemophagocytic syndrome, infection-associated**
Use additional code to identify infectious agent or disease

D76.3   **Other histiocytosis syndromes**
Reticulohistiocytoma (giant-cell)
Sinus histiocytosis with massive lymphadenopathy
Xanthogranuloma

√ **D77**   **Other disorders of blood and blood-forming organs in diseases classified elsewhere**
Code first underlying disease, such as:
amyloidosis (E85.-)
congenital early syphilis (A50.0)
echinococcosis (B67.0-B67.9)
malaria (B50.0-B54)
schistosomiasis [bilharziasis] (B65.0-B65.9)
vitamin C deficiency (E54)
  EXCLUDES 1   rupture of spleen due to Plasmodium vivax malaria (B51.0)
       splenitis, splenomegaly in late syphilis (A52.79)
       splenitis, splenomegaly in tuberculosis (A18.85)

Intraoperative and postprocedural complications of the spleen (D78)

√4ᵗʰ **D78**   **Intraoperative and postprocedural complications of the spleen**

√5ᵗʰ **D78.0**   **Intraoperative hemorrhage and hematoma** of the spleen complicating a procedure
  EXCLUDES 1   intraoperative hemorrhage and hematoma of the spleen due to accidental puncture or laceration during a procedure (D78.1-)

D78.01   **Intraoperative hemorrhage and hematoma of the spleen complicating a** procedure on the spleen

D78.02   **Intraoperative hemorrhage and hematoma of the spleen complicating** other procedure

√5ᵗʰ **D78.1**   **Accidental puncture and laceration** of the spleen during a procedure

D78.11   **Accidental puncture and laceration of the spleen during a** procedure on the spleen

D78.12   **Accidental puncture and laceration of the spleen during** other procedure

√5ᵗʰ **D78.2**   **Postprocedural hemorrhage** of the spleen following a procedure

D78.21   **Postprocedural hemorrhage of the spleen following a** procedure on the spleen

D78.22   **Postprocedural hemorrhage of the spleen following** other procedure

√5ᵗʰ **D78.3**   **Postprocedural hematoma and seroma** of the spleen following a procedure

D78.31   **Postprocedural** hematoma of the spleen following a procedure on the spleen

D78.32   **Postprocedural** hematoma of the spleen following other procedure

D78.33   **Postprocedural** seroma of the spleen following a procedure on the spleen

D78.34   **Postprocedural** seroma of the spleen following other procedure

√5ᵗʰ **D78.8**   **Other** intraoperative and postprocedural complications of the spleen
Use additional code, if applicable, to further specify disorder

D78.81   **Other intraoperative** complications of the spleen

D78.89   **Other postprocedural** complications of the spleen

Certain disorders involving the immune mechanism (D80-D89)
INCLUDES defects in the complement system
immunodeficiency disorders, except human immunodeficiency virus [HIV] disease
sarcoidosis
EXCLUDES 1 autoimmune disease (systemic) NOS (M35.9)
functional disorders of polymorphonuclear neutrophils (D71)
human immunodeficiency virus [HIV] disease (B20)

√4ᵗʰ **D80**   **Immunodeficiency with predominantly antibody defects**

D80.0   **Hereditary** hypogammaglobulinemia
Autosomal recessive agammaglobulinemia (Swiss type)
X-linked agammaglobulinemia [Bruton] (with growth hormone deficiency)

D80.1   **Nonfamilial** hypogammaglobulinemia
Agammaglobulinemia with immunoglobulin-bearing B-lymphocytes
Common variable agammaglobulinemia [CVAgamma]
Hypogammaglobulinemia NOS

D80.2   **Selective deficiency of** immunoglobulin A [IgA]

D80.3   **Selective deficiency of** immunoglobulin G [IgG] subclasses

N Newborn: 0   P Pediatric: 0-17   M Maternity: 12-55   A Adult: 15-124   NRS Nonroutine supply Dx   NCDx Noncancer Dx   PDx Primary Dx   ►◄ Revised Text   ● New Code   ▲ Revised Title

500   ICD-10-CM 2018

D80.4 Selective deficiency of immunoglobulin M **[IgM]**

D80.5 Immunodeficiency with increased immunoglobulin M **[IgM]**

D80.6 Antibody deficiency with near-normal immunoglobulins **or with** hyperimmunoglobulinemia

D80.7 Transient hypogammaglobulinemia of infancy

D80.8 Other immunodeficiencies with predominantly antibody defects
Kappa light chain deficiency

D80.9 Immunodeficiency with predominantly antibody defects, unspecified ▽

✓4ᵗʰ **D81 Combined immunodeficiencies**
EXCLUDES 1 *autosomal recessive agammaglobulinemia (Swiss type) (D80.0)*

D81.0 Severe combined immunodeficiency [SCID] with reticular dysgenesis

D81.1 Severe combined immunodeficiency [SCID] with low T- and B-cell numbers

D81.2 Severe combined immunodeficiency [SCID] with low or normal B-cell numbers

D81.3 Adenosine deaminase [ADA] deficiency

D81.4 Nezelof's syndrome

D81.5 Purine nucleoside phosphorylase [PNP] deficiency

D81.6 Major histocompatibility complex class I deficiency
Bare lymphocyte syndrome

D81.7 Major histocompatibility complex class II deficiency

✓5ᵗʰ **D81.8 Other combined immunodeficiencies**

   ✓6ᵗʰ **D81.81 Biotin-dependent carboxylase deficiency**
   Multiple carboxylase deficiency
   EXCLUDES 1 *biotin-dependent carboxylase deficiency due to dietary deficiency of biotin (E53.8)*

      D81.810 Biotinidase deficiency

      D81.818 Other biotin-dependent carboxylase deficiency
      Holocarboxylase synthetase deficiency
      Other multiple carboxylase deficiency

      D81.819 Biotin-dependent carboxylase deficiency, unspecified ▽
      Multiple carboxylase deficiency, unspecified

   D81.89 Other combined immunodeficiencies

D81.9 Combined immunodeficiency, unspecified ▽
Severe combined immunodeficiency disorder [SCID] NOS

✓4ᵗʰ **D82 Immunodeficiency associated with other major defects**
EXCLUDES 1 *ataxia telangiectasia [Louis-Bar] (G11.3)*

D82.0 Wiskott-Aldrich syndrome
Immunodeficiency with thrombocytopenia and eczema

D82.1 Di George's syndrome
Pharyngeal pouch syndrome
Thymic alymphoplasia
Thymic aplasia or hypoplasia with immunodeficiency

D82.2 Immunodeficiency with short-limbed stature

D82.3 Immunodeficiency following hereditary defective response to Epstein-Barr virus
X-linked lymphoproliferative disease

D82.4 Hyperimmunoglobulin E [IgE] syndrome

D82.8 Immunodeficiency associated with other specified major defects

D82.9 Immunodeficiency associated with major defect, unspecified ▽

✓4ᵗʰ **D83 Common variable immunodeficiency**

D83.0 Common variable immunodeficiency with predominant abnormalities of B-cell numbers and function

D83.1 Common variable immunodeficiency with predominant immunoregulatory T-cell disorders

D83.2 Common variable immunodeficiency with autoantibodies to B- or T-cells

D83.8 Other common variable immunodeficiencies

D83.9 Common variable immunodeficiency, unspecified ▽

✓4ᵗʰ **D84 Other immunodeficiencies**

D84.0 Lymphocyte function antigen-1 [LFA-1] defect

D84.1 Defects in the complement system
C1 esterase inhibitor [C1-INH] deficiency

D84.8 Other specified immunodeficiencies

D84.9 Immunodeficiency, unspecified ▽

✓4ᵗʰ **D86 Sarcoidosis**

D86.0 Sarcoidosis of lung

D86.1 Sarcoidosis of lymph nodes

D86.2 Sarcoidosis of lung with sarcoidosis of lymph nodes

D86.3 Sarcoidosis of skin

✓5ᵗʰ **D86.8 Sarcoidosis of other sites**

   D86.81 Sarcoid meningitis

   D86.82 Multiple cranial nerve palsies in sarcoidosis

   D86.83 Sarcoid iridocyclitis

   D86.84 Sarcoid pyelonephritis
   Tubulo-interstitial nephropathy in sarcoidosis

   D86.85 Sarcoid myocarditis

   D86.86 Sarcoid arthropathy
   Polyarthritis in sarcoidosis

   D86.87 Sarcoid myositis

   D86.89 Sarcoidosis of other sites
   Hepatic granulomaUveoparotid fever [Heerfordt]

D86.9 Sarcoidosis, unspecified ▽

✓4ᵗʰ **D89 Other disorders involving the immune mechanism, not elsewhere classified**
EXCLUDES 1 *hyperglobulinemia NOS (R77.1)*
monoclonal gammopathy (of undetermined significance) (D47.2)
EXCLUDES 2 *transplant failure and rejection (T86.-)*

D89.0 Polyclonal hypergammaglobulinemia
Benign hypergammaglobulinemic purpura
Polyclonal gammopathy NOS

D89.1 Cryoglobulinemia
Cryoglobulinemic purpura
Cryoglobulinemic vasculitis
Essential cryoglobulinemia
Idiopathic cryoglobulinemia
Mixed cryoglobulinemia
Primary cryoglobulinemia
Secondary cryoglobulinemia

D89.2 Hypergammaglobulinemia, unspecified ▽

D89.3 Immune reconstitution syndrome
Immune reconstitution inflammatory syndrome [IRIS]
Use additional code for adverse effect, if applicable, to identify drug (T36-T50 with fifth or sixth character 5)

✓5ᵗʰ **D89.4 Mast cell activation syndrome and related disorders**
EXCLUDES 1 *aggressive systemic mastocytosis ▶(C96.21)◀*
▶congenital cutaneous mastocytosis◀ (Q82.2)
▶(non-congenital) cutaneous mastocytosis (D47.01)
(indolent) systemic mastocytosis (D47.02)
malignant mast cell neoplasm (C96.2-)◀
malignant mastocytoma ▶(C96.29)◀
mast cell leukemia (C94.3-)
▶mast cell sarcoma (C96.22)
mastocytoma NOS (D47.09)
other mast cell neoplasms of uncertain behavior (D47.09)◀
systemic mastocytosis associated with a clonal hematologic non-mast cell lineage disease (SM-AHNMD)▶(D47.02)◀

   D89.40 Mast cell activation, unspecified ▽
   Mast cell activation disorder, unspecified
   Mast cell activation syndrome, NOS

   D89.41 Monoclonal mast cell activation syndrome

   D89.42 Idiopathic mast cell activation syndrome

   D89.43 Secondary mast cell activation
   Secondary mast cell activation syndrome
   Code also underlying etiology, if known

   D89.49 Other mast cell activation disorder
   Other mast cell activation syndrome

Chapter 3. Diseases of the Blood and Blood-forming Organs

☑5ᵗʰ **D89.8** **Other specified disorders involving the immune mechanism, not elsewhere classified**

    ☑6ᵗʰ **D89.81** **Graft-versus-host disease**

Code first underlying cause, such as:
    complications of transplanted organs and tissue (T86.-)
    complications of blood transfusion (T80.89)
Use additional code to identify associated manifestations, such as:
    desquamative dermatitis (L30.8)
    diarrhea (R19.7)
    elevated bilirubin (R17)
    hair loss (L65.9)

      D89.810 **Acute graft-versus-host disease**

      D89.811 **Chronic graft-versus-host disease**

      D89.812 **Acute on chronic graft-versus-host disease**

      D89.813 **Graft-versus-host disease, unspecified** ▽

    D89.82 **Autoimmune lymphoproliferative syndrome [ALPS]**

DEF: Rare genetic alteration of the Fas protein; impairs normal cellular apoptosis (normal cell death), causing abnormal accumulation of lymphocytes in the lymph glands, liver, and spleen; symptoms include neutropenia, anemia, and thrombocytopenia.

    D89.89 **Other specified disorders involving the immune mechanism, not elsewhere classified**

      EXCLUDES 1   *human immunodeficiency virus disease (B20)*

D89.9 **Disorder involving the immune mechanism, unspecified** ▽

Immune disease NOS
AHA: 2015, 3Q, 22

Ⓝ Newborn: 0   Ⓟ Pediatric: 0-17   Ⓜ Maternity: 12-55   Ⓐ Adult: 15-124   NRS Nonroutine supply Dx   NC Dx Noncancer Dx   PDx Primary Dx   ▶◀ Revised Text   ● New Code   ▲ Revised Title

502   ICD-10-CM 2018

Chapter 4. Endocrine, Nutritional and Metabolic Diseases (E00–E89)

Chapter Specific Guidelines with Coding Examples

The chapter specific guidelines from the ICD-10-CM Official Guidelines for Coding and Reporting have been provided below. Along with these guidelines are coding examples, contained in the shaded boxes, that have been developed to help illustrate the coding and/or sequencing guidance found in these guidelines.

a. Diabetes mellitus

The diabetes mellitus codes are combination codes that include the type of diabetes mellitus, the body system affected, and the complications affecting that body system. As many codes within a particular category as are necessary to describe all of the complications of the disease may be used. They should be sequenced based on the reason for a particular encounter. Assign as many codes from categories E08–E13 as needed to identify all of the associated conditions that the patient has.

> Patient is admitted with reported diagnoses of uncontrolled diabetes, type 2, with diabetic polyneuropathy and diabetic retinopathy with macular edema. Endocrinology clinical notes indicate a current HgA1c of 12.4 and "persistent blood glucose elevations over 300."
>
> **E11.65**   **Type 2 diabetes mellitus with hyperglycemia**
>
> **E11.311**   **Type 2 diabetes mellitus with unspecified diabetic retinopathy with macular edema**
>
> **E11.42**   **Type 2 diabetes mellitus with diabetic polyneuropathy**
>
> *Explanation*: Use as many codes to describe the diabetic complications as needed. Many are combination codes that describe more than one condition. "Uncontrolled" may reference hypo- or hyperglycemia, based upon available provider documentation.

1) Type of diabetes

The age of a patient is not the sole determining factor, though most type 1 diabetics develop the condition before reaching puberty. For this reason type 1 diabetes mellitus is also referred to as juvenile diabetes.

> A 45-year-old patient is diagnosed with Type 1 diabetes.
>
> **E10.9**   **Type 1 diabetes mellitus without complications**
>
> *Explanation*: Although most type 1 diabetics are diagnosed in childhood or adolescence, it can also begin in adults.

2) Type of diabetes mellitus not documented

If the type of diabetes mellitus is not documented in the medical record the default is E11.-, Type 2 diabetes mellitus.

> Patient is referred with new diagnoses reported in provider clinical notes as diabetes and hypertension.
>
> **E11.9**   **Type 2 diabetes mellitus without complications**
>
> **I10**   **Essential (primary) hypertension**
>
> *Explanation*: Since the type of diabetes was not documented and no complications were noted, the default code is E11.9.

3) Diabetes mellitus and the use of insulin and oral hypoglycemics

If the documentation in a medical record does not indicate the type of diabetes but does indicate that the patient uses insulin, code E11-, Type 2 diabetes mellitus, should be assigned. **An additional code should be assigned from category Z79 to identify the long-term (current) use of insulin or oral hypoglycemic drugs. If the patient is treated with both oral medications and insulin, only the code for long-term (current) use of insulin should be assigned. Code Z79.4 should not be assigned if insulin is given temporarily to bring a type 2 patient's blood sugar under control during an encounter.**

> Patient is referred with documented provider notes reporting 10-year history of diabetes requiring daily insulin use.
>
> **E11.9**   **Type 2 diabetes mellitus without complication**
>
> **Z79.4**   **Long term (current) use of insulin**
>
> *Explanation*: Do not assume that a patient requiring insulin use must have type 1 diabetes. The default for diabetes without further specification defaults to type 2. Add the code for long-term use of insulin.

4) Diabetes mellitus in pregnancy and gestational diabetes

See Section I.C.15. Diabetes mellitus in pregnancy.

See Section I.C.15. Gestational (pregnancy induced) diabetes

5) Complications due to insulin pump malfunction

(a) Underdose of insulin due to insulin pump failure

An underdose of insulin due to an insulin pump failure should be assigned to a code from subcategory T85.6, Mechanical complication of other specified internal and external prosthetic devices, implants and grafts, that specifies the type of pump malfunction, as the principal or first-listed code, followed by code T38.3X6-, Underdosing of insulin and oral hypoglycemic [antidiabetic] drugs. Additional codes for the type of diabetes mellitus and any associated complications due to the underdosing should also be assigned.

> A 76-year-old male with diabetic ESRD is admitted for rehabilitation and develops hyperglycemia. He has had an implanted insulin pump for 14 years and after returning from the ER, is noted to have experienced hyperglycemia due to a pump malfunction resulting in too little insulin being administered. On return, the blood sugars are resolving.
>
> **T85.614D**   **Breakdown (mechanical) of insulin pump, subsequent encounter**
>
> **T38.3X6D**   **Underdosing of insulin and oral hypoglycemic [antidiabetic] drugs, subsequent encounter**
>
> **E11.65**   **Type 2 diabetes mellitus with hyperglycemia**
>
> **E11.22**   **Type 2 diabetes mellitus with diabetic chronic kidney disease**
>
> **N18.6**   **End stage renal disease**
>
> *Explanation*: The complication code for the mechanical breakdown of the pump is sequenced first, followed by the underdosing code and type of diabetes with complication. If two or more diabetic complications are present, assign all codes needed to capture each complication. The seventh character D is used for a subsequent encounter.

(b) Overdose of insulin due to insulin pump failure

The principal or first-listed code for an encounter due to an insulin pump malfunction resulting in an overdose of insulin, should also be T85.6-, Mechanical complication of other specified internal and external prosthetic devices, implants and grafts, followed by code T38.3X1-, Poisoning by insulin and oral hypoglycemic [antidiabetic] drugs, accidental (unintentional).

> A 70-year-old female with type 2 diabetes is found on the floor and sent to the ER. On her return from the hospital, it is noted that a failure of her insulin pump, resulting in excess insulin administration, caused the hypoglycemia, resulting in her condition.
>
> **T85.614D**   **Breakdown (mechanical) of insulin pump, subsequent encounter**
>
> **T38.3X1D**   **Poisoning by insulin and oral hypoglycemic [antidiabetic] drugs, accidental (unintentional), subsequent encounter**
>
> **E11.649**   **Type 2 diabetes mellitus with hypoglycemia without coma**
>
> *Explanation*: The complication code for the mechanical breakdown of the pump is sequenced first, followed by the code for poisoning and type of diabetes with any associated complications. The seventh character D is used for subsequent encounter.

6) Secondary diabetes mellitus

Codes under categories E08, Diabetes mellitus due to underlying condition, E09, Drug or chemical induced diabetes mellitus, and E13, Other specified diabetes mellitus, identify complications/manifestations associated with secondary diabetes mellitus. Secondary diabetes is always caused by another condition or event (e.g., cystic fibrosis, malignant neoplasm of pancreas, pancreatectomy, adverse effect of drug, or poisoning).

(a) Secondary diabetes mellitus and the use of insulin or oral hypoglycemic drugs

For patients with secondary diabetes mellitus who routinely use insulin or oral hypoglycemic drugs, an additional code from category Z79 should be assigned to identify the long-term (current) use of insulin or oral hypoglycemic drugs. If the patient is treated with both oral medications and insulin, only the code for long-term (current) use of insulin should be assigned. Code Z79.4 should not be assigned if insulin is given temporarily to bring a type 2 patient's blood sugar under control during an encounter.

> Type 2 diabetic with diabetic polyneuropathy on insulin.
>
> **E11.42   Type 2 diabetes mellitus with diabetic polyneuropathy**
>
> **Z79.4   Long-term (current) use of insulin**
>
> *Explanation*: Add the Z code for the long-term use of insulin because the insulin is taken chronically.

(b) Assigning and sequencing secondary diabetes codes and its causes

The sequencing of the secondary diabetes codes in relationship to codes for the cause of the diabetes is based on the Tabular List instructions for categories E08, E09 and E13.

(i) Secondary diabetes mellitus due to pancreatectomy

For postpancreatectomy diabetes mellitus (lack of insulin due to the surgical removal of all or part of the pancreas), assign code E89.1, Postprocedural hypoinsulinemia. Assign a code from category E13 and a code from subcategory Z90.41, Acquired absence of pancreas, as additional codes.

> Patient with newly diagnosed diabetes after surgical removal of part of pancreas. Patient is now insulin-dependent following the procedure.
>
> **E89.1   Postprocedural hypoinsulinemia**
>
> **E13.9   Other specified diabetes mellitus without complications**
>
> **Z90.411   Acquired partial absence of pancreas**
>
> **Z79.4   Long term (current) use of insulin**
>
> *Explanation*: Sequence the postprocedural complication of the hypoinsulinemia due to the partial removal of the pancreas as the first-listed code, followed by the other specified diabetes (NEC) with or without complications and the partial or total acquired absence of the pancreas. Instructional notes at E89.1 specify to "use additional code" for insulin use.

(ii) Secondary diabetes due to drugs

Secondary diabetes may be caused by an adverse effect of correctly administered medications, poisoning or sequela of poisoning.

See section I.C.19.e for coding of adverse effects and poisoning, and section I.C.20 for external cause code reporting.

> Subsequent encounter for corticosteroid-induced diabetes mellitus.
>
> **E09.9   Drug or chemical induced diabetes mellitus without complications**
>
> **T38.0X5D   Adverse effect of glucocorticoids and synthetic analogues, subsequent encounter**
>
> *Explanation*: If the diabetes is caused by an adverse effect of a drug, the diabetic condition is coded first. If it occurs from a poisoning or overdose, the poisoning code causing the diabetes is sequenced first.

Chapter 4. Endocrine, Nutritional and Metabolic Diseases (E00-E89)

NOTE All neoplasms, whether functionally active or not, are classified in Chapter 2. Appropriate codes in this chapter (i.e. E05.8, E07.0, E16-E31, E34-) may be used as additional codes to indicate either functional activity by neoplasms and ectopic endocrine tissue or hyperfunction and hypofunction of endocrine glands associated with neoplasms and other conditions classified elsewhere.

EXCLUDES 1 *transitory endocrine and metabolic disorders specific to newborn (P70-P74)*

This chapter contains the following blocks:

E00-E07 Disorders of thyroid gland
E08-E13 Diabetes mellitus
E15-E16 Other disorders of glucose regulation and pancreatic internal secretion
E20-E35 Disorders of other endocrine glands
E36 Intraoperative complications of endocrine system
E40-E46 Malnutrition
E50-E64 Other nutritional deficiencies
E65-E68 Overweight, obesity and other hyperalimentation
E70-E88 Metabolic disorders
E89 Postprocedural endocrine and metabolic complications and disorders, not elsewhere classified

Disorders of thyroid gland (E00-E07)

✓4ᵗʰ E00 Congenital iodine-deficiency syndrome
Use additional code (F70-F79) to identify associated intellectual disabilities
EXCLUDES 1 *subclinical iodine-deficiency hypothyroidism (E02)*

E00.0 Congenital iodine-deficiency syndrome, neurological type
Endemic cretinism, neurological type

E00.1 Congenital iodine-deficiency syndrome, myxedematous type
Endemic hypothyroid cretinism
Endemic cretinism, myxedematous type

E00.2 Congenital iodine-deficiency syndrome, mixed type
Endemic cretinism, mixed type

E00.9 Congenital iodine-deficiency syndrome, unspecified ▽
Congenital iodine-deficiency hypothyroidism NOS
Endemic cretinism NOS

✓4ᵗʰ E01 Iodine-deficiency related thyroid disorders and allied conditions
EXCLUDES 1 *congenital iodine-deficiency syndrome (E00.-)*
subclinical iodine-deficiency hypothyroidism (E02)

E01.0 Iodine-deficiency related diffuse (endemic) goiter

E01.1 Iodine-deficiency related multinodular (endemic) goiter
Iodine-deficiency related nodular goiter

E01.2 Iodine-deficiency related (endemic) goiter, unspecified ▽
Endemic goiter NOS

E01.8 Other iodine-deficiency related thyroid disorders and allied conditions
Acquired iodine-deficiency hypothyroidism NOS

E02 Subclinical iodine-deficiency hypothyroidism

✓4ᵗʰ E03 Other hypothyroidism
EXCLUDES 1 *iodine-deficiency related hypothyroidism (E00-E02)*
postprocedural hypothyroidism (E89.0)

E03.0 Congenital hypothyroidism with diffuse goiter
Congenital parenchymatous goiter (nontoxic)
Congenital goiter (nontoxic) NOS
EXCLUDES 1 *transitory congenital goiter with normal function (P72.0)*

E03.1 Congenital hypothyroidism without goiter
Aplasia of thyroid (with myxedema)
Congenital atrophy of thyroid
Congenital hypothyroidism NOS

E03.2 Hypothyroidism due to medicaments and other exogenous substances
Code first poisoning due to drug or toxin, if applicable (T36-T65 with fifth or sixth character 1-4 or 6)
Use additional code for adverse effect, if applicable, to identify drug (T36-T50 with fifth or sixth character 5)

E03.3 Postinfectious hypothyroidism

E03.4 Atrophy of thyroid (acquired)
EXCLUDES 1 *congenital atrophy of thyroid (E03.1)*

E03.5 Myxedema coma NC Dx

E03.8 Other specified hypothyroidism

E03.9 Hypothyroidism, unspecified ▽
Myxedema NOS

✓4ᵗʰ E04 Other nontoxic goiter
EXCLUDES 1 *congenital goiter (NOS) (diffuse) (parenchymatous) (E03.0)*
iodine-deficiency related goiter (E00-E02)

E04.0 Nontoxic diffuse goiter
Diffuse (colloid) nontoxic goiter
Simple nontoxic goiter

E04.1 Nontoxic single thyroid nodule
Colloid nodule (cystic) (thyroid)
Nontoxic uninodular goiter
Thyroid (cystic) nodule NOS
DEF: Enlarged thyroid, commonly due to decreased thyroid production, with single nodule; no clinical hypothyroidism.

E04.2 Nontoxic multinodular goiter
Cystic goiter NOS
Multinodular (cystic) goiter NOS
DEF: Enlarged thyroid, commonly due to decreased thyroid production with multiple nodules; no clinical hypothyroidism.

E04.8 Other specified nontoxic goiter

E04.9 Nontoxic goiter, unspecified ▽
Goiter NOS
Nodular goiter (nontoxic) NOS

✓4ᵗʰ E05 Thyrotoxicosis [hyperthyroidism]
EXCLUDES 1 *chronic thyroiditis with transient thyrotoxicosis (E06.2)*
neonatal thyrotoxicosis (P72.1)

✓5ᵗʰ E05.0 Thyrotoxicosis with diffuse goiter
Exophthalmic or toxic goiter NOS
Graves' disease
Toxic diffuse goiter
DEF: Diffuse thyroid enlargement accompanied by hyperthyroidism, bulging eyes, and dermopathy.

E05.00 Thyrotoxicosis with diffuse goiter without thyrotoxic crisis or storm

E05.01 Thyrotoxicosis with diffuse goiter with thyrotoxic crisis or storm

✓5ᵗʰ E05.1 Thyrotoxicosis with toxic single thyroid nodule
Thyrotoxicosis with toxic uninodular goiter
DEF: Symptomatic hyperthyroidism with a single nodule on the enlarged thyroid gland. Abrupt onset of symptoms include extreme nervousness, insomnia, weight loss, tremors, and psychosis or coma.

E05.10 Thyrotoxicosis with toxic single thyroid nodule without thyrotoxic crisis or storm

E05.11 Thyrotoxicosis with toxic single thyroid nodule with thyrotoxic crisis or storm

✓5ᵗʰ E05.2 Thyrotoxicosis with toxic multinodular goiter
Toxic nodular goiter NOS

E05.20 Thyrotoxicosis with toxic multinodular goiter without thyrotoxic crisis or storm

E05.21 Thyrotoxicosis with toxic multinodular goiter with thyrotoxic crisis or storm

✓5ᵗʰ E05.3 Thyrotoxicosis from ectopic thyroid tissue

E05.30 Thyrotoxicosis from ectopic thyroid tissue without thyrotoxic crisis or storm

E05.31 Thyrotoxicosis from ectopic thyroid tissue with thyrotoxic crisis or storm

✓5ᵗʰ E05.4 Thyrotoxicosis factitia

E05.40 Thyrotoxicosis factitia without thyrotoxic crisis or storm

E05.41 Thyrotoxicosis factitia with thyrotoxic crisis or storm

Goiter

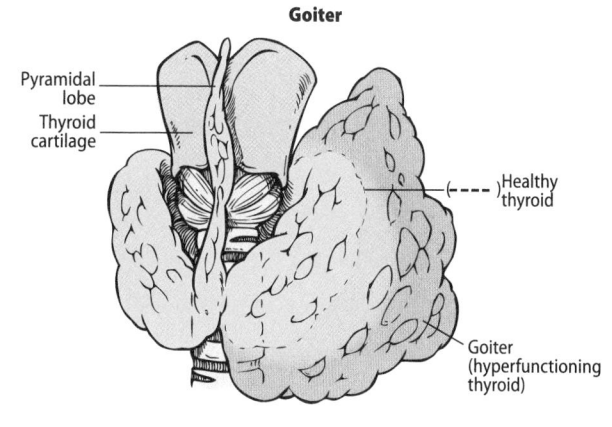

Pyramidal lobe
Thyroid cartilage
Healthy thyroid
Goiter (hyperfunctioning thyroid)

Chapter 4. Endocrine, Nutritional and Metabolic Diseases

E00–E05.41

√5ᵗʰ **E05.8** Other **thyrotoxicosis**
Overproduction of thyroid-stimulating hormone

     E05.80 **Other thyrotoxicosis** without thyrotoxic crisis or storm

     E05.81 **Other thyrotoxicosis** with thyrotoxic crisis or storm

√5ᵗʰ **E05.9** **Thyrotoxicosis,** unspecified
Hyperthyroidism NOS

     E05.90 **Thyrotoxicosis, unspecified** without thyrotoxic crisis or storm ▽

     E05.91 **Thyrotoxicosis, unspecified** with thyrotoxic crisis or storm ▽

√4ᵗʰ **E06** **Thyroiditis**
     EXCLUDES 1   *postpartum thyroiditis (O90.5)*

     E06.0 Acute **thyroiditis**
Abscess of thyroid
Pyogenic thyroiditis
Suppurative thyroiditis
Use additional code (B95-B97) to identify infectious agent

     E06.1 Subacute **thyroiditis**
de Quervain thyroiditis
Giant-cell thyroiditis
Granulomatous thyroiditis
Nonsuppurative thyroiditis
Viral thyroiditis
     EXCLUDES 1   *autoimmune thyroiditis (E06.3)*

     E06.2 Chronic **thyroiditis** with transient thyrotoxicosis
     EXCLUDES 1   *autoimmune thyroiditis (E06.3)*

     E06.3 Autoimmune **thyroiditis**
Hashimoto's thyroiditis
Hashitoxicosis (transient)
Lymphadenoid goiter
Lymphocytic thyroiditis
Struma lymphomatosa

     E06.4 Drug-induced **thyroiditis**
Use additional code for adverse effect, if applicable, to identify drug (T36-T50 with fifth or sixth character 5)

     E06.5 Other chronic **thyroiditis**
Chronic fibrous thyroiditis
Chronic thyroiditis NOS
Ligneous thyroiditis
Riedel thyroiditis

     E06.9 **Thyroiditis,** unspecified ▽

√4ᵗʰ **E07** **Other disorders of thyroid**

     E07.0 **Hypersecretion of calcitonin**
C-cell hyperplasia of thyroid
Hypersecretion of thyrocalcitonin

     E07.1 **Dyshormogenetic goiter**
Familial dyshormogenetic goiter
Pendred's syndrome
     EXCLUDES 1   *transitory congenital goiter with normal function (P72.0)*

√5ᵗʰ **E07.8** **Other specified disorders of thyroid**

     E07.81 **Sick-euthyroid syndrome**
Euthyroid sick-syndrome

     E07.89 **Other specified disorders of thyroid**
Abnormality of thyroid-binding globulin
Hemorrhage of thyroid
Infarction of thyroid

     E07.9 **Disorder of thyroid, unspecified** ▽

Diabetes mellitus (E08-E13)

AHA: 2017, 1Q, 42; 2016, 2Q, 36; 2016, 1Q, 11-13

√4ᵗʰ **E08** **Diabetes mellitus** due to underlying condition
Code first the underlying condition, such as:
     congenital rubella (P35.0)
     cushing's syndrome (E24.-)
     cystic fibrosis (E84.-)
     malignant neoplasm (C00-C96)
     malnutrition (E40-E46)
     pancreatitis and other diseases of the pancreas (K85.-, K86.-)
Use additional code to identify control using:
     insulin (Z79.4)
     oral antidiabetic drugs (Z79.84)
     oral hypoglycemic drugs (Z79.84)
     EXCLUDES 1   *drug or chemical induced diabetes mellitus (E09.-)*
         gestational diabetes (O24.4-)
         neonatal diabetes mellitus (P70.2)
         postpancreatectomy diabetes mellitus (E13.-)
         postprocedural diabetes mellitus (E13.-)
         secondary diabetes mellitus NEC (E13.-)
         type 1 diabetes mellitus (E10.-)
         type 2 diabetes mellitus (E11.-)
     AHA: 2013, 4Q, 114; 2013, 3Q, 20

√5ᵗʰ **E08.0** **Diabetes mellitus due to underlying condition with hyperosmolarity**

     E08.00 *Diabetes mellitus due to underlying condition with hyperosmolarity without nonketotic hyperglycemic-hyperosmolar coma (NKHHC)*

     E08.01 *Diabetes mellitus due to underlying condition with hyperosmolarity with coma*

√5ᵗʰ **E08.1** **Diabetes mellitus due to underlying condition with ketoacidosis**

     E08.10 *Diabetes mellitus due to underlying condition with ketoacidosis without coma*

     E08.11 *Diabetes mellitus due to underlying condition with ketoacidosis with coma*

√5ᵗʰ **E08.2** **Diabetes mellitus due to underlying condition with** kidney complications

     E08.21 *Diabetes mellitus due to underlying condition with diabetic nephropathy*
Diabetes mellitus due to underlying condition with intercapillary glomerulosclerosis
Diabetes mellitus due to underlying condition with intracapillary glomerulonephrosis
Diabetes mellitus due to underlying condition with Kimmelstiel-Wilson disease

     E08.22 *Diabetes mellitus due to underlying condition with diabetic chronic kidney disease*
Use additional code to identify stage of chronic kidney disease (N18.1-N18.6)

     E08.29 *Diabetes mellitus due to underlying condition with other diabetic kidney complication*
Renal tubular degeneration in diabetes mellitus due to underlying condition

√5ᵗʰ **E08.3** **Diabetes mellitus due to underlying condition with** ophthalmic complications

One of the following 7th characters is to be assigned to codes in subcategories E08.32, E08.33, E08.34, E08.35, and E08.37 to designate laterality of the disease:
1   right eye
2   left eye
3   bilateral
9   unspecified eye

√6ᵗʰ **E08.31** **Diabetes mellitus due to underlying condition with unspecified** diabetic retinopathy

     E08.311 *Diabetes mellitus due to underlying condition with unspecified diabetic retinopathy with macular edema* ▽

     E08.319 *Diabetes mellitus due to underlying condition with unspecified diabetic retinopathy without macular edema* ▽

√6ᵗʰ **E08.32** **Diabetes mellitus due to underlying condition with** mild nonproliferative diabetic retinopathy
Diabetes mellitus due to underlying condition with nonproliferative diabetic retinopathy NOS

     √7ᵗʰ **E08.321** *Diabetes mellitus due to underlying condition with mild nonproliferative diabetic retinopathy with macular edema*

N Newborn: 0   P Pediatric: 0-17   M Maternity: 12-55   A Adult: 15-124   NRS Nonroutine supply Dx   NC Dx Noncancer Dx   PDx Primary Dx   ▶◀ Revised Text   ● New Code   ▲ Revised Title

506   ICD-10-CM 2018

✓7th E08.329   *Diabetes mellitus due to underlying condition with mild nonproliferative diabetic retinopathy without macular edema*

✓6th E08.33   **Diabetes mellitus due to underlying condition with** moderate nonproliferative diabetic retinopathy

    ✓7th E08.331   *Diabetes mellitus due to underlying condition with moderate nonproliferative diabetic retinopathy with macular edema*

    ✓7th E08.339   *Diabetes mellitus due to underlying condition with moderate nonproliferative diabetic retinopathy without macular edema*

✓6th E08.34   **Diabetes mellitus due to underlying condition with** severe nonproliferative diabetic retinopathy

    ✓7th E08.341   *Diabetes mellitus due to underlying condition with severe nonproliferative diabetic retinopathy with macular edema*

    ✓7th E08.349   *Diabetes mellitus due to underlying condition with severe nonproliferative diabetic retinopathy without macular edema*

✓6th E08.35   **Diabetes mellitus due to underlying condition with** proliferative diabetic retinopathy

    ✓7th E08.351   *Diabetes mellitus due to underlying condition with proliferative diabetic retinopathy with macular edema*

    ✓7th E08.352   *Diabetes mellitus due to underlying condition with proliferative diabetic retinopathy with traction retinal detachment involving the macula*

    ✓7th E08.353   *Diabetes mellitus due to underlying condition with proliferative diabetic retinopathy with traction retinal detachment not involving the macula*

    ✓7th E08.354   *Diabetes mellitus due to underlying condition with proliferative diabetic retinopathy with combined traction retinal detachment and rhegmatogenous retinal detachment*

    ✓7th E08.355   *Diabetes mellitus due to underlying condition with stable proliferative diabetic retinopathy*

    ✓7th E08.359   *Diabetes mellitus due to underlying condition with proliferative diabetic retinopathy without macular edema*

E08.36   *Diabetes mellitus due to underlying condition with diabetic cataract*
     AHA: 2016, 4Q, 142

✓x7th E08.37   *Diabetes mellitus due to underlying condition with diabetic macular edema, resolved following treatment*

E08.39   *Diabetes mellitus due to underlying condition with other diabetic ophthalmic complication*
     Use additional code to identify manifestation, such as: diabetic glaucoma (H40-H42)

✓5th E08.4   **Diabetes mellitus due to underlying condition with** neurological complications

E08.40   *Diabetes mellitus due to underlying condition with diabetic neuropathy, unspecified* ▽

E08.41   *Diabetes mellitus due to underlying condition with diabetic mononeuropathy*

E08.42   *Diabetes mellitus due to underlying condition with diabetic polyneuropathy*
     Diabetes mellitus due to underlying condition with diabetic neuralgia

E08.43   *Diabetes mellitus due to underlying condition with diabetic autonomic (poly)neuropathy*
     Diabetes mellitus due to underlying condition with diabetic gastroparesis
     AHA: 2013, 4Q, 114

E08.44   *Diabetes mellitus due to underlying condition with diabetic amyotrophy*

E08.49   *Diabetes mellitus due to underlying condition with other diabetic neurological complication*

✓5th E08.5   **Diabetes mellitus due to underlying condition with** circulatory complications

E08.51   *Diabetes mellitus due to underlying condition with diabetic peripheral angiopathy without gangrene*

E08.52   *Diabetes mellitus due to underlying condition with diabetic peripheral angiopathy with gangrene*   **NRS**
     Diabetes mellitus due to underlying condition with diabetic gangrene

E08.59   *Diabetes mellitus due to underlying condition with other circulatory complications*

✓5th E08.6   **Diabetes mellitus due to underlying condition with** other specified complications

✓6th E08.61   **Diabetes mellitus due to underlying condition with** diabetic arthropathy

    E08.610   *Diabetes mellitus due to underlying condition with diabetic neuropathic arthropathy*
      Diabetes mellitus due to underlying condition with Charcôt's joints

    E08.618   *Diabetes mellitus due to underlying condition with other diabetic arthropathy*

✓6th E08.62   **Diabetes mellitus due to underlying condition with** skin complications

    E08.620   *Diabetes mellitus due to underlying condition with diabetic dermatitis*
      Diabetes mellitus due to underlying condition with diabetic necrobiosis lipoidica

    E08.621   *Diabetes mellitus due to underlying condition with foot ulcer*   **NRS**
      Use additional code to identify site of ulcer (L97.4-, L97.5-)
      TIP: Do not assign a code for diabetic ulcer when the ulcer is closed/resolved or to report history of diabetic ulcers; Z86.31 Personal history of diabetic foot ulcer may be assigned.

    E08.622   *Diabetes mellitus due to underlying condition with other skin ulcer*   **NRS**
      Use additional code to identify site of ulcer (L97.1-L97.9, L98.41-L98.49)

    E08.628   *Diabetes mellitus due to underlying condition with other skin complications*

✓6th E08.63   **Diabetes mellitus due to underlying condition with** oral complications

    E08.630   *Diabetes mellitus due to underlying condition with periodontal disease*

    E08.638   *Diabetes mellitus due to underlying condition with other oral complications*

✓6th E08.64   **Diabetes mellitus due to underlying condition with** hypoglycemia

    E08.641   *Diabetes mellitus due to underlying condition with hypoglycemia with coma*

    E08.649   *Diabetes mellitus due to underlying condition with hypoglycemia without coma*
      AHA: 2016, 3Q, 42; 2015, 3Q, 21

E08.65   *Diabetes mellitus due to underlying condition with hyperglycemia*

E08.69   *Diabetes mellitus due to underlying condition with other specified complication*
     Use additional code to identify complication
     AHA: 2016, 4Q, 141; 2016, 1Q, 13

E08.8   *Diabetes mellitus due to underlying condition with unspecified complications* ▽

E08.9   *Diabetes mellitus due to underlying condition without complications*

✓ Additional Character Req   ✓x7th Placeholder Alert   Case-Mix Diagnosis   Manifestation   ▽ Unspecified Dx   *EXCLUDES 1* Not coded here   *EXCLUDES 2* Not included here

ICD-10-CM 2018   **507**

☑4ᵗʰ **E09** **Drug or chemical induced diabetes mellitus**

Code first poisoning due to drug or toxin, if applicable (T36-T65 with fifth or sixth character 1-4 or 6)

Use additional code for adverse effect, if applicable, to identify drug (T36-T50 with fifth or sixth character 5)

Use additional code to identify control using:
  insulin (Z79.4)
  oral antidiabetic drugs (Z79.84)
  oral hypoglycemic drugs (Z79.84)

EXCLUDES 1   diabetes mellitus due to underlying condition (E08.-)
  gestational diabetes (O24.4-)
  neonatal diabetes mellitus (P70.2)
  postpancreatectomy diabetes mellitus (E13.-)
  postprocedural diabetes mellitus (E13.-)
  secondary diabetes mellitus NEC (E13.-)
  type 1 diabetes mellitus (E10.-)
  type 2 diabetes mellitus (E11.-)

AHA: 2013, 4Q, 114; 2013, 3Q, 20

☑5ᵗʰ **E09.0** **Drug or chemical induced diabetes mellitus with hyperosmolarity**

E09.00 **Drug or chemical induced diabetes mellitus with hyperosmolarity without nonketotic hyperglycemic-hyperosmolar coma (NKHHC)**

E09.01 **Drug or chemical induced diabetes mellitus with hyperosmolarity with coma**

☑5ᵗʰ **E09.1** **Drug or chemical induced diabetes mellitus with ketoacidosis**

E09.10 **Drug or chemical induced diabetes mellitus with ketoacidosis without coma**

E09.11 **Drug or chemical induced diabetes mellitus with ketoacidosis with coma**

☑5ᵗʰ **E09.2** **Drug or chemical induced diabetes mellitus with kidney complications**

E09.21 **Drug or chemical induced diabetes mellitus with diabetic nephropathy**
Drug or chemical induced diabetes mellitus with intercapillary glomerulosclerosis
Drug or chemical induced diabetes mellitus with intracapillary glomerulonephrosis
Drug or chemical induced diabetes mellitus with Kimmelstiel-Wilson disease

E09.22 **Drug or chemical induced diabetes mellitus with diabetic chronic kidney disease**
Use additional code to identify stage of chronic kidney disease (N18.1-N18.6)

E09.29 **Drug or chemical induced diabetes mellitus with other diabetic kidney complication**
Drug or chemical induced diabetes mellitus with renal tubular degeneration

☑5ᵗʰ **E09.3** **Drug or chemical induced diabetes mellitus with ophthalmic complications**

One of the following 7th characters is to be assigned to codes in subcategories E09.32, E09.33, E09.34, E09.35, and E09.37 to designate laterality of the disease:
1   right eye
2   left eye
3   bilateral
9   unspecified eye

☑6ᵗʰ **E09.31** **Drug or chemical induced diabetes mellitus with unspecified diabetic retinopathy**

E09.311 **Drug or chemical induced diabetes mellitus with unspecified diabetic retinopathy with macular edema** ▽

E09.319 **Drug or chemical induced diabetes mellitus with unspecified diabetic retinopathy without macular edema** ▽

☑6ᵗʰ **E09.32** **Drug or chemical induced diabetes mellitus with mild nonproliferative diabetic retinopathy**
Drug or chemical induced diabetes mellitus with nonproliferative diabetic retinopathy NOS

☑7ᵗʰ **E09.321** **Drug or chemical induced diabetes mellitus with mild nonproliferative diabetic retinopathy with macular edema**

☑7ᵗʰ **E09.329** **Drug or chemical induced diabetes mellitus with mild nonproliferative diabetic retinopathy without macular edema**

☑6ᵗʰ **E09.33** **Drug or chemical induced diabetes mellitus with moderate nonproliferative diabetic retinopathy**

☑7ᵗʰ **E09.331** **Drug or chemical induced diabetes mellitus with moderate nonproliferative diabetic retinopathy with macular edema**

☑7ᵗʰ **E09.339** **Drug or chemical induced diabetes mellitus with moderate nonproliferative diabetic retinopathy without macular edema**

☑6ᵗʰ **E09.34** **Drug or chemical induced diabetes mellitus with severe nonproliferative diabetic retinopathy**

☑7ᵗʰ **E09.341** **Drug or chemical induced diabetes mellitus with severe nonproliferative diabetic retinopathy with macular edema**

☑7ᵗʰ **E09.349** **Drug or chemical induced diabetes mellitus with severe nonproliferative diabetic retinopathy without macular edema**

☑6ᵗʰ **E09.35** **Drug or chemical induced diabetes mellitus with proliferative diabetic retinopathy**

☑7ᵗʰ **E09.351** **Drug or chemical induced diabetes mellitus with proliferative diabetic retinopathy with macular edema**

☑7ᵗʰ **E09.352** **Drug or chemical induced diabetes mellitus with proliferative diabetic retinopathy with traction retinal detachment involving the macula**

☑7ᵗʰ **E09.353** **Drug or chemical induced diabetes mellitus with proliferative diabetic retinopathy with traction retinal detachment not involving the macula**

☑7ᵗʰ **E09.354** **Drug or chemical induced diabetes mellitus with proliferative diabetic retinopathy with combined traction retinal detachment and rhegmatogenous retinal detachment**

☑7ᵗʰ **E09.355** **Drug or chemical induced diabetes mellitus with stable proliferative diabetic retinopathy**

☑7ᵗʰ **E09.359** **Drug or chemical induced diabetes mellitus with proliferative diabetic retinopathy without macular edema**

E09.36 **Drug or chemical induced diabetes mellitus with diabetic cataract**
AHA: 2016, 4Q, 142

☑x7ᵗʰ **E09.37** **Drug or chemical induced diabetes mellitus with diabetic macular edema, resolved following treatment**

E09.39 **Drug or chemical induced diabetes mellitus with other diabetic ophthalmic complication**
Use additional code to identify manifestation, such as:
diabetic glaucoma (H40-H42)

☑5ᵗʰ **E09.4** **Drug or chemical induced diabetes mellitus with neurological complications**

E09.40 **Drug or chemical induced diabetes mellitus with neurological complications with diabetic neuropathy, unspecified** ▽

E09.41 **Drug or chemical induced diabetes mellitus with neurological complications with diabetic mononeuropathy**

E09.42 **Drug or chemical induced diabetes mellitus with neurological complications with diabetic polyneuropathy**
Drug or chemical induced diabetes mellitus with diabetic neuralgia

E09.43 **Drug or chemical induced diabetes mellitus with neurological complications with diabetic autonomic (poly)neuropathy**
Drug or chemical induced diabetes mellitus with diabetic gastroparesis
AHA: 2013, 4Q, 114

E09.44 **Drug or chemical induced diabetes mellitus with neurological complications with diabetic amyotrophy**

E09.49 **Drug or chemical induced diabetes mellitus with neurological complications with other diabetic neurological complication**

Ⓝ Newborn: 0   Ⓟ Pediatric: 0-17   Ⓜ Maternity: 12-55   Ⓐ Adult: 15-124   NRS Nonroutine supply Dx   NCDx Noncancer Dx   PDx Primary Dx   ▶◀ Revised Text   ● New Code   ▲ Revised Title

508   ICD-10-CM 2018

✓5ᵗʰ E09.5 Drug or chemical induced diabetes mellitus with circulatory complications

    E09.51 Drug or chemical induced diabetes mellitus with diabetic peripheral angiopathy without gangrene

    E09.52 Drug or chemical induced diabetes mellitus **NRS** **with diabetic** peripheral angiopathy with gangrene
        Drug or chemical induced diabetes mellitus with diabetic gangrene

    E09.59 Drug or chemical induced diabetes mellitus with other circulatory complications

✓5ᵗʰ E09.6 Drug or chemical induced diabetes mellitus with other specified complications

    ✓6ᵗʰ E09.61 Drug or chemical induced diabetes mellitus with diabetic arthropathy

        E09.610 Drug or chemical induced diabetes mellitus with diabetic neuropathic arthropathy
            Drug or chemical induced diabetes mellitus with Charcôt's joints

        E09.618 Drug or chemical induced diabetes mellitus with other diabetic arthropathy

    ✓6ᵗʰ E09.62 Drug or chemical induced diabetes mellitus with skin complications

        E09.620 Drug or chemical induced diabetes mellitus with diabetic dermatitis
            Drug or chemical induced diabetes mellitus with diabetic necrobiosis lipoidica

        E09.621 Drug or chemical induced diabetes **NRS** **mellitus with** foot ulcer
            Use additional code to identify site of ulcer (L97.4-, L97.5-)
            TIP: Do not assign a code for diabetic ulcer when the ulcer is closed/resolved or to report history of diabetic ulcers; Z86.31 Personal history of diabetic foot ulcer may be assigned.

        E09.622 Drug or chemical induced diabetes **NRS** **mellitus with** other skin ulcer
            Use additional code to identify site of ulcer (L97.1-L97.9, L98.41-L98.49)

        E09.628 Drug or chemical induced diabetes mellitus with other skin complications

    ✓6ᵗʰ E09.63 Drug or chemical induced diabetes mellitus with oral complications

        E09.630 Drug or chemical induced diabetes mellitus with periodontal disease

        E09.638 Drug or chemical induced diabetes mellitus with other oral complications

    ✓6ᵗʰ E09.64 Drug or chemical induced diabetes mellitus with hypoglycemia

        E09.641 Drug or chemical induced diabetes mellitus with hypoglycemia with coma

        E09.649 Drug or chemical induced diabetes mellitus with hypoglycemia without coma
            AHA: 2016, 3Q, 42; 2015, 3Q, 21

    E09.65 Drug or chemical induced diabetes mellitus with hyperglycemia

    E09.69 Drug or chemical induced diabetes mellitus with other specified complication
        Use additional code to identify complication
        AHA: 2016, 4Q, 141; 2016, 1Q, 13

E09.8 Drug or chemical induced diabetes mellitus with unspecified complications ▽

E09.9 Drug or chemical induced diabetes mellitus without complications

---

✓4ᵗʰ E10 Type 1 diabetes mellitus
    INCLUDES brittle diabetes (mellitus)
         diabetes (mellitus) due to autoimmune process
         diabetes (mellitus) due to immune mediated pancreatic islet beta-cell destruction
         idiopathic diabetes (mellitus)
         juvenile onset diabetes (mellitus)
         ketosis-prone diabetes (mellitus)
    EXCLUDES 1 *diabetes mellitus due to underlying condition (E08.-)*
         drug or chemical induced diabetes mellitus (E09.-)
         gestational diabetes (O24.4-)
         hyperglycemia NOS (R73.9)
         neonatal diabetes mellitus (P70.2)
         postpancreatectomy diabetes mellitus (E13.-)
         postprocedural diabetes mellitus (E13.-)
         secondary diabetes mellitus NEC (E13.-)
         type 2 diabetes mellitus (E11.-)
    AHA: 2013, 4Q, 114; 2013, 3Q, 20

✓5ᵗʰ E10.1 Type 1 diabetes mellitus with ketoacidosis
    AHA: 2013, 3Q, 20

    E10.10 Type 1 diabetes mellitus with ketoacidosis without coma

    E10.11 Type 1 diabetes mellitus with ketoacidosis with coma

✓5ᵗʰ E10.2 Type 1 diabetes mellitus with kidney complications

    E10.21 Type 1 diabetes mellitus with diabetic nephropathy
        Type 1 diabetes mellitus with intercapillary glomerulosclerosis
        Type 1 diabetes mellitus with intracapillary glomerulonephrosis
        Type 1 diabetes mellitus with Kimmelstiel-Wilson disease

    E10.22 Type 1 diabetes mellitus with diabetic chronic kidney disease
        Use additional code to identify stage of chronic kidney disease (N18.1-N18.6)

    E10.29 Type 1 diabetes mellitus with other diabetic kidney complication
        Type 1 diabetes mellitus with renal tubular degeneration
        AHA: 2016, 1Q, 13

✓5ᵗʰ E10.3 Type 1 diabetes mellitus with ophthalmic complications

    One of the following 7th characters is to be assigned to codes in subcategories E10.32, E10.33, E10.34, E10.35, and E10.37 to designate laterality of the disease:
    1   right eye
    2   left eye
    3   bilateral
    9   unspecified eye

    ✓6ᵗʰ E10.31 Type 1 diabetes mellitus with unspecified diabetic retinopathy

        E10.311 Type 1 diabetes mellitus with unspecified diabetic retinopathy with macular edema ▽

        E10.319 Type 1 diabetes mellitus with unspecified diabetic retinopathy without macular edema ▽

    ✓6ᵗʰ E10.32 Type 1 diabetes mellitus with mild nonproliferative diabetic retinopathy
        Type 1 diabetes mellitus with nonproliferative diabetic retinopathy NOS

        ✓7ᵗʰ E10.321 Type 1 diabetes mellitus with mild nonproliferative diabetic retinopathy with macular edema

        ✓7ᵗʰ E10.329 Type 1 diabetes mellitus with mild nonproliferative diabetic retinopathy without macular edema

    ✓6ᵗʰ E10.33 Type 1 diabetes mellitus with moderate nonproliferative **diabetic** retinopathy

        ✓7ᵗʰ E10.331 Type 1 diabetes mellitus with moderate nonproliferative diabetic retinopathy with macular edema

        ✓7ᵗʰ E10.339 Type 1 diabetes mellitus with moderate nonproliferative diabetic retinopathy without macular edema

    ✓6ᵗʰ E10.34 Type 1 diabetes mellitus with severe nonproliferative **diabetic** retinopathy

        ✓7ᵗʰ E10.341 Type 1 diabetes mellitus with severe nonproliferative diabetic retinopathy with macular edema

---

✓ Additional Character Req   ✓x7ᵗʰ Placeholder Alert   Case-Mix Diagnosis   Manifestation   ▽ Unspecified Dx   **EXCLUDES 1** Not coded here   **EXCLUDES 2** Not included here

ICD-10-CM 2018   **509**

√7ᵗʰ **E10.349 Type 1 diabetes mellitus with severe nonproliferative diabetic retinopathy without macular edema**

√6ᵗʰ **E10.35 Type 1 diabetes mellitus with proliferative diabetic retinopathy**

√7ᵗʰ **E10.351 Type 1 diabetes mellitus with proliferative diabetic retinopathy with macular edema**

√7ᵗʰ **E10.352 Type 1 diabetes mellitus with proliferative diabetic retinopathy with traction retinal detachment involving the macula**

√7ᵗʰ **E10.353 Type 1 diabetes mellitus with proliferative diabetic retinopathy with traction retinal detachment not involving the macula**

√7ᵗʰ **E10.354 Type 1 diabetes mellitus with proliferative diabetic retinopathy with combined traction retinal detachment and rhegmatogenous retinal detachment**

√7ᵗʰ **E10.355 Type 1 diabetes mellitus with stable proliferative diabetic retinopathy**

√7ᵗʰ **E10.359 Type 1 diabetes mellitus with proliferative diabetic retinopathy without macular edema**

E10.36 Type 1 diabetes mellitus with diabetic cataract
    AHA: 2016, 4Q, 142

√x7ᵗʰ **E10.37 Type 1 diabetes mellitus with diabetic macular edema, resolved following treatment**

E10.39 Type 1 diabetes mellitus with other diabetic ophthalmic complication
    Use additional code to identify manifestation, such as:
    diabetic glaucoma (H40-H42)

√5ᵗʰ **E10.4 Type 1 diabetes mellitus with neurological complications**

E10.40 Type 1 diabetes mellitus with diabetic neuropathy, unspecified ▽

E10.41 Type 1 diabetes mellitus with diabetic mononeuropathy

E10.42 Type 1 diabetes mellitus with diabetic polyneuropathy
    Type 1 diabetes mellitus with diabetic neuralgia

E10.43 Type 1 diabetes mellitus with diabetic autonomic (poly)neuropathy
    Type 1 diabetes mellitus with diabetic gastroparesis
    AHA: 2013, 4Q, 114

E10.44 Type 1 diabetes mellitus with diabetic amyotrophy

E10.49 Type 1 diabetes mellitus with other diabetic neurological complication

√5ᵗʰ **E10.5 Type 1 diabetes mellitus with circulatory complications**

E10.51 Type 1 diabetes mellitus with diabetic peripheral angiopathy without gangrene

E10.52 Type 1 diabetes mellitus with diabetic peripheral angiopathy with gangrene NRS
    Type 1 diabetes mellitus with diabetic gangrene

E10.59 Type 1 diabetes mellitus with other circulatory complications

√5ᵗʰ **E10.6 Type 1 diabetes mellitus with other specified complications**

√6ᵗʰ **E10.61 Type 1 diabetes mellitus with diabetic arthropathy**

E10.610 Type 1 diabetes mellitus with diabetic neuropathic arthropathy
    Type 1 diabetes mellitus with Charcôt's joints

E10.618 Type 1 diabetes mellitus with other diabetic arthropathy

√6ᵗʰ **E10.62 Type 1 diabetes mellitus with skin complications**

E10.620 Type 1 diabetes mellitus with diabetic dermatitis
    Type 1 diabetes mellitus with diabetic necrobiosis lipoidica

E10.621 Type 1 diabetes mellitus with foot ulcer NRS
    Use additional code to identify site of ulcer (L97.4-, L97.5-)
    TIP: Do not assign a code for diabetic ulcer when the ulcer is closed/resolved or to report history of diabetic ulcers; Z86.31 Personal history of diabetic foot ulcer may be assigned.

E10.622 Type 1 diabetes mellitus with other skin ulcer NRS
    Use additional code to identify site of ulcer (L97.1-L97.9, L98.41-L98.49)

E10.628 Type 1 diabetes mellitus with other skin complications

√6ᵗʰ **E10.63 Type 1 diabetes mellitus with oral complications**

E10.630 Type 1 diabetes mellitus with periodontal disease

E10.638 Type 1 diabetes mellitus with other oral complications

√6ᵗʰ **E10.64 Type 1 diabetes mellitus with hypoglycemia**

E10.641 Type 1 diabetes mellitus with hypoglycemia with coma

E10.649 Type 1 diabetes mellitus with hypoglycemia without coma
    AHA: 2016, 3Q, 42; 2016, 1Q, 13; 2015, 3Q, 21

E10.65 Type 1 diabetes mellitus with hyperglycemia
    AHA: 2013, 3Q, 20

E10.69 Type 1 diabetes mellitus with other specified complication
    Use additional code to identify complication
    AHA: 2016, 4Q, 141; 2016, 1Q, 13

E10.8 Type 1 diabetes mellitus with unspecified complications ▽

E10.9 Type 1 diabetes mellitus without complications

√4ᵗʰ **E11 Type 2 diabetes mellitus**
    INCLUDES   diabetes (mellitus) due to insulin secretory defect
         diabetes NOS
         insulin resistant diabetes (mellitus)
    Use additional code to identify control using:
       insulin (Z79.4)
       oral antidiabetic drugs (Z79.84)
       oral hypoglycemic drugs (Z79.84)
    EXCLUDES 1   *diabetes mellitus due to underlying condition (E08.-)*
         drug or chemical induced diabetes mellitus (E09.-)
         gestational diabetes (O24.4-)
         neonatal diabetes mellitus (P70.2)
         postpancreatectomy diabetes mellitus (E13.-)
         postprocedural diabetes mellitus (E13.-)
         secondary diabetes mellitus NEC (E13.-)
         type 1 diabetes mellitus (E10.-)
    AHA: 2016, 2Q, 10; 2013, 4Q, 114; 2013, 3Q, 20; 2013, 1Q, 26

√5ᵗʰ **E11.0 Type 2 diabetes mellitus with hyperosmolarity**

E11.00 Type 2 diabetes mellitus with hyperosmolarity without nonketotic hyperglycemic-hyperosmolar coma (NKHHC)

E11.01 Type 2 diabetes mellitus with hyperosmolarity with coma

● √5ᵗʰ **E11.1 Type 2 diabetes mellitus with ketoacidosis**

● **E11.10 Type 2 diabetes mellitus with ketoacidosis without coma**

● **E11.11 Type 2 diabetes mellitus with ketoacidosis with coma**

√5ᵗʰ **E11.2 Type 2 diabetes mellitus with kidney complications**

E11.21 Type 2 diabetes mellitus with diabetic nephropathy
    Type 2 diabetes mellitus with intercapillary glomerulosclerosis
    Type 2 diabetes mellitus with intracapillary glomerulonephrosis
    Type 2 diabetes mellitus with Kimmelstiel-Wilson disease

E11.22 Type 2 diabetes mellitus with diabetic chronic kidney disease
    Use additional code to identify stage of chronic kidney disease (N18.1-N18.6)
    AHA: 2016, 1Q, 12

E11.29 Type 2 diabetes mellitus with other diabetic kidney complication
    Type 2 diabetes mellitus with renal tubular degeneration

√5ᵗʰ **E11.3 Type 2 diabetes mellitus with ophthalmic complications**

One of the following 7th characters is to be assigned to codes in subcategories E11.32, E11.33, E11.34, E11.35, and E11.37 to designate laterality of the disease:
1   right eye
2   left eye
3   bilateral
9   unspecified eye

√6ᵗʰ **E11.31 Type 2 diabetes mellitus with unspecified diabetic retinopathy**

E11.311 Type 2 diabetes mellitus with unspecified diabetic retinopathy with macular edema ▽

E11.319 **Type 2 diabetes mellitus with unspecified diabetic retinopathy** without macular edema ▽

√6ᵗʰ E11.32 **Type 2 diabetes mellitus with** mild nonproliferative **diabetic** retinopathy
Type 2 diabetes mellitus with nonproliferative diabetic retinopathy NOS

√7ᵗʰ E11.321 **Type 2 diabetes mellitus with mild nonproliferative diabetic retinopathy with macular edema**

√7ᵗʰ E11.329 **Type 2 diabetes mellitus with mild nonproliferative diabetic retinopathy without macular edema**

√6ᵗʰ E11.33 **Type 2 diabetes mellitus with** moderate nonproliferative **diabetic** retinopathy

√7ᵗʰ E11.331 **Type 2 diabetes mellitus with moderate nonproliferative diabetic retinopathy with macular edema**

√7ᵗʰ E11.339 **Type 2 diabetes mellitus with moderate nonproliferative diabetic retinopathy without macular edema**

√6ᵗʰ E11.34 **Type 2 diabetes mellitus with** severe nonproliferative **diabetic** retinopathy

√7ᵗʰ E11.341 **Type 2 diabetes mellitus with severe nonproliferative diabetic retinopathy with macular edema**

√7ᵗʰ E11.349 **Type 2 diabetes mellitus with severe nonproliferative diabetic retinopathy without macular edema**

√6ᵗʰ E11.35 **Type 2 diabetes mellitus with** proliferative diabetic retinopathy

√7ᵗʰ E11.351 **Type 2 diabetes mellitus with proliferative diabetic retinopathy** with macular edema

√7ᵗʰ E11.352 **Type 2 diabetes mellitus with proliferative diabetic retinopathy** with traction retinal detachment involving the macula

√7ᵗʰ E11.353 **Type 2 diabetes mellitus with proliferative diabetic retinopathy** with traction retinal detachment not involving the macula

√7ᵗʰ E11.354 **Type 2 diabetes mellitus with proliferative diabetic retinopathy** with combined traction retinal detachment and rhegmatogenous retinal detachment

√7ᵗʰ E11.355 **Type 2 diabetes mellitus** with stable proliferative diabetic retinopathy

√7ᵗʰ E11.359 **Type 2 diabetes mellitus with proliferative diabetic retinopathy** without macular edema

E11.36 **Type 2 diabetes mellitus with diabetic** cataract
AHA: 2016, 4Q, 142

√x7ᵗʰ E11.37 **Type 2 diabetes mellitus with diabetic** macular edema, resolved following treatment

E11.39 **Type 2 diabetes mellitus with other diabetic ophthalmic complication**
Use additional code to identify manifestation, such as:
diabetic glaucoma (H40-H42)

√5ᵗʰ E11.4 **Type 2 diabetes mellitus with** neurological complications

E11.40 **Type 2 diabetes mellitus with diabetic** neuropathy, unspecified ▽
AHA: 2013, 4Q, 129

E11.41 **Type 2 diabetes mellitus with diabetic** mononeuropathy

E11.42 **Type 2 diabetes mellitus with diabetic** polyneuropathy
Type 2 diabetes mellitus with diabetic neuralgia
AHA: 2016, 1Q, 12

E11.43 **Type 2 diabetes mellitus with diabetic** autonomic (poly)neuropathy
Type 2 diabetes mellitus with diabetic gastroparesis
AHA: 2013, 4Q, 114

E11.44 **Type 2 diabetes mellitus with diabetic amyotrophy**

E11.49 **Type 2 diabetes mellitus with other diabetic neurological complication**

√5ᵗʰ E11.5 **Type 2 diabetes mellitus with** circulatory complications

E11.51 **Type 2 diabetes mellitus with diabetic** peripheral angiopathy without gangrene

E11.52 **Type 2 diabetes mellitus with diabetic** peripheral angiopathy with gangrene   **NRS**
Type 2 diabetes mellitus with diabetic gangrene

E11.59 **Type 2 diabetes mellitus with other circulatory complications**

√5ᵗʰ E11.6 **Type 2 diabetes mellitus with** other specified complications

√6ᵗʰ E11.61 **Type 2 diabetes mellitus with** diabetic arthropathy

E11.610 **Type 2 diabetes mellitus with diabetic neuropathic arthropathy**
Type 2 diabetes mellitus with Charcôt's joints

E11.618 **Type 2 diabetes mellitus with other diabetic arthropathy**

√6ᵗʰ E11.62 **Type 2 diabetes mellitus with** skin complications

E11.620 **Type 2 diabetes mellitus with diabetic dermatitis**
Type 2 diabetes mellitus with diabetic necrobiosis lipoidica

E11.621 **Type 2 diabetes mellitus with** foot ulcer   **NRS**
Use additional code to identify site of ulcer (L97.4-, L97.5-)
AHA: 2016, 1Q, 12
TIP: Do not assign a code for diabetic ulcer when the ulcer is closed/resolved or to report history of diabetic ulcers; Z86.31 Personal history of diabetic foot ulcer may be assigned.

E11.622 **Type 2 diabetes mellitus with** other skin ulcer   **NRS**
Use additional code to identify site of ulcer (L97.1-L97.9, L98.41-L98.49)

E11.628 **Type 2 diabetes mellitus with other skin complications**

√6ᵗʰ E11.63 **Type 2 diabetes mellitus with** oral complications

E11.630 **Type 2 diabetes mellitus with** periodontal disease

E11.638 **Type 2 diabetes mellitus with other oral complications**

√6ᵗʰ E11.64 **Type 2 diabetes mellitus with** hypoglycemia

E11.641 **Type 2 diabetes mellitus with hypoglycemia** with coma

E11.649 **Type 2 diabetes mellitus with hypoglycemia** without coma
AHA: 2016, 3Q, 42; 2015, 3Q, 21

E11.65 **Type 2 diabetes mellitus with** hyperglycemia
AHA: 2013, 3Q, 20

E11.69 **Type 2 diabetes mellitus with other specified complication**
Use additional code to identify complication
AHA: 2016, 4Q, 141; 2016, 1Q, 13

E11.8 **Type 2 diabetes mellitus with unspecified complications** ▽

E11.9 **Type 2 diabetes mellitus** without complications

√4ᵗʰ E13 Other specified **diabetes mellitus**
INCLUDES   diabetes mellitus due to genetic defects of beta-cell function
diabetes mellitus due to genetic defects in insulin action
postpancreatectomy diabetes mellitus
postprocedural diabetes mellitus
secondary diabetes mellitus NEC
Use additional code to identify control using:
insulin (Z79.4)
oral antidiabetic drugs (Z79.84)
oral hypoglycemic drugs (Z79.84)
EXCLUDES 1   *diabetes (mellitus) due to autoimmune process (E10.-)*
diabetes (mellitus) due to immune mediated pancreatic islet beta-cell destruction (E10.-)
diabetes mellitus due to underlying condition (E08.-)
drug or chemical induced diabetes mellitus (E09.-)
gestational diabetes (O24.4-)
neonatal diabetes mellitus (P70.2)
type 1 diabetes mellitus (E10.-)
~~*type 2 diabetes mellitus (E11.-)*~~
AHA: 2013, 4Q, 114; 2013, 3Q, 20
TIP: Postprocedural hypoinsulinemia (E89.1) identifies diabetes mellitus resulting from pancreatectomy and should be assigned before E13.

√5ᵗʰ E13.0 **Other specified diabetes mellitus with** hyperosmolarity

E13.00 **Other specified diabetes mellitus with hyperosmolarity** without nonketotic hyperglycemic-hyperosmolar coma (NKHHC)
EXCLUDES 2 ▶*type 2 diabetes mellitus (E11.-)*◀

E13.01 **Other specified diabetes mellitus with hyperosmolarity** with coma

E13.1 Other specified diabetes mellitus with ketoacidosis
AHA: 2016, 2Q, 10; 2013, 1Q, 26

E13.10 Other specified diabetes mellitus with ketoacidosis without coma

E13.11 Other specified diabetes mellitus with ketoacidosis with coma

E13.2 Other specified diabetes mellitus with kidney complications

E13.21 Other specified diabetes mellitus with diabetic nephropathy
Other specified diabetes mellitus with intercapillary glomerulosclerosis
Other specified diabetes mellitus with intracapillary glomerulonephrosis
Other specified diabetes mellitus with Kimmelstiel-Wilson disease

E13.22 Other specified diabetes mellitus with diabetic chronic kidney disease
Use additional code to identify stage of chronic kidney disease (N18.1-N18.6)

E13.29 Other specified diabetes mellitus with other diabetic kidney complication
Other specified diabetes mellitus with renal tubular degeneration

E13.3 Other specified diabetes mellitus with ophthalmic complications

One of the following 7th characters is to be assigned to codes in subcategories E13.32, E13.33, E13.34, E13.35, and E13.37 to designate laterality of the disease:
1 right eye
2 left eye
3 bilateral
9 unspecified eye

E13.31 Other specified diabetes mellitus with unspecified diabetic retinopathy

E13.311 Other specified diabetes mellitus with unspecified diabetic retinopathy with macular edema

E13.319 Other specified diabetes mellitus with unspecified diabetic retinopathy without macular edema

E13.32 Other specified diabetes mellitus with mild nonproliferative diabetic retinopathy
Other specified diabetes mellitus with nonproliferative diabetic retinopathy NOS

E13.321 Other specified diabetes mellitus with mild nonproliferative diabetic retinopathy with macular edema

E13.329 Other specified diabetes mellitus with mild nonproliferative diabetic retinopathy without macular edema

E13.33 Other specified diabetes mellitus with moderate nonproliferative diabetic retinopathy

E13.331 Other specified diabetes mellitus with moderate nonproliferative diabetic retinopathy with macular edema

E13.339 Other specified diabetes mellitus with moderate nonproliferative diabetic retinopathy without macular edema

E13.34 Other specified diabetes mellitus with severe nonproliferative diabetic retinopathy

E13.341 Other specified diabetes mellitus with severe nonproliferative diabetic retinopathy with macular edema

E13.349 Other specified diabetes mellitus with severe nonproliferative diabetic retinopathy without macular edema

E13.35 Other specified diabetes mellitus with proliferative diabetic retinopathy

E13.351 Other specified diabetes mellitus with proliferative diabetic retinopathy with macular edema

E13.352 Other specified diabetes mellitus with proliferative diabetic retinopathy with traction retinal detachment involving the macula

E13.353 Other specified diabetes mellitus with proliferative diabetic retinopathy with traction retinal detachment not involving the macula

E13.354 Other specified diabetes mellitus with proliferative diabetic retinopathy with combined traction retinal detachment and rhegmatogenous retinal detachment

E13.355 Other specified diabetes mellitus with stable proliferative diabetic retinopathy

E13.359 Other specified diabetes mellitus with proliferative diabetic retinopathy without macular edema

E13.36 Other specified diabetes mellitus with diabetic cataract
AHA: 2016, 4Q, 142

E13.37 Other specified diabetes mellitus with diabetic macular edema, resolved following treatment

E13.39 Other specified diabetes mellitus with other diabetic ophthalmic complication
Use additional code to identify manifestation, such as:
diabetic glaucoma (H40-H42)

E13.4 Other specified diabetes mellitus with neurological complications

E13.40 Other specified diabetes mellitus with diabetic neuropathy, unspecified

E13.41 Other specified diabetes mellitus with diabetic mononeuropathy

E13.42 Other specified diabetes mellitus with diabetic polyneuropathy
Other specified diabetes mellitus with diabetic neuralgia

E13.43 Other specified diabetes mellitus with diabetic autonomic (poly)neuropathy
Other specified diabetes mellitus with diabetic gastroparesis
AHA: 2013, 4Q, 114

E13.44 Other specified diabetes mellitus with diabetic amyotrophy

E13.49 Other specified diabetes mellitus with other diabetic neurological complication

E13.5 Other specified diabetes mellitus with circulatory complications

E13.51 Other specified diabetes mellitus with diabetic peripheral angiopathy without gangrene

E13.52 Other specified diabetes mellitus with diabetic peripheral angiopathy with gangrene
Other specified diabetes mellitus with diabetic gangrene

E13.59 Other specified diabetes mellitus with other circulatory complications

E13.6 Other specified diabetes mellitus with other specified complications

E13.61 Other specified diabetes mellitus with diabetic arthropathy

E13.610 Other specified diabetes mellitus with diabetic neuropathic arthropathy
Other specified diabetes mellitus with Charcôt's joints

E13.618 Other specified diabetes mellitus with other diabetic arthropathy

E13.62 Other specified diabetes mellitus with skin complications

E13.620 Other specified diabetes mellitus with diabetic dermatitis
Other specified diabetes mellitus with diabetic necrobiosis lipoidica

E13.621 Other specified diabetes mellitus with foot ulcer
Use additional code to identify site of ulcer (L97.4-, L97.5-)
TIP: Do not assign a code for diabetic ulcer when the ulcer is closed/resolved or to report history of diabetic ulcers; Z86.31 Personal history of diabetic foot ulcer may be assigned.

E13.622 Other specified diabetes mellitus with other skin ulcer
Use additional code to identify site of ulcer (L97.1-L97.9, L98.41-L98.49)

E13.628 Other specified diabetes mellitus with other skin complications

N Newborn: 0 P Pediatric: 0-17 M Maternity: 12-55 A Adult: 15-124 NRS Nonroutine supply Dx NC-Dx Noncancer Dx PDx Primary Dx ►◄ Revised Text ● New Code ▲ Revised Title

512 ICD-10-CM 2018

☑6ᵗʰ **E13.63** **Other specified diabetes mellitus with** oral complications

E13.630 **Other specified diabetes mellitus with** periodontal disease

E13.638 **Other specified diabetes mellitus with** other oral complications

☑6ᵗʰ **E13.64** **Other specified diabetes mellitus with** hypoglycemia

E13.641 **Other specified diabetes mellitus with hypoglycemia** with coma

E13.649 **Other specified diabetes mellitus with hypoglycemia** without coma
AHA: 2016, 3Q, 42; 2015, 3Q, 21

E13.65 **Other specified diabetes mellitus with** hyperglycemia

E13.69 **Other specified diabetes mellitus with other specified complication**
Use additional code to identify complication
AHA: 2016, 4Q, 141; 2016, 1Q, 13

E13.8 **Other specified diabetes mellitus with unspecified complications** ▽

E13.9 **Other specified diabetes mellitus** without complications

Other disorders of glucose regulation and pancreatic internal secretion (E15-E16)

E15 **Nondiabetic hypoglycemic coma**
INCLUDES drug-induced insulin coma in nondiabetic
hyperinsulinism with hypoglycemic coma
hypoglycemic coma NOS

☑4ᵗʰ **E16** **Other disorders of pancreatic internal secretion**

E16.0 **Drug-induced hypoglycemia without coma**
Use additional code for adverse effect, if applicable, to identify drug (T36-T50 with fifth or sixth character 5)
EXCLUDES 1 diabetes with hypoglycemia without coma
▶(E09.649)◀

E16.1 **Other hypoglycemia**
Functional hyperinsulinism
Functional nonhyperinsulinemic hypoglycemia
Hyperinsulinism NOS
Hyperplasia of pancreatic islet beta cells NOS
EXCLUDES 1 diabetes with hypoglycemia (E08.649, E10.649, E11.649, E13.649)
hypoglycemia in infant of diabetic mother (P70.1)
neonatal hypoglycemia (P70.4)

E16.2 **Hypoglycemia, unspecified** ▽
EXCLUDES 1 diabetes with hypoglycemia (E08.649, E10.649, E11.649, E13.649)
AHA: 2016, 3Q, 42

E16.3 **Increased secretion of glucagon**
Hyperplasia of pancreatic endocrine cells with glucagon excess

E16.4 **Increased secretion of gastrin**
Hypergastrinemia
Hyperplasia of pancreatic endocrine cells with gastrin excess
Zollinger-Ellison syndrome

E16.8 **Other specified disorders of pancreatic internal secretion**
Increased secretion from endocrine pancreas of growth hormone-releasing hormone
Increased secretion from endocrine pancreas of pancreatic polypeptide
Increased secretion from endocrine pancreas of somatostatin
Increased secretion from endocrine pancreas of vasoactive-intestinal polypeptide

E16.9 **Disorder of pancreatic internal secretion, unspecified** ▽
Islet-cell hyperplasia NOS
Pancreatic endocrine cell hyperplasia NOS

Disorders of other endocrine glands (E20-E35)

EXCLUDES 1 galactorrhea (N64.3)
gynecomastia (N62)

☑4ᵗʰ **E20** **Hypoparathyroidism**
EXCLUDES 1 Di George's syndrome (D82.1)
postprocedural hypoparathyroidism (E89.2)
tetany NOS (R29.0)
transitory neonatal hypoparathyroidism (P71.4)

E20.0 **Idiopathic hypoparathyroidism**
DEF: Abnormally low secretion of parathyroid hormones, with unknown cause, which causes decreased calcium and increased phosphorus in the blood, resulting in muscle cramps, tetany, tingling, or burning in lips, fingers, and toes, and cataracts.

E20.1 **Pseudohypoparathyroidism**

E20.8 **Other hypoparathyroidism**

E20.9 **Hypoparathyroidism, unspecified** ▽
Parathyroid tetany

☑4ᵗʰ **E21** **Hyperparathyroidism and other disorders of parathyroid gland**
EXCLUDES 1 adult osteomalacia (M83.-)
ectopic hyperparathyroidism (E34.2)
familial hypocalciuric hypercalcemia (E83.52)
hungry bone syndrome (E83.81)
infantile and juvenile osteomalacia (E55.0)

E21.0 **Primary hyperparathyroidism**
Hyperplasia of parathyroid
Osteitis fibrosa cystica generalisata [von Recklinghausen's disease of bone]
DEF: Parathyroid dysfunction commonly caused by hyperplasia of two or more glands; characteristic hypercalcemia and increased parathyroid hormone levels.

E21.1 **Secondary hyperparathyroidism, not elsewhere classified**
EXCLUDES 1 secondary hyperparathyroidism of renal origin (N25.81)

E21.2 **Other hyperparathyroidism**
Tertiary hyperparathyroidism
EXCLUDES 1 familial hypocalciuric hypercalcemia (E83.52)

E21.3 **Hyperparathyroidism, unspecified** ▽

E21.4 **Other specified disorders of parathyroid gland**

E21.5 **Disorder of parathyroid gland, unspecified** ▽

☑4ᵗʰ **E22** **Hyperfunction of pituitary gland**
EXCLUDES 1 Cushing's syndrome (E24.-)
Nelson's syndrome (E24.1)
overproduction of ACTH not associated with Cushing's disease (E27.0)
overproduction of pituitary ACTH (E24.0)
overproduction of thyroid-stimulating hormone (E05.8-)

E22.0 **Acromegaly and pituitary gigantism**
Overproduction of growth hormone
EXCLUDES 1 constitutional gigantism (E34.4)
constitutional tall stature (E34.4)
increased secretion from endocrine pancreas of growth hormone-releasing hormone (E16.8)

E22.1 **Hyperprolactinemia**
Use additional code for adverse effect, if applicable, to identify drug (T36-T50 with fifth or sixth character 5)

E22.2 **Syndrome of inappropriate secretion of antidiuretic hormone**

E22.8 **Other hyperfunction of pituitary gland**
Central precocious puberty

E22.9 **Hyperfunction of pituitary gland, unspecified** ▽

☑4ᵗʰ **E23** **Hypofunction and other disorders of the pituitary gland**
INCLUDES the listed conditions whether the disorder is in the pituitary or the hypothalamus
EXCLUDES 1 postprocedural hypopituitarism (E89.3)

E23.0 **Hypopituitarism**
Fertile eunuch syndrome
Hypogonadotropic hypogonadism
Idiopathic growth hormone deficiency
Isolated deficiency of gonadotropin
Isolated deficiency of growth hormone
Isolated deficiency of pituitary hormone
Kallmann's syndrome
Lorain-Levi short stature
Necrosis of pituitary gland (postpartum)
Panhypopituitarism
Pituitary cachexia
Pituitary insufficiency NOS
Pituitary short stature
Sheehan's syndrome
Simmonds' disease

E23.1 **Drug-induced hypopituitarism**
Use additional code for adverse effect, if applicable, to identify drug (T36-T50 with fifth or sixth character 5)

E23.2 **Diabetes insipidus**
EXCLUDES 1 nephrogenic diabetes insipidus (N25.1)

E23.3 **Hypothalamic dysfunction, not elsewhere classified**
EXCLUDES 1 Prader-Willi syndrome (Q87.1)
Russell-Silver syndrome (Q87.1)

E23.6 **Other disorders of pituitary gland**
Abscess of pituitary
Adiposogenital dystrophy

E23.7 **Disorder of pituitary gland, unspecified** ▽

✓4th **E24 Cushing's syndrome**
> EXCLUDES1   congenital adrenal hyperplasia (E25.0)

E24.0 Pituitary-dependent Cushing's disease
> Overproduction of pituitary ACTH
> Pituitary-dependent hypercorticalism

E24.1 Nelson's syndrome

E24.2 Drug-induced Cushing's syndrome
> Use additional code for adverse effect, if applicable, to identify drug (T36-T50 with fifth or sixth character 5)

E24.3 Ectopic ACTH syndrome

E24.4 Alcohol-induced pseudo-Cushing's syndrome

E24.8 Other Cushing's syndrome

E24.9 Cushing's syndrome, unspecified ▽

✓4th **E25 Adrenogenital disorders**
> INCLUDES   adrenogenital syndromes, virilizing or feminizing, whether acquired or due to adrenal hyperplasia
> consequent on inborn enzyme defects in hormone synthesis
> female adrenal pseudohermaphroditism
> female heterosexual precocious pseudopuberty
> male isosexual precocious pseudopuberty
> male macrogenitosomia praecox
> male sexual precocity with adrenal hyperplasia
> male virilization (female)
>
> EXCLUDES1   indeterminate sex and pseudohermaphroditism (Q56)
> chromosomal abnormalities (Q90-Q99)

E25.0 Congenital adrenogenital disorders associated with enzyme deficiency
> Congenital adrenal hyperplasia
> 21-Hydroxylase deficiency
> Salt-losing congenital adrenal hyperplasia

E25.8 Other adrenogenital disorders
> Idiopathic adrenogenital disorder
> Use additional code for adverse effect, if applicable, to identify drug (T36-T50 with fifth or sixth character 5)

E25.9 Adrenogenital disorder, unspecified ▽
> Adrenogenital syndrome NOS

✓4th **E26 Hyperaldosteronism**

✓5th **E26.0 Primary hyperaldosteronism**

E26.01 Conn's syndrome
> Code also adrenal adenoma (D35.0-)

E26.02 Glucocorticoid-remediable aldosteronism
> Familial aldosteronism type I
> **DEF:** Rare autosomal dominant familial form of primary aldosteronism in which the secretion of aldosterone is under the influence of adrenocorticotrophic hormone (ACTH) rather than the renin-angiotensin mechanism; moderate hypersecretion of aldosterone and suppressed plasma renin activity that are rapidly reversed by administration of glucosteroids; symptoms include hypertension and mild hypokalemia.

E26.09 Other primary hyperaldosteronism
> Primary aldosteronism due to adrenal hyperplasia (bilateral)

E26.1 Secondary hyperaldosteronism

✓5th **E26.8 Other hyperaldosteronism**

E26.81 Bartter's syndrome

E26.89 Other hyperaldosteronism

E26.9 Hyperaldosteronism, unspecified ▽
> Aldosteronism NOS
> Hyperaldosteronism NOS

✓4th **E27 Other disorders of adrenal gland**

E27.0 Other adrenocortical overactivity
> Overproduction of ACTH, not associated with Cushing's disease
> Premature adrenarche
> EXCLUDES1   Cushing's syndrome (E24.-)

E27.1 Primary adrenocortical insufficiency
> Addison's disease
> Autoimmune adrenalitis
> EXCLUDES1   Addison only phenotype adrenoleukodystrophy (E71.528)
> amyloidosis (E85.-)
> tuberculous Addison's disease (A18.7)
> Waterhouse-Friderichsen syndrome (A39.1)

E27.2 Addisonian crisis
> Adrenal crisis
> Adrenocortical crisis

E27.3 Drug-induced adrenocortical insufficiency
> Use additional code for adverse effect, if applicable, to identify drug (T36-T50 with fifth or sixth character 5)

✓5th **E27.4 Other and unspecified adrenocortical insufficiency**
> EXCLUDES1   adrenoleukodystrophy [Addison-Schilder] (E71.528)
> Waterhouse-Friderichsen syndrome (A39.1)

E27.40 Unspecified adrenocortical insufficiency ▽
> Adrenocortical insufficiency NOS
> Hypoaldosteronism

E27.49 Other adrenocortical insufficiency
> Adrenal hemorrhage
> Adrenal infarction

E27.5 Adrenomedullary hyperfunction
> Adrenomedullary hyperplasia
> Catecholamine hypersecretion

E27.8 Other specified disorders of adrenal gland
> Abnormality of cortisol-binding globulin

E27.9 Disorder of adrenal gland, unspecified ▽

✓4th **E28 Ovarian dysfunction**
> EXCLUDES1   isolated gonadotropin deficiency (E23.0)
> postprocedural ovarian failure (E89.4-)

E28.0 Estrogen excess ♀
> Use additional code for adverse effect, if applicable, to identify drug (T36-T50 with fifth or sixth character 5)

E28.1 Androgen excess ♀
> Hypersecretion of ovarian androgens
> Use additional code for adverse effect, if applicable, to identify drug (T36-T50 with fifth or sixth character 5)

E28.2 Polycystic ovarian syndrome ♀
> Sclerocystic ovary syndrome
> Stein-Leventhal syndrome

✓5th **E28.3 Primary ovarian failure**
> EXCLUDES1   pure gonadal dysgenesis (Q99.1)
> Turner's syndrome (Q96.-)

✓6th **E28.31 Premature menopause**

E28.310 Symptomatic premature menopause A ♀
> Symptoms such as flushing, sleeplessness, headache, lack of concentration, associated with premature menopause

E28.319 Asymptomatic premature menopause A ♀
> Premature menopause NOS

E28.39 Other primary ovarian failure ♀
> Decreased estrogen
> Resistant ovary syndrome

E28.8 Other ovarian dysfunction ♀
> Ovarian hyperfunction NOS
> EXCLUDES1   postprocedural ovarian failure (E89.4-)

E28.9 Ovarian dysfunction, unspecified ♀ ▽

✓4th **E29 Testicular dysfunction**
> EXCLUDES1   androgen insensitivity syndrome (E34.5-)
> azoospermia or oligospermia NOS (N46.0-N46.1)
> isolated gonadotropin deficiency (E23.0)
> Klinefelter's syndrome (Q98.0-Q98.1, Q98.4)

E29.0 Testicular hyperfunction ♂
> Hypersecretion of testicular hormones

E29.1 Testicular hypofunction ♂
> Defective biosynthesis of testicular androgen NOS
> 5-delta-Reductase deficiency (with male pseudohermaphroditism)
> Testicular hypogonadism NOS
> Use additional code for adverse effect, if applicable, to identify drug (T36-T50 with fifth or sixth character 5)
> EXCLUDES1   postprocedural testicular hypofunction (E89.5)

E29.8 Other testicular dysfunction ♂

E29.9 Testicular dysfunction, unspecified ♂ ▽

✓4th **E30 Disorders of puberty, not elsewhere classified**

E30.0 Delayed puberty
> Constitutional delay of puberty
> Delayed sexual development

E30.1 Precocious puberty P
> Precocious menstruation
> EXCLUDES1   Albright (-McCune) (-Sternberg) syndrome (Q78.1)
> central precocious puberty (E22.8)
> congenital adrenal hyperplasia (E25.0)
> female heterosexual precocious pseudopuberty (E25.-)
> male isosexual precocious pseudopuberty (E25.-)

N Newborn: 0   P Pediatric: 0-17   M Maternity: 12-55   A Adult: 15-124   NRS Nonroutine supply Dx   NCDx Noncancer Dx   PDx Primary Dx   ►◄ Revised Text   ● New Code   ▲ Revised Title

E30.8　**Other disorders of puberty**　　　　🅿
　　　　Premature thelarche

E30.9　**Disorder of puberty, unspecified**　　　▽

✓4th E31　**Polyglandular dysfunction**
　　　　EXCLUDES 1　ataxia telangiectasia [Louis-Bar] (G11.3)
　　　　　　　　dystrophia myotonica [Steinert] (G71.11)
　　　　　　　　pseudohypoparathyroidism (E20.1)

E31.0　**Autoimmune polyglandular failure**
　　　　Schmidt's syndrome

E31.1　**Polyglandular hyperfunction**
　　　　EXCLUDES 1　multiple endocrine adenomatosis (E31.2-)
　　　　　　　　multiple endocrine neoplasia (E31.2-)

✓5th E31.2　**Multiple endocrine neoplasia [MEN] syndromes**
　　　　Multiple endocrine adenomatosis
　　　　Code also any associated malignancies and other conditions
　　　　　associated with the syndromes

　　　E31.20　**Multiple endocrine neoplasia [MEN] syndrome,**　▽
　　　　　　unspecified
　　　　　　Multiple endocrine adenomatosis NOS
　　　　　　Multiple endocrine neoplasia [MEN] syndrome NOS

　　　E31.21　**Multiple endocrine neoplasia [MEN] type I**
　　　　　　Wermer's syndrome

　　　E31.22　**Multiple endocrine neoplasia [MEN] type IIA**
　　　　　　Sipple's syndrome

　　　E31.23　**Multiple endocrine neoplasia [MEN] type IIB**

E31.8　**Other polyglandular dysfunction**

E31.9　**Polyglandular dysfunction, unspecified**　　　▽

✓4th E32　**Diseases of thymus**
　　　　EXCLUDES 1　aplasia or hypoplasia of thymus with immunodeficiency (D82.1)
　　　　　　　　myasthenia gravis (G70.0)

E32.0　**Persistent hyperplasia of thymus**
　　　　Hypertrophy of thymus

E32.1　**Abscess of thymus**

E32.8　**Other diseases of thymus**
　　　　EXCLUDES 1　aplasia or hypoplasia with immunodeficiency (D82.1)
　　　　　　　　thymoma (D15.0)

E32.9　**Disease of thymus, unspecified**　　　▽

✓4th E34　**Other endocrine disorders**
　　　　EXCLUDES 1　pseudohypoparathyroidism (E20.1)

E34.0　**Carcinoid syndrome**
　　　　NOTE　May be used as an additional code to identify
　　　　　　functional activity associated with a carcinoid tumor.

E34.1　**Other hypersecretion of intestinal hormones**

E34.2　**Ectopic hormone secretion, not elsewhere classified**
　　　　EXCLUDES 1　ectopic ACTH syndrome (E24.3)

E34.3　**Short stature due to endocrine disorder**
　　　　Constitutional short stature
　　　　Laron-type short stature
　　　　EXCLUDES 1　achondroplastic short stature (Q77.4)
　　　　　　　　hypochondroplastic short stature (Q77.4)
　　　　　　　　nutritional short stature (E45)
　　　　　　　　pituitary short stature (E23.0)
　　　　　　　　progeria (E34.8)
　　　　　　　　renal short stature (N25.0)
　　　　　　　　Russell-Silver syndrome (Q87.1)
　　　　　　　　short-limbed stature with immunodeficiency (D82.2)
　　　　　　　　short stature in specific dysmorphic syndromes— code
　　　　　　　　　to syndrome—see Alphabetical Index
　　　　　　　　short stature NOS (R62.52)

E34.4　**Constitutional tall stature**
　　　　Constitutional gigantism

✓5th E34.5　**Androgen insensitivity syndrome**

　　　E34.50　**Androgen insensitivity syndrome, unspecified**　▽
　　　　　　Androgen insensitivity NOS

　　　E34.51　**Complete androgen insensitivity syndrome**
　　　　　　Complete androgen insensitivity
　　　　　　de Quervain syndrome
　　　　　　Goldberg-Maxwell syndrome

　　　E34.52　**Partial androgen insensitivity syndrome**
　　　　　　Partial androgen insensitivity
　　　　　　Reifenstein syndrome

E34.8　**Other specified endocrine disorders**
　　　　Pineal gland dysfunction
　　　　Progeria
　　　　EXCLUDES 2　pseudohypoparathyroidism (E20.1)

E34.9　**Endocrine disorder, unspecified**　　　▽
　　　　Endocrine disturbance NOS
　　　　Hormone disturbance NOS

E35　***Disorders of endocrine glands in diseases classified elsewhere***
　　　　Code first underlying disease, such as:
　　　　　late congenital syphilis of thymus gland [Dubois disease] (A50.5)
　　　　Use additional code, if applicable, to identify:
　　　　　sequelae of tuberculosis of other organs (B90.8)
　　　　EXCLUDES 1　Echinococcus granulosus infection of thyroid gland (B67.3)
　　　　　　　　meningococcal hemorrhagic adrenalitis (A39.1)
　　　　　　　　syphilis of endocrine gland (A52.79)
　　　　　　　　tuberculosis of adrenal gland, except calcification (A18.7)
　　　　　　　　tuberculosis of endocrine gland NEC (A18.82)
　　　　　　　　tuberculosis of thyroid gland (A18.81)
　　　　　　　　Waterhouse-Friderichsen syndrome (A39.1)

Intraoperative complications of endocrine system (E36)

✓4th E36　**Intraoperative complications of endocrine system**
　　　　EXCLUDES 2　postprocedural endocrine and metabolic complications and
　　　　　　　　disorders, not elsewhere classified (E89.-)

✓5th E36.0　**Intraoperative hemorrhage and hematoma of an endocrine**
　　　　system organ or structure complicating a procedure
　　　　EXCLUDES 1　intraoperative hemorrhage and hematoma of an
　　　　　　　　endocrine system organ or structure due to
　　　　　　　　accidental puncture or laceration during a
　　　　　　　　procedure (E36.1-)

　　　E36.01　**Intraoperative hemorrhage and hematoma of an**
　　　　　　endocrine system organ or structure complicating
　　　　　　an endocrine system procedure

　　　E36.02　**Intraoperative hemorrhage and hematoma of an**
　　　　　　endocrine system organ or structure complicating
　　　　　　other procedure

✓5th E36.1　**Accidental puncture and laceration of an endocrine system**
　　　　organ or structure during a procedure

　　　E36.11　**Accidental puncture and laceration of an endocrine**
　　　　　　system organ or structure during an endocrine
　　　　　　system procedure

　　　E36.12　**Accidental puncture and laceration of an endocrine**
　　　　　　system organ or structure during other procedure

　　　E36.8　**Other intraoperative complications of endocrine system**
　　　　　　Use additional code, if applicable, to further specify disorder

Malnutrition (E40-E46)

EXCLUDES 1　intestinal malabsorption (K90.-)
　　　　sequelae of protein-calorie malnutrition (E64.0)
EXCLUDES 2　nutritional anemias (D50-D53)
　　　　starvation (T73.0)

E40　**Kwashiorkor**
　　　　Severe malnutrition with nutritional edema with dyspigmentation of
　　　　　skin and hair
　　　　EXCLUDES 1　marasmic kwashiorkor (E42)

E41　**Nutritional marasmus**
　　　　Severe malnutrition with marasmus
　　　　EXCLUDES 1　marasmic kwashiorkor (E42)
　　　　DEF: Protein-calorie malabsorption or malnutrition in children;
　　　　characterized by tissue wasting, dehydration, and subcutaneous fat
　　　　depletion; may occur with infectious disease; also called infantile atrophy.

E42　**Marasmic kwashiorkor**
　　　　Intermediate form severe protein-calorie malnutrition
　　　　Severe protein-calorie malnutrition with signs of both kwashiorkor and
　　　　　marasmus

E43　**Unspecified severe protein-calorie malnutrition**　　　▽
　　　　Starvation edema

✓4th E44　**Protein-calorie malnutrition of moderate and mild degree**

　　　E44.0　**Moderate protein-calorie malnutrition**

　　　E44.1　**Mild protein-calorie malnutrition**

E45　**Retarded development following protein-calorie malnutrition**
　　　　Nutritional short stature
　　　　Nutritional stunting
　　　　Physical retardation due to malnutrition

E46　**Unspecified protein-calorie malnutrition**　　　▽
　　　　Malnutrition NOS
　　　　Protein-calorie imbalance NOS
　　　　EXCLUDES 1　nutritional deficiency NOS (E63.9)

Other nutritional deficiencies (E50-E64)

EXCLUDES 2   *nutritional anemias (D50-D53)*

✓4ᵗʰ E50   Vitamin A deficiency
> *EXCLUDES 1*   *sequelae of vitamin A deficiency (E64.1)*

    E50.0   Vitamin A deficiency with conjunctival xerosis

    E50.1   Vitamin A deficiency with Bitot's spot and conjunctival xerosis
> Bitot's spot in the young child
> **DEF:** Vitamin A deficiency with conjunctival dryness, superficial spots of keratinized epithelium.

    E50.2   Vitamin A deficiency with corneal xerosis

    E50.3   Vitamin A deficiency with corneal ulceration and xerosis

    E50.4   Vitamin A deficiency with keratomalacia
> **DEF:** Vitamin A deficiency creating corneal dryness; progresses to corneal insensitivity, softness, and necrosis; usually bilateral.

    E50.5   Vitamin A deficiency with night blindness

    E50.6   Vitamin A deficiency with xerophthalmic scars of cornea

    E50.7   Other ocular manifestations of vitamin A deficiency
> Xerophthalmia NOS

    E50.8   Other manifestations of vitamin A deficiency
> Follicular keratosis
> Xeroderma

    E50.9   Vitamin A deficiency, unspecified ▽
> Hypovitaminosis A NOS

✓4ᵗʰ E51   Thiamine deficiency
> *EXCLUDES 1*   *sequelae of thiamine deficiency (E64.8)*

    ✓5ᵗʰ E51.1   Beriberi

       E51.11   Dry beriberi
> Beriberi NOS
> Beriberi with polyneuropathy

       E51.12   Wet beriberi
> Beriberi with cardiovascular manifestations
> Cardiovascular beriberi
> Shoshin disease

    E51.2   Wernicke's encephalopathy

    E51.8   Other manifestations of thiamine deficiency

    E51.9   Thiamine deficiency, unspecified ▽

E52   Niacin deficiency [pellagra]
> Niacin (-tryptophan) deficiency
> Nicotinamide deficiency
> Pellagra (alcoholic)
> *EXCLUDES 1*   *sequelae of niacin deficiency (E64.8)*

✓4ᵗʰ E53   Deficiency of other B group vitamins
> *EXCLUDES 1*   *sequelae of vitamin B deficiency (E64.8)*

    E53.0   Riboflavin deficiency
> Ariboflavinosis
> Vitamin B2 deficiency

    E53.1   Pyridoxine deficiency
> Vitamin B6 deficiency
> *EXCLUDES 1*   *pyridoxine-responsive sideroblastic anemia (D64.3)*

    E53.8   Deficiency of other specified B group vitamins
> Biotin deficiency   Folic acid deficiency
> Cyanocobalamin deficiency   Pantothenic acid deficiency
> Folate deficiency   Vitamin B12 deficiency
> *EXCLUDES 1*   *folate deficiency anemia (D52.-)*
>   *vitamin B12 deficiency anemia (D51.-)*

    E53.9   Vitamin B deficiency, unspecified ▽

E54   Ascorbic acid deficiency
> Deficiency of vitamin C
> Scurvy
> *EXCLUDES 1*   *scorbutic anemia (D53.2)*
>   *sequelae of vitamin C deficiency (E64.2)*
> **DEF:** Vitamin C deficiency causing swollen gums, myalgia, weight loss, and weakness.

✓4ᵗʰ E55   Vitamin D deficiency
> *EXCLUDES 1*   *adult osteomalacia (M83.-)*
>   *osteoporosis (M80.-)*
>   *sequelae of rickets (E64.3)*

    E55.0   Rickets, active
> Infantile osteomalacia   Juvenile osteomalacia
> *EXCLUDES 1*   *celiac rickets (K90.0)*
>   *Crohn's rickets (K50.-)*
>   *hereditary vitamin D-dependent rickets (E83.32)*
>   *inactive rickets (E64.3)*
>   *renal rickets (N25.0)*
>   *sequelae of rickets (E64.3)*
>   *vitamin D-resistant rickets (E83.31)*

    E55.9   Vitamin D deficiency, unspecified ▽
> Avitaminosis D

✓4ᵗʰ E56   Other vitamin deficiencies
> *EXCLUDES 1*   *sequelae of other vitamin deficiencies (E64.8)*

    E56.0   Deficiency of vitamin E

    E56.1   Deficiency of vitamin K
> *EXCLUDES 1*   *deficiency of coagulation factor due to vitamin K deficiency (D68.4)*
>   *vitamin K deficiency of newborn (P53)*

    E56.8   Deficiency of other vitamins

    E56.9   Vitamin deficiency, unspecified ▽

E58   Dietary calcium deficiency
> *EXCLUDES 1*   *disorders of calcium metabolism (E83.5-)*
>   *sequelae of calcium deficiency (E64.8)*

E59   Dietary selenium deficiency
> Keshan disease
> *EXCLUDES 1*   *sequelae of selenium deficiency (E64.8)*

E60   Dietary zinc deficiency

✓4ᵗʰ E61   Deficiency of other nutrient elements
> Use additional code for adverse effect, if applicable, to identify drug (T36-T50 with fifth or sixth character 5)
> *EXCLUDES 1*   *disorders of mineral metabolism (E83.-)*
>   *iodine deficiency related thyroid disorders (E00-E02)*
>   *sequelae of malnutrition and other nutritional deficiencies (E64.-)*

    E61.0   Copper deficiency

    E61.1   Iron deficiency
> *EXCLUDES 1*   *iron deficiency anemia (D50.-)*

    E61.2   Magnesium deficiency

    E61.3   Manganese deficiency

    E61.4   Chromium deficiency

    E61.5   Molybdenum deficiency

    E61.6   Vanadium deficiency

    E61.7   Deficiency of multiple nutrient elements

    E61.8   Deficiency of other specified nutrient elements

    E61.9   Deficiency of nutrient element, unspecified ▽

✓4ᵗʰ E63   Other nutritional deficiencies
> *EXCLUDES 1*   *dehydration (E86.0)*
>   *failure to thrive, adult (R62.7)*
>   *failure to thrive, child (R62.51)*
>   *feeding problems in newborn (P92.-)*
>   *sequelae of malnutrition and other nutritional deficiencies (E64.-)*

    E63.0   Essential fatty acid [EFA] deficiency

    E63.1   Imbalance of constituents of food intake

    E63.8   Other specified nutritional deficiencies

    E63.9   Nutritional deficiency, unspecified ▽

✓4ᵗʰ E64   Sequelae of malnutrition and other nutritional deficiencies
> **NOTE**   This category is to be used to indicate conditions in categories E43, E44, E46, E50-E63 as the cause of sequelae, which are themselves classified elsewhere. The 'sequelae' include conditions specified as such; they also include the late effects of diseases classifiable to the above categories if the disease itself is no longer present.
> Code first condition resulting from (sequela) of malnutrition and other nutritional deficiencies

    E64.0   Sequelae of protein-calorie malnutrition
> *EXCLUDES 2*   *retarded development following protein-calorie malnutrition (E45)*

    E64.1   Sequelae of vitamin A deficiency

    E64.2   Sequelae of vitamin C deficiency

    E64.3   Sequelae of rickets

    E64.8   Sequelae of other nutritional deficiencies

    E64.9   Sequelae of unspecified nutritional deficiency ▽

Overweight, obesity and other hyperalimentation (E65-E68)

E65   Localized adiposity
> Fat pad

Ⓝ Newborn: 0   Ⓟ Pediatric: 0-17   Ⓜ Maternity: 12-55   Ⓐ Adult: 15-124   **NRS** Nonroutine supply Dx   **NCDx** Noncancer Dx   **PDx** Primary Dx   ▶◀ Revised Text   ● New Code   ▲ Revised Title

516   ICD-10-CM 2018

☑4ᵗʰ **E66 Overweight and obesity**

Code first obesity complicating pregnancy, childbirth and the puerperium, if applicable (O99.21-)

Use additional code to identify body mass index (BMI), if known (Z68.-)

EXCLUDES 1   adiposogenital dystrophy (E23.6)
        lipomatosis NOS (E88.2)
        lipomatosis dolorosa [Dercum] (E88.2)
        Prader-Willi syndrome (Q87.1)

TIP: BMI may be calculated and assigned as a secondary diagnosis based on documentation of clinicians other than the diagnosing provider.

☑5ᵗʰ **E66.0 Obesity** due to excess calories

E66.01 Morbid (severe) obesity due to excess calories

EXCLUDES 1   morbid (severe) obesity with alveolar hypoventilation (E66.2)

E66.09 Other obesity due to excess calories

E66.1 Drug-induced obesity

Use additional code for adverse effect, if applicable, to identify drug (T36-T50 with fifth or sixth character 5)

E66.2 Morbid (severe) obesity with **alveolar hypoventilation**

Obesity hypoventilation syndrome (OHS)
Pickwickian syndrome

E66.3 Overweight

E66.8 Other obesity

E66.9 Obesity, unspecified   ▽

Obesity NOS

☑4ᵗʰ **E67 Other hyperalimentation**

EXCLUDES 1   hyperalimentation NOS (R63.2)
        sequelae of hyperalimentation (E68)

E67.0 Hypervitaminosis A

E67.1 Hypercarotinemia

E67.2 Megavitamin-B6 syndrome

E67.3 Hypervitaminosis D

E67.8 Other specified hyperalimentation

E68 Sequelae of hyperalimentation

Code first condition resulting from (sequela) of hyperalimentation

Metabolic disorders (E70-E88)

EXCLUDES 1   androgen insensitivity syndrome (E34.5-)
        congenital adrenal hyperplasia (E25.0)
        Ehlers-Danlos syndrome (Q79.6)
        hemolytic anemias attributable to enzyme disorders (D55.-)
        Marfan's syndrome (Q87.0)
        5-alpha-reductase deficiency (E29.1)

☑4ᵗʰ **E70 Disorders of aromatic amino-acid metabolism**

E70.0 Classical phenylketonuria

E70.1 Other hyperphenylalaninemias

☑5ᵗʰ **E70.2 Disorders of tyrosine metabolism**

EXCLUDES 1   transitory tyrosinemia of newborn (P74.5)

E70.20 Disorder of tyrosine metabolism, unspecified   ▽

E70.21 Tyrosinemia

Hypertyrosinemia

E70.29 Other disorders of tyrosine metabolism

Alkaptonuria
Ochronosis

☑5ᵗʰ **E70.3 Albinism**

E70.30 Albinism, unspecified   ▽

☑6ᵗʰ **E70.31 Ocular albinism**

E70.310 X-linked ocular albinism

E70.311 Autosomal recessive ocular albinism

E70.318 Other ocular albinism

E70.319 Ocular albinism, unspecified   ▽

☑6ᵗʰ **E70.32 Oculocutaneous albinism**

EXCLUDES 1   Chediak-Higashi syndrome (E70.330)
        Hermansky-Pudlak syndrome (E70.331)

E70.320 Tyrosinase negative oculocutaneous albinism

Albinism I
Oculocutaneous albinism ty-neg

E70.321 Tyrosinase positive oculocutaneous albinism

Albinism II
Oculocutaneous albinism ty-pos

E70.328 Other oculocutaneous albinism

Cross syndrome

E70.329 Oculocutaneous albinism, unspecified   ▽

☑6ᵗʰ **E70.33 Albinism with hematologic abnormality**

E70.330 Chediak-Higashi syndrome

E70.331 Hermansky-Pudlak syndrome

E70.338 Other albinism with hematologic abnormality

E70.339 Albinism with hematologic abnormality, unspecified   ▽

E70.39 Other specified albinism

Piebaldism

☑5ᵗʰ **E70.4 Disorders of histidine metabolism**

E70.40 Disorders of histidine metabolism, unspecified   ▽

E70.41 Histidinemia

E70.49 Other disorders of histidine metabolism

E70.5 Disorders of tryptophan metabolism

E70.8 Other disorders of aromatic amino-acid metabolism

E70.9 Disorder of aromatic amino-acid metabolism, unspecified   ▽

☑4ᵗʰ **E71 Disorders of branched-chain amino-acid metabolism and fatty-acid metabolism**

E71.0 Maple-syrup-urine disease

☑5ᵗʰ **E71.1 Other disorders of branched-chain amino-acid metabolism**

☑6ᵗʰ **E71.11 Branched-chain organic acidurias**

E71.110 Isovaleric acidemia

E71.111 3-methylglutaconic aciduria

E71.118 Other branched-chain organic acidurias

☑6ᵗʰ **E71.12 Disorders of propionate metabolism**

E71.120 Methylmalonic acidemia

E71.121 Propionic acidemia

E71.128 Other disorders of propionate metabolism

E71.19 Other disorders of branched-chain amino-acid metabolism

Hyperleucine-isoleucinemia
Hypervalinemia

E71.2 Disorder of branched-chain amino-acid metabolism, unspecified   ▽

☑5ᵗʰ **E71.3 Disorders of fatty-acid metabolism**

EXCLUDES 1   peroxisomal disorders (E71.5)
        Refsum's disease (G60.1)
        Schilder's disease (G37.0)

EXCLUDES 2   carnitine deficiency due to inborn error of metabolism (E71.42)

E71.30 Disorder of fatty-acid metabolism, unspecified   ▽

☑6ᵗʰ **E71.31 Disorders of fatty-acid oxidation**

E71.310 Long chain/very long chain acyl CoA dehydrogenase deficiency

LCAD
VLCAD

E71.311 Medium chain acyl CoA dehydrogenase deficiency

MCAD

E71.312 Short chain acyl CoA dehydrogenase deficiency

SCAD

E71.313 Glutaric aciduria type II

Glutaric aciduria type II A
Glutaric aciduria type II B
Glutaric aciduria type II C

EXCLUDES 1   glutaric aciduria (type 1) NOS (E72.3)

E71.314 Muscle carnitine palmitoyltransferase deficiency

E71.318 Other disorders of fatty-acid oxidation

E71.32 Disorders of ketone metabolism

E71.39 Other disorders of fatty-acid metabolism

☑5ᵗʰ **E71.4 Disorders of carnitine metabolism**

EXCLUDES 1   muscle carnitine palmitoyltransferase deficiency (E71.314)

E71.40 Disorder of carnitine metabolism, unspecified   ▽

E71.41 Primary carnitine deficiency

E71.42 Carnitine deficiency due to inborn errors of metabolism

Code also associated inborn error or metabolism

E71.43 Iatrogenic carnitine deficiency

Carnitine deficiency due to hemodialysis
Carnitine deficiency due to Valproic acid therapy

☑ Additional Character Req   ☑x7ᵗʰ Placeholder Alert   Case-Mix Diagnosis   Manifestation   ▽ Unspecified Dx   *EXCLUDES 1* Not coded here   *EXCLUDES 2* Not included here

✓6ᵗʰ **E71.44** **Other secondary** **carnitine deficiency**
   E71.440 **Ruvalcaba-Myhre-Smith syndrome**
   E71.448 **Other secondary carnitine deficiency**

✓5ᵗʰ **E71.5** **Peroxisomal** **disorders**
  EXCLUDES 1 *Schilder's disease (G37.0)*
  E71.50 **Peroxisomal disorder, unspecified** ▽

✓6ᵗʰ **E71.51** **Disorders of peroxisome** **biogenesis**
   Group 1 peroxisomal disorders
   EXCLUDES 1 *Refsum's disease (G60.1)*
   E71.510 **Zellweger syndrome**
   E71.511 **Neonatal adrenoleukodystrophy**
     EXCLUDES 1 *X-linked adrenoleuko- dystrophy (E71.52-)*
   E71.518 **Other disorders of peroxisome biogenesis**

✓6ᵗʰ **E71.52** **X-linked adrenoleukodystrophy**
   E71.520 **Childhood cerebral X-linked adrenoleukodystrophy**
   E71.521 **Adolescent X-linked adrenoleukodystrophy**
   E71.522 **Adrenomyeloneuropathy**
   E71.528 **Other X-linked adrenoleukodystrophy**
     Addison only phenotype adrenoleukodystrophy
     Addison-Schilder adrenoleukodystrophy
   E71.529 **X-linked adrenoleukodystrophy, unspecified type** ▽

  E71.53 **Other** **group 2 peroxisomal disorders**

✓6ᵗʰ **E71.54** **Other** **peroxisomal disorders**
   E71.540 **Rhizomelic chondrodysplasia punctata**
     EXCLUDES 1 *chondrodysplasia punctata NOS (Q77.3)*
   E71.541 **Zellweger-like syndrome**
   E71.542 **Other group 3 peroxisomal disorders**
   E71.548 **Other peroxisomal disorders**

✓4ᵗʰ **E72** **Other disorders of amino-acid metabolism**
  EXCLUDES 1 *disorders of:*
   aromatic amino-acid metabolism (E70.-)
   branched-chain amino-acid metabolism (E71.0-E71.2)
   fatty-acid metabolism (E71.3)
   purine and pyrimidine metabolism (E79.-)
   gout (M1A.-, M10.-)

✓5ᵗʰ **E72.0** **Disorders of amino-acid** **transport**
  EXCLUDES 1 *disorders of tryptophan metabolism (E70.5)*
  E72.00 **Disorders of amino-acid transport, unspecified** ▽
  E72.01 **Cystinuria**
  E72.02 **Hartnup's disease**
  E72.03 **Lowe's syndrome**
   Use additional code for associated glaucoma (H42)
  E72.04 **Cystinosis**
   Fanconi (-de Toni) (-Debré) syndrome with cystinosis
   EXCLUDES 1 *Fanconi (-de Toni) (-Debré) syndrome without cystinosis (E72.09)*
  E72.09 **Other disorders of amino-acid transport**
   Fanconi (-de Toni) (-Debré) syndrome, unspecified

✓5ᵗʰ **E72.1** **Disorders of sulfur-bearing amino-acid metabolism**
  EXCLUDES 1 *cystinosis (E72.04)*
   cystinuria (E72.01)
   transcobalamin II deficiency (D51.2)
  E72.10 **Disorders of sulfur-bearing amino-acid metabolism, unspecified** ▽
  E72.11 **Homocystinuria**
   Cystathionine synthase deficiency
  E72.12 **Methylenetetrahydrofolate reductase deficiency**
  E72.19 **Other disorders of sulfur-bearing amino-acid metabolism**
   Cystathioninuria
   Methioninemia
   Sulfite oxidase deficiency

✓5ᵗʰ **E72.2** **Disorders of urea cycle metabolism**
  EXCLUDES 1 *disorders of ornithine metabolism (E72.4)*
  E72.20 **Disorder of urea cycle metabolism, unspecified** ▽
   Hyperammonemia
   EXCLUDES 1 *hyperammonemia- hyperornithinemia- homocitrullinemia syndrome (E72.4)*
   transient hyperammonemia of newborn (P74.6)

  E72.21 **Argininemia**
  E72.22 **Arginosuccinic aciduria**
  E72.23 **Citrullinemia**
  E72.29 **Other disorders of urea cycle metabolism**

  E72.3 **Disorders of lysine and hydroxylysine metabolism**
   Glutaric aciduria NOS   Hydroxylysinemia
   Glutaric aciduria (type I) Hyperlysinemia
   EXCLUDES 1 *glutaric aciduria type II (E71.313)*
     Refsum's disease (G60.1)
     Zellweger syndrome (E71.510)

  E72.4 **Disorders of ornithine metabolism**
   Hyperammonemia-hyperornithinemia-homocitrullinemia syndrome
   Ornithinemia (types I, II)
   Ornithine transcarbamylase deficiency
   EXCLUDES 1 *hereditary choroidal dystrophy (H31.2-)*

✓5ᵗʰ **E72.5** **Disorders of glycine metabolism**
  E72.50 **Disorder of glycine metabolism, unspecified** ▽
  E72.51 **Non-ketotic hyperglycinemia**
  E72.52 **Trimethylaminuria**
  E72.53 **Hyperoxaluria**
   Oxalosis
   Oxaluria
  E72.59 **Other disorders of glycine metabolism**
   D-glycericacidemia
   Hyperhydroxyprolinemia
   Hyperprolinemia (types I, II)
   Sarcosinemia

  E72.8 **Other specified disorders of amino-acid metabolism**
   Disorders of beta-amino-acid metabolism
   Disorders of gamma-glutamyl cycle

  E72.9 **Disorder of amino-acid metabolism, unspecified** ▽

✓4ᵗʰ **E73** **Lactose intolerance**
  E73.0 **Congenital lactase deficiency**
  E73.1 **Secondary lactase deficiency**
  E73.8 **Other lactose intolerance**
  E73.9 **Lactose intolerance, unspecified** ▽

✓4ᵗʰ **E74** **Other disorders of carbohydrate metabolism**
  EXCLUDES 1 *diabetes mellitus (E08-E13)*
   hypoglycemia NOS (E16.2)
   increased secretion of glucagon (E16.3)
   mucopolysaccharidosis (E76.0-E76.3)

✓5ᵗʰ **E74.0** **Glycogen storage disease** ▽
  E74.00 **Glycogen storage disease, unspecified**
  E74.01 **von Gierke disease**
   Type I glycogen storage disease
  E74.02 **Pompe disease**
   Cardiac glycogenosis
   Type II glycogen storage disease
  E74.03 **Cori disease**
   Forbes disease
   Type III glycogen storage disease
  E74.04 **McArdle disease**
   Type V glycogen storage disease
  E74.09 **Other glycogen storage disease**
   Andersen disease
   Hers disease
   Tauri disease
   Glycogen storage disease, types 0, IV, VI-XI
   Liver phosphorylase deficiency
   Muscle phosphofructokinase deficiency

✓5ᵗʰ **E74.1** **Disorders of fructose metabolism**
  EXCLUDES 1 *muscle phosphofructokinase deficiency (E74.09)*
  E74.10 **Disorder of fructose metabolism, unspecified** ▽
  E74.11 **Essential fructosuria**
   Fructokinase deficiency
  E74.12 **Hereditary fructose intolerance**
   Fructosemia
  E74.19 **Other disorders of fructose metabolism**
   Fructose-1, 6-diphosphatase deficiency

✓5ᵗʰ **E74.2** **Disorders of galactose metabolism**
  E74.20 **Disorders of galactose metabolism, unspecified** ▽
  E74.21 **Galactosemia**
   DEF: Any of three genetic disorders due to defective galactose metabolism; symptoms include failure to thrive in infancy, jaundice, liver and spleen damage, cataracts, and mental retardation.

Ⓝ Newborn: 0 Ⓟ Pediatric: 0-17 Ⓜ Maternity: 12-55 Ⓐ Adult: 15-124 **NRS** Nonroutine supply Dx **NCDx** Noncancer Dx **PDx** Primary Dx ►◄ Revised Text ● New Code ▲ Revised Title

518   ICD-10-CM 2018

E74.29   **Other disorders of galactose metabolism**
Galactokinase deficiency

☑5ᵗʰ   **E74.3**   **Other disorders of** intestinal carbohydrate absorption
    EXCLUDES 2   *lactose intolerance (E73.-)*

E74.31   **Sucrase-isomaltase deficiency**

E74.39   **Other disorders of intestinal carbohydrate absorption**
Disorder of intestinal carbohydrate absorption NOS
Glucose-galactose malabsorption
Sucrase deficiency

E74.4   **Disorders of** pyruvate metabolism and gluconeogenesis
Deficiency of phosphoenolpyruvate carboxykinase
Deficiency of pyruvate carboxylase
Deficiency of pyruvate dehydrogenase
    EXCLUDES 1   *disorders of pyruvate metabolism and*
gluconeogenesis with anemia (D55.-)
Leigh's syndrome (G31.82)

E74.8   **Other specified disorders of carbohydrate metabolism**
Essential pentosuria
Renal glycosuria

E74.9   **Disorder of carbohydrate metabolism, unspecified**   ▽

☑4ᵗʰ   **E75**   **Disorders of** sphingolipid **metabolism and** other lipid storage **disorders**
    EXCLUDES 1   *mucolipidosis, types I-III (E77.0-E77.1)*
Refsum's disease (G60.1)

☑5ᵗʰ   **E75.0**   **GM2 gangliosidosis**

E75.00   **GM2 gangliosidosis, unspecified**   ▽

E75.01   Sandhoff **disease**

E75.02   Tay-Sachs **disease**
DEF: Genetic mutation of the HEXA gene that inhibits
the breakdown of a toxic substance called ganglioside.
The accumulation of ganglioside results in destruction
of the neurons in the brain and spinal cord.

E75.09   **Other GM2 gangliosidosis**
Adult GM2 gangliosidosis
Juvenile GM2 gangliosidosis

☑5ᵗʰ   **E75.1**   **Other and unspecified gangliosidosis**

E75.10   **Unspecified gangliosidosis**   ▽
Gangliosidosis NOS

E75.11   Mucolipidosis IV

E75.19   **Other gangliosidosis**
GM1 gangliosidosis
GM3 gangliosidosis

☑5ᵗʰ   **E75.2**   **Other sphingolipidosis**
    EXCLUDES 1   *adrenoleukodystrophy [Addison-Schilder] (E71.528)*

E75.21   **Fabry (-Anderson) disease**

E75.22   **Gaucher disease**

E75.23   Krabbe disease

☑6ᵗʰ   E75.24   **Niemann-Pick disease**

E75.240   **Niemann-Pick disease** type A

E75.241   **Niemann-Pick disease** type B

E75.242   **Niemann-Pick disease** type C

Tay-Sachs Disease

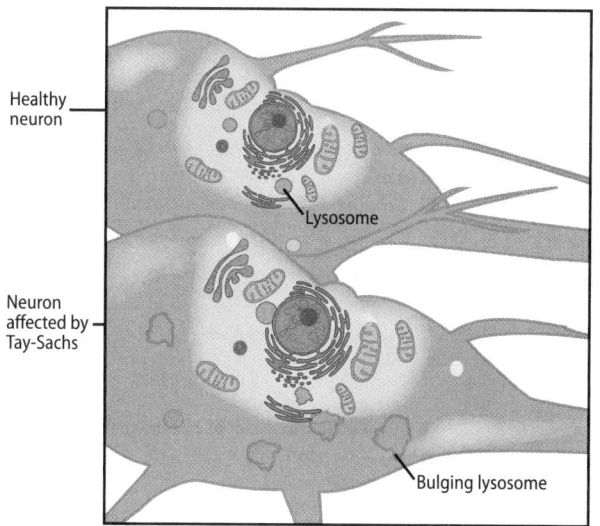

Healthy neuron

Lysosome

Neuron affected by Tay-Sachs

Bulging lysosome

E75.243   **Niemann-Pick disease** type D

E75.248   **Other Niemann-Pick disease**

E75.249   **Niemann-Pick disease, unspecified**   ▽

E75.25   Metachromatic leukodystrophy

E75.29   Other sphingolipidosis
Farber's syndrome
Sulfatase deficiency
Sulfatide lipidosis

E75.3   **Sphingolipidosis, unspecified**   ▽

E75.4   Neuronal ceroid lipofuscinosis
Batten disease
Bielschowsky-Jansky disease
Kufs disease
Spielmeyer-Vogt disease

E75.5   **Other lipid storage disorders**
Cerebrotendinous cholesterosis [van Bogaert-Scherer-Epstein]
Wolman's disease

E75.6   **Lipid storage disorder, unspecified**   ▽

☑4ᵗʰ   **E76**   **Disorders of** glycosaminoglycan **metabolism**

☑5ᵗʰ   **E76.0**   **Mucopolysaccharidosis,** type I

E76.01   Hurler's **syndrome**

E76.02   Hurler-Scheie **syndrome**

E76.03   Scheie's **syndrome**

E76.1   **Mucopolysaccharidosis,** type II
Hunter's syndrome

☑5ᵗʰ   **E76.2**   **Other** mucopolysaccharidoses

☑6ᵗʰ   E76.21   Morquio **mucopolysaccharidoses**

E76.210   **Morquio A mucopolysaccharidoses**
Classic Morquio syndrome
Morquio syndrome A
Mucopolysaccharidosis, type IVA

E76.211   **Morquio B mucopolysaccharidoses**
Morquio-like mucopolysaccharidoses
Morquio-like syndrome
Morquio syndrome B
Mucopolysaccharidosis, type IVB

E76.219   **Morquio mucopolysaccharidoses, unspecified**   ▽
Morquio syndrome
Mucopolysaccharidosis, type IV

E76.22   Sanfilippo **mucopolysaccharidoses**
Mucopolysaccharidosis, type III (A) (B) (C) (D)
Sanfilippo A syndrome
Sanfilippo B syndrome
Sanfilippo C syndrome
Sanfilippo D syndrome

E76.29   **Other mucopolysaccharidoses**
beta-Glucuronidase deficiency
Maroteaux-Lamy (mild) (severe) syndrome
Mucopolysaccharidosis, types VI, VII

E76.3   **Mucopolysaccharidosis, unspecified**   ▽

E76.8   **Other disorders of glucosaminoglycan metabolism**

E76.9   **Glucosaminoglycan metabolism disorder, unspecified**   ▽

☑4ᵗʰ   **E77**   **Disorders of** glycoprotein **metabolism**

E77.0   Defects in post-translational modification of lysosomal enzymes
Mucolipidosis II [I-cell disease]
Mucolipidosis III [pseudo-Hurler polydystrophy]

E77.1   Defects in glycoprotein degradation
Aspartylglucosaminuria
Fucosidosis
Mannosidosis
Sialidosis [mucolipidosis I]

E77.8   **Other disorders of glycoprotein metabolism**

E77.9   **Disorder of glycoprotein metabolism, unspecified**   ▽

☑4ᵗʰ   **E78**   **Disorders of** lipoprotein metabolism and other lipidemias
    EXCLUDES 1   *sphingolipidosis (E75.0-E75.3)*

☑5ᵗʰ   **E78.0**   **Pure hypercholesterolemia**

E78.00   **Pure hypercholesterolemia, unspecified**   ▽
Fredrickson's hyperlipoproteinemia, type IIa
Hyperbetalipoproteinemia
Low-density-lipoprotein-type [LDL]
    hyperlipoproteinemia
▶(Pure) hypercholesterolemia NOS◀

E78.01   **Familial hypercholesterolemia**

E78.1 **Pure hyperglyceridemia**
Elevated fasting triglycerides
Endogenous hyperglyceridemia
Fredrickson's hyperlipoproteinemia, type IV
Hyperlipidemia, group B
Hyperprebetalipoproteinemia
Very-low-density-lipoprotein-type [VLDL] hyperlipoproteinemia

E78.2 **Mixed hyperlipidemia**
Broad- or floating-betalipoproteinemia
Combined hyperlipidemia NOS
Elevated cholesterol with elevated triglycerides NEC
Fredrickson's hyperlipoproteinemia, type IIb or III
Hyperbetalipoproteinemia with prebetalipoproteinemia
Hypercholesteremia with endogenous hyperglyceridemia
Hyperlipidemia, group C
Tubo-eruptive xanthoma
Xanthoma tuberosum
EXCLUDES 1 *cerebrotendinous cholesterosis [van Bogaert-Scherer-Epstein] (E75.5)*
familial combined hyperlipidemia (E78.4)

E78.3 **Hyperchylomicronemia**
Chylomicron retention disease
Fredrickson's hyperlipoproteinemia, type I or V
Hyperlipidemia, group D
Mixed hyperglyceridemia

E78.4 **Other hyperlipidemia**
Familial combined hyperlipidemia

E78.5 **Hyperlipidemia, unspecified** ▽

E78.6 **Lipoprotein deficiency**
Abetalipoproteinemia
Depressed HDL cholesterol
High-density lipoprotein deficiency
Hypoalphalipoproteinemia
Hypobetalipoproteinemia (familial)
Lecithin cholesterol acyltransferase deficiency
Tangier disease

✓5th **E78.7** **Disorders of bile acid and cholesterol metabolism**
EXCLUDES 1 *Niemann-Pick disease type C (E75.242)*

    E78.70 **Disorder of bile acid and cholesterol metabolism, unspecified** ▽

    E78.71 **Barth syndrome**

    E78.72 **Smith-Lemli-Opitz syndrome**

    E78.79 **Other disorders of bile acid and cholesterol metabolism**

✓5th **E78.8** **Other disorders of lipoprotein metabolism**

    E78.81 **Lipoid dermatoarthritis**

    E78.89 **Other lipoprotein metabolism disorders**

E78.9 **Disorder of lipoprotein metabolism, unspecified** ▽

✓4th **E79** **Disorders of purine and pyrimidine metabolism**
EXCLUDES 1 *Ataxia-telangiectasia (Q87.1)*
Bloom's syndrome (Q82.8)
Cockayne's syndrome (Q87.1)
calculus of kidney (N20.0)
combined immunodeficiency disorders (D81.-)
Fanconi's anemia (D61.09)
gout (M1A.-, M10.-)
orotaciduric anemia (D53.0)
progeria (E34.8)
Werner's syndrome (E34.8)
xeroderma pigmentosum (Q82.1)

E79.0 **Hyperuricemia without signs of inflammatory arthritis and tophaceous disease**
Asymptomatic hyperuricemia

E79.1 **Lesch-Nyhan syndrome**
HGPRT deficiency

E79.2 **Myoadenylate deaminase deficiency**

E79.8 **Other disorders of purine and pyrimidine metabolism**
Hereditary xanthinuria

E79.9 **Disorder of purine and pyrimidine metabolism, unspecified** ▽

✓4th **E80** **Disorders of porphyrin and bilirubin metabolism**
INCLUDES defects of catalase and peroxidase

E80.0 **Hereditary erythropoietic porphyria**
Congenital erythropoietic porphyria
Erythropoietic protoporphyria

E80.1 **Porphyria cutanea tarda**

✓5th **E80.2** **Other and unspecified porphyria**

    E80.20 **Unspecified porphyria** ▽
Porphyria NOS

    E80.21 **Acute intermittent (hepatic) porphyria**

    E80.29 **Other porphyria**
Hereditary coproporphyria

E80.3 **Defects of catalase and peroxidase**
Acatalasia [Takahara]

E80.4 **Gilbert syndrome**

E80.5 **Crigler-Najjar syndrome**

E80.6 **Other disorders of bilirubin metabolism**
Dubin-Johnson syndrome
Rotor's syndrome

E80.7 **Disorder of bilirubin metabolism, unspecified** ▽

✓4th **E83** **Disorders of mineral metabolism**
EXCLUDES 1 *dietary mineral deficiency (E58-E61)*
parathyroid disorders (E20-E21)
vitamin D deficiency (E55.-)

✓5th **E83.0** **Disorders of copper metabolism**

    E83.00 **Disorder of copper metabolism, unspecified** ▽

    E83.01 **Wilson's disease**
Code also associated Kayser Fleischer ring (H18.04-)

    E83.09 **Other disorders of copper metabolism**
Menkes' (kinky hair) (steely hair) disease

✓5th **E83.1** **Disorders of iron metabolism**
EXCLUDES 1 *iron deficiency anemia (D50.-)*
sideroblastic anemia (D64.0-D64.3)

    E83.10 **Disorder of iron metabolism, unspecified** ▽

    ✓6th **E83.11** **Hemochromatosis**
EXCLUDES 1 ▶*GALD (P78.84)*
gestational alloimmune liver disease (P78.84)
neonatal hemochromatosis (P78.84)◀

        E83.110 **Hereditary hemochromatosis**
Bronzed diabetes
Pigmentary cirrhosis (of liver)
Primary (hereditary) hemochromatosis

        E83.111 **Hemochromatosis due to repeated red blood cell transfusions**
Iron overload due to repeated red blood cell transfusions
Transfusion (red blood cell) associated hemochromatosis

        E83.118 **Other hemochromatosis**

        E83.119 **Hemochromatosis, unspecified** ▽

    E83.19 **Other disorders of iron metabolism**
Use additional code, if applicable, for idiopathic pulmonary hemosiderosis (J84.03)

E83.2 **Disorders of zinc metabolism**
Acrodermatitis enteropathica

✓5th **E83.3** **Disorders of phosphorus metabolism and phosphatases**
EXCLUDES 1 *adult osteomalacia (M83.-)*
osteoporosis (M80.-)

    E83.30 **Disorder of phosphorus metabolism, unspecified** ▽

    E83.31 **Familial hypophosphatemia**
Vitamin D-resistant osteomalacia
Vitamin D-resistant rickets
EXCLUDES 1 *vitamin D-deficiency rickets (E55.0)*

    E83.32 **Hereditary vitamin D-dependent rickets (type 1) (type 2)**
25-hydroxyvitamin D 1-alpha-hydroxylase deficiency
Pseudovitamin D deficiency
Vitamin D receptor defect

    E83.39 **Other disorders of phosphorus metabolism**
Acid phosphatase deficiency
Hypophosphatasia

✓5th **E83.4** **Disorders of magnesium metabolism**

    E83.40 **Disorders of magnesium metabolism, unspecified** ▽

    E83.41 **Hypermagnesemia**

    E83.42 **Hypomagnesemia**

    E83.49 **Other disorders of magnesium metabolism**

✓5th **E83.5** **Disorders of calcium metabolism**
EXCLUDES 1 *chondrocalcinosis (M11.1-M11.2)*
hungry bone syndrome (E83.81)
hyperparathyroidism (E21.0-E21.3)

    E83.50 **Unspecified disorder of calcium metabolism** ▽

    E83.51 **Hypocalcemia**

    E83.52 **Hypercalcemia**
Familial hypocalciuric hypercalcemia

E83.59   **Other disorders of calcium metabolism**
Idiopathic hypercalciuria

✓5ᵗʰ **E83.8**   **Other disorders of** mineral **metabolism**

E83.81   **Hungry bone syndrome**

E83.89   **Other disorders of mineral metabolism**

E83.9   **Disorder of mineral metabolism, unspecified** ▽

✓4ᵗʰ **E84**   **Cystic fibrosis**
INCLUDES   mucoviscidosis
Code also exocrine pancreatic insufficiency (K86.81)

E84.0   **Cystic fibrosis with** pulmonary manifestations
Use additional code to identify any infectious organism present, such as:
Pseudomonas (B96.5)

✓5ᵗʰ **E84.1**   **Cystic fibrosis with** intestinal manifestations

E84.11   **Meconium ileus in cystic fibrosis**   N
EXCLUDES 1   meconium ileus not due to cystic fibrosis (P76.0)

E84.19   **Cystic fibrosis with** other intestinal manifestations
Distal intestinal obstruction syndrome

E84.8   **Cystic fibrosis with other** manifestations

E84.9   **Cystic fibrosis, unspecified** ▽

✓4ᵗʰ **E85**   **Amyloidosis**
EXCLUDES 1   Alzheimer's disease (G30.0-)
EXCLUDES 2   ▶Alzheimer's disease (G30.0-)◀
DEF: Conditions of diverse etiologies characterized by the accumulation of insoluble fibrillar proteins (amyloid) in various organs and tissues of the body, compromising vital functions.

E85.0   **Non-neuropathic heredofamilial** amyloidosis
Hereditary amyloid nephropathy
▶Code also associated disorders, such as:
autoinflammatory syndromes (M04.-)◀
EXCLUDES 2 ▶transthyretin-related (ATTR) familial amyloid cardiomyopathy (E85.4)◀

E85.1   **Neuropathic heredofamilial** amyloidosis
Amyloid polyneuropathy (Portuguese)
▶Transthyretin-related (ATTR) familial amyloid polyneuropathy◀
AHA: 2012, 4Q, 99

E85.2   **Heredofamilial** amyloidosis, unspecified ▽

E85.3   **Secondary systemic** amyloidosis
Hemodialysis-associated amyloidosis

E85.4   **Organ-limited** amyloidosis
Localized amyloidosis
▶Transthyretin-related (ATTR) familial amyloid cardiomyopathy◀

✓5ᵗʰ **E85.8**   **Other amyloidosis**

●   E85.81   **Light chain (AL)** amyloidosis

●   E85.82   **Wild-type transthyretin-related (ATTR)** amyloidosis
Senile systemic amyloidosis (SSA)

●   E85.89   **Other amyloidosis**

E85.9   **Amyloidosis, unspecified** ▽

✓4ᵗʰ **E86**   **Volume depletion**
Use additional code(s) for any associated disorders of electrolyte and acid-base balance (E87.-)
EXCLUDES 1   dehydration of newborn (P74.1)
hypovolemic shock NOS (R57.1)
postprocedural hypovolemic shock (T81.19)
traumatic hypovolemic shock (T79.4)

E86.0   **Dehydration**
AHA: 2014, 1Q, 7

E86.1   **Hypovolemia**
Depletion of volume of plasma

E86.9   **Volume depletion, unspecified** ▽
DEF: Depletion of total body water (dehydration) and/or contraction of total intravascular plasma (hypovolemia).

✓4ᵗʰ **E87**   **Other disorders of** fluid, electrolyte and acid-base balance
EXCLUDES 1   diabetes insipidus (E23.2)
electrolyte imbalance associated with hyperemesis gravidarum (O21.1)
electrolyte imbalance following ectopic or molar pregnancy (O08.5)
familial periodic paralysis (G72.3)

E87.0   **Hyperosmolality and hypernatremia**
Sodium [Na] excess
Sodium [Na] overload
AHA: 2014, 1Q, 7

E87.1   **Hypo-osmolality and hyponatremia**
Sodium [Na] deficiency
EXCLUDES 1   syndrome of inappropriate secretion of antidiuretic hormone (E22.2)
AHA: 2014, 1Q, 7

E87.2   **Acidosis**
Acidosis NOS
Lactic acidosis
Metabolic acidosis
Respiratory acidosis
EXCLUDES 1   diabetic acidosis—see categories E08-E10, E13 with ketoacidosis

E87.3   **Alkalosis**
Alkalosis NOS
Metabolic alkalosis
Respiratory alkalosis

E87.4   **Mixed disorder of acid-base balance**

E87.5   **Hyperkalemia**
Potassium [K] excess
Potassium [K] overload

E87.6   **Hypokalemia**
Potassium [K] deficiency

✓5ᵗʰ **E87.7**   **Fluid overload**
EXCLUDES 1   edema NOS (R60.9)
fluid retention (R60.9)

E87.70   **Fluid overload, unspecified** ▽

E87.71   **Transfusion associated** circulatory overload
Fluid overload due to transfusion (blood) (blood components)
TACO

E87.79   **Other fluid overload**

E87.8   **Other disorders of electrolyte and fluid balance, not elsewhere classified**
Electrolyte imbalance NOS
Hyperchloremia
Hypochloremia

✓4ᵗʰ **E88**   **Other and unspecified metabolic disorders**
Use additional codes for associated conditions
EXCLUDES 1   histiocytosis X (chronic) (C96.6)

✓5ᵗʰ **E88.0**   **Disorders of plasma-protein metabolism, not elsewhere classified**
EXCLUDES 1   disorder of lipoprotein metabolism (E78.-)
monoclonal gammopathy (of undetermined significance) (D47.2)
polyclonal hypergammaglobulinemia (D89.0)
Waldenström's macroglobulinemia (C88.0)

E88.01   **Alpha-1-antitrypsin deficiency**
AAT deficiency

E88.09   **Other disorders of plasma-protein metabolism, not elsewhere classified**
Bisalbuminemia

E88.1   **Lipodystrophy, not elsewhere classified**
Lipodystrophy NOS
EXCLUDES 1   Whipple's disease (K90.81)

E88.2   **Lipomatosis, not elsewhere classified**
Lipomatosis NOS
Lipomatosis (Check) dolorosa [Dercum]

E88.3   **Tumor lysis syndrome**
Tumor lysis syndrome (spontaneous)
Tumor lysis syndrome following antineoplastic drug chemotherapy
Use additional code for adverse effect, if applicable, to identify drug (T45.1X5)
DEF: A potentially fatal metabolic complication of tumor necrosis caused by either spontaneous or treatment-related accumulation of byproducts from dying cancer cells; symptoms include hyperkalemia, hyperphosphatemia, hypocalcemia, hyperuricemia, and hyperuricosuria.

✓5ᵗʰ **E88.4**   **Mitochondrial metabolism disorders**
EXCLUDES 1   disorders of pyruvate metabolism (E74.4)
Kearns-Sayre syndrome (H49.81)
Leber's disease (H47.22)
Leigh's encephalopathy (G31.82)
Mitochondrial myopathy, NEC (G71.3)
Reye's syndrome (G93.7)

E88.40   **Mitochondrial metabolism disorder, unspecified** ▽

E88.41   **MELAS syndrome**
Mitochondrial myopathy, encephalopathy, lactic acidosis and stroke-like episodes

---

Chapter 4. Endocrine, Nutritional and Metabolic Diseases *(side tab)*

E88.42   **MERRF syndrome**
Myoclonic epilepsy associated with ragged-red fibers
Code also progressive myoclonic epilepsy (G40.3-)

E88.49   **Other mitochondrial metabolism disorders**

✓5ᵗʰ   **E88.8**   **Other specified metabolic disorders**

E88.81   **Metabolic syndrome**
Dysmetabolic syndrome X
Use additional codes for associated manifestations,
such as:
obesity (E66.-)

E88.89   **Other specified metabolic disorders**
Launois-Bensaude adenolipomatosis
EXCLUDES 1   *adult pulmonary Langerhans cell
histiocytosis (J84.82)*

E88.9   **Metabolic disorder, unspecified**   ▽

Postprocedural endocrine and metabolic complications and disorders, not elsewhere classified (E89)

✓4ᵗʰ   **E89**   **Postprocedural endocrine and metabolic complications and disorders, not elsewhere classified**
EXCLUDES 2   *intraoperative complications of endocrine system organ or structure (E36.0-, E36.1-, E36.8)*

E89.0   **Postprocedural hypothyroidism**
Postirradiation hypothyroidism
Postsurgical hypothyroidism

E89.1   **Postprocedural hypoinsulinemia**
Postpancreatectomy hyperglycemia
Postsurgical hypoinsulinemia
Use additional code, if applicable, to identify:
acquired absence of pancreas (Z90.41-)
diabetes mellitus (postpancreatectomy) (postprocedural)
(E13.-)
insulin use (Z79.4)
EXCLUDES 1   *transient postprocedural hyperglycemia (R73.9)
transient postprocedural hypoglycemia (E16.2)*

E89.2   **Postprocedural hypoparathyroidism**
Parathyroprival tetany

E89.3   **Postprocedural hypopituitarism**
Postirradiation hypopituitarism

✓5ᵗʰ   **E89.4**   **Postprocedural ovarian failure**

E89.40   **Asymptomatic postprocedural ovarian failure**   ♀
Postprocedural ovarian failure NOS

E89.41   **Symptomatic postprocedural ovarian failure**   ♀
Symptoms such as flushing, sleeplessness, headache,
lack of concentration, associated with
postprocedural menopause

E89.5   **Postprocedural testicular hypofunction**   ♂

E89.6   **Postprocedural adrenocortical (-medullary) hypofunction**

✓5ᵗʰ   **E89.8**   **Other postprocedural endocrine and metabolic complications and disorders**

✓6ᵗʰ   E89.81   **Postprocedural hemorrhage of an endocrine system organ or structure following a procedure**

E89.810   **Postprocedural hemorrhage of an**   **NRS**
**endocrine system organ or structure
following an endocrine system
procedure**

E89.811   **Postprocedural hemorrhage of an**   **NRS**
**endocrine system organ or structure
following other procedure**

✓6ᵗʰ   E89.82   **Postprocedural hematoma and seroma of an endocrine system organ or structure**

E89.820   **Postprocedural hematoma of an**   **NRS**
**endocrine system organ or structure
following an endocrine system procedure**

E89.821   **Postprocedural hematoma of an**   **NRS**
**endocrine system organ or structure
following other procedure**

E89.822   **Postprocedural seroma of an endocrine
system organ or structure following an
endocrine system procedure**

E89.823   **Postprocedural seroma of an endocrine
system organ or structure following other
procedure**

E89.89   **Other postprocedural endocrine and metabolic
complications and disorders**
Use additional code, if applicable, to further specify
disorder

Ⓝ Newborn: 0   Ⓟ Pediatric: 0-17   Ⓜ Maternity: 12-55   Ⓐ Adult: 15-124   **NRS** Nonroutine supply Dx   **NC Dx** Noncancer Dx   **PDx** Primary Dx   ▶◀ Revised Text   ● New Code   ▲ Revised Title

522   ICD-10-CM 2018

Chapter 5. Mental, Behavioral and Neurodevelopmental Disorders (F01–F99)

Chapter Specific Guidelines with Coding Examples

The chapter specific guidelines from the ICD-10-CM Official Guidelines for Coding and Reporting have been provided below. Along with these guidelines are coding examples, contained in the shaded boxes, that have been developed to help illustrate the coding and/or sequencing guidance found in these guidelines.

a. Pain disorders related to psychological factors

Assign code F45.41, for pain that is exclusively related to psychological disorders. As indicated by the Excludes 1 note under category G89, a code from category G89 should not be assigned with code F45.41.

> Perceived abdominal pain determined to be persistent somatoform pain disorder.
>
> **F45.41**   **Pain disorder exclusively related to psychological factors**
>
> *Explanation:* This pain was diagnosed as being exclusively psychological; therefore, no code from category G89 is added.

Code F45.42, Pain disorders with related psychological factors, should be used with a code from category G89, Pain, not elsewhere classified, if there is documentation of a psychological component for a patient with acute or chronic pain.

See Section I.C.6. Pain

b. Mental and behavioral disorders due to psychoactive substance use

1) In remission

Selection of codes for "in remission" for categories F10-F19, Mental and behavioral disorders due to psychoactive substance use (categories F10-F19 with **-11,** -.21) requires the provider's clinical judgment. The appropriate codes for "in remission" are assigned only on the basis of provider documentation (as defined in the Official Guidelines for Coding and Reporting), **unless otherwise instructed by the classification.**

Mild substance use disorders in early or sustained remission are classified to the appropriate codes for substance abuse in remission, and moderate or severe substance use disorders in early or sustained remission are classified to the appropriate codes for substance dependence in remission.

2) Psychoactive substance use, abuse and dependence

When the provider documentation refers to use, abuse and dependence of the same substance (e.g. alcohol, opioid, cannabis, etc.), only one code should be assigned to identify the pattern of use based on the following hierarchy:

- If both use and abuse are documented, assign only the code for abuse
- If both abuse and dependence are documented, assign only the code for dependence
- If use, abuse and dependence are all documented, assign only the code for dependence
- If both use and dependence are documented, assign only the code for dependence.

> History and physical notes cannabis dependence; progress note says cannabis abuse.
>
> **F12.20**   **Cannabis dependence, uncomplicated**
>
> *Explanation:* In the hierarchy, the dependence code is used if both abuse and dependence are documented.

> Discharge summary says cocaine abuse; progress notes list cocaine use.
>
> **F14.10**   **Cocaine abuse, uncomplicated**
>
> *Explanation:* In the hierarchy, the abuse code is used if both abuse and use are documented.

3) Psychoactive substance use *disorders*

As with all other diagnoses, the codes for psychoactive substance use **disorders** (F10.9-, F11.9-, F12.9-, F13.9-, F14.9-, F15.9-, F16.9-) should only be assigned based on provider documentation and when they meet the definition of a reportable diagnosis (see Section III, Reporting Additional Diagnoses). The codes are to be used only when the psychoactive substance use is associated with a **physical,** mental or behavioral disorder, and such a relationship is documented by the provider.

Chapter 5. Mental, Behavioral and Neurodevelopmental Disorders (F01-F99)

INCLUDES   disorders of psychological development
EXCLUDES 2   *symptoms, signs and abnormal clinical laboratory findings, not elsewhere classified (R00-R99)*

This chapter contains the following blocks:

F01-F09	Mental disorders due to known physiological conditions
F10-F19	Mental and behavioral disorders due to psychoactive substance use
F20-F29	Schizophrenia, schizotypal, delusional, and other non-mood psychotic disorders
F30-F39	Mood [affective] disorders
F40-F48	Anxiety, dissociative, stress-related, somatoform and other nonpsychotic mental disorders
F50-F59	Behavioral syndromes associated with physiological disturbances and physical factors
F60-F69	Disorders of adult personality and behavior
F70-F79	Intellectual disabilities
F80-F89	Pervasive and specific developmental disorders
F90-F98	Behavioral and emotional disorders with onset usually occurring in childhood and adolescence
F99	Unspecified mental disorder

Mental disorders due to known physiological conditions (F01-F09)

NOTE   This block comprises a range of mental disorders grouped together on the basis of their having in common a demonstrable etiology in cerebral disease, brain injury, or other insult leading to cerebral dysfunction. The dysfunction may be primary, as in diseases, injuries, and insults that affect the brain directly and selectively; or secondary, as in systemic diseases and disorders that attack the brain only as one of the multiple organs or systems of the body that are involved.

✓4ᵗʰ F01   Vascular dementia
Vascular dementia as a result of infarction of the brain due to vascular disease, including hypertensive cerebrovascular disease.
INCLUDES   arteriosclerotic dementia
Code first the underlying physiological condition or sequelae of cerebrovascular disease.

  ✓5ᵗʰ F01.5   Vascular dementia

    F01.50   Vascular dementia without behavioral disturbance   A
       Major neurocognitive disorder without behavioral disturbance

    F01.51   Vascular dementia with behavioral disturbance   A
       Major neurocognitive disorder due to vascular disease, with behavioral disturbance
       Major neurocognitive disorder with aggressive behavior
       Major neurocognitive disorder with combative behavior
       Major neurocognitive disorder with violent behavior
       Vascular dementia with aggressive behavior
       Vascular dementia with combative behavior
       Vascular dementia with violent behavior
       Use additional code, if applicable, to identify wandering in vascular dementia (Z91.83)

✓4ᵗʰ F02   Dementia in other diseases classified elsewhere
INCLUDES   major neurocognitive disorder in other diseases classified elsewhere
Code first the underlying physiological condition, such as:
   Alzheimer's (G30.-)
   cerebral lipidosis (E75.4)
   Creutzfeldt-Jakob disease (A81.0-)
   dementia with Lewy bodies (G31.83)
   dementia with Parkinsonism (G31.83)
   epilepsy and recurrent seizures (G40.-)
   frontotemporal dementia (G31.09)
   hepatolenticular degeneration (E83.0)
   human immunodeficiency virus [HIV] disease (B20)
   Huntington's disease (G10)
   hypercalcemia (E83.52)
   hypothyroidism, acquired (E00-E03.-)
   intoxications (T36-T65)
   Jakob-Creutzfeldt disease (A81.0-)
   multiple sclerosis (G35)
   neurosyphilis (A52.17)
   niacin deficiency [pellagra] (E52)
   Parkinson's disease (G20)
   Pick's disease (G31.01)
   polyarteritis nodosa (M30.0)
   prion disease (A81.9)
   systemic lupus erythematosus (M32.-)
   traumatic brain injury (S06.-)
   trypanosomiasis (B56.-, B57.-)
   vitamin B deficiency (E53.8)
EXCLUDES 2   *dementia in alcohol and psychoactive substance disorders (F10-F19, with .17, .27, .97)*
       vascular dementia (F01.5-)

  ✓5ᵗʰ F02.8   Dementia in other diseases classified elsewhere
     AHA: 2017, 2Q, 7; 2016, 4Q, 141; 2016, 2Q, 6
     TIP: Functional quadriplegia (R53.2) is not integral to Alzheimer's dementia and can be separately coded.

    F02.80   Dementia in other diseases classified elsewhere without behavioral disturbance
       Dementia in other diseases classified elsewhere NOS
       Major neurocognitive disorder in other diseases classified elsewhere

    F02.81   Dementia in other diseases classified elsewhere with behavioral disturbance
       Dementia in other diseases classified elsewhere with aggressive behavior
       Dementia in other diseases classified elsewhere with combative behavior
       Dementia in other diseases classified elsewhere with violent behavior
       Major neurocognitive disorder in other diseases classified elsewhere with aggressive behavior
       Major neurocognitive disorder in other diseases classified elsewhere with combative behavior
       Major neurocognitive disorder in other diseases classified elsewhere with violent behavior
       Use additional code, if applicable, to identify wandering in dementia in conditions classified elsewhere (Z91.83)

✓4ᵗʰ F03   Unspecified dementia
   Presenile dementia NOS
   Presenile psychosis NOS
   Primary degenerative dementia NOS
   Senile dementia NOS
   Senile dementia depressed or paranoid type
   Senile psychosis NOS
EXCLUDES 1   *senility NOS (R41.81)*
EXCLUDES 2   *mild memory disturbance due to known physiological condition (F06.8)*
       senile dementia with delirium or acute confusional state (F05)

  ✓5ᵗʰ F03.9   Unspecified dementia

    F03.90   Unspecified dementia without behavioral disturbance   NC Dx   A ▽
       Dementia NOS
       AHA: 2012, 4Q, 92

    F03.91   Unspecified dementia with behavioral disturbance   NC Dx   A ▽
       Unspecified dementia with aggressive behavior
       Unspecified dementia with combative behavior
       Unspecified dementia with violent behavior
       Use additional code, if applicable, to identify wandering in unspecified dementia (Z91.83)

N Newborn: 0   P Pediatric: 0-17   M Maternity: 12-55   A Adult: 15-124   NRS Nonroutine supply Dx   NC Dx Noncancer Dx   PDx Primary Dx   ►◄ Revised Text   ● New Code   ▲ Revised Title

524   ICD-10-CM 2018

F04   Amnestic disorder due to known physiological condition
Korsakov's psychosis or syndrome, nonalcoholic
Code first the underlying physiological condition
EXCLUDES 1   *amnesia NOS (R41.3)*
anterograde amnesia (R41.1)
dissociative amnesia (F44.0)
retrograde amnesia (R41.2)
EXCLUDES 2   *alcohol-induced or unspecified Korsakov's syndrome (F10.26, F10.96)*
Korsakov's syndrome induced by other psychoactive substances (F13.26, F13.96, F19.16, F19.26, F19.96)

F05   Delirium due to known physiological condition
Acute or subacute brain syndrome
Acute or subacute confusional state (nonalcoholic)
Acute or subacute infective psychosis
Acute or subacute organic reaction
Acute or subacute psycho-organic syndrome
Delirium of mixed etiology
Delirium superimposed on dementia
Sundowning
Code first the underlying physiological condition
EXCLUDES 1   *delirium NOS (R41.0)*
EXCLUDES 2   *delirium tremens alcohol-induced or unspecified (F10.231, F10.921)*

✓4ᵗʰ **F06   Other mental disorders due to known physiological condition**
INCLUDES   mental disorders due to endocrine disorder
mental disorders due to exogenous hormone
mental disorders due to exogenous toxic substance
mental disorders due to primary cerebral disease
mental disorders due to somatic illness
mental disorders due to systemic disease affecting the brain
Code first the underlying physiological condition
EXCLUDES 1   *unspecified dementia (F03)*
EXCLUDES 2   *delirium due to known physiological condition (F05)*
dementia as classified in F01-F02
other mental disorders associated with alcohol and other psychoactive substances (F10-F19)

F06.0   Psychotic disorder with hallucinations due to known physiological condition
Organic hallucinatory state (nonalcoholic)
EXCLUDES 2   *hallucinations and perceptual disturbance induced by alcohol and other psychoactive substances (F10-F19 with .151, .251, .951)*
schizophrenia (F20.-)

F06.1   Catatonic disorder due to known physiological condition
Catatonia associated with another mental disorder
Catatonia NOS
EXCLUDES 1   *catatonic stupor (R40.1)*
stupor NOS (R40.1)
EXCLUDES 2   *catatonic schizophrenia (F20.2)*
dissociative stupor (F44.2)

F06.2   Psychotic disorder with delusions due to known physiological condition
Paranoid and paranoid-hallucinatory organic states
Schizophrenia-like psychosis in epilepsy
EXCLUDES 2   *alcohol and drug-induced psychotic disorder (F10-F19 with .150, .250, .950)*
brief psychotic disorder (F23)
delusional disorder (F22)
schizophrenia (F20.-)

✓5ᵗʰ **F06.3   Mood disorder due to known physiological condition**
EXCLUDES 2   *mood disorders due to alcohol and other psychoactive substances (F10-F19 with .14, .24, .94)*
mood disorders, not due to known physiological condition or unspecified (F30-F39)

F06.30   Mood disorder due to known physiological condition, unspecified   ▽

F06.31   Mood disorder due to known physiological condition with depressive features
▶Depressive disorder due to known physiological condition, with depressive features◀

F06.32   Mood disorder due to known physiological condition with major depressive-like episode
▶Depressive disorder due to known physiological condition, with major depressive–like episode◀

F06.33   Mood disorder due to known physiological condition with manic features
▶Bipolar and related disorder due to a known physiological condition, with manic features
Bipolar and related disorder due to known physiological condition, with manic- or hypomanic-like episodes◀

F06.34   Mood disorder due to known physiological condition with mixed features
▶Bipolar and related disorder due to known physiological condition, with mixed features
Depressive disorder due to known physiological condition, with mixed features◀

F06.4   Anxiety disorder due to known physiological condition
EXCLUDES 2   *anxiety disorders due to alcohol and other psychoactive substances (F10-F19 with .180, .280, .980)*
anxiety disorders, not due to known physiological condition or unspecified (F40.-, F41.-)

F06.8   Other specified mental disorders due to known physiological condition
Epileptic psychosis NOS
▶Obsessive-compulsive and related disorder due to a known physiological condition◀
Organic dissociative disorder
Organic emotionally labile [asthenic] disorder

✓4ᵗʰ **F07   Personality and behavioral disorders due to known physiological condition**
Code first the underlying physiological condition

F07.0   Personality change due to known physiological condition
Frontal lobe syndrome
Limbic epilepsy personality syndrome
Lobotomy syndrome
Organic personality disorder
Organic pseudopsychopathic personality
Organic pseudoretarded personality
Postleucotomy syndrome
Code first underlying physiological condition
EXCLUDES 1   *mild cognitive impairment (G31.84)*
postconcussional syndrome (F07.81)
postencephalitic syndrome (F07.89)
signs and symptoms involving emotional state (R45.-)
EXCLUDES 2   *specific personality disorder (F60.-)*

✓5ᵗʰ **F07.8   Other personality and behavioral disorders due to known physiological condition**

F07.81   Postconcussional syndrome
Postcontusional syndrome (encephalopathy)
Post-traumatic brain syndrome, nonpsychotic
Use additional code to identify associated post-traumatic headache, if applicable (G44.3-)
EXCLUDES 1   *current concussion (brain) (S06.0-)*
postencephalitic syndrome (F07.89)

F07.89   Other personality and behavioral disorders due to known physiological condition
Postencephalitic syndrome
Right hemispheric organic affective disorder

F07.9   Unspecified personality and behavioral disorder due to known physiological condition   ▽
Organic psychosyndrome

F09   Unspecified mental disorder due to known physiological condition   ▽
Mental disorder NOS due to known physiological condition
Organic brain syndrome NOS
Organic mental disorder NOS
Organic psychosis NOS
Symptomatic psychosis NOS
Code first the underlying physiological condition
EXCLUDES 1   *psychosis NOS (F29)*

Mental and behavioral disorders due to psychoactive substance use (F10-F19)

AHA: 2017, 2Q, 27

✓4ᵗʰ **F10   Alcohol related disorders**
Use additional code for blood alcohol level, if applicable (Y90.-)

✓5ᵗʰ **F10.1   Alcohol abuse**
EXCLUDES 1   *alcohol dependence (F10.2-)*
alcohol use, unspecified (F10.9-)
AHA: 2015, 2Q, 15

F10.10   Alcohol abuse, uncomplicated
Alcohol use disorder, mild

☑ Additional Character Req   ✓x7ᵗʰ Placeholder Alert   Case-Mix Diagnosis   Manifestation   ▽ Unspecified Dx   EXCLUDES 1 Not coded here   EXCLUDES 2 Not included here

Chapter 5. Mental, Behavioral and Neurodevelopmental Disorders

F10.11–F10.951

F10.11 Alcohol abuse, in remission
Alcohol use disorder, mild, in early remission
Alcohol use disorder, mild, in sustained remission

✓6ᵗʰ **F10.12 Alcohol abuse with intoxication**

F10.120 Alcohol abuse with intoxication, uncomplicated

F10.121 Alcohol abuse with intoxication delirium

F10.129 Alcohol abuse with intoxication, unspecified ▽

F10.14 Alcohol abuse with alcohol-induced mood disorder
Alcohol use disorder, mild, with alcohol-induced bipolar or related disorder
Alcohol use disorder, mild, with alcohol-induced depressive disorder

✓6ᵗʰ **F10.15 Alcohol abuse with alcohol-induced psychotic disorder**

F10.150 Alcohol abuse with alcohol-induced psychotic disorder with delusions

F10.151 Alcohol abuse with alcohol-induced psychotic disorder with hallucinations
DEF: Psychosis lasting less than six months with slight or no clouding of consciousness in which auditory hallucinations predominate.

F10.159 Alcohol abuse with alcohol-induced psychotic disorder, unspecified ▽

✓6ᵗʰ **F10.18 Alcohol abuse with other alcohol-induced disorders**

F10.180 Alcohol abuse with alcohol-induced anxiety disorder

F10.181 Alcohol abuse with alcohol-induced sexual dysfunction

F10.182 Alcohol abuse with alcohol-induced sleep disorder

F10.188 Alcohol abuse with other alcohol-induced disorder

F10.19 Alcohol abuse with unspecified alcohol-induced disorder ▽

✓5ᵗʰ **F10.2 Alcohol dependence**
EXCLUDES 1   alcohol abuse (F10.1-)
     alcohol use, unspecified (F10.9-)
EXCLUDES 2   toxic effect of alcohol (T51.0-)

F10.20 Alcohol dependence, uncomplicated
Alcohol use disorder, moderate
Alcohol use disorder, severe

F10.21 Alcohol dependence, in remission
▶Alcohol use disorder, moderate, in early remission
Alcohol use disorder, moderate, in sustained remission
Alcohol use disorder, severe, in early remission
Alcohol use disorder, severe, in sustained remission◀

✓6ᵗʰ **F10.22 Alcohol dependence with intoxication**
Acute drunkenness (in alcoholism)
EXCLUDES 2   alcohol dependence with withdrawal (F10.23-)

F10.220 Alcohol dependence with intoxication, uncomplicated

F10.221 Alcohol dependence with intoxication delirium

F10.229 Alcohol dependence with intoxication, unspecified ▽

✓6ᵗʰ **F10.23 Alcohol dependence with withdrawal**
EXCLUDES 2   alcohol dependence with intoxication (F10.22-)
AHA: 2015, 2Q, 15

F10.230 Alcohol dependence with withdrawal, uncomplicated

F10.231 Alcohol dependence with withdrawal delirium

F10.232 Alcohol dependence with withdrawal with perceptual disturbance

F10.239 Alcohol dependence with withdrawal, unspecified ▽

F10.24 Alcohol dependence with alcohol-induced mood disorder
Alcohol use disorder, moderate, with alcohol-induced bipolar or related disorder
Alcohol use disorder, moderate, with alcohol-induced depressive disorder
Alcohol use disorder, severe, with alcohol-induced bipolar or related disorder
Alcohol use disorder, severe, with alcohol-induced depressive disorder

✓6ᵗʰ **F10.25 Alcohol dependence with alcohol-induced psychotic disorder**

F10.250 Alcohol dependence with alcohol-induced psychotic disorder with delusions

F10.251 Alcohol dependence with alcohol-induced psychotic disorder with hallucinations

F10.259 Alcohol dependence with alcohol-induced psychotic disorder, unspecified ▽

F10.26 Alcohol dependence with alcohol-induced persisting amnestic disorder
Alcohol use disorder, moderate, with alcohol-induced major neurocognitive disorder, amnestic-confabulatory type
Alcohol use disorder, severe, with alcohol-induced major neurocognitive disorder, amnestic-confabulatory type
DEF: Prominent and lasting reduced memory span, disordered time appreciation and confabulation, occurs in alcoholics as sequel to acute alcoholic psychosis.

F10.27 Alcohol dependence with alcohol-induced persisting dementia
Alcohol use disorder, moderate, with alcohol-induced major neurocognitive disorder, nonamnestic-confabulatory type
Alcohol use disorder, severe, with alcohol-induced major neurocognitive disorder, nonamnestic-confabulatory type

✓6ᵗʰ **F10.28 Alcohol dependence with other alcohol-induced disorders**

F10.280 Alcohol dependence with alcohol-induced anxiety disorder

F10.281 Alcohol dependence with alcohol-induced sexual dysfunction

F10.282 Alcohol dependence with alcohol-induced sleep disorder

F10.288 Alcohol dependence with other alcohol-induced disorder
Alcohol use disorder, moderate, with alcohol-induced mild neurocognitive disorder
Alcohol use disorder, severe, with alcohol-induced mild neurocognitive disorder

F10.29 Alcohol dependence with unspecified alcohol-induced disorder ▽

✓5ᵗʰ **F10.9 Alcohol use, unspecified**
EXCLUDES 1   alcohol abuse (F10.1-)
     alcohol dependence (F10.2-)

✓6ᵗʰ **F10.92 Alcohol use, unspecified with intoxication**

F10.920 Alcohol use, unspecified with intoxication, uncomplicated

F10.921 Alcohol use, unspecified with intoxication delirium

F10.929 Alcohol use, unspecified with intoxication, unspecified ▽

F10.94 Alcohol use, unspecified with alcohol-induced mood disorder
Alcohol induced bipolar or related disorder, without use disorder
Alcohol induced depressive disorder, without use disorder

✓6ᵗʰ **F10.95 Alcohol use, unspecified with alcohol-induced psychotic disorder**

F10.950 Alcohol use, unspecified with alcohol-induced psychotic disorder with delusions

F10.951 Alcohol use, unspecified with alcohol-induced psychotic disorder with hallucinations

Ⓝ Newborn: 0   Ⓟ Pediatric: 0-17   Ⓜ Maternity: 12-55   Ⓐ Adult: 15-124   NRS Nonroutine supply Dx   NC Dx Noncancer Dx   PDx Primary Dx   ▶◀ Revised Text   ● New Code   ▲ Revised Title

526   ICD-10-CM 2018

F10.959 Alcohol use, unspecified with alcohol-induced psychotic disorder, unspecified ▽
Alcohol-induced psychotic disorder without use disorder

F10.96 Alcohol use, unspecified with alcohol-induced persisting amnestic disorder
Alcohol-induced major neurocognitive disorder, amnestic-confabulatory type, without use disorder

F10.97 Alcohol use, unspecified with alcohol-induced persisting dementia
Alcohol-induced major neurocognitive disorder, nonamnestic-confabulatory type, without use disorder

✓6th **F10.98** Alcohol use, unspecified with other alcohol-induced disorders
    F10.980 Alcohol use, unspecified with alcohol-induced anxiety disorder
        Alcohol induced anxiety disorder, without use disorder
    F10.981 Alcohol use, unspecified with alcohol-induced sexual dysfunction
        Alcohol induced sexual dysfunction, without use disorder
    F10.982 Alcohol use, unspecified with alcohol-induced sleep disorder
        Alcohol induced sleep disorder, without use disorder
    F10.988 Alcohol use, unspecified with other alcohol-induced disorder
        Alcohol induced mild neurocognitive disorder, without use disorder

F10.99 Alcohol use, unspecified with unspecified alcohol-induced disorder ▽

✓4th **F11** Opioid related disorders
✓5th **F11.1** Opioid abuse
    EXCLUDES 1 opioid dependence (F11.2-)
                opioid use, unspecified (F11.9-)

    F11.10 Opioid abuse, uncomplicated
        Opioid use disorder, mild

●   **F11.11** Opioid abuse, in remission
        Opioid use disorder, mild, in early remission
        Opioid use disorder, mild, in sustained remission

✓6th   **F11.12** Opioid abuse with intoxication
        F11.120 Opioid abuse with intoxication, uncomplicated
        F11.121 Opioid abuse with intoxication delirium
        F11.122 Opioid abuse with intoxication with perceptual disturbance
        F11.129 Opioid abuse with intoxication, unspecified ▽

    F11.14 Opioid abuse with opioid-induced mood disorder
        Opioid use disorder, mild, with opioid-induced depressive disorder

✓6th   **F11.15** Opioid abuse with opioid-induced psychotic disorder
        F11.150 Opioid abuse with opioid-induced psychotic disorder with delusions
        F11.151 Opioid abuse with opioid-induced psychotic disorder with hallucinations
        F11.159 Opioid abuse with opioid-induced psychotic disorder, unspecified ▽

✓6th   **F11.18** Opioid abuse with other opioid-induced disorder
        F11.181 Opioid abuse with opioid-induced sexual dysfunction
        F11.182 Opioid abuse with opioid-induced sleep disorder
        F11.188 Opioid abuse with other opioid-induced disorder

    F11.19 Opioid abuse with unspecified opioid-induced disorder ▽

✓5th **F11.2** Opioid dependence
    EXCLUDES 1 opioid abuse (F11.1-)
                opioid use, unspecified (F11.9-)
    EXCLUDES 2 opioid poisoning (T40.0-T40.2-)

    F11.20 Opioid dependence, uncomplicated
        Opioid use disorder, moderate
        Opioid use disorder, severe

F11.21 Opioid dependence, in remission
    ▶Opioid use disorder, moderate, in early remission
    Opioid use disorder, moderate, in sustained remission
    Opioid use disorder, severe, in early remission
    Opioid use disorder, severe, in sustained remission◀

✓6th **F11.22** Opioid dependence with intoxication
    EXCLUDES 1 opioid dependence with withdrawal (F11.23)
    F11.220 Opioid dependence with intoxication, uncomplicated
    F11.221 Opioid dependence with intoxication delirium
    F11.222 Opioid dependence with intoxication with perceptual disturbance
    F11.229 Opioid dependence with intoxication, unspecified ▽

F11.23 Opioid dependence with withdrawal
    EXCLUDES 1 opioid dependence with intoxication (F11.22-)

F11.24 Opioid dependence with opioid-induced mood disorder
    Opioid use disorder, moderate, with opioid induced depressive disorder

✓6th **F11.25** Opioid dependence with opioid-induced psychotic disorder
    F11.250 Opioid dependence with opioid-induced psychotic disorder with delusions
    F11.251 Opioid dependence with opioid-induced psychotic disorder with hallucinations
    F11.259 Opioid dependence with opioid-induced psychotic disorder, unspecified ▽

✓6th **F11.28** Opioid dependence with other opioid-induced disorder
    F11.281 Opioid dependence with opioid-induced sexual dysfunction
    F11.282 Opioid dependence with opioid-induced sleep disorder
    F11.288 Opioid dependence with other opioid-induced disorder

F11.29 Opioid dependence with unspecified opioid-induced disorder ▽

✓5th **F11.9** Opioid use, unspecified
    EXCLUDES 1 opioid abuse (F11.1-)
                opioid dependence (F11.2-)

    F11.90 Opioid use, unspecified, uncomplicated

✓6th   **F11.92** Opioid use, unspecified with intoxication
        EXCLUDES 1 opioid use, unspecified with withdrawal (F11.93)
        F11.920 Opioid use, unspecified with intoxication, uncomplicated
        F11.921 Opioid use, unspecified with intoxication delirium
                Opioid-induced delirium
        F11.922 Opioid use, unspecified with intoxication with perceptual disturbance
        F11.929 Opioid use, unspecified with intoxication, unspecified ▽

F11.93 Opioid use, unspecified with withdrawal
    EXCLUDES 1 opioid use, unspecified with intoxication (F11.92-)

F11.94 Opioid use, unspecified with opioid-induced mood disorder
    Opioid induced depressive disorder, without use disorder

✓6th **F11.95** Opioid use, unspecified with opioid-induced psychotic disorder
    F11.950 Opioid use, unspecified with opioid-induced psychotic disorder with delusions
    F11.951 Opioid use, unspecified with opioid-induced psychotic disorder with hallucinations
    F11.959 Opioid use, unspecified with opioid-induced psychotic disorder, unspecified ▽

Chapter 5. Mental, Behavioral and Neurodevelopmental Disorders

F10.959–F11.959

☑ Additional Character Req   ✓×7th Placeholder Alert   Case-Mix Diagnosis   Manifestation   ▽ Unspecified Dx   **EXCLUDES 1** Not coded here   **EXCLUDES 2** Not included here

Chapter 5. Mental, Behavioral and Neurodevelopmental Disorders

✓6th **F11.98** **Opioid use, unspecified with** other **specified opioid-induced disorder**
     F11.981 **Opioid use, unspecified with opioid-induced** sexual dysfunction
         Opioid induced sexual dysfunction, without use disorder
     F11.982 **Opioid use, unspecified with opioid-induced** sleep disorder
         Opioid induced sleep disorder, without use disorder
     F11.988 **Opioid use, unspecified with other opioid-induced disorder**
         Opioid induced anxiety disorder, without use disorder
   F11.99 **Opioid use, unspecified with unspecified opioid-induced disorder** ▽

✓4th **F12** **Cannabis related disorders**
   INCLUDES marijuana

✓5th **F12.1** **Cannabis** abuse
     EXCLUDES 1   cannabis dependence (F12.2-)
           cannabis use, unspecified (F12.9-)
   F12.10 **Cannabis abuse,** uncomplicated
     Cannabis use disorder, mild
   F12.11 **Cannabis abuse,** in remission
     Cannabis use disorder, mild, in early remission
     Cannabis use disorder, mild, in sustained remission
✓6th **F12.12** **Cannabis abuse with** intoxication
     F12.120 **Cannabis abuse with intoxication,** uncomplicated
     F12.121 **Cannabis abuse with intoxication** delirium
     F12.122 **Cannabis abuse with intoxication with** perceptual disturbance
     F12.129 **Cannabis abuse with intoxication, unspecified** ▽
✓6th **F12.15** **Cannabis abuse with** psychotic disorder
     F12.150 **Cannabis abuse with psychotic disorder with** delusions
     F12.151 **Cannabis abuse with psychotic disorder with** hallucinations
     F12.159 **Cannabis abuse with psychotic disorder, unspecified** ▽
✓6th **F12.18** **Cannabis abuse with** other **cannabis-induced disorder**
     F12.180 **Cannabis abuse with cannabis-induced** anxiety disorder
     F12.188 **Cannabis abuse with other cannabis-induced disorder**
         Cannabis use disorder, mild, with cannabis-induced sleep disorder
   F12.19 **Cannabis abuse with unspecified cannabis-induced disorder** ▽

✓5th **F12.2** **Cannabis** dependence
     EXCLUDES 1   cannabis abuse (F12.1-)
           cannabis use, unspecified (F12.9-)
     EXCLUDES 2   cannabis poisoning (T40.7-)
   F12.20 **Cannabis dependence,** uncomplicated
     Cannabis use disorder, moderate
     Cannabis use disorder, severe
   F12.21 **Cannabis dependence,** in remission
     ▶Cannabis use disorder, moderate, in early remission
     Cannabis use disorder, moderate, in sustained remission
     Cannabis use disorder, severe, in early remission
     Cannabis use disorder, severe, in sustained remission◀
✓6th **F12.22** **Cannabis dependence with** intoxication
     F12.220 **Cannabis dependence with intoxication,** uncomplicated
     F12.221 **Cannabis dependence with intoxication** delirium
     F12.222 **Cannabis dependence with intoxication with** perceptual disturbance
     F12.229 **Cannabis dependence with intoxication, unspecified** ▽
✓6th **F12.25** **Cannabis dependence with** psychotic disorder
     F12.250 **Cannabis dependence with psychotic disorder with** delusions
     F12.251 **Cannabis dependence with psychotic disorder with** hallucinations

F12.259 **Cannabis dependence with psychotic disorder, unspecified** ▽
✓6th **F12.28** **Cannabis dependence with** other **cannabis-induced disorder**
     F12.280 **Cannabis dependence with cannabis-induced** anxiety disorder
     F12.288 **Cannabis dependence with other cannabis-induced disorder**
         Cannabis use disorder, moderate, with cannabis-induced sleep disorder
         Cannabis use disorder, severe, with cannabis-induced sleep disorder
         Cannabis withdrawal
   F12.29 **Cannabis dependence with unspecified cannabis-induced disorder** ▽

✓5th **F12.9** **Cannabis use,** unspecified
     EXCLUDES 1   cannabis abuse (F12.1-)
           cannabis dependence (F12.2-)
   F12.90 **Cannabis use, unspecified,** uncomplicated
✓6th **F12.92** **Cannabis use, unspecified with** intoxication
     F12.920 **Cannabis use, unspecified with intoxication,** uncomplicated
     F12.921 **Cannabis use, unspecified with intoxication** delirium
     F12.922 **Cannabis use, unspecified with intoxication with** perceptual disturbance
     F12.929 **Cannabis use, unspecified with intoxication, unspecified** ▽
✓6th **F12.95** **Cannabis use, unspecified with** psychotic disorder
     F12.950 **Cannabis use, unspecified with psychotic disorder with** delusions
     F12.951 **Cannabis use, unspecified with psychotic disorder with** hallucinations
     F12.959 **Cannabis use, unspecified with psychotic disorder, unspecified** ▽
         Cannabis induced psychotic disorder, without use disorder
✓6th **F12.98** **Cannabis use, unspecified with** other **cannabis-induced disorder**
     F12.980 **Cannabis use, unspecified with** anxiety disorder
         Cannabis induced anxiety disorder, without use disorder
     F12.988 **Cannabis use, unspecified with other cannabis-induced disorder**
         Cannabis induced sleep disorder, without use disorder
   F12.99 **Cannabis use, unspecified with unspecified cannabis-induced disorder** ▽

✓4th **F13** **Sedative, hypnotic, or anxiolytic related disorders**
✓5th **F13.1** **Sedative, hypnotic or anxiolytic-related** abuse
     EXCLUDES 1   sedative, hypnotic or anxiolytic-related dependence (F13.2-)
           sedative, hypnotic, or anxiolytic use, unspecified (F13.9-)
   F13.10 **Sedative, hypnotic or anxiolytic abuse,** uncomplicated
     Sedative, hypnotic, or anxiolytic use disorder, mild
   F13.11 **Sedative, hypnotic or anxiolytic abuse,** in remission
     Sedative, hypnotic or anxiolytic use disorder, mild, in early remission
     Sedative, hypnotic or anxiolytic use disorder, mild, in sustained remission
✓6th **F13.12** **Sedative, hypnotic or anxiolytic abuse with** intoxication
     F13.120 **Sedative, hypnotic or anxiolytic abuse with intoxication,** uncomplicated
     F13.121 **Sedative, hypnotic or anxiolytic abuse with intoxication** delirium
     F13.129 **Sedative, hypnotic or anxiolytic abuse with intoxication, unspecified** ▽

N Newborn: 0   P Pediatric: 0-17   M Maternity: 12-55   A Adult: 15-124   NRS Nonroutine supply Dx   NCDx Noncancer Dx   PDx Primary Dx   ▶◀ Revised Text   ● New Code   ▲ Revised Title

528   ICD-10-CM 2018

F13.14 Sedative, hypnotic or anxiolytic abuse with sedative, hypnotic or anxiolytic-induced mood disorder
▶Sedative, hypnotic, or anxiolytic use disorder, mild, with sedative, hypnotic, or anxiolytic-induced bipolar or related disorder
Sedative, hypnotic, or anxiolytic use disorder, mild, with sedative, hypnotic, or anxiolytic-induced depressive disorder◀

✓6th **F13.15 Sedative, hypnotic or anxiolytic abuse with sedative, hypnotic or anxiolytic-induced** psychotic disorder

F13.150 Sedative, hypnotic or anxiolytic abuse with sedative, hypnotic or anxiolytic-induced psychotic disorder with delusions

F13.151 Sedative, hypnotic or anxiolytic abuse with sedative, hypnotic or anxiolytic-induced psychotic disorder with hallucinations

F13.159 Sedative, hypnotic or anxiolytic ▽ **abuse with sedative, hypnotic or anxiolytic-induced psychotic disorder, unspecified**

✓6th **F13.18 Sedative, hypnotic or anxiolytic abuse with** other **sedative, hypnotic or anxiolytic-induced disorders**

F13.180 Sedative, hypnotic or anxiolytic abuse with sedative, hypnotic or anxiolytic-induced anxiety disorder

F13.181 Sedative, hypnotic or anxiolytic abuse with sedative, hypnotic or anxiolytic-induced sexual dysfunction

F13.182 Sedative, hypnotic or anxiolytic abuse with sedative, hypnotic or anxiolytic-induced sleep disorder

F13.188 Sedative, hypnotic or anxiolytic abuse with other sedative, hypnotic or anxiolytic-induced disorder

F13.19 Sedative, hypnotic or anxiolytic abuse with ▽ **unspecified sedative, hypnotic or anxiolytic-induced disorder**

✓5th **F13.2 Sedative, hypnotic or anxiolytic-related** dependence
EXCLUDES 1 *sedative, hypnotic or anxiolytic-related abuse (F13.1-)*
sedative, hypnotic, or anxiolytic use, unspecified (F13.9-)
EXCLUDES 2 *sedative, hypnotic, or anxiolytic poisoning (T42.-)*

F13.20 Sedative, hypnotic or anxiolytic dependence, uncomplicated

F13.21 Sedative, hypnotic or anxiolytic dependence, in remission
▶Sedative, hypnotic or anxiolytic use disorder, moderate, in early remission
Sedative, hypnotic or anxiolytic use disorder, moderate, in sustained remission
Sedative, hypnotic or anxiolytic use disorder, severe, in early remission
Sedative, hypnotic or anxiolytic use disorder, severe, in sustained remission◀

✓6th **F13.22 Sedative, hypnotic or anxiolytic dependence with intoxication**
EXCLUDES 1 *sedative, hypnotic or anxiolytic dependence with withdrawal (F13.23-)*

F13.220 Sedative, hypnotic or anxiolytic dependence with intoxication, uncomplicated

F13.221 Sedative, hypnotic or anxiolytic dependence with intoxication delirium

F13.229 Sedative, hypnotic or anxiolytic ▽ **dependence with intoxication, unspecified**

✓6th **F13.23 Sedative, hypnotic or anxiolytic dependence with** withdrawal
Sedative, hypnotic, or anxiolytic use disorder, moderate
Sedative, hypnotic, or anxiolytic use disorder, severe
EXCLUDES 1 *sedative, hypnotic or anxiolytic dependence with intoxication (F13.22-)*

F13.230 Sedative, hypnotic or anxiolytic dependence with withdrawal, uncomplicated

F13.231 Sedative, hypnotic or anxiolytic dependence with withdrawal delirium

F13.232 Sedative, hypnotic or anxiolytic dependence with withdrawal with perceptual disturbance
Sedative, hypnotic, or anxiolytic withdrawal with perceptual disturbances

F13.239 Sedative, hypnotic or anxiolytic ▽ **dependence with withdrawal, unspecified**
Sedative, hypnotic, or anxiolytic withdrawal without perceptual disturbances

F13.24 Sedative, hypnotic or anxiolytic dependence with sedative, hypnotic or anxiolytic-induced mood disorder
▶Sedative, hypnotic, or anxiolytic use disorder, moderate, with sedative, hypnotic, or anxiolytic-induced bipolar or related disorder
Sedative, hypnotic, or anxiolytic use disorder, moderate, with sedative, hypnotic, or anxiolytic-induced depressive disorder◀
Sedative, hypnotic, or anxiolytic use disorder, severe, with sedative, hypnotic, or anxiolytic-induced bipolar or related disorder
▶Sedative, hypnotic, or anxiolytic use disorder, severe, with sedative, hypnotic, or anxiolytic-induced depressive disorder◀

✓6th **F13.25 Sedative, hypnotic or anxiolytic dependence with sedative, hypnotic or anxiolytic-induced** psychotic disorder

F13.250 Sedative, hypnotic or anxiolytic dependence with sedative, hypnotic or anxiolytic-induced psychotic disorder with delusions

F13.251 Sedative, hypnotic or anxiolytic dependence with sedative, hypnotic or anxiolytic-induced psychotic disorder with hallucinations

F13.259 Sedative, hypnotic or anxiolytic ▽ **dependence with sedative, hypnotic or anxiolytic-induced psychotic disorder, unspecified**

F13.26 Sedative, hypnotic or anxiolytic dependence with sedative, hypnotic or anxiolytic-induced persisting amnestic disorder

F13.27 Sedative, hypnotic or anxiolytic dependence with sedative, hypnotic or anxiolytic-induced persisting dementia
▶Sedative, hypnotic, or anxiolytic use disorder, moderate, with sedative, hypnotic, or anxiolytic-induced major neurocognitive disorder◀
Sedative, hypnotic, or anxiolytic use disorder, severe, with sedative, hypnotic, or anxiolytic-induced major neurocognitive disorder

✓6th **F13.28 Sedative, hypnotic or anxiolytic dependence with** other **sedative, hypnotic or anxiolytic-induced disorders**

F13.280 Sedative, hypnotic or anxiolytic dependence with sedative, hypnotic or anxiolytic-induced anxiety disorder

F13.281 Sedative, hypnotic or anxiolytic dependence with sedative, hypnotic or anxiolytic-induced sexual dysfunction

F13.282 Sedative, hypnotic or anxiolytic dependence with sedative, hypnotic or anxiolytic-induced sleep disorder

F13.288 Sedative, hypnotic or anxiolytic dependence with other sedative, hypnotic or anxiolytic-induced disorder
▶Sedative, hypnotic, or anxiolytic use disorder, moderate, with sedative, hypnotic, or anxiolytic-induced mild neurocognitive disorder
Sedative, hypnotic, or anxiolytic use disorder, severe, with sedative, hypnotic, or anxiolytic-induced mild neurocognitive disorder◀

F13.29 Sedative, hypnotic or anxiolytic dependence ▽ **with unspecified sedative, hypnotic or anxiolytic-induced disorder**

✓ Additional Character Req   ✓x7th Placeholder Alert   Case-Mix Diagnosis   Manifestation   ▽ Unspecified Dx   EXCLUDES 1 Not coded here   EXCLUDES 2 Not included here

ICD-10-CM 2018   **529**

✓5th **F13.9** **Sedative, hypnotic or anxiolytic-related use,** unspecified
> EXCLUDES 1   *sedative, hypnotic or anxiolytic-related abuse (F13.1-)*
> *sedative, hypnotic or anxiolytic-related dependence (F13.2-)*

F13.90 **Sedative, hypnotic, or anxiolytic use, unspecified, uncomplicated**

✓6th **F13.92** **Sedative, hypnotic or anxiolytic use, unspecified with** intoxication
> EXCLUDES 1   *sedative, hypnotic or anxiolytic use, unspecified with withdrawal (F13.93-)*

F13.920 **Sedative, hypnotic or anxiolytic use, unspecified with intoxication, uncomplicated**

F13.921 **Sedative, hypnotic or anxiolytic use, unspecified with intoxication** delirium
Sedative, hypnotic, or anxiolytic-induced delirium

F13.929 **Sedative, hypnotic or anxiolytic use, unspecified with intoxication, unspecified** ▽

✓6th **F13.93** **Sedative, hypnotic or anxiolytic use, unspecified with** withdrawal
> EXCLUDES 1   *sedative, hypnotic or anxiolytic use, unspecified with intoxication (F13.92-)*

F13.930 **Sedative, hypnotic or anxiolytic use, unspecified with withdrawal, uncomplicated**

F13.931 **Sedative, hypnotic or anxiolytic use, unspecified with withdrawal** delirium

F13.932 **Sedative, hypnotic or anxiolytic use, unspecified with withdrawal with** perceptual disturbances

F13.939 **Sedative, hypnotic or anxiolytic use, unspecified with withdrawal, unspecified** ▽

F13.94 **Sedative, hypnotic or anxiolytic use, unspecified with sedative, hypnotic or anxiolytic-induced** mood disorder
Sedative, hypnotic, or anxiolytic-induced bipolar or related disorder, without use disorder
Sedative, hypnotic, or anxiolytic-induced depressive disorder, without use disorder

✓6th **F13.95** **Sedative, hypnotic or anxiolytic use, unspecified with sedative, hypnotic or anxiolytic-induced** psychotic disorder

F13.950 **Sedative, hypnotic or anxiolytic use, unspecified with sedative, hypnotic or anxiolytic-induced psychotic disorder with** delusions

F13.951 **Sedative, hypnotic or anxiolytic use, unspecified with sedative, hypnotic or anxiolytic-induced psychotic disorder with** hallucinations

F13.959 **Sedative, hypnotic or anxiolytic use, unspecified with sedative, hypnotic or anxiolytic-induced psychotic disorder, unspecified** ▽
▶Sedative, hypnotic, or anxiolytic-induced psychotic disorder, without use disorder◀

F13.96 **Sedative, hypnotic or anxiolytic use, unspecified with sedative, hypnotic or anxiolytic-induced** persisting amnestic disorder

F13.97 **Sedative, hypnotic or anxiolytic use, unspecified with sedative, hypnotic or anxiolytic-induced** persisting dementia
▶Sedative, hypnotic, or anxiolytic-induced major neurocognitive disorder, without use disorder◀

✓6th **F13.98** **Sedative, hypnotic or anxiolytic use, unspecified with** other **sedative, hypnotic or anxiolytic-induced disorders**

F13.980 **Sedative, hypnotic or anxiolytic use, unspecified with sedative, hypnotic or anxiolytic-induced** anxiety disorder
▶Sedative, hypnotic, or anxiolytic-induced anxiety disorder, without use disorder◀

F13.981 **Sedative, hypnotic or anxiolytic use, unspecified with sedative, hypnotic or anxiolytic-induced** sexual dysfunction
▶Sedative, hypnotic, or anxiolytic-induced sexual dysfunction disorder, without use disorder◀

F13.982 **Sedative, hypnotic or anxiolytic use, unspecified with sedative, hypnotic or anxiolytic-induced** sleep disorder
▶Sedative, hypnotic, or anxiolytic-induced sleep disorder, without use disorder◀

F13.988 **Sedative, hypnotic or anxiolytic use, unspecified with other sedative, hypnotic or anxiolytic-induced disorder**
▶Sedative, hypnotic, or anxiolytic-induced mild neurocognitive disorder◀

F13.99 **Sedative, hypnotic or anxiolytic use, unspecified with unspecified sedative, hypnotic or anxiolytic-induced disorder** ▽

✓4th **F14** **Cocaine related disorders**
> EXCLUDES 2   *other stimulant-related disorders (F15.-)*

✓5th **F14.1** **Cocaine** abuse
> EXCLUDES 1   *cocaine dependence (F14.2-)*
> *cocaine use, unspecified (F14.9-)*

F14.10 **Cocaine abuse,** uncomplicated
Cocaine use disorder, mild

● **F14.11** **Cocaine abuse,** in remission
Cocaine use disorder, mild, in early remission
Cocaine use disorder, mild, in sustained remission

✓6th **F14.12** **Cocaine abuse with** intoxication

F14.120 **Cocaine abuse with intoxication, uncomplicated**

F14.121 **Cocaine abuse with intoxication with** delirium

F14.122 **Cocaine abuse with intoxication with** perceptual disturbance

F14.129 **Cocaine abuse with intoxication, unspecified** ▽

F14.14 **Cocaine abuse with cocaine-induced** mood disorder
Cocaine use disorder, mild, with cocaine-induced bipolar or related disorder
Cocaine use disorder, mild, with cocaine-induced depressive disorder

✓6th **F14.15** **Cocaine abuse with cocaine-induced** psychotic disorder

F14.150 **Cocaine abuse with cocaine-induced psychotic disorder with** delusions

F14.151 **Cocaine abuse with cocaine-induced psychotic disorder with** hallucinations

F14.159 **Cocaine abuse with cocaine-induced psychotic disorder, unspecified** ▽

✓6th **F14.18** **Cocaine abuse with** other **cocaine-induced disorder**

F14.180 **Cocaine abuse with cocaine-induced** anxiety disorder

F14.181 **Cocaine abuse with cocaine-induced** sexual dysfunction

F14.182 **Cocaine abuse with cocaine-induced** sleep disorder

F14.188 **Cocaine abuse with other cocaine-induced disorder**
Cocaine use disorder, mild, with cocaine-induced obsessive compulsive or related disorder

F14.19 **Cocaine abuse with unspecified cocaine-induced disorder** ▽

✓5th **F14.2** **Cocaine** dependence
> EXCLUDES 1   *cocaine abuse (F14.1-)*
> *cocaine use, unspecified (F14.9-)*
> EXCLUDES 2   *cocaine poisoning (T40.5-)*

F14.20 **Cocaine dependence,** uncomplicated
Cocaine use disorder, moderate
Cocaine use disorder, severe

F14.21 **Cocaine dependence,** in remission
▶Cocaine use disorder, moderate, in early remission
Cocaine use disorder, moderate, in sustained remission
Cocaine use disorder, severe, in early remission
Cocaine use disorder, severe, in sustained remission◀

Ⓝ Newborn: 0   Ⓟ Pediatric: 0-17   Ⓜ Maternity: 12-55   Ⓐ Adult: 15-124   NRS Nonroutine supply Dx   NCDx Noncancer Dx   PDx Primary Dx   ▶◀ Revised Text   ● New Code   ▲ Revised Title

530   ICD-10-CM 2018

✓6ᵗʰ **F14.22 Cocaine dependence with** intoxication
> **EXCLUDES 1** *cocaine dependence with withdrawal (F14.23)*

     F14.220 Cocaine dependence with intoxication, uncomplicated

     F14.221 Cocaine dependence with intoxication delirium

     F14.222 Cocaine dependence with intoxication with perceptual disturbance

     F14.229 Cocaine dependence with intoxication, unspecified ▽

F14.23 Cocaine dependence with withdrawal
> **EXCLUDES 1** *cocaine dependence with intoxication (F14.22-)*

F14.24 Cocaine dependence with cocaine-induced mood disorder
> Cocaine use disorder, moderate, with cocaine-induced bipolar or related disorder
> Cocaine use disorder, moderate, with cocaine-induced depressive disorder
> Cocaine use disorder, severe, with cocaine-induced bipolar or related disorder
> Cocaine use disorder, severe, with cocaine-induced depressive disorder

✓6ᵗʰ **F14.25 Cocaine dependence with cocaine-induced** psychotic disorder

     F14.250 Cocaine dependence with cocaine-induced psychotic disorder with delusions

     F14.251 Cocaine dependence with cocaine-induced psychotic disorder with hallucinations

     F14.259 Cocaine dependence with cocaine-induced psychotic disorder, unspecified ▽

✓6ᵗʰ **F14.28 Cocaine dependence with** other cocaine-induced disorder

     F14.280 Cocaine dependence with cocaine-induced anxiety disorder

     F14.281 Cocaine dependence with cocaine-induced sexual dysfunction

     F14.282 Cocaine dependence with cocaine-induced sleep disorder

     F14.288 Cocaine dependence with other cocaine-induced disorder
> Cocaine use disorder, moderate, with cocaine-induced obsessive compulsive or related disorder
> Cocaine use disorder, severe, with cocaine-induced obsessive compulsive or related disorder

F14.29 Cocaine dependence with unspecified cocaine-induced disorder ▽

✓5ᵗʰ **F14.9 Cocaine use,** unspecified
> **EXCLUDES 1** *cocaine abuse (F14.1-)*
> *cocaine dependence (F14.2-)*

F14.90 Cocaine use, unspecified, uncomplicated

✓6ᵗʰ **F14.92 Cocaine use, unspecified with** intoxication

     F14.920 Cocaine use, unspecified with intoxication, uncomplicated

     F14.921 Cocaine use, unspecified with intoxication delirium

     F14.922 Cocaine use, unspecified with intoxication with perceptual disturbance

     F14.929 Cocaine use, unspecified with intoxication, unspecified ▽

F14.94 Cocaine use, unspecified with cocaine-induced mood disorder
> Cocaine induced bipolar or related disorder, without use disorder
> Cocaine induced depressive disorder, without use disorder

✓6ᵗʰ **F14.95 Cocaine use, unspecified with cocaine-induced** psychotic disorder

     F14.950 Cocaine use, unspecified with cocaine-induced psychotic disorder with delusions

     F14.951 Cocaine use, unspecified with cocaine-induced psychotic disorder with hallucinations

     F14.959 Cocaine use, unspecified with cocaine-induced psychotic disorder, unspecified ▽
> Cocaine induced psychotic disorder, without use disorder

✓6ᵗʰ **F14.98 Cocaine use, unspecified with** other specified cocaine-induced disorder

     F14.980 Cocaine use, unspecified with cocaine-induced anxiety disorder
> Cocaine induced anxiety disorder, without use disorder

     F14.981 Cocaine use, unspecified with cocaine-induced sexual dysfunction
> Cocaine induced sexual dysfunction, without use disorder

     F14.982 Cocaine use, unspecified with cocaine-induced sleep disorder
> Cocaine induced sleep disorder, without use disorder

     F14.988 Cocaine use, unspecified with other cocaine-induced disorder
> Cocaine induced obsessive compulsive or related disorder

     F14.99 Cocaine use, unspecified with unspecified cocaine-induced disorder ▽

✓4ᵗʰ **F15 Other stimulant related disorders**
> **INCLUDES** amphetamine-related disorders
> caffeine
> **EXCLUDES 2** *cocaine-related disorders (F14.-)*

✓5ᵗʰ **F15.1 Other stimulant** abuse
> **EXCLUDES 1** *other stimulant dependence (F15.2-)*
> *other stimulant use, unspecified (F15.9-)*

     F15.10 Other stimulant abuse, uncomplicated
> Amphetamine type substance use disorder, mild
> Other or unspecified stimulant use disorder, mild

●   **F15.11 Other stimulant abuse,** in remission
> Amphetamine type substance use disorder, mild, in early remission
> Amphetamine type substance use disorder, mild, in sustained remission
> Other or unspecified stimulant use disorder, mild, in early remission
> Other or unspecified stimulant use disorder, mild, in sustained remission

✓6ᵗʰ **F15.12 Other stimulant abuse with** intoxication

     F15.120 Other stimulant abuse with intoxication, uncomplicated

     F15.121 Other stimulant abuse with intoxication delirium

     F15.122 Other stimulant abuse with intoxication with perceptual disturbance
> Amphetamine or other stimulant use disorder, mild, with amphetamine or other stimulant intoxication, with perceptual disturbances

     F15.129 Other stimulant abuse with intoxication, unspecified ▽
> Amphetamine or other stimulant use disorder, mild, with amphetamine or other stimulant intoxication, without perceptual disturbances

F15.14 Other stimulant abuse with stimulant-induced mood disorder
> Amphetamine or other stimulant use disorder, mild, with amphetamine or other stimulant induced bipolar or related disorder
> Amphetamine or other stimulant use disorder, mild, with amphetamine or other stimulant induced depressive disorder

✓6ᵗʰ **F15.15 Other stimulant abuse with stimulant-induced** psychotic disorder

     F15.150 Other stimulant abuse with stimulant-induced psychotic disorder with delusions

     F15.151 Other stimulant abuse with stimulant-induced psychotic disorder with hallucinations

---

✔ Additional Character Req   ✔x7ᵗʰ Placeholder Alert   Case-Mix Diagnosis   Manifestation   ▽ Unspecified Dx   **EXCLUDES 1** Not coded here   **EXCLUDES 2** Not included here

ICD-10-CM 2018   531

F15.159   **Other stimulant abuse with stimulant-induced psychotic disorder, unspecified** ▽

✓6ᵗʰ   F15.18   **Other stimulant abuse with** other **stimulant-induced disorder**

F15.18Ø   **Other stimulant abuse with stimulant-induced** anxiety disorder

F15.181   **Other stimulant abuse with stimulant-induced** sexual dysfunction

F15.182   **Other stimulant abuse with stimulant-induced** sleep disorder

F15.188   **Other stimulant abuse with other stimulant-induced disorder**
Amphetamine or other stimulant use disorder, mild, with amphetamine or other stimulant induced obsessive-compulsive or related disorder

F15.19   **Other stimulant abuse with unspecified stimulant-induced disorder** ▽

✓5ᵗʰ   F15.2   **Other stimulant** dependence

> **EXCLUDES 1**   *other stimulant abuse (F15.1-)*
> *other stimulant use, unspecified (F15.9-)*

F15.2Ø   **Other stimulant dependence, uncomplicated**
Amphetamine type substance use disorder, moderate
Amphetamine type substance use disorder, severe
Other or unspecified stimulant use disorder, moderate
Other or unspecified stimulant use disorder, severe

F15.21   **Other stimulant dependence,** in remission
▶Amphetamine type substance use disorder, moderate, in early remission
Amphetamine type substance use disorder, moderate, in sustained remission
Amphetamine type substance use disorder, severe, in early remission
Amphetamine type substance use disorder, severe, in sustained remission
Other or unspecified stimulant use disorder, moderate, in early remission
Other or unspecified stimulant use disorder, moderate, in sustained remission
Other or unspecified stimulant use disorder, severe, in early remission
Other or unspecified stimulant use disorder, severe, in sustained remission◀

✓6ᵗʰ   F15.22   **Other stimulant dependence with** intoxication

> **EXCLUDES 1**   *other stimulant dependence with withdrawal (F15.23)*

F15.22Ø   **Other stimulant dependence with intoxication,** uncomplicated

F15.221   **Other stimulant dependence with intoxication** delirium

F15.222   **Other stimulant dependence with intoxication with** perceptual disturbance
Amphetamine or other stimulant use disorder, moderate, with amphetamine or other stimulant intoxication, with perceptual disturbances
Amphetamine or other stimulant use disorder, severe, with amphetamine or other stimulant intoxication, with perceptual disturbances

F15.229   **Other stimulant dependence with intoxication, unspecified** ▽
Amphetamine or other stimulant use disorder, moderate, with amphetamine or other stimulant intoxication, without perceptual disturbances
Amphetamine or other stimulant use disorder, severe, with amphetamine or other stimulant intoxication, without perceptual disturbances

F15.23   **Other stimulant dependence with** withdrawal
Amphetamine or other stimulant withdrawal

> **EXCLUDES 1**   *other stimulant dependence with intoxication (F15.22-)*

F15.24   **Other stimulant dependence with stimulant-induced** mood disorder
Amphetamine or other stimulant use disorder, moderate, with amphetamine or other stimulant-induced bipolar or related disorder
Amphetamine or other stimulant use disorder, moderate, with amphetamine or other stimulant induced depressive disorder
Amphetamine or other stimulant use disorder, severe, with amphetamine or other stimulant-induced bipolar or related disorder
Amphetamine or other stimulant use disorder, severe, with amphetamine or other stimulant-induced depressive disorder

✓6ᵗʰ   F15.25   **Other stimulant dependence with stimulant-induced** psychotic disorder

F15.25Ø   **Other stimulant dependence with stimulant-induced psychotic disorder with** delusions

F15.251   **Other stimulant dependence with stimulant-induced psychotic disorder with** hallucinations

F15.259   **Other stimulant dependence with stimulant-induced psychotic disorder, unspecified** ▽

✓6ᵗʰ   F15.28   **Other stimulant dependence with** other **stimulant-induced disorder**

F15.28Ø   **Other stimulant dependence with stimulant-induced** anxiety disorder

F15.281   **Other stimulant dependence with stimulant-induced** sexual dysfunction

F15.282   **Other stimulant dependence with stimulant-induced** sleep disorder

F15.288   **Other stimulant dependence with other stimulant-induced disorder**
▶Amphetamine or other stimulant use disorder, moderate, with amphetamine or other stimulant induced obsessive compulsive or related disorder
Amphetamine or other stimulant use disorder, severe, with amphetamine or other stimulant induced obsessive compulsive or related disorder◀

F15.29   **Other stimulant dependence with unspecified stimulant-induced disorder** ▽

✓5ᵗʰ   F15.9   **Other stimulant use,** unspecified

> **EXCLUDES 1**   *other stimulant abuse (F15.1-)*
> *other stimulant dependence (F15.2-)*

F15.9Ø   **Other stimulant use, unspecified,** uncomplicated

✓6ᵗʰ   F15.92   **Other stimulant use, unspecified** with intoxication

> **EXCLUDES 1**   *other stimulant use, unspecified with withdrawal (F15.93)*

F15.92Ø   **Other stimulant use, unspecified with intoxication,** uncomplicated

F15.921   **Other stimulant use, unspecified with intoxication** delirium
Amphetamine or other stimulant-induced delirium

F15.922   **Other stimulant use, unspecified with intoxication with** perceptual disturbance

F15.929   **Other stimulant use, unspecified with intoxication, unspecified** ▽
Caffeine intoxication

F15.93   **Other stimulant use, unspecified with** withdrawal
Caffeine withdrawal

> **EXCLUDES 1**   *other stimulant use, unspecified with intoxication (F15.92-)*

F15.94   **Other stimulant use, unspecified with stimulant-induced** mood disorder
Amphetamine or other stimulant-induced bipolar or related disorder, without use disorder
Amphetamine or other stimulant-induced depressive disorder, without use disorder

✓6ᵗʰ   F15.95   **Other stimulant use, unspecified with stimulant-induced** psychotic disorder

F15.95Ø   **Other stimulant use, unspecified with stimulant-induced psychotic disorder with** delusions

---

Ⓝ Newborn: 0   Ⓟ Pediatric: 0-17   Ⓜ Maternity: 12-55   Ⓐ Adult: 15-124   **NRS** Nonroutine supply Dx   **NC Dx** Noncancer Dx   **PDx** Primary Dx   ▶◀ Revised Text   ● New Code   ▲ Revised Title

532   ICD-10-CM 2018

F15.951 **Other stimulant use, unspecified with stimulant-induced psychotic disorder with** hallucinations

F15.959 **Other stimulant use, unspecified with stimulant-induced psychotic disorder, unspecified** ▽
▶Amphetamine or other stimulant-induced psychotic disorder, without use disorder◀

✓6ᵗʰ **F15.98 Other stimulant use, unspecified with** other **stimulant-induced disorder**

F15.980 **Other stimulant use, unspecified with stimulant-induced** anxiety disorder
Amphetamine or other stimulant-induced anxiety disorder, without use disorder
Caffeine induced anxiety disorder, without use disorder

F15.981 **Other stimulant use, unspecified with stimulant-induced** sexual dysfunction
Amphetamine or other stimulant-induced sexual dysfunction, without use disorder

F15.982 **Other stimulant use, unspecified with stimulant-induced** sleep disorder
Amphetamine or other stimulant-induced sleep disorder, without use disorder
Caffeine induced sleep disorder, without use disorder

F15.988 **Other stimulant use, unspecified with other stimulant-induced disorder**
Amphetamine or other stimulant-induced obsessive compulsive or related disorder, without use disorder

F15.99 **Other stimulant use, unspecified with unspecified stimulant-induced disorder** ▽

✓4ᵗʰ **F16** Hallucinogen **related disorders**
INCLUDES ecstasy
PCP
phencyclidine

✓5ᵗʰ **F16.1 Hallucinogen** abuse
EXCLUDES 1 hallucinogen dependence (F16.2-)
hallucinogen use, unspecified (F16.9-)

F16.10 **Hallucinogen abuse,** uncomplicated
Other hallucinogen use disorder, mild
Phencyclidine use disorder, mild

• F16.11 **Hallucinogen abuse,** in remission
Other hallucinogen use disorder, mild, in early remission
Other hallucinogen use disorder, mild, in sustained remission
Phencyclidine use disorder, mild, in early remission
Phencyclidine use disorder, mild, in sustained remission

✓6ᵗʰ F16.12 **Hallucinogen abuse with** intoxication

F16.120 **Hallucinogen abuse with intoxication,** uncomplicated

F16.121 **Hallucinogen abuse with intoxication with** delirium

F16.122 **Hallucinogen abuse with intoxication with** perceptual disturbance

F16.129 **Hallucinogen abuse with intoxication, unspecified** ▽

F16.14 **Hallucinogen abuse with hallucinogen-induced** mood disorder
Other hallucinogen use disorder, mild, with other hallucinogen induced bipolar or related disorder
Other hallucinogen use disorder, mild, with other hallucinogen induced depressive disorder
Phencyclidine use disorder, mild, with phencyclidine induced bipolar or related disorder
Phencyclidine use disorder, mild, with phencyclidine induced depressive disorder

✓6ᵗʰ F16.15 **Hallucinogen abuse with hallucinogen-induced** psychotic disorder

F16.150 **Hallucinogen abuse with hallucinogen-induced psychotic disorder with** delusions

F16.151 **Hallucinogen abuse with hallucinogen-induced psychotic disorder with** hallucinations

F16.159 **Hallucinogen abuse with hallucinogen-induced psychotic disorder, unspecified** ▽

✓6ᵗʰ F16.18 **Hallucinogen abuse with** other **hallucinogen-induced disorder**

F16.180 **Hallucinogen abuse with hallucinogen-induced** anxiety disorder

F16.183 **Hallucinogen abuse with hallucinogen** persisting perception disorder (flashbacks)

F16.188 **Hallucinogen abuse with other hallucinogen-induced disorder**

F16.19 **Hallucinogen abuse with unspecified hallucinogen-induced disorder** ▽

✓5ᵗʰ **F16.2 Hallucinogen** dependence
EXCLUDES 1 hallucinogen abuse (F16.1-)
hallucinogen use, unspecified (F16.9-)

F16.20 **Hallucinogen dependence,** uncomplicated
Other hallucinogen use disorder, moderate
Other hallucinogen use disorder, severe
Phencyclidine use disorder, moderate
Phencyclidine use disorder, severe

F16.21 **Hallucinogen dependence,** in remission
▶Other hallucinogen use disorder, moderate, in early remission
Other hallucinogen use disorder, moderate, in sustained remission
Other hallucinogen use disorder, severe, in early remission
Other hallucinogen use disorder, severe, in sustained remission
Phencyclidine use disorder, moderate, in early remission
Phencyclidine use disorder, moderate, in sustained remission
Phencyclidine use disorder, severe, in early remission
Phencyclidine use disorder, severe, in sustained remission◀

✓6ᵗʰ F16.22 **Hallucinogen dependence with** intoxication

F16.220 **Hallucinogen dependence with intoxication,** uncomplicated

F16.221 **Hallucinogen dependence with intoxication with** delirium

F16.229 **Hallucinogen dependence with intoxication, unspecified** ▽

F16.24 **Hallucinogen dependence with hallucinogen-induced** mood disorder
Other hallucinogen use disorder, moderate, with other hallucinogen induced bipolar or related disorder
Other hallucinogen use disorder, moderate, with other hallucinogen induced depressive disorder
Other hallucinogen use disorder, severe, with other hallucinogen-induced bipolar or related disorder
Other hallucinogen use disorder, severe, with other hallucinogen-induced depressive disorder
Phencyclidine use disorder, moderate, with phencyclidine induced bipolar or related disorder
Phencyclidine use disorder, moderate, with phencyclidine induced depressive disorder
Phencyclidine use disorder, severe, with phencyclidine induced bipolar or related disorder
Phencyclidine use disorder, severe, with phencyclidine-induced depressive disorder

✓6ᵗʰ F16.25 **Hallucinogen dependence with hallucinogen-induced** psychotic disorder

F16.250 **Hallucinogen dependence with hallucinogen-induced psychotic disorder with** delusions

F16.251 **Hallucinogen dependence with hallucinogen-induced psychotic disorder with** hallucinations

F16.259 **Hallucinogen dependence with hallucinogen-induced psychotic disorder, unspecified** ▽

✓6ᵗʰ F16.28 **Hallucinogen dependence with** other **hallucinogen-induced disorder**

F16.280 **Hallucinogen dependence with hallucinogen-induced** anxiety disorder

F16.283 **Hallucinogen dependence with hallucinogen** persisting perception disorder (flashbacks)

F16.288   Hallucinogen dependence with other hallucinogen-induced disorder

F16.29   Hallucinogen dependence with unspecified hallucinogen-induced disorder ▽

✓5ᵗʰ **F16.9**   Hallucinogen use, unspecified
> EXCLUDES 1   hallucinogen abuse (F16.1-)
> hallucinogen dependence (F16.2-)

F16.90   Hallucinogen use, unspecified, uncomplicated

✓6ᵗʰ **F16.92**   Hallucinogen use, unspecified with intoxication

F16.920   Hallucinogen use, unspecified with intoxication, uncomplicated

F16.921   Hallucinogen use, unspecified with intoxication with delirium
> Other hallucinogen intoxication delirium

F16.929   Hallucinogen use, unspecified with intoxication, unspecified ▽

F16.94   Hallucinogen use, unspecified with hallucinogen-induced mood disorder
> Other hallucinogen induced bipolar or related disorder, without use disorder
> Other hallucinogen induced depressive disorder, without use disorder
> Phencyclidine induced bipolar or related disorder, without use disorder
> Phencyclidine induced depressive disorder, without use disorder

✓6ᵗʰ **F16.95**   Hallucinogen use, unspecified with hallucinogen-induced psychotic disorder

F16.950   Hallucinogen use, unspecified with hallucinogen-induced psychotic disorder with delusions

F16.951   Hallucinogen use, unspecified with hallucinogen-induced psychotic disorder with hallucinations

F16.959   Hallucinogen use, unspecified with hallucinogen-induced psychotic disorder, unspecified ▽
> Other hallucinogen induced psychotic disorder, without use disorder
> Phencyclidine induced psychotic disorder, without use disorder

✓6ᵗʰ **F16.98**   Hallucinogen use, unspecified with other specified hallucinogen-induced disorder

F16.980   Hallucinogen use, unspecified with hallucinogen-induced anxiety disorder
> Other hallucinogen-induced anxiety disorder, without use disorder
> Phencyclidine induced anxiety disorder, without use disorder

F16.983   Hallucinogen use, unspecified with hallucinogen persisting perception disorder (flashbacks)

F16.988   Hallucinogen use, unspecified with other hallucinogen-induced disorder

F16.99   Hallucinogen use, unspecified with unspecified hallucinogen-induced disorder ▽

✓4ᵗʰ **F17**   Nicotine dependence
> EXCLUDES 1   history of tobacco dependence (Z87.891)
> tobacco use NOS (Z72.0)
> EXCLUDES 2   tobacco use (smoking) during pregnancy, childbirth and the puerperium (O99.33-)
> toxic effect of nicotine (T65.2-)

AHA: 2013, 4Q, 108-109
TIP: Provider documentation indicating "smoker" without further specification should be coded to F17.200 Nicotine dependence, unspecified, uncomplicated.

✓5ᵗʰ **F17.2**   Nicotine dependence

✓6ᵗʰ **F17.20**   Nicotine dependence, unspecified

F17.200   Nicotine dependence, unspecified, uncomplicated ▽
> Tobacco use disorder, mild
> Tobacco use disorder, moderate
> Tobacco use disorder, severe
> **AHA:** 2016, 1Q, 36

F17.201   Nicotine dependence, unspecified, in remission ▽
> ▶Tobacco use disorder, mild, in early remission
> Tobacco use disorder, mild, in sustained remission
> Tobacco use disorder, moderate, in early remission
> Tobacco use disorder, moderate, in sustained remission
> Tobacco use disorder, severe, in early remission
> Tobacco use disorder, severe, in sustained remission◀

F17.203   Nicotine dependence unspecified, with withdrawal ▽
> Tobacco withdrawal

F17.208   Nicotine dependence, unspecified, with other nicotine-induced disorders ▽

F17.209   Nicotine dependence, unspecified, with unspecified nicotine-induced disorders ▽

✓6ᵗʰ **F17.21**   Nicotine dependence, cigarettes

F17.210   Nicotine dependence, cigarettes, uncomplicated
> **AHA:** 2017, 2Q, 28-29

F17.211   Nicotine dependence, cigarettes, in remission
> ▶Tobacco use disorder, cigarettes, mild, in early remission
> Tobacco use disorder, cigarettes, mild, in sustained remission
> Tobacco use disorder, cigarettes, moderate, in early remission
> Tobacco use disorder, cigarettes, moderate, in sustained remission
> Tobacco use disorder, cigarettes, severe, in early remission
> Tobacco use disorder, cigarettes, severe, in sustained remission◀

F17.213   Nicotine dependence, cigarettes, with withdrawal

F17.218   Nicotine dependence, cigarettes, with other nicotine-induced disorders

F17.219   Nicotine dependence, cigarettes, with unspecified nicotine-induced disorders ▽

✓6ᵗʰ **F17.22**   Nicotine dependence, chewing tobacco

F17.220   Nicotine dependence, chewing tobacco, uncomplicated

F17.221   Nicotine dependence, chewing tobacco, in remission
> ▶Tobacco use disorder, chewing tobacco, mild, in early remission
> Tobacco use disorder, chewing tobacco, mild, in sustained remission
> Tobacco use disorder, chewing tobacco, moderate, in early remission
> Tobacco use disorder, chewing tobacco, moderate, in sustained remission
> Tobacco use disorder, chewing tobacco, severe, in early remission
> Tobacco use disorder, chewing tobacco, severe, in sustained remission◀

F17.223   Nicotine dependence, chewing tobacco, with withdrawal

F17.228   Nicotine dependence, chewing tobacco, with other nicotine-induced disorders

F17.229   Nicotine dependence, chewing tobacco, with unspecified nicotine-induced disorders ▽

✓6ᵗʰ **F17.29**   Nicotine dependence, other tobacco product

F17.290   Nicotine dependence, other tobacco product, uncomplicated
> **AHA:** 2017, 2Q, 28-29

N Newborn: 0   P Pediatric: 0-17   M Maternity: 12-55   A Adult: 15-124   NRS Nonroutine supply Dx   NCDx Noncancer Dx   PDx Primary Dx   ▶◀ Revised Text   ● New Code   ▲ Revised Title

534   ICD-10-CM 2018

F17.291   **Nicotine dependence, other tobacco product,** in remission
▶Tobacco use disorder, other tobacco product, mild, in early remission
Tobacco use disorder, other tobacco product, mild, in sustained remission
Tobacco use disorder, other tobacco product, moderate, in early remission
Tobacco use disorder, other tobacco product, moderate, in sustained remission
Tobacco use disorder, other tobacco product, severe, in early remission
Tobacco use disorder, other tobacco product, severe, in sustained remission◀

F17.293   **Nicotine dependence, other tobacco product, with** withdrawal

F17.298   **Nicotine dependence, other tobacco product, with other nicotine-induced disorders**

F17.299   **Nicotine dependence, other tobacco product, with unspecified nicotine-induced disorders** ▽

✓4ᵗʰ **F18**   Inhalant **related disorders**
INCLUDES   volatile solvents

✓5ᵗʰ **F18.1**   **Inhalant** abuse
EXCLUDES 1   inhalant dependence (F18.2-)
inhalant use, unspecified (F18.9-)

F18.10   **Inhalant abuse,** uncomplicated
Inhalant use disorder, mild

●   **F18.11**   **Inhalant abuse,** in remission
Inhalant use disorder, mild, in early remission
Inhalant use disorder, mild, in sustained remission

✓6ᵗʰ **F18.12**   **Inhalant abuse with** intoxication
F18.120   **Inhalant abuse with intoxication,** uncomplicated
F18.121   **Inhalant abuse with intoxication** delirium
F18.129   **Inhalant abuse with intoxication, unspecified** ▽

F18.14   **Inhalant abuse with inhalant-induced** mood disorder
Inhalant use disorder, mild, with inhalant induced depressive disorder

✓6ᵗʰ **F18.15**   **Inhalant abuse with inhalant-induced** psychotic disorder
F18.150   **Inhalant abuse with inhalant-induced psychotic disorder with** delusions
F18.151   **Inhalant abuse with inhalant-induced psychotic disorder with** hallucinations
F18.159   **Inhalant abuse with inhalant-induced psychotic disorder, unspecified** ▽

F18.17   **Inhalant abuse with inhalant-induced** dementia
Inhalant use disorder, mild, with inhalant induced major neurocognitive disorder

✓6ᵗʰ **F18.18**   **Inhalant abuse with** other **inhalant-induced disorders**
F18.180   **Inhalant abuse with inhalant-induced** anxiety disorder
F18.188   **Inhalant abuse with other inhalant-induced disorder**
Inhalant use disorder, mild, with inhalant induced mild neurocognitive disorder

F18.19   **Inhalant abuse with unspecified inhalant-induced disorder** ▽

✓5ᵗʰ **F18.2**   **Inhalant** dependence
EXCLUDES 1   inhalant abuse (F18.1-)
inhalant use, unspecified (F18.9-)

F18.20   **Inhalant dependence,** uncomplicated
Inhalant use disorder, moderate
Inhalant use disorder, severe

F18.21   **Inhalant dependence,** in remission
▶Inhalant use disorder, moderate, in early remission
Inhalant use disorder, moderate, in sustained remission
Inhalant use disorder, severe, in early remission
Inhalant use disorder, severe, in sustained remission◀

✓6ᵗʰ **F18.22**   **Inhalant dependence with** intoxication
F18.220   **Inhalant dependence with intoxication, uncomplicated**

F18.221   **Inhalant dependence with intoxication** delirium

F18.229   **Inhalant dependence with intoxication, unspecified** ▽

F18.24   **Inhalant dependence with inhalant-induced** mood disorder
Inhalant use disorder, moderate, with inhalant induced depressive disorder
Inhalant use disorder, severe, with inhalant induced depressive disorder

✓6ᵗʰ **F18.25**   **Inhalant dependence with inhalant-induced** psychotic disorder
F18.250   **Inhalant dependence with inhalant-induced psychotic disorder with** delusions
F18.251   **Inhalant dependence with inhalant-induced psychotic disorder with** hallucinations
F18.259   **Inhalant dependence with inhalant-induced psychotic disorder, unspecified** ▽

F18.27   **Inhalant dependence with inhalant-induced** dementia
Inhalant use disorder, moderate, with inhalant induced major neurocognitive disorder
Inhalant use disorder, severe, with inhalant induced major neurocognitive disorder

✓6ᵗʰ **F18.28**   **Inhalant dependence with** other **inhalant-induced disorders**
F18.280   **Inhalant dependence with inhalant-induced** anxiety disorder
F18.288   **Inhalant dependence with other inhalant-induced disorder**
Inhalant use disorder, moderate, with inhalant-induced mild neurocognitive disorder
Inhalant use disorder, severe, with inhalant-induced mild neurocognitive disorder

F18.29   **Inhalant dependence with unspecified inhalant-induced disorder** ▽

✓5ᵗʰ **F18.9**   **Inhalant use,** unspecified
EXCLUDES 1   inhalant abuse (F18.1-)
inhalant dependence (F18.2-)

F18.90   **Inhalant use, unspecified,** uncomplicated

✓6ᵗʰ **F18.92**   **Inhalant use, unspecified with** intoxication
F18.920   **Inhalant use, unspecified with intoxication,** uncomplicated
F18.921   **Inhalant use, unspecified with intoxication with** delirium
F18.929   **Inhalant use, unspecified with intoxication, unspecified** ▽

F18.94   **Inhalant use, unspecified with inhalant-induced** mood disorder
Inhalant induced depressive disorder

✓6ᵗʰ **F18.95**   **Inhalant use, unspecified with inhalant-induced** psychotic disorder
F18.950   **Inhalant use, unspecified with inhalant-induced psychotic disorder with** delusions
F18.951   **Inhalant use, unspecified with inhalant-induced psychotic disorder with** hallucinations
F18.959   **Inhalant use, unspecified with inhalant-induced psychotic disorder, unspecified** ▽

F18.97   **Inhalant use, unspecified with inhalant-induced** persisting dementia
Inhalant-induced major neurocognitive disorder

✓6ᵗʰ **F18.98**   **Inhalant use, unspecified with** other **inhalant-induced disorders**
F18.980   **Inhalant use, unspecified with inhalant-induced** anxiety disorder
F18.988   **Inhalant use, unspecified with other inhalant-induced disorder**
Inhalant-induced mild neurocognitive disorder

F18.99   **Inhalant use, unspecified with unspecified inhalant-induced disorder** ▽

Chapter 5. Mental, Behavioral and Neurodevelopmental Disorders

✓4ᵗʰ **F19** Other psychoactive substance related disorders
     INCLUDES   polysubstance drug use (indiscriminate drug use)

✓5ᵗʰ **F19.1** Other psychoactive substance abuse
     EXCLUDES 1   *other psychoactive substance dependence (F19.2-)*
             other psychoactive substance use, unspecified (F19.9-)

●   **F19.10** Other psychoactive substance abuse, uncomplicated
       Other (or unknown) substance use disorder, mild

F19.11 Other psychoactive substance abuse, in remission
       Other (or unknown) substance use disorder, mild, in early remission
       Other (or unknown) substance use disorder, mild, in sustained remission

✓6ᵗʰ **F19.12** Other psychoactive substance abuse with intoxication

     F19.120 Other psychoactive substance abuse with intoxication, uncomplicated

     F19.121 Other psychoactive substance abuse with intoxication delirium

     F19.122 Other psychoactive substance abuse with intoxication with perceptual disturbances

     F19.129 Other psychoactive substance abuse with intoxication, unspecified ▽

F19.14 Other psychoactive substance abuse with psychoactive substance-induced mood disorder
       Other (or unknown) substance use disorder, mild, with other (or unknown) substance-induced bipolar or related disorder
       Other (or unknown) substance use disorder, mild, with other (or unknown) substance-induced depressive disorder

✓6ᵗʰ **F19.15** Other psychoactive substance abuse with psychoactive substance-induced psychotic disorder

     F19.150 Other psychoactive substance abuse with psychoactive substance-induced psychotic disorder with delusions

     F19.151 Other psychoactive substance abuse with psychoactive substance-induced psychotic disorder with hallucinations

     F19.159 Other psychoactive substance abuse with psychoactive substance-induced psychotic disorder, unspecified ▽

F19.16 Other psychoactive substance abuse with psychoactive substance-induced persisting amnestic disorder

F19.17 Other psychoactive substance abuse with psychoactive substance-induced persisting dementia
       Other (or unknown) substance use disorder, mild, with other (or unknown) substance-induced major neurocognitive disorder

✓6ᵗʰ **F19.18** Other psychoactive substance abuse with other psychoactive substance-induced disorders

     F19.180 Other psychoactive substance abuse with psychoactive substance-induced anxiety disorder

     F19.181 Other psychoactive substance abuse with psychoactive substance-induced sexual dysfunction

     F19.182 Other psychoactive substance abuse with psychoactive substance-induced sleep disorder

     F19.188 Other psychoactive substance abuse with other psychoactive substance-induced disorder
         Other (or unknown) substance use disorder, mild, with other (or unknown) substance induced mild neurocognitive disorder
         Other (or unknown) substance use disorder, mild, with other (or unknown) substance induced obsessive-compulsive or related disorder

F19.19 Other psychoactive substance abuse with unspecified psychoactive substance-induced disorder ▽

✓5ᵗʰ **F19.2** Other psychoactive substance dependence
     EXCLUDES 1   *other psychoactive substance abuse (F19.1-)*
             other psychoactive substance use, unspecified (F19.9-)

F19.20 Other psychoactive substance dependence, uncomplicated
       Other (or unknown) substance use disorder, moderate
       Other (or unknown) substance use disorder, severe

F19.21 Other psychoactive substance dependence, in remission
     ▶Other (or unknown) substance use disorder, moderate, in early remission
       Other (or unknown) substance use disorder, moderate, in sustained remission
       Other (or unknown) substance use disorder, severe, in early remission
       Other (or unknown) substance use, severe, in sustained remission◀

✓6ᵗʰ **F19.22** Other psychoactive substance dependence with intoxication
     EXCLUDES 1   *other psychoactive substance dependence with withdrawal (F19.23-)*

     F19.220 Other psychoactive substance dependence with intoxication, uncomplicated

     F19.221 Other psychoactive substance dependence with intoxication delirium

     F19.222 Other psychoactive substance dependence with intoxication with perceptual disturbance

     F19.229 Other psychoactive substance dependence with intoxication, unspecified ▽

✓6ᵗʰ **F19.23** Other psychoactive substance dependence with withdrawal
     EXCLUDES 1   *other psychoactive substance dependence with intoxication (F19.22-)*

     F19.230 Other psychoactive substance dependence with withdrawal, uncomplicated

     F19.231 Other psychoactive substance dependence with withdrawal delirium

     F19.232 Other psychoactive substance dependence with withdrawal with perceptual disturbance

     F19.239 Other psychoactive substance dependence with withdrawal, unspecified ▽

F19.24 Other psychoactive substance dependence with psychoactive substance-induced mood disorder
       Other (or unknown) substance use disorder, moderate, with other (or unknown) substance induced bipolar or related disorder
       Other (or unknown) substance use disorder, moderate, with other (or unknown) substance induced depressive disorder
       Other (or unknown) substance use disorder, severe, with other (or unknown) substance induced bipolar or related disorder
       Other (or unknown) substance use disorder, severe, with other (or unknown) substance induced depressive disorder

✓6ᵗʰ **F19.25** Other psychoactive substance dependence with psychoactive substance-induced psychotic disorder

     F19.250 Other psychoactive substance dependence with psychoactive substance-induced psychotic disorder with delusions

     F19.251 Other psychoactive substance dependence with psychoactive substance-induced psychotic disorder with hallucinations

     F19.259 Other psychoactive substance dependence with psychoactive substance-induce d psychotic disorder, unspecified ▽

F19.26 Other psychoactive substance dependence with psychoactive substance-induced persisting amnestic disorder

Ⓝ Newborn: 0   Ⓟ Pediatric: 0-17   Ⓜ Maternity: 12-55   Ⓐ Adult: 15-124   NRS Nonroutine supply Dx   NC Dx Noncancer Dx   PDx Primary Dx   ▶◀ Revised Text   ● New Code   ▲ Revised Title

536   ICD-10-CM 2018

F19.27 **Other psychoactive substance dependence with psychoactive substance-induced** persisting dementia
Other (or unknown) substance use disorder, moderate, with other (or unknown) substance induced major neurocognitive disorder
Other (or unknown) substance use disorder, severe, with other (or unknown) substance induced major neurocognitive disorder

✓6th **F19.28** **Other psychoactive substance dependence with** other psychoactive substance-induced disorders

  F19.280 **Other psychoactive substance dependence with psychoactive substance-induced** anxiety disorder

  F19.281 **Other psychoactive substance dependence with psychoactive substance-induced** sexual dysfunction

  F19.282 **Other psychoactive substance dependence with psychoactive substance-induced** sleep disorder

  F19.288 **Other psychoactive substance dependence with other psychoactive substance-induced disorder**
Other (or unknown) substance use disorder, moderate, with other (or unknown) substance induced mild neurocognitive disorder
Other (or unknown) substance use disorder, severe, with other (or unknown) substance induced mild neurocognitive disorder
Other (or unknown) substance use disorder, moderate, with other (or unknown) substance induced obsessive compulsive or related disorder
Other (or unknown) substance use disorder, severe, with other (or unknown) substance induced obsessive-compulsive or related disorder

F19.29 **Other psychoactive substance dependence with unspecified psychoactive substance-induced disorder** ▽

✓5th **F19.9** **Other psychoactive substance** use, unspecified
EXCLUDES 1   other psychoactive substance abuse (F19.1-)
other psychoactive substance dependence (F19.2-)

F19.90 **Other psychoactive substance use, unspecified,** uncomplicated

✓6th **F19.92** **Other psychoactive substance use, unspecified with** intoxication
EXCLUDES 1   other psychoactive substance use, unspecified with withdrawal (F19.93)

  F19.920 **Other psychoactive substance use, unspecified with intoxication,** uncomplicated

  F19.921 **Other psychoactive substance use, unspecified with intoxication with** delirium
Other (or unknown) substance-induced delirium

  F19.922 **Other psychoactive substance use, unspecified with intoxication with** perceptual disturbance

  F19.929 **Other psychoactive substance use, unspecified with intoxication, unspecified** ▽

✓6th **F19.93** **Other psychoactive substance use, unspecified with** withdrawal
EXCLUDES 1   other psychoactive substance use, unspecified with intoxication (F19.92-)

  F19.930 **Other psychoactive substance use, unspecified with withdrawal,** uncomplicated

  F19.931 **Other psychoactive substance use, unspecified with withdrawal** delirium

  F19.932 **Other psychoactive substance use, unspecified with withdrawal with** perceptual disturbance

  F19.939 **Other psychoactive substance use, unspecified with withdrawal, unspecified** ▽

F19.94 **Other psychoactive substance use, unspecified with psychoactive substance-induced** mood disorder
Other (or unknown) substance-induced bipolar or related disorder, without use disorder
Other (or unknown) substance-induced depressive disorder, without use disorder

✓6th **F19.95** **Other psychoactive substance use, unspecified with psychoactive substance-induced** psychotic disorder

  F19.950 **Other psychoactive substance use, unspecified with psychoactive substance-induced psychotic disorder with** delusions

  F19.951 **Other psychoactive substance use, unspecified with psychoactive substance-induced psychotic disorder with** hallucinations

  F19.959 **Other psychoactive substance use, unspecified with psychoactive substance-induced psychotic disorder, unspecified** ▽
Other or unknown substance-induced psychotic disorder, without use disorder

F19.96 **Other psychoactive substance use, unspecified with psychoactive substance-induced** persisting amnestic disorder

F19.97 **Other psychoactive substance use, unspecified with psychoactive substance-induced** persisting dementia
Other (or unknown) substance-induced major neurocognitive disorder, without use disorder

✓6th **F19.98** **Other psychoactive substance use, unspecified with** other psychoactive substance-induced disorders

  F19.980 **Other psychoactive substance use, unspecified with psychoactive substance-induced** anxiety disorder
Other (or unknown) substance-induced anxiety disorder, without use disorder

  F19.981 **Other psychoactive substance use, unspecified with psychoactive substance-induced** sexual dysfunction
Other (or unknown) substance-induced sexual dysfunction, without use disorder

  F19.982 **Other psychoactive substance use, unspecified with psychoactive substance-induced** sleep disorder
Other (or unknown) substance-induced sleep disorder, without use disorder

  F19.988 **Other psychoactive substance use, unspecified with other psychoactive substance-induced disorder**
Other (or unknown) substance-induced mild neurocognitive disorder, without use disorder
Other (or unknown) substance-induced obsessive-compulsive or related disorder, without use disorder

F19.99 **Other psychoactive substance use, unspecified with unspecified psychoactive substance-induced disorder** ▽

Schizophrenia, schizotypal, delusional, and other non-mood psychotic disorders (F20-F29)

✓4th **F20** **Schizophrenia**
EXCLUDES 1   brief psychotic disorder (F23)
cyclic schizophrenia (F25.0)
mood [affective] disorders with psychotic symptoms (F30.2, F31.2, F31.5, F31.64, F32.3, F33.3)
schizoaffective disorder (F25.-)
schizophrenic reaction NOS (F23)
EXCLUDES 2   schizophrenic reaction in:
alcoholism (F10.15-, F10.25-, F10.95-)
brain disease (F06.2)
epilepsy (F06.2)
psychoactive drug use (F11-F19 with .15. .25, .95)
schizotypal disorder (F21)
DEF: Group of disorders with disturbances in thought (delusions, hallucinations), mood (blunted, flattened, inappropriate affect), sense of self; also bizarre, purposeless behavior, repetitive activity, or inactivity.

F20.0 Paranoid schizophrenia
Paraphrenic schizophrenia
EXCLUDES 1 *involutional paranoid state (F22)*
paranoia (F22)
DEF: Preoccupied with delusional suspicions and auditory hallucinations related to single theme; usually hostile, grandiose, threatening, persecutory, occasionally hypochondriacal.

F20.1 Disorganized schizophrenia
Hebephrenic schizophrenia
Hebephrenia

F20.2 Catatonic schizophrenia
Schizophrenic catalepsy
Schizophrenic catatonia
Schizophrenic flexibilitas cerea
EXCLUDES 1 *catatonic stupor (R40.1)*
DEF: Extreme changes in motor activity; one extreme is decreased response or reaction to the environment and the other is spontaneous activity.

F20.3 Undifferentiated schizophrenia
Atypical schizophrenia
EXCLUDES 1 *acute schizophrenia-like psychotic disorder (F23)*
EXCLUDES 2 *post-schizophrenic depression (F32.89)*

F20.5 Residual schizophrenia
Restzustand (schizophrenic)
Schizophrenic residual state

✓5ᵗʰ F20.8 Other schizophrenia
    F20.81 Schizophreniform disorder
        Schizophreniform psychosis NOS
    F20.89 Other schizophrenia
        Cenesthopathic schizophrenia
        Simple schizophrenia

F20.9 Schizophrenia, unspecified ▽

F21 Schizotypal disorder
Borderline schizophrenia
Latent schizophrenia
Latent schizophrenic reaction
Prepsychotic schizophrenia
Prodromal schizophrenia
Pseudoneurotic schizophrenia
Pseudopsychopathic schizophrenia
Schizotypal personality disorder
EXCLUDES 2 *Asperger's syndrome (F84.5)*
schizoid personality disorder (F60.1)

F22 Delusional disorders
Delusional dysmorphophobia
Involutional paranoid state
Paranoia
Paranoia querulans
Paranoid psychosis
Paranoid state
Paraphrenia (late)
Sensitiver Beziehungswahn
EXCLUDES 1 *mood [affective] disorders with psychotic symptoms (F30.2, F31.2, F31.5, F31.64, F32.3, F33.3)*
paranoid schizophrenia (F20.0)
EXCLUDES 2 *paranoid personality disorder (F60.0)*
paranoid psychosis, psychogenic (F23)
paranoid reaction (F23)

F23 Brief psychotic disorder
Paranoid reaction
Psychogenic paranoid psychosis
EXCLUDES 2 *mood [affective] disorders with psychotic symptoms (F30.2, F31.2, F31.5, F31.64, F32.3, F33.3)*

F24 Shared psychotic disorder
Folie à deux
Induced paranoid disorder
Induced psychotic disorder

✓4ᵗʰ F25 Schizoaffective disorders
EXCLUDES 1 *mood [affective] disorders with psychotic symptoms (F30.2, F31.2, F31.5, F31.64, F32.3, F33.3)*
schizophrenia (F20.-)

F25.0 Schizoaffective disorder, bipolar type
Cyclic schizophrenia
Schizoaffective disorder, manic type
Schizoaffective disorder, mixed type
Schizoaffective psychosis, bipolar type
~~Schizophreniform psychosis, manic type~~

F25.1 Schizoaffective disorder, depressive type
Schizoaffective psychosis, depressive type
~~Schizophreniform psychosis, depressive type~~

F25.8 Other schizoaffective disorders

F25.9 Schizoaffective disorder, unspecified ▽
Schizoaffective psychosis NOS

F28 Other psychotic disorder not due to a substance or known physiological condition
Chronic hallucinatory psychosis
▶Other specified schizophrenia spectrum and other psychotic disorder◀

F29 Unspecified psychosis not due to a substance or known physiological condition ▽
Psychosis NOS
▶Unspecified schizophrenia spectrum and other psychotic disorder◀
EXCLUDES 1 *mental disorder NOS (F99)*
unspecified mental disorder due to known physiological condition (F09)

Mood [affective] disorders (F30-F39)

✓4ᵗʰ F30 Manic episode
INCLUDES bipolar disorder, single manic episode
mixed affective episode
EXCLUDES 1 *bipolar disorder (F31.-)*
major depressive disorder, recurrent (F33.-)
major depressive disorder, single episode (F32.-)

✓5ᵗʰ F30.1 Manic episode without psychotic symptoms
    F30.10 Manic episode without psychotic symptoms, unspecified ▽
    F30.11 Manic episode without psychotic symptoms, mild
    F30.12 Manic episode without psychotic symptoms, moderate
    F30.13 Manic episode, severe, without psychotic symptoms

F30.2 Manic episode, severe with psychotic symptoms
Manic stupor
Mania with mood-congruent psychotic symptoms
Mania with mood-incongruent psychotic symptoms

F30.3 Manic episode in partial remission

F30.4 Manic episode in full remission

F30.8 Other manic episodes
Hypomania

F30.9 Manic episode, unspecified ▽
Mania NOS

✓4ᵗʰ F31 Bipolar disorder
INCLUDES ▶bipolar I disorder
bipolar type I disorder◀
manic-depressive illness
manic-depressive psychosis
manic-depressive reaction
EXCLUDES 1 *bipolar disorder, single manic episode (F30.-)*
major depressive disorder, single episode (F32.-)
major depressive disorder, recurrent (F33.-)
EXCLUDES 2 *cyclothymia (F34.0)*

F31.0 Bipolar disorder, current episode hypomanic

✓5ᵗʰ F31.1 Bipolar disorder, current episode manic without psychotic features
    F31.10 Bipolar disorder, current episode manic without psychotic features, unspecified ▽
    F31.11 Bipolar disorder, current episode manic without psychotic features, mild
    F31.12 Bipolar disorder, current episode manic without psychotic features, moderate
    F31.13 Bipolar disorder, current episode manic without psychotic features, severe

F31.2 Bipolar disorder, current episode manic severe with psychotic features
Bipolar disorder, current episode manic with mood-congruent psychotic symptoms
Bipolar disorder, current episode manic with mood-incongruent psychotic symptoms
▶Bipolar I disorder, current or most recent episode manic with psychotic features◀

✓5ᵗʰ F31.3 Bipolar disorder, current episode depressed, mild or moderate severity
    F31.30 Bipolar disorder, current episode depressed, mild or moderate severity, unspecified ▽
    F31.31 Bipolar disorder, current episode depressed, mild
    F31.32 Bipolar disorder, current episode depressed, moderate

F31.4 Bipolar Disorder, current episode depressed, severe, without psychotic features

Ⓝ Newborn: 0   Ⓟ Pediatric: 0-17   Ⓜ Maternity: 12-55   Ⓐ Adult: 15-124   **NRS** Nonroutine supply Dx   **NCDx** Noncancer Dx   **PDx** Primary Dx   ▶◀ Revised Text   ● New Code   ▲ Revised Title

538   ICD-10-CM 2018

F31.5   Bipolar disorder, current episode depressed, severe, with psychotic features
- Bipolar disorder, current episode depressed with mood-incongruent psychotic symptoms
- Bipolar disorder, current episode depressed with mood-congruent psychotic symptoms
- ▶Bipolar I disorder, current or most recent episode depressed, with psychotic features◀

✓5ᵗʰ **F31.6**   Bipolar disorder, current episode mixed

    F31.60   Bipolar disorder, current episode mixed, unspecified   ▽

    F31.61   Bipolar disorder, current episode mixed, mild

    F31.62   Bipolar disorder, current episode mixed, moderate

    F31.63   Bipolar disorder, current episode mixed, severe, without psychotic features

    F31.64   Bipolar disorder, current episode mixed, severe, with psychotic features
- Bipolar disorder, current episode mixed with mood-congruent psychotic symptoms
- Bipolar disorder, current episode mixed with mood-incongruent psychotic symptoms

✓5ᵗʰ **F31.7**   Bipolar disorder, currently in remission

    F31.70   Bipolar disorder, currently in remission, most recent episode unspecified   ▽

    F31.71   Bipolar disorder, in partial remission, most recent episode hypomanic

    F31.72   Bipolar disorder, in full remission, most recent episode hypomanic

    F31.73   Bipolar disorder, in partial remission, most recent episode manic

    F31.74   Bipolar disorder, in full remission, most recent episode manic

    F31.75   Bipolar disorder, in partial remission, most recent episode depressed

    F31.76   Bipolar disorder, in full remission, most recent episode depressed

    F31.77   Bipolar disorder, in partial remission, most recent episode mixed

    F31.78   Bipolar disorder, in full remission, most recent episode mixed

✓5ᵗʰ **F31.8**   Other bipolar disorders

    F31.81   Bipolar II disorder
- ▶Bipolar disorder, type 2◀

    F31.89   Other bipolar disorder
- Recurrent manic episodes NOS

F31.9   Bipolar disorder, unspecified   ▽
- ▶Manic depression◀

✓4ᵗʰ **F32**   **Major depressive disorder, single episode**
- INCLUDES   single episode of agitated depression
- single episode of depressive reaction
- single episode of major depression
- single episode of psychogenic depression
- single episode of reactive depression
- single episode of vital depression
- EXCLUDES 1   bipolar disorder (F31.-)
- manic episode (F30.-)
- recurrent depressive disorder (F33.-)
- EXCLUDES 2   adjustment disorder (F43.2)
- **DEF:** Mood disorder that produces depression; may exhibit as sadness, low self-esteem, or guilt feelings; other manifestations may be withdrawal from friends and family and interrupted sleep.

F32.0   Major depressive disorder, single episode, mild

F32.1   Major depressive disorder, single episode, moderate

F32.2   Major depressive disorder, single episode, severe without psychotic features

F32.3   Major depressive disorder, single episode, severe with psychotic features
- Single episode of major depression with mood-congruent psychotic symptoms
- Single episode of major depression with mood-incongruent psychotic symptoms
- Single episode of major depression with psychotic symptoms
- Single episode of psychogenic depressive psychosis
- Single episode of psychotic depression
- Single episode of reactive depressive psychosis

F32.4   Major depressive disorder, single episode, in partial remission

F32.5   Major depressive disorder, single episode, in full remission

✓5ᵗʰ **F32.8**   Other depressive episodes

    F32.81   Premenstrual dysphoric disorder   ♀
- EXCLUDES 1   premenstrual tension syndrome (N94.3)

    F32.89   Other specified depressive episodes
- Atypical depression
- Post-schizophrenic depression
- Single episode of 'masked' depression NOS

F32.9   Major depressive disorder, single episode, unspecified   ▽
- Depression NOS
- Depressive disorder NOS
- Major depression NOS
- **AHA:** 2013, 4Q, 107
- **TIP:** Use for chronic depression, not further specified.

✓4ᵗʰ **F33**   **Major depressive disorder, recurrent**
- INCLUDES   recurrent episodes of depressive reaction
- recurrent episodes of endogenous depression
- recurrent episodes of major depression
- recurrent episodes of psychogenic depression
- recurrent episodes of reactive depression
- recurrent episodes of seasonal depressive disorder
- recurrent episodes of vital depression
- EXCLUDES 1   bipolar disorder (F31.-)
- manic episode (F30.-)

F33.0   Major depressive disorder, recurrent, mild

F33.1   Major depressive disorder, recurrent, moderate

F33.2   Major depressive disorder, recurrent, severe without psychotic features

F33.3   Major depressive disorder, recurrent, severe with psychotic symptoms
- Endogenous depression with psychotic symptoms
- ▶Major depressive disorder, recurrent, with psychotic features◀
- Recurrent severe episodes of major depression with mood-congruent psychotic symptoms
- Recurrent severe episodes of major depression with mood-incongruent psychotic symptoms
- Recurrent severe episodes of major depression with psychotic symptoms
- Recurrent severe episodes of psychogenic depressive psychosis
- Recurrent severe episodes of psychotic depression
- Recurrent severe episodes of reactive depressive psychosis

✓5ᵗʰ **F33.4**   Major depressive disorder, recurrent, in remission

    F33.40   Major depressive disorder, recurrent, in remission, unspecified   ▽

    F33.41   Major depressive disorder, recurrent, in partial remission

    F33.42   Major depressive disorder, recurrent, in full remission

F33.8   Other recurrent depressive disorders
- Recurrent brief depressive episodes

F33.9   Major depressive disorder, recurrent, unspecified   ▽
- Monopolar depression NOS

✓4ᵗʰ **F34**   **Persistent mood [affective] disorders**

F34.0   Cyclothymic disorder
- Affective personality disorder
- Cycloid personality
- Cyclothymia
- Cyclothymic personality

F34.1   Dysthymic disorder
- Depressive neurosis
- Depressive personality disorder
- Dysthymia
- Neurotic depression
- Persistent anxiety depression
- Persistent depressive disorder
- EXCLUDES 2   anxiety depression (mild or not persistent) (F41.8)
- **DEF:** Depression without psychosis; less severe but persistent depression; is considered a mild to moderate chronic form of depression.

✓5ᵗʰ **F34.8**   Other persistent mood [affective] disorders

    F34.81   Disruptive mood dysregulation disorder

    F34.89   Other specified persistent mood disorders

F34.9   Persistent mood [affective] disorder, unspecified   ▽

F39   **Unspecified mood [affective] disorder**   ▽
- Affective psychosis NOS

✓ Additional Character Req   ✓x7ᵗʰ Placeholder Alert   Case-Mix Diagnosis   Manifestation   ▽ Unspecified Dx   EXCLUDES 1 Not coded here   EXCLUDES 2 Not included here

Chapter 5. Mental, Behavioral and Neurodevelopmental Disorders

Anxiety, dissociative, stress-related, somatoform and other nonpsychotic mental disorders (F40-F48)

✓4th F40 Phobic anxiety disorders

✓5th F40.0 Agoraphobia
DEF: Profound anxiety or fear of leaving familiar settings like home, or being in unfamiliar locations or with strangers or crowds; may or may not be preceded by recurrent panic attacks.

F40.00 Agoraphobia, unspecified ▽

F40.01 Agoraphobia with panic disorder
Panic disorder with agoraphobia
EXCLUDES 1   *panic disorder without agoraphobia (F41.0)*

F40.02 Agoraphobia without panic disorder

✓5th F40.1 Social phobias
Anthropophobia
►Social anxiety disorder◄
Social anxiety disorder of childhood
Social neurosis

F40.10 Social phobia, unspecified ▽

F40.11 Social phobia, generalized

✓5th F40.2 Specific (isolated) phobias
EXCLUDES 2   *dysmorphophobia (nondelusional) (F45.22)*
            nosophobia (F45.22)

✓6th F40.21 Animal type phobia
F40.210 Arachnophobia
Fear of spiders
F40.218 Other animal type phobia

✓6th F40.22 Natural environment type phobia
F40.220 Fear of thunderstorms
F40.228 Other natural environment type phobia

✓6th F40.23 Blood, injection, injury type phobia
F40.230 Fear of blood
F40.231 Fear of injections and transfusions
F40.232 Fear of other medical care
F40.233 Fear of injury

✓6th F40.24 Situational type phobia
F40.240 Claustrophobia
F40.241 Acrophobia
F40.242 Fear of bridges
F40.243 Fear of flying
F40.248 Other situational type phobia

✓6th F40.29 Other specified phobia
F40.290 Androphobia
Fear of men
F40.291 Gynephobia
Fear of women
F40.298 Other specified phobia

F40.8 Other phobic anxiety disorders
Phobic anxiety disorder of childhood

F40.9 Phobic anxiety disorder, unspecified ▽
Phobia NOS
Phobic state NOS

✓4th F41 Other anxiety disorders
EXCLUDES 2   *anxiety in:*
         acute stress reaction (F43.0)
         transient adjustment reaction (F43.2)
         neurasthenia (F48.8)
         psychophysiologic disorders (F45.-)
         separation anxiety (F93.0)

▲ **F41.0 Panic disorder [episodic paroxysmal anxiety]**
Panic attack
Panic state
EXCLUDES 1   *panic disorder with agoraphobia (F40.01)*
DEF: Neurotic disorder characterized by recurrent panic or anxiety, apprehension, fear, or terror; symptoms include shortness of breath, palpitations, dizziness, shakiness; fear of dying may persist.

F41.1 Generalized anxiety disorder
Anxiety neurosis
Anxiety reaction
Anxiety state
Overanxious disorder
EXCLUDES 2   *neurasthenia (F48.8)*

F41.3 Other mixed anxiety disorders

F41.8 Other specified anxiety disorders
Anxiety depression (mild or not persistent)
Anxiety hysteria
Mixed anxiety and depressive disorder

F41.9 Anxiety disorder, unspecified ▽
Anxiety NOS

✓4th F42 Obsessive-compulsive disorder
EXCLUDES 2   *obsessive-compulsive personality (disorder) (F60.5)*
         obsessive-compulsive symptoms occurring in depression (F32-F33)
         obsessive-compulsive symptoms occurring in schizophrenia (F20.-)

F42.2 Mixed obsessional thoughts and acts

F42.3 Hoarding disorder

F42.4 Excoriation (skin-picking) disorder
EXCLUDES 1   *factitial dermatitis (L98.1)*
         other specified behavioral and emotional disorders with onset usually occurring in early childhood and adolescence (F98.8)

F42.8 Other obsessive-compulsive disorder
Anancastic neurosis
Obsessive-compulsive neurosis

F42.9 Obsessive-compulsive disorder, unspecified ▽

✓4th F43 Reaction to severe stress, and adjustment disorders

F43.0 Acute stress reaction
Acute crisis reaction
Acute reaction to stress
Combat and operational stress reaction
Combat fatigue
Crisis state
Psychic shock

✓5th F43.1 Post-traumatic stress disorder (PTSD)
Traumatic neurosis
DEF: Preoccupation with traumatic events beyond normal experience; i.e., rape, personal assault, etc.; also recurring flashbacks of trauma; symptoms include difficulty remembering, sleeping, or concentrating, and guilt feelings for surviving.

F43.10 Post-traumatic stress disorder, unspecified ▽
F43.11 Post-traumatic stress disorder, acute
F43.12 Post-traumatic stress disorder, chronic

✓5th F43.2 Adjustment disorders
Culture shock
Grief reaction
Hospitalism in children
EXCLUDES 2   *separation anxiety disorder of childhood (F93.0)*

F43.20 Adjustment disorder, unspecified ▽
F43.21 Adjustment disorder with depressed mood
     AHA: 2014, 1Q, 25
F43.22 Adjustment disorder with anxiety
F43.23 Adjustment disorder with mixed anxiety and depressed mood
F43.24 Adjustment disorder with disturbance of conduct
F43.25 Adjustment disorder with mixed disturbance of emotions and conduct
F43.29 Adjustment disorder with other symptoms

F43.8 Other reactions to severe stress
Other specified trauma and stressor-related disorder

F43.9 Reaction to severe stress, unspecified ▽
Trauma and stressor-related disorder, NOS

✓4th F44 Dissociative and conversion disorders
INCLUDES   conversion hysteria
         conversion reaction
         hysteria
         hysterical psychosis
EXCLUDES 2   *malingering [conscious simulation] (Z76.5)*

F44.0 Dissociative amnesia
EXCLUDES 1   *amnesia NOS (R41.3)*
         anterograde amnesia (R41.1)
         dissociative amnesia with dissociative fugue (F44.1)
         retrograde amnesia (R41.2)
EXCLUDES 2   *alcohol-or other psychoactive substance-induced amnestic disorder (F10, F13, F19 with .26, .96)*
         amnestic disorder due to known physiological condition (F04)
         postictal amnesia in epilepsy (G40.-)

F44.1 Dissociative fugue
Dissociative amnesia with dissociative fugue
EXCLUDES 2   *postictal fugue in epilepsy (G40.-)*
DEF: Dissociative hysteria; identified by loss of memory, flight from familiar surroundings to a completely separate environment, episodes may last hours or days; conscious activity is not associated with perception of surroundings and there is no later memory of episode.

Ⓝ Newborn: 0   Ⓟ Pediatric: 0-17   Ⓜ Maternity: 12-55   Ⓐ Adult: 15-124   **NRS** Nonroutine supply Dx   **NC Dx** Noncancer Dx   **PDx** Primary Dx   ►◄ Revised Text   ● New Code   ▲ Revised Title

540   ICD-10-CM 2018

F44.2 Dissociative stupor
> EXCLUDES 1   catatonic stupor (R40.1)
> stupor NOS (R40.1)
> EXCLUDES 2   catatonic disorder due to known physiological
> condition (F06.1)
> depressive stupor (F32, F33)
> manic stupor (F30, F31)

F44.4 Conversion disorder with motor symptom or deficit
> ►Conversion disorder with abnormal movement
> Conversion disorder with speech symptoms
> Conversion disorder with swallowing symptoms
> Conversion disorder with weakness/paralysis◄
> Dissociative motor disorders
> Psychogenic aphonia
> Psychogenic dysphonia

F44.5 Conversion disorder with seizures or convulsions
> ►Conversion disorder with attacks or seizures◄
> Dissociative convulsions

F44.6 Conversion disorder with sensory symptom or deficit
> ►Conversion disorder with anesthesia or sensory loss
> Conversion disorder with special sensory symptoms◄
> Dissociative anesthesia and sensory loss
> Psychogenic deafness

F44.7 Conversion disorder with mixed symptom presentation

✓5ᵗʰ **F44.8 Other dissociative and conversion disorders**

     F44.81 Dissociative identity disorder
> Multiple personality disorder

     F44.89 Other dissociative and conversion disorders
> Ganser's syndrome
> Psychogenic confusion
> Psychogenic twilight state
> Trance and possession disorders

F44.9 Dissociative and conversion disorder, unspecified ▽
> Dissociative disorder NOS

✓4ᵗʰ **F45 Somatoform disorders**
> EXCLUDES 2   dissociative and conversion disorders (F44.-)
> factitious disorders (F68.1-)
> hair-plucking (F63.3)
> lalling (F80.0)
> lisping (F80.0)
> malingering [conscious simulation] (Z76.5)
> nail-biting (F98.8)
> psychological or behavioral factors associated with disorders or
> diseases classified elsewhere (F54)
> sexual dysfunction, not due to a substance or known
> physiological condition (F52.-)
> thumb-sucking (F98.8)
> tic disorders (in childhood and adolescence) (F95.-)
> Tourette's syndrome (F95.2)
> trichotillomania (F63.3)

F45.0 Somatization disorder
> Briquet's disorder
> Multiple psychosomatic disorder

F45.1 Undifferentiated somatoform disorder
> Somatic symptom disorder
> Undifferentiated psychosomatic disorder

✓5ᵗʰ **F45.2 Hypochondriacal disorders**
> EXCLUDES 2   delusional dysmorphophobia (F22)
> fixed delusions about bodily functions or shape (F22)

     F45.20 Hypochondriacal disorder, unspecified ▽
     F45.21 Hypochondriasis
> Hypochondriacal neurosis
> Illness anxiety disorder

     F45.22 Body dysmorphic disorder
> Dysmorphophobia (nondelusional)
> Nosophobia

     F45.29 Other hypochondriacal disorders

✓5ᵗʰ **F45.4 Pain disorders related to psychological factors**
> EXCLUDES 1   pain NOS (R52)

     F45.41 Pain disorder exclusively related to psychological factors
> Somatoform pain disorder (persistent)

     F45.42 Pain disorder with related psychological factors
> Code also associated acute or chronic pain (G89.-)

F45.8 Other somatoform disorders
> Psychogenic dysmenorrhea
> Psychogenic dysphagia, including "globus hystericus"
> Psychogenic pruritus
> Psychogenic torticollis
> Somatoform autonomic dysfunction
> Teeth grinding
> EXCLUDES 1   sleep related teeth grinding (G47.63)

F45.9 Somatoform disorder, unspecified ▽
> Psychosomatic disorder NOS

✓4ᵗʰ **F48 Other nonpsychotic mental disorders**

     F48.1 Depersonalization-derealization syndrome

     F48.2 Pseudobulbar affect
> Involuntary emotional expression disorder
> Code first underlying cause, if known, such as:
> amyotrophic lateral sclerosis (G12.21)
> multiple sclerosis (G35)
> sequelae of cerebrovascular disease (I69.-)
> sequelae of traumatic intracranial injury (S06.-)

     F48.8 Other specified nonpsychotic mental disorders
> Dhat syndrome
> Neurasthenia
> Occupational neurosis, including writer's cramp
> Psychasthenia
> Psychasthenic neurosis
> Psychogenic syncope

     F48.9 Nonpsychotic mental disorder, unspecified ▽
> Neurosis NOS

Behavioral syndromes associated with physiological disturbances and physical factors (F50-F59)

✓4ᵗʰ **F50 Eating disorders**
> EXCLUDES 1   anorexia NOS (R63.0)
> feeding difficulties (R63.3)
> ►feeding problems of newborn (P92.-)◄
> polyphagia (R63.2)
> EXCLUDES 2   feeding disorder in infancy or childhood (F98.2-)

✓5ᵗʰ **F50.0 Anorexia nervosa**
> EXCLUDES 1   loss of appetite (R63.0)
> psychogenic loss of appetite (F50.89)

     F50.00 Anorexia nervosa, unspecified ▽
     F50.01 Anorexia nervosa, restricting type
     F50.02 Anorexia nervosa, binge eating/purging type
> EXCLUDES 1   bulimia nervosa (F50.2)

     F50.2 Bulimia nervosa
> Bulimia NOS
> Hyperorexia nervosa
> EXCLUDES 1   anorexia nervosa, binge eating/purging type (F50.02)

✓5ᵗʰ **F50.8 Other eating disorders**
> EXCLUDES 2   pica of infancy and childhood (F98.3)

     F50.81 Binge eating disorder
●   **F50.82 Avoidant/restrictive food intake disorder**
     F50.89 Other specified eating disorder
> Pica in adults
> Psychogenic loss of appetite

     F50.9 Eating disorder, unspecified ▽
> Atypical anorexia nervosa
> Atypical bulimia nervosa
> ►Feeding or eating disorder, unspecified
> Other specified feeding disorder◄

✓4ᵗʰ **F51 Sleep disorders not due to a substance or known physiological condition**
> EXCLUDES 2   organic sleep disorders (G47.-)

✓5ᵗʰ **F51.0 Insomnia not due to a substance or known physiological condition**
> EXCLUDES 2   alcohol related insomnia (F10.182, F10.282, F10.982)
> drug-related insomnia (F11.182, F11.282, F11.982,
> F13.182, F13.282, F13.982, F14.182, F14.282,
> F14.982, F15.182, F15.282, F15.982, F19.182,
> F19.282, F19.982)
> insomnia NOS (G47.0-)
> insomnia due to known physiological condition
> (G47.0-)
> organic insomnia (G47.0-)
> sleep deprivation (Z72.820)

     F51.01 Primary insomnia
> Idiopathic insomnia

     F51.02 Adjustment insomnia

☑ Additional Character Req   ✓1ᵗ Placeholder Alert   Case-Mix Diagnosis   Manifestation   ▽ Unspecified Dx   EXCLUDES 1 Not coded here   EXCLUDES 2 Not included here

ICD-10-CM 2018   541

F51.03   Paradoxical insomnia

F51.04   Psychophysiologic insomnia

F51.05   Insomnia due to other mental disorder
    Code also associated mental disorder

F51.09   Other insomnia not due to a substance or known physiological condition

✓5ᵗʰ **F51.1**   Hypersomnia not due to a substance or known physiological condition
    EXCLUDES 2   alcohol related hypersomnia (F10.182, F10.282, F10.982)
      drug-related hypersomnia (F11.182, F11.282, F11.982, F13.182, F13.282, F13.982, F14.182, F14.282, F14.982, F15.182, F15.282, F15.982, F19.182, F19.282, F19.982)
      hypersomnia NOS (G47.10)
      hypersomnia due to known physiological condition (G47.10)
      idiopathic hypersomnia (G47.11, G47.12)
      narcolepsy (G47.4-)

F51.11   Primary hypersomnia

F51.12   Insufficient sleep syndrome
    EXCLUDES 1   sleep deprivation (Z72.820)

F51.13   Hypersomnia due to other mental disorder
    Code also associated mental disorder

F51.19   Other hypersomnia not due to a substance or known physiological condition

F51.3   Sleepwalking [somnambulism]
    ▶Non–rapid eye movement sleep arousal disorders, sleepwalking type◀

F51.4   Sleep terrors [night terrors]
    ▶Non–rapid eye movement sleep arousal disorders, sleep terror type◀

F51.5   Nightmare disorder
    Dream anxiety disorder

F51.8   Other sleep disorders not due to a substance or known physiological condition

F51.9   Sleep disorder not due to a substance or known physiological condition, unspecified   ▽
    Emotional sleep disorder NOS

✓4ᵗʰ **F52**   Sexual dysfunction not due to a substance or known physiological condition
    EXCLUDES 2   Dhat syndrome (F48.8)

F52.0   Hypoactive sexual desire disorder
    Lack or loss of sexual desire
    ▶Male hypoactive sexual desire disorder◀
    Sexual anhedonia
    EXCLUDES 1   decreased libido (R68.82)

F52.1   Sexual aversion disorder
    Sexual aversion and lack of sexual enjoyment

✓5ᵗʰ **F52.2**   Sexual arousal disorders
    Failure of genital response

    F52.21   Male erectile disorder   ♂
      ▶Erectile disorder◀
      Psychogenic impotence
      EXCLUDES 1   impotence of organic origin (N52.-)
        impotence NOS (N52.-)

    F52.22   Female sexual arousal disorder   ♀
      ▶Female sexual interest/arousal disorder◀

✓5ᵗʰ **F52.3**   Orgasmic disorder
    Inhibited orgasm
    Psychogenic anorgasmy

    F52.31   Female orgasmic disorder   ♀

    F52.32   Male orgasmic disorder   ♂
      Delayed ejaculation

F52.4   Premature ejaculation   ♂

F52.5   Vaginismus not due to a substance or known physiological condition   ♀
    Psychogenic vaginismus
    EXCLUDES 2   vaginismus (due to a known physiological condition) (N94.2)
    DEF: Psychogenic response resulting in painful contractions of vaginal canal muscles; can be severe enough to prevent sexual intercourse.

F52.6   Dyspareunia not due to a substance or known physiological condition   ♀
    Genito-pelvic pain penetration disorder
    Psychogenic dyspareunia
    EXCLUDES 2   dyspareunia (due to a known physiological condition) (N94.1-)

F52.8   Other sexual dysfunction not due to a substance or known physiological condition
    Excessive sexual drive
    Nymphomania
    Satyriasis

F52.9   Unspecified sexual dysfunction not due to a substance or known physiological condition   ▽
    Sexual dysfunction NOS

F53   Puerperal psychosis   Ⓜ♀
    Postpartum depression
    EXCLUDES 1   mood disorders with psychotic features (F30.2, F31.2, F31.5, F31.64, F32.3, F33.3)
      postpartum dysphoria (O90.6)
      psychosis in schizophrenia, schizotypal, delusional, and other psychotic disorders (F20-F29)

F54   *Psychological and behavioral factors associated with disorders or diseases classified elsewhere*
    Psychological factors affecting physical conditions
    Code first the associated physical disorder, such as:
      asthma (J45.-)
      dermatitis (L23-L25)
      gastric ulcer (K25.-)
      mucous colitis (K58.-)
      ulcerative colitis (K51.-)
      urticaria (L50.-)
    EXCLUDES 2   tension-type headache (G44.2)

✓4ᵗʰ **F55**   Abuse of non-psychoactive substances
    EXCLUDES 2   abuse of psychoactive substances (F10-F19)

    F55.0   Abuse of antacids

    F55.1   Abuse of herbal or folk remedies

    F55.2   Abuse of laxatives

    F55.3   Abuse of steroids or hormones

    F55.4   Abuse of vitamins

    F55.8   Abuse of other non-psychoactive substances

F59   Unspecified behavioral syndromes associated with physiological disturbances and physical factors   ▽
    Psychogenic physiological dysfunction NOS

Disorders of adult personality and behavior (F60-F69)

✓4ᵗʰ **F60**   Specific personality disorders

    F60.0   Paranoid personality disorder
      Expansive paranoid personality (disorder)
      Fanatic personality (disorder)
      Paranoid personality (disorder)
      Querulant personality (disorder)
      Sensitive paranoid personality (disorder)
      EXCLUDES 2   paranoia (F22)
        paranoia querulans (F22)
        paranoid psychosis (F22)
        paranoid schizophrenia (F20.0)
        paranoid state (F22)

    F60.1   Schizoid personality disorder
      EXCLUDES 2   Asperger's syndrome (F84.5)
        delusional disorder (F22)
        schizoid disorder of childhood (F84.5)
        schizophrenia (F20.-)
        schizotypal disorder (F21)

    F60.2   Antisocial personality disorder
      Amoral personality (disorder)
      Asocial personality (disorder)
      Dissocial personality disorder
      Psychopathic personality (disorder)
      Sociopathic personality (disorder)
      EXCLUDES 1   conduct disorders (F91.-)
      EXCLUDES 2   borderline personality disorder (F60.3)

    F60.3   Borderline personality disorder
      Aggressive personality (disorder)
      Emotionally unstable personality (disorder)
      Explosive personality (disorder)
      EXCLUDES 2   antisocial personality disorder (F60.2)

    F60.4   Histrionic personality disorder
      Hysterical personality (disorder)
      Psychoinfantile personality (disorder)

    F60.5   Obsessive-compulsive personality disorder
      Anankastic personality (disorder)
      Compulsive personality (disorder)
      Obsessional personality (disorder)
      EXCLUDES 2   obsessive-compulsive disorder (F42-)

F60.6 **Avoidant personality disorder**
Anxious personality disorder

F60.7 **Dependent personality disorder**
Asthenic personality (disorder)
Inadequate personality (disorder)
Passive personality (disorder)

✓5ᵗʰ **F60.8** **Other specific personality disorders**

    F60.81 **Narcissistic personality disorder**

    F60.89 **Other specific personality disorders**
        Eccentric personality disorder
        "Haltlose" type personality disorder
        Immature personality disorder
        Passive-aggressive personality disorder
        Psychoneurotic personality disorder
        Self-defeating personality disorder

F60.9 **Personality disorder, unspecified**   ▽
Character disorder NOS
Character neurosis NOS
Pathological personality NOS

✓4ᵗʰ **F63** **Impulse disorders**
    EXCLUDES 2   *habitual excessive use of alcohol or psychoactive substances*
                (F10-F19)
                impulse disorders involving sexual behavior (F65.-)

F63.0 **Pathological gambling**
Compulsive gambling
▶Gambling disorder◀
    EXCLUDES 1   *gambling and betting NOS (Z72.6)*
    EXCLUDES 2   *excessive gambling by manic patients (F30, F31)*
                gambling in antisocial personality disorder (F60.2)

F63.1 **Pyromania**
Pathological fire-setting
    EXCLUDES 2   *fire-setting (by) (in):*
                adult with antisocial personality disorder (F60.2)
                alcohol or psychoactive substance intoxication
                  (F10-F19)
                conduct disorders (F91.-)
                mental disorders due to known physiological
                  condition (F01-F09)
                schizophrenia (F20.-)

F63.2 **Kleptomania**
Pathological stealing
    EXCLUDES 1   *shoplifting as the reason for observation for suspected*
                mental disorder (Z03.8)
    EXCLUDES 2   *depressive disorder with stealing (F31-F33)*
                stealing due to underlying mental condition—code to
                  mental condition
                stealing in mental disorders due to known
                  physiological condition (F01-F09)

F63.3 **Trichotillomania**
Hair plucking
    EXCLUDES 2   *other stereotyped movement disorder (F98.4)*

✓5ᵗʰ **F63.8** **Other impulse disorders**

    F63.81 **Intermittent explosive disorder**

    F63.89 **Other impulse disorders**

F63.9 **Impulse disorder, unspecified**   ▽
Impulse control disorder NOS

✓4ᵗʰ **F64** **Gender identity disorders**

F64.0 **Transsexualism**
Gender identity disorder in adolescence and adulthood
Gender dysphoria in adolescents and adults

F64.1 **Dual role transvestism**
Use additional code to identify sex reassignment status
    (Z87.890)
    EXCLUDES 1   *gender identity disorder in childhood (F64.2)*
    EXCLUDES 2   *fetishistic transvestism (F65.1)*

F64.2 **Gender identity disorder of** childhood   P
Gender dysphoria in children
    EXCLUDES 1   *gender identity disorder in adolescence and adulthood*
                (F64.0)
    EXCLUDES 2   *sexual maturation disorder (F66)*

F64.8 **Other gender identity disorders**
▶Other specified gender dysphoria◀

F64.9 **Gender identity disorder, unspecified**   ▽
▶Gender dysphoria, unspecified◀
Gender-role disorder NOS

✓4ᵗʰ **F65** **Paraphilias**

F65.0 **Fetishism**
▶Fetishistic disorder◀

F65.1 **Transvestic fetishism**
Fetishistic transvestism
▶Transvestic disorder◀

F65.2 **Exhibitionism**
▶Exhibitionistic disorder◀

F65.3 **Voyeurism**
▶Voyeuristic disorder◀

F65.4 **Pedophilia**
▶Pedophilic disorder◀

✓5ᵗʰ **F65.5** **Sadomasochism**

    F65.50 **Sadomasochism, unspecified**   ▽

    F65.51 **Sexual masochism**
        ▶Sexual masochism disorder◀

    F65.52 **Sexual sadism**
        ▶Sexual sadism disorder◀

✓5ᵗʰ **F65.8** **Other paraphilias**

    F65.81 **Frotteurism**
        ▶Frotteuristic disorder◀

    F65.89 **Other paraphilias**
        Necrophilia
        ▶Other specified paraphilic disorder◀

F65.9 **Paraphilia, unspecified**   ▽
▶Paraphilic disorder, unspecified◀
Sexual deviation NOS

F66 **Other sexual disorders**
Sexual maturation disorder
Sexual relationship disorder

✓4ᵗʰ **F68** **Other disorders of adult personality and behavior**

✓5ᵗʰ **F68.1** **Factitious disorder**
Compensation neurosis
Elaboration of physical symptoms for psychological reasons
Hospital hopper syndrome
Münchhausen's syndrome
Peregrinating patient
    EXCLUDES 2   *factitial dermatitis (L98.1)*
                person feigning illness (with obvious motivation)
                  (Z76.5)

    F68.10 **Factitious disorder, unspecified**   ▽

    F68.11 **Factitious disorder** with predominantly
        psychological signs and symptoms

    F68.12 **Factitious disorder** with predominantly physical
        signs and symptoms

    F68.13 **Factitious disorder** with combined psychological and
        physical signs and symptoms

    F68.8 **Other specified disorders of adult personality and behavior**

F69 **Unspecified disorder of adult personality and behavior**   🅰▽

Intellectual disabilities (F70-F79)

Code first any associated physical or developmental disorders
EXCLUDES 1   *borderline intellectual functioning, IQ above 70 to 84 (R41.83)*

F70 **Mild intellectual disabilities**
IQ level 50-55 to approximately 70
Mild mental subnormality

F71 **Moderate intellectual disabilities**
IQ level 35-40 to 50-55
Moderate mental subnormality

F72 **Severe intellectual disabilities**
IQ 20-25 to 35-40
Severe mental subnormality

F73 **Profound intellectual disabilities**
IQ level below 20-25
Profound mental subnormality

F78 **Other intellectual disabilities**

F79 **Unspecified intellectual disabilities**   ▽
Mental deficiency NOS
Mental subnormality NOS

✓ Additional Character Req   ✓x7ᵗʰ Placeholder Alert   Case-Mix Diagnosis   Manifestation   ▽ Unspecified Dx   EXCLUDES 1 Not coded here   EXCLUDES 2 Not included here

ICD-10-CM 2018   543

Chapter 5. Mental, Behavioral and Neurodevelopmental Disorders

Pervasive and specific developmental disorders (F80-F89)

✓4th F80 Specific developmental disorders of speech and language

F80.0 Phonological disorder
Dyslalia
Functional speech articulation disorder
Lalling
Lisping
Phonological developmental disorder
Speech articulation developmental disorder
Speech-sound disorder
> **EXCLUDES 1** *speech articulation impairment due to aphasia NOS (R47.01)*
> *speech articulation impairment due to apraxia (R48.2)*
> **EXCLUDES 2** *speech articulation impairment due to hearing loss (F80.4)*
> *speech articulation impairment due to intellectual disabilities (F70-F79)*
> *speech articulation impairment with expressive language developmental disorder (F80.1)*
> *speech articulation impairment with mixed receptive expressive language developmental disorder (F80.2)*

F80.1 Expressive language disorder
Developmental dysphasia or aphasia, expressive type
> **EXCLUDES 1** *dysphasia and aphasia NOS (R47.-)*
> *mixed receptive-expressive language disorder (F80.2)*
> **EXCLUDES 2** *acquired aphasia with epilepsy [Landau-Kleffner] (G40.80-)*
> *intellectual disabilities (F70-F79)*
> *pervasive developmental disorders (F84.-)*
> *selective mutism (F94.0)*

F80.2 Mixed receptive-expressive language disorder
Developmental dysphasia or aphasia, receptive type
Developmental Wernicke's aphasia
> **EXCLUDES 1** *central auditory processing disorder (H93.25)*
> *dysphasia or aphasia NOS (R47.-)*
> *expressive language disorder (F80.1)*
> *expressive type dysphasia or aphasia (F80.1)*
> *word deafness (H93.25)*
> **EXCLUDES 2** *acquired aphasia with epilepsy [Landau-Kleffner] (G40.80-)*
> *intellectual disabilities (F70-F79)*
> *pervasive developmental disorders (F84.-)*
> *selective mutism (F94.0)*

F80.4 Speech and language development delay due to hearing loss
Code also type of hearing loss (H90.-, H91.-)

✓5th F80.8 Other developmental disorders of speech and language
AHA: 2017, 1Q, 27

F80.81 Childhood onset fluency disorder
Cluttering NOS
Stuttering NOS
> **EXCLUDES 1** *adult onset fluency disorder (F98.5)*
> *fluency disorder in conditions classified elsewhere (R47.82)*
> *fluency disorder (stuttering) following cerebrovascular disease (I69. with final characters-23)*

F80.82 Social pragmatic communication disorder
> **EXCLUDES 1** *Asperger's syndrome (F84.5)*
> *autistic disorder (F84.0)*

F80.89 Other developmental disorders of speech and language

F80.9 Developmental disorder of speech and language, unspecified ▽
Communication disorder NOS
Language disorder NOS

✓4th F81 Specific developmental disorders of scholastic skills

F81.0 Specific reading disorder
"Backward reading"
Developmental dyslexia
▶Specific learning disorder, with impairment in reading◀
Specific reading retardation
> **EXCLUDES 1** *alexia NOS (R48.0)*
> *dyslexia NOS (R48.0)*

DEF: Serious impairment of reading skills unexplained in relation to general intelligence and teaching processes.

F81.2 Mathematics disorder
Developmental acalculia
Developmental arithmetical disorder
Developmental Gerstmann's syndrome
▶Specific learning disorder, with impairment in mathmatics◀
> **EXCLUDES 1** *acalculia NOS (R48.8)*
> **EXCLUDES 2** *arithmetical difficulties associated with a reading disorder (F81.0)*
> *arithmetical difficulties associated with a spelling disorder (F81.81)*
> *arithmetical difficulties due to inadequate teaching (Z55.8)*

✓5th F81.8 Other developmental disorders of scholastic skills

F81.81 Disorder of written expression
▶Specific learning disorder, with impairment in written expression◀
Specific spelling disorder

F81.89 Other developmental disorders of scholastic skills

F81.9 Developmental disorder of scholastic skills, unspecified ▽
Knowledge acquisition disability NOS
Learning disability NOS
Learning disorder NOS

F82 Specific developmental disorder of motor function
Clumsy child syndrome
Developmental coordination disorder
Developmental dyspraxia
> **EXCLUDES 1** *abnormalities of gait and mobility (R26.-)*
> *lack of coordination (R27.-)*
> **EXCLUDES 2** *lack of coordination secondary to intellectual disabilities (F70-F79)*

✓4th F84 Pervasive developmental disorders
Use additional code to identify any associated medical condition and intellectual disabilities

F84.0 Autistic disorder
Autism spectrum disorder
Infantile autism
Infantile psychosis
Kanner's syndrome
> **EXCLUDES 1** *Asperger's syndrome (F84.5)*

AHA: 2017, 1Q, 27
TIP: When the encounter is focused on treatment of conditions related to autism spectrum disorder, first assign codes to identify the problem or manifestation of autism receiving therapeutic services.

F84.2 Rett's syndrome
> **EXCLUDES 1** *Asperger's syndrome (F84.5)*
> *autistic disorder (F84.0)*
> *other childhood disintegrative disorder (F84.3)*

F84.3 Other childhood disintegrative disorder P
Dementia infantilis
Disintegrative psychosis
Heller's syndrome
Symbiotic psychosis
Use additional code to identify any associated neurological condition
> **EXCLUDES 1** *Asperger's syndrome (F84.5)*
> *autistic disorder (F84.0)*
> *Rett's syndrome (F84.2)*

F84.5 Asperger's syndrome
Asperger's disorder
Autistic psychopathy
Schizoid disorder of childhood

F84.8 Other pervasive developmental disorders
Overactive disorder associated with intellectual disabilities and stereotyped movements

F84.9 Pervasive developmental disorder, unspecified ▽
Atypical autism

F88 Other disorders of psychological development
Developmental agnosia
Global development delay
Other specified neurodevelopmental disorder

F89 Unspecified disorder of psychological development ▽
Developmental disorder NOS
Neurodevelopmental disorder NOS

Ⓝ Newborn: 0 Ⓟ Pediatric: 0-17 Ⓜ Maternity: 12-55 Ⓐ Adult: 15-124 NRS Nonroutine supply Dx NCDx Noncancer Dx PDx Primary Dx ▶◀ Revised Text ● New Code ▲ Revised Title

544 | ICD-10-CM 2018

Behavioral and emotional disorders with onset usually occurring in childhood and adolescence (F90-F98)

NOTE Codes within categories F90-F98 may be used regardless of the age of a patient. These disorders generally have onset within the childhood or adolescent years, but may continue throughout life or not be diagnosed until adulthood.

✓4ᵗʰ F90 Attention-deficit hyperactivity disorders
INCLUDES attention deficit disorder with hyperactivity
attention deficit syndrome with hyperactivity
EXCLUDES 2 anxiety disorders (F40.-, F41.-)
mood [affective] disorders (F30-F39)
pervasive developmental disorders (F84.-)
schizophrenia (F20.-)

F90.0 Attention-deficit hyperactivity disorder, predominantly inattentive type
▶Attention-deficit/hyperactivity disorder, predominantly inattentive presentation◀

F90.1 Attention-deficit hyperactivity disorder, predominantly hyperactive type
▶Attention-deficit/hyperactivity disorder, predominantly hyperactive impulsive presentation◀

F90.2 Attention-deficit hyperactivity disorder, combined type
▶Attention-deficit/hyperactivity disorder, combined presentation◀

F90.8 Attention-deficit hyperactivity disorder, other type

F90.9 Attention-deficit hyperactivity disorder, unspecified type ▽
Attention-deficit hyperactivity disorder of childhood or adolescence NOS
Attention-deficit hyperactivity disorder NOS

✓4ᵗʰ F91 Conduct disorders
EXCLUDES 1 antisocial behavior (Z72.81-)
antisocial personality disorder (F60.2)
EXCLUDES 2 conduct problems associated with attention-deficit hyperactivity disorder (F90.-)
mood [affective] disorders (F30-F39)
pervasive developmental disorders (F84.-)
schizophrenia (F20.-)

F91.0 Conduct disorder confined to family context

F91.1 Conduct disorder, childhood-onset type
Unsocialized conduct disorder
Conduct disorder, solitary aggressive type
Unsocialized aggressive disorder

F91.2 Conduct disorder, adolescent-onset type
Socialized conduct disorder
Conduct disorder, group type

F91.3 Oppositional defiant disorder

F91.8 Other conduct disorders
Other specified conduct disorder
Other specified disruptive disorder

F91.9 Conduct disorder, unspecified ▽
Behavioral disorder NOS
Conduct disorder NOS
Disruptive behavior disorder NOS
Disruptive disorder NOS

✓4ᵗʰ F93 Emotional disorders with onset specific to childhood

F93.0 Separation anxiety disorder of childhood
EXCLUDES 2 mood [affective] disorders (F30-F39)
nonpsychotic mental disorders (F40-F48)
phobic anxiety disorder of childhood (F40.8)
social phobia (F40.1)

F93.8 Other childhood emotional disorders
Identity disorder
EXCLUDES 2 gender identity disorder of childhood (F64.2)

F93.9 Childhood emotional disorder, unspecified ▽

✓4ᵗʰ F94 Disorders of social functioning with onset specific to childhood and adolescence

F94.0 Selective mutism
Elective mutism
EXCLUDES 2 pervasive developmental disorders (F84.-)
schizophrenia (F20.-)
specific developmental disorders of speech and language (F80.-)
transient mutism as part of separation anxiety in young children (F93.0)

F94.1 Reactive attachment disorder of childhood
Use additional code to identify any associated failure to thrive or growth retardation
EXCLUDES 1 disinhibited attachment disorder of childhood (F94.1)
normal variation in pattern of selective attachment
EXCLUDES 2 Asperger's syndrome (F84.5)
maltreatment syndromes (T74.-)
sexual or physical abuse in childhood, resulting in psychosocial problems (Z62.81-)

F94.2 Disinhibited attachment disorder of childhood
Affectionless psychopathy
Institutional syndrome
EXCLUDES 1 reactive attachment disorder of childhood (F94.1)
EXCLUDES 2 Asperger's syndrome (F84.5)
attention-deficit hyperactivity disorders (F90.-)
hospitalism in children (F43.2-)

F94.8 Other childhood disorders of social functioning

F94.9 Childhood disorder of social functioning, unspecified ▽

✓4ᵗʰ F95 Tic disorder

F95.0 Transient tic disorder
Provisional tic disorder

F95.1 Chronic motor or vocal tic disorder

F95.2 Tourette's disorder
Combined vocal and multiple motor tic disorder [de la Tourette]
Tourette's syndrome

F95.8 Other tic disorders

F95.9 Tic disorder, unspecified ▽
Tic NOS

✓4ᵗʰ F98 Other behavioral and emotional disorders with onset usually occurring in childhood and adolescence
EXCLUDES 2 breath-holding spells (R06.89)
gender identity disorder of childhood (F64.2)
Kleine-Levin syndrome (G47.13)
obsessive-compulsive disorder (F42-)
sleep disorders not due to a substance or known physiological condition (F51.-)

F98.0 Enuresis not due to a substance or known physiological condition
Enuresis (primary) (secondary) of nonorganic origin
Functional enuresis
Psychogenic enuresis
Urinary incontinence of nonorganic origin
EXCLUDES 1 enuresis NOS (R32)

F98.1 Encopresis not due to a substance or known physiological condition
Functional encopresis
Incontinence of feces of nonorganic origin
Psychogenic encopresis
Use additional code to identify the cause of any coexisting constipation
EXCLUDES 1 encopresis NOS (R15.-)

✓5ᵗʰ F98.2 Other feeding disorders of infancy and childhood
EXCLUDES 1 feeding difficulties (R63.3)
EXCLUDES 2 anorexia nervosa and other eating disorders (F50.-)
feeding problems of newborn (P92.-)
pica of infancy or childhood (F98.3)

F98.21 Rumination disorder of infancy

F98.29 Other feeding disorders of infancy and early childhood

F98.3 Pica of infancy and childhood

F98.4 Stereotyped movement disorders
Stereotype/habit disorder
EXCLUDES 1 abnormal involuntary movements (R25.-)
EXCLUDES 2 compulsions in obsessive-compulsive disorder (F42-)
hair plucking (F63.3)
movement disorders of organic origin (G20-G25)
nail-biting (F98.8)
nose-picking (F98.8)
stereotypies that are part of a broader psychiatric condition (F01-F95)
thumb-sucking (F98.8)
tic disorders (F95.-)
trichotillomania (F63.3)

✓ Additional Character Req   ✓x7ᵗʰ Placeholder Alert   Case-Mix Diagnosis   Manifestation   ▽ Unspecified Dx   **EXCLUDES 1** Not coded here   **EXCLUDES 2** Not included here

ICD-10-CM 2018   545

Chapter 5. Mental, Behavioral and Neurodevelopmental Disorders

F98.5   **Adult onset fluency disorder**
> **EXCLUDES 1**   *childhood onset fluency disorder (F80.81)*
> *dysphasia (R47.02)*
> *fluency disorder in conditions classified elsewhere (R47.82)*
> *fluency disorder (stuttering) following cerebrovascular disease (I69. with final characters -23)*
> *tic disorders (F95.-)*

F98.8   **Other specified behavioral and emotional disorders with onset usually occurring in childhood and adolescence**
> Excessive masturbation
> Nail-biting
> Nose-picking
> Thumb-sucking

F98.9   **Unspecified behavioral and emotional disorders with onset usually occurring in childhood and adolescence** ▽

Unspecified mental disorder (F99)

F99   **Mental disorder, not otherwise specified** ▽
> Mental illness NOS
> **EXCLUDES 1**   *unspecified mental disorder due to known physiological condition (F09)*

N Newborn: 0   P Pediatric: 0-17   M Maternity: 12-55   A Adult: 15-124   **NRS** Nonroutine supply Dx   **NC Dx** Noncancer Dx   **PDx** Primary Dx   ▶◀ Revised Text   ● New Code   ▲ Revised Title

546   ICD-10-CM 2018

Chapter 6. Diseases of the Nervous System (G00-G99)

Chapter Specific Guidelines with Coding Examples

The chapter specific guidelines from the ICD-10-CM Official Guidelines for Coding and Reporting have been provided below. Along with these guidelines are coding examples, contained in the shaded boxes, that have been developed to help illustrate the coding and/or sequencing guidance found in these guidelines.

a. Dominant/nondominant side

Codes from category G81, Hemiplegia and hemiparesis, and subcategories G83.1, Monoplegia of lower limb, G83.2, Monoplegia of upper limb, and G83.3, Monoplegia, unspecified, identify whether the dominant or nondominant side is affected. Should the affected side be documented, but not specified as dominant or nondominant, and the classification system does not indicate a default, code selection is as follows:

- For ambidextrous patients, the default should be dominant.
- If the left side is affected, the default is non-dominant.
- If the right side is affected, the default is dominant.

> Hemiplegia affecting left side of ambidextrous patient.
>
> **G81.92　　Hemiplegia, unspecified affecting left dominant side**
>
> *Explanation*: Documentation states that the left side is affected and dominant is used for ambidextrous persons.

> Right spastic hemiplegia, unknown whether patient is right- or left-handed.
>
> **G81.11　　Spastic hemiplegia affecting right dominant side**
>
> *Explanation*: Since it is unknown whether the patient is right- or left-handed, if the right side is affected, the default is dominant.

b. Pain—Category G89

1) General coding information

Codes in category G89, Pain, not elsewhere classified, may be used in conjunction with codes from other categories and chapters to provide more detail about acute or chronic pain and neoplasm-related pain, unless otherwise indicated below.

If the pain is not specified as acute or chronic, post-thoracotomy, postprocedural, or neoplasm-related, do not assign codes from category G89.

A code from category G89 should not be assigned if the underlying (definitive) diagnosis is known, unless the reason for the encounter is pain control/ management and not management of the underlying condition.

When an admission or encounter is for a procedure aimed at treating the underlying condition (e.g., spinal fusion, kyphoplasty), a code for the underlying condition (e.g., vertebral fracture, spinal stenosis) should be assigned as the principal diagnosis. No code from category G89 should be assigned.

(a) Category G89 codes as principal or first-listed diagnosis

Category G89 codes are acceptable as principal diagnosis or the first-listed code:

- When pain control or pain management is the reason for the admission/encounter (e.g., a patient with displaced intervertebral disc, nerve impingement and severe back pain presents for injection of steroid into the spinal canal). The underlying cause of the pain should be reported as an additional diagnosis, if known.

> A patient is admitted for rehabilitation focused on pain management. Provider notes indicate malignant neoplasm of the bone, with associated pain and debility.
>
> **G89.3　　Neoplasm related pain (acute) (chronic)**
>
> **C41.9　　Malignant neoplasm of bone and articular cartilage, unspecified**
>
> *Explanation*: Since the care focuses on controlling neoplasm-related pain, rather than treating the bone cancer, the pain code is sequenced first followed by the code for the underlying condition.

> A patient with severe lumbar spinal stenosis is admitted for physical therapy and nursing for pain management for "chronic back pain" per provider referral documentation.
>
> **G89.29　　Other chronic pain**
>
> **M48.061　　Spinal stenosis, lumbar region, without neurogenic claudication**
>
> *Explanation*: Since the encounter is for control of pain and not treating the underlying condition, the pain code is sequenced first. The M54 code for back pain is not necessary as the underlying condition code (M48.061) represents the specific site.

- When a patient is admitted for the insertion of a neurostimulator for pain control, assign the appropriate pain code as the principal or first-listed diagnosis. When an admission or encounter is for a procedure aimed at treating the underlying condition and a neurostimulator is inserted for pain control during the same admission/encounter, a code for the underlying condition should be assigned as the principal diagnosis and the appropriate pain code should be assigned as a secondary diagnosis.

(b) Use of category G89 codes in conjunction with site specific pain codes

(i) Assigning category G89 and site-specific pain codes

Codes from category G89 may be used in conjunction with codes that identify the site of pain (including codes from chapter 18) if the category G89 code provides additional information. For example, if the code describes the site of the pain, but does not fully describe whether the pain is acute or chronic, then both codes should be assigned.

> Patient is admitted for skilled rehabilitation with physical therapy. Rehabilitative services will focus on chronic lower back pain.
>
> **M54.5　　Low back pain**
>
> **G89.29　　Other chronic pain**
>
> *Explanation*: No underlying cause has been determined for the pain; documentation specifies only the site of the pain and its chronicity. A code describing where the pain is located (site) is sequenced first with an additional G89.- code reported to indicate the chronic nature of the back pain.

(ii) Sequencing of category G89 codes with site-specific pain codes

The sequencing of category G89 codes with site-specific pain codes (including chapter 18 codes), is dependent on the circumstances of the encounter/admission as follows:

- If the encounter is for pain control or pain management, assign the code from category G89 followed by the code identifying the specific site of pain (e.g., encounter for pain management for acute neck pain from trauma is assigned code G89.11, Acute pain due to trauma, followed by code M54.2, Cervicalgia, to identify the site of pain).

> Patient is admitted for rehabilitation following hospitalization for a fall. Provider orders specify rehabilitative therapy services due to acute post-fall right knee pain. Nursing will medically manage pain control.
>
> **G89.11　　Acute pain due to trauma**
>
> **M25.561　　Pain in right knee**
>
> *Explanation*: The focus of the skilled care is rehabilitation for pain management, so code G89.11 is sequenced first. Since this does not fully describe the condition, an additional code to indicate the site of the pain is added.

- If the encounter is for any other reason except pain control or pain management, and a related definitive diagnosis has not been established (confirmed) by the provider, assign the code for the specific site of pain first, followed by the appropriate code from category G89.

2) Pain due to devices, implants and grafts

See Section I.C.19. Pain due to medical devices

Chapter 6. Diseases of the Nervous System

3) Postoperative pain

The provider's documentation should be used to guide the coding of postoperative pain, as well as *Section III. Reporting Additional Diagnoses* and *Section IV. Diagnostic Coding and Reporting in the Outpatient Setting.*

The default for post-thoracotomy and other postoperative pain not specified as acute or chronic is the code for the acute form.

Routine or expected postoperative pain immediately after surgery should not be coded.

Patient is admitted for skilled care following surgery for repair of a large abdominal hernia. He requires skilled nursing for postoperative pain management and observation and home health aide due to unexpected and severe pain that is impacting self-care.

G89.18   **Other acute postprocedural pain**

Z48.815   **Encounter for surgical aftercare following surgery on the digestive system**

Explanation: When acute or chronic is not documented, default to acute. Some postoperative pain is expected, but the above documentation indicates this patient had pain that was unexpected and severe, limiting the patient's ability to return home and necessitating a skilled stay.

(a) Postoperative pain not associated with specific postoperative complication

Postoperative pain not associated with a specific postoperative complication is assigned to the appropriate postoperative pain code in category G89.

(b) Postoperative pain associated with specific postoperative complication

Postoperative pain associated with a specific postoperative complication (such as painful wire sutures) is assigned to the appropriate code(s) found in Chapter 19, Injury, poisoning, and certain other consequences of external causes. If appropriate, use additional code(s) from category G89 to identify acute or chronic pain (G89.18 or G89.28).

4) Chronic pain

Chronic pain is classified to subcategory G89.2. There is no time frame defining when pain becomes chronic pain. The provider's documentation should be used to guide use of these codes.

5) Neoplasm related pain

Code G89.3 is assigned to pain documented as being related, associated or due to cancer, primary or secondary malignancy, or tumor. This code is assigned regardless of whether the pain is acute or chronic.

This code may be assigned as the principal or first-listed code when the stated reason for the admission/encounter is documented as pain control/pain management. The underlying neoplasm should be reported as an additional diagnosis.

Patient with history of primary cancer of the prostate and pain due to bone metastasis is admitted to skilled care for continued pain control post-hospitalization.

G89.3   **Neoplasm related pain (acute)(chronic)**

C79.51   **Secondary malignant neoplasm of bone**

Z85.46   **Personal history of malignant neoplasm of prostate**

Explanation: After hospitalization, the patient was admitted to skilled home health care for continued management of pain secondary to bone metastasis. The neoplasm was not the reason for the skilled care and is sequenced after the code for the neoplasm-related pain. Code G89.3 is used for both acute and chronic cancer-related pain.

When the reason for the admission/encounter is management of the neoplasm and the pain associated with the neoplasm is also documented, code G89.3 may be assigned as an additional diagnosis. It is not necessary to assign an additional code for the site of the pain.

See Section I.C.2 for instructions on the sequencing of neoplasms for all other stated reasons for the admission/encounter (except for pain control/pain management).

Provider notes bone neoplasm with current neoplastic fracture of right femur. The fracture is healing normally, but diffuse pain due to extensive neoplastic bone disease in that lower extremity is documented.

M84.551D   **Pathological fracture in neoplastic disease, right femur, subsequent encounter for fracture with routine healing**

C40.21   **Malignant neoplasm of long bones of right lower limb**

G89.3   **Neoplasm related pain (acute) (chronic)**

Explanation: The reason for the encounter is the treatment of the pathological femur fracture due to bone cancer. Additional codes to identify the neoplasm and neoplastic pain should also be assigned.

---

6) Chronic pain syndrome

Central pain syndrome (G89.0) and chronic pain syndrome (G89.4) are different than the term "chronic pain," and therefore codes should only be used when the provider has specifically documented this condition.

See Section I.C.5. Pain disorders related to psychological factors

Chapter 6. Diseases of the Nervous System (G00-G99)

EXCLUDES 2   *certain conditions originating in the perinatal period (P04-P96)*
certain infectious and parasitic diseases (A00-B99)
complications of pregnancy, childbirth and the puerperium (O00-O9A)
congenital malformations, deformations, and chromosomal abnormalities (Q00-Q99)
endocrine, nutritional and metabolic diseases (E00-E88)
injury, poisoning and certain other consequences of external causes (S00-T88)
neoplasms (C00-D49)
symptoms, signs and abnormal clinical and laboratory findings, not elsewhere classified (R00-R94)

This chapter contains the following blocks:

G00-G09   Inflammatory diseases of the central nervous system
G10-G14   Systemic atrophies primarily affecting the central nervous system
G20-G26   Extrapyramidal and movement disorders
G30-G32   Other degenerative diseases of the nervous system
G35-G37   Demyelinating diseases of the central nervous system
G40-G47   Episodic and paroxysmal disorders
G50-G59   Nerve, nerve root and plexus disorders
G60-G65   Polyneuropathies and other disorders of the peripheral nervous system
G70-G73   Diseases of myoneural junction and muscle
G80-G83   Cerebral palsy and other paralytic syndromes
G89-G99   Other disorders of the nervous system

Inflammatory diseases of the central nervous system (G00-G09)

✓4ᵗʰ G00   Bacterial meningitis, not elsewhere classified
    INCLUDES   bacterial arachnoiditis
             bacterial leptomeningitis
             bacterial meningitis
             bacterial pachymeningitis
    EXCLUDES 1 ► *bacterial meningoencephalitis* ◄ *(G04.2)*
                ► *bacterial meningomyelitis* ◄ *(G04.2)*

G00.0   Hemophilus meningitis
     Meningitis due to Hemophilus influenzae

G00.1   Pneumococcal meningitis
     Meningtitis due to Streptococcal pneumoniae

G00.2   Streptococcal meningitis
     Use additional code to further identify organism (B95.0-B95.5)

G00.3   Staphylococcal meningitis
     Use additional code to further identify organism (B95.61-B95.8)

G00.8   Other bacterial meningitis
     Meningitis due to Escherichia coli
     Meningitis due to Friedländer's bacillus
     Meningitis due to Klebsiella
     Use additional code to further identify organism (B96.-)

G00.9   Bacterial meningitis, unspecified   ▽
     Meningitis due to gram-negative bacteria, unspecified
     Purulent meningitis NOS
     Pyogenic meningitis NOS
     Suppurative meningitis NOS

G01   *Meningitis in bacterial diseases classified elsewhere*
    Code first underlying disease
    EXCLUDES 1   *meningitis (in):*
                gonococcal (A54.81)
                leptospirosis (A27.81)
                listeriosis (A32.11)
                Lyme disease (A69.21)
                meningococcal (A39.0)
                neurosyphilis (A52.13)
                tuberculosis (A17.0)
            meningoencephalitis and meningomyelitis in bacterial diseases classified elsewhere (G05)

G02   *Meningitis in other infectious and parasitic diseases classified elsewhere*
    Code first underlying disease, such as:
     African trypanosomiasis (B56.-)
     poliovirus infection (A80.-)
    EXCLUDES 1   *candidal meningitis (B37.5)*
              coccidioidomycosis meningitis (B38.4)
              cryptococcal meningitis (B45.1)
              herpesviral [herpes simplex] meningitis (B00.3)
              infectious mononucleosis complicated by meningitis (B27.- with fourth character 2)
              measles complicated by meningitis (B05.1)
              meningoencephalitis and meningomyelitis in other infectious and parasitic diseases classified elsewhere (G05)
              mumps meningitis (B26.1)
              rubella meningitis (B06.02)
              varicella [chickenpox] meningitis (B01.0)
              zoster meningitis (B02.1)

✓4ᵗʰ G03   Meningitis due to other and unspecified causes
    INCLUDES   arachnoiditis NOS
             leptomeningitis NOS
             meningitis NOS
             pachymeningitis NOS
    EXCLUDES 1   *meningoencephalitis (G04.-)*
              meningomyelitis (G04.-)

G03.0   Nonpyogenic meningitis
     Aseptic meningitis
     Nonbacterial meningitis

G03.1   Chronic meningitis

G03.2   Benign recurrent meningitis [Mollaret]

G03.8   Meningitis due to other specified causes

G03.9   Meningitis, unspecified   ▽
     Arachnoiditis (spinal) NOS

✓4ᵗʰ G04   Encephalitis, myelitis and encephalomyelitis
    INCLUDES   acute ascending myelitis
             meningoencephalitis
             meningomyelitis
    EXCLUDES 1   *encephalopathy NOS (G93.40)*
    EXCLUDES 2   *acute transverse myelitis (G37.3-)*
              alcoholic encephalopathy (G31.2)
              benign myalgic encephalomyelitis (G93.3)
              multiple sclerosis (G35)
              subacute necrotizing myelitis (G37.4)
              toxic encephalitis (G92)
              toxic encephalopathy (G92)

✓5ᵗʰ G04.0   Acute disseminated encephalitis and encephalomyelitis (ADEM)
     EXCLUDES 1   *acute necrotizing hemorrhagic encephalopathy (G04.3-)*
                other noninfectious acute disseminated encephalomyelitis (noninfectious ADEM) (G04.81)

    G04.00   Acute disseminated encephalitis and   ▽
           encephalomyelitis, unspecified

    G04.01   Postinfectious acute disseminated encephalitis and encephalomyelitis (postinfectious ADEM)
           EXCLUDES 1   *post chickenpox encephalitis (B01.1)*
                    post measles encephalitis (B05.0)
                    post measles myelitis (B05.1)

    G04.02   Postimmunization acute disseminated encephalitis, myelitis and encephalomyelitis
           Encephalitis, postimmunization
           Encephalomyelitis, postimmunization
           Use additional code to identify the vaccine (T50.A-, T50.B-, T50.Z-)

    G04.1   Tropical spastic paraplegia

    G04.2   Bacterial meningoencephalitis and meningomyelitis, not elsewhere classified

✓5ᵗʰ G04.3   Acute necrotizing hemorrhagic encephalopathy
     EXCLUDES 1   *acute disseminated encephalitis and encephalomyelitis (G04.0-)*

    G04.30   Acute necrotizing hemorrhagic encephalopathy,   ▽
           unspecified

    G04.31   Postinfectious acute necrotizing hemorrhagic encephalopathy

    G04.32   Postimmunization acute necrotizing hemorrhagic encephalopathy
           Use additional code to identify the vaccine (T50.A-, T50.B-, T50.Z-)

✓ Additional Character Req   ✓x7ᵗʰ Placeholder Alert   Case-Mix Diagnosis   Manifestation   ▽ Unspecified Dx   **EXCLUDES 1** Not coded here   **EXCLUDES 2** Not included here

ICD-10-CM 2018   **549**

G04.39   **Other acute necrotizing hemorrhagic encephalopathy**
Code also underlying etiology, if applicable

✓5ᵗʰ **G04.8**   **Other encephalitis, myelitis and encephalomyelitis**
Code also any associated seizure (G40.-, R56.9)

G04.81   **Other encephalitis and encephalomyelitis** `NC Dx`
Noninfectious acute disseminated encephalomyelitis (noninfectious ADEM)

G04.89   **Other myelitis** `NC Dx`

✓5ᵗʰ **G04.9**   **Encephalitis, myelitis and encephalomyelitis, unspecified**

G04.90   **Encephalitis and encephalomyelitis, unspecified** ▽
Ventriculitis (cerebral) NOS

G04.91   **Myelitis, unspecified** ▽

✓4ᵗʰ **G05**   **Encephalitis, myelitis and encephalomyelitis in diseases classified elsewhere**
Code first underlying disease, such as:
human immunodeficiency virus [HIV] disease (B20)
poliovirus (A80.-)
suppurative otitis media (H66.01-H66.4)
trichinellosis (B75)

EXCLUDES 1   adenoviral encephalitis, myelitis and encephalomyelitis (A85.1)
congenital toxoplasmosis encephalitis, myelitis and encephalomyelitis (P37.1)
cytomegaloviral encephalitis, myelitis and encephalomyelitis (B25.8)
encephalitis, myelitis and encephalomyelitis (in) measles (B05.0)
encephalitis, myelitis and encephalomyelitis (in) systemic lupus erythematosus (M32.19)
enteroviral encephalitis, myelitis and encephalomyelitis (A85.0)
eosinophilic meningoencephalitis (B83.2)
herpesviral [herpes simplex] encephalitis, myelitis and encephalomyelitis (B00.4)
listerial encephalitis, myelitis and encephalomyelitis (A32.12)
meningococcal encephalitis, myelitis and encephalomyelitis (A39.81)
mumps encephalitis, myelitis and encephalomyelitis (B26.2)
postchickenpox encephalitis, myelitis and encephalomyelitis (B01.1-)
rubella encephalitis, myelitis and encephalomyelitis (B06.01)
toxoplasmosis encephalitis, myelitis and encephalomyelitis (B58.2)
zoster encephalitis, myelitis and encephalomyelitis (B02.0)

G05.3   **Encephalitis and encephalomyelitis in diseases classified elsewhere**
Meningoencephalitis in diseases classified elsewhere

G05.4   **Myelitis in diseases classified elsewhere**
Meningomyelitis in diseases classified elsewhere

✓4ᵗʰ **G06**   **Intracranial and intraspinal abscess and granuloma**
Use additional code (B95-B97) to identify infectious agent

G06.0   **Intracranial abscess and granuloma**
Brain [any part] abscess (embolic)
Cerebellar abscess (embolic)
Cerebral abscess (embolic)
Intracranial epidural abscess or granuloma
Intracranial extradural abscess or granuloma
Intracranial subdural abscess or granuloma
Otogenic abscess (embolic)

EXCLUDES 1   tuberculous intracranial abscess and granuloma (A17.81)

G06.1   **Intraspinal abscess and granuloma**
Abscess (embolic) of spinal cord [any part]
Intraspinal epidural abscess or granuloma
Intraspinal extradural abscess or granuloma
Intraspinal subdural abscess or granuloma

EXCLUDES 1   tuberculous intraspinal abscess and granuloma (A17.81)

G06.2   **Extradural and subdural abscess, unspecified** ▽

G07   **Intracranial and intraspinal abscess and granuloma in diseases classified elsewhere**
Code first underlying disease, such as:
schistosomiasis granuloma of brain (B65.-)

EXCLUDES 1   abscess of brain:
amebic (A06.6)
chromomycotic (B43.1)
gonococcal (A54.82)
tuberculous (A17.81)
tuberculoma of meninges (A17.1)

G08   **Intracranial and intraspinal phlebitis and thrombophlebitis**
Septic embolism of intracranial or intraspinal venous sinuses and veins
Septic endophlebitis of intracranial or intraspinal venous sinuses and veins
Septic phlebitis of intracranial or intraspinal venous sinuses and veins
Septic thrombophlebitis of intracranial or intraspinal venous sinuses and veins
Septic thrombosis of intracranial or intraspinal venous sinuses and veins

EXCLUDES 1   intracranial phlebitis and thrombophlebitis complicating:
abortion, ectopic or molar pregnancy (O00-O07, O08.7)
pregnancy, childbirth and the puerperium (O22.5, O87.3)
nonpyogenic intracranial phlebitis and thrombophlebitis (I67.6)

EXCLUDES 2   intracranial phlebitis and thrombophlebitis complicating nonpyogenic intraspinal phlebitis and thrombophlebitis (G95.1)

DEF: Inflammation and formation of blood clot in a vein within the brain or spine, or their linings.

G09   **Sequelae of inflammatory diseases of central nervous system**
`NOTE`   Category G09 is to be used to indicate conditions whose primary classification is to G00-G08 as the cause of sequelae, themselves classifiable elsewhere. The "sequelae" include conditions specified as residuals.
Code first condition resulting from (sequela) of inflammatory diseases of central nervous system

Systemic atrophies primarily affecting the central nervous system (G10-G14)

G10   **Huntington's disease**
Huntington's chorea
Huntington's dementia
▶Code also dementia in other diseases classified elsewhere without behavioral disturbance (F02.80)◀
DEF: Genetic disease caused by degeneration of nerve cells in the brain, characterized by chronic progressive mental deterioration; dementia and death within 15 to 20 years of onset.

✓4ᵗʰ **G11**   **Hereditary ataxia**
EXCLUDES 2   cerebral palsy (G80.-)
hereditary and idiopathic neuropathy (G60.-)
metabolic disorders (E70-E88)

G11.0   **Congenital nonprogressive ataxia**

G11.1   **Early-onset cerebellar ataxia**
Early-onset cerebellar ataxia with essential tremor
Early-onset cerebellar ataxia with myoclonus [Hunt's ataxia]
Early-onset cerebellar ataxia with retained tendon reflexes
Friedreich's ataxia (autosomal recessive)
X-linked recessive spinocerebellar ataxia

G11.2   **Late-onset cerebellar ataxia** A

G11.3   **Cerebellar ataxia with defective DNA repair**
Ataxia telangiectasia [Louis-Bar]
EXCLUDES 2   Cockayne's syndrome (Q87.1)
other disorders of purine and pyrimidine metabolism (E79.-)
xeroderma pigmentosum (Q82.1)

G11.4   **Hereditary spastic paraplegia**

G11.8   **Other hereditary ataxias**

G11.9   **Hereditary ataxia, unspecified** ▽
Hereditary cerebellar ataxia NOS
Hereditary cerebellar degeneration
Hereditary cerebellar disease
Hereditary cerebellar syndrome

✓4ᵗʰ **G12**   **Spinal muscular atrophy and related syndromes**
G12.0   **Infantile spinal muscular atrophy, type I [Werdnig-Hoffman]**
G12.1   **Other inherited spinal muscular atrophy**
Adult form spinal muscular atrophy
Childhood form, type II spinal muscular atrophy
Distal spinal muscular atrophy
Juvenile form, type III spinal muscular atrophy [Kugelberg-Welander]
Progressive bulbar palsy of childhood [Fazio-Londe]
Scapuloperoneal form spinal muscular atrophy

✓5ᵗʰ **G12.2**   **Motor neuron disease**
G12.20   **Motor neuron disease, unspecified** ▽
G12.21   **Amyotrophic lateral sclerosis** A
~~Progressive spinal muscle atrophy~~
G12.22   **Progressive bulbar palsy**
● **G12.23**   **Primary lateral sclerosis**
● **G12.24**   **Familial motor neuron disease**
● **G12.25**   **Progressive spinal muscle atrophy**

G12.29   **Other motor neuron disease**
       Familial motor neuron disease
       Primary lateral sclerosis

G12.8   **Other spinal muscular atrophies and related syndromes**

G12.9   **Spinal muscular atrophy, unspecified**   ▽

✓4ᵗʰ **G13**   **Systemic atrophies primarily affecting central nervous system in diseases classified elsewhere**

G13.0   *Paraneoplastic neuromyopathy and neuropathy*
     Carcinomatous neuromyopathy
     Sensorial paraneoplastic neuropathy [Denny Brown]
     Code first underlying neoplasm (C00-D49)

G13.1   *Other systemic atrophy primarily affecting central nervous system in neoplastic disease*
     Paraneoplastic limbic encephalopathy
     Code first underlying neoplasm (C00-D49)

G13.2   *Systemic atrophy primarily affecting the central nervous system in myxedema*
     Code first underlying disease, such as:
       hypothyroidism (E03.-)
       myxedematous congenital iodine deficiency (E00.1)

G13.8   *Systemic atrophy primarily affecting central nervous system in other diseases classified elsewhere*
     Code first underlying disease

G14   **Postpolio syndrome**
     INCLUDES   postpolio myelitic syndrome
     EXCLUDES 1   *sequelae of poliomyelitis (B91)*

Extrapyramidal and movement disorders (G20-G26)

G20   **Parkinson's disease**   NC Dx
     Hemiparkinsonism
     Idiopathic Parkinsonism or Parkinson's disease
     Paralysis agitans
     Parkinsonism or Parkinson's disease NOS
     Primary Parkinsonism or Parkinson's disease
     EXCLUDES 1   *dementia with Parkinsonism (G31.83)*
     AHA: 2017, 2Q, 7; 2016, 2Q, 6
     TIP: Repeated falls (R29.6) are not integral to Parkinson's disease and can be separately coded.

✓4ᵗʰ **G21**   **Secondary parkinsonism**
     EXCLUDES 1   *dementia with Parkinsonism (G31.83)*
       Huntington's disease (G10)
       Shy-Drager syndrome (G90.3)
       syphilitic Parkinsonism (A52.19)

G21.0   **Malignant neuroleptic syndrome**
     Use additional code for adverse effect, if applicable, to identify drug (T43.3X5, T43.4X5, T43.505, T43.595)
     EXCLUDES 1   *neuroleptic induced parkinsonism (G21.11)*

✓5ᵗʰ *G21.1*   **Other drug-induced secondary parkinsonism**
     G21.11   **Neuroleptic induced parkinsonism**
       Use additional code for adverse effect, if applicable, to identify drug (T43.3X5, T43.4X5, T43.505, T43.595)
       EXCLUDES 1   *malignant neuroleptic syndrome (G21.0)*

     G21.19   **Other drug induced secondary parkinsonism**
       ▶Other medication-induced parkinsonism◀
       Use additional code for adverse effect, if applicable, to identify drug (T36-T50 with fifth or sixth character 5)

G21.2   **Secondary parkinsonism due to other external agents**
     Code first (T51-T65) to identify external agent

G21.3   **Postencephalitic parkinsonism**

G21.4   **Vascular parkinsonism**

G21.8   **Other secondary parkinsonism**

G21.9   **Secondary parkinsonism, unspecified**   ▽

✓4ᵗʰ **G23**   **Other degenerative diseases of basal ganglia**
     EXCLUDES 2   *multi-system degeneration of the autonomic nervous system (G90.3)*

G23.0   **Hallervorden-Spatz disease**
     Pigmentary pallidal degeneration

G23.1   **Progressive supranuclear ophthalmoplegia [Steele-Richardson-Olszewski]**
     Progressive supranuclear palsy

G23.2   **Striatonigral degeneration**

G23.8   **Other specified degenerative diseases of basal ganglia**
     Calcification of basal ganglia

G23.9   **Degenerative disease of basal ganglia, unspecified**   ▽

✓4ᵗʰ **G24**   **Dystonia**
     INCLUDES   dyskinesia
     EXCLUDES 2   *athetoid cerebral palsy (G80.3)*

✓5ᵗʰ *G24.0*   **Drug induced dystonia**
     Use additional code for adverse effect, if applicable, to identify drug (T36-T50 with fifth or sixth character5)

     G24.01   **Drug induced subacute dyskinesia**
       Drug induced blepharospasm
       Drug induced orofacial dyskinesia
       Neuroleptic induced tardive dyskinesia
       Tardive dyskinesia

     G24.02   **Drug induced acute dystonia**
       Acute dystonic reaction to drugs
       Neuroleptic induced acute dystonia

     G24.09   **Other drug induced dystonia**

G24.1   **Genetic torsion dystonia**
     Dystonia deformans progressiva
     Dystonia musculorum deformans
     Familial torsion dystonia
     Idiopathic familial dystonia
     Idiopathic (torsion) dystonia NOS
     (Schwalbe-) Ziehen-Oppenheim disease

G24.2   **Idiopathic nonfamilial dystonia**

G24.3   **Spasmodic torticollis**
     EXCLUDES 1   *congenital torticollis (Q68.0)*
       hysterical torticollis (F44.4)
       ocular torticollis (R29.891)
       psychogenic torticollis (F45.8)
       torticollis NOS (M43.6)
       traumatic recurrent torticollis (S13.4)

G24.4   **Idiopathic orofacial dystonia**
     Orofacial dyskinesia
     EXCLUDES 1   *drug induced orofacial dyskinesia (G24.01)*

G24.5   **Blepharospasm**
     EXCLUDES 1   *drug induced blepharospasm (G24.01)*

G24.8   **Other dystonia**
     Acquired torsion dystonia NOS

G24.9   **Dystonia, unspecified**   ▽
     Dyskinesia NOS

✓4ᵗʰ **G25**   **Other extrapyramidal and movement disorders**
     EXCLUDES 2   *sleep related movement disorders (G47.6-)*

G25.0   **Essential tremor**
     Familial tremor
     EXCLUDES 1   *tremor NOS (R25.1)*

G25.1   **Drug-induced tremor**
     Use additional code for adverse effect, if applicable, to identify drug (T36-T50 with fifth or sixth character 5)

G25.2   **Other specified forms of tremor**
     Intention tremor

G25.3   **Myoclonus**
     Drug-induced myoclonus
     Palatal myoclonus
     Use additional code for adverse effect, if applicable, to identify drug (T36-T50 with fifth or sixth character 5)
     EXCLUDES 1   *facial myokymia (G51.4)*
       myoclonic epilepsy (G40.-)

G25.4   **Drug-induced chorea**
     Use additional code for adverse effect, if applicable, to identify drug (T36-T50 with fifth or sixth character 5)

G25.5   **Other chorea**
     Chorea NOS
     EXCLUDES 1   *chorea NOS with heart involvement (I02.0)*
       Huntington's chorea (G10)
       rheumatic chorea (I02.-)
       Sydenham's chorea (I02.-)

✓5ᵗʰ *G25.6*   **Drug induced tics and other tics of organic origin**
     G25.61   **Drug induced tics**
       Use additional code for adverse effect, if applicable, to identify drug (T36-T50 with fifth or sixth character 5)

     G25.69   **Other tics of organic origin**
       EXCLUDES 1   *habit spasm (F95.9)*
       tic NOS (F95.9)
       Tourette's syndrome (F95.2)

✓5ᵗʰ *G25.7*   **Other and unspecified drug induced movement disorders**
     Use additional code for adverse effect, if applicable, to identify drug (T36-T50 with fifth or sixth character 5)

     G25.70   **Drug induced movement disorder, unspecified**   ▽

✔ Additional Character Req   ✔x7ᵗʰ Placeholder Alert   Case-Mix Diagnosis   Manifestation   ▽ Unspecified Dx   EXCLUDES 1 Not coded here   EXCLUDES 2 Not included here

Chapter 6. Diseases of the Nervous System

G25.71   Drug induced akathisia
    Drug induced acathisia
    Neuroleptic induced acute akathisia
    ▶Tardive akathisia◀

G25.79   Other drug induced movement disorders

✓5ᵗʰ **G25.8   Other specified extrapyramidal and movement disorders**

G25.81   Restless legs syndrome
    DEF: Neurological disorder of unknown etiology creating an irresistible urge to move the legs, which may temporarily relieve the symptoms; is accompanied by motor restlessness and sensations of pain, burning, prickling, or tingling.

G25.82   Stiff-man syndrome

G25.83   Benign shuddering attacks

G25.89   Other specified extrapyramidal and movement disorders

G25.9   Extrapyramidal and movement disorder, unspecified ▽

G26   *Extrapyramidal and movement disorders in diseases classified elsewhere*
    Code first underlying disease

Other degenerative diseases of the nervous system (G30-G32)

✓4ᵗʰ **G30   Alzheimer's disease**
    INCLUDES   Alzheimer's dementia senile and presenile forms
    Use additional code to identify:
       delirium, if applicable (F05)
       dementia with behavioral disturbance (F02.81)
       dementia without behavioral disturbance (F02.80)
    EXCLUDES 1   *senile degeneration of brain NEC (G31.1)*
          senile dementia NOS (F03)
          senility NOS (R41.81)
    AHA: 2017, 1Q, 43
    TIP: Sundowning (F05) is not integral to Alzheimer's disease and can be coded separately.

G30.0   Alzheimer's disease with early onset   NC Dx

G30.1   Alzheimer's disease with late onset   NC Dx A

G30.8   Other Alzheimer's disease   NC Dx

G30.9   Alzheimer's disease, unspecified   NC Dx ▽
    AHA: 2016, 2Q, 6; 2012, 4Q, 95

✓4ᵗʰ **G31   Other degenerative diseases of nervous system, not elsewhere classified**
    Use additional code to identify:
       dementia with behavioral disturbance (F02.81)
       dementia without behavioral disturbance (F02.80)
    EXCLUDES 2   *Reye's syndrome (G93.7)*

✓5ᵗʰ **G31.0   Frontotemporal dementia**

G31.01   Pick's disease   NC Dx
    Primary progressive aphasia
    Progressive isolated aphasia
    DEF: A progressive frontotemporal dementia with asymmetrical atrophy of the frontal and temporal regions of the cerebral cortex, abnormal rounded brain cells called Pick cells with the presence of abnormal staining of protein (called tau); symptoms include prominent apathy, behavioral changes such as disinhibition and restlessness, echolalia, impairment of language, memory, and intellect, increased carelessness, poor personal hygiene, and decreased attention span.

G31.09   Other frontotemporal dementia   NC Dx
    Frontal dementia

G31.1   Senile degeneration of brain, not elsewhere classified   NC Dx
    EXCLUDES 1   *Alzheimer's disease (G30.-)*
          senility NOS (R41.81)

G31.2   Degeneration of nervous system due to alcohol
    Alcoholic cerebellar ataxia
    Alcoholic cerebellar degeneration
    Alcoholic cerebral degeneration
    Alcoholic encephalopathy
    Dysfunction of the autonomic nervous system due to alcohol
    Code also associated alcoholism (F10.-)

✓5ᵗʰ **G31.8   Other specified degenerative diseases of nervous system**

G31.81   Alpers disease
    Grey-matter degeneration

G31.82   Leigh's disease
    Subacute necrotizing encephalopathy

G31.83   Dementia with Lewy bodies   NC Dx
    Dementia with Parkinsonism
    Lewy body dementia
    Lewy body disease
    AHA: 2017, 2Q, 7; 2016, 4Q, 141
    DEF: A cerebral dementia with neurophysiologic changes, increased hippocampal volume, hypoperfusion in the occipital lobes, beta amyloid deposits with neurofibrillary tangles, and atrophy of cortex and brainstem. Hallmark neuropsychological characteristics include fluctuating cognition with pronounced variation in attention and alertness; recurrent hallucinations; and Parkinsonism.

G31.84   Mild cognitive impairment, so stated
    ▶Mild neurocognitive disorder◀
    EXCLUDES 1   *age related cognitive decline (R41.81)*
          altered mental status (R41.82)
          cerebral degeneration (G31.9)
          change in mental status (R41.82)
          cognitive deficits following (sequelae of) cerebral hemorrhage or infarction (I69.01-, I69.11-, I69.21-, I69.31-, I69.81-, I69.91-)
          cognitive impairment due to intracranial or head injury (S06.-)
          dementia (F01.-, F02.-, F03)
          mild memory disturbance (F06.8)
          neurologic neglect syndrome (R41.4)
          personality change, nonpsychotic (F68.8)

G31.85   Corticobasal degeneration   NC Dx

G31.89   Other specified degenerative diseases of nervous system

G31.9   Degenerative disease of nervous system, unspecified ▽

✓4ᵗʰ **G32   Other degenerative disorders of nervous system in diseases classified elsewhere**

G32.0   *Subacute combined degeneration of spinal cord in diseases classified elsewhere*
    Dana-Putnam syndrome
    Sclerosis of spinal cord (combined) (dorsolateral) (posterolateral)
    Code first underlying disease, such as:
       anemia (D51.9)
       dietary (D51.3)
       pernicious (D51.0)
       vitamin B12 deficiency (E53.8)
    EXCLUDES 1   *syphilitic combined degeneration of spinal cord (A52.11)*

✓5ᵗʰ **G32.8   Other specified degenerative disorders of nervous system in diseases classified elsewhere**
    Code first underlying disease, such as:
       amyloidosis cerebral degeneration (E85.-)
       cerebral degeneration (due to) hypothyroidism (E00.0-E03.9)
       cerebral degeneration (due to) neoplasm (C00-D49)
       cerebral degeneration (due to) vitamin B deficiency, except thiamine (E52-E53.-)
    EXCLUDES 1   *superior hemorrhagic polioencephalitis [Wernicke's encephalopathy] (E51.2)*

G32.81   *Cerebellar ataxia in diseases classified elsewhere*
    Code first underlying disease, such as:
       celiac disease (with gluten ataxia) (K90.0)
       cerebellar ataxia (in) neoplastic disease (paraneoplastic cerebellar degeneration) (C00-D49)
       non-celiac gluten ataxia (M35.9)
    EXCLUDES 1   *systemic atrophy primarily affecting the central nervous system in alcoholic cerebellar ataxia (G31.2)*
          systemic atrophy primarily affecting the central nervous system in myxedema (G13.2)

G32.89   *Other specified degenerative disorders of nervous system in diseases classified elsewhere*
    Degenerative encephalopathy in diseases classified elsewhere

Ⓝ Newborn: 0   Ⓟ Pediatric: 0-17   Ⓜ Maternity: 12-55   Ⓐ Adult: 15-124   NRS Nonroutine supply Dx   NC Dx Noncancer Dx   PDx Primary Dx   ▶◀ Revised Text   ● New Code   ▲ Revised Title

552   ICD-10-CM 2018

Demyelinating diseases of the central nervous system (G35-G37)

G35 Multiple sclerosis `NC Dx`
Disseminated multiple sclerosis
Generalized multiple sclerosis
Multiple sclerosis NOS
Multiple sclerosis of brain stem
Multiple sclerosis of cord

`☑4ᵗʰ` **G36 Other acute disseminated demyelination**
EXCLUDES 1   postinfectious encephalitis and encephalomyelitis NOS (G04.01)

G36.0 Neuromyelitis optica [Devic]
Demyelination in optic neuritis
EXCLUDES 1   optic neuritis NOS (H46)

G36.1 Acute and subacute hemorrhagic leukoencephalitis [Hurst]

G36.8 Other specified acute disseminated demyelination

G36.9 Acute disseminated demyelination, unspecified   ▽

`☑4ᵗʰ` **G37 Other demyelinating diseases of central nervous system**

G37.0 Diffuse sclerosis of central nervous system
Periaxial encephalitis
Schilder's disease
EXCLUDES 1   X linked adrenoleukodystrophy (E71.52-)

G37.1 Central demyelination of corpus callosum

G37.2 Central pontine myelinolysis

G37.3 Acute transverse myelitis in demyelinating disease of central nervous system
Acute transverse myelitis NOS
Acute transverse myelopathy
EXCLUDES 1   multiple sclerosis (G35)
neuromyelitis optica [Devic] (G36.0)

G37.4 Subacute necrotizing myelitis of central nervous system

G37.5 Concentric sclerosis [Balo] of central nervous system

G37.8 Other specified demyelinating diseases of central nervous system

G37.9 Demyelinating disease of central nervous system, unspecified   ▽

Episodic and paroxysmal disorders (G40-G47)

`☑4ᵗʰ` **G40 Epilepsy and recurrent seizures**
`NOTE`   The following terms are to be considered equivalent to intractable: pharmacoresistant (pharmacologically resistant), treatment resistant, refractory (medically) and poorly controlled
EXCLUDES 1   conversion disorder with seizures (F44.5)
convulsions NOS (R56.9)
post traumatic seizures (R56.1)
seizure (convulsive) NOS (R56.9)
seizure of newborn (P90)
EXCLUDES 2   hippocampal sclerosis (G93.81)
mesial temporal sclerosis (G93.81)
temporal sclerosis (G93.81)
Todd's paralysis (G83.84)

`☑5ᵗʰ` **G40.0 Localization-related (focal) (partial) idiopathic epilepsy and epileptic syndromes with** seizures of localized onset
Benign childhood epilepsy with centrotemporal EEG spikes
Childhood epilepsy with occipital EEG paroxysms
EXCLUDES 1   adult onset localization-related epilepsy (G40.1-, G40.2-)

`☑6ᵗʰ` **G40.00 Localization-related (focal) (partial) idiopathic epilepsy and epileptic syndromes with seizures of localized onset,** not intractable
Localization-related (focal) (partial) idiopathic epilepsy and epileptic syndromes with seizures of localized onset without intractability

G40.001 Localization-related (focal) (partial) idiopathic epilepsy and epileptic syndromes with seizures of localized onset, not intractable, with status epilepticus

G40.009 Localization-related (focal) (partial) idiopathic epilepsy and epileptic syndromes with seizures of localized onset, not intractable, without status epilepticus
Localization-related (focal) (partial) idiopathic epilepsy and epileptic syndromes with seizures of localized onset NOS

`☑6ᵗʰ` **G40.01 Localization-related (focal) (partial) idiopathic epilepsy and epileptic syndromes with seizures of localized onset,** intractable

G40.011 Localization-related (focal) (partial) idiopathic epilepsy and epileptic syndromes with seizures of localized onset, intractable, with status epilepticus

G40.019 Localization-related (focal) (partial) idiopathic epilepsy and epileptic syndromes with seizures of localized onset, intractable, without status epilepticus

`☑5ᵗʰ` **G40.1 Localization-related (focal) (partial) symptomatic epilepsy and epileptic syndromes** with simple partial seizures
Attacks without alteration of consciousness
Epilepsia partialis continua [Kozhevnikof]
Simple partial seizures developing into secondarily generalized seizures

`☑6ᵗʰ` **G40.10 Localization-related (focal) (partial) symptomatic epilepsy and epileptic syndromes with simple partial seizures,** not intractable
Localization-related (focal) (partial) symptomatic epilepsy and epileptic syndromes with simple partial seizures without intractability

G40.101 Localization-related (focal) (partial) symptomatic epilepsy and epileptic syndromes with simple partial seizures, not intractable, with status epilepticus

G40.109 Localization-related (focal) (partial) symptomatic epilepsy and epileptic syndromes with simple partial seizures, not intractable, without status epilepticus
Localization-related (focal) (partial) symptomatic epilepsy and epileptic syndromes with simple partial seizures NOS

`☑6ᵗʰ` **G40.11 Localization-related (focal) (partial) symptomatic epilepsy and epileptic syndromes with simple partial seizures,** intractable

G40.111 Localization-related (focal) (partial) symptomatic epilepsy and epileptic syndromes with simple partial seizures, intractable, with status epilepticus

G40.119 Localization-related (focal) (partial) symptomatic epilepsy and epileptic syndromes with simple partial seizures, intractable, without status epilepticus

`☑5ᵗʰ` **G40.2 Localization-related (focal) (partial) symptomatic epilepsy and epileptic syndromes** with complex partial seizures
Attacks with alteration of consciousness, often with automatisms
Complex partial seizures developing into secondarily generalized seizures

`☑6ᵗʰ` **G40.20 Localization-related (focal) (partial) symptomatic epilepsy and epileptic syndromes with complex partial seizures,** not intractable
Localization-related (focal) (partial) symptomatic epilepsy and epileptic syndromes with complex partial seizures without intractability

G40.201 Localization-related (focal) (partial) symptomatic epilepsy and epileptic syndromes with complex partial seizures, not intractable, with status epilepticus

G40.209 Localization-related (focal) (partial) symptomatic epilepsy and epileptic syndromes with complex partial seizures, not intractable, without status epilepticus
Localization-related (focal) (partial) symptomatic epilepsy and epileptic syndromes with complex partial seizures NOS

`☑6ᵗʰ` **G40.21 Localization-related (focal) (partial) symptomatic epilepsy and epileptic syndromes with complex partial seizures,** intractable

G40.211 Localization-related (focal) (partial) symptomatic epilepsy and epileptic syndromes with complex partial seizures, intractable, with status epilepticus

G40.219 Localization-related (focal) (partial) symptomatic epilepsy and epileptic syndromes with complex partial seizures, intractable, without status epilepticus

✓5ᵗʰ **G40.3** Generalized **idiopathic epilepsy and epileptic syndromes**
  Code also MERRF syndrome, if applicable (E88.42)

  ✓6ᵗʰ **G40.30** **Generalized idiopathic epilepsy and epileptic syndromes,** not intractable
    Generalized idiopathic epilepsy and epileptic syndromes without intractability

      G40.301 **Generalized idiopathic epilepsy and epileptic syndromes, not intractable,** with status epilepticus

      G40.309 **Generallzed idiopathic epilepsy and epileptic syndromes, not intractable,** without status epilepticus
        Generalized idiopathic epilepsy and epileptic syndromes NOS

  ✓6ᵗʰ **G40.31** **Generalized idiopathic epilepsy and epileptic syndromes,** intractable

      G40.311 **Generalized idiopathic epilepsy and epileptic syndromes, intractable,** with status epilepticus

      G40.319 **Generalized idiopathic epilepsy and epileptic syndromes, intractable,** without status epilepticus

✓5ᵗʰ **G40.A** Absence **epileptic syndrome**
  Childhood absence epilepsy [pyknolepsy]
  Juvenile absence epilepsy
  Absence epileptic syndrome, NOS

  ✓6ᵗʰ **G40.A0** **Absence epileptic syndrome,** not intractable

      G40.A01 **Absence epileptic syndrome, not intractable,** with status epilepticus

      G40.A09 **Absence epileptic syndrome, not intractable,** without status epilepticus

  ✓6ᵗʰ **G40.A1** **Absence epileptic syndrome,** intractable

      G40.A11 **Absence epileptic syndrome, intractable,** with status epilepticus

      G40.A19 **Absence epileptic syndrome, intractable,** without status epilepticus

✓5ᵗʰ **G40.B** Juvenile myoclonic epilepsy **[impulsive petit mal]**

  ✓6ᵗʰ **G40.B0** **Juvenile myoclonic epilepsy,** not intractable

      G40.B01 **Juvenile myoclonic epilepsy, not intractable,** with status epilepticus

      G40.B09 **Juvenile myoclonic epilepsy, not intractable,** without status epilepticus

  ✓6ᵗʰ **G40.B1** **Juvenile myoclonic epilepsy,** intractable

      G40.B11 **Juvenile myoclonic epilepsy, intractable,** with status epilepticus

      G40.B19 **Juvenile myoclonic epilepsy, intractable,** without status epilepticus

✓5ᵗʰ **G40.4** Other generalized **epilepsy and epileptic syndromes**
  Epilepsy with grand mal seizures on awakening
  Epilepsy with myoclonic absences
  Epilepsy with myoclonic-astatic seizures
  Grand mal seizure NOS
  Nonspecific atonic epileptic seizures
  Nonspecific clonic epileptic seizures
  Nonspecific myoclonic epileptic seizures
  Nonspecific tonic epileptic seizures
  Nonspecific tonic-clonic epileptic seizures
  Symptomatic early myoclonic encephalopathy

  ✓6ᵗʰ **G40.40** **Other generalized epilepsy and epileptic syndromes,** not intractable
    Other generalized epilepsy and epileptic syndromes without intractability
    Other generalized epilepsy and epileptic syndromes NOS

      G40.401 **Other generalized epilepsy and epileptic syndromes, not intractable,** with status epilepticus

      G40.409 **Other generalized epilepsy and epileptic syndromes, not intractable,** without status epilepticus

  ✓6ᵗʰ **G40.41** **Other generalized epilepsy and epileptic syndromes,** intractable

      G40.411 **Other generalized epilepsy and epileptic syndromes, intractable,** with status epilepticus

      G40.419 **Other generalized epilepsy and epileptic syndromes, intractable,** without status epilepticus

✓5ᵗʰ **G40.5** **Epileptic seizures related to** external causes
  Epileptic seizures related to alcohol
  Epileptic seizures related to drugs
  Epileptic seizures related to hormonal changes
  Epileptic seizures related to sleep deprivation
  Epileptic seizures related to stress
  Use additional code for adverse effect, if applicable, to identify drug (T36-T50 with fifth or sixth character 5)
  Code also, if applicable, associated epilepsy and recurrent seizures (G40.-)

  ✓6ᵗʰ **G40.50** **Epileptic seizures related to external causes,** not intractable

      G40.501 **Epileptic seizures related to external causes, not intractable,** with status epilepticus

      G40.509 **Epileptic seizures related to external causes, not intractable,** without status epilepticus
        Epileptic seizures related to external causes, NOS

✓5ᵗʰ **G40.8** **Other epilepsy and recurrent seizures**
  Epilepsies and epileptic syndromes undetermined as to whether they are focal or generalized
  Landau-Kleffner syndrome

  ✓6ᵗʰ **G40.80** **Other epilepsy**

      G40.801 **Other epilepsy, not intractable,** with status epilepticus
        Other epilepsy without intractability with status epilepticus

      G40.802 **Other epilepsy, not intractable,** without status epilepticus
        Other epilepsy without intractability without status epilepticus

      G40.803 **Other epilepsy, intractable,** with status epilepticus

      G40.804 **Other epilepsy, intractable,** without status epilepticus

  ✓6ᵗʰ **G40.81** **Lennox-Gastaut syndrome**

      G40.811 **Lennox-Gastaut syndrome,** not intractable, with status epilepticus

      G40.812 **Lennox-Gastaut syndrome,** not intractable, without status epilepticus

      G40.813 **Lennox-Gastaut syndrome,** intractable, with status epilepticus

      G40.814 **Lennox-Gastaut syndrome,** intractable, without status epilepticus

  ✓6ᵗʰ **G40.82** **Epileptic spasms**
    Infantile spasms
    Salaam attacks
    West's syndrome

      G40.821 **Epileptic spasms,** not intractable, with status epilepticus

      G40.822 **Epileptic spasms,** not intractable, without status epilepticus

      G40.823 **Epileptic spasms,** intractable, with status epilepticus

      G40.824 **Epileptic spasms,** intractable, without status epilepticus

    G40.89 **Other seizures**
        EXCLUDES 1 *post traumatic seizures (R56.1)*
        recurrent seizures NOS (G40.909)
        seizure NOS (R56.9)

✓5ᵗʰ **G40.9** **Epilepsy,** unspecified

  ✓6ᵗʰ **G40.90** **Epilepsy, unspecified,** not intractable
    Epilepsy, unspecified, without intractability

      G40.901 **Epilepsy, unspecified, not intractable,** with status epilepticus ▽

      G40.909 **Epilepsy, unspecified, not intractable,** without status epilepticus ▽
        Epilepsy NOS
        Epileptic convulsions NOS
        Epileptic fits NOS
        Epileptic seizures NOS
        Recurrent seizures NOS
        Seizure disorder NOS

Ⓝ Newborn: 0   Ⓟ Pediatric: 0-17   Ⓜ Maternity: 12-55   Ⓐ Adult: 15-124   **NRS** Nonroutine supply Dx   **NCDx** Noncancer Dx   **PDx** Primary Dx   ►◄ Revised Text   ● New Code   ▲ Revised Title

✓6ᵗʰ **G40.91** **Epilepsy, unspecified,** intractable
Intractable seizure disorder NOS

     G40.911 **Epilepsy, unspecified, intractable,** ▽
with status epilepticus

     G40.919 **Epilepsy, unspecified, intractable,** ▽
without status epilepticus

✓4ᵗʰ **G43** **Migraine**
NOTE The following terms are to be considered equivalent to
intractable: pharmacoresistant (pharmacologically resistant),
treatment resistant, refractory (medically) and poorly
controlled.
Use additional code for adverse effect, if applicable, to identify drug
(T36-T50 with fifth or sixth character 5)
EXCLUDES 1 headache NOS (R51)
lower half migraine (G44.00)
EXCLUDES 2 headache syndromes (G44.-)

✓5ᵗʰ **G43.0** **Migraine** without aura
Common migraine
EXCLUDES 1 chronic migraine without aura (G43.7-)

     ✓6ᵗʰ **G43.00** **Migraine without aura,** not intractable
Migraine without aura without mention of refractory
migraine

     G43.001 **Migraine without aura, not intractable,**
with status migrainosus

     G43.009 **Migraine without aura, not intractable,**
without status migrainosus
Migraine without aura NOS

     ✓6ᵗʰ **G43.01** **Migraine without aura,** intractable
Migraine without aura with refractory migraine

     G43.011 **Migraine without aura, intractable, with**
status migrainosus

     G43.019 **Migraine without aura, intractable,**
without status migrainosus

✓5ᵗʰ **G43.1** **Migraine** with aura
Basilar migraine
Classical migraine
Migraine equivalents
Migraine preceded or accompanied by transient focal
neurological phenomena
Migraine triggered seizures
Migraine with acute-onset aura
Migraine with aura without headache (migraine equivalents)
Migraine with prolonged aura
Migraine with typical aura
Retinal migraine
Code also any associated seizure (G40.-, R56.9)
EXCLUDES 1 persistent migraine aura (G43.5-, G43.6-)

     ✓6ᵗʰ **G43.10** **Migraine with aura,** not intractable
Migraine with aura without mention of refractory
migraine

     G43.101 **Migraine with aura, not intractable, with**
status migrainosus

     G43.109 **Migraine with aura, not intractable,**
without status migrainosus
Migraine with aura NOS

     ✓6ᵗʰ **G43.11** **Migraine with aura,** intractable
Migraine with aura with refractory migraine

     G43.111 **Migraine with aura, intractable, with**
status migrainosus

     G43.119 **Migraine with aura, intractable, without**
status migrainosus

✓5ᵗʰ **G43.4** **Hemiplegic** migraine
Familial migraine
Sporadic migraine

     ✓6ᵗʰ **G43.40** **Hemiplegic migraine,** not intractable
Hemiplegic migraine without refractory migraine

     G43.401 **Hemiplegic migraine, not intractable, with**
status migrainosus

     G43.409 **Hemiplegic migraine, not intractable,**
without status migrainosus
Hemiplegic migraine NOS

     ✓6ᵗʰ **G43.41** **Hemiplegic migraine,** intractable
Hemiplegic migraine with refractory migraine

     G43.411 **Hemiplegic migraine, intractable, with**
status migrainosus

     G43.419 **Hemiplegic migraine, intractable, without**
status migrainosus

✓5ᵗʰ **G43.5** Persistent **migraine** aura without cerebral infarction

     ✓6ᵗʰ **G43.50** **Persistent migraine aura without cerebral infarction,**
not intractable
Persistent migraine aura without cerebral infarction,
without refractory migraine

     G43.501 **Persistent migraine aura without cerebral**
infarction, not intractable, with status
migrainosus

     G43.509 **Persistent migraine aura without cerebral**
infarction, not intractable, without status
migrainosus
Persistent migraine aura NOS

     ✓6ᵗʰ **G43.51** **Persistent migraine aura without cerebral infarction,**
intractable
Persistent migraine aura without cerebral infarction,
with refractory migraine

     G43.511 **Persistent migraine aura without cerebral**
infarction, intractable, with status
migrainosus

     G43.519 **Persistent migraine aura without cerebral**
infarction, intractable, without status
migrainosus

✓5ᵗʰ **G43.6** Persistent **migraine** aura with cerebral infarction
Code also the type of cerebral infarction (I63.-)

     ✓6ᵗʰ **G43.60** **Persistent migraine aura with cerebral infarction,**
not intractable
Persistent migraine aura with cerebral infarction,
without refractory migraine

     G43.601 **Persistent migraine aura with cerebral**
infarction, not intractable, with status
migrainosus

     G43.609 **Persistent migraine aura with cerebral**
infarction, not intractable, without status
migrainosus

     ✓6ᵗʰ **G43.61** **Persistent migraine aura with cerebral infarction,**
intractable
Persistent migraine aura with cerebral infarction, with
refractory migraine

     G43.611 **Persistent migraine aura with cerebral**
infarction, intractable, with status
migrainosus

     G43.619 **Persistent migraine aura with cerebral**
infarction, intractable, without status
migrainosus

✓5ᵗʰ **G43.7** Chronic **migraine** without aura
Transformed migraine
EXCLUDES 1 migraine without aura (G43.0-)

     ✓6ᵗʰ **G43.70** **Chronic migraine without aura,** not intractable
Chronic migraine without aura, without refractory
migraine

     G43.701 **Chronic migraine without aura, not**
intractable, with status migrainosus

     G43.709 **Chronic migraine without aura, not**
intractable, without status migrainosus
Chronic migraine without aura NOS

     ✓6ᵗʰ **G43.71** **Chronic migraine without aura,** intractable
Chronic migraine without aura, with refractory
migraine

     G43.711 **Chronic migraine without aura,**
intractable, with status migrainosus

     G43.719 **Chronic migraine without aura,**
intractable, without status migrainosus

✓5ᵗʰ **G43.A** Cyclical vomiting
TIP: Assign K31.89 Other diseases of stomach and duodenum,
along with the appropriate code from category R11 Nausea and
vomiting, to identify cyclical vomiting not related to migraine.

     G43.A0 **Cyclical vomiting,** not intractable
Cyclical vomiting, without refractory migraine

     G43.A1 **Cyclical vomiting,** intractable
Cyclical vomiting, with refractory migraine

✓5ᵗʰ **G43.B** Ophthalmoplegic **migraine**

     G43.B0 **Ophthalmoplegic migraine,** not intractable
Ophthalmoplegic migraine, without refractory
migraine

     G43.B1 **Ophthalmoplegic migraine,** intractable
Ophthalmoplegic migraine, with refractory migraine

✓ Additional Character Req   ✓x7ᵗʰ Placeholder Alert   Case-Mix Diagnosis   Manifestation   ▽ Unspecified Dx   **EXCLUDES 1** Not coded here   **EXCLUDES 2** Not included here

Chapter 6. Diseases of the Nervous System

G43.C–G44.219

✓5ᵗʰ **G43.C** Periodic headache syndromes in child or adult

     G43.CØ **Periodic headache syndromes in child or adult, not intractable**
         Periodic headache syndromes in child or adult, without refractory migraine

     G43.C1 **Periodic headache syndromes in child or adult, intractable**
         Periodic headache syndromes in child or adult, with refractory migraine

✓5ᵗʰ **G43.D** Abdominal migraine

     G43.DØ **Abdominal migraine, not intractable**
         Abdominal migraine, without refractory migraine

     G43.D1 **Abdominal migraine, intractable**
         Abdominal migraine, with refractory migraine

✓5ᵗʰ **G43.8** Other migraine

     ✓6ᵗʰ **G43.80** Other migraine, not intractable
         Other migraine, without refractory migraine

         G43.801 **Other migraine, not intractable, with status migrainosus**

         G43.809 **Other migraine, not intractable, without status migrainosus**

     ✓6ᵗʰ **G43.81** Other migraine, intractable
         Other migraine, with refractory migraine

         G43.811 **Other migraine, intractable, with status migrainosus**

         G43.819 **Other migraine, intractable, without status migrainosus**

     ✓6ᵗʰ **G43.82** Menstrual migraine, not intractable
         Menstrual headache, not intractable
         Menstrual migraine, without refractory migraine
         Menstrually related migraine, not intractable
         Pre-menstrual headache, not intractable
         Pre-menstrual migraine, not intractable
         Pure menstrual migraine, not intractable
         Code also associated premenstrual tension syndrome (N94.3)

         G43.821 **Menstrual migraine, not intractable, with status migrainosus** ♀

         G43.829 **Menstrual migraine, not intractable, without status migrainosus** ♀
         Menstrual migraine NOS

     ✓6ᵗʰ **G43.83** Menstrual migraine, intractable
         Menstrual headache, intractable
         Menstrual migraine, with refractory migraine
         Menstrually related migraine, intractable
         Pre-menstrual headache, intractable
         Pre-menstrual migraine, intractable
         Pure menstrual migraine, intractable
         Code also associated premenstrual tension syndrome (N94.3)

         G43.831 **Menstrual migraine, intractable, with status migrainosus** ♀

         G43.839 **Menstrual migraine, intractable, without status migrainosus** ♀

✓5ᵗʰ **G43.9** Migraine, unspecified

     ✓6ᵗʰ **G43.90** Migraine, unspecified, not intractable
         Migraine, unspecified, without refractory migraine

         G43.901 **Migraine, unspecified, not intractable, with status migrainosus** ▽
         Status migrainosus NOS

         G43.909 **Migraine, unspecified, not intractable, without status migrainosus** ▽
         Migraine NOS

     ✓6ᵗʰ **G43.91** Migraine, unspecified, intractable
         Migraine, unspecified, with refractory migraine

         G43.911 **Migraine, unspecified, intractable, with status migrainosus** ▽

         G43.919 **Migraine, unspecified, intractable, without status migrainosus** ▽

✓4ᵗʰ **G44** Other headache syndromes

     EXCLUDES 1   headache NOS (R51)
     EXCLUDES 2   atypical facial pain (G50.1)
             headache due to lumbar puncture (G97.1)
             migraines (G43.-)
             trigeminal neuralgia (G50.0)

✓5ᵗʰ **G44.Ø** Cluster headaches and other trigeminal autonomic cephalgias (TAC)

     ✓6ᵗʰ **G44.00** Cluster headache syndrome, unspecified
         Ciliary neuralgia
         Cluster headache NOS
         Histamine cephalgia
         Lower half migraine
         Migrainous neuralgia

         G44.001 **Cluster headache syndrome, unspecified, intractable** ▽

         G44.009 **Cluster headache syndrome, unspecified, not intractable** ▽
         Cluster headache syndrome NOS

     ✓6ᵗʰ **G44.01** Episodic cluster headache

         G44.011 **Episodic cluster headache, intractable**

         G44.019 **Episodic cluster headache, not intractable**
         Episodic cluster headache NOS

     ✓6ᵗʰ **G44.02** Chronic cluster headache

         G44.021 **Chronic cluster headache, intractable**

         G44.029 **Chronic cluster headache, not intractable**
         Chronic cluster headache NOS

     ✓6ᵗʰ **G44.03** Episodic paroxysmal hemicrania
         Paroxysmal hemicrania NOS

         G44.031 **Episodic paroxysmal hemicrania, intractable**

         G44.039 **Episodic paroxysmal hemicrania, not intractable**
         Episodic paroxysmal hemicrania NOS

     ✓6ᵗʰ **G44.04** Chronic paroxysmal hemicrania

         G44.041 **Chronic paroxysmal hemicrania, intractable**

         G44.049 **Chronic paroxysmal hemicrania, not intractable**
         Chronic paroxysmal hemicrania NOS

     ✓6ᵗʰ **G44.05** Short lasting unilateral neuralgiform headache with conjunctival injection and tearing (SUNCT)

         G44.051 **Short lasting unilateral neuralgiform headache with conjunctival injection and tearing (SUNCT), intractable**

         G44.059 **Short lasting unilateral neuralgiform headache with conjunctival injection and tearing (SUNCT), not intractable**
         Short lasting unilateral neuralgiform headache with conjunctival injection and tearing (SUNCT) NOS

     ✓6ᵗʰ **G44.09** Other trigeminal autonomic cephalgias (TAC)

         G44.091 **Other trigeminal autonomic cephalgias (TAC), intractable**

         G44.099 **Other trigeminal autonomic cephalgias syndrome (TAC), not intractable**

     G44.1 Vascular headache, not elsewhere classified
         EXCLUDES 2   cluster headache (G44.0)
             complicated headache syndromes (G44.5-)
             drug-induced headache (G44.4-)
             migraine (G43.-)
             other specified headache syndromes (G44.8-)
             post-traumatic headache (G44.3-)
             tension-type headache (G44.2-)

✓5ᵗʰ **G44.2** Tension-type headache

     ✓6ᵗʰ **G44.20** Tension-type headache, unspecified

         G44.201 **Tension-type headache, unspecified, intractable** ▽

         G44.209 **Tension-type headache, unspecified, not intractable** ▽
         Tension headache NOS

     ✓6ᵗʰ **G44.21** Episodic tension-type headache

         G44.211 **Episodic tension-type headache, intractable**

         G44.219 **Episodic tension-type headache, not intractable**
         Episodic tension-type headache NOS

Ⓝ Newborn: 0   Ⓟ Pediatric: 0-17   Ⓜ Maternity: 12-55   Ⓐ Adult: 15-124   **NRS** Nonroutine supply Dx   **NC Dx** Noncancer Dx   **PDx** Primary Dx   ▶◀ Revised Text   ● New Code   ▲ Revised Title

556   ICD-10-CM 2018

✓6ᵗʰ **G44.22** Chronic **tension-type headache**
　　G44.221 **Chronic tension-type headache,** intractable
　　G44.229 **Chronic tension-type headache,** not intractable
　　　　Chronic tension-type headache NOS

✓5ᵗʰ **G44.3** Post-traumatic **headache**
　✓6ᵗʰ **G44.30** **Post-traumatic headache,** unspecified
　　G44.301 **Post-traumatic headache, unspecified,** intractable　　▽
　　G44.309 **Post-traumatic headache, unspecified,** not intractable　　▽
　　　　Post-traumatic headache NOS

　✓6ᵗʰ **G44.31** Acute **post-traumatic headache**
　　G44.311 **Acute post-traumatic headache,** intractable
　　G44.319 **Acute post-traumatic headache,** not intractable
　　　　Acute post-traumatic headache NOS

　✓6ᵗʰ **G44.32** Chronic **post-traumatic headache**
　　G44.321 **Chronic post-traumatic headache,** intractable
　　G44.329 **Chronic post-traumatic headache,** not intractable
　　　　Chronic post-traumatic headache NOS

✓5ᵗʰ **G44.4** Drug-induced **headache, not elsewhere classified**
　　Medication overuse headache
　　Use additional code for adverse effect, if applicable, to identify drug (T36-T50 with fifth or sixth character 5)
　　G44.40 **Drug-induced headache, not elsewhere classified,** not intractable
　　G44.41 **Drug-induced headache, not elsewhere classified,** intractable

✓5ᵗʰ **G44.5** Complicated **headache syndromes**
　　G44.51 Hemicrania continua
　　G44.52 New daily persistent headache (NDPH)
　　G44.53 Primary thunderclap **headache**
　　G44.59 **Other complicated headache syndrome**

✓5ᵗʰ **G44.8** Other specified **headache syndromes**
　　G44.81 Hypnic **headache**
　　G44.82 **Headache associated with** sexual activity
　　　　Orgasmic headache
　　　　Preorgasmic headache
　　G44.83 Primary cough **headache**
　　G44.84 Primary exertional **headache**
　　G44.85 Primary stabbing **headache**
　　G44.89 **Other headache syndrome**

✓4ᵗʰ **G45** **Transient cerebral ischemic attacks and related syndromes**
　　EXCLUDES 1　neonatal cerebral ischemia (P91.0)
　　　　transient retinal artery occlusion (H34.0-)
　　G45.0 **Vertebro-basilar artery syndrome**
　　G45.1 **Carotid artery syndrome (hemispheric)**
　　G45.2 **Multiple and bilateral precerebral artery syndromes**
　　G45.3 **Amaurosis fugax**
　　G45.4 **Transient global amnesia**
　　　　EXCLUDES 1　amnesia NOS (R41.3)
　　G45.8 **Other transient cerebral ischemic attacks and related syndromes**
　　G45.9 **Transient cerebral ischemic attack, unspecified**　　▽
　　　　Spasm of cerebral artery
　　　　TIA
　　　　Transient cerebral ischemia NOS

✓4ᵗʰ **G46** **Vascular syndromes of brain in cerebrovascular diseases**
　　Code first underlying cerebrovascular disease (I60-I69)
　　G46.0 Middle **cerebral artery syndrome**
　　G46.1 Anterior **cerebral artery syndrome**
　　G46.2 Posterior **cerebral artery syndrome**
　　G46.3 Brain stem stroke **syndrome**
　　　　Benedikt syndrome
　　　　Claude syndrome
　　　　Foville syndrome
　　　　Millard-Gubler syndrome
　　　　Wallenberg syndrome
　　　　Weber syndrome
　　G46.4 Cerebellar stroke **syndrome**

G46.5 Pure motor lacunar **syndrome**
G46.6 Pure sensory lacunar **syndrome**
G46.7 Other lacunar **syndromes**
G46.8 **Other vascular syndromes of brain in cerebrovascular diseases**

✓4ᵗʰ **G47** **Sleep disorders**
　EXCLUDES 2　nightmares (F51.5)
　　nonorganic sleep disorders (F51.-)
　　sleep terrors (F51.4)
　　sleepwalking (F51.3)

✓5ᵗʰ **G47.0** **Insomnia**
　EXCLUDES 2　alcohol related insomnia (F10.182, F10.282, F10.982)
　　drug-related insomnia (F11.182, F11.282, F11.982, F13.182, F13.282, F13.982, F14.182, F14.282, F14.982, F15.182, F15.282, F15.982, F19.182, F19.282, F19.982)
　　idiopathic insomnia (F51.01)
　　insomnia due to a mental disorder (F51.05)
　　insomnia not due to a substance or known physiological condition (F51.0-)
　　nonorganic insomnia (F51.0-)
　　primary insomnia (F51.01)
　　sleep apnea (G47.3-)
　　G47.00 **Insomnia, unspecified**　　▽
　　　　Insomnia NOS
　　G47.01 **Insomnia** due to medical condition
　　　　Code also associated medical condition
　　G47.09 **Other insomnia**

✓5ᵗʰ **G47.1** **Hypersomnia**
　EXCLUDES 2　alcohol-related hypersomnia (F10.182, F10.282, F10.982)
　　drug-related hypersomnia (F11.182, F11.282, F11.982, F13.182, F13.282, F13.982, F14.182, F14.282, F14.982, F15.182, F15.282, F15.982, F19.182, F19.282, F19.982)
　　hypersomnia due to a mental disorder (F51.13)
　　hypersomnia not due to a substance or known physiological condition (F51.1-)
　　primary hypersomnia (F51.11)
　　sleep apnea (G47.3-)
　　G47.10 **Hypersomnia, unspecified**　　▽
　　　　Hypersomnia NOS
　　G47.11 Idiopathic **hypersomnia** with long sleep time
　　　　Idiopathic hypersomnia NOS
　　G47.12 Idiopathic **hypersomnia** without long sleep time
　　G47.13 Recurrent **hypersomnia**
　　　　Kleine-Levin syndrome
　　　　Menstrual related hypersomnia
　　G47.14 **Hypersomnia** due to medical condition
　　　　Code also associated medical condition
　　G47.19 **Other hypersomnia**

✓5ᵗʰ **G47.2** **Circadian rhythm sleep disorders**
　　Disorders of the sleep wake schedule
　　Inversion of nyctohemeral rhythm
　　Inversion of sleep rhythm
　　G47.20 **Circadian rhythm sleep disorder, unspecified type**　　▽
　　　　Sleep wake schedule disorder NOS
　　G47.21 **Circadian rhythm sleep disorder,** delayed sleep phase **type**
　　　　Delayed sleep phase syndrome
　　G47.22 **Circadian rhythm sleep disorder,** advanced sleep phase **type**
　　G47.23 **Circadian rhythm sleep disorder,** irregular sleep wake **type**
　　　　Irregular sleep-wake pattern
　　G47.24 **Circadian rhythm sleep disorder,** free running **type**
　　　　▶Circadian rhythm sleep disorder, non-24-hour sleep-wake type◀
　　G47.25 **Circadian rhythm sleep disorder,** jet lag **type**
　　G47.26 **Circadian rhythm sleep disorder,** shift work **type**
　　G47.27 *Circadian rhythm sleep disorder in conditions classified elsewhere*
　　　　Code first underlying condition
　　G47.29 **Other circadian rhythm sleep disorder**

Chapter 6. Diseases of the Nervous System

G47.3–G53

✓5th **G47.3   Sleep apnea**
    Code also any associated underlying condition
    EXCLUDES 1   apnea NOS (R06.81)
             Cheyne-Stokes breathing (R06.3)
             pickwickian syndrome (E66.2)
             sleep apnea of newborn (P28.3)

    G47.30   Sleep apnea, unspecified ▽
         Sleep apnea NOS

    G47.31   Primary central sleep apnea
         ►Idiopathic central sleep apnea◄

    G47.32   High altitude periodic breathing

    G47.33   Obstructive sleep apnea (adult) (pediatric)
         ►Obstructive sleep apnea hypopnea◄
         EXCLUDES 1   obstructive sleep apnea of newborn (P28.3)

    G47.34   Idiopathic sleep related nonobstructive alveolar hypoventilation
         Sleep related hypoxia

    G47.35   Congenital central alveolar hypoventilation syndrome

    G47.36   Sleep related hypoventilation in conditions classified elsewhere
         Sleep related hypoxemia in conditions classified elsewhere
         Code first underlying condition

    G47.37   Central sleep apnea in conditions classified elsewhere
         Code first underlying condition

    G47.39   Other sleep apnea

✓5th **G47.4   Narcolepsy and cataplexy**

    ✓6th **G47.41   Narcolepsy**
         G47.411   Narcolepsy with cataplexy
         G47.419   Narcolepsy without cataplexy
             Narcolepsy NOS

    ✓6th **G47.42   Narcolepsy in conditions classified elsewhere**
         Code first underlying condition
         G47.421   Narcolepsy in conditions classified elsewhere with cataplexy
         G47.429   Narcolepsy in conditions classified elsewhere without cataplexy

✓5th **G47.5   Parasomnia**
    EXCLUDES 1   alcohol induced parasomnia (F10.182, F10.282, F10.982)
             drug induced parasomnia (F11.182, F11.282, F11.982, F13.182, F13.282, F13.982, F14.182, F14.282, F14.982, F15.182, F15.282, F15.982, F19.182, F19.282, F19.982)
             parasomnia not due to a substance or known physiological condition (F51.8)

    G47.50   Parasomnia, unspecified ▽
         Parasomnia NOS

    G47.51   Confusional arousals

    G47.52   REM sleep behavior disorder

    G47.53   Recurrent isolated sleep paralysis

    G47.54   Parasomnia in conditions classified elsewhere
         Code first underlying condition

    G47.59   Other parasomnia

✓5th **G47.6   Sleep related movement disorders**
    EXCLUDES 2   restless legs syndrome (G25.81)

    G47.61   Periodic limb movement disorder
         ~~Periodic limb movement disorder~~

    G47.62   Sleep related leg cramps

    G47.63   Sleep related bruxism
         EXCLUDES 1   psychogenic bruxism (F45.8)

    G47.69   Other sleep related movement disorders

G47.8   Other sleep disorders
    ►Other specified sleep-wake disorder◄

G47.9   Sleep disorder, unspecified ▽
    Sleep disorder NOS
    ►Unspecified sleep-wake disorder◄

Trigeminal and Facial Nerve Branches

Nerve, nerve root and plexus disorders (G50-G59)

EXCLUDES 1   current traumatic nerve, nerve root and plexus disorders—see Injury, nerve by body region
             neuralgia NOS (M79.2)
             neuritis NOS (M79.2)
             peripheral neuritis in pregnancy (O26.82-)
             radiculitis NOS (M54.1-)

✓4th **G50   Disorders of trigeminal nerve**
    INCLUDES   disorders of 5th cranial nerve

    G50.0   Trigeminal neuralgia
         Syndrome of paroxysmal facial pain
         Tic douloureux

    G50.1   Atypical facial pain

    G50.8   Other disorders of trigeminal nerve

    G50.9   Disorder of trigeminal nerve, unspecified ▽

✓4th **G51   Facial nerve disorders**
    INCLUDES   disorders of 7th cranial nerve

    G51.0   Bell's palsy
         Facial palsy

    G51.1   Geniculate ganglionitis
         EXCLUDES 1   postherpetic geniculate ganglionitis (B02.21)

    G51.2   Melkersson's syndrome
         Melkersson-Rosenthal syndrome

    G51.3   Clonic hemifacial spasm

    G51.4   Facial myokymia

    G51.8   Other disorders of facial nerve

    G51.9   Disorder of facial nerve, unspecified ▽

✓4th **G52   Disorders of other cranial nerves**
    EXCLUDES 2   disorders of acoustic [8th] nerve (H93.3)
             disorders of optic [2nd] nerve (H46, H47.0)
             paralytic strabismus due to nerve palsy (H49.0-H49.2)

    G52.0   Disorders of olfactory nerve
         Disorders of 1st cranial nerve

    G52.1   Disorders of glossopharyngeal nerve
         Disorder of 9th cranial nerve
         Glossopharyngeal neuralgia

    G52.2   Disorders of vagus nerve
         Disorders of pneumogastric [10th] nerve

    G52.3   Disorders of hypoglossal nerve
         Disorders of 12th cranial nerve

    G52.7   Disorders of multiple cranial nerves
         Polyneuritis cranialis

    G52.8   Disorders of other specified cranial nerves

    G52.9   Cranial nerve disorder, unspecified ▽

G53   Cranial nerve disorders in diseases classified elsewhere
    Code first underlying disease, such as:
         neoplasm (C00-D49)
    EXCLUDES 1   multiple cranial nerve palsy in sarcoidosis (D86.82)
             multiple cranial nerve palsy in syphilis (A52.15)
             postherpetic geniculate ganglionitis (B02.21)
             postherpetic trigeminal neuralgia (B02.22)

N Newborn: 0   P Pediatric: 0-17   M Maternity: 12-55   A Adult: 15-124   NRS Nonroutine supply Dx   NCDx Noncancer Dx   PDx Primary Dx   ►◄ Revised Text   ● New Code   ▲ Revised Title

558   ICD-10-CM 2018

✓4ᵗʰ **G54   Nerve root and plexus disorders**

> **EXCLUDES 1** current traumatic nerve root and plexus disorders—see nerve injury by body region
> intervertebral disc disorders (M50-M51)
> neuralgia or neuritis NOS (M79.2)
> neuritis or radiculitis brachial NOS (M54.13)
> neuritis or radiculitis lumbar NOS (M54.16)
> neuritis or radiculitis lumbosacral NOS (M54.17)
> neuritis or radiculitis thoracic NOS (M54.14)
> radiculitis NOS (M54.10)
> radiculopathy NOS (M54.10)
> spondylosis (M47.-)

G54.0   Brachial plexus disorders
Thoracic outlet syndrome
DEF: Acquired disorder affecting the spinal nerves that send signals to the shoulder, arm, and hand; causes corresponding motor and sensory dysfunction; characterized by regional paresthesia, pain, and muscle weakness, and in severe cases paralysis.

G54.1   Lumbosacral plexus disorders

G54.2   Cervical root disorders, not elsewhere classified

G54.3   Thoracic root disorders, not elsewhere classified

G54.4   Lumbosacral root disorders, not elsewhere classified

G54.5   Neuralgic amyotrophy
Parsonage-Aldren-Turner syndrome
Shoulder-girdle neuritis
> **EXCLUDES 1** neuralgic amyotrophy in diabetes mellitus (E08-E13 with .44)

G54.6   Phantom limb syndrome with pain

G54.7   Phantom limb syndrome without pain
Phantom limb syndrome NOS

G54.8   Other nerve root and plexus disorders

G54.9   Nerve root and plexus disorder, unspecified   ▽

G55   Nerve root and plexus compressions in diseases classified elsewhere
Code first underlying disease, such as:
neoplasm (C00-D49)
> **EXCLUDES 1** nerve root compression (due to) (in) ankylosing spondylitis (M45.-)
> nerve root compression (due to) (in) dorsopathies (M53.-, M54.-)
> nerve root compression (due to) (in) intervertebral disc disorders (M50.1-, M51.1-)
> nerve root compression (due to) (in) spondylopathies (M46.-, M48.-)

✓4ᵗʰ **G56   Mononeuropathies of upper limb**
> **EXCLUDES 1** current traumatic nerve disorder—see nerve injury by body region

✓5ᵗʰ **G56.0   Carpal tunnel syndrome**

G56.00   Carpal tunnel syndrome, unspecified upper limb   ▽

G56.01   Carpal tunnel syndrome, right upper limb

Nerves of Upper Limb

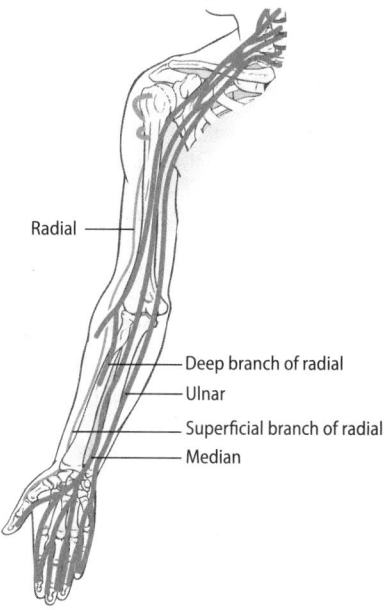

Radial
Deep branch of radial
Ulnar
Superficial branch of radial
Median

G56.02   Carpal tunnel syndrome, left upper limb

G56.03   Carpal tunnel syndrome, bilateral upper limbs

✓5ᵗʰ **G56.1   Other lesions of median nerve**

G56.10   Other lesions of median nerve, unspecified upper limb   ▽

G56.11   Other lesions of median nerve, right upper limb

G56.12   Other lesions of median nerve, left upper limb

G56.13   Other lesions of median nerve, bilateral upper limbs

✓5ᵗʰ **G56.2   Lesion of ulnar nerve**
Tardy ulnar nerve palsy

G56.20   Lesion of ulnar nerve, unspecified upper limb   ▽

G56.21   Lesion of ulnar nerve, right upper limb

G56.22   Lesion of ulnar nerve, left upper limb

G56.23   Lesion of ulnar nerve, bilateral upper limbs

✓5ᵗʰ **G56.3   Lesion of radial nerve**

G56.30   Lesion of radial nerve, unspecified upper limb   ▽

G56.31   Lesion of radial nerve, right upper limb

G56.32   Lesion of radial nerve, left upper limb

G56.33   Lesion of radial nerve, bilateral upper limbs

✓5ᵗʰ **G56.4   Causalgia of upper limb**
Complex regional pain syndrome II of upper limb
> **EXCLUDES 1** complex regional pain syndrome I of lower limb (G90.52-)
> complex regional pain syndrome I of upper limb (G90.51-)
> complex regional pain syndrome II of lower limb (G57.7-)
> reflex sympathetic dystrophy of lower limb (G90.52-)
> reflex sympathetic dystrophy of upper limb (G90.51-)

G56.40   Causalgia of unspecified upper limb   ▽

G56.41   Causalgia of right upper limb

G56.42   Causalgia of left upper limb

G56.43   Causalgia of bilateral upper limbs

✓5ᵗʰ **G56.8   Other specified mononeuropathies of upper limb**
Interdigital neuroma of upper limb

G56.80   Other specified mononeuropathies of unspecified upper limb   ▽

G56.81   Other specified mononeuropathies of right upper limb

G56.82   Other specified mononeuropathies of left upper limb

G56.83   Other specified mononeuropathies of bilateral upper limbs

✓5ᵗʰ **G56.9   Unspecified mononeuropathy of upper limb**

G56.90   Unspecified mononeuropathy of unspecified upper limb   ▽

G56.91   Unspecified mononeuropathy of right upper limb   ▽

G56.92   Unspecified mononeuropathy of left upper limb   ▽

G56.93   Unspecified mononeuropathy of bilateral upper limbs   ▽

✓4ᵗʰ **G57   Mononeuropathies of lower limb**
> **EXCLUDES 1** current traumatic nerve disorder—see nerve injury by body region

✓5ᵗʰ **G57.0   Lesion of sciatic nerve**
> **EXCLUDES 1** sciatica NOS (M54.3-)
> **EXCLUDES 2** sciatica attributed to intervertebral disc disorder (M51.1-)

G57.00   Lesion of sciatic nerve, unspecified lower limb   ▽

G57.01   Lesion of sciatic nerve, right lower limb

G57.02   Lesion of sciatic nerve, left lower limb

G57.03   Lesion of sciatic nerve, bilateral lower limbs

✓5ᵗʰ **G57.1   Meralgia paresthetica**
Lateral cutaneous nerve of thigh syndrome

G57.10   Meralgia paresthetica, unspecified lower limb   ▽

G57.11   Meralgia paresthetica, right lower limb

G57.12   Meralgia paresthetica, left lower limb

G57.13   Meralgia paresthetica, bilateral lower limbs

✓5ᵗʰ **G57.2   Lesion of femoral nerve**

G57.20   Lesion of femoral nerve, unspecified lower limb   ▽

G57.21   Lesion of femoral nerve, right lower limb

G57.22   Lesion of femoral nerve, left lower limb

G57.23   Lesion of femoral nerve, bilateral lower limbs

✓ Additional Character Req   ✓x7ᵗʰ Placeholder Alert   Case-Mix Diagnosis   Manifestation   ▽ Unspecified Dx   **EXCLUDES 1** Not coded here   **EXCLUDES 2** Not included here

Chapter 6. Diseases of the Nervous System

Nerves of Lower Limb

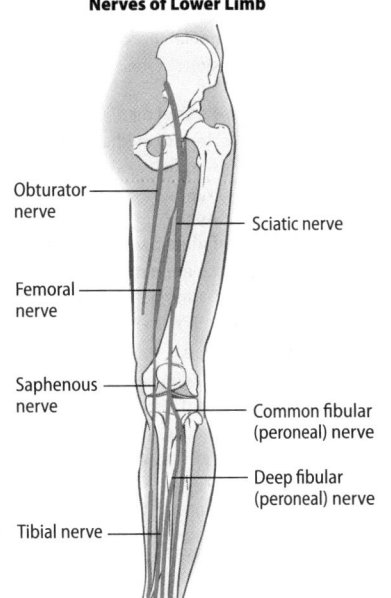

Obturator nerve
Sciatic nerve
Femoral nerve
Saphenous nerve
Common fibular (peroneal) nerve
Deep fibular (peroneal) nerve
Tibial nerve
Superficial fibular (peroneal) nerve

✓5ᵗʰ **G57.3 Lesion of** lateral popliteal nerve
Peroneal nerve palsy
    G57.30 Lesion of lateral popliteal nerve, unspecified lower limb ▽
    G57.31 Lesion of lateral popliteal nerve, right lower limb
    G57.32 Lesion of lateral popliteal nerve, left lower limb
    G57.33 Lesion of lateral popliteal nerve, bilateral lower limbs

✓5ᵗʰ **G57.4 Lesion of** medial popliteal nerve
    G57.40 Lesion of medial popliteal nerve, unspecified lower limb ▽
    G57.41 Lesion of medial popliteal nerve, right lower limb
    G57.42 Lesion of medial popliteal nerve, left lower limb
    G57.43 Lesion of medial popliteal nerve, bilateral lower limbs

✓5ᵗʰ **G57.5 Tarsal tunnel syndrome**
    G57.50 Tarsal tunnel syndrome, unspecified lower limb ▽
    G57.51 Tarsal tunnel syndrome, right lower limb
    G57.52 Tarsal tunnel syndrome, left lower limb
    G57.53 Tarsal tunnel syndrome, bilateral lower limbs

✓5ᵗʰ **G57.6 Lesion of** plantar nerve
Morton's metatarsalgia
    G57.60 Lesion of plantar nerve, unspecified lower limb ▽
    G57.61 Lesion of plantar nerve, right lower limb
    G57.62 Lesion of plantar nerve, left lower limb
    G57.63 Lesion of plantar nerve, bilateral lower limbs

✓5ᵗʰ **G57.7 Causalgia of lower limb**
Complex regional pain syndrome II of lower limb
    EXCLUDES 1 complex regional pain syndrome I of lower limb (G90.52-)
      complex regional pain syndrome I of upper limb (G90.51-)
      complex regional pain syndrome II of upper limb (G56.4-)
      reflex sympathetic dystrophy of lower limb (G90.52-)
      reflex sympathetic dystrophy of upper limb (G90.51-)
    G57.70 Causalgia of unspecified lower limb ▽
    G57.71 Causalgia of right lower limb
    G57.72 Causalgia of left lower limb
    G57.73 Causalgia of bilateral lower limbs

✓5ᵗʰ **G57.8 Other specified mononeuropathies of lower limb**
Interdigital neuroma of lower limb
    G57.80 Other specified mononeuropathies of unspecified lower limb ▽
    G57.81 Other specified mononeuropathies of right lower limb

    G57.82 Other specified mononeuropathies of left lower limb
    G57.83 Other specified mononeuropathies of bilateral lower limbs

✓5ᵗʰ **G57.9 Unspecified mononeuropathy of lower limb**
    G57.90 Unspecified mononeuropathy of unspecified lower limb ▽
    G57.91 Unspecified mononeuropathy of right lower limb ▽
    G57.92 Unspecified mononeuropathy of left lower limb ▽
    G57.93 Unspecified mononeuropathy of bilateral lower limbs

✓4ᵗʰ **G58 Other mononeuropathies**
    G58.0 Intercostal neuropathy
    G58.7 Mononeuritis multiplex
    G58.8 Other specified mononeuropathies
    G58.9 Mononeuropathy, unspecified ▽

G59 Mononeuropathy in diseases classified elsewhere
Code first underlying disease
    EXCLUDES 1 diabetic mononeuropathy (E08-E13 with .41)
      syphilitic nerve paralysis (A52.19)
      syphilitic neuritis (A52.15)
      tuberculous mononeuropathy (A17.83)

Polyneuropathies and other disorders of the peripheral nervous system (G60-G65)

    EXCLUDES 1 neuralgia NOS (M79.2)
      neuritis NOS (M79.2)
      peripheral neuritis in pregnancy (O26.82-)
      radiculitis NOS (M54.10)

✓4ᵗʰ **G60 Hereditary and idiopathic neuropathy**
    G60.0 Hereditary motor and sensory neuropathy
      Charcôt-Marie-Tooth disease
      Déjérine-Sottas disease
      Hereditary motor and sensory neuropathy, types I-IV
      Hypertrophic neuropathy of infancy
      Peroneal muscular atrophy (axonal type) (hypertrophic type)
      Roussy-Levy syndrome
    G60.1 Refsum's disease
      Infantile Refsum disease
      DEF: Genetic disorder of lipid metabolism; characterized by retinitis pigmentosa, degenerative nerve disease, ataxia, and dry, rough, scaly skin.
    G60.2 Neuropathy in association with hereditary ataxia
    G60.3 Idiopathic progressive neuropathy
    G60.8 Other hereditary and idiopathic neuropathies
      Dominantly inherited sensory neuropathy
      Morvan's disease
      Nelaton's syndrome
      Recessively inherited sensory neuropathy
    G60.9 Hereditary and idiopathic neuropathy, unspecified ▽

✓4ᵗʰ **G61 Inflammatory polyneuropathy**
    G61.0 Guillain-Barre syndrome
      Acute (post-)infective polyneuritis
      Miller Fisher syndrome
      AHA: 2014, 2Q, 4
    G61.1 Serum neuropathy
      Use additional code for adverse effect, if applicable, to identify serum (T50.-)
    ✓5ᵗʰ **G61.8 Other inflammatory polyneuropathies**
      G61.81 Chronic inflammatory demyelinating polyneuritis
      G61.82 Multifocal motor neuropathy
       MMN
      G61.89 Other inflammatory polyneuropathies
    G61.9 Inflammatory polyneuropathy, unspecified ▽

✓4ᵗʰ **G62 Other and unspecified polyneuropathies**
    G62.0 Drug-induced polyneuropathy
      Use additional code for adverse effect, if applicable, to identify drug (T36-T50 with fifth or sixth character 5)
    G62.1 Alcoholic polyneuropathy
    G62.2 Polyneuropathy due to other toxic agents
      Code first (T51-T65) to identify toxic agent
    ✓5ᵗʰ **G62.8 Other specified polyneuropathies**
      G62.81 Critical illness polyneuropathy
       Acute motor neuropathy

Ⓝ Newborn: 0   Ⓟ Pediatric: 0-17   Ⓜ Maternity: 12-55   Ⓐ Adult: 15-124   **NRS** Nonroutine supply Dx   **NC Dx** Noncancer Dx   **PDX** Primary Dx   ▶◀ Revised Text   ● New Code   ▲ Revised Title

560   ICD-10-CM 2018

G62.82 Radiation-induced **polyneuropathy**
Use additional external cause code (W88-W90, X39.0-) to identify cause

G62.89 **Other specified polyneuropathies**
AHA: 2016, 2Q, 11

G62.9 **Polyneuropathy, unspecified** ▽
Neuropathy NOS

G63 *Polyneuropathy in diseases classified elsewhere*
Code first underlying disease, such as:
amyloidosis (E85.-)
endocrine disease, except diabetes (E00-E07, E15-E16, E20-E34)
metabolic diseases (E70-E88)
neoplasm (C00-D49)
nutritional deficiency (E40-E64)
EXCLUDES 1   *polyneuropathy (in):*
diabetes mellitus (E08-E13 with .42)
diphtheria (A36.83)
infectious mononucleosis (B27.0-B27.9 with 1)
Lyme disease (A69.22)
mumps (B26.84)
postherpetic (B02.23)
rheumatoid arthritis (M05.33)
scleroderma (M34.83)
systemic lupus erythematosus (M32.19)
AHA: 2012, 4Q, 99

G64 **Other disorders of peripheral nervous system**
Disorder of peripheral nervous system NOS

✓4ᵗʰ **G65** **Sequelae of inflammatory and toxic polyneuropathies**
Code first condition resulting from (sequela) of inflammatory and toxic polyneuropathies

G65.0 **Sequelae of** Guillain-Barré syndrome

G65.1 **Sequelae of other** inflammatory **polyneuropathy**

G65.2 **Sequelae of** toxic **polyneuropathy**

Diseases of myoneural junction and muscle (G70-G73)

✓4ᵗʰ **G70** **Myasthenia gravis and other myoneural disorders**
EXCLUDES 1   *botulism (A05.1, A48.51-A48.52)*
transient neonatal myasthenia gravis (P94.0)

✓5ᵗʰ **G70.0** **Myasthenia gravis**

G70.00 **Myasthenia gravis** without (acute) exacerbation
Myasthenia gravis NOS

G70.01 **Myasthenia gravis** with (acute) exacerbation   NC Dx
Myasthenia gravis in crisis

G70.1 **Toxic myoneural disorders**
Code first (T51-T65) to identify toxic agent

G70.2 **Congenital and developmental myasthenia**

✓5ᵗʰ **G70.8** **Other specified myoneural disorders**

G70.80 **Lambert-Eaton syndrome, unspecified** ▽
Lambert-Eaton syndrome NOS

G70.81 *Lambert-Eaton syndrome in disease classified elsewhere*
Code first underlying disease
EXCLUDES 1   *Lambert-Eaton syndrome in neoplastic disease (G73.1)*

G70.89 **Other specified myoneural disorders**

G70.9 **Myoneural disorder, unspecified** ▽

✓4ᵗʰ **G71** **Primary disorders of muscles**
EXCLUDES 2   *arthrogryposis multiplex congenita (Q74.3)*
metabolic disorders (E70-E88)
myositis (M60.-)

G71.0 **Muscular** dystrophy   NC Dx
Autosomal recessive, childhood type, muscular dystrophy resembling Duchenne or Becker muscular dystrophy
Benign [Becker] muscular dystrophy
Benign scapuloperoneal muscular dystrophy with early contractures [Emery-Dreifuss]
Congenital muscular dystrophy NOS
Congenital muscular dystrophy with specific morphological abnormalities of the muscle fiber
Distal muscular dystrophy
Facioscapulohumeral muscular dystrophy
Limb-girdle muscular dystrophy
Ocular muscular dystrophy
Oculopharyngeal muscular dystrophy
Scapuloperoneal muscular dystrophy
Severe [Duchenne] muscular dystrophy

✓5ᵗʰ **G71.1** Myotonic **disorders**

G71.11 **Myotonic muscular dystrophy**   NC Dx
Dystrophia myotonica [Steinert]
Myotonia atrophica
Myotonic dystrophy
Proximal myotonic myopathy (PROMM)
Steinert disease

G71.12 **Myotonia** congenita
Acetazolamide responsive myotonia congenita
Dominant myotonia congenita [Thomsen disease]
Myotonia levior
Recessive myotonia congenita [Becker disease]

G71.13 **Myotonic** chondrodystrophy
Chondrodystrophic myotonia
Congenital myotonic chondrodystrophy
Schwartz-Jampel disease

G71.14 Drug induced **myotonia**
Use additional code for adverse effect, if applicable, to identify drug (T36-T50 with fifth or sixth character 5)

G71.19 **Other specified myotonic disorders**
Myotonia fluctuans
Myotonia permanens
Neuromyotonia [Isaacs]
Paramyotonia congenita (of von Eulenburg)
Pseudomyotonia
Symptomatic myotonia

G71.2 Congenital myopathies
Central core disease
Fiber-type disproportion
Minicore disease
Multicore disease
Myotubular (centronuclear) myopathy
Nemaline myopathy
EXCLUDES 1   *arthrogryposis multiplex congenita (Q74.3)*

G71.3 Mitochondrial myopathy, **not elsewhere classified**
EXCLUDES 1   *Kearns-Sayre syndrome (H49.81)*
Leber's disease (H47.21)
Leigh's encephalopathy (G31.82)
mitochondrial metabolism disorders (E88.4-)
Reye's syndrome (G93.7)

G71.8 **Other primary disorders of muscles**

G71.9 **Primary disorder of muscle, unspecified** ▽
Hereditary myopathy NOS

✓4ᵗʰ **G72** **Other and unspecified myopathies**
EXCLUDES 1   *arthrogryposis multiplex congenita (Q74.3)*
dermatopolymyositis (M33.-)
ischemic infarction of muscle (M62.2-)
myositis (M60.-)
polymyositis (M33.2-)

G72.0 Drug-induced **myopathy**
Use additional code for adverse effect, if applicable, to identify drug (T36-T50 with fifth or sixth character 5)

G72.1 Alcoholic **myopathy**
Use additional code to identify alcoholism (F10.-)

G72.2 **Myopathy** due to other toxic agents
Code first (T51-T65) to identify toxic agent

G72.3 Periodic paralysis
Familial periodic paralysis
Hyperkalemic periodic paralysis (familial)
Hypokalemic periodic paralysis (familial)
Myotonic periodic paralysis (familial)
Normokalemic paralysis (familial)
Potassium sensitive periodic paralysis
EXCLUDES 1   *paramyotonia congenita (of von Eulenburg) (G71.19)*

✓5ᵗʰ **G72.4** Inflammatory and immune **myopathies, not elsewhere classified**

G72.41 Inclusion body myositis [IBM]

G72.49 **Other inflammatory and immune myopathies, not elsewhere classified**
Inflammatory myopathy NOS

✓5ᵗʰ **G72.8** Other specified **myopathies**

G72.81 Critical illness **myopathy**
Acute necrotizing myopathy
Acute quadriplegic myopathy
Intensive care (ICU) myopathy
Myopathy of critical illness

G72.89 **Other specified myopathies**

G72.9 **Myopathy, unspecified** ▽

✓ Additional Character Req   ✓x7ᵗʰ Placeholder Alert   Case-Mix Diagnosis   Manifestation   ▽ Unspecified Dx   EXCLUDES 1 Not coded here   EXCLUDES 2 Not included here

✓4th **G73** **Disorders of myoneural junction and muscle in diseases classified elsewhere**

     G73.1 *Lambert-Eaton syndrome in neoplastic disease*
         Code first underlying neoplasm (C00-D49)
         EXCLUDES 1   *Lambert-Eaton syndrome not associated with neoplasm (G70.80-G70.81)*

     G73.3 *Myasthenic syndromes in other diseases classified elsewhere*
         Code first underlying disease, such as:
           neoplasm (C00-D49)
           thyrotoxicosis (E05.-)

     G73.7 *Myopathy in diseases classified elsewhere*
         Code first underlying disease, such as:
           hyperparathyroidism (E21.0, E21.3)
           hypoparathyroidism (E20.-)
           glycogen storage disease (E74.0)
           lipid storage disorders (E75.-)
         EXCLUDES 1   *myopathy in:*
           rheumatoid arthritis (M05.4-)
           sarcoidosis (D86.87)
           scleroderma (M34.82)
           sicca syndrome [Sjögren] (M35.03)
           systemic lupus erythematosus (M32.19)

Cerebral palsy and other paralytic syndromes (G80-G83)

✓4th **G80** **Cerebral palsy**
     EXCLUDES 1   *hereditary spastic paraplegia (G11.4)*

     G80.0 Spastic quadriplegic **cerebral palsy**
         Congenital spastic paralysis (cerebral)

     G80.1 Spastic diplegic **cerebral palsy**
         Spastic cerebral palsy NOS

     G80.2 Spastic hemiplegic **cerebral palsy**

     G80.3 Athetoid **cerebral palsy**
         Double athetosis (syndrome)
         Dyskinetic cerebral palsy
         Dystonic cerebral palsy
         Vogt disease

     G80.4 Ataxic **cerebral palsy**

     G80.8 Other **cerebral palsy**
         Mixed cerebral palsy syndromes

     G80.9 **Cerebral palsy, unspecified** ▽
         Cerebral palsy NOS

✓4th **G81** **Hemiplegia and hemiparesis**
     NOTE   This category is to be used only when hemiplegia (complete)(incomplete) is reported without further specification, or is stated to be old or longstanding but of unspecified cause. The category is also for use in multiple coding to identify these types of hemiplegia resulting from any cause.
     EXCLUDES 1   *congenital cerebral palsy (G80.-)*
         hemiplegia and hemiparesis due to sequela of cerebrovascular disease (I69.05-, I69.15-, I69.25-, I69.35-, I69.85-, I69.95-)
     AHA: 2015, 1Q, 25

✓5th   **G81.0** Flaccid **hemiplegia**
       G81.00 **Flaccid hemiplegia affecting unspecified side** ▽
       G81.01 **Flaccid hemiplegia affecting** right dominant **side**
       G81.02 **Flaccid hemiplegia affecting** left dominant **side**
       G81.03 **Flaccid hemiplegia affecting** right nondominant **side**
       G81.04 **Flaccid hemiplegia affecting** left nondominant **side**

✓5th   **G81.1** Spastic **hemiplegia**
       G81.10 **Spastic hemiplegia affecting unspecified side** ▽
       G81.11 **Spastic hemiplegia affecting** right dominant **side**
       G81.12 **Spastic hemiplegia affecting** left dominant **side**
       G81.13 **Spastic hemiplegia affecting** right nondominant **side**
       G81.14 **Spastic hemiplegia affecting** left nondominant **side**

✓5th   **G81.9** Hemiplegia, **unspecified**
       AHA: 2014, 1Q, 23
       G81.90 **Hemiplegia, unspecified affecting unspecified side** ▽
       G81.91 **Hemiplegia, unspecified affecting** right dominant **side** ▽
       G81.92 **Hemiplegia, unspecified affecting** left dominant **side** ▽
       G81.93 **Hemiplegia, unspecified affecting** right nondominant **side** ▽
       G81.94 **Hemiplegia, unspecified affecting** left nondominant **side** ▽

✓4th **G82** **Paraplegia (paraparesis) and quadriplegia (quadriparesis)**
     NOTE   This category is to be used only when the listed conditions are reported without further specification, or are stated to be old or longstanding but of unspecified cause. The category is also for use in multiple coding to identify these conditions resulting from any cause
     EXCLUDES 1   *congenital cerebral palsy (G80.-)*
         functional quadriplegia (R53.2)
         hysterical paralysis (F44.4)

✓5th   **G82.2** Paraplegia
       Paralysis of both lower limbs NOS
       Paraparesis (lower) NOS
       Paraplegia (lower) NOS
       G82.20 **Paraplegia, unspecified** ▽
       G82.21 **Paraplegia,** complete
       G82.22 **Paraplegia,** incomplete

✓5th   **G82.5** Quadriplegia
       G82.50 **Quadriplegia, unspecified** ▽
       G82.51 **Quadriplegia, C1-C4 complete**
       G82.52 **Quadriplegia, C1-C4 incomplete**
       G82.53 **Quadriplegia, C5-C7 complete**
       G82.54 **Quadriplegia, C5-C7 incomplete**

✓4th **G83** **Other paralytic syndromes**
     NOTE   This category is to be used only when the listed conditions are reported without further specification, or are stated to be old or longstanding but of unspecified cause. The category is also for use in multiple coding to identify these conditions resulting from any cause.
     INCLUDES   paralysis (complete) (incomplete), except as in G80-G82

     G83.0 Diplegia **of upper limbs**
         Diplegia (upper)
         Paralysis of both upper limbs

✓5th   **G83.1** Monoplegia **of lower limb**
       Paralysis of lower limb
       EXCLUDES 1   *monoplegia of lower limbs due to sequela of cerebrovascular disease (I69.04-, I69.14-, I69.24-, I69.34-, I69.84-, I69.94-)*
       G83.10 **Monoplegia of lower limb affecting unspecified side** ▽
       G83.11 **Monoplegia of lower limb affecting** right dominant **side**
       G83.12 **Monoplegia of lower limb affecting** left dominant **side**
       G83.13 **Monoplegia of lower limb affecting** right nondominant **side**
       G83.14 **Monoplegia of lower limb affecting** left nondominant **side**

✓5th   **G83.2** Monoplegia **of upper limb**
       Paralysis of upper limb
       EXCLUDES 1   *monoplegia of upper limbs due to sequela of cerebrovascular disease (I69.03-, I69.13-, I69.23-, I69.33-, I69.83-, I69.93-)*
       G83.20 **Monoplegia of upper limb affecting unspecified side** ▽
       G83.21 **Monoplegia of upper limb affecting** right dominant **side**
       G83.22 **Monoplegia of upper limb affecting** left dominant **side**
       G83.23 **Monoplegia of upper limb affecting** right nondominant **side**
       G83.24 **Monoplegia of upper limb affecting** left nondominant **side**

✓5th   **G83.3** Monoplegia, unspecified
       G83.30 **Monoplegia, unspecified affecting unspecified side** ▽
       G83.31 **Monoplegia, unspecified affecting** right dominant **side** ▽
       G83.32 **Monoplegia, unspecified affecting** left dominant **side** ▽
       G83.33 **Monoplegia, unspecified affecting** right nondominant **side** ▽
       G83.34 **Monoplegia, unspecified affecting** left nondominant **side** ▽

     G83.4 Cauda equina syndrome
         Neurogenic bladder due to cauda equina syndrome
         EXCLUDES 1   *cord bladder NOS (G95.89)*
           neurogenic bladder NOS (N31.9)

G83.5 **Locked-in state**

✓5ᵗʰ **G83.8** **Other specified paralytic syndromes**
    EXCLUDES 1 *paralytic syndromes due to current spinal cord injury—code to spinal cord injury (S14, S24, S34)*

    G83.81 **Brown-Séquard syndrome**
    G83.82 **Anterior cord syndrome**
    G83.83 **Posterior cord syndrome**
    G83.84 **Todd's paralysis (postepileptic)**
    G83.89 **Other specified paralytic syndromes**

G83.9 **Paralytic syndrome, unspecified**   ▽

Other disorders of the nervous system (G89-G99)

✓4ᵗʰ **G89** **Pain, not elsewhere classified**
    Code also related psychological factors associated with pain (F45.42)
    EXCLUDES 1 *generalized pain NOS (R52)*
        pain disorders exclusively related to psychological factors (F45.41)
        pain NOS (R52)
    EXCLUDES 2 *atypical face pain (G50.1)*
        headache syndromes (G44.-)
        localized pain, unspecified type—code to pain by site, such as:
            abdomen pain (R10.-)
            back pain (M54.9)
            breast pain (N64.4)
            chest pain (R07.1-R07.9)
            ear pain (H92.0-)
            eye pain (H57.1)
            headache (R51)
            joint pain (M25.5-)
            limb pain (M79.6-)
            lumbar region pain (M54.5)
            painful urination (R30.9)
            pelvic and perineal pain (R10.2)
            renal colic (N23)
            shoulder pain (M25.51-)
            spine pain (M54.-)
            throat pain (R07.0)
            tongue pain (K14.6)
            tooth pain (K08.8)
        migraines (G43.-)
        myalgia (M79.1)
        pain from prosthetic devices, implants, and grafts (T82.84, T83.84, T84.84, T85.84-)
        phantom limb syndrome with pain (G54.6)
        vulvar vestibulitis (N94.810)
        vulvodynia (N94.81-)

    G89.0 **Central pain syndrome**
        Déjérine-Roussy syndrome
        Myelopathic pain syndrome
        Thalamic pain syndrome (hyperesthetic)

    ✓5ᵗʰ **G89.1** **Acute pain, not elsewhere classified**
        G89.11 **Acute pain due to trauma**
        G89.12 **Acute post-thoracotomy pain**
            Post-thoracotomy pain NOS
        G89.18 **Other acute postprocedural pain**
            Postoperative pain NOS
            Postprocedural pain NOS

    ✓5ᵗʰ **G89.2** **Chronic pain, not elsewhere classified**
        EXCLUDES 1 *causalgia, lower limb (G57.7-)*
            causalgia, upper limb (G56.4-)
            central pain syndrome (G89.0)
            chronic pain syndrome (G89.4)
            complex regional pain syndrome II, lower limb (G57.7-)
            complex regional pain syndrome II, upper limb (G56.4-)
            neoplasm related chronic pain (G89.3)
            reflex sympathetic dystrophy (G90.5-)
        G89.21 **Chronic pain due to trauma**
        G89.22 **Chronic post-thoracotomy pain**
        G89.28 **Other chronic postprocedural pain**
            Other chronic postoperative pain
        G89.29 **Other chronic pain**

    G89.3 **Neoplasm related pain (acute) (chronic)**
        Cancer associated pain
        Pain due to malignancy (primary) (secondary)
        Tumor associated pain

    G89.4 **Chronic pain syndrome**
        Chronic pain associated with significant psychosocial dysfunction

✓4ᵗʰ **G90** **Disorders of autonomic nervous system**
    EXCLUDES 1 *dysfunction of the autonomic nervous system due to alcohol (G31.2)*

    ✓5ᵗʰ **G90.0** **Idiopathic peripheral autonomic neuropathy**
        G90.01 **Carotid sinus syncope**
            Carotid sinus syndrome
            DEF: Vagal activation caused by pressure on the carotid sinus baroreceptors; sympathetic nerve impulses may cause sinus arrest or AV block.
        G90.09 **Other idiopathic peripheral autonomic neuropathy**
            Idiopathic peripheral autonomic neuropathy NOS

    G90.1 **Familial dysautonomia [Riley-Day]**

    G90.2 **Horner's syndrome**
        Bernard(-Horner) syndrome
        Cervical sympathetic dystrophy or paralysis

    G90.3 **Multi-system degeneration of the autonomic nervous system**
        Neurogenic orthostatic hypotension [Shy-Drager]
        EXCLUDES 1 *orthostatic hypotension NOS (I95.1)*

    G90.4 **Autonomic dysreflexia**
        Use additional code to identify the cause, such as:
            fecal impaction (K56.41)
            pressure ulcer (pressure area) (L89.-)
            urinary tract infection (N39.0)

    ✓5ᵗʰ **G90.5** **Complex regional pain syndrome I (CRPS I)**
        Reflex sympathetic dystrophy
        EXCLUDES 1 *causalgia of lower limb (G57.7-)*
            causalgia of upper limb (G56.4-)
            complex regional pain syndrome II of lower limb (G57.7-)
            complex regional pain syndrome II of upper limb (G56.4-)
        G90.50 **Complex regional pain syndrome I, unspecified**   ▽
        ✓6ᵗʰ **G90.51** **Complex regional pain syndrome I of upper limb**
            G90.511 **Complex regional pain syndrome I of right upper limb**
            G90.512 **Complex regional pain syndrome I of left upper limb**
            G90.513 **Complex regional pain syndrome I of upper limb, bilateral**
            G90.519 **Complex regional pain syndrome I of unspecified upper limb**   ▽
        ✓6ᵗʰ **G90.52** **Complex regional pain syndrome I of lower limb**
            G90.521 **Complex regional pain syndrome I of right lower limb**
            G90.522 **Complex regional pain syndrome I of left lower limb**
            G90.523 **Complex regional pain syndrome I of lower limb, bilateral**
            G90.529 **Complex regional pain syndrome I of unspecified lower limb**   ▽
        G90.59 **Complex regional pain syndrome I of other specified site**

    G90.8 **Other disorders of autonomic nervous system**
    G90.9 **Disorder of the autonomic nervous system, unspecified**   ▽

✓4ᵗʰ **G91** **Hydrocephalus**
    INCLUDES acquired hydrocephalus
    EXCLUDES 1 *Arnold-Chiari syndrome with hydrocephalus (Q07.-)*
        congenital hydrocephalus (Q03.-)
        spina bifida with hydrocephalus (Q05.-)

    G91.0 **Communicating hydrocephalus**
        Secondary normal pressure hydrocephalus

    G91.1 **Obstructive hydrocephalus**
        DEF: Obstruction of cerebrospinal fluid passage from brain into spinal canal; characterized by headaches, drowsiness, poor coordination, urinary incontinence, nausea, vomiting, and papilledema.

    G91.2 **(Idiopathic) normal pressure hydrocephalus**
        Normal pressure hydrocephalus NOS

    G91.3 **Post-traumatic hydrocephalus, unspecified**   ▽

Hydrocephalus (Acquired)

| Normal ventricles | Hydrocephalic ventricles |

G91.4 Hydrocephalus in diseases classified elsewhere
> Code first underlying condition, such as:
>> congenital syphilis (A50.4-)
>> neoplasm (C00-D49)
>> *EXCLUDES 1* *hydrocephalus due to congenital toxoplasmosis (P37.1)*
>> **AHA:** 2014, 3Q, 3

G91.8 Other hydrocephalus

G91.9 Hydrocephalus, unspecified ▽

G92 Toxic encephalopathy
> Toxic encephalitis
> Toxic metabolic encephalopathy
> ►Code first, if applicable, drug induced (T36-T50)◄
> Code first (T51-T65) to identify toxic agent
> **AHA:** 2017, 1Q, 39-40
> **DEF:** Brain tissue degeneration due to toxic substance.

✓4ᵗʰ G93 Other disorders of brain

G93.0 Cerebral cysts
> Arachnoid cyst
> Porencephalic cyst, acquired
>> *EXCLUDES 1* *acquired periventricular cysts of newborn (P91.1)*
>> *congenital cerebral cysts (Q04.6)*

G93.1 Anoxic brain damage, not elsewhere classified
>> *EXCLUDES 1* *cerebral anoxia due to anesthesia during labor and*
>>> *delivery (O74.3)*
>> *cerebral anoxia due to anesthesia during the*
>>> *puerperium (O89.2)*
>> *neonatal anoxia (P84)*
> **DEF:** Brain injury not resulting from birth trauma that is due to lack of oxygen. Brain cells, when deprived of oxygen, begin to expire after 4 minutes.

G93.2 Benign intracranial hypertension
>> *EXCLUDES 1* *hypertensive encephalopathy (I67.4)*

G93.3 Postviral fatigue syndrome
> Benign myalgic encephalomyelitis
>> *EXCLUDES 1* *chronic fatigue syndrome NOS (R53.82)*

✓5ᵗʰ G93.4 Other and unspecified encephalopathy
>> *EXCLUDES 1* *alcoholic encephalopathy (G31.2)*
>> *encephalopathy in diseases classified elsewhere (G94)*
>> *hypertensive encephalopathy (I67.4)*
>> *toxic (metabolic) encephalopathy (G92)*

> **G93.40 Encephalopathy, unspecified** ▽
>> **AHA:** 2017, 2Q, 8

> **G93.41 Metabolic encephalopathy**
>> Septic encephalopathy
>> **AHA:** 2017, 2Q, 8; 2016, 3Q, 42; 2015, 3Q, 21

> **G93.49 Other encephalopathy**
>> Encephalopathy NEC
>> **AHA:** 2017, 2Q, 9

G93.5 Compression of brain
> Arnold-Chiari type 1 compression of brain
> Compression of brain (stem)
> Herniation of brain (stem)
>> *EXCLUDES 1* *diffuse traumatic compression of brain (S06.2-)*
>> *focal traumatic compression of brain (S06.3-)*

G93.6 Cerebral edema
>> *EXCLUDES 1* *cerebral edema due to birth injury (P11.0)*
>> *traumatic cerebral edema (S06.1-)*

G93.7 Reye's syndrome [P]
> Code first (T39.0-), if salicylates-induced
> ►Code first poisoning due to salicylates, if applicable (T39.0-, with sixth character 1-4)◄
> ►Use additional code for adverse effect due to salicylates, if applicable (T39.0-, with sixth character 5)◄
> **DEF:** Rare childhood illness often developed after a viral upper respiratory infection; characterized by vomiting, elevated serum transaminase, brain swelling, disturbances of consciousness, seizures, and changes in liver and other viscera; can be fatal.

✓5ᵗʰ G93.8 Other specified disorders of brain

> **G93.81 Temporal sclerosis**
>> Hippocampal sclerosis
>> Mesial temporal sclerosis

> **G93.82 Brain death**

> **G93.89 Other specified disorders of brain**
>> Postradiation encephalopathy

G93.9 Disorder of brain, unspecified ▽

G94 *Other disorders of brain in diseases classified elsewhere*
> Code first underlying disease
>> *EXCLUDES 1* *encephalopathy in congenital syphilis (A50.49)*
>> *encephalopathy in influenza (J09.X9, J10.81, J11.81)*
>> *encephalopathy in syphilis (A52.19)*
>> *hydrocephalus in diseases classified elsewhere (G91.4)*

✓4ᵗʰ G95 Other and unspecified diseases of spinal cord
>> *EXCLUDES 2* *myelitis (G04.-)*

G95.0 Syringomyelia and syringobulbia

✓5ᵗʰ G95.1 Vascular myelopathies
>> *EXCLUDES 2* *intraspinal phlebitis and thrombophlebitis, except*
>>> *non-pyogenic (G08)*

> **G95.11 Acute infarction of spinal cord (embolic) (nonembolic)**
>> Anoxia of spinal cord
>> Arterial thrombosis of spinal cord

> **G95.19 Other vascular myelopathies**
>> Edema of spinal cord
>> Hematomyelia
>> Nonpyogenic intraspinal phlebitis and thrombophlebitis
>> Subacute necrotic myelopathy

✓5ᵗʰ G95.2 Other and unspecified cord compression

> **G95.20 Unspecified cord compression** ▽

> **G95.29 Other cord compression**

✓5ᵗʰ G95.8 Other specified diseases of spinal cord
>> *EXCLUDES 1* *neurogenic bladder NOS (N31.9)*
>> *neurogenic bladder due to cauda equina syndrome*
>>> *(G83.4)*
>> *neuromuscular dysfunction of bladder without spinal*
>>> *cord lesion (N31.-)*

> **G95.81 Conus medullaris syndrome**

> **G95.89 Other specified diseases of spinal cord**
>> Cord bladder NOS
>> Drug-induced myelopathy
>> Radiation-induced myelopathy
>>> *EXCLUDES 1* *myelopathy NOS (G95.9)*

G95.9 Disease of spinal cord, unspecified ▽
> Myelopathy NOS

✓4ᵗʰ G96 Other disorders of central nervous system

G96.0 Cerebrospinal fluid leak
>> *EXCLUDES 1* *cerebrospinal fluid leak from spinal puncture (G97.0)*
> **DEF:** Cerebrospinal fluid discharging from the nose or the ear; caused by fracture of frontal bone with tearing of dura mater and arachnoid; characterized by watery drainage usually from only one side of the nose or one ear, headache, vision changes, and hearing loss.

✓5ᵗʰ G96.1 Disorders of meninges, not elsewhere classified

> **G96.11 Dural tear**
>> *EXCLUDES 1* *accidental puncture or laceration of dura*
>>> *during a procedure (G97.41)*
>> **AHA:** 2014, 4Q, 24

> **G96.12 Meningeal adhesions (cerebral) (spinal)**

> **G96.19 Other disorders of meninges, not elsewhere classified**

G96.8 Other specified disorders of central nervous system

G96.9 Disorder of central nervous system, unspecified ▽

Spinal Puncture

- Spinal cord
- Epidural space
- Subarachnoid space
- Vertebra
- Spinal needle

Lumbar area

✓4ᵗʰ G97 Intraoperative and postprocedural complications and disorders of nervous system, not elsewhere classified
> EXCLUDES 2   intraoperative and postprocedural cerebrovascular infarction (I97.81-, I97.82-)

G97.0 Cerebrospinal fluid leak from spinal puncture

G97.1 Other reaction to spinal and lumbar puncture
> Headache due to lumbar puncture

G97.2 Intracranial hypotension following ventricular shunting

✓5ᵗʰ G97.3 Intraoperative hemorrhage and hematoma of a nervous system organ or structure complicating a procedure
> EXCLUDES 1   intraoperative hemorrhage and hematoma of a nervous system organ or structure due to accidental puncture and laceration during a procedure (G97.4-)

    G97.31 Intraoperative hemorrhage and hematoma of a nervous system organ or structure complicating a nervous system procedure

    G97.32 Intraoperative hemorrhage and hematoma of a nervous system organ or structure complicating other procedure

✓5ᵗʰ G97.4 Accidental puncture and laceration of a nervous system organ or structure during a procedure

    G97.41 Accidental puncture or laceration of dura during a procedure
> Incidental (inadvertent) durotomy
> **AHA:** 2014, 4Q, 24

    G97.48 Accidental puncture and laceration of other nervous system organ or structure during a nervous system procedure

    G97.49 Accidental puncture and laceration of other nervous system organ or structure during other procedure

✓5ᵗʰ G97.5 Postprocedural hemorrhage of a nervous system organ or structure following a procedure

    G97.51 Postprocedural hemorrhage of a nervous system organ or structure following a nervous system procedure

    G97.52 Postprocedural hemorrhage of a nervous system organ or structure following other procedure

✓5ᵗʰ G97.6 Postprocedural hematoma and seroma of a nervous system organ or structure following a procedure

    G97.61 Postprocedural hematoma of a nervous system organ or structure following a nervous system procedure

    G97.62 Postprocedural hematoma of a nervous system organ or structure following other procedure

    G97.63 Postprocedural seroma of a nervous system organ or structure following a nervous system procedure

    G97.64 Postprocedural seroma of a nervous system organ or structure following other procedure

✓5ᵗʰ G97.8 Other intraoperative and postprocedural complications and disorders of nervous system
> Use additional code to further specify disorder

    G97.81 Other intraoperative complications of nervous system

    G97.82 Other postprocedural complications and disorders of nervous system

✓4ᵗʰ G98 Other disorders of nervous system not elsewhere classified
> INCLUDES   nervous system disorder NOS

G98.0 Neurogenic arthritis, not elsewhere classified
> Nonsyphilitic neurogenic arthropathy NEC
> Nonsyphilitic neurogenic spondylopathy NEC
> EXCLUDES 1   spondylopathy (in):
>   syringomyelia and syringobulbia (G95.0)
>   tabes dorsalis (A52.11)

G98.8 Other disorders of nervous system
> Nervous system disorder NOS

✓4ᵗʰ G99 Other disorders of nervous system in diseases classified elsewhere

G99.0 Autonomic neuropathy in diseases classified elsewhere
> Code first underlying disease, such as:
>   amyloidosis (E85.-)
>   gout (M1A.-, M10.-)
>   hyperthyroidism (E05.-)
> EXCLUDES 1   diabetic autonomic neuropathy (E08-E13 with .43)

G99.2 Myelopathy in diseases classified elsewhere
> Code first underlying disease, such as:
>   neoplasm (C00-D49)
> EXCLUDES 1   myelopathy in:
>   intervertebral disease (M50.0-, M51.0-)
>   spondylosis (M47.0-, M47.1-)

G99.8 Other specified disorders of nervous system in diseases classified elsewhere
> Code first underlying disorder, such as:
>   amyloidosis (E85.-)
>   avitaminosis (E56.9)
> EXCLUDES 1   nervous system involvement in:
>   cysticercosis (B69.0)
>   rubella (B06.0-)
>   syphilis (A52.1-)

✓ Additional Character Req   ✓x7ᵗʰ Placeholder Alert   Case-Mix Diagnosis   Manifestation   ▽ Unspecified Dx   EXCLUDES 1 Not coded here   EXCLUDES 2 Not included here

ICD-10-CM 2018

565

Chapter 7. Diseases of the Eye and Adnexa (H00–H59)

Chapter Specific Guidelines with Coding Examples

The chapter specific guidelines from the ICD-10-CM Official Guidelines for Coding and Reporting have been provided below. Along with these guidelines are coding examples, contained in the shaded boxes, that have been developed to help illustrate the coding and/or sequencing guidance found in these guidelines.

a. Glaucoma

1) Assigning glaucoma codes

Assign as many codes from category H40, Glaucoma, as needed to identify the type of glaucoma, the affected eye, and the glaucoma stage.

2) Bilateral glaucoma with same type and stage

When a patient has bilateral glaucoma and both eyes are documented as being the same type and stage, and there is a code for bilateral glaucoma, report only the code for the type of glaucoma, bilateral, with the seventh character for the stage.

> Bilateral severe stage pigmentary glaucoma.
>
> **H40.1333   Pigmentary glaucoma, bilateral, severe stage**
>
> *Explanation*: In this scenario, the patient has the same type and stage of glaucoma in both eyes. As this type of glaucoma has a code for bilateral, assign only the code for the bilateral glaucoma with the seventh character for the stage.

When a patient has bilateral glaucoma and both eyes are documented as being the same type and stage, and the classification does not provide a code for bilateral glaucoma (i.e. subcategories H40.10, H40.11 and H40.20) report only one code for the type of glaucoma with the appropriate seventh character for the stage.

> Bilateral open-angle glaucoma; not specified as to type and stage indeterminate in both eyes.
>
> **H40.10X4   Unspecified open-angle glaucoma, indeterminate stage**
>
> *Explanation*: In this scenario, the patient has glaucoma of the same type and stage of both eyes, but there is no code specifically for bilateral glaucoma. Only one code is assigned with the appropriate seventh character for the stage.

3) Bilateral glaucoma stage with different types or stages

When a patient has bilateral glaucoma and each eye is documented as having a different type or stage, and the classification distinguishes laterality, assign the appropriate code for each eye rather than the code for bilateral glaucoma.

> Bilateral chronic angle-closure glaucoma; right eye is documented as mild stage and left eye as moderate stage.
>
> **H40.2211   Chronic angle-closure glaucoma, right eye, mild stage**
>
> **H40.2222   Chronic angle-closure glaucoma, left eye, moderate stage**
>
> *Explanation*: In this scenario the patient has the same type of glaucoma in both eyes, but each eye is at a different stage. Because the subcategory for this condition identifies laterality, one code is assigned for the right eye and one code is assigned for the left eye, each with the appropriate seventh character for the stage appended.

When a patient has bilateral glaucoma and each eye is documented as having a different type, and the classification does not distinguish laterality (i.e. subcategories H40.10, H40.11 and H40.20), assign one code for each type of glaucoma with the appropriate seventh character for the stage.

> Documentation relates mild, unspecified primary angle-closure glaucoma of the left eye with mild unspecified open-angle glaucoma of the right eye.
>
> **H40.20X1   Unspecified primary angle-closure glaucoma, mild stage**
>
> **H40.10X1   Unspecified open-angle glaucoma, mild stage**
>
> *Explanation*: In this scenario the patient has a different type of glaucoma in each eye and the classification does not distinguish laterality. A code for each type of glaucoma is assigned, each with the appropriate seventh character for the stage.

When a patient has bilateral glaucoma and each eye is documented as having the same type, but different stage, and the classification does not distinguish laterality (i.e. subcategories H40.10, H40.11 and H40.20), assign a code for the type of glaucoma for each eye with the seventh character for the specific glaucoma stage documented for each eye.

> Bilateral open-angle glaucoma, not specified as to type; the right eye is documented to be in mild stage and the left eye as being in moderate stage.
>
> **H40.10X2   Unspecified open-angle glaucoma, moderate stage**
>
> **H40.10X1   Unspecified open-angle glaucoma, mild stage**
>
> *Explanation*: In this scenario the patient has the same type of glaucoma in each eye but each eye is at a different stage, and the classification does not distinguish laterality at this subcategory level. Two codes are assigned; both codes represent the same type of glaucoma but each has a different seventh character identifying the appropriate stage for each eye.

4) Patient admitted with glaucoma and stage evolves during the admission

If a patient is admitted with glaucoma and the stage progresses during the admission, assign the code for highest stage documented.

5) Indeterminate stage glaucoma

Assignment of the seventh character "4" for "indeterminate stage" should be based on the clinical documentation. The seventh character "4" is used for glaucomas whose stage cannot be clinically determined. This seventh character should not be confused with the seventh character "0", unspecified, which should be assigned when there is no documentation regarding the stage of the glaucoma.

b. Blindness

If "blindness" or "low vision" of both eyes is documented but the visual impairment category is not documented, assign code H54.3, Unqualified visual loss, both eyes. If "blindness" or "low vision" in one eye is documented but the visual impairment category is not documented, assign a code from H54.6-, Unqualified visual loss, one eye. If "blindness" or "visual loss" is documented without any information about whether one or both eyes are affected, assign code H54.7, Unspecified visual loss.

Chapter 7. Diseases of the Eye and Adnexa (H00–H59)

NOTE   Use an external cause code following the code for the eye condition, if applicable, to identify the cause of the eye condition.

EXCLUDES 2   certain conditions originating in the perinatal period (P04-P96)
certain infectious and parasitic diseases (A00-B99)
complications of pregnancy, childbirth and the puerperium (O00-O9A)
congenital malformations, deformations, and chromosomal abnormalities (Q00-Q99)
diabetes mellitus related eye conditions (E09.3-, E10.3-, E11.3-, E13.3-)
endocrine, nutritional and metabolic diseases (E00-E88)
injury (trauma) of eye and orbit (S05.-)
injury, poisoning and certain other consequences of external causes (S00-T88)
neoplasms (C00-D49)
symptoms, signs and abnormal clinical and laboratory findings, not elsewhere classified (R00-R94)
syphilis related eye disorders (A50.01, A50.3-, A51.43, A52.71)

This chapter contains the following blocks:

H00-H05	Disorders of eyelid, lacrimal system and orbit
H10-H11	Disorders of conjunctiva
H15-H22	Disorders of sclera, cornea, iris and ciliary body
H25-H28	Disorders of lens
H30-H36	Disorders of choroid and retina
H40-H42	Glaucoma
H43-H44	Disorders of vitreous body and globe
H46-H47	Disorders of optic nerve and visual pathways
H49-H52	Disorders of ocular muscles, binocular movement, accommodation and refraction
H53-H54	Visual disturbances and blindness
H55-H57	Other disorders of eye and adnexa
H59	Intraoperative and postprocedural complications and disorders of eye and adnexa, not elsewhere classified

Disorders of eyelid, lacrimal system and orbit (H00-H05)

EXCLUDES 2   open wound of eyelid (S01.1-)
superficial injury of eyelid (S00.1-, S00.2-)

✓4ᵗʰ **H00 Hordeolum and chalazion**

  ✓5ᵗʰ **H00.0** Hordeolum (externum) (internum) of eyelid

    ✓6ᵗʰ **H00.01 Hordeolum externum**
         Hordeolum NOS
         Stye

         H00.011 Hordeolum externum right upper eyelid
         H00.012 Hordeolum externum right lower eyelid
         H00.013 Hordeolum externum right eye, unspecified eyelid ▽
         H00.014 Hordeolum externum left upper eyelid
         H00.015 Hordeolum externum left lower eyelid
         H00.016 Hordeolum externum left eye, unspecified eyelid ▽
         H00.019 Hordeolum externum unspecified eye, unspecified eyelid ▽

    ✓6ᵗʰ **H00.02 Hordeolum internum**
         Infection of meibomian gland

         H00.021 Hordeolum internum right upper eyelid
         H00.022 Hordeolum internum right lower eyelid
         H00.023 Hordeolum internum right eye, unspecified eyelid ▽
         H00.024 Hordeolum internum left upper eyelid
         H00.025 Hordeolum internum left lower eyelid
         H00.026 Hordeolum internum left eye, unspecified eyelid ▽
         H00.029 Hordeolum internum unspecified eye, unspecified eyelid ▽

    ✓6ᵗʰ **H00.03 Abscess of eyelid**
         Furuncle of eyelid

         H00.031 Abscess of right upper eyelid
         H00.032 Abscess of right lower eyelid
         H00.033 Abscess of eyelid right eye, unspecified eyelid ▽
         H00.034 Abscess of left upper eyelid
         H00.035 Abscess of left lower eyelid
         H00.036 Abscess of eyelid left eye, unspecified eyelid ▽
         H00.039 Abscess of eyelid unspecified eye, unspecified eyelid ▽

✓6ᵗʰ **H00.1 Chalazion**
   Meibomian (gland) cyst
   EXCLUDES 2   infected meibomian gland (H00.02-)

   H00.11 Chalazion right upper eyelid
   H00.12 Chalazion right lower eyelid
   H00.13 Chalazion right eye, unspecified eyelid ▽
   H00.14 Chalazion left upper eyelid
   H00.15 Chalazion left lower eyelid
   H00.16 Chalazion left eye, unspecified eyelid ▽
   H00.19 Chalazion unspecified eye, unspecified eyelid ▽

✓4ᵗʰ **H01 Other inflammation of eyelid**

  ✓5ᵗʰ **H01.0 Blepharitis**
     EXCLUDES 1   blepharoconjunctivitis (H10.5-)

    ✓6ᵗʰ **H01.00 Unspecified blepharitis**
         H01.001 Unspecified blepharitis right upper eyelid ▽
         H01.002 Unspecified blepharitis right lower eyelid ▽
         H01.003 Unspecified blepharitis right eye, unspecified eyelid ▽
         H01.004 Unspecified blepharitis left upper eyelid ▽
         H01.005 Unspecified blepharitis left lower eyelid ▽
         H01.006 Unspecified blepharitis left eye, unspecified eyelid ▽
         H01.009 Unspecified blepharitis unspecified eye, unspecified eyelid ▽

    ✓6ᵗʰ **H01.01 Ulcerative blepharitis**
         H01.011 Ulcerative blepharitis right upper eyelid
         H01.012 Ulcerative blepharitis right lower eyelid
         H01.013 Ulcerative blepharitis right eye, unspecified eyelid ▽
         H01.014 Ulcerative blepharitis left upper eyelid
         H01.015 Ulcerative blepharitis left lower eyelid
         H01.016 Ulcerative blepharitis left eye, unspecified eyelid ▽
         H01.019 Ulcerative blepharitis unspecified eye, unspecified eyelid ▽

    ✓6ᵗʰ **H01.02 Squamous blepharitis**
         H01.021 Squamous blepharitis right upper eyelid
         H01.022 Squamous blepharitis right lower eyelid
         H01.023 Squamous blepharitis right eye, unspecified eyelid ▽
         H01.024 Squamous blepharitis left upper eyelid
         H01.025 Squamous blepharitis left lower eyelid
         H01.026 Squamous blepharitis left eye, unspecified eyelid ▽
         H01.029 Squamous blepharitis unspecified eye, unspecified eyelid ▽

  ✓5ᵗʰ **H01.1 Noninfectious dermatoses of eyelid**

    ✓6ᵗʰ **H01.11 Allergic dermatitis of eyelid**
         Contact dermatitis of eyelid
         H01.111 Allergic dermatitis of right upper eyelid
         H01.112 Allergic dermatitis of right lower eyelid
         H01.113 Allergic dermatitis of right eye, unspecified eyelid ▽
         H01.114 Allergic dermatitis of left upper eyelid
         H01.115 Allergic dermatitis of left lower eyelid
         H01.116 Allergic dermatitis of left eye, unspecified eyelid ▽
         H01.119 Allergic dermatitis of unspecified eye, unspecified eyelid ▽

    ✓6ᵗʰ **H01.12 Discoid lupus erythematosus of eyelid**
         H01.121 Discoid lupus erythematosus of right upper eyelid
         H01.122 Discoid lupus erythematosus of right lower eyelid
         H01.123 Discoid lupus erythematosus of right eye, unspecified eyelid ▽
         H01.124 Discoid lupus erythematosus of left upper eyelid
         H01.125 Discoid lupus erythematosus of left lower eyelid

N Newborn: 0   P Pediatric: 0-17   M Maternity: 12-55   A Adult: 15-124   NRS Nonroutine supply Dx   NC Dx Noncancer Dx   PDx Primary Dx   ▶◀ Revised Text   ● New Code   ▲ Revised Title

568   ICD-10-CM 2018

H01.126 Discoid lupus erythematosus of left eye, unspecified eyelid ▽

H01.129 Discoid lupus erythematosus of unspecified eye, unspecified eyelid ▽

✓6ᵗʰ **H01.13** Eczematous dermatitis of eyelid

H01.131 Eczematous dermatitis of right upper eyelid

H01.132 Eczematous dermatitis of right lower eyelid

H01.133 Eczematous dermatitis of right eye, unspecified eyelid ▽

H01.134 Eczematous dermatitis of left upper eyelid

H01.135 Eczematous dermatitis of left lower eyelid

H01.136 Eczematous dermatitis of left eye, unspecified eyelid ▽

H01.139 Eczematous dermatitis of unspecified eye, unspecified eyelid ▽

✓6ᵗʰ **H01.14** Xeroderma of eyelid

H01.141 Xeroderma of right upper eyelid

H01.142 Xeroderma of right lower eyelid

H01.143 Xeroderma of right eye, unspecified eyelid ▽

H01.144 Xeroderma of left upper eyelid

H01.145 Xeroderma of left lower eyelid

H01.146 Xeroderma of left eye, unspecified eyelid ▽

H01.149 Xeroderma of unspecified eye, unspecified eyelid ▽

H01.8 Other specified inflammations of eyelid

H01.9 Unspecified inflammation of eyelid ▽
Inflammation of eyelid NOS

✓4ᵗʰ **H02** Other disorders of eyelid
EXCLUDES 1 congenital malformations of eyelid (Q10.0-Q10.3)

✓5ᵗʰ **H02.0** Entropion and trichiasis of eyelid

✓6ᵗʰ **H02.00** Unspecified entropion of eyelid

H02.001 Unspecified entropion of right upper eyelid ▽

H02.002 Unspecified entropion of right lower eyelid ▽

H02.003 Unspecified entropion of right eye, unspecified eyelid ▽

H02.004 Unspecified entropion of left upper eyelid ▽

H02.005 Unspecified entropion of left lower eyelid ▽

H02.006 Unspecified entropion of left eye, unspecified eyelid ▽

H02.009 Unspecified entropion of unspecified eye, unspecified eyelid ▽

✓6ᵗʰ **H02.01** Cicatricial entropion of eyelid

H02.011 Cicatricial entropion of right upper eyelid

H02.012 Cicatricial entropion of right lower eyelid

H02.013 Cicatricial entropion of right eye, unspecified eyelid ▽

H02.014 Cicatricial entropion of left upper eyelid

H02.015 Cicatricial entropion of left lower eyelid

H02.016 Cicatricial entropion of left eye, unspecified eyelid ▽

H02.019 Cicatricial entropion of unspecified eye, unspecified eyelid ▽

✓6ᵗʰ **H02.02** Mechanical entropion of eyelid

H02.021 Mechanical entropion of right upper eyelid

H02.022 Mechanical entropion of right lower eyelid

H02.023 Mechanical entropion of right eye, unspecified eyelid ▽

H02.024 Mechanical entropion of left upper eyelid

H02.025 Mechanical entropion of left lower eyelid

H02.026 Mechanical entropion of left eye, unspecified eyelid ▽

H02.029 Mechanical entropion of unspecified eye, unspecified eyelid ▽

✓6ᵗʰ **H02.03** Senile entropion of eyelid

H02.031 Senile entropion of right upper eyelid A

H02.032 Senile entropion of right lower eyelid A

H02.033 Senile entropion of right eye, unspecified eyelid A▽

H02.034 Senile entropion of left upper eyelid A

H02.035 Senile entropion of left lower eyelid A

H02.036 Senile entropion of left eye, unspecified eyelid A▽

H02.039 Senile entropion of unspecified eye, unspecified eyelid A▽

✓6ᵗʰ **H02.04** Spastic entropion of eyelid

H02.041 Spastic entropion of right upper eyelid

H02.042 Spastic entropion of right lower eyelid

H02.043 Spastic entropion of right eye, unspecified eyelid ▽

H02.044 Spastic entropion of left upper eyelid

H02.045 Spastic entropion of left lower eyelid

H02.046 Spastic entropion of left eye, unspecified eyelid ▽

H02.049 Spastic entropion of unspecified eye, unspecified eyelid ▽

▲ ✓6ᵗʰ **H02.05** Trichiasis without entropion

▲ **H02.051** Trichiasis without entropion right upper eyelid

▲ **H02.052** Trichiasis without entropion right lower eyelid

▲ **H02.053** Trichiasis without entropion right eye, unspecified eyelid ▽

▲ **H02.054** Trichiasis without entropion left upper eyelid

▲ **H02.055** Trichiasis without entropion left lower eyelid

▲ **H02.056** Trichiasis without entropion left eye, unspecified eyelid ▽

▲ **H02.059** Trichiasis without entropion unspecified eye, unspecified eyelid ▽

✓5ᵗʰ **H02.1** Ectropion of eyelid

✓6ᵗʰ **H02.10** Unspecified ectropion of eyelid

H02.101 Unspecified ectropion of right upper eyelid ▽

H02.102 Unspecified ectropion of right lower eyelid ▽

H02.103 Unspecified ectropion of right eye, unspecified eyelid ▽

H02.104 Unspecified ectropion of left upper eyelid ▽

H02.105 Unspecified ectropion of left lower eyelid ▽

H02.106 Unspecified ectropion of left eye, unspecified eyelid ▽

H02.109 Unspecified ectropion of unspecified eye, unspecified eyelid ▽

Entropion and Ectropion

Normal eyelid   Entropion   Ectropion

✓6th H02.11 Cicatricial ectropion of eyelid
- H02.111 Cicatricial ectropion of right upper eyelid
- H02.112 Cicatricial ectropion of right lower eyelid
- H02.113 Cicatricial ectropion of right eye, unspecified eyelid ▽
- H02.114 Cicatricial ectropion of left upper eyelid
- H02.115 Cicatricial ectropion of left lower eyelid
- H02.116 Cicatricial ectropion of left eye, unspecified eyelid ▽
- H02.119 Cicatricial ectropion of unspecified eye, unspecified eyelid ▽

✓6th H02.12 Mechanical ectropion of eyelid
- H02.121 Mechanical ectropion of right upper eyelid
- H02.122 Mechanical ectropion of right lower eyelid
- H02.123 Mechanical ectropion of right eye, unspecified eyelid ▽
- H02.124 Mechanical ectropion of left upper eyelid
- H02.125 Mechanical ectropion of left lower eyelid
- H02.126 Mechanical ectropion of left eye, unspecified eyelid ▽
- H02.129 Mechanical ectropion of unspecified eye, unspecified eyelid ▽

✓6th H02.13 Senile ectropion of eyelid
- H02.131 Senile ectropion of right upper eyelid 🄰
- H02.132 Senile ectropion of right lower eyelid 🄰
- H02.133 Senile ectropion of right eye, unspecified eyelid 🄰▽
- H02.134 Senile ectropion of left upper eyelid 🄰
- H02.135 Senile ectropion of left lower eyelid 🄰
- H02.136 Senile ectropion of left eye, unspecified eyelid 🄰▽
- H02.139 Senile ectropion of unspecified eye, unspecified eyelid 🄰▽

✓6th H02.14 Spastic ectropion of eyelid
- H02.141 Spastic ectropion of right upper eyelid
- H02.142 Spastic ectropion of right lower eyelid
- H02.143 Spastic ectropion of right eye, unspecified eyelid ▽
- H02.144 Spastic ectropion of left upper eyelid
- H02.145 Spastic ectropion of left lower eyelid
- H02.146 Spastic ectropion of left eye, unspecified eyelid ▽
- H02.149 Spastic ectropion of unspecified eye, unspecified eyelid ▽

✓5th H02.2 Lagophthalmos

✓6th H02.20 Unspecified lagophthalmos
- H02.201 Unspecified lagophthalmos right upper eyelid ▽
- H02.202 Unspecified lagophthalmos right lower eyelid ▽
- H02.203 Unspecified lagophthalmos right eye, unspecified eyelid ▽
- H02.204 Unspecified lagophthalmos left upper eyelid ▽
- H02.205 Unspecified lagophthalmos left lower eyelid ▽
- H02.206 Unspecified lagophthalmos left eye, unspecified eyelid ▽
- H02.209 Unspecified lagophthalmos unspecified eye, unspecified eyelid ▽

✓6th H02.21 Cicatricial lagophthalmos
- H02.211 Cicatricial lagophthalmos right upper eyelid
- H02.212 Cicatricial lagophthalmos right lower eyelid
- H02.213 Cicatricial lagophthalmos right eye, unspecified eyelid ▽
- H02.214 Cicatricial lagophthalmos left upper eyelid
- H02.215 Cicatricial lagophthalmos left lower eyelid
- H02.216 Cicatricial lagophthalmos left eye, unspecified eyelid ▽
- H02.219 Cicatricial lagophthalmos unspecified eye, unspecified eyelid ▽

✓6th H02.22 Mechanical lagophthalmos
- H02.221 Mechanical lagophthalmos right upper eyelid
- H02.222 Mechanical lagophthalmos right lower eyelid
- H02.223 Mechanical lagophthalmos right eye, unspecified eyelid ▽
- H02.224 Mechanical lagophthalmos left upper eyelid
- H02.225 Mechanical lagophthalmos left lower eyelid
- H02.226 Mechanical lagophthalmos left eye, unspecified eyelid ▽
- H02.229 Mechanical lagophthalmos unspecified eye, unspecified eyelid ▽

✓6th H02.23 Paralytic lagophthalmos
- H02.231 Paralytic lagophthalmos right upper eyelid
- H02.232 Paralytic lagophthalmos right lower eyelid
- H02.233 Paralytic lagophthalmos right eye, unspecified eyelid ▽
- H02.234 Paralytic lagophthalmos left upper eyelid
- H02.235 Paralytic lagophthalmos left lower eyelid
- H02.236 Paralytic lagophthalmos left eye, unspecified eyelid ▽
- H02.239 Paralytic lagophthalmos unspecified eye, unspecified eyelid ▽

✓5th H02.3 Blepharochalasis
    Pseudoptosis
- H02.30 Blepharochalasis unspecified eye, unspecified eyelid ▽
- H02.31 Blepharochalasis right upper eyelid
- H02.32 Blepharochalasis right lower eyelid
- H02.33 Blepharochalasis right eye, unspecified eyelid ▽
- H02.34 Blepharochalasis left upper eyelid
- H02.35 Blepharochalasis left lower eyelid
- H02.36 Blepharochalasis left eye, unspecified eyelid ▽

✓5th H02.4 Ptosis of eyelid

✓6th H02.40 Unspecified ptosis of eyelid
- H02.401 Unspecified ptosis of right eyelid ▽
- H02.402 Unspecified ptosis of left eyelid ▽
- H02.403 Unspecified ptosis of bilateral eyelids ▽
- H02.409 Unspecified ptosis of unspecified eyelid ▽

✓6th H02.41 Mechanical ptosis of eyelid
- H02.411 Mechanical ptosis of right eyelid
- H02.412 Mechanical ptosis of left eyelid
- H02.413 Mechanical ptosis of bilateral eyelids
- H02.419 Mechanical ptosis of unspecified eyelid ▽

✓6th H02.42 Myogenic ptosis of eyelid
- H02.421 Myogenic ptosis of right eyelid
- H02.422 Myogenic ptosis of left eyelid
- H02.423 Myogenic ptosis of bilateral eyelids
- H02.429 Myogenic ptosis of unspecified eyelid ▽

✓6th H02.43 Paralytic ptosis of eyelid
    Neurogenic ptosis of eyelid
- H02.431 Paralytic ptosis of right eyelid
- H02.432 Paralytic ptosis of left eyelid
- H02.433 Paralytic ptosis of bilateral eyelids
- H02.439 Paralytic ptosis unspecified eyelid ▽

✓5th H02.5 Other disorders affecting eyelid function
    EXCLUDES 2 *blepharospasm (G24.5)*
    organic tic (G25.69)
    psychogenic tic (F95.-)

✓6th H02.51 Abnormal innervation syndrome
- H02.511 Abnormal innervation syndrome right upper eyelid
- H02.512 Abnormal innervation syndrome right lower eyelid
- H02.513 Abnormal innervation syndrome right eye, unspecified eyelid ▽
- H02.514 Abnormal innervation syndrome left upper eyelid

🄽 Newborn: 0   🄿 Pediatric: 0-17   🄼 Maternity: 12-55   🄰 Adult: 15-124   **NRS** Nonroutine supply Dx   **NCDx** Noncancer Dx   **PDx** Primary Dx   ▶◀ Revised Text   ● New Code   ▲ Revised Title

H02.515   **Abnormal innervation syndrome** left lower **eyelid**

H02.516   **Abnormal innervation syndrome** left eye, **unspecified eyelid** ▽

H02.519   **Abnormal innervation syndrome unspecified eye, unspecified eyelid** ▽

√6ᵗʰ **H02.52   Blepharophimosis**
Ankyloblepharon

H02.521   **Blepharophimosis** right upper **eyelid**

H02.522   **Blepharophimosis** right lower **eyelid**

H02.523   **Blepharophimosis** right eye, **unspecified eyelid** ▽

H02.524   **Blepharophimosis** left upper **eyelid**

H02.525   **Blepharophimosis** left lower **eyelid**

H02.526   **Blepharophimosis** left eye, **unspecified eyelid** ▽

H02.529   **Blepharophimosis unspecified eye, unspecified lid** ▽

√6ᵗʰ **H02.53   Eyelid retraction**
Eyelid lag

H02.531   **Eyelid retraction** right upper **eyelid**

H02.532   **Eyelid retraction** right lower **eyelid**

H02.533   **Eyelid retraction** right eye, **unspecified eyelid** ▽

H02.534   **Eyelid retraction** left upper **eyelid**

H02.535   **Eyelid retraction** left lower **eyelid**

H02.536   **Eyelid retraction** left eye, **unspecified eyelid** ▽

H02.539   **Eyelid retraction unspecified eye, unspecified lid** ▽

H02.59   **Other disorders affecting eyelid function**
Deficient blink reflex
Sensory disorders

√5ᵗʰ **H02.6   Xanthelasma of eyelid**

H02.60   **Xanthelasma of unspecified eye, unspecified eyelid** ▽

H02.61   **Xanthelasma of** right upper **eyelid**

H02.62   **Xanthelasma of** right lower **eyelid**

H02.63   **Xanthelasma of** right eye, **unspecified eyelid** ▽

H02.64   **Xanthelasma of** left upper **eyelid**

H02.65   **Xanthelasma of** left lower **eyelid**

H02.66   **Xanthelasma of** left eye, **unspecified eyelid** ▽

√5ᵗʰ **H02.7   Other and unspecified degenerative disorders of eyelid and periocular area**

H02.70   **Unspecified degenerative disorders of eyelid and periocular area** ▽

√6ᵗʰ **H02.71   Chloasma of eyelid and periocular area**
Dyspigmentation of eyelid
Hyperpigmentation of eyelid

H02.711   **Chloasma of** right upper **eyelid and periocular area**

H02.712   **Chloasma of** right lower **eyelid and periocular area**

H02.713   **Chloasma of** right eye, **unspecified eyelid and periocular area** ▽

H02.714   **Chloasma of** left upper **eyelid and periocular area**

H02.715   **Chloasma of** left lower **eyelid and periocular area**

H02.716   **Chloasma of** left eye, **unspecified eyelid and periocular area** ▽

H02.719   **Chloasma of unspecified eye, unspecified eyelid and periocular area** ▽

√6ᵗʰ **H02.72   Madarosis of eyelid and periocular area**
Hypotrichosis of eyelid

H02.721   **Madarosis of** right upper **eyelid and periocular area**

H02.722   **Madarosis of** right lower **eyelid and periocular area**

H02.723   **Madarosis of** right eye, **unspecified eyelid and periocular area** ▽

H02.724   **Madarosis of** left upper **eyelid and periocular area**

H02.725   **Madarosis of** left lower **eyelid and periocular area**

H02.726   **Madarosis of** left eye, **unspecified eyelid and periocular area** ▽

H02.729   **Madarosis of unspecified eye, unspecified eyelid and periocular area** ▽

√6ᵗʰ **H02.73   Vitiligo of eyelid and periocular area**
Hypopigmentation of eyelid

H02.731   **Vitiligo of** right upper **eyelid and periocular area**

H02.732   **Vitiligo of** right lower **eyelid and periocular area**

H02.733   **Vitiligo of** right eye, **unspecified eyelid and periocular area**

H02.734   **Vitiligo of** left upper **eyelid and periocular area**

H02.735   **Vitiligo of** left lower **eyelid and periocular area**

H02.736   **Vitiligo of** left eye, **unspecified eyelid and periocular area** ▽

H02.739   **Vitiligo of unspecified eye, unspecified eyelid and periocular area** ▽

H02.79   **Other degenerative disorders of eyelid and periocular area**

√5ᵗʰ **H02.8   Other specified disorders of eyelid**

√6ᵗʰ **H02.81   Retained foreign body in eyelid**
Use additional code to identify the type of retained foreign body (Z18.-)

EXCLUDES 1   *laceration of eyelid with foreign body (S01.12-)*
retained intraocular foreign body (H44.6-, H44.7-)
superficial foreign body of eyelid and periocular area (S00.25-)

H02.811   **Retained foreign body in** right upper **eyelid**

H02.812   **Retained foreign body in** right lower **eyelid**

H02.813   **Retained foreign body in** right eye, **unspecified eyelid** ▽

H02.814   **Retained foreign body in** left upper **eyelid**

H02.815   **Retained foreign body in** left lower **eyelid**

H02.816   **Retained foreign body in** left eye, **unspecified eyelid** ▽

H02.819   **Retained foreign body in unspecified eye, unspecified eyelid** ▽

√6ᵗʰ **H02.82   Cysts of eyelid**
Sebaceous cyst of eyelid

H02.821   **Cysts of** right upper **eyelid**

H02.822   **Cysts of** right lower **eyelid**

H02.823   **Cysts of** right eye, **unspecified eyelid** ▽

H02.824   **Cysts of** left upper **eyelid**

H02.825   **Cysts of** left lower **eyelid**

H02.826   **Cysts of** left eye, **unspecified eyelid** ▽

H02.829   **Cysts of unspecified eye, unspecified eyelid** ▽

√6ᵗʰ **H02.83   Dermatochalasis of eyelid**
DEF: Acquired form of connective tissue disorder associated with decreased elastic tissue and abnormal elastin formation, resulting in loss of elasticity of the skin of the eyelid; generally associated with aging.

H02.831   **Dermatochalasis of** right upper **eyelid**

H02.832   **Dermatochalasis of** right lower **eyelid**

H02.833   **Dermatochalasis of** right eye, **unspecified eyelid** ▽

H02.834   **Dermatochalasis of** left upper **eyelid**

H02.835   **Dermatochalasis of** left lower **eyelid**

H02.836   **Dermatochalasis of** left eye, **unspecified eyelid** ▽

H02.839   **Dermatochalasis of unspecified eye, unspecified eyelid** ▽

√6ᵗʰ **H02.84   Edema of eyelid**
Hyperemia of eyelid

H02.841   **Edema of** right upper **eyelid**

H02.842   **Edema of** right lower **eyelid**

H02.843   **Edema of** right eye, **unspecified eyelid** ▽

H02.844   **Edema of** left upper **eyelid**

H02.845   **Edema of** left lower **eyelid**

H02.846   **Edema of** left eye, **unspecified eyelid** ▽

H02.849   **Edema of unspecified eye, unspecified eyelid** ▽

☑ Additional Character Req   √x7ᵗʰ Placeholder Alert   Case-Mix Diagnosis   Manifestation   ▽ Unspecified Dx   **EXCLUDES 1** Not coded here   **EXCLUDES 2** Not included here

✓6ᵗʰ **H02.85** Elephantiasis of eyelid
    H02.851 **Elephantiasis of right upper eyelid**
    H02.852 **Elephantiasis of right lower eyelid**
    H02.853 **Elephantiasis of right eye, unspecified** ▽
        eyelid
    H02.854 **Elephantiasis of left upper eyelid**
    H02.855 **Elephantiasis of left lower eyelid**
    H02.856 **Elephantiasis of left eye, unspecified** ▽
        eyelid
    H02.859 **Elephantiasis of unspecified eye,** ▽
        unspecified eyelid

✓6ᵗʰ **H02.86** Hypertrichosis of eyelid
    H02.861 **Hypertrichosis of right upper eyelid**
    H02.862 **Hypertrichosis of right lower eyelid**
    H02.863 **Hypertrichosis of right eye, unspecified** ▽
        eyelid
    H02.864 **Hypertrichosis of left upper eyelid**
    H02.865 **Hypertrichosis of left lower eyelid**
    H02.866 **Hypertrichosis of left eye, unspecified** ▽
        eyelid
    H02.869 **Hypertrichosis of unspecified eye,** ▽
        unspecified eyelid

✓6ᵗʰ **H02.87** Vascular anomalies of eyelid
    H02.871 **Vascular anomalies of right upper eyelid**
    H02.872 **Vascular anomalies of right lower eyelid**
    H02.873 **Vascular anomalies of right eye,** ▽
        unspecified eyelid
    H02.874 **Vascular anomalies of left upper eyelid**
    H02.875 **Vascular anomalies of left lower eyelid**
    H02.876 **Vascular anomalies of left eye,** ▽
        unspecified eyelid
    H02.879 **Vascular anomalies of unspecified eye,** ▽
        unspecified eyelid

  H02.89 **Other specified disorders of eyelid**
    Hemorrhage of eyelid

  H02.9 **Unspecified disorder of eyelid** ▽
    Disorder of eyelid NOS

✓4ᵗʰ **H04 Disorders of lacrimal system**
    EXCLUDES 1 *congenital malformations of lacrimal system (Q10.4-Q10.6)*

✓5ᵗʰ **H04.0** Dacryoadenitis
  ✓6ᵗʰ **H04.00** Unspecified dacryoadenitis
    H04.001 **Unspecified dacryoadenitis, right** ▽
        lacrimal gland
    H04.002 **Unspecified dacryoadenitis, left** ▽
        lacrimal gland
    H04.003 **Unspecified dacryoadenitis, bilateral** ▽
        lacrimal glands
    H04.009 **Unspecified dacryoadenitis,** ▽
        unspecified lacrimal gland

  ✓6ᵗʰ **H04.01** Acute dacryoadenitis
    H04.011 **Acute dacryoadenitis, right lacrimal gland**
    H04.012 **Acute dacryoadenitis, left lacrimal gland**
    H04.013 **Acute dacryoadenitis, bilateral lacrimal**
        glands
    H04.019 **Acute dacryoadenitis, unspecified** ▽
        lacrimal gland

  ✓6ᵗʰ **H04.02** Chronic dacryoadenitis
    H04.021 **Chronic dacryoadenitis, right lacrimal**
        gland
    H04.022 **Chronic dacryoadenitis, left lacrimal gland**
    H04.023 **Chronic dacryoadenitis, bilateral lacrimal**
        glands
    H04.029 **Chronic dacryoadenitis, unspecified** ▽
        lacrimal gland

  ✓6ᵗʰ **H04.03** Chronic enlargement of lacrimal gland
    H04.031 **Chronic enlargement of right lacrimal**
        gland
    H04.032 **Chronic enlargement of left lacrimal gland**
    H04.033 **Chronic enlargement of bilateral lacrimal**
        glands
    H04.039 **Chronic enlargement of unspecified** ▽
        lacrimal gland

✓5ᵗʰ **H04.1** Other disorders of lacrimal gland
  ✓6ᵗʰ **H04.11** Dacryops
    H04.111 **Dacryops of right lacrimal gland**
    H04.112 **Dacryops of left lacrimal gland**
    H04.113 **Dacryops of bilateral lacrimal glands**
    H04.119 **Dacryops of unspecified lacrimal gland** ▽

  ✓6ᵗʰ **H04.12** Dry eye syndrome
    Tear film insufficiency, NOS
    H04.121 **Dry eye syndrome of right lacrimal gland**
    H04.122 **Dry eye syndrome of left lacrimal gland**
    H04.123 **Dry eye syndrome of bilateral lacrimal**
        glands
    H04.129 **Dry eye syndrome of unspecified** ▽
        lacrimal gland

  ✓6ᵗʰ **H04.13** Lacrimal cyst
    Lacrimal cystic degeneration
    H04.131 **Lacrimal cyst, right lacrimal gland**
    H04.132 **Lacrimal cyst, left lacrimal gland**
    H04.133 **Lacrimal cyst, bilateral lacrimal glands**
    H04.139 **Lacrimal cyst, unspecified lacrimal** ▽
        gland

  ✓6ᵗʰ **H04.14** Primary lacrimal gland atrophy
    H04.141 **Primary lacrimal gland atrophy, right**
        lacrimal gland
    H04.142 **Primary lacrimal gland atrophy, left**
        lacrimal gland
    H04.143 **Primary lacrimal gland atrophy, bilateral**
        lacrimal glands
    H04.149 **Primary lacrimal gland atrophy,** ▽
        unspecified lacrimal gland

  ✓6ᵗʰ **H04.15** Secondary lacrimal gland atrophy
    H04.151 **Secondary lacrimal gland atrophy, right**
        lacrimal gland
    H04.152 **Secondary lacrimal gland atrophy, left**
        lacrimal gland
    H04.153 **Secondary lacrimal gland atrophy,**
        bilateral lacrimal glands
    H04.159 **Secondary lacrimal gland atrophy,** ▽
        unspecified lacrimal gland

  ✓6ᵗʰ **H04.16** Lacrimal gland dislocation
    H04.161 **Lacrimal gland dislocation, right lacrimal**
        gland
    H04.162 **Lacrimal gland dislocation, left lacrimal**
        gland
    H04.163 **Lacrimal gland dislocation, bilateral**
        lacrimal glands
    H04.169 **Lacrimal gland dislocation,** ▽
        unspecified lacrimal gland

  H04.19 **Other specified disorders of lacrimal gland**

✓5ᵗʰ **H04.2** Epiphora
  ✓6ᵗʰ **H04.20** Unspecified epiphora
    H04.201 **Unspecified epiphora, right lacrimal** ▽
        gland
    H04.202 **Unspecified epiphora, left lacrimal** ▽
        gland
    H04.203 **Unspecified epiphora, bilateral** ▽
        lacrimal glands
    H04.209 **Unspecified epiphora, unspecified** ▽
        lacrimal gland

  ✓6ᵗʰ **H04.21** Epiphora due to excess lacrimation
    H04.211 **Epiphora due to excess lacrimation, right**
        lacrimal gland
    H04.212 **Epiphora due to excess lacrimation, left**
        lacrimal gland
    H04.213 **Epiphora due to excess lacrimation,**
        bilateral lacrimal glands
    H04.219 **Epiphora due to excess lacrimation,** ▽
        unspecified lacrimal gland

  ✓6ᵗʰ **H04.22** Epiphora due to insufficient drainage
    H04.221 **Epiphora due to insufficient drainage,**
        right lacrimal gland
    H04.222 **Epiphora due to insufficient drainage,**
        left lacrimal gland

H04.223   Epiphora due to insufficient drainage, bilateral lacrimal glands

H04.229   Epiphora due to insufficient drainage, unspecified lacrimal gland ▽

✓5ᵗʰ **H04.3**   **Acute and unspecified inflammation of lacrimal passages**
EXCLUDES 1   neonatal dacryocystitis (P39.1)

✓6ᵗʰ **H04.30**   Unspecified dacryocystitis

H04.301   Unspecified dacryocystitis of right lacrimal passage ▽

H04.302   Unspecified dacryocystitis of left lacrimal passage ▽

H04.303   Unspecified dacryocystitis of bilateral lacrimal passages ▽

H04.309   Unspecified dacryocystitis of unspecified lacrimal passage ▽

✓6ᵗʰ **H04.31**   Phlegmonous dacryocystitis

H04.311   Phlegmonous dacryocystitis of right lacrimal passage

H04.312   Phlegmonous dacryocystitis of left lacrimal passage

H04.313   Phlegmonous dacryocystitis of bilateral lacrimal passages

H04.319   Phlegmonous dacryocystitis of unspecified lacrimal passage ▽

✓6ᵗʰ **H04.32**   Acute dacryocystitis
Acute dacryopericystitis

H04.321   Acute dacryocystitis of right lacrimal passage

H04.322   Acute dacryocystitis of left lacrimal passage

H04.323   Acute dacryocystitis of bilateral lacrimal passages

H04.329   Acute dacryocystitis of unspecified lacrimal passage ▽

✓6ᵗʰ **H04.33**   Acute lacrimal canaliculitis

H04.331   Acute lacrimal canaliculitis of right lacrimal passage

H04.332   Acute lacrimal canaliculitis of left lacrimal passage

H04.333   Acute lacrimal canaliculitis of bilateral lacrimal passages

H04.339   Acute lacrimal canaliculitis of unspecified lacrimal passage ▽

✓5ᵗʰ **H04.4**   **Chronic inflammation of lacrimal passages**

✓6ᵗʰ **H04.41**   Chronic dacryocystitis

H04.411   Chronic dacryocystitis of right lacrimal passage

H04.412   Chronic dacryocystitis of left lacrimal passage

H04.413   Chronic dacryocystitis of bilateral lacrimal passages

H04.419   Chronic dacryocystitis of unspecified lacrimal passage ▽

✓6ᵗʰ **H04.42**   Chronic lacrimal canaliculitis

H04.421   Chronic lacrimal canaliculitis of right lacrimal passage

H04.422   Chronic lacrimal canaliculitis of left lacrimal passage

H04.423   Chronic lacrimal canaliculitis of bilateral lacrimal passages

H04.429   Chronic lacrimal canaliculitis of unspecified lacrimal passage ▽

✓6ᵗʰ **H04.43**   Chronic lacrimal mucocele

H04.431   Chronic lacrimal mucocele of right lacrimal passage

H04.432   Chronic lacrimal mucocele of left lacrimal passage

H04.433   Chronic lacrimal mucocele of bilateral lacrimal passages

H04.439   Chronic lacrimal mucocele of unspecified lacrimal passage ▽

✓6ᵗʰ **H04.5**   **Stenosis and insufficiency of lacrimal passages**

✓6ᵗʰ **H04.51**   Dacryolith

H04.511   Dacryolith of right lacrimal passage

H04.512   Dacryolith of left lacrimal passage

H04.513   Dacryolith of bilateral lacrimal passages

H04.519   Dacryolith of unspecified lacrimal passage ▽

✓6ᵗʰ **H04.52**   Eversion of lacrimal punctum

H04.521   Eversion of right lacrimal punctum

H04.522   Eversion of left lacrimal punctum

H04.523   Eversion of bilateral lacrimal punctum

H04.529   Eversion of unspecified lacrimal punctum ▽

✓6ᵗʰ **H04.53**   Neonatal obstruction of nasolacrimal duct
EXCLUDES 1   congenital stenosis and stricture of lacrimal duct (Q10.5)

H04.531   Neonatal obstruction of right nasolacrimal duct   N

H04.532   Neonatal obstruction of left nasolacrimal duct   N

H04.533   Neonatal obstruction of bilateral nasolacrimal duct   N

H04.539   Neonatal obstruction of unspecified nasolacrimal duct   N ▽

✓6ᵗʰ **H04.54**   Stenosis of lacrimal canaliculi

H04.541   Stenosis of right lacrimal canaliculi

H04.542   Stenosis of left lacrimal canaliculi

H04.543   Stenosis of bilateral lacrimal canaliculi

H04.549   Stenosis of unspecified lacrimal canaliculi ▽

✓6ᵗʰ **H04.55**   Acquired stenosis of nasolacrimal duct

H04.551   Acquired stenosis of right nasolacrimal duct

H04.552   Acquired stenosis of left nasolacrimal duct

H04.553   Acquired stenosis of bilateral nasolacrimal duct

H04.559   Acquired stenosis of unspecified nasolacrimal duct ▽

✓6ᵗʰ **H04.56**   Stenosis of lacrimal punctum

H04.561   Stenosis of right lacrimal punctum

H04.562   Stenosis of left lacrimal punctum

H04.563   Stenosis of bilateral lacrimal punctum

H04.569   Stenosis of unspecified lacrimal punctum ▽

✓6ᵗʰ **H04.57**   Stenosis of lacrimal sac

H04.571   Stenosis of right lacrimal sac

H04.572   Stenosis of left lacrimal sac

H04.573   Stenosis of bilateral lacrimal sac

H04.579   Stenosis of unspecified lacrimal sac ▽

✓5ᵗʰ **H04.6**   **Other changes of lacrimal passages**

✓6ᵗʰ **H04.61**   Lacrimal fistula

H04.611   Lacrimal fistula right lacrimal passage

H04.612   Lacrimal fistula left lacrimal passage

H04.613   Lacrimal fistula bilateral lacrimal passages

H04.619   Lacrimal fistula unspecified lacrimal passage ▽

H04.69   Other changes of lacrimal passages

✓5ᵗʰ **H04.8**   **Other disorders of lacrimal system**

✓6ᵗʰ **H04.81**   Granuloma of lacrimal passages

H04.811   Granuloma of right lacrimal passage

H04.812   Granuloma of left lacrimal passage

H04.813   Granuloma of bilateral lacrimal passages

H04.819   Granuloma of unspecified lacrimal passage ▽

H04.89   Other disorders of lacrimal system

H04.9   Disorder of lacrimal system, unspecified ▽

✓4ᵗʰ **H05**   **Disorders of orbit**
EXCLUDES 1   congenital malformation of orbit (Q10.7)

✓5ᵗʰ **H05.0**   Acute inflammation of orbit

H05.00   Unspecified acute inflammation of orbit ▽

✓6ᵗʰ **H05.01**   Cellulitis of orbit
Abscess of orbit

H05.011   Cellulitis of right orbit

H05.012   Cellulitis of left orbit

H05.013   Cellulitis of bilateral orbits

H05.019   Cellulitis of unspecified orbit ▽

✓6ᵗʰ **H05.02**   Osteomyelitis of orbit

H05.021   Osteomyelitis of right orbit

✔ Additional Character Req   ✔x7ᵗʰ Placeholder Alert   Case-Mix Diagnosis   Manifestation   ▽ Unspecified Dx   *EXCLUDES 1* Not coded here   *EXCLUDES 2* Not included here

            H05.022   **Osteomyelitis of** left **orbit**
            H05.023   **Osteomyelitis of** bilateral **orbits**
            H05.029   **Osteomyelitis of unspecified orbit** ▽

✓6th   **H05.03**   Periostitis **of orbit**
            H05.031   **Periostitis of** right **orbit**
            H05.032   **Periostitis of** left **orbit**
            H05.033   **Periostitis of** bilateral **orbits**
            H05.039   **Periostitis of unspecified orbit** ▽

✓6th   **H05.04**   Tenonitis **of orbit**
            H05.041   **Tenonitis of** right **orbit**
            H05.042   **Tenonitis of** left **orbit**
            H05.043   **Tenonitis of** bilateral **orbits**
            H05.049   **Tenonitis of unspecified orbit** ▽

✓5th   **H05.1**   Chronic inflammatory **disorders of orbit**
        H05.10   **Unspecified chronic inflammatory disorders** ▽
                 of orbit

✓6th   **H05.11**   Granuloma **of orbit**
            Pseudotumor (inflammatory) of orbit
            H05.111   **Granuloma of** right **orbit**
            H05.112   **Granuloma of** left **orbit**
            H05.113   **Granuloma of** bilateral **orbits**
            H05.119   **Granuloma of unspecified orbit** ▽

✓6th   **H05.12**   **Orbital** myositis
            H05.121   **Orbital myositis,** right **orbit**
            H05.122   **Orbital myositis,** left **orbit**
            H05.123   **Orbital myositis,** bilateral
            H05.129   **Orbital myositis, unspecified orbit** ▽

✓5th   **H05.2**   **Exophthalmic conditions**
        H05.20   **Unspecified exophthalmos** ▽

✓6th   **H05.21**   **Displacement (lateral) of globe**
            H05.211   **Displacement (lateral) of globe,** right **eye**
            H05.212   **Displacement (lateral) of globe,** left **eye**
            H05.213   **Displacement (lateral) of globe,** bilateral
            H05.219   **Displacement (lateral) of globe,** ▽
                  unspecified eye

✓6th   **H05.22**   **Edema of orbit**
            Orbital congestion
            H05.221   **Edema of** right **orbit**
            H05.222   **Edema of** left **orbit**
            H05.223   **Edema of** bilateral **orbit**
            H05.229   **Edema of unspecified orbit** ▽

✓6th   **H05.23**   **Hemorrhage of orbit**
            H05.231   **Hemorrhage of** right **orbit**
            H05.232   **Hemorrhage of** left **orbit**
            H05.233   **Hemorrhage of** bilateral **orbit**
            H05.239   **Hemorrhage of unspecified orbit** ▽

✓6th   **H05.24**   Constant **exophthalmos**
            H05.241   **Constant exophthalmos,** right **eye**
            H05.242   **Constant exophthalmos,** left **eye**
            H05.243   **Constant exophthalmos,** bilateral
            H05.249   **Constant exophthalmos, unspecified** ▽
                  eye

✓6th   **H05.25**   Intermittent **exophthalmos**
            H05.251   **Intermittent exophthalmos,** right **eye**
            H05.252   **Intermittent exophthalmos,** left **eye**
            H05.253   **Intermittent exophthalmos,** bilateral
            H05.259   **Intermittent exophthalmos,** ▽
                  unspecified eye

✓6th   **H05.26**   Pulsating **exophthalmos**
            H05.261   **Pulsating exophthalmos,** right **eye**
            H05.262   **Pulsating exophthalmos,** left **eye**
            H05.263   **Pulsating exophthalmos,** bilateral
            H05.269   **Pulsating exophthalmos, unspecified** ▽
                  eye

✓5th   **H05.3**   **Deformity of orbit**
        EXCLUDES 1   *congenital deformity of orbit (Q10.7)*
                 hypertelorism (Q75.2)
        H05.30   **Unspecified deformity of orbit** ▽

✓6th   **H05.31**   Atrophy **of orbit**
            H05.311   **Atrophy of** right **orbit**
            H05.312   **Atrophy of** left **orbit**
            H05.313   **Atrophy of** bilateral **orbit**

            H05.319   **Atrophy of unspecified orbit** ▽

✓6th   **H05.32**   **Deformity of orbit** due to bone disease
            Code also associated bone disease
            H05.321   **Deformity of** right **orbit due to bone disease**
            H05.322   **Deformity of** left **orbit due to bone disease**
            H05.323   **Deformity of** bilateral **orbits due to bone disease**
            H05.329   **Deformity of unspecified orbit due to** ▽
                  bone disease

✓6th   **H05.33**   **Deformity of orbit** due to trauma or surgery
            H05.331   **Deformity of** right **orbit due to trauma or surgery**
            H05.332   **Deformity of** left **orbit due to trauma or surgery**
            H05.333   **Deformity of** bilateral **orbits due to trauma or surgery**
            H05.339   **Deformity of unspecified orbit due to** ▽
                  trauma or surgery

✓6th   **H05.34**   Enlargement **of orbit**
            H05.341   **Enlargement of** right **orbit**
            H05.342   **Enlargement of** left **orbit**
            H05.343   **Enlargement of** bilateral **orbits**
            H05.349   **Enlargement of unspecified orbit** ▽

✓6th   **H05.35**   Exostosis **of orbit**
            H05.351   **Exostosis of** right **orbit**
            H05.352   **Exostosis of** left **orbit**
            H05.353   **Exostosis of** bilateral **orbits**
            H05.359   **Exostosis of unspecified orbit** ▽

✓5th   **H05.4**   **Enophthalmos**

✓6th   **H05.40**   Unspecified **enophthalmos**
            H05.401   **Unspecified enophthalmos,** right **eye** ▽
            H05.402   **Unspecified enophthalmos,** left **eye** ▽
            H05.403   **Unspecified enophthalmos,** bilateral ▽
            H05.409   **Unspecified enophthalmos,** ▽
                  unspecified eye

✓6th   **H05.41**   **Enophthalmos** due to atrophy of orbital tissue
            H05.411   **Enophthalmos due to atrophy of orbital tissue,** right **eye**
            H05.412   **Enophthalmos due to atrophy of orbital tissue,** left **eye**
            H05.413   **Enophthalmos due to atrophy of orbital tissue,** bilateral
            H05.419   **Enophthalmos due to atrophy of** ▽
                  orbital tissue, unspecified eye

✓6th   **H05.42**   **Enophthalmos** due to trauma or surgery
            H05.421   **Enophthalmos due to trauma or surgery,** right **eye**
            H05.422   **Enophthalmos due to trauma or surgery,** left **eye**
            H05.423   **Enophthalmos due to trauma or surgery,** bilateral
            H05.429   **Enophthalmos due to trauma or** ▽
                  surgery, unspecified eye

✓5th   **H05.5**   **Retained (old) foreign body following penetrating wound of orbit**
        Retrobulbar foreign body
        Use additional code to identify the type of retained foreign body (Z18.-)
        EXCLUDES 1   *current penetrating wound of orbit (S05.4-)*
        EXCLUDES 2   *retained foreign body of eyelid (H02.81-)*
                 retained intraocular foreign body (H44.6-, H44.7-)
        H05.50   **Retained (old) foreign body following** ▽
                 penetrating wound of unspecified orbit
        H05.51   **Retained (old) foreign body following penetrating wound of** right **orbit**
        H05.52   **Retained (old) foreign body following penetrating wound of** left **orbit**
        H05.53   **Retained (old) foreign body following penetrating wound of** bilateral **orbits**

✓5th   **H05.8**   **Other disorders of orbit**

✓6th   **H05.81**   **Cyst of orbit**
            Encephalocele of orbit
            H05.811   **Cyst of** right **orbit**
            H05.812   **Cyst of** left **orbit**

Ⓝ Newborn: 0   Ⓟ Pediatric: 0-17   Ⓜ Maternity: 12-55   Ⓐ Adult: 15-124   NRS Nonroutine supply Dx   NCDx Noncancer Dx   PDx Primary Dx   ▶◀ Revised Text   ● New Code   ▲ Revised Title

574   ICD-10-CM 2018

H05.813   Cyst of bilateral orbits
H05.81   Cyst of unspecified orbit ▽

✓6ᵗʰ H05.82   **Myopathy of extraocular muscles**
    H05.821   Myopathy of extraocular muscles, right orbit
    H05.822   Myopathy of extraocular muscles, left orbit
    H05.823   Myopathy of extraocular muscles, bilateral
    H05.829   Myopathy of extraocular muscles, unspecified orbit ▽

H05.89   Other disorders of orbit
H05.9   Unspecified disorder of orbit ▽

Disorders of conjunctiva (H10-H11)

✓4ᵗʰ **H10 Conjunctivitis**
   EXCLUDES 1   *keratoconjunctivitis (H16.2-)*

✓5ᵗʰ H10.0   **Mucopurulent conjunctivitis**
   ✓6ᵗʰ H10.01   **Acute follicular conjunctivitis**
    H10.011   Acute follicular conjunctivitis, right eye
    H10.012   Acute follicular conjunctivitis, left eye
    H10.013   Acute follicular conjunctivitis, bilateral
    H10.019   Acute follicular conjunctivitis, unspecified eye ▽

   ✓6ᵗʰ H10.02   **Other mucopurulent conjunctivitis**
    H10.021   Other mucopurulent conjunctivitis, right eye
    H10.022   Other mucopurulent conjunctivitis, left eye
    H10.023   Other mucopurulent conjunctivitis, bilateral
    H10.029   Other mucopurulent conjunctivitis, unspecified eye ▽

✓5ᵗʰ H10.1   **Acute atopic conjunctivitis**
   Acute papillary conjunctivitis
   H10.10   Acute atopic conjunctivitis, unspecified eye ▽
   H10.11   Acute atopic conjunctivitis, right eye
   H10.12   Acute atopic conjunctivitis, left eye
   H10.13   Acute atopic conjunctivitis, bilateral

✓5ᵗʰ H10.2   **Other acute conjunctivitis**
   ✓6ᵗʰ H10.21   **Acute toxic conjunctivitis**
    Acute chemical conjunctivitis
    Code first (T51-T65) to identify chemical and intent
    EXCLUDES 1   *burn and corrosion of eye and adnexa (T26.-)*
    H10.211   Acute toxic conjunctivitis, right eye
    H10.212   Acute toxic conjunctivitis, left eye
    H10.213   Acute toxic conjunctivitis, bilateral
    H10.219   Acute toxic conjunctivitis, unspecified eye ▽

   ✓6ᵗʰ H10.22   **Pseudomembranous conjunctivitis**
    H10.221   Pseudomembranous conjunctivitis, right eye
    H10.222   Pseudomembranous conjunctivitis, left eye
    H10.223   Pseudomembranous conjunctivitis, bilateral
    H10.229   Pseudomembranous conjunctivitis, unspecified eye ▽

   ✓6ᵗʰ H10.23   **Serous conjunctivitis, except viral**
    EXCLUDES 1   *viral conjunctivitis (B30.-)*
    H10.231   Serous conjunctivitis, except viral, right eye
    H10.232   Serous conjunctivitis, except viral, left eye
    H10.233   Serous conjunctivitis, except viral, bilateral
    H10.239   Serous conjunctivitis, except viral, unspecified eye ▽

✓5ᵗʰ H10.3   **Unspecified acute conjunctivitis**
   EXCLUDES 1   *ophthalmia neonatorum NOS (P39.1)*
   H10.30   Unspecified acute conjunctivitis, unspecified eye ▽
   H10.31   Unspecified acute conjunctivitis, right eye ▽
   H10.32   Unspecified acute conjunctivitis, left eye ▽
   H10.33   Unspecified acute conjunctivitis, bilateral ▽

✓5ᵗʰ H10.4   **Chronic conjunctivitis**
   ✓6ᵗʰ H10.40   **Unspecified chronic conjunctivitis**
    H10.401   Unspecified chronic conjunctivitis, right eye ▽
    H10.402   Unspecified chronic conjunctivitis, left eye ▽
    H10.403   Unspecified chronic conjunctivitis, bilateral ▽
    H10.409   Unspecified chronic conjunctivitis, unspecified eye ▽

   ✓6ᵗʰ H10.41   **Chronic giant papillary conjunctivitis**
    H10.411   Chronic giant papillary conjunctivitis, right eye
    H10.412   Chronic giant papillary conjunctivitis, left eye
    H10.413   Chronic giant papillary conjunctivitis, bilateral
    H10.419   Chronic giant papillary conjunctivitis, unspecified eye ▽

   ✓6ᵗʰ H10.42   **Simple chronic conjunctivitis**
    H10.421   Simple chronic conjunctivitis, right eye
    H10.422   Simple chronic conjunctivitis, left eye
    H10.423   Simple chronic conjunctivitis, bilateral
    H10.429   Simple chronic conjunctivitis, unspecified eye ▽

   ✓6ᵗʰ H10.43   **Chronic follicular conjunctivitis**
    H10.431   Chronic follicular conjunctivitis, right eye
    H10.432   Chronic follicular conjunctivitis, left eye
    H10.433   Chronic follicular conjunctivitis, bilateral
    H10.439   Chronic follicular conjunctivitis, unspecified eye ▽

   H10.44   **Vernal conjunctivitis**
    EXCLUDES 1   *vernal keratoconjunctivitis with limbar and corneal involvement (H16.26-)*

   H10.45   Other chronic allergic conjunctivitis

✓5ᵗʰ H10.5   **Blepharoconjunctivitis**
   ✓6ᵗʰ H10.50   **Unspecified blepharoconjunctivitis**
    H10.501   Unspecified blepharoconjunctivitis, right eye ▽
    H10.502   Unspecified blepharoconjunctivitis, left eye ▽
    H10.503   Unspecified blepharoconjunctivitis, bilateral ▽
    H10.509   Unspecified blepharoconjunctivitis, unspecified eye ▽

   ✓6ᵗʰ H10.51   **Ligneous conjunctivitis**
    H10.511   Ligneous conjunctivitis, right eye
    H10.512   Ligneous conjunctivitis, left eye
    H10.513   Ligneous conjunctivitis, bilateral
    H10.519   Ligneous conjunctivitis, unspecified eye ▽

   ✓6ᵗʰ H10.52   **Angular blepharoconjunctivitis**
    H10.521   Angular blepharoconjunctivitis, right eye
    H10.522   Angular blepharoconjunctivitis, left eye
    H10.523   Angular blepharoconjunctivitis, bilateral
    H10.529   Angular blepharoconjunctivitis, unspecified eye ▽

   ✓6ᵗʰ H10.53   **Contact blepharoconjunctivitis**
    H10.531   Contact blepharoconjunctivitis, right eye
    H10.532   Contact blepharoconjunctivitis, left eye
    H10.533   Contact blepharoconjunctivitis, bilateral
    H10.539   Contact blepharoconjunctivitis, unspecified eye ▽

✓5ᵗʰ H10.8   **Other conjunctivitis**
   ✓6ᵗʰ H10.81   **Pingueculitis**
    EXCLUDES 1   *pinguecula (H11.15-)*
    H10.811   Pingueculitis, right eye
    H10.812   Pingueculitis, left eye
    H10.813   Pingueculitis, bilateral
    H10.819   Pingueculitis, unspecified eye ▽
   H10.89   Other conjunctivitis
H10.9   Unspecified conjunctivitis ▽

✓ Additional Character Req   ✓×7ᵗʰ Placeholder Alert   Case-Mix Diagnosis   Manifestation   ▽ Unspecified Dx   EXCLUDES 1 Not coded here   EXCLUDES 2 Not included here

ICD-10-CM 2018   575

Chapter 7. Diseases of the Eye and Adnexa

Pterygium

Pterygium

Pinguecula

Pinguecula

✓4ᵗʰ **H11 Other disorders of conjunctiva**
    EXCLUDES 1   *keratoconjunctivitis (H16.2-)*

✓5ᵗʰ **H11.0 Pterygium of eye**
    EXCLUDES 1   *pseudopterygium (H11.81-)*

    ✓6ᵗʰ **H11.00 Unspecified pterygium of eye**
      H11.001   Unspecified pterygium of right eye   ▽
      H11.002   Unspecified pterygium of left eye   ▽
      H11.003   Unspecified pterygium of eye, bilateral   ▽
      H11.009   Unspecified pterygium of unspecified eye   ▽

    ✓6ᵗʰ **H11.01 Amyloid pterygium**
      H11.011   Amyloid pterygium of right eye
      H11.012   Amyloid pterygium of left eye
      H11.013   Amyloid pterygium of eye, bilateral
      H11.019   Amyloid pterygium of unspecified eye   ▽

    ✓6ᵗʰ **H11.02 Central pterygium of eye**
      H11.021   Central pterygium of right eye
      H11.022   Central pterygium of left eye
      H11.023   Central pterygium of eye, bilateral
      H11.029   Central pterygium of unspecified eye   ▽

    ✓6ᵗʰ **H11.03 Double pterygium of eye**
      H11.031   Double pterygium of right eye
      H11.032   Double pterygium of left eye
      H11.033   Double pterygium of eye, bilateral
      H11.039   Double pterygium of unspecified eye   ▽

    ✓6ᵗʰ **H11.04 Peripheral pterygium of eye, stationary**
      H11.041   Peripheral pterygium, stationary, right eye
      H11.042   Peripheral pterygium, stationary, left eye
      H11.043   Peripheral pterygium, stationary, bilateral
      H11.049   Peripheral pterygium, stationary, unspecified eye   ▽

    ✓6ᵗʰ **H11.05 Peripheral pterygium of eye, progressive**
      H11.051   Peripheral pterygium, progressive, right eye
      H11.052   Peripheral pterygium, progressive, left eye
      H11.053   Peripheral pterygium, progressive, bilateral
      H11.059   Peripheral pterygium, progressive, unspecified eye   ▽

    ✓6ᵗʰ **H11.06 Recurrent pterygium of eye**
      H11.061   Recurrent pterygium of right eye
      H11.062   Recurrent pterygium of left eye
      H11.063   Recurrent pterygium of eye, bilateral
      H11.069   Recurrent pterygium of unspecified eye   ▽

✓5ᵗʰ **H11.1 Conjunctival degenerations and deposits**
    EXCLUDES 2   *pseudopterygium (H11.81)*
      H11.10   Unspecified conjunctival degenerations   ▽

    ✓6ᵗʰ **H11.11 Conjunctival deposits**
      H11.111   Conjunctival deposits, right eye
      H11.112   Conjunctival deposits, left eye
      H11.113   Conjunctival deposits, bilateral
      H11.119   Conjunctival deposits, unspecified eye   ▽

    ✓6ᵗʰ **H11.12 Conjunctival concretions**
      H11.121   Conjunctival concretions, right eye
      H11.122   Conjunctival concretions, left eye

     H11.123   Conjunctival concretions, bilateral
     H11.129   Conjunctival concretions, unspecified eye   ▽

    ✓6ᵗʰ **H11.13 Conjunctival pigmentations**
      Conjunctival argyrosis [argyria]
      H11.131   Conjunctival pigmentations, right eye
      H11.132   Conjunctival pigmentations, left eye
      H11.133   Conjunctival pigmentations, bilateral
      H11.139   Conjunctival pigmentations, unspecified eye   ▽

    ✓6ᵗʰ **H11.14 Conjunctival xerosis, unspecified**
      EXCLUDES 1   *xerosis of conjunctiva due to vitamin A deficiency (E50.0, E50.1)*
      DEF: Abnormal dryness of conjunctiva due to lack of insufficient tears or conjunctival secretions.
      H11.141   Conjunctival xerosis, unspecified, right eye   ▽
      H11.142   Conjunctival xerosis , unspecified, left eye   ▽
      H11.143   Conjunctival xerosis, unspecified, bilateral   ▽
      H11.149   Conjunctival xerosis, unspecified, unspecified eye   ▽

    ✓6ᵗʰ **H11.15 Pinguecula**
      EXCLUDES 1   *pingueculitis (H10.81-)*
      H11.151   Pinguecula, right eye
      H11.152   Pinguecula, left eye
      H11.153   Pinguecula, bilateral
      H11.159   Pinguecula, unspecified eye   ▽

✓5ᵗʰ **H11.2 Conjunctival scars**

    ✓6ᵗʰ **H11.21 Conjunctival adhesions and strands (localized)**
      H11.211   Conjunctival adhesions and strands (localized), right eye
      H11.212   Conjunctival adhesions and strands (localized), left eye
      H11.213   Conjunctival adhesions and strands (localized), bilateral
      H11.219   Conjunctival adhesions and strands (localized), unspecified eye   ▽

    ✓6ᵗʰ **H11.22 Conjunctival granuloma**
      H11.221   Conjunctival granuloma, right eye
      H11.222   Conjunctival granuloma, left eye
      H11.223   Conjunctival granuloma, bilateral
      H11.229   Conjunctival granuloma, unspecified   ▽

    ✓6ᵗʰ **H11.23 Symblepharon**
      H11.231   Symblepharon, right eye
      H11.232   Symblepharon, left eye
      H11.233   Symblepharon, bilateral
      H11.239   Symblepharon, unspecified eye   ▽

    ✓6ᵗʰ **H11.24 Scarring of conjunctiva**
      H11.241   Scarring of conjunctiva, right eye
      H11.242   Scarring of conjunctiva, left eye
      H11.243   Scarring of conjunctiva, bilateral
      H11.249   Scarring of conjunctiva, unspecified eye   ▽

Ⓝ Newborn: 0   Ⓟ Pediatric: 0-17   Ⓜ Maternity: 12-55   Ⓐ Adult: 15-124   **NRS** Nonroutine supply Dx   **NCDx** Noncancer Dx   **PDx** Primary Dx   ▶◀ Revised Text   ● New Code   ▲ Revised Title

576   ICD-10-CM 2018

✓5ᵗʰ **H11.3 Conjunctival hemorrhage**
      Subconjunctival hemorrhage
      H11.30 Conjunctival hemorrhage, unspecified eye   ▽
      H11.31 Conjunctival hemorrhage, right eye
      H11.32 Conjunctival hemorrhage, left eye
      H11.33 Conjunctival hemorrhage, bilateral

✓5ᵗʰ **H11.4 Other conjunctival vascular disorders and cysts**
      ✓6ᵗʰ **H11.41 Vascular abnormalities of conjunctiva**
            Conjunctival aneurysm
            H11.411 Vascular abnormalities of conjunctiva, right eye
            H11.412 Vascular abnormalities of conjunctiva, left eye
            H11.413 Vascular abnormalities of conjunctiva, bilateral
            H11.419 Vascular abnormalities of conjunctiva, unspecified eye   ▽
      ✓6ᵗʰ **H11.42 Conjunctival edema**
            H11.421 Conjunctival edema, right eye
            H11.422 Conjunctival edema, left eye
            H11.423 Conjunctival edema, bilateral
            H11.429 Conjunctival edema, unspecified eye   ▽
      ✓6ᵗʰ **H11.43 Conjunctival hyperemia**
            H11.431 Conjunctival hyperemia, right eye
            H11.432 Conjunctival hyperemia, left eye
            H11.433 Conjunctival hyperemia, bilateral
            H11.439 Conjunctival hyperemia, unspecified eye   ▽
      ✓6ᵗʰ **H11.44 Conjunctival cysts**
            H11.441 Conjunctival cysts, right eye
            H11.442 Conjunctival cysts, left eye
            H11.443 Conjunctival cysts, bilateral
            H11.449 Conjunctival cysts, unspecified eye   ▽

✓5ᵗʰ **H11.8 Other specified disorders of conjunctiva**
      ✓6ᵗʰ **H11.81 Pseudopterygium of conjunctiva**
            H11.811 Pseudopterygium of conjunctiva, right eye
            H11.812 Pseudopterygium of conjunctiva, left eye
            H11.813 Pseudopterygium of conjunctiva, bilateral
            H11.819 Pseudopterygium of conjunctiva, unspecified eye   ▽
      ✓6ᵗʰ **H11.82 Conjunctivochalasis**
            H11.821 Conjunctivochalasis, right eye
            H11.822 Conjunctivochalasis, left eye
            H11.823 Conjunctivochalasis, bilateral
            H11.829 Conjunctivochalasis, unspecified eye   ▽
      H11.89 Other specified disorders of conjunctiva
H11.9 Unspecified disorder of conjunctiva   ▽

Disorders of sclera, cornea, iris and ciliary body (H15-H22)

✓4ᵗʰ **H15 Disorders of sclera**
   ✓5ᵗʰ **H15.0 Scleritis**
      ✓6ᵗʰ **H15.00 Unspecified scleritis**
            H15.001 Unspecified scleritis, right eye   ▽
            H15.002 Unspecified scleritis, left eye   ▽
            H15.003 Unspecified scleritis, bilateral   ▽
            H15.009 Unspecified scleritis, unspecified eye   ▽
      ✓6ᵗʰ **H15.01 Anterior scleritis**
            H15.011 Anterior scleritis, right eye
            H15.012 Anterior scleritis, left eye
            H15.013 Anterior scleritis, bilateral
            H15.019 Anterior scleritis, unspecified eye   ▽
      ✓6ᵗʰ **H15.02 Brawny scleritis**
            H15.021 Brawny scleritis, right eye
            H15.022 Brawny scleritis, left eye
            H15.023 Brawny scleritis, bilateral
            H15.029 Brawny scleritis, unspecified eye   ▽

✓6ᵗʰ **H15.03 Posterior scleritis**
      Sclerotenonitis
      H15.031 Posterior scleritis, right eye
      H15.032 Posterior scleritis, left eye
      H15.033 Posterior scleritis, bilateral
      H15.039 Posterior scleritis, unspecified eye   ▽
✓6ᵗʰ **H15.04 Scleritis with corneal involvement**
      H15.041 Scleritis with corneal involvement, right eye
      H15.042 Scleritis with corneal involvement, left eye
      H15.043 Scleritis with corneal involvement, bilateral
      H15.049 Scleritis with corneal involvement, unspecified eye   ▽
✓6ᵗʰ **H15.05 Scleromalacia perforans**
      H15.051 Scleromalacia perforans, right eye
      H15.052 Scleromalacia perforans, left eye
      H15.053 Scleromalacia perforans, bilateral
      H15.059 Scleromalacia perforans, unspecified eye   ▽
✓6ᵗʰ **H15.09 Other scleritis**
      Scleral abscess
      H15.091 Other scleritis, right eye
      H15.092 Other scleritis, left eye
      H15.093 Other scleritis, bilateral
      H15.099 Other scleritis, unspecified eye   ▽

✓5ᵗʰ **H15.1 Episcleritis**
   ✓6ᵗʰ **H15.10 Unspecified episcleritis**
         H15.101 Unspecified episcleritis, right eye   ▽
         H15.102 Unspecified episcleritis, left eye   ▽
         H15.103 Unspecified episcleritis, bilateral   ▽
         H15.109 Unspecified episcleritis, unspecified eye   ▽
   ✓6ᵗʰ **H15.11 Episcleritis periodica fugax**
         H15.111 Episcleritis periodica fugax, right eye
         H15.112 Episcleritis periodica fugax, left eye
         H15.113 Episcleritis periodica fugax, bilateral
         H15.119 Episcleritis periodica fugax, unspecified eye ▽
   ✓6ᵗʰ **H15.12 Nodular episcleritis**
         H15.121 Nodular episcleritis, right eye
         H15.122 Nodular episcleritis, left eye
         H15.123 Nodular episcleritis, bilateral
         H15.129 Nodular episcleritis, unspecified eye   ▽

✓5ᵗʰ **H15.8 Other disorders of sclera**
      EXCLUDES 2 blue sclera (Q13.5)
                  degenerative myopia (H44.2-)
   ✓6ᵗʰ **H15.81 Equatorial staphyloma**
         H15.811 Equatorial staphyloma, right eye
         H15.812 Equatorial staphyloma, left eye
         H15.813 Equatorial staphyloma, bilateral
         H15.819 Equatorial staphyloma, unspecified eye   ▽
   ✓6ᵗʰ **H15.82 Localized anterior staphyloma**
         H15.821 Localized anterior staphyloma, right eye
         H15.822 Localized anterior staphyloma, left eye
         H15.823 Localized anterior staphyloma, bilateral
         H15.829 Localized anterior staphyloma, unspecified eye ▽
   ✓6ᵗʰ **H15.83 Staphyloma posticum**
         H15.831 Staphyloma posticum, right eye
         H15.832 Staphyloma posticum, left eye
         H15.833 Staphyloma posticum, bilateral
         H15.839 Staphyloma posticum, unspecified eye   ▽
   ✓6ᵗʰ **H15.84 Scleral ectasia**
         H15.841 Scleral ectasia, right eye
         H15.842 Scleral ectasia, left eye
         H15.843 Scleral ectasia, bilateral
         H15.849 Scleral ectasia, unspecified eye   ▽

✓6ᵗʰ **H15.85** Ring **staphyloma**
     H15.851 Ring staphyloma, right eye
     H15.852 Ring staphyloma, left eye
     H15.853 Ring staphyloma, bilateral
     H15.859 Ring staphyloma, unspecified eye ▽
     H15.89 Other disorders of sclera
    H15.9 Unspecified disorder of sclera ▽

✓4ᵗʰ **H16 Keratitis**

✓5ᵗʰ   **H16.0** Corneal ulcer

✓6ᵗʰ   **H16.00** Unspecified corneal ulcer
     H16.001 Unspecified corneal ulcer, right eye ▽
     H16.002 Unspecified corneal ulcer, left eye ▽
     H16.003 Unspecified corneal ulcer, bilateral ▽
     H16.009 Unspecified corneal ulcer, unspecified eye ▽

✓6ᵗʰ   **H16.01** Central corneal ulcer
     H16.011 Central corneal ulcer, right eye
     H16.012 Central corneal ulcer, left eye
     H16.013 Central corneal ulcer, bilateral
     H16.019 Central corneal ulcer, unspecified eye ▽

✓6ᵗʰ   **H16.02** Ring corneal ulcer
     H16.021 Ring corneal ulcer, right eye
     H16.022 Ring corneal ulcer, left eye
     H16.023 Ring corneal ulcer, bilateral
     H16.029 Ring corneal ulcer, unspecified eye ▽

✓6ᵗʰ   **H16.03** Corneal ulcer with hypopyon
     H16.031 Corneal ulcer with hypopyon, right eye
     H16.032 Corneal ulcer with hypopyon, left eye
     H16.033 Corneal ulcer with hypopyon, bilateral
     H16.039 Corneal ulcer with hypopyon, unspecified eye ▽

✓6ᵗʰ   **H16.04** Marginal corneal ulcer
     H16.041 Marginal corneal ulcer, right eye
     H16.042 Marginal corneal ulcer, left eye
     H16.043 Marginal corneal ulcer, bilateral
     H16.049 Marginal corneal ulcer, unspecified eye ▽

✓6ᵗʰ   **H16.05** Mooren's corneal ulcer
     H16.051 Mooren's corneal ulcer, right eye
     H16.052 Mooren's corneal ulcer, left eye
     H16.053 Mooren's corneal ulcer, bilateral
     H16.059 Mooren's corneal ulcer, unspecified eye ▽

✓6ᵗʰ   **H16.06** Mycotic corneal ulcer
     H16.061 Mycotic corneal ulcer, right eye
     H16.062 Mycotic corneal ulcer, left eye
     H16.063 Mycotic corneal ulcer, bilateral
     H16.069 Mycotic corneal ulcer, unspecified eye ▽

✓6ᵗʰ   **H16.07** Perforated corneal ulcer
     H16.071 Perforated corneal ulcer, right eye
     H16.072 Perforated corneal ulcer, left eye
     H16.073 Perforated corneal ulcer, bilateral
     H16.079 Perforated corneal ulcer, unspecified eye ▽

✓5ᵗʰ   **H16.1** Other and unspecified superficial keratitis without conjunctivitis

✓6ᵗʰ   **H16.10** Unspecified superficial keratitis
     H16.101 Unspecified superficial keratitis, right eye ▽
     H16.102 Unspecified superficial keratitis, left eye ▽
     H16.103 Unspecified superficial keratitis, bilateral ▽
     H16.109 Unspecified superficial keratitis, unspecified eye ▽

✓6ᵗʰ   **H16.11** Macular keratitis
       Areolar keratitis
       Nummular keratitis
       Stellate keratitis
       Striate keratitis
     H16.111 Macular keratitis, right eye
     H16.112 Macular keratitis, left eye
     H16.113 Macular keratitis, bilateral
     H16.119 Macular keratitis, unspecified eye ▽

✓6ᵗʰ   **H16.12** Filamentary keratitis
     H16.121 Filamentary keratitis, right eye
     H16.122 Filamentary keratitis, left eye
     H16.123 Filamentary keratitis, bilateral
     H16.129 Filamentary keratitis, unspecified eye ▽

✓6ᵗʰ   **H16.13** Photokeratitis
       Snow blindness
       Welders keratitis
     H16.131 Photokeratitis, right eye
     H16.132 Photokeratitis, left eye
     H16.133 Photokeratitis, bilateral
     H16.139 Photokeratitis, unspecified eye ▽

✓6ᵗʰ   **H16.14** Punctate keratitis
     H16.141 Punctate keratitis, right eye
     H16.142 Punctate keratitis, left eye
     H16.143 Punctate keratitis, bilateral
     H16.149 Punctate keratitis, unspecified eye ▽

✓5ᵗʰ   **H16.2** Keratoconjunctivitis

✓6ᵗʰ   **H16.20** Unspecified keratoconjunctivitis
       Superficial keratitis with conjunctivitis NOS
     H16.201 Unspecified keratoconjunctivitis, right eye ▽
     H16.202 Unspecified keratoconjunctivitis, left eye ▽
     H16.203 Unspecified keratoconjunctivitis, bilateral ▽
     H16.209 Unspecified keratoconjunctivitis, unspecified eye ▽

✓6ᵗʰ   **H16.21** Exposure keratoconjunctivitis
     H16.211 Exposure keratoconjunctivitis, right eye
     H16.212 Exposure keratoconjunctivitis, left eye
     H16.213 Exposure keratoconjunctivitis, bilateral
     H16.219 Exposure keratoconjunctivitis, unspecified eye ▽

✓6ᵗʰ   **H16.22** Keratoconjunctivitis sicca, not specified as Sjögren's
       EXCLUDES 1   *Sjögren's syndrome (M35.01)*
     H16.221 Keratoconjunctivitis sicca, not specified as Sjögren's, right eye
     H16.222 Keratoconjunctivitis sicca, not specified as Sjögren's, left eye
     H16.223 Keratoconjunctivitis sicca, not specified as Sjögren's, bilateral
     H16.229 Keratoconjunctivitis sicca, not specified as Sjögren's, unspecified eye ▽

✓6ᵗʰ   **H16.23** Neurotrophic keratoconjunctivitis
     H16.231 Neurotrophic keratoconjunctivitis, right eye
     H16.232 Neurotrophic keratoconjunctivitis, left eye
     H16.233 Neurotrophic keratoconjunctivitis, bilateral
     H16.239 Neurotrophic keratoconjunctivitis, unspecified eye ▽

✓6ᵗʰ   **H16.24** Ophthalmia nodosa
     H16.241 Ophthalmia nodosa, right eye
     H16.242 Ophthalmia nodosa, left eye
     H16.243 Ophthalmia nodosa, bilateral
     H16.249 Ophthalmia nodosa, unspecified eye ▽

✓6ᵗʰ   **H16.25** Phlyctenular keratoconjunctivitis
     H16.251 Phlyctenular keratoconjunctivitis, right eye
     H16.252 Phlyctenular keratoconjunctivitis, left eye
     H16.253 Phlyctenular keratoconjunctivitis, bilateral
     H16.259 Phlyctenular keratoconjunctivitis, unspecified eye ▽

✓6ᵗʰ   **H16.26** Vernal keratoconjunctivitis, with limbar and corneal involvement
       EXCLUDES 1   *vernal conjunctivitis without limbar and corneal involvement (H10.44)*
     H16.261 Vernal keratoconjunctivitis, with limbar and corneal involvement, right eye
     H16.262 Vernal keratoconjunctivitis, with limbar and corneal involvement, left eye
     H16.263 Vernal keratoconjunctivitis, with limbar and corneal involvement, bilateral

---

Ⓝ Newborn: 0   Ⓟ Pediatric: 0-17   Ⓜ Maternity: 12-55   Ⓐ Adult: 15-124   **NRS** Nonroutine supply Dx   **NC Dx** Noncancer Dx   **PDX** Primary Dx   ▶◀ Revised Text   ● New Code   ▲ Revised Title

H16.269 Vernal keratoconjunctivitis, with limbar and corneal involvement, unspecified eye ▽

H16.29 Other keratoconjunctivitis
H16.291 Other keratoconjunctivitis, right eye
H16.292 Other keratoconjunctivitis, left eye
H16.293 Other keratoconjunctivitis, bilateral
H16.299 Other keratoconjunctivitis, unspecified eye ▽

H16.3 Interstitial and deep keratitis

H16.30 Unspecified interstitial keratitis
H16.301 Unspecified interstitial keratitis, right eye ▽
H16.302 Unspecified interstitial keratitis, left eye ▽
H16.303 Unspecified interstitial keratitis, bilateral ▽
H16.309 Unspecified interstitial keratitis, unspecified eye ▽

H16.31 Corneal abscess
H16.311 Corneal abscess, right eye
H16.312 Corneal abscess, left eye
H16.313 Corneal abscess, bilateral
H16.319 Corneal abscess, unspecified eye ▽

H16.32 Diffuse interstitial keratitis
Cogan's syndrome
H16.321 Diffuse interstitial keratitis, right eye
H16.322 Diffuse interstitial keratitis, left eye
H16.323 Diffuse interstitial keratitis, bilateral
H16.329 Diffuse interstitial keratitis, unspecified eye ▽

H16.33 Sclerosing keratitis
H16.331 Sclerosing keratitis, right eye
H16.332 Sclerosing keratitis, left eye
H16.333 Sclerosing keratitis, bilateral
H16.339 Sclerosing keratitis, unspecified eye ▽

H16.39 Other interstitial and deep keratitis
H16.391 Other interstitial and deep keratitis, right eye
H16.392 Other interstitial and deep keratitis, left eye
H16.393 Other interstitial and deep keratitis, bilateral
H16.399 Other interstitial and deep keratitis, unspecified eye ▽

H16.4 Corneal neovascularization

H16.40 Unspecified corneal neovascularization
H16.401 Unspecified corneal neovascularization, right eye ▽
H16.402 Unspecified corneal neovascularization, left eye ▽
H16.403 Unspecified corneal neovascularization, bilateral ▽
H16.409 Unspecified corneal neovascularization, unspecified eye ▽

H16.41 Ghost vessels (corneal)
H16.411 Ghost vessels (corneal), right eye
H16.412 Ghost vessels (corneal), left eye
H16.413 Ghost vessels (corneal), bilateral
H16.419 Ghost vessels (corneal), unspecified eye ▽

H16.42 Pannus (corneal)
H16.421 Pannus (corneal), right eye
H16.422 Pannus (corneal), left eye
H16.423 Pannus (corneal), bilateral
H16.429 Pannus (corneal), unspecified eye ▽

H16.43 Localized vascularization of cornea
H16.431 Localized vascularization of cornea, right eye
H16.432 Localized vascularization of cornea, left eye
H16.433 Localized vascularization of cornea, bilateral
H16.439 Localized vascularization of cornea, unspecified eye ▽

H16.44 Deep vascularization of cornea
H16.441 Deep vascularization of cornea, right eye
H16.442 Deep vascularization of cornea, left eye
H16.443 Deep vascularization of cornea, bilateral
H16.449 Deep vascularization of cornea, unspecified eye ▽

H16.8 Other keratitis
H16.9 Unspecified keratitis ▽

H17 Corneal scars and opacities

H17.0 Adherent leukoma
H17.00 Adherent leukoma, unspecified eye ▽
H17.01 Adherent leukoma, right eye
H17.02 Adherent leukoma, left eye
H17.03 Adherent leukoma, bilateral

H17.1 Central corneal opacity
H17.10 Central corneal opacity, unspecified eye ▽
H17.11 Central corneal opacity, right eye
H17.12 Central corneal opacity, left eye
H17.13 Central corneal opacity, bilateral

H17.8 Other corneal scars and opacities

H17.81 Minor opacity of cornea
Corneal nebula
H17.811 Minor opacity of cornea, right eye
H17.812 Minor opacity of cornea, left eye
H17.813 Minor opacity of cornea, bilateral
H17.819 Minor opacity of cornea, unspecified eye ▽

H17.82 Peripheral opacity of cornea
H17.821 Peripheral opacity of cornea, right eye
H17.822 Peripheral opacity of cornea, left eye
H17.823 Peripheral opacity of cornea, bilateral
H17.829 Peripheral opacity of cornea, unspecified eye ▽

H17.89 Other corneal scars and opacities
H17.9 Unspecified corneal scar and opacity ▽

H18 Other disorders of cornea

H18.0 Corneal pigmentations and deposits

H18.00 Unspecified corneal deposit
H18.001 Unspecified corneal deposit, right eye ▽
H18.002 Unspecified corneal deposit, left eye ▽
H18.003 Unspecified corneal deposit, bilateral ▽
H18.009 Unspecified corneal deposit, unspecified eye ▽

H18.01 Anterior corneal pigmentations
Staehli's line
H18.011 Anterior corneal pigmentations, right eye
H18.012 Anterior corneal pigmentations, left eye
H18.013 Anterior corneal pigmentations, bilateral
H18.019 Anterior corneal pigmentations, unspecified eye ▽

H18.02 Argentous corneal deposits
H18.021 Argentous corneal deposits, right eye
H18.022 Argentous corneal deposits, left eye
H18.023 Argentous corneal deposits, bilateral
H18.029 Argentous corneal deposits, unspecified eye ▽

H18.03 Corneal deposits in metabolic disorders
Code also associated metabolic disorder
H18.031 Corneal deposits in metabolic disorders, right eye
H18.032 Corneal deposits in metabolic disorders, left eye
H18.033 Corneal deposits in metabolic disorders, bilateral
H18.039 Corneal deposits in metabolic disorders, unspecified eye ▽

H18.04 Kayser-Fleischer ring
Code also associated Wilson's disease (E83.01)
H18.041 Kayser-Fleischer ring, right eye
H18.042 Kayser-Fleischer ring, left eye
H18.043 Kayser-Fleischer ring, bilateral
H18.049 Kayser-Fleischer ring, unspecified eye ▽

✓6ᵗʰ **H18.05** **Posterior** corneal pigmentations
Krukenberg's spindle
　H18.051　**Posterior** corneal pigmentations, right eye
　H18.052　**Posterior** corneal pigmentations, left eye
　H18.053　**Posterior** corneal pigmentations, bilateral
　H18.059　**Posterior** corneal pigmentations, ▽
　　　　　unspecified eye

✓6ᵗʰ **H18.06** **Stromal** corneal pigmentations
Hematocornea
　H18.061　**Stromal** corneal pigmentations, right eye
　H18.062　**Stromal** corneal pigmentations, left eye
　H18.063　**Stromal** corneal pigmentations, bilateral
　H18.069　**Stromal** corneal pigmentations, ▽
　　　　　unspecified eye

✓5ᵗʰ **H18.1** **Bullous keratopathy**
DEF: Corneal swelling due to damaged corneal endothelium; characterized by recurring, rupturing epithelial "blisters"; occurs in glaucoma, iridocyclitis and Fuchs dystrophy.
　H18.10　**Bullous keratopathy, unspecified eye**　▽
　H18.11　**Bullous keratopathy, right eye**
　H18.12　**Bullous keratopathy, left eye**
　H18.13　**Bullous keratopathy, bilateral**

✓5ᵗʰ **H18.2** **Other and unspecified corneal edema**
　H18.20　**Unspecified corneal edema**　▽

✓6ᵗʰ **H18.21** **Corneal edema** secondary to contact lens
　　EXCLUDES 2　other corneal disorders due to contact lens (H18.82-)
　H18.211　**Corneal edema secondary to contact lens, right eye**
　H18.212　**Corneal edema secondary to contact lens, left eye**
　H18.213　**Corneal edema secondary to contact lens, bilateral**
　H18.219　**Corneal edema secondary to contact** ▽
　　　　　lens, unspecified eye

✓6ᵗʰ **H18.22** **Idiopathic** corneal edema
　H18.221　**Idiopathic corneal edema, right eye**
　H18.222　**Idiopathic corneal edema, left eye**
　H18.223　**Idiopathic corneal edema, bilateral**
　H18.229　**Idiopathic corneal edema, unspecified** ▽
　　　　　eye

✓6ᵗʰ **H18.23** **Secondary** corneal edema
　H18.231　**Secondary corneal edema, right eye**
　H18.232　**Secondary corneal edema, left eye**
　H18.233　**Secondary corneal edema, bilateral**
　H18.239　**Secondary corneal edema, unspecified** ▽
　　　　　eye

✓5ᵗʰ **H18.3** **Changes of corneal membranes**
　H18.30　**Unspecified corneal membrane change**　▽

✓6ᵗʰ **H18.31** **Folds and rupture in** Bowman's membrane
　H18.311　**Folds and rupture in Bowman's membrane, right eye**
　H18.312　**Folds and rupture in Bowman's membrane, left eye**
　H18.313　**Folds and rupture in Bowman's membrane, bilateral**
　H18.319　**Folds and rupture in Bowman's** ▽
　　　　　membrane, unspecified eye

✓6ᵗʰ **H18.32** **Folds** in Descemet's membrane
　H18.321　**Folds in Descemet's membrane, right eye**
　H18.322　**Folds in Descemet's membrane, left eye**
　H18.323　**Folds in Descemet's membrane, bilateral**
　H18.329　**Folds in Descemet's membrane,** ▽
　　　　　unspecified eye

✓6ᵗʰ **H18.33** **Rupture** in Descemet's membrane
　H18.331　**Rupture in Descemet's membrane, right eye**
　H18.332　**Rupture in Descemet's membrane, left eye**
　H18.333　**Rupture in Descemet's membrane, bilateral**
　H18.339　**Rupture in Descemet's membrane,** ▽
　　　　　unspecified eye

✓5ᵗʰ **H18.4** **Corneal degeneration**
　　EXCLUDES 1　Mooren's ulcer (H16.0-)
　　　　　　recurrent erosion of cornea (H18.83-)
　H18.40　**Unspecified corneal degeneration**　▽

✓6ᵗʰ **H18.41** **Arcus senilis**
Senile corneal changes
　H18.411　**Arcus senilis, right eye**
　H18.412　**Arcus senilis, left eye**
　H18.413　**Arcus senilis, bilateral**
　H18.419　**Arcus senilis, unspecified eye**　▽

✓6ᵗʰ **H18.42** **Band** keratopathy
　H18.421　**Band keratopathy, right eye**
　H18.422　**Band keratopathy, left eye**
　H18.423　**Band keratopathy, bilateral**
　H18.429　**Band keratopathy, unspecified eye**　▽

　H18.43　**Other calcerous corneal degeneration**

✓6ᵗʰ **H18.44** **Keratomalacia**
　　EXCLUDES 1　keratomalacia due to vitamin A deficiency (E50.4)
　H18.441　**Keratomalacia, right eye**
　H18.442　**Keratomalacia, left eye**
　H18.443　**Keratomalacia, bilateral**
　H18.449　**Keratomalacia, unspecified eye**　▽

✓6ᵗʰ **H18.45** **Nodular** corneal degeneration
　H18.451　**Nodular corneal degeneration, right eye**
　H18.452　**Nodular corneal degeneration, left eye**
　H18.453　**Nodular corneal degeneration, bilateral**
　H18.459　**Nodular corneal degeneration,** ▽
　　　　　unspecified eye

✓6ᵗʰ **H18.46** **Peripheral** corneal degeneration
　H18.461　**Peripheral corneal degeneration, right eye**
　H18.462　**Peripheral corneal degeneration, left eye**
　H18.463　**Peripheral corneal degeneration, bilateral**
　H18.469　**Peripheral corneal degeneration,** ▽
　　　　　unspecified eye

　H18.49　**Other corneal degeneration**

✓5ᵗʰ **H18.5** **Hereditary corneal dystrophies**
　H18.50　**Unspecified hereditary corneal dystrophies**　▽
　H18.51　**Endothelial corneal dystrophy**
　　　　　Fuchs' dystrophy
　H18.52　**Epithelial (juvenile) corneal dystrophy**
　H18.53　**Granular corneal dystrophy**
　H18.54　**Lattice corneal dystrophy**
　H18.55　**Macular corneal dystrophy**
　H18.59　**Other hereditary corneal dystrophies**

✓5ᵗʰ **H18.6** **Keratoconus**

✓6ᵗʰ **H18.60** **Keratoconus,** unspecified
　H18.601　**Keratoconus, unspecified, right eye**　▽
　H18.602　**Keratoconus, unspecified, left eye**　▽
　H18.603　**Keratoconus, unspecified, bilateral**　▽
　H18.609　**Keratoconus, unspecified, unspecified** ▽
　　　　　eye

✓6ᵗʰ **H18.61** **Keratoconus,** stable
　H18.611　**Keratoconus, stable, right eye**
　H18.612　**Keratoconus, stable, left eye**
　H18.613　**Keratoconus, stable, bilateral**
　H18.619　**Keratoconus, stable, unspecified eye**　▽

✓6ᵗʰ **H18.62** **Keratoconus,** unstable
　　　　　Acute hydrops
　H18.621　**Keratoconus, unstable, right eye**
　H18.622　**Keratoconus, unstable, left eye**
　H18.623　**Keratoconus, unstable, bilateral**
　H18.629　**Keratoconus, unstable, unspecified eye** ▽

✓5ᵗʰ **H18.7** **Other and unspecified corneal deformities**
　　EXCLUDES 1　congenital malformations of cornea (Q13.3-Q13.4)
　H18.70　**Unspecified corneal deformity**　▽

✓6ᵗʰ **H18.71** **Corneal** ectasia
　H18.711　**Corneal ectasia, right eye**
　H18.712　**Corneal ectasia, left eye**
　H18.713　**Corneal ectasia, bilateral**
　H18.719　**Corneal ectasia, unspecified eye**　▽

Ⓝ Newborn: 0　Ⓟ Pediatric: 0-17　Ⓜ Maternity: 12-55　Ⓐ Adult: 15-124　NRS Nonroutine supply Dx　NC Dx Noncancer Dx　PDx Primary Dx　▶◀ Revised Text　● New Code　▲ Revised Title

580　　　　　　　　　　　　　　　　　　　　　　　　　　　　　　ICD-10-CM 2018

✓6ᵗʰ **H18.72** Corneal staphyloma
    H18.721 Corneal staphyloma, right eye
    H18.722 Corneal staphyloma, left eye
    H18.723 Corneal staphyloma, bilateral
    H18.729 Corneal staphyloma, unspecified eye ▽
✓6ᵗʰ **H18.73** Descemetocele
    H18.731 Descemetocele, right eye
    H18.732 Descemetocele, left eye
    H18.733 Descemetocele, bilateral
    H18.739 Descemetocele, unspecified eye ▽
✓6ᵗʰ **H18.79** Other corneal deformities
    H18.791 Other corneal deformities, right eye
    H18.792 Other corneal deformities, left eye
    H18.793 Other corneal deformities, bilateral
    H18.799 Other corneal deformities, unspecified eye ▽
✓5ᵗʰ **H18.8** Other specified disorders of cornea
✓6ᵗʰ **H18.81** Anesthesia and hypoesthesia of cornea
    H18.811 Anesthesia and hypoesthesia of cornea, right eye
    H18.812 Anesthesia and hypoesthesia of cornea, left eye
    H18.813 Anesthesia and hypoesthesia of cornea, bilateral
    H18.819 Anesthesia and hypoesthesia of cornea, unspecified eye ▽
✓6ᵗʰ **H18.82** Corneal disorder due to contact lens
    EXCLUDES 2 corneal edema due to contact lens (H18.21-)
    H18.821 Corneal disorder due to contact lens, right eye
    H18.822 Corneal disorder due to contact lens, left eye
    H18.823 Corneal disorder due to contact lens, bilateral
    H18.829 Corneal disorder due to contact lens, unspecified eye ▽
✓6ᵗʰ **H18.83** Recurrent erosion of cornea
    H18.831 Recurrent erosion of cornea, right eye
    H18.832 Recurrent erosion of cornea, left eye
    H18.833 Recurrent erosion of cornea, bilateral
    H18.839 Recurrent erosion of cornea, unspecified eye ▽
✓6ᵗʰ **H18.89** Other specified disorders of cornea
    H18.891 Other specified disorders of cornea, right eye
    H18.892 Other specified disorders of cornea, left eye
    H18.893 Other specified disorders of cornea, bilateral
    H18.899 Other specified disorders of cornea, unspecified eye ▽
H18.9 Unspecified disorder of cornea ▽

✓4ᵗʰ **H20** Iridocyclitis
✓5ᵗʰ **H20.0** Acute and subacute iridocyclitis
    Acute anterior uveitis
    Acute cyclitis
    Acute iritis
    Subacute anterior uveitis
    Subacute cyclitis
    Subacute iritis
    EXCLUDES 1 iridocyclitis, iritis, uveitis (due to) (in) diabetes mellitus (E08-E13 with .39)
    iridocyclitis, iritis, uveitis (due to) (in) diphtheria (A36.89)
    iridocyclitis, iritis, uveitis (due to) (in) gonococcal (A54.32)
    iridocyclitis, iritis, uveitis (due to) (in) herpes (simplex) (B00.51)
    iridocyclitis, iritis, uveitis (due to) (in) herpes zoster (B02.32)
    iridocyclitis, iritis, uveitis (due to) (in) late congenital syphilis (A50.39)
    iridocyclitis, iritis, uveitis (due to) (in) late syphilis (A52.71)
    iridocyclitis, iritis, uveitis (due to) (in) sarcoidosis (D86.83)
    iridocyclitis, iritis, uveitis (due to) (in) syphilis (A51.43)
    iridocyclitis, iritis, uveitis (due to) (in) toxoplasmosis (B58.09)
    iridocyclitis, iritis, uveitis (due to) (in) tuberculosis (A18.54)
    H20.00 Unspecified acute and subacute iridocyclitis ▽
✓6ᵗʰ **H20.01** Primary iridocyclitis
    H20.011 Primary iridocyclitis, right eye
    H20.012 Primary iridocyclitis, left eye
    H20.013 Primary iridocyclitis, bilateral
    H20.019 Primary iridocyclitis, unspecified eye ▽
✓6ᵗʰ **H20.02** Recurrent acute iridocyclitis
    H20.021 Recurrent acute iridocyclitis, right eye
    H20.022 Recurrent acute iridocyclitis, left eye
    H20.023 Recurrent acute iridocyclitis, bilateral
    H20.029 Recurrent acute iridocyclitis, unspecified eye ▽
✓6ᵗʰ **H20.03** Secondary infectious iridocyclitis
    H20.031 Secondary infectious iridocyclitis, right eye
    H20.032 Secondary infectious iridocyclitis, left eye
    H20.033 Secondary infectious iridocyclitis, bilateral
    H20.039 Secondary infectious iridocyclitis, unspecified eye ▽
✓6ᵗʰ **H20.04** Secondary noninfectious iridocyclitis
    H20.041 Secondary noninfectious iridocyclitis, right eye
    H20.042 Secondary noninfectious iridocyclitis, left eye
    H20.043 Secondary noninfectious iridocyclitis, bilateral
    H20.049 Secondary noninfectious iridocyclitis, unspecified eye ▽
✓6ᵗʰ **H20.05** Hypopyon
    H20.051 Hypopyon, right eye
    H20.052 Hypopyon, left eye
    H20.053 Hypopyon, bilateral
    H20.059 Hypopyon, unspecified eye ▽
✓5ᵗʰ **H20.1** Chronic iridocyclitis
    Use additional code for any associated cataract (H26.21-)
    EXCLUDES 2 posterior cyclitis (H30.2-)
    H20.10 Chronic iridocyclitis, unspecified eye ▽
    H20.11 Chronic iridocyclitis, right eye
    H20.12 Chronic iridocyclitis, left eye
    H20.13 Chronic iridocyclitis, bilateral
✓5ᵗʰ **H20.2** Lens-induced iridocyclitis
    H20.20 Lens-induced iridocyclitis, unspecified eye ▽
    H20.21 Lens-induced iridocyclitis, right eye
    H20.22 Lens-induced iridocyclitis, left eye
    H20.23 Lens-induced iridocyclitis, bilateral

Chapter 7. Diseases of the Eye and Adnexa

Hyphema

- Iris
- Cornea
- Hyphema

✓5th **H20.8** Other **iridocyclitis**
　　EXCLUDES 2　glaucomatocyclitis crises (H40.4-)
　　　　　　　posterior cyclitis (H30.2-)
　　　　　　　sympathetic uveitis (H44.13-)

　✓6th **H20.81** Fuchs' heterochromic cyclitis
　　　H20.811 Fuchs' heterochromic cyclitis, right eye
　　　H20.812 Fuchs' heterochromic cyclitis, left eye
　　　H20.813 Fuchs' heterochromic cyclitis, bilateral
　　　H20.819 Fuchs' heterochromic cyclitis, unspecified eye ▽

　✓6th **H20.82** Vogt-Koyanagi syndrome
　　　H20.821 Vogt-Koyanagi syndrome, right eye
　　　H20.822 Vogt-Koyanagi syndrome, left eye
　　　H20.823 Vogt-Koyanagi syndrome, bilateral
　　　H20.829 Vogt-Koyanagi syndrome, unspecified eye ▽

H20.9 Unspecified iridocyclitis ▽
　　Uveitis NOS

✓4th **H21** Other disorders of iris and ciliary body
　　EXCLUDES 2　sympathetic uveitis (H44.1-)

✓5th **H21.0** Hyphema
　　EXCLUDES 1　traumatic hyphema (S05.1-)
　　H21.00 Hyphema, unspecified eye ▽
　　H21.01 Hyphema, right eye
　　H21.02 Hyphema, left eye
　　H21.03 Hyphema, bilateral

✓5th **H21.1** Other vascular disorders of iris and ciliary body
　　Neovascularization of iris or ciliary body
　　Rubeosis iridis
　　Rubeosis of iris

　✓6th **H21.1X** Other vascular disorders of iris and ciliary body
　　　H21.1X1 Other vascular disorders of iris and ciliary body, right eye
　　　H21.1X2 Other vascular disorders of iris and ciliary body, left eye
　　　H21.1X3 Other vascular disorders of iris and ciliary body, bilateral
　　　H21.1X9 Other vascular disorders of iris and ciliary body, unspecified eye ▽

✓5th **H21.2** Degeneration of iris and ciliary body

　✓6th **H21.21** Degeneration of chamber angle
　　　H21.211 Degeneration of chamber angle, right eye
　　　H21.212 Degeneration of chamber angle, left eye
　　　H21.213 Degeneration of chamber angle, bilateral
　　　H21.219 Degeneration of chamber angle, unspecified eye ▽

　✓6th **H21.22** Degeneration of ciliary body
　　　H21.221 Degeneration of ciliary body, right eye
　　　H21.222 Degeneration of ciliary body, left eye
　　　H21.223 Degeneration of ciliary body, bilateral
　　　H21.229 Degeneration of ciliary body, unspecified eye ▽

　✓6th **H21.23** Degeneration of iris (pigmentary)
　　　Translucency of iris
　　　H21.231 Degeneration of iris (pigmentary), right eye
　　　H21.232 Degeneration of iris (pigmentary), left eye

　　　H21.233 Degeneration of iris (pigmentary), bilateral
　　　H21.239 Degeneration of iris (pigmentary), unspecified eye ▽

　✓6th **H21.24** Degeneration of pupillary margin
　　　H21.241 Degeneration of pupillary margin, right eye
　　　H21.242 Degeneration of pupillary margin, left eye
　　　H21.243 Degeneration of pupillary margin, bilateral
　　　H21.249 Degeneration of pupillary margin, unspecified eye ▽

　✓6th **H21.25** Iridoschisis
　　　H21.251 Iridoschisis, right eye
　　　H21.252 Iridoschisis, left eye
　　　H21.253 Iridoschisis, bilateral
　　　H21.259 Iridoschisis, unspecified eye ▽

　✓6th **H21.26** Iris atrophy (essential) (progressive)
　　　H21.261 Iris atrophy (essential) (progressive), right eye
　　　H21.262 Iris atrophy (essential) (progressive), left eye
　　　H21.263 Iris atrophy (essential) (progressive), bilateral
　　　H21.269 Iris atrophy (essential) (progressive), unspecified eye ▽

　✓6th **H21.27** Miotic pupillary cyst
　　　H21.271 Miotic pupillary cyst, right eye
　　　H21.272 Miotic pupillary cyst, left eye
　　　H21.273 Miotic pupillary cyst, bilateral
　　　H21.279 Miotic pupillary cyst, unspecified eye ▽

　　H21.29 Other iris atrophy

✓5th **H21.3** Cyst of iris, ciliary body and anterior chamber
　　EXCLUDES 2　miotic pupillary cyst (H21.27-)

　✓6th **H21.30** Idiopathic cysts of iris, ciliary body or anterior chamber
　　　Cyst of iris, ciliary body or anterior chamber NOS
　　　H21.301 Idiopathic cysts of iris, ciliary body or anterior chamber, right eye
　　　H21.302 Idiopathic cysts of iris, ciliary body or anterior chamber, left eye
　　　H21.303 Idiopathic cysts of iris, ciliary body or anterior chamber, bilateral
　　　H21.309 Idiopathic cysts of iris, ciliary body or anterior chamber, unspecified eye ▽

　✓6th **H21.31** Exudative cysts of iris or anterior chamber
　　　H21.311 Exudative cysts of iris or anterior chamber, right eye
　　　H21.312 Exudative cysts of iris or anterior chamber, left eye
　　　H21.313 Exudative cysts of iris or anterior chamber, bilateral
　　　H21.319 Exudative cysts of iris or anterior chamber, unspecified eye ▽

　✓6th **H21.32** Implantation cysts of iris, ciliary body or anterior chamber
　　　H21.321 Implantation cysts of iris, ciliary body or anterior chamber, right eye
　　　H21.322 Implantation cysts of iris, ciliary body or anterior chamber, left eye
　　　H21.323 Implantation cysts of iris, ciliary body or anterior chamber, bilateral
　　　H21.329 Implantation cysts of iris, ciliary body or anterior chamber, unspecified eye ▽

　✓6th **H21.33** Parasitic cyst of iris, ciliary body or anterior chamber
　　　H21.331 Parasitic cyst of iris, ciliary body or anterior chamber, right eye
　　　H21.332 Parasitic cyst of iris, ciliary body or anterior chamber, left eye
　　　H21.333 Parasitic cyst of iris, ciliary body or anterior chamber, bilateral
　　　H21.339 Parasitic cyst of iris, ciliary body or anterior chamber, unspecified eye ▽

N Newborn: 0　P Pediatric: 0-17　M Maternity: 12-55　A Adult: 15-124　NRS Nonroutine supply Dx　NCDx Noncancer Dx　PDx Primary Dx　▶◀ Revised Text　● New Code　▲ Revised Title

582　　　　　ICD-10-CM 2018

✓6ᵗʰ **H21.34 Primary cyst of pars plana**
    H21.341 Primary cyst of pars plana, right eye
    H21.342 Primary cyst of pars plana, left eye
    H21.343 Primary cyst of pars plana, bilateral
    H21.349 Primary cyst of pars plana, unspecified eye ▽

✓6ᵗʰ **H21.35 Exudative cyst of pars plana**
    DEF: Protein, fatty-filled bullous elevation of nonpigmented outermost ciliary epithelium of pars plana; due to fluid leak from blood vessels.
    H21.351 Exudative cyst of pars plana, right eye
    H21.352 Exudative cyst of pars plana, left eye
    H21.353 Exudative cyst of pars plana, bilateral
    H21.359 Exudative cyst of pars plana, unspecified eye ▽

✓5ᵗʰ **H21.4 Pupillary membranes**
    Iris bombé
    Pupillary occlusion
    Pupillary seclusion
    EXCLUDES 1 *congenital pupillary membranes (Q13.8)*
    H21.40 Pupillary membranes, unspecified eye ▽
    H21.41 Pupillary membranes, right eye
    H21.42 Pupillary membranes, left eye
    H21.43 Pupillary membranes, bilateral

✓5ᵗʰ **H21.5 Other and unspecified adhesions and disruptions of iris and ciliary body**
    EXCLUDES 1 *corectopia (Q13.2)*
    ✓6ᵗʰ **H21.50 Unspecified adhesions of iris**
        Synechia (iris) NOS
        H21.501 Unspecified adhesions of iris, right eye ▽
        H21.502 Unspecified adhesions of iris, left eye ▽
        H21.503 Unspecified adhesions of iris, bilateral ▽
        H21.509 Unspecified adhesions of iris and ciliary body, unspecified eye ▽
    ✓6ᵗʰ **H21.51 Anterior synechiae (iris)**
        H21.511 Anterior synechiae (iris), right eye
        H21.512 Anterior synechiae (iris), left eye
        H21.513 Anterior synechiae (iris), bilateral
        H21.519 Anterior synechiae (iris), unspecified eye ▽
    ✓6ᵗʰ **H21.52 Goniosynechiae**
        H21.521 Goniosynechiae, right eye
        H21.522 Goniosynechiae, left eye
        H21.523 Goniosynechiae, bilateral
        H21.529 Goniosynechiae, unspecified eye ▽
    ✓6ᵗʰ **H21.53 Iridodialysis**
        H21.531 Iridodialysis, right eye
        H21.532 Iridodialysis, left eye
        H21.533 Iridodialysis, bilateral
        H21.539 Iridodialysis, unspecified eye ▽
    ✓6ᵗʰ **H21.54 Posterior synechiae (iris)**
        H21.541 Posterior synechiae (iris), right eye
        H21.542 Posterior synechiae (iris), left eye
        H21.543 Posterior synechiae (iris), bilateral
        H21.549 Posterior synechiae (iris), unspecified eye ▽
    ✓6ᵗʰ **H21.55 Recession of chamber angle**
        H21.551 Recession of chamber angle, right eye
        H21.552 Recession of chamber angle, left eye
        H21.553 Recession of chamber angle, bilateral
        H21.559 Recession of chamber angle, unspecified eye ▽
    ✓6ᵗʰ **H21.56 Pupillary abnormalities**
        Deformed pupil
        Ectopic pupil
        Rupture of sphincter, pupil
        EXCLUDES 1 *congenital deformity of pupil (Q13.2-)*
        H21.561 Pupillary abnormality, right eye
        H21.562 Pupillary abnormality, left eye
        H21.563 Pupillary abnormality, bilateral
        H21.569 Pupillary abnormality, unspecified eye ▽

✓5ᵗʰ **H21.8 Other specified disorders of iris and ciliary body**
    H21.81 Floppy iris syndrome
        Intraoperative floppy iris syndrome (IFIS)
        Use additional code for adverse effect, if applicable, to identify drug (T36-T50 with fifth or sixth character 5)
    H21.82 Plateau iris syndrome (post-iridectomy) (postprocedural)
    H21.89 Other specified disorders of iris and ciliary body
    H21.9 Unspecified disorder of iris and ciliary body ▽

H22 Disorders of iris and ciliary body in diseases classified elsewhere
    Code first underlying disease, such as:
        gout (M1A.-, M10.-)
        leprosy (A30.-)
        parasitic disease (B89)

Disorders of lens (H25-H28)

✓4ᵗʰ **H25 Age-related cataract**
    Senile cataract
    EXCLUDES 2 *capsular glaucoma with pseudoexfoliation of lens (H40.1-)*
    ✓5ᵗʰ **H25.0 Age-related incipient cataract**
        ✓6ᵗʰ **H25.01 Cortical age-related cataract**
            H25.011 Cortical age-related cataract, right eye Ⓐ
            H25.012 Cortical age-related cataract, left eye Ⓐ
            H25.013 Cortical age-related cataract, bilateral Ⓐ
            H25.019 Cortical age-related cataract, unspecified eye Ⓐ▽
        ✓6ᵗʰ **H25.03 Anterior subcapsular polar age-related cataract**
            H25.031 Anterior subcapsular polar age-related cataract, right eye Ⓐ
            H25.032 Anterior subcapsular polar age-related cataract, left eye Ⓐ
            H25.033 Anterior subcapsular polar age-related cataract, bilateral Ⓐ
            H25.039 Anterior subcapsular polar age-related cataract, unspecified eye Ⓐ▽
        ✓6ᵗʰ **H25.04 Posterior subcapsular polar age-related cataract**
            H25.041 Posterior subcapsular polar age-related cataract, right eye Ⓐ
            H25.042 Posterior subcapsular polar age-related cataract, left eye Ⓐ
            H25.043 Posterior subcapsular polar age-related cataract, bilateral Ⓐ
            H25.049 Posterior subcapsular polar age-related cataract, unspecified eye Ⓐ▽
        ✓6ᵗʰ **H25.09 Other age-related incipient cataract**
            Coronary age-related cataract
            Punctate age-related cataract
            Water clefts
            H25.091 Other age-related incipient cataract, right eye Ⓐ
            H25.092 Other age-related incipient cataract, left eye Ⓐ
            H25.093 Other age-related incipient cataract, bilateral Ⓐ
            H25.099 Other age-related incipient cataract, unspecified eye Ⓐ▽
    ✓5ᵗʰ **H25.1 Age-related nuclear cataract**
        Cataracta brunescens
        Nuclear sclerosis cataract
        AHA: 2016, 1Q, 32
        H25.10 Age-related nuclear cataract, unspecified eye Ⓐ▽
        H25.11 Age-related nuclear cataract, right eye Ⓐ
        H25.12 Age-related nuclear cataract, left eye Ⓐ
        H25.13 Age-related nuclear cataract, bilateral Ⓐ
    ✓5ᵗʰ **H25.2 Age-related cataract, morgagnian type**
        Age-related hypermature cataract
        H25.20 Age-related cataract, morgagnian type, unspecified eye Ⓐ▽
        H25.21 Age-related cataract, morgagnian type, right eye Ⓐ
        H25.22 Age-related cataract, morgagnian type, left eye Ⓐ
        H25.23 Age-related cataract, morgagnian type, bilateral Ⓐ

✓ Additional Character Req   ✓x7ᵗʰ Placeholder Alert   Case-Mix Diagnosis   Manifestation   ▽ Unspecified Dx   **EXCLUDES 1** Not coded here   **EXCLUDES 2** Not included here

ICD-10-CM 2018   **583**

Chapter 7. Diseases of the Eye and Adnexa

H21.34-H25.23

Chapter 7. Diseases of the Eye and Adnexa

H25.8–H26.229

Cataracts

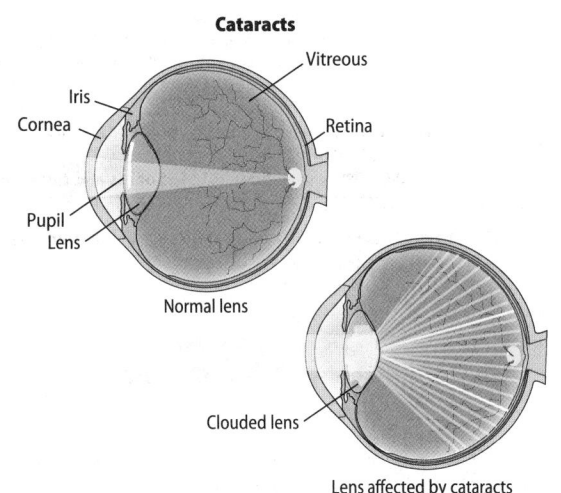

Normal lens

Clouded lens

Lens affected by cataracts

✓5th H25.8 Other age-related cataract

    ✓6th H25.81 Combined forms of age-related cataract

        H25.811   Combined forms of age-related cataract, right eye   A

        H25.812   Combined forms of age-related cataract, left eye   A

        H25.813   Combined forms of age-related cataract, bilateral   A

        H25.819   Combined forms of age-related cataract, unspecified eye   A ▽

    H25.89   Other age-related cataract   A

H25.9 Unspecified age-related cataract   A ▽

✓4th H26 Other cataract

    EXCLUDES 1   congenital cataract (Q12.0)

    ✓5th H26.0 Infantile and juvenile cataract

        ✓6th H26.00 Unspecified infantile and juvenile cataract

            H26.001   Unspecified infantile and juvenile cataract, right eye   P ▽

            H26.002   Unspecified infantile and juvenile cataract, left eye   P ▽

            H26.003   Unspecified infantile and juvenile cataract, bilateral   P ▽

            H26.009   Unspecified infantile and juvenile cataract, unspecified eye   P ▽

        ✓6th H26.01 Infantile and juvenile cortical, lamellar, or zonular cataract

            H26.011   Infantile and juvenile cortical, lamellar, or zonular cataract, right eye   P

            H26.012   Infantile and juvenile cortical, lamellar, or zonular cataract, left eye   P

            H26.013   Infantile and juvenile cortical, lamellar, or zonular cataract, bilateral   P

            H26.019   Infantile and juvenile cortical, lamellar, or zonular cataract, unspecified eye   P ▽

        ✓6th H26.03 Infantile and juvenile nuclear cataract

            H26.031   Infantile and juvenile nuclear cataract, right eye   P

            H26.032   Infantile and juvenile nuclear cataract, left eye   P

            H26.033   Infantile and juvenile nuclear cataract, bilateral   P

            H26.039   Infantile and juvenile nuclear cataract, unspecified eye   P ▽

        ✓6th H26.04 Anterior subcapsular polar infantile and juvenile cataract

            H26.041   Anterior subcapsular polar infantile and juvenile cataract, right eye   P

            H26.042   Anterior subcapsular polar infantile and juvenile cataract, left eye   P

            H26.043   Anterior subcapsular polar infantile and juvenile cataract, bilateral   P

            H26.049   Anterior subcapsular polar infantile and juvenile cataract, unspecified eye   P ▽

        ✓6th H26.05 Posterior subcapsular polar infantile and juvenile cataract

            H26.051   Posterior subcapsular polar infantile and juvenile cataract, right eye   P

            H26.052   Posterior subcapsular polar infantile and juvenile cataract, left eye   P

            H26.053   Posterior subcapsular polar infantile and juvenile cataract, bilateral   P

            H26.059   Posterior subcapsular polar infantile and juvenile cataract, unspecified eye   P ▽

        ✓6th H26.06 Combined forms of infantile and juvenile cataract

            H26.061   Combined forms of infantile and juvenile cataract, right eye   P

            H26.062   Combined forms of infantile and juvenile cataract, left eye   P

            H26.063   Combined forms of infantile and juvenile cataract, bilateral   P

            H26.069   Combined forms of infantile and juvenile cataract, unspecified eye   P ▽

        H26.09   Other infantile and juvenile cataract   P

    ✓5th H26.1 Traumatic cataract

        Use additional code (Chapter 20) to identify external cause

        ✓6th H26.10 Unspecified traumatic cataract

            H26.101   Unspecified traumatic cataract, right eye   ▽

            H26.102   Unspecified traumatic cataract, left eye   ▽

            H26.103   Unspecified traumatic cataract, bilateral   ▽

            H26.109   Unspecified traumatic cataract, unspecified eye   ▽

        ✓6th H26.11 Localized traumatic opacities

            H26.111   Localized traumatic opacities, right eye

            H26.112   Localized traumatic opacities, left eye

            H26.113   Localized traumatic opacities, bilateral

            H26.119   Localized traumatic opacities, unspecified eye   ▽

        ✓6th H26.12 Partially resolved traumatic cataract

            H26.121   Partially resolved traumatic cataract, right eye

            H26.122   Partially resolved traumatic cataract, left eye

            H26.123   Partially resolved traumatic cataract, bilateral

            H26.129   Partially resolved traumatic cataract, unspecified eye   ▽

        ✓6th H26.13 Total traumatic cataract

            H26.131   Total traumatic cataract, right eye

            H26.132   Total traumatic cataract, left eye

            H26.133   Total traumatic cataract, bilateral

            H26.139   Total traumatic cataract, unspecified eye   ▽

    ✓5th H26.2 Complicated cataract

        H26.20 Unspecified complicated cataract   ▽

            Cataracta complicata NOS

        ✓6th H26.21 Cataract with neovascularization

            Code also associated condition, such as: chronic iridocyclitis (H20.1-)

            H26.211   Cataract with neovascularization, right eye

            H26.212   Cataract with neovascularization, left eye

            H26.213   Cataract with neovascularization, bilateral

            H26.219   Cataract with neovascularization, unspecified eye   ▽

        ✓6th H26.22 Cataract secondary to ocular disorders (degenerative) (inflammatory)

            Code also associated ocular disorder

            H26.221   Cataract secondary to ocular disorders (degenerative) (inflammatory), right eye

            H26.222   Cataract secondary to ocular disorders (degenerative) (inflammatory), left eye

            H26.223   Cataract secondary to ocular disorders (degenerative) (inflammatory), bilateral

            H26.229   Cataract secondary to ocular disorders (degenerative) (inflammatory), unspecified eye   ▽

N Newborn: 0   P Pediatric: 0-17   M Maternity: 12-55   A Adult: 15-124   **NRS** Nonroutine supply Dx   **NC Dx** Noncancer Dx   **PDx** Primary Dx   ►◄ Revised Text   ● New Code   ▲ Revised Title

584   ICD-10-CM 2018

☑6ᵗʰ H26.23 Glaucomatous flecks (subcapsular)
Code first underlying glaucoma (H40-H42)
H26.231 Glaucomatous flecks (subcapsular), right eye
H26.232 Glaucomatous flecks (subcapsular), left eye
H26.233 Glaucomatous flecks (subcapsular), bilateral
H26.239 Glaucomatous flecks (subcapsular), unspecified eye ▽

☑5ᵗʰ H26.3 Drug-induced cataract
Toxic cataract
Use additional code for adverse effect, if applicable, to identify drug (T36-T50 with fifth or sixth character 5)
H26.30 Drug-induced cataract, unspecified eye ▽
H26.31 Drug-induced cataract, right eye
H26.32 Drug-induced cataract, left eye
H26.33 Drug-induced cataract, bilateral

☑5ᵗʰ H26.4 Secondary cataract
H26.40 Unspecified secondary cataract ▽
☑6ᵗʰ H26.41 Soemmering's ring
H26.411 Soemmering's ring, right eye
H26.412 Soemmering's ring, left eye
H26.413 Soemmering's ring, bilateral
H26.419 Soemmering's ring, unspecified eye ▽
☑6ᵗʰ H26.49 Other secondary cataract
H26.491 Other secondary cataract, right eye
H26.492 Other secondary cataract, left eye
H26.493 Other secondary cataract, bilateral
H26.499 Other secondary cataract, unspecified eye ▽
H26.8 Other specified cataract
H26.9 Unspecified cataract ▽

☑4ᵗʰ H27 Other disorders of lens
EXCLUDES 1 congenital lens malformations (Q12.-)
mechanical complications of intraocular lens implant (T85.2)
pseudophakia (Z96.1)

☑5ᵗʰ H27.0 Aphakia
Acquired absence of lens
Acquired aphakia
Aphakia due to trauma
EXCLUDES 1 cataract extraction status (Z98.4-)
congenital absence of lens (Q12.3)
congenital aphakia (Q12.3)
H27.00 Aphakia, unspecified eye ▽
H27.01 Aphakia, right eye
H27.02 Aphakia, left eye
H27.03 Aphakia, bilateral

☑5ᵗʰ H27.1 Dislocation of lens
H27.10 Unspecified dislocation of lens ▽
☑6ᵗʰ H27.11 Subluxation of lens
H27.111 Subluxation of lens, right eye
H27.112 Subluxation of lens, left eye
H27.113 Subluxation of lens, bilateral
H27.119 Subluxation of lens, unspecified eye ▽
☑6ᵗʰ H27.12 Anterior dislocation of lens
H27.121 Anterior dislocation of lens, right eye
H27.122 Anterior dislocation of lens, left eye
H27.123 Anterior dislocation of lens, bilateral
H27.129 Anterior dislocation of lens, unspecified eye ▽
☑6ᵗʰ H27.13 Posterior dislocation of lens
H27.131 Posterior dislocation of lens, right eye
H27.132 Posterior dislocation of lens, left eye
H27.133 Posterior dislocation of lens, bilateral
H27.139 Posterior dislocation of lens, unspecified eye ▽
H27.8 Other specified disorders of lens
H27.9 Unspecified disorder of lens ▽

H28 Cataract in diseases classified elsewhere
Code first underlying disease, such as:
hypoparathyroidism (E20.-)
myotonia (G71.1-)
myxedema (E03.-)
protein-calorie malnutrition (E40-E46)
EXCLUDES 1 cataract in diabetes mellitus (E08.36, E09.36, E10.36, E11.36, E13.36)

Disorders of choroid and retina (H30-H36)

☑4ᵗʰ H30 Chorioretinal inflammation
☑5ᵗʰ H30.0 Focal chorioretinal inflammation
Focal chorioretinitis
Focal choroiditis
Focal retinitis
Focal retinochoroiditis
☑6ᵗʰ H30.00 Unspecified focal chorioretinal inflammation
Focal chorioretinitis NOS
Focal choroiditis NOS
Focal retinitis NOS
Focal retinochoroiditis NOS
H30.001 Unspecified focal chorioretinal inflammation, right eye ▽
H30.002 Unspecified focal chorioretinal inflammation, left eye ▽
H30.003 Unspecified focal chorioretinal inflammation, bilateral ▽
H30.009 Unspecified focal chorioretinal inflammation, unspecified eye
☑6ᵗʰ H30.01 Focal chorioretinal inflammation, juxtapapillary
H30.011 Focal chorioretinal inflammation, juxtapapillary, right eye
H30.012 Focal chorioretinal inflammation, juxtapapillary, left eye
H30.013 Focal chorioretinal inflammation, juxtapapillary, bilateral
H30.019 Focal chorioretinal inflammation, juxtapapillary, unspecified eye ▽
☑6ᵗʰ H30.02 Focal chorioretinal inflammation of posterior pole
H30.021 Focal chorioretinal inflammation of posterior pole, right eye
H30.022 Focal chorioretinal inflammation of posterior pole, left eye
H30.023 Focal chorioretinal inflammation of posterior pole, bilateral
H30.029 Focal chorioretinal inflammation of posterior pole, unspecified eye ▽
☑6ᵗʰ H30.03 Focal chorioretinal inflammation, peripheral
H30.031 Focal chorioretinal inflammation, peripheral, right eye
H30.032 Focal chorioretinal inflammation, peripheral, left eye
H30.033 Focal chorioretinal inflammation, peripheral, bilateral
H30.039 Focal chorioretinal inflammation, peripheral, unspecified eye ▽
☑6ᵗʰ H30.04 Focal chorioretinal inflammation, macular or paramacular
H30.041 Focal chorioretinal inflammation, macular or paramacular, right eye
H30.042 Focal chorioretinal inflammation, macular or paramacular, left eye
H30.043 Focal chorioretinal inflammation, macular or paramacular, bilateral
H30.049 Focal chorioretinal inflammation, macular or paramacular, unspecified eye ▽

☑ Additional Character Req   ✓x7ᵗʰ Placeholder Alert   Case-Mix Diagnosis   Manifestation   ▽ Unspecified Dx   EXCLUDES 1 Not coded here   EXCLUDES 2 Not included here

ICD-10-CM 2018   585

Chapter 7. Diseases of the Eye and Adnexa

H30.1–H31.112

✓5ᵗʰ **H30.1** Disseminated **chorioretinal inflammation**
Disseminated chorioretinitis
Disseminated choroiditis
Disseminated retinitis
Disseminated retinochoroiditis
 EXCLUDES 2   *exudative retinopathy (H35.02-)*

  ✓6ᵗʰ **H30.10** Unspecified **disseminated chorioretinal inflammation**
Disseminated chorioretinitis NOS
Disseminated choroiditis NOS
Disseminated retinitis NOS
Disseminated retinochoroiditis NOS

    H30.101   **Unspecified disseminated chorioretinal** ▽
inflammation, right eye

    H30.102   **Unspecified disseminated chorioretinal** ▽
inflammation, left eye

    H30.103   **Unspecified disseminated chorioretinal** ▽
inflammation, bilateral

    H30.109   **Unspecified disseminated chorioretinal** ▽
inflammation, unspecified eye

  ✓6ᵗʰ **H30.11** Disseminated **chorioretinal inflammation of posterior pole**

    H30.111   **Disseminated chorioretinal inflammation of posterior pole, right eye**

    H30.112   **Disseminated chorioretinal inflammation of posterior pole, left eye**

    H30.113   **Disseminated chorioretinal inflammation of posterior pole, bilateral**

    H30.119   **Disseminated chorioretinal** ▽
inflammation of posterior pole, unspecified eye

  ✓6ᵗʰ **H30.12** Disseminated **chorioretinal inflammation, peripheral**

    H30.121   **Disseminated chorioretinal inflammation, peripheral right eye**

    H30.122   **Disseminated chorioretinal inflammation, peripheral, left eye**

    H30.123   **Disseminated chorioretinal inflammation, peripheral, bilateral**

    H30.129   **Disseminated chorioretinal** ▽
inflammation, peripheral, unspecified eye

  ✓6ᵗʰ **H30.13** Disseminated **chorioretinal inflammation, generalized**

    H30.131   **Disseminated chorioretinal inflammation, generalized, right eye**

    H30.132   **Disseminated chorioretinal inflammation, generalized, left eye**

    H30.133   **Disseminated chorioretinal inflammation, generalized, bilateral**

    H30.139   **Disseminated chorioretinal** ▽
inflammation, generalized, unspecified eye

  ✓6ᵗʰ **H30.14** Acute **posterior multifocal placoid pigment epitheliopathy**

    H30.141   **Acute posterior multifocal placoid pigment epitheliopathy, right eye**

    H30.142   **Acute posterior multifocal placoid pigment epitheliopathy, left eye**

    H30.143   **Acute posterior multifocal placoid pigment epitheliopathy, bilateral**

    H30.149   **Acute posterior multifocal placoid** ▽
pigment epitheliopathy, unspecified eye

✓5ᵗʰ **H30.2** Posterior **cyclitis**
Pars planitis

    H30.20   **Posterior cyclitis, unspecified eye** ▽

    H30.21   **Posterior cyclitis, right eye**

    H30.22   **Posterior cyclitis, left eye**

    H30.23   **Posterior cyclitis, bilateral**

✓5ᵗʰ **H30.8** Other **chorioretinal inflammations**

  ✓6ᵗʰ **H30.81** Harada's **disease**

    H30.811   **Harada's disease, right eye**

    H30.812   **Harada's disease, left eye**

    H30.813   **Harada's disease, bilateral**

    H30.819   **Harada's disease, unspecified eye** ▽

  ✓6ᵗʰ **H30.89** Other **chorioretinal inflammations**

    H30.891   **Other chorioretinal inflammations, right eye**

    H30.892   **Other chorioretinal inflammations, left eye**

    H30.893   **Other chorioretinal inflammations, bilateral**

    H30.899   **Other chorioretinal inflammations,** ▽
unspecified eye

✓5ᵗʰ **H30.9** Unspecified **chorioretinal inflammation**
Chorioretinitis NOS
Choroiditis NOS
Neuroretinitis NOS
Retinitis NOS
Retinochoroiditis NOS

    H30.90   **Unspecified chorioretinal inflammation,** ▽
unspecified eye

    H30.91   **Unspecified chorioretinal inflammation, right eye** ▽

    H30.92   **Unspecified chorioretinal inflammation, left eye** ▽

    H30.93   **Unspecified chorioretinal inflammation, bilateral** ▽

✓4ᵗʰ **H31** **Other disorders of choroid**

  ✓5ᵗʰ **H31.0** Chorioretinal **scars**
 EXCLUDES 2   *postsurgical chorioretinal scars (H59.81-)*

  ✓6ᵗʰ **H31.00** Unspecified **chorioretinal scars**

    H31.001   **Unspecified chorioretinal scars, right** ▽
eye

    H31.002   **Unspecified chorioretinal scars, left** ▽
eye

    H31.003   **Unspecified chorioretinal scars,** ▽
bilateral

    H31.009   **Unspecified chorioretinal scars,** ▽
unspecified eye

  ✓6ᵗʰ **H31.01** Macula **scars of posterior pole (postinflammatory) (post-traumatic)**
 EXCLUDES 1   *postprocedural choriorentinal scar (H59.81-)*

    H31.011   **Macula scars of posterior pole (postinflammatory) (post-traumatic), right eye**

    H31.012   **Macula scars of posterior pole (postinflammatory) (post-traumatic), left eye**

    H31.013   **Macula scars of posterior pole (postinflammatory) (post-traumatic), bilateral**

    H31.019   **Macula scars of posterior pole** ▽
(postinflammatory) (post-traumatic), unspecified eye

  ✓6ᵗʰ **H31.02** Solar **retinopathy**

    H31.021   **Solar retinopathy, right eye**

    H31.022   **Solar retinopathy, left eye**

    H31.023   **Solar retinopathy, bilateral**

    H31.029   **Solar retinopathy, unspecified eye** ▽

  ✓6ᵗʰ **H31.09** Other **chorioretinal scars**

    H31.091   **Other chorioretinal scars, right eye**

    H31.092   **Other chorioretinal scars, left eye**

    H31.093   **Other chorioretinal scars, bilateral**

    H31.099   **Other chorioretinal scars, unspecified** ▽
eye

  ✓5ᵗʰ **H31.1** Choroidal **degeneration**
 EXCLUDES 2   *angioid streaks of macula (H35.33)*

  ✓6ᵗʰ **H31.10** Unspecified **choroidal degeneration**
Choroidal sclerosis NOS

    H31.101   **Choroidal degeneration, unspecified,** ▽
right eye

    H31.102   **Choroidal degeneration, unspecified,** ▽
left eye

    H31.103   **Choroidal degeneration, unspecified,** ▽
bilateral

    H31.109   **Choroidal degeneration, unspecified,** ▽
unspecified eye

  ✓6ᵗʰ **H31.11** Age-related **choroidal atrophy**

    H31.111   **Age-related choroidal atrophy,** Ⓐ
right eye

    H31.112   **Age-related choroidal atrophy,** Ⓐ
left eye

Ⓝ Newborn: 0   Ⓟ Pediatric: 0-17   Ⓜ Maternity: 12-55   Ⓐ Adult: 15-124   **NRS** Nonroutine supply Dx   **NCDx** Noncancer Dx   **PDx** Primary Dx   ▶◀ Revised Text   ● New Code   ▲ Revised Title

H31.113 **Age-related choroidal atrophy,** 🅰
bilateral

H31.119 **Age-related choroidal atrophy,** 🅰 ▽
unspecified eye

✓6ᵗʰ **H31.12** Diffuse secondary **atrophy of choroid**

H31.121 **Diffuse secondary atrophy of choroid,**
right eye

H31.122 **Diffuse secondary atrophy of choroid,**
left eye

H31.123 **Diffuse secondary atrophy of choroid,**
bilateral

H31.129 **Diffuse secondary atrophy of choroid,** ▽
unspecified eye

✓5ᵗʰ **H31.2** **Hereditary choroidal dystrophy**

EXCLUDES 2   hyperornithinemia (E72.4)
ornithinemia (E72.4)

H31.20 **Hereditary choroidal dystrophy, unspecified** ▽

H31.21 **Choroideremia**

H31.22 **Choroidal dystrophy (central areolar) (generalized)**
(peripapillary)

H31.23 **Gyrate atrophy, choroid**

H31.29 **Other hereditary choroidal dystrophy**

✓5ᵗʰ **H31.3** **Choroidal** hemorrhage and rupture

✓6ᵗʰ **H31.30** Unspecified **choroidal hemorrhage**

H31.301 **Unspecified choroidal hemorrhage,** ▽
right eye

H31.302 **Unspecified choroidal hemorrhage,** ▽
left eye

H31.303 **Unspecified choroidal hemorrhage,** ▽
bilateral

H31.309 **Unspecified choroidal hemorrhage,** ▽
unspecified eye

✓6ᵗʰ **H31.31** Expulsive **choroidal hemorrhage**

H31.311 **Expulsive choroidal hemorrhage,** right **eye**

H31.312 **Expulsive choroidal hemorrhage,** left **eye**

H31.313 **Expulsive choroidal hemorrhage,** bilateral

H31.319 **Expulsive choroidal hemorrhage,** ▽
unspecified eye

✓6ᵗʰ **H31.32** **Choroidal** rupture

H31.321 **Choroidal rupture,** right **eye**

H31.322 **Choroidal rupture,** left **eye**

H31.323 **Choroidal rupture,** bilateral

H31.329 **Choroidal rupture, unspecified eye** ▽

✓5ᵗʰ **H31.4** **Choroidal** detachment

✓6ᵗʰ **H31.40** Unspecified **choroidal detachment**

H31.401 **Unspecified choroidal detachment,** ▽
right eye

H31.402 **Unspecified choroidal detachment,** ▽
left eye

H31.403 **Unspecified choroidal detachment,** ▽
bilateral

H31.409 **Unspecified choroidal detachment,** ▽
unspecified eye

✓6ᵗʰ **H31.41** Hemorrhagic **choroidal detachment**

H31.411 **Hemorrhagic choroidal detachment,** right
eye

H31.412 **Hemorrhagic choroidal detachment,** left
eye

H31.413 **Hemorrhagic choroidal detachment,**
bilateral

H31.419 **Hemorrhagic choroidal detachment,** ▽
unspecified eye

✓6ᵗʰ **H31.42** Serous **choroidal detachment**

H31.421 **Serous choroidal detachment,** right **eye**

H31.422 **Serous choroidal detachment,** left **eye**

H31.423 **Serous choroidal detachment,** bilateral

H31.429 **Serous choroidal detachment,** ▽
unspecified eye

H31.8 **Other specified disorders of choroid**

H31.9 **Unspecified disorder of choroid** ▽

H32 *Chorioretinal disorders in diseases classified elsewhere*

Code first underlying disease, such as:
congenital toxoplasmosis (P37.1)
histoplasmosis (B39.-)
leprosy (A30.-)

EXCLUDES 1   chorioretinitis (in):
toxoplasmosis (acquired) (B58.01)
tuberculosis (A18.53)

✓4ᵗʰ **H33** **Retinal detachments and breaks**

EXCLUDES 1   detachment of retinal pigment epithelium (H35.72-, H35.73-)

✓5ᵗʰ **H33.0** **Retinal detachment** with retinal break

Rhegmatogenous retinal detachment

EXCLUDES 1   serous retinal detachment (without retinal break)
(H33.2-)

✓6ᵗʰ **H33.00** Unspecified **retinal detachment with retinal break**

H33.001 **Unspecified retinal detachment with** ▽
retinal break, right **eye**

H33.002 **Unspecified retinal detachment with** ▽
retinal break, left **eye**

H33.003 **Unspecified retinal detachment with** ▽
retinal break, bilateral

H33.009 **Unspecified retinal detachment with** ▽
retinal break, unspecified eye

✓6ᵗʰ **H33.01** **Retinal detachment with** single break

H33.011 **Retinal detachment with single break,**
right **eye**

H33.012 **Retinal detachment with single break,**
left **eye**

H33.013 **Retinal detachment with single break,**
bilateral

H33.019 **Retinal detachment with single break,** ▽
unspecified eye

✓6ᵗʰ **H33.02** **Retinal detachment with** multiple breaks

H33.021 **Retinal detachment with multiple breaks,**
right **eye**

H33.022 **Retinal detachment with multiple breaks,**
left **eye**

H33.023 **Retinal detachment with multiple breaks,**
bilateral

H33.029 **Retinal detachment with multiple** ▽
breaks, unspecified eye

✓6ᵗʰ **H33.03** **Retinal detachment with** giant retinal tear

H33.031 **Retinal detachment with giant retinal**
tear, right **eye**

H33.032 **Retinal detachment with giant retinal**
tear, left **eye**

H33.033 **Retinal detachment with giant retinal**
tear, bilateral

H33.039 **Retinal detachment with giant retinal** ▽
tear, unspecified eye

✓6ᵗʰ **H33.04** **Retinal detachment with** retinal dialysis

H33.041 **Retinal detachment with retinal dialysis,**
right **eye**

H33.042 **Retinal detachment with retinal dialysis,**
left **eye**

Retinal Detachment

Lens — Vitreous — Choroid — Area of detachment — Retina — Sclera — Cornea — Iris

✓ Additional Character Req   ✓x7ᵗʰ Placeholder Alert   Case-Mix Diagnosis   Manifestation   ▽ Unspecified Dx   *EXCLUDES 1* Not coded here   *EXCLUDES 2* Not included here

ICD-10-CM 2018   **587**

Chapter 7. Diseases of the Eye and Adnexa

H31.113–H33.042

Chapter 7. Diseases of the Eye and Adnexa

        H33.043   Retinal detachment with retinal dialysis, bilateral

        H33.049   Retinal detachment with retinal dialysis, unspecified eye ▽

✓6ᵗʰ   **H33.05**   Total retinal detachment

        H33.051   Total retinal detachment, right eye

        H33.052   Total retinal detachment, left eye

        H33.053   Total retinal detachment, bilateral

        H33.059   Total retinal detachment, unspecified eye ▽

✓5ᵗʰ   **H33.1**   Retinoschisis and retinal cysts

    EXCLUDES 1   congenital retinoschisis (Q14.1)
            microcystoid degeneration of retina (H35.42-)

✓6ᵗʰ   **H33.10**   Unspecified retinoschisis

        H33.101   Unspecified retinoschisis, right eye ▽

        H33.102   Unspecified retinoschisis, left eye ▽

        H33.103   Unspecified retinoschisis, bilateral ▽

        H33.109   Unspecified retinoschisis, unspecified eye ▽

✓6ᵗʰ   **H33.11**   Cyst of ora serrata

        H33.111   Cyst of ora serrata, right eye

        H33.112   Cyst of ora serrata, left eye

        H33.113   Cyst of ora serrata, bilateral

        H33.119   Cyst of ora serrata, unspecified eye ▽

✓6ᵗʰ   **H33.12**   Parasitic cyst of retina

        H33.121   Parasitic cyst of retina, right eye

        H33.122   Parasitic cyst of retina, left eye

        H33.123   Parasitic cyst of retina, bilateral

        H33.129   Parasitic cyst of retina, unspecified eye ▽

✓6ᵗʰ   **H33.19**   Other retinoschisis and retinal cysts

    Pseudocyst of retina

        H33.191   Other retinoschisis and retinal cysts, right eye

        H33.192   Other retinoschisis and retinal cysts, left eye

        H33.193   Other retinoschisis and retinal cysts, bilateral

        H33.199   Other retinoschisis and retinal cysts, unspecified eye ▽

✓5ᵗʰ   **H33.2**   Serous retinal detachment

    Retinal detachment NOS
    Retinal detachment without retinal break

    EXCLUDES 1   central serous chorioretinopathy (H35.71-)

    H33.20   Serous retinal detachment, unspecified eye ▽

    H33.21   Serous retinal detachment, right eye

    H33.22   Serous retinal detachment, left eye

    H33.23   Serous retinal detachment, bilateral

✓5ᵗʰ   **H33.3**   Retinal breaks without detachment

    EXCLUDES 1   chorioretinal scars after surgery for detachment (H59.81-)
            peripheral retinal degeneration without break (H35.4-)

✓6ᵗʰ   **H33.30**   Unspecified retinal break

        H33.301   Unspecified retinal break, right eye ▽

        H33.302   Unspecified retinal break, left eye ▽

        H33.303   Unspecified retinal break, bilateral ▽

        H33.309   Unspecified retinal break, unspecified eye ▽

✓6ᵗʰ   **H33.31**   Horseshoe tear of retina without detachment

    Operculum of retina without detachment

        H33.311   Horseshoe tear of retina without detachment, right eye

        H33.312   Horseshoe tear of retina without detachment, left eye

        H33.313   Horseshoe tear of retina without detachment, bilateral

        H33.319   Horseshoe tear of retina without detachment, unspecified eye ▽

✓6ᵗʰ   **H33.32**   Round hole of retina without detachment

        H33.321   Round hole, right eye

        H33.322   Round hole, left eye

        H33.323   Round hole, bilateral

        H33.329   Round hole, unspecified eye ▽

✓6ᵗʰ   **H33.33**   Multiple defects of retina without detachment

        H33.331   Multiple defects of retina without detachment, right eye

        H33.332   Multiple defects of retina without detachment, left eye

        H33.333   Multiple defects of retina without detachment, bilateral

        H33.339   Multiple defects of retina without detachment, unspecified eye ▽

✓5ᵗʰ   **H33.4**   Traction detachment of retina

    Proliferative vitreo-retinopathy with retinal detachment

    H33.40   Traction detachment of retina, unspecified eye ▽

    H33.41   Traction detachment of retina, right eye

    H33.42   Traction detachment of retina, left eye

    H33.43   Traction detachment of retina, bilateral

    H33.8   Other retinal detachments

✓4ᵗʰ   **H34**   **Retinal vascular occlusions**

    EXCLUDES 1   amaurosis fugax (G45.3)

✓5ᵗʰ   **H34.0**   Transient retinal artery occlusion

    H34.00   Transient retinal artery occlusion, unspecified eye ▽

    H34.01   Transient retinal artery occlusion, right eye

    H34.02   Transient retinal artery occlusion, left eye

    H34.03   Transient retinal artery occlusion, bilateral

✓5ᵗʰ   **H34.1**   Central retinal artery occlusion

    H34.10   Central retinal artery occlusion, unspecified eye ▽

    H34.11   Central retinal artery occlusion, right eye

    H34.12   Central retinal artery occlusion, left eye

    H34.13   Central retinal artery occlusion, bilateral

✓5ᵗʰ   **H34.2**   Other retinal artery occlusions

✓6ᵗʰ   **H34.21**   Partial retinal artery occlusion

    Hollenhorst's plaque
    Retinal microembolism

        H34.211   Partial retinal artery occlusion, right eye

        H34.212   Partial retinal artery occlusion, left eye

        H34.213   Partial retinal artery occlusion, bilateral

        H34.219   Partial retinal artery occlusion, unspecified eye ▽

✓6ᵗʰ   **H34.23**   Retinal artery branch occlusion

        H34.231   Retinal artery branch occlusion, right eye

        H34.232   Retinal artery branch occlusion, left eye

        H34.233   Retinal artery branch occlusion, bilateral

        H34.239   Retinal artery branch occlusion, unspecified eye ▽

✓5ᵗʰ   **H34.8**   Other retinal vascular occlusions

✓6ᵗʰ   **H34.81**   Central retinal vein occlusion

> One of the following 7th characters is to be assigned to codes in subcategory H34.81 to designate the severity of the occlusion:
> 0   with macular edema
> 1   with retinal neovascularization
> 2   stable
>   old central retinal vein occlusion

    ✓7ᵗʰ   **H34.811**   Central retinal vein occlusion, right eye

    ✓7ᵗʰ   **H34.812**   Central retinal vein occlusion, left eye

    ✓7ᵗʰ   **H34.813**   Central retinal vein occlusion, bilateral

    ✓7ᵗʰ   **H34.819**   Central retinal vein occlusion, unspecified eye ▽

✓6ᵗʰ   **H34.82**   Venous engorgement

    Incipient retinal vein occlusion
    Partial retinal vein occlusion

        H34.821   Venous engorgement, right eye

        H34.822   Venous engorgement, left eye

        H34.823   Venous engorgement, bilateral

        H34.829   Venous engorgement, unspecified eye ▽

Ⓝ Newborn: 0   Ⓟ Pediatric: 0-17   Ⓜ Maternity: 12-55   Ⓐ Adult: 15-124   **NRS** Nonroutine supply Dx   **NC Dx** Noncancer Dx   **PDx** Primary Dx   ►◄ Revised Text   ● New Code   ▲ Revised Title

588   ICD-10-CM 2018

✓6ᵗʰ **H34.83**   **Tributary (branch) retinal vein occlusion**

> One of the following 7th characters is to be assigned to codes in subcategory H34.83 to designate the severity of the occlusion:
> Ø   with macular edema
> 1   with retinal neovascularization
> 2   stable
>   old tributary (branch) retinal vein occlusion

✓7ᵗʰ   **H34.831**   **Tributary (branch) retinal vein occlusion, right eye**

✓7ᵗʰ   **H34.832**   **Tributary (branch) retinal vein occlusion, left eye**

✓7ᵗʰ   **H34.833**   **Tributary (branch) retinal vein occlusion, bilateral**

✓7ᵗʰ   **H34.839**   **Tributary (branch) retinal vein occlusion, unspecified eye** ▽

H34.9   **Unspecified retinal vascular occlusion** ▽

✓4ᵗʰ **H35**   **Other retinal disorders**
    EXCLUDES 2   *diabetic retinal disorders (E08.311- E08.359, E09.311- E09.359, E10.311- E10.359, E11.311- E11.359, E13.311- E13.359)*

✓5ᵗʰ **H35.0**   **Background retinopathy and retinal vascular changes**
    Code also any associated hypertension (I10.-)

    H35.00   **Unspecified background retinopathy** ▽

✓6ᵗʰ **H35.01**   **Changes in retinal vascular appearance**
    Retinal vascular sheathing

    H35.011   **Changes in retinal vascular appearance, right eye**

    H35.012   **Changes in retinal vascular appearance, left eye**

    H35.013   **Changes in retinal vascular appearance, bilateral**

    H35.019   **Changes in retinal vascular appearance, unspecified eye** ▽

✓6ᵗʰ **H35.02**   **Exudative retinopathy**
    Coats retinopathy

    H35.021   **Exudative retinopathy, right eye**
    H35.022   **Exudative retinopathy, left eye**
    H35.023   **Exudative retinopathy, bilateral**
    H35.029   **Exudative retinopathy, unspecified eye** ▽

✓6ᵗʰ **H35.03**   **Hypertensive retinopathy**

    H35.031   **Hypertensive retinopathy, right eye**
    H35.032   **Hypertensive retinopathy, left eye**
    H35.033   **Hypertensive retinopathy, bilateral**
    H35.039   **Hypertensive retinopathy, unspecified eye** ▽

✓6ᵗʰ **H35.04**   **Retinal micro-aneurysms, unspecified**

    H35.041   **Retinal micro-aneurysms, unspecified, right eye** ▽

    H35.042   **Retinal micro-aneurysms, unspecified, left eye** ▽

    H35.043   **Retinal micro-aneurysms, unspecified, bilateral** ▽

    H35.049   **Retinal micro-aneurysms, unspecified, unspecified eye** ▽

✓6ᵗʰ **H35.05**   **Retinal neovascularization, unspecified**

    H35.051   **Retinal neovascularization, unspecified, right eye** ▽

    H35.052   **Retinal neovascularization, unspecified, left eye** ▽

    H35.053   **Retinal neovascularization, unspecified, bilateral** ▽

    H35.059   **Retinal neovascularization, unspecified, unspecified eye** ▽

✓6ᵗʰ **H35.06**   **Retinal vasculitis**
    Eales disease
    Retinal perivasculitis
    DEF: Sight-threatening intraocular inflammation of the retinal blood vessels; causes minimal, partial, or even complete blindness.

    H35.061   **Retinal vasculitis, right eye**
    H35.062   **Retinal vasculitis, left eye**
    H35.063   **Retinal vasculitis, bilateral**
    H35.069   **Retinal vasculitis, unspecified eye**

✓6ᵗʰ **H35.07**   **Retinal telangiectasis**

    H35.071   **Retinal telangiectasis, right eye**
    H35.072   **Retinal telangiectasis, left eye**
    H35.073   **Retinal telangiectasis, bilateral**
    H35.079   **Retinal telangiectasis, unspecified eye** ▽

    H35.09   **Other intraretinal microvascular abnormalities**
       Retinal varices

✓5ᵗʰ **H35.1**   **Retinopathy of prematurity**

✓6ᵗʰ **H35.10**   **Retinopathy of prematurity, unspecified**
    Retinopathy of prematurity NOS

    H35.101   **Retinopathy of prematurity, unspecified, right eye** ▽

    H35.102   **Retinopathy of prematurity, unspecified, left eye** ▽

    H35.103   **Retinopathy of prematurity, unspecified, bilateral** ▽

    H35.109   **Retinopathy of prematurity, unspecified, unspecified eye** ▽

✓6ᵗʰ **H35.11**   **Retinopathy of prematurity, stage Ø**

    H35.111   **Retinopathy of prematurity, stage Ø, right eye**

    H35.112   **Retinopathy of prematurity, stage Ø, left eye**

    H35.113   **Retinopathy of prematurity, stage Ø, bilateral**

    H35.119   **Retinopathy of prematurity, stage Ø, unspecified eye** ▽

✓6ᵗʰ **H35.12**   **Retinopathy of prematurity, stage 1**

    H35.121   **Retinopathy of prematurity, stage 1, right eye**

    H35.122   **Retinopathy of prematurity, stage 1, left eye**

    H35.123   **Retinopathy of prematurity, stage 1, bilateral**

    H35.129   **Retinopathy of prematurity, stage 1, unspecified eye** ▽

✓6ᵗʰ **H35.13**   **Retinopathy of prematurity, stage 2**

    H35.131   **Retinopathy of prematurity, stage 2, right eye**

    H35.132   **Retinopathy of prematurity, stage 2, left eye**

    H35.133   **Retinopathy of prematurity, stage 2, bilateral**

    H35.139   **Retinopathy of prematurity, stage 2, unspecified eye** ▽

✓6ᵗʰ **H35.14**   **Retinopathy of prematurity, stage 3**

    H35.141   **Retinopathy of prematurity, stage 3, right eye**

    H35.142   **Retinopathy of prematurity, stage 3, left eye**

    H35.143   **Retinopathy of prematurity, stage 3, bilateral**

    H35.149   **Retinopathy of prematurity, stage 3, unspecified eye** ▽

✓6ᵗʰ **H35.15**   **Retinopathy of prematurity, stage 4**

    H35.151   **Retinopathy of prematurity, stage 4, right eye**

    H35.152   **Retinopathy of prematurity, stage 4, left eye**

    H35.153   **Retinopathy of prematurity, stage 4, bilateral**

    H35.159   **Retinopathy of prematurity, stage 4, unspecified eye** ▽

✓6ᵗʰ **H35.16**   **Retinopathy of prematurity, stage 5**

    H35.161   **Retinopathy of prematurity, stage 5, right eye**

    H35.162   **Retinopathy of prematurity, stage 5, left eye**

    H35.163   **Retinopathy of prematurity, stage 5, bilateral**

    H35.169   **Retinopathy of prematurity, stage 5, unspecified eye** ▽

✓6ᵗʰ **H35.17**   **Retrolental fibroplasia**

    H35.171   **Retrolental fibroplasia, right eye**
    H35.172   **Retrolental fibroplasia, left eye**
    H35.173   **Retrolental fibroplasia, bilateral**
    H35.179   **Retrolental fibroplasia, unspecified eye** ▽

✔ Additional Character Req   ✓x7ᵗʰ Placeholder Alert   Case-Mix Diagnosis   Manifestation   ▽ Unspecified Dx   EXCLUDES 1 Not coded here   EXCLUDES 2 Not included here

ICD-10-CM 2018   589

Chapter 7. Diseases of the Eye and Adnexa

H34.83–H35.179

Chapter 7. Diseases of the Eye and Adnexa

H35.2–H35.459

✓5ᵗʰ H35.2 Other non-diabetic proliferative retinopathy
Proliferative vitreo-retinopathy
EXCLUDES 1   *proliferative vitreo-retinopathy with retinal detachment (H33.4-)*

     H35.20 Other non-diabetic proliferative retinopathy, unspecified eye ▽

     H35.21 Other non-diabetic proliferative retinopathy, right eye

     H35.22 Other non-diabetic proliferative retinopathy, left eye

     H35.23 Other non-diabetic proliferative retinopathy, bilateral

✓5ᵗʰ H35.3 Degeneration of macula and posterior pole

     H35.30 Unspecified macular degeneration Ⓐ ▽
Age-related macular degeneration

     ✓6ᵗʰ H35.31 Nonexudative age-related macular degeneration
Atrophic age-related macular degeneration
Dry age-related macular degeneration
AHA: 2016, 4Q, 21

One of the following 7th characters is to be assigned to codes in subcategory H35.31 to designate the stage of the disease:
0   stage unspecified
1   early dry stage
2   intermediate dry stage
3   advanced atrophic without subfoveal involvement
    advanced dry stage
4   advanced atrophic with subfoveal involvement

     ✓7ᵗʰ H35.311 Nonexudative age-related macular degeneration, right eye Ⓐ

     ✓7ᵗʰ H35.312 Nonexudative age-related macular degeneration, left eye Ⓐ

     ✓7ᵗʰ H35.313 Nonexudative age-related macular degeneration, bilateral Ⓐ

     ✓7ᵗʰ H35.319 Nonexudative age-related macular degeneration, unspecified eye Ⓐ ▽

     ✓6ᵗʰ H35.32 Exudative age-related macular degeneration
Wet age-related macular degeneration

One of the following 7th characters is to be assigned to codes in subcategory H35.32 to designate the stage of the disease:
0   stage unspecified
1   with active choroidal neovascularization
2   with inactive choroidal neovascularization
    with involuted or regressed neovascularization
3   with inactive scar

     ✓7ᵗʰ H35.321 Exudative age-related macular degeneration, right eye Ⓐ

     ✓7ᵗʰ H35.322 Exudative age-related macular degeneration, left eye Ⓐ

     ✓7ᵗʰ H35.323 Exudative age-related macular degeneration, bilateral Ⓐ

     ✓7ᵗʰ H35.329 Exudative age-related macular degeneration, unspecified eye Ⓐ ▽

     H35.33 Angioid streaks of macula
DEF: Degeneration of choroid; characterized by broad, irregular, dark brown streaks radiating from optic disc; occurs with pseudoxanthoma elasticum or Paget's disease.

     ✓6ᵗʰ H35.34 Macular cyst, hole, or pseudohole

     H35.341 Macular cyst, hole, or pseudohole, right eye

     H35.342 Macular cyst, hole, or pseudohole, left eye

     H35.343 Macular cyst, hole, or pseudohole, bilateral

     H35.349 Macular cyst, hole, or pseudohole, unspecified eye ▽

     ✓6ᵗʰ H35.35 Cystoid macular degeneration
EXCLUDES 1   *cystoid macular edema following cataract surgery (H59.03-)*

     H35.351 Cystoid macular degeneration, right eye

     H35.352 Cystoid macular degeneration, left eye

     H35.353 Cystoid macular degeneration, bilateral

     H35.359 Cystoid macular degeneration, unspecified eye ▽

✓6ᵗʰ H35.36 Drusen (degenerative) of macula
AHA: 2017, 1Q, 51; 2016, 4Q, 21

     H35.361 Drusen (degenerative) of macula, right eye

     H35.362 Drusen (degenerative) of macula, left eye

     H35.363 Drusen (degenerative) of macula, bilateral

     H35.369 Drusen (degenerative) of macula, unspecified eye ▽

✓6ᵗʰ H35.37 Puckering of macula

     H35.371 Puckering of macula, right eye

     H35.372 Puckering of macula, left eye

     H35.373 Puckering of macula, bilateral

     H35.379 Puckering of macula, unspecified eye ▽

✓6ᵗʰ H35.38 Toxic maculopathy
Code first poisoning due to drug or toxin, if applicable (T36-T65 with fifth or sixth character 1-4 or 6)
Use additional code for adverse effect, if applicable, to identify drug (T36-T50 with fifth or sixth character 5)

     H35.381 Toxic maculopathy, right eye

     H35.382 Toxic maculopathy, left eye

     H35.383 Toxic maculopathy, bilateral

     H35.389 Toxic maculopathy, unspecified eye ▽

✓5ᵗʰ H35.4 Peripheral retinal degeneration
EXCLUDES 1   *hereditary retinal degeneration (dystrophy) (H35.5-)*
peripheral retinal degeneration with retinal break (H33.3-)

     H35.40 Unspecified peripheral retinal degeneration ▽

     ✓6ᵗʰ H35.41 Lattice degeneration of retina
Palisade degeneration of retina
DEF: Degeneration of retina; often bilateral, usually benign; characterized by lines intersecting at irregular intervals in peripheral retina; retinal thinning and retinal holes may occur.

     H35.411 Lattice degeneration of retina, right eye

     H35.412 Lattice degeneration of retina, left eye

     H35.413 Lattice degeneration of retina, bilateral

     H35.419 Lattice degeneration of retina, unspecified eye ▽

     ✓6ᵗʰ H35.42 Microcystoid degeneration of retina

     H35.421 Microcystoid degeneration of retina, right eye

     H35.422 Microcystoid degeneration of retina, left eye

     H35.423 Microcystoid degeneration of retina, bilateral

     H35.429 Microcystoid degeneration of retina, unspecified eye ▽

     ✓6ᵗʰ H35.43 Paving stone degeneration of retina

     H35.431 Paving stone degeneration of retina, right eye

     H35.432 Paving stone degeneration of retina, left eye

     H35.433 Paving stone degeneration of retina, bilateral

     H35.439 Paving stone degeneration of retina, unspecified eye ▽

     ✓6ᵗʰ H35.44 Age-related reticular degeneration of retina

     H35.441 Age-related reticular degeneration of retina, right eye Ⓐ

     H35.442 Age-related reticular degeneration of retina, left eye Ⓐ

     H35.443 Age-related reticular degeneration of retina, bilateral Ⓐ

     H35.449 Age-related reticular degeneration of retina, unspecified eye Ⓐ ▽

     ✓6ᵗʰ H35.45 Secondary pigmentary degeneration

     H35.451 Secondary pigmentary degeneration, right eye

     H35.452 Secondary pigmentary degeneration, left eye

     H35.453 Secondary pigmentary degeneration, bilateral

     H35.459 Secondary pigmentary degeneration, unspecified eye ▽

Ⓝ Newborn: 0   Ⓟ Pediatric: 0-17   Ⓜ Maternity: 12-55   Ⓐ Adult: 15-124   **NRS** Nonroutine supply Dx   **NCDx** Noncancer Dx   **PDx** Primary Dx   ►◄ Revised Text   ● New Code   ▲ Revised Title

590   ICD-10-CM 2018

✓6th **H35.46** Secondary vitreoretinal degeneration

     H35.461 Secondary vitreoretinal degeneration, right eye

     H35.462 Secondary vitreoretinal degeneration, left eye

     H35.463 Secondary vitreoretinal degeneration, bilateral

     H35.469 Secondary vitreoretinal degeneration, unspecified eye ▽

✓5th **H35.5** Hereditary retinal dystrophy

     EXCLUDES 1   *dystrophies primarily involving Bruch's membrane (H31.1-)*

     H35.50 Unspecified hereditary retinal dystrophy ▽

     H35.51 Vitreoretinal dystrophy

     H35.52 Pigmentary retinal dystrophy
         Albipunctate retinal dystrophy
         Retinitis pigmentosa
         Tapetoretinal dystrophy

     H35.53 Other dystrophies primarily involving the sensory retina
         Stargardt's disease

     H35.54 Dystrophies primarily involving the retinal pigment epithelium
         Vitelliform retinal dystrophy

✓5th **H35.6** Retinal hemorrhage

     H35.60 Retinal hemorrhage, unspecified eye ▽

     H35.61 Retinal hemorrhage, right eye

     H35.62 Retinal hemorrhage, left eye

     H35.63 Retinal hemorrhage, bilateral

✓5th **H35.7** Separation of retinal layers

     EXCLUDES 1   *retinal detachment (serous) (H33.2-)*
                rhegmatogenous retinal detachment (H33.0-)

     H35.70 Unspecified separation of retinal layers ▽

✓6th **H35.71** Central serous chorioretinopathy

     H35.711 Central serous chorioretinopathy, right eye

     H35.712 Central serous chorioretinopathy, left eye

     H35.713 Central serous chorioretinopathy, bilateral

     H35.719 Central serous chorioretinopathy, unspecified eye ▽

✓6th **H35.72** Serous detachment of retinal pigment epithelium

     H35.721 Serous detachment of retinal pigment epithelium, right eye

     H35.722 Serous detachment of retinal pigment epithelium, left eye

     H35.723 Serous detachment of retinal pigment epithelium, bilateral

     H35.729 Serous detachment of retinal pigment epithelium, unspecified eye ▽

✓6th **H35.73** Hemorrhagic detachment of retinal pigment epithelium

     H35.731 Hemorrhagic detachment of retinal pigment epithelium, right eye

     H35.732 Hemorrhagic detachment of retinal pigment epithelium, left eye

     H35.733 Hemorrhagic detachment of retinal pigment epithelium, bilateral

     H35.739 Hemorrhagic detachment of retinal pigment epithelium, unspecified eye ▽

✓5th **H35.8** Other specified retinal disorders

     EXCLUDES 2   *retinal hemorrhage (H35.6-)*

     H35.81 Retinal edema
         Retinal cotton wool spots

     H35.82 Retinal ischemia

     H35.89 Other specified retinal disorders

H35.9 Unspecified retinal disorder ▽

H36 *Retinal disorders in diseases classified elsewhere*
     Code first underlying disease, such as:
         lipid storage disorders (E75.-)
         sickle-cell disorders (D57.-)
     EXCLUDES 1   *arteriosclerotic retinopathy (H35.0-)*
                diabetic retinopathy (E08.3-, E09.3-, E10.3-, E11.3-, E13.3-)

Glaucoma (H40-H42)

✓4th **H40** Glaucoma

     EXCLUDES 1   *absolute glaucoma (H44.51-)*
                congenital glaucoma (Q15.0)
                traumatic glaucoma due to birth injury (P15.3)

✓5th **H40.0** Glaucoma suspect

     ✓6th **H40.00** Preglaucoma, unspecified

         H40.001 Preglaucoma, unspecified, right eye ▽

         H40.002 Preglaucoma, unspecified, left eye ▽

         H40.003 Preglaucoma, unspecified, bilateral ▽

         H40.009 Preglaucoma, unspecified, unspecified eye ▽

     ✓6th **H40.01** Open angle with borderline findings, low risk
         Open angle, low risk

         H40.011 Open angle with borderline findings, low risk, right eye

         H40.012 Open angle with borderline findings, low risk, left eye

         H40.013 Open angle with borderline findings, low risk, bilateral

         H40.019 Open angle with borderline findings, low risk, unspecified eye ▽

     ✓6th **H40.02** Open angle with borderline findings, high risk
         Open angle, high risk

         H40.021 Open angle with borderline findings, high risk, right eye

         H40.022 Open angle with borderline findings, high risk, left eye

         H40.023 Open angle with borderline findings, high risk, bilateral

         H40.029 Open angle with borderline findings, high risk, unspecified eye ▽

     ✓6th **H40.03** Anatomical narrow angle
         Primary angle closure suspect

         H40.031 Anatomical narrow angle, right eye

         H40.032 Anatomical narrow angle, left eye

         H40.033 Anatomical narrow angle, bilateral

         H40.039 Anatomical narrow angle, unspecified eye ▽

     ✓6th **H40.04** Steroid responder

         H40.041 Steroid responder, right eye

         H40.042 Steroid responder, left eye

         H40.043 Steroid responder, bilateral

         H40.049 Steroid responder, unspecified eye ▽

     ✓6th **H40.05** Ocular hypertension

         H40.051 Ocular hypertension, right eye

         H40.052 Ocular hypertension, left eye

         H40.053 Ocular hypertension, bilateral

         H40.059 Ocular hypertension, unspecified eye ▽

     ✓6th **H40.06** Primary angle closure without glaucoma damage

         H40.061 Primary angle closure without glaucoma damage, right eye

         H40.062 Primary angle closure without glaucoma damage, left eye

         H40.063 Primary angle closure without glaucoma damage, bilateral

         H40.069 Primary angle closure without glaucoma damage, unspecified eye ▽

✓5th **H40.1** Open-angle glaucoma

> One of the following 7th characters is to be assigned to each code in subcategories H40.10, H40.11-, H40.12-, H40.13-, and H40.14- to designate the stage of glaucoma.
> 0   stage unspecified
> 1   mild stage
> 2   moderate stage
> 3   severe stage
> 4   indeterminate stage

     ✓x7th **H40.10** Unspecified open-angle glaucoma ▽

     ✓6th **H40.11** Primary open-angle glaucoma
         Chronic simple glaucoma

         ✓7th **H40.111** Primary open-angle glaucoma, right eye

         ✓7th **H40.112** Primary open-angle glaucoma, left eye

         ✓7th **H40.113** Primary open-angle glaucoma, bilateral

         ✓7th **H40.119** Primary open-angle glaucoma, unspecified eye ▽

☑ Additional Character Req   ✓x7th Placeholder Alert   Case-Mix Diagnosis   Manifestation   ▽ Unspecified Dx   *EXCLUDES 1* Not coded here   *EXCLUDES 2* Not included here

ICD-10-CM 2018   **591**

✓6ᵗʰ **H40.12** Low-tension **glaucoma**
- ✓7ᵗʰ **H40.121** Low-tension glaucoma, **right** eye
- ✓7ᵗʰ **H40.122** Low-tension glaucoma, **left** eye
- ✓7ᵗʰ **H40.123** Low-tension glaucoma, **bilateral**
- ✓7ᵗʰ **H40.129** Low-tension glaucoma, **unspecified eye** ▽

✓6ᵗʰ **H40.13** Pigmentary **glaucoma**
- ✓7ᵗʰ **H40.131** Pigmentary glaucoma, **right** eye
- ✓7ᵗʰ **H40.132** Pigmentary glaucoma, **left** eye
- ✓7ᵗʰ **H40.133** Pigmentary glaucoma, **bilateral**
- ✓7ᵗʰ **H40.139** Pigmentary glaucoma, **unspecified eye** ▽

✓6ᵗʰ **H40.14** Capsular glaucoma with pseudoexfoliation **of lens**
- ✓7ᵗʰ **H40.141** Capsular glaucoma with pseudoexfoliation of lens, **right** eye
- ✓7ᵗʰ **H40.142** Capsular glaucoma with pseudoexfoliation of lens, **left** eye
- ✓7ᵗʰ **H40.143** Capsular glaucoma with pseudoexfoliation of lens, **bilateral**
- ✓7ᵗʰ **H40.149** Capsular glaucoma with pseudoexfoliation of lens, **unspecified eye** ▽

✓6ᵗʰ **H40.15** Residual stage **of open-angle glaucoma**
- **H40.151** Residual stage of open-angle glaucoma, **right** eye
- **H40.152** Residual stage of open-angle glaucoma, **left** eye
- **H40.153** Residual stage of open-angle glaucoma, **bilateral**
- **H40.159** Residual stage of open-angle glaucoma, **unspecified eye** ▽

✓5ᵗʰ **H40.2** Primary angle-closure **glaucoma**

> **EXCLUDES 1**   aqueous misdirection (H40.83-)
> malignant glaucoma (H40.83-)

> One of the following 7th characters is to be assigned to each code in subcategories H40.20 and H40.22- to designate the stage of glaucoma.
> Ø   stage unspecified
> 1   mild stage
> 2   moderate stage
> 3   severe stage
> 4   indeterminate stage

✓x7ᵗʰ **H40.20** Unspecified primary angle-closure **glaucoma** ▽

✓6ᵗʰ **H40.21** Acute **angle-closure glaucoma**
Acute angle-closure glaucoma attack
Acute angle-closure glaucoma crisis
- **H40.211** Acute angle-closure glaucoma, **right** eye
- **H40.212** Acute angle-closure glaucoma, **left** eye
- **H40.213** Acute angle-closure glaucoma, **bilateral**
- **H40.219** Acute angle-closure glaucoma, **unspecified eye** ▽

✓6ᵗʰ **H40.22** Chronic **angle-closure glaucoma**
Chronic primary angle-closure glaucoma
- ✓7ᵗʰ **H40.221** Chronic angle-closure glaucoma, **right** eye
- ✓7ᵗʰ **H40.222** Chronic angle-closure glaucoma, **left** eye
- ✓7ᵗʰ **H40.223** Chronic angle-closure glaucoma, **bilateral**
- ✓7ᵗʰ **H40.229** Chronic angle-closure glaucoma, **unspecified eye** ▽

Open Angle/Angle Closure Glaucoma

✓6ᵗʰ **H40.23** Intermittent **angle-closure glaucoma**
- **H40.231** Intermittent angle-closure glaucoma, **right** eye
- **H40.232** Intermittent angle-closure glaucoma, **left** eye
- **H40.233** Intermittent angle-closure glaucoma, **bilateral**
- **H40.239** Intermittent angle-closure glaucoma, **unspecified eye** ▽

✓6ᵗʰ **H40.24** Residual stage **of angle-closure glaucoma**
- **H40.241** Residual stage of angle-closure glaucoma, **right** eye
- **H40.242** Residual stage of angle-closure glaucoma, **left** eye
- **H40.243** Residual stage of angle-closure glaucoma, **bilateral**
- **H40.249** Residual stage of angle-closure glaucoma, **unspecified eye** ▽

✓5ᵗʰ **H40.3** Glaucoma secondary **to eye** trauma
Code also underlying condition

> One of the following 7th characters is to be assigned to each code in subcategory H40.3- to designate the stage of glaucoma.
> Ø   stage unspecified
> 1   mild stage
> 2   moderate stage
> 3   severe stage
> 4   indeterminate stage

✓x7ᵗʰ **H40.30** Glaucoma secondary to eye trauma, **unspecified eye** ▽

✓x7ᵗʰ **H40.31** Glaucoma secondary to eye trauma, **right** eye

✓x7ᵗʰ **H40.32** Glaucoma secondary to eye trauma, **left** eye

✓x7ᵗʰ **H40.33** Glaucoma secondary to eye trauma, **bilateral**

✓5ᵗʰ **H40.4** Glaucoma secondary **to eye** inflammation
Code also underlying condition

> One of the following 7th characters is to be assigned to each code in subcategory H40.4- to designate the stage of glaucoma.
> Ø   stage unspecified
> 1   mild stage
> 2   moderate stage
> 3   severe stage
> 4   indeterminate stage

✓x7ᵗʰ **H40.40** Glaucoma secondary to eye inflammation, **unspecified eye** ▽

✓x7ᵗʰ **H40.41** Glaucoma secondary to eye inflammation, **right** eye

✓x7ᵗʰ **H40.42** Glaucoma secondary to eye inflammation, **left** eye

✓x7ᵗʰ **H40.43** Glaucoma secondary to eye inflammation, **bilateral**

✓5ᵗʰ **H40.5** Glaucoma secondary **to other** eye disorders
Code also underlying eye disorder

> One of the following 7th characters is to be assigned to each code in subcategory H40.5- to designate the stage of glaucoma.
> Ø   stage unspecified
> 1   mild stage
> 2   moderate stage
> 3   severe stage
> 4   indeterminate stage

✓x7ᵗʰ **H40.50** Glaucoma secondary to other eye disorders, **unspecified eye** ▽

✓x7ᵗʰ **H40.51** Glaucoma secondary to other eye disorders, **right eye**

✓x7ᵗʰ **H40.52** Glaucoma secondary to other eye disorders, **left** eye

✓x7ᵗʰ **H40.53** Glaucoma secondary to other eye disorders, **bilateral**

Ⓝ Newborn: 0   Ⓟ Pediatric: 0-17   Ⓜ Maternity: 12-55   Ⓐ Adult: 15-124   NRS Nonroutine supply Dx   NCDx Noncancer Dx   PDx Primary Dx   ▶◀ Revised Text   ● New Code   ▲ Revised Title

592   ICD-10-CM 2018

☑5ᵗʰ H40.6 Glaucoma secondary to drugs
Use additional code for adverse effect, if applicable, to identify drug (T36-T50 with fifth or sixth character 5)

> One of the following 7th characters is to be assigned to each code in subcategory H40.6- to designate the stage of glaucoma.
> 0   stage unspecified
> 1   mild stage
> 2   moderate stage
> 3   severe stage
> 4   indeterminate stage

    ☑x7ᵗʰ **H40.60** Glaucoma secondary to drugs, unspecified eye ▽
    ☑x7ᵗʰ **H40.61** Glaucoma secondary to drugs, right eye
    ☑x7ᵗʰ **H40.62** Glaucoma secondary to drugs, left eye
    ☑x7ᵗʰ **H40.63** Glaucoma secondary to drugs, bilateral

☑5ᵗʰ H40.8 Other glaucoma
    ☑6ᵗʰ **H40.81** Glaucoma with increased episcleral venous pressure
        H40.811 Glaucoma with increased episcleral venous pressure, right eye
        H40.812 Glaucoma with increased episcleral venous pressure, left eye
        H40.813 Glaucoma with increased episcleral venous pressure, bilateral
        H40.819 Glaucoma with increased episcleral venous pressure, unspecified eye ▽
    ☑6ᵗʰ **H40.82** Hypersecretion glaucoma
        H40.821 Hypersecretion glaucoma, right eye
        H40.822 Hypersecretion glaucoma, left eye
        H40.823 Hypersecretion glaucoma, bilateral
        H40.829 Hypersecretion glaucoma, unspecified eye ▽
    ☑6ᵗʰ **H40.83** Aqueous misdirection
        Malignant glaucoma
        H40.831 Aqueous misdirection, right eye
        H40.832 Aqueous misdirection, left eye
        H40.833 Aqueous misdirection, bilateral
        H40.839 Aqueous misdirection, unspecified eye ▽
    H40.89 Other specified glaucoma
  H40.9 Unspecified glaucoma ▽

H42 Glaucoma in diseases classified elsewhere
Code first underlying condition, such as:
    amyloidosis (E85.-)
    aniridia (Q13.1)
  ▶glaucoma (in) diabetes mellitus (E08.39, E09.39, E10.39, E11.39, E13.39)◀
    Lowe's syndrome (E72.03)
    Reiger's anomaly (Q13.81)
    specified metabolic disorder (E70-E88)
  EXCLUDES 1   glaucoma (in) onchocerciasis (B73.02)
           glaucoma (in) syphilis (A52.71)
           glaucoma (in) tuberculous (A18.59)
  EXCLUDES 2   ~~glaucoma (in) diabetes mellitus (E08.39, E09.39, E10.39, E11.39, E13.39)~~

Disorders of vitreous body and globe (H43-H44)

☑4ᵗʰ H43 Disorders of vitreous body
  ☑5ᵗʰ H43.0 Vitreous prolapse
    EXCLUDES 1   traumatic vitreous prolapse (S05.2-)
           vitreous syndrome following cataract surgery (H59.0-)
    H43.00 Vitreous prolapse, unspecified eye ▽
    H43.01 Vitreous prolapse, right eye
    H43.02 Vitreous prolapse, left eye
    H43.03 Vitreous prolapse, bilateral
  ☑5ᵗʰ H43.1 Vitreous hemorrhage
    H43.10 Vitreous hemorrhage, unspecified eye ▽
    H43.11 Vitreous hemorrhage, right eye
    H43.12 Vitreous hemorrhage, left eye
    H43.13 Vitreous hemorrhage, bilateral
  ☑5ᵗʰ H43.2 Crystalline deposits in vitreous body
    H43.20 Crystalline deposits in vitreous body, unspecified eye ▽
    H43.21 Crystalline deposits in vitreous body, right eye
    H43.22 Crystalline deposits in vitreous body, left eye
    H43.23 Crystalline deposits in vitreous body, bilateral

☑5ᵗʰ H43.3 Other vitreous opacities
  ☑6ᵗʰ **H43.31** Vitreous membranes and strands
    H43.311 Vitreous membranes and strands, right eye
    H43.312 Vitreous membranes and strands, left eye
    H43.313 Vitreous membranes and strands, bilateral
    H43.319 Vitreous membranes and strands, unspecified eye ▽
  ☑6ᵗʰ **H43.39** Other vitreous opacities
    Vitreous floaters
    H43.391 Other vitreous opacities, right eye
    H43.392 Other vitreous opacities, left eye
    H43.393 Other vitreous opacities, bilateral
    H43.399 Other vitreous opacities, unspecified eye ▽

☑5ᵗʰ H43.8 Other disorders of vitreous body
  EXCLUDES 1   proliferative vitreo-retinopathy with retinal detachment (H33.4-)
  EXCLUDES 2   vitreous abscess (H44.02-)
  ☑6ᵗʰ **H43.81** Vitreous degeneration
    Vitreous detachment
    H43.811 Vitreous degeneration, right eye
    H43.812 Vitreous degeneration, left eye
    H43.813 Vitreous degeneration, bilateral
    H43.819 Vitreous degeneration, unspecified eye ▽
  ☑6ᵗʰ **H43.82** Vitreomacular adhesion
    Vitreomacular traction
    H43.821 Vitreomacular adhesion, right eye ⒜
    H43.822 Vitreomacular adhesion, left eye ⒜
    H43.823 Vitreomacular adhesion, bilateral ⒜
    H43.829 Vitreomacular adhesion, unspecified eye ⒜▽
    H43.89 Other disorders of vitreous body
  H43.9 Unspecified disorder of vitreous body ▽

☑4ᵗʰ H44 Disorders of globe
  INCLUDES   disorders affecting multiple structures of eye
  ☑5ᵗʰ H44.0 Purulent endophthalmitis
    Use additional code to identify organism
    EXCLUDES 1   bleb associated endophthalmitis (H59.4-)
  ☑6ᵗʰ **H44.00** Unspecified purulent endophthalmitis
    H44.001 Unspecified purulent endophthalmitis, right eye ▽
    H44.002 Unspecified purulent endophthalmitis, left eye ▽
    H44.003 Unspecified purulent endophthalmitis, bilateral ▽
    H44.009 Unspecified purulent endophthalmitis, unspecified eye ▽
  ☑6ᵗʰ **H44.01** Panophthalmitis (acute)
    H44.011 Panophthalmitis (acute), right eye
    H44.012 Panophthalmitis (acute), left eye
    H44.013 Panophthalmitis (acute), bilateral
    H44.019 Panophthalmitis (acute), unspecified eye ▽
  ☑6ᵗʰ **H44.02** Vitreous abscess (chronic)
    H44.021 Vitreous abscess (chronic), right eye
    H44.022 Vitreous abscess (chronic), left eye
    H44.023 Vitreous abscess (chronic), bilateral
    H44.029 Vitreous abscess (chronic), unspecified eye ▽
  ☑5ᵗʰ H44.1 Other endophthalmitis
    EXCLUDES 1   bleb associated endophthalmitis (H59.4-)
    EXCLUDES 2   ophthalmia nodosa (H16.2-)
  ☑6ᵗʰ **H44.11** Panuveitis
    DEF: Inflammation of all layers of uvea of eye, including choroid, iris, and ciliary body; also typically involves lens, retina, optic nerve, and vitreous; causes reduced vision or blindness.
    H44.111 Panuveitis, right eye
    H44.112 Panuveitis, left eye
    H44.113 Panuveitis, bilateral
    H44.119 Panuveitis, unspecified eye ▽

Chapter 7. Diseases of the Eye and Adnexa

✓6ᵗʰ **H44.12 Parasitic endophthalmitis, unspecified**
    H44.121   Parasitic endophthalmitis, unspecified, ▽ right eye
    H44.122   Parasitic endophthalmitis, unspecified, ▽ left eye
    H44.123   Parasitic endophthalmitis, unspecified, ▽ bilateral
    H44.129   Parasitic endophthalmitis, unspecified, ▽ unspecified eye

✓6ᵗʰ **H44.13 Sympathetic uveitis**
    H44.131   Sympathetic uveitis, right eye
    H44.132   Sympathetic uveitis, left eye
    H44.133   Sympathetic uveitis, bilateral
    H44.139   Sympathetic uveitis, unspecified eye ▽

H44.19 Other endophthalmitis

✓5ᵗʰ **H44.2 Degenerative myopia**
    Malignant myopia
    H44.20 Degenerative myopia, unspecified eye ▽
    H44.21 Degenerative myopia, right eye
    H44.22 Degenerative myopia, left eye
    H44.23 Degenerative myopia, bilateral

● ✓6ᵗʰ **H44.2A Degenerative myopia with choroidal neovascularization**
    Use additional code for any associated choroid disorders (H31.-)
●   H44.2A1   Degenerative myopia with choroidal neovascularization, right eye
●   H44.2A2   Degenerative myopia with choroidal neovascularization, left eye
●   H44.2A3   Degenerative myopia with choroidal neovascularization, bilateral eye
●   H44.2A9   Degenerative myopia with choroidal ▽ neovascularization, unspecified eye

● ✓6ᵗʰ **H44.2B Degenerative myopia with macular hole**
●   H44.2B1   Degenerative myopia with macular hole, right eye
●   H44.2B2   Degenerative myopia with macular hole, left eye
●   H44.2B3   Degenerative myopia with macular hole, bilateral eye
●   H44.2B9   Degenerative myopia with macular ▽ hole, unspecified eye

● ✓6ᵗʰ **H44.2C Degenerative myopia with retinal detachment**
    Use additional code to identify the retinal detachment (H33.-)
●   H44.2C1   Degenerative myopia with retinal detachment, right eye
●   H44.2C2   Degenerative myopia with retinal detachment, left eye
●   H44.2C3   Degenerative myopia with retinal detachment, bilateral eye
●   H44.2C9   Degenerative myopia with retinal ▽ detachment, unspecified eye

● ✓6ᵗʰ **H44.2D Degenerative myopia with foveoschisis**
●   H44.2D1   Degenerative myopia with foveoschisis, right eye
●   H44.2D2   Degenerative myopia with foveoschisis, left eye
●   H44.2D3   Degenerative myopia with foveoschisis, bilateral eye
●   H44.2D9   Degenerative myopia with ▽ foveoschisis, unspecified eye

● ✓6ᵗʰ **H44.2E Degenerative myopia with other maculopathy**
●   H44.2E1   Degenerative myopia with other maculopathy, right eye
●   H44.2E2   Degenerative myopia with other maculopathy, left eye
●   H44.2E3   Degenerative myopia with other maculopathy, bilateral eye
●   H44.2E9   Degenerative myopia with other ▽ maculopathy, unspecified eye

✓5ᵗʰ **H44.3 Other and unspecified degenerative disorders of globe**
    H44.30 Unspecified degenerative disorder of globe ▽
✓6ᵗʰ   **H44.31 Chalcosis**
    H44.311   Chalcosis, right eye
    H44.312   Chalcosis, left eye
    H44.313   Chalcosis, bilateral
    H44.319   Chalcosis, unspecified eye ▽

✓6ᵗʰ **H44.32 Siderosis of eye**
    DEF: Iron pigment deposits within tissue of eyeball; caused by high iron content of blood; characterized by cataract, rust-colored anterior subcapsular deposits, iris heterochromia, pupillary mydriasis, and depressed electroretinogram amplitudes.
    H44.321   Siderosis of eye, right eye
    H44.322   Siderosis of eye, left eye
    H44.323   Siderosis of eye, bilateral
    H44.329   Siderosis of eye, unspecified eye ▽

✓6ᵗʰ **H44.39 Other degenerative disorders of globe**
    H44.391   Other degenerative disorders of globe, right eye
    H44.392   Other degenerative disorders of globe, left eye
    H44.393   Other degenerative disorders of globe, bilateral
    H44.399   Other degenerative disorders of globe, ▽ unspecified eye

✓5ᵗʰ **H44.4 Hypotony of eye**
    H44.40 Unspecified hypotony of eye ▽
✓6ᵗʰ   **H44.41 Flat anterior chamber hypotony of eye**
    H44.411   Flat anterior chamber hypotony of right eye
    H44.412   Flat anterior chamber hypotony of left eye
    H44.413   Flat anterior chamber hypotony of eye, bilateral
    H44.419   Flat anterior chamber hypotony of ▽ unspecified eye

✓6ᵗʰ **H44.42 Hypotony of eye due to ocular fistula**
    H44.421   Hypotony of right eye due to ocular fistula
    H44.422   Hypotony of left eye due to ocular fistula
    H44.423   Hypotony of eye due to ocular fistula, bilateral
    H44.429   Hypotony of unspecified eye due to ▽ ocular fistula

✓6ᵗʰ **H44.43 Hypotony of eye due to other ocular disorders**
    H44.431   Hypotony of eye due to other ocular disorders, right eye
    H44.432   Hypotony of eye due to other ocular disorders, left eye
    H44.433   Hypotony of eye due to other ocular disorders, bilateral
    H44.439   Hypotony of eye due to other ocular ▽ disorders, unspecified eye

✓6ᵗʰ **H44.44 Primary hypotony of eye**
    H44.441   Primary hypotony of right eye
    H44.442   Primary hypotony of left eye
    H44.443   Primary hypotony of eye, bilateral
    H44.449   Primary hypotony of unspecified eye ▽

✓5ᵗʰ **H44.5 Degenerated conditions of globe**
    H44.50 Unspecified degenerated conditions of globe ▽
✓6ᵗʰ   **H44.51 Absolute glaucoma**
    H44.511   Absolute glaucoma, right eye
    H44.512   Absolute glaucoma, left eye
    H44.513   Absolute glaucoma, bilateral
    H44.519   Absolute glaucoma, unspecified eye ▽

✓6ᵗʰ **H44.52 Atrophy of globe**
    Phthisis bulbi
    H44.521   Atrophy of globe, right eye
    H44.522   Atrophy of globe, left eye
    H44.523   Atrophy of globe, bilateral
    H44.529   Atrophy of globe, unspecified eye ▽

✓6ᵗʰ **H44.53 Leucocoria**
    H44.531   Leucocoria, right eye
    H44.532   Leucocoria, left eye
    H44.533   Leucocoria, bilateral
    H44.539   Leucocoria, unspecified eye ▽

Ⓝ Newborn: 0   Ⓟ Pediatric: 0-17   Ⓜ Maternity: 12-55   Ⓐ Adult: 15-124   𝗡𝗥𝗦 Nonroutine supply Dx   𝗡𝗖𝗗𝘅 Noncancer Dx   𝗣𝗗𝘅 Primary Dx   ▶◀ Revised Text   ● New Code   ▲ Revised Title

594   ICD-10-CM 2018

Chapter 7. Diseases of the Eye and Adnexa

✓5ᵗʰ **H44.6** **Retained (old) intraocular foreign body,** magnetic

    Use additional code to identify magnetic foreign body (Z18.11)

    EXCLUDES 1   *current intraocular foreign body (S05.-)*

    EXCLUDES 2   *retained foreign body in eyelid (H02.81-)*

            retained (old) foreign body following penetrating wound of orbit (H05.5-)

            retained (old) intraocular foreign body, nonmagnetic (H44.7-)

✓6ᵗʰ **H44.60** Unspecified **retained (old) intraocular foreign body, magnetic**

    H44.601 **Unspecified retained (old) intraocular foreign body, magnetic,** right **eye** ▽

    H44.602 **Unspecified retained (old) intraocular foreign body, magnetic,** left **eye** ▽

    H44.603 **Unspecified retained (old) intraocular foreign body, magnetic,** bilateral ▽

    H44.609 **Unspecified retained (old) intraocular foreign body, magnetic, unspecified eye** ▽

✓6ᵗʰ **H44.61** **Retained (old) magnetic foreign body in** anterior chamber

    H44.611 **Retained (old) magnetic foreign body in anterior chamber,** right **eye**

    H44.612 **Retained (old) magnetic foreign body in anterior chamber,** left **eye**

    H44.613 **Retained (old) magnetic foreign body in anterior chamber,** bilateral

    H44.619 **Retained (old) magnetic foreign body in anterior chamber, unspecified eye** ▽

✓6ᵗʰ **H44.62** **Retained (old) magnetic foreign body in** iris or ciliary body

    H44.621 **Retained (old) magnetic foreign body in iris or ciliary body,** right **eye**

    H44.622 **Retained (old) magnetic foreign body in iris or ciliary body,** left **eye**

    H44.623 **Retained (old) magnetic foreign body in iris or ciliary body,** bilateral

    H44.629 **Retained (old) magnetic foreign body in iris or ciliary body, unspecified eye** ▽

✓6ᵗʰ **H44.63** **Retained (old) magnetic foreign body in** lens

    H44.631 **Retained (old) magnetic foreign body in lens,** right **eye**

    H44.632 **Retained (old) magnetic foreign body in lens,** left **eye**

    H44.633 **Retained (old) magnetic foreign body in lens,** bilateral

    H44.639 **Retained (old) magnetic foreign body in lens, unspecified eye** ▽

✓6ᵗʰ **H44.64** **Retained (old) magnetic foreign body in** posterior wall of globe

    H44.641 **Retained (old) magnetic foreign body in posterior wall of globe,** right **eye**

    H44.642 **Retained (old) magnetic foreign body in posterior wall of globe,** left **eye**

    H44.643 **Retained (old) magnetic foreign body in posterior wall of globe,** bilateral

    H44.649 **Retained (old) magnetic foreign body in posterior wall of globe, unspecified eye** ▽

✓6ᵗʰ **H44.65** **Retained (old) magnetic foreign body in** vitreous body

    H44.651 **Retained (old) magnetic foreign body in vitreous body,** right **eye**

    H44.652 **Retained (old) magnetic foreign body in vitreous body,** left **eye**

    H44.653 **Retained (old) magnetic foreign body in vitreous body,** bilateral

    H44.659 **Retained (old) magnetic foreign body in vitreous body, unspecified eye** ▽

✓6ᵗʰ **H44.69** **Retained (old) intraocular foreign body, magnetic, in** other or multiple sites

    H44.691 **Retained (old) intraocular foreign body, magnetic, in other or multiple sites,** right **eye**

    H44.692 **Retained (old) intraocular foreign body, magnetic, in other or multiple sites,** left **eye**

    H44.693 **Retained (old) intraocular foreign body, magnetic, in other or multiple sites,** bilateral

    H44.699 **Retained (old) intraocular foreign body, magnetic, in other or multiple sites, unspecified eye** ▽

✓5ᵗʰ **H44.7** **Retained (old) intraocular foreign body,** nonmagnetic

    Use additional code to identify nonmagnetic foreign body (Z18.01-Z18.10, Z18.12, Z18.2-Z18.9)

    EXCLUDES 1   *current intraocular foreign body (S05.-)*

    EXCLUDES 2   *retained foreign body in eyelid (H02.81-)*

            retained (old) foreign body following penetrating wound of orbit (H05.5-)

            retained (old) intraocular foreign body, magnetic (H44.6-)

✓6ᵗʰ **H44.70** Unspecified **retained (old) intraocular foreign body, nonmagnetic**

    H44.701 **Unspecified retained (old) intraocular foreign body, nonmagnetic,** right **eye** ▽

    H44.702 **Unspecified retained (old) intraocular foreign body, nonmagnetic,** left **eye** ▽

    H44.703 **Unspecified retained (old) intraocular foreign body, nonmagnetic,** bilateral ▽

    H44.709 **Unspecified retained (old) intraocular foreign body, nonmagnetic, unspecified eye** ▽

            Retained (old) intraocular foreign body NOS

✓6ᵗʰ **H44.71** **Retained (nonmagnetic) (old) foreign body in** anterior chamber

    H44.711 **Retained (nonmagnetic) (old) foreign body in anterior chamber,** right **eye**

    H44.712 **Retained (nonmagnetic) (old) foreign body in anterior chamber,** left **eye**

    H44.713 **Retained (nonmagnetic) (old) foreign body in anterior chamber,** bilateral

    H44.719 **Retained (nonmagnetic) (old) foreign body in anterior chamber, unspecified eye** ▽

✓6ᵗʰ **H44.72** **Retained (nonmagnetic) (old) foreign body in** iris or ciliary body

    H44.721 **Retained (nonmagnetic) (old) foreign body in iris or ciliary body,** right **eye**

    H44.722 **Retained (nonmagnetic) (old) foreign body in iris or ciliary body,** left **eye**

    H44.723 **Retained (nonmagnetic) (old) foreign body in iris or ciliary body,** bilateral

    H44.729 **Retained (nonmagnetic) (old) foreign body in iris or ciliary body, unspecified eye** ▽

✓6ᵗʰ **H44.73** **Retained (nonmagnetic) (old) foreign body in** lens

    H44.731 **Retained (nonmagnetic) (old) foreign body in lens,** right **eye**

    H44.732 **Retained (nonmagnetic) (old) foreign body in lens,** left **eye**

    H44.733 **Retained (nonmagnetic) (old) foreign body in lens,** bilateral

    H44.739 **Retained (nonmagnetic) (old) foreign body in lens, unspecified eye** ▽

✓6ᵗʰ **H44.74** **Retained (nonmagnetic) (old) foreign body in** posterior wall of globe

    H44.741 **Retained (nonmagnetic) (old) foreign body in posterior wall of globe,** right **eye**

    H44.742 **Retained (nonmagnetic) (old) foreign body in posterior wall of globe,** left **eye**

    H44.743 **Retained (nonmagnetic) (old) foreign body in posterior wall of globe,** bilateral

    H44.749 **Retained (nonmagnetic) (old) foreign body in posterior wall of globe, unspecified eye** ▽

✓6ᵗʰ **H44.75** **Retained (nonmagnetic) (old) foreign body in** vitreous body

    H44.751 **Retained (nonmagnetic) (old) foreign body in vitreous body,** right **eye**

    H44.752 **Retained (nonmagnetic) (old) foreign body in vitreous body,** left **eye**

    H44.753 **Retained (nonmagnetic) (old) foreign body in vitreous body,** bilateral

    H44.759 **Retained (nonmagnetic) (old) foreign body in vitreous body, unspecified eye** ▽

☑ Additional Character Req   ✓x7ᵗʰ Placeholder Alert   Case-Mix Diagnosis   Manifestation   ▽ Unspecified Dx   *EXCLUDES 1* Not coded here   *EXCLUDES 2* Not included here

ICD-10-CM 2018   **595**

Chapter 7. Diseases of the Eye and Adnexa

H44.6–H44.759

✓6ᵗʰ **H44.79** Retained (old) intraocular foreign body, nonmagnetic, in other or multiple sites

     H44.791   Retained (old) intraocular foreign body, nonmagnetic, in other or multiple sites, right eye

     H44.792   Retained (old) intraocular foreign body, nonmagnetic, in other or multiple sites, left eye

     H44.793   Retained (old) intraocular foreign body, nonmagnetic, in other or multiple sites, bilateral

     H44.799   Retained (old) intraocular foreign body, nonmagnetic, in other or multiple sites, unspecified eye   ▽

✓5ᵗʰ **H44.8** Other disorders of globe

   ✓6ᵗʰ **H44.81** Hemophthalmos

     DEF: Pool of blood within eyeball, not from current injury.

     H44.811   Hemophthalmos, right eye

     H44.812   Hemophthalmos, left eye

     H44.813   Hemophthalmos, bilateral

     H44.819   Hemophthalmos, unspecified eye   ▽

   ✓6ᵗʰ **H44.82** Luxation of globe

     H44.821   Luxation of globe, right eye

     H44.822   Luxation of globe, left eye

     H44.823   Luxation of globe, bilateral

     H44.829   Luxation of globe, unspecified eye   ▽

   H44.89 Other disorders of globe

  H44.9 Unspecified disorder of globe   ▽

Disorders of optic nerve and visual pathways (H46-H47)

✓4ᵗʰ **H46** Optic neuritis

     EXCLUDES 2   ischemic optic neuropathy (H47.01-)
                neuromyelitis optica [Devic] (G36.0)

  ✓5ᵗʰ **H46.0** Optic papillitis

     H46.00   Optic papillitis, unspecified eye   ▽

     H46.01   Optic papillitis, right eye

     H46.02   Optic papillitis, left eye

     H46.03   Optic papillitis, bilateral

  ✓5ᵗʰ **H46.1** Retrobulbar neuritis

     Retrobulbar neuritis NOS

     EXCLUDES 1   syphilitic retrobulbar neuritis (A52.15)

     H46.10   Retrobulbar neuritis, unspecified eye   ▽

     H46.11   Retrobulbar neuritis, right eye

     H46.12   Retrobulbar neuritis, left eye

     H46.13   Retrobulbar neuritis, bilateral

  H46.2 Nutritional optic neuropathy

  H46.3 Toxic optic neuropathy

     Code first (T51-T65) to identify cause

  H46.8 Other optic neuritis

  H46.9 Unspecified optic neuritis   ▽

✓4ᵗʰ **H47** Other disorders of optic [2nd] nerve and visual pathways

  ✓5ᵗʰ **H47.0** Disorders of optic nerve, not elsewhere classified

   ✓6ᵗʰ **H47.01** Ischemic optic neuropathy

     H47.011   Ischemic optic neuropathy, right eye

     H47.012   Ischemic optic neuropathy, left eye

     H47.013   Ischemic optic neuropathy, bilateral

     H47.019   Ischemic optic neuropathy, unspecified eye   ▽

   ✓6ᵗʰ **H47.02** Hemorrhage in optic nerve sheath

     H47.021   Hemorrhage in optic nerve sheath, right eye

     H47.022   Hemorrhage in optic nerve sheath, left eye

     H47.023   Hemorrhage in optic nerve sheath, bilateral

     H47.029   Hemorrhage in optic nerve sheath, unspecified eye   ▽

   ✓6ᵗʰ **H47.03** Optic nerve hypoplasia

     H47.031   Optic nerve hypoplasia, right eye

     H47.032   Optic nerve hypoplasia, left eye

     H47.033   Optic nerve hypoplasia, bilateral

     H47.039   Optic nerve hypoplasia, unspecified eye   ▽

   ✓6ᵗʰ **H47.09** Other disorders of optic nerve, not elsewhere classified

     Compression of optic nerve

     H47.091   Other disorders of optic nerve, not elsewhere classified, right eye

     H47.092   Other disorders of optic nerve, not elsewhere classified, left eye

     H47.093   Other disorders of optic nerve, not elsewhere classified, bilateral

     H47.099   Other disorders of optic nerve, not elsewhere classified, unspecified eye   ▽

  ✓5ᵗʰ **H47.1** Papilledema

     H47.10   Unspecified papilledema   ▽

     H47.11   Papilledema associated with increased intracranial pressure

     H47.12   Papilledema associated with decreased ocular pressure

     H47.13   Papilledema associated with retinal disorder

   ✓6ᵗʰ **H47.14** Foster-Kennedy syndrome

     H47.141   Foster-Kennedy syndrome, right eye

     H47.142   Foster-Kennedy syndrome, left eye

     H47.143   Foster-Kennedy syndrome, bilateral

     H47.149   Foster-Kennedy syndrome, unspecified eye   ▽

  ✓5ᵗʰ **H47.2** Optic atrophy

     H47.20   Unspecified optic atrophy   ▽

   ✓6ᵗʰ **H47.21** Primary optic atrophy

     H47.211   Primary optic atrophy, right eye

     H47.212   Primary optic atrophy, left eye

     H47.213   Primary optic atrophy, bilateral

     H47.219   Primary optic atrophy, unspecified eye   ▽

   H47.22 Hereditary optic atrophy

     Leber's optic atrophy

   ✓6ᵗʰ **H47.23** Glaucomatous optic atrophy

     H47.231   Glaucomatous optic atrophy, right eye

     H47.232   Glaucomatous optic atrophy, left eye

     H47.233   Glaucomatous optic atrophy, bilateral

     H47.239   Glaucomatous optic atrophy, unspecified eye   ▽

   ✓6ᵗʰ **H47.29** Other optic atrophy

     Temporal pallor of optic disc

     H47.291   Other optic atrophy, right eye

     H47.292   Other optic atrophy, left eye

     H47.293   Other optic atrophy, bilateral

     H47.299   Other optic atrophy, unspecified eye   ▽

  ✓5ᵗʰ **H47.3** Other disorders of optic disc

   ✓6ᵗʰ **H47.31** Coloboma of optic disc

     H47.311   Coloboma of optic disc, right eye

     H47.312   Coloboma of optic disc, left eye

     H47.313   Coloboma of optic disc, bilateral

     H47.319   Coloboma of optic disc, unspecified eye   ▽

   ✓6ᵗʰ **H47.32** Drusen of optic disc

     H47.321   Drusen of optic disc, right eye

     H47.322   Drusen of optic disc, left eye

     H47.323   Drusen of optic disc, bilateral

     H47.329   Drusen of optic disc, unspecified eye   ▽

   ✓6ᵗʰ **H47.33** Pseudopapilledema of optic disc

     H47.331   Pseudopapilledema of optic disc, right eye

     H47.332   Pseudopapilledema of optic disc, left eye

     H47.333   Pseudopapilledema of optic disc, bilateral

     H47.339   Pseudopapilledema of optic disc, unspecified eye   ▽

   ✓6ᵗʰ **H47.39** Other disorders of optic disc

     H47.391   Other disorders of optic disc, right eye

     H47.392   Other disorders of optic disc, left eye

     H47.393   Other disorders of optic disc, bilateral

     H47.399   Other disorders of optic disc, unspecified eye   ▽

Ⓝ Newborn: 0   Ⓟ Pediatric: 0-17   Ⓜ Maternity: 12-55   Ⓐ Adult: 15-124   **NRS** Nonroutine supply Dx   **NCDx** Noncancer Dx   **PDx** Primary Dx   ▶◀ Revised Text   ● New Code   ▲ Revised Title

596   ICD-10-CM 2018

✓5ᵗʰ H47.4 Disorders of optic chiasm
Code also underlying condition

H47.41 Disorders of optic chiasm in (due to) inflammatory disorders

H47.42 Disorders of optic chiasm in (due to) neoplasm

H47.43 Disorders of optic chiasm in (due to) vascular disorders

H47.49 Disorders of optic chiasm in (due to) other disorders

✓5ᵗʰ H47.5 Disorders of other visual pathways
Disorders of optic tracts, geniculate nuclei and optic radiations
Code also underlying condition

   ✓6ᵗʰ H47.51 Disorders of visual pathways in (due to) inflammatory disorders

      H47.511 Disorders of visual pathways in (due to) inflammatory disorders, right side

      H47.512 Disorders of visual pathways in (due to) inflammatory disorders, left side

      H47.519 Disorders of visual pathways in (due to) inflammatory disorders, unspecified side ▽

   ✓6ᵗʰ H47.52 Disorders of visual pathways in (due to) neoplasm

      H47.521 Disorders of visual pathways in (due to) neoplasm, right side

      H47.522 Disorders of visual pathways in (due to) neoplasm, left side

      H47.529 Disorders of visual pathways in (due to) neoplasm, unspecified side ▽

   ✓6ᵗʰ H47.53 Disorders of visual pathways in (due to) vascular disorders

      H47.531 Disorders of visual pathways in (due to) vascular disorders, right side

      H47.532 Disorders of visual pathways in (due to) vascular disorders, left side

      H47.539 Disorders of visual pathways in (due to) vascular disorders, unspecified side ▽

✓5ᵗʰ H47.6 Disorders of visual cortex
Code also underlying condition
EXCLUDES 1 injury to visual cortex S04.04

   ✓6ᵗʰ H47.61 Cortical blindness

      H47.611 Cortical blindness, right side of brain

      H47.612 Cortical blindness, left side of brain

      H47.619 Cortical blindness, unspecified side of brain ▽

   ✓6ᵗʰ H47.62 Disorders of visual cortex in (due to) inflammatory disorders

      H47.621 Disorders of visual cortex in (due to) inflammatory disorders, right side of brain

      H47.622 Disorders of visual cortex in (due to) inflammatory disorders, left side of brain

      H47.629 Disorders of visual cortex in (due to) inflammatory disorders, unspecified side of brain ▽

   ✓6ᵗʰ H47.63 Disorders of visual cortex in (due to) neoplasm

      H47.631 Disorders of visual cortex in (due to) neoplasm, right side of brain

      H47.632 Disorders of visual cortex in (due to) neoplasm, left side of brain

      H47.639 Disorders of visual cortex in (due to) neoplasm, unspecified side of brain ▽

   ✓6ᵗʰ H47.64 Disorders of visual cortex in (due to) vascular disorders

      H47.641 Disorders of visual cortex in (due to) vascular disorders, right side of brain

      H47.642 Disorders of visual cortex in (due to) vascular disorders, left side of brain

      H47.649 Disorders of visual cortex in (due to) vascular disorders, unspecified side of brain ▽

H47.9 Unspecified disorder of visual pathways ▽

Disorders of ocular muscles, binocular movement, accommodation and refraction (H49-H52)

EXCLUDES 2 nystagmus and other irregular eye movements (H55)

✓4ᵗʰ H49 Paralytic strabismus
EXCLUDES 2 internal ophthalmoplegia (H52.51-)
internuclear ophthalmoplegia (H51.2-)
progressive supranuclear ophthalmoplegia (G23.1)

✓5ᵗʰ H49.0 Third [oculomotor] nerve palsy

   H49.00 Third [oculomotor] nerve palsy, unspecified eye ▽

   H49.01 Third [oculomotor] nerve palsy, right eye

   H49.02 Third [oculomotor] nerve palsy, left eye

   H49.03 Third [oculomotor] nerve palsy, bilateral

✓5ᵗʰ H49.1 Fourth [trochlear] nerve palsy

   H49.10 Fourth [trochlear] nerve palsy, unspecified eye ▽

   H49.11 Fourth [trochlear] nerve palsy, right eye

   H49.12 Fourth [trochlear] nerve palsy, left eye

   H49.13 Fourth [trochlear] nerve palsy, bilateral

✓5ᵗʰ H49.2 Sixth [abducent] nerve palsy

   H49.20 Sixth [abducent] nerve palsy, unspecified eye ▽

   H49.21 Sixth [abducent] nerve palsy, right eye

   H49.22 Sixth [abducent] nerve palsy, left eye

   H49.23 Sixth [abducent] nerve palsy, bilateral

✓5ᵗʰ H49.3 Total (external) ophthalmoplegia

   H49.30 Total (external) ophthalmoplegia, unspecified eye ▽

   H49.31 Total (external) ophthalmoplegia, right eye

   H49.32 Total (external) ophthalmoplegia, left eye

   H49.33 Total (external) ophthalmoplegia, bilateral

✓5ᵗʰ H49.4 Progressive external ophthalmoplegia
EXCLUDES 1 Kearns-Sayre syndrome (H49.81-)

   H49.40 Progressive external ophthalmoplegia, unspecified eye ▽

   H49.41 Progressive external ophthalmoplegia, right eye

   H49.42 Progressive external ophthalmoplegia, left eye

   H49.43 Progressive external ophthalmoplegia, bilateral

✓5ᵗʰ H49.8 Other paralytic strabismus

   ✓6ᵗʰ H49.81 Kearns-Sayre syndrome
Progressive external ophthalmoplegia with pigmentary retinopathy
Use additional code for other manifestation, such as: heart block (I45.9)

      H49.811 Kearns-Sayre syndrome, right eye

      H49.812 Kearns-Sayre syndrome, left eye

      H49.813 Kearns-Sayre syndrome, bilateral

      H49.819 Kearns-Sayre syndrome, unspecified eye ▽

   ✓6ᵗʰ H49.88 Other paralytic strabismus
External ophthalmoplegia NOS

      H49.881 Other paralytic strabismus, right eye

      H49.882 Other paralytic strabismus, left eye

      H49.883 Other paralytic strabismus, bilateral

      H49.889 Other paralytic strabismus, unspecified eye ▽

H49.9 Unspecified paralytic strabismus ▽

✓4ᵗʰ H50 Other strabismus

✓5ᵗʰ H50.0 Esotropia
Convergent concomitant strabismus
EXCLUDES 1 intermittent esotropia (H50.31-, H50.32)

   H50.00 Unspecified esotropia ▽

   ✓6ᵗʰ H50.01 Monocular esotropia

      H50.011 Monocular esotropia, right eye

      H50.012 Monocular esotropia, left eye

   ✓6ᵗʰ H50.02 Monocular esotropia with A pattern

      H50.021 Monocular esotropia with A pattern, right eye

      H50.022 Monocular esotropia with A pattern, left eye

   ✓6ᵗʰ H50.03 Monocular esotropia with V pattern

      H50.031 Monocular esotropia with V pattern, right eye

      H50.032 Monocular esotropia with V pattern, left eye

✓ Additional Character Req   ✓x7ᵗʰ Placeholder Alert   Case-Mix Diagnosis   Manifestation   ▽ Unspecified Dx   *EXCLUDES 1* Not coded here   *EXCLUDES 2* Not included here

Chapter 7. Diseases of the Eye and Adnexa (side margin)

H50.04–H52.219 (side margin)

Eye Muscle Diseases

R.　　　　　L.
Monocular (one eye only) esotropia (inward)

Monocular exotropia (outward)

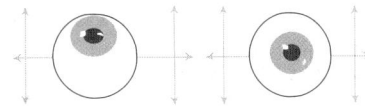

Monocular hypertropia (upward)

✓6ᵗʰ **H50.04** Monocular esotropia with other noncomitancies
　　　　H50.041　Monocular esotropia with other noncomitancies, right eye
　　　　H50.042　Monocular esotropia with other noncomitancies, left eye
H50.05 Alternating esotropia
H50.06 Alternating esotropia with A pattern
H50.07 Alternating esotropia with V pattern
H50.08 Alternating esotropia with other noncomitancies
✓5ᵗʰ **H50.1** Exotropia
　　Divergent concomitant strabismus
　　EXCLUDES 1　intermittent exotropia (H50.33-, H50.34)
H50.10 Unspecified exotropia　▽
✓6ᵗʰ **H50.11** Monocular exotropia
　　　　H50.111　Monocular exotropia, right eye
　　　　H50.112　Monocular exotropia, left eye
✓6ᵗʰ **H50.12** Monocular exotropia with A pattern
　　　　H50.121　Monocular exotropia with A pattern, right eye
　　　　H50.122　Monocular exotropia with A pattern, left eye
✓6ᵗʰ **H50.13** Monocular exotropia with V pattern
　　　　H50.131　Monocular exotropia with V pattern, right eye
　　　　H50.132　Monocular exotropia with V pattern, left eye
✓6ᵗʰ **H50.14** Monocular exotropia with other noncomitancies
　　　　H50.141　Monocular exotropia with other noncomitancies, right eye
　　　　H50.142　Monocular exotropia with other noncomitancies, left eye
H50.15 Alternating exotropia
H50.16 Alternating exotropia with A pattern
H50.17 Alternating exotropia with V pattern
H50.18 Alternating exotropia with other noncomitancies
✓5ᵗʰ **H50.2** Vertical strabismus
　　Hypertropia
H50.21 Vertical strabismus, right eye
H50.22 Vertical strabismus, left eye
✓5ᵗʰ **H50.3** Intermittent heterotropia
H50.30 Unspecified intermittent heterotropia　▽
✓6ᵗʰ **H50.31** Intermittent monocular esotropia
　　　　H50.311　Intermittent monocular esotropia, right eye
　　　　H50.312　Intermittent monocular esotropia, left eye
H50.32 Intermittent alternating esotropia

✓6ᵗʰ **H50.33** Intermittent monocular exotropia
　　　　H50.331　Intermittent monocular exotropia, right eye
　　　　H50.332　Intermittent monocular exotropia, left eye
H50.34 Intermittent alternating exotropia
✓5ᵗʰ **H50.4** Other and unspecified heterotropia
H50.40 Unspecified heterotropia　▽
✓6ᵗʰ **H50.41** Cyclotropia
　　　　H50.411　Cyclotropia, right eye
　　　　H50.412　Cyclotropia, left eye
H50.42 Monofixation syndrome
H50.43 Accommodative component in esotropia
✓5ᵗʰ **H50.5** Heterophoria
H50.50 Unspecified heterophoria　▽
H50.51 Esophoria
H50.52 Exophoria
H50.53 Vertical heterophoria
H50.54 Cyclophoria
H50.55 Alternating heterophoria
✓5ᵗʰ **H50.6** Mechanical strabismus
H50.60 Mechanical strabismus, unspecified　▽
✓6ᵗʰ **H50.61** Brown's sheath syndrome
　　　　H50.611　Brown's sheath syndrome, right eye
　　　　H50.612　Brown's sheath syndrome, left eye
H50.69 Other mechanical strabismus
　　　　Strabismus due to adhesions
　　　　Traumatic limitation of duction of eye muscle
✓5ᵗʰ **H50.8** Other specified strabismus
✓6ᵗʰ **H50.81** Duane's syndrome
　　　　H50.811　Duane's syndrome, right eye
　　　　H50.812　Duane's syndrome, left eye
H50.89 Other specified strabismus
H50.9 Unspecified strabismus　▽
✓4ᵗʰ **H51** Other disorders of binocular movement
H51.0 Palsy (spasm) of conjugate gaze
✓5ᵗʰ **H51.1** Convergence insufficiency and excess
H51.11 Convergence insufficiency
H51.12 Convergence excess
✓5ᵗʰ **H51.2** Internuclear ophthalmoplegia
H51.20 Internuclear ophthalmoplegia, unspecified eye　▽
H51.21 Internuclear ophthalmoplegia, right eye
H51.22 Internuclear ophthalmoplegia, left eye
H51.23 Internuclear ophthalmoplegia, bilateral
H51.8 Other specified disorders of binocular movement
H51.9 Unspecified disorder of binocular movement　▽
✓4ᵗʰ **H52** Disorders of refraction and accommodation
✓5ᵗʰ **H52.0** Hypermetropia
H52.00 Hypermetropia, unspecified eye　▽
H52.01 Hypermetropia, right eye
H52.02 Hypermetropia, left eye
H52.03 Hypermetropia, bilateral
✓5ᵗʰ **H52.1** Myopia
　　EXCLUDES 1　degenerative myopia (H44.2-)
H52.10 Myopia, unspecified eye　▽
H52.11 Myopia, right eye
H52.12 Myopia, left eye
H52.13 Myopia, bilateral
✓5ᵗʰ **H52.2** Astigmatism
✓6ᵗʰ **H52.20** Unspecified astigmatism
　　　　H52.201　Unspecified astigmatism, right eye　▽
　　　　H52.202　Unspecified astigmatism, left eye　▽
　　　　H52.203　Unspecified astigmatism, bilateral　▽
　　　　H52.209　Unspecified astigmatism, unspecified eye　▽
✓6ᵗʰ **H52.21** Irregular astigmatism
　　　　H52.211　Irregular astigmatism, right eye
　　　　H52.212　Irregular astigmatism, left eye
　　　　H52.213　Irregular astigmatism, bilateral
　　　　H52.219　Irregular astigmatism, unspecified eye　▽

✓6ᵗʰ H52.22 Regular astigmatism
- H52.221 Regular astigmatism, right eye
- H52.222 Regular astigmatism, left eye
- H52.223 Regular astigmatism, bilateral
- H52.229 Regular astigmatism, unspecified eye ▽

✓5ᵗʰ H52.3 Anisometropia and aniseikonia
- H52.31 Anisometropia
- H52.32 Aniseikonia

H52.4 Presbyopia

✓5ᵗʰ H52.5 Disorders of accommodation

  ✓6ᵗʰ H52.51 Internal ophthalmoplegia (complete) (total)
- H52.511 Internal ophthalmoplegia (complete) (total), right eye
- H52.512 Internal ophthalmoplegia (complete) (total), left eye
- H52.513 Internal ophthalmoplegia (complete) (total), bilateral
- H52.519 Internal ophthalmoplegia (complete) (total), unspecified eye ▽

  ✓6ᵗʰ H52.52 Paresis of accommodation
- H52.521 Paresis of accommodation, right eye
- H52.522 Paresis of accommodation, left eye
- H52.523 Paresis of accommodation, bilateral
- H52.529 Paresis of accommodation, unspecified eye ▽

  ✓6ᵗʰ H52.53 Spasm of accommodation
- H52.531 Spasm of accommodation, right eye
- H52.532 Spasm of accommodation, left eye
- H52.533 Spasm of accommodation, bilateral
- H52.539 Spasm of accommodation, unspecified eye ▽

H52.6 Other disorders of refraction
H52.7 Unspecified disorder of refraction ▽

Visual disturbances and blindness (H53-H54)

✓4ᵗʰ H53 Visual disturbances

✓5ᵗʰ H53.0 Amblyopia ex anopsia
- EXCLUDES1 amblyopia due to vitamin A deficiency (E50.5)

  ✓6ᵗʰ H53.00 Unspecified amblyopia
- H53.001 Unspecified amblyopia, right eye ▽
- H53.002 Unspecified amblyopia, left eye ▽
- H53.003 Unspecified amblyopia, bilateral ▽
- H53.009 Unspecified amblyopia, unspecified eye ▽

  ✓6ᵗʰ H53.01 Deprivation amblyopia
- H53.011 Deprivation amblyopia, right eye
- H53.012 Deprivation amblyopia, left eye
- H53.013 Deprivation amblyopia, bilateral
- H53.019 Deprivation amblyopia, unspecified eye ▽

  ✓6ᵗʰ H53.02 Refractive amblyopia
- H53.021 Refractive amblyopia, right eye
- H53.022 Refractive amblyopia, left eye
- H53.023 Refractive amblyopia, bilateral
- H53.029 Refractive amblyopia, unspecified eye ▽

  ✓6ᵗʰ H53.03 Strabismic amblyopia
- EXCLUDES1 strabismus (H50.-)
- H53.031 Strabismic amblyopia, right eye
- H53.032 Strabismic amblyopia, left eye
- H53.033 Strabismic amblyopia, bilateral
- H53.039 Strabismic amblyopia, unspecified eye ▽

  ✓6ᵗʰ H53.04 Amblyopia suspect
- H53.041 Amblyopia suspect, right eye
- H53.042 Amblyopia suspect, left eye
- H53.043 Amblyopia suspect, bilateral
- H53.049 Amblyopia suspect, unspecified eye ▽

✓5ᵗʰ H53.1 Subjective visual disturbances
- EXCLUDES1 subjective visual disturbances due to vitamin A deficiency (E50.5)
  - visual hallucinations (R44.1)
- H53.10 Unspecified subjective visual disturbances ▽

H53.11 Day blindness
- Hemeralopia

✓6ᵗʰ H53.12 Transient visual loss
- Scintillating scotoma
- EXCLUDES1 amaurosis fugax (G45.3-)
  - transient retinal artery occlusion (H34.0-)
- H53.121 Transient visual loss, right eye
- H53.122 Transient visual loss, left eye
- H53.123 Transient visual loss, bilateral
- H53.129 Transient visual loss, unspecified eye ▽

✓6ᵗʰ H53.13 Sudden visual loss
- H53.131 Sudden visual loss, right eye
- H53.132 Sudden visual loss, left eye
- H53.133 Sudden visual loss, bilateral
- H53.139 Sudden visual loss, unspecified eye ▽

✓6ᵗʰ H53.14 Visual discomfort
- Asthenopia
- Photophobia
- H53.141 Visual discomfort, right eye
- H53.142 Visual discomfort, left eye
- H53.143 Visual discomfort, bilateral
- H53.149 Visual discomfort, unspecified ▽

H53.15 Visual distortions of shape and size
- Metamorphopsia

H53.16 Psychophysical visual disturbances

H53.19 Other subjective visual disturbances
- Visual halos

H53.2 Diplopia
- Double vision

✓5ᵗʰ H53.3 Other and unspecified disorders of binocular vision
- H53.30 Unspecified disorder of binocular vision ▽
- H53.31 Abnormal retinal correspondence
- H53.32 Fusion with defective stereopsis
- H53.33 Simultaneous visual perception without fusion
- H53.34 Suppression of binocular vision

✓5ᵗʰ H53.4 Visual field defects
- H53.40 Unspecified visual field defects ▽

  ✓6ᵗʰ H53.41 Scotoma involving central area
- Central scotoma
- H53.411 Scotoma involving central area, right eye
- H53.412 Scotoma involving central area, left eye
- H53.413 Scotoma involving central area, bilateral
- H53.419 Scotoma involving central area, unspecified eye ▽

  ✓6ᵗʰ H53.42 Scotoma of blind spot area
- Enlarged blind spot
- H53.421 Scotoma of blind spot area, right eye
- H53.422 Scotoma of blind spot area, left eye
- H53.423 Scotoma of blind spot area, bilateral
- H53.429 Scotoma of blind spot area, unspecified eye ▽

  ✓6ᵗʰ H53.43 Sector or arcuate defects
- Arcuate scotoma
- Bjerrum scotoma
- H53.431 Sector or arcuate defects, right eye
- H53.432 Sector or arcuate defects, left eye
- H53.433 Sector or arcuate defects, bilateral
- H53.439 Sector or arcuate defects, unspecified eye ▽

  ✓6ᵗʰ H53.45 Other localized visual field defect
- Peripheral visual field defect
- Ring scotoma NOS
- Scotoma NOS
- H53.451 Other localized visual field defect, right eye
- H53.452 Other localized visual field defect, left eye
- H53.453 Other localized visual field defect, bilateral
- H53.459 Other localized visual field defect, unspecified eye ▽

✓6ᵗʰ **H53.46** Homonymous **bilateral field defects**
    Homonymous hemianopia   Quadrant anopia
    Homonymous hemianopsia   Quadrant anopsia

     H53.461 Homonymous bilateral field defects, right side

     H53.462 Homonymous bilateral field defects, left side

     H53.469 Homonymous bilateral field defects, ▽ unspecified side
         Homonymous bilateral field defects NOS

H53.47 Heteronymous **bilateral field defects**
     Heteronymous hemianop(s)ia

✓6ᵗʰ **H53.48** Generalized contraction **of visual field**

     H53.481 Generalized contraction of visual field, right eye

     H53.482 Generalized contraction of visual field, left eye

     H53.483 Generalized contraction of visual field, bilateral

     H53.489 Generalized contraction of visual field, ▽ unspecified eye

✓5ᵗʰ **H53.5** Color vision deficiencies
     Color blindness
     EXCLUDES 2   day blindness (H53.11)

     H53.50 Unspecified color vision deficiencies ▽
         Color blindness NOS

     H53.51 Achromatopsia
         DEF: Nonprogressive genetic visual disorder; characterized by complete color blindness, decreased vision, and light sensitivity.

     H53.52 Acquired color vision deficiency

     H53.53 Deuteranomaly
         Deuteranopia
         DEF: Male-only genetic disorder; difficulty in distinguishing green and red, no shortened spectrum.

     H53.54 Protanomaly
         Protanopia

     H53.55 Tritanomaly
         Tritanopia

     H53.59 Other color vision deficiencies

✓5ᵗʰ **H53.6** Night blindness
     EXCLUDES 1   night blindness due to vitamin A deficiency (E50.5)

     H53.60 Unspecified night blindness ▽

     H53.61 Abnormal dark adaptation curve

     H53.62 Acquired night blindness

     H53.63 Congenital night blindness

     H53.69 Other night blindness

✓5ᵗʰ **H53.7** Vision sensitivity deficiencies

     H53.71 Glare sensitivity

     H53.72 Impaired contrast sensitivity

H53.8 Other visual disturbances

H53.9 Unspecified visual disturbance ▽

✓4ᵗʰ **H54** **Blindness and low vision**
     NOTE   For definition of visual impairment categories see table below
     Code first any associated underlying cause of the blindness
     EXCLUDES 1   amaurosis fugax (G45.3)

✓5ᵗʰ **H54.0** Blindness, both eyes
     Visual impairment categories 3, 4, 5 in both eyes.

     ✓6ᵗʰ **H54.0X** Blindness, both eyes, different category levels

     ✓7ᵗʰ **H54.0X3** Blindness right eye, category 3

         H54.0X33 Blindness right eye category 3, blindness left eye category 3

         H54.0X34 Blindness right eye category 3, blindness left eye category 4

         H54.0X35 Blindness right eye category 3, blindness left eye category 5

     ✓7ᵗʰ **H54.0X4** Blindness right eye, category 4

         H54.0X43 Blindness right eye category 4, blindness left eye category 3

         H54.0X44 Blindness right eye category 4, blindness left eye category 4

         H54.0X45 Blindness right eye category 4, blindness left eye category 5

     ✓7ᵗʰ **H54.0X5** Blindness right eye, category 5

         H54.0X53 Blindness right eye category 5, blindness left eye category 3

         H54.0X54 Blindness right eye category 5, blindness left eye category 4

         H54.0X55 Blindness right eye category 5, blindness left eye category 5

✓5ᵗʰ **H54.1** Blindness, one eye, low vision other eye
     Visual impairment categories 3, 4, 5 in one eye, with categories 1 or 2 in the other eye.

     H54.10 Blindness, one eye, low vision other eye, ▽ unspecified eyes

     ✓6ᵗʰ **H54.11** Blindness, right eye, low vision left eye

     ✓7ᵗʰ **H54.113** Blindness right eye category 3, low vision left eye

         H54.1131 Blindness right eye category 3, low vision left eye category 1

         H54.1132 Blindness right eye category 3, low vision left eye category 2

     ✓7ᵗʰ **H54.114** Blindness right eye category 4, low vision left eye

         H54.1141 Blindness right eye category 4, low vision left eye category 1

         H54.1142 Blindness right eye category 4, low vision left eye category 2

     ✓7ᵗʰ **H54.115** Blindness right eye category 5, low vision left eye

         H54.1151 Blindness right eye category 5, low vision left eye category 1

         H54.1152 Blindness right eye category 5, low vision left eye category 2

     ✓6ᵗʰ **H54.12** Blindness, left eye, low vision right eye

     ✓7ᵗʰ **H54.121** Low vision right eye category 1, blindness left eye

         H54.1213 Low vision right eye category 1, blindness left eye category 3

         H54.1214 Low vision right eye category 1, blindness left eye category 4

         H54.1215 Low vision right eye category 1, blindness left eye category 5

     ✓7ᵗʰ **H54.122** Low vision right eye category 2, blindness left eye

         H54.1223 Low vision right eye category 2, blindness left eye category 3

         H54.1224 Low vision right eye category 2, blindness left eye category 4

         H54.1225 Low vision right eye category 2, blindness left eye category 5

✓5ᵗʰ **H54.2** Low vision, both eyes
     Visual impairment categories 1 or 2 in both eyes.

     ✓6ᵗʰ **H54.2X** Low vision, both eyes, different category levels

     ✓7ᵗʰ **H54.2X1** Low vision, right eye, category 1

         H54.2X11 Low vision right eye category 1, low vision left eye category 1

         H54.2X12 Low vision right eye category 1, low vision left eye category 2

     ✓7ᵗʰ **H54.2X2** Low vision, right eye, category 2

         H54.2X21 Low vision right eye category 2, low vision left eye category 1

         H54.2X22 Low vision right eye category 2, low vision left eye category 2

H54.3 Unqualified **visual loss, both eyes**
     Visual impairment category 9 in both eyes.

Ⓝ Newborn: 0   Ⓟ Pediatric: 0-17   Ⓜ Maternity: 12-55   Ⓐ Adult: 15-124   **NRS** Nonroutine supply Dx   **NC Dx** Noncancer Dx   **PDx** Primary Dx   ▶◀ Revised Text   ● New Code   ▲ Revised Title

600   ICD-10-CM 2018

√5ᵗʰ **H54.4** Blindness, one eye
  Visual impairment categories 3, 4, 5 in one eye [normal vision in other eye].

  H54.40 Blindness, one eye, unspecified eye   ▽

√6ᵗʰ **H54.41** Blindness, right eye, normal vision left eye

  ● √7ᵗʰ **H54.413** Blindness, right eye, category 3
  ● **H54.413A** Blindness right eye category 3, normal vision left eye
  ● √7ᵗʰ **H54.414** Blindness, right eye, category 4
  ● **H54.414A** Blindness right eye category 4, normal vision left eye
  ● √7ᵗʰ **H54.415** Blindness, right eye, category 5
  ● **H54.415A** Blindness right eye category 5, normal vision left eye

√6ᵗʰ **H54.42** Blindness, left eye, normal vision right eye

  ● √7ᵗʰ **H54.42A** Blindness, left eye, category 3-5
  ● **H54.42A3** Blindness left eye category 3, normal vision right eye
  ● **H54.42A4** Blindness left eye category 4, normal vision right eye
  ● **H54.42A5** Blindness left eye category 5, normal vision right eye

√5ᵗʰ **H54.5** Low vision, one eye
  Visual impairment categories 1 or 2 in one eye [normal vision in other eye].

  H54.50 Low vision, one eye, unspecified eye   ▽

√6ᵗʰ **H54.51** Low vision, right eye, normal vision left eye

  ● √7ᵗʰ **H54.511** Low vision, right eye, category 1-2
  ● **H54.511A** Low vision right eye category 1, normal vision left eye
  ● **H54.512A** Low vision right eye category 2, normal vision left eye

√6ᵗʰ **H54.52** Low vision, left eye, normal vision right eye

  ● √7ᵗʰ **H54.52A** Low vision, left eye, category 1-2
  ● **H54.52A1** Low vision left eye category 1, normal vision right eye
  ● **H54.52A2** Low vision left eye category 2, normal vision right eye

√5ᵗʰ **H54.6** Unqualified visual loss, one eye
  Visual impairment category 9 in one eye [normal vision in other eye].

  H54.60 Unqualified visual loss, one eye, unspecified   ▽
  H54.61 Unqualified visual loss, right eye, normal vision left eye
  H54.62 Unqualified visual loss, left eye, normal vision right eye

H54.7 Unspecified visual loss   ▽
  Visual impairment category 9 NOS

H54.8 Legal blindness, as defined in USA
  Blindness NOS according to USA definition
  EXCLUDES 1 legal blindness with specification of impairment level (H54.0-H54.7)

NOTE The table below gives a classification of severity of visual impairment recommended by a WHO Study Group on the Prevention of Blindness, Geneva, 6-10 November l972.

The term "low vision" in category H54 comprises categories 1 and 2 of the table, the term "blindness" categories 3, 4 and 5, and the term "unqualified visual loss" category 9.

If the extent of the visual field is taken into account, patients with a field no greater than 10 but greater than 5 around central fixation should be placed in category 3 and patients with a field no greater than 5 around central fixation should be placed in category 4, even if the central acuity is not impaired.

Category of visual impairment	Visual acuity with best possible correction	
	Maximum less than:	**Minimum equal to or better than:**
1	6/18 3/10 (0.3) 20/70	6/60 1/10 (0.1) 20/200
2	6/60 1/10 (0.1) 20/200	3/60 1/20 (0.05) 20/400
3	3/60 1/200 (0.05) 20/400	1/60 (finger counting at one meter) 1/50 (0.02) 5/300 (20/1200)
4	1/60 (finger counting at one meter) 1/50 (0.02) 5/300	Light perception
5	No light perception	
9	Undetermined or unspecified	

Other disorders of eye and adnexa (H55-H57)

√4ᵗʰ **H55** Nystagmus and other irregular eye movements

√5ᵗʰ **H55.0** Nystagmus

  H55.00 Unspecified nystagmus   ▽
  H55.01 Congenital nystagmus
  H55.02 Latent nystagmus
  H55.03 Visual deprivation nystagmus
  H55.04 Dissociated nystagmus
  H55.09 Other forms of nystagmus

√5ᵗʰ **H55.8** Other irregular eye movements

  H55.81 Saccadic eye movements
  H55.89 Other irregular eye movements

√4ᵗʰ **H57** Other disorders of eye and adnexa

√5ᵗʰ **H57.0** Anomalies of pupillary function

  H57.00 Unspecified anomaly of pupillary function   ▽
  H57.01 Argyll Robertson pupil, atypical
    EXCLUDES 1 syphilitic Argyll Robertson pupil (A52.19)
  H57.02 Anisocoria
  H57.03 Miosis
  H57.04 Mydriasis

  √6ᵗʰ **H57.05** Tonic pupil
    H57.051 Tonic pupil, right eye
    H57.052 Tonic pupil, left eye
    H57.053 Tonic pupil, bilateral
    H57.059 Tonic pupil, unspecified eye   ▽
  H57.09 Other anomalies of pupillary function

√5ᵗʰ **H57.1** Ocular pain

  H57.10 Ocular pain, unspecified eye   ▽
  H57.11 Ocular pain, right eye
  H57.12 Ocular pain, left eye
  H57.13 Ocular pain, bilateral

H57.8 Other specified disorders of eye and adnexa
H57.9 Unspecified disorder of eye and adnexa   ▽

☑ Additional Character Req   √x7ᵗʰ Placeholder Alert   Case-Mix Diagnosis   Manifestation   ▽ Unspecified Dx   **EXCLUDES 1** Not coded here   **EXCLUDES 2** Not included here

Intraoperative and postprocedural complications and disorders of eye and adnexa, not elsewhere classified (H59)

✓4ᵗʰ **H59** **Intraoperative and postprocedural complications and disorders of eye and adnexa, not elsewhere classified**

    EXCLUDES 1 *mechanical complication of intraocular lens (T85.2)*
              mechanical complication of other ocular prosthetic devices, implants and grafts (T85.3)
              pseudophakia (Z96.1)
              secondary cataracts (H26.4-)

✓5ᵗʰ **H59.0** **Disorders of the eye following cataract surgery**

  ✓6ᵗʰ **H59.01** **Keratopathy (bullous aphakic) following cataract surgery**
      Vitreal corneal syndrome
      Vitreous (touch) syndrome

    H59.011 **Keratopathy (bullous aphakic) following cataract surgery, right eye**
    H59.012 **Keratopathy (bullous aphakic) following cataract surgery, left eye**
    H59.013 **Keratopathy (bullous aphakic) following cataract surgery, bilateral**
    H59.019 **Keratopathy (bullous aphakic) following cataract surgery, unspecified eye** ▽

  ✓6ᵗʰ **H59.02** **Cataract (lens) fragments in eye following cataract surgery**
    H59.021 **Cataract (lens) fragments in eye following cataract surgery, right eye**
    H59.022 **Cataract (lens) fragments in eye following cataract surgery, left eye**
    H59.023 **Cataract (lens) fragments in eye following cataract surgery, bilateral**
    H59.029 **Cataract (lens) fragments in eye following cataract surgery, unspecified eye** ▽

  ✓6ᵗʰ **H59.03** **Cystoid macular edema following cataract surgery**
    H59.031 **Cystoid macular edema following cataract surgery, right eye**
    H59.032 **Cystoid macular edema following cataract surgery, left eye**
    H59.033 **Cystoid macular edema following cataract surgery, bilateral**
    H59.039 **Cystoid macular edema following cataract surgery, unspecified eye** ▽

  ✓6ᵗʰ **H59.09** **Other disorders of the eye following cataract surgery**
    H59.091 **Other disorders of the right eye following cataract surgery**
    H59.092 **Other disorders of the left eye following cataract surgery**
    H59.093 **Other disorders of the eye following cataract surgery, bilateral**
    H59.099 **Other disorders of unspecified eye following cataract surgery** ▽

✓5ᵗʰ **H59.1** **Intraoperative hemorrhage and hematoma of eye and adnexa complicating a procedure**

    EXCLUDES 1 *intraoperative hemorrhage and hematoma of eye and adnexa due to accidental puncture or laceration during a procedure (H59.2-)*

  ✓6ᵗʰ **H59.11** **Intraoperative hemorrhage and hematoma of eye and adnexa complicating an ophthalmic procedure**
    H59.111 **Intraoperative hemorrhage and hematoma of right eye and adnexa complicating an ophthalmic procedure**
    H59.112 **Intraoperative hemorrhage and hematoma of left eye and adnexa complicating an ophthalmic procedure**
    H59.113 **Intraoperative hemorrhage and hematoma of eye and adnexa complicating an ophthalmic procedure, bilateral**
    H59.119 **Intraoperative hemorrhage and hematoma of unspecified eye and adnexa complicating an ophthalmic procedure** ▽

  ✓6ᵗʰ **H59.12** **Intraoperative hemorrhage and hematoma of eye and adnexa complicating other procedure**
    H59.121 **Intraoperative hemorrhage and hematoma of right eye and adnexa complicating other procedure**
    H59.122 **Intraoperative hemorrhage and hematoma of left eye and adnexa complicating other procedure**
    H59.123 **Intraoperative hemorrhage and hematoma of eye and adnexa complicating other procedure, bilateral**
    H59.129 **Intraoperative hemorrhage and hematoma of unspecified eye and adnexa complicating other procedure** ▽

✓5ᵗʰ **H59.2** **Accidental puncture and laceration of eye and adnexa during a procedure**

  ✓6ᵗʰ **H59.21** **Accidental puncture and laceration of eye and adnexa during an ophthalmic procedure**
    H59.211 **Accidental puncture and laceration of right eye and adnexa during an ophthalmic procedure**
    H59.212 **Accidental puncture and laceration of left eye and adnexa during an ophthalmic procedure**
    H59.213 **Accidental puncture and laceration of eye and adnexa during an ophthalmic procedure, bilateral**
    H59.219 **Accidental puncture and laceration of unspecified eye and adnexa during an ophthalmic procedure** ▽

  ✓6ᵗʰ **H59.22** **Accidental puncture and laceration of eye and adnexa during other procedure**
    H59.221 **Accidental puncture and laceration of right eye and adnexa during other procedure**
    H59.222 **Accidental puncture and laceration of left eye and adnexa during other procedure**
    H59.223 **Accidental puncture and laceration of eye and adnexa during other procedure, bilateral**
    H59.229 **Accidental puncture and laceration of unspecified eye and adnexa during other procedure** ▽

✓5ᵗʰ **H59.3** **Postprocedural hemorrhage, hematoma, and seroma of eye and adnexa following a procedure**

  ✓6ᵗʰ **H59.31** **Postprocedural hemorrhage of eye and adnexa following an ophthalmic procedure**
    H59.311 **Postprocedural hemorrhage of right eye and adnexa following an ophthalmic procedure**
    H59.312 **Postprocedural hemorrhage of left eye and adnexa following an ophthalmic procedure**
    H59.313 **Postprocedural hemorrhage of eye and adnexa following an ophthalmic procedure, bilateral**
    H59.319 **Postprocedural hemorrhage of unspecified eye and adnexa following an ophthalmic procedure** ▽

  ✓6ᵗʰ **H59.32** **Postprocedural hemorrhage of eye and adnexa following other procedure**
    H59.321 **Postprocedural hemorrhage of right eye and adnexa following other procedure**
    H59.322 **Postprocedural hemorrhage of left eye and adnexa following other procedure**
    H59.323 **Postprocedural hemorrhage of eye and adnexa following other procedure, bilateral**
    H59.329 **Postprocedural hemorrhage of unspecified eye and adnexa following other procedure** ▽

  ✓6ᵗʰ **H59.33** **Postprocedural hematoma of eye and adnexa following an ophthalmic procedure**
    H59.331 **Postprocedural hematoma of right eye and adnexa following an ophthalmic procedure**
    H59.332 **Postprocedural hematoma of left eye and adnexa following an ophthalmic procedure**

Ⓝ Newborn: 0 Ⓟ Pediatric: 0-17 Ⓜ Maternity: 12-55 Ⓐ Adult: 15-124 NRS Nonroutine supply Dx NCDx Noncancer Dx PDx Primary Dx ▶◀ Revised Text ● New Code ▲ Revised Title

602   ICD-10-CM 2018

H59.333   Postprocedural hematoma of eye and adnexa following an ophthalmic procedure, bilateral

H59.339   Postprocedural hematoma of unspecified eye and adnexa following an ophthalmic procedure ▽

☑6ᵗʰ H59.34   Postprocedural hematoma of eye and adnexa following other procedure

H59.341   Postprocedural hematoma of right eye and adnexa following other procedure

H59.342   Postprocedural hematoma of left eye and adnexa following other procedure

H59.343   Postprocedural hematoma of eye and adnexa following other procedure, bilateral

H59.349   Postprocedural hematoma of unspecified eye and adnexa following other procedure ▽

☑6ᵗʰ H59.35   Postprocedural seroma of eye and adnexa following an ophthalmic procedure

H59.351   Postprocedural seroma of right eye and adnexa following an ophthalmic procedure

H59.352   Postprocedural seroma of left eye and adnexa following an ophthalmic procedure

H59.353   Postprocedural seroma of eye and adnexa following an ophthalmic procedure, bilateral

H59.359   Postprocedural seroma of unspecified eye and adnexa following an ophthalmic procedure ▽

☑6ᵗʰ H59.36   Postprocedural seroma of eye and adnexa following other procedure

H59.361   Postprocedural seroma of right eye and adnexa following other procedure

H59.362   Postprocedural seroma of left eye and adnexa following other procedure

H59.363   Postprocedural seroma of eye and adnexa following other procedure, bilateral

H59.369   Postprocedural seroma of unspecified eye and adnexa following other procedure ▽

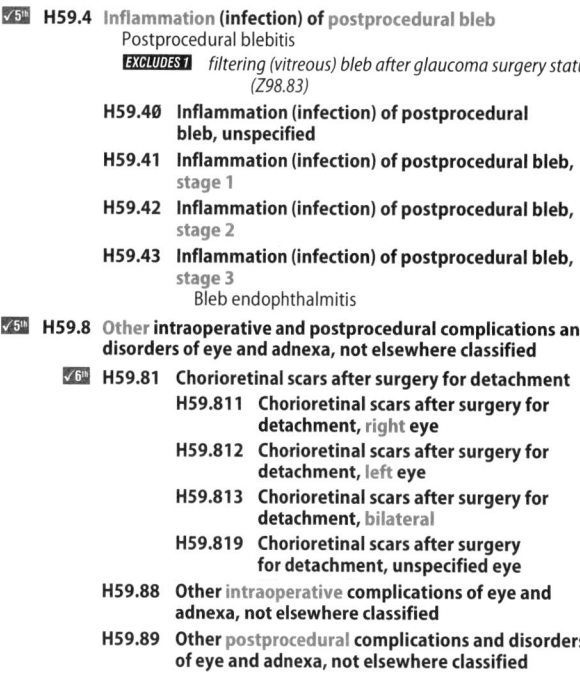

☑5ᵗʰ H59.4   Inflammation (infection) of postprocedural bleb
Postprocedural blebitis
EXCLUDES1   filtering (vitreous) bleb after glaucoma surgery status (Z98.83)

H59.40   Inflammation (infection) of postprocedural bleb, unspecified ▽

H59.41   Inflammation (infection) of postprocedural bleb, stage 1

H59.42   Inflammation (infection) of postprocedural bleb, stage 2

H59.43   Inflammation (infection) of postprocedural bleb, stage 3
Bleb endophthalmitis

☑5ᵗʰ H59.8   Other intraoperative and postprocedural complications and disorders of eye and adnexa, not elsewhere classified

☑6ᵗʰ H59.81   Chorioretinal scars after surgery for detachment

H59.811   Chorioretinal scars after surgery for detachment, right eye

H59.812   Chorioretinal scars after surgery for detachment, left eye

H59.813   Chorioretinal scars after surgery for detachment, bilateral

H59.819   Chorioretinal scars after surgery for detachment, unspecified eye ▽

H59.88   Other intraoperative complications of eye and adnexa, not elsewhere classified

H59.89   Other postprocedural complications and disorders of eye and adnexa, not elsewhere classified

☑ Additional Character Req   ☑x7ᵗʰ Placeholder Alert   Case-Mix Diagnosis   Manifestation   ▽ Unspecified Dx   **EXCLUDES1** Not coded here   **EXCLUDES2** Not included here

ICD-10-CM 2018

603

Chapter 8. Diseases of the Ear and Mastoid Process (H60–H95)

Chapter Specific Coding Guidelines and Examples
Reserved for future guideline expansion.

Chapter 8. Diseases of the Ear and Mastoid Process (H60–H95)

NOTE Use an external cause code following the code for the ear condition, if applicable, to identify the cause of the ear condition.

EXCLUDES 2 certain conditions originating in the perinatal period (P04-P96)
certain infectious and parasitic diseases (A00-B99)
complications of pregnancy, childbirth and the puerperium (O00-O9A)
congenital malformations, deformations and chromosomal abnormalities (Q00-Q99)
endocrine, nutritional and metabolic diseases (E00-E88)
injury, poisoning and certain other consequences of external causes (S00-T88)
neoplasms (C00-D49)
symptoms, signs and abnormal clinical and laboratory findings, not elsewhere classified (R00-R94)

This chapter contains the following blocks:
H60-H62   Diseases of external ear
H65-H75   Diseases of middle ear and mastoid
H80-H83   Diseases of inner ear
H90-H94   Other disorders of ear
H95   Intraoperative and postprocedural complications and disorders of ear and mastoid process, not elsewhere classified

Diseases of external ear (H60-H62)

✓4ᵗʰ H60 Otitis externa

✓5ᵗʰ H60.0 Abscess of external ear
Boil of external ear
Carbuncle of auricle or external auditory canal
Furuncle of external ear
    H60.00 Abscess of external ear, unspecified ear ▽
    H60.01 Abscess of right external ear
    H60.02 Abscess of left external ear
    H60.03 Abscess of external ear, bilateral

✓5ᵗʰ H60.1 Cellulitis of external ear
Cellulitis of auricle
Cellulitis of external auditory canal
    H60.10 Cellulitis of external ear, unspecified ear ▽
    H60.11 Cellulitis of right external ear
    H60.12 Cellulitis of left external ear
    H60.13 Cellulitis of external ear, bilateral

✓5ᵗʰ H60.2 Malignant otitis externa
    H60.20 Malignant otitis externa, unspecified ear ▽
    H60.21 Malignant otitis externa, right ear
    H60.22 Malignant otitis externa, left ear
    H60.23 Malignant otitis externa, bilateral

✓5ᵗʰ H60.3 Other infective otitis externa
   ✓6ᵗʰ H60.31 Diffuse otitis externa
      H60.311 Diffuse otitis externa, right ear
      H60.312 Diffuse otitis externa, left ear
      H60.313 Diffuse otitis externa, bilateral
      H60.319 Diffuse otitis externa, unspecified ear ▽
   ✓6ᵗʰ H60.32 Hemorrhagic otitis externa
      H60.321 Hemorrhagic otitis externa, right ear
      H60.322 Hemorrhagic otitis externa, left ear
      H60.323 Hemorrhagic otitis externa, bilateral
      H60.329 Hemorrhagic otitis externa, unspecified ear ▽
   ✓6ᵗʰ H60.33 Swimmer's ear
      DEF: Otitis externa; commonly occurs when water gets trapped in the ear after swimming.
      H60.331 Swimmer's ear, right ear
      H60.332 Swimmer's ear, left ear
      H60.333 Swimmer's ear, bilateral
      H60.339 Swimmer's ear, unspecified ear ▽
   ✓6ᵗʰ H60.39 Other infective otitis externa
      H60.391 Other infective otitis externa, right ear
      H60.392 Other infective otitis externa, left ear
      H60.393 Other infective otitis externa, bilateral
      H60.399 Other infective otitis externa, unspecified ear ▽

✓5ᵗʰ H60.4 Cholesteatoma of external ear
Keratosis obturans of external ear (canal)
    EXCLUDES 2 cholesteatoma of middle ear (H71.-)
           recurrent cholesteatoma of postmastoidectomy cavity (H95.0-)
    H60.40 Cholesteatoma of external ear, unspecified ear ▽
    H60.41 Cholesteatoma of right external ear
    H60.42 Cholesteatoma of left external ear
    H60.43 Cholesteatoma of external ear, bilateral

✓5ᵗʰ H60.5 Acute noninfective otitis externa
   ✓6ᵗʰ H60.50 Unspecified acute noninfective otitis externa
      Acute otitis externa NOS
      H60.501 Unspecified acute noninfective otitis externa, right ear ▽
      H60.502 Unspecified acute noninfective otitis externa, left ear ▽
      H60.503 Unspecified acute noninfective otitis externa, bilateral ▽
      H60.509 Unspecified acute noninfective otitis externa, unspecified ear ▽
   ✓6ᵗʰ H60.51 Acute actinic otitis externa
      H60.511 Acute actinic otitis externa, right ear
      H60.512 Acute actinic otitis externa, left ear
      H60.513 Acute actinic otitis externa, bilateral
      H60.519 Acute actinic otitis externa, unspecified ear ▽
   ✓6ᵗʰ H60.52 Acute chemical otitis externa
      H60.521 Acute chemical otitis externa, right ear
      H60.522 Acute chemical otitis externa, left ear
      H60.523 Acute chemical otitis externa, bilateral
      H60.529 Acute chemical otitis externa, unspecified ear ▽
   ✓6ᵗʰ H60.53 Acute contact otitis externa
      H60.531 Acute contact otitis externa, right ear
      H60.532 Acute contact otitis externa, left ear
      H60.533 Acute contact otitis externa, bilateral
      H60.539 Acute contact otitis externa, unspecified ear ▽
   ✓6ᵗʰ H60.54 Acute eczematoid otitis externa
      H60.541 Acute eczematoid otitis externa, right ear
      H60.542 Acute eczematoid otitis externa, left ear
      H60.543 Acute eczematoid otitis externa, bilateral
      H60.549 Acute eczematoid otitis externa, unspecified ear ▽
   ✓6ᵗʰ H60.55 Acute reactive otitis externa
      H60.551 Acute reactive otitis externa, right ear
      H60.552 Acute reactive otitis externa, left ear
      H60.553 Acute reactive otitis externa, bilateral
      H60.559 Acute reactive otitis externa, unspecified ear ▽
   ✓6ᵗʰ H60.59 Other noninfective acute otitis externa
      H60.591 Other noninfective acute otitis externa, right ear
      H60.592 Other noninfective acute otitis externa, left ear
      H60.593 Other noninfective acute otitis externa, bilateral
      H60.599 Other noninfective acute otitis externa, unspecified ear ▽

✓5ᵗʰ H60.6 Unspecified chronic otitis externa
    H60.60 Unspecified chronic otitis externa, unspecified ear ▽
    H60.61 Unspecified chronic otitis externa, right ear ▽
    H60.62 Unspecified chronic otitis externa, left ear ▽
    H60.63 Unspecified chronic otitis externa, bilateral ▽

✓5ᵗʰ H60.8 Other otitis externa
   ✓6ᵗʰ H60.8X Other otitis externa
      H60.8X1 Other otitis externa, right ear
      H60.8X2 Other otitis externa, left ear
      H60.8X3 Other otitis externa, bilateral
      H60.8X9 Other otitis externa, unspecified ear ▽

N Newborn: 0   P Pediatric: 0-17   M Maternity: 12-55   A Adult: 15-124   NRS Nonroutine supply Dx   NC Dx Noncancer Dx   PDx Primary Dx   ▶◀ Revised Text   ● New Code   ▲ Revised Title

✓5ᵗʰ H60.9   **Unspecified otitis externa**

     H60.90   Unspecified otitis externa, unspecified ear   ▽
     H60.91   Unspecified otitis externa, right ear   ▽
     H60.92   Unspecified otitis externa, left ear   ▽
     H60.93   Unspecified otitis externa, bilateral   ▽

✓4ᵗʰ H61   **Other disorders of external ear**

   ✓5ᵗʰ H61.0   **Chondritis and perichondritis of external ear**
       Chondrodermatitis nodularis chronica helicis
       Perichondritis of auricle
       Perichondritis of pinna

     ✓6ᵗʰ H61.00   Unspecified perichondritis of external ear
       H61.001   Unspecified perichondritis of right external ear   ▽
       H61.002   Unspecified perichondritis of left external ear   ▽
       H61.003   Unspecified perichondritis of external ear, bilateral   ▽
       H61.009   Unspecified perichondritis of external ear, unspecified ear   ▽

     ✓6ᵗʰ H61.01   Acute perichondritis of external ear
       H61.011   Acute perichondritis of right external ear
       H61.012   Acute perichondritis of left external ear
       H61.013   Acute perichondritis of external ear, bilateral
       H61.019   Acute perichondritis of external ear, unspecified ear   ▽

     ✓6ᵗʰ H61.02   Chronic perichondritis of external ear
       H61.021   Chronic perichondritis of right external ear
       H61.022   Chronic perichondritis of left external ear
       H61.023   Chronic perichondritis of external ear, bilateral
       H61.029   Chronic perichondritis of external ear, unspecified ear   ▽

     ✓6ᵗʰ H61.03   Chondritis of external ear
       Chondritis of auricle
       Chondritis of pinna
       AHA: 2015, 1Q, 18
       DEF: Infection that has progressed into the cartilage; presents as indurated and edematous skin over the pinna; vascular compromise occurs with tissue necrosis and deformity.
       H61.031   Chondritis of right external ear
       H61.032   Chondritis of left external ear
       H61.033   Chondritis of external ear, bilateral
       H61.039   Chondritis of external ear, unspecified ear   ▽

   ✓5ᵗʰ H61.1   **Noninfective disorders of pinna**
       EXCLUDES 2   cauliflower ear (M95.1-)
                 gouty tophi of ear (M1A.-)

     ✓6ᵗʰ H61.10   Unspecified noninfective disorders of pinna
       Disorder of pinna NOS
       H61.101   Unspecified noninfective disorders of pinna, right ear   ▽
       H61.102   Unspecified noninfective disorders of pinna, left ear   ▽
       H61.103   Unspecified noninfective disorders of pinna, bilateral   ▽
       H61.109   Unspecified noninfective disorders of pinna, unspecified ear   ▽

     ✓6ᵗʰ H61.11   Acquired deformity of pinna
       Acquired deformity of auricle
       EXCLUDES 2   cauliflower ear (M95.1-)
       H61.111   Acquired deformity of pinna, right ear
       H61.112   Acquired deformity of pinna, left ear
       H61.113   Acquired deformity of pinna, bilateral
       H61.119   Acquired deformity of pinna, unspecified ear   ▽

     ✓6ᵗʰ H61.12   Hematoma of pinna
       Hematoma of auricle
       H61.121   Hematoma of pinna, right ear
       H61.122   Hematoma of pinna, left ear
       H61.123   Hematoma of pinna, bilateral
       H61.129   Hematoma of pinna, unspecified ear   ▽

     ✓6ᵗʰ H61.19   Other noninfective disorders of pinna
       H61.191   Noninfective disorders of pinna, right ear
       H61.192   Noninfective disorders of pinna, left ear
       H61.193   Noninfective disorders of pinna, bilateral
       H61.199   Noninfective disorders of pinna, unspecified ear   ▽

   ✓5ᵗʰ H61.2   **Impacted cerumen**
       Wax in ear
     H61.20   Impacted cerumen, unspecified ear   ▽
     H61.21   Impacted cerumen, right ear
     H61.22   Impacted cerumen, left ear
     H61.23   Impacted cerumen, bilateral

   ✓5ᵗʰ H61.3   **Acquired stenosis of external ear canal**
       Collapse of external ear canal
       EXCLUDES 1   postprocedural stenosis of external ear canal (H95.81-)

     ✓6ᵗʰ H61.30   Acquired stenosis of external ear canal, unspecified
       H61.301   Acquired stenosis of right external ear canal, unspecified   ▽
       H61.302   Acquired stenosis of left external ear canal, unspecified   ▽
       H61.303   Acquired stenosis of external ear canal, unspecified, bilateral   ▽
       H61.309   Acquired stenosis of external ear canal, unspecified, unspecified ear

     ✓6ᵗʰ H61.31   Acquired stenosis of external ear canal secondary to trauma
       H61.311   Acquired stenosis of right external ear canal secondary to trauma
       H61.312   Acquired stenosis of left external ear canal secondary to trauma
       H61.313   Acquired stenosis of external ear canal secondary to trauma, bilateral
       H61.319   Acquired stenosis of external ear canal secondary to trauma, unspecified ear   ▽

     ✓6ᵗʰ H61.32   Acquired stenosis of external ear canal secondary to inflammation and infection
       DEF: Narrowing of the external ear canal; due to chronic inflammation or infection.
       H61.321   Acquired stenosis of right external ear canal secondary to inflammation and infection
       H61.322   Acquired stenosis of left external ear canal secondary to inflammation and infection
       H61.323   Acquired stenosis of external ear canal secondary to inflammation and infection, bilateral
       H61.329   Acquired stenosis of external ear canal secondary to inflammation and infection, unspecified ear   ▽

     ✓6ᵗʰ H61.39   Other acquired stenosis of external ear canal
       H61.391   Other acquired stenosis of right external ear canal
       H61.392   Other acquired stenosis of left external ear canal
       H61.393   Other acquired stenosis of external ear canal, bilateral
       H61.399   Other acquired stenosis of external ear canal, unspecified ear   ▽

   ✓5ᵗʰ H61.8   **Other specified disorders of external ear**

     ✓6ᵗʰ H61.81   Exostosis of external canal
       H61.811   Exostosis of right external canal
       H61.812   Exostosis of left external canal
       H61.813   Exostosis of external canal, bilateral
       H61.819   Exostosis of external canal, unspecified ear   ▽

     ✓6ᵗʰ H61.89   Other specified disorders of external ear
       H61.891   Other specified disorders of right external ear
       H61.892   Other specified disorders of left external ear
       H61.893   Other specified disorders of external ear, bilateral
       H61.899   Other specified disorders of external ear, unspecified ear   ▽

☑ Additional Character Req   ✓×7ᵗʰ Placeholder Alert   Case-Mix Diagnosis   Manifestation   ▽ Unspecified Dx   EXCLUDES 1 Not coded here   EXCLUDES 2 Not included here

ICD-10-CM 2018   607

Chapter 8. Diseases of the Ear and Mastoid Process

✓5ᵗʰ **H61.9** **Disorder of external ear, unspecified**

    H61.90 **Disorder of external ear, unspecified, unspecified** ▽
        ear

    H61.91 **Disorder of** right **external ear, unspecified** ▽

    H61.92 **Disorder of** left **external ear, unspecified** ▽

    H61.93 **Disorder of external ear, unspecified,** bilateral ▽

✓4ᵗʰ **H62** **Disorders of external ear in diseases classified elsewhere**

✓5ᵗʰ **H62.4** **Otitis externa in other diseases classified elsewhere**
    Code first underlying disease, such as:
      erysipelas (A46)
      impetigo (LØ1.Ø)

    EXCLUDES 1   *otitis externa (in):*
         candidiasis (B37.84)
         herpes viral [herpes simplex] (BØØ.1)
         herpes zoster (BØ2.8)

    H62.40 *Otitis externa in other diseases classified* ▽
        elsewhere, *unspecified* *ear*

    H62.41 *Otitis externa in other diseases classified elsewhere,*
        right *ear*

    H62.42 *Otitis externa in other diseases classified elsewhere,*
        left *ear*

    H62.43 *Otitis externa in other diseases classified elsewhere,*
        bilateral

✓5ᵗʰ **H62.8** **Other disorders of external ear in diseases classified**
    elsewhere
    Code first underlying disease, such as:
      gout (M1A.-, M1Ø.-)

    ✓6ᵗʰ **H62.8X** **Other disorders of external ear in diseases classified**
        elsewhere

        H62.8X1 *Other disorders of* right *external ear in*
            diseases classified elsewhere

        H62.8X2 *Other disorders of* left *external ear in*
            diseases classified elsewhere

        H62.8X3 *Other disorders of external ear in diseases*
            classified elsewhere, *bilateral*

        H62.8X9 *Other disorders of external ear in* ▽
            diseases classified elsewhere,
            unspecified *ear*

Diseases of middle ear and mastoid (H65-H75)

✓4ᵗʰ **H65** **Nonsuppurative otitis media**
    INCLUDES   nonsuppurative otitis media with myringitis
    Use additional code for any associated perforated tympanic membrane
    (H72.-)
    Use additional code to identify:
      exposure to environmental tobacco smoke (Z77.22)
      exposure to tobacco smoke in the perinatal period (P96.81)
      history of tobacco dependence (Z87.891)
      occupational exposure to environmental tobacco smoke (Z57.31)
      tobacco dependence (F17.-)
      tobacco use (Z72.Ø)

✓5ᵗʰ **H65.Ø** **Acute serous otitis media**
    Acute and subacute secretory otitis

    H65.ØØ **Acute serous otitis media, unspecified ear** ▽

    H65.Ø1 **Acute serous otitis media,** right **ear**

    H65.Ø2 **Acute serous otitis media,** left **ear**

    H65.Ø3 **Acute serous otitis media,** bilateral

    H65.Ø4 **Acute serous otitis media,** recurrent, right **ear**

    H65.Ø5 **Acute serous otitis media,** recurrent, left **ear**

    H65.Ø6 **Acute serous otitis media,** recurrent, bilateral

    H65.Ø7 **Acute serous otitis media,** recurrent, ▽
        unspecified ear

✓5ᵗʰ **H65.1** **Other acute** **nonsuppurative otitis media**
    EXCLUDES 1   *otitic barotrauma (T7Ø.Ø)*
         otitis media (acute) NOS (H66.9)

    ✓6ᵗʰ **H65.11** **Acute and subacute allergic otitis media (mucoid)**
        (sanguinous) (serous)

        H65.111 **Acute and subacute allergic otitis media**
            (mucoid) (sanguinous) (serous), right **ear**

        H65.112 **Acute and subacute allergic otitis media**
            (mucoid) (sanguinous) (serous), left **ear**

        H65.113 **Acute and subacute allergic otitis media**
            (mucoid) (sanguinous) (serous), bilateral

        H65.114 **Acute and subacute allergic otitis media**
            (mucoid) (sanguinous) (serous), recurrent,
            right **ear**

        H65.115 **Acute and subacute allergic otitis media**
            (mucoid) (sanguinous) (serous), recurrent,
            left **ear**

        H65.116 **Acute and subacute allergic otitis media**
            (mucoid) (sanguinous) (serous), recurrent,
            bilateral

        H65.117 **Acute and subacute allergic otitis** ▽
            media (mucoid) (sanguinous) (serous),
            recurrent, **unspecified ear**

        H65.119 **Acute and subacute allergic otitis** ▽
            media (mucoid) (sanguinous) (serous),
            unspecified ear

    ✓6ᵗʰ **H65.19** **Other acute** **nonsuppurative otitis media**
        Acute and subacute mucoid otitis media
        Acute and subacute nonsuppurative otitis media NOS
        Acute and subacute sanguinous otitis media
        Acute and subacute seromucinous otitis media

        H65.191 **Other acute nonsuppurative otitis media,**
            right **ear**

        H65.192 **Other acute nonsuppurative otitis media,**
            left **ear**

        H65.193 **Other acute nonsuppurative otitis media,**
            bilateral

        H65.194 **Other acute nonsuppurative otitis media,**
            recurrent, right **ear**

        H65.195 **Other acute nonsuppurative otitis media,**
            recurrent, left **ear**

        H65.196 **Other acute nonsuppurative otitis media,**
            recurrent, bilateral

        H65.197 **Other acute nonsuppurative otitis** ▽
            media recurrent, **unspecified ear**

        H65.199 **Other acute nonsuppurative otitis** ▽
            media, unspecified ear

✓5ᵗʰ **H65.2** **Chronic serous** **otitis media**
    Chronic tubotympanal catarrh

    H65.20 **Chronic serous otitis media, unspecified ear** ▽

    H65.21 **Chronic serous otitis media,** right **ear**

    H65.22 **Chronic serous otitis media,** left **ear**

    H65.23 **Chronic serous otitis media,** bilateral

✓5ᵗʰ **H65.3** **Chronic mucoid** **otitis media**
    Chronic mucinous otitis media
    Chronic secretory otitis media
    Glue ear
    Chronic transudative otitis media
    EXCLUDES 1   *adhesive middle ear disease (H74.1)*

    H65.30 **Chronic mucoid otitis media, unspecified ear** ▽

    H65.31 **Chronic mucoid otitis media,** right **ear**

    H65.32 **Chronic mucoid otitis media,** left **ear**

    H65.33 **Chronic mucoid otitis media,** bilateral

✓5ᵗʰ **H65.4** **Other chronic** **nonsuppurative otitis media**

    ✓6ᵗʰ **H65.41** **Chronic** allergic **otitis media**

        H65.411 **Chronic allergic otitis media,** right **ear**

        H65.412 **Chronic allergic otitis media,** left **ear**

        H65.413 **Chronic allergic otitis media,** bilateral

        H65.419 **Chronic allergic otitis media,** ▽
            unspecified ear

    ✓6ᵗʰ **H65.49** **Other chronic nonsuppurative otitis media**
        Chronic exudative otitis media
        Chronic nonsuppurative otitis media NOS
        Chronic otitis media with effusion (nonpurulent)
        Chronic seromucinous otitis media

        H65.491 **Other chronic nonsuppurative otitis**
            media, right **ear**

        H65.492 **Other chronic nonsuppurative otitis**
            media, left **ear**

        H65.493 **Other chronic nonsuppurative otitis**
            media, bilateral

        H65.499 **Other chronic nonsuppurative otitis** ▽
            media, unspecified ear

✓5ᵗʰ **H65.9** **Unspecified nonsuppurative otitis media**
    Allergic otitis media NOS   Secretory otitis media NOS
    Catarrhal otitis media NOS   Seromucinous otitis media NOS
    Exudative otitis media NOS   Serous otitis media NOS
    Mucoid otitis media NOS   Transudative otitis media NOS
    Otitis media with effusion
      (nonpurulent) NOS

    H65.90 **Unspecified nonsuppurative otitis media,** ▽
        unspecified ear

Ⓝ Newborn: 0   Ⓟ Pediatric: 0-17   Ⓜ Maternity: 12-55   Ⓐ Adult: 15-124   **NRS** Nonroutine supply Dx   **NC Dx** Noncancer Dx   **PDx** Primary Dx   ▶◀ Revised Text   ● New Code   ▲ Revised Title

608   ICD-10-CM 2018

H65.91   **Unspecified nonsuppurative otitis media, right ear** ▽

H65.92   **Unspecified nonsuppurative otitis media, left ear** ▽

H65.93   **Unspecified nonsuppurative otitis media, bilateral** ▽

✓4ᵗʰ **H66**   **Suppurative and unspecified otitis media**
> INCLUDES   suppurative and unspecified otitis media with myringitis
> Use additional code to identify:
>   exposure to environmental tobacco smoke (Z77.22)
>   exposure to tobacco smoke in the perinatal period (P96.81)
>   history of tobacco dependence (Z87.891)
>   occupational exposure to environmental tobacco smoke (Z57.31)
>   tobacco dependence (F17.-)
>   tobacco use (Z72.0)
> AHA: 2016, 1Q, 34

✓5ᵗʰ **H66.0**   **Acute suppurative otitis media**

  ✓6ᵗʰ **H66.00**   **Acute suppurative otitis media without spontaneous rupture of ear drum**

     H66.001   **Acute suppurative otitis media without spontaneous rupture of ear drum, right ear**

     H66.002   **Acute suppurative otitis media without spontaneous rupture of ear drum, left ear**

     H66.003   **Acute suppurative otitis media without spontaneous rupture of ear drum, bilateral**

     H66.004   **Acute suppurative otitis media without spontaneous rupture of ear drum, recurrent, right ear**

     H66.005   **Acute suppurative otitis media without spontaneous rupture of ear drum, recurrent, left ear**

     H66.006   **Acute suppurative otitis media without spontaneous rupture of ear drum, recurrent, bilateral**

     H66.007   **Acute suppurative otitis media without spontaneous rupture of ear drum, recurrent, unspecified ear** ▽

     H66.009   **Acute suppurative otitis media without spontaneous rupture of ear drum, unspecified ear** ▽

  ✓6ᵗʰ **H66.01**   **Acute suppurative otitis media with spontaneous rupture of ear drum**
> **DEF:** Sudden, severe inflammation of middle ear, with pressure causing the perforation of ear drum tissue.

     H66.011   **Acute suppurative otitis media with spontaneous rupture of ear drum, right ear**

     H66.012   **Acute suppurative otitis media with spontaneous rupture of ear drum, left ear**

     H66.013   **Acute suppurative otitis media with spontaneous rupture of ear drum, bilateral**

     H66.014   **Acute suppurative otitis media with spontaneous rupture of ear drum, recurrent, right ear**

     H66.015   **Acute suppurative otitis media with spontaneous rupture of ear drum, recurrent, left ear**

     H66.016   **Acute suppurative otitis media with spontaneous rupture of ear drum, recurrent, bilateral**

     H66.017   **Acute suppurative otitis media with spontaneous rupture of ear drum, recurrent, unspecified ear** ▽

     H66.019   **Acute suppurative otitis media with spontaneous rupture of ear drum, unspecified ear** ▽

✓5ᵗʰ **H66.1**   **Chronic tubotympanic suppurative otitis media**
> Benign chronic suppurative otitis media
> Chronic tubotympanic disease
> Use additional code for any associated perforated tympanic membrane (H72.-)

   H66.10   **Chronic tubotympanic suppurative otitis media, unspecified** ▽

   H66.11   **Chronic tubotympanic suppurative otitis media, right ear**

   H66.12   **Chronic tubotympanic suppurative otitis media, left ear**

   H66.13   **Chronic tubotympanic suppurative otitis media, bilateral**

✓5ᵗʰ **H66.2**   **Chronic atticoantral suppurative otitis media**
> Chronic atticoantral disease
> Use additional code for any associated perforated tympanic membrane (H72.-)

   H66.20   **Chronic atticoantral suppurative otitis media, unspecified ear** ▽

   H66.21   **Chronic atticoantral suppurative otitis media, right ear**

   H66.22   **Chronic atticoantral suppurative otitis media, left ear**

   H66.23   **Chronic atticoantral suppurative otitis media, bilateral**

✓5ᵗʰ **H66.3**   **Other chronic suppurative otitis media**
> Chronic suppurative otitis media NOS
> Use additional code for any associated perforated tympanic membrane (H72.-)
> EXCLUDES 1   tuberculous otitis media (A18.6)

  ✓6ᵗʰ **H66.3X**   **Other chronic suppurative otitis media**

     H66.3X1   **Other chronic suppurative otitis media, right ear**

     H66.3X2   **Other chronic suppurative otitis media, left ear**

     H66.3X3   **Other chronic suppurative otitis media, bilateral**

     H66.3X9   **Other chronic suppurative otitis media, unspecified ear** ▽

✓5ᵗʰ **H66.4**   **Suppurative otitis media, unspecified**
> Purulent otitis media NOS
> Use additional code for any associated perforated tympanic membrane (H72.-)

   H66.40   **Suppurative otitis media, unspecified, unspecified ear** ▽

   H66.41   **Suppurative otitis media, unspecified, right ear**

   H66.42   **Suppurative otitis media, unspecified, left ear**

   H66.43   **Suppurative otitis media, unspecified, bilateral**

✓5ᵗʰ **H66.9**   **Otitis media, unspecified**
> Otitis media NOS
> Acute otitis media NOS
> Chronic otitis media NOS
> Use additional code for any associated perforated tympanic membrane (H72.-)

   H66.90   **Otitis media, unspecified, unspecified ear** ▽

   H66.91   **Otitis media, unspecified, right ear** ▽

   H66.92   **Otitis media, unspecified, left ear** ▽

   H66.93   **Otitis media, unspecified, bilateral** ▽

✓4ᵗʰ **H67**   **Otitis media in diseases classified elsewhere**
> Code first underlying disease, such as:
>   viral disease NEC (B00-B34)
> Use additional code for any associated perforated tympanic membrane (H72.-)
> EXCLUDES 1   otitis media in:
>   influenza (J09.X9, J10.83, J11.83)
>   measles (B05.3)
>   scarlet fever (A38.0)
>   tuberculosis (A18.6)

   H67.1   *Otitis media in diseases classified elsewhere, right ear*

   H67.2   *Otitis media in diseases classified elsewhere, left ear*

   H67.3   *Otitis media in diseases classified elsewhere, bilateral*

   H67.9   *Otitis media in diseases classified elsewhere, unspecified ear* ▽

✓4ᵗʰ **H68**   **Eustachian salpingitis and obstruction**

✓5ᵗʰ **H68.0**   **Eustachian salpingitis**

  ✓6ᵗʰ **H68.00**   **Unspecified Eustachian salpingitis**

     H68.001   **Unspecified Eustachian salpingitis, right ear** ▽

     H68.002   **Unspecified Eustachian salpingitis, left ear** ▽

     H68.003   **Unspecified Eustachian salpingitis, bilateral** ▽

     H68.009   **Unspecified Eustachian salpingitis, unspecified ear** ▽

  ✓6ᵗʰ **H68.01**   **Acute Eustachian salpingitis**

     H68.011   **Acute Eustachian salpingitis, right ear**

     H68.012   **Acute Eustachian salpingitis, left ear**

     H68.013   **Acute Eustachian salpingitis, bilateral**

☑ Additional Character Req   ✓x7ᵗʰ Placeholder Alert   Case-Mix Diagnosis   Manifestation   ▽ Unspecified Dx   EXCLUDES 1 Not coded here   EXCLUDES 2 Not included here

ICD-10-CM 2018   **609**

Chapter 8. Diseases of the Ear and Mastoid Process

      H68.019 Acute Eustachian salpingitis, ▽
unspecified ear

✓6ᵗʰ H68.02 **Chronic** Eustachian salpingitis
      H68.021 Chronic Eustachian salpingitis, right ear
      H68.022 Chronic Eustachian salpingitis, left ear
      H68.023 Chronic Eustachian salpingitis, bilateral
      H68.029 Chronic Eustachian salpingitis, ▽
unspecified ear

✓5ᵗʰ **H68.1** **Obstruction** of Eustachian tube
    Stenosis of Eustachian tube
    Stricture of Eustachian tube

✓6ᵗʰ H68.10 **Unspecified** obstruction of Eustachian tube
      H68.101 Unspecified obstruction of ▽
Eustachian tube, right ear
      H68.102 Unspecified obstruction of ▽
Eustachian tube, left ear
      H68.103 Unspecified obstruction of ▽
Eustachian tube, bilateral
      H68.109 Unspecified obstruction of ▽
Eustachian tube, unspecified ear

✓6ᵗʰ H68.11 **Osseous** obstruction of Eustachian tube
      H68.111 Osseous obstruction of Eustachian tube, right ear
      H68.112 Osseous obstruction of Eustachian tube, left ear
      H68.113 Osseous obstruction of Eustachian tube, bilateral
      H68.119 Osseous obstruction of Eustachian ▽
tube, unspecified ear

✓6ᵗʰ H68.12 **Intrinsic cartilagenous** obstruction of Eustachian tube
      H68.121 Intrinsic cartilagenous obstruction of Eustachian tube, right ear
      H68.122 Intrinsic cartilagenous obstruction of Eustachian tube, left ear
      H68.123 Intrinsic cartilagenous obstruction of Eustachian tube, bilateral
      H68.129 Intrinsic cartilagenous obstruction ▽
of Eustachian tube, unspecified ear

✓6ᵗʰ H68.13 **Extrinsic cartilagenous** obstruction of Eustachian tube
    Compression of Eustachian tube
      H68.131 Extrinsic cartilagenous obstruction of Eustachian tube, right ear
      H68.132 Extrinsic cartilagenous obstruction of Eustachian tube, left ear
      H68.133 Extrinsic cartilagenous obstruction of Eustachian tube, bilateral
      H68.139 Extrinsic cartilagenous obstruction of ▽
Eustachian tube, unspecified ear

✓4ᵗʰ **H69** **Other and unspecified disorders of Eustachian tube**

✓5ᵗʰ **H69.0** **Patulous** Eustachian tube
      H69.00 Patulous Eustachian tube, unspecified ear ▽
      H69.01 Patulous Eustachian tube, right ear
      H69.02 Patulous Eustachian tube, left ear
      H69.03 Patulous Eustachian tube, bilateral

✓5ᵗʰ **H69.8** **Other specified** disorders of Eustachian tube
      H69.80 Other specified disorders of Eustachian tube, ▽
unspecified ear
      H69.81 Other specified disorders of Eustachian tube, right
ear
      H69.82 Other specified disorders of Eustachian tube, left ear
      H69.83 Other specified disorders of Eustachian tube,
bilateral

✓5ᵗʰ **H69.9** **Unspecified** Eustachian tube disorder
      H69.90 Unspecified Eustachian tube disorder, ▽
unspecified ear
      H69.91 Unspecified Eustachian tube disorder, right ear ▽
      H69.92 Unspecified Eustachian tube disorder, left ear ▽
      H69.93 Unspecified Eustachian tube disorder, bilateral ▽

✓4ᵗʰ **H70** **Mastoiditis and related conditions**

✓5ᵗʰ **H70.0** **Acute mastoiditis**
    Abscess of mastoid
    Empyema of mastoid

✓6ᵗʰ H70.00 **Acute mastoiditis** without complications
      H70.001 Acute mastoiditis without complications,
right ear
      H70.002 Acute mastoiditis without complications,
left ear
      H70.003 Acute mastoiditis without complications,
bilateral
      H70.009 Acute mastoiditis without ▽
complications, unspecified ear

✓6ᵗʰ H70.01 **Subperiosteal abscess** of mastoid
      H70.011 Subperiosteal abscess of mastoid, right
ear
      H70.012 Subperiosteal abscess of mastoid, left ear
      H70.013 Subperiosteal abscess of mastoid,
bilateral
      H70.019 Subperiosteal abscess of mastoid, ▽
unspecified ear

✓6ᵗʰ H70.09 **Acute mastoiditis** with other complications
      H70.091 Acute mastoiditis with other
complications, right ear
      H70.092 Acute mastoiditis with other
complications, left ear
      H70.093 Acute mastoiditis with other
complications, bilateral
      H70.099 Acute mastoiditis with other ▽
complications, unspecified ear

✓5ᵗʰ **H70.1** **Chronic mastoiditis**
    Caries of mastoid
    Fistula of mastoid
    EXCLUDES 1 *tuberculous mastoiditis (A18.03)*
      H70.10 Chronic mastoiditis, unspecified ear ▽
      H70.11 Chronic mastoiditis, right ear
      H70.12 Chronic mastoiditis, left ear
      H70.13 Chronic mastoiditis, bilateral

✓5ᵗʰ **H70.2** **Petrositis**
    Inflammation of petrous bone

✓6ᵗʰ H70.20 **Unspecified** petrositis
      H70.201 Unspecified petrositis, right ear ▽
      H70.202 Unspecified petrositis, left ear ▽
      H70.203 Unspecified petrositis, bilateral ▽
      H70.209 Unspecified petrositis, unspecified ear ▽

✓6ᵗʰ H70.21 **Acute petrositis**
    DEF: Sudden, severe inflammation of petrous temporal
bone behind the ear; associated with middle ear
infection.
      H70.211 Acute petrositis, right ear
      H70.212 Acute petrositis, left ear
      H70.213 Acute petrositis, bilateral
      H70.219 Acute petrositis, unspecified ear ▽

✓6ᵗʰ H70.22 **Chronic petrositis**
      H70.221 Chronic petrositis, right ear
      H70.222 Chronic petrositis, left ear
      H70.223 Chronic petrositis, bilateral
      H70.229 Chronic petrositis, unspecified ear ▽

✓5ᵗʰ **H70.8** **Other mastoiditis and related conditions**
    EXCLUDES 1 *preauricular sinus and cyst (Q18.1)*
                  sinus, fistula, and cyst of branchial cleft (Q18.0)

✓6ᵗʰ H70.81 **Postauricular fistula**
      H70.811 Postauricular fistula, right ear
      H70.812 Postauricular fistula, left ear
      H70.813 Postauricular fistula, bilateral
      H70.819 Postauricular fistula, unspecified ear ▽

✓6ᵗʰ H70.89 **Other** mastoiditis and related conditions
      H70.891 Other mastoiditis and related conditions,
right ear
      H70.892 Other mastoiditis and related conditions,
left ear
      H70.893 Other mastoiditis and related conditions,
bilateral
      H70.899 Other mastoiditis and related ▽
conditions, unspecified ear

N Newborn: 0   **P** Pediatric: 0-17   **M** Maternity: 12-55   **A** Adult: 15-124   **NRS** Nonroutine supply Dx   **NCDx** Noncancer Dx   **PDx** Primary Dx   ▶◀ Revised Text   ● New Code   ▲ Revised Title

610   ICD-10-CM 2018

Cholesteatoma of Middle Ear

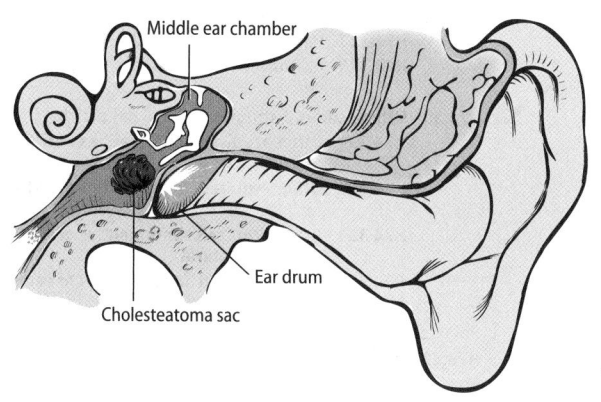

Middle ear chamber

Cholesteatoma sac

Ear drum

✓5ᵗʰ **H70.9** Unspecified **mastoiditis**

    H70.90 Unspecified mastoiditis, unspecified ear ▽

    H70.91 Unspecified mastoiditis, right ear ▽

    H70.92 Unspecified mastoiditis, left ear ▽

    H70.93 Unspecified mastoiditis, bilateral ▽

✓4ᵗʰ **H71** **Cholesteatoma of middle ear**

    EXCLUDES 2 *cholesteatoma of external ear (H60.4-)*

                recurrent cholesteatoma of postmastoidectomy cavity (H95.0-)

✓5ᵗʰ **H71.0** Cholesteatoma of **attic**

    H71.00 Cholesteatoma of attic, unspecified ear ▽

    H71.01 Cholesteatoma of attic, right ear

    H71.02 Cholesteatoma of attic, left ear

    H71.03 Cholesteatoma of attic, bilateral

✓5ᵗʰ **H71.1** Cholesteatoma of **tympanum**

    H71.10 Cholesteatoma of tympanum, unspecified ear ▽

    H71.11 Cholesteatoma of tympanum, right ear

    H71.12 Cholesteatoma of tympanum, left ear

    H71.13 Cholesteatoma of tympanum, bilateral

✓5ᵗʰ **H71.2** Cholesteatoma of **mastoid**

    H71.20 Cholesteatoma of mastoid, unspecified ear ▽

    H71.21 Cholesteatoma of mastoid, right ear

    H71.22 Cholesteatoma of mastoid, left ear

    H71.23 Cholesteatoma of mastoid, bilateral

✓5ᵗʰ **H71.3** Diffuse **cholesteatosis**

    H71.30 Diffuse cholesteatosis, unspecified ear ▽

    H71.31 Diffuse cholesteatosis, right ear

    H71.32 Diffuse cholesteatosis, left ear

    H71.33 Diffuse cholesteatosis, bilateral

✓5ᵗʰ **H71.9** Unspecified **cholesteatoma**

    H71.90 Unspecified cholesteatoma, unspecified ear ▽

    H71.91 Unspecified cholesteatoma, right ear ▽

    H71.92 Unspecified cholesteatoma, left ear ▽

    H71.93 Unspecified cholesteatoma, bilateral ▽

✓4ᵗʰ **H72** **Perforation of tympanic membrane**

    INCLUDES persistent post-traumatic perforation of ear drum

                postinflammatory perforation of ear drum

    Code first any associated otitis media (H65.-, H66.1-, H66.2-, H66.3-, H66.4-, H66.9-, H67.-)

    EXCLUDES 1 *acute suppurative otitis media with rupture of the tympanic membrane (H66.01-)*

                traumatic rupture of ear drum (S09.2-)

✓5ᵗʰ **H72.0** Central **perforation of tympanic membrane**

    H72.00 Central perforation of tympanic membrane, unspecified ear ▽

    H72.01 Central perforation of tympanic membrane, right ear

    H72.02 Central perforation of tympanic membrane, left ear

    H72.03 Central perforation of tympanic membrane, bilateral

✓5ᵗʰ **H72.1** Attic **perforation of tympanic membrane**

    Perforation of pars flaccida

    H72.10 Attic perforation of tympanic membrane, unspecified ear ▽

    H72.11 Attic perforation of tympanic membrane, right ear

    H72.12 Attic perforation of tympanic membrane, left ear

    H72.13 Attic perforation of tympanic membrane, bilateral

✓5ᵗʰ **H72.2** Other marginal perforations of tympanic membrane

    ✓6ᵗʰ **H72.2X** Other marginal **perforations of tympanic membrane**

        H72.2X1 Other marginal perforations of tympanic membrane, right ear

        H72.2X2 Other marginal perforations of tympanic membrane, left ear

        H72.2X3 Other marginal perforations of tympanic membrane, bilateral

        H72.2X9 Other marginal perforations of tympanic membrane, unspecified ear ▽

✓5ᵗʰ **H72.8** Other **perforations of tympanic membrane**

    ✓6ᵗʰ **H72.81** Multiple **perforations of tympanic membrane**

        H72.811 Multiple perforations of tympanic membrane, right ear

        H72.812 Multiple perforations of tympanic membrane, left ear

        H72.813 Multiple perforations of tympanic membrane, bilateral

        H72.819 Multiple perforations of tympanic membrane, unspecified ear ▽

    ✓6ᵗʰ **H72.82** Total **perforations of tympanic membrane**

        H72.821 Total perforations of tympanic membrane, right ear

        H72.822 Total perforations of tympanic membrane, left ear

        H72.823 Total perforations of tympanic membrane, bilateral

        H72.829 Total perforations of tympanic membrane, unspecified ear ▽

✓5ᵗʰ **H72.9** Unspecified **perforation of tympanic membrane**

    H72.90 Unspecified perforation of tympanic membrane, unspecified ear ▽

    H72.91 Unspecified perforation of tympanic membrane, right ear ▽

    H72.92 Unspecified perforation of tympanic membrane, left ear ▽

    H72.93 Unspecified perforation of tympanic membrane, bilateral ▽

✓4ᵗʰ **H73** **Other disorders of tympanic membrane**

✓5ᵗʰ **H73.0** Acute **myringitis**

    EXCLUDES 1 *acute myringitis with otitis media (H65, H66)*

    ✓6ᵗʰ **H73.00** Unspecified **acute myringitis**

        Acute tympanitis NOS

        H73.001 Acute myringitis, right ear

        H73.002 Acute myringitis, left ear

        H73.003 Acute myringitis, bilateral

        H73.009 Acute myringitis, unspecified ear ▽

    ✓6ᵗʰ **H73.01** Bullous **myringitis**

        DEF: Bacterial or viral otitis media; characterized by the appearance of serous or hemorrhagic blebs on the ear drum and sudden onset of severe pain in ear.

        H73.011 Bullous myringitis, right ear

        H73.012 Bullous myringitis, left ear

        H73.013 Bullous myringitis, bilateral

        H73.019 Bullous myringitis, unspecified ear ▽

    ✓6ᵗʰ **H73.09** Other **acute myringitis**

        H73.091 Other acute myringitis, right ear

        H73.092 Other acute myringitis, left ear

        H73.093 Other acute myringitis, bilateral

        H73.099 Other acute myringitis, unspecified ear ▽

✓5ᵗʰ **H73.1** Chronic **myringitis**

    Chronic tympanitis

    EXCLUDES 1 *chronic myringitis with otitis media (H65, H66)*

    H73.10 Chronic myringitis, unspecified ear ▽

    H73.11 Chronic myringitis, right ear

    H73.12 Chronic myringitis, left ear

    H73.13 Chronic myringitis, bilateral

✓ Additional Character Req   ✓x7ᵗʰ Placeholder Alert   Case-Mix Diagnosis   Manifestation   ▽ Unspecified Dx   **EXCLUDES 1** Not coded here   **EXCLUDES 2** Not included here

ICD-10-CM 2018   611

Chapter 8. Diseases of the Ear and Mastoid Process

✓5th **H73.2** Unspecified myringitis

     H73.20 Unspecified myringitis, unspecified ear ▽

     H73.21 Unspecified myringitis, right ear ▽

     H73.22 Unspecified myringitis, left ear ▽

     H73.23 Unspecified myringitis, bilateral ▽

✓5th **H73.8** Other specified disorders of tympanic membrane

     ✓6th **H73.81** Atrophic flaccid tympanic membrane

         H73.811 Atrophic flaccid tympanic membrane, right ear

         H73.812 Atrophic flaccid tympanic membrane, left ear

         H73.813 Atrophic flaccid tympanic membrane, bilateral

         H73.819 Atrophic flaccid tympanic membrane, unspecified ear ▽

     ✓6th **H73.82** Atrophic nonflaccid tympanic membrane

         H73.821 Atrophic nonflaccid tympanic membrane, right ear

         H73.822 Atrophic nonflaccid tympanic membrane, left ear

         H73.823 Atrophic nonflaccid tympanic membrane, bilateral

         H73.829 Atrophic nonflaccid tympanic membrane, unspecified ear ▽

     ✓6th **H73.89** Other specified disorders of tympanic membrane

         H73.891 Other specified disorders of tympanic membrane, right ear

         H73.892 Other specified disorders of tympanic membrane, left ear

         H73.893 Other specified disorders of tympanic membrane, bilateral

         H73.899 Other specified disorders of tympanic membrane, unspecified ear ▽

✓5th **H73.9** Unspecified disorder of tympanic membrane

     H73.90 Unspecified disorder of tympanic membrane, unspecified ear ▽

     H73.91 Unspecified disorder of tympanic membrane, right ear ▽

     H73.92 Unspecified disorder of tympanic membrane, left ear ▽

     H73.93 Unspecified disorder of tympanic membrane, bilateral ▽

✓4th **H74** Other disorders of middle ear mastoid

     EXCLUDES 2 mastoiditis (H70.-)

     ✓5th **H74.0** Tympanosclerosis

         DEF: Calcification of tissue in the ear drum, middle ear bones, and middle ear canal.

         H74.01 Tympanosclerosis, right ear

         H74.02 Tympanosclerosis, left ear

         H74.03 Tympanosclerosis, bilateral

         H74.09 Tympanosclerosis, unspecified ear ▽

     ✓5th **H74.1** Adhesive middle ear disease

         Adhesive otitis

         EXCLUDES 1 glue ear (H65.3-)

         H74.11 Adhesive right middle ear disease

         H74.12 Adhesive left middle ear disease

         H74.13 Adhesive middle ear disease, bilateral

         H74.19 Adhesive middle ear disease, unspecified ear ▽

     ✓5th **H74.2** Discontinuity and dislocation of ear ossicles

         H74.20 Discontinuity and dislocation of ear ossicles, unspecified ear ▽

         H74.21 Discontinuity and dislocation of right ear ossicles

         H74.22 Discontinuity and dislocation of left ear ossicles

         H74.23 Discontinuity and dislocation of ear ossicles, bilateral

     ✓5th **H74.3** Other acquired abnormalities of ear ossicles

         ✓6th **H74.31** Ankylosis of ear ossicles

             H74.311 Ankylosis of ear ossicles, right ear

             H74.312 Ankylosis of ear ossicles, left ear

             H74.313 Ankylosis of ear ossicles, bilateral

             H74.319 Ankylosis of ear ossicles, unspecified ear ▽

         ✓6th **H74.32** Partial loss of ear ossicles

             H74.321 Partial loss of ear ossicles, right ear

             H74.322 Partial loss of ear ossicles, left ear

             H74.323 Partial loss of ear ossicles, bilateral

             H74.329 Partial loss of ear ossicles, unspecified ear ▽

         ✓6th **H74.39** Other acquired abnormalities of ear ossicles

             H74.391 Other acquired abnormalities of right ear ossicles

             H74.392 Other acquired abnormalities of left ear ossicles

             H74.393 Other acquired abnormalities of ear ossicles, bilateral

             H74.399 Other acquired abnormalities of ear ossicles, unspecified ear ▽

     ✓5th **H74.4** Polyp of middle ear

         H74.40 Polyp of middle ear, unspecified ear ▽

         H74.41 Polyp of right middle ear

         H74.42 Polyp of left middle ear

         H74.43 Polyp of middle ear, bilateral

     ✓5th **H74.8** Other specified disorders of middle ear and mastoid

         ✓6th **H74.8X** Other specified disorders of middle ear and mastoid

             H74.8X1 Other specified disorders of right middle ear and mastoid

             H74.8X2 Other specified disorders of left middle ear and mastoid

             H74.8X3 Other specified disorders of middle ear and mastoid, bilateral

             H74.8X9 Other specified disorders of middle ear and mastoid, unspecified ear ▽

     ✓5th **H74.9** Unspecified disorder of middle ear and mastoid

         H74.90 Unspecified disorder of middle ear and mastoid, unspecified ear ▽

         H74.91 Unspecified disorder of right middle ear and mastoid ▽

         H74.92 Unspecified disorder of left middle ear and mastoid ▽

         H74.93 Unspecified disorder of middle ear and mastoid, bilateral ▽

✓4th **H75** Other disorders of middle ear and mastoid in diseases classified elsewhere

     Code first underlying disease

     ✓5th **H75.0** Mastoiditis in infectious and parasitic diseases classified elsewhere

         EXCLUDES 1 mastoiditis (in):

             syphilis (A52.77)

             tuberculosis (A18.03)

         H75.00 *Mastoiditis in infectious and parasitic diseases classified elsewhere, unspecified ear* ▽

         H75.01 *Mastoiditis in infectious and parasitic diseases classified elsewhere, right ear*

         H75.02 *Mastoiditis in infectious and parasitic diseases classified elsewhere, left ear*

         H75.03 *Mastoiditis in infectious and parasitic diseases classified elsewhere, bilateral*

     ✓5th **H75.8** Other specified disorders of middle ear and mastoid in diseases classified elsewhere

         H75.80 *Other specified disorders of middle ear and mastoid in diseases classified elsewhere, unspecified ear* ▽

         H75.81 *Other specified disorders of right middle ear and mastoid in diseases classified elsewhere*

         H75.82 *Other specified disorders of left middle ear and mastoid in diseases classified elsewhere*

         H75.83 *Other specified disorders of middle ear and mastoid in diseases classified elsewhere, bilateral*

Diseases of inner ear (H80-H83)

✓4th **H80** Otosclerosis

     INCLUDES otospongiosis

     ✓5th **H80.0** Otosclerosis involving oval window, nonobliterative

         H80.00 Otosclerosis involving oval window, nonobliterative, unspecified ear ▽

         H80.01 Otosclerosis involving oval window, nonobliterative, right ear

N Newborn: 0   P Pediatric: 0-17   M Maternity: 12-55   A Adult: 15-124   NRS Nonroutine supply Dx   NC Dx Noncancer Dx   PDx Primary Dx   ►◄ Revised Text   ● New Code   ▲ Revised Title

612   ICD-10-CM 2018

H73.2–H80.01

H80.02   Otosclerosis involving oval window, nonobliterative, left ear

H80.03   Otosclerosis involving oval window, nonobliterative, bilateral

✓5ᵗʰ **H80.1**   Otosclerosis involving oval window, obliterative

H80.10   Otosclerosis involving oval window, obliterative, unspecified ear ▽

H80.11   Otosclerosis involving oval window, obliterative, right ear

H80.12   Otosclerosis involving oval window, obliterative, left ear

H80.13   Otosclerosis involving oval window, obliterative, bilateral

✓5ᵗʰ **H80.2**   Cochlear otosclerosis
     Otosclerosis involving otic capsule
     Otosclerosis involving round window

H80.20   Cochlear otosclerosis, unspecified ear ▽

H80.21   Cochlear otosclerosis, right ear

H80.22   Cochlear otosclerosis, left ear

H80.23   Cochlear otosclerosis, bilateral

✓5ᵗʰ **H80.8**   Other otosclerosis

H80.80   Other otosclerosis, unspecified ear ▽

H80.81   Other otosclerosis, right ear

H80.82   Other otosclerosis, left ear

H80.83   Other otosclerosis, bilateral

✓5ᵗʰ **H80.9**   Unspecified otosclerosis

H80.90   Unspecified otosclerosis, unspecified ear ▽

H80.91   Unspecified otosclerosis, right ear ▽

H80.92   Unspecified otosclerosis, left ear ▽

H80.93   Unspecified otosclerosis, bilateral ▽

✓4ᵗʰ **H81**   **Disorders of vestibular function**
     EXCLUDES 1   epidemic vertigo (A88.1)
                 vertigo NOS (R42)

✓5ᵗʰ **H81.0**   Ménière's disease
     Labyrinthine hydrops
     Ménière's syndrome or vertigo

H81.01   Ménière's disease, right ear

H81.02   Ménière's disease, left ear

H81.03   Ménière's disease, bilateral

H81.09   Ménière's disease, unspecified ear ▽

✓5ᵗʰ **H81.1**   Benign paroxysmal vertigo

H81.10   Benign paroxysmal vertigo, unspecified ear ▽

H81.11   Benign paroxysmal vertigo, right ear

H81.12   Benign paroxysmal vertigo, left ear

H81.13   Benign paroxysmal vertigo, bilateral

✓5ᵗʰ **H81.2**   Vestibular neuronitis
     DEF: Transient benign vertigo, caused by inflammation of the vestibular nerve; characterized by response to caloric stimulation on one side, nystagmus with rhythmic movement of eyes; normal auditory function present.

H81.20   Vestibular neuronitis, unspecified ear ▽

H81.21   Vestibular neuronitis, right ear

H81.22   Vestibular neuronitis, left ear

H81.23   Vestibular neuronitis, bilateral

✓5ᵗʰ **H81.3**   Other peripheral vertigo

✓6ᵗʰ **H81.31**   Aural vertigo

H81.311   Aural vertigo, right ear

H81.312   Aural vertigo, left ear

H81.313   Aural vertigo, bilateral

H81.319   Aural vertigo, unspecified ear ▽

✓6ᵗʰ **H81.39**   Other peripheral vertigo
     Lermoyez' syndrome
     Otogenic vertigo
     Peripheral vertigo NOS

H81.391   Other peripheral vertigo, right ear

H81.392   Other peripheral vertigo, left ear

H81.393   Other peripheral vertigo, bilateral

H81.399   Other peripheral vertigo, unspecified ear ▽

✓5ᵗʰ **H81.4**   Vertigo of central origin
     Central positional nystagmus

H81.41   Vertigo of central origin, right ear

H81.42   Vertigo of central origin, left ear

H81.43   Vertigo of central origin, bilateral

H81.49   Vertigo of central origin, unspecified ear ▽

✓5ᵗʰ **H81.8**   Other disorders of vestibular function

✓6ᵗʰ **H81.8X**   Other disorders of vestibular function

H81.8X1   Other disorders of vestibular function, right ear

H81.8X2   Other disorders of vestibular function, left ear

H81.8X3   Other disorders of vestibular function, bilateral

H81.8X9   Other disorders of vestibular function, unspecified ear ▽

✓5ᵗʰ **H81.9**   Unspecified disorder of vestibular function
     Vertiginous syndrome NOS

H81.90   Unspecified disorder of vestibular function, unspecified ear ▽

H81.91   Unspecified disorder of vestibular function, right ear ▽

H81.92   Unspecified disorder of vestibular function, left ear ▽

H81.93   Unspecified disorder of vestibular function, bilateral ▽

✓4ᵗʰ **H82**   **Vertiginous syndromes in diseases classified elsewhere**
     Code first underlying disease
     EXCLUDES 1   epidemic vertigo (A88.1)

H82.1   *Vertiginous syndromes in diseases classified elsewhere, right ear*

H82.2   *Vertiginous syndromes in diseases classified elsewhere, left ear*

H82.3   *Vertiginous syndromes in diseases classified elsewhere, bilateral*

H82.9   *Vertiginous syndromes in diseases classified elsewhere, unspecified ear* ▽

✓4ᵗʰ **H83**   **Other diseases of inner ear**

✓5ᵗʰ **H83.0**   Labyrinthitis
     DEF: Inflammation of the inner ear, or labyrinth; characterized by pus, vertigo, dizziness, nausea, and hearing loss.

H83.01   Labyrinthitis, right ear

H83.02   Labyrinthitis, left ear

H83.03   Labyrinthitis, bilateral

H83.09   Labyrinthitis, unspecified ear ▽

✓5ᵗʰ **H83.1**   Labyrinthine fistula

H83.11   Labyrinthine fistula, right ear

H83.12   Labyrinthine fistula, left ear

H83.13   Labyrinthine fistula, bilateral

H83.19   Labyrinthine fistula, unspecified ear ▽

✓5ᵗʰ **H83.2**   Labyrinthine dysfunction
     Labyrinthine hypersensitivity
     Labyrinthine hypofunction
     Labyrinthine loss of function
     DEF: Decreased function of the labyrinth sensors.

✓6ᵗʰ **H83.2X**   Labyrinthine dysfunction

H83.2X1   Labyrinthine dysfunction, right ear

H83.2X2   Labyrinthine dysfunction, left ear

H83.2X3   Labyrinthine dysfunction, bilateral

H83.2X9   Labyrinthine dysfunction, unspecified ear ▽

✓5ᵗʰ **H83.3**   Noise effects on inner ear
     Acoustic trauma of inner ear
     Noise-induced hearing loss of inner ear

✓6ᵗʰ **H83.3X**   Noise effects on inner ear

H83.3X1   Noise effects on right inner ear

H83.3X2   Noise effects on left inner ear

H83.3X3   Noise effects on inner ear, bilateral

H83.3X9   Noise effects on inner ear, unspecified ear ▽

✓5ᵗʰ **H83.8**   Other specified diseases of inner ear

✓6ᵗʰ **H83.8X**   Other specified diseases of inner ear

H83.8X1   Other specified diseases of right inner ear

H83.8X2   Other specified diseases of left inner ear

H83.8X3   Other specified diseases of inner ear, bilateral

H83.8X9   Other specified diseases of inner ear, unspecified ear ▽

✓ Additional Character Req   ✓ₓ7ᵗʰ Placeholder Alert   Case-Mix Diagnosis   Manifestation   ▽ Unspecified Dx   EXCLUDES 1 Not coded here   EXCLUDES 2 Not included here

✓5th **H83.9 Unspecified disease of inner ear**
     H83.90   Unspecified disease of inner ear, unspecified ear ▽
     H83.91   Unspecified disease of right inner ear ▽
     H83.92   Unspecified disease of left inner ear ▽
     H83.93   Unspecified disease of inner ear, bilateral ▽

Other disorders of ear (H90-H94)

✓4th **H90 Conductive and sensorineural hearing loss**
     EXCLUDES 1   *deaf nonspeaking NEC (H91.3)*
           deafness NOS (H91.9-)
           hearing loss NOS (H91.9-)
           noise-induced hearing loss (H83.3-)
           ototoxic hearing loss (H91.0-)
           sudden (idiopathic) hearing loss (H91.2-)
    AHA: 2015, 2Q, 7

    H90.0 Conductive hearing loss, bilateral

✓5th **H90.1 Conductive hearing loss, unilateral with unrestricted hearing on the contralateral side**
     H90.11   Conductive hearing loss, unilateral, right ear, with unrestricted hearing on the contralateral side
     H90.12   Conductive hearing loss, unilateral, left ear, with unrestricted hearing on the contralateral side

    H90.2 Conductive hearing loss, unspecified ▽
       Conductive deafness NOS

    H90.3 Sensorineural hearing loss, bilateral

✓5th **H90.4 Sensorineural hearing loss, unilateral with unrestricted hearing on the contralateral side**
     H90.41   Sensorineural hearing loss, unilateral, right ear, with unrestricted hearing on the contralateral side
     H90.42   Sensorineural hearing loss, unilateral, left ear, with unrestricted hearing on the contralateral side

    H90.5 Unspecified sensorineural hearing loss ▽
       Central hearing loss NOS
       Congenital deafness NOS
       Neural hearing loss NOS
       Perceptive hearing loss NOS
       Sensorineural deafness NOS
       Sensory hearing loss NOS
       EXCLUDES 1   *abnormal auditory perception (H93.2-)*
               psychogenic deafness (F44.6)

    H90.6 Mixed conductive and sensorineural hearing loss, bilateral
       AHA: 2015, 2Q, 7

✓5th **H90.7 Mixed conductive and sensorineural hearing loss, unilateral with unrestricted hearing on the contralateral side**
     H90.71   Mixed conductive and sensorineural hearing loss, unilateral, right ear, with unrestricted hearing on the contralateral side
     H90.72   Mixed conductive and sensorineural hearing loss, unilateral, left ear, with unrestricted hearing on the contralateral side

    H90.8 Mixed conductive and sensorineural hearing loss, unspecified ▽

✓5th **H90.A Conductive and sensorineural hearing loss with restricted hearing on the contralateral side**
    ✓6th **H90.A1 Conductive hearing loss, unilateral, with restricted hearing on the contralateral side**
       H90.A11   Conductive hearing loss, unilateral, right ear with restricted hearing on the contralateral side
       H90.A12   Conductive hearing loss, unilateral, left ear with restricted hearing on the contralateral side
    ✓6th **H90.A2 Sensorineural hearing loss, unilateral, with restricted hearing on the contralateral side**
       H90.A21   Sensorineural hearing loss, unilateral, right ear, with restricted hearing on the contralateral side
       H90.A22   Sensorineural hearing loss, unilateral, left ear, with restricted hearing on the contralateral side
    ✓6th **H90.A3 Mixed conductive and sensorineural hearing loss, unilateral with restricted hearing on the contralateral side**
       H90.A31   Mixed conductive and sensorineural hearing loss, unilateral, right ear with restricted hearing on the contralateral side

       H90.A32   Mixed conductive and sensorineural hearing loss, unilateral, left ear with restricted hearing on the contralateral side

✓4th **H91 Other and unspecified hearing loss**
     EXCLUDES 1   *abnormal auditory perception (H93.2-)*
              hearing loss as classified in H90-
              impacted cerumen (H61.2-)
              noise-induced hearing loss (H83.3-)
              psychogenic deafness (F44.6)
              transient ischemic deafness (H93.01-)

✓5th **H91.0 Ototoxic hearing loss**
       Code first poisoning due to drug or toxin, if applicable (T36-T65 with fifth or sixth character 1-4 or 6)
       Use additional code for adverse effect, if applicable, to identify drug (T36-T50 with fifth or sixth character 5)
     H91.01   Ototoxic hearing loss, right ear
     H91.02   Ototoxic hearing loss, left ear
     H91.03   Ototoxic hearing loss, bilateral
     H91.09   Ototoxic hearing loss, unspecified ear ▽

✓5th **H91.1 Presbycusis**
       Presbyacusia
     H91.10   Presbycusis, unspecified ear ▽
     H91.11   Presbycusis, right ear
     H91.12   Presbycusis, left ear
     H91.13   Presbycusis, bilateral

✓5th **H91.2 Sudden idiopathic hearing loss**
       Sudden hearing loss NOS
     H91.20   Sudden idiopathic hearing loss, unspecified ear ▽
     H91.21   Sudden idiopathic hearing loss, right ear
     H91.22   Sudden idiopathic hearing loss, left ear
     H91.23   Sudden idiopathic hearing loss, bilateral

    H91.3 Deaf nonspeaking, not elsewhere classified

✓5th **H91.8 Other specified hearing loss**
    ✓6th **H91.8X Other specified hearing loss**
       H91.8X1   Other specified hearing loss, right ear
       H91.8X2   Other specified hearing loss, left ear
       H91.8X3   Other specified hearing loss, bilateral
       H91.8X9   Other specified hearing loss, unspecified ear ▽

✓5th **H91.9 Unspecified hearing loss**
       Deafness NOS
       High frequency deafness
       Low frequency deafness
     H91.90   Unspecified hearing loss, unspecified ear ▽
     H91.91   Unspecified hearing loss, right ear ▽
     H91.92   Unspecified hearing loss, left ear ▽
     H91.93   Unspecified hearing loss, bilateral ▽

✓4th **H92 Otalgia and effusion of ear**
✓5th **H92.0 Otalgia**
     H92.01   Otalgia, right ear
     H92.02   Otalgia, left ear
     H92.03   Otalgia, bilateral
     H92.09   Otalgia, unspecified ear ▽

✓5th **H92.1 Otorrhea**
       EXCLUDES 1   *leakage of cerebrospinal fluid through ear (G96.0)*
     H92.10   Otorrhea, unspecified ear ▽
     H92.11   Otorrhea, right ear
     H92.12   Otorrhea, left ear
     H92.13   Otorrhea, bilateral

✓5th **H92.2 Otorrhagia**
       EXCLUDES 1   *traumatic otorrhagia—code to injury*
     H92.20   Otorrhagia, unspecified ear ▽
     H92.21   Otorrhagia, right ear
     H92.22   Otorrhagia, left ear
     H92.23   Otorrhagia, bilateral

✓4th **H93 Other disorders of ear, not elsewhere classified**
✓5th **H93.0 Degenerative and vascular disorders of ear**
       EXCLUDES 1   *presbycusis (H91.1)*
    ✓6th **H93.01 Transient ischemic deafness**
       H93.011   Transient ischemic deafness, right ear
       H93.012   Transient ischemic deafness, left ear

N Newborn: 0   P Pediatric: 0-17   M Maternity: 12-55   A Adult: 15-124   NRS Nonroutine supply Dx   NC Dx Noncancer Dx   PDx Primary Dx   ►◄ Revised Text   ● New Code   ▲ Revised Title

614   ICD-10-CM 2018

H93.013 Transient ischemic deafness, bilateral

H93.019 Transient ischemic deafness, ▽
          unspecified ear

✓6ᵗʰ H93.09 Unspecified degenerative and vascular disorders of
          ear

H93.091 Unspecified degenerative and ▽
          vascular disorders of right ear

H93.092 Unspecified degenerative and ▽
          vascular disorders of left ear

H93.093 Unspecified degenerative and ▽
          vascular disorders of ear, bilateral

H93.099 Unspecified degenerative and ▽
          vascular disorders of unspecified ear

✓5ᵗʰ H93.1 Tinnitus

H93.11 Tinnitus, right ear

H93.12 Tinnitus, left ear

H93.13 Tinnitus, bilateral

H93.19 Tinnitus, unspecified ear ▽

✓5ᵗʰ H93.A Pulsatile Tinnitus

H93.A1 Pulsatile tinnitus, right ear

H93.A2 Pulsatile tinnitus, left ear

H93.A3 Pulsatile tinnitus, bilateral

H93.A9 Pulsatile tinnitus, unspecified ear ▽

✓5ᵗʰ H93.2 Other abnormal auditory perceptions
          EXCLUDES 2 auditory hallucinations (R44.0)

✓6ᵗʰ H93.21 Auditory recruitment

H93.211 Auditory recruitment, right ear

H93.212 Auditory recruitment, left ear

H93.213 Auditory recruitment, bilateral

H93.219 Auditory recruitment, unspecified ear ▽

✓6ᵗʰ H93.22 Diplacusis

H93.221 Diplacusis, right ear

H93.222 Diplacusis, left ear

H93.223 Diplacusis, bilateral

H93.229 Diplacusis, unspecified ear ▽

✓6ᵗʰ H93.23 Hyperacusis
          DEF: Exceptionally acute sense of hearing caused by
          such conditions as Bell's palsy; this term may also refer
          to painful sensitivity to sounds.

H93.231 Hyperacusis, right ear

H93.232 Hyperacusis, left ear

H93.233 Hyperacusis, bilateral

H93.239 Hyperacusis, unspecified ear ▽

✓6ᵗʰ H93.24 Temporary auditory threshold shift

H93.241 Temporary auditory threshold shift, right
          ear

H93.242 Temporary auditory threshold shift, left
          ear

H93.243 Temporary auditory threshold shift,
          bilateral

H93.249 Temporary auditory threshold shift, ▽
          unspecified ear

H93.25 Central auditory processing disorder
          Congenital auditory imperception
          Word deafness
          EXCLUDES 1 mixed receptive-expressive language
                     disorder (F80.2)

✓6ᵗʰ H93.29 Other abnormal auditory perceptions

H93.291 Other abnormal auditory perceptions,
          right ear

H93.292 Other abnormal auditory perceptions,
          left ear

H93.293 Other abnormal auditory perceptions,
          bilateral

H93.299 Other abnormal auditory perceptions, ▽
          unspecified ear

✓5ᵗʰ H93.3 Disorders of acoustic nerve
          Disorder of 8th cranial nerve
          EXCLUDES 1 acoustic neuroma (D33.3)
                     syphilitic acoustic neuritis (A52.15)

✓6ᵗʰ H93.3X Disorders of acoustic nerve

H93.3X1 Disorders of right acoustic nerve

H93.3X2 Disorders of left acoustic nerve

H93.3X3 Disorders of bilateral acoustic nerves

H93.3X9 Disorders of unspecified acoustic nerve ▽

✓5ᵗʰ H93.8 Other specified disorders of ear

✓6ᵗʰ H93.8X Other specified disorders of ear

H93.8X1 Other specified disorders of right ear

H93.8X2 Other specified disorders of left ear

H93.8X3 Other specified disorders of ear, bilateral

H93.8X9 Other specified disorders of ear, ▽
          unspecified ear

✓5ᵗʰ H93.9 Unspecified disorder of ear

H93.90 Unspecified disorder of ear, unspecified ear ▽

H93.91 Unspecified disorder of right ear ▽

H93.92 Unspecified disorder of left ear ▽

H93.93 Unspecified disorder of ear, bilateral ▽

✓4ᵗʰ H94 Other disorders of ear in diseases classified elsewhere

✓5ᵗʰ H94.0 Acoustic neuritis in infectious and parasitic diseases classified
          elsewhere
          Code first underlying disease, such as:
          parasitic disease (B65-B89)
          EXCLUDES 1 acoustic neuritis (in):
                     herpes zoster (B02.29)
                     syphilis (A52.15)

H94.00 Acoustic neuritis in infectious and parasitic ▽
          diseases classified elsewhere, unspecified ear

H94.01 Acoustic neuritis in infectious and parasitic
          diseases classified elsewhere, right ear

H94.02 Acoustic neuritis in infectious and parasitic
          diseases classified elsewhere, left ear

H94.03 Acoustic neuritis in infectious and parasitic
          diseases classified elsewhere, bilateral

✓5ᵗʰ H94.8 Other specified disorders of ear in diseases classified
          elsewhere
          Code first underlying disease, such as:
          congenital syphilis (A50.0)
          EXCLUDES 1 aural myiasis (B87.4)
                     syphilitic labyrinthitis (A52.79)

H94.80 Other specified disorders of ear in diseases ▽
          classified elsewhere, unspecified ear

H94.81 Other specified disorders of right ear in
          diseases classified elsewhere

H94.82 Other specified disorders of left ear in
          diseases classified elsewhere

H94.83 Other specified disorders of ear in diseases
          classified elsewhere, bilateral

Intraoperative and postprocedural complications and disorders of ear and mastoid process, not elsewhere classified (H95)

✓4ᵗʰ H95 Intraoperative and postprocedural complications and disorders
          of ear and mastoid process, not elsewhere classified

✓5ᵗʰ H95.0 Recurrent cholesteatoma of postmastoidectomy cavity

H95.00 Recurrent cholesteatoma of postmastoidectomy ▽
          cavity, unspecified ear

H95.01 Recurrent cholesteatoma of postmastoidectomy
          cavity, right ear

H95.02 Recurrent cholesteatoma of postmastoidectomy
          cavity, left ear

H95.03 Recurrent cholesteatoma of postmastoidectomy
          cavity, bilateral ears

✓5ᵗʰ H95.1 Other disorders of ear and mastoid process following
          mastoidectomy

✓6ᵗʰ H95.11 Chronic inflammation of postmastoidectomy cavity

H95.111 Chronic inflammation of
          postmastoidectomy cavity, right ear

H95.112 Chronic inflammation of
          postmastoidectomy cavity, left ear

H95.113 Chronic inflammation of
          postmastoidectomy cavity, bilateral ears

H95.119 Chronic inflammation of ▽
          postmastoidectomy cavity,
          unspecified ear

✓6ᵗʰ H95.12 Granulation of postmastoidectomy cavity

H95.121 Granulation of postmastoidectomy cavity,
          right ear

H95.122 Granulation of postmastoidectomy cavity,
          left ear

H95.123 Granulation of postmastoidectomy cavity,
          bilateral ears

✓ Additional Character Req   ✓x7ᵗʰ Placeholder Alert   Case-Mix Diagnosis   Manifestation   ▽ Unspecified Dx   EXCLUDES 1 Not coded here   EXCLUDES 2 Not included here

ICD-10-CM 2018

615

H93.013–H95.123

      H95.129   **Granulation of postmastoidectomy cavity, unspecified ear**   ▽

✓6th   **H95.13**   **Mucosal cyst of postmastoidectomy cavity**

      H95.131   **Mucosal cyst of postmastoidectomy cavity, right ear**

      H95.132   **Mucosal cyst of postmastoidectomy cavity, left ear**

      H95.133   **Mucosal cyst of postmastoidectomy cavity, bilateral ears**

      H95.139   **Mucosal cyst of postmastoidectomy cavity, unspecified ear**   ▽

✓6th   **H95.19**   **Other disorders following mastoidectomy**

      H95.191   **Other disorders following mastoidectomy, right ear**

      H95.192   **Other disorders following mastoidectomy, left ear**

      H95.193   **Other disorders following mastoidectomy, bilateral ears**

      H95.199   **Other disorders following mastoidectomy, unspecified ear**   ▽

✓5th   **H95.2**   **Intraoperative hemorrhage and hematoma of ear and mastoid process complicating a procedure**

      EXCLUDES 1   *intraoperative hemorrhage and hematoma of ear and mastoid process due to accidental puncture or laceration during a procedure (H95.3-)*

      H95.21   **Intraoperative hemorrhage and hematoma of ear and mastoid process complicating a procedure on the ear and mastoid process**

      H95.22   **Intraoperative hemorrhage and hematoma of ear and mastoid process complicating other procedure**

✓5th   **H95.3**   **Accidental puncture and laceration of ear and mastoid process during a procedure**

      H95.31   **Accidental puncture and laceration of the ear and mastoid process during a procedure on the ear and mastoid process**

      H95.32   **Accidental puncture and laceration of the ear and mastoid process during other procedure**

✓5th   **H95.4**   **Postprocedural hemorrhage of ear and mastoid process following a procedure**

      H95.41   **Postprocedural hemorrhage of ear and mastoid process following a procedure on the ear and mastoid process**

      H95.42   **Postprocedural hemorrhage of ear and mastoid process following other procedure**

✓5th   **H95.5**   **Postprocedural hematoma and seroma of ear and mastoid process following a procedure**

      H95.51   **Postprocedural hematoma of ear and mastoid process following a procedure on the ear and mastoid process**

      H95.52   **Postprocedural hematoma of ear and mastoid process following other procedure**

      H95.53   **Postprocedural seroma of ear and mastoid process following a procedure on the ear and mastoid process**

      H95.54   **Postprocedural seroma of ear and mastoid process following other procedure**

✓5th   **H95.8**   **Other intraoperative and postprocedural complications and disorders of the ear and mastoid process, not elsewhere classified**

      EXCLUDES 2   *postprocedural complications and disorders following mastoidectomy (H95.Ø-, H95.1-)*

✓6th   **H95.81**   **Postprocedural stenosis of external ear canal**

      H95.811   **Postprocedural stenosis of right external ear canal**

      H95.812   **Postprocedural stenosis of left external ear canal**

      H95.813   **Postprocedural stenosis of external ear canal, bilateral**

      H95.819   **Postprocedural stenosis of unspecified external ear canal**   ▽

      H95.88   **Other intraoperative complications and disorders of the ear and mastoid process, not elsewhere classified**

        Use additional code, if applicable, to further specify disorder

      H95.89   **Other postprocedural complications and disorders of the ear and mastoid process, not elsewhere classified**

        Use additional code, if applicable, to further specify disorder

Ⓝ Newborn: 0   Ⓟ Pediatric: 0-17   Ⓜ Maternity: 12-55   Ⓐ Adult: 15-124   **NRS** Nonroutine supply Dx   **NCDx** Noncancer Dx   **PDx** Primary Dx   ▶◀ Revised Text   ● New Code   ▲ Revised Title

616   ICD-10-CM 2018

Chapter 9. Diseases of the Circulatory System (I00–I99)

Chapter Specific Guidelines with Coding Examples

The chapter specific guidelines from the ICD-10-CM Official Guidelines for Coding and Reporting have been provided below. Along with these guidelines are coding examples, contained in the shaded boxes, that have been developed to help illustrate the coding and/or sequencing guidance found in these guidelines.

a. Hypertension

The classification presumes a causal relationship between hypertension and heart involvement and between hypertension and kidney involvement, as the two conditions are linked by the term "with" in the Alphabetic Index. These conditions should be coded as related even in the absence of provider documentation explicitly linking them, unless the documentation clearly states the conditions are unrelated.

For hypertension and conditions not specifically linked by relational terms such as "with," "associated with" or "due to" in the classification, provider documentation must link the conditions in order to code them as related.

1) Hypertension with heart disease

Hypertension with heart conditions classified to I50.- or I51.4-I51.9, are assigned to a code from category I11, Hypertensive heart disease. Use additional code(s) from category I50, Heart failure, to identify the type(s) of heart failure in those patients with heart failure.

The same heart conditions (I50.-, I51.4-I51.9) with hypertension are coded separately if the provider has specifically documented a different cause. Sequence according to the circumstances of the admission/encounter.

> Hypertensive heart disease with left heart failure
>
> | | |
> |---|---|
> | **I11.0** | **Hypertensive heart disease with heart failure** |
> | **I50.1** | **Left ventricular failure, unspecified** |
>
> *Explanation*: A causal relationship between hypertension and heart disease must be stated or implied to report codes from category I11 Hypertensive heart disease. Use an additional code to identify type of heart failure (I50.-).

2) Hypertensive chronic kidney disease

Assign codes from category I12, Hypertensive chronic kidney disease, when both hypertension and a condition classifiable to category N18, Chronic kidney disease (CKD), are present. CKD should not be coded as hypertensive if the physician has specifically documented a different cause.

The appropriate code from category N18 should be used as a secondary code with a code from category I12 to identify the stage of chronic kidney disease.

See Section I.C.14. Chronic kidney disease.

If a patient has hypertensive chronic kidney disease and acute renal failure, an additional code for the acute renal failure is required.

> Patient is admitted with stage IV chronic kidney disease (CKD). The physician has also documented hypertension for this patient.
>
> | | |
> |---|---|
> | **I12.9** | **Hypertensive chronic kidney disease with stage 1 through stage 4 chronic kidney disease, or unspecified chronic kidney disease** |
> | **N18.4** | **Chronic kidney disease, stage 4 (severe)** |
>
> *Explanation*: A causal relationship between hypertension and chronic kidney disease (CKD) is assumed unless otherwise documented. Use an additional code to identify the stage of chronic kidney disease.

3) Hypertensive heart and chronic kidney disease

Assign codes from combination category I13, Hypertensive heart and chronic kidney disease, when there is hypertension with both heart and kidney involvement. If heart failure is present, assign an additional code from category I50 to identify the type of heart failure.

The appropriate code from category N18, Chronic kidney disease, should be used as a secondary code with a code from category I13 to identify the stage of chronic kidney disease.

See Section I.C.14. Chronic kidney disease.

The codes in category I13, Hypertensive heart and chronic kidney disease, are combination codes that include hypertension, heart disease and chronic kidney disease. The Includes note at I13 specifies that the conditions included at I11 and I12 are included together in I13. If a patient has hypertension, heart disease and chronic kidney disease then a code

from I13 should be used, not individual codes for hypertension, heart disease and chronic kidney disease, or codes from I11 or I12.

For patients with both acute renal failure and chronic kidney disease an additional code for acute renal failure is required.

> Hypertensive heart and kidney disease with congestive heart failure and stage 2 chronic kidney disease.
>
> | | |
> |---|---|
> | **I13.0** | **Hypertensive heart and chronic kidney disease with heart failure and stage 1 through stage 4 chronic kidney disease, or unspecified chronic kidney disease** |
> | **I50.9** | **Heart failure, unspecified** |
> | **N18.2** | **Chronic kidney disease, stage 2 (mild)** |
>
> *Explanation*: Combination codes in category I13 are used to report conditions classifiable to *both* categories I11 and I12. Do not report conditions classifiable to I11 and I12 separately. Use additional codes to report type of heart failure and stage of CKD.

4) Hypertensive cerebrovascular disease

For hypertensive cerebrovascular disease, first assign the appropriate code from categories I60-I69, followed by the appropriate hypertension code.

5) Hypertensive retinopathy

Subcategory H35.0, Background retinopathy and retinal vascular changes, should be used with a code from category I10 – I15, Hypertensive disease to include the systemic hypertension. The sequencing is based on the reason for the encounter.

> Hypertensive retinopathy of the right eye.
>
> | | |
> |---|---|
> | **H35.031** | **Hypertensive retinopathy, right eye** |
> | **I10** | **Essential (primary) hypertension** |
>
> *Explanation*: Hypertensive retinopathy requires two codes: the appropriate subcategory H35.0 code and a code for the hypertension.

6) Hypertension, secondary

Secondary hypertension is due to an underlying condition. Two codes are required: one to identify the underlying etiology and one from category I15 to identify the hypertension. Sequencing of codes is determined by the reason for admission/encounter.

> Renovascular hypertension due to renal artery atherosclerosis.
>
> | | |
> |---|---|
> | **I15.0** | **Renovascular hypertension** |
> | **I70.1** | **Atherosclerosis of renal artery** |
>
> *Explanation*: Secondary hypertension requires two codes: a code to identify the etiology and the appropriate I15 code.

7) Hypertension, transient

Assign code R03.0, Elevated blood pressure reading without diagnosis of hypertension, unless patient has an established diagnosis of hypertension. Assign code O13.-, Gestational [pregnancy-induced] hypertension without significant proteinuria, or O14.-, Pre-eclampsia, for transient hypertension of pregnancy.

8) Hypertension, controlled

This diagnostic statement usually refers to an existing state of hypertension under control by therapy. Assign the appropriate code from categories I10-I15, Hypertensive diseases.

9) Hypertension, uncontrolled

Uncontrolled hypertension may refer to untreated hypertension or hypertension not responding to current therapeutic regimen. In either case, assign the appropriate code from categories I10-I15, Hypertensive diseases.

10) Hypertensive crisis

Assign a code from category I16, Hypertensive crisis, for documented hypertensive urgency, hypertensive emergency or unspecified hypertensive crisis. Code also any identified hypertensive disease (I10-I15). The sequencing is based on the reason for the encounter.

10) Pulmonary hypertension

Pulmonary hypertension is classified to category I27, Other pulmonary heart diseases. For secondary pulmonary hypertension (I27.1, I27.2-), code also any associated conditions or adverse effects of drugs or toxins. The sequencing is based on the reason for the encounter.

b. Atherosclerotic coronary artery disease and angina

ICD-10-CM has combination codes for atherosclerotic heart disease with angina pectoris. The subcategories for these codes are I25.11, Atherosclerotic heart disease of native coronary artery with angina pectoris and I25.7, Atherosclerosis of coronary artery bypass graft(s) and coronary artery of transplanted heart with angina pectoris.

When using one of these combination codes it is not necessary to use an additional code for angina pectoris. A causal relationship can be assumed in a patient with both atherosclerosis and angina pectoris, unless the documentation indicates the angina is due to something other than the atherosclerosis.

If a patient with coronary artery disease is admitted due to an acute myocardial infarction (AMI), the AMI should be sequenced before the coronary artery disease.

See Section I.C.9. Acute myocardial infarction (AMI)

Patient is being seen for spastic angina pectoris. She also has a documented history of progressive coronary artery disease of the native vessels.

I25.111   Atherosclerotic heart disease of native coronary artery with angina pectoris with documented spasm

Explanation: Report the combination code for atherosclerotic heart disease (coronary artery disease) with angina pectoris. A causal relationship is assumed in a patient with both atherosclerosis and angina pectoris, unless the documentation indicates the angina is due to something other than the atherosclerosis. When using one of these combination codes, it is not necessary to use an additional code for angina pectoris.

c. Intraoperative and postprocedural cerebrovascular accident

Medical record documentation should clearly specify the cause- and- effect relationship between the medical intervention and the cerebrovascular accident in order to assign a code for intraoperative or postprocedural cerebrovascular accident.

Proper code assignment depends on whether it was an infarction or hemorrhage and whether it occurred intraoperatively or postoperatively. If it was a cerebral hemorrhage, code assignment depends on the type of procedure performed.

d. Sequelae of cerebrovascular disease

1) Category I69, Sequelae of cerebrovascular disease

Category I69 is used to indicate conditions classifiable to categories I60-I67 as the causes of sequela (neurologic deficits), themselves classified elsewhere. These "late effects" include neurologic deficits that persist after initial onset of conditions classifiable to categories I60-I67. The neurologic deficits caused by cerebrovascular disease may be present from the onset or may arise at any time after the onset of the condition classifiable to categories I60-I67.

Patient admitted for skilled services following hospital stay for stroke due to thrombosis of posterior cerebral artery. Provider documentation indicates residual memory deficit.

I69.311   Memory deficit following cerebral infarction

I69.392   Facial weakness following cerebral infarction

Explanation: In the post-acute care setting, the residual sequelae of an acute cerebral vascular accident are the focus of care for the encounter. The residual deficits may not be present from the onset and may occur at any time following the initial stroke. All deficits should be coded when documented as related to the cerebrovascular disease, regardless of when they develop. If it is unclear if a condition may be sequelae of cerebrovascular disease, the provider should be queried as to the relationship between the conditions.

Codes from category I69, Sequelae of cerebrovascular disease, that specify hemiplegia, hemiparesis and monoplegia identify whether the dominant or nondominant side is affected. Should the affected side be documented, but not specified as dominant or nondominant, and the classification system does not indicate a default, code selection is as follows:

- For ambidextrous patients, the default should be dominant.
- If the left side is affected, the default is non-dominant.
- If the right side is affected, the default is dominant.

2) Codes from category I69 with codes from I60–I67

Codes from category I69 may be assigned on a health care record with codes from I60-I67, if the patient has a current cerebrovascular disease and deficits from an old cerebrovascular disease.

3) Codes from category I69 and personal history of transient ischemic attack (TIA) and cerebral infarction (Z86.73)

Codes from category I69 should not be assigned if the patient does not have neurologic deficits.

See Section I.C.21. 4. History (of) for use of personal history codes

An 86-year-old female patient was hospitalized due to transient ischemic attack. The patient is now being discharged with orders for home health for skilled nursing and physical therapy. Provider notes also report hypertension and stage III CKD.

I12.9   Hypertensive chronic kidney disease with stage 1 through stage 4 chronic kidney disease, or unspecified chronic kidney disease

N18.3   Chronic kidney disease, stage 3 (moderate)

Z86.73   Personal history of transient ischemic attack (TIA), and cerebral infarction without residual deficits

Explanation: A transient ischemic attack is an event in which blood flow to the brain is blocked temporarily and then restored. Acute symptoms may mimic those of a stroke but, by definition, are transient and therefore resolve quickly and completely. Because no residual deficits are present, code Z86.73 should be assigned to indicate a history of TIA.

e. Acute myocardial infarction (AMI)

1) Type 1 ST elevation myocardial infarction (STEMI) and non-ST elevation myocardial infarction (NSTEMI)

The ICD-10-CM codes for **type 1** acute myocardial infarction (AMI) identify the site, such as anterolateral wall or true posterior wall. Subcategories I21.0-I21.2 and code I21.3 are used for **type 1** ST elevation myocardial infarction (STEMI). Code I21.4, Non-ST elevation (NSTEMI) myocardial infarction, is used for **type 1** non ST elevation myocardial infarction (NSTEMI) and nontransmural MIs.

If **a type 1** NSTEMI evolves to STEMI, assign the STEMI code. If **a type 1** STEMI converts to NSTEMI due to thrombolytic therapy, it is still coded as STEMI.

For encounters occurring while the myocardial infarction is equal to, or less than, four weeks old, including transfers to another acute setting or a postacute setting, and the myocardial infarction meets the definition for "other diagnoses" (see Section III, Reporting Additional Diagnoses), codes from category I21 may continue to be reported. For encounters after the 4 week time frame and the patient is still receiving care related to the myocardial infarction, the appropriate aftercare code should be assigned, rather than a code from category I21. For old or healed myocardial infarctions not requiring further care, code I25.2, Old myocardial infarction, may be assigned.

2) Acute myocardial infarction, unspecified

Code **I21.9, Acute myocardial infarction, unspecified,** is the default for unspecified acute myocardial infarction **or unspecified type**. If only **type 1** STEMI or transmural MI without the site is documented, assign code I21.3, **ST elevation (STEMI) myocardial infarction of unspecified site**.

3) AMI documented as nontransmural or subendocardial but site provided

If an AMI is documented as nontransmural or subendocardial, but the site is provided, it is still coded as a subendocardial AMI.

See Section I.C.21.3 for information on coding status post administration of tPA in a different facility within the last 24 hours.

Acute inferior subendocardial myocardial infarction (NSTEMI).

I21.4   Non-ST elevation (NSTEMI) myocardial infarction

Explanation: An AMI documented as subendocardial or nontransmural is coded as such (I21.4, I22.2), even if the site of infarction is specified.

4) Subsequent acute myocardial infarction

A code from category I22, Subsequent ST elevation (STEMI) and non-ST elevation (NSTEMI) myocardial infarction, is to be used when a patient who has suffered **a type 1 or unspecified** AMI has a new AMI within the 4 week time frame of the initial AMI. A code from category I22 must be used in conjunction with a code from category I21. The sequencing of the I22 and I21 codes depends on the circumstances of the encounter.

Do not assign code I22 for subsequent myocardial infarctions other than type 1 or unspecified. For subsequent type 2 AMI assign only code I21.A1. For subsequent type 4 or type 5 AMI, assign only code I21.A9.

5) Other types of myocardial infarction

The ICD-10-CM provides codes for different types of myocardial infarction. Type 1 myocardial infarctions are assigned to codes I21.0-I21.4.

Type 2 myocardial infarction, and myocardial infarction due to demand ischemia or secondary to ischemic balance, is assigned to code I21.A1, Myocardial infarction type 2 with a code for the underlying cause. Do not assign code I24.8, Other forms of acute ischemic heart disease for the demand ischemia. Sequencing of type 2 AMI or the underlying cause is dependent on the circumstances of admission. When a type 2 AMI code is described as NSTEMI or STEMI, only assign code I21.A1. Codes I21.01-I21.4 should only be assigned for type 1 AMIs.

Acute myocardial infarctions type 3, 4a, 4b, 4c and 5 are assigned to code I21.A9, Other myocardial infarction type.

The "Code also" and "Code first" notes should be followed related to complications, and for coding of postprocedural myocardial infarctions during or following cardiac surgery.

Chapter 9. Diseases of the Circulatory System (I00-I99)

EXCLUDES 2   certain conditions originating in the perinatal period (P04-P96)
certain infectious and parasitic diseases (A00-B99)
complications of pregnancy, childbirth and the puerperium (O00-O9A)
congenital malformations, deformations, and chromosomal abnormalities (Q00-Q99)
endocrine, nutritional and metabolic diseases (E00-E88)
injury, poisoning and certain other consequences of external causes (S00-T88)
neoplasms (C00-D49)
symptoms, signs and abnormal clinical and laboratory findings, not elsewhere classified (R00-R94)
systemic connective tissue disorders (M30-M36)
transient cerebral ischemic attacks and related syndromes (G45.-)

This chapter contains the following blocks:

I00-I02   Acute rheumatic fever
I05-I09   Chronic rheumatic heart diseases
I10-I16   Hypertensive diseases
I20-I25   Ischemic heart diseases
I26-I28   Pulmonary heart disease and diseases of pulmonary circulation
I30-I52   Other forms of heart disease
I60-I69   Cerebrovascular diseases
I70-I79   Diseases of arteries, arterioles and capillaries
I80-I89   Diseases of veins, lymphatic vessels and lymph nodes, not elsewhere classified
I95-I99   Other and unspecified disorders of the circulatory system

Acute rheumatic fever (I00-I02)

I00   **Rheumatic fever without heart involvement**
    INCLUDES   arthritis, rheumatic, acute or subacute
    EXCLUDES 1   rheumatic fever with heart involvement (I01.0-I01.9)

☑4ᵗʰ **I01**   **Rheumatic fever with heart involvement**
    EXCLUDES 1   chronic diseases of rheumatic origin (I05-I09) unless rheumatic fever is also present or there is evidence of reactivation or activity of the rheumatic process.

    I01.0   **Acute rheumatic pericarditis**
       Any condition in I00 with pericarditis
       Rheumatic pericarditis (acute)
       EXCLUDES 1   acute pericarditis not specified as rheumatic (I30.-)

    I01.1   **Acute rheumatic endocarditis**
       Any condition in I00 with endocarditis or valvulitis
       Acute rheumatic valvulitis

    I01.2   **Acute rheumatic myocarditis**
       Any condition in I00 with myocarditis

    I01.8   **Other acute rheumatic heart disease**
       Any condition in I00 with other or multiple types of heart involvement
       Acute rheumatic pancarditis

    I01.9   **Acute rheumatic heart disease, unspecified**   ▽
       Any condition in I00 with unspecified type of heart involvement
       Rheumatic carditis, acute
       Rheumatic heart disease, active or acute

☑4ᵗʰ **I02**   **Rheumatic chorea**
    INCLUDES   Sydenham's chorea
    EXCLUDES 1   chorea NOS (G25.5)
                  Huntington's chorea (G10)

    I02.0   **Rheumatic chorea with heart involvement**
       Chorea NOS with heart involvement
       Rheumatic chorea with heart involvement of any type classifiable under I01-

    I02.9   **Rheumatic chorea without heart involvement**
       Rheumatic chorea NOS

Chronic rheumatic heart diseases (I05-I09)

☑4ᵗʰ **I05**   **Rheumatic mitral valve diseases**
    INCLUDES   conditions classifiable to both I05.0 and I05.2-I05.9, whether specified as rheumatic or not
    EXCLUDES 1   mitral valve disease specified as nonrheumatic (I34.-)
                  mitral valve disease with aortic and/or tricuspid valve involvement (I08.-)

    I05.0   **Rheumatic mitral stenosis**
       Mitral (valve) obstruction (rheumatic)
       DEF: Narrowing of mitral valve between left atrium and left ventricle; due to rheumatic fever; characterized by shortness of breath during or after exercise, fatigue, palpitations, chest discomfort, and swelling of feet or legs.

    I05.1   **Rheumatic mitral insufficiency**
       Rheumatic mitral incompetence
       Rheumatic mitral regurgitation
       EXCLUDES 1   mitral insufficiency not specified as rheumatic (I34.0)

    I05.2   **Rheumatic mitral stenosis with insufficiency**
       Rheumatic mitral stenosis with incompetence or regurgitation

    I05.8   **Other rheumatic mitral valve diseases**
       Rheumatic mitral (valve) failure

    I05.9   **Rheumatic mitral valve disease, unspecified**   ▽
       Rheumatic mitral (valve) disorder (chronic) NOS

☑4ᵗʰ **I06**   **Rheumatic aortic valve diseases**
    EXCLUDES 1   aortic valve disease not specified as rheumatic (I35.-)
                  aortic valve disease with mitral and/or tricuspid valve involvement (I08.-)

    I06.0   **Rheumatic aortic stenosis**
       Rheumatic aortic (valve) obstruction

    I06.1   **Rheumatic aortic insufficiency**
       Rheumatic aortic incompetence
       Rheumatic aortic regurgitation

    I06.2   **Rheumatic aortic stenosis with insufficiency**
       Rheumatic aortic stenosis with incompetence or regurgitation

    I06.8   **Other rheumatic aortic valve diseases**

    I06.9   **Rheumatic aortic valve disease, unspecified**   ▽
       Rheumatic aortic (valve) disease NOS

☑4ᵗʰ **I07**   **Rheumatic tricuspid valve diseases**
    INCLUDES   rheumatic tricuspid valve diseases specified as rheumatic or unspecified
    EXCLUDES 1   tricuspid valve disease specified as nonrheumatic (I36.-)
                  tricuspid valve disease with aortic and/or mitral valve involvement (I08.-)

    I07.0   **Rheumatic tricuspid stenosis**
       Tricuspid (valve) stenosis (rheumatic)

    I07.1   **Rheumatic tricuspid insufficiency**
       Tricuspid (valve) insufficiency (rheumatic)

    I07.2   **Rheumatic tricuspid stenosis and insufficiency**

    I07.8   **Other rheumatic tricuspid valve diseases**

    I07.9   **Rheumatic tricuspid valve disease, unspecified**   ▽
       Rheumatic tricuspid valve disorder NOS

☑4ᵗʰ **I08**   **Multiple valve diseases**
    INCLUDES   multiple valve diseases specified as rheumatic or unspecified
    EXCLUDES 1   endocarditis, valve unspecified (I38)
                  multiple valve disease specified a nonrheumatic (I34.-, I35.-, I36.-, I37.-, I38.-, Q22.-, Q23.-, Q24.8-)
                  rheumatic valve disease NOS (I09.1)

    I08.0   **Rheumatic disorders of both mitral and aortic valves**
       Involvement of both mitral and aortic valves specified as rheumatic or unspecified

    I08.1   **Rheumatic disorders of both mitral and tricuspid valves**

    I08.2   **Rheumatic disorders of both aortic and tricuspid valves**

    I08.3   **Combined rheumatic disorders of mitral, aortic and tricuspid valves**

    I08.8   **Other rheumatic multiple valve diseases**

    I08.9   **Rheumatic multiple valve disease, unspecified**   ▽

☑4ᵗʰ **I09**   **Other rheumatic heart diseases**

    I09.0   **Rheumatic myocarditis**
       EXCLUDES 1   myocarditis not specified as rheumatic (I51.4)

    I09.1   **Rheumatic diseases of endocardium, valve unspecified**   ▽
       Rheumatic endocarditis (chronic)
       Rheumatic valvulitis (chronic)
       EXCLUDES 1   endocarditis, valve unspecified (I38)

    I09.2   **Chronic rheumatic pericarditis**
       Adherent pericardium, rheumatic
       Chronic rheumatic mediastinopericarditis
       Chronic rheumatic myopericarditis
       EXCLUDES 1   chronic pericarditis not specified as rheumatic (I31.-)

☑5ᵗʰ   **I09.8**   **Other specified rheumatic heart diseases**

       I09.81   **Rheumatic heart failure**   NC Dx
          Use additional code to identify type of heart failure (I50.-)
          DEF: Decreased cardiac output, edema, and hypertension; due to rheumatic heart disease.

       I09.89   **Other specified rheumatic heart diseases**
          Rheumatic disease of pulmonary valve

    I09.9   **Rheumatic heart disease, unspecified**   ▽
       Rheumatic carditis
       EXCLUDES 1   rheumatoid carditis (M05.31)

Ⓝ Newborn: 0   Ⓟ Pediatric: 0-17   Ⓜ Maternity: 12-55   Ⓐ Adult: 15-124   **NRS** Nonroutine supply Dx   **NC Dx** Noncancer Dx   **PDx** Primary Dx   ▶◀ Revised Text   ● New Code   ▲ Revised Title

620   ICD-10-CM 2018

Hypertensive diseases (I10-I16)

Use additional code to identify:
  exposure to environmental tobacco smoke (Z77.22)
  history of tobacco dependence (Z87.891)
  occupational exposure to environmental tobacco smoke (Z57.31)
  tobacco dependence (F17.-)
  tobacco use (Z72.0)

EXCLUDES 1   *neonatal hypertension (P29.2)*
     primary pulmonary hypertension (I27.0)
EXCLUDES 2   *hypertensive disease complicating pregnancy, childbirth and the*
     puerperium (O10-O11, O13-O16)

I10   **Essential (primary) hypertension**
    INCLUDES high blood pressure
            hypertension (arterial) (benign) (essential) (malignant)
              (primary) (systemic)
    EXCLUDES 1 *hypertensive disease complicating pregnancy, childbirth and*
            the puerperium (O10-O11, O13-O16)
    EXCLUDES 2 *essential (primary) hypertension involving vessels of brain*
            (I60-I69)
            essential (primary) hypertension involving vessels of eye
            (H35.0-)
    AHA: 2016, 4Q, 27

✓4th I11   **Hypertensive heart disease**
    INCLUDES ▶any condition in I50.-, I51.4-I51.9 due to hypertension◀

    I11.0   **Hypertensive heart disease with heart failure**   NC Dx
        Hypertensive heart failure
        Use additional code to identify type of heart failure (I50.-)
        AHA: 2017, 1Q, 47

    I11.9   **Hypertensive heart disease without heart failure**   ▽
        Hypertensive heart disease NOS

✓4th I12   **Hypertensive chronic kidney disease**
    INCLUDES any condition in N18 and N26- due to hypertension
            arteriosclerosis of kidney
            arteriosclerotic nephritis (chronic) (interstitial)
            hypertensive nephropathy
            nephrosclerosis
    EXCLUDES 1 *hypertension due to kidney disease (I15.0, I15.1)*
            renovascular hypertension (I15.0)
            secondary hypertension (I15.-)
    EXCLUDES 2 *acute kidney failure (N17.-)*
    AHA: 2016, 3Q, 22
    TIP: Do not assign codes I12–I13 to report hypertension when provider
    documentation indicates CKD attributable to another cause.

    I12.0   **Hypertensive chronic kidney disease with stage 5**   NC Dx
        chronic kidney disease or end stage renal disease
        Use additional code to identify the stage of chronic kidney
        disease (N18.5, N18.6)

    I12.9   **Hypertensive chronic kidney disease with stage 1**   ▽
        through stage 4 chronic kidney disease, or unspecified
        chronic kidney disease
        Hypertensive chronic kidney disease NOS
        Hypertensive renal disease NOS
        Use additional code to identify the stage of chronic kidney
        disease (N18.1-N18.4, N18.9)

✓4th I13   **Hypertensive heart and chronic kidney disease**
    INCLUDES any condition in I11.- with any condition in I12.-
            cardiorenal disease
            cardiovascular renal disease
    TIP: Do not assign codes I12–I13 to report hypertension when provider
    documentation indicates CKD attributable to another cause.

    I13.0   **Hypertensive heart and chronic kidney disease with**   NC Dx
        heart failure and stage 1 through stage 4 chronic kidney
        disease, or unspecified chronic kidney disease
        Use additional code to identify type of heart failure (I50.-)
        Use additional code to identify stage of chronic kidney disease
        (N18.1-N18.4, N18.9)

    ✓5th I13.1   **Hypertensive heart and chronic kidney disease without heart**
      failure

        I13.10   **Hypertensive heart and chronic kidney disease**   ▽
            without heart failure, with stage 1 through
            stage 4 chronic kidney disease, or unspecified
            chronic kidney disease
            Hypertensive heart disease and hypertensive chronic
            kidney disease NOS
            Use additional code to identify the stage of chronic
            kidney disease (N18.1-N18.4, N18.9)

        I13.11   **Hypertensive heart and chronic kidney disease**   NC Dx
            without heart failure, with stage 5 chronic
            kidney disease, or end stage renal disease
            Use additional code to identify the stage of chronic
            kidney disease (N18.5, N18.6)

    I13.2   **Hypertensive heart and chronic kidney disease with**   NC Dx
        heart failure and with stage 5 chronic kidney disease,
        or end stage renal disease
        Use additional code to identify type of heart failure (I50.-)
        Use additional code to identify the stage of chronic kidney
        disease (N18.5, N18.6)

✓4th I15   **Secondary hypertension**
    Code also underlying condition
    EXCLUDES 1 *postprocedural hypertension (I97.3)*
    EXCLUDES 2 *secondary hypertension involving vessels of brain (I60-I69)*
            secondary hypertension involving vessels of eye (H35.0-)

    I15.0   **Renovascular hypertension**

    I15.1   **Hypertension secondary to other renal disorders**
        AHA: 2016, 3Q, 22

    I15.2   **Hypertension secondary to endocrine disorders**

    I15.8   **Other secondary hypertension**

    I15.9   **Secondary hypertension, unspecified**   ▽

✓4th I16   **Hypertensive crisis**
    Code also any identified hypertensive disease (I10-I15)
    AHA: 2016, 4Q, 27

    I16.0   **Hypertensive urgency**

    I16.1   **Hypertensive emergency**

    I16.9   **Hypertensive crisis, unspecified**   ▽

Ischemic heart diseases (I20-I25)

Use additional code to identify presence of hypertension (I10-I16)

✓4th I20   **Angina pectoris**
    Use additional code to identify:
      exposure to environmental tobacco smoke (Z77.22)
      history of tobacco dependence (Z87.891)
      occupational exposure to environmental tobacco smoke (Z57.31)
      tobacco dependence (F17.-)
      tobacco use (Z72.0)
    EXCLUDES 1 *angina pectoris with atherosclerotic heart disease of native*
            coronary arteries (I25.1-)
            atherosclerosis of coronary artery bypass graft(s) and coronary
            artery of transplanted heart with angina pectoris (I25.7-)
            postinfarction angina (I23.7)

    I20.0   **Unstable angina**
        Accelerated angina
        Crescendo angina
        De novo effort angina
        Intermediate coronary syndrome
        Preinfarction syndrome
        Worsening effort angina
        DEF: A condition representing an intermediate stage between
        angina of effort and acute myocardial infarction.

    I20.1   **Angina pectoris with documented spasm**
        Angiospastic angina
        Prinzmetal angina
        Spasm-induced angina
        Variant angina

    I20.8   **Other forms of angina pectoris**
        Angina equivalent
        Angina of effort
        Coronary slow flow syndrome
        Stable angina
        Stenocardia
        Use additional code(s) for symptoms associated with angina
        equivalent

    I20.9   **Angina pectoris, unspecified**   ▽
        Angina NOS
        Anginal syndrome
        Cardiac angina
        Ischemic chest pain

✓ Additional Character Req   ✓x7th Placeholder Alert   Case-Mix Diagnosis   Manifestation   ▽ Unspecified Dx   **EXCLUDES 1** Not coded here   **EXCLUDES 2** Not included here

ICD-10-CM 2018   **621**

I10–I20.9

Chapter 9. Diseases of the Circulatory System

▲ ✓4ᵗʰ **I21 Acute myocardial infarction**

INCLUDES   cardiac infarction
coronary (artery) embolism
coronary (artery) occlusion
coronary (artery) rupture
coronary (artery) thrombosis
infarction of heart, myocardium, or ventricle
myocardial infarction specified as acute or with a stated
     duration of 4 weeks (28 days) or less from onset

Use additional code, if applicable, to identify:
exposure to environmental tobacco smoke (Z77.22)
history of tobacco dependence (Z87.891)
occupational exposure to environmental tobacco smoke (Z57.31)
status post administration of tPA (rtPA) in a different facility within
     the last 24 hours prior to admission to current facility (Z92.82)
tobacco dependence (F17.-)
tobacco use (Z72.0)

EXCLUDES 2   old myocardial infarction (I25.2)
postmyocardial infarction syndrome (I24.1)
▶subsequent type 1 myocardial infarction◀ (I22.-)

AHA: 2017, 1Q, 44-45; 2016, 4Q, 140; 2015, 2Q, 16; 2013, 1Q, 25; 2012, 4Q, 96, 102-103

✓5ᵗʰ **I21.0 ST elevation (STEMI) myocardial infarction of anterior wall**
▶Type 1 ST elevation myocardial infarction of anterior wall◀

   I21.01 ST elevation (STEMI) myocardial infarction involving left main coronary artery

   I21.02 ST elevation (STEMI) myocardial infarction involving left anterior descending coronary artery
ST elevation (STEMI) myocardial infarction involving diagonal coronary artery
AHA: 2013, 1Q, 25

   I21.09 ST elevation (STEMI) myocardial infarction involving other coronary artery of anterior wall
Acute transmural myocardial infarction of anterior wall
Anteroapical transmural (Q wave) infarction (acute)
Anterolateral transmural (Q wave) infarction (acute)
Anteroseptal transmural (Q wave) infarction (acute)
Transmural (Q wave) infarction (acute) (of) anterior (wall) NOS
AHA: 2012, 4Q, 102-103

✓5ᵗʰ **I21.1 ST elevation (STEMI) myocardial infarction of inferior wall**
▶Type 1 ST elevation myocardial infarction of inferior wall◀

   I21.11 ST elevation (STEMI) myocardial infarction involving right coronary artery
Inferoposterior transmural (Q wave) infarction (acute)

   I21.19 ST elevation (STEMI) myocardial infarction involving other coronary artery of inferior wall
Acute transmural myocardial infarction of inferior wall
Inferolateral transmural (Q wave) infarction (acute)
Transmural (Q wave) infarction (acute) (of) diaphragmatic wall
Transmural (Q wave) infarction (acute) (of) inferior (wall) NOS
EXCLUDES 2   ST elevation (STEMI) myocardial infarction involving left circumflex coronary artery (I21.21)
AHA: 2012, 4Q, 96

✓5ᵗʰ **I21.2 ST elevation (STEMI) myocardial infarction of other sites**
▶Type 1 ST elevation myocardial infarction of other sites◀

   I21.21 ST elevation (STEMI) myocardial infarction involving left circumflex coronary artery
ST elevation (STEMI) myocardial infarction involving oblique marginal coronary artery

   I21.29 ST elevation (STEMI) myocardial infarction involving other sites
Acute transmural myocardial infarction of other sites
Apical-lateral transmural (Q wave) infarction (acute)
Basal-lateral transmural (Q wave) infarction (acute)
High lateral transmural (Q wave) infarction (acute)
Lateral (wall) NOS transmural (Q wave) infarction (acute)
Posterior (true) transmural (Q wave) infarction (acute)
Posterobasal transmural (Q wave) infarction (acute)
Posterolateral transmural (Q wave) infarction (acute)
Posteroseptal transmural (Q wave) infarction (acute)
Septal transmural (Q wave) infarction (acute) NOS

I21.3 ST elevation (STEMI) myocardial infarction of unspecified site   ▽
Acute transmural myocardial infarction of unspecified site
~~Myocardial infarction (acute) NOS~~
Transmural (Q wave) myocardial infarction NOS
▶Type 1 ST elevation myocardial infarction of unspecified site◀

I21.4 Non-ST elevation (NSTEMI) myocardial infarction
Acute subendocardial myocardial infarction
Non-Q wave myocardial infarction NOS
Nontransmural myocardial infarction NOS
▶Type 1 non-ST elevation myocardial infarction◀
AHA: 2017, 1Q, 44-45

● **I21.9 Acute myocardial infarction, unspecified**   ▽
Myocardial infarction (acute) NOS

● ✓5ᵗʰ **I21.A Other type of myocardial infarction**

●   **I21.A1 Myocardial infarction type 2**
Myocardial infarction due to demand ischemia
Myocardial infarction secondary to ischemic imbalance
Code also the underlying cause, if known and applicable, such as:
anemia (D50.0-D64.9)
chronic obstructive pulmonary disease (J44.-)
heart failure (I50.-)
paroxysmal tachycardia (I47.0-I47.9)
renal failure (N17.0-N19)
shock (R57.0-R57.9)

●   **I21.A9 Other myocardial infarction type**
Myocardial infarction associated with revascularization procedure
Myocardial infarction type 3
Myocardial infarction type 4a
Myocardial infarction type 4b
Myocardial infarction type 4c
Myocardial infarction type 5
Code first, if applicable, postprocedural myocardial infarction following cardiac surgery (I97.190), or postprocedural myocardial infarction during cardiac surgery (I97.790)
Code also complication, if known and applicable, such as:
(acute) stent occlusion (T82.897-)
(acute) stent stenosis (T82.857-)
(acute) stent thrombosis (T82.867-)
cardiac arrest due to underlying cardiac condition (I46.2)
complication of percutaneous coronary intervention (PCI) (I97.89)
occlusion of coronary artery bypass graft (T82.218-)

✓4ᵗʰ **I22 Subsequent ST elevation (STEMI) and non-ST elevation (NSTEMI) myocardial infarction**

INCLUDES   acute myocardial infarction occurring within four weeks (28 days) of a previous acute myocardial infarction, regardless of site
cardiac infarction
coronary (artery) embolism
coronary (artery) occlusion
coronary (artery) rupture
coronary (artery) thrombosis
infarction of heart, myocardium, or ventricle
recurrent myocardial infarction
reinfarction of myocardium
rupture of heart, myocardium, or ventricle
▶subsequent type 1 myocardial infarction◀

Use additional code, if applicable, to identify:
exposure to environmental tobacco smoke (Z77.22)
history of tobacco dependence (Z87.891)
occupational exposure to environmental tobacco smoke (Z57.31)
status post administration of tPA (rtPA) in a different facility within
     the last 24 hours prior to admission to current facility (Z92.82)
tobacco dependence (F17.-)
tobacco use (Z72.0)

EXCLUDES 1 ▶subsequent myocardial infarction, type 2 (I21.A1)
subsequent myocardial infarction of other type (type 3) (type 4) (type 5) (I21.A9)◀

AHA: 2017, 2Q, 11; 2013, 1Q, 25; 2012, 4Q, 97, 102-103

I22.0 Subsequent ST elevation (STEMI) myocardial infarction of anterior wall
Subsequent acute transmural myocardial infarction of anterior wall
Subsequent transmural (Q wave) infarction (acute)(of) anterior (wall) NOS
Subsequent anteroapical transmural (Q wave) infarction (acute)
Subsequent anterolateral transmural (Q wave) infarction (acute)
Subsequent anteroseptal transmural (Q wave) infarction (acute)

N Newborn: 0   P Pediatric: 0-17   M Maternity: 12-55   A Adult: 15-124   NRS Nonroutine supply Dx   NC Dx Noncancer Dx   PDx Primary Dx   ▶◀ Revised Text   ● New Code   ▲ Revised Title

622   ICD-10-CM 2018

Chapter 9. Diseases of the Circulatory System

I22.1 **Subsequent ST elevation (STEMI) myocardial infarction of inferior wall**
Subsequent acute transmural myocardial infarction of inferior wall
Subsequent transmural (Q wave) infarction (acute)(of) diaphragmatic wall
Subsequent transmural (Q wave) infarction (acute)(of) inferior (wall) NOS
Subsequent inferolateral transmural (Q wave) infarction (acute)
Subsequent inferoposterior transmural (Q wave) infarction (acute)
AHA: 2012, 4Q, 102

I22.2 **Subsequent non-ST elevation (NSTEMI) myocardial infarction**
Subsequent acute subendocardial myocardial infarction
Subsequent non-Q wave myocardial infarction NOS
Subsequent nontransmural myocardial infarction NOS

I22.8 **Subsequent ST elevation (STEMI) myocardial infarction of other sites**
Subsequent acute transmural myocardial infarction of other sites
Subsequent apical-lateral transmural (Q wave) myocardial infarction (acute)
Subsequent basal-lateral transmural (Q wave) myocardial infarction (acute)
Subsequent high lateral transmural (Q wave) myocardial infarction (acute)
Subsequent transmural (Q wave) myocardial infarction (acute)(of) lateral (wall) NOS
Subsequent posterior (true)transmural (Q wave) myocardial infarction (acute)
Subsequent posterobasal transmural (Q wave) myocardial infarction (acute)
Subsequent posterolateral transmural (Q wave) myocardial infarction (acute)
Subsequent posteroseptal transmural (Q wave) myocardial infarction (acute)
Subsequent septal NOS transmural (Q wave) myocardial infarction (acute)

I22.9 **Subsequent ST elevation (STEMI) myocardial infarction of unspecified site** ▽
Subsequent acute myocardial infarction of unspecified site
Subsequent myocardial infarction (acute) NOS

✓4ᵗʰ **I23** **Certain current complications following ST elevation (STEMI) and non-ST elevation (NSTEMI) myocardial infarction (within the 28 day period)**
AHA: 2017, 2Q, 11

I23.0 **Hemopericardium as current complication following acute myocardial infarction** 🅰
EXCLUDES 1 *hemopericardium not specified as current complication following acute myocardial infarction (I31.2)*

I23.1 **Atrial septal defect as current complication following acute myocardial infarction** 🅰
EXCLUDES 1 *acquired atrial septal defect not specified as current complication following acute myocardial infarction (I51.0)*

I23.2 **Ventricular septal defect as current complication following acute myocardial infarction** 🅰
EXCLUDES 1 *acquired ventricular septal defect not specified as current complication following acute myocardial infarction (I51.0)*

I23.3 **Rupture of cardiac wall without hemopericardium as current complication following acute myocardial infarction** 🅰

I23.4 **Rupture of chordae tendineae as current complication following acute myocardial infarction**
EXCLUDES 1 *rupture of chordae tendineae not specified as current complication following acute myocardial infarction (I51.1)*

I23.5 **Rupture of papillary muscle as current complication following acute myocardial infarction**
EXCLUDES 1 *rupture of papillary muscle not specified as current complication following acute myocardial infarction (I51.2)*

I23.6 **Thrombosis of atrium, auricular appendage, and ventricle as current complications following acute myocardial infarction** 🅰
EXCLUDES 1 *thrombosis of atrium, auricular appendage, and ventricle not specified as current complication following acute myocardial infarction (I51.3)*

I23.7 **Postinfarction angina** 🅰
AHA: 2015, 2Q, 16

I23.8 **Other current complications following acute myocardial infarction** 🅰

✓4ᵗʰ **I24** **Other acute ischemic heart diseases**
EXCLUDES 1 *angina pectoris (I20.-)*
       transient myocardial ischemia in newborn (P29.4)

I24.0 **Acute coronary thrombosis not resulting in myocardial infarction**
Acute coronary (artery) (vein) embolism not resulting in myocardial infarction
Acute coronary (artery) (vein) occlusion not resulting in myocardial infarction
Acute coronary (artery) (vein) thromboembolism not resulting in myocardial infarction
EXCLUDES 1 *atherosclerotic heart disease (I25.1-)*
AHA: 2013, 1Q, 24

I24.1 **Dressler's syndrome**
Postmyocardial infarction syndrome
EXCLUDES 1 *postinfarction angina (I23.7)*

I24.8 **Other forms of acute ischemic heart disease**
EXCLUDES 1 ▶*myocardial infarction due to demand ischemia (I21.A1)*◀

I24.9 **Acute ischemic heart disease, unspecified** ▽
EXCLUDES 1 *ischemic heart disease (chronic) NOS (I25.9)*

✓4ᵗʰ **I25** **Chronic ischemic heart disease**
Use additional code to identify:
chronic total occlusion of coronary artery (I25.82)
exposure to environmental tobacco smoke (Z77.22)
history of tobacco dependence (Z87.891)
occupational exposure to environmental tobacco smoke (Z57.31)
tobacco dependence (F17.-)
tobacco use (Z72.0)

✓5ᵗʰ **I25.1** **Atherosclerotic heart disease of native coronary artery**
Atherosclerotic cardiovascular disease
Coronary (artery) atheroma
Coronary (artery) atherosclerosis
Coronary (artery) disease
Coronary (artery) sclerosis
Use additional code, if applicable, to identify:
coronary atherosclerosis due to calcified coronary lesion (I25.84)
coronary atherosclerosis due to lipid rich plaque (I25.83)
EXCLUDES 2 *atheroembolism (I75.-)*
     atherosclerosis of coronary artery bypass graft(s) and transplanted heart (I25.7-)

I25.10 **Atherosclerotic heart disease of native coronary artery without angina pectoris** 🅰▽
Atherosclerotic heart disease NOS
AHA: 2015, 2Q, 16; 2012, 4Q, 92

✓6ᵗʰ **I25.11** **Atherosclerotic heart disease of native coronary artery with angina pectoris**

I25.110 **Atherosclerotic heart disease of native coronary artery with unstable angina pectoris** 🅰
EXCLUDES 1 *unstable angina without atherosclerotic heart disease (I20.0)*

I25.111 **Atherosclerotic heart disease of native coronary artery with angina pectoris with documented spasm** 🅰
EXCLUDES 1 *angina pectoris with documented spasm without atherosclerotic heart disease (I20.1)*

Atheromas

Atheromas (fatty tissue and/or plaque)   Lumen

☑ Additional Character Req   ✓ₓ7ᵗʰ Placeholder Alert   Case-Mix Diagnosis   Manifestation   ▽ Unspecified Dx   *EXCLUDES 1* Not coded here   *EXCLUDES 2* Not included here

I25.118 Atherosclerotic heart disease of native coronary artery with other forms of angina pectoris A
> EXCLUDES 1 other forms of angina pectoris without atherosclerotic heart disease (I20.8
> **AHA:** 2015, 2Q, 16

I25.119 Atherosclerotic heart disease of native coronary artery with unspecified angina pectoris A ▽
Atherosclerotic heart disease with angina NOS
Atherosclerotic heart disease with ischemic chest pain
> EXCLUDES 1 unspecified angina pectoris without atherosclerotic heart disease (I20.9)

I25.2 Old myocardial infarction
Healed myocardial infarction
Past myocardial infarction diagnosed by ECG or other investigation, but currently presenting no symptoms

I25.3 Aneurysm of heart NC Dx
Mural aneurysm
Ventricular aneurysm

✓5ᵗʰ **I25.4 Coronary artery aneurysm and dissection**
I25.41 Coronary artery aneurysm NC Dx
Coronary arteriovenous fistula, acquired
> EXCLUDES 1 congenital coronary (artery) aneurysm (Q24.5)

I25.42 Coronary artery dissection NC Dx
DEF: A tear in the intimal arterial wall of a coronary artery resulting in the sudden intrusion of blood within the layers of the wall.

I25.5 Ischemic cardiomyopathy NC Dx
> EXCLUDES 2 coronary atherosclerosis (I25.1-, I25.7-)

I25.6 Silent myocardial ischemia NC Dx

✓5ᵗʰ **I25.7 Atherosclerosis of coronary artery bypass graft(s) and coronary artery of transplanted heart with angina pectoris**
Use additional code, if applicable, to identify:
coronary atherosclerosis due to calcified coronary lesion (I25.84)
coronary atherosclerosis due to lipid rich plaque (I25.83)
> EXCLUDES 1 atherosclerosis of bypass graft(s) of transplanted heart without angina pectoris (I25.812)
> atherosclerosis of coronary artery bypass graft(s) without angina pectoris (I25.810)
> atherosclerosis of native coronary artery of transplanted heart without angina pectoris (I25.811)
> ~~embolism or thrombus of coronary artery bypass graft(s) (T82.8-)~~

✓6ᵗʰ **I25.70 Atherosclerosis of coronary artery bypass graft(s), unspecified, with angina pectoris**
I25.700 Atherosclerosis of coronary artery bypass graft(s), unspecified, with unstable angina pectoris A ▽
> EXCLUDES 1 unstable angina pectoris without atherosclerosis of coronary artery bypass graft (I20.0)

I25.701 Atherosclerosis of coronary artery bypass graft(s), unspecified, with angina pectoris with documented spasm A ▽
> EXCLUDES 1 angina pectoris with documented spasm without atherosclerosis of coronary artery bypass graft (I20.1)

I25.708 Atherosclerosis of coronary artery bypass graft(s), unspecified, with other forms of angina pectoris A ▽
> EXCLUDES 1 other forms of angina pectoris without atherosclerosis of coronary artery bypass graft (I20.8)

I25.709 Atherosclerosis of coronary artery bypass graft(s), unspecified, with unspecified angina pectoris A ▽
> EXCLUDES 1 unspecified angina pectoris without atherosclerosis of coronary artery bypass graft (I20.9)

✓6ᵗʰ **I25.71 Atherosclerosis of autologous vein coronary artery bypass graft(s) with angina pectoris**
I25.710 Atherosclerosis of autologous vein coronary artery bypass graft(s) with unstable angina pectoris A
> EXCLUDES 1 unstable angina without atherosclerosis of autologous vein coronary artery bypass graft(s) (I20.0)
> EXCLUDES 2 ▶embolism or thrombus of coronary artery bypass graft(s) (T82.8-)◀

I25.711 Atherosclerosis of autologous vein coronary artery bypass graft(s) with angina pectoris with documented spasm A
> EXCLUDES 1 angina pectoris with documented spasm without atherosclerosis of autologous vein coronary artery bypass graft(s) (I20.1)

I25.718 Atherosclerosis of autologous vein coronary artery bypass graft(s) with other forms of angina pectoris A
> EXCLUDES 1 other forms of angina pectoris without atherosclerosis of autologous vein coronary artery bypass graft(s) (I20.8)

I25.719 Atherosclerosis of autologous vein coronary artery bypass graft(s) with unspecified angina pectoris A ▽
> EXCLUDES 1 unspecified angina pectoris without atherosclerosis of autologous vein coronary artery bypass graft(s) (I20.9)

✓6ᵗʰ **I25.72 Atherosclerosis of autologous artery coronary artery bypass graft(s) with angina pectoris**
Atherosclerosis of internal mammary artery graft with angina pectoris
I25.720 Atherosclerosis of autologous artery coronary artery bypass graft(s) with unstable angina pectoris A
> EXCLUDES 1 unstable angina without atherosclerosis of autologous artery coronary artery bypass graft(s) (I20.0)

I25.721 Atherosclerosis of autologous artery coronary artery bypass graft(s) with angina pectoris with documented spasm A
> EXCLUDES 1 angina pectoris with documented spasm without atherosclerosis of autologous artery coronary artery bypass graft(s) (I20.1)

I25.728 Atherosclerosis of autologous artery coronary artery bypass graft(s) with other forms of angina pectoris A
> EXCLUDES 1 other forms of angina pectoris without atherosclerosis of autologous artery coronary artery bypass graft(s) (I20.8)

I25.729 Atherosclerosis of autologous artery coronary artery bypass graft(s) with unspecified angina pectoris A ▽
> EXCLUDES 1 unspecified angina pectoris without atherosclerosis of autologous artery coronary artery bypass graft(s) (I20.9)

✓6ᵗʰ **I25.73 Atherosclerosis of nonautologous biological coronary artery bypass graft(s) with angina pectoris**
I25.730 Atherosclerosis of nonautologous biological coronary artery bypass graft(s) with unstable angina pectoris A
> EXCLUDES 1 unstable angina without atherosclerosis of nonautologous biological coronary artery bypass graft(s) (I20.0)

I25.731   **Atherosclerosis of nonautologous biological coronary artery bypass graft(s) with angina pectoris with documented spasm**   A
> EXCLUDES 1   *angina pectoris with documented spasm without atherosclerosis of nonautologous biological coronary artery bypass graft(s) (I20.1)*

I25.738   **Atherosclerosis of nonautologous biological coronary artery bypass graft(s) with other forms of angina pectoris**   A
> EXCLUDES 1   *other forms of angina pectoris without atherosclerosis of nonautologous biological coronary artery bypass graft(s) (I20.8)*

I25.739   **Atherosclerosis of nonautologous biological coronary artery bypass graft(s) with unspecified angina pectoris**   A ▽
> EXCLUDES 1   *unspecified angina pectoris without atherosclerosis of nonautologous biological coronary artery bypass graft(s) (I20.9)*

✓6ᵗʰ   **I25.75**   **Atherosclerosis of native coronary artery of transplanted heart with angina pectoris**
> EXCLUDES 1   *atherosclerosis of native coronary artery of transplanted heart without angina pectoris (I25.811)*

I25.750   **Atherosclerosis of native coronary artery of transplanted heart with unstable angina**

I25.751   **Atherosclerosis of native coronary artery of transplanted heart with angina pectoris with documented spasm**

I25.758   **Atherosclerosis of native coronary artery of transplanted heart with other forms of angina pectoris**

I25.759   **Atherosclerosis of native coronary artery of transplanted heart with unspecified angina pectoris**   ▽

✓6ᵗʰ   **I25.76**   **Atherosclerosis of bypass graft of coronary artery of transplanted heart with angina pectoris**
> EXCLUDES 1   *atherosclerosis of bypass graft of coronary artery of transplanted heart without angina pectoris (I25.812)*

I25.760   **Atherosclerosis of bypass graft of coronary artery of transplanted heart with unstable angina**   A

I25.761   **Atherosclerosis of bypass graft of coronary artery of transplanted heart with angina pectoris with documented spasm**   A

I25.768   **Atherosclerosis of bypass graft of coronary artery of transplanted heart with other forms of angina pectoris**   A

I25.769   **Atherosclerosis of bypass graft of coronary artery of transplanted heart with unspecified angina pectoris**   A ▽

✓6ᵗʰ   **I25.79**   **Atherosclerosis of other coronary artery bypass graft(s) with angina pectoris**

I25.790   **Atherosclerosis of other coronary artery bypass graft(s) with unstable angina pectoris**   A
> EXCLUDES 1   *unstable angina without atherosclerosis of other coronary artery bypass graft(s) (I20.0)*

I25.791   **Atherosclerosis of other coronary artery bypass graft(s) with angina pectoris with documented spasm**   A
> EXCLUDES 1   *angina pectoris with documented spasm without atherosclerosis of other coronary artery bypass graft(s) (I20.1)*

I25.798   **Atherosclerosis of other coronary artery bypass graft(s) with other forms of angina pectoris**   A
> EXCLUDES 1   *other forms of angina pectoris without atherosclerosis of other coronary artery bypass graft(s) (I20.8)*

I25.799   **Atherosclerosis of other coronary artery bypass graft(s) with unspecified angina pectoris**   A ▽
> EXCLUDES 1   *unspecified angina pectoris without atherosclerosis of other coronary artery bypass graft(s) (I20.9)*

✓5ᵗʰ   **I25.8**   **Other forms of chronic ischemic heart disease**

✓6ᵗʰ   **I25.81**   **Atherosclerosis of other coronary vessels without angina pectoris**
> Use additional code, if applicable, to identify:
> coronary atherosclerosis due to calcified coronary lesion (I25.84)
> coronary atherosclerosis due to lipid rich plaque (I25.83)
> EXCLUDES 1   *atherosclerotic heart disease of native coronary artery without angina pectoris (I25.10)*

I25.810   **Atherosclerosis of coronary artery bypass graft(s) without angina pectoris**   A
> Atherosclerosis of coronary artery bypass graft NOS
> EXCLUDES 1   *atherosclerosis of coronary bypass graft(s) with angina pectoris (I25.70--I25.73-, I25.79-)*

I25.811   **Atherosclerosis of native coronary artery of transplanted heart without angina pectoris**
> Atherosclerosis of native coronary artery of transplanted heart NOS
> EXCLUDES 1   *atherosclerosis of native coronary artery of transplanted heart with angina pectoris (I25.75-)*

I25.812   **Atherosclerosis of bypass graft of coronary artery of transplanted heart without angina pectoris**   A
> Atherosclerosis of bypass graft of transplanted heart NOS
> EXCLUDES 1   *atherosclerosis of bypass graft of transplanted heart with angina pectoris (I25.76)*

I25.82   **Chronic total occlusion of coronary artery**
> Complete occlusion of coronary artery
> Total occlusion of coronary artery
> Code first coronary atherosclerosis (I25.1-, I25.7-, I25.81-)
> EXCLUDES 1   ▶*acute coronary occlusion with myocardial infarction (I21.0-I21.9, I22.-)*◀
> ▶*acute coronary occlusion without myocardial infarction*◀ *(I24.0)*
> **DEF:** Complete blockage of coronary artery due to plaque accumulation over an extended period of time; results in substantial reduction of blood flow; characterized by angina or chest pain.

I25.83   **Coronary atherosclerosis due to lipid rich plaque**   A
> Code first coronary atherosclerosis (I25.1-, I25.7-, I25.81-)

I25.84   **Coronary atherosclerosis due to calcified coronary lesion**
> Coronary atherosclerosis due to severely calcified coronary lesion
> Code first coronary atherosclerosis (I25.1-, I25.7-, I25.81-)

I25.89   **Other forms of chronic ischemic heart disease**   NC Dx

I25.9   **Chronic ischemic heart disease, unspecified**   NC Dx ▽
> Ischemic heart disease (chronic) NOS

☑ Additional Character Req   ✓x7ᵗʰ Placeholder Alert   Case-Mix Diagnosis   Manifestation   ▽ Unspecified Dx   EXCLUDES 1 Not coded here   EXCLUDES 2 Not included here

ICD-10-CM 2018   625

I25.731–I25.9

Pulmonary heart disease and diseases of pulmonary circulation (I26-I28)

✓4th **I26 Pulmonary embolism**
INCLUDES pulmonary (acute) (artery)(vein) infarction
pulmonary (acute) (artery)(vein) thromboembolism
pulmonary (acute) (artery)(vein) thrombosis
EXCLUDES 2 chronic pulmonary embolism (I27.82)
personal history of pulmonary embolism (Z86.711)
pulmonary embolism due to trauma (T79.0, T79.1)
pulmonary embolism due to complications of surgical and medical care (T80.0, T81.7-, T82.8-)
pulmonary embolism complicating abortion, ectopic or molar pregnancy (O00-O07, O08.2)
pulmonary embolism complicating pregnancy, childbirth and the puerperium (O88.-)
septic (non-pulmonary) arterial embolism (I76)

✓5th **I26.0 Pulmonary embolism with acute cor pulmonale**

I26.01 Septic pulmonary embolism with acute cor pulmonale
Code first underlying infection

I26.02 Saddle embolus of pulmonary artery with acute cor pulmonale NC Dx

I26.09 Other pulmonary embolism with acute cor pulmonale NC Dx
Acute cor pulmonale NOS
AHA: 2014, 4Q, 21

✓5th **I26.9 Pulmonary embolism without acute cor pulmonale**

I26.90 Septic pulmonary embolism without acute cor pulmonale
Code first underlying infection

I26.92 Saddle embolus of pulmonary artery without acute cor pulmonale NC Dx

I26.99 Other pulmonary embolism without acute cor pulmonale NC Dx
Acute pulmonary embolism NOS
Pulmonary embolism NOS

✓4th **I27 Other pulmonary heart diseases**

I27.0 Primary pulmonary hypertension NC Dx
▶Heritable pulmonary arterial hypertension
Idiopathic pulmonary arterial hypertension
Primary group 1 pulmonary hypertension
Primary pulmonary arterial hypertension◀
EXCLUDES 1 ▶persistent pulmonary hypertension of newborn (P29.30)◀
pulmonary hypertension NOS ▶(I27.20)◀
▶secondary pulmonary arterial hypertension (I27.21)◀
secondary pulmonary hypertension ▶(I27.29)◀

I27.1 Kyphoscoliotic heart disease NC Dx

✓5th **I27.2 Other secondary pulmonary hypertension** NC Dx
Pulmonary hypertension NOS
Code also associated underlying condition
EXCLUDES 1 ▶Eisenmenger's syndrome (I27.83)◀
AHA: 2014, 4Q, 21

I27.20 Pulmonary hypertension, unspecified ▽
Pulmonary hypertension NOS

I27.21 Secondary pulmonary arterial hypertension
(Associated) (drug-induced) (toxin-induced) pulmonary arterial hypertension NOS
(Associated) (drug-induced) (toxin-induced) (secondary) group 1 pulmonary hypertension
Code also associated conditions if applicable, or adverse effects of drugs or toxins, such as:
adverse effect of appetite depressants (T50.5X5)
congenital heart disease (Q20-Q28)
human immunodeficiency virus [HIV] disease (B20)
polymyositis (M33.2-)
portal hypertension (K76.6)
rheumatoid arthritis (M05.-)
schistosomiasis (B65.-)
Sjögren syndrome (M35.0-)
systemic sclerosis (M34.-)

I27.22 Pulmonary hypertension due to left heart disease
Group 2 pulmonary hypertension
Code also associated left heart disease, if known, such as:
multiple valve disease (I08.-)
rheumatic mitral valve diseases (I05.-)
rheumatic aortic valve diseases (I06.-)

I27.23 Pulmonary hypertension due to lung diseases and hypoxia
Group 3 pulmonary hypertension
Code also associated lung disease, if known, such as:
bronchiectasis (J47.-)
cystic fibrosis with pulmonary manifestations (E84.0)
interstitial lung disease (J84.-)
pleural effusion (J90)
sleep apnea (G47.3-)

I27.24 Chronic thromboembolic pulmonary hypertension
Group 4 pulmonary hypertension
Code also associated pulmonary embolism, if applicable (I26.-, I27.82)

I27.29 Other secondary pulmonary hypertension
Group 5 pulmonary hypertension
Pulmonary hypertension with unclear multifactorial mechanisms
Pulmonary hypertension due to hematologic disorders
Pulmonary hypertension due to metabolic disorders
Pulmonary hypertension due to other systemic disorders
Code also other associated disorders, if known, such as:
chronic myeloid leukemia (C92.10- C92.22)
essential thrombocythemia (D47.3)
Gaucher disease (E75.22)
hypertensive chronic kidney disease with end stage renal disease (I12.0, I12.11, I13.2)
hyperthyroidism (E05.-)
hypothyroidism (E00-E03)
polycythemia vera (D45)
sarcoidosis (D86.-)
AHA: 2016, 2Q, 8

✓5th **I27.8 Other specified pulmonary heart diseases**

I27.81 Cor pulmonale (chronic) NC Dx
Cor pulmonale NOS
EXCLUDES 1 acute cor pulmonale (I26.0-)
AHA: 2014, 4Q, 21

I27.82 Chronic pulmonary embolism NC Dx
Use additional code, if applicable, for associated long-term (current) use of anticoagulants (Z79.01)
EXCLUDES 1 personal history of pulmonary embolism (Z86.711)
DEF: A long-standing condition commonly associated with pulmonary hypertension in which small blood clots travel to the lungs repeatedly over many weeks, months, or years, requiring continuation of established anticoagulant or thrombolytic therapy.

I27.83 Eisenmenger's syndrome NC Dx
Eisenmenger's complex
(Irreversible) Eisenmenger's disease
Pulmonary hypertension with right to left shunt related to congenital heart disease
Code also underlying heart defect, if known, such as:
atrial septal defect (Q21.1)
Eisenmenger's defect (Q21.8)
patent ductus arteriosus (Q25.0)
ventricular septal defect (Q21.0)

I27.89 Other specified pulmonary heart diseases
Eisenmenger's complex
Eisenmenger's syndrome
EXCLUDES 1 Eisenmenger's defect (Q21.8)

I27.9 Pulmonary heart disease, unspecified NC Dx ▽
Chronic cardiopulmonary disease

✓4th **I28 Other diseases of pulmonary vessels**

I28.0 Arteriovenous fistula of pulmonary vessels NC Dx
EXCLUDES 1 congenital arteriovenous fistula (Q25.72)

I28.1 Aneurysm of pulmonary artery NC Dx
EXCLUDES 1 congenital aneurysm (Q25.79)
congenital arteriovenous aneurysm (Q25.72)

I28.8 Other diseases of pulmonary vessels
Pulmonary arteritis
Pulmonary endarteritis
Rupture of pulmonary vessels
Stenosis of pulmonary vessels
Stricture of pulmonary vessels

I28.9 Disease of pulmonary vessels, unspecified ▽

N Newborn: 0   P Pediatric: 0-17   M Maternity: 12-55   A Adult: 15-124   NRS Nonroutine supply Dx   NC Dx Noncancer Dx   PDx Primary Dx   ▶◀ Revised Text   ● New Code   ▲ Revised Title

626   ICD-10-CM 2018

I26–I28.9

Other forms of heart disease (I30-I52)

☑4ᵗʰ I30 Acute pericarditis

INCLUDES acute mediastinopericarditis
acute myopericarditis
acute pericardial effusion
acute pleuropericarditis
acute pneumopericarditis

EXCLUDES 1 *Dressler's syndrome (I24.1)*
rheumatic pericarditis (acute) (I01.0)
▶*viral pericarditis due to Coxsakie virus (B33.23)*◀

I30.0 Acute nonspecific idiopathic pericarditis

I30.1 Infective pericarditis
Pneumococcal pericarditis
Pneumopyopericardium
Purulent pericarditis
Pyopericarditis
Pyopericardium
Pyopneumopericardium
Staphylococcal pericarditis
Streptococcal pericarditis
Suppurative pericarditis
Viral pericarditis
Use additional code (B95-B97) to identify infectious agent

I30.8 Other forms of acute pericarditis

I30.9 Acute pericarditis, unspecified ▽

☑4ᵗʰ I31 Other diseases of pericardium

EXCLUDES 1 *diseases of pericardium specified as rheumatic (I09.2)*
postcardiotomy syndrome (I97.0)
traumatic injury to pericardium (S26.-)

I31.0 Chronic adhesive pericarditis
Accretio cordis
Adherent pericardium
Adhesive mediastinopericarditis

I31.1 Chronic constrictive pericarditis
Concretio cordis
Pericardial calcification

I31.2 Hemopericardium, not elsewhere classified
EXCLUDES 1 *hemopericardium as current complication following acute myocardial infarction (I23.0)*
DEF: Presence of blood in the pericardial sac (pericardium). It can lead to potentially fatal cardiac tamponade if enough blood enters the pericardial cavity.

I31.3 Pericardial effusion (noninflammatory)
Chylopericardium
EXCLUDES 1 *acute pericardial effusion (I30.9)*

I31.4 Cardiac tamponade
Code first underlying cause

I31.8 Other specified diseases of pericardium
Epicardial plaques
Focal pericardial adhesions

I31.9 Disease of pericardium, unspecified ▽
Pericarditis (chronic) NOS

Cardiac Tamponade

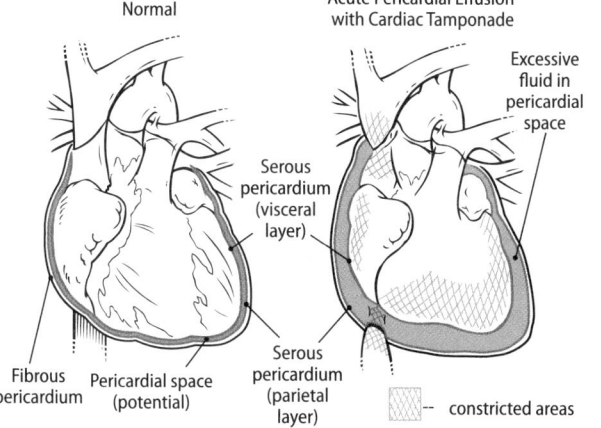

Normal

Acute Pericardial Effusion with Cardiac Tamponade

Excessive fluid in pericardial space

Serous pericardium (visceral layer)

Serous pericardium (parietal layer)

Fibrous pericardium Pericardial space (potential)

▨ -- constricted areas

I32 Pericarditis in diseases classified elsewhere
Code first underlying disease
EXCLUDES 1 *pericarditis (in):*
coxsackie (virus) (B33.23)
gonococcal (A54.83)
meningococcal (A39.53)
rheumatoid (arthritis) (M05.31)
syphilitic (A52.06)
systemic lupus erythematosus (M32.12)
tuberculosis (A18.84)

I33 Acute and subacute endocarditis
EXCLUDES 1 *acute rheumatic endocarditis (I01.1)*
endocarditis NOS (I38)

I33.0 Acute and subacute infective endocarditis
Bacterial endocarditis (acute) (subacute)
Infective endocarditis (acute) (subacute) NOS
Endocarditis lenta (acute) (subacute)
Malignant endocarditis (acute) (subacute)
Purulent endocarditis (acute) (subacute)
Septic endocarditis (acute) (subacute)
Ulcerative endocarditis (acute) (subacute)
Vegetative endocarditis (acute) (subacute)
Use additional code (B95-B97) to identify infectious agent

I33.9 Acute and subacute endocarditis, unspecified ▽
Acute endocarditis NOS
Acute myoendocarditis NOS
Acute periendocarditis NOS
Subacute endocarditis NOS
Subacute myoendocarditis NOS
Subacute periendocarditis NOS

☑4ᵗʰ I34 Nonrheumatic mitral valve disorders
EXCLUDES 1 *mitral valve disease (I05.9)*
mitral valve failure (I05.8)
mitral valve stenosis (I05.0)
mitral valve disorder of unspecified cause with diseases of aortic and/or tricuspid valve(s) (I08.-)
mitral valve disorder of unspecified cause with mitral stenosis or obstruction (I05.0)
mitral valve disorder specified as congenital ▶(Q23.2, Q23.9)◀
mitral valve disorder specified as rheumatic (I05.-)

I34.0 Nonrheumatic mitral (valve) insufficiency
Nonrheumatic mitral (valve) incompetence NOS
Nonrheumatic mitral (valve) regurgitation NOS

I34.1 Nonrheumatic mitral (valve) prolapse
Floppy nonrheumatic mitral valve syndrome
EXCLUDES 1 *Marfan's syndrome (Q87.4-)*

I34.2 Nonrheumatic mitral (valve) stenosis

I34.8 Other nonrheumatic mitral valve disorders

I34.9 Nonrheumatic mitral valve disorder, unspecified ▽

☑4ᵗʰ I35 Nonrheumatic aortic valve disorders
EXCLUDES 1 *aortic valve disorder of unspecified cause but with diseases of mitral and/or tricuspid valve(s) (I08.-)*
aortic valve disorder specified as congenital (Q23.0, Q23.1)
aortic valve disorder specified as rheumatic (I06.-)
hypertrophic subaortic stenosis (I42.1)

I35.0 Nonrheumatic aortic (valve) stenosis

I35.1 Nonrheumatic aortic (valve) insufficiency
Nonrheumatic aortic (valve) incompetence NOS
Nonrheumatic aortic (valve) regurgitation NOS

I35.2 Nonrheumatic aortic (valve) stenosis with insufficiency

I35.8 Other nonrheumatic aortic valve disorders

I35.9 Nonrheumatic aortic valve disorder, unspecified ▽

☑4ᵗʰ I36 Nonrheumatic tricuspid valve disorders
EXCLUDES 1 *tricuspid valve disorders of unspecified cause (I07.-)*
tricuspid valve disorders specified as congenital (Q22.4, Q22.8, Q22.9)
tricuspid valve disorders specified as rheumatic (I07.-)
tricuspid valve disorders with aortic and/or mitral valve involvement (I08.-)

I36.0 Nonrheumatic tricuspid (valve) stenosis

I36.1 Nonrheumatic tricuspid (valve) insufficiency
Nonrheumatic tricuspid (valve) incompetence
Nonrheumatic tricuspid (valve) regurgitation

I36.2 Nonrheumatic tricuspid (valve) stenosis with insufficiency

I36.8 Other nonrheumatic tricuspid valve disorders

I36.9 Nonrheumatic tricuspid valve disorder, unspecified ▽

☑4ᵗʰ I37   Nonrheumatic pulmonary valve disorders
> **EXCLUDES 1**   pulmonary valve disorder specified as congenital (Q22.1, Q22.2, Q22.3)
> pulmonary valve disorder specified as rheumatic (I09.89)

I37.0   Nonrheumatic pulmonary valve stenosis

I37.1   Nonrheumatic pulmonary valve insufficiency
Nonrheumatic pulmonary valve incompetence
Nonrheumatic pulmonary valve regurgitation

I37.2   Nonrheumatic pulmonary valve stenosis with insufficiency

I37.8   Other nonrheumatic pulmonary valve disorders

I37.9   Nonrheumatic pulmonary valve disorder, unspecified ▽

I38   Endocarditis, valve unspecified ▽
> **INCLUDES**   endocarditis (chronic) NOS
> valvular incompetence NOS
> valvular insufficiency NOS
> valvular regurgitation NOS
> valvular stenosis NOS
> valvulitis (chronic) NOS

> **EXCLUDES 1**   congenital insufficiency of cardiac valve NOS (Q24.8)
> congenital stenosis of cardiac valve NOS (Q24.8)
> endocardial fibroelastosis (I42.4)
> endocarditis specified as rheumatic (I09.1)

I39   *Endocarditis and heart valve disorders in diseases classified elsewhere*
> Code first underlying disease, such as:
> Q fever (A78)

> **EXCLUDES 1**   endocardial involvement in:
> candidiasis (B37.6)
> gonococcal infection (A54.83)
> Libman-Sacks disease (M32.11)
> listerosis (A32.82)
> meningococcal infection (A39.51)
> rheumatoid arthritis (M05.31)
> syphilis (A52.03)
> tuberculosis (A18.84)
> typhoid fever (A01.02)

☑4ᵗʰ I40   Acute myocarditis
> **INCLUDES**   subacute myocarditis
> **EXCLUDES 1**   acute rheumatic myocarditis (I01.2)

I40.0   Infective myocarditis
Septic myocarditis
Use additional code (B95-B97) to identify infectious agent

I40.1   Isolated myocarditis
Fiedler's myocarditis
Giant cell myocarditis
Idiopathic myocarditis

I40.8   Other acute myocarditis

I40.9   Acute myocarditis, unspecified ▽

I41   *Myocarditis in diseases classified elsewhere*
> Code first underlying disease, such as:
> typhus (A75.0-A75.9)

> **EXCLUDES 1**   myocarditis (in):
> Chagas' disease (chronic) (B57.2)
> acute (B57.0)
> coxsackie (virus) infection (B33.22)
> diphtheritic (A36.81)
> gonococcal (A54.83)
> influenzal (J09.X9, J10.82, J11.82)
> meningococcal (A39.52)
> mumps (B26.82)
> rheumatoid arthritis (M05.31)
> sarcoid (D86.85)
> syphilis (A52.06)
> toxoplasmosis (B58.81)
> tuberculous (A18.84)

☑4ᵗʰ I42   Cardiomyopathy
> **INCLUDES**   myocardiopathy
> Code first pre-existing cardiomyopathy complicating pregnancy and puerperium (O99.4)
> **EXCLUDES 2**   ischemic cardiomyopathy (I25.5)
> peripartum cardiomyopathy (O90.3)
> ventricular hypertrophy (I51.7)

I42.0   Dilated cardiomyopathy
Congestive cardiomyopathy

I42.1   Obstructive hypertrophic cardiomyopathy
Hypertrophic subaortic stenosis (idiopathic)
DEF: Cardiomyopathy marked by left ventricle hypertrophy, enlarged septum; results in obstructed blood flow, arrhythmias, mitral regurgitation, and sudden cardiac death.

I42.2   Other hypertrophic cardiomyopathy
Nonobstructive hypertrophic cardiomyopathy

I42.3   Endomyocardial (eosinophilic) disease
Endomyocardial (tropical) fibrosis
Löffler's endocarditis

I42.4   Endocardial fibroelastosis
Congenital cardiomyopathy
Elastomyofibrosis

I42.5   Other restrictive cardiomyopathy
Constrictive cardiomyopathy NOS

I42.6   Alcoholic cardiomyopathy
Code also presence of alcoholism (F10.-)

I42.7   Cardiomyopathy due to drug and external agent
Code first poisoning due to drug or toxin, if applicable (T36-T65 with fifth or sixth character 1-4 or 6)
Use additional code for adverse effect, if applicable, to identify drug (T36-T50 with fifth or sixth character 5)

I42.8   Other cardiomyopathies

I42.9   Cardiomyopathy, unspecified ▽
Cardiomyopathy (primary) (secondary) NOS

I43   *Cardiomyopathy in diseases classified elsewhere*
> Code first underlying disease, such as:
> amyloidosis (E85.-)
> glycogen storage disease (E74.0)
> gout (M10.0-)
> thyrotoxicosis (E05.0-E05.9-)

> **EXCLUDES 1**   cardiomyopathy (in):
> coxsackie (virus) (B33.24)
> diphtheria (A36.81)
> sarcoidosis (D86.85)
> tuberculosis (A18.84)

☑4ᵗʰ I44   Atrioventricular and left bundle-branch block

I44.0   Atrioventricular block, first degree

I44.1   Atrioventricular block, second degree
Atrioventricular block, type I and II
Möbitz block, type I and II
Second degree block, type I and II
Wenckebach's block

I44.2   Atrioventricular block, complete
Complete heart block NOS
Third degree block

☑5ᵗʰ I44.3   Other and unspecified atrioventricular block
Atrioventricular block NOS

    I44.30   Unspecified atrioventricular block ▽

    I44.39   Other atrioventricular block

I44.4   Left anterior fascicular block

I44.5   Left posterior fascicular block

☑5ᵗʰ I44.6   Other and unspecified fascicular block

    I44.60   Unspecified fascicular block ▽
Left bundle-branch hemiblock NOS

    I44.69   Other fascicular block

I44.7   Left bundle-branch block, unspecified ▽

☑4ᵗʰ I45   Other conduction disorders

I45.0   Right fascicular block

☑5ᵗʰ I45.1   Other and unspecified right bundle-branch block

    I45.10   Unspecified right bundle-branch block ▽
Right bundle-branch block NOS

    I45.19   Other right bundle-branch block

I45.2   Bifascicular block

I45.3   Trifascicular block

I45.4   Nonspecific intraventricular block
Bundle-branch block NOS

I45.5   Other specified heart block
Sinoatrial block
Sinoauricular block
> **EXCLUDES 1**   heart block NOS (I45.9)

I45.6   Pre-excitation syndrome
Accelerated atrioventricular conduction
Accessory atrioventricular conduction
Anomalous atrioventricular excitation
Lown-Ganong-Levine syndrome
Pre-excitation atrioventricular conduction
Wolff-Parkinson-White syndrome

Conduction Disorders

Sinoatrial node (pacemaker)

Internodal tracts:
Anterior
Middle
Posterior

Bachmann's bundle

Left bundle branch block

Atrioventricular node

Atrioventricular bundle (of His)

Left bundle branch:
Anterior fascicle
Posterior fascicle

Atrioventricular block

Accessory bundle (of Kent)

Left bundle branch hemiblock

Right bundle branch

Right bundle branch block

Moderator band

Purkinje fibers

✓5th **I45.8**   **Other specified conduction disorders**

     I45.81   **Long QT syndrome**
         DEF: Condition characterized by recurrent syncope, malignant arrhythmias, and sudden death; characteristic prolonged Q-T interval on electrocardiogram.

     I45.89   **Other specified conduction disorders**
         Atrioventricular [AV] dissociation
         Interference dissociation
         Isorhythmic dissociation
         Nonparoxysmal AV nodal tachycardia
         AHA: 2013, 2Q, 31

     I45.9   **Conduction disorder, unspecified**   ▽
         Heart block NOS
         Stokes-Adams syndrome

✓4th **I46**   **Cardiac arrest**
     EXCLUDES 1   cardiogenic shock (R57.0)

     I46.2   **Cardiac arrest due to underlying cardiac condition**
         Code first underlying cardiac condition

     I46.8   **Cardiac arrest due to other underlying condition**
         Code first underlying condition

     I46.9   **Cardiac arrest, cause unspecified**   ▽

✓4th **I47**   **Paroxysmal tachycardia**
     Code first tachycardia complicating:
       abortion or ectopic or molar pregnancy (O00-O07, O08.8)
       obstetric surgery and procedures (O75.4)
     EXCLUDES 1   tachycardia NOS (R00.0)
              sinoauricular tachycardia NOS (R00.0)
              sinus [sinusal] tachycardia NOS (R00.0)

     I47.0   **Re-entry ventricular arrhythmia**

     I47.1   **Supraventricular tachycardia**
         Atrial (paroxysmal) tachycardia
         Atrioventricular [AV] (paroxysmal) tachycardia
         Atrioventricular re-entrant (nodal) tachycardia [AVNRT] [AVRT]
         Junctional (paroxysmal) tachycardia
         Nodal (paroxysmal) tachycardia

     I47.2   **Ventricular tachycardia**
         AHA: 2013, 3Q, 23

     I47.9   **Paroxysmal tachycardia, unspecified**   ▽
         Bouveret (-Hoffman) syndrome

✓4th **I48**   **Atrial fibrillation and flutter**

     I48.0   **Paroxysmal atrial fibrillation**

     I48.1   **Persistent atrial fibrillation**

     I48.2   **Chronic atrial fibrillation**
         Permanent atrial fibrillation

     I48.3   **Typical atrial flutter**
         Type I atrial flutter

     I48.4   **Atypical atrial flutter**
         Type II atrial flutter

✓5th   **I48.9**   **Unspecified atrial fibrillation and atrial flutter**
       I48.91   **Unspecified atrial fibrillation**   ▽
       I48.92   **Unspecified atrial flutter**   ▽

✓4th **I49**   **Other cardiac arrhythmias**
     Code first cardiac arrhythmia complicating:
       abortion or ectopic or molar pregnancy (O00-O07, O08.8)
       obstetric surgery and procedures (O75.4)
     EXCLUDES 1   bradycardia NOS (R00.1)
              neonatal dysrhythmia (P29.1-)
              sinoatrial bradycardia (R00.1)
              sinus bradycardia (R00.1)
              vagal bradycardia (R00.1)
     EXCLUDES 2   ▶bradycardia NOS (R00.1)◀

✓5th   **I49.0**   **Ventricular fibrillation and flutter**
       I49.01   **Ventricular fibrillation**
       I49.02   **Ventricular flutter**

     I49.1   **Atrial premature depolarization**
         Atrial premature beats

     I49.2   **Junctional premature depolarization**

     I49.3   **Ventricular premature depolarization**

✓5th   **I49.4**   **Other and unspecified premature depolarization**
       I49.40   **Unspecified premature depolarization**   ▽
           Premature beats NOS
           I49.49

           Other premature depolarization
           Ectopic beats
           Extrasystoles
           Extrasystolic arrhythmias
           Premature contractions

     I49.5   **Sick sinus syndrome**
         Tachycardia-bradycardia syndrome

     I49.8   **Other specified cardiac arrhythmias**
         ▶Brugada syndrome◀
         Coronary sinus rhythm disorder
         Ectopic rhythm disorder
         Nodal rhythm disorder

     I49.9   **Cardiac arrhythmia, unspecified**   ▽
         Arrhythmia (cardiac) NOS

✓4th **I50**   **Heart failure**
     Code first:
       heart failure complicating abortion or ectopic or molar pregnancy (O00-O07, O08.8)
       heart failure following surgery (I97.13-)
       heart failure due to hypertension (I11.0)
       heart failure due to hypertension with chronic kidney disease (I13.-)
       obstetric surgery and procedures (O75.4)
       rheumatic heart failure (I09.81)
     EXCLUDES 1   neonatal cardiac failure (P29.0)
     EXCLUDES 2   cardiac arrest (I46.-)
     AHA: 2017, 1Q, 47; 2014, 1Q, 25; 2013, 2Q, 33

▲   **I50.1**   **Left ventricular failure, unspecified**   NC Dx   ▽
         Cardiac asthma
         Edema of lung with heart disease NOS
         Edema of lung with heart failure
         Left heart failure
         Pulmonary edema with heart disease NOS
         Pulmonary edema with heart failure
       EXCLUDES 1   edema of lung without heart disease or heart failure (J81.-)
               pulmonary edema without heart disease or failure (J81.-)

✓5th   **I50.2**   **Systolic (congestive) heart failure**
       ▶Heart failure with reduced ejection fraction [HFrEF]
       Systolic left ventricular heart failure◀
       ▶Code also end stage heart failure, if applicable (I50.84)◀
       EXCLUDES 1   combined systolic (congestive) and diastolic (congestive) heart failure (I50.4-)
       AHA: 2017, 1Q, 46; 2016, 1Q, 10
       [8]   **I50.20**   **Unspecified systolic (congestive) heart failure**   ▽
       I50.21   **Acute systolic (congestive) heart failure**   NC Dx
       I50.22   **Chronic systolic (congestive) heart failure**   NC Dx
       I50.23   **Acute on chronic systolic (congestive) heart failure**   NC Dx

---

[8]   Hospice questionable admission diagnosis.

✅ Additional Character Req   ✓x7th Placeholder Alert   Case-Mix Diagnosis   Manifestation   ▽ Unspecified Dx   EXCLUDES 1 Not coded here   EXCLUDES 2 Not included here

ICD-10-CM 2018   629

Chapter 9. Diseases of the Circulatory System

I50.3   ✓5th   **Diastolic (congestive) heart failure**
▶Diastolic left ventricular heart failure
Heart failure with normal ejection fraction
Heart failure with preserved ejection fraction [HFpEF]◄
▶Code also end stage heart failure, if applicable (I50.84)◄
EXCLUDES 1   combined systolic (congestive) and diastolic
(congestive) heart failure (I50.4-)
AHA: 2017, 1Q, 46; 2016, 1Q, 10

   8   **I50.30**   Unspecified diastolic (congestive) heart failure   ▽

      I50.31   Acute diastolic (congestive) heart failure   NC Dx

      I50.32   Chronic diastolic (congestive) heart failure   NC Dx

      I50.33   Acute on chronic diastolic (congestive) heart failure   NC Dx

I50.4   ✓5th   **Combined systolic (congestive) and diastolic (congestive) heart failure**
▶Combined systolic and diastolic left ventricular heart failure
Heart failure with reduced ejection fraction and diastolic dysfunction◄
▶Code also end stage heart failure, if applicable (I50.84)◄
AHA: 2017, 1Q, 46; 2016, 1Q, 10

   8   **I50.40**   Unspecified combined systolic (congestive) and diastolic (congestive) heart failure   ▽

      I50.41   Acute combined systolic (congestive) and diastolic (congestive) heart failure   NC Dx

      I50.42   Chronic combined systolic (congestive) and diastolic (congestive) heart failure   NC Dx

      I50.43   Acute on chronic combined systolic (congestive) and diastolic (congestive) heart failure   NC Dx

●   ✓5th   **I50.8**   **Other heart failure**

●   ✓6th   **I50.81**   **Right heart failure**
Right ventricular failure

●   **I50.810**   Right heart failure, unspecified   NC Dx ▽
Right heart failure without mention of left heart failure
Right ventricular failure NOS

●   **I50.811**   Acute right heart failure   NC Dx
Acute isolated right heart failure
Acute (isolated) right ventricular failure

●   **I50.812**   Chronic right heart failure   NC Dx
Chronic isolated right heart failure
Chronic (isolated) right ventricular failure

●   **I50.813**   Acute on chronic right heart failure   NC Dx
Acute on chronic isolated right heart failure
Acute on chronic (isolated) right ventricular failure
Acute decompensation of chronic (isolated) right ventricular failure
Acute exacerbation of chronic (isolated) right ventricular failure

●   **I50.814**   Right heart failure due to left heart failure   NC Dx
Right ventricular failure secondary to left ventricular failure
Code also the type of left ventricular failure, if known (I50.2-I50.43)
EXCLUDES 1   right heart failure with but not due to left heart failure (I50.82)

●   **I50.82**   **Biventricular heart failure**   NC Dx
Code also the type of left ventricular failure as systolic, diastolic, or combined, if known (I50.2-I50.43)

●   **I50.83**   **High output heart failure**   NC Dx

●   **I50.84**   **End stage heart failure**   NC Dx
Stage D heart failure
Code also the type of heart failure as systolic, diastolic, or combined, if known (I50.2-I50.43)

●   **I50.89**   **Other heart failure**

   8   **I50.9**   **Heart failure, unspecified**   ▽
Biventricular (heart) failure NOS
Cardiac, heart or myocardial failure NOS
Congestive heart disease
Congestive heart failure NOS
Right ventricular failure (secondary to left heart failure)
EXCLUDES 2   fluid overload (E87.70)
AHA: 2017, 1Q, 45-46; 2014, 4Q, 21; 2012, 4Q, 92

I51   ✓4th   **Complications and ill-defined descriptions of heart disease**
EXCLUDES 1   any condition in I51.4-I51.9 due to hypertension (I11.-)
any condition in I51.4-I51.9 due to hypertension and chronic kidney disease (I13.-)
heart disease specified as rheumatic (I00-I09)

I51.0   **Cardiac septal defect, acquired**   A
Acquired septal atrial defect (old)
Acquired septal auricular defect (old)
Acquired septal ventricular defect (old)
EXCLUDES 1   cardiac septal defect as current complication following acute myocardial infarction (I23.1, I23.2)
DEF: Abnormal communication between opposite heart chambers due to defect of septum; not present at birth.

I51.1   **Rupture of chordae tendineae, not elsewhere classified**   NC Dx
EXCLUDES 1   rupture of chordae tendineae as current complication following acute myocardial infarction (I23.4)

I51.2   **Rupture of papillary muscle, not elsewhere classified**   NC Dx
EXCLUDES 1   rupture of papillary muscle as current complication following acute myocardial infarction (I23.5)

I51.3   **Intracardiac thrombosis, not elsewhere classified**   NC Dx
Apical thrombosis (old)
Atrial thrombosis (old)
Auricular thrombosis (old)
Mural thrombosis (old)
Ventricular thrombosis (old)
EXCLUDES 1   intracardiac thrombosis as current complication following acute myocardial infarction (I23.6)
AHA: 2013, 1Q, 24

I51.4   **Myocarditis, unspecified**   NC Dx ▽
Chronic (interstitial) myocarditis
Myocardial fibrosis
Myocarditis NOS
EXCLUDES 1   acute or subacute myocarditis (I40.-)

I51.5   **Myocardial degeneration**   NC Dx
Fatty degeneration of heart or myocardium
Myocardial disease
Senile degeneration of heart or myocardium

I51.7   **Cardiomegaly**
Cardiac dilatation
Cardiac hypertrophy
Ventricular dilatation

✓5th   **I51.8**   **Other ill-defined heart diseases**

   I51.81   **Takotsubo syndrome**
Reversible left ventricular dysfunction following sudden emotional stress
Stress induced cardiomyopathy
Takotsubo cardiomyopathy
Transient left ventricular apical ballooning syndrome

   I51.89   **Other ill-defined heart diseases**
Carditis (acute)(chronic)
Pancarditis (acute)(chronic)

I51.9   **Heart disease, unspecified**   ▽

I52   *Other heart disorders in diseases classified elsewhere*
Code first underlying disease, such as:
congenital syphilis (A50.5)
mucopolysaccharidosis (E76.3)
schistosomiasis (B65.0-B65.9)
EXCLUDES 1   heart disease (in):
gonococcal infection (A54.83)
meningococcal infection (A39.50)
rheumatoid arthritis (M05.31)
syphilis (A52.06)

---

8   Hospice questionable admission diagnosis.

N Newborn: 0   P Pediatric: 0-17   M Maternity: 12-55   A Adult: 15-124   NRS Nonroutine supply Dx   NC Dx Noncancer Dx   PDx Primary Dx   ▶◄ Revised Text   ● New Code   ▲ Revised Title

630   ICD-10-CM 2018

Cerebrovascular diseases (I60-I69)

Use additional code to identify presence of:
alcohol abuse and dependence (F10.-)
exposure to environmental tobacco smoke (Z77.22)
history of tobacco dependence (Z87.891)
hypertension (I10-I15)
occupational exposure to environmental tobacco smoke (Z57.31)
tobacco dependence (F17.-)
tobacco use (Z72.0)
> *EXCLUDES 1*   *transient cerebral ischemic attacks and related syndromes (G45.-)*
> *traumatic intracranial hemorrhage (S06.-)*
AHA: 2014, 3Q, 5; 2012, 4Q, 91-92

✓4ᵗʰ **I60**   **Nontraumatic subarachnoid hemorrhage**
> INCLUDES   ruptured cerebral aneurysm
> *EXCLUDES 1*   *syphilitic ruptured cerebral aneurysm (A52.05)*
> *EXCLUDES 2*   *sequelae of subarachnoid hemorrhage (I69.0-)*

   ✓5ᵗʰ **I60.0**   **Nontraumatic subarachnoid hemorrhage from** carotid siphon and bifurcation
     I60.00   **Nontraumatic subarachnoid hemorrhage** `NCDx` ▽ **from unspecified carotid siphon and bifurcation**
     I60.01   **Nontraumatic subarachnoid hemorrhage from** `NCDx` right **carotid siphon and bifurcation**
     I60.02   **Nontraumatic subarachnoid hemorrhage from** `NCDx` left **carotid siphon and bifurcation**

   ✓5ᵗʰ **I60.1**   **Nontraumatic subarachnoid hemorrhage from** middle cerebral artery
     I60.10   **Nontraumatic subarachnoid hemorrhage** `NCDx` ▽ **from unspecified middle cerebral artery**
     I60.11   **Nontraumatic subarachnoid hemorrhage from** `NCDx` right **middle cerebral artery**
     I60.12   **Nontraumatic subarachnoid hemorrhage from** `NCDx` left **middle cerebral artery**

   I60.2   **Nontraumatic subarachnoid hemorrhage from** anterior `NCDx` communicating artery

   ✓5ᵗʰ **I60.3**   **Nontraumatic subarachnoid hemorrhage from** posterior communicating artery
     I60.30   **Nontraumatic subarachnoid hemorrhage** `NCDx` ▽ **from unspecified posterior communicating artery**
     I60.31   **Nontraumatic subarachnoid hemorrhage from** `NCDx` right **posterior communicating artery**
     I60.32   **Nontraumatic subarachnoid hemorrhage from** `NCDx` left **posterior communicating artery**

   I60.4   **Nontraumatic subarachnoid hemorrhage from** basilar `NCDx` artery

   ✓5ᵗʰ **I60.5**   **Nontraumatic subarachnoid hemorrhage from** vertebral artery
     I60.50   **Nontraumatic subarachnoid hemorrhage** `NCDx` ▽ **from unspecified vertebral artery**
     I60.51   **Nontraumatic subarachnoid hemorrhage from** `NCDx` right **vertebral artery**
     I60.52   **Nontraumatic subarachnoid hemorrhage from** `NCDx` left **vertebral artery**

   I60.6   **Nontraumatic subarachnoid hemorrhage from other** `NCDx` intracranial arteries

   I60.7   **Nontraumatic subarachnoid hemorrhage from** `NCDx` ▽ **unspecified intracranial artery**
Ruptured (congenital) berry aneurysm
Ruptured (congenital) cerebral aneurysm
Subarachnoid hemorrhage (nontraumatic) from cerebral artery NOS
Subarachnoid hemorrhage (nontraumatic) from communicating artery NOS
> *EXCLUDES 1*   *berry aneurysm, nonruptured (I67.1)*

   I60.8   **Other nontraumatic subarachnoid hemorrhage** `NCDx`
Meningeal hemorrhage
Rupture of cerebral arteriovenous malformation

   I60.9   **Nontraumatic subarachnoid hemorrhage, unspecified** `NCDx` ▽

✓4ᵗʰ **I61**   **Nontraumatic intracerebral hemorrhage**
> *EXCLUDES 2*   *sequelae of intracerebral hemorrhage (I69.1-)*
AHA: 2017, 2Q, 9-10

   I61.0   **Nontraumatic intracerebral hemorrhage in** hemisphere, `NCDx` subcortical
Deep intracerebral hemorrhage (nontraumatic)

   I61.1   **Nontraumatic intracerebral hemorrhage in** hemisphere, `NCDx` cortical
Cerebral lobe hemorrhage (nontraumatic)
Superficial intracerebral hemorrhage (nontraumatic)

   I61.2   **Nontraumatic intracerebral hemorrhage in** `NCDx` ▽ hemisphere, **unspecified**

   I61.3   **Nontraumatic intracerebral hemorrhage in** brain stem `NCDx`

   I61.4   **Nontraumatic intracerebral hemorrhage in** cerebellum `NCDx`

   I61.5   **Nontraumatic intracerebral hemorrhage,** `NCDx` **intraventricular**

   I61.6   **Nontraumatic intracerebral hemorrhage,** multiple `NCDx` localized

   I61.8   **Other nontraumatic intracerebral hemorrhage** `NCDx`

   I61.9   **Nontraumatic intracerebral hemorrhage, unspecified** `NCDx` ▽

✓4ᵗʰ **I62**   **Other and unspecified nontraumatic intracranial hemorrhage**
> *EXCLUDES 2*   *sequelae of intracranial hemorrhage (I69.2)*

   ✓5ᵗʰ **I62.0**   **Nontraumatic** subdural **hemorrhage**
     I62.00   **Nontraumatic subdural hemorrhage,** `NCDx` ▽ **unspecified**
     I62.01   **Nontraumatic** acute **subdural hemorrhage** `NCDx`
     I62.02   **Nontraumatic** subacute **subdural hemorrhage** `NCDx`
     I62.03   **Nontraumatic** chronic **subdural hemorrhage** `NCDx`

   I62.1   **Nontraumatic** extradural **hemorrhage** `NCDx`
Nontraumatic epidural hemorrhage

   I62.9   **Nontraumatic intracranial hemorrhage, unspecified** `NCDx` ▽

✓4ᵗʰ **I63**   **Cerebral infarction**
> INCLUDES   occlusion and stenosis of cerebral and precerebral arteries, resulting in cerebral infarction
Use additional code, if applicable, to identify status post administration of tPA (rtPA) in a different facility within the last 24 hours prior to admission to current facility (Z92.82)
Use additional code, if known, to indicate National Institutes of Health Stroke Scale (NIHSS) score (R29.7-)
> *EXCLUDES 2*   *sequelae of cerebral infarction (I69.3-)*
AHA: 2017, 2Q, 9-10; 2014, 1Q, 23

   ✓5ᵗʰ **I63.0**   **Cerebral infarction due to** thrombosis **of** precerebral **arteries**
     I63.00   **Cerebral infarction due to thrombosis of** `NCDx` ▽ **unspecified precerebral artery**
     ✓6ᵗʰ **I63.01**   **Cerebral infarction due to thrombosis of** vertebral **artery**
       I63.011   **Cerebral infarction due to thrombosis** `NCDx` **of** right **vertebral artery**
       I63.012   **Cerebral infarction due to thrombosis of** left **vertebral artery** `NCDx`
       I63.013   **Cerebral infarction due to thrombosis** `NCDx` **of** bilateral **vertebral arteries**
       I63.019   **Cerebral infarction due to** `NCDx` ▽ **thrombosis of unspecified vertebral artery**
     I63.02   **Cerebral infarction due to thrombosis of** `NCDx` basilar **artery**
     ✓6ᵗʰ **I63.03**   **Cerebral infarction due to thrombosis of** carotid **artery**
       I63.031   **Cerebral infarction due to thrombosis** `NCDx` **of** right **carotid artery**
       I63.032   **Cerebral infarction due to thrombosis** `NCDx` **of** left **carotid artery**
       I63.033   **Cerebral infarction due to thrombosis** `NCDx` **of** bilateral **carotid arteries**
       I63.039   **Cerebral infarction due to** `NCDx` ▽ **thrombosis of unspecified carotid artery**
     I63.09   **Cerebral infarction due to thrombosis of other** `NCDx` precerebral **artery**

   ✓5ᵗʰ **I63.1**   **Cerebral infarction due to** embolism **of** precerebral **arteries**
     I63.10   **Cerebral infarction due to embolism of** `NCDx` ▽ **precerebral artery**
     ✓6ᵗʰ **I63.11**   **Cerebral infarction due to embolism of** vertebral **artery**
       I63.111   **Cerebral infarction due to embolism** `NCDx` **of** right **vertebral artery**
       I63.112   **Cerebral infarction due to embolism** `NCDx` **of** left **vertebral artery**
       I63.113   **Cerebral infarction due to embolism** `NCDx` **of** bilateral **vertebral arteries**
       I63.119   **Cerebral infarction due to** `NCDx` ▽ **embolism of unspecified vertebral artery**
     I63.12   **Cerebral infarction due to embolism of** `NCDx` basilar **artery**

☑ Additional Character Req   ✓x7ᵗʰ Placeholder Alert   Case-Mix Diagnosis   Manifestation   ▽ Unspecified Dx   *EXCLUDES 1* Not coded here   *EXCLUDES 2* Not included here

ICD-10-CM 2018   **631**

I60–I63.12

✓6th **I63.13** **Cerebral infarction due to embolism of** carotid **artery**

    I63.131 **Cerebral infarction due to embolism of** right **carotid artery** NC Dx

    I63.132 **Cerebral infarction due to embolism of** left **carotid artery** NC Dx

    I63.133 **Cerebral infarction due to embolism of** bilateral **carotid arteries** NC Dx

    I63.139 **Cerebral infarction due to embolism of unspecified carotid artery** NC Dx ▽

I63.19 **Cerebral infarction due to embolism of other precerebral artery** NC Dx

✓5th **I63.2** **Cerebral infarction due to** unspecified occlusion or stenosis **of** precerebral **arteries**

    I63.20 **Cerebral infarction due to unspecified occulision or stenosis of unspecified precerebral arteries** NC Dx ▽

    ✓6th **I63.21** **Cerebral infarction due to unspecified occlusion or stenosis of** vertebral **arteries**

        I63.211 **Cerebral infarction due to unspecified occlusion or stenosis of** right **vertebral artery** NC Dx

        I63.212 **Cerebral infarction due to unspecified occlusion or stenosis of** left **vertebral artery** NC Dx

        I63.213 **Cerebral infarction due to unspecified occlusion or stenosis of** bilateral **vertebral arteries** NC Dx

        I63.219 **Cerebral infarction due to unspecified occlusion or stenosis of unspecified vertebral arteries** NC Dx ▽

    I63.22 **Cerebral infarction due to unspecified occlusion or stenosis of** basilar **artery** NC Dx

    ✓6th **I63.23** **Cerebral infarction due to unspecified occlusion or stenosis of** carotid **arteries**

        I63.231 **Cerebral infarction due to unspecified occlusion or stenosis of** right **carotid arteries** NC Dx

        I63.232 **Cerebral infarction due to unspecified occlusion or stenosis of** left **carotid arteries** NC Dx

        I63.233 **Cerebral infarction due to unspecified occlusion or stenosis of** bilateral **carotid arteries** NC Dx

        I63.239 **Cerebral infarction due to unspecified occlusion or stenosis of unspecified carotid arteries** NC Dx ▽

    I63.29 **Cerebral infarction due to unspecified occulision or stenosis of other precerebral arteries** NC Dx

✓5th **I63.3** **Cerebral infarction due to** thrombosis **of** cerebral **arteries**

    I63.30 **Cerebral infarction due to thrombosis of unspecified cerebral artery** NC Dx ▽

    ✓6th **I63.31** **Cerebral infarction due to thrombosis of** middle **cerebral artery**

        I63.311 **Cerebral infarction due to thrombosis of** right **middle cerebral artery** NC Dx

        I63.312 **Cerebral infarction due to thrombosisof** left **middle cerebral artery** NC Dx

        I63.313 **Cerebral infarction due to thrombosis of** bilateral **middle cerebral arteries** NC Dx

        I63.319 **Cerebral infarction due to thrombosisof unspecified middle cerebral artery** NC Dx ▽

    ✓6th **I63.32** **Cerebral infarction due to thrombosis of** anterior **cerebral artery**

        I63.321 **Cerebral infarction due to thrombosis of** right **anterior cerebral artery** NC Dx

        I63.322 **Cerebral infarction due to thrombosis of** left **anterior cerebral artery** NC Dx

        I63.323 **Cerebral infarction due to thrombosis of** bilateral **anterior cerebral arteries** NC Dx

        I63.329 **Cerebral infarction due to thrombosis of unspecified anterior cerebral artery** NC Dx ▽

✓6th **I63.33** **Cerebral infarction due to thrombosis of** posterior **cerebral artery**

    I63.331 **Cerebral infarction due to thrombosis of** right **posterior cerebral artery** NC Dx

    I63.332 **Cerebral infarction due to thrombosis of** left **posterior cerebral artery** NC Dx

    I63.333 **Cerebral infarction to thrombosis of** bilateral **posterior cerebral arteries** NC Dx

    I63.339 **Cerebral infarction due to thrombosisof unspecified posterior cerebral artery** NC Dx ▽

✓6th **I63.34** **Cerebral infarction due to thrombosis of** cerebellar **artery**

    I63.341 **Cerebral infarction due to thrombosis of** right **cerebellar artery** NC Dx

    I63.342 **Cerebral infarction due to thrombosis of** left **cerebellar artery** NC Dx

    I63.343 **Cerebral infarction to thrombosis of** bilateral **cerebellar arteries** NC Dx

    I63.349 **Cerebral infarction due to thrombosis of unspecified cerebellar artery** NC Dx ▽

I63.39 **Cerebral infarction due to thrombosis of other cerebral artery** NC Dx

✓5th **I63.4** **Cerebral infarction due to** embolism **of** cerebral **arteries**

    I63.40 **Cerebral infarction due to embolism of unspecified cerebral artery** NC Dx ▽

    ✓6th **I63.41** **Cerebral infarction due to embolism of** middle **cerebral artery**

        I63.411 **Cerebral infarction due to embolism of** right **middle cerebral artery** NC Dx

        I63.412 **Cerebral infarction due to embolism of** left **middle cerebral artery** NC Dx

        I63.413 **Cerebral infarction due to embolism of** bilateral **middle cerebral arteries** NC Dx

        I63.419 **Cerebral infarction due to embolism of unspecified middle cerebral artery** NC Dx ▽

    ✓6th **I63.42** **Cerebral infarction due to embolism of** anterior **cerebral artery**

        I63.421 **Cerebral infarction due to embolism of** right **anterior cerebral artery** NC Dx

        I63.422 **Cerebral infarction due to embolism of** left **anterior cerebral artery** NC Dx

        I63.423 **Cerebral infarction due to embolism of** bilateral **anterior cerebral arteries** NC Dx

        I63.429 **Cerebral infarction due to embolism of unspecified anterior cerebral artery** NC Dx ▽

    ✓6th **I63.43** **Cerebral infarction due to embolism of** posterior **cerebral artery**

        I63.431 **Cerebral infarction due to embolism of** right **posterior cerebral artery** NC Dx

        I63.432 **Cerebral infarction due to embolism of** left **posterior cerebral artery** NC Dx

        I63.433 **Cerebral infarction due to embolism of** bilateral **posterior cerebral arteries** NC Dx

        I63.439 **Cerebral infarction due to embolism of unspecified posterior cerebral artery** NC Dx ▽

    ✓6th **I63.44** **Cerebral infarction due to embolism of** cerebellar **artery**

        I63.441 **Cerebral infarction due to embolism of** right **cerebellar artery** NC Dx

        I63.442 **Cerebral infarction due to embolism of** left **cerebellar artery** NC Dx

        I63.443 **Cerebral infarction due to embolism of** bilateral **cerebellar arteries** NC Dx

        I63.449 **Cerebral infarction due to embolism of unspecified cerebellar artery** NC Dx ▽

I63.49 **Cerebral infarction due to embolism of other cerebral artery** NC Dx

N Newborn: 0   P Pediatric: 0-17   M Maternity: 12-55   A Adult: 15-124   NRS Nonroutine supply Dx   NC Dx Noncancer Dx   PDx Primary Dx   ▶◀ Revised Text   ● New Code   ▲ Revised Title

632   ICD-10-CM 2018

☑5ᵗʰ **I63.5** **Cerebral infarction due to** unspecified occlusion or stenosis of cerebral **arteries**

     I63.50 **Cerebral infarction due to unspecified occlusion or stenosis of unspecified cerebral artery** `NC Dx` ▽

     ☑6ᵗʰ **I63.51** **Cerebral infarction due to unspecified occlusion or stenosis of** middle **cerebral artery**

         I63.511 **Cerebral infarction due to unspecified occlusion or stenosis of** right **middle cerebral artery** `NC Dx`

         I63.512 **Cerebral infarction due to unspecified occlusion or stenosis of** left **middle cerebral artery** `NC Dx`

▲   **I63.513** **Cerebral infarction due to unspecified occlusion or stenosis of** bilateral **middle cerebral arteries** `NC Dx`

         I63.519 **Cerebral infarction due to unspecified occlusion or stenosis of unspecified middle cerebral artery** `NC Dx` ▽

     ☑6ᵗʰ **I63.52** **Cerebral infarction due to unspecified occlusion or stenosis of** anterior **cerebral artery**

         I63.521 **Cerebral infarction due to unspecified occlusion or stenosis of** right **anterior cerebral artery** `NC Dx`

         I63.522 **Cerebral infarction due to unspecified occlusion or stenosis of** left **anterior cerebral artery** `NC Dx`

▲   **I63.523** **Cerebral infarction due to unspecified occlusion or stenosis of** bilateral **anterior cerebral arteries** `NC Dx`

         I63.529 **Cerebral infarction due to unspecified occlusion or stenosis of unspecified anterior cerebral artery** `NC Dx` ▽

     ☑6ᵗʰ **I63.53** **Cerebral infarction due to unspecified occlusion or stenosis of** posterior **cerebral artery**

         I63.531 **Cerebral infarction due to unspecified occlusion or stenosis of** right **posterior cerebral artery** `NC Dx`

         I63.532 **Cerebral infarction due to unspecified occlusion or stenosis of** left **posterior cerebral artery** `NC Dx`

▲   **I63.533** **Cerebral infarction due to unspecified occlusion or stenosis of** bilateral **posterior cerebral arteries** `NC Dx`

         I63.539 **Cerebral infarction due to unspecified occlusion or stenosis of unspecified posterior cerebral artery** `NC Dx` ▽

     ☑6ᵗʰ **I63.54** **Cerebral infarction due to unspecified occlusion or stenosis of** cerebellar **artery**

         I63.541 **Cerebral infarction due to unspecified occlusion or stenosis of** right **cerebellar artery** `NC Dx`

         I63.542 **Cerebral infarction due to unspecified occlusion or stenosis of** left **cerebellar artery** `NC Dx`

         I63.543 **Cerebral infarction due to unspecified occlusion or stenosis of** bilateral **cerebellar arteries** `NC Dx`

         I63.549 **Cerebral infarction due to unspecified occlusion or stenosis of unspecified cerebellar artery** `NC Dx` ▽

     I63.59 **Cerebral infarction due to unspecified occlusion or stenosis of other cerebral artery** `NC Dx`

I63.6 **Cerebral infarction due to** cerebral venous thrombosis, **nonpyogenic** `NC Dx`

I63.8 **Other cerebral infarction** `NC Dx`

I63.9 **Cerebral infarction, unspecified** `NC Dx` ▽
     Stroke NOS
     EXCLUDES 2 ▶transient cerebral ischemic attacks and related syndromes (G45.-)◀
     AHA: 2015, 1Q, 25

☑4ᵗʰ **I65** **Occlusion and stenosis of** precerebral **arteries,** not resulting in cerebral infarction
     `INCLUDES` embolism of precerebral artery
         narrowing of precerebral artery
         obstruction (complete) (partial) of precerebral artery
         thrombosis of precerebral artery
     EXCLUDES 1 insufficiency, NOS, of precerebral artery (G45.-)
         insufficiency of precerebral arteries causing cerebral infarction (I63.0-I63.2)

     ☑5ᵗʰ **I65.0** **Occlusion and stenosis of** vertebral **artery**

         I65.01 **Occlusion and stenosis of** right **vertebral artery**

         I65.02 **Occlusion and stenosis of** left **vertebral artery**

         I65.03 **Occlusion and stenosis of** bilateral **vertebral arteries**

         I65.09 **Occlusion and stenosis of unspecified vertebra artery** ▽

     I65.1 **Occlusion and stenosis of** basilar **artery**

     ☑5ᵗʰ **I65.2** **Occlusion and stenosis of** carotid **artery**

         I65.21 **Occlusion and stenosis of** right **carotid artery**

         I65.22 **Occlusion and stenosis of** left **carotid artery**

         I65.23 **Occlusion and stenosis of** bilateral **carotid arteries**

         I65.29 **Occlusion and stenosis of unspecified carotid artery** ▽

     I65.8 **Occlusion and stenosis of other precerebral arteries**

     I65.9 **Occlusion and stenosis of unspecified precerebral artery** ▽
     Occlusion and stenosis of precerebral artery NOS

☑4ᵗʰ **I66** **Occlusion and stenosis of** cerebral **arteries,** not resulting in cerebral infarction
     `INCLUDES` embolism of cerebral artery
         narrowing of cerebral artery
         obstruction (complete) (partial) of cerebral artery
         thrombosis of cerebral artery
     EXCLUDES 1 occlusion and stenosis of cerebral artery causing cerebral infarction (I63.3-I63.5)

     ☑5ᵗʰ **I66.0** **Occlusion and stenosis of** middle **cerebral artery**

         I66.01 **Occlusion and stenosis of** right **middle cerebral artery**

         I66.02 **Occlusion and stenosis of** left **middle cerebral artery**

         I66.03 **Occlusion and stenosis of** bilateral **middle cerebral arteries**

         I66.09 **Occlusion and stenosis of unspecified middle cerebral artery** ▽

     ☑5ᵗʰ **I66.1** **Occlusion and stenosis of** anterior **cerebral artery**

         I66.11 **Occlusion and stenosis of** right **anterior cerebral artery**

         I66.12 **Occlusion and stenosis of** left **anterior cerebral artery**

         I66.13 **Occlusion and stenosis of** bilateral **anterior cerebral arteries**

         I66.19 **Occlusion and stenosis of unspecified anterior cerebral artery** ▽

     ☑5ᵗʰ **I66.2** **Occlusion and stenosis of** posterior **cerebral artery**

         I66.21 **Occlusion and stenosis of** right **posterior cerebral artery**

         I66.22 **Occlusion and stenosis of** left **posterior cerebral artery**

         I66.23 **Occlusion and stenosis of** bilateral **posterior cerebral arteries**

         I66.29 **Occlusion and stenosis of unspecified posterior cerebral artery** ▽

     I66.3 **Occlusion and stenosis of** cerebellar **arteries**

     I66.8 **Occlusion and stenosis of other cerebral arteries**
     Occlusion and stenosis of perforating arteries

     I66.9 **Occlusion and stenosis of unspecified cerebral artery** ▽

☑4ᵗʰ **I67** **Other cerebrovascular diseases**
     EXCLUDES 2 sequelae of the listed conditions (I69.8)

     I67.0 **Dissection of cerebral arteries, nonruptured**
         EXCLUDES 1 ruptured cerebral arteries (I60.7)

☑ Additional Character Req   ✓x7ᵗʰ Placeholder Alert   Case-Mix Diagnosis   Manifestation   ▽ Unspecified Dx   *EXCLUDES 1* Not coded here   *EXCLUDES 2* Not included here

ICD-10-CM 2018   **633**

Chapter 9. Diseases of the Circulatory System

I67.1–I69.Ø31

Berry Aneurysm

Berry aneurysms form at the site of a weakness in an arterial wall, often at a junction

Berry aneurysm

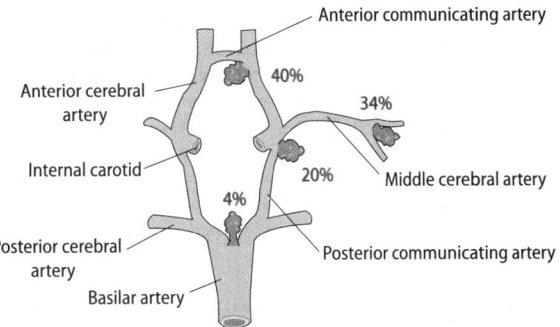

Anterior communicating artery

Anterior cerebral artery

Internal carotid

40%

34%

20%

Middle cerebral artery

4%

Posterior cerebral artery

Posterior communicating artery

Basilar artery

I67.1 Cerebral aneurysm, nonruptured
Cerebral aneurysm NOS
Cerebral arteriovenous fistula, acquired
Internal carotid artery aneurysm, intracranial portion
Internal carotid artery aneurysm, NOS
> EXCLUDES 1   *congenital cerebral aneurysm, nonruptured (Q28.-)*
> *ruptured cerebral aneurysm (I60.7)*

I67.2 Cerebral atherosclerosis   NC Dx A
Atheroma of cerebral and precerebral arteries

I67.3 Progressive vascular leukoencephalopathy
Binswanger's disease

I67.4 Hypertensive encephalopathy   NC Dx
> EXCLUDES 2   ►*insufficiency, NOS, of precerebral arteries (G45.2)*◄

I67.5 Moyamoya disease   NC Dx
DEF: Cerebrovascular ischemia; vessels occlude and rupture, causing tiny hemorrhages at base of brain; affects predominantly Japanese people.

I67.6 Nonpyogenic thrombosis of intracranial venous system   NC Dx
Nonpyogenic thrombosis of cerebral vein
Nonpyogenic thrombosis of intracranial venous sinus
> EXCLUDES 1   *nonpyogenic thrombosis of intracranial venous system causing infarction (I63.6)*

I67.7 Cerebral arteritis, not elsewhere classified   NC Dx
Granulomatous angiitis of the nervous system
> EXCLUDES 1   *allergic granulomatous angiitis (M3Ø.1)*

✓5th **I67.8 Other specified cerebrovascular diseases**

    I67.81 Acute cerebrovascular insufficiency   NC Dx
Acute cerebrovascular insufficiency unspecified as to location or reversibility

    I67.82 Cerebral ischemia   NC Dx
Chronic cerebral ischemia

    I67.83 Posterior reversible encephalopathy syndrome
PRES

    ✓6th **I67.84 Cerebral vasospasm and vasoconstriction**

       I67.841 Reversible cerebrovascular vasoconstriction syndrome
Call-Fleming syndrome
Code first underlying condition, if applicable, such as eclampsia (O15.ØØ-O15.9)

       I67.848 Other cerebrovascular vasospasm and vasoconstriction

    I67.89 Other cerebrovascular disease   NC Dx

8 **I67.9 Cerebrovascular disease, unspecified**   ▽

✓4th **I68 Cerebrovascular disorders in diseases classified elsewhere**

I68.Ø Cerebral amyloid angiopathy
Code first underlying amyloidosis (E85.-)

I68.2 Cerebral arteritis in other diseases classified elsewhere
Code first underlying disease
> EXCLUDES 1   *cerebral arteritis (in):*
> *listerosis (A32.89)*
> *systemic lupus erythematosus (M32.19)*
> *syphilis (A52.Ø4)*
> *tuberculosis (A18.89)*

I68.8 Other cerebrovascular disorders in diseases classified elsewhere
Code first underlying disease
> EXCLUDES 1   *syphilitic cerebral aneurysm (A52.Ø5)*

✓4th **I69 Sequelae of cerebrovascular disease**
> NOTE   Category I69 is to be used to indicate conditions in I6Ø-I67 as the cause of sequelae. The "sequelae" include conditions specified as such or as residuals which may occur at any time after the onset of the causal condition
> EXCLUDES 1   *personal history of cerebral infarction without residual deficit (Z86.73)*
> *personal history of prolonged reversible ischemic neurologic deficit (PRIND) (Z86.73)*
> *personal history of reversible ischemic neurolgeic deficit (RIND) (Z86.73)*
> *sequelae of traumatic intracranial injury (SØ6.-)*
> ~~*transient ischemic attack (TIA) (G45.9)*~~

AHA: 2017, 1Q, 47; 2015, 1Q, 25; 2012, 4Q, 106
TIP: Unilateral weakness (including upper or lower limb weakness), when indicated by provider documentation as related to an old or recent CVA, is synonymous with hemiplegia/hemiparesis as a sequela of CVA.

✓5th **I69.Ø Sequelae of nontraumatic subarachnoid hemorrhage**

    I69.ØØ Unspecified sequelae of nontraumatic subarachnoid hemorrhage   ▽

    ✓6th **I69.Ø1 Cognitive deficits following nontraumatic subarachnoid hemorrhage**

       I69.Ø1Ø Attention and concentration deficit following nontraumatic subarachnoid hemorrhage

       I69.Ø11 Memory deficit following nontraumatic subarachnoid hemorrhage

       I69.Ø12 Visuospatial deficit and spatial neglect following nontraumatic subarachnoid hemorrhage

       I69.Ø13 Psychomotor deficit following nontraumatic subarachnoid hemorrhage

       I69.Ø14 Frontal lobe and executive function deficit following nontraumatic subarachnoid hemorrhage

       I69.Ø15 Cognitive social or emotional deficit following nontraumatic subarachnoid hemorrhage

       I69.Ø18 Other symptoms and signs involving cognitive functions following nontraumatic subarachnoid hemorrhage

       I69.Ø19 Unspecified symptoms and signs involving cognitive functions following nontraumatic subarachnoid hemorrhage   ▽

    ✓6th **I69.Ø2 Speech and language deficits following nontraumatic subarachnoid hemorrhage**

       I69.Ø2Ø Aphasia following nontraumatic subarachnoid hemorrhage

       I69.Ø21 Dysphasia following nontraumatic subarachnoid hemorrhage

       I69.Ø22 Dysarthria following nontraumatic subarachnoid hemorrhage

       I69.Ø23 Fluency disorder following nontraumatic subarachnoid hemorrhage
Stuttering following nontraumatic subarachnoid hemorrhage

       I69.Ø28 Other speech and language deficits following nontraumatic subarachnoid hemorrhage

    ✓6th **I69.Ø3 Monoplegia of upper limb following nontraumatic subarachnoid hemorrhage**
AHA: 2017, 1Q, 47

       I69.Ø31 Monoplegia of upper limb following nontraumatic subarachnoid hemorrhage affecting right dominant side

---

8 Hospice questionable admission diagnosis.

N Newborn: 0   P Pediatric: 0-17   M Maternity: 12-55   A Adult: 15-124   NRS Nonroutine supply Dx   NC Dx Noncancer Dx   PDx Primary Dx   ►◄ Revised Text   ● New Code   ▲ Revised Title

634   ICD-10-CM 2018

I69.032 Monoplegia of upper limb following nontraumatic subarachnoid hemorrhage affecting left dominant side

I69.033 Monoplegia of upper limb following nontraumatic subarachnoid hemorrhage affecting right non-dominant side

I69.034 Monoplegia of upper limb following nontraumatic subarachnoid hemorrhage affecting left non-dominant side

I69.039 Monoplegia of upper limb following nontraumatic subarachnoid hemorrhage affecting unspecified side ▽

✓6ᵗʰ **I69.04** Monoplegia of lower limb following nontraumatic subarachnoid hemorrhage
AHA: 2017, 1Q, 47

I69.041 Monoplegia of lower limb following nontraumatic subarachnoid hemorrhage affecting right dominant side

I69.042 Monoplegia of lower limb following nontraumatic subarachnoid hemorrhage affecting left dominant side

I69.043 Monoplegia of lower limb following nontraumatic subarachnoid hemorrhage affecting right non-dominant side

I69.044 Monoplegia of lower limb following nontraumatic subarachnoid hemorrhage affecting left non-dominant side

I69.049 Monoplegia of lower limb following nontraumatic subarachnoid hemorrhage affecting unspecified side ▽

✓6ᵗʰ **I69.05** Hemiplegia and hemiparesis following nontraumatic subarachnoid hemorrhage
AHA: 2015, 1Q, 25

I69.051 Hemiplegia and hemiparesis following nontraumatic subarachnoid hemorrhage affecting right dominant side

I69.052 Hemiplegia and hemiparesis following nontraumatic subarachnoid hemorrhage affecting left dominant side

I69.053 Hemiplegia and hemiparesis following nontraumatic subarachnoid hemorrhage affecting right non-dominant side

I69.054 Hemiplegia and hemiparesis following nontraumatic subarachnoid hemorrhage affecting left non-dominant side

I69.059 Hemiplegia and hemiparesis following nontraumatic subarachnoid hemorrhage affecting unspecified side ▽

✓6ᵗʰ **I69.06** Other paralytic syndrome following nontraumatic subarachnoid hemorrhage
Use additional code to identify type of paralytic syndrome, such as:
locked-in state (G83.5)
quadriplegia (G82.5-)
EXCLUDES 1 *hemiplegia/hemiparesis following nontraumatic subarachnoid hemorrhage (I69.05-)*
monoplegia of lower limb following nontraumatic subarachnoid hemorrhage (I69.04-)
monoplegia of upper limb following nontraumatic subarachnoid hemorrhage (I69.03-)

I69.061 Other paralytic syndrome following nontraumatic subarachnoid hemorrhage affecting right dominant side

I69.062 Other paralytic syndrome following nontraumatic subarachnoid hemorrhage affecting left dominant side

I69.063 Other paralytic syndrome following nontraumatic subarachnoid hemorrhage affecting right non-dominant side

I69.064 Other paralytic syndrome following nontraumatic subarachnoid hemorrhage affecting left non-dominant side

I69.065 Other paralytic syndrome following nontraumatic subarachnoid hemorrhage, bilateral

I69.069 Other paralytic syndrome following nontraumatic subarachnoid hemorrhage affecting unspecified side ▽

✓6ᵗʰ **I69.09** Other sequelae of nontraumatic subarachnoid hemorrhage

I69.090 Apraxia following nontraumatic subarachnoid hemorrhage

I69.091 Dysphagia following nontraumatic subarachnoid hemorrhage
Use additional code to identify the type of dysphagia, if known (R13.1-)

I69.092 Facial weakness following nontraumatic subarachnoid hemorrhage
Facial droop following nontraumatic subarachnoid hemorrhage

I69.093 Ataxia following nontraumatic subarachnoid hemorrhage

I69.098 Other sequelae following nontraumatic subarachnoid hemorrhage
Alterations of sensation following nontraumatic subarachnoid hemorrhage
Disturbance of vision following nontraumatic subarachnoid hemorrhage
Use additional code to identify the sequelae

✓5ᵗʰ **I69.1** Sequelae of nontraumatic intracerebral hemorrhage

I69.10 Unspecified sequelae of nontraumatic intracerebral hemorrhage ▽

✓6ᵗʰ **I69.11** Cognitive deficits following nontraumatic intracerebral hemorrhage

I69.110 Attention and concentration deficit following nontraumatic intracerebral hemorrhage

I69.111 Memory deficit following nontraumatic intracerebral hemorrhage

I69.112 Visuospatial deficit and spatial neglect following nontraumatic intracerebral hemorrhage

I69.113 Psychomotor deficit following nontraumatic intracerebral hemorrhage

I69.114 Frontal lobe and executive function deficit following nontraumatic intracerebral hemorrhage

I69.115 Cognitive social or emotional deficit following nontraumatic intracerebral hemorrhage

I69.118 Other symptoms and signs involving cognitive functions following nontraumatic intracerebral hemorrhage

I69.119 Unspecified symptoms and signs involving cognitive functions following nontraumatic intracerebral hemorrhage ▽

✓6ᵗʰ **I69.12** Speech and language deficits following nontraumatic intracerebral hemorrhage

I69.120 Aphasia following nontraumatic intracerebral hemorrhage

I69.121 Dysphasia following nontraumatic intracerebral hemorrhage

I69.122 Dysarthria following nontraumatic intracerebral hemorrhage

I69.123 Fluency disorder following nontraumatic intracerebral hemorrhage
Stuttering following nontraumatic intracerebral hemorrhage

I69.128 Other speech and language deficits following nontraumatic intracerebral hemorrhage

✓6ᵗʰ **I69.13** Monoplegia of upper limb following nontraumatic intracerebral hemorrhage
AHA: 2017, 1Q, 47

I69.131 Monoplegia of upper limb following nontraumatic intracerebral hemorrhage affecting right dominant side

I69.132 Monoplegia of upper limb following nontraumatic intracerebral hemorrhage affecting left dominant side

I69.133 Monoplegia of upper limb following nontraumatic intracerebral hemorrhage affecting right non-dominant side

I69.134 Monoplegia of upper limb following nontraumatic intracerebral hemorrhage affecting left non-dominant side

✔ Additional Character Req   ✔x7ᵗʰ Placeholder Alert   Case-Mix Diagnosis   Manifestation   ▽ Unspecified Dx   *EXCLUDES 1* Not coded here   *EXCLUDES 2* Not included here

ICD-10-CM 2018   635

Chapter 9. Diseases of the Circulatory System

I69.032–I69.134

I69.139   **Monoplegia of upper limb following nontraumatic intracerebral hemorrhage affecting unspecified side** ▽

✓6ᵗʰ I69.14   Monoplegia of lower limb following nontraumatic intracerebral hemorrhage
AHA: 2017, 1Q, 47

    I69.141   **Monoplegia of lower limb following nontraumatic intracerebral hemorrhage affecting right dominant side**

    I69.142   **Monoplegia of lower limb following nontraumatic intracerebral hemorrhage affecting left dominant side**

    I69.143   **Monoplegia of lower limb following nontraumatic intracerebral hemorrhage affecting right non-dominant side**

    I69.144   **Monoplegia of lower limb following nontraumatic intracerebral hemorrhage affecting left non-dominant side**

    I69.149   **Monoplegia of lower limb following nontraumatic intracerebral hemorrhage affecting unspecified side** ▽

✓6ᵗʰ I69.15   Hemiplegia and hemiparesis following nontraumatic intracerebral hemorrhage
AHA: 2015, 1Q, 25

    I69.151   **Hemiplegia and hemiparesis following nontraumatic intracerebral hemorrhage affecting right dominant side**

    I69.152   **Hemiplegia and hemiparesis following nontraumatic intracerebral hemorrhage affecting left dominant side**

    I69.153   **Hemiplegia and hemiparesis following nontraumatic intracerebral hemorrhage affecting right non-dominant side**

    I69.154   **Hemiplegia and hemiparesis following nontraumatic intracerebral hemorrhage affecting left non-dominant side**

    I69.159   **Hemiplegia and hemiparesis following nontraumatic intracerebral hemorrhage affecting unspecified side** ▽

✓6ᵗʰ I69.16   Other paralytic syndrome following nontraumatic intracerebral hemorrhage
Use additional code to identify type of paralytic syndrome, such as:
locked-in state (G83.5)
quadriplegia (G82.5-)
    EXCLUDES 1   *hemiplegia/hemiparesis following nontraumatic intracerebral hemorrhage (I69.15-)*
monoplegia of lower limb following nontraumatic intracerebral hemorrhage (I69.14-)
monoplegia of upper limb following nontraumatic intracerebral hemorrhage (I69.13-)

    I69.161   **Other paralytic syndrome following nontraumatic intracerebral hemorrhage affecting right dominant side**

    I69.162   **Other paralytic syndrome following nontraumatic intracerebral hemorrhage affecting left dominant side**

    I69.163   **Other paralytic syndrome following nontraumatic intracerebral hemorrhage affecting right non-dominant side**

    I69.164   **Other paralytic syndrome following nontraumatic intracerebral hemorrhage affecting left non-dominant side**

    I69.165   **Other paralytic syndrome following nontraumatic intracerebral hemorrhage, bilateral**

    I69.169   **Other paralytic syndrome following nontraumatic intracerebral hemorrhage affecting unspecified side** ▽

✓6ᵗʰ I69.19   Other sequelae of nontraumatic intracerebral hemorrhage

    I69.190   **Apraxia following nontraumatic intracerebral hemorrhage**

    I69.191   **Dysphagia following nontraumatic intracerebral hemorrhage**
Use additional code to identify the type of dysphagia, if known (R13.1-)

I69.192   **Facial weakness following nontraumatic intracerebral hemorrhage**
Facial droop following nontraumatic intracerebral hemorrhage

I69.193   **Ataxia following nontraumatic intracerebral hemorrhage**

I69.198   **Other sequelae of nontraumatic intracerebral hemorrhage**
Alteration of sensations following nontraumatic intracerebral hemorrhage
Disturbance of vision following nontraumatic intracerebral hemorrhage
Use additional code to identify the sequelae

✓5ᵗʰ I69.2   Sequelae of other nontraumatic intracranial hemorrhage

    I69.20   **Unspecified sequelae of other nontraumatic intracranial hemorrhage** ▽

✓6ᵗʰ I69.21   Cognitive deficits following other nontraumatic intracranial hemorrhage

    I69.210   **Attention and concentration deficit following other nontraumatic intracranial hemorrhage**

    I69.211   **Memory deficit following other nontraumatic intracranial hemorrhage**

    I69.212   **Visuospatial deficit and spatial neglect following other nontraumatic intracranial hemorrhage**

    I69.213   **Psychomotor deficit following other nontraumatic intracranial hemorrhage**

    I69.214   **Frontal lobe and executive function deficit following other nontraumatic intracranial hemorrhage**

    I69.215   **Cognitive social or emotional deficit following other nontraumatic intracranial hemorrhage**

    I69.218   **Other symptoms and signs involving cognitive functions following other nontraumatic intracranial hemorrhage**

    I69.219   **Unspecified symptoms and signs involving cognitive functions following other nontraumatic intracranial hemorrhage** ▽

✓6ᵗʰ I69.22   Speech and language deficits following other nontraumatic intracranial hemorrhage

    I69.220   **Aphasia following other nontraumatic intracranial hemorrhage**

    I69.221   **Dysphasia following other nontraumatic intracranial hemorrhage**

    I69.222   **Dysarthria following other nontraumatic intracranial hemorrhage**

    I69.223   **Fluency disorder following other nontraumatic intracranial hemorrhage**
Stuttering following other nontraumatic intracranial hemorrhage

    I69.228   **Other speech and language deficits following other nontraumatic intracranial hemorrhage**

✓6ᵗʰ I69.23   Monoplegia of upper limb following other nontraumatic intracranial hemorrhage
AHA: 2017, 1Q, 47

    I69.231   **Monoplegia of upper limb following other nontraumatic intracranial hemorrhage affecting right dominant side**

    I69.232   **Monoplegia of upper limb following other nontraumatic intracranial hemorrhage affecting left dominant side**

    I69.233   **Monoplegia of upper limb following other nontraumatic intracranial hemorrhage affecting right non-dominant side**

    I69.234   **Monoplegia of upper limb following other nontraumatic intracranial hemorrhage affecting left non-dominant side**

    I69.239   **Monoplegia of upper limb following other nontraumatic intracranial hemorrhage affecting unspecified side** ▽

N Newborn: 0   P Pediatric: 0-17   M Maternity: 12-55   A Adult: 15-124   **NRS** Nonroutine supply Dx   **NCDx** Noncancer Dx   **PDx** Primary Dx   ▶◀ Revised Text   ● New Code   ▲ Revised Title

636   ICD-10-CM 2018

✓6th **I69.24** Monoplegia of lower limb following other nontraumatic intracranial hemorrhage
AHA: 2017, 1Q, 47

     I69.241 Monoplegia of lower limb following other nontraumatic intracranial hemorrhage affecting right dominant side

     I69.242 Monoplegia of lower limb following other nontraumatic intracranial hemorrhage affecting left dominant side

     I69.243 Monoplegia of lower limb following other nontraumatic intracranial hemorrhage affecting right non-dominant side

     I69.244 Monoplegia of lower limb following other nontraumatic intracranial hemorrhage affecting left non-dominant side

     I69.249 Monoplegia of lower limb following other nontraumatic intracranial hemorrhage affecting unspecified side ▽

✓6th **I69.25** Hemiplegia and hemiparesis following other nontraumatic intracranial hemorrhage
AHA: 2015, 1Q, 25

     I69.251 Hemiplegia and hemiparesis following other nontraumatic intracranial hemorrhage affecting right dominant side

     I69.252 Hemiplegia and hemiparesis following other nontraumatic intracranial hemorrhage affecting left dominant side

     I69.253 Hemiplegia and hemiparesis following other nontraumatic intracranial hemorrhage affecting right non-dominant side

     I69.254 Hemiplegia and hemiparesis following other nontraumatic intracranial hemorrhage affecting left non-dominant side

     I69.259 Hemiplegia and hemiparesis following other nontraumatic intracranial hemorrhage affecting unspecified side ▽

✓6th **I69.26** Other paralytic syndrome following other nontraumatic intracranial hemorrhage
Use additional code to identify type of paralytic syndrome, such as:
locked-in state (G83.5)
quadriplegia (G82.5-)
EXCLUDES 1   *hemiplegia/hemiparesis following other nontraumatic intracranial hemorrhage (I69.25-)*
monoplegia of lower limb following other nontraumatic intracranial hemorrhage (I69.24-)
monoplegia of upper limb following other nontraumatic intracranial hemorrhage (I69.23-)

     I69.261 Other paralytic syndrome following other nontraumatic intracranial hemorrhage affecting right dominant side

     I69.262 Other paralytic syndrome following other nontraumatic intracranial hemorrhage affecting left dominant side

     I69.263 Other paralytic syndrome following other nontraumatic intracranial hemorrhage affecting right non-dominant side

     I69.264 Other paralytic syndrome following other nontraumatic intracranial hemorrhage affecting left non-dominant side

     I69.265 Other paralytic syndrome following other nontraumatic intracranial hemorrhage, bilateral

     I69.269 Other paralytic syndrome following other nontraumatic intracranial hemorrhage affecting unspecified side ▽

✓6th **I69.29** Other sequelae of other nontraumatic intracranial hemorrhage

     I69.290 Apraxia following other nontraumatic intracranial hemorrhage

     I69.291 Dysphagia following other nontraumatic intracranial hemorrhage
Use additional code to identify the type of dysphagia, if known (R13.1-)

     I69.292 Facial weakness following other nontraumatic intracranial hemorrhage
Facial droop following other nontraumatic intracranial hemorrhage

     I69.293 Ataxia following other nontraumatic intracranial hemorrhage

     I69.298 Other sequelae of other nontraumatic intracranial hemorrhage
Alteration of sensation following other nontraumatic intracranial hemorrhage
Disturbance of vision following other nontraumatic intracranial hemorrhage
Use additional code to identify the sequelae

✓5th **I69.3** Sequelae of cerebral infarction
Sequelae of stroke NOS
AHA: 2013, 4Q, 127-128; 2012, 4Q, 92, 94

     I69.30 Unspecified sequelae of cerebral infarction ▽

✓6th **I69.31** Cognitive deficits following cerebral infarction

     I69.310 Attention and concentration deficit following cerebral infarction

     I69.311 Memory deficit following cerebral infarction

     I69.312 Visuospatial deficit and spatial neglect following cerebral infarction

     I69.313 Psychomotor deficit following cerebral infarction

     I69.314 Frontal lobe and executive function deficit following cerebral infarction

     I69.315 Cognitive social or emotional deficit following cerebral infarction

     I69.318 Other symptoms and signs involving cognitive functions following cerebral infarction

     I69.319 Unspecified symptoms and signs involving cognitive functions following cerebral infarction ▽

✓6th **I69.32** Speech and language deficits following cerebral infarction

     I69.320 Aphasia following cerebral infarction

     I69.321 Dysphasia following cerebral infarction
AHA: 2012, 4Q, 91

     I69.322 Dysarthria following cerebral infarction
EXCLUDES 2 ▶*transient ischemic attack (TIA) (G45.9)*◀

     I69.323 Fluency disorder following cerebral infarction
Stuttering following cerebral infarction

     I69.328 Other speech and language deficits following cerebral infarction

✓6th **I69.33** Monoplegia of upper limb following cerebral infarction
AHA: 2017, 1Q, 47

     I69.331 Monoplegia of upper limb following cerebral infarction affecting right dominant side

     I69.332 Monoplegia of upper limb following cerebral infarction affecting left dominant side

     I69.333 Monoplegia of upper limb following cerebral infarction affecting right non-dominant side

     I69.334 Monoplegia of upper limb following cerebral infarction affecting left non-dominant side

     I69.339 Monoplegia of upper limb following cerebral infarction affecting unspecified side ▽

✓6th **I69.34** Monoplegia of lower limb following cerebral infarction
AHA: 2017, 1Q, 47

     I69.341 Monoplegia of lower limb following cerebral infarction affecting right dominant side

     I69.342 Monoplegia of lower limb following cerebral infarction affecting left dominant side

     I69.343 Monoplegia of lower limb following cerebral infarction affecting right non-dominant side

Chapter 9. Diseases of the Circulatory System

I69.344   **Monoplegia of lower limb following cerebral infarction affecting** left non-dominant **side**

I69.349   **Monoplegia of lower limb following cerebral infarction affecting unspecified side** ▽

✓6ᵗʰ   I69.35   **Hemiplegia and hemiparesis following cerebral infarction**
AHA: 2015, 1Q, 25

     I69.351   **Hemiplegia and hemiparesis following cerebral infarction affecting** right dominant **side**
         EXCLUDES 2 ▶transient ischemic attack (TIA) (G45.9)◀

     I69.352   **Hemiplegia and hemiparesis following cerebral infarction affecting** left dominant **side**

     I69.353   **Hemiplegia and hemiparesis following cerebral infarction affecting** right non-dominant **side**

     I69.354   **Hemiplegia and hemiparesis following cerebral infarction affecting** left non-dominant **side**
         AHA: 2012, 4Q, 91

     I69.359   **Hemiplegia and hemiparesis following** ▽ **cerebral infarction affecting unspecified side**

✓6ᵗʰ   I69.36   **Other paralytic syndrome following cerebral infarction**
Use additional code to identify type of paralytic syndrome, such as:
     locked-in state (G83.5)
     quadriplegia (G82.5-)
EXCLUDES 1 hemiplegia/hemiparesis following cerebral infarction (I69.35-)
     monoplegia of lower limb following cerebral infarction (I69.34-)
     monoplegia of upper limb following cerebral infarction (I69.33-)

     I69.361   **Other paralytic syndrome following cerebral infarction affecting** right dominant **side**

     I69.362   **Other paralytic syndrome following cerebral infarction affecting** left dominant **side**

     I69.363   **Other paralytic syndrome following cerebral infarction affecting** right non-dominant **side**

     I69.364   **Other paralytic syndrome following cerebral infarction affecting** left non-dominant **side**

     I69.365   **Other paralytic syndrome following cerebral infarction,** bilateral

     I69.369   **Other paralytic syndrome following** ▽ **cerebral infarction affecting unspecified side**

✓6ᵗʰ   I69.39   **Other sequelae of cerebral infarction**

     I69.390   Apraxia **following cerebral infarction**

     I69.391   Dysphagia **following cerebral infarction**
         Use additional code to identify the type of dysphagia, if known (R13.1-)

     I69.392   Facial weakness **following cerebral infarction**
         Facial droop following cerebral infarction

     I69.393   Ataxia **following cerebral infarction**

     I69.398   **Other sequelae of cerebral infarction**
         Alteration of sensation following cerebral infarction
         Disturbance of vision following cerebral infarction
         Use additional code to identify the sequelae

✓5ᵗʰ   **I69.8**   **Sequelae of** other cerebrovascular diseases
     EXCLUDES 1 sequelae of traumatic intracranial injury (S06.-)

     I69.80   **Unspecified sequelae of other cerebrovascular** ▽ **disease**

✓6ᵗʰ   I69.81   **Cognitive deficits following other cerebrovascular disease**

     I69.810   Attention and concentration **deficit following other cerebrovascular disease**

I69.811   Memory **deficit following other cerebrovascular disease**

I69.812   Visuospatial **deficit and** spatial neglect **following other cerebrovascular disease**

I69.813   Psychomotor **deficit following other cerebrovascular disease**

I69.814   Frontal lobe and executive function **deficit following other cerebrovascular disease**

I69.815   Cognitive social or emotional **deficit following other cerebrovascular disease**

I69.818   Other **symptoms and signs involving cognitive functions following other cerebrovascular disease**

I69.819   **Unspecified symptoms and signs** ▽ **involving cognitive functions following other cerebrovascular disease**

✓6ᵗʰ   I69.82   **Speech and** language deficits **following other cerebrovascular disease**

     I69.820   Aphasia **following other cerebrovascular disease**

     I69.821   Dysphasia **following other cerebrovascular disease**

     I69.822   Dysarthria **following other cerebrovascular disease**

     I69.823   Fluency **disorder following other cerebrovascular disease**
         Stuttering following other cerebrovascular disease

     I69.828   **Other speech and language deficits following other cerebrovascular disease**

✓6ᵗʰ   I69.83   **Monoplegia of** upper limb **following other cerebrovascular disease**
AHA: 2017, 1Q, 47

     I69.831   **Monoplegia of upper limb following other cerebrovascular disease affecting** right dominant **side**

     I69.832   **Monoplegia of upper limb following other cerebrovascular disease affecting** left dominant **side**

     I69.833   **Monoplegia of upper limb following other cerebrovascular disease affecting** right non-dominant **side**

     I69.834   **Monoplegia of upper limb following other cerebrovascular disease affecting** left non-dominant **side**

     I69.839   **Monoplegia of upper limb following** ▽ **other cerebrovascular disease affecting unspecified side**

✓6ᵗʰ   I69.84   **Monoplegia of** lower limb **following other cerebrovascular disease**
AHA: 2017, 1Q, 47

     I69.841   **Monoplegia of lower limb following other cerebrovascular disease affecting** right dominant **side**

     I69.842   **Monoplegia of lower limb following other cerebrovascular disease affecting** left dominant **side**

     I69.843   **Monoplegia of lower limb following other cerebrovascular disease affecting** right non-dominant **side**

     I69.844   **Monoplegia of lower limb following other cerebrovascular disease affecting** left non-dominant **side**

     I69.849   **Monoplegia of lower limb following** ▽ **other cerebrovascular disease affecting unspecified side**

✓6ᵗʰ   I69.85   **Hemiplegia and** hemiparesis **following other cerebrovascular disease**
AHA: 2015, 1Q, 25

     I69.851   **Hemiplegia and hemiparesis following other cerebrovascular disease affecting** right dominant **side**

     I69.852   **Hemiplegia and hemiparesis following other cerebrovascular disease affecting** left dominant **side**

     I69.853   **Hemiplegia and hemiparesis following other cerebrovascular disease affecting** right non-dominant **side**

     I69.854   **Hemiplegia and hemiparesis following other cerebrovascular disease affecting** left non-dominant **side**

Ⓝ Newborn: 0   Ⓟ Pediatric: 0-17   Ⓜ Maternity: 12-55   Ⓐ Adult: 15-124   **NRS** Nonroutine supply Dx   **NCDx** Noncancer Dx   **PDx** Primary Dx   ▶◀ Revised Text   ● New Code   ▲ Revised Title

638   ICD-10-CM 2018

I69.859 Hemiplegia and hemiparesis following other cerebrovascular disease affecting unspecified side ▽

✓6ᵗʰ **I69.86** Other paralytic syndrome following other cerebrovascular disease
 Use additional code to identify type of paralytic syndrome, such as:
 locked-in state (G83.5)
 quadriplegia (G82.5-)
 EXCLUDES 1 *hemiplegia/hemiparesis following other cerebrovascular disease (I69.85-)*
 monoplegia of lower limb following other cerebrovascular disease (I69.84-)
 monoplegia of upper limb following other cerebrovascular disease (I69.83-)

I69.861 Other paralytic syndrome following other cerebrovascular disease affecting right dominant side

I69.862 Other paralytic syndrome following other cerebrovascular disease affecting left dominant side

I69.863 Other paralytic syndrome following other cerebrovascular disease affecting right non-dominant side

I69.864 Other paralytic syndrome following other cerebrovascular disease affecting left non-dominant side

I69.865 Other paralytic syndrome following other cerebrovascular disease, bilateral

I69.869 Other paralytic syndrome following other cerebrovascular disease affecting unspecified side ▽

✓6ᵗʰ **I69.89** Other sequelae of other cerebrovascular disease

I69.890 Apraxia following other cerebrovascular disease

I69.891 Dysphagia following other cerebrovascular disease
 Use additional code to identify the type of dysphagia, if known (R13.1-)

I69.892 Facial weakness following other cerebrovascular disease
 Facial droop following other cerebrovascular disease

I69.893 Ataxia following other cerebrovascular disease

I69.898 Other sequelae of other cerebrovascular disease
 Alteration of sensation following other cerebrovascular disease
 Disturbance of vision following other cerebrovascular disease
 Use additional code to identify the sequelae

✓5ᵗʰ **I69.9** Sequelae of unspecified cerebrovascular diseases
 EXCLUDES 1 *sequelae of stroke (I69.3)*
 sequelae of traumatic intracranial injury (S06.-)

⁸ **I69.90** Unspecified sequelae of unspecified cerebrovascular disease ▽

✓6ᵗʰ **I69.91** Cognitive deficits following unspecified cerebrovascular disease

I69.910 Attention and concentration deficit following unspecified cerebrovascular disease

I69.911 Memory deficit following unspecified cerebrovascular disease

I69.912 Visuospatial deficit and spatial neglect following unspecified cerebrovascular disease

I69.913 Psychomotor deficit following unspecified cerebrovascular disease

I69.914 Frontal lobe and executive function deficit following unspecified cerebrovascular disease

I69.915 Cognitive social or emotional deficit following unspecified cerebrovascular disease

I69.918 Other symptoms and signs involving cognitive functions following unspecified cerebrovascular disease

I69.919 Unspecified symptoms and signs involving cognitive functions following unspecified cerebrovascular disease ▽

✓6ᵗʰ **I69.92** Speech and language deficits following unspecified cerebrovascular disease

I69.920 Aphasia following unspecified cerebrovascular disease ▽

I69.921 Dysphasia following unspecified cerebrovascular disease ▽

I69.922 Dysarthria following unspecified cerebrovascular disease ▽

I69.923 Fluency disorder following unspecified cerebrovascular disease ▽
 Stuttering following unspecified cerebrovascular disease

I69.928 Other speech and language deficits following unspecified cerebrovascular disease ▽

✓6ᵗʰ **I69.93** Monoplegia of upper limb following unspecified cerebrovascular disease
 AHA: 2017, 1Q, 47

I69.931 Monoplegia of upper limb following unspecified cerebrovascular disease affecting right dominant side ▽

I69.932 Monoplegia of upper limb following unspecified cerebrovascular disease affecting left dominant side ▽

I69.933 Monoplegia of upper limb following unspecified cerebrovascular disease affecting right non-dominant side ▽

I69.934 Monoplegia of upper limb following unspecified cerebrovascular disease affecting left non-dominant side ▽

I69.939 Monoplegia of upper limb following unspecified cerebrovascular disease affecting unspecified side ▽

✓6ᵗʰ **I69.94** Monoplegia of lower limb following unspecified cerebrovascular disease
 AHA: 2017, 1Q, 47

I69.941 Monoplegia of lower limb following unspecified cerebrovascular disease affecting right dominant side ▽

I69.942 Monoplegia of lower limb following unspecified cerebrovascular disease affecting left dominant side ▽

I69.943 Monoplegia of lower limb following unspecified cerebrovascular disease affecting right non-dominant side ▽

I69.944 Monoplegia of lower limb following unspecified cerebrovascular disease affecting left non-dominant side ▽

I69.949 Monoplegia of lower limb following unspecified cerebrovascular disease affecting unspecified side ▽

✓6ᵗʰ **I69.95** Hemiplegia and hemiparesis following unspecified cerebrovascular disease
 AHA: 2015, 1Q, 25

I69.951 Hemiplegia and hemiparesis following unspecified cerebrovascular disease affecting right dominant side ▽

I69.952 Hemiplegia and hemiparesis following unspecified cerebrovascular disease affecting left dominant side ▽

I69.953 Hemiplegia and hemiparesis following unspecified cerebrovascular disease affecting right non-dominant side ▽

I69.954 Hemiplegia and hemiparesis following unspecified cerebrovascular disease affecting left non-dominant side ▽

I69.959 Hemiplegia and hemiparesis following unspecified cerebrovascular disease affecting unspecified side ▽

---

⁸ Hospice questionable admission diagnosis.

✓6ᵗʰ I69.96 Other paralytic syndrome following unspecified cerebrovascular disease
Use additional code to identify type of paralytic syndrome, such as:
locked-in state (G83.5)
quadriplegia (G82.5-)
EXCLUDES 1 hemiplegia/hemiparesis following unspecified cerebrovascular disease (I69.95-)
monoplegia of lower limb following unspecified cerebrovascular disease (I69.94-)
monoplegia of upper limb following unspecified cerebrovascular disease (I69.93-)

I69.961 Other paralytic syndrome following unspecified cerebrovascular disease affecting right dominant side ▽

I69.962 Other paralytic syndrome following unspecified cerebrovascular disease affecting left dominant side ▽

I69.963 Other paralytic syndrome following unspecified cerebrovascular disease affecting right non-dominant side ▽

I69.964 Other paralytic syndrome following unspecified cerebrovascular disease affecting left non-dominant side ▽

I69.965 Other paralytic syndrome following unspecified cerebrovascular disease, bilateral ▽

I69.969 Other paralytic syndrome following unspecified cerebrovascular disease affecting unspecified side ▽

✓6ᵗʰ I69.99 Other sequelae of unspecified cerebrovascular disease

I69.990 Apraxia following unspecified cerebrovascular disease ▽

I69.991 Dysphagia following unspecified cerebrovascular disease ▽
Use additional code to identify the type of dysphagia, if known (R13.1-)

I69.992 Facial weakness following unspecified cerebrovascular disease ▽
Facial droop following unspecified cerebrovascular disease

I69.993 Ataxia following unspecified cerebrovascular disease ▽

I69.998 Other sequelae following unspecified cerebrovascular disease ▽
Alteration in sensation following unspecified cerebrovascular disease
Disturbance of vision following unspecified cerebrovascular disease
Use additional code to identify the sequelae

Diseases of arteries, arterioles and capillaries (I70-I79)

✓4ᵗʰ I70 Atherosclerosis
INCLUDES arteriolosclerosis
arterial degeneration
arteriosclerosis
arteriosclerotic vascular disease
arteriovascular degeneration
atheroma
endarteritis deformans or obliterans
senile arteritis
senile endarteritis
vascular degeneration
Use additional code to identify:
exposure to environmental tobacco smoke (Z77.22)
history of tobacco dependence (Z87.891)
occupational exposure to environmental tobacco smoke (Z57.31)
tobacco dependence (F17.-)
tobacco use (Z72.0)
EXCLUDES 2 arteriosclerotic cardiovascular disease (I25.1-)
arteriosclerotic heart disease (I25.1-)
atheroembolism (I75.-)
cerebral atherosclerosis (I67.2)
coronary atherosclerosis (I25.1-)
mesenteric atherosclerosis (K55.1)
precerebral atherosclerosis (I67.2)
primary pulmonary atherosclerosis (I27.0)

I70.0 Atherosclerosis of aorta 🄰

I70.1 Atherosclerosis of renal artery 🄰
Goldblatt's kidney
EXCLUDES 2 atherosclerosis of renal arterioles (I12.-)

✓5ᵗʰ I70.2 Atherosclerosis of native arteries of the extremities
Mönckeberg's (medial) sclerosis
Use additional code, if applicable, to identify chronic total occlusion of artery of extremity (I70.92)
EXCLUDES 2 atherosclerosis of bypass graft of extremities (I70.30-I70.79)

✓6ᵗʰ I70.20 Unspecified atherosclerosis of native arteries of extremities
I70.201 Unspecified atherosclerosis of native arteries of extremities, right leg 🄰▽
I70.202 Unspecified atherosclerosis of native arteries of extremities, left leg 🄰▽
I70.203 Unspecified atherosclerosis of native arteries of extremities, bilateral legs 🄰▽
I70.208 Unspecified atherosclerosis of native arteries of extremities, other extremity 🄰▽
I70.209 Unspecified atherosclerosis of native arteries of extremities, unspecified extremity 🄰▽

✓6ᵗʰ I70.21 Atherosclerosis of native arteries of extremities with intermittent claudication
I70.211 Atherosclerosis of native arteries of extremities with intermittent claudication, right leg 🄰
I70.212 Atherosclerosis of native arteries of extremities with intermittent claudication, left leg 🄰
I70.213 Atherosclerosis of native arteries of extremities with intermittent claudication, bilateral legs 🄰
I70.218 Atherosclerosis of native arteries of extremities with intermittent claudication, other extremity 🄰
I70.219 Atherosclerosis of native arteries of extremities with intermittent claudication, unspecified extremity 🄰▽

✓6ᵗʰ I70.22 Atherosclerosis of native arteries of extremities with rest pain
INCLUDES any condition classifiable to I70.21-
I70.221 Atherosclerosis of native arteries of extremities with rest pain, right leg 🄰
I70.222 Atherosclerosis of native arteries of extremities with rest pain, left leg 🄰
I70.223 Atherosclerosis of native arteries of extremities with rest pain, bilateral legs 🄰
I70.228 Atherosclerosis of native arteries of extremities with rest pain, other extremity 🄰
I70.229 Atherosclerosis of native arteries of extremities with rest pain, unspecified extremity 🄰▽

✓6ᵗʰ I70.23 Atherosclerosis of native arteries of right leg with ulceration
INCLUDES any condition classifiable to I70.211 and I70.221
Use additional code to identify severity of ulcer (L97.-)
I70.231 Atherosclerosis of native arteries of right leg with ulceration of thigh 🅽🆁🆂 🄰
I70.232 Atherosclerosis of native arteries of right leg with ulceration of calf 🅽🆁🆂 🄰
I70.233 Atherosclerosis of native arteries of right leg with ulceration of ankle 🅽🆁🆂 🄰
I70.234 Atherosclerosis of native arteries of right leg with ulceration of heel and midfoot 🅽🆁🆂 🄰
Atherosclerosis of native arteries of right leg with ulceration of plantar surface of midfoot
I70.235 Atherosclerosis of native arteries of right leg with ulceration of other part of foot 🅽🆁🆂 🄰
Atherosclerosis of native arteries of right leg extremities with ulceration of toe
I70.238 Atherosclerosis of native arteries of right leg with ulceration of other part of lower right leg 🅽🆁🆂 🄰

I70.239 Atherosclerosis of native arteries of right leg with ulceration of unspecified site 🅐▽

✓6ᵗʰ **I70.24** Atherosclerosis of native arteries of left leg with ulceration
> INCLUDES any condition classifiable to I70.212 and I70.222
> Use additional code to identify severity of ulcer (L97.-)

I70.241 Atherosclerosis of native arteries of left leg with ulceration of thigh NRS 🅐

I70.242 Atherosclerosis of native arteries of left leg with ulceration of calf NRS 🅐

I70.243 Atherosclerosis of native arteries of left leg with ulceration of ankle NRS 🅐

I70.244 Atherosclerosis of native arteries of left leg with ulceration of heel and midfoot NRS 🅐
> Atherosclerosis of native arteries of left leg with ulceration of plantar surface of midfoot

I70.245 Atherosclerosis of native arteries of left leg with ulceration of other part of foot NRS 🅐
> Atherosclerosis of native arteries of left leg extremities with ulceration of toe

I70.248 Atherosclerosis of native arteries of left leg with ulceration of other part of lower left leg NRS 🅐

I70.249 Atherosclerosis of native arteries of left leg with ulceration of unspecified site NRS 🅐▽

I70.25 Atherosclerosis of native arteries of other extremities with ulceration NRS 🅐
> INCLUDES any condition classifiable to I70.218 and I70.228
> Use additional code to identify the severity of the ulcer (L98.49-)

✓6ᵗʰ **I70.26** Atherosclerosis of native arteries of extremities with gangrene
> INCLUDES any condition classifiable to I70.21-, I70.22-, I70.23-, I70.24-, and I70.25-
> Use additional code to identify the severity of any ulcer (L97.-, L98.49-), if applicable

I70.261 Atherosclerosis of native arteries of extremities with gangrene, right leg NRS 🅐

I70.262 Atherosclerosis of native arteries of extremities with gangrene, left leg NRS 🅐

I70.263 Atherosclerosis of native arteries of extremities with gangrene, bilateral legs NRS 🅐

I70.268 Atherosclerosis of native arteries of extremities with gangrene, other extremity NRS 🅐

I70.269 Atherosclerosis of native arteries of extremities with gangrene, unspecified extremity 🅐▽

✓6ᵗʰ **I70.29** Other atherosclerosis of native arteries of extremities

I70.291 Other atherosclerosis of native arteries of extremities, right leg 🅐

I70.292 Other atherosclerosis of native arteries of extremities, left leg 🅐

I70.293 Other atherosclerosis of native arteries of extremities, bilateral legs 🅐

I70.298 Other atherosclerosis of native arteries of extremities, other extremity 🅐

I70.299 Other atherosclerosis of native arteries of extremities, unspecified extremity 🅐▽

✓5ᵗʰ **I70.3** Atherosclerosis of unspecified type of bypass graft(s) of the extremities
> Use additional code, if applicable, to identify chronic total occlusion of artery of extremity (I70.92)
> EXCLUDES 1 embolism or thrombus of bypass graft(s) of extremities (T82.8-)

✓6ᵗʰ **I70.30** Unspecified atherosclerosis of unspecified type of bypass graft(s) of the extremities

I70.301 Unspecified atherosclerosis of unspecified type of bypass graft(s) of the extremities, right leg 🅐▽

I70.302 Unspecified atherosclerosis of unspecified type of bypass graft(s) of the extremities, left leg 🅐▽

I70.303 Unspecified atherosclerosis of unspecified type of bypass graft(s) of the extremities, bilateral legs 🅐▽

I70.308 Unspecified atherosclerosis of unspecified type of bypass graft(s) of the extremities, other extremity 🅐▽

I70.309 Unspecified atherosclerosis of unspecified type of bypass graft(s) of the extremities, unspecified extremity 🅐▽

✓6ᵗʰ **I70.31** Atherosclerosis of unspecified type of bypass graft(s) of the extremities with intermittent claudication

I70.311 Atherosclerosis of unspecified type of bypass graft(s) of the extremities with intermittent claudication, right leg 🅐

I70.312 Atherosclerosis of unspecified type of bypass graft(s) of the extremities with intermittent claudication, left leg 🅐

I70.313 Atherosclerosis of unspecified type of bypass graft(s) of the extremities with intermittent claudication, bilateral legs 🅐

I70.318 Atherosclerosis of unspecified type of bypass graft(s) of the extremities with intermittent claudication, other extremity 🅐

I70.319 Atherosclerosis of unspecified type of bypass graft(s) of the extremities with intermittent claudication, unspecified extremity 🅐▽

✓6ᵗʰ **I70.32** Atherosclerosis of unspecified type of bypass graft(s) of the extremities with rest pain
> INCLUDES any condition classifiable to I70.31-

I70.321 Atherosclerosis of unspecified type of bypass graft(s) of the extremities with rest pain, right leg 🅐

I70.322 Atherosclerosis of unspecified type of bypass graft(s) of the extremities with rest pain, left leg 🅐

I70.323 Atherosclerosis of unspecified type of bypass graft(s) of the extremities with rest pain, bilateral legs 🅐

I70.328 Atherosclerosis of unspecified type of bypass graft(s) of the extremities with rest pain, other extremity 🅐

I70.329 Atherosclerosis of unspecified type of bypass graft(s) of the extremities with rest pain, unspecified extremity 🅐▽

✓6ᵗʰ **I70.33** Atherosclerosis of unspecified type of bypass graft(s) of the right leg with ulceration
> INCLUDES any condition classifiable to I70.311 and I70.321
> Use additional code to identify severity of ulcer (L97.-)

I70.331 Atherosclerosis of unspecified type of bypass graft(s) of the right leg with ulceration of thigh NRS 🅐

I70.332 Atherosclerosis of unspecified type of bypass graft(s) of the right leg with ulceration of calf NRS 🅐

I70.333 Atherosclerosis of unspecified type of bypass graft(s) of the right leg with ulceration of ankle NRS 🅐

I70.334 Atherosclerosis of unspecified type of bypass graft(s) of the right leg with ulceration of heel and midfoot NRS 🅐
> Atherosclerosis of unspecified type of bypass graft(s) of right leg with ulceration of plantar surface of midfoot

I70.335 Atherosclerosis of unspecified type of bypass graft(s) of the right leg with ulceration of other part of foot NRS 🅐
> Atherosclerosis of unspecified type of bypass graft(s) of the right leg with ulceration of toe

I70.338 Atherosclerosis of unspecified type of bypass graft(s) of the right leg with ulceration of other part of lower leg NRS 🅐

☑ Additional Character Req   ✓7ᵗʰ Placeholder Alert   Case-Mix Diagnosis   Manifestation   ▽ Unspecified Dx   EXCLUDES 1 Not coded here   EXCLUDES 2 Not included here

ICD-10-CM 2018   641

I70.339   Atherosclerosis of unspecified type of bypass graft(s) of the right leg with ulceration of unspecified site   A▽

✓6ᵗʰ I70.34   **Atherosclerosis of unspecified type of bypass graft(s) of the left leg with ulceration**
INCLUDES   any condition classifiable to I70.312 and I70.322
Use additional code to identify severity of ulcer (L97.-)

    I70.341   **Atherosclerosis of unspecified type of bypass graft(s) of the left leg with ulceration of thigh**   NRS A

    I70.342   **Atherosclerosis of unspecified type of bypass graft(s) of the left leg with ulceration of calf**   NRS A

    I70.343   **Atherosclerosis of unspecified type of bypass graft(s) of the left leg with ulceration of ankle**   NRS A

    I70.344   **Atherosclerosis of unspecified type of bypass graft(s) of the left leg with ulceration of heel and midfoot**   NRS A
      Atherosclerosis of unspecified type of bypass graft(s) of left leg with ulceration of plantar surface of midfoot

    I70.345   **Atherosclerosis of unspecified type of bypass graft(s) of the left leg with ulceration of other part of foot**   NRS A
      Atherosclerosis of unspecified type of bypass graft(s) of the left leg with ulceration of toe

    I70.348   **Atherosclerosis of unspecified type of bypass graft(s) of the left leg with ulceration of other part of lower leg**   NRS A

    I70.349   **Atherosclerosis of unspecified type of bypass graft(s) of the left leg with ulceration of unspecified site**   A▽

I70.35   **Atherosclerosis of unspecified type of bypass graft(s) of other extremity with ulceration**   NRS A
INCLUDES   any condition classifiable to I70.318 and I70.328
Use additional code to identify severity of ulcer (L98.49-)

✓6ᵗʰ I70.36   **Atherosclerosis of unspecified type of bypass graft(s) of the extremities with gangrene**
INCLUDES   any condition classifiable to I70.31-, I70.32-, I70.33-, I70.34-, I70.35
Use additional code to identify the severity of any ulcer (L97.-, L98.49-), if applicable

    I70.361   **Atherosclerosis of unspecified type of bypass graft(s) of the extremities with gangrene, right leg**   NRS A

    I70.362   **Atherosclerosis of unspecified type of bypass graft(s) of the extremities with gangrene, left leg**   NRS A

    I70.363   **Atherosclerosis of unspecified type of bypass graft(s) of the extremities with gangrene, bilateral legs**   NRS A

    I70.368   **Atherosclerosis of unspecified type of bypass graft(s) of the extremities with gangrene, other extremity**   NRS A

    I70.369   **Atherosclerosis of unspecified type of bypass graft(s) of the extremities with gangrene, unspecified extremity**   A▽

✓6ᵗʰ I70.39   **Other atherosclerosis of unspecified type of bypass graft(s) of the extremities**

    I70.391   **Other atherosclerosis of unspecified type of bypass graft(s) of the extremities, right leg**   A

    I70.392   **Other atherosclerosis of unspecified type of bypass graft(s) of the extremities, left leg**   A

    I70.393   **Other atherosclerosis of unspecified type of bypass graft(s) of the extremities, bilateral legs**   A

    I70.398   **Other atherosclerosis of unspecified type of bypass graft(s) of the extremities, other extremity**   A

    I70.399   **Other atherosclerosis of unspecified type of bypass graft(s) of the extremities, unspecified extremity**   A▽

✓5ᵗʰ I70.4   **Atherosclerosis of autologous vein bypass graft(s) of the extremities**
Use additional code, if applicable, to identify chronic total occlusion of artery of extremity (I70.92)

✓6ᵗʰ I70.40   **Unspecified atherosclerosis of autologous vein bypass graft(s) of the extremities**

    I70.401   **Unspecified atherosclerosis of autologous vein bypass graft(s) of the extremities, right leg**   A▽

    I70.402   **Unspecified atherosclerosis of autologous vein bypass graft(s) of the extremities, left leg**   A▽

    I70.403   **Unspecified atherosclerosis of autologous vein bypass graft(s) of the extremities, bilateral legs**   A▽

    I70.408   **Unspecified atherosclerosis of autologous vein bypass graft(s) of the extremities, other extremity**   A▽

    I70.409   **Unspecified atherosclerosis of autologous vein bypass graft(s) of the extremities, unspecified extremity**   A▽

✓6ᵗʰ I70.41   **Atherosclerosis of autologous vein bypass graft(s) of the extremities with intermittent claudication**

    I70.411   **Atherosclerosis of autologous vein bypass graft(s) of the extremities with intermittent claudication, right leg**   A

    I70.412   **Atherosclerosis of autologous vein bypass graft(s) of the extremities with intermittent claudication, left leg**   A

    I70.413   **Atherosclerosis of autologous vein bypass graft(s) of the extremities with intermittent claudication, bilateral legs**   A

    I70.418   **Atherosclerosis of autologous vein bypass graft(s) of the extremities with intermittent claudication, other extremity**   A

    I70.419   **Atherosclerosis of autologous vein bypass graft(s) of the extremities with intermittent claudication, unspecified extremity**   A▽

✓6ᵗʰ I70.42   **Atherosclerosis of autologous vein bypass graft(s) of the extremities with rest pain**
INCLUDES   any condition classifiable to I70.41-

    I70.421   **Atherosclerosis of autologous vein bypass graft(s) of the extremities with rest pain, right leg**   A

    I70.422   **Atherosclerosis of autologous vein bypass graft(s) of the extremities with rest pain, left leg**   A

    I70.423   **Atherosclerosis of autologous vein bypass graft(s) of the extremities with rest pain, bilateral legs**   A

    I70.428   **Atherosclerosis of autologous vein bypass graft(s) of the extremities with rest pain, other extremity**   A

    I70.429   **Atherosclerosis of autologous vein bypass graft(s) of the extremities with rest pain, unspecified extremity**   A▽

✓6ᵗʰ I70.43   **Atherosclerosis of autologous vein bypass graft(s) of the right leg with ulceration**
INCLUDES   any condition classifiable to I70.411 and I70.421
Use additional code to identify severity of ulcer (L97.-)

    I70.431   **Atherosclerosis of autologous vein bypass graft(s) of the right leg with ulceration of thigh**   NRS A

    I70.432   **Atherosclerosis of autologous vein bypass graft(s) of the right leg with ulceration of calf**   NRS A

    I70.433   **Atherosclerosis of autologous vein bypass graft(s) of the right leg with ulceration of ankle**   NRS A

    I70.434   **Atherosclerosis of autologous vein bypass graft(s) of the right leg with ulceration of heel and midfoot**   NRS A
      Atherosclerosis of autologous vein bypass graft(s) of right leg with ulceration of plantar surface of midfoot

N Newborn: 0   P Pediatric: 0-17   M Maternity: 12-55   A Adult: 15-124   NRS Nonroutine supply Dx   NCDx Noncancer Dx   PDx Primary Dx   ▶◀ Revised Text   ● New Code   ▲ Revised Title

642   ICD-10-CM 2018

I70.435   **Atherosclerosis of autologous vein** `NRS` `A` **bypass graft(s) of the right leg with ulceration of other** part of foot

Atherosclerosis of autologous vein bypass graft(s) of right leg with ulceration of toe

I70.438   **Atherosclerosis of autologous vein** `NRS` `A` **bypass graft(s) of the right leg with ulceration of other** part of lower leg

I70.439   **Atherosclerosis of autologous vein** `A` `▽` **bypass graft(s) of the right leg with ulceration of unspecified site**

`✓6ᵗʰ` **I70.44**   **Atherosclerosis of autologous vein bypass graft(s) of the** left leg with **ulceration**

`INCLUDES`   any condition classifiable to I70.412 and I70.422

Use additional code to identify severity of ulcer (L97.-)

I70.441   **Atherosclerosis of autologous vein** `NRS` `A` **bypass graft(s) of the left leg with ulceration of** thigh

I70.442   **Atherosclerosis of autologous vein** `NRS` `A` **bypass graft(s) of the left leg with ulceration of** calf

I70.443   **Atherosclerosis of autologous vein** `NRS` `A` **bypass graft(s) of the left leg with ulceration of** ankle

I70.444   **Atherosclerosis of autologous vein** `NRS` `A` **bypass graft(s) of the left leg with ulceration of** heel and midfoot

Atherosclerosis of autologous vein bypass graft(s) of left leg with ulceration of plantar surface of midfoot

I70.445   **Atherosclerosis of autologous vein** `NRS` `A` **bypass graft(s) of the left leg with ulceration of other** part of foot

Atherosclerosis of autologous vein bypass graft(s) of left leg with ulceration of toe

I70.448   **Atherosclerosis of autologous vein** `NRS` `A` **bypass graft(s) of the left leg with ulceration of other** part of lower leg

I70.449   **Atherosclerosis of autologous vein** `A` `▽` **bypass graft(s) of the left leg with ulceration of unspecified site**

I70.45   **Atherosclerosis of autologous vein bypass** `NRS` `A` **graft(s) of other extremity with** ulceration

`INCLUDES`   any condition classifiable to I70.418, I70.428, and I70.438

Use additional code to identify severity of ulcer (L98.49)

`✓6ᵗʰ` **I70.46**   **Atherosclerosis of autologous vein bypass graft(s) of the extremities with** gangrene

`INCLUDES`   any condition classifiable to I70.41-, I70.42-, and I70.43-, I70.44-, I70.45

Use additional code to identify the severity of any ulcer (L97.-, L98.49-), if applicable

I70.461   **Atherosclerosis of autologous vein** `NRS` `A` **bypass graft(s) of the extremities with gangrene,** right leg

I70.462   **Atherosclerosis of autologous vein** `NRS` `A` **bypass graft(s) of the extremities with gangrene,** left leg

I70.463   **Atherosclerosis of autologous vein** `NRS` `A` **bypass graft(s) of the extremities with gangrene,** bilateral legs

I70.468   **Atherosclerosis of autologous vein** `NRS` `A` **bypass graft(s) of the extremities with gangrene, other extremity**

I70.469   **Atherosclerosis of autologous vein** `A` `▽` **bypass graft(s) of the extremities with gangrene, unspecified extremity**

`✓6ᵗʰ` **I70.49**   Other **atherosclerosis of autologous vein bypass graft(s) of the extremities**

I70.491   **Other atherosclerosis of autologous** `A` **vein bypass graft(s) of the extremities,** right leg

I70.492   **Other atherosclerosis of autologous** `A` **vein bypass graft(s) of the extremities,** left leg

I70.493   **Other atherosclerosis of autologous** `A` **vein bypass graft(s) of the extremities,** bilateral legs

I70.498   **Other atherosclerosis of autologous** `A` **vein bypass graft(s) of the extremities, other extremity**

I70.499   **Other atherosclerosis of autologous** `A` `▽` **vein bypass graft(s) of the extremities, unspecified extremity**

`✓5ᵗʰ` **I70.5**   **Atherosclerosis of** nonautologous biological bypass graft(s) **of the** extremities

Use additional code, if applicable, to identify chronic total occlusion of artery of extremity (I70.92)

`✓6ᵗʰ` **I70.50**   Unspecified **atherosclerosis of nonautologous biological bypass graft(s) of the extremities**

I70.501   **Unspecified atherosclerosis of** `A` `▽` **nonautologous biological bypass graft(s) of the extremities,** right leg

I70.502   **Unspecified atherosclerosis of** `A` `▽` **nonautologous biological bypass graft(s) of the extremities,** left leg

I70.503   **Unspecified atherosclerosis of** `A` `▽` **nonautologous biological bypass graft(s) of the extremities,** bilateral legs

I70.508   **Unspecified atherosclerosis of** `A` `▽` **nonautologous biological bypass graft(s) of the extremities, other extremity**

I70.509   **Unspecified atherosclerosis of** `A` `▽` **nonautologous biological bypass graft(s) of the extremities, unspecified extremity**

`✓6ᵗʰ` **I70.51**   **Atherosclerosis of nonautologous biological bypass graft(s) of the extremities** intermittent claudication

I70.511   **Atherosclerosis of nonautologous** `A` **biological bypass graft(s) of the extremities with intermittent claudication,** right leg

I70.512   **Atherosclerosis of nonautologous** `A` **biological bypass graft(s) of the extremities with intermittent claudication,** left leg

I70.513   **Atherosclerosis of nonautologous** `A` **biological bypass graft(s) of the extremities with intermittent claudication,** bilateral legs

I70.518   **Atherosclerosis of nonautologous** `A` **biological bypass graft(s) of the extremities with intermittent claudication, other extremity**

I70.519   **Atherosclerosis of nonautologous** `A` `▽` **biological bypass graft(s) of the extremities with intermittent claudication, unspecified extremity**

`✓6ᵗʰ` **I70.52**   **Atherosclerosis of nonautologous biological bypass graft(s) of the extremities with** rest pain

`INCLUDES`   any condition classifiable to I70.51-

I70.521   **Atherosclerosis of nonautologous** `A` **biological bypass graft(s) of the extremities with rest pain,** right leg

I70.522   **Atherosclerosis of nonautologous** `A` **biological bypass graft(s) of the extremities with rest pain,** left leg

I70.523   **Atherosclerosis of nonautologous** `A` **biological bypass graft(s) of the extremities with rest pain,** bilateral legs

I70.528   **Atherosclerosis of nonautologous** `A` **biological bypass graft(s) of the extremities with rest pain, other extremity**

I70.529   **Atherosclerosis of nonautologous** `A` `▽` **biological bypass graft(s) of the extremities with rest pain, unspecified extremity**

`✓6ᵗʰ` **I70.53**   **Atherosclerosis of nonautologous biological bypass graft(s) of the** right leg with ulceration

`INCLUDES`   any condition classifiable to I70.511 and I70.521

Use additional code to identify severity of ulcer (L97.-)

I70.531   **Atherosclerosis of nonautologous** `NRS` `A` **biological bypass graft(s) of the right leg with ulceration of** thigh

I70.532   **Atherosclerosis of nonautologous** `NRS` `A` **biological bypass graft(s) of the right leg with ulceration of** calf

☑ Additional Character Req   `✓x7ᵗʰ` Placeholder Alert   Case-Mix Diagnosis   Manifestation   ▽ Unspecified Dx   `EXCLUDES 1` Not coded here   `EXCLUDES 2` Not included here

ICD-10-CM 2018   643

Chapter 9. Diseases of the Circulatory System

I70.533 Atherosclerosis of nonautologous biological bypass graft(s) of the right leg with ulceration of ankle [NRS] [A]

I70.534 Atherosclerosis of nonautologous biological bypass graft(s) of the right leg with ulceration of heel and midfoot [NRS] [A]
Atherosclerosis of nonautologous biological bypass graft(s) of right leg with ulceration of plantar surface of midfoot

I70.535 Atherosclerosis of nonautologous biological bypass graft(s) of the right leg with ulceration of other part of foot [NRS] [A]
Atherosclerosis of nonautologous biological bypass graft(s) of the right leg with ulceration of toe

I70.538 Atherosclerosis of nonautologous biological bypass graft(s) of the right leg with ulceration of other part of lower leg [NRS] [A]

I70.539 Atherosclerosis of nonautologous biological bypass graft(s) of the right leg with ulceration of unspecified site [A] [▽]

✓6th I70.54 Atherosclerosis of nonautologous biological bypass graft(s) of the left leg with ulceration
INCLUDES any condition classifiable to I70.512 and I70.522
Use additional code to identify severity of ulcer (L97.-)

I70.541 Atherosclerosis of nonautologous biological bypass graft(s) of the left leg with ulceration of thigh [NRS] [A]

I70.542 Atherosclerosis of nonautologous biological bypass graft(s) of the left leg with ulceration of calf [NRS] [A]

I70.543 Atherosclerosis of nonautologous biological bypass graft(s) of the left leg with ulceration of ankle [NRS] [A]

I70.544 Atherosclerosis of nonautologous biological bypass graft(s) of the left leg with ulceration of heel and midfoot [NRS] [A]
Atherosclerosis of nonautologous biological bypass graft(s) of left leg with ulceration of plantar surface of midfoot

I70.545 Atherosclerosis of nonautologous biological bypass graft(s) of the left leg with ulceration of other part of foot [NRS] [A]
Atherosclerosis of nonautologous biological bypass graft(s) of the left leg with ulceration of toe

I70.548 Atherosclerosis of nonautologous biological bypass graft(s) of the left leg with ulceration of other part of lower leg [NRS] [A]

I70.549 Atherosclerosis of nonautologous biological bypass graft(s) of the left leg with ulceration of unspecified site [A] [▽]

I70.55 Atherosclerosis of nonautologous biological bypass graft(s) of other extremity with ulceration [NRS] [A]
INCLUDES any condition classifiable to I70.518, I70.528, and I70.538
Use additional code to identify severity of ulcer (L98.49)

✓6th I70.56 Atherosclerosis of nonautologous biological bypass graft(s) of the extremities with gangrene
INCLUDES any condition classifiable to I70.51-, I70.52-, and I70.53-, I70.54-, I70.55
Use additional code to identify the severity of any ulcer (L97.-, L98.49-), if applicable

I70.561 Atherosclerosis of nonautologous biological bypass graft(s) of the extremities with gangrene, right leg [NRS] [A]

I70.562 Atherosclerosis of nonautologous biological bypass graft(s) of the extremities with gangrene, left leg [NRS] [A]

I70.563 Atherosclerosis of nonautologous biological bypass graft(s) of the extremities with gangrene, bilateral legs [NRS] [A]

I70.568 Atherosclerosis of nonautologous biological bypass graft(s) of the extremities with gangrene, other extremity [NRS] [A]

I70.569 Atherosclerosis of nonautologous biological bypass graft(s) of the extremities with gangrene, unspecified extremity [A] [▽]

✓6th I70.59 Other atherosclerosis of nonautologous biological bypass graft(s) of the extremities

I70.591 Other atherosclerosis of nonautologous biological bypass graft(s) of the extremities, right leg [A]

I70.592 Other atherosclerosis of nonautologous biological bypass graft(s) of the extremities, left leg [A]

I70.593 Other atherosclerosis of nonautologous biological bypass graft(s) of the extremities, bilateral legs [A]

I70.598 Other atherosclerosis of nonautologous biological bypass graft(s) of the extremities, other extremity [A]

I70.599 Other atherosclerosis of nonautologous biological bypass graft(s) of the extremities, unspecified extremity [A] [▽]

✓5th I70.6 Atherosclerosis of nonbiological bypass graft(s) of the extremities
Use additional code, if applicable, to identify chronic total occlusion of artery of extremity (I70.92)

✓6th I70.60 Unspecified atherosclerosis of nonbiological bypass graft(s) of the extremities

I70.601 Unspecified atherosclerosis of nonbiological bypass graft(s) of the extremities, right leg [A] [▽]

I70.602 Unspecified atherosclerosis of nonbiological bypass graft(s) of the extremities, left leg [A] [▽]

I70.603 Unspecified atherosclerosis of nonbiological bypass graft(s) of the extremities, bilateral legs [A] [▽]

I70.608 Unspecified atherosclerosis of nonbiological bypass graft(s) of the extremities, other extremity [A] [▽]

I70.609 Unspecified atherosclerosis of nonbiological bypass graft(s) of the extremities, unspecified extremity [A] [▽]

✓6th I70.61 Atherosclerosis of nonbiological bypass graft(s) of the extremities with intermittent claudication

I70.611 Atherosclerosis of nonbiological bypass graft(s) of the extremities with intermittent claudication, right leg [A]

I70.612 Atherosclerosis of nonbiological bypass graft(s) of the extremities with intermittent claudication, left leg [A]

I70.613 Atherosclerosis of nonbiological bypass graft(s) of the extremities with intermittent claudication, bilateral legs [A]

I70.618 Atherosclerosis of nonbiological bypass graft(s) of the extremities with intermittent claudication, other extremity [A]

I70.619 Atherosclerosis of nonbiological bypass graft(s) of the extremities with intermittent claudication, unspecified extremity [A] [▽]

✓6th I70.62 Atherosclerosis of nonbiological bypass graft(s) of the extremities with rest pain
INCLUDES any condition classifiable to I70.61-

I70.621 Atherosclerosis of nonbiological bypass graft(s) of the extremities with rest pain, right leg [A]

I70.622 Atherosclerosis of nonbiological bypass graft(s) of the extremities with rest pain, left leg [A]

I70.623 Atherosclerosis of nonbiological bypass graft(s) of the extremities with rest pain, bilateral legs [A]

I70.628 Atherosclerosis of nonbiological bypass graft(s) of the extremities with rest pain, other extremity [A]

I70.629 Atherosclerosis of nonbiological bypass graft(s) of the extremities with rest pain, unspecified extremity [A] [▽]

[N] Newborn: 0   [P] Pediatric: 0-17   [M] Maternity: 12-55   [A] Adult: 15-124   [NRS] Nonroutine supply Dx   [NCDx] Noncancer Dx   [PDx] Primary Dx   ►◄ Revised Text   ● New Code   ▲ Revised Title

644   ICD-10-CM 2018

✓6ᵗʰ **I70.63** **Atherosclerosis of nonbiological bypass graft(s) of the right leg with ulceration**
> INCLUDES   any condition classifiable to I70.611 and I70.621
> Use additional code to identify severity of ulcer (L97.-)

I70.631 **Atherosclerosis of nonbiological bypass graft(s) of the right leg with ulceration of thigh** NRS A

I70.632 **Atherosclerosis of nonbiological bypass graft(s) of the right leg with ulceration of calf** NRS A

I70.633 **Atherosclerosis of nonbiological bypass graft(s) of the right leg with ulceration of ankle** NRS A

I70.634 **Atherosclerosis of nonbiological bypass graft(s) of the right leg with ulceration of heel and midfoot** NRS A
> Atherosclerosis of nonbiological bypass graft(s) of right leg with ulceration of plantar surface of midfoot

I70.635 **Atherosclerosis of nonbiological bypassgraft(s) of the right leg with ulceration of other part of foot** NRS A
> Atherosclerosis of nonbiological bypass graft(s) of the right leg with ulceration of toe

I70.638 **Atherosclerosis of nonbiological bypassgraft(s) of the right leg with ulceration of other part of lower leg** NRS A

I70.639 **Atherosclerosis of nonbiological bypass graft(s) of the right leg with ulceration of unspecified site** A ▽

✓6ᵗʰ **I70.64** **Atherosclerosis of nonbiological bypass graft(s) of the left leg with ulceration**
> INCLUDES   any condition classifiable to I70.612 and I70.622
> Use additional code to identify severity of ulcer (L97.-)

I70.641 **Atherosclerosis of nonbiological bypass graft(s) of the left leg with ulceration of thigh** NRS A

I70.642 **Atherosclerosis of nonbiological bypass graft(s) of the left leg with ulceration of calf** NRS A

I70.643 **Atherosclerosis of nonbiological bypass graft(s) of the left leg with ulceration of ankle** NRS A

I70.644 **Atherosclerosis of nonbiological bypass graft(s) of the left leg with ulceration of heel and midfoot** NRS A
> Atherosclerosis of nonbiological bypass graft(s) of left leg with ulceration of plantar surface of midfoot

I70.645 **Atherosclerosis of nonbiological bypass graft(s) of the left leg with ulceration of other part of foot** NRS A
> Atherosclerosis of nonbiological bypass graft(s) of the left leg with ulceration of toe

I70.648 **Atherosclerosis of nonbiological bypass graft(s) of the left leg with ulceration of other part of lower leg** NRS A

I70.649 **Atherosclerosis of nonbiological bypass graft(s) of the left leg with ulceration of unspecified site** A ▽

I70.65 **Atherosclerosis of nonbiological bypass graft(s) of other extremity with ulceration** NRS A
> INCLUDES   any condition classifiable to I70.618 and I70.628
> Use additional code to identify severity of ulcer (L98.49)

✓6ᵗʰ **I70.66** **Atherosclerosis of nonbiological bypass graft(s) of the extremities with gangrene**
> INCLUDES   any condition classifiable to I70.61-, I70.62-, I70.63-, I70.64-, I70.65
> Use additional code to identify the severity of any ulcer (L97.-, L98.49-), if applicable

I70.661 **Atherosclerosis of nonbiological bypass graft(s) of the extremities with gangrene, right leg** NRS A

I70.662 **Atherosclerosis of nonbiological bypass graft(s) of the extremities with gangrene, left leg** NRS A

I70.663 **Atherosclerosis of nonbiological bypass graft(s) of the extremities with gangrene, bilateral legs** NRS A

I70.668 **Atherosclerosis of nonbiological bypass graft(s) of the extremities with gangrene, other extremity** NRS A

I70.669 **Atherosclerosis of nonbiological bypass graft(s) of the extremities with gangrene, unspecified extremity** A ▽

✓6ᵗʰ **I70.69** **Other atherosclerosis of nonbiological bypass graft(s) of the extremities**

I70.691 **Other atherosclerosis of nonbiological bypass graft(s) of the extremities, right leg** A

I70.692 **Other atherosclerosis of nonbiological bypass graft(s) of the extremities, left leg** A

I70.693 **Other atherosclerosis of nonbiological bypass graft(s) of the extremities, bilateral legs** A

I70.698 **Other atherosclerosis of nonbiological bypass graft(s) of the extremities, other extremity** A

I70.699 **Other atherosclerosis of nonbiological bypass graft(s) of the extremities, unspecified extremity** A ▽

✓5ᵗʰ **I70.7** **Atherosclerosis of other type of bypass graft(s) of the extremities**
> Use additional code, if applicable, to identify chronic total occlusion of artery of extremity (I70.92)

✓6ᵗʰ **I70.70** **Unspecified atherosclerosis of other type of bypass graft(s) of the extremities**

I70.701 **Unspecified atherosclerosis of other type of bypass graft(s) of the extremities, right leg** A ▽

I70.702 **Unspecified atherosclerosis of other type of bypass graft(s) of the extremities, left leg** A ▽

I70.703 **Unspecified atherosclerosis of other type of bypass graft(s) of the extremities, bilateral legs** A ▽

I70.708 **Unspecified atherosclerosis of other type of bypass graft(s) of the extremities, other extremity** A ▽

I70.709 **Unspecified atherosclerosis of other type of bypass graft(s) of the extremities, unspecified extremity** A ▽

✓6ᵗʰ **I70.71** **Atherosclerosis of other type of bypass graft(s) of the extremities with intermittent claudication**

I70.711 **Atherosclerosis of other type of bypass graft(s) of the extremities with intermittent claudication, right leg** A

I70.712 **Atherosclerosis of other type of bypass graft(s) of the extremities with intermittent claudication, left leg** A

I70.713 **Atherosclerosis of other type of bypass graft(s) of the extremities with intermittent claudication, bilateral legs** A

I70.718 **Atherosclerosis of other type of bypass graft(s) of the extremities with intermittent claudication, other extremity** A

I70.719 **Atherosclerosis of other type of graft(s) bypass of the extremities with intermittent claudication, unspecified extremity** A ▽

✓6ᵗʰ **I70.72** **Atherosclerosis of other type of bypass graft(s) of the extremities with rest pain**
> INCLUDES   any condition classifiable to I70.71-

I70.721 **Atherosclerosis of other type of bypass graft(s) of the extremities with rest pain, right leg** A

I70.722 **Atherosclerosis of other type of bypass graft(s) of the extremities with rest pain, left leg** A

I70.723 **Atherosclerosis of other type of bypass graft(s) of the extremities with rest pain, bilateral legs** A

I70.728 **Atherosclerosis of other type of bypass graft(s) of the extremities with rest pain, other extremity** A

✓ Additional Character Req   ✓ᴬ7ᵗʰ Placeholder Alert   Case-Mix Diagnosis   Manifestation   ▽ Unspecified Dx   EXCLUDES1 Not coded here   EXCLUDES2 Not included here

ICD-10-CM 2018   645

Chapter 9. Diseases of the Circulatory System

I70.729   Atherosclerosis of other type of bypass graft(s) of the extremities with rest pain, unspecified extremity   A ▽

✓6ᵗʰ **I70.73**   Atherosclerosis of other type of bypass graft(s) of the right leg with ulceration
   INCLUDES   any condition classifiable to I70.711 and I70.721
   Use additional code to identify severity of ulcer (L97.-)

I70.731   Atherosclerosis of other type of bypass graft(s) of the right leg with ulceration of thigh   NRS A

I70.732   Atherosclerosis of other type of bypass graft(s) of the right leg with ulceration of calf   NRS A

I70.733   Atherosclerosis of other type of bypass graft(s) of the right leg with ulceration of ankle   NRS A

I70.734   Atherosclerosis of other type of bypass graft(s) of the right leg with ulceration of heel and midfoot   NRS A
   Atherosclerosis of other type of bypass graft(s) of right leg with ulceration of plantar surface of midfoot

I70.735   Atherosclerosis of other type of bypass graft(s) of the right leg with ulceration of other part of foot   NRS A
   Atherosclerosis of other type of bypass graft(s) of right leg with ulceration of toe

I70.738   Atherosclerosis of other type of bypass graft(s) of the right leg with ulceration of other part of lower leg   NRS A

I70.739   Atherosclerosis of other type of bypass graft(s) of the right leg with ulceration of unspecified site   A ▽

✓6ᵗʰ **I70.74**   Atherosclerosis of other type of bypass graft(s) of the left leg with ulceration
   INCLUDES   any condition classifiable to I70.712 and I70.722
   Use additional code to identify severity of ulcer (L97.-)

I70.741   Atherosclerosis of other type of bypass graft(s) of the left leg with ulceration of thigh   NRS A

I70.742   Atherosclerosis of other type of bypass graft(s) of the left leg with ulceration of calf   NRS A

I70.743   Atherosclerosis of other type of bypass graft(s) of the left leg with ulceration of ankle   NRS A

I70.744   Atherosclerosis of other type of bypass graft(s) of the left leg with ulceration of heel and midfoot   NRS A
   Atherosclerosis of other type of bypass graft(s) of left leg with ulceration of plantar surface of midfoot

I70.745   Atherosclerosis of other type of bypass graft(s) of the left leg with ulceration of other part of foot   NRS A
   Atherosclerosis of other type of bypass graft(s) of left leg with ulceration of toe

I70.748   Atherosclerosis of other type of bypass graft(s) of the left leg with ulceration of other part of lower leg   NRS A

I70.749   Atherosclerosis of other type of bypass graft(s) of the left leg with ulceration of unspecified site   A ▽

I70.75   Atherosclerosis of other type of bypass graft(s) of other extremity with ulceration   NRS A
   INCLUDES   any condition classifiable to I70.718 and I70.728
   Use additional code to identify severity of ulcer (L98.49)

✓6ᵗʰ **I70.76**   Atherosclerosis of other type of bypass graft(s) of the extremities with gangrene
   INCLUDES   any condition classifiable to I70.71-, I70.72-, I70.73-, I70.74-, I70.75
   Use additional code to identify the severity of any ulcer (L97.-, L98.49-), if applicable

I70.761   Atherosclerosis of other type of bypassgraft(s) of the extremities with gangrene, right leg   NRS A

I70.762   Atherosclerosis of other type of bypassgraft(s) of the extremities with gangrene, left leg   NRS A

I70.763   Atherosclerosis of other type of bypassgraft(s) of the extremities with gangrene, bilateral legs   NRS A

I70.768   Atherosclerosis of other type of bypassgraft(s) of the extremities with gangrene, other extremity   NRS A

I70.769   Atherosclerosis of other type of bypass graft(s) of the extremities with gangrene, unspecified extremity   A ▽

✓6ᵗʰ **I70.79**   Other atherosclerosis of other type of bypass graft(s) of the extremities

I70.791   Other atherosclerosis of other type of bypass graft(s) of the extremities, right leg   A

I70.792   Other atherosclerosis of other type of bypass graft(s) of the extremities, left leg   A

I70.793   Other atherosclerosis of other type of bypass graft(s) of the extremities, bilateral legs   A

I70.798   Other atherosclerosis of other type of bypass graft(s) of the extremities, other extremity   A

I70.799   Other atherosclerosis of other type of bypass graft(s) of the extremities, unspecified extremity   A ▽

I70.8   Atherosclerosis of other arteries   A
   TIP: Arteriosclerosis of the iliac arteries is coded here.

✓5ᵗʰ **I70.9**   Other and unspecified atherosclerosis

I70.90   Unspecified atherosclerosis   A ▽

I70.91   Generalized atherosclerosis   A

I70.92   Chronic total occlusion of artery of the extremities   A
   Complete occlusion of artery of the extremities
   Total occlusion of artery of the extremities
   Code first atherosclerosis of arteries of the extremities (I70.2-, I70.3-, I70.4-, I70.5-, I70.6-, I70.7-)

✓4ᵗʰ **I71**   **Aortic aneurysm and dissection**
   EXCLUDES 1   aortic ectasia (I77.81-)
       syphilitic aortic aneurysm (A52.01)
       traumatic aortic aneurysm (S25.09, S35.09)

✓5ᵗʰ **I71.0**   Dissection of aorta

I71.00   Dissection of unspecified site of aorta   ▽

I71.01   Dissection of thoracic aorta

I71.02   Dissection of abdominal aorta

I71.03   Dissection of thoracoabdominal aorta

I71.1   Thoracic aortic aneurysm, ruptured

I71.2   Thoracic aortic aneurysm, without rupture

I71.3   Abdominal aortic aneurysm, ruptured

I71.4   Abdominal aortic aneurysm, without rupture

I71.5   Thoracoabdominal aortic aneurysm, ruptured

I71.6   Thoracoabdominal aortic aneurysm, without rupture

I71.8   Aortic aneurysm of unspecified site, ruptured   ▽
   Rupture of aorta NOS

I71.9   Aortic aneurysm of unspecified site, without rupture   ▽
   Aneurysm of aorta
   Dilatation of aorta
   Hyaline necrosis of aorta

Ⓝ Newborn: 0   Ⓟ Pediatric: 0-17   Ⓜ Maternity: 12-55   Ⓐ Adult: 15-124   **NRS** Nonroutine supply Dx   **NCDx** Noncancer Dx   **PDx** Primary Dx   ▶◀ Revised Text   ● New Code   ▲ Revised Title

646   ICD-10-CM 2018

Aneurysm

Layers of muscular and elastic tissue

Outer layer

Inner layer

Aneurysm

Aneurysm

☑4ᵗʰ I72   Other aneurysm
INCLUDES aneurysm (cirsoid) (false) (ruptured)
EXCLUDES 2 *acquired aneurysm (I77.0)*
aneurysm (of) aorta (I71.-)
aneurysm (of) arteriovenous NOS (Q27.3-)
carotid artery dissection (I77.71)
cerebral (nonruptured) aneurysm (I67.1)
coronary aneurysm (I25.4)
coronary artery dissection (I25.42)
dissection of artery NEC (I77.79)
dissection of precerebral artery, congenital (nonruptured) (Q28.1)
heart aneurysm (I25.3)
iliac artery dissection (I77.72)
▶*precerebral artery, congenital (nonruptured) (Q28.1)*◀
pulmonary artery aneurysm (I28.1)
renal artery dissection (I77.73)
retinal aneurysm (H35.0)
ruptured cerebral aneurysm (I60.7)
varicose aneurysm (I77.0)
vertebral artery dissection (I77.74)

I72.0   Aneurysm of carotid artery
Aneurysm of common carotid artery
Aneurysm of external carotid artery
Aneurysm of internal carotid artery, extracranial portion
EXCLUDES 1 *aneurysm of internal carotid artery, intracranial portion (I67.1)*
aneurysm of internal carotid artery NOS (I67.1)

I72.1   Aneurysm of artery of upper extremity

I72.2   Aneurysm of renal artery

I72.3   Aneurysm of iliac artery

I72.4   Aneurysm of artery of lower extremity

I72.5   Aneurysm of other precerebral arteries
Aneurysm of basilar artery (trunk)
EXCLUDES 2 *aneurysm of carotid artery (I72.0)*
aneurysm of vertebral artery (I72.6)
dissection of carotid artery (I77.71)
dissection of other precerebral arteries (I77.75)
dissection of vertebral artery (I77.74)

I72.6   Aneurysm of vertebral artery
EXCLUDES 2 *dissection of vertebral artery (I77.74)*

I72.8   Aneurysm of other specified arteries

I72.9   Aneurysm of unspecified site   ▽

☑4ᵗʰ I73   Other peripheral vascular diseases
EXCLUDES 2 *chilblains (T69.1)*
frostbite (T33- T34)
immersion hand or foot (T69.0-)
spasm of cerebral artery (G45.9)

☑5ᵗʰ I73.0   Raynaud's syndrome
Raynaud's disease
Raynaud's phenomenon (secondary)
I73.00   Raynaud's syndrome without gangrene
I73.01   Raynaud's syndrome with gangrene   NRS

I73.1   Thromboangiitis obliterans [Buerger's disease]
DEF: Inflammatory disease of extremity blood vessels, mainly the lower; associated with heavy tobacco use; arteries are more affected than veins; occurs primarily in young men and leads to tissue ischemia and gangrene.

☑5ᵗʰ I73.8   Other specified peripheral vascular diseases
EXCLUDES 1 *diabetic (peripheral) angiopathy (E08-E13 with .51-.52)*
I73.81   Erythromelalgia

I73.89   Other specified peripheral vascular diseases
Acrocyanosis
Erythrocyanosis
Simple acroparesthesia [Schultze's type]
Vasomotor acroparesthesia [Nothnagel's type]

I73.9   Peripheral vascular disease, unspecified   ▽
Intermittent claudication
Peripheral angiopathy NOS
Spasm of artery
EXCLUDES 1 *atherosclerosis of the extremities (I70.2--I70.7-)*

☑4ᵗʰ I74   Arterial embolism and thrombosis
INCLUDES embolic infarction
embolic occlusion
thrombotic infarction
thrombotic occlusion
Code first:
embolism and thrombosis complicating abortion or ectopic or molar pregnancy (O00-O07, O08.2)
embolism and thrombosis complicating pregnancy, childbirth and the puerperium (O88.-)
EXCLUDES 2 *atheroembolism (I75.-)*
basilar embolism and thrombosis (I63.0-I63.2, I65.1)
carotid embolism and thrombosis (I63.0-I63.2, I65.2)
cerebral embolism and thrombosis (I63.3-I63.5, I66-)
coronary embolism and thrombosis (I21-I25)
mesenteric embolism and thrombosis (K55.0-)
ophthalmic embolism and thrombosis (H34.-)
precerebral embolism and thrombosis NOS (I63.0-I63.2, I65.9)
pulmonary embolism and thrombosis (I26.-)
renal embolism and thrombosis (N28.0)
retinal embolism and thrombosis (H34.-)
septic embolism and thrombosis (I76)
vertebral embolism and thrombosis (I63.0-I63.2, I65.0)

☑5ᵗʰ I74.0   Embolism and thrombosis of abdominal aorta
I74.01   Saddle embolus of abdominal aorta
I74.09   Other arterial embolism and thrombosis of abdominal aorta
Aortic bifurcation syndrome
Aortoiliac obstruction
Leriche's syndrome

☑5ᵗʰ I74.1   Embolism and thrombosis of other and unspecified parts of aorta
I74.10   Embolism and thrombosis of unspecified parts of aorta   ▽
I74.11   Embolism and thrombosis of thoracic aorta
I74.19   Embolism and thrombosis of other parts of aorta

I74.2   Embolism and thrombosis of arteries of the upper extremities

I74.3   Embolism and thrombosis of arteries of the lower extremities

I74.4   Embolism and thrombosis of arteries of extremities, unspecified   ▽
Peripheral arterial embolism NOS

I74.5   Embolism and thrombosis of iliac artery

I74.8   Embolism and thrombosis of other arteries

I74.9   Embolism and thrombosis of unspecified artery   ▽

☑4ᵗʰ I75   Atheroembolism
INCLUDES atherothrombotic microembolism
cholesterol embolism

☑5ᵗʰ I75.0   Atheroembolism of extremities
☑6ᵗʰ I75.01   Atheroembolism of upper extremity
I75.011   Atheroembolism of right upper extremity
I75.012   Atheroembolism of left upper extremity
I75.013   Atheroembolism of bilateral upper extremities
I75.019   Atheroembolism of unspecified upper extremity   ▽
☑6ᵗʰ I75.02   Atheroembolism of lower extremity
I75.021   Atheroembolism of right lower extremity
I75.022   Atheroembolism of left lower extremity
I75.023   Atheroembolism of bilateral lower extremities
I75.029   Atheroembolism of unspecified lower extremity   ▽

☑5ᵗʰ I75.8   Atheroembolism of other sites
I75.81   Atheroembolism of kidney
Use additional code for any associated acute kidney failure and chronic kidney disease (N17.-, N18.-)
I75.89   Atheroembolism of other site

☑ Additional Character Req   ☑x7ᵗʰ Placeholder Alert   Case-Mix Diagnosis   Manifestation   ▽ Unspecified Dx   **EXCLUDES 1** Not coded here   **EXCLUDES 2** Not included here

Chapter 9. Diseases of the Circulatory System

I76   **Septic arterial embolism**
Code first underlying infection, such as:
    infective endocarditis (I33.0)
    lung abscess (J85.-)
Use additional code to identify the site of the embolism (I74.-)
    EXCLUDES 2   *septic pulmonary embolism (I26.01, I26.90)*

✓4ᵗʰ I77   **Other disorders of arteries and arterioles**
    EXCLUDES 2   *collagen (vascular) diseases (M30-M36)*
         hypersensitivity angiitis (M31.0)
         pulmonary artery (I28.-)

   I77.0   **Arteriovenous fistula, acquired**
Aneurysmal varix
Arteriovenous aneurysm, acquired
    EXCLUDES 1   *arteriovenous aneurysm NOS (Q27.3-)*
         presence of arteriovenous shunt (fistula) for dialysis (Z99.2)
         traumatic—see injury of blood vessel by body region
    EXCLUDES 2   *cerebral (I67.1)*
         coronary (I25.4)
    DEF: Communication between an artery and vein; caused by trauma or invasive procedures.

   I77.1   **Stricture of artery**
Narrowing of artery

   I77.2   **Rupture of artery**
Erosion of artery
Fistula of artery
Ulcer of artery
    EXCLUDES 1   *traumatic rupture of artery—see injury of blood vessel by body region*

   I77.3   **Arterial fibromuscular dysplasia**
Fibromuscular hyperplasia (of) carotid artery
Fibromuscular hyperplasia (of) renal artery

   I77.4   **Celiac artery compression syndrome**

   I77.5   **Necrosis of artery**

   I77.6   **Arteritis, unspecified**   ▽
Aortitis NOS
Endarteritis NOS
    EXCLUDES 1   *arteritis or endarteritis:*
         aortic arch (M31.4)
         cerebral NEC (I67.7)
         coronary (I25.89)
         deformans (I70.-)
         giant cell (M31.5., M31.6)
         obliterans (I70.-)
         senile (I70.-)

   ✓5ᵗʰ I77.7   **Other arterial dissection**
    EXCLUDES 2   *dissection of aorta (I71.0-)*
         dissection of coronary artery (I25.42)

     I77.70   **Dissection of unspecified artery**   ▽

     I77.71   **Dissection of carotid artery**

     I77.72   **Dissection of iliac artery**

     I77.73   **Dissection of renal artery**

     I77.74   **Dissection of vertebral artery**
        EXCLUDES 2   *aneurysm of vertebral artery (I72.6)*

     I77.75   **Dissection of other precerebral arteries**
Dissection of basilar artery (trunk)
        EXCLUDES 2   *aneurysm of carotid artery (I72.0)*
             aneurysm of other precerebral arteries (I72.5)
             aneurysm of vertebral artery (I72.6)
             dissection of carotid artery (I77.71)
             dissection of vertebral artery (I77.74)

     I77.76   **Dissection of artery of upper extremity**

     I77.77   **Dissection of artery of lower extremity**

     I77.79   **Dissection of other specified artery**

   ✓5ᵗʰ I77.8   **Other specified disorders of arteries and arterioles**

     ✓6ᵗʰ I77.81   **Aortic ectasia**
Ectasis aorta
        EXCLUDES 1   *aortic aneurysm and dissection (I71.0-)*

         I77.810   **Thoracic aortic ectasia**

         I77.811   **Abdominal aortic ectasia**

         I77.812   **Thoracoabdominal aortic ectasia**

         I77.819   **Aortic ectasia, unspecified site**   ▽

     I77.89   **Other specified disorders of arteries and arterioles**

   I77.9   **Disorder of arteries and arterioles, unspecified**   ▽

✓4ᵗʰ I78   **Diseases of capillaries**

   I78.0   **Hereditary hemorrhagic telangiectasia**
Rendu-Osler-Weber disease

   I78.1   **Nevus, non-neoplastic**
Araneus nevus
Senile nevus
Spider nevus
Stellar nevus
    EXCLUDES 1   *nevus NOS (D22.-)*
         vascular NOS (Q82.5)
    EXCLUDES 2   *blue nevus (D22.-)*
         flammeus nevus (Q82.5)
         hairy nevus (D22.-)
         melanocytic nevus (D22.-)
         pigmented nevus (D22.-)
         portwine nevus (Q82.5)
         sanguineous nevus (Q82.5)
         strawberry nevus (Q82.5)
         verrucous nevus (Q82.5)

   I78.8   **Other diseases of capillaries**

   I78.9   **Disease of capillaries, unspecified**   ▽

✓4ᵗʰ I79   **Disorders of arteries, arterioles and capillaries in diseases classified elsewhere**

   I79.0   ***Aneurysm of aorta in diseases classified elsewhere***
Code first underlying disease
    EXCLUDES 1   *syphilitic aneurysm (A52.01)*

   I79.1   ***Aortitis in diseases classified elsewhere***
Code first underlying disease
    EXCLUDES 1   *syphilitic aortitis (A52.02)*

   I79.8   ***Other disorders of arteries, arterioles and capillaries in diseases classified elsewhere***
Code first underlying disease, such as:
    amyloidosis (E85.-)
    EXCLUDES 1   *diabetic (peripheral) angiopathy (E08-E13 with .51-.52)*
         syphilitic endarteritis (A52.09)
         tuberculous endarteritis (A18.89)

Diseases of veins, lymphatic vessels and lymph nodes, not elsewhere classified (I80-I89)

✓4ᵗʰ I80   **Phlebitis and thrombophlebitis**
    INCLUDES   endophlebitis
         inflammation, vein
         periphlebitis
         suppurative phlebitis
Code first:
    phlebitis and thrombophlebitis complicating abortion, ectopic or molar pregnancy (O00-O07, O08.7)
    phlebitis and thrombophlebitis complicating pregnancy, childbirth and the puerperium (O22.-, O87.-)
    EXCLUDES 1   *venous embolism and thrombosis of lower extremities ((I82.4-, I82.5-, I82.81-)*

   ✓5ᵗʰ I80.0   **Phlebitis and thrombophlebitis of superficial vessels of lower extremities**
Phlebitis and thrombophlebitis of femoropopliteal vein

     I80.00   **Phlebitis and thrombophlebitis of superficial vessels of unspecified lower extremity**   ▽

     I80.01   **Phlebitis and thrombophlebitis of superficial vessels of right lower extremity**

     I80.02   **Phlebitis and thrombophlebitis of superficial vessels of left lower extremity**

     I80.03   **Phlebitis and thrombophlebitis of superficial vessels of lower extremities, bilateral**

   ✓5ᵗʰ I80.1   **Phlebitis and thrombophlebitis of femoral vein**

     I80.10   **Phlebitis and thrombophlebitis of unspecified femoral vein**   ▽

     I80.11   **Phlebitis and thrombophlebitis of right femoral vein**

     I80.12   **Phlebitis and thrombophlebitis of left femoral vein**

     I80.13   **Phlebitis and thrombophlebitis of femoral vein, bilateral**

   ✓5ᵗʰ I80.2   **Phlebitis and thrombophlebitis of other and unspecified deep vessels of lower extremities**

     ✓6ᵗʰ I80.20   **Phlebitis and thrombophlebitis of unspecified deep vessels of lower extremities**

         I80.201   **Phlebitis and thrombophlebitis of unspecified deep vessels of right lower extremity**

N Newborn: 0   P Pediatric: 0-17   M Maternity: 12-55   A Adult: 15-124   **NRS** Nonroutine supply Dx   **NCDx** Noncancer Dx   **PDx** Primary Dx   ►◄ Revised Text   ● New Code   ▲ Revised Title

648   ICD-10-CM 2018

I80.202   **Phlebitis and thrombophlebitis of unspecified deep vessels of** left **lower extremity**

I80.203   **Phlebitis and thrombophlebitis of unspecified deep vessels of lower extremities,** bilateral

I80.209   **Phlebitis and thrombophlebitis of unspecified deep vessels of unspecified lower extremity** ▽

☑6ᵗʰ **I80.21**   **Phlebitis and thrombophlebitis of** iliac vein

I80.211   **Phlebitis and thrombophlebitis of** right **iliac vein**

I80.212   **Phlebitis and thrombophlebitis of** left **iliac vein**

I80.213   **Phlebitis and thrombophlebitis of iliac vein,** bilateral

I80.219   **Phlebitis and thrombophlebitis of unspecified iliac vein** ▽

☑6ᵗʰ **I80.22**   **Phlebitis and thrombophlebitis of** popliteal vein

I80.221   **Phlebitis and thrombophlebitis of** right **popliteal vein**

I80.222   **Phlebitis and thrombophlebitis of** left **popliteal vein**

I80.223   **Phlebitis and thrombophlebitis of popliteal vein,** bilateral

I80.229   **Phlebitis and thrombophlebitis of unspecified popliteal vein** ▽

☑6ᵗʰ **I80.23**   **Phlebitis and thrombophlebitis of** tibial vein

I80.231   **Phlebitis and thrombophlebitis of** right **tibial vein**

I80.232   **Phlebitis and thrombophlebitis of** left **tibial vein**

I80.233   **Phlebitis and thrombophlebitis of tibial vein,** bilateral

I80.239   **Phlebitis and thrombophlebitis of unspecified tibial vein** ▽

☑6ᵗʰ **I80.29**   **Phlebitis and thrombophlebitis of** other **deep vessels of lower extremities**

I80.291   **Phlebitis and thrombophlebitis of other deep vessels of** right **lower extremity**

I80.292   **Phlebitis and thrombophlebitis of other deep vessels of** left **lower extremity**

I80.293   **Phlebitis and thrombophlebitis of other deep vessels of lower extremity,** bilateral

I80.299   **Phlebitis and thrombophlebitis of other deep vessels of unspecified lower extremity** ▽

I80.3   **Phlebitis and thrombophlebitis of lower extremities, unspecified** ▽

I80.8   **Phlebitis and thrombophlebitis of other sites**

I80.9   **Phlebitis and thrombophlebitis of unspecified site** ▽

I81   **Portal vein thrombosis**
Portal (vein) obstruction
EXCLUDES 2   *hepatic vein thrombosis (I82.0)*
           phlebitis of portal vein (K75.1)

☑4ᵗʰ **I82**   **Other venous embolism and thrombosis**
Code first venous embolism and thrombosis complicating:
     abortion, ectopic or molar pregnancy (O00-O07, O08.7)
     pregnancy, childbirth and the puerperium (O22.-, O87.-)
EXCLUDES 2   *venous embolism and thrombosis (of):*
           cerebral (I63.6, I67.6)
           coronary (I21-I25)
           intracranial and intraspinal, septic or NOS (G08)
           intracranial, nonpyogenic (I67.6)
           intraspinal, nonpyogenic (G95.1)
           mesenteric (K55.0-)
           portal (I81)
           pulmonary (I26.-)

I82.0   **Budd-Chiari syndrome**
Hepatic vein thrombosis
DEF: Thrombosis or other obstruction of hepatic veins; symptoms include enlarged liver, extensive collateral vessels, intractable ascites, and severe portal hypertension.

I82.1   **Thrombophlebitis migrans**

☑5ᵗʰ **I82.2**   **Embolism and thrombosis of** vena cava **and** other thoracic veins

☑6ᵗʰ **I82.21**   **Embolism and thrombosis of** superior vena cava

I82.210   **Acute embolism and thrombosis of superior vena cava**
Embolism and thrombosis of superior vena cava NOS

I82.211   **Chronic embolism and thrombosis of superior vena cava**

☑6ᵗʰ **I82.22**   **Embolism and thrombosis of** inferior vena cava

I82.220   **Acute embolism and thrombosis of inferior vena cava**
Embolism and thrombosis of inferior vena cava NOS

I82.221   **Chronic embolism and thrombosis of inferior vena cava**

☑6ᵗʰ **I82.29**   **Embolism and thrombosis of** other thoracic veins
Embolism and thrombosis of brachiocephalic (innominate) vein

I82.290   **Acute embolism and thrombosis of other thoracic veins**

I82.291   **Chronic embolism and thrombosis of other thoracic veins**

I82.3   **Embolism and thrombosis of** renal vein

☑5ᵗʰ **I82.4**   Acute **embolism and thrombosis of** deep veins of lower extremity

☑6ᵗʰ **I82.40**   **Acute embolism and thrombosis of** unspecified **deep veins of** lower extremity
Deep vein thrombosis NOS
DVT NOS
EXCLUDES 1   *acute embolism and thrombosis of unspecified deep veins of distal lower extremity (I82.4Z-)*
           acute embolism and thrombosis of unspecified deep veins of proximal lower extremity (I82.4Y-)

I82.401   **Acute embolism and thrombosis of unspecified deep veins of** right **lower extremity** ▽

I82.402   **Acute embolism and thrombosis of unspecified deep veins of** left **lower extremity** ▽

I82.403   **Acute embolism and thrombosis of unspecified deep veins of lower extremity,** bilateral ▽

I82.409   **Acute embolism and thrombosis of unspecified deep veins of unspecified lower extremity** ▽

☑6ᵗʰ **I82.41**   **Acute embolism and thrombosis of** femoral vein

I82.411   **Acute embolism and thrombosis of** right **femoral vein**

I82.412   **Acute embolism and thrombosis of** left **femoral vein**

I82.413   **Acute embolism and thrombosis of femoral vein,** bilateral

I82.419   **Acute embolism and thrombosis of unspecified femoral vein** ▽

☑6ᵗʰ **I82.42**   **Acute embolism and thrombosis of** iliac vein

I82.421   **Acute embolism and thrombosis of** right **iliac vein**

I82.422   **Acute embolism and thrombosis of** left **iliac vein**

I82.423   **Acute embolism and thrombosis of iliac vein,** bilateral

I82.429   **Acute embolism and thrombosis of unspecified iliac vein** ▽

☑6ᵗʰ **I82.43**   **Acute embolism and thrombosis of** popliteal vein

I82.431   **Acute embolism and thrombosis of** right **popliteal vein**

I82.432   **Acute embolism and thrombosis of** left **popliteal vein**

I82.433   **Acute embolism and thrombosis of popliteal vein,** bilateral

I82.439   **Acute embolism and thrombosis of unspecified popliteal vein** ▽

☑6ᵗʰ **I82.44**   **Acute embolism and thrombosis of** tibial vein

I82.441   **Acute embolism and thrombosis of** right **tibial vein**

☑ Additional Character Req   ☑x7ᵗʰ Placeholder Alert   Case-Mix Diagnosis   Manifestation   ▽ Unspecified Dx   EXCLUDES 1 Not coded here   EXCLUDES 2 Not included here

I82.442 Acute embolism and thrombosis of left tibial vein

I82.443 Acute embolism and thrombosis of tibial vein, bilateral

I82.449 Acute embolism and thrombosis of unspecified tibial vein ▽

✓6ᵗʰ I82.49 Acute embolism and thrombosis of other specified deep vein of lower extremity

I82.491 Acute embolism and thrombosis of other specified deep vein of right lower extremity

I82.492 Acute embolism and thrombosis of other specified deep vein of left lower extremity

I82.493 Acute embolism and thrombosis of other specified deep vein of lower extremity, bilateral

I82.499 Acute embolism and thrombosis of other specified deep vein of unspecified lower extremity ▽

✓6ᵗʰ I82.4Y Acute embolism and thrombosis of unspecified deep veins of proximal lower extremity
Acute embolism and thrombosis of deep vein of thigh NOS
Acute embolism and thrombosis of deep vein of upper leg NOS

I82.4Y1 Acute embolism and thrombosis of unspecified deep veins of right proximal lower extremity

I82.4Y2 Acute embolism and thrombosis of unspecified deep veins of left proximal lower extremity

I82.4Y3 Acute embolism and thrombosis of unspecified deep veins of proximal lower extremity, bilateral

I82.4Y9 Acute embolism and thrombosis of unspecified deep veins of unspecified proximal lower extremity ▽

✓6ᵗʰ I82.4Z Acute embolism and thrombosis of unspecified deep veins of distal lower extremity
Acute embolism and thrombosis of deep vein of calf NOS
Acute embolism and thrombosis of deep vein of lower leg NOS

I82.4Z1 Acute embolism and thrombosis of unspecified deep veins of right distal lower extremity

I82.4Z2 Acute embolism and thrombosis of unspecified deep veins of left distal lower extremity

I82.4Z3 Acute embolism and thrombosis of unspecified deep veins of distal lower extremity, bilateral

I82.4Z9 Acute embolism and thrombosis of unspecified deep veins of unspecified distal lower extremity ▽

✓5ᵗʰ I82.5 Chronic embolism and thrombosis of deep veins of lower extremity
Use additional code, if applicable, for associated long-term (current) use of anticoagulants (Z79.01)
EXCLUDES 1 personal history of venous embolism and thrombosis (Z86.718)

✓6ᵗʰ I82.50 Chronic embolism and thrombosis of unspecified deep veins of lower extremity
EXCLUDES 1 chronic embolism and thrombosis of unspecified deep veins of distal lower extremity (I82.5Z-)
chronic embolism and thrombosis of unspecified deep veins of proximal lower extremity (I82.5Y-)

I82.501 Chronic embolism and thrombosis of unspecified deep veins of right lower extremity ▽

I82.502 Chronic embolism and thrombosis of unspecified deep veins of left lower extremity ▽

I82.503 Chronic embolism and thrombosis of unspecified deep veins of lower extremity, bilateral ▽

I82.509 Chronic embolism and thrombosis of unspecified deep veins of unspecified lower extremity ▽

✓6ᵗʰ I82.51 Chronic embolism and thrombosis of femoral vein

I82.511 Chronic embolism and thrombosis of right femoral vein

I82.512 Chronic embolism and thrombosis of left femoral vein

I82.513 Chronic embolism and thrombosis of femoral vein, bilateral

I82.519 Chronic embolism and thrombosis of unspecified femoral vein ▽

✓6ᵗʰ I82.52 Chronic embolism and thrombosis of iliac vein

I82.521 Chronic embolism and thrombosis of right iliac vein

I82.522 Chronic embolism and thrombosis of left iliac vein

I82.523 Chronic embolism and thrombosis of iliac vein, bilateral

I82.529 Chronic embolism and thrombosis of unspecified iliac vein ▽

✓6ᵗʰ I82.53 Chronic embolism and thrombosis of popliteal vein

I82.531 Chronic embolism and thrombosis of right popliteal vein

I82.532 Chronic embolism and thrombosis of left popliteal vein

I82.533 Chronic embolism and thrombosis of popliteal vein, bilateral

I82.539 Chronic embolism and thrombosis of unspecified popliteal vein ▽

✓6ᵗʰ I82.54 Chronic embolism and thrombosis of tibial vein

I82.541 Chronic embolism and thrombosis of right tibial vein

I82.542 Chronic embolism and thrombosis of left tibial vein

I82.543 Chronic embolism and thrombosis of tibial vein, bilateral

I82.549 Chronic embolism and thrombosis of unspecified tibial vein ▽

✓6ᵗʰ I82.59 Chronic embolism and thrombosis of other specified deep vein of lower extremity

I82.591 Chronic embolism and thrombosis of other specified deep vein of right lower extremity

I82.592 Chronic embolism and thrombosis of other specified deep vein of left lower extremity

I82.593 Chronic embolism and thrombosis of other specified deep vein of lower extremity, bilateral

I82.599 Chronic embolism and thrombosis of other specified deep vein of unspecified lower extremity ▽

✓6ᵗʰ I82.5Y Chronic embolism and thrombosis of unspecified deep veins of proximal lower extremity
Chronic embolism and thrombosis of deep veins of thigh NOS
Chronic embolism and thrombosis of deep veins of upper leg NOS

I82.5Y1 Chronic embolism and thrombosis of unspecified deep veins of right proximal lower extremity

I82.5Y2 Chronic embolism and thrombosis of unspecified deep veins of left proximal lower extremity

I82.5Y3 Chronic embolism and thrombosis of unspecified deep veins of proximal lower extremity, bilateral

I82.5Y9 Chronic embolism and thrombosis of unspecified deep veins of unspecified proximal lower extremity ▽

✓6ᵗʰ I82.5Z Chronic embolism and thrombosis of unspecified deep veins of distal lower extremity
Chronic embolism and thrombosis of deep veins of calf NOS
Chronic embolism and thrombosis of deep veins of lower leg NOS

I82.5Z1 Chronic embolism and thrombosis of unspecified deep veins of right distal lower extremity

I82.5Z2 Chronic embolism and thrombosis of unspecified deep veins of left distal lower extremity

I82.5Z3   Chronic embolism and thrombosis of unspecified deep veins of distal lower extremity, bilateral

I82.5Z9   Chronic embolism and thrombosis of unspecified deep veins of unspecified distal lower extremity ▽

✓5ᵗʰ **I82.6**   Acute embolism and thrombosis of veins of upper extremity

   ✓6ᵗʰ **I82.60**   Acute embolism and thrombosis of unspecified veins of upper extremity

     I82.601   Acute embolism and thrombosis of unspecified veins of right upper extremity ▽

     I82.602   Acute embolism and thrombosis of unspecified veins of left upper extremity ▽

     I82.603   Acute embolism and thrombosis of unspecified veins of upper extremity, bilateral ▽

     I82.609   Acute embolism and thrombosis of unspecified veins of unspecified upper extremity ▽

   ✓6ᵗʰ **I82.61**   Acute embolism and thrombosis of superficial veins of upper extremity
Acute embolism and thrombosis of antecubital vein
Acute embolism and thrombosis of basilic vein
Acute embolism and thrombosis of cephalic vein

     I82.611   Acute embolism and thrombosis of superficial veins of right upper extremity

     I82.612   Acute embolism and thrombosis of superficial veins of left upper extremity

     I82.613   Acute embolism and thrombosis of superficial veins of upper extremity, bilateral

     I82.619   Acute embolism and thrombosis of superficial veins of unspecified upper extremity ▽

   ✓6ᵗʰ **I82.62**   Acute embolism and thrombosis of deep veins of upper extremity
Acute embolism and thrombosis of brachial vein
Acute embolism and thrombosis of radial vein
Acute embolism and thrombosis of ulnar vein

     I82.621   Acute embolism and thrombosis of deep veins of right upper extremity

     I82.622   Acute embolism and thrombosis of deep veins of left upper extremity

     I82.623   Acute embolism and thrombosis of deep veins of upper extremity, bilateral

     I82.629   Acute embolism and thrombosis of deep veins of unspecified upper extremity ▽

✓5ᵗʰ **I82.7**   Chronic embolism and thrombosis of veins of upper extremity
Use additional code, if applicable, for associated long-term (current) use of anticoagulants (Z79.01)
EXCLUDES 1   personal history of venous embolism and thrombosis (Z86.718)

   ✓6ᵗʰ **I82.70**   Chronic embolism and thrombosis of unspecified veins of upper extremity

     I82.701   Chronic embolism and thrombosis of unspecified veins of right upper extremity ▽

     I82.702   Chronic embolism and thrombosis of unspecified veins of left upper extremity ▽

     I82.703   Chronic embolism and thrombosis of unspecified veins of upper extremity, bilateral ▽

     I82.709   Chronic embolism and thrombosis of unspecified veins of unspecified upper extremity ▽

   ✓6ᵗʰ **I82.71**   Chronic embolism and thrombosis of superficial veins of upper extremity
Chronic embolism and thrombosis of antecubital vein
Chronic embolism and thrombosis of basilic vein
Chronic embolism and thrombosis of cephalic vein

     I82.711   Chronic embolism and thrombosis of superficial veins of right upper extremity

     I82.712   Chronic embolism and thrombosis of superficial veins of left upper extremity

     I82.713   Chronic embolism and thrombosis of superficial veins of upper extremity, bilateral

     I82.719   Chronic embolism and thrombosis of superficial veins of unspecified upper extremity ▽

   ✓6ᵗʰ **I82.72**   Chronic embolism and thrombosis of deep veins of upper extremity
Chronic embolism and thrombosis of brachial vein
Chronic embolism and thrombosis of radial vein
Chronic embolism and thrombosis of ulnar vein

     I82.721   Chronic embolism and thrombosis of deep veins of right upper extremity

     I82.722   Chronic embolism and thrombosis of deep veins of left upper extremity

     I82.723   Chronic embolism and thrombosis of deep veins of upper extremity, bilateral

     I82.729   Chronic embolism and thrombosis of deep veins of unspecified upper extremity ▽

✓5ᵗʰ **I82.A**   Embolism and thrombosis of axillary vein

   ✓6ᵗʰ **I82.A1**   Acute embolism and thrombosis of axillary vein

     I82.A11   Acute embolism and thrombosis of right axillary vein

     I82.A12   Acute embolism and thrombosis of left axillary vein

     I82.A13   Acute embolism and thrombosis of axillary vein, bilateral

     I82.A19   Acute embolism and thrombosis of unspecified axillary vein ▽

   ✓6ᵗʰ **I82.A2**   Chronic embolism and thrombosis of axillary vein

     I82.A21   Chronic embolism and thrombosis of right axillary vein

     I82.A22   Chronic embolism and thrombosis of left axillary vein

     I82.A23   Chronic embolism and thrombosis of axillary vein, bilateral

     I82.A29   Chronic embolism and thrombosis of unspecified axillary vein ▽

✓5ᵗʰ **I82.B**   Embolism and thrombosis of subclavian vein

   ✓6ᵗʰ **I82.B1**   Acute embolism and thrombosis of subclavian vein

     I82.B11   Acute embolism and thrombosis of right subclavian vein

     I82.B12   Acute embolism and thrombosis of left subclavian vein

     I82.B13   Acute embolism and thrombosis of subclavian vein, bilateral

     I82.B19   Acute embolism and thrombosis of unspecified subclavian vein ▽

   ✓6ᵗʰ **I82.B2**   Chronic embolism and thrombosis of subclavian vein

     I82.B21   Chronic embolism and thrombosis of right subclavian vein

     I82.B22   Chronic embolism and thrombosis of left subclavian vein

     I82.B23   Chronic embolism and thrombosis of subclavian vein, bilateral

     I82.B29   Chronic embolism and thrombosis of unspecified subclavian vein ▽

✓5ᵗʰ **I82.C**   Embolism and thrombosis of internal jugular vein

   ✓6ᵗʰ **I82.C1**   Acute embolism and thrombosis of internal jugular vein

     I82.C11   Acute embolism and thrombosis of right internal jugular vein

     I82.C12   Acute embolism and thrombosis of left internal jugular vein

     I82.C13   Acute embolism and thrombosis of internal jugular vein, bilateral

     I82.C19   Acute embolism and thrombosis of unspecified internal jugular vein ▽

   ✓6ᵗʰ **I82.C2**   Chronic embolism and thrombosis of internal jugular vein

     I82.C21   Chronic embolism and thrombosis of right internal jugular vein

     I82.C22   Chronic embolism and thrombosis of left internal jugular vein

     I82.C23   Chronic embolism and thrombosis of internal jugular vein, bilateral

     I82.C29   Chronic embolism and thrombosis of unspecified internal jugular vein ▽

✔ Additional Character Req   ✔x7ᵗʰ Placeholder Alert   Case-Mix Diagnosis   Manifestation   ▽ Unspecified Dx   EXCLUDES 1 Not coded here   EXCLUDES 2 Not included here

ICD-10-CM 2018   **651**

Chapter 9. Diseases of the Circulatory System

✓5ᵗʰ **I82.8**   **Embolism and thrombosis of other** specified veins
> Use additional code, if applicable, for associated long-term (current) use of anticoagulants (Z79.01)

✓6ᵗʰ   **I82.81**   **Embolism and thrombosis of superficial veins of lower extremities**
> Embolism and thrombosis of saphenous vein (greater) (lesser)

▲   **I82.811**   **Embolism and thrombosis of superficial veins of** right **lower extremity**

▲   **I82.812**   **Embolism and thrombosis of superficial veins of** left **lower extremity**

     I82.813   **Embolism and thrombosis of superficial veins of lower extremities,** bilateral

▲   **I82.819**   **Embolism and thrombosis of superficial** ▽ **veins of unspecified lower extremity**

✓6ᵗʰ   **I82.89**   **Embolism and thrombosis of** other **specified veins**

     I82.890   Acute **embolism and thrombosis of other specified veins**

     I82.891   Chronic **embolism and thrombosis of other specified veins**

✓5ᵗʰ **I82.9**   **Embolism and thrombosis of** unspecified **vein**

     I82.90   Acute **embolism and thrombosis of unspecified** ▽ **vein**
> Embolism of vein NOS
> Thrombosis (vein) NOS

     I82.91   Chronic **embolism and thrombosis of** ▽ **unspecified vein**

✓4ᵗʰ **I83**   **Varicose veins of lower extremities**
> EXCLUDES 1   varicose veins complicating pregnancy (O22.0-)
> varicose veins complicating the puerperium (O87.4)

✓5ᵗʰ **I83.0**   **Varicose veins of lower extremities with** ulcer
> Use additional code to identify severity of ulcer (L97.-)

✓6ᵗʰ   **I83.00**   **Varicose veins of** unspecified **lower extremity with ulcer**

     I83.001   **Varicose veins of unspecified lower** 🅐▽ **extremity with ulcer of** thigh

     I83.002   **Varicose veins of unspecified lower** 🅐▽ **extremity with ulcer of** calf

     I83.003   **Varicose veins of unspecified lower** 🅐▽ **extremity with ulcer of** ankle

     I83.004   **Varicose veins of unspecified lower** 🅐▽ **extremity with ulcer of** heel and midfoot
> Varicose veins of unspecified lower extremity with ulcer of plantar surface of midfoot

     I83.005   **Varicose veins of unspecified lower** 🅐▽ **extremity with ulcer other** part of foot
> Varicose veins of unspecified lower extremity with ulcer of toe

     I83.008   **Varicose veins of unspecified lower** 🅐▽ **extremity with ulcer other** part of lower leg

     I83.009   **Varicose veins of unspecified lower** 🅐▽ **extremity with ulcer of unspecified site**

✓6ᵗʰ   **I83.01**   **Varicose veins of** right **lower extremity with ulcer**

     I83.011   **Varicose veins of right lower extremity** 🅐 **with ulcer of** thigh

     I83.012   **Varicose veins of right lower extremity** 🅐 **with ulcer of** calf

     I83.013   **Varicose veins of right lower extremity** 🅐 **with ulcer of** ankle

     I83.014   **Varicose veins of right lower extremity** 🅐 **with ulcer of** heel and midfoot
> Varicose veins of right lower extremity with ulcer of plantar surface of midfoot

     I83.015   **Varicose veins of right lower extremity** 🅐 **with ulcer other** part of foot
> Varicose veins of right lower extremity with ulcer of toe

     I83.018   **Varicose veins of right lower extremity** 🅐 **with ulcer other** part of lower leg

     I83.019   **Varicose veins of right lower** 🅐▽ **extremity with ulcer of unspecified site**

✓6ᵗʰ   **I83.02**   **Varicose veins of** left **lower extremity with ulcer**

     I83.021   **Varicose veins of left lower extremity** 🅐 **with ulcer of** thigh

     I83.022   **Varicose veins of left lower extremity** 🅐 **with ulcer of** calf

     I83.023   **Varicose veins of left lower extremity** 🅐 **with ulcer of** ankle

     I83.024   **Varicose veins of left lower extremity** 🅐 **with ulcer of** heel and midfoot
> Varicose veins of left lower extremity with ulcer of plantar surface of midfoot

     I83.025   **Varicose veins of left lower extremity** 🅐 **with ulcer other** part of foot
> Varicose veins of left lower extremity with ulcer of toe

     I83.028   **Varicose veins of left lower extremity** 🅐 **with ulcer other** part of lower leg

     I83.029   **Varicose veins of left lower** 🅐▽ **extremity with ulcer of unspecified site**

✓5ᵗʰ **I83.1**   **Varicose veins of lower extremities with** inflammation

     I83.10   **Varicose veins of unspecified lower extremity** 🅐▽ **with inflammation**

     I83.11   **Varicose veins of** right **lower extremity with** 🅐 **inflammation**

     I83.12   **Varicose veins of** left **lower extremity with** 🅐 **inflammation**

✓5ᵗʰ **I83.2**   **Varicose veins of lower extremities with both** ulcer and inflammation
> Use additional code to identify severity of ulcer (L97.-)

✓6ᵗʰ   **I83.20**   **Varicose veins of** unspecified **lower extremity with both ulcer and inflammation**

     I83.201   **Varicose veins of unspecified lower** 🅐▽ **extremity with both ulcer of** thigh **and inflammation**

     I83.202   **Varicose veins of unspecified lower** 🅐▽ **extremity with both ulcer of** calf **and inflammation**

     I83.203   **Varicose veins of unspecified lower** 🅐▽ **extremity with both ulcer of** ankle **and inflammation**

     I83.204   **Varicose veins of unspecified lower** 🅐▽ **extremity with both ulcer of** heel and midfoot **and inflammation**
> Varicose veins of unspecified lower extremity with both ulcer of plantar surface of midfoot and inflammation

     I83.205   **Varicose veins of unspecified lower** 🅐▽ **extremity with both ulcer of other** part of foot **and inflammation**
> Varicose veins of unspecified lower extremity with both ulcer of toe and inflammation

     I83.208   **Varicose veins of unspecified lower** 🅐▽ **extremity with both ulcer of other** part of lower extremity **and inflammation**

     I83.209   **Varicose veins of unspecified lower** 🅐▽ **extremity with both ulcer of unspecified site and inflammation**

✓6ᵗʰ   **I83.21**   **Varicose veins of** right **lower extremity with both ulcer and inflammation**

     I83.211   **Varicose veins of right lower extremity** 🅐 **with both ulcer of** thigh **and inflammation**

     I83.212   **Varicose veins of right lower extremity** 🅐 **with both ulcer of** calf **and inflammation**

     I83.213   **Varicose veins of right lower extremity** 🅐 **with both ulcer of** ankle **and inflammation**

     I83.214   **Varicose veins of right lower extremity** 🅐 **with both ulcer of** heel and midfoot **and inflammation**
> Varicose veins of right lower extremity with both ulcer of plantar surface of midfoot and inflammation

     I83.215   **Varicose veins of right lower extremity** 🅐 **with both ulcer other** part of foot **and inflammation**
> Varicose veins of right lower extremity with both ulcer of toe and inflammation

     I83.218   **Varicose veins of right lower extremity** 🅐 **with both ulcer of other** part of lower extremity **and inflammation**

     I83.219   **Varicose veins of right lower** 🅐▽ **extremity with both ulcer of unspecified site and inflammation**

� Newborn: 0   🅿 Pediatric: 0-17   Ⓜ Maternity: 12-55   🅐 Adult: 15-124   **NRS** Nonroutine supply Dx   **NCDx** Noncancer Dx   **PDx** Primary Dx   ▶◀ Revised Text   ● New Code   ▲ Revised Title

652   ICD-10-CM 2018

✓6ᵗʰ **I83.22** **Varicose veins of** left **lower extremity with both ulcer and inflammation**

     I83.221 **Varicose veins of left lower extremity** 🅰 **with both ulcer of** thigh **and inflammation**

     I83.222 **Varicose veins of left lower extremity** 🅰 **with both ulcer of** calf **and inflammation**

     I83.223 **Varicose veins of left lower extremity** 🅰 **with both ulcer of** ankle **and inflammation**

     I83.224 **Varicose veins of left lower extremity** 🅰 **with both ulcer of** heel and midfoot **and inflammation**
         Varicose veins of left lower extremity with both ulcer of plantar surface of midfoot and inflammation

     I83.225 **Varicose veins of left lower extremity** 🅰 **with both ulcer other** part of foot **and inflammation**
         Varicose veins of left lower extremity with both ulcer of toe and inflammation

     I83.228 **Varicose veins of left lower extremity** 🅰 **with both ulcer of other** part of lower extremity **and inflammation**

     I83.229 **Varicose veins of left lower extremity** 🅰 ▽ **with both ulcer of unspecified site and inflammation**

✓5ᵗʰ **I83.8** **Varicose veins of lower extremities with** other complications

     ✓6ᵗʰ **I83.81** **Varicose veins of lower extremities with** pain

▲   **I83.811** **Varicose veins of** right **lower** 🅰 **extremity with pain**

▲   **I83.812** **Varicose veins of** left **lower extremity** 🅰 **with pain**

     I83.813 **Varicose veins of** bilateral **lower** 🅰 **extremities with pain**

▲   **I83.819** **Varicose veins of unspecified lower** 🅰 ▽ **extremity with pain**

     ✓6ᵗʰ **I83.89** **Varicose veins of lower extremities with** other **complications**
         Varicose veins of lower extremities with edema
         Varicose veins of lower extremities with swelling

▲   **I83.891** **Varicose veins of** right **lower** 🅰 **extremity with other complications**

▲   **I83.892** **Varicose veins of** left **lower extremity** 🅰 **with other complications**

     I83.893 **Varicose veins of** bilateral **lower** 🅰 **extremities with other complications**

▲   **I83.899** **Varicose veins of unspecified lower** 🅰 ▽ **extremity with other complications**

✓5ᵗʰ **I83.9** Asymptomatic **varicose veins of lower extremities**
     Phlebectasia of lower extremities
     Varicose veins of lower extremities
     Varix of lower extremities

     I83.90 **Asymptomatic varicose veins of unspecified** 🅰 ▽ **lower extremity**
         Varicose veins NOS

     I83.91 **Asymptomatic varicose veins of** right **lower** 🅰 **extremity**

     I83.92 **Asymptomatic varicose veins of** left **lower** 🅰 **extremity**

     I83.93 **Asymptomatic varicose veins of** bilateral **lower** 🅰 **extremities**

✓4ᵗʰ **I85** **Esophageal varices**
     Use additional code to identify:
         alcohol abuse and dependence (F10.-)

     ✓5ᵗʰ **I85.0** **Esophageal varices**
         Idiopathic esophageal varices
         Primary esophageal varices

         I85.00 **Esophageal varices** without bleeding
             Esophageal varices NOS

         I85.01 **Esophageal varices** with bleeding

     ✓5ᵗʰ **I85.1** **Secondary esophageal varices**
         Esophageal varices secondary to alcoholic liver disease
         Esophageal varices secondary to cirrhosis of liver
         Esophageal varices secondary to schistosomiasis
         Esophageal varices secondary to toxic liver disease
         Code first underlying disease

         I85.10 **Secondary esophageal varices** without bleeding

         I85.11 **Secondary esophageal varices** with bleeding

✓4ᵗʰ **I86** **Varicose veins of other sites**
     EXCLUDES 1 *varicose veins of unspecified site (I83.9-)*
     EXCLUDES 2 *retinal varices (H35.0-)*

     I86.0 Sublingual **varices**
         DEF: Distended, tortuous veins beneath tongue.

     I86.1 Scrotal **varices** ♂
         Varicocele

     I86.2 Pelvic **varices**

     I86.3 Vulval **varices** ♀
         EXCLUDES 1 *vulval varices complicating childbirth and the puerperium (O87.8)*
                  vulval varices complicating pregnancy (O22.1-)

     I86.4 Gastric **varices**

     I86.8 **Varicose veins of other specified sites** 🅰
         Varicose ulcer of nasal septum

✓4ᵗʰ **I87** **Other disorders of veins**

     ✓5ᵗʰ **I87.0** **Postthrombotic syndrome**
         Chronic venous hypertension due to deep vein thrombosis
         Postphlebitic syndrome
         EXCLUDES 1 *chronic venous hypertension without deep vein thrombosis (I87.3-)*

         ✓6ᵗʰ **I87.00** **Postthrombotic syndrome** without complications
             Asymptomatic postthrombotic syndrome

             I87.001 **Postthrombotic syndrome without complications of** right lower **extremity**

             I87.002 **Postthrombotic syndrome without complications of** left lower **extremity**

             I87.003 **Postthrombotic syndrome without complications of** bilateral lower **extremity**

             I87.009 **Postthrombotic syndrome without** ▽ **complications of unspecified extremity**
                 Postthrombotic syndrome NOS

         ✓6ᵗʰ **I87.01** **Postthrombotic syndrome with** ulcer
             Use additional code to specify site and severity of ulcer (L97.-)

             I87.011 **Postthrombotic syndrome with ulcer of** right lower **extremity**

             I87.012 **Postthrombotic syndrome with ulcer of** left lower **extremity**

             I87.013 **Postthrombotic syndrome with ulcer of** bilateral lower **extremity**

             I87.019 **Postthrombotic syndrome with ulcer** ▽ **of unspecified lower extremity**

         ✓6ᵗʰ **I87.02** **Postthrombotic syndrome with** inflammation

             I87.021 **Postthrombotic syndrome with inflammation of** right lower **extremity**

             I87.022 **Postthrombotic syndrome with inflammation of** left lower **extremity**

             I87.023 **Postthrombotic syndrome with inflammation of** bilateral lower **extremity**

             I87.029 **Postthrombotic syndrome with** ▽ **inflammation of unspecified lower extremity**

         ✓6ᵗʰ **I87.03** **Postthrombotic syndrome with** ulcer and inflammation
             Use additional code to specify site and severity of ulcer (L97.-)

             I87.031 **Postthrombotic syndrome with ulcer and inflammation of** right lower **extremity**

             I87.032 **Postthrombotic syndrome with ulcer and inflammation of** left lower **extremity**

             I87.033 **Postthrombotic syndrome with ulcer and inflammation of** bilateral lower **extremity**

             I87.039 **Postthrombotic syndrome with ulcer** ▽ **and inflammation of unspecified lower extremity**

         ✓6ᵗʰ **I87.09** **Postthrombotic syndrome with** other complications

             I87.091 **Postthrombotic syndrome with other complications of** right lower **extremity**

             I87.092 **Postthrombotic syndrome with other complications of** left lower **extremity**

             I87.093 **Postthrombotic syndrome with other complications of** bilateral lower **extremity**

             I87.099 **Postthrombotic syndrome with other** ▽ **complications of unspecified lower extremity**

☑ Additional Character Req   ✓ₓ7ᵗʰ Placeholder Alert   Case-Mix Diagnosis   Manifestation   ▽ Unspecified Dx   **EXCLUDES 1** Not coded here   **EXCLUDES 2** Not included here

ICD-10-CM 2018   **653**

I87.1 **Compression of vein**
Stricture of vein
Vena cava syndrome (inferior) (superior)
EXCLUDES 2   *compression of pulmonary vein (I28.8)*

I87.2 **Venous insufficiency (chronic) (peripheral)**
Stasis dermatitis
EXCLUDES 1   *stasis dermatitis with varicose veins of lower extremities (I83.1-, I83.2-)*
DEF: Insufficient drainage of venous blood in any part of body; results in edema or dermatosis.

✓5th **I87.3** **Chronic venous hypertension (idiopathic)**
Stasis edema
EXCLUDES 1   *chronic venous hypertension due to deep vein thrombosis (I87.0-)*
varicose veins of lower extremities (I83.-)

✓6th **I87.30** **Chronic venous hypertension (idiopathic) without complications**
Asymptomatic chronic venous hypertension (idiopathic)

I87.301 **Chronic venous hypertension (idiopathic) without complications of right lower extremity**

I87.302 **Chronic venous hypertension (idiopathic) without complications of left lower extremity**

I87.303 **Chronic venous hypertension (idiopathic) without complications of bilateral lower extremity**

I87.309 **Chronic venous hypertension (idiopathic) without complications of unspecified lower extremity** ▽
Chronic venous hypertension NOS

✓6th **I87.31** **Chronic venous hypertension (idiopathic) with ulcer**
Use additional code to specify site and severity of ulcer (L97.-)

I87.311 **Chronic venous hypertension (idiopathic) with ulcer of right lower extremity**

I87.312 **Chronic venous hypertension (idiopathic) with ulcer of left lower extremity**

I87.313 **Chronic venous hypertension (idiopathic) with ulcer of bilateral lower extremity**

I87.319 **Chronic venous hypertension (idiopathic) with ulcer of unspecified lower extremity** ▽

✓6th **I87.32** **Chronic venous hypertension (idiopathic) with inflammation**

I87.321 **Chronic venous hypertension (idiopathic) with inflammation of right lower extremity**

I87.322 **Chronic venous hypertension (idiopathic) with inflammation of left lower extremity**

I87.323 **Chronic venous hypertension (idiopathic) with inflammation of bilateral lower extremity**

I87.329 **Chronic venous hypertension (idiopathic) with inflammation of unspecified lower extremity** ▽

✓6th **I87.33** **Chronic venous hypertension (idiopathic) with ulcer and inflammation**
Use additional code to specify site and severity of ulcer (L97.-)

I87.331 **Chronic venous hypertension (idiopathic) with ulcer and inflammation of right lower extremity**

I87.332 **Chronic venous hypertension (idiopathic) with ulcer and inflammation of left lower extremity**

I87.333 **Chronic venous hypertension (idiopathic) with ulcer and inflammation of bilateral lower extremity**

I87.339 **Chronic venous hypertension (idiopathic) with ulcer and inflammation of unspecified lower extremity** ▽

✓6th **I87.39** **Chronic venous hypertension (idiopathic) with other complications**

I87.391 **Chronic venous hypertension (idiopathic) with other complications of right lower extremity**

I87.392 **Chronic venous hypertension (idiopathic) with other complications of left lower extremity**

I87.393 **Chronic venous hypertension (idiopathic) with other complications of bilateral lower extremity**

I87.399 **Chronic venous hypertension (idiopathic) with other complications of unspecified lower extremity** ▽

I87.8 **Other specified disorders of veins**
Phlebosclerosis
Venofibrosis

I87.9 **Disorder of vein, unspecified** ▽

✓4th **I88** **Nonspecific lymphadenitis**
EXCLUDES 1   *acute lymphadenitis, except mesenteric (L04.-)*
enlarged lymph nodes NOS (R59.-)
human immunodeficiency virus [HIV] disease resulting in generalized lymphadenopathy (B20)

I88.0 **Nonspecific mesenteric lymphadenitis**
Mesenteric lymphadenitis (acute)(chronic)

I88.1 **Chronic lymphadenitis, except mesenteric**
Adenitis
Lymphadenitis

I88.8 **Other nonspecific lymphadenitis**

I88.9 **Nonspecific lymphadenitis, unspecified** ▽
Lymphadenitis NOS

✓4th **I89** **Other noninfective disorders of lymphatic vessels and lymph nodes**
EXCLUDES 1   *chylocele, tunica vaginalis (nonfilarial) NOS (N50.89)*
enlarged lymph nodes NOS (R59.-)
filarial chylocele (B74.-)
hereditary lymphedema (Q82.0)

I89.0 **Lymphedema, not elsewhere classified**
Elephantiasis (nonfilarial) NOS
Lymphangiectasis
Obliteration, lymphatic vessel
Praecox lymphedema
Secondary lymphedema
EXCLUDES 1   *postmastectomy lymphedema (I97.2)*

I89.1 **Lymphangitis**
Chronic lymphangitis
Lymphangitis NOS
Subacute lymphangitis
EXCLUDES 1   *acute lymphangitis (L03.-)*

I89.8 **Other specified noninfective disorders of lymphatic vessels and lymph nodes**
Chylocele (nonfilarial)
Chylous ascites
Chylous cyst
Lipomelanotic reticulosis
Lymph node or vessel fistula
Lymph node or vessel infarction
Lymph node or vessel rupture

I89.9 **Noninfective disorder of lymphatic vessels and lymph nodes, unspecified** ▽
Disease of lymphatic vessels NOS

Other and unspecified disorders of the circulatory system (I95-I99)

✓4th **I95** **Hypotension**
EXCLUDES 1   *cardiovascular collapse (R57.9)*
maternal hypotension syndrome (O26.5-)
nonspecific low blood pressure reading NOS (R03.1)

I95.0 **Idiopathic hypotension**

I95.1 **Orthostatic hypotension**
Hypotension, postural
EXCLUDES 1   *neurogenic orthostatic hypotension [Shy-Drager] (G90.3)*
orthostatic hypotension due to drugs (I95.2)

I95.2 **Hypotension due to drugs**
Orthostatic hypotension due to drugs
Use additional code for adverse effect, if applicable, to identify drug (T36-T50 with fifth or sixth character 5)

I95.3 **Hypotension of hemodialysis**
Intra-dialytic hypotension

✓5th **I95.8** **Other hypotension**

I95.81 **Postprocedural hypotension**

I95.89 **Other hypotension**
Chronic hypotension

N Newborn: 0   P Pediatric: 0-17   M Maternity: 12-55   A Adult: 15-124   NRS Nonroutine supply Dx   NC Dx Noncancer Dx   PDx Primary Dx   ►◄ Revised Text   ● New Code   ▲ Revised Title

654   ICD-10-CM 2018

I95.9 **Hypotension, unspecified** ▽

I96 Gangrene, not elsewhere classified `NRS`
Gangrenous cellulitis
EXCLUDES 1 gangrene in atherosclerosis of native arteries of the extremities (I70.26)
~~gangrene in diabetes mellitus (E08-E13 with .52)~~
gangrene in hernia (K40.1, K40.4, K41.1, K41.4, K42.1, K43.1-, K44.1, K45.1, K46.1)
gangrene in other peripheral vascular diseases (I73.-)
gangrene of certain specified sites—see Alphabetical Index
gas gangrene (A48.0)
pyoderma gangrenosum (L88)
EXCLUDES 2 ▶gangrene in diabetes mellitus (E08-E13 with .52)◀
AHA: 2013, 2Q, 34

✓4th I97 Intraoperative and postprocedural complications and disorders of circulatory system, not elsewhere classified
EXCLUDES 2 postprocedural shock (T81.1-)

I97.0 Postcardiotomy syndrome

✓5th I97.1 Other postprocedural cardiac functional disturbances
EXCLUDES 2 acute pulmonary insufficiency following thoracic surgery (J95.1)
intraoperative cardiac functional disturbances (I97.7-)

✓6th **I97.11 Postprocedural cardiac insufficiency**
I97.110 Postprocedural cardiac insufficiency following cardiac surgery
I97.111 Postprocedural cardiac insufficiency following other surgery

✓6th **I97.12 Postprocedural cardiac arrest**
I97.120 Postprocedural cardiac arrest following cardiac surgery
I97.121 Postprocedural cardiac arrest following other surgery

✓6th **I97.13 Postprocedural heart failure**
Use additional code to identify the heart failure (I50.-)
I97.130 Postprocedural heart failure following cardiac surgery
I97.131 Postprocedural heart failure following other surgery

✓6th **I97.19 Other postprocedural cardiac functional disturbances**
Use additional code, if applicable, to further specify disorder
I97.190 Other postprocedural cardiac functional disturbances following cardiac surgery
▶Use additional code, if applicable, for type 4 or type 5 myocardial infarction, to further specify disorder◀
I97.191 Other postprocedural cardiac functional disturbances following other surgery

I97.2 Postmastectomy lymphedema syndrome `A`
Elephantiasis due to mastectomy
Obliteration of lymphatic vessels

I97.3 Postprocedural hypertension

✓5th I97.4 Intraoperative hemorrhage and hematoma of a circulatory system organ or structure complicating a procedure
EXCLUDES 1 intraoperative hemorrhage and hematoma of a circulatory system organ or structure due to accidental puncture and laceration during a procedure (I97.5-)
EXCLUDES 2 intraoperative cerebrovascular hemorrhage complicating a procedure (G97.3-)

✓6th **I97.41 Intraoperative hemorrhage and hematoma of a circulatory system organ or structure complicating a circulatory system procedure**
I97.410 Intraoperative hemorrhage and hematoma of a circulatory system organ or structure complicating a cardiac catheterization
I97.411 Intraoperative hemorrhage and hematoma of a circulatory system organ or structure complicating a cardiac bypass
I97.418 Intraoperative hemorrhage and hematoma of a circulatory system organ or structure complicating other circulatory system procedure

I97.42 Intraoperative hemorrhage and hematoma of a circulatory system organ or structure complicating other procedure

✓5th I97.5 Accidental puncture and laceration of a circulatory system organ or structure during a procedure
EXCLUDES 2 accidental puncture and laceration of brain during a procedure (G97.4-)

I97.51 Accidental puncture and laceration of a circulatory system organ or structure during a circulatory system procedure
I97.52 Accidental puncture and laceration of a circulatory system organ or structure during other procedure

✓5th I97.6 Postprocedural hemorrhage, hematoma and seroma of a circulatory system organ or structure following a procedure
EXCLUDES 2 postprocedural cerebrovascular hemorrhage complicating a procedure (G97.5-)

✓6th **I97.61 Postprocedural hemorrhage of a circulatory system organ or structure following a circulatory system procedure**
I97.610 Postprocedural hemorrhage of a circulatory system organ or structure following a cardiac catheterization
I97.611 Postprocedural hemorrhage of a circulatory system organ or structure following cardiac bypass
I97.618 Postprocedural hemorrhage of a circulatory system organ or structure following other circulatory system procedure

✓6th **I97.62 Postprocedural hemorrhage, hematoma and seroma of a circulatory system organ or structure following other procedure**
I97.620 Postprocedural hemorrhage of a circulatory system organ or structure following other procedure
I97.621 Postprocedural hematoma of a circulatory system organ or structure following other procedure
I97.622 Postprocedural seroma of a circulatory system organ or structure following procedure

✓6th **I97.63 Postprocedural hematoma of a circulatory system organ or structure following a circulatory system procedure**
I97.630 Postprocedural hematoma of a circulatory system organ or structure following a cardiac catheterization
I97.631 Postprocedural hematoma of a circulatory system organ or structure following cardiac bypass
I97.638 Postprocedural hematoma of a circulatory system organ or structure following other circulatory system procedure

✓6th **I97.64 Postprocedural seroma of a circulatory system organ or structure following a circulatory system procedure**
I97.640 Postprocedural seroma of a circulatory system organ or structure following a cardiac catheterization
I97.641 Postprocedural seroma of a circulatory system organ or structure following cardiac bypass
I97.648 Postprocedural seroma of a circulatory system organ or structure following other circulatory system procedure

✓5th I97.7 Intraoperative cardiac functional disturbances
EXCLUDES 2 acute pulmonary insufficiency following thoracic surgery (J95.1)
postprocedural cardiac functional disturbances (I97.1-)

✓6th **I97.71 Intraoperative cardiac arrest**
I97.710 Intraoperative cardiac arrest during cardiac surgery
I97.711 Intraoperative cardiac arrest during other surgery

✓6ᵗʰ **I97.79**   Other **intraoperative cardiac functional disturbances**
Use additional code, if applicable, to further specify disorder

     I97.790   **Other intraoperative cardiac functional disturbances during** cardiac surgery

     I97.791   **Other intraoperative cardiac functional disturbances during** other surgery

✓5ᵗʰ **I97.8**   Other **intraoperative and postprocedural complications and disorders of the circulatory system, not elsewhere classified**
Use additional code, if applicable, to further specify disorder

     ✓6ᵗʰ **I97.81**   Intraoperative **cerebrovascular infarction**

         I97.810   **Intraoperative cerebrovascular infarction during** cardiac surgery

         I97.811   **Intraoperative cerebrovascular infarction during** other surgery

✓6ᵗʰ **I97.82**   Postprocedural **cerebrovascular infarction**

     I97.820   **Postprocedural cerebrovascular infarction following** cardiac surgery

     I97.821   **Postprocedural cerebrovascular infarction following** other surgery

     I97.88   **Other** intraoperative **complications of the circulatory system, not elsewhere classified**

     I97.89   **Other** postprocedural **complications and disorders of the circulatory system, not elsewhere classified**

✓4ᵗʰ **I99**   **Other and unspecified disorders of circulatory system**

     I99.8   **Other disorder of circulatory system**

     I99.9   **Unspecified disorder of circulatory system**   ▽

Ⓝ Newborn: 0   Ⓟ Pediatric: 0-17   Ⓜ Maternity: 12-55   Ⓐ Adult: 15-124   **NRS** Nonroutine supply Dx   **NC Dx** Noncancer Dx   **PDx** Primary Dx   ▶◀ Revised Text   ● New Code   ▲ Revised Title

656   ICD-10-CM 2018

Chapter 10. Diseases of the Respiratory System (J00–J99)

Chapter Specific Guidelines with Coding Examples

The chapter specific guidelines from the ICD-10-CM Official Guidelines for Coding and Reporting have been provided below. Along with these guidelines are coding examples, contained in the shaded boxes, that have been developed to help illustrate the coding and/or sequencing guidance found in these guidelines.

a. Chronic obstructive pulmonary disease [COPD] and asthma

1) Acute exacerbation of chronic obstructive bronchitis and asthma

The codes in categories J44 and J45 distinguish between uncomplicated cases and those in acute exacerbation. An acute exacerbation is a worsening or a decompensation of a chronic condition. An acute exacerbation is not equivalent to an infection superimposed on a chronic condition, though an exacerbation may be triggered by an infection.

Patient is admitted for continued IV antibiotic administration and physical therapy with diagnoses of MRSA pneumonia with acute exacerbation of COPD. Provider documentation indicates comorbid moderate persistent asthma.

J15.212	**Pneumonia due to Methicillin resistant Staphylococcus aureus**
J44.0	**Chronic obstructive pulmonary disease with acute lower respiratory infection**
J44.1	**Chronic obstructive pulmonary disease with (acute) exacerbation**
J45.40	**Moderate persistent asthma, uncomplicated**

Explanation: ICD-10-CM uses combination codes to create organism-specific classifications for many types of pneumonia. Category J44 distinguishes between COPD that is exacerbated, COPD with acute lower respiratory infection, and COPD without mention of a complication (unspecified). When a lower respiratory infection is present and COPD is diagnosed, two codes would be required, J44.0 and the code for the infection. Sequencing will be dependent on the condition that is the focus of treatment upon admission to the post-acute setting, which in this case is the MRSA pneumonia.

An acute exacerbation is a worsening or decompensation of a chronic condition and must be specified by the provider as such. When both COPD and asthma are diagnosed and the provider reports an acute exacerbation of COPD, an acute exacerbation of asthma cannot be assumed unless specifically stated by the provider.

Exacerbation of moderate persistent asthma with status asthmaticus.

J45.42	**Moderate persistent asthma with status asthmaticus**

Explanation: Category J45 Asthma includes severity-specific subcategories and fifth-character codes to distinguish between uncomplicated cases, those in acute exacerbation, and those with status asthmaticus.

b. Acute respiratory failure

1) Acute respiratory failure as principal diagnosis

A code from subcategory J96.0, Acute respiratory failure, or subcategory J96.2, Acute and chronic respiratory failure, may be assigned as a principal diagnosis when it is the condition established after study to be chiefly responsible for occasioning the admission to the hospital, and the selection is supported by the Alphabetic Index and Tabular List. However, chapter-specific coding guidelines (such as obstetrics, poisoning, HIV, newborn) that provide sequencing direction take precedence.

2) Acute respiratory failure as secondary diagnosis

Respiratory failure may be listed as a secondary diagnosis if it occurs after admission, or if it is present on admission, but does not meet the definition of principal diagnosis.

Acute pneumococcal pneumonia with subsequent development of acute respiratory failure.

J13	**Pneumonia due to Streptococcus pneumoniae**
J96.00	**Acute respiratory failure, unspecified whether with hypoxia or hypercapnia**

Explanation: Acute respiratory failure may be listed as a secondary diagnosis if it occurs after admission, or if it is present on admission but does not meet the definition of principal diagnosis.

3) Sequencing of acute respiratory failure and another acute condition

When a patient is admitted with respiratory failure and another acute condition, (e.g., myocardial infarction, cerebrovascular accident, aspiration pneumonia), the principal diagnosis will not be the same in every situation. This applies whether the other acute condition is a respiratory or nonrespiratory condition. Selection of the principal diagnosis will be dependent on the circumstances of admission. If both the respiratory failure and the other acute condition are equally responsible for occasioning the admission to the hospital, and there are no chapter-specific sequencing rules, the guideline regarding two or more diagnoses that equally meet the definition for principal diagnosis (Section II, C.) may be applied in these situations.

If the documentation is not clear as to whether acute respiratory failure and another condition are equally responsible for occasioning the admission, query the provider for clarification.

c. Influenza due to certain identified influenza viruses

Code only confirmed cases of influenza due to certain identified influenza viruses (category J09), and due to other identified influenza virus (category J10). This is an exception to the hospital inpatient guideline Section II, H. (Uncertain Diagnosis).

In this context, "confirmation" does not require documentation of positive laboratory testing specific for avian or other novel influenza A or other identified influenza virus. However, coding should be based on the provider's diagnostic statement that the patient has avian influenza, or other novel influenza A, for category J09, or has another particular identified strain of influenza, such as H1N1 or H3N2, but not identified as novel or variant, for category J10.

If the provider records "suspected" or "possible" or "probable" avian influenza, or novel influenza, or other identified influenza, then the appropriate influenza code from category J11, Influenza due to unidentified influenza virus, should be assigned. A code from category J09, Influenza due to certain identified influenza viruses, should not be assigned nor should a code from category J10, Influenza due to other identified influenza virus.

Influenza due to avian influenza virus with pneumonia.

J09.X1	**Influenza due to identified novel influenza A virus with pneumonia**

Explanation: Codes in category J09 Influenza due to certain identified influenza viruses should be assigned only for confirmed cases. "Confirmation" does not require positive laboratory testing of a specific influenza virus but does need to be based on the provider's diagnostic statement, which should not include terms such as "possible," "probable," or "suspected."

d. Ventilator associated pneumonia

1) Documentation of ventilator associated pneumonia

As with all procedural or postprocedural complications, code assignment is based on the provider's documentation of the relationship between the condition and the procedure.

Code J95.851, Ventilator associated pneumonia, should be assigned only when the provider has documented ventilator associated pneumonia (VAP). An additional code to identify the organism (e.g., Pseudomonas aeruginosa, code B96.5) should also be assigned. Do not assign an additional code from categories J12-J18 to identify the type of pneumonia.

Code J95.851 should not be assigned for cases where the patient has pneumonia and is on a mechanical ventilator and the provider has not specifically stated that the pneumonia is ventilator-associated pneumonia. If the documentation is unclear as to whether the patient has a pneumonia that is a complication attributable to the mechanical ventilator, query the provider.

Chapter 10. Diseases of the Respiratory System

2) Ventilator associated pneumonia develops after admission

A patient may be admitted with one type of pneumonia (e.g., code J13, Pneumonia due to Streptococcus pneumonia) and subsequently develop VAP. In this instance, the principal diagnosis would be the appropriate code from categories J12-J18 for the pneumonia diagnosed at the time of admission. Code J95.851, Ventilator associated pneumonia, would be assigned as an additional diagnosis when the provider has also documented the presence of ventilator associated pneumonia.

Patient with pneumonia due to *Klebsiella pneumoniae* develops superimposed MRSA ventilator-associated pneumonia.

J15.Ø	**Pneumonia due to Klebsiella pneumoniae**
J95.851	**Ventilator associated pneumonia**
B95.62	**Methicillin resistant Staphylococcus aureus infection as the cause of diseases classified elsewhere**

Explanation: Code assignment for ventilator-associated pneumonia is based on the provider's documentation of the relationship between the condition and the procedure and is reported only when the provider has documented ventilator-associated pneumonia (VAP).

A patient may be admitted with one type of pneumonia and subsequently develop VAP. In this example, the principal diagnosis code describes the pneumonia diagnosed at the time of admission, with code J95.851 Ventilator associated pneumonia, assigned as secondary.

Chapter 10. Diseases of the Respiratory System (J00-J99)

NOTE   When a respiratory condition is described as occurring in more than one site and is not specifically indexed, it should be classified to the lower anatomic site (e.g. tracheobronchitis to bronchitis in J40).

Use additional code, where applicable, to identify:
   exposure to environmental tobacco smoke (Z77.22)
   exposure to tobacco smoke in the perinatal period (P96.81)
   history of tobacco dependence (Z87.891)
   occupational exposure to environmental tobacco smoke (Z57.31)
   tobacco dependence (F17.-)
   tobacco use (Z72.0)

EXCLUDES 2 *certain conditions originating in the perinatal period (P04-P96)*
certain infectious and parasitic diseases (A00-B99)
complications of pregnancy, childbirth and the puerperium (O00-O9A)
congenital malformations, deformations and chromosomal abnormalities (Q00-Q99)
endocrine, nutritional and metabolic diseases (E00-E88)
injury, poisoning and certain other consequences of external causes (S00-T88)
neoplasms (C00-D49)
smoke inhalation (T59.81-)
symptoms, signs and abnormal clinical and laboratory findings, not elsewhere classified (R00-R94)

This chapter contains the following blocks:

J00-J06   Acute upper respiratory infections
J09-J18   Influenza and pneumonia
J20-J22   Other acute lower respiratory infections
J30-J39   Other diseases of upper respiratory tract
J40-J47   Chronic lower respiratory diseases
J60-J70   Lung diseases due to external agents
J80-J84   Other respiratory diseases principally affecting the interstitium
J85-J86   Suppurative and necrotic conditions of the lower respiratory tract
J90-J94   Other diseases of the pleura
J95   Intraoperative and postprocedural complications and disorders of respiratory system, not elsewhere classified
J96-J99   Other diseases of the respiratory system

Acute upper respiratory infections (J00-J06)

EXCLUDES 1 *chronic obstructive pulmonary disease with acute lower respiratory infection (J44.0)*
influenza virus with other respiratory manifestations (J09.X2, J10.1, J11.1)

J00   **Acute nasopharyngitis [common cold]**
   Acute rhinitis
   Coryza (acute)
   Infective nasopharyngitis NOS
   Infective rhinitis
   Nasal catarrh, acute
   Nasopharyngitis NOS
   EXCLUDES 1 *acute pharyngitis (J02.-)*
acute sore throat NOS (J02.9)
pharyngitis NOS (J02.9)
rhinitis NOS (J31.0)
sore throat NOS (J02.9)
   EXCLUDES 2 *allergic rhinitis (J30.1-J30.9)*
chronic pharyngitis (J31.2)
chronic rhinitis (J31.0)
chronic sore throat (J31.2)
nasopharyngitis, chronic (J31.1)
vasomotor rhinitis (J30.0)
   DEF: Acute inflammation of mucous membranes; extends from nares to pharynx; characterized by nasal obstruction, sneezing, runny nose, and sore throat.

✓4th J01   **Acute sinusitis**
   INCLUDES   acute abscess of sinus
     acute empyema of sinus
     acute infection of sinus
     acute inflammation of sinus
     acute suppuration of sinus
   Use additional code (B95-B97) to identify infectious agent
   EXCLUDES 1 *sinusitis NOS (J32.9)*
   EXCLUDES 2 *chronic sinusitis (J32.0-J32.8)*

   ✓5th J01.0   **Acute maxillary sinusitis**
     Acute antritis
     J01.00   **Acute maxillary sinusitis, unspecified**   ▽
     J01.01   **Acute recurrent maxillary sinusitis**

   ✓5th J01.1   **Acute frontal sinusitis**
     J01.10   **Acute frontal sinusitis, unspecified**   ▽
     J01.11   **Acute recurrent frontal sinusitis**

   ✓5th J01.2   **Acute ethmoidal sinusitis**
     J01.20   **Acute ethmoidal sinusitis, unspecified**   ▽
     J01.21   **Acute recurrent ethmoidal sinusitis**

   ✓5th J01.3   **Acute sphenoidal sinusitis**
     J01.30   **Acute sphenoidal sinusitis, unspecified**   ▽
     J01.31   **Acute recurrent sphenoidal sinusitis**

   ✓5th J01.4   **Acute pansinusitis**
     J01.40   **Acute pansinusitis, unspecified**   ▽
     J01.41   **Acute recurrent pansinusitis**

   ✓5th J01.8   **Other acute sinusitis**
     J01.80   **Other acute sinusitis**
      Acute sinusitis involving more than one sinus but not pansinusitis
     J01.81   **Other acute recurrent sinusitis**
      Acute recurrent sinusitis involving more than one sinus but not pansinusitis

   ✓5th J01.9   **Acute sinusitis, unspecified**
     J01.90   **Acute sinusitis, unspecified**   ▽
     J01.91   **Acute recurrent sinusitis, unspecified**   ▽

✓4th J02   **Acute pharyngitis**
   INCLUDES   acute sore throat
   EXCLUDES 1 *acute laryngopharyngitis (J06.0)*
peritonsillar abscess (J36)
pharyngeal abscess (J39.1)
retropharyngeal abscess (J39.0)
   EXCLUDES 2 *chronic pharyngitis (J31.2)*

   J02.0   **Streptococcal pharyngitis**
     Septic pharyngitis
     Streptococcal sore throat
     EXCLUDES 2 *scarlet fever (A38.-)*

   J02.8   **Acute pharyngitis due to other specified organisms**
     Use additional code (B95-B97) to identify infectious agent
     EXCLUDES 1 *acute pharyngitis due to coxsackie virus (B08.5)*
acute pharyngitis due to gonococcus (A54.5)
acute pharyngitis due to herpes [simplex] virus (B00.2)
acute pharyngitis due to infectious mononucleosis (B27.-)
enteroviral vesicular pharyngitis (B08.5)

   J02.9   **Acute pharyngitis, unspecified**   ▽
     Gangrenous pharyngitis (acute)
     Infective pharyngitis (acute) NOS
     Pharyngitis (acute) NOS
     Sore throat (acute) NOS
     Suppurative pharyngitis (acute)
     Ulcerative pharyngitis (acute)

✓4th J03   **Acute tonsillitis**
   EXCLUDES 1 *acute sore throat (J02.-)*
hypertrophy of tonsils (J35.1)
peritonsillar abscess (J36)
sore throat NOS (J02.9)
streptococcal sore throat (J02.0)
   EXCLUDES 2 *chronic tonsillitis (J35.0)*

   ✓5th J03.0   **Streptococcal tonsillitis**
     J03.00   **Acute streptococcal tonsillitis, unspecified**   ▽
     J03.01   **Acute recurrent streptococcal tonsillitis**

   ✓5th J03.8   **Acute tonsillitis due to other specified organisms**
     Use additional code (B95-B97) to identify infectious agent
     EXCLUDES 1 *diphtheritic tonsillitis (A36.0)*
herpesviral pharyngotonsillitis (B00.2)
streptococcal tonsillitis (J03.0)
tuberculous tonsillitis (A15.8)
Vincent's tonsillitis (A69.1)
     J03.80   **Acute tonsillitis due to other specified organisms**
     J03.81   **Acute recurrent tonsillitis due to other specified organisms**

   ✓5th J03.9   **Acute tonsillitis, unspecified**
     Follicular tonsillitis (acute)
     Gangrenous tonsillitis (acute)
     Infective tonsillitis (acute)
     Tonsillitis (acute) NOS
     Ulcerative tonsillitis (acute)
     J03.90   **Acute tonsillitis, unspecified**   ▽
     J03.91   **Acute recurrent tonsillitis, unspecified**   ▽

✓ Additional Character Req   ✓x7th Placeholder Alert   Case-Mix Diagnosis   Manifestation   ▽ Unspecified Dx   **EXCLUDES 1** Not coded here   **EXCLUDES 2** Not included here

ICD-10-CM 2018   659

Chapter 10. Diseases of the Respiratory System

J04–J11.00

☑4ᵗʰ **J04 Acute laryngitis and tracheitis**
Use additional code (B95-B97) to identify infectious agent
EXCLUDES 1   *acute obstructive laryngitis [croup] and epiglottitis (J05.-)*
EXCLUDES 2   *laryngismus (stridulus) (J38.5)*

    J04.0 Acute laryngitis
Edematous laryngitis (acute)
Laryngitis (acute) NOS
Subglottic laryngitis (acute)
Suppurative laryngitis (acute)
Ulcerative laryngitis (acute)
EXCLUDES 1   *acute obstructive laryngitis (J05.0)*
EXCLUDES 2   *chronic laryngitis (J37.0)*

☑5ᵗʰ   **J04.1 Acute tracheitis**
Acute viral tracheitis
Catarrhal tracheitis (acute)
Tracheitis (acute) NOS
EXCLUDES 2   *chronic tracheitis (J42)*

     J04.10 Acute tracheitis without obstruction

     J04.11 Acute tracheitis with obstruction

    J04.2 Acute laryngotracheitis
Laryngotracheitis NOS
Tracheitis (acute) with laryngitis (acute)
EXCLUDES 1   *acute obstructive laryngotracheitis (J05.0)*
EXCLUDES 2   *chronic laryngotracheitis (J37.1)*

☑5ᵗʰ   **J04.3 Supraglottitis, unspecified**

     J04.30 Supraglottitis, unspecified, without obstruction ▽

     J04.31 Supraglottitis, unspecified, with obstruction ▽

☑4ᵗʰ **J05 Acute obstructive laryngitis [croup] and epiglottitis**
Use additional code (B95-B97) to identify infectious agent

    J05.0 Acute obstructive laryngitis [croup]
Obstructive laryngitis (acute) NOS
Obstructive laryngotracheitis NOS
DEF: Acute laryngeal obstruction due to allergy, foreign body, or in the majority of cases a viral infection; symptoms include harsh, barking cough, hoarseness, and persistent high-pitched respiratory sound (stridor).

☑5ᵗʰ   **J05.1 Acute epiglottitis**
EXCLUDES 2   *epiglottitis, chronic (J37.0)*

     J05.10 Acute epiglottitis without obstruction
Epiglottitis NOS

     J05.11 Acute epiglottitis with obstruction

☑4ᵗʰ **J06 Acute upper respiratory infections of multiple and unspecified sites**
EXCLUDES 1   *acute respiratory infection NOS (J22)*
                streptococcal pharyngitis (J02.0)

    J06.0 Acute laryngopharyngitis

    J06.9 Acute upper respiratory infection, unspecified ▽
Upper respiratory disease, acute
Upper respiratory infection NOS

Influenza and pneumonia (J09-J18)

EXCLUDES 2   *allergic or eosinophilic pneumonia (J82)*
                aspiration pneumonia NOS (J69.0)
                congenital pneumonia (P23.9)
                lipid pneumonia (J69.1)
                meconium pneumonia (P24.01)
                neonatal aspiration pneumonia (P24.-)
                pneumonia due to solids and liquids (J69.-)
                rheumatic pneumonia (I00)
                ventilator associated pneumonia (J95.851)

☑4ᵗʰ **J09 Influenza due to certain identified influenza viruses**
EXCLUDES 1 ►*influenza A/H1N1 (J10.-)*◄
                influenza due to other identified influenza virus (J10.-)
                influenza due to unidentified influenza virus (J11.-)
                seasonal influenza due to other identified influenza virus (J10.-)
                seasonal influenza due to unidentified influenza virus (J11.-)

☑5ᵗʰ   **J09.X Influenza due to identified novel influenza A virus**
Avian influenza
Bird influenza
Influenza A/H5N1
Influenza of other animal origin, not bird or swine
Swine influenza virus (viruses that normally cause infections in pigs)
AHA: 2016, 3Q, 10

     J09.X1 Influenza due to identified novel influenza A virus with pneumonia
Code also, if applicable, associated:
lung abscess (J85.1)
other specified type of pneumonia

     J09.X2 Influenza due to identified novel influenza A virus with other respiratory manifestations
Influenza due to identified novel influenza A virus NOS
Influenza due to identified novel influenza A virus with laryngitis
Influenza due to identified novel influenza A virus with pharyngitis
Influenza due to identified novel influenza A virus with upper respiratory symptoms
Use additional code, if applicable, for associated:
pleural effusion (J91.8)
sinusitis (J01.-)

     J09.X3 Influenza due to identified novel influenza A virus with gastrointestinal manifestations
Influenza due to identified novel influenza A virus gastroenteritis
EXCLUDES 1   *'intestinal flu' [viral gastroenteritis] (A08.-)*

     J09.X9 Influenza due to identified novel influenza A virus with other manifestations
Influenza due to identified novel influenza A virus with encephalopathy
Influenza due to identified novel influenza A virus with myocarditis
Influenza due to identified novel influenza A virus with otitis media
Use additional code to identify manifestation

☑4ᵗʰ **J10 Influenza due to other identified influenza virus**
EXCLUDES 1   *influenza due to avian influenza virus (J09.X-)*
                influenza due to swine flu (J09.X-)
                influenza due to unidentifed influenza virus (J11.-)

☑5ᵗʰ   **J10.0 Influenza due to other identified influenza virus with pneumonia**
Code also associated lung abscess, if applicable (J85.1)

     J10.00 Influenza due to other identified influenza virus ▽ **with unspecified type of pneumonia**

     J10.01 Influenza due to other identified influenza virus with the same other identified influenza virus pneumonia

     J10.08 Influenza due to other identified influenza virus with other specified pneumonia
Code also other specified type of pneumonia

    J10.1 Influenza due to other identified influenza virus with other respiratory manifestations
Influenza due to other identified influenza virus NOS
Influenza due to other identified influenza virus with laryngitis
Influenza due to other identified influenza virus with pharyngitis
Influenza due to other identified influenza virus with upper respiratory symptoms
Use additional code for associated pleural effusion, if applicable (J91.8)
Use additional code for associated sinusitis, if applicable (J01.-)
AHA: 2016, 3Q, 10-11

    J10.2 Influenza due to other identified influenza virus with gastrointestinal manifestations
Influenza due to other identified influenza virus gastroenteritis
EXCLUDES 1   *'intestinal flu' [viral gastroenteritis] (A08.-)*

☑5ᵗʰ   **J10.8 Influenza due to other identified influenza virus with other manifestations**

     J10.81 Influenza due to other identified influenza virus with encephalopathy

     J10.82 Influenza due to other identified influenza virus with myocarditis

     J10.83 Influenza due to other identified influenza virus with otitis media
Use additional code for any associated perforated tympanic membrane (H72.-)

     J10.89 Influenza due to other identified influenza virus with other manifestations
Use additional codes to identify the manifestations

☑4ᵗʰ **J11 Influenza due to unidentified influenza virus**

☑5ᵗʰ   **J11.0 Influenza due to unidentified influenza virus with pneumonia**
Code also associated lung abscess, if applicable (J85.1)
AHA: 2016, 3Q, 11

     J11.00 Influenza due to unidentified influenza virus ▽ **with unspecified type of pneumonia**
Influenza with pneumonia NOS

Ⓝ Newborn: 0   Ⓟ Pediatric: 0-17   Ⓜ Maternity: 12-55   Ⓐ Adult: 15-124   **NRS** Nonroutine supply Dx   **NCDx** Noncancer Dx   **PDx** Primary Dx   ►◄ Revised Text   ● New Code   ▲ Revised Title

660   ICD-10-CM 2018

J11.08 Influenza due to unidentified influenza virus with specified pneumonia
Code also other specified type of pneumonia

J11.1 Influenza due to unidentified influenza virus with other respiratory manifestations
Influenza NOS
Influenzal laryngitis NOS
Influenzal pharyngitis NOS
Influenza with upper respiratory symptoms NOS
Use additional code for associated pleural effusion, if applicable (J91.8)
Use additional code for associated sinusitis, if applicable (J01.-)

J11.2 Influenza due to unidentified influenza virus with gastrointestinal manifestations
Influenza gastroenteritis NOS
EXCLUDES 1 'intestinal flu' [viral gastroenteritis] (A08.-)

✓5ᵗʰ **J11.8 Influenza due to unidentified influenza virus with other manifestations**

J11.81 Influenza due to unidentified influenza virus with encephalopathy
Influenzal encephalopathy NOS

J11.82 Influenza due to unidentified influenza virus with myocarditis
Influenzal myocarditis NOS

J11.83 Influenza due to unidentified influenza virus with otitis media
Influenzal otitis media NOS
Use additional code for any associated perforated tympanic membrane (H72.-)

J11.89 Influenza due to unidentified influenza virus with other manifestations
Use additional codes to identify the manifestations

✓4ᵗʰ **J12 Viral pneumonia, not elsewhere classified**
INCLUDES bronchopneumonia due to viruses other than influenza viruses
Code first associated influenza, if applicable (J09.X1, J10.0-, J11.0-)
Code also associated abscess, if applicable (J85.1)
EXCLUDES 1 aspiration pneumonia due to anesthesia during labor and delivery (O74.0)
aspiration pneumonia due to anesthesia during pregnancy (O29)
aspiration pneumonia due to anesthesia during puerperium (O89.0)
aspiration pneumonia due to solids and liquids (J69.-)
aspiration pneumonia NOS (J69.0)
congenital pneumonia (P23.0)
congenital rubella pneumonitis (P35.0)
interstitial pneumonia NOS (J84.9)
lipid pneumonia (J69.1)
neonatal aspiration pneumonia (P24.-)
AHA: 2016, 3Q, 15; 2013, 4Q, 118

J12.0 Adenoviral pneumonia

J12.1 Respiratory syncytial virus pneumonia

J12.2 Parainfluenza virus pneumonia

J12.3 Human metapneumovirus pneumonia

✓5ᵗʰ **J12.8 Other viral pneumonia**

J12.81 Pneumonia due to SARS-associated coronavirus
Severe acute respiratory syndrome NOS
DEF: A severe adult respiratory syndrome caused by the coronavirus, specified as inflammation of the lungs with consolidation.

J12.89 Other viral pneumonia

J12.9 Viral pneumonia, unspecified ▽

J13 Pneumonia due to Streptococcus pneumoniae
Bronchopneumonia due to S. pneumoniae
Code first associated influenza, if applicable (J09.X1, J10.0-, J11.0-)
Code also associated lung abscess, if applicable (J85.1)
EXCLUDES 1 congenital pneumonia due to S. pneumoniae (P23.6)
lobar pneumonia, unspecified organism (J18.1)
pneumonia due to other streptococci (J15.3-J15.4)
AHA: 2016, 3Q, 15; 2013, 4Q, 118

J14 Pneumonia due to Hemophilus influenzae
Bronchopneumonia due to H. influenzae
Code first associated influenza, if applicable (J09.X1, J10.0-, J11.0-)
Code also associated lung abscess, if applicable (J85.1)
EXCLUDES 1 congenital pneumonia due to H. influenzae (P23.6)
AHA: 2016, 3Q, 15; 2013, 4Q, 118

✓4ᵗʰ **J15 Bacterial pneumonia, not elsewhere classified**
INCLUDES bronchopneumonia due to bacteria other than S. pneumoniae and H. influenzae
Code first associated influenza, if applicable (J09.X1, J10.0-, J11.0-)
Code also associated lung abscess, if applicable (J85.1)
EXCLUDES 1 chlamydial pneumonia (J16.0)
congenital pneumonia (P23.-)
Legionnaires' disease (A48.1)
spirochetal pneumonia (A69.8)
AHA: 2016, 3Q, 15; 2013, 4Q, 118

J15.0 Pneumonia due to Klebsiella pneumoniae

J15.1 Pneumonia due to Pseudomonas

✓5ᵗʰ **J15.2 Pneumonia due to staphylococcus**

J15.20 Pneumonia due to staphylococcus, unspecified ▽

✓6ᵗʰ **J15.21 Pneumonia due to Staphylococcus aureus**

J15.211 Pneumonia due to Methicillin susceptible Staphylococcus aureus
MSSA pneumonia
Pneumonia due to Staphylococcus aureus NOS

J15.212 Pneumonia due to Methicillin resistant Staphylococcus aureus

J15.29 Pneumonia due to other staphylococcus

J15.3 Pneumonia due to streptococcus, group B

J15.4 Pneumonia due to other streptococci
EXCLUDES 1 pneumonia due to streptococcus, group B (J15.3)
pneumonia due to Streptococcus pneumoniae (J13)

J15.5 Pneumonia due to Escherichia coli

▲ **J15.6 Pneumonia due to other Gram-negative bacteria**
▶Pneumonia due to other aerobic Gram-negative bacteria◀
Pneumonia due to Serratia marcescens

J15.7 Pneumonia due to Mycoplasma pneumoniae

J15.8 Pneumonia due to other specified bacteria

J15.9 Unspecified bacterial pneumonia ▽
Pneumonia due to gram-positive bacteria

✓4ᵗʰ **J16 Pneumonia due to other infectious organisms, not elsewhere classified**
Code first associated influenza, if applicable (J09.X1, J10.0-, J11.0-)
Code also associated lung abscess, if applicable (J85.1)
EXCLUDES 1 congenital pneumonia (P23.-)
ornithosis (A70)
pneumocystosis (B59)
pneumonia NOS (J18.9)
AHA: 2016, 3Q, 15; 2013, 4Q, 118

J16.0 Chlamydial pneumonia

J16.8 Pneumonia due to other specified infectious organisms

J17 Pneumonia in diseases classified elsewhere
Code first underlying disease, such as:
Q fever (A78)
rheumatic fever (I00)
schistosomiasis (B65.0-B65.9)
EXCLUDES 1 candidial pneumonia (B37.1)
chlamydial pneumonia (J16.0)
gonorrheal pneumonia (A54.84)
histoplasmosis pneumonia (B39.0-B39.2)
measles pneumonia (B05.2)
nocardiosis pneumonia (A43.0)
pneumocystosis (B59)
pneumonia due to Pneumocystis carinii (B59)
pneumonia due to Pneumocystis jiroveci (B59)
pneumonia in actinomycosis (A42.0)
pneumonia in anthrax (A22.1)
pneumonia in ascariasis (B77.81)
pneumonia in aspergillosis (B44.0-B44.1)
pneumonia in coccidioidomycosis (B38.0-B38.2)
pneumonia in cytomegalovirus disease (B25.0)
pneumonia in toxoplasmosis (B58.3)
rubella pneumonia (B06.81)
salmonella pneumonia (A02.22)
spirochetal infection NEC with pneumonia (A69.8)
tularemia pneumonia (A21.2)
typhoid fever with pneumonia (A01.03)
varicella pneumonia (B01.2)
whooping cough with pneumonia (A37 with fifth-character 1)
AHA: 2016, 3Q, 15; 2013, 4Q, 118

☑ Additional Character Req   ☑x7ᵗʰ Placeholder Alert   Case-Mix Diagnosis   Manifestation   ▽ Unspecified Dx   *EXCLUDES 1* Not coded here   *EXCLUDES 2* Not included here

✓4ᵗʰ **J18**   **Pneumonia, unspecified organism**

Code first associated influenza, if applicable (J09.X1, J10.0-, J11.0-)

EXCLUDES 1   *abscess of lung with pneumonia (J85.1)*
aspiration pneumonia due to anesthesia during labor and delivery (O74.0)
aspiration pneumonia due to anesthesia during pregnancy (O29)
aspiration pneumonia due to anesthesia during puerperium (O89.0)
aspiration pneumonia due to solids and liquids (J69.-)
aspiration pneumonia NOS (J69.0)
congenital pneumonia (P23.0)
drug-induced interstitial lung disorder (J70.2-J70.4)
interstitial pneumonia NOS (J84.9)
lipid pneumonia (J69.1)
neonatal aspiration pneumonia (P24.-)
pneumonitis due to external agents (J67-J70)
pneumonitis due to fumes and vapors (J68.0)
usual interstitial pneumonia (J84.17)

AHA: 2016, 3Q, 15; 2013, 4Q, 118
TIP: Hemoptysis (R04.2) is not integral to pneumonia and can be coded separately.

J18.0   **Bronchopneumonia, unspecified organism**   ▽

EXCLUDES 1   *hypostatic bronchopneumonia (J18.2)*
lipid pneumonia (J69.1)

EXCLUDES 2   *acute bronchiolitis (J21.-)*
chronic bronchiolitis (J44.9)

J18.1   **Lobar pneumonia, unspecified organism**   ▽

J18.2   **Hypostatic pneumonia, unspecified organism**   ▽
Hypostatic bronchopneumonia
Passive pneumonia

J18.8   **Other pneumonia, unspecified organism**   ▽

J18.9   **Pneumonia, unspecified organism**   ▽
AHA: 2014, 3Q, 4; 2013, 4Q, 119; 2012, 4Q, 94

Other acute lower respiratory infections (J20-J22)

EXCLUDES 2   *chronic obstructive pulmonary disease with acute lower respiratory infection (J44.0)*

✓4ᵗʰ **J20**   **Acute bronchitis**

INCLUDES   acute and subacute bronchitis (with) bronchospasm
acute and subacute bronchitis (with) tracheitis
acute and subacute bronchitis (with) tracheobronchitis, acute
acute and subacute fibrinous bronchitis
acute and subacute membranous bronchitis
acute and subacute purulent bronchitis
acute and subacute septic bronchitis

EXCLUDES 1   *bronchitis NOS (J40)*
tracheobronchitis NOS (J40)

EXCLUDES 2   *acute bronchitis with bronchiectasis (J47.0)*
acute bronchitis with chronic obstructive asthma (J44.0)
acute bronchitis with chronic obstructive pulmonary disease (J44.0)
allergic bronchitis NOS (J45.909)
bronchitis due to chemicals, fumes and vapors (J68.0)
chronic bronchitis NOS (J42)
chronic mucopurulent bronchitis (J41.1)
chronic obstructive bronchitis (J44.-)
chronic obstructive tracheobronchitis (J44.-)
chronic simple bronchitis (J41.0)
chronic tracheobronchitis (J42)

AHA: 2016, 3Q, 10, 16
DEF: Acute inflammation of main branches of bronchial tree due to infectious or irritant agents; symptoms include cough with a varied production of sputum, fever, substernal soreness, and lung rales; usually last for three to 10 days.

J20.0   **Acute bronchitis due to Mycoplasma pneumoniae**

J20.1   **Acute bronchitis due to Hemophilus influenzae**

J20.2   **Acute bronchitis due to streptococcus**

J20.3   **Acute bronchitis due to coxsackievirus**

J20.4   **Acute bronchitis due to parainfluenza virus**

J20.5   **Acute bronchitis due to respiratory syncytial virus**

J20.6   **Acute bronchitis due to rhinovirus**

J20.7   **Acute bronchitis due to echovirus**

J20.8   **Acute bronchitis due to other specified organisms**

J20.9   **Acute bronchitis, unspecified**   ▽

✓4ᵗʰ **J21**   **Acute bronchiolitis**

INCLUDES   acute bronchiolitis with bronchospasm

EXCLUDES 2   *respiratory bronchiolitis interstitial lung disease (J84.115)*

J21.0   **Acute bronchiolitis due to respiratory syncytial virus**

J21.1   **Acute bronchiolitis due to human metapneumovirus**

J21.8   **Acute bronchiolitis due to other specified organisms**

J21.9   **Acute bronchiolitis, unspecified**   ▽
Bronchiolitis (acute)

EXCLUDES 1   *chronic bronchiolitis (J44.-)*

J22   **Unspecified acute lower respiratory infection**   ▽
Acute (lower) respiratory (tract) infection NOS

EXCLUDES 1   *upper respiratory infection (acute) (J06.9)*

Other diseases of upper respiratory tract (J30-J39)

✓4ᵗʰ **J30**   **Vasomotor and allergic rhinitis**

INCLUDES   spasmodic rhinorrhea

EXCLUDES 1   *allergic rhinitis with asthma (bronchial) (J45.909)*
rhinitis NOS (J31.0)

J30.0   **Vasomotor rhinitis**

J30.1   **Allergic rhinitis due to pollen**
Allergy NOS due to pollen
Hay fever
Pollinosis

J30.2   **Other seasonal allergic rhinitis**

J30.5   **Allergic rhinitis due to food**

✓5ᵗʰ **J30.8**   **Other allergic rhinitis**

J30.81   **Allergic rhinitis due to animal (cat) (dog) hair and dander**

J30.89   **Other allergic rhinitis**
Perennial allergic rhinitis

J30.9   **Allergic rhinitis, unspecified**   ▽

✓4ᵗʰ **J31**   **Chronic rhinitis, nasopharyngitis and pharyngitis**

Use additional code to identify:
exposure to environmental tobacco smoke (Z77.22)
exposure to tobacco smoke in the perinatal period (P96.81)
history of tobacco dependence (Z87.891)
occupational exposure to environmental tobacco smoke (Z57.31)
tobacco dependence (F17.-)
tobacco use (Z72.0)

J31.0   **Chronic rhinitis**
Atrophic rhinitis (chronic)
Granulomatous rhinitis (chronic)
Hypertrophic rhinitis (chronic)
Obstructive rhinitis (chronic)
Ozena
Purulent rhinitis (chronic)
Rhinitis (chronic) NOS
Ulcerative rhinitis (chronic)

EXCLUDES 1   *allergic rhinitis (J30.1-J30.9)*
vasomotor rhinitis (J30.0)

DEF: Persistent inflammation of mucous membranes of nose; characterized by postnasal drip.

J31.1   **Chronic nasopharyngitis**

EXCLUDES 2   *acute nasopharyngitis (J00)*

DEF: Persistent inflammation of mucous membranes extending from nares to pharynx; characterized by constant irritation in nasopharynx and postnasal drip.

J31.2   **Chronic pharyngitis**
Atrophic pharyngitis (chronic)
Chronic sore throat
Granular pharyngitis (chronic)
Hypertrophic pharyngitis (chronic)

EXCLUDES 2   *acute pharyngitis (J02.9)*

Ⓝ Newborn: 0   Ⓟ Pediatric: 0-17   Ⓜ Maternity: 12-55   Ⓐ Adult: 15-124   **NRS** Nonroutine supply Dx   **NCDx** Noncancer Dx   **PDx** Primary Dx   ▶◀ Revised Text   ● New Code   ▲ Revised Title

662   ICD-10-CM 2018

☑4ᵗʰ **J32 Chronic sinusitis**

INCLUDES   sinus abscess
sinus empyema
sinus infection
sinus suppuration

Use additional code to identify:
exposure to environmental tobacco smoke (Z77.22)
exposure to tobacco smoke in the perinatal period (P96.81)
history of tobacco dependence (Z87.891)
infectious agent (B95-B97)
occupational exposure to environmental tobacco smoke (Z57.31)
tobacco dependence (F17.-)
tobacco use (Z72.0)

EXCLUDES 2   *acute sinusitis (J01.-)*

J32.0 Chronic maxillary sinusitis
Antritis (chronic)
Maxillary sinusitis NOS

J32.1 Chronic frontal sinusitis
Frontal sinusitis NOS

J32.2 Chronic ethmoidal sinusitis
Ethmoidal sinusitis NOS
EXCLUDES 1   *Woakes' ethmoiditis (J33.1)*

J32.3 Chronic sphenoidal sinusitis
Sphenoidal sinusitis NOS

J32.4 Chronic pansinusitis
Pansinusitis NOS

J32.8 Other chronic sinusitis
Sinusitis (chronic) involving more than one sinus but not pansinusitis

J32.9 Chronic sinusitis, unspecified   ▽
Sinusitis (chronic) NOS

☑4ᵗʰ **J33 Nasal polyp**

Use additional code to identify:
exposure to environmental tobacco smoke (Z77.22)
exposure to tobacco smoke in the perinatal period (P96.81)
history of tobacco dependence (Z87.891)
occupational exposure to environmental tobacco smoke (Z57.31)
tobacco dependence (F17.-)
tobacco use (Z72.0)

EXCLUDES 1   *adenomatous polyps (D14.0)*

J33.0 Polyp of nasal cavity
Choanal polyp
Nasopharyngeal polyp

J33.1 Polypoid sinus degeneration
Woakes' syndrome or ethmoiditis

J33.8 Other polyp of sinus
Accessory polyp of sinus
Ethmoidal polyp of sinus
Maxillary polyp of sinus
Sphenoidal polyp of sinus

J33.9 Nasal polyp, unspecified   ▽

☑4ᵗʰ **J34 Other and unspecified disorders of nose and nasal sinuses**
EXCLUDES 2   *varicose ulcer of nasal septum (I86.8)*

J34.0 Abscess, furuncle and carbuncle of nose
Cellulitis of nose
Necrosis of nose
Ulceration of nose

J34.1 Cyst and mucocele of nose and nasal sinus

J34.2 Deviated nasal septum
Deflection or deviation of septum (nasal) (acquired)
EXCLUDES 1   *congenital deviated nasal septum (Q67.4)*

J34.3 Hypertrophy of nasal turbinates

☑5ᵗʰ **J34.8 Other specified disorders of nose and nasal sinuses**

J34.81 Nasal mucositis (ulcerative)
Code also type of associated therapy, such as:
antineoplastic and immunosuppressive drugs (T45.1X-)
radiological procedure and radiotherapy (Y84.2)
EXCLUDES 2   *gastrointestinal mucositis (ulcerative) (K92.81)*
mucositis (ulcerative) of vagina and vulva (N76.81)
oral mucositis (ulcerative) (K12.3-)

J34.89 Other specified disorders of nose and nasal sinuses
Perforation of nasal septum NOS
Rhinolith

J34.9 Unspecified disorder of nose and nasal sinuses   ▽

☑4ᵗʰ **J35 Chronic diseases of tonsils and adenoids**

Use additional code to identify:
exposure to environmental tobacco smoke (Z77.22)
exposure to tobacco smoke in the perinatal period (P96.81)
history of tobacco dependence (Z87.891)
occupational exposure to environmental tobacco smoke (Z57.31)
tobacco dependence (F17.-)
tobacco use (Z72.0)

☑5ᵗʰ **J35.0 Chronic tonsillitis and adenoiditis**
EXCLUDES 2   *acute tonsillitis (J03.-)*

J35.01 Chronic tonsillitis

J35.02 Chronic adenoiditis

J35.03 Chronic tonsillitis and adenoiditis

J35.1 Hypertrophy of tonsils
Enlargement of tonsils
EXCLUDES 1   *hypertrophy of tonsils with tonsillitis (J35.0-)*

J35.2 Hypertrophy of adenoids
Enlargement of adenoids
EXCLUDES 1   *hypertrophy of adenoids with adenoiditis (J35.0-)*

J35.3 Hypertrophy of tonsils with hypertrophy of adenoids
EXCLUDES 1   *hypertrophy of tonsils and adenoids with tonsillitis and adenoiditis (J35.03)*

J35.8 Other chronic diseases of tonsils and adenoids
Adenoid vegetations
Amygdalolith
Calculus, tonsil
Cicatrix of tonsil (and adenoid)
Tonsillar tag
Ulcer of tonsil

J35.9 Chronic disease of tonsils and adenoids, unspecified   ▽
Disease (chronic) of tonsils and adenoids NOS

J36 Peritonsillar abscess

INCLUDES   abscess of tonsil
peritonsillar cellulitis
quinsy

Use additional code (B95-B97) to identify infectious agent
EXCLUDES 1   *acute tonsillitis (J03.-)*
chronic tonsillitis (J35.0)
retropharyngeal abscess (J39.0)
tonsillitis NOS (J03.9-)

☑4ᵗʰ **J37 Chronic laryngitis and laryngotracheitis**

Use additional code to identify:
exposure to environmental tobacco smoke (Z77.22)
exposure to tobacco smoke in the perinatal period (P96.81)
history of tobacco dependence (Z87.891)
infectious agent (B95-B97)
occupational exposure to environmental tobacco smoke (Z57.31)
tobacco dependence (F17.-)
tobacco use (Z72.0)

J37.0 Chronic laryngitis
Catarrhal laryngitis
Hypertrophic laryngitis
Sicca laryngitis
EXCLUDES 2   *acute laryngitis (J04.0)*
obstructive (acute) laryngitis (J05.0)

J37.1 Chronic laryngotracheitis
Laryngitis, chronic, with tracheitis (chronic)
Tracheitis, chronic, with laryngitis
EXCLUDES 1   *chronic tracheitis (J42)*
EXCLUDES 2   *acute laryngotracheitis (J04.2)*
acute tracheitis (J04.1)

Chapter 10. Diseases of the Respiratory System

✓4th **J38 Diseases of vocal cords and larynx, not elsewhere classified**
　Use additional code to identify:
　　exposure to environmental tobacco smoke (Z77.22)
　　exposure to tobacco smoke in the perinatal period (P96.81)
　　history of tobacco dependence (Z87.891)
　　occupational exposure to environmental tobacco smoke (Z57.31)
　　tobacco dependence (F17.-)
　　tobacco use (Z72.0)
　　EXCLUDES 1　*congenital laryngeal stridor (P28.89)*
　　　　obstructive laryngitis (acute) (J05.0)
　　　　postprocedural subglottic stenosis (J95.5)
　　　　stridor (R06.1)
　　　　ulcerative laryngitis (J04.0)

✓5th **J38.0 Paralysis of vocal cords and larynx**
　Laryngoplegia
　Paralysis of glottis
　　J38.00 Paralysis of vocal cords and larynx, unspecified　▽
　　J38.01 Paralysis of vocal cords and larynx, unilateral
　　J38.02 Paralysis of vocal cords and larynx, bilateral

J38.1 Polyp of vocal cord and larynx
　　EXCLUDES 1　*adenomatous polyps (D14.1)*

J38.2 Nodules of vocal cords
　Chorditis (fibrinous)(nodosa)(tuberosa)
　Singer's nodes
　Teacher's nodes

J38.3 Other diseases of vocal cords
　Abscess of vocal cords
　Cellulitis of vocal cords
　Granuloma of vocal cords
　Leukokeratosis of vocal cords
　Leukoplakia of vocal cords

J38.4 Edema of larynx
　Edema (of) glottis
　Subglottic edema
　Supraglottic edema
　　EXCLUDES 1　*acute obstructive laryngitis [croup] (J05.0)*
　　　　edematous laryngitis (J04.0)

J38.5 Laryngeal spasm
　Laryngismus (stridulus)

J38.6 Stenosis of larynx

J38.7 Other diseases of larynx
　Abscess of larynx　　　　Pachyderma of larynx
　Cellulitis of larynx　　　 Perichondritis of larynx
　Disease of larynx NOS　　Ulcer of larynx
　Necrosis of larynx

✓4th **J39 Other diseases of upper respiratory tract**
　　EXCLUDES 1　*acute respiratory infection NOS (J22)*
　　　　acute upper respiratory infection (J06.9)
　　　　upper respiratory inflammation due to chemicals, gases, fumes or vapors (J68.2)

J39.0 Retropharyngeal and parapharyngeal abscess
　Peripharyngeal abscess
　　EXCLUDES 1　*peritonsillar abscess (J36)*
　DEF: Purulent infection behind pharynx and front of precerebral fascia; characterized by neck stiffness, cervical lymphadenopathy, sore throat, fever, and stridor.

J39.1 Other abscess of pharynx
　Cellulitis of pharynx
　Nasopharyngeal abscess

J39.2 Other diseases of pharynx
　Cyst of pharynx
　Edema of pharynx
　　EXCLUDES 2　*chronic pharyngitis (J31.2)*
　　　　ulcerative pharyngitis (J02.9)

J39.3 Upper respiratory tract hypersensitivity reaction, site unspecified　▽
　　EXCLUDES 1　*hypersensitivity reaction of upper respiratory tract, such as:*
　　　　extrinsic allergic alveolitis (J67.9)
　　　　pneumoconiosis (J60-J67.9)

J39.8 Other specified diseases of upper respiratory tract

J39.9 Disease of upper respiratory tract, unspecified　▽

Chronic lower respiratory diseases (J40-J47)

EXCLUDES 1　*bronchitis due to chemicals, gases, fumes and vapors (J68.0)*
EXCLUDES 2　*cystic fibrosis (E84.-)*

J40 Bronchitis, not specified as acute or chronic　▽
　Bronchitis NOS
　Bronchitis with tracheitis NOS
　Catarrhal bronchitis
　Tracheobronchitis NOS
　Use additional code to identify:
　　exposure to environmental tobacco smoke (Z77.22)
　　exposure to tobacco smoke in the perinatal period (P96.81)
　　history of tobacco dependence (Z87.891)
　　occupational exposure to environmental tobacco smoke (Z57.31)
　　tobacco dependence (F17.-)
　　tobacco use (Z72.0)
　　EXCLUDES 1　*acute bronchitis (J20.-)*
　　　　allergic bronchitis NOS (J45.909)
　　　　asthmatic bronchitis NOS (J45.9-)
　　　　bronchitis due to chemicals, gases, fumes and vapors (J68.0)

✓4th **J41 Simple and mucopurulent chronic bronchitis**
　Use additional code to identify:
　　exposure to environmental tobacco smoke (Z77.22)
　　exposure to tobacco smoke in the perinatal period (P96.81)
　　history of tobacco dependence (Z87.891)
　　occupational exposure to environmental tobacco smoke (Z57.31)
　　tobacco dependence (F17.-)
　　tobacco use (Z72.0)
　　EXCLUDES 1　*chronic bronchitis NOS (J42)*
　　　　chronic obstructive bronchitis (J44.-)

　J41.0 Simple chronic bronchitis
　J41.1 Mucopurulent chronic bronchitis
　J41.8 Mixed simple and mucopurulent chronic bronchitis

J42 Unspecified chronic bronchitis　▽
　Chronic bronchitis NOS
　Chronic tracheitis
　Chronic tracheobronchitis
　Use additional code to identify:
　　exposure to environmental tobacco smoke (Z77.22)
　　exposure to tobacco smoke in the perinatal period (P96.81)
　　history of tobacco dependence (Z87.891)
　　occupational exposure to environmental tobacco smoke (Z57.31)
　　tobacco dependence (F17.-)
　　tobacco use (Z72.0)
　　EXCLUDES 1　*chronic asthmatic bronchitis (J44.-)*
　　　　chronic bronchitis with airways obstruction (J44.-)
　　　　chronic emphysematous bronchitis (J44.-)
　　　　chronic obstructive pulmonary disease NOS (J44.9)
　　　　simple and mucopurulent chronic bronchitis (J41.-)

✓4th **J43 Emphysema**
　Use additional code to identify:
　　exposure to environmental tobacco smoke (Z77.22)
　　history of tobacco dependence (Z87.891)
　　occupational exposure to environmental tobacco smoke (Z57.31)
　　tobacco dependence (F17.-)
　　tobacco use (Z72.0)
　　EXCLUDES 1　*compensatory emphysema (J98.3)*
　　　　emphysema due to inhalation of chemicals, gases, fumes or vapors (J68.4)
　　　　emphysema with chronic (obstructive) bronchitis (J44.-)
　　　　emphysematous (obstructive) bronchitis (J44.-)
　　　　interstitial emphysema (J98.2)
　　　　mediastinal emphysema (J98.2)
　　　　neonatal interstitial emphysema (P25.0)
　　　　surgical (subcutaneous) emphysema (T81.82)
　　　　traumatic subcutaneous emphysema (T79.7)

　J43.0 Unilateral pulmonary emphysema [MacLeod's syndrome]
　Swyer-James syndrome
　Unilateral emphysema
　Unilateral hyperlucent lung
　Unilateral pulmonary artery functional hypoplasia
　Unilateral transparency of lung

　J43.1 Panlobular emphysema
　Panacinar emphysema

　J43.2 Centrilobular emphysema

　J43.8 Other emphysema

　J43.9 Emphysema, unspecified　▽
　Bullous emphysema (lung)(pulmonary)
　Emphysema (lung)(pulmonary) NOS
　Emphysematous bleb
　Vesicular emphysema (lung)(pulmonary)

N Newborn: 0　P Pediatric: 0-17　M Maternity: 12-55　A Adult: 15-124　NRS Nonroutine supply Dx　NCDx Noncancer Dx　PDx Primary Dx　▶◀ Revised Text　● New Code　▲ Revised Title

Emphysema

Asthma

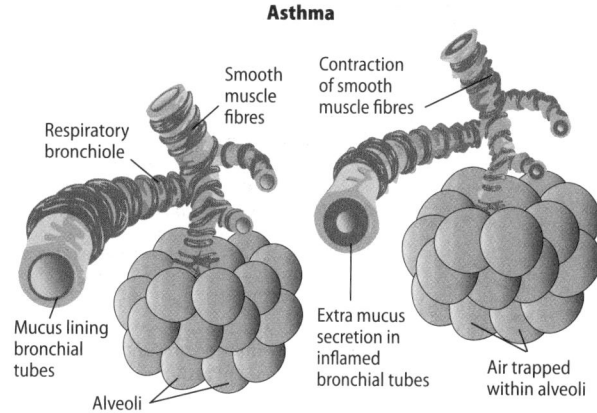

Normal alveoli   Asthmatic alveoli

☑4th **J44   Other chronic obstructive pulmonary disease**

INCLUDES   asthma with chronic obstructive pulmonary disease
chronic asthmatic (obstructive) bronchitis
chronic bronchitis with airways obstruction
chronic bronchitis with emphysema
chronic emphysematous bronchitis
chronic obstructive asthma
chronic obstructive bronchitis
chronic obstructive tracheobronchitis

Code also type of asthma, if applicable (J45.-)
Use additional code to identify:
exposure to environmental tobacco smoke (Z77.22)
history of tobacco dependence (Z87.891)
occupational exposure to environmental tobacco smoke (Z57.31)
tobacco dependence (F17.-)
tobacco use (Z72.0)

EXCLUDES 1   *bronchiectasis (J47.-)*
chronic bronchitis NOS (J42)
chronic simple and mucopurulent bronchitis (J41.-)
chronic tracheitis (J42)
chronic tracheobronchitis (J42)
emphysema without chronic bronchitis (J43.-)

EXCLUDES 2   *lung diseases due to external agents (J60-J70)*

AHA: 2017, 1Q, 25-26; 2016, 3Q, 15-16; 2013, 4Q, 109

J44.0   Chronic obstructive pulmonary disease with acute lower respiratory infection   NC Dx

▶Code also to identify the infection◀
~~Use additional code to identify the infection~~
AHA: 2017, 1Q, 24-25

J44.1   Chronic obstructive pulmonary disease with (acute) exacerbation   NC Dx

Decompensated COPD
Decompensated COPD with (acute) exacerbation

EXCLUDES 2   *chronic obstructive pulmonary disease [COPD] with acute bronchitis (J44.0)*
▶*lung diseases due to external agents (J60-J70)*◀

AHA: 2017, 1Q, 26; 2016, 1Q, 35
TIP: Assign only when provider documentation specifies exacerbation or decompensation of COPD. Exacerbation of COPD should not be assumed based upon worsening of other pulmonary disease or identification of COPD as "end-stage."

J44.9   Chronic obstructive pulmonary disease, unspecified   NC Dx ▽

Chronic obstructive airway disease NOS
Chronic obstructive lung disease NOS

EXCLUDES 2   ▶*lung diseases due to external agents (J60-J70)*◀
AHA: 2016, 1Q, 36; 2014, 4Q, 21; 2013, 4Q, 109

☑4th **J45   Asthma**

INCLUDES   allergic (predominantly) asthma
allergic bronchitis NOS
allergic rhinitis with asthma
atopic asthma
extrinsic allergic asthma
hay fever with asthma
idiosyncratic asthma
intrinsic nonallergic asthma
nonallergic asthma

Use additional code to identify:
exposure to environmental tobacco smoke (Z77.22)
exposure to tobacco smoke in the perinatal period (P96.81)
history of tobacco dependence (Z87.891)
occupational exposure to environmental tobacco smoke (Z57.31)
tobacco dependence (F17.-)
tobacco use (Z72.0)

EXCLUDES 1   *detergent asthma (J69.8)*
eosinophilic asthma (J82)
~~*lung diseases due to external agents (J60-J70)*~~
miner's asthma (J60)
wheezing NOS (R06.2)
wood asthma (J67.8)

EXCLUDES 2   *asthma with chronic obstructive pulmonary disease (J44.9)*
chronic asthmatic (obstructive) bronchitis (J44.9)
chronic obstructive asthma (J44.9)

AHA: 2017, 1Q, 25-26; 2012, 4Q, 99
DEF: Status asthmaticus: Severe, intractable episode of asthma that is unresponsive to normal therapeutic measures.
TIP: When asthma is present concurrent to COPD but not specified as to type or current exacerbation, assign only a code from J44.

☑5th **J45.2   Mild intermittent asthma**

J45.20   Mild intermittent asthma, uncomplicated
Mild intermittent asthma NOS

J45.21   Mild intermittent asthma with (acute) exacerbation

J45.22   Mild intermittent asthma with status asthmaticus

☑5th **J45.3   Mild persistent asthma**

J45.30   Mild persistent asthma, uncomplicated
Mild persistent asthma NOS

J45.31   Mild persistent asthma with (acute) exacerbation
AHA: 2016, 1Q, 35

J45.32   Mild persistent asthma with status asthmaticus

☑5th **J45.4   Moderate persistent asthma**

J45.40   Moderate persistent asthma, uncomplicated
Moderate persistent asthma NOS

J45.41   Moderate persistent asthma with (acute) exacerbation
AHA: 2017, 1Q, 26

J45.42   Moderate persistent asthma with status asthmaticus

☑5th **J45.5   Severe persistent asthma**

J45.50   Severe persistent asthma, uncomplicated
Severe persistent asthma NOS

J45.51   Severe persistent asthma with (acute) exacerbation

J45.52   Severe persistent asthma with status asthmaticus

Chapter 10. Diseases of the Respiratory System (side margin)

✓5th **J45.9** Other and unspecified **asthma**

  ✓6th **J45.90** Unspecified **asthma**
       Asthmatic bronchitis NOS
       Childhood asthma NOS
       Late onset asthma

       J45.901 **Unspecified asthma with (acute) exacerbation** ▽

       J45.902 **Unspecified asthma with status asthmaticus** ▽

       J45.909 **Unspecified asthma, uncomplicated** ▽
         Asthma NOS
         EXCLUDES 2 ▶*lung diseases due to external agents (J60-J70)*◀
         AHA: 2017, 1Q, 25

  ✓6th **J45.99** Other **asthma**

       J45.990 **Exercise induced bronchospasm**

       J45.991 **Cough variant asthma**

       J45.998 **Other asthma**

✓4th **J47** **Bronchiectasis**
   INCLUDES bronchiolectasis
   Use additional code to identify:
     exposure to environmental tobacco smoke (Z77.22)
     exposure to tobacco smoke in the perinatal period (P96.81)
     history of tobacco dependence (Z87.891)
     occupational exposure to environmental tobacco smoke (Z57.31)
     tobacco dependence (F17.-)
     tobacco use (Z72.0)
   EXCLUDES 1 *congenital bronchiectasis (Q33.4)*
       tuberculous bronchiectasis (current disease) (A15.0)

   J47.0 **Bronchiectasis with acute lower respiratory infection**
     Bronchiectasis with acute bronchitis
     Use additional code to identify the infection

   J47.1 **Bronchiectasis with (acute) exacerbation**

   J47.9 **Bronchiectasis, uncomplicated** ▽
     Bronchiectasis NOS

Lung diseases due to external agents (J60-J70)
EXCLUDES 2 *asthma (J45.-)*
     malignant neoplasm of bronchus and lung (C34.-)

J60 **Coalworker's pneumoconiosis** 🅰
   Anthracosilicosis
   Anthracosis
   Black lung disease
   Coalworker's lung
   EXCLUDES 1 *coalworker pneumoconiosis with tuberculosis, any type in A15 (J65)*

J61 **Pneumoconiosis due to asbestos and other mineral fibers** 🅰
   Asbestosis
   EXCLUDES 1 *pleural plaque with asbestosis (J92.0)*
     pneumoconiosis with tuberculosis, any type in A15 (J65)

✓4th **J62** **Pneumoconiosis due to dust containing silica**
   INCLUDES silicotic fibrosis (massive) of lung
   EXCLUDES 1 *pneumoconiosis with tuberculosis, any type in A15 (J65)*

   J62.0 **Pneumoconiosis due to talc dust**

   J62.8 **Pneumoconiosis due to other dust containing silica**
     Silicosis NOS

✓4th **J63** **Pneumoconiosis due to other inorganic dusts**
   EXCLUDES 1 *pneumoconiosis with tuberculosis, any type in A15 (J65)*

   J63.0 **Aluminosis (of lung)**

   J63.1 **Bauxite fibrosis (of lung)**

   J63.2 **Berylliosis**

   J63.3 **Graphite fibrosis (of lung)**

   J63.4 **Siderosis**

   J63.5 **Stannosis**

   J63.6 **Pneumoconiosis due to other specified inorganic dusts**

J64 **Unspecified pneumoconiosis** ▽
   EXCLUDES 1 *pneumonoconiosis with tuberculosis, any type in A15 (J65)*

J65 **Pneumoconiosis associated with tuberculosis**
   Any condition in J60-J64 with tuberculosis, any type in A15
   Silicotuberculosis

✓4th **J66** **Airway disease due to specific organic dust**
   EXCLUDES 2 *allergic alveolitis (J67.-)*
     asbestosis (J61)
     bagassosis (J67.1)
     farmer's lung (J67.0)
     hypersensitivity pneumonitis due to organic dust (J67.-)
     reactive airways dysfunction syndrome (J68.3)

   J66.0 **Byssinosis**
     Airway disease due to cotton dust

   J66.1 **Flax-dressers' disease**

   J66.2 **Cannabinosis**

   J66.8 **Airway disease due to other specific organic dusts**

✓4th **J67** **Hypersensitivity pneumonitis due to organic dust**
   INCLUDES allergic alveolitis and pneumonitis due to inhaled organic dust and particles of fungal, actinomycetic or other origin
   EXCLUDES 1 *pneumonitis due to inhalation of chemicals, gases, fumes or vapors (J68.0)*

   J67.0 **Farmer's lung**
     Harvester's lung
     Haymaker's lung
     Moldy hay disease

   J67.1 **Bagassosis**
     Bagasse disease
     Bagasse pneumonitis

   J67.2 **Bird fancier's lung**
     Budgerigar fancier's disease or lung
     Pigeon fancier's disease or lung

   J67.3 **Suberosis**
     Corkhandler's disease or lung
     Corkworker's disease or lung

   J67.4 **Maltworker's lung**
     Alveolitis due to Aspergillus clavatus

   J67.5 **Mushroom-worker's lung**

   J67.6 **Maple-bark-stripper's lung**
     Alveolitis due to Cryptostroma corticale
     Cryptostromosis

   J67.7 **Air conditioner and humidifier lung**
     Allergic alveolitis due to fungal, thermophilic actinomycetes and other organisms growing in ventilation [air conditioning] systems

   J67.8 **Hypersensitivity pneumonitis due to other organic dusts**
     Cheese-washer's lung   Furrier's lung
     Coffee-worker's lung   Sequoiosis
     Fish-meal worker's lung

   J67.9 **Hypersensitivity pneumonitis due to unspecified organic dust** ▽
     Allergic alveolitis (extrinsic) NOS
     Hypersensitivity pneumonitis NOS

✓4th **J68** **Respiratory conditions due to inhalation of chemicals, gases, fumes and vapors**
   Code first (T51-T65) to identify cause
   Use additional code to identify associated respiratory conditions, such as:
     acute respiratory failure (J96.0-)

   J68.0 **Bronchitis and pneumonitis due to chemicals, gases, fumes and vapors**
     Chemical bronchitis (acute)

   J68.1 **Pulmonary edema due to chemicals, gases, fumes and vapors**
     Chemical pulmonary edema (acute) (chronic)
     EXCLUDES 1 *pulmonary edema (acute) (chronic) NOS (J81.-)*

   J68.2 **Upper respiratory inflammation due to chemicals, gases, fumes and vapors, not elsewhere classified**

   J68.3 **Other acute and subacute respiratory conditions due to chemicals, gases, fumes and vapors**
     Reactive airways dysfunction syndrome

   J68.4 **Chronic respiratory conditions due to chemicals, gases, fumes and vapors**
     Emphysema (diffuse) (chronic) due to inhalation of chemicals, gases, fumes and vapors
     Obliterative bronchiolitis (chronic) (subacute) due to inhalation of chemicals, gases, fumes and vapors
     Pulmonary fibrosis (chronic) due to inhalation of chemicals, gases, fumes and vapors
     EXCLUDES 1 *chronic pulmonary edema due to chemicals, gases, fumes and vapors (J68.1)*

   J68.8 **Other respiratory conditions due to chemicals, gases, fumes and vapors**

🆖 Newborn: 0   🅿 Pediatric: 0-17   🅼 Maternity: 12-55   🅰 Adult: 15-124   **NRS** Nonroutine supply Dx   **NCDx** Noncancer Dx   **PDx** Primary Dx   ▶◀ Revised Text   ● New Code   ▲ Revised Title

666   ICD-10-CM 2018

J68.9   **Unspecified respiratory condition due to chemicals, gases, fumes and vapors**

☑4ᵗʰ **J69**   **Pneumonitis due to solids and liquids**
> EXCLUDES 1   *neonatal aspiration syndromes (P24.-)*
>   *postprocedural pneumonitis (J95.4)*
> **AHA:** 2017, 1Q, 24

J69.0   **Pneumonitis due to inhalation of food and vomit**
Aspiration pneumonia NOS
Aspiration pneumonia (due to) food (regurgitated)
Aspiration pneumonia (due to) gastric secretions
Aspiration pneumonia (due to) milk
Aspiration pneumonia (due to) vomit
Code also any associated foreign body in respiratory tract (T17.-)
> EXCLUDES 1   *chemical pneumonitis due to anesthesia (J95.4)*
>   *obstetric aspiration pneumonitis (O74.0)*

TIP: Aspiration pneumonia is not classified to respiratory infection codes and does not warrant the assignment of J44.0 Chronic obstructive pulmonary disease with acute lower respiratory infection, when present concurrently with COPD.

J69.1   **Pneumonitis due to inhalation of oils and essences**
Exogenous lipoid pneumonia
Lipid pneumonia NOS
Code first (T51-T65) to identify substance
> EXCLUDES 1   *endogenous lipoid pneumonia (J84.89)*

J69.8   **Pneumonitis due to inhalation of other solids and liquids**
Pneumonitis due to aspiration of blood
Pneumonitis due to aspiration of detergent
Code first (T51-T65) to identify substance

☑4ᵗʰ **J70**   **Respiratory conditions due to other external agents**

J70.0   **Acute pulmonary manifestations due to radiation**
Radiation pneumonitis
Use additional code (W88-W90, X39.0-) to identify the external cause

J70.1   **Chronic and other pulmonary manifestations due to radiation**
Fibrosis of lung following radiation
Use additional code (W88-W90, X39.0-) to identify the external cause

J70.2   **Acute drug-induced interstitial lung disorders**
Use additional code for adverse effect, if applicable, to identify drug (T36-T50 with fifth or sixth character 5)
> EXCLUDES 1   *interstitial pneumonia NOS (J84.9)*
>   *lymphoid interstitial pneumonia (J84.2)*

J70.3   **Chronic drug-induced interstitial lung disorders**
Use additional code for adverse effect, if applicable, to identify drug (T36-T50 with fifth or sixth character 5)
> EXCLUDES 1   *interstitial pneumonia NOS (J84.9)*
>   *lymphoid interstitial pneumonia (J84.2)*

J70.4   **Drug-induced interstitial lung disorders, unspecified** ▽
Use additional code for adverse effect, if applicable, to identify drug (T36-T50 with fifth or sixth character 5)
> EXCLUDES 1   *interstitial pneumonia NOS (J84.9)*
>   *lymphoid interstitial pneumonia (J84.2)*

J70.5   **Respiratory conditions due to smoke inhalation**
Smoke inhalation NOS
> EXCLUDES 1   *smoke inhalation due to chemicals, gases, fumes and vapors (J68.9)*
> **AHA:** 2013, 4Q, 121

J70.8   **Respiratory conditions due to other specified external agents**
Code first (T51-T65) to identify the external agent

J70.9   **Respiratory conditions due to unspecified external agent** ▽
Code first (T51-T65) to identify the external agent

Other respiratory diseases principally affecting the interstitium (J80-J84)

J80   **Acute respiratory distress syndrome**
Acute respiratory distress syndrome in adult or child
Adult hyaline membrane disease
> EXCLUDES 1   *respiratory distress syndrome in newborn (perinatal) (P22.0)*
> **AHA:** 2017, 1Q, 26

TIP: J80 should be assigned only when acute respiratory distress *syndrome* (ARDS) is specified. When provider documentation indicates only "respiratory distress," assign R06.00 Dyspnea for unspecified respiratory distress in an adult or child.

☑4ᵗʰ **J81**   **Pulmonary edema**
Use additional code to identify:
exposure to environmental tobacco smoke (Z77.22)
history of tobacco dependence (Z87.891)
occupational exposure to environmental tobacco smoke (Z57.31)
tobacco dependence (F17.-)
tobacco use (Z72.0)
> EXCLUDES 1   *chemical (acute) pulmonary edema (J68.1)*
>   *hypostatic pneumonia (J18.2)*
>   *passive pneumonia (J18.2)*
>   *pulmonary edema due to external agents (J60-J70)*
>   *pulmonary edema with heart disease NOS (I50.1)*
>   *pulmonary edema with heart failure (I50.1)*

J81.0   **Acute pulmonary edema**
Acute edema of lung

J81.1   **Chronic pulmonary edema**
Pulmonary congestion (chronic) (passive)
Pulmonary edema NOS

J82   **Pulmonary eosinophilia, not elsewhere classified**
Allergic pneumonia
Eosinophilic asthma
Eosinophilic pneumonia
Löffler's pneumonia
Tropical (pulmonary) eosinophilia NOS
> EXCLUDES 1   *pulmonary eosinophilia due to aspergillosis (B44.-)*
>   *pulmonary eosinophilia due to drugs (J70.2-J70.4)*
>   *pulmonary eosinophilia due to specified parasitic infection (B50-B83)*
>   *pulmonary eosinophilia due to systemic connective tissue disorders (M30-M36)*
>   *pulmonary infiltrate NOS (R91.8)*

☑4ᵗʰ **J84**   **Other interstitial pulmonary diseases**
> EXCLUDES 1   *drug-induced interstitial lung disorders (J70.2-J70.4)*
>   *interstitial emphysema (J98.2)*
>   ~~*lung diseases due to external agents (J60-J70)*~~
> EXCLUDES 2   ▶*lung diseases due to external agents (J60-J70)*◀

☑5ᵗʰ J84.0   **Alveolar and parieto-alveolar conditions**

J84.01   **Alveolar proteinosis**
> **DEF:** Reduced ventilation due to proteinaceous deposits on alveoli; symptoms include dyspnea, cough, chest pain, weakness, weight loss, and hemoptysis.

J84.02   **Pulmonary alveolar microlithiasis**

J84.03   ***Idiopathic pulmonary hemosiderosis***
Essential brown induration of lung
Code first underlying disease, such as:
disorders of iron metabolism (E83.1-)
> EXCLUDES 1   *acute idiopathic pulmonary hemorrhage in infants [AIPHI] (R04.81)*
> **DEF:** Fibrosis of alveolar walls; marked by abnormal accumulation of iron as hemosiderin in lungs; primarily affects children; symptoms include anemia, fluid in lungs, and blood in sputum; etiology unknown.

J84.09   **Other alveolar and parieto-alveolar conditions**

☑5ᵗʰ J84.1   **Other interstitial pulmonary diseases with fibrosis**
> EXCLUDES 1   *pulmonary fibrosis (chronic) due to inhalation of chemicals, gases, fumes or vapors (J68.4)*
>   *pulmonary fibrosis (chronic) following radiation (J70.1)*

J84.10   **Pulmonary fibrosis, unspecified** ▽
Capillary fibrosis of lung
Cirrhosis of lung (chronic) NOS
Fibrosis of lung (atrophic) (chronic) (confluent) (massive) (perialveolar) (peribronchial) NOS
Induration of lung (chronic) NOS
Postinflammatory pulmonary fibrosis

☑6ᵗʰ J84.11   **Idiopathic interstitial pneumonia**
> EXCLUDES 1   *lymphoid interstitial pneumonia (J84.2)*
>   *pneumocystis pneumonia (B59)*

J84.111   **Idiopathic interstitial pneumonia, not otherwise specified** ▽

J84.112   **Idiopathic pulmonary fibrosis**
Cryptogenic fibrosing alveolitis
Idiopathic fibrosing alveolitis

J84.113   **Idiopathic non-specific interstitial pneumonitis**
> EXCLUDES 1   *non-specific interstitial pneumonia NOS, or due to known underlying cause (J84.89)*

☑ Additional Character Req   ✓x7ᵗʰ Placeholder Alert   Case-Mix Diagnosis   Manifestation   ▽ Unspecified Dx   EXCLUDES 1 Not coded here   EXCLUDES 2 Not included here

ICD-10-CM 2018   **667**

J84.114 Acute interstitial **pneumonitis**
Hamman-Rich syndrome
EXCLUDES 1 *pneumocystis pneumonia (B59)*

J84.115 Respiratory bronchiolitis interstitial **lung disease**

J84.116 Cryptogenic organizing **pneumonia**
EXCLUDES 1 *organizing pneumonia NOS, or due to known underlying cause (J84.89)*

J84.117 Desquamative **interstitial pneumonia**

J84.17 Other interstitial pulmonary diseases with fibrosis in diseases classified elsewhere
Interstitial pneumonia (nonspecific) (usual) due to collagen vascular disease
Interstitial pneumonia (nonspecific) (usual) in diseases classified elsewhere
Organizing pneumonia due to collagen vascular disease
Organizing pneumonia in diseases classified elsewhere
Code first underlying disease, such as:
progressive systemic sclerosis (M34.0)
rheumatoid arthritis (M05.00-M06.9)
systemic lupus erythematosis (M32.0-M32.9)

J84.2 **Lymphoid interstitial pneumonia**
Lymphoid interstitial pneumonitis

☑5ᵗʰ **J84.8** Other specified **interstitial pulmonary diseases**
EXCLUDES 1 *exogenous lipoid pneumonia (J69.1)*
unspecified lipoid pneumonia (J69.1)

J84.81 **Lymphangioleiomyomatosis** ♀
Lymphangiomyomatosis

J84.82 **Adult pulmonary Langerhans cell histiocytosis** Ⓐ
Adult PLCH

J84.83 **Surfactant mutations of the lung**
DEF: Genetic disorder resulting in insufficient secretion of a complex mixture of phospholipids and proteins that reduce surface tension in the alveoli following the onset of breathing to facilitate lung expansion in the newborn; leading indication for pediatric lung transplantation.

☑6ᵗʰ **J84.84** Other interstitial lung diseases of childhood
J84.841 **Neuroendocrine cell hyperplasia of infancy**
J84.842 **Pulmonary interstitial glycogenosis**
J84.843 **Alveolar capillary dysplasia with vein misalignment**
J84.848 **Other interstitial lung diseases of childhood**

J84.89 **Other specified interstitial pulmonary diseases**
Endogenous lipoid pneumonia
Interstitial pneumonitis
Non-specific interstitial pneumonitis NOS
Organizing pneumonia NOS
Code first, if applicable:
poisoning due to drug or toxin (T51-T65 with fifth or sixth character to indicate intent), for toxic pneumonopathy
underlying cause of pneumonopathy, if known
Use additional code, for adverse effect, to identify drug (T36-T50 with fifth or sixth character 5), if drug-induced
EXCLUDES 1 *cryptogenic organizing pneumonia (J84.116)*
idiopathic non-specific interstitial pneumonitis (J84.113)
lipoid pneumonia, exogenous or unspecified (J69.1)
lymphoid interstitial pneumonia (J84.2)

J84.9 **Interstitial pulmonary disease, unspecified** ▽
Interstitial pneumonia NOS

Suppurative and necrotic conditions of the lower respiratory tract (J85-J86)

☑4ᵗʰ **J85** **Abscess of lung and mediastinum**
Use additional code (B95-B97) to identify infectious agent.
J85.0 **Gangrene** and **necrosis of lung**
J85.1 **Abscess of lung** with pneumonia
Code also the type of pneumonia
J85.2 **Abscess of lung** without pneumonia
Abscess of lung NOS
J85.3 **Abscess of mediastinum**

☑4ᵗʰ **J86** **Pyothorax**
Use additional code (B95-B97) to identify infectious agent
EXCLUDES 1 *abscess of lung (J85.-)*
pyothorax due to tuberculosis (A15.6)

J86.0 **Pyothorax** with fistula
Bronchocutaneous fistula
Bronchopleural fistula
Hepatopleural fistula
Mediastinal fistula
Pleural fistula
Thoracic fistula
Any condition classifiable to J86.9 with fistula
DEF: Purulent infection of respiratory cavity, with communication from cavity to another structure.

J86.9 **Pyothorax** without fistula
Abscess of pleura
Abscess of thorax
Empyema (chest) (lung) (pleura)
Fibrinopurulent pleurisy
Purulent pleurisy
Pyopneumothorax
Septic pleurisy
Seropurulent pleurisy
Suppurative pleurisy

Other diseases of the pleura (J90-J94)

J90 **Pleural effusion, not elsewhere classified**
Encysted pleurisy
Pleural effusion NOS
Pleurisy with effusion (exudative) (serous)
EXCLUDES 1 *chylous (pleural) effusion (J94.0)*
malignant pleural effusion (J91.0))
pleurisy NOS (R09.1)
tuberculous pleural effusion (A15.6)

☑4ᵗʰ **J91** **Pleural effusion in conditions classified elsewhere**
EXCLUDES 2 *pleural effusion in heart failure (I50.-)*
pleural effusion in systemic lupus erythematosus (M32.13)

J91.0 Malignant pleural effusion
Code first underlying neoplasm

J91.8 Pleural effusion in other conditions classified elsewhere
Code first underlying disease, such as:
filariasis (B74.0-B74.9)
influenza (J09.X2, J10.1, J11.1)
AHA: 2015, 2Q, 15

☑4ᵗʰ **J92** **Pleural plaque**
INCLUDES pleural thickening
J92.0 **Pleural plaque** with presence of asbestos
J92.9 **Pleural plaque** without asbestos
Pleural plaque NOS

Pleural Effusion

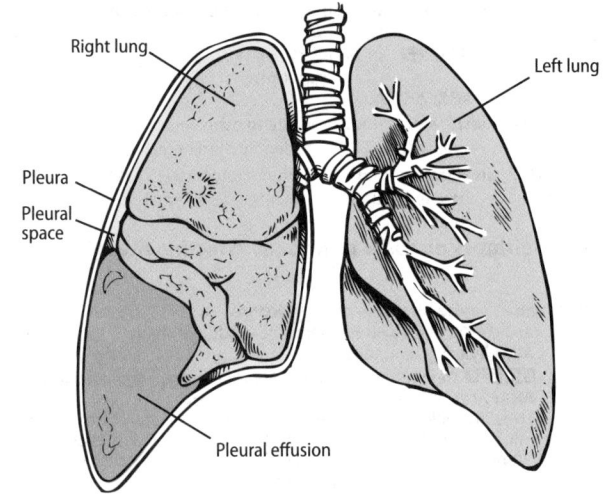

Right lung
Left lung
Pleura
Pleural space
Pleural effusion

☑4ᵗʰ **J93**   **Pneumothorax and air leak**

> **EXCLUDES 1**   *congenital or perinatal pneumothorax (P25.1)*
> *postprocedural air leak (J95.812)*
> *postprocedural pneumothorax (J95.811)*
> *traumatic pneumothorax (S27.0)*
> *tuberculous (current disease) pneumothorax (A15.-)*
> *pyopneumothorax (J86.-)*

     J93.0   **Spontaneous tension pneumothorax**
         DEF: Leaking air from lung into lining, causing collapse.

☑5ᵗʰ   **J93.1**   **Other spontaneous pneumothorax**

         J93.11   **Primary spontaneous pneumothorax**

         J93.12   **Secondary spontaneous pneumothorax**
             Code first underlying condition, such as:
                 catamenial pneumothorax due to endometriosis
                    (N80.8)
                 cystic fibrosis (E84.-)
                 eosinophilic pneumonia (J82)
                 lymphangioleiomyomatosis (J84.81)
                 malignant neoplasm of bronchus and lung (C34.-)
                 Marfan's syndrome (Q87.4)
                 pneumonia due to Pneumocystis carinii (B59)
                 secondary malignant neoplasm of lung (C78.0-)
                 spontaneous rupture of the esophagus (K22.3)

☑5ᵗʰ   **J93.8**   **Other pneumothorax and air leak**

         J93.81   **Chronic pneumothorax**

         J93.82   **Other air leak**
             Persistent air leak

         J93.83   **Other pneumothorax**
             Acute pneumothorax
             Spontaneous pneumothorax NOS

     J93.9   **Pneumothorax, unspecified**   ▽
         Pneumothorax NOS

☑4ᵗʰ **J94**   **Other pleural conditions**

> **EXCLUDES 1**   *pleurisy NOS (R09.1)*
> *traumatic hemopneumothorax (S27.2)*
> *traumatic hemothorax (S27.1)*
> *tuberculous pleural conditions (current disease) (A15.-)*

     J94.0   **Chylous effusion**
         Chyliform effusion

     J94.1   **Fibrothorax**

     J94.2   **Hemothorax**
         Hemopneumothorax

     J94.8   **Other specified pleural conditions**
         Hydropneumothorax
         Hydrothorax

     J94.9   **Pleural condition, unspecified**   ▽

Tracheostomy

Tracheostomy
in place

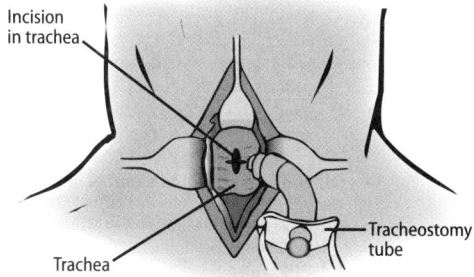

Incision
in trachea

Trachea

Tracheostomy
tube

Intraoperative and postprocedural complications and disorders of respiratory system, not elsewhere classified (J95)

☑4ᵗʰ **J95**   **Intraoperative and postprocedural complications and disorders of respiratory system, not elsewhere classified**

> **EXCLUDES 2**   *aspiration pneumonia (J69.-)*
> *emphysema (subcutaneous) resulting from a procedure (T81.82)*
> *hypostatic pneumonia (J18.2)*
> *pulmonary manifestations due to radiation (J70.0- J70.1)*

☑5ᵗʰ   **J95.0**   **Tracheostomy complications**

         J95.00   **Unspecified tracheostomy complication**   ▽

         J95.01   **Hemorrhage from tracheostomy stoma**

         J95.02   **Infection of tracheostomy stoma**
             Use additional code to identify type of infection,
                 such as:
                    cellulitis of neck ▶(L03.221)◀
                    sepsis (A40, A41.-)

         J95.03   **Malfunction of tracheostomy stoma**
             Mechanical complication of tracheostomy stoma
             Obstruction of tracheostomy airway
             Tracheal stenosis due to tracheostomy

         J95.04   **Tracheo-esophageal fistula following tracheostomy**

         J95.09   **Other tracheostomy complication**

     J95.1   **Acute pulmonary insufficiency following thoracic surgery**

> **EXCLUDES 2**   *functional disturbances following cardiac surgery (I97.0, I97.1-)*

     J95.2   **Acute pulmonary insufficiency following nonthoracic surgery**

> **EXCLUDES 2**   *functional disturbances following cardiac surgery (I97.0, I97.1-)*

     J95.3   **Chronic pulmonary insufficiency following surgery**

> **EXCLUDES 2**   *functional disturbances following cardiac surgery (I97.0, I97.1-)*

     J95.4   **Chemical pneumonitis due to anesthesia**
         Mendelson's syndrome
         Postprocedural aspiration pneumonia
         Use additional code for adverse effect, if applicable, to identify
             drug (T41.- with fifth or sixth character 5)

> **EXCLUDES 1**   *aspiration pneumonitis due to anesthesia*
> *complicating labor and delivery (O74.0)*
> *aspiration pneumonitis due to anesthesia*
> *complicating pregnancy (O29)*
> *aspiration pneumonitis due to anesthesia*
> *complicating the puerperium (O89.01)*

     J95.5   **Postprocedural subglottic stenosis**

☑5ᵗʰ   **J95.6**   **Intraoperative hemorrhage and hematoma of a respiratory system organ or structure complicating a procedure**

> **EXCLUDES 1**   *intraoperative hemorrhage and hematoma of a respiratory system organ or structure due to accidental puncture and laceration during procedure (J95.7-)*

         J95.61   **Intraoperative hemorrhage and hematoma of a respiratory system organ or structure complicating a respiratory system procedure**

         J95.62   **Intraoperative hemorrhage and hematoma of a respiratory system organ or structure complicating other procedure**

☑5ᵗʰ   **J95.7**   **Accidental puncture and laceration of a respiratory system organ or structure during a procedure**

> **EXCLUDES 2**   *postprocedural pneumothorax (J95.811)*

         J95.71   **Accidental puncture and laceration of a respiratory system organ or structure during a respiratory system procedure**

         J95.72   **Accidental puncture and laceration of a respiratory system organ or structure during other procedure**

☑5ᵗʰ   **J95.8**   **Other intraoperative and postprocedural complications and disorders of respiratory system, not elsewhere classified**

         ☑6ᵗʰ   **J95.81**   **Postprocedural pneumothorax and air leak**

             J95.811   **Postprocedural pneumothorax**

             J95.812   **Postprocedural air leak**

         ☑6ᵗʰ   **J95.82**   **Postprocedural respiratory failure**

> **EXCLUDES 1**   *respiratory failure in other conditions (J96.-)*

             J95.821   **Acute postprocedural respiratory failure**
                 Postprocedural respiratory failure NOS

             J95.822   **Acute and chronic postprocedural respiratory failure**

☑ Additional Character Req   ☑x7ᵗʰ Placeholder Alert   Case-Mix Diagnosis   Manifestation   ▽ Unspecified Dx   **EXCLUDES 1** Not coded here   **EXCLUDES 2** Not included here

ICD-10-CM 2018   **669**

Chapter 10. Diseases of the Respiratory System

✓6ᵗʰ **J95.83** Postprocedural hemorrhage of a respiratory system organ or structure following a procedure

  J95.830 Postprocedural hemorrhage of a respiratory system organ or structure following a respiratory system procedure

  J95.831 Postprocedural hemorrhage of a respiratory system organ or structure following other procedure

  J95.84 Transfusion-related acute lung injury (TRALI)
    DEF: A relatively rare, but serious, pulmonary complication of blood transfusion, with acute respiratory distress, noncardiogenic pulmonary edema, cyanosis, hypoxemia, hypotension, fever, and chills.

✓6ᵗʰ **J95.85** Complication of respirator [ventilator]

  J95.850 Mechanical complication of respirator
    EXCLUDES 1   encounter for respirator [ventilator] dependence during power failure (Z99.12)

  J95.851 Ventilator associated pneumonia
    Ventilator associated pneumonitis
    Use additional code to identify the organism, if known (B95.-, B96.-, B97.-)
    EXCLUDES 1   ventilator lung in newborn (P27.8)
    AHA: 2017, 1Q, 25

  J95.859 Other complication of respirator [ventilator]

✓6ᵗʰ **J95.86** Postprocedural hematoma and seroma of a respiratory system organ or structure following a procedure

  J95.860 Postprocedural hematoma of a respiratory system organ or structure following a respiratory system procedure

  J95.861 Postprocedural hematoma of a respiratory system organ or structure following other procedure

  J95.862 Postprocedural seroma of a respiratory system organ or structure following a respiratory system procedure

  J95.863 Postprocedural seroma of a respiratory system organ or structure following other procedure

  J95.88 Other intraoperative complications of respiratory system, not elsewhere classified

  J95.89 Other postprocedural complications and disorders of respiratory system, not elsewhere classified
    Use additional code to identify disorder, such as:
    aspiration pneumonia (J69.-)
    bacterial or viral pneumonia (J12-J18)
    EXCLUDES 2   acute pulmonary insufficiency following thoracic surgery (J95.1)
    postprocedural subglottic stenosis (J95.5)

Other diseases of the respiratory system (J96-J99)

✓4ᵗʰ **J96** Respiratory failure, not elsewhere classified
  EXCLUDES 1   acute respiratory distress syndrome (J80)
    cardiorespiratory failure (R09.2)
    newborn respiratory distress syndrome (P22.0)
    postprocedural respiratory failure (J95.82-)
    respiratory arrest (R09.2)
    respiratory arrest of newborn (P28.81)
    respiratory failure of newborn (P28.5)

✓5ᵗʰ **J96.0** Acute respiratory failure

  J96.00 Acute respiratory failure, unspecified whether with hypoxia or hypercapnia ▽
    AHA: 2016, 3Q, 14; 2013, 4Q, 121

  J96.01 Acute respiratory failure with hypoxia

  J96.02 Acute respiratory failure with hypercapnia

✓5ᵗʰ **J96.1** Chronic respiratory failure

  J96.10 Chronic respiratory failure, unspecified whether with hypoxia or hypercapnia ▽
    AHA: 2016, 1Q, 38; 2015, 1Q, 21

  J96.11 Chronic respiratory failure with hypoxia
    AHA: 2013, 4Q, 129

  J96.12 Chronic respiratory failure with hypercapnia

✓5ᵗʰ **J96.2** Acute and chronic respiratory failure
  Acute on chronic respiratory failure

  J96.20 Acute and chronic respiratory failure, unspecified whether with hypoxia or hypercapnia ▽

  J96.21 Acute and chronic respiratory failure with hypoxia

  J96.22 Acute and chronic respiratory failure with hypercapnia

✓5ᵗʰ **J96.9** Respiratory failure, unspecified

  J96.90 Respiratory failure, unspecified, unspecified whether with hypoxia or hypercapnia ▽

  J96.91 Respiratory failure, unspecified with hypoxia ▽

  J96.92 Respiratory failure, unspecified with hypercapnia ▽

✓4ᵗʰ **J98** Other respiratory disorders
  Use additional code to identify:
    exposure to environmental tobacco smoke (Z77.22)
    exposure to tobacco smoke in the perinatal period (P96.81)
    history of tobacco dependence (Z87.891)
    occupational exposure to environmental tobacco smoke (Z57.31)
    tobacco dependence (F17.-)
    tobacco use (Z72.0)
  EXCLUDES 1   newborn apnea (P28.4)
    newborn sleep apnea (P28.3)
  EXCLUDES 2   apnea NOS (R06.81)
    sleep apnea (G47.3-)

✓5ᵗʰ **J98.0** Diseases of bronchus, not elsewhere classified

  J98.01 Acute bronchospasm
    EXCLUDES 1   acute bronchiolitis with bronchospasm (J21.-)
    acute bronchitis with bronchospasm (J20.-)
    asthma (J45.-)
    exercise induced bronchospasm (J45.990)

  J98.09 Other diseases of bronchus, not elsewhere classified
    Broncholithiasis
    Calcification of bronchus
    Stenosis of bronchus
    Tracheobronchial collapse
    Tracheobronchial dyskinesia
    Ulcer of bronchus

✓5ᵗʰ **J98.1** Pulmonary collapse
  EXCLUDES 1   therapeutic collapse of lung status (Z98.3)

  J98.11 Atelectasis
    EXCLUDES 1   newborn atelectasis
    tuberculous atelectasis (current disease) (A15)

  J98.19 Other pulmonary collapse

  J98.2 Interstitial emphysema
    Mediastinal emphysema
    EXCLUDES 1   emphysema NOS (J43.9)
    emphysema in newborn (P25.0)
    surgical emphysema (subcutaneous) (T81.82)
    traumatic subcutaneous emphysema (T79.7)

  J98.3 Compensatory emphysema
    DEF: Distention of all or part of the lung caused by disease processes or surgical intervention that decreased volume in another part of the lung; overcompensation reaction to the loss of capacity in another part of the lung; occurs in association with pneumonias, pleural effusions, atelectasis, empyema, and pneumothorax.

  J98.4 Other disorders of lung
    Calcification of lung
    Cystic lung disease (acquired)
    Lung disease NOS
    Pulmolithiasis
    EXCLUDES 1   acute interstitial pneumonitis (J84.114)
    pulmonary insufficiency following surgery (J95.1-J95.2)

✓5ᵗʰ **J98.5** Diseases of mediastinum, not elsewhere classified
  EXCLUDES 2   abscess of mediastinum (J85.3)

  J98.51 Mediastinitis
    Code first: underlying condition, if applicable, such as postoperative mediastinitis (T81.-)

  J98.59 Other diseases of mediastinum, not elsewhere classified
    Fibrosis of mediastinum
    Hernia of mediastinum
    Retraction of mediastinum

N Newborn: 0   P Pediatric: 0-17   M Maternity: 12-55   A Adult: 15-124   NRS Nonroutine supply Dx   NCDx Noncancer Dx   PDx Primary Dx   ►◄ Revised Text   ● New Code   ▲ Revised Title

670   ICD-10-CM 2018

J98.6 **Disorders of diaphragm**
Diaphragmatitis
Paralysis of diaphragm
Relaxation of diaphragm
> **EXCLUDES 1**   *congenital malformation of diaphragm NEC (Q79.1)*
> *congenital diaphragmatic hernia (Q79.0)*
> **EXCLUDES 2**   *diaphragmatic hernia (K44.-)*

J98.8 **Other specified respiratory disorders**

J98.9 **Respiratory disorder, unspecified**   ▽
Respiratory disease (chronic) NOS

J99   ***Respiratory disorders in diseases classified elsewhere***
Code first underlying disease, such as:
amyloidosis (E85.-)
ankylosing spondylitis (M45)
congenital syphilis (A50.5)
cryoglobulinemia (D89.1)
early congenital syphilis (A50.0)
schistosomiasis (B65.0-B65.9)
> **EXCLUDES 1**   *respiratory disorders in:*
> *amebiasis (A06.5)*
> *blastomycosis (B40.0-B40.2)*
> *candidiasis (B37.1)*
> *coccidioidomycosis (B38.0-B38.2)*
> *cystic fibrosis with pulmonary manifestations (E84.0)*
> *dermatomyositis (M33.01, M33.11)*
> *histoplasmosis (B39.0-B39.2)*
> *late syphilis (A52.72, A52.73)*
> *polymyositis (M33.21)*
> *sicca syndrome (M35.02)*
> *systemic lupus erythematosus (M32.13)*
> *systemic sclerosis (M34.81)*
> *Wegener's granulomatosis (M31.30-M31.31)*

☑ Additional Character Req   ✓x7ᵗ Placeholder Alert   Case-Mix Diagnosis   Manifestation   ▽ Unspecified Dx   **EXCLUDES 1** Not coded here   **EXCLUDES 2** Not included here

Chapter 11. Diseases of the Digestive System (KØØ–K95)

Chapter Specific Coding Guidelines and Examples
Reserved for future guideline expansion.

Chapter 11. Diseases of the Digestive System

Chapter 11. Diseases of the Digestive System (K00-K95)

EXCLUDES 2   certain conditions originating in the perinatal period (P04-P96)
certain infectious and parasitic diseases (A00-B99)
complications of pregnancy, childbirth and the puerperium (O00-O9A)
congenital malformations, deformations and chromosomal abnormalities (Q00-Q99)
endocrine, nutritional and metabolic diseases (E00-E88)
injury, poisoning and certain other consequences of external causes (S00-T88)
neoplasms (C00-D49)
symptoms, signs and abnormal clinical and laboratory findings, not elsewhere classified (R00-R94)

This chapter contains the following blocks:

K00-K14 Diseases of oral cavity and salivary glands
K20-K31 Diseases of esophagus, stomach and duodenum
K35-K38 Diseases of appendix
K40-K46 Hernia
K50-K52 Noninfective enteritis and colitis
K55-K64 Other diseases of intestines
K65-K68 Diseases of peritoneum and retroperitoneum
K70-K77 Diseases of liver
K80-K87 Disorders of gallbladder, biliary tract and pancreas
K90-K95 Other diseases of the digestive system

Diseases of oral cavity and salivary glands (K00-K14)

✓4ᵗʰ **K00 Disorders of tooth development and eruption**
EXCLUDES 2   embedded and impacted teeth (K01.-)

K00.0 Anodontia
Hypodontia
Oligodontia
EXCLUDES 1   acquired absence of teeth (K08.1-)

K00.1 Supernumerary teeth
Distomolar
Fourth molar
Mesiodens
Paramolar
Supplementary teeth
EXCLUDES 2   supernumerary roots (K00.2)

K00.2 Abnormalities of size and form of teeth
Concrescence of teeth
Dens evaginatus
Dens in dente
Dens invaginatus
Enamel pearls
Fusion of teeth
Gemination of teeth
Macrodontia
Microdontia
Peg-shaped [conical] teeth
Supernumerary roots
Taurodontism
Tuberculum paramolare
EXCLUDES 1   abnormalities of teeth due to congenital syphilis (A50.5)
tuberculum Carabelli, which is regarded as a normal variation and should not be coded

Tooth Anatomy

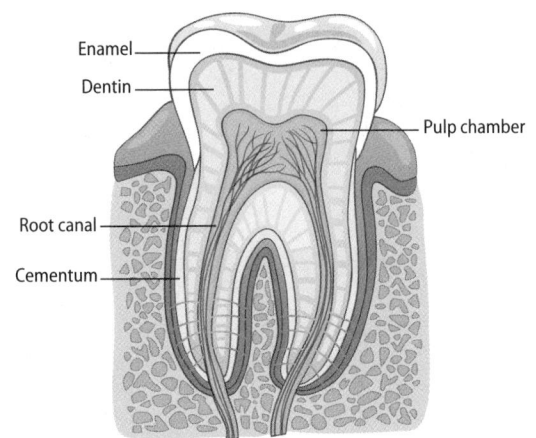

Enamel
Dentin
Pulp chamber
Root canal
Cementum

K00.3 Mottled teeth
Dental fluorosis
Mottling of enamel
Nonfluoride enamel opacities
EXCLUDES 2   deposits [accretions] on teeth (K03.6)

K00.4 Disturbances in tooth formation
Aplasia and hypoplasia of cementum
Dilaceration of tooth
Enamel hypoplasia (neonatal) (postnatal) (prenatal)
Regional odontodysplasia
Turner's tooth
EXCLUDES 1   Hutchinson's teeth and mulberry molars in congenital syphilis (A50.5)
EXCLUDES 2   mottled teeth (K00.3)

K00.5 Hereditary disturbances in tooth structure, not elsewhere classified
Amelogenesis imperfecta
Dentinogenesis imperfecta
Odontogenesis imperfecta
Dentinal dysplasia
Shell teeth

K00.6 Disturbances in tooth eruption
Dentia praecox
Natal tooth
Neonatal tooth
Premature eruption of tooth
Premature shedding of primary [deciduous] tooth
Prenatal teeth
Retained [persistent] primary tooth
EXCLUDES 2   embedded and impacted teeth (K01.-)

K00.7 Teething syndrome

K00.8 Other disorders of tooth development
Color changes during tooth formation
Intrinsic staining of teeth NOS
EXCLUDES 2   posteruptive color changes (K03.7)

K00.9 Disorder of tooth development, unspecified   ▽
Disorder of odontogenesis NOS

✓4ᵗʰ **K01 Embedded and impacted teeth**
EXCLUDES 1   abnormal position of fully erupted teeth (M26.3-)

K01.0 Embedded teeth

K01.1 Impacted teeth

✓4ᵗʰ **K02 Dental caries**
INCLUDES   caries of dentine
dental cavities
early childhood caries
pre-eruptive caries
recurrent caries (dentino enamel junction) (enamel) (to the pulp)
tooth decay

K02.3 Arrested dental caries
Arrested coronal and root caries

✓5ᵗʰ **K02.5 Dental caries on pit and fissure surface**
Dental caries on chewing surface of tooth

K02.51 Dental caries on pit and fissure surface limited to enamel
White spot lesions [initial caries] on pit and fissure surface of tooth

K02.52 Dental caries on pit and fissure surface penetrating into dentin
Primary dental caries, cervical origin

K02.53 Dental caries on pit and fissure surface penetrating into pulp

✓5ᵗʰ **K02.6 Dental caries on smooth surface**

K02.61 Dental caries on smooth surface limited to enamel
White spot lesions [initial caries] on smooth surface of tooth

K02.62 Dental caries on smooth surface penetrating into dentin

K02.63 Dental caries on smooth surface penetrating into pulp

K02.7 Dental root caries

K02.9 Dental caries, unspecified   ▽

✓4ᵗʰ **K03 Other diseases of hard tissues of teeth**
EXCLUDES 2   bruxism (F45.8)
dental caries (K02.-)
teeth-grinding NOS (F45.8)

K03.0 Excessive attrition of teeth
Approximal wear of teeth
Occlusal wear of teeth

Ⓝ Newborn: 0 Ⓟ Pediatric: 0-17 Ⓜ Maternity: 12-55 Ⓐ Adult: 15-124 NRS Nonroutine supply Dx NCDx Noncancer Dx PDx Primary Dx ►◄ Revised Text ● New Code ▲ Revised Title

674   ICD-10-CM 2018

K00-K03.0

K03.1 Abrasion of teeth
    Dentifrice abrasion of teeth
    Habitual abrasion of teeth
    Occupational abrasion of teeth
    Ritual abrasion of teeth
    Traditional abrasion of teeth
    Wedge defect NOS

K03.2 Erosion of teeth
    Erosion of teeth due to diet
    Erosion of teeth due to drugs and medicaments
    Erosion of teeth due to persistent vomiting
    Erosion of teeth NOS
    Idiopathic erosion of teeth
    Occupational erosion of teeth

K03.3 Pathological resorption of teeth
    Internal granuloma of pulp
    Resorption of teeth (external)

K03.4 Hypercementosis
    Cementation hyperplasia

K03.5 Ankylosis of teeth

K03.6 Deposits [accretions] on teeth
    Betel deposits [accretions] on teeth
    Black deposits [accretions] on teeth
    Extrinsic staining of teeth NOS
    Green deposits [accretions] on teeth
    Materia alba deposits [accretions] on teeth
    Orange deposits [accretions] on teeth
    Staining of teeth NOS
    Subgingival dental calculus
    Supragingival dental calculus
    Tobacco deposits [accretions] on teeth

K03.7 Posteruptive color changes of dental hard tissues
    EXCLUDES 2   *deposits [accretions] on teeth (K03.6)*

✓5ᵗʰ **K03.8 Other specified diseases of hard tissues of teeth**
    K03.81 Cracked tooth
       EXCLUDES 1   *asymptomatic craze lines in enamel—omit code*
          broken or fractured tooth due to trauma (S02.5)
    K03.89 Other specified diseases of hard tissues of teeth

K03.9 Disease of hard tissues of teeth, unspecified   ▽

✓4ᵗʰ **K04 Diseases of pulp and periapical tissues**

✓5ᵗʰ **K04.0 Pulpitis**
    Acute pulpitis
    Chronic (hyperplastic) (ulcerative) pulpitis
    K04.01 Reversible pulpitis
    K04.02 Irreversible pulpitis

K04.1 Necrosis of pulp
    Pulpal gangrene

K04.2 Pulp degeneration
    Denticles
    Pulpal calcifications
    Pulpal stones

K04.3 Abnormal hard tissue formation in pulp
    Secondary or irregular dentine

K04.4 Acute apical periodontitis of pulpal origin
    Acute apical periodontitis NOS
    EXCLUDES 1   *acute periodontitis (K05.2-)*
    DEF: Severe inflammation of the area surrounding the tip of a tooth's root; often secondary to infection or trauma.

K04.5 Chronic apical periodontitis
    Apical or periapical granuloma
    Apical periodontitis NOS
    EXCLUDES 1   *chronic periodontitis (K05.3-)*

K04.6 Periapical abscess with sinus
    Dental abscess with sinus
    Dentoalveolar abscess with sinus

K04.7 Periapical abscess without sinus
    Dental abscess without sinus
    Dentoalveolar abscess without sinus
    ~~Periapical abscess without sinus~~

K04.8 Radicular cyst
    Apical (periodontal) cyst
    Periapical cyst
    Residual radicular cyst
    EXCLUDES 2   *lateral periodontal cyst (K09.0)*
    DEF: Most common odontogenic cyst in tissue around tooth apex due to chronic inflammation of dental pulp.

✓5ᵗʰ **K04.9 Other and unspecified diseases of pulp and periapical tissues**
    K04.90 Unspecified diseases of pulp and periapical tissues   ▽
    K04.99 Other diseases of pulp and periapical tissues

✓4ᵗʰ **K05 Gingivitis and periodontal diseases**
    Use additional code to identify:
      alcohol abuse and dependence (F10.-)
      exposure to environmental tobacco smoke (Z77.22)
      exposure to tobacco smoke in the perinatal period (P96.81)
      history of tobacco dependence (Z87.891)
      occupational exposure to environmental tobacco smoke (Z57.31)
      tobacco dependence (F17.-)
      tobacco use (Z72.0)

✓5ᵗʰ **K05.0 Acute gingivitis**
    EXCLUDES 1   *acute necrotizing ulcerative gingivitis (A69.1)*
          herpesviral [herpes simplex] gingivostomatitis (B00.2)
    K05.00 Acute gingivitis, plaque induced
      Acute gingivitis NOS
      Plaque induced gingival disease
    K05.01 Acute gingivitis, non-plaque induced

✓5ᵗʰ **K05.1 Chronic gingivitis**
    Desquamative gingivitis (chronic)
    Gingivitis (chronic) NOS
    Hyperplastic gingivitis (chronic)
    Pregnancy associated gingivitis
    Simple marginal gingivitis (chronic)
    Ulcerative gingivitis (chronic)
    Code first, if applicable, diseases of the digestive system complicating pregnancy (O99.61-)
    K05.10 Chronic gingivitis, plaque induced
      Chronic gingivitis NOS
      Gingivitis NOS
    K05.11 Chronic gingivitis, non-plaque induced

✓5ᵗʰ **K05.2 Aggressive periodontitis**
    Acute pericoronitis
    EXCLUDES 1   *acute apical periodontitis (K04.4)*
          periapical abscess (K04.7)
          periapical abscess with sinus (K04.6)
    K05.20 Aggressive periodontitis, unspecified   ▽
    ✓6ᵗʰ **K05.21 Aggressive periodontitis, localized**
      Periodontal abscess
      K05.211 Aggressive periodontitis, localized, slight
      K05.212 Aggressive periodontitis, localized, moderate
      K05.213 Aggressive periodontitis, localized, severe
      K05.219 Aggressive periodontitis, localized, unspecified severity   ▽
    ✓6ᵗʰ **K05.22 Aggressive periodontitis, generalized**
      K05.221 Aggressive periodontitis, generalized, slight
      K05.222 Aggressive periodontitis, generalized, moderate
      K05.223 Aggressive periodontitis, generalized, severe
      K05.229 Aggressive periodontitis, generalized, unspecified severity   ▽

✓5ᵗʰ **K05.3 Chronic periodontitis**
    Chronic pericoronitis
    Complex periodontitis
    Periodontitis NOS
    Simplex periodontitis
    EXCLUDES 1   *chronic apical periodontitis (K04.5)*
    K05.30 Chronic periodontitis, unspecified   ▽
    ✓6ᵗʰ **K05.31 Chronic periodontitis, localized**
      K05.311 Chronic periodontitis, localized, slight
      K05.312 Chronic periodontitis, localized, moderate
      K05.313 Chronic periodontitis, localized, severe
      K05.319 Chronic periodontitis, localized, unspecified severity   ▽

✓ Additional Character Req   ✓7ᵗʰ Placeholder Alert   Case-Mix Diagnosis   Manifestation   ▽ Unspecified Dx   EXCLUDES 1 Not coded here   EXCLUDES 2 Not included here

Chapter 11. Diseases of the Digestive System

K05.32–K08.404

✓6ᵗʰ **K05.32** **Chronic periodontitis,** generalized

     K05.321 **Chronic periodontitis, generalized,** slight

     K05.322 **Chronic periodontitis, generalized,** moderate

     K05.323 **Chronic periodontitis, generalized,** severe

     K05.329 **Chronic periodontitis, generalized,** unspecified **severity** ▽

K05.4 **Periodontosis**
     Juvenile periodontosis

K05.5 **Other periodontal diseases**
     Combined periodontic-endodontic lesion
     Narrow gingival width (of periodontal soft tissue)
     EXCLUDES 2   *leukoplakia of gingiva (K13.21)*

K05.6 **Periodontal disease, unspecified** ▽

✓4ᵗʰ **K06** **Other disorders of gingiva and edentulous alveolar ridge**
     EXCLUDES 2   *acute gingivitis (K05.0)*
              atrophy of edentulous alveolar ridge (K08.2)
              chronic gingivitis (K05.1)
              gingivitis NOS (K05.1)

✓5ᵗʰ **K06.0** **Gingival** recession
     ▶Gingival recession (postinfective) (postprocedural)◀

● ✓6ᵗʰ **K06.01** **Gingival recession,** localized
●
     K06.010 **Localized gingival recession, unspecified** ▽
            Localized gingival recession, NOS

●   **K06.011** **Localized gingival recession,** minimal

●   **K06.012** **Localized gingival recession,** moderate

●   **K06.013** **Localized gingival recession,** severe

● ✓6ᵗʰ **K06.02** **Gingival recession,** generalized
●
     K06.020 **Generalized gingival recession, unspecified** ▽
            Generalized gingival recession, NOS

●   **K06.021** **Generalized gingival recession,** minimal

●   **K06.022** **Generalized gingival recession,** moderate

●   **K06.023** **Generalized gingival recession,** severe

K06.1 **Gingival** enlargement
     Gingival fibromatosis

K06.2 **Gingival and edentulous alveolar ridge lesions associated with** trauma
     Irritative hyperplasia of edentulous ridge [denture hyperplasia]
     Use additional code (Chapter 20) to identify external cause or denture status (Z97.2)

K06.3 **Horizontal alveolar bone loss**

K06.8 **Other specified disorders of gingiva and edentulous alveolar ridge**
     Fibrous epulis
     Flabby alveolar ridge
     Giant cell epulis
     Peripheral giant cell granuloma of gingiva
     Pyogenic granuloma of gingiva
     Vertical ridge deficiency
     EXCLUDES 2   *gingival cyst (K09.0)*

K06.9 **Disorder of gingiva and edentulous alveolar ridge, unspecified** ▽

✓4ᵗʰ **K08** **Other disorders of teeth and supporting structures**
     EXCLUDES 2   *dentofacial anomalies [including malocclusion] (M26.-)*
              disorders of jaw (M27.-)

K08.0 **Exfoliation of teeth due to systemic causes**
     Code also underlying systemic condition

✓5ᵗʰ **K08.1** **Complete loss of teeth**
     Acquired loss of teeth, complete
     EXCLUDES 1   *congenital absence of teeth (K00.0)*
              exfoliation of teeth due to systemic causes (K08.0)
              partial loss of teeth (K08.4-)

     ✓6ᵗʰ **K08.10** **Complete loss of teeth,** unspecified cause

         K08.101 **Complete loss of teeth, unspecified cause,** class I ▽

         K08.102 **Complete loss of teeth, unspecified cause,** class II ▽

         K08.103 **Complete loss of teeth, unspecified cause,** class III ▽

         K08.104 **Complete loss of teeth, unspecified cause,** class IV ▽

K08.109 **Complete loss of teeth, unspecified cause, unspecified class** ▽
     Edentulism NOS

✓6ᵗʰ **K08.11** **Complete loss of teeth** due to trauma

     K08.111 **Complete loss of teeth due to trauma,** class I

     K08.112 **Complete loss of teeth due to trauma,** class II

     K08.113 **Complete loss of teeth due to trauma,** class III

     K08.114 **Complete loss of teeth due to trauma,** class IV

     K08.119 **Complete loss of teeth due to trauma,** unspecified class ▽

✓6ᵗʰ **K08.12** **Complete loss of teeth due to** periodontal diseases

     K08.121 **Complete loss of teeth due to periodontal diseases,** class I

     K08.122 **Complete loss of teeth due to periodontal diseases,** class II

     K08.123 **Complete loss of teeth due to periodontal diseases,** class III

     K08.124 **Complete loss of teeth due to periodontal diseases,** class IV

     K08.129 **Complete loss of teeth due to periodontal diseases, unspecified class** ▽

✓6ᵗʰ **K08.13** **Complete loss of teeth due to** caries

     K08.131 **Complete loss of teeth due to caries,** class I

     K08.132 **Complete loss of teeth due to caries,** class II

     K08.133 **Complete loss of teeth due to caries,** class III

     K08.134 **Complete loss of teeth due to caries,** class IV

     K08.139 **Complete loss of teeth due to caries, unspecified class** ▽

✓6ᵗʰ **K08.19** **Complete loss of teeth due to** other specified **cause**

     K08.191 **Complete loss of teeth due to other specified cause,** class I

     K08.192 **Complete loss of teeth due to other specified cause,** class II

     K08.193 **Complete loss of teeth due to other specified cause,** class III

     K08.194 **Complete loss of teeth due to other specified cause,** class IV

     K08.199 **Complete loss of teeth due to other specified cause, unspecified class** ▽

✓5ᵗʰ **K08.2** **Atrophy of edentulous alveolar ridge**

     K08.20 **Unspecified atrophy of edentulous alveolar ridge** ▽
         Atrophy of the mandible NOS
         Atrophy of the maxilla NOS

     K08.21 Minimal **atrophy of the** mandible
         Minimal atrophy of the edentulous mandible

     K08.22 Moderate **atrophy of the** mandible
         Moderate atrophy of the edentulous mandible

     K08.23 Severe **atrophy of the** mandible
         Severe atrophy of the edentulous mandible

     K08.24 Minimal **atrophy of** maxilla
         Minimal atrophy of the edentulous maxilla

     K08.25 Moderate **atrophy of the** maxilla
         Moderate atrophy of the edentulous maxilla

     K08.26 Severe **atrophy of the** maxilla
         Severe atrophy of the edentulous maxilla

K08.3 **Retained dental root**

✓5ᵗʰ **K08.4** **Partial loss of teeth**
     Acquired loss of teeth, partial
     EXCLUDES 1   *complete loss of teeth (K08.1-)*
              congenital absence of teeth (K00.0)
     EXCLUDES 2   *exfoliation of teeth due to systemic causes (K08.0)*

     ✓6ᵗʰ **K08.40** **Partial loss of teeth,** unspecified cause

         K08.401 **Partial loss of teeth, unspecified cause,** class I ▽

         K08.402 **Partial loss of teeth, unspecified cause,** class II ▽

         K08.403 **Partial loss of teeth, unspecified cause,** class III ▽

         K08.404 **Partial loss of teeth, unspecified cause,** class IV ▽

Ⓝ Newborn: 0   Ⓟ Pediatric: 0-17   Ⓜ Maternity: 12-55   Ⓐ Adult: 15-124   **NRS** Nonroutine supply Dx   **NC Dx** Noncancer Dx   **PDx** Primary Dx   ▶◀ Revised Text   ● New Code   ▲ Revised Title

676   ICD-10-CM 2018

K08.409   **Partial loss of teeth, unspecified cause, unspecified class** ▽
    Tooth extraction status NOS

√6ᵗʰ K08.41   **Partial loss of teeth due to trauma**

K08.411   **Partial loss of teeth due to trauma, class I**
K08.412   **Partial loss of teeth due to trauma, class II**
K08.413   **Partial loss of teeth due to trauma, class III**
K08.414   **Partial loss of teeth due to trauma, class IV**
K08.419   **Partial loss of teeth due to trauma, unspecified class** ▽

√6ᵗʰ K08.42   **Partial loss of teeth due to periodontal diseases**

K08.421   **Partial loss of teeth due to periodontal diseases, class I**
K08.422   **Partial loss of teeth due to periodontal diseases, class II**
K08.423   **Partial loss of teeth due to periodontal diseases, class III**
K08.424   **Partial loss of teeth due to periodontal diseases, class IV**
K08.429   **Partial loss of teeth due to periodontal diseases, unspecified class** ▽

√6ᵗʰ K08.43   **Partial loss of teeth due to caries**

K08.431   **Partial loss of teeth due to caries, class I**
K08.432   **Partial loss of teeth due to caries, class II**
K08.433   **Partial loss of teeth due to caries, class III**
K08.434   **Partial loss of teeth due to caries, class IV**
K08.439   **Partial loss of teeth due to caries, unspecified class** ▽

√6ᵗʰ K08.49   **Partial loss of teeth due to other specified cause**

K08.491   **Partial loss of teeth due to other specified cause, class I**
K08.492   **Partial loss of teeth due to other specified cause, class II**
K08.493   **Partial loss of teeth due to other specified cause, class III**
K08.494   **Partial loss of teeth due to other specified cause, class IV**
K08.499   **Partial loss of teeth due to other specified cause, unspecified class** ▽

√5ᵗʰ K08.5   **Unsatisfactory restoration of tooth**
    Defective bridge, crown, filling
    Defective dental restoration
    EXCLUDES 1   *dental restoration status (Z98.811)*
    EXCLUDES 2   *endosseous dental implant failure (M27.6-)*
            unsatisfactory endodontic treatment (M27.5-)

K08.50   **Unsatisfactory restoration of tooth, unspecified** ▽
    Defective dental restoration NOS

K08.51   **Open restoration margins of tooth**
    Dental restoration failure of marginal integrity
    Open margin on tooth restoration
    Poor gingival margin to tooth restoration

K08.52   **Unrepairable overhanging of dental restorative materials**
    Overhanging of tooth restoration

√6ᵗʰ K08.53   **Fractured dental restorative material**
    EXCLUDES 1   *cracked tooth (K03.81)*
            traumatic fracture of tooth (S02.5)

K08.530   **Fractured dental restorative material without loss of material**
K08.531   **Fractured dental restorative material with loss of material**
K08.539   **Fractured dental restorative material, unspecified** ▽

K08.54   **Contour of existing restoration of tooth biologically incompatible with oral health**
    Dental restoration failure of periodontal anatomical integrity
    Unacceptable contours of existing restoration of tooth
    Unacceptable morphology of existing restoration of tooth

K08.55   **Allergy to existing dental restorative material**
    Use additional code to identify the specific type of allergy

K08.56   **Poor aesthetic of existing restoration of tooth**
    Dental restoration aesthetically inadequate or displeasing

K08.59   **Other unsatisfactory restoration of tooth**
    Other defective dental restoration

√5ᵗʰ K08.8   **Other specified disorders of teeth and supporting structures**

K08.81   **Primary occlusal trauma**
K08.82   **Secondary occlusal trauma**
K08.89   **Other specified disorders of teeth and supporting structures**
    Enlargement of alveolar ridge NOS
    Insufficient anatomic crown height
    Insufficient clinical crown length
    Irregular alveolar process
    Toothache NOS

K08.9   **Disorder of teeth and supporting structures, unspecified** ▽

√4ᵗʰ **K09**   **Cysts of oral region, not elsewhere classified**
    INCLUDES   lesions showing histological features both of aneurysmal cyst and of another fibro-osseous lesion
    EXCLUDES 2   *cysts of jaw (M27.0-, M27.4-)*
            radicular cyst (K04.8)

K09.0   **Developmental odontogenic cysts**
    Dentigerous cyst
    Eruption cyst
    Follicular cyst
    Gingival cyst
    Lateral periodontal cyst
    Primordial cyst
    EXCLUDES 2   *keratocysts (D16.4, D16.5)*
            odontogenic keratocystic tumors (D16.4, D16.5)

K09.1   **Developmental (nonodontogenic) cysts of oral region**
    Cyst (of) incisive canal
    Cyst (of) palatine of papilla
    Globulomaxillary cyst
    Median palatal cyst
    Nasoalveolar cyst
    Nasolabial cyst
    Nasopalatine duct cyst

K09.8   **Other cysts of oral region, not elsewhere classified**
    Dermoid cyst
    Epidermoid cyst
    Lymphoepithelial cyst
    Epstein's pearl

K09.9   **Cyst of oral region, unspecified** ▽

√4ᵗʰ **K11**   **Diseases of salivary glands**
    Use additional code to identify:
    alcohol abuse and dependence (F10.-)
    exposure to environmental tobacco smoke (Z77.22)
    exposure to tobacco smoke in the perinatal period (P96.81)
    whistory of tobacco dependence (Z87.891)
    occupational exposure to environmental tobacco smoke (Z57.31)
    tobacco dependence (F17.-)
    tobacco use (Z72.0)

K11.0   **Atrophy of salivary gland**

K11.1   **Hypertrophy of salivary gland**
    DEF: Overgrowth of or enlarged salivary gland tissue; caused by infection, salivary duct blockage, autoimmune diseases, and benign and malignant tumors.

√5ᵗʰ K11.2   **Sialoadenitis**
    Parotitis
    EXCLUDES 1   *epidemic parotitis (B26.-)*
            mumps (B26.-)
            uveoparotid fever [Heerfordt] (D86.89)

K11.20   **Sialoadenitis, unspecified** ▽
K11.21   **Acute sialoadenitis**
    EXCLUDES 1   *acute recurrent sialoadenitis (K11.22)*
K11.22   **Acute recurrent sialoadenitis**
K11.23   **Chronic sialoadenitis**

K11.3   **Abscess of salivary gland**

K11.4   **Fistula of salivary gland**
    EXCLUDES 1   *congenital fistula of salivary gland (Q38.4)*

K11.5   **Sialolithiasis**
    Calculus of salivary gland or duct
    Stone of salivary gland or duct

K11.6   **Mucocele of salivary gland**
    Mucous extravasation cyst of salivary gland
    Mucous retention cyst of salivary gland
    Ranula

K11.7   **Disturbances of salivary secretion**
    Hypoptyalism
    Ptyalism
    Xerostomia
    EXCLUDES 2   *dry mouth NOS (R68.2)*

☑ Additional Character Req   √x7ᵗʰ Placeholder Alert   Case-Mix Diagnosis   Manifestation   ▽ Unspecified Dx   EXCLUDES 1 Not coded here   EXCLUDES 2 Not included here

Chapter 11. Diseases of the Digestive System

K11.8   **Other diseases of salivary glands**
   Benign lymphoepithelial lesion of salivary gland
   Mikulicz' disease
   Necrotizing sialometaplasia
   Sialectasia
   Stenosis of salivary duct
   Stricture of salivary duct
   EXCLUDES 1   *sicca syndrome [Sjögren] (M35.0-)*

K11.9   **Disease of salivary gland, unspecified**   ▽
   Sialoadenopathy NOS

✓4ᵗʰ **K12**   **Stomatitis and related lesions**
   Use additional code to identify:
   alcohol abuse and dependence (F10.-)
   exposure to environmental tobacco smoke (Z77.22)
   exposure to tobacco smoke in the perinatal period (P96.81)
   history of tobacco dependence (Z87.891)
   occupational exposure to environmental tobacco smoke (Z57.31)
   tobacco dependence (F17.-)
   tobacco use (Z72.0)
   EXCLUDES 1   *cancrum oris (A69.0)*
        cheilitis (K13.0)
        gangrenous stomatitis (A69.0)
        herpesviral [herpes simplex] gingivostomatitis (B00.2)
        noma (A69.0)

K12.0   **Recurrent oral aphthae**
   Aphthous stomatitis (major) (minor)
   Bednar's aphthae
   Periadenitis mucosa necrotica recurrens
   Recurrent aphthous ulcer
   Stomatitis herpetiformis
   DEF: Disorder of unknown etiology with small oval or round painful ulcers of the mouth marked by a grayish exudate and a red halo effect.

K12.1   **Other forms of stomatitis**
   Stomatitis NOS
   Denture stomatitis
   Ulcerative stomatitis
   Vesicular stomatitis
   EXCLUDES 1   *acute necrotizing ulcerative stomatitis (A69.1)*
        Vincent's stomatitis (A69.1)

K12.2   **Cellulitis and abscess of mouth**   **NRS**
   Cellulitis of mouth (floor)
   Submandibular abscess
   EXCLUDES 2   *abscess of salivary gland (K11.3)*
        abscess of tongue (K14.0)
        periapical abscess (K04.6-K04.7)
        periodontal abscess (K05.21)
        peritonsillar abscess (J36)

✓5ᵗʰ **K12.3**   **Oral mucositis (ulcerative)**
   Mucositis (oral) (oropharyneal)
   EXCLUDES 2   *gastrointestinal mucositis (ulcerative) (K92.81)*
        mucositis (ulcerative) of vagina and vulva (N76.81)
        nasal mucositis (ulcerative) (J34.81)

   K12.30   **Oral mucositis (ulcerative), unspecified** ▽

   K12.31   **Oral mucositis (ulcerative) due to antineoplastic therapy**
     Use additional code for adverse effect, if applicable, to identify antineoplastic and immunosuppressive drugs (T45.1X5)
     Use additional code for other antineoplastic therapy, such as:
       radiological procedure and radiotherapy (Y84.2)

   K12.32   **Oral mucositis (ulcerative) due to other drugs**
     Use additional code for adverse effect, if applicable, to identify drug (T36-T50 with fifth or sixth character 5)

   K12.33   **Oral mucositis (ulcerative) due to radiation**
     Use additional external cause code (W88-W90, X39.0-) to identify cause

   K12.39   **Other oral mucositis (ulcerative)**
     Viral oral mucositis (ulcerative)

✓4ᵗʰ **K13**   **Other diseases of lip and oral mucosa**
   INCLUDES   epithelial disturbances of tongue
   Use additional code to identify:
   alcohol abuse and dependence (F10.-)
   exposure to environmental tobacco smoke (Z77.22)
   exposure to tobacco smoke in the perinatal period (P96.81)
   history of tobacco dependence (Z87.891)
   occupational exposure to environmental tobacco smoke (Z57.31)
   tobacco dependence (F17.-)
   tobacco use (Z72.0)
   EXCLUDES 2   *certain disorders of gingiva and edentulous alveolar ridge (K05-K06)*
        cysts of oral region (K09.-)
        diseases of tongue (K14.-)
        stomatitis and related lesions (K12.-)

K13.0   **Diseases of lips**
   Abscess of lips   Exfoliative cheilitis
   Angular cheilitis   Fistula of lips
   Cellulitis of lips   Glandular cheilitis
   Cheilitis NOS   Hypertrophy of lips
   Cheilodynia   Perlèche NEC
   Cheilosis
   EXCLUDES 1   *ariboflavinosis (E53.0)*
        cheilitis due to radiation-related disorders (L55-L59)
        congenital fistula of lips (Q38.0)
        congenital hypertrophy of lips (Q18.6)
        Perlèche due to candidiasis (B37.83)
        Perlèche due to riboflavin deficiency (E53.0)

K13.1   **Cheek and lip biting**

✓5ᵗʰ **K13.2**   **Leukoplakia and other disturbances of oral epithelium, including tongue**
   EXCLUDES 1   *carcinoma in situ of oral epithelium (D00.0-)*
        hairy leukoplakia (K13.3)

   K13.21   **Leukoplakia of oral mucosa, including tongue**
     Leukokeratosis of oral mucosa
     Leukoplakia of gingiva, lips, tongue
     EXCLUDES 1   *hairy leukoplakia (K13.3)*
         leukokeratosis nicotina palati (K13.24)

   K13.22   **Minimal keratinized residual ridge mucosa**
     Minimal keratinization of alveolar ridge mucosa

   K13.23   **Excessive keratinized residual ridge mucosa**
     Excessive keratinization of alveolar ridge mucosa

   K13.24   **Leukokeratosis nicotina palati**
     Smoker's palate

   K13.29   **Other disturbances of oral epithelium, including tongue**
     Erythroplakia of mouth or tongue
     Focal epithelial hyperplasia of mouth or tongue
     Leukoedema of mouth or tongue
     Other oral epithelium disturbances

K13.3   **Hairy leukoplakia**

K13.4   **Granuloma and granuloma-like lesions of oral mucosa**
   Eosinophilic granuloma
   Granuloma pyogenicum
   Verrucous xanthoma

K13.5   **Oral submucous fibrosis**
   Submucous fibrosis of tongue

K13.6   **Irritative hyperplasia of oral mucosa**
   EXCLUDES 2   *irritative hyperplasia of edentulous ridge [denture hyperplasia] (K06.2)*

✓5ᵗʰ **K13.7**   **Other and unspecified lesions of oral mucosa**
   K13.70   **Unspecified lesions of oral mucosa**   ▽
   K13.79   **Other lesions of oral mucosa**
     Focal oral mucinosis

N Newborn: 0   P Pediatric: 0-17   M Maternity: 12-55   A Adult: 15-124   NRS Nonroutine supply Dx   NCDx Noncancer Dx   PDx Primary Dx   ▶◀ Revised Text   ● New Code   ▲ Revised Title

678   ICD-10-CM 2018

☑4ᵗʰ K14   Diseases of tongue
Use additional code to identify:
alcohol abuse and dependence (F10.-)
exposure to environmental tobacco smoke (Z77.22)
history of tobacco dependence (Z87.891)
occupational exposure to environmental tobacco smoke (Z57.31)
tobacco dependence (F17.-)
tobacco use (Z72.0)
EXCLUDES 2 *erythroplakia (K13.29)*
focal epithelial hyperplasia (K13.29)
leukedema of tongue (K13.29)
leukoplakia of tongue (K13.21)
hairy leukoplakia (K13.3)
macroglossia (congenital) (Q38.2)
submucous fibrosis of tongue (K13.5)

K14.0   Glossitis
Abscess of tongue
Ulceration (traumatic) of tongue
EXCLUDES 1 *atrophic glossitis (K14.4)*

K14.1   Geographic tongue
Benign migratory glossitis
Glossitis areata exfoliativa

K14.2   Median rhomboid glossitis

K14.3   Hypertrophy of tongue papillae
Black hairy tongue
Coated tongue
Hypertrophy of foliate papillae
Lingua villosa nigra

K14.4   Atrophy of tongue papillae
Atrophic glossitis

K14.5   Plicated tongue
Fissured tongue
Furrowed tongue
Scrotal tongue
EXCLUDES 1 *fissured tongue, congenital (Q38.3)*

K14.6   Glossodynia
Glossopyrosis
Painful tongue

K14.8   Other diseases of tongue
Atrophy of tongue
Crenated tongue
Enlargement of tongue
Glossocele
Glossoptosis
Hypertrophy of tongue

K14.9   Disease of tongue, unspecified   ▽
Glossopathy NOS

Diseases of esophagus, stomach and duodenum (K20-K31)
EXCLUDES 2 *hiatus hernia (K44.-)*

☑4ᵗʰ K20   Esophagitis
Use additional code to identify:
alcohol abuse and dependence (F10.-)
EXCLUDES 1 *erosion of esophagus (K22.1-)*
esophagitis with gastro-esophageal reflux disease (K21.0)
reflux esophagitis (K21.0)
ulcerative esophagitis (K22.1-)
EXCLUDES 2 *eosinophilic gastritis or gastroenteritis (K52.81)*

K20.0   Eosinophilic esophagitis
K20.8   Other esophagitis
Abscess of esophagus
K20.9   Esophagitis, unspecified   ▽
Esophagitis NOS

☑4ᵗʰ K21   Gastro-esophageal reflux disease
EXCLUDES 1 *newborn esophageal reflux (P78.83)*

K21.0   Gastro-esophageal reflux disease with esophagitis
Reflux esophagitis

K21.9   Gastro-esophageal reflux disease without esophagitis
Esophageal reflux NOS
AHA: 2016, 1Q, 18

☑4ᵗʰ K22   Other diseases of esophagus
EXCLUDES 2 *esophageal varices (I85.-)*

K22.0   Achalasia of cardia
Achalasia NOS
Cardiospasm
EXCLUDES 1 *congenital cardiospasm (Q39.5)*
DEF: Esophageal motility disorder; caused by absence of esophageal peristalsis and impaired relaxation of lower esophageal sphincter; characterized by dysphagia, regurgitation, and heartburn.

☑5ᵗʰ K22.1   Ulcer of esophagus
Barrett's ulcer
Erosion of esophagus
Fungal ulcer of esophagus
Peptic ulcer of esophagus
Ulcer of esophagus due to ingestion of chemicals
Ulcer of esophagus due to ingestion of drugs and medicaments
Ulcerative esophagitis
Code first poisoning due to drug or toxin, if applicable (T36-T65 with fifth or sixth character 1-4 or 6)
Use additional code for adverse effect, if applicable, to identify drug (T36-T50 with fifth or sixth character 5)
EXCLUDES 1 *Barrett's esophagus (K22.7-)*

K22.10   Ulcer of esophagus without bleeding
Ulcer of esophagus NOS

K22.11   Ulcer of esophagus with bleeding
EXCLUDES 2 *bleeding esophageal varices (I85.01, I85.11)*

K22.2   Esophageal obstruction
Compression of esophagus
Constriction of esophagus
Stenosis of esophagus
Stricture of esophagus
EXCLUDES 1 *congenital stenosis or stricture of esophagus (Q39.3)*

K22.3   Perforation of esophagus
Rupture of esophagus
EXCLUDES 1 *traumatic perforation of (thoracic) esophagus (S27.8-)*

K22.4   Dyskinesia of esophagus
Corkscrew esophagus
Diffuse esophageal spasm
Spasm of esophagus
EXCLUDES 1 *cardiospasm (K22.0)*

K22.5   Diverticulum of esophagus, acquired
Esophageal pouch, acquired
EXCLUDES 1 *diverticulum of esophagus (congenital) (Q39.6)*

K22.6   Gastro-esophageal laceration-hemorrhage syndrome
Mallory-Weiss syndrome

☑5ᵗʰ K22.7   Barrett's esophagus
Barrett's disease
Barrett's syndrome
EXCLUDES 1 *Barrett's ulcer (K22.1)*
malignant neoplasm of esophagus (C15.-)
DEF: A metaplastic disorder in which specialized columnar epithelial cells replace the normal squamous epithelial cells; secondary to chronic gastroesophageal reflux damage to the mucosa; increases risk of developing adenocarcinoma.

K22.70   Barrett's esophagus without dysplasia
Barrett's esophagus NOS

☑6ᵗʰ K22.71   Barrett's esophagus with dysplasia
K22.710   Barrett's esophagus with low grade dysplasia
K22.711   Barrett's esophagus with high grade dysplasia
K22.719   Barrett's esophagus with dysplasia, unspecified   ▽

K22.8   Other specified diseases of esophagus
Hemorrhage of esophagus NOS
EXCLUDES 2 *esophageal varices (I85.-)*
Paterson-Kelly syndrome (D50.1)

K22.9   Disease of esophagus, unspecified   ▽

☑ Additional Character Req   ✓x7ᵗʰ Placeholder Alert   Case-Mix Diagnosis   Manifestation   ▽ Unspecified Dx   **EXCLUDES 1** Not coded here   **EXCLUDES 2** Not included here

Chapter 11. Diseases of the Digestive System

K23–K29.71

Gastrointestinal Ulcers

Esophagus

Esophageal ulcer

Stomach

Duodenal ulcer

Gastric ulcer

Small intestine

K23 Disorders of esophagus in diseases classified elsewhere
Code first underlying disease, such as:
congenital syphilis (A50.5)
> EXCLUDES 1   late syphilis (A52.79)
> megaesophagus due to Chagas' disease (B57.31)
> tuberculosis (A18.83)

☑4ᵗʰ K25 Gastric ulcer
INCLUDES   erosion (acute) of stomach
pylorus ulcer (peptic)
stomach ulcer (peptic)
Use additional code to identify:
alcohol abuse and dependence (F10.-)
> EXCLUDES 1   acute gastritis (K29.0-)
> peptic ulcer NOS (K27.-)

K25.0   Acute gastric ulcer with hemorrhage
K25.1   Acute gastric ulcer with perforation
K25.2   Acute gastric ulcer with both hemorrhage and perforation
K25.3   Acute gastric ulcer without hemorrhage or perforation
K25.4   Chronic or unspecified gastric ulcer with hemorrhage
K25.5   Chronic or unspecified gastric ulcer with perforation
K25.6   Chronic or unspecified gastric ulcer with both hemorrhage and perforation
K25.7   Chronic gastric ulcer without hemorrhage or perforation
K25.9   Gastric ulcer, unspecified as acute or chronic, without   ▽
hemorrhage or perforation

☑4ᵗʰ K26 Duodenal ulcer
INCLUDES   erosion (acute) of duodenum
duodenum ulcer (peptic)
postpyloric ulcer (peptic)
Use additional code to identify:
alcohol abuse and dependence (F10.-)
> EXCLUDES 1   peptic ulcer NOS (K27.-)

K26.0   Acute duodenal ulcer with hemorrhage
K26.1   Acute duodenal ulcer with perforation
K26.2   Acute duodenal ulcer with both hemorrhage and perforation
K26.3   Acute duodenal ulcer without hemorrhage or perforation
K26.4   Chronic or unspecified duodenal ulcer with hemorrhage
> AHA: 2016, 1Q, 14
> TIP: Use for bleeding duodenal ulcer resulting from anticoagulant therapy. When the adverse effect of an anticoagulant is the cause of such bleeding, additional codes D68.32 Hemorrhagic disorder due to extrinsic circulating anticoagulant, and T45.515- Adverse effect of anticoagulants, should be assigned.

K26.5   Chronic or unspecified duodenal ulcer with perforation
K26.6   Chronic or unspecified duodenal ulcer with both hemorrhage and perforation
K26.7   Chronic duodenal ulcer without hemorrhage or perforation
K26.9   Duodenal ulcer, unspecified as acute or chronic, without   ▽
hemorrhage or perforation

☑4ᵗʰ K27 Peptic ulcer, site unspecified
INCLUDES   gastroduodenal ulcer NOS
peptic ulcer NOS
Use additional code to identify:
alcohol abuse and dependence (F10.-)
> EXCLUDES 1   peptic ulcer of newborn (P78.82)

K27.0   Acute peptic ulcer, site unspecified, with hemorrhage
K27.1   Acute peptic ulcer, site unspecified, with perforation

K27.2   Acute peptic ulcer, site unspecified, with both hemorrhage and perforation
K27.3   Acute peptic ulcer, site unspecified, without hemorrhage or perforation
K27.4   Chronic or unspecified peptic ulcer, site unspecified, with hemorrhage
K27.5   Chronic or unspecified peptic ulcer, site unspecified, with perforation
K27.6   Chronic or unspecified peptic ulcer, site unspecified, with both hemorrhage and perforation
K27.7   Chronic peptic ulcer, site unspecified, without hemorrhage or perforation
K27.9   Peptic ulcer, site unspecified, unspecified as acute or   ▽
chronic, without hemorrhage or perforation

☑4ᵗʰ K28 Gastrojejunal ulcer
INCLUDES   anastomotic ulcer (peptic) or erosion
gastrocolic ulcer (peptic) or erosion
gastrointestinal ulcer (peptic) or erosion
gastrojejunal ulcer (peptic) or erosion
jejunal ulcer (peptic) or erosion
marginal ulcer (peptic) or erosion
stomal ulcer (peptic) or erosion
Use additional code to identify:
alcohol abuse and dependence (F10.-)
> EXCLUDES 1   primary ulcer of small intestine (K63.3)

K28.0   Acute gastrojejunal ulcer with hemorrhage
K28.1   Acute gastrojejunal ulcer with perforation
K28.2   Acute gastrojejunal ulcer with both hemorrhage and perforation
K28.3   Acute gastrojejunal ulcer without hemorrhage or perforation
K28.4   Chronic or unspecified gastrojejunal ulcer with hemorrhage
K28.5   Chronic or unspecified gastrojejunal ulcer with perforation
K28.6   Chronic or unspecified gastrojejunal ulcer with both hemorrhage and perforation
K28.7   Chronic gastrojejunal ulcer without hemorrhage or perforation
K28.9   Gastrojejunal ulcer, unspecified as acute or chronic,   ▽
without hemorrhage or perforation

☑4ᵗʰ K29 Gastritis and duodenitis
> EXCLUDES 1   eosinophilic gastritis or gastroenteritis (K52.81)
> Zollinger-Ellison syndrome (E16.4)

☑5ᵗʰ   **K29.0   Acute gastritis**
Use additional code to identify:
alcohol abuse and dependence (F10.-)
> EXCLUDES 1   erosion (acute) of stomach (K25.-)
> K29.00   Acute gastritis without bleeding
> K29.01   Acute gastritis with bleeding

☑5ᵗʰ   **K29.2   Alcoholic gastritis**
Use additional code to identify:
alcohol abuse and dependence (F10.-)
> K29.20   Alcoholic gastritis without bleeding
> K29.21   Alcoholic gastritis with bleeding

☑5ᵗʰ   **K29.3   Chronic superficial gastritis**
> K29.30   Chronic superficial gastritis without bleeding
> K29.31   Chronic superficial gastritis with bleeding

☑5ᵗʰ   **K29.4   Chronic atrophic gastritis**
Gastric atrophy
> K29.40   Chronic atrophic gastritis without bleeding
> K29.41   Chronic atrophic gastritis with bleeding

☑5ᵗʰ   **K29.5   Unspecified chronic gastritis**
Chronic antral gastritis
Chronic fundal gastritis
> K29.50   Unspecified chronic gastritis without bleeding   ▽
> K29.51   Unspecified chronic gastritis with bleeding   ▽

☑5ᵗʰ   **K29.6   Other gastritis**
Giant hypertrophic gastritis
Granulomatous gastritis
Ménétrier's disease
> K29.60   Other gastritis without bleeding
> K29.61   Other gastritis with bleeding

☑5ᵗʰ   **K29.7   Gastritis, unspecified**
> K29.70   Gastritis, unspecified, without bleeding   ▽
> K29.71   Gastritis, unspecified, with bleeding   ▽

Ⓝ Newborn: 0   Ⓟ Pediatric: 0-17   Ⓜ Maternity: 12-55   Ⓐ Adult: 15-124   NRS Nonroutine supply Dx   NC Dx Noncancer Dx   PDx Primary Dx   ▶◀ Revised Text   ● New Code   ▲ Revised Title

680   ICD-10-CM 2018

✓5ᵗʰ **K29.8** Duodenitis

    K29.80 **Duodenitis** without bleeding

    K29.81 **Duodenitis** with bleeding

✓5ᵗʰ **K29.9** Gastroduodenitis, unspecified

    K29.90 **Gastroduodenitis, unspecified,** without bleeding ▽

    K29.91 **Gastroduodenitis, unspecified, with bleeding** ▽

K30 **Functional dyspepsia**

    Indigestion

    EXCLUDES 1   dyspepsia NOS (R10.13)
             heartburn (R12)
             nervous dyspepsia (F45.8)
             neurotic dyspepsia (F45.8)
             psychogenic dyspepsia (F45.8)

✓4ᵗʰ **K31** **Other diseases of stomach and duodenum**

    INCLUDES   functional disorders of stomach

    EXCLUDES 2   diabetic gastroparesis (E08.43, E09.43, E10.43, E11.43, E13.43)
             diverticulum of duodenum (K57.00-K57.13)

    K31.0 **Acute dilatation of stomach**
             Acute distention of stomach

    K31.1 **Adult hypertrophic pyloric stenosis**   Ⓐ
             Pyloric stenosis NOS
             EXCLUDES 1   congenital or infantile pyloric stenosis (Q40.0)

    K31.2 **Hourglass stricture and stenosis of stomach**
             EXCLUDES 1   congenital hourglass stomach (Q40.2)
                        hourglass contraction of stomach (K31.89)

    K31.3 **Pylorospasm, not elsewhere classified**
             EXCLUDES 1   congenital or infantile pylorospasm (Q40.0)
                        neurotic pylorospasm (F45.8)
                        psychogenic pylorospasm (F45.8)

    K31.4 **Gastric diverticulum**
             EXCLUDES 1   congenital diverticulum of stomach (Q40.2)

    K31.5 **Obstruction of duodenum**
             Constriction of duodenum
             Duodenal ileus (chronic)
             Stenosis of duodenum
             Stricture of duodenum
             Volvulus of duodenum
             EXCLUDES 1   congenital stenosis of duodenum (Q41.0)

    K31.6 **Fistula of stomach and duodenum**
             Gastrocolic fistula
             Gastrojejunocolic fistula

    K31.7 **Polyp of stomach and duodenum**
             EXCLUDES 1   adenomatous polyp of stomach (D13.1)

✓5ᵗʰ   **K31.8** **Other specified diseases of stomach and duodenum**

    ✓6ᵗʰ **K31.81** **Angiodysplasia of stomach and duodenum**

        K31.811 **Angiodysplasia of stomach and duodenum with bleeding**

        K31.819 **Angiodysplasia of stomach and duodenum** without bleeding
                 Angiodysplasia of stomach and duodenum NOS

    K31.82 **Dieulafoy lesion (hemorrhagic) of stomach and duodenum**
             EXCLUDES 2   Dieulafoy lesion of intestine (K63.81)

    K31.83 **Achlorhydria**
             DEF: Absence of hydrochloric acid in gastric secretions due to gastric mucosa atrophy; unresponsive to histamines; also known as gastric anacidity.

    K31.84 **Gastroparesis**
             Gastroparalysis
             Code first underlying disease, if known, such as:
                anorexia nervosa (F50.0-)
                diabetes mellitus (E08.43, E09.43, E10.43, E11.43, E13.43)
                scleroderma (M34.-)
             AHA: 2013, 4Q, 114

    K31.89 **Other diseases of stomach and duodenum**
             AHA: 2017, 1Q, 28
             TIP: Use for cyclical vomiting not related to migraine, along with a code from category R11 Nausea and vomiting.

    K31.9 **Disease of stomach and duodenum, unspecified** ▽

Diseases of appendix (K35-K38)

✓4ᵗʰ **K35** Acute **appendicitis**

    K35.2 **Acute appendicitis** with generalized peritonitis
             Appendicitis (acute) with generalized (diffuse) peritonitis following rupture or perforation of appendix
             Perforated appendix NOS
             Ruptured appendix NOS

    K35.3 **Acute appendicitis** with localized peritonitis
             Acute appendicitis with or without perforation or rupture with peritonitis NOS
             Acute appendicitis with or without perforation or rupture with localized peritonitis
             Acute appendicitis with peritoneal abscess

✓5ᵗʰ   **K35.8** Other and unspecified acute appendicitis

    K35.80 **Unspecified acute appendicitis** ▽
             Acute appendicitis NOS
             Acute appendicitis without (localized) (generalized) peritonitis

    K35.89 **Other acute appendicitis**

K36 **Other appendicitis**
     Chronic appendicitis
     Recurrent appendicitis

K37 **Unspecified appendicitis** ▽
     EXCLUDES 1   unspecified appendicitis with peritonitis (K35.2-K35.3)

✓4ᵗʰ **K38** **Other diseases of appendix**

    K38.0 **Hyperplasia of appendix**

    K38.1 **Appendicular concretions**
             Fecalith of appendix
             Stercolith of appendix

    K38.2 **Diverticulum of appendix**

    K38.3 **Fistula of appendix**

    K38.8 **Other specified diseases of appendix**
             Intussusception of appendix

    K38.9 **Disease of appendix, unspecified** ▽

Hernia (K40-K46)

NOTE   Hernia with both gangrene and obstruction is classified to hernia with gangrene.

INCLUDES   acquired hernia
             congenital [except diaphragmatic or hiatus] hernia
             recurrent hernia

✓4ᵗʰ **K40** Inguinal **hernia**
    INCLUDES   bubonocele
             direct inguinal hernia
             double inguinal hernia
             indirect inguinal hernia
             inguinal hernia NOS
             oblique inguinal hernia
             scrotal hernia

✓5ᵗʰ   **K40.0** Bilateral **inguinal hernia,** with obstruction, without gangrene
             Inguinal hernia (bilateral) causing obstruction without gangrene
             Incarcerated inguinal hernia (bilateral) without gangrene
             Irreducible inguinal hernia (bilateral) without gangrene
             Strangulated inguinal hernia (bilateral) without gangrene

    K40.00 **Bilateral inguinal hernia, with obstruction, without gangrene,** not specified as recurrent
             Bilateral inguinal hernia, with obstruction, without gangrene NOS

    K40.01 **Bilateral inguinal hernia, with obstruction, without gangrene,** recurrent

Hernia Sites

Abdominal ring; Indirect inguinal hernia; Anterior inguinal wall; Direct inguinal hernia; Spermatic cord; Femoral hernia; Inguinal ligament; Femoral sheath; Epigastric hernia; Paraumbilical hernia; Inguinal hernias; Femoral hernia

✓ Additional Character Req   ✓x7ᵗʰ Placeholder Alert   Case-Mix Diagnosis   Manifestation   ▽ Unspecified Dx   EXCLUDES 1 Not coded here   EXCLUDES 2 Not included here

ICD-10-CM 2018   681

Chapter 11. Diseases of the Digestive System

✓5ᵗʰ **K40.1** Bilateral **inguinal hernia,** with gangrene

    K40.10 **Bilateral inguinal hernia, with gangrene,** not specified as recurrent
        Bilateral inguinal hernia, with gangrene NOS

    K40.11 **Bilateral inguinal hernia, with gangrene, recurrent**

✓5ᵗʰ **K40.2** Bilateral **inguinal hernia,** without obstruction or gangrene

    K40.20 **Bilateral inguinal hernia, without obstruction or gangrene,** not specified as recurrent
        Bilateral inguinal hernia NOS

    K40.21 **Bilateral inguinal hernia, without obstruction or gangrene, recurrent**

✓5ᵗʰ **K40.3** Unilateral **inguinal hernia,** with obstruction, without gangrene
    Inguinal hernia (unilateral) causing obstruction without gangrene
    Incarcerated inguinal hernia (unilateral) without gangrene
    Irreducible inguinal hernia (unilateral) without gangrene
    Strangulated inguinal hernia (unilateral) without gangrene

    K40.30 **Unilateral inguinal hernia, with obstruction, without gangrene,** not specified as recurrent
        Inguinal hernia, with obstruction NOS
        Unilateral inguinal hernia, with obstruction, without gangrene NOS

    K40.31 **Unilateral inguinal hernia, with obstruction, without gangrene, recurrent**

✓5ᵗʰ **K40.4** Unilateral **inguinal hernia,** with gangrene

    K40.40 **Unilateral inguinal hernia, with gangrene,** not specified as recurrent
        Inguinal hernia with gangrene NOS
        Unilateral inguinal hernia with gangrene NOS

    K40.41 **Unilateral inguinal hernia, with gangrene, recurrent**

✓5ᵗʰ **K40.9** Unilateral **inguinal hernia,** without obstruction or gangrene

    K40.90 **Unilateral inguinal hernia, without obstruction or gangrene,** not specified as recurrent
        Inguinal hernia NOS
        Unilateral inguinal hernia NOS

    K40.91 **Unilateral inguinal hernia, without obstruction or gangrene, recurrent**

✓4ᵗʰ **K41** **Femoral hernia**

✓5ᵗʰ **K41.0** Bilateral **femoral hernia,** with obstruction, without gangrene
    Femoral hernia (bilateral) causing obstruction, without gangrene
    Incarcerated femoral hernia (bilateral), without gangrene
    Irreducible femoral hernia (bilateral), without gangrene
    Strangulated femoral hernia (bilateral), without gangrene

    K41.00 **Bilateral femoral hernia, with obstruction, without gangrene,** not specified as recurrent
        Bilateral femoral hernia, with obstruction, without gangrene NOS

    K41.01 **Bilateral femoral hernia, with obstruction, without gangrene, recurrent**

✓5ᵗʰ **K41.1** Bilateral **femoral hernia,** with gangrene

    K41.10 **Bilateral femoral hernia, with gangrene,** not specified as recurrent
        Bilateral femoral hernia, with gangrene NOS

    K41.11 **Bilateral femoral hernia, with gangrene, recurrent**

✓5ᵗʰ **K41.2** Bilateral **femoral hernia,** without obstruction or gangrene

    K41.20 **Bilateral femoral hernia, without obstruction or gangrene,** not specified as recurrent
        Bilateral femoral hernia NOS

    K41.21 **Bilateral femoral hernia, without obstruction or gangrene, recurrent**

✓5ᵗʰ **K41.3** Unilateral **femoral hernia,** with obstruction, without gangrene
    Femoral hernia (unilateral) causing obstruction, without gangrene
    Incarcerated femoral hernia (unilateral), without gangrene
    Irreducible femoral hernia (unilateral), without gangrene
    Strangulated femoral hernia (unilateral), without gangrene

    K41.30 **Unilateral femoral hernia, with obstruction, without gangrene,** not specified as recurrent
        Femoral hernia, with obstruction NOS
        Unilateral femoral hernia, with obstruction NOS

    K41.31 **Unilateral femoral hernia, with obstruction, without gangrene, recurrent**

✓5ᵗʰ **K41.4** Unilateral **femoral hernia,** with gangrene

    K41.40 **Unilateral femoral hernia, with gangrene,** not specified as recurrent
        Femoral hernia, with gangrene NOS
        Unilateral femoral hernia, with gangrene NOS

    K41.41 **Unilateral femoral hernia, with gangrene, recurrent**

✓5ᵗʰ **K41.9** Unilateral **femoral hernia,** without obstruction or gangrene

    K41.90 **Unilateral femoral hernia, without obstruction or gangrene,** not specified as recurrent
        Femoral hernia NOS
        Unilateral femoral hernia NOS

    K41.91 **Unilateral femoral hernia, without obstruction or gangrene, recurrent**

✓4ᵗʰ **K42** **Umbilical hernia**
    INCLUDES paraumbilical hernia
    EXCLUDES 1 *omphalocele (Q79.2)*

  K42.0 **Umbilical hernia** with obstruction, without gangrene
    Umbilical hernia causing obstruction, without gangrene
    Incarcerated umbilical hernia, without gangrene
    Irreducible umbilical hernia, without gangrene
    Strangulated umbilical hernia, without gangrene

  K42.1 **Umbilical hernia** with gangrene
    Gangrenous umbilical hernia

  K42.9 **Umbilical hernia** without obstruction or gangrene
    Umbilical hernia NOS

✓4ᵗʰ **K43** **Ventral hernia**

  K43.0 Incisional **hernia with obstruction,** without gangrene
    Incisional hernia causing obstruction, without gangrene
    Incarcerated incisional hernia, without gangrene
    Irreducible incisional hernia, without gangrene
    Strangulated incisional hernia, without gangrene

  K43.1 Incisional **hernia with gangrene**
    Gangrenous incisional hernia

  K43.2 Incisional **hernia without obstruction or gangrene**
    Incisional hernia NOS

  K43.3 Parastomal **hernia with obstruction,** without gangrene
    Incarcerated parastomal hernia, without gangrene
    Irreducible parastomal hernia, without gangrene
    Parastomal hernia causing obstruction, without gangrene
    Strangulated parastomal hernia, without gangrene

  K43.4 Parastomal **hernia with gangrene**
    Gangrenous parastomal hernia

  K43.5 Parastomal **hernia without obstruction or gangrene**
    Parastomal hernia NOS

  K43.6 **Other and unspecified ventral hernia with obstruction,** without gangrene ▽
    Epigastric hernia causing obstruction, without gangrene
    Hypogastric hernia causing obstruction, without gangrene
    Incarcerated epigastric hernia without gangrene
    Incarcerated hypogastric hernia without gangrene
    Incarcerated midline hernia without gangrene
    Incarcerated spigelian hernia without gangrene
    Incarcerated subxiphoid hernia without gangrene
    Irreducible epigastric hernia without gangrene
    Irreducible hypogastric hernia without gangrene
    Irreducible midline hernia without gangrene
    Irreducible spigelian hernia without gangrene
    Irreducible subxiphoid hernia without gangrene
    Midline hernia causing obstruction, without gangrene
    Spigelian hernia causing obstruction, without gangrene
    Strangulated epigastric hernia without gangrene
    Strangulated hypogastric hernia without gangrene
    Strangulated midline hernia without gangrene
    Strangulated spigelian hernia without gangrene
    Strangulated subxiphoid hernia without gangrene
    Subxiphoid hernia causing obstruction, without gangrene

  K43.7 **Other and unspecified ventral hernia** with gangrene ▽
    Any condition listed under K43.6 specified as gangrenous

  K43.9 **Ventral hernia** without obstruction or gangrene ▽
    Epigastric hernia
    Ventral hernia NOS

Ⓝ Newborn: 0   Ⓟ Pediatric: 0-17   Ⓜ Maternity: 12-55   Ⓐ Adult: 15-124   NRS Nonroutine supply Dx   NC Dx Noncancer Dx   PD Dx Primary Dx   ▶◀ Revised Text   ● New Code   ▲ Revised Title

682   ICD-10-CM 2018

Chapter 11. Diseases of the Digestive System

Hiatal Hernia

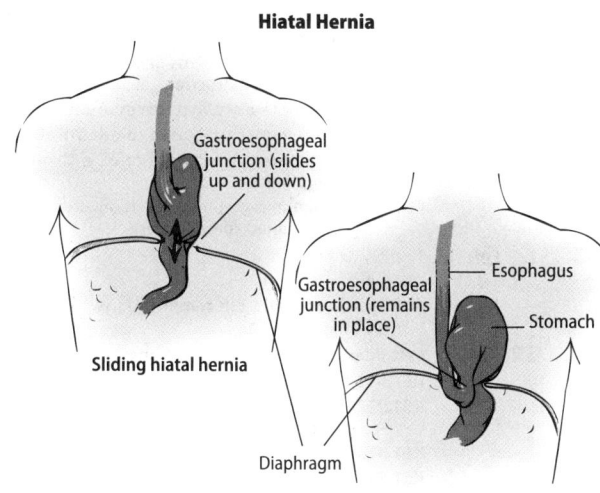

Gastroesophageal junction (slides up and down)

Sliding hiatal hernia

Gastroesophageal junction (remains in place)

Esophagus

Stomach

Diaphragm

Paraesophageal hiatal hernia

✓4ᵗʰ **K44** Diaphragmatic **hernia**
  INCLUDES   hiatus hernia (esophageal) (sliding)
    paraesophageal hernia
  EXCLUDES 1   *congenital diaphragmatic hernia (Q79.0)*
    congenital hiatus hernia (Q40.1)

  K44.0 Diaphragmatic hernia with obstruction, without gangrene
    Diaphragmatic hernia causing obstruction
    Incarcerated diaphragmatic hernia
    Irreducible diaphragmatic hernia
    Strangulated diaphragmatic hernia

  K44.1 Diaphragmatic hernia with gangrene
    Gangrenous diaphragmatic hernia

  K44.9 Diaphragmatic hernia without obstruction or gangrene
    Diaphragmatic hernia NOS

✓4ᵗʰ **K45** Other abdominal **hernia**
  INCLUDES   abdominal hernia, specified site NEC
    lumbar hernia
    obturator hernia
    pudendal hernia
    retroperitoneal hernia
    sciatic hernia

  K45.0 Other specified abdominal hernia with obstruction, without gangrene
    Other specified abdominal hernia causing obstruction
    Other specified incarcerated abdominal hernia
    Other specified irreducible abdominal hernia
    Other specified strangulated abdominal hernia

  K45.1 Other specified abdominal hernia with gangrene
    Any condition listed under K45 specified as gangrenous

  K45.8 Other specified abdominal hernia without obstruction or gangrene

✓4ᵗʰ **K46** Unspecified abdominal **hernia**
  INCLUDES   enterocele
    epiplocele
    hernia NOS
    interstitial hernia
    intestinal hernia
    intra-abdominal hernia
  EXCLUDES 1   *vaginal enterocele (N81.5)*

  K46.0 Unspecified abdominal hernia with obstruction, without gangrene   ▽
    Unspecified abdominal hernia causing obstruction
    Unspecified incarcerated abdominal hernia
    Unspecified irreducible abdominal hernia
    Unspecified strangulated abdominal hernia

  K46.1 Unspecified abdominal hernia with gangrene   ▽
    Any condition listed under K46 specified as gangrenous

  K46.9 Unspecified abdominal hernia without obstruction or gangrene   ▽
    Abdominal hernia NOS

Noninfective enteritis and colitis (K50-K52)

INCLUDES   noninfective inflammatory bowel disease
EXCLUDES 1   *irritable bowel syndrome (K58.-)*
  megacolon (K59.3-)

✓4ᵗʰ **K50** Crohn's disease [regional enteritis]
  INCLUDES   granulomatous enteritis
  Use additional code to identify manifestations, such as:
    pyoderma gangrenosum (L88)
  EXCLUDES 1   *ulcerative colitis (K51.-)*
  AHA: 2012, 4Q, 104

  ✓5ᵗʰ **K50.0** Crohn's disease of small intestine
    Crohn's disease [regional enteritis] of duodenum
    Crohn's disease [regional enteritis] of ileum
    Crohn's disease [regional enteritis] of jejunum
    Regional ileitis
    Terminal ileitis
    EXCLUDES 1   *Crohn's disease of both small and large intestine (K50.8-)*

    K50.00 Crohn's disease of small intestine without complications

    ✓6ᵗʰ **K50.01** Crohn's disease of small intestine with complications
      K50.011 Crohn's disease of small intestine with rectal bleeding
      K50.012 Crohn's disease of small intestine with intestinal obstruction
      K50.013 Crohn's disease of small intestine with fistula
      K50.014 Crohn's disease of small intestine with abscess   NRS
        AHA: 2012, 4Q, 104
      K50.018 Crohn's disease of small intestine with other complication
      K50.019 Crohn's disease of small intestine with unspecified complications   ▽

  ✓5ᵗʰ **K50.1** Crohn's disease of large intestine
    Crohn's disease [regional enteritis] of colon
    Crohn's disease [regional enteritis] of large bowel
    Crohn's disease [regional enteritis] of rectum
    Granulomatous colitis
    Regional colitis
    EXCLUDES 1   *Crohn's disease of both small and large intestine (K50.8)*

    K50.10 Crohn's disease of large intestine without complications

    ✓6ᵗʰ **K50.11** Crohn's disease of large intestine with complications
      K50.111 Crohn's disease of large intestine with rectal bleeding
      K50.112 Crohn's disease of large intestine with intestinal obstruction
      K50.113 Crohn's disease of large intestine with fistula
      K50.114 Crohn's disease of large intestine with abscess   NRS
      K50.118 Crohn's disease of large intestine with other complication
      K50.119 Crohn's disease of large intestine with unspecified complications   ▽

  ✓5ᵗʰ **K50.8** Crohn's disease of both small and large intestine
    K50.80 Crohn's disease of both small and large intestine without complications

    ✓6ᵗʰ **K50.81** Crohn's disease of both small and large intestine with complications
      K50.811 Crohn's disease of both small and large intestine with rectal bleeding
      K50.812 Crohn's disease of both small and large intestine with intestinal obstruction
      K50.813 Crohn's disease of both small and large intestine with fistula
      K50.814 Crohn's disease of both small and large intestine with abscess   NRS
      K50.818 Crohn's disease of both small and large intestine with other complication
      K50.819 Crohn's disease of both small and large intestine with unspecified complications   ▽

☑ Additional Character Req   ✓x7ᵗʰ Placeholder Alert   Case-Mix Diagnosis   Manifestation   ▽ Unspecified Dx   EXCLUDES 1 Not coded here   EXCLUDES 2 Not included here

ICD-10-CM 2018   683

Chapter 11. Diseases of the Digestive System

K50.9   Crohn's disease, unspecified ✓5th

   K50.90   Crohn's disease, unspecified, without complications ▽
     Crohn's disease NOS
     Regional enteritis NOS

   ✓6th **K50.91   Crohn's disease, unspecified, with complications**

     K50.911   Crohn's disease, unspecified, with rectal bleeding ▽

     K50.912   Crohn's disease, unspecified, with intestinal obstruction ▽

     K50.913   Crohn's disease, unspecified, with fistula ▽

     K50.914   Crohn's disease, unspecified, with abscess NRS ▽

     K50.918   Crohn's disease, unspecified, with other complication ▽

     K50.919   Crohn's disease, unspecified, with unspecified complications ▽

K51   Ulcerative colitis ✓4th
   Use additional code to identify manifestations, such as:
     pyoderma gangrenosum (L88)
   EXCLUDES 1   Crohn's disease [regional enteritis] (K50.-)

   ✓5th **K51.0   Ulcerative (chronic) pancolitis**
     Backwash ileitis

     K51.00   Ulcerative (chronic) pancolitis without complications
       Ulcerative (chronic) pancolitis NOS

     ✓6th **K51.01   Ulcerative (chronic) pancolitis with complications**

       K51.011   Ulcerative (chronic) pancolitis with rectal bleeding

       K51.012   Ulcerative (chronic) pancolitis with intestinal obstruction

       K51.013   Ulcerative (chronic) pancolitis with fistula

       K51.014   Ulcerative (chronic) pancolitis with abscess

       K51.018   Ulcerative (chronic) pancolitis with other complication

       K51.019   Ulcerative (chronic) pancolitis with unspecified complications ▽

   ✓5th **K51.2   Ulcerative (chronic) proctitis**

     K51.20   Ulcerative (chronic) proctitis without complications
       Ulcerative (chronic) proctitis NOS

     ✓6th **K51.21   Ulcerative (chronic) proctitis with complications**

       K51.211   Ulcerative (chronic) proctitis with rectal bleeding

       K51.212   Ulcerative (chronic) proctitis with intestinal obstruction

       K51.213   Ulcerative (chronic) proctitis with fistula

       K51.214   Ulcerative (chronic) proctitis with abscess

       K51.218   Ulcerative (chronic) proctitis with other complication

       K51.219   Ulcerative (chronic) proctitis with unspecified complications ▽

   ✓5th **K51.3   Ulcerative (chronic) rectosigmoiditis**

     K51.30   Ulcerative (chronic) rectosigmoiditis without complications
       Ulcerative (chronic) rectosigmoiditis NOS

     ✓6th **K51.31   Ulcerative (chronic) rectosigmoiditis with complications**

       K51.311   Ulcerative (chronic) rectosigmoiditis with rectal bleeding

       K51.312   Ulcerative (chronic) rectosigmoiditis with intestinal obstruction

       K51.313   Ulcerative (chronic) rectosigmoiditis with fistula

       K51.314   Ulcerative (chronic) rectosigmoiditis with abscess

       K51.318   Ulcerative (chronic) rectosigmoiditis with other complication

       K51.319   Ulcerative (chronic) rectosigmoiditis with unspecified complications ▽

   ✓5th **K51.4   Inflammatory polyps of colon**
     EXCLUDES 1   adenomatous polyp of colon (D12.6)
       polyposis of colon (D12.6)
       polyps of colon NOS (K63.5)

     K51.40   Inflammatory polyps of colon without complications
       Inflammatory polyps of colon NOS

   ✓6th **K51.41   Inflammatory polyps of colon with complications**

     K51.411   Inflammatory polyps of colon with rectal bleeding

     K51.412   Inflammatory polyps of colon with intestinal obstruction

     K51.413   Inflammatory polyps of colon with fistula

     K51.414   Inflammatory polyps of colon with abscess

     K51.418   Inflammatory polyps of colon with other complication

     K51.419   Inflammatory polyps of colon with unspecified complications ▽

   ✓5th **K51.5   Left sided colitis**
     Left hemicolitis

     K51.50   Left sided colitis without complications
       Left sided colitis NOS

     ✓6th **K51.51   Left sided colitis with complications**

       K51.511   Left sided colitis with rectal bleeding

       K51.512   Left sided colitis with intestinal obstruction

       K51.513   Left sided colitis with fistula

       K51.514   Left sided colitis with abscess

       K51.518   Left sided colitis with other complication

       K51.519   Left sided colitis with unspecified complications ▽

   ✓5th **K51.8   Other ulcerative colitis**

     K51.80   Other ulcerative colitis without complications

     ✓6th **K51.81   Other ulcerative colitis with complications**

       K51.811   Other ulcerative colitis with rectal bleeding

       K51.812   Other ulcerative colitis with intestinal obstruction

       K51.813   Other ulcerative colitis with fistula

       K51.814   Other ulcerative colitis with abscess

       K51.818   Other ulcerative colitis with other complication

       K51.819   Other ulcerative colitis with unspecified complications ▽

   ✓5th **K51.9   Ulcerative colitis, unspecified**

     K51.90   Ulcerative colitis, unspecified, without complications ▽

     ✓6th **K51.91   Ulcerative colitis, unspecified, with complications**

       K51.911   Ulcerative colitis, unspecified with rectal bleeding ▽

       K51.912   Ulcerative colitis, unspecified with intestinal obstruction ▽

       K51.913   Ulcerative colitis, unspecified with fistula ▽

       K51.914   Ulcerative colitis, unspecified with abscess ▽

       K51.918   Ulcerative colitis, unspecified with other complication ▽

       K51.919   Ulcerative colitis, unspecified with unspecified complications ▽

K52   Other and unspecified noninfective gastroenteritis and colitis ✓4th

   K52.0   Gastroenteritis and colitis due to radiation

   K52.1   Toxic gastroenteritis and colitis
     Drug-induced gastroenteritis and colitis
     Code first (T51-T65) to identify toxic agent
     Use additional code for adverse effect, if applicable, to identify drug (T36-T50 with fifth or sixth character 5)

   ✓5th **K52.2   Allergic and dietetic gastroenteritis and colitis**
     Use additional code to identify type of food allergy (Z91.01-, Z91.02-)
     EXCLUDES 2   allergic eosinophilic colitis (K52.82)
       allergic eosinophilic esophagitis (K20.0)
       allergic eosinophilic gastritis (K52.81)
       allergic eosinophilic gastroenteritis (K52.81)
       food protein-induced proctocolitis (K52.82)
     DEF: True immunoglobulin E (IgE)-mediated allergic reaction of the lining of the stomach, intestines, or colon to food proteins; causes nausea, vomiting, diarrhea, and abdominal cramping.

     K52.21   Food protein-induced enterocolitis syndrome
       Use additional code for hypovolemic shock, if present (R57.1)

     K52.22   Food protein-induced enteropathy

N Newborn: 0   P Pediatric: 0-17   M Maternity: 12-55   A Adult: 15-124   NRS Nonroutine supply Dx   NC Dx Noncancer Dx   PDx Primary Dx   ▶◀ Revised Text   ● New Code   ▲ Revised Title

684   ICD-10-CM 2018

K52.29 Other **allergic and dietetic gastroenteritis and colitis**
Food hypersensitivity gastroenteritis or colitis
Immediate gastrointestinal hypersensitivity

K52.3 **Indeterminate colitis**
Colonic inflammatory bowel disease unclassified (IBDU)
EXCLUDES 1 *unspecified colitis (K52.9)*

✓5th **K52.8** **Other specified noninfective gastroenteritis and colitis**

K52.81 **Eosinophilic gastritis or gastroenteritis**
Eosinophilic enteritis
EXCLUDES 2 *eosinophilic esophagitis (K20.0)*

K52.82 **Eosinophilic colitis**
Allergic proctocolitis
Food-induced eosinophilic proctocolitis
Food protein-induced proctocolitis
Milk protein-induced proctocolitis

✓6th **K52.83** **Microscopic colitis**
K52.831 Collagenous **colitis**
K52.832 Lymphocytic **colitis**
K52.838 Other **microscopic colitis**
K52.839 **Microscopic colitis, unspecified** ▽

K52.89 **Other specified noninfective gastroenteritis and colitis**

K52.9 **Noninfective gastroenteritis and colitis, unspecified** ▽
Colitis NOS
Enteritis NOS
Gastroenteritis NOS
Ileitis NOS
Jejunitis NOS
Sigmoiditis NOS
EXCLUDES 1 *diarrhea NOS (R19.7)*
functional diarrhea (K59.1)
infectious gastroenteritis and colitis NOS (A09)
neonatal diarrhea (noninfective) (P78.3)
psychogenic diarrhea (F45.8)

Other diseases of intestines (K55-K64)

✓4th **K55** **Vascular disorders of intestine**
EXCLUDES 1 *necrotizing enterocolitis of newborn (P77.-)*

✓5th **K55.0** Acute **vascular disorders of intestine**
Infarction of appendices epiploicae
Mesenteric (artery) (vein) embolism
Mesenteric (artery) (vein) infarction
Mesenteric (artery) (vein) thrombosis

✓6th **K55.01** **Acute (reversible) ischemia of small intestine**
K55.011 Focal (segmental) acute (reversible) **ischemia of small intestine**
K55.012 Diffuse **acute (reversible) ischemia of small intestine**
K55.019 **Acute (reversible) ischemia of small** ▽ **intestine, extent unspecified**

✓6th **K55.02** **Acute infarction of small intestine**
Gangrene of small intestine
Necrosis of small intestine
K55.021 Focal (segmental) acute infarction of small **intestine**
K55.022 Diffuse **acute infarction of small intestine**
K55.029 **Acute infarction of small intestine,** ▽ **extent unspecified**

✓6th **K55.03** **Acute (reversible) ischemia of large intestine**
Acute fulminant ischemic colitis
Subacute ischemic colitis
K55.031 Focal (segmental) acute (reversible) **ischemia of large intestine**
K55.032 Diffuse **acute (reversible) ischemia of large intestine**
K55.039 **Acute (reversible) ischemia of large** ▽ **intestine, extent unspecified**

✓6th **K55.04** **Acute infarction of large intestine**
Gangrene of large intestine
Necrosis of large intestine
K55.041 Focal (segmental) acute infarction of large **intestine**
K55.042 Diffuse **acute infarction of large intestine**
K55.049 **Acute infarction of large intestine,** ▽ **extent unspecified**

✓6th **K55.05** **Acute (reversible) ischemia of intestine, part unspecified**
K55.051 Focal (segmental) acute (reversible) **ischemia of intestine, part unspecified**
K55.052 Diffuse **acute (reversible) ischemia of intestine, part unspecified**
K55.059 **Acute (reversible) ischemia of** ▽ **intestine, part and extent unspecified**

✓6th **K55.06** **Acute infarction of intestine, part unspecified**
Acute intestinal infarction
Gangrene of intestine
Necrosis of intestine
K55.061 Focal (segmental) acute infarction of ▽ **intestine, part unspecified**
K55.062 Diffuse **acute infarction of intestine,** ▽ **part unspecified**
K55.069 **Acute infarction of intestine, part** ▽ **and extent unspecified**

K55.1 Chronic **vascular disorders of intestine**
Chronic ischemic colitis
Chronic ischemic enteritis
Chronic ischemic enterocolitis
Ischemic stricture of intestine
Mesenteric atherosclerosis
Mesenteric vascular insufficiency

✓5th **K55.2** Angiodysplasia **of colon**
K55.20 **Angiodysplasia of colon** without hemorrhage
K55.21 **Angiodysplasia of colon** with hemorrhage
DEF: Small vascular abnormalities due to fragile blood vessels in the colon; results in blood loss from the gastrointestinal (GI) tract.

✓5th **K55.3** **Necrotizing enterocolitis**
EXCLUDES 1 *necrotizing enterocolitis of newborn (P77.-)*
EXCLUDES 2 *necrotizing enterocolitis due to Clostridium difficile* ►*(A04.7-)*◄
K55.30 **Necrotizing enterocolitis,** unspecified ▽
Necrotizing enterocolitis, NOS
K55.31 Stage 1 **necrotizing enterocolitis**
Necrotizing enterocolitis without pneumatosis, without perforation
K55.32 Stage 2 **necrotizing enterocolitis**
Necrotizing enterocolitis with pneumatosis, without perforation
K55.33 Stage 3 **necrotizing enterocolitis**
Necrotizing enterocolitis with perforation
Necrotizing enterocolitis with pneumatosis and perforation

K55.8 **Other vascular disorders of intestine**
K55.9 **Vascular disorder of intestine, unspecified** ▽
Ischemic colitis
Ischemic enteritis
Ischemic enterocolitis

✓4th **K56** **Paralytic ileus and intestinal obstruction without hernia**
EXCLUDES 1 *congenital stricture or stenosis of intestine (Q41-Q42)*
cystic fibrosis with meconium ileus (E84.11)
intestinal obstruction with hernia (K40-K46)
ischemic stricture of intestine (K55.1)
meconium ileus NOS (P76.0)
neonatal intestinal obstructions classifiable to P76-
obstruction of duodenum (K31.5)
postprocedural intestinal obstruction ►*(K91.3-)*◄
stenosis of anus or rectum (K62.4)

K56.0 **Paralytic ileus**
Paralysis of bowel
Paralysis of colon
Paralysis of intestine
EXCLUDES 1 *gallstone ileus (K56.3)*
ileus NOS (K56.7)
obstructive ileus NOS ►*(K56.69-)*◄

K56.1 **Intussusception**
Intussusception or invagination of bowel
Intussusception or invagination of colon
Intussusception or invagination of intestine
Intussusception or invagination of rectum
EXCLUDES 2 *intussusception of appendix (K38.8)*
DEF: Intestinal obstruction due to prolapse of a bowel section into adjacent section; occurs primarily in children; symptoms include acute abdominal pain, vomiting, and passage of blood and mucus from rectum.

✓ Additional Character Req   ✓x7th Placeholder Alert   Case-Mix Diagnosis   Manifestation   ▽ Unspecified Dx   *EXCLUDES 1* Not coded here   *EXCLUDES 2* Not included here

ICD-10-CM 2018   **685**

Chapter 11. Diseases of the Digestive System

K56.2 Volvulus
Strangulation of colon or intestine
Torsion of colon or intestine
Twist of colon or intestine
EXCLUDES 2 volvulus of duodenum (K31.5)

K56.3 Gallstone ileus
Obstruction of intestine by gallstone

✓5th **K56.4 Other impaction of intestine**

K56.41 Fecal impaction
EXCLUDES 1 constipation (K59.0-)
incomplete defecation (R15.0)

K56.49 Other impaction of intestine

▲ ✓5th **K56.5 Intestinal adhesions [bands] with obstruction (postinfection)**
Abdominal hernia due to adhesions with obstruction
▶Peritoneal adhesions [bands] with intestinal obstruction (postinfection)◀
AHA: 2017, 2Q, 12

● **K56.50 Intestinal adhesions [bands], unspecified as to partial versus complete obstruction** ▽
Intestinal adhesions with obstruction NOS

● **K56.51 Intestinal adhesions [bands], with partial obstruction**
Intestinal adhesions with incomplete obstruction

● **K56.52 Intestinal adhesions [bands] with complete obstruction**

✓5th **K56.6 Other and unspecified intestinal obstruction**
AHA: 2017, 2Q, 12

✓6th **K56.60 Unspecified intestinal obstruction**
~~Intestinal obstruction NOS~~
EXCLUDES 1 intestinal obstruction due to specified condition—code to condition

● **K56.600 Partial intestinal obstruction, unspecified as to cause** ▽
Incomplete intestinal obstruction, NOS

● **K56.601 Complete intestinal obstruction, unspecified as to cause** ▽

● **K56.609 Unspecified intestinal obstruction, unspecified as to partial versus complete obstruction** ▽
Intestinal obstruction NOS

✓6th **K56.69 Other intestinal obstruction**
Enterostenosis NOS
Obstructive ileus NOS
Occlusion of colon or intestine NOS
Stenosis of colon or intestine NOS
Stricture of colon or intestine NOS
EXCLUDES 1 intestinal obstruction due to specified condition—code to condition

● **K56.690 Other partial intestinal obstruction**
Other incomplete intestinal obstruction

● **K56.691 Other complete intestinal obstruction**

● **K56.699 Other intestinal obstruction unspecified as to partial versus complete obstruction** ▽
Other intestinal obstruction, NEC

K56.7 Ileus, unspecified ▽
EXCLUDES 1 obstructive ileus ▶(K56.69-)◀
EXCLUDES 2 ▶intestinal obstruction with hernia (K40-K46)◀
AHA: 2017, 1Q, 40

✓4th **K57 Diverticular disease of intestine**
EXCLUDES 1 congenital diverticulum of intestine (Q43.8)
Meckel's diverticulum (Q43.0)
EXCLUDES 2 diverticulum of appendix (K38.2)

✓5th **K57.0 Diverticulitis of small intestine with perforation and abscess**
Diverticulitis of small intestine with peritonitis
EXCLUDES 1 diverticulitis of both small and large intestine with perforation and abscess (K57.4-)

K57.00 Diverticulitis of small intestine with perforation and abscess without bleeding

K57.01 Diverticulitis of small intestine with perforation and abscess with bleeding

Volvulus

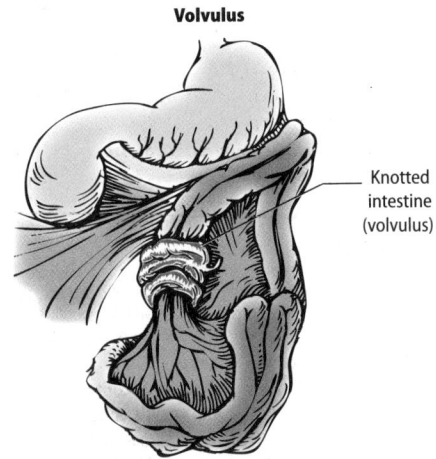

Knotted intestine (volvulus)

✓5th **K57.1 Diverticular disease of small intestine without perforation or abscess**
EXCLUDES 1 diverticular disease of both small and large intestine without perforation or abscess (K57.5-)

K57.10 Diverticulosis of small intestine without perforation or abscess without bleeding
Diverticular disease of small intestine NOS

K57.11 Diverticulosis of small intestine without perforation or abscess with bleeding

K57.12 Diverticulitis of small intestine without perforation or abscess without bleeding

K57.13 Diverticulitis of small intestine without perforation or abscess with bleeding

✓5th **K57.2 Diverticulitis of large intestine with perforation and abscess**
Diverticulitis of colon with peritonitis
EXCLUDES 1 diverticulitis of both small and large intestine with perforation and abscess (K57.4-)

K57.20 Diverticulitis of large intestine with perforation and abscess without bleeding

K57.21 Diverticulitis of large intestine with perforation and abscess with bleeding

✓5th **K57.3 Diverticular disease of large intestine without perforation or abscess**
EXCLUDES 1 diverticular disease of both small and large intestine without perforation or abscess (K57.5-)

K57.30 Diverticulosis of large intestine without perforation or abscess without bleeding
Diverticular disease of colon NOS

K57.31 Diverticulosis of large intestine without perforation or abscess with bleeding

K57.32 Diverticulitis of large intestine without perforation or abscess without bleeding

K57.33 Diverticulitis of large intestine without perforation or abscess with bleeding

✓5th **K57.4 Diverticulitis of both small and large intestine with perforation and abscess**
Diverticulitis of both small and large intestine with peritonitis

K57.40 Diverticulitis of both small and large intestine with perforation and abscess without bleeding

K57.41 Diverticulitis of both small and large intestine with perforation and abscess with bleeding

✓5th **K57.5 Diverticular disease of both small and large intestine without perforation or abscess**

K57.50 Diverticulosis of both small and large intestine without perforation or abscess without bleeding
Diverticular disease of both small and large intestine NOS

K57.51 Diverticulosis of both small and large intestine without perforation or abscess with bleeding

K57.52 Diverticulitis of both small and large intestine without perforation or abscess without bleeding

K57.53 Diverticulitis of both small and large intestine without perforation or abscess with bleeding

✓5th **K57.8 Diverticulitis of intestine, part unspecified, with perforation and abscess**
Diverticulitis of intestine NOS with peritonitis

K57.80 Diverticulitis of intestine, part unspecified, with perforation and abscess without bleeding ▽

N Newborn: 0   P Pediatric: 0-17   M Maternity: 12-55   A Adult: 15-124   NRS Nonroutine supply Dx   NC Dx Noncancer Dx   PDx Primary Dx   ▶◀ Revised Text   ● New Code   ▲ Revised Title

686   ICD-10-CM 2018

K57.81 Diverticulitis of intestine, part unspecified, with perforation and abscess with bleeding ▽

✓5ᵗʰ **K57.9** Diverticular disease of intestine, part unspecified, without perforation or abscess

K57.90 Diverticulosis of intestine, part unspecified, without perforation or abscess without bleeding ▽
Diverticular disease of intestine NOS

K57.91 Diverticulosis of intestine, part unspecified, without perforation or abscess with bleeding ▽

K57.92 Diverticulitis of intestine, part unspecified, without perforation or abscess without bleeding ▽

K57.93 Diverticulitis of intestine, part unspecified, without perforation or abscess with bleeding ▽

✓4ᵗʰ **K58** Irritable bowel syndrome
INCLUDES irritable colon
spastic colon

K58.0 Irritable bowel syndrome with diarrhea
K58.1 Irritable bowel syndrome with constipation
K58.2 Mixed irritable bowel syndrome
K58.8 Other irritable bowel syndrome
K58.9 Irritable bowel syndrome without diarrhea
Irritable bowel syndrome NOS

✓4ᵗʰ **K59** Other functional intestinal disorders
EXCLUDES1 change in bowel habit NOS (R19.4)
intestinal malabsorption (K90.-)
psychogenic intestinal disorders (F45.8)
EXCLUDES2 functional disorders of stomach (K31.-)

✓5ᵗʰ **K59.0** Constipation
Use additional code for adverse effect, if applicable, to identify drug (T36-T50 with fifth or sixth character 5)
EXCLUDES1 fecal impaction (K56.41)
incomplete defecation (R15.0)

K59.00 Constipation, unspecified ▽
K59.01 Slow transit constipation
DEF: Delay in the transit of fecal material through the colon secondary to smooth muscle dysfunction or decreased peristaltic contractions along the colon: also called colonic inertia or delayed transit.

K59.02 Outlet dysfunction constipation
K59.03 Drug induced constipation
Use additional code for adverse effect, if applicable, to identify drug (T36-T50 with fifth or sixth character 5)

K59.04 Chronic idiopathic constipation
Functional constipation

K59.09 Other constipation
Chronic constipation

K59.1 Functional diarrhea
EXCLUDES1 diarrhea NOS (R19.7)
irritable bowel syndrome with diarrhea (K58.0)

K59.2 Neurogenic bowel, not elsewhere classified
DEF: Disorder of bowel due to spinal cord lesion due to injury or as a complication of conditions such as multiple sclerosis (MS) or spina bifida; loss of bowel control is the primary symptom, manifested as constipation or bowel incontinence.

✓5ᵗʰ **K59.3** Megacolon, not elsewhere classified
Dilatation of colon
Code first, if applicable (T51-T65) to identify toxic agent
EXCLUDES1 congenital megacolon (aganglionic) (Q43.1)
megacolon (due to) (in) Chagas' disease (B57.32)
megacolon (due to) (in) Clostridium difficile
▶(A04.7-)◀
megacolon (due to) (in) Hirschsprung's disease (Q43.1)

K59.31 Toxic megacolon
K59.39 Other megacolon
Megacolon NOS

K59.4 Anal spasm
Proctalgia fugax

K59.8 Other specified functional intestinal disorders
Atony of colon
Pseudo-obstruction (acute) (chronic) of intestine

K59.9 Functional intestinal disorder, unspecified ▽

✓4ᵗʰ **K60** Fissure and fistula of anal and rectal regions
EXCLUDES1 fissure and fistula of anal and rectal regions with abscess or cellulitis (K61.-)
EXCLUDES2 anal sphincter tear (healed) (nontraumatic) (old) (K62.81)

K60.0 Acute anal fissure NRS

K60.1 Chronic anal fissure NRS
K60.2 Anal fissure, unspecified NRS ▽
K60.3 Anal fistula NRS
K60.4 Rectal fistula NRS
Fistula of rectum to skin
EXCLUDES1 rectovaginal fistula (N82.3)
vesicorectal fistual (N32.1)
K60.5 Anorectal fistula NRS

✓4ᵗʰ **K61** Abscess of anal and rectal regions
INCLUDES abscess of anal and rectal regions
cellulitis of anal and rectal regions

K61.0 Anal abscess NRS
Perianal abscess
EXCLUDES1 intrasphincteric abscess (K61.4)

K61.1 Rectal abscess NRS
Perirectal abscess
EXCLUDES1 ischiorectal abscess (K61.3)
AHA: 2012, 4Q, 104

K61.2 Anorectal abscess NRS
K61.3 Ischiorectal abscess NRS
Abscess of ischiorectal fossa
K61.4 Intrasphincteric abscess NRS

✓4ᵗʰ **K62** Other diseases of anus and rectum
INCLUDES anal canal
EXCLUDES2 colostomy and enterostomy malfunction (K94.0-, K94.1-)
fecal incontinence (R15.-)
hemorrhoids (K64.-)

K62.0 Anal polyp
K62.1 Rectal polyp
EXCLUDES1 adenomatous polyp (D12.8)

K62.2 Anal prolapse
Prolapse of anal canal

K62.3 Rectal prolapse
Prolapse of rectal mucosa

K62.4 Stenosis of anus and rectum
Stricture of anus (sphincter)

K62.5 Hemorrhage of anus and rectum
EXCLUDES1 gastrointestinal bleeding NOS (K92.2)
melena (K92.1)
neonatal rectal hemorrhage (P54.2)

K62.6 Ulcer of anus and rectum
Solitary ulcer of anus and rectum
Stercoral ulcer of anus and rectum
EXCLUDES1 fissure and fistula of anus and rectum (K60.-)
ulcerative colitis (K51.-)

K62.7 Radiation proctitis
Use additional code to identify the type of radiation (W90.-)

✓5ᵗʰ **K62.8** Other specified diseases of anus and rectum
EXCLUDES2 ulcerative proctitis (K51.2)

K62.81 Anal sphincter tear (healed) (nontraumatic) (old)
Tear of anus, nontraumatic
Use additional code for any associated fecal incontinence (R15.-)
EXCLUDES2 anal fissure (K60.-)
anal sphincter tear (healed) (old) complicating delivery (O34.7-)
traumatic tear of anal sphincter (S31.831)

K62.82 Dysplasia of anus
Anal intraepithelial neoplasia I and II (AIN I and II) (histologically confirmed)
Dysplasia of anus NOS
Mild and moderate dysplasia of anus (histologically confirmed)
EXCLUDES1 abnormal results from anal cytologic examination without histologic confirmation (R85.61-)
anal intraepithelial neoplasia III (D01.3)
carcinoma in situ of anus (D01.3)
HGSIL of anus (R85.613)
severe dysplasia of anus (D01.3)

K62.89 Other specified diseases of anus and rectum
Proctitis NOS
Use additional code for any associated fecal incontinence (R15.-)

K62.9 Disease of anus and rectum, unspecified ▽

✓ Additional Character Req   ✓x7ᵗʰ Placeholder Alert   Case-Mix Diagnosis   Manifestation   ▽ Unspecified Dx   EXCLUDES1 Not coded here   EXCLUDES2 Not included here

Chapter 11. Diseases of the Digestive System *(side tab)*

☑4ᵗʰ **K63 Other diseases of intestine**

K63.0 Abscess of intestine
     EXCLUDES 1   abscess of intestine with Crohn's disease (K50.014, K50.114, K50.814, K50.914)
            abscess of intestine with diverticular disease (K57.0, K57.2, K57.4, K57.8)
            abscess of intestine with ulcerative colitis (K51.014, K51.214, K51.314, K51.414, K51.514, K51.814, K51.914)
     EXCLUDES 2   abscess of anal and rectal regions (K61.-)
            abscess of appendix (K35.3)

K63.1 Perforation of intestine (nontraumatic)
     Perforation (nontraumatic) of rectum
     EXCLUDES 1   perforation (nontraumatic) of duodenum (K26.-)
            perforation (nontraumatic) of intestine with diverticular disease (K57.0, K57.2, K57.4, K57.8)
     EXCLUDES 2   perforation (nontraumatic) of appendix (K35.2, K35.3)

K63.2 Fistula of intestine
     EXCLUDES 1   fistula of duodenum (K31.6)
            fistula of intestine with Crohn's disease (K50.013, K50.113, K50.813, K50.913)
            fistula of intestine with ulcerative colitis (K51.013, K51.213, K51.313, K51.413, K51.513, K51.813, K51.913)
     EXCLUDES 2   fistula of anal and rectal regions (K60.-)
            fistula of appendix (K38.3)
            intestinal-genital fistula, female (N82.2-N82.4)
            vesicointestinal fistula (N32.1)

K63.3 Ulcer of intestine
     Primary ulcer of small intestine
     EXCLUDES 1   duodenal ulcer (K26.-)
            gastrointestinal ulcer (K28.-)
            gastrojejunal ulcer (K28.-)
            jejunal ulcer (K28.-)
            peptic ulcer, site unspecified (K27.-)
            ulcer of intestine with perforation (K63.1)
            ulcer of anus or rectum (K62.6)
            ulcerative colitis (K51.-)

K63.4 Enteroptosis

K63.5 Polyp of colon
     EXCLUDES 1   adenomatous polyp of colon (D12.6)
            inflammatory polyp of colon (K51.4-)
            polyposis of colon (D12.6)
     AHA: 2017, 1Q, 15; 2015, 2Q, 14

☑5ᵗʰ **K63.8 Other specified diseases of intestine**

     K63.81 Dieulafoy lesion of intestine
         EXCLUDES 2   Dieulafoy lesion of stomach and duodenum (K31.82)

     K63.89 Other specified diseases of intestine
         AHA: 2013, 2Q, 31

K63.9 Disease of intestine, unspecified   ▽

☑4ᵗʰ **K64 Hemorrhoids and perianal venous thrombosis**
     INCLUDES piles
     EXCLUDES 1   hemorrhoids complicating childbirth and the puerperium (O87.2)
            hemorrhoids complicating pregnancy (O22.4)

K64.0 First degree hemorrhoids
     Grade/stage I hemorrhoids
     Hemorrhoids (bleeding) without prolapse outside of anal canal

K64.1 Second degree hemorrhoids
     Grade/stage II hemorrhoids
     Hemorrhoids (bleeding) that prolapse with straining, but retract spontaneously

K64.2 Third degree hemorrhoids
     Grade/stage III hemorrhoids
     Hemorrhoids (bleeding) that prolapse with straining and require manual replacement back inside anal canal

K64.3 Fourth degree hemorrhoids
     Grade/stage IV hemorrhoids
     Hemorrhoids (bleeding) with prolapsed tissue that cannot be manually replaced

K64.4 Residual hemorrhoidal skin tags
     External hemorrhoids, NOS
     Skin tags of anus

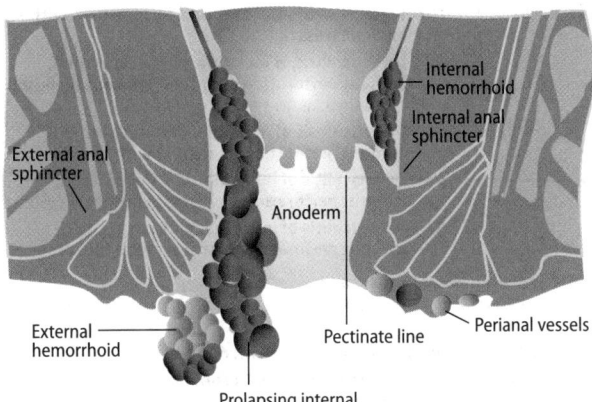

Hemorrhoids

Internal hemorrhoid
Internal anal sphincter
External anal sphincter
Anoderm
External hemorrhoid
Pectinate line
Perianal vessels
Prolapsing internal hemorrhoid

K64.5 Perianal venous thrombosis
     External hemorrhoids with thrombosis
     Perianal hematoma
     Thrombosed hemorrhoids NOS

K64.8 Other hemorrhoids
     Internal hemorrhoids, without mention of degree
     Prolapsed hemorrhoids, degree not specified

K64.9 Unspecified hemorrhoids   ▽
     Hemorrhoids (bleeding) NOS
     Hemorrhoids (bleeding) without mention of degree

Diseases of peritoneum and retroperitoneum (K65-K68)

☑4ᵗʰ **K65 Peritonitis**
     Use additional code (B95-B97), to identify infectious agent
     EXCLUDES 1   acute appendicitis with generalized peritonitis (K35.2)
            aseptic peritonitis (T81.6)
            benign paroxysmal peritonitis (E85.0)
            chemical peritonitis (T81.6)
            diverticulitis of both small and large intestine with peritonitis (K57.4-)
            diverticulitis of colon with peritonitis (K57.2-)
            diverticulitis of intestine, NOS, with peritonitis (K57.8-)
            diverticulitis of small intestine with peritonitis (K57.0-)
            gonococcal peritonitis (A54.85)
            neonatal peritonitis (P78.0-P78.1)
            pelvic peritonitis, female (N73.3-N73.5)
            periodic familial peritonitis (E85.0)
            peritonitis due to talc or other foreign substance (T81.6)
            peritonitis in chlamydia (A74.81)
            peritonitis in diphtheria (A36.89)
            peritonitis in syphilis (late) (A52.74)
            peritonitis in tuberculosis (A18.31)
            peritonitis with or following abortion or ectopic or molar pregnancy (O00-O07, O08.0)
            peritonitis with or following appendicitis (K35.-)
            peritonitis with or following diverticular disease of intestine (K57.-)
            puerperal peritonitis (O85)
            retroperitoneal infections (K68.-)

K65.0 Generalized (acute) peritonitis
     Pelvic peritonitis (acute), male
     Subphrenic peritonitis (acute)
     Suppurative peritonitis (acute)

K65.1 Peritoneal abscess
     Abdominopelvic abscess   Subdiaphragmatic abscess
     Abscess (of) omentum   Subhepatic abscess
     Abscess (of) peritoneum   Subphrenic abscess
     Mesenteric abscess
     Retrocecal abscess

K65.2 Spontaneous bacterial peritonitis
     EXCLUDES 1   bacterial peritonitis NOS (K65.9)

K65.3 Choleperitonitis
     Peritonitis due to bile
     DEF: Inflammation of the peritoneum due to leakage of bile into the peritoneal cavity resulting from rupture of the bile passages or gallbladder.

Ⓝ Newborn: 0   Ⓟ Pediatric: 0-17   Ⓜ Maternity: 12-55   Ⓐ Adult: 15-124   **NRS** Nonroutine supply Dx   **NC Dx** Noncancer Dx   **PD Dx** Primary Dx   ▶◀ Revised Text   ● New Code   ▲ Revised Title

688   ICD-10-CM 2018

K63–K65.3 *(side tab)*

K65.4 ~~Sclerosing mesenteritis~~
    Fat necrosis of peritoneum
    (Idiopathic) sclerosing mesenteric fibrosis
    Mesenteric lipodystrophy
    Mesenteric panniculitis
    Retractile mesenteritis

K65.8 **Other peritonitis**
    Chronic proliferative peritonitis
    Peritonitis due to urine

K65.9 **Peritonitis, unspecified** ▽
    Bacterial peritonitis NOS
    AHA: 2013, 2Q, 31

√4ᵗʰ **K66** **Other disorders of peritoneum**
    EXCLUDES 2   ascites (R18.-)
                  peritoneal effusion (chronic) (R18.8)

    K66.0 **Peritoneal adhesions (postprocedural) (postinfection)**
        Adhesions (of) abdominal (wall)   Adhesions (of) omentum
        Adhesions (of) diaphragm   Adhesions (of) stomach
        Adhesions (of) intestine   Adhesive bands
        Adhesions (of) male pelvis   Mesenteric adhesions
        EXCLUDES 1   female pelvic adhesions [bands] (N73.6)
                    peritoneal adhesions with intestinal obstruction
                   ▶(K56.5-)◀

    K66.1 **Hemoperitoneum**
        EXCLUDES 1   traumatic hemoperitoneum (S36.8-)

    K66.8 **Other specified disorders of peritoneum**

    K66.9 **Disorder of peritoneum, unspecified** ▽

K67 *Disorders of peritoneum in infectious diseases classified elsewhere*
    Code first underlying disease, such as:
        congenital syphilis (A50.0)
        helminthiasis (B65.0-B83.9)
    EXCLUDES 1   peritonitis in chlamydia (A74.81)
                peritonitis in diphtheria (A36.89)
                peritonitis in gonococcal (A54.85)
                peritonitis in syphilis (late) (A52.74)
                peritonitis in tuberculosis (A18.31)

√4ᵗʰ **K68** **Disorders of retroperitoneum**
    √5ᵗʰ **K68.1** **Retroperitoneal abscess**
        K68.11 ~~Postprocedural~~ **retroperitoneal abscess** NRS
        K68.12 ~~Psoas muscle~~ **abscess**
        K68.19 **Other retroperitoneal abscess**
    K68.9 **Other disorders of retroperitoneum**

Diseases of liver (K70-K77)

EXCLUDES 1   jaundice NOS (R17)
EXCLUDES 2   hemochromatosis (E83.11-)
            Reye's syndrome (G93.7)
            viral hepatitis (B15-B19)
            Wilson's disease (E83.0)

√4ᵗʰ **K70** **Alcoholic liver disease**
    Use additional code to identify:
        alcohol abuse and dependence (F10.-)

    K70.0 **Alcoholic** ~~fatty liver~~   A

    √5ᵗʰ **K70.1** **Alcoholic** ~~hepatitis~~
        K70.10 **Alcoholic hepatitis** ~~without ascites~~   A
        K70.11 **Alcoholic hepatitis** ~~with ascites~~   A

    K70.2 **Alcoholic** ~~fibrosis and sclerosis~~ **of liver**   NC Dx A

    √5ᵗʰ **K70.3** **Alcoholic** ~~cirrhosis~~ **of liver**
        Alcoholic cirrhosis NOS
        K70.30 **Alcoholic cirrhosis of liver** ~~without ascites~~   NC Dx A
        K70.31 **Alcoholic cirrhosis of liver** ~~with ascites~~   NC Dx A

    √5ᵗʰ **K70.4** **Alcoholic** ~~hepatic failure~~
        Acute alcoholic hepatic failure
        Alcoholic hepatic failure NOS
        Chronic alcoholic hepatic failure
        Subacute alcoholic hepatic failure
        K70.40 **Alcoholic hepatic failure** ~~without coma~~   NC Dx A
        K70.41 **Alcoholic hepatic failure** ~~with coma~~   NC Dx A

    K70.9 **Alcoholic liver disease, unspecified**   A ▽

√4ᵗʰ **K71** **Toxic liver disease**
    INCLUDES   drug-induced idiosyncratic (unpredictable) liver disease
                  drug-induced toxic (predictable) liver disease
    Code first poisoning due to drug or toxin, if applicable (T36-T65 with fifth or sixth character 1-4 or 6)
    Use additional code for adverse effect, if applicable, to identify drug (T36-T50 with fifth or sixth character 5)
    EXCLUDES 2   alcoholic liver disease (K70.-)
                Budd-Chiari syndrome (I82.0)

    K71.0 **Toxic liver disease with** ~~cholestasis~~   NC Dx
        Cholestasis with hepatocyte injury
        "Pure" cholestasis

    √5ᵗʰ **K71.1** **Toxic liver disease with** ~~hepatic necrosis~~
        Hepatic failure (acute) (chronic) due to drugs
        K71.10 **Toxic liver disease with hepatic necrosis,** ~~without coma~~   NC Dx
        K71.11 **Toxic liver disease with hepatic necrosis,** ~~with coma~~   NC Dx

    K71.2 **Toxic liver disease with** ~~acute hepatitis~~   NC Dx
    K71.3 **Toxic liver disease with** ~~chronic persistent hepatitis~~   NC Dx
    K71.4 **Toxic liver disease with** ~~chronic lobular hepatitis~~   NC Dx

    √5ᵗʰ **K71.5** **Toxic liver disease with** ~~chronic active hepatitis~~
        Toxic liver disease with lupoid hepatitis
        K71.50 **Toxic liver disease with chronic active hepatitis** ~~without ascites~~   NC Dx
        K71.51 **Toxic liver disease with chronic active hepatitis** ~~with ascites~~   NC Dx

    K71.6 **Toxic liver disease with** ~~hepatitis, not elsewhere~~ **classified**   NC Dx
    K71.7 **Toxic liver disease with** ~~fibrosis and cirrhosis~~ **of liver**   NC Dx
    K71.8 **Toxic liver disease with other disorders of liver**   NC Dx
        Toxic liver disease with focal nodular hyperplasia
        Toxic liver disease with hepatic granulomas
        Toxic liver disease with peliosis hepatis
        Toxic liver disease with veno-occlusive disease of liver

    K71.9 **Toxic liver disease, unspecified**   NC Dx ▽

√4ᵗʰ **K72** **Hepatic failure, not elsewhere classified**
    INCLUDES   fulminant hepatitis NEC, with hepatic failure
                  hepatic encephalopathy NOS
                  liver (cell) necrosis with hepatic failure
                  malignant hepatitis NEC, with hepatic failure
                  yellow liver atrophy or dystrophy
    EXCLUDES 1   alcoholic hepatic failure (K70.4)
                hepatic failure with toxic liver disease (K71.1-)
                icterus of newborn (P55-P59)
                postprocedural hepatic failure (K91.82)
    EXCLUDES 2   hepatic failure complicating abortion or ectopic or molar pregnancy (O00-O07, O08.8)
                hepatic failure complicating pregnancy, childbirth and the puerperium (O26.6-)
                viral hepatitis with hepatic coma (B15-B19)
    AHA: 2017, 1Q, 41

    √5ᵗʰ **K72.0** ~~Acute and subacute~~ **hepatic failure**
        Acute non-viral hepatitis NOS
        AHA: 2015, 2Q, 17; 2014, 2Q, 13
        K72.00 **Acute and subacute hepatic failure** ~~without coma~~   NC Dx
        K72.01 **Acute and subacute hepatic failure** ~~with coma~~   NC Dx

    √5ᵗʰ **K72.1** ~~Chronic~~ **hepatic failure**
        K72.10 **Chronic hepatic failure** ~~without coma~~   NC Dx
        K72.11 **Chronic hepatic failure** ~~with coma~~   NC Dx

    √5ᵗʰ **K72.9** **Hepatic failure,** ~~unspecified~~
        K72.90 **Hepatic failure, unspecified** ~~without coma~~   NC Dx ▽
            AHA: 2016, 2Q, 35
        K72.91 **Hepatic failure, unspecified** ~~with coma~~   NC Dx ▽
            Hepatic coma NOS

√4ᵗʰ **K73** **Chronic hepatitis, not elsewhere classified**
    EXCLUDES 1   alcoholic hepatitis (chronic) (K70.1-)
                drug-induced hepatitis (chronic) (K71.-)
                granulomatous hepatitis (chronic) NEC (K75.3)
                reactive, nonspecific hepatitis (chronic) (K75.2)
                viral hepatitis (chronic) (B15-B19)

    K73.0 **Chronic** ~~persistent~~ **hepatitis, not elsewhere classified**   NC Dx
    K73.1 **Chronic** ~~lobular~~ **hepatitis, not elsewhere classified**   NC Dx
    K73.2 **Chronic** ~~active~~ **hepatitis, not elsewhere classified**   NC Dx
    K73.8 **Other chronic hepatitis, not elsewhere classified**   NC Dx
    K73.9 **Chronic hepatitis, unspecified**   NC Dx ▽

✔ Additional Character Req   √7ᵗʰ Placeholder Alert   Case-Mix Diagnosis   Manifestation   ▽ Unspecified Dx   *EXCLUDES 1* Not coded here   *EXCLUDES 2* Not included here

ICD-10-CM 2018   **689**

Chapter 11. Diseases of the Digestive System

☑4ᵗʰ **K74 Fibrosis and cirrhosis of liver**
Code also, if applicable, viral hepatitis (acute) (chronic) (B15-B19)
> EXCLUDES 1   *alcoholic cirrhosis (of liver) (K70.3)*
> *alcoholic fibrosis of liver (K70.2)*
> *cardiac sclerosis of liver (K76.1)*
> *cirrhosis (of liver) with toxic liver disease (K71.7)*
> *congenital cirrhosis (of liver) (P78.81)*
> *pigmentary cirrhosis (of liver) (E83.110)*

K74.0 Hepatic fibrosis   NC Dx
K74.1 Hepatic sclerosis   NC Dx
K74.2 Hepatic fibrosis with hepatic sclerosis   NC Dx
K74.3 Primary biliary cirrhosis   NC Dx
Chronic nonsuppurative destructive cholangitis
K74.4 Secondary biliary cirrhosis   NC Dx
K74.5 Biliary cirrhosis, unspecified   NC Dx ▽

☑5ᵗʰ **K74.6 Other and unspecified cirrhosis of liver**
    K74.60 Unspecified cirrhosis of liver   NC Dx ▽
       Cirrhosis (of liver) NOS
    K74.69 Other cirrhosis of liver   NC Dx
       Cryptogenic cirrhosis (of liver)
       Macronodular cirrhosis (of liver)
       Micronodular cirrhosis (of liver)
       Mixed type cirrhosis (of liver)
       Portal cirrhosis (of liver)
       Postnecrotic cirrhosis (of liver)

☑4ᵗʰ **K75 Other inflammatory liver diseases**
> EXCLUDES 2   *toxic liver disease (K71.-)*

K75.0 Abscess of liver
Cholangitic hepatic abscess
Hematogenic hepatic abscess
Hepatic abscess NOS
Lymphogenic hepatic abscess
Pylephlebitic hepatic abscess
> EXCLUDES 1   *amebic liver abscess (A06.4)*
> *cholangitis without liver abscess (K83.0)*
> *pylephlebitis without liver abscess (K75.1)*
> EXCLUDES 2   *acute or subacute hepatitis NOS (B17.9)*
> *acute or subacute non-viral hepatitis (K72.0)*
> *chronic hepatitis NEC (K73.8)*

K75.1 Phlebitis of portal vein
Pylephlebitis
> EXCLUDES 1   *pylephlebitic liver abscess (K75.0)*
> **DEF:** Inflammation of portal vein or branches; may be due to diverticulitis, perforated appendicitis, or peritonitis; symptoms include fever, chills, jaundice, sweating, and abscess in various body parts.

K75.2 Nonspecific reactive hepatitis   NC Dx
> EXCLUDES 1   *acute or subacute hepatitis (K72.0-)*
> *chronic hepatitis NEC (K73.-)*
> *viral hepatitis (B15-B19)*

K75.3 Granulomatous hepatitis, not elsewhere classified   NC Dx
> EXCLUDES 1   *acute or subacute hepatitis (K72.0-)*
> *chronic hepatitis NEC (K73.-)*
> *viral hepatitis (B15-B19)*

K75.4 Autoimmune hepatitis   NC Dx
Lupoid hepatitis NEC

☑5ᵗʰ **K75.8 Other specified inflammatory liver diseases**
    K75.81 Nonalcoholic steatohepatitis (NASH)   NC Dx
    K75.89 Other specified inflammatory liver diseases   NC Dx

K75.9 Inflammatory liver disease, unspecified   NC Dx ▽
Hepatitis NOS
> EXCLUDES 1   *acute or subacute hepatitis (K72.0-)*
> *chronic hepatitis NEC (K73.-)*
> *viral hepatitis (B15-B19)*
> **AHA:** 2015, 2Q, 17

☑4ᵗʰ **K76 Other diseases of liver**
> EXCLUDES 2   *alcoholic liver disease (K70.-)*
> *amyloid degeneration of liver (E85.-)*
> *cystic disease of liver (congenital) (Q44.6)*
> *hepatic vein thrombosis (I82.0)*
> *hepatomegaly NOS (R16.0)*
> *pigmentary cirrhosis (of liver) (E83.110)*
> *portal vein thrombosis (I81)*
> *toxic liver disease (K71.-)*

K76.0 Fatty (change of) liver, not elsewhere classified
Nonalcoholic fatty liver disease (NAFLD)
> EXCLUDES 1   *nonalcoholic steatohepatitis (NASH) (K75.81)*

K76.1 Chronic passive congestion of liver
Cardiac cirrhosis
Cardiac sclerosis

K76.2 Central hemorrhagic necrosis of liver
> EXCLUDES 1   *liver necrosis with hepatic failure (K72.-)*

K76.3 Infarction of liver

K76.4 Peliosis hepatis   NC Dx
Hepatic angiomatosis

K76.5 Hepatic veno-occlusive disease
> EXCLUDES 1   *Budd-Chiari syndrome (I82.0)*

K76.6 Portal hypertension
Use additional code for any associated complications, such as:
   portal hypertensive gastropathy (K31.89)

K76.7 Hepatorenal syndrome   NC Dx
> EXCLUDES 1   *hepatorenal syndrome following labor and delivery (O90.4)*
> *postprocedural hepatorenal syndrome (K91.83)*

☑5ᵗʰ **K76.8 Other specified diseases of liver**
    K76.81 Hepatopulmonary syndrome
       Code first underlying liver disease, such as:
       alcoholic cirrhosis of liver (K70.3-)
       cirrhosis of liver without mention of alcohol (K74.6-)
    K76.89 Other specified diseases of liver
       Cyst (simple) of liver
       Focal nodular hyperplasia of liver
       Hepatoptosis

K76.9 Liver disease, unspecified   ▽

K77 Liver disorders in diseases classified elsewhere
Code first underlying disease, such as:
   amyloidosis (E85.-)
   congenital syphilis (A50.0, A50.5)
   congenital toxoplasmosis (P37.1)
   schistosomiasis (B65.0-B65.9)
> EXCLUDES 1   *alcoholic hepatitis (K70.1-)*
> *alcoholic liver disease (K70-.)*
> *cytomegaloviral hepatitis (B25.1)*
> *herpesviral [herpes simplex] hepatitis (B00.81)*
> *infectious mononucleosis with liver disease (B27.0-B27.9 with .9)*
> *mumps hepatitis (B26.81)*
> *sarcoidosis with liver disease (D86.89)*
> *secondary syphilis with liver disease (A51.45)*
> *syphilis (late) with liver disease (A52.74)*
> *toxoplasmosis (acquired) hepatitis (B58.1)*
> *tuberculosis with liver disease (A18.83)*

Disorders of gallbladder, biliary tract and pancreas (K80-K87)

☑4ᵗʰ **K80 Cholelithiasis**
> EXCLUDES 1   *retained cholelithiasis following cholecystectomy (K91.86)*

☑5ᵗʰ **K80.0 Calculus of gallbladder with acute cholecystitis**
Any condition listed in K80.2 with acute cholecystitis
    K80.00 Calculus of gallbladder with acute cholecystitis without obstruction
    K80.01 Calculus of gallbladder with acute cholecystitis with obstruction

☑5ᵗʰ **K80.1 Calculus of gallbladder with other cholecystitis**
    K80.10 Calculus of gallbladder with chronic cholecystitis without obstruction
       Cholelithiasis with cholecystitis NOS
    K80.11 Calculus of gallbladder with chronic cholecystitis with obstruction
    K80.12 Calculus of gallbladder with acute and chronic cholecystitis without obstruction
    K80.13 Calculus of gallbladder with acute and chronic cholecystitis with obstruction
    K80.18 Calculus of gallbladder with other cholecystitis without obstruction
    K80.19 Calculus of gallbladder with other cholecystitis with obstruction

☑5ᵗʰ **K80.2 Calculus of gallbladder without cholecystitis**
Cholecystolithiasis without cholecystitis
Cholelithiasis (without cholecystitis)
Colic (recurrent) of gallbladder (without cholecystitis)
Gallstone (impacted) of cystic duct (without cholecystitis)
Gallstone (impacted) of gallbladder (without cholecystitis)
    K80.20 Calculus of gallbladder without cholecystitis without obstruction

Ⓝ Newborn: 0   Ⓟ Pediatric: 0-17   Ⓜ Maternity: 12-55   Ⓐ Adult: 15-124   NRS Nonroutine supply Dx   NC Dx Noncancer Dx   PDx Primary Dx   ▶◀ Revised Text   ● New Code   ▲ Revised Title

690   ICD-10-CM 2018

K74–K80.20

Chapter 11. Diseases of the Digestive System

Cholelithiasis

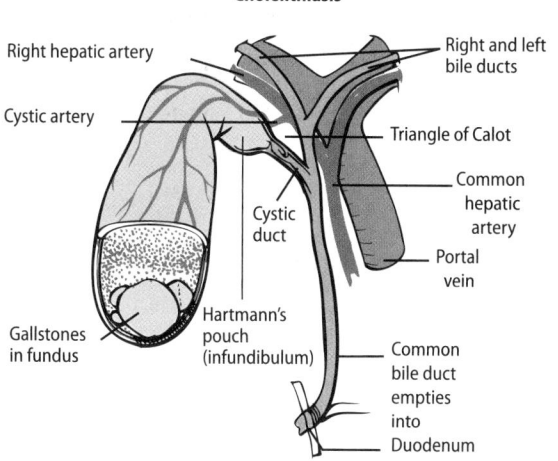

Right hepatic artery

Cystic artery

Right and left bile ducts

Triangle of Calot

Common hepatic artery

Portal vein

Cystic duct

Gallstones in fundus

Hartmann's pouch (infundibulum)

Common bile duct empties into Duodenum

K80.21   Calculus of gallbladder without cholecystitis with obstruction

✓5th **K80.3   Calculus of** bile duct with cholangitis
Any condition listed in K80.5 with cholangitis

K80.30   Calculus of bile duct with cholangitis, unspecified, without obstruction ▽

K80.31   Calculus of bile duct with cholangitis, unspecified, with obstruction ▽

K80.32   Calculus of bile duct with acute **cholangitis** without obstruction

K80.33   Calculus of bile duct with acute **cholangitis** with obstruction

K80.34   Calculus of bile duct with chronic **cholangitis** without obstruction

K80.35   Calculus of bile duct with chronic **cholangitis** with obstruction

K80.36   Calculus of bile duct with acute and chronic cholangitis without obstruction

K80.37   Calculus of bile duct with acute and chronic cholangitis with obstruction

✓5th **K80.4   Calculus of** bile duct with cholecystitis
Any condition listed in K80.5 with cholecystitis (with cholangitis)

K80.40   Calculus of bile duct with cholecystitis, unspecified, without obstruction ▽

K80.41   Calculus of bile duct with cholecystitis, unspecified, with obstruction ▽

K80.42   Calculus of bile duct with acute **cholecystitis** without obstruction

K80.43   Calculus of bile duct with acute **cholecystitis** with obstruction

K80.44   Calculus of bile duct with chronic **cholecystitis** without obstruction

K80.45   Calculus of bile duct with chronic **cholecystitis** with obstruction

K80.46   Calculus of bile duct with acute and chronic **cholecystitis** without obstruction

K80.47   Calculus of bile duct with acute and chronic **cholecystitis** with obstruction

✓5th **K80.5   Calculus of** bile duct without cholangitis or cholecystitis
Choledocholithiasis (without cholangitis or cholecystitis)
Gallstone (impacted) of bile duct NOS (without cholangitis or cholecystitis)
Gallstone (impacted) of common duct (without cholangitis or cholecystitis)
Gallstone (impacted) of hepatic duct (without cholangitis or cholecystitis)
Hepatic cholelithiasis (without cholangitis or cholecystitis)
Hepatic colic (recurrent) (without cholangitis or cholecystitis)

K80.50   Calculus of bile duct without cholangitis or cholecystitis without obstruction

K80.51   Calculus of bile duct without cholangitis or cholecystitis with obstruction

✓5th **K80.6   Calculus of** gallbladder and bile duct with cholecystitis

K80.60   Calculus of gallbladder and bile duct with cholecystitis, unspecified, without obstruction ▽

K80.61   Calculus of gallbladder and bile duct with cholecystitis, unspecified, with obstruction ▽

K80.62   Calculus of gallbladder and bile duct with acute **cholecystitis** without obstruction

K80.63   Calculus of gallbladder and bile duct with acute **cholecystitis** with obstruction

K80.64   Calculus of gallbladder and bile duct with chronic **cholecystitis** without obstruction

K80.65   Calculus of gallbladder and bile duct with chronic **cholecystitis** with obstruction

K80.66   Calculus of gallbladder and bile duct with acute and chronic **cholecystitis** without obstruction

K80.67   Calculus of gallbladder and bile duct with acute and chronic **cholecystitis** with obstruction

✓5th **K80.7   Calculus of** gallbladder and bile duct without cholecystitis

K80.70   Calculus of gallbladder and bile duct without cholecystitis without obstruction

K80.71   Calculus of gallbladder and bile duct without cholecystitis with obstruction

✓5th **K80.8   Other** cholelithiasis

K80.80   Other cholelithiasis without obstruction

K80.81   Other cholelithiasis with obstruction

✓4th **K81   Cholecystitis**
EXCLUDES 1   cholecystitis with cholelithiasis (K80.-)

K81.0   Acute cholecystitis
Abscess of gallbladder
Angiocholecystitis
Emphysematous (acute) cholecystitis
Empyema of gallbladder
Gangrene of gallbladder
Gangrenous cholecystitis
Suppurative cholecystitis

K81.1   Chronic cholecystitis

K81.2   Acute cholecystitis with chronic **cholecystitis**

K81.9   Cholecystitis, unspecified ▽

✓4th **K82   Other diseases of gallbladder**
EXCLUDES 1   nonvisualization of gallbladder (R93.2)
postcholecystectomy syndrome (K91.5)

K82.0   Obstruction of gallbladder
Occlusion of cystic duct or gallbladder without cholelithiasis
Stenosis of cystic duct or gallbladder without cholelithiasis
Stricture of cystic duct or gallbladder without cholelithiasis
EXCLUDES 1   obstruction of gallbladder with cholelithiasis (K80.-)

K82.1   Hydrops of gallbladder
Mucocele of gallbladder

K82.2   Perforation of gallbladder
Rupture of cystic duct or gallbladder

K82.3   Fistula of gallbladder
Cholecystocolic fistula
Cholecystoduodenal fistula

K82.4   Cholesterolosis of gallbladder
Strawberry gallbladder
EXCLUDES 1   cholesterolosis of gallbladder with cholecystitis (K81.-)
cholesterolosis of gallbladder with cholelithiasis (K80.-)

K82.8   Other specified diseases of gallbladder
Adhesions of cystic duct or gallbladder
Atrophy of cystic duct or gallbladder
Cyst of cystic duct or gallbladder
Dyskinesia of cystic duct or gallbladder
Hypertrophy of cystic duct or gallbladder
Nonfunctioning of cystic duct or gallbladder
Ulcer of cystic duct or gallbladder

K82.9   Disease of gallbladder, unspecified ▽

☑ Additional Character Req   ✓x7th Placeholder Alert   Case-Mix Diagnosis   Manifestation   ▽ Unspecified Dx   **EXCLUDES 1** Not coded here   **EXCLUDES 2** Not included here

ICD-10-CM 2018

691

Chapter 11. Diseases of the Digestive System

K83–K90.41

✓4ᵗʰ **K83** **Other diseases of biliary tract**
> EXCLUDES 1   *postcholecystectomy syndrome (K91.5)*
> EXCLUDES 2   *conditions involving the gallbladder (K81-K82)*
>   *conditions involving the cystic duct (K81-K82)*

K83.0 **Cholangitis**
Ascending cholangitis
Cholangitis NOS
Primary cholangitis
Recurrent cholangitis
Sclerosing cholangitis
Secondary cholangitis
Stenosing cholangitis
Suppurative cholangitis
> EXCLUDES 1   *cholangitic liver abscess (K75.0)*
>   *cholangitis with choledocholithiasis (K80.3-, K80.4-)*
>   *chronic nonsuppurative destructive cholangitis (K74.3)*

K83.1 **Obstruction of bile duct**
Occlusion of bile duct without cholelithiasis
Stenosis of bile duct without cholelithiasis
Stricture of bile duct without cholelithiasis
> EXCLUDES 1   *congenital obstruction of bile duct (Q44.3)*
>   *obstruction of bile duct with cholelithiasis (K80.-)*

AHA: 2016, 1Q, 18

K83.2 **Perforation of bile duct**
Rupture of bile duct

K83.3 **Fistula of bile duct**
Choledochoduodenal fistula

K83.4 **Spasm of sphincter of Oddi**

K83.5 **Biliary cyst**

K83.8 **Other specified diseases of biliary tract**
Adhesions of biliary tract
Atrophy of biliary tract
Hypertrophy of biliary tract
Ulcer of biliary tract

K83.9 **Disease of biliary tract, unspecified**   ▽

✓4ᵗʰ **K85** **Acute pancreatitis**
> INCLUDES   acute (recurrent) pancreatitis
>   subacute pancreatitis

✓5ᵗʰ **K85.0** **Idiopathic** acute pancreatitis
K85.00 **Idiopathic acute pancreatitis** without necrosis or infection
K85.01 **Idiopathic acute pancreatitis** with uninfected necrosis
K85.02 **Idiopathic acute pancreatitis** with infected necrosis

✓5ᵗʰ **K85.1** **Biliary** acute pancreatitis
Gallstone pancreatitis
K85.10 **Biliary acute pancreatitis** without necrosis or infection
K85.11 **Biliary acute pancreatitis** with uninfected necrosis
K85.12 **Biliary acute pancreatitis** with infected necrosis

✓5ᵗʰ **K85.2** **Alcohol induced** acute pancreatitis
> EXCLUDES 2   *alcohol induced chronic pancreatitis (K86.0)*
K85.20 **Alcohol induced acute pancreatitis** without necrosis or infection
K85.21 **Alcohol induced acute pancreatitis** with uninfected necrosis
K85.22 **Alcohol induced acute pancreatitis** with infected necrosis

✓5ᵗʰ **K85.3** **Drug induced** acute pancreatitis
Use additional code for adverse effect, if applicable, to identify drug (T36-T50 with fifth or sixth character 5)
Use additional code to identify drug abuse and dependence (F11. – F17.-)
K85.30 **Drug induced acute pancreatitis** without necrosis or infection
K85.31 **Drug induced acute pancreatitis** with uninfected necrosis
K85.32 **Drug induced acute pancreatitis** with infected necrosis

✓5ᵗʰ **K85.8** **Other** acute pancreatitis
K85.80 **Other acute pancreatitis** without necrosis or infection
K85.81 **Other acute pancreatitis** with uninfected necrosis
K85.82 **Other acute pancreatitis** with infected necrosis

✓5ᵗʰ **K85.9** **Acute pancreatitis,** unspecified
Pancreatitis NOS
K85.90 **Acute pancreatitis** without necrosis or infection, unspecified   ▽
K85.91 **Acute pancreatitis** with uninfected necrosis, unspecified   ▽
K85.92 **Acute pancreatitis** with infected necrosis, unspecified   ▽

✓4ᵗʰ **K86** **Other diseases of pancreas**
> EXCLUDES 2   *fibrocystic disease of pancreas (E84.-)*
>   *islet cell tumor (of pancreas) (D13.7)*
>   *pancreatic steatorrhea (K90.3)*

K86.0 **Alcohol-induced chronic pancreatitis**
Use additional code to identify:
alcohol abuse and dependence (F10.-)
Code also exocrine pancreatic insufficiency (K86.81)
> EXCLUDES 2   *alcohol induced acute pancreatitis (K85.2-)*

K86.1 **Other chronic pancreatitis**
Chronic pancreatitis NOS
Infectious chronic pancreatitis
Recurrent chronic pancreatitis
Relapsing chronic pancreatitis
Code also exocrine pancreatic insufficiency (K86.81)

K86.2 **Cyst of pancreas**

K86.3 **Pseudocyst of pancreas**

✓5ᵗʰ **K86.8** **Other specified diseases of pancreas**
K86.81 **Exocrine pancreatic insufficiency**
K86.89 **Other specified diseases of pancreas**
Aseptic pancreatic necrosis, unrelated to acute pancreatitis
Atrophy of pancreas
Calculus of pancreas
Cirrhosis of pancreas
Fibrosis of pancreas
Pancreatic fat necrosis, unrelated to acute pancreatitis
Pancreatic infantilism
Pancreatic necrosis NOS, unrelated to acute pancreatitis

K86.9 **Disease of pancreas, unspecified**   ▽

K87 **Disorders of gallbladder, biliary tract and pancreas in diseases classified elsewhere**
Code first underlying disease
> EXCLUDES 1   *cytomegaloviral pancreatitis (B25.2)*
>   *mumps pancreatitis (B26.3)*
>   *syphilitic gallbladder (A52.74)*
>   *syphilitic pancreas (A52.74)*
>   *tuberculosis of gallbladder (A18.83)*
>   *tuberculosis of pancreas (A18.83)*

Other diseases of the digestive system (K90-K95)

✓4ᵗʰ **K90** **Intestinal malabsorption**
> EXCLUDES 1   *intestinal malabsorption following gastrointestinal surgery (K91.2)*

K90.0 **Celiac disease**
Celiac disease with steatorrhea
▶Celiac gluten-sensitive enteropathy◀
Nontropical sprue
Use additional code for associated disorders including:
dermatitis herpetiformis (L13.0)
gluten ataxia (G32.81)
Code also exocrine pancreatic insufficiency (K86.81)
DEF: Malabsorption syndrome due to gluten consumption; symptoms include fetid, bulky, frothy, oily stools, distended abdomen, gas, asthenia, electrolyte depletion, and vitamin B, D, and K deficiency.

K90.1 **Tropical sprue**
Sprue NOS
Tropical steatorrhea

K90.2 **Blind loop syndrome, not elsewhere classified**
Blind loop syndrome NOS
> EXCLUDES 1   *congenital blind loop syndrome (Q43.8)*
>   *postsurgical blind loop syndrome (K91.2)*

K90.3 **Pancreatic steatorrhea**

✓5ᵗʰ **K90.4** **Other malabsorption due to intolerance**
> EXCLUDES 2   ▶*celiac gluten-sensitive enteropathy*◀ *(K90.0)*
>   *lactose intolerance (E73.-)*

K90.41 **Non-celiac gluten sensitivity**
Gluten sensitivity NOS
Non-celiac gluten sensitive enteropathy

Ⓝ Newborn: 0   Ⓟ Pediatric: 0-17   Ⓜ Maternity: 12-55   Ⓐ Adult: 15-124   NRS Nonroutine supply Dx   NC Dx Noncancer Dx   PDx Primary Dx   ▶◀ Revised Text   ● New Code   ▲ Revised Title

692   ICD-10-CM 2018

K90.49 **Malabsorption due to intolerance, not elsewhere classified**
     Malabsorption due to intolerance to carbohydrate
     Malabsorption due to intolerance to fat
     Malabsorption due to intolerance to protein
     Malabsorption due to intolerance to starch

✓5ᵗʰ K90.8 **Other intestinal malabsorption**

K90.81 **Whipple's disease**

K90.89 **Other intestinal malabsorption**

K90.9 **Intestinal malabsorption, unspecified**   ▽

✓4ᵗʰ **K91 Intraoperative and postprocedural complications and disorders of digestive system, not elsewhere classified**

> EXCLUDES 2   complications of artificial opening of digestive system (K94.-)
> complications of bariatric procedures (K95.-)
> gastrojejunal ulcer (K28.-)
> postprocedural (radiation) retroperitoneal abscess (K68.11)
> radiation colitis (K52.0)
> radiation gastroenteritis (K52.0)
> radiation proctitis (K62.7)

K91.0 **Vomiting following gastrointestinal surgery**

K91.1 **Postgastric surgery syndromes**
     Dumping syndrome
     Postgastrectomy syndrome
     Postvagotomy syndrome

K91.2 **Postsurgical malabsorption, not elsewhere classified**
     Postsurgical blind loop syndrome
> EXCLUDES 1   malabsorption osteomalacia in adults (M83.2)
> malabsorption osteoporosis, postsurgical (M80.8-, M81.8)

✓5ᵗʰ K91.3 **Postprocedural intestinal obstruction**
     AHA: 2017, 1Q, 40

●   K91.30 **Postprocedural intestinal obstruction, unspecified as to partial versus complete**   ▽
       Postprocedural intestinal obstruction NOS

●   K91.31 **Postprocedural partial intestinal obstruction**
       Postprocedural incomplete intestinal obstruction

●   K91.32 **Postprocedural complete intestinal obstruction**

K91.5 **Postcholecystectomy syndrome**

✓5ᵗʰ K91.6 **Intraoperative hemorrhage and hematoma of a digestive system organ or structure complicating a procedure**
> EXCLUDES 1   intraoperative hemorrhage and hematoma of a digestive system organ or structure due to accidental puncture and laceration during a procedure (K91.7-)

K91.61 **Intraoperative hemorrhage and hematoma of a digestive system organ or structure complicating a digestive system procedure**

K91.62 **Intraoperative hemorrhage and hematoma of a digestive system organ or structure complicating other procedure**

✓5ᵗʰ K91.7 **Accidental puncture and laceration of a digestive system organ or structure during a procedure**

K91.71 **Accidental puncture and laceration of a digestive system organ or structure during a digestive system procedure**

K91.72 **Accidental puncture and laceration of a digestive system organ or structure during other procedure**

✓5ᵗʰ K91.8 **Other intraoperative and postprocedural complications and disorders of digestive system**

K91.81 **Other intraoperative complications of digestive system**

K91.82 **Postprocedural hepatic failure**

K91.83 **Postprocedural hepatorenal syndrome**

✓6ᵗʰ K91.84 **Postprocedural hemorrhage of a digestive system organ or structure following a procedure**

K91.840 **Postprocedural hemorrhage of a digestive system organ or structure following a digestive system procedure**
       AHA: 2016, 1Q, 15

K91.841 **Postprocedural hemorrhage of a digestive system organ or structure following other procedure**

✓6ᵗʰ K91.85 **Complications of intestinal pouch**

K91.850 **Pouchitis**
       Inflammation of internal ileoanal pouch
       DEF: Inflammatory complication of an existing surgically created ileoanal pouch, resulting in multiple GI complaints, including diarrhea, abdominal pain, rectal bleeding, fecal urgency, or incontinence.

K91.858 **Other complications of intestinal pouch**

K91.86 **Retained cholelithiasis following cholecystectomy**

✓6ᵗʰ K91.87 **Postprocedural hematoma and seroma of a digestive system organ or structure following a procedure**

K91.870 **Postprocedural hematoma of a digestive system organ or structure following a digestive system procedure**

K91.871 **Postprocedural hematoma of a digestive system organ or structure following other procedure**

K91.872 **Postprocedural seroma of a digestive system organ or structure following a digestive system procedure**

K91.873 **Postprocedural seroma of a digestive system organ or structure following other procedure**

K91.89 **Other postprocedural complications and disorders of digestive system**
     Use additional code, if applicable, to further specify disorder
> EXCLUDES 2   postprocedural retroperitoneal abscess (K68.11)

     AHA: 2017, 1Q, 40

✓4ᵗʰ **K92 Other diseases of digestive system**
> EXCLUDES 1   neonatal gastrointestinal hemorrhage (P54.0-P54.3)

K92.0 **Hematemesis**

K92.1 **Melena**
> EXCLUDES 1   occult blood in feces (R19.5)

K92.2 **Gastrointestinal hemorrhage, unspecified**   ▽
     Gastric hemorrhage NOS
     Intestinal hemorrhage NOS
> EXCLUDES 1   acute hemorrhagic gastritis (K29.01)
> hemorrhage of anus and rectum (K62.5)
> angiodysplasia of stomach with hemorrhage (K31.811)
> diverticular disease with hemorrhage (K57.-)
> gastritis and duodenitis with hemorrhage (K29.-)
> peptic ulcer with hemorrhage (K25-K28)

✓5ᵗʰ K92.8 **Other specified diseases of the digestive system**

K92.81 **Gastrointestinal mucositis (ulcerative)**
     Code also type of associated therapy, such as:
       antineoplastic and immunosuppressive drugs (T45.1X-)
       radiological procedure and radiotherapy (Y84.2)
> EXCLUDES 2   mucositis (ulcerative) of vagina and vulva (N76.81)
> nasal mucositis (ulcerative) (J34.81)
> oral mucositis (ulcerative) (K12.3-)

K92.89 **Other specified diseases of the digestive system**

K92.9 **Disease of digestive system, unspecified**   ▽

✓4ᵗʰ **K94 Complications of artificial openings of the digestive system**

✓5ᵗʰ K94.0 **Colostomy complications**

K94.00 **Colostomy complication, unspecified**   ▽

K94.01 **Colostomy hemorrhage**

K94.02 **Colostomy infection**
     Use additional code to specify type of infection, such as:
       cellulitis of abdominal wall (L03.311)
       sepsis (A40-, A41-)

K94.03 **Colostomy malfunction**
     Mechanical complication of colostomy

K94.09 **Other complications of colostomy**

✓5ᵗʰ K94.1 **Enterostomy complications**

K94.10 **Enterostomy complication, unspecified**   ▽

K94.11 **Enterostomy hemorrhage**

K94.12 **Enterostomy infection**
     Use additional code to specify type of infection, such as:
       cellulitis of abdominal wall (L03.311)
       sepsis (A40-, A41-)

☑ Additional Character Req   ✓x7ᵗʰ Placeholder Alert   Case-Mix Diagnosis   Manifestation   ▽ Unspecified Dx   EXCLUDES 1 Not coded here   EXCLUDES 2 Not included here

ICD-10-CM 2018   **693**

Chapter 11. Diseases of the Digestive System

K94.13   **Enterostomy malfunction**
Mechanical complication of enterostomy

K94.19   **Other complications of enterostomy**

✓5ᵗʰ **K94.2**   Gastrostomy complications

K94.20   **Gastrostomy complication, unspecified** ▽

K94.21   **Gastrostomy hemorrhage**

K94.22   **Gastrostomy infection**
Use additional code to specify type of infection,
such as:
cellulitis of abdominal wall (LØ3.311)
sepsis (A4Ø-, A41-)

K94.23   **Gastrostomy malfunction**
Mechanical complication of gastrostomy

K94.29   **Other complications of gastrostomy**

✓5ᵗʰ **K94.3**   Esophagostomy complications

K94.30   **Esophagostomy complications, unspecified** ▽

K94.31   **Esophagostomy hemorrhage**

K94.32   **Esophagostomy infection**
Use additional code to identify the infection

K94.33   **Esophagostomy malfunction**
Mechanical complication of esophagostomy

K94.39   **Other complications of esophagostomy**

✓4ᵗʰ **K95**   **Complications of bariatric procedures**

✓5ᵗʰ **K95.Ø**   **Complications of gastric band procedure**

K95.Ø1   **Infection due to gastric band procedure**
Use additional code to specify type of infection or
organism, such as:
bacterial and viral infectious agents (B95.-, B96.-)
cellulitis of abdominal wall (LØ3.311)
sepsis (A4Ø.-, A41.-)

K95.Ø9   **Other complications of gastric band procedure**
Use additional code, if applicable, to further specify
complication

✓5ᵗʰ **K95.8**   **Complications of other bariatric procedure**
EXCLUDES 1   complications of gastric band surgery (K95.Ø-)

K95.81   **Infection due to other bariatric procedure**
Use additional code to specify type of infection or
organism, such as:
bacterial and viral infectious agents (B95.-, B96.-)
cellulitis of abdominal wall (LØ3.311)
sepsis (A4Ø.-, A41.-)

K95.89   **Other complications of other bariatric procedure**
Use additional code, if applicable, to further specify
complication

N Newborn: 0   P Pediatric: 0-17   M Maternity: 12-55   A Adult: 15-124   NRS Nonroutine supply Dx   NC Dx Noncancer Dx   PDx Primary Dx   ▶◀ Revised Text   ● New Code   ▲ Revised Title

694   ICD-10-CM 2018

Chapter 12. Diseases of the Skin and Subcutaneous Tissue (LØØ–L99)

Chapter Specific Guidelines with Coding Examples

The chapter specific guidelines from the ICD-10-CM Official Guidelines for Coding and Reporting have been provided below. Along with these guidelines are coding examples, contained in the shaded boxes, that have been developed to help illustrate the coding and/or sequencing guidance found in these guidelines.

a. Pressure ulcer stage codes

1) Pressure ulcer stages

Codes from category L89, Pressure ulcer, are combination codes that identify the site of the pressure ulcer as well as the stage of the ulcer.

The ICD-10-CM classifies pressure ulcer stages based on severity, which is designated by stages 1-4, unspecified stage and unstageable.

Assign as many codes from category L89 as needed to identify all the pressure ulcers the patient has, if applicable.

> Stage 4 pressure ulcer right heel, 9 x 10 cm that invades the muscle and fascia; stage 2 pressure ulcer of left elbow.
>
> **L89.614**   **Pressure ulcer of right heel, stage 4**
>
> **L89.022**   **Pressure ulcer of left elbow, stage 2**
>
> *Explanation:* Patient has a right heel pressure ulcer documented as stage 4 and a left elbow pressure ulcer documented as stage 2. Combination codes from category L89 Pressure ulcer, identify the site of the pressure ulcer as well as the stage. Assign as many codes from category L89 as needed to identify all the pressure ulcers the patient has.

2) Unstageable pressure ulcers

Assignment of the code for unstageable pressure ulcer (L89.--Ø) should be based on the clinical documentation. These codes are used for pressure ulcers whose stage cannot be clinically determined (e.g., the ulcer is covered by eschar or has been treated with a skin or muscle graft) and pressure ulcers that are documented as deep tissue injury but not documented as due to trauma. This code should not be confused with the codes for unspecified stage (L89.--9). When there is no documentation regarding the stage of the pressure ulcer, assign the appropriate code for unspecified stage (L89.--9).

> Pressure ulcer of the right lower back documented as unstageable due to the presence of thick eschar covering the ulcer.
>
> **L89.130**   **Pressure ulcer of right lower back, unstageable**
>
> *Explanation:* Codes for unstageable pressure ulcers are assigned when the stage cannot be clinically determined (e.g., the ulcer is covered by eschar or has been treated with a skin or muscle graft).

3) Documented pressure ulcer stage

Assignment of the pressure ulcer stage code should be guided by clinical documentation of the stage or documentation of the terms found in the Alphabetic Index. For clinical terms describing the stage that are not found in the Alphabetic Index, and there is no documentation of the stage, the provider should be queried.

> Left heel pressure ulcer with partial thickness skin loss involving the dermis.
>
> **L89.622**   **Pressure ulcer of left heel, stage 2**
>
> *Explanation:* Code assignment for the pressure ulcer stage should be guided by either the clinical documentation of the stage or the documentation of terms found in the Alphabetic Index. The clinical documentation describing the left heel pressure ulcer "partial thickness skin loss involving the dermis" matches the ICD-10-CM index parenthetical description for stage 2 "(abrasion, blister, partial thickness skin loss involving epidermis and/or dermis)."

4) Patients admitted with pressure ulcers documented as healed

No code is assigned if the documentation states that the pressure ulcer is completely healed.

> Patient is admitted for a second skilled home health admission within one year and is known to previously have had a pressure ulcer of the left heel during last admission 8 months prior. The area is observed and is currently healed with no signs of tissue breakdown.
>
> **Z87.2**   **Personal history of diseases of the skin and subcutaneous tissue**
>
> *Explanation:* Assign only code Z87.2 indicating a history of pressure ulcer. This code includes conditions classifiable to LØØ–L99 such as pressure ulcers. Code L89 should not be assigned for a pressure ulcer that is reported to be healed.

5) Patients admitted with pressure ulcers documented as healing

Pressure ulcers described as healing should be assigned the appropriate pressure ulcer stage code based on the documentation in the medical record. If the documentation does not provide information about the stage of the healing pressure ulcer, assign the appropriate code for unspecified stage.

If the documentation is unclear as to whether the patient has a current (new) pressure ulcer or if the patient is being treated for a healing pressure ulcer, query the provider.

For ulcers that were present on admission but healed at the time of discharge, assign the code for the site and stage of the pressure ulcer at the time of admission.

6) Patient admitted with pressure ulcer evolving into another stage during the admission

If a patient is admitted **to an inpatient hospital** with a pressure ulcer at one stage and it progresses to a higher stage, two separate codes should be assigned: one code for the site and stage of the ulcer on admission and a second code for the same ulcer site and the highest stage reported during the stay.

b. Non-pressure chronic ulcers

1) Patients admitted with non-pressure ulcers documented as healed

No code is assigned if the documentation states that the non-pressure ulcer is completely healed.

2) Patients admitted with non-pressure ulcers documented as healing

Non-pressure ulcers described as healing should be assigned the appropriate non-pressure ulcer code based on the documentation in the medical record. If the documentation does not provide information about the severity of the healing non-pressure ulcer, assign the appropriate code for unspecified severity.

If the documentation is unclear as to whether the patient has a current (new) non-pressure ulcer or if the patient is being treated for a healing non-pressure ulcer, query the provider.

For ulcers that were present on admission but healed at the time of discharge, assign the code for the site and severity of the non-pressure ulcer at the time of admission.

3) Patient admitted with non-pressure ulcer that progresses to another severity level during the admission

If a patient is admitted to an inpatient hospital with a non-pressure ulcer at one severity level and it progresses to a higher severity level, two separate codes should be assigned: one code for the site and severity level of the ulcer on admission and a second code for the same ulcer site and the highest severity level reported during the stay.

Chapter 12. Diseases of the Skin and Subcutaneous Tissue (L00-L99)

> EXCLUDES 2   *certain conditions originating in the perinatal period (P04-P96)*
> *certain infectious and parasitic diseases (A00-B99)*
> *complications of pregnancy, childbirth and the puerperium (O00-O9A)*
> *congenital malformations, deformations, and chromosomal abnormalities (Q00-Q99)*
> *endocrine, nutritional and metabolic diseases (E00-E88)*
> *lipomelanotic reticulosis (I89.8)*
> *neoplasms (C00-D49)*
> *symptoms, signs and abnormal clinical and laboratory findings, not elsewhere classified (R00-R94)*
> *systemic connective tissue disorders (M30-M36)*
> *viral warts (B07.-)*

This chapter contains the following blocks:

L00-L08	Infections of the skin and subcutaneous tissue
L10-L14	Bullous disorders
L20-L30	Dermatitis and eczema
L40-L45	Papulosquamous disorders
L49-L54	Urticaria and erythema
L55-L59	Radiation-related disorders of the skin and subcutaneous tissue
L60-L75	Disorders of skin appendages
L76	Intraoperative and postprocedural complications of skin and subcutaneous tissue
L80-L99	Other disorders of the skin and subcutaneous tissue

Infections of the skin and subcutaneous tissue (L00-L08)

Use additional code (B95-B97) to identify infectious agent

> EXCLUDES 2   *hordeolum (H00.0)*
> *infective dermatitis (L30.3)*
> *local infections of skin classified in Chapter 1*
> *lupus panniculitis (L93.2)*
> *panniculitis NOS (M79.3)*
> *panniculitis of neck and back (M54.0-)*
> *Perlèche NOS (K13.0)*
> *Perlèche due to candidiasis (B37.0)*
> *Perlèche due to riboflavin deficiency (E53.0)*
> *pyogenic granuloma (L98.0)*
> *relapsing panniculitis [Weber-Christian] (M35.6)*
> *viral warts (B07.-)*
> *zoster (B02.-)*

L00   Staphylococcal scalded skin syndrome
    Ritter's disease
    Use additional code to identify percentage of skin exfoliation (L49.-)
> EXCLUDES 1   *bullous impetigo (L01.03)*
> *pemphigus neonatorum (L01.03) (L51.2)*
> *toxic epidermal necrolysis [Lyell] (L51.2)*

    DEF: Infectious skin disease of children younger than 5 years marked by eruptions ranging from a few localized blisters to widespread, easily ruptured, fine vesicles and bullae affecting almost the entire body; results in exfoliation of large planes of skin and leaves raw areas.

✓4ᵗʰ **L01   Impetigo**
> EXCLUDES 1   *impetigo herpetiformis (L40.1)*

✓5ᵗʰ **L01.0   Impetigo**
      Impetigo contagiosa
      Impetigo vulgaris

     L01.00   Impetigo, unspecified   ▽
        Impetigo NOS

     L01.01   Non-bullous impetigo

     L01.02   Bockhart's impetigo
        Impetigo follicularis
        Perifolliculitis NOS
        Superficial pustular perifolliculitis

     L01.03   Bullous impetigo
        Impetigo neonatorum   Pemphigus neonatorum

     L01.09   Other impetigo
        Ulcerative impetigo

   L01.1   Impetiginization of other dermatoses

✓4ᵗʰ **L02   Cutaneous abscess, furuncle and carbuncle**
    Use additional code to identify organism (B95-B96)
> EXCLUDES 2   *abscess of anus and rectal regions (K61.-)*
> *abscess of female genital organs (external) (N76.4)*
> *abscess of male genital organs (external) (N48.2, N49-)*

✓5ᵗʰ **L02.0   Cutaneous abscess, furuncle and carbuncle of face**
> EXCLUDES 2   *abscess of ear, external (H60.0)*
> *abscess of eyelid (H00.0)*
> *abscess of head [any part, except face] (L02.8)*
> *abscess of lacrimal gland (H04.0)*
> *abscess of lacrimal passages (H04.3)*
> *abscess of mouth (K12.2)*
> *abscess of nose (J34.0)*
> *abscess of orbit (H05.0)*
> *submandibular abscess (K12.2)*

     L02.01   Cutaneous abscess of face   NRS
     L02.02   Furuncle of face   NRS
        Boil of face
        Folliculitis of face
     L02.03   Carbuncle of face   NRS

✓5ᵗʰ **L02.1   Cutaneous abscess, furuncle and carbuncle of neck**
     L02.11   Cutaneous abscess of neck   NRS
     L02.12   Furuncle of neck   NRS
        Boil of neck
        Folliculitis of neck
     L02.13   Carbuncle of neck   NRS

✓5ᵗʰ **L02.2   Cutaneous abscess, furuncle and carbuncle of trunk**
> EXCLUDES 1   *non-newborn omphalitis (L08.82)*
> *omphalitis of newborn (P38.-)*
> EXCLUDES 2   *abscess of breast (N61.1)*
> *abscess of buttocks (L02.3)*
> *abscess of female external genital organs (N76.4)*
> *abscess of hip (L02.4)*
> *abscess of male external genital organs (N48.2, N49-)*

✓6ᵗʰ   **L02.21   Cutaneous abscess of trunk**
     L02.211   Cutaneous abscess of abdominal wall   NRS
     L02.212   Cutaneous abscess of back [any part, except buttock]   NRS
     L02.213   Cutaneous abscess of chest wall   NRS
     L02.214   Cutaneous abscess of groin   NRS
     L02.215   Cutaneous abscess of perineum   NRS
     L02.216   Cutaneous abscess of umbilicus   NRS
     L02.219   Cutaneous abscess of trunk, unspecified   NRS ▽

✓6ᵗʰ   **L02.22   Furuncle of trunk**
       Boil of trunk
       Folliculitis of trunk
     L02.221   Furuncle of abdominal wall   NRS
     L02.222   Furuncle of back [any part, except buttock]   NRS
     L02.223   Furuncle of chest wall   NRS
     L02.224   Furuncle of groin   NRS
     L02.225   Furuncle of perineum   NRS
     L02.226   Furuncle of umbilicus   NRS
     L02.229   Furuncle of trunk, unspecified   ▽

✓6ᵗʰ   **L02.23   Carbuncle of trunk**
     L02.231   Carbuncle of abdominal wall   NRS
     L02.232   Carbuncle of back [any part, except buttock]   NRS
     L02.233   Carbuncle of chest wall   NRS
     L02.234   Carbuncle of groin   NRS
     L02.235   Carbuncle of perineum   NRS
     L02.236   Carbuncle of umbilicus   NRS
     L02.239   Carbuncle of trunk, unspecified   ▽

✓5ᵗʰ **L02.3   Cutaneous abscess, furuncle and carbuncle of buttock**
> EXCLUDES 1   *pilonidal cyst with abscess (L05.01)*

     L02.31   Cutaneous abscess of buttock   NRS
        Cutaneous abscess of gluteal region

     L02.32   Furuncle of buttock   NRS
        Boil of buttock
        Folliculitis of buttock
        Furuncle of gluteal region

     L02.33   Carbuncle of buttock   NRS
        Carbuncle of gluteal region

Ⓝ Newborn: 0   Ⓟ Pediatric: 0-17   Ⓜ Maternity: 12-55   Ⓐ Adult: 15-124   **NRS** Nonroutine supply Dx   **NC Dx** Noncancer Dx   **PDx** Primary Dx   ▶◀ Revised Text   ● New Code   ▲ Revised Title

696   ICD-10-CM 2018

✓5th **L02.4 Cutaneous abscess, furuncle and carbuncle of** limb

> EXCLUDES 2   *cutaneous abscess, furuncle and carbuncle of groin (L02.214, L02.224, L02.234)*
> *cutaneous abscess, furuncle and carbuncle of hand (L02.5-)*
> *cutaneous abscess, furuncle and carbuncle of foot (L02.6-)*

✓6th **L02.41 Cutaneous abscess of** limb

     L02.411 **Cutaneous abscess of** right axilla   NRS
     L02.412 **Cutaneous abscess of** left axilla   NRS
     L02.413 **Cutaneous abscess of** right upper **limb**   NRS
     L02.414 **Cutaneous abscess of** left upper **limb**   NRS
     L02.415 **Cutaneous abscess of** right lower **limb**   NRS
     L02.416 **Cutaneous abscess of** left lower **limb**   NRS
     L02.419 **Cutaneous abscess of limb, unspecified** ▽

✓6th **L02.42 Furuncle of** limb
     Boil of limb
     Folliculitis of limb

     L02.421 **Furuncle of** right axilla   NRS
     L02.422 **Furuncle of** left axilla   NRS
     L02.423 **Furuncle of** right upper **limb**   NRS
     L02.424 **Furuncle of** left upper **limb**   NRS
     L02.425 **Furuncle of** right lower **limb**   NRS
     L02.426 **Furuncle of** left lower **limb**   NRS
     L02.429 **Furuncle of limb, unspecified** ▽

✓6th **L02.43 Carbuncle of** limb

     L02.431 **Carbuncle of** right axilla   NRS
     L02.432 **Carbuncle of** left axilla   NRS
     L02.433 **Carbuncle of** right upper **limb**   NRS
     L02.434 **Carbuncle of** left upper **limb**   NRS
     L02.435 **Carbuncle of** right lower **limb**   NRS
     L02.436 **Carbuncle of** left lower **limb**   NRS
     L02.439 **Carbuncle of limb, unspecified** ▽

✓5th **L02.5 Cutaneous abscess, furuncle and carbuncle of** hand

✓6th **L02.51 Cutaneous abscess of** hand

     L02.511 **Cutaneous abscess of** right **hand**   NRS
     L02.512 **Cutaneous abscess of** left **hand**   NRS
     L02.519 **Cutaneous abscess of unspecified hand** ▽

✓6th **L02.52 Furuncle** hand
     Boil of hand
     Folliculitis of hand

     L02.521 **Furuncle** right **hand**   NRS
     L02.522 **Furuncle** left **hand**   NRS
     L02.529 **Furuncle unspecified hand** ▽

✓6th **L02.53 Carbuncle of** hand

     L02.531 **Carbuncle of** right **hand**   NRS
     L02.532 **Carbuncle of** left **hand**   NRS
     L02.539 **Carbuncle of unspecified hand** ▽

✓5th **L02.6 Cutaneous abscess, furuncle and carbuncle of** foot

✓6th **L02.61 Cutaneous abscess of** foot

     L02.611 **Cutaneous abscess of** right **foot**   NRS
     L02.612 **Cutaneous abscess of** left **foot**   NRS
     L02.619 **Cutaneous abscess of unspecified foot** ▽

✓6th **L02.62 Furuncle of** foot
     Boil of foot
     Folliculitis of foot

     L02.621 **Furuncle of** right **foot**   NRS
     L02.622 **Furuncle of** left **foot**   NRS
     L02.629 **Furuncle of unspecified foot** ▽

✓6th **L02.63 Carbuncle of** foot

     L02.631 **Carbuncle of** right **foot**   NRS
     L02.632 **Carbuncle of** left **foot**   NRS
     L02.639 **Carbuncle of unspecified foot** ▽

✓5th **L02.8 Cutaneous abscess, furuncle and carbuncle of** other sites

✓6th **L02.81 Cutaneous abscess of** other sites

     L02.811 **Cutaneous abscess of** head **[any part, except face]**   NRS
     L02.818 **Cutaneous abscess of other sites**   NRS

✓6th **L02.82 Furuncle of** other sites
     Boil of other sites
     Folliculitis of other sites

     L02.821 **Furuncle of** head **[any part, except face]**   NRS
     L02.828 **Furuncle of other sites**   NRS

✓6th **L02.83 Carbuncle of** other sites

     L02.831 **Carbuncle of** head **[any part, except face]**   NRS
     L02.838 **Carbuncle of other sites**   NRS

✓5th **L02.9 Cutaneous abscess, furuncle and carbuncle, unspecified**

     L02.91 **Cutaneous abscess, unspecified** ▽
     L02.92 **Furuncle, unspecified** ▽
         Boil NOS
         Furunculosis NOS
     L02.93 **Carbuncle, unspecified** ▽

✓4th **L03 Cellulitis and acute lymphangitis**

> EXCLUDES 2   *cellulitis of anal and rectal region (K61.-)*
> *cellulitis of external auditory canal (H60.1)*
> *cellulitis of eyelid (H00.03-)*
> *cellulitis of female external genital organs (N76.4)*
> *cellulitis of lacrimal apparatus (H04.3)*
> *cellulitis of male external genital organs (N48.2, N49-)*
> *cellulitis of mouth (K12.2)*
> *cellulitis of nose (J34.0)*
> *eosinophilic cellulitis [Wells] (L98.3)*
> *febrile neutrophilic dermatosis [Sweet] (L98.2)*
> *lymphangitis (chronic) (subacute) (I89.1)*

✓5th **L03.0 Cellulitis and acute lymphangitis of** finger and toe
     Infection of nail
     Onychia
     Paronychia
     Perionychia

✓6th **L03.01 Cellulitis of** finger
     Felon
     Whitlow
     EXCLUDES 1   *herpetic whitlow (B00.89)*
     DEF: Felon: Superficial bacterial skin infection at the tip of the finger.

     L03.011 **Cellulitis of** right **finger**   NRS
     L03.012 **Cellulitis of** left **finger**   NRS
     L03.019 **Cellulitis of unspecified finger** ▽

✓6th **L03.02 Acute lymphangitis of** finger
     Hangnail with lymphangitis of finger

     L03.021 **Acute lymphangitis of** right **finger**   NRS
     L03.022 **Acute lymphangitis of** left **finger**   NRS
     L03.029 **Acute lymphangitis of unspecified finger** ▽

✓6th **L03.03 Cellulitis of** toe

     L03.031 **Cellulitis of** right **toe**   NRS
     L03.032 **Cellulitis of** left **toe**   NRS
     L03.039 **Cellulitis of unspecified toe** ▽

✓6th **L03.04 Acute lymphangitis of** toe
     Hangnail with lymphangitis of toe

     L03.041 **Acute lymphangitis of** right **toe**   NRS
     L03.042 **Acute lymphangitis of** left **toe**   NRS
     L03.049 **Acute lymphangitis of unspecified toe** ▽

✓5th **L03.1 Cellulitis and acute lymphangitis of** other parts **of limb**

✓6th **L03.11 Cellulitis of** other parts **of limb**
     EXCLUDES 2   *cellulitis of fingers (L03.01-)*
         cellulitis of toes (L03.03-)
         groin (L03.314)

     L03.111 **Cellulitis of** right axilla   NRS
     L03.112 **Cellulitis of** left axilla   NRS
     L03.113 **Cellulitis of** right upper **limb**   NRS
     L03.114 **Cellulitis of** left upper **limb**   NRS
     L03.115 **Cellulitis of** right lower **limb**   NRS
     L03.116 **Cellulitis of** left lower **limb**   NRS
     L03.119 **Cellulitis of unspecified part of limb** ▽

✓6th **L03.12 Acute lymphangitis of** other parts **of limb**
     EXCLUDES 2   *acute lymphangitis of fingers (L03.02-)*
         acute lymphangitis of groin (L03.324)
         acute lymphangitis of toes (L03.04-)

     L03.121 **Acute lymphangitis of** right axilla   NRS
     L03.122 **Acute lymphangitis of** left axilla   NRS
     L03.123 **Acute lymphangitis of** right upper **limb**   NRS
     L03.124 **Acute lymphangitis of** left upper **limb**   NRS
     L03.125 **Acute lymphangitis of** right lower **limb**   NRS

✓ Additional Character Req   ✓x7th Placeholder Alert   Case-Mix Diagnosis   Manifestation   ▽ Unspecified Dx   EXCLUDES 1 Not coded here   EXCLUDES 2 Not included here

ICD-10-CM 2018   697

Chapter 12. Diseases of the Skin and Subcutaneous Tissue

L02.4–L03.125

L03.126   **Acute lymphangitis of** left lower limb   NRS

L03.129   **Acute lymphangitis of unspecified part of limb**   ▽

✓5ᵗʰ **L03.2**   **Cellulitis and acute lymphangitis of** face and neck

   ✓6ᵗʰ **L03.21**   **Cellulitis and acute lymphangitis of** face

     L03.211   Cellulitis of face   NRS

       EXCLUDES 2   abscess of orbit (H05.01-)

         cellulitis of ear (H60.1-)

         cellulitis of eyelid (H00.03-)

         cellulitis of head (L03.811)

         cellulitis of lacrimal apparatus (H04.3)

         cellulitis of lip (K13.0)

         cellulitis of mouth (K12.2)

         cellulitis of nose (internal) (J34.0)

         cellulitis of orbit (H05.01-)

         cellulitis of scalp (L03.811)

       AHA: 2013, 4Q, 123

     L03.212   Acute lymphangitis of face   NRS

     L03.213   Periorbital cellulitis   NRS

       Preseptal cellulitis

   ✓6ᵗʰ **L03.22**   **Cellulitis and acute lymphangitis of** neck

     L03.221   Cellulitis of neck   NRS

     L03.222   Acute lymphangitis of neck   NRS

✓5ᵗʰ **L03.3**   **Cellulitis and acute lymphangitis of** trunk

   ✓6ᵗʰ **L03.31**   **Cellulitis of** trunk

       EXCLUDES 2   cellulitis of anal and rectal regions (K61.-)

         cellulitis of breast NOS (N61.0)

         cellulitis of female external genital organs (N76.4)

         cellulitis of male external genital organs (N48.2, N49-)

         omphalitis of newborn (P38.-)

         puerperal cellulitis of breast (O91.2)

     L03.311   Cellulitis of abdominal wall   NRS

       EXCLUDES 2   cellulitis of umbilicus (L03.316)

         cellulitis of groin (L03.314)

     L03.312   Cellulitis of back [any part except buttock]   NRS

     L03.313   Cellulitis of chest wall   NRS

     L03.314   Cellulitis of groin   NRS

     L03.315   Cellulitis of perineum   NRS

     L03.316   Cellulitis of umbilicus   NRS

     L03.317   Cellulitis of buttock   NRS

     L03.319   Cellulitis of trunk, unspecified   NRS ▽

   ✓6ᵗʰ **L03.32**   **Acute lymphangitis of** trunk

     L03.321   Acute lymphangitis of abdominal wall   NRS

     L03.322   Acute lymphangitis of back [any part except buttock]   NRS

     L03.323   Acute lymphangitis of chest wall   NRS

     L03.324   Acute lymphangitis of groin   NRS

     L03.325   Acute lymphangitis of perineum   NRS

     L03.326   Acute lymphangitis of umbilicus   NRS

     L03.327   Acute lymphangitis of buttock   NRS

     L03.329   Acute lymphangitis of trunk, unspecified   NRS ▽

✓5ᵗʰ **L03.8**   **Cellulitis and acute lymphangitis of** other sites

   ✓6ᵗʰ **L03.81**   **Cellulitis of** other sites

     L03.811   Cellulitis of head [any part, except face]   NRS

       Cellulitis of scalp

       EXCLUDES 2   cellulitis of face (L03.211)

     L03.818   Cellulitis of other sites   NRS

   ✓6ᵗʰ **L03.89**   **Acute lymphangitis of** other sites

     L03.891   Acute lymphangitis of head [any part, except face]   NRS

     L03.898   Acute lymphangitis of other sites   NRS

✓5ᵗʰ **L03.9**   **Cellulitis and acute lymphangitis, unspecified**

     L03.90   Cellulitis, unspecified   ▽

     L03.91   Acute lymphangitis, unspecified   ▽

       EXCLUDES 1   lymphangitis NOS (I89.1)

✓4ᵗʰ **L04**   **Acute lymphadenitis**

   INCLUDES   abscess (acute) of lymph nodes, except mesenteric

     acute lymphadenitis, except mesenteric

   EXCLUDES 1   chronic or subacute lymphadenitis, except mesenteric (I88.1)

     enlarged lymph nodes (R59.-)

     human immunodeficiency virus [HIV] disease resulting in generalized lymphadenopathy (B20)

     lymphadenitis NOS (I88.9)

     nonspecific mesenteric lymphadenitis (I88.0)

   L04.0   **Acute lymphadenitis of** face, head and neck   NRS

   L04.1   **Acute lymphadenitis of** trunk   NRS

   L04.2   **Acute lymphadenitis of** upper limb   NRS

     Acute lymphadenitis of axilla

     Acute lymphadenitis of shoulder

   L04.3   **Acute lymphadenitis of** lower limb   NRS

     Acute lymphadenitis of hip

     EXCLUDES 2   acute lymphadenitis of groin (L04.1)

   L04.8   **Acute lymphadenitis of** other sites   NRS

   L04.9   **Acute lymphadenitis, unspecified**   ▽

✓4ᵗʰ **L05**   **Pilonidal cyst and sinus**

   ✓5ᵗʰ **L05.0**   **Pilonidal cyst and sinus** with abscess

     L05.01   Pilonidal cyst with abscess   NRS

       Pilonidal abscess

       Pilonidal dimple with abscess

       Postanal dimple with abscess

       EXCLUDES 2   congenital sacral dimple (Q82.6)

         parasacral dimple (Q82.6)

     L05.02   Pilonidal sinus with abscess   NRS

       Coccygeal fistula with abscess

       Coccygeal sinus with abscess

       Pilonidal fistula with abscess

   ✓5ᵗʰ **L05.9**   **Pilonidal cyst and sinus** without abscess

     L05.91   Pilonidal cyst without abscess   NRS

       Pilonidal dimple

       Postanal dimple

       Pilonidal cyst NOS

       EXCLUDES 2   congenital sacral dimple (Q82.6)

         parasacral dimple (Q82.6)

     L05.92   Pilonidal sinus without abscess   NRS

       Coccygeal fistula

       Coccygeal sinus without abscess

       Pilonidal fistula

✓4ᵗʰ **L08**   **Other local infections of skin and subcutaneous tissue**

   L08.0   **Pyoderma**   NRS

     Dermatitis gangrenosa

     Purulent dermatitis

     Septic dermatitis

     Suppurative dermatitis

     EXCLUDES 1   pyoderma gangrenosum (L88)

       pyoderma vegetans (L08.81)

   L08.1   **Erythrasma**

   ✓5ᵗʰ **L08.8**   **Other specified local infections of the skin and subcutaneous tissue**

     L08.81   Pyoderma vegetans   NRS

       EXCLUDES 1   pyoderma gangrenosum (L88)

       pyoderma NOS (L08.0)

Pilonidal Cyst

Skin

Fistula

Pilonidal cyst

Fat

Bone

Ⓝ Newborn: 0   Ⓟ Pediatric: 0-17   Ⓜ Maternity: 12-55   Ⓐ Adult: 15-124   NRS Nonroutine supply Dx   NC Dx Noncancer Dx   PD Dx Primary Dx   ►◄ Revised Text   ● New Code   ▲ Revised Title

698   ICD-10-CM 2018

L08.82 Omphalitis not of newborn `NRS`
  EXCLUDES 1 omphalitis of newborn (P38.-)

L08.89 Other specified local infections of the skin and subcutaneous tissue `NRS`

L08.9 Local infection of the skin and subcutaneous tissue, unspecified `NRS` ▽

Bullous disorders (L10-L14)

EXCLUDES 1 benign familial pemphigus [Hailey-Hailey] (Q82.8)
staphylococcal scalded skin syndrome (L00)
toxic epidermal necrolysis [Lyell] (L51.2)

✓4th **L10 Pemphigus**
  EXCLUDES 1 pemphigus neonatorum (L01.03)

L10.0 Pemphigus vulgaris

L10.1 Pemphigus vegetans

L10.2 Pemphigus foliaceous

L10.3 Brazilian pemphigus [fogo selvagem]

L10.4 Pemphigus erythematosus
  Senear-Usher syndrome

L10.5 Drug-induced pemphigus
  Use additional code for adverse effect, if applicable, to identify drug (T36-T50 with fifth or sixth character 5)

✓5th **L10.8 Other pemphigus**

  L10.81 Paraneoplastic pemphigus

  L10.89 Other pemphigus

L10.9 Pemphigus, unspecified ▽

✓4th **L11 Other acantholytic disorders**

L11.0 Acquired keratosis follicularis
  EXCLUDES 1 keratosis follicularis (congenital) [Darier-White] (Q82.8)

L11.1 Transient acantholytic dermatosis [Grover]

L11.8 Other specified acantholytic disorders

L11.9 Acantholytic disorder, unspecified ▽

✓4th **L12 Pemphigoid**
  EXCLUDES 1 herpes gestationis (O26.4-)
    impetigo herpetiformis (L40.1)

L12.0 Bullous pemphigoid

L12.1 Cicatricial pemphigoid
  Benign mucous membrane pemphigoid
  DEF: Chronic autoimmune disease characterized by subepidermal blistering lesions of mucosa, including the conjunctiva; seen predominantly in the elderly; produces adhesions and scarring.

L12.2 Chronic bullous disease of childhood `P`
  Juvenile dermatitis herpetiformis

✓5th **L12.3 Acquired epidermolysis bullosa**
  EXCLUDES 1 epidermolysis bullosa (congenital) (Q81.-)

  L12.30 Acquired epidermolysis bullosa, unspecified ▽

  L12.31 Epidermolysis bullosa due to drug
    Use additional code for adverse effect, if applicable, to identify drug (T36-T50 with fifth or sixth character 5)

  L12.35 Other acquired epidermolysis bullosa

L12.8 Other pemphigoid

L12.9 Pemphigoid, unspecified ▽

✓4th **L13 Other bullous disorders**

L13.0 Dermatitis herpetiformis
  Duhring's disease
  Hydroa herpetiformis
  EXCLUDES 1 juvenile dermatitis herpetiformis (L12.2)
    senile dermatitis herpetiformis (L12.0)
  DEF: Skin disease to which people are genetically predisposed resulting from an immunological response to gluten; seen as an extremely pruritic eruption of various lesions that frequently heal, leaving hyperpigmentation or hypopigmentation and occasionally scarring; usually associated with an asymptomatic gluten-sensitive enteropathy.

L13.1 Subcorneal pustular dermatitis
  Sneddon-Wilkinson disease

L13.8 Other specified bullous disorders

L13.9 Bullous disorder, unspecified ▽

L14 **Bullous disorders in diseases classified elsewhere**
  Code first underlying disease

Dermatitis and eczema (L20-L30)

`NOTE` In this block the terms dermatitis and eczema are used synonymously and interchangeably.

EXCLUDES 2 chronic (childhood) granulomatous disease (D71)
dermatitis gangrenosa (L08.0)
dermatitis herpetiformis (L13.0)
dry skin dermatitis (L85.3)
factitial dermatitis (L98.1)
perioral dermatitis (L71.0)
radiation-related disorders of the skin and subcutaneous tissue (L55-L59)
stasis dermatitis (I87.2)

✓4th **L20 Atopic dermatitis**

L20.0 Besnier's prurigo

✓5th **L20.8 Other atopic dermatitis**
  EXCLUDES 2 circumscribed neurodermatitis (L28.0)

  L20.81 Atopic neurodermatitis
    Diffuse neurodermatitis

  L20.82 Flexural eczema

  L20.83 Infantile (acute) (chronic) eczema `P`

  L20.84 Intrinsic (allergic) eczema

  L20.89 Other atopic dermatitis

L20.9 Atopic dermatitis, unspecified ▽

✓4th **L21 Seborrheic dermatitis**
  EXCLUDES 2 infective dermatitis (L30.3)
    seborrheic keratosis (L82.-)

L21.0 Seborrhea capitis `P`
  Cradle cap

L21.1 Seborrheic infantile dermatitis `P`

L21.8 Other seborrheic dermatitis

L21.9 Seborrheic dermatitis, unspecified ▽
  Seborrhea NOS

L22 Diaper dermatitis
  Diaper erythema
  Diaper rash
  Psoriasiform diaper rash

✓4th **L23 Allergic contact dermatitis**
  EXCLUDES 1 allergy NOS (T78.40)
    contact dermatitis NOS (L25.9)
    dermatitis NOS (L30.9)
  EXCLUDES 2 dermatitis due to substances taken internally (L27.-)
    dermatitis of eyelid (H01.1-)
    diaper dermatitis (L22)
    eczema of external ear (H60.5-)
    irritant contact dermatitis (L24.-)
    perioral dermatitis (L71.0)
    radiation-related disorders of the skin and subcutaneous tissue (L55-L59)

L23.0 Allergic contact dermatitis due to metals
  Allergic contact dermatitis due to chromium
  Allergic contact dermatitis due to nickel

L23.1 Allergic contact dermatitis due to adhesives

L23.2 Allergic contact dermatitis due to cosmetics

L23.3 Allergic contact dermatitis due to drugs in contact with skin
  Use additional code for adverse effect, if applicable, to identify drug (T36-T50 with fifth or sixth character 5)
  EXCLUDES 2 dermatitis due to ingested drugs and medicaments (L27.0-L27.1)

L23.4 Allergic contact dermatitis due to dyes

L23.5 Allergic contact dermatitis due to other chemical products
  Allergic contact dermatitis due to cement
  Allergic contact dermatitis due to insecticide
  Allergic contact dermatitis due to plastic
  Allergic contact dermatitis due to rubber

L23.6 Allergic contact dermatitis due to food in contact with the skin
  EXCLUDES 2 dermatitis due to ingested food (L27.2)

L23.7 Allergic contact dermatitis due to plants, except food
  EXCLUDES 2 allergy NOS due to pollen (J30.1)

✓5th **L23.8 Allergic contact dermatitis due to other agents**

  L23.81 Allergic contact dermatitis due to animal (cat) (dog) dander
    Allergic contact dermatitis due to animal (cat) (dog) hair

  L23.89 Allergic contact dermatitis due to other agents

L23.9   **Allergic contact dermatitis, unspecified cause** ▽
       Allergic contact eczema NOS

✓4ᵗʰ **L24**   **Irritant contact dermatitis**
     EXCLUDES 1   *allergy NOS (T78.40)*
               contact dermatitis NOS (L25.9)
               dermatitis NOS (L30.9)
     EXCLUDES 2   *allergic contact dermatitis (L23.-)*
               dermatitis due to substances taken internally (L27.-)
               dermatitis of eyelid (H01.1-)
               diaper dermatitis (L22)
               eczema of external ear (H60.5-)
               perioral dermatitis (L71.0)
               radiation-related disorders of the skin and subcutaneous tissue (L55-L59)

    L24.0   **Irritant contact dermatitis due to** detergents
    L24.1   **Irritant contact dermatitis due to** oils and greases
    L24.2   **Irritant contact dermatitis due to** solvents
          Irritant contact dermatitis due to chlorocompound
          Irritant contact dermatitis due to cyclohexane
          Irritant contact dermatitis due to ester
          Irritant contact dermatitis due to glycol
          Irritant contact dermatitis due to hydrocarbon
          Irritant contact dermatitis due to ketone
    L24.3   **Irritant contact dermatitis due to** cosmetics
    L24.4   **Irritant contact dermatitis due to** drugs in contact with skin
          Use additional code for adverse effect, if applicable, to identify drug (T36-T50 with fifth or sixth character 5)
    L24.5   **Irritant contact dermatitis due to** other chemical products
          Irritant contact dermatitis due to cement
          Irritant contact dermatitis due to insecticide
          Irritant contact dermatitis due to plastic
          Irritant contact dermatitis due to rubber
    L24.6   **Irritant contact dermatitis due to** food in contact with skin
       EXCLUDES 2   *dermatitis due to ingested food (L27.2)*
    L24.7   **Irritant contact dermatitis due to** plants, except food
       EXCLUDES 2   *allergy NOS to pollen (J30.1)*
    ✓5ᵗʰ **L24.8**   **Irritant contact dermatitis due to** other agents
       L24.81   **Irritant contact dermatitis due to** metals
            Irritant contact dermatitis due to chromium
            Irritant contact dermatitis due to nickel
       L24.89   **Irritant contact dermatitis due to other agents**
            Irritant contact dermatitis due to dyes
    L24.9   **Irritant contact dermatitis, unspecified cause** ▽
          Irritant contact eczema NOS

✓4ᵗʰ **L25**   **Unspecified contact dermatitis**
     EXCLUDES 1   *allergic contact dermatitis (L23.-)*
               allergy NOS (T78.40)
               dermatitis NOS (L30.9)
               irritant contact dermatitis (L24.-)
     EXCLUDES 2   *dermatitis due to ingested substances (L27.-)*
               dermatitis of eyelid (H01.1-)
               eczema of external ear (H60.5-)
               perioral dermatitis (L71.0)
               radiation-related disorders of the skin and subcutaneous tissue (L55-L59)

    L25.0   **Unspecified contact dermatitis due to** cosmetics ▽
    L25.1   **Unspecified contact dermatitis due to** drugs in contact with skin ▽
          Use additional code for adverse effect, if applicable, to identify drug (T36-T50 with fifth or sixth character 5)
       EXCLUDES 2   *dermatitis due to ingested drugs and medicaments (L27.0-L27.1)*
    L25.2   **Unspecified contact dermatitis due to** dyes ▽
    L25.3   **Unspecified contact dermatitis due to** other chemical products ▽
          Unspecified contact dermatitis due to cement
          Unspecified contact dermatitis due to insecticide
    L25.4   **Unspecified contact dermatitis due to** food in contact with skin ▽
       EXCLUDES 2   *dermatitis due to ingested food (L27.2)*
    L25.5   **Unspecified contact dermatitis due to** plants, except food ▽
       EXCLUDES 1   *nettle rash (L50.9)*
       EXCLUDES 2   *allergy NOS due to pollen (J30.1)*
    L25.8   **Unspecified contact dermatitis due to other** agents ▽
    L25.9   **Unspecified contact dermatitis, unspecified cause** ▽
          Contact dermatitis (occupational) NOS
          Contact eczema (occupational) NOS

L26   **Exfoliative dermatitis**
          Hebra's pityriasis
     EXCLUDES 1   *Ritter's disease (L00)*

✓4ᵗʰ **L27**   **Dermatitis due to substances taken internally**
     EXCLUDES 1   *allergy NOS (T78.40)*
     EXCLUDES 2   *adverse food reaction, except dermatitis (T78.0-T78.1)*
               contact dermatitis (L23-L25)
               drug photoallergic response (L56.1)
               drug phototoxic response (L56.0)
               urticaria (L50.-)

    L27.0   **Generalized skin eruption due to drugs and medicaments taken internally**
          Use additional code for adverse effect, if applicable, to identify drug (T36-T50 with fifth or sixth character 5)
    L27.1   **Localized skin eruption due to drugs and medicaments taken internally**
          Use additional code for adverse effect, if applicable, to identify drug (T36-T50 with fifth or sixth character 5)
    L27.2   **Dermatitis due to ingested** food
       EXCLUDES 2   *dermatitis due to food in contact with skin (L23.6, L24.6, L25.4)*
    L27.8   **Dermatitis due to other substances taken internally**
    L27.9   **Dermatitis due to unspecified substance taken internally** ▽

✓4ᵗʰ **L28**   **Lichen simplex chronicus and prurigo**
    L28.0   **Lichen simplex chronicus**
          Circumscribed neurodermatitis
          Lichen NOS
    L28.1   **Prurigo nodularis**
    L28.2   **Other prurigo**
          Prurigo NOS
          Prurigo Hebra
          Prurigo mitis
          Urticaria papulosa

✓4ᵗʰ **L29**   **Pruritus**
     EXCLUDES 1   *neurotic excoriation (L98.1)*
               psychogenic pruritus (F45.8)
    L29.0   **Pruritus** ani
    L29.1   **Pruritus** scroti   ♂
    L29.2   **Pruritus** vulvae   ♀
    L29.3   **Anogenital pruritus, unspecified** ▽
    L29.8   **Other pruritus**
    L29.9   **Pruritus, unspecified** ▽
          Itch NOS

✓4ᵗʰ **L30**   **Other and unspecified dermatitis**
     EXCLUDES 2   *contact dermatitis (L23-L25)*
               dry skin dermatitis (L85.3)
               small plaque parapsoriasis (L41.3)
               stasis dermatitis (I87.2)
    L30.0   **Nummular dermatitis**
    L30.1   **Dyshidrosis [pompholyx]**
    L30.2   **Cutaneous autosensitization**
          Candidid [levurid]
          Dermatophytid
          Eczematid
    L30.3   **Infective dermatitis**
          Infectious eczematoid dermatitis
    L30.4   **Erythema intertrigo**
    L30.5   **Pityriasis alba**
    L30.8   **Other specified dermatitis**
    L30.9   **Dermatitis, unspecified** ▽
          Eczema NOS

Papulosquamous disorders (L40-L45)

✓4ᵗʰ **L40**   **Psoriasis**
    L40.0   **Psoriasis** vulgaris
          Nummular psoriasis
          Plaque psoriasis
    L40.1   **Generalized pustular psoriasis**
          Impetigo herpetiformis
          Von Zumbusch's disease
    L40.2   **Acrodermatitis continua**
    L40.3   **Pustulosis palmaris et plantaris**
    L40.4   **Guttate psoriasis**

Ⓝ Newborn: 0   Ⓟ Pediatric: 0-17   Ⓜ Maternity: 12-55   Ⓐ Adult: 15-124   **NRS** Nonroutine supply Dx   **NC Dx** Noncancer Dx   **PDx** Primary Dx   ►◄ Revised Text   ● New Code   ▲ Revised Title

700   ICD-10-CM 2018

✓5ᵗʰ **L40.5** Arthropathic **psoriasis**

    L40.50 Arthropathic **psoriasis, unspecified** ▽

    L40.51 Distal interphalangeal **psoriatic arthropathy**

    L40.52 **Psoriatic arthritis** mutilans

    L40.53 **Psoriatic** spondylitis

    L40.54 **Psoriatic** juvenile **arthropathy**

    L40.59 Other **psoriatic arthropathy**

L40.8 Other **psoriasis**
    Flexural psoriasis

L40.9 **Psoriasis, unspecified** ▽

✓4ᵗʰ **L41** **Parapsoriasis**
    EXCLUDES 1   poikiloderma vasculare atrophicans (L94.5)

L41.0 **Pityriasis lichenoides et varioliformis acuta**
    Mucha-Habermann disease

L41.1 **Pityriasis lichenoides chronica**

L41.3 Small plaque **parapsoriasis**

L41.4 Large plaque **parapsoriasis**

L41.5 Retiform **parapsoriasis**

L41.8 Other **parapsoriasis**

L41.9 **Parapsoriasis, unspecified** ▽

L42 **Pityriasis rosea**

✓4ᵗʰ **L43** **Lichen planus**
    EXCLUDES 1   lichen planopilaris (L66.1)

L43.0 Hypertrophic **lichen planus**

L43.1 Bullous **lichen planus**

L43.2 **Lichenoid** drug reaction
    Use additional code for adverse effect, if applicable, to identify drug (T36-T50 with fifth or sixth character 5)

L43.3 Subacute **(active) lichen planus**
    Lichen planus tropicus

L43.8 Other **lichen planus**

L43.9 **Lichen planus, unspecified** ▽

✓4ᵗʰ **L44** Other **papulosquamous disorders**

L44.0 **Pityriasis rubra pilaris**

L44.1 **Lichen nitidus**
    DEF: Chronic, inflammatory, asymptomatic skin disorder, characterized by numerous glistening, flat-topped, discrete, skin-colored micropapules, most often on the penis, lower abdomen, inner thighs, wrists, forearms, breasts and buttocks.

L44.2 **Lichen striatus**

L44.3 **Lichen ruber moniliformis**

L44.4 **Infantile papular acrodermatitis [Gianotti-Crosti]** ℗

L44.8 Other specified **papulosquamous disorders**

L44.9 **Papulosquamous disorder, unspecified** ▽

L45 *Papulosquamous disorders in diseases classified elsewhere*
    Code first underlying disease

Urticaria and erythema (L49-L54)

EXCLUDES 1   Lyme disease (A69.2-)
    rosacea (L71.-)

✓4ᵗʰ **L49** **Exfoliation due to erythematous conditions according to extent of body surface involved**
    Code first erythematous condition causing exfoliation, such as:
    Ritter's disease (L00)
    (Staphylococcal) scalded skin syndrom (L00)
    Stevens-Johnson syndrome (L51.1)
    Stevens-Johnson syndrome-toxic epidermal necrolysis overlap syndrome (L51.3)
    toxic epidermal necrolysis (L51.2)

L49.0 **Exfoliation due to erythematous condition involving** less than 10 percent **of body surface**
    Exfoliation due to erythematous condition NOS

L49.1 **Exfoliation due to erythematous condition involving** 10-19 percent **of body surface**

L49.2 **Exfoliation due to erythematous condition involving** 20-29 percent **of body surface**

L49.3 **Exfoliation due to erythematous condition involving** 30-39 percent **of body surface**

L49.4 **Exfoliation due to erythematous condition involving** 40-49 percent **of body surface**

L49.5 **Exfoliation due to erythematous condition involving** 50-59 percent **of body surface**

L49.6 **Exfoliation due to erythematous condition involving** 60-69 percent **of body surface**

L49.7 **Exfoliation due to erythematous condition involving** 70-79 percent **of body surface**

L49.8 **Exfoliation due to erythematous condition involving** 80-89 percent **of body surface**

L49.9 **Exfoliation due to erythematous condition involving** 90 or more percent **of body surface**

✓4ᵗʰ **L50** **Urticaria**
    EXCLUDES 1   *allergic contact dermatitis (L23.-)*
    angioneurotic edema (T78.3)
    giant urticaria (T78.3)
    hereditary angio-edema (D84.1)
    Quincke's edema (T78.3)
    serum urticaria (T80.6-)
    solar urticaria (L56.3)
    urticaria neonatorum (P83.8)
    urticaria papulosa (L28.2)
    urticaria pigmentosa (Q82.2)

L50.0 Allergic **urticaria**

L50.1 Idiopathic **urticaria**

L50.2 **Urticaria due to** cold and heat
    EXCLUDES 2   familial cold urticaria (M04.2)

L50.3 Dermatographic **urticaria**

L50.4 Vibratory **urticaria**

L50.5 Cholinergic **urticaria**

L50.6 Contact **urticaria**

L50.8 Other **urticaria**
    Chronic urticaria
    Recurrent periodic urticaria

L50.9 **Urticaria, unspecified** ▽

✓4ᵗʰ **L51** **Erythema** multiforme
    Use additional code for adverse effect, if applicable, to identify drug (T36-T50 with fifth or sixth character 5)
    Use additional code to identify associated manifestations, such as:
    arthropathy associated with dermatological disorders (M14.8-)
    conjunctival edema (H11.42)
    conjunctivitis (H10.22-)
    corneal scars and opacities (H17.-)
    corneal ulcer (H16.0-)
    edema of eyelid (H02.84)
    inflammation of eyelid (H01.8)
    keratoconjunctivitis sicca (H16.22-)
    mechanical lagophthalmos (H02.22-)
    stomatitis (K12.-)
    symblepharon (H11.23-)
    Use additional code to identify percentage of skin exfoliation (L49.-)
    EXCLUDES 1   staphylococcal scalded skin syndrome (L00)
    Ritter's disease (L00)

L51.0 Nonbullous **erythema multiforme**

L51.1 **Stevens-Johnson syndrome**

L51.2 **Toxic epidermal necrolysis [Lyell]**

L51.3 **Stevens-Johnson syndrome-toxic epidermal necrolysis overlap syndrome**
    SJS-TEN overlap syndrome

L51.8 Other **erythema multiforme**

L51.9 **Erythema multiforme, unspecified** ▽
    Erythema iris
    Erythema multiforme major NOS
    Erythema multiforme minor NOS
    Herpes iris

L52 **Erythema** nodosum
    EXCLUDES 1   tuberculous erythema nodosum (A18.4)
    DEF: A form of panniculitis (inflammation of the fat layer beneath the skin) of particularly women, usually seen as a hypersensitivity reaction to infections, drugs, sarcoidosis, and specific enteropathies; the acute stage is associated with fever, malaise, and arthralgia; the lesions are pink to blue in color as tender nodules and are found on the front of the legs below the knees.

✓4ᵗʰ **L53** Other **erythematous conditions**
    EXCLUDES 1   erythema ab igne (L59.0)
    erythema due to external agents in contact with skin (L23-L25)
    erythema intertrigo (L30.4)

L53.0 **Toxic erythema**
    Code first poisoning due to drug or toxin, if applicable (T36-T65 with fifth or sixth character 1-4 or 6)
    Use additional code for adverse effect, if applicable, to identify drug (T36-T50 with fifth or sixth character 5)
    EXCLUDES 1   neonatal erythema toxicum (P83.1)

✓ Additional Character Req   ✓x7ᵗʰ Placeholder Alert   Case-Mix Diagnosis   Manifestation   ▽ Unspecified Dx   EXCLUDES 1 Not coded here   EXCLUDES 2 Not included here

ICD-10-CM 2018

701

L40.5–L53.0

Chapter 12. Diseases of the Skin and Subcutaneous Tissue

L53.1–L66.9

L53.1 Erythema annulare centrifugum

L53.2 Erythema marginatum

L53.3 Other chronic figurate **erythema**

L53.8 Other specified erythematous conditions

L53.9 Erythematous condition, unspecified ▽
  Erythema NOS
  Erythroderma NOS

L54 Erythema in diseases classified elsewhere
  Code first underlying disease

Radiation-related disorders of the skin and subcutaneous tissue (L55-L59)

☑4th **L55 Sunburn**

L55.0 Sunburn of first degree

L55.1 Sunburn of second degree

L55.2 Sunburn of third degree

L55.9 Sunburn, unspecified ▽

☑4th **L56 Other acute skin changes due to ultraviolet radiation**
  Use additional code to identify the source of the ultraviolet radiation (W89, X32)

L56.0 Drug phototoxic response
  Use additional code for adverse effect, if applicable, to identify drug (T36-T50 with fifth or sixth character 5)

L56.1 Drug photoallergic response
  Use additional code for adverse effect, if applicable, to identify drug (T36-T50 with fifth or sixth character 5)

L56.2 Photocontact dermatitis [berloque dermatitis]

L56.3 Solar urticaria

L56.4 Polymorphous light eruption

L56.5 Disseminated superficial actinic porokeratosis (DSAP)
  DEF: Autosomal dominant skin condition occurring in sun-exposed areas of the skin (particularly the arms and legs); characterized by superficial annular, keratotic, brownish-red spots or thickenings with depressed centers and sharp, ridged borders; may evolve into squamous cell carcinoma.

L56.8 Other specified acute skin changes due to ultraviolet radiation

L56.9 Acute skin change due to ultraviolet radiation, unspecified ▽

☑4th **L57 Skin changes due to chronic exposure to nonionizing radiation**
  Use additional code to identify the source of the ultraviolet radiation
  ▶(W89)◀

L57.0 Actinic keratosis
  Keratosis NOS
  Senile keratosis
  Solar keratosis

L57.1 Actinic reticuloid

L57.2 Cutis rhomboidalis nuchae

L57.3 Poikiloderma of Civatte

L57.4 Cutis laxa senilis
  Elastosis senilis

L57.5 Actinic granuloma

L57.8 Other skin changes due to chronic exposure to nonionizing radiation
  Farmer's skin
  Sailor's skin
  Solar dermatitis

L57.9 Skin changes due to chronic exposure to nonionizing radiation, unspecified ▽

☑4th **L58 Radiodermatitis**
  Use additional code to identify the source of the radiation (W88, W90)

L58.0 Acute radiodermatitis

L58.1 Chronic radiodermatitis

L58.9 Radiodermatitis, unspecified ▽

☑4th **L59 Other disorders of skin and subcutaneous tissue related to radiation**

L59.0 Erythema ab igne [dermatitis ab igne]

L59.8 Other specified disorders of the skin and subcutaneous tissue related to radiation
  AHA: 2017, 1Q, 33

L59.9 Disorder of the skin and subcutaneous tissue related to radiation, unspecified ▽

Nail Disorders

Normal

Koilonychia

Beau's Lines

Disorders of skin appendages (L60-L75)

EXCLUDES 1 congenital malformations of integument (Q84.-)

☑4th **L60 Nail disorders**
  EXCLUDES 2 clubbing of nails (R68.3)
  onychia and paronychia (L03.0-)

L60.0 Ingrowing nail

L60.1 Onycholysis

L60.2 Onychogryphosis

L60.3 Nail dystrophy

L60.4 Beau's lines

L60.5 Yellow nail syndrome

L60.8 Other nail disorders

L60.9 Nail disorder, unspecified ▽

L62 Nail disorders in diseases classified elsewhere
  Code first underlying disease, such as:
  pachydermoperiostosis (M89.4-)

☑4th **L63 Alopecia areata**

L63.0 Alopecia (capitis) totalis

L63.1 Alopecia universalis

L63.2 Ophiasis

L63.8 Other alopecia areata

L63.9 Alopecia areata, unspecified ▽

☑4th **L64 Androgenic alopecia**
  INCLUDES male-pattern baldness

L64.0 Drug-induced androgenic alopecia
  Use additional code for adverse effect, if applicable, to identify drug (T36-T50 with fifth or sixth character 5)

L64.8 Other androgenic alopecia

L64.9 Androgenic alopecia, unspecified ▽

☑4th **L65 Other nonscarring hair loss**
  Use additional code for adverse effect, if applicable, to identify drug (T36-T50 with fifth or sixth character 5)
  EXCLUDES 1 trichotillomania (F63.3)

L65.0 Telogen effluvium
  DEF: A form of nonscarring alopecia characterized by shedding of hair from premature telogen development in follicles due to stress, including shock, childbirth, surgery, drugs, or weight loss.

L65.1 Anagen effluvium

L65.2 Alopecia mucinosa

L65.8 Other specified nonscarring hair loss

L65.9 Nonscarring hair loss, unspecified ▽
  Alopecia NOS

☑4th **L66 Cicatricial alopecia [scarring hair loss]**

L66.0 Pseudopelade

L66.1 Lichen planopilaris
  Follicular lichen planus

L66.2 Folliculitis decalvans

L66.3 Perifolliculitis capitis abscedens

L66.4 Folliculitis ulerythematosa reticulata

L66.8 Other cicatricial alopecia
  AHA: 2015, 1Q, 19

L66.9 Cicatricial alopecia, unspecified ▽

Ⓝ Newborn: 0   Ⓟ Pediatric: 0-17   Ⓜ Maternity: 12-55   Ⓐ Adult: 15-124   **NRS** Nonroutine supply Dx   **NCDx** Noncancer Dx   **PDx** Primary Dx   ▶◀ Revised Text   ● New Code   ▲ Revised Title

702   ICD-10-CM 2018

✓4ᵗʰ L67   Hair color and hair shaft abnormalities

EXCLUDES 1   monilethrix (Q84.1)
pili annulati (Q84.1)
telogen effluvium (L65.0)

L67.0   Trichorrhexis nodosa

L67.1   Variations in hair color
Canities
Greyness, hair (premature)
Heterochromia of hair
Poliosis circumscripta, acquired
Poliosis NOS

L67.8   Other hair color and hair shaft abnormalities
Fragilitas crinium

L67.9   Hair color and hair shaft abnormality, unspecified ▽

✓4ᵗʰ L68   Hypertrichosis

INCLUDES   excess hair

EXCLUDES 1   congenital hypertrichosis (Q84.2)
persistent lanugo (Q84.2)

L68.0   Hirsutism

L68.1   Acquired hypertrichosis lanuginosa

L68.2   Localized hypertrichosis

L68.3   Polytrichia

L68.8   Other hypertrichosis

L68.9   Hypertrichosis, unspecified ▽

✓4ᵗʰ L70   Acne

EXCLUDES 2   acne keloid (L73.0)

L70.0   Acne vulgaris

L70.1   Acne conglobata

L70.2   Acne varioliformis
Acne necrotica miliaris
DEF: Rare form of acne characterized by development of persistent brown papulo-pustules followed by scar formation; usually on the brow and temporoparietal part of the scalp.

L70.3   Acne tropica

L70.4   Infantile acne   ℙ

L70.5   Acné excoriée
Acné excoriée des jeunes filles
Picker's acne

L70.8   Other acne

L70.9   Acne, unspecified ▽

✓4ᵗʰ L71   Rosacea

Use additional code for adverse effect, if applicable, to identify drug (T36-T50 with fifth or sixth character 5)

L71.0   Perioral dermatitis

L71.1   Rhinophyma

L71.8   Other rosacea

L71.9   Rosacea, unspecified ▽

✓4ᵗʰ L72   Follicular cysts of skin and subcutaneous tissue

L72.0   Epidermal cyst

✓5ᵗʰ L72.1   Pilar and trichodermal cyst

     L72.11   Pilar cyst

     L72.12   Trichodermal cyst
Trichilemmal (proliferating) cyst

L72.2   Steatocystoma multiplex

L72.3   Sebaceous cyst
EXCLUDES 2   pilar cyst (L72.11)
trichilemmal (proliferating) cyst (L72.12)

L72.8   Other follicular cysts of the skin and subcutaneous tissue

L72.9   Follicular cyst of the skin and subcutaneous tissue, unspecified ▽

✓4ᵗʰ L73   Other follicular disorders

L73.0   Acne keloid

L73.1   Pseudofolliculitis barbae

L73.2   Hidradenitis suppurativa

L73.8   Other specified follicular disorders
Sycosis barbae

L73.9   Follicular disorder, unspecified ▽

✓4ᵗʰ L74   Eccrine sweat disorders

EXCLUDES 2   generalized hyperhidrosis (R61)

L74.0   Miliaria rubra

L74.1   Miliaria crystallina

L74.2   Miliaria profunda
Miliaria tropicalis

L74.3   Miliaria, unspecified ▽

L74.4   Anhidrosis
Hypohidrosis

✓5ᵗʰ L74.5   Focal hyperhidrosis

   ✓6ᵗʰ L74.51   Primary focal hyperhidrosis

     L74.510   Primary focal hyperhidrosis, axilla

     L74.511   Primary focal hyperhidrosis, face

     L74.512   Primary focal hyperhidrosis, palms

     L74.513   Primary focal hyperhidrosis, soles

     L74.519   Primary focal hyperhidrosis, unspecified ▽

   L74.52   Secondary focal hyperhidrosis
Frey's syndrome

L74.8   Other eccrine sweat disorders

L74.9   Eccrine sweat disorder, unspecified ▽
Sweat gland disorder NOS

✓4ᵗʰ L75   Apocrine sweat disorders

EXCLUDES 1   dyshidrosis (L30.1)
hidradenitis suppurativa (L73.2)

L75.0   Bromhidrosis

L75.1   Chromhidrosis

L75.2   Apocrine miliaria
Fox-Fordyce disease
DEF: Chronic, usually pruritic disease evidenced by small follicular papular eruptions, especially in the axillary and pubic areas; develops from the closure and rupture of the affected apocrine glands' intraepidermal portion of the ducts.

L75.8   Other apocrine sweat disorders

L75.9   Apocrine sweat disorder, unspecified ▽

Intraoperative and postprocedural complications of skin and subcutaneous tissue (L76)

✓4ᵗʰ L76   Intraoperative and postprocedural complications of skin and subcutaneous tissue

✓5ᵗʰ L76.0   Intraoperative hemorrhage and hematoma of skin and subcutaneous tissue complicating a procedure

EXCLUDES 1   intraoperative hemorrhage and hematoma of skin and subcutaneous tissue due to accidental puncture and laceration during a procedure (L76.1-)

   L76.01   Intraoperative hemorrhage and hematoma of skin and subcutaneous tissue complicating a dermatologic procedure

   L76.02   Intraoperative hemorrhage and hematoma of skin and subcutaneous tissue complicating other procedure

✓5ᵗʰ L76.1   Accidental puncture and laceration of skin and subcutaneous tissue during a procedure

   L76.11   Accidental puncture and laceration of skin and subcutaneous tissue during a dermatologic procedure

   L76.12   Accidental puncture and laceration of skin and subcutaneous tissue during other procedure

✓5ᵗʰ L76.2   Postprocedural hemorrhage of skin and subcutaneous tissue following a procedure

   L76.21   Postprocedural hemorrhage of skin and subcutaneous tissue following a dermatologic procedure

   L76.22   Postprocedural hemorrhage of skin and subcutaneous tissue following other procedure

✓5ᵗʰ L76.3   Postprocedural hematoma and seroma of skin and subcutaneous tissue following a procedure

   L76.31   Postprocedural hematoma of skin and subcutaneous tissue following a dermatologic procedure

   L76.32   Postprocedural hematoma of skin and subcutaneous tissue following other procedure

   L76.33   Postprocedural seroma of skin and subcutaneous tissue following a dermatologic procedure

   L76.34   Postprocedural seroma of skin and subcutaneous tissue following other procedure

✓5ᵗʰ L76.8   Other intraoperative and postprocedural complications of skin and subcutaneous tissue

Use additional code, if applicable, to further specify disorder

   L76.81   Other intraoperative complications of skin and subcutaneous tissue

   L76.82   Other postprocedural complications of skin and subcutaneous tissue

---

✓ Additional Character Req   ✓x7ᵗʰ Placeholder Alert   Case-Mix Diagnosis   Manifestation   ▽ Unspecified Dx   **EXCLUDES 1** Not coded here   **EXCLUDES 2** Not included here

Chapter 12. Diseases of the Skin and Subcutaneous Tissue

Other disorders of the skin and subcutaneous tissue (L80-L99)

L80   Vitiligo
> EXCLUDES 2   vitiligo of eyelids (H02.73-)
>   vitiligo of vulva (N90.89)
> **DEF:** Persistent, progressive development of nonpigmented white patches on otherwise normal skin.

✓4th L81   Other disorders of pigmentation
> EXCLUDES 1   birthmark NOS (Q82.5)
>   Peutz-Jeghers syndrome (Q85.8)
> EXCLUDES 2   nevus—see Alphabetical Index

- **L81.0**   Postinflammatory hyperpigmentation
- **L81.1**   Chloasma
- **L81.2**   Freckles
- **L81.3**   Café au lait spots
- **L81.4**   Other melanin hyperpigmentation
  > Lentigo
- **L81.5**   Leukoderma, not elsewhere classified
- **L81.6**   Other disorders of diminished melanin formation
- **L81.7**   Pigmented purpuric dermatosis
  > Angioma serpiginosum
- **L81.8**   Other specified disorders of pigmentation
  > Iron pigmentation
  > Tattoo pigmentation
- **L81.9**   Disorder of pigmentation, unspecified   ▽

✓4th L82   Seborrheic keratosis
> INCLUDES   basal cell papilloma
>   dermatosis papulosa nigra
>   Leser-Trélat disease
> EXCLUDES 2   seborrheic dermatitis (L21.-)

- **L82.0**   **Inflamed** seborrheic keratosis
- **L82.1**   Other seborrheic keratosis
  > Seborrheic keratosis NOS

L83   Acanthosis nigricans
> Confluent and reticulated papillomatosis
> **DEF:** Diffuse, velvety hyperplasia of the spinous skin layer of the axilla and other body folds marked by gray, brown, or black pigmentation; in adult form often associated with malignant acanthosis nigricans in a benign, nevoid form relatively generalized.

L84   Corns and callosities
> Callus
> Clavus

✓4th L85   Other epidermal thickening
> EXCLUDES 2   hypertrophic disorders of the skin (L91.-)

- **L85.0**   Acquired ichthyosis
  > EXCLUDES 1   congenital ichthyosis (Q80.-)
- **L85.1**   Acquired keratosis [keratoderma] palmaris et plantaris
  > EXCLUDES 1   inherited keratosis palmaris et plantaris (Q82.8)
- **L85.2**   Keratosis punctata (palmaris et plantaris)
- **L85.3**   Xerosis cutis
  > Dry skin dermatitis
- **L85.8**   Other specified epidermal thickening
  > Cutaneous horn
- **L85.9**   Epidermal thickening, unspecified   ▽

L86   *Keratoderma in diseases classified elsewhere*
> Code first underlying disease, such as:
>   Reiter's disease (M02.3-)
> EXCLUDES 1   gonococcal keratoderma (A54.89)
>   gonococcal keratosis (A54.89)
>   keratoderma due to vitamin A deficiency (E50.8)
>   keratosis due to vitamin A deficiency (E50.8)
>   xeroderma due to vitamin A deficiency (E50.8)

✓4th L87   Transepidermal elimination disorders
> EXCLUDES 1   granuloma annulare (perforating) (L92.0)

- **L87.0**   Keratosis follicularis et parafollicularis in cutem penetrans
  > Hyperkeratosis follicularis penetrans
  > Kyrle disease
- **L87.1**   Reactive perforating collagenosis
- **L87.2**   Elastosis perforans serpiginosa
- **L87.8**   Other transepidermal elimination disorders
- **L87.9**   Transepidermal elimination disorder, unspecified   ▽

L88   Pyoderma gangrenosum   NRS
> Phagedenic pyoderma
> EXCLUDES 1   dermatitis gangrenosa (L08.0)
> **DEF:** Persistent debilitating skin disease characterized by irregular, boggy, blue-red ulcerations, with central healing and undermined edges.

Four Stages of Pressure Ulcer

Stage 1
Persistent focal erythema

Stage 2
Abrasion, blister, partial thickness skin loss involving epidermis and/or dermis

Stage 3
Full thickness skin loss involving damage or necrosis of subcutaneous tissue

Stage 4
Necrosis of soft tissues through to underlying muscle, tendon, or bone

✓4th L89   Pressure ulcer
> INCLUDES   bed sore
>   decubitus ulcer
>   plaster ulcer
>   pressure area
>   pressure sore
> Code first any associated gangrene (I96)
> EXCLUDES 2   decubitus (trophic) ulcer of cervix (uteri) (N86)
>   diabetic ulcers (E08.621, E08.622, E09.621, E09.622, E10.621, E10.622, E11.621, E11.622, E13.621, E13.622)
>   non-pressure chronic ulcer of skin (L97.-)
>   skin infections (L00-L08)
>   varicose ulcer (I83.0, I83.2)
> **AHA:** 2017, 1Q, 49; 2016, 4Q, 143

✓5th L89.0   Pressure ulcer of **elbow**

✓6th L89.00   Pressure ulcer of **unspecified elbow**

- **L89.000**   Pressure ulcer of unspecified elbow, **unstageable**   ▽
- **L89.001**   Pressure ulcer of unspecified elbow, **stage 1**   ▽
  > Healing pressure ulcer of unspecified elbow, stage 1
  > Pressure pre-ulcer skin changes limited to persistent focal edema, unspecified elbow
- **L89.002**   Pressure ulcer of unspecified elbow, **stage 2**   ▽
  > Healing pressure ulcer of unspecified elbow, stage 2
  > Pressure ulcer with abrasion, blister, partial thickness skin loss involving epidermis and/or dermis, unspecified elbow
- **L89.003**   Pressure ulcer of unspecified elbow, **stage 3**   ▽
  > Healing pressure ulcer of unspecified elbow, stage 3
  > Pressure ulcer with full thickness skin loss involving damage or necrosis of subcutaneous tissue, unspecified elbow
- **L89.004**   Pressure ulcer of unspecified elbow, **stage 4**   ▽
  > Healing pressure ulcer of unspecified elbow, stage 4
  > Pressure ulcer with necrosis of soft tissues through to underlying muscle, tendon, or bone, unspecified elbow
- **L89.009**   Pressure ulcer of unspecified elbow, **unspecified stage**   ▽
  > Healing pressure ulcer of elbow NOS
  > Healing pressure ulcer of unspecified elbow, unspecified stage

Labels on figures: Epidermis, Dermis, Subcutaneous tissue, Superficial fascia, Muscle, Deep fascia, Bone

---

Ⓝ Newborn: 0   Ⓟ Pediatric: 0-17   Ⓜ Maternity: 12-55   Ⓐ Adult: 15-124   NRS Nonroutine supply Dx   NCDx Noncancer Dx   PDx Primary Dx   ◄► Revised Text   ● New Code   ▲ Revised Title

704   ICD-10-CM 2018

✓6ᵗʰ **L89.01** **Pressure ulcer of** right elbow
  L89.010 **Pressure ulcer of right elbow,** unstageable
  L89.011 **Pressure ulcer of right elbow,** stage 1
    Healing pressure ulcer of right elbow, stage 1
    Pressure pre-ulcer skin changes limited to persistent focal edema, right elbow
  L89.012 **Pressure ulcer of right elbow,** stage 2
    Healing pressure ulcer of right elbow, stage 2
    Pressure ulcer with abrasion, blister, partial thickness skin loss involving epidermis and/or dermis, right elbow
  L89.013 **Pressure ulcer of right elbow,** stage 3
    Healing pressure ulcer of right elbow, stage 3
    Pressure ulcer with full thickness skin loss involving damage or necrosis of subcutaneous tissue, right elbow
  L89.014 **Pressure ulcer of right elbow,** stage 4
    Healing pressure ulcer of right elbow, stage 4
    Pressure ulcer with necrosis of soft tissues through to underlying muscle, tendon, or bone, right elbow
  L89.019 **Pressure ulcer of right elbow, unspecified stage** ▽
    Healing pressure right of elbow NOS
    ▶Healing pressure ulcer of right elbow, unspecified stage◀

✓6ᵗʰ **L89.02** **Pressure ulcer of** left elbow
  L89.020 **Pressure ulcer of left elbow,** unstageable
  L89.021 **Pressure ulcer of left elbow,** stage 1
    Healing pressure ulcer of left elbow, stage 1
    Pressure pre-ulcer skin changes limited to persistent focal edema, left elbow
  L89.022 **Pressure ulcer of left elbow,** stage 2
    Healing pressure ulcer of left elbow, stage 2
    Pressure ulcer with abrasion, blister, partial thickness skin loss involving epidermis and/or dermis, left elbow
  L89.023 **Pressure ulcer of left elbow,** stage 3
    Healing pressure ulcer of left elbow, stage 3
    Pressure ulcer with full thickness skin loss involving damage or necrosis of subcutaneous tissue, left elbow
  L89.024 **Pressure ulcer of left elbow,** stage 4
    Healing pressure ulcer of left elbow, stage 4
    Pressure ulcer with necrosis of soft tissues through to underlying muscle, tendon, or bone, left elbow
  L89.029 **Pressure ulcer of left elbow, unspecified stage** ▽
    Healing pressure ulcer of left elbow NOS
    ▶Healing pressure ulcer of left elbow, unspecified stage◀

✓5ᵗʰ **L89.1** **Pressure ulcer of** back
  ✓6ᵗʰ **L89.10** **Pressure ulcer of** unspecified part of back
    L89.100 **Pressure ulcer of unspecified part of back,** unstageable ▽
    L89.101 **Pressure ulcer of unspecified part of back,** stage 1 ▽
      Healing pressure ulcer of unspecified part of back, stage 1
      Pressure pre-ulcer skin changes limited to persistent focal edema, unspecified part of back
    L89.102 **Pressure ulcer of unspecified part of back,** stage 2 ▽
      Healing pressure ulcer of unspecified part of back, stage 2
      Pressure ulcer with abrasion, blister, partial thickness skin loss involving epidermis and/or dermis, unspecified part of back
    L89.103 **Pressure ulcer of unspecified part of back,** stage 3 ▽
      Healing pressure ulcer of unspecified part of back, stage 3
      Pressure ulcer with full thickness skin loss involving damage or necrosis of subcutaneous tissue, unspecified part of back

    L89.104 **Pressure ulcer of unspecified part of back,** stage 4 ▽
      Healing pressure ulcer of unspecified part of back, stage 4
      Pressure ulcer with necrosis of soft tissues through to underlying muscle, tendon, or bone, unspecified part of back
    L89.109 **Pressure ulcer of unspecified part of back, unspecified stage** ▽
      Healing pressure ulcer of unspecified part of back NOS
      Healing pressure ulcer of unspecified part of back, unspecified stage

✓6ᵗʰ **L89.11** **Pressure ulcer of** right upper back
  Pressure ulcer of right shoulder blade
  L89.110 **Pressure ulcer of right upper back,** unstageable
  L89.111 **Pressure ulcer of right upper back,** stage 1
    Healing pressure ulcer of right upper back, stage 1
    Pressure pre-ulcer skin changes limited to persistent focal edema, right upper back
  L89.112 **Pressure ulcer of right upper back,** stage 2
    Healing pressure ulcer of right upper back, stage 2
    Pressure ulcer with abrasion, blister, partial thickness skin loss involving epidermis and/or dermis, right upper back
  L89.113 **Pressure ulcer of right upper back,** stage 3
    Healing pressure ulcer of right upper back, stage 3
    Pressure ulcer with full thickness skin loss involving damage or necrosis of subcutaneous tissue, right upper back
  L89.114 **Pressure ulcer of right upper back,** stage 4
    Healing pressure ulcer of right upper back, stage 4
    Pressure ulcer with necrosis of soft tissues through to underlying muscle, tendon, or bone, right upper back
  L89.119 **Pressure ulcer of right upper back, unspecified stage** ▽
    Healing pressure ulcer of right upper back NOS
    Healing pressure ulcer of right upper back, unspecified stage

✓6ᵗʰ **L89.12** **Pressure ulcer of** left upper back
  Pressure ulcer of left shoulder blade
  L89.120 **Pressure ulcer of left upper back,** unstageable
  L89.121 **Pressure ulcer of left upper back,** stage 1
    Healing pressure ulcer of left upper back, stage 1
    Pressure pre-ulcer skin changes limited to persistent focal edema, left upper back
  L89.122 **Pressure ulcer of left upper back,** stage 2
    Healing pressure ulcer of left upper back, stage 2
    Pressure ulcer with abrasion, blister, partial thickness skin loss involving epidermis and/or dermis, left upper back
  L89.123 **Pressure ulcer of left upper back,** stage 3
    Healing pressure ulcer of left upper back, stage 3
    Pressure ulcer with full thickness skin loss involving damage or necrosis of subcutaneous tissue, left upper back
  L89.124 **Pressure ulcer of left upper back,** stage 4
    Healing pressure ulcer of left upper back, stage 4
    Pressure ulcer with necrosis of soft tissues through to underlying muscle, tendon, or bone, left upper back
  L89.129 **Pressure ulcer of left upper back, unspecified stage** ▽
    Healing pressure ulcer of left upper back NOS
    Healing pressure ulcer of left upper back, unspecified stage

✓6ᵗʰ **L89.13** Pressure ulcer of right lower back

L89.130 **Pressure ulcer of right lower back, unstageable**

L89.131 **Pressure ulcer of right lower back, stage 1**
Healing pressure ulcer of right lower back, stage 1
Pressure pre-ulcer skin changes limited to persistent focal edema, right lower back

L89.132 **Pressure ulcer of right lower back, stage 2**
Healing pressure ulcer of right lower back, stage 2
Pressure ulcer with abrasion, blister, partial thickness skin loss involving epidermis and/or dermis, right lower back

L89.133 **Pressure ulcer of right lower back, stage 3**
Healing pressure ulcer of right lower back, stage 3
Pressure ulcer with full thickness skin loss involving damage or necrosis of subcutaneous tissue, right lower back

L89.134 **Pressure ulcer of right lower back, stage 4**
Healing pressure ulcer of right lower back, stage 4
Pressure ulcer with necrosis of soft tissues through to underlying muscle, tendon, or bone, right lower back

L89.139 **Pressure ulcer of right lower back, unspecified stage** ▽
Healing pressure ulcer of right lower back NOS
Healing pressure ulcer of right lower back, unspecified stage

✓6ᵗʰ **L89.14** Pressure ulcer of left lower back

L89.140 **Pressure ulcer of left lower back, unstageable**

L89.141 **Pressure ulcer of left lower back, stage 1**
Healing pressure ulcer of left lower back, stage 1
Pressure pre-ulcer skin changes limited to persistent focal edema, left lower back

L89.142 **Pressure ulcer of left lower back, stage 2**
Healing pressure ulcer of left lower back, stage 2
Pressure ulcer with abrasion, blister, partial thickness skin loss involving epidermis and/or dermis, left lower back

L89.143 **Pressure ulcer of left lower back, stage 3**
Healing pressure ulcer of left lower back, stage 3
Pressure ulcer with full thickness skin loss involving damage or necrosis of subcutaneous tissue, left lower back

L89.144 **Pressure ulcer of left lower back, stage 4**
Healing pressure ulcer of left lower back, stage 4
Pressure ulcer with necrosis of soft tissues through to underlying muscle, tendon, or bone, left lower back

L89.149 **Pressure ulcer of left lower back, unspecified stage** ▽
Healing pressure ulcer of left lower back NOS
Healing pressure ulcer of left lower back, unspecified stage

✓6ᵗʰ **L89.15** Pressure ulcer of sacral region
Pressure ulcer of coccyx
Pressure ulcer of tailbone

L89.150 **Pressure ulcer of sacral region, unstageable**

L89.151 **Pressure ulcer of sacral region, stage 1**
Healing pressure ulcer of sacral region, stage 1
Pressure pre-ulcer skin changes limited to persistent focal edema, sacral region

L89.152 **Pressure ulcer of sacral region, stage 2**
Healing pressure ulcer of sacral region, stage 2
Pressure ulcer with abrasion, blister, partial thickness skin loss involving epidermis and/or dermis, sacral region

L89.153 **Pressure ulcer of sacral region, stage 3**
Healing pressure ulcer of sacral region, stage 3
Pressure ulcer with full thickness skin loss involving damage or necrosis of subcutaneous tissue, sacral region

L89.154 **Pressure ulcer of sacral region, stage 4**
Healing pressure ulcer of sacral region, stage 4
Pressure ulcer with necrosis of soft tissues through to underlying muscle, tendon, or bone, sacral region

L89.159 **Pressure ulcer of sacral region, unspecified stage** ▽
Healing pressure ulcer of sacral region NOS
Healing pressure ulcer of sacral region, unspecified stage

✓5ᵗʰ **L89.2** Pressure ulcer of hip

✓6ᵗʰ **L89.20** Pressure ulcer of unspecified hip

L89.200 **Pressure ulcer of unspecified hip, unstageable** ▽

L89.201 **Pressure ulcer of unspecified hip, stage 1** ▽
Healing pressure ulcer of unspecified hip, stage 1
Pressure pre-ulcer skin changes limited to persistent focal edema, unspecified hip

L89.202 **Pressure ulcer of unspecified hip, stage 2** ▽
Healing pressure ulcer of unspecified hip, stage 2
Pressure ulcer with abrasion, blister, partial thickness skin loss involving epidermis and/or dermis, unspecified hip

L89.203 **Pressure ulcer of unspecified hip, stage 3** ▽
Healing pressure ulcer of unspecified hip, stage 3
Pressure ulcer with full thickness skin loss involving damage or necrosis of subcutaneous tissue, unspecified hip

L89.204 **Pressure ulcer of unspecified hip, stage 4** ▽
Healing pressure ulcer of unspecified hip, stage 4
Pressure ulcer with necrosis of soft tissues through to underlying muscle, tendon, or bone, unspecified hip

L89.209 **Pressure ulcer of unspecified hip, unspecified stage** ▽
Healing pressure ulcer of unspecified hip NOS
Healing pressure ulcer of unspecified hip, unspecified stage

✓6ᵗʰ **L89.21** Pressure ulcer of right hip

L89.210 **Pressure ulcer of right hip, unstageable**

L89.211 **Pressure ulcer of right hip, stage 1**
Healing pressure ulcer of right hip, stage 1
Pressure pre-ulcer skin changes limited to persistent focal edema, right hip

L89.212 **Pressure ulcer of right hip, stage 2**
Healing pressure ulcer of right hip, stage 2
Pressure ulcer with abrasion, blister, partial thickness skin loss involving epidermis and/or dermis, right hip

L89.213 **Pressure ulcer of right hip, stage 3**
Healing pressure ulcer of right hip, stage 3
Pressure ulcer with full thickness skin loss involving damage or necrosis of subcutaneous tissue, right hip

L89.214 **Pressure ulcer of right hip, stage 4**
Healing pressure ulcer of right hip, stage 4
Pressure ulcer with necrosis of soft tissues through to underlying muscle, tendon, or bone, right hip

L89.219 **Pressure ulcer of right hip, unspecified stage** ▽
Healing pressure ulcer of right hip NOS
Healing pressure ulcer of right hip, unspecified stage

☑6ᵗʰ **L89.22** **Pressure ulcer of** left hip

    L89.220 **Pressure ulcer of left hip,** unstageable

    L89.221 **Pressure ulcer of left hip,** stage 1
        Healing pressure ulcer of left hip, stage 1
        Pressure pre-ulcer skin changes limited to persistent focal edema, left hip

    L89.222 **Pressure ulcer of left hip,** stage 2
        Healing pressure ulcer of left hip, stage 2
        Pressure ulcer with abrasion, blister, partial thickness skin loss involving epidermis and/or dermis, left hip

    L89.223 **Pressure ulcer of left hip,** stage 3
        Healing pressure ulcer of left hip, stage 3
        Pressure ulcer with full thickness skin loss involving damage or necrosis of subcutaneous tissue, left hip

    L89.224 **Pressure ulcer of left hip,** stage 4
        Healing pressure ulcer of left hip, stage 4
        Pressure ulcer with necrosis of soft tissues through to underlying muscle, tendon, or bone, left hip

    L89.229 **Pressure ulcer of left hip, unspecified stage** ▽
        Healing pressure ulcer of left hip NOS
        Healing pressure ulcer of left hip, unspecified stage

☑5ᵗʰ **L89.3** **Pressure ulcer of** buttock

  ☑6ᵗʰ **L89.30** **Pressure ulcer of** unspecified buttock

    L89.300 **Pressure ulcer of unspecified buttock, unstageable** ▽

    L89.301 **Pressure ulcer of unspecified buttock, stage 1** ▽
        Healing pressure ulcer of unspecified buttock, stage 1
        Pressure pre-ulcer skin changes limited to persistent focal edema, unspecified buttock

    L89.302 **Pressure ulcer of unspecified buttock, stage 2** ▽
        Healing pressure ulcer of unspecified buttock, stage 2
        Pressure ulcer with abrasion, blister, partial thickness skin loss involving epidermis and/or dermis, unspecified buttock

    L89.303 **Pressure ulcer of unspecified buttock, stage 3** ▽
        Healing pressure ulcer of unspecified buttock, stage 3
        Pressure ulcer with full thickness skin loss involving damage or necrosis of subcutaneous tissue, unspecified buttock

    L89.304 **Pressure ulcer of unspecified buttock, stage 4** ▽
        Healing pressure ulcer of unspecified buttock, stage 4
        Pressure ulcer with necrosis of soft tissues through to underlying muscle, tendon, or bone, unspecified buttock

    L89.309 **Pressure ulcer of unspecified buttock, unspecified stage** ▽
        Healing pressure ulcer of unspecified buttock NOS
        Healing pressure ulcer of unspecified buttock, unspecified stage

  ☑6ᵗʰ **L89.31** **Pressure ulcer of** right buttock

    L89.310 **Pressure ulcer of right buttock, unstageable**

    L89.311 **Pressure ulcer of right buttock,** stage 1
        Healing pressure ulcer of right buttock, stage 1
        Pressure pre-ulcer skin changes limited to persistent focal edema, right buttock

    L89.312 **Pressure ulcer of right buttock,** stage 2
        Healing pressure ulcer of right buttock, stage 2
        Pressure ulcer with abrasion, blister, partial thickness skin loss involving epidermis and/or dermis, right buttock

    L89.313 **Pressure ulcer of right buttock,** stage 3
        Healing pressure ulcer of right buttock, stage 3
        Pressure ulcer with full thickness skin loss involving damage or necrosis of subcutaneous tissue, right buttock

    L89.314 **Pressure ulcer of right buttock,** stage 4
        Healing pressure ulcer of right buttock, stage 4
        Pressure ulcer with necrosis of soft tissues through to underlying muscle, tendon, or bone, right buttock

    L89.319 **Pressure ulcer of right buttock, unspecified stage** ▽
        Healing pressure ulcer of right buttock NOS
        Healing pressure ulcer of right buttock, unspecified stage

  ☑6ᵗʰ **L89.32** **Pressure ulcer of** left buttock

    L89.320 **Pressure ulcer of left buttock,** unstageable

    L89.321 **Pressure ulcer of left buttock,** stage 1
        Healing pressure ulcer of left buttock, stage 1
        Pressure pre-ulcer skin changes limited to persistent focal edema, left buttock

    L89.322 **Pressure ulcer of left buttock,** stage 2
        Healing pressure ulcer of left buttock, stage 2
        Pressure ulcer with abrasion, blister, partial thickness skin loss involving epidermis and/or dermis, left buttock

    L89.323 **Pressure ulcer of left buttock,** stage 3
        Healing pressure ulcer of left buttock, stage 3
        Pressure ulcer with full thickness skin loss involving damage or necrosis of subcutaneous tissue, left buttock

    L89.324 **Pressure ulcer of left buttock,** stage 4
        Healing pressure ulcer of left buttock, stage 4
        Pressure ulcer with necrosis of soft tissues through to underlying muscle, tendon, or bone, left buttock

    L89.329 **Pressure ulcer of left buttock, unspecified stage** ▽
        Healing pressure ulcer of left buttock NOS
        Healing pressure ulcer of left buttock, unspecified stage

☑5ᵗʰ **L89.4** **Pressure ulcer of contiguous site of** back, buttock and hip

    L89.40 **Pressure ulcer of contiguous site of back, buttock and hip, unspecified stage** ▽
        Healing pressure ulcer of contiguous site of back, buttock and hip NOS
        Healing pressure ulcer of contiguous site of back, buttock and hip, unspecified stage

    L89.41 **Pressure ulcer of contiguous site of back, buttock and hip,** stage 1
        Healing pressure ulcer of contiguous site of back, buttock and hip, stage 1
        Pressure pre-ulcer skin changes limited to persistent focal edema, contiguous site of back, buttock and hip

    L89.42 **Pressure ulcer of contiguous site of back, buttock and hip,** stage 2
        Healing pressure ulcer of contiguous site of back, buttock and hip, stage 2
        Pressure ulcer with abrasion, blister, partial thickness skin loss involving epidermis and/or dermis, contiguous site of back, buttock and hip

    L89.43 **Pressure ulcer of contiguous site of back, buttock and hip,** stage 3
        Healing pressure ulcer of contiguous site of back, buttock and hip, stage 3
        Pressure ulcer with full thickness skin loss involving damage or necrosis of subcutaneous tissue, contiguous site of back, buttock and hip

    L89.44 **Pressure ulcer of contiguous site of back, buttock and hip,** stage 4
        Healing pressure ulcer of contiguous site of back, buttock and hip, stage 4
        Pressure ulcer with necrosis of soft tissues through to underlying muscle, tendon, or bone, contiguous site of back, buttock and hip

---

☑ Additional Character Req   ✓ₓ7ᵗʰ Placeholder Alert   Case-Mix Diagnosis   Manifestation   ▽ Unspecified Dx   **EXCLUDES 1** Not coded here   **EXCLUDES 2** Not included here

Chapter 12. Diseases of the Skin and Subcutaneous Tissue

L89.45 Pressure ulcer of contiguous site of back, buttock and hip, unstageable

✓5th **L89.5 Pressure ulcer of ankle**

  ✓6th **L89.50 Pressure ulcer of unspecified ankle**

    L89.500 Pressure ulcer of unspecified ankle, unstageable ▽

    L89.501 Pressure ulcer of unspecified ankle, stage 1 ▽
Healing pressure ulcer of unspecified ankle, stage 1
Pressure pre-ulcer skin changes limited to persistent focal edema, unspecified ankle

    L89.502 Pressure ulcer of unspecified ankle, stage 2 ▽
Healing pressure ulcer of unspecified ankle, stage 2
Pressure ulcer with abrasion, blister, partial thickness skin loss involving epidermis and/or dermis, unspecified ankle

    L89.503 Pressure ulcer of unspecified ankle, stage 3 ▽
Healing pressure ulcer of unspecified ankle, stage 3
Pressure ulcer with full thickness skin loss involving damage or necrosis of subcutaneous tissue, unspecified ankle

    L89.504 Pressure ulcer of unspecified ankle, stage 4 ▽
Healing pressure ulcer of unspecified ankle, stage 4
Pressure ulcer with necrosis of soft tissues through to underlying muscle, tendon, or bone, unspecified ankle

    L89.509 Pressure ulcer of unspecified ankle, unspecified stage ▽
Healing pressure ulcer of unspecified ankle NOS
Healing pressure ulcer of unspecified ankle, unspecified stage

  ✓6th **L89.51 Pressure ulcer of right ankle**

    L89.510 Pressure ulcer of right ankle, unstageable

    L89.511 Pressure ulcer of right ankle, stage 1
Healing pressure ulcer of right ankle, stage 1
Pressure pre-ulcer skin changes limited to persistent focal edema, right ankle

    L89.512 Pressure ulcer of right ankle, stage 2
Healing pressure ulcer of right ankle, stage 2
Pressure ulcer with abrasion, blister, partial thickness skin loss involving epidermis and/or dermis, right ankle

    L89.513 Pressure ulcer of right ankle, stage 3
Healing pressure ulcer of right ankle, stage 3
Pressure ulcer with full thickness skin loss involving damage or necrosis of subcutaneous tissue, right ankle

    L89.514 Pressure ulcer of right ankle, stage 4
Healing pressure ulcer of right ankle, stage 4
Pressure ulcer with necrosis of soft tissues through to underlying muscle, tendon, or bone, right ankle

    L89.519 Pressure ulcer of right ankle, unspecified stage ▽
Healing pressure ulcer of right ankle NOS
Healing pressure ulcer of right ankle, unspecified stage

  ✓6th **L89.52 Pressure ulcer of left ankle**

    L89.520 Pressure ulcer of left ankle, unstageable

    L89.521 Pressure ulcer of left ankle, stage 1
Healing pressure ulcer of left ankle, stage 1
Pressure pre-ulcer skin changes limited to persistent focal edema, left ankle

    L89.522 Pressure ulcer of left ankle, stage 2
Healing pressure ulcer of left ankle, stage 2
Pressure ulcer with abrasion, blister, partial thickness skin loss involving epidermis and/or dermis, left ankle

    L89.523 Pressure ulcer of left ankle, stage 3
Healing pressure ulcer of left ankle, stage 3
Pressure ulcer with full thickness skin loss involving damage or necrosis of subcutaneous tissue, left ankle

    L89.524 Pressure ulcer of left ankle, stage 4
Healing pressure ulcer of left ankle, stage 4
Pressure ulcer with necrosis of soft tissues through to underlying muscle, tendon, or bone, left ankle

    L89.529 Pressure ulcer of left ankle, unspecified stage ▽
Healing pressure ulcer of left ankle NOS
Healing pressure ulcer of left ankle, unspecified stage

✓5th **L89.6 Pressure ulcer of heel**

  ✓6th **L89.60 Pressure ulcer of unspecified heel**

    L89.600 Pressure ulcer of unspecified heel, unstageable ▽

    L89.601 Pressure ulcer of unspecified heel, stage 1 ▽
Healing pressure ulcer of unspecified heel, stage 1
Pressure pre-ulcer skin changes limited to persistent focal edema, unspecified heel

    L89.602 Pressure ulcer of unspecified heel, stage 2 ▽
Healing pressure ulcer of unspecified heel, stage 2
Pressure ulcer with abrasion, blister, partial thickness skin loss involving epidermis and/or dermis, unspecified heel

    L89.603 Pressure ulcer of unspecified heel, stage 3 ▽
Healing pressure ulcer of unspecified heel, stage 3
Pressure ulcer with full thickness skin loss involving damage or necrosis of subcutaneous tissue, unspecified heel

    L89.604 Pressure ulcer of unspecified heel, stage 4 ▽
Healing pressure ulcer of unspecified heel, stage 4
Pressure ulcer with necrosis of soft tissues through to underlying muscle, tendon, or bone, unspecified heel

    L89.609 Pressure ulcer of unspecified heel, unspecified stage ▽
Healing pressure ulcer of unspecified heel NOS
Healing pressure ulcer of unspecified heel, unspecified stage

  ✓6th **L89.61 Pressure ulcer of right heel**

    L89.610 Pressure ulcer of right heel, unstageable

    L89.611 Pressure ulcer of right heel, stage 1
Healing pressure ulcer of right heel, stage 1
Pressure pre-ulcer skin changes limited to persistent focal edema, right heel

    L89.612 Pressure ulcer of right heel, stage 2
Healing pressure ulcer of right heel, stage 2
Pressure ulcer with abrasion, blister, partial thickness skin loss involving epidermis and/or dermis, right heel

    L89.613 Pressure ulcer of right heel, stage 3
Healing pressure ulcer of right heel, stage 3
Pressure ulcer with full thickness skin loss involving damage or necrosis of subcutaneous tissue, right heel

    L89.614 Pressure ulcer of right heel, stage 4
Healing pressure ulcer of right heel, stage 4
Pressure ulcer with necrosis of soft tissues through to underlying muscle, tendon, or bone, right heel

    L89.619 Pressure ulcer of right heel, unspecified stage ▽
Healing pressure ulcer of right heel NOS
▶Healing pressure ulcer of right heel, unspecified stage◀

Ⓝ Newborn: 0 Ⓟ Pediatric: 0-17 Ⓜ Maternity: 12-55 Ⓐ Adult: 15-124 **NRS** Nonroutine supply Dx **NCDx** Noncancer Dx **PDx** Primary Dx ▶◀ Revised Text ● New Code ▲ Revised Title

708 ICD-10-CM 2018

✓6ᵗʰ L89.62 Pressure ulcer of left heel

L89.620 Pressure ulcer of left heel, unstageable

L89.621 Pressure ulcer of left heel, stage 1
Healing pressure ulcer of left heel, stage 1
Pressure pre-ulcer skin changes limited to persistent focal edema, left heel

L89.622 Pressure ulcer of left heel, stage 2
Healing pressure ulcer of left heel, stage 2
Pressure ulcer with abrasion, blister, partial thickness skin loss involving epidermis and/or dermis, left heel

L89.623 Pressure ulcer of left heel, stage 3
Healing pressure ulcer of left heel, stage 3
Pressure ulcer with full thickness skin loss involving damage or necrosis of subcutaneous tissue, left heel

L89.624 Pressure ulcer of left heel, stage 4
Healing pressure ulcer of left heel, stage 4
Pressure ulcer with necrosis of soft tissues through to underlying muscle, tendon, or bone, left heel

L89.629 Pressure ulcer of left heel, unspecified stage ▽
Healing pressure ulcer of left heel NOS
Healing pressure ulcer of left heel, unspecified stage

✓5ᵗʰ L89.8 Pressure ulcer of other site

✓6ᵗʰ L89.81 Pressure ulcer of head
Pressure ulcer of face

L89.810 Pressure ulcer of head, unstageable

L89.811 Pressure ulcer of head, stage 1
Healing pressure ulcer of head, stage 1
Pressure pre-ulcer skin changes limited to persistent focal edema, head

L89.812 Pressure ulcer of head, stage 2
Healing pressure ulcer of head, stage 2
Pressure ulcer with abrasion, blister, partial thickness skin loss involving epidermis and/or dermis, head

L89.813 Pressure ulcer of head, stage 3
Healing pressure ulcer of head, stage 3
Pressure ulcer with full thickness skin loss involving damage or necrosis of subcutaneous tissue, head

L89.814 Pressure ulcer of head, stage 4
Healing pressure ulcer of head, stage 4
Pressure ulcer with necrosis of soft tissues through to underlying muscle, tendon, or bone, head

L89.819 Pressure ulcer of head, unspecified stage ▽
Healing pressure ulcer of head NOS
Healing pressure ulcer of head, unspecified stage

✓6ᵗʰ L89.89 Pressure ulcer of other site

L89.890 Pressure ulcer of other site, unstageable

L89.891 Pressure ulcer of other site, stage 1
Healing pressure ulcer of other site, stage 1
Pressure pre-ulcer skin changes limited to persistent focal edema, other site

L89.892 Pressure ulcer of other site, stage 2
Healing pressure ulcer of other site, stage 2
Pressure ulcer with abrasion, blister, partial thickness skin loss involving epidermis and/or dermis, other site

L89.893 Pressure ulcer of other site, stage 3
Healing pressure ulcer of other site, stage 3
Pressure ulcer with full thickness skin loss involving damage or necrosis of subcutaneous tissue, other site

L89.894 Pressure ulcer of other site, stage 4
Healing pressure ulcer of other site, stage 4
Pressure ulcer with necrosis of soft tissues through to underlying muscle, tendon, or bone, other site

L89.899 Pressure ulcer of other site, unspecified stage ▽
Healing pressure ulcer of other site NOS
Healing pressure ulcer of other site, unspecified stage

✓5ᵗʰ L89.9 Pressure ulcer of unspecified site

L89.90 Pressure ulcer of unspecified site, unspecified stage ▽
Healing pressure ulcer of unspecified site NOS
Healing pressure ulcer of unspecified site, unspecified stage

L89.91 Pressure ulcer of unspecified site, stage 1 ▽
Healing pressure ulcer of unspecified site, stage 1
Pressure pre-ulcer skin changes limited to persistent focal edema, unspecified site

L89.92 Pressure ulcer of unspecified site, stage 2 ▽
Healing pressure ulcer of unspecified site, stage 2
Pressure ulcer with abrasion, blister, partial thickness skin loss involving epidermis and/or dermis, unspecified site

L89.93 Pressure ulcer of unspecified site, stage 3 ▽
Healing pressure ulcer of unspecified site, stage 3
Pressure ulcer with full thickness skin loss involving damage or necrosis of subcutaneous tissue, unspecified site

L89.94 Pressure ulcer of unspecified site, stage 4 ▽
Healing pressure ulcer of unspecified site, stage 4
Pressure ulcer with necrosis of soft tissues through to underlying muscle, tendon, or bone, unspecified site

L89.95 Pressure ulcer of unspecified site, unstageable ▽

✓4ᵗʰ L90 Atrophic disorders of skin

L90.0 Lichen sclerosus et atrophicus
EXCLUDES 2 lichen sclerosus of external female genital organs (N90.4)
lichen sclerosus of external male genital organs (N48.0)

L90.1 Anetoderma of Schweninger-Buzzi

L90.2 Anetoderma of Jadassohn-Pellizzari

L90.3 Atrophoderma of Pasini and Pierini

L90.4 Acrodermatitis chronica atrophicans

L90.5 Scar conditions and fibrosis of skin
Adherent scar (skin)
Cicatrix
Disfigurement of skin due to scar
Fibrosis of skin NOS
Scar NOS
EXCLUDES 2 hypertrophic scar (L91.0)
keloid scar (L91.0)
AHA: 2016, 2Q, 5; 2015, 1Q, 19

L90.6 Striae atrophicae

L90.8 Other atrophic disorders of skin

L90.9 Atrophic disorder of skin, unspecified ▽

✓4ᵗʰ L91 Hypertrophic disorders of skin

L91.0 Hypertrophic scar
Keloid
Keloid scar
EXCLUDES 2 acne keloid (L73.0)
scar NOS (L90.5)
DEF: Overgrowth of scar tissue due to excess amounts of collagen during connective tissue repair; occurs mainly on upper trunk, face.

L91.8 Other hypertrophic disorders of the skin

L91.9 Hypertrophic disorder of the skin, unspecified ▽

✓4ᵗʰ L92 Granulomatous disorders of skin and subcutaneous tissue
EXCLUDES 2 actinic granuloma (L57.5)

L92.0 Granuloma annulare
Perforating granuloma annulare

L92.1 Necrobiosis lipoidica, not elsewhere classified
EXCLUDES 1 necrobiosis lipoidica associated with diabetes mellitus (E08-E13 with .620)

L92.2 Granuloma faciale [eosinophilic granuloma of skin]

L92.3 Foreign body granuloma of the skin and subcutaneous tissue
Use additional code to identify the type of retained foreign body (Z18.-)

L92.8 Other granulomatous disorders of the skin and subcutaneous tissue NRS

L92.9 Granulomatous disorder of the skin and subcutaneous tissue, unspecified ▽
EXCLUDES 2 ▶umbilical granuloma (P83.81)◀

☑4ᵗʰ **L93   Lupus erythematosus**

Use additional code for adverse effect, if applicable, to identify drug (T36-T50 with fifth or sixth character 5)

EXCLUDES 1   lupus exedens (A18.4)
lupus vulgaris (A18.4)
scleroderma (M34.-)
systemic lupus erythematosus (M32.-)

L93.0   Discoid lupus erythematosus
Lupus erythematosus NOS

L93.1   Subacute cutaneous lupus erythematosus

L93.2   Other local lupus erythematosus
Lupus erythematosus profundus
Lupus panniculitis

☑4ᵗʰ **L94   Other localized connective tissue disorders**
EXCLUDES 1   systemic connective tissue disorders (M30-M36)

L94.0   Localized scleroderma [morphea]
Circumscribed scleroderma

L94.1   Linear scleroderma
En coup de sabre lesion

L94.2   Calcinosis cutis

L94.3   Sclerodactyly

L94.4   Gottron's papules

L94.5   Poikiloderma vasculare atrophicans

L94.6   Ainhum

L94.8   Other specified localized connective tissue disorders

L94.9   Localized connective tissue disorder, unspecified ▽

☑4ᵗʰ **L95   Vasculitis limited to skin, not elsewhere classified**
EXCLUDES 1   angioma serpiginosum (L81.7)
Henoch(-Schönlein) purpura (D69.0)
hypersensitivity angiitis (M31.0)
lupus panniculitis (L93.2)
panniculitis NOS (M79.3)
panniculitis of neck and back (M54.0-)
polyarteritis nodosa (M30.0)
relapsing panniculitis (M35.6)
rheumatoid vasculitis (M05.2)
serum sickness (T80.6-)
urticaria (L50.-)
Wegener's granulomatosis (M31.3-)

L95.0   Livedoid vasculitis
Atrophie blanche (en plaque)

L95.1   Erythema elevatum diutinum

L95.8   Other vasculitis limited to the skin

L95.9   Vasculitis limited to the skin, unspecified ▽

☑4ᵗʰ **L97   Non-pressure chronic ulcer of lower limb, not elsewhere classified**
INCLUDES   chronic ulcer of skin of lower limb NOS
non-healing ulcer of skin
non-infected sinus of skin
trophic ulcer NOS
tropical ulcer NOS
ulcer of skin of lower limb NOS

Code first any associated underlying condition, such as:
any associated gangrene (I96)
atherosclerosis of the lower extremities (I70.23-, I70.24-, I70.33-, I70.34-, I70.43-, I70.44-, I70.53-, I70.54-, I70.63-, I70.64-, I70.73-, I70.74-)
chronic venous hypertension (I87.31-, I87.33-)
diabetic ulcers (E08.621, E08.622, E09.621, E09.622, E10.621, E10.622, E11.621, E11.622, E13.621, E13.622)
postphlebitic syndrome (I87.01-, I87.03-)
postthrombotic syndrome (I87.01-, I87.03-)
varicose ulcer (I83.0-, I83.2-)

EXCLUDES 2   pressure ulcer (pressure area) (L89.-)
skin infections (L00-L08)
specific infections classified to A00-B99

TIP: Code assignment for the severity of non-pressure chronic ulcers may be based on medical record documentation from clinicians who are not the patient's provider.

☑5ᵗʰ **L97.1   Non-pressure chronic ulcer of thigh**

☑6ᵗʰ **L97.10   Non-pressure chronic ulcer of unspecified thigh**

L97.101   Non-pressure chronic ulcer of unspecified thigh limited to breakdown of skin ▽

L97.102   Non-pressure chronic ulcer of unspecified thigh with fat layer exposed ▽

L97.103   Non-pressure chronic ulcer of unspecified thigh with necrosis of muscle ▽

L97.104   Non-pressure chronic ulcer of unspecified thigh with necrosis of bone ▽

L97.105   Non-pressure chronic ulcer of unspecified thigh with muscle involvement without evidence of necrosis ▽

L97.106   Non-pressure chronic ulcer of unspecified thigh with bone involvement without evidence of necrosis ▽

L97.108   Non-pressure chronic ulcer of unspecified thigh with other specified severity ▽

L97.109   Non-pressure chronic ulcer of unspecified thigh with unspecified severity ▽

☑6ᵗʰ **L97.11   Non-pressure chronic ulcer of right thigh**

L97.111   Non-pressure chronic ulcer of right thigh limited to breakdown of skin   NRS

L97.112   Non-pressure chronic ulcer of right thigh with fat layer exposed   NRS

L97.113   Non-pressure chronic ulcer of right thigh with necrosis of muscle   NRS

L97.114   Non-pressure chronic ulcer of right thigh with necrosis of bone   NRS

L97.115   Non-pressure chronic ulcer of right thigh with muscle involvement without evidence of necrosis

L97.116   Non-pressure chronic ulcer of right thigh with bone involvement without evidence of necrosis

L97.118   Non-pressure chronic ulcer of right thigh with other specified severity

L97.119   Non-pressure chronic ulcer of right thigh with unspecified severity   NRS ▽

☑6ᵗʰ **L97.12   Non-pressure chronic ulcer of left thigh**

L97.121   Non-pressure chronic ulcer of left thigh limited to breakdown of skin   NRS

L97.122   Non-pressure chronic ulcer of left thigh with fat layer exposed   NRS

L97.123   Non-pressure chronic ulcer of left thigh with necrosis of muscle   NRS

L97.124   Non-pressure chronic ulcer of left thigh with necrosis of bone   NRS

L97.125   Non-pressure chronic ulcer of left thigh with muscle involvement without evidence of necrosis

L97.126   Non-pressure chronic ulcer of left thigh with bone involvement without evidence of necrosis

L97.128   Non-pressure chronic ulcer of left thigh with other specified severity

L97.129   Non-pressure chronic ulcer of left thigh with unspecified severity   NRS ▽

☑5ᵗʰ **L97.2   Non-pressure chronic ulcer of calf**

☑6ᵗʰ **L97.20   Non-pressure chronic ulcer of unspecified calf**

L97.201   Non-pressure chronic ulcer of unspecified calf limited to breakdown of skin ▽

L97.202   Non-pressure chronic ulcer of unspecified calf with fat layer exposed ▽

L97.203   Non-pressure chronic ulcer of unspecified calf with necrosis of muscle ▽

L97.204   Non-pressure chronic ulcer of unspecified calf with necrosis of bone ▽

L97.205   Non-pressure chronic ulcer of unspecified calf with muscle involvement without evidence of necrosis ▽

L97.206   Non-pressure chronic ulcer of unspecified calf with bone involvement without evidence of necrosis ▽

L97.208   Non-pressure chronic ulcer of unspecified calf with other specified severity ▽

L97.209   Non-pressure chronic ulcer of unspecified calf with unspecified severity ▽

✓6th L97.21   Non-pressure chronic ulcer of right calf

L97.211   Non-pressure chronic ulcer of right calf limited to breakdown of skin   NRS

L97.212   Non-pressure chronic ulcer of right calf with fat layer exposed   NRS

L97.213   Non-pressure chronic ulcer of right calf with necrosis of muscle   NRS

L97.214   Non-pressure chronic ulcer of right calf with necrosis of bone   NRS

L97.215   Non-pressure chronic ulcer of right calf with muscle involvement without evidence of necrosis

L97.216   Non-pressure chronic ulcer of right calf with bone involvement without evidence of necrosis

L97.218   Non-pressure chronic ulcer of right calf with other specified severity

L97.219   Non-pressure chronic ulcer of right calf with unspecified severity   NRS ▽

✓6th L97.22   Non-pressure chronic ulcer of left calf

L97.221   Non-pressure chronic ulcer of left calf limited to breakdown of skin   NRS

L97.222   Non-pressure chronic ulcer of left calf with fat layer exposed   NRS

L97.223   Non-pressure chronic ulcer of left calf with necrosis of muscle   NRS

L97.224   Non-pressure chronic ulcer of left calf with necrosis of bone   NRS

L97.225   Non-pressure chronic ulcer of left calf with muscle involvement without evidence of necrosis

L97.226   Non-pressure chronic ulcer of left calf with bone involvement without evidence of necrosis

L97.228   Non-pressure chronic ulcer of left calf with other specified severity

L97.229   Non-pressure chronic ulcer of left calf with unspecified severity   NRS ▽

✓5th L97.3   Non-pressure chronic ulcer of ankle

✓6th L97.30   Non-pressure chronic ulcer of unspecified ankle

L97.301   Non-pressure chronic ulcer of unspecified ankle limited to breakdown of skin ▽

L97.302   Non-pressure chronic ulcer of unspecified ankle with fat layer exposed ▽

L97.303   Non-pressure chronic ulcer of unspecified ankle with necrosis of muscle ▽

L97.304   Non-pressure chronic ulcer of unspecified ankle with necrosis of bone ▽

L97.305   Non-pressure chronic ulcer of unspecified ankle with muscle involvement without evidence of necrosis ▽

L97.306   Non-pressure chronic ulcer of unspecified ankle with bone involvement without evidence of necrosis ▽

L97.308   Non-pressure chronic ulcer of unspecified ankle with other specified severity ▽

L97.309   Non-pressure chronic ulcer of unspecified ankle with unspecified severity ▽

✓6th L97.31   Non-pressure chronic ulcer of right ankle

L97.311   Non-pressure chronic ulcer of right ankle limited to breakdown of skin   NRS

L97.312   Non-pressure chronic ulcer of right ankle with fat layer exposed   NRS

L97.313   Non-pressure chronic ulcer of right ankle with necrosis of muscle   NRS

L97.314   Non-pressure chronic ulcer of right ankle with necrosis of bone   NRS

L97.315   Non-pressure chronic ulcer of right ankle with muscle involvement without evidence of necrosis

L97.316   Non-pressure chronic ulcer of right ankle with bone involvement without evidence of necrosis

L97.318   Non-pressure chronic ulcer of right ankle with other specified severity

L97.319   Non-pressure chronic ulcer of right ankle with unspecified severity   NRS ▽

✓6th L97.32   Non-pressure chronic ulcer of left ankle

L97.321   Non-pressure chronic ulcer of left ankle limited to breakdown of skin   NRS

L97.322   Non-pressure chronic ulcer of left ankle with fat layer exposed   NRS

L97.323   Non-pressure chronic ulcer of left ankle with necrosis of muscle   NRS

L97.324   Non-pressure chronic ulcer of left ankle with necrosis of bone   NRS

L97.325   Non-pressure chronic ulcer of left ankle with muscle involvement without evidence of necrosis

L97.326   Non-pressure chronic ulcer of left ankle with bone involvement without evidence of necrosis

L97.328   Non-pressure chronic ulcer of left ankle with other specified severity

L97.329   Non-pressure chronic ulcer of left ankle with unspecified severity   NRS ▽

✓5th L97.4   Non-pressure chronic ulcer of heel and midfoot
Non-pressure chronic ulcer of plantar surface of midfoot

✓6th L97.40   Non-pressure chronic ulcer of unspecified heel and midfoot

L97.401   Non-pressure chronic ulcer of unspecified heel and midfoot limited to breakdown of skin ▽

L97.402   Non-pressure chronic ulcer of unspecified heel and midfoot with fat layer exposed ▽

L97.403   Non-pressure chronic ulcer of unspecified heel and midfoot with necrosis of muscle ▽

L97.404   Non-pressure chronic ulcer of unspecified heel and midfoot with necrosis of bone ▽

L97.405   Non-pressure chronic ulcer of unspecified heel and midfoot with muscle involvement without evidence of necrosis ▽

L97.406   Non-pressure chronic ulcer of unspecified heel and midfoot with bone involvement without evidence of necrosis ▽

L97.408   Non-pressure chronic ulcer of unspecified heel and midfoot with other specified severity ▽

L97.409   Non-pressure chronic ulcer of unspecified heel and midfoot with unspecified severity ▽

✓6th L97.41   Non-pressure chronic ulcer of right heel and midfoot

L97.411   Non-pressure chronic ulcer of right heel and midfoot limited to breakdown of skin   NRS

L97.412   Non-pressure chronic ulcer of right heel and midfoot with fat layer exposed   NRS

L97.413   Non-pressure chronic ulcer of right heel and midfoot with necrosis of muscle   NRS

L97.414   Non-pressure chronic ulcer of right heel and midfoot with necrosis of bone   NRS

L97.415   Non-pressure chronic ulcer of right heel and midfoot with muscle involvement without evidence of necrosis

L97.416   Non-pressure chronic ulcer of right heel and midfoot with bone involvement without evidence of necrosis

L97.418   Non-pressure chronic ulcer of right heel and midfoot with other specified severity

L97.419   Non-pressure chronic ulcer of right heel and midfoot with unspecified severity   NRS ▽

☑ Additional Character Req   ✓x7th Placeholder Alert   Case-Mix Diagnosis   Manifestation   ▽ Unspecified Dx   EXCLUDES 1 Not coded here   EXCLUDES 2 Not included here

ICD-10-CM 2018   711

Chapter 12. Diseases of the Skin and Subcutaneous Tissue

✓6ᵗʰ **L97.42** **Non-pressure chronic ulcer of** left heel and midfoot

L97.421 **Non-pressure chronic ulcer of left heel and midfoot** limited to breakdown of skin [NRS]

    AHA: 2016, 1Q, 12

L97.422 **Non-pressure chronic ulcer of left heel and midfoot** with fat layer exposed [NRS]

L97.423 **Non-pressure chronic ulcer of left heel and midfoot** with necrosis of muscle [NRS]

L97.424 **Non-pressure chronic ulcer of left heel and midfoot** with necrosis of bone [NRS]

L97.425 **Non-pressure chronic ulcer of left heel and midfoot** with muscle involvement without evidence of necrosis

L97.426 **Non-pressure chronic ulcer of left heel and midfoot** with bone involvement without evidence of necrosis

L97.428 **Non-pressure chronic ulcer of left heel and midfoot** with other specified severity

L97.429 **Non-pressure chronic ulcer of left heel and midfoot with unspecified severity** [NRS] ▽

✓5ᵗʰ **L97.5** **Non-pressure chronic ulcer of** other part of foot
Non-pressure chronic ulcer of toe

✓6ᵗʰ **L97.50** **Non-pressure chronic ulcer of** other part of unspecified foot

L97.501 **Non-pressure chronic ulcer of other part of unspecified foot** limited to breakdown of skin ▽

L97.502 **Non-pressure chronic ulcer of other part of unspecified foot** with fat layer exposed ▽

L97.503 **Non-pressure chronic ulcer of other part of unspecified foot** with necrosis of muscle ▽

L97.504 **Non-pressure chronic ulcer of other part of unspecified foot** with necrosis of bone ▽

L97.505 **Non-pressure chronic ulcer of other part of unspecified foot** with muscle involvement without evidence of necrosis ▽

L97.506 **Non-pressure chronic ulcer of other part of unspecified foot** with bone involvement without evidence of necrosis ▽

L97.508 **Non-pressure chronic ulcer of other part of unspecified foot** with other specified severity ▽

L97.509 **Non-pressure chronic ulcer of other part of unspecified foot** with unspecified severity ▽

✓6ᵗʰ **L97.51** **Non-pressure chronic ulcer of** other part of right foot

L97.511 **Non-pressure chronic ulcer of other part of right foot** limited to breakdown of skin [NRS]

L97.512 **Non-pressure chronic ulcer of other part of right foot** with fat layer exposed [NRS]

L97.513 **Non-pressure chronic ulcer of other part of right foot** with necrosis of muscle [NRS]

L97.514 **Non-pressure chronic ulcer of other part of right foot** with necrosis of bone [NRS]

L97.515 **Non-pressure chronic ulcer of other part of right foot** with muscle involvement without evidence of necrosis

L97.516 **Non-pressure chronic ulcer of other part of right foot** with bone involvement without evidence of necrosis

L97.518 **Non-pressure chronic ulcer of other part of right foot** with other specified severity

L97.519 **Non-pressure chronic ulcer of other part of right foot** with unspecified severity [NRS] ▽

✓6ᵗʰ **L97.52** **Non-pressure chronic ulcer of** other part of left foot

L97.521 **Non-pressure chronic ulcer of other part of left foot** limited to breakdown of skin [NRS]

L97.522 **Non-pressure chronic ulcer of other part of left foot** with fat layer exposed [NRS]

L97.523 **Non-pressure chronic ulcer of other part of left foot** with necrosis of muscle [NRS]

L97.524 **Non-pressure chronic ulcer of other part of left foot** with necrosis of bone [NRS]

L97.525 **Non-pressure chronic ulcer of other part of left foot** with muscle involvement without evidence of necrosis

L97.526 **Non-pressure chronic ulcer of other part of left foot** with bone involvement without evidence of necrosis

L97.528 **Non-pressure chronic ulcer of other part of left foot** with other specified severity

L97.529 **Non-pressure chronic ulcer of other part of left foot** with unspecified severity [NRS] ▽

✓5ᵗʰ **L97.8** **Non-pressure chronic ulcer of** other part of lower leg

✓6ᵗʰ **L97.80** **Non-pressure chronic ulcer of** other part of unspecified lower leg

L97.801 **Non-pressure chronic ulcer of other part of unspecified lower leg** limited to breakdown of skin ▽

L97.802 **Non-pressure chronic ulcer of other part of unspecified lower leg** with fat layer exposed ▽

L97.803 **Non-pressure chronic ulcer of other part of unspecified lower leg** with necrosis of muscle ▽

L97.804 **Non-pressure chronic ulcer of other part of unspecified lower leg** with necrosis of bone ▽

L97.805 **Non-pressure chronic ulcer of other part of unspecified lower leg** with muscle involvement without evidence of necrosis ▽

L97.806 **Non-pressure chronic ulcer of other part of unspecified lower leg** with bone involvement without evidence of necrosis ▽

L97.808 **Non-pressure chronic ulcer of other part of unspecified lower leg** with other specified severity ▽

L97.809 **Non-pressure chronic ulcer of other part of unspecified lower leg** with unspecified severity ▽

✓6ᵗʰ **L97.81** **Non-pressure chronic ulcer of** other part of right lower leg

L97.811 **Non-pressure chronic ulcer of other part of right lower leg** limited to breakdown of skin [NRS]

L97.812 **Non-pressure chronic ulcer of other part of right lower leg** with fat layer exposed [NRS]

L97.813 **Non-pressure chronic ulcer of other part of right lower leg** with necrosis of muscle [NRS]

L97.814 **Non-pressure chronic ulcer of other part of right lower leg** with necrosis of bone [NRS]

L97.815 **Non-pressure chronic ulcer of other part of right lower leg** with muscle involvement without evidence of necrosis

L97.816 **Non-pressure chronic ulcer of other part of right lower leg** with bone involvement without evidence of necrosis

L97.818 **Non-pressure chronic ulcer of other part of right lower leg** with other specified severity

L97.819 **Non-pressure chronic ulcer of other part of right lower leg** with unspecified severity [NRS] ▽

✓6ᵗʰ **L97.82** **Non-pressure chronic ulcer of** other part of left lower leg

L97.821 **Non-pressure chronic ulcer of other part of left lower leg** limited to breakdown of skin [NRS]

L97.822 **Non-pressure chronic ulcer of other part of left lower leg** with fat layer exposed [NRS]

N Newborn: 0   P Pediatric: 0-17   M Maternity: 12-55   A Adult: 15-124   NRS Nonroutine supply Dx   NC Dx Noncancer Dx   PDx Primary Dx   ►◄ Revised Text   ● New Code   ▲ Revised Title

712   ICD-10-CM 2018

L97.823   **Non-pressure chronic ulcer of other part of left lower leg** with necrosis of muscle   **NRS**

L97.824   **Non-pressure chronic ulcer of other part of left lower leg** with necrosis of bone   **NRS**

L97.825   **Non-pressure chronic ulcer of other part of left lower leg** with muscle involvement without evidence of necrosis

L97.826   **Non-pressure chronic ulcer of other part of left lower leg** with bone involvement without evidence of necrosis

L97.828   **Non-pressure chronic ulcer of other part of left lower leg with other specified severity**

L97.829   **Non-pressure chronic ulcer of other part of left lower leg with unspecified severity**   **NRS** ▽

√5ᵗʰ **L97.9**   **Non-pressure chronic ulcer of** unspecified part of lower leg

   √6ᵗʰ **L97.90**   **Non-pressure chronic ulcer of** unspecified part of unspecified lower leg

      L97.901   **Non-pressure chronic ulcer of unspecified part of unspecified lower leg** limited to breakdown of skin   **NRS** ▽

      L97.902   **Non-pressure chronic ulcer of unspecified part of unspecified lower leg** with fat layer exposed   **NRS** ▽

      L97.903   **Non-pressure chronic ulcer of unspecified part of unspecified lower leg** with necrosis of muscle   **NRS** ▽

      L97.904   **Non-pressure chronic ulcer of unspecified part of unspecified lower leg** with necrosis of bone   **NRS** ▽

      L97.905   **Non-pressure chronic ulcer of unspecified part of unspecified lower leg** with muscle involvement without evidence of necrosis   ▽

      L97.906   **Non-pressure chronic ulcer of unspecified part of unspecified lower leg** with bone involvement without evidence of necrosis   ▽

      L97.908   **Non-pressure chronic ulcer of unspecified part of unspecified lower leg with other specified severity**   ▽

      L97.909   **Non-pressure chronic ulcer of unspecified part of unspecified lower leg with unspecified severity**   **NRS** ▽

   √6ᵗʰ **L97.91**   **Non-pressure chronic ulcer of** unspecified part of right lower leg

      L97.911   **Non-pressure chronic ulcer of unspecified part of right lower leg** limited to breakdown of skin   **NRS** ▽

      L97.912   **Non-pressure chronic ulcer of unspecified part of right lower leg** with fat layer exposed   **NRS** ▽

      L97.913   **Non-pressure chronic ulcer of unspecified part of right lower leg** with necrosis of muscle   **NRS** ▽

      L97.914   **Non-pressure chronic ulcer of unspecified part of right lower leg** with necrosis of bone   **NRS** ▽

      L97.915   **Non-pressure chronic ulcer of unspecified part of right lower leg** with muscle involvement without evidence of necrosis   ▽

      L97.916   **Non-pressure chronic ulcer of unspecified part of right lower leg** with bone involvement without evidence of necrosis   ▽

      L97.918   **Non-pressure chronic ulcer of unspecified part of right lower leg with other specified severity**   ▽

      L97.919   **Non-pressure chronic ulcer of unspecified part of right lower leg with unspecified severity**   **NRS** ▽

   √6ᵗʰ **L97.92**   **Non-pressure chronic ulcer of** unspecified part of left lower leg

      L97.921   **Non-pressure chronic ulcer of unspecified part of left lower leg** limited to breakdown of skin   **NRS** ▽

L97.922   **Non-pressure chronic ulcer of unspecified part of left lower leg with fat layer exposed**   **NRS** ▽

L97.923   **Non-pressure chronic ulcer of unspecified part of left lower leg** with necrosis of muscle   **NRS** ▽

L97.924   **Non-pressure chronic ulcer of unspecified part of left lower leg** with necrosis of bone   **NRS** ▽

L97.925   **Non-pressure chronic ulcer of unspecified part of left lower leg** with muscle involvement without evidence of necrosis   ▽

L97.926   **Non-pressure chronic ulcer of unspecified part of left lower leg** with bone involvement without evidence of necrosis   ▽

L97.928   **Non-pressure chronic ulcer of unspecified part of left lower leg with other specified severity**   ▽

L97.929   **Non-pressure chronic ulcer of unspecified part of left lower leg with unspecified severity**   **NRS** ▽

√4ᵗʰ **L98**   **Other disorders of skin and subcutaneous tissue, not elsewhere classified**

L98.0   **Pyogenic granuloma**   **NRS**

   EXCLUDES 2   pyogenic granuloma of gingiva (K06.8)
          pyogenic granuloma of maxillary alveolar ridge (K04.5)
          pyogenic granuloma of oral mucosa (K13.4)

   DEF: Solitary polypoid capillary hemangioma often associated with local irritation, trauma, and superimposed inflammation; located on the skin and gingival or oral mucosa; they bleed easily and may ulcerate and form crusted sores.

L98.1   **Factitial dermatitis**

   Neurotic excoriation

   EXCLUDES 1   excoriation (skin-picking) disorder (F42.4)

   DEF: Self-inflicted skin lesions to satisfy an unconscious psychological or emotional need; methods used to injure the skin include deep excoriations with a sharp instrument, scarification with a knife, or the application of caustic chemicals and burning, sometimes with a cigarette.

L98.2   **Febrile neutrophilic dermatosis [Sweet]**

L98.3   **Eosinophilic cellulitis [Wells]**   **NRS**

√5ᵗʰ **L98.4**   **Non-pressure chronic ulcer of skin, not elsewhere classified**

   Chronic ulcer of skin NOS
   Tropical ulcer NOS
   Ulcer of skin NOS

   EXCLUDES 2   pressure ulcer (pressure area) (L89.-)
          gangrene (I96)
          skin infections (L00-L08)
          specific infections classified to A00-B99
          ulcer of lower limb NEC (L97.-)
          varicose ulcer (I83.0-I82.2)

   TIP: Code assignment for the severity of non-pressure chronic ulcers may be based on medical record documentation from clinicians who are not the patient's provider.

   √6ᵗʰ **L98.41**   **Non-pressure chronic ulcer of** buttock

      L98.411   **Non-pressure chronic ulcer of buttock limited to breakdown of skin**   **NRS**

      L98.412   **Non-pressure chronic ulcer of buttock with fat layer exposed**   **NRS**

      L98.413   **Non-pressure chronic ulcer of buttock with necrosis of muscle**   **NRS**

      L98.414   **Non-pressure chronic ulcer of buttock with necrosis of bone**   **NRS**

      L98.415   **Non-pressure chronic ulcer of buttock** with muscle involvement without evidence of necrosis

      L98.416   **Non-pressure chronic ulcer of buttock** with bone involvement without evidence of necrosis

      L98.418   **Non-pressure chronic ulcer of buttock** with other specified severity

      L98.419   **Non-pressure chronic ulcer of buttock with unspecified severity**   **NRS** ▽

   √6ᵗʰ **L98.42**   **Non-pressure chronic ulcer of** back

      L98.421   **Non-pressure chronic ulcer of back limited to breakdown of skin**   **NRS**

☑ Additional Character Req   √x7ᵗʰ Placeholder Alert   Case-Mix Diagnosis   Manifestation   ▽ Unspecified Dx   *EXCLUDES 1* Not coded here   *EXCLUDES 2* Not included here

L98.422 Non-pressure chronic ulcer of back with fat layer exposed `NRS`

L98.423 Non-pressure chronic ulcer of back with necrosis of muscle `NRS`

L98.424 Non-pressure chronic ulcer of back with necrosis of bone `NRS`

L98.425 Non-pressure chronic ulcer of back with muscle involvement without evidence of necrosis

L98.426 Non-pressure chronic ulcer of back with bone involvement without evidence of necrosis

L98.428 Non-pressure chronic ulcer of back with other specified severity

L98.429 Non-pressure chronic ulcer of back with unspecified severity `NRS` ▽

✓6ᵗʰ **L98.49** Non-pressure chronic ulcer of skin of other sites
Non-pressure chronic ulcer of skin NOS

L98.491 Non-pressure chronic ulcer of skin of other sites limited to breakdown of skin `NRS`

L98.492 Non-pressure chronic ulcer of skin of other sites with fat layer exposed `NRS`

L98.493 Non-pressure chronic ulcer of skin of other sites with necrosis of muscle `NRS`

L98.494 Non-pressure chronic ulcer of skin of other sites with necrosis of bone `NRS`

L98.495 Non-pressure chronic ulcer of other sites with muscle involvement without evidence of necrosis

L98.496 Non-pressure chronic ulcer of other sites with bone involvement without evidence of necrosis

L98.498 Non-pressure chronic ulcer of other sites with other specified severity

L98.499 Non-pressure chronic ulcer of skin of other sites with unspecified severity `NRS` ▽

L98.5 Mucinosis of the skin
Focal mucinosis
Lichen myxedematosus
Reticular erythematous mucinosis
EXCLUDES 1   *focal oral mucinosis (K13.79)*
myxedema (E03.9)

L98.6 Other infiltrative disorders of the skin and subcutaneous tissue
EXCLUDES 1   *hyalinosis cutis et mucosae (E78.89)*

L98.7 Excessive and redundant skin and subcutaneous tissue
Loose or sagging skin following bariatric surgery weight loss
Loose or sagging skin following dietary weight loss
Loose or sagging skin, NOS
EXCLUDES 2   *acquired excess or redundant skin of eyelid (H02.3-)*
congenital excess or redundant skin of eyelid (Q10.3)
skin changes due to chronic exposure to nonionizing radiation (L57.-)

L98.8 Other specified disorders of the skin and subcutaneous tissue
AHA: 2013, 2Q, 32

L98.9 Disorder of the skin and subcutaneous tissue, unspecified ▽

L99 *Other disorders of skin and subcutaneous tissue in diseases classified elsewhere*
Code first underlying disease, such as:
amyloidosis (E85.-)
EXCLUDES 1   *skin disorders in diabetes (E08-E13 with .62)*
skin disorders in gonorrhea (A54.89)
skin disorders in syphilis (A51.31, A52.79)

Ⓝ Newborn: 0   Ⓟ Pediatric: 0-17   Ⓜ Maternity: 12-55   Ⓐ Adult: 15-124   `NRS` Nonroutine supply Dx   `NCDx` Noncancer Dx   `PDx` Primary Dx   ►◄ Revised Text   ● New Code   ▲ Revised Title

714   ICD-10-CM 2018

Chapter 13. Diseases of the Musculoskeletal System and Connective Tissue (M00–M99)

Chapter Specific Guidelines with Coding Examples

The chapter specific guidelines from the ICD-10-CM Official Guidelines for Coding and Reporting have been provided below. Along with these guidelines are coding examples, contained in the shaded boxes, that have been developed to help illustrate the coding and/or sequencing guidance found in these guidelines.

a. Site and laterality

Most of the codes within Chapter 13 have site and laterality designations. The site represents the bone, joint or the muscle involved. For some conditions where more than one bone, joint or muscle is usually involved, such as osteoarthritis, there is a "multiple sites" code available. For categories where no multiple site code is provided and more than one bone, joint or muscle is involved, multiple codes should be used to indicate the different sites involved.

> Right elbow infective bursitis
>
> **M71.121　　Other infective bursitis, right elbow**
>
> *Explanation:* Most of the codes within chapter 13 have site and laterality designations. The site represents the bone, joint, or the muscle involved.

> Rheumatoid arthritis of multiple sites without rheumatoid factor
>
> **M06.09　　Rheumatoid arthritis without rheumatoid factor, multiple sites**
>
> *Explanation:* For some conditions where more than one bone, joint or muscle is usually involved, such as osteoarthritis, there is a "multiple sites" code available.

> Osteomyelitis of the fourth thoracic and second lumbar vertebrae
>
> **M46.24　　Osteomyelitis of vertebra, thoracic region**
>
> **M46.26　　Osteomyelitis of vertebra, lumbar region**
>
> *Explanation:* For categories without a multiple site code and more than one bone, joint, or muscle is involved, multiple codes should be used to indicate the different sites involved.

1) Bone versus joint

For certain conditions, the bone may be affected at the upper or lower end, (e.g., avascular necrosis of bone, M87, Osteoporosis, M80, M81). Though the portion of the bone affected may be at the joint, the site designation will be the bone, not the joint.

> Idiopathic avascular necrosis of the femoral head of the left hip joint
>
> **M87.052　　Idiopathic aseptic necrosis of left femur**
>
> *Explanation:* For certain conditions such as avascular necrosis, the bone may be affected at the joint, but the site designation is the bone, not the joint.

b. Acute traumatic versus chronic or recurrent musculoskeletal conditions

Many musculoskeletal conditions are a result of previous injury or trauma to a site, or are recurrent conditions. Bone, joint or muscle conditions that are the result of a healed injury are usually found in chapter 13. Recurrent bone, joint or muscle conditions are also usually found in chapter 13. Any current, acute injury should be coded to the appropriate injury code from chapter 19. Chronic or recurrent conditions should generally be coded with a code from chapter 13. If it is difficult to determine from the documentation in the record which code is best to describe a condition, query the provider.

> Old bucket handle tear of right medial meniscus
>
> **M23.203　　Derangement of unspecified medial meniscus due to old tear or injury, right knee**
>
> *Explanation:* Chronic or recurrent conditions should generally be coded with a code from chapter 13.

c. Coding of pathologic fractures

7th character A is for use as long as the patient is receiving active treatment for the fracture. Examples of active treatment are: surgical treatment, emergency department encounter, evaluation and continuing treatment by the same or a different physician. While the patient may be seen by a new or different provider over the course of treatment for a pathological fracture, assignment of the 7th character is based on whether the patient is undergoing active treatment and not whether the provider is seeing the patient for the first time.

7th character D is to be used for encounters after the patient has completed active treatment **for the fracture and is receiving routine care for the fracture during the healing or recovery phase.** The other 7th characters, listed under each subcategory in the Tabular List, are to be used for subsequent encounters for treatment of problems associated with the healing, such as malunions, nonunions, and sequelae.

> Following a hospital and inpatient rehabilitation stay for treatment of a pathological fracture of the right femur, a 72-year-old woman is admitted to home health for continued physical therapy and pain management.
>
> **M84.451D　　Pathological fracture, right femur, subsequent encounter for fracture with routine healing**
>
> *Explanation:* The use of seventh character D is appropriate when the patient is receiving routine care for the fracture during the healing and recovery phase. Depending on the category/subcategory, other seventh characters are available to designate subsequent care related to complications associated with the healing phase. For subcategory M84.4- these include delayed healing (seventh character G), nonunion (seventh character K), malunion (seventh character P), and sequela (seventh character S).

Care for complications of surgical treatment for fracture repairs during the healing or recovery phase should be coded with the appropriate complication codes.

See Section I.C.19. Coding of traumatic fractures.

d. Osteoporosis

Osteoporosis is a systemic condition, meaning that all bones of the musculoskeletal system are affected. Therefore, site is not a component of the codes under category M81, Osteoporosis without current pathological fracture. The site codes under category M80, Osteoporosis with current pathological fracture, identify the site of the fracture, not the osteoporosis.

1) Osteoporosis without pathological fracture

Category M81, Osteoporosis without current pathological fracture, is for use for patients with osteoporosis who do not currently have a pathologic fracture due to the osteoporosis, even if they have had a fracture in the past. For patients with a history of osteoporosis fractures, status code Z87.310, Personal history of (healed) osteoporosis fracture, should follow the code from M81.

> Age-related osteoporosis with healed osteoporotic fracture of the lumbar vertebra
>
> **M81.0　　Age-related osteoporosis without current pathological fracture**
>
> **Z87.310　　Personal history of (healed) osteoporosis fracture**
>
> *Explanation:* Category M81 is used for patients with osteoporosis who do not currently have a pathologic fracture due to the osteoporosis. To report a previous (healed) fracture, status code Z87.310 Personal history of (healed) osteoporosis fracture, should follow the code from M81.

2) Osteoporosis with current pathological fracture

Category M80, Osteoporosis with current pathological fracture, is for patients who have a current pathological fracture at the time of an encounter. The codes under M80 identify the site of the fracture. A code from category M80, not a traumatic fracture code, should be used for any patient with known osteoporosis who suffers a fracture, even if the patient had a minor fall or trauma, if that fall or trauma would not usually break a normal, healthy bone.

> Disuse osteoporosis with current fracture of right shoulder sustained lifting a grocery bag, subsequent encounter
>
> **M80.811D　　Other osteoporosis with current pathological fracture, right shoulder, subsequent encounter for fracture with routine healing**
>
> *Explanation:* A code from category M80, not a traumatic fracture code, should be used for any patient with known osteoporosis who suffers a fracture, even if the patient had a minor fall or trauma, if that fall or trauma would not usually break a normal, healthy bone.

Muscle/Tendon Table

ICD-10-CM categorizes certain muscles and tendons in the upper and lower extremities by their action (e.g., extension, flexion), their anatomical location (e.g., posterior, anterior), and/or whether they are intrinsic or extrinsic to a certain anatomical area. The Muscle/Tendon Table is provided at the beginning of chapters 13 and 19 as a resource to help users when code selection depends on one or more of these characteristics. Please note that this table is not all-inclusive, and proper code assignment should be based on the provider's documentation.

Body Region	Muscle	Extensor Tendon	Flexor Tendon	Other Tendon
Shoulder				
	Deltoid	Posterior deltoid	Anterior deltoid	
	Rotator cuff			
	Infraspinatus			Infraspinatus
	Subscapularis			Subscapularis
	Supraspinatus			Supraspinatus
	Teres minor			Teres minor
	Teres major	Teres major		
Upper arm				
	Anterior muscles			
	Biceps brachii — long head		Biceps brachii — long head	
	Biceps brachii — short head		Biceps brachii — short head	
	Brachialis		Brachialis	
	Coracobrachialis		Coracobrachialis	
	Posterior muscles			
	Triceps brachii	Triceps brachii		
Forearm				
	Anterior muscles			
	Flexors			
	Deep			
	Flexor digitorum profundus		Flexor digitorum profundus	
	Flexor pollicis longus		Flexor pollicis longus	
	Intermediate			
	Flexor digitorum superficialis		Flexor digitorum superficialis	
	Superficial			
	Flexor carpi radialis		Flexor carpi radialis	
	Flexor carpi ulnaris		Flexor carpi ulnaris	
	Palmaris longus		Palmaris longus	
	Pronators			
	Pronator quadratus			Pronator quadratus
	Pronator teres			Pronator teres
	Posterior muscles			
	Extensors			
	Deep			
	Abductor pollicis longus			Abductor pollicis longus
	Extensor indicis	Extensor indicis		
	Extensor pollicis brevis	Extensor pollicis brevis		
	Extensor pollicis longus	Extensor pollicis longus		
	Superficial			
	Brachioradialis			Brachioradialis
	Extensor carpi radialis brevis	Extensor carpi radialis brevis		
	Extensor carpi radialis longus	Extensor carpi radialis longus		
	Extensor carpi ulnaris	Extensor carpi ulnaris		
	Extensor digiti minimi	Extensor digiti minimi		
	Extensor digitorum	Extensor digitorum		
	Anconeus	Anconeus		
	Supinator			Supinator

Body Region	Muscle	Extensor Tendon	Flexor Tendon	Other Tendon
Hand				
Extrinsic — attach to a site in the forearm as well as a site in the hand with action related to hand movement at the wrist				
	Extensor carpi radialis brevis	Extensor carpi radialis brevis		
	Extensor carpi radialis longus	Extensor carpie radialis longus		
	Extensor carpi ulnaris	Extensor carpi ulnaris		
	Flexor carpi radialis		Flexor carpi radialis	
	Flexor carpi ulnaris		Flexor carpi ulnaris	
	Flexor digitorum superficialis		Flexor digitorum superficialis	
	Palmaris longus		Palmaris longus	
Extrinsic — attach to a site in the forearm as well as a site in the hand with action in the hand related to finger movement				
	Adductor pollicis longus			Adductor pollicis longus
	Extensor digiti minimi	Extensor digiti minimi		
	Extensor digitorum	Extensor digitorum		
	Extensor indicis	Extensor indicis		
	Flexor digitorum profundus		Flexor digitorum profundus	
	Flexor digitorum superficialis		Flexor digitorum superficialis	
Extrinsic — attach to a site in the forearm as well as a site in the hand with action in the hand related to thumb movement				
	Extensor pollicis brevis	Extensor pollicis brevis		
	Extensor pollicis longus	Extensor pollicis longus		
	Flexor pollicis longus		Flexor pollicis longus	
Intrinsic — found within the hand only				
	Adductor pollicis			Adductor pollicis
	Dorsal interossei	Dorsal interossei	Dorsal interossei	
	Lumbricals	Lumbricals	Lumbricals	
	Palmaris brevis			Palmaris brevis
	Palmar interossei	Palmar interossei	Palmar interossei	
	Hypothenar muscles			
	Abductor digiti minimi			Abductor digiti minimi
	Flexor digiti minimi brevis		Flexor digiti minimi brevis	
	Oppenens digiti minimi		Oppenens digiti minimi	
	Thenar muscles			
	Abductor pollicis brevis			Abductor pollicis brevis
	Flexor pollicis brevis		Flexor pollicis brevis	
	Oppenens pollicis		Oppenens pollicis	
Thigh				
	Anterior muscles			
	Iliopsoas		Iliopsoas	
	Pectineus		Pectineus	
	Quadriceps	Quadriceps		
	Rectus femoris	Rectus femoris — Extends knee	Rectus femoris — Flexes hip	
	Vastus intermedius	Vastus intermedius		
	Vastus lateralis	Vastus lateralis		
	Vastus medialis	Vastus medialis		
	Sartorius		Sartorius	
	Medial muscles			
	Adductor brevis			Adductor brevis
	Adductor longus			Adductor longus
	Adductor magnus			Adductor magnus
	Gracilis			Gracilis
	Obturator externus			Obturator externus
	Posterior muscles			
	Hamstring	Hamstring — Extends hip	Hamstring — Flexes knee	
	Biceps femoris	Biceps femoris	Biceps femoris	
	Semimembranosus	Semimembranosus	Semimembranosus	
	Semitendinosus	Semitendinosus	Semitendinosus	

Body Region	Muscle	Extensor Tendon	Flexor Tendon	Other Tendon
Lower leg				
	Anterior muscles			
	Extensor digitorum longus	Extensor digitorum longus		
	Extensor hallucis longus	Extensor hallucis longus		
	Fibularis (peroneus) tertius	Fibularis (peroneus) tertius		
	Tibialis anterior	Tibialis anterior		Tibialis anterior
	Lateral muscles			
	Fibularis (peroneus) brevis		Fibularis (peroneus) brevis	
	Fibularis (peroneus) longus		Fibularis (peroneus) longus	
	Posterior muscles			
	Deep			
	Flexor digitorum longus		Flexor digitorum longus	
	Flexor hallucis longus		Flexor hallucis longus	
	Popliteus		Popliteus	
	Tibialis posterior		Tibialis posterior	
	Superficial			
	Gastrocnemius		Gastrocnemius	
	Plantaris		Plantaris	
	Soleus		Soleus	
				Calcaneal (Achilles)
Ankle/Foot				
Extrinsic — attach to a site in the lower leg as well as a site in the foot with action related to foot movement at the ankle				
	Plantaris		Plantaris	
	Soleus		Soleus	
	Tibialis anterior	Tibialis anterior		
	Tibialis posterior		Tibialis posterior	
Extrinsic — attach to a site in the lower leg as well as a site in the foot with action in the foot related to toe movement				
	Extensor digitorum longus	Extensor digitorum longus		
	Extensor hallicus longus	Extensor hallicus longus		
	Flexor digitorum longus		Flexor digitorum longus	
	Flexor hallucis longus		Flexor hallucis longus	
Intrinsic — found within the ankle/foot only				
	Dorsal muscles			
	Extensor digitorum brevis	Extensor digitorum brevis		
	Extensor hallucis brevis	Extensor hallucis brevis		
	Plantar muscles			
	Abductor digiti minimi		Abductor digiti minimi	
	Abductor hallucis		Abductor hallucis	
	Dorsal interossei	Dorsal interossei	Dorsal interossei	
	Flexor digiti minimi brevis		Flexor digiti minimi brevis	
	Flexor digitorum brevis		Flexor digitorum brevis	
	Flexor hallucis brevis		Flexor hallucis brevis	
	Lumbricals	Lumbricals	Lumbricals	
	Quadratus plantae		Quadratus plantae	
	Plantar interossei	Plantar interossei	Plantar interossei	

Chapter 13. Diseases of the Musculoskeletal System and Connective Tissue (M00-M99)

NOTE Use an external cause code following the code for the musculoskeletal condition, if applicable, to identify the cause of the musculoskeletal condition.

EXCLUDES 2 arthropathic psoriasis (L40.5-)
certain conditions originating in the perinatal period (P04-P96)
certain infectious and parasitic diseases (A00-B99)
compartment syndrome (traumatic) (T79.A-)
complications of pregnancy, childbirth and the puerperium (O00-O9A)
congenital malformations, deformations, and chromosomal abnormalities (Q00-Q99)
endocrine, nutritional and metabolic diseases (E00-E88)
injury, poisoning and certain other consequences of external causes (S00-T88)
neoplasms (C00-D49)
symptoms, signs and abnormal clinical and laboratory findings, not elsewhere classified (R00-R94)

This chapter contains the following blocks:

M00-M02 Infectious arthropathies
M04   ~~Autoinflammatory syndromes~~
M05-M14 Inflammatory polyarthropathies
M15-M19 Osteoarthritis
M20-M25 Other joint disorders
M26-M27 Dentofacial anomalies [including malocclusion] and other disorders of jaw
M30-M36 Systemic connective tissue disorders
M40-M43 Deforming dorsopathies
M45-M49 Spondylopathies
M50-M54 Other dorsopathies
M60-M63 Disorders of muscles
M65-M67 Disorders of synovium and tendon
M70-M79 Other soft tissue disorders
M80-M85 Disorders of bone density and structure
M86-M90 Other osteopathies
M91-M94 Chondropathies
M95   Other disorders of the musculoskeletal system and connective tissue
M96   Intraoperative and postprocedural complications and disorders of musculoskeletal system, not elsewhere classified
M97   ~~Periprosthetic fracture around internal prosthetic joint~~
M99   Biomechanical lesions, not elsewhere classified

ARTHROPATHIES (M00-M25)

INCLUDES disorders affecting predominantly peripheral (limb) joints

Infectious arthropathies (M00-M02)

NOTE This block comprises arthropathies due to microbiological agents. Distinction is made between the following types of etiological relationship:

a) direct infection of joint, where organisms invade synovial tissue and microbial antigen is present in the joint;
b) indirect infection, which may be of two types: a reactive arthropathy, where microbial infection of the body is established but neither organisms nor antigens can be identified in the joint, and a postinfective arthropathy, where microbial antigen is present but recovery of an organism is inconstant and evidence of local multiplication is lacking.

✓4th **M00 Pyogenic arthritis**

✓5th   **M00.0 Staphylococcal arthritis and polyarthritis**
Use additional code (B95.61-B95.8) to identify bacterial agent
EXCLUDES 2 infection and inflammatory reaction due to internal joint prosthesis (T84.5-)

M00.00 Staphylococcal arthritis, unspecified joint ▽

✓6th   M00.01 Staphylococcal arthritis, shoulder
M00.011 Staphylococcal arthritis, right shoulder
M00.012 Staphylococcal arthritis, left shoulder
M00.019 Staphylococcal arthritis, unspecified shoulder ▽

✓6th   M00.02 Staphylococcal arthritis, elbow
M00.021 Staphylococcal arthritis, right elbow
M00.022 Staphylococcal arthritis, left elbow
M00.029 Staphylococcal arthritis, unspecified elbow ▽

✓6th   M00.03 Staphylococcal arthritis, wrist
Staphylococcal arthritis of carpal bones
M00.031 Staphylococcal arthritis, right wrist
M00.032 Staphylococcal arthritis, left wrist

M00.039 Staphylococcal arthritis, unspecified wrist ▽

✓6th   M00.04 Staphylococcal arthritis, hand
Staphylococcal arthritis of metacarpus and phalanges
M00.041 Staphylococcal arthritis, right hand
M00.042 Staphylococcal arthritis, left hand
M00.049 Staphylococcal arthritis, unspecified hand ▽

✓6th   M00.05 Staphylococcal arthritis, hip
M00.051 Staphylococcal arthritis, right hip
M00.052 Staphylococcal arthritis, left hip
M00.059 Staphylococcal arthritis, unspecified hip ▽

✓6th   M00.06 Staphylococcal arthritis, knee
M00.061 Staphylococcal arthritis, right knee
M00.062 Staphylococcal arthritis, left knee
M00.069 Staphylococcal arthritis, unspecified knee ▽

✓6th   M00.07 Staphylococcal arthritis, ankle and foot
Staphylococcal arthritis, tarsus, metatarsus and phalanges
M00.071 Staphylococcal arthritis, right ankle and foot
M00.072 Staphylococcal arthritis, left ankle and foot
M00.079 Staphylococcal arthritis, unspecified ankle and foot ▽

M00.08 Staphylococcal arthritis, vertebrae

M00.09 Staphylococcal polyarthritis

✓5th   **M00.1 Pneumococcal arthritis and polyarthritis**
M00.10 Pneumococcal arthritis, unspecified joint ▽

✓6th   M00.11 Pneumococcal arthritis, shoulder
M00.111 Pneumococcal arthritis, right shoulder
M00.112 Pneumococcal arthritis, left shoulder
M00.119 Pneumococcal arthritis, unspecified shoulder ▽

✓6th   M00.12 Pneumococcal arthritis, elbow
M00.121 Pneumococcal arthritis, right elbow
M00.122 Pneumococcal arthritis, left elbow
M00.129 Pneumococcal arthritis, unspecified elbow ▽

✓6th   M00.13 Pneumococcal arthritis, wrist
Pneumococcal arthritis of carpal bones
M00.131 Pneumococcal arthritis, right wrist
M00.132 Pneumococcal arthritis, left wrist
M00.139 Pneumococcal arthritis, unspecified wrist ▽

✓6th   M00.14 Pneumococcal arthritis, hand
Pneumococcal arthritis of metacarpus and phalanges
M00.141 Pneumococcal arthritis, right hand
M00.142 Pneumococcal arthritis, left hand
M00.149 Pneumococcal arthritis, unspecified hand ▽

✓6th   M00.15 Pneumococcal arthritis, hip
M00.151 Pneumococcal arthritis, right hip
M00.152 Pneumococcal arthritis, left hip
M00.159 Pneumococcal arthritis, unspecified hip ▽

✓6th   M00.16 Pneumococcal arthritis, knee
M00.161 Pneumococcal arthritis, right knee
M00.162 Pneumococcal arthritis, left knee
M00.169 Pneumococcal arthritis, unspecified knee ▽

✓6th   M00.17 Pneumococcal arthritis, ankle and foot
Pneumococcal arthritis, tarsus, metatarsus and phalanges
M00.171 Pneumococcal arthritis, right ankle and foot
M00.172 Pneumococcal arthritis, left ankle and foot
M00.179 Pneumococcal arthritis, unspecified ankle and foot ▽

M00.18 Pneumococcal arthritis, vertebrae

M00.19 Pneumococcal polyarthritis

✓5ᵗʰ **M00.2 Other streptococcal arthritis and polyarthritis**
Use additional code (B95.0-B95.2, B95.4-B95.5) to identify bacterial agent

  M00.20 Other streptococcal arthritis, unspecified joint ▽

✓6ᵗʰ **M00.21** Other streptococcal arthritis, shoulder
  M00.211 Other streptococcal arthritis, right shoulder
  M00.212 Other streptococcal arthritis, left shoulder
  M00.219 Other streptococcal arthritis, unspecified shoulder ▽

✓6ᵗʰ **M00.22** Other streptococcal arthritis, elbow
  M00.221 Other streptococcal arthritis, right elbow
  M00.222 Other streptococcal arthritis, left elbow
  M00.229 Other streptococcal arthritis, unspecified elbow ▽

✓6ᵗʰ **M00.23** Other streptococcal arthritis, wrist
Other streptococcal arthritis of carpal bones
  M00.231 Other streptococcal arthritis, right wrist
  M00.232 Other streptococcal arthritis, left wrist
  M00.239 Other streptococcal arthritis, unspecified wrist ▽

✓6ᵗʰ **M00.24** Other streptococcal arthritis, hand
Other streptococcal arthritis metacarpus and phalanges
  M00.241 Other streptococcal arthritis, right hand
  M00.242 Other streptococcal arthritis, left hand
  M00.249 Other streptococcal arthritis, unspecified hand ▽

✓6ᵗʰ **M00.25** Other streptococcal arthritis, hip
  M00.251 Other streptococcal arthritis, right hip
  M00.252 Other streptococcal arthritis, left hip
  M00.259 Other streptococcal arthritis, unspecified hip ▽

✓6ᵗʰ **M00.26** Other streptococcal arthritis, knee
  M00.261 Other streptococcal arthritis, right knee
  M00.262 Other streptococcal arthritis, left knee
  M00.269 Other streptococcal arthritis, unspecified knee ▽

✓6ᵗʰ **M00.27** Other streptococcal arthritis, ankle and foot
Other streptococcal arthritis, tarsus, metatarsus and phalanges
  M00.271 Other streptococcal arthritis, right ankle and foot
  M00.272 Other streptococcal arthritis, left ankle and foot
  M00.279 Other streptococcal arthritis, unspecified ankle and foot ▽

  M00.28 Other streptococcal arthritis, vertebrae
  M00.29 Other streptococcal polyarthritis

✓5ᵗʰ **M00.8 Arthritis and polyarthritis due to other bacteria**
Use additional code (B96) to identify bacteria

  M00.80 Arthritis due to other bacteria, unspecified joint ▽

✓6ᵗʰ **M00.81** Arthritis due to other bacteria, shoulder
  M00.811 Arthritis due to other bacteria, right shoulder
  M00.812 Arthritis due to other bacteria, left shoulder
  M00.819 Arthritis due to other bacteria, unspecified shoulder ▽

✓6ᵗʰ **M00.82** Arthritis due to other bacteria, elbow
  M00.821 Arthritis due to other bacteria, right elbow
  M00.822 Arthritis due to other bacteria, left elbow
  M00.829 Arthritis due to other bacteria, unspecified elbow ▽

✓6ᵗʰ **M00.83** Arthritis due to other bacteria, wrist
Arthritis due to other bacteria, carpal bones
  M00.831 Arthritis due to other bacteria, right wrist
  M00.832 Arthritis due to other bacteria, left wrist
  M00.839 Arthritis due to other bacteria, unspecified wrist ▽

✓6ᵗʰ **M00.84** Arthritis due to other bacteria, hand
Arthritis due to other bacteria, metacarpus and phalanges
  M00.841 Arthritis due to other bacteria, right hand
  M00.842 Arthritis due to other bacteria, left hand

  M00.849 Arthritis due to other bacteria, unspecified hand ▽

✓6ᵗʰ **M00.85** Arthritis due to other bacteria, hip
  M00.851 Arthritis due to other bacteria, right hip
  M00.852 Arthritis due to other bacteria, left hip
  M00.859 Arthritis due to other bacteria, unspecified hip ▽

✓6ᵗʰ **M00.86** Arthritis due to other bacteria, knee
  M00.861 Arthritis due to other bacteria, right knee
  M00.862 Arthritis due to other bacteria, left knee
  M00.869 Arthritis due to other bacteria, unspecified knee ▽

✓6ᵗʰ **M00.87** Arthritis due to other bacteria, ankle and foot
Arthritis due to other bacteria, tarsus, metatarsus, and phalanges
  M00.871 Arthritis due to other bacteria, right ankle and foot
  M00.872 Arthritis due to other bacteria, left ankle and foot
  M00.879 Arthritis due to other bacteria, unspecified ankle and foot ▽

  M00.88 Arthritis due to other bacteria, vertebrae
  M00.89 Polyarthritis due to other bacteria

M00.9 Pyogenic arthritis, unspecified ▽
Infective arthritis NOS

✓4ᵗʰ **M01 Direct infections of joint in infectious and parasitic diseases classified elsewhere**
Code first underlying disease, such as:
leprosy [Hansen's disease] (A30.-)
mycoses (B35-B49)
O'nyong-nyong fever (A92.1)
paratyphoid fever (A01.1-A01.4)

EXCLUDES 1 arthropathy in Lyme disease (A69.23)
gonococcal arthritis (A54.42)
meningococcal arthritis (A39.83)
mumps arthritis (B26.85)
postinfective arthropathy (M02.-)
postmeningococcal arthritis (A39.84)
reactive arthritis (M02.3)
rubella arthritis (B06.82)
sarcoidosis arthritis (D86.86)
typhoid fever arthritis (A01.04)
tuberculosis arthritis (A18.01-A18.02)

✓5ᵗʰ **M01.X Direct infection of joint in infectious and parasitic diseases classified elsewhere**

  M01.X0 Direct infection of unspecified joint in infectious and parasitic diseases classified elsewhere ▽

✓6ᵗʰ **M01.X1** Direct infection of shoulder joint in infectious and parasitic diseases classified elsewhere
  M01.X11 Direct infection of right shoulder in infectious and parasitic diseases classified elsewhere
  M01.X12 Direct infection of left shoulder in infectious and parasitic diseases classified elsewhere
  M01.X19 Direct infection of unspecified shoulder in infectious and parasitic diseases classified elsewhere ▽

✓6ᵗʰ **M01.X2** Direct infection of elbow in infectious and parasitic diseases classified elsewhere
  M01.X21 Direct infection of right elbow in infectious and parasitic diseases classified elsewhere
  M01.X22 Direct infection of left elbow in infectious and parasitic diseases classified elsewhere
  M01.X29 Direct infection of unspecified elbow in infectious and parasitic diseases classified elsewhere

✓6ᵗʰ **M01.X3** Direct infection of wrist in infectious and parasitic diseases classified elsewhere
Direct infection of carpal bones in infectious and parasitic diseases classified elsewhere
  M01.X31 Direct infection of right wrist in infectious and parasitic diseases classified elsewhere
  M01.X32 Direct infection of left wrist in infectious and parasitic diseases classified elsewhere
  M01.X39 Direct infection of unspecified wrist in infectious and parasitic diseases classified elsewhere ▽

Ⓝ Newborn: 0   Ⓟ Pediatric: 0-17   Ⓜ Maternity: 12-55   Ⓐ Adult: 15-124   **NRS** Nonroutine supply Dx   **NCDx** Noncancer Dx   **PDx** Primary Dx   ►◄ Revised Text   ● New Code   ▲ Revised Title

720   ICD-10-CM 2018

✓6ᵗʰ **M01.X4** **Direct infection of** hand **in infectious and parasitic diseases classified elsewhere**
  Direct infection of metacarpus and phalanges in infectious and parasitic diseases classified elsewhere

    M01.X41   *Direct infection of right hand in infectious and parasitic diseases classified elsewhere*

    M01.X42   *Direct infection of left hand in infectious and parasitic diseases classified elsewhere*

    M01.X49   *Direct infection of unspecified hand in infectious and parasitic diseases classified elsewhere*   ▽

✓6ᵗʰ **M01.X5** **Direct infection of** hip **in infectious and parasitic diseases classified elsewhere**

    M01.X51   *Direct infection of right hip in infectious and parasitic diseases classified elsewhere*

    M01.X52   *Direct infection of left hip in infectious and parasitic diseases classified elsewhere*

    M01.X59   *Direct infection of unspecified hip in infectious and parasitic diseases classified elsewhere*   ▽

✓6ᵗʰ **M01.X6** **Direct infection of** knee **in infectious and parasitic diseases classified elsewhere**

    M01.X61   *Direct infection of right knee in infectious and parasitic diseases classified elsewhere*

    M01.X62   *Direct infection of left knee in infectious and parasitic diseases classified elsewhere*

    M01.X69   *Direct infection of unspecified knee in infectious and parasitic diseases classified elsewhere*   ▽

✓6ᵗʰ **M01.X7** **Direct infection of** ankle and foot **in infectious and parasitic diseases classified elsewhere**
  Direct infection of tarsus, metatarsus and phalanges in infectious and parasitic diseases classified elsewhere

    M01.X71   *Direct infection of right ankle and foot in infectious and parasitic diseases classified elsewhere*

    M01.X72   *Direct infection of left ankle and foot in infectious and parasitic diseases classified elsewhere*

    M01.X79   *Direct infection of unspecified ankle and foot in infectious and parasitic diseases classified elsewhere*   ▽

    M01.X8   *Direct infection of vertebrae in infectious and parasitic diseases classified elsewhere*

    M01.X9   *Direct infection of multiple joints in infectious and parasitic diseases classified elsewhere*

✓4ᵗʰ **M02 Postinfective and reactive arthropathies**

Code first underlying disease, such as:
  congenital syphilis [Clutton's joints] (A50.5)
  enteritis due to Yersinia enterocolitica (A04.6)
  infective endocarditis (I33.0)
  viral hepatitis (B15-B19)

EXCLUDES 1   Behçet's disease (M35.2)
  direct infections of joint in infectious and parasitic diseases classified elsewhere (M01.-)
  postmeningococcal arthritis (A39.84)
  mumps arthritis (B26.85)
  rheumatic fever (I00)
  rubella arthritis (B06.82)
  syphilis arthritis (late) (A52.77)
  tabetic arthropathy [Charcôt's] (A52.16)

✓5ᵗʰ **M02.0** **Arthropathy** following intestinal bypass

    M02.00   **Arthropathy following intestinal bypass, unspecified site**   ▽

✓6ᵗʰ   **M02.01**   **Arthropathy following intestinal bypass,** shoulder

      M02.011   **Arthropathy following intestinal bypass, right shoulder**

      M02.012   **Arthropathy following intestinal bypass, left shoulder**

      M02.019   **Arthropathy following intestinal bypass, unspecified shoulder**   ▽

✓6ᵗʰ   **M02.02**   **Arthropathy following intestinal bypass,** elbow

      M02.021   **Arthropathy following intestinal bypass, right elbow**

      M02.022   **Arthropathy following intestinal bypass, left elbow**

      M02.029   **Arthropathy following intestinal bypass, unspecified elbow**

✓6ᵗʰ   **M02.03**   **Arthropathy following intestinal bypass,** wrist
  Arthropathy following intestinal bypass, carpal bones

      M02.031   **Arthropathy following intestinal bypass, right wrist**

      M02.032   **Arthropathy following intestinal bypass, left wrist**

      M02.039   **Arthropathy following intestinal bypass, unspecified wrist**   ▽

✓6ᵗʰ   **M02.04**   **Arthropathy following intestinal bypass,** hand
  Arthropathy following intestinal bypass, metacarpals and phalanges

      M02.041   **Arthropathy following intestinal bypass, right hand**

      M02.042   **Arthropathy following intestinal bypass, left hand**

      M02.049   **Arthropathy following intestinal bypass, unspecified hand**   ▽

✓6ᵗʰ   **M02.05**   **Arthropathy following intestinal bypass,** hip

      M02.051   **Arthropathy following intestinal bypass, right hip**

      M02.052   **Arthropathy following intestinal bypass, left hip**

      M02.059   **Arthropathy following intestinal bypass, unspecified hip**   ▽

✓6ᵗʰ   **M02.06**   **Arthropathy following intestinal bypass,** knee

      M02.061   **Arthropathy following intestinal bypass, right knee**

      M02.062   **Arthropathy following intestinal bypass, left knee**

      M02.069   **Arthropathy following intestinal bypass, unspecified knee**   ▽

✓6ᵗʰ   **M02.07**   **Arthropathy following intestinal bypass,** ankle and foot
  Arthropathy following intestinal bypass, tarsus, metatarsus and phalanges

      M02.071   **Arthropathy following intestinal bypass, right ankle and foot**

      M02.072   **Arthropathy following intestinal bypass, left ankle and foot**

      M02.079   **Arthropathy following intestinal bypass, unspecified ankle and foot**   ▽

    M02.08   **Arthropathy following intestinal bypass,** vertebrae

    M02.09   **Arthropathy following intestinal bypass,** multiple sites

✓5ᵗʰ **M02.1** Postdysenteric **arthropathy**

    M02.10   **Postdysenteric arthropathy, unspecified site**   ▽

✓6ᵗʰ   **M02.11**   **Postdysenteric arthropathy,** shoulder

      M02.111   **Postdysenteric arthropathy, right shoulder**

      M02.112   **Postdysenteric arthropathy, left shoulder**

      M02.119   **Postdysenteric arthropathy, unspecified shoulder**   ▽

✓6ᵗʰ   **M02.12**   **Postdysenteric arthropathy,** elbow

      M02.121   **Postdysenteric arthropathy, right elbow**

      M02.122   **Postdysenteric arthropathy, left elbow**

      M02.129   **Postdysenteric arthropathy, unspecified elbow**   ▽

✓6ᵗʰ   **M02.13**   **Postdysenteric arthropathy,** wrist
  Postdysenteric arthropathy, carpal bones

      M02.131   **Postdysenteric arthropathy, right wrist**

      M02.132   **Postdysenteric arthropathy, left wrist**

      M02.139   **Postdysenteric arthropathy, unspecified wrist**

✓6ᵗʰ   **M02.14**   **Postdysenteric arthropathy,** hand
  Postdysenteric arthropathy, metacarpus and phalanges

      M02.141   **Postdysenteric arthropathy, right hand**

      M02.142   **Postdysenteric arthropathy, left hand**

      M02.149   **Postdysenteric arthropathy, unspecified hand**   ▽

✓6ᵗʰ   **M02.15**   **Postdysenteric arthropathy,** hip

      M02.151   **Postdysenteric arthropathy, right hip**

      M02.152   **Postdysenteric arthropathy, left hip**

      M02.159   **Postdysenteric arthropathy, unspecified hip**   ▽

✓ Additional Character Req   ✓7ᵗʰ Placeholder Alert   Case-Mix Diagnosis   Manifestation   ▽ Unspecified Dx   **EXCLUDES 1** Not coded here   **EXCLUDES 2** Not included here

✓6ᵗʰ **M02.16 Postdysenteric arthropathy,** knee
     M02.161 Postdysenteric arthropathy, right knee
     M02.162 Postdysenteric arthropathy, left knee
     M02.169 Postdysenteric arthropathy, ▽
              unspecified knee

✓6ᵗʰ **M02.17 Postdysenteric arthropathy,** ankle and foot
     Postdysenteric arthropathy, tarsus, metatarsus and phalanges
     M02.171 Postdysenteric arthropathy, right ankle and foot
     M02.172 Postdysenteric arthropathy, left ankle and foot
     M02.179 Postdysenteric arthropathy, ▽
              unspecified ankle and foot

     M02.18 Postdysenteric arthropathy, vertebrae
     M02.19 Postdysenteric arthropathy, multiple sites

✓5ᵗʰ **M02.2 Postimmunization arthropathy**
     M02.20 Postimmunization arthropathy, unspecified site ▽

✓6ᵗʰ **M02.21 Postimmunization arthropathy,** shoulder
     M02.211 Postimmunization arthropathy, right shoulder
     M02.212 Postimmunization arthropathy, left shoulder
     M02.219 Postimmunization arthropathy, ▽
              unspecified shoulder

✓6ᵗʰ **M02.22 Postimmunization arthropathy,** elbow
     M02.221 Postimmunization arthropathy, right elbow
     M02.222 Postimmunization arthropathy, left elbow
     M02.229 Postimmunization arthropathy, ▽
              unspecified elbow

✓6ᵗʰ **M02.23 Postimmunization arthropathy,** wrist
     Postimmunization arthropathy, carpal bones
     M02.231 Postimmunization arthropathy, right wrist
     M02.232 Postimmunization arthropathy, left wrist
     M02.239 Postimmunization arthropathy, ▽
              unspecified wrist

✓6ᵗʰ **M02.24 Postimmunization arthropathy,** hand
     Postimmunization arthropathy, metacarpus and phalanges
     M02.241 Postimmunization arthropathy, right hand
     M02.242 Postimmunization arthropathy, left hand
     M02.249 Postimmunization arthropathy, ▽
              unspecified hand

✓6ᵗʰ **M02.25 Postimmunization arthropathy,** hip
     M02.251 Postimmunization arthropathy, right hip
     M02.252 Postimmunization arthropathy, left hip
     M02.259 Postimmunization arthropathy, unspecified hip

✓6ᵗʰ **M02.26 Postimmunization arthropathy,** knee
     M02.261 Postimmunization arthropathy, right knee
     M02.262 Postimmunization arthropathy, left knee
     M02.269 Postimmunization arthropathy, ▽
              unspecified knee

✓6ᵗʰ **M02.27 Postimmunization arthropathy,** ankle and foot
     Postimmunization arthropathy, tarsus, metatarsus and phalanges
     M02.271 Postimmunization arthropathy, right ankle and foot
     M02.272 Postimmunization arthropathy, left ankle and foot
     M02.279 Postimmunization arthropathy, ▽
              unspecified ankle and foot

     M02.28 Postimmunization arthropathy, vertebrae
     M02.29 Postimmunization arthropathy, multiple sites

✓5ᵗʰ **M02.3 Reiter's disease**
     Reactive arthritis
     M02.30 Reiter's disease, unspecified site ▽

✓6ᵗʰ **M02.31 Reiter's disease,** shoulder
     M02.311 Reiter's disease, right shoulder
     M02.312 Reiter's disease, left shoulder
     M02.319 Reiter's disease, unspecified shoulder ▽

✓6ᵗʰ **M02.32 Reiter's disease,** elbow
     M02.321 Reiter's disease, right elbow
     M02.322 Reiter's disease, left elbow
     M02.329 Reiter's disease, unspecified elbow ▽

✓6ᵗʰ **M02.33 Reiter's disease,** wrist
     Reiter's disease, carpal bones
     M02.331 Reiter's disease, right wrist
     M02.332 Reiter's disease, left wrist
     M02.339 Reiter's disease, unspecified wrist ▽

✓6ᵗʰ **M02.34 Reiter's disease,** hand
     Reiter's disease, metacarpus and phalanges
     M02.341 Reiter's disease, right hand
     M02.342 Reiter's disease, left hand
     M02.349 Reiter's disease, unspecified hand ▽

✓6ᵗʰ **M02.35 Reiter's disease,** hip
     M02.351 Reiter's disease, right hip
     M02.352 Reiter's disease, left hip
     M02.359 Reiter's disease, unspecified hip ▽

✓6ᵗʰ **M02.36 Reiter's disease,** knee
     M02.361 Reiter's disease, right knee
     M02.362 Reiter's disease, left knee
     M02.369 Reiter's disease, unspecified knee ▽

✓6ᵗʰ **M02.37 Reiter's disease,** ankle and foot
     Reiter's disease, tarsus, metatarsus and phalanges
     M02.371 Reiter's disease, right ankle and foot
     M02.372 Reiter's disease, left ankle and foot
     M02.379 Reiter's disease, unspecified ankle ▽
              and foot

     M02.38 Reiter's disease, vertebrae
     M02.39 Reiter's disease, multiple sites

✓5ᵗʰ **M02.8 Other reactive arthropathies**
     M02.80 Other reactive arthropathies, unspecified site ▽

✓6ᵗʰ **M02.81 Other reactive arthropathies,** shoulder
     M02.811 Other reactive arthropathies, right shoulder
     M02.812 Other reactive arthropathies, left shoulder
     M02.819 Other reactive arthropathies, ▽
              unspecified shoulder

✓6ᵗʰ **M02.82 Other reactive arthropathies,** elbow
     M02.821 Other reactive arthropathies, right elbow
     M02.822 Other reactive arthropathies, left elbow
     M02.829 Other reactive arthropathies, ▽
              unspecified elbow

✓6ᵗʰ **M02.83 Other reactive arthropathies,** wrist
     Other reactive arthropathies, carpal bones
     M02.831 Other reactive arthropathies, right wrist
     M02.832 Other reactive arthropathies, left wrist
     M02.839 Other reactive arthropathies, ▽
              unspecified wrist

✓6ᵗʰ **M02.84 Other reactive arthropathies,** hand
     Other reactive arthropathies, metacarpus and phalanges
     M02.841 Other reactive arthropathies, right hand
     M02.842 Other reactive arthropathies, left hand
     M02.849 Other reactive arthropathies, ▽
              unspecified hand

✓6ᵗʰ **M02.85 Other reactive arthropathies,** hip
     M02.851 Other reactive arthropathies, right hip
     M02.852 Other reactive arthropathies, left hip
     M02.859 Other reactive arthropathies, ▽
              unspecified hip

✓6ᵗʰ **M02.86 Other reactive arthropathies,** knee
     M02.861 Other reactive arthropathies, right knee
     M02.862 Other reactive arthropathies, left knee
     M02.869 Other reactive arthropathies, ▽
              unspecified knee

✓6ᵗʰ **M02.87 Other reactive arthropathies,** ankle and foot
     Other reactive arthropathies, tarsus, metatarsus and phalanges
     M02.871 Other reactive arthropathies, right ankle and foot
     M02.872 Other reactive arthropathies, left ankle and foot
     M02.879 Other reactive arthropathies, ▽
              unspecified ankle and foot

Ⓝ Newborn: 0   Ⓟ Pediatric: 0-17   Ⓜ Maternity: 12-55   Ⓐ Adult: 15-124   NRS Nonroutine supply Dx   NCDx Noncancer Dx   PDx Primary Dx   ▶◀ Revised Text   ● New Code   ▲ Revised Title

722   ICD-10-CM 2018

M02.88   *Other reactive arthropathies, vertebrae*

M02.89   *Other reactive arthropathies, multiple sites*

M02.9   *Reactive arthropathy, unspecified* ▽

Autoinflammatory syndromes (M04)

✓4th M04   Autoinflammatory syndromes
EXCLUDES 2   *Crohn's disease (K50.-)*

M04.1   Periodic fever syndromes
Familial Mediterranean fever
Hyperimmunoglobin D syndrome
Mevalonate kinase deficiency
Tumor necrosis factor receptor associated periodic syndrome [TRAPS]

M04.2   Cryopyrin-associated periodic syndromes
Chronic infantile neurological, cutaneous and articular syndrome [CINCA]
Familial cold autoinflammatory syndrome
Familial cold urticaria
Muckle-Wells syndrome
Neonatal onset multisystemic inflammatory disorder [NOMID]

M04.8   Other autoinflammatory syndromes
Blau syndrome
Deficiency of interleukin 1 receptor antagonist [DIRA]
Majeed syndrome
Periodic fever, aphthous stomatitis, pharyngitis, and adenopathy syndrome [PFAPA]
Pyogenic arthritis, pyoderma gangrenosum, and acne syndrome [PAPA]

M04.9   Autoinflammatory syndrome, unspecified ▽

Inflammatory polyarthropathies (M05-M14)

✓4th M05   Rheumatoid arthritis with rheumatoid factor
EXCLUDES 1   *rheumatic fever (I00)*
juvenile rheumatoid arthritis (M08.-)
rheumatoid arthritis of spine (M45.-)
DEF: Rheumatoid arthritis: Autoimmune systemic disease that causes chronic inflammation of joints and other areas of the body, manifested by inflammatory changes in articular structures and synovial membranes, atrophy, and loss in bone density.

✓5th M05.0   Felty's syndrome
Rheumatoid arthritis with splenoadenomegaly and leukopenia

M05.00   Felty's syndrome, unspecified site ▽

✓6th M05.01   Felty's syndrome, shoulder
M05.011   Felty's syndrome, right shoulder
M05.012   Felty's syndrome, left shoulder
M05.019   Felty's syndrome, unspecified shoulder ▽

✓6th M05.02   Felty's syndrome, elbow
M05.021   Felty's syndrome, right elbow
M05.022   Felty's syndrome, left elbow
M05.029   Felty's syndrome, unspecified elbow ▽

✓6th M05.03   Felty's syndrome, wrist
Felty's syndrome, carpal bones
M05.031   Felty's syndrome, right wrist
M05.032   Felty's syndrome, left wrist
M05.039   Felty's syndrome, unspecified wrist ▽

✓6th M05.04   Felty's syndrome, hand
Felty's syndrome, metacarpus and phalanges
M05.041   Felty's syndrome, right hand
M05.042   Felty's syndrome, left hand
M05.049   Felty's syndrome, unspecified hand ▽

✓6th M05.05   Felty's syndrome, hip
M05.051   Felty's syndrome, right hip
M05.052   Felty's syndrome, left hip
M05.059   Felty's syndrome, unspecified hip ▽

✓6th M05.06   Felty's syndrome, knee
M05.061   Felty's syndrome, right knee
M05.062   Felty's syndrome, left knee
M05.069   Felty's syndrome, unspecified knee ▽

✓6th M05.07   Felty's syndrome, ankle and foot
Felty's syndrome, tarsus, metatarsus and phalanges
M05.071   Felty's syndrome, right ankle and foot
M05.072   Felty's syndrome, left ankle and foot
M05.079   Felty's syndrome, unspecified ankle and foot ▽

M05.09   Felty's syndrome, multiple sites

✓5th M05.1   Rheumatoid lung disease with rheumatoid arthritis
DEF: Lung disorders associated with rheumatoid arthritis.

M05.10   Rheumatoid lung disease with rheumatoid arthritis of unspecified site ▽

✓6th M05.11   Rheumatoid lung disease with rheumatoid arthritis of shoulder
M05.111   Rheumatoid lung disease with rheumatoid arthritis of right shoulder
M05.112   Rheumatoid lung disease with rheumatoid arthritis of left shoulder
M05.119   Rheumatoid lung disease with rheumatoid arthritis of unspecified shoulder ▽

✓6th M05.12   Rheumatoid lung disease with rheumatoid arthritis of elbow
M05.121   Rheumatoid lung disease with rheumatoid arthritis of right elbow
M05.122   Rheumatoid lung disease with rheumatoid arthritis of left elbow
M05.129   Rheumatoid lung disease with rheumatoid arthritis of unspecified elbow ▽

✓6th M05.13   Rheumatoid lung disease with rheumatoid arthritis of wrist
Rheumatoid lung disease with rheumatoid arthritis, carpal bones
M05.131   Rheumatoid lung disease with rheumatoid arthritis of right wrist
M05.132   Rheumatoid lung disease with rheumatoid arthritis of left wrist
M05.139   Rheumatoid lung disease with rheumatoid arthritis of unspecified wrist ▽

✓6th M05.14   Rheumatoid lung disease with rheumatoid arthritis of hand
Rheumatoid lung disease with rheumatoid arthritis, metacarpus and phalanges
M05.141   Rheumatoid lung disease with rheumatoid arthritis of right hand
M05.142   Rheumatoid lung disease with rheumatoid arthritis of left hand
M05.149   Rheumatoid lung disease with rheumatoid arthritis of unspecified hand ▽

✓6th M05.15   Rheumatoid lung disease with rheumatoid arthritis of hip
M05.151   Rheumatoid lung disease with rheumatoid arthritis of right hip
M05.152   Rheumatoid lung disease with rheumatoid arthritis of left hip
M05.159   Rheumatoid lung disease with rheumatoid arthritis of unspecified hip ▽

✓6th M05.16   Rheumatoid lung disease with rheumatoid arthritis of knee
M05.161   Rheumatoid lung disease with rheumatoid arthritis of right knee
M05.162   Rheumatoid lung disease with rheumatoid arthritis of left knee
M05.169   Rheumatoid lung disease with rheumatoid arthritis of unspecified knee ▽

✓6th M05.17   Rheumatoid lung disease with rheumatoid arthritis of ankle and foot
Rheumatoid lung disease with rheumatoid arthritis, tarsus, metatarsus and phalanges
M05.171   Rheumatoid lung disease with rheumatoid arthritis of right ankle and foot
M05.172   Rheumatoid lung disease with rheumatoid arthritis of left ankle and foot
M05.179   Rheumatoid lung disease with rheumatoid arthritis of unspecified ankle and foot ▽

M05.19   Rheumatoid lung disease with rheumatoid arthritis of multiple sites

✓5th M05.2   Rheumatoid vasculitis with rheumatoid arthritis

M05.20   Rheumatoid vasculitis with rheumatoid arthritis of unspecified site ▽

✓6th M05.21   Rheumatoid vasculitis with rheumatoid arthritis of shoulder
M05.211   Rheumatoid vasculitis with rheumatoid arthritis of right shoulder

✓ Additional Character Req   ✓x7th Placeholder Alert   Case-Mix Diagnosis   Manifestation   ▽ Unspecified Dx   EXCLUDES 1 Not coded here   EXCLUDES 2 Not included here

ICD-10-CM 2018   723

M02.88–M05.211

M05.212 Rheumatoid vasculitis with rheumatoid arthritis of left shoulder

M05.219 ▽ Rheumatoid vasculitis with rheumatoid arthritis of unspecified shoulder

✓6ᵗʰ M05.22 Rheumatoid vasculitis with rheumatoid arthritis of elbow

M05.221 Rheumatoid vasculitis with rheumatoid arthritis of right elbow

M05.222 Rheumatoid vasculitis with rheumatoid arthritis of left elbow

M05.229 ▽ Rheumatoid vasculitis with rheumatoid arthritis of unspecified elbow

✓6ᵗʰ M05.23 Rheumatoid vasculitis with rheumatoid arthritis of wrist

Rheumatoid vasculitis with rheumatoid arthritis, carpal bones

M05.231 Rheumatoid vasculitis with rheumatoid arthritis of right wrist

M05.232 Rheumatoid vasculitis with rheumatoid arthritis of left wrist

M05.239 ▽ Rheumatoid vasculitis with rheumatoid arthritis of unspecified wrist

✓6ᵗʰ M05.24 Rheumatoid vasculitis with rheumatoid arthritis of hand

Rheumatoid vasculitis with rheumatoid arthritis, metacarpus and phalanges

M05.241 Rheumatoid vasculitis with rheumatoid arthritis of right hand

M05.242 Rheumatoid vasculitis with rheumatoid arthritis of left hand

M05.249 ▽ Rheumatoid vasculitis with rheumatoid arthritis of unspecified hand

✓6ᵗʰ M05.25 Rheumatoid vasculitis with rheumatoid arthritis of hip

M05.251 Rheumatoid vasculitis with rheumatoid arthritis of right hip

M05.252 Rheumatoid vasculitis with rheumatoid arthritis of left hip

M05.259 ▽ Rheumatoid vasculitis with rheumatoid arthritis of unspecified hip

✓6ᵗʰ M05.26 Rheumatoid vasculitis with rheumatoid arthritis of knee

M05.261 Rheumatoid vasculitis with rheumatoid arthritis of right knee

M05.262 Rheumatoid vasculitis with rheumatoid arthritis of left knee

M05.269 ▽ Rheumatoid vasculitis with rheumatoid arthritis of unspecified knee

✓6ᵗʰ M05.27 Rheumatoid vasculitis with rheumatoid arthritis of ankle and foot

Rheumatoid vasculitis with rheumatoid arthritis, tarsus, metatarsus and phalanges

M05.271 Rheumatoid vasculitis with rheumatoid arthritis of right ankle and foot

M05.272 Rheumatoid vasculitis with rheumatoid arthritis of left ankle and foot

M05.279 ▽ Rheumatoid vasculitis with rheumatoid arthritis of unspecified ankle and foot

M05.29 Rheumatoid vasculitis with rheumatoid arthritis of multiple sites

✓5ᵗʰ M05.3 Rheumatoid heart disease with rheumatoid arthritis

Rheumatoid carditis   Rheumatoid myocarditis
Rheumatoid endocarditis   Rheumatoid pericarditis

M05.30 ▽ Rheumatoid heart disease with rheumatoid arthritis of unspecified site

✓6ᵗʰ M05.31 Rheumatoid heart disease with rheumatoid arthritis of shoulder

M05.311 Rheumatoid heart disease with rheumatoid arthritis of right shoulder

M05.312 Rheumatoid heart disease with rheumatoid arthritis of left shoulder

M05.319 ▽ Rheumatoid heart disease with rheumatoid arthritis of unspecified shoulder

✓6ᵗʰ M05.32 Rheumatoid heart disease with rheumatoid arthritis of elbow

M05.321 Rheumatoid heart disease with rheumatoid arthritis of right elbow

M05.322 Rheumatoid heart disease with rheumatoid arthritis of left elbow

M05.329 ▽ Rheumatoid heart disease with rheumatoid arthritis of unspecified elbow

✓6ᵗʰ M05.33 Rheumatoid heart disease with rheumatoid arthritis of wrist

Rheumatoid heart disease with rheumatoid arthritis, carpal bones

M05.331 Rheumatoid heart disease with rheumatoid arthritis of right wrist

M05.332 Rheumatoid heart disease with rheumatoid arthritis of left wrist

M05.339 ▽ Rheumatoid heart disease with rheumatoid arthritis of unspecified wrist

✓6ᵗʰ M05.34 Rheumatoid heart disease with rheumatoid arthritis of hand

Rheumatoid heart disease with rheumatoid arthritis, metacarpus and phalanges

M05.341 Rheumatoid heart disease with rheumatoid arthritis of right hand

M05.342 Rheumatoid heart disease with rheumatoid arthritis of left hand

M05.349 ▽ Rheumatoid heart disease with rheumatoid arthritis of unspecified hand

✓6ᵗʰ M05.35 Rheumatoid heart disease with rheumatoid arthritis of hip

M05.351 Rheumatoid heart disease with rheumatoid arthritis of right hip

M05.352 Rheumatoid heart disease with rheumatoid arthritis of left hip

M05.359 ▽ Rheumatoid heart disease with rheumatoid arthritis of unspecified hip

✓6ᵗʰ M05.36 Rheumatoid heart disease with rheumatoid arthritis of knee

M05.361 Rheumatoid heart disease with rheumatoid arthritis of right knee

M05.362 Rheumatoid heart disease with rheumatoid arthritis of left knee

M05.369 ▽ Rheumatoid heart disease with rheumatoid arthritis of unspecified knee

✓6ᵗʰ M05.37 Rheumatoid heart disease with rheumatoid arthritis of ankle and foot

Rheumatoid heart disease with rheumatoid arthritis, tarsus, metatarsus and phalanges

M05.371 Rheumatoid heart disease with rheumatoid arthritis of right ankle and foot

M05.372 Rheumatoid heart disease with rheumatoid arthritis of left ankle and foot

M05.379 ▽ Rheumatoid heart disease with rheumatoid arthritis of unspecified ankle and foot

M05.39 Rheumatoid heart disease with rheumatoid arthritis of multiple sites

✓5ᵗʰ M05.4 Rheumatoid myopathy with rheumatoid arthritis

M05.40 ▽ Rheumatoid myopathy with rheumatoid arthritis of unspecified site

✓6ᵗʰ M05.41 Rheumatoid myopathy with rheumatoid arthritis of shoulder

M05.411 Rheumatoid myopathy with rheumatoid arthritis of right shoulder

M05.412 Rheumatoid myopathy with rheumatoid arthritis of left shoulder

M05.419 ▽ Rheumatoid myopathy with rheumatoid arthritis of unspecified shoulder

✓6ᵗʰ M05.42 Rheumatoid myopathy with rheumatoid arthritis of elbow

M05.421 Rheumatoid myopathy with rheumatoid arthritis of right elbow

M05.422 Rheumatoid myopathy with rheumatoid arthritis of left elbow

M05.429 ▽ Rheumatoid myopathy with rheumatoid arthritis of unspecified elbow

Ⓝ Newborn: 0   Ⓟ Pediatric: 0-17   Ⓜ Maternity: 12-55   Ⓐ Adult: 15-124   NRS Nonroutine supply Dx   NCDx Noncancer Dx   PDx Primary Dx   ▶◀ Revised Text   ● New Code   ▲ Revised Title

724   ICD-10-CM 2018

✓6th **M05.43 Rheumatoid myopathy with rheumatoid arthritis of** wrist
Rheumatoid myopathy with rheumatoid arthritis, carpal bones

     M05.431 **Rheumatoid myopathy with rheumatoid arthritis of** right **wrist**

     M05.432 **Rheumatoid myopathy with rheumatoid arthritis of** left **wrist**

     M05.439 **Rheumatoid myopathy with rheumatoid arthritis of unspecified wrist** ▽

✓6th **M05.44 Rheumatoid myopathy with rheumatoid arthritis of** hand
Rheumatoid myopathy with rheumatoid arthritis, metacarpus and phalanges

     M05.441 **Rheumatoid myopathy with rheumatoid arthritis of** right **hand**

     M05.442 **Rheumatoid myopathy with rheumatoid arthritis of** left **hand**

     M05.449 **Rheumatoid myopathy with rheumatoid arthritis of unspecified hand** ▽

✓6th **M05.45 Rheumatoid myopathy with rheumatoid arthritis of** hip

     M05.451 **Rheumatoid myopathy with rheumatoid arthritis of** right **hip**

     M05.452 **Rheumatoid myopathy with rheumatoid arthritis of** left **hip**

     M05.459 **Rheumatoid myopathy with rheumatoid arthritis of unspecified hip** ▽

✓6th **M05.46 Rheumatoid myopathy with rheumatoid arthritis of** knee

     M05.461 **Rheumatoid myopathy with rheumatoid arthritis of** right **knee**

     M05.462 **Rheumatoid myopathy with rheumatoid arthritis of** left **knee**

     M05.469 **Rheumatoid myopathy with rheumatoid arthritis of unspecified knee** ▽

✓6th **M05.47 Rheumatoid myopathy with rheumatoid arthritis of** ankle and foot
Rheumatoid myopathy with rheumatoid arthritis, tarsus, metatarsus and phalanges

     M05.471 **Rheumatoid myopathy with rheumatoid arthritis of** right **ankle and foot**

     M05.472 **Rheumatoid myopathy with rheumatoid arthritis of** left **ankle and foot**

     M05.479 **Rheumatoid myopathy with rheumatoid arthritis of unspecified ankle and foot** ▽

     M05.49 **Rheumatoid myopathy with rheumatoid arthritis of multiple sites**

✓5th **M05.5 Rheumatoid** polyneuropathy with rheumatoid arthritis

     M05.50 **Rheumatoid polyneuropathy with rheumatoid arthritis of unspecified site** ▽

✓6th **M05.51 Rheumatoid polyneuropathy with rheumatoid arthritis of** shoulder

     M05.511 **Rheumatoid polyneuropathy with rheumatoid arthritis of** right **shoulder**

     M05.512 **Rheumatoid polyneuropathy with rheumatoid arthritis of** left **shoulder**

     M05.519 **Rheumatoid polyneuropathy with rheumatoid arthritis of unspecified shoulder** ▽

✓6th **M05.52 Rheumatoid polyneuropathy with rheumatoid arthritis of** elbow

     M05.521 **Rheumatoid polyneuropathy with rheumatoid arthritis of** right **elbow**

     M05.522 **Rheumatoid polyneuropathy with rheumatoid arthritis of** left **elbow**

     M05.529 **Rheumatoid polyneuropathy with rheumatoid arthritis of unspecified elbow** ▽

✓6th **M05.53 Rheumatoid polyneuropathy with rheumatoid arthritis of** wrist
Rheumatoid polyneuropathy with rheumatoid arthritis, carpal bones

     M05.531 **Rheumatoid polyneuropathy with rheumatoid arthritis of** right **wrist**

     M05.532 **Rheumatoid polyneuropathy with rheumatoid arthritis of** left **wrist**

     M05.539 **Rheumatoid polyneuropathy with rheumatoid arthritis of unspecified wrist** ▽

✓6th **M05.54 Rheumatoid polyneuropathy with rheumatoid arthritis of** hand
Rheumatoid polyneuropathy with rheumatoid arthritis, metacarpus and phalanges

     M05.541 **Rheumatoid polyneuropathy with rheumatoid arthritis of** right **hand**

     M05.542 **Rheumatoid polyneuropathy with rheumatoid arthritis of** left **hand**

     M05.549 **Rheumatoid polyneuropathy with rheumatoid arthritis of unspecified hand** ▽

✓6th **M05.55 Rheumatoid polyneuropathy with rheumatoid arthritis of** hip

     M05.551 **Rheumatoid polyneuropathy with rheumatoid arthritis of** right **hip**

     M05.552 **Rheumatoid polyneuropathy with rheumatoid arthritis of** left **hip**

     M05.559 **Rheumatoid polyneuropathy with rheumatoid arthritis of unspecified hip** ▽

✓6th **M05.56 Rheumatoid polyneuropathy with rheumatoid arthritis of** knee

     M05.561 **Rheumatoid polyneuropathy with rheumatoid arthritis of** right **knee**

     M05.562 **Rheumatoid polyneuropathy with rheumatoid arthritis of** left **knee**

     M05.569 **Rheumatoid polyneuropathy with rheumatoid arthritis of unspecified knee** ▽

✓6th **M05.57 Rheumatoid polyneuropathy with rheumatoid arthritis of** ankle and foot
Rheumatoid polyneuropathy with rheumatoid arthritis, tarsus, metatarsus and phalanges

     M05.571 **Rheumatoid polyneuropathy with rheumatoid arthritis of** right **ankle and foot**

     M05.572 **Rheumatoid polyneuropathy with rheumatoid arthritis of** left **ankle and foot**

     M05.579 **Rheumatoid polyneuropathy with rheumatoid arthritis of unspecified ankle and foot** ▽

     M05.59 **Rheumatoid polyneuropathy with rheumatoid arthritis of multiple sites**

✓5th **M05.6 Rheumatoid arthritis** with involvement of other organs and systems

     M05.60 **Rheumatoid arthritis of unspecified site with involvement of other organs and systems** ▽

✓6th **M05.61 Rheumatoid arthritis of** shoulder **with involvement of other organs and systems**

     M05.611 **Rheumatoid arthritis of** right **shoulder with involvement of other organs and systems**

     M05.612 **Rheumatoid arthritis of** left **shoulder with involvement of other organs and systems**

     M05.619 **Rheumatoid arthritis of unspecified shoulder with involvement of other organs and systems** ▽

✓6th **M05.62 Rheumatoid arthritis of** elbow **with involvement of other organs and systems**

     M05.621 **Rheumatoid arthritis of** right **elbow with involvement of other organs and systems**

     M05.622 **Rheumatoid arthritis of** left **elbow with involvement of other organs and systems**

     M05.629 **Rheumatoid arthritis of unspecified elbow with involvement of other organs and systems** ▽

✓6th **M05.63 Rheumatoid arthritis of** wrist **with involvement of other organs and systems**
Rheumatoid arthritis of carpal bones with involvement of other organs and systems

     M05.631 **Rheumatoid arthritis of** right **wrist with involvement of other organs and systems**

     M05.632 **Rheumatoid arthritis of** left **wrist with involvement of other organs and systems**

     M05.639 **Rheumatoid arthritis of unspecified wrist with involvement of other organs and systems** ▽

✓ Additional Character Req   ✓x7th Placeholder Alert   Case-Mix Diagnosis   Manifestation   ▽ Unspecified Dx   *EXCLUDES 1* Not coded here   *EXCLUDES 2* Not included here

✓6ᵗʰ **M05.64** Rheumatoid arthritis of hand with involvement of other organs and systems
Rheumatoid arthritis of metacarpus and phalanges with involvement of other organs and systems

M05.641 Rheumatoid arthritis of right hand with involvement of other organs and systems

M05.642 Rheumatoid arthritis of left hand with involvement of other organs and systems

M05.649 Rheumatoid arthritis of unspecified ▽ hand with involvement of other organs and systems

✓6ᵗʰ **M05.65** Rheumatoid arthritis of hip with involvement of other organs and systems

M05.651 Rheumatoid arthritis of right hip with involvement of other organs and systems

M05.652 Rheumatoid arthritis of left hip with involvement of other organs and systems

M05.659 Rheumatoid arthritis of unspecified hip ▽ with involvement of other organs and systems

✓6ᵗʰ **M05.66** Rheumatoid arthritis of knee with involvement of other organs and systems

M05.661 Rheumatoid arthritis of right knee with involvement of other organs and systems

M05.662 Rheumatoid arthritis of left knee with involvement of other organs and systems

M05.669 Rheumatoid arthritis of unspecified ▽ knee with involvement of other organs and systems

✓6ᵗʰ **M05.67** Rheumatoid arthritis of ankle and foot with involvement of other organs and systems
Rheumatoid arthritis of tarsus, metatarsus and phalanges with involvement of other organs and systems

M05.671 Rheumatoid arthritis of right ankle and foot with involvement of other organs and systems

M05.672 Rheumatoid arthritis of left ankle and foot with involvement of other organs and systems

M05.679 Rheumatoid arthritis of unspecified ▽ ankle and foot with involvement of other organs and systems

M05.69 Rheumatoid arthritis of multiple sites with involvement of other organs and systems

✓5ᵗʰ **M05.7** Rheumatoid arthritis with rheumatoid factor without organ or systems involvement

M05.70 Rheumatoid arthritis with rheumatoid factor of ▽ unspecified site without organ or systems involvement

✓6ᵗʰ **M05.71** Rheumatoid arthritis with rheumatoid factor of shoulder without organ or systems involvement

M05.711 Rheumatoid arthritis with rheumatoid factor of right shoulder without organ or systems involvement

M05.712 Rheumatoid arthritis with rheumatoid factor of left shoulder without organ or systems involvement

M05.719 Rheumatoid arthritis with rheumatoid ▽ factor of unspecified shoulder without organ or systems involvement

✓6ᵗʰ **M05.72** Rheumatoid arthritis with rheumatoid factor of elbow without organ or systems involvement

M05.721 Rheumatoid arthritis with rheumatoid factor of right elbow without organ or systems involvement

M05.722 Rheumatoid arthritis with rheumatoid factor of left elbow without organ or systems involvement

M05.729 Rheumatoid arthritis with rheumatoid ▽ factor of unspecified elbow without organ or systems involvement

✓6ᵗʰ **M05.73** Rheumatoid arthritis with rheumatoid factor of wrist without organ or systems involvement

M05.731 Rheumatoid arthritis with rheumatoid factor of right wrist without organ or systems involvement

M05.732 Rheumatoid arthritis with rheumatoid factor of left wrist without organ or systems involvement

M05.739 Rheumatoid arthritis with rheumatoid ▽ factor of unspecified wrist without organ or systems involvement

✓6ᵗʰ **M05.74** Rheumatoid arthritis with rheumatoid factor of hand without organ or systems involvement

M05.741 Rheumatoid arthritis with rheumatoid factor of right hand without organ or systems involvement

M05.742 Rheumatoid arthritis with rheumatoid factor of left hand without organ or systems involvement

M05.749 Rheumatoid arthritis with rheumatoid ▽ factor of unspecified hand without organ or systems involvement

✓6ᵗʰ **M05.75** Rheumatoid arthritis with rheumatoid factor of hip without organ or systems involvement

M05.751 Rheumatoid arthritis with rheumatoid factor of right hip without organ or systems involvement

M05.752 Rheumatoid arthritis with rheumatoid factor of left hip without organ or systems involvement

M05.759 Rheumatoid arthritis with rheumatoid ▽ factor of unspecified hip without organ or systems involvement

✓6ᵗʰ **M05.76** Rheumatoid arthritis with rheumatoid factor of knee without organ or systems involvement

M05.761 Rheumatoid arthritis with rheumatoid factor of right knee without organ or systems involvement

M05.762 Rheumatoid arthritis with rheumatoid factor of left knee without organ or systems involvement

M05.769 Rheumatoid arthritis with rheumatoid ▽ factor of unspecified knee without organ or systems involvement

✓6ᵗʰ **M05.77** Rheumatoid arthritis with rheumatoid factor of ankle and foot without organ or systems involvement

M05.771 Rheumatoid arthritis with rheumatoid factor of right ankle and foot without organ or systems involvement

M05.772 Rheumatoid arthritis with rheumatoid factor of left ankle and foot without organ or systems involvement

M05.779 Rheumatoid arthritis with rheumatoid ▽ factor of unspecified ankle and foot without organ or systems involvement

M05.79 Rheumatoid arthritis with rheumatoid factor of multiple sites without organ or systems involvement

✓5ᵗʰ **M05.8** Other rheumatoid arthritis with rheumatoid factor

M05.80 Other rheumatoid arthritis with rheumatoid ▽ factor of unspecified site

✓6ᵗʰ **M05.81** Other rheumatoid arthritis with rheumatoid factor of shoulder

M05.811 Other rheumatoid arthritis with rheumatoid factor of right shoulder

M05.812 Other rheumatoid arthritis with rheumatoid factor of left shoulder

M05.819 Other rheumatoid arthritis with ▽ rheumatoid factor of unspecified shoulder

✓6ᵗʰ **M05.82** Other rheumatoid arthritis with rheumatoid factor of elbow

M05.821 Other rheumatoid arthritis with rheumatoid factor of right elbow

M05.822 Other rheumatoid arthritis with rheumatoid factor of left elbow

M05.829 Other rheumatoid arthritis with ▽ rheumatoid factor of unspecified elbow

✓6ᵗʰ **M05.83** Other rheumatoid arthritis with rheumatoid factor of wrist

M05.831 Other rheumatoid arthritis with rheumatoid factor of right wrist

M05.832 Other rheumatoid arthritis with rheumatoid factor of left wrist

M05.839 Other rheumatoid arthritis with ▽ rheumatoid factor of unspecified wrist

N Newborn: 0   P Pediatric: 0-17   M Maternity: 12-55   A Adult: 15-124   **NRS** Nonroutine supply Dx   **NCDx** Noncancer Dx   **PDx** Primary Dx   ▶◀ Revised Text   ● New Code   ▲ Revised Title

726 ICD-10-CM 2018

✓6th **M05.84** **Other rheumatoid arthritis with rheumatoid factor of** hand

    M05.841 **Other rheumatoid arthritis with rheumatoid factor of** right **hand**

    M05.842 **Other rheumatoid arthritis with rheumatoid factor of** left **hand**

    M05.849 **Other rheumatoid arthritis with rheumatoid factor of unspecified hand** ▽

✓6th **M05.85** **Other rheumatoid arthritis with rheumatoid factor of** hip

    M05.851 **Other rheumatoid arthritis with rheumatoid factor of** right **hip**

    M05.852 **Other rheumatoid arthritis with rheumatoid factor of** left **hip**

    M05.859 **Other rheumatoid arthritis with rheumatoid factor of unspecified hip** ▽

✓6th **M05.86** **Other rheumatoid arthritis with rheumatoid factor of** knee

    M05.861 **Other rheumatoid arthritis with rheumatoid factor of** right **knee**

    M05.862 **Other rheumatoid arthritis with rheumatoid factor of** left **knee**

    M05.869 **Other rheumatoid arthritis with rheumatoid factor of unspecified knee** ▽

✓6th **M05.87** **Other rheumatoid arthritis with rheumatoid factor of** ankle and foot

    M05.871 **Other rheumatoid arthritis with rheumatoid factor of** right **ankle and foot**

    M05.872 **Other rheumatoid arthritis with rheumatoid factor of** left **ankle and foot**

    M05.879 **Other rheumatoid arthritis with rheumatoid factor of unspecified ankle and foot** ▽

    M05.89 **Other rheumatoid arthritis with rheumatoid factor of** multiple sites

M05.9 **Rheumatoid arthritis with rheumatoid factor, unspecified** ▽

✓4th **M06** **Other rheumatoid arthritis**

DEF: Rheumatoid arthritis: Autoimmune systemic disease that causes chronic inflammation of joints and other areas of the body, manifested by inflammatory changes in articular structures and synovial membranes, atrophy, and loss in bone density.

✓5th **M06.0** **Rheumatoid arthritis** without rheumatoid factor

    M06.00 **Rheumatoid arthritis without rheumatoid factor, unspecified site** ▽

✓6th **M06.01** **Rheumatoid arthritis without rheumatoid factor,** shoulder

    M06.011 **Rheumatoid arthritis without rheumatoid factor,** right **shoulder**

    M06.012 **Rheumatoid arthritis without rheumatoid factor,** left **shoulder**

    M06.019 **Rheumatoid arthritis without rheumatoid factor, unspecified shoulder** ▽

✓6th **M06.02** **Rheumatoid arthritis without rheumatoid factor,** elbow

    M06.021 **Rheumatoid arthritis without rheumatoid factor,** right **elbow**

    M06.022 **Rheumatoid arthritis without rheumatoid factor,** left **elbow**

    M06.029 **Rheumatoid arthritis without rheumatoid factor, unspecified elbow** ▽

✓6th **M06.03** **Rheumatoid arthritis without rheumatoid factor,** wrist

    M06.031 **Rheumatoid arthritis without rheumatoid factor,** right **wrist**

    M06.032 **Rheumatoid arthritis without rheumatoid factor,** left **wrist**

    M06.039 **Rheumatoid arthritis without rheumatoid factor, unspecified wrist** ▽

✓6th **M06.04** **Rheumatoid arthritis without rheumatoid factor,** hand

    M06.041 **Rheumatoid arthritis without rheumatoid factor,** right **hand**

    M06.042 **Rheumatoid arthritis without rheumatoid factor,** left **hand**

    M06.049 **Rheumatoid arthritis without rheumatoid factor, unspecified hand** ▽

✓6th **M06.05** **Rheumatoid arthritis without rheumatoid factor,** hip

    M06.051 **Rheumatoid arthritis without rheumatoid factor,** right **hip**

    M06.052 **Rheumatoid arthritis without rheumatoid factor,** left **hip**

    M06.059 **Rheumatoid arthritis without rheumatoid factor, unspecified hip** ▽

✓6th **M06.06** **Rheumatoid arthritis without rheumatoid factor,** knee

    M06.061 **Rheumatoid arthritis without rheumatoid factor,** right **knee**

    M06.062 **Rheumatoid arthritis without rheumatoid factor,** left **knee**

    M06.069 **Rheumatoid arthritis without rheumatoid factor, unspecified knee** ▽

✓6th **M06.07** **Rheumatoid arthritis without rheumatoid factor,** ankle and foot

    M06.071 **Rheumatoid arthritis without rheumatoid factor,** right **ankle and foot**

    M06.072 **Rheumatoid arthritis without rheumatoid factor,** left **ankle and foot**

    M06.079 **Rheumatoid arthritis without rheumatoid factor, unspecified ankle and foot** ▽

    M06.08 **Rheumatoid arthritis without rheumatoid factor,** vertebrae

    M06.09 **Rheumatoid arthritis without rheumatoid factor,** multiple sites

M06.1 **Adult-onset Still's disease**   Ⓐ

    EXCLUDES 1   *Still's disease NOS (M08.2-)*

✓5th **M06.2** **Rheumatoid bursitis**

    M06.20 **Rheumatoid bursitis, unspecified site** ▽

✓6th **M06.21** **Rheumatoid bursitis,** shoulder

    M06.211 **Rheumatoid bursitis,** right **shoulder**

    M06.212 **Rheumatoid bursitis,** left **shoulder**

    M06.219 **Rheumatoid bursitis, unspecified shoulder** ▽

✓6th **M06.22** **Rheumatoid bursitis,** elbow

    M06.221 **Rheumatoid bursitis,** right **elbow**

    M06.222 **Rheumatoid bursitis,** left **elbow**

    M06.229 **Rheumatoid bursitis, unspecified elbow** ▽

✓6th **M06.23** **Rheumatoid bursitis,** wrist

    M06.231 **Rheumatoid bursitis,** right **wrist**

    M06.232 **Rheumatoid bursitis,** left **wrist**

    M06.239 **Rheumatoid bursitis, unspecified wrist** ▽

✓6th **M06.24** **Rheumatoid bursitis,** hand

    M06.241 **Rheumatoid bursitis,** right **hand**

    M06.242 **Rheumatoid bursitis,** left **hand**

    M06.249 **Rheumatoid bursitis, unspecified hand** ▽

✓6th **M06.25** **Rheumatoid bursitis,** hip

    M06.251 **Rheumatoid bursitis,** right **hip**

    M06.252 **Rheumatoid bursitis,** left **hip**

    M06.259 **Rheumatoid bursitis, unspecified hip** ▽

✓6th **M06.26** **Rheumatoid bursitis,** knee

    M06.261 **Rheumatoid bursitis,** right **knee**

    M06.262 **Rheumatoid bursitis,** left **knee**

    M06.269 **Rheumatoid bursitis, unspecified knee** ▽

✓6th **M06.27** **Rheumatoid bursitis,** ankle and foot

    M06.271 **Rheumatoid bursitis,** right **ankle and foot**

    M06.272 **Rheumatoid bursitis,** left **ankle and foot**

    M06.279 **Rheumatoid bursitis, unspecified ankle and foot** ▽

    M06.28 **Rheumatoid bursitis,** vertebrae

    M06.29 **Rheumatoid bursitis,** multiple sites

✓5th **M06.3** **Rheumatoid nodule**

    M06.30 **Rheumatoid nodule, unspecified site** ▽

✓6th **M06.31** **Rheumatoid nodule,** shoulder

    M06.311 **Rheumatoid nodule,** right **shoulder**

    M06.312 **Rheumatoid nodule,** left **shoulder**

    M06.319 **Rheumatoid nodule, unspecified shoulder** ▽

✓ Additional Character Req   ✓x7th Placeholder Alert   Case-Mix Diagnosis   Manifestation   ▽ Unspecified Dx   EXCLUDES 1 Not coded here   EXCLUDES 2 Not included here

ICD-10-CM 2018   727

Chapter 13. Diseases of the Musculoskeletal System and Connective Tissue

M06.32–M08.012

✓6ᵗʰ **M06.32** Rheumatoid nodule, elbow
     M06.321 Rheumatoid nodule, right elbow
     M06.322 Rheumatoid nodule, left elbow
     M06.329 Rheumatoid nodule, unspecified elbow ▽

✓6ᵗʰ **M06.33** Rheumatoid nodule, wrist
     M06.331 Rheumatoid nodule, right wrist
     M06.332 Rheumatoid nodule, left wrist
     M06.339 Rheumatoid nodule, unspecified wrist ▽

✓6ᵗʰ **M06.34** Rheumatoid nodule, hand
     M06.341 Rheumatoid nodule, right hand
     M06.342 Rheumatoid nodule, left hand
     M06.349 Rheumatoid nodule, unspecified hand ▽

✓6ᵗʰ **M06.35** Rheumatoid nodule, hip
     M06.351 Rheumatoid nodule, right hip
     M06.352 Rheumatoid nodule, left hip
     M06.359 Rheumatoid nodule, unspecified hip ▽

✓6ᵗʰ **M06.36** Rheumatoid nodule, knee
     M06.361 Rheumatoid nodule, right knee
     M06.362 Rheumatoid nodule, left knee
     M06.369 Rheumatoid nodule, unspecified knee ▽

✓6ᵗʰ **M06.37** Rheumatoid nodule, ankle and foot
     M06.371 Rheumatoid nodule, right ankle and foot
     M06.372 Rheumatoid nodule, left ankle and foot
     M06.379 Rheumatoid nodule, unspecified ankle and foot ▽

     M06.38 Rheumatoid nodule, vertebrae
     M06.39 Rheumatoid nodule, multiple sites

M06.4 Inflammatory polyarthropathy
     EXCLUDES 1   polyarthritis NOS (M13.0)

✓5ᵗʰ **M06.8** Other specified rheumatoid arthritis
     M06.80 Other specified rheumatoid arthritis, unspecified ▽ site

✓6ᵗʰ **M06.81** Other specified rheumatoid arthritis, shoulder
     M06.811 Other specified rheumatoid arthritis, right shoulder
     M06.812 Other specified rheumatoid arthritis, left shoulder
     M06.819 Other specified rheumatoid arthritis, unspecified shoulder ▽

✓6ᵗʰ **M06.82** Other specified rheumatoid arthritis, elbow
     M06.821 Other specified rheumatoid arthritis, right elbow
     M06.822 Other specified rheumatoid arthritis, left elbow
     M06.829 Other specified rheumatoid arthritis, unspecified elbow ▽

✓6ᵗʰ **M06.83** Other specified rheumatoid arthritis, wrist
     M06.831 Other specified rheumatoid arthritis, right wrist
     M06.832 Other specified rheumatoid arthritis, left wrist
     M06.839 Other specified rheumatoid arthritis, unspecified wrist ▽

✓6ᵗʰ **M06.84** Other specified rheumatoid arthritis, hand
     M06.841 Other specified rheumatoid arthritis, right hand
     M06.842 Other specified rheumatoid arthritis, left hand
     M06.849 Other specified rheumatoid arthritis, unspecified hand ▽

✓6ᵗʰ **M06.85** Other specified rheumatoid arthritis, hip
     M06.851 Other specified rheumatoid arthritis, right hip
     M06.852 Other specified rheumatoid arthritis, left hip
     M06.859 Other specified rheumatoid arthritis, unspecified hip ▽

✓6ᵗʰ **M06.86** Other specified rheumatoid arthritis, knee
     M06.861 Other specified rheumatoid arthritis, right knee
     M06.862 Other specified rheumatoid arthritis, left knee
     M06.869 Other specified rheumatoid arthritis, unspecified knee ▽

✓6ᵗʰ **M06.87** Other specified rheumatoid arthritis, ankle and foot
     M06.871 Other specified rheumatoid arthritis, right ankle and foot
     M06.872 Other specified rheumatoid arthritis, left ankle and foot
     M06.879 Other specified rheumatoid arthritis, unspecified ankle and foot ▽

     M06.88 Other specified rheumatoid arthritis, vertebrae
     M06.89 Other specified rheumatoid arthritis, multiple sites

M06.9 Rheumatoid arthritis, unspecified ▽

✓4ᵗʰ **M07** Enteropathic arthropathies
     Code also associated enteropathy, such as:
       regional enteritis [Crohn's disease] (K50.-)
       ulcerative colitis (K51.-)
     EXCLUDES 1   psoriatic arthropathies (L40.5-)

✓5ᵗʰ **M07.6** Enteropathic arthropathies
     M07.60 Enteropathic arthropathies, unspecified site ▽

✓6ᵗʰ **M07.61** Enteropathic arthropathies, shoulder
     M07.611 Enteropathic arthropathies, right shoulder
     M07.612 Enteropathic arthropathies, left shoulder
     M07.619 Enteropathic arthropathies, unspecified shoulder ▽

✓6ᵗʰ **M07.62** Enteropathic arthropathies, elbow
     M07.621 Enteropathic arthropathies, right elbow
     M07.622 Enteropathic arthropathies, left elbow
     M07.629 Enteropathic arthropathies, unspecified elbow ▽

✓6ᵗʰ **M07.63** Enteropathic arthropathies, wrist
     M07.631 Enteropathic arthropathies, right wrist
     M07.632 Enteropathic arthropathies, left wrist
     M07.639 Enteropathic arthropathies, unspecified wrist ▽

✓6ᵗʰ **M07.64** Enteropathic arthropathies, hand
     M07.641 Enteropathic arthropathies, right hand
     M07.642 Enteropathic arthropathies, left hand
     M07.649 Enteropathic arthropathies, unspecified hand ▽

✓6ᵗʰ **M07.65** Enteropathic arthropathies, hip
     M07.651 Enteropathic arthropathies, right hip
     M07.652 Enteropathic arthropathies, left hip
     M07.659 Enteropathic arthropathies, unspecified hip ▽

✓6ᵗʰ **M07.66** Enteropathic arthropathies, knee
     M07.661 Enteropathic arthropathies, right knee
     M07.662 Enteropathic arthropathies, left knee
     M07.669 Enteropathic arthropathies, unspecified knee ▽

✓6ᵗʰ **M07.67** Enteropathic arthropathies, ankle and foot
     M07.671 Enteropathic arthropathies, right ankle and foot
     M07.672 Enteropathic arthropathies, left ankle and foot
     M07.679 Enteropathic arthropathies, unspecified ankle and foot ▽

     M07.68 Enteropathic arthropathies, vertebrae
     M07.69 Enteropathic arthropathies, multiple sites

✓4ᵗʰ **M08** Juvenile arthritis
     Code also any associated underlying condition, such as:
       regional enteritis [Crohn's disease] (K50.-)
       ulcerative colitis (K51.-)
     EXCLUDES 1   arthropathy in Whipple's disease (M14.8)
               Felty's syndrome (M05.0)
               juvenile dermatomyositis (M33.0-)
               psoriatic juvenile arthropathy (L40.54)

✓5ᵗʰ **M08.0** Unspecified juvenile rheumatoid arthritis
     Juvenile rheumatoid arthritis with or without rheumatoid factor
     M08.00 Unspecified juvenile rheumatoid arthritis of unspecified site ▽

✓6ᵗʰ **M08.01** Unspecified juvenile rheumatoid arthritis, shoulder
     M08.011 Unspecified juvenile rheumatoid arthritis, right shoulder ▽
     M08.012 Unspecified juvenile rheumatoid arthritis, left shoulder ▽

Ⓝ Newborn: 0   Ⓟ Pediatric: 0-17   Ⓜ Maternity: 12-55   Ⓐ Adult: 15-124   NRS Nonroutine supply Dx   NC Dx Noncancer Dx   PDx Primary Dx   ▶◀ Revised Text   ● New Code   ▲ Revised Title

728   ICD-10-CM 2018

M08.019 Unspecified juvenile rheumatoid arthritis, unspecified shoulder ▽

✓6ᵗʰ M08.02 Unspecified juvenile rheumatoid arthritis of elbow

    M08.021 **Unspecified juvenile rheumatoid arthritis, right elbow** ▽

    M08.022 **Unspecified juvenile rheumatoid arthritis, left elbow** ▽

    M08.029 Unspecified juvenile rheumatoid arthritis, unspecified elbow ▽

✓6ᵗʰ M08.03 Unspecified juvenile rheumatoid arthritis, wrist

    M08.031 **Unspecified juvenile rheumatoid arthritis, right wrist** ▽

    M08.032 **Unspecified juvenile rheumatoid arthritis, left wrist** ▽

    M08.039 Unspecified juvenile rheumatoid arthritis, unspecified wrist ▽

✓6ᵗʰ M08.04 Unspecified juvenile rheumatoid arthritis, hand

    M08.041 **Unspecified juvenile rheumatoid arthritis, right hand** ▽

    M08.042 **Unspecified juvenile rheumatoid arthritis, left hand** ▽

    M08.049 Unspecified juvenile rheumatoid arthritis, unspecified hand ▽

✓6ᵗʰ M08.05 Unspecified juvenile rheumatoid arthritis, hip

    M08.051 **Unspecified juvenile rheumatoid arthritis, right hip** ▽

    M08.052 **Unspecified juvenile rheumatoid arthritis, left hip** ▽

    M08.059 Unspecified juvenile rheumatoid arthritis, unspecified hip ▽

✓6ᵗʰ M08.06 Unspecified juvenile rheumatoid arthritis, knee

    M08.061 **Unspecified juvenile rheumatoid arthritis, right knee** ▽

    M08.062 **Unspecified juvenile rheumatoid arthritis, left knee** ▽

    M08.069 Unspecified juvenile rheumatoid arthritis, unspecified knee ▽

✓6ᵗʰ M08.07 Unspecified juvenile rheumatoid arthritis, ankle and foot

    M08.071 **Unspecified juvenile rheumatoid arthritis, right ankle and foot** ▽

    M08.072 **Unspecified juvenile rheumatoid arthritis, left ankle and foot** ▽

    M08.079 Unspecified juvenile rheumatoid arthritis, unspecified ankle and foot ▽

    M08.08 **Unspecified juvenile rheumatoid arthritis, vertebrae** ▽

    M08.09 **Unspecified juvenile rheumatoid arthritis, multiple sites** ▽

M08.1 **Juvenile ankylosing spondylitis**

    EXCLUDES 1 ankylosing spondylitis in adults (M45.0-)

✓5ᵗʰ M08.2 **Juvenile rheumatoid arthritis** with systemic onset

    Still's disease NOS

    EXCLUDES 1 adult-onset Still's disease (M06.1-)

    M08.20 Juvenile rheumatoid arthritis with systemic onset, unspecified site ▽

✓6ᵗʰ M08.21 Juvenile rheumatoid arthritis with systemic onset, shoulder

    M08.211 **Juvenile rheumatoid arthritis with systemic onset, right shoulder**

    M08.212 **Juvenile rheumatoid arthritis with systemic onset, left shoulder**

    M08.219 Juvenile rheumatoid arthritis with systemic onset, unspecified shoulder ▽

✓6ᵗʰ M08.22 Juvenile rheumatoid arthritis with systemic onset, elbow

    M08.221 **Juvenile rheumatoid arthritis with systemic onset, right elbow**

    M08.222 **Juvenile rheumatoid arthritis with systemic onset, left elbow**

    M08.229 Juvenile rheumatoid arthritis with systemic onset, unspecified elbow ▽

✓6ᵗʰ M08.23 Juvenile rheumatoid arthritis with systemic onset, wrist

    M08.231 **Juvenile rheumatoid arthritis with systemic onset, right wrist**

    M08.232 **Juvenile rheumatoid arthritis with systemic onset, left wrist**

    M08.239 Juvenile rheumatoid arthritis with systemic onset, unspecified wrist ▽

✓6ᵗʰ M08.24 Juvenile rheumatoid arthritis with systemic onset, hand

    M08.241 **Juvenile rheumatoid arthritis with systemic onset, right hand**

    M08.242 **Juvenile rheumatoid arthritis with systemic onset, left hand**

    M08.249 Juvenile rheumatoid arthritis with systemic onset, unspecified hand ▽

✓6ᵗʰ M08.25 Juvenile rheumatoid arthritis with systemic onset, hip

    M08.251 **Juvenile rheumatoid arthritis with systemic onset, right hip**

    M08.252 **Juvenile rheumatoid arthritis with systemic onset, left hip**

    M08.259 Juvenile rheumatoid arthritis with systemic onset, unspecified hip ▽

✓6ᵗʰ M08.26 Juvenile rheumatoid arthritis with systemic onset, knee

    M08.261 **Juvenile rheumatoid arthritis with systemic onset, right knee**

    M08.262 **Juvenile rheumatoid arthritis with systemic onset, left knee**

    M08.269 Juvenile rheumatoid arthritis with systemic onset, unspecified knee ▽

✓6ᵗʰ M08.27 Juvenile rheumatoid arthritis with systemic onset, ankle and foot

    M08.271 **Juvenile rheumatoid arthritis with systemic onset, right ankle and foot**

    M08.272 **Juvenile rheumatoid arthritis with systemic onset, left ankle and foot**

    M08.279 Juvenile rheumatoid arthritis with systemic onset, unspecified ankle and foot ▽

    M08.28 **Juvenile rheumatoid arthritis with systemic onset, vertebrae**

    M08.29 **Juvenile rheumatoid arthritis with systemic onset, multiple sites**

M08.3 **Juvenile rheumatoid polyarthritis (seronegative)**

✓5ᵗʰ M08.4 **Pauciarticular juvenile rheumatoid arthritis**

    M08.40 Pauciarticular juvenile rheumatoid arthritis, unspecified site ▽

✓6ᵗʰ M08.41 Pauciarticular juvenile rheumatoid arthritis, shoulder

    M08.411 **Pauciarticular juvenile rheumatoid arthritis, right shoulder**

    M08.412 **Pauciarticular juvenile rheumatoid arthritis, left shoulder**

    M08.419 Pauciarticular juvenile rheumatoid arthritis, unspecified shoulder ▽

✓6ᵗʰ M08.42 Pauciarticular juvenile rheumatoid arthritis, elbow

    M08.421 **Pauciarticular juvenile rheumatoid arthritis, right elbow**

    M08.422 **Pauciarticular juvenile rheumatoid arthritis, left elbow**

    M08.429 Pauciarticular juvenile rheumatoid arthritis, unspecified elbow ▽

✓6ᵗʰ M08.43 Pauciarticular juvenile rheumatoid arthritis, wrist

    M08.431 **Pauciarticular juvenile rheumatoid arthritis, right wrist**

    M08.432 **Pauciarticular juvenile rheumatoid arthritis, left wrist**

    M08.439 Pauciarticular juvenile rheumatoid arthritis, unspecified wrist ▽

✓6ᵗʰ M08.44 Pauciarticular juvenile rheumatoid arthritis, hand

    M08.441 **Pauciarticular juvenile rheumatoid arthritis, right hand**

    M08.442 **Pauciarticular juvenile rheumatoid arthritis, left hand**

    M08.449 Pauciarticular juvenile rheumatoid arthritis, unspecified hand ▽

✓6ᵗʰ M08.45 Pauciarticular juvenile rheumatoid arthritis, hip

    M08.451 **Pauciarticular juvenile rheumatoid arthritis, right hip**

☑ Additional Character Req   ✓x7ᵗʰ Placeholder Alert   Case-Mix Diagnosis   Manifestation   ▽ Unspecified Dx   **EXCLUDES 1** Not coded here   **EXCLUDES 2** Not included here

ICD-10-CM 2018

729

Chapter 13. Diseases of the Musculoskeletal System and Connective Tissue

M08.452–M1A.039

      M08.452 **Pauciarticular juvenile rheumatoid arthritis, left hip**

      M08.459 **Pauciarticular juvenile rheumatoid arthritis, unspecified hip** ▽

✓6ᵗʰ M08.46 **Pauciarticular juvenile rheumatoid arthritis, knee**

      M08.461 **Pauciarticular juvenile rheumatoid arthritis, right knee**

      M08.462 **Pauciarticular juvenile rheumatoid arthritis, left knee**

      M08.469 **Pauciarticular juvenile rheumatoid arthritis, unspecified knee** ▽

✓6ᵗʰ M08.47 **Pauciarticular juvenile rheumatoid arthritis, ankle and foot**

      M08.471 **Pauciarticular juvenile rheumatoid arthritis, right ankle and foot**

      M08.472 **Pauciarticular juvenile rheumatoid arthritis, left ankle and foot**

      M08.479 **Pauciarticular juvenile rheumatoid arthritis, unspecified ankle and foot** ▽

      M08.48 **Pauciarticular juvenile rheumatoid arthritis, vertebrae**

✓5ᵗʰ M08.8 **Other juvenile arthritis**

      M08.80 **Other juvenile arthritis, unspecified site** ▽

✓6ᵗʰ M08.81 **Other juvenile arthritis, shoulder**

      M08.811 **Other juvenile arthritis, right shoulder**

      M08.812 **Other juvenile arthritis, left shoulder**

      M08.819 **Other juvenile arthritis, unspecified shoulder** ▽

✓6ᵗʰ M08.82 **Other juvenile arthritis, elbow**

      M08.821 **Other juvenile arthritis, right elbow**

      M08.822 **Other juvenile arthritis, left elbow**

      M08.829 **Other juvenile arthritis, unspecified elbow** ▽

✓6ᵗʰ M08.83 **Other juvenile arthritis, wrist**

      M08.831 **Other juvenile arthritis, right wrist**

      M08.832 **Other juvenile arthritis, left wrist**

      M08.839 **Other juvenile arthritis, unspecified wrist** ▽

✓6ᵗʰ M08.84 **Other juvenile arthritis, hand**

      M08.841 **Other juvenile arthritis, right hand**

      M08.842 **Other juvenile arthritis, left hand**

      M08.849 **Other juvenile arthritis, unspecified hand** ▽

✓6ᵗʰ M08.85 **Other juvenile arthritis, hip**

      M08.851 **Other juvenile arthritis, right hip**

      M08.852 **Other juvenile arthritis, left hip**

      M08.859 **Other juvenile arthritis, unspecified hip** ▽

✓6ᵗʰ M08.86 **Other juvenile arthritis, knee**

      M08.861 **Other juvenile arthritis, right knee**

      M08.862 **Other juvenile arthritis, left knee**

      M08.869 **Other juvenile arthritis, unspecified knee** ▽

✓6ᵗʰ M08.87 **Other juvenile arthritis, ankle and foot**

      M08.871 **Other juvenile arthritis, right ankle and foot**

      M08.872 **Other juvenile arthritis, left ankle and foot**

      M08.879 **Other juvenile arthritis, unspecified ankle and foot** ▽

      M08.88 **Other juvenile arthritis, other specified site**
           Other juvenile arthritis, vertebrae

      M08.89 **Other juvenile arthritis, multiple sites**

✓5ᵗʰ M08.9 **Juvenile arthritis, unspecified**

      EXCLUDES 1 *juvenile rheumatoid arthritis, unspecified (M08.0-)*

      M08.90 **Juvenile arthritis, unspecified, unspecified site** ▽

✓6ᵗʰ M08.91 **Juvenile arthritis, unspecified, shoulder**

      M08.911 **Juvenile arthritis, unspecified, right shoulder** ▽

      M08.912 **Juvenile arthritis, unspecified, left shoulder** ▽

      M08.919 **Juvenile arthritis, unspecified, unspecified shoulder** ▽

✓6ᵗʰ M08.92 **Juvenile arthritis, unspecified, elbow**

      M08.921 **Juvenile arthritis, unspecified, right elbow** ▽

      M08.922 **Juvenile arthritis, unspecified, left elbow** ▽

      M08.929 **Juvenile arthritis, unspecified, unspecified elbow** ▽

✓6ᵗʰ M08.93 **Juvenile arthritis, unspecified, wrist**

      M08.931 **Juvenile arthritis, unspecified, right wrist** ▽

      M08.932 **Juvenile arthritis, unspecified, left wrist** ▽

      M08.939 **Juvenile arthritis, unspecified, unspecified wrist** ▽

✓6ᵗʰ M08.94 **Juvenile arthritis, unspecified, hand**

      M08.941 **Juvenile arthritis, unspecified, right hand** ▽

      M08.942 **Juvenile arthritis, unspecified, left hand** ▽

      M08.949 **Juvenile arthritis, unspecified, unspecified hand** ▽

✓6ᵗʰ M08.95 **Juvenile arthritis, unspecified, hip**

      M08.951 **Juvenile arthritis, unspecified, right hip** ▽

      M08.952 **Juvenile arthritis, unspecified, left hip** ▽

      M08.959 **Juvenile arthritis, unspecified, unspecified hip** ▽

✓6ᵗʰ M08.96 **Juvenile arthritis, unspecified, knee**

      M08.961 **Juvenile arthritis, unspecified, right knee** ▽

      M08.962 **Juvenile arthritis, unspecified, left knee** ▽

      M08.969 **Juvenile arthritis, unspecified, unspecified knee** ▽

✓6ᵗʰ M08.97 **Juvenile arthritis, unspecified, ankle and foot** ▽

      M08.971 **Juvenile arthritis, unspecified, right ankle and foot** ▽

      M08.972 **Juvenile arthritis, unspecified, left ankle and foot** ▽

      M08.979 **Juvenile arthritis, unspecified, unspecified ankle and foot** ▽

      M08.98 **Juvenile arthritis, unspecified, vertebrae** ▽

      M08.99 **Juvenile arthritis, unspecified, multiple sites** ▽

✓4ᵗʰ **M1A Chronic gout**

     Use additional code to identify:
       autonomic neuropathy in diseases classified elsewhere (G99.0)
       calculus of urinary tract in diseases classified elsewhere (N22)
       cardiomyopathy in diseases classified elsewhere (I43)
       disorders of external ear in diseases classified elsewhere (H61.1-, H62.8-)
       disorders of iris and ciliary body in diseases classified elsewhere (H22)
       glomerular disorders in diseases classified elsewhere (N08)

     EXCLUDES 1 *gout NOS (M10.-)*

     EXCLUDES 2 *acute gout (M10.-)*

     The appropriate 7th character is to be added to each code from category M1A.
     0   without tophus (tophi)
     1   with tophus (tophi)

✓5ᵗʰ **M1A.0 Idiopathic chronic gout**
       Chronic gouty bursitis
       Primary chronic gout

     ✓x7ᵗʰ M1A.00 **Idiopathic chronic gout, unspecified site** ▽

     ✓6ᵗʰ M1A.01 **Idiopathic chronic gout, shoulder**

       ✓7ᵗʰ M1A.011 **Idiopathic chronic gout, right shoulder**

       ✓7ᵗʰ M1A.012 **Idiopathic chronic gout, left shoulder**

       ✓7ᵗʰ M1A.019 **Idiopathic chronic gout, unspecified shoulder** ▽

     ✓6ᵗʰ M1A.02 **Idiopathic chronic gout, elbow**

       ✓7ᵗʰ M1A.021 **Idiopathic chronic gout, right elbow**

       ✓7ᵗʰ M1A.022 **Idiopathic chronic gout, left elbow**

       ✓7ᵗʰ M1A.029 **Idiopathic chronic gout, unspecified elbow** ▽

     ✓6ᵗʰ M1A.03 **Idiopathic chronic gout, wrist**

       ✓7ᵗʰ M1A.031 **Idiopathic chronic gout, right wrist**

       ✓7ᵗʰ M1A.032 **Idiopathic chronic gout, left wrist**

       ✓7ᵗʰ M1A.039 **Idiopathic chronic gout, unspecified wrist** ▽

N Newborn: 0   P Pediatric: 0-17   M Maternity: 12-55   A Adult: 15-124   **NRS** Nonroutine supply Dx   **NCDx** Noncancer Dx   **PDx** Primary Dx   ▶◀ Revised Text   ● New Code   ▲ Revised Title

730   ICD-10-CM 2018

Chapter 13. Diseases of the Musculoskeletal System and Connective Tissue

✓6ᵗʰ **M1A.04 Idiopathic chronic gout,** hand
  ✓7ᵗʰ **M1A.041 Idiopathic chronic gout,** right **hand**
  ✓7ᵗʰ **M1A.042 Idiopathic chronic gout,** left **hand**
  ✓7ᵗʰ **M1A.049 Idiopathic chronic gout, unspecified hand** ▽

✓6ᵗʰ **M1A.05 Idiopathic chronic gout,** hip
  ✓7ᵗʰ **M1A.051 Idiopathic chronic gout,** right **hip**
  ✓7ᵗʰ **M1A.052 Idiopathic chronic gout,** left **hip**
  ✓7ᵗʰ **M1A.059 Idiopathic chronic gout, unspecified hip** ▽

✓6ᵗʰ **M1A.06 Idiopathic chronic gout,** knee
  ✓7ᵗʰ **M1A.061 Idiopathic chronic gout,** right **knee**
  ✓7ᵗʰ **M1A.062 Idiopathic chronic gout,** left **knee**
  ✓7ᵗʰ **M1A.069 Idiopathic chronic gout, unspecified knee** ▽

✓6ᵗʰ **M1A.07 Idiopathic chronic gout,** ankle and foot
  ✓7ᵗʰ **M1A.071 Idiopathic chronic gout,** right **ankle and foot**
  ✓7ᵗʰ **M1A.072 Idiopathic chronic gout,** left **ankle and foot**
  ✓7ᵗʰ **M1A.079 Idiopathic chronic gout, unspecified ankle and foot** ▽

✓x7ᵗʰ **M1A.08 Idiopathic chronic gout,** vertebrae
✓x7ᵗʰ **M1A.09 Idiopathic chronic gout,** multiple sites

✓5ᵗʰ **M1A.1 Lead-induced** chronic gout
  Code first toxic effects of lead and its compounds (T56.0-)

✓x7ᵗʰ **M1A.10 Lead-induced chronic gout, unspecified site** ▽

✓6ᵗʰ **M1A.11 Lead-induced chronic gout,** shoulder
  ✓7ᵗʰ **M1A.111 Lead-induced chronic gout,** right **shoulder**
  ✓7ᵗʰ **M1A.112 Lead-induced chronic gout,** left **shoulder**
  ✓7ᵗʰ **M1A.119 Lead-induced chronic gout, unspecified shoulder** ▽

✓6ᵗʰ **M1A.12 Lead-induced chronic gout,** elbow
  ✓7ᵗʰ **M1A.121 Lead-induced chronic gout,** right **elbow**
  ✓7ᵗʰ **M1A.122 Lead-induced chronic gout,** left **elbow**
  ✓7ᵗʰ **M1A.129 Lead-induced chronic gout, unspecified elbow** ▽

✓6ᵗʰ **M1A.13 Lead-induced chronic gout,** wrist
  ✓7ᵗʰ **M1A.131 Lead-induced chronic gout,** right **wrist**
  ✓7ᵗʰ **M1A.132 Lead-induced chronic gout,** left **wrist**
  ✓7ᵗʰ **M1A.139 Lead-induced chronic gout, unspecified wrist** ▽

✓6ᵗʰ **M1A.14 Lead-induced chronic gout,** hand
  ✓7ᵗʰ **M1A.141 Lead-induced chronic gout,** right **hand**
  ✓7ᵗʰ **M1A.142 Lead-induced chronic gout,** left **hand**
  ✓7ᵗʰ **M1A.149 Lead-induced chronic gout, unspecified hand** ▽

✓6ᵗʰ **M1A.15 Lead-induced chronic gout,** hip
  ✓7ᵗʰ **M1A.151 Lead-induced chronic gout,** right **hip**
  ✓7ᵗʰ **M1A.152 Lead-induced chronic gout,** left **hip**
  ✓7ᵗʰ **M1A.159 Lead-induced chronic gout, unspecified hip** ▽

✓6ᵗʰ **M1A.16 Lead-induced chronic gout,** knee
  ✓7ᵗʰ **M1A.161 Lead-induced chronic gout,** right **knee**
  ✓7ᵗʰ **M1A.162 Lead-induced chronic gout,** left **knee**
  ✓7ᵗʰ **M1A.169 Lead-induced chronic gout, unspecified knee** ▽

✓6ᵗʰ **M1A.17 Lead-induced chronic gout,** ankle and foot
  ✓7ᵗʰ **M1A.171 Lead-induced chronic gout,** right **ankle and foot**
  ✓7ᵗʰ **M1A.172 Lead-induced chronic gout,** left **ankle and foot**
  ✓7ᵗʰ **M1A.179 Lead-induced chronic gout, unspecified ankle and foot** ▽

✓x7ᵗʰ **M1A.18 Lead-induced chronic gout,** vertebrae
✓x7ᵗʰ **M1A.19 Lead-induced chronic gout,** multiple sites

✓5ᵗʰ **M1A.2 Drug-induced** chronic gout
  Use additional code for adverse effect, if applicable, to identify drug (T36-T50 with fifth or sixth character 5)

✓x7ᵗʰ **M1A.20 Drug-induced chronic gout, unspecified site** ▽

✓6ᵗʰ **M1A.21 Drug-induced chronic gout,** shoulder
  ✓7ᵗʰ **M1A.211 Drug-induced chronic gout,** right **shoulder**
  ✓7ᵗʰ **M1A.212 Drug-induced chronic gout,** left **shoulder**
  ✓7ᵗʰ **M1A.219 Drug-induced chronic gout, unspecified shoulder** ▽

✓6ᵗʰ **M1A.22 Drug-induced chronic gout,** elbow
  ✓7ᵗʰ **M1A.221 Drug-induced chronic gout,** right **elbow**
  ✓7ᵗʰ **M1A.222 Drug-induced chronic gout,** left **elbow**
  ✓7ᵗʰ **M1A.229 Drug-induced chronic gout, unspecified elbow** ▽

✓6ᵗʰ **M1A.23 Drug-induced chronic gout,** wrist
  ✓7ᵗʰ **M1A.231 Drug-induced chronic gout,** right **wrist**
  ✓7ᵗʰ **M1A.232 Drug-induced chronic gout,** left **wrist**
  ✓7ᵗʰ **M1A.239 Drug-induced chronic gout, unspecified wrist** ▽

✓6ᵗʰ **M1A.24 Drug-induced chronic gout,** hand
  ✓7ᵗʰ **M1A.241 Drug-induced chronic gout,** right **hand**
  ✓7ᵗʰ **M1A.242 Drug-induced chronic gout,** left **hand**
  ✓7ᵗʰ **M1A.249 Drug-induced chronic gout, unspecified hand** ▽

✓6ᵗʰ **M1A.25 Drug-induced chronic gout,** hip
  ✓7ᵗʰ **M1A.251 Drug-induced chronic gout,** right **hip**
  ✓7ᵗʰ **M1A.252 Drug-induced chronic gout,** left **hip**
  ✓7ᵗʰ **M1A.259 Drug-induced chronic gout, unspecified hip** ▽

✓6ᵗʰ **M1A.26 Drug-induced chronic gout,** knee
  ✓7ᵗʰ **M1A.261 Drug-induced chronic gout,** right **knee**
  ✓7ᵗʰ **M1A.262 Drug-induced chronic gout,** left **knee**
  ✓7ᵗʰ **M1A.269 Drug-induced chronic gout, unspecified knee** ▽

✓6ᵗʰ **M1A.27 Drug-induced chronic gout,** ankle and foot
  ✓7ᵗʰ **M1A.271 Drug-induced chronic gout,** right **ankle and foot**
  ✓7ᵗʰ **M1A.272 Drug-induced chronic gout,** left **ankle and foot**
  ✓7ᵗʰ **M1A.279 Drug-induced chronic gout, unspecified ankle and foot** ▽

✓x7ᵗʰ **M1A.28 Drug-induced chronic gout,** vertebrae
✓x7ᵗʰ **M1A.29 Drug-induced chronic gout,** multiple sites

✓5ᵗʰ **M1A.3 Chronic gout** due to renal impairment
  Code first associated renal disease

✓x7ᵗʰ **M1A.30 Chronic gout due to renal impairment, unspecified site** ▽

✓6ᵗʰ **M1A.31 Chronic gout due to renal impairment,** shoulder
  ✓7ᵗʰ **M1A.311 Chronic gout due to renal impairment,** right **shoulder**
  ✓7ᵗʰ **M1A.312 Chronic gout due to renal impairment,** left **shoulder**
  ✓7ᵗʰ **M1A.319 Chronic gout due to renal impairment, unspecified shoulder** ▽

✓6ᵗʰ **M1A.32 Chronic gout due to renal impairment,** elbow
  ✓7ᵗʰ **M1A.321 Chronic gout due to renal impairment,** right **elbow**
  ✓7ᵗʰ **M1A.322 Chronic gout due to renal impairment,** left **elbow**
  ✓7ᵗʰ **M1A.329 Chronic gout due to renal impairment, unspecified elbow** ▽

✓6ᵗʰ **M1A.33 Chronic gout due to renal impairment,** wrist
  ✓7ᵗʰ **M1A.331 Chronic gout due to renal impairment,** right **wrist**
  ✓7ᵗʰ **M1A.332 Chronic gout due to renal impairment,** left **wrist**
  ✓7ᵗʰ **M1A.339 Chronic gout due to renal impairment, unspecified wrist** ▽

✓6ᵗʰ **M1A.34 Chronic gout due to renal impairment,** hand
  ✓7ᵗʰ **M1A.341 Chronic gout due to renal impairment,** right **hand**
  ✓7ᵗʰ **M1A.342 Chronic gout due to renal impairment,** left **hand**
  ✓7ᵗʰ **M1A.349 Chronic gout due to renal impairment, unspecified hand** ▽

✓ Additional Character Req   ✓x7ᵗʰ Placeholder Alert   Case-Mix Diagnosis   Manifestation   ▽ Unspecified Dx   **EXCLUDES 1** Not coded here   **EXCLUDES 2** Not included here

Chapter 13. Diseases of the Musculoskeletal System and Connective Tissue

M1A.35–M10.149

✓6ᵗʰ **M1A.35 Chronic gout due to renal impairment, hip**

     ✓7ᵗʰ **M1A.351 Chronic gout due to renal impairment, right hip**

     ✓7ᵗʰ **M1A.352 Chronic gout due to renal impairment, left hip**

     ✓7ᵗʰ **M1A.359 Chronic gout due to renal impairment, unspecified hip** ▽

✓6ᵗʰ **M1A.36 Chronic gout due to renal impairment, knee**

     ✓7ᵗʰ **M1A.361 Chronic gout due to renal impairment, right knee**

     ✓7ᵗʰ **M1A.362 Chronic gout due to renal impairment, left knee**

     ✓7ᵗʰ **M1A.369 Chronic gout due to renal impairment, unspecified knee** ▽

✓6ᵗʰ **M1A.37 Chronic gout due to renal impairment, ankle and foot**

     ✓7ᵗʰ **M1A.371 Chronic gout due to renal impairment, right ankle and foot**

     ✓7ᵗʰ **M1A.372 Chronic gout due to renal impairment, left ankle and foot**

     ✓7ᵗʰ **M1A.379 Chronic gout due to renal impairment, unspecified ankle and foot** ▽

✓x7ᵗʰ **M1A.38 Chronic gout due to renal impairment, vertebrae**

✓x7ᵗʰ **M1A.39 Chronic gout due to renal impairment, multiple sites**

✓5ᵗʰ **M1A.4 Other secondary chronic gout**

     Code first associated condition

✓x7ᵗʰ **M1A.40 Other secondary chronic gout, unspecified site** ▽

✓6ᵗʰ **M1A.41 Other secondary chronic gout, shoulder**

     ✓7ᵗʰ **M1A.411 Other secondary chronic gout, right shoulder**

     ✓7ᵗʰ **M1A.412 Other secondary chronic gout, left shoulder**

     ✓7ᵗʰ **M1A.419 Other secondary chronic gout, unspecified shoulder** ▽

✓6ᵗʰ **M1A.42 Other secondary chronic gout, elbow**

     ✓7ᵗʰ **M1A.421 Other secondary chronic gout, right elbow**

     ✓7ᵗʰ **M1A.422 Other secondary chronic gout, left elbow**

     ✓7ᵗʰ **M1A.429 Other secondary chronic gout, unspecified elbow** ▽

✓6ᵗʰ **M1A.43 Other secondary chronic gout, wrist**

     ✓7ᵗʰ **M1A.431 Other secondary chronic gout, right wrist**

     ✓7ᵗʰ **M1A.432 Other secondary chronic gout, left wrist**

     ✓7ᵗʰ **M1A.439 Other secondary chronic gout, unspecified wrist** ▽

✓6ᵗʰ **M1A.44 Other secondary chronic gout, hand**

     ✓7ᵗʰ **M1A.441 Other secondary chronic gout, right hand**

     ✓7ᵗʰ **M1A.442 Other secondary chronic gout, left hand**

     ✓7ᵗʰ **M1A.449 Other secondary chronic gout, unspecified hand** ▽

✓6ᵗʰ **M1A.45 Other secondary chronic gout, hip**

     ✓7ᵗʰ **M1A.451 Other secondary chronic gout, right hip**

     ✓7ᵗʰ **M1A.452 Other secondary chronic gout, left hip**

     ✓7ᵗʰ **M1A.459 Other secondary chronic gout, unspecified hip** ▽

✓6ᵗʰ **M1A.46 Other secondary chronic gout, knee**

     ✓7ᵗʰ **M1A.461 Other secondary chronic gout, right knee**

     ✓7ᵗʰ **M1A.462 Other secondary chronic gout, left knee**

     ✓7ᵗʰ **M1A.469 Other secondary chronic gout, unspecified knee** ▽

✓6ᵗʰ **M1A.47 Other secondary chronic gout, ankle and foot**

     ✓7ᵗʰ **M1A.471 Other secondary chronic gout, right ankle and foot**

     ✓7ᵗʰ **M1A.472 Other secondary chronic gout, left ankle and foot**

     ✓7ᵗʰ **M1A.479 Other secondary chronic gout, unspecified ankle and foot** ▽

✓x7ᵗʰ **M1A.48 Other secondary chronic gout, vertebrae**

✓x7ᵗʰ **M1A.49 Other secondary chronic gout, multiple sites**

✓x7ᵗʰ **M1A.9 Chronic gout, unspecified** ▽

✓4ᵗʰ **M10 Gout**

Acute gout
Gout attack
Gout flare
Podagra

Use additional code to identify:
autonomic neuropathy in diseases classified elsewhere (G99.0)
calculus of urinary tract in diseases classified elsewhere (N22)
cardiomyopathy in diseases classified elsewhere (I43)
disorders of external ear in diseases classified elsewhere (H61.1-, H62.8-)
disorders of iris and ciliary body in diseases classified elsewhere (H22)
glomerular disorders in diseases classified elsewhere (N08)

EXCLUDES 2   chronic gout (M1A.-)

DEF: Purine and pyrimidine metabolic disorders; manifested by hyperuricemia and recurrent acute inflammatory arthritis; monosodium urate or monohydrate crystals may be deposited in and around the joints, leading to joint destruction and severe crippling.

✓5ᵗʰ **M10.0 Idiopathic gout**

Gouty bursitis
Primary gout

     M10.00 Idiopathic gout, unspecified site ▽

✓6ᵗʰ **M10.01 Idiopathic gout, shoulder**

     M10.011 Idiopathic gout, right shoulder

     M10.012 Idiopathic gout, left shoulder

     M10.019 Idiopathic gout, unspecified shoulder ▽

✓6ᵗʰ **M10.02 Idiopathic gout, elbow**

     M10.021 Idiopathic gout, right elbow

     M10.022 Idiopathic gout, left elbow

     M10.029 Idiopathic gout, unspecified elbow ▽

✓6ᵗʰ **M10.03 Idiopathic gout, wrist**

     M10.031 Idiopathic gout, right wrist

     M10.032 Idiopathic gout, left wrist

     M10.039 Idiopathic gout, unspecified wrist ▽

✓6ᵗʰ **M10.04 Idiopathic gout, hand**

     M10.041 Idiopathic gout, right hand

     M10.042 Idiopathic gout, left hand

     M10.049 Idiopathic gout, unspecified hand ▽

✓6ᵗʰ **M10.05 Idiopathic gout, hip**

     M10.051 Idiopathic gout, right hip

     M10.052 Idiopathic gout, left hip

     M10.059 Idiopathic gout, unspecified hip ▽

✓6ᵗʰ **M10.06 Idiopathic gout, knee**

     M10.061 Idiopathic gout, right knee

     M10.062 Idiopathic gout, left knee

     M10.069 Idiopathic gout, unspecified knee ▽

✓6ᵗʰ **M10.07 Idiopathic gout, ankle and foot**

     M10.071 Idiopathic gout, right ankle and foot

     M10.072 Idiopathic gout, left ankle and foot

     M10.079 Idiopathic gout, unspecified ankle and foot ▽

     M10.08 Idiopathic gout, vertebrae

     M10.09 Idiopathic gout, multiple sites

✓5ᵗʰ **M10.1 Lead-induced gout**

     Code first toxic effects of lead and its compounds (T56.0-)

     M10.10 Lead-induced gout, unspecified site ▽

✓6ᵗʰ **M10.11 Lead-induced gout, shoulder**

     M10.111 Lead-induced gout, right shoulder

     M10.112 Lead-induced gout, left shoulder

     M10.119 Lead-induced gout, unspecified shoulder ▽

✓6ᵗʰ **M10.12 Lead-induced gout, elbow**

     M10.121 Lead-induced gout, right elbow

     M10.122 Lead-induced gout, left elbow

     M10.129 Lead-induced gout, unspecified elbow ▽

✓6ᵗʰ **M10.13 Lead-induced gout, wrist**

     M10.131 Lead-induced gout, right wrist

     M10.132 Lead-induced gout, left wrist

     M10.139 Lead-induced gout, unspecified wrist ▽

✓6ᵗʰ **M10.14 Lead-induced gout, hand**

     M10.141 Lead-induced gout, right hand

     M10.142 Lead-induced gout, left hand

     M10.149 Lead-induced gout, unspecified hand ▽

Ⓝ Newborn: 0   Ⓟ Pediatric: 0-17   Ⓜ Maternity: 12-55   Ⓐ Adult: 15-124   **NRS** Nonroutine supply Dx   **NC Dx** Noncancer Dx   **PDx** Primary Dx   ▶◀ Revised Text   ● New Code   ▲ Revised Title

732   ICD-10-CM 2018

✓6th **M10.15 Lead-induced gout,** hip
    M10.151 Lead-induced gout, right hip
    M10.152 Lead-induced gout, left hip
    M10.159 Lead-induced gout, unspecified hip ▽

✓6th **M10.16 Lead-induced gout,** knee
    M10.161 Lead-induced gout, right knee
    M10.162 Lead-induced gout, left knee
    M10.169 Lead-induced gout, unspecified knee ▽

✓6th **M10.17 Lead-induced gout,** ankle and foot
    M10.171 Lead-induced gout, right ankle and foot
    M10.172 Lead-induced gout, left ankle and foot
    M10.179 Lead-induced gout, unspecified ankle and foot ▽

    M10.18 Lead-induced gout, vertebrae
    M10.19 Lead-induced gout, multiple sites

✓5th **M10.2 Drug-induced** gout
    Use additional code for adverse effect, if applicable, to identify drug (T36-T50 with fifth or sixth character 5)

    M10.20 Drug-induced gout, unspecified site ▽

✓6th **M10.21 Drug-induced gout,** shoulder
    M10.211 Drug-induced gout, right shoulder
    M10.212 Drug-induced gout, left shoulder
    M10.219 Drug-induced gout, unspecified shoulder ▽

✓6th **M10.22 Drug-induced gout,** elbow
    M10.221 Drug-induced gout, right elbow
    M10.222 Drug-induced gout, left elbow
    M10.229 Drug-induced gout, unspecified elbow ▽

✓6th **M10.23 Drug-induced gout,** wrist
    M10.231 Drug-induced gout, right wrist
    M10.232 Drug-induced gout, left wrist
    M10.239 Drug-induced gout, unspecified wrist ▽

✓6th **M10.24 Drug-induced gout,** hand
    M10.241 Drug-induced gout, right hand
    M10.242 Drug-induced gout, left hand
    M10.249 Drug-induced gout, unspecified hand ▽

✓6th **M10.25 Drug-induced gout,** hip
    M10.251 Drug-induced gout, right hip
    M10.252 Drug-induced gout, left hip
    M10.259 Drug-induced gout, unspecified hip ▽

✓6th **M10.26 Drug-induced gout,** knee
    M10.261 Drug-induced gout, right knee
    M10.262 Drug-induced gout, left knee
    M10.269 Drug-induced gout, unspecified knee ▽

✓6th **M10.27 Drug-induced gout,** ankle and foot
    M10.271 Drug-induced gout, right ankle and foot
    M10.272 Drug-induced gout, left ankle and foot
    M10.279 Drug-induced gout, unspecified ankle and foot ▽

    M10.28 Drug-induced gout, vertebrae
    M10.29 Drug-induced gout, multiple sites

✓5th **M10.3 Gout due to** renal impairment
    Code first associated renal disease

    M10.30 Gout due to renal impairment, unspecified site ▽

✓6th **M10.31 Gout due to renal impairment,** shoulder
    M10.311 Gout due to renal impairment, right shoulder
    M10.312 Gout due to renal impairment, left shoulder
    M10.319 Gout due to renal impairment, unspecified shoulder ▽

✓6th **M10.32 Gout due to renal impairment,** elbow
    M10.321 Gout due to renal impairment, right elbow
    M10.322 Gout due to renal impairment, left elbow
    M10.329 Gout due to renal impairment, unspecified elbow ▽

✓6th **M10.33 Gout due to renal impairment,** wrist
    M10.331 Gout due to renal impairment, right wrist
    M10.332 Gout due to renal impairment, left wrist
    M10.339 Gout due to renal impairment, unspecified wrist ▽

✓6th **M10.34 Gout due to renal impairment,** hand
    M10.341 Gout due to renal impairment, right hand
    M10.342 Gout due to renal impairment, left hand
    M10.349 Gout due to renal impairment, unspecified hand ▽

✓6th **M10.35 Gout due to renal impairment,** hip
    M10.351 Gout due to renal impairment, right hip
    M10.352 Gout due to renal impairment, left hip
    M10.359 Gout due to renal impairment, unspecified hip ▽

✓6th **M10.36 Gout due to renal impairment,** knee
    M10.361 Gout due to renal impairment, right knee
    M10.362 Gout due to renal impairment, left knee
    M10.369 Gout due to renal impairment, unspecified knee ▽

✓6th **M10.37 Gout due to renal impairment,** ankle and foot
    M10.371 Gout due to renal impairment, right ankle and foot
    M10.372 Gout due to renal impairment, left ankle and foot
    M10.379 Gout due to renal impairment, unspecified ankle and foot ▽

    M10.38 Gout due to renal impairment, vertebrae
    M10.39 Gout due to renal impairment, multiple sites

✓5th **M10.4 Other secondary** gout
    Code first associated condition

    M10.40 Other secondary gout, unspecified site ▽

✓6th **M10.41 Other secondary gout,** shoulder
    M10.411 Other secondary gout, right shoulder
    M10.412 Other secondary gout, left shoulder
    M10.419 Other secondary gout, unspecified shoulder ▽

✓6th **M10.42 Other secondary gout,** elbow
    M10.421 Other secondary gout, right elbow
    M10.422 Other secondary gout, left elbow
    M10.429 Other secondary gout, unspecified elbow ▽

✓6th **M10.43 Other secondary gout,** wrist
    M10.431 Other secondary gout, right wrist
    M10.432 Other secondary gout, left wrist
    M10.439 Other secondary gout, unspecified wrist ▽

✓6th **M10.44 Other secondary gout,** hand
    M10.441 Other secondary gout, right hand
    M10.442 Other secondary gout, left hand
    M10.449 Other secondary gout, unspecified hand ▽

✓6th **M10.45 Other secondary gout,** hip
    M10.451 Other secondary gout, right hip
    M10.452 Other secondary gout, left hip
    M10.459 Other secondary gout, unspecified hip ▽

✓6th **M10.46 Other secondary gout,** knee
    M10.461 Other secondary gout, right knee
    M10.462 Other secondary gout, left knee
    M10.469 Other secondary gout, unspecified knee ▽

✓6th **M10.47 Other secondary gout,** ankle and foot
    M10.471 Other secondary gout, right ankle and foot
    M10.472 Other secondary gout, left ankle and foot
    M10.479 Other secondary gout, unspecified ankle and foot ▽

    M10.48 Other secondary gout, vertebrae
    M10.49 Other secondary gout, multiple sites

    M10.9 Gout, unspecified ▽
    Gout NOS

✓4th **M11 Other crystal arthropathies**

✓5th **M11.0 Hydroxyapatite deposition disease**
    M11.00 Hydroxyapatite deposition disease, unspecified site ▽

✓6th **M11.01 Hydroxyapatite deposition disease,** shoulder
    M11.011 **Hydroxyapatite deposition disease, right shoulder**

☑ Additional Character Req   ✓x7th Placeholder Alert   Case-Mix Diagnosis   Manifestation   ▽ Unspecified Dx   **EXCLUDES 1** Not coded here   **EXCLUDES 2** Not included here

ICD-10-CM 2018   733

Chapter 13. Diseases of the Musculoskeletal System and Connective Tissue

M11.Ø12–M11.829

M11.Ø12 **Hydroxyapatite deposition disease, left shoulder**

M11.Ø19 Hydroxyapatite deposition disease, unspecified shoulder ▽

✓6ᵗʰ M11.Ø2 Hydroxyapatite deposition disease, elbow

M11.Ø21 **Hydroxyapatite deposition disease, right elbow**

M11.Ø22 **Hydroxyapatite deposition disease, left elbow**

M11.Ø29 Hydroxyapatite deposition disease, unspecified elbow ▽

✓6ᵗʰ M11.Ø3 Hydroxyapatite deposition disease, wrist

M11.Ø31 **Hydroxyapatite deposition disease, right wrist**

M11.Ø32 **Hydroxyapatite deposition disease, left wrist**

M11.Ø39 Hydroxyapatite deposition disease, unspecified wrist ▽

✓6ᵗʰ M11.Ø4 Hydroxyapatite deposition disease, hand

M11.Ø41 **Hydroxyapatite deposition disease, right hand**

M11.Ø42 **Hydroxyapatite deposition disease, left hand**

M11.Ø49 Hydroxyapatite deposition disease, unspecified hand ▽

✓6ᵗʰ M11.Ø5 Hydroxyapatite deposition disease, hip

M11.Ø51 **Hydroxyapatite deposition disease, right hip**

M11.Ø52 **Hydroxyapatite deposition disease, left hip**

M11.Ø59 Hydroxyapatite deposition disease, unspecified hip ▽

✓6ᵗʰ M11.Ø6 Hydroxyapatite deposition disease, knee

M11.Ø61 **Hydroxyapatite deposition disease, right knee**

M11.Ø62 **Hydroxyapatite deposition disease, left knee**

M11.Ø69 Hydroxyapatite deposition disease, unspecified knee ▽

✓6ᵗʰ M11.Ø7 Hydroxyapatite deposition disease, ankle and foot

M11.Ø71 **Hydroxyapatite deposition disease, right ankle and foot**

M11.Ø72 **Hydroxyapatite deposition disease, left ankle and foot**

M11.Ø79 Hydroxyapatite deposition disease, unspecified ankle and foot ▽

M11.Ø8 Hydroxyapatite deposition disease, vertebrae

M11.Ø9 Hydroxyapatite deposition disease, multiple sites

✓5ᵗʰ M11.1 Familial chondrocalcinosis

M11.1Ø Familial chondrocalcinosis, unspecified site ▽

✓6ᵗʰ M11.11 Familial chondrocalcinosis, shoulder

M11.111 **Familial chondrocalcinosis, right shoulder**

M11.112 **Familial chondrocalcinosis, left shoulder**

M11.119 Familial chondrocalcinosis, unspecified shoulder ▽

✓6ᵗʰ M11.12 Familial chondrocalcinosis, elbow

M11.121 **Familial chondrocalcinosis, right elbow**

M11.122 **Familial chondrocalcinosis, left elbow**

M11.129 Familial chondrocalcinosis, unspecified elbow ▽

✓6ᵗʰ M11.13 Familial chondrocalcinosis, wrist

M11.131 **Familial chondrocalcinosis, right wrist**

M11.132 **Familial chondrocalcinosis, left wrist**

M11.139 Familial chondrocalcinosis, unspecified wrist ▽

✓6ᵗʰ M11.14 Familial chondrocalcinosis, hand

M11.141 **Familial chondrocalcinosis, right hand**

M11.142 **Familial chondrocalcinosis, left hand**

M11.149 Familial chondrocalcinosis, unspecified hand ▽

✓6ᵗʰ M11.15 Familial chondrocalcinosis, hip

M11.151 **Familial chondrocalcinosis, right hip**

M11.152 **Familial chondrocalcinosis, left hip**

M11.159 Familial chondrocalcinosis, unspecified hip ▽

✓6ᵗʰ M11.16 Familial chondrocalcinosis, knee

M11.161 **Familial chondrocalcinosis, right knee**

M11.162 **Familial chondrocalcinosis, left knee**

M11.169 Familial chondrocalcinosis, unspecified knee ▽

✓6ᵗʰ M11.17 Familial chondrocalcinosis, ankle and foot

M11.171 **Familial chondrocalcinosis, right ankle and foot**

M11.172 **Familial chondrocalcinosis, left ankle and foot**

M11.179 Familial chondrocalcinosis, unspecified ankle and foot ▽

M11.18 Familial chondrocalcinosis, vertebrae

M11.19 Familial chondrocalcinosis, multiple sites

✓5ᵗʰ M11.2 Other chondrocalcinosis
Chondrocalcinosis NOS

M11.2Ø Other chondrocalcinosis, unspecified site ▽

✓6ᵗʰ M11.21 Other chondrocalcinosis, shoulder

M11.211 **Other chondrocalcinosis, right shoulder**

M11.212 **Other chondrocalcinosis, left shoulder**

M11.219 Other chondrocalcinosis, unspecified shoulder ▽

✓6ᵗʰ M11.22 Other chondrocalcinosis, elbow

M11.221 **Other chondrocalcinosis, right elbow**

M11.222 **Other chondrocalcinosis, left elbow**

M11.229 Other chondrocalcinosis, unspecified elbow ▽

✓6ᵗʰ M11.23 Other chondrocalcinosis, wrist

M11.231 **Other chondrocalcinosis, right wrist**

M11.232 **Other chondrocalcinosis, left wrist**

M11.239 Other chondrocalcinosis, unspecified wrist ▽

✓6ᵗʰ M11.24 Other chondrocalcinosis, hand

M11.241 **Other chondrocalcinosis, right hand**

M11.242 **Other chondrocalcinosis, left hand**

M11.249 Other chondrocalcinosis, unspecified hand ▽

✓6ᵗʰ M11.25 Other chondrocalcinosis, hip

M11.251 **Other chondrocalcinosis, right hip**

M11.252 **Other chondrocalcinosis, left hip**

M11.259 Other chondrocalcinosis, unspecified hip ▽

✓6ᵗʰ M11.26 Other chondrocalcinosis, knee

M11.261 **Other chondrocalcinosis, right knee**

M11.262 **Other chondrocalcinosis, left knee**

M11.269 Other chondrocalcinosis, unspecified knee ▽

✓6ᵗʰ M11.27 Other chondrocalcinosis, ankle and foot

M11.271 **Other chondrocalcinosis, right ankle and foot**

M11.272 **Other chondrocalcinosis, left ankle and foot**

M11.279 Other chondrocalcinosis, unspecified ankle and foot ▽

M11.28 Other chondrocalcinosis, vertebrae

M11.29 Other chondrocalcinosis, multiple sites

✓5ᵗʰ M11.8 Other specified crystal arthropathies

M11.8Ø Other specified crystal arthropathies, unspecified site ▽

✓6ᵗʰ M11.81 Other specified crystal arthropathies, shoulder

M11.811 **Other specified crystal arthropathies, right shoulder**

M11.812 **Other specified crystal arthropathies, left shoulder**

M11.819 Other specified crystal arthropathies, unspecified shoulder ▽

✓6ᵗʰ M11.82 Other specified crystal arthropathies, elbow

M11.821 **Other specified crystal arthropathies, right elbow**

M11.822 **Other specified crystal arthropathies, left elbow**

M11.829 Other specified crystal arthropathies, unspecified elbow ▽

Ⓝ Newborn: 0   Ⓟ Pediatric: 0-17   Ⓜ Maternity: 12-55   Ⓐ Adult: 15-124   **NRS** Nonroutine supply Dx   **NCDx** Noncancer Dx   **PDx** Primary Dx   ▶◀ Revised Text   ● New Code   ▲ Revised Title

734   ICD-10-CM 2018

√6ᵗʰ **M11.83 Other specified crystal arthropathies,** wrist
     M11.831 **Other specified crystal arthropathies, right wrist**
     M11.832 **Other specified crystal arthropathies, left wrist**
     M11.839 Other specified crystal arthropathies, unspecified wrist ▽

√6ᵗʰ **M11.84 Other specified crystal arthropathies,** hand
     M11.841 **Other specified crystal arthropathies, right hand**
     M11.842 **Other specified crystal arthropathies, left hand**
     M11.849 Other specified crystal arthropathies, unspecified hand ▽

√6ᵗʰ **M11.85 Other specified crystal arthropathies,** hip
     M11.851 **Other specified crystal arthropathies, right hip**
     M11.852 **Other specified crystal arthropathies, left hip**
     M11.859 Other specified crystal arthropathies, unspecified hip ▽

√6ᵗʰ **M11.86 Other specified crystal arthropathies,** knee
     M11.861 **Other specified crystal arthropathies, right knee**
     M11.862 **Other specified crystal arthropathies, left knee**
     M11.869 Other specified crystal arthropathies, unspecified knee ▽

√6ᵗʰ **M11.87 Other specified crystal arthropathies,** ankle and foot
     M11.871 **Other specified crystal arthropathies, right ankle and foot**
     M11.872 **Other specified crystal arthropathies, left ankle and foot**
     M11.879 Other specified crystal arthropathies, unspecified ankle and foot ▽

   M11.88 **Other specified crystal arthropathies,** vertebrae
   M11.89 **Other specified crystal arthropathies,** multiple sites

M11.9 **Crystal arthropathy, unspecified** ▽

√4ᵗʰ **M12 Other and unspecified arthropathy**
     EXCLUDES 1   arthrosis (M15-M19)
           cricoarytenoid arthropathy (J38.7)

√5ᵗʰ **M12.0 Chronic postrheumatic arthropathy [Jaccoud]**
     M12.00 **Chronic postrheumatic arthropathy [Jaccoud], unspecified site** ▽

√6ᵗʰ **M12.01 Chronic postrheumatic arthropathy [Jaccoud],** shoulder
     M12.011 **Chronic postrheumatic arthropathy [Jaccoud], right shoulder**
     M12.012 **Chronic postrheumatic arthropathy [Jaccoud], left shoulder**
     M12.019 **Chronic postrheumatic arthropathy [Jaccoud], unspecified shoulder** ▽

√6ᵗʰ **M12.02 Chronic postrheumatic arthropathy [Jaccoud],** elbow
     M12.021 **Chronic postrheumatic arthropathy [Jaccoud], right elbow**
     M12.022 **Chronic postrheumatic arthropathy [Jaccoud], left elbow**
     M12.029 **Chronic postrheumatic arthropathy [Jaccoud], unspecified elbow** ▽

√6ᵗʰ **M12.03 Chronic postrheumatic arthropathy [Jaccoud],** wrist
     M12.031 **Chronic postrheumatic arthropathy [Jaccoud], right wrist**
     M12.032 **Chronic postrheumatic arthropathy [Jaccoud], left wrist**
     M12.039 **Chronic postrheumatic arthropathy [Jaccoud], unspecified wrist** ▽

√6ᵗʰ **M12.04 Chronic postrheumatic arthropathy [Jaccoud],** hand
     M12.041 **Chronic postrheumatic arthropathy [Jaccoud], right hand**
     M12.042 **Chronic postrheumatic arthropathy [Jaccoud], left hand**
     M12.049 **Chronic postrheumatic arthropathy [Jaccoud], unspecified hand** ▽

√6ᵗʰ **M12.05 Chronic postrheumatic arthropathy [Jaccoud],** hip
     M12.051 **Chronic postrheumatic arthropathy [Jaccoud], right hip**

M12.052 **Chronic postrheumatic arthropathy [Jaccoud], left hip**
M12.059 Chronic postrheumatic arthropathy [Jaccoud], unspecified hip ▽

√6ᵗʰ **M12.06 Chronic postrheumatic arthropathy [Jaccoud],** knee
     M12.061 **Chronic postrheumatic arthropathy [Jaccoud], right knee**
     M12.062 **Chronic postrheumatic arthropathy [Jaccoud], left knee**
     M12.069 Chronic postrheumatic arthropathy [Jaccoud], unspecified knee ▽

√6ᵗʰ **M12.07 Chronic postrheumatic arthropathy [Jaccoud],** ankle and foot
     M12.071 **Chronic postrheumatic arthropathy [Jaccoud], right ankle and foot**
     M12.072 **Chronic postrheumatic arthropathy [Jaccoud], left ankle and foot**
     M12.079 Chronic postrheumatic arthropathy [Jaccoud], unspecified ankle and foot ▽

   M12.08 **Chronic postrheumatic arthropathy [Jaccoud], other specified site**
     Chronic postrheumatic arthropathy [Jaccoud], vertebrae

   M12.09 **Chronic postrheumatic arthropathy [Jaccoud],** multiple sites

√5ᵗʰ **M12.1 Kaschin-Beck disease**
     Osteochondroarthrosis deformans endemica
   M12.10 **Kaschin-Beck disease, unspecified site** ▽

√6ᵗʰ **M12.11 Kaschin-Beck disease,** shoulder
     M12.111 **Kaschin-Beck disease, right shoulder**
     M12.112 **Kaschin-Beck disease, left shoulder**
     M12.119 **Kaschin-Beck disease, unspecified shoulder** ▽

√6ᵗʰ **M12.12 Kaschin-Beck disease,** elbow
     M12.121 **Kaschin-Beck disease, right elbow**
     M12.122 **Kaschin-Beck disease, left elbow**
     M12.129 **Kaschin-Beck disease, unspecified elbow** ▽

√6ᵗʰ **M12.13 Kaschin-Beck disease,** wrist
     M12.131 **Kaschin-Beck disease, right wrist**
     M12.132 **Kaschin-Beck disease, left wrist**
     M12.139 Kaschin-Beck disease, unspecified wrist ▽

√6ᵗʰ **M12.14 Kaschin-Beck disease,** hand
     M12.141 **Kaschin-Beck disease, right hand**
     M12.142 **Kaschin-Beck disease, left hand**
     M12.149 Kaschin-Beck disease, unspecified hand ▽

√6ᵗʰ **M12.15 Kaschin-Beck disease,** hip
     M12.151 **Kaschin-Beck disease, right hip**
     M12.152 **Kaschin-Beck disease, left hip**
     M12.159 Kaschin-Beck disease, unspecified hip ▽

√6ᵗʰ **M12.16 Kaschin-Beck disease,** knee
     M12.161 **Kaschin-Beck disease, right knee**
     M12.162 **Kaschin-Beck disease, left knee**
     M12.169 Kaschin-Beck disease, unspecified knee ▽

√6ᵗʰ **M12.17 Kaschin-Beck disease,** ankle and foot
     M12.171 **Kaschin-Beck disease, right ankle and foot**
     M12.172 **Kaschin-Beck disease, left ankle and foot**
     M12.179 **Kaschin-Beck disease, unspecified ankle and foot** ▽

   M12.18 **Kaschin-Beck disease,** vertebrae
   M12.19 **Kaschin-Beck disease,** multiple sites

√5ᵗʰ **M12.2 Villonodular synovitis (pigmented)**
   M12.20 **Villonodular synovitis (pigmented), unspecified site** ▽

√6ᵗʰ **M12.21 Villonodular synovitis (pigmented),** shoulder
     M12.211 **Villonodular synovitis (pigmented), right shoulder**
     M12.212 **Villonodular synovitis (pigmented), left shoulder**
     M12.219 **Villonodular synovitis (pigmented), unspecified shoulder** ▽

√6ᵗʰ **M12.22 Villonodular synovitis (pigmented),** elbow
     M12.221 **Villonodular synovitis (pigmented), right elbow**

☑ Additional Character Req   √x7ᵗʰ Placeholder Alert   Case-Mix Diagnosis   Manifestation   ▽ Unspecified Dx   **EXCLUDES 1** Not coded here   **EXCLUDES 2** Not included here

M12.222 **Villonodular synovitis (pigmented),** left elbow

M12.229 Villonodular synovitis (pigmented), unspecified elbow ▽

✓6ᵗʰ **M12.23** Villonodular synovitis (pigmented), wrist

M12.231 **Villonodular synovitis (pigmented),** right wrist

M12.232 **Villonodular synovitis (pigmented),** left wrist

M12.239 Villonodular synovitis (pigmented), unspecified wrist ▽

✓6ᵗʰ **M12.24** Villonodular synovitis (pigmented), hand

M12.241 **Villonodular synovitis (pigmented),** right hand

M12.242 **Villonodular synovitis (pigmented),** left hand

M12.249 Villonodular synovitis (pigmented), unspecified hand ▽

✓6ᵗʰ **M12.25** Villonodular synovitis (pigmented), hip

M12.251 **Villonodular synovitis (pigmented),** right hip

M12.252 **Villonodular synovitis (pigmented),** left hip

M12.259 Villonodular synovitis (pigmented), unspecified hip ▽

✓6ᵗʰ **M12.26** Villonodular synovitis (pigmented), knee

M12.261 **Villonodular synovitis (pigmented),** right knee

M12.262 **Villonodular synovitis (pigmented),** left knee

M12.269 Villonodular synovitis (pigmented), unspecified knee ▽

✓6ᵗʰ **M12.27** Villonodular synovitis (pigmented), ankle and foot

M12.271 **Villonodular synovitis (pigmented),** right ankle and foot

M12.272 **Villonodular synovitis (pigmented),** left ankle and foot

M12.279 Villonodular synovitis (pigmented), unspecified ankle and foot ▽

M12.28 **Villonodular synovitis (pigmented), other specified site**
Villonodular synovitis (pigmented), vertebrae

M12.29 **Villonodular synovitis (pigmented),** multiple sites

✓5ᵗʰ **M12.3** Palindromic rheumatism

M12.30 Palindromic rheumatism, unspecified site ▽

✓6ᵗʰ **M12.31** Palindromic rheumatism, shoulder

M12.311 **Palindromic rheumatism,** right shoulder

M12.312 **Palindromic rheumatism,** left shoulder

M12.319 Palindromic rheumatism, unspecified shoulder ▽

✓6ᵗʰ **M12.32** Palindromic rheumatism, elbow

M12.321 **Palindromic rheumatism,** right elbow

M12.322 **Palindromic rheumatism,** left elbow

M12.329 Palindromic rheumatism, unspecified elbow ▽

✓6ᵗʰ **M12.33** Palindromic rheumatism, wrist

M12.331 **Palindromic rheumatism,** right wrist

M12.332 **Palindromic rheumatism,** left wrist

M12.339 Palindromic rheumatism, unspecified wrist ▽

✓6ᵗʰ **M12.34** Palindromic rheumatism, hand

M12.341 **Palindromic rheumatism,** right hand

M12.342 **Palindromic rheumatism,** left hand

M12.349 Palindromic rheumatism, unspecified hand ▽

✓6ᵗʰ **M12.35** Palindromic rheumatism, hip

M12.351 **Palindromic rheumatism,** right hip

M12.352 **Palindromic rheumatism,** left hip

M12.359 Palindromic rheumatism, unspecified hip ▽

✓6ᵗʰ **M12.36** Palindromic rheumatism, knee

M12.361 **Palindromic rheumatism,** right knee

M12.362 **Palindromic rheumatism,** left knee

M12.369 Palindromic rheumatism, unspecified knee ▽

✓6ᵗʰ **M12.37** Palindromic rheumatism, ankle and foot

M12.371 **Palindromic rheumatism,** right ankle and foot

M12.372 **Palindromic rheumatism,** left ankle and foot

M12.379 Palindromic rheumatism, unspecified ankle and foot ▽

M12.38 **Palindromic rheumatism, other specified site**
Palindromic rheumatism, vertebrae

M12.39 **Palindromic rheumatism,** multiple sites

✓5ᵗʰ **M12.4** Intermittent hydrarthrosis

M12.40 Intermittent hydrarthrosis, unspecified site ▽

✓6ᵗʰ **M12.41** Intermittent hydrarthrosis, shoulder

M12.411 **Intermittent hydrarthrosis,** right shoulder

M12.412 **Intermittent hydrarthrosis,** left shoulder

M12.419 Intermittent hydrarthrosis, unspecified shoulder ▽

✓6ᵗʰ **M12.42** Intermittent hydrarthrosis, elbow

M12.421 **Intermittent hydrarthrosis,** right elbow

M12.422 **Intermittent hydrarthrosis,** left elbow

M12.429 Intermittent hydrarthrosis, unspecified elbow ▽

✓6ᵗʰ **M12.43** Intermittent hydrarthrosis, wrist

M12.431 **Intermittent hydrarthrosis,** right wrist

M12.432 **Intermittent hydrarthrosis,** left wrist

M12.439 Intermittent hydrarthrosis, unspecified wrist ▽

✓6ᵗʰ **M12.44** Intermittent hydrarthrosis, hand

M12.441 **Intermittent hydrarthrosis,** right hand

M12.442 **Intermittent hydrarthrosis,** left hand

M12.449 Intermittent hydrarthrosis, unspecified hand ▽

✓6ᵗʰ **M12.45** Intermittent hydrarthrosis, hip

M12.451 **Intermittent hydrarthrosis,** right hip

M12.452 **Intermittent hydrarthrosis,** left hip

M12.459 Intermittent hydrarthrosis, unspecified hip ▽

✓6ᵗʰ **M12.46** Intermittent hydrarthrosis, knee

M12.461 **Intermittent hydrarthrosis,** right knee

M12.462 **Intermittent hydrarthrosis,** left knee

M12.469 Intermittent hydrarthrosis, unspecified knee ▽

✓6ᵗʰ **M12.47** Intermittent hydrarthrosis, ankle and foot

M12.471 **Intermittent hydrarthrosis,** right ankle and foot

M12.472 **Intermittent hydrarthrosis,** left ankle and foot

M12.479 Intermittent hydrarthrosis, unspecified ankle and foot ▽

M12.48 **Intermittent hydrarthrosis, other site**

M12.49 **Intermittent hydrarthrosis,** multiple sites

✓5ᵗʰ **M12.5** Traumatic arthropathy

EXCLUDES 1 *current injury–see Alphabetic Index*
post-traumatic osteoarthritis NOS (M19.1-)
post-traumatic osteoarthritis of first carpometacarpal joint (M18.2-M18.3)
post-traumatic osteoarthritis of hip (M16.4-M16.5)
post-traumatic osteoarthritis of knee (M17.2-M17.3)
post-traumatic osteoarthritis of other single joints (M19.1-)

AHA: 2015, 1Q, 17

M12.50 Traumatic arthropathy, unspecified site ▽

✓6ᵗʰ **M12.51** Traumatic arthropathy, shoulder

M12.511 **Traumatic arthropathy,** right shoulder

M12.512 **Traumatic arthropathy,** left shoulder

M12.519 Traumatic arthropathy, unspecified shoulder ▽

✓6ᵗʰ **M12.52** Traumatic arthropathy, elbow

M12.521 **Traumatic arthropathy,** right elbow

M12.522 **Traumatic arthropathy,** left elbow

M12.529 Traumatic arthropathy, unspecified elbow ▽

✓6ᵗʰ **M12.53** Traumatic arthropathy, wrist

M12.531 **Traumatic arthropathy,** right wrist

M12.532 **Traumatic arthropathy,** left wrist

Ⓝ Newborn: 0 Ⓟ Pediatric: 0-17 Ⓜ Maternity: 12-55 Ⓐ Adult: 15-124 **NRS** Nonroutine supply Dx **NCDx** Noncancer Dx **PDx** Primary Dx ►◄ Revised Text ● New Code ▲ Revised Title

736   ICD-10-CM 2018

M12.539   Traumatic arthropathy, unspecified wrist ▽

✓6ᵗʰ M12.54   Traumatic arthropathy, hand
    M12.541   Traumatic arthropathy, right hand
    M12.542   Traumatic arthropathy, left hand
    M12.549   Traumatic arthropathy, unspecified hand

✓6ᵗʰ M12.55   Traumatic arthropathy, hip
    M12.551   Traumatic arthropathy, right hip
    M12.552   Traumatic arthropathy, left hip
    M12.559   Traumatic arthropathy, unspecified hip ▽

✓6ᵗʰ M12.56   Traumatic arthropathy, knee
    M12.561   Traumatic arthropathy, right knee
    M12.562   Traumatic arthropathy, left knee
    M12.569   Traumatic arthropathy, unspecified knee ▽

✓6ᵗʰ M12.57   Traumatic arthropathy, ankle and foot
    M12.571   Traumatic arthropathy, right ankle and foot
    M12.572   Traumatic arthropathy, left ankle and foot
    M12.579   Traumatic arthropathy, unspecified ankle and foot ▽

M12.58   Traumatic arthropathy, other specified site
    Traumatic arthropathy, vertebrae

M12.59   Traumatic arthropathy, multiple sites

✓5ᵗʰ M12.8   Other specific arthropathies, not elsewhere classified
    Transient arthropathy

M12.80   Other specific arthropathies, not elsewhere classified, unspecified site ▽

✓6ᵗʰ M12.81   Other specific arthropathies, not elsewhere classified, shoulder
    M12.811   Other specific arthropathies, not elsewhere classified, right shoulder
    M12.812   Other specific arthropathies, not elsewhere classified, left shoulder
    M12.819   Other specific arthropathies, not elsewhere classified, unspecified shoulder

✓6ᵗʰ M12.82   Other specific arthropathies, not elsewhere classified, elbow
    M12.821   Other specific arthropathies, not elsewhere classified, right elbow
    M12.822   Other specific arthropathies, not elsewhere classified, left elbow
    M12.829   Other specific arthropathies, not elsewhere classified, unspecified elbow ▽

✓6ᵗʰ M12.83   Other specific arthropathies, not elsewhere classified, wrist
    M12.831   Other specific arthropathies, not elsewhere classified, right wrist
    M12.832   Other specific arthropathies, not elsewhere classified, left wrist
    M12.839   Other specific arthropathies, not elsewhere classified, unspecified wrist ▽

✓6ᵗʰ M12.84   Other specific arthropathies, not elsewhere classified, hand
    M12.841   Other specific arthropathies, not elsewhere classified, right hand
    M12.842   Other specific arthropathies, not elsewhere classified, left hand
    M12.849   Other specific arthropathies, not elsewhere classified, unspecified hand ▽

✓6ᵗʰ M12.85   Other specific arthropathies, not elsewhere classified, hip
    M12.851   Other specific arthropathies, not elsewhere classified, right hip
    M12.852   Other specific arthropathies, not elsewhere classified, left hip
    M12.859   Other specific arthropathies, not elsewhere classified, unspecified hip ▽

✓6ᵗʰ M12.86   Other specific arthropathies, not elsewhere classified, knee
    M12.861   Other specific arthropathies, not elsewhere classified, right knee
    M12.862   Other specific arthropathies, not elsewhere classified, left knee

M12.869   Other specific arthropathies, not elsewhere classified, unspecified knee ▽

✓6ᵗʰ M12.87   Other specific arthropathies, not elsewhere classified, ankle and foot
    M12.871   Other specific arthropathies, not elsewhere classified, right ankle and foot
    M12.872   Other specific arthropathies, not elsewhere classified, left ankle and foot
    M12.879   Other specific arthropathies, not elsewhere classified, unspecified ankle and foot ▽

M12.88   Other specific arthropathies, not elsewhere classified, other specified site
    Other specific arthropathies, not elsewhere classified, vertebrae

M12.89   Other specific arthropathies, not elsewhere classified, multiple sites

M12.9   Arthropathy, unspecified ▽

✓4ᵗʰ **M13   Other arthritis**
    EXCLUDES 1   arthrosis (M15-M19)
              osteoarthritis (M15-M19)

M13.0   Polyarthritis, unspecified ▽

✓5ᵗʰ M13.1   Monoarthritis, not elsewhere classified
    M13.10   Monoarthritis, not elsewhere classified, unspecified site ▽

✓6ᵗʰ M13.11   Monoarthritis, not elsewhere classified, shoulder
    M13.111   Monoarthritis, not elsewhere classified, right shoulder
    M13.112   Monoarthritis, not elsewhere classified, left shoulder
    M13.119   Monoarthritis, not elsewhere classified, unspecified shoulder ▽

✓6ᵗʰ M13.12   Monoarthritis, not elsewhere classified, elbow
    M13.121   Monoarthritis, not elsewhere classified, right elbow
    M13.122   Monoarthritis, not elsewhere classified, left elbow
    M13.129   Monoarthritis, not elsewhere classified, unspecified elbow ▽

✓6ᵗʰ M13.13   Monoarthritis, not elsewhere classified, wrist
    M13.131   Monoarthritis, not elsewhere classified, right wrist
    M13.132   Monoarthritis, not elsewhere classified, left wrist
    M13.139   Monoarthritis, not elsewhere classified, unspecified wrist ▽

✓6ᵗʰ M13.14   Monoarthritis, not elsewhere classified, hand
    M13.141   Monoarthritis, not elsewhere classified, right hand
    M13.142   Monoarthritis, not elsewhere classified, left hand
    M13.149   Monoarthritis, not elsewhere classified, unspecified hand ▽

✓6ᵗʰ M13.15   Monoarthritis, not elsewhere classified, hip
    M13.151   Monoarthritis, not elsewhere classified, right hip
    M13.152   Monoarthritis, not elsewhere classified, left hip
    M13.159   Monoarthritis, not elsewhere classified, unspecified hip ▽

✓6ᵗʰ M13.16   Monoarthritis, not elsewhere classified, knee
    M13.161   Monoarthritis, not elsewhere classified, right knee
    M13.162   Monoarthritis, not elsewhere classified, left knee
    M13.169   Monoarthritis, not elsewhere classified, unspecified knee ▽

✓6ᵗʰ M13.17   Monoarthritis, not elsewhere classified, ankle and foot
    M13.171   Monoarthritis, not elsewhere classified, right ankle and foot
    M13.172   Monoarthritis, not elsewhere classified, left ankle and foot
    M13.179   Monoarthritis, not elsewhere classified, unspecified ankle and foot ▽

✓ Additional Character Req   ✓x7ᵗʰ Placeholder Alert   Case-Mix Diagnosis   Manifestation   ▽ Unspecified Dx   **EXCLUDES 1** Not coded here   **EXCLUDES 2** Not included here

ICD-10-CM 2018   737

Chapter 13. Diseases of the Musculoskeletal System and Connective Tissue

M13.8–M14.869

☑5ᵗʰ **M13.8 Other specified arthritis**
Allergic arthritis
EXCLUDES 1 osteoarthritis (M15-M19)

     M13.80 Other specified arthritis, unspecified site ▽

☑6ᵗʰ **M13.81 Other specified arthritis, shoulder**
     M13.811 Other specified arthritis, right shoulder
     M13.812 Other specified arthritis, left shoulder ▽
     M13.819 Other specified arthritis, unspecified shoulder

☑6ᵗʰ **M13.82 Other specified arthritis, elbow**
     M13.821 Other specified arthritis, right elbow
     M13.822 Other specified arthritis, left elbow ▽
     M13.829 Other specified arthritis, unspecified elbow

☑6ᵗʰ **M13.83 Other specified arthritis, wrist**
     M13.831 Other specified arthritis, right wrist
     M13.832 Other specified arthritis, left wrist ▽
     M13.839 Other specified arthritis, unspecified wrist

☑6ᵗʰ **M13.84 Other specified arthritis, hand**
     M13.841 Other specified arthritis, right hand
     M13.842 Other specified arthritis, left hand ▽
     M13.849 Other specified arthritis, unspecified hand

☑6ᵗʰ **M13.85 Other specified arthritis, hip**
     M13.851 Other specified arthritis, right hip
     M13.852 Other specified arthritis, left hip ▽
     M13.859 Other specified arthritis, unspecified hip

☑6ᵗʰ **M13.86 Other specified arthritis, knee**
     M13.861 Other specified arthritis, right knee
     M13.862 Other specified arthritis, left knee ▽
     M13.869 Other specified arthritis, unspecified knee

☑6ᵗʰ **M13.87 Other specified arthritis, ankle and foot**
     M13.871 Other specified arthritis, right ankle and foot
     M13.872 Other specified arthritis, left ankle and foot ▽
     M13.879 Other specified arthritis, unspecified ankle and foot

     M13.88 Other specified arthritis, other site
     M13.89 Other specified arthritis, multiple sites

☑4ᵗʰ **M14 Arthropathies in other diseases classified elsewhere**
EXCLUDES 1 arthropathy in:
     diabetes mellitus (E08-E13 with .61-)
     hematological disorders (M36.2-M36.3)
     hypersensitivity reactions (M36.4)
     neoplastic disease (M36.1)
     neurosyphillis (A52.16)
     sarcoidosis (D86.86)
     enteropathic arthropathies (M07.-)
     juvenile psoriatic arthropathy (L40.54)
     lipoid dermatoarthritis (E78.81)

☑5ᵗʰ **M14.6 Charcôt's joint**
Neuropathic arthropathy
EXCLUDES 1 Charcôt's joint in diabetes mellitus (E08-E13 with .610)
     Charcôt's joint in tabes dorsalis (A52.16)

     M14.60 Charcôt's joint, unspecified site ▽

☑6ᵗʰ **M14.61 Charcôt's joint, shoulder**
     M14.611 Charcôt's joint, right shoulder
     M14.612 Charcôt's joint, left shoulder
     M14.619 Charcôt's joint, unspecified shoulder ▽

☑6ᵗʰ **M14.62 Charcôt's joint, elbow**
     M14.621 Charcôt's joint, right elbow
     M14.622 Charcôt's joint, left elbow
     M14.629 Charcôt's joint, unspecified elbow ▽

☑6ᵗʰ **M14.63 Charcôt's joint, wrist**
     M14.631 Charcôt's joint, right wrist
     M14.632 Charcôt's joint, left wrist
     M14.639 Charcôt's joint, unspecified wrist ▽

☑6ᵗʰ **M14.64 Charcôt's joint, hand**
     M14.641 Charcôt's joint, right hand
     M14.642 Charcôt's joint, left hand

     M14.649 Charcôt's joint, unspecified hand ▽

☑6ᵗʰ **M14.65 Charcôt's joint, hip**
     M14.651 Charcôt's joint, right hip
     M14.652 Charcôt's joint, left hip
     M14.659 Charcôt's joint, unspecified hip ▽

☑6ᵗʰ **M14.66 Charcôt's joint, knee**
     M14.661 Charcôt's joint, right knee
     M14.662 Charcôt's joint, left knee
     M14.669 Charcôt's joint, unspecified knee ▽

☑6ᵗʰ **M14.67 Charcôt's joint, ankle and foot**
     M14.671 Charcôt's joint, right ankle and foot
     M14.672 Charcôt's joint, left ankle and foot
     M14.679 Charcôt's joint, unspecified ankle and foot ▽

     M14.68 Charcôt's joint, vertebrae
     M14.69 Charcôt's joint, multiple sites

☑5ᵗʰ **M14.8 Arthropathies in other specified diseases classified elsewhere**
Code first underlying disease, such as:
     amyloidosis (E85.-)
     erythema multiforme (L51.-)
     erythema nodosum (L52)
     hemochromatosis (E83.11-)
     hyperparathyroidism (E21.-)
     hypothyroidism (E00-E03)
     sickle-cell disorders (D57.-)
     thyrotoxicosis [hyperthyroidism] (E05.-)
     Whipple's disease (K90.81)

     M14.80 Arthropathies in other specified diseases classified elsewhere, unspecified site ▽

☑6ᵗʰ **M14.81 Arthropathies in other specified diseases classified elsewhere, shoulder**
     M14.811 Arthropathies in other specified diseases classified elsewhere, right shoulder
     M14.812 Arthropathies in other specified diseases classified elsewhere, left shoulder
     M14.819 Arthropathies in other specified diseases classified elsewhere, unspecified shoulder ▽

☑6ᵗʰ **M14.82 Arthropathies in other specified diseases classified elsewhere, elbow**
     M14.821 Arthropathies in other specified diseases classified elsewhere, right elbow
     M14.822 Arthropathies in other specified diseases classified elsewhere, left elbow
     M14.829 Arthropathies in other specified diseases classified elsewhere, unspecified elbow ▽

☑6ᵗʰ **M14.83 Arthropathies in other specified diseases classified elsewhere, wrist**
     M14.831 Arthropathies in other specified diseases classified elsewhere, right wrist
     M14.832 Arthropathies in other specified diseases classified elsewhere, left wrist
     M14.839 Arthropathies in other specified diseases classified elsewhere, unspecified wrist ▽

☑6ᵗʰ **M14.84 Arthropathies in other specified diseases classified elsewhere, hand**
     M14.841 Arthropathies in other specified diseases classified elsewhere, right hand
     M14.842 Arthropathies in other specified diseases classified elsewhere, left hand
     M14.849 Arthropathies in other specified diseases classified elsewhere, unspecified hand ▽

☑6ᵗʰ **M14.85 Arthropathies in other specified diseases classified elsewhere, hip**
     M14.851 Arthropathies in other specified diseases classified elsewhere, right hip
     M14.852 Arthropathies in other specified diseases classified elsewhere, left hip
     M14.859 Arthropathies in other specified diseases classified elsewhere, unspecified hip ▽

☑6ᵗʰ **M14.86 Arthropathies in other specified diseases classified elsewhere, knee**
     M14.861 Arthropathies in other specified diseases classified elsewhere, right knee
     M14.862 Arthropathies in other specified diseases classified elsewhere, left knee
     M14.869 Arthropathies in other specified diseases classified elsewhere, unspecified knee ▽

Ⓝ Newborn: 0   Ⓟ Pediatric: 0-17   Ⓜ Maternity: 12-55   Ⓐ Adult: 15-124   **NRS** Nonroutine supply Dx   **NCDx** Noncancer Dx   **PDx** Primary Dx   ►◄ Revised Text   ● New Code   ▲ Revised Title

738   ICD-10-CM 2018

✓6th **M14.87 Arthropathies in other specified diseases classified elsewhere,** ankle and foot

    M14.871   *Arthropathies in other specified diseases classified elsewhere,* right *ankle and foot*

    M14.872   *Arthropathies in other specified diseases classified elsewhere,* left *ankle and foot*

    M14.879   *Arthropathies in other specified diseases classified elsewhere,* unspecified *ankle and foot* ▽

   M14.88   *Arthropathies in other specified diseases classified elsewhere,* vertebrae

   M14.89   *Arthropathies in other specified diseases classified elsewhere,* multiple sites

Osteoarthritis (M15-M19)

EXCLUDES 2   osteoarthritis of spine (M47.-)

✓4th **M15 Polyosteoarthritis**

   INCLUDES   arthritis of multiple sites

   EXCLUDES 1   bilateral involvement of single joint (M16-M19)

   M15.0 Primary generalized (osteo)arthritis

   M15.1 Heberden's nodes (with arthropathy)
     Interphalangeal distal osteoarthritis

   M15.2 Bouchard's nodes (with arthropathy)
     Juxtaphalangeal distal osteoarthritis

   M15.3 Secondary multiple arthritis
     Post-traumatic polyosteoarthritis

   M15.4 Erosive (osteo)arthritis

   M15.8 Other polyosteoarthritis

   M15.9 Polyosteoarthritis, unspecified ▽
     Generalized osteoarthritis NOS

✓4th **M16 Osteoarthritis of** hip
   AHA: 2016, 4Q, 146

   M16.0 Bilateral primary osteoarthritis of hip

✓5th   **M16.1 Unilateral primary osteoarthritis of hip**
     Primary osteoarthritis of hip NOS

     M16.10 Unilateral primary osteoarthritis, unspecified hip ▽
     M16.11 Unilateral primary osteoarthritis, right hip
     M16.12 Unilateral primary osteoarthritis, left hip

   M16.2 Bilateral osteoarthritis resulting from hip dysplasia

✓5th   **M16.3 Unilateral osteoarthritis resulting from hip dysplasia**
     Dysplastic osteoarthritis of hip NOS

     M16.30 Unilateral osteoarthritis resulting from hip dysplasia, unspecified hip ▽
     M16.31 Unilateral osteoarthritis resulting from hip dysplasia, right hip
     M16.32 Unilateral osteoarthritis resulting from hip dysplasia, left hip

   M16.4 Bilateral post-traumatic osteoarthritis of hip

✓5th   **M16.5 Unilateral post-traumatic osteoarthritis of hip**
     Post-traumatic osteoarthritis of hip NOS

     M16.50 Unilateral post-traumatic osteoarthritis, unspecified hip ▽
     M16.51 Unilateral post-traumatic osteoarthritis, right hip
     M16.52 Unilateral post-traumatic osteoarthritis, left hip

   M16.6 Other bilateral secondary osteoarthritis of hip

   M16.7 Other unilateral secondary osteoarthritis of hip
     Secondary osteoarthritis of hip NOS

   M16.9 Osteoarthritis of hip, unspecified ▽

✓4th **M17 Osteoarthritis of** knee
   AHA: 2016, 4Q, 146-147

   M17.0 Bilateral primary osteoarthritis of knee

✓5th   **M17.1 Unilateral primary osteoarthritis of knee**
     Primary osteoarthritis of knee NOS

     M17.10 Unilateral primary osteoarthritis, unspecified knee ▽
     M17.11 Unilateral primary osteoarthritis, right knee
     M17.12 Unilateral primary osteoarthritis, left knee

   M17.2 Bilateral post-traumatic osteoarthritis of knee

✓5th   **M17.3 Unilateral post-traumatic osteoarthritis of knee**
     Post-traumatic osteoarthritis of knee NOS

     M17.30 Unilateral post-traumatic osteoarthritis, unspecified knee ▽
     M17.31 Unilateral post-traumatic osteoarthritis, right knee
     M17.32 Unilateral post-traumatic osteoarthritis, left knee

   M17.4 Other bilateral secondary osteoarthritis of knee

   M17.5 Other unilateral secondary osteoarthritis of knee
     Secondary osteoarthritis of knee NOS

   M17.9 Osteoarthritis of knee, unspecified ▽

✓4th **M18 Osteoarthritis of** first carpometacarpal joint

   M18.0 Bilateral primary osteoarthritis of first carpometacarpal joints

✓5th   **M18.1 Unilateral primary osteoarthritis of first carpometacarpal joint**
     Primary osteoarthritis of first carpometacarpal joint NOS

     M18.10 Unilateral primary osteoarthritis of first carpometacarpal joint, unspecified hand ▽
     M18.11 Unilateral primary osteoarthritis of first carpometacarpal joint, right hand
     M18.12 Unilateral primary osteoarthritis of first carpometacarpal joint, left hand

   M18.2 Bilateral post-traumatic osteoarthritis of first carpometacarpal joints

✓5th   **M18.3 Unilateral post-traumatic osteoarthritis of first carpometacarpal joint**
     Post-traumatic osteoarthritis of first carpometacarpal joint NOS

     M18.30 Unilateral post-traumatic osteoarthritis of first carpometacarpal joint, unspecified hand ▽
     M18.31 Unilateral post-traumatic osteoarthritis of first carpometacarpal joint, right hand
     M18.32 Unilateral post-traumatic osteoarthritis of first carpometacarpal joint, left hand

   M18.4 Other bilateral secondary osteoarthritis of first carpometacarpal joints

✓5th   **M18.5 Other unilateral secondary osteoarthritis of first carpometacarpal joint**
     Secondary osteoarthritis of first carpometacarpal joint NOS

     M18.50 Other unilateral secondary osteoarthritis of first carpometacarpal joint, unspecified hand ▽
     M18.51 Other unilateral secondary osteoarthritis of first carpometacarpal joint, right hand
     M18.52 Other unilateral secondary osteoarthritis of first carpometacarpal joint, left hand

   M18.9 Osteoarthritis of first carpometacarpal joint, unspecified ▽

✓4th **M19 Other and unspecified osteoarthritis**

   EXCLUDES 1   polyarthritis (M15.-)

   EXCLUDES 2   arthrosis of spine (M47.-)
     hallux rigidus (M20.2)
     osteoarthritis of spine (M47.-)

✓5th   **M19.0 Primary osteoarthritis of other joints**
     AHA: 2016, 4Q, 145

✓6th   **M19.01 Primary osteoarthritis, shoulder**
       M19.011 Primary osteoarthritis, right shoulder
       M19.012 Primary osteoarthritis, left shoulder
       M19.019 Primary osteoarthritis, unspecified shoulder ▽

✓6th   **M19.02 Primary osteoarthritis, elbow**
       M19.021 Primary osteoarthritis, right elbow
       M19.022 Primary osteoarthritis, left elbow
       M19.029 Primary osteoarthritis, unspecified elbow ▽

✓6th   **M19.03 Primary osteoarthritis, wrist**
       M19.031 Primary osteoarthritis, right wrist
       M19.032 Primary osteoarthritis, left wrist
       M19.039 Primary osteoarthritis, unspecified wrist ▽

✓6th   **M19.04 Primary osteoarthritis, hand**
       EXCLUDES 2   primary osteoarthritis of first carpometacarpal joint (M18.0-, M18.1-)
       M19.041 Primary osteoarthritis, right hand
       M19.042 Primary osteoarthritis, left hand
       M19.049 Primary osteoarthritis, unspecified hand ▽

✓6th   **M19.07 Primary osteoarthritis ankle and foot**
       M19.071 Primary osteoarthritis, right ankle and foot
       M19.072 Primary osteoarthritis, left ankle and foot
       M19.079 Primary osteoarthritis, unspecified ankle and foot ▽

☑ Additional Character Req   ✓x7th Placeholder Alert   Case-Mix Diagnosis   Manifestation   ▽ Unspecified Dx   EXCLUDES 1 Not coded here   EXCLUDES 2 Not included here

Chapter 13. Diseases of the Musculoskeletal System and Connective Tissue

✓5ᵗʰ **M19.1** Post-traumatic osteoarthritis of other joints
  ✓6ᵗʰ **M19.11** Post-traumatic osteoarthritis, shoulder
  M19.111 Post-traumatic osteoarthritis, right shoulder
  M19.112 Post-traumatic osteoarthritis, left shoulder
  M19.119 Post-traumatic osteoarthritis, unspecified shoulder ▽
  ✓6ᵗʰ **M19.12** Post-traumatic osteoarthritis, elbow
  M19.121 Post-traumatic osteoarthritis, right elbow
  M19.122 Post-traumatic osteoarthritis, left elbow
  M19.129 Post-traumatic osteoarthritis, unspecified elbow ▽
  ✓6ᵗʰ **M19.13** Post-traumatic osteoarthritis, wrist
  M19.131 Post-traumatic osteoarthritis, right wrist
  M19.132 Post-traumatic osteoarthritis, left wrist
  M19.139 Post-traumatic osteoarthritis, unspecified wrist ▽
  ✓6ᵗʰ **M19.14** Post-traumatic osteoarthritis, hand
  EXCLUDES 2 *post-traumatic osteoarthritis of first carpometacarpal joint (M18.2-, M18.3-)*
  M19.141 Post-traumatic osteoarthritis, right hand
  M19.142 Post-traumatic osteoarthritis, left hand
  M19.149 Post-traumatic osteoarthritis, unspecified hand ▽
  ✓6ᵗʰ **M19.17** Post-traumatic osteoarthritis, ankle and foot
  M19.171 Post-traumatic osteoarthritis, right ankle and foot
  M19.172 Post-traumatic osteoarthritis, left ankle and foot
  M19.179 Post-traumatic osteoarthritis, unspecified ankle and foot ▽

✓5ᵗʰ **M19.2** Secondary osteoarthritis of other joints
  ✓6ᵗʰ **M19.21** Secondary osteoarthritis, shoulder
  M19.211 Secondary osteoarthritis, right shoulder
  M19.212 Secondary osteoarthritis, left shoulder
  M19.219 Secondary osteoarthritis, unspecified shoulder ▽
  ✓6ᵗʰ **M19.22** Secondary osteoarthritis, elbow
  M19.221 Secondary osteoarthritis, right elbow
  M19.222 Secondary osteoarthritis, left elbow
  M19.229 Secondary osteoarthritis, unspecified elbow ▽
  ✓6ᵗʰ **M19.23** Secondary osteoarthritis, wrist
  M19.231 Secondary osteoarthritis, right wrist
  M19.232 Secondary osteoarthritis, left wrist
  M19.239 Secondary osteoarthritis, unspecified wrist ▽
  ✓6ᵗʰ **M19.24** Secondary osteoarthritis, hand
  M19.241 Secondary osteoarthritis, right hand
  M19.242 Secondary osteoarthritis, left hand
  M19.249 Secondary osteoarthritis, unspecified hand ▽
  ✓6ᵗʰ **M19.27** Secondary osteoarthritis, ankle and foot
  M19.271 Secondary osteoarthritis, right ankle and foot
  M19.272 Secondary osteoarthritis, left ankle and foot
  M19.279 Secondary osteoarthritis, unspecified ankle and foot ▽

✓5ᵗʰ **M19.9** Osteoarthritis, unspecified site
  M19.90 Unspecified osteoarthritis, unspecified site ▽
  Arthrosis NOS   Osteoarthritis NOS
  Arthritis NOS
  AHA: 2016, 4Q, 147
  M19.91 Primary osteoarthritis, unspecified site ▽
  Primary osteoarthritis NOS
  M19.92 Post-traumatic osteoarthritis, unspecified site ▽
  Post-traumatic osteoarthritis NOS
  M19.93 Secondary osteoarthritis, unspecified site ▽
  Secondary osteoarthritis NOS

Other joint disorders (M20-M25)

EXCLUDES 2 *joints of the spine (M40-M54)*

✓4ᵗʰ **M20** Acquired deformities of fingers and toes
  EXCLUDES 1 *acquired absence of fingers and toes (Z89.-)*
  congenital absence of fingers and toes (Q71.3-, Q72.3-)
  congenital deformities and malformations of fingers and toes (Q66-, Q68-Q70, Q74-)
  ✓5ᵗʰ **M20.0** Deformity of finger(s)
  EXCLUDES 1 *clubbing of fingers (R68.3)*
  palmar fascial fibromatosis [Dupuytren] (M72.0)
  trigger finger (M65.3)
  ✓6ᵗʰ **M20.00** Unspecified deformity of finger(s)
  M20.001 Unspecified deformity of right finger(s) ▽
  M20.002 Unspecified deformity of left finger(s) ▽
  M20.009 Unspecified deformity of unspecified finger(s) ▽
  ✓6ᵗʰ **M20.01** Mallet finger
  M20.011 Mallet finger of right finger(s)
  M20.012 Mallet finger of left finger(s)
  M20.019 Mallet finger of unspecified finger(s) ▽
  ✓6ᵗʰ **M20.02** Boutonnière deformity
  DEF: A deformity of the finger caused by flexion of the proximal interphalangeal joint and hyperextension of the distal joint; results from rheumatoid arthritis, osteoarthritis, or injury; also called buttonhole deformity.
  M20.021 Boutonnière deformity of right finger(s)
  M20.022 Boutonnière deformity of left finger(s)
  M20.029 Boutonnière deformity of unspecified finger(s) ▽
  ✓6ᵗʰ **M20.03** Swan-neck deformity
  DEF: Flexed distal and hyperextended proximal interphalangeal joint; most commonly caused by rheumatoid arthritis.
  M20.031 Swan-neck deformity of right finger(s)
  M20.032 Swan-neck deformity of left finger(s)
  M20.039 Swan-neck deformity of unspecified finger(s) ▽
  ✓6ᵗʰ **M20.09** Other deformity of finger(s)
  M20.091 Other deformity of right finger(s)
  M20.092 Other deformity of left finger(s)
  M20.099 Other deformity of finger(s), unspecified finger(s) ▽
  ✓5ᵗʰ **M20.1** Hallux valgus (acquired)
  EXCLUDES 2 *bunion (M21.6-)*
  M20.10 Hallux valgus (acquired), unspecified foot ▽
  M20.11 Hallux valgus (acquired), right foot
  M20.12 Hallux valgus (acquired), left foot

Hallux Valgus

Hallux valgus

Medial eminence of metatarsal bone

Right foot

Ⓝ Newborn: 0   Ⓟ Pediatric: 0-17   Ⓜ Maternity: 12-55   Ⓐ Adult: 15-124   NRS Nonroutine supply Dx   NCDx Noncancer Dx   PDx Primary Dx   ▶◀ Revised Text   ● New Code   ▲ Revised Title

740   ICD-10-CM 2018

☑5ᵗʰ M20.2 Hallux rigidus
     M20.20 Hallux rigidus, unspecified foot ▽
     M20.21 Hallux rigidus, right foot
     M20.22 Hallux rigidus, left foot

☑5ᵗʰ M20.3 Hallux varus (acquired)
     M20.30 Hallux varus (acquired), unspecified foot ▽
     M20.31 Hallux varus (acquired), right foot
     M20.32 Hallux varus (acquired), left foot

☑5ᵗʰ M20.4 Other hammer toe(s) (acquired)
     M20.40 Other hammer toe(s) (acquired), unspecified foot ▽
     M20.41 Other hammer toe(s) (acquired), right foot
     M20.42 Other hammer toe(s) (acquired), left foot

☑5ᵗʰ M20.5 Other deformities of toe(s) (acquired)
     ☑6ᵗʰ M20.5X Other deformities of toe(s) (acquired)
       M20.5X1 Other deformities of toe(s) (acquired), right foot
       M20.5X2 Other deformities of toe(s) (acquired), left foot
       M20.5X9 Other deformities of toe(s) (acquired), unspecified foot ▽

☑5ᵗʰ M20.6 Acquired deformities of toe(s), unspecified
     M20.60 Acquired deformities of toe(s), unspecified, unspecified foot ▽
     M20.61 Acquired deformities of toe(s), unspecified, right foot ▽
     M20.62 Acquired deformities of toe(s), unspecified, left foot ▽

☑4ᵗʰ M21 Other acquired deformities of limbs
     EXCLUDES 1   acquired absence of limb (Z89.-)
        congenital absence of limbs (Q71-Q73)
        congenital deformities and malformations of limbs (Q65-Q66, Q68-Q74)
     EXCLUDES 2   acquired deformities of fingers or toes (M20.-)
        coxa plana (M91.2)

☑5ᵗʰ M21.0 Valgus deformity, not elsewhere classified
     EXCLUDES 1   metatarsus valgus (Q66.6)
        talipes calcaneovalgus (Q66.4)
     M21.00 Valgus deformity, not elsewhere classified, unspecified site ▽
     ☑6ᵗʰ M21.02 Valgus deformity, not elsewhere classified, elbow
       Cubitus valgus
       M21.021 Valgus deformity, not elsewhere classified, right elbow
       M21.022 Valgus deformity, not elsewhere classified, left elbow
       M21.029 Valgus deformity, not elsewhere classified, unspecified elbow ▽
     ☑6ᵗʰ M21.05 Valgus deformity, not elsewhere classified, hip
       M21.051 Valgus deformity, not elsewhere classified, right hip
       M21.052 Valgus deformity, not elsewhere classified, left hip
       M21.059 Valgus deformity, not elsewhere classified, unspecified hip ▽
     ☑6ᵗʰ M21.06 Valgus deformity, not elsewhere classified, knee
       Genu valgum
       Knock knee
       M21.061 Valgus deformity, not elsewhere classified, right knee
       M21.062 Valgus deformity, not elsewhere classified, left knee
       M21.069 Valgus deformity, not elsewhere classified, unspecified knee ▽
     ☑6ᵗʰ M21.07 Valgus deformity, not elsewhere classified, ankle
       M21.071 Valgus deformity, not elsewhere classified, right ankle
       M21.072 Valgus deformity, not elsewhere classified, left ankle
       M21.079 Valgus deformity, not elsewhere classified, unspecified ankle ▽

☑5ᵗʰ M21.1 Varus deformity, not elsewhere classified
     EXCLUDES 1   metatarsus varus (Q66.22)
        tibia vara (M92.5)
     M21.10 Varus deformity, not elsewhere classified, unspecified site ▽

Genu Valga (knock-knee)

☑6ᵗʰ M21.12 Varus deformity, not elsewhere classified, elbow
     Cubitus varus, elbow
     M21.121 Varus deformity, not elsewhere classified, right elbow
     M21.122 Varus deformity, not elsewhere classified, left elbow
     M21.129 Varus deformity, not elsewhere classified, unspecified elbow ▽

☑6ᵗʰ M21.15 Varus deformity, not elsewhere classified, hip
     M21.151 Varus deformity, not elsewhere classified, right hip
     M21.152 Varus deformity, not elsewhere classified, left hip
     M21.159 Varus deformity, not elsewhere classified, unspecified ▽

☑6ᵗʰ M21.16 Varus deformity, not elsewhere classified, knee
     Bow leg
     Genu varum
     M21.161 Varus deformity, not elsewhere classified, right knee
     M21.162 Varus deformity, not elsewhere classified, left knee
     M21.169 Varus deformity, not elsewhere classified, unspecified knee ▽

☑6ᵗʰ M21.17 Varus deformity, not elsewhere classified, ankle
     M21.171 Varus deformity, not elsewhere classified, right ankle
     M21.172 Varus deformity, not elsewhere classified, left ankle

Genu Varus (bowleg)

☑ Additional Character Req   ☑7ᵗʰ Placeholder Alert   Case-Mix Diagnosis   Manifestation   ▽ Unspecified Dx   **EXCLUDES 1** Not coded here   **EXCLUDES 2** Not included here

        M21.179   Varus deformity, not elsewhere classified, unspecified ankle ▽

✓5ᵗʰ   **M21.2**   Flexion deformity
        M21.20   Flexion deformity, unspecified site ▽
   ✓6ᵗʰ   **M21.21**   Flexion deformity, shoulder
        M21.211   Flexion deformity, right shoulder
        M21.212   Flexion deformity, left shoulder
        M21.219   Flexion deformity, unspecified shoulder ▽
   ✓6ᵗʰ   **M21.22**   Flexion deformity, elbow
        M21.221   Flexion deformity, right elbow
        M21.222   Flexion deformity, left elbow
        M21.229   Flexion deformity, unspecified elbow ▽
   ✓6ᵗʰ   **M21.23**   Flexion deformity, wrist
        M21.231   Flexion deformity, right wrist
        M21.232   Flexion deformity, left wrist
        M21.239   Flexion deformity, unspecified wrist ▽
   ✓6ᵗʰ   **M21.24**   Flexion deformity, finger joints
        M21.241   Flexion deformity, right finger joints
        M21.242   Flexion deformity, left finger joints
        M21.249   Flexion deformity, unspecified finger joints ▽
   ✓6ᵗʰ   **M21.25**   Flexion deformity, hip
        M21.251   Flexion deformity, right hip
        M21.252   Flexion deformity, left hip
        M21.259   Flexion deformity, unspecified hip ▽
   ✓6ᵗʰ   **M21.26**   Flexion deformity, knee
        M21.261   Flexion deformity, right knee
        M21.262   Flexion deformity, left knee
        M21.269   Flexion deformity, unspecified knee ▽
   ✓6ᵗʰ   **M21.27**   Flexion deformity, ankle and toes
        M21.271   Flexion deformity, right ankle and toes
        M21.272   Flexion deformity, left ankle and toes
        M21.279   Flexion deformity, unspecified ankle and toes ▽

✓5ᵗʰ   **M21.3**   Wrist or foot drop (acquired)
   ✓6ᵗʰ   **M21.33**   Wrist drop (acquired)
        M21.331   Wrist drop, right wrist
        M21.332   Wrist drop, left wrist
        M21.339   Wrist drop, unspecified wrist ▽
   ✓6ᵗʰ   **M21.37**   Foot drop (acquired)
        M21.371   Foot drop, right foot
        M21.372   Foot drop, left foot
        M21.379   Foot drop, unspecified foot ▽

✓5ᵗʰ   **M21.4**   Flat foot [pes planus] (acquired)
     EXCLUDES 1   congenital pes planus (Q66.5-)
        M21.40   Flat foot [pes planus] (acquired), unspecified foot ▽
        M21.41   Flat foot [pes planus] (acquired), right foot
        M21.42   Flat foot [pes planus] (acquired), left foot

✓5ᵗʰ   **M21.5**   Acquired clawhand, clubhand, clawfoot and clubfoot
     EXCLUDES 1   clubfoot, not specified as acquired (Q66.89)
   ✓6ᵗʰ   **M21.51**   Acquired clawhand
        M21.511   Acquired clawhand, right hand
        M21.512   Acquired clawhand, left hand
        M21.519   Acquired clawhand, unspecified hand ▽
   ✓6ᵗʰ   **M21.52**   Acquired clubhand
        M21.521   Acquired clubhand, right hand
        M21.522   Acquired clubhand, left hand
        M21.529   Acquired clubhand, unspecified hand ▽
   ✓6ᵗʰ   **M21.53**   Acquired clawfoot
        DEF: High foot arch with hyperextended toes at metatarsophalangeal joint and flexed toes at distal joints
        M21.531   Acquired clawfoot, right foot
        M21.532   Acquired clawfoot, left foot
        M21.539   Acquired clawfoot, unspecified foot ▽
   ✓6ᵗʰ   **M21.54**   Acquired clubfoot
        M21.541   Acquired clubfoot, right foot
        M21.542   Acquired clubfoot, left foot
        M21.549   Acquired clubfoot, unspecified foot ▽

✓5ᵗʰ   **M21.6**   Other acquired deformities of foot
     EXCLUDES 2   deformities of toe (acquired) (M20.1-M20.6-)
   ✓6ᵗʰ   **M21.61**   Bunion
        M21.611   Bunion of right foot
        M21.612   Bunion of left foot
        M21.619   Bunion of unspecified foot ▽
   ✓6ᵗʰ   **M21.62**   Bunionette
        M21.621   Bunionette of right foot
        M21.622   Bunionette of left foot
        M21.629   Bunionette of unspecified foot ▽
   ✓6ᵗʰ   **M21.6X**   Other acquired deformities of foot
        M21.6X1   Other acquired deformities of right foot
        M21.6X2   Other acquired deformities of left foot
        M21.6X9   Other acquired deformities of unspecified foot ▽

✓5ᵗʰ   **M21.7**   Unequal limb length (acquired)
     NOTE   The site used should correspond to the shorter limb.
        M21.70   Unequal limb length (acquired), unspecified site ▽
   ✓6ᵗʰ   **M21.72**   Unequal limb length (acquired), humerus
        M21.721   Unequal limb length (acquired), right humerus
        M21.722   Unequal limb length (acquired), left humerus
        M21.729   Unequal limb length (acquired), unspecified humerus ▽
   ✓6ᵗʰ   **M21.73**   Unequal limb length (acquired), ulna and radius
        M21.731   Unequal limb length (acquired), right ulna
        M21.732   Unequal limb length (acquired), left ulna
        M21.733   Unequal limb length (acquired), right radius
        M21.734   Unequal limb length (acquired), left radius
        M21.739   Unequal limb length (acquired), unspecified ulna and radius ▽
   ✓6ᵗʰ   **M21.75**   Unequal limb length (acquired), femur
        M21.751   Unequal limb length (acquired), right femur
        M21.752   Unequal limb length (acquired), left femur
        M21.759   Unequal limb length (acquired), unspecified femur ▽
   ✓6ᵗʰ   **M21.76**   Unequal limb length (acquired), tibia and fibula
        M21.761   Unequal limb length (acquired), right tibia
        M21.762   Unequal limb length (acquired), left tibia
        M21.763   Unequal limb length (acquired), right fibula
        M21.764   Unequal limb length (acquired), left fibula
        M21.769   Unequal limb length (acquired), unspecified tibia and fibula ▽

✓5ᵗʰ   **M21.8**   Other specified acquired deformities of limbs
     EXCLUDES 2   coxa plana (M91.2)
        M21.80   Other specified acquired deformities of unspecified limb ▽
   ✓6ᵗʰ   **M21.82**   Other specified acquired deformities of upper arm
        M21.821   Other specified acquired deformities of right upper arm
        M21.822   Other specified acquired deformities of left upper arm
        M21.829   Other specified acquired deformities of unspecified upper arm ▽
   ✓6ᵗʰ   **M21.83**   Other specified acquired deformities of forearm
        M21.831   Other specified acquired deformities of right forearm
        M21.832   Other specified acquired deformities of left forearm
        M21.839   Other specified acquired deformities of unspecified forearm ▽
   ✓6ᵗʰ   **M21.85**   Other specified acquired deformities of thigh
        M21.851   Other specified acquired deformities of right thigh
        M21.852   Other specified acquired deformities of left thigh
        M21.859   Other specified acquired deformities of unspecified thigh ▽

Ⓝ Newborn: 0   Ⓟ Pediatric: 0-17   Ⓜ Maternity: 12-55   Ⓐ Adult: 15-124   **NRS** Nonroutine supply Dx   **NCDx** Noncancer Dx   **PDx** Primary Dx   ▶◀ Revised Text   ● New Code   ▲ Revised Title

742   ICD-10-CM 2018

✓6ᵗʰ **M21.86**   Other specified acquired deformities of lower leg

     M21.861   Other specified acquired deformities of right lower leg

     M21.862   Other specified acquired deformities of left lower leg

     M21.869   Other specified acquired deformities of ▽ unspecified lower leg

✓5ᵗʰ **M21.9**   Unspecified acquired deformity of limb and hand

     M21.90   Unspecified acquired deformity of unspecified ▽ limb

   ✓6ᵗʰ **M21.92**   Unspecified acquired deformity of upper arm

     M21.921   Unspecified acquired deformity of ▽ right upper arm

     M21.922   Unspecified acquired deformity of ▽ left upper arm

     M21.929   Unspecified acquired deformity of ▽ unspecified upper arm

   ✓6ᵗʰ **M21.93**   Unspecified acquired deformity of forearm

     M21.931   Unspecified acquired deformity of ▽ right forearm

     M21.932   Unspecified acquired deformity of ▽ left forearm

     M21.939   Unspecified acquired deformity of ▽ unspecified forearm

   ✓6ᵗʰ **M21.94**   Unspecified acquired deformity of hand

     M21.941   Unspecified acquired deformity of ▽ hand, right hand

     M21.942   Unspecified acquired deformity of ▽ hand, left hand

     M21.949   Unspecified acquired deformity of ▽ hand, unspecified hand

   ✓6ᵗʰ **M21.95**   Unspecified acquired deformity of thigh

     M21.951   Unspecified acquired deformity of ▽ right thigh

     M21.952   Unspecified acquired deformity of ▽ left thigh

     M21.959   Unspecified acquired deformity of ▽ unspecified thigh

   ✓6ᵗʰ **M21.96**   Unspecified acquired deformity of lower leg

     M21.961   Unspecified acquired deformity of ▽ right lower leg

     M21.962   Unspecified acquired deformity of ▽ left lower leg

     M21.969   Unspecified acquired deformity of ▽ unspecified lower leg

✓4ᵗʰ **M22**   **Disorder of patella**

   EXCLUDES 1   traumatic dislocation of patella (S83.Ø-)

✓5ᵗʰ **M22.Ø**   Recurrent dislocation of patella

     M22.ØØ   Recurrent dislocation of patella, unspecified knee ▽

     M22.Ø1   Recurrent dislocation of patella, right knee

     M22.Ø2   Recurrent dislocation of patella, left knee

✓5ᵗʰ **M22.1**   Recurrent subluxation of patella

     Incomplete dislocation of patella

     M22.1Ø   Recurrent subluxation of patella, unspecified ▽ knee

     M22.11   Recurrent subluxation of patella, right knee

     M22.12   Recurrent subluxation of patella, left knee

✓5ᵗʰ **M22.2**   Patellofemoral disorders

   ✓6ᵗʰ **M22.2X**   Patellofemoral disorders

     M22.2X1   Patellofemoral disorders, right knee

     M22.2X2   Patellofemoral disorders, left knee

     M22.2X9   Patellofemoral disorders, unspecified ▽ knee

✓5ᵗʰ **M22.3**   Other derangements of patella

   ✓6ᵗʰ **M22.3X**   Other derangements of patella

     M22.3X1   Other derangements of patella, right knee

     M22.3X2   Other derangements of patella, left knee

     M22.3X9   Other derangements of patella, ▽ unspecified knee

✓5ᵗʰ **M22.4**   Chondromalacia patellae

     M22.4Ø   Chondromalacia patellae, unspecified knee ▽

     M22.41   Chondromalacia patellae, right knee

     M22.42   Chondromalacia patellae, left knee

✓5ᵗʰ **M22.8**   Other disorders of patella

   ✓6ᵗʰ **M22.8X**   Other disorders of patella

     M22.8X1   Other disorders of patella, right knee

     M22.8X2   Other disorders of patella, left knee

     M22.8X9   Other disorders of patella, unspecified ▽ knee

✓5ᵗʰ **M22.9**   Unspecified disorder of patella

     M22.9Ø   Unspecified disorder of patella, unspecified knee ▽

     M22.91   Unspecified disorder of patella, right knee ▽

     M22.92   Unspecified disorder of patella, left knee ▽

✓4ᵗʰ **M23**   **Internal derangement of knee**

   EXCLUDES 1   ankylosis (M24.66)

     current injury—see injury of knee and lower leg (S8Ø-S89)

     deformity of knee (M21.-)

     osteochondritis dissecans (M93.2)

     recurrent dislocation or subluxation of joints (M24.4)

     recurrent dislocation or subluxation of patella (M22.Ø-M22.1)

✓5ᵗʰ **M23.Ø**   Cystic meniscus

   ✓6ᵗʰ **M23.ØØ**   Cystic meniscus, unspecified meniscus

     Cystic meniscus, unspecified lateral meniscus

     Cystic meniscus, unspecified medial meniscus

     M23.ØØØ   Cystic meniscus, unspecified lateral meniscus, right knee

     M23.ØØ1   Cystic meniscus, unspecified lateral meniscus, left knee

     M23.ØØ2   Cystic meniscus, unspecified lateral ▽ meniscus, unspecified knee

     M23.ØØ3   Cystic meniscus, unspecified medial meniscus, right knee

     M23.ØØ4   Cystic meniscus, unspecified medial meniscus, left knee

     M23.ØØ5   Cystic meniscus, unspecified medial ▽ meniscus, unspecified knee

     M23.ØØ6   Cystic meniscus, unspecified meniscus, right knee

     M23.ØØ7   Cystic meniscus, unspecified meniscus, left knee

     M23.ØØ9   Cystic meniscus, unspecified meniscus, ▽ unspecified knee

   ✓6ᵗʰ **M23.Ø1**   Cystic meniscus, anterior horn of medial meniscus

     M23.Ø11   Cystic meniscus, anterior horn of medial meniscus, right knee

     M23.Ø12   Cystic meniscus, anterior horn of medial meniscus, left knee

     M23.Ø19   Cystic meniscus, anterior horn of ▽ medial meniscus, unspecified knee

   ✓6ᵗʰ **M23.Ø2**   Cystic meniscus, posterior horn of medial meniscus

     M23.Ø21   Cystic meniscus, posterior horn of medial meniscus, right knee

     M23.Ø22   Cystic meniscus, posterior horn of medial meniscus, left knee

     M23.Ø29   Cystic meniscus, posterior horn of ▽ medial meniscus, unspecified knee

   ✓6ᵗʰ **M23.Ø3**   Cystic meniscus, other medial meniscus

     M23.Ø31   Cystic meniscus, other medial meniscus, right knee

     M23.Ø32   Cystic meniscus, other medial meniscus, left knee

     M23.Ø39   Cystic meniscus, other medial ▽ meniscus, unspecified knee

   ✓6ᵗʰ **M23.Ø4**   Cystic meniscus, anterior horn of lateral meniscus

     M23.Ø41   Cystic meniscus, anterior horn of lateral meniscus, right knee

     M23.Ø42   Cystic meniscus, anterior horn of lateral meniscus, left knee

     M23.Ø49   Cystic meniscus, anterior horn of ▽ lateral meniscus, unspecified knee

   ✓6ᵗʰ **M23.Ø5**   Cystic meniscus, posterior horn of lateral meniscus

     M23.Ø51   Cystic meniscus, posterior horn of lateral meniscus, right knee

     M23.Ø52   Cystic meniscus, posterior horn of lateral meniscus, left knee

     M23.Ø59   Cystic meniscus, posterior horn of ▽ lateral meniscus, unspecified knee

---

✓ Additional Character Req   ✓x7ᵗʰ Placeholder Alert   Case-Mix Diagnosis   Manifestation   ▽ Unspecified Dx   EXCLUDES 1 Not coded here   EXCLUDES 2 Not included here

Derangement of Meniscus

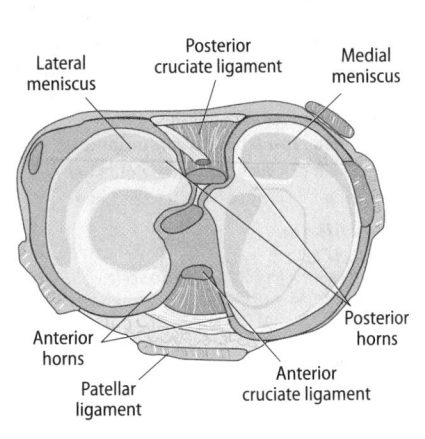

Overhead view of right knee

Bucket handle tear

Radial tear

Meniscus

✓6ᵗʰ M23.06 Cystic meniscus, other lateral meniscus
   M23.061 Cystic meniscus, other lateral meniscus, right knee
   M23.062 Cystic meniscus, other lateral meniscus, left knee
   M23.069 Cystic meniscus, other lateral meniscus, unspecified knee ▽

✓5ᵗʰ M23.2 Derangement of meniscus due to old tear or injury
   Old bucket-handle tear

✓6ᵗʰ M23.20 Derangement of unspecified meniscus due to old tear or injury
   Derangement of unspecified lateral meniscus due to old tear or injury
   Derangement of unspecified medial meniscus due to old tear or injury
   M23.200 Derangement of unspecified lateral meniscus due to old tear or injury, right knee
   M23.201 Derangement of unspecified lateral meniscus due to old tear or injury, left knee
   M23.202 Derangement of unspecified lateral meniscus due to old tear or injury, unspecified knee ▽
   M23.203 Derangement of unspecified medial meniscus due to old tear or injury, right knee
   M23.204 Derangement of unspecified medial meniscus due to old tear or injury, left knee
   M23.205 Derangement of unspecified medial meniscus due to old tear or injury, unspecified knee ▽
   M23.206 Derangement of unspecified meniscus due to old tear or injury, right knee
   M23.207 Derangement of unspecified meniscus due to old tear or injury, left knee
   M23.209 Derangement of unspecified meniscus due to old tear or injury, unspecified knee ▽

✓6ᵗʰ M23.21 Derangement of anterior horn of medial meniscus due to old tear or injury
   M23.211 Derangement of anterior horn of medial meniscus due to old tear or injury, right knee
   M23.212 Derangement of anterior horn of medial meniscus due to old tear or injury, left knee
   M23.219 Derangement of anterior horn of medial meniscus due to old tear or injury, unspecified knee ▽

✓6ᵗʰ M23.22 Derangement of posterior horn of medial meniscus due to old tear or injury
   M23.221 Derangement of posterior horn of medial meniscus due to old tear or injury, right knee
   M23.222 Derangement of posterior horn of medial meniscus due to old tear or injury, left knee
   M23.229 Derangement of posterior horn of medial meniscus due to old tear or injury, unspecified knee ▽

✓6ᵗʰ M23.23 Derangement of other medial meniscus due to old tear or injury
   M23.231 Derangement of other medial meniscus due to old tear or injury, right knee
   M23.232 Derangement of other medial meniscus due to old tear or injury, left knee
   M23.239 Derangement of other medial meniscus due to old tear or injury, unspecified knee ▽

✓6ᵗʰ M23.24 Derangement of anterior horn of lateral meniscus due to old tear or injury
   M23.241 Derangement of anterior horn of lateral meniscus due to old tear or injury, right knee
   M23.242 Derangement of anterior horn of lateral meniscus due to old tear or injury, left knee
   M23.249 Derangement of anterior horn of lateral meniscus due to old tear or injury, unspecified knee ▽

✓6ᵗʰ M23.25 Derangement of posterior horn of lateral meniscus due to old tear or injury
   M23.251 Derangement of posterior horn of lateral meniscus due to old tear or injury, right knee
   M23.252 Derangement of posterior horn of lateral meniscus due to old tear or injury, left knee
   M23.259 Derangement of posterior horn of lateral meniscus due to old tear or injury, unspecified knee ▽

✓6ᵗʰ M23.26 Derangement of other lateral meniscus due to old tear or injury
   M23.261 Derangement of other lateral meniscus due to old tear or injury, right knee
   M23.262 Derangement of other lateral meniscus due to old tear or injury, left knee
   M23.269 Derangement of other lateral meniscus due to old tear or injury, unspecified knee ▽

✓5ᵗʰ M23.3 Other meniscus derangements
   Degenerate meniscus
   Detached meniscus
   Retained meniscus

✓6ᵗʰ M23.30 Other meniscus derangements, unspecified meniscus
   Other meniscus derangements, unspecified lateral meniscus
   Other meniscus derangements, unspecified medial meniscus
   M23.300 Other meniscus derangements, unspecified lateral meniscus, right knee ▽
   M23.301 Other meniscus derangements, unspecified lateral meniscus, left knee ▽
   M23.302 Other meniscus derangements, unspecified lateral meniscus, unspecified knee ▽
   M23.303 Other meniscus derangements, unspecified medial meniscus, right knee ▽
   M23.304 Other meniscus derangements, unspecified medial meniscus, left knee ▽
   M23.305 Other meniscus derangements, unspecified medial meniscus, unspecified knee ▽
   M23.306 Other meniscus derangements, unspecified meniscus, right knee ▽
   M23.307 Other meniscus derangements, unspecified meniscus, left knee ▽

Ⓝ Newborn: 0   Ⓟ Pediatric: 0-17   Ⓜ Maternity: 12-55   Ⓐ Adult: 15-124   **NRS** Nonroutine supply Dx   **NCDx** Noncancer Dx   **PDx** Primary Dx   ▶◀ Revised Text   ● New Code   ▲ Revised Title

744   ICD-10-CM 2018

      M23.309   Other meniscus derangements, unspecified meniscus, unspecified knee ▽

☑6ᵗʰ M23.31   Other meniscus derangements, anterior horn of medial meniscus

      M23.311   Other meniscus derangements, anterior horn of medial meniscus, right knee

      M23.312   Other meniscus derangements, anterior horn of medial meniscus, left knee

      M23.319   Other meniscus derangements, anterior horn of medial meniscus, unspecified knee ▽

☑6ᵗʰ M23.32   Other meniscus derangements, posterior horn of medial meniscus

      M23.321   Other meniscus derangements, posterior horn of medial meniscus, right knee

      M23.322   Other meniscus derangements, posterior horn of medial meniscus, left knee

      M23.329   Other meniscus derangements, posterior horn of medial meniscus, unspecified knee ▽

☑6ᵗʰ M23.33   Other meniscus derangements, other medial meniscus

      M23.331   Other meniscus derangements, other medial meniscus, right knee

      M23.332   Other meniscus derangements, other medial meniscus, left knee

      M23.339   Other meniscus derangements, other medial meniscus, unspecified knee ▽

☑6ᵗʰ M23.34   Other meniscus derangements, anterior horn of lateral meniscus

      M23.341   Other meniscus derangements, anterior horn of lateral meniscus, right knee

      M23.342   Other meniscus derangements, anterior horn of lateral meniscus, left knee

      M23.349   Other meniscus derangements, anterior▽ horn of lateral meniscus, unspecified knee

☑6ᵗʰ M23.35   Other meniscus derangements, posterior horn of lateral meniscus

      M23.351   Other meniscus derangements, posterior horn of lateral meniscus, right knee

      M23.352   Other meniscus derangements, posterior horn of lateral meniscus, left knee

      M23.359   Other meniscus derangements, posterior horn of lateral meniscus, unspecified knee ▽

☑6ᵗʰ M23.36   Other meniscus derangements, other lateral meniscus

      M23.361   Other meniscus derangements, other lateral meniscus, right knee

      M23.362   Other meniscus derangements, other lateral meniscus, left knee

      M23.369   Other meniscus derangements, other lateral meniscus, unspecified knee ▽

☑5ᵗʰ M23.4   Loose body in knee

      M23.40   Loose body in knee, unspecified knee ▽

      M23.41   Loose body in knee, right knee

      M23.42   Loose body in knee, left knee

☑5ᵗʰ M23.5   Chronic instability of knee

      M23.50   Chronic instability of knee, unspecified knee ▽

      M23.51   Chronic instability of knee, right knee

      M23.52   Chronic instability of knee, left knee

☑5ᵗʰ M23.6   Other spontaneous disruption of ligament(s) of knee

☑6ᵗʰ M23.60   Other spontaneous disruption of unspecified ligament of knee

      M23.601   Other spontaneous disruption of ▽ unspecified ligament of right knee

      M23.602   Other spontaneous disruption of ▽ unspecified ligament of left knee

      M23.609   Other spontaneous disruption of ▽ unspecified ligament of unspecified knee

☑6ᵗʰ M23.61   Other spontaneous disruption of anterior cruciate ligament of knee

      M23.611   Other spontaneous disruption of anterior cruciate ligament of right knee

      M23.612   Other spontaneous disruption of anterior cruciate ligament of left knee

      M23.619   Other spontaneous disruption of ▽ anterior cruciate ligament of unspecified knee

☑6ᵗʰ M23.62   Other spontaneous disruption of posterior cruciate ligament of knee

      M23.621   Other spontaneous disruption of posterior cruciate ligament of right knee

      M23.622   Other spontaneous disruption of posterior cruciate ligament of left knee

      M23.629   Other spontaneous disruption of ▽ posterior cruciate ligament of unspecified knee

☑6ᵗʰ M23.63   Other spontaneous disruption of medial collateral ligament of knee

      M23.631   Other spontaneous disruption of medial collateral ligament of right knee

      M23.632   Other spontaneous disruption of medial collateral ligament of left knee

      M23.639   Other spontaneous disruption of ▽ medial collateral ligament of unspecified knee

☑6ᵗʰ M23.64   Other spontaneous disruption of lateral collateral ligament of knee

      M23.641   Other spontaneous disruption of lateral collateral ligament of right knee

      M23.642   Other spontaneous disruption of lateral collateral ligament of left knee

      M23.649   Other spontaneous disruption of ▽ lateral collateral ligament of unspecified knee

☑6ᵗʰ M23.67   Other spontaneous disruption of capsular ligament of knee

      M23.671   Other spontaneous disruption of capsular ligament of right knee

      M23.672   Other spontaneous disruption of capsular ligament of left knee

      M23.679   Other spontaneous disruption of ▽ capsular ligament of unspecified knee

☑5ᵗʰ M23.8   Other internal derangements of knee
      Laxity of ligament of knee
      Snapping knee

☑6ᵗʰ M23.8X   Other internal derangements of knee

      M23.8X1   Other internal derangements of right knee

      M23.8X2   Other internal derangements of left knee

      M23.8X9   Other internal derangements of ▽ unspecified knee

☑5ᵗʰ M23.9   Unspecified internal derangement of knee

      M23.90   Unspecified internal derangement of unspecified ▽ knee

      M23.91   Unspecified internal derangement of right knee ▽

      M23.92   Unspecified internal derangement of left knee ▽

☑4ᵗʰ M24   Other specific joint derangements

   EXCLUDES 1   current injury—see injury of joint by body region
   EXCLUDES 2   ganglion (M67.4)
         snapping knee (M23.8-)
         temporomandibular joint disorders (M26.6-)

☑5ᵗʰ M24.0   Loose body in joint
   EXCLUDES 2   loose body in knee (M23.4)

      M24.00   Loose body in unspecified joint ▽

☑6ᵗʰ M24.01   Loose body in shoulder

      M24.011   Loose body in right shoulder

      M24.012   Loose body in left shoulder

      M24.019   Loose body in unspecified shoulder ▽

☑6ᵗʰ M24.02   Loose body in elbow

      M24.021   Loose body in right elbow

      M24.022   Loose body in left elbow

      M24.029   Loose body in unspecified elbow ▽

☑6ᵗʰ M24.03   Loose body in wrist

      M24.031   Loose body in right wrist

      M24.032   Loose body in left wrist

      M24.039   Loose body in unspecified wrist ▽

☑6ᵗʰ M24.04   Loose body in finger joints

      M24.041   Loose body in right finger joint(s)

      M24.042   Loose body in left finger joint(s)

☑ Additional Character Req   ✓ₓ7ᵗʰ Placeholder Alert   Case-Mix Diagnosis   Manifestation   ▽ Unspecified Dx   *EXCLUDES 1* Not coded here   *EXCLUDES 2* Not included here

M24.049   Loose body in unspecified finger joint(s) ▽

✓6ᵗʰ M24.05   Loose body in hip
    M24.051   Loose body in right hip
    M24.052   Loose body in left hip
    M24.059   Loose body in unspecified hip ▽

✓6ᵗʰ M24.07   Loose body in ankle and toe joints
    M24.071   Loose body in right ankle
    M24.072   Loose body in left ankle
    M24.073   Loose body in unspecified ankle ▽
    M24.074   Loose body in right toe joint(s)
    M24.075   Loose body in left toe joint(s)
    M24.076   Loose body in unspecified toe joints ▽

    M24.08   Loose body, other site

✓5ᵗʰ M24.1   Other articular cartilage disorders
    EXCLUDES 2   chondrocalcinosis (M11.1, M11.2-)
                internal derangement of knee (M23.-)
                metastatic calcification (E83.5)
                ochronosis (E70.2)

    M24.10   Other articular cartilage disorders, unspecified site ▽

✓6ᵗʰ M24.11   Other articular cartilage disorders, shoulder
    M24.111   Other articular cartilage disorders, right shoulder
    M24.112   Other articular cartilage disorders, left shoulder
    M24.119   Other articular cartilage disorders, unspecified shoulder ▽

✓6ᵗʰ M24.12   Other articular cartilage disorders, elbow
    M24.121   Other articular cartilage disorders, right elbow
    M24.122   Other articular cartilage disorders, left elbow
    M24.129   Other articular cartilage disorders, unspecified elbow ▽

✓6ᵗʰ M24.13   Other articular cartilage disorders, wrist
    M24.131   Other articular cartilage disorders, right wrist
    M24.132   Other articular cartilage disorders, left wrist
    M24.139   Other articular cartilage disorders, unspecified wrist ▽

✓6ᵗʰ M24.14   Other articular cartilage disorders, hand
    M24.141   Other articular cartilage disorders, right hand
    M24.142   Other articular cartilage disorders, left hand
    M24.149   Other articular cartilage disorders, unspecified hand ▽

✓6ᵗʰ M24.15   Other articular cartilage disorders, hip
    M24.151   Other articular cartilage disorders, right hip
    M24.152   Other articular cartilage disorders, left hip
    M24.159   Other articular cartilage disorders, unspecified hip ▽

✓6ᵗʰ M24.17   Other articular cartilage disorders, ankle and foot
    M24.171   Other articular cartilage disorders, right ankle
    M24.172   Other articular cartilage disorders, left ankle
    M24.173   Other articular cartilage disorders, unspecified ankle ▽
    M24.174   Other articular cartilage disorders, right foot
    M24.175   Other articular cartilage disorders, left foot
    M24.176   Other articular cartilage disorders, unspecified foot ▽

✓5ᵗʰ M24.2   Disorder of ligament
    Instability secondary to old ligament injury
    Ligamentous laxity NOS
    EXCLUDES 1   familial ligamentous laxity (M35.7)
    EXCLUDES 2   internal derangement of knee (M23.5-M23.89)

    M24.20   Disorder of ligament, unspecified site ▽

✓6ᵗʰ M24.21   Disorder of ligament, shoulder
    M24.211   Disorder of ligament, right shoulder

    M24.212   Disorder of ligament, left shoulder
    M24.219   Disorder of ligament, unspecified shoulder ▽

✓6ᵗʰ M24.22   Disorder of ligament, elbow
    M24.221   Disorder of ligament, right elbow
    M24.222   Disorder of ligament, left elbow
    M24.229   Disorder of ligament, unspecified elbow ▽

✓6ᵗʰ M24.23   Disorder of ligament, wrist
    M24.231   Disorder of ligament, right wrist
    M24.232   Disorder of ligament, left wrist
    M24.239   Disorder of ligament, unspecified wrist ▽

✓6ᵗʰ M24.24   Disorder of ligament, hand
    M24.241   Disorder of ligament, right hand
    M24.242   Disorder of ligament, left hand
    M24.249   Disorder of ligament, unspecified hand ▽

✓6ᵗʰ M24.25   Disorder of ligament, hip
    M24.251   Disorder of ligament, right hip
    M24.252   Disorder of ligament, left hip
    M24.259   Disorder of ligament, unspecified hip ▽

✓6ᵗʰ M24.27   Disorder of ligament, ankle and foot
    M24.271   Disorder of ligament, right ankle
    M24.272   Disorder of ligament, left ankle
    M24.273   Disorder of ligament, unspecified ankle ▽
    M24.274   Disorder of ligament, right foot
    M24.275   Disorder of ligament, left foot
    M24.276   Disorder of ligament, unspecified foot ▽

    M24.28   Disorder of ligament, vertebrae

✓5ᵗʰ M24.3   Pathological dislocation of joint, not elsewhere classified
    EXCLUDES 1   congenital dislocation or displacement of joint—see congenital malformations and deformations of the musculoskeletal system (Q65-Q79)
                current injury—see injury of joints and ligaments by body region
                recurrent dislocation of joint (M24.4-)

    M24.30   Pathological dislocation of unspecified joint, not elsewhere classified ▽

✓6ᵗʰ M24.31   Pathological dislocation of shoulder, not elsewhere classified
    M24.311   Pathological dislocation of right shoulder, not elsewhere classified
    M24.312   Pathological dislocation of left shoulder, not elsewhere classified
    M24.319   Pathological dislocation of unspecified shoulder, not elsewhere classified ▽

✓6ᵗʰ M24.32   Pathological dislocation of elbow, not elsewhere classified
    M24.321   Pathological dislocation of right elbow, not elsewhere classified
    M24.322   Pathological dislocation of left elbow, not elsewhere classified
    M24.329   Pathological dislocation of unspecified elbow, not elsewhere classified ▽

✓6ᵗʰ M24.33   Pathological dislocation of wrist, not elsewhere classified
    M24.331   Pathological dislocation of right wrist, not elsewhere classified
    M24.332   Pathological dislocation of left wrist, not elsewhere classified
    M24.339   Pathological dislocation of unspecified wrist, not elsewhere classified ▽

✓6ᵗʰ M24.34   Pathological dislocation of hand, not elsewhere classified
    M24.341   Pathological dislocation of right hand, not elsewhere classified
    M24.342   Pathological dislocation of left hand, not elsewhere classified
    M24.349   Pathological dislocation of unspecified hand, not elsewhere classified ▽

✓6ᵗʰ M24.35   Pathological dislocation of hip, not elsewhere classified
    M24.351   Pathological dislocation of right hip, not elsewhere classified
    M24.352   Pathological dislocation of left hip, not elsewhere classified

N Newborn: 0   P Pediatric: 0-17   M Maternity: 12-55   A Adult: 15-124   NRS Nonroutine supply Dx   NCDx Noncancer Dx   PDx Primary Dx   ▶◀ Revised Text   ● New Code   ▲ Revised Title

746   ICD-10-CM 2018

     M24.359   Pathological dislocation of unspecified ▽
hip, not elsewhere classified

✓6ᵗʰ M24.36   Pathological dislocation of knee, not elsewhere
classified

     M24.361   **Pathological dislocation of right knee,
not elsewhere classified**

     M24.362   **Pathological dislocation of left knee,
not elsewhere classified**

     M24.369   Pathological dislocation of unspecified ▽
knee, not elsewhere classified

✓6ᵗʰ M24.37   Pathological dislocation of ankle and foot, not
elsewhere classified

     M24.371   **Pathological dislocation of right ankle,
not elsewhere classified**

     M24.372   **Pathological dislocation of left ankle, not
elsewhere classified**

     M24.373   Pathological dislocation of unspecified ▽
ankle, not elsewhere classified

     M24.374   **Pathological dislocation of right foot, not
elsewhere classified**

     M24.375   **Pathological dislocation of left foot, not
elsewhere classified**

     M24.376   Pathological dislocation of unspecified ▽
foot, not elsewhere classified

✓5ᵗʰ M24.4   **Recurrent dislocation of joint**
Recurrent subluxation of joint
EXCLUDES 2   *recurrent dislocation of patella (M22.0-M22.1)*
recurrent vertebral dislocation (M43.3-, M43.4, M43.5-)

     M24.40   Recurrent dislocation, unspecified joint   ▽

✓6ᵗʰ M24.41   Recurrent dislocation, shoulder

     M24.411   **Recurrent dislocation, right shoulder**
     M24.412   **Recurrent dislocation, left shoulder**
     M24.419   Recurrent dislocation, unspecified   ▽
shoulder

✓6ᵗʰ M24.42   Recurrent dislocation, elbow

     M24.421   **Recurrent dislocation, right elbow**
     M24.422   **Recurrent dislocation, left elbow**
     M24.429   Recurrent dislocation, unspecified   ▽
elbow

✓6ᵗʰ M24.43   Recurrent dislocation, wrist

     M24.431   **Recurrent dislocation, right wrist**
     M24.432   **Recurrent dislocation, left wrist**
     M24.439   Recurrent dislocation, unspecified wrist ▽

✓6ᵗʰ M24.44   Recurrent dislocation, hand and finger(s)

     M24.441   **Recurrent dislocation, right hand**
     M24.442   **Recurrent dislocation, left hand**
     M24.443   Recurrent dislocation, unspecified hand ▽
     M24.444   Recurrent dislocation, right finger
     M24.445   Recurrent dislocation, left finger
     M24.446   Recurrent dislocation, unspecified   ▽
finger

✓6ᵗʰ M24.45   Recurrent dislocation, hip

     M24.451   **Recurrent dislocation, right hip**
     M24.452   **Recurrent dislocation, left hip**
     M24.459   Recurrent dislocation, unspecified hip ▽

✓6ᵗʰ M24.46   Recurrent dislocation, knee

     M24.461   **Recurrent dislocation, right knee**
     M24.462   **Recurrent dislocation, left knee**
     M24.469   Recurrent dislocation, unspecified   ▽
knee

✓6ᵗʰ M24.47   Recurrent dislocation, ankle, foot and toes

     M24.471   **Recurrent dislocation, right ankle**
     M24.472   **Recurrent dislocation, left ankle**
     M24.473   Recurrent dislocation, unspecified   ▽
ankle
     M24.474   **Recurrent dislocation, right foot**
     M24.475   **Recurrent dislocation, left foot**
     M24.476   Recurrent dislocation, unspecified foot ▽
     M24.477   **Recurrent dislocation, right toe(s)**
     M24.478   **Recurrent dislocation, left toe(s)**
     M24.479   Recurrent dislocation, unspecified   ▽
toe(s)

✓5ᵗʰ M24.5   **Contracture of joint**

EXCLUDES 1   *contracture of muscle without contracture of joint
(M62.4-)*
*contracture of tendon (sheath) without contracture of
joint (M62.4-)*
Dupuytren's contracture (M72.0)
EXCLUDES 2   *acquired deformities of limbs (M20-M21)*
AHA: 2016, 2Q, 6

     M24.50   Contracture, unspecified joint   ▽

✓6ᵗʰ M24.51   Contracture, shoulder

     M24.511   **Contracture, right shoulder**
     M24.512   **Contracture, left shoulder**
     M24.519   Contracture, unspecified shoulder   ▽

✓6ᵗʰ M24.52   Contracture, elbow

     M24.521   **Contracture, right elbow**
     M24.522   **Contracture, left elbow**
     M24.529   Contracture, unspecified elbow   ▽

✓6ᵗʰ M24.53   Contracture, wrist

     M24.531   **Contracture, right wrist**
     M24.532   **Contracture, left wrist**
     M24.539   Contracture, unspecified wrist   ▽

✓6ᵗʰ M24.54   Contracture, hand

     M24.541   **Contracture, right hand**
     M24.542   **Contracture, left hand**
     M24.549   Contracture, unspecified hand   ▽

✓6ᵗʰ M24.55   Contracture, hip

     M24.551   **Contracture, right hip**
     M24.552   **Contracture, left hip**
     M24.559   Contracture, unspecified hip   ▽

✓6ᵗʰ M24.56   Contracture, knee

     M24.561   **Contracture, right knee**
     M24.562   **Contracture, left knee**
     M24.569   Contracture, unspecified knee   ▽

✓6ᵗʰ M24.57   Contracture, ankle and foot

     M24.571   **Contracture, right ankle**
     M24.572   **Contracture, left ankle**
     M24.573   Contracture, unspecified ankle   ▽
     M24.574   **Contracture, right foot**
     M24.575   **Contracture, left foot**
     M24.576   Contracture, unspecified foot   ▽

✓5ᵗʰ M24.6   **Ankylosis of joint**

EXCLUDES 1   *stiffness of joint without ankylosis (M25.6-)*
EXCLUDES 2   *spine (M43.2-)*

     M24.60   Ankylosis, unspecified joint   ▽

✓6ᵗʰ M24.61   Ankylosis, shoulder

     M24.611   **Ankylosis, right shoulder**
     M24.612   **Ankylosis, left shoulder**
     M24.619   Ankylosis, unspecified shoulder   ▽

✓6ᵗʰ M24.62   Ankylosis, elbow

     M24.621   **Ankylosis, right elbow**
     M24.622   **Ankylosis, left elbow**
     M24.629   Ankylosis, unspecified elbow   ▽

✓6ᵗʰ M24.63   Ankylosis, wrist

     M24.631   **Ankylosis, right wrist**
     M24.632   **Ankylosis, left wrist**
     M24.639   Ankylosis, unspecified wrist   ▽

✓6ᵗʰ M24.64   Ankylosis, hand

     M24.641   **Ankylosis, right hand**
     M24.642   **Ankylosis, left hand**
     M24.649   Ankylosis, unspecified hand   ▽

✓6ᵗʰ M24.65   Ankylosis, hip

     M24.651   **Ankylosis, right hip**
     M24.652   **Ankylosis, left hip**
     M24.659   Ankylosis, unspecified hip   ▽

✓6ᵗʰ M24.66   Ankylosis, knee

     M24.661   **Ankylosis, right knee**
     M24.662   **Ankylosis, left knee**
     M24.669   Ankylosis, unspecified knee   ▽

✓6ᵗʰ M24.67   Ankylosis, ankle and foot

     M24.671   **Ankylosis, right ankle**
     M24.672   **Ankylosis, left ankle**
     M24.673   Ankylosis, unspecified ankle   ▽

☑ Additional Character Req   ✓ˣ⁷ᵗʰ Placeholder Alert   Case-Mix Diagnosis   Manifestation   ▽ Unspecified Dx   EXCLUDES 1 Not coded here   EXCLUDES 2 Not included here

M24.674 **Ankylosis, right foot**
M24.675 **Ankylosis, left foot**
M24.676 Ankylosis, unspecified foot ▽

M24.7 Protrusio acetabuli

✓5th **M24.8 Other specific joint derangements, not elsewhere classified**
  EXCLUDES 2 *iliotibial band syndrome (M76.3)*

M24.80 **Other specific joint derangements of unspecified joint, not elsewhere classified** ▽

✓6th M24.81 **Other specific joint derangements of shoulder, not elsewhere classified**
  M24.811 Other specific joint derangements of right shoulder, not elsewhere classified
  M24.812 Other specific joint derangements of left shoulder, not elsewhere classified
  M24.819 Other specific joint derangements of unspecified shoulder, not elsewhere classified ▽

✓6th M24.82 **Other specific joint derangements of elbow, not elsewhere classified**
  M24.821 Other specific joint derangements of right elbow, not elsewhere classified
  M24.822 Other specific joint derangements of left elbow, not elsewhere classified
  M24.829 Other specific joint derangements of unspecified elbow, not elsewhere classified

✓6th M24.83 **Other specific joint derangements of wrist, not elsewhere classified**
  M24.831 Other specific joint derangements of right wrist, not elsewhere classified
  M24.832 Other specific joint derangements of left wrist, not elsewhere classified
  M24.839 Other specific joint derangements of unspecified wrist, not elsewhere classified ▽

✓6th M24.84 **Other specific joint derangements of hand, not elsewhere classified**
  M24.841 Other specific joint derangements of right hand, not elsewhere classified
  M24.842 Other specific joint derangements of left hand, not elsewhere classified
  M24.849 Other specific joint derangements of unspecified hand, not elsewhere classified ▽

✓6th M24.85 **Other specific joint derangements of hip, not elsewhere classified**
  Irritable hip
  M24.851 Other specific joint derangements of right hip, not elsewhere classified
  M24.852 Other specific joint derangements of left hip, not elsewhere classified
  M24.859 Other specific joint derangements of unspecified hip, not elsewhere classified ▽

✓6th M24.87 **Other specific joint derangements of ankle and foot, not elsewhere classified**
  M24.871 Other specific joint derangements of right ankle, not elsewhere classified
  M24.872 Other specific joint derangements of left ankle, not elsewhere classified
  M24.873 Other specific joint derangements of unspecified ankle, not elsewhere classified ▽
  M24.874 Other specific joint derangements of right foot, not elsewhere classified
  M24.875 Other specific joint derangements left foot, not elsewhere classified
  M24.876 Other specific joint derangements of unspecified foot, not elsewhere classified ▽

M24.9 **Joint derangement, unspecified** ▽

✓4th **M25 Other joint disorder, not elsewhere classified**
  EXCLUDES 2 *abnormality of gait and mobility (R26.-)*
    acquired deformities of limb (M20-M21)
    calcification of bursa (M71.4-)
    calcification of shoulder (joint) (M75.3)
    calcification of tendon (M65.2-)
    difficulty in walking (R26.2)
    temporomandibular joint disorder (M26.6-)

✓5th **M25.0 Hemarthrosis**
  EXCLUDES 1 *current injury—see injury of joint by body region*
    hemophilic arthropathy (M36.2)
  M25.00 Hemarthrosis, unspecified joint ▽
✓6th M25.01 Hemarthrosis, shoulder
  M25.011 **Hemarthrosis, right shoulder**
  M25.012 **Hemarthrosis, left shoulder**
  M25.019 Hemarthrosis, unspecified shoulder ▽
✓6th M25.02 Hemarthrosis, elbow
  M25.021 **Hemarthrosis, right elbow**
  M25.022 **Hemarthrosis, left elbow**
  M25.029 Hemarthrosis, unspecified elbow ▽
✓6th M25.03 Hemarthrosis, wrist
  M25.031 **Hemarthrosis, right wrist**
  M25.032 **Hemarthrosis, left wrist**
  M25.039 Hemarthrosis, unspecified wrist ▽
✓6th M25.04 Hemarthrosis, hand
  M25.041 **Hemarthrosis, right hand**
  M25.042 **Hemarthrosis, left hand**
  M25.049 Hemarthrosis, unspecified hand ▽
✓6th M25.05 Hemarthrosis, hip
  M25.051 **Hemarthrosis, right hip**
  M25.052 **Hemarthrosis, left hip**
  M25.059 Hemarthrosis, unspecified hip ▽
✓6th M25.06 Hemarthrosis, knee
  M25.061 **Hemarthrosis, right knee**
  M25.062 **Hemarthrosis, left knee**
  M25.069 Hemarthrosis, unspecified knee ▽
✓6th M25.07 Hemarthrosis, ankle and foot
  M25.071 **Hemarthrosis, right ankle**
  M25.072 **Hemarthrosis, left ankle**
  M25.073 Hemarthrosis, unspecified ankle ▽
  M25.074 **Hemarthrosis, right foot**
  M25.075 **Hemarthrosis, left foot**
  M25.076 Hemarthrosis, unspecified foot ▽
M25.08 **Hemarthrosis, other specified site**
  Hemarthrosis, vertebrae

✓5th **M25.1 Fistula of joint**
  M25.10 Fistula, unspecified joint ▽
✓6th M25.11 Fistula, shoulder
  M25.111 Fistula, right shoulder
  M25.112 Fistula, left shoulder
  M25.119 Fistula, unspecified shoulder ▽
✓6th M25.12 Fistula, elbow
  M25.121 Fistula, right elbow
  M25.122 Fistula, left elbow
  M25.129 Fistula, unspecified elbow ▽
✓6th M25.13 Fistula, wrist
  M25.131 Fistula, right wrist
  M25.132 Fistula, left wrist
  M25.139 Fistula, unspecified wrist ▽
✓6th M25.14 Fistula, hand
  M25.141 Fistula, right hand
  M25.142 Fistula, left hand
  M25.149 Fistula, unspecified hand ▽
✓6th M25.15 Fistula, hip
  M25.151 Fistula, right hip
  M25.152 Fistula, left hip
  M25.159 Fistula, unspecified hip ▽
✓6th M25.16 Fistula, knee
  M25.161 Fistula, right knee
  M25.162 Fistula, left knee
  M25.169 Fistula, unspecified knee ▽
✓6th M25.17 Fistula, ankle and foot
  M25.171 Fistula, right ankle
  M25.172 Fistula, left ankle
  M25.173 Fistula, unspecified ankle ▽
  M25.174 Fistula, right foot
  M25.175 Fistula, left foot
  M25.176 Fistula, unspecified foot ▽

N Newborn: 0 P Pediatric: 0-17 M Maternity: 12-55 A Adult: 15-124 NRS Nonroutine supply Dx NCDx Noncancer Dx PDx Primary Dx ▶◀ Revised Text ● New Code ▲ Revised Title

748   ICD-10-CM 2018

M25.18   **Fistula, other specified site**
     Fistula, vertebrae

✓5ᵗʰ **M25.2**   **Flail joint**

     M25.20   Flail joint, unspecified joint   ▽

     ✓6ᵗʰ **M25.21**   Flail joint, shoulder
         M25.211   Flail joint, right shoulder
         M25.212   Flail joint, left shoulder
         M25.219   Flail joint, unspecified shoulder   ▽

     ✓6ᵗʰ **M25.22**   Flail joint, elbow
         M25.221   Flail joint, right elbow
         M25.222   Flail joint, left elbow
         M25.229   Flail joint, unspecified elbow   ▽

     ✓6ᵗʰ **M25.23**   Flail joint, wrist
         M25.231   Flail joint, right wrist
         M25.232   Flail joint, left wrist
         M25.239   Flail joint, unspecified wrist   ▽

     ✓6ᵗʰ **M25.24**   Flail joint, hand
         M25.241   Flail joint, right hand
         M25.242   Flail joint, left hand
         M25.249   Flail joint, unspecified hand   ▽

     ✓6ᵗʰ **M25.25**   Flail joint, hip
         M25.251   Flail joint, right hip
         M25.252   Flail joint, left hip
         M25.259   Flail joint, unspecified hip   ▽

     ✓6ᵗʰ **M25.26**   Flail joint, knee
         M25.261   Flail joint, right knee
         M25.262   Flail joint, left knee
         M25.269   Flail joint, unspecified knee   ▽

     ✓6ᵗʰ **M25.27**   Flail joint, ankle and foot
         M25.271   Flail joint, right ankle and foot
         M25.272   Flail joint, left ankle and foot
         M25.279   Flail joint, unspecified ankle and foot   ▽

     M25.28   Flail joint, other site

✓5ᵗʰ **M25.3**   **Other instability of joint**
     EXCLUDES 1   instability of joint secondary to old ligament injury (M24.2-)
         instability of joint secondary to removal of joint prosthesis (M96.8-)
     EXCLUDES 2   spinal instabilities (M53.2-)

     M25.30   Other instability, unspecified joint   ▽

     ✓6ᵗʰ **M25.31**   Other instability, shoulder
         M25.311   Other instability, right shoulder
         M25.312   Other instability, left shoulder
         M25.319   Other instability, unspecified shoulder   ▽

     ✓6ᵗʰ **M25.32**   Other instability, elbow
         M25.321   Other instability, right elbow
         M25.322   Other instability, left elbow
         M25.329   Other instability, unspecified elbow   ▽

     ✓6ᵗʰ **M25.33**   Other instability, wrist
         M25.331   Other instability, right wrist
         M25.332   Other instability, left wrist
         M25.339   Other instability, unspecified wrist   ▽

     ✓6ᵗʰ **M25.34**   Other instability, hand
         M25.341   Other instability, right hand
         M25.342   Other instability, left hand
         M25.349   Other instability, unspecified hand   ▽

     ✓6ᵗʰ **M25.35**   Other instability, hip
         M25.351   Other instability, right hip
         M25.352   Other instability, left hip
         M25.359   Other instability, unspecified hip   ▽

     ✓6ᵗʰ **M25.36**   Other instability, knee
         M25.361   Other instability, right knee
         M25.362   Other instability, left knee
         M25.369   Other instability, unspecified knee   ▽

     ✓6ᵗʰ **M25.37**   Other instability, ankle and foot
         M25.371   Other instability, right ankle
         M25.372   Other instability, left ankle
         M25.373   Other instability, unspecified ankle   ▽
         M25.374   Other instability, right foot
         M25.375   Other instability, left foot
         M25.376   Other instability, unspecified foot   ▽

✓5ᵗʰ **M25.4**   **Effusion of joint**
     EXCLUDES 1   hydrarthrosis in yaws (A66.6)
         intermittent hydrarthrosis (M12.4-)
         other infective (teno)synovitis (M65.1-)

     M25.40   Effusion, unspecified joint   ▽

     ✓6ᵗʰ **M25.41**   Effusion, shoulder
         M25.411   Effusion, right shoulder
         M25.412   Effusion, left shoulder
         M25.419   Effusion, unspecified shoulder   ▽

     ✓6ᵗʰ **M25.42**   Effusion, elbow
         M25.421   Effusion, right elbow
         M25.422   Effusion, left elbow
         M25.429   Effusion, unspecified elbow   ▽

     ✓6ᵗʰ **M25.43**   Effusion, wrist
         M25.431   Effusion, right wrist
         M25.432   Effusion, left wrist
         M25.439   Effusion, unspecified wrist   ▽

     ✓6ᵗʰ **M25.44**   Effusion, hand
         M25.441   Effusion, right hand
         M25.442   Effusion, left hand
         M25.449   Effusion, unspecified hand   ▽

     ✓6ᵗʰ **M25.45**   Effusion, hip
         M25.451   Effusion, right hip
         M25.452   Effusion, left hip
         M25.459   Effusion, unspecified hip   ▽

     ✓6ᵗʰ **M25.46**   Effusion, knee
         M25.461   Effusion, right knee
         M25.462   Effusion, left knee
         M25.469   Effusion, unspecified knee   ▽

     ✓6ᵗʰ **M25.47**   Effusion, ankle and foot
         M25.471   Effusion, right ankle
         M25.472   Effusion, left ankle
         M25.473   Effusion, unspecified ankle   ▽
         M25.474   Effusion, right foot
         M25.475   Effusion, left foot
         M25.476   Effusion, unspecified foot   ▽

     M25.48   Effusion, other site

✓5ᵗʰ **M25.5**   **Pain in joint**
     EXCLUDES 2   pain in hand (M79.64-)
         pain in fingers (M79.64-)
         pain in foot (M79.67-)
         pain in limb (M79.6-)
         pain in toes (M79.67-)

     M25.50   Pain in unspecified joint   ▽

     ✓6ᵗʰ **M25.51**   Pain in shoulder
         M25.511   Pain in right shoulder
         M25.512   Pain in left shoulder
         M25.519   Pain in unspecified shoulder   ▽

     ✓6ᵗʰ **M25.52**   Pain in elbow
         M25.521   Pain in right elbow
         M25.522   Pain in left elbow
         M25.529   Pain in unspecified elbow   ▽

     ✓6ᵗʰ **M25.53**   Pain in wrist
         M25.531   Pain in right wrist
         M25.532   Pain in left wrist
         M25.539   Pain in unspecified wrist   ▽

     ✓6ᵗʰ **M25.54**   Pain in joints of hand
         M25.541   Pain in joints of right hand
         M25.542   Pain in joints of left hand
         M25.549   Pain in joints of unspecified hand   ▽
             Pain in joints of hand NOS

     ✓6ᵗʰ **M25.55**   Pain in hip
         M25.551   Pain in right hip
         M25.552   Pain in left hip
         M25.559   Pain in unspecified hip   ▽

     ✓6ᵗʰ **M25.56**   Pain in knee
         M25.561   Pain in right knee
         M25.562   Pain in left knee
         M25.569   Pain in unspecified knee   ▽

✔ Additional Character Req   ✔x7ᵗʰ Placeholder Alert   Case-Mix Diagnosis   Manifestation   ▽ Unspecified Dx   **EXCLUDES 1** Not coded here   **EXCLUDES 2** Not included here

Chapter 13. Diseases of the Musculoskeletal System and Connective Tissue

M25.57–M25.9

√6ᵗʰ **M25.57 Pain in** ankle and joints of foot
     M25.571 Pain in right **ankle and joints of right foot**
     M25.572 Pain in left **ankle and joints of left foot**
     M25.579 Pain in unspecified ankle and joints of ▽
             unspecified foot

√5ᵗʰ **M25.6 Stiffness of joint, not elsewhere classified**
     EXCLUDES 1   ankylosis of joint (M24.6-)
               contracture of joint (M24.5-)
     M25.60 Stiffness of unspecified joint, not elsewhere ▽
             classified

√6ᵗʰ **M25.61 Stiffness of** shoulder, **not elsewhere classified**
     M25.611 Stiffness of right **shoulder, not elsewhere**
             classified
     M25.612 Stiffness of left **shoulder, not elsewhere**
             classified
     M25.619 Stiffness of unspecified shoulder, not ▽
             elsewhere classified

√6ᵗʰ **M25.62 Stiffness of** elbow, **not elsewhere classified**
     M25.621 Stiffness of right **elbow, not elsewhere**
             classified
     M25.622 Stiffness of left **elbow, not elsewhere**
             classified
     M25.629 Stiffness of unspecified elbow, not ▽
             elsewhere classified

√6ᵗʰ **M25.63 Stiffness of** wrist, **not elsewhere classified**
     M25.631 Stiffness of right **wrist, not elsewhere**
             classified
     M25.632 Stiffness of left **wrist, not elsewhere**
             classified
     M25.639 Stiffness of unspecified wrist, not ▽
             elsewhere classified

√6ᵗʰ **M25.64 Stiffness of** hand, **not elsewhere classified**
     M25.641 Stiffness of right **hand, not elsewhere**
             classified
     M25.642 Stiffness of left **hand, not elsewhere**
             classified
     M25.649 Stiffness of unspecified hand, not ▽
             elsewhere classified

√6ᵗʰ **M25.65 Stiffness of** hip, **not elsewhere classified**
     M25.651 Stiffness of right **hip, not elsewhere**
             classified
     M25.652 Stiffness of left **hip, not elsewhere**
             classified
     M25.659 Stiffness of unspecified hip, not ▽
             elsewhere classified

√6ᵗʰ **M25.66 Stiffness of** knee, **not elsewhere classified**
     M25.661 Stiffness of right **knee, not elsewhere**
             classified
     M25.662 Stiffness of left **knee, not elsewhere**
             classified
     M25.669 Stiffness of unspecified knee, not ▽
             elsewhere classified

√6ᵗʰ **M25.67 Stiffness of** ankle and foot, **not elsewhere classified**
     M25.671 Stiffness of right **ankle, not elsewhere**
             classified
     M25.672 Stiffness of left **ankle, not elsewhere**
             classified
     M25.673 Stiffness of unspecified ankle, not ▽
             elsewhere classified
     M25.674 Stiffness of right **foot, not elsewhere**
             classified
     M25.675 Stiffness of left **foot, not elsewhere**
             classified
     M25.676 Stiffness of unspecified foot, not ▽
             elsewhere classified

√5ᵗʰ **M25.7 Osteophyte**
     M25.70 Osteophyte, unspecified joint ▽

√6ᵗʰ **M25.71 Osteophyte,** shoulder
     M25.711 Osteophyte, right **shoulder**
     M25.712 Osteophyte, left **shoulder**
     M25.719 Osteophyte, unspecified shoulder ▽

√6ᵗʰ **M25.72 Osteophyte,** elbow
     M25.721 Osteophyte, right **elbow**
     M25.722 Osteophyte, left **elbow**
     M25.729 Osteophyte, unspecified elbow ▽

√6ᵗʰ **M25.73 Osteophyte,** wrist
     M25.731 Osteophyte, right **wrist**
     M25.732 Osteophyte, left **wrist**
     M25.739 Osteophyte, unspecified wrist ▽

√6ᵗʰ **M25.74 Osteophyte,** hand
     M25.741 Osteophyte, right **hand**
     M25.742 Osteophyte, left **hand**
     M25.749 Osteophyte, unspecified hand ▽

√6ᵗʰ **M25.75 Osteophyte,** hip
     M25.751 Osteophyte, right **hip**
     M25.752 Osteophyte, left **hip**
     M25.759 Osteophyte, unspecified hip ▽

√6ᵗʰ **M25.76 Osteophyte,** knee
     M25.761 Osteophyte, right **knee**
     M25.762 Osteophyte, left **knee**
     M25.769 Osteophyte, unspecified knee ▽

√6ᵗʰ **M25.77 Osteophyte,** ankle and foot
     M25.771 Osteophyte, right **ankle**
     M25.772 Osteophyte, left **ankle**
     M25.773 Osteophyte, unspecified ankle ▽
     M25.774 Osteophyte, right **foot**
     M25.775 Osteophyte, left **foot**
     M25.776 Osteophyte, unspecified foot ▽
     M25.78 Osteophyte, vertebrae

√5ᵗʰ **M25.8 Other specified joint disorders**
     M25.80 Other specified joint disorders, unspecified joint ▽

√6ᵗʰ **M25.81 Other specified joint disorders,** shoulder
     M25.811 Other specified joint disorders, right
             shoulder
     M25.812 Other specified joint disorders, left
             shoulder
     M25.819 Other specified joint disorders, ▽
             unspecified shoulder

√6ᵗʰ **M25.82 Other specified joint disorders,** elbow
     M25.821 Other specified joint disorders, right
             elbow
     M25.822 Other specified joint disorders, left **elbow**
     M25.829 Other specified joint disorders, ▽
             unspecified elbow

√6ᵗʰ **M25.83 Other specified joint disorders,** wrist
     M25.831 Other specified joint disorders, right **wrist**
     M25.832 Other specified joint disorders, left **wrist**
     M25.839 Other specified joint disorders, ▽
             unspecified wrist

√6ᵗʰ **M25.84 Other specified joint disorders,** hand
     M25.841 Other specified joint disorders, right **hand**
     M25.842 Other specified joint disorders, left **hand**
     M25.849 Other specified joint disorders, ▽
             unspecified hand

√6ᵗʰ **M25.85 Other specified joint disorders,** hip
     AHA: 2014, 4Q, 25
     M25.851 Other specified joint disorders, right **hip**
     M25.852 Other specified joint disorders, left **hip**
     M25.859 Other specified joint disorders, ▽
             unspecified hip

√6ᵗʰ **M25.86 Other specified joint disorders,** knee
     M25.861 Other specified joint disorders, right **knee**
     M25.862 Other specified joint disorders, left **knee**
     M25.869 Other specified joint disorders, ▽
             unspecified knee

√6ᵗʰ **M25.87 Other specified joint disorders,** ankle and foot
     M25.871 Other specified joint disorders, right **ankle**
             and foot
     M25.872 Other specified joint disorders, left **ankle**
             and foot
     M25.879 Other specified joint disorders, ▽
             unspecified ankle and foot

     M25.9 Joint disorder, unspecified ▽

N Newborn: 0   P Pediatric: 0-17   M Maternity: 12-55   A Adult: 15-124   **NRS** Nonroutine supply Dx   **NCDx** Noncancer Dx   **PDx** Primary Dx   ▶◀ Revised Text   ● New Code   ▲ Revised Title

750   ICD-10-CM 2018

Dentofacial anomalies [including malocclusion] and other disorders of jaw (M26-M27)

EXCLUDES 1   hemifacial atrophy or hypertrophy (Q67.4)
unilateral condylar hyperplasia or hypoplasia (M27.8)

✓4ᵗʰ **M26 Dentofacial anomalies [including malocclusion]**

✓5ᵗʰ **M26.0 Major anomalies of jaw size**
    EXCLUDES 1   acromegaly (E22.0)
       Robin's syndrome (Q87.0)

   M26.00 Unspecified anomaly of jaw size ▽
   M26.01 Maxillary hyperplasia
   M26.02 Maxillary hypoplasia
     AHA: 2014, 3Q, 23
   M26.03 Mandibular hyperplasia
   M26.04 Mandibular hypoplasia
   M26.05 Macrogenia
   M26.06 Microgenia
   M26.07 Excessive tuberosity of jaw
     Entire maxillary tuberosity
   M26.09 Other specified anomalies of jaw size

✓5ᵗʰ **M26.1 Anomalies of jaw-cranial base relationship**
   M26.10 Unspecified anomaly of jaw-cranial base relationship ▽
   M26.11 Maxillary asymmetry
   M26.12 Other jaw asymmetry
   M26.19 Other specified anomalies of jaw-cranial base relationship

✓5ᵗʰ **M26.2 Anomalies of dental arch relationship**
   M26.20 Unspecified anomaly of dental arch relationship ▽
   ✓6ᵗʰ **M26.21 Malocclusion, Angle's class**
     M26.211 Malocclusion, Angle's class I
       Neutro-occlusion
     M26.212 Malocclusion, Angle's class II
       Disto-occlusion Division I
       Disto-occlusion Division II
     M26.213 Malocclusion, Angle's class III
       Mesio-occlusion
     M26.219 Malocclusion, Angle's class, unspecified ▽
   ✓6ᵗʰ **M26.22 Open occlusal relationship**
     M26.220 Open anterior occlusal relationship
       Anterior openbite
     M26.221 Open posterior occlusal relationship
       Posterior openbite
   M26.23 Excessive horizontal overlap
     Excessive horizontal overjet
   M26.24 Reverse articulation
     Crossbite (anterior) (posterior)
   M26.25 Anomalies of interarch distance
   M26.29 Other anomalies of dental arch relationship
     Midline deviation of dental arch
     Overbite (excessive) deep
     Overbite (excessive) horizontal
     Overbite (excessive) vertical
     Posterior lingual occlusion of mandibular teeth

✓5ᵗʰ **M26.3 Anomalies of tooth position of fully erupted tooth or teeth**
   EXCLUDES 2   embedded and impacted teeth (K01.-)

   M26.30 Unspecified anomaly of tooth position of fully erupted tooth or teeth ▽
     Abnormal spacing of fully erupted tooth or teeth NOS
     Displacement of fully erupted tooth or teeth NOS
     Transposition of fully erupted tooth or teeth NOS
   M26.31 Crowding of fully erupted teeth
   M26.32 Excessive spacing of fully erupted teeth
     Diastema of fully erupted tooth or teeth NOS
   M26.33 Horizontal displacement of fully erupted tooth or teeth
     Tipped tooth or teeth
     Tipping of fully erupted tooth
   M26.34 Vertical displacement of fully erupted tooth or teeth
     Extruded tooth
     Infraeruption of tooth or teeth
     Supraeruption of tooth or teeth
   M26.35 Rotation of fully erupted tooth or teeth
   M26.36 Insufficient interocclusal distance of fully erupted teeth (ridge)
     Lack of adequate intermaxillary vertical dimension of fully erupted teeth

   M26.37 Excessive interocclusal distance of fully erupted teeth
     Excessive intermaxillary vertical dimension of fully erupted teeth
     Loss of occlusal vertical dimension of fully erupted teeth
   M26.39 Other anomalies of tooth position of fully erupted tooth or teeth

   M26.4 Malocclusion, unspecified ▽

✓5ᵗʰ **M26.5 Dentofacial functional abnormalities**
   EXCLUDES 1   bruxism (F45.8)
       teeth-grinding NOS (F45.8)

   M26.50 Dentofacial functional abnormalities, unspecified ▽
   M26.51 Abnormal jaw closure
   M26.52 Limited mandibular range of motion
   M26.53 Deviation in opening and closing of the mandible
   M26.54 Insufficient anterior guidance
     Insufficient anterior occlusal guidance
   M26.55 Centric occlusion maximum intercuspation discrepancy
     EXCLUDES 1   centric occlusion NOS (M26.59)
   M26.56 Non-working side interference
     Balancing side interference
   M26.57 Lack of posterior occlusal support
   M26.59 Other dentofacial functional abnormalities
     Centric occlusion (of teeth) NOS
     Malocclusion due to abnormal swallowing
     Malocclusion due to mouth breathing
     Malocclusion due to tongue, lip or finger habits

✓5ᵗʰ **M26.6 Temporomandibular joint disorders**
   EXCLUDES 2   current temporomandibular joint dislocation (S03.0)
       current temporomandibular joint sprain (S03.4)

   ✓6ᵗʰ **M26.60 Temporomandibular joint disorder, unspecified**
     M26.601 Right temporomandibular joint disorder, unspecified ▽
     M26.602 Left temporomandibular joint disorder, unspecified ▽
     M26.603 Bilateral temporomandibular joint disorder, unspecified
     M26.609 Unspecified temporomandibular joint disorder, unspecified side ▽
       Temporomandibular joint disorder NOS
   ✓6ᵗʰ **M26.61 Adhesions and ankylosis of temporomandibular joint**
     M26.611 Adhesions and ankylosis of right temporomandibular joint
     M26.612 Adhesions and ankylosis of left temporomandibular joint
     M26.613 Adhesions and ankylosis of bilateral temporomandibular joint
     M26.619 Adhesions and ankylosis of temporomandibular joint, unspecified side ▽
   ✓6ᵗʰ **M26.62 Arthralgia of temporomandibular joint**
     M26.621 Arthralgia of right temporomandibular joint
     M26.622 Arthralgia of left temporomandibular joint
     M26.623 Arthralgia of bilateral temporomandibular joint
     M26.629 Arthralgia of temporomandibular joint, unspecified side ▽

Temporomandibular Joint

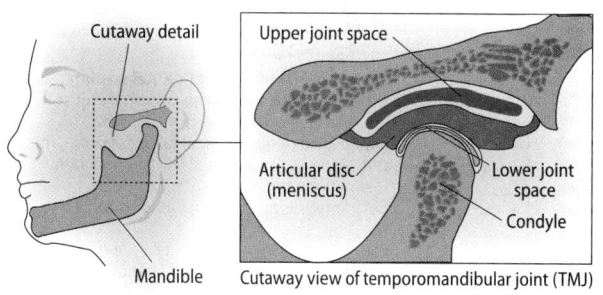

Cutaway detail

Upper joint space

Articular disc (meniscus)

Lower joint space

Condyle

Mandible

Cutaway view of temporomandibular joint (TMJ)

✓ Additional Character Req   ✓x7ᵗʰ Placeholder Alert   Case-Mix Diagnosis   Manifestation   ▽ Unspecified Dx   **EXCLUDES 1** Not coded here   **EXCLUDES 2** Not included here

✓6ᵗʰ **M26.63** Articular disc disorder **of temporomandibular joint**

    M26.631 Articular disc disorder of right temporomandibular joint

    M26.632 Articular disc disorder of left temporomandibular joint

    M26.633 Articular disc disorder of bilateral temporomandibular joint

    M26.639 Articular disc disorder of ▽ temporomandibular joint, unspecified **side**

M26.69 Other specified disorders of temporomandibular joint

✓5ᵗʰ **M26.7 Dental alveolar anomalies**

    M26.70 Unspecified alveolar anomaly   ▽

    M26.71 Alveolar maxillary hyperplasia

    M26.72 Alveolar mandibular hyperplasia

    M26.73 Alveolar maxillary hypoplasia

    M26.74 Alveolar mandibular hypoplasia

    M26.79 Other specified alveolar anomalies

✓5ᵗʰ **M26.8 Other dentofacial anomalies**

    M26.81 Anterior **soft tissue impingement**
        Anterior soft tissue impingement on teeth

    M26.82 Posterior **soft tissue impingement**
        Posterior soft tissue impingement on teeth

    M26.89 Other dentofacial anomalies

M26.9 Dentofacial anomaly, unspecified   ▽

✓4ᵗʰ **M27 Other diseases of jaws**

M27.0 Developmental disorders of jaws
    Latent bone cyst of jaw
    Stafne's cyst
    Torus mandibularis
    Torus palatinus

M27.1 Giant cell granuloma, central
    Giant cell granuloma NOS
    EXCLUDES 1 *peripheral giant cell granuloma (K06.8)*

M27.2 Inflammatory conditions of jaws
    Osteitis of jaw(s)
    Osteomyelitis (neonatal) jaw(s)
    Osteoradionecrosis jaw(s)
    Periostitis jaw(s)
    Sequestrum of jaw bone
    Use additional code (W88-W90, X39.0) to identify radiation, if radiation-induced
    EXCLUDES 2 *osteonecrosis of jaw due to drug (M87.180)*

M27.3 Alveolitis of jaws
    Alveolar osteitis
    Dry socket

✓5ᵗʰ **M27.4 Other and unspecified cysts of jaw**
    EXCLUDES 1 *cysts of oral region (K09.-)*
        latent bone cyst of jaw (M27.0)
        Stafne's cyst (M27.0)

    M27.40 Unspecified cyst of jaw   ▽
        Cyst of jaw NOS

    M27.49 Other cysts of jaw
        Aneurysmal cyst of jaw
        Hemorrhagic cyst of jaw
        Traumatic cyst of jaw

✓5ᵗʰ **M27.5 Periradicular pathology associated with previous endodontic treatment**

    M27.51 Perforation of root canal space due to endodontic treatment

    M27.52 Endodontic overfill

    M27.53 Endodontic underfill

    M27.59 Other periradicular pathology associated with previous endodontic treatment

✓5ᵗʰ **M27.6 Endosseous dental implant failure**

    M27.61 Osseointegration **failure of dental implant**
        Hemorrhagic complications of dental implant placement
        Iatrogenic osseointegration failure of dental implant
        Osseointegration failure of dental implant due to complications of systemic disease
        Osseointegration failure of dental implant due to poor bone quality
        Pre-integration failure of dental implant NOS
        Pre-osseointegration failure of dental implant

    M27.62 Post-osseointegration biological **failure of dental implant**
        Failure of dental implant due to lack of attached gingiva
        Failure of dental implant due to occlusal trauma (caused by poor prosthetic design)
        Failure of dental implant due to parafunctional habits
        Failure of dental implant due to periodontal infection (peri-implantitis)
        Failure of dental implant due to poor oral hygiene
        Iatrogenic post-osseointegration failure of dental implant
        Post-osseointegration failure of dental implant due to complications of systemic disease

    M27.63 Post-osseointegration mechanical **failure of dental implant**
        Failure of dental prosthesis causing loss of dental implant
        Fracture of dental implant
        EXCLUDES 2 *cracked tooth (K03.81)*
            fractured dental restorative material with loss of material (K08.531)
            fractured dental restorative material without loss of material (K08.530)
            fractured tooth (S02.5)

    M27.69 Other endosseous dental implant failure
        Dental implant failure NOS

M27.8 Other specified diseases of jaws

Cherubism	Unilateral condylar hyperplasia
Exostosis	Unilateral condylar hypoplasia
Fibrous dysplasia	

    EXCLUDES 1 *jaw pain (R68.84)*

M27.9 Disease of jaws, unspecified   ▽

Systemic connective tissue disorders (M30-M36)

INCLUDES autoimmune disease NOS
    collagen (vascular) disease NOS
    systemic autoimmune disease
    systemic collagen (vascular) disease

EXCLUDES 1 *autoimmune disease, single organ or single cell-type—code to relevant condition category*

✓4ᵗʰ **M30 Polyarteritis nodosa and related conditions**
    EXCLUDES 1 *microscopic polyarteritis (M31.7)*

M30.0 Polyarteritis nodosa

M30.1 Polyarteritis with lung involvement [Churg-Strauss]
    Allergic granulomatous angiitis

M30.2 Juvenile polyarteritis

M30.3 Mucocutaneous lymph node syndrome [Kawasaki]

M30.8 Other conditions related to polyarteritis nodosa
    Polyangiitis overlap syndrome

✓4ᵗʰ **M31 Other necrotizing vasculopathies**

M31.0 Hypersensitivity angiitis
    Goodpasture's syndrome

M31.1 Thrombotic microangiopathy
    Thrombotic thrombocytopenic purpura

M31.2 Lethal midline granuloma

✓5ᵗʰ **M31.3 Wegener's granulomatosis**
    Necrotizing respiratory granulomatosis

    M31.30 Wegener's granulomatosis without renal involvement
        Wegener's granulomatosis NOS

    M31.31 Wegener's granulomatosis with renal involvement

M31.4 Aortic arch syndrome [Takayasu]

M31.5 Giant cell arteritis with polymyalgia rheumatica

M31.6 Other giant cell arteritis

M31.7 Microscopic polyangiitis
    Microscopic polyarteritis
    EXCLUDES 1 *polyarteritis nodosa (M30.0)*

M31.8 Other specified necrotizing vasculopathies
    Hypocomplementemic vasculitis
    Septic vasculitis

M31.9 Necrotizing vasculopathy, unspecified   ▽

✓4ᵗʰ **M32 Systemic lupus erythematosus (SLE)**
    EXCLUDES 1 *lupus erythematosus (discoid) (NOS) (L93.0)*

M32.0 Drug-induced systemic lupus erythematosus
    Use additional code for adverse effect, if applicable, to identify drug (T36-T50 with fifth or sixth character 5)

Ⓝ Newborn: 0   Ⓟ Pediatric: 0-17   Ⓜ Maternity: 12-55   Ⓐ Adult: 15-124   NRS Nonroutine supply Dx   NC Dx Noncancer Dx   PDx Primary Dx   ▶◀ Revised Text   ● New Code   ▲ Revised Title

752   ICD-10-CM 2018

√5ᵗʰ **M32.1 Systemic lupus erythematosus** with organ or system involvement

  M32.10 Systemic lupus erythematosus, organ or system involvement unspecified ▽

  M32.11 Endocarditis in systemic lupus erythematosus
    Libman-Sacks disease

  M32.12 Pericarditis in systemic lupus erythematosus
    Lupus pericarditis

  M32.13 Lung involvement in systemic lupus erythematosus
    Pleural effusion due to systemic lupus erythematosus

  M32.14 Glomerular disease in systemic lupus erythematosus
    Lupus renal disease NOS
    AHA: 2013, 4Q, 125

  M32.15 Tubulo-interstitial nephropathy in systemic lupus erythematosus

  M32.19 Other organ or system involvement in systemic lupus erythematosus

M32.8 Other forms of systemic lupus erythematosus

M32.9 Systemic lupus erythematosus, unspecified ▽
  SLE NOS
  Systemic lupus erythematosus NOS
  Systemic lupus erythematosus without organ involvement

√4ᵗʰ **M33 Dermatopolymyositis**

▲ √5ᵗʰ **M33.0 Juvenile dermatomyositis**

▲   **M33.00 Juvenile dermatomyositis, organ involvement unspecified** ▽

▲   **M33.01 Juvenile dermatomyositis with respiratory involvement**

▲   **M33.02 Juvenile dermatomyositis with myopathy**

●   **M33.03 Juvenile dermatomyositis without myopathy**

▲   **M33.09 Juvenile dermatomyositis with other organ involvement**

▲ √5ᵗʰ **M33.1 Other dermatomyositis**
  ▶Adult dermatomyositis◀

▲   **M33.10 Other dermatomyositis, organ involvement unspecified** ▽

▲   **M33.11 Other dermatomyositis with respiratory involvement**

▲   **M33.12 Other dermatomyositis with myopathy**

●   **M33.13 Other dermatomyositis without myopathy**
    Dermatomyositis NOS

▲   **M33.19 Other dermatomyositis with other organ involvement**

√5ᵗʰ **M33.2 Polymyositis**

  M33.20 Polymyositis, organ involvement unspecified ▽

  M33.21 Polymyositis with respiratory involvement

  M33.22 Polymyositis with myopathy

  M33.29 Polymyositis with other organ involvement

√5ᵗʰ **M33.9 Dermatopolymyositis, unspecified**

  M33.90 Dermatopolymyositis, unspecified, organ involvement unspecified ▽

  M33.91 Dermatopolymyositis, unspecified with respiratory involvement ▽

  M33.92 Dermatopolymyositis, unspecified with myopathy ▽

●   **M33.93 Dermatopolymyositis, unspecified without myopathy** ▽

  M33.99 Dermatopolymyositis, unspecified with other organ involvement ▽

√4ᵗʰ **M34 Systemic sclerosis [scleroderma]**
  EXCLUDES1 circumscribed scleroderma (L94.0)
    neonatal scleroderma (P83.8)

M34.0 Progressive systemic sclerosis

M34.1 CR(E)ST syndrome
  Combination of calcinosis, Raynaud's phenomenon, esophageal dysfunction, sclerodactyly, telangiectasia

M34.2 Systemic sclerosis induced by drug and chemical
  Code first poisoning due to drug or toxin, if applicable (T36-T65 with fifth or sixth character 1-4 or 6)
  Use additional code for adverse effect, if applicable, to identify drug (T36-T50 with fifth or sixth character 5)

√5ᵗʰ **M34.8 Other forms of systemic sclerosis**

  M34.81 Systemic sclerosis with lung involvement

  M34.82 Systemic sclerosis with myopathy

  M34.83 Systemic sclerosis with polyneuropathy

  M34.89 Other systemic sclerosis

M34.9 Systemic sclerosis, unspecified ▽

√4ᵗʰ **M35 Other systemic involvement of connective tissue**
  EXCLUDES1 reactive perforating collagenosis (L87.1)

√5ᵗʰ **M35.0 Sicca syndrome [Sjögren]**
  DEF: Autoimmune disease; associated with keratoconjunctivitis, laryngopharyngitis, rhinitis, dry mouth, enlarged parotid gland, and chronic polyarthritis.

  M35.00 Sicca syndrome, unspecified ▽

  M35.01 Sicca syndrome with keratoconjunctivitis

  M35.02 Sicca syndrome with lung involvement

  M35.03 Sicca syndrome with myopathy

  M35.04 Sicca syndrome with tubulo-interstitial nephropathy
    Renal tubular acidosis in sicca syndrome

  M35.09 Sicca syndrome with other organ involvement

M35.1 Other overlap syndromes
  Mixed connective tissue disease
  EXCLUDES1 polyangiitis overlap syndrome (M30.8)

M35.2 Behçet's disease

M35.3 Polymyalgia rheumatica
  EXCLUDES1 polymyalgia rheumatica with giant cell arteritis (M31.5)

M35.4 Diffuse (eosinophilic) fasciitis

M35.5 Multifocal fibrosclerosis

M35.6 Relapsing panniculitis [Weber-Christian]
  EXCLUDES1 lupus panniculitis (L93.2)
    panniculitis NOS (M79.3-)

M35.7 Hypermobility syndrome
  Familial ligamentous laxity
  EXCLUDES1 Ehlers-Danlos syndrome (Q79.6)
    ligamentous laxity, NOS (M24.2-)

M35.8 Other specified systemic involvement of connective tissue

M35.9 Systemic involvement of connective tissue, unspecified ▽
  Autoimmune disease (systemic) NOS
  Collagen (vascular) disease NOS

√4ᵗʰ **M36 Systemic disorders of connective tissue in diseases classified elsewhere**
  EXCLUDES2 arthropathies in diseases classified elsewhere (M14.-)

M36.0 Dermato(poly)myositis in neoplastic disease
  Code first underlying neoplasm (C00-D49)

M36.1 Arthropathy in neoplastic disease
  Code first underlying neoplasm, such as:
    leukemia (C91-C95)
    malignant histiocytosis (C96.A)
    multiple myeloma (C90.0)

M36.2 Hemophilic arthropathy
  Hemarthrosis in hemophilic arthropathy
  Code first underlying disease, such as:
    factor VIII deficiency (D66)
      with vascular defect (D68.0)
    factor IX deficiency (D67)
    hemophilia (classical) (D66)
    hemophilia B (D67)
    hemophilia C (D68.1)

M36.3 Arthropathy in other blood disorders

M36.4 Arthropathy in hypersensitivity reactions classified elsewhere
  Code first underlying disease, such as:
    Henoch (-Schönlein) purpura (D69.0)
    serum sickness (T80.6-)

M36.8 Systemic disorders of connective tissue in other diseases classified elsewhere
  Code first underlying disease, such as:
    alkaptonuria (E70.2)
    hypogammaglobulinemia (D80.-)
    ochronosis (E70.2)

✔ Additional Character Req √x7ᵗʰ Placeholder Alert Case-Mix Diagnosis Manifestation ▽ Unspecified Dx EXCLUDES1 Not coded here EXCLUDES2 Not included here

ICD-10-CM 2018   753

Chapter 13. Diseases of the Musculoskeletal System and Connective Tissue

DORSOPATHIES (M40-M54)

Deforming dorsopathies (M40-M43)

✓4th M40 Kyphosis and lordosis
> **EXCLUDES 1**   *congenital kyphosis and lordosis (Q76.4)*
> *kyphoscoliosis (M41.-)*
> *postprocedural kyphosis and lordosis (M96.-)*

✓5th M40.0 Postural kyphosis
> **EXCLUDES 1**   *osteochondrosis of spine (M42.-)*

     M40.00   **Postural kyphosis, site unspecified** ▽
     M40.03   **Postural kyphosis, cervicothoracic region**
     M40.04   **Postural kyphosis, thoracic region**
     M40.05   **Postural kyphosis, thoracolumbar region**

✓5th M40.1 Other secondary kyphosis

     M40.10   **Other secondary kyphosis, site unspecified** ▽
     M40.12   **Other secondary kyphosis, cervical region**
     M40.13   **Other secondary kyphosis, cervicothoracic region**
     M40.14   **Other secondary kyphosis, thoracic region**
     M40.15   **Other secondary kyphosis, thoracolumbar region**

✓5th M40.2 Other and unspecified kyphosis

   ✓6th M40.20 Unspecified kyphosis
     M40.202   **Unspecified kyphosis, cervical region** ▽
     M40.203   **Unspecified kyphosis, cervicothoracic region** ▽
     M40.204   **Unspecified kyphosis, thoracic region** ▽
     M40.205   **Unspecified kyphosis, thoracolumbar region** ▽
     M40.209   **Unspecified kyphosis, site unspecified** ▽

   ✓6th M40.29 Other kyphosis
     M40.292   **Other kyphosis, cervical region**
     M40.293   **Other kyphosis, cervicothoracic region**
     M40.294   **Other kyphosis, thoracic region**
     M40.295   **Other kyphosis, thoracolumbar region**
     M40.299   **Other kyphosis, site unspecified** ▽

✓5th M40.3 Flatback syndrome

     M40.30   **Flatback syndrome, site unspecified** ▽
     M40.35   **Flatback syndrome, thoracolumbar region**
     M40.36   **Flatback syndrome, lumbar region**
     M40.37   **Flatback syndrome, lumbosacral region**

✓5th M40.4 Postural lordosis
> Acquired lordosis

     M40.40   **Postural lordosis, site unspecified** ▽
     M40.45   **Postural lordosis, thoracolumbar region**
     M40.46   **Postural lordosis, lumbar region**
     M40.47   **Postural lordosis, lumbosacral region**

✓5th M40.5 Lordosis, unspecified

     M40.50   **Lordosis, unspecified, site unspecified** ▽
     M40.55   **Lordosis, unspecified, thoracolumbar region**
     M40.56   **Lordosis, unspecified, lumbar region**
     M40.57   **Lordosis, unspecified, lumbosacral region**

Kyphosis and Lordosis

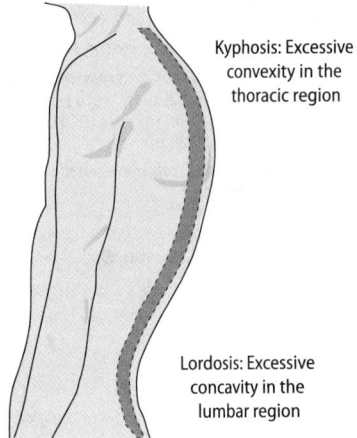

Kyphosis: Excessive convexity in the thoracic region

Lordosis: Excessive concavity in the lumbar region

Scoliosis

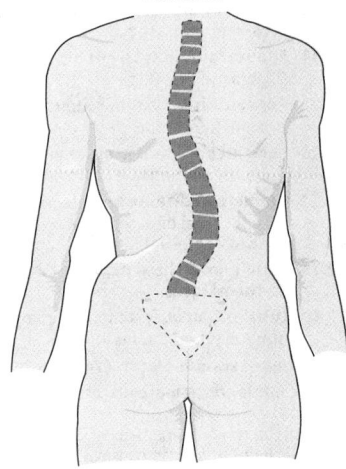

Lateral curvature of spine

✓4th M41 Scoliosis
> **INCLUDES**   kyphoscoliosis
> **EXCLUDES 1**   *congenital scoliosis due to bony malformation (Q76.3)*
> *congenital scoliosis NOS (Q67.5)*
> *kyphoscoliotic heart disease (I27.1)*
> *postprocedural scoliosis (M96.-)*
> *postural congenital scoliosis (Q67.5)*

✓5th M41.0 Infantile idiopathic scoliosis
> **AHA:** 2014, 4Q, 26

     M41.00   **Infantile idiopathic scoliosis, site unspecified** ▽
     M41.02   **Infantile idiopathic scoliosis, cervical region**
     M41.03   **Infantile idiopathic scoliosis, cervicothoracic region**
     M41.04   **Infantile idiopathic scoliosis, thoracic region**
     M41.05   **Infantile idiopathic scoliosis, thoracolumbar region**
     M41.06   **Infantile idiopathic scoliosis, lumbar region**
     M41.07   **Infantile idiopathic scoliosis, lumbosacral region**
     M41.08   **Infantile idiopathic scoliosis, sacral and sacrococcygeal region**

✓5th M41.1 Juvenile and adolescent idiopathic scoliosis

   ✓6th M41.11 Juvenile idiopathic scoliosis
> **AHA:** 2014, 4Q, 28
     M41.112   **Juvenile idiopathic scoliosis, cervical region**
     M41.113   **Juvenile idiopathic scoliosis, cervicothoracic region**
     M41.114   **Juvenile idiopathic scoliosis, thoracic region**
     M41.115   **Juvenile idiopathic scoliosis, thoracolumbar region**
     M41.116   **Juvenile idiopathic scoliosis, lumbar region**
     M41.117   **Juvenile idiopathic scoliosis, lumbosacral region**
     M41.119   **Juvenile idiopathic scoliosis, site unspecified** ▽

   ✓6th M41.12 Adolescent scoliosis
     M41.122   **Adolescent idiopathic scoliosis, cervical region**
     M41.123   **Adolescent idiopathic scoliosis, cervicothoracic region**
     M41.124   **Adolescent idiopathic scoliosis, thoracic region**
     M41.125   **Adolescent idiopathic scoliosis, thoracolumbar region**
     M41.126   **Adolescent idiopathic scoliosis, lumbar region**
     M41.127   **Adolescent idiopathic scoliosis, lumbosacral region**
     M41.129   **Adolescent idiopathic scoliosis, site unspecified** ▽

✓5th M41.2 Other idiopathic scoliosis

     M41.20   **Other idiopathic scoliosis, site unspecified** ▽

Ⓝ Newborn: 0   Ⓟ Pediatric: 0-17   Ⓜ Maternity: 12-55   Ⓐ Adult: 15-124   **NRS** Nonroutine supply Dx   **NC Dx** Noncancer Dx   **PDx** Primary Dx   ►◄ Revised Text   ● New Code   ▲ Revised Title

754   ICD-10-CM 2018

M41.22 **Other idiopathic scoliosis,** cervical **region**

M41.23 **Other idiopathic scoliosis,** cervicothoracic **region**

M41.24 **Other idiopathic scoliosis,** thoracic **region**

M41.25 **Other idiopathic scoliosis,** thoracolumbar **region**

M41.26 **Other idiopathic scoliosis,** lumbar **region**

M41.27 **Other idiopathic scoliosis,** lumbosacral **region**

✓5ᵗʰ **M41.3** Thoracogenic **scoliosis**

M41.30 **Thoracogenic scoliosis, site unspecified** ▽

M41.34 **Thoracogenic scoliosis,** thoracic **region**

M41.35 **Thoracogenic scoliosis,** thoracolumbar **region**

✓5ᵗʰ **M41.4** Neuromuscular **scoliosis**

Scoliosis secondary to cerebral palsy, Friedreich's ataxia, poliomyelitis and other neuromuscular disorders

Code also underlying condition

AHA: 2014, 4Q, 27

M41.40 **Neuromuscular scoliosis, site unspecified** ▽

M41.41 **Neuromuscular scoliosis,** occipito-atlanto-axial **region**

M41.42 **Neuromuscular scoliosis,** cervical **region**

M41.43 **Neuromuscular scoliosis,** cervicothoracic **region**

M41.44 **Neuromuscular scoliosis,** thoracic **region**

M41.45 **Neuromuscular scoliosis,** thoracolumbar **region**

M41.46 **Neuromuscular scoliosis,** lumbar **region**

M41.47 **Neuromuscular scoliosis,** lumbosacral **region**

✓5ᵗʰ **M41.5** Other secondary **scoliosis**

M41.50 **Other secondary scoliosis, site unspecified** ▽

M41.52 **Other secondary scoliosis,** cervical **region**

M41.53 **Other secondary scoliosis,** cervicothoracic **region**

M41.54 **Other secondary scoliosis,** thoracic **region**

M41.55 **Other secondary scoliosis,** thoracolumbar **region**

M41.56 **Other secondary scoliosis,** lumbar **region**

M41.57 **Other secondary scoliosis,** lumbosacral **region**

✓5ᵗʰ **M41.8** Other **forms of scoliosis**

M41.80 **Other forms of scoliosis, site unspecified** ▽

M41.82 **Other forms of scoliosis,** cervical **region**

M41.83 **Other forms of scoliosis,** cervicothoracic **region**

M41.84 **Other forms of scoliosis,** thoracic **region**

M41.85 **Other forms of scoliosis,** thoracolumbar **region**

M41.86 **Other forms of scoliosis,** lumbar **region**

M41.87 **Other forms of scoliosis,** lumbosacral **region**

M41.9 **Scoliosis, unspecified** ▽

✓4ᵗʰ **M42** **Spinal osteochondrosis**

✓5ᵗʰ **M42.0** Juvenile **osteochondrosis of spine**

Calvé's disease

Scheuermann's disease

EXCLUDES 1 *postural kyphosis (M40.0)*

M42.00 **Juvenile osteochondrosis of spine, site unspecified** ▽

M42.01 **Juvenile osteochondrosis of spine, occipito-atlanto-axial region**

M42.02 **Juvenile osteochondrosis of spine,** cervical **region**

M42.03 **Juvenile osteochondrosis of spine,** cervicothoracic **region**

M42.04 **Juvenile osteochondrosis of spine,** thoracic **region**

M42.05 **Juvenile osteochondrosis of spine,** thoracolumbar **region**

M42.06 **Juvenile osteochondrosis of spine,** lumbar **region**

M42.07 **Juvenile osteochondrosis of spine,** lumbosacral **region**

M42.08 **Juvenile osteochondrosis of spine,** sacral and sacrococcygeal **region**

M42.09 **Juvenile osteochondrosis of spine,** multiple sites **in spine**

✓5ᵗʰ **M42.1** Adult **osteochondrosis of spine**

M42.10 **Adult osteochondrosis of spine, site unspecified** A ▽

M42.11 **Adult osteochondrosis of spine, occipito-atlanto-axial region** A

M42.12 **Adult osteochondrosis of spine,** cervical **region** A

M42.13 **Adult osteochondrosis of spine,** cervicothoracic **region** A

M42.14 **Adult osteochondrosis of spine,** thoracic **region** A

M42.15 **Adult osteochondrosis of spine,** thoracolumbar **region** A

M42.16 **Adult osteochondrosis of spine,** lumbar **region** A

M42.17 **Adult osteochondrosis of spine,** lumbosacral **region** A

M42.18 **Adult osteochondrosis of spine,** sacral and sacrococcygeal **region** A

M42.19 **Adult osteochondrosis of spine,** multiple sites **in spine** A

M42.9 **Spinal osteochondrosis, unspecified** ▽

✓4ᵗʰ **M43** **Other deforming dorsopathies**

EXCLUDES 1 *congenital spondylolysis and spondylolisthesis (Q76.2)*
hemivertebra (Q76.3-Q76.4)
Klippel-Feil syndrome (Q76.1)
lumbarization and sacralization (Q76.4)
platyspondylisis (Q76.4)
spina bifida occulta (Q76.0)
spinal curvature in osteoporosis (M80.-)
spinal curvature in Paget's disease of bone [osteitis deformans] (M88.-)

✓5ᵗʰ **M43.0** **Spondylolysis**

EXCLUDES 1 *congenital spondylolysis (Q76.2)*
spondylolisthesis (M43.1)

M43.00 **Spondylolysis, site unspecified** ▽

M43.01 **Spondylolysis,** occipito-atlanto-axial **region**

M43.02 **Spondylolysis,** cervical **region**

M43.03 **Spondylolysis,** cervicothoracic **region**

M43.04 **Spondylolysis,** thoracic **region**

M43.05 **Spondylolysis,** thoracolumbar **region**

M43.06 **Spondylolysis,** lumbar **region**

M43.07 **Spondylolysis,** lumbosacral **region**

M43.08 **Spondylolysis,** sacral and sacrococcygeal **region**

M43.09 **Spondylolysis,** multiple sites **in spine**

✓5ᵗʰ **M43.1** **Spondylolisthesis**

EXCLUDES 1 *acute traumatic of lumbosacral region (S33.1)*
acute traumatic of sites other than lumbosacral—code to Fracture, vertebra, by region
congenital spondylolisthesis (Q76.2)

M43.10 **Spondylolisthesis, site unspecified** ▽

M43.11 **Spondylolisthesis,** occipito-atlanto-axial **region**

M43.12 **Spondylolisthesis,** cervical **region**

M43.13 **Spondylolisthesis,** cervicothoracic **region**

M43.14 **Spondylolisthesis,** thoracic **region**

M43.15 **Spondylolisthesis,** thoracolumbar **region**

M43.16 **Spondylolisthesis,** lumbar **region**

M43.17 **Spondylolisthesis,** lumbosacral **region**

M43.18 **Spondylolisthesis,** sacral and sacrococcygeal **region**

M43.19 **Spondylolisthesis,** multiple sites **in spine**

✓5ᵗʰ **M43.2** **Fusion of spine**

Ankylosis of spinal joint

EXCLUDES 1 *ankylosing spondylitis (M45.0-)*
congenital fusion of spine (Q76.4)

EXCLUDES 2 *arthrodesis status (Z98.1)*
pseudoarthrosis after fusion or arthrodesis (M96.0)

M43.20 **Fusion of spine, site unspecified** ▽

M43.21 **Fusion of spine,** occipito-atlanto-axial **region**

M43.22 **Fusion of spine,** cervical **region**

M43.23 **Fusion of spine,** cervicothoracic **region**

M43.24 **Fusion of spine,** thoracic **region**

M43.25 **Fusion of spine,** thoracolumbar **region**

M43.26 **Fusion of spine,** lumbar **region**

M43.27 **Fusion of spine,** lumbosacral **region**

M43.28 **Fusion of spine,** sacral and sacrococcygeal **region**

M43.3 **Recurrent atlantoaxial dislocation with myelopathy**

M43.4 **Other recurrent atlantoaxial dislocation**

✓5ᵗʰ **M43.5** **Other recurrent vertebral dislocation**

EXCLUDES 1 *biomechanical lesions NEC (M99.-)*

✓6ᵗʰ **M43.5X** **Other recurrent vertebral dislocation**

M43.5X2 **Other recurrent vertebral dislocation,** cervical **region**

M43.5X3 **Other recurrent vertebral dislocation,** cervicothoracic **region**

M43.5X4 **Other recurrent vertebral dislocation,** thoracic **region**

✓ Additional Character Req   ✓x7ᵗʰ Placeholder Alert   Case-Mix Diagnosis   Manifestation   ▽ Unspecified Dx   EXCLUDES 1 Not coded here   EXCLUDES 2 Not included here

ICD-10-CM 2018   755

M43.5X5 Other recurrent vertebral dislocation, thoracolumbar region

M43.5X6 Other recurrent vertebral dislocation, lumbar region

M43.5X7 Other recurrent vertebral dislocation, lumbosacral region

M43.5X8 Other recurrent vertebral dislocation, sacral and sacrococcygeal region

M43.5X9 Other recurrent vertebral dislocation, site unspecified ▽

M43.6 Torticollis
> EXCLUDES 1 *congenital (sternomastoid) torticollis (Q68.0)*
> *current injury—see Injury, of spine, by body region*
> *ocular torticollis (R29.891)*
> *psychogenic torticollis (F45.8)*
> *spasmodic torticollis (G24.3)*
> *torticollis due to birth injury (P15.2)*

✓5th **M43.8 Other specified deforming dorsopathies**
> EXCLUDES 2 *kyphosis and lordosis (M40.-)*
> *scoliosis (M41.-)*

✓6th **M43.8X Other specified deforming dorsopathies**

M43.8X1 Other specified deforming dorsopathies, occipito-atlanto-axial region

M43.8X2 Other specified deforming dorsopathies, cervical region

M43.8X3 Other specified deforming dorsopathies, cervicothoracic region

M43.8X4 Other specified deforming dorsopathies, thoracic region

M43.8X5 Other specified deforming dorsopathies, thoracolumbar region

M43.8X6 Other specified deforming dorsopathies, lumbar region

M43.8X7 Other specified deforming dorsopathies, lumbosacral region

M43.8X8 Other specified deforming dorsopathies, sacral and sacrococcygeal region

M43.8X9 Other specified deforming dorsopathies, site unspecified ▽

M43.9 Deforming dorsopathy, unspecified ▽
> Curvature of spine NOS

Spondylopathies (M45-M49)

✓4th **M45 Ankylosing spondylitis**
> Rheumatoid arthritis of spine
> EXCLUDES 1 *arthropathy in Reiter's disease (M02.3-)*
> *juvenile (ankylosing) spondylitis (M08.1)*
> EXCLUDES 2 *Behçet's disease (M35.2)*

M45.0 Ankylosing spondylitis of multiple sites in spine

M45.1 Ankylosing spondylitis of occipito-atlanto-axial region

M45.2 Ankylosing spondylitis of cervical region

M45.3 Ankylosing spondylitis of cervicothoracic region

M45.4 Ankylosing spondylitis of thoracic region

M45.5 Ankylosing spondylitis of thoracolumbar region

M45.6 Ankylosing spondylitis lumbar region

M45.7 Ankylosing spondylitis of lumbosacral region

M45.8 Ankylosing spondylitis sacral and sacrococcygeal region

M45.9 Ankylosing spondylitis of unspecified sites in spine ▽

✓4th **M46 Other inflammatory spondylopathies**

✓5th **M46.0 Spinal enthesopathy**
> Disorder of ligamentous or muscular attachments of spine

M46.00 Spinal enthesopathy, site unspecified ▽

M46.01 Spinal enthesopathy, occipito-atlanto-axial region

M46.02 Spinal enthesopathy, cervical region

M46.03 Spinal enthesopathy, cervicothoracic region

M46.04 Spinal enthesopathy, thoracic region

M46.05 Spinal enthesopathy, thoracolumbar region

M46.06 Spinal enthesopathy, lumbar region

M46.07 Spinal enthesopathy, lumbosacral region

M46.08 Spinal enthesopathy, sacral and sacrococcygeal region

M46.09 Spinal enthesopathy, multiple sites in spine

M46.1 Sacroiliitis, not elsewhere classified
> **DEF:** Inflammation of sacroiliac joint (situated at juncture of sacrum and hip); characterized by pain in buttocks or lower back that can extend down one or both legs.

✓5th **M46.2 Osteomyelitis of vertebra**

M46.20 Osteomyelitis of vertebra, site unspecified ▽

M46.21 Osteomyelitis of vertebra, occipito-atlanto-axial region

M46.22 Osteomyelitis of vertebra, cervical region

M46.23 Osteomyelitis of vertebra, cervicothoracic region

M46.24 Osteomyelitis of vertebra, thoracic region

M46.25 Osteomyelitis of vertebra, thoracolumbar region

M46.26 Osteomyelitis of vertebra, lumbar region

M46.27 Osteomyelitis of vertebra, lumbosacral region

M46.28 Osteomyelitis of vertebra, sacral and sacrococcygeal region

✓5th **M46.3 Infection of intervertebral disc (pyogenic)**
> Use additional code (B95-B97) to identify infectious agent

M46.30 Infection of intervertebral disc (pyogenic), site unspecified ▽

M46.31 Infection of intervertebral disc (pyogenic), occipito-atlanto-axial region

M46.32 Infection of intervertebral disc (pyogenic), cervical region

M46.33 Infection of intervertebral disc (pyogenic), cervicothoracic region

M46.34 Infection of intervertebral disc (pyogenic), thoracic region

M46.35 Infection of intervertebral disc (pyogenic), thoracolumbar region

M46.36 Infection of intervertebral disc (pyogenic), lumbar region

M46.37 Infection of intervertebral disc (pyogenic), lumbosacral region

M46.38 Infection of intervertebral disc (pyogenic), sacral and sacrococcygeal region

M46.39 Infection of intervertebral disc (pyogenic), multiple sites in spine

✓5th **M46.4 Discitis, unspecified**

M46.40 Discitis, unspecified, site unspecified ▽

M46.41 Discitis, unspecified, occipito-atlanto-axial region ▽

M46.42 Discitis, unspecified, cervical region ▽

M46.43 Discitis, unspecified, cervicothoracic region ▽

M46.44 Discitis, unspecified, thoracic region ▽

M46.45 Discitis, unspecified, thoracolumbar region ▽

M46.46 Discitis, unspecified, lumbar region ▽

M46.47 Discitis, unspecified, lumbosacral region ▽

M46.48 Discitis, unspecified, sacral and sacrococcygeal region ▽

M46.49 Discitis, unspecified, multiple sites in spine ▽

✓5th **M46.5 Other infective spondylopathies**

M46.50 Other infective spondylopathies, site unspecified ▽

M46.51 Other infective spondylopathies, occipito-atlanto-axial region

M46.52 Other infective spondylopathies, cervical region

M46.53 Other infective spondylopathies, cervicothoracic region

M46.54 Other infective spondylopathies, thoracic region

M46.55 Other infective spondylopathies, thoracolumbar region

M46.56 Other infective spondylopathies, lumbar region

M46.57 Other infective spondylopathies, lumbosacral region

M46.58 Other infective spondylopathies, sacral and sacrococcygeal region

M46.59 Other infective spondylopathies, multiple sites in spine

✓5th **M46.8 Other specified inflammatory spondylopathies**

M46.80 Other specified inflammatory spondylopathies, site unspecified ▽

M46.81 Other specified inflammatory spondylopathies, occipito-atlanto-axial region

M46.82 Other specified inflammatory spondylopathies, cervical region

Ⓝ Newborn: 0   Ⓟ Pediatric: 0-17   Ⓜ Maternity: 12-55   Ⓐ Adult: 15-124   **NRS** Nonroutine supply Dx   **NC Dx** Noncancer Dx   **PDx** Primary Dx   ▶◀ Revised Text   ● New Code   ▲ Revised Title

756   ICD-10-CM 2018

M46.83 **Other specified inflammatory spondylopathies, cervicothoracic region**

M46.84 **Other specified inflammatory spondylopathies, thoracic region**

M46.85 **Other specified inflammatory spondylopathies, thoracolumbar region**

M46.86 **Other specified inflammatory spondylopathies, lumbar region**

M46.87 **Other specified inflammatory spondylopathies, lumbosacral region**

M46.88 **Other specified inflammatory spondylopathies, sacral and sacrococcygeal region**

M46.89 **Other specified inflammatory spondylopathies, multiple sites in spine**

✓5ᵗʰ M46.9 **Unspecified inflammatory spondylopathy**

M46.90 **Unspecified inflammatory spondylopathy, site unspecified** ▽

M46.91 **Unspecified inflammatory spondylopathy, occipito-atlanto-axial region** ▽

M46.92 **Unspecified inflammatory spondylopathy, cervical region** ▽

M46.93 **Unspecified inflammatory spondylopathy, cervicothoracic region** ▽

M46.94 **Unspecified inflammatory spondylopathy, thoracic region** ▽

M46.95 **Unspecified inflammatory spondylopathy, thoracolumbar region** ▽

M46.96 **Unspecified inflammatory spondylopathy, lumbar region** ▽

M46.97 **Unspecified inflammatory spondylopathy, lumbosacral region** ▽

M46.98 **Unspecified inflammatory spondylopathy, sacral and sacrococcygeal region** ▽

M46.99 **Unspecified inflammatory spondylopathy, multiple sites in spine** ▽

✓4ᵗʰ **M47 Spondylosis**
     INCLUDES   arthrosis or osteoarthritis of spine
                   degeneration of facet joints

✓5ᵗʰ M47.0 **Anterior spinal and vertebral artery** compression syndromes

✓6ᵗʰ M47.01 **Anterior spinal artery** compression syndromes

M47.011 **Anterior spinal artery compression syndromes, occipito-atlanto-axial region**

M47.012 **Anterior spinal artery compression syndromes, cervical region**

M47.013 **Anterior spinal artery compression syndromes, cervicothoracic region**

M47.014 **Anterior spinal artery compression syndromes, thoracic region**

M47.015 **Anterior spinal artery compression syndromes, thoracolumbar region**

M47.016 **Anterior spinal artery compression syndromes, lumbar region**

M47.019 **Anterior spinal artery compression syndromes, site unspecified** ▽

✓6ᵗʰ M47.02 **Vertebral artery** compression syndromes

M47.021 **Vertebral artery compression syndromes, occipito-atlanto-axial region**

M47.022 **Vertebral artery compression syndromes, cervical region**

M47.029 **Vertebral artery compression syndromes, site unspecified** ▽

✓5ᵗʰ M47.1 **Other spondylosis** with myelopathy
     Spondylogenic compression of spinal cord
     EXCLUDES 1   *vertebral subluxation (M43.3-M43.5X9)*

M47.10 **Other spondylosis with myelopathy, site unspecified** ▽

M47.11 **Other spondylosis with myelopathy, occipito-atlanto-axial region**

M47.12 **Other spondylosis with myelopathy, cervical region**

M47.13 **Other spondylosis with myelopathy, cervicothoracic region**

M47.14 **Other spondylosis with myelopathy, thoracic region**

M47.15 **Other spondylosis with myelopathy, thoracolumbar region**

M47.16 **Other spondylosis with myelopathy, lumbar region**

✓5ᵗʰ M47.2 **Other spondylosis** with radiculopathy

M47.20 **Other spondylosis with radiculopathy, site unspecified** ▽

M47.21 **Other spondylosis with radiculopathy, occipito-atlanto-axial region**

M47.22 **Other spondylosis with radiculopathy, cervical region**

M47.23 **Other spondylosis with radiculopathy, cervicothoracic region**

M47.24 **Other spondylosis with radiculopathy, thoracic region**

M47.25 **Other spondylosis with radiculopathy, thoracolumbar region**

M47.26 **Other spondylosis with radiculopathy, lumbar region**

M47.27 **Other spondylosis with radiculopathy, lumbosacral region**

M47.28 **Other spondylosis with radiculopathy, sacral and sacrococcygeal region**

✓5ᵗʰ M47.8 **Other** spondylosis

✓6ᵗʰ M47.81 **Spondylosis** without myelopathy or radiculopathy

M47.811 **Spondylosis without myelopathy or radiculopathy, occipito-atlanto-axial region**

M47.812 **Spondylosis without myelopathy or radiculopathy, cervical region**

M47.813 **Spondylosis without myelopathy or radiculopathy, cervicothoracic region**

M47.814 **Spondylosis without myelopathy or radiculopathy, thoracic region**

M47.815 **Spondylosis without myelopathy or radiculopathy, thoracolumbar region**

M47.816 **Spondylosis without myelopathy or radiculopathy, lumbar region**

M47.817 **Spondylosis without myelopathy or radiculopathy, lumbosacral region**

M47.818 **Spondylosis without myelopathy or radiculopathy, sacral and sacrococcygeal region**

M47.819 **Spondylosis without myelopathy or radiculopathy, site unspecified** ▽

✓6ᵗʰ M47.89 **Other** spondylosis

M47.891 **Other spondylosis, occipito-atlanto-axial region**

M47.892 **Other spondylosis, cervical region**

M47.893 **Other spondylosis, cervicothoracic region**

M47.894 **Other spondylosis, thoracic region**

M47.895 **Other spondylosis, thoracolumbar region**

M47.896 **Other spondylosis, lumbar region**

M47.897 **Other spondylosis, lumbosacral region**

M47.898 **Other spondylosis, sacral and sacrococcygeal region**

M47.899 **Other spondylosis, site unspecified** ▽

M47.9 **Spondylosis, unspecified** ▽

✓4ᵗʰ **M48 Other spondylopathies**

✓5ᵗʰ M48.0 **Spinal stenosis**
     Caudal stenosis

M48.00 **Spinal stenosis, site unspecified** ▽

M48.01 **Spinal stenosis, occipito-atlanto-axial region**

M48.02 **Spinal stenosis, cervical region**

M48.03 **Spinal stenosis, cervicothoracic region**

M48.04 **Spinal stenosis, thoracic region**

M48.05 **Spinal stenosis, thoracolumbar region**

✓6ᵗʰ M48.06 **Spinal stenosis, lumbar region**
     DEF: Spinal canal narrowing in the lumbar area with nerve root compression, causing muscle pain, fatigue, and weakness during extension of the lumbar spine; pain is relieved by sitting or bending.

● M48.061 **Spinal stenosis, lumbar region** without neurogenic claudication
     Spinal stenosis, lumbar region NOS

● M48.062 **Spinal stenosis, lumbar region** with neurogenic claudication

M48.07 **Spinal stenosis, lumbosacral region**

M48.08 **Spinal stenosis, sacral and sacrococcygeal region**

✓ Additional Character Req   ✓7ᵗʰ Placeholder Alert   Case-Mix Diagnosis   Manifestation   ▽ Unspecified Dx   EXCLUDES 1 Not coded here   EXCLUDES 2 Not included here

ICD-10-CM 2018   757

✓5ᵗʰ **M48.1 Ankylosing hyperostosis [Forestier]**
Diffuse idiopathic skeletal hyperostosis [DISH]

   M48.10 Ankylosing hyperostosis [Forestier], site unspecified ▽

   M48.11 Ankylosing hyperostosis [Forestier], occipito-atlanto-axial region

   M48.12 Ankylosing hyperostosis [Forestier], cervical region

   M48.13 Ankylosing hyperostosis [Forestier], cervicothoracic region

   M48.14 Ankylosing hyperostosis [Forestier], thoracic region

   M48.15 Ankylosing hyperostosis [Forestier], thoracolumbar region

   M48.16 Ankylosing hyperostosis [Forestier], lumbar region

   M48.17 Ankylosing hyperostosis [Forestier], lumbosacral region

   M48.18 Ankylosing hyperostosis [Forestier], sacral and sacrococcygeal region

   M48.19 Ankylosing hyperostosis [Forestier], multiple sites in spine

✓5ᵗʰ **M48.2 Kissing spine**

   M48.20 Kissing spine, site unspecified ▽

   M48.21 Kissing spine, occipito-atlanto-axial region

   M48.22 Kissing spine, cervical region

   M48.23 Kissing spine, cervicothoracic region

   M48.24 Kissing spine, thoracic region

   M48.25 Kissing spine, thoracolumbar region

   M48.26 Kissing spine, lumbar region

   M48.27 Kissing spine, lumbosacral region

✓5ᵗʰ **M48.3 Traumatic spondylopathy**

   M48.30 Traumatic spondylopathy, site unspecified ▽

   M48.31 Traumatic spondylopathy, occipito-atlanto-axial region

   M48.32 Traumatic spondylopathy, cervical region

   M48.33 Traumatic spondylopathy, cervicothoracic region

   M48.34 Traumatic spondylopathy, thoracic region

   M48.35 Traumatic spondylopathy, thoracolumbar region

   M48.36 Traumatic spondylopathy, lumbar region

   M48.37 Traumatic spondylopathy, lumbosacral region

   M48.38 Traumatic spondylopathy, sacral and sacrococcygeal region

✓5ᵗʰ **M48.4 Fatigue fracture of vertebra**
Stress fracture of vertebra

   EXCLUDES 1   *pathological fracture NOS (M84.4-)*
     pathological fracture of vertebra due to neoplasm (M84.58)
     pathological fracture of vertebra due to other diagnosis (M84.68)
     pathological fracture of vertebra due to osteoporosis (M80.-)
     traumatic fracture of vertebrae (S12.0-S12.3-, S22.0-, S32.0-)

The appropriate 7th character is to be added to each code from subcategory M48.4.
A   initial encounter for fracture
D   subsequent encounter for fracture with routine healing
G   subsequent encounter for fracture with delayed healing
S   sequela of fracture

  ✓x7ᵗʰ **M48.40 Fatigue fracture of vertebra, site unspecified** ▽

  ✓x7ᵗʰ **M48.41 Fatigue fracture of vertebra, occipito-atlanto-axial region**

  ✓x7ᵗʰ **M48.42 Fatigue fracture of vertebra, cervical region**

  ✓x7ᵗʰ **M48.43 Fatigue fracture of vertebra, cervicothoracic region**

  ✓x7ᵗʰ **M48.44 Fatigue fracture of vertebra, thoracic region**

  ✓x7ᵗʰ **M48.45 Fatigue fracture of vertebra, thoracolumbar region**

  ✓x7ᵗʰ **M48.46 Fatigue fracture of vertebra, lumbar region**

  ✓x7ᵗʰ **M48.47 Fatigue fracture of vertebra, lumbosacral region**

  ✓x7ᵗʰ **M48.48 Fatigue fracture of vertebra, sacral and sacrococcygeal region**

✓5ᵗʰ **M48.5 Collapsed vertebra, not elsewhere classified**
Collapsed vertebra NOS
Compression fracture of vertebra NOS
Wedging of vertebra NOS

   EXCLUDES 1   *current injury—see Injury of spine, by body region*
     fatigue fracture of vertebra (M48.4)
     pathological fracture of vertebra due to neoplasm (M84.58)
     pathological fracture of vertebra due to other diagnosis (M84.68)
     pathological fracture of vertebra due to osteoporosis (M80.-)
     pathological fracture NOS (M84.4-)
     stress fracture of vertebra (M48.4-)
     traumatic fracture of vertebra (S12-, S22-, S32-)

The appropriate 7th character is to be added to each code from subcategory M48.5.
A   initial encounter for fracture
D   subsequent encounter for fracture with routine healing
G   subsequent encounter for fracture with delayed healing
S   sequela of fracture

  1 ✓x7ᵗʰ **M48.50 Collapsed vertebra, not elsewhere classified, site unspecified** ▽

  1 ✓x7ᵗʰ **M48.51 Collapsed vertebra, not elsewhere classified, occipito-atlanto-axial region**

  1 ✓x7ᵗʰ **M48.52 Collapsed vertebra, not elsewhere classified, cervical region**

  1 ✓x7ᵗʰ **M48.53 Collapsed vertebra, not elsewhere classified, cervicothoracic region**

  1 ✓x7ᵗʰ **M48.54 Collapsed vertebra, not elsewhere classified, thoracic region**

  1 ✓x7ᵗʰ **M48.55 Collapsed vertebra, not elsewhere classified, thoracolumbar region**

  1 ✓x7ᵗʰ **M48.56 Collapsed vertebra, not elsewhere classified, lumbar region**

  1 ✓x7ᵗʰ **M48.57 Collapsed vertebra, not elsewhere classified, lumbosacral region**

  1 ✓x7ᵗʰ **M48.58 Collapsed vertebra, not elsewhere classified, sacral and sacrococcygeal region**

✓5ᵗʰ **M48.8 Other specified spondylopathies**
Ossification of posterior longitudinal ligament

  ✓6ᵗʰ **M48.8X Other specified spondylopathies**

    M48.8X1 Other specified spondylopathies, occipito-atlanto-axial region

    M48.8X2 Other specified spondylopathies, cervical region

    M48.8X3 Other specified spondylopathies, cervicothoracic region

    M48.8X4 Other specified spondylopathies, thoracic region

    M48.8X5 Other specified spondylopathies, thoracolumbar region

    M48.8X6 Other specified spondylopathies, lumbar region

    M48.8X7 Other specified spondylopathies, lumbosacral region

    M48.8X8 Other specified spondylopathies, sacral and sacrococcygeal region

    M48.8X9 Other specified spondylopathies, site unspecified ▽

 M48.9 Spondylopathy, unspecified ▽

---

1   Case-mix diagnosis with 7th character indicating subsequent encounter.

Ⓝ Newborn: 0   Ⓟ Pediatric: 0-17   Ⓜ Maternity: 12-55   Ⓐ Adult: 15-124   **NRS** Nonroutine supply Dx   **NCDx** Noncancer Dx   **PDx** Primary Dx   ▶◀ Revised Text   ● New Code   ▲ Revised Title

758   ICD-10-CM 2018

✔4ᵗʰ M49 Spondylopathies in diseases classified elsewhere

INCLUDES curvature of spine in diseases classified elsewhere
deformity of spine in diseases classified elsewhere
kyphosis in diseases classified elsewhere
scoliosis in diseases classified elsewhere
spondylopathy in diseases classified elsewhere

Code first underlying disease, such as:
brucellosis (A23.-)
Charcôt-Marie-Tooth disease (G60.0)
enterobacterial infections (A01-A04)
osteitis fibrosa cystica (E21.0)

EXCLUDES 1 curvature of spine in tuberculosis [Pott's] (A18.01)
enteropathic arthropathies (M07.-)
gonococcal spondylitis (A54.41)
neuropathic [tabes dorsalis] spondylitis (A52.11)
neuropathic spondylopathy in syringomyelia (G95.0)
neuropathic spondylopathy in tabes dorsalis (A52.11)
nonsyphilitic neuropathic spondylopathy NEC (G98.0)
spondylitis in syphilis (acquired) (A52.77)
tuberculous spondylitis (A18.01)
typhoid fever spondylitis (A01.05)

✔5ᵗʰ M49.8 Spondylopathy in diseases classified elsewhere

M49.80 *Spondylopathy in diseases classified elsewhere, site unspecified* ▽

M49.81 *Spondylopathy in diseases classified elsewhere, occipito-atlanto-axial region*

M49.82 *Spondylopathy in diseases classified elsewhere, cervical region*

M49.83 *Spondylopathy in diseases classified elsewhere, cervicothoracic region*

M49.84 *Spondylopathy in diseases classified elsewhere, thoracic region*

M49.85 *Spondylopathy in diseases classified elsewhere, thoracolumbar region*

M49.86 *Spondylopathy in diseases classified elsewhere, lumbar region*

M49.87 *Spondylopathy in diseases classified elsewhere, lumbosacral region*

M49.88 *Spondylopathy in diseases classified elsewhere, sacral and sacrococcygeal region*

M49.89 *Spondylopathy in diseases classified elsewhere, multiple sites in spine*

Other dorsopathies (M50-M54)

EXCLUDES 1 current injury—see injury of spine by body region
discitis NOS (M46.4-)

✔4ᵗʰ M50 Cervical disc disorders

NOTE Code to the most superior level of disorder.
INCLUDES cervicothoracic disc disorders with cervicalgia
cervicothoracic disc disorders
AHA: 2016, 1Q, 17

✔5ᵗʰ M50.0 Cervical disc disorder with myelopathy

M50.00 **Cervical disc disorder with myelopathy, unspecified cervical region** ▽

M50.01 **Cervical disc disorder with myelopathy, high cervical region**
C2-C3 disc disorder with myelopathy
C3-C4 disc disorder with myelopathy

✔6ᵗʰ M50.02 Cervical disc disorder with myelopathy, mid-cervical region

M50.020 **Cervical disc disorder with myelopathy, mid-cervical region, unspecified level** ▽

M50.021 **Cervical disc disorder at C4-C5 level with myelopathy**
C4-C5 disc disorder with myelopathy

M50.022 **Cervical disc disorder at C5-C6 level with myelopathy**
C5-C6 disc disorder with myelopathy

M50.023 **Cervical disc disorder at C6-C7 level with myelopathy**
C6-C7 disc disorder with myelopathy

M50.03 **Cervical disc disorder with myelopathy, cervicothoracic region**
C7-T1 disc disorder with myelopathy

✔5ᵗʰ M50.1 Cervical disc disorder with radiculopathy

EXCLUDES 2 brachial radiculitis NOS (M54.13)

M50.10 **Cervical disc disorder with radiculopathy, unspecified cervical region** ▽

M50.11 **Cervical disc disorder with radiculopathy, high cervical region**
C2-C3 disc disorder with radiculopathy
C3 radiculopathy due to disc disorder
C3-C4 disc disorder with radiculopathy
C4 radiculopathy due to disc disorder

✔6ᵗʰ M50.12 Cervical disc disorder with radiculopathy, mid-cervical region

M50.120 **Mid-cervical disc disorder, unspecified** ▽

M50.121 **Cervical disc disorder at C4-C5 level with radiculopathy**
C4-C5 disc disorder with radiculopathy
C5 radiculopathy due to disc disorder

M50.122 **Cervical disc disorder at C5-C6 level with radiculopathy**
C5-C6 disc disorder with radiculopathy
C6 radiculopathy due to disc disorder

M50.123 **Cervical disc disorder at C6-C7 level with radiculopathy**
C6-C7 disc disorder with radiculopathy
C7 radiculopathy due to disc disorder

M50.13 **Cervical disc disorder with radiculopathy, cervicothoracic region**
C7-T1 disc disorder with radiculopathy
C8 radiculopathy due to disc disorder

✔5ᵗʰ M50.2 Other cervical disc displacement

M50.20 **Other cervical disc displacement, unspecified cervical region** ▽

M50.21 **Other cervical disc displacement, high cervical region**
Other C2-C3 cervical disc displacement
Other C3-C4 cervical disc displacement

✔6ᵗʰ M50.22 Other cervical disc displacement, mid-cervical region

M50.220 **Other cervical disc displacement, mid-cervical region, unspecified level** ▽

M50.221 **Other cervical disc displacement at C4-C5 level**
Other C4-C5 cervical disc displacement

M50.222 **Other cervical disc displacement at C5-C6 level**
Other C5-C6 cervical disc displacement

M50.223 **Other cervical disc displacement at C6-C7 level**
Other C6-C7 cervical disc displacement

M50.23 **Other cervical disc displacement, cervicothoracic region**
Other C7-T1 cervical disc displacement

✔5ᵗʰ M50.3 Other cervical disc degeneration

M50.30 **Other cervical disc degeneration, unspecified cervical region** ▽

M50.31 **Other cervical disc degeneration, high cervical region**
Other C2-C3 cervical disc degeneration
Other C3-C4 cervical disc degeneration

✔6ᵗʰ M50.32 Other cervical disc degeneration, mid-cervical region

M50.320 **Other cervical disc degeneration, mid-cervical region, unspecified level** ▽

M50.321 **Other cervical disc degeneration at C4-C5 level**
Other C4-C5 cervical disc degeneration

M50.322 **Other cervical disc degeneration at C5-C6 level**
Other C5-C6 cervical disc degeneration

M50.323 **Other cervical disc degeneration at C6-C7 level**
Other C6-C7 cervical disc degeneration

M50.33 **Other cervical disc degeneration, cervicothoracic region**
Other C7-T1 cervical disc degeneration

✔5ᵗʰ M50.8 Other cervical disc disorders

M50.80 **Other cervical disc disorders, unspecified cervical region** ▽

M50.81 **Other cervical disc disorders, high cervical region**
Other C2-C3 cervical disc disorders
Other C3-C4 cervical disc disorders

✔ Additional Character Req   ✔7ᵗʰ Placeholder Alert   Case-Mix Diagnosis   Manifestation   ▽ Unspecified Dx   **EXCLUDES 1** Not coded here   **EXCLUDES 2** Not included here

Chapter 13. Diseases of the Musculoskeletal System and Connective Tissue

 ✓6ᵗʰ **M50.82** **Other cervical disc disorders, mid-cervical region**

    M50.820 **Other cervical disc disorders, mid-cervical region, unspecified level** ▽

    M50.821 **Other cervical disc disorders at C4-C5 level**
        Other C4-C5 cervical disc disorders

    M50.822 **Other cervical disc disorders at C5-C6 level**
        Other C5-C6 cervical disc disorders

    M50.823 **Other cervical disc disorders at C6-C7 level**
        Other C6-C7 cervical disc disorders

 M50.83 **Other cervical disc disorders, cervicothoracic region**
    Other C7-T1 cervical disc disorders

 ✓5ᵗʰ **M50.9** **Cervical disc disorder, unspecified**

    M50.90 **Cervical disc disorder, unspecified, unspecified cervical region** ▽

    M50.91 **Cervical disc disorder, unspecified, high cervical region** ▽
        C2-C3 cervical disc disorder, unspecified
        C3-C4 cervical disc disorder, unspecified

 ✓6ᵗʰ **M50.92** **Cervical disc disorder, unspecified, mid-cervical region**

    M50.920 **Unspecified cervical disc disorder, mid-cervical region, unspecified level** ▽

    M50.921 **Unspecified cervical disc disorder at C4-C5 level** ▽
        Unspecified C4-C5 cervical disc disorder

    M50.922 **Unspecified cervical disc disorder at C5-C6 level** ▽
        Unspecified C5-C6 cervical disc disorder

    M50.923 **Unspecified cervical disc disorder at C6-C7 level** ▽
        Unspecified C6-C7 cervical disc disorder

 M50.93 **Cervical disc disorder, unspecified, cervicothoracic region** ▽
    C7-T1 cervical disc disorder, unspecified

 ✓4ᵗʰ **M51** **Thoracic, thoracolumbar, and lumbosacral intervertebral disc disorders**
    EXCLUDES 2 cervical and cervicothoracic disc disorders (M50.-)
        sacral and sacrococcygeal disorders (M53.3)

 ✓5ᵗʰ **M51.0** **Thoracic, thoracolumbar and lumbosacral intervertebral disc disorders with myelopathy**

    M51.04 **Intervertebral disc disorders with myelopathy, thoracic region**

    M51.05 **Intervertebral disc disorders with myelopathy, thoracolumbar region**

    M51.06 **Intervertebral disc disorders with myelopathy, lumbar region**

 ✓5ᵗʰ **M51.1** **Thoracic, thoracolumbar and lumbosacral intervertebral disc disorders with radiculopathy**
    Sciatica due to intervertebral disc disorder
    EXCLUDES 1 lumbar radiculitis NOS (M54.16)
        sciatica NOS (M54.3)

    M51.14 **Intervertebral disc disorders with radiculopathy, thoracic region**

    M51.15 **Intervertebral disc disorders with radiculopathy, thoracolumbar region**

    M51.16 **Intervertebral disc disorders with radiculopathy, lumbar region**

    M51.17 **Intervertebral disc disorders with radiculopathy, lumbosacral region**

 ✓5ᵗʰ **M51.2** **Other thoracic, thoracolumbar and lumbosacral intervertebral disc displacement**
    Lumbago due to displacement of intervertebral disc

    M51.24 **Other intervertebral disc displacement, thoracic region**

    M51.25 **Other intervertebral disc displacement, thoracolumbar region**

    M51.26 **Other intervertebral disc displacement, lumbar region**

    M51.27 **Other intervertebral disc displacement, lumbosacral region**

Displacement Intervertebral Disc

Normal Top View — Lamina, Ligamentum flavum, Disc annulus, Nucleus pulposus

Herniated Top View — Nucleus pulposus, Spinal cord, Herniates through annulus, Spinal nerve

 ✓5ᵗʰ **M51.3** **Other thoracic, thoracolumbar and lumbosacral intervertebral disc degeneration**
    AHA: 2013, 3Q, 22

    M51.34 **Other intervertebral disc degeneration, thoracic region**

    M51.35 **Other intervertebral disc degeneration, thoracolumbar region**

    M51.36 **Other intervertebral disc degeneration, lumbar region**

    M51.37 **Other intervertebral disc degeneration, lumbosacral region**

 ✓5ᵗʰ **M51.4** **Schmorl's nodes**
    DEF: Irregular bone defect in the margin of the vertebral body; causes herniation into end plate of vertebral body.

    M51.44 **Schmorl's nodes, thoracic region**

    M51.45 **Schmorl's nodes, thoracolumbar region**

    M51.46 **Schmorl's nodes, lumbar region**

    M51.47 **Schmorl's nodes, lumbosacral region**

 ✓5ᵗʰ **M51.8** **Other thoracic, thoracolumbar and lumbosacral intervertebral disc disorders**

    M51.84 **Other intervertebral disc disorders, thoracic region**

    M51.85 **Other intervertebral disc disorders, thoracolumbar region**

    M51.86 **Other intervertebral disc disorders, lumbar region**

    M51.87 **Other intervertebral disc disorders, lumbosacral region**

 M51.9 **Unspecified thoracic, thoracolumbar and lumbosacral intervertebral disc disorder** ▽

 ✓4ᵗʰ **M53** **Other and unspecified dorsopathies, not elsewhere classified**

 M53.0 **Cervicocranial syndrome**
    Posterior cervical sympathetic syndrome

 M53.1 **Cervicobrachial syndrome**
    EXCLUDES 2 cervical disc disorder (M50.-)
        thoracic outlet syndrome (G54.0)

 ✓5ᵗʰ **M53.2** **Spinal instabilities**

  ✓6ᵗʰ **M53.2X** **Spinal instabilities**

    M53.2X1 **Spinal instabilities, occipito-atlanto-axial region**

    M53.2X2 **Spinal instabilities, cervical region**

    M53.2X3 **Spinal instabilities, cervicothoracic region**

    M53.2X4 **Spinal instabilities, thoracic region**

    M53.2X5 **Spinal instabilities, thoracolumbar region**

    M53.2X6 **Spinal instabilities, lumbar region**

    M53.2X7 **Spinal instabilities, lumbosacral region**

    M53.2X8 **Spinal instabilities, sacral and sacrococcygeal region**

    M53.2X9 **Spinal instabilities, site unspecified** ▽

 M53.3 **Sacrococcygeal disorders, not elsewhere classified**
    Coccygodynia

 ✓5ᵗʰ **M53.8** **Other specified dorsopathies**

    M53.80 **Other specified dorsopathies, site unspecified** ▽

    M53.81 **Other specified dorsopathies, occipito-atlanto-axial region**

    M53.82 **Other specified dorsopathies, cervical region**

N Newborn: 0   P Pediatric: 0-17   M Maternity: 12-55   A Adult: 15-124   NRS Nonroutine supply Dx   NC Dx Noncancer Dx   PDx Primary Dx   ►◄ Revised Text   ● New Code   ▲ Revised Title

760   ICD-10-CM 2018

M53.83 Other specified dorsopathies, cervicothoracic region

M53.84 Other specified dorsopathies, thoracic region

M53.85 Other specified dorsopathies, thoracolumbar region

M53.86 Other specified dorsopathies, lumbar region

M53.87 Other specified dorsopathies, lumbosacral region

M53.88 Other specified dorsopathies, sacral and sacrococcygeal region

M53.9 Dorsopathy, unspecified   ▽

✓4ᵗʰ **M54 Dorsalgia**
> EXCLUDES 1   *psychogenic dorsalgia (F45.41)*

✓5ᵗʰ **M54.0 Panniculitis affecting regions of neck and back**
> EXCLUDES 1   *lupus panniculitis (L93.2)*
> *panniculitis NOS (M79.3)*
> *relapsing [Weber-Christian] panniculitis (M35.6)*

M54.00 Panniculitis affecting regions of neck and back, site unspecified   ▽

M54.01 Panniculitis affecting regions of neck and back, occipito-atlanto-axial region

M54.02 Panniculitis affecting regions of neck and back, cervical region

M54.03 Panniculitis affecting regions of neck and back, cervicothoracic region

M54.04 Panniculitis affecting regions of neck and back, thoracic region

M54.05 Panniculitis affecting regions of neck and back, thoracolumbar region

M54.06 Panniculitis affecting regions of neck and back, lumbar region

M54.07 Panniculitis affecting regions of neck and back, lumbosacral region

M54.08 Panniculitis affecting regions of neck and back, sacral and sacrococcygeal region

M54.09 Panniculitis affecting regions, neck and back, multiple sites in spine

✓5ᵗʰ **M54.1 Radiculopathy**
> Brachial neuritis or radiculitis NOS
> Lumbar neuritis or radiculitis NOS
> Lumbosacral neuritis or radiculitis NOS
> Thoracic neuritis or radiculitis NOS
> Radiculitis NOS
> EXCLUDES 1   *neuralgia and neuritis NOS (M79.2)*
> *radiculopathy with cervical disc disorder (M50.1)*
> *radiculopathy with lumbar and other intervertebral disc disorder (M51.1-)*
> *radiculopathy with spondylosis (M47.2-)*

M54.10 Radiculopathy, site unspecified   ▽

M54.11 Radiculopathy, occipito-atlanto-axial region

M54.12 Radiculopathy, cervical region

M54.13 Radiculopathy, cervicothoracic region

M54.14 Radiculopathy, thoracic region

M54.15 Radiculopathy, thoracolumbar region

M54.16 Radiculopathy, lumbar region

M54.17 Radiculopathy, lumbosacral region

M54.18 Radiculopathy, sacral and sacrococcygeal region

M54.2 Cervicalgia
> EXCLUDES 1   *cervicalgia due to intervertebral cervical disc disorder (M50.-)*

✓5ᵗʰ **M54.3 Sciatica**
> EXCLUDES 1   *lesion of sciatic nerve (G57.0)*
> *sciatica due to intervertebral disc disorder (M51.1-)*
> *sciatica with lumbago (M54.4-)*

M54.30 Sciatica, unspecified side   ▽

M54.31 Sciatica, right side

M54.32 Sciatica, left side

✓5ᵗʰ **M54.4 Lumbago with sciatica**
> EXCLUDES 1   *lumbago with sciatica due to intervertebral disc disorder (M51.1-)*
> AHA: 2016, 2Q, 7

M54.40 Lumbago with sciatica, unspecified side   ▽

M54.41 Lumbago with sciatica, right side

M54.42 Lumbago with sciatica, left side

M54.5 Low back pain
> Loin pain
> Lumbago NOS
> EXCLUDES 1   *low back strain (S39.012)*
> *lumbago due to intervertebral disc displacement (M51.2-)*
> *lumbago with sciatica (M54.4-)*

M54.6 Pain in thoracic spine
> EXCLUDES 1   *pain in thoracic spine due to intervertebral disc disorder (M51.-)*

✓5ᵗʰ **M54.8 Other dorsalgia**
> EXCLUDES 1   *dorsalgia in thoracic region (M54.6)*
> *low back pain (M54.5)*

M54.81 Occipital neuralgia

M54.89 Other dorsalgia

M54.9 Dorsalgia, unspecified   ▽
> Backache NOS   Back pain NOS

SOFT TISSUE DISORDERS (M60-M79)

Disorders of muscles (M60-M63)
> EXCLUDES 1   *dermatopolymyositis (M33.-)*
> *muscular dystrophies and myopathies (G71-G72)*
> *myopathy in amyloidosis (E85.-)*
> *myopathy in polyarteritis nodosa (M30.0)*
> *myopathy in rheumatoid arthritis (M05.32)*
> *myopathy in scleroderma (M34.-)*
> *myopathy in Sjögren's syndrome (M35.03)*
> *myopathy in systemic lupus erythematosus (M32.-)*

✓4ᵗʰ **M60 Myositis**
> EXCLUDES 2   *inclusion body myositis [IBM] (G72.41)*

✓5ᵗʰ **M60.0 Infective myositis**
> Tropical pyomyositis
> Use additional code (B95-B97) to identify infectious agent

✓6ᵗʰ **M60.00** Infective myositis, unspecified site

M60.000 Infective myositis, unspecified right arm
> Infective myositis, right upper limb NOS

M60.001 Infective myositis, unspecified left arm
> Infective myositis, left upper limb NOS

M60.002 Infective myositis, unspecified arm   ▽
> Infective myositis, upper limb NOS

M60.003 Infective myositis, unspecified right leg
> Infective myositis, right lower limb NOS

M60.004 Infective myositis, unspecified left leg
> Infective myositis, left lower limb NOS

M60.005 Infective myositis, unspecified leg   ▽
> Infective myositis, lower limb NOS

M60.009 Infective myositis, unspecified site   ▽

✓6ᵗʰ **M60.01** Infective myositis, shoulder

M60.011 Infective myositis, right shoulder

M60.012 Infective myositis, left shoulder

M60.019 Infective myositis, unspecified shoulder   ▽

✓6ᵗʰ **M60.02** Infective myositis, upper arm

M60.021 Infective myositis, right upper arm

M60.022 Infective myositis, left upper arm

M60.029 Infective myositis, unspecified upper arm   ▽

✓6ᵗʰ **M60.03** Infective myositis, forearm

M60.031 Infective myositis, right forearm

M60.032 Infective myositis, left forearm

M60.039 Infective myositis, unspecified forearm   ▽

✓6ᵗʰ **M60.04** Infective myositis, hand and fingers

M60.041 Infective myositis, right hand

M60.042 Infective myositis, left hand

M60.043 Infective myositis, unspecified hand   ▽

M60.044 Infective myositis, right finger(s)

M60.045 Infective myositis, left finger(s)

M60.046 Infective myositis, unspecified finger(s)   ▽

✓6ᵗʰ **M60.05** Infective myositis, thigh

M60.051 Infective myositis, right thigh

M60.052 Infective myositis, left thigh

M60.059 Infective myositis, unspecified thigh   ▽

✓6ᵗʰ **M60.06** Infective myositis, lower leg

M60.061 Infective myositis, right lower leg

✓ Additional Character Req   ✓x7ᵗʰ Placeholder Alert   Case-Mix Diagnosis   Manifestation   ▽ Unspecified Dx   EXCLUDES 1 Not coded here   EXCLUDES 2 Not included here

ICD-10-CM 2018   761

M60.062 Infective myositis, left lower leg
M60.069 Infective myositis, unspecified lower leg ▽

✓6ᵗʰ M60.07 Infective myositis, ankle, foot and toes
M60.070 Infective myositis, right ankle
M60.071 Infective myositis, left ankle
M60.072 Infective myositis, unspecified ankle ▽
M60.073 Infective myositis, right foot
M60.074 Infective myositis, left foot
M60.075 Infective myositis, unspecified foot ▽
M60.076 Infective myositis, right toe(s)
M60.077 Infective myositis, left toe(s)
M60.078 Infective myositis, unspecified toe(s) ▽
M60.08 Infective myositis, other site
M60.09 Infective myositis, multiple sites

✓5ᵗʰ M60.1 Interstitial myositis
M60.10 Interstitial myositis of unspecified site ▽

✓6ᵗʰ M60.11 Interstitial myositis, shoulder
M60.111 Interstitial myositis, right shoulder
M60.112 Interstitial myositis, left shoulder
M60.119 Interstitial myositis, unspecified shoulder ▽

✓6ᵗʰ M60.12 Interstitial myositis, upper arm
M60.121 Interstitial myositis, right upper arm
M60.122 Interstitial myositis, left upper arm
M60.129 Interstitial myositis, unspecified upper arm ▽

✓6ᵗʰ M60.13 Interstitial myositis, forearm
M60.131 Interstitial myositis, right forearm
M60.132 Interstitial myositis, left forearm
M60.139 Interstitial myositis, unspecified forearm ▽

✓6ᵗʰ M60.14 Interstitial myositis, hand
M60.141 Interstitial myositis, right hand
M60.142 Interstitial myositis, left hand
M60.149 Interstitial myositis, unspecified hand ▽

✓6ᵗʰ M60.15 Interstitial myositis, thigh
M60.151 Interstitial myositis, right thigh
M60.152 Interstitial myositis, left thigh
M60.159 Interstitial myositis, unspecified thigh ▽

✓6ᵗʰ M60.16 Interstitial myositis, lower leg
M60.161 Interstitial myositis, right lower leg
M60.162 Interstitial myositis, left lower leg
M60.169 Interstitial myositis, unspecified lower leg ▽

✓6ᵗʰ M60.17 Interstitial myositis, ankle and foot
M60.171 Interstitial myositis, right ankle and foot
M60.172 Interstitial myositis, left ankle and foot
M60.179 Interstitial myositis, unspecified ankle and foot ▽
M60.18 Interstitial myositis, other site
M60.19 Interstitial myositis, multiple sites

✓5ᵗʰ M60.2 Foreign body granuloma of soft tissue, not elsewhere classified
Use additional code to identify the type of retained foreign body (Z18.-)
EXCLUDES 1   foreign body granuloma of skin and subcutaneous tissue (L92.3)

M60.20 Foreign body granuloma of soft tissue, not elsewhere classified, unspecified site ▽

✓6ᵗʰ M60.21 Foreign body granuloma of soft tissue, not elsewhere classified, shoulder
M60.211 Foreign body granuloma of soft tissue, not elsewhere classified, right shoulder
M60.212 Foreign body granuloma of soft tissue, not elsewhere classified, left shoulder
M60.219 Foreign body granuloma of soft tissue, not elsewhere classified, unspecified shoulder ▽

✓6ᵗʰ M60.22 Foreign body granuloma of soft tissue, not elsewhere classified, upper arm
M60.221 Foreign body granuloma of soft tissue, not elsewhere classified, right upper arm

M60.222 Foreign body granuloma of soft tissue, not elsewhere classified, left upper arm
M60.229 Foreign body granuloma of soft tissue, not elsewhere classified, unspecified upper arm ▽

✓6ᵗʰ M60.23 Foreign body granuloma of soft tissue, not elsewhere classified, forearm
M60.231 Foreign body granuloma of soft tissue, not elsewhere classified, right forearm
M60.232 Foreign body granuloma of soft tissue, not elsewhere classified, left forearm
M60.239 Foreign body granuloma of soft tissue, not elsewhere classified, unspecified forearm ▽

✓6ᵗʰ M60.24 Foreign body granuloma of soft tissue, not elsewhere classified, hand
M60.241 Foreign body granuloma of soft tissue, not elsewhere classified, right hand
M60.242 Foreign body granuloma of soft tissue, not elsewhere classified, left hand
M60.249 Foreign body granuloma of soft tissue, not elsewhere classified, unspecified hand ▽

✓6ᵗʰ M60.25 Foreign body granuloma of soft tissue, not elsewhere classified, thigh
M60.251 Foreign body granuloma of soft tissue, not elsewhere classified, right thigh
M60.252 Foreign body granuloma of soft tissue, not elsewhere classified, left thigh
M60.259 Foreign body granuloma of soft tissue, not elsewhere classified, unspecified thigh ▽

✓6ᵗʰ M60.26 Foreign body granuloma of soft tissue, not elsewhere classified, lower leg
M60.261 Foreign body granuloma of soft tissue, not elsewhere classified, right lower leg
M60.262 Foreign body granuloma of soft tissue, not elsewhere classified, left lower leg
M60.269 Foreign body granuloma of soft tissue, not elsewhere classified, unspecified lower leg ▽

✓6ᵗʰ M60.27 Foreign body granuloma of soft tissue, not elsewhere classified, ankle and foot
M60.271 Foreign body granuloma of soft tissue, not elsewhere classified, right ankle and foot
M60.272 Foreign body granuloma of soft tissue, not elsewhere classified, left ankle and foot
M60.279 Foreign body granuloma of soft tissue, not elsewhere classified, unspecified ankle and foot ▽
M60.28 Foreign body granuloma of soft tissue, not elsewhere classified, other site

✓5ᵗʰ M60.8 Other myositis
M60.80 Other myositis, unspecified site ▽

✓6ᵗʰ M60.81 Other myositis shoulder
M60.811 Other myositis, right shoulder
M60.812 Other myositis, left shoulder
M60.819 Other myositis, unspecified shoulder ▽

✓6ᵗʰ M60.82 Other myositis, upper arm
M60.821 Other myositis, right upper arm
M60.822 Other myositis, left upper arm
M60.829 Other myositis, unspecified upper arm ▽

✓6ᵗʰ M60.83 Other myositis, forearm
M60.831 Other myositis, right forearm
M60.832 Other myositis, left forearm
M60.839 Other myositis, unspecified forearm ▽

✓6ᵗʰ M60.84 Other myositis, hand
M60.841 Other myositis, right hand
M60.842 Other myositis, left hand
M60.849 Other myositis, unspecified hand ▽

✓6ᵗʰ M60.85 Other myositis, thigh
M60.851 Other myositis, right thigh
M60.852 Other myositis, left thigh
M60.859 Other myositis, unspecified thigh ▽

✓6ᵗʰ M60.86 Other myositis, lower leg
M60.861 Other myositis, right lower leg
M60.862 Other myositis, left lower leg
M60.869 Other myositis, unspecified lower leg ▽

Ⓝ Newborn: 0   Ⓟ Pediatric: 0-17   Ⓜ Maternity: 12-55   Ⓐ Adult: 15-124   NRS Nonroutine supply Dx   NC Dx Noncancer Dx   PDx Primary Dx   ►◄ Revised Text   ● New Code   ▲ Revised Title

762   ICD-10-CM 2018

☑6ᵗʰ **M60.87** Other myositis, ankle and foot

M60.871 Other myositis, right ankle and foot

M60.872 Other myositis, left ankle and foot

M60.879 Other myositis, unspecified ankle and foot ▽

M60.88 Other myositis, other site

M60.89 Other myositis, multiple sites

M60.9 Myositis, unspecified ▽

☑4ᵗʰ **M61** **Calcification and ossification of muscle**

☑5ᵗʰ **M61.0** Myositis ossificans traumatica

M61.00 Myositis ossificans traumatica, unspecified site ▽

☑6ᵗʰ **M61.01** Myositis ossificans traumatica, shoulder

M61.011 Myositis ossificans traumatica, right shoulder

M61.012 Myositis ossificans traumatica, left shoulder

M61.019 Myositis ossificans traumatica, unspecified shoulder ▽

☑6ᵗʰ **M61.02** Myositis ossificans traumatica, upper arm

M61.021 Myositis ossificans traumatica, right upper arm

M61.022 Myositis ossificans traumatica, left upper arm

M61.029 Myositis ossificans traumatica, unspecified upper arm ▽

☑6ᵗʰ **M61.03** Myositis ossificans traumatica, forearm

M61.031 Myositis ossificans traumatica, right forearm

M61.032 Myositis ossificans traumatica, left forearm

M61.039 Myositis ossificans traumatica, unspecified forearm ▽

☑6ᵗʰ **M61.04** Myositis ossificans traumatica, hand

M61.041 Myositis ossificans traumatica, right hand

M61.042 Myositis ossificans traumatica, left hand

M61.049 Myositis ossificans traumatica, unspecified hand ▽

☑6ᵗʰ **M61.05** Myositis ossificans traumatica, thigh

M61.051 Myositis ossificans traumatica, right thigh

M61.052 Myositis ossificans traumatica, left thigh

M61.059 Myositis ossificans traumatica, unspecified thigh ▽

☑6ᵗʰ **M61.06** Myositis ossificans traumatica, lower leg

M61.061 Myositis ossificans traumatica, right lower leg

M61.062 Myositis ossificans traumatica, left lower leg

M61.069 Myositis ossificans traumatica, unspecified lower leg ▽

☑6ᵗʰ **M61.07** Myositis ossificans traumatica, ankle and foot

M61.071 Myositis ossificans traumatica, right ankle and foot

M61.072 Myositis ossificans traumatica, left ankle and foot

M61.079 Myositis ossificans traumatica, unspecified ankle and foot ▽

M61.08 Myositis ossificans traumatica, other site

M61.09 Myositis ossificans traumatica, multiple sites

☑5ᵗʰ **M61.1** Myositis ossificans progressiva
Fibrodysplasia ossificans progressiva

M61.10 Myositis ossificans progressiva, unspecified site ▽

☑6ᵗʰ **M61.11** Myositis ossificans progressiva, shoulder

M61.111 Myositis ossificans progressiva, right shoulder

M61.112 Myositis ossificans progressiva, left shoulder

M61.119 Myositis ossificans progressiva, unspecified shoulder ▽

☑6ᵗʰ **M61.12** Myositis ossificans progressiva, upper arm

M61.121 Myositis ossificans progressiva, right upper arm

M61.122 Myositis ossificans progressiva, left upper arm

M61.129 Myositis ossificans progressiva, unspecified arm ▽

☑6ᵗʰ **M61.13** Myositis ossificans progressiva, forearm

M61.131 Myositis ossificans progressiva, right forearm

M61.132 Myositis ossificans progressiva, left forearm

M61.139 Myositis ossificans progressiva, unspecified forearm ▽

☑6ᵗʰ **M61.14** Myositis ossificans progressiva, hand and finger(s)

M61.141 Myositis ossificans progressiva, right hand

M61.142 Myositis ossificans progressiva, left hand

M61.143 Myositis ossificans progressiva, unspecified hand ▽

M61.144 Myositis ossificans progressiva, right finger(s)

M61.145 Myositis ossificans progressiva, left finger(s)

M61.146 Myositis ossificans progressiva, unspecified finger(s) ▽

☑6ᵗʰ **M61.15** Myositis ossificans progressiva, thigh

M61.151 Myositis ossificans progressiva, right thigh

M61.152 Myositis ossificans progressiva, left thigh

M61.159 Myositis ossificans progressiva, unspecified thigh ▽

☑6ᵗʰ **M61.16** Myositis ossificans progressiva, lower leg

M61.161 Myositis ossificans progressiva, right lower leg

M61.162 Myositis ossificans progressiva, left lower leg

M61.169 Myositis ossificans progressiva, unspecified lower leg ▽

☑6ᵗʰ **M61.17** Myositis ossificans progressiva, ankle, foot and toe(s)

M61.171 Myositis ossificans progressiva, right ankle

M61.172 Myositis ossificans progressiva, left ankle

M61.173 Myositis ossificans progressiva, unspecified ankle ▽

M61.174 Myositis ossificans progressiva, right foot

M61.175 Myositis ossificans progressiva, left foot

M61.176 Myositis ossificans progressiva, unspecified foot ▽

M61.177 Myositis ossificans progressiva, right toe(s)

M61.178 Myositis ossificans progressiva, left toe(s)

M61.179 Myositis ossificans progressiva, unspecified toe(s) ▽

M61.18 Myositis ossificans progressiva, other site

M61.19 Myositis ossificans progressiva, multiple sites

☑5ᵗʰ **M61.2** Paralytic calcification and ossification of muscle
Myositis ossificans associated with quadriplegia or paraplegia

M61.20 Paralytic calcification and ossification of muscle, unspecified site ▽

☑6ᵗʰ **M61.21** Paralytic calcification and ossification of muscle, shoulder

M61.211 Paralytic calcification and ossification of muscle, right shoulder

M61.212 Paralytic calcification and ossification of muscle, left shoulder

M61.219 Paralytic calcification and ossification of muscle, unspecified shoulder ▽

☑6ᵗʰ **M61.22** Paralytic calcification and ossification of muscle, upper arm

M61.221 Paralytic calcification and ossification of muscle, right upper arm

M61.222 Paralytic calcification and ossification of muscle, left upper arm

M61.229 Paralytic calcification and ossification of muscle, unspecified upper arm ▽

☑6ᵗʰ **M61.23** Paralytic calcification and ossification of muscle, forearm

M61.231 Paralytic calcification and ossification of muscle, right forearm

M61.232 Paralytic calcification and ossification of muscle, left forearm

M61.239 Paralytic calcification and ossification of muscle, unspecified forearm ▽

☑ Additional Character Req   ☑x7ᵗʰ Placeholder Alert   Case-Mix Diagnosis   Manifestation   ▽ Unspecified Dx   **EXCLUDES 1** Not coded here   **EXCLUDES 2** Not included here

√6th **M61.24 Paralytic calcification and ossification of muscle, hand**

     M61.241 Paralytic calcification and ossification of muscle, right hand

     M61.242 Paralytic calcification and ossification of muscle, left hand

     M61.249 Paralytic calcification and ossification of muscle, unspecified hand ▽

√6th **M61.25 Paralytic calcification and ossification of muscle, thigh**

     M61.251 Paralytic calcification and ossification of muscle, right thigh

     M61.252 Paralytic calcification and ossification of muscle, left thigh

     M61.259 Paralytic calcification and ossification of muscle, unspecified thigh ▽

√6th **M61.26 Paralytic calcification and ossification of muscle, lower leg**

     M61.261 Paralytic calcification and ossification of muscle, right lower leg

     M61.262 Paralytic calcification and ossification of muscle, left lower leg

     M61.269 Paralytic calcification and ossification of muscle, unspecified lower leg ▽

√6th **M61.27 Paralytic calcification and ossification of muscle, ankle and foot**

     M61.271 Paralytic calcification and ossification of muscle, right ankle and foot

     M61.272 Paralytic calcification and ossification of muscle, left ankle and foot

     M61.279 Paralytic calcification and ossification of muscle, unspecified ankle and foot ▽

M61.28 Paralytic calcification and ossification of muscle, other site

M61.29 Paralytic calcification and ossification of muscle, multiple sites

√5th **M61.3 Calcification and ossification of muscles associated with burns**

     Myositis ossificans associated with burns

     M61.30 Calcification and ossification of muscles associated with burns, unspecified site ▽

√6th **M61.31 Calcification and ossification of muscles associated with burns, shoulder**

     M61.311 Calcification and ossification of muscles associated with burns, right shoulder

     M61.312 Calcification and ossification of muscles associated with burns, left shoulder

     M61.319 Calcification and ossification of muscles associated with burns, unspecified shoulder ▽

√6th **M61.32 Calcification and ossification of muscles associated with burns, upper arm**

     M61.321 Calcification and ossification of muscles associated with burns, right upper arm

     M61.322 Calcification and ossification of muscles associated with burns, left upper arm

     M61.329 Calcification and ossification of muscles associated with burns, unspecified upper arm ▽

√6th **M61.33 Calcification and ossification of muscles associated with burns, forearm**

     M61.331 Calcification and ossification of muscles associated with burns, right forearm

     M61.332 Calcification and ossification of muscles associated with burns, left forearm

     M61.339 Calcification and ossification of muscles associated with burns, unspecified forearm ▽

√6th **M61.34 Calcification and ossification of muscles associated with burns, hand**

     M61.341 Calcification and ossification of muscles associated with burns, right hand

     M61.342 Calcification and ossification of muscles associated with burns, left hand

     M61.349 Calcification and ossification of muscles associated with burns, unspecified hand ▽

√6th **M61.35 Calcification and ossification of muscles associated with burns, thigh**

     M61.351 Calcification and ossification of muscles associated with burns, right thigh

     M61.352 Calcification and ossification of muscles associated with burns, left thigh

     M61.359 Calcification and ossification of muscles associated with burns, unspecified thigh ▽

√6th **M61.36 Calcification and ossification of muscles associated with burns, lower leg**

     M61.361 Calcification and ossification of muscles associated with burns, right lower leg

     M61.362 Calcification and ossification of muscles associated with burns, left lower leg

     M61.369 Calcification and ossification of muscles associated with burns, unspecified lower leg ▽

√6th **M61.37 Calcification and ossification of muscles associated with burns, ankle and foot**

     M61.371 Calcification and ossification of muscles associated with burns, right ankle and foot

     M61.372 Calcification and ossification of muscles associated with burns, left ankle and foot

     M61.379 Calcification and ossification of muscles associated with burns, unspecified ankle and foot ▽

M61.38 Calcification and ossification of muscles associated with burns, other site

M61.39 Calcification and ossification of muscles associated with burns, multiple sites

√5th **M61.4 Other calcification of muscle**

     EXCLUDES 1   calcific tendinitis NOS (M65.2-)
                 calcific tendinitis of shoulder (M75.3)

     M61.40 Other calcification of muscle, unspecified site ▽

√6th **M61.41 Other calcification of muscle, shoulder**

     M61.411 Other calcification of muscle, right shoulder

     M61.412 Other calcification of muscle, left shoulder

     M61.419 Other calcification of muscle, unspecified shoulder ▽

√6th **M61.42 Other calcification of muscle, upper arm**

     M61.421 Other calcification of muscle, right upper arm

     M61.422 Other calcification of muscle, left upper arm

     M61.429 Other calcification of muscle, unspecified upper arm ▽

√6th **M61.43 Other calcification of muscle, forearm**

     M61.431 Other calcification of muscle, right forearm

     M61.432 Other calcification of muscle, left forearm

     M61.439 Other calcification of muscle, unspecified forearm ▽

√6th **M61.44 Other calcification of muscle, hand**

     M61.441 Other calcification of muscle, right hand

     M61.442 Other calcification of muscle, left hand

     M61.449 Other calcification of muscle, unspecified hand ▽

√6th **M61.45 Other calcification of muscle, thigh**

     M61.451 Other calcification of muscle, right thigh

     M61.452 Other calcification of muscle, left thigh

     M61.459 Other calcification of muscle, unspecified thigh ▽

√6th **M61.46 Other calcification of muscle, lower leg**

     M61.461 Other calcification of muscle, right lower leg

     M61.462 Other calcification of muscle, left lower leg

     M61.469 Other calcification of muscle, unspecified lower leg ▽

√6th **M61.47 Other calcification of muscle, ankle and foot**

     M61.471 Other calcification of muscle, right ankle and foot

     M61.472 Other calcification of muscle, left ankle and foot

M61.479 **Other calcification of muscle, unspecified ankle and foot** ▽
M61.48 **Other calcification of muscle, other site**
M61.49 **Other calcification of muscle, multiple sites**

✓5ᵗʰ **M61.5 Other ossification of muscle**
M61.50 **Other ossification of muscle, unspecified site** ▽
✓6ᵗʰ M61.51 **Other ossification of muscle, shoulder**
M61.511 **Other ossification of muscle, right shoulder**
M61.512 **Other ossification of muscle, left shoulder**
M61.519 **Other ossification of muscle, unspecified shoulder** ▽
✓6ᵗʰ M61.52 **Other ossification of muscle, upper arm**
M61.521 **Other ossification of muscle, right upper arm**
M61.522 **Other ossification of muscle, left upper arm**
M61.529 **Other ossification of muscle, unspecified upper arm** ▽
✓6ᵗʰ M61.53 **Other ossification of muscle, forearm**
M61.531 **Other ossification of muscle, right forearm**
M61.532 **Other ossification of muscle, left forearm**
M61.539 **Other ossification of muscle, unspecified forearm** ▽
✓6ᵗʰ M61.54 **Other ossification of muscle, hand**
M61.541 **Other ossification of muscle, right hand**
M61.542 **Other ossification of muscle, left hand**
M61.549 **Other ossification of muscle, unspecified hand** ▽
✓6ᵗʰ M61.55 **Other ossification of muscle, thigh**
M61.551 **Other ossification of muscle, right thigh**
M61.552 **Other ossification of muscle, left thigh**
M61.559 **Other ossification of muscle, unspecified thigh**
✓6ᵗʰ M61.56 **Other ossification of muscle, lower leg**
M61.561 **Other ossification of muscle, right lower leg**
M61.562 **Other ossification of muscle, left lower leg**
M61.569 **Other ossification of muscle, unspecified lower leg** ▽
✓6ᵗʰ M61.57 **Other ossification of muscle, ankle and foot**
M61.571 **Other ossification of muscle, right ankle and foot**
M61.572 **Other ossification of muscle, left ankle and foot**
M61.579 **Other ossification of muscle, unspecified ankle and foot** ▽
M61.58 **Other ossification of muscle, other site**
M61.59 **Other ossification of muscle, multiple sites**
M61.9 **Calcification and ossification of muscle, unspecified** ▽

✓4ᵗʰ **M62 Other disorders of muscle**
EXCLUDES 1   alcoholic myopathy (G72.1)
cramp and spasm (R25.2)
drug-induced myopathy (G72.0)
myalgia (M79.1)
stiff-man syndrome (G25.82)
EXCLUDES 2   nontraumatic hematoma of muscle (M79.81)

✓5ᵗʰ **M62.0 Separation of muscle (nontraumatic)**
Diastasis of muscle
EXCLUDES 1   diastasis recti complicating pregnancy, labor and delivery (O71.8)
traumatic separation of muscle—see strain of muscle by body region
M62.00 **Separation of muscle (nontraumatic), unspecified site** ▽
✓6ᵗʰ M62.01 **Separation of muscle (nontraumatic), shoulder**
M62.011 **Separation of muscle (nontraumatic), right shoulder**
M62.012 **Separation of muscle (nontraumatic), left shoulder**
M62.019 **Separation of muscle (nontraumatic), unspecified shoulder** ▽
✓6ᵗʰ M62.02 **Separation of muscle (nontraumatic), upper arm**
M62.021 **Separation of muscle (nontraumatic), right upper arm**

M62.022 **Separation of muscle (nontraumatic), left upper arm**
M62.029 **Separation of muscle (nontraumatic), unspecified upper arm** ▽
✓6ᵗʰ M62.03 **Separation of muscle (nontraumatic), forearm**
M62.031 **Separation of muscle (nontraumatic), right forearm**
M62.032 **Separation of muscle (nontraumatic), left forearm**
M62.039 **Separation of muscle (nontraumatic), unspecified forearm** ▽
✓6ᵗʰ M62.04 **Separation of muscle (nontraumatic), hand**
M62.041 **Separation of muscle (nontraumatic), right hand**
M62.042 **Separation of muscle (nontraumatic), left hand**
M62.049 **Separation of muscle (nontraumatic), unspecified hand** ▽
✓6ᵗʰ M62.05 **Separation of muscle (nontraumatic), thigh**
M62.051 **Separation of muscle (nontraumatic), right thigh**
M62.052 **Separation of muscle (nontraumatic), left thigh**
M62.059 **Separation of muscle (nontraumatic), unspecified thigh** ▽
✓6ᵗʰ M62.06 **Separation of muscle (nontraumatic), lower leg**
M62.061 **Separation of muscle (nontraumatic), right lower leg**
M62.062 **Separation of muscle (nontraumatic), left lower leg**
M62.069 **Separation of muscle (nontraumatic), unspecified lower leg** ▽
✓6ᵗʰ M62.07 **Separation of muscle (nontraumatic), ankle and foot**
M62.071 **Separation of muscle (nontraumatic), right ankle and foot**
M62.072 **Separation of muscle (nontraumatic), left ankle and foot**
M62.079 **Separation of muscle (nontraumatic), unspecified ankle and foot** ▽
M62.08 **Separation of muscle (nontraumatic), other site**

✓5ᵗʰ **M62.1 Other rupture of muscle (nontraumatic)**
EXCLUDES 1   traumatic rupture of muscle—see strain of muscle by body region
EXCLUDES 2   rupture of tendon (M66.-)
M62.10 **Other rupture of muscle (nontraumatic), unspecified site** ▽
✓6ᵗʰ M62.11 **Other rupture of muscle (nontraumatic), shoulder**
M62.111 **Other rupture of muscle (nontraumatic), right shoulder**
M62.112 **Other rupture of muscle (nontraumatic), left shoulder**
M62.119 **Other rupture of muscle (nontraumatic), unspecified shoulder** ▽
✓6ᵗʰ M62.12 **Other rupture of muscle (nontraumatic), upper arm**
M62.121 **Other rupture of muscle (nontraumatic), right upper arm**
M62.122 **Other rupture of muscle (nontraumatic), left upper arm**
M62.129 **Other rupture of muscle (nontraumatic), unspecified upper arm** ▽
✓6ᵗʰ M62.13 **Other rupture of muscle (nontraumatic), forearm**
M62.131 **Other rupture of muscle (nontraumatic), right forearm**
M62.132 **Other rupture of muscle (nontraumatic), left forearm**
M62.139 **Other rupture of muscle (nontraumatic), unspecified forearm** ▽
✓6ᵗʰ M62.14 **Other rupture of muscle (nontraumatic), hand**
M62.141 **Other rupture of muscle (nontraumatic), right hand**
M62.142 **Other rupture of muscle (nontraumatic), left hand**
M62.149 **Other rupture of muscle (nontraumatic), unspecified hand** ▽

✓6ᵗʰ **M62.15 Other rupture of muscle (nontraumatic),** thigh
     M62.151 Other rupture of muscle (nontraumatic), right **thigh**
     M62.152 Other rupture of muscle (nontraumatic), left **thigh**
     M62.159 Other rupture of muscle (nontraumatic), unspecified thigh ▽

✓6ᵗʰ **M62.16 Other rupture of muscle (nontraumatic),** lower leg
     M62.161 Other rupture of muscle (nontraumatic), right **lower leg**
     M62.162 Other rupture of muscle (nontraumatic), left **lower leg**
     M62.169 Other rupture of muscle (nontraumatic), unspecified lower leg ▽

✓6ᵗʰ **M62.17 Other rupture of muscle (nontraumatic),** ankle and foot
     M62.171 Other rupture of muscle (nontraumatic), right **ankle and foot**
     M62.172 Other rupture of muscle (nontraumatic), left **ankle and foot**
     M62.179 Other rupture of muscle (nontraumatic), unspecified ankle and foot ▽

     M62.18 Other rupture of muscle (nontraumatic), other site

✓5ᵗʰ **M62.2 Nontraumatic ischemic infarction of muscle**
     EXCLUDES 1   *compartment syndrome (traumatic) (T79.A-)*
         nontraumatic compartment syndrome (M79.A-)
         rhabdomyolysis (M62.82)
         traumatic ischemia of muscle (T79.6)
         Volkmann's ischemic contracture (T79.6)

     M62.20 Nontraumatic ischemic infarction of muscle, unspecified site ▽

✓6ᵗʰ **M62.21 Nontraumatic ischemic infarction of muscle,** shoulder
     M62.211 Nontraumatic ischemic infarction of muscle, right **shoulder**
     M62.212 Nontraumatic ischemic infarction of muscle, left **shoulder**
     M62.219 Nontraumatic ischemic infarction of muscle, unspecified shoulder ▽

✓6ᵗʰ **M62.22 Nontraumatic ischemic infarction of muscle,** upper arm
     M62.221 Nontraumatic ischemic infarction of muscle, right **upper arm**
     M62.222 Nontraumatic ischemic infarction of muscle, left **upper arm**
     M62.229 Nontraumatic ischemic infarction of muscle, unspecified upper arm ▽

✓6ᵗʰ **M62.23 Nontraumatic ischemic infarction of muscle,** forearm
     M62.231 Nontraumatic ischemic infarction of muscle, right **forearm**
     M62.232 Nontraumatic ischemic infarction of muscle, left **forearm**
     M62.239 Nontraumatic ischemic infarction of muscle, unspecified forearm ▽

✓6ᵗʰ **M62.24 Nontraumatic ischemic infarction of muscle,** hand
     M62.241 Nontraumatic ischemic infarction of muscle, right **hand**
     M62.242 Nontraumatic ischemic infarction of muscle, left **hand**
     M62.249 Nontraumatic ischemic infarction of muscle, unspecified hand ▽

✓6ᵗʰ **M62.25 Nontraumatic ischemic infarction of muscle,** thigh
     M62.251 Nontraumatic ischemic infarction of muscle, right **thigh**
     M62.252 Nontraumatic ischemic infarction of muscle, left **thigh**
     M62.259 Nontraumatic ischemic infarction of muscle, unspecified thigh ▽

✓6ᵗʰ **M62.26 Nontraumatic ischemic infarction of muscle,** lower leg
     M62.261 Nontraumatic ischemic infarction of muscle, right **lower leg**
     M62.262 Nontraumatic ischemic infarction of muscle, left **lower leg**
     M62.269 Nontraumatic ischemic infarction of muscle, unspecified lower leg ▽

✓6ᵗʰ **M62.27 Nontraumatic ischemic infarction of muscle,** ankle and foot
     M62.271 Nontraumatic ischemic infarction of muscle, right **ankle and foot**
     M62.272 Nontraumatic ischemic infarction of muscle, left **ankle and foot**
     M62.279 Nontraumatic ischemic infarction of muscle, unspecified ankle and foot ▽

     M62.28 Nontraumatic ischemic infarction of muscle, other site

M62.3 Immobility syndrome (paraplegic)

✓5ᵗʰ **M62.4 Contracture of muscle**
     Contracture of tendon (sheath)
     EXCLUDES 1   *contracture of joint (M24.5-)*

     M62.40 Contracture of muscle, unspecified site ▽

✓6ᵗʰ **M62.41 Contracture of muscle,** shoulder
     M62.411 Contracture of muscle, right **shoulder**
     M62.412 Contracture of muscle, left **shoulder**
     M62.419 Contracture of muscle, unspecified shoulder ▽

✓6ᵗʰ **M62.42 Contracture of muscle,** upper arm
     M62.421 Contracture of muscle, right **upper arm**
     M62.422 Contracture of muscle, left **upper arm**
     M62.429 Contracture of muscle, unspecified upper arm ▽

✓6ᵗʰ **M62.43 Contracture of muscle,** forearm
     M62.431 Contracture of muscle, right **forearm**
     M62.432 Contracture of muscle, left **forearm**
     M62.439 Contracture of muscle, unspecified forearm ▽

✓6ᵗʰ **M62.44 Contracture of muscle,** hand
     M62.441 Contracture of muscle, right **hand**
     M62.442 Contracture of muscle, left **hand**
     M62.449 Contracture of muscle, unspecified hand ▽

✓6ᵗʰ **M62.45 Contracture of muscle,** thigh
     M62.451 Contracture of muscle, right **thigh**
     M62.452 Contracture of muscle, left **thigh**
     M62.459 Contracture of muscle, unspecified thigh ▽

✓6ᵗʰ **M62.46 Contracture of muscle,** lower leg
     M62.461 Contracture of muscle, right **lower leg**
     M62.462 Contracture of muscle, left **lower leg**
     M62.469 Contracture of muscle, unspecified lower leg ▽

✓6ᵗʰ **M62.47 Contracture of muscle,** ankle and foot
     M62.471 Contracture of muscle, right **ankle and foot**
     M62.472 Contracture of muscle, left **ankle and foot**
     M62.479 Contracture of muscle, unspecified ankle and foot ▽

     M62.48 Contracture of muscle, other site

     M62.49 Contracture of muscle, multiple sites

✓5ᵗʰ **M62.5 Muscle wasting and atrophy, not elsewhere classified**
     Disuse atrophy NEC
     EXCLUDES 1   *neuralgic amyotrophy (G54.5)*
         progressive muscular atrophy ▶*(G12.21)*◀
         sarcopenia (M62.84)
     EXCLUDES 2   *pelvic muscle wasting (N81.84)*

     M62.50 Muscle wasting and atrophy, not elsewhere classified, unspecified site ▽

✓6ᵗʰ **M62.51 Muscle wasting and atrophy, not elsewhere classified,** shoulder
     M62.511 Muscle wasting and atrophy, not elsewhere classified, right **shoulder**
     M62.512 Muscle wasting and atrophy, not elsewhere classified, left **shoulder**
     M62.519 Muscle wasting and atrophy, not elsewhere classified, unspecified shoulder ▽

✓6ᵗʰ **M62.52 Muscle wasting and atrophy, not elsewhere classified,** upper arm
     M62.521 Muscle wasting and atrophy, not elsewhere classified, right **upper arm**

Ⓝ Newborn: 0   Ⓟ Pediatric: 0-17   Ⓜ Maternity: 12-55   Ⓐ Adult: 15-124   **NRS** Nonroutine supply Dx   **NC Dx** Noncancer Dx   **PDx** Primary Dx   ▶◀ Revised Text   ● New Code   ▲ Revised Title

766   ICD-10-CM 2018

M62.522 Muscle wasting and atrophy, not elsewhere classified, left upper arm

M62.529 Muscle wasting and atrophy, not elsewhere classified, unspecified upper arm ▽

✓6ᵗʰ **M62.53** Muscle wasting and atrophy, not elsewhere classified, forearm

M62.531 Muscle wasting and atrophy, not elsewhere classified, right forearm

M62.532 Muscle wasting and atrophy, not elsewhere classified, left forearm

M62.539 Muscle wasting and atrophy, not elsewhere classified, unspecified forearm ▽

✓6ᵗʰ **M62.54** Muscle wasting and atrophy, not elsewhere classified, hand

M62.541 Muscle wasting and atrophy, not elsewhere classified, right hand

M62.542 Muscle wasting and atrophy, not elsewhere classified, left hand

M62.549 Muscle wasting and atrophy, not elsewhere classified, unspecified hand ▽

✓6ᵗʰ **M62.55** Muscle wasting and atrophy, not elsewhere classified, thigh

M62.551 Muscle wasting and atrophy, not elsewhere classified, right thigh

M62.552 Muscle wasting and atrophy, not elsewhere classified, left thigh

M62.559 Muscle wasting and atrophy, not elsewhere classified, unspecified thigh ▽

✓6ᵗʰ **M62.56** Muscle wasting and atrophy, not elsewhere classified, lower leg

M62.561 Muscle wasting and atrophy, not elsewhere classified, right lower leg

M62.562 Muscle wasting and atrophy, not elsewhere classified, left lower leg

M62.569 Muscle wasting and atrophy, not elsewhere classified, unspecified lower leg ▽

✓6ᵗʰ **M62.57** Muscle wasting and atrophy, not elsewhere classified, ankle and foot

M62.571 Muscle wasting and atrophy, not elsewhere classified, right ankle and foot

M62.572 Muscle wasting and atrophy, not elsewhere classified, left ankle and foot

M62.579 Muscle wasting and atrophy, not elsewhere classified, unspecified ankle and foot ▽

M62.58 Muscle wasting and atrophy, not elsewhere classified, other site

M62.59 Muscle wasting and atrophy, not elsewhere classified, multiple sites

✓5ᵗʰ **M62.8** Other specified disorders of muscle
EXCLUDES 2 nontraumatic hematoma of muscle (M79.81)

M62.81 Muscle weakness (generalized)
EXCLUDES 1 muscle weakness in sarcopenia (M62.84)

M62.82 Rhabdomyolysis
EXCLUDES 1 traumatic rhabdomyolysis (T79.6)
DEF: Rapid disintegration or destruction of skeletal muscle caused by direct or indirect injury; resulting in the excretion of muscle protein myoglobin into the urine.

✓6ᵗʰ **M62.83** Muscle spasm

M62.830 Muscle spasm of back

M62.831 Muscle spasm of calf
Charley-horse

M62.838 Other muscle spasm

M62.84 Sarcopenia
Age-related sarcopenia
Code first underlying disease, if applicable, such as:
disorders of myoneural junction and muscle disease in diseases classified elsewhere (G73.-)
other and unspecified myopathies (G72.-)
primary disorders of muscles (G71.-)

M62.89 Other specified disorders of muscle
Muscle (sheath) hernia

M62.9 Disorder of muscle, unspecified ▽

✓4ᵗʰ **M63** **Disorders of muscle in diseases classified elsewhere**
Code first underlying disease, such as:
leprosy (A30.-)
neoplasm (C49-, C79.89, D21-, D48.1)
schistosomiasis (B65.-)
trichinellosis (B75)
EXCLUDES 1 myopathy in cysticercosis (B69.81)
myopathy in endocrine diseases (G73.7)
myopathy in metabolic diseases (G73.7)
myopathy in sarcoidosis (D86.87)
myopathy in secondary syphilis (A51.49)
myopathy in syphilis (late) (A52.78)
myopathy in toxoplasmosis (B58.82)
myopathy in tuberculosis (A18.09)

✓5ᵗʰ **M63.8** Disorders of muscle in diseases classified elsewhere

M63.80 *Disorders of muscle in diseases classified elsewhere, unspecified site* ▽

✓6ᵗʰ *M63.81* *Disorders of muscle in diseases classified elsewhere, shoulder*

M63.811 *Disorders of muscle in diseases classified elsewhere, right shoulder*

M63.812 *Disorders of muscle in diseases classified elsewhere, left shoulder*

M63.819 *Disorders of muscle in diseases classified elsewhere, unspecified shoulder* ▽

✓6ᵗʰ *M63.82* *Disorders of muscle in diseases classified elsewhere, upper arm*

M63.821 *Disorders of muscle in diseases classified elsewhere, right upper arm*

M63.822 *Disorders of muscle in diseases classified elsewhere, left upper arm*

M63.829 *Disorders of muscle in diseases classified elsewhere, unspecified upper arm* ▽

✓6ᵗʰ *M63.83* *Disorders of muscle in diseases classified elsewhere, forearm*

M63.831 *Disorders of muscle in diseases classified elsewhere, right forearm*

M63.832 *Disorders of muscle in diseases classified elsewhere, left forearm*

M63.839 *Disorders of muscle in diseases classified elsewhere, unspecified forearm* ▽

✓6ᵗʰ *M63.84* *Disorders of muscle in diseases classified elsewhere, hand*

M63.841 *Disorders of muscle in diseases classified elsewhere, right hand*

M63.842 *Disorders of muscle in diseases classified elsewhere, left hand*

M63.849 *Disorders of muscle in diseases classified elsewhere, unspecified hand* ▽

✓6ᵗʰ *M63.85* *Disorders of muscle in diseases classified elsewhere, thigh*

M63.851 *Disorders of muscle in diseases classified elsewhere, right thigh*

M63.852 *Disorders of muscle in diseases classified elsewhere, left thigh*

M63.859 *Disorders of muscle in diseases classified elsewhere, unspecified thigh* ▽

✓6ᵗʰ *M63.86* *Disorders of muscle in diseases classified elsewhere, lower leg*

M63.861 *Disorders of muscle in diseases classified elsewhere, right lower leg*

M63.862 *Disorders of muscle in diseases classified elsewhere, left lower leg*

M63.869 *Disorders of muscle in diseases classified elsewhere, unspecified lower leg* ▽

✓6ᵗʰ *M63.87* *Disorders of muscle in diseases classified elsewhere, ankle and foot*

M63.871 *Disorders of muscle in diseases classified elsewhere, right ankle and foot*

M63.872 *Disorders of muscle in diseases classified elsewhere, left ankle and foot*

M63.879 *Disorders of muscle in diseases classified elsewhere, unspecified ankle and foot* ▽

M63.88 *Disorders of muscle in diseases classified elsewhere, other site*

M63.89 *Disorders of muscle in diseases classified elsewhere, multiple sites*

✓ Additional Character Req   ✓x7ᵗʰ Placeholder Alert   Case-Mix Diagnosis   Manifestation   ▽ Unspecified Dx   EXCLUDES 1 Not coded here   EXCLUDES 2 Not included here

Disorders of synovium and tendon (M65-M67)

√4ᵗʰ M65 Synovitis and tenosynovitis

EXCLUDES 1   *chronic crepitant synovitis of hand and wrist (M70.0-)*
current injury—see injury of ligament or tendon by body region
soft tissue disorders related to use, overuse and pressure (M70.-)

√5ᵗʰ M65.0 Abscess of tendon sheath
     Use additional code (B95-B96) to identify bacterial agent.

   M65.00   Abscess of tendon sheath, unspecified site ▽

√6ᵗʰ M65.01 Abscess of tendon sheath, shoulder
     M65.011   Abscess of tendon sheath, right shoulder
     M65.012   Abscess of tendon sheath, left shoulder
     M65.019   Abscess of tendon sheath, unspecified ▽ shoulder

√6ᵗʰ M65.02 Abscess of tendon sheath, upper arm
     M65.021   Abscess of tendon sheath, right upper arm
     M65.022   Abscess of tendon sheath, left upper arm
     M65.029   Abscess of tendon sheath, unspecified ▽ upper arm

√6ᵗʰ M65.03 Abscess of tendon sheath, forearm
     M65.031   Abscess of tendon sheath, right forearm
     M65.032   Abscess of tendon sheath, left forearm
     M65.039   Abscess of tendon sheath, unspecified ▽ forearm

√6ᵗʰ M65.04 Abscess of tendon sheath, hand
     M65.041   Abscess of tendon sheath, right hand
     M65.042   Abscess of tendon sheath, left hand
     M65.049   Abscess of tendon sheath, unspecified ▽ hand

√6ᵗʰ M65.05 Abscess of tendon sheath, thigh
     M65.051   Abscess of tendon sheath, right thigh
     M65.052   Abscess of tendon sheath, left thigh
     M65.059   Abscess of tendon sheath, unspecified ▽ thigh

√6ᵗʰ M65.06 Abscess of tendon sheath, lower leg
     M65.061   Abscess of tendon sheath, right lower leg
     M65.062   Abscess of tendon sheath, left lower leg
     M65.069   Abscess of tendon sheath, unspecified ▽ lower leg

√6ᵗʰ M65.07 Abscess of tendon sheath, ankle and foot
     M65.071   Abscess of tendon sheath, right ankle and foot
     M65.072   Abscess of tendon sheath, left ankle and foot
     M65.079   Abscess of tendon sheath, unspecified ▽ ankle and foot

   M65.08   Abscess of tendon sheath, other site

√5ᵗʰ M65.1 Other infective (teno)synovitis
   M65.10   Other infective (teno)synovitis, unspecified site ▽

√6ᵗʰ M65.11 Other infective (teno)synovitis, shoulder
     M65.111   Other infective (teno)synovitis, right shoulder
     M65.112   Other infective (teno)synovitis, left shoulder
     M65.119   Other infective (teno)synovitis, unspecified shoulder ▽

√6ᵗʰ M65.12 Other infective (teno)synovitis, elbow
     M65.121   Other infective (teno)synovitis, right elbow
     M65.122   Other infective (teno)synovitis, left elbow
     M65.129   Other infective (teno)synovitis, unspecified elbow ▽

√6ᵗʰ M65.13 Other infective (teno)synovitis, wrist
     M65.131   Other infective (teno)synovitis, right wrist
     M65.132   Other infective (teno)synovitis, left wrist
     M65.139   Other infective (teno)synovitis, unspecified wrist ▽

√6ᵗʰ M65.14 Other infective (teno)synovitis, hand
     M65.141   Other infective (teno)synovitis, right hand
     M65.142   Other infective (teno)synovitis, left hand
     M65.149   Other infective (teno)synovitis, unspecified hand ▽

√6ᵗʰ M65.15 Other infective (teno)synovitis, hip
     M65.151   Other infective (teno)synovitis, right hip

     M65.152   Other infective (teno)synovitis, left hip
     M65.159   Other infective (teno)synovitis, unspecified hip ▽

√6ᵗʰ M65.16 Other infective (teno)synovitis, knee
     M65.161   Other infective (teno)synovitis, right knee
     M65.162   Other infective (teno)synovitis, left knee
     M65.169   Other infective (teno)synovitis, unspecified knee ▽

√6ᵗʰ M65.17 Other infective (teno)synovitis, ankle and foot
     M65.171   Other infective (teno)synovitis, right ankle and foot
     M65.172   Other infective (teno)synovitis, left ankle and foot
     M65.179   Other infective (teno)synovitis, unspecified ankle and foot ▽

   M65.18   Other infective (teno)synovitis, other site
   M65.19   Other infective (teno)synovitis, multiple sites

√5ᵗʰ M65.2 Calcific tendinitis

EXCLUDES 1   *tendinitis as classified in M75-M77*
calcified tendinitis of shoulder (M75.3)

   M65.20   Calcific tendinitis, unspecified site ▽

√6ᵗʰ M65.22 Calcific tendinitis, upper arm
     M65.221   Calcific tendinitis, right upper arm
     M65.222   Calcific tendinitis, left upper arm
     M65.229   Calcific tendinitis, unspecified upper ▽ arm

√6ᵗʰ M65.23 Calcific tendinitis, forearm
     M65.231   Calcific tendinitis, right forearm
     M65.232   Calcific tendinitis, left forearm
     M65.239   Calcific tendinitis, unspecified ▽ forearm

√6ᵗʰ M65.24 Calcific tendinitis, hand
     M65.241   Calcific tendinitis, right hand
     M65.242   Calcific tendinitis, left hand
     M65.249   Calcific tendinitis, unspecified hand ▽

√6ᵗʰ M65.25 Calcific tendinitis, thigh
     M65.251   Calcific tendinitis, right thigh
     M65.252   Calcific tendinitis, left thigh
     M65.259   Calcific tendinitis, unspecified thigh ▽

√6ᵗʰ M65.26 Calcific tendinitis, lower leg
     M65.261   Calcific tendinitis, right lower leg
     M65.262   Calcific tendinitis, left lower leg
     M65.269   Calcific tendinitis, unspecified lower ▽ leg

√6ᵗʰ M65.27 Calcific tendinitis, ankle and foot
     M65.271   Calcific tendinitis, right ankle and foot
     M65.272   Calcific tendinitis, left ankle and foot
     M65.279   Calcific tendinitis, unspecified ankle ▽ and foot

   M65.28   Calcific tendinitis, other site
   M65.29   Calcific tendinitis, multiple sites

√5ᵗʰ M65.3 Trigger finger
     Nodular tendinous disease

   M65.30   Trigger finger, unspecified finger ▽

√6ᵗʰ M65.31 Trigger thumb
     M65.311   Trigger thumb, right thumb
     M65.312   Trigger thumb, left thumb
     M65.319   Trigger thumb, unspecified thumb ▽

√6ᵗʰ M65.32 Trigger finger, index finger
     M65.321   Trigger finger, right index finger
     M65.322   Trigger finger, left index finger
     M65.329   Trigger finger, unspecified index ▽ finger

√6ᵗʰ M65.33 Trigger finger, middle finger
     M65.331   Trigger finger, right middle finger
     M65.332   Trigger finger, left middle finger
     M65.339   Trigger finger, unspecified middle ▽ finger

√6ᵗʰ M65.34 Trigger finger, ring finger
     M65.341   Trigger finger, right ring finger
     M65.342   Trigger finger, left ring finger
     M65.349   Trigger finger, unspecified ring finger ▽

◻ Newborn: 0   ◻ Pediatric: 0-17   ◻ Maternity: 12-55   ◻ Adult: 15-124   **NRS** Nonroutine supply Dx   **NCDx** Noncancer Dx   **PDx** Primary Dx   ►◄ Revised Text   ● New Code   ▲ Revised Title

768   ICD-10-CM 2018

✓6ᵗʰ **M65.35 Trigger finger,** little finger
     M65.351 Trigger finger, right **little finger**
     M65.352 Trigger finger, left **little finger**
     M65.359 Trigger finger, unspecified little finger ▽

M65.4 Radial styloid tenosynovitis [de Quervain]

✓5ᵗʰ **M65.8 Other synovitis and tenosynovitis**
     M65.80 Other synovitis and tenosynovitis, unspecified ▽
         site

     ✓6ᵗʰ **M65.81 Other synovitis and tenosynovitis,** shoulder
         M65.811 Other synovitis and tenosynovitis,
             right **shoulder**
         M65.812 Other synovitis and tenosynovitis,
             left **shoulder**
         M65.819 Other synovitis and tenosynovitis, ▽
             unspecified shoulder

     ✓6ᵗʰ **M65.82 Other synovitis and tenosynovitis,** upper arm
         M65.821 Other synovitis and tenosynovitis,
             right **upper arm**
         M65.822 Other synovitis and tenosynovitis,
             left **upper arm**
         M65.829 Other synovitis and tenosynovitis, ▽
             unspecified upper arm

     ✓6ᵗʰ **M65.83 Other synovitis and tenosynovitis,** forearm
         M65.831 Other synovitis and tenosynovitis,
             right **forearm**
         M65.832 Other synovitis and tenosynovitis,
             left **forearm**
         M65.839 Other synovitis and tenosynovitis, ▽
             unspecified forearm

     ✓6ᵗʰ **M65.84 Other synovitis and tenosynovitis,** hand
         M65.841 Other synovitis and tenosynovitis, right
             hand
         M65.842 Other synovitis and tenosynovitis, left
             hand
         M65.849 Other synovitis and tenosynovitis, ▽
             unspecified hand

     ✓6ᵗʰ **M65.85 Other synovitis and tenosynovitis,** thigh
         M65.851 Other synovitis and tenosynovitis, right
             thigh
         M65.852 Other synovitis and tenosynovitis, left
             thigh
         M65.859 Other synovitis and tenosynovitis, ▽
             unspecified thigh

     ✓6ᵗʰ **M65.86 Other synovitis and tenosynovitis,** lower leg
         M65.861 Other synovitis and tenosynovitis,
             right **lower leg**
         M65.862 Other synovitis and tenosynovitis,
             left **lower leg**
         M65.869 Other synovitis and tenosynovitis, ▽
             unspecified lower leg

     ✓6ᵗʰ **M65.87 Other synovitis and tenosynovitis,** ankle and foot
         M65.871 Other synovitis and tenosynovitis,
             right **ankle and foot**
         M65.872 Other synovitis and tenosynovitis,
             left **ankle and foot**
         M65.879 Other synovitis and tenosynovitis, ▽
             unspecified ankle and foot

     M65.88 Other synovitis and tenosynovitis, other site
     M65.89 Other synovitis and tenosynovitis, multiple sites
M65.9 Synovitis and tenosynovitis, unspecified ▽

✓4ᵗʰ **M66 Spontaneous rupture of synovium and tendon**
     INCLUDES   rupture that occurs when a normal force is applied to tissues
             that are inferred to have less than normal strength
     EXCLUDES 2   rotator cuff syndrome (M75.1-)
             rupture where an abnormal force is applied to normal
             tissue—see injury of tendon by body region

M66.0 Rupture of popliteal cyst

✓5ᵗʰ **M66.1 Rupture of** synovium
     Rupture of synovial cyst
     EXCLUDES 2   rupture of popliteal cyst (M66.0)
     M66.10 Rupture of synovium, unspecified joint ▽
     ✓6ᵗʰ **M66.11 Rupture of synovium,** shoulder
         M66.111 Rupture of synovium, right **shoulder**
         M66.112 Rupture of synovium, left **shoulder**

         M66.119 Rupture of synovium, unspecified ▽
             shoulder

     ✓6ᵗʰ **M66.12 Rupture of synovium,** elbow
         M66.121 Rupture of synovium, right **elbow**
         M66.122 Rupture of synovium, left **elbow**
         M66.129 Rupture of synovium, unspecified ▽
             elbow

     ✓6ᵗʰ **M66.13 Rupture of synovium,** wrist
         M66.131 Rupture of synovium, right **wrist**
         M66.132 Rupture of synovium, left **wrist**
         M66.139 Rupture of synovium, unspecified wrist ▽

     ✓6ᵗʰ **M66.14 Rupture of synovium,** hand and fingers
         M66.141 Rupture of synovium, right **hand**
         M66.142 Rupture of synovium, left **hand**
         M66.143 Rupture of synovium, unspecified hand ▽
         M66.144 Rupture of synovium, right **finger(s)**
         M66.145 Rupture of synovium, left **finger(s)**
         M66.146 Rupture of synovium, unspecified ▽
             finger(s)

     ✓6ᵗʰ **M66.15 Rupture of synovium,** hip
         M66.151 Rupture of synovium, right **hip**
         M66.152 Rupture of synovium, left **hip**
         M66.159 Rupture of synovium, unspecified hip ▽

     ✓6ᵗʰ **M66.17 Rupture of synovium,** ankle, foot and toes
         M66.171 Rupture of synovium, right **ankle**
         M66.172 Rupture of synovium, left **ankle**
         M66.173 Rupture of synovium, unspecified ▽
             ankle
         M66.174 Rupture of synovium, right **foot**
         M66.175 Rupture of synovium, left **foot**
         M66.176 Rupture of synovium, unspecified foot ▽
         M66.177 Rupture of synovium, right **toe(s)**
         M66.178 Rupture of synovium, left **toe(s)**
         M66.179 Rupture of synovium, unspecified ▽
             toe(s)

     M66.18 Rupture of synovium, other site

✓5ᵗʰ **M66.2 Spontaneous rupture of** extensor tendons
     TIP: Refer to the Muscle/Tendon table at the beginning of this
     chapter.
     M66.20 Spontaneous rupture of extensor tendons, ▽
         unspecified site

     ✓6ᵗʰ **M66.21 Spontaneous rupture of extensor tendons,** shoulder
         M66.211 Spontaneous rupture of extensor
             tendons, right **shoulder**
         M66.212 Spontaneous rupture of extensor
             tendons, left **shoulder**
         M66.219 Spontaneous rupture of extensor ▽
             tendons, unspecified shoulder

     ✓6ᵗʰ **M66.22 Spontaneous rupture of extensor tendons,** upper
         arm
         M66.221 Spontaneous rupture of extensor tendons,
             right **upper arm**
         M66.222 Spontaneous rupture of extensor tendons,
             left **upper arm**
         M66.229 Spontaneous rupture of extensor ▽
             tendons, unspecified upper arm

     ✓6ᵗʰ **M66.23 Spontaneous rupture of extensor tendons,** forearm
         M66.231 Spontaneous rupture of extensor tendons,
             right **forearm**
         M66.232 Spontaneous rupture of extensor tendons,
             left **forearm**
         M66.239 Spontaneous rupture of extensor ▽
             tendons, unspecified forearm

     ✓6ᵗʰ **M66.24 Spontaneous rupture of extensor tendons,** hand
         M66.241 Spontaneous rupture of extensor tendons,
             right **hand**
         M66.242 Spontaneous rupture of extensor tendons,
             left **hand**
         M66.249 Spontaneous rupture of extensor ▽
             tendons, unspecified hand

     ✓6ᵗʰ **M66.25 Spontaneous rupture of extensor tendons,** thigh
         M66.251 Spontaneous rupture of extensor
             tendons, right **thigh**
         M66.252 Spontaneous rupture of extensor
             tendons, left **thigh**

☑ Additional Character Req   ✓x7ᵗʰ Placeholder Alert   Case-Mix Diagnosis   Manifestation   ▽ Unspecified Dx   EXCLUDES 1 Not coded here   EXCLUDES 2 Not included here

ICD-10-CM 2018   **769**

M66.259 Spontaneous rupture of extensor tendons, unspecified thigh ▽

✓6ᵗʰ **M66.26** Spontaneous rupture of extensor tendons, lower leg

   M66.261 Spontaneous rupture of extensor tendons, right lower leg

   M66.262 Spontaneous rupture of extensor tendons, left lower leg

   M66.269 Spontaneous rupture of extensor tendons, unspecified lower leg ▽

✓6ᵗʰ **M66.27** Spontaneous rupture of extensor tendons, ankle and foot

   M66.271 Spontaneous rupture of extensor tendons, right ankle and foot

   M66.272 Spontaneous rupture of extensor tendons, left ankle and foot

   M66.279 Spontaneous rupture of extensor tendons, unspecified ankle and foot ▽

M66.28 Spontaneous rupture of extensor tendons, other site

M66.29 Spontaneous rupture of extensor tendons, multiple sites

✓5ᵗʰ **M66.3** Spontaneous rupture of flexor tendons

   TIP: Refer to the Muscle/Tendon table at the beginning of this chapter.

   M66.3Ø Spontaneous rupture of flexor tendons, unspecified site ▽

✓6ᵗʰ **M66.31** Spontaneous rupture of flexor tendons, shoulder

   M66.311 Spontaneous rupture of flexor tendons, right shoulder

   M66.312 Spontaneous rupture of flexor tendons, left shoulder

   M66.319 Spontaneous rupture of flexor tendons, unspecified shoulder ▽

✓6ᵗʰ **M66.32** Spontaneous rupture of flexor tendons, upper arm

   M66.321 Spontaneous rupture of flexor tendons, right upper arm

   M66.322 Spontaneous rupture of flexor tendons, left upper arm

   M66.329 Spontaneous rupture of flexor tendons, unspecified upper arm ▽

✓6ᵗʰ **M66.33** Spontaneous rupture of flexor tendons, forearm

   M66.331 Spontaneous rupture of flexor tendons, right forearm

   M66.332 Spontaneous rupture of flexor tendons, left forearm

   M66.339 Spontaneous rupture of flexor tendons, unspecified forearm ▽

✓6ᵗʰ **M66.34** Spontaneous rupture of flexor tendons, hand

   M66.341 Spontaneous rupture of flexor tendons, right hand

   M66.342 Spontaneous rupture of flexor tendons, left hand

   M66.349 Spontaneous rupture of flexor tendons, unspecified hand ▽

✓6ᵗʰ **M66.35** Spontaneous rupture of flexor tendons, thigh

   M66.351 Spontaneous rupture of flexor tendons, right thigh

   M66.352 Spontaneous rupture of flexor tendons, left thigh

   M66.359 Spontaneous rupture of flexor tendons, unspecified thigh ▽

✓6ᵗʰ **M66.36** Spontaneous rupture of flexor tendons, lower leg

   M66.361 Spontaneous rupture of flexor tendons, right lower leg

   M66.362 Spontaneous rupture of flexor tendons, left lower leg

   M66.369 Spontaneous rupture of flexor tendons, unspecified lower leg ▽

✓6ᵗʰ **M66.37** Spontaneous rupture of flexor tendons, ankle and foot

   M66.371 Spontaneous rupture of flexor tendons, right ankle and foot

   M66.372 Spontaneous rupture of flexor tendons, left ankle and foot

   M66.379 Spontaneous rupture of flexor tendons, unspecified ankle and foot ▽

M66.38 Spontaneous rupture of flexor tendons, other site

M66.39 Spontaneous rupture of flexor tendons, multiple sites

✓5ᵗʰ **M66.8** Spontaneous rupture of other tendons

   TIP: Refer to the Muscle/Tendon table at the beginning of this chapter.

   M66.8Ø Spontaneous rupture of other tendons, unspecified site ▽

✓6ᵗʰ **M66.81** Spontaneous rupture of other tendons, shoulder

   M66.811 Spontaneous rupture of other tendons, right shoulder

   M66.812 Spontaneous rupture of other tendons, left shoulder

   M66.819 Spontaneous rupture of other tendons, unspecified shoulder ▽

✓6ᵗʰ **M66.82** Spontaneous rupture of other tendons, upper arm

   M66.821 Spontaneous rupture of other tendons, right upper arm

   M66.822 Spontaneous rupture of other tendons, left upper arm

   M66.829 Spontaneous rupture of other tendons, unspecified upper arm ▽

✓6ᵗʰ **M66.83** Spontaneous rupture of other tendons, forearm

   M66.831 Spontaneous rupture of other tendons, right forearm

   M66.832 Spontaneous rupture of other tendons, left forearm

   M66.839 Spontaneous rupture of other tendons, unspecified forearm ▽

✓6ᵗʰ **M66.84** Spontaneous rupture of other tendons, hand

   M66.841 Spontaneous rupture of other tendons, right hand

   M66.842 Spontaneous rupture of other tendons, left hand

   M66.849 Spontaneous rupture of other tendons, unspecified hand ▽

✓6ᵗʰ **M66.85** Spontaneous rupture of other tendons, thigh

   M66.851 Spontaneous rupture of other tendons, right thigh

   M66.852 Spontaneous rupture of other tendons, left thigh

   M66.859 Spontaneous rupture of other tendons, unspecified thigh ▽

✓6ᵗʰ **M66.86** Spontaneous rupture of other tendons, lower leg

   M66.861 Spontaneous rupture of other tendons, right lower leg

   M66.862 Spontaneous rupture of other tendons, left lower leg

   M66.869 Spontaneous rupture of other tendons, unspecified lower leg ▽

✓6ᵗʰ **M66.87** Spontaneous rupture of other tendons, ankle and foot

   M66.871 Spontaneous rupture of other tendons, right ankle and foot

   M66.872 Spontaneous rupture of other tendons, left ankle and foot

   M66.879 Spontaneous rupture of other tendons, unspecified ankle and foot ▽

M66.88 Spontaneous rupture of other tendons, other

M66.89 Spontaneous rupture of other tendons, multiple sites

M66.9 Spontaneous rupture of unspecified tendon ▽
   Rupture at musculotendinous junction, nontraumatic

✓4ᵗʰ **M67** Other disorders of synovium and tendon
   EXCLUDES 1 palmar fascial fibromatosis [Dupuytren] (M72.Ø)
   tendinitis NOS (M77.9-)
   xanthomatosis localized to tendons (E78.2)

✓5ᵗʰ **M67.Ø** Short Achilles tendon (acquired)

   M67.ØØ Short Achilles tendon (acquired), unspecified ankle ▽

   M67.Ø1 Short Achilles tendon (acquired), right ankle

   M67.Ø2 Short Achilles tendon (acquired), left ankle

✓5ᵗʰ **M67.2** Synovial hypertrophy, not elsewhere classified
   EXCLUDES 1 villonodular synovitis (pigmented) (M12.2-)

   M67.2Ø Synovial hypertrophy, not elsewhere classified, unspecified site ▽

N Newborn: 0   P Pediatric: 0-17   M Maternity: 12-55   A Adult: 15-124   NRS Nonroutine supply Dx   NCDx Noncancer Dx   PDx Primary Dx   ►◄ Revised Text   ● New Code   ▲ Revised Title

770   ICD-10-CM 2018

☑6ᵗʰ **M67.21** Synovial hypertrophy, not elsewhere classified, shoulder
- **M67.211** Synovial hypertrophy, not elsewhere classified, right shoulder
- **M67.212** Synovial hypertrophy, not elsewhere classified, left shoulder
- **M67.219** Synovial hypertrophy, not elsewhere classified, unspecified shoulder ▽

☑6ᵗʰ **M67.22** Synovial hypertrophy, not elsewhere classified, upper arm
- **M67.221** Synovial hypertrophy, not elsewhere classified, right upper arm
- **M67.222** Synovial hypertrophy, not elsewhere classified, left upper arm
- **M67.229** Synovial hypertrophy, not elsewhere classified, unspecified upper arm ▽

☑6ᵗʰ **M67.23** Synovial hypertrophy, not elsewhere classified, forearm
- **M67.231** Synovial hypertrophy, not elsewhere classified, right forearm
- **M67.232** Synovial hypertrophy, not elsewhere classified, left forearm
- **M67.239** Synovial hypertrophy, not elsewhere classified, unspecified forearm ▽

☑6ᵗʰ **M67.24** Synovial hypertrophy, not elsewhere classified, hand
- **M67.241** Synovial hypertrophy, not elsewhere classified, right hand
- **M67.242** Synovial hypertrophy, not elsewhere classified, left hand
- **M67.249** Synovial hypertrophy, not elsewhere classified, unspecified hand ▽

☑6ᵗʰ **M67.25** Synovial hypertrophy, not elsewhere classified, thigh
- **M67.251** Synovial hypertrophy, not elsewhere classified, right thigh
- **M67.252** Synovial hypertrophy, not elsewhere classified, left thigh
- **M67.259** Synovial hypertrophy, not elsewhere classified, unspecified thigh ▽

☑6ᵗʰ **M67.26** Synovial hypertrophy, not elsewhere classified, lower leg
- **M67.261** Synovial hypertrophy, not elsewhere classified, right lower leg
- **M67.262** Synovial hypertrophy, not elsewhere classified, left lower leg
- **M67.269** Synovial hypertrophy, not elsewhere classified, unspecified lower leg ▽

☑6ᵗʰ **M67.27** Synovial hypertrophy, not elsewhere classified, ankle and foot
- **M67.271** Synovial hypertrophy, not elsewhere classified, right ankle and foot
- **M67.272** Synovial hypertrophy, not elsewhere classified, left ankle and foot
- **M67.279** Synovial hypertrophy, not elsewhere classified, unspecified ankle and foot ▽

M67.28 Synovial hypertrophy, not elsewhere classified, other site

M67.29 Synovial hypertrophy, not elsewhere classified, multiple sites

☑5ᵗʰ **M67.3** Transient synovitis
Toxic synovitis
EXCLUDES 1　palindromic rheumatism (M12.3-)

M67.30 Transient synovitis, unspecified site ▽

☑6ᵗʰ **M67.31** Transient synovitis, shoulder
- **M67.311** Transient synovitis, right shoulder
- **M67.312** Transient synovitis, left shoulder
- **M67.319** Transient synovitis, unspecified shoulder ▽

☑6ᵗʰ **M67.32** Transient synovitis, elbow
- **M67.321** Transient synovitis, right elbow
- **M67.322** Transient synovitis, left elbow
- **M67.329** Transient synovitis, unspecified elbow ▽

☑6ᵗʰ **M67.33** Transient synovitis, wrist
- **M67.331** Transient synovitis, right wrist
- **M67.332** Transient synovitis, left wrist
- **M67.339** Transient synovitis, unspecified wrist ▽

☑6ᵗʰ **M67.34** Transient synovitis, hand
- **M67.341** Transient synovitis, right hand
- **M67.342** Transient synovitis, left hand
- **M67.349** Transient synovitis, unspecified hand ▽

☑6ᵗʰ **M67.35** Transient synovitis, hip
- **M67.351** Transient synovitis, right hip
- **M67.352** Transient synovitis, left hip
- **M67.359** Transient synovitis, unspecified hip ▽

☑6ᵗʰ **M67.36** Transient synovitis, knee
- **M67.361** Transient synovitis, right knee
- **M67.362** Transient synovitis, left knee
- **M67.369** Transient synovitis, unspecified knee ▽

☑6ᵗʰ **M67.37** Transient synovitis, ankle and foot
- **M67.371** Transient synovitis, right ankle and foot
- **M67.372** Transient synovitis, left ankle and foot
- **M67.379** Transient synovitis, unspecified ankle and foot ▽

M67.38 Transient synovitis, other site

M67.39 Transient synovitis, multiple sites

☑5ᵗʰ **M67.4** Ganglion
Ganglion of joint or tendon (sheath)
EXCLUDES 1　ganglion in yaws (A66.6)
EXCLUDES 2　cyst of bursa (M71.2-M71.3)
　　　　　　　cyst of synovium (M71.2-M71.3)

M67.40 Ganglion, unspecified site ▽

☑6ᵗʰ **M67.41** Ganglion, shoulder
- **M67.411** Ganglion, right shoulder
- **M67.412** Ganglion, left shoulder
- **M67.419** Ganglion, unspecified shoulder ▽

☑6ᵗʰ **M67.42** Ganglion, elbow
- **M67.421** Ganglion, right elbow
- **M67.422** Ganglion, left elbow
- **M67.429** Ganglion, unspecified elbow ▽

☑6ᵗʰ **M67.43** Ganglion, wrist
- **M67.431** Ganglion, right wrist
- **M67.432** Ganglion, left wrist
- **M67.439** Ganglion, unspecified wrist ▽

☑6ᵗʰ **M67.44** Ganglion, hand
- **M67.441** Ganglion, right hand
- **M67.442** Ganglion, left hand
- **M67.449** Ganglion, unspecified hand ▽

☑6ᵗʰ **M67.45** Ganglion, hip
- **M67.451** Ganglion, right hip
- **M67.452** Ganglion, left hip
- **M67.459** Ganglion, unspecified hip ▽

☑6ᵗʰ **M67.46** Ganglion, knee
- **M67.461** Ganglion, right knee
- **M67.462** Ganglion, left knee
- **M67.469** Ganglion, unspecified knee ▽

Ganglion of Wrist

Extensor tendon sheaths

Ganglion of wrist (fluid-filled sac)

☑ Additional Character Req　　☑x7ᵗʰ Placeholder Alert　　Case-Mix Diagnosis　　Manifestation　　▽ Unspecified Dx　　*EXCLUDES 1* Not coded here　　*EXCLUDES 2* Not included here

Chapter 13. Diseases of the Musculoskeletal System and Connective Tissue

✓6ᵗʰ **M67.47 Ganglion,** ankle and foot
     M67.471 Ganglion, right ankle and foot
     M67.472 Ganglion, left ankle and foot
     M67.479 Ganglion, unspecified ankle and foot ▽
   M67.48 Ganglion, other site
   M67.49 Ganglion, multiple sites

✓5ᵗʰ **M67.5 Plica syndrome**
     Plica knee
   M67.50 Plica syndrome, unspecified knee ▽
   M67.51 Plica syndrome, right knee
   M67.52 Plica syndrome, left knee

✓5ᵗʰ **M67.8 Other specified disorders of synovium and tendon**
   M67.80 Other specified disorders of synovium and ▽
     tendon, unspecified site
   ✓6ᵗʰ **M67.81 Other specified disorders of synovium and tendon,** shoulder
     M67.811 Other specified disorders of synovium, right shoulder
     M67.812 Other specified disorders of synovium, left shoulder
     M67.813 Other specified disorders of tendon, right shoulder
     M67.814 Other specified disorders of tendon, left shoulder
     M67.819 Other specified disorders of synovium ▽ **and tendon, unspecified shoulder**
   ✓6ᵗʰ **M67.82 Other specified disorders of synovium and tendon,** elbow
     M67.821 Other specified disorders of synovium, right elbow
     M67.822 Other specified disorders of synovium, left elbow
     M67.823 Other specified disorders of tendon, right elbow
     M67.824 Other specified disorders of tendon, left elbow
     M67.829 Other specified disorders of synovium ▽ **and tendon, unspecified elbow**
   ✓6ᵗʰ **M67.83 Other specified disorders of synovium and tendon,** wrist
     M67.831 Other specified disorders of synovium, right wrist
     M67.832 Other specified disorders of synovium, left wrist
     M67.833 Other specified disorders of tendon, right wrist
     M67.834 Other specified disorders of tendon, left wrist
     M67.839 Other specified disorders of synovium ▽ **and tendon, unspecified forearm**
   ✓6ᵗʰ **M67.84 Other specified disorders of synovium and tendon,** hand
     M67.841 Other specified disorders of synovium, right hand
     M67.842 Other specified disorders of synovium, left hand
     M67.843 Other specified disorders of tendon, right hand
     M67.844 Other specified disorders of tendon, left hand
     M67.849 Other specified disorders of synovium ▽ **and tendon, unspecified hand**
   ✓6ᵗʰ **M67.85 Other specified disorders of synovium and tendon,** hip
     M67.851 Other specified disorders of synovium, right hip
     M67.852 Other specified disorders of synovium, left hip
     M67.853 Other specified disorders of tendon, right hip
     M67.854 Other specified disorders of tendon, left hip
     M67.859 Other specified disorders of synovium ▽ **and tendon, unspecified hip**

✓6ᵗʰ **M67.86 Other specified disorders of synovium and tendon,** knee
     M67.861 Other specified disorders of synovium, right knee
     M67.862 Other specified disorders of synovium, left knee
     M67.863 Other specified disorders of tendon, right knee
     M67.864 Other specified disorders of tendon, left knee
     M67.869 Other specified disorders of synovium ▽ **and tendon, unspecified knee**
✓6ᵗʰ **M67.87 Other specified disorders of synovium and tendon,** ankle and foot
     M67.871 Other specified disorders of synovium, right ankle and foot
     M67.872 Other specified disorders of synovium, left ankle and foot
     M67.873 Other specified disorders of tendon, right ankle and foot
     M67.874 Other specified disorders of tendon, left ankle and foot
     M67.879 Other specified disorders of synovium ▽ **and tendon, unspecified ankle and foot**
   M67.88 Other specified disorders of synovium and tendon, other site
   M67.89 Other specified disorders of synovium and tendon, multiple sites
✓5ᵗʰ **M67.9 Unspecified disorder of synovium and tendon**
   M67.90 Unspecified disorder of synovium and tendon, ▽ **unspecified site**
   ✓6ᵗʰ **M67.91 Unspecified disorder of synovium and tendon,** shoulder
     M67.911 Unspecified disorder of synovium and ▽ **tendon, right shoulder**
     M67.912 Unspecified disorder of synovium and ▽ **tendon, left shoulder**
     M67.919 Unspecified disorder of synovium and ▽ **tendon, unspecified shoulder**
   ✓6ᵗʰ **M67.92 Unspecified disorder of synovium and tendon,** upper arm
     M67.921 Unspecified disorder of synovium and ▽ **tendon, right upper arm**
     M67.922 Unspecified disorder of synovium and ▽ **tendon, left upper arm**
     M67.929 Unspecified disorder of synovium ▽ **and tendon, unspecified upper arm**
   ✓6ᵗʰ **M67.93 Unspecified disorder of synovium and tendon,** forearm
     M67.931 Unspecified disorder of synovium ▽ **and tendon, right forearm**
     M67.932 Unspecified disorder of synovium ▽ **and tendon, left forearm**
     M67.939 Unspecified disorder of synovium ▽ **and tendon, unspecified forearm**
   ✓6ᵗʰ **M67.94 Unspecified disorder of synovium and tendon,** hand
     M67.941 Unspecified disorder of synovium ▽ **and tendon, right hand**
     M67.942 Unspecified disorder of synovium ▽ **and tendon, left hand**
     M67.949 Unspecified disorder of synovium ▽ **and tendon, unspecified hand**
   ✓6ᵗʰ **M67.95 Unspecified disorder of synovium and tendon,** thigh
     M67.951 Unspecified disorder of synovium ▽ **and tendon, right thigh**
     M67.952 Unspecified disorder of synovium ▽ **and tendon, left thigh**
     M67.959 Unspecified disorder of synovium ▽ **and tendon, unspecified thigh**
   ✓6ᵗʰ **M67.96 Unspecified disorder of synovium and tendon,** lower leg
     M67.961 Unspecified disorder of synovium ▽ **and tendon, right lower leg**
     M67.962 Unspecified disorder of synovium ▽ **and tendon, left lower leg**

Ⓝ Newborn: 0   Ⓟ Pediatric: 0-17   Ⓜ Maternity: 12-55   Ⓐ Adult: 15-124   **NRS** Nonroutine supply Dx   **NC Dx** Noncancer Dx   **PDx** Primary Dx   ▶◀ Revised Text   ● New Code   ▲ Revised Title

772   ICD-10-CM 2018

M67.969 Unspecified disorder of synovium and tendon, unspecified lower leg ▽

✓6ᵗʰ M67.97 Unspecified disorder of synovium and tendon, ankle and foot

M67.971 Unspecified disorder of synovium and tendon, right ankle and foot ▽

M67.972 Unspecified disorder of synovium and tendon, left ankle and foot ▽

M67.979 Unspecified disorder of synovium and tendon, unspecified ankle and foot ▽

M67.98 Unspecified disorder of synovium and tendon, other site ▽

M67.99 Unspecified disorder of synovium and tendon, multiple sites ▽

Other soft tissue disorders (M70-M79)

✓4ᵗʰ M70 Soft tissue disorders related to use, overuse and pressure
INCLUDES soft tissue disorders of occupational origin
Use additional external cause code to identify activity causing disorder (Y93.-)
EXCLUDES 1 bursitis NOS (M71.9-)
EXCLUDES 2 bursitis of shoulder (M75.5)
    enthesopathies (M76-M77)
    pressure ulcer (pressure area) (L89.-)

✓5ᵗʰ M70.0 Crepitant synovitis (acute) (chronic) of hand and wrist

✓6ᵗʰ M70.03 Crepitant synovitis (acute) (chronic), wrist

M70.031 Crepitant synovitis (acute) (chronic), right wrist

M70.032 Crepitant synovitis (acute) (chronic), left wrist

M70.039 Crepitant synovitis (acute) (chronic), unspecified wrist ▽

✓6ᵗʰ M70.04 Crepitant synovitis (acute) (chronic), hand

M70.041 Crepitant synovitis (acute) (chronic), right hand

M70.042 Crepitant synovitis (acute) (chronic), left hand

M70.049 Crepitant synovitis (acute) (chronic), unspecified hand ▽

✓5ᵗʰ M70.1 Bursitis of hand

M70.10 Bursitis, unspecified hand ▽

M70.11 Bursitis, right hand

M70.12 Bursitis, left hand

✓5ᵗʰ M70.2 Olecranon bursitis

M70.20 Olecranon bursitis, unspecified elbow ▽

M70.21 Olecranon bursitis, right elbow

M70.22 Olecranon bursitis, left elbow

✓5ᵗʰ M70.3 Other bursitis of elbow

M70.30 Other bursitis of elbow, unspecified elbow ▽

M70.31 Other bursitis of elbow, right elbow

M70.32 Other bursitis of elbow, left elbow

Knee Bursae

✓5ᵗʰ M70.4 Prepatellar bursitis

M70.40 Prepatellar bursitis, unspecified knee ▽

M70.41 Prepatellar bursitis, right knee

M70.42 Prepatellar bursitis, left knee

✓5ᵗʰ M70.5 Other bursitis of knee

M70.50 Other bursitis of knee, unspecified knee ▽

M70.51 Other bursitis of knee, right knee

M70.52 Other bursitis of knee, left knee

✓5ᵗʰ M70.6 Trochanteric bursitis
Trochanteric tendinitis

M70.60 Trochanteric bursitis, unspecified hip ▽

M70.61 Trochanteric bursitis, right hip

M70.62 Trochanteric bursitis, left hip

✓5ᵗʰ M70.7 Other bursitis of hip
Ischial bursitis

M70.70 Other bursitis of hip, unspecified hip ▽

M70.71 Other bursitis of hip, right hip

M70.72 Other bursitis of hip, left hip

✓5ᵗʰ M70.8 Other soft tissue disorders related to use, overuse and pressure

M70.80 Other soft tissue disorders related to use, overuse and pressure of unspecified site ▽

✓6ᵗʰ M70.81 Other soft tissue disorders related to use, overuse and pressure of shoulder

M70.811 Other soft tissue disorders related to use, overuse and pressure, right shoulder

M70.812 Other soft tissue disorders related to use, overuse and pressure, left shoulder

M70.819 Other soft tissue disorders related to use, overuse and pressure, unspecified shoulder ▽

✓6ᵗʰ M70.82 Other soft tissue disorders related to use, overuse and pressure of upper arm

M70.821 Other soft tissue disorders related to use, overuse and pressure, right upper arm

M70.822 Other soft tissue disorders related to use, overuse and pressure, left upper arm

M70.829 Other soft tissue disorders related to use, overuse and pressure, unspecified upper arms ▽

✓6ᵗʰ M70.83 Other soft tissue disorders related to use, overuse and pressure of forearm

M70.831 Other soft tissue disorders related to use, overuse and pressure, right forearm

M70.832 Other soft tissue disorders related to use, overuse and pressure, left forearm

M70.839 Other soft tissue disorders related to use, overuse and pressure, unspecified forearm ▽

✓6ᵗʰ M70.84 Other soft tissue disorders related to use, overuse and pressure of hand

M70.841 Other soft tissue disorders related to use, overuse and pressure, right hand

M70.842 Other soft tissue disorders related to use, overuse and pressure, left hand

M70.849 Other soft tissue disorders related to use, overuse and pressure, unspecified hand ▽

✓6ᵗʰ M70.85 Other soft tissue disorders related to use, overuse and pressure of thigh

M70.851 Other soft tissue disorders related to use, overuse and pressure, right thigh

M70.852 Other soft tissue disorders related to use, overuse and pressure, left thigh

M70.859 Other soft tissue disorders related to use, overuse and pressure, unspecified thigh ▽

✓6ᵗʰ M70.86 Other soft tissue disorders related to use, overuse and pressure lower leg

M70.861 Other soft tissue disorders related to use, overuse and pressure, right lower leg

M70.862 Other soft tissue disorders related to use, overuse and pressure, left lower leg

M70.869 Other soft tissue disorders related to use, overuse and pressure, unspecified leg ▽

✓ Additional Character Req   ✓x7ᵗʰ Placeholder Alert   Case-Mix Diagnosis   Manifestation   ▽ Unspecified Dx   EXCLUDES 1 Not coded here   EXCLUDES 2 Not included here

Chapter 13. Diseases of the Musculoskeletal System and Connective Tissue

✓6ᵗʰ **M70.87 Other soft tissue disorders related to use, overuse and pressure of** ankle and foot

     M70.871 Other soft tissue disorders related to use, overuse and pressure, right **ankle and foot**

     M70.872 Other soft tissue disorders related to use, overuse and pressure, left **ankle and foot**

     M70.879 Other soft tissue disorders related to use, overuse and pressure, unspecified ankle and foot ▽

M70.88 Other soft tissue disorders related to use, overuse and pressure other site

M70.89 Other soft tissue disorders related to use, overuse and pressure multiple sites

✓5ᵗʰ **M70.9 Unspecified soft tissue disorder related to use, overuse and pressure**

     M70.90 Unspecified soft tissue disorder related to use, overuse and pressure of unspecified site ▽

✓6ᵗʰ **M70.91 Unspecified soft tissue disorder related to use, overuse and pressure of** shoulder

     M70.911 Unspecified soft tissue disorder related to use, overuse and pressure, right **shoulder** ▽

     M70.912 Unspecified soft tissue disorder related to use, overuse and pressure, left **shoulder** ▽

     M70.919 Unspecified soft tissue disorder related to use, overuse and pressure, unspecified shoulder ▽

✓6ᵗʰ **M70.92 Unspecified soft tissue disorder related to use, overuse and pressure of** upper arm

     M70.921 Unspecified soft tissue disorder related to use, overuse and pressure, right **upper arm** ▽

     M70.922 Unspecified soft tissue disorder related to use, overuse and pressure, left **upper arm** ▽

     M70.929 Unspecified soft tissue disorder related to use, overuse and pressure, unspecified upper arm ▽

✓6ᵗʰ **M70.93 Unspecified soft tissue disorder related to use, overuse and pressure of** forearm

     M70.931 Unspecified soft tissue disorder related to use, overuse and pressure, right **forearm** ▽

     M70.932 Unspecified soft tissue disorder related to use, overuse and pressure, left **forearm** ▽

     M70.939 Unspecified soft tissue disorder related to use, overuse and pressure, unspecified forearm ▽

✓6ᵗʰ **M70.94 Unspecified soft tissue disorder related to use, overuse and pressure of** hand

     M70.941 Unspecified soft tissue disorder related to use, overuse and pressure, right **hand** ▽

     M70.942 Unspecified soft tissue disorder related to use, overuse and pressure, left **hand** ▽

     M70.949 Unspecified soft tissue disorder related to use, overuse and pressure, unspecified hand ▽

✓6ᵗʰ **M70.95 Unspecified soft tissue disorder related to use, overuse and pressure of** thigh

     M70.951 Unspecified soft tissue disorder related to use, overuse and pressure, right **thigh** ▽

     M70.952 Unspecified soft tissue disorder related to use, overuse and pressure, left **thigh** ▽

     M70.959 Unspecified soft tissue disorder related to use, overuse and pressure, unspecified thigh ▽

✓6ᵗʰ **M70.96 Unspecified soft tissue disorder related to use, overuse and pressure** lower leg

     M70.961 Unspecified soft tissue disorder related to use, overuse and pressure, right **lower leg** ▽

     M70.962 Unspecified soft tissue disorder related to use, overuse and pressure, left **lower leg** ▽

     M70.969 Unspecified soft tissue disorder related to use, overuse and pressure, unspecified lower leg ▽

✓6ᵗʰ **M70.97 Unspecified soft tissue disorder related to use, overuse and pressure of** ankle and foot

     M70.971 Unspecified soft tissue disorder related to use, overuse and pressure, right **ankle and foot** ▽

     M70.972 Unspecified soft tissue disorder related to use, overuse and pressure, left **ankle and foot** ▽

     M70.979 Unspecified soft tissue disorder related to use, overuse and pressure, unspecified ankle and foot ▽

M70.98 Unspecified soft tissue disorder related to use, overuse and pressure other ▽

M70.99 Unspecified soft tissue disorder related to use, overuse and pressure multiple sites ▽

✓4ᵗʰ **M71 Other bursopathies**

EXCLUDES 1   bunion (M20.1)
     bursitis related to use, overuse or pressure (M70.-)
     enthesopathies (M76-M77)

✓5ᵗʰ **M71.0 Abscess of bursa**

     Use additional code (B95.-, B96.-) to identify causative organism

     M71.00 Abscess of bursa, unspecified site ▽

✓6ᵗʰ **M71.01 Abscess of bursa,** shoulder

     M71.011 Abscess of bursa, right **shoulder**

     M71.012 Abscess of bursa, left **shoulder**

     M71.019 Abscess of bursa, unspecified shoulder ▽

✓6ᵗʰ **M71.02 Abscess of bursa,** elbow

     M71.021 Abscess of bursa, right **elbow**

     M71.022 Abscess of bursa, left **elbow**

     M71.029 Abscess of bursa, unspecified elbow ▽

✓6ᵗʰ **M71.03 Abscess of bursa,** wrist

     M71.031 Abscess of bursa, right **wrist**

     M71.032 Abscess of bursa, left **wrist**

     M71.039 Abscess of bursa, unspecified wrist ▽

✓6ᵗʰ **M71.04 Abscess of bursa,** hand

     M71.041 Abscess of bursa, right **hand**

     M71.042 Abscess of bursa, left **hand**

     M71.049 Abscess of bursa, unspecified hand ▽

✓6ᵗʰ **M71.05 Abscess of bursa,** hip

     M71.051 Abscess of bursa, right **hip**

     M71.052 Abscess of bursa, left **hip**

     M71.059 Abscess of bursa, unspecified hip ▽

✓6ᵗʰ **M71.06 Abscess of bursa,** knee

     M71.061 Abscess of bursa, right **knee**

     M71.062 Abscess of bursa, left **knee**

     M71.069 Abscess of bursa, unspecified knee ▽

✓6ᵗʰ **M71.07 Abscess of bursa,** ankle and foot

     M71.071 Abscess of bursa, right **ankle and foot**

     M71.072 Abscess of bursa, left **ankle and foot**

     M71.079 Abscess of bursa, unspecified ankle and foot ▽

M71.08 Abscess of bursa, other site

M71.09 Abscess of bursa, multiple sites

✓5ᵗʰ **M71.1 Other infective bursitis**

     Use additional code (B95.-, B96.-) to identify causative organism

     M71.10 Other infective bursitis, unspecified site ▽

✓6ᵗʰ **M71.11 Other infective bursitis,** shoulder

     M71.111 Other infective bursitis, right **shoulder**

     M71.112 Other infective bursitis, left **shoulder**

     M71.119 Other infective bursitis, unspecified shoulder ▽

✓6ᵗʰ **M71.12 Other infective bursitis,** elbow

     M71.121 Other infective bursitis, right **elbow**

     M71.122 Other infective bursitis, left **elbow**

     M71.129 Other infective bursitis, unspecified elbow ▽

✓6ᵗʰ **M71.13 Other infective bursitis,** wrist

     M71.131 Other infective bursitis, right **wrist**

     M71.132 Other infective bursitis, left **wrist**

     M71.139 Other infective bursitis, unspecified wrist ▽

✓6ᵗʰ **M71.14 Other infective bursitis,** hand

     M71.141 Other infective bursitis, right **hand**

N Newborn: 0   P Pediatric: 0-17   M Maternity: 12-55   A Adult: 15-124   NRS Nonroutine supply Dx   NC Dx Noncancer Dx   PDx Primary Dx   ▶◀ Revised Text   ● New Code   ▲ Revised Title

774   ICD-10-CM 2018

M71.142   Other infective bursitis, left hand
M71.149   Other infective bursitis, unspecified hand   ▽

✓6ᵗʰ M71.15   Other infective bursitis, hip
     M71.151   Other infective bursitis, right hip
     M71.152   Other infective bursitis, left hip
     M71.159   Other infective bursitis, unspecified hip ▽

✓6ᵗʰ M71.16   Other infective bursitis, knee
     M71.161   Other infective bursitis, right knee
     M71.162   Other infective bursitis, left knee
     M71.169   Other infective bursitis, unspecified knee   ▽

✓6ᵗʰ M71.17   Other infective bursitis, ankle and foot
     M71.171   Other infective bursitis, right ankle and foot
     M71.172   Other infective bursitis, left ankle and foot
     M71.179   Other infective bursitis, unspecified ankle and foot   ▽

M71.18   Other infective bursitis, other site
M71.19   Other infective bursitis, multiple sites

✓5ᵗʰ M71.2   Synovial cyst of popliteal space [Baker]
     EXCLUDES 1   synovial cyst of popliteal space with rupture (M66.0)
     M71.20   Synovial cyst of popliteal space [Baker], unspecified knee   ▽
     M71.21   Synovial cyst of popliteal space [Baker], right knee
     M71.22   Synovial cyst of popliteal space [Baker], left knee

✓5ᵗʰ M71.3   Other bursal cyst
     Synovial cyst NOS
     EXCLUDES 1   synovial cyst with rupture (M66.1-)
     M71.30   Other bursal cyst, unspecified site   ▽

✓6ᵗʰ M71.31   Other bursal cyst, shoulder
     M71.311   Other bursal cyst, right shoulder
     M71.312   Other bursal cyst, left shoulder
     M71.319   Other bursal cyst, unspecified shoulder ▽

✓6ᵗʰ M71.32   Other bursal cyst, elbow
     M71.321   Other bursal cyst, right elbow
     M71.322   Other bursal cyst, left elbow
     M71.329   Other bursal cyst, unspecified elbow   ▽

✓6ᵗʰ M71.33   Other bursal cyst, wrist
     M71.331   Other bursal cyst, right wrist
     M71.332   Other bursal cyst, left wrist
     M71.339   Other bursal cyst, unspecified wrist   ▽

✓6ᵗʰ M71.34   Other bursal cyst, hand
     M71.341   Other bursal cyst, right hand
     M71.342   Other bursal cyst, left hand
     M71.349   Other bursal cyst, unspecified hand   ▽

✓6ᵗʰ M71.35   Other bursal cyst, hip
     M71.351   Other bursal cyst, right hip
     M71.352   Other bursal cyst, left hip
     M71.359   Other bursal cyst, unspecified hip   ▽

Baker's Cyst

Baker's cyst connected to knee joint synovial cavity

✓6ᵗʰ M71.37   Other bursal cyst, ankle and foot
     M71.371   Other bursal cyst, right ankle and foot
     M71.372   Other bursal cyst, left ankle and foot
     M71.379   Other bursal cyst, unspecified ankle and foot   ▽

M71.38   Other bursal cyst, other site
M71.39   Other bursal cyst, multiple sites

✓5ᵗʰ M71.4   Calcium deposit in bursa
     EXCLUDES 2   calcium deposit in bursa of shoulder (M75.3)
     M71.40   Calcium deposit in bursa, unspecified site   ▽

✓6ᵗʰ M71.42   Calcium deposit in bursa, elbow
     M71.421   Calcium deposit in bursa, right elbow
     M71.422   Calcium deposit in bursa, left elbow
     M71.429   Calcium deposit in bursa, unspecified elbow   ▽

✓6ᵗʰ M71.43   Calcium deposit in bursa, wrist
     M71.431   Calcium deposit in bursa, right wrist
     M71.432   Calcium deposit in bursa, left wrist
     M71.439   Calcium deposit in bursa, unspecified wrist   ▽

✓6ᵗʰ M71.44   Calcium deposit in bursa, hand
     M71.441   Calcium deposit in bursa, right hand
     M71.442   Calcium deposit in bursa, left hand
     M71.449   Calcium deposit in bursa, unspecified hand   ▽

✓6ᵗʰ M71.45   Calcium deposit in bursa, hip
     M71.451   Calcium deposit in bursa, right hip
     M71.452   Calcium deposit in bursa, left hip
     M71.459   Calcium deposit in bursa, unspecified hip   ▽

✓6ᵗʰ M71.46   Calcium deposit in bursa, knee
     M71.461   Calcium deposit in bursa, right knee
     M71.462   Calcium deposit in bursa, left knee
     M71.469   Calcium deposit in bursa, unspecified knee   ▽

✓6ᵗʰ M71.47   Calcium deposit in bursa, ankle and foot
     M71.471   Calcium deposit in bursa, right ankle and foot
     M71.472   Calcium deposit in bursa, left ankle and foot
     M71.479   Calcium deposit in bursa, unspecified ankle and foot   ▽

M71.48   Calcium deposit in bursa, other site
M71.49   Calcium deposit in bursa, multiple sites

✓5ᵗʰ M71.5   Other bursitis, not elsewhere classified
     EXCLUDES 1   bursitis NOS (M71.9-)
     EXCLUDES 2   bursitis of shoulder (M75.5)
             bursitis of tibial collateral [Pellegrini-Stieda] (M76.4-)
     M71.50   Other bursitis, not elsewhere classified, unspecified site   ▽

✓6ᵗʰ M71.52   Other bursitis, not elsewhere classified, elbow
     M71.521   Other bursitis, not elsewhere classified, right elbow
     M71.522   Other bursitis, not elsewhere classified, left elbow
     M71.529   Other bursitis, not elsewhere classified, unspecified elbow   ▽

✓6ᵗʰ M71.53   Other bursitis, not elsewhere classified, wrist
     M71.531   Other bursitis, not elsewhere classified, right wrist
     M71.532   Other bursitis, not elsewhere classified, left wrist
     M71.539   Other bursitis, not elsewhere classified, unspecified wrist   ▽

✓6ᵗʰ M71.54   Other bursitis, not elsewhere classified, hand
     M71.541   Other bursitis, not elsewhere classified, right hand
     M71.542   Other bursitis, not elsewhere classified, left hand
     M71.549   Other bursitis, not elsewhere classified, unspecified hand   ▽

✓6ᵗʰ M71.55   Other bursitis, not elsewhere classified, hip
     M71.551   Other bursitis, not elsewhere classified, right hip

---

✓ Additional Character Req   ✓ₓ7ᵗʰ Placeholder Alert   Case-Mix Diagnosis   Manifestation   ▽ Unspecified Dx   *EXCLUDES 1* Not coded here   *EXCLUDES 2* Not included here

M71.552   Other bursitis, not elsewhere classified, left hip

M71.559   Other bursitis, not elsewhere classified, ▽ unspecified hip

✓6ᵗʰ **M71.56**   Other bursitis, not elsewhere classified, knee

M71.561   Other bursitis, not elsewhere classified, right knee

M71.562   Other bursitis, not elsewhere classified, left knee

M71.569   Other bursitis, not elsewhere classified, ▽ unspecified knee

✓6ᵗʰ **M71.57**   Other bursitis, not elsewhere classified, ankle and foot

M71.571   Other bursitis, not elsewhere classified, right ankle and foot

M71.572   Other bursitis, not elsewhere classified, left ankle and foot

M71.579   Other bursitis, not elsewhere classified, ▽ unspecified ankle and foot

M71.58   Other bursitis, not elsewhere classified, other site

✓5ᵗʰ **M71.8**   **Other specified bursopathies**

M71.80   Other specified bursopathies, unspecified site ▽

✓6ᵗʰ **M71.81**   Other specified bursopathies, shoulder

M71.811   Other specified bursopathies, right shoulder

M71.812   Other specified bursopathies, left shoulder

M71.819   Other specified bursopathies, ▽ unspecified shoulder

✓6ᵗʰ **M71.82**   Other specified bursopathies, elbow

M71.821   Other specified bursopathies, right elbow

M71.822   Other specified bursopathies, left elbow

M71.829   Other specified bursopathies, ▽ unspecified elbow

✓6ᵗʰ **M71.83**   Other specified bursopathies, wrist

M71.831   Other specified bursopathies, right wrist

M71.832   Other specified bursopathies, left wrist

M71.839   Other specified bursopathies, ▽ unspecified wrist

✓6ᵗʰ **M71.84**   Other specified bursopathies, hand

M71.841   Other specified bursopathies, right hand

M71.842   Other specified bursopathies, left hand

M71.849   Other specified bursopathies, ▽ unspecified hand

✓6ᵗʰ **M71.85**   Other specified bursopathies, hip

M71.851   Other specified bursopathies, right hip

M71.852   Other specified bursopathies, left hip

M71.859   Other specified bursopathies, ▽ unspecified hip

✓6ᵗʰ **M71.86**   Other specified bursopathies, knee

M71.861   Other specified bursopathies, right knee

M71.862   Other specified bursopathies, left knee

M71.869   Other specified bursopathies, ▽ unspecified knee

✓6ᵗʰ **M71.87**   Other specified bursopathies, ankle and foot

M71.871   Other specified bursopathies, right ankle and foot

M71.872   Other specified bursopathies, left ankle and foot

M71.879   Other specified bursopathies, ▽ unspecified ankle and foot

M71.88   Other specified bursopathies, other site

M71.89   Other specified bursopathies, multiple sites

M71.9   **Bursopathy, unspecified** ▽
Bursitis NOS

✓4ᵗʰ **M72**   **Fibroblastic disorders**
EXCLUDES 2   retroperitoneal fibromatosis (D48.3)

M72.0   **Palmar fascial fibromatosis [Dupuytren]** 🄰
DEF: Dupuytren's contracture: Flexion deformity of finger, due to shortened, thickened fibrosing of palmar fascia; cause unknown; associated with long-standing epilepsy.

M72.1   **Knuckle pads**

M72.2   **Plantar fascial fibromatosis**
Plantar fasciitis
DEF: Rapid-growing and multiplanar nodular swellings and pain in the foot; not associated with contractures.

M72.4   **Pseudosarcomatous fibromatosis**
Nodular fasciitis

M72.6   **Necrotizing fasciitis**
Use additional code (B95.-, B96.-) to identify causative organism

M72.8   **Other fibroblastic disorders**
Abscess of fascia
Fasciitis NEC
Other infective fasciitis
Use additional code to (B95.-, B96.-) identify causative organism
EXCLUDES 1   diffuse (eosinophilic) fasciitis (M35.4)
necrotizing fasciitis (M72.6)
nodular fasciitis (M72.4)
perirenal fasciitis NOS (N13.5)
perirenal fasciitis with infection (N13.6)
plantar fasciitis (M72.2)

M72.9   **Fibroblastic disorder, unspecified** ▽
Fasciitis NOS
Fibromatosis NOS

✓4ᵗʰ **M75**   **Shoulder lesions**
EXCLUDES 2   shoulder-hand syndrome (M89.0-)

✓5ᵗʰ **M75.0**   **Adhesive capsulitis of shoulder**
Frozen shoulder
Periarthritis of shoulder
AHA: 2015, 2Q, 23

M75.00   Adhesive capsulitis of unspecified shoulder ▽

M75.01   Adhesive capsulitis of right shoulder

M75.02   Adhesive capsulitis of left shoulder

✓5ᵗʰ **M75.1**   **Rotator cuff tear or rupture, not specified as traumatic**
Rotator cuff syndrome
Supraspinatus syndrome
Supraspinatus tear or rupture, not specified as traumatic
EXCLUDES 1   tear of rotator cuff, traumatic (S46.01-)

✓6ᵗʰ **M75.10**   Unspecified rotator cuff tear or rupture, not specified as traumatic

M75.100   Unspecified rotator cuff tear or rupture ▽ of unspecified shoulder, not specified as traumatic

M75.101   Unspecified rotator cuff tear or rupture ▽ of right shoulder, not specified as traumatic

M75.102   Unspecified rotator cuff tear or rupture ▽ of left shoulder, not specified as traumatic

✓6ᵗʰ **M75.11**   Incomplete rotator cuff tear or rupture not specified as traumatic

M75.110   Incomplete rotator cuff tear or rupture ▽ of unspecified shoulder, not specified as traumatic

M75.111   Incomplete rotator cuff tear or rupture of right shoulder, not specified as traumatic

M75.112   Incomplete rotator cuff tear or rupture of left shoulder, not specified as traumatic

✓6ᵗʰ **M75.12**   Complete rotator cuff tear or rupture not specified as traumatic

M75.120   Complete rotator cuff tear or rupture ▽ of unspecified shoulder, not specified as traumatic

M75.121   Complete rotator cuff tear or rupture of right shoulder, not specified as traumatic

M75.122   Complete rotator cuff tear or rupture of left shoulder, not specified as traumatic

✓5ᵗʰ **M75.2**   **Bicipital tendinitis**

M75.20   Bicipital tendinitis, unspecified shoulder ▽

M75.21   Bicipital tendinitis, right shoulder

M75.22   Bicipital tendinitis, left shoulder

✓5ᵗʰ **M75.3**   **Calcific tendinitis of shoulder**
Calcified bursa of shoulder

M75.30   Calcific tendinitis of unspecified shoulder ▽

M75.31   Calcific tendinitis of right shoulder

M75.32   Calcific tendinitis of left shoulder

✓5ᵗʰ **M75.4**   **Impingement syndrome of shoulder**

M75.40   Impingement syndrome of unspecified ▽ shoulder

M75.41   Impingement syndrome of right shoulder

M75.42   Impingement syndrome of left shoulder

🄽 Newborn: 0   🄿 Pediatric: 0-17   🄼 Maternity: 12-55   🄰 Adult: 15-124   **NRS** Nonroutine supply Dx   **NCDx** Noncancer Dx   **PDx** Primary Dx   ▶◀ Revised Text   ● New Code   ▲ Revised Title

776   ICD-10-CM 2018

✓5ᵗʰ **M75.5 Bursitis of shoulder**
    M75.50 Bursitis of unspecified shoulder ▽
    M75.51 Bursitis of right shoulder
    M75.52 Bursitis of left shoulder

✓5ᵗʰ **M75.8 Other shoulder lesions**
    M75.80 Other shoulder lesions, unspecified shoulder ▽
    M75.81 Other shoulder lesions, right shoulder
    M75.82 Other shoulder lesions, left shoulder

✓5ᵗʰ **M75.9 Shoulder lesion, unspecified**
    M75.90 Shoulder lesion, unspecified, unspecified shoulder ▽
    M75.91 Shoulder lesion, unspecified, right shoulder ▽
    M75.92 Shoulder lesion, unspecified, left shoulder ▽

✓4ᵗʰ **M76 Enthesopathies, lower limb, excluding foot**
    EXCLUDES 2   bursitis due to use, overuse and pressure (M70.-)
          enthesopathies of ankle and foot (M77.5-)

✓5ᵗʰ **M76.0 Gluteal tendinitis**
    M76.00 Gluteal tendinitis, unspecified hip ▽
    M76.01 Gluteal tendinitis, right hip
    M76.02 Gluteal tendinitis, left hip

✓5ᵗʰ **M76.1 Psoas tendinitis**
    M76.10 Psoas tendinitis, unspecified hip ▽
    M76.11 Psoas tendinitis, right hip
    M76.12 Psoas tendinitis, left hip

✓5ᵗʰ **M76.2 Iliac crest spur**
    M76.20 Iliac crest spur, unspecified hip ▽
    M76.21 Iliac crest spur, right hip
    M76.22 Iliac crest spur, left hip

✓5ᵗʰ **M76.3 Iliotibial band syndrome**
    M76.30 Iliotibial band syndrome, unspecified leg ▽
    M76.31 Iliotibial band syndrome, right leg
    M76.32 Iliotibial band syndrome, left leg

✓5ᵗʰ **M76.4 Tibial collateral bursitis [Pellegrini-Stieda]**
    M76.40 Tibial collateral bursitis [Pellegrini-Stieda], unspecified leg ▽
    M76.41 Tibial collateral bursitis [Pellegrini-Stieda], right leg
    M76.42 Tibial collateral bursitis [Pellegrini-Stieda], left leg

✓5ᵗʰ **M76.5 Patellar tendinitis**
    M76.50 Patellar tendinitis, unspecified knee ▽
    M76.51 Patellar tendinitis, right knee
    M76.52 Patellar tendinitis, left knee

✓5ᵗʰ **M76.6 Achilles tendinitis**
    Achilles bursitis
    M76.60 Achilles tendinitis, unspecified leg ▽
    M76.61 Achilles tendinitis, right leg
    M76.62 Achilles tendinitis, left leg

✓5ᵗʰ **M76.7 Peroneal tendinitis**
    M76.70 Peroneal tendinitis, unspecified leg ▽
    M76.71 Peroneal tendinitis, right leg
    M76.72 Peroneal tendinitis, left leg

✓5ᵗʰ **M76.8 Other specified enthesopathies of lower limb, excluding foot**
    ✓6ᵗʰ **M76.81 Anterior tibial syndrome**
       M76.811 Anterior tibial syndrome, right leg
       M76.812 Anterior tibial syndrome, left leg
       M76.819 Anterior tibial syndrome, unspecified leg ▽
    ✓6ᵗʰ **M76.82 Posterior tibial tendinitis**
       M76.821 Posterior tibial tendinitis, right leg
       M76.822 Posterior tibial tendinitis, left leg
       M76.829 Posterior tibial tendinitis, unspecified leg ▽
    ✓6ᵗʰ **M76.89 Other specified enthesopathies of lower limb, excluding foot**
       M76.891 Other specified enthesopathies of right lower limb, excluding foot
       M76.892 Other specified enthesopathies of left lower limb, excluding foot
       M76.899 Other specified enthesopathies of unspecified lower limb, excluding foot ▽

M76.9 Unspecified enthesopathy, lower limb, excluding foot ▽

✓4ᵗʰ **M77 Other enthesopathies**
    EXCLUDES 1   bursitis NOS (M71.9-)
    EXCLUDES 2   bursitis due to use, overuse and pressure (M70.-)
          osteophyte (M25.7)
          spinal enthesopathy (M46.0-)

✓5ᵗʰ **M77.0 Medial epicondylitis**
    M77.00 Medial epicondylitis, unspecified elbow ▽
    M77.01 Medial epicondylitis, right elbow
    M77.02 Medial epicondylitis, left elbow

✓5ᵗʰ **M77.1 Lateral epicondylitis**
    Tennis elbow
    M77.10 Lateral epicondylitis, unspecified elbow ▽
    M77.11 Lateral epicondylitis, right elbow
    M77.12 Lateral epicondylitis, left elbow

✓5ᵗʰ **M77.2 Periarthritis of wrist**
    M77.20 Periarthritis, unspecified wrist ▽
    M77.21 Periarthritis, right wrist
    M77.22 Periarthritis, left wrist

✓5ᵗʰ **M77.3 Calcaneal spur**
    DEF: Overgrowth of calcaneus bone on underside of the heel; causes pain on walking; due to chronic avulsion injury of plantar fascia from calcaneus.
    M77.30 Calcaneal spur, unspecified foot ▽
    M77.31 Calcaneal spur, right foot
    M77.32 Calcaneal spur, left foot

✓5ᵗʰ **M77.4 Metatarsalgia**
    EXCLUDES 1   Morton's metatarsalgia (G57.6)
    M77.40 Metatarsalgia, unspecified foot ▽
    M77.41 Metatarsalgia, right foot
    M77.42 Metatarsalgia, left foot

✓5ᵗʰ **M77.5 Other enthesopathy of foot**
    M77.50 Other enthesopathy of unspecified foot ▽
    M77.51 Other enthesopathy of right foot
    M77.52 Other enthesopathy of left foot

M77.8 Other enthesopathies, not elsewhere classified

M77.9 Enthesopathy, unspecified ▽
    Bone spur NOS   Periarthritis NOS
    Capsulitis NOS   Tendinitis NOS

✓4ᵗʰ **M79 Other and unspecified soft tissue disorders, not elsewhere classified**
    EXCLUDES 1   psychogenic rheumatism (F45.8)
          soft tissue pain, psychogenic (F45.41)

M79.0 Rheumatism, unspecified ▽
    EXCLUDES 1   fibromyalgia (M79.7)
          palindromic rheumatism (M12.3-)

M79.1 Myalgia
    Myofascial pain syndrome
    EXCLUDES 1   fibromyalgia (M79.7)
          myositis (M60.-)

M79.2 Neuralgia and neuritis, unspecified ▽
    EXCLUDES 1   brachial radiculitis NOS (M54.1)
          lumbosacral radiculitis NOS (M54.1)
          mononeuropathies (G56-G58)
          radiculitis NOS (M54.1)
          sciatica (M54.3-M54.4)

M79.3 Panniculitis, unspecified ▽
    EXCLUDES 1   lupus panniculitis (L93.2)
          neck and back panniculitis (M54.0-)
          relapsing [Weber-Christian] panniculitis (M35.6)

M79.4 Hypertrophy of (infrapatellar) fat pad

M79.5 Residual foreign body in soft tissue
    EXCLUDES 1   foreign body granuloma of skin and subcutaneous tissue (L92.3)
          foreign body granuloma of soft tissue (M60.2-)

✓5ᵗʰ **M79.6 Pain in limb, hand, foot, fingers and toes**
    EXCLUDES 2   pain in joint (M25.5-)
    ✓6ᵗʰ **M79.60 Pain in limb, unspecified**
       M79.601 Pain in right arm
          Pain in right upper limb NOS
       M79.602 Pain in left arm
          Pain in left upper limb NOS
       M79.603 Pain in arm, unspecified ▽
          Pain in upper limb NOS
       M79.604 Pain in right leg
          Pain in right lower limb NOS

☑ Additional Character Req   ✓x7ᵗʰ Placeholder Alert   Case-Mix Diagnosis   Manifestation   ▽ Unspecified Dx   *EXCLUDES 1* Not coded here   *EXCLUDES 2* Not included here

M79.605   **Pain in** left leg
Pain in left lower limb NOS

M79.606   **Pain in** leg, unspecified   ▽
Pain in lower limb NOS

M79.609   **Pain in** unspecified limb   ▽
Pain in limb NOS

✓6ᵗʰ **M79.62**   **Pain in** upper arm
Pain in axillary region

M79.621   **Pain in** right upper arm

M79.622   **Pain in** left upper arm

M79.629   **Pain in** unspecified upper arm   ▽

✓6ᵗʰ **M79.63**   **Pain in** forearm

M79.631   **Pain in** right forearm

M79.632   **Pain in** left forearm

M79.639   **Pain in** unspecified forearm   ▽

✓6ᵗʰ **M79.64**   **Pain in** hand and fingers

M79.641   **Pain in** right hand

M79.642   **Pain in** left hand

M79.643   **Pain in** unspecified hand   ▽

M79.644   **Pain in** right finger(s)

M79.645   **Pain in** left finger(s)

M79.646   **Pain in** unspecified finger(s)   ▽

✓6ᵗʰ **M79.65**   **Pain in** thigh

M79.651   **Pain in** right thigh

M79.652   **Pain in** left thigh

M79.659   **Pain in** unspecified thigh   ▽

✓6ᵗʰ **M79.66**   **Pain in** lower leg

M79.661   **Pain in** right lower leg

M79.662   **Pain in** left lower leg

M79.669   **Pain in** unspecified lower leg   ▽

✓6ᵗʰ **M79.67**   **Pain in** foot and toes

M79.671   **Pain in** right foot

M79.672   **Pain in** left foot

M79.673   **Pain in** unspecified foot   ▽

M79.674   **Pain in** right toe(s)

M79.675   **Pain in** left toe(s)

M79.676   **Pain in** unspecified toe(s)   ▽

M79.7   **Fibromyalgia**
Fibromyositis
Fibrositis
Myofibrositis

✓5ᵗʰ **M79.A**   **Nontraumatic compartment syndrome**
Code first, if applicable, associated postprocedural complication

EXCLUDES 1   compartment syndrome NOS (T79.A-)
fibromyalgia (M79.7)
nontraumatic ischemic infarction of muscle (M62.2-)
traumatic compartment syndrome (T79.A-)

✓6ᵗʰ **M79.A1**   **Nontraumatic compartment syndrome of** upper
extremity
Nontraumatic compartment syndrome of shoulder, arm, forearm, wrist, hand, and fingers

M79.A11   **Nontraumatic compartment syndrome of** right **upper extremity**

M79.A12   **Nontraumatic compartment syndrome of** left **upper extremity**

M79.A19   **Nontraumatic compartment syndrome** ▽ **of unspecified upper extremity**

✓6ᵗʰ **M79.A2**   **Nontraumatic compartment syndrome of** lower
extremity
Nontraumatic compartment syndrome of hip, buttock, thigh, leg, foot, and toes

M79.A21   **Nontraumatic compartment syndrome of** right **lower extremity**

M79.A22   **Nontraumatic compartment syndrome of** left **lower extremity**

M79.A29   **Nontraumatic compartment syndrome** ▽ **of unspecified lower extremity**

M79.A3   **Nontraumatic compartment syndrome of** abdomen

M79.A9   **Nontraumatic compartment syndrome of other sites**

✓5ᵗʰ **M79.8**   **Other specified soft tissue disorders**

M79.81   **Nontraumatic hematoma of soft tissue**
Nontraumatic hematoma of muscle
Nontraumatic seroma of muscle and soft tissue

M79.89   **Other specified soft tissue disorders**
Polyalgia

M79.9   **Soft tissue disorder, unspecified**   ▽

OSTEOPATHIES AND CHONDROPATHIES (M80-M94)

Disorders of bone density and structure (M80-M85)

✓4ᵗʰ **M80**   **Osteoporosis** with current pathological fracture

INCLUDES   osteoporosis with current fragility fracture

Use additional code to identify major osseous defect, if applicable (M89.7-)

EXCLUDES 1   collapsed vertebra NOS (M48.5)
pathological fracture NOS (M84.4)
wedging of vertebra NOS (M48.5)

EXCLUDES 2   personal history of (healed) osteoporosis fracture (Z87.310)

TIP: The term "improper alignment" is not synonymous with malunion or nonunion of a fracture when noted in provider documentation.

> The appropriate 7th character is to be added to each code from category M80.
> A   initial encounter for fracture
> D   subsequent encounter for fracture with routine healing
> G   subsequent encounter for fracture with delayed healing
> K   subsequent encounter for fracture with nonunion
> P   subsequent encounter for fracture with malunion
> S   sequela

✓5ᵗʰ **M80.0**   **Age-related** osteoporosis with current pathological fracture
Involutional osteoporosis with current pathological fracture
Osteoporosis NOS with current pathological fracture
Postmenopausal osteoporosis with current pathological fracture
Senile osteoporosis with current pathological fracture

✓x7ᵗʰ **M80.00**   **Age-related osteoporosis with current** 🅰▽ **pathological fracture, unspecified site**

✓6ᵗʰ **M80.01**   **Age-related osteoporosis with current pathological fracture,** shoulder

1 ✓7ᵗʰ **M80.011**   **Age-related osteoporosis with current** 🅰 **pathological fracture, right shoulder**

1 ✓7ᵗʰ **M80.012**   **Age-related osteoporosis with current** 🅰 **pathological fracture, left shoulder**

✓7ᵗʰ **M80.019**   **Age-related osteoporosis with** 🅰▽ **current pathological fracture, unspecified shoulder**

✓6ᵗʰ **M80.02**   **Age-related osteoporosis with current pathological fracture,** humerus

1 ✓7ᵗʰ **M80.021**   **Age-related osteoporosis with current** 🅰 **pathological fracture, right humerus**

1 ✓7ᵗʰ **M80.022**   **Age-related osteoporosis with current** 🅰 **pathological fracture, left humerus**

✓7ᵗʰ **M80.029**   **Age-related osteoporosis with** 🅰▽ **current pathological fracture, unspecified humerus**

✓6ᵗʰ **M80.03**   **Age-related osteoporosis with current pathological fracture,** forearm
Age-related osteoporosis with current pathological fracture of wrist

1 ✓7ᵗʰ **M80.031**   **Age-related osteoporosis with current** 🅰 **pathological fracture, right forearm**

1 ✓7ᵗʰ **M80.032**   **Age-related osteoporosis with current** 🅰 **pathological fracture, left forearm**

✓7ᵗʰ **M80.039**   **Age-related osteoporosis with** 🅰▽ **current pathological fracture, unspecified forearm**

✓6ᵗʰ **M80.04**   **Age-related osteoporosis with current pathological fracture,** hand

1 ✓7ᵗʰ **M80.041**   **Age-related osteoporosis with current** 🅰 **pathological fracture, right hand**

1 ✓7ᵗʰ **M80.042**   **Age-related osteoporosis with current** 🅰 **pathological fracture, left hand**

✓7ᵗʰ **M80.049**   **Age-related osteoporosis with** 🅰▽ **current pathological fracture, unspecified hand**

✓6ᵗʰ **M80.05**   **Age-related osteoporosis with current pathological fracture,** femur
Age-related osteoporosis with current pathological fracture of hip

1 ✓7ᵗʰ **M80.051**   **Age-related osteoporosis with current** 🅰 **pathological fracture, right femur**

---

1   Case-mix diagnosis with 7th character indicating subsequent encounter.

Ⓝ Newborn: 0   Ⓟ Pediatric: 0-17   Ⓜ Maternity: 12-55   🅰 Adult: 15-124   **NRS** Nonroutine supply Dx   **NC Dx** Noncancer Dx   **PDx** Primary Dx   ▶◀ Revised Text   ● New Code   ▲ Revised Title

778   ICD-10-CM 2018

Chapter 13. Diseases of the Musculoskeletal System and Connective Tissue

M80.052 Age-related osteoporosis with current pathological fracture, left femur △

M80.059 Age-related osteoporosis with current pathological fracture, unspecified femur △▽

M80.06 Age-related osteoporosis with current pathological fracture, lower leg

M80.061 Age-related osteoporosis with current pathological fracture, right lower leg △

M80.062 Age-related osteoporosis with current pathological fracture, left lower leg △

M80.069 Age-related osteoporosis with current pathological fracture, unspecified lower leg △▽

M80.07 Age-related osteoporosis with current pathological fracture, ankle and foot

M80.071 Age-related osteoporosis with current pathological fracture, right ankle and foot △

M80.072 Age-related osteoporosis with current pathological fracture, left ankle and foot △

M80.079 Age-related osteoporosis with current pathological fracture, unspecified ankle and foot △▽

M80.08 Age-related osteoporosis with current pathological fracture, vertebra(e) △

M80.8 Other osteoporosis with current pathological fracture
Drug-induced osteoporosis with current pathological fracture
Idiopathic osteoporosis with current pathological fracture
Osteoporosis of disuse with current pathological fracture
Postoophorectomy osteoporosis with current pathological fracture
Postsurgical malabsorption osteoporosis with current pathological fracture
Post-traumatic osteoporosis with current pathological fracture
Use additional code for adverse effect, if applicable, to identify drug (T36-T50 with fifth or sixth character 5)

M80.80 Other osteoporosis with current pathological fracture, unspecified site ▽

M80.81 Other osteoporosis with pathological fracture, shoulder

M80.811 Other osteoporosis with current pathological fracture, right shoulder

M80.812 Other osteoporosis with current pathological fracture, left shoulder

M80.819 Other osteoporosis with current pathological fracture, unspecified shoulder ▽

M80.82 Other osteoporosis with current pathological fracture, humerus

M80.821 Other osteoporosis with current pathological fracture, right humerus

M80.822 Other osteoporosis with current pathological fracture, left humerus

M80.829 Other osteoporosis with current pathological fracture, unspecified humerus ▽

M80.83 Other osteoporosis with current pathological fracture, forearm
Other osteoporosis with current pathological fracture of wrist

M80.831 Other osteoporosis with current pathological fracture, right forearm

M80.832 Other osteoporosis with current pathological fracture, left forearm

M80.839 Other osteoporosis with current pathological fracture, unspecified forearm ▽

M80.84 Other osteoporosis with current pathological fracture, hand

M80.841 Other osteoporosis with current pathological fracture, right hand

M80.842 Other osteoporosis with current pathological fracture, left hand

M80.849 Other osteoporosis with current pathological fracture, unspecified hand ▽

M80.85 Other osteoporosis with current pathological fracture, femur
Other osteoporosis with current pathological fracture of hip

M80.851 Other osteoporosis with current pathological fracture, right femur

M80.852 Other osteoporosis with current pathological fracture, left femur

M80.859 Other osteoporosis with current pathological fracture, unspecified femur ▽

M80.86 Other osteoporosis with current pathological fracture, lower leg

M80.861 Other osteoporosis with current pathological fracture, right lower leg

M80.862 Other osteoporosis with current pathological fracture, left lower leg

M80.869 Other osteoporosis with current pathological fracture, unspecified lower leg

M80.87 Other osteoporosis with current pathological fracture, ankle and foot

M80.871 Other osteoporosis with current pathological fracture, right ankle and foot

M80.872 Other osteoporosis with current pathological fracture, left ankle and foot

M80.879 Other osteoporosis with current pathological fracture, unspecified ankle and foot ▽

M80.88 Other osteoporosis with current pathological fracture, vertebra(e)

M81 Osteoporosis without current pathological fracture
Use additional code to identify:
major osseous defect, if applicable (M89.7-)
personal history of (healed) osteoporosis fracture, if applicable (Z87.310)
EXCLUDES 1   osteoporosis with current pathological fracture (M80.-)
Sudeck's atrophy (M89.0)

M81.0 Age-related osteoporosis without current pathological fracture △
Involutional osteoporosis without current pathological fracture
Osteoporosis NOS
Postmenopausal osteoporosis without current pathological fracture
Senile osteoporosis without current pathological fracture

M81.6 Localized osteoporosis [Lequesne]
EXCLUDES 1   Sudeck's atrophy (M89.0)

M81.8 Other osteoporosis without current pathological fracture
Drug-induced osteoporosis without current pathological fracture
Idiopathic osteoporosis without current pathological fracture
Osteoporosis of disuse without current pathological fracture
Postoophorectomy osteoporosis without current pathological fracture
Postsurgical malabsorption osteoporosis without current pathological fracture
Post-traumatic osteoporosis without current pathological fracture
Use additional code for adverse effect, if applicable, to identify drug (T36-T50 with fifth or sixth character 5)

M83 Adult osteomalacia
EXCLUDES 1   infantile and juvenile osteomalacia (E55.0)
renal osteodystrophy (N25.0)
rickets (active) (E55.0)
rickets (active) sequelae (E64.3)
vitamin D-resistant osteomalacia (E83.3)
vitamin D-resistant rickets (active) (E83.3)

M83.0 Puerperal osteomalacia   M♀

M83.1 Senile osteomalacia   △

M83.2 Adult osteomalacia due to malabsorption   △
Postsurgical malabsorption osteomalacia in adults

M83.3 Adult osteomalacia due to malnutrition   △

M83.4 Aluminum bone disease

M83.5 Other drug-induced osteomalacia in adults   △
Use additional code for adverse effect, if applicable, to identify drug (T36-T50 with fifth or sixth character 5)

M83.8 Other adult osteomalacia   △

M83.9 Adult osteomalacia, unspecified   △▽

---

1   Case-mix diagnosis with 7th character indicating subsequent encounter.

☑ Additional Character Req   ✓x7ᵗʰ Placeholder Alert   Case-Mix Diagnosis   Manifestation   ▽ Unspecified Dx   EXCLUDES 1 Not coded here   EXCLUDES 2 Not included here

✓4ᵗʰ M84 Disorder of continuity of bone

> **EXCLUDES 2**   traumatic fracture of bone-see fracture, by site
>
> **TIP:** The term "improper alignment" is not synonymous with malunion or nonunion of a fracture when noted in provider documentation.

✓5ᵗʰ M84.3 Stress fracture

> Fatigue fracture   Stress fracture NOS
> March fracture   Stress reaction
>
> Use additional external cause code(s) to identify the cause of the stress fracture
>
> **EXCLUDES 1**   pathological fracture NOS (M84.4-)
>   pathological fracture due to osteoporosis (M80.-)
>   traumatic fracture (S12-, S22-, S32-, S42-, S52-, S62-, S72-, S82-, S92-)
>
> **EXCLUDES 2**   personal history of (healed) stress (fatigue) fracture (Z87.312)
>   stress fracture of vertebra (M48.4-)

> The appropriate 7th character is to be added to each code from subcategory M84.3-.
> A   initial encounter for fracture
> D   subsequent encounter for fracture with routine healing
> G   subsequent encounter for fracture with delayed healing
> K   subsequent encounter for fracture with nonunion
> P   subsequent encounter for fracture with malunion
> S   sequela

✓x7ᵗʰ M84.30 Stress fracture, unspecified site ▽

✓6ᵗʰ M84.31 Stress fracture, shoulder
- **✓7ᵗʰ M84.311 Stress fracture, right shoulder**
- **✓7ᵗʰ M84.312 Stress fracture, left shoulder**
- **✓7ᵗʰ M84.319 Stress fracture, unspecified shoulder** ▽

✓6ᵗʰ M84.32 Stress fracture, humerus
- **✓7ᵗʰ M84.321 Stress fracture, right humerus**
- **✓7ᵗʰ M84.322 Stress fracture, left humerus**
- **✓7ᵗʰ M84.329 Stress fracture, unspecified humerus** ▽

✓6ᵗʰ M84.33 Stress fracture, ulna and radius
- **✓7ᵗʰ M84.331 Stress fracture, right ulna**
- **✓7ᵗʰ M84.332 Stress fracture, left ulna**
- **✓7ᵗʰ M84.333 Stress fracture, right radius**
- **✓7ᵗʰ M84.334 Stress fracture, left radius**
- **✓7ᵗʰ M84.339 Stress fracture, unspecified ulna and radius** ▽

✓6ᵗʰ M84.34 Stress fracture, hand and fingers
- **✓7ᵗʰ M84.341 Stress fracture, right hand**
- **✓7ᵗʰ M84.342 Stress fracture, left hand**
- **✓7ᵗʰ M84.343 Stress fracture, unspecified hand** ▽
- **✓7ᵗʰ M84.344 Stress fracture, right finger(s)**
- **✓7ᵗʰ M84.345 Stress fracture, left finger(s)**
- **✓7ᵗʰ M84.346 Stress fracture, unspecified finger(s)** ▽

✓6ᵗʰ M84.35 Stress fracture, pelvis and femur
> Stress fracture, hip
- **✓7ᵗʰ M84.350 Stress fracture, pelvis**
- **✓7ᵗʰ M84.351 Stress fracture, right femur**
- **✓7ᵗʰ M84.352 Stress fracture, left femur**
- **✓7ᵗʰ M84.353 Stress fracture, unspecified femur** ▽
- **✓7ᵗʰ M84.359 Stress fracture, hip, unspecified** ▽

✓6ᵗʰ M84.36 Stress fracture, tibia and fibula
- **✓7ᵗʰ M84.361 Stress fracture, right tibia**
- **✓7ᵗʰ M84.362 Stress fracture, left tibia**
- **✓7ᵗʰ M84.363 Stress fracture, right fibula**
- **✓7ᵗʰ M84.364 Stress fracture, left fibula**
- **✓7ᵗʰ M84.369 Stress fracture, unspecified tibia and fibula** ▽

✓6ᵗʰ M84.37 Stress fracture, ankle, foot and toes
- **✓7ᵗʰ M84.371 Stress fracture, right ankle**
- **✓7ᵗʰ M84.372 Stress fracture, left ankle**
- **✓7ᵗʰ M84.373 Stress fracture, unspecified ankle** ▽
- **✓7ᵗʰ M84.374 Stress fracture, right foot**
- **✓7ᵗʰ M84.375 Stress fracture, left foot**
- **✓7ᵗʰ M84.376 Stress fracture, unspecified foot** ▽
- **✓7ᵗʰ M84.377 Stress fracture, right toe(s)**
- **✓7ᵗʰ M84.378 Stress fracture, left toe(s)**
- **✓7ᵗʰ M84.379 Stress fracture, unspecified toe(s)** ▽

✓x7ᵗʰ M84.38 Stress fracture, other site
> **EXCLUDES 2**   stress fracture of vertebra (M48.4-)

✓5ᵗʰ M84.4 Pathological fracture, not elsewhere classified

> Chronic fracture
> Pathological fracture NOS
>
> **EXCLUDES 1**   collapsed vertebra NEC (M48.5)
>   pathological fracture in neoplastic disease (M84.5-)
>   pathological fracture in osteoporosis (M80.-)
>   pathological fracture in other disease (M84.6-)
>   stress fracture (M84.3-)
>   traumatic fracture (S12.-, S22.-, S32.-, S42.-, S52.-, S62.-, S72.-, S82.-, S92.-)
>
> **EXCLUDES 2**   personal history of (healed) pathological fracture (Z87.311)

> The appropriate 7th character is to be added to each code from subcategory M84.4-.
> A   initial encounter for fracture
> D   subsequent encounter for fracture with routine healing
> G   subsequent encounter for fracture with delayed healing
> K   subsequent encounter for fracture with nonunion
> P   subsequent encounter for fracture with malunion
> S   sequela

✓x7ᵗʰ M84.40 Pathological fracture, unspecified site ▽

✓6ᵗʰ M84.41 Pathological fracture, shoulder
- [1] **✓7ᵗʰ M84.411 Pathological fracture, right shoulder**
- [1] **✓7ᵗʰ M84.412 Pathological fracture, left shoulder**
- **✓7ᵗʰ M84.419 Pathological fracture, unspecified shoulder** ▽

✓6ᵗʰ M84.42 Pathological fracture, humerus
- [1] **✓7ᵗʰ M84.421 Pathological fracture, right humerus**
- [1] **✓7ᵗʰ M84.422 Pathological fracture, left humerus**
- **✓7ᵗʰ M84.429 Pathological fracture, unspecified humerus** ▽

✓6ᵗʰ M84.43 Pathological fracture, ulna and radius
- [1] **✓7ᵗʰ M84.431 Pathological fracture, right ulna**
- [1] **✓7ᵗʰ M84.432 Pathological fracture, left ulna**
- [1] **✓7ᵗʰ M84.433 Pathological fracture, right radius**
- [1] **✓7ᵗʰ M84.434 Pathological fracture, left radius**
- **✓7ᵗʰ M84.439 Pathological fracture, unspecified ulna and radius** ▽

✓6ᵗʰ M84.44 Pathological fracture, hand and fingers
- [1] **✓7ᵗʰ M84.441 Pathological fracture, right hand**
- [1] **✓7ᵗʰ M84.442 Pathological fracture, left hand**
- **✓7ᵗʰ M84.443 Pathological fracture, unspecified hand** ▽
- **✓7ᵗʰ M84.444 Pathological fracture, right finger(s)**
- **✓7ᵗʰ M84.445 Pathological fracture, left finger(s)**
- **✓7ᵗʰ M84.446 Pathological fracture, unspecified finger(s)** ▽

✓6ᵗʰ M84.45 Pathological fracture, femur and pelvis
- [1] **✓7ᵗʰ M84.451 Pathological fracture, right femur**
- [1] **✓7ᵗʰ M84.452 Pathological fracture, left femur**
- **✓7ᵗʰ M84.453 Pathological fracture, unspecified femur** ▽
- [1] **✓7ᵗʰ M84.454 Pathological fracture, pelvis**
- **✓7ᵗʰ M84.459 Pathological fracture, hip, unspecified** ▽

✓6ᵗʰ M84.46 Pathological fracture, tibia and fibula
- [1] **✓7ᵗʰ M84.461 Pathological fracture, right tibia**
- [1] **✓7ᵗʰ M84.462 Pathological fracture, left tibia**
- [1] **✓7ᵗʰ M84.463 Pathological fracture, right fibula**
- [1] **✓7ᵗʰ M84.464 Pathological fracture, left fibula**
- **✓7ᵗʰ M84.469 Pathological fracture, unspecified tibia and fibula** ▽

✓6ᵗʰ M84.47 Pathological fracture, ankle, foot and toes
- [1] **✓7ᵗʰ M84.471 Pathological fracture, right ankle**
- [1] **✓7ᵗʰ M84.472 Pathological fracture, left ankle**
- **✓7ᵗʰ M84.473 Pathological fracture, unspecified ankle** ▽
- [1] **✓7ᵗʰ M84.474 Pathological fracture, right foot**
- [1] **✓7ᵗʰ M84.475 Pathological fracture, left foot**

---

[1]   Case-mix diagnosis with 7th character indicating subsequent encounter.

Ⓝ Newborn: 0   Ⓟ Pediatric: 0-17   Ⓜ Maternity: 12-55   Ⓐ Adult: 15-124   **NRS** Nonroutine supply Dx   **NCDx** Noncancer Dx   **PDx** Primary Dx   ▶◀ Revised Text   ● New Code   ▲ Revised Title

780   ICD-10-CM 2018

☑7ᵗʰ **M84.476** Pathological fracture, unspecified foot ▽
¹ ☑7ᵗʰ **M84.477** **Pathological fracture, right toe(s)**
¹ ☑7ᵗʰ **M84.478** **Pathological fracture, left toe(s)**
☑7ᵗʰ **M84.479** Pathological fracture, unspecified ▽
     toe(s)
¹ ✓x7ᵗʰ **M84.48** **Pathological fracture, other site**

☑5ᵗʰ **M84.5** Pathological fracture in neoplastic disease
     Code also underlying neoplasm

> The appropriate 7th character is to be added to each code
> from subcategory M84.5-.
> A   initial encounter for fracture
> D   subsequent encounter for fracture with routine healing
> G   subsequent encounter for fracture with delayed healing
> K   subsequent encounter for fracture with nonunion
> P   subsequent encounter for fracture with malunion
> S   sequela

✓x7ᵗʰ **M84.50** Pathological fracture in neoplastic disease, ▽
     unspecified site
✓6ᵗʰ **M84.51** Pathological fracture in neoplastic disease, shoulder
¹ ☑7ᵗʰ **M84.511** **Pathological fracture in neoplastic**
     disease, right shoulder
¹ ☑7ᵗʰ **M84.512** **Pathological fracture in neoplastic**
     disease, left shoulder
☑7ᵗʰ **M84.519** Pathological fracture in neoplastic ▽
     disease, unspecified shoulder
✓6ᵗʰ **M84.52** Pathological fracture in neoplastic disease, humerus
¹ ☑7ᵗʰ **M84.521** **Pathological fracture in neoplastic**
     disease, right humerus
¹ ☑7ᵗʰ **M84.522** **Pathological fracture in neoplastic**
     disease, left humerus
☑7ᵗʰ **M84.529** Pathological fracture in neoplastic ▽
     disease, unspecified humerus
✓6ᵗʰ **M84.53** Pathological fracture in neoplastic disease,
     ulna and radius
¹ ☑7ᵗʰ **M84.531** **Pathological fracture in neoplastic**
     disease, right ulna
¹ ☑7ᵗʰ **M84.532** **Pathological fracture in neoplastic**
     disease, left ulna
¹ ☑7ᵗʰ **M84.533** **Pathological fracture in neoplastic**
     disease, right radius
¹ ☑7ᵗʰ **M84.534** **Pathological fracture in neoplastic**
     disease, left radius
☑7ᵗʰ **M84.539** Pathological fracture in neoplastic ▽
     disease, unspecified ulna and radius
✓6ᵗʰ **M84.54** Pathological fracture in neoplastic disease, hand
¹ ☑7ᵗʰ **M84.541** **Pathological fracture in neoplastic**
     disease, right hand
¹ ☑7ᵗʰ **M84.542** **Pathological fracture in neoplastic**
     disease, left hand
☑7ᵗʰ **M84.549** Pathological fracture in neoplastic ▽
     disease, unspecified hand
✓6ᵗʰ **M84.55** Pathological fracture in neoplastic disease,
     pelvis and femur
¹ ☑7ᵗʰ **M84.550** **Pathological fracture in neoplastic**
     disease, pelvis
¹ ☑7ᵗʰ **M84.551** **Pathological fracture in neoplastic**
     disease, right femur
¹ ☑7ᵗʰ **M84.552** **Pathological fracture in neoplastic**
     disease, left femur
☑7ᵗʰ **M84.553** Pathological fracture in neoplastic ▽
     disease, unspecified femur
☑7ᵗʰ **M84.559** Pathological fracture in neoplastic ▽
     disease, hip, unspecified
✓6ᵗʰ **M84.56** Pathological fracture in neoplastic disease,
     tibia and fibula
¹ ☑7ᵗʰ **M84.561** **Pathological fracture in neoplastic**
     disease, right tibia
¹ ☑7ᵗʰ **M84.562** **Pathological fracture in neoplastic**
     disease, left tibia
¹ ☑7ᵗʰ **M84.563** **Pathological fracture in neoplastic**
     disease, right fibula
¹ ☑7ᵗʰ **M84.564** **Pathological fracture in neoplastic**
     disease, left fibula

☑7ᵗʰ **M84.569** Pathological fracture in neoplastic ▽
     disease, unspecified tibia and fibula
✓6ᵗʰ **M84.57** Pathological fracture in neoplastic disease, ankle
     and foot
¹ ☑7ᵗʰ **M84.571** **Pathological fracture in neoplastic**
     disease, right ankle
¹ ☑7ᵗʰ **M84.572** **Pathological fracture in neoplastic**
     disease, left ankle
☑7ᵗʰ **M84.573** Pathological fracture in neoplastic ▽
     disease, unspecified ankle
¹ ☑7ᵗʰ **M84.574** **Pathological fracture in neoplastic**
     disease, right foot
¹ ☑7ᵗʰ **M84.575** **Pathological fracture in neoplastic**
     disease, left foot
☑7ᵗʰ **M84.576** Pathological fracture in neoplastic ▽
     disease, unspecified foot
¹ ✓x7ᵗʰ **M84.58** **Pathological fracture in neoplastic disease, other**
     specified site
     Pathological fracture in neoplastic disease, vertebrae

✓5ᵗʰ **M84.6** Pathological fracture in other disease
     Code also underlying condition
     EXCLUDES 1   pathological fracture in osteoporosis (M80.-)

> The appropriate 7th character is to be added to each code
> from subcategory M84.6-.
> A   initial encounter for fracture
> D   subsequent encounter for fracture with routine healing
> G   subsequent encounter for fracture with delayed healing
> K   subsequent encounter for fracture with nonunion
> P   subsequent encounter for fracture with malunion
> S   sequela

✓x7ᵗʰ **M84.60** Pathological fracture in other disease, ▽
     unspecified site
✓6ᵗʰ **M84.61** Pathological fracture in other disease, shoulder
¹ ☑7ᵗʰ **M84.611** **Pathological fracture in other disease,**
     right shoulder
¹ ☑7ᵗʰ **M84.612** **Pathological fracture in other disease,**
     left shoulder
☑7ᵗʰ **M84.619** Pathological fracture in other disease, ▽
     unspecified shoulder
✓6ᵗʰ **M84.62** Pathological fracture in other disease, humerus
¹ ☑7ᵗʰ **M84.621** **Pathological fracture in other disease,**
     right humerus
¹ ☑7ᵗʰ **M84.622** **Pathological fracture in other disease,**
     left humerus
☑7ᵗʰ **M84.629** Pathological fracture in other disease, ▽
     unspecified humerus
✓6ᵗʰ **M84.63** Pathological fracture in other disease, ulna and
     radius
¹ ☑7ᵗʰ **M84.631** **Pathological fracture in other disease,**
     right ulna
¹ ☑7ᵗʰ **M84.632** **Pathological fracture in other disease,**
     left ulna
¹ ☑7ᵗʰ **M84.633** **Pathological fracture in other disease,**
     right radius
¹ ☑7ᵗʰ **M84.634** **Pathological fracture in other disease,**
     left radius
☑7ᵗʰ **M84.639** Pathological fracture in other disease, ▽
     unspecified ulna and radius
✓6ᵗʰ **M84.64** Pathological fracture in other disease, hand
¹ ☑7ᵗʰ **M84.641** **Pathological fracture in other disease,**
     right hand
¹ ☑7ᵗʰ **M84.642** **Pathological fracture in other disease,**
     left hand
☑7ᵗʰ **M84.649** Pathological fracture in other disease, ▽
     unspecified hand
✓6ᵗʰ **M84.65** Pathological fracture in other disease, pelvis and
     femur
¹ ☑7ᵗʰ **M84.650** **Pathological fracture in other disease,**
     pelvis
¹ ☑7ᵗʰ **M84.651** **Pathological fracture in other disease,**
     right femur
¹ ☑7ᵗʰ **M84.652** **Pathological fracture in other disease,**
     left femur

---

¹   Case-mix diagnosis with 7th character indicating subsequent encounter.

☑ Additional Character Req   ✓x7ᵗʰ Placeholder Alert   Case-Mix Diagnosis   Manifestation   ▽ Unspecified Dx   *EXCLUDES 1* Not coded here   *EXCLUDES 2* Not included here

✓7ᵗʰ **M84.653** Pathological fracture in other disease, unspecified femur ▽

✓7ᵗʰ **M84.659** Pathological fracture in other disease, hip, unspecified ▽

✓6ᵗʰ **M84.66** Pathological fracture in other disease, tibia and fibula

1 ✓7ᵗʰ **M84.661** Pathological fracture in other disease, right tibia

1 ✓7ᵗʰ **M84.662** Pathological fracture in other disease, left tibia

1 ✓7ᵗʰ **M84.663** Pathological fracture in other disease, right fibula

1 ✓7ᵗʰ **M84.664** Pathological fracture in other disease, left fibula

✓7ᵗʰ **M84.669** Pathological fracture in other disease, unspecified tibia and fibula ▽

✓6ᵗʰ **M84.67** Pathological fracture in other disease, ankle and foot

1 ✓7ᵗʰ **M84.671** Pathological fracture in other disease, right ankle

1 ✓7ᵗʰ **M84.672** Pathological fracture in other disease, left ankle

✓7ᵗʰ **M84.673** Pathological fracture in other disease, unspecified ankle ▽

1 ✓7ᵗʰ **M84.674** Pathological fracture in other disease, right foot

1 ✓7ᵗʰ **M84.675** Pathological fracture in other disease, left foot

✓7ᵗʰ **M84.676** Pathological fracture in other disease, unspecified foot ▽

1 ✓x7ᵗʰ **M84.68** Pathological fracture in other disease, other site

✓5ᵗʰ **M84.7** Nontraumatic fracture, not elsewhere classified

✓6ᵗʰ **M84.75** Atypical femoral fracture

> The appropriate 7th character is to be added to each code from subcategory M84.75-.
> A   initial encounter for fracture
> D   subsequent encounter for fracture with routine healing
> G   subsequent encounter for fracture with delayed healing
> K   subsequent encounter for fracture with nonunion
> P   subsequent encounter for fracture with malunion
> S   sequela

✓7ᵗʰ **M84.750** Atypical femoral fracture, unspecified ▽

2 ✓7ᵗʰ **M84.751** Incomplete atypical femoral fracture, right leg

2 ✓7ᵗʰ **M84.752** Incomplete atypical femoral fracture, left leg

✓7ᵗʰ **M84.753** Incomplete atypical femoral fracture, unspecified leg ▽

2 ✓7ᵗʰ **M84.754** Complete transverse atypical femoral fracture, right leg

2 ✓7ᵗʰ **M84.755** Complete transverse atypical femoral fracture, left leg

✓7ᵗʰ **M84.756** Complete transverse atypical femoral fracture, unspecified leg ▽

2 ✓7ᵗʰ **M84.757** Complete oblique atypical femoral fracture, right leg

2 ✓7ᵗʰ **M84.758** Complete oblique atypical femoral fracture, left leg

✓7ᵗʰ **M84.759** Complete oblique atypical femoral fracture, unspecified leg ▽

✓5ᵗʰ **M84.8** Other disorders of continuity of bone

M84.80 Other disorders of continuity of bone, unspecified site ▽

✓6ᵗʰ **M84.81** Other disorders of continuity of bone, shoulder

M84.811 Other disorders of continuity of bone, right shoulder

M84.812 Other disorders of continuity of bone, left shoulder

M84.819 Other disorders of continuity of bone, unspecified shoulder ▽

✓6ᵗʰ **M84.82** Other disorders of continuity of bone, humerus

M84.821 Other disorders of continuity of bone, right humerus

M84.822 Other disorders of continuity of bone, left humerus

M84.829 Other disorders of continuity of bone, unspecified humerus ▽

✓6ᵗʰ **M84.83** Other disorders of continuity of bone, ulna and radius

M84.831 Other disorders of continuity of bone, right ulna

M84.832 Other disorders of continuity of bone, left ulna

M84.833 Other disorders of continuity of bone, right radius

M84.834 Other disorders of continuity of bone, left radius

M84.839 Other disorders of continuity of bone, unspecified ulna and radius ▽

✓6ᵗʰ **M84.84** Other disorders of continuity of bone, hand

M84.841 Other disorders of continuity of bone, right hand

M84.842 Other disorders of continuity of bone, left hand

M84.849 Other disorders of continuity of bone, unspecified hand ▽

✓6ᵗʰ **M84.85** Other disorders of continuity of bone, pelvic region and thigh

M84.851 Other disorders of continuity of bone, right pelvic region and thigh

M84.852 Other disorders of continuity of bone, left pelvic region and thigh

M84.859 Other disorders of continuity of bone, unspecified pelvic region and thigh ▽

✓6ᵗʰ **M84.86** Other disorders of continuity of bone, tibia and fibula

M84.861 Other disorders of continuity of bone, right tibia

M84.862 Other disorders of continuity of bone, left tibia

M84.863 Other disorders of continuity of bone, right fibula

M84.864 Other disorders of continuity of bone, left fibula

M84.869 Other disorders of continuity of bone, unspecified tibia and fibula ▽

✓6ᵗʰ **M84.87** Other disorders of continuity of bone, ankle and foot

M84.871 Other disorders of continuity of bone, right ankle and foot

M84.872 Other disorders of continuity of bone, left ankle and foot

M84.879 Other disorders of continuity of bone, unspecified ankle and foot ▽

M84.88 Other disorders of continuity of bone, other site

M84.9 Disorder of continuity of bone, unspecified ▽

✓4ᵗʰ **M85** Other disorders of bone density and structure

EXCLUDES 1   osteogenesis imperfecta (Q78.0)
osteopetrosis (Q78.2)
osteopoikilosis (Q78.8)
polyostotic fibrous dysplasia (Q78.1)

✓5ᵗʰ **M85.0** Fibrous dysplasia (monostotic)

EXCLUDES 2   fibrous dysplasia of jaw (M27.8)

M85.00 Fibrous dysplasia (monostotic), unspecified site ▽

✓6ᵗʰ **M85.01** Fibrous dysplasia (monostotic), shoulder

M85.011 Fibrous dysplasia (monostotic), right shoulder

M85.012 Fibrous dysplasia (monostotic), left shoulder

M85.019 Fibrous dysplasia (monostotic), unspecified shoulder ▽

✓6ᵗʰ **M85.02** Fibrous dysplasia (monostotic), upper arm

M85.021 Fibrous dysplasia (monostotic), right upper arm

---

1   Case-mix diagnosis with 7th character indicating subsequent encounter.
2   Case-mix diagnosis only when the 7th character signifies subsequent encounter.

Ⓝ Newborn: 0   Ⓟ Pediatric: 0-17   Ⓜ Maternity: 12-55   Ⓐ Adult: 15-124   NRS Nonroutine supply Dx   NCDx Noncancer Dx   PDx Primary Dx   ►◄ Revised Text   ● New Code   ▲ Revised Title

782   ICD-10-CM 2018

       M85.022   Fibrous dysplasia (monostotic), left upper arm

       M85.029   Fibrous dysplasia (monostotic), unspecified upper arm ▽

✓6ᵗʰ M85.03   Fibrous dysplasia (monostotic), forearm

       M85.031   Fibrous dysplasia (monostotic), right forearm

       M85.032   Fibrous dysplasia (monostotic), left forearm

       M85.039   Fibrous dysplasia (monostotic), unspecified forearm ▽

✓6ᵗʰ M85.04   Fibrous dysplasia (monostotic), hand

       M85.041   Fibrous dysplasia (monostotic), right hand

       M85.042   Fibrous dysplasia (monostotic), left hand

       M85.049   Fibrous dysplasia (monostotic), unspecified hand ▽

✓6ᵗʰ M85.05   Fibrous dysplasia (monostotic), thigh

       M85.051   Fibrous dysplasia (monostotic), right thigh

       M85.052   Fibrous dysplasia (monostotic), left thigh

       M85.059   Fibrous dysplasia (monostotic), unspecified thigh ▽

✓6ᵗʰ M85.06   Fibrous dysplasia (monostotic), lower leg

       M85.061   Fibrous dysplasia (monostotic), right lower leg

       M85.062   Fibrous dysplasia (monostotic), left lower leg

       M85.069   Fibrous dysplasia (monostotic), unspecified lower leg ▽

✓6ᵗʰ M85.07   Fibrous dysplasia (monostotic), ankle and foot

       M85.071   Fibrous dysplasia (monostotic), right ankle and foot

       M85.072   Fibrous dysplasia (monostotic), left ankle and foot

       M85.079   Fibrous dysplasia (monostotic), unspecified ankle and foot ▽

    M85.08   Fibrous dysplasia (monostotic), other site

    M85.09   Fibrous dysplasia (monostotic), multiple sites

✓5ᵗʰ M85.1   Skeletal fluorosis

    M85.10   Skeletal fluorosis, unspecified site ▽

✓6ᵗʰ M85.11   Skeletal fluorosis, shoulder

       M85.111   Skeletal fluorosis, right shoulder

       M85.112   Skeletal fluorosis, left shoulder

       M85.119   Skeletal fluorosis, unspecified shoulder ▽

✓6ᵗʰ M85.12   Skeletal fluorosis, upper arm

       M85.121   Skeletal fluorosis, right upper arm

       M85.122   Skeletal fluorosis, left upper arm

       M85.129   Skeletal fluorosis, unspecified upper arm ▽

✓6ᵗʰ M85.13   Skeletal fluorosis, forearm

       M85.131   Skeletal fluorosis, right forearm

       M85.132   Skeletal fluorosis, left forearm

       M85.139   Skeletal fluorosis, unspecified forearm ▽

✓6ᵗʰ M85.14   Skeletal fluorosis, hand

       M85.141   Skeletal fluorosis, right hand

       M85.142   Skeletal fluorosis, left hand

       M85.149   Skeletal fluorosis, unspecified hand ▽

✓6ᵗʰ M85.15   Skeletal fluorosis, thigh

       M85.151   Skeletal fluorosis, right thigh

       M85.152   Skeletal fluorosis, left thigh

       M85.159   Skeletal fluorosis, unspecified thigh ▽

✓6ᵗʰ M85.16   Skeletal fluorosis, lower leg

       M85.161   Skeletal fluorosis, right lower leg

       M85.162   Skeletal fluorosis, left lower leg

       M85.169   Skeletal fluorosis, unspecified lower leg ▽

✓6ᵗʰ M85.17   Skeletal fluorosis, ankle and foot

       M85.171   Skeletal fluorosis, right ankle and foot

       M85.172   Skeletal fluorosis, left ankle and foot

       M85.179   Skeletal fluorosis, unspecified ankle and foot ▽

    M85.18   Skeletal fluorosis, other site

    M85.19   Skeletal fluorosis, multiple sites

M85.2   Hyperostosis of skull

    DEF: Abnormal bone growth on inner aspect of cranial bones.

✓5ᵗʰ M85.3   Osteitis condensans

    M85.30   Osteitis condensans, unspecified site ▽

✓6ᵗʰ M85.31   Osteitis condensans, shoulder

       M85.311   Osteitis condensans, right shoulder

       M85.312   Osteitis condensans, left shoulder

       M85.319   Osteitis condensans, unspecified shoulder ▽

✓6ᵗʰ M85.32   Osteitis condensans, upper arm

       M85.321   Osteitis condensans, right upper arm

       M85.322   Osteitis condensans, left upper arm

       M85.329   Osteitis condensans, unspecified upper arm ▽

✓6ᵗʰ M85.33   Osteitis condensans, forearm

       M85.331   Osteitis condensans, right forearm

       M85.332   Osteitis condensans, left forearm

       M85.339   Osteitis condensans, unspecified forearm ▽

✓6ᵗʰ M85.34   Osteitis condensans, hand

       M85.341   Osteitis condensans, right hand

       M85.342   Osteitis condensans, left hand

       M85.349   Osteitis condensans, unspecified hand ▽

✓6ᵗʰ M85.35   Osteitis condensans, thigh

       M85.351   Osteitis condensans, right thigh

       M85.352   Osteitis condensans, left thigh

       M85.359   Osteitis condensans, unspecified thigh ▽

✓6ᵗʰ M85.36   Osteitis condensans, lower leg

       M85.361   Osteitis condensans, right lower leg

       M85.362   Osteitis condensans, left lower leg

       M85.369   Osteitis condensans, unspecified lower leg ▽

✓6ᵗʰ M85.37   Osteitis condensans, ankle and foot

       M85.371   Osteitis condensans, right ankle and foot

       M85.372   Osteitis condensans, left ankle and foot

       M85.379   Osteitis condensans, unspecified ankle and foot ▽

    M85.38   Osteitis condensans, other site

    M85.39   Osteitis condensans, multiple sites

✓5ᵗʰ M85.4   Solitary bone cyst

    EXCLUDES 2   solitary cyst of jaw (M27.4)

    M85.40   Solitary bone cyst, unspecified site ▽

✓6ᵗʰ M85.41   Solitary bone cyst, shoulder

       M85.411   Solitary bone cyst, right shoulder

       M85.412   Solitary bone cyst, left shoulder

       M85.419   Solitary bone cyst, unspecified shoulder ▽

✓6ᵗʰ M85.42   Solitary bone cyst, humerus

       M85.421   Solitary bone cyst, right humerus

       M85.422   Solitary bone cyst, left humerus

       M85.429   Solitary bone cyst, unspecified humerus ▽

✓6ᵗʰ M85.43   Solitary bone cyst, ulna and radius

       M85.431   Solitary bone cyst, right ulna and radius

       M85.432   Solitary bone cyst, left ulna and radius

       M85.439   Solitary bone cyst, unspecified ulna and radius ▽

✓6ᵗʰ M85.44   Solitary bone cyst, hand

       M85.441   Solitary bone cyst, right hand

       M85.442   Solitary bone cyst, left hand

       M85.449   Solitary bone cyst, unspecified hand ▽

✓6ᵗʰ M85.45   Solitary bone cyst, pelvis

       M85.451   Solitary bone cyst, right pelvis

       M85.452   Solitary bone cyst, left pelvis

       M85.459   Solitary bone cyst, unspecified pelvis ▽

✓6ᵗʰ M85.46   Solitary bone cyst, tibia and fibula

       M85.461   Solitary bone cyst, right tibia and fibula

       M85.462   Solitary bone cyst, left tibia and fibula

       M85.469   Solitary bone cyst, unspecified tibia and fibula ▽

✓6ᵗʰ M85.47   Solitary bone cyst, ankle and foot

       M85.471   Solitary bone cyst, right ankle and foot

✓ Additional Character Req   √x7ᵗʰ Placeholder Alert   Case-Mix Diagnosis   Manifestation   ▽ Unspecified Dx   EXCLUDES 1 Not coded here   EXCLUDES 2 Not included here

M85.472 Solitary bone cyst, left ankle and foot
M85.479 Solitary bone cyst, unspecified ankle ▽
          and foot
M85.48 Solitary bone cyst, other site
✓5ᵗʰ M85.5 Aneurysmal bone cyst
      EXCLUDES 2 aneurysmal cyst of jaw (M27.4)
      DEF: Solitary bone lesion, bulges into periosteum; marked by calcified rim.
M85.50 Aneurysmal bone cyst, unspecified site ▽
✓6ᵗʰ M85.51 Aneurysmal bone cyst, shoulder
      M85.511 Aneurysmal bone cyst, right shoulder
      M85.512 Aneurysmal bone cyst, left shoulder
      M85.519 Aneurysmal bone cyst, unspecified ▽
               shoulder
✓6ᵗʰ M85.52 Aneurysmal bone cyst, upper arm
      M85.521 Aneurysmal bone cyst, right upper arm
      M85.522 Aneurysmal bone cyst, left upper arm
      M85.529 Aneurysmal bone cyst, unspecified ▽
               upper arm
✓6ᵗʰ M85.53 Aneurysmal bone cyst, forearm
      M85.531 Aneurysmal bone cyst, right forearm
      M85.532 Aneurysmal bone cyst, left forearm
      M85.539 Aneurysmal bone cyst, unspecified ▽
               forearm
✓6ᵗʰ M85.54 Aneurysmal bone cyst, hand
      M85.541 Aneurysmal bone cyst, right hand
      M85.542 Aneurysmal bone cyst, left hand
      M85.549 Aneurysmal bone cyst, unspecified ▽
               hand
✓6ᵗʰ M85.55 Aneurysmal bone cyst, thigh
      M85.551 Aneurysmal bone cyst, right thigh
      M85.552 Aneurysmal bone cyst, left thigh
      M85.559 Aneurysmal bone cyst, unspecified ▽
               thigh
✓6ᵗʰ M85.56 Aneurysmal bone cyst, lower leg
      M85.561 Aneurysmal bone cyst, right lower leg
      M85.562 Aneurysmal bone cyst, left lower leg
      M85.569 Aneurysmal bone cyst, unspecified ▽
               lower leg
✓6ᵗʰ M85.57 Aneurysmal bone cyst, ankle and foot
      M85.571 Aneurysmal bone cyst, right ankle and foot
      M85.572 Aneurysmal bone cyst, left ankle and foot
      M85.579 Aneurysmal bone cyst, unspecified ▽
               ankle and foot
M85.58 Aneurysmal bone cyst, other site
M85.59 Aneurysmal bone cyst, multiple sites
✓5ᵗʰ M85.6 Other cyst of bone
      EXCLUDES 1 cyst of jaw NEC (M27.4)
                  osteitis fibrosa cystica generalisata [von
                  Recklinghausen's disease of bone] (E21.0)
M85.60 Other cyst of bone, unspecified site ▽
✓6ᵗʰ M85.61 Other cyst of bone, shoulder
      M85.611 Other cyst of bone, right shoulder
      M85.612 Other cyst of bone, left shoulder
      M85.619 Other cyst of bone, unspecified ▽
               shoulder
✓6ᵗʰ M85.62 Other cyst of bone, upper arm
      M85.621 Other cyst of bone, right upper arm
      M85.622 Other cyst of bone, left upper arm
      M85.629 Other cyst of bone, unspecified upper ▽
               arm
✓6ᵗʰ M85.63 Other cyst of bone, forearm
      M85.631 Other cyst of bone, right forearm
      M85.632 Other cyst of bone, left forearm
      M85.639 Other cyst of bone, unspecified forearm ▽
✓6ᵗʰ M85.64 Other cyst of bone, hand
      M85.641 Other cyst of bone, right hand
      M85.642 Other cyst of bone, left hand
      M85.649 Other cyst of bone, unspecified hand ▽
✓6ᵗʰ M85.65 Other cyst of bone, thigh
      M85.651 Other cyst of bone, right thigh
      M85.652 Other cyst of bone, left thigh

M85.659 Other cyst of bone, unspecified thigh ▽
✓6ᵗʰ M85.66 Other cyst of bone, lower leg
      M85.661 Other cyst of bone, right lower leg
      M85.662 Other cyst of bone, left lower leg
      M85.669 Other cyst of bone, unspecified lower ▽
               leg
✓6ᵗʰ M85.67 Other cyst of bone, ankle and foot
      M85.671 Other cyst of bone, right ankle and foot
      M85.672 Other cyst of bone, left ankle and foot
      M85.679 Other cyst of bone, unspecified ankle ▽
               and foot
M85.68 Other cyst of bone, other site
M85.69 Other cyst of bone, multiple sites
✓5ᵗʰ M85.8 Other specified disorders of bone density and structure
      Hyperostosis of bones, except skull
      Osteosclerosis, acquired
      EXCLUDES 1 diffuse idiopathic skeletal hyperostosis [DISH] (M48.1)
                  osteosclerosis congenita (Q77.4)
                  osteosclerosis fragilitas (generalista) (Q78.2)
                  osteosclerosis myelofibrosis (D75.81)
M85.80 Other specified disorders of bone density and ▽
        structure, unspecified site
✓6ᵗʰ M85.81 Other specified disorders of bone density and
            structure, shoulder
      M85.811 Other specified disorders of bone density
               and structure, right shoulder
      M85.812 Other specified disorders of bone density
               and structure, left shoulder
      M85.819 Other specified disorders of bone ▽
               density and structure, unspecified
               shoulder
✓6ᵗʰ M85.82 Other specified disorders of bone density and
            structure, upper arm
      M85.821 Other specified disorders of bone density
               and structure, right upper arm
      M85.822 Other specified disorders of bone density
               and structure, left upper arm
      M85.829 Other specified disorders of bone ▽
               density and structure, unspecified
               upper arm
✓6ᵗʰ M85.83 Other specified disorders of bone density and
            structure, forearm
      M85.831 Other specified disorders of bone density
               and structure, right forearm
      M85.832 Other specified disorders of bone density
               and structure, left forearm
      M85.839 Other specified disorders of bone ▽
               density and structure, unspecified
               forearm
✓6ᵗʰ M85.84 Other specified disorders of bone density and
            structure, hand
      M85.841 Other specified disorders of bone density
               and structure, right hand
      M85.842 Other specified disorders of bone density
               and structure, left hand
      M85.849 Other specified disorders of bone ▽
               density and structure, unspecified hand
✓6ᵗʰ M85.85 Other specified disorders of bone density and
            structure, thigh
      M85.851 Other specified disorders of bone density
               and structure, right thigh
      M85.852 Other specified disorders of bone density
               and structure, left thigh
      M85.859 Other specified disorders of bone ▽
               density and structure, unspecified thigh
✓6ᵗʰ M85.86 Other specified disorders of bone density and
            structure, lower leg
      M85.861 Other specified disorders of bone density
               and structure, right lower leg
      M85.862 Other specified disorders of bone density
               and structure, left lower leg
      M85.869 Other specified disorders of bone ▽
               density and structure, unspecified
               lower leg
✓6ᵗʰ M85.87 Other specified disorders of bone density and
            structure, ankle and foot
      M85.871 Other specified disorders of bone density
               and structure, right ankle and foot

Ⓝ Newborn: 0 Ⓟ Pediatric: 0-17 Ⓜ Maternity: 12-55 Ⓐ Adult: 15-124 NRS Nonroutine supply Dx NC Dx Noncancer Dx PDx Primary Dx ▶◀ Revised Text ● New Code ▲ Revised Title

784   ICD-10-CM 2018

M85.872   Other specified disorders of bone density and structure, left ankle and foot

M85.879   Other specified disorders of bone density and structure, unspecified ankle and foot ▽

M85.88   Other specified disorders of bone density and structure, other site

M85.89   Other specified disorders of bone density and structure, multiple sites

M85.9   Disorder of bone density and structure, unspecified ▽

Other osteopathies (M86-M90)

EXCLUDES 1   postprocedural osteopathies (M96.-)

✓4th M86 Osteomyelitis

Use additional code (B95-B97) to identify infectious agent

Use additional code to identify major osseous defect, if applicable (M89.7-)

EXCLUDES 1   osteomyelitis due to:
echinococcus (B67.2)
gonococcus (A54.43)
salmonella (A02.24)

EXCLUDES 2   ostemyelitis of:
orbit (H05.0-)
petrous bone (H70.2-)
vertebra (M46.2-)

✓5th M86.0   Acute hematogenous osteomyelitis

M86.00   Acute hematogenous osteomyelitis, unspecified site ▽

✓6th M86.01   Acute hematogenous osteomyelitis, shoulder

M86.011   Acute hematogenous osteomyelitis, right shoulder

M86.012   Acute hematogenous osteomyelitis, left shoulder

M86.019   Acute hematogenous osteomyelitis, unspecified shoulder ▽

✓6th M86.02   Acute hematogenous osteomyelitis, humerus

M86.021   Acute hematogenous osteomyelitis, right humerus

M86.022   Acute hematogenous osteomyelitis, left humerus

M86.029   Acute hematogenous osteomyelitis, unspecified humerus ▽

✓6th M86.03   Acute hematogenous osteomyelitis, radius and ulna

M86.031   Acute hematogenous osteomyelitis, right radius and ulna

M86.032   Acute hematogenous osteomyelitis, left radius and ulna

M86.039   Acute hematogenous osteomyelitis, unspecified radius and ulna ▽

✓6th M86.04   Acute hematogenous osteomyelitis, hand

M86.041   Acute hematogenous osteomyelitis, right hand

M86.042   Acute hematogenous osteomyelitis, left hand

M86.049   Acute hematogenous osteomyelitis, unspecified hand ▽

✓6th M86.05   Acute hematogenous osteomyelitis, femur

M86.051   Acute hematogenous osteomyelitis, right femur

M86.052   Acute hematogenous osteomyelitis, left femur

M86.059   Acute hematogenous osteomyelitis, unspecified femur ▽

✓6th M86.06   Acute hematogenous osteomyelitis, tibia and fibula

M86.061   Acute hematogenous osteomyelitis, right tibia and fibula

M86.062   Acute hematogenous osteomyelitis, left tibia and fibula

M86.069   Acute hematogenous osteomyelitis, unspecified tibia and fibula ▽

✓6th M86.07   Acute hematogenous osteomyelitis, ankle and foot

M86.071   Acute hematogenous osteomyelitis, right ankle and foot

M86.072   Acute hematogenous osteomyelitis, left ankle and foot

M86.079   Acute hematogenous osteomyelitis, unspecified ankle and foot ▽

M86.08   Acute hematogenous osteomyelitis, other sites

M86.09   Acute hematogenous osteomyelitis, multiple sites

✓5th M86.1   Other acute osteomyelitis

M86.10   Other acute osteomyelitis, unspecified site ▽

✓6th M86.11   Other acute osteomyelitis, shoulder

M86.111   Other acute osteomyelitis, right shoulder

M86.112   Other acute osteomyelitis, left shoulder

M86.119   Other acute osteomyelitis, unspecified shoulder ▽

✓6th M86.12   Other acute osteomyelitis, humerus

M86.121   Other acute osteomyelitis, right humerus

M86.122   Other acute osteomyelitis, left humerus

M86.129   Other acute osteomyelitis, unspecified humerus ▽

✓6th M86.13   Other acute osteomyelitis, radius and ulna

M86.131   Other acute osteomyelitis, right radius and ulna

M86.132   Other acute osteomyelitis, left radius and ulna

M86.139   Other acute osteomyelitis, unspecified radius and ulna ▽

✓6th M86.14   Other acute osteomyelitis, hand

M86.141   Other acute osteomyelitis, right hand

M86.142   Other acute osteomyelitis, left hand

M86.149   Other acute osteomyelitis, unspecified hand ▽

✓6th M86.15   Other acute osteomyelitis, femur

M86.151   Other acute osteomyelitis, right femur

M86.152   Other acute osteomyelitis, left femur

M86.159   Other acute osteomyelitis, unspecified femur ▽

✓6th M86.16   Other acute osteomyelitis, tibia and fibula

M86.161   Other acute osteomyelitis, right tibia and fibula

M86.162   Other acute osteomyelitis, left tibia and fibula

M86.169   Other acute osteomyelitis, unspecified tibia and fibula ▽

✓6th M86.17   Other acute osteomyelitis, ankle and foot

M86.171   Other acute osteomyelitis, right ankle and foot

M86.172   Other acute osteomyelitis, left ankle and foot

M86.179   Other acute osteomyelitis, unspecified ankle and foot ▽

M86.18   Other acute osteomyelitis, other site

M86.19   Other acute osteomyelitis, multiple sites

✓5th M86.2   Subacute osteomyelitis

M86.20   Subacute osteomyelitis, unspecified site ▽

✓6th M86.21   Subacute osteomyelitis, shoulder

M86.211   Subacute osteomyelitis, right shoulder

M86.212   Subacute osteomyelitis, left shoulder

M86.219   Subacute osteomyelitis, unspecified shoulder ▽

✓6th M86.22   Subacute osteomyelitis, humerus

M86.221   Subacute osteomyelitis, right humerus

M86.222   Subacute osteomyelitis, left humerus

M86.229   Subacute osteomyelitis, unspecified humerus ▽

✓6th M86.23   Subacute osteomyelitis, radius and ulna

M86.231   Subacute osteomyelitis, right radius and ulna

M86.232   Subacute osteomyelitis, left radius and ulna

M86.239   Subacute osteomyelitis, unspecified radius and ulna ▽

✓6th M86.24   Subacute osteomyelitis, hand

M86.241   Subacute osteomyelitis, right hand

M86.242   Subacute osteomyelitis, left hand

M86.249   Subacute osteomyelitis, unspecified hand ▽

✓6th M86.25   Subacute osteomyelitis, femur

M86.251   Subacute osteomyelitis, right femur

M86.252   Subacute osteomyelitis, left femur

✓ Additional Character Req   ✓x7th Placeholder Alert   Case-Mix Diagnosis   Manifestation   ▽ Unspecified Dx   EXCLUDES 1 Not coded here   EXCLUDES 2 Not included here

M86.259　Subacute osteomyelitis, unspecified femur ▽

✓6th M86.26　Subacute osteomyelitis, tibia and fibula
　　　M86.261　Subacute osteomyelitis, right tibia and fibula
　　　M86.262　Subacute osteomyelitis, left tibia and fibula
　　　M86.269　Subacute osteomyelitis, unspecified tibia and fibula ▽

✓6th M86.27　Subacute osteomyelitis, ankle and foot
　　　M86.271　Subacute osteomyelitis, right ankle and foot
　　　M86.272　Subacute osteomyelitis, left ankle and foot
　　　M86.279　Subacute osteomyelitis, unspecified ankle and foot ▽

M86.28　Subacute osteomyelitis, other site
M86.29　Subacute osteomyelitis, multiple sites

✓5th M86.3　Chronic multifocal osteomyelitis
M86.30　Chronic multifocal osteomyelitis, unspecified site ▽

✓6th M86.31　Chronic multifocal osteomyelitis, shoulder
　　　M86.311　Chronic multifocal osteomyelitis, right shoulder
　　　M86.312　Chronic multifocal osteomyelitis, left shoulder
　　　M86.319　Chronic multifocal osteomyelitis, unspecified shoulder ▽

✓6th M86.32　Chronic multifocal osteomyelitis, humerus
　　　M86.321　Chronic multifocal osteomyelitis, right humerus
　　　M86.322　Chronic multifocal osteomyelitis, left humerus
　　　M86.329　Chronic multifocal osteomyelitis, unspecified humerus ▽

✓6th M86.33　Chronic multifocal osteomyelitis, radius and ulna
　　　M86.331　Chronic multifocal osteomyelitis, right radius and ulna
　　　M86.332　Chronic multifocal osteomyelitis, left radius and ulna
　　　M86.339　Chronic multifocal osteomyelitis, unspecified radius and ulna ▽

✓6th M86.34　Chronic multifocal osteomyelitis, hand
　　　M86.341　Chronic multifocal osteomyelitis, right hand
　　　M86.342　Chronic multifocal osteomyelitis, left hand
　　　M86.349　Chronic multifocal osteomyelitis, unspecified hand ▽

✓6th M86.35　Chronic multifocal osteomyelitis, femur
　　　M86.351　Chronic multifocal osteomyelitis, right femur
　　　M86.352　Chronic multifocal osteomyelitis, left femur
　　　M86.359　Chronic multifocal osteomyelitis, unspecified femur ▽

✓6th M86.36　Chronic multifocal osteomyelitis, tibia and fibula
　　　M86.361　Chronic multifocal osteomyelitis, right tibia and fibula
　　　M86.362　Chronic multifocal osteomyelitis, left tibia and fibula
　　　M86.369　Chronic multifocal osteomyelitis, unspecified tibia and fibula ▽

✓6th M86.37　Chronic multifocal osteomyelitis, ankle and foot
　　　M86.371　Chronic multifocal osteomyelitis, right ankle and foot
　　　M86.372　Chronic multifocal osteomyelitis, left ankle and foot
　　　M86.379　Chronic multifocal osteomyelitis, unspecified ankle and foot ▽

M86.38　Chronic multifocal osteomyelitis, other site
M86.39　Chronic multifocal osteomyelitis, multiple sites

✓5th M86.4　Chronic osteomyelitis with draining sinus
M86.40　Chronic osteomyelitis with draining sinus, unspecified site ▽

✓6th M86.41　Chronic osteomyelitis with draining sinus, shoulder
　　　M86.411　Chronic osteomyelitis with draining sinus, right shoulder
　　　M86.412　Chronic osteomyelitis with draining sinus, left shoulder
　　　M86.419　Chronic osteomyelitis with draining sinus, unspecified shoulder ▽

✓6th M86.42　Chronic osteomyelitis with draining sinus, humerus
　　　M86.421　Chronic osteomyelitis with draining sinus, right humerus
　　　M86.422　Chronic osteomyelitis with draining sinus, left humerus
　　　M86.429　Chronic osteomyelitis with draining sinus, unspecified humerus ▽

✓6th M86.43　Chronic osteomyelitis with draining sinus, radius and ulna
　　　M86.431　Chronic osteomyelitis with draining sinus, right radius and ulna
　　　M86.432　Chronic osteomyelitis with draining sinus, left radius and ulna
　　　M86.439　Chronic osteomyelitis with draining sinus, unspecified radius and ulna ▽

✓6th M86.44　Chronic osteomyelitis with draining sinus, hand
　　　M86.441　Chronic osteomyelitis with draining sinus, right hand
　　　M86.442　Chronic osteomyelitis with draining sinus, left hand
　　　M86.449　Chronic osteomyelitis with draining sinus, unspecified hand ▽

✓6th M86.45　Chronic osteomyelitis with draining sinus, femur
　　　M86.451　Chronic osteomyelitis with draining sinus, right femur
　　　M86.452　Chronic osteomyelitis with draining sinus, left femur
　　　M86.459　Chronic osteomyelitis with draining sinus, unspecified femur ▽

✓6th M86.46　Chronic osteomyelitis with draining sinus, tibia and fibula
　　　M86.461　Chronic osteomyelitis with draining sinus, right tibia and fibula
　　　M86.462　Chronic osteomyelitis with draining sinus, left tibia and fibula
　　　M86.469　Chronic osteomyelitis with draining sinus, unspecified tibia and fibula ▽

✓6th M86.47　Chronic osteomyelitis with draining sinus, ankle and foot
　　　M86.471　Chronic osteomyelitis with draining sinus, right ankle and foot
　　　M86.472　Chronic osteomyelitis with draining sinus, left ankle and foot
　　　M86.479　Chronic osteomyelitis with draining sinus, unspecified ankle and foot ▽

M86.48　Chronic osteomyelitis with draining sinus, other site
M86.49　Chronic osteomyelitis with draining sinus, multiple sites

✓5th M86.5　Other chronic hematogenous osteomyelitis
M86.50　Other chronic hematogenous osteomyelitis, unspecified site ▽

✓6th M86.51　Other chronic hematogenous osteomyelitis, shoulder
　　　M86.511　Other chronic hematogenous osteomyelitis, right shoulder
　　　M86.512　Other chronic hematogenous osteomyelitis, left shoulder
　　　M86.519　Other chronic hematogenous osteomyelitis, unspecified shoulder ▽

✓6th M86.52　Other chronic hematogenous osteomyelitis, humerus
　　　M86.521　Other chronic hematogenous osteomyelitis, right humerus
　　　M86.522　Other chronic hematogenous osteomyelitis, left humerus
　　　M86.529　Other chronic hematogenous osteomyelitis, unspecified humerus ▽

✓6th M86.53　Other chronic hematogenous osteomyelitis, radius and ulna
　　　M86.531　Other chronic hematogenous osteomyelitis, right radius and ulna
　　　M86.532　Other chronic hematogenous osteomyelitis, left radius and ulna

M86.539 Other chronic hematogenous osteomyelitis, unspecified radius and ulna ▽

✓6ᵗʰ **M86.54** Other chronic hematogenous osteomyelitis, hand
M86.541 **Other chronic hematogenous osteomyelitis, right hand**
M86.542 **Other chronic hematogenous osteomyelitis, left hand**
M86.549 Other chronic hematogenous osteomyelitis, unspecified hand ▽

✓6ᵗʰ **M86.55** Other chronic hematogenous osteomyelitis, femur
M86.551 **Other chronic hematogenous osteomyelitis, right femur**
M86.552 **Other chronic hematogenous osteomyelitis, left femur**
M86.559 Other chronic hematogenous osteomyelitis, unspecified femur ▽

✓6ᵗʰ **M86.56** Other chronic hematogenous osteomyelitis, tibia and fibula
M86.561 **Other chronic hematogenous osteomyelitis, right tibia and fibula**
M86.562 **Other chronic hematogenous osteomyelitis, left tibia and fibula**
M86.569 Other chronic hematogenous osteomyelitis, unspecified tibia and fibula ▽

✓6ᵗʰ **M86.57** Other chronic hematogenous osteomyelitis, ankle and foot
M86.571 **Other chronic hematogenous osteomyelitis, right ankle and foot**
M86.572 **Other chronic hematogenous osteomyelitis, left ankle and foot**
M86.579 Other chronic hematogenous osteomyelitis, unspecified ankle and foot ▽

M86.58 Other chronic hematogenous osteomyelitis, other site
M86.59 Other chronic hematogenous osteomyelitis, multiple sites

✓5ᵗʰ **M86.6** Other chronic osteomyelitis
M86.60 Other chronic osteomyelitis, unspecified site ▽

✓6ᵗʰ **M86.61** Other chronic osteomyelitis, shoulder
M86.611 **Other chronic osteomyelitis, right shoulder**
M86.612 **Other chronic osteomyelitis, left shoulder**
M86.619 Other chronic osteomyelitis, unspecified shoulder ▽

✓6ᵗʰ **M86.62** Other chronic osteomyelitis, humerus
M86.621 **Other chronic osteomyelitis, right humerus**
M86.622 **Other chronic osteomyelitis, left humerus**
M86.629 Other chronic osteomyelitis, unspecified humerus ▽

✓6ᵗʰ **M86.63** Other chronic osteomyelitis, radius and ulna
M86.631 **Other chronic osteomyelitis, right radius and ulna**
M86.632 **Other chronic osteomyelitis, left radius and ulna**
M86.639 Other chronic osteomyelitis, unspecified radius and ulna ▽

✓6ᵗʰ **M86.64** Other chronic osteomyelitis, hand
M86.641 **Other chronic osteomyelitis, right hand**
M86.642 **Other chronic osteomyelitis, left hand**
M86.649 Other chronic osteomyelitis, unspecified hand ▽

✓6ᵗʰ **M86.65** Other chronic osteomyelitis, thigh
M86.651 **Other chronic osteomyelitis, right thigh**
M86.652 **Other chronic osteomyelitis, left thigh**
M86.659 Other chronic osteomyelitis, unspecified thigh ▽

✓6ᵗʰ **M86.66** Other chronic osteomyelitis, tibia and fibula
M86.661 **Other chronic osteomyelitis, right tibia and fibula**
M86.662 **Other chronic osteomyelitis, left tibia and fibula**
M86.669 Other chronic osteomyelitis, unspecified tibia and fibula ▽

✓6ᵗʰ **M86.67** Other chronic osteomyelitis, ankle and foot
M86.671 **Other chronic osteomyelitis, right ankle and foot**
AHA: 2016, 1Q, 13
M86.672 **Other chronic osteomyelitis, left ankle and foot**
M86.679 Other chronic osteomyelitis, unspecified ankle and foot ▽

M86.68 Other chronic osteomyelitis, other site
M86.69 Other chronic osteomyelitis, multiple sites

✓5ᵗʰ **M86.8** Other osteomyelitis
Brodie's abscess
✓6ᵗʰ **M86.8X** Other osteomyelitis
M86.8X0 Other osteomyelitis, multiple sites
M86.8X1 Other osteomyelitis, shoulder
M86.8X2 Other osteomyelitis, upper arm
M86.8X3 Other osteomyelitis, forearm
M86.8X4 Other osteomyelitis, hand
M86.8X5 Other osteomyelitis, thigh
M86.8X6 Other osteomyelitis, lower leg
M86.8X7 Other osteomyelitis, ankle and foot
M86.8X8 Other osteomyelitis, other site
M86.8X9 Other osteomyelitis, unspecified sites ▽

M86.9 Osteomyelitis, unspecified ▽
Infection of bone NOS
Periostitis without osteomyelitis

✓4ᵗʰ **M87 Osteonecrosis**
INCLUDES avascular necrosis of bone
Use additional code to identify major osseous defect, if applicable (M89.7-)
EXCLUDES 1 juvenile osteonecrosis (M91-M92)
osteochondropathies (M90-M93)

✓5ᵗʰ **M87.0** Idiopathic aseptic necrosis of bone
M87.00 Idiopathic aseptic necrosis of unspecified bone ▽
✓6ᵗʰ **M87.01** Idiopathic aseptic necrosis of shoulder
Idiopathic aseptic necrosis of clavicle and scapula
M87.011 Idiopathic aseptic necrosis of right shoulder
M87.012 Idiopathic aseptic necrosis of left shoulder
M87.019 Idiopathic aseptic necrosis of unspecified shoulder ▽

✓6ᵗʰ **M87.02** Idiopathic aseptic necrosis of humerus
M87.021 Idiopathic aseptic necrosis of right humerus
M87.022 Idiopathic aseptic necrosis of left humerus
M87.029 Idiopathic aseptic necrosis of unspecified humerus ▽

✓6ᵗʰ **M87.03** Idiopathic aseptic necrosis of radius, ulna and carpus
M87.031 Idiopathic aseptic necrosis of right radius
M87.032 Idiopathic aseptic necrosis of left radius
M87.033 Idiopathic aseptic necrosis of unspecified radius ▽
M87.034 Idiopathic aseptic necrosis of right ulna
M87.035 Idiopathic aseptic necrosis of left ulna
M87.036 Idiopathic aseptic necrosis of unspecified ulna ▽
M87.037 Idiopathic aseptic necrosis of right carpus
M87.038 Idiopathic aseptic necrosis of left carpus
M87.039 Idiopathic aseptic necrosis of unspecified carpus ▽

✓6ᵗʰ **M87.04** Idiopathic aseptic necrosis of hand and fingers
Idiopathic aseptic necrosis of metacarpals and phalanges of hands
M87.041 Idiopathic aseptic necrosis of right hand
M87.042 Idiopathic aseptic necrosis of left hand
M87.043 Idiopathic aseptic necrosis of unspecified hand ▽
M87.044 Idiopathic aseptic necrosis of right finger(s)
M87.045 Idiopathic aseptic necrosis of left finger(s)
M87.046 Idiopathic aseptic necrosis of unspecified finger(s) ▽

✓6ᵗʰ **M87.05** Idiopathic aseptic necrosis of pelvis and femur
M87.050 Idiopathic aseptic necrosis of pelvis
M87.051 **Idiopathic aseptic necrosis of right femur**

Chapter 13. Diseases of the Musculoskeletal System and Connective Tissue

      M87.052 **Idiopathic aseptic necrosis of** left femur

      M87.059 **Idiopathic aseptic necrosis of unspecified femur** ▽
            Idiopathic aseptic necrosis of hip NOS

✓6ᵗʰ M87.06 **Idiopathic aseptic necrosis of** tibia and fibula

      M87.061 **Idiopathic aseptic necrosis of** right tibia

      M87.062 **Idiopathic aseptic necrosis of** left tibia

      M87.063 **Idiopathic aseptic necrosis of unspecified tibia** ▽

      M87.064 **Idiopathic aseptic necrosis of** right fibula

      M87.065 **Idiopathic aseptic necrosis of** left fibula

      M87.066 **Idiopathic aseptic necrosis of unspecified fibula** ▽

✓6ᵗʰ M87.07 **Idiopathic aseptic necrosis of** ankle, foot and toes
         Idiopathic aseptic necrosis of metatarsus, tarsus, and phalanges of toes

      M87.071 **Idiopathic aseptic necrosis of** right ankle

      M87.072 **Idiopathic aseptic necrosis of** left ankle

      M87.073 **Idiopathic aseptic necrosis of unspecified ankle** ▽

      M87.074 **Idiopathic aseptic necrosis of** right foot

      M87.075 **Idiopathic aseptic necrosis of** left foot

      M87.076 **Idiopathic aseptic necrosis of unspecified foot** ▽

      M87.077 **Idiopathic aseptic necrosis of** right toe(s)

      M87.078 **Idiopathic aseptic necrosis of** left toe(s)

      M87.079 **Idiopathic aseptic necrosis of unspecified toe(s)** ▽

    M87.08 **Idiopathic aseptic necrosis of bone, other site**

    M87.09 **Idiopathic aseptic necrosis of bone,** multiple sites

✓5ᵗʰ M87.1 **Osteonecrosis** due to drugs
    Use additional code for adverse effect, if applicable, to identify drug (T36-T50 with fifth or sixth character 5)

    M87.10 **Osteonecrosis due to drugs, unspecified bone** ▽

✓6ᵗʰ M87.11 **Osteonecrosis due to drugs,** shoulder

      M87.111 **Osteonecrosis due to drugs, right shoulder**

      M87.112 **Osteonecrosis due to drugs, left shoulder**

      M87.119 **Osteonecrosis due to drugs, unspecified shoulder** ▽

✓6ᵗʰ M87.12 **Osteonecrosis due to drugs,** humerus

      M87.121 **Osteonecrosis due to drugs, right humerus**

      M87.122 **Osteonecrosis due to drugs, left humerus**

      M87.129 **Osteonecrosis due to drugs, unspecified humerus** ▽

✓6ᵗʰ M87.13 **Osteonecrosis due to drugs of** radius, ulna and carpus

      M87.131 **Osteonecrosis due to drugs of** right radius

      M87.132 **Osteonecrosis due to drugs of** left radius

      M87.133 **Osteonecrosis due to drugs of unspecified radius** ▽

      M87.134 **Osteonecrosis due to drugs of** right ulna

      M87.135 **Osteonecrosis due to drugs of** left ulna

      M87.136 **Osteonecrosis due to drugs of unspecified ulna** ▽

      M87.137 **Osteonecrosis due to drugs of** right carpus

      M87.138 **Osteonecrosis due to drugs of** left carpus

      M87.139 **Osteonecrosis due to drugs of unspecified carpus** ▽

✓6ᵗʰ M87.14 **Osteonecrosis due to drugs,** hand and fingers

      M87.141 **Osteonecrosis due to drugs,** right hand

      M87.142 **Osteonecrosis due to drugs,** left hand

      M87.143 **Osteonecrosis due to drugs, unspecified hand** ▽

      M87.144 **Osteonecrosis due to drugs,** right finger(s)

      M87.145 **Osteonecrosis due to drugs,** left finger(s)

      M87.146 **Osteonecrosis due to drugs, unspecified finger(s)** ▽

✓6ᵗʰ M87.15 **Osteonecrosis due to drugs,** pelvis and femur

      M87.150 **Osteonecrosis due to drugs,** pelvis

      M87.151 **Osteonecrosis due to drugs,** right femur

      M87.152 **Osteonecrosis due to drugs,** left femur

      M87.159 **Osteonecrosis due to drugs, unspecified femur** ▽

✓6ᵗʰ M87.16 **Osteonecrosis due to drugs,** tibia and fibula

      M87.161 **Osteonecrosis due to drugs,** right tibia

      M87.162 **Osteonecrosis due to drugs,** left tibia

      M87.163 **Osteonecrosis due to drugs, unspecified tibia** ▽

      M87.164 **Osteonecrosis due to drugs,** right fibula

      M87.165 **Osteonecrosis due to drugs,** left fibula

      M87.166 **Osteonecrosis due to drugs, unspecified fibula** ▽

✓6ᵗʰ M87.17 **Osteonecrosis due to drugs,** ankle, foot and toes

      M87.171 **Osteonecrosis due to drugs,** right ankle

      M87.172 **Osteonecrosis due to drugs,** left ankle

      M87.173 **Osteonecrosis due to drugs, unspecified ankle** ▽

      M87.174 **Osteonecrosis due to drugs,** right foot

      M87.175 **Osteonecrosis due to drugs,** left foot

      M87.176 **Osteonecrosis due to drugs, unspecified foot** ▽

      M87.177 **Osteonecrosis due to drugs,** right toe(s)

      M87.178 **Osteonecrosis due to drugs,** left toe(s)

      M87.179 **Osteonecrosis due to drugs, unspecified toe(s)** ▽

✓6ᵗʰ M87.18 **Osteonecrosis due to drugs,** other site

      M87.180 **Osteonecrosis due to drugs,** jaw

      M87.188 **Osteonecrosis due to drugs, other site**

    M87.19 **Osteonecrosis due to drugs,** multiple sites

✓5ᵗʰ M87.2 **Osteonecrosis** due to previous trauma

    M87.20 **Osteonecrosis due to previous trauma, unspecified bone** ▽

✓6ᵗʰ M87.21 **Osteonecrosis due to previous trauma,** shoulder

      M87.211 **Osteonecrosis due to previous trauma, right shoulder**

      M87.212 **Osteonecrosis due to previous trauma, left shoulder**

      M87.219 **Osteonecrosis due to previous trauma, unspecified shoulder** ▽

✓6ᵗʰ M87.22 **Osteonecrosis due to previous trauma,** humerus

      M87.221 **Osteonecrosis due to previous trauma, right humerus**

      M87.222 **Osteonecrosis due to previous trauma, left humerus**

      M87.229 **Osteonecrosis due to previous trauma, unspecified humerus** ▽

✓6ᵗʰ M87.23 **Osteonecrosis due to previous trauma of** radius, ulna and carpus

      M87.231 **Osteonecrosis due to previous trauma of** right radius

      M87.232 **Osteonecrosis due to previous trauma of** left radius

      M87.233 **Osteonecrosis due to previous trauma of unspecified radius** ▽

      M87.234 **Osteonecrosis due to previous trauma of** right ulna

      M87.235 **Osteonecrosis due to previous trauma of** left ulna

      M87.236 **Osteonecrosis due to previous trauma of unspecified ulna** ▽

      M87.237 **Osteonecrosis due to previous trauma of** right carpus

      M87.238 **Osteonecrosis due to previous trauma of** left carpus

      M87.239 **Osteonecrosis due to previous trauma of unspecified carpus** ▽

✓6ᵗʰ M87.24 **Osteonecrosis due to previous trauma,** hand and fingers

      M87.241 **Osteonecrosis due to previous trauma, right hand**

      M87.242 **Osteonecrosis due to previous trauma, left hand**

      M87.243 **Osteonecrosis due to previous trauma, unspecified hand** ▽

      M87.244 **Osteonecrosis due to previous trauma, right finger(s)**

      M87.245 **Osteonecrosis due to previous trauma, left finger(s)**

      M87.246 **Osteonecrosis due to previous trauma, unspecified finger(s)** ▽

Ⓝ Newborn: 0   Ⓟ Pediatric: 0-17   Ⓜ Maternity: 12-55   Ⓐ Adult: 15-124   NRS Nonroutine supply Dx   NCDx Noncancer Dx   PDx Primary Dx   ►◄ Revised Text   ● New Code   ▲ Revised Title

788   ICD-10-CM 2018

M87.25 Osteonecrosis due to previous trauma, pelvis and femur
M87.250 Osteonecrosis due to previous trauma, pelvis
M87.251 Osteonecrosis due to previous trauma, right femur
M87.252 Osteonecrosis due to previous trauma, left femur
M87.256 Osteonecrosis due to previous trauma, unspecified femur ▽

M87.26 Osteonecrosis due to previous trauma, tibia and fibula
M87.261 Osteonecrosis due to previous trauma, right tibia
M87.262 Osteonecrosis due to previous trauma, left tibia
M87.263 Osteonecrosis due to previous trauma, unspecified tibia ▽
M87.264 Osteonecrosis due to previous trauma, right fibula
M87.265 Osteonecrosis due to previous trauma, left fibula
M87.266 Osteonecrosis due to previous trauma, unspecified fibula ▽

M87.27 Osteonecrosis due to previous trauma, ankle, foot and toes
M87.271 Osteonecrosis due to previous trauma, right ankle
M87.272 Osteonecrosis due to previous trauma, left ankle
M87.273 Osteonecrosis due to previous trauma, unspecified ankle ▽
M87.274 Osteonecrosis due to previous trauma, right foot
M87.275 Osteonecrosis due to previous trauma, left foot
M87.276 Osteonecrosis due to previous trauma, unspecified foot ▽
M87.277 Osteonecrosis due to previous trauma, right toe(s)
M87.278 Osteonecrosis due to previous trauma, left toe(s)
M87.279 Osteonecrosis due to previous trauma, unspecified toe(s) ▽

M87.28 Osteonecrosis due to previous trauma, other site
M87.29 Osteonecrosis due to previous trauma, multiple sites

M87.3 Other secondary osteonecrosis
M87.30 Other secondary osteonecrosis, unspecified bone ▽

M87.31 Other secondary osteonecrosis, shoulder
M87.311 Other secondary osteonecrosis, right shoulder
M87.312 Other secondary osteonecrosis, left shoulder
M87.319 Other secondary osteonecrosis, unspecified shoulder ▽

M87.32 Other secondary osteonecrosis, humerus
M87.321 Other secondary osteonecrosis, right humerus
M87.322 Other secondary osteonecrosis, left humerus
M87.329 Other secondary osteonecrosis, unspecified humerus ▽

M87.33 Other secondary osteonecrosis of radius, ulna and carpus
M87.331 Other secondary osteonecrosis of right radius
M87.332 Other secondary osteonecrosis of left radius
M87.333 Other secondary osteonecrosis of unspecified radius ▽
M87.334 Other secondary osteonecrosis of right ulna
M87.335 Other secondary osteonecrosis of left ulna
M87.336 Other secondary osteonecrosis of unspecified ulna ▽
M87.337 Other secondary osteonecrosis of right carpus
M87.338 Other secondary osteonecrosis of left carpus
M87.339 Other secondary osteonecrosis of unspecified carpus ▽

M87.34 Other secondary osteonecrosis, hand and fingers
M87.341 Other secondary osteonecrosis, right hand
M87.342 Other secondary osteonecrosis, left hand
M87.343 Other secondary osteonecrosis, unspecified hand ▽
M87.344 Other secondary osteonecrosis, right finger(s)
M87.345 Other secondary osteonecrosis, left finger(s)
M87.346 Other secondary osteonecrosis, unspecified finger(s) ▽

M87.35 Other secondary osteonecrosis, pelvis and femur
M87.350 Other secondary osteonecrosis, pelvis
M87.351 Other secondary osteonecrosis, right femur
M87.352 Other secondary osteonecrosis, left femur
M87.353 Other secondary osteonecrosis, unspecified femur ▽

M87.36 Other secondary osteonecrosis, tibia and fibula
M87.361 Other secondary osteonecrosis, right tibia
M87.362 Other secondary osteonecrosis, left tibia
M87.363 Other secondary osteonecrosis, unspecified tibia ▽
M87.364 Other secondary osteonecrosis, right fibula
M87.365 Other secondary osteonecrosis, left fibula
M87.366 Other secondary osteonecrosis, unspecified fibula ▽

M87.37 Other secondary osteonecrosis, ankle and foot
M87.371 Other secondary osteonecrosis, right ankle
M87.372 Other secondary osteonecrosis, left ankle
M87.373 Other secondary osteonecrosis, unspecified ankle ▽
M87.374 Other secondary osteonecrosis, right foot
M87.375 Other secondary osteonecrosis, left foot
M87.376 Other secondary osteonecrosis, unspecified foot ▽
M87.377 Other secondary osteonecrosis, right toe(s)
M87.378 Other secondary osteonecrosis, left toe(s)
M87.379 Other secondary osteonecrosis, unspecified toe(s) ▽

M87.38 Other secondary osteonecrosis, other site
M87.39 Other secondary osteonecrosis, multiple sites

M87.8 Other osteonecrosis
M87.80 Other osteonecrosis, unspecified bone ▽

M87.81 Other osteonecrosis, shoulder
M87.811 Other osteonecrosis, right shoulder
M87.812 Other osteonecrosis, left shoulder
M87.819 Other osteonecrosis, unspecified shoulder ▽

M87.82 Other osteonecrosis, humerus
M87.821 Other osteonecrosis, right humerus
M87.822 Other osteonecrosis, left humerus
M87.829 Other osteonecrosis, unspecified humerus ▽

M87.83 Other osteonecrosis of radius, ulna and carpus
M87.831 Other osteonecrosis of right radius
M87.832 Other osteonecrosis of left radius
M87.833 Other osteonecrosis of unspecified radius ▽
M87.834 Other osteonecrosis of right ulna
M87.835 Other osteonecrosis of left ulna
M87.836 Other osteonecrosis of unspecified ulna ▽
M87.837 Other osteonecrosis of right carpus
M87.838 Other osteonecrosis of left carpus
M87.839 Other osteonecrosis of unspecified carpus ▽

Chapter 13. Diseases of the Musculoskeletal System and Connective Tissue

☑6ᵗʰ **M87.84** Other osteonecrosis, hand and fingers
     M87.841 Other osteonecrosis, right hand
     M87.842 Other osteonecrosis, left hand
     M87.843 Other osteonecrosis, unspecified hand ▽
     M87.844 Other osteonecrosis, right finger(s)
     M87.845 Other osteonecrosis, left finger(s)
     M87.849 Other osteonecrosis, unspecified ▽
               finger(s)

☑6ᵗʰ **M87.85** Other osteonecrosis, pelvis and femur
     M87.850 Other osteonecrosis, pelvis
     M87.851 Other osteonecrosis, right femur
     M87.852 Other osteonecrosis, left femur
     M87.859 Other osteonecrosis, unspecified femur ▽

☑6ᵗʰ **M87.86** Other osteonecrosis, tibia and fibula
     M87.861 Other osteonecrosis, right tibia
     M87.862 Other osteonecrosis, left tibia
     M87.863 Other osteonecrosis, unspecified tibia ▽
     M87.864 Other osteonecrosis, right fibula
     M87.865 Other osteonecrosis, left fibula
     M87.869 Other osteonecrosis, unspecified fibula ▽

☑6ᵗʰ **M87.87** Other osteonecrosis, ankle, foot and toes
     M87.871 Other osteonecrosis, right ankle
     M87.872 Other osteonecrosis, left ankle
     M87.873 Other osteonecrosis, unspecified ankle ▽
     M87.874 Other osteonecrosis, right foot
     M87.875 Other osteonecrosis, left foot
     M87.876 Other osteonecrosis, unspecified foot ▽
     M87.877 Other osteonecrosis, right toe(s)
     M87.878 Other osteonecrosis, left toe(s)
     M87.879 Other osteonecrosis, unspecified toe(s) ▽

     M87.88 Other osteonecrosis, other site
     M87.89 Other osteonecrosis, multiple sites

M87.9 Osteonecrosis, unspecified ▽
     Necrosis of bone NOS

☑4ᵗʰ **M88** Osteitis deformans [Paget's disease of bone]
     EXCLUDES 1 osteitis deformans in neoplastic disease (M90.6)

M88.0 Osteitis deformans of skull

M88.1 Osteitis deformans of vertebrae

☑5ᵗʰ **M88.8** Osteitis deformans of other bones
    ☑6ᵗʰ **M88.81** Osteitis deformans of shoulder
     M88.811 Osteitis deformans of right shoulder
     M88.812 Osteitis deformans of left shoulder
     M88.819 Osteitis deformans of unspecified ▽
               shoulder

    ☑6ᵗʰ **M88.82** Osteitis deformans of upper arm
     M88.821 Osteitis deformans of right upper arm
     M88.822 Osteitis deformans of left upper arm
     M88.829 Osteitis deformans of unspecified ▽
               upper arm

    ☑6ᵗʰ **M88.83** Osteitis deformans of forearm
     M88.831 Osteitis deformans of right forearm
     M88.832 Osteitis deformans of left forearm
     M88.839 Osteitis deformans of unspecified ▽
               forearm

    ☑6ᵗʰ **M88.84** Osteitis deformans of hand
     M88.841 Osteitis deformans of right hand
     M88.842 Osteitis deformans of left hand
     M88.849 Osteitis deformans of unspecified hand ▽

    ☑6ᵗʰ **M88.85** Osteitis deformans of thigh
     M88.851 Osteitis deformans of right thigh
     M88.852 Osteitis deformans of left thigh
     M88.859 Osteitis deformans of unspecified thigh ▽

    ☑6ᵗʰ **M88.86** Osteitis deformans of lower leg
     M88.861 Osteitis deformans of right lower leg
     M88.862 Osteitis deformans of left lower leg
     M88.869 Osteitis deformans of unspecified ▽
               lower leg

    ☑6ᵗʰ **M88.87** Osteitis deformans of ankle and foot
     M88.871 Osteitis deformans of right ankle and foot
     M88.872 Osteitis deformans of left ankle and foot
     M88.879 Osteitis deformans of unspecified ▽
               ankle and foot

M88.88 Osteitis deformans of other bones
     EXCLUDES 2 osteitis deformans of skull (M88.0)
                     osteitis deformans of vertebrae (M88.1)

     M88.89 Osteitis deformans of multiple sites

M88.9 Osteitis deformans of unspecified bone ▽

☑4ᵗʰ **M89** Other disorders of bone

☑5ᵗʰ **M89.0** Algoneurodystrophy
     Shoulder-hand syndrome
     Sudeck's atrophy
     EXCLUDES 1 causalgia, lower limb (G57.7-)
                     causalgia, upper limb (G56.4-)
                     complex regional pain syndrome II, lower limb (G57.7-)
                     complex regional pain syndrome II, upper limb (G56.4-)
                     reflex sympathetic dystrophy (G90.5-)

     M89.00 Algoneurodystrophy, unspecified site ▽

    ☑6ᵗʰ **M89.01** Algoneurodystrophy, shoulder
     M89.011 Algoneurodystrophy, right shoulder
     M89.012 Algoneurodystrophy, left shoulder
     M89.019 Algoneurodystrophy, unspecified ▽
               shoulder

    ☑6ᵗʰ **M89.02** Algoneurodystrophy, upper arm
     M89.021 Algoneurodystrophy, right upper arm
     M89.022 Algoneurodystrophy, left upper arm
     M89.029 Algoneurodystrophy, unspecified ▽
               upper arm

    ☑6ᵗʰ **M89.03** Algoneurodystrophy, forearm
     M89.031 Algoneurodystrophy, right forearm
     M89.032 Algoneurodystrophy, left forearm
     M89.039 Algoneurodystrophy, unspecified ▽
               forearm

    ☑6ᵗʰ **M89.04** Algoneurodystrophy, hand
     M89.041 Algoneurodystrophy, right hand
     M89.042 Algoneurodystrophy, left hand
     M89.049 Algoneurodystrophy, unspecified hand ▽

    ☑6ᵗʰ **M89.05** Algoneurodystrophy, thigh
     M89.051 Algoneurodystrophy, right thigh
     M89.052 Algoneurodystrophy, left thigh
     M89.059 Algoneurodystrophy, unspecified thigh ▽

    ☑6ᵗʰ **M89.06** Algoneurodystrophy, lower leg
     M89.061 Algoneurodystrophy, right lower leg
     M89.062 Algoneurodystrophy, left lower leg
     M89.069 Algoneurodystrophy, unspecified ▽
               lower leg

    ☑6ᵗʰ **M89.07** Algoneurodystrophy, ankle and foot
     M89.071 Algoneurodystrophy, right ankle and foot
     M89.072 Algoneurodystrophy, left ankle and foot
     M89.079 Algoneurodystrophy, unspecified ankle ▽
               and foot

     M89.08 Algoneurodystrophy, other site
     M89.09 Algoneurodystrophy, multiple sites

☑5ᵗʰ **M89.1** Physeal arrest
     Arrest of growth plate
     Epiphyseal arrest
     Growth plate arrest

    ☑6ᵗʰ **M89.12** Physeal arrest, humerus
     M89.121 Complete physeal arrest, right proximal humerus
     M89.122 Complete physeal arrest, left proximal humerus
     M89.123 Partial physeal arrest, right proximal humerus
     M89.124 Partial physeal arrest, left proximal humerus
     M89.125 Complete physeal arrest, right distal humerus
     M89.126 Complete physeal arrest, left distal humerus
     M89.127 Partial physeal arrest, right distal humerus
     M89.128 Partial physeal arrest, left distal humerus
     M89.129 Physeal arrest, humerus, unspecified ▽

    ☑6ᵗʰ **M89.13** Physeal arrest, forearm
     M89.131 Complete physeal arrest, right distal radius
     M89.132 Complete physeal arrest, left distal radius

M89.133 Partial physeal arrest, right distal radius
M89.134 Partial physeal arrest, left distal radius
M89.138 Other physeal arrest of forearm
M89.139 Physeal arrest, forearm, unspecified ▽

✓6ᵗʰ M89.15 Physeal arrest, femur
M89.151 Complete physeal arrest, right proximal femur
M89.152 Complete physeal arrest, left proximal femur
M89.153 Partial physeal arrest, right proximal femur
M89.154 Partial physeal arrest, left proximal femur
M89.155 Complete physeal arrest, right distal femur
M89.156 Complete physeal arrest, left distal femur
M89.157 Partial physeal arrest, right distal femur
M89.158 Partial physeal arrest, left distal femur
M89.159 Physeal arrest, femur, unspecified ▽

✓6ᵗʰ M89.16 Physeal arrest, lower leg
M89.160 Complete physeal arrest, right proximal tibia
M89.161 Complete physeal arrest, left proximal tibia
M89.162 Partial physeal arrest, right proximal tibia
M89.163 Partial physeal arrest, left proximal tibia
M89.164 Complete physeal arrest, right distal tibia
M89.165 Complete physeal arrest, left distal tibia
M89.166 Partial physeal arrest, right distal tibia
M89.167 Partial physeal arrest, left distal tibia
M89.168 Other physeal arrest of lower leg
M89.169 Physeal arrest, lower leg, unspecified ▽

M89.18 Physeal arrest, other site

✓5ᵗʰ M89.2 Other disorders of bone development and growth
M89.20 Other disorders of bone development and growth, unspecified site ▽

✓6ᵗʰ M89.21 Other disorders of bone development and growth, shoulder
M89.211 Other disorders of bone development and growth, right shoulder
M89.212 Other disorders of bone development and growth, left shoulder
M89.219 Other disorders of bone development and growth, unspecified shoulder ▽

✓6ᵗʰ M89.22 Other disorders of bone development and growth, humerus
M89.221 Other disorders of bone development and growth, right humerus
M89.222 Other disorders of bone development and growth, left humerus
M89.229 Other disorders of bone development and growth, unspecified humerus ▽

✓6ᵗʰ M89.23 Other disorders of bone development and growth, ulna and radius
M89.231 Other disorders of bone development and growth, right ulna
M89.232 Other disorders of bone development and growth, left ulna
M89.233 Other disorders of bone development and growth, right radius
M89.234 Other disorders of bone development and growth, left radius
M89.239 Other disorders of bone development and growth, unspecified ulna and radius ▽

✓6ᵗʰ M89.24 Other disorders of bone development and growth, hand
M89.241 Other disorders of bone development and growth, right hand
M89.242 Other disorders of bone development and growth, left hand
M89.249 Other disorders of bone development and growth, unspecified hand ▽

✓6ᵗʰ M89.25 Other disorders of bone development and growth, femur
M89.251 Other disorders of bone development and growth, right femur

M89.252 Other disorders of bone development and growth, left femur
M89.259 Other disorders of bone development and growth, unspecified femur ▽

✓6ᵗʰ M89.26 Other disorders of bone development and growth, tibia and fibula
M89.261 Other disorders of bone development and growth, right tibia
M89.262 Other disorders of bone development and growth, left tibia
M89.263 Other disorders of bone development and growth, right fibula
M89.264 Other disorders of bone development and growth, left fibula
M89.269 Other disorders of bone development and growth, unspecified lower leg ▽

✓6ᵗʰ M89.27 Other disorders of bone development and growth, ankle and foot
M89.271 Other disorders of bone development and growth, right ankle and foot
M89.272 Other disorders of bone development and growth, left ankle and foot
M89.279 Other disorders of bone development and growth, unspecified ankle and foot ▽

M89.28 Other disorders of bone development and growth, other site
M89.29 Other disorders of bone development and growth, multiple sites

✓5ᵗʰ M89.3 Hypertrophy of bone
M89.30 Hypertrophy of bone, unspecified site ▽

✓6ᵗʰ M89.31 Hypertrophy of bone, shoulder
M89.311 Hypertrophy of bone, right shoulder
M89.312 Hypertrophy of bone, left shoulder
M89.319 Hypertrophy of bone, unspecified shoulder ▽

✓6ᵗʰ M89.32 Hypertrophy of bone, humerus
M89.321 Hypertrophy of bone, right humerus
M89.322 Hypertrophy of bone, left humerus
M89.329 Hypertrophy of bone, unspecified humerus ▽

✓6ᵗʰ M89.33 Hypertrophy of bone, ulna and radius
M89.331 Hypertrophy of bone, right ulna
M89.332 Hypertrophy of bone, left ulna
M89.333 Hypertrophy of bone, right radius
M89.334 Hypertrophy of bone, left radius
M89.339 Hypertrophy of bone, unspecified ulna and radius ▽

✓6ᵗʰ M89.34 Hypertrophy of bone, hand
M89.341 Hypertrophy of bone, right hand
M89.342 Hypertrophy of bone, left hand
M89.349 Hypertrophy of bone, unspecified hand ▽

✓6ᵗʰ M89.35 Hypertrophy of bone, femur
M89.351 Hypertrophy of bone, right femur
M89.352 Hypertrophy of bone, left femur
M89.359 Hypertrophy of bone, unspecified femur ▽

✓6ᵗʰ M89.36 Hypertrophy of bone, tibia and fibula
M89.361 Hypertrophy of bone, right tibia
M89.362 Hypertrophy of bone, left tibia
M89.363 Hypertrophy of bone, right fibula
M89.364 Hypertrophy of bone, left fibula
M89.369 Hypertrophy of bone, unspecified tibia ▽ and fibula

✓6ᵗʰ M89.37 Hypertrophy of bone, ankle and foot
M89.371 Hypertrophy of bone, right ankle and foot
M89.372 Hypertrophy of bone, left ankle and foot
M89.379 Hypertrophy of bone, unspecified ▽ ankle and foot

M89.38 Hypertrophy of bone, other site
M89.39 Hypertrophy of bone, multiple sites

Chapter 13. Diseases of the Musculoskeletal System and Connective Tissue

✓5ᵗʰ **M89.4 Other hypertrophic osteoarthropathy**
Marie-Bamberger disease
Pachydermoperiostosis

     M89.40 Other hypertrophic osteoarthropathy, unspecified site ▽

✓6ᵗʰ **M89.41 Other hypertrophic osteoarthropathy, shoulder**
     M89.411 Other hypertrophic osteoarthropathy, right shoulder
     M89.412 Other hypertrophic osteoarthropathy, left shoulder
     M89.419 Other hypertrophic osteoarthropathy, unspecified shoulder ▽

✓6ᵗʰ **M89.42 Other hypertrophic osteoarthropathy, upper arm**
     M89.421 Other hypertrophic osteoarthropathy, right upper arm
     M89.422 Other hypertrophic osteoarthropathy, left upper arm
     M89.429 Other hypertrophic osteoarthropathy, unspecified upper arm ▽

✓6ᵗʰ **M89.43 Other hypertrophic osteoarthropathy, forearm**
     M89.431 Other hypertrophic osteoarthropathy, right forearm
     M89.432 Other hypertrophic osteoarthropathy, left forearm
     M89.439 Other hypertrophic osteoarthropathy, unspecified forearm ▽

✓6ᵗʰ **M89.44 Other hypertrophic osteoarthropathy, hand**
     M89.441 Other hypertrophic osteoarthropathy, right hand
     M89.442 Other hypertrophic osteoarthropathy, left hand
     M89.449 Other hypertrophic osteoarthropathy, unspecified hand ▽

✓6ᵗʰ **M89.45 Other hypertrophic osteoarthropathy, thigh**
     M89.451 Other hypertrophic osteoarthropathy, right thigh
     M89.452 Other hypertrophic osteoarthropathy, left thigh
     M89.459 Other hypertrophic osteoarthropathy, unspecified thigh ▽

✓6ᵗʰ **M89.46 Other hypertrophic osteoarthropathy, lower leg**
     M89.461 Other hypertrophic osteoarthropathy, right lower leg
     M89.462 Other hypertrophic osteoarthropathy, left lower leg
     M89.469 Other hypertrophic osteoarthropathy, unspecified lower leg ▽

✓6ᵗʰ **M89.47 Other hypertrophic osteoarthropathy, ankle and foot**
     M89.471 Other hypertrophic osteoarthropathy, right ankle and foot
     M89.472 Other hypertrophic osteoarthropathy, left ankle and foot
     M89.479 Other hypertrophic osteoarthropathy, unspecified ankle and foot ▽

     M89.48 Other hypertrophic osteoarthropathy, other site
     M89.49 Other hypertrophic osteoarthropathy, multiple sites

✓5ᵗʰ **M89.5 Osteolysis**
Use additional code to identify major osseous defect, if applicable (M89.7-)
EXCLUDES 2 periprosthetic osteolysis of internal prosthetic joint (T84.05-)

     M89.50 Osteolysis, unspecified site ▽

✓6ᵗʰ **M89.51 Osteolysis, shoulder**
     M89.511 Osteolysis, right shoulder
     M89.512 Osteolysis, left shoulder
     M89.519 Osteolysis, unspecified shoulder ▽

✓6ᵗʰ **M89.52 Osteolysis, upper arm**
     M89.521 Osteolysis, right upper arm
     M89.522 Osteolysis, left upper arm
     M89.529 Osteolysis, unspecified upper arm ▽

✓6ᵗʰ **M89.53 Osteolysis, forearm**
     M89.531 Osteolysis, right forearm
     M89.532 Osteolysis, left forearm
     M89.539 Osteolysis, unspecified forearm ▽

✓6ᵗʰ **M89.54 Osteolysis, hand**
     M89.541 Osteolysis, right hand
     M89.542 Osteolysis, left hand
     M89.549 Osteolysis, unspecified hand ▽

✓6ᵗʰ **M89.55 Osteolysis, thigh**
     M89.551 Osteolysis, right thigh
     M89.552 Osteolysis, left thigh
     M89.559 Osteolysis, unspecified thigh ▽

✓6ᵗʰ **M89.56 Osteolysis, lower leg**
     M89.561 Osteolysis, right lower leg
     M89.562 Osteolysis, left lower leg
     M89.569 Osteolysis, unspecified lower leg ▽

✓6ᵗʰ **M89.57 Osteolysis, ankle and foot**
     M89.571 Osteolysis, right ankle and foot
     M89.572 Osteolysis, left ankle and foot
     M89.579 Osteolysis, unspecified ankle and foot ▽

     M89.58 Osteolysis, other site
     M89.59 Osteolysis, multiple sites

✓5ᵗʰ **M89.6 Osteopathy after poliomyelitis**
Use additional code (B91) to identify previous poliomyelitis
EXCLUDES 1 postpolio syndrome (G14)

     M89.60 Osteopathy after poliomyelitis, unspecified site ▽

✓6ᵗʰ **M89.61 Osteopathy after poliomyelitis, shoulder**
     M89.611 Osteopathy after poliomyelitis, right shoulder
     M89.612 Osteopathy after poliomyelitis, left shoulder
     M89.619 Osteopathy after poliomyelitis, unspecified shoulder ▽

✓6ᵗʰ **M89.62 Osteopathy after poliomyelitis, upper arm**
     M89.621 Osteopathy after poliomyelitis, right upper arm
     M89.622 Osteopathy after poliomyelitis, left upper arm
     M89.629 Osteopathy after poliomyelitis, unspecified upper arm ▽

✓6ᵗʰ **M89.63 Osteopathy after poliomyelitis, forearm**
     M89.631 Osteopathy after poliomyelitis, right forearm
     M89.632 Osteopathy after poliomyelitis, left forearm
     M89.639 Osteopathy after poliomyelitis, unspecified forearm ▽

✓6ᵗʰ **M89.64 Osteopathy after poliomyelitis, hand**
     M89.641 Osteopathy after poliomyelitis, right hand
     M89.642 Osteopathy after poliomyelitis, left hand
     M89.649 Osteopathy after poliomyelitis, unspecified hand ▽

✓6ᵗʰ **M89.65 Osteopathy after poliomyelitis, thigh**
     M89.651 Osteopathy after poliomyelitis, right thigh
     M89.652 Osteopathy after poliomyelitis, left thigh
     M89.659 Osteopathy after poliomyelitis, unspecified thigh ▽

✓6ᵗʰ **M89.66 Osteopathy after poliomyelitis, lower leg**
     M89.661 Osteopathy after poliomyelitis, right lower leg
     M89.662 Osteopathy after poliomyelitis, left lower leg
     M89.669 Osteopathy after poliomyelitis, unspecified lower leg ▽

✓6ᵗʰ **M89.67 Osteopathy after poliomyelitis, ankle and foot**
     M89.671 Osteopathy after poliomyelitis, right ankle and foot
     M89.672 Osteopathy after poliomyelitis, left ankle and foot
     M89.679 Osteopathy after poliomyelitis, unspecified ankle and foot ▽

     M89.68 Osteopathy after poliomyelitis, other site
     M89.69 Osteopathy after poliomyelitis, multiple sites

Ⓝ Newborn: 0   Ⓟ Pediatric: 0-17   Ⓜ Maternity: 12-55   Ⓐ Adult: 15-124   **NRS** Nonroutine supply Dx   **NC Dx** Noncancer Dx   **PDx** Primary Dx   ▶◀ Revised Text   ● New Code   ▲ Revised Title

792   ICD-10-CM 2018

✓5ᵗʰ **M89.7 Major osseous defect**

Code first underlying disease, if known, such as:
- aseptic necrosis of bone (M87.-)
- malignant neoplasm of bone (C40.-)
- osteolysis (M89.5)
- osteomyelitis (M86.-)
- osteonecrosis (M87.-)
- osteoporosis (M80.-, M81.-)
- periprosthetic osteolysis (T84.05-)

M89.70   Major osseous defect, unspecified site   ▽

✓6ᵗʰ **M89.71**   Major osseous defect, shoulder region
Major osseous defect clavicle or scapula

M89.711   Major osseous defect, right shoulder region

M89.712   Major osseous defect, left shoulder region

M89.719   Major osseous defect, unspecified shoulder region   ▽

✓6ᵗʰ **M89.72**   Major osseous defect, humerus

M89.721   Major osseous defect, right humerus

M89.722   Major osseous defect, left humerus

M89.729   Major osseous defect, unspecified humerus   ▽

✓6ᵗʰ **M89.73**   Major osseous defect, forearm
Major osseous defect of radius and ulna

M89.731   Major osseous defect, right forearm

M89.732   Major osseous defect, left forearm

M89.739   Major osseous defect, unspecified forearm   ▽

✓6ᵗʰ **M89.74**   Major osseous defect, hand
Major osseous defect of carpus, fingers, metacarpus

M89.741   Major osseous defect, right hand

M89.742   Major osseous defect, left hand

M89.749   Major osseous defect, unspecified hand ▽

✓6ᵗʰ **M89.75**   Major osseous defect, pelvic region and thigh
Major osseous defect of femur and pelvis

M89.751   Major osseous defect, right pelvic region and thigh

M89.752   Major osseous defect, left pelvic region and thigh

M89.759   Major osseous defect, unspecified pelvic region and thigh   ▽

✓6ᵗʰ **M89.76**   Major osseous defect, lower leg
Major osseous defect of fibula and tibia

M89.761   Major osseous defect, right lower leg

M89.762   Major osseous defect, left lower leg

M89.769   Major osseous defect, unspecified lower leg   ▽

✓6ᵗʰ **M89.77**   Major osseous defect, ankle and foot
Major osseous defect of metatarsus, tarsus, toes

M89.771   Major osseous defect, right ankle and foot

M89.772   Major osseous defect, left ankle and foot

M89.779   Major osseous defect, unspecified ankle and foot   ▽

M89.78   Major osseous defect, other site

M89.79   Major osseous defect, multiple sites

✓5ᵗʰ **M89.8 Other specified disorders of bone**
Infantile cortical hyperostoses
Post-traumatic subperiosteal ossification

✓6ᵗʰ **M89.8X**   Other specified disorders of bone

M89.8X0   Other specified disorders of bone, multiple sites

M89.8X1   Other specified disorders of bone, shoulder

M89.8X2   Other specified disorders of bone, upper arm

M89.8X3   Other specified disorders of bone, forearm

M89.8X4   Other specified disorders of bone, hand

M89.8X5   Other specified disorders of bone, thigh

M89.8X6   Other specified disorders of bone, lower leg

M89.8X7   Other specified disorders of bone, ankle and foot

M89.8X8   Other specified disorders of bone, other site

M89.8X9   Other specified disorders of bone, unspecified site   ▽

M89.9 Disorder of bone, unspecified   ▽

✓4ᵗʰ **M90 Osteopathies in diseases classified elsewhere**

EXCLUDES1   osteochondritis, osteomyelitis, and osteopathy (in):
- cryptococcosis (B45.3)
- diabetes mellitus (E08-E13 with .69-)x
- gonococcal (A54.43)
- neurogenic syphilis (A52.11)
- renal osteodystrophy (N25.0)
- salmonellosis (A02.24)
- secondary syphilis (A51.46)
- syphilis (late) (A52.77)

✓5ᵗʰ **M90.5 Osteonecrosis in diseases classified elsewhere**

Code first underlying disease, such as:
- caisson disease (T70.3)
- hemoglobinopathy (D50-D64)

M90.50   *Osteonecrosis in diseases classified elsewhere, unspecified site*   ▽

✓6ᵗʰ **M90.51**   Osteonecrosis in diseases classified elsewhere, shoulder

M90.511   *Osteonecrosis in diseases classified elsewhere, right shoulder*

M90.512   *Osteonecrosis in diseases classified elsewhere, left shoulder*

M90.519   *Osteonecrosis in diseases classified elsewhere, unspecified shoulder*   ▽

✓6ᵗʰ **M90.52**   Osteonecrosis in diseases classified elsewhere, upper arm

M90.521   *Osteonecrosis in diseases classified elsewhere, right upper arm*

M90.522   *Osteonecrosis in diseases classified elsewhere, left upper arm*

M90.529   *Osteonecrosis in diseases classified elsewhere, unspecified upper arm*   ▽

✓6ᵗʰ **M90.53**   Osteonecrosis in diseases classified elsewhere, forearm

M90.531   *Osteonecrosis in diseases classified elsewhere, right forearm*

M90.532   *Osteonecrosis in diseases classified elsewhere, left forearm*

M90.539   *Osteonecrosis in diseases classified elsewhere, unspecified forearm*   ▽

✓6ᵗʰ **M90.54**   Osteonecrosis in diseases classified elsewhere, hand

M90.541   *Osteonecrosis in diseases classified elsewhere, right hand*

M90.542   *Osteonecrosis in diseases classified elsewhere, left hand*

M90.549   *Osteonecrosis in diseases classified elsewhere, unspecified hand*   ▽

✓6ᵗʰ **M90.55**   Osteonecrosis in diseases classified elsewhere, thigh

M90.551   *Osteonecrosis in diseases classified elsewhere, right thigh*

M90.552   *Osteonecrosis in diseases classified elsewhere, left thigh*

M90.559   *Osteonecrosis in diseases classified elsewhere, unspecified thigh*   ▽

✓6ᵗʰ **M90.56**   Osteonecrosis in diseases classified elsewhere, lower leg

M90.561   *Osteonecrosis in diseases classified elsewhere, right lower leg*

M90.562   *Osteonecrosis in diseases classified elsewhere, left lower leg*

M90.569   *Osteonecrosis in diseases classified elsewhere, unspecified lower leg*   ▽

✓6ᵗʰ **M90.57**   Osteonecrosis in diseases classified elsewhere, ankle and foot

M90.571   *Osteonecrosis in diseases classified elsewhere, right ankle and foot*

M90.572   *Osteonecrosis in diseases classified elsewhere, left ankle and foot*

M90.579   *Osteonecrosis in diseases classified elsewhere, unspecified ankle and foot*   ▽

M90.58   *Osteonecrosis in diseases classified elsewhere, other site*

M90.59   *Osteonecrosis in diseases classified elsewhere, multiple sites*

✔ Additional Character Req   ✓x7ᵗʰ Placeholder Alert   Case-Mix Diagnosis   Manifestation   ▽ Unspecified Dx   EXCLUDES1 Not coded here   EXCLUDES2 Not included here

✓5ᵗʰ **M90.6 Osteitis deformans in neoplastic diseases**
Osteitis deformans in malignant neoplasm of bone
Code first the neoplasm (C40-, C41-)
EXCLUDES 1 osteitis deformans [Paget's disease of bone] (M88.-)

M90.60 *Osteitis deformans in neoplastic diseases,* ▽
unspecified site

✓6ᵗʰ **M90.61 Osteitis deformans in neoplastic diseases,** shoulder
M90.611 *Osteitis deformans in neoplastic diseases,*
right shoulder
M90.612 *Osteitis deformans in neoplastic diseases,*
left shoulder
M90.619 *Osteitis deformans in neoplastic* ▽
diseases, unspecified shoulder

✓6ᵗʰ **M90.62 Osteitis deformans in neoplastic diseases,** upper arm
M90.621 *Osteitis deformans in neoplastic diseases,*
right upper arm
M90.622 *Osteitis deformans in neoplastic diseases,*
left upper arm
M90.629 *Osteitis deformans in neoplastic* ▽
diseases, unspecified upper arm

✓6ᵗʰ **M90.63 Osteitis deformans in neoplastic diseases,** forearm
M90.631 *Osteitis deformans in neoplastic diseases,*
right forearm
M90.632 *Osteitis deformans in neoplastic diseases,*
left forearm
M90.639 *Osteitis deformans in neoplastic* ▽
diseases, unspecified forearm

✓6ᵗʰ **M90.64 Osteitis deformans in neoplastic diseases,** hand
M90.641 *Osteitis deformans in neoplastic diseases,*
right hand
M90.642 *Osteitis deformans in neoplastic diseases,*
left hand
M90.649 *Osteitis deformans in neoplastic* ▽
diseases, unspecified hand

✓6ᵗʰ **M90.65 Osteitis deformans in neoplastic diseases,** thigh
M90.651 *Osteitis deformans in neoplastic diseases,*
right thigh
M90.652 *Osteitis deformans in neoplastic diseases,*
left thigh
M90.659 *Osteitis deformans in neoplastic* ▽
diseases, unspecified thigh

✓6ᵗʰ **M90.66 Osteitis deformans in neoplastic diseases,** lower leg
M90.661 *Osteitis deformans in neoplastic diseases,*
right lower leg
M90.662 *Osteitis deformans in neoplastic diseases,*
left lower leg
M90.669 *Osteitis deformans in neoplastic* ▽
diseases, unspecified lower leg

✓6ᵗʰ **M90.67 Osteitis deformans in neoplastic diseases,** ankle and
foot
M90.671 *Osteitis deformans in neoplastic diseases,*
right ankle and foot
M90.672 *Osteitis deformans in neoplastic diseases,*
left ankle and foot
M90.679 *Osteitis deformans in neoplastic* ▽
diseases, unspecified ankle and foot

M90.68 *Osteitis deformans in neoplastic diseases, other site*
M90.69 *Osteitis deformans in neoplastic diseases, multiple*
sites

✓5ᵗʰ **M90.8 Osteopathy in diseases classified elsewhere**
Code first underlying disease, such as:
rickets (E55.0)
vitamin-D-resistant rickets (E83.3)

M90.80 *Osteopathy in diseases classified elsewhere,* ▽
unspecified site

✓6ᵗʰ **M90.81 Osteopathy in diseases classified elsewhere,**
shoulder
M90.811 *Osteopathy in diseases classified elsewhere,*
right shoulder
M90.812 *Osteopathy in diseases classified elsewhere,*
left shoulder
M90.819 *Osteopathy in diseases classified* ▽
elsewhere, unspecified shoulder

✓6ᵗʰ **M90.82 Osteopathy in diseases classified elsewhere,** upper
arm
M90.821 *Osteopathy in diseases classified elsewhere,*
right upper arm

M90.822 *Osteopathy in diseases classified elsewhere,*
left upper arm
M90.829 *Osteopathy in diseases classified* ▽
elsewhere, unspecified upper arm

✓6ᵗʰ **M90.83 Osteopathy in diseases classified elsewhere,** forearm
M90.831 *Osteopathy in diseases classified elsewhere,*
right forearm
M90.832 *Osteopathy in diseases classified elsewhere,*
left forearm
M90.839 *Osteopathy in diseases classified* ▽
elsewhere, unspecified forearm

✓6ᵗʰ **M90.84 Osteopathy in diseases classified elsewhere,** hand
M90.841 *Osteopathy in diseases classified elsewhere,*
right hand
M90.842 *Osteopathy in diseases classified elsewhere,*
left hand
M90.849 *Osteopathy in diseases classified* ▽
elsewhere, unspecified hand

✓6ᵗʰ **M90.85 Osteopathy in diseases classified elsewhere,** thigh
M90.851 *Osteopathy in diseases classified elsewhere,*
right thigh
M90.852 *Osteopathy in diseases classified elsewhere,*
left thigh
M90.859 *Osteopathy in diseases classified* ▽
elsewhere, unspecified thigh

✓6ᵗʰ **M90.86 Osteopathy in diseases classified elsewhere,** lower
leg
M90.861 *Osteopathy in diseases classified elsewhere,*
right lower leg
M90.862 *Osteopathy in diseases classified elsewhere,*
left lower leg
M90.869 *Osteopathy in diseases classified* ▽
elsewhere, unspecified lower leg

✓6ᵗʰ **M90.87 Osteopathy in diseases classified elsewhere,** ankle
and foot
M90.871 *Osteopathy in diseases classified elsewhere,*
right ankle and foot
M90.872 *Osteopathy in diseases classified elsewhere,*
left ankle and foot
M90.879 *Osteopathy in diseases classified* ▽
elsewhere, unspecified ankle and foot

M90.88 *Osteopathy in diseases classified elsewhere, other site*
M90.89 *Osteopathy in diseases classified elsewhere, multiple*
sites

Chondropathies (M91-M94)
EXCLUDES 1 postprocedural chondropathies (M96.-)

✓4ᵗʰ **M91 Juvenile osteochondrosis of hip and pelvis**
EXCLUDES 1 slipped upper femoral epiphysis (nontraumatic) (M93.0)

M91.0 Juvenile osteochondrosis of pelvis
Osteochondrosis (juvenile) of acetabulum
Osteochondrosis (juvenile) of iliac crest [Buchanan]
Osteochondrosis (juvenile) of ischiopubic synchondrosis [van
Neck]
Osteochondrosis (juvenile) of symphysis pubis [Pierson]

✓5ᵗʰ **M91.1 Juvenile osteochondrosis of head of femur**
[Legg-Calvé-Perthes]
M91.10 Juvenile osteochondrosis of head of femur ▽
[Legg-Calvé-Perthes], unspecified leg
M91.11 Juvenile osteochondrosis of head of femur
[Legg-Calvé-Perthes], right leg
M91.12 Juvenile osteochondrosis of head of femur
[Legg-Calvé-Perthes], left leg

✓5ᵗʰ **M91.2 Coxa plana**
Hip deformity due to previous juvenile osteochondrosis
M91.20 Coxa plana, unspecified hip ▽
M91.21 Coxa plana, right hip
M91.22 Coxa plana, left hip

✓5ᵗʰ **M91.3 Pseudocoxalgia**
M91.30 Pseudocoxalgia, unspecified hip ▽
M91.31 Pseudocoxalgia, right hip
M91.32 Pseudocoxalgia, left hip

✓5ᵗʰ **M91.4 Coxa magna**
M91.40 Coxa magna, unspecified hip ▽
M91.41 Coxa magna, right hip
M91.42 Coxa magna, left hip

✓5ᵗʰ **M91.8 Other juvenile osteochondrosis of hip and pelvis**
Juvenile osteochondrosis after reduction of congenital dislocation of hip

M91.80 Other juvenile osteochondrosis of hip and pelvis, unspecified leg ▽

M91.81 Other juvenile osteochondrosis of hip and pelvis, right leg

M91.82 Other juvenile osteochondrosis of hip and pelvis, left leg

✓5ᵗʰ **M91.9 Juvenile osteochondrosis of hip and pelvis, unspecified**

M91.90 Juvenile osteochondrosis of hip and pelvis, unspecified, unspecified leg ▽

M91.91 Juvenile osteochondrosis of hip and pelvis, unspecified, right leg ▽

M91.92 Juvenile osteochondrosis of hip and pelvis, unspecified, left leg ▽

✓4ᵗʰ **M92 Other juvenile osteochondrosis**

✓5ᵗʰ **M92.0 Juvenile osteochondrosis of humerus**
Osteochondrosis (juvenile) of capitulum of humerus [Panner]
Osteochondrosis (juvenile) of head of humerus [Haas]

M92.00 Juvenile osteochondrosis of humerus, unspecified arm ▽

M92.01 Juvenile osteochondrosis of humerus, right arm

M92.02 Juvenile osteochondrosis of humerus, left arm

✓5ᵗʰ **M92.1 Juvenile osteochondrosis of radius and ulna**
Osteochondrosis (juvenile) of lower ulna [Burns]
Osteochondrosis (juvenile) of radial head [Brailsford]

M92.10 Juvenile osteochondrosis of radius and ulna, unspecified arm ▽

M92.11 Juvenile osteochondrosis of radius and ulna, right arm

M92.12 Juvenile osteochondrosis of radius and ulna, left arm

✓5ᵗʰ **M92.2 Juvenile osteochondrosis, hand**

✓6ᵗʰ **M92.20 Unspecified juvenile osteochondrosis, hand**

M92.201 Unspecified juvenile osteochondrosis, right hand ▽

M92.202 Unspecified juvenile osteochondrosis, left hand ▽

M92.209 Unspecified juvenile osteochondrosis, unspecified hand ▽

✓6ᵗʰ **M92.21 Osteochondrosis (juvenile) of carpal lunate [Kienböck]**

M92.211 Osteochondrosis (juvenile) of carpal lunate [Kienböck], right hand

M92.212 Osteochondrosis (juvenile) of carpal lunate [Kienböck], left hand

M92.219 Osteochondrosis (juvenile) of carpal lunate [Kienböck], unspecified hand ▽

✓6ᵗʰ **M92.22 Osteochondrosis (juvenile) of metacarpal heads [Mauclaire]**

M92.221 Osteochondrosis (juvenile) of metacarpal heads [Mauclaire], right hand

M92.222 Osteochondrosis (juvenile) of metacarpal heads [Mauclaire], left hand

M92.229 Osteochondrosis (juvenile) of metacarpal heads [Mauclaire], unspecified hand ▽

✓6ᵗʰ **M92.29 Other juvenile osteochondrosis, hand**

M92.291 Other juvenile osteochondrosis, right hand

M92.292 Other juvenile osteochondrosis, left hand

M92.299 Other juvenile osteochondrosis, unspecified hand ▽

✓5ᵗʰ **M92.3 Other juvenile osteochondrosis, upper limb**

M92.30 Other juvenile osteochondrosis, unspecified upper limb ▽

M92.31 Other juvenile osteochondrosis, right upper limb

M92.32 Other juvenile osteochondrosis, left upper limb

✓5ᵗʰ **M92.4 Juvenile osteochondrosis of patella**
Osteochondrosis (juvenile) of primary patellar center [Köhler]
Osteochondrosis (juvenile) of secondary patellar centre [Sinding Larsen]

M92.40 Juvenile osteochondrosis of patella, unspecified knee ▽

M92.41 Juvenile osteochondrosis of patella, right knee

M92.42 Juvenile osteochondrosis of patella, left knee

✓5ᵗʰ **M92.5 Juvenile osteochondrosis of tibia and fibula**
Osteochondrosis (juvenile) of proximal tibia [Blount]
Osteochondrosis (juvenile) of tibial tubercle [Osgood-Schlatter]
Tibia vara

M92.50 Juvenile osteochondrosis of tibia and fibula, unspecified leg ▽

M92.51 Juvenile osteochondrosis of tibia and fibula, right leg

M92.52 Juvenile osteochondrosis of tibia and fibula, left leg

✓5ᵗʰ **M92.6 Juvenile osteochondrosis of tarsus**
Osteochondrosis (juvenile) of calcaneum [Sever]
Osteochondrosis (juvenile) of os tibiale externum [Haglund]
Osteochondrosis (juvenile) of talus [Diaz]
Osteochondrosis (juvenile) of tarsal navicular [Köhler]

M92.60 Juvenile osteochondrosis of tarsus, unspecified ankle ▽

M92.61 Juvenile osteochondrosis of tarsus, right ankle

M92.62 Juvenile osteochondrosis of tarsus, left ankle

✓5ᵗʰ **M92.7 Juvenile osteochondrosis of metatarsus**
Osteochondrosis (juvenile) of fifth metatarsus [Iselin]
Osteochondrosis (juvenile) of second metatarsus [Freiberg]

M92.70 Juvenile osteochondrosis of metatarsus, unspecified foot ▽

M92.71 Juvenile osteochondrosis of metatarsus, right foot

M92.72 Juvenile osteochondrosis of metatarsus, left foot

M92.8 Other specified juvenile osteochondrosis
Calcaneal apophysitis

M92.9 Juvenile osteochondrosis, unspecified ▽
Juvenile apophysitis NOS
Juvenile epiphysitis NOS
Juvenile osteochondritis NOS
Juvenile osteochondrosis NOS

✓4ᵗʰ **M93 Other osteochondropathies**
EXCLUDES 2   osteochondrosis of spine (M42.-)

✓5ᵗʰ **M93.0 Slipped upper femoral epiphysis (nontraumatic)**
Use additional code for associated chondrolysis (M94.3)

✓6ᵗʰ **M93.00 Unspecified slipped upper femoral epiphysis (nontraumatic)**

M93.001 Unspecified slipped upper femoral epiphysis (nontraumatic), right hip ▽

M93.002 Unspecified slipped upper femoral epiphysis (nontraumatic), left hip ▽

M93.003 Unspecified slipped upper femoral epiphysis (nontraumatic), unspecified hip ▽

✓6ᵗʰ **M93.01 Acute slipped upper femoral epiphysis (nontraumatic)**

M93.011 Acute slipped upper femoral epiphysis (nontraumatic), right hip

M93.012 Acute slipped upper femoral epiphysis (nontraumatic), left hip

M93.013 Acute slipped upper femoral epiphysis (nontraumatic), unspecified hip ▽

✓6ᵗʰ **M93.02 Chronic slipped upper femoral epiphysis (nontraumatic)**

M93.021 Chronic slipped upper femoral epiphysis (nontraumatic), right hip

M93.022 Chronic slipped upper femoral epiphysis (nontraumatic), left hip

M93.023 Chronic slipped upper femoral epiphysis (nontraumatic), unspecified hip ▽

✓6ᵗʰ **M93.03 Acute on chronic slipped upper femoral epiphysis (nontraumatic)**

M93.031 Acute on chronic slipped upper femoral epiphysis (nontraumatic), right hip

M93.032 Acute on chronic slipped upper femoral epiphysis (nontraumatic), left hip

M93.033 Acute on chronic slipped upper femoral epiphysis (nontraumatic), unspecified hip ▽

M93.1 Kienböck's disease of adults Ⓐ
Adult osteochondrosis of carpal lunates

✓5ᵗʰ **M93.2 Osteochondritis dissecans**

M93.20 Osteochondritis dissecans of unspecified site ▽

✓ Additional Character Req   ✓x7ᵗʰ Placeholder Alert   Case-Mix Diagnosis   Manifestation   ▽ Unspecified Dx   *EXCLUDES 1* Not coded here   *EXCLUDES 2* Not included here

√6ᵗʰ **M93.21** Osteochondritis dissecans of shoulder
- **M93.211** Osteochondritis dissecans, right shoulder
- **M93.212** Osteochondritis dissecans, left shoulder
- **M93.219** Osteochondritis dissecans, unspecified shoulder ▽

√6ᵗʰ **M93.22** Osteochondritis dissecans of elbow
- **M93.221** Osteochondritis dissecans, right elbow
- **M93.222** Osteochondritis dissecans, left elbow
- **M93.229** Osteochondritis dissecans, unspecified elbow ▽

√6ᵗʰ **M93.23** Osteochondritis dissecans of wrist
- **M93.231** Osteochondritis dissecans, right wrist
- **M93.232** Osteochondritis dissecans, left wrist
- **M93.239** Osteochondritis dissecans, unspecified wrist ▽

√6ᵗʰ **M93.24** Osteochondritis dissecans of joints of hand
- **M93.241** Osteochondritis dissecans, joints of right hand
- **M93.242** Osteochondritis dissecans, joints of left hand
- **M93.249** Osteochondritis dissecans, joints of unspecified hand ▽

√6ᵗʰ **M93.25** Osteochondritis dissecans of hip
- **M93.251** Osteochondritis dissecans, right hip
- **M93.252** Osteochondritis dissecans, left hip
- **M93.259** Osteochondritis dissecans, unspecified hip ▽

√6ᵗʰ **M93.26** Osteochondritis dissecans knee
- **M93.261** Osteochondritis dissecans, right knee
- **M93.262** Osteochondritis dissecans, left knee
- **M93.269** Osteochondritis dissecans, unspecified knee ▽

√6ᵗʰ **M93.27** Osteochondritis dissecans of ankle and joints of foot
- **M93.271** Osteochondritis dissecans, right ankle and joints of right foot
- **M93.272** Osteochondritis dissecans, left ankle and joints of left foot
- **M93.279** Osteochondritis dissecans, unspecified ankle and joints of foot ▽

- **M93.28** Osteochondritis dissecans other site
- **M93.29** Osteochondritis dissecans multiple sites

√5ᵗʰ **M93.8** Other specified osteochondropathies
- **M93.80** Other specified osteochondropathies of unspecified site ▽

√6ᵗʰ **M93.81** Other specified osteochondropathies of shoulder
- **M93.811** Other specified osteochondropathies, right shoulder
- **M93.812** Other specified osteochondropathies, left shoulder
- **M93.819** Other specified osteochondropathies, unspecified shoulder ▽

√6ᵗʰ **M93.82** Other specified osteochondropathies of upper arm
- **M93.821** Other specified osteochondropathies, right upper arm
- **M93.822** Other specified osteochondropathies, left upper arm
- **M93.829** Other specified osteochondropathies, unspecified upper arm ▽

√6ᵗʰ **M93.83** Other specified osteochondropathies of forearm
- **M93.831** Other specified osteochondropathies, right forearm
- **M93.832** Other specified osteochondropathies, left forearm
- **M93.839** Other specified osteochondropathies, unspecified forearm ▽

√6ᵗʰ **M93.84** Other specified osteochondropathies of hand
- **M93.841** Other specified osteochondropathies, right hand
- **M93.842** Other specified osteochondropathies, left hand
- **M93.849** Other specified osteochondropathies, unspecified hand ▽

√6ᵗʰ **M93.85** Other specified osteochondropathies of thigh
- **M93.851** Other specified osteochondropathies, right thigh
- **M93.852** Other specified osteochondropathies, left thigh
- **M93.859** Other specified osteochondropathies, unspecified thigh ▽

√6ᵗʰ **M93.86** Other specified osteochondropathies lower leg
- **M93.861** Other specified osteochondropathies, right lower leg
- **M93.862** Other specified osteochondropathies, left lower leg
- **M93.869** Other specified osteochondropathies, unspecified lower leg ▽

√6ᵗʰ **M93.87** Other specified osteochondropathies of ankle and foot
- **M93.871** Other specified osteochondropathies, right ankle and foot
- **M93.872** Other specified osteochondropathies, left ankle and foot
- **M93.879** Other specified osteochondropathies, unspecified ankle and foot ▽

- **M93.88** Other specified osteochondropathies other site
- **M93.89** Other specified osteochondropathies multiple sites

√5ᵗʰ **M93.9** Osteochondropathy, unspecified
Apophysitis NOS
Epiphysitis NOS
Osteochondritis NOS
Osteochondrosis NOS
- **M93.90** Osteochondropathy, unspecified of unspecified site ▽

√6ᵗʰ **M93.91** Osteochondropathy, unspecified of shoulder
- **M93.911** Osteochondropathy, unspecified, right shoulder ▽
- **M93.912** Osteochondropathy, unspecified, left shoulder ▽
- **M93.919** Osteochondropathy, unspecified, unspecified shoulder ▽

√6ᵗʰ **M93.92** Osteochondropathy, unspecified of upper arm
- **M93.921** Osteochondropathy, unspecified, right upper arm ▽
- **M93.922** Osteochondropathy, unspecified, left upper arm ▽
- **M93.929** Osteochondropathy, unspecified, unspecified upper arm ▽

√6ᵗʰ **M93.93** Osteochondropathy, unspecified of forearm
- **M93.931** Osteochondropathy, unspecified, right forearm ▽
- **M93.932** Osteochondropathy, unspecified, left forearm ▽
- **M93.939** Osteochondropathy, unspecified, unspecified forearm ▽

√6ᵗʰ **M93.94** Osteochondropathy, unspecified of hand
- **M93.941** Osteochondropathy, unspecified, right hand ▽
- **M93.942** Osteochondropathy, unspecified, left hand ▽
- **M93.949** Osteochondropathy, unspecified, unspecified hand ▽

√6ᵗʰ **M93.95** Osteochondropathy, unspecified of thigh
- **M93.951** Osteochondropathy, unspecified, right thigh ▽
- **M93.952** Osteochondropathy, unspecified, left thigh ▽
- **M93.959** Osteochondropathy, unspecified, unspecified thigh ▽

√6ᵗʰ **M93.96** Osteochondropathy, unspecified lower leg
- **M93.961** Osteochondropathy, unspecified, right lower leg ▽
- **M93.962** Osteochondropathy, unspecified, left lower leg ▽
- **M93.969** Osteochondropathy, unspecified, unspecified lower leg ▽

√6ᵗʰ **M93.97** Osteochondropathy, unspecified of ankle and foot
- **M93.971** Osteochondropathy, unspecified, right ankle and foot ▽
- **M93.972** Osteochondropathy, unspecified, left ankle and foot ▽
- **M93.979** Osteochondropathy, unspecified, unspecified ankle and foot ▽

N Newborn: 0   P Pediatric: 0-17   M Maternity: 12-55   A Adult: 15-124   NRS Nonroutine supply Dx   NC Dx Noncancer Dx   PDx Primary Dx   ▶◀ Revised Text   ● New Code   ▲ Revised Title

796   ICD-10-CM 2018

M93.98   **Osteochondropathy, unspecified other site**   ▽
M93.99   **Osteochondropathy, unspecified** multiple sites   ▽

✓4th **M94   Other disorders of cartilage**

M94.0   **Chondrocostal junction syndrome [Tietze]**
Costochondritis

M94.1   **Relapsing polychondritis**

✓5th   **M94.2   Chondromalacia**
EXCLUDES 1   chondromalacia patellae (M22.4)

M94.20   **Chondromalacia, unspecified site**   ▽

✓6th   **M94.21   Chondromalacia, shoulder**
M94.211   **Chondromalacia, right shoulder**
M94.212   **Chondromalacia, left shoulder**
M94.219   **Chondromalacia, unspecified shoulder**   ▽

✓6th   **M94.22   Chondromalacia, elbow**
M94.221   **Chondromalacia, right elbow**
M94.222   **Chondromalacia, left elbow**
M94.229   **Chondromalacia, unspecified elbow**   ▽

✓6th   **M94.23   Chondromalacia, wrist**
M94.231   **Chondromalacia, right wrist**
M94.232   **Chondromalacia, left wrist**
M94.239   **Chondromalacia, unspecified wrist**   ▽

✓6th   **M94.24   Chondromalacia, joints of hand**
M94.241   **Chondromalacia, joints of right hand**
M94.242   **Chondromalacia, joints of left hand**
M94.249   **Chondromalacia, joints of unspecified hand**   ▽

✓6th   **M94.25   Chondromalacia, hip**
M94.251   **Chondromalacia, right hip**
M94.252   **Chondromalacia, left hip**
M94.259   **Chondromalacia, unspecified hip**   ▽

✓6th   **M94.26   Chondromalacia, knee**
M94.261   **Chondromalacia, right knee**
M94.262   **Chondromalacia, left knee**
M94.269   **Chondromalacia, unspecified knee**   ▽

✓6th   **M94.27   Chondromalacia, ankle and joints of foot**
M94.271   **Chondromalacia, right ankle and joints of right foot**
M94.272   **Chondromalacia, left ankle and joints of left foot**
M94.279   **Chondromalacia, unspecified ankle and joints of foot**   ▽

M94.28   **Chondromalacia, other site**

M94.29   **Chondromalacia, multiple sites**

✓5th   **M94.3   Chondrolysis**
Code first any associated slipped upper femoral epiphysis (nontraumatic) (M93.0-)

✓6th   **M94.35   Chondrolysis, hip**
M94.351   **Chondrolysis, right hip**
M94.352   **Chondrolysis, left hip**
M94.359   **Chondrolysis, unspecified hip**   ▽

✓5th   **M94.8   Other specified disorders of cartilage**

✓6th   **M94.8X   Other specified disorders of cartilage**
M94.8X0   **Other specified disorders of cartilage, multiple sites**
M94.8X1   **Other specified disorders of cartilage, shoulder**
M94.8X2   **Other specified disorders of cartilage, upper arm**
M94.8X3   **Other specified disorders of cartilage, forearm**
M94.8X4   **Other specified disorders of cartilage, hand**
M94.8X5   **Other specified disorders of cartilage, thigh**
M94.8X6   **Other specified disorders of cartilage, lower leg**
M94.8X7   **Other specified disorders of cartilage, ankle and foot**
M94.8X8   **Other specified disorders of cartilage, other site**
M94.8X9   **Other specified disorders of cartilage, unspecified sites**   ▽

M94.9   **Disorder of cartilage, unspecified**   ▽

Other disorders of the musculoskeletal system and connective tissue (M95)

✓4th **M95   Other acquired deformities of musculoskeletal system and connective tissue**
EXCLUDES 2   acquired absence of limbs and organs (Z89-Z90)
acquired deformities of limbs (M20-M21)
congenital malformations and deformations of the musculoskeletal system (Q65-Q79)
deforming dorsopathies (M40-M43)
dentofacial anomalies [including malocclusion] (M26.-)
postprocedural musculoskeletal disorders (M96.-)

M95.0   **Acquired deformity of nose**
EXCLUDES 2   deviated nasal septum (J34.2)

✓5th   **M95.1   Cauliflower ear**
EXCLUDES 2   other acquired deformities of ear (H61.1)
DEF: Acquired deformity of the external ear; due to injury, subsequent perichondritis.

M95.10   **Cauliflower ear, unspecified ear**   ▽
M95.11   **Cauliflower ear, right ear**
M95.12   **Cauliflower ear, left ear**

M95.2   **Other acquired deformity of head**

M95.3   **Acquired deformity of neck**

M95.4   **Acquired deformity of chest and rib**
AHA: 2014, 4Q, 26-27

M95.5   **Acquired deformity of pelvis**
EXCLUDES 1   maternal care for known or suspected disproportion (O33.-)

M95.8   **Other specified acquired deformities of musculoskeletal system**

M95.9   **Acquired deformity of musculoskeletal system, unspecified**   ▽

Intraoperative and postprocedural complications and disorders of musculoskeletal system, not elsewhere classified (M96)

✓4th **M96   Intraoperative and postprocedural complications and disorders of musculoskeletal system, not elsewhere classified**
EXCLUDES 2   arthropathy following intestinal bypass (M02.0-)
complications of internal orthopedic prosthetic devices, implants and grafts (T84.-)
disorders associated with osteoporosis (M80)
periprosthetic fracture around internal prosthetic joint (M97.-)
presence of functional implants and other devices (Z96-Z97)

M96.0   **Pseudarthrosis after fusion or arthrodesis**

M96.1   **Postlaminectomy syndrome, not elsewhere classified**

M96.2   **Postradiation kyphosis**

M96.3   **Postlaminectomy kyphosis**

M96.4   **Postsurgical lordosis**

M96.5   **Postradiation scoliosis**

✓5th   **M96.6   Fracture of bone following insertion of orthopedic implant, joint prosthesis, or bone plate**
Intraoperative fracture of bone during insertion of orthopedic implant, joint prosthesis, or bone plate
EXCLUDES 2   complication of internal orthopedic devices, implants or grafts (T84.-)

✓6th   **M96.62   Fracture of humerus following insertion of orthopedic implant, joint prosthesis, or bone plate**
M96.621   **Fracture of humerus following insertion of orthopedic implant, joint prosthesis, or bone plate, right arm**
M96.622   **Fracture of humerus following insertion of orthopedic implant, joint prosthesis, or bone plate, left arm**
M96.629   **Fracture of humerus following insertion of orthopedic implant, joint prosthesis, or bone plate, unspecified arm**   ▽

✓6th   **M96.63   Fracture of radius or ulna following insertion of orthopedic implant, joint prosthesis, or bone plate**
M96.631   **Fracture of radius or ulna following insertion of orthopedic implant, joint prosthesis, or bone plate, right arm**
M96.632   **Fracture of radius or ulna following insertion of orthopedic implant, joint prosthesis, or bone plate, left arm**
M96.639   **Fracture of radius or ulna following insertion of orthopedic implant, joint prosthesis, or bone plate, unspecified arm**   ▽

☑ Additional Character Req   ✓x7th Placeholder Alert   Case-Mix Diagnosis   Manifestation   ▽ Unspecified Dx   *EXCLUDES 1* Not coded here   *EXCLUDES 2* Not included here

M96.65 Fracture of pelvis following insertion of orthopedic implant, joint prosthesis, or bone plate

✓6ᵗʰ **M96.66** Fracture of femur following insertion of orthopedic implant, joint prosthesis, or bone plate

     M96.661 Fracture of femur following insertion of orthopedic implant, joint prosthesis, or bone plate, right leg

     M96.662 Fracture of femur following insertion of orthopedic implant, joint prosthesis, or bone plate, left leg

     M96.669 Fracture of femur following insertion of orthopedic implant, joint prosthesis, or bone plate, unspecified leg ▽

✓6ᵗʰ **M96.67** Fracture of tibia or fibula following insertion of orthopedic implant, joint prosthesis, or bone plate

     M96.671 Fracture of tibia or fibula following insertion of orthopedic implant, joint prosthesis, or bone plate, right leg

     M96.672 Fracture of tibia or fibula following insertion of orthopedic implant, joint prosthesis, or bone plate, left leg

     M96.679 Fracture of tibia or fibula following insertion of orthopedic implant, joint prosthesis, or bone plate, unspecified leg ▽

M96.69 Fracture of other bone following insertion of orthopedic implant, joint prosthesis, or bone plate

✓5ᵗʰ **M96.8** Other intraoperative and postprocedural complications and disorders of musculoskeletal system, not elsewhere classified

✓6ᵗʰ **M96.81** Intraoperative hemorrhage and hematoma of a musculoskeletal structure complicating a procedure

     EXCLUDES 1   intraoperative hemorrhage and hematoma of a musculoskeletal structure due to accidental puncture and laceration during a procedure (M96.82-)

     M96.810 Intraoperative hemorrhage and hematoma of a musculoskeletal structure complicating a musculoskeletal system procedure

     M96.811 Intraoperative hemorrhage and hematoma of a musculoskeletal structure complicating other procedure

✓6ᵗʰ **M96.82** Accidental puncture and laceration of a musculoskeletal structure during a procedure

     M96.820 Accidental puncture and laceration of a musculoskeletal structure during a musculoskeletal system procedure

     M96.821 Accidental puncture and laceration of a musculoskeletal structure during other procedure

✓6ᵗʰ **M96.83** Postprocedural hemorrhage of a musculoskeletal structure following a procedure

     M96.830 Postprocedural hemorrhage of a musculoskeletal structure following a musculoskeletal system procedure

     M96.831 Postprocedural hemorrhage of a musculoskeletal structure following other procedure

✓6ᵗʰ **M96.84** Postprocedural hematoma and seroma of a musculoskeletal structure following a procedure

     M96.840 Postprocedural hematoma of a musculoskeletal structure following a musculoskeletal system procedure

     M96.841 Postprocedural hematoma of a musculoskeletal structure following other procedure

     M96.842 Postprocedural seroma of a musculoskeletal structure following a musculoskeletal system procedure

     M96.843 Postprocedural seroma of a musculoskeletal structure following other procedure

M96.89 Other intraoperative and postprocedural complications and disorders of the musculoskeletal system

     Instability of joint secondary to removal of joint prosthesis

     Use additional code, if applicable, to further specify disorder

Periprosthetic fracture around internal prosthetic joint (M97)

✓4ᵗʰ **M97** Periprosthetic fracture around internal prosthetic joint

     EXCLUDES 2   breakage (fracture) of prosthetic joint (T84.01-)

           fracture of bone following insertion of orthopedic implant, joint prosthesis or bone plate (M96.6-)

     The appropriate 7th character is to be added to each code from category M97.
     A   initial encounter
     D   subsequent encounter
     S   sequela

✓5ᵗʰ **M97.0** Periprosthetic fracture around internal prosthetic hip joint

     ✓x7ᵗʰ **M97.01** Periprosthetic fracture around internal prosthetic right hip joint

     ✓x7ᵗʰ **M97.02** Periprosthetic fracture around internal prosthetic left hip joint

✓5ᵗʰ **M97.1** Periprosthetic fracture around internal prosthetic knee joint

     ✓x7ᵗʰ **M97.11** Periprosthetic fracture around internal prosthetic right knee joint

     ✓x7ᵗʰ **M97.12** Periprosthetic fracture around internal prosthetic left knee joint

✓5ᵗʰ **M97.2** Periprosthetic fracture around internal prosthetic ankle joint

     ✓x7ᵗʰ **M97.21** Periprosthetic fracture around internal prosthetic right ankle joint

     ✓x7ᵗʰ **M97.22** Periprosthetic fracture around internal prosthetic left ankle joint

✓5ᵗʰ **M97.3** Periprosthetic fracture around internal prosthetic shoulder joint

     ✓x7ᵗʰ **M97.31** Periprosthetic fracture around internal prosthetic right shoulder joint

     ✓x7ᵗʰ **M97.32** Periprosthetic fracture around internal prosthetic left shoulder joint

✓5ᵗʰ **M97.4** Periprosthetic fracture around internal prosthetic elbow joint

     ✓x7ᵗʰ **M97.41** Periprosthetic fracture around internal prosthetic right elbow joint

     ✓x7ᵗʰ **M97.42** Periprosthetic fracture around internal prosthetic left elbow joint

✓x7ᵗʰ **M97.8** Periprosthetic fracture around other internal prosthetic joint

     Periprosthetic fracture around internal prosthetic finger joint
     Periprosthetic fracture around internal prosthetic spinal joint
     Periprosthetic fracture around internal prosthetic toe joint
     Periprosthetic fracture around internal prosthetic wrist joint
     Use additional code to identify the joint (Z96.6-)

✓x7ᵗʰ **M97.9** Periprosthetic fracture around unspecified internal prosthetic joint ▽

Biomechanical lesions, not elsewhere classified (M99)

✓4ᵗʰ **M99** Biomechanical lesions, not elsewhere classified

     NOTE   This category should not be used if the condition can be classified elsewhere.

✓5ᵗʰ **M99.0** Segmental and somatic dysfunction

     M99.00 Segmental and somatic dysfunction of head region

     M99.01 Segmental and somatic dysfunction of cervical region

     M99.02 Segmental and somatic dysfunction of thoracic region

     M99.03 Segmental and somatic dysfunction of lumbar region

     M99.04 Segmental and somatic dysfunction of sacral region

     M99.05 Segmental and somatic dysfunction of pelvic region

     M99.06 Segmental and somatic dysfunction of lower extremity

     M99.07 Segmental and somatic dysfunction of upper extremity

     M99.08 Segmental and somatic dysfunction of rib cage

     M99.09 Segmental and somatic dysfunction of abdomen and other regions

✓5ᵗʰ **M99.1** Subluxation complex (vertebral)

     M99.10 Subluxation complex (vertebral) of head region

     M99.11 Subluxation complex (vertebral) of cervical region

     M99.12 Subluxation complex (vertebral) of thoracic region

     M99.13 Subluxation complex (vertebral) of lumbar region

     M99.14 Subluxation complex (vertebral) of sacral region

     M99.15 Subluxation complex (vertebral) of pelvic region

Ⓝ Newborn: 0   Ⓟ Pediatric: 0-17   Ⓜ Maternity: 12-55   Ⓐ Adult: 15-124   **NRS** Nonroutine supply Dx   **NCDx** Noncancer Dx   **PDx** Primary Dx   ►◄ Revised Text   ● New Code   ▲ Revised Title

798   ICD-10-CM 2018

M99.16   Subluxation complex (vertebral) of lower extremity

M99.17   Subluxation complex (vertebral) of upper extremity

M99.18   Subluxation complex (vertebral) of rib cage

M99.19   Subluxation complex (vertebral) of abdomen and other regions

✓5ᵗʰ **M99.2 Subluxation stenosis of neural canal**

M99.20   **Subluxation stenosis of neural canal of head region**

M99.21   **Subluxation stenosis of neural canal of cervical region**

M99.22   **Subluxation stenosis of neural canal of thoracic region**

M99.23   **Subluxation stenosis of neural canal of lumbar region**

M99.24   **Subluxation stenosis of neural canal of sacral region**

M99.25   **Subluxation stenosis of neural canal of pelvic region**

M99.26   **Subluxation stenosis of neural canal of lower extremity**

M99.27   **Subluxation stenosis of neural canal of upper extremity**

M99.28   **Subluxation stenosis of neural canal of rib cage**

M99.29   **Subluxation stenosis of neural canal of abdomen and other regions**

✓5ᵗʰ **M99.3 Osseous stenosis of neural canal**

M99.30   **Osseous stenosis of neural canal of head region**

M99.31   **Osseous stenosis of neural canal of cervical region**

M99.32   **Osseous stenosis of neural canal of thoracic region**

M99.33   **Osseous stenosis of neural canal of lumbar region**

M99.34   **Osseous stenosis of neural canal of sacral region**

M99.35   **Osseous stenosis of neural canal of pelvic region**

M99.36   **Osseous stenosis of neural canal of lower extremity**

M99.37   **Osseous stenosis of neural canal of upper extremity**

M99.38   **Osseous stenosis of neural canal of rib cage**

M99.39   **Osseous stenosis of neural canal of abdomen and other regions**

✓5ᵗʰ **M99.4 Connective tissue stenosis of neural canal**

M99.40   **Connective tissue stenosis of neural canal of head region**

M99.41   **Connective tissue stenosis of neural canal of cervical region**

M99.42   **Connective tissue stenosis of neural canal of thoracic region**

M99.43   **Connective tissue stenosis of neural canal of lumbar region**

M99.44   **Connective tissue stenosis of neural canal of sacral region**

M99.45   **Connective tissue stenosis of neural canal of pelvic region**

M99.46   **Connective tissue stenosis of neural canal of lower extremity**

M99.47   **Connective tissue stenosis of neural canal of upper extremity**

M99.48   **Connective tissue stenosis of neural canal of rib cage**

M99.49   **Connective tissue stenosis of neural canal of abdomen and other regions**

✓5ᵗʰ **M99.5 Intervertebral disc stenosis of neural canal**

M99.50   **Intervertebral disc stenosis of neural canal of head region**

M99.51   **Intervertebral disc stenosis of neural canal of cervical region**

M99.52   **Intervertebral disc stenosis of neural canal of thoracic region**

M99.53   **Intervertebral disc stenosis of neural canal of lumbar region**

M99.54   **Intervertebral disc stenosis of neural canal of sacral region**

M99.55   **Intervertebral disc stenosis of neural canal of pelvic region**

M99.56   **Intervertebral disc stenosis of neural canal of lower extremity**

M99.57   **Intervertebral disc stenosis of neural canal of upper extremity**

M99.58   **Intervertebral disc stenosis of neural canal of rib cage**

M99.59   **Intervertebral disc stenosis of neural canal of abdomen and other regions**

✓5ᵗʰ **M99.6 Osseous and subluxation stenosis of intervertebral foramina**

M99.60   **Osseous and subluxation stenosis of intervertebral foramina of head region**

M99.61   **Osseous and subluxation stenosis of intervertebral foramina of cervical region**

M99.62   **Osseous and subluxation stenosis of intervertebral foramina of thoracic region**

M99.63   **Osseous and subluxation stenosis of intervertebral foramina of lumbar region**

M99.64   **Osseous and subluxation stenosis of intervertebral foramina of sacral region**

M99.65   **Osseous and subluxation stenosis of intervertebral foramina of pelvic region**

M99.66   **Osseous and subluxation stenosis of intervertebral foramina of lower extremity**

M99.67   **Osseous and subluxation stenosis of intervertebral foramina of upper extremity**

M99.68   **Osseous and subluxation stenosis of intervertebral foramina of rib cage**

M99.69   **Osseous and subluxation stenosis of intervertebral foramina of abdomen and other regions**

✓5ᵗʰ **M99.7 Connective tissue and disc stenosis of intervertebral foramina**

M99.70   **Connective tissue and disc stenosis of intervertebral foramina of head region**

M99.71   **Connective tissue and disc stenosis of intervertebral foramina of cervical region**

M99.72   **Connective tissue and disc stenosis of intervertebral foramina of thoracic region**

M99.73   **Connective tissue and disc stenosis of intervertebral foramina of lumbar region**

M99.74   **Connective tissue and disc stenosis of intervertebral foramina of sacral region**

M99.75   **Connective tissue and disc stenosis of intervertebral foramina of pelvic region**

M99.76   **Connective tissue and disc stenosis of intervertebral foramina of lower extremity**

M99.77   **Connective tissue and disc stenosis of intervertebral foramina of upper extremity**

M99.78   **Connective tissue and disc stenosis of intervertebral foramina of rib cage**

M99.79   **Connective tissue and disc stenosis of intervertebral foramina of abdomen and other regions**

✓5ᵗʰ **M99.8 Other biomechanical lesions**

M99.80   **Other biomechanical lesions of head region**

M99.81   **Other biomechanical lesions of cervical region**

M99.82   **Other biomechanical lesions of thoracic region**

M99.83   **Other biomechanical lesions of lumbar region**

M99.84   **Other biomechanical lesions of sacral region**

M99.85   **Other biomechanical lesions of pelvic region**

M99.86   **Other biomechanical lesions of lower extremity**

M99.87   **Other biomechanical lesions of upper extremity**

M99.88   **Other biomechanical lesions of rib cage**

M99.89   **Other biomechanical lesions of abdomen and other regions**

M99.9   **Biomechanical lesion, unspecified**   ▽

☑ Additional Character Req   ✓7ᵗʰ Placeholder Alert   Case-Mix Diagnosis   Manifestation   ▽ Unspecified Dx   **EXCLUDES 1** Not coded here   **EXCLUDES 2** Not included here

Chapter 14. Diseases of Genitourinary System (N00–N99)

Chapter Specific Guidelines with Coding Examples

The chapter specific guidelines from the ICD-10-CM Official Guidelines for Coding and Reporting have been provided below. Along with these guidelines are coding examples, contained in the shaded boxes, that have been developed to help illustrate the coding and/or sequencing guidance found in these guidelines.

a. Chronic kidney disease

1) Stages of chronic kidney disease (CKD)

The ICD-10-CM classifies CKD based on severity. The severity of CKD is designated by stages 1-5. Stage 2, code N18.2, equates to mild CKD; stage 3, code N18.3, equates to moderate CKD; and stage 4, code N18.4, equates to severe CKD. Code N18.6, End stage renal disease (ESRD), is assigned when the provider has documented end-stage-renal disease (ESRD).

If both a stage of CKD and ESRD are documented, assign code N18.6 only.

Stage 5 chronic kidney disease with ESRD requiring chronic dialysis	
N18.6	**End stage renal disease**
Z99.2	**Dependence on renal dialysis**

Explanation: The diagnostic statement indicates the patient has chronic kidney disease, documented both as stage 5 and as ESRD requiring chronic dialysis. Code N18.6 End stage renal disease (ESRD), is assigned when the provider has documented end-stage-renal disease (ESRD). If both a stage of CKD and ESRD are documented, assign code N18.6 only.

2) Chronic kidney disease and kidney transplant status

Patients who have undergone kidney transplant may still have some form of chronic kidney disease (CKD) because the kidney transplant may not fully restore kidney function. Therefore, the presence of CKD alone does not constitute a transplant complication. Assign the appropriate N18 code for the patient's stage of CKD and code Z94.0, Kidney transplant status. If a transplant complication such as failure or rejection or other transplant complication is documented, see section I.C.19.g for information on coding complications of a kidney transplant. If the documentation is unclear as to whether the patient has a complication of the transplant, query the provider.

Patient with residual chronic kidney disease stage 1 after kidney transplant	
N18.1	**Chronic kidney disease, stage 1**
Z94.0	**Kidney transplant status**

Explanation: Patients who have undergone kidney transplant may still have some form of chronic kidney disease (CKD) because the kidney transplant may not fully restore kidney function. The presence of CKD alone does not constitute a transplant complication. Assign the appropriate N18 code for the patient's stage of CKD and code Z94.0 Kidney transplant status.

3) Chronic kidney disease with other conditions

Patients with CKD may also suffer from other serious conditions, most commonly diabetes mellitus and hypertension. The sequencing of the CKD code in relationship to codes for other contributing conditions is based on the conventions in the Tabular List.

See I.C.9. Hypertensive chronic kidney disease.

See I.C.19. Chronic kidney disease and kidney transplant complications.

Type 1 diabetic chronic kidney disease, stage 2	
E10.22	**Type 1 diabetes mellitus with diabetic chronic kidney disease**
N18.2	**Chronic kidney disease, stage 2 (mild)**

Explanation: Patients with CKD may also suffer from other serious conditions such as diabetes mellitus. The sequencing of the CKD code in relationship to codes for other contributing conditions is based on the conventions in the Tabular List. Diabetic CKD code E10.22 includes an instructional note to "Use additional code to identify stage of chronic kidney disease (N18.1–N18.6)," thus providing sequencing direction.

Chapter 14. Diseases of the Genitourinary System (N00-N99)

EXCLUDES 2   certain conditions originating in the perinatal period (P04-P96)
certain infectious and parasitic diseases (A00-B99)
complications of pregnancy, childbirth and the puerperium (O00-O9A)
congenital malformations, deformations and chromosomal abnormalities (Q00-Q99)
endocrine, nutritional and metabolic diseases (E00-E88)
injury, poisoning and certain other consequences of external causes (S00-T88)
neoplasms (C00-D49)
symptoms, signs and abnormal clinical and laboratory findings, not elsewhere classified (R00-R94)

This chapter contains the following blocks:

N00-N08   Glomerular diseases
N10-N16   Renal tubulo-interstitial diseases
N17-N19   Acute kidney failure and chronic kidney disease
N20-N23   Urolithiasis
N25-N29   Other disorders of kidney and ureter
N30-N39   Other diseases of the urinary system
N40-N53   Diseases of male genital organs
N60-N65   Disorders of breast
N70-N77   Inflammatory diseases of female pelvic organs
N80-N98   Noninflammatory disorders of female genital tract
N99   Intraoperative and postprocedural complications and disorders of genitourinary system, not elsewhere classified

Glomerular diseases (N00-N08)

Code also any associated kidney failure (N17-N19).
EXCLUDES 1   hypertensive chronic kidney disease (I12.-)

✓4th **N00   Acute nephritic syndrome**
INCLUDES   acute glomerular disease
acute glomerulonephritis
acute nephritis
EXCLUDES 1   acute tubulo-interstitial nephritis (N10)
nephritic syndrome NOS (N05.-)

N00.0   Acute nephritic syndrome with minor glomerular abnormality
Acute nephritic syndrome with minimal change lesion

N00.1   Acute nephritic syndrome with focal and segmental glomerular lesions
Acute nephritic syndrome with focal and segmental hyalinosis
Acute nephritic syndrome with focal and segmental sclerosis
Acute nephritic syndrome with focal glomerulonephritis

N00.2   Acute nephritic syndrome with diffuse membranous glomerulonephritis

N00.3   Acute nephritic syndrome with diffuse mesangial proliferative glomerulonephritis

N00.4   Acute nephritic syndrome with diffuse endocapillary proliferative glomerulonephritis

N00.5   Acute nephritic syndrome with diffuse mesangiocapillary glomerulonephritis
Acute nephritic syndrome with membranoproliferative glomerulonephritis, types 1 and 3, or NOS

N00.6   Acute nephritic syndrome with dense deposit disease
Acute nephritic syndrome with membranoproliferative glomerulonephritis, type 2

N00.7   Acute nephritic syndrome with diffuse crescentic glomerulonephritis
Acute nephritic syndrome with extracapillary glomerulonephritis

N00.8   Acute nephritic syndrome with other morphologic changes
Acute nephritic syndrome with proliferative glomerulonephritis NOS

N00.9   Acute nephritic syndrome with unspecified morphologic changes   ▽

✓4th **N01   Rapidly progressive nephritic syndrome**
INCLUDES   rapidly progressive glomerular disease
rapidly progressive glomerulonephritis
rapidly progressive nephritis
EXCLUDES 1   nephritic syndrome NOS (N05.-)

N01.0   Rapidly progressive nephritic syndrome with minor glomerular abnormality
Rapidly progressive nephritic syndrome with minimal change lesion

N01.1   Rapidly progressive nephritic syndrome with focal and segmental glomerular lesions
Rapidly progressive nephritic syndrome with focal and segmental hyalinosis
Rapidly progressive nephritic syndrome with focal and segmental sclerosis
Rapidly progressive nephritic syndrome with focal glomerulonephritis

N01.2   Rapidly progressive nephritic syndrome with diffuse membranous glomerulonephritis

N01.3   Rapidly progressive nephritic syndrome with diffuse mesangial proliferative glomerulonephritis

N01.4   Rapidly progressive nephritic syndrome with diffuse endocapillary proliferative glomerulonephritis

N01.5   Rapidly progressive nephritic syndrome with diffuse mesangiocapillary glomerulonephritis
Rapidly progressive nephritic syndrome with membranoproliferative glomerulonephritis, types 1 and 3, or NOS

N01.6   Rapidly progressive nephritic syndrome with dense deposit disease
Rapidly progressive nephritic syndrome with membranoproliferative glomerulonephritis, type 2

N01.7   Rapidly progressive nephritic syndrome with diffuse crescentic glomerulonephritis
Rapidly progressive nephritic syndrome with extracapillary glomerulonephritis

N01.8   Rapidly progressive nephritic syndrome with other morphologic changes
Rapidly progressive nephritic syndrome with proliferative glomerulonephritis NOS

N01.9   Rapidly progressive nephritic syndrome with unspecified morphologic changes   ▽

✓4th **N02   Recurrent and persistent hematuria**
EXCLUDES 1   acute cystitis with hematuria (N30.01)
hematuria NOS (R31.9)
hematuria not associated with specified morphologic lesions (R31.-)

N02.0   Recurrent and persistent hematuria with minor glomerular abnormality
Recurrent and persistent hematuria with minimal change lesion

N02.1   Recurrent and persistent hematuria with focal and segmental glomerular lesions
Recurrent and persistent hematuria with focal and segmental hyalinosis
Recurrent and persistent hematuria with focal and segmental sclerosis
Recurrent and persistent hematuria with focal glomerulonephritis

N02.2   Recurrent and persistent hematuria with diffuse membranous glomerulonephritis

N02.3   Recurrent and persistent hematuria with diffuse mesangial proliferative glomerulonephritis

N02.4   Recurrent and persistent hematuria with diffuse endocapillary proliferative glomerulonephritis

N02.5   Recurrent and persistent hematuria with diffuse mesangiocapillary glomerulonephritis
Recurrent and persistent hematuria with membranoproliferative glomerulonephritis, types 1 and 3, or NOS

N02.6   Recurrent and persistent hematuria with dense deposit disease
Recurrent and persistent hematuria with membranoproliferative glomerulonephritis, type 2

N02.7   Recurrent and persistent hematuria with diffuse crescentic glomerulonephritis
Recurrent and persistent hematuria with extracapillary glomerulonephritis

N02.8   Recurrent and persistent hematuria with other morphologic changes
Recurrent and persistent hematuria with proliferative glomerulonephritis NOS

N02.9   Recurrent and persistent hematuria with unspecified morphologic changes   ▽
AHA: 2017, 2Q, 5

✓4ᵗʰ N03 Chronic nephritic syndrome

INCLUDES chronic glomerular disease
    chronic glomerulonephritis
    chronic nephritis

EXCLUDES 1 *chronic tubulo-interstitial nephritis (N11.-)*
    diffuse sclerosing glomerulonephritis (N05.8-)
    nephritic syndrome NOS (N05.-)

DEF: Slow, progressive type of nephritis characterized by inflammation of the capillary loops in the glomeruli of the kidney, which leads to renal failure.

N03.0 Chronic nephritic syndrome with minor glomerular abnormality
    Chronic nephritic syndrome with minimal change lesion

N03.1 Chronic nephritic syndrome with focal and segmental glomerular lesions
    Chronic nephritic syndrome with focal and segmental hyalinosis
    Chronic nephritic syndrome with focal and segmental sclerosis
    Chronic nephritic syndrome with focal glomerulonephritis

N03.2 Chronic nephritic syndrome with diffuse membranous glomerulonephritis

N03.3 Chronic nephritic syndrome with diffuse mesangial proliferative glomerulonephritis

N03.4 Chronic nephritic syndrome with diffuse endocapillary proliferative glomerulonephritis

N03.5 Chronic nephritic syndrome with diffuse mesangiocapillary glomerulonephritis
    Chronic nephritic syndrome with membranoproliferative glomerulonephritis, types 1 and 3, or NOS

N03.6 Chronic nephritic syndrome with dense deposit disease
    Chronic nephritic syndrome with membranoproliferative glomerulonephritis, type 2

N03.7 Chronic nephritic syndrome with diffuse crescentic glomerulonephritis
    Chronic nephritic syndrome with extracapillary glomerulonephritis

N03.8 Chronic nephritic syndrome with other morphologic changes
    Chronic nephritic syndrome with proliferative glomerulonephritis NOS

N03.9 Chronic nephritic syndrome with unspecified morphologic changes ▽

✓4ᵗʰ N04 Nephrotic syndrome

INCLUDES congenital nephrotic syndrome
    lipoid nephrosis

N04.0 Nephrotic syndrome with minor glomerular abnormality
    Nephrotic syndrome with minimal change lesion

N04.1 Nephrotic syndrome with focal and segmental glomerular lesions
    Nephrotic syndrome with focal and segmental hyalinosis
    Nephrotic syndrome with focal and segmental sclerosis
    Nephrotic syndrome with focal glomerulonephritis

N04.2 Nephrotic syndrome with diffuse membranous glomerulonephritis

N04.3 Nephrotic syndrome with diffuse mesangial proliferative glomerulonephritis

N04.4 Nephrotic syndrome with diffuse endocapillary proliferative glomerulonephritis

N04.5 Nephrotic syndrome with diffuse mesangiocapillary glomerulonephritis
    Nephrotic syndrome with membranoproliferative glomerulonephritis, types 1 and 3, or NOS

N04.6 Nephrotic syndrome with dense deposit disease
    Nephrotic syndrome with membranoproliferative glomerulonephritis, type 2

N04.7 Nephrotic syndrome with diffuse crescentic glomerulonephritis
    Nephrotic syndrome with extracapillary glomerulonephritis

N04.8 Nephrotic syndrome with other morphologic changes
    Nephrotic syndrome with proliferative glomerulonephritis NOS

N04.9 Nephrotic syndrome with unspecified morphologic changes ▽

✓4ᵗʰ N05 Unspecified nephritic syndrome

INCLUDES glomerular disease NOS
    glomerulonephritis NOS
    nephritis NOS
    nephropathy NOS and renal disease NOS with morphological lesion specified in .0-.8

EXCLUDES 1 *nephropathy NOS with no stated morphological lesion (N28.9)*
    renal disease NOS with no stated morphological lesion (N28.9)
    tubulo-interstitial nephritis NOS (N12)

N05.0 Unspecified nephritic syndrome with minor glomerular abnormality ▽
    Unspecified nephritic syndrome with minimal change lesion

N05.1 Unspecified nephritic syndrome with focal and segmental glomerular lesions ▽
    Unspecified nephritic syndrome with focal and segmental hyalinosis
    Unspecified nephritic syndrome with focal and segmental sclerosis
    Unspecified nephritic syndrome with focal glomerulonephritis

N05.2 Unspecified nephritic syndrome with diffuse membranous glomerulonephritis ▽

N05.3 Unspecified nephritic syndrome with diffuse mesangial proliferative glomerulonephritis ▽

N05.4 Unspecified nephritic syndrome with diffuse endocapillary proliferative glomerulonephritis ▽

N05.5 Unspecified nephritic syndrome with diffuse mesangiocapillary glomerulonephritis ▽
    Unspecified nephritic syndrome with membranoproliferative glomerulonephritis, types 1 and 3, or NOS

N05.6 Unspecified nephritic syndrome with dense deposit disease ▽
    Unspecified nephritic syndrome with membranoproliferative glomerulonephritis, type 2

N05.7 Unspecified nephritic syndrome with diffuse crescentic glomerulonephritis ▽
    Unspecified nephritic syndrome with extracapillary glomerulonephritis

N05.8 Unspecified nephritic syndrome with other morphologic changes ▽
    Unspecified nephritic syndrome with proliferative glomerulonephritis NOS

N05.9 Unspecified nephritic syndrome with unspecified morphologic changes ▽

✓4ᵗʰ N06 Isolated proteinuria with specified morphological lesion

EXCLUDES 1 *proteinuria not associated with specific morphologic lesions (R80.0)*

N06.0 Isolated proteinuria with minor glomerular abnormality
    Isolated proteinuria with minimal change lesion

N06.1 Isolated proteinuria with focal and segmental glomerular lesions
    Isolated proteinuria with focal and segmental hyalinosis
    Isolated proteinuria with focal and segmental sclerosis
    Isolated proteinuria with focal glomerulonephritis

N06.2 Isolated proteinuria with diffuse membranous glomerulonephritis

N06.3 Isolated proteinuria with diffuse mesangial proliferative glomerulonephritis

N06.4 Isolated proteinuria with diffuse endocapillary proliferative glomerulonephritis

N06.5 Isolated proteinuria with diffuse mesangiocapillary glomerulonephritis
    Isolated proteinuria with membranoproliferative glomerulonephritis, types 1 and 3, or NOS

N06.6 Isolated proteinuria with dense deposit disease
    Isolated proteinuria with membranoproliferative glomerulonephritis, type 2

N06.7 Isolated proteinuria with diffuse crescentic glomerulonephritis
    Isolated proteinuria with extracapillary glomerulonephritis

N06.8 Isolated proteinuria with other morphologic lesion
    Isolated proteinuria with proliferative glomerulonephritis NOS

N06.9 Isolated proteinuria with unspecified morphologic lesion ▽

✓4ᵗʰ N07 Hereditary nephropathy, not elsewhere classified

EXCLUDES 2 *Alport's syndrome (Q87.81-)*
    hereditary amyloid nephropathy (E85.-)
    nail patella syndrome (Q87.2)
    non-neuropathic heredofamilial amyloidosis (E85.-)

N07.0 Hereditary nephropathy, not elsewhere classified with minor glomerular abnormality
    Hereditary nephropathy, not elsewhere classified with minimal change lesion

N07.1 Hereditary nephropathy, not elsewhere classified with focal and segmental glomerular lesions
    Hereditary nephropathy, not elsewhere classified with focal and segmental hyalinosis
    Hereditary nephropathy, not elsewhere classified with focal and segmental sclerosis
    Hereditary nephropathy, not elsewhere classified with focal glomerulonephritis

---

✓ Additional Character Req   ✓x7ᵗʰ Placeholder Alert   Case-Mix Diagnosis   Manifestation   ▽ Unspecified Dx   EXCLUDES 1 Not coded here   EXCLUDES 2 Not included here

N07.2 Hereditary nephropathy, not elsewhere classified with diffuse membranous glomerulonephritis

N07.3 Hereditary nephropathy, not elsewhere classified with diffuse mesangial proliferative glomerulonephritis

N07.4 Hereditary nephropathy, not elsewhere classified with diffuse endocapillary proliferative glomerulonephritis

N07.5 Hereditary nephropathy, not elsewhere classified with diffuse mesangiocapillary glomerulonephritis
> Hereditary nephropathy, not elsewhere classified with membranoproliferative glomerulonephritis, types 1 and 3, or NOS

N07.6 Hereditary nephropathy, not elsewhere classified with dense deposit disease
> Hereditary nephropathy, not elsewhere classified with membranoproliferative glomerulonephritis, type 2

N07.7 Hereditary nephropathy, not elsewhere classified with diffuse crescentic glomerulonephritis
> Hereditary nephropathy, not elsewhere classified with extracapillary glomerulonephritis

N07.8 Hereditary nephropathy, not elsewhere classified with other morphologic lesions
> Hereditary nephropathy, not elsewhere classified with proliferative glomerulonephritis NOS

N07.9 Hereditary nephropathy, not elsewhere classified with unspecified morphologic lesions ▽

N08 *Glomerular disorders in diseases classified elsewhere*
> Glomerulonephritis
> Nephritis
> Nephropathy
> Code first underlying disease, such as:
>> amyloidosis (E85.-)
>> congenital syphilis (A50.5)
>> cryoglobulinemia (D89.1)
>> disseminated intravascular coagulation (D65)
>> gout (M1A.-, M10.-)
>> microscopic polyangiitis (M31.7)
>> multiple myeloma (C90.0-)
>> sepsis (A40.0-A41.9)
>> sickle-cell disease (D57.0-D57.8)
>
> **EXCLUDES 1** *glomerulonephritis, nephritis and nephropathy (in):*
>> *antiglomerular basement membrane disease (M31.0)*
>> *diabetes (E08-E13 with .21)*
>> *gonococcal (A54.21)*
>> *Goodpasture's syndrome (M31.0)*
>> *hemolytic-uremic syndrome (D59.3)*
>> *lupus (M32.14)*
>> *mumps (B26.83)*
>> *syphilis (A52.75)*
>> *systemic lupus erythematosus (M32.14)*
>> *Wegener's granulomatosis (M31.31)*
>> *pyelonephritis in diseases classified elsewhere (N16)*
>> *renal tubulo-interstitial disorders classified elsewhere (N16)*

Renal tubulo-interstitial diseases (N10-N16)

INCLUDES pyelonephritis
EXCLUDES 1 *pyeloureteritis cystica (N28.85)*

N10 Acute pyelonephritis
> Acute infectious interstitial nephritis
> Acute pyelitis
> Acute tubulo-interstitial nephritis
> Hemoglobin nephrosis
> Myoglobin nephrosis
> Use additional code (B95-B97), to identify infectious agent

✓4ᵗʰ N11 Chronic tubulo-interstitial nephritis
> **INCLUDES** chronic infectious interstitial nephritis
> chronic pyelitis
> chronic pyelonephritis
> Use additional code (B95-B97), to identify infectious agent

N11.0 Nonobstructive reflux-associated chronic pyelonephritis
> Pyelonephritis (chronic) associated with (vesicoureteral) reflux
> **EXCLUDES 1** *vesicoureteral reflux NOS (N13.70)*

N11.1 Chronic obstructive pyelonephritis
> Pyelonephritis (chronic) associated with anomaly of pelviureteric junction
> Pyelonephritis (chronic) associated with anomaly of pyeloureteric junction
> Pyelonephritis (chronic) associated with crossing of vessel
> Pyelonephritis (chronic) associated with kinking of ureter
> Pyelonephritis (chronic) associated with obstruction of ureter
> Pyelonephritis (chronic) associated with stricture of pelviureteric junction
> Pyelonephritis (chronic) associated with stricture of ureter
> **EXCLUDES 1** *calculous pyelonephritis (N20.9)*
>> *obstructive uropathy (N13.-)*

N11.8 Other chronic tubulo-interstitial nephritis
> Nonobstructive chronic pyelonephritis NOS

N11.9 Chronic tubulo-interstitial nephritis, unspecified ▽
> Chronic interstitial nephritis NOS
> Chronic pyelitis NOS
> Chronic pyelonephritis NOS

N12 Tubulo-interstitial nephritis, not specified as acute or chronic
> Interstitial nephritis NOS
> Pyelitis NOS
> Pyelonephritis NOS
> **EXCLUDES 1** *calculous pyelonephritis (N20.9)*

✓4ᵗʰ N13 Obstructive and reflux uropathy
> **EXCLUDES 2** *calculus of kidney and ureter without hydronephrosis (N20.-)*
>> *congenital obstructive defects of renal pelvis and ureter (Q62.0-Q62.3)*
>> *hydronephrosis with ureteropelvic junction obstruction ▶(Q62.11)◀*
>> *obstructive pyelonephritis (N11.1)*

N13.0 Hydronephrosis with ureteropelvic junction obstruction
> Hydronephrosis due to acquired occlusion of ureteropelvic junction
> **EXCLUDES 2** *hydronephrosis with ureteropelvic junction obstruction due to calculus (N13.2)*

N13.1 Hydronephrosis with ureteral stricture, not elsewhere classified
> **EXCLUDES 1** *hydronephrosis with ureteral stricture with infection (N13.6)*

N13.2 Hydronephrosis with renal and ureteral calculous obstruction
> **EXCLUDES 1** *hydronephrosis with renal and ureteral calculous obstruction with infection (N13.6)*

N13.4 Hydroureter
> **EXCLUDES 1** *congenital hydroureter (Q62.3-)*
>> *hydroureter with infection (N13.6)*
>> *vesicoureteral-reflux with hydroureter (N13.73-)*

✓5ᵗʰ N13.3 Other and unspecified hydronephrosis
> **EXCLUDES 1** *hydronephrosis with infection (N13.6)*
>
> **N13.30 Unspecified hydronephrosis** ▽
>
> **N13.39 Other hydronephrosis**

Hydronephrosis/UPJ Obstruction

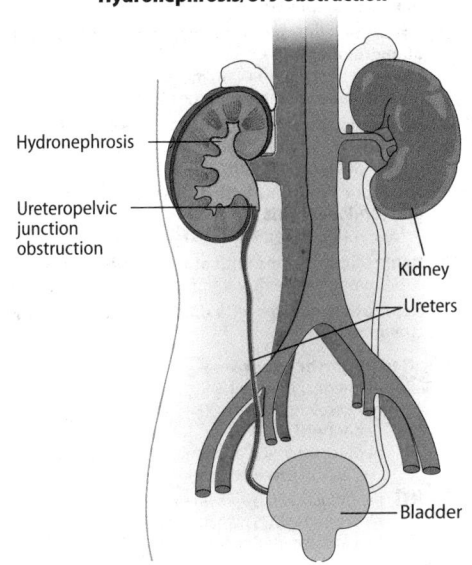

Hydronephrosis

Ureteropelvic junction obstruction

Kidney

Ureters

Bladder

N Newborn: 0   **P** Pediatric: 0-17   **M** Maternity: 12-55   **A** Adult: 15-124   **NRS** Nonroutine supply Dx   **NC Dx** Noncancer Dx   **PDx** Primary Dx   ▶◀ Revised Text   ● New Code   ▲ Revised Title

804   ICD-10-CM 2018

Vesicoureteral Reflux

Normal flow of urine   Urine flowing the wrong way (VUR)

N13.5 Crossing vessel and stricture of ureter without hydronephrosis
Kinking and stricture of ureter without hydronephrosis
EXCLUDES 1   crossing vessel and stricture of ureter without hydronephrosis with infection (N13.6)

N13.6 Pyonephrosis
Conditions in N13.0-N13.5 with infection
Obstructive uropathy with infection
Use additional code (B95-B97), to identify infectious agent

✓5ᵗʰ **N13.7 Vesicoureteral-reflux**
EXCLUDES 1   reflux-associated pyelonephritis (N11.0)

N13.70 Vesicoureteral-reflux, unspecified ▽
Vesicoureteral-reflux NOS

N13.71 Vesicoureteral-reflux without reflux nephropathy

✓6ᵗʰ **N13.72 Vesicoureteral-reflux with reflux nephropathy without hydroureter**

N13.721 Vesicoureteral-reflux with reflux nephropathy without hydroureter, unilateral

N13.722 Vesicoureteral-reflux with reflux nephropathy without hydroureter, bilateral

N13.729 Vesicoureteral-reflux with reflux nephropathy without hydroureter, unspecified ▽

✓6ᵗʰ **N13.73 Vesicoureteral-reflux with reflux nephropathy with hydroureter**

N13.731 Vesicoureteral-reflux with reflux nephropathy with hydroureter, unilateral

N13.732 Vesicoureteral-reflux with reflux nephropathy with hydroureter, bilateral

N13.739 Vesicoureteral-reflux with reflux nephropathy with hydroureter, unspecified ▽

N13.8 Other obstructive and reflux uropathy
Urinary tract obstruction due to specified cause
Code first, if applicable, any causal condition, such as:
enlarged prostate (N40.1)

N13.9 Obstructive and reflux uropathy, unspecified ▽
Urinary tract obstruction NOS

✓4ᵗʰ **N14 Drug- and heavy-metal-induced tubulo-interstitial and tubular conditions**
Code first poisoning due to drug or toxin, if applicable (T36-T65 with fifth or sixth character 1-4 or 6)
Use additional code for adverse effect, if applicable, to identify drug (T36-T50 with fifth or sixth character 5)

N14.0 Analgesic nephropathy

N14.1 Nephropathy induced by other drugs, medicaments and biological substances

N14.2 Nephropathy induced by unspecified drug, medicament or biological substance ▽

N14.3 Nephropathy induced by heavy metals

N14.4 Toxic nephropathy, not elsewhere classified

✓4ᵗʰ **N15 Other renal tubulo-interstitial diseases**

N15.0 Balkan nephropathy
Balkan endemic nephropathy

N15.1 Renal and perinephric abscess

N15.8 Other specified renal tubulo-interstitial diseases

N15.9 Renal tubulo-interstitial disease, unspecified ▽
Infection of kidney NOS
EXCLUDES 1   urinary tract infection NOS (N39.0)

N16 Renal tubulo-interstitial disorders in diseases classified elsewhere
Pyelonephritis   Tubulo-interstitial nephritis
Code first underlying disease, such as:
brucellosis (A23.0-A23.9)
cryoglobulinemia (D89.1)
glycogen storage disease (E74.0)
leukemia (C91-C95)
lymphoma (C81.0-C85.9, C96.0-C96.9)
multiple myeloma (C90.0-)
sepsis (A40.0-A41.9)
Wilson's disease (E83.0)
EXCLUDES 1   diphtheritic pyelonephritis and tubulo-interstitial nephritis (A36.84)
pyelonephritis and tubulo-interstitial nephritis in candidiasis (B37.49)
pyelonephritis and tubulo-interstitial nephritis in cystinosis (E72.04)
pyelonephritis and tubulo-interstitial nephritis in salmonella infection (A02.25)
pyelonephritis and tubulo-interstitial nephritis in sarcoidosis (D86.84)
pyelonephritis and tubulo-interstitial nephritis in sicca syndrome [Sjogren's] (M35.04)
pyelonephritis and tubulo-interstitial nephritis in systemic lupus erythematosus (M32.15)
pyelonephritis and tubulo-interstitial nephritis in toxoplasmosis (B58.83)
renal tubular degeneration in diabetes (E08-E13 with .29)
syphilitic pyelonephritis and tubulo-interstitial nephritis (A52.75)

Acute kidney failure and chronic kidney disease (N17-N19)

EXCLUDES 2   congenital renal failure (P96.0)
drug- and heavy-metal-induced tubulo-interstitial and tubular conditions (N14.-)
extrarenal uremia (R39.2)
hemolytic-uremic syndrome (D59.3)
hepatorenal syndrome (K76.7)
postpartum hepatorenal syndrome (O90.4)
posttraumatic renal failure (T79.5)
prerenal uremia (R39.2)
renal failure complicating abortion or ectopic or molar pregnancy (O00-O07, O08.4)
renal failure following labor and delivery (O90.4)
renal failure postprocedural (N99.0)

✓4ᵗʰ **N17 Acute kidney failure**
Code also associated underlying condition
EXCLUDES 1   posttraumatic renal failure (T79.5)
AHA: 2013, 4Q, 124

N17.0 Acute kidney failure with tubular necrosis   NC Dx
Acute tubular necrosis
Renal tubular necrosis
Tubular necrosis NOS

N17.1 Acute kidney failure with acute cortical necrosis   NC Dx
Acute cortical necrosis
Cortical necrosis NOS
Renal cortical necrosis

N17.2 Acute kidney failure with medullary necrosis   NC Dx
Medullary [papillary] necrosis NOS
Acute medullary [papillary] necrosis
Renal medullary [papillary] necrosis

N17.8 Other acute kidney failure   NC Dx

N17.9 Acute kidney failure, unspecified   NC Dx ▽
Acute kidney injury (nontraumatic)
EXCLUDES 2   traumatic kidney injury (S37.0-)

☑ Additional Character Req   ✓x7ᵗʰ Placeholder Alert   Case-Mix Diagnosis   Manifestation   ▽ Unspecified Dx   EXCLUDES 1 Not coded here   EXCLUDES 2 Not included here

ICD-10-CM 2018   805

✔4ᵗʰ N18 Chronic kidney disease (CKD)

Code first any associated:
diabetic chronic kidney disease (E08.22, E09.22, E10.22, E11.22, E13.22)
hypertensive chronic kidney disease (I12-, I13-)
Use additional code to identify kidney transplant status, if applicable, (Z94.0)

AHA: 2013, 1Q, 24

TIP: CKD/ESRD occurring in an individual with a history of kidney transplant should not be assumed to be a transplant complication unless specifically indicated as such by provider documentation.

TIP: The term "chronic renal impairment" should not be interpreted as CKD or chronic renal insufficiency and should be coded as N28.9.

N18.1 Chronic kidney disease, stage 1

N18.2 Chronic kidney disease, stage 2 (mild)

N18.3 Chronic kidney disease, stage 3 (moderate)

N18.4 Chronic kidney disease, stage 4 (severe)

N18.5 Chronic kidney disease, stage
> EXCLUDES 1 — chronic kidney disease, stage 5 requiring chronic dialysis (N18.6)

DEF: End-stage renal disease (ESRD) with GFR value of 15 ml/min or less not yet requiring chronic dialysis.

N18.6 End stage renal disease   NC Dx
Chronic kidney disease requiring chronic dialysis
Use additional code to identify dialysis status (Z99.2)
AHA: 2016, 3Q, 22; 2016, 1Q, 12; 2013, 4Q, 124-125

⁸ N18.9 Chronic kidney disease, unspecified ▽
Chronic renal disease
Chronic renal failure NOS
Chronic renal insufficiency
▶Chronic uremia NOS
Diffuse sclerosing glomerulonephritis NOS◀

⁸ N19 Unspecified kidney failure ▽
Uremia NOS
> EXCLUDES 1 — acute kidney failure (N17.-)
> chronic kidney disease (N18.-)
> chronic uremia (N18.9)
> extrarenal uremia (R39.2)
> prerenal uremia (R39.2)
> renal insufficiency (acute) (N28.9)
> uremia of newborn (P96.0)

Urolithiasis (N20-N23)

AHA: 2017, 1Q, 5; 2015, 2Q, 8

✔4ᵗʰ N20 Calculus of kidney and ureter

Calculous pyelonephritis
> EXCLUDES 1 — nephrocalcinosis (E83.5)
> that with hydronephrosis (N13.2)

N20.0 Calculus of kidney
Nephrolithiasis NOS
Renal calculus
Renal stone
Staghorn calculus
Stone in kidney

N20.1 Calculus of ureter
Ureteric stone
AHA: 2016, 3Q, 22

N20.2 Calculus of kidney with calculus of ureter

N20.9 Urinary calculus, unspecified ▽

✔4ᵗʰ N21 Calculus of lower urinary tract

> INCLUDES — calculus of lower urinary tract with cystitis and urethritis

N21.0 Calculus in bladder
Calculus in diverticulum of bladder
Urinary bladder stone
> EXCLUDES 2 — staghorn calculus (N20.0)

N21.1 Calculus in urethra
> EXCLUDES 2 — calculus of prostate (N42.0)

N21.8 Other lower urinary tract calculus

N21.9 Calculus of lower urinary tract, unspecified ▽
> EXCLUDES 1 — calculus of urinary tract NOS (N20.9)

N22 Calculus of urinary tract in diseases classified elsewhere

Code first underlying disease, such as:
gout (M1A.-, M10.-)
schistosomiasis (B65.0-B65.9)

N23 Unspecified renal colic ▽

Other disorders of kidney and ureter (N25-N29)

> EXCLUDES 2 — disorders of kidney and ureter with urolithiasis (N20-N23)

✔4ᵗʰ N25 Disorders resulting from impaired renal tubular function

> EXCLUDES 1 — ~~metabolic disorders classifiable to E70-E88~~

N25.0 Renal osteodystrophy
Azotemic osteodystrophy
Phosphate-losing tubular disorders
Renal rickets
Renal short stature
> EXCLUDES 2 ▶metabolic disorders classifiable to E70-E88◀

N25.1 Nephrogenic diabetes insipidus
> EXCLUDES 1 — diabetes insipidus NOS (E23.2)

DEF: Type of diabetes due to inability of renal tubules to reabsorb water back into the body; not responsive to vasopressin (antidiuretic hormone); characterized by excessive thirst and excessive urine production; may develop into chronic renal insufficiency.

✔5ᵗʰ N25.8 Other disorders resulting from impaired renal tubular function

N25.81 Secondary hyperparathyroidism of renal origin
> EXCLUDES 2 ▶metabolic disorders classifiable to E70-E88◀

DEF: Parathyroid dysfunction caused by chronic renal failure; phosphate clearance is impaired, phosphate is released from bone, vitamin D is not produced, intestinal calcium absorption is low, and blood levels of calcium are lowered, causing excessive production of parathyroid hormone.

N25.89 Other disorders resulting from impaired renal tubular function
Hypokalemic nephropathy
Lightwood-Albright syndrome
Renal tubular acidosis NOS

N25.9 Disorder resulting from impaired renal tubular function, unspecified ▽

✔4ᵗʰ N26 Unspecified contracted kidney

> EXCLUDES 1 — contracted kidney due to hypertension (I12.-)
> diffuse sclerosing glomerulonephritis (N05.8-)
> hypertensive nephrosclerosis (arteriolar) (arteriosclerotic) (I12.-)
> small kidney of unknown cause (N27.-)

N26.1 Atrophy of kidney (terminal)

N26.2 Page kidney

N26.9 Renal sclerosis, unspecified ▽

✔4ᵗʰ N27 Small kidney of unknown cause

> INCLUDES — oligonephronia

N27.0 Small kidney, unilateral

N27.1 Small kidney, bilateral

N27.9 Small kidney, unspecified ▽

✔4ᵗʰ N28 Other disorders of kidney and ureter, not elsewhere classified

N28.0 Ischemia and infarction of kidney
Renal artery embolism   Renal artery thrombosis
Renal artery obstruction   Renal infarct
Renal artery occlusion
> EXCLUDES 1 — atherosclerosis of renal artery (extrarenal part) (I70.1)
> congenital stenosis of renal artery (Q27.1)
> Goldblatt's kidney (I70.1)

N28.1 Cyst of kidney, acquired
▶Cyst (multiple) (solitary) of kidney (acquired)◀
> EXCLUDES 1 — cystic kidney disease (congenital) (Q61.-)

✔5ᵗʰ N28.8 Other specified disorders of kidney and ureter

> EXCLUDES 1 — hydroureter (N13.4)
> ureteric stricture with hydronephrosis (N13.1)
> ureteric stricture without hydronephrosis (N13.5)

N28.81 Hypertrophy of kidney

N28.82 Megaloureter

N28.83 Nephroptosis

N28.84 Pyelitis cystica

N28.85 Pyeloureteritis cystica

N28.86 Ureteritis cystica

N28.89 Other specified disorders of kidney and ureter

---

⁸ Hospice questionable admission diagnosis.

Ⓝ Newborn: 0 Ⓟ Pediatric: 0-17 Ⓜ Maternity: 12-55 Ⓐ Adult: 15-124 NRS Nonroutine supply Dx NC Dx Noncancer Dx PDx Primary Dx ▶◀ Revised Text ● New Code ▲ Revised Title

806

ICD-10-CM 2018

N18–N28.89

N28.9 Disorder of kidney and ureter, unspecified
Nephropathy NOS
Renal disease (acute) NOS
Renal insufficiency (acute)
> **EXCLUDES 1** chronic renal insufficiency (N18.9)
> unspecified nephritic syndrome (N05.-)

AHA: 2016, 1Q, 13
TIP: The term "chronic renal impairment" should not be interpreted as CKD or chronic renal insufficiency and should be coded as N28.9.

N29 Other disorders of kidney and ureter in diseases classified elsewhere
Code first underlying disease, such as:
amyloidosis (E85.-)
nephrocalcinosis (E83.5)
schistosomiasis (B65.0-B65.9)
> **EXCLUDES 1** disorders of kidney and ureter in:
> cystinosis (E72.0)
> gonorrhea (A54.21)
> syphilis (A52.75)
> tuberculosis (A18.11)

Other diseases of the urinary system (N30-N39)
> **EXCLUDES 1** urinary infection (complicating):
> abortion or ectopic or molar pregnancy (O00-O07, O08.8)
> pregnancy, childbirth and the puerperium (O23-, O75.3, O86.2-)

✓4th N30 Cystitis
Use additional code to identify infectious agent (B95-B97)
> **EXCLUDES 1** prostatocystitis (N41.3)

AHA: 2017, 1Q, 6

✓5th N30.0 Acute cystitis
> **EXCLUDES 1** irradiation cystitis (N30.4-)
> trigonitis (N30.3-)

N30.00 Acute cystitis without hematuria
N30.01 Acute cystitis with hematuria

✓5th N30.1 Interstitial cystitis (chronic)
N30.10 Interstitial cystitis (chronic) without hematuria
N30.11 Interstitial cystitis (chronic) with hematuria

✓5th N30.2 Other chronic cystitis
N30.20 Other chronic cystitis without hematuria
N30.21 Other chronic cystitis with hematuria

✓5th N30.3 Trigonitis
Urethrotrigonitis
N30.30 Trigonitis without hematuria
N30.31 Trigonitis with hematuria

✓5th N30.4 Irradiation cystitis
N30.40 Irradiation cystitis without hematuria
N30.41 Irradiation cystitis with hematuria

✓5th N30.8 Other cystitis
Abscess of bladder
N30.80 Other cystitis without hematuria
N30.81 Other cystitis with hematuria

✓5th N30.9 Cystitis, unspecified
N30.90 Cystitis, unspecified without hematuria ▽
N30.91 Cystitis, unspecified with hematuria ▽

✓4th N31 Neuromuscular dysfunction of bladder, not elsewhere classified
Use additional code to identify any associated urinary incontinence (N39.3-N39.4-)
> **EXCLUDES 1** cord bladder NOS (G95.89)
> neurogenic bladder due to cauda equina syndrome (G83.4)
> neuromuscular dysfunction due to spinal cord lesion (G95.89)

N31.0 Uninhibited neuropathic bladder, not elsewhere classified
N31.1 Reflex neuropathic bladder, not elsewhere classified
N31.2 Flaccid neuropathic bladder, not elsewhere classified
Atonic (motor) (sensory) neuropathic bladder
Autonomous neuropathic bladder
Nonreflex neuropathic bladder
N31.8 Other neuromuscular dysfunction of bladder
N31.9 Neuromuscular dysfunction of bladder, unspecified ▽
Neurogenic bladder dysfunction NOS

✓4th N32 Other disorders of bladder
> **EXCLUDES 2** calculus of bladder (N21.0)
> cystocele (N81.1-)
> hernia or prolapse of bladder, female (N81.1-)

N32.0 Bladder-neck obstruction
Bladder-neck stenosis (acquired)
> **EXCLUDES 1** congenital bladder-neck obstruction (Q64.3-)

DEF: Bladder outlet and vesicourethral obstruction; occurs as a consequence of benign prostatic hypertrophy or prostatic cancer; may also occur in either sex due to strictures, radiation, cystoscopy, catheterization, injury, infection, blood clots, bladder cancer, impaction, or other disease that compresses the bladder neck.

N32.1 Vesicointestinal fistula
Vesicorectal fistula

N32.2 Vesical fistula, not elsewhere classified
> **EXCLUDES 1** fistula between bladder and female genital tract (N82.0-N82.1)

N32.3 Diverticulum of bladder
> **EXCLUDES 1** congenital diverticulum of bladder (Q64.6)
> diverticulitis of bladder (N30.8-)

✓5th N32.8 Other specified disorders of bladder
N32.81 Overactive bladder
Detrusor muscle hyperactivity
> **EXCLUDES 1** frequent urination due to specified bladder condition—code to condition

DEF: Sudden involuntary contractions of the muscular wall of bladder; results in sudden, strong urge to urinate.

N32.89 Other specified disorders of bladder
Bladder hemorrhage
Bladder hypertrophy
Calcified bladder
Contracted bladder

N32.9 Bladder disorder, unspecified ▽

N33 Bladder disorders in diseases classified elsewhere
Code first underlying disease, such as:
schistosomiasis (B65.0-B65.9)
> **EXCLUDES 1** bladder disorder in syphilis (A52.76)
> bladder disorder in tuberculosis (A18.12)
> candidal cystitis (B37.41)
> chlamydial cystitis (A56.01)
> cystitis in gonorrhea (A54.01)
> cystitis in neurogenic bladder (N31.-)
> diphtheritic cystitis (A36.85)
> neurogenic bladder (N31.-)
> syphilitic cystitis (A52.76)
> trichomonal cystitis (A59.03)

✓4th N34 Urethritis and urethral syndrome
Use additional code (B95-B97), to identify infectious agent
> **EXCLUDES 2** Reiter's disease (M02.3-)
> urethritis in diseases with a predominantly sexual mode of transmission (A50-A64)
> urethrotrigonitis (N30.3-)

AHA: 2017, 1Q, 6

N34.0 Urethral abscess
Abscess (of) Cowper's gland
Abscess (of) Littrés gland
Abscess (of) urethral (gland)
Periurethral abscess
> **EXCLUDES 1** urethral caruncle (N36.2)

N34.1 Nonspecific urethritis
Nongonococcal urethritis
Nonvenereal urethritis

N34.2 Other urethritis
Meatitis, urethral
Postmenopausal urethritis
Ulcer of urethra (meatus)
Urethritis NOS

N34.3 Urethral syndrome, unspecified ▽

✓4th N35 Urethral stricture
> **EXCLUDES 1** congenital urethral stricture (Q64.3-)
> postprocedural urethral stricture (N99.1-)

✓5th N35.0 Post-traumatic urethral stricture
Urethral stricture due to injury
> **EXCLUDES 1** postprocedural urethral stricture (N99.1-)

✓6th N35.01 Post-traumatic urethral stricture, male
N35.010 Post-traumatic urethral stricture, male, meatal ♂
N35.011 Post-traumatic bulbous urethral stricture

✓ Additional Character Req | ✓x7th Placeholder Alert | Case-Mix Diagnosis | Manifestation | ▽ Unspecified Dx | **EXCLUDES 1** Not coded here | **EXCLUDES 2** Not included here

ICD-10-CM 2018

807

N35.012 Post-traumatic membranous urethral stricture

N35.013 Post-traumatic anterior urethral stricture

N35.014 Post-traumatic urethral stricture, male, unspecified   ♂▽

✓6ᵗʰ **N35.02** Post-traumatic urethral stricture, female

N35.021 Urethral stricture due to childbirth ♀

N35.028 Other post-traumatic urethral stricture, female ♀

✓5ᵗʰ **N35.1** Postinfective urethral stricture, not elsewhere classified

> EXCLUDES 1   urethral stricture associated with schistosomiasis (B65-, N29)
> gonococcal urethral stricture (A54.01)
> syphilitic urethral stricture (A52.76)

✓6ᵗʰ **N35.11** Postinfective urethral stricture, not elsewhere classified, male

N35.111 Postinfective urethral stricture, not elsewhere classified, male, meatal   ♂

▲   **N35.112** Postinfective bulbous urethral stricture, not elsewhere classified, male

▲   **N35.113** Postinfective membranous urethral stricture, not elsewhere classified, male

▲   **N35.114** Postinfective anterior urethral stricture, not elsewhere classified, male

N35.119 Postinfective urethral stricture, not elsewhere classified, male, unspecified   ♂▽

N35.12 Postinfective urethral stricture, not elsewhere classified, female   ♀

N35.8 Other urethral stricture

> EXCLUDES 1   postprocedural urethral stricture (N99.1-)

N35.9 Urethral stricture, unspecified ▽

✓4ᵗʰ **N36** Other disorders of urethra

N36.0 Urethral fistula
Urethroperineal fistula
Urethrorectal fistula
Urinary fistula NOS

> EXCLUDES 1   urethroscrotal fistula (N50.89)
> urethrovaginal fistula (N82.1)
> urethrovesicovaginal fistula (N82.1)

N36.1 Urethral diverticulum

N36.2 Urethral caruncle

✓5ᵗʰ **N36.4** Urethral functional and muscular disorders
Use additional code to identify associated urinary stress incontinence (N39.3)

N36.41 Hypermobility of urethra

N36.42 Intrinsic sphincter deficiency (ISD)

N36.43 Combined hypermobility of urethra and intrinsic sphincter deficiency

N36.44 Muscular disorders of urethra
Bladder sphincter dyssynergy

N36.5 Urethral false passage

N36.8 Other specified disorders of urethra

> EXCLUDES 1   congenital urethrocele (Q64.7)
> female urethrocele (N81.0)

N36.9 Urethral disorder, unspecified ▽

N37   *Urethral disorders in diseases classified elsewhere*
Code first underlying disease

> EXCLUDES 1   urethritis (in):
> candidal infection (B37.41)
> chlamydial (A56.01)
> gonorrhea (A54.01)
> syphilis (A52.76)
> trichomonal infection (A59.03)
> tuberculosis (A18.13)

✓4ᵗʰ **N39** Other disorders of urinary system

> EXCLUDES 2   hematuria NOS (R31.-)
> recurrent or persistent hematuria (N02.-)
> recurrent or persistent hematuria with specified morphological lesion (N02.-)
> proteinuria NOS (R80.-)

N39.0 Urinary tract infection, site not specified ▽
Use additional code (B95-B97), to identify infectious agent

> EXCLUDES 1   candidiasis of urinary tract (B37.4-)
> neonatal urinary tract infection (P39.3)
> urinary tract infection of specified site, such as:
> cystitis (N30.-)
> urethritis (N34.-)

AHA: 2017, 1Q, 6; 2012, 4Q, 94
TIP: Do not assign code based solely on laboratory results indicating positive bacterial growth unless such results have been interpreted by the provider, who confirmed a UTI diagnosis.

N39.3 Stress incontinence (female) (male)
Code also any associated overactive bladder (N32.81)

> EXCLUDES 1   mixed incontinence (N39.46)

✓5ᵗʰ **N39.4** Other specified urinary incontinence
Code also any associated overactive bladder (N32.81)

> EXCLUDES 1   enuresis NOS (R32)
> functional urinary incontinence (R39.81)
> urinary incontinence associated with cognitive impairment (R39.81)
> urinary incontinence NOS (R32)
> urinary incontinence of nonorganic origin (F98.0)

N39.41 Urge incontinence

> EXCLUDES 1   mixed incontinence (N39.46)

N39.42 Incontinence without sensory awareness
Insensible (urinary) incontinence

N39.43 Post-void dribbling

N39.44 Nocturnal enuresis

N39.45 Continuous leakage

N39.46 Mixed incontinence
Urge and stress incontinence

✓6ᵗʰ **N39.49** Other specified urinary incontinence

N39.490 Overflow incontinence

N39.491 Coital incontinence

N39.492 Postural (urinary) incontinence

N39.498 Other specified urinary incontinence
Reflex incontinence
Total incontinence

N39.8 Other specified disorders of urinary system

N39.9 Disorder of urinary system, unspecified ▽

Diseases of male genital organs (N40-N53)

✓4ᵗʰ **N40** Benign prostatic hyperplasia

> INCLUDES   adenofibromatous hypertrophy of prostate
> benign hypertrophy of the prostate
> benign prostatic hypertrophy
> BPH
> enlarged prostate
> nodular prostate
> polyp of prostate

> EXCLUDES 1   benign neoplasms of prostate (adenoma, benign) (fibroadenoma) (fibroma) (myoma) (D29.1)

> EXCLUDES 2   malignant neoplasm of prostate (C61)

N40.0 Benign prostatic hyperplasia without lower urinary tract symptoms   🅰♂
Enlarged prostate NOS
Enlarged prostate without LUTS

N40.1 Benign prostatic hyperplasia with lower urinary tract symptoms   🅰♂
Enlarged prostate with LUTS
Use additional code for associated symptoms, when specified:
incomplete bladder emptying (R39.14)
nocturia (R35.1)
straining on urination (R39.16)
urinary frequency (R35.0)
urinary hesitancy (R39.11)
urinary incontinence (N39.4-)
urinary obstruction (N13.8)
urinary retention (R33.8)
urinary urgency (R39.15)
weak urinary stream (R39.12)

N40.2 Nodular prostate without lower urinary tract symptoms   🅰♂
Nodular prostate without LUTS

N40.3 Nodular prostate with lower urinary tract symptoms A♂
　　Use additional code for associated symptoms, when specified:
　　　incomplete bladder emptying (R39.14)
　　　nocturia (R35.1)
　　　straining on urination (R39.16)
　　　urinary frequency (R35.0)
　　　urinary hesitancy (R39.11)
　　　urinary incontinence (N39.4-)
　　　urinary obstruction (N13.8)
　　　urinary retention (R33.8)
　　　urinary urgency (R39.15)
　　　weak urinary stream (R39.12)

✓4th **N41 Inflammatory diseases of prostate**
　　Use additional code (B95-B97), to identify infectious agent
　　N41.0 Acute prostatitis A♂
　　N41.1 Chronic prostatitis A♂
　　N41.2 Abscess of prostate A♂
　　N41.3 Prostatocystitis A♂
　　N41.4 Granulomatous prostatitis A♂
　　N41.8 Other inflammatory diseases of prostate A♂
　　N41.9 Inflammatory disease of prostate, unspecified A♂▽
　　　　Prostatitis NOS

✓4th **N42 Other and unspecified disorders of prostate**
　　N42.0 Calculus of prostate A♂
　　　　Prostatic stone
　　　　DEF: Formation of small, solid stone often composed of calcium
　　　　carbonate or calcium phosphate in the prostate gland.
　　N42.1 Congestion and hemorrhage of prostate A♂
　　　　EXCLUDES 1　enlarged prostate (N40.-)
　　　　　　　　　hematuria (R31.-)
　　　　　　　　　hyperplasia of prostate (N40.-)
　　　　　　　　　inflammatory diseases of prostate (N41.-)
　✓5th **N42.3 Dysplasia of prostate**
　　　N42.30 Unspecified dysplasia of prostate ♂▽
　　　N42.31 Prostatic intraepithelial neoplasia ♂
　　　　　PIN
　　　　　Prostatic intraepithelial neoplasia I (PIN I)
　　　　　Prostatic intraepithelial neoplasia II (PIN II)
　　　　　EXCLUDES 1　prostatic intraepithelial neoplasia III (PIN III)
　　　　　　　　　　(D07.5)
　　　　　DEF: Abnormality of shape and size of the intraepithelial
　　　　　tissues of the prostate; premalignant condition
　　　　　characterized by stalks and absence of a basilar cell
　　　　　layer; synonyms are intraductal dysplasia, large acinar
　　　　　atypical hyperplasia, atypical primary hyperplasia,
　　　　　hyperplasia with malignant changes, marked atypia, or
　　　　　duct-acinar dysplasia.
　　　N42.32 Atypical small acinar proliferation of prostate ♂
　　　N42.39 Other dysplasia of prostate ♂
　✓5th **N42.8 Other specified disorders of prostate**
　　　N42.81 Prostatodynia syndrome A♂
　　　　　Painful prostate syndrome
　　　N42.82 Prostatosis syndrome A♂
　　　N42.83 Cyst of prostate A♂
　　　N42.89 Other specified disorders of prostate A♂
　　N42.9 Disorder of prostate, unspecified A♂▽

✓4th **N43 Hydrocele and spermatocele**
　　INCLUDES　hydrocele of spermatic cord, testis or tunica vaginalis
　　EXCLUDES 1　congenital hydrocele (P83.5)
　　N43.0 Encysted hydrocele ♂
　　N43.1 Infected hydrocele ♂
　　　　Use additional code (B95-B97), to identify infectious agent
　　N43.2 Other hydrocele ♂
　　N43.3 Hydrocele, unspecified ♂▽
　✓5th **N43.4 Spermatocele of epididymis**
　　　　Spermatic cyst
　　　N43.40 Spermatocele of epididymis, unspecified ♂▽
　　　N43.41 Spermatocele of epididymis, single ♂
　　　N43.42 Spermatocele of epididymis, multiple ♂

Hydrocele

Normal　　Noncommunicating hydrocele　　Communicating hydrocele　　Hydrocele of the cord

Testicle
Scrotum

✓4th **N44 Noninflammatory disorders of testis**
　✓5th **N44.0 Torsion of testis**
　　　N44.00 Torsion of testis, unspecified ♂▽
　　　N44.01 Extravaginal torsion of spermatic cord ♂
　　　　　DEF: Torsion of the spermatic cord just below the tunica
　　　　　vaginalis attachments.
　　　N44.02 Intravaginal torsion of spermatic cord ♂
　　　　　Torsion of spermatic cord NOS
　　　N44.03 Torsion of appendix testis ♂
　　　N44.04 Torsion of appendix epididymis ♂
　　N44.1 Cyst of tunica albuginea testis ♂
　　N44.2 Benign cyst of testis ♂
　　N44.8 Other noninflammatory disorders of the testis ♂

✓4th **N45 Orchitis and epididymitis**
　　Use additional code (B95-B97), to identify infectious agent
　　N45.1 Epididymitis ♂
　　N45.2 Orchitis ♂
　　N45.3 Epididymo-orchitis ♂
　　N45.4 Abscess of epididymis or testis ♂

✓4th **N46 Male infertility**
　　EXCLUDES 1　vasectomy status (Z98.52)
　✓5th **N46.0 Azoospermia**
　　　　Absolute male infertility
　　　　Male infertility due to germinal (cell) aplasia
　　　　Male infertility due to spermatogenic arrest (complete)
　　　N46.01 Organic azoospermia A♂
　　　　　Azoospermia NOS
　　✓6th **N46.02 Azoospermia due to extratesticular causes**
　　　　　Code also associated cause
　　　　N46.021 Azoospermia due to drug therapy A♂
　　　　N46.022 Azoospermia due to infection A♂
　　　　N46.023 Azoospermia due to obstruction of efferent ducts A♂
　　　　N46.024 Azoospermia due to radiation A♂
　　　　N46.025 Azoospermia due to systemic disease A♂
　　　　N46.029 Azoospermia due to other extratesticular causes A♂
　✓5th **N46.1 Oligospermia**
　　　　Male infertility due to germinal cell desquamation
　　　　Male infertility due to hypospermatogenesis
　　　　Male infertility due to incomplete spermatogenic arrest
　　　N46.11 Organic oligospermia A♂
　　　　　Oligospermia NOS
　　✓6th **N46.12 Oligospermia due to extratesticular causes**
　　　　　Code also associated cause
　　　　N46.121 Oligospermia due to drug therapy A♂
　　　　N46.122 Oligospermia due to infection A♂
　　　　N46.123 Oligospermia due to obstruction of efferent ducts A♂
　　　　N46.124 Oligospermia due to radiation A♂
　　　　N46.125 Oligospermia due to systemic disease A♂
　　　　N46.129 Oligospermia due to other extratesticular causes A♂
　　N46.8 Other male infertility A♂
　　N46.9 Male infertility, unspecified A♂▽

✓4ᵗʰ **N47 Disorders of prepuce**

    N47.0 Adherent prepuce, newborn   N ♂

    N47.1 Phimosis   ♂

    N47.2 Paraphimosis   ♂

    N47.3 Deficient foreskin   ♂

    N47.4 Benign cyst of prepuce   ♂

    N47.5 Adhesions of prepuce and glans penis   ♂

    N47.6 Balanoposthitis   ♂
        Use additional code (B95-B97), to identify infectious agent
           EXCLUDES 1   *balanitis (N48.1)*

    N47.7 Other inflammatory diseases of prepuce   ♂
        Use additional code (B95-B97), to identify infectious agent

    N47.8 Other disorders of prepuce   ♂

✓4ᵗʰ **N48 Other disorders of penis**

    N48.0 Leukoplakia of penis   ♂
        Balanitis xerotica obliterans
        Kraurosis of penis
        Lichen sclerosus of external male genital organs
           EXCLUDES 1   *carcinoma in situ of penis (D07.4)*

    N48.1 Balanitis   ♂
        Use additional code (B95-B97), to identify infectious agent
           EXCLUDES 1   *amebic balanitis (A06.8)*
                   balanitis xerotica obliterans (N48.0)
                   candidal balanitis (B37.42)
                   gonococcal balanitis (A54.23)
                   herpesviral [herpes simplex] balanitis (A60.01)

✓5ᵗʰ   **N48.2 Other inflammatory disorders of penis**
        Use additional code (B95-B97), to identify infectious agent
           EXCLUDES 1   *balanitis (N48.1)*
                   balanitis xerotica obliterans (N48.0)
                   balanoposthitis (N47.6)

        N48.21 Abscess of corpus cavernosum and penis   ♂

        N48.22 Cellulitis of corpus cavernosum and penis   ♂

        N48.29 Other inflammatory disorders of penis   ♂

✓5ᵗʰ   **N48.3 Priapism**
        Painful erection
        Code first underlying cause

        N48.30 Priapism, unspecified   ♂ ▽

        N48.31 Priapism due to trauma   ♂

        N48.32 *Priapism due to disease classified elsewhere*   ♂

        N48.33 Priapism, drug-induced   ♂

        N48.39 Other priapism   ♂

    N48.5 Ulcer of penis   ♂

    N48.6 Induration penis plastica   ♂
        Peyronie's disease
        Plastic induration of penis

✓5ᵗʰ   **N48.8 Other specified disorders of penis**

        N48.81 Thrombosis of superficial vein of penis   ♂

        N48.82 Acquired torsion of penis   ♂
           Acquired torsion of penis NOS
           EXCLUDES 1   *congenital torsion of penis (Q55.63)*

        N48.83 Acquired buried penis   ♂
           EXCLUDES 1   *congenital hidden penis (Q55.64)*

        N48.89 Other specified disorders of penis   ♂

    N48.9 Disorder of penis, unspecified   ♂ ▽

✓4ᵗʰ **N49 Inflammatory disorders of male genital organs, not elsewhere classified**
        Use additional code (B95-B97), to identify infectious agent
           EXCLUDES 1   *inflammation of penis (N48.1, N48.2-)*
                   orchitis and epididymitis (N45.-)

    N49.0 Inflammatory disorders of seminal vesicle   ♂
        Vesiculitis NOS

    N49.1 Inflammatory disorders of spermatic cord, tunica vaginalis and vas deferens   ♂
        Vasitis

    N49.2 Inflammatory disorders of scrotum   ♂

    N49.3 Fournier gangrene   ♂

    N49.8 Inflammatory disorders of other specified male genital organs   ♂
        Inflammation of multiple sites in male genital organs

    N49.9 Inflammatory disorder of unspecified male genital organ   ♂ ▽
        Abscess of unspecified male genital organ
        Boil of unspecified male genital organ
        Carbuncle of unspecified male genital organ
        Cellulitis of unspecified male genital organ

✓4ᵗʰ **N50 Other and unspecified disorders of male genital organs**
        EXCLUDES 2   *torsion of testis (N44.0-)*

    N50.0 Atrophy of testis   ♂

    N50.1 Vascular disorders of male genital organs   ♂
        Hematocele, NOS, of male genital organs
        Hemorrhage of male genital organs
        Thrombosis of male genital organs

    N50.3 Cyst of epididymis   ♂

✓5ᵗʰ   **N50.8 Other specified disorders of male genital organs**

    ✓6ᵗʰ **N50.81 Testicular pain**

        N50.811 Right testicular pain   ♂

        N50.812 Left testicular pain   ♂

        N50.819 Testicular pain, unspecified   ♂ ▽

        N50.82 Scrotal pain   ♂

        N50.89 Other specified disorders of the male genital organs   ♂
           Atrophy of scrotum, seminal vesicle, spermatic cord, tunica vaginalis and vas deferens
           Chylocele, tunica vaginalis (nonfilarial) NOS
           Edema of scrotum, seminal vesicle, spermatic cord, tunica vaginalis and vas deferens
           Hypertrophy of scrotum, seminal vesicle, spermatic cord, tunica vaginalis and vas deferens
           Stricture of spermatic cord, tunica vaginalis, and vas deferens
           Ulcer of scrotum, seminal vesicle, spermatic cord, testis, tunica vaginalis and vas deferens
           Urethroscrotal fistula

    N50.9 Disorder of male genital organs, unspecified   ♂ ▽

N51   ***Disorders of male genital organs in diseases classified elsewhere***   ♂
        Code first underlying disease, such as:
           filariasis (B74.0-B74.9)
           EXCLUDES 1   *amebic balanitis (A06.8)*
                   candidal balanitis (B37.42)
                   gonococcal balanitis (A54.23)
                   gonococcal prostatitis (A54.22)
                   herpesviral [herpes simplex] balanitis (A60.01)
                   trichomonal prostatitis (A59.02)
                   tuberculous prostatitis (A18.14)

✓4ᵗʰ **N52 Male erectile dysfunction**
        EXCLUDES 1   *psychogenic impotence (F52.21)*

✓5ᵗʰ   **N52.0 Vasculogenic erectile dysfunction**

        N52.01 Erectile dysfunction due to arterial insufficiency   A ♂

        N52.02 Corporo-venous occlusive erectile dysfunction   A ♂

        N52.03 Combined arterial insufficiency and corporo-venous occlusive erectile dysfunction   A ♂

    N52.1 *Erectile dysfunction due to diseases classified elsewhere*   A ♂
        Code first underlying disease

    N52.2 Drug-induced erectile dysfunction   A ♂

✓5ᵗʰ   **N52.3 Postprocedural erectile dysfunction**

        N52.31 Erectile dysfunction following radical prostatectomy   A ♂

        N52.32 Erectile dysfunction following radical cystectomy   A ♂

        N52.33 Erectile dysfunction following urethral surgery   A ♂

        N52.34 Erectile dysfunction following simple prostatectomy   A ♂

        N52.35 Erectile dysfunction following radiation therapy   A ♂

        N52.36 Erectile dysfunction following interstitial seed therapy   A ♂

        N52.37 Erectile dysfunction following prostate ablative therapy   A ♂
           Erectile dysfunction following cryotherapy
           Erectile dysfunction following other prostate ablative therapies
           Erectile dysfunction following ultrasound ablative therapies

        N52.39 Other and unspecified postprocedural erectile dysfunction   A ♂ ▽

N52.8   Other male erectile dysfunction   A♂

N52.9   Male erectile dysfunction, unspecified   A♂▽
     Impotence NOS

✓4ᵗʰ **N53   Other male sexual dysfunction**
     EXCLUDES 1   *psychogenic sexual dysfunction (F52.-)*

   ✓5ᵗʰ **N53.1   Ejaculatory dysfunction**
     EXCLUDES 1   *premature ejaculation (F52.4)*

     N53.11   Retarded ejaculation   ♂

     N53.12   Painful ejaculation   ♂

     N53.13   Anejaculatory orgasm   ♂

     N53.14   Retrograde ejaculation   ♂
       DEF: A form of male sexual dysfunction in which the semen enters the bladder instead of going out through the urethra during ejaculation.

     N53.19   Other ejaculatory dysfunction   ♂
       Ejaculatory dysfunction NOS

   N53.8   Other male sexual dysfunction   ♂

   N53.9   Unspecified male sexual dysfunction   ♂▽

Disorders of breast (N60-N65)

EXCLUDES 1   *disorders of breast associated with childbirth (O91-O92)*

✓4ᵗʰ **N60   Benign mammary dysplasia**
     INCLUDES   fibrocystic mastopathy

   ✓5ᵗʰ **N60.0   Solitary cyst of breast**
     Cyst of breast

     N60.01   Solitary cyst of right breast

     N60.02   Solitary cyst of left breast

     N60.09   Solitary cyst of unspecified breast   ▽

   ✓5ᵗʰ **N60.1   Diffuse cystic mastopathy**
     Cystic breast
     Fibrocystic disease of breast
     EXCLUDES 1   *diffuse cystic mastopathy with epithelial proliferation (N60.3-)*

     N60.11   Diffuse cystic mastopathy of right breast   A

     N60.12   Diffuse cystic mastopathy of left breast   A

     N60.19   Diffuse cystic mastopathy of unspecified breast   A▽

   ✓5ᵗʰ **N60.2   Fibroadenosis of breast**
     Adenofibrosis of breast
     EXCLUDES 2   *fibroadenoma of breast (D24.-)*

     N60.21   Fibroadenosis of right breast

     N60.22   Fibroadenosis of left breast

     N60.29   Fibroadenosis of unspecified breast   ▽

   ✓5ᵗʰ **N60.3   Fibrosclerosis of breast**
     Cystic mastopathy with epithelial proliferation

     N60.31   Fibrosclerosis of right breast

     N60.32   Fibrosclerosis of left breast

     N60.39   Fibrosclerosis of unspecified breast   ▽

   ✓5ᵗʰ **N60.4   Mammary duct ectasia**

     N60.41   Mammary duct ectasia of right breast

     N60.42   Mammary duct ectasia of left breast

     N60.49   Mammary duct ectasia of unspecified breast   ▽

   ✓5ᵗʰ **N60.8   Other benign mammary dysplasias**

     N60.81   Other benign mammary dysplasias of right breast

     N60.82   Other benign mammary dysplasias of left breast

     N60.89   Other benign mammary dysplasias of unspecified breast   ▽

   ✓5ᵗʰ **N60.9   Unspecified benign mammary dysplasia**

     N60.91   Unspecified benign mammary dysplasia of right breast   ▽

     N60.92   Unspecified benign mammary dysplasia of left breast   ▽

     N60.99   Unspecified benign mammary dysplasia of unspecified breast   ▽

✓4ᵗʰ **N61   Inflammatory disorders of breast**
     EXCLUDES 1   *inflammatory carcinoma of breast (C50.9)*
       inflammatory disorder of breast associated with childbirth (O91.-)
       neonatal infective mastitis (P39.0)
       thrombophlebitis of breast [Mondor's disease] (I80.8)

N61.0   Mastitis without abscess
     Infective mastitis (acute) (nonpuerperal) (subacute)
     Mastitis (acute) (nonpuerperal) (subacute) NOS
     Cellulitis (acute) (nonpuerperal) (subacute) of breast NOS
     Cellulitis (acute) (nonpuerperal) (subacute) of nipple NOS

N61.1   Abscess of the breast and nipple
     Abscess (acute) (chronic) (nonpuerperal) of areola
     Abscess (acute) (chronic) (nonpuerperal) of breast
     Carbuncle of breast
     Mastitis with abscess

N62   Hypertrophy of breast
     Gynecomastia
     Hypertrophy of breast NOS
     Massive pubertal hypertrophy of breast
     EXCLUDES 1   *breast engorgement of newborn (P83.4)*
       disproportion of reconstructed breast (N65.1)

✓4ᵗʰ **N63   Unspecified lump in breast**
     Nodule(s) NOS in breast

●   **N63.0   Unspecified lump in unspecified breast**   ▽

●   ✓5ᵗʰ **N63.1   Unspecified lump in the right breast**

●   **N63.10   Unspecified lump in the right breast, unspecified quadrant**   ▽

●   **N63.11   Unspecified lump in the right breast, upper outer quadrant**   ▽

●   **N63.12   Unspecified lump in the right breast, upper inner quadrant**   ▽

●   **N63.13   Unspecified lump in the right breast, lower outer quadrant**   ▽

●   **N63.14   Unspecified lump in the right breast, lower inner quadrant**   ▽

●   ✓5ᵗʰ **N63.2   Unspecified lump in the left breast**

●   **N63.20   Unspecified lump in the left breast, unspecified quadrant**   ▽

●   **N63.21   Unspecified lump in the left breast, upper outer quadrant**   ▽

●   **N63.22   Unspecified lump in the left breast, upper inner quadrant**   ▽

●   **N63.23   Unspecified lump in the left breast, lower outer quadrant**   ▽

●   **N63.24   Unspecified lump in the left breast, lower inner quadrant**   ▽

●   ✓5ᵗʰ **N63.3   Unspecified lump in axillary tail**

●   **N63.31   Unspecified lump in axillary tail of the right breast**   ▽

●   **N63.32   Unspecified lump in axillary tail of the left breast**   ▽

●   ✓5ᵗʰ **N63.4   Unspecified lump in breast, subareolar**

●   **N63.41   Unspecified lump in right breast, subareolar**   ▽

●   **N63.42   Unspecified lump in left breast, subareolar**   ▽

✓4ᵗʰ **N64   Other disorders of breast**
     EXCLUDES 2   *mechanical complication of breast prosthesis and implant (T85.4-)*

N64.0   Fissure and fistula of nipple

N64.1   Fat necrosis of breast
     Fat necrosis (segmental) of breast
     Code first breast necrosis due to breast graft (T85.898)

N64.2   Atrophy of breast

N64.3   Galactorrhea not associated with childbirth

N64.4   Mastodynia

   ✓5ᵗʰ **N64.5   Other signs and symptoms in breast**
     EXCLUDES 2   *abnormal findings on diagnostic imaging of breast (R92.-)*

     N64.51   Induration of breast

     N64.52   Nipple discharge
       EXCLUDES 1   *abnormal findings in nipple discharge (R89.-)*

     N64.53   Retraction of nipple

     N64.59   Other signs and symptoms in breast

   ✓5ᵗʰ **N64.8   Other specified disorders of breast**

     N64.81   Ptosis of breast   A
       EXCLUDES 1   *ptosis of native breast in relation to reconstructed breast (N65.1)*

✔ Additional Character Req   ✔x7ᵗʰ Placeholder Alert   Case-Mix Diagnosis   Manifestation   ▽ Unspecified Dx   EXCLUDES 1 Not coded here   EXCLUDES 2 Not included here

ICD-10-CM 2018   811

N52.8–N64.81

N64.82 Hypoplasia of breast   A
Micromastia
EXCLUDES 1   *congenital absence of breast (Q83.0)*
hypoplasia of native breast in relation to reconstructed breast (N65.1)

N64.89 Other specified disorders of breast
Galactocele
Subinvolution of breast (postlactational)

N64.9 Disorder of breast, unspecified   ▽

✓4ᵗʰ **N65 Deformity and disproportion of reconstructed breast**

N65.0 Deformity of reconstructed breast   A
Contour irregularity in reconstructed breast
Excess tissue in reconstructed breast
Misshapen reconstructed breast

N65.1 Disproportion of reconstructed breast   A
Breast asymmetry between native breast and reconstructed breast
Disproportion between native breast and reconstructed breast

Inflammatory diseases of female pelvic organs (N70-N77)

EXCLUDES 1   *inflammatory diseases of female pelvic organs complicating:*
abortion or ectopic or molar pregnancy (O00-O07, O08.0)
pregnancy, childbirth and the puerperium (O23-, O75.3, O85, O86-)

✓4ᵗʰ **N70 Salpingitis and oophoritis**
INCLUDES   abscess (of) fallopian tube
abscess (of) ovary
pyosalpinx
salpingo-oophoritis
tubo-ovarian abscess
tubo-ovarian inflammatory disease
Use additional code (B95-B97), to identify infectious agent
EXCLUDES 1   *gonococcal infection (A54.24)*
tuberculous infection (A18.17)

✓5ᵗʰ **N70.0 Acute salpingitis and oophoritis**
   N70.01 Acute salpingitis   ♀
   N70.02 Acute oophoritis   ♀
   N70.03 Acute salpingitis and oophoritis   ♀

✓5ᵗʰ **N70.1 Chronic salpingitis and oophoritis**
Hydrosalpinx
   N70.11 Chronic salpingitis   ♀
   N70.12 Chronic oophoritis   ♀
   N70.13 Chronic salpingitis and oophoritis   ♀

✓5ᵗʰ **N70.9 Salpingitis and oophoritis, unspecified**
   N70.91 Salpingitis, unspecified   ♀ ▽
   N70.92 Oophoritis, unspecified   ♀ ▽
   N70.93 Salpingitis and oophoritis, unspecified   ♀ ▽

✓4ᵗʰ **N71 Inflammatory disease of uterus, except cervix**
INCLUDES   endo (myo) metritis
metritis
myometritis
pyometra
uterine abscess
Use additional code (B95-B97), to identify infectious agent
EXCLUDES 1   *hyperplastic endometritis (N85.0-)*
infection of uterus following delivery (O85, O86.-)

N71.0 Acute inflammatory disease of uterus   ♀
N71.1 Chronic inflammatory disease of uterus   ♀
N71.9 Inflammatory disease of uterus, unspecified   ♀ ▽

N72 Inflammatory disease of cervix uteri   ♀
INCLUDES   cervicitis (with or without erosion or ectropion)
endocervicitis (with or without erosion or ectropion)
exocervicitis (with or without erosion or ectropion)
Use additional code (B95-B97), to identify infectious agent
EXCLUDES 1   *erosion and ectropion of cervix without cervicitis (N86)*

✓4ᵗʰ **N73 Other female pelvic inflammatory diseases**
Use additional code (B95-B97), to identify infectious agent

N73.0 Acute parametritis and pelvic cellulitis   ♀
Abscess of broad ligament
Abscess of parametrium
Pelvic cellulitis, female
DEF: Parametritis: Inflammation of the parametrium; pelvic cellulitis is a synonym for parametritis.

N73.1 Chronic parametritis and pelvic cellulitis   ♀
Any condition in N73.0 specified as chronic
EXCLUDES 1   *tuberculous parametritis and pelvic cellulitis (A18.17)*

N73.2 Unspecified parametritis and pelvic cellulitis   ♀ ▽
Any condition in N73.0 unspecified whether acute or chronic

N73.3 Female acute pelvic peritonitis   ♀
N73.4 Female chronic pelvic peritonitis   ♀
EXCLUDES 1   *tuberculous pelvic (female) peritonitis (A18.17)*

N73.5 Female pelvic peritonitis, unspecified   ♀ ▽
N73.6 Female pelvic peritoneal adhesions (postinfective)   ♀
EXCLUDES 2   *postprocedural pelvic peritoneal adhesions (N99.4)*
AHA: 2014, 1Q, 6

N73.8 Other specified female pelvic inflammatory diseases   ♀
N73.9 Female pelvic inflammatory disease, unspecified   ♀ ▽
Female pelvic infection or inflammation NOS

N74 Female pelvic inflammatory disorders in diseases classified elsewhere   ♀
Code first underlying disease
EXCLUDES 1   *chlamydial cervicitis (A56.02)*
chlamydial pelvic inflammatory disease (A56.11)
gonococcal cervicitis (A54.03)
gonococcal pelvic inflammatory disease (A54.24)
herpesviral [herpes simplex] cervicitis (A60.03)
herpesviral [herpes simplex] pelvic inflammatory disease (A60.09)
syphilitic cervicitis (A52.76)
syphilitic pelvic inflammatory disease (A52.76)
trichomonal cervicitis (A59.09)
tuberculous cervicitis (A18.16)
tuberculous pelvic inflammatory disease (A18.17)

✓4ᵗʰ **N75 Diseases of Bartholin's gland**
N75.0 Cyst of Bartholin's gland   ♀
N75.1 Abscess of Bartholin's gland   ♀
N75.8 Other diseases of Bartholin's gland   ♀
Bartholinitis
N75.9 Disease of Bartholin's gland, unspecified   ♀ ▽

✓4ᵗʰ **N76 Other inflammation of vagina and vulva**
Use additional code (B95-B97), to identify infectious agent
EXCLUDES 2   *senile (atrophic) vaginitis (N95.2)*
vulvar vestibulitis (N94.810)

N76.0 Acute vaginitis   ♀
Acute vulvovaginitis
Vaginitis NOS
Vulvovaginitis NOS

N76.1 Subacute and chronic vaginitis   ♀
Chronic vulvovaginitis
Subacute vulvovaginitis

N76.2 Acute vulvitis   ♀
Vulvitis NOS

N76.3 Subacute and chronic vulvitis   ♀
N76.4 Abscess of vulva   ♀
Furuncle of vulva
N76.5 Ulceration of vagina   ♀
N76.6 Ulceration of vulva   ♀

✓5ᵗʰ **N76.8 Other specified inflammation of vagina and vulva**
   N76.81 Mucositis (ulcerative) of vagina and vulva   ♀
Code also type of associated therapy, such as:
antineoplastic and immunosuppressive drugs (T45.1X-)
radiological procedure and radiotherapy (Y84.2)
EXCLUDES 2   *gastrointestinal mucositis (ulcerative) (K92.81)*
nasal mucositis (ulcerative) (J34.81)
oral mucositis (ulcerative) (K12.3-)

   N76.89 Other specified inflammation of vagina and vulva   ♀

✓4ᵗʰ **N77 Vulvovaginal ulceration and inflammation in diseases classified elsewhere**
N77.0 Ulceration of vulva in diseases classified elsewhere   ♀
Code first underlying disease, such as:
Behçet's disease (M35.2)
EXCLUDES 1   *ulceration of vulva in gonococcal infection (A54.02)*
ulceration of vulva in herpesviral [herpes simplex] infection (A60.04)
ulceration of vulva in syphilis (A51.0)
ulceration of vulva in tuberculosis (A18.18)

N Newborn: 0   P Pediatric: 0-17   M Maternity: 12-55   A Adult: 15-124   NRS Nonroutine supply Dx   NC Dx Noncancer Dx   PD Dx Primary Dx   ▶◀ Revised Text   ● New Code   ▲ Revised Title

812   ICD-10-CM 2018

N77.1   *Vaginitis, vulvitis and vulvovaginitis in diseases classified elsewhere*   ♀

> Code first underlying disease, such as:
> pinworm (B80)
>
> EXCLUDES 1   *candidal vulvovaginitis (B37.3)*
> *chlamydial vulvovaginitis (A56.02)*
> *gonococcal vulvovaginitis (A54.02)*
> *herpesviral [herpes simplex] vulvovaginitis (A60.04)*
> *trichomonal vulvovaginitis (A59.01)*
> *tuberculous vulvovaginitis (A18.18)*
> *vulvovaginitis in early syphilis (A51.0)*
> *vulvovaginitis in late syphilis (A52.76)*

Noninflammatory disorders of female genital tract (N80-N98)

✓4ᵗʰ **N80**   **Endometriosis**

N80.0   **Endometriosis of** uterus
> Adenomyosis
> EXCLUDES 1   *stromal endometriosis (D39.0)*

N80.1   **Endometriosis of** ovary   ♀

N80.2   **Endometriosis of** fallopian tube   ♀

N80.3   **Endometriosis of** pelvic peritoneum   ♀

N80.4   **Endometriosis of** rectovaginal septum and vagina   ♀

N80.5   **Endometriosis of** intestine   ♀

N80.6   **Endometriosis in** cutaneous scar   ♀

N80.8   **Other endometriosis**   ♀
> ▶Endometriosis of thorax◀

N80.9   **Endometriosis, unspecified**   ♀ ▽

✓4ᵗʰ **N81**   **Female genital prolapse**

> EXCLUDES 1   *genital prolapse complicating pregnancy, labor or delivery (O34.5-)*
> *prolapse and hernia of ovary and fallopian tube (N83.4-)*
> *prolapse of vaginal vault after hysterectomy (N99.3)*

N81.0   **Urethrocele**   ♀
> EXCLUDES 1   *urethrocele with cystocele (N81.1-)*
> *urethrocele with prolapse of uterus (N81.2-N81.4)*

✓5ᵗʰ **N81.1**   **Cystocele**
> Cystocele with urethrocele
> Cystourethrocele
> EXCLUDES 1   *cystocele with prolapse of uterus (N81.2-N81.4)*

N81.10   **Cystocele, unspecified**   ♀ ▽
> Prolapse of (anterior) vaginal wall NOS

N81.11   **Cystocele, midline**   ♀

N81.12   **Cystocele, lateral**   ♀
> Paravaginal cystocele
> **DEF:** Detachment of the lateral support connections of the vagina at the arcus tendineus fasciae pelvis (ATFP) results in bladder drop; bladder herniates into the vagina laterally.

N81.2   **Incomplete** uterovaginal prolapse   ♀
> First degree uterine prolapse
> Prolapse of cervix NOS
> Second degree uterine prolapse
> EXCLUDES 1   ▶cervical stump prolapse◀ (N81.85)

N81.3   **Complete** uterovaginal prolapse   ♀
> Procidentia (uteri) NOS
> Third degree uterine prolapse

N81.4   **Uterovaginal prolapse, unspecified**   ♀ ▽
> Prolapse of uterus NOS

N81.5   **Vaginal enterocele**   ♀
> EXCLUDES 1   *enterocele with prolapse of uterus (N81.2-N81.4)*

N81.6   **Rectocele**   ♀
> Prolapse of posterior vaginal wall
> Use additional code for any associated fecal incontinence, if applicable (R15.-)
> EXCLUDES 2   *perineocele (N81.81)*
> *rectal prolapse (K62.3)*
> *rectocele with prolapse of uterus (N81.2-N81.4)*

✓5ᵗʰ **N81.8**   **Other female genital prolapse**

N81.81   **Perineocele**   ♀

N81.82   **Incompetence or weakening of** pubocervical tissue   ♀

N81.83   **Incompetence or weakening of** rectovaginal tissue   ♀

N81.84   **Pelvic muscle wasting**   ♀
> Disuse atrophy of pelvic muscles and anal sphincter

N81.85   **Cervical stump prolapse**   ♀

Types of Pelvic Organ Prolapse

Urethrocele

Cystocele

Rectocele

Enterocele

N81.89   **Other female genital prolapse**   ♀
> Deficient perineum
> Old laceration of muscles of pelvic floor

N81.9   **Female genital prolapse, unspecified**   ♀ ▽

✓4ᵗʰ **N82**   **Fistulae involving female genital tract**
> EXCLUDES 1   *vesicointestinal fistulae (N32.1)*

N82.0   **Vesicovaginal** fistula   ♀

N82.1   **Other female urinary-genital tract fistulae**   ♀
> Cervicovesical fistula
> Ureterovaginal fistula
> Urethrovaginal fistula
> Uteroureteric fistula
> Uterovesical fistula

N82.2   **Fistula of vagina to** small **intestine**   ♀

N82.3   **Fistula of vagina to** large **intestine**   ♀
> Rectovaginal fistula

N82.4   **Other female intestinal-genital tract fistulae**   ♀
> Intestinouterine fistula

N82.5   **Female** genital tract-skin **fistulae**   ♀
> Uterus to abdominal wall fistula
> Vaginoperineal fistula

N82.8   **Other female genital tract fistulae**   ♀

N82.9   **Female genital tract fistula, unspecified**   ♀ ▽

✓4ᵗʰ **N83**   **Noninflammatory disorders of ovary, fallopian tube and broad ligament**
> EXCLUDES 2   *hydrosalpinx (N70.1-)*

✓5ᵗʰ **N83.0**   **Follicular cyst of ovary**
> Cyst of graafian follicle
> Hemorrhagic follicular cyst (of ovary)

N83.00   **Follicular cyst of ovary, unspecified side**   ♀ ▽

N83.01   **Follicular cyst of** right **ovary**   ♀

N83.02   **Follicular cyst of** left **ovary**   ♀

✓5ᵗʰ **N83.1**   **Corpus luteum cyst**
> Hemorrhagic corpus luteum cyst

N83.10   **Corpus luteum cyst of ovary, unspecified side**   ♀ ▽

N83.11   **Corpus luteum cyst of** right **ovary**   ♀

N83.12   **Corpus luteum cyst of** left **ovary**   ♀

✓5ᵗʰ **N83.2**   **Other and unspecified ovarian cysts**
> EXCLUDES 1   *developmental ovarian cyst (Q50.1)*
> *neoplastic ovarian cyst (D27.-)*
> *polycystic ovarian syndrome (E28.2)*
> *Stein-Leventhal syndrome (E28.2)*

✓6ᵗʰ **N83.20**   **Unspecified ovarian cysts**

N83.201   **Unspecified ovarian cyst,** right **side**   ♀ ▽

N83.202   **Unspecified ovarian cyst,** left **side**   ♀ ▽

N83.209   **Unspecified ovarian cyst, unspecified side**   ♀ ▽
> Ovarian cyst, NOS

☑ Additional Character Req   ✓ˣ7ᵗʰ Placeholder Alert   Case-Mix Diagnosis   Manifestation   ▽ Unspecified Dx   EXCLUDES 1 Not coded here   EXCLUDES 2 Not included here

✓6ᵗʰ N83.29 Other ovarian cysts
Retention cyst of ovary
Simple cyst of ovary

N83.291 Other ovarian cyst, right side ♀
N83.292 Other ovarian cyst, left side ♀
N83.299 Other ovarian cyst, unspecified side ♀▽

✓5ᵗʰ N83.3 Acquired atrophy of ovary and fallopian tube

✓6ᵗʰ N83.31 Acquired atrophy of ovary
N83.311 Acquired atrophy of right ovary ♀
N83.312 Acquired atrophy of left ovary ♀
N83.319 Acquired atrophy of ovary, unspecified side ♀▽
Acquired atrophy of ovary, NOS

✓6ᵗʰ N83.32 Acquired atrophy of fallopian tube
N83.321 Acquired atrophy of right fallopian tube ♀
N83.322 Acquired atrophy of left fallopian tube ♀
N83.329 Acquired atrophy of fallopian tube, unspecified side ♀▽
Acquired atrophy of fallopian tube, NOS

✓6ᵗʰ N83.33 Acquired atrophy of ovary and fallopian tube
N83.331 Acquired atrophy of right ovary and fallopian tube ♀
N83.332 Acquired atrophy of left ovary and fallopian tube ♀
N83.339 Acquired atrophy of ovary and fallopian tube, unspecified side ♀▽
Acquired atrophy of ovary and fallopian tube, NOS

✓5ᵗʰ N83.4 Prolapse and hernia of ovary and fallopian tube
N83.40 Prolapse and hernia of ovary and fallopian tube, unspecified side ♀▽
Prolapse and hernia of ovary and fallopian tube, NOS
N83.41 Prolapse and hernia of right ovary and fallopian tube ♀
N83.42 Prolapse and hernia of left ovary and fallopian tube ♀

✓5ᵗʰ N83.5 Torsion of ovary, ovarian pedicle and fallopian tube
Torsion of accessory tube

✓6ᵗʰ N83.51 Torsion of ovary and ovarian pedicle
N83.511 Torsion of right ovary and ovarian pedicle ♀
N83.512 Torsion of left ovary and ovarian pedicle ♀
N83.519 Torsion of ovary and ovarian pedicle, unspecified side ♀▽
Torsion of ovary and ovarian pedicle, NOS

✓6ᵗʰ N83.52 Torsion of fallopian tube
Torsion of hydatid of Morgagni
N83.521 Torsion of right fallopian tube ♀
N83.522 Torsion of left fallopian tube ♀
N83.529 Torsion of fallopian tube, unspecified side ♀▽
Torsion of fallopian tube, NOS

N83.53 Torsion of ovary, ovarian pedicle and fallopian tube ♀

N83.6 Hematosalpinx ♀
EXCLUDES 1 hematosalpinx (with) (in):
hematocolpos (N89.7)
hematometra (N85.7)
tubal pregnancy (O00.1-)

N83.7 Hematoma of broad ligament ♀

N83.8 Other noninflammatory disorders of ovary, fallopian tube and broad ligament ♀
Broad ligament laceration syndrome [Allen-Masters]

N83.9 Noninflammatory disorder of ovary, fallopian tube and broad ligament, unspecified ♀▽

✓4ᵗʰ N84 Polyp of female genital tract
EXCLUDES 1 adenomatous polyp (D28.-)
placental polyp (O90.89)

N84.0 Polyp of corpus uteri ♀
Polyp of endometrium
Polyp of uterus NOS
EXCLUDES 1 polypoid endometrial hyperplasia (N85.0-)

N84.1 Polyp of cervix uteri ♀
Mucous polyp of cervix

N84.2 Polyp of vagina ♀

Inversion of Uterus

Uterus

N84.3 Polyp of vulva ♀
Polyp of labia

N84.8 Polyp of other parts of female genital tract ♀

N84.9 Polyp of female genital tract, unspecified ♀▽

✓4ᵗʰ N85 Other noninflammatory disorders of uterus, except cervix
EXCLUDES 1 endometriosis (N80.-)
inflammatory diseases of uterus (N71.-)
noninflammatory disorders of cervix, except malposition (N86-N88)
polyp of corpus uteri (N84.0)
uterine prolapse (N81.-)

✓5ᵗʰ N85.0 Endometrial hyperplasia
N85.00 Endometrial hyperplasia, unspecified ♀▽
Hyperplasia (adenomatous) (cystic) (glandular) of endometrium
Hyperplastic endometritis
N85.01 Benign endometrial hyperplasia ♀
Endometrial hyperplasia (complex) (simple) without atypia
N85.02 Endometrial intraepithelial neoplasia [EIN] ♀
Endometrial hyperplasia with atypia
EXCLUDES 1 malignant neoplasm of endometrium (with endometrial intraepithelial neoplasia [EIN]) (C54.1)

N85.2 Hypertrophy of uterus ♀
Bulky or enlarged uterus
EXCLUDES 1 puerperal hypertrophy of uterus (O90.89)

N85.3 Subinvolution of uterus ♀
EXCLUDES 1 puerperal subinvolution of uterus (O90.89)

N85.4 Malposition of uterus ♀
Anteversion of uterus
Retroflexion of uterus
Retroversion of uterus
EXCLUDES 1 malposition of uterus complicating pregnancy, labor or delivery (O34.5-, O65.5)

N85.5 Inversion of uterus ♀
EXCLUDES 1 current obstetric trauma (O71.2)
postpartum inversion of uterus (O71.2)

N85.6 Intrauterine synechiae ♀

N85.7 Hematometra ♀
Hematosalpinx with hematometra
EXCLUDES 1 hematometra with hematocolpos (N89.7)
DEF: Accumulation of blood within the uterus.

N85.8 Other specified noninflammatory disorders of uterus ♀
Atrophy of uterus, acquired
Fibrosis of uterus NOS

N85.9 Noninflammatory disorder of uterus, unspecified ♀▽
Disorder of uterus NOS

N86 Erosion and ectropion of cervix uteri ♀
Decubitus (trophic) ulcer of cervix
Eversion of cervix
EXCLUDES 1 erosion and ectropion of cervix with cervicitis (N72)

✓4ᵗʰ N87 Dysplasia of cervix uteri
EXCLUDES 1 abnormal results from cervical cytologic examination without histologic confirmation (R87.61-)
carcinoma in situ of cervix uteri (D06.-)
cervical intraepithelial neoplasia III [CIN III] (D06.-)
HGSIL of cervix (R87.613)
severe dysplasia of cervix uteri (D06.-)

Ⓝ Newborn: 0 Ⓟ Pediatric: 0-17 Ⓜ Maternity: 12-55 Ⓐ Adult: 15-124 NRS Nonroutine supply Dx NCDx Noncancer Dx PDx Primary Dx ►◄ Revised Text ● New Code ▲ Revised Title

814   ICD-10-CM 2018

N87.Ø   Mild **cervical dysplasia**   ♀
     Cervical intraepithelial neoplasia I [CIN I]

N87.1   Moderate **cervical dysplasia**   ♀
     Cervical intraepithelial neoplasia II [CIN II]

N87.9   **Dysplasia of cervix uteri, unspecified**   ♀▽
     Anaplasia of cervix
     Cervical atypism
     Cervical dysplasia NOS

✓4ᵗʰ **N88**   **Other noninflammatory disorders of cervix uteri**
     EXCLUDES 2   inflammatory disease of cervix (N72)
               polyp of cervix (N84.1)

N88.Ø   **Leukoplakia of cervix uteri**   ♀

N88.1   **Old laceration of cervix uteri**   ♀
     Adhesions of cervix
     EXCLUDES 1   current obstetric trauma (O71.3)

N88.2   **Stricture and stenosis of cervix uteri**   ♀
     EXCLUDES 1   stricture and stenosis of cervix uteri complicating labor
               (O65.5)

N88.3   **Incompetence of cervix uteri**   ♀
     Investigation and management of (suspected) cervical
       incompetence in a nonpregnant woman
     EXCLUDES 1   cervical incompetence complicating pregnancy
               (O34.3-)

N88.4   **Hypertrophic elongation of cervix uteri**   ♀

N88.8   **Other specified noninflammatory disorders of cervix uteri**   ♀
     EXCLUDES 1   current obstetric trauma (O71.3)

N88.9   **Noninflammatory disorder of cervix uteri, unspecified**   ♀▽

✓4ᵗʰ **N89**   **Other noninflammatory disorders of vagina**
     EXCLUDES 1   abnormal results from vaginal cytologic examination without
               histologic confirmation (R87.62-)
               carcinoma in situ of vagina (DØ7.2)
               HGSIL of vagina (R87.623)
               inflammation of vagina (N76.-)
               senile (atrophic) vaginitis (N95.2)
               severe dysplasia of vagina (DØ7.2)
               trichomonal leukorrhea (A59.ØØ)
               vaginal intraepithelial neoplasia [VAIN], grade III (DØ7.2)

N89.Ø   Mild **vaginal dysplasia**   ♀
     Vaginal intraepithelial neoplasia [VAIN], grade I

N89.1   Moderate **vaginal dysplasia**   ♀
     Vaginal intraepithelial neoplasia [VAIN], grade II

N89.3   **Dysplasia of vagina, unspecified**   ♀▽

N89.4   **Leukoplakia of vagina**   ♀

N89.5   **Stricture and atresia of vagina**   ♀
     Vaginal adhesions
     Vaginal stenosis
     EXCLUDES 1   congenital atresia or stricture (Q52.4)
               postprocedural adhesions of vagina (N99.2)

N89.6   **Tight hymenal ring**   ♀
     Rigid hymen
     Tight introitus
     EXCLUDES 1   imperforate hymen (Q52.3)

N89.7   **Hematocolpos**   ♀
     Hematocolpos with hematometra or hematosalpinx

N89.8   **Other specified noninflammatory disorders of vagina**   ♀
     Leukorrhea NOS
     Old vaginal laceration
     Pessary ulcer of vagina
     EXCLUDES 1   current obstetric trauma (O7Ø-, O71.4, O71.7-O71.8)
               old laceration involving muscles of pelvic floor (N81.8)

N89.9   **Noninflammatory disorder of vagina, unspecified**   ♀▽

✓4ᵗʰ **N9Ø**   **Other noninflammatory disorders of vulva and perineum**
     EXCLUDES 1   anogenital (venereal) warts (A63.Ø)
               carcinoma in situ of vulva (DØ7.1)
               condyloma acuminatum (A63.Ø)
               current obstetric trauma (O7Ø-, O71.7-O71.8)
               inflammation of vulva (N76.-)
               severe dysplasia of vulva (DØ7.1)
               vulvar intraepithelial neoplasm III [VIN III] (DØ7.1)

N9Ø.Ø   Mild **vulvar dysplasia**   ♀
     Vulvar intraepithelial neoplasia [VIN], grade I

N9Ø.1   Moderate **vulvar dysplasia**   ♀
     Vulvar intraepithelial neoplasia [VIN], grade II

N9Ø.3   **Dysplasia of vulva, unspecified**   ♀▽

N9Ø.4   **Leukoplakia of vulva**   ♀
     Dystrophy of vulva
     Kraurosis of vulva
     Lichen sclerosus of external female genital organs

N9Ø.5   **Atrophy of vulva**   ♀
     Stenosis of vulva

✓5ᵗʰ **N9Ø.6**   **Hypertrophy of vulva**

     N9Ø.6Ø   **Unspecified hypertrophy of vulva**   ♀▽
         Unspecified hypertrophy of labia

     N9Ø.61   **Childhood asymmetric labium majus enlargement**   ♀
         CALME

     N9Ø.69   **Other specified hypertrophy of vulva**   ♀
         Other specified hypertrophy of labia

N9Ø.7   **Vulvar cyst**   ♀

✓5ᵗʰ **N9Ø.8**   **Other specified noninflammatory disorders of vulva and perineum**

     ✓6ᵗʰ **N9Ø.81**   **Female genital mutilation status**
         Female genital cutting status

         N9Ø.81Ø   **Female genital mutilation status, unspecified**   ♀▽
             Female genital cutting status, unspecified
             Female genital mutilation status NOS

         N9Ø.811   **Female genital mutilation Type I status**   ♀
             Clitorectomy status
             Female genital cutting Type I status

         N9Ø.812   **Female genital mutilation Type II status** ♀
             Clitorectomy with excision of labia minora status
             Female genital cutting Type II status

         N9Ø.813   **Female genital mutilation Type III status** ♀
             Female genital cutting Type III status
             Infibulation status

         N9Ø.818   **Other female genital mutilation status**   ♀
             Female genital cutting Type IV status
             Female genital mutilation Type IV status
             Other female genital cutting status

     N9Ø.89   **Other specified noninflammatory disorders of vulva and perineum**   ♀
         Adhesions of vulva
         Hypertrophy of clitoris

N9Ø.9   **Noninflammatory disorder of vulva and perineum, unspecified**   ♀▽

✓4ᵗʰ **N91**   **Absent, scanty and rare menstruation**
     EXCLUDES 1   ovarian dysfunction (E28.-)

N91.Ø   **Primary amenorrhea**   ♀

N91.1   **Secondary amenorrhea**   ♀

N91.2   **Amenorrhea, unspecified**   ♀▽

N91.3   **Primary oligomenorrhea**   ♀

N91.4   **Secondary oligomenorrhea**   ♀

N91.5   **Oligomenorrhea, unspecified**   ♀▽
     Hypomenorrhea NOS

✓4ᵗʰ **N92**   **Excessive, frequent and irregular menstruation**
     EXCLUDES 1   postmenopausal bleeding (N95.Ø)
               precocious puberty (menstruation) (E3Ø.1)

N92.Ø   **Excessive and frequent menstruation with regular cycle**   ♀
     Heavy periods NOS
     Menorrhagia NOS
     Polymenorrhea

N92.1   **Excessive and frequent menstruation with irregular cycle**   ♀
     Irregular intermenstrual bleeding
     Irregular, shortened intervals between menstrual bleeding
     Menometrorrhagia
     Metrorrhagia

N92.2   **Excessive menstruation at puberty**   P♀
     Excessive bleeding associated with onset of menstrual periods
     Pubertal menorrhagia
     Puberty bleeding

N92.3   **Ovulation bleeding**   ♀
     Regular intermenstrual bleeding

N92.4   **Excessive bleeding in the premenopausal period**   ♀
     Climacteric menorrhagia or metrorrhagia
     Menopausal menorrhagia or metrorrhagia
     Preclimacteric menorrhagia or metrorrhagia
     Premenopausal menorrhagia or metrorrhagia

N92.5   **Other specified irregular menstruation**   ♀

✓ Additional Character Req   ✓x7ᵗʰ Placeholder Alert   Case-Mix Diagnosis   Manifestation   ▽ Unspecified Dx   EXCLUDES 1 Not coded here   EXCLUDES 2 Not included here

N92.6 Irregular menstruation, unspecified ♀▽
Irregular bleeding NOS
Irregular periods NOS
EXCLUDES 1 irregular menstruation with:
lengthened intervals or scanty bleeding
(N91.3-N91.5)
shortened intervals or excessive bleeding (N92.1)

☑4ᵗʰ **N93 Other abnormal uterine and vaginal bleeding**
EXCLUDES 1 neonatal vaginal hemorrhage (P54.6)
precocious puberty (menstruation) (E30.1)
pseudomenses (P54.6)

N93.0 Postcoital and contact bleeding ♀
N93.1 Pre-pubertal vaginal bleeding ♀
N93.8 Other specified abnormal uterine and vaginal bleeding ♀
Dysfunctional or functional uterine or vaginal bleeding NOS
N93.9 Abnormal uterine and vaginal bleeding, unspecified ♀▽

☑4ᵗʰ **N94 Pain and other conditions associated with female genital organs and menstrual cycle**
N94.0 Mittelschmerz ♀
DEF: One-sided, lower abdominal pain occurring between menstrual periods; associated with ovulation.

☑5ᵗʰ **N94.1 Dyspareunia**
EXCLUDES 1 psychogenic dyspareunia (F52.6)
N94.10 Unspecified dyspareunia ♀▽
N94.11 Superficial (introital) dyspareunia ♀
N94.12 Deep dyspareunia ♀
N94.19 Other specified dyspareunia ♀

N94.2 Vaginismus ♀
EXCLUDES 1 psychogenic vaginismus (F52.5)

N94.3 Premenstrual tension syndrome ♀
~~Premenstrual dysphoric disorder~~
Code also associated menstrual migraine (G43.82-, G43.83-)
EXCLUDES 1 premenstrual dysphoric disorder (F32.81)

N94.4 Primary dysmenorrhea ♀
N94.5 Secondary dysmenorrhea ♀
N94.6 Dysmenorrhea, unspecified ♀▽
EXCLUDES 1 psychogenic dysmenorrhea (F45.8)

☑5ᵗʰ **N94.8 Other specified conditions associated with female genital organs and menstrual cycle**
☑6ᵗʰ **N94.81 Vulvodynia**
N94.810 Vulvar vestibulitis ♀
N94.818 Other vulvodynia ♀
N94.819 Vulvodynia, unspecified ♀▽
Vulvodynia NOS
N94.89 Other specified conditions associated with female genital organs and menstrual cycle ♀
N94.9 Unspecified condition associated with female genital organs and menstrual cycle ♀▽

☑4ᵗʰ **N95 Menopausal and other perimenopausal disorders**
Menopausal and other perimenopausal disorders due to naturally occurring (age-related) menopause and perimenopause
EXCLUDES 1 excessive bleeding in the premenopausal period (N92.4)
menopausal and perimenopausal disorders due to artificial or premature menopause (E89.4-, E28.31-)
premature menopause (E28.31-)
EXCLUDES 2 postmenopausal osteoporosis (M81.0-)
postmenopausal osteoporosis with current pathological fracture (M80.0-)
postmenopausal urethritis (N34.2)

N95.0 Postmenopausal bleeding ♀
N95.1 Menopausal and female climacteric states ♀
Symptoms such as flushing, sleeplessness, headache, lack of concentration, associated with natural (age-related) menopause
Use additional code for associated symptoms
EXCLUDES 1 asymptomatic menopausal state (Z78.0)
symptoms associated with artificial menopause (E89.41)
symptoms associated with premature menopause (E28.310)
N95.2 Postmenopausal atrophic vaginitis ♀
Senile (atrophic) vaginitis
N95.8 Other specified menopausal and perimenopausal disorders ♀
N95.9 Unspecified menopausal and perimenopausal disorder ♀▽

N96 Recurrent pregnancy loss ♀
Investigation or care in a nonpregnant woman with history of recurrent pregnancy loss
EXCLUDES 1 recurrent pregnancy loss with current pregnancy (O26.2-)

☑4ᵗʰ **N97 Female infertility**
INCLUDES inability to achieve a pregnancy
sterility, female NOS
EXCLUDES 1 female infertility associated with:
hypopituitarism (E23.0)
Stein-Leventhal syndrome (E28.2)
EXCLUDES 2 incompetence of cervix uteri (N88.3)
DEF: Infertility: Inability to conceive for at least one year with regular intercourse.
DEF: Primary infertility: Infertility occurring in patients who have never conceived.
DEF: Secondary infertility: Infertility occurring in patients who have previously conceived.

N97.0 Female infertility associated with anovulation ♀
N97.1 Female infertility of tubal origin ♀
Female infertility associated with congenital anomaly of tube
Female infertility due to tubal block
Female infertility due to tubal occlusion
Female infertility due to tubal stenosis
N97.2 Female infertility of uterine origin ♀
Female infertility associated with congenital anomaly of uterus
Female infertility due to nonimplantation of ovum
N97.8 Female infertility of other origin ♀
N97.9 Female infertility, unspecified ♀▽

☑4ᵗʰ **N98 Complications associated with artificial fertilization**
N98.0 Infection associated with artificial insemination ♀
N98.1 Hyperstimulation of ovaries ♀
Hyperstimulation of ovaries NOS
Hyperstimulation of ovaries associated with induced ovulation
N98.2 Complications of attempted introduction of fertilized ovum following in vitro fertilization ♀
N98.3 Complications of attempted introduction of embryo in embryo transfer ♀
N98.8 Other complications associated with artificial fertilization ♀
N98.9 Complication associated with artificial fertilization, unspecified ♀▽

Intraoperative and postprocedural complications and disorders of genitourinary system, not elsewhere classified (N99)

☑4ᵗʰ **N99 Intraoperative and postprocedural complications and disorders of genitourinary system, not elsewhere classified**
EXCLUDES 2 irradiation cystitis (N30.4-)
postoophorectomy osteoporosis with current pathological fracture (M80.8-)
postoophorectomy osteoporosis without current pathological fracture (M81.8)

N99.0 Postprocedural (acute) (chronic) kidney failure
Use additional code to type of kidney disease

☑5ᵗʰ **N99.1 Postprocedural urethral stricture**
Postcatheterization urethral stricture
☑6ᵗʰ **N99.11 Postprocedural urethral stricture, male**
N99.110 Postprocedural urethral stricture, male, meatal ♂
▲ **N99.111 Postprocedural bulbous urethral stricture, male** ♂
▲ **N99.112 Postprocedural membranous urethral stricture, male** ♂
▲ **N99.113 Postprocedural anterior bulbous urethral stricture, male** ♂
N99.114 Postprocedural urethral stricture, male, unspecified ♂▽
N99.115 Postprocedural fossa navicularis urethral stricture
N99.12 Postprocedural urethral stricture, female ♀
N99.2 Postprocedural adhesions of vagina ♀
N99.3 Prolapse of vaginal vault after hysterectomy ♀
N99.4 Postprocedural pelvic peritoneal adhesions
EXCLUDES 2 pelvic peritoneal adhesions NOS (N73.6)
postinfective pelvic peritoneal adhesions (N73.6)

Ⓝ Newborn: 0　Ⓟ Pediatric: 0-17　Ⓜ Maternity: 12-55　Ⓐ Adult: 15-124　**NRS** Nonroutine supply Dx　**NCDx** Noncancer Dx　**PDx** Primary Dx　▶◀ Revised Text　● New Code　▲ Revised Title

816　　　　　　　　　　　　　　　　　　　　　　　　　　　　　　　　　　　ICD-10-CM 2018

✓5ᵗʰ **N99.5 Complications of stoma of urinary tract**

> EXCLUDES 2   mechanical complication of urinary catheter (T83.0-)

✓6ᵗʰ **N99.51 Complication of** cystostomy

     N99.510 Cystostomy hemorrhage

     N99.511 Cystostomy infection

     N99.512 Cystostomy malfunction

     N99.518 Other cystostomy complication

✓6ᵗʰ **N99.52 Complication of** incontinent external stoma **of urinary tract**

     N99.520 Hemorrhage **of incontinent external stoma of urinary tract**

     N99.521 Infection **of incontinent external stoma of urinary tract**

     N99.522 Malfunction **of incontinent external stoma of urinary tract**

     N99.523 Herniation **of incontinent stoma of urinary tract**

     N99.524 Stenosis **of incontinent stoma of urinary tract**

     N99.528 Other **complication of incontinent external stoma of urinary tract**

✓6ᵗʰ **N99.53 Complication of** continent stoma **of urinary tract**

     N99.530 Hemorrhage **of continent stoma of urinary tract**

     N99.531 Infection **of continent stoma of urinary tract**

     N99.532 Malfunction **of continent stoma of urinary tract**

     N99.533 Herniation **of continent stoma of urinary tract**

     N99.534 Stenosis **of continent stoma of urinary tract**

     N99.538 Other **complication of continent stoma of urinary tract**

✓5ᵗʰ **N99.6** Intraoperative hemorrhage and hematoma **of a genitourinary system organ or structure complicating a procedure**

> EXCLUDES 1   intraoperative hemorrhage and hematoma of a genitourinary system organ or structure due to accidental puncture or laceration during a procedure (N99.7-)

     N99.61 Intraoperative hemorrhage and hematoma of a genitourinary system organ or structure complicating a genitourinary system procedure

     N99.62 Intraoperative hemorrhage and hematoma of a genitourinary system organ or structure complicating other procedure

✓5ᵗʰ **N99.7** Accidental puncture and laceration **of a genitourinary system organ or structure during a procedure**

     N99.71 Accidental puncture and laceration of a genitourinary system organ or structure during a genitourinary system procedure

     N99.72 Accidental puncture and laceration of a genitourinary system organ or structure during other procedure

✓5ᵗʰ **N99.8** Other **intraoperative and postprocedural complications and disorders of genitourinary system**

     N99.81 Other intraoperative complications **of genitourinary system**

✓6ᵗʰ **N99.82** Postprocedural hemorrhage **of a genitourinary system organ or structure following a procedure**

     N99.820 Postprocedural hemorrhage of a genitourinary system organ or structure following a genitourinary system procedure

     N99.821 Postprocedural hemorrhage of a genitourinary system organ or structure following other procedure

     N99.83 Residual ovary syndrome   ♀

✓6ᵗʰ **N99.84** Postprocedural hematoma and seroma **of a genitourinary system organ or structure following a procedure**

     N99.840 Postprocedural hematoma **of a genitourinary system organ or structure following a** genitourinary system procedure

     N99.841 Postprocedural hematoma **of a genitourinary system organ or structure following** other procedure

     N99.842 Postprocedural seroma **of a genitourinary system organ or structure following a** genitourinary system procedure

     N99.843 Postprocedural seroma **of a genitourinary system organ or structure following** other procedure

     N99.89 Other postprocedural complications and disorders of genitourinary system

---

☑ Additional Character Req   ✓✗7ᵗʰ Placeholder Alert   Case-Mix Diagnosis   Manifestation   ▽ Unspecified Dx   EXCLUDES 1 Not coded here   EXCLUDES 2 Not included here

Chapter 15. Pregnancy, Childbirth and the Puerperium (O00–O9A)

Chapter Specific Guidelines with Coding Examples

The chapter specific guidelines from the ICD-10-CM Official Guidelines for Coding and Reporting have been provided below. Along with these guidelines are coding examples, contained in the shaded boxes, that have been developed to help illustrate the coding and/or sequencing guidance found in these guidelines.

a. General rules for obstetric cases

1) Codes from chapter 15 and sequencing priority

Obstetric cases require codes from chapter 15, codes in the range O00–O9A, Pregnancy, Childbirth, and the Puerperium. Chapter 15 codes have sequencing priority over codes from other chapters. Additional codes from other chapters may be used in conjunction with chapter 15 codes to further specify conditions. Should the provider document that the pregnancy is incidental to the encounter, then code Z33.1, Pregnant state, incidental, should be used in place of any chapter 15 codes. It is the provider's responsibility to state that the condition being treated is not affecting the pregnancy.

	Bladder abscess in pregnant patient at 25 weeks' gestation
O23.12	Infections of bladder in pregnancy, second trimester
N30.80	Other cystitis without hematuria
Z3A.25	25 weeks gestation of pregnancy

Explanation: The documentation does not indicate that the pregnancy is incidental or in any way unaffected by the bladder abscess; therefore, an obstetrics code should be sequenced first. An additional code was provided to identify the specific bladder condition as this information is not called out specifically in the obstetrics code.

2) Chapter 15 codes used only on the maternal record

Chapter 15 codes are to be used only on the maternal record, never on the record of the newborn.

3) Final character for trimester

The majority of codes in Chapter 15 have a final character indicating the trimester of pregnancy. The timeframes for the trimesters are indicated at the beginning of the chapter. If trimester is not a component of a code, it is because the condition always occurs in a specific trimester, or the concept of trimester of pregnancy is not applicable. Certain codes have characters for only certain trimesters because the condition does not occur in all trimesters, but it may occur in more than just one.

Assignment of the final character for trimester should be based on the provider's documentation of the trimester (or number of weeks) for the current admission/encounter. This applies to the assignment of trimester for pre-existing conditions as well as those that develop during or are due to the pregnancy. The provider's documentation of the number of weeks may be used to assign the appropriate code identifying the trimester.

Whenever delivery occurs during the current admission, and there is an "in childbirth" option for the obstetric complication being coded, the "in childbirth" code should be assigned.

	Pregnant patient at 21 weeks' gestation admitted with excessive vomiting
O21.2	Late vomiting of pregnancy
Z3A.21	21 weeks gestation of pregnancy

Explanation: Category O21 classifies vomiting in pregnancy. Although code selection is based on whether the vomiting is before or after 20 completed weeks, these codes are not further classified by trimester. If vomiting only in the second trimester was documented, the provider should be queried for the specific week of gestation, as this will affect code selection.

4) Selection of trimester for inpatient admissions that encompass more than one trimester

In instances when a patient is admitted to a hospital for complications of pregnancy during one trimester and remains in the hospital into a subsequent trimester, the trimester character for the antepartum complication code should be assigned on the basis of the trimester when the complication developed, not the trimester of the discharge. If the condition developed prior to the current admission/encounter or represents a pre-existing condition, the trimester character for the trimester at the time of the admission/encounter should be assigned.

5) Unspecified trimester

Each category that includes codes for trimester has a code for "unspecified trimester." The "unspecified trimester" code should rarely be used, such as when the documentation in the record is insufficient to determine the trimester and it is not possible to obtain clarification.

6) 7th character for fetus identification

Where applicable, a 7th character is to be assigned for certain categories (O31, O32, O33.3 - O33.6, O35, O36, O40, O41, O60.1, O60.2, O64, and O69) to identify the fetus for which the complication code applies.

Assign 7th character "0":

- For single gestations
- When the documentation in the record is insufficient to determine the fetus affected and it is not possible to obtain clarification.
- When it is not possible to clinically determine which fetus is affected.

b. Selection of OB principal or first-listed diagnosis

1) Routine outpatient prenatal visits

For routine outpatient prenatal visits when no complications are present, a code from category Z34, Encounter for supervision of normal pregnancy, should be used as the first-listed diagnosis. These codes should not be used in conjunction with chapter 15 codes.

2) Supervision of high-risk pregnancy

Codes from category O09, Supervision of high-risk pregnancy, are intended for use only during the prenatal period. For complications during the labor or delivery episode as a result of a high-risk pregnancy, assign the applicable complication codes from Chapter 15. If there are no complications during the labor or delivery episode, assign code O80, Encounter for full-term uncomplicated delivery.

For routine prenatal outpatient visits for patients with high-risk pregnancies, a code from category O09, Supervision of high-risk pregnancy, should be used as the first-listed diagnosis. Secondary chapter 15 codes may be used in conjunction with these codes if appropriate.

3) Episodes when no delivery occurs

In episodes when no delivery occurs, the principal diagnosis should correspond to the principal complication of the pregnancy which necessitated the encounter. Should more than one complication exist, all of which are treated or monitored, any of the complications codes may be sequenced first.

4) When a delivery occurs

When an obstetric patient is admitted and delivers during that admission, the condition that prompted the admission should be sequenced as the principal diagnosis. If multiple conditions prompted the admission, sequence the one most related to the delivery as the principal diagnosis. A code for any complication of the delivery should be assigned as an additional diagnosis. In cases of cesarean delivery, if the patient was admitted with a condition that resulted in the performance of a cesarean procedure, that condition should be selected as the principal diagnosis. If the reason for the admission was unrelated to the condition resulting in the cesarean delivery, the condition related to the reason for the admission should be selected as the principal diagnosis.

5) Outcome of delivery

A code from category Z37, Outcome of delivery, should be included on every maternal record when a delivery has occurred. These codes are not to be used on subsequent records or on the newborn record.

c. Pre-existing conditions versus conditions due to the pregnancy

Certain categories in Chapter 15 distinguish between conditions of the mother that existed prior to pregnancy (pre-existing) and those that are a direct result of pregnancy. When assigning codes from Chapter 15, it is important to assess if a condition was pre-existing prior to pregnancy or developed during or due to the pregnancy in order to assign the correct code.

Categories that do not distinguish between pre-existing and pregnancy-related conditions may be used for either. It is acceptable to use codes specifically for the puerperium with codes complicating pregnancy and childbirth if a condition arises postpartum during the delivery encounter.

Chapter 15. Pregnancy, Childbirth and the Puerperium *(vertical sidebar)*

d. Pre-existing hypertension in pregnancy

Category O10, Pre-existing hypertension complicating pregnancy, childbirth and the puerperium, includes codes for hypertensive heart and hypertensive chronic kidney disease. When assigning one of the O10 codes that includes hypertensive heart disease or hypertensive chronic kidney disease, it is necessary to add a secondary code from the appropriate hypertension category to specify the type of heart failure or chronic kidney disease.

See Section I.C.9. Hypertension.

e. Fetal conditions affecting the management of the mother

1) Codes from categories O35 and O36

Codes from categories O35, Maternal care for known or suspected fetal abnormality and damage, and O36, Maternal care for other fetal problems, are assigned only when the fetal condition is actually responsible for modifying the management of the mother, i.e., by requiring diagnostic studies, additional observation, special care, or termination of pregnancy. The fact that the fetal condition exists does not justify assigning a code from this series to the mother's record.

2) In utero surgery

In cases when surgery is performed on the fetus, a diagnosis code from category O35, Maternal care for known or suspected fetal abnormality and damage, should be assigned identifying the fetal condition. Assign the appropriate procedure code for the procedure performed.

No code from Chapter 16, the perinatal codes, should be used on the mother's record to identify fetal conditions. Surgery performed in utero on a fetus is still to be coded as an obstetric encounter.

f. HIV infection in pregnancy, childbirth and the puerperium

During pregnancy, childbirth or the puerperium, a patient admitted because of an HIV-related illness should receive a principal diagnosis from subcategory O98.7-, Human immunodeficiency [HIV] disease complicating pregnancy, childbirth and the puerperium, followed by the code(s) for the HIV-related illness(es).

Patients with asymptomatic HIV infection status admitted during pregnancy, childbirth, or the puerperium should receive codes of O98.7- and Z21, Asymptomatic human immunodeficiency virus [HIV] infection status.

An HIV-positive female, age 42, with a history of Down syndrome is admitted for skilled nursing care, medication management, and observation due to worsening HIV-associated nephritis during her pregnancy. Current provider reports indicate she is 13 weeks pregnant.

O98.711	Human immunodeficiency virus [HIV] disease complicating pregnancy, first trimester
B20	Human immunodeficiency virus [HIV] disease
N08	Glomerular disorders in diseases classified elsewhere
O99.89	Other specified diseases and conditions complicating pregnancy, childbirth and the puerperium
Q90.9	Down syndrome, unspecified
Z3A.13	13 weeks gestation of pregnancy

Explanation: When HIV and associated complications require treatment during the course of a pregnancy, a code from subcategory O98.7- must be assigned, followed by the codes for the HIV infection and any manifestation(s) related to the HIV. Code Z3A.13 should also be used in this scenario to report the current gestation.

---

g. Diabetes mellitus in pregnancy

Diabetes mellitus is a significant complicating factor in pregnancy. Pregnant women who are diabetic should be assigned a code from category O24, Diabetes mellitus in pregnancy, childbirth, and the puerperium, first, followed by the appropriate diabetes code(s) (E08-E13) from Chapter 4.

h. Long term use of insulin and oral hypoglycemics

See section I.C.4.a.3 for information on the long term use of insulin and oral hypoglycemic.

i. Gestational (pregnancy induced) diabetes

Gestational (pregnancy induced) diabetes can occur during the second and third trimester of pregnancy in women who were not diabetic prior to pregnancy. Gestational diabetes can cause complications in the pregnancy similar to those of pre-existing diabetes mellitus. It also puts the woman at greater risk of developing diabetes after the pregnancy. Codes for gestational diabetes are in subcategory O24.4, Gestational diabetes mellitus. No other code from category O24, Diabetes mellitus in pregnancy, childbirth, and the puerperium, should be used with a code from O24.4.

The codes under subcategory O24.4 include diet controlled, insulin controlled, and controlled by oral hypoglycemic drugs. If a patient with gestational diabetes is treated with both diet and insulin, only the code for insulin-controlled is required. If a patient with gestational diabetes is treated with both diet and oral hypoglycemic medications, only the code for "controlled by oral hypoglycemic drugs" is required. Code Z79.4, Long-term (current) use of insulin or code Z79.84, Long-term (current) use of oral hypoglycemic drugs, should not be assigned with codes from subcategory O24.4.

An abnormal glucose tolerance in pregnancy is assigned a code from subcategory O99.81, Abnormal glucose complicating pregnancy, childbirth, and the puerperium.

j. Sepsis and septic shock complicating abortion, pregnancy, childbirth and the puerperium

When assigning a chapter 15 code for sepsis complicating abortion, pregnancy, childbirth, and the puerperium, a code for the specific type of infection should be assigned as an additional diagnosis. If severe sepsis is present, a code from subcategory R65.2, Severe sepsis, and code(s) for associated organ dysfunction(s) should also be assigned as additional diagnoses.

Patient is admitted to the skilled home health nursing for an extended course of intravenous antibiotic administration due to MSSA sepsis that resulted from a miscarriage 1 week ago.

O03.87	Sepsis following complete or unspecified spontaneous abortion
B95.61	Methicillin susceptible Staphylococcus aureus infection as the cause of diseases classified elsewhere

Explanation: The type of infection that caused this patient to become septic was methicillin susceptible *Staphylococcus aureus* (MSSA), which as a secondary code helps capture all aspects related to this patient's septic condition.

---

k. Puerperal sepsis

Code O85, Puerperal sepsis, should be assigned with a secondary code to identify the causal organism (e.g., for a bacterial infection, assign a code from category B95-B96, Bacterial infections in conditions classified elsewhere). A code from category A40, Streptococcal sepsis, or A41, Other sepsis, should not be used for puerperal sepsis. If applicable, use additional codes to identify severe sepsis (R65.2-) and any associated acute organ dysfunction.

l. Alcohol and tobacco use during pregnancy, childbirth and the puerperium

1) Alcohol use during pregnancy, childbirth and the puerperium

Codes under subcategory O99.31, Alcohol use complicating pregnancy, childbirth, and the puerperium, should be assigned for any pregnancy case when a mother uses alcohol during the pregnancy or postpartum. A secondary code from category F10, Alcohol related disorders, should also be assigned to identify manifestations of the alcohol use.

2) Tobacco use during pregnancy, childbirth and the puerperium

Codes under subcategory O99.33, Smoking (tobacco) complicating pregnancy, childbirth, and the puerperium, should be assigned for any pregnancy case when a mother uses any type of tobacco product during the pregnancy or postpartum. A secondary code from category F17, Nicotine dependence, should also be assigned to identify the type of nicotine dependence.

m. Poisoning, toxic effects, adverse effects and underdosing in a pregnant patient

A code from subcategory O9A.2, Injury, poisoning and certain other consequences of external causes complicating pregnancy, childbirth, and the puerperium, should be sequenced first, followed by the appropriate injury, poisoning, toxic effect, adverse effect or underdosing code, and then the additional code(s) that specifies the condition caused by the poisoning, toxic effect, adverse effect or underdosing.

See Section I.C.19. Adverse effects, poisoning, underdosing and toxic effects.

An 18-week pregnant female, who is wheelchair-bound due to paraplegia, is admitted for skilled nursing care with medication instruction after developing severe hypotension due to taking an incorrect dose of nifedipine. The drug was ordered to control her transient hypertension during the pregnancy, and she remains on the drug now with the correct dose administered.

O9A.212	Injury, poisoning and certain other consequences of external causes complicating pregnancy, second trimester
T46.1X1D	Poisoning by calcium-channel blockers, accidental (unintentional), subsequent encounter
I95.2	Hypotension due to drugs
O13.2	Gestational [pregnancy-induced] hypertension without significant proteinuria, second trimester
O99.352	Diseases of the nervous system complicating pregnancy, second trimester
G82.20	Paraplegia, unspecified
Z3A.18	18 weeks gestation of pregnancy

Explanation: Although the poisoning with resulting hypotension is the reason for admission, a code from the obstetrics chapter must first be assigned. Codes from chapter 15 have sequencing priority over codes from other chapters.

n. Normal delivery, code O80

1) Encounter for full term uncomplicated delivery
Code O80 should be assigned when a woman is admitted for a full-term normal delivery and delivers a single, healthy infant without any complications antepartum, during the delivery, or postpartum during the delivery episode. Code O80 is always a principal diagnosis. It is not to be used if any other code from chapter 15 is needed to describe a current complication of the antenatal, delivery, or perinatal period. Additional codes from other chapters may be used with code O80 if they are not related to or are in any way complicating the pregnancy.

2) Uncomplicated delivery with resolved antepartum complication
Code O80 may be used if the patient had a complication at some point during the pregnancy, but the complication is not present at the time of the admission for delivery.

3) Outcome of delivery for O80
Z37.0, Single live birth, is the only outcome of delivery code appropriate for use with O80.

o. The peripartum and postpartum periods

1) Peripartum and postpartum periods
The postpartum period begins immediately after delivery and continues for six weeks following delivery. The peripartum period is defined as the last month of pregnancy to five months postpartum.

2) Peripartum and postpartum complication
A postpartum complication is any complication occurring within the six-week period.

3) Pregnancy-related complications after 6 week period
Chapter 15 codes may also be used to describe pregnancy-related complications after the peripartum or postpartum period if the provider documents that a condition is pregnancy related.

A 46-year-old woman had a baby boy 7 weeks ago. Following delivery, she quickly developed severe pseudomonas pyelonephritis, necessitating IV antibiotic therapy. She is referred to home health where she will be continued on antibiotics via PICC line. The physician reports "puerperal pseudomonas pyelonephritis."

O86.21	Infection of kidney following delivery
B96.5	Pseudomonas (aeruginosa) (mallei) (pseudomallei) as the cause of diseases classified elsewhere
Z45.2	Encounter for adjustment and management of vascular access device
Z79.2	Long term (current) use of antibiotics

Explanation: While not all infections of the urinary tract occurring after delivery are related directly to the delivery, in this case the physician reports "puerperal" in reference to the pyelonephritis. This indicates a need to assign a code from chapter 15 for the infection.

4) Admission for routine postpartum care following delivery outside hospital
When the mother delivers outside the hospital prior to admission and is admitted for routine postpartum care and no complications are noted,

code Z39.0, Encounter for care and examination of mother immediately after delivery, should be assigned as the principal diagnosis.

5) Pregnancy associated cardiomyopathy
Pregnancy associated cardiomyopathy, code O90.3, is unique in that it may be diagnosed in the third trimester of pregnancy but may continue to progress months after delivery. For this reason, it is referred to as peripartum cardiomyopathy. Code O90.3 is only for use when the cardiomyopathy develops as a result of pregnancy in a woman who did not have pre-existing heart disease.

A 36-year-old woman with no pre-existing conditions started experiencing heart failure symptoms late in the 3rd trimester of her second pregnancy. After an extensive workup she was diagnosed with nonobstructive hypertrophic cardiomyopathy. She made it through the delivery without any further complications but was referred to home health for observation of her condition and physical therapy to address reduced endurance. The cardiologist reports that the cardiomyopathy was directly related to the pregnancy and remains unresolved.

| O90.3 | Peripartum cardiomyopathy |
| I42.2 | Other hypertrophic cardiomyopathy |

Explanation: Because this patient has no cardiac history and no other conditions were found to be the cause of her cardiomyopathy, code O90.3 is most appropriate. An additional code for the specific type of cardiomyopathy may also be assigned, according to the inclusion term at code O90.3 as well as the Excludes 2 note at category I42.

Since this patient has no cardiac history, continues to experience cardiomyopathy in the postpartum period, and was diagnosed during the pregnancy, code O90.3 must be used. Also assign a code sequenced after O90.3 to specify the specific type of cardiomyopathy, as peripartum cardiomyopathy and codes from category I42 are listed as Excludes 2 conditions.

p. Code O94, Sequelae of complication of pregnancy, childbirth, and the puerperium

1) Code O94
Code O94, Sequelae of complication of pregnancy, childbirth, and the puerperium, is for use in those cases when an initial complication of a pregnancy develops a sequelae requiring care or treatment at a future date.

2) After the initial postpartum period
This code may be used at any time after the initial postpartum period.

3) Sequencing of code O94
This code, like all sequela codes, is to be sequenced following the code describing the sequelae of the complication.

q. Termination of pregnancy and spontaneous abortions

1) Abortion with liveborn fetus
When an attempted termination of pregnancy results in a liveborn fetus, assign code Z33.2, Encounter for elective termination of pregnancy and a code from category Z37, Outcome of Delivery.

2) Retained products of conception following an abortion
Subsequent encounters for retained products of conception following a spontaneous abortion or elective termination of pregnancy, **without complications** are assigned O03.4, **Incomplete spontaneous,** abortion **without complication,** or codes O07.4, Failed attempted termination of pregnancy without complication. This advice is appropriate even when the patient was discharged previously with a discharge diagnosis of complete abortion. **If the patient has a specific complication associated with the spontaneous abortion or elective termination of pregnancy in addition to retained products of conception, assign the appropriate complication in category O03 or O07 instead of code O03.4 or O07.4**

3) Complications leading to abortion
Codes from Chapter 15 may be used as additional codes to identify any documented complications of the pregnancy in conjunction with codes in categories in **O04,** O07 and O08.

r. Abuse in a pregnant patient
For suspected or confirmed cases of abuse of a pregnant patient, a code(s) from subcategories O9A.3, Physical abuse complicating pregnancy, childbirth, and the puerperium, O9A.4, Sexual abuse complicating pregnancy, childbirth, and the puerperium, and O9A.5, Psychological abuse complicating pregnancy, childbirth, and the puerperium, should be sequenced first, followed by the appropriate codes (if applicable) to identify any associated current injury due to physical abuse, sexual abuse, and the perpetrator of abuse.

See Section I.C.19. Adult and child abuse, neglect and other maltreatment.

Chapter 15. Pregnancy, Childbirth and the Puerperium (O00-O9A)

NOTE CODES FROM THIS CHAPTER ARE FOR USE ONLY ON MATERNAL RECORDS, NEVER ON NEWBORN RECORDS.

Codes from this chapter are for use for conditions related to or aggravated by the pregnancy, childbirth, or by the puerperium (maternal causes or obstetric causes).

NOTE Trimesters are counted from the first day of the last menstrual period. They are defined as follows:

1st trimester- less than 14 weeks 0 days
2nd trimester- 14 weeks 0 days to less than 28 weeks 0 days
3rd trimester- 28 weeks 0 days until delivery.

Use additional code from category Z3A, Weeks of gestation, to identify the specific week of the pregnancy, if known

EXCLUDES 1 *supervision of normal pregnancy (Z34.-)*
EXCLUDES 2 *mental and behavioral disorders associated with the puerperium (F53)*
obstetrical tetanus (A34)
postpartum necrosis of pituitary gland (E23.0)
puerperal osteomalacia (M83.0)

AHA: 2016, 1Q, 3-5; 2014, 3Q, 17

This chapter contains the following blocks:

O00-O08   Pregnancy with abortive outcome
O09   Supervision of high risk pregnancy
O10-O16   Edema, proteinuria and hypertensive disorders in pregnancy, childbirth and the puerperium
O20-O29   Other maternal disorders predominantly related to pregnancy
O30-O48   Maternal care related to the fetus and amniotic cavity and possible delivery problems
O60-O77   Complications of labor and delivery
O80, O82   Encounter for delivery
O85-O92   Complications predominantly related to the puerperium
O94-O9A   Other obstetric conditions, not elsewhere classified

Pregnancy with abortive outcome (O00-O08)

EXCLUDES 1 *continuing pregnancy in multiple gestation after abortion of one fetus or more (O31.1-, O31.3-)*

√4ᵗʰ **O00 Ectopic pregnancy**
   INCLUDES ruptured ectopic pregnancy
   Use additional code from category O08 to identify any associated complication
   AHA: 2014, 3Q, 17
   DEF: Implantation of fertilized egg outside the uterus, usually in fallopian tube or abdomen; requires emergency treatment.

√5ᵗʰ **O00.0 Abdominal pregnancy**
   EXCLUDES 1 *maternal care for viable fetus in abdominal pregnancy (O36.7-)*

     O00.00 Abdominal pregnancy without intrauterine pregnancy   🅜♀
       Abdominal pregnancy NOS

     O00.01 Abdominal pregnancy with intrauterine pregnancy   🅜♀

Ectopic Pregnancy

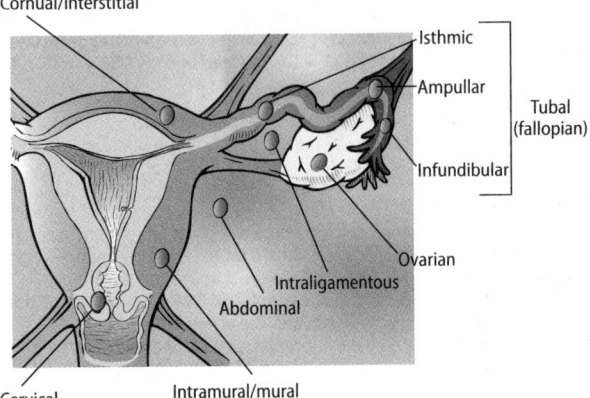

Cornual/interstitial
Isthmic
Ampullar
Tubal (fallopian)
Infundibular
Ovarian
Intraligamentous
Abdominal
Cervical
Intramural/mural

√5ᵗʰ **O00.1 Tubal pregnancy**
   Fallopian pregnancy
   Rupture of (fallopian) tube due to pregnancy
   Tubal abortion

   √6ᵗʰ **O00.10 Tubal pregnancy** without intrauterine pregnancy
     Tubal pregnancy NOS

     O00.101 Right tubal pregnancy without intrauterine pregnancy

     O00.102 Left tubal pregnancy without intrauterine pregnancy

     O00.109 Unspecified tubal pregnancy without intrauterine pregnancy ▽

   √6ᵗʰ **O00.11 Tubal pregnancy** with intrauterine pregnancy

     O00.111 Right tubal pregnancy with intrauterine pregnancy

     O00.112 Left tubal pregnancy with intrauterine pregnancy

     O00.119 Unspecified tubal pregnancy with intrauterine pregnancy ▽

√5ᵗʰ **O00.2 Ovarian pregnancy**

   √6ᵗʰ **O00.20 Ovarian pregnancy** without intrauterine pregnancy
     Ovarian pregnancy NOS

     O00.201 Right ovarian pregnancy without intrauterine pregnancy

     O00.202 Left ovarian pregnancy without intrauterine pregnancy

     O00.209 Unspecified ovarian pregnancy without intrauterine pregnancy ▽

   √6ᵗʰ **O00.21 Ovarian pregnancy** with intrauterine pregnancy

     O00.211 Right ovarian pregnancy with intrauterine pregnancy

     O00.212 Left ovarian pregnancy with intrauterine pregnancy

     O00.219 Unspecified ovarian pregnancy with intrauterine pregnancy ▽

√5ᵗʰ **O00.8 Other ectopic pregnancy**
   Cervical pregnancy
   Cornual pregnancy
   Intraligamentous pregnancy
   Mural pregnancy

     O00.80 Other ectopic pregnancy without intrauterine pregnancy   🅜♀
       Other ectopic pregnancy NOS

     O00.81 Other ectopic pregnancy with intrauterine pregnancy   🅜♀

√5ᵗʰ **O00.9 Ectopic pregnancy, unspecified**

     O00.90 Unspecified ectopic pregnancy without intrauterine pregnancy   🅜♀▽
       Ectopic pregnancy NOS

     O00.91 Unspecified ectopic pregnancy with intrauterine pregnancy   🅜♀

√4ᵗʰ **O01 Hydatidiform mole**
   Use additional code from category O08 to identify any associated complication
   EXCLUDES 1 *chorioadenoma (destruens) (D39.2)*
     malignant hydatidiform mole (D39.2)
   AHA: 2014, 3Q, 17
   DEF: Abnormal product of pregnancy; marked by mass of cysts resembling bunch of grapes due to chorionic villi proliferation and dissolution; must be surgically removed.

   O01.0 Classical hydatidiform mole   🅜♀
     Complete hydatidiform mole

   O01.1 Incomplete and partial hydatidiform mole   🅜♀

   O01.9 Hydatidiform mole, unspecified   🅜♀▽
     Trophoblastic disease NOS
     Vesicular mole NOS

√4ᵗʰ **O02 Other abnormal products of conception**
   Use additional code from category O08 to identify any associated complication
   EXCLUDES 1 *papyraceous fetus (O31.0-)*
   AHA: 2014, 3Q, 17

   O02.0 Blighted ovum and nonhydatidiform mole   🅜♀
     Carneous mole
     Fleshy mole
     Intrauterine mole NOS
     Molar pregnancy NEC
     Pathological ovum

O02.1 Missed abortion   Ⓜ♀
     Early fetal death, before completion of 20 weeks of gestation, with retention of dead fetus
     EXCLUDES 1   *failed induced abortion (O07.-)*
         fetal death (intrauterine) (late) (O36.4)
         missed abortion with blighted ovum (O02.0)
         missed abortion with hydatidiform mole (O01.-)
         missed abortion with nonhydatidiform (O02.0)
         missed abortion with other abnormal products of conception (O02.8-)
         missed delivery (O36.4)
         stillbirth (P95)

✓5ᵗʰ **O02.8 Other specified abnormal products of conception**
     EXCLUDES 1   *abnormal products of conception with blighted ovum (O02.0)*
         abnormal products of conception with hydatidiform mole (O01.-)
         abnormal products of conception with nonhydatidiform mole (O02.0)

     O02.81 Inappropriate change in quantitative human chorionic gonadotropin (hCG) in early pregnancy   Ⓜ♀
         Biochemical pregnancy
         Chemical pregnancy
         Inappropriate level of quantitative human chorionic gonadotropin (hCG) for gestational age in early pregnancy

     O02.89 Other abnormal products of conception   Ⓜ♀

     O02.9 Abnormal product of conception, unspecified   Ⓜ♀▽

✓4ᵗʰ **O03 Spontaneous abortion**
     NOTE   Incomplete abortion includes retained products of conception following spontaneous abortion
     INCLUDES   miscarriage

O03.0 Genital tract and pelvic infection following incomplete spontaneous abortion   Ⓜ♀
     Endometritis following incomplete spontaneous abortion
     Oophoritis following incomplete spontaneous abortion
     Parametritis following incomplete spontaneous abortion
     Pelvic peritonitis following incomplete spontaneous abortion
     Salpingitis following incomplete spontaneous abortion
     Salpingo-oophoritis following incomplete spontaneous abortion
     EXCLUDES 1   *sepsis following incomplete spontaneous abortion (O03.37)*
         urinary tract infection following incomplete spontaneous abortion (O03.38)

O03.1 Delayed or excessive hemorrhage following incomplete spontaneous abortion   Ⓜ♀
     Afibrinogenemia following incomplete spontaneous abortion
     Defibrination syndrome following incomplete spontaneous abortion
     Hemolysis following incomplete spontaneous abortion
     Intravascular coagulation following incomplete spontaneous abortion

O03.2 Embolism following incomplete spontaneous abortion   Ⓜ♀
     Air embolism following incomplete spontaneous abortion
     Amniotic fluid embolism following incomplete spontaneous abortion
     Blood-clot embolism following incomplete spontaneous abortion
     Embolism NOS following incomplete spontaneous abortion
     Fat embolism following incomplete spontaneous abortion
     Pulmonary embolism following incomplete spontaneous abortion
     Pyemic embolism following incomplete spontaneous abortion
     Septic or septicopyemic embolism following incomplete spontaneous abortion
     Soap embolism following incomplete spontaneous abortion

✓5ᵗʰ **O03.3 Other and unspecified complications following incomplete spontaneous abortion**

     O03.30 Unspecified complication following incomplete spontaneous abortion   Ⓜ♀▽

     O03.31 Shock following incomplete spontaneous abortion   Ⓜ♀
         Circulatory collapse following incomplete spontaneous abortion
         Shock (postprocedural) following incomplete spontaneous abortion
         EXCLUDES 1   *shock due to infection following incomplete spontaneous abortion (O03.37)*

O03.32 Renal failure following incomplete spontaneous abortion   Ⓜ♀
     Kidney failure (acute) following incomplete spontaneous abortion
     Oliguria following incomplete spontaneous abortion
     Renal shutdown following incomplete spontaneous abortion
     Renal tubular necrosis following incomplete spontaneous abortion
     Uremia following incomplete spontaneous abortion

O03.33 Metabolic disorder following incomplete spontaneous abortion   Ⓜ♀

O03.34 Damage to pelvic organs following incomplete spontaneous abortion   Ⓜ♀
     Laceration, perforation, tear or chemical damage of bladder following incomplete spontaneous abortion
     Laceration, perforation, tear or chemical damage of bowel following incomplete spontaneous abortion
     Laceration, perforation, tear or chemical damage of broad ligament following incomplete spontaneous abortion
     Laceration, perforation, tear or chemical damage of cervix following incomplete spontaneous abortion
     Laceration, perforation, tear or chemical damage of periurethral tissue following incomplete spontaneous abortion
     Laceration, perforation, tear or chemical damage of uterus following incomplete spontaneous abortion
     Laceration, perforation, tear or chemical damage of vagina following incomplete spontaneous abortion

O03.35 Other venous complications following incomplete spontaneous abortion   Ⓜ♀

O03.36 Cardiac arrest following incomplete spontaneousabortion   Ⓜ♀

O03.37 Sepsis following incomplete spontaneous abortion   Ⓜ♀
     Use additional code to identify infectious agent (B95-B97)
     Use additional code to identify severe sepsis, if applicable (R65.2-)
     EXCLUDES 1   *septic or septicopyemic embolism following incomplete spontaneous abortion (O03.2)*

O03.38 Urinary tract infection following incomplete spontaneous abortion   Ⓜ♀
     Cystitis following incomplete spontaneous abortion

O03.39 Incomplete spontaneous abortion with other complications   Ⓜ♀

O03.4 Incomplete spontaneous abortion without complication   Ⓜ♀

O03.5 Genital tract and pelvic infection following complete or unspecified spontaneous abortion   Ⓜ♀
     Endometritis following complete or unspecified spontaneous abortion
     Oophoritis following complete or unspecified spontaneous abortion
     Parametritis following complete or unspecified spontaneous abortion
     Pelvic peritonitis following complete or unspecified spontaneous abortion
     Salpingitis following complete or unspecified spontaneous abortion
     Salpingo-oophoritis following complete or unspecified spontaneous abortion
     EXCLUDES 1   *sepsis following complete or unspecified spontaneous abortion (O03.87)*
         urinary tract infection following complete or unspecified spontaneous abortion (O03.88)

O03.6 Delayed or excessive hemorrhage following complete or unspecified spontaneous abortion   Ⓜ♀
     Afibrinogenemia following complete or unspecified spontaneous abortion
     Defibrination syndrome following complete or unspecified spontaneous abortion
     Hemolysis following complete or unspecified spontaneous abortion
     Intravascular coagulation following complete or unspecified spontaneous abortion

Chapter 15. Pregnancy, Childbirth and the Puerperium

O03.7 **Embolism following** complete or unspecified **spontaneous abortion** ＭＱ

Air embolism following complete or unspecified spontaneous abortion

Amniotic fluid embolism following complete or unspecified spontaneous abortion

Blood-clot embolism following complete or unspecified spontaneous abortion

Embolism NOS following complete or unspecified spontaneous abortion

Fat embolism following complete or unspecified spontaneous abortion

Pulmonary embolism following complete or unspecified spontaneous abortion

Pyemic embolism following complete or unspecified spontaneous abortion

Septic or septicopyemic embolism following complete or unspecified spontaneous abortion

Soap embolism following complete or unspecified spontaneous abortion

✓5ᵗʰ **O03.8** **Other** and unspecified complications **following** complete or unspecified **spontaneous abortion**

O03.80 **Unspecified complication following complete or unspecified spontaneous abortion** ＭＱ▽

O03.81 **Shock following complete or unspecified spontaneous abortion** ＭＱ

Circulatory collapse following complete or unspecified spontaneous abortion

Shock (postprocedural) following complete or unspecified spontaneous abortion

EXCLUDES 1 *shock due to infection following complete or unspecified spontaneous abortion (O03.87)*

O03.82 **Renal failure following complete or unspecified spontaneous abortion** ＭＱ

Kidney failure (acute) following complete or unspecified spontaneous abortion

Oliguria following complete or unspecified spontaneous abortion

Renal shutdown following complete or unspecified spontaneous abortion

Renal tubular necrosis following complete or unspecified spontaneous abortion

Uremia following complete or unspecified spontaneous abortion

O03.83 **Metabolic disorder following complete or unspecified spontaneous abortion** ＭＱ

O03.84 **Damage to pelvic organs following complete or unspecified spontaneous abortion** ＭＱ

Laceration, perforation, tear or chemical damage of bladder following complete or unspecified spontaneous abortion

Laceration, perforation, tear or chemical damage of bowel following complete or unspecified spontaneous abortion

Laceration, perforation, tear or chemical damage of broad ligament following complete or unspecified spontaneous abortion

Laceration, perforation, tear or chemical damage of cervix following complete or unspecified spontaneous abortion

Laceration, perforation, tear or chemical damage of periurethral tissue following complete or unspecified spontaneous abortion

Laceration, perforation, tear or chemical damage of uterus following complete or unspecified spontaneous abortion

Laceration, perforation, tear or chemical damage of vagina following complete or unspecified spontaneous abortion

O03.85 **Other** venous **complications following complete or unspecified spontaneous abortion** ＭＱ

O03.86 **Cardiac arrest following complete or unspecified spontaneous abortion** ＭＱ

O03.87 **Sepsis following complete or unspecified spontaneous abortion** ＭＱ

Use additional code to identify infectious agent (B95-B97)

Use additional code to identify severe sepsis, if applicable (R65.2-)

EXCLUDES 1 *septic or septicopyemic embolism following complete or unspecified spontaneous abortion (O03.7)*

O03.88 **Urinary tract infection following complete or unspecified spontaneous abortion** ＭＱ

Cystitis following complete or unspecified spontaneous abortion

O03.89 **Complete or unspecified spontaneous abortion with other complications** ＭＱ

O03.9 **Complete or unspecified spontaneous abortion** without complication ＭＱ▽

Miscarriage NOS

Spontaneous abortion NOS

✓4ᵗʰ **O04** **Complications following (induced) termination of pregnancy**

INCLUDES   complications following (induced) termination of pregnancy

EXCLUDES 1   *encounter for elective termination of pregnancy, uncomplicated (Z33.2)*

failed attempted termination of pregnancy (O07.-)

O04.5 **Genital tract and pelvic infection following (induced) termination of pregnancy** ＭＱ

Endometritis following (induced) termination of pregnancy

Oophoritis following (induced) termination of pregnancy

Parametritis following (induced) termination of pregnancy

Pelvic peritonitis following (induced) termination of pregnancy

Salpingitis following (induced) termination of pregnancy

Salpingo-oophoritis following (induced) termination of pregnancy

EXCLUDES 1 *sepsis following (induced) termination of pregnancy (O04.87)*

urinary tract infection following (induced) termination of pregnancy (O04.88)

O04.6 **Delayed or excessive hemorrhage following (induced) termination of pregnancy** ＭＱ

Afibrinogenemia following (induced) termination of pregnancy

Defibrination syndrome following (induced) termination of pregnancy

Hemolysis following (induced) termination of pregnancy

Intravascular coagulation following (induced) termination of pregnancy

O04.7 **Embolism following (induced) termination of pregnancy** ＭＱ

Air embolism following (induced) termination of pregnancy

Amniotic fluid embolism following (induced) termination of pregnancy

Blood-clot embolism following (induced) termination of pregnancy

Embolism NOS following (induced) termination of pregnancy

Fat embolism following (induced) termination of pregnancy

Pulmonary embolism following (induced) termination of pregnancy

Pyemic embolism following (induced) termination of pregnancy

Septic or septicopyemic embolism following (induced) termination of pregnancy

Soap embolism following (induced) termination of pregnancy

✓5ᵗʰ **O04.8** **(Induced) termination of pregnancy with** other and unspecified **complications**

O04.80 **(Induced) termination of pregnancy with unspecified complications** ＭＱ▽

O04.81 **Shock following (induced) termination of pregnancy** ＭＱ

Circulatory collapse following (induced) termination of pregnancy

Shock (postprocedural) following (induced) termination of pregnancy

EXCLUDES 1 *shock due to infection following (induced) termination of pregnancy (O04.87)*

O04.82 **Renal failure following (induced) termination of pregnancy** ＭＱ

Kidney failure (acute) following (induced) termination of pregnancy

Oliguria following (induced) termination of pregnancy

Renal shutdown following (induced) termination of pregnancy

Renal tubular necrosis following (induced) termination of pregnancy

Uremia following (induced) termination of pregnancy

O04.83 **Metabolic disorder following (induced) termination of pregnancy** ＭＱ

Ⓝ Newborn: 0   Ⓟ Pediatric: 0-17   Ⓜ Maternity: 12-55   Ⓐ Adult: 15-124   NRS Nonroutine supply Dx   NCDx Noncancer Dx   PDx Primary Dx   ▶◀ Revised Text   ● New Code   ▲ Revised Title

824   ICD-10-CM 2018

O04.84   **Damage to pelvic organs following (induced)** Ⓜ♀
    termination of pregnancy
     Laceration, perforation, tear or chemical damage of
      bladder following (induced) termination of
      pregnancy
     Laceration, perforation, tear or chemical damage of
      bowel following (induced) termination of
      pregnancy
     Laceration, perforation, tear or chemical damage of
      broad ligament following (induced) termination
      of pregnancy
     Laceration, perforation, tear or chemical damage of
      cervix following (induced) termination of
      pregnancy
     Laceration, perforation, tear or chemical damage of
      periurethral tissue following (induced)
      termination of pregnancy
     Laceration, perforation, tear or chemical damage of
      uterus following (induced) termination of
      pregnancy
     Laceration, perforation, tear or chemical damage of
      vagina following (induced) termination of
      pregnancy

O04.85   **Other venous complications following (induced)** Ⓜ♀
    termination of pregnancy

O04.86   **Cardiac arrest following (induced) termination** Ⓜ♀
    of pregnancy

O04.87   **Sepsis following (induced) termination of** Ⓜ♀
    pregnancy
     Use additional code to identify infectious agent
      (B95-B97)
     Use additional code to identify severe sepsis, if
      applicable (R65.2-)
     EXCLUDES 1   *septic or septicopyemic embolism following*
       (induced) termination of pregnancy
       (O04.7)

O04.88   **Urinary tract infection following (induced)** Ⓜ♀
    termination of pregnancy
     Cystitis following (induced) termination of pregnancy

O04.89   **(Induced) termination of pregnancy with other** Ⓜ♀
    complications

✓4ᵗʰ **O07**   **Failed attempted termination of pregnancy**
    INCLUDES   failure of attempted induction of termination of pregnancy
       incomplete elective abortion
    EXCLUDES 1   *incomplete spontaneous abortion (O03.0-)*

O07.0   **Genital tract and pelvic infection following failed** Ⓜ♀
    attempted termination of pregnancy
     Endometritis following failed attempted termination of
      pregnancy
     Oophoritis following failed attempted termination of pregnancy
     Parametritis following failed attempted termination of
      pregnancy
     Pelvic peritonitis following failed attempted termination of
      pregnancy
     Salpingitis following failed attempted termination of pregnancy
     Salpingo-oophoritis following failed attempted termination of
      pregnancy
     EXCLUDES 1   *sepsis following failed attempted termination of*
       pregnancy (O07.37)
       urinary tract infection following failed attempted
       termination of pregnancy (O07.38)

O07.1   **Delayed or excessive hemorrhage following failed** Ⓜ♀
    attempted termination of pregnancy
     Afibrinogenemia following failed attempted termination of
      pregnancy
     Defibrination syndrome following failed attempted termination
      of pregnancy
     Hemolysis following failed attempted termination of pregnancy
     Intravascular coagulation following failed attempted
      termination of pregnancy

O07.2   **Embolism following failed attempted termination of** Ⓜ♀
    pregnancy
     Air embolism following failed attempted termination of
      pregnancy
     Amniotic fluid embolism following failed attempted termination
      of pregnancy
     Blood-clot embolism following failed attempted termination of
      pregnancy
     Embolism NOS following failed attempted termination of
      pregnancy
     Fat embolism following failed attempted termination of
      pregnancy
     Pulmonary embolism following failed attempted termination of
      pregnancy
     Pyemic embolism following failed attempted termination of
      pregnancy
     Septic or septicopyemic embolism following failed attempted
      termination of pregnancy
     Soap embolism following failed attempted termination of
      pregnancy

✓5ᵗʰ **O07.3**   **Failed attempted termination of pregnancy with other and**
    unspecified complications

O07.30   **Failed attempted termination of pregnancy** Ⓜ♀▽
     with unspecified complications

O07.31   **Shock following failed attempted termination** Ⓜ♀
     of pregnancy
      Circulatory collapse following failed attempted
       termination of pregnancy
      Shock (postprocedural) following failed attempted
       termination of pregnancy
      EXCLUDES 1   *shock due to infection following failed*
        attempted termination of pregnancy
        (O07.37)

O07.32   **Renal failure following failed attempted** Ⓜ♀
     termination of pregnancy
      Kidney failure (acute) following failed attempted
       termination of pregnancy
      Oliguria following failed attempted termination of
       pregnancy
      Renal shutdown following failed attempted
       termination of pregnancy
      Renal tubular necrosis following failed attempted
       termination of pregnancy
      Uremia following failed attempted termination of
       pregnancy

O07.33   **Metabolic disorder following failed attempted** Ⓜ♀
     termination of pregnancy

O07.34   **Damage to pelvic organs following failed** Ⓜ♀
     attempted termination of pregnancy
      Laceration, perforation, tear or chemical damage of
       bladder following failed attempted termination
       of pregnancy
      Laceration, perforation, tear or chemical damage of
       bowel following failed attempted termination of
       pregnancy
      Laceration, perforation, tear or chemical damage of
       broad ligament following failed attempted
       termination of pregnancy
      Laceration, perforation, tear or chemical damage of
       cervix following failed attempted termination of
       pregnancy
      Laceration, perforation, tear or chemical damage of
       periurethral tissue following failed attempted
       termination of pregnancy
      Laceration, perforation, tear or chemical damage of
       uterus following failed attempted termination of
       pregnancy
      Laceration, perforation, tear or chemical damage of
       vagina following failed attempted termination of
       pregnancy

O07.35   **Other venous complications following failed** Ⓜ♀
     attempted termination of pregnancy

O07.36   **Cardiac arrest following failed attempted** Ⓜ♀
     termination of pregnancy

O07.37   **Sepsis following failed attempted termination** Ⓜ♀
     of pregnancy
      Use additional code to identify infectious agent
       (B95-B97)
      Use additional code to identify severe sepsis, if
       applicable (R65.2-)
      EXCLUDES 1   *septic or septicopyemic embolism following*
        failed attempted termination of
        pregnancy (O07.2)

☑ Additional Character Req   ✓ₓ7ᵗʰ Placeholder Alert   Case-Mix Diagnosis   Manifestation   ▽ Unspecified Dx   **EXCLUDES 1** Not coded here   **EXCLUDES 2** Not included here

ICD-10-CM 2018   825

O07.38 **Urinary tract infection** following failed attempted termination of pregnancy   Ⓜ♀
Cystitis following failed attempted termination of pregnancy

O07.39 **Failed attempted termination of pregnancy with other complications**   Ⓜ♀

O07.4 **Failed attempted termination of pregnancy** without complication   Ⓜ♀

✓4ᵗʰ **O08** **Complications following ectopic and molar pregnancy**
This category is for use with categories O00-O02 to identify any associated complications

O08.0 **Genital tract and pelvic infection following ectopic and molar pregnancy**   Ⓜ♀
Endometritis following ectopic and molar pregnancy
Oophoritis following ectopic and molar pregnancy
Parametritis following ectopic and molar pregnancy
Pelvic peritonitis following ectopic and molar pregnancy
Salpingitis following ectopic and molar pregnancy
Salpingo-oophoritis following ectopic and molar pregnancy
EXCLUDES 1 *sepsis following ectopic and molar pregnancy (O08.82)*
urinary tract infection (O08.83)

O08.1 **Delayed or excessive hemorrhage following ectopic and molar pregnancy**   Ⓜ♀
Afibrinogenemia following ectopic and molar pregnancy
Defibrination syndrome following ectopic and molar pregnancy
Hemolysis following ectopic and molar pregnancy
Intravascular coagulation following ectopic and molar pregnancy
EXCLUDES 1 *delayed or excessive hemorrhage due to incomplete abortion (O03.1)*

O08.2 **Embolism following ectopic and molar pregnancy**   Ⓜ♀
Air embolism following ectopic and molar pregnancy
Amniotic fluid embolism following ectopic and molar pregnancy
Blood-clot embolism following ectopic and molar pregnancy
Embolism NOS following ectopic and molar pregnancy
Fat embolism following ectopic and molar pregnancy
Pulmonary embolism following ectopic and molar pregnancy
Pyemic embolism following ectopic and molar pregnancy
Septic or septicopyemic embolism following ectopic and molar pregnancy
Soap embolism following ectopic and molar pregnancy

O08.3 **Shock following ectopic and molar pregnancy**   Ⓜ♀
Circulatory collapse following ectopic and molar pregnancy
Shock (postprocedural) following ectopic and molar pregnancy
EXCLUDES 1 *shock due to infection following ectopic and molar pregnancy (O08.82)*

O08.4 **Renal failure following ectopic and molar pregnancy**   Ⓜ♀
Kidney failure (acute) following ectopic and molar pregnancy
Oliguria following ectopic and molar pregnancy
Renal shutdown following ectopic and molar pregnancy
Renal tubular necrosis following ectopic and molar pregnancy
Uremia following ectopic and molar pregnancy

O08.5 **Metabolic disorders following an ectopic and molar pregnancy**   Ⓜ♀

O08.6 **Damage to pelvic organs and tissues following an ectopic and molar pregnancy**   Ⓜ♀
Laceration, perforation, tear or chemical damage of bladder following an ectopic and molar pregnancy
Laceration, perforation, tear or chemical damage of bowel following an ectopic and molar pregnancy
Laceration, perforation, tear or chemical damage of broad ligament following an ectopic and molar pregnancy
Laceration, perforation, tear or chemical damage of cervix following an ectopic and molar pregnancy
Laceration, perforation, tear or chemical damage of periurethral tissue following an ectopic and molar pregnancy
Laceration, perforation, tear or chemical damage of uterus following an ectopic and molar pregnancy
Laceration, perforation, tear or chemical damage of vagina following an ectopic and molar pregnancy

O08.7 **Other venous complications following an ectopic and molar pregnancy**   Ⓜ♀

✓5ᵗʰ **O08.8** **Other complications following an ectopic and molar pregnancy**   Ⓜ♀
O08.81 **Cardiac arrest following an ectopic and molar pregnancy**   Ⓜ♀

O08.82 **Sepsis following ectopic and molar pregnancy**   Ⓜ♀
Use additional code to identify infectious agent (B95-B97)
Use additional code to identify severe sepsis, if applicable (R65.2-)
EXCLUDES 1 *septic or septicopyemic embolism following ectopic and molar pregnancy (O08.2)*

O08.83 **Urinary tract infection following an ectopic and molar pregnancy**   Ⓜ♀
Cystitis following an ectopic and molar pregnancy

O08.89 **Other complications following an ectopic and molar pregnancy**   Ⓜ♀

O08.9 **Unspecified complication following an ectopic and molar pregnancy**   Ⓜ♀▽

Supervision of high risk pregnancy (O09)

✓4ᵗʰ **O09** **Supervision of high risk pregnancy**
AHA: 2016, 4Q, 150

✓5ᵗʰ **O09.0** **Supervision of pregnancy with history of infertility**
O09.00 **Supervision of pregnancy with history of infertility, unspecified trimester**   Ⓜ♀▽
O09.01 **Supervision of pregnancy with history of infertility, first trimester**   Ⓜ♀
O09.02 **Supervision of pregnancy with history of infertility, second trimester**   Ⓜ♀
O09.03 **Supervision of pregnancy with history of infertility, third trimester**   Ⓜ♀

✓5ᵗʰ **O09.1** **Supervision of pregnancy with history of ectopic pregnancy**
O09.10 **Supervision of pregnancy with history of ectopic pregnancy, unspecified trimester**   Ⓜ♀▽
O09.11 **Supervision of pregnancy with history of ectopic pregnancy, first trimester**   Ⓜ♀
O09.12 **Supervision of pregnancy with history of ectopic pregnancy, second trimester**   Ⓜ♀
O09.13 **Supervision of pregnancy with history of ectopic pregnancy, third trimester**   Ⓜ♀

✓5ᵗʰ **O09.A** **Supervision of pregnancy with history of molar pregnancy**
O09.A0 **Supervision of pregnancy with history of molar pregnancy, unspecified trimester**   Ⓜ♀▽
O09.A1 **Supervision of pregnancy with history of molar pregnancy, first trimester**   Ⓜ♀
O09.A2 **Supervision of pregnancy with history of molar pregnancy, second trimester**   Ⓜ♀
O09.A3 **Supervision of pregnancy with history of molar pregnancy, third trimester**   Ⓜ♀

✓5ᵗʰ **O09.2** **Supervision of pregnancy with other poor reproductive or obstetric history**
EXCLUDES 2 *pregnancy care for patient with history of recurrent pregnancy loss (O26.2-)*

✓6ᵗʰ **O09.21** **Supervision of pregnancy with history of pre-term labor**
O09.211 **Supervision of pregnancy with history of pre-term labor, first trimester**   Ⓜ♀
O09.212 **Supervision of pregnancy with history of pre-term labor, second trimester**   Ⓜ♀
O09.213 **Supervision of pregnancy with history of pre-term labor, third trimester**   Ⓜ♀
O09.219 **Supervision of pregnancy with history of pre-term labor, unspecified trimester**   Ⓜ♀▽

✓6ᵗʰ **O09.29** **Supervision of pregnancy with other poor reproductive or obstetric history**
Supervision of pregnancy with history of neonatal death
Supervision of pregnancy with history of stillbirth
O09.291 **Supervision of pregnancy with other poor reproductive or obstetric history, first trimester**   Ⓜ♀
O09.292 **Supervision of pregnancy with other poor reproductive or obstetric history, second trimester**   Ⓜ♀
O09.293 **Supervision of pregnancy with other poor reproductive or obstetric history, third trimester**   Ⓜ♀
O09.299 **Supervision of pregnancy with other poor reproductive or obstetric history, unspecified trimester**   Ⓜ♀▽

Ⓝ Newborn: 0 Ⓟ Pediatric: 0-17 Ⓜ Maternity: 12-55 Ⓐ Adult: 15-124 ⁿᴿˢ Nonroutine supply Dx ᴺᶜᴰˣ Noncancer Dx ᴾᴰˣ Primary Dx ►◄ Revised Text ● New Code ▲ Revised Title

826   ICD-10-CM 2018

✓5ᵗʰ **O09.3 Supervision of pregnancy with** insufficient antenatal care
Supervision of concealed pregnancy
Supervision of hidden pregnancy

    O09.30 Supervision of pregnancy with insufficient Ⓜ♀▽
antenatal care, unspecified trimester

    O09.31 Supervision of pregnancy with insufficient Ⓜ♀
antenatal care, first trimester

    O09.32 Supervision of pregnancy with insufficient Ⓜ♀
antenatal care, second trimester

    O09.33 Supervision of pregnancy with insufficient Ⓜ♀
antenatal care, third trimester

✓5ᵗʰ **O09.4 Supervision of pregnancy with** grand multiparity

    O09.40 Supervision of pregnancy with grand Ⓜ♀▽
multiparity, unspecified trimester

    O09.41 Supervision of pregnancy with grand Ⓜ♀
multiparity, first trimester

    O09.42 Supervision of pregnancy with grand Ⓜ♀
multiparity, second trimester

    O09.43 Supervision of pregnancy with grand Ⓜ♀
multiparity, third trimester

✓5ᵗʰ **O09.5 Supervision of** elderly primigravida and multigravida
Pregnancy for a female 35 years and older at expected date of
delivery

  ✓6ᵗʰ **O09.51 Supervision of** elderly primigravida

    O09.511 Supervision of elderly primigravida, Ⓜ♀
first trimester

    O09.512 Supervision of elderly primigravida, Ⓜ♀
second trimester

    O09.513 Supervision of elderly primigravida, Ⓜ♀
third trimester

    O09.519 Supervision of elderly primigravida, Ⓜ♀▽
unspecified trimester

  ✓6ᵗʰ **O09.52 Supervision of** elderly multigravida

    O09.521 Supervision of elderly multigravida, Ⓜ♀
first trimester

    O09.522 Supervision of elderly multigravida, Ⓜ♀
second trimester

    O09.523 Supervision of elderly multigravida, Ⓜ♀
third trimester

    O09.529 Supervision of elderly multigravida, Ⓜ♀▽
unspecified trimester

✓5ᵗʰ **O09.6 Supervision of** young primigravida and multigravida
Supervision of pregnancy for a female less than 16 years old at
expected date of delivery

  ✓6ᵗʰ **O09.61 Supervision of young** primigravida

    O09.611 Supervision of young primigravida, Ⓜ♀
first trimester

    O09.612 Supervision of young primigravida, Ⓜ♀
second trimester

    O09.613 Supervision of young primigravida, Ⓜ♀
third trimester

    O09.619 Supervision of young primigravida, Ⓜ♀▽
unspecified trimester

  ✓6ᵗʰ **O09.62 Supervision of young** multigravida

    O09.621 Supervision of young multigravida, Ⓜ♀
first trimester

    O09.622 Supervision of young multigravida, Ⓜ♀
second trimester

    O09.623 Supervision of young multigravida, Ⓜ♀
third trimester

    O09.629 Supervision of young multigravida, Ⓜ♀▽
unspecified trimester

✓5ᵗʰ **O09.7 Supervision of high risk pregnancy due to** social problems

    O09.70 Supervision of high risk pregnancy due to Ⓜ♀▽
social problems, unspecified trimester

    O09.71 Supervision of high risk pregnancy due to Ⓜ♀
social problems, first trimester

    O09.72 Supervision of high risk pregnancy due to Ⓜ♀
social problems, second trimester

    O09.73 Supervision of high risk pregnancy due to Ⓜ♀
social problems, third trimester

✓5ᵗʰ **O09.8 Supervision of** other high risk pregnancies

  ✓6ᵗʰ **O09.81 Supervision of pregnancy** resulting from assisted
reproductive technology
Supervision of pregnancy resulting from in-vitro
fertilization
EXCLUDES 2 gestational carrier status (Z33.3)

    O09.811 Supervision of pregnancy resulting Ⓜ♀
from assisted reproductive technology,
first trimester

    O09.812 Supervision of pregnancy resulting Ⓜ♀
from assisted reproductive technology,
second trimester

    O09.813 Supervision of pregnancy resulting Ⓜ♀
from assisted reproductive technology,
third trimester

    O09.819 Supervision of pregnancy resulting Ⓜ♀▽
from assisted reproductive technology,
unspecified trimester

  ✓6ᵗʰ **O09.82 Supervision of pregnancy with** history of in utero
procedure during previous pregnancy

    O09.821 Supervision of pregnancy with history Ⓜ♀
of in utero procedure during previous
pregnancy, first trimester

    O09.822 Supervision of pregnancy with history Ⓜ♀
of in utero procedure during previous
pregnancy, second trimester

    O09.823 Supervision of pregnancy with history Ⓜ♀
of in utero procedure during previous
pregnancy, third trimester

    O09.829 Supervision of pregnancy with Ⓜ♀▽
history of in utero procedure during
previous pregnancy, unspecified
trimester
EXCLUDES 1 supervision of pregnancy affected
by in utero procedure during
current pregnancy (O35.7)

  ✓6ᵗʰ **O09.89 Supervision of** other high risk pregnancies

    O09.891 Supervision of other high risk Ⓜ♀
pregnancies, first trimester

    O09.892 Supervision of other high risk Ⓜ♀
pregnancies, second trimester

    O09.893 Supervision of other high risk Ⓜ♀
pregnancies, third trimester

    O09.899 Supervision of other high risk Ⓜ♀▽
pregnancies, unspecified trimester

✓5ᵗʰ **O09.9 Supervision of high risk pregnancy,** unspecified

    O09.90 Supervision of high risk pregnancy, Ⓜ♀▽
unspecified, unspecified trimester

    O09.91 Supervision of high risk pregnancy, Ⓜ♀▽
unspecified, first trimester

    O09.92 Supervision of high risk pregnancy, Ⓜ♀▽
unspecified, second trimester

    O09.93 Supervision of high risk pregnancy, Ⓜ♀▽
unspecified, third trimester

Edema, proteinuria and hypertensive disorders in pregnancy, childbirth and the puerperium (O10-O16)

✓4ᵗʰ **O10 Pre-existing hypertension complicating pregnancy, childbirth and the puerperium**
INCLUDES pre-existing hypertension with pre-existing proteinuria
complicating pregnancy, childbirth and the puerperium
EXCLUDES 2 pre-existing hypertension with superimposed pre-eclampsia
complicating pregnancy, childbirth and the puerperium
(O11.-)

  ✓5ᵗʰ **O10.0 Pre-existing** essential **hypertension complicating pregnancy, childbirth and the puerperium**
Any condition in I10 specified as a reason for obstetric care
during pregnancy, childbirth or the puerperium

  ✓6ᵗʰ **O10.01 Pre-existing essential hypertension complicating** pregnancy

    O10.011 Pre-existing essential hypertension Ⓜ♀
complicating pregnancy, first
trimester

    O10.012 Pre-existing essential hypertension Ⓜ♀
complicating pregnancy, second
trimester

    O10.013 Pre-existing essential hypertension Ⓜ♀
complicating pregnancy, third
trimester

    O10.019 Pre-existing essential hypertension Ⓜ♀▽
complicating pregnancy, unspecified
trimester

    O10.02 Pre-existing essential hypertension Ⓜ♀
complicating childbirth

☑ Additional Character Req   ✓x7ᵗʰ Placeholder Alert   Case-Mix Diagnosis   Manifestation   ▽ Unspecified Dx   *EXCLUDES 1* Not coded here   *EXCLUDES 2* Not included here

ICD-10-CM 2018   **827**

O10.03   Pre-existing essential hypertension complicating the puerperium   Ⓜ♀

✓5ᵗʰ **O10.1   Pre-existing hypertensive** heart disease **complicating pregnancy, childbirth and the puerperium**
Any condition in I11 specified as a reason for obstetric care during pregnancy, childbirth or the puerperium
Use additional code from I11 to identify the type of hypertensive heart disease

    ✓6ᵗʰ **O10.11   Pre-existing hypertensive heart disease complicating** pregnancy

       O10.111   Pre-existing hypertensive heart disease complicating pregnancy, first trimester   Ⓜ♀

       O10.112   Pre-existing hypertensive heart disease complicating pregnancy, second trimester   Ⓜ♀

       O10.113   Pre-existing hypertensive heart disease complicating pregnancy, third trimester   Ⓜ♀

       O10.119   Pre-existing hypertensive heart disease complicating pregnancy, unspecified trimester   Ⓜ♀▽

    O10.12   Pre-existing hypertensive heart disease complicating childbirth   Ⓜ♀

    O10.13   Pre-existing hypertensive heart disease complicating the puerperium   Ⓜ♀

✓5ᵗʰ **O10.2   Pre-existing hypertensive** chronic kidney disease **complicating pregnancy, childbirth and the puerperium**
Any condition in I12 specified as a reason for obstetric care during pregnancy, childbirth or the puerperium
Use additional code from I12 to identify the type of hypertensive chronic kidney disease

    ✓6ᵗʰ **O10.21   Pre-existing hypertensive chronic kidney disease complicating** pregnancy

       O10.211   Pre-existing hypertensive chronic kidney disease complicating pregnancy, first trimester   Ⓜ♀

       O10.212   Pre-existing hypertensive chronic kidney disease complicating pregnancy, second trimester   Ⓜ♀

       O10.213   Pre-existing hypertensive chronic kidney disease complicating pregnancy, third trimester   Ⓜ♀

       O10.219   Pre-existing hypertensive chronic kidney disease complicating pregnancy, unspecified trimester   Ⓜ♀▽

    O10.22   Pre-existing hypertensive chronic kidney disease complicating childbirth   Ⓜ♀

    O10.23   Pre-existing hypertensive chronic kidney disease complicating the puerperium   Ⓜ♀

✓5ᵗʰ **O10.3   Pre-existing hypertensive** heart and chronic kidney disease **complicating pregnancy, childbirth and the puerperium**
Any condition in I13 specified as a reason for obstetric care during pregnancy, childbirth or the puerperium
Use additional code from I13 to identify the type of hypertensive heart and chronic kidney disease

    ✓6ᵗʰ **O10.31   Pre-existing hypertensive heart and chronic kidney disease complicating** pregnancy

       O10.311   Pre-existing hypertensive heart and chronic kidney disease complicating pregnancy, first trimester   Ⓜ♀

       O10.312   Pre-existing hypertensive heart and chronic kidney disease complicating pregnancy, second trimester   Ⓜ♀

       O10.313   Pre-existing hypertensive heart and chronic kidney disease complicating pregnancy, third trimester   Ⓜ♀

       O10.319   Pre-existing hypertensive heart and chronic kidney disease complicating pregnancy, unspecified trimester   Ⓜ♀▽

    O10.32   Pre-existing hypertensive heart and chronic kidney disease complicating childbirth   Ⓜ♀

    O10.33   Pre-existing hypertensive heart and chronic kidney disease complicating the puerperium   Ⓜ♀

✓5ᵗʰ **O10.4   Pre-existing** secondary **hypertension complicating pregnancy, childbirth and the puerperium**
Any condition in I15 specified as a reason for obstetric care during pregnancy, childbirth or the puerperium
Use additional code from I15 to identify the type of secondary hypertension

    ✓6ᵗʰ **O10.41   Pre-existing secondary hypertension complicating** pregnancy

       O10.411   Pre-existing secondary hypertension complicating pregnancy, first trimester   Ⓜ♀

       O10.412   Pre-existing secondary hypertension complicating pregnancy, second trimester   Ⓜ♀

       O10.413   Pre-existing secondary hypertension complicating pregnancy, third trimester   Ⓜ♀

       O10.419   Pre-existing secondary hypertension complicating pregnancy, unspecified trimester   Ⓜ♀▽

    O10.42   Pre-existing secondary hypertension complicating childbirth   Ⓜ♀

    O10.43   Pre-existing secondary hypertension complicating the puerperium   Ⓜ♀

✓5ᵗʰ **O10.9 ** Unspecified **pre-existing hypertension complicating pregnancy, childbirth and the puerperium**

    ✓6ᵗʰ **O10.91   Unspecified pre-existing hypertension complicating** pregnancy

       O10.911   Unspecified pre-existing hypertension complicating pregnancy, first trimester   Ⓜ♀▽

       O10.912   Unspecified pre-existing hypertension complicating pregnancy, second trimester   Ⓜ♀▽

       O10.913   Unspecified pre-existing hypertension complicating pregnancy, third trimester   Ⓜ♀▽

       O10.919   Unspecified pre-existing hypertension complicating pregnancy, unspecified trimester   Ⓜ♀▽

    O10.92   Unspecified pre-existing hypertension complicating childbirth   Ⓜ♀▽

    O10.93   Unspecified pre-existing hypertension complicating the puerperium   Ⓜ♀▽

✓4ᵗʰ **O11 ** Pre-existing **hypertension with** pre-eclampsia
    INCLUDES   conditions in O10 complicated by pre-eclampsia
              pre-eclampsia superimposed pre-existing hypertension
    Use additional code from O10 to identify the type of hypertension

    O11.1   Pre-existing hypertension with pre-eclampsia, first trimester   Ⓜ♀

    O11.2   Pre-existing hypertension with pre-eclampsia, second trimester   Ⓜ♀

    O11.3   Pre-existing hypertension with pre-eclampsia, third trimester   Ⓜ♀

    O11.4   Pre-existing hypertension with pre-eclampsia, complicating childbirth   Ⓜ♀

    O11.5   Pre-existing hypertension with pre-eclampsia, complicating the puerperium   Ⓜ♀

    O11.9   Pre-existing hypertension with pre-eclampsia, unspecified trimester   Ⓜ♀▽

✓4ᵗʰ **O12 ** Gestational **[pregnancy-induced] edema and proteinuria without hypertension**

    ✓5ᵗʰ **O12.0   Gestational** edema

       O12.00   Gestational edema, unspecified trimester   Ⓜ♀▽

       O12.01   Gestational edema, first trimester   Ⓜ♀

       O12.02   Gestational edema, second trimester   Ⓜ♀

       O12.03   Gestational edema, third trimester   Ⓜ♀

       O12.04   Gestational edema, complicating childbirth   Ⓜ♀

       O12.05   Gestational edema, complicating the puerperium   Ⓜ♀

    ✓5ᵗʰ **O12.1   Gestational** proteinuria

       O12.10   Gestational proteinuria, unspecified trimester   Ⓜ♀▽

       O12.11   Gestational proteinuria, first trimester   Ⓜ♀

       O12.12   Gestational proteinuria, second trimester   Ⓜ♀

       O12.13   Gestational proteinuria, third trimester   Ⓜ♀

Ⓝ Newborn: 0   Ⓟ Pediatric: 0-17   Ⓜ Maternity: 12-55   Ⓐ Adult: 15-124   NRS Nonroutine supply Dx   NC Dx Noncancer Dx   PDx Primary Dx   ▶◀ Revised Text   ● New Code   ▲ Revised Title

O12.14   **Gestational proteinuria, complicating** childbirth   Ⓜ♀

O12.15   **Gestational proteinuria, complicating the** puerperium   Ⓜ♀

☑5ᵗʰ **O12.2**   **Gestational** edema with proteinuria

O12.20   **Gestational edema with proteinuria, unspecified trimester**   Ⓜ♀▽

O12.21   **Gestational edema with proteinuria,** first trimester   Ⓜ♀

O12.22   **Gestational edema with proteinuria,** second trimester   Ⓜ♀

O12.23   **Gestational edema with proteinuria,** third trimester   Ⓜ♀

O12.24   **Gestational edema with proteinuria, complicating** childbirth   Ⓜ♀

O12.25   **Gestational edema with proteinuria, complicating the** puerperium   Ⓜ♀

☑4ᵗʰ **O13**   Gestational **[pregnancy-induced] hypertension without significant proteinuria**
     INCLUDES   gestational hypertension NOS
         transient hypertension of pregnancy
     AHA: 2016, 1Q, 5

O13.1   **Gestational [pregnancy-induced] hypertension without significant proteinuria,** first trimester   Ⓜ♀

O13.2   **Gestational [pregnancy-induced] hypertension without significant proteinuria,** second trimester   Ⓜ♀

O13.3   **Gestational [pregnancy-induced] hypertension without significant proteinuria,** third trimester   Ⓜ♀

O13.4   **Gestational [pregnancy-induced] hypertension without significant proteinuria, complicating** childbirth   Ⓜ♀

O13.5   **Gestational [pregnancy-induced] hypertension without significant proteinuria, complicating the** puerperium   Ⓜ♀

O13.9   **Gestational [pregnancy-induced] hypertension without significant proteinuria, unspecified trimester**   Ⓜ♀▽

☑4ᵗʰ **O14**   Pre-eclampsia
     EXCLUDES 1   pre-existing hypertension with pre-eclampsia (O11)

☑5ᵗʰ **O14.0**   Mild to moderate **pre-eclampsia**

O14.00   **Mild to moderate pre-eclampsia, unspecified** trimester   Ⓜ♀▽

O14.02   **Mild to moderate pre-eclampsia,** second trimester   Ⓜ♀

O14.03   **Mild to moderate pre-eclampsia,** third trimester   Ⓜ♀

O14.04   **Mild to moderate pre-eclampsia, complicating** childbirth   Ⓜ♀

O14.05   **Mild to moderate pre-eclampsia, complicating the** puerperium   Ⓜ♀

☑5ᵗʰ **O14.1**   Severe **pre-eclampsia**
     EXCLUDES 1   HELLP syndrome (O14.2-)

O14.10   **Severe pre-eclampsia, unspecified trimester**   Ⓜ♀▽

O14.12   **Severe pre-eclampsia,** second trimester   Ⓜ♀

O14.13   **Severe pre-eclampsia,** third trimester   Ⓜ♀

O14.14   **Severe pre-eclampsia complicating** childbirth   Ⓜ♀

O14.15   **Severe pre-eclampsia, complicating the** puerperium   Ⓜ♀

☑5ᵗʰ **O14.2**   HELLP syndrome
     Severe pre-eclampsia with hemolysis, elevated liver enzymes and low platelet count (HELLP)

O14.20   **HELLP syndrome (HELLP), unspecified trimester**   Ⓜ♀▽

O14.22   **HELLP syndrome (HELLP),** second trimester   Ⓜ♀

O14.23   **HELLP syndrome (HELLP),** third trimester   Ⓜ♀

O14.24   **HELLP syndrome, complicating** childbirth   Ⓜ♀

O14.25   **HELLP syndrome, complicating the** puerperium   Ⓜ♀

☑5ᵗʰ **O14.9**   Unspecified **pre-eclampsia**

O14.90   **Unspecified pre-eclampsia, unspecified trimester**   Ⓜ♀▽

O14.92   **Unspecified pre-eclampsia,** second trimester   Ⓜ♀▽

O14.93   **Unspecified pre-eclampsia,** third trimester   Ⓜ♀▽

O14.94   **Unspecified pre-eclampsia, complicating** childbirth   Ⓜ♀▽

O14.95   **Unspecified pre-eclampsia, complicating the** puerperium   Ⓜ♀▽

☑4ᵗʰ **O15**   Eclampsia
     INCLUDES   convulsions following conditions in O10-O14 and O16

☑5ᵗʰ **O15.0**   Eclampsia complicating pregnancy

O15.00   **Eclampsia complicating pregnancy, unspecified trimester**   Ⓜ♀▽

O15.02   **Eclampsia complicating pregnancy,** second trimester   Ⓜ♀

O15.03   **Eclampsia complicating pregnancy,** third trimester   Ⓜ♀

O15.1   **Eclampsia complicating** labor   Ⓜ♀

O15.2   **Eclampsia complicating the** puerperium   Ⓜ♀

O15.9   **Eclampsia, unspecified as to time period**   Ⓜ♀▽
     Eclampsia NOS

☑4ᵗʰ **O16**   Unspecified maternal hypertension

O16.1   **Unspecified maternal hypertension,** first trimester   Ⓜ♀▽

O16.2   **Unspecified maternal hypertension,** second trimester   Ⓜ♀▽

O16.3   **Unspecified maternal hypertension,** third trimester   Ⓜ♀▽

O16.4   **Unspecified maternal hypertension, complicating** childbirth   Ⓜ♀▽

O16.5   **Unspecified maternal hypertension, complicating the** puerperium   Ⓜ♀▽

O16.9   **Unspecified maternal hypertension, unspecified trimester**   Ⓜ♀▽

Other maternal disorders predominantly related to pregnancy (O20-O29)

     EXCLUDES 2   maternal care related to the fetus and amniotic cavity and possible delivery problems (O30-O48)
         maternal diseases classifiable elsewhere but complicating pregnancy, labor and delivery, and the puerperium (O98-O99)

☑4ᵗʰ **O20**   **Hemorrhage in early pregnancy**
     Hemorrhage before completion of 20 weeks gestation
     EXCLUDES 1   pregnancy with abortive outcome (O00-O08)

O20.0   **Threatened abortion**   Ⓜ♀
     Hemorrhage specified as due to threatened abortion
     DEF: Bloody discharge during pregnancy; cervix may be dilated and pregnancy threatened, but the pregnancy is not terminated.

O20.8   **Other hemorrhage in early pregnancy**   Ⓜ♀

O20.9   **Hemorrhage in early pregnancy, unspecified**   Ⓜ♀▽

☑4ᵗʰ **O21**   **Excessive vomiting in pregnancy**

O21.0   Mild **hyperemesis gravidarum**   Ⓜ♀
     Hyperemesis gravidarum, mild or unspecified, starting before the end of the 20th week of gestation

O21.1   **Hyperemesis gravidarum with** metabolic disturbance   Ⓜ♀
     Hyperemesis gravidarum, starting before the end of the 20th week of gestation, with metabolic disturbance such as carbohydrate depletion
     Hyperemesis gravidarum, starting before the end of the 20th week of gestation, with metabolic disturbance such as dehydration
     Hyperemesis gravidarum, starting before the end of the 20th week of gestation, with metabolic disturbance such as electrolyte imbalance

O21.2   Late **vomiting of pregnancy**   Ⓜ♀
     Excessive vomiting starting after 20 completed weeks of gestation

O21.8   **Other vomiting complicating pregnancy**   Ⓜ♀
     Vomiting due to diseases classified elsewhere, complicating pregnancy
     Use additional code, to identify cause

O21.9   **Vomiting of pregnancy, unspecified**   Ⓜ♀▽

O22   **Venous complications and hemorrhoids in pregnancy**
     EXCLUDES 1   venous complications of:
         abortion NOS (O03.9)
         ectopic or molar pregnancy (O08.7)
         failed attempted abortion (O07.35)
         induced abortion (O04.85)
         spontaneous abortion (O03.89)
     EXCLUDES 2   obstetric pulmonary embolism (O88.-)
         venous complications and hemorrhoids of childbirth and the puerperium (O87.-)

☑5ᵗʰ **O22.0**   Varicose veins of lower extremity **in pregnancy**
     Varicose veins NOS in pregnancy
     DEF: Distended, tortuous veins of lower extremities associated with pregnancy.

O22.00   **Varicose veins of lower extremity in pregnancy, unspecified trimester**   Ⓜ♀▽

☑ Additional Character Req   ✔x7ᵗʰ Placeholder Alert   Case-Mix Diagnosis   Manifestation   ▽ Unspecified Dx   EXCLUDES 1 Not coded here   EXCLUDES 2 Not included here

ICD-10-CM 2018   829

O22.01 Varicose veins of lower extremity in pregnancy, first trimester Ⓜ♀

O22.02 Varicose veins of lower extremity in pregnancy, second trimester Ⓜ♀

O22.03 Varicose veins of lower extremity in pregnancy, third trimester Ⓜ♀

✓5ᵗʰ **O22.1 Genital varices in pregnancy**
Perineal varices in pregnancy
Vaginal varices in pregnancy
Vulval varices in pregnancy

O22.10 Genital varices in pregnancy, unspecified trimester Ⓜ♀▽

O22.11 Genital varices in pregnancy, first trimester Ⓜ♀

O22.12 Genital varices in pregnancy, second trimester Ⓜ♀

O22.13 Genital varices in pregnancy, third trimester Ⓜ♀

✓5ᵗʰ **O22.2 Superficial thrombophlebitis in pregnancy**
Phlebitis in pregnancy NOS
Thrombophlebitis of legs in pregnancy
Thrombosis in pregnancy NOS
Use additional code to identify the superficial thrombophlebitis (I80.0-)

O22.20 Superficial thrombophlebitis in pregnancy, unspecified trimester Ⓜ♀▽

O22.21 Superficial thrombophlebitis in pregnancy, first trimester Ⓜ♀

O22.22 Superficial thrombophlebitis in pregnancy, second trimester Ⓜ♀

O22.23 Superficial thrombophlebitis in pregnancy, third trimester Ⓜ♀

✓5ᵗʰ **O22.3 Deep phlebothrombosis in pregnancy**
Deep vein thrombosis, antepartum
Use additional code to identify the deep vein thrombosis (I82.4-, I82.5-, I82.62-. I82.72-)
Use additional code, if applicable, for associated long-term (current) use of anticoagulants (Z79.01)

O22.30 Deep phlebothrombosis in pregnancy, unspecified trimester Ⓜ♀▽

O22.31 Deep phlebothrombosis in pregnancy, first trimester Ⓜ♀

O22.32 Deep phlebothrombosis in pregnancy, second trimester Ⓜ♀

O22.33 Deep phlebothrombosis in pregnancy, third trimester Ⓜ♀

✓5ᵗʰ **O22.4 Hemorrhoids in pregnancy**

O22.40 Hemorrhoids in pregnancy, unspecified trimester Ⓜ♀▽

O22.41 Hemorrhoids in pregnancy, first trimester Ⓜ♀

O22.42 Hemorrhoids in pregnancy, second trimester Ⓜ♀

O22.43 Hemorrhoids in pregnancy, third trimester Ⓜ♀

✓5ᵗʰ **O22.5 Cerebral venous thrombosis in pregnancy**
Cerebrovenous sinus thrombosis in pregnancy

O22.50 Cerebral venous thrombosis in pregnancy, unspecified trimester Ⓜ♀▽

O22.51 Cerebral venous thrombosis in pregnancy, first trimester Ⓜ♀

O22.52 Cerebral venous thrombosis in pregnancy, second trimester Ⓜ♀

O22.53 Cerebral venous thrombosis in pregnancy, third trimester Ⓜ♀

✓5ᵗʰ **O22.8 Other venous complications in pregnancy**

✓6ᵗʰ **O22.8X Other venous complications in pregnancy**

O22.8X1 Other venous complications in pregnancy, first trimester Ⓜ♀

O22.8X2 Other venous complications in pregnancy, second trimester Ⓜ♀

O22.8X3 Other venous complications in pregnancy, third trimester Ⓜ♀

O22.8X9 Other venous complications in pregnancy, unspecified trimester Ⓜ♀▽

✓5ᵗʰ **O22.9 Venous complication in pregnancy, unspecified**
Gestational phlebitis NOS
Gestational phlebopathy NOS
Gestational thrombosis NOS

O22.90 Venous complication in pregnancy, unspecified, unspecified trimester Ⓜ♀▽

O22.91 Venous complication in pregnancy, unspecified, first trimester Ⓜ♀▽

O22.92 Venous complication in pregnancy, unspecified, second trimester Ⓜ♀▽

O22.93 Venous complication in pregnancy, unspecified, third trimester Ⓜ♀▽

✓4ᵗʰ **O23 Infections of genitourinary tract in pregnancy**
Use additional code to identify organism (B95.-, B96.-)

EXCLUDES 2 gonococcal infections complicating pregnancy, childbirth and the puerperium (O98.2)
infections with a predominantly sexual mode of transmission NOS complicating pregnancy, childbirth and the puerperium (O98.3)
syphilis complicating pregnancy, childbirth and the puerperium (O98.1)
tuberculosis of genitourinary system complicating pregnancy, childbirth and the puerperium (O98.0)
venereal disease NOS complicating pregnancy, childbirth and the puerperium (O98.3)

✓5ᵗʰ **O23.0 Infections of kidney in pregnancy**
Pyelonephritis in pregnancy

O23.00 Infections of kidney in pregnancy, unspecified trimester Ⓜ♀▽

O23.01 Infections of kidney in pregnancy, first trimester Ⓜ♀

O23.02 Infections of kidney in pregnancy, second trimester Ⓜ♀

O23.03 Infections of kidney in pregnancy, third trimester Ⓜ♀

✓5ᵗʰ **O23.1 Infections of bladder in pregnancy**

O23.10 Infections of bladder in pregnancy, unspecified trimester Ⓜ♀▽

O23.11 Infections of bladder in pregnancy, first trimester Ⓜ♀

O23.12 Infections of bladder in pregnancy, second trimester Ⓜ♀

O23.13 Infections of bladder in pregnancy, third trimester Ⓜ♀

✓5ᵗʰ **O23.2 Infections of urethra in pregnancy**

O23.20 Infections of urethra in pregnancy, unspecified trimester Ⓜ♀▽

O23.21 Infections of urethra in pregnancy, first trimester Ⓜ♀

O23.22 Infections of urethra in pregnancy, second trimester Ⓜ♀

O23.23 Infections of urethra in pregnancy, third trimester Ⓜ♀

✓5ᵗʰ **O23.3 Infections of other parts of urinary tract in pregnancy**

O23.30 Infections of other parts of urinary tract in pregnancy, unspecified trimester Ⓜ♀▽

O23.31 Infections of other parts of urinary tract in pregnancy, first trimester Ⓜ♀

O23.32 Infections of other parts of urinary tract in pregnancy, second trimester Ⓜ♀

O23.33 Infections of other parts of urinary tract in pregnancy, third trimester Ⓜ♀

✓5ᵗʰ **O23.4 Unspecified infection of urinary tract in pregnancy**

O23.40 Unspecified infection of urinary tract in pregnancy, unspecified trimester Ⓜ♀▽

O23.41 Unspecified infection of urinary tract in pregnancy, first trimester Ⓜ♀▽

O23.42 Unspecified infection of urinary tract in pregnancy, second trimester Ⓜ♀▽

O23.43 Unspecified infection of urinary tract in pregnancy, third trimester Ⓜ♀▽

✓5ᵗʰ **O23.5 Infections of the genital tract in pregnancy**

✓6ᵗʰ **O23.51 Infection of cervix in pregnancy**

O23.511 Infections of cervix in pregnancy, first trimester Ⓜ♀

O23.512 Infections of cervix in pregnancy, second trimester Ⓜ♀

O23.513 Infections of cervix in pregnancy, third trimester Ⓜ♀

O23.519 Infections of cervix in pregnancy, unspecified trimester Ⓜ♀▽

✓6ᵗʰ **O23.52 Salpingo-oophoritis in pregnancy**
Oophoritis in pregnancy
Salpingitis in pregnancy

O23.521 Salpingo-oophoritis in pregnancy, first trimester Ⓜ♀

O23.522   **Salpingo-oophoritis in pregnancy, second trimester**   Ⓜ♀

O23.523   **Salpingo-oophoritis in pregnancy, third trimester**   Ⓜ♀

O23.529   **Salpingo-oophoritis in pregnancy, unspecified trimester**   Ⓜ♀▽

√6ᵗʰ **O23.59**   **Infection of** other part **of genital tract in pregnancy**

O23.591   **Infection of other part of genital tract in pregnancy,** first trimester   Ⓜ♀

O23.592   **Infection of other part of genital tract in pregnancy,** second trimester   Ⓜ♀

O23.593   **Infection of other part of genital tract in pregnancy,** third trimester   Ⓜ♀

O23.599   **Infection of other part of genital tract in pregnancy, unspecified trimester**   Ⓜ♀▽

√5ᵗʰ **O23.9**   Unspecified **genitourinary tract infection in pregnancy**
Genitourinary tract infection in pregnancy NOS

O23.90   **Unspecified genitourinary tract infection in pregnancy, unspecified trimester**   Ⓜ♀▽

O23.91   **Unspecified genitourinary tract infection in pregnancy,** first trimester   Ⓜ♀▽

O23.92   **Unspecified genitourinary tract infection in pregnancy,** second trimester   Ⓜ♀▽

O23.93   **Unspecified genitourinary tract infection in pregnancy,** third trimester   Ⓜ♀▽

√4ᵗʰ **O24**   Diabetes mellitus **in pregnancy, childbirth, and the puerperium**

√5ᵗʰ **O24.0**   Pre-existing type 1 **diabetes mellitus, in pregnancy, childbirth and the puerperium**
Juvenile onset diabetes mellitus, in pregnancy, childbirth and the puerperium
Ketosis-prone diabetes mellitus in pregnancy, childbirth and the puerperium
Use additional code from category E10 to further identify any manifestations

√6ᵗʰ **O24.01**   **Pre-existing type 1 diabetes mellitus, in** pregnancy

O24.011   **Pre-existing type 1 diabetes mellitus, in pregnancy,** first trimester   Ⓜ♀

O24.012   **Pre-existing type 1 diabetes mellitus, in pregnancy,** second trimester   Ⓜ♀

O24.013   **Pre-existing type 1 diabetes mellitus, in pregnancy,** third trimester   Ⓜ♀

O24.019   **Pre-existing type 1 diabetes mellitus, in pregnancy, unspecified trimester**   Ⓜ♀▽

O24.02   **Pre-existing type 1 diabetes mellitus, in** childbirth   Ⓜ♀

O24.03   **Pre-existing type 1 diabetes mellitus, in the** puerperium   Ⓜ♀

√5ᵗʰ **O24.1**   Pre-existing type 2 **diabetes mellitus, in pregnancy, childbirth and the puerperium**
Insulin-resistant diabetes mellitus in pregnancy, childbirth and the puerperium
Use additional code (for):
   from category E11 to further identify any manifestations
   long-term (current) use of insulin (Z79.4)

√6ᵗʰ **O24.11**   **Pre-existing type 2 diabetes mellitus, in** pregnancy

O24.111   **Pre-existing type 2 diabetes mellitus, in pregnancy,** first trimester   Ⓜ♀

O24.112   **Pre-existing type 2 diabetes mellitus, in pregnancy,** second trimester   Ⓜ♀

O24.113   **Pre-existing type 2 diabetes mellitus, in pregnancy,** third trimester   Ⓜ♀

O24.119   **Pre-existing type 2 diabetes mellitus, in pregnancy, unspecified trimester**   Ⓜ♀▽

O24.12   **Pre-existing type 2 diabetes mellitus, in** childbirth   Ⓜ♀

O24.13   **Pre-existing type 2 diabetes mellitus, in the** puerperium   Ⓜ♀

√5ᵗʰ **O24.3**   Unspecified pre-existing **diabetes mellitus in pregnancy, childbirth and the puerperium**
Use additional code (for):
   from category E11 to further identify any manifestation
   long-term (current) use of insulin (Z79.4)

√6ᵗʰ **O24.31**   Unspecified **pre-existing diabetes mellitus in pregnancy**

O24.311   **Unspecified pre-existing diabetes mellitus in pregnancy,** first trimester   Ⓜ♀▽

O24.312   **Unspecified pre-existing diabetes mellitus in pregnancy,** second trimester   Ⓜ♀▽

O24.313   **Unspecified pre-existing diabetes mellitus in pregnancy,** third trimester   Ⓜ♀▽

O24.319   **Unspecified pre-existing diabetes mellitus in pregnancy, unspecified trimester**   Ⓜ♀▽

O24.32   **Unspecified pre-existing diabetes mellitus in** childbirth   Ⓜ♀▽

O24.33   **Unspecified pre-existing diabetes mellitus in the** puerperium   Ⓜ♀▽

√5ᵗʰ **O24.4**   Gestational **diabetes mellitus**
Diabetes mellitus arising in pregnancy
Gestational diabetes mellitus NOS

√6ᵗʰ **O24.41**   **Gestational diabetes mellitus in** pregnancy

O24.410   **Gestational diabetes mellitus in pregnancy, diet controlled**   Ⓜ♀

O24.414   **Gestational diabetes mellitus in pregnancy, insulin controlled**   Ⓜ♀

O24.415   **Gestational diabetes mellitus in pregnancy, controlled by oral hypoglycemic drugs**   Ⓜ♀
Gestational diabetes mellitus in pregnancy, controlled by oral antidiabetic drugs

O24.419   **Gestational diabetes mellitus in pregnancy, unspecified control**   Ⓜ♀▽
AHA: 2015, 4Q, 34

√6ᵗʰ **O24.42**   **Gestational diabetes mellitus in** childbirth
AHA: 2016, 1Q, 5

O24.420   **Gestational diabetes mellitus in childbirth, diet controlled**   Ⓜ♀

O24.424   **Gestational diabetes mellitus in childbirth, insulin controlled**   Ⓜ♀

O24.425   **Gestational diabetes mellitus in childbirth, controlled by oral hypoglycemic drugs**   Ⓜ♀
Gestational diabetes mellitus in childbirth, controlled by oral antidiabetic drugs

O24.429   **Gestational diabetes mellitus in childbirth, unspecified control**   Ⓜ♀▽
AHA: 2015, 4Q, 34

√6ᵗʰ **O24.43**   **Gestational diabetes mellitus in the** puerperium

O24.430   **Gestational diabetes mellitus in the puerperium, diet controlled**   Ⓜ♀

O24.434   **Gestational diabetes mellitus in the puerperium, insulin controlled**   Ⓜ♀

O24.435   **Gestational diabetes mellitus in puerperium, controlled by oral hypoglycemic drugs**   Ⓜ♀
Gestational diabetes mellitus in puerperium, controlled by oral antidiabetic drugs

O24.439   **Gestational diabetes mellitus in the puerperium, unspecified control**   Ⓜ♀▽
AHA: 2015, 4Q, 34

√5ᵗʰ **O24.8**   Other pre-existing **diabetes mellitus in pregnancy, childbirth, and the puerperium**
Use additional code (for):
   from categories E08, E09 and E13 to further identify any manifestation
   long-term (current) use of insulin (Z79.4)

√6ᵗʰ **O24.81**   **Other pre-existing diabetes mellitus in** pregnancy

O24.811   **Other pre-existing diabetes mellitus in pregnancy,** first trimester   Ⓜ♀

O24.812   **Other pre-existing diabetes mellitus in pregnancy,** second trimester   Ⓜ♀

O24.813   **Other pre-existing diabetes mellitus in pregnancy,** third trimester   Ⓜ♀

O24.819   **Other pre-existing diabetes mellitus in pregnancy, unspecified trimester**   Ⓜ♀▽

O24.82   **Other pre-existing diabetes mellitus in** childbirth   Ⓜ♀

O24.83   **Other pre-existing diabetes mellitus in the** puerperium   Ⓜ♀

Chapter 15. Pregnancy, Childbirth and the Puerperium

✓5th **O24.9** **Unspecified diabetes mellitus in pregnancy, childbirth and the puerperium**
Use additional code for long-term (current) use of insulin (Z79.4)

     ✓6th **O24.91** **Unspecified diabetes mellitus in** pregnancy
       O24.911 **Unspecified diabetes mellitus in pregnancy,** first trimester   Ⓜ♀▽
       O24.912 **Unspecified diabetes mellitus in pregnancy,** second trimester   Ⓜ♀▽
       O24.913 **Unspecified diabetes mellitus in pregnancy,** third trimester   Ⓜ♀▽
       O24.919 **Unspecified diabetes mellitus in pregnancy,** unspecified trimester   Ⓜ♀▽
     O24.92 **Unspecified diabetes mellitus in** childbirth   Ⓜ♀▽
     O24.93 **Unspecified diabetes mellitus in the** puerperium   Ⓜ♀▽

✓4th **O25** **Malnutrition in pregnancy, childbirth and the puerperium**

     ✓5th **O25.1** **Malnutrition in** pregnancy
       O25.10 **Malnutrition in pregnancy, unspecified trimester**   Ⓜ♀▽
       O25.11 **Malnutrition in pregnancy,** first trimester   Ⓜ♀
       O25.12 **Malnutrition in pregnancy,** second trimester   Ⓜ♀
       O25.13 **Malnutrition in pregnancy,** third trimester   Ⓜ♀
     O25.2 **Malnutrition in** childbirth   Ⓜ♀
     O25.3 **Malnutrition in the** puerperium   Ⓜ♀

✓4th **O26** **Maternal care for other conditions predominantly related to pregnancy**

     ✓5th **O26.0** **Excessive weight gain in pregnancy**
       EXCLUDES 2   gestational edema (O12.0, O12.2)
       O26.00 **Excessive weight gain in pregnancy, unspecified trimester**   Ⓜ♀▽
       O26.01 **Excessive weight gain in pregnancy,** first trimester   Ⓜ♀
       O26.02 **Excessive weight gain in pregnancy,** second trimester   Ⓜ♀
       O26.03 **Excessive weight gain in pregnancy,** third trimester   Ⓜ♀

     ✓5th **O26.1** **Low weight gain in pregnancy**
       O26.10 **Low weight gain in pregnancy, unspecified trimester**   Ⓜ♀▽
       O26.11 **Low weight gain in pregnancy,** first trimester   Ⓜ♀
       O26.12 **Low weight gain in pregnancy,** second trimester   Ⓜ♀
       O26.13 **Low weight gain in pregnancy,** third trimester   Ⓜ♀

     ✓5th **O26.2** **Pregnancy care for patient with recurrent pregnancy loss**
       O26.20 **Pregnancy care for patient with recurrent pregnancy loss, unspecified trimester**   Ⓜ♀▽
       O26.21 **Pregnancy care for patient with recurrent pregnancy loss,** first trimester   Ⓜ♀
       O26.22 **Pregnancy care for patient with recurrent pregnancy loss,** second trimester   Ⓜ♀
       O26.23 **Pregnancy care for patient with recurrent pregnancy loss,** third trimester   Ⓜ♀

     ✓5th **O26.3** **Retained intrauterine contraceptive device in pregnancy**
       O26.30 **Retained intrauterine contraceptive device in pregnancy, unspecified trimester**   Ⓜ♀▽
       O26.31 **Retained intrauterine contraceptive device in pregnancy,** first trimester   Ⓜ♀
       O26.32 **Retained intrauterine contraceptive device in pregnancy,** second trimester   Ⓜ♀
       O26.33 **Retained intrauterine contraceptive device in pregnancy,** third trimester   Ⓜ♀

     ✓5th **O26.4** **Herpes gestationis**
       O26.40 **Herpes gestationis, unspecified trimester**   Ⓜ♀▽
       O26.41 **Herpes gestationis,** first trimester   Ⓜ♀
       O26.42 **Herpes gestationis,** second trimester   Ⓜ♀
       O26.43 **Herpes gestationis,** third trimester   Ⓜ♀

     ✓5th **O26.5** **Maternal hypotension syndrome**
       Supine hypotensive syndrome
       O26.50 **Maternal hypotension syndrome, unspecified trimester**   Ⓜ♀▽
       O26.51 **Maternal hypotension syndrome,** first trimester   Ⓜ♀
       O26.52 **Maternal hypotension syndrome,** second trimester   Ⓜ♀
       O26.53 **Maternal hypotension syndrome,** third trimester   Ⓜ♀

✓5th **O26.6** **Liver and biliary tract disorders in pregnancy, childbirth and the puerperium**
Use additional code to identify the specific disorder
     EXCLUDES 2   hepatorenal syndrome following labor and delivery (O90.4)

     ✓6th **O26.61** **Liver and biliary tract disorders in** pregnancy
       O26.611 **Liver and biliary tract disorders in pregnancy,** first trimester   Ⓜ♀
       O26.612 **Liver and biliary tract disorders in pregnancy,** second trimester   Ⓜ♀
       O26.613 **Liver and biliary tract disorders in pregnancy,** third trimester   Ⓜ♀
       O26.619 **Liver and biliary tract disorders in pregnancy,** unspecified trimester   Ⓜ♀▽
     O26.62 **Liver and biliary tract disorders in** childbirth   Ⓜ♀
     O26.63 **Liver and biliary tract disorders in the** puerperium   Ⓜ♀

✓5th **O26.7** **Subluxation of symphysis (pubis) in pregnancy, childbirth and the puerperium**
     EXCLUDES 1   traumatic separation of symphysis (pubis) during childbirth (O71.6)

     ✓6th **O26.71** **Subluxation of symphysis (pubis) in** pregnancy
       O26.711 **Subluxation of symphysis (pubis) in pregnancy,** first trimester   Ⓜ♀
       O26.712 **Subluxation of symphysis (pubis) in pregnancy,** second trimester   Ⓜ♀
       O26.713 **Subluxation of symphysis (pubis) in pregnancy,** third trimester   Ⓜ♀
       O26.719 **Subluxation of symphysis (pubis) in pregnancy,** unspecified trimester   Ⓜ♀▽
     O26.72 **Subluxation of symphysis (pubis) in** childbirth   Ⓜ♀
     O26.73 **Subluxation of symphysis (pubis) in the** puerperium   Ⓜ♀

✓5th **O26.8** **Other specified pregnancy related conditions**

     ✓6th **O26.81** **Pregnancy related exhaustion and fatigue**
       O26.811 **Pregnancy related exhaustion and fatigue,** first trimester   Ⓜ♀
       O26.812 **Pregnancy related exhaustion and fatigue,** second trimester   Ⓜ♀
       O26.813 **Pregnancy related exhaustion and fatigue,** third trimester   Ⓜ♀
       O26.819 **Pregnancy related exhaustion and fatigue, unspecified trimester**   Ⓜ♀▽

     ✓6th **O26.82** **Pregnancy related peripheral neuritis**
       O26.821 **Pregnancy related peripheral neuritis,** first trimester   Ⓜ♀
       O26.822 **Pregnancy related peripheral neuritis,** second trimester   Ⓜ♀
       O26.823 **Pregnancy related peripheral neuritis,** third trimester   Ⓜ♀
       O26.829 **Pregnancy related peripheral neuritis, unspecified trimester**   Ⓜ♀▽

     ✓6th **O26.83** **Pregnancy related renal disease**
       Use additional code to identify the specific disorder
       O26.831 **Pregnancy related renal disease,** first trimester   Ⓜ♀
       O26.832 **Pregnancy related renal disease,** second trimester   Ⓜ♀
       O26.833 **Pregnancy related renal disease,** third trimester   Ⓜ♀
       O26.839 **Pregnancy related renal disease, unspecified trimester**   Ⓜ♀▽

     ✓6th **O26.84** **Uterine size-date discrepancy complicating pregnancy**
       EXCLUDES 1   encounter for suspected problem with fetal growth ruled out (Z03.74)
       O26.841 **Uterine size-date discrepancy,** first trimester   Ⓜ♀
       O26.842 **Uterine size-date discrepancy,** second trimester   Ⓜ♀
       O26.843 **Uterine size-date discrepancy,** third trimester   Ⓜ♀
       O26.849 **Uterine size-date discrepancy, unspecified trimester**   Ⓜ♀▽

     ✓6th **O26.85** **Spotting complicating pregnancy**
       O26.851 **Spotting complicating pregnancy,** first trimester   Ⓜ♀

Ⓝ Newborn: 0   Ⓟ Pediatric: 0-17   Ⓜ Maternity: 12-55   Ⓐ Adult: 15-124   NRS Nonroutine supply Dx   NC Dx Noncancer Dx   PDx Primary Dx   ►◄ Revised Text   ● New Code   ▲ Revised Title

832   ICD-10-CM 2018

O26.852 Spotting complicating pregnancy, second trimester Ⓜ♀

O26.853 Spotting complicating pregnancy, third trimester Ⓜ♀

O26.859 Spotting complicating pregnancy, unspecified trimester Ⓜ♀▽

O26.86 Pruritic urticarial papules and plaques of pregnancy (PUPPP) Ⓜ♀
Polymorphic eruption of pregnancy

✓6ᵗʰ **O26.87** Cervical shortening
EXCLUDES1 encounter for suspected cervical shortening ruled out (Z03.75)
DEF: A cervix that has shortened to < 25 mm before the 24th week of pregnancy; warning sign for impending premature delivery; treated by cervical cerclage placement or progesterone.

O26.872 Cervical shortening, second trimester Ⓜ♀

O26.873 Cervical shortening, third trimester Ⓜ♀

O26.879 Cervical shortening, unspecified trimester Ⓜ♀▽

✓6ᵗʰ **O26.89** Other specified pregnancy related conditions
AHA: 2015, 3Q, 40

O26.891 Other specified pregnancy related conditions, first trimester Ⓜ♀

O26.892 Other specified pregnancy related conditions, second trimester Ⓜ♀

O26.893 Other specified pregnancy related conditions, third trimester Ⓜ♀

O26.899 Other specified pregnancy related conditions, unspecified trimester Ⓜ♀▽

✓5ᵗʰ **O26.9** Pregnancy related conditions, unspecified

O26.90 Pregnancy related conditions, unspecified, unspecified trimester Ⓜ♀▽

O26.91 Pregnancy related conditions, unspecified, first trimester Ⓜ♀▽

O26.92 Pregnancy related conditions, unspecified, second trimester Ⓜ♀▽

O26.93 Pregnancy related conditions, unspecified, third trimester Ⓜ♀▽

✓4ᵗʰ **O28** **Abnormal findings on antenatal screening of mother**
EXCLUDES1 diagnostic findings classified elsewhere—see Alphabetical Index

O28.0 Abnormal hematological finding on antenatal screening of mother Ⓜ♀

O28.1 Abnormal biochemical finding on antenatal screening of mother Ⓜ♀

O28.2 Abnormal cytological finding on antenatal screening of mother Ⓜ♀

O28.3 Abnormal ultrasonic finding on antenatal screening of mother Ⓜ♀

O28.4 Abnormal radiological finding on antenatal screening of mother Ⓜ♀

O28.5 Abnormal chromosomal and genetic finding on antenatal screening of mother Ⓜ♀

O28.8 Other abnormal findings on antenatal screening of mother Ⓜ♀

O28.9 Unspecified abnormal findings on antenatal screening of mother Ⓜ♀▽

✓4ᵗʰ **O29** **Complications of anesthesia during pregnancy**
INCLUDES maternal complications arising from the administration of a general, regional or local anesthetic, analgesic or other sedation during pregnancy
Use additional code, if necessary, to identify the complication
EXCLUDES2 complications of anesthesia during labor and delivery (O74.-)
complications of anesthesia during the puerperium (O89.-)

✓5ᵗʰ **O29.0** Pulmonary complications of anesthesia during pregnancy

✓6ᵗʰ **O29.01** Aspiration pneumonitis due to anesthesia during pregnancy
Inhalation of stomach contents or secretions NOS due to anesthesia during pregnancy
Mendelson's syndrome due to anesthesia during pregnancy

O29.011 Aspiration pneumonitis due to anesthesia during pregnancy, first trimester Ⓜ♀

O29.012 Aspiration pneumonitis due to anesthesia during pregnancy, second trimester Ⓜ♀

O29.013 Aspiration pneumonitis due to anesthesia during pregnancy, third trimester Ⓜ♀

O29.019 Aspiration pneumonitis due to anesthesia during pregnancy, unspecified trimester Ⓜ♀▽

✓6ᵗʰ **O29.02** Pressure collapse of lung due to anesthesia during pregnancy

O29.021 Pressure collapse of lung due to anesthesia during pregnancy, first trimester Ⓜ♀

O29.022 Pressure collapse of lung due to anesthesia during pregnancy, second trimester Ⓜ♀

O29.023 Pressure collapse of lung due to anesthesia during pregnancy, third trimester Ⓜ♀

O29.029 Pressure collapse of lung due to anesthesia during pregnancy, unspecified trimester Ⓜ♀▽

✓6ᵗʰ **O29.09** Other pulmonary complications of anesthesia during pregnancy

O29.091 Other pulmonary complications of anesthesia during pregnancy, first trimester Ⓜ♀

O29.092 Other pulmonary complications of anesthesia during pregnancy, second trimester Ⓜ♀

O29.093 Other pulmonary complications of anesthesia during pregnancy, third trimester Ⓜ♀

O29.099 Other pulmonary complications of anesthesia during pregnancy, unspecified trimester Ⓜ♀▽

✓5ᵗʰ **O29.1** Cardiac complications of anesthesia during pregnancy

✓6ᵗʰ **O29.11** Cardiac arrest due to anesthesia during pregnancy

O29.111 Cardiac arrest due to anesthesia during pregnancy, first trimester Ⓜ♀

O29.112 Cardiac arrest due to anesthesia during pregnancy, second trimester Ⓜ♀

O29.113 Cardiac arrest due to anesthesia during pregnancy, third trimester Ⓜ♀

O29.119 Cardiac arrest due to anesthesia during pregnancy, unspecified trimester Ⓜ♀▽

✓6ᵗʰ **O29.12** Cardiac failure due to anesthesia during pregnancy

O29.121 Cardiac failure due to anesthesia during pregnancy, first trimester Ⓜ♀

O29.122 Cardiac failure due to anesthesia during pregnancy, second trimester Ⓜ♀

O29.123 Cardiac failure due to anesthesia during pregnancy, third trimester Ⓜ♀

O29.129 Cardiac failure due to anesthesia during pregnancy, unspecified trimester Ⓜ♀▽

✓6ᵗʰ **O29.19** Other cardiac complications of anesthesia during pregnancy

O29.191 Other cardiac complications of anesthesia during pregnancy, first trimester Ⓜ♀

O29.192 Other cardiac complications of anesthesia during pregnancy, second trimester Ⓜ♀

O29.193 Other cardiac complications of anesthesia during pregnancy, third trimester Ⓜ♀

O29.199 Other cardiac complications of anesthesia during pregnancy, unspecified trimester Ⓜ♀▽

✓5ᵗʰ **O29.2** Central nervous system complications of anesthesia during pregnancy

✓6ᵗʰ **O29.21** Cerebral anoxia due to anesthesia during pregnancy

O29.211 Cerebral anoxia due to anesthesia during pregnancy, first trimester Ⓜ♀

O29.212 Cerebral anoxia due to anesthesia during pregnancy, second trimester Ⓜ♀

O29.213 Cerebral anoxia due to anesthesia during pregnancy, third trimester Ⓜ♀

O29.219 Cerebral anoxia due to anesthesia during pregnancy, unspecified trimester Ⓜ♀▽

✓6ᵗʰ O29.29 Other central nervous system **complications of anesthesia during pregnancy**

     O29.291   Other central nervous system complications of anesthesia during pregnancy, first trimester   Ⓜ♀

     O29.292   Other central nervous system complications of anesthesia during pregnancy, second trimester   Ⓜ♀

     O29.293   Other central nervous system complications of anesthesia during pregnancy, third trimester   Ⓜ♀

     O29.299   Other central nervous system complications of anesthesia during pregnancy, unspecified trimester   Ⓜ♀▽

✓5ᵗʰ O29.3 Toxic reaction **to local anesthesia during pregnancy**

   ✓6ᵗʰ O29.3X   **Toxic reaction to local anesthesia during pregnancy**

     O29.3X1   Toxic reaction to local anesthesia during pregnancy, first trimester   Ⓜ♀

     O29.3X2   Toxic reaction to local anesthesia during pregnancy, second trimester   Ⓜ♀

     O29.3X3   Toxic reaction to local anesthesia during pregnancy, third trimester   Ⓜ♀

     O29.3X9   Toxic reaction to local anesthesia during pregnancy, unspecified trimester   Ⓜ♀▽

✓5ᵗʰ O29.4 Spinal and epidural anesthesia induced headache **during pregnancy**

     O29.40   Spinal and epidural anesthesia induced headache during pregnancy, unspecified trimester   Ⓜ♀▽

     O29.41   Spinal and epidural anesthesia induced headache during pregnancy, first trimester   Ⓜ♀

     O29.42   Spinal and epidural anesthesia induced headache during pregnancy, second trimester   Ⓜ♀

     O29.43   Spinal and epidural anesthesia induced headache during pregnancy, third trimester   Ⓜ♀

✓5ᵗʰ O29.5 Other **complications of** spinal and epidural anesthesia during pregnancy

   ✓6ᵗʰ O29.5X   **Other complications of spinal and epidural anesthesia during pregnancy**

     O29.5X1   Other complications of spinal and epidural anesthesia during pregnancy, first trimester   Ⓜ♀

     O29.5X2   Other complications of spinal and epidural anesthesia during pregnancy, second trimester   Ⓜ♀

     O29.5X3   Other complications of spinal and epidural anesthesia during pregnancy, third trimester   Ⓜ♀

     O29.5X9   Other complications of spinal and epidural anesthesia during pregnancy, unspecified trimester   Ⓜ♀▽

✓5ᵗʰ O29.6 Failed or difficult intubation **for anesthesia during pregnancy**

     O29.60   Failed or difficult intubation for anesthesia during pregnancy, unspecified trimester   Ⓜ♀▽

     O29.61   Failed or difficult intubation for anesthesia during pregnancy, first trimester   Ⓜ♀

     O29.62   Failed or difficult intubation for anesthesia during pregnancy, second trimester   Ⓜ♀

     O29.63   Failed or difficult intubation for anesthesia during pregnancy, third trimester   Ⓜ♀

✓5ᵗʰ O29.8 Other complications of anesthesia during pregnancy

   ✓6ᵗʰ O29.8X   **Other complications of anesthesia during pregnancy**

     O29.8X1   Other complications of anesthesia during pregnancy, first trimester   Ⓜ♀

     O29.8X2   Other complications of anesthesia during pregnancy, second trimester   Ⓜ♀

     O29.8X3   Other complications of anesthesia during pregnancy, third trimester   Ⓜ♀

     O29.8X9   Other complications of anesthesia during pregnancy, unspecified trimester   Ⓜ♀▽

✓5ᵗʰ O29.9 Unspecified **complication of anesthesia during pregnancy**

     O29.90   Unspecified complication of anesthesia during pregnancy, unspecified trimester   Ⓜ♀▽

     O29.91   Unspecified complication of anesthesia duringpregnancy, first trimester   Ⓜ♀▽

     O29.92   Unspecified complication of anesthesia duringpregnancy, second trimester   Ⓜ♀▽

     O29.93   Unspecified complication of anesthesia duringpregnancy, third trimester   Ⓜ♀▽

Maternal care related to the fetus and amniotic cavity and possible delivery problems (O3Ø-O48)

✓4ᵗʰ O3Ø Multiple gestation

     Code also any complications specific to multiple gestation

   ✓5ᵗʰ O3Ø.Ø   Twin pregnancy

     ✓6ᵗʰ O3Ø.ØØ   **Twin pregnancy, unspecified number of placenta and unspecified number of amniotic sacs**

       O3Ø.ØØ1   Twin pregnancy, unspecified number of placenta and unspecified number of amniotic sacs, first trimester   Ⓜ♀▽

       O3Ø.ØØ2   Twin pregnancy, unspecified number of placenta and unspecified number of amniotic sacs, second trimester   Ⓜ♀▽

       O3Ø.ØØ3   Twin pregnancy, unspecified number of placenta and unspecified number of amniotic sacs, third trimester   Ⓜ♀▽

       O3Ø.ØØ9   Twin pregnancy, unspecified number of placenta and unspecified number of amniotic sacs, unspecified trimester   Ⓜ♀▽

     ✓6ᵗʰ O3Ø.Ø1   Twin pregnancy, monochorionic/monoamniotic

       Twin pregnancy, one placenta, one amniotic sac

       EXCLUDES 1   conjoined twins (O3Ø.Ø2-)

       O3Ø.Ø11   Twin pregnancy, monochorionic/monoamniotic, first trimester   Ⓜ♀

       O3Ø.Ø12   Twin pregnancy, monochorionic/monoamniotic, second trimester   Ⓜ♀

       O3Ø.Ø13   Twin pregnancy, monochorionic/monoamniotic, third trimester   Ⓜ♀

       O3Ø.Ø19   Twin pregnancy, monochorionic/monoamniotic, unspecified trimester   Ⓜ♀▽

     ✓6ᵗʰ O3Ø.Ø2   Conjoined twin pregnancy

       O3Ø.Ø21   Conjoined twin pregnancy, first trimester   Ⓜ♀

       O3Ø.Ø22   Conjoined twin pregnancy, second trimester   Ⓜ♀

       O3Ø.Ø23   Conjoined twin pregnancy, third trimester   Ⓜ♀

       O3Ø.Ø29   Conjoined twin pregnancy, unspecified trimester   Ⓜ♀▽

Twin Gestation – Monochorionic/Monoamniotic

1 Chorionic sac
1 Amniotic sac
2 Fetuses
2 Umbilical cords
1 Placenta

Ⓝ Newborn: 0   Ⓟ Pediatric: 0-17   Ⓜ Maternity: 12-55   Ⓐ Adult: 15-124   NRS Nonroutine supply Dx   NCDx Noncancer Dx   PDx Primary Dx   ►◄ Revised Text   ● New Code   ▲ Revised Title

834   ICD-10-CM 2018

Twin Gestation – Monochorionic/Diamniotic

- 1 Chorionic sac
- 2 Amniotic sacs
- 2 Fetuses
- 2 Umbilical cords
- 1 Placenta

Twin Gestation – Dichorionic/Diamniotic

- 2 Chorionic sacs
- 2 Amniotic sacs
- 2 Fetuses
- 2 Umbilical cords
- 2 Placentas

✓6ᵗʰ **O30.03**   **Twin pregnancy, monochorionic/diamniotic**
Twin pregnancy, one placenta, two amniotic sacs

     O30.031   Twin pregnancy, monochorionic/diamniotic, **first trimester**   Ⓜ♀

     O30.032   Twin pregnancy, monochorionic/diamniotic, **second trimester**   Ⓜ♀

     O30.033   Twin pregnancy, monochorionic/diamniotic, **third trimester**   Ⓜ♀

     O30.039   Twin pregnancy, monochorionic/diamniotic, **unspecified trimester**   Ⓜ♀▽

✓6ᵗʰ **O30.04**   **Twin pregnancy, dichorionic/diamniotic**
Twin pregnancy, two placentae, two amniotic sacs

     O30.041   Twin pregnancy, dichorionic/diamniotic, **first trimester**   Ⓜ♀

     O30.042   Twin pregnancy, dichorionic/diamniotic, **second trimester**   Ⓜ♀

     O30.043   Twin pregnancy, dichorionic/diamniotic, **third trimester**   Ⓜ♀

     O30.049   Twin pregnancy, dichorionic/diamniotic, **unspecified trimester**   Ⓜ♀▽

✓6ᵗʰ **O30.09**   **Twin pregnancy, unable to determine number** of placenta and number of amniotic sacs

     O30.091   Twin pregnancy, unable to determine number of placenta and number of amniotic sacs, **first trimester**   Ⓜ♀

     O30.092   Twin pregnancy, unable to determine number of placenta and number of amniotic sacs, **second trimester**   Ⓜ♀

     O30.093   Twin pregnancy, unable to determine number of placenta and number of amniotic sacs, **third trimester**   Ⓜ♀

     O30.099   Twin pregnancy, unable to determine number of placenta and number of amniotic sacs, **unspecified trimester**   Ⓜ♀▽

✓5ᵗʰ **O30.1**   **Triplet pregnancy**

     ✓6ᵗʰ **O30.10**   **Triplet pregnancy, unspecified number** of placenta and **unspecified number** of amniotic sacs
AHA: 2016, 2Q, 8

         O30.101   Triplet pregnancy, unspecified number of placenta and unspecified number of amniotic sacs, **first trimester**   Ⓜ♀▽

         O30.102   Triplet pregnancy, unspecified number of placenta and unspecified number of amniotic sacs, **second trimester**   Ⓜ♀▽

         O30.103   Triplet pregnancy, unspecified number of placenta and unspecified number of amniotic sacs, **third trimester**   Ⓜ♀▽

         O30.109   Triplet pregnancy, unspecified number of placenta and unspecified number of amniotic sacs, unspecified trimester   Ⓜ♀▽

     ✓6ᵗʰ **O30.11**   **Triplet pregnancy with two or more monochorionic fetuses**

         O30.111   Triplet pregnancy with two or more monochorionic fetuses, **first trimester**   Ⓜ♀

         O30.112   Triplet pregnancy with two or more monochorionic fetuses, **second trimester**   Ⓜ♀

         O30.113   Triplet pregnancy with two or more monochorionic fetuses, **third trimester**   Ⓜ♀

         O30.119   Triplet pregnancy with two or more monochorionic fetuses, unspecified trimester   Ⓜ♀▽

     ✓6ᵗʰ **O30.12**   **Triplet pregnancy with two or more monoamniotic fetuses**

         O30.121   Triplet pregnancy with two or more monoamniotic fetuses, **first trimester**   Ⓜ♀

         O30.122   Triplet pregnancy with two or more monoamniotic fetuses, **second trimester**   Ⓜ♀

         O30.123   Triplet pregnancy with two or more monoamniotic fetuses, **third trimester**   Ⓜ♀

         O30.129   Triplet pregnancy with two or more monoamniotic fetuses, unspecified trimester   Ⓜ♀▽

     ✓6ᵗʰ **O30.19**   **Triplet pregnancy, unable to determine number** of placenta and number of amniotic sacs

         O30.191   Triplet pregnancy, unable to determine number of placenta and number of amniotic sacs, **first trimester**   Ⓜ♀

         O30.192   Triplet pregnancy, unable to determine number of placenta and number of amniotic sacs, **second trimester**   Ⓜ♀

         O30.193   Triplet pregnancy, unable to determine number of placenta and number of amniotic sacs, **third trimester**   Ⓜ♀

         O30.199   Triplet pregnancy, unable to determine number of placenta and number of amniotic sacs, **unspecified trimester**   Ⓜ♀▽

✓6ᵗʰ **O30.2**   **Quadruplet pregnancy**

     ✓6ᵗʰ **O30.20**   **Quadruplet pregnancy, unspecified number of** placenta and **unspecified number of** amniotic sacs

         O30.201   Quadruplet pregnancy, unspecified number of placenta and unspecified number of amniotic sacs, **first trimester**   Ⓜ♀▽

         O30.202   Quadruplet pregnancy, unspecified number of placenta and unspecified number of amniotic sacs, **second trimester**   Ⓜ♀▽

         O30.203   Quadruplet pregnancy, unspecified number of placenta and unspecified number of amniotic sacs, **third trimester**   Ⓜ♀▽

         O30.209   Quadruplet pregnancy, unspecified number of placenta and unspecified number of amniotic sacs, unspecified trimester   Ⓜ♀▽

     ✓6ᵗʰ **O30.21**   **Quadruplet pregnancy with two or more monochorionic fetuses**

         O30.211   Quadruplet pregnancy with two or more monochorionic fetuses, **first trimester**   Ⓜ♀

✓ Additional Character Req   ✓x7ᵗʰ Placeholder Alert   Case-Mix Diagnosis   Manifestation   ▽ Unspecified Dx   *EXCLUDES 1* Not coded here   *EXCLUDES 2* Not included here

Chapter 15. Pregnancy, Childbirth and the Puerperium

O30.212–O31.21

O30.212 Quadruplet pregnancy with two or more monochorionic fetuses, second trimester   Ⓜ♀

O30.213 Quadruplet pregnancy with two or more monochorionic fetuses, third trimester   Ⓜ♀

O30.219 Quadruplet pregnancy with two or more monochorionic fetuses, unspecified trimester   Ⓜ♀▽

✓6ᵗʰ **O30.22** Quadruplet pregnancy with two or more monoamniotic fetuses

O30.221 Quadruplet pregnancy with two or more monoamniotic fetuses, first trimester   Ⓜ♀

O30.222 Quadruplet pregnancy with two or more monoamniotic fetuses, second trimester   Ⓜ♀

O30.223 Quadruplet pregnancy with two or more monoamniotic fetuses, third trimester   Ⓜ♀

O30.229 Quadruplet pregnancy with two or more monoamniotic fetuses, unspecified trimester   Ⓜ♀▽

✓6ᵗʰ **O30.29** Quadruplet pregnancy, unable to determine number of placenta and number of amniotic sacs

O30.291 Quadruplet pregnancy, unable to determine number of placenta and number of amniotic sacs, first trimester   Ⓜ♀

O30.292 Quadruplet pregnancy, unable to determine number of placenta and number of amniotic sacs, second trimester   Ⓜ♀

O30.293 Quadruplet pregnancy, unable to determine number of placenta and number of amniotic sacs, third trimester   Ⓜ♀

O30.299 Quadruplet pregnancy, unable to determine number of placenta and number of amniotic sacs, unspecified   Ⓜ♀▽

✓5ᵗʰ **O30.8** Other specified multiple gestation
Multiple gestation pregnancy greater than quadruplets

✓6ᵗʰ **O30.80** Other specified multiple gestation, unspecified number of placenta and unspecified number of amniotic sacs

O30.801 Other specified multiple gestation, unspecified number of placenta and unspecified number of amniotic sacs, first trimester   Ⓜ♀▽

O30.802 Other specified multiple gestation, unspecified number of placenta and unspecified number of amniotic sacs, second trimester   Ⓜ♀▽

O30.803 Other specified multiple gestation, unspecified number of placenta and unspecified number of amniotic sacs, third trimester   Ⓜ♀▽

O30.809 Other specified multiple gestation, unspecified number of placenta and unspecified number of amniotic sacs, unspecified trimester   Ⓜ♀▽

✓6ᵗʰ **O30.81** Other specified multiple gestation with two or more monochorionic fetuses

O30.811 Other specified multiple gestation with two or more monochorionic fetuses, first trimester   Ⓜ♀

O30.812 Other specified multiple gestation with two or more monochorionic fetuses, second trimester   Ⓜ♀

O30.813 Other specified multiple gestation with two or more monochorionic fetuses, third trimester   Ⓜ♀

O30.819 Other specified multiple gestation with two or more monochorionic fetuses, unspecified trimester   Ⓜ♀▽

✓6ᵗʰ **O30.82** Other specified multiple gestation with two or more monoamniotic fetuses

O30.821 Other specified multiple gestation with two or more monoamniotic fetuses, first trimester   Ⓜ♀

O30.822 Other specified multiple gestation with two or more monoamniotic fetuses, second trimester   Ⓜ♀

O30.823 Other specified multiple gestation with two or more monoamniotic fetuses, third trimester   Ⓜ♀

O30.829 Other specified multiple gestation with two or more monoamniotic fetuses, unspecified trimester   Ⓜ♀▽

✓6ᵗʰ **O30.89** Other specified multiple gestation, unable to determine number of placenta and number of amniotic sacs

O30.891 Other specified multiple gestation, unable to determine number of placenta and number of amniotic sacs, first trimester   Ⓜ♀

O30.892 Other specified multiple gestation, unable to determine number of placenta and number of amniotic sacs, second trimester   Ⓜ♀

O30.893 Other specified multiple gestation, unable to determine number of placenta and number of amniotic sacs, third trimester   Ⓜ♀

O30.899 Other specified multiple gestation, unable to determine number of placenta and number of amniotic sacs, unspecified trimester   Ⓜ♀▽

✓5ᵗʰ **O30.9** Multiple gestation, unspecified
Multiple pregnancy NOS

O30.90 Multiple gestation, unspecified, unspecified trimester   Ⓜ♀▽

O30.91 Multiple gestation, unspecified, first trimester   Ⓜ♀▽

O30.92 Multiple gestation, unspecified, second trimester   Ⓜ♀▽

O30.93 Multiple gestation, unspecified, third trimester   Ⓜ♀▽

✓4ᵗʰ **O31** **Complications specific to multiple gestation**

EXCLUDES 2   delayed delivery of second twin, triplet, etc. (O63.2)
malpresentation of one fetus or more (O32.9)
placental transfusion syndromes (O43.0-)

AHA: 2012, 4Q, 107

One of the following 7th characters is to be assigned to each code under category O31. 7th character 0 is for single gestations and multiple gestations where the fetus is unspecified. 7th characters 1 through 9 are for cases of multiple gestations to identify the fetus for which the code applies. The appropriate code from category O30, Multiple gestation, must also be assigned when assigning a code from category O31 that has a 7th character of 1 through 9.

0   not applicable or unspecified   4   fetus 4
1   fetus 1   5   fetus 5
2   fetus 2   9   other fetus
3   fetus 3

✓5ᵗʰ **O31.0** Papyraceous fetus
Fetus compressus

✓x7ᵗʰ **O31.00** Papyraceous fetus, unspecified trimester   Ⓜ♀▽

✓x7ᵗʰ **O31.01** Papyraceous fetus, first trimester   Ⓜ♀

✓x7ᵗʰ **O31.02** Papyraceous fetus, second trimester   Ⓜ♀

✓x7ᵗʰ **O31.03** Papyraceous fetus, third trimester   Ⓜ♀

✓5ᵗʰ **O31.1** Continuing pregnancy after spontaneous abortion of one fetus or more

✓x7ᵗʰ **O31.10** Continuing pregnancy after spontaneous abortion of one fetus or more, unspecified trimester   Ⓜ♀▽

✓x7ᵗʰ **O31.11** Continuing pregnancy after spontaneous abortion of one fetus or more, first trimester   Ⓜ♀

✓x7ᵗʰ **O31.12** Continuing pregnancy after spontaneous abortion of one fetus or more, second trimester   Ⓜ♀

✓x7ᵗʰ **O31.13** Continuing pregnancy after spontaneous abortion of one fetus or more, third trimester   Ⓜ♀

✓5ᵗʰ **O31.2** Continuing pregnancy after intrauterine death of one fetus or more

✓x7ᵗʰ **O31.20** Continuing pregnancy after intrauterine death of one fetus or more, unspecified trimester   Ⓜ♀▽

✓x7ᵗʰ **O31.21** Continuing pregnancy after intrauterine death of one fetus or more, first trimester   Ⓜ♀

Ⓝ Newborn: 0   Ⓟ Pediatric: 0-17   Ⓜ Maternity: 12-55   Ⓐ Adult: 15-124   NRS Nonroutine supply Dx   NCDx Noncancer Dx   PDx Primary Dx   ▶◀ Revised Text   ● New Code   ▲ Revised Title

836   ICD-10-CM 2018

√x7ᵗʰ **O31.22** **Continuing pregnancy after intrauterine death of one fetus or more,** second trimester Ⓜ♀

√x7ᵗʰ **O31.23** **Continuing pregnancy after intrauterine death of one fetus or more,** third trimester Ⓜ♀

√5ᵗʰ **O31.3** **Continuing pregnancy after** elective fetal reduction of one fetus or more
Continuing pregnancy after selective termination of one fetus or more

√x7ᵗʰ **O31.30** **Continuing pregnancy after elective fetal reduction of one fetus or more,** unspecified trimester Ⓜ♀▽

√x7ᵗʰ **O31.31** **Continuing pregnancy after elective fetal reduction of one fetus or more,** first trimester Ⓜ♀

√x7ᵗʰ **O31.32** **Continuing pregnancy after elective fetal reduction of one fetus or more,** second trimester Ⓜ♀

√x7ᵗʰ **O31.33** **Continuing pregnancy after elective fetal reduction of one fetus or more,** third trimester Ⓜ♀

√5ᵗʰ **O31.8** **Other complications specific to multiple gestation**

√6ᵗʰ **O31.8X** **Other complications specific to multiple gestation**

√7ᵗʰ **O31.8X1** **Other complications specific to multiple gestation,** first trimester Ⓜ♀

√7ᵗʰ **O31.8X2** **Other complications specific to multiple gestation,** second trimester Ⓜ♀

√7ᵗʰ **O31.8X3** **Other complications specific to multiple gestation,** third trimester Ⓜ♀

√7ᵗʰ **O31.8X9** **Other complications specific to multiple gestation,** unspecified trimester Ⓜ♀▽

√4ᵗʰ **O32** **Maternal care for malpresentation of fetus**
INCLUDES the listed conditions as a reason for observation, hospitalization or other obstetric care of the mother, or for cesarean delivery before onset of labor
EXCLUDES 1 malpresentation of fetus with obstructed labor (O64.-)
AHA: 2012, 4Q, 107

> One of the following 7th characters is to be assigned to each code under category O32. 7th character Ø is for single gestations and multiple gestations where the fetus is unspecified. 7th characters 1 through 9 are for cases of multiple gestations to identify the fetus for which the code applies. The appropriate code from category O30, Multiple gestation, must also be assigned when assigning a code from category O32 that has a 7th character of 1 through 9.
> Ø not applicable or unspecified   4 fetus 4
> 1 fetus 1   5 fetus 5
> 2 fetus 2   9 other fetus
> 3 fetus 3

√x7ᵗʰ **O32.0** **Maternal care for** unstable lie Ⓜ♀

√x7ᵗʰ **O32.1** **Maternal care for** breech presentation Ⓜ♀
Maternal care for buttocks presentation
Maternal care for complete breech
Maternal care for frank breech
EXCLUDES 1 footling presentation (O32.8)
incomplete breech (O32.8)
DEF: Fetus presentation in a longitudinal lie with the buttocks or feet closest to birth canal; may require external cephalic version or cesarean delivery.

√x7ᵗʰ **O32.2** **Maternal care for** transverse and oblique lie Ⓜ♀
Maternal care for oblique presentation
Maternal care for transverse presentation

√x7ᵗʰ **O32.3** **Maternal care for** face, brow and chin presentation Ⓜ♀

√x7ᵗʰ **O32.4** **Maternal care for** high head at term Ⓜ♀
Maternal care for failure of head to enter pelvic brim

√x7ᵗʰ **O32.6** **Maternal care for** compound presentation Ⓜ♀

√x7ᵗʰ **O32.8** **Maternal care for other** malpresentation of fetus Ⓜ♀
Maternal care for footling presentation
Maternal care for incomplete breech

√x7ᵗʰ **O32.9** **Maternal care for malpresentation of fetus,** unspecified Ⓜ♀▽

√4ᵗʰ **O33** **Maternal care for disproportion**
INCLUDES the listed conditions as a reason for observation, hospitalization or other obstetric care of the mother, or for cesarean delivery before onset of labor
EXCLUDES 1 disproportion with obstructed labor (O65-O66)

O33.0 **Maternal care for disproportion due to** deformity of maternal pelvic bones Ⓜ♀
Maternal care for disproportion due to pelvic deformity causing disproportion NOS

O33.1 **Maternal care for disproportion due to** generally contracted pelvis Ⓜ♀
Maternal care for disproportion due to contracted pelvis NOS causing disproportion

O33.2 **Maternal care for disproportion due to** inlet contraction of pelvis Ⓜ♀
Maternal care for disproportion due to inlet contraction (pelvis) causing disproportion

√x7ᵗʰ **O33.3** **Maternal care for disproportion due to** outlet contraction of pelvis Ⓜ♀
Maternal care for disproportion due to mid-cavity contraction (pelvis)
Maternal care for disproportion due to outlet contraction (pelvis)

> One of the following 7th characters is to be assigned to code O33.3. 7th character Ø is for single gestations and multiple gestations where the fetus is unspecified. 7th characters 1 through 9 are for cases of multiple gestations to identify the fetus for which the code applies. The appropriate code from category O30, Multiple gestation, must also be assigned when assigning code O33.3 with a 7th character of 1 through 9.
> Ø not applicable or unspecified   4 fetus 4
> 1 fetus 1   5 fetus 5
> 2 fetus 2   9 other fetus
> 3 fetus 3

√x7ᵗʰ **O33.4** **Maternal care for disproportion of mixed maternal and fetal origin** Ⓜ♀

> One of the following 7th characters is to be assigned to code O33.4. 7th character Ø is for single gestations and multiple gestations where the fetus is unspecified. 7th characters 1 through 9 are for cases of multiple gestations to identify the fetus for which the code applies. The appropriate code from category O30, Multiple gestation, must also be assigned when assigning code O33.4 with a 7th character of 1 through 9.
> Ø not applicable or unspecified   4 fetus 4
> 1 fetus 1   5 fetus 5
> 2 fetus 2   9 other fetus
> 3 fetus 3

√x7ᵗʰ **O33.5** **Maternal care for disproportion due to unusually large fetus** Ⓜ♀
Maternal care for disproportion due to disproportion of fetal origin with normally formed fetus
Maternal care for disproportion due to fetal disproportion NOS

> One of the following 7th characters is to be assigned to code O33.5. 7th character Ø is for single gestations and multiple gestations where the fetus is unspecified. 7th characters 1 through 9 are for cases of multiple gestations to identify the fetus for which the code applies. The appropriate code from category O30, Multiple gestation, must also be assigned when assigning code O33.5 with a 7th character of 1 through 9.
> Ø not applicable or unspecified   4 fetus 4
> 1 fetus 1   5 fetus 5
> 2 fetus 2   9 other fetus
> 3 fetus 3

Fetal Malpresentation
Breech
Shoulder (arm prolapse)
Mother's pelvis
Face (mentum)
Compound (extremity together with head)
Oblique

√x7ᵗʰ O33.6 Maternal care for disproportion due to hydrocephalic fetus Ⓜ♀

> One of the following 7th characters is to be assigned to code O33.6. 7th character Ø is for single gestations and multiple gestations where the fetus is unspecified. 7th characters 1 through 9 are for cases of multiple gestations to identify the fetus for which the code applies. The appropriate code from category O3Ø, Multiple gestation, must also be assigned when assigning code O33.6 with a 7th character of 1 through 9.
>
> Ø   not applicable or unspecified   4   fetus 4
> 1   fetus 1   5   fetus 5
> 2   fetus 2   9   other fetus
> 3   fetus 3

√x7ᵗʰ O33.7 Maternal care for disproportion due to other fetal deformities Ⓜ♀
> Maternal care for disproportion due to fetal ascites
> Maternal care for disproportion due to fetal hydrops
> Maternal care for disproportion due to fetal meningomyelocele
> Maternal care for disproportion due to fetal sacral teratoma
> Maternal care for disproportion due to fetal tumor
> **EXCLUDES 1**   *obstructed labor due to other fetal deformities (O66.3)*

> One of the following 7th characters is to be assigned to code O33.7. 7th character Ø is for single gestations and multiple gestations where the fetus is unspecified. 7th characters 1 through 9 are for cases of multiple gestations to identify the fetus for which the code applies. The appropriate code from category O3Ø, Multiple gestation, must also be assigned when assigning code O33.7 with a 7th character of 1 through 9.
>
> Ø   not applicable or unspecified   4   fetus 4
> 1   fetus 1   5   fetus 5
> 2   fetus 2   9   other fetus
> 3   fetus 3

O33.8 Maternal care for disproportion of other origin Ⓜ♀

O33.9 Maternal care for disproportion, unspecified Ⓜ♀▽
> Maternal care for disproportion due to cephalopelvic disproportion NOS
> Maternal care for disproportion due to fetopelvic disproportion NOS

√4ᵗʰ O34 Maternal care for abnormality of pelvic organs
> **INCLUDES**   the listed conditions as a reason for hospitalization or other obstetric care of the mother, or for cesarean delivery before onset of labor

Code first any associated obstructed labor (O65.5)
Use additional code for specific condition

√5ᵗʰ O34.Ø Maternal care for congenital malformation of uterus
> Maternal care for double uterus
> Maternal care for uterus bicornis

   O34.ØØ Maternal care for unspecified congenital malformation of uterus, unspecified trimester Ⓜ♀▽

   O34.Ø1 Maternal care for unspecified congenital malformation of uterus, first trimester Ⓜ♀▽

   O34.Ø2 Maternal care for unspecified congenital malformation of uterus, second trimester Ⓜ♀▽

   O34.Ø3 Maternal care for unspecified congenital malformation of uterus, third trimester Ⓜ♀▽

√5ᵗʰ O34.1 Maternal care for benign tumor of corpus uteri
> **EXCLUDES 2**   *maternal care for benign tumor of cervix (O34.4-)*
> *maternal care for malignant neoplasm of uterus (O9A.1-)*

   O34.1Ø Maternal care for benign tumor of corpus uteri, unspecified trimester Ⓜ♀▽

   O34.11 Maternal care for benign tumor of corpus uteri, first trimester Ⓜ♀

   O34.12 Maternal care for benign tumor of corpus uteri, second trimester Ⓜ♀

   O34.13 Maternal care for benign tumor of corpus uteri, third trimester Ⓜ♀

√5ᵗʰ O34.2 Maternal care due to uterine scar from previous surgery

   √6ᵗʰ O34.21 Maternal care for scar from previous cesarean delivery

      O34.211 Maternal care for low transverse scar from previous cesarean delivery Ⓜ♀

      O34.212 Maternal care for vertical scar from previous cesarean delivery Ⓜ♀
> Maternal care for classical scar from previous cesarean delivery

      O34.219 Maternal care for unspecified type scar from previous cesarean delivery Ⓜ♀▽

   O34.29 Maternal care due to uterine scar from other previous surgery Ⓜ♀
> Maternal care due to uterine scar from other transmural uterine incision

√5ᵗʰ O34.3 Maternal care for cervical incompetence
> Maternal care for cerclage with or without cervical incompetence
> Maternal care for Shirodkar suture with or without cervical incompetence

   O34.3Ø Maternal care for cervical incompetence, unspecified trimester Ⓜ♀▽

   O34.31 Maternal care for cervical incompetence, first trimester Ⓜ♀

   O34.32 Maternal care for cervical incompetence, second trimester Ⓜ♀

   O34.33 Maternal care for cervical incompetence, third trimester Ⓜ♀

√5ᵗʰ O34.4 Maternal care for other abnormalities of cervix

   O34.4Ø Maternal care for other abnormalities of cervix, unspecified trimester Ⓜ♀▽

   O34.41 Maternal care for other abnormalities of cervix, first trimester Ⓜ♀

   O34.42 Maternal care for other abnormalities of cervix, second trimester Ⓜ♀

   O34.43 Maternal care for other abnormalities of cervix, third trimester Ⓜ♀

√5ᵗʰ O34.5 Maternal care for other abnormalities of gravid uterus

   √6ᵗʰ O34.51 Maternal care for incarceration of gravid uterus

      O34.511 Maternal care for incarceration of gravid uterus, first trimester Ⓜ♀

      O34.512 Maternal care for incarceration of gravid uterus, second trimester Ⓜ♀

      O34.513 Maternal care for incarceration of gravid uterus, third trimester Ⓜ♀

      O34.519 Maternal care for incarceration of gravid uterus, unspecified trimester Ⓜ♀▽

   √6ᵗʰ O34.52 Maternal care for prolapse of gravid uterus

      O34.521 Maternal care for prolapse of gravid uterus, first trimester Ⓜ♀

      O34.522 Maternal care for prolapse of gravid uterus, second trimester Ⓜ♀

      O34.523 Maternal care for prolapse of gravid uterus, third trimester Ⓜ♀

      O34.529 Maternal care for prolapse of gravid uterus, unspecified trimester Ⓜ♀▽

   √6ᵗʰ O34.53 Maternal care for retroversion of gravid uterus

      O34.531 Maternal care for retroversion of gravid uterus, first trimester Ⓜ♀

      O34.532 Maternal care for retroversion of gravid uterus, second trimester Ⓜ♀

      O34.533 Maternal care for retroversion of gravid uterus, third trimester Ⓜ♀

      O34.539 Maternal care for retroversion of gravid uterus, unspecified trimester Ⓜ♀▽

   √6ᵗʰ O34.59 Maternal care for other abnormalities of gravid uterus

      O34.591 Maternal care for other abnormalities of gravid uterus, first trimester Ⓜ♀

      O34.592 Maternal care for other abnormalities of gravid uterus, second trimester Ⓜ♀

      O34.593 Maternal care for other abnormalities of gravid uterus, third trimester Ⓜ♀

      O34.599 Maternal care for other abnormalities of gravid uterus, unspecified trimester Ⓜ♀▽

√5ᵗʰ O34.6 Maternal care for abnormality of vagina
> **EXCLUDES 2**   *maternal care for vaginal varices in pregnancy (O22.1-)*

   O34.6Ø Maternal care for abnormality of vagina, unspecified trimester Ⓜ♀▽

   O34.61 Maternal care for abnormality of vagina, first trimester Ⓜ♀

   O34.62 Maternal care for abnormality of vagina, second trimester Ⓜ♀

   O34.63 Maternal care for abnormality of vagina, third trimester Ⓜ♀

Ⓝ Newborn: 0   Ⓟ Pediatric: 0-17   Ⓜ Maternity: 12-55   Ⓐ Adult: 15-124   **NRS** Nonroutine supply Dx   **NCDx** Noncancer Dx   **PDx** Primary Dx   ►◄ Revised Text   ● New Code   ▲ Revised Title

✓5th **O34.7 Maternal care for** abnormality of vulva and perineum

     EXCLUDES 2   *maternal care for perineal and vulval varices in pregnancy (O22.1-)*

     O34.70 Maternal care for abnormality of vulva and perineum, unspecified trimester   Ⓜ♀▽

     O34.71 Maternal care for abnormality of vulva and perineum, first trimester   Ⓜ♀

     O34.72 Maternal care for abnormality of vulva and perineum, second trimester   Ⓜ♀

     O34.73 Maternal care for abnormality of vulva and perineum, third trimester   Ⓜ♀

✓5th **O34.8 Maternal care for** other abnormalities of pelvic organs

     O34.80 Maternal care for other abnormalities of pelvic organs, unspecified trimester   Ⓜ♀▽

     O34.81 Maternal care for other abnormalities of pelvic organs, first trimester   Ⓜ♀

     O34.82 Maternal care for other abnormalities of pelvic organs, second trimester   Ⓜ♀

     O34.83 Maternal care for other abnormalities of pelvic organs, third trimester   Ⓜ♀

✓5th **O34.9 Maternal care for abnormality of pelvic organ,** unspecified

     O34.90 Maternal care for abnormality of pelvic organ, unspecified, unspecified trimester   Ⓜ♀▽

     O34.91 Maternal care for abnormality of pelvic organ, unspecified, first trimester   Ⓜ♀▽

     O34.92 Maternal care for abnormality of pelvic organ, unspecified, second trimester   Ⓜ♀▽

     O34.93 Maternal care for abnormality of pelvic organ, unspecified, third trimester   Ⓜ♀▽

✓4th **O35 Maternal care for known or suspected fetal abnormality and damage**

     INCLUDES   the listed conditions in the fetus as a reason for hospitalization or other obstetric care to the mother, or for termination of pregnancy

     Code also any associated maternal condition

     EXCLUDES 1   *encounter for suspected maternal and fetal conditions ruled out (Z03.7-)*

> One of the following 7th characters is to be assigned to each code under category O35. 7th character 0 is for single gestations and multiple gestations where the fetus is unspecified. 7th characters 1 through 9 are for cases of multiple gestations to identify the fetus for which the code applies. The appropriate code from category O30, Multiple gestation, must also be assigned when assigning a code from category O35 that has a 7th character of 1 through 9.
> | 0 | not applicable or unspecified | 4 | fetus 4 |
> |---|---|---|---|
> | 1 | fetus 1 | 5 | fetus 5 |
> | 2 | fetus 2 | 9 | other fetus |
> | 3 | fetus 3 | | |

✓x7th **O35.0 Maternal care for (suspected)** central nervous system malformation in fetus   Ⓜ♀

     Maternal care for fetal anencephaly
     Maternal care for fetal hydrocephalus
     Maternal care for fetal spina bifida
     EXCLUDES 2   *chromosomal abnormality in fetus (O35.1)*

✓x7th **O35.1 Maternal care for (suspected)** chromosomal abnormality in fetus   Ⓜ♀

✓x7th **O35.2 Maternal care for (suspected)** hereditary disease in fetus   Ⓜ♀

     EXCLUDES 2   *chromosomal abnormality in fetus (O35.1)*

✓x7th **O35.3 Maternal care for (suspected)** damage to fetus from viral disease in mother   Ⓜ♀

     Maternal care for damage to fetus from maternal cytomegalovirus infection
     Maternal care for damage to fetus from maternal rubella

✓x7th **O35.4 Maternal care for (suspected)** damage to fetus from alcohol   Ⓜ♀

✓x7th **O35.5 Maternal care for (suspected)** damage to fetus by drugs   Ⓜ♀

     Maternal care for damage to fetus from drug addiction

✓x7th **O35.6 Maternal care for (suspected)** damage to fetus by radiation   Ⓜ♀

✓x7th **O35.7 Maternal care for (suspected)** damage to fetus by other medical procedures   Ⓜ♀

     Maternal care for damage to fetus by amniocentesis
     Maternal care for damage to fetus by biopsy procedures
     Maternal care for damage to fetus by hematological investigation
     Maternal care for damage to fetus by intrauterine contraceptive device
     Maternal care for damage to fetus by intrauterine surgery

✓x7th **O35.8 Maternal care for other (suspected) fetal abnormality and damage**   Ⓜ♀

     Maternal care for damage to fetus from maternal listeriosis
     Maternal care for damage to fetus from maternal toxoplasmosis

✓x7th **O35.9 Maternal care for (suspected)** fetal abnormality and damage, **unspecified**   Ⓜ♀▽

✓4th **O36 Maternal care for other fetal problems**

     INCLUDES   the listed conditions in the fetus as a reason for hospitalization or other obstetric care of the mother, or for termination of pregnancy

     EXCLUDES 1   *encounter for suspected maternal and fetal conditions ruled out (Z03.7-)*
                 placental transfusion syndromes (O43.0-)

     EXCLUDES 2   *labor and delivery complicated by fetal stress (O77.-)*
     AHA: 2015, 3Q, 40

> One of the following 7th characters is to be assigned to each code under category O36. 7th character 0 is for single gestations and multiple gestations where the fetus is unspecified. 7th characters 1 through 9 are for cases of multiple gestations to identify the fetus for which the code applies. The appropriate code from category O30, Multiple gestation, must also be assigned when assigning a code from category O36 that has a 7th character of 1 through 9.
> | 0 | not applicable or unspecified | 4 | fetus 4 |
> |---|---|---|---|
> | 1 | fetus 1 | 5 | fetus 5 |
> | 2 | fetus 2 | 9 | other fetus |
> | 3 | fetus 3 | | |

✓5th **O36.0 Maternal care for rhesus isoimmunization**

     Maternal care for Rh incompatibility (with hydrops fetalis)

     ✓6th **O36.01 Maternal care for** anti-D [Rh] antibodies

         AHA: 2014, 4Q, 17

         ✓7th **O36.011 Maternal care for anti-D [Rh] antibodies,** first trimester   Ⓜ♀

         ✓7th **O36.012 Maternal care for anti-D [Rh] antibodies,** second trimester   Ⓜ♀

         ✓7th **O36.013 Maternal care for anti-D [Rh] antibodies,** third trimester   Ⓜ♀

         ✓7th **O36.019 Maternal care for anti-D [Rh] antibodies, unspecified trimester**   Ⓜ♀▽

     ✓6th **O36.09 Maternal care for** other rhesus isoimmunization

         ✓7th **O36.091 Maternal care for other rhesus isoimmunization,** first trimester   Ⓜ♀

         ✓7th **O36.092 Maternal care for other rhesus isoimmunization,** second trimester   Ⓜ♀

         ✓7th **O36.093 Maternal care for other rhesus isoimmunization,** third trimester   Ⓜ♀

         ✓7th **O36.099 Maternal care for other rhesus isoimmunization, unspecified trimester**   Ⓜ♀▽

✓5th **O36.1 Maternal care for other isoimmunization**

     Maternal care for ABO isoimmunization

     ✓6th **O36.11 Maternal care for** Anti-A sensitization

         Maternal care for isoimmunization NOS (with hydrops fetalis)

         ✓7th **O36.111 Maternal care for Anti-A sensitization,** first trimester   Ⓜ♀

         ✓7th **O36.112 Maternal care for Anti-A sensitization,** second trimester   Ⓜ♀

         ✓7th **O36.113 Maternal care for Anti-A sensitization,** third trimester   Ⓜ♀

         ✓7th **O36.119 Maternal care for Anti-A sensitization, unspecified trimester**   Ⓜ♀▽

     ✓6th **O36.19 Maternal care for** other isoimmunization

         Maternal care for Anti-B sensitization

         ✓7th **O36.191 Maternal care for other isoimmunization,** first trimester   Ⓜ♀

         ✓7th **O36.192 Maternal care for other isoimmunization,** second trimester   Ⓜ♀

         ✓7th **O36.193 Maternal care for other isoimmunization,** third trimester   Ⓜ♀

✓ Additional Character Req   ✓x7th Placeholder Alert   Case-Mix Diagnosis   Manifestation   ▽ Unspecified Dx   EXCLUDES 1 Not coded here   EXCLUDES 2 Not included here

ICD-10-CM 2018   839

   ✓7ᵗʰ **O36.199** **Maternal care for other** Ⓜ♀▽
      isoimmunization, unspecified trimester

✓5ᵗʰ **O36.2** **Maternal care for hydrops fetalis**
   Maternal care for hydrops fetalis NOS
   Maternal care for hydrops fetalis not associated with
    isoimmunization
    EXCLUDES 1   *hydrops fetalis associated with ABO isoimmunization*
      (O36.1-)
      hydrops fetalis associated with rhesus
      isoimmunization (O36.0-)

   ✓x7ᵗʰ **O36.20** **Maternal care for hydrops fetalis, unspecified** Ⓜ♀▽
      trimester

   ✓x7ᵗʰ **O36.21** **Maternal care for hydrops fetalis, first** Ⓜ♀
      trimester

   ✓x7ᵗʰ **O36.22** **Maternal care for hydrops fetalis, second** Ⓜ♀
      trimester

   ✓x7ᵗʰ **O36.23** **Maternal care for hydrops fetalis, third** Ⓜ♀
      trimester

✓x7ᵗʰ **O36.4** **Maternal care for intrauterine death** Ⓜ♀
   Maternal care for intrauterine fetal death NOS
   Maternal care for intrauterine fetal death after completion of 20
    weeks of gestation
   Maternal care for late fetal death
   Maternal care for missed delivery
    EXCLUDES 1   *missed abortion (O02.1)*
      stillbirth (P95)

✓5ᵗʰ **O36.5** **Maternal care for known or suspected poor fetal growth**
   ✓6ᵗʰ **O36.51** **Maternal care for known or suspected placental**
      insufficiency
     ✓7ᵗʰ **O36.511** **Maternal care for known or suspected** Ⓜ♀
       placental insufficiency, first trimester
     ✓7ᵗʰ **O36.512** **Maternal care for known or suspected** Ⓜ♀
       placental insufficiency, second trimester
     ✓7ᵗʰ **O36.513** **Maternal care for known or suspected** Ⓜ♀
       placental insufficiency, third trimester
     ✓7ᵗʰ **O36.519** **Maternal care for known or** Ⓜ♀▽
       suspected placental insufficiency,
       unspecified trimester

   ✓6ᵗʰ **O36.59** **Maternal care for other known or suspected poor**
      fetal growth
     Maternal care for known or suspected light-for-dates
      NOS
     Maternal care for known or suspected small-for-dates
      NOS
     ✓7ᵗʰ **O36.591** **Maternal care for other known or** Ⓜ♀
       suspected poor fetal growth, first
       trimester
     ✓7ᵗʰ **O36.592** **Maternal care for other known or** Ⓜ♀
       suspected poor fetal growth, second
       trimester
     ✓7ᵗʰ **O36.593** **Maternal care for other known or** Ⓜ♀
       suspected poor fetal growth, third
       trimester
     ✓7ᵗʰ **O36.599** **Maternal care for other known or** Ⓜ♀▽
       suspected poor fetal growth,
       unspecified trimester

✓5ᵗʰ **O36.6** **Maternal care for excessive fetal growth**
   Maternal care for known or suspected large-for-dates
   ✓x7ᵗʰ **O36.60** **Maternal care for excessive fetal growth,** Ⓜ♀▽
      unspecified trimester
   ✓x7ᵗʰ **O36.61** **Maternal care for excessive fetal growth,** Ⓜ♀
      first trimester
   ✓x7ᵗʰ **O36.62** **Maternal care for excessive fetal growth,** Ⓜ♀
      second trimester
   ✓x7ᵗʰ **O36.63** **Maternal care for excessive fetal growth,** Ⓜ♀
      third trimester

✓5ᵗʰ **O36.7** **Maternal care for viable fetus in abdominal pregnancy**
   ✓x7ᵗʰ **O36.70** **Maternal care for viable fetus in abdominal** Ⓜ♀▽
      pregnancy, unspecified trimester
   ✓x7ᵗʰ **O36.71** **Maternal care for viable fetus in abdominal** Ⓜ♀
      pregnancy, first trimester
   ✓x7ᵗʰ **O36.72** **Maternal care for viable fetus in abdominal** Ⓜ♀
      pregnancy, second trimester
   ✓x7ᵗʰ **O36.73** **Maternal care for viable fetus in abdominal** Ⓜ♀
      pregnancy, third trimester

✓5ᵗʰ **O36.8** **Maternal care for other specified fetal problems**
   ✓x7ᵗʰ **O36.80** **Pregnancy with inconclusive fetal viability** Ⓜ♀
     Encounter to determine fetal viability of pregnancy

   ✓6ᵗʰ **O36.81** **Decreased fetal movements**
     ✓7ᵗʰ **O36.812** **Decreased fetal movements, second** Ⓜ♀
       trimester
     ✓7ᵗʰ **O36.813** **Decreased fetal movements, third** Ⓜ♀
       trimester
     ✓7ᵗʰ **O36.819** **Decreased fetal movements,** Ⓜ♀▽
       unspecified trimester

   ✓6ᵗʰ **O36.82** **Fetal anemia and thrombocytopenia**
     ✓7ᵗʰ **O36.821** **Fetal anemia and thrombocytopenia,** Ⓜ♀
       first trimester
     ✓7ᵗʰ **O36.822** **Fetal anemia and thrombocytopenia,** Ⓜ♀
       second trimester
     ✓7ᵗʰ **O36.823** **Fetal anemia and thrombocytopenia,** Ⓜ♀
       third trimester
     ✓7ᵗʰ **O36.829** **Fetal anemia and** Ⓜ♀▽
       thrombocytopenia, unspecified
       trimester

   ✓6ᵗʰ **O36.83** **Maternal care for abnormalities of the fetal heart**
      rate or rhythm
     ✓7ᵗʰ **O36.831** **Maternal care for abnormalities of the**
       fetal heart rate or rhythm, first trimester
     ✓7ᵗʰ **O36.832** **Maternal care for abnormalities of the**
       fetal heart rate or rhythm, second
       trimester
     ✓7ᵗʰ **O36.833** **Maternal care for abnormalities of the**
       fetal heart rate or rhythm, third trimester
     ✓7ᵗʰ **O36.839** **Maternal care for abnormalities of the** ▽
       fetal heart rate or rhythm, unspecified
       trimester

   ✓6ᵗʰ **O36.89** **Maternal care for other specified fetal problems**
     ✓7ᵗʰ **O36.891** **Maternal care for other specified** Ⓜ♀
       fetal problems, first trimester
     ✓7ᵗʰ **O36.892** **Maternal care for other specified** Ⓜ♀
       fetal problems, second trimester
     ✓7ᵗʰ **O36.893** **Maternal care for other specified** Ⓜ♀
       fetal problems, third trimester
     ✓7ᵗʰ **O36.899** **Maternal care for other specified** Ⓜ♀▽
       fetal problems, unspecified trimester

✓5ᵗʰ **O36.9** **Maternal care for fetal problem, unspecified**
   ✓x7ᵗʰ **O36.90** **Maternal care for fetal problem, unspecified,** Ⓜ♀▽
      unspecified trimester
   ✓x7ᵗʰ **O36.91** **Maternal care for fetal problem, unspecified,** Ⓜ♀▽
      first trimester
   ✓x7ᵗʰ **O36.92** **Maternal care for fetal problem, unspecified,** Ⓜ♀▽
      second trimester
   ✓x7ᵗʰ **O36.93** **Maternal care for fetal problem, unspecified,** Ⓜ♀▽
      third trimester

✓4ᵗʰ **O40** **Polyhydramnios**
   INCLUDES   hydramnios
   EXCLUDES 1   *encounter for suspected maternal and fetal conditions ruled out*
      (Z03.7-)
   AHA: 2016, 1Q, 4

> One of the following 7th characters is to be assigned to each code
> under category O40. 7th character 0 is for single gestations and
> multiple gestations where the fetus is unspecified. 7th characters 1
> through 9 are for cases of multiple gestations to identify the fetus
> for which the code applies. The appropriate code from category
> O30, Multiple gestation, must also be assigned when assigning a
> code from category O40 that has a 7th character of 1 through 9.
>   0   not applicable or unspecified   4   fetus 4
>   1   fetus 1   5   fetus 5
>   2   fetus 2   9   other fetus
>   3   fetus 3

✓x7ᵗʰ **O40.1** **Polyhydramnios, first trimester** Ⓜ♀
✓x7ᵗʰ **O40.2** **Polyhydramnios, second trimester** Ⓜ♀
✓x7ᵗʰ **O40.3** **Polyhydramnios, third trimester** Ⓜ♀
✓x7ᵗʰ **O40.9** **Polyhydramnios, unspecified trimester** Ⓜ♀▽

✓4ᵗʰ O41 Other disorders of amniotic fluid and membranes

> **EXCLUDES1** encounter for suspected maternal and fetal conditions ruled out (Z03.7-)

> One of the following 7th characters is to be assigned to each code under category O41. 7th character Ø is for single gestations and multiple gestations where the fetus is unspecified. 7th characters 1 through 9 are for cases of multiple gestations to identify the fetus for which the code applies. The appropriate code from category O30, Multiple gestation, must also be assigned when assigning a code from category O41 that has a 7th character of 1 through 9.
> Ø   not applicable or unspecified   4   fetus 4
> 1   fetus 1   5   fetus 5
> 2   fetus 2   9   other fetus
> 3   fetus 3

✓5ᵗʰ O41.0 Oligohydramnios
    Oligohydramnios without rupture of membranes

  ✓x7ᵗʰ O41.00 Oligohydramnios, unspecified trimester Ⓜ♀▽

  ✓x7ᵗʰ O41.01 Oligohydramnios, first trimester Ⓜ♀

  ✓x7ᵗʰ O41.02 Oligohydramnios, second trimester Ⓜ♀

  ✓x7ᵗʰ O41.03 Oligohydramnios, third trimester Ⓜ♀

✓5ᵗʰ O41.1 Infection of amniotic sac and membranes

  ✓6ᵗʰ O41.10 Infection of amniotic sac and membranes, unspecified

    ✓7ᵗʰ O41.101 Infection of amniotic sac and membranes, unspecified, first trimester Ⓜ♀▽

    ✓7ᵗʰ O41.102 Infection of amniotic sac and membranes, unspecified, second trimester Ⓜ♀▽

    ✓7ᵗʰ O41.103 Infection of amniotic sac and membranes, unspecified, third trimester Ⓜ♀▽

    ✓7ᵗʰ O41.109 Infection of amniotic sac and membranes, unspecified, unspecified trimester Ⓜ♀▽

  ✓6ᵗʰ O41.12 Chorioamnionitis

    ✓7ᵗʰ O41.121 Chorioamnionitis, first trimester Ⓜ♀

    ✓7ᵗʰ O41.122 Chorioamnionitis, second trimester Ⓜ♀

    ✓7ᵗʰ O41.123 Chorioamnionitis, third trimester Ⓜ♀

    ✓7ᵗʰ O41.129 Chorioamnionitis, unspecified trimester Ⓜ♀▽

  ✓6ᵗʰ O41.14 Placentitis

    ✓7ᵗʰ O41.141 Placentitis, first trimester Ⓜ♀

    ✓7ᵗʰ O41.142 Placentitis, second trimester Ⓜ♀

    ✓7ᵗʰ O41.143 Placentitis, third trimester Ⓜ♀

    ✓7ᵗʰ O41.149 Placentitis, unspecified trimester Ⓜ♀▽

✓5ᵗʰ O41.8 Other specified disorders of amniotic fluid and membranes

  ✓6ᵗʰ O41.8X Other specified disorders of amniotic fluid and membranes

    ✓7ᵗʰ O41.8X1 Other specified disorders of amniotic fluid and membranes, first trimester Ⓜ♀

    ✓7ᵗʰ O41.8X2 Other specified disorders of amniotic fluid and membranes, second trimester Ⓜ♀

    ✓7ᵗʰ O41.8X3 Other specified disorders of amniotic fluid and membranes, third trimester Ⓜ♀

    ✓7ᵗʰ O41.8X9 Other specified disorders of amniotic fluid and membranes, unspecified trimester Ⓜ♀▽

✓5ᵗʰ O41.9 Disorder of amniotic fluid and membranes, unspecified

  ✓x7ᵗʰ O41.90 Disorder of amniotic fluid and membranes, unspecified, unspecified trimester Ⓜ♀▽

  ✓x7ᵗʰ O41.91 Disorder of amniotic fluid and membranes, unspecified, first trimester Ⓜ♀▽

  ✓x7ᵗʰ O41.92 Disorder of amniotic fluid and membranes, unspecified, second trimester Ⓜ♀▽

  ✓x7ᵗʰ O41.93 Disorder of amniotic fluid and membranes, unspecified, third trimester Ⓜ♀▽

✓4ᵗʰ O42 Premature rupture of membranes
    AHA: 2016, 1Q, 3

✓5ᵗʰ O42.0 Premature rupture of membranes, onset of labor within 24 hours of rupture

  O42.00 Premature rupture of membranes, onset of labor within 24 hours of rupture, unspecified weeks of gestation Ⓜ♀▽

  ✓6ᵗʰ O42.01 Preterm premature rupture of membranes, onset of labor within 24 hours of rupture
    Premature rupture of membranes before 37 completed weeks of gestation

    O42.011 Preterm premature rupture of membranes, onset of labor within 24 hours of rupture, first trimester Ⓜ♀

    O42.012 Preterm premature rupture of membranes, onset of labor within 24 hours of rupture, second trimester Ⓜ♀

    O42.013 Preterm premature rupture of membranes, onset of labor within 24 hours of rupture, third trimester Ⓜ♀

    O42.019 Preterm premature rupture of membranes, onset of labor within 24 hours of rupture, unspecified trimester Ⓜ♀▽

  O42.02 Full-term premature rupture of membranes, onset of labor within 24 hours of rupture Ⓜ♀
    Premature rupture of membranes at or after 37 completed weeks of gestation, onset of labor within 24 hours of rupture

✓5ᵗʰ O42.1 Premature rupture of membranes, onset of labor more than 24 hours following rupture
    AHA: 2016, 1Q, 5

  O42.10 Premature rupture of membranes, onset of labor more than 24 hours following rupture, unspecified weeks of gestation Ⓜ♀▽

  ✓6ᵗʰ O42.11 Preterm premature rupture of membranes, onset of labor more than 24 hours following rupture
    Premature rupture of membranes before 37 completed weeks of gestation

    O42.111 Preterm premature rupture of membranes, onset of labor more than 24 hours following rupture, first trimester Ⓜ♀

    O42.112 Preterm premature rupture of membranes, onset of labor more than 24 hours following rupture, second trimester Ⓜ♀

    O42.113 Preterm premature rupture of membranes, onset of labor more than 24 hours following rupture, third trimester Ⓜ♀

    O42.119 Preterm premature rupture of membranes, onset of labor more than 24 hours following rupture, unspecified trimester Ⓜ♀▽

  O42.12 Full-term premature rupture of membranes, onset of labor more than 24 hours following rupture Ⓜ♀
    Premature rupture of membranes at or after 37 completed weeks of gestation, onset of labor more than 24 hours following rupture

✓5ᵗʰ O42.9 Premature rupture of membranes, unspecified as to length of time between rupture and onset of labor

  O42.90 Premature rupture of membranes, unspecified as to length of time between rupture and onset of labor, unspecified weeks of gestation Ⓜ♀▽

  ✓6ᵗʰ O42.91 Preterm premature rupture of membranes, unspecified as to length of time between rupture and onset of labor
    Premature rupture of membranes before 37 completed weeks of gestation

    O42.911 Preterm premature rupture of membranes, unspecified as to length of time between rupture and onset of labor, first trimester Ⓜ♀▽

    O42.912 Preterm premature rupture of membranes, unspecified as to length of time between rupture and onset of labor, second trimester Ⓜ♀▽

    O42.913 Preterm premature rupture of membranes, unspecified as to length of time between rupture and onset of labor, third trimester Ⓜ♀▽

    O42.919 Preterm premature rupture of membranes, unspecified as to length of time between rupture and onset of labor, unspecified trimester Ⓜ♀▽

✓ Additional Character Req   ✓x7ᵗʰ Placeholder Alert   Case-Mix Diagnosis   Manifestation   ▽ Unspecified Dx   **EXCLUDES1** Not coded here   **EXCLUDES2** Not included here

ICD-10-CM 2018   **841**

O42.92 Full-term **premature rupture of membranes,** unspecified as to length of time between rupture and onset of labor
> Premature rupture of membranes at or after 37 completed weeks of gestation, unspecified as to length of time between rupture and onset of labor

✓4ᵗʰ **O43 Placental disorders**
> EXCLUDES 2   maternal care for poor fetal growth due to placental insufficiency (O36.5-)
> placenta previa (O44.-)
> placental polyp (O90.89)
> placentitis (O41.14-)
> premature separation of placenta [abruptio placentae] (O45.-)

✓5ᵗʰ **O43.0 Placental transfusion syndromes**

✓6ᵗʰ **O43.01** Fetomaternal **placental transfusion syndrome**
> Maternofetal placental transfusion syndrome

O43.011 **Fetomaternal placental transfusion syndrome,** first trimester   Ⓜ♀

O43.012 **Fetomaternal placental transfusion syndrome,** second trimester   Ⓜ♀

O43.013 **Fetomaternal placental transfusion syndrome,** third trimester   Ⓜ♀

O43.019 **Fetomaternal placental transfusion syndrome,** unspecified trimester   Ⓜ♀▽

✓6ᵗʰ **O43.02** Fetus-to-fetus **placental transfusion syndrome**

O43.021 **Fetus-to-fetus placental transfusion syndrome,** first trimester   Ⓜ♀

O43.022 **Fetus-to-fetus placental transfusion syndrome,** second trimester   Ⓜ♀

O43.023 **Fetus-to-fetus placental transfusion syndrome,** third trimester   Ⓜ♀

O43.029 **Fetus-to-fetus placental transfusion syndrome,** unspecified trimester   Ⓜ♀▽

✓5ᵗʰ **O43.1 Malformation of placenta**

✓6ᵗʰ **O43.10** **Malformation of placenta,** unspecified
> Abnormal placenta NOS

O43.101 **Malformation of placenta, unspecified,** first trimester   Ⓜ♀▽

O43.102 **Malformation of placenta, unspecified,** second trimester   Ⓜ♀▽

O43.103 **Malformation of placenta, unspecified,** third trimester   Ⓜ♀▽

O43.109 **Malformation of placenta, unspecified, unspecified trimester**   Ⓜ♀▽

✓6ᵗʰ **O43.11** Circumvallate **placenta**

O43.111 **Circumvallate placenta,** first trimester   Ⓜ♀

O43.112 **Circumvallate placenta,** second trimester   Ⓜ♀

O43.113 **Circumvallate placenta,** third trimester Ⓜ♀

O43.119 **Circumvallate placenta,** unspecified trimester   Ⓜ♀▽

✓6ᵗʰ **O43.12** Velamentous insertion of umbilical cord

O43.121 **Velamentous insertion of umbilical cord,** first trimester   Ⓜ♀

O43.122 **Velamentous insertion of umbilical cord,** second trimester   Ⓜ♀

O43.123 **Velamentous insertion of umbilical cord,** third trimester   Ⓜ♀

Twin to Twin Transfusion Syndrome (TTTS)

Healthy twins   Twins with TTTS

O43.129 **Velamentous insertion of umbilical cord, unspecified trimester**   Ⓜ♀▽

✓6ᵗʰ **O43.19** Other malformation of placenta

O43.191 **Other malformation of placenta,** first trimester   Ⓜ♀

O43.192 **Other malformation of placenta,** second trimester   Ⓜ♀

O43.193 **Other malformation of placenta,** third trimester   Ⓜ♀

O43.199 **Other malformation of placenta, unspecified trimester**   Ⓜ♀▽

✓5ᵗʰ **O43.2 Morbidly adherent placenta**
> Code also associated third stage postpartum hemorrhage, if applicable (O72.0)
> EXCLUDES 1   retained placenta (O73.-)

✓6ᵗʰ **O43.21** Placenta accreta

O43.211 **Placenta accreta,** first trimester   Ⓜ♀
O43.212 **Placenta accreta,** second trimester   Ⓜ♀
O43.213 **Placenta accreta,** third trimester   Ⓜ♀
O43.219 **Placenta accreta, unspecified trimester**   Ⓜ♀▽

✓6ᵗʰ **O43.22** Placenta increta

O43.221 **Placenta increta,** first trimester   Ⓜ♀
O43.222 **Placenta increta,** second trimester   Ⓜ♀
O43.223 **Placenta increta,** third trimester   Ⓜ♀
O43.229 **Placenta increta, unspecified trimester**   Ⓜ♀▽

✓6ᵗʰ **O43.23** Placenta percreta

O43.231 **Placenta percreta,** first trimester   Ⓜ♀
O43.232 **Placenta percreta,** second trimester   Ⓜ♀
O43.233 **Placenta percreta,** third trimester   Ⓜ♀
O43.239 **Placenta percreta, unspecified trimester**   Ⓜ♀▽

✓5ᵗʰ **O43.8 Other placental disorders**

✓6ᵗʰ **O43.81** Placental infarction

O43.811 **Placental infarction,** first trimester   Ⓜ♀
O43.812 **Placental infarction,** second trimester Ⓜ♀
O43.813 **Placental infarction,** third trimester   Ⓜ♀
O43.819 **Placental infarction, unspecified trimester**   Ⓜ♀▽

✓6ᵗʰ **O43.89** Other placental disorders
> Placental dysfunction

O43.891 **Other placental disorders,** first trimester   Ⓜ♀
O43.892 **Other placental disorders,** second trimester   Ⓜ♀
O43.893 **Other placental disorders,** third trimester   Ⓜ♀
O43.899 **Other placental disorders, unspecified trimester**   Ⓜ♀▽

✓5ᵗʰ **O43.9 Unspecified placental disorder**

O43.90 **Unspecified placental disorder, unspecified trimester**   Ⓜ♀▽
O43.91 **Unspecified placental disorder,** first trimester   Ⓜ♀▽
O43.92 **Unspecified placental disorder,** second trimester   Ⓜ♀▽
O43.93 **Unspecified placental disorder,** third trimester   Ⓜ♀▽

✓4ᵗʰ **O44 Placenta previa**
> DEF: Placenta implanted in lower segment of uterus; commonly causes hemorrhage in the last trimester of pregnancy.

✓5ᵗʰ **O44.0** Complete **placenta previa NOS or** without hemorrhage
> Placenta previa NOS

O44.00 **Complete placenta previa NOS or without hemorrhage, unspecified trimester**   Ⓜ♀▽
O44.01 **Complete placenta previa NOS or without hemorrhage,** first trimester   Ⓜ♀
O44.02 **Complete placenta previa NOS or without hemorrhage,** second trimester   Ⓜ♀
O44.03 **Complete placenta previa NOS or without hemorrhage,** third trimester   Ⓜ♀

Ⓝ Newborn: 0   Ⓟ Pediatric: 0-17   Ⓜ Maternity: 12-55   Ⓐ Adult: 15-124   NRS Nonroutine supply Dx   NCDx Noncancer Dx   PDx Primary Dx   ►◄ Revised Text   ● New Code   ▲ Revised Title

842   ICD-10-CM 2018

✓5ᵗʰ **O44.1 Complete placenta previa with hemorrhage**
> EXCLUDES 1   *labor and delivery complicated by hemorrhage from vasa previa (O69.4)*

     O44.10 Complete placenta previa with hemorrhage, unspecified trimester   Ⓜ♀▽

     O44.11 Complete placenta previa with hemorrhage, first trimester   Ⓜ♀

     O44.12 Complete placenta previa with hemorrhage, second trimester   Ⓜ♀

     O44.13 Complete placenta previa with hemorrhage, third trimester   Ⓜ♀

✓5ᵗʰ **O44.2 Partial placenta previa without hemorrhage**
Marginal placenta previa, NOS or without hemorrhage

     O44.20 Partial placenta previa NOS or without hemorrhage, unspecified trimester   Ⓜ♀▽

     O44.21 Partial placenta previa NOS or without hemorrhage, first trimester   Ⓜ♀

     O44.22 Partial placenta previa NOS or without hemorrhage, second trimester   Ⓜ♀

     O44.23 Partial placenta previa NOS or without hemorrhage, third trimester   Ⓜ♀

✓5ᵗʰ **O44.3 Partial placenta previa with hemorrhage**
Marginal placenta previa with hemorrhage

     O44.30 Partial placenta previa with hemorrhage, unspecified trimester   Ⓜ♀▽

     O44.31 Partial placenta previa with hemorrhage, first trimester   Ⓜ♀

     O44.32 Partial placenta previa with hemorrhage, second trimester   Ⓜ♀

     O44.33 Partial placenta previa with hemorrhage, third trimester   Ⓜ♀

✓5ᵗʰ **O44.4 Low lying placenta NOS or without hemorrhage**
Low implantation of placenta NOS or without hemorrhage

     O44.40 Low lying placenta NOS or without hemorrhage, unspecified trimester   Ⓜ♀▽

     O44.41 Low lying placenta NOS or without hemorrhage, first trimester   Ⓜ♀

     O44.42 Low lying placenta NOS or without hemorrhage, second trimester   Ⓜ♀

     O44.43 Low lying placenta NOS or without hemorrhage, third trimester   Ⓜ♀

✓5ᵗʰ **O44.5 Low lying placenta with hemorrhage**
Low implantation of placenta with hemorrhage

     O44.50 Low lying placenta with hemorrhage, unspecified trimester   Ⓜ♀▽

     O44.51 Low lying placenta with hemorrhage, first trimester   Ⓜ♀

     O44.52 Low lying placenta with hemorrhage, second trimester   Ⓜ♀

     O44.53 Low lying placenta with hemorrhage, third trimester   Ⓜ♀

✓4ᵗʰ **O45 Premature separation of placenta [abruptio placentae]**

✓5ᵗʰ **O45.0 Premature separation of placenta with coagulation defect**

   ✓6ᵗʰ **O45.00 Premature separation of placenta with coagulation defect, unspecified**

     O45.001 Premature separation of placenta with coagulation defect, unspecified, first trimester   Ⓜ♀▽

     O45.002 Premature separation of placenta with coagulation defect, unspecified, second trimester   Ⓜ♀▽

     O45.003 Premature separation of placenta with coagulation defect, unspecified, third trimester   Ⓜ♀▽

     O45.009 Premature separation of placenta with coagulation defect, unspecified, unspecified trimester   Ⓜ♀▽

   ✓6ᵗʰ **O45.01 Premature separation of placenta with afibrinogenemia**
Premature separation of placenta with hypofibrinogenemia

     O45.011 Premature separation of placenta with afibrinogenemia, first trimester   Ⓜ♀

     O45.012 Premature separation of placenta with afibrinogenemia, second trimester   Ⓜ♀

     O45.013 Premature separation of placenta with afibrinogenemia, third trimester   Ⓜ♀

     O45.019 Premature separation of placenta with afibrinogenemia, unspecified trimester   Ⓜ♀▽

   ✓6ᵗʰ **O45.02 Premature separation of placenta with disseminated intravascular coagulation**

     O45.021 Premature separation of placenta with disseminated intravascular coagulation, first trimester   Ⓜ♀

     O45.022 Premature separation of placenta with disseminated intravascular coagulation, second trimester   Ⓜ♀

     O45.023 Premature separation of placenta with disseminated intravascular coagulation, third trimester   Ⓜ♀

     O45.029 Premature separation of placenta with disseminated intravascular coagulation, unspecified trimester   Ⓜ♀▽

   ✓6ᵗʰ **O45.09 Premature separation of placenta with other coagulation defect**

     O45.091 Premature separation of placenta with other coagulation defect, first trimester   Ⓜ♀

     O45.092 Premature separation of placenta with other coagulation defect, second trimester   Ⓜ♀

     O45.093 Premature separation of placenta with other coagulation defect, third trimester   Ⓜ♀

     O45.099 Premature separation of placenta with other coagulation defect, unspecified trimester   Ⓜ♀▽

✓5ᵗʰ **O45.8 Other premature separation of placenta**

   ✓6ᵗʰ **O45.8X Other premature separation of placenta**

     O45.8X1 Other premature separation of placenta, first trimester   Ⓜ♀

     O45.8X2 Other premature separation of placenta, second trimester   Ⓜ♀

     O45.8X3 Other premature separation of placenta, third trimester   Ⓜ♀

     O45.8X9 Other premature separation of placenta, unspecified trimester   Ⓜ♀▽

✓5ᵗʰ **O45.9 Premature separation of placenta, unspecified**
Abruptio placentae NOS

     O45.90 Premature separation of placenta, unspecified, unspecified trimester   Ⓜ♀▽

     O45.91 Premature separation of placenta, unspecified, first trimester   Ⓜ♀▽

     O45.92 Premature separation of placenta, unspecified, second trimester   Ⓜ♀▽

     O45.93 Premature separation of placenta, unspecified, third trimester   Ⓜ♀▽

✓4ᵗʰ **O46 Antepartum hemorrhage, not elsewhere classified**
> EXCLUDES 1   *hemorrhage in early pregnancy (O20.-)*
> *intrapartum hemorrhage NEC (O67.-)*
> *placenta previa (O44.-)*
> *premature separation of placenta [abruptio placentae] (O45.-)*

DEF: Uterine hemorrhage prior to delivery; not related to placenta previa or abruptio placentae.

✓5ᵗʰ **O46.0 Antepartum hemorrhage with coagulation defect**

   ✓6ᵗʰ **O46.00 Antepartum hemorrhage with coagulation defect, unspecified**

     O46.001 Antepartum hemorrhage with coagulation defect, unspecified, first trimester   Ⓜ♀▽

     O46.002 Antepartum hemorrhage with coagulation defect, unspecified, second trimester   Ⓜ♀▽

     O46.003 Antepartum hemorrhage with coagulation defect, unspecified, third trimester   Ⓜ♀▽

     O46.009 Antepartum hemorrhage with coagulation defect, unspecified, unspecified trimester   Ⓜ♀▽

   ✓6ᵗʰ **O46.01 Antepartum hemorrhage with afibrinogenemia**
Antepartum hemorrhage with hypofibrinogenemia

     O46.011 Antepartum hemorrhage with afibrinogenemia, first trimester   Ⓜ♀

     O46.012 Antepartum hemorrhage with afibrinogenemia, second trimester   Ⓜ♀

✓ Additional Character Req   ✓x7ᵗʰ Placeholder Alert   Case-Mix Diagnosis   Manifestation   ▽ Unspecified Dx   EXCLUDES 1 Not coded here   EXCLUDES 2 Not included here

O46.013   Antepartum hemorrhage with afibrinogenemia, third trimester   M♀

O46.019   Antepartum hemorrhage with afibrinogenemia, unspecified trimester   M♀▽

√6ᵗʰ **O46.02   Antepartum hemorrhage with disseminated intravascular coagulation**

O46.021   Antepartum hemorrhage with disseminated intravascular coagulation, first trimester   M♀

O46.022   Antepartum hemorrhage with disseminated intravascular coagulation, second trimester   M♀

O46.023   Antepartum hemorrhage with disseminated intravascular coagulation, third trimester   M♀

O46.029   Antepartum hemorrhage with disseminated intravascular coagulation, unspecified trimester   M♀▽

√6ᵗʰ **O46.09   Antepartum hemorrhage with other coagulation defect**

O46.091   Antepartum hemorrhage with other coagulation defect, first trimester   M♀

O46.092   Antepartum hemorrhage with other coagulation defect, second trimester   M♀

O46.093   Antepartum hemorrhage with other coagulation defect, third trimester   M♀

O46.099   Antepartum hemorrhage with other coagulation defect, unspecified trimester   M♀▽

√5ᵗʰ **O46.8   Other antepartum hemorrhage**

√6ᵗʰ **O46.8X   Other antepartum hemorrhage**

O46.8X1   Other antepartum hemorrhage, first trimester   M♀

O46.8X2   Other antepartum hemorrhage, second trimester   M♀

O46.8X3   Other antepartum hemorrhage, third trimester   M♀

O46.8X9   Other antepartum hemorrhage, unspecified trimester   M♀▽

√5ᵗʰ **O46.9   Antepartum hemorrhage, unspecified**

O46.90   Antepartum hemorrhage, unspecified, unspecified trimester   M♀▽

O46.91   Antepartum hemorrhage, unspecified, first trimester   M♀▽

O46.92   Antepartum hemorrhage, unspecified, second trimester   M♀▽

O46.93   Antepartum hemorrhage, unspecified, third trimester   M♀▽

√4ᵗʰ **O47   False labor**

INCLUDES   Braxton Hicks contractions
threatened labor
EXCLUDES 1   *preterm labor (O60.-)*

√5ᵗʰ **O47.0   False labor before 37 completed weeks of gestation**

O47.00   False labor before 37 completed weeks of gestation, unspecified trimester   M♀▽

O47.02   False labor before 37 completed weeks of gestation, second trimester   M♀

O47.03   False labor before 37 completed weeks of gestation, third trimester   M♀

O47.1   False labor at or after 37 completed weeks of gestation   M♀

O47.9   False labor, unspecified   M♀▽

√4ᵗʰ **O48   Late pregnancy**

O48.0   Post-term pregnancy   M♀
Pregnancy over 40 completed weeks to 42 completed weeks gestation

O48.1   Prolonged pregnancy   M♀
Pregnancy which has advanced beyond 42 completed weeks gestation
AHA: 2016, 1Q, 5

Complications of labor and delivery (O60-O77)

√4ᵗʰ **O60   Preterm labor**

INCLUDES   onset (spontaneous) of labor before 37 completed weeks of gestation
EXCLUDES 1   *false labor (O47.0-)*
threatened labor NOS (O47.0-)

√5ᵗʰ **O60.0   Preterm labor without delivery**

O60.00   Preterm labor without delivery, unspecified trimester   M♀▽

O60.02   Preterm labor without delivery, second trimester   M♀

O60.03   Preterm labor without delivery, third trimester   M♀

√5ᵗʰ **O60.1   Preterm labor with preterm delivery**
AHA: 2016, 2Q, 10

> One of the following 7th characters is to be assigned to each code under subcategory O60.1. 7th character 0 is for single gestations and multiple gestations where the fetus is unspecified. 7th characters 1 through 9 are for cases of multiple gestations to identify the fetus for which the code applies. The appropriate code from category O30, Multiple gestation, must also be assigned when assigning a code from subcategory O60.1 that has a 7th character of 1 through 9.
> | | | | |
> |---|---|---|---|
> | 0 | not applicable or unspecified | 4 | fetus 4 |
> | 1 | fetus 1 | 5 | fetus 5 |
> | 2 | fetus 2 | 9 | other fetus |
> | 3 | fetus 3 | | |

√x7ᵗʰ **O60.10   Preterm labor with preterm delivery, unspecified trimester**   M♀▽
Preterm labor with delivery NOS

√x7ᵗʰ **O60.12   Preterm labor second trimester with preterm delivery second trimester**   M♀

√x7ᵗʰ **O60.13   Preterm labor second trimester with preterm delivery third trimester**   M♀

√x7ᵗʰ **O60.14   Preterm labor third trimester with preterm delivery third trimester**   M♀

√5ᵗʰ **O60.2   Term delivery with preterm labor**

> One of the following 7th characters is to be assigned to each code under subcategory O60.2. 7th character 0 is for single gestations and multiple gestations where the fetus is unspecified. 7th characters 1 through 9 are for cases of multiple gestations to identify the fetus for which the code applies. The appropriate code from category O30, Multiple gestation, must also be assigned when assigning a code from subcategory O60.2 that has a 7th character of 1 through 9.
> | | | | |
> |---|---|---|---|
> | 0 | not applicable or unspecified | 4 | fetus 4 |
> | 1 | fetus 1 | 5 | fetus 5 |
> | 2 | fetus 2 | 9 | other fetus |
> | 3 | fetus 3 | | |

√x7ᵗʰ **O60.20   Term delivery with preterm labor, unspecified trimester**   M♀▽

√x7ᵗʰ **O60.22   Term delivery with preterm labor, second trimester**   M♀

√x7ᵗʰ **O60.23   Term delivery with preterm labor, third trimester**   M♀

√4ᵗʰ **O61   Failed induction of labor**

O61.0   Failed medical induction of labor   M♀
Failed induction (of labor) by oxytocin
Failed induction (of labor) by prostaglandins

O61.1   Failed instrumental induction of labor   M♀
Failed mechanical induction (of labor)
Failed surgical induction (of labor)

O61.8   Other failed induction of labor   M♀

O61.9   Failed induction of labor, unspecified   M♀▽

√4ᵗʰ **O62   Abnormalities of forces of labor**

O62.0   Primary inadequate contractions   M♀
Failure of cervical dilatation
Primary hypotonic uterine dysfunction
Uterine inertia during latent phase of labor

O62.1   Secondary uterine inertia   M♀
Arrested active phase of labor
Secondary hypotonic uterine dysfunction

N Newborn: 0   P Pediatric: 0-17   M Maternity: 12-55   A Adult: 15-124   NRS Nonroutine supply Dx   NCDx Noncancer Dx   PDx Primary Dx   ▶◀ Revised Text   ● New Code   ▲ Revised Title

844   ICD-10-CM 2018

O62.2 Other uterine inertia   Ⓜ♀

Atony of uterus without hemorrhage
Atony of uterus NOS
Desultory labor
Hypotonic uterine dysfunction NOS
Irregular labor
Poor contractions
Slow slope active phase of labor
Uterine inertia NOS

EXCLUDES 1   atony of uterus with hemorrhage (postpartum) (O72.1)
postpartum atony of uterus without hemorrhage (O75.89)

O62.3 Precipitate labor   Ⓜ♀

O62.4 Hypertonic, incoordinate, and prolonged uterine contractions   Ⓜ♀

Cervical spasm
Contraction ring dystocia
Dyscoordinate labor
Hour-glass contraction of uterus
Hypertonic uterine dysfunction
Incoordinate uterine action

Tetanic contractions
Uterine dystocia NOS
Uterine spasm

EXCLUDES 1   dystocia (fetal) (maternal) NOS (O66.9)

O62.8 Other abnormalities of forces of labor   Ⓜ♀

O62.9 Abnormality of forces of labor, unspecified   Ⓜ♀ ▽

✓4ᵗʰ **O63 Long labor**

O63.0 Prolonged first stage (of labor)   Ⓜ♀

O63.1 Prolonged second stage (of labor)   Ⓜ♀

O63.2 Delayed delivery of second twin, triplet, etc.   Ⓜ♀

O63.9 Long labor, unspecified   Ⓜ♀ ▽
Prolonged labor NOS

✓4ᵗʰ **O64 Obstructed labor due to malposition and malpresentation of fetus**

One of the following 7th characters is to be assigned to each code under category O64. 7th character 0 is for single gestations and multiple gestations where the fetus is unspecified. 7th characters 1 through 9 are for cases of multiple gestations to identify the fetus for which the code applies. The appropriate code from category O30, Multiple gestation, must also be assigned when assigning a code from category O64 that has a 7th character of 1 through 9.

0	not applicable or unspecified	4	fetus 4
1	fetus 1	5	fetus 5
2	fetus 2	9	other fetus
3	fetus 3		

✓x7ᵗʰ **O64.0 Obstructed labor due to incomplete rotation of fetal head**   Ⓜ♀

Deep transverse arrest
Obstructed labor due to persistent occipitoiliac (position)
Obstructed labor due to persistent occipitoposterior (position)
Obstructed labor due to persistent occipitosacral (position)
Obstructed labor due to persistent occipitotransverse (position)

✓x7ᵗʰ **O64.1 Obstructed labor due to breech presentation**   Ⓜ♀
Obstructed labor due to buttocks presentation
Obstructed labor due to complete breech presentation
Obstructed labor due to frank breech presentation

✓x7ᵗʰ **O64.2 Obstructed labor due to face presentation**   Ⓜ♀
Obstructed labor due to chin presentation

✓x7ᵗʰ **O64.3 Obstructed labor due to brow presentation**   Ⓜ♀

Fetal Malposition

Breech

Shoulder
(arm prolapse)

Mother's pelvis

Face
(mentum)

Compound
(extremity together with head)

Oblique

✓x7ᵗʰ **O64.4 Obstructed labor due to shoulder presentation**   Ⓜ♀
Prolapsed arm
EXCLUDES 1   impacted shoulders (O66.0)
shoulder dystocia (O66.0)
g

O64.5 Obstructed labor due to compound presentation   Ⓜ♀

✓x7ᵗʰ **O64.8 Obstructed labor due to other malposition and malpresentation**   Ⓜ♀
Obstructed labor due to footling presentation
Obstructed labor due to incomplete breech presentation

✓x7ᵗʰ **O64.9 Obstructed labor due to malposition and malpresentation, unspecified**   Ⓜ♀ ▽

✓4ᵗʰ **O65 Obstructed labor due to maternal pelvic abnormality**

O65.0 Obstructed labor due to deformed pelvis   Ⓜ♀

O65.1 Obstructed labor due to generally contracted pelvis   Ⓜ♀

O65.2 Obstructed labor due to pelvic inlet contraction   Ⓜ♀

O65.3 Obstructed labor due to pelvic outlet and mid-cavity contraction   Ⓜ♀

O65.4 Obstructed labor due to fetopelvic disproportion, unspecified   Ⓜ♀ ▽
EXCLUDES 1   dystocia due to abnormality of fetus (O66.2-O66.3)

O65.5 Obstructed labor due to abnormality of maternal pelvic organs   Ⓜ♀
Obstructed labor due to conditions listed in O34-
Use additional code to identify abnormality of pelvic organs (O34.-)

O65.8 Obstructed labor due to other maternal pelvic abnormalities   Ⓜ♀

O65.9 Obstructed labor due to maternal pelvic abnormality, unspecified   Ⓜ♀ ▽

✓4ᵗʰ **O66 Other obstructed labor**

O66.0 Obstructed labor due to shoulder dystocia   Ⓜ♀
Impacted shoulders
DEF: Obstructed labor due to impacted fetal shoulders; emergency condition that may require cesarean section, forceps delivery, vacuum extraction, or simphysiotomy.

O66.1 Obstructed labor due to locked twins   Ⓜ♀

O66.2 Obstructed labor due to unusually large fetus   Ⓜ♀

O66.3 Obstructed labor due to other abnormalities of fetus   Ⓜ♀
Dystocia due to fetal ascites
Dystocia due to fetal hydrops
Dystocia due to fetal meningomyelocele
Dystocia due to fetal sacral teratoma
Dystocia due to fetal tumor
Dystocia due to hydrocephalic fetus
Use additional code to identify cause of obstruction

✓5ᵗʰ **O66.4 Failed trial of labor**

O66.40 Failed trial of labor, unspecified   Ⓜ♀ ▽

O66.41 Failed attempted vaginal birth after previous cesarean delivery   Ⓜ♀
Code first rupture of uterus, if applicable (O71.0-, O71.1)

O66.5 Attempted application of vacuum extractor and forceps   Ⓜ♀
Attempted application of vacuum or forceps, with subsequent delivery by forceps or cesarean delivery

O66.6 Obstructed labor due to other multiple fetuses   Ⓜ♀

O66.8 Other specified obstructed labor   Ⓜ♀
Use additional code to identify cause of obstruction

O66.9 Obstructed labor, unspecified   Ⓜ♀ ▽
Dystocia NOS
Fetal dystocia NOS
Maternal dystocia NOS

✓4ᵗʰ **O67 Labor and delivery complicated by intrapartum hemorrhage, not elsewhere classified**
EXCLUDES 1   antepartum hemorrhage NEC (O46.-)
placenta previa (O44.-)
premature separation of placenta [abruptio placentae] (O45.-)
EXCLUDES 2   postpartum hemorrhage (O72.-)

O67.0 Intrapartum hemorrhage with coagulation defect   Ⓜ♀
Intrapartum hemorrhage (excessive) associated with afibrinogenemia
Intrapartum hemorrhage (excessive) associated with disseminated intravascular coagulation
Intrapartum hemorrhage (excessive) associated with hyperfibrinolysis
Intrapartum hemorrhage (excessive) associated with hypofibrinogenemia

✓ Additional Character Req   ✓x7ᵗʰ Placeholder Alert   Case-Mix Diagnosis   Manifestation   ▽ Unspecified Dx   EXCLUDES 1 Not coded here   EXCLUDES 2 Not included here

ICD-10-CM 2018   845

Chapter 15. Pregnancy, Childbirth and the Puerperium

O62.2–O67.0

O67.8 Other intrapartum hemorrhage   Ⓜ♀
> Excessive intrapartum hemorrhage

O67.9 Intrapartum hemorrhage, unspecified   Ⓜ♀ ▽

O68 Labor and delivery complicated by abnormality of fetal acid-base balance   Ⓜ♀
> Fetal acidemia complicating labor and delivery
> Fetal acidosis complicating labor and delivery
> Fetal alkalosis complicating labor and delivery
> Fetal metabolic acidemia complicating labor and delivery
> **EXCLUDES 1**   *fetal stress NOS (O77.9)*
> *labor and delivery complicated by electrocardiographic evidence of fetal stress (O77.8)*
> *labor and delivery complicated by ultrasonic evidence of fetal stress (O77.8)*
> **EXCLUDES 2**   *abnormality in fetal heart rate or rhythm (O76)*
> *labor and delivery complicated by meconium in amniotic fluid (O77.0)*

✓4ᵗʰ O69 Labor and delivery complicated by umbilical cord complications
> AHA: 2016, 1Q, 5

> One of the following 7th characters is to be assigned to each code under category O69. 7th character Ø is for single gestations and multiple gestations where the fetus is unspecified. 7th characters 1 through 9 are for cases of multiple gestations to identify the fetus for which the code applies. The appropriate code from category O30, Multiple gestation, must also be assigned when assigning a code from category O69 that has a 7th character of 1 through 9.
> | Ø | not applicable or unspecified | 3 | fetus 3 |
> |---|---|---|---|
> | | | 4 | fetus 4 |
> | 1 | fetus 1 | 5 | fetus 5 |
> | 2 | fetus 2 | 9 | other fetus |

✓x7ᵗʰ O69.0 Labor and delivery complicated by prolapse of cord   Ⓜ♀
> **DEF:** Abnormal presentation of fetus; marked by protruding umbilical cord during labor; can cause fetal death.

✓x7ᵗʰ O69.1 Labor and delivery complicated by cord around neck, with compression   Ⓜ♀
> **EXCLUDES 1**   *labor and delivery complicated by cord around neck, without compression (O69.81)*

✓x7ᵗʰ O69.2 Labor and delivery complicated by other cord entanglement, with compression   Ⓜ♀
> Labor and delivery complicated by compression of cord NOS
> Labor and delivery complicated by entanglement of cords of twins in monoamniotic sac
> Labor and delivery complicated by knot in cord
> **EXCLUDES 1**   *labor and delivery complicated by other cord entanglement, without compression (O69.82)*

✓x7ᵗʰ O69.3 Labor and delivery complicated by short cord   Ⓜ♀

✓x7ᵗʰ O69.4 Labor and delivery complicated by vasa previa   Ⓜ♀
> Labor and delivery complicated by hemorrhage from vasa previa

✓x7ᵗʰ O69.5 Labor and delivery complicated by vascular lesion of cord   Ⓜ♀
> Labor and delivery complicated by cord bruising
> Labor and delivery complicated by cord hematoma
> Labor and delivery complicated by thrombosis of umbilical vessels

✓5ᵗʰ O69.8 Labor and delivery complicated by other cord complications
> **✓x7ᵗʰ O69.81 Labor and delivery complicated by cord around neck, without compression**   Ⓜ♀
> > AHA: 2016, 1Q, 5

> **✓x7ᵗʰ O69.82 Labor and delivery complicated by other cord entanglement, without compression**   Ⓜ♀

> **✓x7ᵗʰ O69.89 Labor and delivery complicated by other cord complications**   Ⓜ♀

✓x7ᵗʰ O69.9 Labor and delivery complicated by cord complication, unspecified   Ⓜ♀ ▽

✓4ᵗʰ O70 Perineal laceration during delivery
> **INCLUDES**   episiotomy extended by laceration
> **EXCLUDES 1**   *obstetric high vaginal laceration alone (O71.4)*
> AHA: 2016, 2Q, 34; 2016, 1Q, 3-4, 5

> **O70.0 First degree perineal laceration during delivery**   Ⓜ♀
> > Perineal laceration, rupture or tear involving fourchette during delivery
> > Perineal laceration, rupture or tear involving labia during delivery
> > Perineal laceration, rupture or tear involving skin during delivery
> > Perineal laceration, rupture or tear involving vagina during delivery
> > Perineal laceration, rupture or tear involving vulva during delivery
> > Slight perineal laceration, rupture or tear during delivery

O70.1 Second degree perineal laceration during delivery   Ⓜ♀
> Perineal laceration, rupture or tear during delivery as in O70.0, also involving pelvic floor
> Perineal laceration, rupture or tear during delivery as in O70.0, also involving perineal muscles
> Perineal laceration, rupture or tear during delivery as in O70.0, also involving vaginal muscles
> **EXCLUDES 1**   *perineal laceration involving anal sphincter (O70.2)*

✓5ᵗʰ O70.2 Third degree perineal laceration during delivery
> Perineal laceration, rupture or tear during delivery as in O70.1, also involving anal sphincter
> Perineal laceration, rupture or tear during delivery as in O70.1, also involving rectovaginal septum
> Perineal laceration, rupture or tear during delivery as in O70.1, also involving sphincter NOS
> **EXCLUDES 1**   *anal sphincter tear during delivery without third degree perineal laceration (O70.4)*
> *perineal laceration involving anal or rectal mucosa (O70.3)*

> **O70.20 Third degree perineal laceration during delivery, unspecified**   Ⓜ♀ ▽

> **O70.21 Third degree perineal laceration during delivery, IIIa**   Ⓜ♀
> > Third degree perineal laceration during delivery with less than 50% of external anal sphincter (EAS) thickness torn

> **O70.22 Third degree perineal laceration during delivery, IIIb**   Ⓜ♀
> > Third degree perineal laceration during delivery with more than 50% external anal sphincter (EAS) thickness torn

> **O70.23 Third degree perineal laceration during delivery, IIIc**   Ⓜ♀
> > Third degree perineal laceration during delivery with both external anal sphincter (EAS) and internal anal sphincter (IAS) torn

O70.3 Fourth degree perineal laceration during delivery   Ⓜ♀
> Perineal laceration, rupture or tear during delivery as in O70.2, also involving anal mucosa
> Perineal laceration, rupture or tear during delivery as in O70.2, also involving rectal mucosa

O70.4 Anal sphincter tear complicating delivery, not associated with third degree laceration   Ⓜ♀
> **EXCLUDES 1**   *anal sphincter tear with third degree perineal laceration (O70.2)*

O70.9 Perineal laceration during delivery, unspecified   Ⓜ♀ ▽

✓4ᵗʰ O71 Other obstetric trauma
> Obstetric damage from instruments

> **✓5ᵗʰ O71.0 Rupture of uterus (spontaneous) before onset of labor**
> > **EXCLUDES 1**   *disruption of (current) cesarean delivery wound (O90.0)*
> > *laceration of uterus, NEC (O71.81)*

> > **O71.00 Rupture of uterus before onset of labor, unspecified trimester**   Ⓜ♀ ▽

> > **O71.02 Rupture of uterus before onset of labor, second trimester**   Ⓜ♀

> > **O71.03 Rupture of uterus before onset of labor, third trimester**   Ⓜ♀

> **O71.1 Rupture of uterus during labor**   Ⓜ♀
> > Rupture of uterus not stated as occurring before onset of labor
> > **EXCLUDES 1**   *disruption of cesarean delivery wound (O90.0)*
> > *laceration of uterus, NEC (O71.81)*

> **O71.2 Postpartum inversion of uterus**   Ⓜ♀

> **O71.3 Obstetric laceration of cervix**   Ⓜ♀
> > Annular detachment of cervix

> **O71.4 Obstetric high vaginal laceration alone**   Ⓜ♀
> > Laceration of vaginal wall without perineal laceration
> > **EXCLUDES 1**   *obstetric high vaginal laceration with perineal laceration (O70.-)*
> > AHA: 2016, 1Q, 5

> **O71.5 Other obstetric injury to pelvic organs**   Ⓜ♀
> > Obstetric injury to bladder
> > Obstetric injury to urethra
> > **EXCLUDES 2**   *obstetric periurethral trauma (O71.82)*
> > AHA: 2014, 4Q, 18

> **O71.6 Obstetric damage to pelvic joints and ligaments**   Ⓜ♀
> > Obstetric avulsion of inner symphyseal cartilage
> > Obstetric damage to coccyx
> > Obstetric traumatic separation of symphysis (pubis)

Ⓝ Newborn: 0   Ⓟ Pediatric: 0-17   Ⓜ Maternity: 12-55   Ⓐ Adult: 15-124   **NRS** Nonroutine supply Dx   **NCDx** Noncancer Dx   **PDx** Primary Dx   ▶◀ Revised Text   ● New Code   ▲ Revised Title

846   ICD-10-CM 2018

O71.7 **Obstetric** hematoma of pelvis   ⓜ♀
     Obstetric hematoma of perineum
     Obstetric hematoma of vagina
     Obstetric hematoma of vulva

✓5ᵗʰ **O71.8** **Other specified obstetric trauma**

     O71.81 **Laceration of uterus, not elsewhere classified**   ⓜ♀

     O71.82 **Other specified trauma to perineum and vulva**   ⓜ♀
         Obstetric periurethral trauma
         AHA: 2016, 1Q, 4; 2014, 4Q, 18

     O71.89 **Other specified obstetric trauma**   ⓜ♀

     O71.9 **Obstetric trauma, unspecified**   ⓜ♀▽

✓4ᵗʰ **O72 Postpartum hemorrhage**
     INCLUDES   hemorrhage after delivery of fetus or infant

     O72.0 **Third-stage** hemorrhage   ⓜ♀
         Hemorrhage associated with retained, trapped or adherent
             placenta
         Retained placenta NOS
         Code also type of adherent placenta (O43.2-)

     O72.1 **Other** immediate **postpartum hemorrhage**   ⓜ♀
         Hemorrhage following delivery of placenta
         Postpartum hemorrhage (atonic) NOS
         Uterine atony with hemorrhage
         EXCLUDES 1   uterine atony NOS (O62.2)
                     uterine atony without hemorrhage (O62.2)
                     postpartum atony of uterus without hemorrhage
                       (O75.89)
         AHA: 2016, 1Q, 4

     O72.2 **Delayed and secondary postpartum hemorrhage**   ⓜ♀
         Hemorrhage associated with retained portions of placenta or
             membranes after the first 24 hours following delivery of
             placenta
         Retained products of conception NOS, following delivery

     O72.3 **Postpartum** coagulation defects   ⓜ♀
         Postpartum afibrinogenemia
         Postpartum fibrinolysis

✓4ᵗʰ **O73 Retained placenta and membranes, without hemorrhage**
     EXCLUDES 1   placenta accreta (O43.21-)
                  placenta increta (O43.22-)
                  placenta percreta (O43.23-)
     DEF: Postpartum condition resulting from failure to expel placental
     membrane tissues due to failed contractions of uterine wall.

     O73.0 **Retained** placenta **without hemorrhage**   ⓜ♀
         Adherent placenta, without hemorrhage
         Trapped placenta without hemorrhage

     O73.1 **Retained** portions of placenta and membranes, **without**   ⓜ♀
     hemorrhage
         Retained products of conception following delivery, without
             hemorrhage

✓4ᵗʰ **O74 Complications of anesthesia during labor and delivery**
     INCLUDES   maternal complications arising from the administration of a
                     general, regional or local anesthetic, analgesic or other
                     sedation during labor and delivery
     Use additional code, if applicable, to identify specific complication

     O74.0 **Aspiration pneumonitis** due to anesthesia during labor   ⓜ♀
     and delivery
         Inhalation of stomach contents or secretions NOS due to
             anesthesia during labor and delivery
         Mendelson's syndrome due to anesthesia during labor and
             delivery

     O74.1 **Other** pulmonary **complications of anesthesia during**   ⓜ♀
     labor and delivery

     O74.2 **Cardiac complications of anesthesia during labor and**   ⓜ♀
     delivery

     O74.3 **Central nervous system complications of anesthesia**   ⓜ♀
     during labor and delivery

     O74.4 **Toxic reaction to local anesthesia during labor and**   ⓜ♀
     delivery

     O74.5 **Spinal and epidural anesthesia-induced headache**   ⓜ♀
     during labor and delivery

     O74.6 **Other complications of** spinal and epidural anesthesia   ⓜ♀
     during labor and delivery

     O74.7 **Failed or difficult intubation for anesthesia during**   ⓜ♀
     labor and delivery

     O74.8 **Other complications of anesthesia during labor and**   ⓜ♀
     delivery

     O74.9 **Complication of anesthesia during labor and delivery,**   ⓜ♀▽
     unspecified

✓4ᵗʰ **O75 Other complications of labor and delivery, not elsewhere classified**
     EXCLUDES 2   puerperal (postpartum) infection (O86.-)
                  puerperal (postpartum) sepsis (O85)

     O75.0 **Maternal distress during labor and delivery**   ⓜ♀

     O75.1 **Shock during or following labor and delivery**   ⓜ♀
         Obstetric shock following labor and delivery

     O75.2 **Pyrexia during labor, not elsewhere classified**   ⓜ♀

     O75.3 **Other infection during labor**   ⓜ♀
         Sepsis during labor
         Use additional code (B95-B97), to identify infectious agent

     O75.4 **Other complications of obstetric surgery and procedures**   ⓜ♀
         Cardiac arrest following obstetric surgery or procedures
         Cardiac failure following obstetric surgery or procedures
         Cerebral anoxia following obstetric surgery or procedures
         Pulmonary edema following obstetric surgery or procedures
         Use additional code to identify specific complication
         EXCLUDES 2   complications of anesthesia during labor and delivery
                     (O74.-)
                  disruption of obstetrical (surgical) wound
                     (O90.0-O90.1)
                  hematoma of obstetrical (surgical) wound (O90.2)
                  infection of obstetrical (surgical) wound (O86.0)

     O75.5 **Delayed delivery after artificial rupture of membranes**   ⓜ♀

✓5ᵗʰ   **O75.8** **Other specified complications of labor and delivery**

         O75.81 **Maternal exhaustion complicating labor**   ⓜ♀
         and delivery

         O75.82 **Onset (spontaneous) of labor after 37**   ⓜ♀
         completed weeks of gestation but before 39
         completed weeks gestation, with delivery by
         (planned) cesarean section
             Delivery by (planned) cesarean section occurring after
                 37 completed weeks of gestation but before 39
                 completed weeks gestation due to (spontaneous)
                 onset of labor
             Code first to specify reason for planned cesarean
                 section such as:
                 cephalopelvic disproportion (normally formed
                    fetus) (O33.9)
                 previous cesarean delivery (O34.21)

         O75.89 **Other specified complications of labor**   ⓜ♀
         and delivery

     O75.9 **Complication of labor and delivery, unspecified**   ⓜ♀▽

O76 Abnormality in fetal heart rate and rhythm complicating   ⓜ♀
labor and delivery
     Depressed fetal heart rate tones complicating labor and delivery
     Fetal bradycardia complicating labor and delivery
     Fetal heart rate abnormal variability complicating labor and delivery
     Fetal heart rate decelerations complicating labor and delivery
     Fetal heart rate irregularity complicating labor and delivery
     Fetal tachycardia complicating labor and delivery
     Non-reassuring fetal heart rate or rhythm complicating labor and
         delivery
     EXCLUDES 1   fetal stress NOS (O77.9)
                  labor and delivery complicated by electrocardiographic
                     evidence of fetal stress (O77.8)
                  labor and delivery complicated by ultrasonic evidence of fetal
                     stress (O77.8)
     EXCLUDES 2   fetal metabolic acidemia (O68)
                  other fetal stress (O77.0-O77.1)
     AHA: 2013, 4Q, 118

✓4ᵗʰ **O77 Other fetal stress complicating labor and delivery**

     O77.0 **Labor and delivery complicated by meconium in**   ⓜ♀
     amniotic fluid
         AHA: 2013, 4Q, 117-118

     O77.1 **Fetal stress in labor or delivery due to drug**   ⓜ♀
     administration

     O77.8 **Labor and delivery complicated by other evidence of**   ⓜ♀
     fetal stress
         Labor and delivery complicated by electrocardiographic
             evidence of fetal stress
         Labor and delivery complicated by ultrasonic evidence of fetal
             stress
         EXCLUDES 1   abnormality in fetal heart rate or rhythm (O76)
                     abnormality of fetal acid-base balance (O68)
                     fetal metabolic acidemia (O68)

     O77.9 **Labor and delivery complicated by fetal stress,**   ⓜ♀▽
     unspecified
         EXCLUDES 1   abnormality in fetal heart rate or rhythm (O76)
                     abnormality of fetal acid-base balance (O68)
                     fetal metabolic acidemia (O68)

☑ Additional Character Req   ✓×7ᵗʰ Placeholder Alert   Case-Mix Diagnosis   Manifestation   ▽ Unspecified Dx   EXCLUDES 1 Not coded here   EXCLUDES 2 Not included here

Chapter 15. Pregnancy, Childbirth and the Puerperium

Encounter for delivery (O80–O82)

O80 Encounter for full-term uncomplicated delivery   Ⓜ♀
> **NOTE**   Delivery requiring minimal or no assistance, with or without episiotomy, without fetal manipulation [e.g., rotation version] or instrumentation [forceps] of a spontaneous, cephalic, vaginal, full-term, single, live-born infant. This code is for use as a single diagnosis code and is not to be used with any other code from chapter 15.
> Use additional code to indicate outcome of delivery (Z37.0)
> **AHA:** 2016, 4Q, 150; 2014, 2Q, 9

O82 Encounter for cesarean delivery without indication   Ⓜ♀
> Use additional code to indicate outcome of delivery (Z37.0)

Complications predominantly related to the puerperium (O85–O92)

> **EXCLUDES 2**   mental and behavioral disorders associated with the puerperium (F53)
> obstetrical tetanus (A34)
> puerperal osteomalacia (M83.0)

O85 Puerperal sepsis   Ⓜ♀
> Postpartum sepsis
> Puerperal peritonitis
> Puerperal pyemia
> Use additional code (B95-B97), to identify infectious agent
> Use additional code (R65.2-) to identify severe sepsis, if applicable
> **EXCLUDES 1**   fever of unknown origin following delivery (O86.4)
> genital tract infection following delivery (O86.1-)
> obstetric pyemic and septic embolism (O88.3-)
> puerperal septic thrombophlebitis (O86.81)
> urinary tract infection following delivery (O86.2-)
> **EXCLUDES 2**   sepsis during labor (O75.3)

✓4ᵗʰ O86 Other puerperal infections
> Use additional code (B95-B97), to identify infectious agent
> **EXCLUDES 2**   infection during labor (O75.3)
> obstetrical tetanus (A34)

   O86.0 Infection of obstetric surgical wound   Ⓜ♀
> Infected cesarean delivery wound following delivery
> Infected perineal repair following delivery

   ✓5ᵗʰ O86.1 Other infection of genital tract following delivery
     O86.11 Cervicitis following delivery   Ⓜ♀
     O86.12 Endometritis following delivery   Ⓜ♀
     O86.13 Vaginitis following delivery   Ⓜ♀
     O86.19 Other infection of genital tract following delivery   Ⓜ♀

   ✓5ᵗʰ O86.2 Urinary tract infection following delivery
     O86.20 Urinary tract infection following delivery, unspecified   Ⓜ♀▽
       Puerperal urinary tract infection NOS
     O86.21 Infection of kidney following delivery   Ⓜ♀
     O86.22 Infection of bladder following delivery   Ⓜ♀
       Infection of urethra following delivery
     O86.29 Other urinary tract infection following delivery   Ⓜ♀

   O86.4 Pyrexia of unknown origin following delivery   Ⓜ♀
> Puerperal infection NOS following delivery
> Puerperal pyrexia NOS following delivery
> **EXCLUDES 2**   pyrexia during labor (O75.2)
> **DEF:** Fever of unknown origin experienced by the mother after childbirth.

   ✓5ᵗʰ O86.8 Other specified puerperal infections
     O86.81 Puerperal septic thrombophlebitis   Ⓜ♀
     O86.89 Other specified puerperal infections   Ⓜ♀

✓4ᵗʰ O87 Venous complications and hemorrhoids in the puerperium
> **INCLUDES**   venous complications in labor, delivery and the puerperium
> **EXCLUDES 2**   obstetric embolism (O88.-)
> puerperal septic thrombophlebitis (O86.81)
> venous complications in pregnancy (O22.-)

   O87.0 Superficial thrombophlebitis in the puerperium   Ⓜ♀
> Puerperal phlebitis NOS
> Puerperal thrombosis NOS

   O87.1 Deep phlebothrombosis in the puerperium   Ⓜ♀
> Deep vein thrombosis, postpartum
> Pelvic thrombophlebitis, postpartum
> Use additional code to identify the deep vein thrombosis (I82.4-, I82.5-, I82.62-. I82.72-)
> Use additional code, if applicable, for associated long-term (current) use of anticoagulants (Z79.01)

   O87.2 Hemorrhoids in the puerperium   Ⓜ♀

   O87.3 Cerebral venous thrombosis in the puerperium   Ⓜ♀
> Cerebrovenous sinus thrombosis in the puerperium

   O87.4 Varicose veins of lower extremity in the puerperium   Ⓜ♀

   O87.8 Other venous complications in the puerperium   Ⓜ♀
> Genital varices in the puerperium

   O87.9 Venous complication in the puerperium, unspecified   Ⓜ♀▽
> Puerperal phlebopathy NOS

✓4ᵗʰ O88 Obstetric embolism
> **EXCLUDES 1**   embolism complicating abortion NOS (O03.2)
> embolism complicating ectopic or molar pregnancy (O08.2)
> embolism complicating failed attempted abortion (O07.2)
> embolism complicating induced abortion (O04.7)
> embolism complicating spontaneous abortion (O03.2, O03.7)

   ✓5ᵗʰ O88.0 Obstetric air embolism
> **DEF:** Sudden blocking of pulmonary artery or right ventricle with air or nitrogen bubbles.

     ✓6ᵗʰ O88.01 Obstetric air embolism in pregnancy
       O88.011 Air embolism in pregnancy, first trimester   Ⓜ♀
       O88.012 Air embolism in pregnancy, second trimester   Ⓜ♀
       O88.013 Air embolism in pregnancy, third trimester   Ⓜ♀
       O88.019 Air embolism in pregnancy, unspecified trimester   Ⓜ♀▽
     O88.02 Air embolism in childbirth   Ⓜ♀
     O88.03 Air embolism in the puerperium   Ⓜ♀

   ✓5ᵗʰ O88.1 Amniotic fluid embolism
> Anaphylactoid syndrome in pregnancy

     ✓6ᵗʰ O88.11 Amniotic fluid embolism in pregnancy
       O88.111 Amniotic fluid embolism in pregnancy, first trimester   Ⓜ♀
       O88.112 Amniotic fluid embolism in pregnancy, second trimester   Ⓜ♀
       O88.113 Amniotic fluid embolism in pregnancy, third trimester   Ⓜ♀
       O88.119 Amniotic fluid embolism in pregnancy, unspecified trimester   Ⓜ♀▽
     O88.12 Amniotic fluid embolism in childbirth   Ⓜ♀
     O88.13 Amniotic fluid embolism in the puerperium   Ⓜ♀

   ✓5ᵗʰ O88.2 Obstetric thromboembolism
     ✓6ᵗʰ O88.21 Thromboembolism in pregnancy
       Obstetric (pulmonary) embolism NOS
       O88.211 Thromboembolism in pregnancy, first trimester   Ⓜ♀
       O88.212 Thromboembolism in pregnancy, second trimester   Ⓜ♀
       O88.213 Thromboembolism in pregnancy, third trimester   Ⓜ♀
       O88.219 Thromboembolism in pregnancy, unspecified trimester   Ⓜ♀▽
     O88.22 Thromboembolism in childbirth   Ⓜ♀
     O88.23 Thromboembolism in the puerperium   Ⓜ♀
       Puerperal (pulmonary) embolism NOS

   ✓5ᵗʰ O88.3 Obstetric pyemic and septic embolism
     ✓6ᵗʰ O88.31 Pyemic and septic embolism in pregnancy
       O88.311 Pyemic and septic embolism in pregnancy, first trimester   Ⓜ♀
       O88.312 Pyemic and septic embolism in pregnancy, second trimester   Ⓜ♀
       O88.313 Pyemic and septic embolism in pregnancy, third trimester   Ⓜ♀
       O88.319 Pyemic and septic embolism in pregnancy, unspecified trimester   Ⓜ♀▽
     O88.32 Pyemic and septic embolism in childbirth   Ⓜ♀
     O88.33 Pyemic and septic embolism in the puerperium   Ⓜ♀

   ✓5ᵗʰ O88.8 Other obstetric embolism
> Obstetric fat embolism

     ✓6ᵗʰ O88.81 Other embolism in pregnancy
       O88.811 Other embolism in pregnancy, first trimester   Ⓜ♀
       O88.812 Other embolism in pregnancy, second trimester   Ⓜ♀
       O88.813 Other embolism in pregnancy, third trimester   Ⓜ♀

Ⓝ Newborn: 0   Ⓟ Pediatric: 0-17   Ⓜ Maternity: 12-55   Ⓐ Adult: 15-124   **NRS** Nonroutine supply Dx   **NCDx** Noncancer Dx   **PDx** Primary Dx   ►◄ Revised Text   ● New Code   ▲ Revised Title

O80–O88.813

848   ICD-10-CM 2018

O88.819   **Other embolism in pregnancy, unspecified trimester**   ⓜ♀▽

O88.82   **Other embolism in** childbirth   ⓜ♀

O88.83   **Other embolism in the** puerperium   ⓜ♀

✓4ᵗʰ **O89   Complications of anesthesia during the puerperium**
> INCLUDES   maternal complications arising from the administration of a general, regional or local anesthetic, analgesic or other sedation during the puerperium
>
> Use additional code, if applicable, to identify specific complication

✓5ᵗʰ **O89.0   Pulmonary complications of anesthesia during the puerperium**

    O89.01   **Aspiration pneumonitis due to anesthesia during the puerperium**   ⓜ♀
> Inhalation of stomach contents or secretions NOS due to anesthesia during the puerperium
> Mendelson's syndrome due to anesthesia during the puerperium

    O89.09   **Other pulmonary complications of anesthesia during the puerperium**   ⓜ♀

   O89.1   **Cardiac complications of anesthesia during the puerperium**   ⓜ♀

   O89.2   **Central nervous system complications of anesthesia during the puerperium**   ⓜ♀

   O89.3   **Toxic reaction to local anesthesia during the puerperium**   ⓜ♀

   O89.4   **Spinal and epidural anesthesia-induced headache during the puerperium**   ⓜ♀

   O89.5   **Other complications of spinal and epidural anesthesia during the puerperium**   ⓜ♀

   O89.6   **Failed or difficult intubation for anesthesia during the puerperium**   ⓜ♀

   O89.8   **Other complications of anesthesia during the puerperium**   ⓜ♀

   O89.9   **Complication of anesthesia during the puerperium, unspecified**   ⓜ♀▽

✓4ᵗʰ **O90   Complications of the puerperium, not elsewhere classified**

   O90.0   **Disruption of cesarean delivery wound**   ⓜ♀
> Dehiscence of cesarean delivery wound
> EXCLUDES 1   rupture of uterus (spontaneous) before onset of labor (O71.0-)
>   rupture of uterus during labor (O71.1)

   O90.1   **Disruption of perineal obstetric wound**   ⓜ♀
> Disruption of wound of episiotomy
> Disruption of wound of perineal laceration
> Secondary perineal tear

   O90.2   **Hematoma of obstetric wound**   ⓜ♀

   O90.3   **Peripartum cardiomyopathy**   ⓜ♀
> Conditions in I42- arising during pregnancy and the puerperium
> EXCLUDES 1   pre-existing heart disease complicating pregnancy and the puerperium (O99.4-)
> **DEF:** Any structural or functional abnormality of the ventricular myocardium, noninflammatory disease of obscure or unknown etiology with onset during the postpartum period.

   O90.4   **Postpartum acute kidney failure**   ⓜ♀
> Hepatorenal syndrome following labor and delivery

   O90.5   **Postpartum thyroiditis**   ⓜ♀

   O90.6   **Postpartum mood disturbance**   ⓜ♀
> Postpartum blues
> Postpartum dysphoria
> Postpartum sadness
> EXCLUDES 1   postpartum depression (F53)
>   puerperal psychosis (F53)

✓5ᵗʰ **O90.8   Other complications of the puerperium, not elsewhere classified**

    O90.81   **Anemia of the puerperium**   ⓜ♀
> Postpartum anemia NOS
> EXCLUDES 1   pre-existing anemia complicating the puerperium (O99.03)

    O90.89   **Other complications of the puerperium, not elsewhere classified**   ⓜ♀
> Placental polyp

   O90.9   **Complication of the puerperium, unspecified**   ⓜ♀▽

✓4ᵗʰ **O91   Infections of breast associated with pregnancy, the puerperium and lactation**
> Use additional code to identify infection

✓5ᵗʰ **O91.0   Infection of nipple associated with pregnancy, the puerperium and lactation**

   ✓6ᵗʰ   O91.01   **Infection of nipple associated with** pregnancy
> Gestational abscess of nipple

      O91.011   **Infection of nipple associated with pregnancy, first trimester**   ⓜ♀

      O91.012   **Infection of nipple associated with pregnancy, second trimester**   ⓜ♀

      O91.013   **Infection of nipple associated with pregnancy, third trimester**   ⓜ♀

      O91.019   **Infection of nipple associated with pregnancy, unspecified trimester**   ⓜ♀▽

    O91.02   **Infection of nipple associated with the** puerperium   ⓜ♀
> Puerperal abscess of nipple

    O91.03   **Infection of nipple associated with** lactation   ⓜ♀
> Abscess of nipple associated with lactation

✓5ᵗʰ **O91.1   Abscess of breast associated with pregnancy, the puerperium and lactation**

   ✓6ᵗʰ   O91.11   **Abscess of breast associated with** pregnancy
> Gestational mammary abscess
> Gestational purulent mastitis
> Gestational subareolar abscess

      O91.111   **Abscess of breast associated with pregnancy, first trimester**   ⓜ♀

      O91.112   **Abscess of breast associated with pregnancy, second trimester**   ⓜ♀

      O91.113   **Abscess of breast associated with pregnancy, third trimester**   ⓜ♀

      O91.119   **Abscess of breast associated with pregnancy, unspecified trimester**   ⓜ♀▽

    O91.12   **Abscess of breast associated with the** puerperium   ⓜ♀
> Puerperal mammary abscess
> Puerperal purulent mastitis
> Puerperal subareolar abscess

    O91.13   **Abscess of breast associated with** lactation   ⓜ♀
> Mammary abscess associated with lactation
> Purulent mastitis associated with lactation
> Subareolar abscess associated with lactation

✓5ᵗʰ **O91.2   Nonpurulent mastitis associated with pregnancy, the puerperium and lactation**

   ✓6ᵗʰ   O91.21   **Nonpurulent mastitis associated with** pregnancy
> Gestational interstitial mastitis
> Gestational lymphangitis of breast
> Gestational mastitis NOS
> Gestational parenchymatous mastitis

      O91.211   **Nonpurulent mastitis associated with pregnancy, first trimester**   ⓜ♀

      O91.212   **Nonpurulent mastitis associated with pregnancy, second trimester**   ⓜ♀

      O91.213   **Nonpurulent mastitis associated with pregnancy, third trimester**   ⓜ♀

      O91.219   **Nonpurulent mastitis associated with pregnancy, unspecified trimester**   ⓜ♀▽

    O91.22   **Nonpurulent mastitis associated with the** puerperium   ⓜ♀
> Puerperal interstitial mastitis
> Puerperal lymphangitis of breast
> Puerperal mastitis NOS
> Puerperal parenchymatous mastitis

    O91.23   **Nonpurulent mastitis associated with** lactation   ⓜ♀
> Interstitial mastitis associated with lactation
> Lymphangitis of breast associated with lactation
> Mastitis NOS associated with lactation
> Parenchymatous mastitis associated with lactation

✓4ᵗʰ **O92   Other disorders of breast and disorders of lactation associated with pregnancy and the puerperium**

✓5ᵗʰ **O92.0   Retracted nipple associated with pregnancy, the puerperium, and lactation**

   ✓6ᵗʰ   O92.01   **Retracted nipple associated with** pregnancy

      O92.011   **Retracted nipple associated with pregnancy, first trimester**   ⓜ♀

      O92.012   **Retracted nipple associated with pregnancy, second trimester**   ⓜ♀

☑ Additional Character Req   ✓x7ᵗʰ Placeholder Alert   Case-Mix Diagnosis   Manifestation   ▽ Unspecified Dx   EXCLUDES 1 Not coded here   EXCLUDES 2 Not included here

ICD-10-CM 2018   849

O92.013   **Retracted nipple associated with pregnancy,** third trimester   Ⓜ♀

O92.019   **Retracted nipple associated with pregnancy, unspecified trimester**   Ⓜ♀▽

O92.02   **Retracted nipple associated with the** puerperium   Ⓜ♀

O92.03   **Retracted nipple associated with** lactation   Ⓜ♀

✓5ᵗʰ **O92.1   Cracked nipple associated with pregnancy, the puerperium, and lactation**
Fissure of nipple, gestational or puerperal

   ✓6ᵗʰ **O92.11   Cracked nipple associated with** pregnancy

     O92.111   **Cracked nipple associated with pregnancy,** first trimester   Ⓜ♀

     O92.112   **Cracked nipple associated with pregnancy,** second trimester   Ⓜ♀

     O92.113   **Cracked nipple associated with pregnancy,** third trimester   Ⓜ♀

     O92.119   **Cracked nipple associated with pregnancy, unspecified trimester**   Ⓜ♀▽

   O92.12   **Cracked nipple associated with the** puerperium   Ⓜ♀

   O92.13   **Cracked nipple associated with** lactation   Ⓜ♀

✓5ᵗʰ **O92.2   Other and unspecified disorders of breast associated with pregnancy and the puerperium**

   O92.20   **Unspecified disorder of breast associated with pregnancy and the puerperium**   Ⓜ♀▽

   O92.29   **Other disorders of breast associated with pregnancy and the puerperium**   Ⓜ♀

O92.3   Agalactia   Ⓜ♀
Primary agalactia
   EXCLUDES 1   elective agalactia (O92.5)
     secondary agalactia (O92.5)
     therapeutic agalactia (O92.5)
   DEF: Absence of milk secretion in a female after delivery.

O92.4   Hypogalactia   Ⓜ♀

O92.5   Suppressed lactation   Ⓜ♀
Elective agalactia
Secondary agalactia
Therapeutic agalactia
   EXCLUDES 1   primary agalactia (O92.3)

O92.6   Galactorrhea   Ⓜ♀
   DEF: Excessive or persistent milk secretion by breast; may occur in absence of nursing.

✓5ᵗʰ **O92.7   Other and unspecified disorders of lactation**

   O92.70   **Unspecified disorders of lactation**   Ⓜ♀▽

   O92.79   **Other disorders of lactation**   Ⓜ♀
     Puerperal galactocele

Other obstetric conditions, not elsewhere classified (O94-O9A)

O94   Sequelae of complication of pregnancy, childbirth, and the puerperium   Ⓜ♀
   NOTE   This category is to be used to indicate conditions in O00-O77.-, O85-O94 and O98-O9A.- as the cause of late effects. The sequelae include conditions specified as such, or as late effects, which may occur at any time after the puerperium.
   Code first condition resulting from (sequela) of complication of pregnancy, childbirth, and the puerperium

✓4ᵗʰ **O98   Maternal infectious and parasitic diseases classifiable elsewhere but complicating pregnancy, childbirth and the puerperium**
   INCLUDES   the listed conditions when complicating the pregnant state, when aggravated by the pregnancy, or as a reason for obstetric care
   Use additional code (Chapter 1), to identify specific infectious or parasitic disease
   EXCLUDES 2   herpes gestationis (O26.4-)
     infectious carrier state (O99.82-, O99.83-)
     obstetrical tetanus (A34)
     puerperal infection (O86.-)
     puerperal sepsis (O85)
     when the reason for maternal care is that the disease is known or suspected to have affected the fetus (O35-O36)

   ✓5ᵗʰ **O98.0   Tuberculosis complicating pregnancy, childbirth and the puerperium**
     Conditions in A15-A19

     ✓6ᵗʰ **O98.01   Tuberculosis complicating** pregnancy

       O98.011   **Tuberculosis complicating pregnancy,** Ⓜ♀
         first trimester

       O98.012   **Tuberculosis complicating pregnancy,** Ⓜ♀
         second trimester

       O98.013   **Tuberculosis complicating pregnancy,** Ⓜ♀
         third trimester

       O98.019   **Tuberculosis complicating pregnancy, unspecified trimester**   Ⓜ♀▽

     O98.02   **Tuberculosis complicating** childbirth   Ⓜ♀

     O98.03   **Tuberculosis complicating the** puerperium   Ⓜ♀

   ✓5ᵗʰ **O98.1   Syphilis complicating pregnancy, childbirth and the puerperium**
     Conditions in A50-A53

     ✓6ᵗʰ **O98.11   Syphilis complicating** pregnancy

       O98.111   **Syphilis complicating pregnancy,** first Ⓜ♀
         trimester

       O98.112   **Syphilis complicating pregnancy,** Ⓜ♀
         second trimester

       O98.113   **Syphilis complicating pregnancy,** Ⓜ♀
         third trimester

       O98.119   **Syphilis complicating pregnancy, unspecified trimester**   Ⓜ♀▽

     O98.12   **Syphilis complicating** childbirth   Ⓜ♀

     O98.13   **Syphilis complicating the** puerperium   Ⓜ♀

   ✓5ᵗʰ **O98.2   Gonorrhea complicating pregnancy, childbirth and the puerperium**
     Conditions in A54-

     ✓6ᵗʰ **O98.21   Gonorrhea complicating** pregnancy

       O98.211   **Gonorrhea complicating pregnancy,** Ⓜ♀
         first trimester

       O98.212   **Gonorrhea complicating pregnancy,** Ⓜ♀
         second trimester

       O98.213   **Gonorrhea complicating pregnancy,** Ⓜ♀
         third trimester

       O98.219   **Gonorrhea complicating pregnancy, unspecified trimester**   Ⓜ♀▽

     O98.22   **Gonorrhea complicating** childbirth   Ⓜ♀

     O98.23   **Gonorrhea complicating the** puerperium   Ⓜ♀

   ✓5ᵗʰ **O98.3   Other infections with a predominantly sexual mode of transmission complicating pregnancy, childbirth and the puerperium**
     Conditions in A55-A64

     ✓6ᵗʰ **O98.31   Other infections with a predominantly sexual mode of transmission complicating** pregnancy

       O98.311   **Other infections with a predominantly sexual mode of transmission complicating pregnancy, first trimester**   Ⓜ♀

       O98.312   **Other infections with a predominantly sexual mode of transmission complicating pregnancy, second trimester**   Ⓜ♀

       O98.313   **Other infections with a predominantly sexual mode of transmission complicating pregnancy, third trimester**   Ⓜ♀

       O98.319   **Other infections with a predominantly sexual mode of transmission complicating pregnancy, unspecified trimester**   Ⓜ♀▽

     O98.32   **Other infections with a predominantly sexual mode of transmission complicating** childbirth   Ⓜ♀

     O98.33   **Other infections with a predominantly sexual mode of transmission complicating the** puerperium   Ⓜ♀

   ✓5ᵗʰ **O98.4   Viral hepatitis complicating pregnancy, childbirth and the puerperium**
     Conditions in B15-B19

     ✓6ᵗʰ **O98.41   Viral hepatitis complicating** pregnancy

       O98.411   **Viral hepatitis complicating pregnancy,** first trimester   Ⓜ♀

       O98.412   **Viral hepatitis complicating pregnancy,** second trimester   Ⓜ♀

       O98.413   **Viral hepatitis complicating pregnancy,** third trimester   Ⓜ♀

       O98.419   **Viral hepatitis complicating pregnancy, unspecified trimester**   Ⓜ♀▽

     O98.42   **Viral hepatitis complicating** childbirth   Ⓜ♀

     O98.43   **Viral hepatitis complicating the** puerperium   Ⓜ♀

Ⓝ Newborn: 0   Ⓟ Pediatric: 0-17   Ⓜ Maternity: 12-55   Ⓐ Adult: 15-124   **NRS** Nonroutine supply Dx   **NC Dx** Noncancer Dx   **PDx** Primary Dx   ▶◀ Revised Text   ● New Code   ▲ Revised Title

850   ICD-10-CM 2018

✓5th **O98.5** Other viral diseases **complicating pregnancy, childbirth and the puerperium**
     Conditions in A80-B09, B25-B34, R87.81-, R87.82-
     EXCLUDES 1   *human immunodeficiency virus [HIV] disease complicating pregnancy, childbirth and the puerperium (O98.7-)*

    ✓6th **O98.51** **Other viral diseases complicating** pregnancy
       O98.511 **Other viral diseases complicating pregnancy,** first trimester   Ⓜ♀
       O98.512 **Other viral diseases complicating pregnancy,** second trimester   Ⓜ♀
       O98.513 **Other viral diseases complicating pregnancy,** third trimester   Ⓜ♀
       O98.519 **Other viral diseases complicating pregnancy,** unspecified trimester   Ⓜ♀▽

    O98.52 **Other viral diseases complicating** childbirth   Ⓜ♀
    O98.53 **Other viral diseases complicating the** puerperium   Ⓜ♀

✓5th **O98.6** Protozoal diseases **complicating pregnancy, childbirth and the puerperium**
     Conditions in B50-B64

    ✓6th **O98.61** **Protozoal diseases complicating** pregnancy
       O98.611 **Protozoal diseases complicating pregnancy,** first trimester   Ⓜ♀
       O98.612 **Protozoal diseases complicating pregnancy,** second trimester   Ⓜ♀
       O98.613 **Protozoal diseases complicating pregnancy,** third trimester   Ⓜ♀
       O98.619 **Protozoal diseases complicating pregnancy,** unspecified trimester   Ⓜ♀▽

    O98.62 **Protozoal diseases complicating** childbirth   Ⓜ♀
    O98.63 **Protozoal diseases complicating the** puerperium   Ⓜ♀

✓5th **O98.7** Human immunodeficiency virus [HIV] disease **complicating pregnancy, childbirth and the puerperium**
     Use additional code to identify the type of HIV disease:
       acquired immune deficiency syndrome (AIDS) (B20)
       asymptomatic HIV status (Z21)
       HIV positive NOS (Z21)
       symptomatic HIV disease (B20)

    ✓6th **O98.71** **Human immunodeficiency virus [HIV] disease complicating** pregnancy
       O98.711 **Human immunodeficiency virus [HIV] disease complicating pregnancy,** first trimester   Ⓜ♀
       O98.712 **Human immunodeficiency virus [HIV] disease complicating pregnancy,** second trimester   Ⓜ♀
       O98.713 **Human immunodeficiency virus [HIV] disease complicating pregnancy,** third trimester   Ⓜ♀
       O98.719 **Human immunodeficiency virus [HIV] disease complicating pregnancy,** unspecified trimester   Ⓜ♀▽

    O98.72 **Human immunodeficiency virus [HIV] disease complicating** childbirth   Ⓜ♀
    O98.73 **Human immunodeficiency virus [HIV] disease complicating the** puerperium   Ⓜ♀

✓5th **O98.8** Other maternal infectious and parasitic diseases **complicating pregnancy, childbirth and the puerperium**

    ✓6th **O98.81** **Other maternal infectious and parasitic diseases complicating** pregnancy
       O98.811 **Other maternal infectious and parasitic diseases complicating pregnancy,** first trimester   Ⓜ♀
       O98.812 **Other maternal infectious and parasitic diseases complicating pregnancy,** second trimester   Ⓜ♀
       O98.813 **Other maternal infectious and parasitic diseases complicating pregnancy,** third trimester   Ⓜ♀
       O98.819 **Other maternal infectious and parasitic diseases complicating pregnancy,** unspecified trimester   Ⓜ♀▽

    O98.82 **Other maternal infectious and parasitic diseases complicating** childbirth   Ⓜ♀
    O98.83 **Other maternal infectious and parasitic diseases complicating the** puerperium   Ⓜ♀

✓5th **O98.9** Unspecified **maternal infectious and parasitic disease complicating pregnancy, childbirth and the puerperium**

    ✓6th **O98.91** **Unspecified maternal infectious and parasitic disease complicating** pregnancy
       O98.911 **Unspecified maternal infectious and parasitic disease complicating pregnancy,** first trimester   Ⓜ♀▽
       O98.912 **Unspecified maternal infectious and parasitic disease complicating pregnancy,** second trimester   Ⓜ♀▽
       O98.913 **Unspecified maternal infectious and parasitic disease complicating pregnancy,** third trimester   Ⓜ♀▽
       O98.919 **Unspecified maternal infectious and parasitic disease complicating pregnancy,** unspecified trimester   Ⓜ♀▽

    O98.92 **Unspecified maternal infectious and parasitic disease complicating** childbirth   Ⓜ♀▽
    O98.93 **Unspecified maternal infectious and parasitic disease complicating the** puerperium   Ⓜ♀▽

✓4th **O99** **Other maternal diseases classifiable elsewhere but complicating pregnancy, childbirth and the puerperium**
     INCLUDES   conditions which complicate the pregnant state, are aggravated by the pregnancy or are a main reason for obstetric care
     Use additional code to identify specific condition
     EXCLUDES 2   *when the reason for maternal care is that the condition is known or suspected to have affected the fetus (O35-O36)*

✓5th **O99.0** Anemia **complicating pregnancy, childbirth and the puerperium**
     Conditions in D50-D64
     EXCLUDES 1   *anemia arising in the puerperium (O90.81)*
              postpartum anemia NOS (O90.81)

    ✓6th **O99.01** **Anemia complicating** pregnancy
       AHA: 2016, 1Q, 4
       O99.011 **Anemia complicating pregnancy,** first trimester   Ⓜ♀
       O99.012 **Anemia complicating pregnancy,** second trimester   Ⓜ♀
       O99.013 **Anemia complicating pregnancy,** third trimester   Ⓜ♀
       O99.019 **Anemia complicating pregnancy,** unspecified trimester   Ⓜ♀▽

    O99.02 **Anemia complicating** childbirth   Ⓜ♀
    O99.03 **Anemia complicating the** puerperium   Ⓜ♀
       EXCLUDES 1   *postpartum anemia not pre-existing prior to delivery (O90.81)*

✓5th **O99.1** Other diseases of the blood and blood-forming organs and certain disorders involving the immune mechanism **complicating pregnancy, childbirth and the puerperium**
     Conditions in D65-D89
     EXCLUDES 1   ▶*hemorrhage with coagulation defects (O45.-, O46.0-, O67.0, O72.3)*◀
     EXCLUDES 2   *hemorrhage with coagulation defects (O45.-, O46.0-, O67.0, O72.3)*

    ✓6th **O99.11** **Other diseases of the blood and blood-forming organs and certain disorders involving the immune mechanism complicating** pregnancy
       O99.111 **Other diseases of the blood and blood-forming organs and certain disorders involving the immune mechanism complicating pregnancy,** first trimester   Ⓜ♀
       O99.112 **Other diseases of the blood and blood-forming organs and certain disorders involving the immune mechanism complicating pregnancy,** second trimester   Ⓜ♀
       O99.113 **Other diseases of the blood and blood-forming organs and certain disorders involving the immune mechanism complicating pregnancy,** third trimester   Ⓜ♀
       O99.119 **Other diseases of the blood and blood-forming organs and certain disorders involving the immune mechanism complicating pregnancy,** unspecified trimester   Ⓜ♀▽

Chapter 15. Pregnancy, Childbirth and the Puerperium

O99.12   Other diseases of the blood and blood-forming organs and certain disorders involving the immune mechanism complicating childbirth   Ⓜ♀

O99.13   Other diseases of the blood and blood-forming organs and certain disorders involving the immune mechanism complicating the puerperium   Ⓜ♀

✓5ᵗʰ **O99.2**   Endocrine, nutritional and metabolic diseases complicating pregnancy, childbirth and the puerperium

Conditions in E00-E88

EXCLUDES 2   diabetes mellitus (O24.-)
malnutrition (O25.-)
postpartum thyroiditis (O90.5)

✓6ᵗʰ **O99.21**   Obesity complicating pregnancy, childbirth, and the puerperium

Use additional code to identify the type of obesity (E66.-)

O99.210   Obesity complicating pregnancy, unspecified trimester   Ⓜ♀ ▽

O99.211   Obesity complicating pregnancy, first trimester   Ⓜ♀

O99.212   Obesity complicating pregnancy, second trimester   Ⓜ♀

O99.213   Obesity complicating pregnancy, third trimester   Ⓜ♀

O99.214   Obesity complicating childbirth   Ⓜ♀

O99.215   Obesity complicating the puerperium   Ⓜ♀

✓6ᵗʰ **O99.28**   Other endocrine, nutritional and metabolic diseases complicating pregnancy, childbirth and the puerperium

O99.280   Endocrine, nutritional and metabolic diseases complicating pregnancy, unspecified trimester   Ⓜ♀ ▽

O99.281   Endocrine, nutritional and metabolic diseases complicating pregnancy, first trimester   Ⓜ♀

O99.282   Endocrine, nutritional and metabolic diseases complicating pregnancy, second trimester   Ⓜ♀

O99.283   Endocrine, nutritional and metabolic diseases complicating pregnancy, third trimester   Ⓜ♀

O99.284   Endocrine, nutritional and metabolic diseases complicating childbirth   Ⓜ♀

O99.285   Endocrine, nutritional and metabolic diseases complicating the puerperium   Ⓜ♀

✓5ᵗʰ **O99.3**   Mental disorders and diseases of the nervous system complicating pregnancy, childbirth and the puerperium

✓6ᵗʰ **O99.31**   Alcohol use complicating pregnancy, childbirth, and the puerperium

Use additional code(s) from F10 to identify manifestations of the alcohol use

O99.310   Alcohol use complicating pregnancy, unspecified trimester   Ⓜ♀ ▽

O99.311   Alcohol use complicating pregnancy, first trimester   Ⓜ♀

O99.312   Alcohol use complicating pregnancy, second trimester   Ⓜ♀

O99.313   Alcohol use complicating pregnancy, third trimester   Ⓜ♀

O99.314   Alcohol use complicating childbirth   Ⓜ♀

O99.315   Alcohol use complicating the puerperium   Ⓜ♀

✓6ᵗʰ **O99.32**   Drug use complicating pregnancy, childbirth, and the puerperium

Use additional code(s) from F11-F16 and F18-F19 to identify manifestations of the drug use

O99.320   Drug use complicating pregnancy, unspecified trimester   Ⓜ♀ ▽

O99.321   Drug use complicating pregnancy, first trimester   Ⓜ♀

O99.322   Drug use complicating pregnancy, second trimester   Ⓜ♀

O99.323   Drug use complicating pregnancy, third trimester   Ⓜ♀

O99.324   Drug use complicating childbirth   Ⓜ♀

O99.325   Drug use complicating the puerperium   Ⓜ♀

✓6ᵗʰ **O99.33**   Tobacco use disorder complicating pregnancy, childbirth, and the puerperium

Smoking complicating pregnancy, childbirth, and the puerperium

Use additional code from category F17 to identify type of tobacco nicotine dependence

O99.330   Smoking (tobacco) complicating pregnancy, unspecified trimester   Ⓜ♀ ▽

O99.331   Smoking (tobacco) complicating pregnancy, first trimester   Ⓜ♀

O99.332   Smoking (tobacco) complicating pregnancy, second trimester   Ⓜ♀

O99.333   Smoking (tobacco) complicating pregnancy, third trimester   Ⓜ♀

O99.334   Smoking (tobacco) complicating childbirth   Ⓜ♀

O99.335   Smoking (tobacco) complicating the puerperium   Ⓜ♀

✓6ᵗʰ **O99.34**   Other mental disorders complicating pregnancy, childbirth, and the puerperium

Conditions in F01-F09 and F20-F99

EXCLUDES 2   postpartum mood disturbance (O90.6)
postnatal psychosis (F53)
puerperal psychosis (F53)

O99.340   Other mental disorders complicating pregnancy, unspecified trimester   Ⓜ♀ ▽

O99.341   Other mental disorders complicating pregnancy, first trimester   Ⓜ♀

O99.342   Other mental disorders complicating pregnancy, second trimester   Ⓜ♀

O99.343   Other mental disorders complicating pregnancy, third trimester   Ⓜ♀

O99.344   Other mental disorders complicating childbirth   Ⓜ♀

O99.345   Other mental disorders complicating the puerperium   Ⓜ♀

✓6ᵗʰ **O99.35**   Diseases of the nervous system complicating pregnancy, childbirth, and the puerperium

Conditions in G00-G99

EXCLUDES 2   pregnancy related peripheral neuritis (O26.8-)

O99.350   Diseases of the nervous system complicating pregnancy, unspecified trimester   Ⓜ♀ ▽

O99.351   Diseases of the nervous system complicating pregnancy, first trimester   Ⓜ♀

O99.352   Diseases of the nervous system complicating pregnancy, second trimester   Ⓜ♀

O99.353   Diseases of the nervous system complicating pregnancy, third trimester   Ⓜ♀

O99.354   Diseases of the nervous system complicating childbirth   Ⓜ♀

O99.355   Diseases of the nervous system complicating the puerperium   Ⓜ♀

✓5ᵗʰ **O99.4**   Diseases of the circulatory system complicating pregnancy, childbirth and the puerperium

Conditions in I00-I99

EXCLUDES 1   peripartum cardiomyopathy (O90.3)

EXCLUDES 2   hypertensive disorders (O10-O16)
obstetric embolism (O88.-)
venous complications and cerebrovenous sinus thrombosis in labor, childbirth and the puerperium (O87.-)
venous complications and cerebrovenous sinus thrombosis in pregnancy (O22.-)

AHA: 2016, 2Q, 8

✓6ᵗʰ **O99.41**   Diseases of the circulatory system complicating pregnancy

O99.411   Diseases of the circulatory system complicating pregnancy, first trimester   Ⓜ♀

O99.412   Diseases of the circulatory system complicating pregnancy, second trimester   Ⓜ♀

O99.413   Diseases of the circulatory system complicating pregnancy, third trimester   Ⓜ♀

Ⓝ Newborn: 0   Ⓟ Pediatric: 0-17   Ⓜ Maternity: 12-55   Ⓐ Adult: 15-124   NRS Nonroutine supply Dx   NC Dx Noncancer Dx   PDx Primary Dx   ▶◀ Revised Text   ● New Code   ▲ Revised Title

O99.419   Diseases of the circulatory system complicating pregnancy, unspecified trimester   Ⓜ♀▽

O99.42   Diseases of the circulatory system complicating childbirth   Ⓜ♀

O99.43   Diseases of the circulatory system complicating the puerperium   Ⓜ♀

✓5th **O99.5**   Diseases of the respiratory system complicating pregnancy, childbirth and the puerperium
Conditions in J00-J99

   ✓6th **O99.51**   Diseases of the respiratory system complicating pregnancy

     O99.511   Diseases of the respiratory system complicating pregnancy, first trimester   Ⓜ♀

     O99.512   Diseases of the respiratory system complicating pregnancy, second trimester   Ⓜ♀

     O99.513   Diseases of the respiratory system complicating pregnancy, third trimester   Ⓜ♀

     O99.519   Diseases of the respiratory system complicating pregnancy, unspecified trimester   Ⓜ♀▽

   O99.52   Diseases of the respiratory system complicating childbirth   Ⓜ♀

   O99.53   Diseases of the respiratory system complicating the puerperium   Ⓜ♀

✓5th **O99.6**   Diseases of the digestive system complicating pregnancy, childbirth and the puerperium
Conditions in K00-K93
> EXCLUDES 2   hemorrhoids in pregnancy (O22.4-)
> liver and biliary tract disorders in pregnancy, childbirth and the puerperium (O26.6-)

   ✓6th **O99.61**   Diseases of the digestive system complicating pregnancy
AHA: 2016, 1Q, 4

     O99.611   Diseases of the digestive system complicating pregnancy, first trimester   Ⓜ♀

     O99.612   Diseases of the digestive system complicating pregnancy, second trimester   Ⓜ♀

     O99.613   Diseases of the digestive system complicating pregnancy, third trimester   Ⓜ♀

     O99.619   Diseases of the digestive system complicating pregnancy, unspecified trimester   Ⓜ♀▽

   O99.62   Diseases of the digestive system complicating childbirth   Ⓜ♀

   O99.63   Diseases of the digestive system complicating the puerperium   Ⓜ♀

✓5th **O99.7**   Diseases of the skin and subcutaneous tissue complicating pregnancy, childbirth and the puerperium
Conditions in L00-L99
> EXCLUDES 2   herpes gestationis (O26.4)
> pruritic urticarial papules and plaques of pregnancy (PUPPP) (O26.86)

   ✓6th **O99.71**   Diseases of the skin and subcutaneous tissue complicating pregnancy

     O99.711   Diseases of the skin and subcutaneous tissue complicating pregnancy, first trimester   Ⓜ♀

     O99.712   Diseases of the skin and subcutaneous tissue complicating pregnancy, second trimester   Ⓜ♀

     O99.713   Diseases of the skin and subcutaneous tissue complicating pregnancy, third trimester   Ⓜ♀

     O99.719   Diseases of the skin and subcutaneous tissue complicating pregnancy, unspecified trimester   Ⓜ♀▽

   O99.72   Diseases of the skin and subcutaneous tissue complicating childbirth   Ⓜ♀

   O99.73   Diseases of the skin and subcutaneous tissue complicating the puerperium   Ⓜ♀

✓5th **O99.8**   Other specified diseases and conditions complicating pregnancy, childbirth and the puerperium
Conditions in D00-D48, H00-H95, M00-N99, and Q00-Q99
Use additional code to identify condition
> EXCLUDES 2   genitourinary infections in pregnancy (O23.-)
> infection of genitourinary tract following delivery (O86.1-O86.3)
> malignant neoplasm complicating pregnancy, childbirth and the puerperium (O9A.1-)
> maternal care for known or suspected abnormality of maternal pelvic organs (O34.-)
> postpartum acute kidney failure (O90.4)
> traumatic injuries in pregnancy (O9A.2)

   ✓6th **O99.81**   Abnormal glucose complicating pregnancy, childbirth and the puerperium
> EXCLUDES 1   gestational diabetes (O24.4-)
AHA: 2016, 1Q, 4

     O99.810   Abnormal glucose complicating pregnancy   Ⓜ♀

     O99.814   Abnormal glucose complicating childbirth   Ⓜ♀

     O99.815   Abnormal glucose complicating the puerperium   Ⓜ♀

   ✓6th **O99.82**   Streptococcus B carrier state complicating pregnancy, childbirth and the puerperium
> EXCLUDES 1   carrier of streptococcus group B (GBS) in a nonpregnant woman (Z22.330)

     O99.820   Streptococcus B carrier state complicating pregnancy   Ⓜ♀

     O99.824   Streptococcus B carrier state complicating childbirth   Ⓜ♀

     O99.825   Streptococcus B carrier state complicating the puerperium   Ⓜ♀

   ✓6th **O99.83**   Other infection carrier state complicating pregnancy, childbirth and the puerperium
Use additional code to identify the carrier state (Z22.-)

     O99.830   Other infection carrier state complicating pregnancy   Ⓜ♀

     O99.834   Other infection carrier state complicating childbirth   ♀

     O99.835   Other infection carrier state complicating the puerperium   Ⓜ♀

   ✓6th **O99.84**   Bariatric surgery status complicating pregnancy, childbirth and the puerperium
Gastric banding status complicating pregnancy, childbirth and the puerperium
Gastric bypass status for obesity complicating pregnancy, childbirth and the puerperium
Obesity surgery status complicating pregnancy, childbirth and the puerperium

     O99.840   Bariatric surgery status complicating pregnancy, unspecified trimester   Ⓜ♀▽

     O99.841   Bariatric surgery status complicating pregnancy, first trimester   Ⓜ♀

     O99.842   Bariatric surgery status complicating pregnancy, second trimester   Ⓜ♀

     O99.843   Bariatric surgery status complicating pregnancy, third trimester   Ⓜ♀

     O99.844   Bariatric surgery status complicating childbirth   Ⓜ♀

     O99.845   Bariatric surgery status complicating the puerperium   Ⓜ♀

   O99.89   Other specified diseases and conditions complicating pregnancy, childbirth and the puerperium   Ⓜ♀

✓4th **O9A**   Maternal malignant neoplasms, traumatic injuries and abuse classifiable elsewhere but complicating pregnancy, childbirth and the puerperium

   ✓5th **O9A.1**   Malignant neoplasm complicating pregnancy, childbirth and the puerperium
Conditions in C00-C96
Use additional code to identify neoplasm
> EXCLUDES 2   maternal care for benign tumor of corpus uteri (O34.1-)
> maternal care for benign tumor of cervix (O34.4-)
AHA: 2015, 3Q, 19

     ✓6th **O9A.11**   Malignant neoplasm complicating pregnancy

       O9A.111   Malignant neoplasm complicating pregnancy, first trimester   Ⓜ♀

☑ Additional Character Req   ✓x7th Placeholder Alert   Case-Mix Diagnosis   Manifestation   ▽ Unspecified Dx   EXCLUDES 1 Not coded here   EXCLUDES 2 Not included here

ICD-10-CM 2018   853

Chapter 15. Pregnancy, Childbirth and the Puerperium

    O9A.112 Malignant neoplasm complicating Ⓜ♀
    pregnancy, second trimester

    O9A.113 Malignant neoplasm complicating Ⓜ♀
    pregnancy, third trimester

    O9A.119 Malignant neoplasm complicating Ⓜ♀▽
    pregnancy, unspecified trimester

  O9A.12 Malignant neoplasm complicating childbirth Ⓜ♀

  O9A.13 Malignant neoplasm complicating the Ⓜ♀
  puerperium

✓5th **O9A.2** Injury, poisoning and certain other consequences of external causes **complicating pregnancy, childbirth and the puerperium**
    Conditions in S00-T88, except T74 and T76
    Use additional code(s) to identify the injury or poisoning
    EXCLUDES 2   *physical, sexual and psychological abuse complicating pregnancy, childbirth and the puerperium (O9A.3-, O9A.4-, O9A.5-)*

  ✓6th **O9A.21** Injury, poisoning and certain other consequences of external causes complicating pregnancy

    O9A.211 Injury, poisoning and certain other Ⓜ♀
    consequences of external causes complicating pregnancy, first trimester

    O9A.212 Injury, poisoning and certain other Ⓜ♀
    consequences of external causes complicating pregnancy, second trimester

    O9A.213 Injury, poisoning and certain other Ⓜ♀
    consequences of external causes complicating pregnancy, third rimester

    O9A.219 Injury, poisoning and certain other Ⓜ♀▽
    consequences of external causes complicating pregnancy, unspecified trimester

  O9A.22 Injury, poisoning and certain other Ⓜ♀
  consequences of external causes complicating childbirth

  O9A.23 Injury, poisoning and certain other Ⓜ♀
  consequencesof external causes complicating the puerperium

✓5th **O9A.3** Physical abuse **complicating pregnancy, childbirth and the puerperium**
    Conditions in T74.11 or T76.11
    Use additional code (if applicable):
      to identify any associated current injury due to physical abuse
      to identify the perpetrator of abuse (Y07.-)
    EXCLUDES 2   *sexual abuse complicating pregnancy, childbirth and the puerperium (O9A.4)*

  ✓6th **O9A.31** Physical abuse complicating pregnancy

    O9A.311 Physical abuse complicating Ⓜ♀
    pregnancy, first trimester

    O9A.312 Physical abuse complicating Ⓜ♀
    pregnancy,second trimester

    O9A.313 Physical abuse complicating Ⓜ♀
    pregnancy, third trimester

    O9A.319 Physical abuse complicating Ⓜ♀▽
    pregnancy,unspecified trimester

  O9A.32 Physical abuse complicating childbirth Ⓜ♀

  O9A.33 Physical abuse complicating the puerperium Ⓜ♀

✓5th **O9A.4** Sexual abuse **complicating pregnancy, childbirth and the puerperium**
    Conditions in T74.21 or T76.21
    Use additional code (if applicable):
      to identify any associated current injury due to sexual abuse
      to identify the perpetrator of abuse (Y07.-)

  ✓6th **O9A.41** Sexual abuse complicating pregnancy

    O9A.411 Sexual abuse complicating pregnancy, Ⓜ♀
    first trimester

    O9A.412 Sexual abuse complicating pregnancy, Ⓜ♀
    second trimester

    O9A.413 Sexual abuse complicating pregnancy, Ⓜ♀
    third trimester

    O9A.419 Sexual abuse complicating Ⓜ♀▽
    pregnancy, unspecified trimester

  O9A.42 Sexual abuse complicating childbirth Ⓜ♀

  O9A.43 Sexual abuse complicating the puerperium Ⓜ♀

✓5th **O9A.5** Psychological abuse **complicating pregnancy, childbirth and the puerperium**
    Conditions in T74.31 or T76.31
    Use additional code to identify the perpetrator of abuse (Y07.-)

  ✓6th **O9A.51** Psychological abuse complicating pregnancy

    O9A.511 Psychological abuse complicating Ⓜ♀
    pregnancy, first trimester

    O9A.512 Psychological abuse complicating Ⓜ♀
    pregnancy, second trimester

    O9A.513 Psychological abuse complicating Ⓜ♀
    pregnancy, third trimester

    O9A.519 Psychological abuse complicating Ⓜ♀▽
    pregnancy, unspecified trimester

  O9A.52 Psychological abuse complicating childbirth Ⓜ♀

  O9A.53 Psychological abuse complicating the Ⓜ♀
  puerperium

Ⓝ Newborn: 0   Ⓟ Pediatric: 0-17   Ⓜ Maternity: 12-55   Ⓐ Adult: 15-124   **NRS** Nonroutine supply Dx   **NC Dx** Noncancer Dx   **PDx** Primary Dx   ▶◀ Revised Text   ● New Code   ▲ Revised Title

854   ICD-10-CM 2018

Chapter 16. Certain Conditions Originating in the Perinatal Period (P00–P96)

Chapter Specific Guidelines with Coding Examples

The chapter specific guidelines from the ICD-10-CM Official Guidelines for Coding and Reporting have been provided below. Along with these guidelines are coding examples, contained in the shaded boxes, that have been developed to help illustrate the coding and/or sequencing guidance found in these guidelines.

For coding and reporting purposes the perinatal period is defined as before birth through the 28th day following birth. The following guidelines are provided for reporting purposes

a. General Perinatal Rules

1) Use of chapter 16 codes

Codes in this chapter are <u>never</u> for use on the maternal record. Codes from Chapter 15, the obstetric chapter, are never permitted on the newborn record. Chapter 16 codes may be used throughout the life of the patient if the condition is still present.

2) Principal diagnosis for birth record

When coding the birth episode in a newborn record, assign a code from category Z38, Liveborn infants according to place of birth and type of delivery, as the principal diagnosis. A code from category Z38 is assigned only once, to a newborn at the time of birth. If a newborn is transferred to another institution, a code from category Z38 should not be used at the receiving hospital.

A code from category Z38 is used only on the newborn record, not on the mother's record.

3) Use of codes from other chapters with codes from chapter 16

Codes from other chapters may be used with codes from chapter 16 if the codes from the other chapters provide more specific detail. Codes for signs and symptoms may be assigned when a definitive diagnosis has not been established. If the reason for the encounter is a perinatal condition, the code from chapter 16 should be sequenced first.

4) Use of chapter 16 codes after the perinatal period

Should a condition originate in the perinatal period, and continue throughout the life of the patient, the perinatal code should continue to be used regardless of the patient's age.

> A 7-year-old patient with history of birth injury that resulted in Erb's palsy is seen for subscapularis release.
>
> **P14.0   Erb's paralysis due to birth injury**
>
> *Explanation:* Although in this instance Erb's palsy is specifically related to a birth injury, it has not resolved and continues to be a health concern. A perinatal code is appropriate even though this patient is beyond the perinatal period.

5) Birth process or community acquired conditions

If a newborn has a condition that may be either due to the birth process or community acquired and the documentation does not indicate which it is, the default is due to the birth process and the code from Chapter 16 should be used. If the condition is community-acquired, a code from Chapter 16 should not be assigned.

6) Code all clinically significant conditions

All clinically significant conditions noted on routine newborn examination should be coded. A condition is clinically significant if it requires:

clinical evaluation; or

therapeutic treatment; or

diagnostic procedures; or

extended length of hospital stay; or

increased nursing care and/or monitoring; or

has implications for future health care needs

Note: The perinatal guidelines listed above are the same as the general coding guidelines for "additional diagnoses", except for the final point regarding implications for future health care needs. Codes should be assigned for conditions that have been specified by the provider as having implications for future health care needs.

b. Observation and Evaluation of Newborns for Suspected Conditions not Found

1) *Use of Z05 codes*

Assign a code from category Z05, Observation and evaluation of newborns and infants for suspected conditions ruled out, to identify those instances when a healthy newborn is evaluated for a suspected condition that is determined after study not to be present. Do not use a code from category Z05 when the patient has identified signs or symptoms of a suspected problem; in such cases code the sign or symptom.

2) *Z05 on other than the birth record*

A code from category Z05 may also be assigned as a principal or first-listed code for readmissions or encounters when the code from category Z38 code no longer applies. Codes from category Z05 are for use only for healthy newborns and infants for which no condition after study is found to be present.

3) *Z05 on a birth record*

A code from category Z05 is to be used as a secondary code after the code from category Z38, Liveborn infants according to place of birth and type of delivery.

c. Coding additional perinatal diagnoses

1) Assigning codes for conditions that require treatment

Assign codes for conditions that require treatment or further investigation, prolong the length of stay, or require resource utilization.

2) Codes for conditions specified as having implications for future health care needs

Assign codes for conditions that have been specified by the provider as having implications for future health care needs.

Note: This guideline should not be used for adult patients.

d. Prematurity and fetal growth retardation

Providers utilize different criteria in determining prematurity. A code for prematurity should not be assigned unless it is documented. Assignment of codes in categories P05, Disorders of newborn related to slow fetal growth and fetal malnutrition, and P07, Disorders of newborn related to short gestation and low birth weight, not elsewhere classified, should be based on the recorded birth weight and estimated gestational age.

When both birth weight and gestational age are available, two codes from category P07 should be assigned, with the code for birth weight sequenced before the code for gestational age.

e. Low birth weight and immaturity status

Codes from category P07, Disorders of newborn related to short gestation and low birth weight, not elsewhere classified, are for use for a child or adult who was premature or had a low birth weight as a newborn and this is affecting the patient's current health status.

See Section I.C.21. Factors influencing health status and contact with health services, Status.

> A 35-year-old patient, who weighed 659 grams at birth, is seen for heart disease documented as being a consequence of the low birth weight.
>
> **I51.9   Heart disease, unspecified**
>
> **P07.02   Extremely low birth weight newborn, 500–749 grams**
>
> *Explanation:* A code from subcategories P07.0- and P07.1- is appropriate, regardless of the age of the patient, as long as the documentation provides a clear link between the patient's current illness and the low birth weight.

f. **Bacterial sepsis of newborn**

Category P36, Bacterial sepsis of newborn, includes congenital sepsis. If a perinate is documented as having sepsis without documentation of congenital or community acquired, the default is congenital and a code from category P36 should be assigned. If the P36 code includes the causal organism, an additional code from category B95, Streptococcus, Staphylococcus, and Enterococcus as the cause of diseases classified elsewhere, or B96, Other bacterial agents as the cause of diseases classified elsewhere, should not be assigned. If the P36 code does not include the causal organism, assign an additional code from category B96. If applicable, use additional codes to identify severe sepsis (R65.2-) and any associated acute organ dysfunction.

A full-term infant born 7 days ago developed severe sepsis within 48 hours of discharge. The infant was readmitted. Cultures were taken, which came back positive for *E. coli*. The infant was stabilized and will now be transferred to a pediatric home health agency for an additional 2 weeks of IV antibiotic therapy administration.

P36.4   **Sepsis of newborn due to Escherichia coli**

R65.20   **Severe sepsis without septic shock**

Explanation: When the provider documentation does not specify whether sepsis in the newborn/perinate is congenital or community-acquired, the default code is from category P36 and the condition is assumed to be congenital. A code from chapter 1, "Certain Infectious and Parasitic Diseases," is not required as the sepsis code is a combination code that includes the organism.

g. **Stillbirth**

Code P95, Stillbirth, is only for use in institutions that maintain separate records for stillbirths. No other code should be used with P95. Code P95 should not be used on the mother's record.

Chapter 16. Certain Conditions Originating in the Perinatal Period (P00-P96)

> **NOTE**   Codes from this chapter are for use on newborn records only, never on maternal records.
>
> **INCLUDES**   conditions that have their origin in the fetal or perinatal period (before birth through the first 28 days after birth) even if morbidity occurs later
>
> **EXCLUDES 2**   congenital malformations, deformations and chromosomal abnormalities (Q00-Q99)
> endocrine, nutritional and metabolic diseases (E00-E88)
> injury, poisoning and certain other consequences of external causes (S00-T88)
> neoplasms (C00-D49)
> tetanus neonatorum (A33)

This chapter contains the following blocks:

P00-P04	Newborn affected by maternal factors and by complications of pregnancy, labor, and delivery
P05-P08	Disorders of newborn related to length of gestation and fetal growth
P09	Abnormal findings on neonatal screening
P10-P15	Birth trauma
P19-P29	Respiratory and cardiovascular disorders specific to the perinatal period
P35-P39	Infections specific to the perinatal period
P50-P61	Hemorrhagic and hematological disorders of newborn
P70-P74	Transitory endocrine and metabolic disorders specific to newborn
P76-P78	Digestive system disorders of newborn
P80-P83	Conditions involving the integument and temperature regulation of newborn
P84	Other problems with newborn
P90-P96	Other disorders originating in the perinatal period

Newborn affected by maternal factors and by complications of pregnancy, labor, and delivery (P00-P04)

> **NOTE**   These codes are for use when the listed maternal conditions are specified as the cause of confirmed morbidity or potential morbidity which have their origin in the perinatal period (before birth through the first 28 days after birth).

✓4th **P00**   **Newborn affected by** maternal conditions **that may be unrelated to present pregnancy**

> Code first any current condition in newborn
>
> **EXCLUDES 2**   encounter for observation of newborn for suspected diseases and conditions ruled out (Z05.-)
> newborn affected by maternal complications of pregnancy (P01.-)
> newborn affected by maternal endocrine and metabolic disorders (P70-P74)
> newborn affected by noxious substances transmitted via placenta or breast milk (P04.-)

   P00.0   **Newborn affected by maternal** hypertensive **disorders**
Newborn affected by maternal conditions classifiable to O10-O11, O13-O16

   P00.1   **Newborn affected by maternal** renal and urinary tract **diseases**
Newborn affected by maternal conditions classifiable to N00-N39

   P00.2   **Newborn affected by maternal** infectious and parasitic **diseases**
Newborn affected by maternal infectious disease classifiable to A00-B99, J09 and J10

> **EXCLUDES 1**   ~~infections specific to the perinatal period (P35-P39)~~
> maternal genital tract or other localized infections (P00.8)
>
> **EXCLUDES 2**   ►infections specific to the perinatal period (P35-P39)◄
> **AHA:** 2015, 3Q, 20

   P00.3   **Newborn affected by other maternal** circulatory and respiratory **diseases**
Newborn affected by maternal conditions classifiable to I00-I99, J00-J99, Q20-Q34 and not included in P00.0, P00.2

   P00.4   **Newborn affected by maternal** nutritional **disorders**
Newborn affected by maternal disorders classifiable to E40-E64
Maternal malnutrition NOS

   P00.5   **Newborn affected by maternal** injury
Newborn affected by maternal conditions classifiable to O9A.2-

   P00.6   **Newborn affected by** surgical procedure on mother
Newborn affected by amniocentesis

> **EXCLUDES 1**   Cesarean delivery for present delivery (P03.4)
> damage to placenta from amniocentesis, Cesarean delivery or surgical induction (P02.1)
> previous surgery to uterus or pelvic organs (P03.89)
>
> **EXCLUDES 2**   newborn affected by complication of (fetal) intrauterine procedure (P96.5)

   P00.7   **Newborn affected by** other medical procedures on mother**, not elsewhere classified**
Newborn affected by radiation to mother

> **EXCLUDES 1**   damage to placenta from amniocentesis, cesarean delivery or surgical induction (P02.1)
> newborn affected by other complications of labor and delivery (P03.-)

✓5th   **P00.8**   **Newborn affected by other maternal conditions**

     P00.81   **Newborn affected by** periodontal disease **in mother**

     P00.89   **Newborn affected by** other **maternal conditions**
Newborn affected by conditions classifiable to T80-T88
Newborn affected by maternal genital tract or other localized infections
Newborn affected by maternal systemic lupus erythematosus

   P00.9   **Newborn affected by** unspecified **maternal condition** ▽

✓4th **P01**   **Newborn affected by** maternal complications of pregnancy

> Code first any current condition in newborn
>
> **EXCLUDES 2**   encounter for observation of newborn for suspected diseases and conditions ruled out (Z05.-)

   P01.0   **Newborn affected by** incompetent cervix

   P01.1   **Newborn affected by** premature rupture of membranes

   P01.2   **Newborn affected by** oligohydramnios

> **EXCLUDES 1**   oligohydramnios due to premature rupture of membranes (P01.1)
> **DEF:** Low amniotic fluid level, resulting in underdeveloped organs in the fetus.

   P01.3   **Newborn affected by** polyhydramnios
Newborn affected by hydramnios

   P01.4   **Newborn affected by** ectopic pregnancy
Newborn affected by abdominal pregnancy

   P01.5   **Newborn affected by** multiple pregnancy
Newborn affected by triplet (pregnancy)
Newborn affected by twin (pregnancy)

   P01.6   **Newborn affected by** maternal death

   P01.7   **Newborn affected by** malpresentation before labor
Newborn affected by breech presentation before labor
Newborn affected by external version before labor
Newborn affected by face presentation before labor
Newborn affected by transverse lie before labor
Newborn affected by unstable lie before labor

   P01.8   **Newborn affected by** other **maternal complications of pregnancy**

   P01.9   **Newborn affected by maternal complication of pregnancy,** unspecified ▽

✓4th **P02**   **Newborn affected by complications of** placenta, cord and membranes

> Code first any current condition in newborn
>
> **EXCLUDES 2**   encounter for observation of newborn for suspected diseases and conditions ruled out (Z05.-)

   P02.0   **Newborn affected by** placenta previa
DEF: Placenta developed in lower segment of uterus; can cause hemorrhaging leading to preterm delivery.

   P02.1   **Newborn affected by other forms of placental** separation and hemorrhage
Newborn affected by abruptio placenta
Newborn affected by accidental hemorrhage
Newborn affected by antepartum hemorrhage
Newborn affected by damage to placenta from amniocentesis, cesarean delivery or surgical induction
Newborn affected by maternal blood loss
Newborn affected by premature separation of placenta

✓5th   **P02.2**   **Newborn affected by other and unspecified** morphological and functional abnormalities **of placenta**

     P02.20   **Newborn affected by** unspecified morphological ▽ **and functional abnormalities of placenta**

     P02.29   **Newborn affected by** other **morphological and functional** abnormalities **of placenta**
Newborn affected by placental dysfunction
Newborn affected by placental infarction
Newborn affected by placental insufficiency

☑ Additional Character Req   ✓x7th Placeholder Alert   Case-Mix Diagnosis   Manifestation   ▽ Unspecified Dx   **EXCLUDES 1** Not coded here   **EXCLUDES 2** Not included here

P02.3 Newborn affected by placental transfusion syndromes
     Newborn affected by placental and cord abnormalities resulting in twin-to-twin or other transplacental transfusion

P02.4 Newborn affected by prolapsed cord

P02.5 Newborn affected by other compression of umbilical cord
     Newborn affected by umbilical cord (tightly) around neck
     Newborn affected by entanglement of umbilical cord
     Newborn affected by knot in umbilical cord

✓5ᵗʰ **P02.6 Newborn affected by other and unspecified** conditions of umbilical cord

     P02.60 Newborn affected by unspecified conditions of umbilical cord ▽

     P02.69 Newborn affected by other conditions of umbilical cord
         Newborn affected by short umbilical cord
         Newborn affected by vasa previa
         EXCLUDES 1 *newborn affected by single umbilical artery (Q27.0)*

P02.7 Newborn affected by chorioamnionitis
     Newborn affected by amnionitis
     Newborn affected by membranitis
     Newborn affected by placentitis
     DEF: Inflammation of the fetal membranes due to maternal infection; characterized by fetal tachycardia, respiratory distress, apnea, weak cries, and poor sucking.

P02.8 Newborn affected by other abnormalities of membranes

P02.9 Newborn affected by abnormality of membranes, unspecified ▽

✓4ᵗʰ **P03 Newborn affected by other complications of** labor and delivery
     Code first any current condition in newborn
     EXCLUDES 2 *encounter for observation of newborn for suspected diseases and conditions ruled out (Z05.-)*

P03.0 Newborn affected by breech delivery and extraction

P03.1 Newborn affected by other malpresentation, malposition and disproportion **during labor and delivery**
     Newborn affected by contracted pelvis
     Newborn affected by conditions classifiable to O64-O66
     Newborn affected by persistent occipitoposterior
     Newborn affected by transverse lie

P03.2 Newborn affected by forceps delivery

P03.3 Newborn affected by delivery by vacuum extractor **[ventouse]**

Forceps Assisted Birth

Forceps extractor

Vacuum Assisted Birth

Vacuum extractor

P03.4 Newborn affected by Cesarean delivery

P03.5 Newborn affected by precipitate delivery
     Newborn affected by rapid second stage

P03.6 Newborn affected by abnormal uterine contractions
     Newborn affected by conditions classifiable to O62.-, except O62.3
     Newborn affected by hypertonic labor
     Newborn affected by uterine inertia

✓5ᵗʰ **P03.8 Newborn affected by other specified complications of labor and delivery**

     ✓6ᵗʰ **P03.81 Newborn affected by** abnormality in fetal (intrauterine) heart rate or rhythm
         EXCLUDES 1 *neonatal cardiac dysrhythmia (P29.1-)*

         P03.810 Newborn affected by abnormality in fetal (intrauterine) heart rate or rhythm before the onset of labor

         P03.811 Newborn affected by abnormality in fetal (intrauterine) heart rate or rhythm during labor

         P03.819 Newborn affected by abnormality in fetal (intrauterine) heart rate or rhythm, unspecified as to time of onset ▽

     P03.82 Meconium passage **during delivery**
         EXCLUDES 1 *meconium aspiration (P24.00, P24.01)*
                  meconium staining (P96.83)
         DEF: Fetal intestinal activity that increases in response to a fetomaternal distressed state during delivery; the anal sphincter relaxes, and meconium is passed into the amniotic fluid.

     P03.89 Newborn affected by other specified complications of labor and delivery
         Newborn affected by abnormality of maternal soft tissues
         Newborn affected by conditions classifiable to O60-O75 and by procedures used in labor and delivery not included in P02.- and P03.0-P03.6
         Newborn affected by induction of labor

P03.9 Newborn affected by complication of labor and delivery, unspecified ▽

✓4ᵗʰ **P04 Newborn affected by** noxious substances transmitted via placenta or breast milk
     INCLUDES nonteratogenic effects of substances transmitted via placenta
     EXCLUDES 2 *congenital malformations (Q00-Q99)*
                  encounter for observation of newborn for suspected diseases and conditions ruled out (Z05.-)
                  neonatal jaundice from excessive hemolysis due to drugs or toxins transmitted from mother (P58.4)
                  newborn in contact with and (suspected) exposures hazardous to health not transmitted via placenta or breast milk (Z77.-)

P04.0 Newborn affected by maternal anesthesia and analgesia **in pregnancy, labor and delivery**
     Newborn affected by reactions and intoxications from maternal opiates and tranquilizers administered during labor and delivery

P04.1 Newborn affected by other maternal medication
     Newborn affected by cancer chemotherapy
     Newborn affected by cytotoxic drugs
     EXCLUDES 1 *dysmorphism due to warfarin (Q86.2)*
                  fetal hydantoin syndrome (Q86.1)
                  maternal use of drugs of addiction (P04.4-)

P04.2 Newborn affected by maternal use of tobacco
     Newborn affected by exposure in utero to tobacco smoke
     EXCLUDES 2 *newborn exposure to environmental tobacco smoke (P96.81)*

P04.3 Newborn affected by maternal use of alcohol
     EXCLUDES 1 *fetal alcohol syndrome (Q86.0)*

✓5ᵗʰ **P04.4 Newborn affected by maternal use of** drugs of addiction

     P04.41 Newborn affected by maternal use of cocaine
         "Crack baby"

     P04.49 Newborn affected by maternal use of other drugs of addiction
         EXCLUDES 2 *newborn affected by maternal anesthesia and analgesia (P04.0)*
                  withdrawal symptoms from maternal use of drugs of addiction (P96.1)

P04.5 Newborn affected by maternal use of nutritional chemical substances

P04.6 Newborn affected by maternal exposure to environmental chemical substances

P04.8   Newborn affected by other maternal noxious substances

P04.9   Newborn affected by maternal noxious substance, unspecified ▽

Disorders of newborn related to length of gestation and fetal growth (P05-P08)

✓4ᵗʰ P05   Disorders of newborn related to slow fetal growth and fetal malnutrition

✓5ᵗʰ P05.0   Newborn light for gestational age
Newborn light-for-dates
Weight below but length above 10th percentile for gestational age

P05.00   Newborn light for gestational age, unspecified weight ▽

P05.01   Newborn light for gestational age, less than 500 grams

P05.02   Newborn light for gestational age, 500-749 grams

P05.03   Newborn light for gestational age, 750-999 grams

P05.04   Newborn light for gestational age, 1000-1249 grams

P05.05   Newborn light for gestational age, 1250-1499 grams

P05.06   Newborn light for gestational age, 1500-1749 grams

P05.07   Newborn light for gestational age, 1750-1999 grams

P05.08   Newborn light for gestational age, 2000-2499 grams

P05.09   Newborn light for gestational age, 2500 grams and over
Newborn light for gestational age, other

✓5ᵗʰ P05.1   Newborn small for gestational age
Newborn small-and-light-for-gestational age
Newborn small-for-dates
Weight and length below 10th percentile for gestational age

P05.10   Newborn small for gestational age, unspecified weight ▽

P05.11   Newborn small for gestational age, less than 500 grams

P05.12   Newborn small for gestational age, 500-749 grams

P05.13   Newborn small for gestational age, 750-999 grams

P05.14   Newborn small for gestational age, 1000-1249 grams

P05.15   Newborn small for gestational age, 1250-1499 grams

P05.16   Newborn small for gestational age, 1500-1749 grams

P05.17   Newborn small for gestational age, 1750-1999 grams

P05.18   Newborn small for gestational age, 2000-2499 grams

P05.19   Newborn small for gestational age, other
Newborn small for gestational age, 2500 grams and over

P05.2   Newborn affected by fetal (intrauterine) malnutrition not light or small for gestational age
Infant, not light or small for gestational age, showing signs of fetal malnutrition, such as dry, peeling skin and loss of subcutaneous tissue
EXCLUDES 1   newborn affected by fetal malnutrition with light for gestational age (P05.0-)
newborn affected by fetal malnutrition with small for gestational age (P05.1-)

P05.9   Newborn affected by slow intrauterine growth, unspecified ▽
Newborn affected by fetal growth retardation NOS

✓4ᵗʰ P07   Disorders of newborn related to short gestation and low birth weight, not elsewhere classified
NOTE   When both birth weight and gestational age of the newborn are available, both should be coded with birth weight sequenced before gestational age
INCLUDES   the listed conditions, without further specification, as the cause of morbidity or additional care, in newborn

✓5ᵗʰ P07.0   Extremely low birth weight newborn
Newborn birth weight 999 g. or less
EXCLUDES 1   low birth weight due to slow fetal growth and fetal malnutrition (P05.-)

P07.00   Extremely low birth weight newborn, unspecified weight ▽

P07.01   Extremely low birth weight newborn, less than 500 grams

P07.02   Extremely low birth weight newborn, 500-749 grams

P07.03   Extremely low birth weight newborn, 750-999 grams

✓5ᵗʰ P07.1   Other low birth weight newborn
Newborn birth weight 1000-2499 g.
EXCLUDES 1   low birth weight due to slow fetal growth and fetal malnutrition (P05.-)

P07.10   Other low birth weight newborn, unspecified weight ▽

P07.14   Other low birth weight newborn, 1000-1249 grams

P07.15   Other low birth weight newborn, 1250-1499 grams

P07.16   Other low birth weight newborn, 1500-1749 grams

P07.17   Other low birth weight newborn, 1750-1999 grams

P07.18   Other low birth weight newborn, 2000-2499 grams

✓5ᵗʰ P07.2   Extreme immaturity of newborn
Less than 28 completed weeks (less than 196 completed days) of gestation.

P07.20   Extreme immaturity of newborn, unspecified weeks of gestation ▽
Gestational age less than 28 completed weeks NOS

P07.21   Extreme immaturity of newborn, gestational age less than 23 completed weeks
Extreme immaturity of newborn, gestational age less than 23 weeks, 0 days

P07.22   Extreme immaturity of newborn, gestational age 23 completed weeks
Extreme immaturity of newborn, gestational age 23 weeks, 0 days through 23 weeks, 6 days

P07.23   Extreme immaturity of newborn, gestational age 24 completed weeks
Extreme immaturity of newborn, gestational age 24 weeks, 0 days through 24 weeks, 6 days

P07.24   Extreme immaturity of newborn, gestational age 25 completed weeks
Extreme immaturity of newborn, gestational age 25 weeks, 0 days through 25 weeks, 6 days

P07.25   Extreme immaturity of newborn, gestational age 26 completed weeks
Extreme immaturity of newborn, gestational age 26 weeks, 0 days through 26 weeks, 6 days

P07.26   Extreme immaturity of newborn, gestational age 27 completed weeks
Extreme immaturity of newborn, gestational age 27 weeks, 0 days through 27 weeks, 6 days

✓5ᵗʰ P07.3   Preterm [premature] newborn [other]
28 completed weeks or more but less than 37 completed weeks (196 completed days but less than 259 completed days) of gestation
Prematurity NOS

P07.30   Preterm newborn, unspecified weeks of gestation ▽

P07.31   Preterm newborn, gestational age 28 completed weeks
Preterm newborn, gestational age 28 weeks, 0 days through 28 weeks, 6 days

P07.32   Preterm newborn, gestational age 29 completed weeks
Preterm newborn, gestational age 29 weeks, 0 days through 29 weeks, 6 days

☑ Additional Character Req   ✓x7ᵗʰ Placeholder Alert   Case-Mix Diagnosis   Manifestation   ▽ Unspecified Dx   *EXCLUDES 1* Not coded here   *EXCLUDES 2* Not included here

ICD-10-CM 2018   **859**

P07.33 **Preterm newborn, gestational age** 30 completed weeks
Preterm newborn, gestational age 30 weeks, 0 days through 30 weeks, 6 days

P07.34 **Preterm newborn, gestational age** 31 completed weeks
Preterm newborn, gestational age 31 weeks, 0 days through 31 weeks, 6 days

P07.35 **Preterm newborn, gestational age** 32 completed weeks
Preterm newborn, gestational age 32 weeks, 0 days through 32 weeks, 6 days

P07.36 **Preterm newborn, gestational age** 33 completed weeks
Preterm newborn, gestational age 33 weeks, 0 days through 33 weeks, 6 days

P07.37 **Preterm newborn, gestational age** 34 completed weeks
Preterm newborn, gestational age 34 weeks, 0 days through 34 weeks, 6 days

P07.38 **Preterm newborn, gestational age** 35 completed weeks
Preterm newborn, gestational age 35 weeks, 0 days through 35 weeks, 6 days

P07.39 **Preterm newborn, gestational age** 36 completed weeks
Preterm newborn, gestational age 36 weeks, 0 days through 36 weeks, 6 days

P08 Disorders of newborn related to long gestation and high birth weight
NOTE When both birth weight and gestational age of the newborn are available, priority of assignment should be given to birth weight
INCLUDES the listed conditions, without further specification, as causes of morbidity or additional care, in newborn

P08.0 **Exceptionally large newborn baby**
Usually implies a birth weight of 4500 g. or more
EXCLUDES 1 syndrome of infant of diabetic mother (P70.1)
syndrome of infant of mother with gestational diabetes (P70.0)

P08.1 **Other heavy for gestational age newborn**
Other newborn heavy- or large-for-dates regardless of period of gestation
Usually implies a birth weight of 4000 g. to 4499 g.
EXCLUDES 1 newborn with a birth weight of 4500 or more (P08.0)
syndrome of infant of diabetic mother (P70.1)
syndrome of infant of mother with gestational diabetes (P70.0).

P08.2 **Late newborn, not heavy for gestational age**
AHA: 2014, 1Q, 14

P08.21 **Post-term newborn**
Newborn with gestation period over 40 completed weeks to 42 completed weeks

P08.22 **Prolonged gestation of newborn**
Newborn with gestation period over 42 completed weeks (294 days or more), not heavy- or large-for-dates.
Postmaturity NOS

Abnormal findings on neonatal screening (P09)

P09 Abnormal findings on neonatal screening
Use additional code to identify signs, symptoms and conditions associated with the screening
EXCLUDES 2 nonspecific serologic evidence of human immunodeficiency virus [HIV] (R75)

Birth trauma (P10-P15)

P10 Intracranial laceration and hemorrhage due to birth injury
EXCLUDES 1 intracranial hemorrhage of newborn NOS (P52.9)
intracranial hemorrhage of newborn due to anoxia or hypoxia (P52.-)
nontraumatic intracranial hemorrhage of newborn (P52.-)

P10.0 **Subdural hemorrhage due to birth injury**
Subdural hematoma (localized) due to birth injury
EXCLUDES 1 subdural hemorrhage accompanying tentorial tear (P10.4)

P10.1 **Cerebral hemorrhage due to birth injury**
P10.2 **Intraventricular hemorrhage due to birth injury**
P10.3 **Subarachnoid hemorrhage due to birth injury**

Birth Injuries to Scalp

P10.4 **Tentorial tear due to birth injury**
P10.8 **Other intracranial lacerations and hemorrhages due to birth injury**
P10.9 **Unspecified intracranial laceration and hemorrhage due to birth injury**

P11 Other birth injuries to central nervous system
P11.0 **Cerebral edema due to birth injury**
P11.1 **Other specified brain damage due to birth injury**
P11.2 **Unspecified brain damage due to birth injury**
P11.3 **Birth injury to facial nerve**
Facial palsy due to birth injury
P11.4 **Birth injury to other cranial nerves**
P11.5 **Birth injury to spine and spinal cord**
Fracture of spine due to birth injury
P11.9 **Birth injury to central nervous system, unspecified**

P12 Birth injury to scalp
P12.0 **Cephalhematoma due to birth injury**
P12.1 **Chignon (from vacuum extraction) due to birth injury**
P12.2 **Epicranial subaponeurotic hemorrhage due to birth injury**
Subgaleal hemorrhage
P12.3 **Bruising of scalp due to birth injury**
P12.4 **Injury of scalp of newborn due to monitoring equipment**
Sampling incision of scalp of newborn
Scalp clip (electrode) injury of newborn

P12.8 **Other birth injuries to scalp**
P12.81 **Caput succedaneum**
P12.89 **Other birth injuries to scalp**
P12.9 **Birth injury to scalp, unspecified**

P13 Birth injury to skeleton
EXCLUDES 2 birth injury to spine (P11.5)
P13.0 **Fracture of skull due to birth injury**
P13.1 **Other birth injuries to skull**
EXCLUDES 1 cephalhematoma (P12.0)
P13.2 **Birth injury to femur**
P13.3 **Birth injury to other long bones**
P13.4 **Fracture of clavicle due to birth injury**
P13.8 **Birth injuries to other parts of skeleton**
P13.9 **Birth injury to skeleton, unspecified**

P14 Birth injury to peripheral nervous system
P14.0 **Erb's paralysis due to birth injury**
P14.1 **Klumpke's paralysis due to birth injury**
P14.2 **Phrenic nerve paralysis due to birth injury**
P14.3 **Other brachial plexus birth injuries**
P14.8 **Birth injuries to other parts of peripheral nervous system**
P14.9 **Birth injury to peripheral nervous system, unspecified**

P15 Other birth injuries
P15.0 **Birth injury to liver**
Rupture of liver due to birth injury
P15.1 **Birth injury to spleen**
Rupture of spleen due to birth injury
P15.2 **Sternomastoid injury due to birth injury**

P15.3   **Birth injury to** eye
Subconjunctival hemorrhage due to birth injury
Traumatic glaucoma due to birth injury

P15.4   **Birth injury to** face
Facial congestion due to birth injury

P15.5   **Birth injury to** external genitalia

P15.6   **Subcutaneous fat necrosis** due to birth injury

P15.8   **Other specified birth injuries**
TIP: Use for any injury of newborn from scalpel.

P15.9   **Birth injury, unspecified**   ▽

Respiratory and cardiovascular disorders specific to the perinatal period (P19-P29)

✓4ᵗʰ **P19**   **Metabolic acidemia in newborn**
INCLUDES   metabolic acidemia in newborn

P19.0   **Metabolic acidemia in newborn first noted** before onset of labor

P19.1   **Metabolic acidemia in newborn first noted** during labor

P19.2   **Metabolic acidemia noted** at birth

P19.9   **Metabolic acidemia, unspecified**   ▽

✓4ᵗʰ **P22**   **Respiratory distress of newborn**
EXCLUDES 1   respiratory arrest of newborn (P28.81)
respiratory failure of newborn NOS (P28.5)

P22.0   **Respiratory distress syndrome of newborn**
Cardiorespiratory distress syndrome of newborn
Hyaline membrane disease
Idiopathic respiratory distress syndrome [IRDS or RDS] of newborn
Pulmonary hypoperfusion syndrome
Respiratory distress syndrome, type I
DEF: Severe chest contractions upon air intake and expiratory grunting; infant appears blue due to oxygen deficiency and has rapid respiratory rate; formerly called hyaline membrane disease.

P22.1   **Transient tachypnea of newborn**
Idiopathic tachypnea of newborn
Respiratory distress syndrome, type II
Wet lung syndrome
DEF: Rapid, labored breathing of newborn; short-term problem that begins after birth and lasts about three days.

P22.8   **Other respiratory distress of newborn**

P22.9   **Respiratory distress of newborn, unspecified**   ▽

✓4ᵗʰ **P23**   **Congenital pneumonia**
INCLUDES   infective pneumonia acquired in utero or during birth
EXCLUDES 1   neonatal pneumonia resulting from aspiration (P24.-)

P23.0   **Congenital pneumonia due to** viral agent
Use additional code (B97) to identify organism
EXCLUDES 1   congenital rubella pneumonitis (P35.0)

P23.1   **Congenital pneumonia due to** Chlamydia

P23.2   **Congenital pneumonia due to** staphylococcus

P23.3   **Congenital pneumonia due to** streptococcus, group B

P23.4   **Congenital pneumonia due to** Escherichia coli

P23.5   **Congenital pneumonia due to** Pseudomonas

P23.6   **Congenital pneumonia due to other** bacterial agents
Congenital pneumonia due to Hemophilus influenzae
Congenital pneumonia due to Klebsiella pneumoniae
Congenital pneumonia due to Mycoplasma
Congenital pneumonia due to Streptococcus, except group B
Use additional code (B95-B96) to identify organism

P23.8   **Congenital pneumonia due to other** organisms

P23.9   **Congenital pneumonia, unspecified**   ▽

✓4ᵗʰ **P24**   **Neonatal aspiration**
INCLUDES   aspiration in utero and during delivery

✓5ᵗʰ **P24.0**   **Meconium** aspiration
EXCLUDES 1   meconium passage (without aspiration) during delivery (P03.82)
meconium staining (P96.83)

P24.00   **Meconium aspiration** without respiratory symptoms
Meconium aspiration NOS

P24.01   **Meconium aspiration** with respiratory symptoms
Meconium aspiration pneumonia
Meconium aspiration pneumonitis
Meconium aspiration syndrome NOS
Use additional code to identify any secondary pulmonary hypertension, if applicable ▶(I27.2-)◀
DEF: Aspiration of fetal intestinal material during or prior to delivery; usually a complication of placental insufficiency, causing pneumonitis and bronchial obstruction (inflammatory reaction of lungs).

✓5ᵗʰ **P24.1**   **Neonatal aspiration of** (clear) amniotic fluid and mucus
Neonatal aspiration of liquor (amnii)

P24.10   **Neonatal aspiration of (clear) amniotic fluid and mucus** without respiratory symptoms
Neonatal aspiration of amniotic fluid and mucus NOS

P24.11   **Neonatal aspiration of (clear) amniotic fluid and mucus** with respiratory symptoms
Neonatal aspiration of amniotic fluid and mucus with pneumonia
Neonatal aspiration of amniotic fluid and mucus with pneumonitis
Use additional code to identify any secondary pulmonary hypertension, if applicable ▶(I27.2-)◀

✓5ᵗʰ **P24.2**   **Neonatal aspiration of** blood

P24.20   **Neonatal aspiration of blood** without respiratory symptoms
Neonatal aspiration of blood NOS

P24.21   **Neonatal aspiration of blood** with respiratory symptoms
Neonatal aspiration of blood with pneumonia
Neonatal aspiration of blood with pneumonitis
Use additional code to identify any secondary pulmonary hypertension, if applicable ▶(I27.2-)◀

✓5ᵗʰ **P24.3**   **Neonatal aspiration of** milk and regurgitated food
Neonatal aspiration of stomach contents

P24.30   **Neonatal aspiration of milk and regurgitated food** without respiratory symptoms
Neonatal aspiration of milk and regurgitated food NOS

P24.31   **Neonatal aspiration of milk and regurgitated food** with respiratory symptoms
Neonatal aspiration of milk and regurgitated food with pneumonia
Neonatal aspiration of milk and regurgitated food with pneumonitis
Use additional code to identify any secondary pulmonary hypertension, if applicable ▶(I27.2-)◀

✓5ᵗʰ **P24.8**   **Other** neonatal aspiration

P24.80   **Other neonatal aspiration** without respiratory symptoms
Neonatal aspiration NEC

P24.81   **Other neonatal aspiration** with respiratory symptoms
Neonatal aspiration pneumonia NEC
Neonatal aspiration with pneumonitis NEC
Neonatal aspiration with pneumonia NOS
Neonatal aspiration with pneumonitis NOS
Use additional code to identify any secondary pulmonary hypertension, if applicable ▶(I27.2-)◀

P24.9   **Neonatal aspiration, unspecified**   ▽

✓4ᵗʰ **P25**   **Interstitial emphysema and related conditions originating in the perinatal period**

P25.0   **Interstitial emphysema** originating in the perinatal period

P25.1   **Pneumothorax** originating in the perinatal period

P25.2   **Pneumomediastinum** originating in the perinatal period

P25.3   **Pneumopericardium** originating in the perinatal period

P25.8   **Other conditions related to interstitial emphysema** originating in the perinatal period

✓4ᵗʰ **P26**   **Pulmonary hemorrhage originating in the perinatal period**
EXCLUDES 1   acute idiopathic hemorrhage in infants over 28 days old (R04.81)

P26.0   **Tracheobronchial** hemorrhage originating in the perinatal period

P26.1   **Massive pulmonary** hemorrhage originating in the perinatal period

P26.8   **Other pulmonary hemorrhages originating in the perinatal period**

P26.9   **Unspecified pulmonary hemorrhage originating in the perinatal period**   ▽

✓ Additional Character Req   ✓x7ᵗʰ Placeholder Alert   Case-Mix Diagnosis   Manifestation   ▽ Unspecified Dx   EXCLUDES 1 Not coded here   EXCLUDES 2 Not included here

ICD-10-CM 2018   861

✓4ᵗʰ **P27 Chronic respiratory disease originating in the perinatal period**
EXCLUDES1   *respiratory distress of newborn (P22.0–P22.9)*
EXCLUDES2 ▶*respiratory distress of newborn (P22.0–P22.9)*◀

P27.0 Wilson-Mikity syndrome
Pulmonary dysmaturity

P27.1 Bronchopulmonary dysplasia originating in the perinatal period

P27.8 Other chronic respiratory diseases originating in the perinatal period
Congenital pulmonary fibrosis
Ventilator lung in newborn

P27.9 Unspecified chronic respiratory disease originating in the perinatal period ▽

✓4ᵗʰ **P28 Other respiratory conditions originating in the perinatal period**
EXCLUDES1   *congenital malformations of the respiratory system (Q30–Q34)*

P28.0 Primary atelectasis of newborn
Primary failure to expand terminal respiratory units
Pulmonary hypoplasia associated with short gestation
Pulmonary immaturity NOS

✓5ᵗʰ **P28.1 Other and unspecified atelectasis of newborn**

P28.10 Unspecified atelectasis of newborn ▽
Atelectasis of newborn NOS

P28.11 Resorption atelectasis without respiratory distress syndrome
EXCLUDES1   *resorption atelectasis with respiratory distress syndrome (P22.0)*

P28.19 Other atelectasis of newborn
Partial atelectasis of newborn
Secondary atelectasis of newborn

P28.2 Cyanotic attacks of newborn
EXCLUDES1   *apnea of newborn (P28.3-P28.4)*
EXCLUDES1   *apnea of newborn (P28.3-P28.4)*

P28.3 Primary sleep apnea of newborn
Central sleep apnea of newborn
Obstructive sleep apnea of newborn
Sleep apnea of newborn NOS
DEF: Unexplained cessation of breathing when a neonate makes no respiratory effort for 20 seconds or longer, or when neonate's breathing cessation is accompanied by cyanosis, bradycardia, or hypotonia.

P28.4 Other apnea of newborn
Apnea of prematurity
Obstructive apnea of newborn
EXCLUDES1   *obstructive sleep apnea of newborn (P28.3)*

P28.5 Respiratory failure of newborn
EXCLUDES1   *respiratory arrest of newborn (P28.81)*
respiratory distress of newborn (P22.0-)

✓5ᵗʰ **P28.8 Other specified respiratory conditions of newborn**

P28.81 Respiratory arrest of newborn

P28.89 Other specified respiratory conditions of newborn
Congenital laryngeal stridor
Sniffles in newborn
Snuffles in newborn
EXCLUDES1   *early congenital syphilitic rhinitis (A50.05)*

P28.9 Respiratory condition of newborn, unspecified ▽
Respiratory depression in newborn

✓4ᵗʰ **P29 Cardiovascular disorders originating in the perinatal period**
EXCLUDES1   *congenital malformations of the circulatory system (Q20–Q28)*

P29.0 Neonatal cardiac failure

✓5ᵗʰ **P29.1 Neonatal cardiac dysrhythmia**

P29.11 Neonatal tachycardia

P29.12 Neonatal bradycardia

P29.2 Neonatal hypertension

✓5ᵗʰ **P29.3 Persistent fetal circulation**
~~Delayed closure of ductus arteriosus~~
~~(Persistent) pulmonary hypertension of newborn~~

● **P29.30 Pulmonary hypertension of newborn**
Persistent pulmonary hypertension of newborn

● **P29.38 Other persistent fetal circulation**
Delayed closure of ductus arteriosus

P29.4 Transient myocardial ischemia in newborn

✓5ᵗʰ **P29.8 Other cardiovascular disorders originating in the perinatal period**

P29.81 Cardiac arrest of newborn

P29.89 Other cardiovascular disorders originating in the perinatal period
AHA: 2014, 4Q, 23

P29.9 Cardiovascular disorder originating in the perinatal period, unspecified ▽

Infections specific to the perinatal period (P35-P39)
Infections acquired in utero, during birth via the umbilicus, or during the first 28 days after birth
EXCLUDES2   *asymptomatic human immunodeficiency virus [HIV] infection status (Z21)*
congenital gonococcal infection (A54.-)
congenital pneumonia (P23.-)
congenital syphilis (A50.-)
human immunodeficiency virus [HIV] disease (B20)
infant botulism (A48.51)
infectious diseases not specific to the perinatal period (A00-B99, J09, J10-)
intestinal infectious disease (A00-A09)
laboratory evidence of human immunodeficiency virus [HIV] (R75)
tetanus neonatorum (A33)

✓4ᵗʰ **P35 Congenital viral diseases**
INCLUDES   infections acquired in utero or during birth

P35.0 Congenital rubella syndrome
Congenital rubella pneumonitis

P35.1 Congenital cytomegalovirus infection

P35.2 Congenital herpesviral [herpes simplex] infection

P35.3 Congenital viral hepatitis

P35.8 Other congenital viral diseases
Congenital varicella [chickenpox]

P35.9 Congenital viral disease, unspecified ▽

✓4ᵗʰ **P36 Bacterial sepsis of newborn**
INCLUDES   congenital sepsis
Use additional code(s), if applicable, to identify severe sepsis (R65.2-) and associated acute organ dysfunction(s)

P36.0 Sepsis of newborn due to streptococcus, group B

✓5ᵗʰ **P36.1 Sepsis of newborn due to other and unspecified streptococci**

P36.10 Sepsis of newborn due to unspecified streptococci ▽

P36.19 Sepsis of newborn due to other streptococci

P36.2 Sepsis of newborn due to Staphylococcus aureus

✓5ᵗʰ **P36.3 Sepsis of newborn due to other and unspecified staphylococci**

P36.30 Sepsis of newborn due to unspecified staphylococci ▽

P36.39 Sepsis of newborn due to other staphylococci

P36.4 Sepsis of newborn due to Escherichia coli

P36.5 Sepsis of newborn due to anaerobes

P36.8 Other bacterial sepsis of newborn
Use additional code from category B96 to identify organism

P36.9 Bacterial sepsis of newborn, unspecified ▽

✓4ᵗʰ **P37 Other congenital infectious and parasitic diseases**
EXCLUDES2   *congenital syphilis (A50.-)*
infectious neonatal diarrhea (A00-A09)
necrotizing enterocolitis in newborn (P77.-)
noninfectious neonatal diarrhea (P78.3)
ophthalmia neonatorum due to gonococcus (A54.31)
tetanus neonatorum (A33)

P37.0 Congenital tuberculosis

P37.1 Congenital toxoplasmosis
Hydrocephalus due to congenital toxoplasmosis

P37.2 Neonatal (disseminated) listeriosis

P37.3 Congenital falciparum malaria

P37.4 Other congenital malaria

P37.5 Neonatal candidiasis

P37.8 Other specified congenital infectious and parasitic diseases

P37.9 Congenital infectious or parasitic disease, unspecified ▽

✓4ᵗʰ **P38 Omphalitis of newborn**
EXCLUDES1   *omphalitis not of newborn (L08.82)*
tetanus omphalitis (A33)
umbilical hemorrhage of newborn (P51.-)

P38.1 Omphalitis with mild hemorrhage

N Newborn: 0   P Pediatric: 0-17   M Maternity: 12-55   A Adult: 15-124   NRS Nonroutine supply Dx   NC Dx Noncancer Dx   PDx Primary Dx   ▶◀ Revised Text   ● New Code   ▲ Revised Title

P38.9   **Omphalitis** without hemorrhage
         Omphalitis of newborn NOS

☑4ᵗʰ P39   **Other infections specific to the perinatal period**
         Use additional code to identify organism or specific infection

P39.0   **Neonatal infective** mastitis
         EXCLUDES 1   breast engorgement of newborn (P83.4)
                       noninfective mastitis of newborn (P83.4)

P39.1   **Neonatal** conjunctivitis and dacryocystitis
         Neonatal chlamydial conjunctivitis
         Ophthalmia neonatorum NOS
         EXCLUDES 1   gonococcal conjunctivitis (A54.31)

P39.2   **Intra-amniotic** infection affecting newborn, not elsewhere classified

P39.3   **Neonatal** urinary tract **infection**

P39.4   **Neonatal** skin **infection**
         Neonatal pyoderma
         EXCLUDES 1   pemphigus neonatorum (L00)
                       staphylococcal scalded skin syndrome (L00)

P39.8   **Other specified infections specific to the perinatal period**

P39.9   **Infection specific to the perinatal period, unspecified**   ▽

Hemorrhagic and hematological disorders of newborn (P50-P61)

EXCLUDES 1   congenital stenosis and stricture of bile ducts (Q44.3)
              Crigler-Najjar syndrome (E80.5)
              Dubin-Johnson syndrome (E80.6)
              Gilbert syndrome (E80.4)
              hereditary hemolytic anemias (D55-D58)

☑4ᵗʰ P50   **Newborn affected by intrauterine (fetal)** blood loss
         EXCLUDES 1   congenital anemia from intrauterine (fetal) blood loss (P61.3)

P50.0   **Newborn affected by intrauterine (fetal) blood loss from vasa previa**

P50.1   **Newborn affected by intrauterine (fetal) blood loss from ruptured cord**

P50.2   **Newborn affected by intrauterine (fetal) blood loss from placenta**

P50.3   **Newborn affected by hemorrhage into** co-twin

P50.4   **Newborn affected by hemorrhage into** maternal circulation

P50.5   **Newborn affected by intrauterine (fetal) blood loss from** cut end of co-twin's cord

P50.8   **Newborn affected by other intrauterine (fetal) blood loss**

P50.9   **Newborn affected by intrauterine (fetal) blood loss, unspecified**   ▽
         Newborn affected by fetal hemorrhage NOS

☑4ᵗʰ P51   **Umbilical** hemorrhage of newborn
         EXCLUDES 1   omphalitis with mild hemorrhage (P38.1)
                       umbilical hemorrhage from cut end of co-twins cord (P50.5)

P51.0   **Massive** umbilical hemorrhage of newborn

P51.8   **Other umbilical hemorrhages of newborn**
         Slipped umbilical ligature NOS

P51.9   **Umbilical hemorrhage of newborn, unspecified**   ▽

☑4ᵗʰ P52   **Intracranial nontraumatic hemorrhage of newborn**
         INCLUDES   intracranial hemorrhage due to anoxia or hypoxia
         EXCLUDES 1   intracranial hemorrhage due to birth injury (P10.-)
                       intracranial hemorrhage due to other injury (S06.-)

P52.0   **Intraventricular (nontraumatic) hemorrhage,** grade 1, **of newborn**
         Subependymal hemorrhage (without intraventricular extension)
         Bleeding into germinal matrix

P52.1   **Intraventricular (nontraumatic) hemorrhage,** grade 2, **of newborn**
         Subependymal hemorrhage with intraventricular extension
         Bleeding into ventricle

☑5ᵗʰ P52.2   **Intraventricular (nontraumatic) hemorrhage, grade 3 and grade 4, of newborn**

P52.21   **Intraventricular (nontraumatic) hemorrhage,** grade 3, **of newborn**
          Subependymal hemorrhage with intraventricular extension with enlargement of ventricle

P52.22   **Intraventricular (nontraumatic) hemorrhage,** grade 4, **of newborn**
          Bleeding into cerebral cortex
          Subependymal hemorrhage with intracerebral extension

P52.3   **Unspecified intraventricular (nontraumatic) hemorrhage of newborn**   ▽

P52.4   **Intracerebral (nontraumatic) hemorrhage of newborn**

P52.5   **Subarachnoid (nontraumatic) hemorrhage of newborn**

P52.6   **Cerebellar (nontraumatic) and posterior fossa hemorrhage of newborn**

P52.8   **Other intracranial (nontraumatic) hemorrhages of newborn**

P52.9   **Intracranial (nontraumatic) hemorrhage of newborn, unspecified**   ▽

P53   **Hemorrhagic disease of newborn**
       Vitamin K deficiency of newborn

☑4ᵗʰ P54   **Other** neonatal hemorrhages
         EXCLUDES 1   newborn affected by (intrauterine) blood loss (P50.-)
                       pulmonary hemorrhage originating in the perinatal period (P26.-)

P54.0   **Neonatal hematemesis**
         EXCLUDES 1   neonatal hematemesis due to swallowed maternal blood (P78.2)

P54.1   **Neonatal melena**
         EXCLUDES 1   neonatal melena due to swallowed maternal blood (P78.2)

P54.2   **Neonatal rectal hemorrhage**

P54.3   **Other neonatal gastrointestinal hemorrhage**

P54.4   **Neonatal adrenal hemorrhage**

P54.5   **Neonatal cutaneous hemorrhage**
         Neonatal bruising
         Neonatal ecchymoses
         Neonatal petechiae
         Neonatal superficial hematomata
         EXCLUDES 2   bruising of scalp due to birth injury (P12.3)
                       cephalhematoma due to birth injury (P12.0)

P54.6   **Neonatal vaginal hemorrhage**   ♀
         Neonatal pseudomenses

P54.8   **Other specified neonatal hemorrhages**

P54.9   **Neonatal hemorrhage, unspecified**   ▽

☑4ᵗʰ P55   **Hemolytic disease of newborn**

P55.0   Rh **isoimmunization of newborn**
         DEF: Incompatible Rh fetal-maternal blood grouping; prematurely destroys red blood cells; characterized by jaundice, asphyxia, pulmonary hypertension, edema, respiratory distress, kernicterus, and coagulopathies; detected by Coombs test.

P55.1   ABO **isoimmunization of newborn**
         AHA: 2015, 3Q, 20

P55.8   **Other hemolytic diseases of newborn**

P55.9   **Hemolytic disease of newborn, unspecified**   ▽

☑4ᵗʰ P56   **Hydrops fetalis due to hemolytic disease**
         EXCLUDES 1   hydrops fetalis NOS (P83.2)

P56.0   **Hydrops fetalis due to** isoimmunization

☑5ᵗʰ P56.9   **Hydrops fetalis due to** other and unspecified **hemolytic disease**

P56.90   **Hydrops fetalis due to unspecified hemolytic disease**   ▽

P56.99   **Hydrops fetalis due to other hemolytic disease**

☑4ᵗʰ P57   **Kernicterus**

P57.0   **Kernicterus due to** isoimmunization
         DEF: Complication of erythroblastosis fetalis associated with severe neural symptoms, high blood bilirubin levels and nerve cell destruction; results in bilirubin-pigmented gray matter of central nervous system.

P57.8   **Other specified kernicterus**
         EXCLUDES 1   Crigler-Najjar syndrome (E80.5)

P57.9   **Kernicterus, unspecified**   ▽

☑4ᵗʰ P58   **Neonatal jaundice due to other excessive hemolysis**
         EXCLUDES 1   jaundice due to isoimmunization (P55-P57)

P58.0   **Neonatal jaundice due to** bruising

P58.1   **Neonatal jaundice due to** bleeding

P58.2   **Neonatal jaundice due to** infection

P58.3   **Neonatal jaundice due to** polycythemia

☑5ᵗʰ P58.4   **Neonatal jaundice due to** drugs or toxins **transmitted from mother or given to newborn**
         Code first poisoning due to drug or toxin, if applicable (T36-T65 with fifth or sixth character 1-4 or 6)
         Use additional code for adverse effect, if applicable, to identify drug (T36-T50 with fifth or sixth character 5)

P58.41   **Neonatal jaundice due to drugs or toxins** transmitted from mother

☑ Additional Character Req   ✓x7ᵗʰ Placeholder Alert   Case-Mix Diagnosis   Manifestation   ▽ Unspecified Dx   EXCLUDES 1 Not coded here   EXCLUDES 2 Not included here

ICD-10-CM 2018   **863**

P58.42   **Neonatal jaundice due to drugs or toxins given to newborn**

P58.5   **Neonatal jaundice due to** swallowed maternal blood

P58.8   **Neonatal jaundice due to other specified excessive hemolysis**

P58.9   **Neonatal jaundice due to excessive hemolysis, unspecified** ▽

✓4ᵗʰ **P59**   **Neonatal jaundice from other and unspecified causes**
> EXCLUDES1   *jaundice due to inborn errors of metabolism (E70-E88)*
>   *kernicterus (P57.-)*

P59.0   **Neonatal jaundice associated with** preterm delivery
> Hyperbilirubinemia of prematurity
> Jaundice due to delayed conjugation associated with preterm delivery

P59.1   Inspissated bile syndrome

✓5ᵗʰ **P59.2**   **Neonatal jaundice from other and unspecified** hepatocellular damage
> EXCLUDES1   *congenital viral hepatitis (P35.3)*

     P59.20   **Neonatal jaundice from unspecified hepatocellular damage** ▽

     P59.29   **Neonatal jaundice from other hepatocellular damage**
> Neonatal giant cell hepatitis
> Neonatal (idiopathic) hepatitis

P59.3   **Neonatal jaundice from** breast milk inhibitor

P59.8   **Neonatal jaundice from other specified causes**

P59.9   **Neonatal jaundice, unspecified** ▽
> Neonatal physiological jaundice (intense)(prolonged) NOS
> **AHA:** 2015, 3Q, 20

P60   **Disseminated intravascular coagulation of newborn**
> Defibrination syndrome of newborn

✓4ᵗʰ **P61**   **Other perinatal hematological disorders**
> EXCLUDES1   *transient hypogammaglobulinemia of infancy (D80.7)*

P61.0   **Transient neonatal thrombocytopenia**
> Neonatal thrombocytopenia due to exchange transfusion
> Neonatal thrombocytopenia due to idiopathic maternal thrombocytopenia
> Neonatal thrombocytopenia due to isoimmunization
> **DEF:** Temporary decrease in blood platelets of newborn; secondary to placental insufficiency.

P61.1   **Polycythemia neonatorum**
> **DEF:** Abnormal increase of total red blood cells of newborn; results in hyperviscosity, which slows the flow of blood through small blood vessels.

P61.2   **Anemia of prematurity**

P61.3   **Congenital anemia from fetal blood loss**

P61.4   **Other congenital anemias, not elsewhere classified**
> Congenital anemia NOS

P61.5   **Transient neonatal neutropenia**
> EXCLUDES1   *congenital neutropenia (nontransient) (D70.0)*
> **DEF:** Low blood neutrophil counts of newborn; occurs due to maternal hypertension, sepsis, twin-twin transfusion, alloimmunization, and hemolytic disease.

P61.6   **Other transient neonatal disorders of coagulation**

P61.8   **Other specified perinatal hematological disorders**

P61.9   **Perinatal hematological disorder, unspecified** ▽

Transitory endocrine and metabolic disorders specific to newborn (P70-P74)

> INCLUDES   transitory endocrine and metabolic disturbances caused by the infant's response to maternal endocrine and metabolic factors, or its adjustment to extrauterine environment

✓4ᵗʰ **P70**   **Transitory disorders of** carbohydrate metabolism **specific to newborn**

P70.0   **Syndrome of infant of mother with** gestational diabetes
> Newborn (with hypoglycemia) affected by maternal gestational diabetes
> EXCLUDES1   *newborn (with hypoglycemia) affected by maternal (pre-existing) diabetes mellitus (P70.1)*
>   *syndrome of infant of a diabetic mother (P70.1)*

P70.1   **Syndrome of infant of a** diabetic mother
> Newborn (with hypoglycemia) affected by maternal (pre-existing) diabetes mellitus
> EXCLUDES1   *newborn (with hypoglycemia) affected by maternal gestational diabetes (P70.0)*
>   *syndrome of infant of mother with gestational diabetes (P70.0)*

P70.2   **Neonatal** diabetes mellitus

P70.3   Iatrogenic **neonatal** hypoglycemia

P70.4   **Other neonatal hypoglycemia**
> Transitory neonatal hypoglycemia

P70.8   **Other transitory disorders of carbohydrate metabolism of newborn**

P70.9   **Transitory disorder of carbohydrate metabolism of newborn, unspecified** ▽

✓4ᵗʰ **P71**   **Transitory neonatal disorders of** calcium and magnesium metabolism

P71.0   **Cow's milk hypocalcemia in newborn**

P71.1   **Other neonatal hypocalcemia**
> EXCLUDES1   *neonatal hypoparathyroidism (P71.4)*

P71.2   **Neonatal** hypomagnesemia

P71.3   **Neonatal** tetany without calcium or magnesium deficiency
> Neonatal tetany NOS

P71.4   **Transitory neonatal** hypoparathyroidism

P71.8   **Other transitory neonatal disorders of calcium and magnesium metabolism**

P71.9   **Transitory neonatal disorder of calcium and magnesium metabolism, unspecified** ▽

✓4ᵗʰ **P72**   **Other transitory neonatal** endocrine disorders
> EXCLUDES1   *congenital hypothyroidism with or without goiter (E03.0-E03.1)*
>   *dyshormogenetic goiter (E07.1)*
>   *Pendred's syndrome (E07.1)*

P72.0   **Neonatal goiter, not elsewhere classified**
> Transitory congenital goiter with normal functioning

P72.1   Transitory **neonatal** hyperthyroidism
> Neonatal thyrotoxicosis

P72.2   **Other transitory neonatal disorders of** thyroid function, not elsewhere classified
> Transitory neonatal hypothyroidism

P72.8   **Other specified transitory neonatal endocrine disorders**

P72.9   **Transitory neonatal endocrine disorder, unspecified** ▽

✓4ᵗʰ **P74**   **Other transitory neonatal** electrolyte and metabolic disturbances

P74.0   Late metabolic acidosis **of newborn**
> EXCLUDES1   *(fetal) metabolic acidosis of newborn (P19)*

P74.1   Dehydration **of newborn**

P74.2   **Disturbances of** sodium balance **of newborn**

P74.3   **Disturbances of** potassium balance **of newborn**

P74.4   **Other transitory electrolyte disturbances of newborn**

P74.5   **Transitory** tyrosinemia **of newborn**

P74.6   **Transitory** hyperammonemia **of newborn**

P74.8   **Other transitory metabolic disturbances of newborn**
> Amino-acid metabolic disorders described as transitory

P74.9   **Transitory metabolic disturbance of newborn, unspecified** ▽

Digestive system disorders of newborn (P76-P78)

✓4ᵗʰ **P76**   **Other intestinal obstruction of newborn**

P76.0   **Meconium plug syndrome**
> Meconium ileus NOS
> EXCLUDES1   *meconium ileus in cystic fibrosis (E84.11)*

P76.1   **Transitory ileus of newborn**
> EXCLUDES1   *Hirschsprung's disease (Q43.1)*

P76.2   **Intestinal obstruction due to inspissated milk**

P76.8   **Other specified intestinal obstruction of newborn**
> EXCLUDES1   *intestinal obstruction classifiable to K56-*

P76.9   **Intestinal obstruction of newborn, unspecified** ▽

✓4ᵗʰ **P77**   Necrotizing enterocolitis **of newborn**
> **DEF:** Serious intestinal infection and inflammation in preterm infants; severity is measured by stages and may progress to life-threatening perforation or peritonitis; resection surgical treatment may be necessary.

P77.1   Stage 1 **necrotizing enterocolitis in newborn**
> Necrotizing enterocolitis without pneumatosis, without perforation
> **DEF:** Broad-spectrum symptoms with nonspecific signs, including feeding intolerance, abdominal distention, bradycardia, and metabolic abnormalities.

P77.2   Stage 2 **necrotizing enterocolitis in newborn**
> Necrotizing enterocolitis with pneumatosis, without perforation
> **DEF:** Radiographic confirmation of necrotizing enterocolitis showing intestinal dilatation, fixed loops of bowels, pneumatosis intestinalis, metabolic acidosis, and thrombocytopenia.

N Newborn: 0   P Pediatric: 0-17   M Maternity: 12-55   A Adult: 15-124   **NRS** Nonroutine supply Dx   **NCDx** Noncancer Dx   **PDx** Primary Dx   ▶◀ Revised Text   ● New Code   ▲ Revised Title

P77.3   **Stage 3** **necrotizing enterocolitis in newborn**
Necrotizing enterocolitis with perforation
Necrotizing enterocolitis with pneumatosis and perforation
DEF: Advanced stage in which infant demonstrates signs of bowel perforation, septic shock, metabolic acidosis, ascites, disseminated intravascular coagulopathy, neutropenia.

P77.9   **Necrotizing enterocolitis in newborn, unspecified** ▽
Necrotizing enterocolitis in newborn, NOS

☑4ᵗʰ **P78**   **Other perinatal digestive system disorders**
EXCLUDES 1   cystic fibrosis (E84.0-E84.9)
neonatal gastrointestinal hemorrhages (P54.0-P54.3)

P78.0   **Perinatal intestinal perforation**
Meconium peritonitis

P78.1   **Other neonatal peritonitis**
Neonatal peritonitis NOS

P78.2   **Neonatal hematemesis and melena due to swallowed maternal blood**

P78.3   **Noninfective neonatal diarrhea**
Neonatal diarrhea NOS

☑5ᵗʰ **P78.8**   **Other specified perinatal digestive system disorders**

P78.81   **Congenital cirrhosis (of liver)**

P78.82   **Peptic ulcer of newborn**

P78.83   **Newborn esophageal reflux**
Neonatal esophageal reflux

●   **P78.84**   **Gestational alloimmune liver disease**
GALD
Neonatal hemochromatosis
EXCLUDES 1   hemochromatosis (E83.11-)

P78.89   **Other specified perinatal digestive system disorders**

P78.9   **Perinatal digestive system disorder, unspecified** ▽

Conditions involving the integument and temperature regulation of newborn (P80-P83)

☑4ᵗʰ **P80**   **Hypothermia of newborn**

P80.0   **Cold injury syndrome**
Severe and usually chronic hypothermia associated with a pink flushed appearance, edema and neurological and biochemical abnormalities.
EXCLUDES 1   mild hypothermia of newborn (P80.8)

P80.8   **Other hypothermia of newborn**
Mild hypothermia of newborn

P80.9   **Hypothermia of newborn, unspecified** ▽

☑4ᵗʰ **P81**   **Other disturbances of temperature regulation of newborn**

P81.0   **Environmental hyperthermia of newborn**

P81.8   **Other specified disturbances of temperature regulation of newborn**

P81.9   **Disturbance of temperature regulation of newborn, unspecified** ▽
Fever of newborn NOS

☑4ᵗʰ **P83**   **Other conditions of integument specific to newborn**
EXCLUDES 1   congenital malformations of skin and integument (Q80-Q84)
hydrops fetalis due to hemolytic disease (P56.-)
neonatal skin infection (P39.4)
staphylococcal scalded skin syndrome (L00)
EXCLUDES 2   cradle cap (L21.0)
diaper [napkin] dermatitis (L22)

P83.0   **Sclerema neonatorum**
DEF: Diffuse, rapidly progressing white, waxy, nonpitting hardening of tissue, usually of legs and feet that is life-threatening; found in preterm or debilitated infants; unknown etiology.

P83.1   **Neonatal erythema toxicum**

P83.2   **Hydrops fetalis not due to hemolytic disease**
Hydrops fetalis NOS
DEF: Severe, life-threatening problem of newborn characterized by severe edema of entire body; unrelated to immune response.

☑5ᵗʰ **P83.3**   **Other and unspecified edema specific to newborn**

P83.30   **Unspecified edema specific to newborn** ▽

P83.39   **Other edema specific to newborn**

P83.4   **Breast engorgement of newborn**
Noninfective mastitis of newborn

P83.5   **Congenital hydrocele** ♂

P83.6   **Umbilical polyp of newborn**

☑5ᵗʰ **P83.8**   **Other specified conditions of integument specific to newborn**
~~Bronze baby syndrome~~
~~Neonatal scleroderma~~
~~Urticaria neonatorum~~

●   **P83.81**   **Umbilical granuloma**
EXCLUDES 2   granulomatous disorder of the skin and subcutaneous tissue, unspecified (L92.9)

●   **P83.88**   **Other specified conditions of integument specific to newborn**
Bronze baby syndrome
Neonatal scleroderma
Urticaria neonatorum

P83.9   **Condition of the integument specific to newborn, unspecified** ▽

Other problems with newborn (P84)

P84   **Other problems with newborn**
Acidemia of newborn   Hypoxemia of newborn
Acidosis of newborn   Hypoxia of newborn NOS
Anoxia of newborn NOS   Mixed metabolic and respiratory
Asphyxia of newborn NOS   acidosis of newborn
Hypercapnia of newborn
EXCLUDES 1   intracranial hemorrhage due to anoxia or hypoxia (P52.-)
hypoxic ischemic encephalopathy [HIE] (P91.6-)
late metabolic acidosis of newborn (P74.0)

Other disorders originating in the perinatal period (P90-P96)

P90   **Convulsions of newborn**
EXCLUDES 1   benign myoclonic epilepsy in infancy (G40.3-)
benign neonatal convulsions (familial) (G40.3-)

☑4ᵗʰ **P91**   **Other disturbances of cerebral status of newborn**

P91.0   **Neonatal cerebral ischemia**

P91.1   **Acquired periventricular cysts of newborn**

P91.2   **Neonatal cerebral leukomalacia**
Periventricular leukomalacia

P91.3   **Neonatal cerebral irritability**

P91.4   **Neonatal cerebral depression**

P91.5   **Neonatal coma**

☑5ᵗʰ **P91.6**   **Hypoxic ischemic encephalopathy [HIE]**
EXCLUDES 1   ►neonatal cerebral depression (P91.4)
neonatal cerebral irritability (P91.3)
neonatal coma (P91.5)◄

P91.60   **Hypoxic ischemic encephalopathy [HIE], unspecified** ▽

P91.61   **Mild hypoxic ischemic encephalopathy [HIE]**

P91.62   **Moderate hypoxic ischemic encephalopathy [HIE]**

P91.63   **Severe hypoxic ischemic encephalopathy [HIE]**

☑5ᵗʰ **P91.8**   **Other specified disturbances of cerebral status of newborn**

●   ☑6ᵗʰ **P91.81**   **Neonatal encephalopathy**

●   **P91.811**   **Neonatal encephalopathy in diseases classified elsewhere**
Code first underlying condition, if known, such as:
congenital cirrhosis (of liver) (P78.71)
intracranial nontraumatic hemorrhage of newborn (P52.-)
kernicterus (P57.-)

●   **P91.819**   **Neonatal encephalopathy, unspecified** ▽

●   **P91.88**   **Other specified disturbances of cerebral status of newborn**

P91.9   **Disturbance of cerebral status of newborn, unspecified** ▽

☑4ᵗʰ **P92**   **Feeding problems of newborn**
EXCLUDES 1   ►eating disorders (F50.-)◄
feeding problems in child over 28 days old (R63.3)
AHA: 2016, 3Q, 19

☑5ᵗʰ **P92.0**   **Vomiting of newborn**
EXCLUDES 1   vomiting of child over 28 days old (R11.-)

P92.01   **Bilious vomiting of newborn**
EXCLUDES 1   bilious vomiting in child over 28 days old (R11.14)

P92.09   **Other vomiting of newborn**
EXCLUDES 1   regurgitation of food in newborn (P92.1)

P92.1   **Regurgitation and rumination of newborn**

P92.2   **Slow feeding of newborn**

☑ Additional Character Req   ᵛˣ⁷ᵗʰ Placeholder Alert   Case-Mix Diagnosis   Manifestation   ▽ Unspecified Dx   *EXCLUDES 1* Not coded here   *EXCLUDES 2* Not included here

ICD-10-CM 2018   **865**

Chapter 16. Certain Conditions Originating in the Perinatal Period *(side tab)*

P92.3 Underfeeding of newborn

P92.4 Overfeeding of newborn

P92.5 Neonatal difficulty in feeding at breast
     AHA: 2017, 1Q, 28

P92.6 Failure to thrive in newborn
     EXCLUDES 1   failure to thrive in child over 28 days old (R62.51)

P92.8 Other feeding problems of newborn

P92.9 Feeding problem of newborn, unspecified   ▽

✓4ᵗʰ **P93** Reactions and intoxications due to drugs administered to newborn
     INCLUDES   reactions and intoxications due to drugs administered to fetus affecting newborn
     EXCLUDES 1   jaundice due to drugs or toxins transmitted from mother or given to newborn (P58.4-)
           reactions and intoxications from maternal opiates, tranquilizers and other medication (P04.0-P04.1, P04.4)
           withdrawal symptoms from maternal use of drugs of addiction (P96.1)
           withdrawal symptoms from therapeutic use of drugs in newborn (P96.2)

P93.0 Grey baby syndrome
     Grey syndrome from chloramphenicol administration in newborn

P93.8 Other reactions and intoxications due to drugs administered to newborn
     Use additional code for adverse effect, if applicable, to identify drug (T36-T50 with fifth or sixth character 5)

✓4ᵗʰ **P94** Disorders of muscle tone of newborn

P94.0 Transient neonatal myasthenia gravis
     EXCLUDES 1   myasthenia gravis (G70.0)

P94.1 Congenital hypertonia

P94.2 Congenital hypotonia
     Floppy baby syndrome, unspecified

P94.8 Other disorders of muscle tone of newborn

P94.9 Disorder of muscle tone of newborn, unspecified   ▽

P95 Stillbirth
     Deadborn fetus NOS
     Fetal death of unspecified cause
     Stillbirth NOS
     EXCLUDES 1   maternal care for intrauterine death (O36.4)
           missed abortion (O02.1)
           outcome of delivery, stillbirth (Z37.1, Z37.3, Z37.4, Z37.7)

✓4ᵗʰ **P96** Other conditions originating in the perinatal period

P96.0 Congenital renal failure
     Uremia of newborn

P96.1 Neonatal withdrawal symptoms from maternal use of drugs of addiction
     Drug withdrawal syndrome in infant of dependent mother
     Neonatal abstinence syndrome
     EXCLUDES 1   reactions and intoxications from maternal opiates and tranquilizers administered during labor and delivery (P04.0)

P96.2 Withdrawal symptoms from therapeutic use of drugs in newborn

P96.3 Wide cranial sutures of newborn
     Neonatal craniotabes

P96.5 Complication to newborn due to (fetal) intrauterine procedure
     EXCLUDES 2   newborn affected by amniocentesis (P00.6)

✓5ᵗʰ **P96.8** Other specified conditions originating in the perinatal period

P96.81 Exposure to (parental) (environmental) tobacco smoke in the perinatal period
     EXCLUDES 2   newborn affected by in utero exposure to tobacco (P04.2)
           exposure to environmental tobacco smoke after the perinatal period (Z77.22)

P96.82 Delayed separation of umbilical cord

P96.83 Meconium staining
     EXCLUDES 1   meconium aspiration (P24.00, P24.01)
           meconium passage during delivery (P03.82)

P96.89 Other specified conditions originating in the perinatal period
     Use additional code to specify condition

P96.9 Condition originating in the perinatal period, unspecified   ▽
     Congenital debility NOS

Ⓝ Newborn: 0   Ⓟ Pediatric: 0-17   Ⓜ Maternity: 12-55   Ⓐ Adult: 15-124   NRS Nonroutine supply Dx   NCDx Noncancer Dx   PDx Primary Dx   ▶◀ Revised Text   ● New Code   ▲ Revised Title

866   ICD-10-CM 2018

P92.3–P96.9 *(side tab, bottom)*

Chapter 17. Congenital Malformations, Deformations and Chromosomal Abnormalities (Q00–Q99)

Chapter Specific Guidelines with Coding Examples

The chapter specific guidelines from the ICD-10-CM Official Guidelines for Coding and Reporting have been provided below. Along with these guidelines are coding examples, contained in the shaded boxes, that have been developed to help illustrate the coding and/or sequencing guidance found in these guidelines.

Assign an appropriate code(s) from categories Q00-Q99, Congenital malformations, deformations, and chromosomal abnormalities when a malformation/deformation or chromosomal abnormality is documented. A malformation/deformation/or chromosomal abnormality may be the principal/first-listed diagnosis on a record or a secondary diagnosis.

When a malformation/deformation/or chromosomal abnormality does not have a unique code assignment, assign additional code(s) for any manifestations that may be present.

When the code assignment specifically identifies the malformation/deformation/or chromosomal abnormality, manifestations that are an inherent component of the anomaly should not be coded separately. Additional codes should be assigned for manifestations that are not an inherent component.

8-day-old infant with tetralogy of Fallot and pulmonary stenosis

Q21.3   Tetralogy of Fallot

Explanation: Pulmonary stenosis is inherent in the disease process of tetralogy of Fallot. When the code assignment specifically identifies the malformation/deformation/or chromosomal abnormality, manifestations that are inherent components of the anomaly should not be coded separately.

7-month-old infant with Down syndrome and common atrioventricular canal

Q90.9   Down syndrome, unspecified

Q21.2   Atrioventricular septal defect

Explanation: While a common atrioventricular canal is often associated with patients with Down syndrome, this manifestation is not an inherent component and may be reported separately. When the code assignment specifically identifies the anomaly, manifestations that are inherent components of the condition should not be coded separately. Additional codes should be assigned for manifestations that are not inherent components.

Codes from Chapter 17 may be used throughout the life of the patient. If a congenital malformation or deformity has been corrected, a personal history code should be used to identify the history of the malformation or deformity. Although present at birth, malformation/deformation/or chromosomal abnormality may not be identified until later in life. Whenever the condition is diagnosed by the physician, it is appropriate to assign a code from codes Q00-Q99. For the birth admission, the appropriate code from category Z38, Liveborn infants, according to place of birth and type of delivery, should be sequenced as the principal diagnosis, followed by any congenital anomaly codes, Q00- Q99.

Three-year-old with history of corrected ventricular septal defect

Z87.74   Personal history of (corrected) congenital malformations of heart and circulatory system

Explanation: If a congenital malformation or deformity has been corrected, a personal history code should be used to identify the history of the malformation or deformity.

Forty-year-old man with headaches diagnosed with congenital arteriovenous malformation by brain scan

Q28.2   Arteriovenous malformation of cerebral vessels

Explanation: Although present at birth, malformations may not be identified until later in life. Whenever the condition is diagnosed by the physician, it is appropriate to assign a code from the range Q00–Q99.

Chapter 17. Congenital Malformations, Deformations and Chromosomal Abnormalities(Q00-Q99)

NOTE   Codes from this chapter are not for use on maternal or fetal records.

EXCLUDES 2 *inborn errors of metabolism (E70-E88)*

This chapter contains the following blocks:

Q00-Q07   Congenital malformations of the nervous system
Q10-Q18   Congenital malformations of eye, ear, face and neck
Q20-Q28   Congenital malformations of the circulatory system
Q30-Q34   Congenital malformations of the respiratory system
Q35-Q37   Cleft lip and cleft palate
Q38-Q45   Other congenital malformations of the digestive system
Q50-Q56   Congenital malformations of genital organs
Q60-Q64   Congenital malformations of the urinary system
Q65-Q79   Congenital malformations and deformations of the
           musculoskeletal system
Q80-Q89   Other congenital malformations
Q90-Q99   Chromosomal abnormalities, not elsewhere classified

Congenital malformations of the nervous system (Q00-Q07)

✓4ᵗʰ Q00 Anencephaly and similar malformations

   Q00.0 Anencephaly
      Acephaly
      Acrania
      Amyelencephaly
      Hemianencephaly
      Hemicephaly

   Q00.1 Craniorachischisis

   Q00.2 Iniencephaly

✓4ᵗʰ Q01 Encephalocele
   INCLUDES   Arnold-Chiari syndrome, type III
      encephalocystocele
      encephalomyelocele
      hydroencephalocele
      hydromeningocele, cranial
      meningocele, cerebral
      meningoencephalocele
      EXCLUDES 1 Meckel-Gruber syndrome (Q61.9)

   Q01.0 Frontal encephalocele

   Q01.1 Nasofrontal encephalocele

   Q01.2 Occipital encephalocele

   Q01.8 Encephalocele of other sites

   Q01.9 Encephalocele, unspecified   ▽

   Q02 Microcephaly
      INCLUDES   hydromicrocephaly
         micrencephalon
         EXCLUDES 1 Meckel-Gruber syndrome (Q61.9)

✓4ᵗʰ Q03 Congenital hydrocephalus
      INCLUDES   hydrocephalus in newborn
      EXCLUDES 1 Arnold-Chiari syndrome, type II (Q07.0-)
         acquired hydrocephalus (G91.-)
         hydrocephalus due to congenital toxoplasmosis (P37.1)
         hydrocephalus with spina bifida (Q05.0-Q05.4)

   Q03.0 Malformations of aqueduct of Sylvius
      Anomaly of aqueduct of Sylvius
      Obstruction of aqueduct of Sylvius, congenital
      Stenosis of aqueduct of Sylvius

Congenital Hydrocephalus

Normal ventricles   Hydrocephalic ventricles

Q03.1 Atresia of foramina of Magendie and Luschka
      Dandy-Walker syndrome

Q03.8 Other congenital hydrocephalus

Q03.9 Congenital hydrocephalus, unspecified   ▽

✓4ᵗʰ Q04 Other congenital malformations of brain
      EXCLUDES 1 cyclopia (Q87.0)
         macrocephaly (Q75.3)

   Q04.0 Congenital malformations of corpus callosum
      Agenesis of corpus callosum

   Q04.1 Arhinencephaly

   Q04.2 Holoprosencephaly

   Q04.3 Other reduction deformities of brain
      Absence of part of brain   Hypoplasia of part of brain
      Agenesis of part of brain   Lissencephaly
      Agyria   Microgyria
      Aplasia of part of brain   Pachygyria
      Hydranencephaly
      EXCLUDES 1 congenital malformations of corpus callosum (Q04.0)

   Q04.4 Septo-optic dysplasia of brain

   Q04.5 Megalencephaly

   Q04.6 Congenital cerebral cysts
      Porencephaly
      Schizencephaly
      EXCLUDES 1 acquired porencephalic cyst (G93.0)

   Q04.8 Other specified congenital malformations of brain
      Arnold-Chiari syndrome, type IV
      Macrogyria

   Q04.9 Congenital malformation of brain, unspecified   ▽
      Congenital anomaly NOS of brain
      Congenital deformity NOS of brain
      Congenital disease or lesion NOS of brain
      Multiple anomalies NOS of brain, congenital

✓4ᵗʰ Q05 Spina bifida
      Hydromeningocele (spinal)
      Meningocele (spinal)
      Meningomyelocele
      Myelocele
      Myelomeningocele
      Rachischisis
      Spina bifida (aperta)(cystica)
      Syringomyelocele
      Use additional code for any associated paraplegia (paraparesis) (G82.2-)
      EXCLUDES 1 Arnold-Chiari syndrome, type II (Q07.0-)
         spina bifida occulta (Q76.0)

   Q05.0 Cervical spina bifida with hydrocephalus

   Q05.1 Thoracic spina bifida with hydrocephalus
      Dorsal spina bifida with hydrocephalus
      Thoracolumbar spina bifida with hydrocephalus

   Q05.2 Lumbar spina bifida with hydrocephalus
      Lumbosacral spina bifida with hydrocephalus

   Q05.3 Sacral spina bifida with hydrocephalus

   Q05.4 Unspecified spina bifida with hydrocephalus   ▽

   Q05.5 Cervical spina bifida without hydrocephalus

   Q05.6 Thoracic spina bifida without hydrocephalus
      Dorsal spina bifida NOS
      Thoracolumbar spina bifida NOS

   Q05.7 Lumbar spina bifida without hydrocephalus
      Lumbosacral spina bifida NOS

   Q05.8 Sacral spina bifida without hydrocephalus

   Q05.9 Spina bifida, unspecified   ▽

Spina Bifida

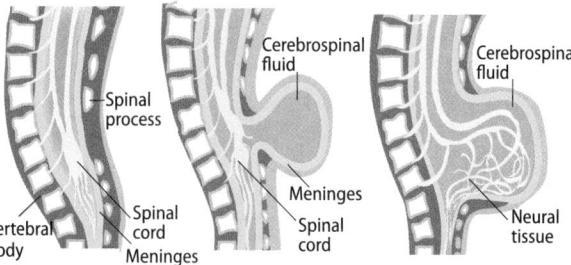

Spina bifida occulta   Meningocele   Myelomeningocele

Ⓝ Newborn: 0 🄿 Pediatric: 0-17 Ⓜ Maternity: 12-55 🄰 Adult: 15-124 **NRS** Nonroutine supply Dx **NC Dx** Noncancer Dx **PDx** Primary Dx ►◄ Revised Text ● New Code ▲ Revised Title

868   ICD-10-CM 2018

✓4th Q06   Other congenital malformations of spinal cord

Q06.0   Amyelia

Q06.1   Hypoplasia and dysplasia of spinal cord
Atelomyelia
Myelatelia
Myelodysplasia of spinal cord

Q06.2   Diastematomyelia
DEF: Rare congenital anomaly often associated with spina bifida; the spinal cord is separated into longitudinal halves by a bony, cartilaginous or fibrous septum, each half surrounded by a dural sac.

Q06.3   Other congenital cauda equina malformations

Q06.4   Hydromyelia
Hydrorachis

Q06.8   Other specified congenital malformations of spinal cord

Q06.9   Congenital malformation of spinal cord, unspecified   ▽
Congenital anomaly NOS of spinal cord
Congenital deformity NOS of spinal cord
Congenital disease or lesion NOS of spinal cord

✓4th Q07   Other congenital malformations of nervous system
    EXCLUDES 2   congenital central alveolar hypoventilation syndrome (G47.35)
                 familial dysautonomia [Riley-Day] (G90.1)
                 neurofibromatosis (nonmalignant) (Q85.0-)

✓5th Q07.0   Arnold-Chiari syndrome
Arnold-Chiari syndrome, type II
    EXCLUDES 1   Arnold-Chiari syndrome, type III (Q01.-)
                 Arnold-Chiari syndrome, type IV (Q04.8)

     Q07.00   Arnold-Chiari syndrome without spina bifida or hydrocephalus

     Q07.01   Arnold-Chiari syndrome with spina bifida

     Q07.02   Arnold-Chiari syndrome with hydrocephalus

     Q07.03   Arnold-Chiari syndrome with spina bifida and hydrocephalus

Q07.8   Other specified congenital malformations of nervous system
Agenesis of nerve
Displacement of brachial plexus
Jaw-winking syndrome
Marcus Gunn's syndrome

Q07.9   Congenital malformation of nervous system, unspecified   ▽
Congenital anomaly NOS of nervous system
Congenital deformity NOS of nervous system
Congenital disease or lesion NOS of nervous system

Congenital malformations of eye, ear, face and neck (Q10-Q18)
    EXCLUDES 2   cleft lip and cleft palate (Q35-Q37)
                 congenital malformation of cervical spine (Q05.0, Q05.5, Q67.5, Q76.0-Q76.4)
                 congenital malformation of larynx (Q31.-)
                 congenital malformation of lip NEC (Q38.0)
                 congenital malformation of nose (Q30.-)
                 congenital malformation of parathyroid gland (Q89.2)
                 congenital malformation of thyroid gland (Q89.2)

✓4th Q10   Congenital malformations of eyelid, lacrimal apparatus and orbit
    EXCLUDES 1   cryptophthalmos NOS (Q11.2)
                 cryptophthalmos syndrome (Q87.0)

Q10.0   Congenital ptosis
DEF: Congenital drooping of eyelid; mostly idiopathic, but may occur genetically.

Q10.1   Congenital ectropion

Q10.2   Congenital entropion

Q10.3   Other congenital malformations of eyelid
Ablepharon
Blepharophimosis, congenital
Coloboma of eyelid
Congenital absence or agenesis of cilia
Congenital absence or agenesis of eyelid
Congenital accessory eyelid
Congenital accessory eye muscle
Congenital malformation of eyelid NOS

Q10.4   Absence and agenesis of lacrimal apparatus
Congenital absence of punctum lacrimale

Q10.5   Congenital stenosis and stricture of lacrimal duct

Q10.6   Other congenital malformations of lacrimal apparatus
Congenital malformation of lacrimal apparatus NOS

Q10.7   Congenital malformation of orbit

Q14.9   Congenital malformation of posterior segment of eye,   ▽

Coloboma of Lens

Coloboma

✓4th Q11   Anophthalmos, microphthalmos and macrophthalmos

Q11.0   Cystic eyeball

Q11.1   Other anophthalmos
Anophthalmos NOS
Agenesis of eye
Aplasia of eye

Q11.2   Microphthalmos
Cryptophthalmos NOS   Hypoplasia of eye
Dysplasia of eye   Rudimentary eye
    EXCLUDES 1   cryptophthalmos syndrome (Q87.0)

Q11.3   Macrophthalmos
    EXCLUDES 1   macrophthalmos in congenital glaucoma (Q15.0)

✓4th Q12   Congenital lens malformations

Q12.0   Congenital cataract

Q12.1   Congenital displaced lens

Q12.2   Coloboma of lens

Q12.3   Congenital aphakia

Q12.4   Spherophakia

Q12.8   Other congenital lens malformations
Microphakia

Q12.9   Congenital lens malformation, unspecified   ▽

✓4th Q13   Congenital malformations of anterior segment of eye

Q13.0   Coloboma of iris
Coloboma NOS

Q13.1   Absence of iris
Aniridia
Use additional code for associated glaucoma (H42)
DEF: Incompletely formed or absent iris; affects both eyes; dominant trait.

Q13.2   Other congenital malformations of iris
Anisocoria, congenital
Atresia of pupil
Congenital malformation of iris NOS
Corectopia

Q13.3   Congenital corneal opacity

Q13.4   Other congenital corneal malformations
Congenital malformation of cornea NOS
Microcornea
Peter's anomaly

Q13.5   Blue sclera

✓5th Q13.8   Other congenital malformations of anterior segment of eye

     Q13.81   Rieger's anomaly
         Use additional code for associated glaucoma (H42)

     Q13.89   Other congenital malformations of anterior segment of eye

Q13.9   Congenital malformation of anterior segment of eye, unspecified   ▽

✓4th Q14   Congenital malformations of posterior segment of eye
    EXCLUDES 2   optic nerve hypoplasia (H47.03-)

Q14.0   Congenital malformation of vitreous humor
Congenital vitreous opacity

Q14.1   Congenital malformation of retina
Congenital retinal aneurysm

Q14.2   Congenital malformation of optic disc
Coloboma of optic disc

Q14.3   Congenital malformation of choroid

Q14.8   Other congenital malformations of posterior segment of eye
Coloboma of the fundus

unspecified

✓ Additional Character Req   ✓x7th Placeholder Alert   Case-Mix Diagnosis   Manifestation   ▽ Unspecified Dx   *EXCLUDES 1* Not coded here   *EXCLUDES 2* Not included here

Chapter 17. Congenital Malformations, Deformations and Chromosomal Abnormalities

Q15–Q21.0

✓4th Q15 Other congenital malformations of eye
EXCLUDES 1   congenital nystagmus (H55.01)
     ocular albinism (E70.31-)
     optic nerve hypoplasia (H47.03-)
     retinitis pigmentosa (H35.52)

Q15.0 Congenital glaucoma
Axenfeld's anomaly
Buphthalmos
Glaucoma of childhood
Glaucoma of newborn
Hydrophthalmos
Keratoglobus, congenital, with glaucoma
Macrocornea with glaucoma
Macrophthalmos in congenital glaucoma
Megalocornea with glaucoma

Q15.8 Other specified congenital malformations of eye

Q15.9 Congenital malformation of eye, unspecified ▽
Congenital anomaly of eye
Congenital deformity of eye

✓4th Q16 Congenital malformations of ear causing impairment of hearing
EXCLUDES 1   congenital deafness (H90.-)

Q16.0 Congenital absence of (ear) auricle

Q16.1 Congenital absence, atresia and stricture of auditory canal (external)
Congenital atresia or stricture of osseous meatus

Q16.2 Absence of eustachian tube

Q16.3 Congenital malformation of ear ossicles
Congenital fusion of ear ossicles

Q16.4 Other congenital malformations of middle ear
Congenital malformation of middle ear NOS

Q16.5 Congenital malformation of inner ear
Congenital anomaly of membranous labyrinth
Congenital anomaly of organ of Corti

Q16.9 Congenital malformation of ear causing impairment of hearing, unspecified ▽
Congenital absence of ear NOS

✓4th Q17 Other congenital malformations of ear
EXCLUDES 1   congenital malformations of ear with impairment of hearing (Q16.0- Q16.9)
     preauricular sinus (Q18.1)

Q17.0 Accessory auricle
Accessory tragus
Polyotia
Preauricular appendage or tag
Supernumerary ear
Supernumerary lobule

Q17.1 Macrotia
DEF: Birth defect characterized by abnormal enlargement of the pinna of the ear.

Q17.2 Microtia

Q17.3 Other misshapen ear
Pointed ear

Q17.4 Misplaced ear
Low-set ears
EXCLUDES 1   cervical auricle (Q18.2)

Q17.5 Prominent ear
Bat ear

Q17.8 Other specified congenital malformations of ear
Congenital absence of lobe of ear

Q17.9 Congenital malformation of ear, unspecified ▽
Congenital anomaly of ear NOS

✓4th Q18 Other congenital malformations of face and neck
EXCLUDES 1   cleft lip and cleft palate (Q35-Q37)
     conditions classified to Q67.0-Q67.4
     congenital malformations of skull and face bones (Q75.-)
     cyclopia (Q87.0)
     dentofacial anomalies [including malocclusion] (M26.-)
     malformation syndromes affecting facial appearance (Q87.0)
     persistent thyroglossal duct (Q89.2)

Q18.0 Sinus, fistula and cyst of branchial cleft
Branchial vestige

Q18.1 Preauricular sinus and cyst
Fistula of auricle, congenital
Cervicoaural fistula

Q18.2 Other branchial cleft malformations
Branchial cleft malformation NOS
Cervical auricle
Otocephaly

Q18.3 Webbing of neck
Pterygium colli
DEF: Congenital malformation characterized by thick, triangular skinfold that stretches from the lateral side of the neck across the shoulder; associated with genetic conditions Turner's and Noonan's syndromes.

Q18.4 Macrostomia
DEF: Rare congenital craniofacial bilateral or unilateral anomaly of mouth due to malformed maxillary and mandibular processes; results in abnormally large mouth extending towards ear.

Q18.5 Microstomia

Q18.6 Macrocheilia
Hypertrophy of lip, congenital

Q18.7 Microcheilia

Q18.8 Other specified congenital malformations of face and neck
Medial cyst of face and neck
Medial fistula of face and neck
Medial sinus of face and neck

Q18.9 Congenital malformation of face and neck, unspecified ▽
Congenital anomaly NOS of face and neck

Congenital malformations of the circulatory system (Q20-Q28)

✓4th Q20 Congenital malformations of cardiac chambers and connections
EXCLUDES 1   dextrocardia with situs inversus (Q89.3)
     mirror-image atrial arrangement with situs inversus (Q89.3)

Q20.0 Common arterial trunk
Persistent truncus arteriosus
EXCLUDES 1   aortic septal defect (Q21.4)

Q20.1 Double outlet right ventricle
Taussig-Bing syndrome

Q20.2 Double outlet left ventricle

Q20.3 Discordant ventriculoarterial connection
Dextrotransposition of aorta
Transposition of great vessels (complete)

Q20.4 Double inlet ventricle
Common ventricle
Cor triloculare biatriatum
Single ventricle

Q20.5 Discordant atrioventricular connection
Corrected transposition
Levotransposition
Ventricular inversion

Q20.6 Isomerism of atrial appendages
Isomerism of atrial appendages with asplenia or polysplenia

Q20.8 Other congenital malformations of cardiac chambers and connections
Cor binoculare

Q20.9 Congenital malformation of cardiac chambers and connections, unspecified ▽

✓4th Q21 Congenital malformations of cardiac septa
EXCLUDES 1   acquired cardiac septal defect (I51.0)

Q21.0 Ventricular septal defect
Roger's disease

Atrial Septal Defect

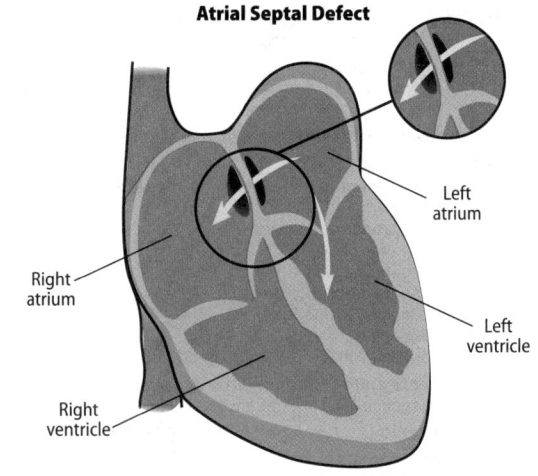

Left atrium

Right atrium

Left ventricle

Right ventricle

N Newborn: 0   P Pediatric: 0-17   M Maternity: 12-55   A Adult: 15-124   NRS Nonroutine supply Dx   NCDx Noncancer Dx   PDx Primary Dx   ▶◀ Revised Text   ● New Code   ▲ Revised Title

870   ICD-10-CM 2018

Atrioventricular Septal Defect

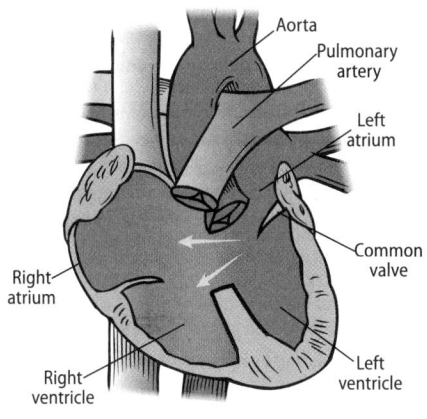

Q21.1 Atrial septal defect
Coronary sinus defect
Patent or persistent foramen ovale
Patent or persistent ostium secundum defect (type II)
Patent or persistent sinus venosus defect

Q21.2 Atrioventricular septal defect
Common atrioventricular canal
Endocardial cushion defect
Ostium primum atrial septal defect (type I)

Q21.3 Tetralogy of Fallot
Ventricular septal defect with pulmonary stenosis or atresia, dextroposition of aorta and hypertrophy of right ventricle.
AHA: 2014, 3Q, 16
TIP: Do not assign an additional code for obstruction of right ventricular outflow tract muscle bundles in a patient with tetralogy of Fallot, as this is an inherent component of the disease.

Q21.4 Aortopulmonary septal defect
Aortic septal defect
Aortopulmonary window

Q21.8 Other congenital malformations of cardiac septa
Eisenmenger's defect
Pentalogy of Fallot
▶Code also if applicable:
Eisenmenger's complex (I27.83)
Eisenmenger's syndrome (I27.83)◀
EXCLUDES 1 *Eisenmenger's complex (I27.8)*
Eisenmenger's syndrome (I27.8)

Q21.9 Congenital malformation of cardiac septum, unspecified ▽
Septal (heart) defect NOS

✓4ᵗʰ Q22 Congenital malformations of pulmonary and tricuspid valves

Q22.0 Pulmonary valve atresia

Q22.1 Congenital pulmonary valve stenosis
DEF: Stenosis of opening between pulmonary artery and right ventricle; causes obstructed blood outflow from right ventricle.

Q22.2 Congenital pulmonary valve insufficiency
Congenital pulmonary valve regurgitation

Q22.3 Other congenital malformations of pulmonary valve
Congenital malformation of pulmonary valve NOS
Supernumerary cusps of pulmonary valve

Q22.4 Congenital tricuspid stenosis
Congenital tricuspid atresia

Q22.5 Ebstein's anomaly
DEF: Malformation of the tricuspid valve characterized by septal and posterior leaflets attaching to the wall of the right ventricle; causes the right ventricle to fuse with the atrium into a large right atrium and a small ventricle; leads to heart failure and abnormal cardiac rhythm.

Q22.6 Hypoplastic right heart syndrome

Q22.8 Other congenital malformations of tricuspid valve

Q22.9 Congenital malformation of tricuspid valve, unspecified ▽

✓4ᵗʰ Q23 Congenital malformations of aortic and mitral valves

Q23.0 Congenital stenosis of aortic valve
Congenital aortic atresia
Congenital aortic stenosis NOS
EXCLUDES 1 *congenital stenosis of aortic valve in hypoplastic left heart syndrome (Q23.4)*
congenital subaortic stenosis (Q24.4)
supravalvular aortic stenosis (congenital) (Q25.3)

Q23.1 Congenital insufficiency of aortic valve
Bicuspid aortic valve
Congenital aortic insufficiency

Q23.2 Congenital mitral stenosis
Congenital mitral atresia
DEF: Congenital stenosis of mitral valve orifice between left atrium and ventricle; at the supravalvular, valvular, or subvalvular levels; causes obstruction to left ventricular filling.

Q23.3 Congenital mitral insufficiency

Q23.4 Hypoplastic left heart syndrome

Q23.8 Other congenital malformations of aortic and mitral valves

Q23.9 Congenital malformation of aortic and mitral valves, unspecified ▽

✓4ᵗʰ Q24 Other congenital malformations of heart
EXCLUDES 1 *endocardial fibroelastosis (I42.4)*

Q24.0 Dextrocardia
EXCLUDES 1 *dextrocardia with situs inversus (Q89.3)*
isomerism of atrial appendages (with asplenia or polysplenia) (Q20.6)
mirror-image atrial arrangement with situs inversus (Q89.3)

Q24.1 Levocardia

Q24.2 Cor triatriatum

Q24.3 Pulmonary infundibular stenosis
Subvalvular pulmonic stenosis

Q24.4 Congenital subaortic stenosis
DEF: Congenital heart defect characterized by stenosis of left ventricular outflow tract due to fibrous tissue ring or septal hypertrophy below aortic valve.

Q24.5 Malformation of coronary vessels
Congenital coronary (artery) aneurysm

Q24.6 Congenital heart block

Q24.8 Other specified congenital malformations of heart
Congenital diverticulum of left ventricle
Congenital malformation of myocardium
Congenital malformation of pericardium
Malposition of heart
Uhl's disease

Q24.9 Congenital malformation of heart, unspecified ▽
Congenital anomaly of heart
Congenital disease of heart

✓4ᵗʰ Q25 Congenital malformations of great arteries

Q25.0 Patent ductus arteriosus
Patent ductus Botallo
Persistent ductus arteriosus

Q25.1 Coarctation of aorta
Coarctation of aorta (preductal) (postductal)
Stenosis of aorta

✓5ᵗʰ Q25.2 Atresia of aorta

Patent Ductus Arteriosus

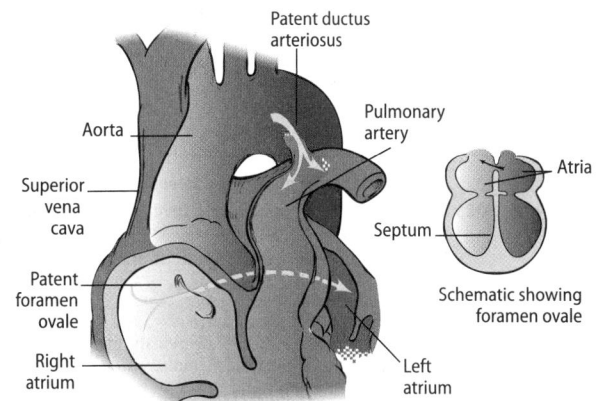

Schematic showing foramen ovale

✓ Additional Character Req   ✓ₓ7ᵗʰ Placeholder Alert   Case-Mix Diagnosis   Manifestation   ▽ Unspecified Dx   **EXCLUDES 1** Not coded here   **EXCLUDES 2** Not included here

Aortic Arch Anomalies

Aortic arch — Esophagus — Trachea

Normal aortic arch

Double aortic arch　　　　Right aortic arch

Q25.21　Interruption of aortic arch
Atresia of aortic arch

Q25.29　Other atresia of aorta
Atresia of aorta

Q25.3　Supravalvular aortic stenosis
EXCLUDES 1　*congenital aortic stenosis NOS (Q23.0)*
congenital stenosis of aortic valve (Q23.0)

✓5th **Q25.4　Other congenital malformations of aorta**
EXCLUDES 1　*hypoplasia of aorta in hypoplastic left heart syndrome (Q23.4)*

Q25.40　Congenital malformation of aorta unspecified ▽

Q25.41　Absence and aplasia of aorta

Q25.42　Hypoplasia of aorta

Q25.43　Congenital aneurysm of aorta
Congenital aneurysm of aortic root
Congenital aneurysm of aortic sinus

Q25.44　Congenital dilation of aorta

Q25.45　Double aortic arch
Vascular ring of aorta

Q25.46　Tortuous aortic arch
Persistent convolutions of aortic arch

Q25.47　Right aortic arch
Persistent right aortic arch

Q25.48　Anomalous origin of subclavian artery

Q25.49　Other congenital malformations of aorta
▶Aortic arch◀
Bovine arch◀

Q25.5　Atresia of pulmonary artery

Q25.6　Stenosis of pulmonary artery
Supravalvular pulmonary stenosis

✓5th **Q25.7　Other congenital malformations of pulmonary artery**

Q25.71　Coarctation of pulmonary artery

Q25.72　Congenital pulmonary arteriovenous malformation
Congenital pulmonary arteriovenous aneurysm

Q25.79　Other congenital malformations of pulmonary artery
Aberrant pulmonary artery
Agenesis of pulmonary artery
Congenital aneurysm of pulmonary artery
Congenital anomaly of pulmonary artery
Hypoplasia of pulmonary artery

Q25.8　Other congenital malformations of other great arteries

Q25.9　Congenital malformation of great arteries, unspecified ▽

✓4th **Q26　Congenital malformations of great veins**

Q26.0　Congenital stenosis of vena cava
Congenital stenosis of vena cava (inferior)(superior)

Q26.1　Persistent left superior vena cava

Q26.2　Total anomalous pulmonary venous connection
Total anomalous pulmonary venous return [TAPVR], subdiaphragmatic
Total anomalous pulmonary venous return [TAPVR], supradiaphragmatic

Q26.3　Partial anomalous pulmonary venous connection
Partial anomalous pulmonary venous return

Q26.4　Anomalous pulmonary venous connection, unspecified ▽

Q26.5　Anomalous portal venous connection

Q26.6　Portal vein-hepatic artery fistula

Q26.8　Other congenital malformations of great veins
Absence of vena cava (inferior) (superior)
Azygos continuation of inferior vena cava
Persistent left posterior cardinal vein
Scimitar syndrome

Q26.9　Congenital malformation of great vein, unspecified ▽
Congenital anomaly of vena cava (inferior) (superior) NOS

✓4th **Q27　Other congenital malformations of peripheral vascular system**
EXCLUDES 2　*anomalies of cerebral and precerebral vessels (Q28.0-Q28.3)*
anomalies of coronary vessels (Q24.5)
anomalies of pulmonary artery (Q25.5-Q25.7)
congenital retinal aneurysm (Q14.1)
hemangioma and lymphangioma (D18.-)

Q27.0　Congenital absence and hypoplasia of umbilical artery
Single umbilical artery

Q27.1　Congenital renal artery stenosis

Q27.2　Other congenital malformations of renal artery
Congenital malformation of renal artery NOS
Multiple renal arteries

✓5th **Q27.3　Arteriovenous malformation (peripheral)**
Arteriovenous aneurysm
EXCLUDES 1　*acquired arteriovenous aneurysm (I77.0)*
EXCLUDES 2　*arteriovenous malformation of cerebral vessels (Q28.2)*
arteriovenous malformation of precerebral vessels (Q28.0)

Q27.30　Arteriovenous malformation, site unspecified ▽

Q27.31　Arteriovenous malformation of vessel of upper limb

Q27.32　Arteriovenous malformation of vessel of lower limb

Q27.33　Arteriovenous malformation of digestive system vessel

Q27.34　Arteriovenous malformation of renal vessel

Q27.39　Arteriovenous malformation, other site

Q27.4　Congenital phlebectasia

Q27.8　Other specified congenital malformations of peripheral vascular system
Absence of peripheral vascular system
Atresia of peripheral vascular system
Congenital aneurysm (peripheral)
Congenital stricture, artery
Congenital varix
EXCLUDES 1　*arteriovenous malformation (Q27.3-)*

Q27.9　Congenital malformation of peripheral vascular system, unspecified ▽
Anomaly of artery or vein NOS

✓4th **Q28　Other congenital malformations of circulatory system**
EXCLUDES 1　*congenital aneurysm NOS (Q27.8)*
congenital coronary aneurysm (Q24.5)
ruptured cerebral arteriovenous malformation (I60.8)
ruptured malformation of precerebral vessels (I72.0)
EXCLUDES 2　*congenital peripheral aneurysm (Q27.8)*
congenital pulmonary aneurysm (Q25.79)
congenital retinal aneurysm (Q14.1)

Q28.0　Arteriovenous malformation of precerebral vessels
Congenital arteriovenous precerebral aneurysm (nonruptured)

Q28.1　Other malformations of precerebral vessels
Congenital malformation of precerebral vessels NOS
Congenital precerebral aneurysm (nonruptured)

Q28.2　Arteriovenous malformation of cerebral vessels
Arteriovenous malformation of brain NOS
Congenital arteriovenous cerebral aneurysm (nonruptured)

Q28.3　Other malformations of cerebral vessels
Congenital cerebral aneurysm (nonruptured)
Congenital malformation of cerebral vessels NOS
Developmental venous anomaly

Q28.8　Other specified congenital malformations of circulatory system
Congenital aneurysm, specified site NEC
Spinal vessel anomaly

Q28.9 **Congenital malformation of circulatory system, unspecified** ▽

Congenital malformations of the respiratory system (Q30-Q34)

✓4ᵗʰ **Q30 Congenital malformations of** nose
     EXCLUDES 1 *congenital deviation of nasal septum (Q67.4)*

Q30.0 Choanal atresia
     Atresia of nares (anterior) (posterior)
     Congenital stenosis of nares (anterior) (posterior)

Q30.1 Agenesis and underdevelopment of nose
     Congenital absent of nose

Q30.2 Fissured, notched and cleft nose

Q30.3 Congenital perforated nasal septum

Q30.8 Other congenital malformations of nose
     Accessory nose
     Congenital anomaly of nasal sinus wall

Q30.9 Congenital malformation of nose, unspecified ▽

✓4ᵗʰ **Q31 Congenital malformations of** larynx
     EXCLUDES 1 *congenital laryngeal stridor NOS (P28.89)*

Q31.0 Web of larynx
     Glottic web of larynx
     Subglottic web of larynx
     Web of larynx NOS
     DEF: Congenital malformation of larynx; marked by thin, translucent, or thick, fibrotic membrane-like structure between vocal folds; characterized by shortness of breath, and stridor.

Q31.1 Congenital subglottic stenosis

Q31.2 Laryngeal hypoplasia

Q31.3 Laryngocele

Q31.5 Congenital laryngomalacia

Q31.8 Other congenital malformations of larynx
     Absence of larynx
     Agenesis of larynx
     Atresia of larynx
     Congenital cleft thyroid cartilage
     Congenital fissure of epiglottis
     Congenital stenosis of larynx NEC
     Posterior cleft of cricoid cartilage

Q31.9 Congenital malformation of larynx, unspecified ▽

✓4ᵗʰ **Q32 Congenital malformations of** trachea and bronchus
     EXCLUDES 1 *congenital bronchiectasis (Q33.4)*

Q32.0 Congenital tracheomalacia

Q32.1 Other congenital malformations of trachea
     Atresia of trachea
     Congenital anomaly of tracheal cartilage
     Congenital dilatation of trachea
     Congenital malformation of trachea
     Congenital stenosis of trachea
     Congenital tracheocele

Q32.2 Congenital bronchomalacia

Q32.3 Congenital stenosis of bronchus

Q32.4 Other congenital malformations of bronchus
     Absence of bronchus
     Agenesis of bronchus
     Atresia of bronchus
     Congenital diverticulum of bronchus
     Congenital malformation of bronchus NOS

✓4ᵗʰ **Q33 Congenital malformations of** lung

Q33.0 Congenital cystic lung
     Congenital cystic lung disease
     Congenital honeycomb lung
     Congenital polycystic lung disease
     EXCLUDES 1 *cystic fibrosis (E84.0)*
                 cystic lung disease, acquired or unspecified (J98.4)

Q33.1 Accessory lobe of lung
     Azygos lobe (fissured), lung

Q33.2 Sequestration of lung

Q33.3 Agenesis of lung
     Congenital absence of lung (lobe)

Q33.4 Congenital bronchiectasis

Q33.5 Ectopic tissue in lung

Q33.6 Congenital hypoplasia and dysplasia of lung
     EXCLUDES 1 *pulmonary hypoplasia associated with short gestation (P28.0)*

Q33.8 Other congenital malformations of lung

Q33.9 Congenital malformation of lung, unspecified ▽

✓4ᵗʰ **Q34 Other congenital malformations of respiratory system**
     EXCLUDES 2 *congenital central alveolar hypoventilation syndrome (G47.35)*

Q34.0 Anomaly of pleura

Q34.1 Congenital cyst of mediastinum

Q34.8 Other specified congenital malformations of respiratory system
     Atresia of nasopharynx

Q34.9 Congenital malformation of respiratory system, unspecified ▽
     Congenital absence of respiratory system
     Congenital anomaly of respiratory system NOS

Cleft lip and cleft palate (Q35-Q37)

Use additional code to identify associated malformation of the nose (Q30.2)
EXCLUDES 1 *Robin's syndrome (Q87.0)*

✓4ᵗʰ **Q35 Cleft palate**
     INCLUDES   fissure of palate
               palatoschisis
     EXCLUDES 1 *cleft palate with cleft lip (Q37.-)*

Q35.1 Cleft hard palate

Q35.3 Cleft soft palate

Q35.5 Cleft hard palate with cleft soft palate

Q35.7 Cleft uvula

Q35.9 Cleft palate, unspecified ▽
     Cleft palate NOS

✓4ᵗʰ **Q36 Cleft lip**
     INCLUDES   cheiloschisis
               congenital fissure of lip
               harelip
               labium leporinum
     EXCLUDES 1 *cleft lip with cleft palate (Q37.-)*

Q36.0 Cleft lip, bilateral

Q36.1 Cleft lip, median

Q36.9 Cleft lip, unilateral
     Cleft lip NOS

✓4ᵗʰ **Q37 Cleft palate with cleft lip**
     INCLUDES   cheilopalatoschisis

Q37.0 Cleft hard palate with bilateral cleft lip

Q37.1 Cleft hard palate with unilateral cleft lip
     Cleft hard palate with cleft lip NOS

Q37.2 Cleft soft palate with bilateral cleft lip

Q37.3 Cleft soft palate with unilateral cleft lip
     Cleft soft palate with cleft lip NOS

Q37.4 Cleft hard and soft palate with bilateral cleft lip

Q37.5 Cleft hard and soft palate with unilateral cleft lip
     Cleft hard and soft palate with cleft lip NOS

Q37.8 Unspecified cleft palate with bilateral cleft lip ▽

Q37.9 Unspecified cleft palate with unilateral cleft lip ▽
     Cleft palate with cleft lip NOS

Cleft Palate

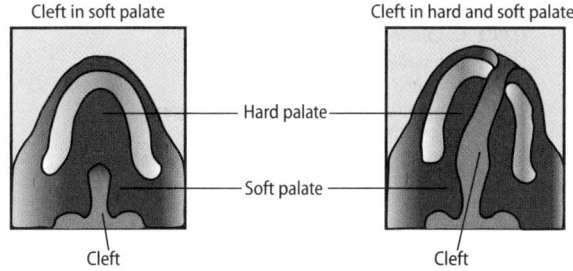

Cleft in soft palate   Cleft in hard and soft palate
Hard palate
Soft palate
Cleft   Cleft

Cleft Lip

Unilateral incomplete   Unilateral complete   Bilateral complete

---

✓ Additional Character Req   ✓x7ᵗʰ Placeholder Alert   Case-Mix Diagnosis   Manifestation   ▽ Unspecified Dx   EXCLUDES 1 Not coded here   EXCLUDES 2 Not included here

Other congenital malformations of the digestive system (Q38-Q45)

✓4ᵗʰ Q38 Other congenital malformations of tongue, mouth and pharynx
> **EXCLUDES 1** dentofacial anomalies (M26.-)
> macrostomia (Q18.4)
> microstomia (Q18.5)

Q38.0 Congenital malformations of lips, not elsewhere classified
Congenital fistula of lip
Congenital malformation of lip NOS
Van der Woude's syndrome
> **EXCLUDES 1** cleft lip (Q36.-)
> cleft lip with cleft palate (Q37.-)
> macrocheilia (Q18.6)
> microcheilia (Q18.7)

Q38.1 Ankyloglossia
Tongue tie

Q38.2 Macroglossia
Congenital hypertrophy of tongue

Q38.3 Other congenital malformations of tongue
Aglossia
Bifid tongue
Congenital adhesion of tongue
Congenital fissure of tongue
Congenital malformation of tongue NOS
Double tongue
Hypoglossia
Hypoplasia of tongue
Microglossia

Q38.4 Congenital malformations of salivary glands and ducts
Atresia of salivary glands and ducts
Congenital absence of salivary glands and ducts
Congenital accessory salivary glands and ducts
Congenital fistula of salivary gland

Q38.5 Congenital malformations of palate, not elsewhere classified
Congenital absence of uvula
Congenital malformation of palate NOS
Congenital high arched palate
> **EXCLUDES 1** cleft palate (Q35.-)
> cleft palate with cleft lip (Q37.-)

Q38.6 Other congenital malformations of mouth
Congenital malformation of mouth NOS

Q38.7 Congenital pharyngeal pouch
Congenital diverticulum of pharynx
> **EXCLUDES 1** pharyngeal pouch syndrome (D82.1)

Q38.8 Other congenital malformations of pharynx
Congenital malformation of pharynx NOS
Imperforate pharynx

✓4ᵗʰ Q39 Congenital malformations of esophagus

Q39.0 Atresia of esophagus without fistula
Atresia of esophagus NOS

Q39.1 Atresia of esophagus with tracheo-esophageal fistula
Atresia of esophagus with broncho-esophageal fistula

Q39.2 Congenital tracheo-esophageal fistula without atresia
Congenital tracheo-esophageal fistula NOS

Q39.3 Congenital stenosis and stricture of esophagus

Q39.4 Esophageal web

Q39.5 Congenital dilatation of esophagus
Congenital cardiospasm

Q39.6 Congenital diverticulum of esophagus
Congenital esophageal pouch

Q39.8 Other congenital malformations of esophagus
Congenital absence of esophagus
Congenital displacement of esophagus
Congenital duplication of esophagus

Q39.9 Congenital malformation of esophagus, unspecified ▽

✓4ᵗʰ Q40 Other congenital malformations of upper alimentary tract

Q40.0 Congenital hypertrophic pyloric stenosis
Congenital or infantile constriction
Congenital or infantile hypertrophy
Congenital or infantile spasm
Congenital or infantile stenosis
Congenital or infantile stricture

Q40.1 Congenital hiatus hernia
Congenital displacement of cardia through esophageal hiatus
> **EXCLUDES 1** congenital diaphragmatic hernia (Q79.0)

Q40.2 Other specified congenital malformations of stomach
Congenital displacement of stomach
Congenital diverticulum of stomach
Congenital hourglass stomach
Congenital duplication of stomach
Megalogastria
Microgastria

Q40.3 Congenital malformation of stomach, unspecified ▽

Q40.8 Other specified congenital malformations of upper alimentary tract

Q40.9 Congenital malformation of upper alimentary tract, unspecified ▽
Congenital anomaly of upper alimentary tract
Congenital deformity of upper alimentary tract

✓4ᵗʰ Q41 Congenital absence, atresia and stenosis of small intestine
> **INCLUDES** congenital obstruction, occlusion or stricture of small intestine or intestine NOS
> **EXCLUDES 1** cystic fibrosis with intestinal manifestation (E84.11)
> meconium ileus NOS (without cystic fibrosis) (P76.0)

Q41.0 Congenital absence, atresia and stenosis of duodenum

Q41.1 Congenital absence, atresia and stenosis of jejunum
Apple peel syndrome
Imperforate jejunum

Q41.2 Congenital absence, atresia and stenosis of ileum

Q41.8 Congenital absence, atresia and stenosis of other specified parts of small intestine

Q41.9 Congenital absence, atresia and stenosis of small intestine, part unspecified ▽
Congenital absence, atresia and stenosis of intestine NOS

✓4ᵗʰ Q42 Congenital absence, atresia and stenosis of large intestine
> **INCLUDES** congenital obstruction, occlusion and stricture of large intestine

Q42.0 Congenital absence, atresia and stenosis of rectum with fistula

Q42.1 Congenital absence, atresia and stenosis of rectum without fistula
Imperforate rectum

Q42.2 Congenital absence, atresia and stenosis of anus with fistula

Q42.3 Congenital absence, atresia and stenosis of anus without fistula
Imperforate anus

Q42.8 Congenital absence, atresia and stenosis of other parts of large intestine

Q42.9 Congenital absence, atresia and stenosis of large intestine, part unspecified ▽

✓4ᵗʰ Q43 Other congenital malformations of intestine

Q43.0 Meckel's diverticulum (displaced) (hypertrophic)
Persistent omphalomesenteric duct
Persistent vitelline duct

Q43.1 Hirschsprung's disease
Aganglionosis
Congenital (aganglionic) megacolon

Q43.2 Other congenital functional disorders of colon
Congenital dilatation of colon

Q43.3 Congenital malformations of intestinal fixation
Congenital omental, anomalous adhesions [bands]
Congenital peritoneal adhesions [bands]
Incomplete rotation of cecum and colon
Insufficient rotation of cecum and colon
Jackson's membrane
Malrotation of colon
Rotation failure of cecum and colon
Universal mesentery

Q43.4 Duplication of intestine

Q43.5 Ectopic anus

Q43.6 Congenital fistula of rectum and anus
> **EXCLUDES 1** congenital fistula of anus with absence, atresia and stenosis (Q42.2)
> congenital fistula of rectum with absence, atresia and stenosis (Q42.0)
> congenital rectovaginal fistula (Q52.2)
> congenital urethrorectal fistula (Q64.73)
> pilonidal fistula or sinus (L05.-)

Q43.7 Persistent cloaca
Cloaca NOS

Q43.8 Other specified congenital malformations of intestine
Congenital blind loop syndrome
Congenital diverticulitis, colon
Congenital diverticulum, intestine
Dolichocolon
Megaloappendix
Megaloduodenum
Microcolon
Transposition of appendix
Transposition of colon
Transposition of intestine
AHA: 2013, 2Q, 31

Q43.9 Congenital malformation of intestine, unspecified ▽

☑4ᵗʰ **Q44 Congenital malformations of** gallbladder, bile ducts and liver

Q44.0 Agenesis, aplasia and hypoplasia of gallbladder
Congenital absence of gallbladder

Q44.1 Other congenital malformations of gallbladder
Congenital malformation of gallbladder NOS
Intrahepatic gallbladder

Q44.2 Atresia of bile ducts

Q44.3 Congenital stenosis and stricture of bile ducts

Q44.4 Choledochal cyst

Q44.5 Other congenital malformations of bile ducts
Accessory hepatic duct
Biliary duct duplication
Congenital malformation of bile duct NOS
Cystic duct duplication

Q44.6 Cystic disease of liver
Fibrocystic disease of liver

Q44.7 Other congenital malformations of liver
Accessory liver
Alagille's syndrome
Congenital absence of liver
Congenital hepatomegaly
Congenital malformation of liver NOS

☑4ᵗʰ **Q45 Other congenital malformations of** digestive system
EXCLUDES 2   congenital diaphragmatic hernia (Q79.0)
    congenital hiatus hernia (Q40.1)

Q45.0 Agenesis, aplasia and hypoplasia of pancreas
Congenital absence of pancreas

Q45.1 Annular pancreas

Q45.2 Congenital pancreatic cyst

Q45.3 Other congenital malformations of pancreas and pancreatic duct
Accessory pancreas
Congenital malformation of pancreas or pancreatic duct NOS
EXCLUDES 1   congenital diabetes mellitus (E10.-)
    cystic fibrosis (E84.0-E84.9)
    fibrocystic disease of pancreas (E84.-)
    neonatal diabetes mellitus (P70.2)

Q45.8 Other specified congenital malformations of digestive system
Absence (complete) (partial) of alimentary tract NOS
Duplication of digestive system
Malposition, congenital of digestive system

Q45.9 Congenital malformation of digestive system, unspecified ▽
Congenital anomaly of digestive system
Congenital deformity of digestive system

Congenital malformations of genital organs (Q50-Q56)

EXCLUDES 1   androgen insensitivity syndrome (E34.5-)
    syndromes associated with anomalies in the number and form of
    chromosomes (Q90-Q99)

☑4ᵗʰ **Q50 Congenital malformations of** ovaries, fallopian tubes and broad ligaments

☑5ᵗʰ **Q50.0 Congenital absence of** ovary
EXCLUDES 1   Turner's syndrome (Q96.-)

    Q50.01 Congenital absence of ovary, unilateral ♀

    Q50.02 Congenital absence of ovary, bilateral ♀

Q50.1 Developmental ovarian cyst ♀

Q50.2 Congenital torsion of ovary ♀

☑5ᵗʰ **Q50.3 Other congenital malformations of** ovary

    Q50.31 Accessory ovary ♀

    Q50.32 Ovarian streak ♀
       46, XX with streak gonads

    Q50.39 Other congenital malformation of ovary ♀
       Congenital malformation of ovary NOS

Q50.4 Embryonic cyst of fallopian tube ♀
Fimbrial cyst

Q50.5 Embryonic cyst of broad ligament ♀
Epoophoron cyst
Parovarian cyst

Q50.6 Other congenital malformations of fallopian tube and broad ligament ♀
Absence of fallopian tube and broad ligament
Accessory fallopian tube and broad ligament
Atresia of fallopian tube and broad ligament
Congenital malformation of fallopian tube or broad ligament NOS

☑4ᵗʰ **Q51 Congenital malformations of** uterus and cervix

Q51.0 Agenesis and aplasia of uterus ♀
Congenital absence of uterus

☑5ᵗʰ **Q51.1 Doubling of uterus with doubling of cervix and vagina**

    Q51.10 Doubling of uterus with doubling of cervix and vagina without obstruction ♀
       Doubling of uterus with doubling of cervix and vagina NOS

    Q51.11 Doubling of uterus with doubling of cervix and vagina with obstruction ♀

Q51.2 Other doubling of uterus ♀
Doubling of uterus NOS
Septate uterus, complete or partial

Q51.3 Bicornate uterus ♀
Bicornate uterus, complete or partial

Q51.4 Unicornate uterus ♀
Unicornate uterus with or without a separate uterine horn
Uterus with only one functioning horn

Q51.5 Agenesis and aplasia of cervix ♀
Congenital absence of cervix

Q51.6 Embryonic cyst of cervix ♀

Q51.7 Congenital fistulae between uterus and digestive and urinary tracts ♀

☑5ᵗʰ **Q51.8 Other congenital malformations of uterus and cervix**

    ☑6ᵗʰ **Q51.81 Other congenital malformations of** uterus

       Q51.810 Arcuate uterus ♀
          Arcuatus uterus

       Q51.811 Hypoplasia of uterus ♀

       Q51.818 Other congenital malformations of uterus ♀
          Müllerian anomaly of uterus NEC

    ☑6ᵗʰ **Q51.82 Other congenital malformations of** cervix

       Q51.820 Cervical duplication ♀

       Q51.821 Hypoplasia of cervix ♀

       Q51.828 Other congenital malformations of cervix ♀

Q51.9 Congenital malformation of uterus and cervix, unspecified ♀▽

☑4ᵗʰ **Q52 Other congenital malformations of** female genitalia

Q52.0 Congenital absence of vagina ♀
Vaginal agenesis, total or partial

☑5ᵗʰ **Q52.1 Doubling of vagina**
EXCLUDES 1   doubling of vagina with doubling of uterus and cervix (Q51.1-)

    Q52.10 Doubling of vagina, unspecified ♀▽
       Septate vagina NOS

    Q52.11 Transverse vaginal septum ♀

    ☑6ᵗʰ **Q52.12 Longitudinal vaginal septum**

       Q52.120 Longitudinal vaginal septum, nonobstructing ♀

       Q52.121 Longitudinal vaginal septum, obstructing, right side ♀

       Q52.122 Longitudinal vaginal septum, obstructing, left side ♀

       Q52.123 Longitudinal vaginal septum, microperforate, right side ♀

       Q52.124 Longitudinal vaginal septum, microperforate, left side ♀

       Q52.129 Other and unspecified longitudinal vaginal septum ♀▽

Q52.2 Congenital rectovaginal fistula ♀
EXCLUDES 1   cloaca (Q43.7)

☑ Additional Character Req   ✓x7ᵗʰ Placeholder Alert   Case-Mix Diagnosis   Manifestation   ▽ Unspecified Dx   *EXCLUDES 1* Not coded here   *EXCLUDES 2* Not included here

Q52.3 Imperforate hymen ♀
> **DEF:** Obstructive anomaly of vagina, characterized by complete closure of membranous fold around external opening of vagina, obstructing the vaginal introitus.

Q52.4 Other congenital malformations of vagina ♀
> Canal of Nuck cyst, congenital
> Congenital malformation of vagina NOS
> Embryonic vaginal cyst
> Gartner's duct cyst

Q52.5 Fusion of labia ♀

Q52.6 Congenital malformation of clitoris ♀

√5ᵗʰ **Q52.7 Other and unspecified congenital malformations of vulva**
> **Q52.70 Unspecified congenital malformations of vulva** ♀▽
> > Congenital malformation of vulva NOS
> **Q52.71 Congenital absence of vulva** ♀
> **Q52.79 Other congenital malformations of vulva** ♀
> > Congenital cyst of vulva

Q52.8 Other specified congenital malformations of female genitalia ♀

Q52.9 Congenital malformation of female genitalia, unspecified ♀▽

√4ᵗʰ **Q53 Undescended and ectopic testicle**
> √5ᵗʰ **Q53.0 Ectopic testis**
> > **Q53.00 Ectopic testis, unspecified** ♂▽
> > **Q53.01 Ectopic testis, unilateral** ♂
> > **Q53.02 Ectopic testes, bilateral** ♂
> √5ᵗʰ **Q53.1 Undescended testicle, unilateral**
> > **Q53.10 Unspecified undescended testicle, unilateral** ♂▽
> > √6ᵗʰ **Q53.11 Abdominal testis, unilateral**
> > > • **Q53.111 Unilateral intraabdominal testis**
> > > • **Q53.112 Unilateral inguinal testis**
> > • **Q53.12 Ectopic perineal testis, unilateral** ♂
> > • **Q53.13 Unilateral high scrotal testis**
> √5ᵗʰ **Q53.2 Undescended testicle, bilateral**
> > **Q53.20 Undescended testicle, unspecified, bilateral** ♂▽
> > √6ᵗʰ **Q53.21 Abdominal testis, bilateral**
> > > • **Q53.211 Bilateral intraabdominal testes**
> > > • **Q53.212 Bilateral inguinal testes**
> > • **Q53.22 Ectopic perineal testis, bilateral** ♂
> > • **Q53.23 Bilateral high scrotal testes**
> **Q53.9 Undescended testicle, unspecified** ♂▽
> > Cryptorchism NOS

√4ᵗʰ **Q54 Hypospadias**
> EXCLUDES 1 *epispadias (Q64.0)*
> **DEF:** Abnormal opening of urethra on the ventral (underside) surface of the penis.
> **Q54.0 Hypospadias, balanic** ♂
> > Hypospadias, coronal
> > Hypospadias, glandular
> **Q54.1 Hypospadias, penile** ♂
> **Q54.2 Hypospadias, penoscrotal** ♂
> **Q54.3 Hypospadias, perineal** ♂
> **Q54.4 Congenital chordee** ♂
> > Chordee without hypospadias
> **Q54.8 Other hypospadias** ♂
> > Hypospadias with intersex state
> **Q54.9 Hypospadias, unspecified** ♂▽

Hypospadias and Epispadias

Balanic (glanular, coronal) hypospadias
Subcoronal hypospadias
Penile hypospadias
Penile raphe
Penoscrotal hypospadius
Scrotal hypospadias
Scrotum
Scrotal raphe
Perineal hypospadias
Hypospadias (ventral view)

Normal external urethral orifice
Glans penis
Foreskin (retracted)
Epispadias
Epispadias (dorsal view)

√4ᵗʰ **Q55 Other congenital malformations of male genital organs**
> EXCLUDES 1 *congenital hydrocele (P83.5)*
> *hypospadias (Q54.-)*
> **Q55.0 Absence and aplasia of testis** ♂
> > Monorchism
> **Q55.1 Hypoplasia of testis and scrotum** ♂
> > Fusion of testes
> √5ᵗʰ **Q55.2 Other and unspecified congenital malformations of testis and scrotum**
> > **Q55.20 Unspecified congenital malformations of testis and scrotum** ♂▽
> > > Congenital malformation of testis or scrotum NOS
> > **Q55.21 Polyorchism** ♂
> > **Q55.22 Retractile testis** ♂
> > **Q55.23 Scrotal transposition** ♂
> > **Q55.29 Other congenital malformations of testis and scrotum** ♂
> **Q55.3 Atresia of vas deferens** ♂
> > Code first any associated cystic fibrosis (E84.-)
> **Q55.4 Other congenital malformations of vas deferens, epididymis, seminal vesicles and prostate** ♂
> > Absence or aplasia of prostate
> > Absence or aplasia of spermatic cord
> > Congenital malformation of vas deferens, epididymis, seminal vesicles or prostate NOS
> **Q55.5 Congenital absence and aplasia of penis** ♂
> √5ᵗʰ **Q55.6 Other congenital malformations of penis**
> > **Q55.61 Curvature of penis (lateral)** ♂
> > **Q55.62 Hypoplasia of penis** ♂
> > > Micropenis
> > **Q55.63 Congenital torsion of penis** ♂
> > > EXCLUDES 1 *acquired torsion of penis (N48.82)*
> > **Q55.64 Hidden penis** ♂
> > > Buried penis
> > > Concealed penis
> > > EXCLUDES 1 *acquired buried penis (N48.83)*
> > **Q55.69 Other congenital malformation of penis** ♂
> > > Congenital malformation of penis NOS
> **Q55.7 Congenital vasocutaneous fistula** ♂
> **Q55.8 Other specified congenital malformations of male genital organs** ♂
> **Q55.9 Congenital malformation of male genital organ, unspecified** ♂▽
> > Congenital anomaly of male genital organ
> > Congenital deformity of male genital organ

√4ᵗʰ **Q56 Indeterminate sex and pseudohermaphroditism**
> EXCLUDES 1 *46, XX true hermaphrodite (Q99.1)*
> *androgen insensitivity syndrome (E34.5-)*
> *chimera 46, XX/46, XY true hermaphrodite (Q99.0)*
> *female pseudohermaphroditism with adrenocortical disorder (E25.-)*
> *pseudohermaphroditism with specified chromosomal anomaly (Q96-Q99)*
> *pure gonadal dysgenesis (Q99.1)*
> **Q56.0 Hermaphroditism, not elsewhere classified**
> > Ovotestis
> **Q56.1 Male pseudohermaphroditism, not elsewhere classified** ♂
> > 46, XY with streak gonads
> > Male pseudohermaphroditism NOS
> **Q56.2 Female pseudohermaphroditism, not elsewhere classified** ♀
> > Female pseudohermaphroditism NOS
> **Q56.3 Pseudohermaphroditism, unspecified** ▽
> **Q56.4 Indeterminate sex, unspecified** ▽
> > Ambiguous genitalia

Congenital malformations of the urinary system (Q60-Q64)

√4ᵗʰ **Q60 Renal agenesis and other reduction defects of kidney**
> INCLUDES congenital absence of kidney
> congenital atrophy of kidney
> infantile atrophy of kidney
> **Q60.0 Renal agenesis, unilateral**
> **Q60.1 Renal agenesis, bilateral**
> **Q60.2 Renal agenesis, unspecified** ▽
> **Q60.3 Renal hypoplasia, unilateral**
> **Q60.4 Renal hypoplasia, bilateral**

N Newborn: 0   P Pediatric: 0-17   M Maternity: 12-55   A Adult: 15-124   NRS Nonroutine supply Dx   NCDx Noncancer Dx   PDx Primary Dx   ▶◀ Revised Text   ● New Code   ▲ Revised Title

876   ICD-10-CM 2018

Q60.5 **Renal hypoplasia, unspecified** ▽

Q60.6 Potter's syndrome

✓4ᵗʰ **Q61 Cystic kidney disease**
> **EXCLUDES 1** acquired cyst of kidney (N28.1)
> Potter's syndrome (Q60.6)

  ✓5ᵗʰ Q61.0 **Congenital renal** cyst

   Q61.00 **Congenital renal cyst, unspecified** ▽
    Cyst of kidney NOS (congenital)

   Q61.01 **Congenital** single **renal cyst**

   Q61.02 **Congenital** multiple **renal cysts**

  ✓5ᵗʰ Q61.1 Polycystic **kidney,** infantile type
    Polycystic kidney, autosomal recessive

   Q61.11 **Cystic dilatation of collecting ducts**

   Q61.19 **Other polycystic kidney, infantile type**

  Q61.2 Polycystic **kidney,** adult type
    Polycystic kidney, autosomal dominant

  Q61.3 **Polycystic kidney, unspecified** ▽
    AHA: 2016, 3Q, 22

  Q61.4 **Renal** dysplasia
    Multicystic dysplastic kidney
    Multicystic kidney (development)
    Multicystic kidney disease
    Multicystic renal dysplasia
    EXCLUDES 1 polycystic kidney disease (Q61.11-Q61.3)

  Q61.5 Medullary cystic **kidney**
    Nephronopthisis
    Sponge kidney NOS
    DEF: Sponge kidney: Dilated collecting tubules; usually asymptomatic but calcinosis in tubules may cause renal insufficiency.

  Q61.8 **Other cystic kidney diseases**
    Fibrocystic kidney
    Fibrocystic renal degeneration or disease

  Q61.9 **Cystic kidney disease, unspecified** ▽
    Meckel-Gruber syndrome

✓4ᵗʰ **Q62 Congenital obstructive defects of** renal pelvis **and congenital malformations of** ureter

  Q62.0 **Congenital** hydronephrosis

  ✓5ᵗʰ Q62.1 **Congenital** occlusion of ureter
    Atresia and stenosis of ureter

   Q62.10 **Congenital occlusion of ureter, unspecified** ▽

   Q62.11 **Congenital occlusion of** ureteropelvic junction

   Q62.12 **Congenital occlusion of** ureterovesical orifice

  Q62.2 **Congenital** megaureter
    Congenital dilatation of ureter

  ✓5ᵗʰ Q62.3 Other **obstructive defects of renal pelvis and ureter**

   Q62.31 **Congenital** ureterocele, orthotopic

   Q62.32 Cecoureterocele
    Ectopic ureterocele

   Q62.39 **Other obstructive defects of renal pelvis and ureter**
    Ureteropelvic junction obstruction NOS

  Q62.4 Agenesis **of ureter**
    Congenital absence ureter

  Q62.5 Duplication of ureter
    Accessory ureter
    Double ureter

  ✓5ᵗʰ Q62.6 Malposition of ureter

   Q62.60 **Malposition of ureter, unspecified** ▽

   Q62.61 Deviation **of ureter**

   Q62.62 Displacement **of ureter**

   Q62.63 Anomalous implantation **of ureter**
    Ectopia of ureter
    Ectopic ureter

   Q62.69 **Other malposition of ureter**

  Q62.7 **Congenital** vesico-uretero-renal reflux

  Q62.8 **Other congenital malformations of ureter**
    Anomaly of ureter NOS

✓4ᵗʰ **Q63 Other congenital malformations of** kidney
> **EXCLUDES 1** congenital nephrotic syndrome (N04.-)

  Q63.0 Accessory **kidney**

  Q63.1 **Lobulated, fused and horseshoe kidney**

Q63.2 Ectopic **kidney**
    Congenital displaced kidney
    Malrotation of kidney

Q63.3 Hyperplastic and giant **kidney**
    Compensatory hypertrophy of kidney

Q63.8 **Other specified congenital malformations of kidney**
    Congenital renal calculi

Q63.9 **Congenital malformation of kidney, unspecified** ▽

✓4ᵗʰ **Q64 Other congenital malformations of** urinary system

  Q64.0 **Epispadias** ♂
> **EXCLUDES 1** hypospadias (Q54.-)

  ✓5ᵗʰ Q64.1 **Exstrophy of** urinary bladder

   Q64.10 **Exstrophy of urinary bladder, unspecified** ▽
    Ectopia vesicae

   Q64.11 Supravesical fissure **of urinary bladder**

   Q64.12 Cloacal exstrophy **of urinary bladder**

   Q64.19 **Other exstrophy of urinary bladder**
    Extroversion of bladder

  Q64.2 **Congenital** posterior urethral valves

  ✓6ᵗʰ Q64.3 **Other atresia and stenosis of** urethra and bladder neck

   Q64.31 **Congenital** bladder neck obstruction
    Congenital obstruction of vesicourethral orifice

   Q64.32 **Congenital** stricture of urethra

   Q64.33 **Congenital** stricture of urinary meatus

   Q64.39 **Other atresia and stenosis of urethra and bladder neck**
    Atresia and stenosis of urethra and bladder neck NOS

  Q64.4 **Malformation of** urachus
    Cyst of urachus
    Patent urachus
    Prolapse of urachus

  Q64.5 **Congenital** absence of bladder and urethra

  Q64.6 **Congenital** diverticulum of bladder

  ✓5ᵗʰ Q64.7 Other and unspecified **congenital malformations of bladder and urethra**
> **EXCLUDES 1** congenital prolapse of bladder (mucosa) (Q79.4)

   Q64.70 **Unspecified congenital malformation of bladder** ▽ **and urethra**
    Malformation of bladder or urethra NOS

   Q64.71 **Congenital** prolapse of urethra

   Q64.72 **Congenital** prolapse of urinary meatus

   Q64.73 **Congenital** urethrorectal fistula

   Q64.74 **Double urethra**

   Q64.75 Double urinary meatus

   Q64.79 **Other congenital malformations of bladder and urethra**

  Q64.8 **Other specified congenital malformations of urinary system**

  Q64.9 **Congenital malformation of urinary system, unspecified** ▽
    Congenital anomaly NOS of urinary system
    Congenital deformity NOS of urinary system

Congenital malformations and deformations of the musculoskeletal system (Q65-Q79)

✓4ᵗʰ **Q65 Congenital deformities of** hip
> **EXCLUDES 1** clicking hip (R29.4)

  ✓5ᵗʰ Q65.0 **Congenital** dislocation of hip, unilateral

   Q65.00 **Congenital dislocation of unspecified hip,** ▽ **unilateral**

   Q65.01 **Congenital dislocation of** right **hip, unilateral**

   Q65.02 **Congenital dislocation of** left **hip, unilateral**

  Q65.1 **Congenital** dislocation of hip, bilateral

  Q65.2 **Congenital dislocation of hip, unspecified** ▽

  ✓5ᵗʰ Q65.3 **Congenital** partial dislocation of hip, unilateral

   Q65.30 **Congenital partial dislocation of unspecified hip,** ▽ **unilateral**

   Q65.31 **Congenital partial dislocation of** right **hip, unilateral**

   Q65.32 **Congenital partial dislocation of** left **hip, unilateral**

  Q65.4 **Congenital** partial dislocation of hip, bilateral

  Q65.5 **Congenital partial dislocation of hip, unspecified** ▽

  Q65.6 **Congenital** unstable **hip**
    Congenital dislocatable hip

▲

✓ Additional Character Req ✓x7ᵗʰ Placeholder Alert Case-Mix Diagnosis Manifestation ▽ Unspecified Dx **EXCLUDES 1** Not coded here **EXCLUDES 2** Not included here

ICD-10-CM 2018 877

Chapter 17. Congenital Malformations, Deformations and Chromosomal Abnormalities

Q60.5–Q65.6

✓5ᵗʰ **Q65.8 Other** congenital deformities of hip
  Q65.81 Congenital coxa valga
  Q65.82 Congenital coxa vara
  Q65.89 Other specified congenital deformities of hip
    Anteversion of femoral neck
    Congenital acetabular dysplasia
Q65.9 Congenital deformity of hip, unspecified ▽

✓4ᵗʰ **Q66 Congenital deformities of** feet
  EXCLUDES 1 reduction defects of feet (Q72.-)
    valgus deformities (acquired) (M21.0-)
    varus deformities (acquired) (M21.1-)
Q66.0 Congenital talipes equinovarus
Q66.1 Congenital talipes calcaneovarus
✓5ᵗʰ **Q66.2 Congenital metatarsus (primus) varus**
  Q66.21 Congenital metatarsus primus varus
  Q66.22 Congenital metatarsus adductus
    Congenital metatarsus varus
Q66.3 Other congenital varus deformities of feet
    Hallux varus, congenital
Q66.4 Congenital talipes calcaneovalgus
✓5ᵗʰ **Q66.5 Congenital** pes planus
    Congenital flat foot
    Congenital rigid flat foot
    Congenital spastic (everted) flat foot
    EXCLUDES 1 pes planus, acquired (M21.4)
  Q66.50 Congenital pes planus, unspecified foot ▽
  Q66.51 Congenital pes planus, right foot
  Q66.52 Congenital pes planus, left foot
Q66.6 Other congenital valgus deformities of feet
    Congenital metatarsus valgus
Q66.7 Congenital pes cavus
✓5ᵗʰ **Q66.8 Other** congenital deformities of feet
  Q66.80 Congenital vertical talus deformity, unspecified foot ▽
  Q66.81 Congenital vertical talus deformity, right foot
  Q66.82 Congenital vertical talus deformity, left foot
  Q66.89 Other specified congenital deformities of feet
    Congenital asymmetric talipes
    Congenital clubfoot NOS
    Congenital talipes NOS
    Congenital tarsal coalition
    Hammer toe, congenital
Q66.9 Congenital deformity of feet, unspecified ▽

✓4ᵗʰ **Q67 Congenital musculoskeletal deformities of** head, face, spine and chest
  EXCLUDES 1 congenital malformation syndromes classified to Q87-
    Potter's syndrome (Q60.6)
Q67.0 Congenital facial asymmetry
Q67.1 Congenital compression facies
Q67.2 Dolichocephaly
Q67.3 Plagiocephaly
Q67.4 Other congenital deformities of skull, face and jaw
    Congenital depressions in skull
    Congenital hemifacial atrophy or hypertrophy
    Deviation of nasal septum, congenital
    Squashed or bent nose, congenital
    EXCLUDES 1 dentofacial anomalies [including malocclusion]
      (M26.-)
      syphilitic saddle nose (A50.5)
Q67.5 Congenital deformity of spine
    Congenital postural scoliosis
    Congenital scoliosis NOS
    EXCLUDES 1 infantile idiopathic scoliosis (M41.0)
      scoliosis due to congenital bony malformation (Q76.3)
    AHA: 2014, 4Q, 26
Q67.6 Pectus excavatum
    Congenital funnel chest
Q67.7 Pectus carinatum
    Congenital pigeon chest
Q67.8 Other congenital deformities of chest
    Congenital deformity of chest wall NOS

✓4ᵗʰ **Q68 Other** congenital musculoskeletal deformities
  EXCLUDES 1 reduction defects of limb(s) (Q71-Q73)
  EXCLUDES 2 congenital myotonic chondrodystrophy (G71.13)
Q68.0 Congenital deformity of sternocleidomastoid muscle
    Congenital contracture of sternocleidomastoid (muscle)
    Congenital (sternomastoid) torticollis
    Sternomastoid tumor (congenital)
Q68.1 Congenital deformity of finger(s) and hand
    Congenital clubfinger
    Spade-like hand (congenital)
Q68.2 Congenital deformity of knee
    Congenital dislocation of knee
    Congenital genu recurvatum
Q68.3 Congenital bowing of femur
    EXCLUDES 1 anteversion of femur (neck) (Q65.89)
Q68.4 Congenital bowing of tibia and fibula
Q68.5 Congenital bowing of long bones of leg, unspecified ▽
Q68.6 Discoid meniscus
Q68.8 Other specified congenital musculoskeletal deformities
    Congenital deformity of clavicle
    Congenital deformity of elbow
    Congenital deformity of forearm
    Congenital deformity of scapula
    Congenital deformity of wrist
    Congenital dislocation of elbow
    Congenital dislocation of shoulder
    Congenital dislocation of wrist

✓4ᵗʰ **Q69 Polydactyly**
Q69.0 Accessory finger(s)
Q69.1 Accessory thumb(s)
Q69.2 Accessory toe(s)
    Accessory hallux
Q69.9 Polydactyly, unspecified ▽
    Supernumerary digit(s) NOS

✓4ᵗʰ **Q70 Syndactyly**
✓5ᵗʰ **Q70.0 Fused fingers**
    Complex syndactyly of fingers with synostosis
  Q70.00 Fused fingers, unspecified hand ▽
  Q70.01 Fused fingers, right hand
  Q70.02 Fused fingers, left hand
  Q70.03 Fused fingers, bilateral
✓5ᵗʰ **Q70.1 Webbed fingers**
    Simple syndactyly of fingers without synostosis
  Q70.10 Webbed fingers, unspecified hand ▽
  Q70.11 Webbed fingers, right hand
  Q70.12 Webbed fingers, left hand
  Q70.13 Webbed fingers, bilateral
✓5ᵗʰ **Q70.2 Fused toes**
    Complex syndactyly of toes with synostosis
  Q70.20 Fused toes, unspecified foot ▽
  Q70.21 Fused toes, right foot
  Q70.22 Fused toes, left foot
  Q70.23 Fused toes, bilateral
✓5ᵗʰ **Q70.3 Webbed toes**
    Simple syndactyly of toes without synostosis
  Q70.30 Webbed toes, unspecified foot ▽
  Q70.31 Webbed toes, right foot
  Q70.32 Webbed toes, left foot
  Q70.33 Webbed toes, bilateral
Q70.4 Polysyndactyly, unspecified ▽
    EXCLUDES 1 specified syndactyly of hand and feet—code to
      specified conditions (Q70.0-Q70.3-)
Q70.9 Syndactyly, unspecified ▽
    Symphalangy NOS

✓4ᵗʰ **Q71 Reduction defects of** upper limb
✓5ᵗʰ **Q71.0 Congenital** complete absence of upper limb
  Q71.00 Congenital complete absence of unspecified upper limb ▽
  Q71.01 Congenital complete absence of right upper limb
  Q71.02 Congenital complete absence of left upper limb
  Q71.03 Congenital complete absence of upper limb, bilateral

Chapter 17. Congenital Malformations, Deformations and Chromosomal Abnormalities (vertical right margin)

✓5ᵗʰ **Q71.1** **Congenital** absence of upper arm and forearm with hand present

    Q71.10 **Congenital absence of unspecified upper arm and forearm with hand present** ▽

    Q71.11 **Congenital absence of** right **upper arm and forearm with hand present**

    Q71.12 **Congenital absence of** left **upper arm and forearm with hand present**

    Q71.13 **Congenital absence of upper arm and forearm with hand present,** bilateral

✓5ᵗʰ **Q71.2** **Congenital** absence of both forearm and hand

    Q71.20 **Congenital absence of both forearm and hand, unspecified upper limb** ▽

    Q71.21 **Congenital absence of both forearm and hand,** right **upper limb**

    Q71.22 **Congenital absence of both forearm and hand,** left **upper limb**

    Q71.23 **Congenital absence of both forearm and hand,** bilateral

✓5ᵗʰ **Q71.3** **Congenital** absence of hand and finger

    Q71.30 **Congenital absence of unspecified hand and finger** ▽

    Q71.31 **Congenital absence of** right **hand and finger**

    Q71.32 **Congenital absence of** left **hand and finger**

    Q71.33 **Congenital absence of hand and finger,** bilateral

✓5ᵗʰ **Q71.4** **Longitudinal reduction defect of** radius
    Clubhand (congenital)
    Radial clubhand

    Q71.40 **Longitudinal reduction defect of unspecified radius** ▽

    Q71.41 **Longitudinal reduction defect of** right **radius**

    Q71.42 **Longitudinal reduction defect of** left **radius**

    Q71.43 **Longitudinal reduction defect of radius,** bilateral

✓5ᵗʰ **Q71.5** **Longitudinal reduction defect of ulna**

    Q71.50 **Longitudinal reduction defect of unspecified ulna** ▽

    Q71.51 **Longitudinal reduction defect of** right **ulna**

    Q71.52 **Longitudinal reduction defect of** left **ulna**

    Q71.53 **Longitudinal reduction defect of ulna,** bilateral

✓5ᵗʰ **Q71.6** Lobster-claw hand

    Q71.60 **Lobster-claw hand, unspecified hand** ▽

    Q71.61 **Lobster-claw** right **hand**

    Q71.62 **Lobster-claw** left **hand**

    Q71.63 **Lobster-claw hand,** bilateral

✓5ᵗʰ **Q71.8** **Other reduction defects of** upper limb

    ✓6ᵗʰ **Q71.81** **Congenital** shortening **of upper limb**

      Q71.811 **Congenital shortening of** right **upper limb**

      Q71.812 **Congenital shortening of** left **upper limb**

      Q71.813 **Congenital shortening of upper limb,** bilateral

      Q71.819 **Congenital shortening of unspecified upper limb** ▽

    ✓6ᵗʰ **Q71.89** Other **reduction defects of upper limb**

      Q71.891 **Other reduction defects of** right **upper limb**

      Q71.892 **Other reduction defects of** left **upper limb**

      Q71.893 **Other reduction defects of upper limb,** bilateral

      Q71.899 **Other reduction defects of unspecified upper limb** ▽

✓5ᵗʰ **Q71.9** Unspecified **reduction defect of upper limb**

    Q71.90 **Unspecified reduction defect of unspecified upper limb** ▽

    Q71.91 **Unspecified reduction defect of** right **upper limb** ▽

    Q71.92 **Unspecified reduction defect of** left **upper limb** ▽

    Q71.93 **Unspecified reduction defect of upper limb,** bilateral ▽

✓4ᵗʰ **Q72** **Reduction defects of** lower limb

  ✓5ᵗʰ **Q72.0** **Congenital** complete absence **of lower limb**

    Q72.00 **Congenital complete absence of unspecified lower limb** ▽

    Q72.01 **Congenital complete absence of** right **lower limb**

    Q72.02 **Congenital complete absence of** left **lower limb**

    Q72.03 **Congenital complete absence of lower limb,** bilateral

✓5ᵗʰ **Q72.1** **Congenital** absence of thigh and lower leg with foot present

    Q72.10 **Congenital absence of unspecified thigh and lower leg with foot present** ▽

    Q72.11 **Congenital absence of** right **thigh and lower leg with foot present**

    Q72.12 **Congenital absence of** left **thigh and lower leg with foot present**

    Q72.13 **Congenital absence of thigh and lower leg with foot present,** bilateral

✓5ᵗʰ **Q72.2** **Congenital** absence of both lower leg and foot

    Q72.20 **Congenital absence of both lower leg and foot, unspecified lower limb** ▽

    Q72.21 **Congenital absence of both lower leg and foot,** right **lower limb**

    Q72.22 **Congenital absence of both lower leg and foot,** left **lower limb**

    Q72.23 **Congenital absence of both lower leg and foot,** bilateral

✓5ᵗʰ **Q72.3** **Congenital** absence of foot and toe(s)

    Q72.30 **Congenital absence of unspecified foot and toe(s)** ▽

    Q72.31 **Congenital absence of** right **foot and toe(s)**

    Q72.32 **Congenital absence of** left **foot and toe(s)**

    Q72.33 **Congenital absence of foot and toe(s),** bilateral

✓5ᵗʰ **Q72.4** **Longitudinal reduction defect of** femur
    Proximal femoral focal deficiency

    Q72.40 **Longitudinal reduction defect of unspecified femur** ▽

    Q72.41 **Longitudinal reduction defect of** right **femur**

    Q72.42 **Longitudinal reduction defect of** left **femur**

    Q72.43 **Longitudinal reduction defect of femur,** bilateral

✓5ᵗʰ **Q72.5** **Longitudinal reduction defect of** tibia

    Q72.50 **Longitudinal reduction defect of unspecified tibia** ▽

    Q72.51 **Longitudinal reduction defect of** right **tibia**

    Q72.52 **Longitudinal reduction defect of** left **tibia**

    Q72.53 **Longitudinal reduction defect of tibia,** bilateral

✓5ᵗʰ **Q72.6** **Longitudinal reduction defect of** fibula

    Q72.60 **Longitudinal reduction defect of unspecified fibula** ▽

    Q72.61 **Longitudinal reduction defect of** right **fibula**

    Q72.62 **Longitudinal reduction defect of** left **fibula**

    Q72.63 **Longitudinal reduction defect of fibula,** bilateral

✓5ᵗʰ **Q72.7** Split foot

    Q72.70 **Split foot, unspecified lower limb** ▽

    Q72.71 **Split foot,** right **lower limb**

    Q72.72 **Split foot,** left **lower limb**

    Q72.73 **Split foot,** bilateral

✓5ᵗʰ **Q72.8** Other **reduction defects of lower limb**

    ✓6ᵗʰ **Q72.81** **Congenital** shortening **of lower limb**

      Q72.811 **Congenital shortening of** right **lower limb**

      Q72.812 **Congenital shortening of** left **lower limb**

      Q72.813 **Congenital shortening of lower limb,** bilateral

      Q72.819 **Congenital shortening of unspecified lower limb** ▽

    ✓6ᵗʰ **Q72.89** Other **reduction defects of lower limb**

      Q72.891 **Other reduction defects of** right **lower limb**

      Q72.892 **Other reduction defects of** left **lower limb**

      Q72.893 **Other reduction defects of lower limb,** bilateral

      Q72.899 **Other reduction defects of unspecified lower limb** ▽

✓5ᵗʰ **Q72.9** Unspecified **reduction defect of lower limb**

    Q72.90 **Unspecified reduction defect of unspecified lower limb** ▽

    Q72.91 **Unspecified reduction defect of** right **lower limb** ▽

    Q72.92 **Unspecified reduction defect of** left **lower limb** ▽

    Q72.93 **Unspecified reduction defect of lower limb,** bilateral ▽

✓4ᵗʰ **Q73** **Reduction defects of** unspecified limb

  Q73.0 **Congenital absence of unspecified limb(s)** ▽
    Amelia NOS

✓ Additional Character Req   ✓x7ᵗʰ Placeholder Alert   Case-Mix Diagnosis   Manifestation   ▽ Unspecified Dx   EXCLUDES 1 Not coded here   EXCLUDES 2 Not included here

Q73.1 Phocomelia, unspecified limb(s) ▽
Phocomelia NOS

Q73.8 Other reduction defects of unspecified limb(s) ▽
Longitudinal reduction deformity of unspecified limb(s)
Ectromelia of limb NOS
Hemimelia of limb NOS
Reduction defect of limb NOS

✓4ᵗʰ **Q74** Other congenital malformations of limb(s)
EXCLUDES 1   polydactyly (Q69.-)
reduction defect of limb (Q71-Q73)
syndactyly (Q70.-)

Q74.0 Other congenital malformations of upper limb(s), including shoulder girdle
Accessory carpal bones
Cleidocranial dysostosis
Congenital pseudarthrosis of clavicle
Macrodactylia (fingers)
Madelung's deformity
Radioulnar synostosis
Sprengel's deformity
Triphalangeal thumb

Q74.1 Congenital malformation of knee
Congenital absence of patella
Congenital dislocation of patella
Congenital genu valgum
Congenital genu varum
Rudimentary patella
EXCLUDES 1   congenital dislocation of knee (Q68.2)
congenital genu recurvatum (Q68.2)
nail patella syndrome (Q87.2)

Q74.2 Other congenital malformations of lower limb(s), including pelvic girdle
Congenital fusion of sacroiliac joint
Congenital malformation of ankle joint
Congenital malformation of sacroiliac joint
EXCLUDES 1   anteversion of femur (neck) (Q65.89)

Q74.3 Arthrogryposis multiplex congenita

Q74.8 Other specified congenital malformations of limb(s)

Q74.9 Unspecified congenital malformation of limb(s) ▽
Congenital anomaly of limb(s) NOS

✓4ᵗʰ **Q75** Other congenital malformations of skull and face bones
EXCLUDES 1   congenital malformation of face NOS (Q18.-)
congenital malformation syndromes classified to Q87.-
dentofacial anomalies [including malocclusion] (M26.-)
musculoskeletal deformities of head and face (Q67.0-Q67.4)
skull defects associated with congenital anomalies of brain such
    as:
    anencephaly (Q00.0)
    encephalocele (Q01.-)
    hydrocephalus (Q03.-)
    microcephaly (Q02)

Q75.0 Craniosynostosis
Acrocephaly
Imperfect fusion of skull
Oxycephaly
Trigonocephaly

Q75.1 Craniofacial dysostosis
Crouzon's disease

Q75.2 Hypertelorism

Q75.3 Macrocephaly

Q75.4 Mandibulofacial dysostosis
Franceschetti syndrome
Treacher Collins syndrome

Q75.5 Oculomandibular dysostosis

Q75.8 Other specified congenital malformations of skull and face bones
Absence of skull bone, congenital
Congenital deformity of forehead
Platybasia

Q75.9 Congenital malformation of skull and face bones, unspecified ▽
Congenital anomaly of face bones NOS
Congenital anomaly of skull NOS

✓4ᵗʰ **Q76** Congenital malformations of spine and bony thorax
EXCLUDES 1   congenital musculoskeletal deformities of spine and chest
    (Q67.5-Q67.8)

Q76.0 Spina bifida occulta
EXCLUDES 1   meningocele (spinal) (Q05.-)
spina bifida (aperta) (cystica) (Q05.-)

Q76.1 Klippel-Feil syndrome
Cervical fusion syndrome

Q76.2 Congenital spondylolisthesis
Congenital spondylolysis
EXCLUDES 1   spondylolisthesis (acquired) (M43.1-)
spondylolysis (acquired) (M43.0-)

Q76.3 Congenital scoliosis due to congenital bony malformation
Hemivertebra fusion or failure of segmentation with scoliosis

✓5ᵗʰ **Q76.4** Other congenital malformations of spine, not associated with scoliosis

  ✓6ᵗʰ **Q76.41** Congenital kyphosis

    Q76.411 Congenital kyphosis, occipito-atlanto-axial region

    Q76.412 Congenital kyphosis, cervical region

    Q76.413 Congenital kyphosis, cervicothoracic region

    Q76.414 Congenital kyphosis, thoracic region

    Q76.415 Congenital kyphosis, thoracolumbar region

    Q76.419 Congenital kyphosis, unspecified region ▽

  ✓6ᵗʰ **Q76.42** Congenital lordosis

    Q76.425 Congenital lordosis, thoracolumbar region

    Q76.426 Congenital lordosis, lumbar region

    Q76.427 Congenital lordosis, lumbosacral region

    Q76.428 Congenital lordosis, sacral and sacrococcygeal region

    Q76.429 Congenital lordosis, unspecified region ▽

  Q76.49 Other congenital malformations of spine, not associated with scoliosis
Congenital absence of vertebra NOS
Congenital fusion of spine NOS
Congenital malformation of lumbosacral (joint) (region) NOS
Congenital malformation of spine NOS
Hemivertebra NOS
Malformation of spine NOS
Platyspondylisis NOS
Supernumerary vertebra NOS

Q76.5 Cervical rib
Supernumerary rib in cervical region

Q76.6 Other congenital malformations of ribs
Accessory rib
Congenital absence of rib
Congenital fusion of ribs
Congenital malformation of ribs NOS
EXCLUDES 1   short rib syndrome (Q77.2)

Q76.7 Congenital malformation of sternum
Congenital absence of sternum
Sternum bifidum

Q76.8 Other congenital malformations of bony thorax

Q76.9 Congenital malformation of bony thorax, unspecified ▽

✓4ᵗʰ **Q77** Osteochondrodysplasia with defects of growth of tubular bones and spine
EXCLUDES 1   mucopolysaccharidosis (E76.0-E76.3)
EXCLUDES 2   congenital myotonic chondrodystrophy (G71.13)

Q77.0 Achondrogenesis
Hypochondrogenesis

Q77.1 Thanatophoric short stature

Q77.2 Short rib syndrome
Asphyxiating thoracic dysplasia [Jeune]

Q77.3 Chondrodysplasia punctata
EXCLUDES 1   Rhizomelic chondrodysplasia punctata (E71.43)

Q77.4 Achondroplasia
Hypochondroplasia
Osteosclerosis congenita

Q77.5 Diastrophic dysplasia

Q77.6 Chondroectodermal dysplasia
Ellis-van Creveld syndrome

Q77.7 Spondyloepiphyseal dysplasia

Q77.8 Other osteochondrodysplasia with defects of growth of tubular bones and spine

Q77.9 Osteochondrodysplasia with defects of growth of tubular ▽ bones and spine, unspecified

☑4th **Q78 Other osteochondrodysplasias**
     EXCLUDES 2 *congenital myotonic chondrodystrophy (G71.13)*

Q78.0 Osteogenesis imperfecta
Fragilitas ossium
Osteopsathyrosis

Q78.1 Polyostotic fibrous dysplasia
Albright(-McCune)(-Sternberg) syndrome

Q78.2 Osteopetrosis
Albers-Schönberg syndrome
Osteosclerosis NOS

Q78.3 Progressive diaphyseal dysplasia
Camurati-Engelmann syndrome

Q78.4 Enchondromatosis
Maffucci's syndrome
Ollier's disease

Q78.5 Metaphyseal dysplasia
Pyle's syndrome

Q78.6 Multiple congenital exostoses
Diaphyseal aclasis

Q78.8 Other specified osteochondrodysplasias
Osteopoikilosis

Q78.9 Osteochondrodysplasia, unspecified ▽
Chondrodystrophy NOS
Osteodystrophy NOS

☑4th **Q79 Congenital malformations of musculoskeletal system, not elsewhere classified**
     EXCLUDES 2 *congenital (sternomastoid) torticollis (Q68.0)*

Q79.0 Congenital diaphragmatic hernia
     EXCLUDES 1 *congenital hiatus hernia (Q40.1)*

Q79.1 Other congenital malformations of diaphragm
Absence of diaphragm
Congenital malformation of diaphragm NOS
Eventration of diaphragm

Q79.2 Exomphalos
Omphalocele
     EXCLUDES 1 *umbilical hernia (K42.-)*

Q79.3 Gastroschisis

Q79.4 Prune belly syndrome
Congenital prolapse of bladder mucosa
Eagle-Barrett syndrome

☑5th **Q79.5 Other congenital malformations of abdominal wall**
     EXCLUDES 1 *umbilical hernia (K42.-)*

     Q79.51 Congenital hernia of bladder

     Q79.59 Other congenital malformations of abdominal wall

Q79.6 Ehlers-Danlos syndrome
DEF: Connective tissue disorder that causes hyperextended skin and joints; results in fragile blood vessels with bleeding, poor wound healing, and subcutaneous pseudotumors.

Q79.8 Other congenital malformations of musculoskeletal system
Absence of muscle   Congenital constricting bands
Absence of tendon   Congenital shortening of tendon
Accessory muscle   Poland syndrome
Amyotrophia congenita

Q79.9 Congenital malformation of musculoskeletal system, unspecified ▽
Congenital anomaly of musculoskeletal system NOS
Congenital deformity of musculoskeletal system NOS

Gastroschisis

distal

Herniated small bowel
(gastroschisis)

Rectus
abdominus m.

Umbilicus

skin

proximal

Defect

Other congenital malformations (Q80-Q89)

☑4th **Q80 Congenital ichthyosis**
     EXCLUDES 1 *Refsum's disease (G60.1)*

Q80.0 Ichthyosis vulgaris

Q80.1 X-linked ichthyosis

Q80.2 Lamellar ichthyosis
Collodion baby

Q80.3 Congenital bullous ichthyosiform erythroderma

Q80.4 Harlequin fetus

Q80.8 Other congenital ichthyosis

Q80.9 Congenital ichthyosis, unspecified ▽

☑4th **Q81 Epidermolysis bullosa**

Q81.0 Epidermolysis bullosa simplex
     EXCLUDES 1 *Cockayne's syndrome (Q87.1)*

Q81.1 Epidermolysis bullosa letalis
Herlitz' syndrome

Q81.2 Epidermolysis bullosa dystrophica

Q81.8 Other epidermolysis bullosa

Q81.9 Epidermolysis bullosa, unspecified ▽

☑4th **Q82 Other congenital malformations of skin**
     EXCLUDES 1 *acrodermatitis enteropathica (E83.2)*
     congenital erythropoietic porphyria (E80.0)
     pilonidal cyst or sinus (L05.-)
     Sturge-Weber (-Dimitri) syndrome (Q85.8)

Q82.0 Hereditary lymphedema

Q82.1 Xeroderma pigmentosum

▲ **Q82.2 Congenital cutaneous mastocytosis**
▶Congenital diffuse cutaneous mastocytosis
Congenital maculopapular cutaneous mastocytosis
Congenital urticaria pigmentosa◀
~~Urticaria pigmentosa~~
     EXCLUDES 1 ▶*cutaneous mastocytosis NOS (D47.01)*
     diffuse cutaneous mastocytosis (with onset after newborn period) (D47.01)◀
     malignant mastocytosis ▶*(C96.2-)*◀
     ▶*systemic mastocytosis (D47.02)*
     urticaria pigmentosa (non-congenital) (with onset after newborn period) (D47.01)◀

Q82.3 Incontinentia pigmenti

Q82.4 Ectodermal dysplasia (anhidrotic)
     EXCLUDES 1 *Ellis-van Creveld syndrome (Q77.6)*

Q82.5 Congenital non-neoplastic nevus
Birthmark NOS
Flammeus Nevus
Portwine Nevus
Sanguineous Nevus
Strawberry Nevus
Vascular Nevus NOS
Verrucous Nevus
     EXCLUDES 2 *araneus nevus (I78.1)*
     café au lait spots (L81.3)
     lentigo (L81.4)
     melanocytic nevus (D22.-)
     nevus NOS (D22.-)
     pigmented nevus (D22.-)
     spider nevus (I78.1)
     stellar nevus (I78.1)

Q82.6 Congenital sacral dimple
Parasacral dimple
     EXCLUDES 2 *pilonidal cyst with abscess (L05.01)*
     pilonidal cyst without abscess (L05.91)

Q82.8 Other specified congenital malformations of skin
Abnormal palmar creases
Accessory skin tags
Benign familial pemphigus [Hailey-Hailey]
Congenital poikiloderma
Cutis laxa (hyperelastica)
Dermatoglyphic anomalies
Inherited keratosis palmaris et plantaris
Keratosis follicularis [Darier-White]
     EXCLUDES 1 *Ehlers-Danlos syndrome (Q79.6)*
     AHA: 2016, 1Q, 17

Q82.9 Congenital malformation of skin, unspecified ▽

☑ Additional Character Req   ☑7th Placeholder Alert   Case-Mix Diagnosis   Manifestation   ▽ Unspecified Dx   **EXCLUDES 1** Not coded here   **EXCLUDES 2** Not included here

ICD-10-CM 2018   **881**

✓4ᵗʰ **Q83 Congenital malformations of breast**
> **EXCLUDES 2**   absence of pectoral muscle (Q79.8)
> hypoplasia of breast (N64.82)
> micromastia (N64.82)

Q83.0 Congenital absence of breast with absent nipple

Q83.1 Accessory breast
> Supernumerary breast

Q83.2 Absent nipple

Q83.3 Accessory nipple
> Supernumerary nipple

Q83.8 Other congenital malformations of breast

Q83.9 Congenital malformation of breast, unspecified ▽

✓4ᵗʰ **Q84 Other congenital malformations of integument**

Q84.0 Congenital alopecia
> Congenital atrichosis

Q84.1 Congenital morphological disturbances of hair, not elsewhere classified
> Beaded hair
> Monilethrix
> Pili annulati
> **EXCLUDES 1**   Menkes' kinky hair syndrome (E83.0)

Q84.2 Other congenital malformations of hair
> Congenital hypertrichosis
> Congenital malformation of hair NOS
> Persistent lanugo

Q84.3 Anonychia
> **EXCLUDES 1**   nail patella syndrome (Q87.2)

Q84.4 Congenital leukonychia

Q84.5 Enlarged and hypertrophic nails
> Congenital onychauxis
> Pachyonychia

Q84.6 Other congenital malformations of nails
> Congenital clubnail
> Congenital koilonychia
> Congenital malformation of nail NOS

Q84.8 Other specified congenital malformations of integument
> Aplasia cutis congenita

Q84.9 Congenital malformation of integument, unspecified ▽
> Congenital anomaly of integument NOS
> Congenital deformity of integument NOS

✓4ᵗʰ **Q85 Phakomatoses, not elsewhere classified**
> **EXCLUDES 1**   ataxia telangiectasia [Louis-Bar] (G11.3)
> familial dysautonomia [Riley-Day] (G90.1)

✓5ᵗʰ **Q85.0 Neurofibromatosis (nonmalignant)**

Q85.00 Neurofibromatosis, unspecified ▽

Q85.01 Neurofibromatosis, type 1
> Von Recklinghausen disease

Q85.02 Neurofibromatosis, type 2
> Acoustic neurofibromatosis
> **DEF:** Inherited condition with cutaneous lesions, benign tumors of peripheral nerves, and bilateral 8th nerve masses.

Q85.03 Schwannomatosis
> **DEF:** A genetic mutation (SMARCB1/INI1) causing multiple benign tumors along nerve pathways; characterized by the exception of 8th cranial nerve involvement.

Q85.09 Other neurofibromatosis

Q85.1 Tuberous sclerosis
> Bourneville's disease
> Epiloia

Q85.8 Other phakomatoses, not elsewhere classified
> Peutz-Jeghers Syndrome
> Sturge-Weber(-Dimitri) syndrome
> von Hippel-Lindau syndrome
> **EXCLUDES 1**   Meckel-Gruber syndrome (Q61.9)

Q85.9 Phakomatosis, unspecified ▽
> Hamartosis NOS

✓4ᵗʰ **Q86 Congenital malformation syndromes due to known exogenous causes, not elsewhere classified**
> **EXCLUDES 2**   iodine-deficiency-related hypothyroidism (E00-E02)
> nonteratogenic effects of substances transmitted via placenta or breast milk (P04.-)

Q86.0 Fetal alcohol syndrome (dysmorphic)

Q86.1 Fetal hydantoin syndrome
> Meadow's syndrome

Q86.2 Dysmorphism due to warfarin

Q86.8 Other congenital malformation syndromes due to known exogenous causes

✓4ᵗʰ **Q87 Other specified congenital malformation syndromes affecting multiple systems**
> Use additional code(s) to identify all associated manifestations

Q87.0 Congenital malformation syndromes predominantly affecting facial appearance
> Acrocephalopolysyndactyly
> Acrocephalosyndactyly [Apert]
> Cryptophthalmos syndrome
> Cyclopia
> Goldenhar syndrome
> Moebius syndrome
> Oro-facial-digital syndrome
> Robin syndrome
> Whistling face

Q87.1 Congenital malformation syndromes predominantly associated with short stature
> Aarskog syndrome
> Cockayne syndrome
> De Lange syndrome
> Dubowitz syndrome
> Noonan syndrome
> Prader-Willi syndrome
> Robinow-Silverman-Smith syndrome
> Russell-Silver syndrome
> Seckel syndrome
> **EXCLUDES 1**   Ellis-van Creveld syndrome (Q77.6)
> Smith-Lemli-Opitz syndrome (E78.72)

Q87.2 Congenital malformation syndromes predominantly involving limbs
> Holt-Oram syndrome
> Klippel-Trenaunay-Weber syndrome
> Nail patella syndrome
> Rubinstein-Taybi syndrome
> Sirenomelia syndrome
> Thrombocytopenia with absent radius [TAR] syndrome
> VATER syndrome

Q87.3 Congenital malformation syndromes involving early overgrowth
> Beckwith-Wiedemann syndrome
> Sotos syndrome
> Weaver syndrome

✓5ᵗʰ **Q87.4 Marfan's syndrome**

Q87.40 Marfan's syndrome, unspecified ▽

✓6ᵗʰ **Q87.41 Marfan's syndrome with cardiovascular manifestations**

Q87.410 Marfan's syndrome with aortic dilation

Q87.418 Marfan's syndrome with other cardiovascular manifestations

Q87.42 Marfan's syndrome with ocular manifestations

Q87.43 Marfan's syndrome with skeletal manifestation

Q87.5 Other congenital malformation syndromes with other skeletal changes

✓5ᵗʰ **Q87.8 Other specified congenital malformation syndromes, not elsewhere classified**
> **EXCLUDES 1**   Zellweger syndrome (E71.510)

Q87.81 Alport syndrome
> Use additional code to identify stage of chronic kidney disease (N18.1-N18.6)

Q87.82 Arterial tortuosity syndrome

Q87.89 Other specified congenital malformation syndromes, not elsewhere classified
> Laurence-Moon (-Bardet)-Biedl syndrome

✓4ᵗʰ **Q89 Other congenital malformations, not elsewhere classified**

✓5ᵗʰ **Q89.0 Congenital absence and malformations of spleen**
> **EXCLUDES 1**   isomerism of atrial appendages (with asplenia or polysplenia) (Q20.6)

Q89.01 Asplenia (congenital)

Q89.09 Congenital malformations of spleen
> Congenital splenomegaly

Q89.1 Congenital malformations of adrenal gland
> **EXCLUDES 1**   adrenogenital disorders (E25.-)
> congenital adrenal hyperplasia (E25.0)

Q89.2 Congenital malformations of other endocrine glands
Congenital malformation of parathyroid or thyroid gland
Persistent thyroglossal duct
Thyroglossal cyst
EXCLUDES 1 *congenital goiter (E03.0)*
congenital hypothyroidism (E03.1)

Q89.3 Situs inversus
Dextrocardia with situs inversus
Mirror-image atrial arrangement with situs inversus
Situs inversus or transversus abdominalis
Situs inversus or transversus thoracis
Transposition of abdominal viscera
Transposition of thoracic viscera
EXCLUDES 1 *dextrocardia NOS (Q24.0)*

Q89.4 Conjoined twins
Craniopagus
Dicephaly
Pygopagus
Thoracopagus

Q89.7 Multiple congenital malformations, not elsewhere classified
Multiple congenital anomalies NOS
Multiple congenital deformities NOS
EXCLUDES 1 *congenital malformation syndromes affecting multiple systems (Q87.-)*

Q89.8 Other specified congenital malformations
Use additional code(s) to identify all associated manifestations

Q89.9 Congenital malformation, unspecified ▽
Congenital anomaly NOS
Congenital deformity NOS

Chromosomal abnormalities, not elsewhere classified (Q90-Q99)
EXCLUDES 2 *mitochondrial metabolic disorders (E88.4-)*

✓4ᵗʰ **Q90 Down syndrome**
Use additional code(s) to identify any associated physical conditions and degree of intellectual disabilities (F70-F79)

Q90.0 Trisomy 21, nonmosaicism (meiotic nondisjunction)

Q90.1 Trisomy 21, mosaicism (mitotic nondisjunction)

Q90.2 Trisomy 21, translocation

Q90.9 Down syndrome, unspecified ▽
Trisomy 21 NOS

✓4ᵗʰ **Q91 Trisomy 18 and Trisomy 13**

Q91.0 Trisomy 18, nonmosaicism (meiotic nondisjunction)

Q91.1 Trisomy 18, mosaicism (mitotic nondisjunction)

Q91.2 Trisomy 18, translocation

Q91.3 Trisomy 18, unspecified ▽

Q91.4 Trisomy 13, nonmosaicism (meiotic nondisjunction)

Q91.5 Trisomy 13, mosaicism (mitotic nondisjunction)

Q91.6 Trisomy 13, translocation

Q91.7 Trisomy 13, unspecified ▽

✓4ᵗʰ **Q92 Other trisomies and partial trisomies of the autosomes, not elsewhere classified**
INCLUDES unbalanced translocations and insertions
EXCLUDES 1 *trisomies of chromosomes 13, 18, 21 (Q90-Q91)*

Q92.0 Whole chromosome trisomy, nonmosaicism (meiotic nondisjunction)

Q92.1 Whole chromosome trisomy, mosaicism (mitotic nondisjunction)

Q92.2 Partial trisomy
Less than whole arm duplicated
Whole arm or more duplicated
EXCLUDES 1 *partial trisomy due to unbalanced translocation (Q92.5)*

Q92.5 Duplications with other complex rearrangements
Partial trisomy due to unbalanced translocations
Code also any associated deletions due to unbalanced translocations, inversions and insertions (Q93.7)

✓5ᵗʰ **Q92.6 Marker chromosomes**
Trisomies due to dicentrics
Trisomies due to extra rings
Trisomies due to isochromosomes
Individual with marker heterochromatin

Q92.61 Marker chromosomes in normal individual

Q92.62 Marker chromosomes in abnormal individual

Q92.7 Triploidy and polyploidy

Q92.8 Other specified trisomies and partial trisomies of autosomes
Duplications identified by fluorescence in situ hybridization (FISH)
Duplications identified by in situ hybridization (ISH)
Duplications seen only at prometaphase

Q92.9 Trisomy and partial trisomy of autosomes, unspecified ▽

✓4ᵗʰ **Q93 Monosomies and deletions from the autosomes, not elsewhere classified**

Q93.0 Whole chromosome monosomy, nonmosaicism (meiotic nondisjunction)

Q93.1 Whole chromosome monosomy, mosaicism (mitotic nondisjunction)

Q93.2 Chromosome replaced with ring, dicentric or isochromosome

Q93.3 Deletion of short arm of chromosome 4
Wolff-Hirschorn syndrome

Q93.4 Deletion of short arm of chromosome 5
Cri-du-chat syndrome

Q93.5 Other deletions of part of a chromosome
Angelman syndrome

Q93.7 Deletions with other complex rearrangements
Deletions due to unbalanced translocations, inversions and insertions
Code also any associated duplications due to unbalanced translocations, inversions and insertions (Q92.5)

✓5ᵗʰ **Q93.8 Other deletions from the autosomes**

Q93.81 Velo-cardio-facial syndrome
Deletion 22q11.2
DEF: Microdeletion syndrome affecting multiple organs; characteristic cleft palate, heart defects, elongated face with almond-shaped eyes, wide nose, small ears, weak immune system, weak musculature, hypothyroidism, short stature, and scoliosis; deletion at q11.2 on the long arm of the chromosome 22.

Q93.88 Other microdeletions
Miller-Dieker syndrome
Smith-Magenis syndrome

Q93.89 Other deletions from the autosomes
Deletions identified by fluorescence in situ hybridization (FISH)
Deletions identified by in situ hybridization (ISH)
Deletions seen only at prometaphase

Q93.9 Deletion from autosomes, unspecified ▽

✓4ᵗʰ **Q95 Balanced rearrangements and structural markers, not elsewhere classified**
INCLUDES Robertsonian and balanced reciprocal translocations and insertions

Q95.0 Balanced translocation and insertion in normal individual

Q95.1 Chromosome inversion in normal individual

Q95.2 Balanced autosomal rearrangement in abnormal individual

Q95.3 Balanced sex/autosomal rearrangement in abnormal individual

Q95.5 Individual with autosomal fragile site

Q95.8 Other balanced rearrangements and structural markers

Q95.9 Balanced rearrangement and structural marker, unspecified ▽

✓4ᵗʰ **Q96 Turner's syndrome**
EXCLUDES 1 *Noonan syndrome (Q87.1)*

Q96.0 Karyotype 45, X ♀

Q96.1 Karyotype 46, X iso (Xq) ♀
Karyotype 46, isochromosome Xq

Q96.2 Karyotype 46, X with abnormal sex chromosome, except iso (Xq) ♀
Karyotype 46, X with abnormal sex chromosome, except isochromosome Xq

Q96.3 Mosaicism, 45, X/46, XX or XY ♀

Q96.4 Mosaicism, 45, X/other cell line(s) with abnormal sex chromosome ♀

Q96.8 Other variants of Turner's syndrome ♀

Q96.9 Turner's syndrome, unspecified ♀▽

✓4ᵗʰ **Q97 Other sex chromosome abnormalities, female phenotype, not elsewhere classified**
EXCLUDES 1 *Turner's syndrome (Q96.-)*

Q97.0 Karyotype 47, XXX ♀

Q97.1 Female with more than three X chromosomes ♀

Q97.2 Mosaicism, lines with various numbers of X chromosomes ♀

Q97.3 Female with 46, XY karyotype ♀

✓ Additional Character Req   ✓×7ᵗʰ Placeholder Alert   Case-Mix Diagnosis   Manifestation   ▽ Unspecified Dx   **EXCLUDES 1** Not coded here   **EXCLUDES 2** Not included here

Q97.8 **Other specified sex chromosome abnormalities, female phenotype** ♀

Q97.9 **Sex chromosome abnormality, female phenotype, unspecified** ♀▽

✓4ᵗʰ **Q98 Other sex chromosome abnormalities, male phenotype, not elsewhere classified**

Q98.0 **Klinefelter syndrome karyotype 47, XXY** ♂

Q98.1 **Klinefelter syndrome, male with more than two X chromosomes** ♂

Q98.3 **Other male with 46, XX karyotype** ♂

Q98.4 **Klinefelter syndrome, unspecified** ♂▽

Q98.5 **Karyotype 47, XYY**

Q98.6 **Male with structurally abnormal sex chromosome** ♂

Q98.7 **Male with sex chromosome mosaicism** ♂

Q98.8 **Other specified sex chromosome abnormalities, male phenotype** ♂

Q98.9 **Sex chromosome abnormality, male phenotype, unspecified** ♂▽

✓4ᵗʰ **Q99 Other chromosome abnormalities, not elsewhere classified**

Q99.0 **Chimera 46, XX/46, XY**
   Chimera 46, XX/46, XY true hermaphrodite

Q99.1 **46, XX true hermaphrodite**
   46, XX with streak gonads
   46, XY with streak gonads
   Pure gonadal dysgenesis

Q99.2 **Fragile X chromosome**
   Fragile X syndrome

Q99.8 **Other specified chromosome abnormalities**

Q99.9 **Chromosomal abnormality, unspecified** ▽

Ⓝ Newborn: 0   Ⓟ Pediatric: 0-17   Ⓜ Maternity: 12-55   Ⓐ Adult: 15-124   **NRS** Nonroutine supply Dx   **NC Dx** Noncancer Dx   **PDx** Primary Dx   ▶◀ Revised Text   ● New Code   ▲ Revised Title

884   ICD-10-CM 2018

Chapter 18. Symptoms, Signs and Abnormal Clinical and Laboratory Findings, Not Elsewhere Classified (R00–R99)

Chapter Specific Guidelines with Coding Examples

The chapter specific guidelines from the ICD-10-CM Official Guidelines for Coding and Reporting have been provided below. Along with these guidelines are coding examples, contained in the shaded boxes, that have been developed to help illustrate the coding and/or sequencing guidance found in these guidelines.

Chapter 18 includes symptoms, signs, abnormal results of clinical or other investigative procedures, and ill-defined conditions regarding which no diagnosis classifiable elsewhere is recorded. Signs and symptoms that point to a specific diagnosis have been assigned to a category in other chapters of the classification.

a. Use of symptom codes

Codes that describe symptoms and signs are acceptable for reporting purposes when a related definitive diagnosis has not been established (confirmed) by the provider.

Chest pain of unknown origin

R07.9   Chest pain, unspecified

Explanation: Codes that describe symptoms such as chest pain are acceptable for reporting purposes when the provider has not established (confirmed) a related definitive diagnosis.

b. Use of a symptom code with a definitive diagnosis code

Codes for signs and symptoms may be reported in addition to a related definitive diagnosis when the sign or symptom is not routinely associated with that diagnosis, such as the various signs and symptoms associated with complex syndromes. The definitive diagnosis code should be sequenced before the symptom code.

Signs or symptoms that are associated routinely with a disease process should not be assigned as additional codes, unless otherwise instructed by the classification.

Pneumonia with hemoptysis

J18.9   Pneumonia, unspecified organism

R04.2   Hemoptysis

Explanation: Codes for signs and symptoms may be reported in addition to a related definitive diagnosis when the sign or symptom is not routinely associated with that diagnosis.

Parkinson's disease noted with shuffling gait and weakness

G20   Parkinson's disease

Explanation: Codes for signs and symptoms routinely associated with a disease process should not be assigned unless the classification instructs otherwise. Shuffling or abnormal gait patterns as well as weakness are inherent symptoms of Parkinson's disease.

c. Combination codes that include symptoms

ICD-10-CM contains a number of combination codes that identify both the definitive diagnosis and common symptoms of that diagnosis. When using one of these combination codes, an additional code should not be assigned for the symptom.

Acute gastritis with hemorrhage

K29.01   Acute gastritis with bleeding

Explanation: When a combination code identifies both the definitive diagnosis and the symptom, an additional code should not be assigned for the symptom.

d. Repeated falls

Code R29.6, Repeated falls, is for use for encounters when a patient has recently fallen and the reason for the fall is being investigated.

Code Z91.81, History of falling, is for use when a patient has fallen in the past and is at risk for future falls. When appropriate, both codes R29.6 and Z91.81 may be assigned together.

e. Coma scale

The coma scale codes (R40.2-) can be used in conjunction with traumatic brain injury codes, acute cerebrovascular disease or sequelae of cerebrovascular disease codes. These codes are primarily for use by trauma registries, but they may be used in any setting where this information is collected. The coma scale may also be used to assess the status of the central nervous system for other non-trauma conditions, such as monitoring patients in the intensive care unit regardless of medical condition. The coma scale codes should be sequenced after the diagnosis code(s).

These codes, one from each subcategory, are needed to complete the scale. The 7th character indicates when the scale was recorded. The 7th character should match for all three codes.

At a minimum, report the initial score documented on presentation at your facility. This may be a score from the emergency medicine technician (EMT) or in the emergency department. If desired, a facility may choose to capture multiple coma scale scores.

Assign code R40.24, Glasgow coma scale, total score, when only the total score is documented in the medical record and not the individual score(s).

A 23-year-old male was found unresponsive due to a skull fracture with concussion and loss of consciousness of unknown duration resulting from an unidentified injury. He was admitted to the hospital, placed on ventilator support, and remained unresponsive. Four weeks following the event, he is sent home with home care and on a home ventilator. He remains unresponsive to all stimuli.

S02.0XXD   Fracture of vault of skull, subsequent encounter for fracture with routine healing

S06.0X9D   Concussion with loss of consciousness of unspecified duration, subsequent encounter

R40.2114   Coma scale, eyes open, never, 24 hours or more after hospital admission

R40.2214   Coma scale, best verbal response, none, 24 hours or more after hospital admission

R40.2314   Coma scale, best motor response, none, 24 hours or more after hospital admission

Z99.11   Dependence on respirator [ventilator] status

Explanation: When individual scores for the Glasgow coma scale are documented, codes from each category are needed to complete the scale. The seventh character 4 indicates that the scores were recorded 24 hours or more after hospital admission. Assign a code from subcategory R40.24- Glasgow coma scale, total score, when only the total and not individual score(s) is documented. Coma scale scores, when coded, should be sequenced after any associated fracture of the skull or intracranial injury.

f. Functional quadriplegia
GUIDELINE HAS BEEN DELETED EFFECTIVE OCTOBER 1, 2017

g. SIRS due to non-infectious process

The systemic inflammatory response syndrome (SIRS) can develop as a result of certain non-infectious disease processes, such as trauma, malignant neoplasm, or pancreatitis. When SIRS is documented with a noninfectious condition, and no subsequent infection is documented, the code for the underlying condition, such as an injury, should be assigned, followed by code R65.10, Systemic inflammatory response syndrome (SIRS) of non-infectious origin without acute organ dysfunction, or code R65.11, Systemic inflammatory response syndrome (SIRS) of non-infectious origin with acute organ dysfunction. If an associated acute organ dysfunction is documented, the appropriate code(s) for the specific type of organ dysfunction(s) should be assigned in addition to code R65.11. If acute organ dysfunction is documented, but it cannot be determined if the acute organ dysfunction is associated with SIRS or due to another condition (e.g., directly due to the trauma), the provider should be queried

Systemic inflammatory response syndrome (SIRS) due to acute gallstone pancreatitis

K85.10   **Biliary acute pancreatitis without necrosis or infection**

R65.10   **Systemic inflammatory response syndrome (SIRS) of noninfectious origin without acute organ dysfunction**

Explanation: When SIRS is documented with a noninfectious condition without subsequent infection documented, the code for the underlying condition such as pancreatitis should be assigned followed by the appropriate code for SIRS of noninfectious origin, either with or without associated organ dysfunction.

h.   Death NOS

Code R99, Ill-defined and unknown cause of mortality, is only for use in the very limited circumstance when a patient who has already died is brought into an emergency department or other healthcare facility and is pronounced dead upon arrival. It does not represent the discharge disposition of death.

i.   NIHSS stroke scale

The NIH stroke scale (NIHSS) codes (R29.7- -) can be used in conjunction with acute stroke codes (I63) to identify the patient's neurological status and the severity of the stroke. The stroke scale codes should be sequenced after the acute stroke diagnosis code(s).

At a minimum, report the initial score documented. If desired, a facility may choose to capture multiple stroke scale scores.

See Section I.B.14. for information concerning the medical record documentation that may be used for assignment of the NIHSS codes.

Chapter 18. Symptoms, Signs and Abnormal Clinical and Laboratory Findings, Not Elsewhere Classified (R00-R99)

NOTE This chapter includes symptoms, signs, abnormal results of clinical or other investigative procedures, and ill-defined conditions regarding which no diagnosis classifiable elsewhere is recorded.

Signs and symptoms that point rather definitely to a given diagnosis have been assigned to a category in other chapters of the classification. In general, categories in this chapter include the less well-defined conditions and symptoms that, without the necessary study of the case to establish a final diagnosis, point perhaps equally to two or more diseases or to two or more systems of the body. Practically all categories in the chapter could be designated "not otherwise specified", "unknown etiology" or "transient". The Alphabetical Index should be consulted to determine which symptoms and signs are to be allocated here and which to other chapters. The residual subcategories, numbered .8, are generally provided for other relevant symptoms that cannot be allocated elsewhere in the classification.

The conditions and signs or symptoms included in categories R00-R94 consist of:

(a) cases for which no more specific diagnosis can be made even after all the facts bearing on the case have been investigated;

(b) signs or symptoms existing at the time of initial encounter that proved to be transient and whose causes could not be determined;

(c) provisional diagnosis in a patient who failed to return for further investigation or care;

(d) cases referred elsewhere for investigation or treatment before the diagnosis was made;

(e) cases in which a more precise diagnosis was not available for any other reason;

(f) certain symptoms, for which supplementary information is provided, that represent important problems in medical care in their own right.

EXCLUDES 2 *abnormal findings on antenatal screening of mother (O28.-)*
certain conditions originating in the perinatal period (P04-P96)
signs and symptoms classified in the body system chapters
signs and symptoms of breast (N63, N64.5)

AHA: 2017, 1Q, 6, 7

This chapter contains the following blocks:

R00-R09	Symptoms and signs involving the circulatory and respiratory systems
R10-R19	Symptoms and signs involving the digestive system and abdomen
R20-R23	Symptoms and signs involving the skin and subcutaneous tissue
R25-R29	Symptoms and signs involving the nervous and musculoskeletal systems
R30-R39	Symptoms and signs involving the genitourinary system
R40-R46	Symptoms and signs involving cognition, perception, emotional state and behavior
R47-R49	Symptoms and signs involving speech and voice
R50-R69	General symptoms and signs
R70-R79	Abnormal findings on examination of blood, without diagnosis
R80-R82	Abnormal findings on examination of urine, without diagnosis
R83-R89	Abnormal findings on examination of other body fluids, substances and tissues, without diagnosis
R90-R94	Abnormal findings on diagnostic imaging and in function studies, without diagnosis
R97	Abnormal tumor markers
R99	Ill-defined and unknown cause of mortality

Symptoms and signs involving the circulatory and respiratory systems (R00-R09)

✓4ᵗʰ R00 Abnormalities of heart beat
> **EXCLUDES 1** *abnormalities originating in the perinatal period (P29.1-)*
> **EXCLUDES 2** *specified arrhythmias (I47-I49)*

    R00.0 Tachycardia, unspecified ▽
> Rapid heart beat
> Sinoauricular tachycardia NOS
> Sinus [sinusal] tachycardia NOS
> > **EXCLUDES 1** *neonatal tachycardia (P29.11)*
> > *paroxysmal tachycardia (I47.-)*
> > **DEF:** Excessively rapid heart rate of more than 100 beats per minute.

    R00.1 Bradycardia, unspecified ▽
> Sinoatrial bradycardia
> Sinus bradycardia
> Slow heart beat
> Vagal bradycardia
> Use additional code for adverse effect, if applicable, to identify drug (T36-T50 with fifth or sixth character 5)
> > **EXCLUDES 1** *neonatal bradycardia (P29.12)*

    R00.2 Palpitations
> Awareness of heart beat

    R00.8 Other abnormalities of heart beat

    R00.9 Unspecified abnormalities of heart beat ▽

✓4ᵗʰ R01 Cardiac murmurs and other cardiac sounds
> **EXCLUDES 1** *cardiac murmurs and sounds originating in the perinatal period (P29.8)*

    R01.0 Benign and innocent cardiac murmurs
> Functional cardiac murmur

    R01.1 Cardiac murmur, unspecified ▽
> Cardiac bruit NOS
> Heart murmur NOS
> Systolic murmur NOS

    R01.2 Other cardiac sounds
> Cardiac dullness, increased or decreased
> Precordial friction

✓4ᵗʰ R03 Abnormal blood-pressure reading, without diagnosis

    R03.0 Elevated blood-pressure reading, without diagnosis of hypertension
> **NOTE** This category is to be used to record an episode of elevated blood pressure in a patient in whom no formal diagnosis of hypertension has been made, or as an isolated incidental finding.

    R03.1 Nonspecific low blood-pressure reading
> **EXCLUDES 1** *hypotension (I95.-)*
> *maternal hypotension syndrome (O26.5-)*
> *neurogenic orthostatic hypotension (G90.3)*

✓4ᵗʰ R04 Hemorrhage from respiratory passages

    R04.0 Epistaxis
> Hemorrhage from nose
> Nosebleed

    R04.1 Hemorrhage from throat
> **EXCLUDES 2** *hemoptysis (R04.2)*

    R04.2 Hemoptysis
> Blood-stained sputum
> Cough with hemorrhage
> **AHA:** 2013, 4Q, 118

✓6ᵗʰ R04.8 Hemorrhage from other sites in respiratory passages

      R04.81 Acute idiopathic pulmonary hemorrhage in infants [P]
> AIPHI
> Acute idiopathic hemorrhage in infants over 28 days old
> > **EXCLUDES 1** *perinatal pulmonary hemorrhage (P26.-)*
> > *von Willebrand's disease (D68.0)*

      R04.89 Hemorrhage from other sites in respiratory passages
> Pulmonary hemorrhage NOS

    R04.9 Hemorrhage from respiratory passages, unspecified ▽

R05 Cough
> **EXCLUDES 1** *cough with hemorrhage (R04.2)*
> *smoker's cough (J41.0)*
> **AHA:** 2016, 2Q, 33

✓4ᵗʰ R06 Abnormalities of breathing
> **EXCLUDES 1** *acute respiratory distress syndrome (J80)*
> *respiratory arrest (R09.2)*
> *respiratory arrest of newborn (P28.81)*
> *respiratory distress syndrome of newborn (P22.-)*
> *respiratory failure (J96.-)*
> *respiratory failure of newborn (P28.5)*

✓5ᵗʰ R06.0 Dyspnea
> **EXCLUDES 1** *tachypnea NOS (R06.82)*
> *transient tachypnea of newborn (P22.1)*

      R06.00 Dyspnea, unspecified ▽
> **AHA:** 2017, 1Q, 26

      R06.01 Orthopnea

      R06.02 Shortness of breath

      ● **R06.03 Acute respiratory distress**

      R06.09 Other forms of dyspnea

✓ Additional Character Req   ✓x7ᵗʰ Placeholder Alert   Case-Mix Diagnosis   Manifestation   ▽ Unspecified Dx   **EXCLUDES 1** Not coded here   **EXCLUDES 2** Not included here

ICD-10-CM 2018

887

Chapter 18. Symptoms, Signs and Abnormal Clinical and Laboratory Findings, Not Elsewhere Classified

R06.1 Stridor
> EXCLUDES 1   *congenital laryngeal stridor (P28.89)*
> *laryngismus (stridulus) (J38.5)*

R06.2 Wheezing
> EXCLUDES 1   *asthma (J45.-)*
> **AHA:** 2016, 2Q, 33
> **DEF:** High-pitched whistling sound during breathing due to stenosis of respiratory passageway; associated with asthma, sleep apnea, bronchiectasis, bronchiolitis, COPD, and pleural effusion.

R06.3 Periodic breathing
> Cheyne-Stokes breathing

R06.4 Hyperventilation
> EXCLUDES 1   *psychogenic hyperventilation (F45.8)*

R06.5 Mouth breathing
> EXCLUDES 2   *dry mouth NOS (R68.2)*

R06.6 Hiccough
> EXCLUDES 1   *psychogenic hiccough (F45.8)*

R06.7 Sneezing

✓5th **R06.8 Other abnormalities of breathing**

     R06.81 Apnea, not elsewhere classified
> Apnea NOS
> EXCLUDES 1   *apnea (of) newborn (P28.4)*
> *sleep apnea (G47.3-)*
> *sleep apnea of newborn (primary) (P28.3)*

     R06.82 Tachypnea, not elsewhere classified
> Tachypnea NOS
> EXCLUDES 1   *transitory tachypnea of newborn (P22.1)*

     R06.83 Snoring

     R06.89 Other abnormalities of breathing
> Breath-holding (spells)
> Sighing

R06.9 Unspecified abnormalities of breathing ▽

✓4th **R07 Pain in throat and chest**
> EXCLUDES 1   *epidemic myalgia (B33.0)*
> EXCLUDES 2   *jaw pain (R68.84)*
> *pain in breast (N64.4)*

     R07.0 Pain in throat
> EXCLUDES 1   *chronic sore throat (J31.2)*
> *sore throat (acute) NOS (J02.9)*
> EXCLUDES 2   *dysphagia (R13.1-)*
> *pain in neck (M54.2)*

     R07.1 Chest pain on breathing
> Painful respiration

     R07.2 Precordial pain

✓5th **R07.8 Other chest pain**

     R07.81 Pleurodynia
> Pleurodynia NOS
> EXCLUDES 1   *epidemic pleurodynia (B33.0)*

     R07.82 Intercostal pain

     R07.89 Other chest pain
> Anterior chest-wall pain NOS

     R07.9 Chest pain, unspecified ▽

✓4th **R09 Other symptoms and signs involving the circulatory and respiratory system**
> EXCLUDES 1   *acute respiratory distress syndrome (J80)*
> *respiratory arrest of newborn (P28.81)*
> *respiratory distress syndrome of newborn (P22.0)*
> *respiratory failure (J96.-)*
> *respiratory failure of newborn (P28.5)*

✓5th **R09.0 Asphyxia and hypoxemia**
> EXCLUDES 1   *asphyxia due to carbon monoxide (T58.-)*
> *asphyxia due to foreign body in respiratory tract (T17.-)*
> *birth (intrauterine) asphyxia (P84)*
> *hypercapnia (R06.4)*
> *hyperventilation (R06.4)*
> *traumatic asphyxia (T71.-)*
> EXCLUDES 2   ▶*hypercapnia (R06.89)*◀

     R09.01 Asphyxia

     R09.02 Hypoxemia

     R09.1 Pleurisy
> EXCLUDES 1   *pleurisy with effusion (J90)*

R09.2 Respiratory arrest
> Cardiorespiratory failure
> EXCLUDES 1   *cardiac arrest (I46.-)*
> *respiratory arrest of newborn (P28.81)*
> *respiratory distress of newborn (P22.0)*
> *respiratory failure (J96.-)*
> *respiratory failure of newborn (P28.5)*
> *respiratory insufficiency (R06.89)*
> *respiratory insufficiency of newborn (P28.5)*

R09.3 Abnormal sputum
> Abnormal amount of sputum
> Abnormal color of sputum
> Abnormal odor of sputum
> Excessive sputum
> EXCLUDES 1   *blood-stained sputum (R04.2)*

✓5th **R09.8 Other specified symptoms and signs involving the circulatory and respiratory systems**

     R09.81 Nasal congestion

     R09.82 Postnasal drip

     R09.89 Other specified symptoms and signs involving the circulatory and respiratory systems
> Abnormal chest percussion
> Bruit (arterial)
> Chest tympany
> Choking sensation
> Feeling of foreign body in throat
> Friction sounds in chest
> Rales
> Weak pulse
> EXCLUDES 2   *foreign body in throat (T17.2-)*
> *wheezing (R06.2)*

Symptoms and signs involving the digestive system and abdomen (R10-R19)

> EXCLUDES 2   *congenital or infantile pylorospasm (Q40.0)*
> *gastrointestinal hemorrhage (K92.0-K92.2)*
> *intestinal obstruction (K56.-)*
> *newborn gastrointestinal hemorrhage (P54.0-P54.3)*
> *newborn intestinal obstruction (P76.-)*
> *pylorospasm (K31.3)*
> *signs and symptoms involving the urinary system (R30-R39)*
> *symptoms referable to female genital organs (N94.-)*
> *symptoms referable to male genital organs (N48-N50)*

✓4th **R10 Abdominal and pelvic pain**
> EXCLUDES 1   *renal colic (N23)*
> EXCLUDES 2   *dorsalgia (M54.-)*
> *flatulence and related conditions (R14.-)*
> **TIP:** Codes from category R10 may be assigned concurrently with a G89 code for pain if needed to describe the site of the pain.

     R10.0 Acute abdomen
> Severe abdominal pain (generalized) (with abdominal rigidity)
> EXCLUDES 1   *abdominal rigidity NOS (R19.3)*
> *generalized abdominal pain NOS (R10.84)*
> *localized abdominal pain (R10.1-R10.3-)*

✓5th **R10.1 Pain localized to upper abdomen**

     R10.10 Upper abdominal pain, unspecified ▽

     R10.11 Right upper quadrant pain

     R10.12 Left upper quadrant pain

     R10.13 Epigastric pain
> Dyspepsia
> EXCLUDES 1   *functional dyspepsia (K30)*

     R10.2 Pelvic and perineal pain
> EXCLUDES 1   *vulvodynia (N94.81)*

✓5th **R10.3 Pain localized to other parts of lower abdomen**

     R10.30 Lower abdominal pain, unspecified ▽

     R10.31 Right lower quadrant pain

     R10.32 Left lower quadrant pain

     R10.33 Periumbilical pain

✓5th **R10.8 Other abdominal pain**

     ✓6th **R10.81 Abdominal tenderness**
> Abdominal tenderness NOS

         R10.811 Right upper quadrant abdominal tenderness

         R10.812 Left upper quadrant abdominal tenderness

         R10.813 Right lower quadrant abdominal tenderness

N Newborn: 0   P Pediatric: 0-17   M Maternity: 12-55   A Adult: 15-124   NRS Nonroutine supply Dx   NC Dx Noncancer Dx   PD Primary Dx   ▶◀ Revised Text   ● New Code   ▲ Revised Title

R06.1–R10.813

888   ICD-10-CM 2018

Abdominal Pain

Right upper quadrant (RUQ)
Left upper quadrant (LUQ)
Epigastric
Periumbilical
Right lower quadrant (RLQ)
Left lower quadrant (LLQ)

Swallowing Function

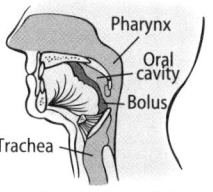

Soft palate — Bolus — Palatine tonsil
Oral phase

Pharynx — Oral cavity — Bolus — Trachea
Oropharyngeal phase

Tongue — Bolus — Epiglottis — Esophagus
Pharyngeal phase

Bolus — Epiglottis — Trachea
Pharyngoesophageal phase

R10.814 Left lower quadrant abdominal tenderness
R10.815 Periumbilic abdominal tenderness
R10.816 Epigastric abdominal tenderness
R10.817 Generalized abdominal tenderness
R10.819 Abdominal tenderness, unspecified site ▽

✓6ᵗʰ **R10.82** Rebound abdominal tenderness
R10.821 Right upper quadrant rebound abdominal tenderness
R10.822 Left upper quadrant rebound abdominal tenderness
R10.823 Right lower quadrant rebound abdominal tenderness
R10.824 Left lower quadrant rebound abdominal tenderness
R10.825 Periumbilic rebound abdominal tenderness
R10.826 Epigastric rebound abdominal tenderness
R10.827 Generalized rebound abdominal tenderness
R10.829 Rebound abdominal tenderness, unspecified site ▽

R10.83 Colic P
Colic NOS   Infantile colic
DEF: Inconsolable crying in an otherwise well-fed and healthy infant for more than three hours a day, three days a week, for more than three weeks.
EXCLUDES 1 *colic in adult and child over 12 months old (R10.84)*

R10.84 Generalized abdominal pain
EXCLUDES 1 *generalized abdominal pain associated with acute abdomen (R10.0)*

R10.9 Unspecified abdominal pain ▽

✓4ᵗʰ **R11** Nausea and vomiting
EXCLUDES 1 *cyclical vomiting associated with migraine (G43.A-)*
excessive vomiting in pregnancy (O21.-)
hematemesis (K92.0)
neonatal hematemesis (P54.0)
newborn vomiting (P92.0-)
psychogenic vomiting (F50.89)
vomiting associated with bulimia nervosa (F50.2)
vomiting following gastrointestinal surgery (K91.0)
AHA: 2017, 1Q, 28
TIP: Assign along with K31.89 Other diseases of stomach and duodenum, to describe cyclical vomiting not due to migraine.
R11.0 Nausea
Nausea NOS
Nausea without vomiting

✓5ᵗʰ **R11.1** Vomiting
R11.10 Vomiting, unspecified ▽
Vomiting NOS
R11.11 Vomiting without nausea
R11.12 Projectile vomiting
R11.13 Vomiting of fecal matter
R11.14 Bilious vomiting
Bilious emesis

R11.2 Nausea with vomiting, unspecified ▽
Persistent nausea with vomiting NOS

R12 Heartburn
EXCLUDES 1 *dyspepsia NOS (R10.13)*
functional dyspepsia (K30)

✓4ᵗʰ **R13** Aphagia and dysphagia
R13.0 Aphagia
Inability to swallow
EXCLUDES 1 *psychogenic aphagia (F50.9)*

✓5ᵗʰ **R13.1** Dysphagia
Code first, if applicable, dysphagia following cerebrovascular disease (I69. with final characters -91)
EXCLUDES 1 *psychogenic dysphagia (F45.8)*
R13.10 Dysphagia, unspecified ▽
Difficulty in swallowing NOS
R13.11 Dysphagia, oral phase
R13.12 Dysphagia, oropharyngeal phase
R13.13 Dysphagia, pharyngeal phase
R13.14 Dysphagia, pharyngoesophageal phase
R13.19 Other dysphagia
Cervical dysphagia
Neurogenic dysphagia

✓4ᵗʰ **R14** Flatulence and related conditions
EXCLUDES 1 *psychogenic aerophagy (F45.8)*
R14.0 Abdominal distension (gaseous)
Bloating
Tympanites (abdominal) (intestinal)
R14.1 Gas pain
R14.2 Eructation
R14.3 Flatulence

✓4ᵗʰ **R15** Fecal incontinence
INCLUDES encopresis NOS
EXCLUDES 1 *fecal incontinence of nonorganic origin (F98.1)*
R15.0 Incomplete defecation
EXCLUDES 1 *constipation (K59.0-)*
fecal impaction (K56.41)
R15.1 Fecal smearing
Fecal soiling
R15.2 Fecal urgency
R15.9 Full incontinence of feces
Fecal incontinence NOS

✓4ᵗʰ **R16** Hepatomegaly and splenomegaly, not elsewhere classified
R16.0 Hepatomegaly, not elsewhere classified
Hepatomegaly NOS
R16.1 Splenomegaly, not elsewhere classified
Splenomegaly NOS
R16.2 Hepatomegaly with splenomegaly, not elsewhere classified
Hepatosplenomegaly NOS

R17 Unspecified jaundice ▽
EXCLUDES 1 *neonatal jaundice (P55, P57-P59)*

✓ Additional Character Req   ✓x7ᵗʰ Placeholder Alert   Case-Mix Diagnosis   Manifestation   ▽ Unspecified Dx   **EXCLUDES 1** Not coded here   **EXCLUDES 2** Not included here

✓4ᵗʰ R18   Ascites

INCLUDES   fluid in peritoneal cavity
EXCLUDES 1   *ascites in alcoholic cirrhosis (K70.31)*
ascites in alcoholic hepatitis (K70.11)
ascites in toxic liver disease with chronic active hepatitis (K71.51)

R18.0   **Malignant** ascites

Code first malignancy, such as:
    malignant neoplasm of ovary (C56.-)
    secondary malignant neoplasm of retroperitoneum and
    peritoneum (C78.6)

R18.8   **Other ascites**

Ascites NOS
Peritoneal effusion (chronic)

✓4ᵗʰ R19   Other symptoms and signs involving the digestive system and abdomen

EXCLUDES 1   *acute abdomen (R10.0)*

✓5ᵗʰ R19.0   Intra-abdominal and pelvic swelling, mass and lump

EXCLUDES 1   *abdominal distension (gaseous) (R14.-)*
ascites (R18.-)

R19.00   **Intra-abdominal and pelvic swelling, mass and lump, unspecified site** ▽

R19.01   **Right upper quadrant** abdominal swelling, mass and lump

R19.02   **Left upper quadrant** abdominal swelling, mass and lump

R19.03   **Right lower quadrant** abdominal swelling, mass and lump

R19.04   **Left lower quadrant** abdominal swelling, mass and lump

R19.05   **Periumbilic** swelling, mass or lump
    Diffuse or generalized umbilical swelling or mass

R19.06   **Epigastric** swelling, mass or lump

R19.07   **Generalized** intra-abdominal and pelvic swelling, mass and lump
    Diffuse or generalized intra-abdominal swelling or mass NOS
    Diffuse or generalized pelvic swelling or mass NOS

R19.09   **Other intra-abdominal and pelvic swelling, mass and lump**

✓5ᵗʰ R19.1   Abnormal bowel sounds

R19.11   **Absent** bowel sounds

R19.12   **Hyperactive** bowel sounds

R19.15   **Other abnormal bowel sounds**
    Abnormal bowel sounds NOS

R19.2   Visible peristalsis

Hyperperistalsis
DEF: Visible movements of muscular attempts to move food through the digestive tract; due to pyloric obstruction, stomach obstruction, or intestinal obstruction.

✓5ᵗʰ R19.3   Abdominal rigidity

EXCLUDES 1   *abdominal rigidity with severe abdominal pain (R10.0)*

R19.30   **Abdominal rigidity, unspecified site** ▽

R19.31   **Right upper quadrant** abdominal rigidity

R19.32   **Left upper quadrant** abdominal rigidity

R19.33   **Right lower quadrant** abdominal rigidity

R19.34   **Left lower quadrant** abdominal rigidity

R19.35   **Periumbilic** abdominal rigidity

R19.36   **Epigastric** abdominal rigidity

R19.37   **Generalized** abdominal rigidity

R19.4   Change in bowel habit

EXCLUDES 1   *constipation (K59.0-)*
functional diarrhea (K59.1)

R19.5   Other fecal abnormalities

Abnormal stool color   Occult blood in feces
Bulky stools   Occult blood in stools
Mucus in stools
EXCLUDES 1   *melena (K92.1)*
neonatal melena (P54.1)

R19.6   Halitosis

R19.7   Diarrhea, unspecified ▽

Diarrhea NOS
EXCLUDES 1   *functional diarrhea (K59.1)*
neonatal diarrhea (P78.3)
psychogenic diarrhea (F45.8)

R19.8   Other specified symptoms and signs involving the digestive system and abdomen

---

Symptoms and signs involving the skin and subcutaneous tissue (R20-R23)

EXCLUDES 2   *symptoms relating to breast (N64.4-N64.5)*

✓4ᵗʰ R20   Disturbances of skin sensation

EXCLUDES 1   *dissociative anesthesia and sensory loss (F44.6)*
psychogenic disturbances (F45.8)

R20.0   Anesthesia **of skin**

R20.1   Hypoesthesia **of skin**

R20.2   Paresthesia **of skin**

Formication
Pins and needles
Tingling skin
EXCLUDES 1   *acroparesthesia (I73.8)*

R20.3   Hyperesthesia

R20.8   Other disturbances of skin sensation

R20.9   Unspecified disturbances of skin sensation ▽

R21   Rash and other nonspecific skin eruption

INCLUDES   rash NOS
EXCLUDES 1   *specified type of rash—code to condition*
vesicular eruption (R23.8)

✓4ᵗʰ R22   Localized swelling, mass and lump of skin and subcutaneous tissue

INCLUDES   subcutaneous nodules (localized)(superficial)
EXCLUDES 1   *abnormal findings on diagnostic imaging (R90-R93)*
edema (R60.-)
enlarged lymph nodes (R59.-)
localized adiposity (E65)
swelling of joint (M25.4-)

R22.0   Localized swelling, mass and lump, **head**

R22.1   Localized swelling, mass and lump, **neck**

R22.2   Localized swelling, mass and lump, **trunk**

EXCLUDES 1   *intra-abdominal or pelvic mass and lump (R19.0-)*
intra-abdominal or pelvic swelling (R19.0-)
EXCLUDES 2   *breast mass and lump (N63)*

✓5ᵗʰ R22.3   Localized swelling, mass and lump, **upper limb**

R22.30   **Localized swelling, mass and lump, unspecified upper limb** ▽

R22.31   **Localized swelling, mass and lump, right upper limb**

R22.32   **Localized swelling, mass and lump, left upper limb**

R22.33   **Localized swelling, mass and lump, upper limb, bilateral**

✓5ᵗʰ R22.4   Localized swelling, mass and lump, **lower limb**

R22.40   **Localized swelling, mass and lump, unspecified lower limb** ▽

R22.41   **Localized swelling, mass and lump, right lower limb**

R22.42   **Localized swelling, mass and lump, left lower limb**

R22.43   **Localized swelling, mass and lump, lower limb, bilateral**

R22.9   Localized swelling, mass and lump, unspecified ▽

✓4ᵗʰ R23   Other skin changes

R23.0   Cyanosis

EXCLUDES 1   *acrocyanosis (I73.8)*
cyanotic attacks of newborn (P28.2)
DEF: Bluish or purplish discoloration of the skin due to inadequate oxygen level of blood.

R23.1   Pallor

Clammy skin

R23.2   Flushing

Excessive blushing
Code first, if applicable, menopausal and female climacteric states (N95.1)

R23.3   Spontaneous ecchymoses

Petechiae
EXCLUDES 1   *ecchymoses of newborn (P54.5)*
purpura (D69.-)

R23.4   Changes in skin texture

Desquamation of skin
Induration of skin
Scaling of skin
EXCLUDES 1   *epidermal thickening NOS (L85.9)*

R23.8   Other skin changes

R23.9   Unspecified skin changes ▽

Symptoms and signs involving the nervous and musculoskeletal systems (R25-R29)

✓4ᵗʰ R25 Abnormal involuntary movements

> **EXCLUDES 1** specific movement disorders (G20-G26)
> stereotyped movement disorders (F98.4)
> tic disorders (F95.-)

R25.0 Abnormal head movements

R25.1 Tremor, unspecified ▽

> **EXCLUDES 1** chorea NOS (G25.5)
> essential tremor (G25.0)
> hysterical tremor (F44.4)
> intention tremor (G25.2)

R25.2 Cramp and spasm

> **EXCLUDES 2** carpopedal spasm (R29.0)
> charley-horse (M62.831)
> infantile spasms (G40.4-)
> muscle spasm of back (M62.830)
> muscle spasm of calf (M62.831)

R25.3 Fasciculation
Twitching NOS

R25.8 Other abnormal involuntary movements

R25.9 Unspecified abnormal involuntary movements ▽

✓4ᵗʰ R26 Abnormalities of gait and mobility

> **EXCLUDES 1** ataxia NOS (R27.0)
> hereditary ataxia (G11.-)
> locomotor (syphilitic) ataxia (A52.11)
> immobility syndrome (paraplegic) (M62.3)

TIP: Assign when the abnormality of gait or mobility is not integral to a known diagnosis.

R26.0 Ataxic gait
Staggering gait

R26.1 Paralytic gait
Spastic gait

R26.2 Difficulty in walking, not elsewhere classified

> **EXCLUDES 1** falling (R29.6)
> unsteadiness on feet (R26.81)

AHA: 2016, 2Q, 7

✓5ᵗʰ R26.8 Other abnormalities of gait and mobility

R26.81 Unsteadiness on feet

R26.89 Other abnormalities of gait and mobility

R26.9 Unspecified abnormalities of gait and mobility ▽

✓4ᵗʰ R27 Other lack of coordination

> **EXCLUDES 1** ataxic gait (R26.0)
> hereditary ataxia (G11.-)
> vertigo NOS (R42)

R27.0 Ataxia, unspecified ▽

> **EXCLUDES 1** ataxia following cerebrovascular disease (I69. with final characters -93)

R27.8 Other lack of coordination

R27.9 Unspecified lack of coordination ▽

✓4ᵗʰ R29 Other symptoms and signs involving the nervous and musculoskeletal systems

R29.0 Tetany
Carpopedal spasm

> **EXCLUDES 1** hysterical tetany (F44.5)
> neonatal tetany (P71.3)
> parathyroid tetany (E20.9)
> post-thyroidectomy tetany (E89.2)

R29.1 Meningismus

R29.2 Abnormal reflex

> **EXCLUDES 2** abnormal pupillary reflex (H57.0)
> hyperactive gag reflex (J39.2)
> vasovagal reaction or syncope (R55)

R29.3 Abnormal posture

R29.4 Clicking hip

> **EXCLUDES 1** congenital deformities of hip (Q65.-)

R29.5 Transient paralysis
Code first any associated spinal cord injury (S14.0, S14.1-, S24.0, S24.1-, S34.0-, S34.1-)

> **EXCLUDES 1** transient ischemic attack (G45.9)

R29.6 Repeated falls
Falling
Tendency to fall

> **EXCLUDES 2** at risk for falling (Z91.81)
> history of falling (Z91.81)

AHA: 2016, 2Q, 6

✓5ᵗʰ R29.7 National Institutes of Health Stroke Scale (NIHSS) score
Code first the type of cerebral infarction (I63.-)

✓6ᵗʰ R29.70 NIHSS score 0-9

R29.700	NIHSS score 0
R29.701	NIHSS score 1
R29.702	NIHSS score 2
R29.703	NIHSS score 3
R29.704	NIHSS score 4
R29.705	NIHSS score 5
R29.706	NIHSS score 6
R29.707	NIHSS score 7
R29.708	NIHSS score 8
R29.709	NIHSS score 9

✓6ᵗʰ R29.71 NIHSS score 10-19

R29.710	NIHSS score 10
R29.711	NIHSS score 11
R29.712	NIHSS score 12
R29.713	NIHSS score 13
R29.714	NIHSS score 14
R29.715	NIHSS score 15
R29.716	NIHSS score 16
R29.717	NIHSS score 17
R29.718	NIHSS score 18
R29.719	NIHSS score 19

✓6ᵗʰ R29.72 NIHSS score 20-29

R29.720	NIHSS score 20
R29.721	NIHSS score 21
R29.722	NIHSS score 22
R29.723	NIHSS score 23
R29.724	NIHSS score 24
R29.725	NIHSS score 25
R29.726	NIHSS score 26
R29.727	NIHSS score 27
R29.728	NIHSS score 28
R29.729	NIHSS score 29

✓6ᵗʰ R29.73 NIHSS score 30-39

R29.730	NIHSS score 30
R29.731	NIHSS score 31
R29.732	NIHSS score 32
R29.733	NIHSS score 33
R29.734	NIHSS score 34
R29.735	NIHSS score 35
R29.736	NIHSS score 36
R29.737	NIHSS score 37
R29.738	NIHSS score 38
R29.739	NIHSS score 39

✓6ᵗʰ R29.74 NIHSS score 40-42

R29.740	NIHSS score 40
R29.741	NIHSS score 41
R29.742	NIHSS score 42

✓5ᵗʰ R29.8 Other symptoms and signs involving the nervous and musculoskeletal systems

✓6ᵗʰ R29.81 Other symptoms and signs involving the nervous system

R29.810 Facial weakness
Facial droop

> **EXCLUDES 1** Bell's palsy (G51.0)
> facial weakness following cerebrovascular disease (I69. with final characters -92)

R29.818 Other symptoms and signs involving the nervous system

✓6ᵗʰ R29.89 Other symptoms and signs involving the musculoskeletal system

> **EXCLUDES 2** pain in limb (M79.6-)

R29.890 Loss of height

> **EXCLUDES 1** osteoporosis (M80-M81)

✓ Additional Character Req   ✓x7ᵗʰ Placeholder Alert   Case-Mix Diagnosis   Manifestation   ▽ Unspecified Dx   **EXCLUDES 1** Not coded here   **EXCLUDES 2** Not included here

R29.891 **Ocular torticollis**
EXCLUDES1   *congenital (sternomastoid)*
torticollis Q68.0
psychogenic torticollis (F45.8)
spasmodic torticollis (G24.3)
torticollis due to birth injury
(P15.8)
torticollis NOS M43.6
DEF: Abnormal head posture as a result of a
contracted state of cervical muscles to
correct a visual disturbance, either double
vision or a visual field defect.

R29.898 **Other symptoms and signs involving the**
musculoskeletal system

√5th R29.9 **Unspecified symptoms and signs involving the nervous and**
musculoskeletal systems

R29.90 **Unspecified symptoms and signs involving the** ▽
nervous system

R29.91 **Unspecified symptoms and signs involving the** ▽
musculoskeletal system

Symptoms and signs involving
the genitourinary system (R30-R39)

√4th R30 **Pain associated with micturition**
EXCLUDES1   *psychogenic pain associated with micturition (F45.8)*

R30.0 **Dysuria**
Strangury

R30.1 **Vesical tenesmus**

R30.9 **Painful micturition, unspecified** ▽
Painful urination NOS

√4th R31 **Hematuria**
EXCLUDES1   *hematuria included with underlying conditions, such as:*
acute cystitis with hematuria (N30.01)
recurrent and persistent hematuria in glomerular diseases
(N02.-)
AHA: 2017, 1Q, 17

R31.0 **Gross hematuria**

R31.1 **Benign essential microscopic hematuria**

√5th R31.2 **Other microscopic hematuria**
R31.21 **Asymptomatic microscopic hematuria**
AMH
R31.29 **Other microscopic hematuria**

R31.9 **Hematuria, unspecified** ▽

R32 **Unspecified urinary incontinence** ▽
Enuresis NOS
EXCLUDES1   *functional urinary incontinence (R39.81)*
nonorganic enuresis (F98.0)
stress incontinence and other specified urinary incontinence
(N39.3-N39.4-)
urinary incontinence associated with cognitive impairment
(R39.81)

√4th R33 **Retention of urine**
EXCLUDES1   *psychogenic retention of urine (F45.8)*

R33.0 **Drug induced retention of urine**
Use additional code for adverse effect, if applicable, to identify
drug (T36-T50 with fifth or sixth character 5)

R33.8 **Other retention of urine**
Code first, if applicable, any causal condition, such as:
enlarged prostate (N40.1)

R33.9 **Retention of urine, unspecified** ▽

R34 **Anuria and oliguria**
EXCLUDES1   *anuria and oliguria complicating abortion or ectopic or molar*
pregnancy (O00-O07, O08.4)
anuria and oliguria complicating pregnancy (O26.83-)
anuria and oliguria complicating the puerperium (O90.4)

√4th R35 **Polyuria**
Code first, if applicable, any causal condition, such as:
enlarged prostate (N40.1)
EXCLUDES1   *psychogenic polyuria (F45.8)*

R35.0 **Frequency of micturition**

R35.1 **Nocturia**

R35.8 **Other polyuria**
Polyuria NOS

√4th R36 **Urethral discharge**

R36.0 **Urethral discharge without blood**

R36.1 **Hematospermia** ♂

R36.9 **Urethral discharge, unspecified** ▽
Penile discharge NOS
Urethrorrhea

R37 **Sexual dysfunction, unspecified** ▽

√4th R39 **Other and unspecified symptoms and signs involving the**
genitourinary system

R39.0 **Extravasation of urine**

√5th R39.1 **Other difficulties with micturition**
Code first, if applicable, any causal condition, such as:
enlarged prostate (N40.1)

R39.11 **Hesitancy of micturition**

R39.12 **Poor urinary stream**
Weak urinary steam

R39.13 **Splitting of urinary stream**

R39.14 **Feeling of incomplete bladder emptying**

R39.15 **Urgency of urination**
EXCLUDES1   *urge incontinence (N39.41, N39.46)*

R39.16 **Straining to void**

√6th R39.19 **Other difficulties with micturition**
R39.191 **Need to immediately re-void**
R39.192 **Position dependent micturition**
R39.198 **Other difficulties with micturition**

R39.2 **Extrarenal uremia**
Prerenal uremia
EXCLUDES1   *uremia NOS (N19)*

√5th R39.8 **Other symptoms and signs involving the genitourinary**
system

R39.81 **Functional urinary incontinence**
Urinary incontinence due to cognitive impairment, or
severe physical disability or immobility
EXCLUDES1   *stress incontinence and other specified*
urinary incontinence (N39.3-N39.4-)
urinary incontinence NOS (R32)

R39.82 **Chronic bladder pain**

● R39.83 **Unilateral non-palpable testicle**

● R39.84 **Bilateral non-palpable testicles**

R39.89 **Other symptoms and signs involving the**
genitourinary system

R39.9 **Unspecified symptoms and signs involving the** ▽
genitourinary system

Symptoms and signs involving cognition, perception,
emotional state and behavior (R40-R46)

EXCLUDES2   *symptoms and signs constituting part of a pattern of mental disorder*
(F01-F99)

√4th R40 **Somnolence, stupor and coma**
EXCLUDES1   *neonatal coma (P91.5)*
somnolence, stupor and coma in diabetes (E08-E13)
somnolence, stupor and coma in hepatic failure (K72.-)
somnolence, stupor and coma in hypoglycemia (nondiabetic)
(E15)

R40.0 **Somnolence**
Drowsiness
EXCLUDES1   *coma (R40.2-)*

R40.1 **Stupor**
Catatonic stupor
Semicoma
EXCLUDES1   *catatonic schizophrenia (F20.2)*
coma (R40.2-)
depressive stupor (F31-F33)
dissociative stupor (F44.2)
manic stupor (F30.2)

N Newborn: 0   P Pediatric: 0-17   M Maternity: 12-55   A Adult: 15-124   NRS Nonroutine supply Dx   NCDx Noncancer Dx   PDx Primary Dx   ►◄ Revised Text   ● New Code   ▲ Revised Title

892   ICD-10-CM 2018

✓5ᵗʰ **R40.2 Coma**
Code first any associated:
  fracture of skull (S02.-)
  intracranial injury (S06.-)
> **NOTE** One code from each subcategory, R40.21-R40.23, is required to complete the coma scale

AHA: 2015, 2Q, 17; 2014, 1Q, 19

  8 R40.20 Unspecified coma   ▽
      Coma NOS
      Unconsciousness NOS

✓6ᵗʰ **R40.21 Coma scale,** eyes open

> The following appropriate 7th character is to be added to subcategories R40.21-, R40.22-, R40.23-, and R40.24-.
> Ø unspecified time
> 1 in the field [EMT or ambulance]
> 2 at arrival to emergency department
> 3 at hospital admission
> 4 24 hours or more after hospital admission

  ✓7ᵗʰ **R40.211 Coma scale, eyes open,** never
  ✓7ᵗʰ **R40.212 Coma scale, eyes open,** to pain
  ✓7ᵗʰ **R40.213 Coma scale, eyes open,** to sound
  ✓7ᵗʰ **R40.214 Coma scale, eyes open,** spontaneous

✓6ᵗʰ **R40.22 Coma scale,** best verbal response
  ✓7ᵗʰ **R40.221 Coma scale, best verbal response,** none
  ✓7ᵗʰ **R40.222 Coma scale, best verbal response, incomprehensible words**
      ▶Incomprehensible sounds
        (2-5 years of age)
      Moans/grunts to pain; restless
        (< 2 years old)◀
  ✓7ᵗʰ **R40.223 Coma scale, best verbal response, inappropriate words**
      ▶Inappropriate crying or screaming
        (< 2 years of age)
      Screaming (2-5 years of age)◀
  ✓7ᵗʰ **R40.224 Coma scale, best verbal response, confused conversation**
      ▶Inappropriate words (2-5 years of age)
      Irritable cries (< 2 years of age)◀
  ✓7ᵗʰ **R40.225 Coma scale, best verbal response, oriented**
      ▶Cooing or babbling or crying appropriately
        (< 2 years of age)
      Uses appropriate words (2- 5 years of age)◀

✓6ᵗʰ **R40.23 Coma scale,** best motor response
  ✓7ᵗʰ **R40.231 Coma scale, best motor response,** none
  ✓7ᵗʰ **R40.232 Coma scale, best motor response, extension**
      ▶Abnormal extensor posturing to pain or
        noxious stimuli (< 2 years of age)
      Extensor posturing to pain or noxious
        stimuli (2-5 years of age)◀
  ✓7ᵗʰ **R40.233 Coma scale, best motor response, abnormal**
      ▶Abnormal flexure posturing to pain or
        noxious stimuli (0-5 years of age)
      Flexion/decorticate posturing (< 2 years of age)◀
  ✓7ᵗʰ **R40.234 Coma scale, best motor response,** flexion withdrawal
      ▶Withdraws from pain or noxious stimuli
        (0-5 years of age)◀
  ✓7ᵗʰ **R40.235 Coma scale, best motor response,** localizes pain
      ▶Localizes pain (2-5 years of age)
      Withdraws to touch (< 2 years of age)◀
  ✓7ᵗʰ **R40.236 Coma scale, best motor response,** obeys commands
      ▶Normal or spontaneous movement (< 2 years of age)
      Obeys commands (2-5 years of age)◀

✓6ᵗʰ **R40.24 Glasgow coma scale, total score**
> **NOTE** Assign a code from subcategory R40.24, when only the total coma score is documented

  ✓7ᵗʰ **R40.241 Glasgow coma scale** score 13-15
  ✓7ᵗʰ **R40.242 Glasgow coma scale** score 9-12
  ✓7ᵗʰ **R40.243 Glasgow coma scale** score 3-8
  ✓7ᵗʰ **R40.244 Other coma, without documented Glasgow coma scale score, or with partial score reported**

R40.3 Persistent vegetative state
  DEF: Persistent wakefulness without consciousness due to nonfunctioning cerebral cortex.

R40.4 Transient alteration of awareness

✓4ᵗʰ **R41 Other symptoms and signs involving cognitive functions and awareness**
> **EXCLUDES 1** *dissociative [conversion] disorders (F44.-)*
>   *mild cognitive impairment, so stated (G31.84)*

  R41.0 Disorientation, unspecified   ▽
      Confusion NOS
      Delirium NOS

  R41.1 Anterograde amnesia

  R41.2 Retrograde amnesia

  R41.3 Other amnesia
      Amnesia NOS
      Memory loss NOS
> **EXCLUDES 1** *amnestic disorder due to known physiologic condition (F04)*
>   *amnestic syndrome due to psychoactive substance use (F10-F19 with 5th character .6)*
>   *mild memory disturbance due to known physiological condition (F06.8)*
>   *transient global amnesia (G45.4)*

  R41.4 Neurologic neglect syndrome
    Asomatognosia   Left-sided neglect
    Hemi-akinesia   Sensory neglect
    Hemi-inattention   Visuospatial neglect
    Hemispatial neglect
> **EXCLUDES 1** *visuospatial deficit (R41.842)*

✓5ᵗʰ **R41.8 Other symptoms and signs involving cognitive functions and awareness**
  R41.81 Age-related cognitive decline   A
      Senility NOS
  R41.82 Altered mental status, unspecified   ▽
      Change in mental status NOS
> **EXCLUDES 1** *altered level of consciousness (R40.-)*
>   *altered mental status due to known condition—code to condition*
>   *delirium NOS (R41.0)*

    AHA: 2012, 4Q, 97

  R41.83 Borderline intellectual functioning
      IQ level 71 to 84
> **EXCLUDES 1** *intellectual disabilities (F70-F79)*

✓6ᵗʰ **R41.84 Other specified cognitive deficit**
> **EXCLUDES 1** *cognitive deficits as sequelae of cerebrovascular disease (I69.01-, I69.11-, I69.21-, I69.31-, I69.81-, I69.91-)*

  R41.840 Attention and concentration deficit
> **EXCLUDES 1** *attention-deficit hyperactivity disorders (F90.-)*

  R41.841 Cognitive communication deficit
  R41.842 Visuospatial deficit
  R41.843 Psychomotor deficit
  R41.844 Frontal lobe and executive function deficit

  R41.89 Other symptoms and signs involving cognitive functions and awareness
      Anosognosia

  R41.9 Unspecified symptoms and signs involving cognitive functions and awareness   ▽
      ▶Unspecified neurocognitive disorder◀

R42 Dizziness and giddiness
  Light-headedness
  Vertigo NOS
> **EXCLUDES 1** *vertiginous syndromes (H81.-)*
>   *vertigo from infrasound (T75.23)*

✓4ᵗʰ **R43 Disturbances of smell and taste**
  R43.0 Anosmia
  R43.1 Parosmia
  R43.2 Parageusia

---

8 Hospice questionable admission diagnosis.

| ✓ Additional Character Req | ✓7ᵗʰ Placeholder Alert | Case-Mix Diagnosis | Manifestation | ▽ Unspecified Dx | EXCLUDES 1 Not coded here | EXCLUDES 2 Not included here |

Chapter 18. Symptoms, Signs and Abnormal Clinical and Laboratory Findings, Not Elsewhere Classified

R43.8   **Other disturbances of smell and taste**
Mixed disturbance of smell and taste

R43.9   **Unspecified disturbances of smell and taste** ▽

✓4th **R44**   **Other symptoms and signs involving general sensations and perceptions**
   EXCLUDES 1   alcoholic hallucinations (F1.5)
     hallucinations in drug psychosis (F11-F19 with .5)
     hallucinations in mood disorders with psychotic symptoms (F30.2, F31.5, F32.3, F33.3)
     hallucinations in schizophrenia, schizotypal and delusional disorders (F20-F29)
   EXCLUDES 2   disturbances of skin sensation (R20.-)

R44.0   **Auditory** hallucinations

R44.1   **Visual** hallucinations

R44.2   **Other hallucinations**

R44.3   **Hallucinations, unspecified** ▽

R44.8   **Other symptoms and signs involving general sensations and perceptions**

R44.9   **Unspecified symptoms and signs involving general sensations and perceptions** ▽

✓4th **R45**   **Symptoms and signs involving emotional state**

R45.0   **Nervousness**
Nervous tension

R45.1   **Restlessness and agitation**

R45.2   **Unhappiness**

R45.3   **Demoralization and apathy**
   EXCLUDES 1   anhedonia (R45.84)

R45.4   **Irritability and anger**

R45.5   **Hostility**

R45.6   **Violent behavior**

R45.7   **State of emotional shock and stress, unspecified** ▽

✓5th **R45.8**   **Other symptoms and signs involving emotional state**

   R45.81   **Low self-esteem**

   R45.82   **Worries**

   R45.83   **Excessive crying of child, adolescent or adult**
     EXCLUDES 1   excessive crying of infant (baby) R68.11

   R45.84   **Anhedonia**

   ✓6th **R45.85**   **Homicidal and suicidal ideations**
     EXCLUDES 1   suicide attempt (T14.91)

     R45.850   **Homicidal** ideations

     R45.851   **Suicidal** ideations
      DEF: Thoughts of committing suicide; no actual attempt of suicide has been made.

   R45.86   **Emotional lability**

   R45.87   **Impulsiveness**

   R45.89   **Other symptoms and signs involving emotional state**

✓4th **R46**   **Symptoms and signs involving appearance and behavior**
   EXCLUDES 1   appearance and behavior in schizophrenia, schizotypal and delusional disorders (F20-F29)
     mental and behavioral disorders (F01-F99)

R46.0   **Very low level of personal hygiene**

R46.1   **Bizarre personal appearance**

R46.2   **Strange and inexplicable behavior**

R46.3   **Overactivity**

R46.4   **Slowness and poor responsiveness**
   EXCLUDES 1   stupor (R40.1)

R46.5   **Suspiciousness and marked evasiveness**

R46.6   **Undue concern and preoccupation with stressful events**

R46.7   **Verbosity and circumstantial detail obscuring reason for contact**

✓5th **R46.8**   **Other symptoms and signs involving appearance and behavior**

   R46.81   **Obsessive-compulsive behavior**
     EXCLUDES 1   obsessive-compulsive disorder (F42-)

   R46.89   **Other symptoms and signs involving appearance and behavior**

Symptoms and signs involving speech and voice (R47-R49)

✓4th **R47**   **Speech disturbances, not elsewhere classified**
   EXCLUDES 1   autism (F84.0)
     cluttering (F80.81)
     specific developmental disorders of speech and language (F80.-)
     stuttering (F80.81)

✓5th **R47.0**   **Dysphasia and aphasia**

   R47.01   **Aphasia**
     EXCLUDES 1   aphasia following cerebrovascular disease (I69. with final characters -20)
     progressive isolated aphasia (G31.01)

   R47.02   **Dysphasia**
     EXCLUDES 1   dysphasia following cerebrovascular disease (I69. with final characters -21)

R47.1   **Dysarthria and anarthria**
   EXCLUDES 1   dysarthria following cerebrovascular disease (I69. with final characters -22)

✓5th **R47.8**   **Other speech disturbances**
   EXCLUDES 1   dysarthria following cerebrovascular disease (I69. with final characters -28)

   R47.81   **Slurred speech**

   R47.82   *Fluency disorder in conditions classified elsewhere*
     Stuttering in conditions classified elsewhere
     Code first underlying disease or condition, such as:
     Parkinson's disease (G20)
     EXCLUDES 1   adult onset fluency disorder (F98.5)
     childhood onset fluency disorder (F80.81)
     fluency disorder (stuttering) following cerebrovascular disease (I69. with final characters-23)

   R47.89   **Other speech disturbances**

R47.9   **Unspecified speech disturbances** ▽

✓4th **R48**   **Dyslexia and other symbolic dysfunctions, not elsewhere classified**
   EXCLUDES 1   specific developmental disorders of scholastic skills (F81.-)

R48.0   **Dyslexia and alexia**

R48.1   **Agnosia**
Astereognosia (astereognosis)
Autotopagnosia
   EXCLUDES 1   visual object agnosia (R48.3)

R48.2   **Apraxia**
   EXCLUDES 1   apraxia following cerebrovascular disease (I69. with final characters -90)

R48.3   **Visual agnosia**
Prosopagnosia
Simultanagnosia (asimultagnosia)

R48.8   **Other symbolic dysfunctions**
Acalculia
Agraphia
AHA: 2017, 1Q, 27
TIP: Assign to indicate echolalia. May be assigned along with F84.0 Autistic disorder, to provide additional information about symptoms being addressed by treatment that are not integral to autism.

R48.9   **Unspecified symbolic dysfunctions** ▽

✓4th **R49**   **Voice and resonance disorders**
   EXCLUDES 1   psychogenic voice and resonance disorders (F44.4)

R49.0   **Dysphonia**
Hoarseness

R49.1   **Aphonia**
Loss of voice

✓5th **R49.2**   **Hypernasality and hyponasality**

   R49.21   **Hypernasality**

   R49.22   **Hyponasality**

R49.8   **Other voice and resonance disorders**

R49.9   **Unspecified voice and resonance disorder** ▽
Change in voice NOS
Resonance disorder NOS

N Newborn: 0   P Pediatric: 0-17   M Maternity: 12-55   A Adult: 15-124   NRS Nonroutine supply Dx   NCDx Noncancer Dx   PDx Primary Dx   ►◄ Revised Text   ● New Code   ▲ Revised Title

894   ICD-10-CM 2018

General symptoms and signs (R50-R69)

✓4ᵗʰ R50　Fever of other and unknown origin
　　EXCLUDES 1　chills without fever (R68.83)
　　　　febrile convulsions (R56.0-)
　　　　fever of unknown origin during labor (O75.2)
　　　　fever of unknown origin in newborn (P81.9)
　　　　hypothermia due to illness (R68.0)
　　　　malignant hyperthermia due to anesthesia (T88.3)
　　　　puerperal pyrexia NOS (O86.4)

　R50.2　Drug induced fever
　　　Use additional code for adverse effect, if applicable, to identify drug (T36-T50 with fifth or sixth character 5)
　　　EXCLUDES 1　postvaccination (postimmunization) fever (R50.83)

　✓5ᵗʰ R50.8　Other specified fever
　　R50.81　Fever presenting with conditions classified elsewhere
　　　　Code first underlying condition when associated fever is present, such as with:
　　　　　leukemia (C91-C95)
　　　　　neutropenia (D70.-)
　　　　　sickle-cell disease (D57.-)
　　　　AHA: 2014, 4Q, 22

　　R50.82　Postprocedural fever
　　　　EXCLUDES 1　postprocedural infection (T81.4-)
　　　　　posttransfusion fever (R50.84)
　　　　　postvaccination (postimmunization) fever (R50.83)

　　R50.83　Postvaccination fever
　　　　Postimmunization fever

　　R50.84　Febrile nonhemolytic transfusion reaction
　　　　FNHTR
　　　　Posttransfusion fever

　R50.9　Fever, unspecified　　　　▽
　　　Fever NOS
　　　Fever of unknown origin [FUO]
　　　Fever with chills
　　　Fever with rigors
　　　Hyperpyrexia NOS
　　　Persistent fever
　　　Pyrexia NOS

R51　Headache
　　Facial pain NOS
　　EXCLUDES 1　atypical face pain (G50.1)
　　　　migraine and other headache syndromes (G43-G44)
　　　　trigeminal neuralgia (G50.0)

R52　Pain, unspecified　　　　▽
　　Acute pain NOS
　　Generalized pain NOS
　　Pain NOS
　　EXCLUDES 1　acute and chronic pain, not elsewhere classified (G89.-)
　　　　localized pain, unspecified type—code to pain by site, such as:
　　　　　abdomen pain (R10.-)
　　　　　back pain (M54.9)
　　　　　breast pain (N64.4)
　　　　　chest pain (R07.1-R07.9)
　　　　　ear pain (H92.0-)
　　　　　eye pain (H57.1)
　　　　　headache (R51)
　　　　　joint pain (M25.5-)
　　　　　limb pain (M79.6-)
　　　　　lumbar region pain (M54.5)
　　　　　pelvic and perineal pain (R10.2)
　　　　　renal colic (N23)
　　　　　shoulder pain (M25.51-)
　　　　　spine pain (M54.-)
　　　　　throat pain (R07.0)
　　　　　tongue pain (K14.6)
　　　　　tooth pain (K08.8)
　　　　pain disorders exclusively related to psychological factors (F45.41)

✓4ᵗʰ R53　Malaise and fatigue
　R53.0　Neoplastic (malignant) related fatigue
　　　Code first associated neoplasm

　R53.1　Weakness
　　　Asthenia NOS
　　　EXCLUDES 1　age-related weakness (R54)
　　　　muscle weakness (M62.8-)
　　　　sarcopenia (M62.84)
　　　　senile asthenia (R54)
　　　AHA: 2017, 1Q, 7; 2015, 1Q, 25

　R53.2　Functional quadriplegia
　　　Complete immobility due to severe physical disability or frailty
　　　EXCLUDES 1　frailty NOS (R54)
　　　　hysterical paralysis (F44.4)
　　　　immobility syndrome (M62.3)
　　　　neurologic quadriplegia (G82.5-)
　　　　quadriplegia (G82.50)
　　　AHA: 2016, 2Q, 6
　　　DEF: Inability to move due to a nonphysiological condition, such as dementia; no mental ability to move independently; typically found in severely demented patients.
　　　TIP: Functional quadriplegia is not considered an integral component of Alzheimer's dementia and may be coded with G30 and F02.80-.

　✓5ᵗʰ R53.8　Other malaise and fatigue
　　　EXCLUDES 1　combat exhaustion and fatigue (F43.0)
　　　　congenital debility (P96.9)
　　　　~~exhaustion and fatigue due to depressive episode (F32.-)~~
　　　　exhaustion and fatigue due to excessive exertion (T73.3)
　　　　exhaustion and fatigue due to exposure (T73.2)
　　　　exhaustion and fatigue due to heat (T67.-)
　　　　exhaustion and fatigue due to pregnancy (O26.8-)
　　　　exhaustion and fatigue due to recurrent depressive episode (F33)
　　　　exhaustion and fatigue due to senile debility (R54)

　　8 R53.81　Other malaise
　　　　Chronic debility
　　　　Debility NOS
　　　　General physical deterioration
　　　　Malaise NOS
　　　　Nervous debility
　　　　EXCLUDES 1　age-related physical debility (R54)

　　R53.82　Chronic fatigue, unspecified　　　▽
　　　　Chronic fatigue syndrome NOS
　　　　EXCLUDES 1　postviral fatigue syndrome (G93.3)

　　R53.83　Other fatigue
　　　　Fatigue NOS
　　　　Lack of energy
　　　　Lethargy
　　　　Tiredness
　　　　EXCLUDES 2　►exhaustion and fatigue due to depressive episode (F32.-)◄

8 R54　Age-related physical debility　　　　Ⓐ
　　Frailty　　　　Senile asthenia
　　Old age　　　Senile debility
　　Senescence
　　EXCLUDES 1　age-related cognitive decline (R41.81)
　　　　sarcopenia (M62.84)
　　　　senile psychosis (F03)
　　　　senility NOS (R41.81)

R55　Syncope and collapse
　　Blackout
　　Fainting
　　Vasovagal attack
　　EXCLUDES 1　cardiogenic shock (R57.0)
　　　　carotid sinus syncope (G90.01)
　　　　heat syncope (T67.1)
　　　　neurocirculatory asthenia (F45.8)
　　　　neurogenic orthostatic hypotension (G90.3)
　　　　orthostatic hypotension (I95.1)
　　　　postprocedural shock (T81.1-)
　　　　psychogenic syncope (F48.8)
　　　　shock NOS (R57.9)
　　　　shock complicating or following abortion or ectopic or molar pregnancy (O00-O07, O08.3)
　　　　shock complicating or following labor and delivery (O75.1)
　　　　Stokes-Adams attack (I45.9)
　　　　unconsciousness NOS (R40.2-)

✓4ᵗʰ R56　Convulsions, not elsewhere classified
　　EXCLUDES 1　dissociative convulsions and seizures (F44.5)
　　　　epileptic convulsions and seizures (G40.-)
　　　　newborn convulsions and seizures (P90)

　✓5ᵗʰ R56.0　Febrile convulsions
　　R56.00　Simple febrile convulsions
　　　　Febrile convulsion NOS
　　　　Febrile seizure NOS

8　Hospice questionable admission diagnosis.

☑ Additional Character Req　　✓7ᵗʰ Placeholder Alert　　Case-Mix Diagnosis　　Manifestation　　▽ Unspecified Dx　　*EXCLUDES 1* Not coded here　　*EXCLUDES 2* Not included here

Chapter 18. Symptoms, Signs and Abnormal Clinical and Laboratory Findings, Not Elsewhere Classified

R56.01   **Complex febrile convulsions**
Atypical febrile seizure
Complex febrile seizure
Complicated febrile seizure
EXCLUDES 1   *status epilepticus (G40.901)*

R56.1   **Post traumatic seizures**
EXCLUDES 1   *post traumatic epilepsy (G40.-)*

R56.9   **Unspecified convulsions** ▽
Convulsion disorder
Fit NOS
Recurrent convulsions
Seizure(s) (convulsive) NOS

✓4ᵗʰ **R57**   **Shock, not elsewhere classified**
EXCLUDES 1   *anaphylactic shock NOS (T78.2)*
anaphylactic reaction or shock due to adverse food reaction (T78.0-)
anaphylactic shock due to adverse effect of correct drug or medicament properly administered (T88.6)
anaphylactic shock due to serum (T80.5-)
anesthetic shock (T88.3)
electric shock (T75.4)
obstetric shock (O75.1)
postprocedural shock (T81.1-)
psychic shock (F43.0)
~~septic shock (R65.21)~~
shock complicating or following ectopic or molar pregnancy (O00–O07, O08.3)
shock due to lightning (T75.01)
traumatic shock (T79.4)
toxic shock syndrome (A48.3)

R57.0   **Cardiogenic shock**
EXCLUDES 2   ▶*septic shock (R65.21)*◀
DEF: Associated with myocardial infarction, cardiac tamponade, and massive pulmonary embolism; symptoms include mental confusion, reduced blood pressure, tachycardia, pallor, and cold, clammy skin.

R57.1   **Hypovolemic shock**

R57.8   **Other shock**

R57.9   **Shock, unspecified** ▽
Failure of peripheral circulation NOS

R58   **Hemorrhage, not elsewhere classified**
Hemorrhage NOS
EXCLUDES 1   *hemorrhage included with underlying conditions, such as:*
acute duodenal ulcer with hemorrhage (K26.0)
acute gastritis with bleeding (K29.01)
ulcerative enterocolitis with rectal bleeding (K51.01)

✓4ᵗʰ **R59**   **Enlarged lymph nodes**
INCLUDES   swollen glands
EXCLUDES 1   *acute lymphadenitis (L04.-)*
chronic lymphadenitis (I88.1)
lymphadenitis NOS (I88.9)
mesenteric (acute) (chronic) lymphadenitis (I88.0)

R59.0   **Localized enlarged lymph nodes**

R59.1   **Generalized enlarged lymph nodes**
Lymphadenopathy NOS

R59.9   **Enlarged lymph nodes, unspecified** ▽

✓4ᵗʰ **R60**   **Edema, not elsewhere classified**
EXCLUDES 1   *angioneurotic edema (T78.3)*
ascites (R18.-)
cerebral edema (G93.6)
cerebral edema due to birth injury (P11.0)
edema of larynx (J38.4)
edema of nasopharynx (J39.2)
edema of pharynx (J39.2)
gestational edema (O12.0-)
hereditary edema (Q82.0)
hydrops fetalis NOS (P83.2)
hydrothorax (J94.8)
~~nutritional edema (E40-E46)~~
hydrops fetalis NOS (P83.2)
newborn edema (P83.3)
pulmonary edema (J81.-)

R60.0   **Localized edema**

R60.1   **Generalized edema**
EXCLUDES 2   ▶*nutritional edema (E40-E46)*◀

R60.9   **Edema, unspecified** ▽
Fluid retention NOS

R61   **Generalized hyperhidrosis**
Excessive sweating
Night sweats
Secondary hyperhidrosis
Code first, if applicable, menopausal and female climacteric states (N95.1)
EXCLUDES 1   *focal (primary) (secondary) hyperhidrosis (L74.5-)*
Frey's syndrome (L74.52)
localized (primary) (secondary) hyperhidrosis (L74.5-)

✓4ᵗʰ **R62**   **Lack of expected normal physiological development in childhood and adults**
EXCLUDES 1   *delayed puberty (E30.0)*
gonadal dysgenesis (Q99.1)
hypopituitarism (E23.0)

R62.0   **Delayed milestone in childhood** P
Delayed attainment of expected physiological developmental stage
Late talker
Late walker

✓5ᵗʰ **R62.5**   **Other and unspecified lack of expected normal physiological development in childhood**
EXCLUDES 1   *HIV disease resulting in failure to thrive (B20)*
physical retardation due to malnutrition (E45)

R62.50   **Unspecified lack of expected normal physiological development in childhood** ▽
Infantilism NOS

R62.51   **Failure to thrive (child)** P
Failure to gain weight
EXCLUDES 1   *failure to thrive in child under 28 days old (P92.6)*
DEF: Organic failure to thrive (FTT): Acute or chronic illness that interferes with nutritional intake, absorption, metabolism excretion, and energy requirements; nonorganic FTT is a symptom of neglect or abuse.

R62.52   **Short stature (child)**
Lack of growth
Physical retardation
Short stature NOS
EXCLUDES 1   *short stature due to endocrine disorder (E34.3)*

R62.59   **Other lack of expected normal physiological development in childhood**

R62.7   **Adult failure to thrive** NC Dx   A

✓4ᵗʰ **R63**   **Symptoms and signs concerning food and fluid intake**
EXCLUDES 1   *bulimia NOS (F50.2)*
eating disorders of nonorganic origin (F50.-)
malnutrition (E40-E46)

R63.0   **Anorexia**
Loss of appetite
EXCLUDES 1   *anorexia nervosa (F50.0-)*
loss of appetite of nonorganic origin (F50.89)

R63.1   **Polydipsia**
Excessive thirst

R63.2   **Polyphagia**
Excessive eating
Hyperalimentation NOS

R63.3   **Feeding difficulties**
Feeding problem (elderly) (infant) NOS
▶Picky eater◀
EXCLUDES 1   ▶*eating disorders (F50.-)*◀
feeding problems of newborn (P92.-)
infant feeding disorder of nonorganic origin (F98.2-)
AHA: 2017, 1Q, 28; 2016, 3Q, 19

R63.4   **Abnormal weight loss**

R63.5   **Abnormal weight gain**
EXCLUDES 1   *excessive weight gain in pregnancy (O26.0-)*
obesity (E66.-)

R63.6   **Underweight**
Use additional code to identify body mass index (BMI), if known (Z68.-)
EXCLUDES 1   *abnormal weight loss (R63.4)*
anorexia nervosa (F50.0-)
malnutrition (E40-E46)

R63.8   **Other symptoms and signs concerning food and fluid intake**

R64   **Cachexia**
Wasting syndrome
Code first underlying condition, if known
EXCLUDES 1   *abnormal weight loss (R63.4)*
nutritional marasmus (E41)

N Newborn: 0   P Pediatric: 0-17   M Maternity: 12-55   A Adult: 15-124   NRS Nonroutine supply Dx   NC Dx Noncancer Dx   PDx Primary Dx   ▶◀ Revised Text   ● New Code   ▲ Revised Title

896   ICD-10-CM 2018

✓4ᵗʰ **R65   Symptoms and signs specifically associated with systemic inflammation and infection**
TIP: ICD-10-CM does not specify a code for SIRS of infectious origin. When provider documentation reports SIRS due to an infectious process, assign only the code for the infection.

✓5ᵗʰ **R65.1   Systemic inflammatory response syndrome [SIRS] of non-infectious origin**
Code first underlying condition, such as:
heatstroke (T67.0)
injury and trauma (S00-T88)
EXCLUDES 1 *sepsis—code to infection*
severe sepsis (R65.2)

R65.10   Systemic inflammatory response syndrome [SIRS] of non-infectious origin without acute organ dysfunction
Systemic inflammatory response syndrome (SIRS) NOS

R65.11   Systemic inflammatory response syndrome [SIRS] of non-infectious origin with acute organ dysfunction
Use additional code to identify specific acute organ dysfunction, such as:
acute kidney failure (N17.-)
acute respiratory failure (J96.0-)
critical illness myopathy (G72.81)
critical illness polyneuropathy (G62.81)
disseminated intravascular coagulopathy [DIC] (D65)
encephalopathy (metabolic) (septic) (G93.41)
hepatic failure (K72.0-)

✓5ᵗʰ **R65.2   Severe sepsis**
Infection with associated acute organ dysfunction
Sepsis with acute organ dysfunction
Sepsis with multiple organ dysfunction
Systemic inflammatory response syndrome due to infectious process with acute organ dysfunction
Code first underlying infection, such as:
infection following a procedure (T81.4-)
infections following infusion, transfusion and therapeutic injection (T80.2-)
puerperal sepsis (O85)
sepsis following complete or unspecified spontaneous abortion (O03.87)
sepsis following ectopic and molar pregnancy (O08.82)
sepsis following incomplete spontaneous abortion (O03.37)
sepsis following (induced) termination of pregnancy (O04.87)
sepsis NOS (A41.9)
Use additional code to identify specific acute organ dysfunction, such as:
acute kidney failure (N17.-)
acute respiratory failure (J96.0-)
critical illness myopathy (G72.81)
critical illness polyneuropathy (G62.81)
disseminated intravascular coagulopathy [DIC] (D65)
encephalopathy (metabolic) (septic) (G93.41)
hepatic failure (K72.0-)
AHA: 2016, 3Q, 8

R65.20   Severe sepsis without septic shock
Severe sepsis NOS
AHA: 2016, 3Q, 14; 2013, 4Q, 119

R65.21   Severe sepsis with septic shock

✓4ᵗʰ **R68   Other general symptoms and signs**

R68.0   Hypothermia, not associated with low environmental temperature
EXCLUDES 1 *hypothermia due to anesthesia (T88.51)*
hypothermia due to low environmental temperature (T68)
hypothermia NOS (accidental) (T68)
newborn hypothermia (P80.-)

✓5ᵗʰ **R68.1   Nonspecific symptoms peculiar to infancy**
EXCLUDES 1 *colic, infantile (R10.83)*
neonatal cerebral irritability (P91.3)
teething syndrome (K00.7)

R68.11   Excessive crying of infant (baby)   ℗
EXCLUDES 1 *excessive crying of child, adolescent, or adult (R45.83)*

R68.12   Fussy infant (baby)   ℗
Irritable infant

R68.13   Apparent life threatening event in infant (ALTE)   ℗
Apparent life threatening event in newborn
▶Brief resolved unexplained event (BRUE)◀
Code first confirmed diagnosis, if known
Use additional code(s) for associated signs and symptoms if no confirmed diagnosis established, or if signs and symptoms are not associated routinely with confirmed diagnosis, or provide additional information for cause of ALTE

R68.19   Other nonspecific symptoms peculiar to infancy   ℗

R68.2   Dry mouth, unspecified   ▽
EXCLUDES 1 *dry mouth due to dehydration (E86.0)*
dry mouth due to sicca syndrome [Sjögren] (M35.0-)
salivary gland hyposecretion (K11.7)

R68.3   Clubbing of fingers
Clubbing of nails
EXCLUDES 1 *congenital clubfinger (Q68.1)*
DEF: Enlarged soft tissue of distal fingers; usually occurs in heart and lung diseases.

✓5ᵗʰ **R68.8   Other general symptoms and signs**

R68.81   Early satiety
DEF: The premature feeling of being full after eating only a small amount of food; mechanism of satiety is multifactorial.

R68.82   Decreased libido   A
Decreased sexual desire

R68.83   Chills (without fever)
Chills NOS
EXCLUDES 1 *chills with fever (R50.9)*

R68.84   Jaw pain
Mandibular pain
Maxilla pain
EXCLUDES 1 *temporomandibular joint arthralgia (M26.62-)*

R68.89   Other general symptoms and signs

R69   Illness, unspecified   ▽
Unknown and unspecified cases of morbidity

Abnormal findings on examination of blood, without diagnosis (R70-R79)

EXCLUDES 2 *abnormal findings on antenatal screening of mother (O28.-)*
abnormalities of lipids (E78.-)
abnormalities of platelets and thrombocytes (D69.-)
abnormalities of white blood cells classified elsewhere (D70-D72)
coagulation hemorrhagic disorders (D65-D68)
diagnostic abnormal findings classified elsewhere—see Alphabetical Index
hemorrhagic and hematological disorders of newborn (P50-P61)

✓4ᵗʰ **R70   Elevated erythrocyte sedimentation rate and abnormality of plasma viscosity**

R70.0   Elevated erythrocyte sedimentation rate

R70.1   Abnormal plasma viscosity

✓4ᵗʰ **R71   Abnormality of red blood cells**
EXCLUDES 1 *anemias (D50-D64)*
anemia of premature infant (P61.2)
benign (familial) polycythemia (D75.0)
congenital anemias (P61.2-P61.4)
newborn anemia due to isoimmunization (P55.-)
polycythemia neonatorum (P61.1)
polycythemia NOS (D75.1)
polycythemia vera (D45)
secondary polycythemia (D75.1)

R71.0   Precipitous drop in hematocrit
Drop (precipitous) in hemoglobin
Drop in hematocrit

R71.8   Other abnormality of red blood cells
Abnormal red-cell morphology NOS
Abnormal red-cell volume NOS
Anisocytosis
Poikilocytosis

Chapter 18. Symptoms, Signs and Abnormal Clinical and Laboratory Findings, Not Elsewhere Classified

☑4th R73 Elevated blood glucose level

EXCLUDES 1   diabetes mellitus (E08-E13)
diabetes mellitus in pregnancy, childbirth and the puerperium (O24.-)
neonatal disorders (P70.0-P70.2)
postsurgical hypoinsulinemia (E89.1)

☑5th R73.0 Abnormal glucose

EXCLUDES 1   abnormal glucose in pregnancy (O99.81-)
diabetes mellitus (E08-E13)
dysmetabolic syndrome X (E88.81)
gestational diabetes (O24.4-)
glycosuria (R81)
hypoglycemia (E16.2)

R73.01 Impaired fasting glucose
Elevated fasting glucose

R73.02 Impaired glucose tolerance (oral)
Elevated glucose tolerance

R73.03 Prediabetes
Latent diabetes

R73.09 Other abnormal glucose
Abnormal glucose NOS
Abnormal non-fasting glucose tolerance

R73.9 Hyperglycemia, unspecified ▽

☑4th R74 Abnormal serum enzyme levels

R74.0 Nonspecific elevation of levels of transaminase and lactic acid dehydrogenase [LDH]

R74.8 Abnormal levels of other serum enzymes
Abnormal level of acid phosphatase
Abnormal level of alkaline phosphatase
Abnormal level of amylase
Abnormal level of lipase [triacylglycerol lipase]

R74.9 Abnormal serum enzyme level, unspecified ▽

R75 Inconclusive laboratory evidence of human immunodeficiency virus [HIV]
Nonconclusive HIV-test finding in infants

EXCLUDES 1   asymptomatic human immunodeficiency virus [HIV] infection status (Z21)
human immunodeficiency virus [HIV] disease (B20)

☑4th R76 Other abnormal immunological findings in serum

R76.0 Raised antibody titer

EXCLUDES 1   isoimmunization in pregnancy (O36.0-O36.1)
isoimmunization affecting newborn (P55.-)

☑5th R76.1 Nonspecific reaction to test for tuberculosis

R76.11 Nonspecific reaction to tuberculin skin test without active tuberculosis
Abnormal result of Mantoux test
PPD positive
Tuberculin (skin test) positive
Tuberculin (skin test) reactor

EXCLUDES 1   nonspecific reaction to cell mediated immunity measurement of gamma interferon antigen response without active tuberculosis (R76.12)

R76.12 Nonspecific reaction to cell mediated immunity measurement of gamma interferon antigen response without active tuberculosis
Nonspecific reaction to QuantiFERON-TB test (QFT) without active tuberculosis

EXCLUDES 1   nonspecific reaction to tuberculin skin test without active tuberculosis (R76.11)
positive tuberculin skin test (R76.11)

R76.8 Other specified abnormal immunological findings in serum
Raised level of immunoglobulins NOS

R76.9 Abnormal immunological finding in serum, unspecified ▽

☑4th R77 Other abnormalities of plasma proteins

EXCLUDES 1   disorders of plasma-protein metabolism (E88.0)

R77.0 Abnormality of albumin

R77.1 Abnormality of globulin
Hyperglobulinemia NOS

R77.2 Abnormality of alphafetoprotein

R77.8 Other specified abnormalities of plasma proteins

R77.9 Abnormality of plasma protein, unspecified ▽

☑4th R78 Findings of drugs and other substances, not normally found in blood
Use additional code to identify any retained foreign body, if applicable (Z18.-)

EXCLUDES 1   mental or behavioral disorders due to psychoactive substance use (F10-F19)

R78.0 Finding of alcohol in blood
Use additional external cause code (Y90.-), for detail regarding alcohol level

R78.1 Finding of opiate drug in blood

R78.2 Finding of cocaine in blood

R78.3 Finding of hallucinogen in blood

R78.4 Finding of other drugs of addictive potential in blood

R78.5 Finding of other psychotropic drug in blood

R78.6 Finding of steroid agent in blood

☑5th R78.7 Finding of abnormal level of heavy metals in blood

R78.71 Abnormal lead level in blood

EXCLUDES 1   lead poisoning (T56.0-)

R78.79 Finding of abnormal level of heavy metals in blood

☑5th R78.8 Finding of other specified substances, not normally found in blood

R78.81 Bacteremia

EXCLUDES 1   sepsis—code to specified infection
DEF: Laboratory finding of bacteria in the blood in the absence of two or more signs of sepsis; transient in nature, it progresses to septicemia with severe infectious process.

R78.89 Finding of other specified substances, not normally found in blood
Finding of abnormal level of lithium in blood

R78.9 Finding of unspecified substance, not normally found in blood ▽

☑4th R79 Other abnormal findings of blood chemistry
Use additional code to identify any retained foreign body, if applicable (Z18.-)

EXCLUDES 1   abnormality of fluid, electrolyte or acid-base balance (E86-E87)
asymptomatic hyperuricemia (E79.0)
hyperglycemia NOS (R73.9)
hypoglycemia NOS (E16.2)
neonatal hypoglycemia (P70.3-P70.4)
specific findings indicating disorder of amino-acid metabolism (E70-E72)
specific findings indicating disorder of carbohydrate metabolism (E73-E74)
specific findings indicating disorder of lipid metabolism (E75.-)

R79.0 Abnormal level of blood mineral
Abnormal blood level of cobalt
Abnormal blood level of copper
Abnormal blood level of iron
Abnormal blood level of magnesium
Abnormal blood level of mineral NEC
Abnormal blood level of zinc

EXCLUDES 1   abnormal level of lithium (R78.89)
disorders of mineral metabolism (E83.-)
neonatal hypomagnesemia (P71.2)
nutritional mineral deficiency (E58-E61)

R79.1 Abnormal coagulation profile
Abnormal or prolonged bleeding time
Abnormal or prolonged coagulation time
Abnormal or prolonged partial thromboplastin time [PTT]
Abnormal or prolonged prothrombin time [PT]

EXCLUDES 1   coagulation defects (D68.-)

EXCLUDES 2   ▶abnormality of fluid, electrolyte or acid-base balance (E86-E87)◀

☑5th R79.8 Other specified abnormal findings of blood chemistry

R79.81 Abnormal blood-gas level

R79.82 Elevated C-reactive protein [CRP]

R79.89 Other specified abnormal findings of blood chemistry

R79.9 Abnormal finding of blood chemistry, unspecified ▽

N Newborn: 0   P Pediatric: 0-17   M Maternity: 12-55   A Adult: 15-124   NRS Nonroutine supply Dx   NC Dx Noncancer Dx   PDx Primary Dx   ▶◀ Revised Text   ● New Code   ▲ Revised Title

898   ICD-10-CM 2018

Abnormal findings on examination of urine, without diagnosis (R80-R82)

EXCLUDES 1 *abnormal findings on antenatal screening of mother (O28.-)*
diagnostic abnormal findings classified elsewhere—see Alphabetical Index
specific findings indicating disorder of amino-acid metabolism (E70-E72)
specific findings indicating disorder of carbohydrate metabolism (E73-E74)

✓4ᵗʰ **R80   Proteinuria**
  EXCLUDES 1 *gestational proteinuria (O12.1-)*

  R80.0   Isolated proteinuria
    Idiopathic proteinuria
    EXCLUDES 1 *isolated proteinuria with specific morphological lesion (N06.-)*

  R80.1   Persistent proteinuria, unspecified ▽

  R80.2   Orthostatic proteinuria, unspecified ▽
    Postural proteinuria

  R80.3   Bence Jones proteinuria

  R80.8   Other proteinuria

  R80.9   Proteinuria, unspecified ▽
    Albuminuria NOS

R81   Glycosuria
  EXCLUDES 1 *renal glycosuria (E74.8)*

✓4ᵗʰ **R82   Other and unspecified abnormal findings in urine**
  INCLUDES chromoabnormalities in urine
  Use additional code to identify any retained foreign body, if applicable (Z18.-)
  EXCLUDES 2 *hematuria (R31.-)*

  R82.0   Chyluria
    EXCLUDES 1 *filarial chyluria (B74.-)*

  R82.1   Myoglobinuria

  R82.2   Biliuria

  R82.3   Hemoglobinuria
    EXCLUDES 1 *hemoglobinuria due to hemolysis from external causes NEC (D59.6)*
    hemoglobinuria due to paroxysmal nocturnal [Marchiafava-Micheli] (D59.5)
    DEF: Free hemoglobin in blood due to rapid hemolysis of red blood cells; causes include burns, crushed injury, sickle cell anemia, thalassemia, parasitic infections, or kidney infections.

  R82.4   Acetonuria
    Ketonuria
    DEF: Excessive excretion of acetone in urine; commonly occurs in diabetic acidosis.

  R82.5   Elevated urine levels of drugs, medicaments and biological substances
    Elevated urine levels of catecholamines
    Elevated urine levels of indoleacetic acid
    Elevated urine levels of 17-ketosteroids
    Elevated urine levels of steroids

  R82.6   Abnormal urine levels of substances chiefly nonmedicinal as to source
    Abnormal urine level of heavy metals

  ✓5ᵗʰ **R82.7   Abnormal findings on microbiological examination of urine**
    EXCLUDES 1 *colonization status (Z22.-)*

    R82.71   Bacteriuria

    R82.79   Other abnormal findings on microbiological examination of urine
      Positive culture findings of urine

  R82.8   Abnormal findings on cytological and histological examination of urine

  ✓5ᵗʰ **R82.9   Other and unspecified abnormal findings in urine**

    R82.90   Unspecified abnormal findings in urine ▽

    R82.91   Other chromoabnormalities of urine
      Chromoconversion (dipstick)
      Idiopathic dipstick converts positive for blood with no cellular forms in sediment
      EXCLUDES 1 *hemoglobinuria (R82.3)*
      myoglobinuria (R82.1)

    R82.99   Other abnormal findings in urine
      Cells and casts in urine
      Crystalluria
      Melanuria

Abnormal findings on examination of other body fluids, substances and tissues, without diagnosis (R83-R89)

EXCLUDES 1 *abnormal findings on antenatal screening of mother (O28.-)*
diagnostic abnormal findings classified elsewhere—see Alphabetical Index
EXCLUDES 2 *abnormal findings on examination of blood, without diagnosis (R70-R79)*
abnormal findings on examination of urine, without diagnosis (R80-R82)
abnormal tumor markers (R97.-)

✓4ᵗʰ **R83   Abnormal findings in cerebrospinal fluid**

  R83.0   Abnormal level of enzymes in cerebrospinal fluid

  R83.1   Abnormal level of hormones in cerebrospinal fluid

  R83.2   Abnormal level of other drugs, medicaments and biological substances in cerebrospinal fluid

  R83.3   Abnormal level of substances chiefly nonmedicinal as to source in cerebrospinal fluid

  R83.4   Abnormal immunological findings in cerebrospinal fluid

  R83.5   Abnormal microbiological findings in cerebrospinal fluid
    Positive culture findings in cerebrospinal fluid
    EXCLUDES 1 *colonization status (Z22.-)*

  R83.6   Abnormal cytological findings in cerebrospinal fluid

  R83.8   Other abnormal findings in cerebrospinal fluid
    Abnormal chromosomal findings in cerebrospinal fluid

  R83.9   Unspecified abnormal finding in cerebrospinal fluid ▽

✓4ᵗʰ **R84   Abnormal findings in specimens from respiratory organs and thorax**
  INCLUDES abnormal findings in bronchial washings
    abnormal findings in nasal secretions
    abnormal findings in pleural fluid
    abnormal findings in sputum
    abnormal findings in throat scrapings
  EXCLUDES 1 *blood-stained sputum (R04.2)*

  R84.0   Abnormal level of enzymes in specimens from respiratory organs and thorax

  R84.1   Abnormal level of hormones in specimens from respiratory organs and thorax

  R84.2   Abnormal level of other drugs, medicaments and biological substances in specimens from respiratory organs and thorax

  R84.3   Abnormal level of substances chiefly nonmedicinal as to source in specimens from respiratory organs and thorax

  R84.4   Abnormal immunological findings in specimens from respiratory organs and thorax

Cerebrospinal Fluid

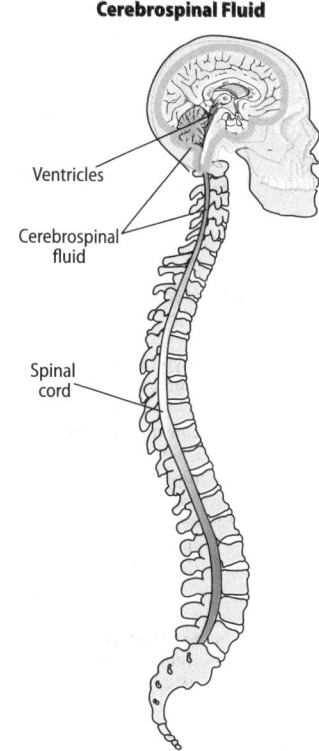

Ventricles

Cerebrospinal fluid

Spinal cord

✔ Additional Character Req   ✔x7ᵗʰ Placeholder Alert   Case-Mix Diagnosis   Manifestation   ▽ Unspecified Dx   **EXCLUDES 1** Not coded here   **EXCLUDES 2** Not included here

R84.5 **Abnormal microbiological findings in specimens from respiratory organs and thorax**
Positive culture findings in specimens from respiratory organs and thorax
EXCLUDES 1　*colonization status (Z22.-)*

R84.6 **Abnormal cytological findings in specimens from respiratory organs and thorax**

R84.7 **Abnormal histological findings in specimens from respiratory organs and thorax**

R84.8 **Other abnormal findings in specimens from respiratory organs and thorax**
Abnormal chromosomal findings in specimens from respiratory organs and thorax

R84.9 **Unspecified abnormal finding in specimens from respiratory organs and thorax** ▽

✓4ᵗʰ **R85** **Abnormal findings in specimens from digestive organs and abdominal cavity**
INCLUDES　abnormal findings in peritoneal fluid
abnormal findings in saliva
EXCLUDES 1　*cloudy peritoneal dialysis effluent (R88.0)*
fecal abnormalities (R19.5)

R85.0 **Abnormal level of enzymes in specimens from digestive organs and abdominal cavity**

R85.1 **Abnormal level of hormones in specimens from digestive organs and abdominal cavity**

R85.2 **Abnormal level of other drugs, medicaments and biological substances in specimens from digestive organs and abdominal cavity**

R85.3 **Abnormal level of substances chiefly nonmedicinal as to source in specimens from digestive organs and abdominal cavity**

R85.4 **Abnormal immunological findings in specimens from digestive organs and abdominal cavity**

R85.5 **Abnormal microbiological findings in specimens from digestive organs and abdominal cavity**
Positive culture findings in specimens from digestive organs and abdominal cavity
EXCLUDES 1　*colonization status (Z22.-)*

✓5ᵗʰ **R85.6** **Abnormal cytological findings in specimens from digestive organs and abdominal cavity**

✓6ᵗʰ **R85.61** **Abnormal cytologic smear of anus**
EXCLUDES 1　*abnormal cytological findings in specimens from other digestive organs and abdominal cavity (R85.69)*
anal intraepithelial neoplasia I [AIN I] (K62.82)
anal intraepithelial neoplasia II [AIN II] (K62.82)
anal intraepithelial neoplasia III [AIN III] (D01.3)
carcinoma in situ of anus (histologically confirmed) (D01.3)
dysplasia (mild) (moderate) of anus (histologically confirmed) (K62.82)
severe dysplasia of anus (histologically confirmed) (D01.3)
EXCLUDES 2　*anal high risk human papillomavirus (HPV) DNA test positive (R85.81)*
anal low risk human papillomavirus (HPV) DNA test positive (R85.82)

R85.610 **Atypical squamous cells of undetermined significance on cytologic smear of anus [ASC-US]**

R85.611 **Atypical squamous cells cannot exclude high grade squamous intraepithelial lesion on cytologic smear of anus [ASC-H]**

R85.612 **Low grade squamous intraepithelial lesion on cytologic smear of anus [LGSIL]**

R85.613 **High grade squamous intraepithelial lesion on cytologic smear of anus [HGSIL]**

R85.614 **Cytologic evidence of malignancy on smear of anus**

R85.615 **Unsatisfactory cytologic smear of anus**
Inadequate sample of cytologic smear of anus

R85.616 **Satisfactory anal smear but lacking transformation zone**

R85.618 **Other abnormal cytological findings on specimens from anus**

R85.619 **Unspecified abnormal cytological findings in specimens from anus** ▽
Abnormal anal cytology NOS
Atypical glandular cells of anus NOS

R85.69 **Abnormal cytological findings in specimens from other digestive organs and abdominal cavity**

R85.7 **Abnormal histological findings in specimens from digestive organs and abdominal cavity**

✓5ᵗʰ **R85.8** **Other abnormal findings in specimens from digestive organs and abdominal cavity**

R85.81 **Anal high risk human papillomavirus [HPV] DNA test positive**
EXCLUDES 1　*anogenital warts due to human papillomavirus (HPV) (A63.0)*
condyloma acuminatum (A63.0)

R85.82 **Anal low risk human papillomavirus [HPV] DNA test positive**
Use additional code for associated human papillomavirus (B97.7)

R85.89 **Other abnormal findings in specimens from digestive organs and abdominal cavity**
Abnormal chromosomal findings in specimens from digestive organs and abdominal cavity

R85.9 **Unspecified abnormal finding in specimens from digestive organs and abdominal cavity** ▽

✓4ᵗʰ **R86** **Abnormal findings in specimens from male genital organs**
INCLUDES　abnormal findings in prostatic secretions
abnormal findings in semen, seminal fluid
abnormal spermatozoa
EXCLUDES 1　*azoospermia (N46.0-)*
oligospermia (N46.1-)

R86.0 **Abnormal level of enzymes in specimens from male genital organs** ♂

R86.1 **Abnormal level of hormones in specimens from male genital organs** ♂

R86.2 **Abnormal level of other drugs, medicaments and biological substances in specimens from male genital organs** ♂

R86.3 **Abnormal level of substances chiefly nonmedicinal as to source in specimens from male genital organs** ♂

R86.4 **Abnormal immunological findings in specimens from male genital organs** ♂

R86.5 **Abnormal microbiological findings in specimens from male genital organs** ♂
Positive culture findings in specimens from male genital organs
EXCLUDES 1　*colonization status (Z22.-)*

R86.6 **Abnormal cytological findings in specimens from male genital organs** ♂

R86.7 **Abnormal histological findings in specimens from male genital organs** ♂

R86.8 **Other abnormal findings in specimens from male genital organs** ♂
Abnormal chromosomal findings in specimens from male genital organs

R86.9 **Unspecified abnormal finding in specimens from male genital organs** ♂▽

✓4ᵗʰ **R87** **Abnormal findings in specimens from female genital organs**
INCLUDES　abnormal findings in secretion and smears from cervix uteri
abnormal findings in secretion and smears from vagina
abnormal findings in secretion and smears from vulva

R87.0 **Abnormal level of enzymes in specimens from female genital organs** ♀

R87.1 **Abnormal level of hormones in specimens from female genital organs** ♀

R87.2 **Abnormal level of other drugs, medicaments and biological substances in specimens from female genital organs** ♀

R87.3 **Abnormal level of substances chiefly nonmedicinal as to source in specimens from female genital organs** ♀

R87.4 **Abnormal immunological findings in specimens from female genital organs** ♀

R87.5 **Abnormal microbiological findings in specimens from female genital organs** ♀
Positive culture findings in specimens from female genital organs
EXCLUDES 1　*colonization status (Z22.-)*

Ⓝ Newborn: 0　Ⓟ Pediatric: 0-17　Ⓜ Maternity: 12-55　Ⓐ Adult: 15-124　NRS Nonroutine supply Dx　NCDx Noncancer Dx　PDx Primary Dx　►◄ Revised Text　● New Code　▲ Revised Title

900　　　ICD-10-CM 2018

✓5ᵗʰ **R87.6 Abnormal** cytological **findings in specimens from female genital organs**

  ✓6ᵗʰ **R87.61 Abnormal cytological findings in specimens from** cervix uteri

    EXCLUDES 1 *abnormal cytological findings in specimens from other female genital organs (R87.69)*

        abnormal cytological findings in specimens from vagina (R87.62-)

        carcinoma in situ of cervix uteri (histologically confirmed) (D06.-)

        cervical intraepithelial neoplasia I [CIN I] (N87.0)

        cervical intraepithelial neoplasia II [CIN II] (N87.1)

        cervical intraepithelial neoplasia III [CIN III] (D06.-)

        dysplasia (mild) (moderate) of cervix uteri (histologically confirmed) (N87.-)

        severe dysplasia of cervix uteri (histologically confirmed) (D06.-)

    EXCLUDES 2 *cervical high risk human papillomavirus (HPV) DNA test positive (R87.810)*

        cervical low risk human papillomavirus (HPV) DNA test positive (R87.820)

    R87.610 Atypical squamous cells of undetermined significance on cytologic smear of cervix [ASC-US] ♀

    R87.611 Atypical squamous cells cannot exclude high grade squamous intraepithelial lesion on cytologic smear of cervix [ASC-H] ♀

    R87.612 Low grade squamous intraepithelial lesion on cytologic smear of cervix [LGSIL] ♀

    R87.613 High grade squamous intraepithelial lesion on cytologic smear of cervix [HGSIL] ♀

    R87.614 Cytologic evidence of malignancy on smear of cervix ♀

    R87.615 Unsatisfactory cytologic smear of cervix ♀
        Inadequate sample of cytologic smear of cervix

    R87.616 Satisfactory cervical smear but lacking transformation zone ♀

    R87.618 Other abnormal cytological findings on specimens from cervix uteri ♀

    R87.619 Unspecified abnormal cytological findings in specimens from cervix uteri ♀▽
        Abnormal cervical cytology NOS
        Abnormal Papanicolaou smear of cervix NOS
        Abnormal thin preparation smear of cervix NOS
        Atypical endocervical cells of cervix NOS
        Atypical endometrial cells of cervix NOS
        Atypical glandular cells of cervix NOS

  ✓6ᵗʰ **R87.62 Abnormal cytological findings in specimens from** vagina
    Use additional code to identify acquired absence of uterus and cervix, if applicable (Z90.71-)

    EXCLUDES 1 *abnormal cytological findings in specimens from cervix uteri (R87.61-)*

        abnormal cytological findings in specimens from other female genital organs (R87.69)

        carcinoma in situ of vagina (histologically confirmed) (D07.2)

        dysplasia (mild) (moderate) of vagina (histologically confirmed) (N89.-)

        severe dysplasia of vagina (histologically confirmed) (D07.2)

        vaginal intraepithelial neoplasia I [VAIN I] (N89.0)

        vaginal intraepithelial neoplasia II [VAIN II] (N89.1)

        vaginal intraepithelial neoplasia III [VAIN III] (D07.2)

    EXCLUDES 2 *vaginal high risk human papillomavirus (HPV) DNA test positive (R87.811)*

        vaginal low risk human papillomavirus (HPV) DNA test positive (R87.821)

    R87.620 Atypical squamous cells of undetermined significance on cytologic smear of vagina [ASC-US] ♀

    R87.621 Atypical squamous cells cannot exclude high grade squamous intraepithelial lesion on cytologic smear of vagina [ASC-H] ♀

    R87.622 Low grade squamous intraepithelial lesion on cytologic smear of vagina [LGSIL] ♀

    R87.623 High grade squamous intraepithelial lesion on cytologic smear of vagina [HGSIL] ♀

    R87.624 Cytologic evidence of malignancy on smear of vagina ♀

    R87.625 Unsatisfactory cytologic smear of vagina ♀
        Inadequate sample of cytologic smear of vagina

    R87.628 Other abnormal cytological findings on specimens from vagina ♀

    R87.629 Unspecified abnormal cytological findings in specimens from vagina ♀▽
        Abnormal Papanicolaou smear of vagina NOS
        Abnormal thin preparation smear of vagina NOS
        Abnormal vaginal cytology NOS
        Atypical endocervical cells of vagina NOS
        Atypical endometrial cells of vagina NOS
        Atypical glandular cells of vagina NOS

  R87.69 Abnormal cytological findings in specimens from other female genital organs ♀
    Abnormal cytological findings in specimens from female genital organs NOS

    EXCLUDES 1 *dysplasia of vulva (histologically confirmed) (N90.0-N90.3)*

R87.7 Abnormal histological findings in specimens from female genital organs ♀

  EXCLUDES 1 *carcinoma in situ (histologically confirmed) of female genital organs (D06-D07.3)*

    cervical intraepithelial neoplasia I [CIN I] (N87.0)

    cervical intraepithelial neoplasia II [CIN II] (N87.1)

    cervical intraepithelial neoplasia III [CIN III] (D06.-)

    dysplasia (mild) (moderate) of cervix uteri (histologically confirmed) (N87.-)

    dysplasia (mild) (moderate) of vagina (histologically confirmed) (N89.-)

    severe dysplasia of cervix uteri (histologically confirmed) (D06.-)

    severe dysplasia of vagina (histologically confirmed) (D07.2)

    vaginal intraepithelial neoplasia I [VAIN I] (N89.0)

    vaginal intraepithelial neoplasia II [VAIN II] (N89.1)

    vaginal intraepithelial neoplasia III [VAIN III] (D07.2)

✓5ᵗʰ **R87.8 Other abnormal findings in specimens from female genital organs**

  ✓6ᵗʰ **R87.81 High risk human papillomavirus [HPV] DNA test positive from female genital organs**

    EXCLUDES 1 *anogenital warts due to human papillomavirus (HPV) (A63.0)*

        condyloma acuminatum (A63.0)

    R87.810 Cervical high risk human papillomavirus [HPV] DNA test positive ♀

    R87.811 Vaginal high risk human papillomavirus [HPV] DNA test positive ♀

  ✓6ᵗʰ **R87.82 Low risk human papillomavirus [HPV] DNA test positive from female genital organs**
    Use additional code for associated human papillomavirus (B97.7)

    R87.820 Cervical low risk human papillomavirus [HPV] DNA test positive ♀

    R87.821 Vaginal low risk human papillomavirus [HPV] DNA test positive ♀

  R87.89 Other abnormal findings in specimens from female genital organs ♀
    Abnormal chromosomal findings in specimens from female genital organs

R87.9 Unspecified abnormal finding in specimens from female genital organs ♀▽

✓4ᵗʰ **R88 Abnormal findings in other body fluids and substances**

  R88.0 Cloudy (hemodialysis) (peritoneal) dialysis effluent

  R88.8 Abnormal findings in other body fluids and substances

☑ Additional Character Req   ✓x7ᵗʰ Placeholder Alert   Case-Mix Diagnosis   Manifestation   ▽ Unspecified Dx   EXCLUDES 1 Not coded here   EXCLUDES 2 Not included here

ICD-10-CM 2018   901

✓4ᵗʰ **R89 Abnormal findings in specimens from** other organs, systems and tissues

     INCLUDES   abnormal findings in nipple discharge
                     abnormal findings in synovial fluid
                     abnormal findings in wound secretions

     R89.Ø Abnormal level of enzymes **in specimens from other organs, systems and tissues**

     R89.1 Abnormal level of hormones **in specimens from other organs, systems and tissues**

     R89.2 Abnormal level of other drugs, medicaments and biological substances in specimens from other organs, systems and tissues

     R89.3 Abnormal level of substances chiefly nonmedicinal **as to source in specimens from other organs, systems and tissues**

     R89.4 Abnormal immunological **findings in specimens from other organs, systems and tissues**

     R89.5 Abnormal microbiological **findings in specimens from other organs, systems and tissues**
         Positive culture findings in specimens from other organs, systems and tissues
         EXCLUDES 1   colonization status (Z22.-)

     R89.6 Abnormal cytological **findings in specimens from other organs, systems and tissues**

     R89.7 Abnormal histological **findings in specimens from other organs, systems and tissues**

     R89.8 Other abnormal findings in specimens from other organs, systems and tissues
         Abnormal chromosomal findings in specimens from other organs, systems and tissues

     R89.9 Unspecified abnormal finding in specimens from other organs, systems and tissues ▽

Abnormal findings on diagnostic imaging and in function studies, without diagnosis (R9Ø-R94)

     INCLUDES   nonspecific abnormal findings on diagnostic imaging by computerized axial tomography [CAT scan]
                     nonspecific abnormal findings on diagnostic imaging by magnetic resonance imaging [MRI][NMR]
                     nonspecific abnormal findings on diagnostic imaging by positron emission tomography [PET scan]
                     nonspecific abnormal findings on diagnostic imaging by thermography
                     nonspecific abnormal findings on diagnostic imaging by ultrasound [echogram]
                     nonspecific abnormal findings on diagnostic imaging by X-ray examination
     EXCLUDES 1   abnormal findings on antenatal screening of mother (O28.-)
                     diagnostic abnormal findings classified elsewhere—see Alphabetical Index

✓4ᵗʰ **R9Ø Abnormal findings on** diagnostic imaging of central nervous system

     R9Ø.Ø Intracranial **space-occupying lesion found on diagnostic imaging of central nervous system**

     ✓5ᵗʰ **R9Ø.8 Other abnormal findings on diagnostic imaging of** central nervous system

         R9Ø.81 Abnormal echoencephalogram

         R9Ø.82 White matter disease, unspecified ▽

         R9Ø.89 Other abnormal findings on diagnostic imaging of central nervous system
                 Other cerebrovascular abnormality found on diagnostic imaging of central nervous system

✓4ᵗʰ **R91 Abnormal findings on diagnostic imaging of** lung

     R91.1 Solitary pulmonary nodule
         Coin lesion lung
         Solitary pulmonary nodule, subsegmental branch of the bronchial tree

     R91.8 Other nonspecific abnormal finding of lung field
         Lung mass NOS found on diagnostic imaging of lung
         Pulmonary infiltrate NOS
         Shadow, lung

✓4ᵗʰ **R92 Abnormal and inconclusive findings on diagnostic imaging of** breast

     R92.Ø Mammographic microcalcification **found on diagnostic imaging of breast**
         EXCLUDES 2   mammographic calcification (calculus) found on diagnostic imaging of breast (R92.1)
         DEF: Calcium and cellular debris deposits in the breast that cannot be felt but can be detected on a mammogram; can be a sign of cancer, benign conditions, or changes in the breast tissue as a result of inflammation, injury, or obstructed duct.

     R92.1 Mammographic calcification **found on diagnostic imaging of breast**
         Mammographic calculus found on diagnostic imaging of breast

     R92.2 Inconclusive **mammogram**
         Dense breasts NOS
         Inconclusive mammogram NEC
         Inconclusive mammography due to dense breasts
         Inconclusive mammography NEC
         AHA: 2015, 1Q, 24

     R92.8 Other abnormal and inconclusive findings on diagnostic imaging of breast

✓4ᵗʰ **R93 Abnormal findings on diagnostic imaging of** other body structures

     R93.Ø Abnormal findings on diagnostic imaging of skull and head, **not elsewhere classified**
         EXCLUDES 1   intracranial space-occupying lesion found on diagnostic imaging (R9Ø.Ø)

     R93.1 Abnormal findings on diagnostic imaging of heart and coronary **circulation**
         Abnormal echocardiogram NOS
         Abnormal heart shadow

     R93.2 Abnormal findings on diagnostic imaging of liver and biliary **tract**
         Nonvisualization of gallbladder

     R93.3 Abnormal findings on diagnostic imaging of other parts of digestive tract

     ✓5ᵗʰ **R93.4 Abnormal findings on diagnostic imaging of** urinary organs
         EXCLUDES 2   hypertrophy of kidney (N28.81)

         R93.41 Abnormal radiologic findings on diagnostic imaging of renal pelvis, ureter, or bladder
                 Filling defect of bladder found on diagnostic imaging
                 Filling defect of renal pelvis found on diagnostic imaging
                 Filling defect of ureter found on diagnostic imaging

         ✓6ᵗʰ **R93.42 Abnormal radiologic findings on diagnostic imaging of** kidney

             R93.421 Abnormal radiologic findings on diagnostic imaging of right **kidney**

             R93.422 Abnormal radiologic findings on diagnostic imaging of left **kidney**

             R93.429 Abnormal radiologic findings on diagnostic imaging of unspecified kidney ▽

         R93.49 Abnormal radiologic findings on diagnostic imaging of other urinary organs

     R93.5 Abnormal findings on diagnostic imaging of other abdominal regions, including retroperitoneum

     R93.6 Abnormal findings on diagnostic imaging of limbs
         EXCLUDES 2   abnormal finding in skin and subcutaneous tissue (R93.8)

     R93.7 Abnormal findings on diagnostic imaging of other parts of musculoskeletal system
         EXCLUDES 2   abnormal findings on diagnostic imaging of skull (R93.Ø)

     R93.8 Abnormal findings on diagnostic imaging of other specified body structures
         Abnormal finding by radioisotope localization of placenta
         Abnormal radiological finding in skin and subcutaneous tissue
         Mediastinal shift

     R93.9 Diagnostic imaging inconclusive due to excess body fat **of patient**

✓4ᵗʰ **R94 Abnormal results of function studies**

     INCLUDES   abnormal results of radionuclide [radioisotope] uptake studies
                     abnormal results of scintigraphy

     ✓5ᵗʰ **R94.Ø Abnormal results of function studies of** central nervous system

         R94.Ø1 Abnormal electroencephalogram [EEG]

         R94.Ø2 Abnormal brain scan

R94.09   **Abnormal results of other function studies of central nervous system**

✓5ᵗʰ **R94.1** **Abnormal results of function studies of** peripheral nervous system and special senses

  ✓6ᵗʰ **R94.11** **Abnormal results of function studies of** eye

    R94.110   **Abnormal** electro-oculogram **[EOG]**

    R94.111   **Abnormal** electroretinogram **[ERG]**
         Abnormal retinal function study

    R94.112   **Abnormal** visually evoked potential **[VEP]**

    R94.113   **Abnormal** oculomotor **study**

    R94.118   **Abnormal results of other function studies of eye**

  ✓6ᵗʰ **R94.12** **Abnormal results of function studies of** ear and other special senses
       AHA: 2016, 3Q, 17

    R94.120   **Abnormal** auditory **function study**

    R94.121   **Abnormal** vestibular **function study**

    R94.128   **Abnormal results of other function studies of ear and other special senses**

  ✓6ᵗʰ **R94.13** **Abnormal results of function studies of** peripheral nervous system

    R94.130   **Abnormal response to nerve stimulation, unspecified** ▽

    R94.131   Abnormal electromyogram **[EMG]**
         EXCLUDES 1 *electromyogram of eye (R94.113)*

    R94.138   **Abnormal results of other function studies of peripheral nervous system**

R94.2 **Abnormal results of** pulmonary function **studies**
   Reduced ventilatory capacity
   Reduced vital capacity

✓5ᵗʰ **R94.3** **Abnormal results of** cardiovascular function **studies**

  R94.30   **Abnormal result of cardiovascular function study, unspecified** ▽

  R94.31   **Abnormal** electrocardiogram **[ECG] [EKG]**
     EXCLUDES 1 *long QT syndrome (I45.81)*

  R94.39   **Abnormal result of other cardiovascular function study**
     Abnormal electrophysiological intracardiac studies
     Abnormal phonocardiogram
     Abnormal vectorcardiogram

R94.4 **Abnormal results of** kidney function **studies**
   Abnormal renal function test

R94.5 **Abnormal results of** liver function **studies**

R94.6 **Abnormal results of** thyroid function **studies**

R94.7 **Abnormal results of other endocrine function studies**
   EXCLUDES 2 *abnormal glucose (R73.0-)*

R94.8 **Abnormal results of function studies of** other organs and systems
   Abnormal basal metabolic rate [BMR]
   Abnormal bladder function test
   Abnormal splenic function test

Abnormal tumor markers (R97)

✓4ᵗʰ **R97** **Abnormal tumor markers**
   Elevated tumor associated antigens [TAA]
   Elevated tumor specific antigens [TSA]

  R97.0 **Elevated carcinoembryonic antigen [CEA]**

  R97.1 **Elevated cancer antigen 125 [CA 125]**   ♀

✓5ᵗʰ **R97.2** **Elevated prostate specific antigen [PSA]**

    R97.20   **Elevated prostate specific antigen [PSA]**   A♂

    R97.21   **Rising PSA following treatment for malignant neoplasm of prostate**   A♂

  R97.8 **Other abnormal tumor markers**

Ill-defined and unknown cause of mortality (R99)

R99 **Ill-defined and unknown cause of mortality**   ▽
   Death (unexplained) NOS
   Unspecified cause of mortality

✓ Additional Character Req   ✓x7ᵗʰ Placeholder Alert   Case-Mix Diagnosis   Manifestation   ▽ Unspecified Dx   **EXCLUDES 1** Not coded here   **EXCLUDES 2** Not included here

ICD-10-CM 2018

903

Chapter 19. Injury, Poisoning and Certain Other Consequences of External Causes (SØØ–T88)

Chapter Specific Guidelines with Coding Examples

The chapter specific guidelines from the ICD-10-CM Official Guidelines for Coding and Reporting have been provided below. Along with these guidelines are coding examples, contained in the shaded boxes, that have been developed to help illustrate the coding and/or sequencing guidance found in these guidelines.

a. Application of 7th characters in Chapter 19

Most categories in chapter 19 have a 7th character requirement for each applicable code. Most categories in this chapter have three 7th character values (with the exception of fractures): A, initial encounter, D, subsequent encounter and S, sequela. Categories for traumatic fractures have additional 7th character values. While the patient may be seen by a new or different provider over the course of treatment for an injury, assignment of the 7th character is based on whether the patient is undergoing active treatment and not whether the provider is seeing the patient for the first time.

For complication codes, active treatment refers to treatment for the condition described by the code, even though it may be related to an earlier precipitating problem. For example, code T84.50XA, Infection and inflammatory reaction due to unspecified internal joint prosthesis, initial encounter, is used when active treatment is provided for the infection, even though the condition relates to the prosthetic device, implant or graft that was placed at a previous encounter.

7th character "A", initial encounter is used for each encounter where the patient is receiving active treatment for the condition.

7th character "D" subsequent encounter is used for encounters after the patient has completed active treatment of the condition and is receiving routine care for the condition during the healing or recovery phase.

> Patient was admitted to home health for continued therapy following acute care stay to treat a nondisplaced fracture to the distal pole of the right scaphoid bone due to a fall from skateboard onto the sidewalk.
>
> **S62.Ø14D   Nondisplaced fracture of the distal pole of navicular [scaphoid] bone of right wrist, subsequent encounter for fracture with routine healing**
>
> **VØØ.131D   Fall from skateboard, subsequent encounter**
>
> *Explanation:* The fracture is coded with the seventh character D, as routine care is being provided in the recovery phase within this home health setting. The external cause code, VØØ.131D, describes the cause of the injury and may be applied for each encounter involving treatment for the fracture. Activity codes, place-of-occurrence codes, and external cause status codes are used only once, at the initial encounter for treatment, and are not required for this environment.

The aftercare Z codes should not be used for aftercare for conditions such as injuries or poisonings, where 7th characters are provided to identify subsequent care. For example, for aftercare of an injury, assign the acute injury code with the 7th character "D" (subsequent encounter).

7th character "S", sequela, is for use for complications or conditions that arise as a direct result of a condition, such as scar formation after a burn. The scars are sequelae of the burn. When using 7th character "S", it is necessary to use both the injury code that precipitated the sequela and the code for the sequela itself. The "S" is added only to the injury code, not the sequela code. The 7th character "S" identifies the injury responsible for the sequela. The specific type of sequela (e.g. scar) is sequenced first, followed by the injury code.

See Section I.B.1Ø Sequelae, (Late Effects)

> Patient with a history of a nondisplaced fracture to the distal pole of the right scaphoid bone due to a fall from a skateboard is admitted for evaluation of arthritis to the right wrist that has developed as a consequence of the traumatic fracture.
>
> **M12.531   Traumatic arthropathy, right wrist**
>
> **S62.Ø14S   Nondisplaced fracture of distal pole of navicular [scaphoid] bone of right wrist, sequela**
>
> **VØØ.131S   Fall from skateboard, sequela**
>
> *Explanation:* The code identifying the specific sequela condition (traumatic arthritis) should be coded first followed by the injury that instigated the development of the sequela (fracture). The scaphoid fracture injury code is given a 7th character S for sequela to represent its role as the inciting injury. The fracture has healed and is not being managed or treated on this admit and therefore is not applicable as a first listed or principal diagnosis. However, it is directly related to the development of the arthritis and should be appended as a secondary code to signify this cause and effect relationship.

b. Coding of injuries

When coding injuries, assign separate codes for each injury unless a combination code is provided, in which case the combination code is assigned. **Codes from category** TØ7, Unspecified multiple injuries should not be assigned in the inpatient setting unless information for a more specific code is not available. Traumatic injury codes (SØØ-T14.9) are not to be used for normal, healing surgical wounds or to identify complications of surgical wounds.

> A 76-year-old man fell from a ladder, resulting in a right humerus fracture, laceration of the right forearm, and laceration of the left shin. Lacerations required sutures, and the humerus fracture was casted. All injuries are healing well.
>
> **S42.3Ø1D   Unspecified fracture of shaft of humerus, right arm, subsequent encounter for fracture with routine healing**
>
> **S51.811D   Laceration without foreign body of right forearm, subsequent encounter**
>
> **S81.812D   Laceration without foreign body, left lower leg, subsequent encounter**
>
> **W11.XXXD   Fall on and from ladder, subsequent encounter**
>
> *Explanation:* Each injury is coded separately. The seventh character D should be assigned for the fracture, which is healing in the recovery phase. The lacerations are coded with the seventh character D as these wounds are not complicated and are healing well, requiring no wound care. An external cause code reports the cause of the injuries.

The code for the most serious injury, as determined by the provider and the focus of treatment, is sequenced first.

1) Superficial injuries

Superficial injuries such as abrasions or contusions are not coded when associated with more severe injuries of the same site.

2) Primary injury with damage to nerves/blood vessels

When a primary injury results in minor damage to peripheral nerves or blood vessels, the primary injury is sequenced first with additional code(s) for injuries to nerves and spinal cord (such as category SØ4), and/or injury to blood vessels (such as category S15). When the primary injury is to the blood vessels or nerves, that injury should be sequenced first.

c. Coding of traumatic fractures

The principles of multiple coding of injuries should be followed in coding fractures. Fractures of specified sites are coded individually by site in accordance with both the provisions within categories SØ2, S12, S22, S32, S42, S49, S52, S59, S62, S72, S79, S82, S89, S92 and the level of detail furnished by medical record content.

A fracture not indicated as open or closed should be coded to closed. A fracture not indicated whether displaced or not displaced should be coded to displaced.

More specific guidelines are as follows:

1) Initial vs. subsequent encounter for fractures

Traumatic fractures are coded using the appropriate 7th character for initial encounter (A, B, C) for each encounter where the patient is receiving active treatment for the fracture. The appropriate 7th character for initial encounter should also be assigned for a patient who delayed seeking treatment for the fracture or nonunion.

Fractures are coded using the appropriate 7th character for subsequent care for encounters after the patient has completed active treatment of the fracture and is receiving routine care for the fracture during the healing or recovery phase.

Care for complications of surgical treatment for fracture repairs during the healing or recovery phase should be coded with the appropriate complication codes.

Care of complications of fractures, such as malunion and nonunion, should be reported with the appropriate 7th character for subsequent care with nonunion (K, M, N,) or subsequent care with malunion (P, Q, R).

Malunion/nonunion: The appropriate 7th character for initial encounter should also be assigned for a patient who delayed seeking treatment for the fracture or nonunion.

> Female patient fell during a hiking excursion almost six months ago and until recently did not feel she needed to seek medical attention for her left ankle pain; x-rays show nonunion of lateral malleolus and surgery has been scheduled
>
> **S82.62XA**   Displaced fracture of lateral malleolus of left fibula, initial encounter for closed fracture
>
> **W01.0XXA**   Fall on same level from slipping, tripping and stumbling without subsequent striking against object, initial encounter
>
> **Y92.821**   Forest as place of occurrence of the external cause
>
> **Y93.01**   Activity, walking, marching and hiking
>
> **Y99.8**   Other external cause status
>
> *Explanation:* A seventh character of A is used for the lateral malleolus nonunion fracture to signify that the fracture is receiving active treatment. The delayed care for the fracture has resulted in a nonunion, but capturing the nonunion in the seventh character is trumped by the provision of active care.

The open fracture designations in the assignment of the 7th character for fractures of the forearm, femur and lower leg, including ankle are based on the Gustilo open fracture classification. When the Gustilo classification type is not specified for an open fracture, the 7th character for open fracture type I or II should be assigned (B, E, H, M, Q).

A code from category M80, not a traumatic fracture code, should be used for any patient with known osteoporosis who suffers a fracture, even if the patient had a minor fall or trauma, if that fall or trauma would not usually break a normal, healthy bone.

See Section I.C.13. Osteoporosis.

The aftercare Z codes should not be used for aftercare for traumatic fractures. For aftercare of a traumatic fracture, assign the acute fracture code with the appropriate 7th character.

2) Multiple fractures sequencing

Multiple fractures are sequenced in accordance with the severity of the fracture.

d. Coding of burns and corrosions

The ICD-10-CM makes a distinction between burns and corrosions. The burn codes are for thermal burns, except sunburns, that come from a heat source, such as a fire or hot appliance. The burn codes are also for burns resulting from electricity and radiation. Corrosions are burns due to chemicals. The guidelines are the same for burns and corrosions.

Current burns (T20-T25) are classified by depth, extent and by agent (X code). Burns are classified by depth as first degree (erythema), second degree (blistering), and third degree (full-thickness involvement). Burns of the eye and internal organs (T26-T28) are classified by site, but not by degree.

1) Sequencing of burn and related condition codes

Sequence first the code that reflects the highest degree of burn when more than one burn is present.

    a.   When the reason for the admission or encounter is for treatment of external multiple burns, sequence first the code that reflects the burn of the highest degree.

    b.   When a patient has both internal and external burns, the circumstances of admission govern the selection of the principal diagnosis or first-listed diagnosis.

    c.   When a patient is admitted for burn injuries and other related conditions such as smoke inhalation and/or respiratory failure, the circumstances of admission govern the selection of the principal or first-listed diagnosis

> Patient is admitted following hospitalization for multiple third-degree burns to both hands and severe smoke inhalation when a candle lit her bedroom curtains on fire. The burns require frequent and complex wound care three times a day. The patient continues with shortness of breath and poor endurance due to smoke inhalation. She is recovering well from the smoke inhalation with normal SpO2 levels, nebulizer treatments, and use of oxygen.
>
> **T23.391A**   Burn of third degree of multiple sites of right wrist and hand, initial encounter
>
> **T23.392A**   Burn of third degree of multiple sites of left wrist and hand, initial encounter
>
> **X08.8XXA**   Exposure to other specified smoke, fire and flames, initial encounter
>
> **T59.811D**   Toxic effect of smoke, accidental (unintentional), initial encounter
>
> **J70.5**   Respiratory conditions due to smoke inhalation
>
> *Explanation:* Based upon provider orders and documentation, the burns are complex and require the most intense care and therefore are coded first. The seventh character A is used for both burns as they remain open with complex active treatment. Because the respiratory condition resulting from smoke inhalation is resolving well and the patient is now in the recovery phase for this condition, the seventh character D is assigned for subsequent episode for the toxic-effect code. For the external cause code X08.8-, the seventh character A is assigned because the resulting burns remain an initial encounter.

2) Burns of the same local site

Classify burns of the same local site (three-character category level, T20-T28) but of different degrees to the subcategory identifying the highest degree recorded in the diagnosis.

> 10-year-old male patient is admitted for third-degree burns of his right palm and second-degree burns of multiple right fingers; right thumb not affected. The burns require complex and frequent dressing changes three times a day, and the patient continues visits to the burn center for debridement.
>
> **T23.351A**   Burn of third degree of right palm, initial encounter
>
> *Explanation:* Although there is a code for second-degree burns of multiple fingers, not including the thumb (T23.131-), this code falls in the same three-digit category that the third-degree burn of the right palm falls under, category T23. Only the subcategory identifying the highest degree is captured when different burn degrees are classified to a single category. The seventh character A is used as the burns continue to require active treatment with complex, frequent wound care and debridement.

> Patient is admitted with third-degree burns of the scalp as well as second-degree burns to the back of the right hand. The burns continue to drain heavily with frequent need for debridement.
>
> **T20.35XA**   Burn of third degree of scalp [any part], initial encounter
>
> **T23.261A**   Burn of second degree of back of right hand, initial encounter
>
> *Explanation:* Since burns to the hand and scalp are classified to two different three-digit categories, both burns may be reported as they represent distinct sites. The seventh character A is used as the burns continue to require active treatment with heavy drainage present and a need for frequent debridement.

3) Non-healing burns

Non-healing burns are coded as acute burns.

Necrosis of burned skin should be coded as a non-healed burn.

4) Infected burn

For any documented infected burn site, use an additional code for the infection.

> Patient is admitted and has a third-degree burn to the left anterior thigh, which the provider reports is infected with pseudomonas. The patient is ordered 4 weeks of IV antibiotics.
>
> | T24.312A | Burn of third degree of left thigh, initial encounter |
> |---|---|
> | B96.5 | Pseudomonas (aeruginosa) (mallei) (pseudomallei) as the cause of diseases classified elsewhere |
> | Z45.2 | Encounter for adjustment and management of vascular access device |
> | Z79.2 | Long term (current) use of antibiotics |
>
> *Explanation:* This burn is infected, and the organism is identified as pseudomonas. ICD-10-CM guidelines indicate to code first the burn and use an additional code to report the infection. Because active treatment, in the form of antibiotic administration, is being provided for the infected burn, the seventh character A is appropriate for this encounter.

5) Assign separate codes for each burn site

When coding burns, assign separate codes for each burn site. Category T30, Burn and corrosion, body region unspecified is extremely vague and should rarely be used.

6) Burns and corrosions classified according to extent of body surface involved

Assign codes from category T31, Burns classified according to extent of body surface involved, or T32, Corrosions classified according to extent of body surface involved, when the site of the burn is not specified or when there is a need for additional data. It is advisable to use category T31 as additional coding when needed to provide data for evaluating burn mortality, such as that needed by burn units. It is also advisable to use category T31 as an additional code for reporting purposes when there is mention of a third-degree burn involving 20 percent or more of the body surface.

Categories T31 and T32 are based on the classic "rule of nines" in estimating body surface involved: head and neck are assigned nine percent, each arm nine percent, each leg 18 percent, the anterior trunk 18 percent, posterior trunk 18 percent, and genitalia one percent. Providers may change these percentage assignments where necessary to accommodate infants and children who have proportionately larger heads than adults, and patients who have large buttocks, thighs, or abdomen that involve burns.

> Patient seen for dressing change after he accidentally spilled acetic acid on himself two days ago. The second-degree burns to his right thigh, covering about 3 percent of his body surface, are healing appropriately.
>
> | T54.2X1D | Toxic effect of corrosive acids and acid-like substances, accidental (unintentional), subsequent encounter |
> |---|---|
> | T24.611D | Corrosion of second degree of right thigh, subsequent encounter |
> | T32.0 | Corrosions involving less than 10% of body surface |
>
> *Explanation:* Code T32.0 provides additional information as to how much of the patient's body was affected by the corrosive substance.

7) Encounters for treatment of sequela of burns

Encounters for the treatment of the late effects of burns or corrosions (i.e., scars or joint contractures) should be coded with a burn or corrosion code with the 7th character "S" for sequela.

8) Sequelae with a late effect code and current burn

When appropriate, both a code for a current burn or corrosion with 7th character "A" or "D" and a burn or corrosion code with 7th character "S" may be assigned on the same record (when both a current burn and sequelae of an old burn exist). Burns and corrosions do not heal at the same rate and a current healing wound may still exist with sequela of a healed burn or corrosion.

See Section I.B.10 Sequela (Late Effects)

> Female patient seen for second-degree burn to the left ear; that is healing well with no current treatment orders. She also has significant scarring on her left elbow from a third-degree burn from childhood.
>
> | T20.212D | Burn of second degree of left ear [any part, except ear drum], subsequent encounter |
> |---|---|
> | L90.5 | Scar conditions and fibrosis of skin |
> | T22.322S | Burn of third degree of left elbow, sequela |
>
> *Explanation:* The patient is being seen for management of a current second-degree burn, which is reflected in the code by appending the seventh character D, indicating that active treatment is no longer needed and the burn is in the recovery phase of healing. The elbow scarring is a sequela of a previous third-degree burn. The sequela condition precedes the original burn injury, which is appended with a seventh character of S.

9) Use of an external cause code with burns and corrosions

An external cause code should be used with burns and corrosions to identify the source and intent of the burn, as well as the place where it occurred.

e. Adverse effects, poisoning, underdosing and toxic effects

Codes in categories T36-T65 are combination codes that include the substance that was taken as well as the intent. No additional external cause code is required for poisonings, toxic effects, adverse effects and underdosing codes.

1) Do not code directly from the Table of Drugs

Do not code directly from the Table of Drugs and Chemicals. Always refer back to the Tabular List.

2) Use as many codes as necessary to describe

Use as many codes as necessary to describe completely all drugs, medicinal or biological substances.

3) If the same code would describe the causative agent

If the same code would describe the causative agent for more than one adverse reaction, poisoning, toxic effect or underdosing, assign the code only once.

4) If two or more drugs, medicinal or biological substances

If two or more drugs, medicinal or biological substances are reported, code each individually unless a combination code is listed in the Table of Drugs and Chemicals.

5) The occurrence of drug toxicity is classified in ICD-10-CM as follows:

(a) Adverse effect

When coding an adverse effect of a drug that has been correctly prescribed and properly administered, assign the appropriate code for the nature of the adverse effect followed by the appropriate code for the adverse effect of the drug (T36-T50). The code for the drug should have a 5th or 6th character "5" (for example T36.0X5-) Examples of the nature of an adverse effect are tachycardia, delirium, gastrointestinal hemorrhaging, vomiting, hypokalemia, hepatitis, renal failure, or respiratory failure.

> A patient with hyperthyroidism is now reported to have jaundice, RUQ abdominal pain, and elevated liver function studies resulting from prescribed treatment with methimazole. The physician has reduced the dose and ordered continued labs and monitoring of the patient's condition.
>
> | R10.11 | Right upper quadrant pain |
> |---|---|
> | R94.5 | Abnormal results of liver function studies |
> | T38.2X5D | Adverse effect off antithyroid drugs, subsequent encounter |
> | E05.90 | Thyrotoxicosis, unspecified without thyrotoxic crisis or storm |
>
> *Explanation:* The side-effects of the drug are coded first, followed by the code for the adverse effect of the drug to identify the drug responsible. The follow-up monitoring of the condition by the home health agency is captured with the use of seventh character D.

(b) Poisoning

When coding a poisoning or reaction to the improper use of a medication (e.g., overdose, wrong substance given or taken in error, wrong route of administration), first assign the appropriate code from categories T36-T50. The poisoning codes have an associated intent as their 5th or 6th character (accidental, intentional self-harm, assault and undetermined. If the intent of the poisoning is unknown or unspecified, code the intent as accidental intent. The undetermined intent is only for use if the documentation in the record specifies that the intent cannot be determined. Use additional code(s) for all manifestations of poisonings.

If there is also a diagnosis of abuse or dependence of the substance, the abuse or dependence is assigned as an additional code.

Examples of poisoning include:

(i) Error was made in drug prescription

Errors made in drug prescription or in the administration of the drug by provider, nurse, patient, or other person.

(ii) Overdose of a drug intentionally taken

If an overdose of a drug was intentionally taken or administered and resulted in drug toxicity, it would be coded as a poisoning.

(iii) Nonprescribed drug taken with correctly prescribed and properly administered drug

If a nonprescribed drug or medicinal agent was taken in combination with a correctly prescribed and properly administered drug, any drug toxicity or other reaction resulting from the interaction of the two drugs would be classified as a poisoning.

(iv) Interaction of drug(s) and alcohol

When a reaction results from the interaction of a drug(s) and alcohol, this would be classified as poisoning.

See Section I.C.4. if poisoning is the result of insulin pump malfunctions.

(c) Underdosing

Underdosing refers to taking less of a medication than is prescribed by a provider or a manufacturer's instruction. For underdosing, assign the code from categories T36-T50 (fifth or sixth character "6").

Codes for underdosing should never be assigned as principal or first-listed codes. If a patient has a relapse or exacerbation of the medical condition for which the drug is prescribed because of the reduction in dose, then the medical condition itself should be coded.

Noncompliance (Z91.12-, Z91.13-) or complication of care (Y63.6-Y63.9) codes are to be used with an underdosing code to indicate intent, if known.

Patient admitted for atrial fibrillation with history of chronic atrial fibrillation for which she is prescribed amiodarone. Financial concerns have left the patient unable to pay for her prescriptions and she has been skipping her amiodarone dose every other day to offset the cost.

I48.2	Chronic atrial fibrillation
T46.2X6A	Underdosing of other antidysrhythmic drugs, initial encounter
Z91.120	Patient's intentional underdosing of medication regimen due to financial hardship

Explanation: By skipping her amiodarone pill every other day, the patient's atrial fibrillation returned. The condition for which the drug was being taken is reported first, followed by an underdosing code to show that the patient was not adhering to her prescription regiment. The Z code helps elaborate on the patient's social and/or economic circumstances that led to the patient taking less then what she was prescribed.

(d) Toxic effects

When a harmful substance is ingested or comes in contact with a person, this is classified as a toxic effect. The toxic effect codes are in categories T51-T65.

Toxic effect codes have an associated intent: accidental, intentional self-harm, assault and undetermined.

f. Adult and child abuse, neglect and other maltreatment

Sequence first the appropriate code from categories T74.- (Adult and child abuse, neglect and other maltreatment, confirmed) or T76.- (Adult and child abuse, neglect and other maltreatment, suspected) for abuse, neglect and other maltreatment, followed by any accompanying mental health or injury code(s).

If the documentation in the medical record states abuse or neglect it is coded as confirmed (T74.-). It is coded as suspected if it is documented as suspected (T76.-).

For cases of confirmed abuse or neglect an external cause code from the assault section (X92-Y09) should be added to identify the cause of any

physical injuries. A perpetrator code (Y07) should be added when the perpetrator of the abuse is known. For suspected cases of abuse or neglect, do not report external cause or perpetrator code.

If a suspected case of abuse, neglect or mistreatment is ruled out during an encounter code Z04.71, Encounter for examination and observation following alleged physical adult abuse, ruled out, or code Z04.72, Encounter for examination and observation following alleged child physical abuse, ruled out, should be used, not a code from T76.

If a suspected case of alleged rape or sexual abuse is ruled out during an encounter code Z04.41, Encounter for examination and observation following alleged adult rape or code Z04.42, Encounter for examination and observation following alleged child rape, should be used, not a code from T76.

See Section I.C.15. Abuse in a pregnant patient.

g. Complications of care

1) General guidelines for complications of care

(a) Documentation of complications of care

See Section I.B.16. for information on documentation of complications of care.

2) Pain due to medical devices

Pain associated with devices, implants or grafts left in a surgical site (for example painful hip prosthesis) is assigned to the appropriate code(s) found in Chapter 19, Injury, poisoning, and certain other consequences of external causes. Specific codes for pain due to medical devices are found in the T code section of the ICD-10-CM. Use additional code(s) from category G89 to identify acute or chronic pain due to presence of the device, implant or graft (G89.18 or G89.28).

A patient with multiple sclerosis has an implanted pain pump in the upper right buttock. The provider notes indicate chronic pain of the lower back due to placement of pain pump.

T85.848D	Pain due to other internal prosthetic devices, implants and grafts, subsequent encounter
M54.5	Low back pain
G89.28	Other chronic postprocedural pain
G35	Multiple sclerosis

Explanation: As the pain is a complication of the implanted pain pump, the complication code is sequenced first. The seventh character D is used, as caregivers in the post-acute care setting will be monitoring this chronic pain condition but not providing active treatment. The T code does not fully describe the site or type of pain, and additional codes should be assigned for these.

3) Transplant complications

(a) Transplant complications other than kidney

Codes under category T86, Complications of transplanted organs and tissues, are for use for both complications and rejection of transplanted organs. A transplant complication code is only assigned if the complication affects the function of the transplanted organ. Two codes are required to fully describe a transplant complication: the appropriate code from category T86 and a secondary code that identifies the complication.

Pre-existing conditions or conditions that develop after the transplant are not coded as complications unless they affect the function of the transplanted organs.

See I.C.21. for transplant organ removal status

See I.C.2. for malignant neoplasm associated with transplanted organ.

(b) Kidney transplant complications

Patients who have undergone kidney transplant may still have some form of chronic kidney disease (CKD) because the kidney transplant may not fully restore kidney function. Code T86.1- should be assigned for documented complications of a kidney transplant, such as transplant failure or rejection or other transplant complication. Code T86.1- should not be assigned for post kidney transplant patients who have chronic kidney (CKD) unless a transplant complication such as transplant failure or rejection is documented. If the documentation is unclear as to whether the patient has a complication of the transplant, query the provider.

Conditions that affect the function of the transplanted kidney, other than CKD, should be assigned a code from subcategory T86.1, Complications of transplanted organ, Kidney, and a secondary code that identifies the complication.

For patients with CKD following a kidney transplant, but who do not have a complication such as failure or rejection, *see section I.C.14. Chronic kidney disease and kidney transplant status.*

Patient seen for chronic kidney disease stage 2; history of successful kidney transplant with no complications identified

N18.2   **Chronic kidney disease, stage 2 (mild)**

Z94.Ø   **Kidney transplant status**

Explanation: This patient's stage 2 CKD is not indicated as being due to the transplanted kidney but instead is just the residual disease the patient had prior to the transplant.

---

4) Complication codes that include the external cause

As with certain other T codes, some of the complications of care codes have the external cause included in the code. The code includes the nature of the complication as well as the type of procedure that caused the complication. No external cause code indicating the type of procedure is necessary for these codes.

5) Complications of care codes within the body system chapters

Intraoperative and postprocedural complication codes are found within the body system chapters with codes specific to the organs and structures of that body system. These codes should be sequenced first, followed by a code(s) for the specific complication, if applicable.

A patient with a history of bilateral ovarian cancer is admitted following a total abdominal hysterectomy. The patient has a Foley catheter with active hematuria and continues with radiation for the neoplastic disease. The provider notes indicate that the bladder was nicked during the hysterectomy procedure.

N99.71   **Accidental puncture and laceration of a genitourinary system organ or structure during a genitourinary system procedure**

R31.9   **Hematuria, unspecified**

C56.1   **Malignant neoplasm of right ovary**

C56.2   **Malignant neoplasm of left ovary**

Z46.6   **Encounter for fitting and adjustment of urinary device**

Explanation: The accidental puncture of the bladder is specifically due to a procedure and is categorized to the genitourinary chapter rather than coded using an injury code from chapter 19.

Muscle/Tendon Table

ICD-10-CM categorizes certain muscles and tendons in the upper and lower extremities by their action (e.g., extension, flexion), their anatomical location (e.g., posterior, anterior), and/or whether they are intrinsic or extrinsic to a certain anatomical area. The Muscle/Tendon Table is provided at the beginning of chapters 13 and 19 as a resource to help users when code selection depends on one or more of these characteristics. Please note that this table is not all-inclusive, and proper code assignment should be based on the provider's documentation.

Body Region	Muscle	Extensor Tendon	Flexor Tendon	Other Tendon
Shoulder				
	Deltoid	Posterior deltoid	Anterior deltoid	
	Rotator cuff			
	Infraspinatus			Infraspinatus
	Subscapularis			Subscapularis
	Supraspinatus			Supraspinatus
	Teres minor			Teres minor
	Teres major	Teres major		
Upper arm				
	Anterior muscles			
	Biceps brachii — long head		Biceps brachii — long head	
	Biceps brachii — short head		Biceps brachii — short head	
	Brachialis		Brachialis	
	Coracobrachialis		Coracobrachialis	
	Posterior muscles			
	Triceps brachii	Triceps brachii		
Forearm				
	Anterior muscles			
	Flexors			
	Deep			
	Flexor digitorum profundus		Flexor digitorum profundus	
	Flexor pollicis longus		Flexor pollicis longus	
	Intermediate			
	Flexor digitorum superficialis		Flexor digitorum superficialis	
	Superficial			
	Flexor carpi radialis		Flexor carpi radialis	
	Flexor carpi ulnaris		Flexor carpi ulnaris	
	Palmaris longus		Palmaris longus	
	Pronators			
	Pronator quadratus			Pronator quadratus
	Pronator teres			Pronator teres
	Posterior muscles			
	Extensors			
	Deep			
	Abductor pollicis longus			Abductor pollicis longus
	Extensor indicis	Extensor indicis		
	Extensor pollicis brevis	Extensor pollicis brevis		
	Extensor pollicis longus	Extensor pollicis longus		
	Superficial			
	Brachioradialis			Brachioradialis
	Extensor carpi radialis brevis	Extensor carpi radialis brevis		
	Extensor carpi radialis longus	Extensor carpi radialis longus		
	Extensor carpi ulnaris	Extensor carpi ulnaris		
	Extensor digiti minimi	Extensor digiti minimi		
	Extensor digitorum	Extensor digitorum		
	Anconeus	Anconeus		
	Supinator			Supinator

Body Region	Muscle	Extensor Tendon	Flexor Tendon	Other Tendon
Hand				
Extrinsic — attach to a site in the forearm as well as a site in the hand with action related to hand movement at the wrist				
	Extensor carpi radialis brevis	Extensor carpi radialis brevis		
	Extensor carpi radialis longus	Extensor carpie radialis longus		
	Extensor carpi ulnaris	Extensor carpi ulnaris		
	Flexor carpi radialis		Flexor carpi radialis	
	Flexor carpi ulnaris		Flexor carpi ulnaris	
	Flexor digitorum superficialis		Flexor digitorum superficialis	
	Palmaris longus		Palmaris longus	
Extrinsic — attach to a site in the forearm as well as a site in the hand with action in the hand related to finger movement				
	Adductor pollicis longus			Adductor pollicis longus
	Extensor digiti minimi	Extensor digiti minimi		
	Extensor digitorum	Extensor digitorum		
	Extensor indicis	Extensor indicis		
	Flexor digitorum profundus		Flexor digitorum profundus	
	Flexor digitorum superficialis		Flexor digitorum superficialis	
Extrinsic — attach to a site in the forearm as well as a site in the hand with action in the hand related to thumb movement				
	Extensor pollicis brevis	Extensor pollicis brevis		
	Extensor pollicis longus	Extensor pollicis longus		
	Flexor pollicis longus		Flexor pollicis longus	
Intrinsic — found within the hand only				
	Adductor pollicis			Adductor pollicis
	Dorsal interossei	Dorsal interossei	Dorsal interossei	
	Lumbricals	Lumbricals	Lumbricals	
	Palmaris brevis			Palmaris brevis
	Palmar interossei	Palmar interossei	Palmar interossei	
	Hypothenar muscles			
	Abductor digiti minimi			Abductor digiti minimi
	Flexor digiti minimi brevis		Flexor digiti minimi brevis	
	Oppenens digiti minimi		Oppenens digiti minimi	
	Thenar muscles			
	Abductor pollicis brevis			Abductor pollicis brevis
	Flexor pollicis brevis		Flexor pollicis brevis	
	Oppenens pollicis		Oppenens pollicis	
Thigh				
	Anterior muscles			
	Iliopsoas		Iliopsoas	
	Pectineus		Pectineus	
	Quadriceps	Quadriceps		
	Rectus femoris	Rectus femoris — Extends knee	Rectus femoris — Flexes hip	
	Vastus intermedius	Vastus intermedius		
	Vastus lateralis	Vastus lateralis		
	Vastus medialis	Vastus medialis		
	Sartorius		Sartorius	
	Medial muscles			
	Adductor brevis			Adductor brevis
	Adductor longus			Adductor longus
	Adductor magnus			Adductor magnus
	Gracilis			Gracilis
	Obturator externus			Obturator externus
	Posterior muscles			
	Hamstring	Hamstring — Extends hip	Hamstring — Flexes knee	
	Biceps femoris	Biceps femoris	Biceps femoris	
	Semimembranosus	Semimembranosus	Semimembranosus	
	Semitendinosus	Semitendinosus	Semitendinosus	

Chapter 19. Injury, Poisoning and Certain Other Consequences of External Causes

Body Region	Muscle	Extensor Tendon	Flexor Tendon	Other Tendon
Lower leg				
	Anterior muscles			
	Extensor digitorum longus	Extensor digitorum longus		
	Extensor hallucis longus	Extensor hallucis longus		
	Fibularis (peroneus) tertius	Fibularis (peroneus) tertius		
	Tibialis anterior	Tibialis anterior		Tibialis anterior
	Lateral muscles			
	Fibularis (peroneus) brevis		Fibularis (peroneus) brevis	
	Fibularis (peroneus) longus		Fibularis (peroneus) longus	
	Posterior muscles			
	Deep			
	Flexor digitorum longus		Flexor digitorum longus	
	Flexor hallucis longus		Flexor hallucis longus	
	Popliteus		Popliteus	
	Tibialis posterior		Tibialis posterior	
	Superficial			
	Gastrocnemius		Gastrocnemius	
	Plantaris		Plantaris	
	Soleus		Soleus	
				Calcaneal (Achilles)
Ankle/Foot				
Extrinsic — attach to a site in the lower leg as well as a site in the foot with action related to foot movement at the ankle				
	Plantaris		Plantaris	
	Soleus		Soleus	
	Tibialis anterior	Tibialis anterior		
	Tibialis posterior		Tibialis posterior	
Extrinsic — attach to a site in the lower leg as well as a site in the foot with action in the foot related to toe movement				
	Extensor digitorum longus	Extensor digitorum longus		
	Extensor hallucis longus	Extensor hallucis longus		
	Flexor digitorum longus		Flexor digitorum longus	
	Flexor hallucis longus		Flexor hallucis longus	
Intrinsic — found within the ankle/foot only				
	Dorsal muscles			
	Extensor digitorum brevis	Extensor digitorum brevis		
	Extensor hallucis brevis	Extensor hallucis brevis		
	Plantar muscles			
	Abductor digiti minimi		Abductor digiti minimi	
	Abductor hallucis		Abductor hallucis	
	Dorsal interossei	Dorsal interossei	Dorsal interossei	
	Flexor digiti minimi brevis		Flexor digiti minimi brevis	
	Flexor digitorum brevis		Flexor digitorum brevis	
	Flexor hallucis brevis		Flexor hallucis brevis	
	Lumbricals	Lumbricals	Lumbricals	
	Quadratus plantae		Quadratus plantae	
	Plantar interossei	Plantar interossei	Plantar interossei	

Chapter 19. Injury, Poisoning and Certain Other Consequences of External Causes (S00-T88)

NOTE Use secondary code(s) from Chapter 20, External causes of morbidity, to indicate cause of injury. Codes within the T section that include the external cause do not require an additional external cause code.

Use additional code to identify any retained foreign body, if applicable (Z18.-)

EXCLUDES 1 birth trauma (P10-P15)
obstetric trauma (O70-O71)

NOTE The chapter uses the S-section for coding different types of injuries related to single body regions and the T-section to cover injuries to unspecified body regions as well as poisoning and certain other consequences of external causes.

AHA: 2016, 2Q, 3-7; 2015, 4Q, 35-38; 2015, 3Q, 37-39, 40; 2015, 2Q, 6; 2015, 1Q, 3-21

This chapter contains the following blocks:

S00-S09	Injuries to the head
S10-S19	Injuries to the neck
S20-S29	Injuries to the thorax
S30-S39	Injuries to the abdomen, lower back, lumbar spine, pelvis and external genitals
S40-S49	Injuries to the shoulder and upper arm
S50-S59	Injuries to the elbow and forearm
S60-S69	Injuries to the wrist, hand and fingers
S70-S79	Injuries to the hip and thigh
S80-S89	Injuries to the knee and lower leg
S90-S99	Injuries to the ankle and foot
T07	Injuries involving multiple body regions
T14	Injury of unspecified body region
T15-T19	Effects of foreign body entering through natural orifice
T20-T25	Burns and corrosions of external body surface, specified by site
T26-T28	Burns and corrosions confined to eye and internal organs
T30-T32	Burns and corrosions of multiple and unspecified body regions
T33-T34	Frostbite
T36-T50	Poisoning by, adverse effect of and underdosing of drugs, medicaments and biological substances
T51-T65	Toxic effects of substances chiefly nonmedicinal as to source
T66-T78	Other and unspecified effects of external causes
T79	Certain early complications of trauma
T80-T88	Complications of surgical and medical care, not elsewhere classified

Injuries to the head (S00-S09)

INCLUDES injuries of ear
injuries of eye
injuries of face [any part]
injuries of gum
injuries of jaw
injuries of oral cavity
injuries of palate
injuries of periocular area
injuries of scalp
injuries of temporomandibular joint area
injuries of tongue
injuries of tooth

Code also for any associated infection

EXCLUDES 2 burns and corrosions (T20-T32)
effects of foreign body in ear (T16)
effects of foreign body in larynx (T17.3)
effects of foreign body in mouth NOS (T18.0)
effects of foreign body in nose (T17.0-T17.1)
effects of foreign body in pharynx (T17.2)
effects of foreign body on external eye (T15.-)
frostbite (T33-T34)
insect bite or sting, venomous (T63.4)

✓4th S00 Superficial injury of head
   EXCLUDES 1 diffuse cerebral contusion (S06.2-)
        focal cerebral contusion (S06.3-)
        injury of eye and orbit (S05.-)
        open wound of head (S01.-)

> The appropriate 7th character is to be added to each code from categories S00.
> A   initial encounter
> D   subsequent encounter
> S   sequela

✓5th S00.0 Superficial injury of scalp
  ✓x7th S00.00 Unspecified superficial injury of scalp ▽
  ✓x7th S00.01 Abrasion of scalp
  ✓x7th S00.02 Blister (nonthermal) of scalp

✓x7th S00.03 Contusion of scalp
  Bruise of scalp
  Hematoma of scalp

✓x7th S00.04 External constriction of part of scalp

✓x7th S00.05 Superficial foreign body of scalp
  Splinter in the scalp

✓x7th S00.06 Insect bite (nonvenomous) of scalp

✓x7th S00.07 Other superficial bite of scalp
  EXCLUDES 1 open bite of scalp (S01.05)

✓5th S00.1 Contusion of eyelid and periocular area
  Black eye
  EXCLUDES 2 contusion of eyeball and orbital tissues (S05.1)

  ✓x7th S00.10 Contusion of unspecified eyelid and periocular area ▽
  ✓x7th S00.11 Contusion of right eyelid and periocular area
  ✓x7th S00.12 Contusion of left eyelid and periocular area

✓5th S00.2 Other and unspecified superficial injuries of eyelid and periocular area
  EXCLUDES 2 superficial injury of conjunctiva and cornea (S05.0-)

  ✓6th S00.20 Unspecified superficial injury of eyelid and periocular area
    ✓7th S00.201 Unspecified superficial injury of right eyelid and periocular area ▽
    ✓7th S00.202 Unspecified superficial injury of left eyelid and periocular area ▽
    ✓7th S00.209 Unspecified superficial injury of unspecified eyelid and periocular area ▽

  ✓6th S00.21 Abrasion of eyelid and periocular area
    ✓7th S00.211 Abrasion of right eyelid and periocular area
    ✓7th S00.212 Abrasion of left eyelid and periocular area
    ✓7th S00.219 Abrasion of unspecified eyelid and periocular area ▽

  ✓6th S00.22 Blister (nonthermal) of eyelid and periocular area
    ✓7th S00.221 Blister (nonthermal) of right eyelid and periocular area
    ✓7th S00.222 Blister (nonthermal) of left eyelid and periocular area
    ✓7th S00.229 Blister (nonthermal) of unspecified eyelid and periocular area ▽

  ✓6th S00.24 External constriction of eyelid and periocular area
    ✓7th S00.241 External constriction of right eyelid and periocular area
    ✓7th S00.242 External constriction of left eyelid and periocular area
    ✓7th S00.249 External constriction of unspecified eyelid and periocular area ▽

  ✓6th S00.25 Superficial foreign body of eyelid and periocular area
    Splinter of eyelid and periocular area
    EXCLUDES 2 retained foreign body in eyelid (H02.81-)
    ✓7th S00.251 Superficial foreign body of right eyelid and periocular area
    ✓7th S00.252 Superficial foreign body of left eyelid and periocular area
    ✓7th S00.259 Superficial foreign body of unspecified eyelid and periocular area ▽

  ✓6th S00.26 Insect bite (nonvenomous) of eyelid and periocular area
    ✓7th S00.261 Insect bite (nonvenomous) of right eyelid and periocular area
    ✓7th S00.262 Insect bite (nonvenomous) of left eyelid and periocular area
    ✓7th S00.269 Insect bite (nonvenomous) of unspecified eyelid and periocular area ▽

  ✓6th S00.27 Other superficial bite of eyelid and periocular area
    EXCLUDES 1 open bite of eyelid and periocular area (S01.15)
    ✓7th S00.271 Other superficial bite of right eyelid and periocular area
    ✓7th S00.272 Other superficial bite of left eyelid and periocular area
    ✓7th S00.279 Other superficial bite of unspecified eyelid and periocular area ▽

☑ Additional Character Req   ✓x7th Placeholder Alert   Case-Mix Diagnosis   Manifestation   ▽ Unspecified Dx   **EXCLUDES 1** Not coded here   **EXCLUDES 2** Not included here

ICD-10-CM 2018   **913**

Chapter 19. Injury, Poisoning and Certain Other Consequences of External Causes

S00.3–S01.00

✓5ᵗʰ **S00.3** Superficial injury of nose

     ✓ˣ7ᵗʰ **S00.30** Unspecified superficial injury of nose ▽

     ✓ˣ7ᵗʰ **S00.31** Abrasion of nose

     ✓ˣ7ᵗʰ **S00.32** Blister (nonthermal) of nose

     ✓ˣ7ᵗʰ **S00.33** Contusion of nose
             Bruise of nose
             Hematoma of nose

     ✓ˣ7ᵗʰ **S00.34** External constriction of nose

     ✓ˣ7ᵗʰ **S00.35** Superficial foreign body of nose
             Splinter in the nose

     ✓ˣ7ᵗʰ **S00.36** Insect bite (nonvenomous) of nose

     ✓ˣ7ᵗʰ **S00.37** Other superficial bite of nose
             EXCLUDES 1 *open bite of nose (S01.25)*

✓5ᵗʰ **S00.4** Superficial injury of ear

     ✓6ᵗʰ **S00.40** Unspecified superficial injury of ear

         ✓7ᵗʰ **S00.401** Unspecified superficial injury of right ear ▽

         ✓7ᵗʰ **S00.402** Unspecified superficial injury of left ear ▽

         ✓7ᵗʰ **S00.409** Unspecified superficial injury of unspecified ear ▽

     ✓6ᵗʰ **S00.41** Abrasion of ear

         ✓7ᵗʰ **S00.411** Abrasion of right ear

         ✓7ᵗʰ **S00.412** Abrasion of left ear

         ✓7ᵗʰ **S00.419** Abrasion of unspecified ear ▽

     ✓6ᵗʰ **S00.42** Blister (nonthermal) of ear

         ✓7ᵗʰ **S00.421** Blister (nonthermal) of right ear

         ✓7ᵗʰ **S00.422** Blister (nonthermal) of left ear

         ✓7ᵗʰ **S00.429** Blister (nonthermal) of unspecified ear ▽

     ✓6ᵗʰ **S00.43** Contusion of ear
         Bruise of ear
         Hematoma of ear

         ✓7ᵗʰ **S00.431** Contusion of right ear

         ✓7ᵗʰ **S00.432** Contusion of left ear

         ✓7ᵗʰ **S00.439** Contusion of unspecified ear ▽

     ✓6ᵗʰ **S00.44** External constriction of ear

         ✓7ᵗʰ **S00.441** External constriction of right ear

         ✓7ᵗʰ **S00.442** External constriction of left ear

         ✓7ᵗʰ **S00.449** External constriction of unspecified ear ▽

     ✓6ᵗʰ **S00.45** Superficial foreign body of ear
         Splinter in the ear

         ✓7ᵗʰ **S00.451** Superficial foreign body of right ear

         ✓7ᵗʰ **S00.452** Superficial foreign body of left ear

         ✓7ᵗʰ **S00.459** Superficial foreign body of unspecified ear ▽

     ✓6ᵗʰ **S00.46** Insect bite (nonvenomous) of ear

         ✓7ᵗʰ **S00.461** Insect bite (nonvenomous) of right ear

         ✓7ᵗʰ **S00.462** Insect bite (nonvenomous) of left ear

         ✓7ᵗʰ **S00.469** Insect bite (nonvenomous) of unspecified ear ▽

     ✓6ᵗʰ **S00.47** Other superficial bite of ear
         EXCLUDES 1 *open bite of ear (S01.35)*

         ✓7ᵗʰ **S00.471** Other superficial bite of right ear

         ✓7ᵗʰ **S00.472** Other superficial bite of left ear

         ✓7ᵗʰ **S00.479** Other superficial bite of unspecified ear ▽

✓5ᵗʰ **S00.5** Superficial injury of lip and oral cavity

     ✓6ᵗʰ **S00.50** Unspecified superficial injury of lip and oral cavity

         ✓7ᵗʰ **S00.501** Unspecified superficial injury of lip ▽

         ✓7ᵗʰ **S00.502** Unspecified superficial injury of oral cavity ▽

     ✓6ᵗʰ **S00.51** Abrasion of lip and oral cavity

         ✓7ᵗʰ **S00.511** Abrasion of lip

         ✓7ᵗʰ **S00.512** Abrasion of oral cavity

     ✓6ᵗʰ **S00.52** Blister (nonthermal) of lip and oral cavity

         ✓7ᵗʰ **S00.521** Blister (nonthermal) of lip

         ✓7ᵗʰ **S00.522** Blister (nonthermal) of oral cavity

---

     ✓6ᵗʰ **S00.53** Contusion of lip and oral cavity

         ✓7ᵗʰ **S00.531** Contusion of lip
             Bruise of lip
             ►Hematoma of lip◄

         ✓7ᵗʰ **S00.532** Contusion of oral cavity
             ►Bruise of oral cavity◄
             Hematoma of oral cavity

     ✓6ᵗʰ **S00.54** External constriction of lip and oral cavity

         ✓7ᵗʰ **S00.541** External constriction of lip

         ✓7ᵗʰ **S00.542** External constriction of oral cavity

     ✓6ᵗʰ **S00.55** Superficial foreign body of lip and oral cavity

         ✓7ᵗʰ **S00.551** Superficial foreign body of lip
             Splinter of lip and oral cavity

         ✓7ᵗʰ **S00.552** Superficial foreign body of oral cavity
             Splinter of lip and oral cavity

     ✓6ᵗʰ **S00.56** Insect bite (nonvenomous) of lip and oral cavity

         ✓7ᵗʰ **S00.561** Insect bite (nonvenomous) of lip

         ✓7ᵗʰ **S00.562** Insect bite (nonvenomous) of oral cavity

     ✓6ᵗʰ **S00.57** Other superficial bite of lip and oral cavity

         ✓7ᵗʰ **S00.571** Other superficial bite of lip
             EXCLUDES 1 *open bite of lip (S01.551)*

         ✓7ᵗʰ **S00.572** Other superficial bite of oral cavity
             EXCLUDES 1 *open bite of oral cavity (S01.552)*

✓5ᵗʰ **S00.8** Superficial injury of other parts of head
     Superficial injuries of face [any part]

     ✓ˣ7ᵗʰ **S00.80** Unspecified superficial injury of other part of head ▽

     ✓ˣ7ᵗʰ **S00.81** Abrasion of other part of head

     ✓ˣ7ᵗʰ **S00.82** Blister (nonthermal) of other part of head

     ✓ˣ7ᵗʰ **S00.83** Contusion of other part of head
         Bruise of other part of head
         Hematoma of other part of head

     ✓ˣ7ᵗʰ **S00.84** External constriction of other part of head

     ✓ˣ7ᵗʰ **S00.85** Superficial foreign body of other part of head
         Splinter in other part of head

     ✓ˣ7ᵗʰ **S00.86** Insect bite (nonvenomous) of other part of head

     ✓ˣ7ᵗʰ **S00.87** Other superficial bite of other part of head
         EXCLUDES 1 *open bite of other part of head (S01.85)*

✓5ᵗʰ **S00.9** Superficial injury of unspecified part of head

     ✓ˣ7ᵗʰ **S00.90** Unspecified superficial injury of unspecified part of head ▽

     ✓ˣ7ᵗʰ **S00.91** Abrasion of unspecified part of head ▽

     ✓ˣ7ᵗʰ **S00.92** Blister (nonthermal) of unspecified part of head ▽

     ✓ˣ7ᵗʰ **S00.93** Contusion of unspecified part of head ▽
         Bruise of head
         Hematoma of head

     ✓ˣ7ᵗʰ **S00.94** External constriction of unspecified part of head ▽

     ✓ˣ7ᵗʰ **S00.95** Superficial foreign body of unspecified part of head ▽
         Splinter of head

     ✓ˣ7ᵗʰ **S00.96** Insect bite (nonvenomous) of unspecified part of head ▽

     ✓ˣ7ᵗʰ **S00.97** Other superficial bite of unspecified part of head ▽
         EXCLUDES 1 *open bite of head (S01.95)*

✓4ᵗʰ **S01** Open wound of head
     Code also any associated:
         injury of cranial nerve (S04.-)
         injury of muscle and tendon of head (S09.1-)
         intracranial injury (S06.-)
         wound infection
     EXCLUDES 1 *open skull fracture (S02- with 7th character B)*
     EXCLUDES 2 *injury of eye and orbit (S05.-)*
                   traumatic amputation of part of head (S08.-)

     The appropriate 7th character is to be added to each code from category S01.
     A   initial encounter
     D   subsequent encounter
     S   sequela

✓5ᵗʰ **S01.0** Open wound of scalp
     EXCLUDES 1 *avulsion of scalp (S08.0)*

     ⁵ ✓ˣ7ᵗʰ **S01.00** Unspecified open wound of scalp   **NRS** ▽

---

⁵ NRS supply diagnosis with 7th character indicating initial or subsequent encounter.

Ⓝ Newborn: 0   Ⓟ Pediatric: 0-17   Ⓜ Maternity: 12-55   Ⓐ Adult: 15-124   **NRS** Nonroutine supply Dx   **NCDx** Noncancer Dx   **PDx** Primary Dx   ►◄ Revised Text   ● New Code   ▲ Revised Title

914   ICD-10-CM 2018

4,5 ✓x7th **S01.01** Laceration without foreign body of scalp   NRS

4,5 ✓x7th **S01.02** Laceration with foreign body of scalp   NRS

4,5 ✓x7th **S01.03** Puncture wound without foreign body of scalp   NRS

4,5 ✓x7th **S01.04** Puncture wound with foreign body of scalp   NRS

4,5 ✓x7th **S01.05** Open bite of scalp   NRS
    Bite of scalp NOS
    EXCLUDES 1 *superficial bite of scalp (S00.06, S00.07-)*

✓5th **S01.1** **Open wound of** eyelid and periocular area
    Open wound of eyelid and periocular area with or without
    involvement of lacrimal passages

   ✓6th **S01.10** Unspecified **open wound of eyelid and periocular area**

     5 ✓7th **S01.101** Unspecified open wound of right eyelid and periocular area   NRS ▽

     5 ✓7th **S01.102** Unspecified open wound of left eyelid and periocular area   NRS ▽

     ✓7th **S01.109** Unspecified open wound of unspecified eyelid and periocular area   ▽

   ✓6th **S01.11** Laceration without foreign body **of eyelid and periocular area**

     4,5 ✓7th **S01.111** **Laceration without foreign body of right eyelid and periocular area**   NRS

     4,5 ✓7th **S01.112** **Laceration without foreign body of left eyelid and periocular area**   NRS

     ✓7th **S01.119** Laceration without foreign body of unspecified eyelid and periocular area   ▽

   ✓6th **S01.12** Laceration with foreign body **of eyelid and periocular area**

     4,5 ✓7th **S01.121** **Laceration with foreign body of right eyelid and periocular area**   NRS

     4,5 ✓7th **S01.122** **Laceration with foreign body of left eyelid and periocular area**   NRS

     ✓7th **S01.129** Laceration with foreign body of unspecified eyelid and periocular area   ▽

   ✓6th **S01.13** Puncture wound without foreign body **of eyelid and periocular area**

     4,5 ✓7th **S01.131** **Puncture wound without foreign body of right eyelid and periocular area**   NRS

     4,5 ✓7th **S01.132** **Puncture wound without foreign body of left eyelid and periocular area**   NRS

     ✓7th **S01.139** Puncture wound without foreign body of unspecified eyelid and periocular area   ▽

   ✓6th **S01.14** Puncture wound with foreign body **of eyelid and periocular area**

     4,5 ✓7th **S01.141** **Puncture wound with foreign body of right eyelid and periocular area**   NRS

     4,5 ✓7th **S01.142** **Puncture wound with foreign body of left eyelid and periocular area**   NRS

     ✓7th **S01.149** Puncture wound with foreign body of unspecified eyelid and periocular area   ▽

   ✓6th **S01.15** Open bite **of eyelid and periocular area**
     Bite of eyelid and periocular area NOS
     EXCLUDES 1 *superficial bite of eyelid and periocular area (S00.26, S00.27)*

     4,5 ✓7th **S01.151** **Open bite of right eyelid and periocular area**   NRS

     4,5 ✓7th **S01.152** **Open bite of left eyelid and periocular area**   NRS

     ✓7th **S01.159** Open bite of unspecified eyelid and periocular area   ▽

✓5th **S01.2** **Open wound of** nose

   5 ✓x7th **S01.20** Unspecified open wound of nose   NRS ▽

   4,5 ✓x7th **S01.21** Laceration without foreign body of nose   NRS

   4,5 ✓x7th **S01.22** Laceration with foreign body of nose   NRS

   4,5 ✓x7th **S01.23** Puncture wound without foreign body of nose   NRS

   4,5 ✓x7th **S01.24** Puncture wound with foreign body of nose   NRS

   4,5 ✓x7th **S01.25** Open bite of nose   NRS
     Bite of nose NOS
     EXCLUDES 1 *superficial bite of nose (S00.36, S00.37)*

✓5th **S01.3** **Open wound of** ear

   ✓6th **S01.30** Unspecified **open wound of ear**

     5 ✓7th **S01.301** Unspecified open wound of right ear   NRS ▽

     5 ✓7th **S01.302** Unspecified open wound of left ear   NRS ▽

     ✓7th **S01.309** Unspecified open wound of unspecified ear   ▽

   ✓6th **S01.31** Laceration without foreign body **of ear**

     4,5 ✓7th **S01.311** **Laceration without foreign body of right ear**   NRS

     4,5 ✓7th **S01.312** **Laceration without foreign body of left ear**   NRS

     ✓7th **S01.319** Laceration without foreign body of unspecified ear   ▽

   ✓6th **S01.32** Laceration with foreign body **of ear**

     4,5 ✓7th **S01.321** **Laceration with foreign body of right ear**   NRS

     4,5 ✓7th **S01.322** **Laceration with foreign body of left ear**   NRS

     ✓7th **S01.329** Laceration with foreign body of unspecified ear   ▽

   ✓6th **S01.33** Puncture wound without foreign body **of ear**

     4,5 ✓7th **S01.331** **Puncture wound without foreign body of right ear**   NRS

     4,5 ✓7th **S01.332** **Puncture wound without foreign body of left ear**   NRS

     ✓7th **S01.339** Puncture wound without foreign body of unspecified ear   ▽

   ✓6th **S01.34** Puncture wound with foreign body **of ear**

     4,5 ✓7th **S01.341** **Puncture wound with foreign body of right ear**   NRS

     4,5 ✓7th **S01.342** **Puncture wound with foreign body of left ear**   NRS

     ✓7th **S01.349** Puncture wound with foreign body of unspecified ear   ▽

   ✓6th **S01.35** Open bite **of ear**
     Bite of ear NOS
     EXCLUDES 1 *superficial bite of ear (S00.46, S00.47)*

     4,5 ✓7th **S01.351** **Open bite of right ear**   NRS

     4,5 ✓7th **S01.352** **Open bite of left ear**   NRS

     ✓7th **S01.359** Open bite of unspecified ear   ▽

✓5th **S01.4** **Open wound of** cheek and temporomandibular area

   ✓6th **S01.40** Unspecified **open wound of cheek and temporomandibular area**

     4,5 ✓7th **S01.401** **Unspecified open wound of right cheek and temporomandibular area**   NRS ▽

     4,5 ✓7th **S01.402** **Unspecified open wound of left cheek and temporomandibular area**   NRS ▽

     ✓7th **S01.409** Unspecified open wound of unspecified cheek and temporomandibular area   ▽

   ✓6th **S01.41** Laceration without foreign body **of cheek and temporomandibular area**

     4,5 ✓7th **S01.411** **Laceration without foreign body of right cheek and temporomandibular area**   NRS

     4,5 ✓7th **S01.412** **Laceration without foreign body of left cheek and temporomandibular area**   NRS

     ✓7th **S01.419** Laceration without foreign body of unspecified cheek and temporomandibular area   ▽

   ✓6th **S01.42** Laceration with foreign body **of cheek and temporomandibular area**

     4,5 ✓7th **S01.421** **Laceration with foreign body of right cheek and temporomandibular area**   NRS

     4,5 ✓7th **S01.422** **Laceration with foreign body of left cheek and temporomandibular area**   NRS

     ✓7th **S01.429** Laceration with foreign body of unspecified cheek and temporomandibular area   ▽

---

4   Case-mix diagnosis with 7th character indicating initial or subsequent encounter.
5   NRS supply diagnosis with 7th character indicating initial or subsequent encounter.

✓ Additional Character Req   ✓x7th Placeholder Alert   Case-Mix Diagnosis   Manifestation   ▽ Unspecified Dx   **EXCLUDES 1** Not coded here   **EXCLUDES 2** Not included here

☑6ᵗʰ **S01.43** Puncture wound without foreign body of cheek and temporomandibular area

     4,5 ☑7ᵗʰ **S01.431** **Puncture wound without foreign body of right cheek and temporomandibular area** NRS

     4,5 ☑7ᵗʰ **S01.432** **Puncture wound without foreign body of left cheek and temporomandibular area** NRS

     ☑7ᵗʰ **S01.439** **Puncture wound without foreign body of unspecified cheek and temporomandibular area** ▽

☑6ᵗʰ **S01.44** Puncture wound with foreign body of cheek and temporomandibular area

     4,5 ☑7ᵗʰ **S01.441** **Puncture wound with foreign body of right cheek and temporomandibular area** NRS

     4,5 ☑7ᵗʰ **S01.442** **Puncture wound with foreign body of left cheek and temporomandibular area** NRS

     ☑7ᵗʰ **S01.449** **Puncture wound with foreign body of unspecified cheek and temporomandibular area** ▽

☑6ᵗʰ **S01.45** Open bite of cheek and temporomandibular area
     Bite of cheek and temporomandibular area NOS
     EXCLUDES 2 superficial bite of cheek and temporomandibular area (S00.86, S00.87)

     4,5 ☑7ᵗʰ **S01.451** **Open bite of right cheek and temporomandibular area** NRS

     4,5 ☑7ᵗʰ **S01.452** **Open bite of left cheek and temporomandibular area** NRS

     ☑7ᵗʰ **S01.459** **Open bite of unspecified cheek and temporomandibular area** ▽

☑5ᵗʰ **S01.5** Open wound of lip and oral cavity
     EXCLUDES 2 tooth dislocation (S03.2)
     tooth fracture (S02.5)

☑6ᵗʰ **S01.50** Unspecified open wound of lip and oral cavity

     5 ☑7ᵗʰ **S01.501** **Unspecified open wound of lip** NRS ▽

     5 ☑7ᵗʰ **S01.502** **Unspecified open wound of oral cavity** NRS ▽

☑6ᵗʰ **S01.51** Laceration of lip and oral cavity without foreign body

     4,5 ☑7ᵗʰ **S01.511** **Laceration without foreign body of lip** NRS

     4,5 ☑7ᵗʰ **S01.512** **Laceration without foreign body of oral cavity** NRS

☑6ᵗʰ **S01.52** Laceration of lip and oral cavity with foreign body

     4,5 ☑7ᵗʰ **S01.521** **Laceration with foreign body of lip** NRS

     4,5 ☑7ᵗʰ **S01.522** **Laceration with foreign body of oral cavity** NRS

☑6ᵗʰ **S01.53** Puncture wound of lip and oral cavity without foreign body

     4,5 ☑7ᵗʰ **S01.531** **Puncture wound without foreign body of lip** NRS

     4,5 ☑7ᵗʰ **S01.532** **Puncture wound without foreign body of oral cavity** NRS

☑6ᵗʰ **S01.54** Puncture wound of lip and oral cavity with foreign body

     4,5 ☑7ᵗʰ **S01.541** **Puncture wound with foreign body of lip** NRS

     4,5 ☑7ᵗʰ **S01.542** **Puncture wound with foreign body of oral cavity** NRS

☑6ᵗʰ **S01.55** Open bite of lip and oral cavity

     4,5 ☑7ᵗʰ **S01.551** **Open bite of lip** NRS
         Bite of lip NOS
         EXCLUDES 1 superficial bite of lip (S00.571)

     4,5 ☑7ᵗʰ **S01.552** **Open bite of oral cavity** NRS
         Bite of oral cavity NOS
         EXCLUDES 1 superficial bite of oral cavity (S00.572)

☑5ᵗʰ **S01.8** Open wound of other parts of head

     5 ☑7ᵗʰ **S01.80** **Unspecified open wound of other part of head** NRS ▽

     4,5 ☑7ᵗʰ **S01.81** **Laceration without foreign body of other part of head** NRS

     4,5 ☑7ᵗʰ **S01.82** **Laceration with foreign body of other part of head** NRS

     4,5 ☑7ᵗʰ **S01.83** **Puncture wound without foreign body of other part of head** NRS

     4,5 ☑7ᵗʰ **S01.84** **Puncture wound with foreign body of other part of head** NRS

     4,5 ☑7ᵗʰ **S01.85** **Open bite of other part of head** NRS
         Bite of other part of head NOS
         EXCLUDES 1 superficial bite of other part of head ▶(S00.87)◀

☑5ᵗʰ **S01.9** Open wound of unspecified part of head

     ☑x7ᵗʰ **S01.90** **Unspecified open wound of unspecified part of head** ▽

     ☑x7ᵗʰ **S01.91** **Laceration without foreign body of unspecified part of head** ▽

     ☑x7ᵗʰ **S01.92** **Laceration with foreign body of unspecified part of head** ▽

     ☑x7ᵗʰ **S01.93** **Puncture wound without foreign body of unspecified part of head** ▽

     ☑x7ᵗʰ **S01.94** **Puncture wound with foreign body of unspecified part of head** ▽

     ☑x7ᵗʰ **S01.95** **Open bite of unspecified part of head** ▽
         Bite of head NOS
         EXCLUDES 1 superficial bite of head NOS (S00.97)

☑4ᵗʰ **S02** **Fracture of skull and facial bones**
     NOTE A fracture not indicated as open or closed should be coded to closed.
     Code also any associated intracranial injury (S06.-).
     AHA: 2017, 1Q, 42

     The appropriate 7th character is to be added to each code from category S02.
     A   initial encounter for closed fracture
     B   initial encounter for open fracture
     D   subsequent encounter for fracture with routine healing
     G   subsequent encounter for fracture with delayed healing
     K   subsequent encounter for fracture with nonunion
     S   sequela

1 ☑x7ᵗʰ **S02.0** **Fracture of vault of skull**
     Fracture of frontal bone
     Fracture of parietal bone

☑5ᵗʰ **S02.1** **Fracture of base of skull**
     EXCLUDES 1 orbit NOS (S02.8)
     EXCLUDES 2 orbital floor (S02.3-)

     ☑6ᵗʰ **S02.10** Unspecified fracture of base of skull

         1 ☑7ᵗʰ **S02.101** **Fracture of base of skull, right side**

         1 ☑7ᵗʰ **S02.102** **Fracture of base of skull, left side**

         ☑7ᵗʰ **S02.109** **Fracture of base of skull, unspecified side** ▽

     ☑6ᵗʰ **S02.11** Fracture of occiput

         ☑7ᵗʰ **S02.110** **Type I occipital condyle fracture, unspecified side** ▽

         ☑7ᵗʰ **S02.111** **Type II occipital condyle fracture, unspecified side** ▽

         ☑7ᵗʰ **S02.112** **Type III occipital condyle fracture, unspecified side** ▽

         1 ☑7ᵗʰ **S02.113** **Unspecified occipital condyle fracture** ▽

         ☑7ᵗʰ **S02.118** **Other fracture of occiput, unspecified side** ▽

         1 ☑7ᵗʰ **S02.119** **Unspecified fracture of occiput** ▽

         1 ☑7ᵗʰ **S02.11A** **Type I occipital condyle fracture, right side**

         1 ☑7ᵗʰ **S02.11B** **Type I occipital condyle fracture, left side**

         1 ☑7ᵗʰ **S02.11C** **Type II occipital condyle fracture, right side**

         1 ☑7ᵗʰ **S02.11D** **Type II occipital condyle fracture, left side**

         1 ☑7ᵗʰ **S02.11E** **Type III occipital condyle fracture, right side**

         1 ☑7ᵗʰ **S02.11F** **Type III occipital condyle fracture, left side**

         1 ☑7ᵗʰ **S02.11G** **Other fracture of occiput, right side**

         1 ☑7ᵗʰ **S02.11H** **Other fracture of occiput, left side**

---

1   Case-mix diagnosis with 7th character indicating subsequent encounter.
4   Case-mix diagnosis with 7th character indicating initial or subsequent encounter.
5   NRS supply diagnosis with 7th character indicating initial or subsequent encounter.

Ⓝ Newborn: 0   Ⓟ Pediatric: 0-17   Ⓜ Maternity: 12-55   Ⓐ Adult: 15-124   NRS Nonroutine supply Dx   NC Dx Noncancer Dx   PDx Primary Dx   ▶◀ Revised Text   ● New Code   ▲ Revised Title

916   ICD-10-CM 2018

¹ ✓x7ᵗʰ **S02.19 Other fracture of base of skull**
Fracture of anterior fossa of base of skull
Fracture of ethmoid sinus
Fracture of frontal sinus
Fracture of middle fossa of base of skull
Fracture of orbital roof
Fracture of posterior fossa of base of skull
Fracture of sphenoid
Fracture of temporal bone

¹ ✓x7ᵗʰ **S02.2 Fracture of nasal bones**

✓5ᵗʰ **S02.3 Fracture of orbital floor**
> *EXCLUDES 1* orbit NOS (S02.8)
> *EXCLUDES 2* orbital roof (S02.1-)

✓x7ᵗʰ **S02.30 Fracture of orbital floor, unspecified side** ▽
¹ ✓x7ᵗʰ **S02.31 Fracture of orbital floor, right side**
¹ ✓x7ᵗʰ **S02.32 Fracture of orbital floor, left side**

✓5ᵗʰ **S02.4 Fracture of malar, maxillary and zygoma bones**
Fracture of superior maxilla
Fracture of upper jaw (bone)
Fracture of zygomatic process of temporal bone

✓6ᵗʰ **S02.40 Fracture of malar, maxillary and zygoma bones, unspecified**
✓7ᵗʰ **S02.400 Malar fracture, unspecified side** ▽
✓7ᵗʰ **S02.401 Maxillary fracture, unspecified side** ▽
✓7ᵗʰ **S02.402 Zygomatic fracture, unspecified side** ▽
¹ ✓7ᵗʰ **S02.40A Malar fracture, right side**
¹ ✓7ᵗʰ **S02.40B Malar fracture, left side**
¹ ✓7ᵗʰ **S02.40C Maxillary fracture, right side**
¹ ✓7ᵗʰ **S02.40D Maxillary fracture, left side**
¹ ✓7ᵗʰ **S02.40E Zygomatic fracture, right side**
¹ ✓7ᵗʰ **S02.40F Zygomatic fracture, left side**

✓6ᵗʰ **S02.41 LeFort fracture**
¹ ✓7ᵗʰ **S02.411 LeFort I fracture**
¹ ✓7ᵗʰ **S02.412 LeFort II fracture**
¹ ✓7ᵗʰ **S02.413 LeFort III fracture**

¹ ✓x7ᵗʰ **S02.42 Fracture of alveolus of maxilla**

✓x7ᵗʰ **S02.5 Fracture of tooth (traumatic)**
Broken tooth
> *EXCLUDES 1* cracked tooth (nontraumatic) (K03.81)

✓5ᵗʰ **S02.6 Fracture of mandible**
Fracture of lower jaw (bone)

✓6ᵗʰ **S02.60 Fracture of mandible, unspecified**
✓7ᵗʰ **S02.600 Fracture of unspecified part of body of mandible, unspecified side** ▽

✓6ᵗʰ **S02.61 Fracture of condylar process of mandible**
✓7ᵗʰ **S02.610 Fracture of condylar process of mandible, unspecified side** ▽
¹ ✓7ᵗʰ **S02.601 Fracture of unspecified part of body of right mandible** ▽

LeFort Fracture Types

Type III
Type II
Type I

Frontal bone Nasal bone Orbital floor

Maxilla

Zygomatic bone (malar) and arch

¹ ✓7ᵗʰ **S02.602 Fracture of unspecified part of body of left mandible** ▽
¹ ✓7ᵗʰ **S02.609 Fracture of mandible, unspecified** ▽
¹ ✓7ᵗʰ **S02.611 Fracture of condylar process of right mandible**
¹ ✓7ᵗʰ **S02.612 Fracture of condylar process of left mandible**

✓6ᵗʰ **S02.62 Fracture of subcondylar process of mandible**
¹ ✓7ᵗʰ **S02.620 Fracture of subcondylar process of mandible, unspecified side** ▽
¹ ✓7ᵗʰ **S02.621 Fracture of subcondylar process of right mandible**
¹ ✓7ᵗʰ **S02.622 Fracture of subcondylar process of left mandible**

✓6ᵗʰ **S02.63 Fracture of coronoid process of mandible**
✓7ᵗʰ **S02.630 Fracture of coronoid process of mandible, unspecified side** ▽
¹ ✓7ᵗʰ **S02.631 Fracture of coronoid process of right mandible**
¹ ✓7ᵗʰ **S02.632 Fracture of coronoid process of left mandible**

✓6ᵗʰ **S02.64 Fracture of ramus of mandible**
✓7ᵗʰ **S02.640 Fracture of ramus of mandible, unspecified side** ▽
¹ ✓7ᵗʰ **S02.641 Fracture of ramus of right mandible**
¹ ✓7ᵗʰ **S02.642 Fracture of ramus of left mandible**

✓6ᵗʰ **S02.65 Fracture of angle of mandible**
✓7ᵗʰ **S02.650 Fracture of angle of mandible, unspecified side** ▽
¹ ✓7ᵗʰ **S02.651 Fracture of angle of right mandible**
¹ ✓7ᵗʰ **S02.652 Fracture of angle of left mandible**

¹ ✓x7ᵗʰ **S02.66 Fracture of symphysis of mandible**

✓6ᵗʰ **S02.67 Fracture of alveolus of mandible**
✓7ᵗʰ **S02.670 Fracture of alveolus of mandible, unspecified side** ▽
¹ ✓7ᵗʰ **S02.671 Fracture of alveolus of right mandible**
¹ ✓7ᵗʰ **S02.672 Fracture of alveolus of left mandible**

¹ ✓x7ᵗʰ **S02.69 Fracture of mandible of other specified site**

✓5ᵗʰ **S02.8 Fractures of other specified skull and facial bones**
Fracture of orbit NOS
Fracture of palate
> *EXCLUDES 1* fracture of orbital floor (S02.3-)
> fracture of orbital roof (S02.1-)

✓x7ᵗʰ **S02.80 Fracture of other specified skull and facial bones, unspecified side** ▽
¹ ✓x7ᵗʰ **S02.81 Fracture of other specified skull and facial bones, right side**
¹ ✓x7ᵗʰ **S02.82 Fracture of other specified skull and facial bones, left side**

✓5ᵗʰ **S02.9 Fracture of unspecified skull and facial bones**
¹ ✓x7ᵗʰ **S02.91 Unspecified fracture of skull** ▽
¹ ✓x7ᵗʰ **S02.92 Unspecified fracture of facial bones** ▽

✓4ᵗʰ **S03 Dislocation and sprain of joints and ligaments of head**
> *INCLUDES* avulsion of joint (capsule) or ligament of head
> laceration of cartilage, joint (capsule) or ligament of head
> sprain of cartilage, joint (capsule) or ligament of head
> traumatic hemarthrosis of joint or ligament of head
> traumatic rupture of joint or ligament of head
> traumatic subluxation of joint or ligament of head
> traumatic tear of joint or ligament of head

Code also any associated open wound
> *EXCLUDES 2* strain of muscle or tendon of head (S09.1)

> The appropriate 7th character is to be added to each code from category S03.
> A initial encounter
> D subsequent encounter
> S sequela

✓5ᵗʰ **S03.0 Dislocation of jaw**
Dislocation of jaw (cartilage) (meniscus)
Dislocation of mandible
Dislocation of temporomandibular (joint)

✓7ᵗʰ **S03.00 Dislocation of jaw, unspecified side** ▽

---

¹ Case-mix diagnosis with 7th character indicating subsequent encounter.

✓7ᵗʰ	S03.01	Dislocation of jaw, right side
✓7ᵗʰ	S03.02	Dislocation of jaw, left side
✓7ᵗʰ	S03.03	Dislocation of jaw, bilateral
✓x7ᵗʰ	S03.1	Dislocation of septal cartilage of nose
✓x7ᵗʰ	S03.2	Dislocation of tooth
✓5ᵗʰ	S03.4	Sprain of jaw

Sprain of temporomandibular (joint) (ligament)

✓7ᵗʰ	S03.40	Sprain of jaw, unspecified side	▽
✓7ᵗʰ	S03.41	Sprain of jaw, right side	
✓7ᵗʰ	S03.42	Sprain of jaw, left side	
✓7ᵗʰ	S03.43	Sprain of jaw, bilateral	
✓x7ᵗʰ	S03.8	Sprain of joints and ligaments of other parts of head	
✓x7ᵗʰ	S03.9	Sprain of joints and ligaments of unspecified parts of head	▽

✓4ᵗʰ **S04 Injury of cranial nerve**

The selection of side should be based on the side of the body being affected

Code first any associated intracranial injury (S06.-)

Code also any associated:
  open wound of head (S01.-)
  skull fracture (S02.-)

The appropriate 7th character is to be added to each code from category S04.
A   initial encounter
D   subsequent encounter
S   sequela

✓5ᵗʰ **S04.0 Injury of optic nerve and pathways**

Use additional code to identify any visual field defect or blindness ▶(H53.4-, H54.-)◀

✓6ᵗʰ	S04.01	Injury of optic nerve	
		Injury of 2nd cranial nerve	
2 ✓7ᵗʰ	S04.011	Injury of optic nerve, right eye	
2 ✓7ᵗʰ	S04.012	Injury of optic nerve, left eye	
✓7ᵗʰ	S04.019	Injury of optic nerve, unspecified eye	▽
		Injury of optic nerve NOS	
3 ✓x7ᵗʰ	S04.02	Injury of optic chiasm	
✓6ᵗʰ	S04.03	Injury of optic tract and pathways	
		Injury of optic radiation	
▲ 3 ✓7ᵗʰ	S04.031	Injury of optic tract and pathways, right side	
▲ 3 ✓7ᵗʰ	S04.032	Injury of optic tract and pathways, left side	
▲ ✓7ᵗʰ	S04.039	Injury of optic tract and pathways, unspecified side	▽
		Injury of optic tract and pathways NOS	
✓6ᵗʰ	S04.04	Injury of visual cortex	
▲ 3 ✓7ᵗʰ	S04.041	Injury of visual cortex, right side	
▲ 3 ✓7ᵗʰ	S04.042	Injury of visual cortex, left side	
▲ ✓7ᵗʰ	S04.049	Injury of visual cortex, unspecified side	▽
		Injury of visual cortex NOS	

✓5ᵗʰ	S04.1	Injury of oculomotor nerve	
		Injury of 3rd cranial nerve	
✓x7ᵗʰ	S04.10	Injury of oculomotor nerve, unspecified side	▽
2 ✓x7ᵗʰ	S04.11	Injury of oculomotor nerve, right side	
2 ✓x7ᵗʰ	S04.12	Injury of oculomotor nerve, left side	
✓5ᵗʰ	S04.2	Injury of trochlear nerve	
		Injury of 4th cranial nerve	
✓x7ᵗʰ	S04.20	Injury of trochlear nerve, unspecified side	▽
2 ✓x7ᵗʰ	S04.21	Injury of trochlear nerve, right side	
2 ✓x7ᵗʰ	S04.22	Injury of trochlear nerve, left side	
✓5ᵗʰ	S04.3	Injury of trigeminal nerve	
		Injury of 5th cranial nerve	
3 ✓x7ᵗʰ	S04.30	Injury of trigeminal nerve, unspecified side	▽
2 ✓x7ᵗʰ	S04.31	Injury of trigeminal nerve, right side	
2 ✓x7ᵗʰ	S04.32	Injury of trigeminal nerve, left side	

✓5ᵗʰ	S04.4	Injury of abducent nerve	
		Injury of 6th cranial nerve	
✓x7ᵗʰ	S04.40	Injury of abducent nerve, unspecified side	▽
2 ✓x7ᵗʰ	S04.41	Injury of abducent nerve, right side	
2 ✓x7ᵗʰ	S04.42	Injury of abducent nerve, left side	
✓5ᵗʰ	S04.5	Injury of facial nerve	
		Injury of 7th cranial nerve	
✓x7ᵗʰ	S04.50	Injury of facial nerve, unspecified side	▽
2 ✓x7ᵗʰ	S04.51	Injury of facial nerve, right side	
2 ✓x7ᵗʰ	S04.52	Injury of facial nerve, left side	
✓5ᵗʰ	S04.6	Injury of acoustic nerve	
		Injury of auditory nerve Injury of 8th cranial nerve	
✓x7ᵗʰ	S04.60	Injury of acoustic nerve, unspecified side	▽
2 ✓x7ᵗʰ	S04.61	Injury of acoustic nerve, right side	
2 ✓x7ᵗʰ	S04.62	Injury of acoustic nerve, left side	
✓5ᵗʰ	S04.7	Injury of accessory nerve	
		Injury of 11th cranial nerve	
✓x7ᵗʰ	S04.70	Injury of accessory nerve, unspecified side	▽
2 ✓x7ᵗʰ	S04.71	Injury of accessory nerve, right side	
2 ✓x7ᵗʰ	S04.72	Injury of accessory nerve, left side	
✓5ᵗʰ	S04.8	Injury of other cranial nerves	
✓6ᵗʰ	S04.81	Injury of olfactory [1st] nerve	
2 ✓7ᵗʰ	S04.811	Injury of olfactory [1st] nerve, right side	
2 ✓7ᵗʰ	S04.812	Injury of olfactory [1st] nerve, left side	
✓7ᵗʰ	S04.819	Injury of olfactory [1st] nerve, unspecified side	▽
✓6ᵗʰ	S04.89	Injury of other cranial nerves	
		Injury of vagus [10th] nerve	
2 ✓7ᵗʰ	S04.891	Injury of other cranial nerves, right side	
2 ✓7ᵗʰ	S04.892	Injury of other cranial nerves, left side	
✓7ᵗʰ	S04.899	Injury of other cranial nerves, unspecified side	▽
2 ✓x7ᵗʰ	S04.9	Injury of unspecified cranial nerve	▽

✓4ᵗʰ **S05 Injury of eye and orbit**

INCLUDES open wound of eye and orbit

EXCLUDES 2 2nd cranial [optic] nerve injury (S04.0-)
3rd cranial [oculomotor] nerve injury (S04.1-)
open wound of eyelid and periocular area (S01.1-)
orbital bone fracture (S02.1-, S02.3-, S02.8-)
superficial injury of eyelid (S00.1-S00.2)

The appropriate 7th character is to be added to each code from category S05.
A   initial encounter
D   subsequent encounter
S   sequela

✓5ᵗʰ **S05.0 Injury of conjunctiva and corneal abrasion without foreign body**

EXCLUDES 1 foreign body in conjunctival sac (T15.1)
foreign body in cornea (T15.0)

✓x7ᵗʰ	S05.00	Injury of conjunctiva and corneal abrasion without foreign body, unspecified eye	▽
✓x7ᵗʰ	S05.01	Injury of conjunctiva and corneal abrasion without foreign body, right eye	
✓x7ᵗʰ	S05.02	Injury of conjunctiva and corneal abrasion without foreign body, left eye	

✓5ᵗʰ **S05.1 Contusion of eyeball and orbital tissues**

Traumatic hyphema

EXCLUDES 2 black eye NOS (S00.1)
contusion of eyelid and periocular area (S00.1)

✓x7ᵗʰ	S05.10	Contusion of eyeball and orbital tissues, unspecified eye	▽
✓x7ᵗʰ	S05.11	Contusion of eyeball and orbital tissues, right eye	
✓x7ᵗʰ	S05.12	Contusion of eyeball and orbital tissues, left eye	

✓6ᵗʰ **S05.2 Ocular laceration and rupture with prolapse or loss of intraocular tissue**

✓x7ᵗʰ	S05.20	Ocular laceration and rupture with prolapse or loss of intraocular tissue, unspecified eye	▽

---

2 Case-mix diagnosis with 7th character indicating subsequent encounter or sequela.
3 Case-mix diagnosis with 7th character indicating sequela.

Ⓝ Newborn: 0   Ⓟ Pediatric: 0-17   Ⓜ Maternity: 12-55   Ⓐ Adult: 15-124   NRS Nonroutine supply Dx   NCDx Noncancer Dx   PDx Primary Dx   ▶◀ Revised Text   ● New Code   ▲ Revised Title

918   ICD-10-CM 2018

√x7ᵗʰ **S05.21** **Ocular laceration and rupture with prolapse or loss of intraocular tissue, right eye**

√x7ᵗʰ **S05.22** **Ocular laceration and rupture with prolapse or loss of intraocular tissue, left eye**

√5ᵗʰ **S05.3** **Ocular laceration** without prolapse or loss of intraocular tissue
Laceration of eye NOS
DEF: Tear in ocular tissue without displacing structures; due to blunt trauma; characterized by pain, redness, and decreased vision.

√x7ᵗʰ **S05.30** **Ocular laceration without prolapse or loss of intraocular tissue, unspecified eye** ▽

√x7ᵗʰ **S05.31** **Ocular laceration without prolapse or loss of intraocular tissue, right eye**

√x7ᵗʰ **S05.32** **Ocular laceration without prolapse or loss of intraocular tissue, left eye**

√5ᵗʰ **S05.4** **Penetrating wound** of orbit with or without foreign body
EXCLUDES 2   retained (old) foreign body following penetrating wound in orbit (H05.5-)

√x7ᵗʰ **S05.40** **Penetrating wound of orbit with or without foreign body, unspecified eye** ▽

1, 6 √x7ᵗʰ **S05.41** **Penetrating wound of orbit with or without foreign body, right eye** NRS

1, 6 √x7ᵗʰ **S05.42** **Penetrating wound of orbit with or without foreign body, left eye** NRS

√5ᵗʰ **S05.5** **Penetrating wound with foreign body** of eyeball
EXCLUDES 2   retained (old) intraocular foreign body (H44.6-, H44.7)

√x7ᵗʰ **S05.50** **Penetrating wound with foreign body of unspecified eyeball** ▽

√x7ᵗʰ **S05.51** **Penetrating wound with foreign body of** right **eyeball**

√x7ᵗʰ **S05.52** **Penetrating wound with foreign body of** left **eyeball**

√5ᵗʰ **S05.6** **Penetrating wound without foreign body** of eyeball
Ocular penetration NOS

√x7ᵗʰ **S05.60** **Penetrating wound without foreign body of unspecified eyeball** ▽

√x7ᵗʰ **S05.61** **Penetrating wound without foreign body of** right **eyeball**

√x7ᵗʰ **S05.62** **Penetrating wound without foreign body of** left **eyeball**

√5ᵗʰ **S05.7** **Avulsion of eye**
Traumatic enucleation

√x7ᵗʰ **S05.70** **Avulsion of unspecified eye** ▽

√x7ᵗʰ **S05.71** **Avulsion of** right **eye**

√x7ᵗʰ **S05.72** **Avulsion of** left **eye**

√5ᵗʰ **S05.8** **Other injuries of eye and orbit**
Lacrimal duct injury

√6ᵗʰ **S05.8X** **Other** injuries of eye and orbit

√7ᵗʰ **S05.8X1** **Other injuries of** right **eye and orbit**

√7ᵗʰ **S05.8X2** **Other injuries of** left **eye and orbit**

√7ᵗʰ **S05.8X9** **Other injuries of unspecified eye and orbit** ▽

√5ᵗʰ **S05.9** **Unspecified** injury of eye and orbit
Injury of eye NOS

√x7ᵗʰ **S05.90** **Unspecified injury of unspecified eye and orbit** ▽

√x7ᵗʰ **S05.91** **Unspecified injury of** right **eye and orbit** ▽

√x7ᵗʰ **S05.92** **Unspecified injury of** left **eye and orbit** ▽

√4ᵗʰ **S06** **Intracranial injury**
NOTE ▶ 7th characters D and S do not apply to codes in category S06 with 6th character 7 – death due to brain injury prior to regaining consciousness, or 8 – death due to other cause prior to regaining consciousness◀
INCLUDES   traumatic brain injury
Code also any associated:
  open wound of head (S01.-)
  skull fracture (S02.-)
EXCLUDES 1   head injury NOS (S09.90)
AHA: 2017, 1Q, 42; 2015, 3Q, 37
TIP: When residual conditions persist as a result of intracranial injury, assign codes to identify the residual deficits, followed by the appropriate S06 code to identify the intracranial injury using 7th character S to identify sequelae. Do not assign Z87.820 Personal history of traumatic brain injury, when residual conditions are present.

The appropriate 7th character is to be added to each code from category S06.
A   initial encounter
D   subsequent encounter
S   sequela

√5ᵗʰ **S06.0** **Concussion**
Commotio cerebri
EXCLUDES 1   concussion with other intracranial injuries classified in subcategories S06.1- to S06.6-, S06.81- and S06.82- code to specified intracranial injury

√6ᵗʰ **S06.0X** **Concussion**

3 √7ᵗʰ **S06.0X0** **Concussion** without loss of consciousness

3 √7ᵗʰ **S06.0X1** **Concussion with loss of consciousness of** 30 minutes or less

3 √7ᵗʰ **S06.0X9** **Concussion with loss of consciousness of** unspecified duration ▽
Concussion NOS

√5ᵗʰ **S06.1** **Traumatic cerebral edema**
Diffuse traumatic cerebral edema
Focal traumatic cerebral edema

√6ᵗʰ **S06.1X** **Traumatic** cerebral edema

2 √7ᵗʰ **S06.1X0** **Traumatic cerebral edema** without loss of consciousness

2 √7ᵗʰ **S06.1X1** **Traumatic cerebral edema with loss of consciousness of** 30 minutes or less

2 √7ᵗʰ **S06.1X2** **Traumatic cerebral edema with loss of consciousness of** 31 minutes to 59 minutes

2 √7ᵗʰ **S06.1X3** **Traumatic cerebral edema with loss of consciousness of** 1 hour to 5 hours 59 minutes

2 √7ᵗʰ **S06.1X4** **Traumatic cerebral edema with loss of consciousness of** 6 hours to 24 hours

2 √7ᵗʰ **S06.1X5** **Traumatic cerebral edema with loss of consciousness** greater than 24 hours with return to pre-existing conscious level

2, 7 √7ᵗʰ **S06.1X6** **Traumatic cerebral edema with loss** NC Dx **of consciousness** greater than 24 hours without return to pre-existing conscious level with patient surviving

√7ᵗʰ **S06.1X7** **Traumatic cerebral edema with loss of consciousness of** any duration with death due to brain injury prior to regaining consciousness

√7ᵗʰ **S06.1X8** **Traumatic cerebral edema with loss of consciousness of** any duration with death due to other cause prior to regaining consciousness

2 √7ᵗʰ **S06.1X9** **Traumatic cerebral edema with loss of consciousness of** unspecified duration ▽
Traumatic cerebral edema NOS

√5ᵗʰ **S06.2** **Diffuse traumatic brain injury**
Diffuse axonal brain injury
EXCLUDES 1   traumatic diffuse cerebral edema (S06.1X-)

√6ᵗʰ **S06.2X** **Diffuse traumatic brain injury**

2 √7ᵗʰ **S06.2X0** **Diffuse traumatic brain injury** without loss of consciousness

2 √7ᵗʰ **S06.2X1** **Diffuse traumatic brain injury with loss of consciousness of** 30 minutes or less

---

1   Case-mix diagnosis with 7th character indicating subsequent encounter.
2   Case-mix diagnosis with 7th character indicating subsequent encounter or sequela.
3   Case-mix diagnosis with 7th character indicating sequela.
6   NRS supply diagnosis with 7th character indicating subsequent encounter.
7   Hospice non-cancer diagnosis with 7th character indicating subsequent encounter.

☑ Additional Character Req   √x7ᵗʰ Placeholder Alert   Case-Mix Diagnosis   Manifestation   ▽ Unspecified Dx   EXCLUDES 1 Not coded here   EXCLUDES 2 Not included here

2 ✓7th **S06.2X2** **Diffuse traumatic brain injury with loss of consciousness of** 31 minutes to 59 minutes

2 ✓7th **S06.2X3** **Diffuse traumatic brain injury with loss of consciousness of** 1 hour to 5 hours 59 minutes

2 ✓7th **S06.2X4** **Diffuse traumatic brain injury with loss of consciousness of** 6 hours to 24 hours

2 ✓7th **S06.2X5** **Diffuse traumatic brain injury with loss of consciousness** greater than 24 hours with return to pre-existing conscious levels

2, 7 ✓7th **S06.2X6** **Diffuse traumatic brain injury with** NC Dx **loss of consciousness** greater than 24 hours without return to pre-existing conscious level with patient surviving

✓7th **S06.2X7** **Diffuse traumatic brain injury with loss of consciousness of** any duration with death due to brain injury prior to regaining consciousness

✓7th **S06.2X8** **Diffuse traumatic brain injury with loss of consciousness of** any duration with death due to **other** cause prior to regaining consciousness

2 ✓7th **S06.2X9** **Diffuse traumatic brain injury with loss** ▽ **of consciousness of** unspecified duration
Diffuse traumatic brain injury NOS

✓5th **S06.3** Focal traumatic brain injury
     EXCLUDES 1 *any condition classifiable to S06.4–S06.6 focal cerebral edema (S06.1)*

✓6th **S06.30** Unspecified **focal traumatic brain injury**

2 ✓7th **S06.300** **Unspecified focal traumatic brain** ▽ **injury** without loss of consciousness

2 ✓7th **S06.301** **Unspecified focal traumatic brain injury** ▽ **with loss of consciousness of** 30 minutes or less

2 ✓7th **S06.302** **Unspecified focal traumatic brain injury** ▽ **with loss of consciousness of** 31 minutes to 59 minutes

2 ✓7th **S06.303** **Unspecified focal traumatic brain injury** ▽ **with loss of consciousness of** 1 hour to 5 hours 59 minutes

2 ✓7th **S06.304** **Unspecified focal traumatic brain injury** ▽ **with loss of consciousness of** 6 hours to 24 hours

2 ✓7th **S06.305** **Unspecified focal traumatic brain injury** ▽ **with loss of consciousness** greater than 24 hours with return to pre-existing conscious level

2, 7 ✓7th **S06.306** **Unspecified focal traumatic brain** NC Dx ▽ **injury with loss of consciousness** greater than 24 hours without return to pre-existing conscious levell with patient surviving

✓7th **S06.307** **Unspecified focal traumatic brain injury** ▽ **with loss of consciousness of** any duration with death due to brain injury prior to regaining consciousness

✓7th **S06.308** **Unspecified focal traumatic brain injury** ▽ **with loss of consciousness of** any duration with death due to **other** cause prior to regaining consciousness

2 ✓7th **S06.309** **Unspecified focal traumatic brain injury** ▽ **with loss of consciousness of unspecified duration**
Unspecified focal traumatic brain injury NOS

✓6th **S06.31** Contusion and laceration of right cerebrum

2 ✓7th **S06.310** **Contusion and laceration of right cerebrum** without loss of consciousness

2 ✓7th **S06.311** **Contusion and laceration of right cerebrum with loss of consciousness of** 30 minutes or less

2 ✓7th **S06.312** **Contusion and laceration of right cerebrum with loss of consciousness of** 31 minutes to 59 minutes

2 ✓7th **S06.313** **Contusion and laceration of right cerebrum with loss of consciousness of** 1 hour to 5 hours 59 minutes

2 ✓7th **S06.314** **Contusion and laceration of right cerebrum with loss of consciousness of** 6 hours to 24 hours

2 ✓7th **S06.315** **Contusion and laceration of right cerebrum with loss of consciousness** greater than 24 hours with return to pre-existing conscious level

2, 7e **S06.316** **Contusion and laceration of right** NC Dx **cerebrum with loss of consciousness** greater than 24 hours without return to pre-existing conscious level with patient surviving

✓7th **S06.317** **Contusion and laceration of right cerebrum with loss of consciousness of** any duration with death due to brain injury prior to regaining consciousness

✓7th **S06.318** **Contusion and laceration of right cerebrum with loss of consciousness of** any duration with death due to **other** cause prior to regaining consciousness

2 ✓7th **S06.319** **Contusion and laceration of right** ▽ **cerebrum with loss of consciousness of unspecified duration**
Contusion and laceration of right cerebrum NOS

✓6th **S06.32** Contusion and laceration of left cerebrum

2 ✓7th **S06.320** **Contusion and laceration of left cerebrum** without loss of consciousness

2 ✓7th **S06.321** **Contusion and laceration of left cerebrum with loss of consciousness of** 30 minutes or less

2 ✓7th **S06.322** **Contusion and laceration of left cerebrum with loss of consciousness of** 31 minutes to 59 minutes

2 ✓7th **S06.323** **Contusion and laceration of left cerebrum with loss of consciousness of** 1 hour to 5 hours 59 minutes

2 ✓7th **S06.324** **Contusion and laceration of left cerebrum with loss of consciousness of** 6 hours to 24 hours

2 ✓7th **S06.325** **Contusion and laceration of left cerebrum with loss of consciousness** greater than 24 hours with return to pre-existing conscious level

2, 7 ✓7th **S06.326** **Contusion and laceration of left** NC Dx **cerebrum with loss of consciousness** greater than 24 hours without return to pre-existing conscious level with patient surviving

✓7th **S06.327** **Contusion and laceration of left cerebrum with loss of consciousness of** any duration with death due to brain injury prior to regaining consciousness

✓7th **S06.328** **Contusion and laceration of left cerebrum with loss of consciousness of** any duration with death due to **other** cause prior to regaining consciousness

2 ✓7th **S06.329** **Contusion and laceration of left** ▽ **cerebrum with loss of consciousness of unspecified duration**
Contusion and laceration of left cerebrum NOS

✓6th **S06.33** Contusion and laceration of cerebrum, unspecified

2 ✓7th **S06.330** **Contusion and laceration of cerebrum,** ▽ **unspecified,** without loss of consciousness

2 ✓7th **S06.331** **Contusion and laceration of cerebrum,** ▽ **unspecified, with loss of consciousness of** 30 minutes or less

2 ✓7th **S06.332** **Contusion and laceration of cerebrum,** ▽ **unspecified, with loss of consciousness of** 31 minutes to 59 minutes

2 ✓7th **S06.333** **Contusion and laceration of cerebrum,** ▽ **unspecified, with loss of consciousness of** 1 hour to 5 hours 59 minutes

2 ✓7th **S06.334** **Contusion and laceration of cerebrum,** ▽ **unspecified, with loss of consciousness of** 6 hours to 24 hours

---

2   Case-mix diagnosis with 7th character indicating subsequent encounter or sequela.
7   Hospice non-cancer diagnosis with 7th character indicating subsequent encounter.

N Newborn: 0   P Pediatric: 0-17   M Maternity: 12-55   A Adult: 15-124   NRS Nonroutine supply Dx   NC Dx Noncancer Dx   PDx Primary Dx   ▶◀ Revised Text   ● New Code   ▲ Revised Title

920   ICD-10-CM 2018

2 ✓7ᵗʰ **S06.335** **Contusion and laceration of cerebrum,** ▽ **unspecified, with loss of consciousness** greater than 24 hours with return to pre-existing conscious level

2, 7 ✓7ᵗʰ **S06.336** **Contusion and laceration of** NC Dx ▽ **cerebrum, unspecified, with loss of consciousness** greater than 24 hours without return to pre-existing conscious level with patient surviving

✓7ᵗʰ **S06.337** **Contusion and laceration of cerebrum,** ▽ **unspecified, with loss of consciousness of** any duration with death due to brain injury prior to regaining consciousness

✓7ᵗʰ **S06.338** **Contusion and laceration of cerebrum,** ▽ **unspecified, with loss of consciousness of** any duration with death due to **other** cause prior to regaining consciousness

2 ✓7ᵗʰ **S06.339** **Contusion and laceration of cerebrum,** ▽ **unspecified, with loss of consciousness of unspecified duration**
Contusion and laceration of cerebrum NOS

✓6ᵗʰ **S06.34** **Traumatic hemorrhage of** right cerebrum
Traumatic intracerebral hemorrhage and hematoma of right cerebrum

2 ✓7ᵗʰ **S06.340** **Traumatic hemorrhage of right cerebrum** without loss of consciousness

2 ✓7ᵗʰ **S06.341** **Traumatic hemorrhage of right cerebrum with loss of consciousness of** 30 minutes or less

2 ✓7ᵗʰ **S06.342** **Traumatic hemorrhage of right cerebrum with loss of consciousness of** 31 minutes to 59 minutes

2 ✓7ᵗʰ **S06.343** **Traumatic hemorrhage of right cerebrum with loss of consciousness of** 1 hours to 5 hours 59 minutes

2 ✓7ᵗʰ **S06.344** **Traumatic hemorrhage of right cerebrum with loss of consciousness of** 6 hours to 24 hours

2 ✓7ᵗʰ **S06.345** **Traumatic hemorrhage of right cerebrum with loss of consciousness** greater than 24 hours with return to pre-existing conscious level

2, 7 ✓7ᵗʰ **S06.346** **Traumatic hemorrhage of right** NC Dx **cerebrum with loss of consciousness** greater than 24 hours without return to pre-existing conscious level with patient surviving

✓7ᵗʰ **S06.347** **Traumatic hemorrhage of right cerebrum with loss of consciousness of** any duration with death due to brain injury prior to regaining consciousness

✓7ᵗʰ **S06.348** **Traumatic hemorrhage of right cerebrum with loss of consciousness of** any duration with death due to **other** cause prior to regaining consciousness

2 ✓7ᵗʰ **S06.349** **Traumatic hemorrhage of right** ▽ **cerebrum with loss of consciousness of unspecified duration**
Traumatic hemorrhage of right cerebrum NOS

✓6ᵗʰ **S06.35** **Traumatic hemorrhage of** left cerebrum
Traumatic intracerebral hemorrhage and hematoma of left cerebrum

2 ✓7ᵗʰ **S06.350** **Traumatic hemorrhage of left cerebrum** without loss of consciousness

2 ✓7ᵗʰ **S06.351** **Traumatic hemorrhage of left cerebrum with loss of consciousness of** 30 minutes or less

2 ✓7ᵗʰ **S06.352** **Traumatic hemorrhage of left cerebrum with loss of consciousness of** 31 minutes to 59 minutes

2 ✓7ᵗʰ **S06.353** **Traumatic hemorrhage of left cerebrum with loss of consciousness of** 1 hours to 5 hours 59 minutes

2 ✓7ᵗʰ **S06.354** **Traumatic hemorrhage of left cerebrum with loss of consciousness of** 6 hours to 24 hours

2 ✓7ᵗʰ **S06.355** **Traumatic hemorrhage of left cerebrum with loss of consciousness** greater than 24 hours with return to pre-existing conscious level

2, 7 ✓7ᵗʰ **S06.356** **Traumatic hemorrhage of left** NC Dx **cerebrum with loss of consciousness** greater than 24 hours without return to pre-existing conscious level with patient surviving

✓7ᵗʰ **S06.357** **Traumatic hemorrhage of left cerebrum with loss of consciousness of** any duration with death due to brain injury prior to regaining consciousness

✓7ᵗʰ **S06.358** **Traumatic hemorrhage of left cerebrum with loss of consciousness of** any duration with death due to **other** cause prior to regaining consciousness

2 ✓7ᵗʰ **S06.359** **Traumatic hemorrhage of left cerebrum** ▽ **with loss of consciousness of unspecified duration**
Traumatic hemorrhage of left cerebrum NOS

✓6ᵗʰ **S06.36** **Traumatic hemorrhage of** cerebrum, unspecified
Traumatic intracerebral hemorrhage and hematoma, unspecified

2 ✓7ᵗʰ **S06.360** **Traumatic hemorrhage of cerebrum,** ▽ **unspecified,** without loss of consciousness

2 ✓7ᵗʰ **S06.361** **Traumatic hemorrhage of cerebrum,** ▽ **unspecified, with loss of consciousness of** 30 minutes or less

2 ✓7ᵗʰ **S06.362** **Traumatic hemorrhage of cerebrum,** ▽ **unspecified, with loss of consciousness of** 31 minutes to 59 minutes

2 ✓7ᵗʰ **S06.363** **Traumatic hemorrhage of cerebrum,** ▽ **unspecified, with loss of consciousness of** 1 hours to 5 hours 59 minutes

2 ✓7ᵗʰ **S06.364** **Traumatic hemorrhage of cerebrum,** ▽ **unspecified, with loss of consciousness of** 6 hours to 24 hours

2 ✓7ᵗʰ **S06.365** **Traumatic hemorrhage of cerebrum,** ▽ **unspecified, with loss of consciousness of** greater than 24 hours with return to pre-existing conscious level

2, 7 ✓7ᵗʰ **S06.366** **Traumatic hemorrhage of** NC Dx ▽ **cerebrum, unspecified, with loss of consciousness of** greater than 24 hours without return to pre-existing conscious level with patient surviving

1 ✓7ᵗʰ **S06.367** **Traumatic hemorrhage of cerebrum,** ▽ **unspecified, with loss of consciousness of** any duration with death due to brain injury prior to regaining consciousness

1 ✓7ᵗʰ **S06.368** **Traumatic hemorrhage of cerebrum,** ▽ **unspecified, with loss of consciousness of** any duration with death due to **other** cause prior to regaining consciousness

2 ✓7ᵗʰ **S06.369** **Traumatic hemorrhage of cerebrum,** ▽ **unspecified, with loss of consciousness of unspecified duration**
Traumatic hemorrhage of cerebrum NOS

✓6ᵗʰ **S06.37** **Contusion, laceration, and hemorrhage of** cerebellum

2 ✓7ᵗʰ **S06.370** **Contusion, laceration, and hemorrhage of cerebellum** without loss of consciousness

2 ✓7ᵗʰ **S06.371** **Contusion, laceration, and hemorrhage of cerebellum with loss of consciousness of** 30 minutes or less

2 ✓7ᵗʰ **S06.372** **Contusion, laceration, and hemorrhage of cerebellum with loss of consciousness of** 31 minutes to 59 minutes

2 ✓7ᵗʰ **S06.373** **Contusion, laceration, and hemorrhage of cerebellum with loss of consciousness of** 1 hour to 5 hours 59 minutes

2 ✓7ᵗʰ **S06.374** **Contusion, laceration, and hemorrhage of cerebellum with loss of consciousness of** 6 hours to 24 hours

---

1 Case-mix diagnosis with 7th character indicating subsequent encounter.
2 Case-mix diagnosis with 7th character indicating subsequent encounter or sequela.
7 Hospice non-cancer diagnosis with 7th character indicating subsequent encounter.

☑ Additional Character Req   ✓x7ᵗʰ Placeholder Alert   Case-Mix Diagnosis   Manifestation   ▽ Unspecified Dx   *EXCLUDES 1* Not coded here   *EXCLUDES 2* Not included here

Chapter 19. Injury, Poisoning and Certain Other Consequences of External Causes

2 ✓7th **S06.375** **Contusion, laceration, and hemorrhage of cerebellum with loss of consciousness** greater than 24 hours with return to pre-existing conscious level

2,7 ✓7th **S06.376** **Contusion, laceration, and hemorrhage of cerebellum with loss of consciousness** greater than 24 hours without return to pre-existing conscious level with patient surviving   NC Dx

1 ✓7th **S06.377** **Contusion, laceration, and hemorrhage of cerebellum with loss of consciousness of** any duration with death due to brain injury prior to regaining consciousness

✓7th **S06.378** **Contusion, laceration, and hemorrhage of cerebellum with loss of consciousness of** any duration with death due to **other** cause prior to regaining consciousness

2 ✓7th **S06.379** **Contusion, laceration, and hemorrhage ▽ of cerebellum with loss of consciousness of unspecified duration**
Contusion, laceration, and hemorrhage of cerebellum NOS

✓6th **S06.38** **Contusion, laceration, and hemorrhage of** brainstem

2 ✓7th **S06.380** **Contusion, laceration, and hemorrhage of brainstem** without loss of consciousness

2 ✓7th **S06.381** **Contusion, laceration, and hemorrhage of brainstem with loss of consciousness of** 30 minutes or less

2 ✓7th **S06.382** **Contusion, laceration, and hemorrhage of brainstem with loss of consciousness of** 31 minutes to 59 minutes

2 ✓7th **S06.383** **Contusion, laceration, and hemorrhage of brainstem with loss of consciousness of** 1 hour to 5 hours 59 minutes

2 ✓7th **S06.384** **Contusion, laceration, and hemorrhage of brainstem with loss of consciousness of** 6 hours to 24 hours

2 ✓7th **S06.385** **Contusion, laceration, and hemorrhage of brainstem with loss of consciousness** greater than 24 hours with return to pre-existing conscious level

2,7 ✓7th **S06.386** **Contusion, laceration, and hemorrhage of brainstem with loss of consciousness** greater than 24 hours without return to pre-existing conscious level with patient surviving   NC Dx

✓7th **S06.387** **Contusion, laceration, and hemorrhage of brainstem with loss of consciousness of** any duration with death due to brain injury prior to regaining consciousness

✓7th **S06.388** **Contusion, laceration, and hemorrhage of brainstem with loss of consciousness of** any duration with death due to **other** cause prior to regaining consciousness

2 ✓7th **S06.389** **Contusion, laceration, and hemorrhage ▽ of brainstem with loss of consciousness of unspecified duration**
Contusion, laceration, and hemorrhage of brainstem NOS

✓5th **S06.4** **Epidural** hemorrhage
Extradural hemorrhage NOS
Extradural hemorrhage (traumatic)

✓6th **S06.4X** **Epidural hemorrhage**

2 ✓7th **S06.4X0** **Epidural hemorrhage** without loss of consciousness

2 ✓7th **S06.4X1** **Epidural hemorrhage with loss of consciousness of** 30 minutes or less

2 ✓7th **S06.4X2** **Epidural hemorrhage with loss of consciousness of** 31 minutes to 59 minutes

2 ✓7th **S06.4X3** **Epidural hemorrhage with loss of consciousness of** 1 hour to 5 hours 59 minutes

2 ✓7th **S06.4X4** **Epidural hemorrhage with loss of consciousness of** 6 hours to 24 hours

2 ✓7th **S06.4X5** **Epidural hemorrhage with loss of consciousness** greater than 24 hours with return to pre-existing conscious level

2,7 ✓7th **S06.4X6** **Epidural hemorrhage with loss of consciousness** greater than 24 hours without return to pre-existing conscious level with patient surviving   NC Dx

✓7th **S06.4X7** **Epidural hemorrhage with loss of consciousness of** any duration with death due to brain injury prior to regaining consciousness

✓7th **S06.4X8** **Epidural hemorrhage with loss of consciousness of** any duration with death due to **other** causes prior to regaining consciousness

2 ✓7th **S06.4X9** **Epidural hemorrhage with loss of ▽ consciousness of unspecified duration**
Epidural hemorrhage NOS

✓5th **S06.5** **Traumatic** subdural **hemorrhage**

✓6th **S06.5X** **Traumatic** subdural **hemorrhage**

✓7th **S06.5X0** **Traumatic subdural hemorrhage** without loss of consciousness

✓7th **S06.5X1** **Traumatic subdural hemorrhage with loss of consciousness of** 30 minutes or less

✓7th **S06.5X2** **Traumatic subdural hemorrhage with loss of consciousness of** 31 minutes to 59 minutes

✓7th **S06.5X3** **Traumatic subdural hemorrhage with loss of consciousness of** 1 hour to 5 hours 59 minutes

✓7th **S06.5X4** **Traumatic subdural hemorrhage with loss of consciousness of** 6 hours to 24 hours

✓7th **S06.5X5** **Traumatic subdural hemorrhage with loss of consciousness** greater than 24 hours with return to pre-existing conscious level

7 ✓7th **S06.5X6** **Traumatic subdural hemorrhage**   NC Dx **with loss of consciousness** greater than 24 hours without return to pre-existing conscious level with patient surviving

✓7th **S06.5X7** **Traumatic subdural hemorrhage with loss of consciousness of** any duration with death due to brain injury before regaining consciousness

✓7th **S06.5X8** **Traumatic subdural hemorrhage with loss of consciousness of** any duration with death due to **other** cause before regaining consciousness

✓7th **S06.5X9** **Traumatic subdural hemorrhage with ▽ loss of consciousness of unspecified duration**
Traumatic subdural hemorrhage NOS

✓5th **S06.6** **Traumatic** subarachnoid **hemorrhage**

✓6th **S06.6X** **Traumatic subarachnoid hemorrhage**

✓7th **S06.6X0** **Traumatic subarachnoid hemorrhage** without loss of consciousness

✓7th **S06.6X1** **Traumatic subarachnoid hemorrhage with loss of consciousness of** 30 minutes or less

✓7th **S06.6X2** **Traumatic subarachnoid hemorrhage with loss of consciousness of** 31 minutes to 59 minutes

✓7th **S06.6X3** **Traumatic subarachnoid hemorrhage with loss of consciousness of** 1 hour to 5 hours 59 minutes

✓7th **S06.6X4** **Traumatic subarachnoid hemorrhage with loss of consciousness of** 6 hours to 24 hours

✓7th **S06.6X5** **Traumatic subarachnoid hemorrhage with loss of consciousness** greater than 24 hours with return to pre-existing conscious level

7 ✓7th **S06.6X6** **Traumatic subarachnoid hemorrhage**   NC Dx **with loss of consciousness** greater than 24 hours without return to pre-existing conscious level with patient surviving

✓7th **S06.6X7** **Traumatic subarachnoid hemorrhage with loss of consciousness of** any duration with death due to brain injury prior to regaining consciousness

---

1   Case–mix diagnosis with 7th character indicating subsequent encounter.
2   Case–mix diagnosis with 7th character indicating subsequent encounter or sequela.
7   Hospice non-cancer diagnosis with 7th character indicating subsequent encounter.

Ⓝ Newborn: 0   Ⓟ Pediatric: 0-17   Ⓜ Maternity: 12-55   Ⓐ Adult: 15-124   NRS Nonroutine supply Dx   NC Dx Noncancer Dx   PDx Primary Dx   ▶◀ Revised Text   ● New Code   ▲ Revised Title

☑7ᵗʰ **S06.6X8** **Traumatic subarachnoid hemorrhage with loss of consciousness of** any duration with death due to **other** cause prior to regaining consciousness

☑7ᵗʰ **S06.6X9** **Traumatic subarachnoid hemorrhage with loss of consciousness of unspecified duration** ▽
Traumatic subarachnoid hemorrhage NOS

☑5ᵗʰ **S06.8** **Other specified intracranial injuries**

☑6ᵗʰ **S06.81** **Injury of** right internal carotid artery, **intracranial portion, not elsewhere classified**

2 ☑7ᵗʰ **S06.810** **Injury of right internal carotid artery, intracranial portion, not elsewhere classified** without loss of consciousness

2 ☑7ᵗʰ **S06.811** **Injury of right internal carotid artery, intracranial portion, not elsewhere classified with loss of consciousness of** 30 minutes or less

2 ☑7ᵗʰ **S06.812** **Injury of right internal carotid artery, intracranial portion, not elsewhere classified with loss of consciousness of** 31 minutes to 59 minutes

2 ☑7ᵗʰ **S06.813** **Injury of right internal carotid artery, intracranial portion, not elsewhere classified with loss of consciousness of** 1 hour to 5 hours 59 minutes

2 ☑7ᵗʰ **S06.814** **Injury of right internal carotid artery, intracranial portion, not elsewhere classified with loss of consciousness of** 6 hours to 24 hours

2 ☑7ᵗʰ **S06.815** **Injury of right internal carotid artery, intracranial portion, not elsewhere classified with loss of consciousness** greater than 24 hours with return to pre-existing conscious level

2, 7 ☑7ᵗʰ **S06.816** **Injury of right internal carotid artery,** NC Dx **intracranial portion, not elsewhere classified with loss of consciousness** greater than 24 hours without return to pre-existing conscious level with patient surviving

☑7ᵗʰ **S06.817** **Injury of right internal carotid artery, intracranial portion, not elsewhere classified with loss of consciousness of** any duration with death due to brain injury prior to regaining consciousness

☑7ᵗʰ **S06.818** **Injury of right internal carotid artery, intracranial portion, not elsewhere classified with loss of consciousness of** any duration with death due to **other** cause prior to regaining consciousness

2 ☑7ᵗʰ **S06.819** **Injury of right internal carotid artery,** ▽ **intracranial portion, not elsewhere classified with loss of consciousness of unspecified duration**
Injury of right internal carotid artery, intracranial portion, not elsewhere classified NOS

☑6ᵗʰ **S06.82** **Injury of** left internal carotid artery, **intracranial portion, not elsewhere classified**

2 ☑7ᵗʰ **S06.820** **Injury of left internal carotid artery, intracranial portion, not elsewhere classified** without loss of consciousness

2 ☑7ᵗʰ **S06.821** **Injury of left internal carotid artery, intracranial portion, not elsewhere classified with loss of consciousness of** 30 minutes or less

2 ☑7ᵗʰ **S06.822** **Injury of left internal carotid artery, intracranial portion, not elsewhere classified with loss of consciousness of** 31 minutes to 59 minutes

2 ☑7ᵗʰ **S06.823** **Injury of left internal carotid artery, intracranial portion, not elsewhere classified with loss of consciousness of** 1 hour to 5 hours 59 minutes

2 ☑7ᵗʰ **S06.824** **Injury of left internal carotid artery, intracranial portion, not elsewhere classified with loss of consciousness of** 6 hours to 24 hours

2 ☑7ᵗʰ **S06.825** **Injury of left internal carotid artery, intracranial portion, not elsewhere classified with loss of consciousness** greater than 24 hours with return to pre-existing conscious level

2, 7 ☑7ᵗʰ **S06.826** **Injury of left internal carotid artery,** NC Dx **intracranial portion, not elsewhere classified with loss of consciousness** greater than 24 hours without return to pre-existing conscious level with patient surviving

☑7ᵗʰ **S06.827** **Injury of left internal carotid artery, intracranial portion, not elsewhere classified with loss of consciousness of** any duration with death due to brain injury prior to regaining consciousness

☑7ᵗʰ **S06.828** **Injury of left internal carotid artery, intracranial portion, not elsewhere classified with loss of consciousness of** any duration with death due to **other** cause prior to regaining consciousness

2 ☑7ᵗʰ **S06.829** **Injury of left internal carotid artery,** ▽ **intracranial portion, not elsewhere classified with loss of consciousness of unspecified duration**
Injury of left internal carotid artery, intracranial portion, not elsewhere classified NOS

☑6ᵗʰ **S06.89** **Other** specified intracranial injury
EXCLUDES 1 concussion (S06.0X-)

2 ☑7ᵗʰ **S06.890** **Other specified intracranial injury** without loss of consciousness

2 ☑7ᵗʰ **S06.891** **Other specified intracranial injury with loss of consciousness of** 30 minutes or less

2 ☑7ᵗʰ **S06.892** **Other specified intracranial injury with loss of consciousness of** 31 minutes to 59 minutes

2 ☑7ᵗʰ **S06.893** **Other specified intracranial injury with loss of consciousness of** 1 hour to 5 hours 59 minutes

2 ☑7ᵗʰ **S06.894** **Other specified intracranial injury with loss of consciousness of** 6 hours to 24 hours

2 ☑7ᵗʰ **S06.895** **Other specified intracranial injury with loss of consciousness** greater than 24 hours with return to pre-existing conscious level

2, 7 ☑7ᵗʰ **S06.896** **Other specified intracranial injury** NC Dx **with loss of consciousness** greater than 24 hours without return to pre-existing conscious level with patient surviving

☑7ᵗʰ **S06.897** **Other specified intracranial injury with loss of consciousness of** any duration with death due to brain injury prior to regaining consciousness

☑7ᵗʰ **S06.898** **Other specified intracranial injury with loss of consciousness of** any duration with death due to **other** cause prior to regaining consciousness

2 ☑7ᵗʰ **S06.899** **Other specified intracranial injury with** ▽ **loss of consciousness of unspecified duration**

☑5ᵗʰ **S06.9** **Unspecified intracranial injury**
Brain injury NOS
Head injury NOS with loss of consciousness
Traumatic brain injury NOS
EXCLUDES 1 conditions classifiable to S06.0- to S06.8- code to specified intracranial injury
head injury NOS (S09.90)

☑6ᵗʰ **S06.9X** Unspecified intracranial injury

2 ☑7ᵗʰ **S06.9X0** **Unspecified intracranial injury** without ▽ loss of consciousness

2 ☑7ᵗʰ **S06.9X1** **Unspecified intracranial injury with** ▽ **loss of consciousness of** 30 minutes or less

2 Case-mix diagnosis with 7th character indicating subsequent encounter or sequela.
7 Hospice non-cancer diagnosis with 7th character indicating subsequent encounter.

☑ Additional Character Req   ☑ˣ⁷ᵗʰ Placeholder Alert   Case-Mix Diagnosis   Manifestation   ▽ Unspecified Dx   **EXCLUDES 1** Not coded here   **EXCLUDES 2** Not included here

2 ✓7ᵗʰ S06.9X2 Unspecified intracranial injury with loss of consciousness of 31 minutes to 59 minutes ▽

2 ✓7ᵗʰ S06.9X3 Unspecified intracranial injury with loss of consciousness of 1 hour to 5 hours 59 minutes ▽

2 ✓7ᵗʰ S06.9X4 Unspecified intracranial injury with loss of consciousness of 6 hours to 24 hours ▽

2 ✓7ᵗʰ S06.9X5 Unspecified intracranial injury with loss of consciousness greater than 24 hours with return to pre-existing conscious level ▽

2, 7 ✓7ᵗʰ S06.9X6 Unspecified intracranial injury with loss of consciousness greater than 24 hours without return to pre-existing conscious level with patient surviving NC Dx ▽

✓7ᵗʰ S06.9X7 Unspecified intracranial injury with loss of consciousness of any duration with death due to brain injury prior to regaining consciousness

✓7ᵗʰ S06.9X8 Unspecified intracranial injury with loss of consciousness of any duration with death due to other cause prior to regaining consciousness ▽

2 ✓7ᵗʰ S06.9X9 Unspecified intracranial injury with loss of consciousness of unspecified duration ▽

✓4ᵗʰ S07 Crushing injury of head
Use additional code for all associated injuries, such as:
    intracranial injuries (S06.-)
    skull fractures (S02.-)

The appropriate 7th character is to be added to each code from category S07.
A   initial encounter
D   subsequent encounter
S   sequela

✓x7ᵗʰ S07.0 Crushing injury of face

✓x7ᵗʰ S07.1 Crushing injury of skull

✓x7ᵗʰ S07.8 Crushing injury of other parts of head

✓x7ᵗʰ S07.9 Crushing injury of head, part unspecified ▽

✓4ᵗʰ S08 Avulsion and traumatic amputation of part of head
An amputation not identified as partial or complete should be coded to complete.

The appropriate 7th character is to be added to each code from category S08.
A   initial encounter
D   subsequent encounter
S   sequela

4,5 ✓x7ᵗʰ S08.0 Avulsion of scalp NRS

✓5ᵗʰ S08.1 Traumatic amputation of ear

✓6ᵗʰ S08.11 Complete traumatic amputation of ear

4,5 ✓7ᵗʰ S08.111 Complete traumatic amputation of right ear NRS

4,5 ✓7ᵗʰ S08.112 Complete traumatic amputation of left ear NRS

✓7ᵗʰ S08.119 Complete traumatic amputation of unspecified ear ▽

✓6ᵗʰ S08.12 Partial traumatic amputation of ear

4,5 ✓7ᵗʰ S08.121 Partial traumatic amputation of right ear NRS

4,5 ✓7ᵗʰ S08.122 Partial traumatic amputation of left ear NRS

✓7ᵗʰ S08.129 Partial traumatic amputation of unspecified ear ▽

✓5ᵗʰ S08.8 Traumatic amputation of other parts of head

✓6ᵗʰ S08.81 Traumatic amputation of nose

4,5 ✓7ᵗʰ S08.811 Complete traumatic amputation of nose NRS

4,5 ✓7ᵗʰ S08.812 Partial traumatic amputation of nose NRS

4,5 ✓x7ᵗʰ S08.89 Traumatic amputation of other parts of head NRS

✓4ᵗʰ S09 Other and unspecified injuries of head

The appropriate 7th character is to be added to each code from category S09.
A   initial encounter
D   subsequent encounter
S   sequela

✓x7ᵗʰ S09.0 Injury of blood vessels of head, not elsewhere classified
EXCLUDES 1   injury of cerebral blood vessels (S06.-)
    injury of precerebral blood vessels (S15.-)

✓5ᵗʰ S09.1 Injury of muscle and tendon of head
Code also any associated open wound (S01.-)
EXCLUDES 2   sprain to joints and ligament of head (S03.9)

✓x7ᵗʰ S09.10 Unspecified injury of muscle and tendon of head ▽
Injury of muscle and tendon of head NOS

✓x7ᵗʰ S09.11 Strain of muscle and tendon of head

4,6 ✓x7ᵗʰ S09.12 Laceration of muscle and tendon of head NRS

✓x7ᵗʰ S09.19 Other specified injury of muscle and tendon of head

✓5ᵗʰ S09.2 Traumatic rupture of ear drum
EXCLUDES 1   traumatic rupture of ear drum due to blast injury (S09.31-)

✓x7ᵗʰ S09.20 Traumatic rupture of unspecified ear drum ▽

1,6 ✓x7ᵗʰ S09.21 Traumatic rupture of right ear drum NRS

1,6 ✓x7ᵗʰ S09.22 Traumatic rupture of left ear drum NRS

✓5ᵗʰ S09.3 Other specified and unspecified injury of middle and inner ear
EXCLUDES 1   injury to ear NOS (S09.91-)
EXCLUDES 2   injury to external ear (S00.4-, S01.3-, S08.1-)

✓6ᵗʰ S09.30 Unspecified injury of middle and inner ear

1,5 ✓7ᵗʰ S09.301 Unspecified injury of right middle and inner ear NRS ▽

1,5 ✓7ᵗʰ S09.302 Unspecified injury of left middle and inner ear NRS ▽

✓7ᵗʰ S09.309 Unspecified injury of unspecified middle and inner ear ▽

✓6ᵗʰ S09.31 Primary blast injury of ear
Blast injury of ear NOS

4,5 ✓7ᵗʰ S09.311 Primary blast injury of right ear NRS

4,5 ✓7ᵗʰ S09.312 Primary blast injury of left ear NRS

4,5 ✓7ᵗʰ S09.313 Primary blast injury of ear, bilateral NRS

✓7ᵗʰ S09.319 Primary blast injury of unspecified ear ▽

✓6ᵗʰ S09.39 Other specified injury of middle and inner ear
Secondary blast injury to ear

1,5 ✓7ᵗʰ S09.391 Other specified injury of right middle and inner ear NRS

1,5 ✓7ᵗʰ S09.392 Other specified injury of left middle and inner ear NRS

✓7ᵗʰ S09.399 Other specified injury of unspecified middle and inner ear ▽

4,5 ✓x7ᵗʰ S09.8 Other specified injuries of head NRS

✓5ᵗʰ S09.9 Unspecified injury of face and head

✓x7ᵗʰ S09.90 Unspecified injury of head ▽
Head injury NOS
EXCLUDES 1   brain injury NOS (S06.9-)
    head injury NOS with loss of consciousness (S06.9-)
    intracranial injury NOS (S06.9-)

✓x7ᵗʰ S09.91 Unspecified injury of ear ▽
Injury of ear NOS

✓x7ᵗʰ S09.92 Unspecified injury of nose ▽
Injury of nose NOS

✓x7ᵗʰ S09.93 Unspecified injury of face ▽
Injury of face NOS

---

1 Case-mix diagnosis with 7th character indicating subsequent encounter.
2 Case-mix diagnosis with 7th character indicating subsequent encounter or sequela.
4 Case-mix diagnosis with 7th character indicating initial or subsequent encounter.
5 NRS supply diagnosis with 7th character indicating initial or subsequent encounter.
6 NRS supply diagnosis with 7th character indicating subsequent encounter.
7 Hospice non-cancer diagnosis with 7th character indicating subsequent encounter.

N Newborn: 0   P Pediatric: 0-17   M Maternity: 12-55   A Adult: 15-124   NRS Nonroutine supply Dx   NC Dx Noncancer Dx   PDx Primary Dx   ▶◀ Revised Text   ● New Code   ▲ Revised Title

924   ICD-10-CM 2018

Injuries to the neck (S10-S19)

INCLUDES   injuries of nape
       injuries of supraclavicular region
       injuries of throat
EXCLUDES 2   *burns and corrosions (T20-T32)*
       effects of foreign body in esophagus (T18.1)
       effects of foreign body in larynx (T17.3)
       effects of foreign body in pharynx (T17.2)
       effects of foreign body in trachea (T17.4)
       frostbite (T33-T34)
       insect bite or sting, venomous (T63.4)

✓4th S10 Superficial injury of neck

The appropriate 7th character is to be added to each code from category S10.
A   initial encounter
D   subsequent encounter
S   sequela

✓x7th **S10.0 Contusion of throat**
       Contusion of cervical esophagus
       Contusion of larynx
       Contusion of pharynx
       Contusion of trachea

✓5th **S10.1 Other and unspecified superficial injuries of throat**
   ✓x7th S10.10 **Unspecified superficial injuries of throat** ▽
   ✓x7th S10.11 **Abrasion** of throat
   ✓x7th S10.12 **Blister (nonthermal)** of throat
   ✓x7th S10.14 **External constriction** of part of throat
   ✓x7th S10.15 **Superficial** foreign body of throat
       Splinter in the throat
   ✓x7th S10.16 **Insect bite (nonvenomous)** of throat
   ✓x7th S10.17 **Other superficial** bite of throat
       EXCLUDES 1 *open bite of throat (S11.85)*

✓5th **S10.8 Superficial injury of** other specified parts of neck
   ✓x7th S10.80 **Unspecified superficial injury of other specified** ▽ **part of neck**
   ✓x7th S10.81 **Abrasion of other specified part of neck**
   ✓x7th S10.82 **Blister (nonthermal) of other specified part of neck**
   ✓x7th S10.83 **Contusion of other specified part of neck**
   ✓x7th S10.84 **External constriction of other specified part of neck**
   ✓x7th S10.85 **Superficial** foreign body **of other specified part of neck**
       Splinter in other specified part of neck
   ✓x7th S10.86 **Insect bite of other specified part of neck**
   ✓x7th S10.87 **Other superficial** bite **of other specified part of neck**
       EXCLUDES 1 *open bite of other specified parts of neck (S11.85)*

✓5th **S10.9 Superficial injury of** unspecified part of neck
   ✓x7th S10.90 **Unspecified superficial injury of unspecified** ▽ **part of neck**
   ✓x7th S10.91 **Abrasion of unspecified part of neck** ▽
   ✓x7th S10.92 **Blister (nonthermal) of unspecified part of neck** ▽
   ✓x7th S10.93 **Contusion of unspecified part of neck** ▽
   ✓x7th S10.94 **External constriction of unspecified part of neck** ▽
   ✓x7th S10.95 **Superficial** foreign body **of unspecified part of** ▽ **neck**
   ✓x7th S10.96 **Insect bite of unspecified part of neck** ▽
   ✓x7th S10.97 **Other superficial** bite **of unspecified part of neck** ▽

✓4th S11 Open wound of neck

Code also any associated:
       spinal cord injury (S14.0, S14.1-)
       wound infection
EXCLUDES 2   *open fracture of vertebra (S12- with 7th character B)*

The appropriate 7th character is to be added to each code from category S11.
A   initial encounter
D   subsequent encounter
S   sequela

✓5th **S11.0 Open wound of larynx and trachea**
   ✓6th **S11.01 Open wound of** larynx
       EXCLUDES 2 *open wound of vocal cord (S11.03)*
      1, 6 ✓7th S11.011 **Laceration without foreign body** NRS **of larynx**
      1, 6 ✓7th S11.012 **Laceration with foreign body of** NRS **larynx**
      1, 6 ✓7th S11.013 **Puncture wound without foreign** NRS **body of larynx**
      1, 6 ✓7th S11.014 **Puncture wound with foreign body** NRS **of larynx**
      1, 6 ✓7th S11.015 **Open bite of larynx** NRS
       Bite of larynx NOS
      6 ✓7th S11.019 **Unspecified open wound of larynx** NRS ▽

   ✓6th **S11.02 Open wound of** trachea
       Open wound of cervical trachea
       Open wound of trachea NOS
       EXCLUDES 2 *open wound of thoracic trachea (S27.5-)*
      1, 6 ✓7th S11.021 **Laceration without foreign body of** NRS **trachea**
      1, 6 ✓7th S11.022 **Laceration with foreign body of** NRS **trachea**
      1, 6 ✓7th S11.023 **Puncture wound without foreign** NRS **body of trachea**
      1, 6 ✓7th S11.024 **Puncture wound with foreign body** NRS **of trachea**
      1, 6 ✓7th S11.025 **Open bite of trachea** NRS
       Bite of trachea NOS
      6 ✓7th S11.029 **Unspecified open wound of trachea** NRS ▽

   ✓6th **S11.03 Open wound of** vocal cord
      1, 6 ✓7th S11.031 **Laceration without foreign body of** NRS **vocal cord**
      1, 6 ✓7th S11.032 **Laceration with foreign body of** NRS **vocal cord**
      1, 6 ✓7th S11.033 **Puncture wound without foreign** NRS **body of vocal cord**
      1, 6 ✓7th S11.034 **Puncture wound with foreign body** NRS **of vocal cord**
      1, 6 ✓7th S11.035 **Open bite of vocal cord** NRS
       Bite of vocal cord NOS
      6 ✓7th S11.039 **Unspecified open wound of vocal** NRS ▽ **cord**

✓5th **S11.1 Open wound of** thyroid gland
      6 ✓x7th S11.10 **Unspecified open wound of thyroid gland** NRS ▽
      1, 6 ✓x7th S11.11 **Laceration without foreign body of thyroid** NRS **gland**
      1, 6 ✓x7th S11.12 **Laceration with foreign body of thyroid gland** NRS
      1, 6 ✓x7th S11.13 **Puncture wound without foreign body of** NRS **thyroid gland**
      1, 6 ✓x7th S11.14 **Puncture wound with foreign body of thyroid** NRS **gland**
      1, 6 ✓x7th S11.15 **Open bite of thyroid gland** NRS
       Bite of thyroid gland NOS

✓5th **S11.2 Open wound of** pharynx and cervical esophagus
       EXCLUDES 1 *open wound of esophagus NOS (S27.8-)*
      6 ✓x7th S11.20 **Unspecified open wound of pharynx and** NRS ▽ **cervical esophagus**
      1, 6 ✓x7th S11.21 **Laceration without foreign body of pharynx** NRS **and cervical esophagus**
      1, 6 ✓x7th S11.22 **Laceration with foreign body of pharynx and** NRS **cervical esophagus**
      1, 6 ✓x7th S11.23 **Puncture wound without foreign body of** NRS **pharynx and cervical esophagus**

---

1   Case-mix diagnosis with 7th character indicating subsequent encounter.
6   NRS supply diagnosis with 7th character indicating subsequent encounter.

✓ Additional Character Req   ✓x7th Placeholder Alert   Case-Mix Diagnosis   Manifestation   ▽ Unspecified Dx   EXCLUDES 1 Not coded here   EXCLUDES 2 Not included here

1, 6 ✓x7ᵗʰ **S11.24** Puncture wound with foreign body of pharynx and cervical esophagus **NRS**

1, 6 ✓x7ᵗʰ **S11.25** Open bite of pharynx and cervical esophagus **NRS**
Bite of pharynx and cervical esophagus NOS

✓5ᵗʰ **S11.8 Open wound of other specified parts of neck**

5 ✓x7ᵗʰ **S11.80** Unspecified open wound of other specified part of neck **NRS** ▽

4,5 ✓x7ᵗʰ **S11.81** Laceration without foreign body of other specified part of neck **NRS**

4,5 ✓x7ᵗʰ **S11.82** Laceration with foreign body of other specified part of neck **NRS**

4,5 ✓x7ᵗʰ **S11.83** Puncture wound without foreign body of other specified part of neck **NRS**

4,5 ✓x7ᵗʰ **S11.84** Puncture wound with foreign body of other specified part of neck **NRS**

4,5 ✓x7ᵗʰ **S11.85** Open bite of other specified part of neck **NRS**
Bite of other specified part of neck NOS
EXCLUDES 1 superficial bite of other specified part of neck (S10.87)

4,5 ✓x7ᵗʰ **S11.89** Other open wound of other specified part of neck **NRS**

✓5ᵗʰ **S11.9 Open wound of unspecified part of neck**

5 ✓x7ᵗʰ **S11.90** Unspecified open wound of unspecified part of neck **NRS** ▽

4,5 ✓x7ᵗʰ **S11.91** Laceration without foreign body of unspecified part of neck **NRS** ▽

4,5 ✓x7ᵗʰ **S11.92** Laceration with foreign body of unspecified part of neck **NRS** ▽

4,5 ✓x7ᵗʰ **S11.93** Puncture wound without foreign body of unspecified part of neck **NRS** ▽

4,5 ✓x7ᵗʰ **S11.94** Puncture wound with foreign body of unspecified part of neck **NRS** ▽

4,5 ✓x7ᵗʰ **S11.95** Open bite of unspecified part of neck **NRS** ▽
Bite of neck NOS
EXCLUDES 1 superficial bite of neck (S10.97)

✓4ᵗʰ **S12 Fracture of cervical vertebra and other parts of neck**
NOTE A fracture not indicated as nondisplaced or displaced should be coded to displaced.
A fracture not indicated as open or closed should be coded to closed.
INCLUDES fracture of cervical neural arch
fracture of cervical spine
fracture of cervical spinous process
fracture of cervical transverse process
fracture of cervical vertebral arch
fracture of neck
Code first any associated cervical spinal cord injury (S14.0, S14.1-)
AHA: 2015, 3Q, 37-39
TIP: The term "improper alignment" is not synonymous with malunion or nonunion of a fracture when noted in provider documentation.

The appropriate 7th character is to be added to each code from subcategories S12.0-S12.6.
A   initial encounter for closed fracture
B   initial encounter for open fracture
D   subsequent encounter for fracture with routine healing
G   subsequent encounter for fracture with delayed healing
K   subsequent encounter for fracture with nonunion
S   sequela

✓5ᵗʰ **S12.0 Fracture of first cervical vertebra**
Atlas

✓6ᵗʰ **S12.00** Unspecified fracture of first cervical vertebra

1 ✓7ᵗʰ **S12.000** Unspecified displaced fracture of first cervical vertebra ▽

1 ✓7ᵗʰ **S12.001** Unspecified nondisplaced fracture of first cervical vertebra ▽

1 ✓x7ᵗʰ **S12.01** Stable burst fracture of first cervical vertebra

1 ✓x7ᵗʰ **S12.02** Unstable burst fracture of first cervical vertebra

✓6ᵗʰ **S12.03** Posterior arch fracture of first cervical vertebra

1 ✓7ᵗʰ **S12.030** Displaced posterior arch fracture of first cervical vertebra

1 ✓7ᵗʰ **S12.031** Nondisplaced posterior arch fracture of first cervical vertebra

✓6ᵗʰ **S12.04** Lateral mass fracture of first cervical vertebra

1 ✓7ᵗʰ **S12.040** Displaced lateral mass fracture of first cervical vertebra

1 ✓7ᵗʰ **S12.041** Nondisplaced lateral mass fracture of first cervical vertebra

✓6ᵗʰ **S12.09** Other fracture of first cervical vertebra

1 ✓7ᵗʰ **S12.090** Other displaced fracture of first cervical vertebra

1 ✓7ᵗʰ **S12.091** Other nondisplaced fracture of first cervical vertebra

✓5ᵗʰ **S12.1 Fracture of second cervical vertebra**
Axis

✓6ᵗʰ **S12.10** Unspecified fracture of second cervical vertebra

1 ✓7ᵗʰ **S12.100** Unspecified displaced fracture of second cervical vertebra ▽

1 ✓7ᵗʰ **S12.101** Unspecified nondisplaced fracture of second cervical vertebra ▽

✓6ᵗʰ **S12.11** Type II dens fracture

1 ✓7ᵗʰ **S12.110** Anterior displaced Type II dens fracture

1 ✓7ᵗʰ **S12.111** Posterior displaced Type II dens fracture

1 ✓7ᵗʰ **S12.112** Nondisplaced Type II dens fracture

✓6ᵗʰ **S12.12** Other dens fracture

1 ✓7ᵗʰ **S12.120** Other displaced dens fracture

1 ✓7ᵗʰ **S12.121** Other nondisplaced dens fracture

✓6ᵗʰ **S12.13** Unspecified traumatic spondylolisthesis of second cervical vertebra

1 ✓7ᵗʰ **S12.130** Unspecified traumatic displaced spondylolisthesis of second cervical vertebra ▽

1 ✓7ᵗʰ **S12.131** Unspecified traumatic nondisplaced spondylolisthesis of second cervical vertebra ▽

1 ✓x7ᵗʰ **S12.14** Type III traumatic spondylolisthesis of second cervical vertebra

✓6ᵗʰ **S12.15** Other traumatic spondylolisthesis of second cervical vertebra

1 ✓7ᵗʰ **S12.150** Other traumatic displaced spondylolisthesis of second cervical vertebra

1 ✓7ᵗʰ **S12.151** Other traumatic nondisplaced spondylolisthesis of second cervical vertebra

✓6ᵗʰ **S12.19** Other fracture of second cervical vertebra

1 ✓7ᵗʰ **S12.190** Other displaced fracture of second cervical vertebra

1 ✓7ᵗʰ **S12.191** Other nondisplaced fracture of second cervical vertebra

✓5ᵗʰ **S12.2 Fracture of third cervical vertebra**

✓6ᵗʰ **S12.20** Unspecified fracture of third cervical vertebra

1 ✓7ᵗʰ **S12.200** Unspecified displaced fracture of third cervical vertebra ▽

1 ✓7ᵗʰ **S12.201** Unspecified nondisplaced fracture of third cervical vertebra ▽

✓6ᵗʰ **S12.23** Unspecified traumatic spondylolisthesis of third cervical vertebra

1 ✓7ᵗʰ **S12.230** Unspecified traumatic displaced spondylolisthesis of third cervical vertebra ▽

1 ✓7ᵗʰ **S12.231** Unspecified traumatic nondisplaced spondylolisthesis of third cervical vertebra ▽

1 ✓x7ᵗʰ **S12.24** Type III traumatic spondylolisthesis of third cervical vertebra

✓6ᵗʰ **S12.25** Other traumatic spondylolisthesis of third cervical vertebra

1 ✓7ᵗʰ **S12.250** Other traumatic displaced spondylolisthesis of third cervical vertebra

1 ✓7ᵗʰ **S12.251** Other traumatic nondisplaced spondylolisthesis of third cervical vertebra

---

1   Case-mix diagnosis with 7th character indicating subsequent encounter.
4   Case-mix diagnosis with 7th character indicating initial or subsequent encounter.
5   NRS supply diagnosis with 7th character indicating initial or subsequent encounter.
6   NRS supply diagnosis with 7th character indicating subsequent encounter.

N Newborn: 0   P Pediatric: 0-17   M Maternity: 12-55   A Adult: 15-124   NRS Nonroutine supply Dx   NC Dx Noncancer Dx   PDx Primary Dx   ▶◀ Revised Text   ● New Code   ▲ Revised Title

926   ICD-10-CM 2018

✓6ᵗʰ **S12.29** Other fracture of third cervical vertebra

1 ✓7ᵗʰ   **S12.290** **Other displaced fracture of third cervical vertebra**

1 ✓7ᵗʰ   **S12.291** **Other nondisplaced fracture of third cervical vertebra**

✓5ᵗʰ **S12.3** Fracture of fourth cervical vertebra

✓6ᵗʰ   **S12.30** Unspecified fracture of fourth cervical vertebra

1 ✓7ᵗʰ   **S12.300** **Unspecified displaced fracture of fourth cervical vertebra** ▽

1 ✓7ᵗʰ   **S12.301** **Unspecified nondisplaced fracture of fourth cervical vertebra** ▽

✓6ᵗʰ   **S12.33** Unspecified traumatic spondylolisthesis of fourth cervical vertebra

1 ✓7ᵗʰ   **S12.330** **Unspecified traumatic displaced spondylolisthesis of fourth cervical vertebra** ▽

1 ✓7ᵗʰ   **S12.331** **Unspecified traumatic nondisplaced spondylolisthesis of fourth cervical vertebra** ▽

1 ✓x7ᵗʰ   **S12.34** Type III traumatic spondylolisthesis of fourth cervical vertebra

✓6ᵗʰ   **S12.35** Other traumatic spondylolisthesis of fourth cervical vertebra

1 ✓7ᵗʰ   **S12.350** **Other traumatic displaced spondylolisthesis of fourth cervical vertebra**

1 ✓7ᵗʰ   **S12.351** **Other traumatic nondisplaced spondylolisthesis of fourth cervical vertebra**

✓6ᵗʰ   **S12.39** Other fracture of fourth cervical vertebra

1 ✓7ᵗʰ   **S12.390** **Other displaced fracture of fourth cervical vertebra**

1 ✓7ᵗʰ   **S12.391** **Other nondisplaced fracture of fourth cervical vertebra**

✓5ᵗʰ **S12.4** Fracture of fifth cervical vertebra

✓6ᵗʰ   **S12.40** Unspecified fracture of fifth cervical vertebra

1 ✓7ᵗʰ   **S12.400** **Unspecified displaced fracture of fifth cervical vertebra** ▽

1 ✓7ᵗʰ   **S12.401** **Unspecified nondisplaced fracture of fifth cervical vertebra** ▽

✓6ᵗʰ   **S12.43** Unspecified traumatic spondylolisthesis of fifth cervical vertebra

1 ✓7ᵗʰ   **S12.430** **Unspecified traumatic displaced spondylolisthesis of fifth cervical vertebra** ▽

1 ✓7ᵗʰ   **S12.431** **Unspecified traumatic nondisplaced spondylolisthesis of fifth cervical vertebra** ▽

1 ✓x7ᵗʰ   **S12.44** Type III traumatic spondylolisthesis of fifth cervical vertebra

✓6ᵗʰ   **S12.45** Other traumatic spondylolisthesis of fifth cervical vertebra

1 ✓7ᵗʰ   **S12.450** **Other traumatic displaced spondylolisthesis of fifth cervical vertebra**

1 ✓7ᵗʰ   **S12.451** **Other traumatic nondisplaced spondylolisthesis of fifth cervical vertebra**

✓6ᵗʰ   **S12.49** Other fracture of fifth cervical vertebra

1 ✓7ᵗʰ   **S12.490** **Other displaced fracture of fifth cervical vertebra**

1 ✓7ᵗʰ   **S12.491** **Other nondisplaced fracture of fifth cervical vertebra**

✓5ᵗʰ **S12.5** Fracture of sixth cervical vertebra

✓6ᵗʰ   **S12.50** Unspecified fracture of sixth cervical vertebra

1 ✓7ᵗʰ   **S12.500** **Unspecified displaced fracture of sixth cervical vertebra** ▽

1 ✓7ᵗʰ   **S12.501** **Unspecified nondisplaced fracture of sixth cervical vertebra** ▽

✓6ᵗʰ   **S12.53** Unspecified traumatic spondylolisthesis of sixth cervical vertebra

1 ✓7ᵗʰ   **S12.530** **Unspecified traumatic displaced spondylolisthesis of sixth cervical vertebra** ▽

1 ✓7ᵗʰ   **S12.531** **Unspecified traumatic nondisplaced spondylolisthesis of sixth cervical vertebra** ▽

1 ✓x7ᵗʰ   **S12.54** Type III traumatic spondylolisthesis of sixth cervical vertebra

✓6ᵗʰ   **S12.55** Other traumatic spondylolisthesis of sixth cervical vertebra

1 ✓7ᵗʰ   **S12.550** **Other traumatic displaced spondylolisthesis of sixth cervical vertebra**

1 ✓7ᵗʰ   **S12.551** **Other traumatic nondisplaced spondylolisthesis of sixth cervical vertebra**

✓6ᵗʰ   **S12.59** Other fracture of sixth cervical vertebra

1 ✓7ᵗʰ   **S12.590** **Other displaced fracture of sixth cervical vertebra**

1 ✓7ᵗʰ   **S12.591** **Other nondisplaced fracture of sixth cervical vertebra**

✓5ᵗʰ **S12.6** Fracture of seventh cervical vertebra

✓6ᵗʰ   **S12.60** Unspecified fracture of seventh cervical vertebra

1 ✓7ᵗʰ   **S12.600** **Unspecified displaced fracture of seventh cervical vertebra** ▽

1 ✓7ᵗʰ   **S12.601** **Unspecified nondisplaced fracture of seventh cervical vertebra** ▽

✓6ᵗʰ   **S12.63** Unspecified traumatic spondylolisthesis of seventh cervical vertebra

1 ✓7ᵗʰ   **S12.630** **Unspecified traumatic displaced spondylolisthesis of seventh cervical vertebra** ▽

1 ✓7ᵗʰ   **S12.631** **Unspecified traumatic nondisplaced spondylolisthesis of seventh cervical vertebra** ▽

1 ✓x7ᵗʰ   **S12.64** Type III traumatic spondylolisthesis of seventh cervical vertebra

✓6ᵗʰ   **S12.65** Other traumatic spondylolisthesis of seventh cervical vertebra

1 ✓7ᵗʰ   **S12.650** **Other traumatic displaced spondylolisthesis of seventh cervical vertebra**

1 ✓7ᵗʰ   **S12.651** **Other traumatic nondisplaced spondylolisthesis of seventh cervical vertebra**

✓6ᵗʰ   **S12.69** Other fracture of seventh cervical vertebra

1 ✓7ᵗʰ   **S12.690** **Other displaced fracture of seventh cervical vertebra**

1 ✓7ᵗʰ   **S12.691** **Other nondisplaced fracture of seventh cervical vertebra**

1 ✓x7ᵗʰ **S12.8** **Fracture of other parts of neck**

Hyoid bone   Thyroid cartilage
Larynx   Trachea

The appropriate 7th character is to be added to code S12.8.
A   initial encounter
D   subsequent encounter
S   sequela

1 ✓x7ᵗʰ **S12.9** **Fracture of neck, unspecified** ▽

Fracture of cervical spine NOS
Fracture of cervical vertebra NOS
Fracture of neck NOS

The appropriate 7th character is to be added to code S12.9.
A   initial encounter
D   subsequent encounter
S   sequela

---

1   Case-mix diagnosis with 7th character indicating subsequent encounter.

✓ Additional Character Req   ✓x7ᵗʰ Placeholder Alert   Case-Mix Diagnosis   Manifestation   ▽ Unspecified Dx   *EXCLUDES 1* Not coded here   *EXCLUDES 2* Not included here

✓4ᵗʰ S13   Dislocation and sprain of joints and ligaments at neck level

> **INCLUDES**   avulsion of joint or ligament at neck level
> laceration of cartilage, joint or ligament at neck level
> sprain of cartilage, joint or ligament at neck level
> traumatic hemarthrosis of joint or ligament at neck level
> traumatic rupture of joint or ligament at neck level
> traumatic subluxation of joint or ligament at neck level
> traumatic tear of joint or ligament at neck level

> Code also any associated open wound

> **EXCLUDES 2**   strain of muscle or tendon at neck level (S16.1)

> The appropriate 7th character is to be added to each code from category S13.
> A   initial encounter
> D   subsequent encounter
> S   sequela

✓x7ᵗʰ S13.0   Traumatic rupture of cervical intervertebral disc

> **EXCLUDES 1**   rupture or displacement (nontraumatic) of cervical intervertebral disc NOS (M50.-)

✓5ᵗʰ S13.1   Subluxation and dislocation of cervical vertebrae

> Code also any associated:
> open wound of neck (S11.-)
> spinal cord injury (S14.1-)

> **EXCLUDES 2**   fracture of cervical vertebrae (S12.0--S12.3-)

> **✓6ᵗʰ S13.10   Subluxation and dislocation of unspecified cervical vertebrae**
>> **✓7ᵗʰ S13.100   Subluxation of unspecified cervical vertebrae** ▽
>> **✓7ᵗʰ S13.101   Dislocation of unspecified cervical vertebrae** ▽

> **✓6ᵗʰ S13.11   Subluxation and dislocation of C0/C1 cervical vertebrae**
>> Subluxation and dislocation of atlantooccipital joint
>> Subluxation and dislocation of atloidooccipital joint
>> Subluxation and dislocation of occipitoatloid joint
>> **✓7ᵗʰ S13.110   Subluxation of C0/C1 cervical vertebrae**
>> **✓7ᵗʰ S13.111   Dislocation of C0/C1 cervical vertebrae**

> **✓6ᵗʰ S13.12   Subluxation and dislocation of C1/C2 cervical vertebrae**
>> Subluxation and dislocation of atlantoaxial joint
>> **✓7ᵗʰ S13.120   Subluxation of C1/C2 cervical vertebrae**
>> **✓7ᵗʰ S13.121   Dislocation of C1/C2 cervical vertebrae**

> **✓6ᵗʰ S13.13   Subluxation and dislocation of C2/C3 cervical vertebrae**
>> **✓7ᵗʰ S13.130   Subluxation of C2/C3 cervical vertebrae**
>> **✓7ᵗʰ S13.131   Dislocation of C2/C3 cervical vertebrae**

> **✓6ᵗʰ S13.14   Subluxation and dislocation of C3/C4 cervical vertebrae**
>> **✓7ᵗʰ S13.140   Subluxation of C3/C4 cervical vertebrae**
>> **✓7ᵗʰ S13.141   Dislocation of C3/C4 cervical vertebrae**

> **✓6ᵗʰ S13.15   Subluxation and dislocation of C4/C5 cervical vertebrae**
>> **✓7ᵗʰ S13.150   Subluxation of C4/C5 cervical vertebrae**
>> **✓7ᵗʰ S13.151   Dislocation of C4/C5 cervical vertebrae**

> **✓6ᵗʰ S13.16   Subluxation and dislocation of C5/C6 cervical vertebrae**
>> **✓7ᵗʰ S13.160   Subluxation of C5/C6 cervical vertebrae**
>> **✓7ᵗʰ S13.161   Dislocation of C5/C6 cervical vertebrae**

> **✓6ᵗʰ S13.17   Subluxation and dislocation of C6/C7 cervical vertebrae**
>> **✓7ᵗʰ S13.170   Subluxation of C6/C7 cervical vertebrae**
>> **✓7ᵗʰ S13.171   Dislocation of C6/C7 cervical vertebrae**

> **✓6ᵗʰ S13.18   Subluxation and dislocation of C7/T1 cervical vertebrae**
>> **✓7ᵗʰ S13.180   Subluxation of C7/T1 cervical vertebrae**
>> **✓7ᵗʰ S13.181   Dislocation of C7/T1 cervical vertebrae**

✓5ᵗʰ S13.2   Dislocation of other and unspecified parts of neck
> **✓x7ᵗʰ S13.20   Dislocation of unspecified parts of neck** ▽
> **✓x7ᵗʰ S13.29   Dislocation of other parts of neck**

4 ✓x7ᵗʰ S13.4   Sprain of ligaments of cervical spine
> Sprain of anterior longitudinal (ligament), cervical
> Sprain of atlanto-axial (joints)
> Sprain of atlanto-occipital (joints)
> Whiplash injury of cervical spine

✓x7ᵗʰ S13.5   Sprain of thyroid region
> Sprain of cricoarytenoid (joint) (ligament)
> Sprain of cricothyroid (joint) (ligament)
> Sprain of thyroid cartilage

4 ✓x7ᵗʰ S13.8   Sprain of joints and ligaments of other parts of neck

4 ✓x7ᵗʰ S13.9   Sprain of joints and ligaments of unspecified parts of neck ▽

✓4ᵗʰ S14   Injury of nerves and spinal cord at neck level

> **NOTE**   Code to highest level of cervical cord injury.

> Code also any associated:
> fracture of cervical vertebra (S12.0- -S12.6-)
> open wound of neck (S11.-)
> transient paralysis (R29.5)

> The appropriate 7th character is to be added to each code from category S14.
> A   initial encounter
> D   subsequent encounter
> S   sequela

2 ✓x7ᵗʰ S14.0   Concussion and edema of cervical spinal cord

✓5ᵗʰ S14.1   Other and unspecified injuries of cervical spinal cord

> **✓6ᵗʰ S14.10   Unspecified injury of cervical spinal cord**
>> **2 ✓7ᵗʰ S14.101   Unspecified injury at C1 level of cervical spinal cord** ▽
>> **2 ✓7ᵗʰ S14.102   Unspecified injury at C2 level of cervical spinal cord** ▽
>> **2 ✓7ᵗʰ S14.103   Unspecified injury at C3 level of cervical spinal cord** ▽
>> **2 ✓7ᵗʰ S14.104   Unspecified injury at C4 level of cervical spinal cord** ▽
>> **2 ✓7ᵗʰ S14.105   Unspecified injury at C5 level of cervical spinal cord** ▽
>> **2 ✓7ᵗʰ S14.106   Unspecified injury at C6 level of cervical spinal cord** ▽
>> **2 ✓7ᵗʰ S14.107   Unspecified injury at C7 level of cervical spinal cord** ▽
>> **2 ✓7ᵗʰ S14.108   Unspecified injury at C8 level of cervical spinal cord** ▽
>> **2 ✓7ᵗʰ S14.109   Unspecified injury at unspecified level of cervical spinal cord** ▽
>>> Injury of cervical spinal cord NOS

> **✓6ᵗʰ S14.11   Complete lesion of cervical spinal cord**
>> **2 ✓7ᵗʰ S14.111   Complete lesion at C1 level of cervical spinal cord**
>> **2 ✓7ᵗʰ S14.112   Complete lesion at C2 level of cervical spinal cord**
>> **2 ✓7ᵗʰ S14.113   Complete lesion at C3 level of cervical spinal cord**
>> **2 ✓7ᵗʰ S14.114   Complete lesion at C4 level of cervical spinal cord**
>> **2 ✓7ᵗʰ S14.115   Complete lesion at C5 level of cervical spinal cord**
>> **2 ✓7ᵗʰ S14.116   Complete lesion at C6 level of cervical spinal cord**
>> **2 ✓7ᵗʰ S14.117   Complete lesion at C7 level of cervical spinal cord**
>> **2 ✓7ᵗʰ S14.118   Complete lesion at C8 level of cervical spinal cord**
>> **2 ✓7ᵗʰ S14.119   Complete lesion at unspecified level of cervical spinal cord** ▽

> **✓6ᵗʰ S14.12   Central cord syndrome of cervical spinal cord**
>> **2 ✓7ᵗʰ S14.121   Central cord syndrome at C1 level of cervical spinal cord**
>> **2 ✓7ᵗʰ S14.122   Central cord syndrome at C2 level of cervical spinal cord**
>> **2 ✓7ᵗʰ S14.123   Central cord syndrome at C3 level of cervical spinal cord**
>> **2 ✓7ᵗʰ S14.124   Central cord syndrome at C4 level of cervical spinal cord**

---

2   Case-mix diagnosis with 7th character indicating subsequent encounter or sequela.
4   Case-mix diagnosis with 7th character indicating initial or subsequent encounter.

Ⓝ Newborn: 0   Ⓟ Pediatric: 0-17   Ⓜ Maternity: 12-55   Ⓐ Adult: 15-124   **NRS** Nonroutine supply Dx   **NCDx** Noncancer Dx   **PDx** Primary Dx   ▶◀ Revised Text   ● New Code   ▲ Revised Title

928   ICD-10-CM 2018

2 ✓7ᵗʰ **S14.125** **Central cord syndrome at** C5 level **of cervical spinal cord**

2 ✓7ᵗʰ **S14.126** **Central cord syndrome at** C6 level **of cervical spinal cord**

2 ✓7ᵗʰ **S14.127** **Central cord syndrome at** C7 level **of cervical spinal cord**

2 ✓7ᵗʰ **S14.128** **Central cord syndrome at** C8 level **of cervical spinal cord**

2 ✓7ᵗʰ **S14.129** **Central cord syndrome at unspecified level of cervical spinal cord** ▽

✓6ᵗʰ **S14.13** Anterior cord syndrome **of cervical spinal cord**

2 ✓7ᵗʰ **S14.131** **Anterior cord syndrome at** C1 level **of cervical spinal cord**

2 ✓7ᵗʰ **S14.132** **Anterior cord syndrome at** C2 level **of cervical spinal cord**

2 ✓7ᵗʰ **S14.133** **Anterior cord syndrome at** C3 level **of cervical spinal cord**

2 ✓7ᵗʰ **S14.134** **Anterior cord syndrome at** C4 level **of cervical spinal cord**

2 ✓7ᵗʰ **S14.135** **Anterior cord syndrome at** C5 level **of cervical spinal cord**

2 ✓7ᵗʰ **S14.136** **Anterior cord syndrome at** C6 level **of cervical spinal cord**

2 ✓7ᵗʰ **S14.137** **Anterior cord syndrome at** C7 level **of cervical spinal cord**

2 ✓7ᵗʰ **S14.138** **Anterior cord syndrome at** C8 level **of cervical spinal cord**

2 ✓7ᵗʰ **S14.139** **Anterior cord syndrome at unspecified level of cervical spinal cord** ▽

✓6ᵗʰ **S14.14** Brown-Séquard syndrome **of cervical spinal cord**

2 ✓7ᵗʰ **S14.141** **Brown-Séquard syndrome at** C1 level **of cervical spinal cord**

2 ✓7ᵗʰ **S14.142** **Brown-Séquard syndrome at** C2 level **of cervical spinal cord**

2 ✓7ᵗʰ **S14.143** **Brown-Séquard syndrome at** C3 level **of cervical spinal cord**

2 ✓7ᵗʰ **S14.144** **Brown-Séquard syndrome at** C4 level **of cervical spinal cord**

2 ✓7ᵗʰ **S14.145** **Brown-Séquard syndrome at** C5 level **of cervical spinal cord**

2 ✓7ᵗʰ **S14.146** **Brown-Séquard syndrome at** C6 level **of cervical spinal cord**

2 ✓7ᵗʰ **S14.147** **Brown-Séquard syndrome at** C7 level **of cervical spinal cord**

2 ✓7ᵗʰ **S14.148** **Brown-Séquard syndrome at** C8 level **of cervical spinal cord**

2 ✓7ᵗʰ **S14.149** **Brown-Séquard syndrome at unspecified level of cervical spinal cord** ▽

✓6ᵗʰ **S14.15** Other incomplete lesions **of cervical spinal cord**
Incomplete lesion of cervical spinal cord NOS
Posterior cord syndrome of cervical spinal cord

2 ✓7ᵗʰ **S14.151** **Other incomplete lesion at** C1 level **of cervical spinal cord**

2 ✓7ᵗʰ **S14.152** **Other incomplete lesion at** C2 level **of cervical spinal cord**

2 ✓7ᵗʰ **S14.153** **Other incomplete lesion at** C3 level **of cervical spinal cord**

2 ✓7ᵗʰ **S14.154** **Other incomplete lesion at** C4 level **of cervical spinal cord**

2 ✓7ᵗʰ **S14.155** **Other incomplete lesion at** C5 level **of cervical spinal cord**

2 ✓7ᵗʰ **S14.156** **Other incomplete lesion at** C6 level **of cervical spinal cord**

2 ✓7ᵗʰ **S14.157** **Other incomplete lesion at** C7 level **of cervical spinal cord**

2 ✓7ᵗʰ **S14.158** **Other incomplete lesion at** C8 level **of cervical spinal cord**

2 ✓7ᵗʰ **S14.159** **Other incomplete lesion at unspecified level of cervical spinal cord** ▽

2 ✓x7ᵗʰ **S14.2** **Injury of** nerve root of cervical spine

2 ✓x7ᵗʰ **S14.3** **Injury of** brachial plexus

2 ✓x7ᵗʰ **S14.4** **Injury of** peripheral nerves of neck

2 ✓x7ᵗʰ **S14.5** **Injury of** cervical sympathetic nerves

2 ✓x7ᵗʰ **S14.8** **Injury of other specified nerves of neck**

2 ✓x7ᵗʰ **S14.9** **Injury of unspecified nerves of neck** ▽

✓4ᵗʰ **S15** **Injury of blood vessels at neck level**
Code also any associated open wound (S11.-)

> The appropriate 7th character is to be added to each code from category S15.
> A   initial encounter
> D   subsequent encounter
> S   sequela

✓5ᵗʰ **S15.0** **Injury of** carotid artery **of neck**
Injury of carotid artery (common) (external) (internal, extracranial portion)
Injury of carotid artery NOS
EXCLUDES 1   injury of internal carotid artery, intracranial portion (S06.8)

✓6ᵗʰ **S15.00** Unspecified **injury of carotid artery**

✓7ᵗʰ **S15.001** **Unspecified injury of** right **carotid artery** ▽

✓7ᵗʰ **S15.002** **Unspecified injury of** left **carotid artery** ▽

✓7ᵗʰ **S15.009** **Unspecified injury of unspecified carotid artery** ▽

✓6ᵗʰ **S15.01** Minor laceration **of carotid artery**
Incomplete transection of carotid artery
Laceration of carotid artery NOS
Superficial laceration of carotid artery

✓7ᵗʰ **S15.011** **Minor laceration of** right **carotid artery**

✓7ᵗʰ **S15.012** **Minor laceration of** left **carotid artery**

✓7ᵗʰ **S15.019** **Minor laceration of unspecified carotid artery** ▽

✓6ᵗʰ **S15.02** Major laceration **of carotid artery**
Complete transection of carotid artery
Traumatic rupture of carotid artery

✓7ᵗʰ **S15.021** **Major laceration of** right **carotid artery**

✓7ᵗʰ **S15.022** **Major laceration of** left **carotid artery**

✓7ᵗʰ **S15.029** **Major laceration of unspecified carotid artery** ▽

✓6ᵗʰ **S15.09** Other **specified injury of carotid artery**

✓7ᵗʰ **S15.091** **Other specified injury of** right **carotid artery**

✓7ᵗʰ **S15.092** **Other specified injury of** left **carotid artery**

✓7ᵗʰ **S15.099** **Other specified injury of unspecified carotid artery** ▽

✓5ᵗʰ **S15.1** **Injury of** vertebral artery

✓6ᵗʰ **S15.10** Unspecified **injury of vertebral artery**

✓7ᵗʰ **S15.101** **Unspecified injury of** right **vertebral artery** ▽

✓7ᵗʰ **S15.102** **Unspecified injury of** left **vertebral artery** ▽

✓7ᵗʰ **S15.109** **Unspecified injury of unspecified vertebral artery** ▽

✓6ᵗʰ **S15.11** Minor laceration **of vertebral artery**
Incomplete transection of vertebral artery
Laceration of vertebral artery NOS
Superficial laceration of vertebral artery

✓7ᵗʰ **S15.111** **Minor laceration of** right **vertebral artery**

✓7ᵗʰ **S15.112** **Minor laceration of** left **vertebral artery**

✓7ᵗʰ **S15.119** **Minor laceration of unspecified vertebral artery** ▽

✓6ᵗʰ **S15.12** Major laceration **of vertebral artery**
Complete transection of vertebral artery
Traumatic rupture of vertebral artery

✓7ᵗʰ **S15.121** **Major laceration of** right **vertebral artery**

✓7ᵗʰ **S15.122** **Major laceration of** left **vertebral artery**

✓7ᵗʰ **S15.129** **Major laceration of unspecified vertebral artery** ▽

✓6ᵗʰ **S15.19** Other **specified injury of vertebral artery**

✓7ᵗʰ **S15.191** **Other specified injury of** right **vertebral artery**

---

2   Case-mix diagnosis with 7th character indicating subsequent encounter or sequela.

✓ Additional Character Req   ✓x7ᵗʰ Placeholder Alert   Case-Mix Diagnosis   Manifestation   ▽ Unspecified Dx   *EXCLUDES 1* Not coded here   *EXCLUDES 2* Not included here

ICD-10-CM 2018   **929**

   ✓7ᵗʰ **S15.192** Other specified injury of **left** vertebral artery

   ✓7ᵗʰ **S15.199** Other specified injury of unspecified vertebral artery ▽

✓5ᵗʰ **S15.2 Injury of external jugular vein**

  ✓6ᵗʰ **S15.20 Unspecified** injury of external jugular vein

   ✓7ᵗʰ **S15.201** Unspecified injury of **right** external jugular vein ▽

   ✓7ᵗʰ **S15.202** Unspecified injury of **left** external jugular vein ▽

   ✓7ᵗʰ **S15.209** Unspecified injury of unspecified external jugular vein ▽

  ✓6ᵗʰ **S15.21 Minor laceration** of external jugular vein

Incomplete transection of external jugular vein
Laceration of external jugular vein NOS
Superficial laceration of external jugular vein

   ✓7ᵗʰ **S15.211** Minor laceration of **right** external jugular vein

   ✓7ᵗʰ **S15.212** Minor laceration of **left** external jugular vein

   ✓7ᵗʰ **S15.219** Minor laceration of unspecified external jugular vein ▽

  ✓6ᵗʰ **S15.22 Major laceration** of external jugular vein

Complete transection of external jugular vein
Traumatic rupture of external jugular vein

   ✓7ᵗʰ **S15.221** Major laceration of **right** external jugular vein

   ✓7ᵗʰ **S15.222** Major laceration of **left** external jugular vein

   ✓7ᵗʰ **S15.229** Major laceration of unspecified external jugular vein ▽

  ✓6ᵗʰ **S15.29 Other** specified injury of external jugular vein

   ✓7ᵗʰ **S15.291** Other specified injury of **right** external jugular vein

   ✓7ᵗʰ **S15.292** Other specified injury of **left** external jugular vein

   ✓7ᵗʰ **S15.299** Other specified injury of unspecified external jugular vein ▽

✓5ᵗʰ **S15.3 Injury of internal jugular vein**

  ✓6ᵗʰ **S15.30 Unspecified** injury of internal jugular vein

   ✓7ᵗʰ **S15.301** Unspecified injury of **right** internal jugular vein ▽

   ✓7ᵗʰ **S15.302** Unspecified injury of **left** internal jugular vein ▽

   ✓7ᵗʰ **S15.309** Unspecified injury of unspecified internal jugular vein ▽

  ✓6ᵗʰ **S15.31 Minor laceration** of internal jugular vein

Incomplete transection of internal jugular vein
Laceration of internal jugular vein NOS
Superficial laceration of internal jugular vein

   ✓7ᵗʰ **S15.311** Minor laceration of **right** internal jugular vein

   ✓7ᵗʰ **S15.312** Minor laceration of **left** internal jugular vein

   ✓7ᵗʰ **S15.319** Minor laceration of unspecified internal jugular vein ▽

  ✓6ᵗʰ **S15.32 Major laceration** of internal jugular vein

Complete transection of internal jugular vein
Traumatic rupture of internal jugular vein

   ✓7ᵗʰ **S15.321** Major laceration of **right** internal jugular vein

   ✓7ᵗʰ **S15.322** Major laceration of **left** internal jugular vein

   ✓7ᵗʰ **S15.329** Major laceration of unspecified internal jugular vein ▽

  ✓6ᵗʰ **S15.39 Other** specified injury of internal jugular vein

   ✓7ᵗʰ **S15.391** Other specified injury of **right** internal jugular vein

   ✓7ᵗʰ **S15.392** Other specified injury of **left** internal jugular vein

   ✓7ᵗʰ **S15.399** Other specified injury of unspecified internal jugular vein ▽

 ✓x7ᵗʰ **S15.8 Injury of other specified blood vessels at neck level**

 ✓x7ᵗʰ **S15.9 Injury of unspecified blood vessel at neck level** ▽

✓4ᵗʰ **S16 Injury of muscle, fascia and tendon at neck level**

Code also any associated open wound (S11.-)

EXCLUDES 2   sprain of joint or ligament at neck level (S13.9)

The appropriate 7th character is to be added to each code from category S16.
A   initial encounter
D   subsequent encounter
S   sequela

4 ✓x7ᵗʰ **S16.1 Strain of muscle, fascia and tendon at neck level**

4,5 ✓x7ᵗʰ **S16.2 Laceration of muscle, fascia and tendon at neck level** 🅽🆁🆂

 ✓x7ᵗʰ **S16.8 Other specified injury of muscle, fascia and tendon at neck level**

 ✓x7ᵗʰ **S16.9 Unspecified injury of muscle, fascia and tendon neck level** ▽

✓4ᵗʰ **S17 Crushing injury of neck**

Use additional code for all associated injuries, such as:
  injury of blood vessels (S15.-)
  open wound of neck (S11.-)
  spinal cord injury (S14.0, S14.1-)
  vertebral fracture (S12.0- -S12.3-)

The appropriate 7th character is to be added to each code from category S17.
A   initial encounter
D   subsequent encounter
S   sequela

 ✓x7ᵗʰ **S17.0 Crushing injury of larynx and trachea**

 ✓x7ᵗʰ **S17.8 Crushing injury of other specified parts of neck**

 ✓x7ᵗʰ **S17.9 Crushing injury of neck, part unspecified** ▽

✓4ᵗʰ **S19 Other specified and unspecified injuries of neck**

The appropriate 7th character is to be added to each code from category S19.
A   initial encounter
D   subsequent encounter
S   sequela

 ✓5ᵗʰ **S19.8 Other specified injuries of neck**

  ✓x7ᵗʰ **S19.80** Other specified injuries of unspecified part of neck ▽

  ✓x7ᵗʰ **S19.81** Other specified injuries of **larynx**

  ✓x7ᵗʰ **S19.82** Other specified injuries of cervical **trachea**

EXCLUDES 2   other specified injury of thoracic trachea (S27.5-)

  ✓x7ᵗʰ **S19.83** Other specified injuries of **vocal cord**

  ✓x7ᵗʰ **S19.84** Other specified injuries of **thyroid gland**

  ✓x7ᵗʰ **S19.85** Other specified injuries of **pharynx and cervical esophagus**

  ✓x7ᵗʰ **S19.89** Other specified injuries of other specified part of neck

 ✓x7ᵗʰ **S19.9 Unspecified injury of neck** ▽

Injuries to the thorax (S20-S29)

INCLUDES   injuries of breast
           injuries of chest (wall)
           injuries of interscapular area

EXCLUDES 2   burns and corrosions (T20-T32)
           effects of foreign body in bronchus (T17.5)
           effects of foreign body in esophagus (T18.1)
           effects of foreign body in lung (T17.8)
           effects of foreign body in trachea (T17.4)
           frostbite (T33-T34)
           injuries of axilla
           injuries of clavicle
           injuries of scapular region
           injuries of shoulder
           insect bite or sting, venomous (T63.4)

✓4ᵗʰ **S20 Superficial injury of thorax**

The appropriate 7th character is to be added to each code from category S20.
A   initial encounter
D   subsequent encounter
S   sequela

 ✓5ᵗʰ **S20.0 Contusion of breast**

  ✓x7ᵗʰ **S20.00** Contusion of breast, unspecified breast ▽

  ✓x7ᵗʰ **S20.01** Contusion of **right** breast

---

4   Case-mix diagnosis with 7th character indicating initial or subsequent encounter.
5   NRS supply diagnosis with 7th character indicating initial or subsequent encounter.

🅽 Newborn: 0   🅿 Pediatric: 0-17   🅼 Maternity: 12-55   🅰 Adult: 15-124   🅽🆁🆂 Nonroutine supply Dx   🅽🅲🅳🆇 Noncancer Dx   🅿🅳🆇 Primary Dx   ▶◀ Revised Text   ● New Code   ▲ Revised Title

930   ICD-10-CM 2018

✓x7ᵗʰ **S20.02**　Contusion of left breast

✓5ᵗʰ **S20.1**　**Other and unspecified superficial injuries of breast**

　✓6ᵗʰ **S20.10**　Unspecified superficial injuries of breast

　　✓7ᵗʰ **S20.101**　Unspecified superficial injuries of breast, right breast　▽

　　✓7ᵗʰ **S20.102**　Unspecified superficial injuries of breast, left breast　▽

　　✓7ᵗʰ **S20.109**　Unspecified superficial injuries of breast, unspecified breast　▽

　✓6ᵗʰ **S20.11**　Abrasion of breast

　　✓7ᵗʰ **S20.111**　Abrasion of breast, right breast

　　✓7ᵗʰ **S20.112**　Abrasion of breast, left breast

　　✓7ᵗʰ **S20.119**　Abrasion of breast, unspecified breast　▽

　✓6ᵗʰ **S20.12**　Blister (nonthermal) of breast

　　✓7ᵗʰ **S20.121**　Blister (nonthermal) of breast, right breast

　　✓7ᵗʰ **S20.122**　Blister (nonthermal) of breast, left breast

　　✓7ᵗʰ **S20.129**　Blister (nonthermal) of breast, unspecified breast　▽

　✓6ᵗʰ **S20.14**　External constriction of part of breast

　　✓7ᵗʰ **S20.141**　External constriction of part of breast, right breast

　　✓7ᵗʰ **S20.142**　External constriction of part of breast, left breast

　　✓7ᵗʰ **S20.149**　External constriction of part of breast, unspecified breast　▽

　✓6ᵗʰ **S20.15**　Superficial foreign body of breast
　　　　　Splinter in the breast

　　✓7ᵗʰ **S20.151**　Superficial foreign body of breast, right breast

　　✓7ᵗʰ **S20.152**　Superficial foreign body of breast, left breast

　　✓7ᵗʰ **S20.159**　Superficial foreign body of breast, unspecified breast　▽

　✓6ᵗʰ **S20.16**　Insect bite (nonvenomous) of breast

　　✓7ᵗʰ **S20.161**　Insect bite (nonvenomous) of breast, right breast

　　✓7ᵗʰ **S20.162**　Insect bite (nonvenomous) of breast, left breast

　　✓7ᵗʰ **S20.169**　Insect bite (nonvenomous) of breast, unspecified breast　▽

　✓6ᵗʰ **S20.17**　Other superficial bite of breast
　　　　　EXCLUDES 1　open bite of breast (S21.05-)

　　✓7ᵗʰ **S20.171**　Other superficial bite of breast, right breast

　　✓7ᵗʰ **S20.172**　Other superficial bite of breast, left breast

　　✓7ᵗʰ **S20.179**　Other superficial bite of breast, unspecified breast　▽

✓5ᵗʰ **S20.2**　**Contusion of thorax**

　✓x7ᵗʰ **S20.20**　Contusion of thorax, unspecified　▽

　✓6ᵗʰ **S20.21**　Contusion of front wall of thorax

　　✓7ᵗʰ **S20.211**　Contusion of right front wall of thorax

　　✓7ᵗʰ **S20.212**　Contusion of left front wall of thorax

　　✓7ᵗʰ **S20.219**　Contusion of unspecified front wall of thorax　▽

　✓6ᵗʰ **S20.22**　Contusion of back wall of thorax

　　✓7ᵗʰ **S20.221**　Contusion of right back wall of thorax

　　✓7ᵗʰ **S20.222**　Contusion of left back wall of thorax

　　✓7ᵗʰ **S20.229**　Contusion of unspecified back wall of thorax　▽

✓5ᵗʰ **S20.3**　**Other and unspecified superficial injuries of front wall of thorax**

　✓6ᵗʰ **S20.30**　Unspecified superficial injuries of front wall of thorax

　　✓7ᵗʰ **S20.301**　Unspecified superficial injuries of right front wall of thorax　▽

　　✓7ᵗʰ **S20.302**　Unspecified superficial injuries of left front wall of thorax　▽

　　✓7ᵗʰ **S20.309**　Unspecified superficial injuries of unspecified front wall of thorax　▽

　✓6ᵗʰ **S20.31**　Abrasion of front wall of thorax

　　✓7ᵗʰ **S20.311**　Abrasion of right front wall of thorax

　　✓7ᵗʰ **S20.312**　Abrasion of left front wall of thorax

　　✓7ᵗʰ **S20.319**　Abrasion of unspecified front wall of thorax　▽

　✓6ᵗʰ **S20.32**　Blister (nonthermal) of front wall of thorax

　　✓7ᵗʰ **S20.321**　Blister (nonthermal) of right front wall of thorax

　　✓7ᵗʰ **S20.322**　Blister (nonthermal) of left front wall of thorax

　　✓7ᵗʰ **S20.329**　Blister (nonthermal) of unspecified front wall of thorax　▽

　✓6ᵗʰ **S20.34**　External constriction of front wall of thorax

　　✓7ᵗʰ **S20.341**　External constriction of right front wall of thorax

　　✓7ᵗʰ **S20.342**　External constriction of left front wall of thorax

　　✓7ᵗʰ **S20.349**　External constriction of unspecified front wall of thorax　▽

　✓6ᵗʰ **S20.35**　Superficial foreign body of front wall of thorax
　　　　　Splinter in front wall of thorax

　　✓7ᵗʰ **S20.351**　Superficial foreign body of right front wall of thorax

　　✓7ᵗʰ **S20.352**　Superficial foreign body of left front wall of thorax

　　✓7ᵗʰ **S20.359**　Superficial foreign body of unspecified front wall of thorax　▽

　✓6ᵗʰ **S20.36**　Insect bite (nonvenomous) of front wall of thorax

　　✓7ᵗʰ **S20.361**　Insect bite (nonvenomous) of right front wall of thorax

　　✓7ᵗʰ **S20.362**　Insect bite (nonvenomous) of left front wall of thorax

　　✓7ᵗʰ **S20.369**　Insect bite (nonvenomous) of unspecified front wall of thorax　▽

　✓6ᵗʰ **S20.37**　Other superficial bite of front wall of thorax
　　　　　EXCLUDES 1　open bite of front wall of thorax (S21.14)

　　✓7ᵗʰ **S20.371**　Other superficial bite of right front wall of thorax

　　✓7ᵗʰ **S20.372**　Other superficial bite of left front wall of thorax

　　✓7ᵗʰ **S20.379**　Other superficial bite of unspecified front wall of thorax　▽

✓5ᵗʰ **S20.4**　**Other and unspecified superficial injuries of back wall of thorax**

　✓6ᵗʰ **S20.40**　Unspecified superficial injuries of back wall of thorax

　　✓7ᵗʰ **S20.401**　Unspecified superficial injuries of right back wall of thorax　▽

　　✓7ᵗʰ **S20.402**　Unspecified superficial injuries of left back wall of thorax　▽

　　✓7ᵗʰ **S20.409**　Unspecified superficial injuries of unspecified back wall of thorax　▽

　✓6ᵗʰ **S20.41**　Abrasion of back wall of thorax

　　✓7ᵗʰ **S20.411**　Abrasion of right back wall of thorax

　　✓7ᵗʰ **S20.412**　Abrasion of left back wall of thorax

　　✓7ᵗʰ **S20.419**　Abrasion of unspecified back wall of thorax　▽

　✓6ᵗʰ **S20.42**　Blister (nonthermal) of back wall of thorax

　　✓7ᵗʰ **S20.421**　Blister (nonthermal) of right back wall of thorax

　　✓7ᵗʰ **S20.422**　Blister (nonthermal) of left back wall of thorax

　　✓7ᵗʰ **S20.429**　Blister (nonthermal) of unspecified back wall of thorax　▽

　✓6ᵗʰ **S20.44**　External constriction of back wall of thorax

　　✓7ᵗʰ **S20.441**　External constriction of right back wall of thorax

　　✓7ᵗʰ **S20.442**　External constriction of left back wall of thorax

　　✓7ᵗʰ **S20.449**　External constriction of unspecified back wall of thorax　▽

　✓6ᵗʰ **S20.45**　Superficial foreign body of back wall of thorax
　　　　　Splinter of back wall of thorax

　　✓7ᵗʰ **S20.451**　Superficial foreign body of right back wall of thorax

　　✓7ᵗʰ **S20.452**　Superficial foreign body of left back wall of thorax

✓ Additional Character Req　　✓x7ᵗʰ Placeholder Alert　　Case-Mix Diagnosis　　Manifestation　　▽ Unspecified Dx　　**EXCLUDES 1** Not coded here　　**EXCLUDES 2** Not included here

ICD-10-CM 2018

931

✓7th **S20.459** Superficial foreign body of unspecified back wall of thorax   ▽

✓6th **S20.46** Insect bite (nonvenomous) of back wall of thorax

  ✓7th **S20.461** Insect bite (nonvenomous) of right back wall of thorax

  ✓7th **S20.462** Insect bite (nonvenomous) of left back wall of thorax

  ✓7th **S20.469** Insect bite (nonvenomous) of unspecified back wall of thorax   ▽

✓6th **S20.47** Other superficial bite of back wall of thorax
    EXCLUDES 1   open bite of back wall of thorax (S21.24)

  ✓7th **S20.471** Other superficial bite of right back wall of thorax

  ✓7th **S20.472** Other superficial bite of left back wall of thorax

  ✓7th **S20.479** Other superficial bite of unspecified back wall of thorax   ▽

✓5th **S20.9** Superficial injury of unspecified parts of thorax
    EXCLUDES 1   contusion of thorax NOS (S20.20)

  ✓x7th **S20.90** Unspecified superficial injury of unspecified parts of thorax   ▽
      Superficial injury of thoracic wall NOS

  ✓x7th **S20.91** Abrasion of unspecified parts of thorax   ▽

  ✓x7th **S20.92** Blister (nonthermal) of unspecified parts of thorax   ▽

  ✓x7th **S20.94** External constriction of unspecified parts of thorax   ▽

  ✓x7th **S20.95** Superficial foreign body of unspecified parts of thorax   ▽
      Splinter in thorax NOS

  ✓x7th **S20.96** Insect bite (nonvenomous) of unspecified parts of thorax   ▽

  ✓x7th **S20.97** Other superficial bite of unspecified parts of thorax   ▽
    EXCLUDES 1   open bite of thorax NOS (S21.95)

✓4th **S21** Open wound of thorax
Code also any associated injury such as:
  injury of heart (S26.-)
  injury of intrathoracic organs (S27.-)
  rib fracture (S22.3-, S22.4-)
  spinal cord injury (S24.0-, S24.1-)
  traumatic hemopneumothorax (S27.3)
  traumatic hemothorax (S27.1)
  traumatic pneumothorax (S27.0)
  wound infection
  EXCLUDES 1   traumatic amputation (partial) of thorax (S28.1)

The appropriate 7th character is to be added to each code from category S21.
A   initial encounter
D   subsequent encounter
S   sequela

✓5th **S21.0** Open wound of breast

✓6th **S21.00** Unspecified open wound of breast

  5 ✓7th **S21.001** Unspecified open wound of right breast   NRS ▽

  5 ✓7th **S21.002** Unspecified open wound of left breast   NRS ▽

  ✓7th **S21.009** Unspecified open wound of unspecified breast   ▽

✓6th **S21.01** Laceration without foreign body of breast

  4,5 ✓7th **S21.011** Laceration without foreign body of right breast   NRS

  4,5 ✓7th **S21.012** Laceration without foreign body of left breast   NRS

  ✓7th **S21.019** Laceration without foreign body of unspecified breast   ▽

✓6th **S21.02** Laceration with foreign body of breast

  4,5 ✓7th **S21.021** Laceration with foreign body of right breast   NRS

  4,5 ✓7th **S21.022** Laceration with foreign body of left breast   NRS

  ✓7th **S21.029** Laceration with foreign body of unspecified breast   ▽

✓6th **S21.03** Puncture wound without foreign body of breast

  4,5 ✓7th **S21.031** Puncture wound without foreign body of right breast   NRS

  4,5 ✓7th **S21.032** Puncture wound without foreign body of left breast   NRS

  ✓7th **S21.039** Puncture wound without foreign body of unspecified breast   ▽

✓6th **S21.04** Puncture wound with foreign body of breast

  4,5 ✓7th **S21.041** Puncture wound with foreign body of right breast   NRS

  4,5 ✓7th **S21.042** Puncture wound with foreign body of left breast   NRS

  ✓7th **S21.049** Puncture wound with foreign body of unspecified breast   ▽

✓6th **S21.05** Open bite of breast
    Bite of breast NOS
    EXCLUDES 1   superficial bite of breast (S20.17)

  4,5 ✓7th **S21.051** Open bite of right breast   NRS

  4,5 ✓7th **S21.052** Open bite of left breast   NRS

  ✓7th **S21.059** Open bite of unspecified breast   ▽

✓5th **S21.1** Open wound of front wall of thorax without penetration into thoracic cavity
Open wound of chest without penetration into thoracic cavity

✓6th **S21.10** Unspecified open wound of front wall of thorax without penetration into thoracic cavity

  5 ✓7th **S21.101** Unspecified open wound of right front wall of thorax without penetration into thoracic cavity   NRS ▽

  5 ✓7th **S21.102** Unspecified open wound of left front wall of thorax without penetration into thoracic cavity   NRS ▽

  ✓7th **S21.109** Unspecified open wound of unspecified front wall of thorax without penetration into thoracic cavity   ▽

✓6th **S21.11** Laceration without foreign body of front wall of thorax without penetration into thoracic cavity

  4,5 ✓7th **S21.111** Laceration without foreign body of right front wall of thorax without penetration into thoracic cavity   NRS

  4,5 ✓7th **S21.112** Laceration without foreign body of left front wall of thorax without penetration into thoracic cavity   NRS

  ✓7th **S21.119** Laceration without foreign body of unspecified front wall of thorax without penetration into thoracic cavity   ▽

✓6th **S21.12** Laceration with foreign body of front wall of thorax without penetration into thoracic cavity

  4,5 ✓7th **S21.121** Laceration with foreign body of right front wall of thorax without penetration into thoracic cavity   NRS

  4,5 ✓7th **S21.122** Laceration with foreign body of left front wall of thorax without penetration into thoracic cavity   NRS

  ✓7th **S21.129** Laceration with foreign body of unspecified front wall of thorax without penetration into thoracic cavity   ▽

✓6th **S21.13** Puncture wound without foreign body of front wall of thorax without penetration into thoracic cavity

  4,5 ✓7th **S21.131** Puncture wound without foreign body of right front wall of thorax without penetration into thoracic cavity   NRS

  4,5 ✓7th **S21.132** Puncture wound without foreign body of left front wall of thorax without penetration into thoracic cavity   NRS

  ✓7th **S21.139** Puncture wound without foreign body of unspecified front wall of thorax without penetration into thoracic cavity   ▽

✓6th **S21.14** Puncture wound with foreign body of front wall of thorax without penetration into thoracic cavity

  4,5 ✓7th **S21.141** Puncture wound with foreign body of right front wall of thorax without penetration into thoracic cavity   NRS

  4,5 ✓7th **S21.142** Puncture wound with foreign body of left front wall of thorax without penetration into thoracic cavity   NRS

---

4   Case-mix diagnosis with 7th character indicating initial or subsequent encounter.
5   NRS supply diagnosis with 7th character indicating initial or subsequent encounter.

N Newborn: 0   P Pediatric: 0-17   M Maternity: 12-55   A Adult: 15-124   NRS Nonroutine supply Dx   NC Dx Noncancer Dx   PDx Primary Dx   ▶◀ Revised Text   ● New Code   ▲ Revised Title

932   ICD-10-CM 2018

√7ᵗʰ **S21.149** Puncture wound with foreign body of ▽
unspecified front wall of thorax without
penetration into thoracic cavity

√6ᵗʰ **S21.15** Open bite of front wall of thorax without
penetration into thoracic cavity
Bite of front wall of thorax NOS
EXCLUDES 1 superficial bite of front wall of thorax (S20.37)

4,5 √7ᵗʰ **S21.151** Open bite of right front wall of thorax NRS
without penetration into thoracic cavity

4,5 √7ᵗʰ **S21.152** Open bite of left front wall of thorax NRS
without penetration into thoracic cavity

√7ᵗʰ **S21.159** Open bite of unspecified front wall of ▽
thorax without penetration into thoracic
cavity

√5ᵗʰ **S21.2** Open wound of back wall of thorax without penetration into
thoracic cavity

√6ᵗʰ **S21.20** Unspecified open wound of back wall of thorax
without penetration into thoracic cavity

5 √7ᵗʰ **S21.201** Unspecified open wound of right NRS ▽
back wall of thorax without
penetration into thoracic cavity

5 √7ᵗʰ **S21.202** Unspecified open wound of left NRS ▽
back wall of thorax without
penetration into thoracic cavity

√7ᵗʰ **S21.209** Unspecified open wound of ▽
unspecified back wall of thorax
without penetration into thoracic cavity

√6ᵗʰ **S21.21** Laceration without foreign body of back wall of
thorax without penetration into thoracic cavity

4,5 √7ᵗʰ **S21.211** Laceration without foreign body of NRS
right back wall of thorax without
penetration into thoracic cavity

4,5 √7ᵗʰ **S21.212** Laceration without foreign body of NRS
left back wall of thorax without
penetration into thoracic cavity

√7ᵗʰ **S21.219** Laceration without foreign body of ▽
unspecified back wall of thorax without
penetration into thoracic cavity

√6ᵗʰ **S21.22** Laceration with foreign body of back wall of thorax
without penetration into thoracic cavity

4,5 √7ᵗʰ **S21.221** Laceration with foreign body of right NRS
back wall of thorax without
penetration into thoracic cavity

4,5 √7ᵗʰ **S21.222** Laceration with foreign body of left NRS
back wall of thorax without
penetration into thoracic cavity

√7ᵗʰ **S21.229** Laceration with foreign body of ▽
unspecified back wall of thorax without
penetration into thoracic cavity

√6ᵗʰ **S21.23** Puncture wound without foreign body of back wall
of thorax without penetration into thoracic cavity

4,5 √7ᵗʰ **S21.231** Puncture wound without foreign body NRS
of right back wall of thorax without
penetration into thoracic cavity

4,5 √7ᵗʰ **S21.232** Puncture wound without foreign body NRS
of left back wall of thorax without
penetration into thoracic cavity

√7ᵗʰ **S21.239** Puncture wound without foreign body ▽
of unspecified back wall of thorax without
penetration into thoracic cavity

√6ᵗʰ **S21.24** Puncture wound with foreign body of back wall of
thorax without penetration into thoracic cavity

4,5 √7ᵗʰ **S21.241** Puncture wound with foreign body of NRS
right back wall of thorax without
penetration into thoracic cavity

4,5 √7ᵗʰ **S21.242** Puncture wound with foreign body of NRS
left back wall of thorax without
penetration into thoracic cavity

√7ᵗʰ **S21.249** Puncture wound with foreign body of ▽
unspecified back wall of thorax without
penetration into thoracic cavity

√6ᵗʰ **S21.25** Open bite of back wall of thorax without penetration
into thoracic cavity
Bite of back wall of thorax NOS
EXCLUDES 1 superficial bite of back wall of thorax (S20.47)

4,5 √7ᵗʰ **S21.251** Open bite of right back wall of thorax NRS
without penetration into thoracic cavity

4,5 √7ᵗʰ **S21.252** Open bite of left back wall of thorax NRS
without penetration into thoracic cavity

√7ᵗʰ **S21.259** Open bite of unspecified back wall of ▽
thorax without penetration into thoracic
cavity

√5ᵗʰ **S21.3** Open wound of front wall of thorax with penetration into
thoracic cavity
Open wound of chest with penetration into thoracic cavity

√6ᵗʰ **S21.30** Unspecified open wound of front wall of thorax with
penetration into thoracic cavity

√7ᵗʰ **S21.301** Unspecified open wound of right front ▽
wall of thorax with penetration into
thoracic cavity

√7ᵗʰ **S21.302** Unspecified open wound of left front ▽
wall of thorax with penetration into
thoracic cavity

√7ᵗʰ **S21.309** Unspecified open wound of ▽
unspecified front wall of thorax with
penetration into thoracic cavity

√6ᵗʰ **S21.31** Laceration without foreign body of front wall of
thorax with penetration into thoracic cavity

√7ᵗʰ **S21.311** Laceration without foreign body of right
front wall of thorax with penetration into
thoracic cavity

√7ᵗʰ **S21.312** Laceration without foreign body of left
front wall of thorax with penetration into
thoracic cavity

√7ᵗʰ **S21.319** Laceration without foreign body of ▽
unspecified front wall of thorax with
penetration into thoracic cavity

√6ᵗʰ **S21.32** Laceration with foreign body of front wall of thorax
with penetration into thoracic cavity

√7ᵗʰ **S21.321** Laceration with foreign body of right front
wall of thorax with penetration into
thoracic cavity

√7ᵗʰ **S21.322** Laceration with foreign body of left front
wall of thorax with penetration into
thoracic cavity

√7ᵗʰ **S21.329** Laceration with foreign body of ▽
unspecified front wall of thorax with
penetration into thoracic cavity

√6ᵗʰ **S21.33** Puncture wound without foreign body of front wall
of thorax with penetration into thoracic cavity

√7ᵗʰ **S21.331** Puncture wound without foreign body of
right front wall of thorax with penetration
into thoracic cavity

√7ᵗʰ **S21.332** Puncture wound without foreign body of
left front wall of thorax with penetration
into thoracic cavity

√7ᵗʰ **S21.339** Puncture wound without foreign body ▽
of unspecified front wall of thorax with
penetration into thoracic cavity

√6ᵗʰ **S21.34** Puncture wound with foreign body of front wall of
thorax with penetration into thoracic cavity

√7ᵗʰ **S21.341** Puncture wound with foreign body of
right front wall of thorax with penetration
into thoracic cavity

√7ᵗʰ **S21.342** Puncture wound with foreign body of left
front wall of thorax with penetration into
thoracic cavity

√7ᵗʰ **S21.349** Puncture wound with foreign body of ▽
unspecified front wall of thorax with
penetration into thoracic cavity

---

4 Case-mix diagnosis with 7th character indicating initial or subsequent encounter.
5 NRS supply diagnosis with 7th character indicating initial or subsequent encounter.

☑ Additional Character Req   ✓ˣ⁷ᵗʰ Placeholder Alert   Case-Mix Diagnosis   Manifestation   ▽ Unspecified Dx   *EXCLUDES 1* Not coded here   *EXCLUDES 2* Not included here

✓6ᵗʰ S21.35　Open bite of front wall of thorax with penetration into thoracic cavity
　　　EXCLUDES 1　superficial bite of front wall of thorax (S20.37)

　　✓7ᵗʰ **S21.351**　**Open bite** of **right** front wall of thorax with penetration into thoracic cavity

　　✓7ᵗʰ **S21.352**　**Open bite** of **left** front wall of thorax with penetration into thoracic cavity

　　✓7ᵗʰ **S21.359**　**Open bite** of unspecified front wall of thorax with penetration into thoracic cavity　▽

✓5ᵗʰ S21.4　Open wound of back wall of thorax with penetration into thoracic cavity

　✓6ᵗʰ S21.40　Unspecified open wound of back wall of thorax with penetration into thoracic cavity

　　✓7ᵗʰ **S21.401**　**Unspecified open wound** of **right** back wall of thorax with penetration into thoracic cavity　▽

　　✓7ᵗʰ **S21.402**　**Unspecified open wound** of **left** back wall of thorax with penetration into thoracic cavity　▽

　　✓7ᵗʰ **S21.409**　**Unspecified open wound** of unspecified back wall of thorax with penetration into thoracic cavity　▽

　✓6ᵗʰ S21.41　Laceration without foreign body of back wall of thorax with penetration into thoracic cavity

　　✓7ᵗʰ **S21.411**　**Laceration without foreign body** of **right** back wall of thorax with penetration into thoracic cavity

　　✓7ᵗʰ **S21.412**　**Laceration without foreign body** of **left** back wall of thorax with penetration into thoracic cavity

　　✓7ᵗʰ **S21.419**　**Laceration without foreign body** of unspecified back wall of thorax with penetration into thoracic cavity　▽

　✓6ᵗʰ S21.42　Laceration with foreign body of back wall of thorax with penetration into thoracic cavity

　　✓7ᵗʰ **S21.421**　**Laceration with foreign body** of **right** back wall of thorax with penetration into thoracic cavity

　　✓7ᵗʰ **S21.422**　**Laceration with foreign body** of **left** back wall of thorax with penetration into thoracic cavity

　　✓7ᵗʰ **S21.429**　**Laceration with foreign body** of unspecified back wall of thorax with penetration into thoracic cavity　▽

　✓6ᵗʰ S21.43　Puncture wound without foreign body of back wall of thorax with penetration into thoracic cavity

　　✓7ᵗʰ **S21.431**　**Puncture wound without foreign body** of **right** back wall of thorax with penetration into thoracic cavity

　　✓7ᵗʰ **S21.432**　**Puncture wound without foreign body** of **left** back wall of thorax with penetration into thoracic cavity

　　✓7ᵗʰ **S21.439**　**Puncture wound without foreign body** of unspecified back wall of thorax with penetration into thoracic cavity　▽

　✓6ᵗʰ S21.44　Puncture wound with foreign body of back wall of thorax with penetration into thoracic cavity

　　✓7ᵗʰ **S21.441**　**Puncture wound with foreign body** of **right** back wall of thorax with penetration into thoracic cavity

　　✓7ᵗʰ **S21.442**　**Puncture wound with foreign body** of **left** back wall of thorax with penetration into thoracic cavity

　　✓7ᵗʰ **S21.449**　**Puncture wound with foreign body** of unspecified back wall of thorax with penetration into thoracic cavity　▽

　✓6ᵗʰ S21.45　Open bite of back wall of thorax with penetration into thoracic cavity
　　　Bite of back wall of thorax NOS
　　　EXCLUDES 1　superficial bite of back wall of thorax (S20.47)

　　✓7ᵗʰ **S21.451**　**Open bite** of **right** back wall of thorax with penetration into thoracic cavity

　　✓7ᵗʰ **S21.452**　**Open bite** of **left** back wall of thorax with penetration into thoracic cavity

　　✓7ᵗʰ **S21.459**　**Open bite** of unspecified back wall of thorax with penetration into thoracic cavity　▽

✓5ᵗʰ S21.9　Open wound of unspecified part of thorax
　　　Open wound of thoracic wall NOS

　✓x7ᵗʰ **S21.90**　**Unspecified open wound of unspecified part of thorax**　▽

　4 ✓x7ᵗʰ **S21.91**　**Laceration without foreign body** of unspecified part of thorax　▽

　✓x7ᵗʰ **S21.92**　**Laceration with foreign body** of unspecified part of thorax　▽

　4 ✓x7ᵗʰ **S21.93**　**Puncture wound without foreign body** of unspecified part of thorax　▽

　✓x7ᵗʰ **S21.94**　**Puncture wound with foreign body** of unspecified part of thorax　▽

　✓x7ᵗʰ **S21.95**　**Open bite** of unspecified part of thorax　▽
　　　EXCLUDES 1　superficial bite of thorax (S20.97)

✓4ᵗʰ S22　Fracture of rib(s), sternum and thoracic spine
　NOTE　A fracture not indicated as nondisplaced or displaced should be coded to displaced.
　　　A fracture not indicated as open or closed should be coded to closed.
　INCLUDES　fracture of thoracic neural arch
　　　fracture of thoracic spinous process
　　　fracture of thoracic transverse process
　　　fracture of thoracic vertebra
　　　fracture of thoracic vertebral arch

Code first any associated:
　injury of intrathoracic organ (S27.-)
　spinal cord injury (S24.0-, S24.1-)
　EXCLUDES 1　transection of thorax (S28.1)
　EXCLUDES 2　fracture of clavicle (S42.0-)
　　　fracture of scapula (S42.1-)
AHA: 2015, 3Q, 37-39
TIP: The term "improper alignment" is not synonymous with malunion or nonunion of a fracture when noted in provider documentation.

The appropriate 7th character is to be added to each code from category S22.
A　initial encounter for closed fracture
B　initial encounter for open fracture
D　subsequent encounter for fracture with routine healing
G　subsequent encounter for fracture with delayed healing
K　subsequent encounter for fracture with nonunion
S　sequela

✓5ᵗʰ S22.0　Fracture of thoracic vertebra

　✓6ᵗʰ S22.00　Fracture of unspecified thoracic vertebra

　　1 ✓7ᵗʰ **S22.000**　**Wedge compression fracture of** unspecified thoracic vertebra　▽

　　1 ✓7ᵗʰ **S22.001**　**Stable burst fracture of** unspecified thoracic vertebra　▽

　　1 ✓7ᵗʰ **S22.002**　**Unstable burst fracture of** unspecified thoracic vertebra　▽

　　1 ✓7ᵗʰ **S22.008**　**Other fracture of** unspecified thoracic vertebra　▽

　　1 ✓7ᵗʰ **S22.009**　**Unspecified fracture of** unspecified thoracic vertebra　▽

　✓6ᵗʰ S22.01　Fracture of first thoracic vertebra

　　1 ✓7ᵗʰ **S22.010**　**Wedge compression fracture of** first thoracic vertebra

　　1 ✓7ᵗʰ **S22.011**　**Stable burst fracture of** first thoracic vertebra

　　1 ✓7ᵗʰ **S22.012**　**Unstable burst fracture of** first thoracic vertebra

　　1 ✓7ᵗʰ **S22.018**　**Other fracture of** first thoracic vertebra

　　1 ✓7ᵗʰ **S22.019**　**Unspecified fracture of** first thoracic vertebra　▽

　✓6ᵗʰ S22.02　Fracture of second thoracic vertebra

　　1 ✓7ᵗʰ **S22.020**　**Wedge compression fracture of** second thoracic vertebra

　　1 ✓7ᵗʰ **S22.021**　**Stable burst fracture of** second thoracic vertebra

　　1 ✓7ᵗʰ **S22.022**　**Unstable burst fracture of** second thoracic vertebra

　　1 ✓7ᵗʰ **S22.028**　**Other fracture of** second thoracic vertebra

---

1　Case-mix diagnosis with 7th character indicating subsequent encounter.
4　Case-mix diagnosis with 7th character indicating initial or subsequent encounter.

N Newborn: 0　P Pediatric: 0-17　M Maternity: 12-55　A Adult: 15-124　NRS Nonroutine supply Dx　NC Dx Noncancer Dx　PDx Primary Dx　▶◀ Revised Text　● New Code　▲ Revised Title

934　　　　　　　　　　　　　　　　　　　　　　　　　　　　　　　　　ICD-10-CM 2018

¹ √7ᵗʰ **S22.029** **Unspecified fracture of second** ▽
thoracic vertebra

√6ᵗʰ **S22.03** **Fracture of** third **thoracic vertebra**

¹ √7ᵗʰ **S22.030** Wedge compression **fracture of third**
thoracic vertebra

¹ √7ᵗʰ **S22.031** Stable burst **fracture of third thoracic**
vertebra

¹ √7ᵗʰ **S22.032** Unstable burst **fracture of third thoracic**
vertebra

¹ √7ᵗʰ **S22.038** **Other fracture of third thoracic vertebra**

¹ √7ᵗʰ **S22.039** **Unspecified fracture of third thoracic** ▽
vertebra

√6ᵗʰ **S22.04** **Fracture of** fourth **thoracic vertebra**

¹ √7ᵗʰ **S22.040** Wedge compression **fracture of fourth**
thoracic vertebra

¹ √7ᵗʰ **S22.041** Stable burst **fracture of fourth thoracic**
vertebra

¹ √7ᵗʰ **S22.042** Unstable burst **fracture of fourth thoracic**
vertebra

¹ √7ᵗʰ **S22.048** **Other fracture of fourth thoracic vertebra**

¹ √7ᵗʰ **S22.049** **Unspecified fracture of fourth thoracic** ▽
vertebra

√6ᵗʰ **S22.05** **Fracture of** T5-T6 **vertebra**

¹ √7ᵗʰ **S22.050** Wedge compression **fracture of T5-T6**
vertebra

¹ √7ᵗʰ **S22.051** Stable burst **fracture of T5-T6 vertebra**

¹ √7ᵗʰ **S22.052** Unstable burst **fracture of T5-T6 vertebra**

¹ √7ᵗʰ **S22.058** **Other fracture of T5-T6 vertebra**

¹ √7ᵗʰ **S22.059** **Unspecified fracture of T5-T6 vertebra** ▽

√6ᵗʰ **S22.06** **Fracture of** T7-T8 **vertebra**

¹ √7ᵗʰ **S22.060** Wedge compression **fracture of T7-T8**
vertebra

¹ √7ᵗʰ **S22.061** Stable burst **fracture of T7-T8 vertebra**

¹ √7ᵗʰ **S22.062** Unstable burst **fracture of T7-T8 vertebra**

¹ √7ᵗʰ **S22.068** **Other fracture of T7-T8 thoracic vertebra**

¹ √7ᵗʰ **S22.069** **Unspecified fracture of T7-T8 vertebra** ▽

√6ᵗʰ **S22.07** **Fracture of** T9-T10 **vertebra**

¹ √7ᵗʰ **S22.070** Wedge compression **fracture of T9-T10**
vertebra

¹ √7ᵗʰ **S22.071** Stable burst **fracture of T9-T10 vertebra**

¹ √7ᵗʰ **S22.072** Unstable burst **fracture of T9-T10 vertebra**

¹ √7ᵗʰ **S22.078** **Other fracture of T9-T10 vertebra**

¹ √7ᵗʰ **S22.079** **Unspecified fracture of T9-T10 vertebra** ▽

√6ᵗʰ **S22.08** **Fracture of** T11-T12 **vertebra**

¹ √7ᵗʰ **S22.080** Wedge compression fracture **of T11-T12**
vertebra

¹ √7ᵗʰ **S22.081** Stable burst **fracture of T11-T12 vertebra**

¹ √7ᵗʰ **S22.082** Unstable burst **fracture of T11-T12**
vertebra

¹ √7ᵗʰ **S22.088** **Other fracture of T11-T12 vertebra**

¹ √7ᵗʰ **S22.089** **Unspecified fracture of T11-T12** ▽
vertebra

√5ᵗʰ **S22.2** **Fracture of** sternum
DEF: Break in flat bone (breast bone) in anterior thorax; caused by
blunt trauma to anterior chest.

√x7ᵗʰ **S22.20** **Unspecified fracture of sternum** ▽

¹ √x7ᵗʰ **S22.21** **Fracture of** manubrium

¹ √x7ᵗʰ **S22.22** **Fracture of** body **of sternum**

¹ √x7ᵗʰ **S22.23** **Sternal** manubrial dissociation

¹ √x7ᵗʰ **S22.24** **Fracture of** xiphoid process

√5ᵗʰ **S22.3** **Fracture of** one rib

¹ √x7ᵗʰ **S22.31** **Fracture of one rib,** right **side**

¹ √x7ᵗʰ **S22.32** **Fracture of one rib,** left **side**

√x7ᵗʰ **S22.39** **Fracture of one rib, unspecified side** ▽

√5ᵗʰ **S22.4** Multiple fractures of ribs
Fractures of two or more ribs
EXCLUDES 1 flail chest (S22.5-)

¹ √x7ᵗʰ **S22.41** **Multiple fractures of ribs,** right **side**

¹ √x7ᵗʰ **S22.42** **Multiple fractures of ribs,** left **side**

¹ √x7ᵗʰ **S22.43** **Multiple fractures of ribs,** bilateral

√x7ᵗʰ **S22.49** **Multiple fractures of ribs, unspecified side** ▽

¹ √x7ᵗʰ **S22.5** **Flail chest**

¹ √x7ᵗʰ **S22.9** **Fracture of bony thorax, part unspecified** ▽

√4ᵗʰ **S23** **Dislocation and sprain of joints and ligaments of thorax**
INCLUDES avulsion of joint or ligament of thorax
laceration of cartilage, joint or ligament of thorax
sprain of cartilage, joint or ligament of thorax
traumatic hemarthrosis of joint or ligament of thorax
traumatic rupture of joint or ligament of thorax
traumatic subluxation of joint or ligament of thorax
traumatic tear of joint or ligament of thorax
Code also any associated open wound
EXCLUDES 2 dislocation, sprain of sternoclavicular joint (S43.2, S43.6)
strain of muscle or tendon of thorax (S29.01-)

The appropriate 7th character is to be added to each code from
category S23.
A   initial encounter
D   subsequent encounter
S   sequela

√x7ᵗʰ **S23.0** **Traumatic rupture of thoracic intervertebral disc**
EXCLUDES 1 rupture or displacement (nontraumatic) of thoracic
intervertebral disc NOS (M51- with fifth
character 4)

√5ᵗʰ **S23.1** **Subluxation and dislocation of thoracic vertebra**
Code also any associated
open wound of thorax (S21.-)
spinal cord injury (S24.0-, S24.1-)
EXCLUDES 2 fracture of thoracic vertebrae (S22.0-)

√6ᵗʰ **S23.10** **Subluxation and dislocation of** unspecified **thoracic**
vertebra

√7ᵗʰ **S23.100** Subluxation **of unspecified thoracic** ▽
vertebra

√7ᵗʰ **S23.101** Dislocation **of unspecified thoracic** ▽
vertebra

√6ᵗʰ **S23.11** **Subluxation and dislocation of** T1/T2 **thoracic**
vertebra

√7ᵗʰ **S23.110** Subluxation **of T1/T2 thoracic vertebra**

√7ᵗʰ **S23.111** Dislocation **of T1/T2 thoracic vertebra**

√6ᵗʰ **S23.12** **Subluxation and dislocation of** T2/T3-T3/T4 **thoracic**
vertebra

√7ᵗʰ **S23.120** Subluxation **of T2/T3 thoracic vertebra**

√7ᵗʰ **S23.121** Dislocation **of T2/T3 thoracic vertebra**

√7ᵗʰ **S23.122** Subluxation **of T3/T4 thoracic vertebra**

√7ᵗʰ **S23.123** Dislocation **of T3/T4 thoracic vertebra**

√6ᵗʰ **S23.13** **Subluxation and dislocation of** T4/T5-T5/T6 **thoracic**
vertebra

√7ᵗʰ **S23.130** Subluxation **of T4/T5 thoracic vertebra**

√7ᵗʰ **S23.131** Dislocation **of T4/T5 thoracic vertebra**

√7ᵗʰ **S23.132** Subluxation **of T5/T6 thoracic vertebra**

√7ᵗʰ **S23.133** Dislocation **of T5/T6 thoracic vertebra**

√6ᵗʰ **S23.14** **Subluxation and dislocation of** T6/T7-T7/T8 **thoracic**
vertebra

√7ᵗʰ **S23.140** Subluxation **of T6/T7 thoracic vertebra**

√7ᵗʰ **S23.141** Dislocation **of T6/T7 thoracic vertebra**

√7ᵗʰ **S23.142** Subluxation **of T7/T8 thoracic vertebra**

√7ᵗʰ **S23.143** Dislocation **of T7/T8 thoracic vertebra**

√6ᵗʰ **S23.15** **Subluxation and dislocation of** T8/T9-T9/T10
thoracic vertebra

√7ᵗʰ **S23.150** Subluxation **of T8/T9 thoracic vertebra**

√7ᵗʰ **S23.151** Dislocation **of T8/T9 thoracic vertebra**

√7ᵗʰ **S23.152** Subluxation **of T9/T10 thoracic vertebra**

√7ᵗʰ **S23.153** Dislocation **of T9/T10 thoracic vertebra**

√6ᵗʰ **S23.16** **Subluxation and dislocation of** T10/T11-T11/T12
thoracic vertebra

√7ᵗʰ **S23.160** Subluxation **of T10/T11 thoracic vertebra**

√7ᵗʰ **S23.161** Dislocation **of T10/T11 thoracic vertebra**

√7ᵗʰ **S23.162** Subluxation **of T11/T12 thoracic vertebra**

√7ᵗʰ **S23.163** Dislocation **of T11/T12 thoracic vertebra**

---

¹   Case-mix diagnosis with 7th character indicating subsequent encounter.

✔ Additional Character Req   √x7ᵗʰ Placeholder Alert   Case-Mix Diagnosis   Manifestation   ▽ Unspecified Dx   **EXCLUDES 1** Not coded here   **EXCLUDES 2** Not included here

✓6ᵗʰ **S23.17** **Subluxation and dislocation of T12/L1 thoracic vertebra**
- ✓7ᵗʰ **S23.170** **Subluxation of T12/L1 thoracic vertebra**
- ✓7ᵗʰ **S23.171** **Dislocation of T12/L1 thoracic vertebra**

✓5ᵗʰ **S23.2** **Dislocation of other and unspecified parts of thorax**
- ✓x7ᵗʰ **S23.20** **Dislocation of unspecified part of thorax** ▽
- ✓x7ᵗʰ **S23.29** **Dislocation of other parts of thorax**

4 ✓x7ᵗʰ **S23.3** **Sprain of ligaments of thoracic spine**

✓5ᵗʰ **S23.4** **Sprain of ribs and sternum**
- ✓x7ᵗʰ **S23.41** **Sprain of ribs**
- ✓6ᵗʰ **S23.42** **Sprain of sternum**
  - ✓7ᵗʰ **S23.420** **Sprain of sternoclavicular (joint) (ligament)**
  - ✓7ᵗʰ **S23.421** **Sprain of chondrosternal joint**
  - ✓7ᵗʰ **S23.428** **Other sprain of sternum**
  - ✓7ᵗʰ **S23.429** **Unspecified sprain of sternum** ▽

4 ✓x7ᵗʰ **S23.8** **Sprain of other specified parts of thorax**

4 ✓x7ᵗʰ **S23.9** **Sprain of unspecified parts of thorax** ▽

✓4ᵗʰ **S24** **Injury of nerves and spinal cord at thorax level**
> **NOTE** Code to highest level of thoracic spinal cord injury.
> Injuries to the spinal cord (S24.0 and S24.1) refer to the cord level and not bone level injury, and can affect nerve roots at and below the level given.
>
> Code also any associated:
> fracture of thoracic vertebra (S22.0-)
> open wound of thorax (S21.-)
> transient paralysis (R29.5)
> **EXCLUDES 2** *injury of brachial plexus (S14.3)*

> The appropriate 7th character is to be added to each code from category S24.
> A   initial encounter
> D   subsequent encounter
> S   sequela

✓x7ᵗʰ **S24.0** **Concussion and edema of thoracic spinal cord**

✓5ᵗʰ **S24.1** **Other and unspecified injuries of thoracic spinal cord**
- ✓6ᵗʰ **S24.10** **Unspecified injury of thoracic spinal cord**
  - 2 ✓7ᵗʰ **S24.101** **Unspecified injury at T1 level of thoracic spinal cord** ▽
  - 2 ✓7ᵗʰ **S24.102** **Unspecified injury at T2-T6 level of thoracic spinal cord** ▽
  - 2 ✓7ᵗʰ **S24.103** **Unspecified injury at T7-T10 level of thoracic spinal cord** ▽
  - 2 ✓7ᵗʰ **S24.104** **Unspecified injury at T11-T12 level of thoracic spinal cord** ▽
  - 2 ✓7ᵗʰ **S24.109** **Unspecified injury at unspecified level of thoracic spinal cord** ▽
    Injury of thoracic spinal cord NOS
- ✓6ᵗʰ **S24.11** **Complete lesion of thoracic spinal cord**
  - 2 ✓7ᵗʰ **S24.111** **Complete lesion at T1 level of thoracic spinal cord**
  - 2 ✓7ᵗʰ **S24.112** **Complete lesion at T2-T6 level of thoracic spinal cord**
  - 2 ✓7ᵗʰ **S24.113** **Complete lesion at T7-T10 level of thoracic spinal cord**
  - 2 ✓7ᵗʰ **S24.114** **Complete lesion at T11-T12 level of thoracic spinal cord**
  - 2 ✓7ᵗʰ **S24.119** **Complete lesion at unspecified level of thoracic spinal cord** ▽
- ✓6ᵗʰ **S24.13** **Anterior cord syndrome of thoracic spinal cord**
  - 2 ✓7ᵗʰ **S24.131** **Anterior cord syndrome at T1 level of thoracic spinal cord**
  - 2 ✓7ᵗʰ **S24.132** **Anterior cord syndrome at T2-T6 level of thoracic spinal cord**
  - 2 ✓7ᵗʰ **S24.133** **Anterior cord syndrome at T7-T10 level of thoracic spinal cord**
  - 2 ✓7ᵗʰ **S24.134** **Anterior cord syndrome at T11-T12 level of thoracic spinal cord**
  - 2 ✓7ᵗʰ **S24.139** **Anterior cord syndrome at unspecified level of thoracic spinal cord** ▽

✓6ᵗʰ **S24.14** **Brown-Séquard syndrome of thoracic spinal cord**
- 2 ✓7ᵗʰ **S24.141** **Brown-Séquard syndrome at T1 level of thoracic spinal cord**
- 2 ✓7ᵗʰ **S24.142** **Brown-Séquard syndrome at T2-T6 level of thoracic spinal cord**
- 2 ✓7ᵗʰ **S24.143** **Brown-Séquard syndrome at T7-T10 level of thoracic spinal cord**
- 2 ✓7ᵗʰ **S24.144** **Brown-Séquard syndrome at T11-T12 level of thoracic spinal cord**
- 2 ✓7ᵗʰ **S24.149** **Brown-Séquard syndrome at unspecified level of thoracic spinal cord** ▽

✓6ᵗʰ **S24.15** **Other incomplete lesions of thoracic spinal cord**
Incomplete lesion of thoracic spinal cord NOS
Posterior cord syndrome of thoracic spinal cord
- 2 ✓7ᵗʰ **S24.151** **Other incomplete lesion at T1 level of thoracic spinal cord**
- 2 ✓7ᵗʰ **S24.152** **Other incomplete lesion at T2-T6 level of thoracic spinal cord**
- 2 ✓7ᵗʰ **S24.153** **Other incomplete lesion at T7-T10 level of thoracic spinal cord**
- 2 ✓7ᵗʰ **S24.154** **Other incomplete lesion at T11-T12 level of thoracic spinal cord**
- 2 ✓7ᵗʰ **S24.159** **Other incomplete lesion at unspecified level of thoracic spinal cord** ▽

2 ✓x7ᵗʰ **S24.2** **Injury of nerve root of thoracic spine**

2 ✓x7ᵗʰ **S24.3** **Injury of peripheral nerves of thorax**

2 ✓x7ᵗʰ **S24.4** **Injury of thoracic sympathetic nervous system**
Injury of cardiac plexus
Injury of esophageal plexus
Injury of pulmonary plexus
Injury of stellate ganglion
Injury of thoracic sympathetic ganglion

2 ✓x7ᵗʰ **S24.8** **Injury of other specified nerves of thorax**

2 ✓x7ᵗʰ **S24.9** **Injury of unspecified nerve of thorax** ▽

✓4ᵗʰ **S25** **Injury of blood vessels of thorax**
Code also any associated open wound (S21.-)

> The appropriate 7th character is to be added to each code from category S25.
> A   initial encounter
> D   subsequent encounter
> S   sequela

✓5ᵗʰ **S25.0** **Injury of thoracic aorta**
Injury of aorta NOS
- ✓x7ᵗʰ **S25.00** **Unspecified injury of thoracic aorta** ▽
- ✓x7ᵗʰ **S25.01** **Minor laceration of thoracic aorta**
  Incomplete transection of thoracic aorta
  Laceration of thoracic aorta NOS
  Superficial laceration of thoracic aorta
- ✓x7ᵗʰ **S25.02** **Major laceration of thoracic aorta**
  Complete transection of thoracic aorta
  Traumatic rupture of thoracic aorta
- ✓x7ᵗʰ **S25.09** **Other specified injury of thoracic aorta**

✓5ᵗʰ **S25.1** **Injury of innominate or subclavian artery**
- ✓6ᵗʰ **S25.10** **Unspecified injury of innominate or subclavian artery**
  - ✓7ᵗʰ **S25.101** **Unspecified injury of right innominate or subclavian artery** ▽
  - ✓7ᵗʰ **S25.102** **Unspecified injury of left innominate or subclavian artery** ▽
  - ✓7ᵗʰ **S25.109** **Unspecified injury of unspecified innominate or subclavian artery** ▽
- ✓6ᵗʰ **S25.11** **Minor laceration of innominate or subclavian artery**
  Incomplete transection of innominate or subclavian artery
  Laceration of innominate or subclavian artery NOS
  Superficial laceration of innominate or subclavian artery
  - ✓7ᵗʰ **S25.111** **Minor laceration of right innominate or subclavian artery**
  - ✓7ᵗʰ **S25.112** **Minor laceration of left innominate or subclavian artery**

---

2 Case-mix diagnosis with 7th character indicating subsequent encounter or sequela.
4 Case-mix diagnosis with 7th character indicating initial or subsequent encounter.

Ⓝ Newborn: 0   Ⓟ Pediatric: 0-17   Ⓜ Maternity: 12-55   Ⓐ Adult: 15-124   **NRS** Nonroutine supply Dx   **NCDx** Noncancer Dx   **PDx** Primary Dx   ▶◀ Revised Text   ● New Code   ▲ Revised Title

√7ᵗʰ **S25.119** Minor laceration of unspecified innominate or subclavian artery ▽

√6ᵗʰ **S25.12** Major laceration of innominate or subclavian artery
Complete transection of innominate or subclavian artery
Traumatic rupture of innominate or subclavian artery

√7ᵗʰ **S25.121** Major laceration of right innominate or subclavian artery

√7ᵗʰ **S25.122** Major laceration of left innominate or subclavian artery

√7ᵗʰ **S25.129** Major laceration of unspecified innominate or subclavian artery ▽

√6ᵗʰ **S25.19** Other specified injury of innominate or subclavian artery

√7ᵗʰ **S25.191** Other specified injury of right innominate or subclavian artery

√7ᵗʰ **S25.192** Other specified injury of left innominate or subclavian artery

√7ᵗʰ **S25.199** Other specified injury of unspecified innominate or subclavian artery ▽

√5ᵗʰ **S25.2** Injury of superior vena cava
Injury of vena cava NOS

√x7ᵗʰ **S25.20** Unspecified injury of superior vena cava ▽

√x7ᵗʰ **S25.21** Minor laceration of superior vena cava
Incomplete transection of superior vena cava
Laceration of superior vena cava NOS
Superficial laceration of superior vena cava

√x7ᵗʰ **S25.22** Major laceration of superior vena cava
Complete transection of superior vena cava
Traumatic rupture of superior vena cava

√x7ᵗʰ **S25.29** Other specified injury of superior vena cava

√5ᵗʰ **S25.3** Injury of innominate or subclavian vein

√6ᵗʰ **S25.30** Unspecified injury of innominate or subclavian vein

√7ᵗʰ **S25.301** Unspecified injury of right innominate or subclavian vein ▽

√7ᵗʰ **S25.302** Unspecified injury of left innominate or subclavian vein ▽

√7ᵗʰ **S25.309** Unspecified injury of unspecified innominate or subclavian vein ▽

√6ᵗʰ **S25.31** Minor laceration of innominate or subclavian vein
Incomplete transection of innominate or subclavian vein
Laceration of innominate or subclavian vein NOS
Superficial laceration of innominate or subclavian vein

√7ᵗʰ **S25.311** Minor laceration of right innominate or subclavian vein

√7ᵗʰ **S25.312** Minor laceration of left innominate or subclavian vein

√7ᵗʰ **S25.319** Minor laceration of unspecified innominate or subclavian vein ▽

√6ᵗʰ **S25.32** Major laceration of innominate or subclavian vein
Complete transection of innominate or subclavian vein
Traumatic rupture of innominate or subclavian vein

√7ᵗʰ **S25.321** Major laceration of right innominate or subclavian vein

√7ᵗʰ **S25.322** Major laceration of left innominate or subclavian vein

√7ᵗʰ **S25.329** Major laceration of unspecified innominate or subclavian vein ▽

√6ᵗʰ **S25.39** Other specified injury of innominate or subclavian vein

√7ᵗʰ **S25.391** Other specified injury of right innominate or subclavian vein

√7ᵗʰ **S25.392** Other specified injury of left innominate or subclavian vein

√7ᵗʰ **S25.399** Other specified injury of unspecified innominate or subclavian vein ▽

√5ᵗʰ **S25.4** Injury of pulmonary blood vessels

√6ᵗʰ **S25.40** Unspecified injury of pulmonary blood vessels

√7ᵗʰ **S25.401** Unspecified injury of right pulmonary blood vessels ▽

√7ᵗʰ **S25.402** Unspecified injury of left pulmonary blood vessels ▽

√7ᵗʰ **S25.409** Unspecified injury of unspecified pulmonary blood vessels ▽

√6ᵗʰ **S25.41** Minor laceration of pulmonary blood vessels
Incomplete transection of pulmonary blood vessels
Laceration of pulmonary blood vessels NOS
Superficial laceration of pulmonary blood vessels

√7ᵗʰ **S25.411** Minor laceration of right pulmonary blood vessels

√7ᵗʰ **S25.412** Minor laceration of left pulmonary blood vessels

√7ᵗʰ **S25.419** Minor laceration of unspecified pulmonary blood vessels ▽

√6ᵗʰ **S25.42** Major laceration of pulmonary blood vessels
Complete transection of pulmonary blood vessels
Traumatic rupture of pulmonary blood vessels

√7ᵗʰ **S25.421** Major laceration of right pulmonary blood vessels

√7ᵗʰ **S25.422** Major laceration of left pulmonary blood vessels

√7ᵗʰ **S25.429** Major laceration of unspecified pulmonary blood vessels ▽

√6ᵗʰ **S25.49** Other specified injury of pulmonary blood vessels

√7ᵗʰ **S25.491** Other specified injury of right pulmonary blood vessels

√7ᵗʰ **S25.492** Other specified injury of left pulmonary blood vessels

√7ᵗʰ **S25.499** Other specified injury of unspecified pulmonary blood vessels ▽

√5ᵗʰ **S25.5** Injury of intercostal blood vessels

√6ᵗʰ **S25.50** Unspecified injury of intercostal blood vessels

√7ᵗʰ **S25.501** Unspecified injury of intercostal blood vessels, right side ▽

√7ᵗʰ **S25.502** Unspecified injury of intercostal blood vessels, left side ▽

√7ᵗʰ **S25.509** Unspecified injury of intercostal blood vessels, unspecified side ▽

√6ᵗʰ **S25.51** Laceration of intercostal blood vessels

√7ᵗʰ **S25.511** Laceration of intercostal blood vessels, right side

√7ᵗʰ **S25.512** Laceration of intercostal blood vessels, left side

√7ᵗʰ **S25.519** Laceration of intercostal blood vessels, unspecified side ▽

√6ᵗʰ **S25.59** Other specified injury of intercostal blood vessels

√7ᵗʰ **S25.591** Other specified injury of intercostal blood vessels, right side

√7ᵗʰ **S25.592** Other specified injury of intercostal blood vessels, left side

√7ᵗʰ **S25.599** Other specified injury of intercostal blood vessels, unspecified side ▽

√5ᵗʰ **S25.8** Injury of other blood vessels of thorax
Injury of azygos vein
Injury of mammary artery or vein

√6ᵗʰ **S25.80** Unspecified injury of other blood vessels of thorax

√7ᵗʰ **S25.801** Unspecified injury of other blood vessels of thorax, right side ▽

√7ᵗʰ **S25.802** Unspecified injury of other blood vessels of thorax, left side ▽

√7ᵗʰ **S25.809** Unspecified injury of other blood vessels of thorax, unspecified side ▽

√6ᵗʰ **S25.81** Laceration of other blood vessels of thorax

√7ᵗʰ **S25.811** Laceration of other blood vessels of thorax, right side

√7ᵗʰ **S25.812** Laceration of other blood vessels of thorax, left side

√7ᵗʰ **S25.819** Laceration of other blood vessels of thorax, unspecified side ▽

√6ᵗʰ **S25.89** Other specified injury of other blood vessels of thorax

√7ᵗʰ **S25.891** Other specified injury of other blood vessels of thorax, right side

√7ᵗʰ **S25.892** Other specified injury of other blood vessels of thorax, left side

√7ᵗʰ **S25.899** Other specified injury of other blood vessels of thorax, unspecified side ▽

☑ Additional Character Req   √x7ᵗʰ Placeholder Alert   Case-Mix Diagnosis   Manifestation   ▽ Unspecified Dx   *EXCLUDES 1* Not coded here   *EXCLUDES 2* Not included here

ICD-10-CM 2018   937

√5ᵗʰ **S25.9   Injury of** unspecified blood vessel **of thorax**

　√ₓ7ᵗʰ **S25.90   Unspecified injury of unspecified blood vessel of thorax**   ▽

　√ₓ7ᵗʰ **S25.91   Laceration of unspecified blood vessel of thorax**   ▽

　√ₓ7ᵗʰ **S25.99   Other specified injury of unspecified blood vessel of thorax**   ▽

√4ᵗʰ **S26   Injury of heart**
Code also any associated:
　open wound of thorax (S21.-)
　traumatic hemopneumothorax (S27.2)
　traumatic hemothorax (S27.1)
　traumatic pneumothorax (S27.0)

The appropriate 7th character is to be added to each code from category S26.
A   initial encounter
D   subsequent encounter
S   sequela

√5ᵗʰ **S26.0   Injury of heart** with hemopericardium
TIP: Do not assign for hemopericardium that is not due to trauma or that has occurred as a result of an intra- or postoperative complication.

　√ₓ7ᵗʰ **S26.00   Unspecified injury of heart with hemopericardium** ▽

　√ₓ7ᵗʰ **S26.01   Contusion of heart with hemopericardium**

　√6ᵗʰ **S26.02   Laceration of heart with hemopericardium**

　　√7ᵗʰ **S26.020   Mild laceration of heart with hemopericardium**
Laceration of heart without penetration of heart chamber

　　√7ᵗʰ **S26.021   Moderate laceration of heart with hemopericardium**
Laceration of heart with penetration of heart chamber

　　√7ᵗʰ **S26.022   Major laceration of heart with hemopericardium**
Laceration of heart with penetration of multiple heart chambers

　√ₓ7ᵗʰ **S26.09   Other injury of heart with hemopericardium**

√5ᵗʰ **S26.1   Injury of heart** without hemopericardium

　√ₓ7ᵗʰ **S26.10   Unspecified injury of heart without hemopericardium**   ▽

　√ₓ7ᵗʰ **S26.11   Contusion of heart without hemopericardium**

　√ₓ7ᵗʰ **S26.12   Laceration of heart without hemopericardium**

　√ₓ7ᵗʰ **S26.19   Other injury of heart without hemopericardium**

√5ᵗʰ **S26.9   Injury of heart,** unspecified with or without hemopericardium

　√ₓ7ᵗʰ **S26.90   Unspecified injury of heart, unspecified with or without hemopericardium**   ▽

　√ₓ7ᵗʰ **S26.91   Contusion of heart, unspecified with or without hemopericardium**   ▽
DEF: Bruising within the heart muscle with no mention of open wound; usually caused by blunt chest trauma in motor vehicle accidents, falling from great heights, or receiving CPR.

　√ₓ7ᵗʰ **S26.92   Laceration of heart, unspecified with or without hemopericardium**   ▽
Laceration of heart NOS

　√ₓ7ᵗʰ **S26.99   Other injury of heart, unspecified with or without hemopericardium**   ▽

√4ᵗʰ **S27   Injury of other and unspecified intrathoracic organs**
Code also any associated open wound of thorax (S21.-)
EXCLUDES 2   injury of cervical esophagus (S10-S19)
　injury of trachea (cervical) (S10-S19)

The appropriate 7th character is to be added to each code from category S27.
A   initial encounter
D   subsequent encounter
S   sequela

√ₓ7ᵗʰ **S27.0   Traumatic pneumothorax**
EXCLUDES 1   spontaneous pneumothorax (J93.-)

√ₓ7ᵗʰ **S27.1   Traumatic hemothorax**

√ₓ7ᵗʰ **S27.2   Traumatic hemopneumothorax**

√5ᵗʰ **S27.3   Other and unspecified injuries of** lung

　√6ᵗʰ **S27.30   Unspecified injury of lung**

　　√7ᵗʰ **S27.301   Unspecified injury of lung,** unilateral   ▽

　　√7ᵗʰ **S27.302   Unspecified injury of lung,** bilateral   ▽

　　√7ᵗʰ **S27.309   Unspecified injury of lung, unspecified**   ▽

　√6ᵗʰ **S27.31   Primary blast injury of lung**
Blast injury of lung NOS

　　√7ᵗʰ **S27.311   Primary blast injury of lung,** unilateral

　　√7ᵗʰ **S27.312   Primary blast injury of lung,** bilateral

　　√7ᵗʰ **S27.319   Primary blast injury of lung, unspecified**   ▽

　√6ᵗʰ **S27.32   Contusion of lung**
DEF: Bruising of lung without mention of open wound.

　　√7ᵗʰ **S27.321   Contusion of lung,** unilateral

　　√7ᵗʰ **S27.322   Contusion of lung,** bilateral

　　√7ᵗʰ **S27.329   Contusion of lung, unspecified**   ▽

　√6ᵗʰ **S27.33   Laceration of lung**

　　√7ᵗʰ **S27.331   Laceration of lung,** unilateral

　　√7ᵗʰ **S27.332   Laceration of lung,** bilateral

　　√7ᵗʰ **S27.339   Laceration of lung, unspecified**   ▽

　√6ᵗʰ **S27.39   Other injuries of lung**
Secondary blast injury of lung

　　√7ᵗʰ **S27.391   Other injuries of lung,** unilateral

　　√7ᵗʰ **S27.392   Other injuries of lung,** bilateral

　　√7ᵗʰ **S27.399   Other injuries of lung, unspecified**   ▽

√5ᵗʰ **S27.4   Injury of** bronchus

　√6ᵗʰ **S27.40   Unspecified injury of bronchus**

　　√7ᵗʰ **S27.401   Unspecified injury of bronchus, unilateral**   ▽

　　√7ᵗʰ **S27.402   Unspecified injury of bronchus, bilateral**   ▽

　　√7ᵗʰ **S27.409   Unspecified injury of bronchus, unspecified**   ▽

　√6ᵗʰ **S27.41   Primary blast injury of bronchus**
Blast injury of bronchus NOS

　　√7ᵗʰ **S27.411   Primary blast injury of bronchus, unilateral**

　　√7ᵗʰ **S27.412   Primary blast injury of bronchus,** bilateral

　　√7ᵗʰ **S27.419   Primary blast injury of bronchus, unspecified**   ▽

　√6ᵗʰ **S27.42   Contusion of bronchus**

　　√7ᵗʰ **S27.421   Contusion of bronchus,** unilateral

　　√7ᵗʰ **S27.422   Contusion of bronchus,** bilateral

　　√7ᵗʰ **S27.429   Contusion of bronchus, unspecified**   ▽

　√6ᵗʰ **S27.43   Laceration of bronchus**

　　√7ᵗʰ **S27.431   Laceration of bronchus,** unilateral

　　√7ᵗʰ **S27.432   Laceration of bronchus,** bilateral

　　√7ᵗʰ **S27.439   Laceration of bronchus, unspecified**   ▽

　√6ᵗʰ **S27.49   Other injury of bronchus**
Secondary blast injury of bronchus

　　√7ᵗʰ **S27.491   Other injury of bronchus,** unilateral

　　√7ᵗʰ **S27.492   Other injury of bronchus,** bilateral

　　√7ᵗʰ **S27.499   Other injury of bronchus, unspecified**   ▽

√5ᵗʰ **S27.5   Injury of** thoracic trachea

　√ₓ7ᵗʰ **S27.50   Unspecified injury of thoracic trachea**   ▽

　√ₓ7ᵗʰ **S27.51   Primary blast injury of thoracic trachea**
Blast injury of thoracic trachea NOS

　√ₓ7ᵗʰ **S27.52   Contusion of thoracic trachea**

　√ₓ7ᵗʰ **S27.53   Laceration of thoracic trachea**

　√ₓ7ᵗʰ **S27.59   Other injury of thoracic trachea**
Secondary blast injury of thoracic trachea

√5ᵗʰ **S27.6   Injury of** pleura

　√ₓ7ᵗʰ **S27.60   Unspecified injury of pleura**   ▽

　√ₓ7ᵗʰ **S27.63   Laceration of pleura**

　√ₓ7ᵗʰ **S27.69   Other injury of pleura**

√5ᵗʰ **S27.8   Injury of** other specified intrathoracic organs

　√6ᵗʰ **S27.80   Injury of diaphragm**

　　√7ᵗʰ **S27.802   Contusion of diaphragm**

　　√7ᵗʰ **S27.803   Laceration of diaphragm**

　　√7ᵗʰ **S27.808   Other injury of diaphragm**

　　√7ᵗʰ **S27.809   Unspecified injury of diaphragm**   ▽

√6ᵗʰ **S27.81** Injury of esophagus (thoracic part)

　√7ᵗʰ **S27.812** Contusion of esophagus (thoracic part)

　√7ᵗʰ **S27.813** Laceration of esophagus (thoracic part)

　√7ᵗʰ **S27.818** Other injury of esophagus (thoracic part)

　√7ᵗʰ **S27.819** Unspecified injury of esophagus ▽
(thoracic part)

√6ᵗʰ **S27.89** Injury of other specified intrathoracic organs
Injury of lymphatic thoracic duct
Injury of thymus gland

　√7ᵗʰ **S27.892** Contusion of other specified intrathoracic organs

　√7ᵗʰ **S27.893** Laceration of other specified intrathoracic organs

　√7ᵗʰ **S27.898** Other injury of other specified intrathoracic organs

　√7ᵗʰ **S27.899** Unspecified injury of other specified ▽
intrathoracic organs

√x7ᵗʰ **S27.9** Injury of unspecified intrathoracic organ ▽

√4ᵗʰ **S28** **Crushing injury of thorax, and traumatic amputation of part of thorax**

> The appropriate 7th character is to be added to each code from category S28.
> A　initial encounter
> D　subsequent encounter
> S　sequela

√x7ᵗʰ **S28.0** **Crushed chest**
Use additional code for all associated injuries
EXCLUDES 1 flail chest (S22.5)

1,5 √x7ᵗʰ **S28.1** **Traumatic amputation (partial) of part of thorax, except** NRS
breast

√5ᵗʰ **S28.2** **Traumatic amputation of breast**

√6ᵗʰ **S28.21** Complete traumatic amputation of breast
Traumatic amputation of breast NOS

1,5 √7ᵗʰ **S28.211** **Complete traumatic amputation of** NRS
right breast

1,5 √7ᵗʰ **S28.212** **Complete traumatic amputation of** NRS
left breast

　√7ᵗʰ **S28.219** **Complete traumatic amputation of** ▽
unspecified breast

√6ᵗʰ **S28.22** Partial traumatic amputation of breast

1,5 √7ᵗʰ **S28.221** **Partial traumatic amputation of** right NRS
breast

1,5 √7ᵗʰ **S28.222** **Partial traumatic amputation of** left NRS
breast

　√7ᵗʰ **S28.229** **Partial traumatic amputation of** ▽
unspecified breast

√4ᵗʰ **S29** **Other and unspecified injuries of thorax**
Code also any associated open wound (S21.-)

> The appropriate 7th character is to be added to each code from category S29.
> A　initial encounter
> D　subsequent encounter
> S　sequela

√5ᵗʰ **S29.0** **Injury of muscle and tendon at thorax level**

√6ᵗʰ **S29.00** Unspecified injury of muscle and tendon of thorax

　√7ᵗʰ **S29.001** **Unspecified injury of muscle and** ▽
tendon of front wall of thorax

　√7ᵗʰ **S29.002** **Unspecified injury of muscle and** ▽
tendon of back wall of thorax

　√7ᵗʰ **S29.009** **Unspecified injury of muscle and** ▽
tendon of unspecified wall of thorax

√6ᵗʰ **S29.01** Strain of muscle and tendon of thorax

　√7ᵗʰ **S29.011** **Strain of muscle and tendon of** front **wall**
of thorax

　√7ᵗʰ **S29.012** **Strain of muscle and tendon of** back **wall**
of thorax

　√7ᵗʰ **S29.019** **Strain of muscle and tendon of** ▽
unspecified wall of thorax

√6ᵗʰ **S29.02** Laceration of muscle and tendon of thorax

4,5 √7ᵗʰ **S29.021** **Laceration of muscle and tendon of** NRS
front **wall of thorax**

4,5 √7ᵗʰ **S29.022** **Laceration of muscle and tendon of** NRS
back **wall of thorax**

4 √7ᵗʰ **S29.029** **Laceration of muscle and tendon of** ▽
unspecified wall of thorax

√6ᵗʰ **S29.09** Other injury of muscle and tendon of thorax

　√7ᵗʰ **S29.091** **Other injury of muscle and tendon of** front
wall of thorax

　√7ᵗʰ **S29.092** **Other injury of muscle and tendon of** back
wall of thorax

　√7ᵗʰ **S29.099** **Other injury of muscle and tendon of** ▽
unspecified wall of thorax

√x7ᵗʰ **S29.8** **Other specified injuries of thorax**

√x7ᵗʰ **S29.9** **Unspecified injury of thorax** ▽

Injuries to the abdomen, lower back, lumbar spine, pelvis and external genitals (S30-S39)

INCLUDES injuries to the abdominal wall
injuries to the anus
injuries to the buttock
injuries to the external genitalia
injuries to the flank
injuries to the groin

EXCLUDES 2 burns and corrosions (T20-T32)
effects of foreign body in anus and rectum (T18.5)
effects of foreign body in genitourinary tract (T19.-)
effects of foreign body in stomach, small intestine and colon(T18.2-T18.4)
frostbite (T33-T34)
insect bite or sting, venomous (T63.4)

√4ᵗʰ **S30** **Superficial injury of abdomen, lower back, pelvis and external genitals**
EXCLUDES 2 superficial injury of hip (S70.-)

> The appropriate 7th character is to be added to each code from category S30.
> A　initial encounter
> D　subsequent encounter
> S　sequela

√x7ᵗʰ **S30.0** **Contusion of lower back and pelvis**
Contusion of buttock

√x7ᵗʰ **S30.1** **Contusion of abdominal wall**
Contusion of flank
Contusion of groin

√5ᵗʰ **S30.2** **Contusion of** external genital organs

√6ᵗʰ **S30.20** Contusion of unspecified external genital organ

　√7ᵗʰ **S30.201** **Contusion of unspecified external** ♂▽
genital organ, male

　√7ᵗʰ **S30.202** **Contusion of unspecified external** ♀▽
genital organ, female

√x7ᵗʰ **S30.21** **Contusion of** penis ♂

√x7ᵗʰ **S30.22** **Contusion of** scrotum and testes ♂

√x7ᵗʰ **S30.23** **Contusion of** vagina and vulva ♀

√x7ᵗʰ **S30.3** **Contusion of** anus

√5ᵗʰ **S30.8** **Other superficial injuries of abdomen, lower back, pelvis and external genitals**

√6ᵗʰ **S30.81** Abrasion of abdomen, lower back, pelvis and external genitals

　√7ᵗʰ **S30.810** **Abrasion of** lower back and pelvis

　√7ᵗʰ **S30.811** **Abrasion of** abdominal wall

　√7ᵗʰ **S30.812** **Abrasion of** penis ♂

　√7ᵗʰ **S30.813** **Abrasion of** scrotum and testes ♂

　√7ᵗʰ **S30.814** **Abrasion of** vagina and vulva ♀

　√7ᵗʰ **S30.815** **Abrasion of unspecified** external ♂▽
genital organs, male

　√7ᵗʰ **S30.816** **Abrasion of unspecified** external ♀▽
genital organs, female

　√7ᵗʰ **S30.817** **Abrasion of** anus

---

¹ Case-mix diagnosis with 7th character indicating subsequent encounter.
⁴ Case-mix diagnosis with 7th character indicating initial or subsequent encounter.
⁵ NRS supply diagnosis with 7th character indicating initial or subsequent encounter.

✓ Additional Character Req　　√x7ᵗʰ Placeholder Alert　　Case-Mix Diagnosis　　Manifestation　　▽ Unspecified Dx　　**EXCLUDES 1** Not coded here　　**EXCLUDES 2** Not included here

✓6th **S30.82** Blister (nonthermal) of abdomen, lower back, pelvis and external genitals

  ✓7th **S30.820** Blister (nonthermal) of lower back and pelvis

  ✓7th **S30.821** Blister (nonthermal) of abdominal wall

  ✓7th **S30.822** Blister (nonthermal) of penis ♂

  ✓7th **S30.823** Blister (nonthermal) of scrotum and testes ♂

  ✓7th **S30.824** Blister (nonthermal) of vagina and vulva ♀

  ✓7th **S30.825** Blister (nonthermal) of unspecified external genital organs, male ♂▽

  ✓7th **S30.826** Blister (nonthermal) of unspecified external genital organs, female ♀▽

  ✓7th **S30.827** Blister (nonthermal) of anus

✓6th **S30.84** External constriction of abdomen, lower back, pelvis and external genitals

  ✓7th **S30.840** External constriction of lower back and pelvis

  ✓7th **S30.841** External constriction of abdominal wall

  ✓7th **S30.842** External constriction of penis ♂
    Hair tourniquet syndrome of penis
    Use additional cause code to identify the constricting item (W49.0-)

  ✓7th **S30.843** External constriction of scrotum and testes ♂

  ✓7th **S30.844** External constriction of vagina and vulva ♀

  ✓7th **S30.845** External constriction of unspecified external genital organs, male ♂▽

  ✓7th **S30.846** External constriction of unspecified external genital organs, female ♀▽

✓6th **S30.85** Superficial foreign body of abdomen, lower back, pelvis and external genitals
    Splinter in the abdomen, lower back, pelvis and external genitals

  ✓7th **S30.850** Superficial foreign body of lower back and pelvis

  ✓7th **S30.851** Superficial foreign body of abdominal wall

  ✓7th **S30.852** Superficial foreign body of penis ♂

  ✓7th **S30.853** Superficial foreign body of scrotum and testes ♂

  ✓7th **S30.854** Superficial foreign body of vagina and vulva ♀

  ✓7th **S30.855** Superficial foreign body of unspecified external genital organs, male ♂▽

  ✓7th **S30.856** Superficial foreign body of unspecified external genital organs, female ♀▽

  ✓7th **S30.857** Superficial foreign body of anus

✓6th **S30.86** Insect bite (nonvenomous) of abdomen, lower back, pelvis and external genitals

  ✓7th **S30.860** Insect bite (nonvenomous) of lower back and pelvis

  ✓7th **S30.861** Insect bite (nonvenomous) of abdominal wall

  ✓7th **S30.862** Insect bite (nonvenomous) of penis ♂

  ✓7th **S30.863** Insect bite (nonvenomous) of scrotum and testes ♂

  ✓7th **S30.864** Insect bite (nonvenomous) of vagina and vulva ♀

  ✓7th **S30.865** Insect bite (nonvenomous) of unspecified external genital organs, male ♂▽

  ✓7th **S30.866** Insect bite (nonvenomous) of unspecified external genital organs, female ♀▽

  ✓7th **S30.867** Insect bite (nonvenomous) of anus

✓6th **S30.87** Other superficial bite of abdomen, lower back, pelvis and external genitals
  EXCLUDES 1 open bite of abdomen, lower back, pelvis and external genitals (S31.05, S31.15, S31.25, S31.35, S31.45, S31.55)

  ✓7th **S30.870** Other superficial bite of lower back and pelvis

  ✓7th **S30.871** Other superficial bite of abdominal wall

  ✓7th **S30.872** Other superficial bite of penis ♂

  ✓7th **S30.873** Other superficial bite of scrotum and testes ♂

  ✓7th **S30.874** Other superficial bite of vagina and vulva ♀

  ✓7th **S30.875** Other superficial bite of unspecified external genital organs, male ♂▽

  ✓7th **S30.876** Other superficial bite of unspecified external genital organs, female ♀▽

  ✓7th **S30.877** Other superficial bite of anus

✓5th **S30.9** Unspecified superficial injury of abdomen, lower back, pelvis and external genitals

  ✓x7th **S30.91** Unspecified superficial injury of lower back and pelvis ▽

  ✓x7th **S30.92** Unspecified superficial injury of abdominal wall ▽

  ✓x7th **S30.93** Unspecified superficial injury of penis ♂▽

  ✓x7th **S30.94** Unspecified superficial injury of scrotum and testes ♂▽

  ✓x7th **S30.95** Unspecified superficial injury of vagina and vulva ♀▽

  ✓x7th **S30.96** Unspecified superficial injury of unspecified external genital organs, male ♂▽

  ✓x7th **S30.97** Unspecified superficial injury of unspecified external genital organs, female ♀▽

  ✓x7th **S30.98** Unspecified superficial injury of anus ▽

✓4th **S31** Open wound of abdomen, lower back, pelvis and external genitals
  Code also any associated:
    spinal cord injury (S24.0, S24.1-, S34.0-, S34.1-)
    wound infection
  EXCLUDES 1 traumatic amputation of part of abdomen, lower back and pelvis (S38.2-, S38.3)
  EXCLUDES 2 open wound of hip (S71.00-S71.02)
    open fracture of pelvis (S32.1- -S32.9 with 7th character B)

> The appropriate 7th character is to be added to each code from category S31.
> A   initial encounter
> D   subsequent encounter
> S   sequela

✓5th **S31.0** Open wound of lower back and pelvis

  ✓6th **S31.00** Unspecified open wound of lower back and pelvis

    5 ✓7th **S31.000** Unspecified open wound of lower back and pelvis without penetration into retroperitoneum NRS ▽
      Unspecified open wound of lower back and pelvis NOS

    ✓7th **S31.001** Unspecified open wound of lower back and pelvis with penetration into retroperitoneum ▽

  ✓6th **S31.01** Laceration without foreign body of lower back and pelvis

    4,5 ✓7th **S31.010** Laceration without foreign body of lower back and pelvis without penetration into retroperitoneum NRS
      Laceration without foreign body of lower back and pelvis NOS

    ✓7th **S31.011** Laceration without foreign body of lower back and pelvis with penetration into retroperitoneum

---

4 Case-mix diagnosis with 7th character indicating initial or subsequent encounter.
5 NRS supply diagnosis with 7th character indicating initial or subsequent encounter.

✓6th **S31.02** Laceration with foreign body of lower back and pelvis

     4,5 ✓7th **S31.020** **Laceration with foreign body of lower back and pelvis** without penetration into retroperitoneum   **NRS**
         Laceration with foreign body of lower back and pelvis NOS

     ✓7th **S31.021** **Laceration with foreign body of lower back and pelvis** with penetration into retroperitoneum

✓6th **S31.03** Puncture wound without foreign body of lower back and pelvis

     4,5 ✓7th **S31.030** **Puncture wound without foreign body of lower back and pelvis** without penetration into retroperitoneum   **NRS**
         Puncture wound without foreign body of lower back and pelvis NOS

     ✓7th **S31.031** **Puncture wound without foreign body of lower back and pelvis** with penetration into retroperitoneum

✓6th **S31.04** Puncture wound with foreign body of lower back and pelvis

     4,5 ✓7th **S31.040** **Puncture wound with foreign body of lower back and pelvis** without penetration into retroperitoneum   **NRS**
         Puncture wound with foreign body of lower back and pelvis NOS

     ✓7th **S31.041** **Puncture wound with foreign body of lower back and pelvis** with penetration into retroperitoneum

✓6th **S31.05** Open bite of lower back and pelvis
     Bite of lower back and pelvis NOS
     EXCLUDES 1 *superficial bite of lower back and pelvis (S30.860, S30.870)*

     4,5 ✓7th **S31.050** **Open bite of lower back and pelvis** without penetration into retroperitoneum   **NRS**
         Open bite of lower back and pelvis NOS

     ✓7th **S31.051** **Open bite of lower back and pelvis** with penetration into retroperitoneum

✓5th **S31.1** Open wound of abdominal wall without penetration into peritoneal cavity
     Open wound of abdominal wall NOS
     EXCLUDES 2 *open wound of abdominal wall with penetration into peritoneal cavity (S31.6-)*

✓6th **S31.10** Unspecified open wound of abdominal wall without penetration into peritoneal cavity

     5 ✓7th **S31.100** **Unspecified open wound of abdominal wall,** right upper quadrant without penetration into peritoneal cavity   **NRS** ▽

     5 ✓7th **S31.101** **Unspecified open wound of abdominal wall,** left upper quadrant without penetration into peritoneal cavity   **NRS** ▽

     5 ✓7th **S31.102** **Unspecified open wound of abdominal wall,** epigastric region without penetration into peritoneal cavity   **NRS** ▽

     5 ✓7th **S31.103** **Unspecified open wound of abdominal wall,** right lower quadrant without penetration into peritoneal cavity   **NRS** ▽

     5 ✓7th **S31.104** **Unspecified open wound of abdominal wall,** left lower quadrant without penetration into peritoneal cavity   **NRS** ▽

     5 ✓7th **S31.105** **Unspecified open wound of abdominal wall,** periumbilic region without penetration into peritoneal cavity   **NRS** ▽

     ✓7th **S31.109** **Unspecified open wound of abdominal wall, unspecified quadrant without penetration into peritoneal cavity** ▽
         Unspecified open wound of abdominal wall NOS

✓6th **S31.11** Laceration without foreign body of abdominal wall without penetration into peritoneal cavity

     4,5 ✓7th **S31.110** **Laceration without foreign body of abdominal wall,** right upper quadrant without penetration into peritoneal cavity   **NRS**

     4,5 ✓7th **S31.111** **Laceration without foreign body of abdominal wall,** left upper quadrant without penetration into peritoneal cavity   **NRS**

     4,5 ✓7th **S31.112** **Laceration without foreign body of abdominal wall,** epigastric region without penetration into peritoneal cavity   **NRS**

     4,5 ✓7th **S31.113** **Laceration without foreign body of abdominal wall,** right lower quadrant without penetration into peritoneal cavity   **NRS**

     4,5 ✓7th **S31.114** **Laceration without foreign body of abdominal wall,** left lower quadrant without penetration into peritoneal cavity   **NRS**

     4,5 ✓7th **S31.115** **Laceration without foreign body of abdominal wall,** periumbilic region without penetration into peritoneal cavity   **NRS**

     ✓7th **S31.119** **Laceration without foreign body of abdominal wall, unspecified quadrant without penetration into peritoneal cavity** ▽

✓6th **S31.12** Laceration with foreign body of abdominal wall without penetration into peritoneal cavity

     4,5 ✓7th **S31.120** **Laceration of abdominal wall with foreign body,** right upper quadrant without penetration into peritoneal cavity   **NRS**

     4,5 ✓7th **S31.121** **Laceration of abdominal wall with foreign body,** left upper quadrant without penetration into peritoneal cavity   **NRS**

     4,5 ✓7th **S31.122** **Laceration of abdominal wall with foreign body,** epigastric region without penetration into peritoneal cavity   **NRS**

     4,5 ✓7th **S31.123** **Laceration of abdominal wall with foreign body,** right lower quadrant without penetration into peritoneal cavity   **NRS**

     4,5 ✓7th **S31.124** **Laceration of abdominal wall with foreign body,** left lower quadrant without penetration into peritoneal cavity   **NRS**

     4,5 ✓7th **S31.125** **Laceration of abdominal wall with foreign body,** periumbilic region without penetration into peritoneal cavity   **NRS**

     ✓7th **S31.129** **Laceration of abdominal wall with foreign body, unspecified quadrant without penetration into peritoneal cavity** ▽

✓6th **S31.13** Puncture wound of abdominal wall without foreign body without penetration into peritoneal cavity

     4,5 ✓7th **S31.130** **Puncture wound of abdominal wall without foreign body,** right upper quadrant without penetration into peritoneal cavity   **NRS**

     4,5 ✓7th **S31.131** **Puncture wound of abdominal wall without foreign body,** left upper quadrant without penetration into peritoneal cavity   **NRS**

     4,5 ✓7th **S31.132** **Puncture wound of abdominal wall without foreign body,** epigastric region without penetration into peritoneal cavity   **NRS**

     4,5 ✓7th **S31.133** **Puncture wound of abdominal wall without foreign body,** right lower quadrant without penetration into peritoneal cavity   **NRS**

     4,5 ✓7th **S31.134** **Puncture wound of abdominal wall without foreign body,** left lower quadrant without penetration into peritoneal cavity   **NRS**

     4,5 ✓7th **S31.135** **Puncture wound of abdominal wall without foreign body,** periumbilic region without penetration into peritoneal cavity   **NRS**

     ✓7th **S31.139** **Puncture wound of abdominal wall without foreign body, unspecified quadrant without penetration into peritoneal cavity** ▽

✓6th **S31.14** Puncture wound of abdominal wall with foreign body without penetration into peritoneal cavity

     4,5 ✓7th **S31.140** **Puncture wound of abdominal wall with foreign body,** right upper quadrant without penetration into peritoneal cavity   **NRS**

     4,5 ✓7th **S31.141** **Puncture wound of abdominal wall with foreign body,** left upper quadrant without penetration into peritoneal cavity   **NRS**

---

4   Case-mix diagnosis with 7th character indicating initial or subsequent encounter.
5   NRS supply diagnosis with 7th character indicating initial or subsequent encounter

---

✓ Additional Character Req   ✓x7th Placeholder Alert   Case-Mix Diagnosis   Manifestation   ▽ Unspecified Dx   **EXCLUDES 1** Not coded here   **EXCLUDES 2** Not included here

Chapter 19. Injury, Poisoning and Certain Other Consequences of External Causes

4,5 √7ᵗʰ **S31.142** Puncture wound of abdominal wall with foreign body, epigastric region without penetration into peritoneal cavity   NRS

4,5 √7ᵗʰ **S31.143** Puncture wound of abdominal wall with foreign body, right lower quadrant without penetration into peritoneal cavity   NRS

4,5 √7ᵗʰ **S31.144** Puncture wound of abdominal wall with foreign body, left lower quadrant without penetration into peritoneal cavity   NRS

4,5 √7ᵗʰ **S31.145** Puncture wound of abdominal wall with foreign body, periumbilic region without penetration into peritoneal cavity   NRS

√7ᵗʰ **S31.149** Puncture wound of abdominal wall with foreign body, unspecified quadrant without penetration into peritoneal cavity   ▽

√6ᵗʰ **S31.15** Open bite of abdominal wall without penetration into peritoneal cavity
    Bite of abdominal wall NOS
    EXCLUDES 1   superficial bite of abdominal wall (S30.871)

4,5 √7ᵗʰ **S31.150** Open bite of abdominal wall, right upper quadrant without penetration into peritoneal cavity   NRS

4,5 √7ᵗʰ **S31.151** Open bite of abdominal wall, left upper quadrant without penetration into peritoneal cavity   NRS

4,5 √7ᵗʰ **S31.152** Open bite of abdominal wall, epigastric region without penetration into peritoneal cavity   NRS

4,5 √7ᵗʰ **S31.153** Open bite of abdominal wall, right lower quadrant without penetration into peritoneal cavity   NRS

4,5 √7ᵗʰ **S31.154** Open bite of abdominal wall, left lower quadrant without penetration into peritoneal cavity   NRS

4,5 √7ᵗʰ **S31.155** Open bite of abdominal wall, periumbilic region without penetration into peritoneal cavity   NRS

√7ᵗʰ **S31.159** Open bite of abdominal wall, unspecified quadrant without penetration into peritoneal cavity   ▽

√5ᵗʰ **S31.2** Open wound of penis

5 √x7ᵗʰ **S31.20** Unspecified open wound of penis   NRS ♂ ▽

4,5 √x7ᵗʰ **S31.21** Laceration without foreign body of penis   NRS ♂

4,5 √x7ᵗʰ **S31.22** Laceration with foreign body of penis   NRS ♂

4,5 √x7ᵗʰ **S31.23** Puncture wound without foreign body of penis   NRS ♂

4,5 √x7ᵗʰ **S31.24** Puncture wound with foreign body of penis   NRS ♂

4,5 √x7ᵗʰ **S31.25** Open bite of penis   NRS ♂
    Bite of penis NOS
    EXCLUDES 1   superficial bite of penis (S30.862, S30.872)

√5ᵗʰ **S31.3** Open wound of scrotum and testes

5 √x7ᵗʰ **S31.30** Unspecified open wound of scrotum and testes   NRS ♂ ▽

4,5 √x7ᵗʰ **S31.31** Laceration without foreign body of scrotum and testes   NRS ♂

4,5 √x7ᵗʰ **S31.32** Laceration with foreign body of scrotum and testes   NRS ♂

4,5 √x7ᵗʰ **S31.33** Puncture wound without foreign body of scrotum and testes   NRS ♂

4,5 √x7ᵗʰ **S31.34** Puncture wound with foreign body of scrotum and testes   NRS ♂

4,5 √x7ᵗʰ **S31.35** Open bite of scrotum and testes   NRS ♂
    Bite of scrotum and testes NOS
    EXCLUDES 1   superficial bite of scrotum and testes (S30.863, S30.873)

√5ᵗʰ **S31.4** Open wound of vagina and vulva
    EXCLUDES 1   injury to vagina and vulva during delivery (O70-, O71.4)

5 √x7ᵗʰ **S31.40** Unspecified open wound of vagina and vulva   NRS ♀ ▽

4,5 √x7ᵗʰ **S31.41** Laceration without foreign body of vagina and vulva   NRS ♀

4,5 √x7ᵗʰ **S31.42** Laceration with foreign body of vagina and vulva   NRS ♀

4,5 √x7ᵗʰ **S31.43** Puncture wound without foreign body of vagina and vulva   NRS ♀

4,5 √x7ᵗʰ **S31.44** Puncture wound with foreign body of vagina and vulva   NRS ♀

4,5 √x7ᵗʰ **S31.45** Open bite of vagina and vulva   NRS ♀
    Bite of vagina and vulva NOS
    EXCLUDES 1   superficial bite of vagina and vulva (S30.864, S30.874)

√5ᵗʰ **S31.5** Open wound of unspecified external genital organs
    EXCLUDES 1   traumatic amputation of external genital organs (S38.21, S38.22)

√6ᵗʰ **S31.50** Unspecified open wound of unspecified external genital organs

5 √7ᵗʰ **S31.501** Unspecified open wound of unspecified external genital organs, male   NRS ♂ ▽

5 √7ᵗʰ **S31.502** Unspecified open wound of unspecified external genital organs, female   NRS ♀ ▽

√6ᵗʰ **S31.51** Laceration without foreign body of unspecified external genital organs

4,5 √7ᵗʰ **S31.511** Laceration without foreign body of unspecified external genital organs, male   NRS ♂ ▽

4,5 √7ᵗʰ **S31.512** Laceration without foreign body of unspecified external genital organs, female   NRS ♀ ▽

√6ᵗʰ **S31.52** Laceration with foreign body of unspecified external genital organs

4,5 √7ᵗʰ **S31.521** Laceration with foreign body of unspecified external genital organs, male   NRS ♂ ▽

4,5 √7ᵗʰ **S31.522** Laceration with foreign body of unspecified external genital organs, female   NRS ♀ ▽

√6ᵗʰ **S31.53** Puncture wound without foreign body of unspecified external genital organs

4,5 √7ᵗʰ **S31.531** Puncture wound without foreign body of unspecified external genital organs, male   NRS ♂ ▽

4,5 √7ᵗʰ **S31.532** Puncture wound without foreign body of unspecified external genital organs, female   NRS ♀ ▽

√6ᵗʰ **S31.54** Puncture wound with foreign body of unspecified external genital organs

4,5 √7ᵗʰ **S31.541** Puncture wound with foreign body of unspecified external genital organs, male   NRS ♂ ▽

4,5 √7ᵗʰ **S31.542** Puncture wound with foreign body of unspecified external genital organs, female   NRS ♀ ▽

√6ᵗʰ **S31.55** Open bite of unspecified external genital organs
    Bite of unspecified external genital organs NOS
    EXCLUDES 1   superficial bite of unspecified external genital organs (S30.865, S30.866, S30.875, S30.876)

4,5 √7ᵗʰ **S31.551** Open bite of unspecified external genital organs, male   NRS ♂ ▽

4,5 √7ᵗʰ **S31.552** Open bite of unspecified external genital organs, female   NRS ♀ ▽

√5ᵗʰ **S31.6** Open wound of abdominal wall with penetration into peritoneal cavity

√6ᵗʰ **S31.60** Unspecified open wound of abdominal wall with penetration into peritoneal cavity

√7ᵗʰ **S31.600** Unspecified open wound of abdominal wall, right upper quadrant with penetration into peritoneal cavity   ▽

√7ᵗʰ **S31.601** Unspecified open wound of abdominal wall, left upper quadrant with penetration into peritoneal cavity   ▽

√7ᵗʰ **S31.602** Unspecified open wound of abdominal wall, epigastric region with penetration into peritoneal cavity   ▽

√7ᵗʰ **S31.603** Unspecified open wound of abdominal wall, right lower quadrant with penetration into peritoneal cavity   ▽

---

4   Case-mix diagnosis with 7th character indicating initial or subsequent encounter.
5   NRS supply diagnosis with 7th character indicating initial or subsequent encounter.

Ⓝ Newborn: 0   Ⓟ Pediatric: 0-17   Ⓜ Maternity: 12-55   Ⓐ Adult: 15-124   NRS Nonroutine supply Dx   NC Dx Noncancer Dx   PDx Primary Dx   ▶◀ Revised Text   ● New Code   ▲ Revised Title

942   ICD-10-CM 2018

√7ᵗʰ **S31.604** Unspecified open wound of abdominal ▽
wall, left lower quadrant with penetration
into peritoneal cavity

√7ᵗʰ **S31.605** Unspecified open wound of abdominal ▽
wall, periumbilic region with penetration
into peritoneal cavity

√7ᵗʰ **S31.609** Unspecified open wound of abdominal ▽
wall, unspecified quadrant with
penetration into peritoneal cavity

√6ᵗʰ **S31.61** Laceration without foreign body of abdominal wall
with penetration into peritoneal cavity

√7ᵗʰ **S31.610** Laceration without foreign body of
abdominal wall, right upper quadrant
with penetration into peritoneal cavity

√7ᵗʰ **S31.611** Laceration without foreign body of
abdominal wall, left upper quadrant with
penetration into peritoneal cavity

√7ᵗʰ **S31.612** Laceration without foreign body of
abdominal wall, epigastric region with
penetration into peritoneal cavity

√7ᵗʰ **S31.613** Laceration without foreign body of
abdominal wall, right lower quadrant with
penetration into peritoneal cavity

√7ᵗʰ **S31.614** Laceration without foreign body of
abdominal wall, left lower quadrant with
penetration into peritoneal cavity

√7ᵗʰ **S31.615** Laceration without foreign body of
abdominal wall, periumbilic region with
penetration into peritoneal cavity

√7ᵗʰ **S31.619** Laceration without foreign body of ▽
abdominal wall, unspecified quadrant
with penetration into peritoneal cavity

√6ᵗʰ **S31.62** Laceration with foreign body of abdominal wall with
penetration into peritoneal cavity

√7ᵗʰ **S31.620** Laceration with foreign body of
abdominal wall, right upper quadrant
with penetration into peritoneal cavity

√7ᵗʰ **S31.621** Laceration with foreign body of
abdominal wall, left upper quadrant with
penetration into peritoneal cavity

√7ᵗʰ **S31.622** Laceration with foreign body of
abdominal wall, epigastric region with
penetration into peritoneal cavity

√7ᵗʰ **S31.623** Laceration with foreign body of
abdominal wall, right lower quadrant with
penetration into peritoneal cavity

√7ᵗʰ **S31.624** Laceration with foreign body of
abdominal wall, left lower quadrant with
penetration into peritoneal cavity

√7ᵗʰ **S31.625** Laceration with foreign body of
abdominal wall, periumbilic region with
penetration into peritoneal cavity

√7ᵗʰ **S31.629** Laceration with foreign body of ▽
abdominal wall, unspecified quadrant
with penetration into peritoneal cavity

√6ᵗʰ **S31.63** Puncture wound without foreign body of abdominal
wall with penetration into peritoneal cavity

√7ᵗʰ **S31.630** Puncture wound without foreign body of
abdominal wall, right upper quadrant
with penetration into peritoneal cavity

√7ᵗʰ **S31.631** Puncture wound without foreign body of
abdominal wall, left upper quadrant with
penetration into peritoneal cavity

√7ᵗʰ **S31.632** Puncture wound without foreign body of
abdominal wall, epigastric region with
penetration into peritoneal cavity

√7ᵗʰ **S31.633** Puncture wound without foreign body of
abdominal wall, right lower quadrant with
penetration into peritoneal cavity

√7ᵗʰ **S31.634** Puncture wound without foreign body of
abdominal wall, left lower quadrant with
penetration into peritoneal cavity

√7ᵗʰ **S31.635** Puncture wound without foreign body of
abdominal wall, periumbilic region with
penetration into peritoneal cavity

√7ᵗʰ **S31.639** Puncture wound without foreign body ▽
of abdominal wall, unspecified quadrant
with penetration into peritoneal cavity

√6ᵗʰ **S31.64** Puncture wound with foreign body of abdominal
wall with penetration into peritoneal cavity

√7ᵗʰ **S31.640** Puncture wound with foreign body of
abdominal wall, right upper quadrant
with penetration into peritoneal cavity

√7ᵗʰ **S31.641** Puncture wound with foreign body of
abdominal wall, left upper quadrant with
penetration into peritoneal cavity

√7ᵗʰ **S31.642** Puncture wound with foreign body of
abdominal wall, epigastric region with
penetration into peritoneal cavity

√7ᵗʰ **S31.643** Puncture wound with foreign body of
abdominal wall, right lower quadrant with
penetration into peritoneal cavity

√7ᵗʰ **S31.644** Puncture wound with foreign body of
abdominal wall, left lower quadrant with
penetration into peritoneal cavity

√7ᵗʰ **S31.645** Puncture wound with foreign body of
abdominal wall, periumbilic region with
penetration into peritoneal cavity

√7ᵗʰ **S31.649** Puncture wound with foreign body of ▽
abdominal wall, unspecified quadrant
with penetration into peritoneal cavity

√6ᵗʰ **S31.65** Open bite of abdominal wall with penetration into
peritoneal cavity

> **EXCLUDES 1** superficial bite of abdominal wall (S30.861,
> S30.871)

√7ᵗʰ **S31.650** Open bite of abdominal wall, right upper
quadrant with penetration into peritoneal
cavity

√7ᵗʰ **S31.651** Open bite of abdominal wall, left upper
quadrant with penetration into peritoneal
cavity

√7ᵗʰ **S31.652** Open bite of abdominal wall, epigastric
region with penetration into peritoneal
cavity

√7ᵗʰ **S31.653** Open bite of abdominal wall, right lower
quadrant with penetration into peritoneal
cavity

√7ᵗʰ **S31.654** Open bite of abdominal wall, left lower
quadrant with penetration into peritoneal
cavity

√7ᵗʰ **S31.655** Open bite of abdominal wall, periumbilic
region with penetration into peritoneal
cavity

√7ᵗʰ **S31.659** Open bite of abdominal wall, ▽
unspecified quadrant with
penetration into peritoneal cavity

√5ᵗʰ **S31.8** Open wound of other parts of abdomen, lower back and
pelvis

√6ᵗʰ **S31.80** Open wound of unspecified buttock

√7ᵗʰ **S31.801** Laceration without foreign body of ▽
unspecified buttock

√7ᵗʰ **S31.802** Laceration with foreign body of ▽
unspecified buttock

√7ᵗʰ **S31.803** Puncture wound without foreign body ▽
of unspecified buttock

√7ᵗʰ **S31.804** Puncture wound with foreign body of ▽
unspecified buttock

√7ᵗʰ **S31.805** Open bite of unspecified buttock ▽
Bite of buttock NOS
> **EXCLUDES 1** superficial bite of buttock
> (S30.870)

√7ᵗʰ **S31.809** Unspecified open wound of ▽
unspecified buttock

√6ᵗʰ **S31.81** Open wound of right buttock

4,5 √7ᵗʰ **S31.811** Laceration without foreign body NRS
of right buttock

4,5 √7ᵗʰ **S31.812** Laceration with foreign body NRS
of right buttock

4,5 √7ᵗʰ **S31.813** Puncture wound without foreign NRS
body of right buttock

---

4   Case-mix diagnosis with 7th character indicating initial or subsequent encounter.
5   NRS supply diagnosis with 7th character indicating initial or subsequent encounter.

☑ Additional Character Req   √x7ᵗʰ Placeholder Alert   Case-Mix Diagnosis   Manifestation   ▽ Unspecified Dx   **EXCLUDES 1** Not coded here   **EXCLUDES 2** Not included here

Chapter 19. Injury, Poisoning and Certain Other Consequences of External Causes

4,5 ✓7th **S31.814** Puncture wound with foreign body of right buttock   NRS

4,5 ✓7th **S31.815** Open bite of right buttock   NRS
     Bite of right buttock NOS
     EXCLUDES 1   superficial bite of buttock (S30.870)

5 ✓7th **S31.819** Unspecified open wound of right buttock   NRS ▽

✓6th **S31.82** Open wound of left buttock

4,5 ✓7th **S31.821** Laceration without foreign body of left buttock   NRS

4,5 ✓7th **S31.822** Laceration with foreign body of left buttock   NRS

4,5 ✓7th **S31.823** Puncture wound without foreign body of left buttock   NRS

4,5 ✓7th **S31.824** Puncture wound with foreign body of left buttock   NRS

4,5 ✓7th **S31.825** Open bite of left buttock   NRS
     Bite of left buttock NOS
     EXCLUDES 1   superficial bite of buttock (S30.870)

5 ✓7th **S31.829** Unspecified open wound of left buttock   NRS ▽

✓6th **S31.83** Open wound of anus

4,5 ✓7th **S31.831** Laceration without foreign body of anus   NRS

4,5 ✓7th **S31.832** Laceration with foreign body of anus   NRS

4,5 ✓7th **S31.833** Puncture wound without foreign body of anus   NRS

4,5 ✓7th **S31.834** Puncture wound with foreign body of anus   NRS

4,5 ✓7th **S31.835** Open bite of anus   NRS
     Bite of anus NOS
     EXCLUDES 1   superficial bite of anus (S30.877)

5 ✓7th **S31.839** Unspecified open wound of anus   NRS ▽

✓4th **S32** **Fracture of lumbar spine and pelvis**
     NOTE   A fracture not indicated as displaced or nondisplaced should be coded to displaced.
     A fracture not indicated as opened or closed should be coded to closed.
     INCLUDES   fracture of lumbosacral neural arch
     fracture of lumbosacral spinous process
     fracture of lumbosacral transverse process
     fracture of lumbosacral vertebra
     fracture of lumbosacral vertebral arch

Code first any associated spinal cord and spinal nerve injury (S34.-)
     EXCLUDES 1   transection of abdomen (S38.3)
     EXCLUDES 2   fracture of hip NOS (S72.0-)
AHA: 2015, 3Q, 37-39; 2012, 4Q, 93
TIP: The term "improper alignment" is not synonymous with malunion or nonunion of a fracture when noted in provider documentation.

The appropriate 7th character is to be added to each code from category S32.
A   initial encounter for closed fracture
B   initial encounter for open fracture
D   subsequent encounter for fracture with routine healing
G   subsequent encounter for fracture with delayed healing
K   subsequent encounter for fracture with nonunion
S   sequela

✓5th **S32.0** **Fracture of lumbar vertebra**
     Fracture of lumbar spine NOS

✓6th **S32.00** **Fracture of unspecified lumbar vertebra**

1 ✓7th **S32.000** Wedge compression fracture of unspecified lumbar vertebra ▽

1 ✓7th **S32.001** Stable burst fracture of unspecified lumbar vertebra ▽

1 ✓7th **S32.002** Unstable burst fracture of unspecified lumbar vertebra ▽

1 ✓7th **S32.008** Other fracture of unspecified lumbar vertebra ▽

1 ✓7th **S32.009** Unspecified fracture of unspecified lumbar vertebra ▽

✓6th **S32.01** **Fracture of first lumbar vertebra**

1 ✓7th **S32.010** Wedge compression fracture of first lumbar vertebra

1 ✓7th **S32.011** Stable burst fracture of first lumbar vertebra

1 ✓7th **S32.012** Unstable burst fracture of first lumbar vertebra

1 ✓7th **S32.018** Other fracture of first lumbar vertebra

1 ✓7th **S32.019** Unspecified fracture of first lumbar vertebra ▽

✓6th **S32.02** **Fracture of second lumbar vertebra**

1 ✓7th **S32.020** Wedge compression fracture of second lumbar vertebra

1 ✓7th **S32.021** Stable burst fracture of second lumbar vertebra

1 ✓7th **S32.022** Unstable burst fracture of second lumbar vertebra

1 ✓7th **S32.028** Other fracture of second lumbar vertebra

1 ✓7th **S32.029** Unspecified fracture of second lumbar vertebra ▽

✓6th **S32.03** **Fracture of third lumbar vertebra**

1 ✓7th **S32.030** Wedge compression fracture of third lumbar vertebra

1 ✓7th **S32.031** Stable burst fracture of third lumbar vertebra

1 ✓7th **S32.032** Unstable burst fracture of third lumbar vertebra

1 ✓7th **S32.038** Other fracture of third lumbar vertebra

1 ✓7th **S32.039** Unspecified fracture of third lumbar vertebra ▽

✓6th **S32.04** **Fracture of fourth lumbar vertebra**

1 ✓7th **S32.040** Wedge compression fracture of fourth lumbar vertebra

1 ✓7th **S32.041** Stable burst fracture of fourth lumbar vertebra

1 ✓7th **S32.042** Unstable burst fracture of fourth lumbar vertebra

1 ✓7th **S32.048** Other fracture of fourth lumbar vertebra

1 ✓7th **S32.049** Unspecified fracture of fourth lumbar vertebra ▽

✓6th **S32.05** **Fracture of fifth lumbar vertebra**

1 ✓7th **S32.050** Wedge compression fracture of fifth lumbar vertebra

1 ✓7th **S32.051** Stable burst fracture of fifth lumbar vertebra

1 ✓7th **S32.052** Unstable burst fracture of fifth lumbar vertebra

1 ✓7th **S32.058** Other fracture of fifth lumbar vertebra

1 ✓7th **S32.059** Unspecified fracture of fifth lumbar vertebra ▽

✓5th **S32.1** **Fracture of sacrum**
     NOTE   For vertical fractures, code to most medial fracture extension.
     Use two codes if both a vertical and transverse fracture are present.
Code also any associated fracture of pelvic ring (S32.8-)

1 ✓x7th **S32.10** Unspecified fracture of sacrum ▽

✓6th **S32.11** **Zone I fracture of sacrum**
     Vertical sacral ala fracture of sacrum

1 ✓7th **S32.110** Nondisplaced Zone I fracture of sacrum

1 ✓7th **S32.111** Minimally displaced Zone I fracture of sacrum

1 ✓7th **S32.112** Severely displaced Zone I fracture of sacrum

1 ✓7th **S32.119** Unspecified Zone I fracture of sacrum ▽

✓6th **S32.12** **Zone II fracture of sacrum**
     Vertical foraminal region fracture of sacrum

1 ✓7th **S32.120** Nondisplaced Zone II fracture of sacrum

1 ✓7th **S32.121** Minimally displaced Zone II fracture of sacrum

1 ✓7th **S32.122** Severely displaced Zone II fracture of sacrum

1 ✓7th **S32.129** Unspecified Zone II fracture of sacrum ▽

---

1   Case-mix diagnosis with 7th character indicating subsequent encounter.
4   Case-mix diagnosis with 7th character indicating initial or subsequent encounter.
5   NRS supply diagnosis with 7th character indicating initial or subsequent encounter.

N Newborn: 0   P Pediatric: 0-17   M Maternity: 12-55   A Adult: 15-124   NRS Nonroutine supply Dx   NC Dx Noncancer Dx   PDx Primary Dx   ►◄ Revised Text   ● New Code   ▲ Revised Title

944   ICD-10-CM 2018

Vertical Sacral Fracture Zones

Zones: ① ② ③

Transverse Sacral Fracture Types

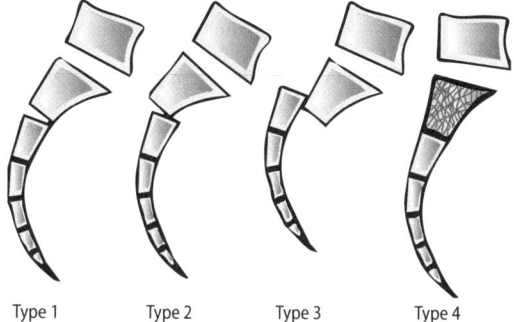

Type 1   Type 2   Type 3   Type 4

✓6th **S32.13** Zone III fracture of sacrum
    Vertical fracture into spinal canal region of sacrum
    1 ✓7th **S32.130** Nondisplaced Zone III fracture of sacrum
    1 ✓7th **S32.131** Minimally displaced Zone III fracture of sacrum
    1 ✓7th **S32.132** Severely displaced Zone III fracture of sacrum
    1 ✓7th **S32.139** Unspecified Zone III fracture of sacrum ▽

1 ✓x7th **S32.14** Type 1 fracture of sacrum
    Transverse flexion fracture of sacrum without displacement

1 ✓x7th **S32.15** Type 2 fracture of sacrum
    Transverse flexion fracture of sacrum with posterior displacement

1 ✓x7th **S32.16** Type 3 fracture of sacrum
    Transverse extension fracture of sacrum with anterior displacement

1 ✓x7th **S32.17** Type 4 fracture of sacrum
    Transverse segmental comminution of upper sacrum

1 ✓x7th **S32.19** Other fracture of sacrum

1 ✓x7th **S32.2** **Fracture of coccyx**

✓5th **S32.3** **Fracture of ilium**
    EXCLUDES 1 fracture of ilium with associated disruption of pelvic ring (S32.8-)

  ✓6th **S32.30** Unspecified fracture of ilium
    1 ✓7th **S32.301** Unspecified fracture of right ilium ▽
    1 ✓7th **S32.302** Unspecified fracture of left ilium ▽
    ✓7th **S32.309** Unspecified fracture of unspecified ilium ▽

  ✓6th **S32.31** Avulsion fracture of ilium
    1 ✓7th **S32.311** Displaced avulsion fracture of right ilium
    1 ✓7th **S32.312** Displaced avulsion fracture of left ilium
    ✓7th **S32.313** Displaced avulsion fracture of unspecified ilium ▽
    1 ✓7th **S32.314** Nondisplaced avulsion fracture of right ilium
    1 ✓7th **S32.315** Nondisplaced avulsion fracture of left ilium
    ✓7th **S32.316** Nondisplaced avulsion fracture of unspecified ilium ▽

  ✓6th **S32.39** Other fracture of ilium
    1 ✓7th **S32.391** Other fracture of right ilium
    1 ✓7th **S32.392** Other fracture of left ilium
    ✓7th **S32.399** Other fracture of unspecified ilium ▽

✓5th **S32.4** **Fracture of acetabulum**
    Code also any associated fracture of pelvic ring (S32.8-)
    AHA: 2016, 3Q, 16

  ✓6th **S32.40** Unspecified fracture of acetabulum
    1 ✓7th **S32.401** Unspecified fracture of right acetabulum ▽
    1 ✓7th **S32.402** Unspecified fracture of left acetabulum ▽
    ✓7th **S32.409** Unspecified fracture of unspecified acetabulum ▽

  ✓6th **S32.41** Fracture of anterior wall of acetabulum
    1 ✓7th **S32.411** Displaced fracture of anterior wall of right acetabulum
    1 ✓7th **S32.412** Displaced fracture of anterior wall of left acetabulum
    1 ✓7th **S32.413** Displaced fracture of anterior wall of unspecified acetabulum ▽
    1 ✓7th **S32.414** Nondisplaced fracture of anterior wall of right acetabulum
    1 ✓7th **S32.415** Nondisplaced fracture of anterior wall of left acetabulum
    ✓7th **S32.416** Nondisplaced fracture of anterior wall of unspecified acetabulum ▽

  ✓6th **S32.42** Fracture of posterior wall of acetabulum
    1 ✓7th **S32.421** Displaced fracture of posterior wall of right acetabulum
    1 ✓7th **S32.422** Displaced fracture of posterior wall of left acetabulum
    ✓7th **S32.423** Displaced fracture of posterior wall of unspecified acetabulum ▽
    1 ✓7th **S32.424** Nondisplaced fracture of posterior wall of right acetabulum
    1 ✓7th **S32.425** Nondisplaced fracture of posterior wall of left acetabulum
    ✓7th **S32.426** Nondisplaced fracture of posterior wall of unspecified acetabulum ▽

  ✓6th **S32.43** Fracture of anterior column [iliopubic] of acetabulum
    1 ✓7th **S32.431** Displaced fracture of anterior column [iliopubic] of right acetabulum
    1 ✓7th **S32.432** Displaced fracture of anterior column [iliopubic] of left acetabulum
    ✓7th **S32.433** Displaced fracture of anterior column [iliopubic] of unspecified acetabulum ▽
    1 ✓7th **S32.434** Nondisplaced fracture of anterior column [iliopubic] of right acetabulum
    1 ✓7th **S32.435** Nondisplaced fracture of anterior column [iliopubic] of left acetabulum
    ✓7th **S32.436** Nondisplaced fracture of anterior column [iliopubic] of unspecified acetabulum ▽

  ✓6th **S32.44** Fracture of posterior column [ilioischial] of acetabulum
    1 ✓7th **S32.441** Displaced fracture of posterior column [ilioischial] of right acetabulum
    1 ✓7th **S32.442** Displaced fracture of posterior column [ilioischial] of left acetabulum
    ✓7th **S32.443** Displaced fracture of posterior column [ilioischial] of unspecified acetabulum ▽
    1 ✓7th **S32.444** Nondisplaced fracture of posterior column [ilioischial] of right acetabulum
    1 ✓7th **S32.445** Nondisplaced fracture of posterior column [ilioischial] of left acetabulum
    ✓7th **S32.446** Nondisplaced fracture of posterior column [ilioischial] of unspecified acetabulum ▽

  ✓6th **S32.45** Transverse fracture of acetabulum
    1 ✓7th **S32.451** Displaced transverse fracture of right acetabulum

---

1 Case-mix diagnosis with 7th character indicating subsequent encounter.

✓ Additional Character Req   ✓7th Placeholder Alert   Case-Mix Diagnosis   Manifestation   ▽ Unspecified Dx   *EXCLUDES 1* Not coded here   *EXCLUDES 2* Not included here

ICD-10-CM 2018   **945**

¹ ✓7ᵗʰ **S32.452** Displaced transverse fracture of left acetabulum

✓7ᵗʰ **S32.453** Displaced transverse fracture of unspecified acetabulum ▽

¹ ✓7ᵗʰ **S32.454** Nondisplaced transverse fracture of right acetabulum

¹ ✓7ᵗʰ **S32.455** Nondisplaced transverse fracture of left acetabulum

✓7ᵗʰ **S32.456** Nondisplaced transverse fracture of unspecified acetabulum ▽

✓6ᵗʰ **S32.46** Associated transverse-posterior fracture of acetabulum

¹ ✓7ᵗʰ **S32.461** Displaced associated transverse-posterior fracture of right acetabulum

¹ ✓7ᵗʰ **S32.462** Displaced associated transverse-posterior fracture of left acetabulum

✓7ᵗʰ **S32.463** Displaced associated transverse-posterior fracture of unspecified acetabulum ▽

¹ ✓7ᵗʰ **S32.464** Nondisplaced associated transverse-posterior fracture of right acetabulum

¹ ✓7ᵗʰ **S32.465** Nondisplaced associated transverse-posterior fracture of left acetabulum

✓7ᵗʰ **S32.466** Nondisplaced associated transverse-posterior fracture of unspecified acetabulum ▽

✓6ᵗʰ **S32.47** Fracture of medial wall of acetabulum

¹ ✓7ᵗʰ **S32.471** Displaced fracture of medial wall of right acetabulum

¹ ✓7ᵗʰ **S32.472** Displaced fracture of medial wall of left acetabulum

✓7ᵗʰ **S32.473** Displaced fracture of medial wall of unspecified acetabulum ▽

¹ ✓7ᵗʰ **S32.474** Nondisplaced fracture of medial wall of right acetabulum

¹ ✓7ᵗʰ **S32.475** Nondisplaced fracture of medial wall of left acetabulum

✓7ᵗʰ **S32.476** Nondisplaced fracture of medial wall of unspecified acetabulum ▽

✓6ᵗʰ **S32.48** Dome fracture of acetabulum

¹ ✓7ᵗʰ **S32.481** Displaced dome fracture of right acetabulum

¹ ✓7ᵗʰ **S32.482** Displaced dome fracture of left acetabulum

✓7ᵗʰ **S32.483** Displaced dome fracture of unspecified acetabulum ▽

¹ ✓7ᵗʰ **S32.484** Nondisplaced dome fracture of right acetabulum

¹ ✓7ᵗʰ **S32.485** Nondisplaced dome fracture of left acetabulum

✓7ᵗʰ **S32.486** Nondisplaced dome fracture of unspecified acetabulum ▽

✓6ᵗʰ **S32.49** Other specified fracture of acetabulum

¹ ✓7ᵗʰ **S32.491** Other specified fracture of right acetabulum

¹ ✓7ᵗʰ **S32.492** Other specified fracture of left acetabulum

✓7ᵗʰ **S32.499** Other specified fracture of unspecified acetabulum ▽

✓5ᵗʰ **S32.5 Fracture of pubis**

 EXCLUDES 1 *fracture of pubis with associated disruption of pelvic ring (S32.8-)*

✓6ᵗʰ **S32.50** Unspecified fracture of pubis

¹ ✓7ᵗʰ **S32.501** Unspecified fracture of right pubis ▽

¹ ✓7ᵗʰ **S32.502** Unspecified fracture of left pubis ▽

✓7ᵗʰ **S32.509** Unspecified fracture of unspecified pubis ▽

✓6ᵗʰ **S32.51** Fracture of superior rim of pubis

¹ ✓7ᵗʰ **S32.511** Fracture of superior rim of right pubis

¹ ✓7ᵗʰ **S32.512** Fracture of superior rim of left pubis

✓7ᵗʰ **S32.519** Fracture of superior rim of unspecified pubis ▽

✓6ᵗʰ **S32.59** Other specified fracture of pubis

¹ ✓7ᵗʰ **S32.591** Other specified fracture of right pubis

¹ ✓7ᵗʰ **S32.592** Other specified fracture of left pubis

✓7ᵗʰ **S32.599** Other specified fracture of unspecified pubis ▽

✓5ᵗʰ **S32.6 Fracture of ischium**

 EXCLUDES 1 *fracture of ischium with associated disruption of pelvic ring (S32.8-)*

✓6ᵗʰ **S32.60** Unspecified fracture of ischium

¹ ✓7ᵗʰ **S32.601** Unspecified fracture of right ischium ▽

¹ ✓7ᵗʰ **S32.602** Unspecified fracture of left ischium ▽

✓7ᵗʰ **S32.609** Unspecified fracture of unspecified ischium ▽

✓6ᵗʰ **S32.61** Avulsion fracture of ischium

¹ ✓7ᵗʰ **S32.611** Displaced avulsion fracture of right ischium

¹ ✓7ᵗʰ **S32.612** Displaced avulsion fracture of left ischium

✓7ᵗʰ **S32.613** Displaced avulsion fracture of unspecified ischium ▽

¹ ✓7ᵗʰ **S32.614** Nondisplaced avulsion fracture of right ischium

¹ ✓7ᵗʰ **S32.615** Nondisplaced avulsion fracture of left ischium

✓7ᵗʰ **S32.616** Nondisplaced avulsion fracture of unspecified ischium ▽

✓6ᵗʰ **S32.69** Other specified fracture of ischium

¹ ✓7ᵗʰ **S32.691** Other specified fracture of right ischium

¹ ✓7ᵗʰ **S32.692** Other specified fracture of left ischium

✓7ᵗʰ **S32.699** Other specified fracture of unspecified ischium ▽

✓5ᵗʰ **S32.8 Fracture of other parts of pelvis**

 Code also any associated:
 fracture of acetabulum (S32.4-)
 sacral fracture (S32.1-)

✓6ᵗʰ **S32.81** Multiple fractures of pelvis with disruption of pelvic ring

 Multiple pelvic fractures with disruption of pelvic circle

¹ ✓7ᵗʰ **S32.810** Multiple fractures of pelvis with stable disruption of pelvic ring

¹ ✓7ᵗʰ **S32.811** Multiple fractures of pelvis with unstable disruption of pelvic ring

¹ ✓x7ᵗʰ **S32.82** Multiple fractures of pelvis without disruption of pelvic ring

 Multiple pelvic fractures without disruption of pelvic circle

¹ ✓x7ᵗʰ **S32.89** Fracture of other parts of pelvis

¹ ✓x7ᵗʰ **S32.9 Fracture of unspecified parts of lumbosacral spine and pelvis** ▽

 Fracture of lumbosacral spine NOS
 Fracture of pelvis NOS
 AHA: 2012, 4Q, 93

Fractures Disrupting Pelvic Circle

Stable

Unstable
(two-place fracture)

Iliac crest
Anterior superior iliac spine
Ischial spine
Acetabulum
Femur
Pelvic circle
Ilium
L5
Sacrum
Coccyx
Pubis
Ischium
Pubic symphysis

Pelvic Bones

---

¹ Case-mix diagnosis with 7th character indicating subsequent encounter.

Ⓝ Newborn: 0 Ⓟ Pediatric: 0-17 Ⓜ Maternity: 12-55 Ⓐ Adult: 15-124 NRS Nonroutine supply Dx NC Dx Noncancer Dx PDx Primary Dx ►◄ Revised Text ● New Code ▲ Revised Title

946 ICD-10-CM 2018

☑️4ᵗʰ **S33 Dislocation and sprain of joints and ligaments of lumbar spine and pelvis**

     INCLUDES   avulsion of joint or ligament of lumbar spine and pelvis

         laceration of cartilage, joint or ligament of lumbar spine and pelvis

         sprain of cartilage, joint or ligament of lumbar spine and pelvis

         traumatic hemarthrosis of joint or ligament of lumbar spine and pelvis

         traumatic rupture of joint or ligament of lumbar spine and pelvis

         traumatic subluxation of joint or ligament of lumbar spine and pelvis

         traumatic tear of joint or ligament of lumbar spine and pelvis

     Code also any associated open wound

     EXCLUDES 1   *nontraumatic rupture or displacement of lumbar intervertebral disc NOS (M51.-)*

         obstetric damage to pelvic joints and ligaments (O71.6)

     EXCLUDES 2   *dislocation and sprain of joints and ligaments of hip (S73.-)*

         strain of muscle of lower back and pelvis (S39.01-)

> The appropriate 7th character is to be added to each code from category S33.
> A   initial encounter
> D   subsequent encounter
> S   sequela

   ☑️x7ᵗʰ **S33.0 Traumatic rupture of lumbar intervertebral disc**

     EXCLUDES 1   *rupture or displacement (nontraumatic) of lumbar intervertebral disc NOS (M51- with fifth character 6)*

   ☑️5ᵗʰ **S33.1 Subluxation and dislocation of lumbar vertebra**

     Code also any associated:

         open wound of abdomen, lower back and pelvis (S31)

         spinal cord injury (S24.0, S24.1-, S34.0-, S34.1-)

     EXCLUDES 2   *fracture of lumbar vertebrae (S32.0-)*

     ☑️6ᵗʰ **S33.10 Subluxation and dislocation of unspecified lumbar vertebra**

         ☑️7ᵗʰ **S33.100** Subluxation of unspecified lumbar vertebra ▽

         ☑️7ᵗʰ **S33.101** Dislocation of unspecified lumbar vertebra ▽

     ☑️6ᵗʰ **S33.11 Subluxation and dislocation of L1/L2 lumbar vertebra**

         ☑️7ᵗʰ **S33.110** Subluxation of L1/L2 lumbar vertebra

         ☑️7ᵗʰ **S33.111** Dislocation of L1/L2 lumbar vertebra

     ☑️6ᵗʰ **S33.12 Subluxation and dislocation of L2/L3 lumbar vertebra**

         ☑️7ᵗʰ **S33.120** Subluxation of L2/L3 lumbar vertebra

         ☑️7ᵗʰ **S33.121** Dislocation of L2/L3 lumbar vertebra

     ☑️6ᵗʰ **S33.13 Subluxation and dislocation of L3/L4 lumbar vertebra**

         ☑️7ᵗʰ **S33.130** Subluxation of L3/L4 lumbar vertebra

         ☑️7ᵗʰ **S33.131** Dislocation of L3/L4 lumbar vertebra

     ☑️6ᵗʰ **S33.14 Subluxation and dislocation of L4/L5 lumbar vertebra**

         ☑️7ᵗʰ **S33.140** Subluxation of L4/L5 lumbar vertebra

         ☑️7ᵗʰ **S33.141** Dislocation of L4/L5 lumbar vertebra

   ☑️x7ᵗʰ **S33.2 Dislocation of sacroiliac and sacrococcygeal joint**

   ☑️5ᵗʰ **S33.3 Dislocation of other and unspecified parts of lumbar spine and pelvis**

     ☑️x7ᵗʰ **S33.30 Dislocation of unspecified parts of lumbar spine and pelvis** ▽

     ☑️x7ᵗʰ **S33.39 Dislocation of other parts of lumbar spine and pelvis**

   ☑️x7ᵗʰ **S33.4 Traumatic rupture of symphysis pubis**

   4 ☑️x7ᵗʰ **S33.5 Sprain of ligaments of lumbar spine**

   4 ☑️x7ᵗʰ **S33.6 Sprain of sacroiliac joint**

   4 ☑️x7ᵗʰ **S33.8 Sprain of other parts of lumbar spine and pelvis**

   4 ☑️x7ᵗʰ **S33.9 Sprain of unspecified parts of lumbar spine and pelvis** ▽

☑️4ᵗʰ **S34 Injury of lumbar and sacral spinal cord and nerves at abdomen, lower back and pelvis level**

     NOTE   Code to highest level of lumbar cord injury.

         Injuries to the spinal cord (S34.0 and S34.1) refer to the cord level and not bone level injury, and can affect nerve roots at and below the level given.

     Code also any associated:

         fracture of vertebra (S22.0-, S32.0-)

         open wound of abdomen, lower back and pelvis (S31.-)

         transient paralysis (R29.5)

> The appropriate 7th character is to be added to each code from category S34.
> A   initial encounter
> D   subsequent encounter
> S   sequela

   ☑️5ᵗʰ **S34.0 Concussion and edema of lumbar and sacral spinal cord**

     2 ☑️x7ᵗʰ **S34.01 Concussion and edema of lumbar spinal cord**

     2 ☑️x7ᵗʰ **S34.02 Concussion and edema of sacral spinal cord**

         Concussion and edema of conus medullaris

   ☑️5ᵗʰ **S34.1 Other and unspecified injury of lumbar and sacral spinal cord**

     ☑️6ᵗʰ **S34.10 Unspecified injury to lumbar spinal cord**

         2 ☑️7ᵗʰ **S34.101 Unspecified injury to L1 level of lumbar spinal cord** ▽

         Unspecified injury to lumbar spinal cord level 1

         2 ☑️7ᵗʰ **S34.102 Unspecified injury to L2 level of lumbar spinal cord** ▽

         Unspecified injury to lumbar spinal cord level 2

         2 ☑️7ᵗʰ **S34.103 Unspecified injury to L3 level of lumbar spinal cord** ▽

         Unspecified injury to lumbar spinal cord level 3

         2 ☑️7ᵗʰ **S34.104 Unspecified injury to L4 level of lumbar spinal cord** ▽

         Unspecified injury to lumbar spinal cord level 4

         2 ☑️7ᵗʰ **S34.105 Unspecified injury to L5 level of lumbar spinal cord** ▽

         Unspecified injury to lumbar spinal cord level 5

         2 ☑️7ᵗʰ **S34.109 Unspecified injury to unspecified level of lumbar spinal cord** ▽

     ☑️6ᵗʰ **S34.11 Complete lesion of lumbar spinal cord**

         2 ☑️7ᵗʰ **S34.111 Complete lesion of L1 level of lumbar spinal cord**

         Complete lesion of lumbar spinal cord level 1

         2 ☑️7ᵗʰ **S34.112 Complete lesion of L2 level of lumbar spinal cord**

         Complete lesion of lumbar spinal cord level 2

         2 ☑️7ᵗʰ **S34.113 Complete lesion of L3 level of lumbar spinal cord**

         Complete lesion of lumbar spinal cord level 3

         2 ☑️7ᵗʰ **S34.114 Complete lesion of L4 level of lumbar spinal cord**

         Complete lesion of lumbar spinal cord level 4

         2 ☑️7ᵗʰ **S34.115 Complete lesion of L5 level of lumbar spinal cord**

         Complete lesion of lumbar spinal cord level 5

         2 ☑️7ᵗʰ **S34.119 Complete lesion of unspecified level of lumbar spinal cord** ▽

     ☑️6ᵗʰ **S34.12 Incomplete lesion of lumbar spinal cord**

         2 ☑️7ᵗʰ **S34.121 Incomplete lesion of L1 level of lumbar spinal cord**

         Incomplete lesion of lumbar spinal cord level 1

         2 ☑️7ᵗʰ **S34.122 Incomplete lesion of L2 level of lumbar spinal cord**

         Incomplete lesion of lumbar spinal cord level 2

---

2   Case-mix diagnosis with 7th character indicating subsequent encounter or sequela.
4   Case-mix diagnosis with 7th character indicating initial or subsequent encounter.

☑️ Additional Character Req   ☑️x7ᵗʰ Placeholder Alert   Case-Mix Diagnosis   Manifestation   ▽ Unspecified Dx   **EXCLUDES 1** Not coded here   **EXCLUDES 2** Not included here

2 √7ᵗʰ **S34.123** **Incomplete lesion of L3 level of lumbar spinal cord**
Incomplete lesion of lumbar spinal cord level 3

2 √7ᵗʰ **S34.124** **Incomplete lesion of L4 level of lumbar spinal cord**
Incomplete lesion of lumbar spinal cord level 4

2 √7ᵗʰ **S34.125** **Incomplete lesion of L5 level of lumbar spinal cord**
Incomplete lesion of lumbar spinal cord level 5

2 √7ᵗʰ **S34.129** **Incomplete lesion of unspecified level of lumbar spinal cord** ▽

√6ᵗʰ **S34.13** **Other and unspecified injury to sacral spinal cord**
Other injury to conus medullaris

2 √7ᵗʰ **S34.131** **Complete lesion of sacral spinal cord**
Complete lesion of conus medullaris

2 √7ᵗʰ **S34.132** **Incomplete lesion of sacral spinal cord**
Incomplete lesion of conus medullaris

2 √7ᵗʰ **S34.139** **Unspecified injury to sacral spinal cord** ▽
Unspecified injury of conus medullaris

√5ᵗʰ **S34.2** **Injury of nerve root of lumbar and sacral spine**

2 √x7ᵗʰ **S34.21** **Injury of nerve root of lumbar spine**

2 √x7ᵗʰ **S34.22** **Injury of nerve root of sacral spine**

2 √x7ᵗʰ **S34.3** **Injury of cauda equina**

2 √x7ᵗʰ **S34.4** **Injury of lumbosacral plexus**

2 √x7ᵗʰ **S34.5** **Injury of lumbar, sacral and pelvic sympathetic nerves**
Injury of celiac ganglion or plexus
Injury of hypogastric plexus
Injury of mesenteric plexus (inferior) (superior)
Injury of splanchnic nerve

2 √x7ᵗʰ **S34.6** **Injury of peripheral nerve(s) at abdomen, lower back and pelvis level**

2 √x7ᵗʰ **S34.8** **Injury of other nerves at abdomen, lower back and pelvis level**

2 √x7ᵗʰ **S34.9** **Injury of unspecified nerves at abdomen, lower back and pelvis level** ▽

√4ᵗʰ **S35** **Injury of blood vessels at abdomen, lower back and pelvis level**
Code also any associated open wound (S31.-)

> The appropriate 7th character is to be added to each code from category S35.
> A initial encounter
> D subsequent encounter
> S sequela

√5ᵗʰ **S35.0** **Injury of abdominal aorta**
EXCLUDES 1 injury of aorta NOS (S25.0)

√x7ᵗʰ **S35.00** **Unspecified injury of abdominal aorta** ▽

√x7ᵗʰ **S35.01** **Minor laceration of abdominal aorta**
Incomplete transection of abdominal aorta
Laceration of abdominal aorta NOS
Superficial laceration of abdominal aorta

√x7ᵗʰ **S35.02** **Major laceration of abdominal aorta**
Complete transection of abdominal aorta
Traumatic rupture of abdominal aorta

√x7ᵗʰ **S35.09** **Other injury of abdominal aorta**

√5ᵗʰ **S35.1** **Injury of inferior vena cava**
Injury of hepatic vein
EXCLUDES 1 injury of vena cava NOS (S25.2)

√x7ᵗʰ **S35.10** **Unspecified injury of inferior vena cava** ▽

√x7ᵗʰ **S35.11** **Minor laceration of inferior vena cava**
Incomplete transection of inferior vena cava
Laceration of inferior vena cava NOS
Superficial laceration of inferior vena cava

√x7ᵗʰ **S35.12** **Major laceration of inferior vena cava**
Complete transection of inferior vena cava
Traumatic rupture of inferior vena cava

√x7ᵗʰ **S35.19** **Other injury of inferior vena cava**

√5ᵗʰ **S35.2** **Injury of celiac or mesenteric artery and branches**

√6ᵗʰ **S35.21** **Injury of celiac artery**

√7ᵗʰ **S35.211** **Minor laceration of celiac artery**
Incomplete transection of celiac artery
Laceration of celiac artery NOS
Superficial laceration of celiac artery

√7ᵗʰ **S35.212** **Major laceration of celiac artery**
Complete transection of celiac artery
Traumatic rupture of celiac artery

√7ᵗʰ **S35.218** **Other injury of celiac artery**

√7ᵗʰ **S35.219** **Unspecified injury of celiac artery** ▽

√6ᵗʰ **S35.22** **Injury of superior mesenteric artery**

√7ᵗʰ **S35.221** **Minor laceration of superior mesenteric artery**
Incomplete transection of superior mesenteric artery
Laceration of superior mesenteric artery NOS
Superficial laceration of superior mesenteric artery

√7ᵗʰ **S35.222** **Major laceration of superior mesenteric artery**
Complete transection of superior mesenteric artery
Traumatic rupture of superior mesenteric artery

√7ᵗʰ **S35.228** **Other injury of superior mesenteric artery**

√7ᵗʰ **S35.229** **Unspecified injury of superior mesenteric artery** ▽

√6ᵗʰ **S35.23** **Injury of inferior mesenteric artery**

√7ᵗʰ **S35.231** **Minor laceration of inferior mesenteric artery**
Incomplete transection of inferior mesenteric artery
Laceration of inferior mesenteric artery NOS
Superficial laceration of inferior mesenteric artery

√7ᵗʰ **S35.232** **Major laceration of inferior mesenteric artery**
Complete transection of inferior mesenteric artery
Traumatic rupture of inferior mesenteric artery

√7ᵗʰ **S35.238** **Other injury of inferior mesenteric artery**

√7ᵗʰ **S35.239** **Unspecified injury of inferior mesenteric artery** ▽

√6ᵗʰ **S35.29** **Injury of branches of celiac and mesenteric artery**
Injury of gastric artery
Injury of gastroduodenal artery
Injury of hepatic artery
Injury of splenic artery

√7ᵗʰ **S35.291** **Minor laceration of branches of celiac and mesenteric artery**
Incomplete transection of branches of celiac and mesenteric artery
Laceration of branches of celiac and mesenteric artery NOS
Superficial laceration of branches of celiac and mesenteric artery

√7ᵗʰ **S35.292** **Major laceration of branches of celiac and mesenteric artery**
Complete transection of branches of celiac and mesenteric artery
Traumatic rupture of branches of celiac and mesenteric artery

√7ᵗʰ **S35.298** **Other injury of branches of celiac and mesenteric artery**

√7ᵗʰ **S35.299** **Unspecified injury of branches of celiac and mesenteric artery** ▽

√5ᵗʰ **S35.3** **Injury of portal or splenic vein and branches**

√6ᵗʰ **S35.31** **Injury of portal vein**

√7ᵗʰ **S35.311** **Laceration of portal vein**

√7ᵗʰ **S35.318** **Other specified injury of portal vein**

√7ᵗʰ **S35.319** **Unspecified injury of portal vein** ▽

√6ᵗʰ **S35.32** **Injury of splenic vein**

√7ᵗʰ **S35.321** **Laceration of splenic vein**

√7ᵗʰ **S35.328** **Other specified injury of splenic vein**

√7ᵗʰ **S35.329** **Unspecified injury of splenic vein** ▽

√6ᵗʰ **S35.33** **Injury of superior mesenteric vein**

√7ᵗʰ **S35.331** **Laceration of superior mesenteric vein**

√7ᵗʰ **S35.338** **Other specified injury of superior mesenteric vein**

---

2 Case-mix diagnosis with 7th character indicating subsequent encounter or sequela.

N Newborn: 0   P Pediatric: 0-17   M Maternity: 12-55   A Adult: 15-124   NRS Nonroutine supply Dx   NC Dx Noncancer Dx   PDx Primary Dx   ▶◀ Revised Text   ● New Code   ▲ Revised Title

948   ICD-10-CM 2018

☑7ᵗʰ **S35.339** Unspecified injury of superior mesenteric vein ▽

☑6ᵗʰ **S35.34** Injury of inferior mesenteric vein

☑7ᵗʰ **S35.341** Laceration of inferior mesenteric vein

☑7ᵗʰ **S35.348** Other specified injury of inferior mesenteric vein

☑7ᵗʰ **S35.349** Unspecified injury of inferior mesenteric vein ▽

☑5ᵗʰ **S35.4** Injury of renal blood vessels

☑6ᵗʰ **S35.40** Unspecified injury of renal blood vessel

☑7ᵗʰ **S35.401** Unspecified injury of right renal artery ▽

☑7ᵗʰ **S35.402** Unspecified injury of left renal artery ▽

☑7ᵗʰ **S35.403** Unspecified injury of unspecified renal artery ▽

☑7ᵗʰ **S35.404** Unspecified injury of right renal vein ▽

☑7ᵗʰ **S35.405** Unspecified injury of left renal vein ▽

☑7ᵗʰ **S35.406** Unspecified injury of unspecified renal vein ▽

☑6ᵗʰ **S35.41** Laceration of renal blood vessel

☑7ᵗʰ **S35.411** Laceration of right renal artery

☑7ᵗʰ **S35.412** Laceration of left renal artery

☑7ᵗʰ **S35.413** Laceration of unspecified renal artery ▽

☑7ᵗʰ **S35.414** Laceration of right renal vein

☑7ᵗʰ **S35.415** Laceration of left renal vein

☑7ᵗʰ **S35.416** Laceration of unspecified renal vein ▽

☑6ᵗʰ **S35.49** Other specified injury of renal blood vessel

☑7ᵗʰ **S35.491** Other specified injury of right renal artery

☑7ᵗʰ **S35.492** Other specified injury of left renal artery

☑7ᵗʰ **S35.493** Other specified injury of unspecified renal artery ▽

☑7ᵗʰ **S35.494** Other specified injury of right renal vein

☑7ᵗʰ **S35.495** Other specified injury of left renal vein

☑7ᵗʰ **S35.496** Other specified injury of unspecified renal vein ▽

☑5ᵗʰ **S35.5** Injury of iliac blood vessels

☑ₓ7ᵗʰ **S35.50** Injury of unspecified iliac blood vessel(s) ▽

☑6ᵗʰ **S35.51** Injury of iliac artery or vein
Injury of hypogastric artery or vein

☑7ᵗʰ **S35.511** Injury of right iliac artery

☑7ᵗʰ **S35.512** Injury of left iliac artery

☑7ᵗʰ **S35.513** Injury of unspecified iliac artery ▽

☑7ᵗʰ **S35.514** Injury of right iliac vein

☑7ᵗʰ **S35.515** Injury of left iliac vein

☑7ᵗʰ **S35.516** Injury of unspecified iliac vein ▽

☑6ᵗʰ **S35.53** Injury of uterine artery or vein

☑7ᵗʰ **S35.531** Injury of right uterine artery ♀

☑7ᵗʰ **S35.532** Injury of left uterine artery ♀

☑7ᵗʰ **S35.533** Injury of unspecified uterine artery ♀▽

☑7ᵗʰ **S35.534** Injury of right uterine vein ♀

☑7ᵗʰ **S35.535** Injury of left uterine vein ♀

☑7ᵗʰ **S35.536** Injury of unspecified uterine vein ♀▽

☑ₓ7ᵗʰ **S35.59** Injury of other iliac blood vessels

☑5ᵗʰ **S35.8** Injury of other blood vessels at abdomen, lower back and pelvis level
Injury of ovarian artery or vein

☑6ᵗʰ **S35.8X** Injury of other blood vessels at abdomen, lower back and pelvis level

☑7ᵗʰ **S35.8X1** Laceration of other blood vessels at abdomen, lower back and pelvis level

☑7ᵗʰ **S35.8X8** Other specified injury of other blood vessels at abdomen, lower back and pelvis level

☑7ᵗʰ **S35.8X9** Unspecified injury of other blood vessels at abdomen, lower back and pelvis level ▽

☑5ᵗʰ **S35.9** Injury of unspecified blood vessel at abdomen, lower back and pelvis level

☑ₓ7ᵗʰ **S35.90** Unspecified injury of unspecified blood vessel at abdomen, lower back and pelvis level ▽

☑ₓ7ᵗʰ **S35.91** Laceration of unspecified blood vessel at abdomen, lower back and pelvis level ▽

☑ₓ7ᵗʰ **S35.99** Other specified injury of unspecified blood vessel at abdomen, lower back and pelvis level ▽

☑4ᵗʰ **S36** Injury of intra-abdominal organs
Code also any associated open wound (S31.-)

> The appropriate 7th character is to be added to each code from category S36.
> A   initial encounter
> D   subsequent encounter
> S   sequela

TIP: Code only the most severe injury reported when assigning a code for intra-abdominal injury; a laceration is more severe than a contusion.

☑5ᵗʰ **S36.0** Injury of spleen
AHA: 2015, 2Q, 36; 2015, 1Q, 10

☑ₓ7ᵗʰ **S36.00** Unspecified injury of spleen ▽

☑6ᵗʰ **S36.02** Contusion of spleen

☑7ᵗʰ **S36.020** Minor contusion of spleen
Contusion of spleen less than 2 cm

☑7ᵗʰ **S36.021** Major contusion of spleen
Contusion of spleen greater than 2 cm

☑7ᵗʰ **S36.029** Unspecified contusion of spleen ▽

☑6ᵗʰ **S36.03** Laceration of spleen

☑7ᵗʰ **S36.030** Superficial (capsular) laceration of spleen
Laceration of spleen less than 1cm
Minor laceration of spleen

☑7ᵗʰ **S36.031** Moderate laceration of spleen
Laceration of spleen 1 to 3 cm

☑7ᵗʰ **S36.032** Major laceration of spleen
Avulsion of spleen
Laceration of spleen greater than 3 cm
Massive laceration of spleen
Multiple moderate lacerations of spleen
Stellate laceration of spleen

☑7ᵗʰ **S36.039** Unspecified laceration of spleen ▽

☑ₓ7ᵗʰ **S36.09** Other injury of spleen

☑5ᵗʰ **S36.1** Injury of liver and gallbladder and bile duct

☑6ᵗʰ **S36.11** Injury of liver

☑7ᵗʰ **S36.112** Contusion of liver

☑7ᵗʰ **S36.113** Laceration of liver, unspecified degree ▽

☑7ᵗʰ **S36.114** Minor laceration of liver
Laceration involving capsule only, or, without significant involvement of hepatic parenchyma [i.e., less than 1cm deep]

☑7ᵗʰ **S36.115** Moderate laceration of liver
Laceration involving parenchyma but without major disruption of parenchyma [i.e., less than 10 cm long and less than 3 cm deep]

☑7ᵗʰ **S36.116** Major laceration of liver
Laceration with significant disruption of hepatic parenchyma [i.e., greater than 10 cm long and 3 cm deep]
Multiple moderate lacerations, with or without hematoma
Stellate laceration of liver

☑7ᵗʰ **S36.118** Other injury of liver

☑7ᵗʰ **S36.119** Unspecified injury of liver ▽

☑6ᵗʰ **S36.12** Injury of gallbladder

☑7ᵗʰ **S36.122** Contusion of gallbladder

☑7ᵗʰ **S36.123** Laceration of gallbladder

☑7ᵗʰ **S36.128** Other injury of gallbladder

☑7ᵗʰ **S36.129** Unspecified injury of gallbladder ▽

☑ₓ7ᵗʰ **S36.13** Injury of bile duct

☑5ᵗʰ **S36.2** Injury of pancreas

☑6ᵗʰ **S36.20** Unspecified injury of pancreas

☑7ᵗʰ **S36.200** Unspecified injury of head of pancreas ▽

☑7ᵗʰ **S36.201** Unspecified injury of body of pancreas ▽

☑7ᵗʰ **S36.202** Unspecified injury of tail of pancreas ▽

☑7ᵗʰ **S36.209** Unspecified injury of unspecified part of pancreas ▽

☑6ᵗʰ **S36.22** Contusion of pancreas

☑7ᵗʰ **S36.220** Contusion of head of pancreas

☑7ᵗʰ **S36.221** Contusion of body of pancreas

☑ Additional Character Req   ☑ₓ7ᵗʰ Placeholder Alert   Case-Mix Diagnosis   Manifestation   ▽ Unspecified Dx   EXCLUDES 1 Not coded here   EXCLUDES 2 Not included here

ICD-10-CM 2018   949

√7th **S36.222** Contusion of tail of pancreas
√7th **S36.229** Contusion of unspecified part of pancreas
√6th **S36.23** Laceration of pancreas, unspecified degree
√7th **S36.230** Laceration of head of pancreas, unspecified degree
√7th **S36.231** Laceration of body of pancreas, unspecified degree
√7th **S36.232** Laceration of tail of pancreas, unspecified degree
√7th **S36.239** Laceration of unspecified part of pancreas, unspecified degree
√6th **S36.24** Minor laceration of pancreas
√7th **S36.240** Minor laceration of head of pancreas
√7th **S36.241** Minor laceration of body of pancreas
√7th **S36.242** Minor laceration of tail of pancreas
√7th **S36.249** Minor laceration of unspecified part of pancreas
√6th **S36.25** Moderate laceration of pancreas
√7th **S36.250** Moderate laceration of head of pancreas
√7th **S36.251** Moderate laceration of body of pancreas
√7th **S36.252** Moderate laceration of tail of pancreas
√7th **S36.259** Moderate laceration of unspecified part of pancreas
√6th **S36.26** Major laceration of pancreas
√7th **S36.260** Major laceration of head of pancreas
√7th **S36.261** Major laceration of body of pancreas
√7th **S36.262** Major laceration of tail of pancreas
√7th **S36.269** Major laceration of unspecified part of pancreas
√6th **S36.29** Other injury of pancreas
√7th **S36.290** Other injury of head of pancreas
√7th **S36.291** Other injury of body of pancreas
√7th **S36.292** Other injury of tail of pancreas
√7th **S36.299** Other injury of unspecified part of pancreas
√5th **S36.3** Injury of stomach
√x7th **S36.30** Unspecified injury of stomach
√x7th **S36.32** Contusion of stomach
√x7th **S36.33** Laceration of stomach
√x7th **S36.39** Other injury of stomach
√5th **S36.4** Injury of small intestine
√6th **S36.40** Unspecified injury of small intestine
√7th **S36.400** Unspecified injury of duodenum
√7th **S36.408** Unspecified injury of other part of small intestine
√7th **S36.409** Unspecified injury of unspecified part of small intestine
√6th **S36.41** Primary blast injury of small intestine
Blast injury of small intestine NOS
√7th **S36.410** Primary blast injury of duodenum
√7th **S36.418** Primary blast injury of other part of small intestine
√7th **S36.419** Primary blast injury of unspecified part of small intestine
√6th **S36.42** Contusion of small intestine
√7th **S36.420** Contusion of duodenum
√7th **S36.428** Contusion of other part of small intestine
√7th **S36.429** Contusion of unspecified part of small intestine
√6th **S36.43** Laceration of small intestine
√7th **S36.430** Laceration of duodenum
√7th **S36.438** Laceration of other part of small intestine
√7th **S36.439** Laceration of unspecified part of small intestine
√6th **S36.49** Other injury of small intestine
√7th **S36.490** Other injury of duodenum
√7th **S36.498** Other injury of other part of small intestine
√7th **S36.499** Other injury of unspecified part of small intestine

√5th **S36.5** Injury of colon
EXCLUDES 2 injury of rectum (S36.6-)
√6th **S36.50** Unspecified injury of colon
√7th **S36.500** Unspecified injury of ascending [right] colon
√7th **S36.501** Unspecified injury of transverse colon
√7th **S36.502** Unspecified injury of descending [left] colon
√7th **S36.503** Unspecified injury of sigmoid colon
√7th **S36.508** Unspecified injury of other part of colon
√7th **S36.509** Unspecified injury of unspecified part of colon
√6th **S36.51** Primary blast injury of colon
Blast injury of colon NOS
√7th **S36.510** Primary blast injury of ascending [right] colon
√7th **S36.511** Primary blast injury of transverse colon
√7th **S36.512** Primary blast injury of descending [left] colon
√7th **S36.513** Primary blast injury of sigmoid colon
√7th **S36.518** Primary blast injury of other part of colon
√7th **S36.519** Primary blast injury of unspecified part of colon
√6th **S36.52** Contusion of colon
√7th **S36.520** Contusion of ascending [right] colon
√7th **S36.521** Contusion of transverse colon
√7th **S36.522** Contusion of descending [left] colon
√7th **S36.523** Contusion of sigmoid colon
√7th **S36.528** Contusion of other part of colon
√7th **S36.529** Contusion of unspecified part of colon
√6th **S36.53** Laceration of colon
√7th **S36.530** Laceration of ascending [right] colon
√7th **S36.531** Laceration of transverse colon
√7th **S36.532** Laceration of descending [left] colon
√7th **S36.533** Laceration of sigmoid colon
√7th **S36.538** Laceration of other part of colon
√7th **S36.539** Laceration of unspecified part of colon
√6th **S36.59** Other injury of colon
Secondary blast injury of colon
√7th **S36.590** Other injury of ascending [right] colon
√7th **S36.591** Other injury of transverse colon
√7th **S36.592** Other injury of descending [left] colon
√7th **S36.593** Other injury of sigmoid colon
√7th **S36.598** Other injury of other part of colon
√7th **S36.599** Other injury of unspecified part of colon
√5th **S36.6** Injury of rectum
√x7th **S36.60** Unspecified injury of rectum
√x7th **S36.61** Primary blast injury of rectum
Blast injury of rectum NOS
√x7th **S36.62** Contusion of rectum
√x7th **S36.63** Laceration of rectum
√x7th **S36.69** Other injury of rectum
Secondary blast injury of rectum
√5th **S36.8** Injury of other intra-abdominal organs
√x7th **S36.81** Injury of peritoneum
√6th **S36.89** Injury of other intra-abdominal organs
Injury of retroperitoneum
√7th **S36.892** Contusion of other intra-abdominal organs
√7th **S36.893** Laceration of other intra-abdominal organs
√7th **S36.898** Other injury of other intra-abdominal organs
√7th **S36.899** Unspecified injury of other intra-abdominal organs
√5th **S36.9** Injury of unspecified intra-abdominal organ
√x7th **S36.90** Unspecified injury of unspecified intra-abdominal organ
√x7th **S36.92** Contusion of unspecified intra-abdominal organ
√x7th **S36.93** Laceration of unspecified intra-abdominal organ

✓x7ᵗʰ **S36.99** **Other injury of unspecified intra-abdominal organ** ▽

✓4ᵗʰ **S37** **Injury of urinary and pelvic organs**
Code also any associated open wound (S31.-)
EXCLUDES 1 *obstetric trauma to pelvic organs (O71.-)*
EXCLUDES 2 *injury of peritoneum (S36.81)*
injury of retroperitoneum (S36.89-)

The appropriate 7th character is to be added to each code from category S37.
A   initial encounter
D   subsequent encounter
S   sequela

✓5ᵗʰ **S37.0** **Injury of kidney**
EXCLUDES 2 *acute kidney injury (nontraumatic) (N17.9)*

✓6ᵗʰ **S37.00** **Unspecified injury of kidney**
✓7ᵗʰ **S37.001** **Unspecified injury of right kidney** ▽
✓7ᵗʰ **S37.002** **Unspecified injury of left kidney** ▽
✓7ᵗʰ **S37.009** **Unspecified injury of unspecified kidney** ▽

✓6ᵗʰ **S37.01** **Minor contusion of kidney**
Contusion of kidney less than 2 cm
Contusion of kidney NOS
✓7ᵗʰ **S37.011** **Minor contusion of right kidney**
✓7ᵗʰ **S37.012** **Minor contusion of left kidney**
✓7ᵗʰ **S37.019** **Minor contusion of unspecified kidney** ▽

✓6ᵗʰ **S37.02** **Major contusion of kidney**
Contusion of kidney greater than 2 cm
✓7ᵗʰ **S37.021** **Major contusion of right kidney**
✓7ᵗʰ **S37.022** **Major contusion of left kidney**
✓7ᵗʰ **S37.029** **Major contusion of unspecified kidney** ▽

✓6ᵗʰ **S37.03** **Laceration of kidney, unspecified degree**
✓7ᵗʰ **S37.031** **Laceration of right kidney, unspecified degree** ▽
✓7ᵗʰ **S37.032** **Laceration of left kidney, unspecified degree** ▽
✓7ᵗʰ **S37.039** **Laceration of unspecified kidney, unspecified degree** ▽

✓6ᵗʰ **S37.04** **Minor laceration of kidney**
Laceration of kidney less than 1 cm
✓7ᵗʰ **S37.041** **Minor laceration of right kidney**
✓7ᵗʰ **S37.042** **Minor laceration of left kidney**
✓7ᵗʰ **S37.049** **Minor laceration of unspecified kidney** ▽

✓6ᵗʰ **S37.05** **Moderate laceration of kidney**
Laceration of kidney 1 to 3 cm
✓7ᵗʰ **S37.051** **Moderate laceration of right kidney**
✓7ᵗʰ **S37.052** **Moderate laceration of left kidney**
✓7ᵗʰ **S37.059** **Moderate laceration of unspecified kidney** ▽

✓6ᵗʰ **S37.06** **Major laceration of kidney**
Avulsion of kidney
Laceration of kidney greater than 3 cm
Massive laceration of kidney
Multiple moderate lacerations of kidney
Stellate laceration of kidney
✓7ᵗʰ **S37.061** **Major laceration of right kidney**
✓7ᵗʰ **S37.062** **Major laceration of left kidney**
✓7ᵗʰ **S37.069** **Major laceration of unspecified kidney** ▽

✓6ᵗʰ **S37.09** **Other injury of kidney**
✓7ᵗʰ **S37.091** **Other injury of right kidney**
✓7ᵗʰ **S37.092** **Other injury of left kidney**
✓7ᵗʰ **S37.099** **Other injury of unspecified kidney** ▽

✓5ᵗʰ **S37.1** **Injury of ureter**
✓x7ᵗʰ **S37.10** **Unspecified injury of ureter** ▽
✓x7ᵗʰ **S37.12** **Contusion of ureter**
✓x7ᵗʰ **S37.13** **Laceration of ureter**
✓x7ᵗʰ **S37.19** **Other injury of ureter**

✓5ᵗʰ **S37.2** **Injury of bladder**
✓x7ᵗʰ **S37.20** **Unspecified injury of bladder** ▽
✓x7ᵗʰ **S37.22** **Contusion of bladder**
✓x7ᵗʰ **S37.23** **Laceration of bladder**
✓x7ᵗʰ **S37.29** **Other injury of bladder**

✓5ᵗʰ **S37.3** **Injury of urethra**
✓x7ᵗʰ **S37.30** **Unspecified injury of urethra** ▽
✓x7ᵗʰ **S37.32** **Contusion of urethra**
✓x7ᵗʰ **S37.33** **Laceration of urethra**
✓x7ᵗʰ **S37.39** **Other injury of urethra**

✓5ᵗʰ **S37.4** **Injury of ovary**
✓6ᵗʰ **S37.40** **Unspecified injury of ovary**
✓7ᵗʰ **S37.401** **Unspecified injury of ovary, unilateral** ♀▽
✓7ᵗʰ **S37.402** **Unspecified injury of ovary, bilateral** ♀▽
✓7ᵗʰ **S37.409** **Unspecified injury of ovary, unspecified** ♀▽

✓6ᵗʰ **S37.42** **Contusion of ovary**
✓7ᵗʰ **S37.421** **Contusion of ovary, unilateral** ♀
✓7ᵗʰ **S37.422** **Contusion of ovary, bilateral** ♀
✓7ᵗʰ **S37.429** **Contusion of ovary, unspecified** ♀▽

✓6ᵗʰ **S37.43** **Laceration of ovary**
✓7ᵗʰ **S37.431** **Laceration of ovary, unilateral** ♀
✓7ᵗʰ **S37.432** **Laceration of ovary, bilateral** ♀
✓7ᵗʰ **S37.439** **Laceration of ovary, unspecified** ♀▽

✓6ᵗʰ **S37.49** **Other injury of ovary**
✓7ᵗʰ **S37.491** **Other injury of ovary, unilateral** ♀
✓7ᵗʰ **S37.492** **Other injury of ovary, bilateral** ♀
✓7ᵗʰ **S37.499** **Other injury of ovary, unspecified** ♀▽

✓5ᵗʰ **S37.5** **Injury of fallopian tube**
S37.50 **Unspecified injury of fallopian tube**
✓7ᵗʰ **S37.501** **Unspecified injury of fallopian tube, unilateral** ♀▽
✓7ᵗʰ **S37.502** **Unspecified injury of fallopian tube, bilateral** ♀▽
✓7ᵗʰ **S37.509** **Unspecified injury of fallopian tube, unspecified** ♀▽

✓6ᵗʰ **S37.51** **Primary blast injury of fallopian tube**
Blast injury of fallopian tube NOS
✓7ᵗʰ **S37.511** **Primary blast injury of fallopian tube, unilateral** ♀
✓7ᵗʰ **S37.512** **Primary blast injury of fallopian tube, bilateral** ♀
✓7ᵗʰ **S37.519** **Primary blast injury of fallopian tube, unspecified** ♀▽

✓6ᵗʰ **S37.52** **Contusion of fallopian tube**
✓7ᵗʰ **S37.521** **Contusion of fallopian tube, unilateral** ♀
✓7ᵗʰ **S37.522** **Contusion of fallopian tube, bilateral** ♀
✓7ᵗʰ **S37.529** **Contusion of fallopian tube, unspecified** ♀▽

✓6ᵗʰ **S37.53** **Laceration of fallopian tube**
✓7ᵗʰ **S37.531** **Laceration of fallopian tube, unilateral** ♀
✓7ᵗʰ **S37.532** **Laceration of fallopian tube, bilateral** ♀
✓7ᵗʰ **S37.539** **Laceration of fallopian tube, unspecified** ♀▽

✓6ᵗʰ **S37.59** **Other injury of fallopian tube**
Secondary blast injury of fallopian tube
✓7ᵗʰ **S37.591** **Other injury of fallopian tube, unilateral** ♀
✓7ᵗʰ **S37.592** **Other injury of fallopian tube, bilateral** ♀
✓7ᵗʰ **S37.599** **Other injury of fallopian tube, unspecified** ♀▽

✓5ᵗʰ **S37.6** **Injury of uterus**
EXCLUDES 1 *injury to gravid uterus (O9A.2-)*
injury to uterus during delivery (O71.-)
✓x7ᵗʰ **S37.60** **Unspecified injury of uterus** ♀▽
✓x7ᵗʰ **S37.62** **Contusion of uterus** ♀
✓x7ᵗʰ **S37.63** **Laceration of uterus** ♀
✓x7ᵗʰ **S37.69** **Other injury of uterus** ♀

✓5ᵗʰ **S37.8** **Injury of other urinary and pelvic organs**
✓6ᵗʰ **S37.81** **Injury of adrenal gland**
✓7ᵗʰ **S37.812** **Contusion of adrenal gland**
✓7ᵗʰ **S37.813** **Laceration of adrenal gland**
✓7ᵗʰ **S37.818** **Other injury of adrenal gland**
✓7ᵗʰ **S37.819** **Unspecified injury of adrenal gland** ▽

✓ Additional Character Req ✓x7ᵗʰ Placeholder Alert Case-Mix Diagnosis Manifestation ▽ Unspecified Dx EXCLUDES 1 Not coded here EXCLUDES 2 Not included here

✓6ᵗʰ **S37.82** Injury of prostate

    ✓7ᵗʰ **S37.822** Contusion of prostate   ♂

    ✓7ᵗʰ **S37.823** Laceration of prostate   ♂

    ✓7ᵗʰ **S37.828** Other injury of prostate   ♂

    ✓7ᵗʰ **S37.829** Unspecified injury of prostate   ♂▽

✓6ᵗʰ **S37.89** Injury of other urinary and pelvic organ

    ✓7ᵗʰ **S37.892** Contusion of other urinary and pelvic organ

    ✓7ᵗʰ **S37.893** Laceration of other urinary and pelvic organ

    ✓7ᵗʰ **S37.898** Other injury of other urinary and pelvic organ

    ✓7ᵗʰ **S37.899** Unspecified injury of other urinary and pelvic organ ▽

✓5ᵗʰ **S37.9** Injury of unspecified urinary and pelvic organ

    ✓ₓ7ᵗʰ **S37.90** Unspecified injury of unspecified urinary and pelvic organ ▽

    ✓ₓ7ᵗʰ **S37.92** Contusion of unspecified urinary and pelvic organ ▽

    ✓ₓ7ᵗʰ **S37.93** Laceration of unspecified urinary and pelvic organ ▽

    ✓ₓ7ᵗʰ **S37.99** Other injury of unspecified urinary and pelvic organ ▽

✓4ᵗʰ **S38** Crushing injury and traumatic amputation of abdomen, lower back, pelvis and external genitals

An amputation not identified as partial or complete should be coded to complete.

> The appropriate 7th character is to be added to each code from category S38.
> A   initial encounter
> D   subsequent encounter
> S   sequela

✓5ᵗʰ **S38.0** Crushing injury of external genital organs

Use additional code for any associated injuries

    ✓6ᵗʰ **S38.00** Crushing injury of unspecified external genital organs

        ✓7ᵗʰ **S38.001** Crushing injury of unspecified external genital organs, male ♂▽

        ✓7ᵗʰ **S38.002** Crushing injury of unspecified external genital organs, female ♀▽

    ✓ₓ7ᵗʰ **S38.01** Crushing injury of penis ♂

    ✓ₓ7ᵗʰ **S38.02** Crushing injury of scrotum and testis ♂

    ✓ₓ7ᵗʰ **S38.03** Crushing injury of vulva ♀

✓ₓ7ᵗʰ **S38.1** Crushing injury of abdomen, lower back, and pelvis

Use additional code for all associated injuries, such as:
fracture of thoracic or lumbar spine and pelvis (S22.0-, S32.-)
injury to intra-abdominal organs (S36.-)
injury to urinary and pelvic organs (S37.-)
open wound of abdominal wall (S31.-)
spinal cord injury (S34.0, S34.1-)

EXCLUDES 2 crushing injury of external genital organs (S38.0-)

✓5ᵗʰ **S38.2** Traumatic amputation of external genital organs

    ✓6ᵗʰ **S38.21** Traumatic amputation of female external genital organs

Traumatic amputation of clitoris
Traumatic amputation of labium (majus) (minus)
Traumatic amputation of vulva

        1,5 ✓7ᵗʰ **S38.211** Complete traumatic amputation of female external genital organs NRS♀

        1,5 ✓7ᵗʰ **S38.212** Partial traumatic amputation of female external genital organs NRS♀

    ✓6ᵗʰ **S38.22** Traumatic amputation of penis

        1,5 ✓7ᵗʰ **S38.221** Complete traumatic amputation of penis NRS♂

        1,5 ✓7ᵗʰ **S38.222** Partial traumatic amputation of penis NRS♂

    ✓6ᵗʰ **S38.23** Traumatic amputation of scrotum and testis

        1,5 ✓7ᵗʰ **S38.231** Complete traumatic amputation of scrotum and testis NRS♂

        1,5 ✓7ᵗʰ **S38.232** Partial traumatic amputation of scrotum and testis NRS♂

1,5 ✓ₓ7ᵗʰ **S38.3** Transection (partial) of abdomen NRS

✓4ᵗʰ **S39** Other and unspecified injuries of abdomen, lower back, pelvis and external genitals

Code also any associated open wound (S31.-)

EXCLUDES 2 sprain of joints and ligaments of lumbar spine and pelvis (S33.-)

> The appropriate 7th character is to be added to each code from category S39.
> A   initial encounter
> D   subsequent encounter
> S   sequela

✓5ᵗʰ **S39.0** Injury of muscle, fascia and tendon of abdomen, lower back and pelvis

    ✓6ᵗʰ **S39.00** Unspecified injury of muscle, fascia and tendon of abdomen, lower back and pelvis

        ✓7ᵗʰ **S39.001** Unspecified injury of muscle, fascia and tendon of abdomen ▽

        ✓7ᵗʰ **S39.002** Unspecified injury of muscle, fascia and tendon of lower back ▽

        ✓7ᵗʰ **S39.003** Unspecified injury of muscle, fascia and tendon of pelvis ▽

    ✓6ᵗʰ **S39.01** Strain of muscle, fascia and tendon of abdomen, lower back and pelvis

        ✓7ᵗʰ **S39.011** Strain of muscle, fascia and tendon of abdomen

        ✓7ᵗʰ **S39.012** Strain of muscle, fascia and tendon of lower back

        ✓7ᵗʰ **S39.013** Strain of muscle, fascia and tendon of pelvis

    ✓6ᵗʰ **S39.02** Laceration of muscle, fascia and tendon of abdomen, lower back and pelvis

        4,5 ✓7ᵗʰ **S39.021** Laceration of muscle, fascia and tendon of abdomen NRS

        4,5 ✓7ᵗʰ **S39.022** Laceration of muscle, fascia and tendon of lower back NRS

        4,5 ✓7ᵗʰ **S39.023** Laceration of muscle, fascia and tendon of pelvis NRS

    ✓6ᵗʰ **S39.09** Other injury of muscle, fascia and tendon of abdomen, lower back and pelvis

        ✓7ᵗʰ **S39.091** Other injury of muscle, fascia and tendon of abdomen

        ✓7ᵗʰ **S39.092** Other injury of muscle, fascia and tendon of lower back

        ✓7ᵗʰ **S39.093** Other injury of muscle, fascia and tendon of pelvis

✓5ᵗʰ **S39.8** Other specified injuries of abdomen, lower back, pelvis and external genitals

    ✓ₓ7ᵗʰ **S39.81** Other specified injuries of abdomen

    ✓ₓ7ᵗʰ **S39.82** Other specified injuries of lower back

    ✓ₓ7ᵗʰ **S39.83** Other specified injuries of pelvis

    ✓6ᵗʰ **S39.84** Other specified injuries of external genitals

        ✓7ᵗʰ **S39.840** Fracture of corpus cavernosum penis ♂

        ✓7ᵗʰ **S39.848** Other specified injuries of external genitals

✓5ᵗʰ **S39.9** Unspecified injury of abdomen, lower back, pelvis and external genitals

    ✓ₓ7ᵗʰ **S39.91** Unspecified injury of abdomen ▽

    ✓ₓ7ᵗʰ **S39.92** Unspecified injury of lower back ▽

    ✓ₓ7ᵗʰ **S39.93** Unspecified injury of pelvis ▽

    ✓ₓ7ᵗʰ **S39.94** Unspecified injury of external genitals ▽

---

1 Case-mix diagnosis with 7th character indicating subsequent encounter.
4 Case-mix diagnosis with 7th character indicating initial or subsequent encounter.
5 NRS supply diagnosis with 7th character indicating initial or subsequent encounter.

N Newborn: 0 P Pediatric: 0-17 M Maternity: 12-55 A Adult: 15-124 NRS Nonroutine supply Dx NCDx Noncancer Dx PDx Primary Dx ►◄ Revised Text ● New Code ▲ Revised Title

Injuries to the shoulder and upper arm (S40-S49)

INCLUDES injuries of axilla
injuries of scapular region
EXCLUDES 2 burns and corrosions (T20-T32)
frostbite (T33-T34)
injuries of elbow (S50-S59)
insect bite or sting, venomous (T63.4)

✔4ᵗʰ **S40 Superficial injury of shoulder and upper arm**

The appropriate 7th character is to be added to each code from
category S40.
A   initial encounter
D   subsequent encounter
S   sequela

✔5ᵗʰ **S40.0 Contusion of shoulder and upper arm**

✔6ᵗʰ **S40.01 Contusion of shoulder**

✔7ᵗʰ **S40.011 Contusion of right shoulder**
✔7ᵗʰ **S40.012 Contusion of left shoulder**
✔7ᵗʰ **S40.019 Contusion of unspecified shoulder** ▽

✔6ᵗʰ **S40.02 Contusion of upper arm**

✔7ᵗʰ **S40.021 Contusion of right upper arm**
✔7ᵗʰ **S40.022 Contusion of left upper arm**
✔7ᵗʰ **S40.029 Contusion of unspecified upper arm** ▽

✔5ᵗʰ **S40.2 Other superficial injuries of shoulder**

✔6ᵗʰ **S40.21 Abrasion of shoulder**

✔7ᵗʰ **S40.211 Abrasion of right shoulder**
✔7ᵗʰ **S40.212 Abrasion of left shoulder**
✔7ᵗʰ **S40.219 Abrasion of unspecified shoulder** ▽

✔6ᵗʰ **S40.22 Blister (nonthermal) of shoulder**

✔7ᵗʰ **S40.221 Blister (nonthermal) of right shoulder**
✔7ᵗʰ **S40.222 Blister (nonthermal) of left shoulder**
✔7ᵗʰ **S40.229 Blister (nonthermal) of unspecified shoulder** ▽

✔6ᵗʰ **S40.24 External constriction of shoulder**

✔7ᵗʰ **S40.241 External constriction of right shoulder**
✔7ᵗʰ **S40.242 External constriction of left shoulder**
✔7ᵗʰ **S40.249 External constriction of unspecified shoulder** ▽

✔6ᵗʰ **S40.25 Superficial foreign body of shoulder**
Splinter in the shoulder

✔7ᵗʰ **S40.251 Superficial foreign body of right shoulder**
✔7ᵗʰ **S40.252 Superficial foreign body of left shoulder**
✔7ᵗʰ **S40.259 Superficial foreign body of unspecified shoulder** ▽

✔6ᵗʰ **S40.26 Insect bite (nonvenomous) of shoulder**

✔7ᵗʰ **S40.261 Insect bite (nonvenomous) of right shoulder**
✔7ᵗʰ **S40.262 Insect bite (nonvenomous) of left shoulder**
✔7ᵗʰ **S40.269 Insect bite (nonvenomous) of unspecified shoulder** ▽

✔6ᵗʰ **S40.27 Other superficial bite of shoulder**
EXCLUDES 1 open bite of shoulder (S41.05)

✔7ᵗʰ **S40.271 Other superficial bite of right shoulder**
✔7ᵗʰ **S40.272 Other superficial bite of left shoulder**
✔7ᵗʰ **S40.279 Other superficial bite of unspecified shoulder** ▽

✔5ᵗʰ **S40.8 Other superficial injuries of upper arm**

✔6ᵗʰ **S40.81 Abrasion of upper arm**

✔7ᵗʰ **S40.811 Abrasion of right upper arm**
✔7ᵗʰ **S40.812 Abrasion of left upper arm**
✔7ᵗʰ **S40.819 Abrasion of unspecified upper arm** ▽

✔6ᵗʰ **S40.82 Blister (nonthermal) of upper arm**

✔7ᵗʰ **S40.821 Blister (nonthermal) of right upper arm**
✔7ᵗʰ **S40.822 Blister (nonthermal) of left upper arm**
✔7ᵗʰ **S40.829 Blister (nonthermal) of unspecified upper arm** ▽

✔6ᵗʰ **S40.84 External constriction of upper arm**

✔7ᵗʰ **S40.841 External constriction of right upper arm**

✔7ᵗʰ **S40.842 External constriction of left upper arm**
✔7ᵗʰ **S40.849 External constriction of unspecified upper arm** ▽

✔6ᵗʰ **S40.85 Superficial foreign body of upper arm**
Splinter in the upper arm

✔7ᵗʰ **S40.851 Superficial foreign body of right upper arm**
✔7ᵗʰ **S40.852 Superficial foreign body of left upper arm**
✔7ᵗʰ **S40.859 Superficial foreign body of unspecified upper arm** ▽

✔6ᵗʰ **S40.86 Insect bite (nonvenomous) of upper arm**

✔7ᵗʰ **S40.861 Insect bite (nonvenomous) of right upper arm**
✔7ᵗʰ **S40.862 Insect bite (nonvenomous) of left upper arm**
✔7ᵗʰ **S40.869 Insect bite (nonvenomous) of unspecified upper arm** ▽

✔6ᵗʰ **S40.87 Other superficial bite of upper arm**
EXCLUDES 1 open bite of upper arm (S41.14)
EXCLUDES 2 other superficial bite of shoulder (S40.27-)

✔7ᵗʰ **S40.871 Other superficial bite of right upper arm**
✔7ᵗʰ **S40.872 Other superficial bite of left upper arm**
✔7ᵗʰ **S40.879 Other superficial bite of unspecified upper arm** ▽

✔5ᵗʰ **S40.9 Unspecified superficial injury of shoulder and upper arm**

✔6ᵗʰ **S40.91 Unspecified superficial injury of shoulder**

✔7ᵗʰ **S40.911 Unspecified superficial injury of right shoulder** ▽
✔7ᵗʰ **S40.912 Unspecified superficial injury of left shoulder** ▽
✔7ᵗʰ **S40.919 Unspecified superficial injury of unspecified shoulder** ▽

✔6ᵗʰ **S40.92 Unspecified superficial injury of upper arm**

✔7ᵗʰ **S40.921 Unspecified superficial injury of right upper arm** ▽
✔7ᵗʰ **S40.922 Unspecified superficial injury of left upper arm** ▽
✔7ᵗʰ **S40.929 Unspecified superficial injury of unspecified upper arm** ▽

✔4ᵗʰ **S41 Open wound of shoulder and upper arm**
Code also any associated wound infection
EXCLUDES 1 traumatic amputation of shoulder and upper arm (S48.-)
EXCLUDES 2 open fracture of shoulder and upper arm (S42.- with 7th character B or C)

The appropriate 7th character is to be added to each code from
category S41.
A   initial encounter
D   subsequent encounter
S   sequela

✔5ᵗʰ **S41.0 Open wound of shoulder**

✔6ᵗʰ **S41.00 Unspecified open wound of shoulder**

5 ✔7ᵗʰ **S41.001 Unspecified open wound of right shoulder** NRS ▽
5 ✔7ᵗʰ **S41.002 Unspecified open wound of left shoulder** NRS ▽
5 ✔7ᵗʰ **S41.009 Unspecified open wound of unspecified shoulder** NRS ▽

✔6ᵗʰ **S41.01 Laceration without foreign body of shoulder**

4,5 ✔7ᵗʰ **S41.011 Laceration without foreign body of right shoulder** NRS
4,5 ✔7ᵗʰ **S41.012 Laceration without foreign body of left shoulder** NRS
✔7ᵗʰ **S41.019 Laceration without foreign body of unspecified shoulder** ▽

✔6ᵗʰ **S41.02 Laceration with foreign body of shoulder**

4,5 ✔7ᵗʰ **S41.021 Laceration with foreign body of right shoulder** NRS
4,5 ✔7ᵗʰ **S41.022 Laceration with foreign body of left shoulder** NRS
✔7ᵗʰ **S41.029 Laceration with foreign body of unspecified shoulder** ▽

---

4 Case-mix diagnosis with 7th character indicating initial or subsequent encounter.
5 NRS supply diagnosis with 7th character indicating initial or subsequent encounter.

☑ Additional Character Req   ✔x7ᵗʰ Placeholder Alert   Case-Mix Diagnosis   Manifestation   ▽ Unspecified Dx   **EXCLUDES 1** Not coded here   **EXCLUDES 2** Not included here

✓6ᵗʰ S41.03   Puncture wound without foreign body of shoulder

> 4,5 ✓7ᵗʰ **S41.031**   **Puncture wound without foreign body of right shoulder**   NRS
>
> 4,5 ✓7ᵗʰ **S41.032**   **Puncture wound without foreign body of left shoulder**   NRS
>
> 4,5 ✓7ᵗʰ **S41.039**   **Puncture wound without foreign body of unspecified shoulder**   ▽

✓6ᵗʰ S41.04   Puncture wound with foreign body of shoulder

> 4,5 ✓7ᵗʰ **S41.041**   **Puncture wound with foreign body of right shoulder**   NRS
>
> 4,5 ✓7ᵗʰ **S41.042**   **Puncture wound with foreign body of left shoulder**   NRS
>
> ✓7ᵗʰ **S41.049**   **Puncture wound with foreign body of unspecified shoulder**   ▽

✓6ᵗʰ S41.05   Open bite of shoulder
> Bite of shoulder NOS
> *EXCLUDES 1*   superficial bite of shoulder (S40.27)
>
> 4,5 ✓7ᵗʰ **S41.051**   **Open bite of right shoulder**   NRS
>
> 4,5 ✓7ᵗʰ **S41.052**   **Open bite of left shoulder**   NRS
>
> ✓7ᵗʰ **S41.059**   **Open bite of unspecified shoulder**   ▽

✓5ᵗʰ S41.1   Open wound of upper arm

✓6ᵗʰ S41.10   Unspecified open wound of upper arm
> AHA: 2016, 3Q, 24
>
> 5 ✓7ᵗʰ **S41.101**   **Unspecified open wound of right upper arm**   NRS ▽
>
> 5 ✓7ᵗʰ **S41.102**   **Unspecified open wound of left upper arm**   NRS ▽
>
> 5 ✓7ᵗʰ **S41.109**   **Unspecified open wound of unspecified upper arm**   NRS ▽

✓6ᵗʰ S41.11   Laceration without foreign body of upper arm

> 4,5 ✓7ᵗʰ **S41.111**   **Laceration without foreign body of right upper arm**   NRS
>
> 4,5 ✓7ᵗʰ **S41.112**   **Laceration without foreign body of left upper arm**   NRS
>
> ✓7ᵗʰ **S41.119**   **Laceration without foreign body of unspecified upper arm**   ▽

✓6ᵗʰ S41.12   Laceration with foreign body of upper arm

> 4,5 ✓7ᵗʰ **S41.121**   **Laceration with foreign body of right upper arm**   NRS
>
> 4,5 ✓7ᵗʰ **S41.122**   **Laceration with foreign body of left upper arm**   NRS
>
> ✓7ᵗʰ **S41.129**   **Laceration with foreign body of unspecified upper arm**   ▽

✓6ᵗʰ S41.13   Puncture wound without foreign body of upper arm
> AHA: 2016, 3Q, 24
>
> 4,5 ✓7ᵗʰ **S41.131**   **Puncture wound without foreign body of right upper arm**   NRS
>
> 4,5 ✓7ᵗʰ **S41.132**   **Puncture wound without foreign body of left upper arm**   NRS
>
> 4 ✓7ᵗʰ **S41.139**   **Puncture wound without foreign body of unspecified upper arm**   ▽

✓6ᵗʰ S41.14   Puncture wound with foreign body of upper arm
> AHA: 2016, 3Q, 24
>
> 4,5 ✓7ᵗʰ **S41.141**   **Puncture wound with foreign body of right upper arm**   NRS
>
> 4,5 ✓7ᵗʰ **S41.142**   **Puncture wound with foreign body of left upper arm**   NRS
>
> ✓7ᵗʰ **S41.149**   **Puncture wound with foreign body of unspecified upper arm**   ▽

✓6ᵗʰ S41.15   Open bite of upper arm
> Bite of upper arm NOS
> *EXCLUDES 1*   superficial bite of upper arm (S40.87)
>
> 4,5 ✓7ᵗʰ **S41.151**   **Open bite of right upper arm**   NRS
>
> 4,5 ✓7ᵗʰ **S41.152**   **Open bite of left upper arm**   NRS
>
> 5 ✓7ᵗʰ **S41.159**   **Open bite of unspecified upper arm**   NRS ▽

✓4ᵗʰ S42   **Fracture of shoulder and upper arm**
> NOTE   A fracture not indicated as displaced or nondisplaced should be coded to displaced.
> A fracture not indicated as open or closed should be coded to closed.
>
> *EXCLUDES 1*   traumatic amputation of shoulder and upper arm (S48.-)
> **AHA:** 2015, 3Q, 37-39
> **TIP:** The term "improper alignment" is not synonymous with malunion or nonunion of a fracture when noted in provider documentation.

> The appropriate 7th character is to be added to all codes from category S42 [unless otherwise indicated].
> A   initial encounter for closed fracture
> B   initial encounter for open fracture
> D   subsequent encounter for fracture with routine healing
> G   subsequent encounter for fracture with delayed healing
> K   subsequent encounter for fracture with nonunion
> P   subsequent encounter for fracture with malunion
> S   sequela

✓5ᵗʰ S42.0   **Fracture of clavicle**

✓6ᵗʰ S42.00   Fracture of unspecified part of clavicle

> 1 ✓7ᵗʰ **S42.001**   **Fracture of unspecified part of right clavicle**   ▽
>
> 1 ✓7ᵗʰ **S42.002**   **Fracture of unspecified part of left clavicle**   ▽
>
> ✓7ᵗʰ **S42.009**   **Fracture of unspecified part of unspecified clavicle**   ▽
> AHA: 2012, 4Q, 93

✓6ᵗʰ S42.01   Fracture of sternal end of clavicle

> 1 ✓7ᵗʰ **S42.011**   **Anterior displaced fracture of sternal end of right clavicle**
>
> 1 ✓7ᵗʰ **S42.012**   **Anterior displaced fracture of sternal end of left clavicle**
>
> 1 ✓7ᵗʰ **S42.013**   **Anterior displaced fracture of sternal end of unspecified clavicle**   ▽
> Displaced fracture of sternal end of clavicle NOS
>
> 1 ✓7ᵗʰ **S42.014**   **Posterior displaced fracture of sternal end of right clavicle**
>
> 1 ✓7ᵗʰ **S42.015**   **Posterior displaced fracture of sternal end of left clavicle**
>
> ✓7ᵗʰ **S42.016**   **Posterior displaced fracture of sternal end of unspecified clavicle**   ▽
>
> 1 ✓7ᵗʰ **S42.017**   **Nondisplaced fracture of sternal end of right clavicle**
>
> 1 ✓7ᵗʰ **S42.018**   **Nondisplaced fracture of sternal end of left clavicle**
>
> ✓7ᵗʰ **S42.019**   **Nondisplaced fracture of sternal end of unspecified clavicle**   ▽

✓6ᵗʰ S42.02   Fracture of shaft of clavicle

> 1 ✓7ᵗʰ **S42.021**   **Displaced fracture of shaft of right clavicle**
>
> 1 ✓7ᵗʰ **S42.022**   **Displaced fracture of shaft of left clavicle**
>
> ✓7ᵗʰ **S42.023**   **Displaced fracture of shaft of unspecified clavicle**   ▽
>
> 1 ✓7ᵗʰ **S42.024**   **Nondisplaced fracture of shaft of right clavicle**
>
> 1 ✓7ᵗʰ **S42.025**   **Nondisplaced fracture of shaft of left clavicle**
>
> ✓7ᵗʰ **S42.026**   **Nondisplaced fracture of shaft of unspecified clavicle**   ▽

✓6ᵗʰ S42.03   Fracture of lateral end of clavicle
> Fracture of acromial end of clavicle
>
> 1 ✓7ᵗʰ **S42.031**   **Displaced fracture of lateral end of right clavicle**
>
> 1 ✓7ᵗʰ **S42.032**   **Displaced fracture of lateral end of left clavicle**
>
> ✓7ᵗʰ **S42.033**   **Displaced fracture of lateral end of unspecified clavicle**   ▽
>
> 1 ✓7ᵗʰ **S42.034**   **Nondisplaced fracture of lateral end of right clavicle**
>
> 1 ✓7ᵗʰ **S42.035**   **Nondisplaced fracture of lateral end of left clavicle**
>
> ✓7ᵗʰ **S42.036**   **Nondisplaced fracture of lateral end of unspecified clavicle**   ▽

---

1   Case-mix diagnosis with 7th character indicating subsequent encounter.
4   Case-mix diagnosis with 7th character indicating initial or subsequent encounter.
5   NRS supply diagnosis with 7th character indicating initial or subsequent encounter.

Ⓝ Newborn: 0   Ⓟ Pediatric: 0-17   Ⓜ Maternity: 12-55   Ⓐ Adult: 15-124   NRS Nonroutine supply Dx   NCDx Noncancer Dx   PDx Primary Dx   ▶◀ Revised Text   ● New Code   ▲ Revised Title

✓5th **S42.1**   **Fracture of** scapula

   ✓6th **S42.10**   **Fracture of** unspecified **part of scapula**

     1 ✓7th **S42.101**   **Fracture of unspecified part of scapula,** right **shoulder** ▽

     1 ✓7th **S42.102**   **Fracture of unspecified part of scapula,** left **shoulder** ▽

     ✓7th **S42.109**   **Fracture of unspecified part of scapula,** unspecified shoulder ▽

   ✓6th **S42.11**   **Fracture of** body **of scapula**

     1 ✓7th **S42.111**   Displaced **fracture of body of scapula,** right **shoulder**

     1 ✓7th **S42.112**   Displaced **fracture of body of scapula,** left **shoulder**

     ✓7th **S42.113**   Displaced **fracture of body of scapula,** unspecified shoulder ▽

     1 ✓7th **S42.114**   Nondisplaced **fracture of body of scapula,** right **shoulder**

     1 ✓7th **S42.115**   Nondisplaced **fracture of body of scapula,** left **shoulder**

     ✓7th **S42.116**   Nondisplaced **fracture of body of scapula, unspecified shoulder** ▽

   ✓6th **S42.12**   **Fracture of** acromial process

     1 ✓7th **S42.121**   Displaced **fracture of acromial process,** right **shoulder**

     1 ✓7th **S42.122**   Displaced **fracture of acromial process,** left **shoulder**

     ✓7th **S42.123**   Displaced **fracture of acromial process,** unspecified shoulder ▽

     1 ✓7th **S42.124**   Nondisplaced **fracture of acromial process, right shoulder**

     1 ✓7th **S42.125**   Nondisplaced **fracture of acromial process,** left **shoulder**

     ✓7th **S42.126**   Nondisplaced **fracture of acromial process, unspecified shoulder** ▽

   ✓6th **S42.13**   **Fracture of** coracoid process

     1 ✓7th **S42.131**   Displaced **fracture of coracoid process,** right **shoulder**

     1 ✓7th **S42.132**   Displaced **fracture of coracoid process,** left **shoulder**

     ✓7th **S42.133**   Displaced **fracture of coracoid process,** unspecified shoulder ▽

     1 ✓7th **S42.134**   Nondisplaced **fracture of coracoid process, right shoulder**

     1 ✓7th **S42.135**   Nondisplaced **fracture of coracoid process,** left **shoulder**

     ✓7th **S42.136**   Nondisplaced **fracture of coracoid process, unspecified shoulder** ▽

   ✓6th **S42.14**   **Fracture of** glenoid cavity **of scapula**

     1 ✓7th **S42.141**   Displaced **fracture of glenoid cavity of scapula,** right **shoulder**

     1 ✓7th **S42.142**   Displaced **fracture of glenoid cavity of scapula,** left **shoulder**

     ✓7th **S42.143**   Displaced **fracture of glenoid cavity of scapula, unspecified shoulder** ▽

     1 ✓7th **S42.144**   Nondisplaced **fracture of glenoid cavity of scapula,** right **shoulder**

     1 ✓7th **S42.145**   Nondisplaced **fracture of glenoid cavity of scapula,** left **shoulder**

     ✓7th **S42.146**   Nondisplaced **fracture of glenoid cavity of scapula, unspecified shoulder** ▽

   ✓6th **S42.15**   **Fracture of** neck **of scapula**

     1 ✓7th **S42.151**   Displaced **fracture of neck of scapula,** right **shoulder**

     1 ✓7th **S42.152**   Displaced **fracture of neck of scapula,** left **shoulder**

     ✓7th **S42.153**   Displaced **fracture of neck of scapula, unspecified shoulder** ▽

     1 ✓7th **S42.154**   Nondisplaced **fracture of neck of scapula, right shoulder**

     1 ✓7th **S42.155**   Nondisplaced **fracture of neck of scapula,** left **shoulder**

     ✓7th **S42.156**   Nondisplaced **fracture of neck of scapula, unspecified shoulder** ▽

   ✓6th **S42.19**   **Fracture of** other **part of scapula**

     1 ✓7th **S42.191**   **Fracture of other part of scapula,** right **shoulder**

     1 ✓7th **S42.192**   **Fracture of other part of scapula,** left **shoulder**

     ✓7th **S42.199**   **Fracture of other part of scapula, unspecified shoulder** ▽

✓5th **S42.2**   **Fracture of** upper end of humerus

   Fracture of proximal end of humerus

   EXCLUDES 2   *fracture of shaft of humerus (S42.3-)*
            physeal fracture of upper end of humerus (S49.0-)

   ✓6th **S42.20**   Unspecified **fracture of upper end of humerus**

     1 ✓7th **S42.201**   **Unspecified fracture of upper end of** right **humerus** ▽

     1 ✓7th **S42.202**   **Unspecified fracture of upper end of** left **humerus** ▽

     ✓7th **S42.209**   **Unspecified fracture of upper end of unspecified humerus**

   ✓6th **S42.21**   Unspecified **fracture of** surgical neck **of humerus**

     Fracture of neck of humerus NOS

     1 ✓7th **S42.211**   **Unspecified** displaced **fracture of surgical neck of** right **humerus** ▽

     1 ✓7th **S42.212**   **Unspecified** displaced **fracture of surgical neck of** left **humerus** ▽

     ✓7th **S42.213**   **Unspecified** displaced **fracture of surgical neck of unspecified humerus** ▽

     1 ✓7th **S42.214**   **Unspecified** nondisplaced **fracture of surgical neck of** right **humerus** ▽

     1 ✓7th **S42.215**   **Unspecified** nondisplaced **fracture of surgical neck of** left **humerus** ▽

     ✓7th **S42.216**   **Unspecified** nondisplaced **fracture of surgical neck of unspecified humerus** ▽

   ✓6th **S42.22**   2-part **fracture of** surgical neck **of humerus**

     1 ✓7th **S42.221**   **2-part** displaced **fracture of surgical neck of** right **humerus**

     1 ✓7th **S42.222**   **2-part** displaced **fracture of surgical neck of** left **humerus**

     ✓7th **S42.223**   **2-part** displaced **fracture of surgical neck of unspecified humerus** ▽

     1 ✓7th **S42.224**   **2-part** nondisplaced **fracture of surgical neck of** right **humerus**

     1 ✓7th **S42.225**   **2-part** nondisplaced **fracture of surgical neck of** left **humerus**

     ✓7th **S42.226**   **2-part** nondisplaced **fracture of surgical neck of unspecified humerus** ▽

   ✓6th **S42.23**   3-part **fracture of** surgical neck **of humerus**

     1 ✓7th **S42.231**   **3-part fracture of surgical neck of** right **humerus**

     1 ✓7th **S42.232**   **3-part fracture of surgical neck of** left **humerus**

     ✓7th **S42.239**   **3-part fracture of surgical neck of unspecified humerus** ▽

   ✓6th **S42.24**   4-part **fracture of** surgical neck **of humerus**

     1 ✓7th **S42.241**   **4-part fracture of surgical neck of** right **humerus**

     1 ✓7th **S42.242**   **4-part fracture of surgical neck of** left **humerus**

     ✓7th **S42.249**   **4-part fracture of surgical neck of unspecified humerus** ▽

   ✓6th **S42.25**   **Fracture of** greater tuberosity **of humerus**

     1 ✓7th **S42.251**   Displaced **fracture of greater tuberosity of** right **humerus**

     1 ✓7th **S42.252**   Displaced **fracture of greater tuberosity of** left **humerus**

     ✓7th **S42.253**   Displaced **fracture of greater tuberosity of unspecified humerus** ▽

     1 ✓7th **S42.254**   Nondisplaced **fracture of greater tuberosity of** right **humerus**

     1 ✓7th **S42.255**   Nondisplaced **fracture of greater tuberosity of** left **humerus**

     ✓7th **S42.256**   Nondisplaced **fracture of greater tuberosity of unspecified humerus** ▽

---

1   Case-mix diagnosis with 7th character indicating subsequent encounter.

✓ Additional Character Req   ✓x7th Placeholder Alert   Case-Mix Diagnosis   Manifestation   ▽ Unspecified Dx   EXCLUDES 1 Not coded here   EXCLUDES 2 Not included here

√6ᵗʰ **S42.26** Fracture of lester tuberosity of humerus

¹ √7ᵗʰ **S42.261** Displaced fracture of lesser tuberosity of right humerus

¹ √7ᵗʰ **S42.262** Displaced fracture of lesser tuberosity of left humerus

√7ᵗʰ **S42.263** Displaced fracture of lesser tuberosity of unspecified humerus ▽

¹ √7ᵗʰ **S42.264** Nondisplaced fracture of lesser tuberosity of right humerus

¹ √7ᵗʰ **S42.265** Nondisplaced fracture of lesser tuberosity of left humerus

√7ᵗʰ **S42.266** Nondisplaced fracture of lesser tuberosity of unspecified humerus ▽

√6ᵗʰ **S42.27** Torus fracture of upper end of humerus

> The appropriate 7th character is to be added to all codes in subcategory S42.27.
> A   initial encounter for closed fracture
> D   subsequent encounter for fracture with routine healing
> G   subsequent encounter for fracture with delayed healing
> K   subsequent encounter for fracture with nonunion
> P   subsequent encounter for fracture with malunion
> S   sequela

¹ √7ᵗʰ **S42.271** Torus fracture of upper end of right humerus

¹ √7ᵗʰ **S42.272** Torus fracture of upper end of left humerus

√7ᵗʰ **S42.279** Torus fracture of upper end of unspecified humerus ▽

√6ᵗʰ **S42.29** Other fracture of upper end of humerus
Fracture of anatomical neck of humerus
Fracture of articular head of humerus

¹ √7ᵗʰ **S42.291** Other displaced fracture of upper end of right humerus

¹ √7ᵗʰ **S42.292** Other displaced fracture of upper end of left humerus

√7ᵗʰ **S42.293** Other displaced fracture of upper end of unspecified humerus ▽

¹ √7ᵗʰ **S42.294** Other nondisplaced fracture of upper end of right humerus

¹ √7ᵗʰ **S42.295** Other nondisplaced fracture of upper end of left humerus

√7ᵗʰ **S42.296** Other nondisplaced fracture of upper end of unspecified humerus ▽

√5ᵗʰ **S42.3** Fracture of shaft of humerus
Fracture of humerus NOS
Fracture of upper arm NOS
EXCLUDES 2   physeal fractures of upper end of humerus (S49.0-)
        physeal fractures of lower end of humerus (S49.1-)

√6ᵗʰ **S42.30** Unspecified fracture of shaft of humerus

¹ √7ᵗʰ **S42.301** Unspecified fracture of shaft of humerus, right arm ▽

¹ √7ᵗʰ **S42.302** Unspecified fracture of shaft of humerus, left arm ▽

√7ᵗʰ **S42.309** Unspecified fracture of shaft of humerus, unspecified arm ▽

√6ᵗʰ **S42.31** Greenstick fracture of shaft of humerus

> The appropriate 7th character is to be added to all codes in subcategory S42.31.
> A   initial encounter for closed fracture
> D   subsequent encounter for fracture with routine healing
> G   subsequent encounter for fracture with delayed healing
> K   subsequent encounter for fracture with nonunion
> P   subsequent encounter for fracture with malunion
> S   sequela

¹ √7ᵗʰ **S42.311** Greenstick fracture of shaft of humerus, right arm

¹ √7ᵗʰ **S42.312** Greenstick fracture of shaft of humerus, left arm

√7ᵗʰ **S42.319** Greenstick fracture of shaft of humerus, unspecified arm ▽

√6ᵗʰ **S42.32** Transverse fracture of shaft of humerus

¹ √7ᵗʰ **S42.321** Displaced transverse fracture of shaft of humerus, right arm

¹ √7ᵗʰ **S42.322** Displaced transverse fracture of shaft of humerus, left arm

√7ᵗʰ **S42.323** Displaced transverse fracture of shaft of humerus, unspecified arm ▽

¹ √7ᵗʰ **S42.324** Nondisplaced transverse fracture of shaft of humerus, right arm

¹ √7ᵗʰ **S42.325** Nondisplaced transverse fracture of shaft of humerus, left arm

√7ᵗʰ **S42.326** Nondisplaced transverse fracture of shaft of humerus, unspecified arm ▽

√6ᵗʰ **S42.33** Oblique fracture of shaft of humerus

¹ √7ᵗʰ **S42.331** Displaced oblique fracture of shaft of humerus, right arm

¹ √7ᵗʰ **S42.332** Displaced oblique fracture of shaft of humerus, left arm

√7ᵗʰ **S42.333** Displaced oblique fracture of shaft of humerus, unspecified arm ▽

¹ √7ᵗʰ **S42.334** Nondisplaced oblique fracture of shaft of humerus, right arm

¹ √7ᵗʰ **S42.335** Nondisplaced oblique fracture of shaft of humerus, left arm

√7ᵗʰ **S42.336** Nondisplaced oblique fracture of shaft of humerus, unspecified arm ▽

√6ᵗʰ **S42.34** Spiral fracture of shaft of humerus

¹ √7ᵗʰ **S42.341** Displaced spiral fracture of shaft of humerus, right arm

¹ √7ᵗʰ **S42.342** Displaced spiral fracture of shaft of humerus, left arm

√7ᵗʰ **S42.343** Displaced spiral fracture of shaft of humerus, unspecified arm ▽

¹ √7ᵗʰ **S42.344** Nondisplaced spiral fracture of shaft of humerus, right arm

¹ √7ᵗʰ **S42.345** Nondisplaced spiral fracture of shaft of humerus, left arm

√7ᵗʰ **S42.346** Nondisplaced spiral fracture of shaft of humerus, unspecified arm ▽

√6ᵗʰ **S42.35** Comminuted fracture of shaft of humerus

¹ √7ᵗʰ **S42.351** Displaced comminuted fracture of shaft of humerus, right arm

¹ √7ᵗʰ **S42.352** Displaced comminuted fracture of shaft of humerus, left arm

√7ᵗʰ **S42.353** Displaced comminuted fracture of shaft of humerus, unspecified arm ▽

¹ √7ᵗʰ **S42.354** Nondisplaced comminuted fracture of shaft of humerus, right arm

¹ √7ᵗʰ **S42.355** Nondisplaced comminuted fracture of shaft of humerus, left arm

√7ᵗʰ **S42.356** Nondisplaced comminuted fracture of shaft of humerus, unspecified arm ▽

√6ᵗʰ **S42.36** Segmental fracture of shaft of humerus

¹ √7ᵗʰ **S42.361** Displaced segmental fracture of shaft of humerus, right arm

¹ √7ᵗʰ **S42.362** Displaced segmental fracture of shaft of humerus, left arm

√7ᵗʰ **S42.363** Displaced segmental fracture of shaft of humerus, unspecified arm ▽

¹ √7ᵗʰ **S42.364** Nondisplaced segmental fracture of shaft of humerus, right arm

¹ √7ᵗʰ **S42.365** Nondisplaced segmental fracture of shaft of humerus, left arm

√7ᵗʰ **S42.366** Nondisplaced segmental fracture of shaft of humerus, unspecified arm ▽

√6ᵗʰ **S42.39** Other fracture of shaft of humerus

¹ √7ᵗʰ **S42.391** Other fracture of shaft of right humerus ▽

¹ √7ᵗʰ **S42.392** Other fracture of shaft of left humerus ▽

√7ᵗʰ **S42.399** Other fracture of shaft of unspecified humerus ▽

---

¹   Case-mix diagnosis with 7th character indicating subsequent encounter.

N Newborn: 0   **P** Pediatric: 0-17   **M** Maternity: 12-55   **A** Adult: 15-124   **NRS** Nonroutine supply Dx   **NCDx** Noncancer Dx   **PDx** Primary Dx   ▶◀ Revised Text   ● New Code   ▲ Revised Title

✓5ᵗʰ **S42.4** **Fracture of** lower end **of humerus**
Fracture of distal end of humerus
EXCLUDES 2   *fracture of shaft of humerus (S42.3-)*
physeal fracture of lower end of humerus (S49.1-)

✓6ᵗʰ **S42.40** Unspecified **fracture of lower end of humerus**
Fracture of elbow NOS

   1 ✓7ᵗʰ **S42.401** Unspecified **fracture of lower end of** right **humerus** ▽

   1 ✓7ᵗʰ **S42.402** Unspecified **fracture of lower end of** left **humerus** ▽

   ✓7ᵗʰ **S42.409** Unspecified **fracture of lower end of unspecified humerus** ▽

✓6ᵗʰ **S42.41** Simple supracondylar **fracture** without intercondylar **fracture of humerus**

   1 ✓7ᵗʰ **S42.411** Displaced **simple supracondylar fracture without intercondylar fracture of** right **humerus**

   1 ✓7ᵗʰ **S42.412** Displaced **simple supracondylar fracture without intercondylar fracture of** left **humerus**

   ✓7ᵗʰ **S42.413** Displaced **simple supracondylar fracture without intercondylar fracture of unspecified humerus** ▽

   1 ✓7ᵗʰ **S42.414** Nondisplaced **simple supracondylar fracture without intercondylar fracture of** right **humerus**

   1 ✓7ᵗʰ **S42.415** Nondisplaced **simple supracondylar fracture without intercondylar fracture of** left **humerus**

   ✓7ᵗʰ **S42.416** Nondisplaced **simple supracondylar fracture without intercondylar fracture of unspecified humerus** ▽

✓6ᵗʰ **S42.42** Comminuted supracondylar **fracture** without intercondylar **fracture of humerus**

   1 ✓7ᵗʰ **S42.421** Displaced **comminuted supracondylar fracture without intercondylar fracture of** right **humerus**

   1 ✓7ᵗʰ **S42.422** Displaced **comminuted supracondylar fracture without intercondylar fracture of** left **humerus**

   ✓7ᵗʰ **S42.423** Displaced **comminuted supracondylar fracture without intercondylar fracture of unspecified humerus** ▽

   1 ✓7ᵗʰ **S42.424** Nondisplaced **comminuted supracondylar fracture without intercondylar fracture of** right **humerus**

   1 ✓7ᵗʰ **S42.425** Nondisplaced **comminuted supracondylar fracture without intercondylar fracture of** left **humerus**

   ✓7ᵗʰ **S42.426** Nondisplaced **comminuted supracondylar fracture without intercondylar fracture of unspecified humerus** ▽

✓6ᵗʰ **S42.43** Fracture (avulsion) of lateral epicondyle **of humerus**

   1 ✓7ᵗʰ **S42.431** Displaced **fracture (avulsion) of lateral epicondyle of** right **humerus**

   1 ✓7ᵗʰ **S42.432** Displaced **fracture (avulsion) of lateral epicondyle of** left **humerus**

   ✓7ᵗʰ **S42.433** Displaced **fracture (avulsion) of lateral epicondyle of unspecified humerus** ▽

   1 ✓7ᵗʰ **S42.434** Nondisplaced **fracture (avulsion) of lateral epicondyle of** right **humerus**

   1 ✓7ᵗʰ **S42.435** Nondisplaced **fracture (avulsion) of lateral epicondyle of** left **humerus**

   ✓7ᵗʰ **S42.436** Nondisplaced **fracture (avulsion) of lateral epicondyle of unspecified humerus** ▽

✓6ᵗʰ **S42.44** Fracture (avulsion) of medial epicondyle **of humerus**

   1 ✓7ᵗʰ **S42.441** Displaced **fracture (avulsion) of medial epicondyle of** right **humerus**

   1 ✓7ᵗʰ **S42.442** Displaced **fracture (avulsion) of medial epicondyle of** left **humerus**

   ✓7ᵗʰ **S42.443** Displaced **fracture (avulsion) of medial epicondyle of unspecified humerus** ▽

   1 ✓7ᵗʰ **S42.444** Nondisplaced **fracture (avulsion) of medial epicondyle of** right **humerus**

   1 ✓7ᵗʰ **S42.445** Nondisplaced **fracture (avulsion) of medial epicondyle of** left **humerus**

   ✓7ᵗʰ **S42.446** Nondisplaced **fracture (avulsion) of medial epicondyle of unspecified humerus** ▽

   1 ✓7ᵗʰ **S42.447** Incarcerated **fracture (avulsion) of medial epicondyle of** right **humerus**

   1 ✓7ᵗʰ **S42.448** Incarcerated **fracture (avulsion) of medial epicondyle of** left **humerus**

   ✓7ᵗʰ **S42.449** Incarcerated **fracture (avulsion) of medial epicondyle of unspecified humerus** ▽

✓6ᵗʰ **S42.45** Fracture of lateral condyle **of humerus**
Fracture of capitellum of humerus

   1 ✓7ᵗʰ **S42.451** Displaced **fracture of lateral condyle of** right **humerus**

   1 ✓7ᵗʰ **S42.452** Displaced **fracture of lateral condyle of** left **humerus**

   ✓7ᵗʰ **S42.453** Displaced **fracture of lateral condyle of unspecified humerus** ▽

   1 ✓7ᵗʰ **S42.454** Nondisplaced **fracture of lateral condyle of** right **humerus**

   1 ✓7ᵗʰ **S42.455** Nondisplaced **fracture of lateral condyle of** left **humerus**

   ✓7ᵗʰ **S42.456** Nondisplaced **fracture of lateral condyle of unspecified humerus** ▽

✓6ᵗʰ **S42.46** Fracture of medial condyle **of humerus**
Trochlea fracture of humerus

   1 ✓7ᵗʰ **S42.461** Displaced **fracture of medial condyle of** right **humerus**

   1 ✓7ᵗʰ **S42.462** Displaced **fracture of medial condyle of** left **humerus**

   ✓7ᵗʰ **S42.463** Displaced **fracture of medial condyle of unspecified humerus** ▽

   1 ✓7ᵗʰ **S42.464** Nondisplaced **fracture of medial condyle of** right **humerus**

   1 ✓7ᵗʰ **S42.465** Nondisplaced **fracture of medial condyle of** left **humerus**

   ✓7ᵗʰ **S42.466** Nondisplaced **fracture of medial condyle of unspecified humerus** ▽

✓6ᵗʰ **S42.47** Transcondylar **fracture of humerus**

   1 ✓7ᵗʰ **S42.471** Displaced **transcondylar fracture of** right **humerus**

   1 ✓7ᵗʰ **S42.472** Displaced **transcondylar fracture of** left **humerus**

   ✓7ᵗʰ **S42.473** Displaced **transcondylar fracture of unspecified humerus** ▽

   1 ✓7ᵗʰ **S42.474** Nondisplaced **transcondylar fracture of** right **humerus**

   1 ✓7ᵗʰ **S42.475** Nondisplaced **transcondylar fracture of** left **humerus**

   ✓7ᵗʰ **S42.476** Nondisplaced **transcondylar fracture of unspecified humerus** ▽

✓6ᵗʰ **S42.48** Torus **fracture of lower end of humerus**

> The appropriate 7th character is to be added to all codes in subcategory S42.48.
> A   initial encounter for closed fracture
> D   subsequent encounter for fracture with routine healing
> G   subsequent encounter for fracture with delayed healing
> K   subsequent encounter for fracture with nonunion
> P   subsequent encounter for fracture with malunion
> S   sequela

   1 ✓7ᵗʰ **S42.481** Torus fracture of lower end of right **humerus**

   1 ✓7ᵗʰ **S42.482** Torus fracture of lower end of left **humerus**

   ✓7ᵗʰ **S42.489** Torus fracture of lower end of unspecified humerus ▽

✓6ᵗʰ **S42.49** Other **fracture of lower end of humerus**

   1 ✓7ᵗʰ **S42.491** Other displaced **fracture of lower end of** right **humerus**

   1 ✓7ᵗʰ **S42.492** Other displaced **fracture of lower end of** left **humerus**

---

1   Case-mix diagnosis with 7th character indicating subsequent encounter.

✓ Additional Character Req   ✓x7ᵗʰ Placeholder Alert   Case-Mix Diagnosis   Manifestation   ▽ Unspecified Dx   EXCLUDES 1 Not coded here   EXCLUDES 2 Not included here

√7ᵗʰ S42.493 Other displaced fracture of lower end of unspecified humerus ▽

1 √7ᵗʰ S42.494 Other nondisplaced fracture of lower end of right humerus

1 √7ᵗʰ S42.495 Other nondisplaced fracture of lower end of left humerus

√7ᵗʰ S42.496 Other nondisplaced fracture of lower end of unspecified humerus ▽

√5ᵗʰ S42.9 Fracture of shoulder girdle, part unspecified
Fracture of shoulder NOS

√×7ᵗʰ S42.90 Fracture of unspecified shoulder girdle, part unspecified ▽

1 √×7ᵗʰ S42.91 Fracture of right shoulder girdle, part unspecified ▽

1 √×7ᵗʰ S42.92 Fracture of left shoulder girdle, part unspecified ▽

√4ᵗʰ S43 Dislocation and sprain of joints and ligaments of shoulder girdle

     INCLUDES   avulsion of joint or ligament of shoulder girdle
laceration of cartilage, joint or ligament of shoulder girdle
sprain of cartilage, joint or ligament of shoulder girdle
traumatic hemarthrosis of joint or ligament of shoulder girdle
traumatic rupture of joint or ligament of shoulder girdle
traumatic subluxation of joint or ligament of shoulder girdle
traumatic tear of joint or ligament of shoulder girdle

Code also any associated open wound
     EXCLUDES 2   strain of muscle, fascia and tendon of shoulder and upper arm (S46.-)

The appropriate 7th character is to be added to each code from category S43.
A   initial encounter
D   subsequent encounter
S   sequela

√5ᵗʰ S43.0 Subluxation and dislocation of shoulder joint
Dislocation of glenohumeral joint
Subluxation of glenohumeral joint

√6ᵗʰ S43.00 Unspecified subluxation and dislocation of shoulder joint
Dislocation of humerus NOS
Subluxation of humerus NOS

1 √7ᵗʰ S43.001 Unspecified subluxation of right shoulder joint ▽

1 √7ᵗʰ S43.002 Unspecified subluxation of left shoulder joint ▽

√7ᵗʰ S43.003 Unspecified subluxation of unspecified shoulder joint ▽

1 √7ᵗʰ S43.004 Unspecified dislocation of right shoulder joint ▽

1 √7ᵗʰ S43.005 Unspecified dislocation of left shoulder joint ▽

√7ᵗʰ S43.006 Unspecified dislocation of unspecified shoulder joint ▽

√6ᵗʰ S43.01 Anterior subluxation and dislocation of humerus

1 √7ᵗʰ S43.011 Anterior subluxation of right humerus

1 √7ᵗʰ S43.012 Anterior subluxation of left humerus

√7ᵗʰ S43.013 Anterior subluxation of unspecified humerus ▽

1 √7ᵗʰ S43.014 Anterior dislocation of right humerus

1 √7ᵗʰ S43.015 Anterior dislocation of left humerus

√7ᵗʰ S43.016 Anterior dislocation of unspecified humerus ▽

√6ᵗʰ S43.02 Posterior subluxation and dislocation of humerus

1 √7ᵗʰ S43.021 Posterior subluxation of right humerus

1 √7ᵗʰ S43.022 Posterior subluxation of left humerus

√7ᵗʰ S43.023 Posterior subluxation of unspecified humerus ▽

1 √7ᵗʰ S43.024 Posterior dislocation of right humerus

1 √7ᵗʰ S43.025 Posterior dislocation of left humerus

√7ᵗʰ S43.026 Posterior dislocation of unspecified humerus ▽

√6ᵗʰ S43.03 Inferior subluxation and dislocation of humerus

1 √7ᵗʰ S43.031 Inferior subluxation of right humerus

1 √7ᵗʰ S43.032 Inferior subluxation of left humerus

√7ᵗʰ S43.033 Inferior subluxation of unspecified humerus ▽

1 √7ᵗʰ S43.034 Inferior dislocation of right humerus

1 √7ᵗʰ S43.035 Inferior dislocation of left humerus

√7ᵗʰ S43.036 Inferior dislocation of unspecified humerus ▽

√6ᵗʰ S43.08 Other subluxation and dislocation of shoulder joint

1 √7ᵗʰ S43.081 Other subluxation of right shoulder joint

1 √7ᵗʰ S43.082 Other subluxation of left shoulder joint

√7ᵗʰ S43.083 Other subluxation of unspecified shoulder joint ▽

1 √7ᵗʰ S43.084 Other dislocation of right shoulder joint

1 √7ᵗʰ S43.085 Other dislocation of left shoulder joint

√7ᵗʰ S43.086 Other dislocation of unspecified shoulder joint ▽

√5ᵗʰ S43.1 Subluxation and dislocation of acromioclavicular joint

√6ᵗʰ S43.10 Unspecified dislocation of acromioclavicular joint

1 √7ᵗʰ S43.101 Unspecified dislocation of right acromioclavicular joint ▽

1 √7ᵗʰ S43.102 Unspecified dislocation of left acromioclavicular joint ▽

√7ᵗʰ S43.109 Unspecified dislocation of unspecified acromioclavicular joint ▽

√6ᵗʰ S43.11 Subluxation of acromioclavicular joint

1 √7ᵗʰ S43.111 Subluxation of right acromioclavicular joint

1 √7ᵗʰ S43.112 Subluxation of left acromioclavicular joint

√7ᵗʰ S43.119 Subluxation of unspecified acromioclavicular joint ▽

√6ᵗʰ S43.12 Dislocation of acromioclavicular joint, 100%-200% displacement

1 √7ᵗʰ S43.121 Dislocation of right acromioclavicular joint, 100%-200% displacement

1 √7ᵗʰ S43.122 Dislocation of left acromioclavicular joint, 100%-200% displacement

√7ᵗʰ S43.129 Dislocation of unspecified acromioclavicular joint, 100%-200% displacement ▽

√6ᵗʰ S43.13 Dislocation of acromioclavicular joint, greater than 200% displacement

1 √7ᵗʰ S43.131 Dislocation of right acromioclavicular joint, greater than 200% displacement

1 √7ᵗʰ S43.132 Dislocation of left acromioclavicular joint, greater than 200% displacement

√7ᵗʰ S43.139 Dislocation of unspecified acromioclavicular joint, greater than 200% displacement ▽

√6ᵗʰ S43.14 Inferior dislocation of acromioclavicular joint

1 √7ᵗʰ S43.141 Inferior dislocation of right acromioclavicular joint

1 √7ᵗʰ S43.142 Inferior dislocation of left acromioclavicular joint

√7ᵗʰ S43.149 Inferior dislocation of unspecified acromioclavicular joint ▽

√6ᵗʰ S43.15 Posterior dislocation of acromioclavicular joint

1 √7ᵗʰ S43.151 Posterior dislocation of right acromioclavicular joint

1 √7ᵗʰ S43.152 Posterior dislocation of left acromioclavicular joint

√7ᵗʰ S43.159 Posterior dislocation of unspecified acromioclavicular joint ▽

√5ᵗʰ S43.2 Subluxation and dislocation of sternoclavicular joint

√6ᵗʰ S43.20 Unspecified subluxation and dislocation of sternoclavicular joint

√7ᵗʰ S43.201 Unspecified subluxation of right sternoclavicular joint ▽

√7ᵗʰ S43.202 Unspecified subluxation of left sternoclavicular joint ▽

√7ᵗʰ S43.203 Unspecified subluxation of unspecified sternoclavicular joint ▽

√7ᵗʰ S43.204 Unspecified dislocation of right sternoclavicular joint ▽

√7ᵗʰ S43.205 Unspecified dislocation of left sternoclavicular joint ▽

√7ᵗʰ S43.206 Unspecified dislocation of unspecified sternoclavicular joint ▽

---

1   Case-mix diagnosis with 7th character indicating subsequent encounter.

Ⓝ Newborn: 0   Ⓟ Pediatric: 0-17   Ⓜ Maternity: 12-55   Ⓐ Adult: 15-124   **NRS** Nonroutine supply Dx   **NCDx** Noncancer Dx   **PDx** Primary Dx   ►◄ Revised Text   ● New Code   ▲ Revised Title

958   ICD-10-CM 2018

√6ᵗʰ **S43.21** Anterior subluxation and dislocation of sternoclavicular joint

   √7ᵗʰ **S43.211** Anterior subluxation of right sternoclavicular joint

   √7ᵗʰ **S43.212** Anterior subluxation of left sternoclavicular joint

   √7ᵗʰ **S43.213** Anterior subluxation of unspecified sternoclavicular joint　▽

   √7ᵗʰ **S43.214** Anterior dislocation of right sternoclavicular joint

   √7ᵗʰ **S43.215** Anterior dislocation of left sternoclavicular joint

   √7ᵗʰ **S43.216** Anterior dislocation of unspecified sternoclavicular joint　▽

√6ᵗʰ **S43.22** Posterior subluxation and dislocation of sternoclavicular joint

   √7ᵗʰ **S43.221** Posterior subluxation of right sternoclavicular joint

   √7ᵗʰ **S43.222** Posterior subluxation of left sternoclavicular joint

   √7ᵗʰ **S43.223** Posterior subluxation of unspecified sternoclavicular joint　▽

   √7ᵗʰ **S43.224** Posterior dislocation of right sternoclavicular joint

   √7ᵗʰ **S43.225** Posterior dislocation of left sternoclavicular joint

   √7ᵗʰ **S43.226** Posterior dislocation of unspecified sternoclavicular joint　▽

√5ᵗʰ **S43.3** Subluxation and dislocation of other and unspecified parts of shoulder girdle

√6ᵗʰ **S43.30** Subluxation and dislocation of unspecified parts of shoulder girdle
     Dislocation of shoulder girdle NOS
     Subluxation of shoulder girdle NOS

   [1] √7ᵗʰ **S43.301** Subluxation of unspecified parts of right shoulder girdle

   [1] √7ᵗʰ **S43.302** Subluxation of unspecified parts of left shoulder girdle

   √7ᵗʰ **S43.303** Subluxation of unspecified parts of unspecified shoulder girdle　▽

   [1] √7ᵗʰ **S43.304** Dislocation of unspecified parts of right shoulder girdle

   [1] √7ᵗʰ **S43.305** Dislocation of unspecified parts of left shoulder girdle

   √7ᵗʰ **S43.306** Dislocation of unspecified parts of unspecified shoulder girdle　▽

√6ᵗʰ **S43.31** Subluxation and dislocation of scapula

   [1] √7ᵗʰ **S43.311** Subluxation of right scapula

   [1] √7ᵗʰ **S43.312** Subluxation of left scapula

   √7ᵗʰ **S43.313** Subluxation of unspecified scapula　▽

   [1] √7ᵗʰ **S43.314** Dislocation of right scapula

   [1] √7ᵗʰ **S43.315** Dislocation of left scapula

   √7ᵗʰ **S43.316** Dislocation of unspecified scapula　▽

√6ᵗʰ **S43.39** Subluxation and dislocation of other parts of shoulder girdle

   [1] √7ᵗʰ **S43.391** Subluxation of other parts of right shoulder girdle

   [1] √7ᵗʰ **S43.392** Subluxation of other parts of left shoulder girdle

   √7ᵗʰ **S43.393** Subluxation of other parts of unspecified shoulder girdle　▽

   [1] √7ᵗʰ **S43.394** Dislocation of other parts of right shoulder girdle

   [1] √7ᵗʰ **S43.395** Dislocation of other parts of left shoulder girdle

   √7ᵗʰ **S43.396** Dislocation of other parts of unspecified shoulder girdle　▽

√5ᵗʰ **S43.4** Sprain of shoulder joint

√6ᵗʰ **S43.40** Unspecified sprain of shoulder joint

   √7ᵗʰ **S43.401** Unspecified sprain of right shoulder joint　▽

   √7ᵗʰ **S43.402** Unspecified sprain of left shoulder joint　▽

   √7ᵗʰ **S43.409** Unspecified sprain of unspecified shoulder joint　▽

√6ᵗʰ **S43.41** Sprain of coracohumeral (ligament)

   √7ᵗʰ **S43.411** Sprain of right coracohumeral (ligament)

   √7ᵗʰ **S43.412** Sprain of left coracohumeral (ligament)

   √7ᵗʰ **S43.419** Sprain of unspecified coracohumeral (ligament)　▽

√6ᵗʰ **S43.42** Sprain of rotator cuff capsule
     EXCLUDES 1　rotator cuff syndrome (complete) (incomplete), not specified as traumatic (M75.1-)
     EXCLUDES 2　injury of tendon of rotator cuff (S46.0-)

   √7ᵗʰ **S43.421** Sprain of right rotator cuff capsule

   √7ᵗʰ **S43.422** Sprain of left rotator cuff capsule

   √7ᵗʰ **S43.429** Sprain of unspecified rotator cuff capsule　▽

√6ᵗʰ **S43.43** Superior glenoid labrum lesion
     SLAP lesion
     DEF: Detachment injury of the superior aspect of the glenoid labrum, which is the ring of fibrocartilage attached to the rim of the glenoid cavity of the scapula.

   √7ᵗʰ **S43.431** Superior glenoid labrum lesion of right shoulder

   √7ᵗʰ **S43.432** Superior glenoid labrum lesion of left shoulder

   √7ᵗʰ **S43.439** Superior glenoid labrum lesion of unspecified shoulder　▽

√6ᵗʰ **S43.49** Other sprain of shoulder joint

   √7ᵗʰ **S43.491** Other sprain of right shoulder joint

   √7ᵗʰ **S43.492** Other sprain of left shoulder joint

   √7ᵗʰ **S43.499** Other sprain of unspecified shoulder joint　▽

√5ᵗʰ **S43.5** Sprain of acromioclavicular joint
     Sprain of acromioclavicular ligament

   √x7ᵗʰ **S43.50** Sprain of unspecified acromioclavicular joint　▽

   √x7ᵗʰ **S43.51** Sprain of right acromioclavicular joint

   √x7ᵗʰ **S43.52** Sprain of left acromioclavicular joint

√5ᵗʰ **S43.6** Sprain of sternoclavicular joint

   √x7ᵗʰ **S43.60** Sprain of unspecified sternoclavicular joint　▽

   √x7ᵗʰ **S43.61** Sprain of right sternoclavicular joint

   √x7ᵗʰ **S43.62** Sprain of left sternoclavicular joint

√5ᵗʰ **S43.8** Sprain of other specified parts of shoulder girdle

   √x7ᵗʰ **S43.80** Sprain of other specified parts of unspecified shoulder girdle　▽

   √x7ᵗʰ **S43.81** Sprain of other specified parts of right shoulder girdle

   √x7ᵗʰ **S43.82** Sprain of other specified parts of left shoulder girdle

√5ᵗʰ **S43.9** Sprain of unspecified parts of shoulder girdle

   √x7ᵗʰ **S43.90** Sprain of unspecified parts of unspecified shoulder girdle　▽
     Sprain of shoulder girdle NOS

   √x7ᵗʰ **S43.91** Sprain of unspecified parts of right shoulder girdle　▽

   √x7ᵗʰ **S43.92** Sprain of unspecified parts of left shoulder girdle　▽

√4ᵗʰ **S44** Injury of nerves at shoulder and upper arm level
   Code also any associated open wound (S41.-)
   EXCLUDES 2　injury of brachial plexus (S14.3-)

   The appropriate 7th character is to be added to each code from category S44.
   A　initial encounter
   D　subsequent encounter
   S　sequela

√5ᵗʰ **S44.0** Injury of ulnar nerve at upper arm level
     EXCLUDES 1　ulnar nerve NOS (S54.0)

   √x7ᵗʰ **S44.00** Injury of ulnar nerve at upper arm level, unspecified arm　▽

   [2] √x7ᵗʰ **S44.01** Injury of ulnar nerve at upper arm level, right arm

   [2] √x7ᵗʰ **S44.02** Injury of ulnar nerve at upper arm level, left arm

---

[1]　Case-mix diagnosis with 7th character indicating subsequent encounter.
[2]　Case-mix diagnosis with 7th character indicating subsequent encounter or sequela.

☑ Additional Character Req　　√x7ᵗʰ Placeholder Alert　　Case-Mix Diagnosis　　Manifestation　　▽ Unspecified Dx　　EXCLUDES 1 Not coded here　　EXCLUDES 2 Not included here

✓5ᵗʰ **S44.1　Injury of** median nerve **at upper arm level**
　　EXCLUDES 1　*median nerve NOS (S54.1)*

　✓x7ᵗʰ **S44.10　Injury of median nerve at upper arm level, unspecified arm** ▽

2 ✓x7ᵗʰ **S44.11　Injury of median nerve at upper arm level,** right **arm**

2 ✓x7ᵗʰ **S44.12　Injury of median nerve at upper arm level,** left **arm**

✓5ᵗʰ **S44.2　Injury of** radial nerve **at upper arm level**
　　EXCLUDES 1　*radial nerve NOS (S54.2)*

　✓x7ᵗʰ **S44.20　Injury of radial nerve at upper arm level, unspecified arm** ▽

2 ✓x7ᵗʰ **S44.21　Injury of radial nerve at upper arm level,** right **arm**

2 ✓x7ᵗʰ **S44.22　Injury of radial nerve at upper arm level,** left **arm**

✓5ᵗʰ **S44.3　Injury of** axillary nerve

　✓x7ᵗʰ **S44.30　Injury of axillary nerve, unspecified arm** ▽

2 ✓x7ᵗʰ **S44.31　Injury of axillary nerve,** right **arm**

2 ✓x7ᵗʰ **S44.32　Injury of axillary nerve,** left **arm**

✓5ᵗʰ **S44.4　Injury of** musculocutaneous nerve

　✓x7ᵗʰ **S44.40　Injury of musculocutaneous nerve, unspecified arm** ▽

2 ✓x7ᵗʰ **S44.41　Injury of musculocutaneous nerve,** right **arm**

2 ✓x7ᵗʰ **S44.42　Injury of musculocutaneous nerve,** left **arm**

✓5ᵗʰ **S44.5　Injury of** cutaneous sensory nerve **at shoulder and upper arm level**

　✓x7ᵗʰ **S44.50　Injury of cutaneous sensory nerve at shoulder and upper arm level, unspecified arm** ▽

2 ✓x7ᵗʰ **S44.51　Injury of cutaneous sensory nerve at shoulder and upper arm level,** right **arm**

2 ✓x7ᵗʰ **S44.52　Injury of cutaneous sensory nerve at shoulder and upper arm level,** left **arm**

✓5ᵗʰ **S44.8　Injury of other nerves at shoulder and upper arm level**

　✓6ᵗʰ **S44.8X　Injury of** other nerves **at shoulder and upper arm level**

　　2 ✓7ᵗʰ **S44.8X1　Injury of other nerves at shoulder and upper arm level,** right **arm**

　　2 ✓7ᵗʰ **S44.8X2　Injury of other nerves at shoulder and upper arm level,** left **arm**

　　✓7ᵗʰ **S44.8X9　Injury of other nerves at shoulder and upper arm level, unspecified arm** ▽

✓5ᵗʰ **S44.9　Injury of** unspecified **nerve at shoulder and upper arm level**

　✓x7ᵗʰ **S44.90　Injury of unspecified nerve at shoulder and upper arm level, unspecified arm** ▽

2 ✓x7ᵗʰ **S44.91　Injury of unspecified nerve at shoulder and upper arm level,** right **arm** ▽

2 ✓x7ᵗʰ **S44.92　Injury of unspecified nerve at shoulder and upper arm level,** left **arm** ▽

✓4ᵗʰ **S45　Injury of blood vessels at shoulder and upper arm level**
　　Code also any associated open wound (S41.-)
　　EXCLUDES 2　*injury of subclavian artery (S25.1)*
　　　　　　　injury of subclavian vein (S25.3)

　　The appropriate 7th character is to be added to each code from category S45.
　　A　initial encounter
　　D　subsequent encounter
　　S　sequela

✓5ᵗʰ **S45.0　Injury of** axillary artery

　✓6ᵗʰ **S45.00　Unspecified injury of axillary artery**

　　✓7ᵗʰ **S45.001　Unspecified injury of axillary artery,** right **side** ▽

　　✓7ᵗʰ **S45.002　Unspecified injury of axillary artery,** left **side** ▽

　　✓7ᵗʰ **S45.009　Unspecified injury of axillary artery, unspecified side** ▽

　✓6ᵗʰ **S45.01　Laceration of axillary artery**

　　✓7ᵗʰ **S45.011　Laceration of axillary artery,** right **side**

　　✓7ᵗʰ **S45.012　Laceration of axillary artery,** left **side**

　　✓7ᵗʰ **S45.019　Laceration of axillary artery, unspecified side** ▽

　✓6ᵗʰ **S45.09　Other specified injury of axillary artery**

　　✓7ᵗʰ **S45.091　Other specified injury of axillary artery,** right **side**

　　✓7ᵗʰ **S45.092　Other specified injury of axillary artery,** left **side**

　　✓7ᵗʰ **S45.099　Other specified injury of axillary artery, unspecified side** ▽

✓5ᵗʰ **S45.1　Injury of** brachial artery

　✓6ᵗʰ **S45.10　Unspecified injury of brachial artery**

　　✓7ᵗʰ **S45.101　Unspecified injury of brachial artery,** right **side** ▽

　　✓7ᵗʰ **S45.102　Unspecified injury of brachial artery,** left **side** ▽

　　✓7ᵗʰ **S45.109　Unspecified injury of brachial artery, unspecified side** ▽

　✓6ᵗʰ **S45.11　Laceration of brachial artery**

　　✓7ᵗʰ **S45.111　Laceration of brachial artery,** right **side**

　　✓7ᵗʰ **S45.112　Laceration of brachial artery,** left **side**

　　✓7ᵗʰ **S45.119　Laceration of brachial artery, unspecified side** ▽

　✓6ᵗʰ **S45.19　Other specified injury of brachial artery**

　　✓7ᵗʰ **S45.191　Other specified injury of brachial artery,** right **side**

　　✓7ᵗʰ **S45.192　Other specified injury of brachial artery,** left **side**

　　✓7ᵗʰ **S45.199　Other specified injury of brachial artery, unspecified side** ▽

✓5ᵗʰ **S45.2　Injury of** axillary or brachial vein

　✓6ᵗʰ **S45.20　Unspecified injury of axillary or brachial vein**

　　✓7ᵗʰ **S45.201　Unspecified injury of axillary or brachial vein,** right **side** ▽

　　✓7ᵗʰ **S45.202　Unspecified injury of axillary or brachial vein,** left **side** ▽

　　✓7ᵗʰ **S45.209　Unspecified injury of axillary or brachial vein, unspecified side** ▽

　✓6ᵗʰ **S45.21　Laceration of axillary or brachial vein**

　　✓7ᵗʰ **S45.211　Laceration of axillary or brachial vein,** right **side**

　　✓7ᵗʰ **S45.212　Laceration of axillary or brachial vein,** left **side**

　　✓7ᵗʰ **S45.219　Laceration of axillary or brachial vein, unspecified side** ▽

　✓6ᵗʰ **S45.29　Other specified injury of axillary or brachial vein**

　　✓7ᵗʰ **S45.291　Other specified injury of axillary or brachial vein,** right **side**

　　✓7ᵗʰ **S45.292　Other specified injury of axillary or brachial vein,** left **side**

　　✓7ᵗʰ **S45.299　Other specified injury of axillary or brachial vein, unspecified side** ▽

✓5ᵗʰ **S45.3　Injury of** superficial vein **at shoulder and upper arm level**

　✓6ᵗʰ **S45.30　Unspecified injury of superficial vein at shoulder and upper arm level**

　　✓7ᵗʰ **S45.301　Unspecified injury of superficial vein at shoulder and upper arm level,** right **arm** ▽

　　✓7ᵗʰ **S45.302　Unspecified injury of superficial vein at shoulder and upper arm level,** left **arm** ▽

　　✓7ᵗʰ **S45.309　Unspecified injury of superficial vein at shoulder and upper arm level, unspecified arm** ▽

　✓6ᵗʰ **S45.31　Laceration of superficial vein at shoulder and upper arm level**

　　✓7ᵗʰ **S45.311　Laceration of superficial vein at shoulder and upper arm level,** right **arm**

　　✓7ᵗʰ **S45.312　Laceration of superficial vein at shoulder and upper arm level,** left **arm**

　　✓7ᵗʰ **S45.319　Laceration of superficial vein at shoulder and upper arm level, unspecified arm** ▽

　✓6ᵗʰ **S45.39　Other specified injury of superficial vein at shoulder and upper arm level**

　　✓7ᵗʰ **S45.391　Other specified injury of superficial vein at shoulder and upper arm level,** right **arm**

　　✓7ᵗʰ **S45.392　Other specified injury of superficial vein at shoulder and upper arm level,** left **arm**

2　Case-mix diagnosis with 7th character indicating subsequent encounter or sequela.

Ⓝ Newborn: 0　Ⓟ Pediatric: 0-17　Ⓜ Maternity: 12-55　Ⓐ Adult: 15-124　NRS Nonroutine supply Dx　NC Dx Noncancer Dx　PDx Primary Dx　▶◀ Revised Text　● New Code　▲ Revised Title

960　　　ICD-10-CM 2018

☑7ᵗʰ **S45.399** Other specified injury of superficial vein at shoulder and upper arm level, unspecified arm ▽

✓5ᵗʰ **S45.8** **Injury of** other specified blood vessels **at shoulder and upper arm level**

  ✓6ᵗʰ **S45.80** Unspecified **injury of other specified blood vessels at shoulder and upper arm level**

    ☑7ᵗʰ **S45.801** Unspecified injury of other specified blood vessels at shoulder and upper arm level, right arm ▽

    ☑7ᵗʰ **S45.802** Unspecified injury of other specified blood vessels at shoulder and upper arm level, left arm ▽

    ☑7ᵗʰ **S45.809** Unspecified injury of other specified blood vessels at shoulder and upper arm level, unspecified arm ▽

  ✓6ᵗʰ **S45.81** Laceration **of other specified blood vessels at shoulder and upper arm level**

    ☑7ᵗʰ **S45.811** Laceration of other specified blood vessels at shoulder and upper arm level, right arm

    ☑7ᵗʰ **S45.812** Laceration of other specified blood vessels at shoulder and upper arm level, left arm

    ☑7ᵗʰ **S45.819** Laceration of other specified blood vessels at shoulder and upper arm level, unspecified arm ▽

  ✓6ᵗʰ **S45.89** Other **specified injury of other specified blood vessels at shoulder and upper arm level**

    ☑7ᵗʰ **S45.891** Other specified injury of other specified blood vessels at shoulder and upper arm level, right arm

    ☑7ᵗʰ **S45.892** Other specified injury of other specified blood vessels at shoulder and upper arm level, left arm

    ☑7ᵗʰ **S45.899** Other specified injury of other specified blood vessels at shoulder and upper arm level, unspecified arm ▽

✓5ᵗʰ **S45.9** **Injury of** unspecified blood vessel **at shoulder and upper arm level**

  ✓6ᵗʰ **S45.90** Unspecified **injury of unspecified blood vessel at shoulder and upper arm level**

    ☑7ᵗʰ **S45.901** Unspecified injury of unspecified blood vessel at shoulder and upper arm level, right arm ▽

    ☑7ᵗʰ **S45.902** Unspecified injury of unspecified blood vessel at shoulder and upper arm level, left arm ▽

    ☑7ᵗʰ **S45.909** Unspecified injury of unspecified blood vessel at shoulder and upper arm level, unspecified arm ▽

  ✓6ᵗʰ **S45.91** Laceration **of unspecified blood vessel at shoulder and upper arm level**

    ☑7ᵗʰ **S45.911** Laceration of unspecified blood vessel at shoulder and upper arm level, right arm ▽

    ☑7ᵗʰ **S45.912** Laceration of unspecified blood vessel at shoulder and upper arm level, left arm ▽

    ☑7ᵗʰ **S45.919** Laceration of unspecified blood vessel at shoulder and upper arm level, unspecified arm ▽

  ✓6ᵗʰ **S45.99** Other **specified injury of unspecified blood vessel at shoulder and upper arm level**

    ☑7ᵗʰ **S45.991** Other specified injury of unspecified blood vessel at shoulder and upper arm level, right arm ▽

    ☑7ᵗʰ **S45.992** Other specified injury of unspecified blood vessel at shoulder and upper arm level, left arm ▽

    ☑7ᵗʰ **S45.999** Other specified injury of unspecified blood vessel at shoulder and upper arm level, unspecified arm ▽

✓4ᵗʰ **S46** **Injury of muscle, fascia and tendon at shoulder and upper arm level**

  Code also any associated open wound (S41.-)
  EXCLUDES 2 injury of muscle, fascia and tendon at elbow (S56.-)
  sprain of joints and ligaments of shoulder girdle (S43.9)
  TIP: Refer to the Muscle/Tendon table at the beginning of this chapter.

  The appropriate 7th character is to be added to each code from category S46.
  A   initial encounter
  D   subsequent encounter
  S   sequela

✓5ᵗʰ **S46.0** **Injury of muscle(s) and tendon(s) of the** rotator cuff **of shoulder**

  ✓6ᵗʰ **S46.00** Unspecified **injury of muscle(s) and tendon(s) of the rotator cuff of shoulder**

    ☑7ᵗʰ **S46.001** Unspecified injury of muscle(s) and tendon(s) of the rotator cuff of right shoulder ▽

    ☑7ᵗʰ **S46.002** Unspecified injury of muscle(s) and tendon(s) of the rotator cuff of left shoulder ▽

    ☑7ᵗʰ **S46.009** Unspecified injury of muscle(s) and tendon(s) of the rotator cuff of unspecified shoulder ▽

  ✓6ᵗʰ **S46.01** Strain **of muscle(s) and tendon(s) of the rotator cuff of shoulder**

    ☑7ᵗʰ **S46.011** Strain of muscle(s) and tendon(s) of the rotator cuff of right shoulder

    ☑7ᵗʰ **S46.012** Strain of muscle(s) and tendon(s) of the rotator cuff of left shoulder

    ☑7ᵗʰ **S46.019** Strain of muscle(s) and tendon(s) of the rotator cuff of unspecified shoulder ▽

  ✓6ᵗʰ **S46.02** Laceration **of muscle(s) and tendon(s) of the rotator cuff of shoulder**

    4,5 ☑7ᵗʰ **S46.021** Laceration of muscle(s) and tendon(s) of the rotator cuff of right shoulder **NRS**

    4,5 ☑7ᵗʰ **S46.022** Laceration of muscle(s) and tendon(s) of the rotator cuff of left shoulder **NRS**

    ☑7ᵗʰ **S46.029** Laceration of muscle(s) and tendon(s) of the rotator cuff of unspecified shoulder ▽

  ✓6ᵗʰ **S46.09** Other **injury of muscle(s) and tendon(s) of the rotator cuff of shoulder**

    ☑7ᵗʰ **S46.091** Other injury of muscle(s) and tendon(s) of the rotator cuff of right shoulder

    ☑7ᵗʰ **S46.092** Other injury of muscle(s) and tendon(s) of the rotator cuff of left shoulder

    ☑7ᵗʰ **S46.099** Other injury of muscle(s) and tendon(s) of the rotator cuff of unspecified shoulder ▽

✓5ᵗʰ **S46.1** **Injury of muscle, fascia and tendon of** long head of biceps

  ✓6ᵗʰ **S46.10** Unspecified **injury of muscle, fascia and tendon of long head of biceps**

    ☑7ᵗʰ **S46.101** Unspecified injury of muscle, fascia and tendon of long head of biceps, right arm ▽

    ☑7ᵗʰ **S46.102** Unspecified injury of muscle, fascia and tendon of long head of biceps, left arm ▽

    ☑7ᵗʰ **S46.109** Unspecified injury of muscle, fascia and tendon of long head of biceps, unspecified arm ▽

  ✓6ᵗʰ **S46.11** Strain **of muscle, fascia and tendon of long head of biceps**

    ☑7ᵗʰ **S46.111** Strain of muscle, fascia and tendon of long head of biceps, right arm

    ☑7ᵗʰ **S46.112** Strain of muscle, fascia and tendon of long head of biceps, left arm

    ☑7ᵗʰ **S46.119** Strain of muscle, fascia and tendon of long head of biceps, unspecified arm ▽

  ✓6ᵗʰ **S46.12** Laceration **of muscle, fascia and tendon of long head of biceps**

    4,5 ☑7ᵗʰ **S46.121** Laceration of muscle, fascia and tendon of long head of biceps, right arm **NRS**

    4,5 ☑7ᵗʰ **S46.122** Laceration of muscle, fascia and tendon of long head of biceps, left arm **NRS**

---

4 Case-mix diagnosis with 7th character indicating initial or subsequent encounter.
5 NRS supply diagnosis with 7th character indicating initial or subsequent encounter.

☑ Additional Character Req   ☑×7ᵗʰ Placeholder Alert   Case-Mix Diagnosis   Manifestation   ▽ Unspecified Dx   *EXCLUDES 1* Not coded here   *EXCLUDES 2* Not included here

√7ᵗʰ **S46.129** Laceration of muscle, fascia and tendon ▽ of long head of biceps, unspecified arm

√6ᵗʰ **S46.19** Other injury of muscle, fascia and tendon of long head of biceps

√7ᵗʰ **S46.191** Other injury of muscle, fascia and tendon of long head of biceps, right arm

√7ᵗʰ **S46.192** Other injury of muscle, fascia and tendon of long head of biceps, left arm

√7ᵗʰ **S46.199** Other injury of muscle, fascia and ▽ tendon of long head of biceps, unspecified arm

√5ᵗʰ **S46.2** Injury of muscle, fascia and tendon of other parts of biceps

√6ᵗʰ **S46.20** Unspecified injury of muscle, fascia and tendon of other parts of biceps

√7ᵗʰ **S46.201** Unspecified injury of muscle, fascia and ▽ tendon of other parts of biceps, right arm

√7ᵗʰ **S46.202** Unspecified injury of muscle, fascia and ▽ tendon of other parts of biceps, left arm

√7ᵗʰ **S46.209** Unspecified injury of muscle, fascia and tendon of other parts of biceps, unspecified arm

√6ᵗʰ **S46.21** Strain of muscle, fascia and tendon of other parts of biceps

√7ᵗʰ **S46.211** Strain of muscle, fascia and tendon of other parts of biceps, right arm

√7ᵗʰ **S46.212** Strain of muscle, fascia and tendon of other parts of biceps, left arm

√7ᵗʰ **S46.219** Strain of muscle, fascia and tendon of ▽ other parts of biceps, unspecified arm

√6ᵗʰ **S46.22** Laceration of muscle, fascia and tendon of other parts of biceps

4,5 √7ᵗʰ **S46.221** Laceration of muscle, fascia and   **NRS** tendon of other parts of biceps, right arm

4,5 √7ᵗʰ **S46.222** Laceration of muscle, fascia and   **NRS** tendon of other parts of biceps, left arm

√7ᵗʰ **S46.229** Laceration of muscle, fascia and tendon ▽ of other parts of biceps, unspecified arm

√6ᵗʰ **S46.29** Other injury of muscle, fascia and tendon of other parts of biceps

√7ᵗʰ **S46.291** Other injury of muscle, fascia and tendon of other parts of biceps, right arm

√7ᵗʰ **S46.292** Other injury of muscle, fascia and tendon of other parts of biceps, left arm

√7ᵗʰ **S46.299** Other injury of muscle, fascia and ▽ tendon of other parts of biceps, unspecified arm

√5ᵗʰ **S46.3** Injury of muscle, fascia and tendon of triceps

√6ᵗʰ **S46.30** Unspecified injury of muscle, fascia and tendon of triceps

√7ᵗʰ **S46.301** Unspecified injury of muscle, fascia ▽ and tendon of triceps, right arm

√7ᵗʰ **S46.302** Unspecified injury of muscle, fascia ▽ and tendon of triceps, left arm

√7ᵗʰ **S46.309** Unspecified injury of muscle, fascia ▽ and tendon of triceps, unspecified arm

√6ᵗʰ **S46.31** Strain of muscle, fascia and tendon of triceps

√7ᵗʰ **S46.311** Strain of muscle, fascia and tendon of triceps, right arm

√7ᵗʰ **S46.312** Strain of muscle, fascia and tendon of triceps, left arm

√7ᵗʰ **S46.319** Strain of muscle, fascia and tendon of ▽ triceps, unspecified arm

√6ᵗʰ **S46.32** Laceration of muscle, fascia and tendon of triceps

4,5 √7ᵗʰ **S46.321** Laceration of muscle, fascia and   **NRS** tendon of triceps, right arm

4,5 √7ᵗʰ **S46.322** Laceration of muscle, fascia and   **NRS** tendon of triceps, left arm

√7ᵗʰ **S46.329** Laceration of muscle, fascia and ▽ tendon of triceps, unspecified arm

√6ᵗʰ **S46.39** Other injury of muscle, fascia and tendon of triceps

√7ᵗʰ **S46.391** Other injury of muscle, fascia and tendon of triceps, right arm

√7ᵗʰ **S46.392** Other injury of muscle, fascia and tendon of triceps, left arm

√7ᵗʰ **S46.399** Other injury of muscle, fascia and ▽ tendon of triceps, unspecified arm

√5ᵗʰ **S46.8** Injury of other muscles, fascia and tendons at shoulder and upper arm level

√6ᵗʰ **S46.80** Unspecified injury of other muscles, fascia and tendons at shoulder and upper arm level

√7ᵗʰ **S46.801** Unspecified injury of other muscles, ▽ fascia and tendons at shoulder and upper arm level, right arm

√7ᵗʰ **S46.802** Unspecified injury of other muscles, ▽ fascia and tendons at shoulder and upper arm level, left arm

√7ᵗʰ **S46.809** Unspecified injury of other muscles, ▽ fascia and tendons at shoulder and upper arm level, unspecified arm

√6ᵗʰ **S46.81** Strain of other muscles, fascia and tendons at shoulder and upper arm level

√7ᵗʰ **S46.811** Strain of other muscles, fascia and tendons at shoulder and upper arm level, right arm

√7ᵗʰ **S46.812** Strain of other muscles, fascia and tendons at shoulder and upper arm level, left arm

√7ᵗʰ **S46.819** Strain of other muscles, fascia and ▽ tendons at shoulder and upper arm level, unspecified arm

√6ᵗʰ **S46.82** Laceration of other muscles, fascia and tendons at shoulder and upper arm level

4,5 √7ᵗʰ **S46.821** Laceration of other muscles, fascia   **NRS** and tendons at shoulder and upper arm level, right arm

4,5 √7ᵗʰ **S46.822** Laceration of other muscles, fascia   **NRS** and tendons at shoulder and upper arm level, left arm

√7ᵗʰ **S46.829** Laceration of other muscles, fascia and ▽ tendons at shoulder and upper arm level, unspecified arm

√6ᵗʰ **S46.89** Other injury of other muscles, fascia and tendons at shoulder and upper arm level

√7ᵗʰ **S46.891** Other injury of other muscles, fascia and tendons at shoulder and upper arm level, right arm

√7ᵗʰ **S46.892** Other injury of other muscles, fascia and tendons at shoulder and upper arm level, left arm

√7ᵗʰ **S46.899** Other injury of other muscles, fascia ▽ and tendons at shoulder and upper arm level, unspecified arm

√5ᵗʰ **S46.9** Injury of unspecified muscle, fascia and tendon at shoulder and upper arm level

√6ᵗʰ **S46.90** Unspecified injury of unspecified muscle, fascia and tendon at shoulder and upper arm level

√7ᵗʰ **S46.901** Unspecified injury of unspecified ▽ muscle, fascia and tendon at shoulder and upper arm level, right arm

√7ᵗʰ **S46.902** Unspecified injury of unspecified ▽ muscle, fascia and tendon at shoulder and upper arm level, left arm

√7ᵗʰ **S46.909** Unspecified injury of unspecified ▽ muscle, fascia and tendon at shoulder and upper arm level, unspecified arm

√6ᵗʰ **S46.91** Strain of unspecified muscle, fascia and tendon at shoulder and upper arm level

√7ᵗʰ **S46.911** Strain of unspecified muscle, fascia ▽ and tendon at shoulder and upper arm level, right arm

√7ᵗʰ **S46.912** Strain of unspecified muscle, fascia ▽ and tendon at shoulder and upper arm level, left arm

---

4 Case-mix diagnosis with 7th character indicating initial or subsequent encounter.
5 NRS supply diagnosis with 7th character indicating initial or subsequent encounter.

✓7ᵗʰ **S46.919** Strain of unspecified muscle, fascia and tendon at shoulder and upper arm level, unspecified arm ▽

✓6ᵗʰ **S46.92** Laceration of unspecified muscle, fascia and tendon at shoulder and upper arm level

    4,5 ✓7ᵗʰ **S46.921** Laceration of unspecified muscle, fascia and tendon at shoulder and upper arm level, right arm **NRS** ▽

    4,5 ✓7ᵗʰ **S46.922** Laceration of unspecified muscle, fascia and tendon at shoulder and upper arm level, left arm **NRS** ▽

    ✓7ᵗʰ **S46.929** Laceration of unspecified muscle, fascia and tendon at shoulder and upper arm level, unspecified arm ▽

✓6ᵗʰ **S46.99** Other injury of unspecified muscle, fascia and tendon at shoulder and upper arm level

    ✓7ᵗʰ **S46.991** Other injury of unspecified muscle, fascia and tendon at shoulder and upper arm level, right arm ▽

    ✓7ᵗʰ **S46.992** Other injury of unspecified muscle, fascia and tendon at shoulder and upper arm level, left arm ▽

    ✓7ᵗʰ **S46.999** Other injury of unspecified muscle, fascia and tendon at shoulder and upper arm level, unspecified arm ▽

✓4ᵗʰ **S47** Crushing injury **of shoulder and upper arm**

    Use additional code for all associated injuries

    EXCLUDES 2 crushing injury of elbow (S57.0-)

    The appropriate 7th character is to be added to each code from category S47.
    A   initial encounter
    D   subsequent encounter
    S   sequela

4 ✓x7ᵗʰ **S47.1** Crushing injury of **right** shoulder and upper arm

4 ✓x7ᵗʰ **S47.2** Crushing injury of **left** shoulder and upper arm

✓x7ᵗʰ **S47.9** Crushing injury of shoulder and upper arm, unspecified arm ▽

✓4ᵗʰ **S48** Traumatic amputation **of shoulder and upper arm**

    An amputation not identified as partial or complete should be coded to complete.

    EXCLUDES 1 traumatic amputation at elbow level (S58.0)

    The appropriate 7th character is to be added to each code from category S48.
    A   initial encounter
    D   subsequent encounter
    S   sequela

✓5ᵗʰ **S48.0** Traumatic amputation at shoulder joint

    ✓6ᵗʰ **S48.01** Complete traumatic amputation at shoulder joint

        4,5 ✓7ᵗʰ **S48.011** Complete traumatic amputation at right shoulder joint **NRS**

        4,5 ✓7ᵗʰ **S48.012** Complete traumatic amputation at left shoulder joint **NRS**

        ✓7ᵗʰ **S48.019** Complete traumatic amputation at unspecified shoulder joint ▽

    ✓6ᵗʰ **S48.02** Partial traumatic amputation at shoulder joint

        4,5 ✓7ᵗʰ **S48.021** Partial traumatic amputation at right shoulder joint **NRS**

        4,5 ✓7ᵗʰ **S48.022** Partial traumatic amputation at left shoulder joint **NRS**

        ✓7ᵗʰ **S48.029** Partial traumatic amputation at unspecified shoulder joint ▽

✓5ᵗʰ **S48.1** Traumatic amputation at level between shoulder and elbow

    ✓6ᵗʰ **S48.11** Complete traumatic amputation at level between shoulder and elbow

        4,5 ✓7ᵗʰ **S48.111** Complete traumatic amputation at level between right shoulder and elbow **NRS**

        4,5 ✓7ᵗʰ **S48.112** Complete traumatic amputation at level between left shoulder and elbow **NRS**

        ✓7ᵗʰ **S48.119** Complete traumatic amputation at level between unspecified shoulder and elbow ▽

✓6ᵗʰ **S48.12** Partial traumatic amputation at level between shoulder and elbow

    4,5 ✓7ᵗʰ **S48.121** Partial traumatic amputation at level between right shoulder and elbow **NRS**

    4,5 ✓7ᵗʰ **S48.122** Partial traumatic amputation at level between left shoulder and elbow **NRS**

    ✓7ᵗʰ **S48.129** Partial traumatic amputation at level between unspecified shoulder and elbow ▽

✓5ᵗʰ **S48.9** Traumatic amputation of shoulder and upper arm, level unspecified

    ✓6ᵗʰ **S48.91** Complete traumatic amputation of shoulder and upper arm, level unspecified

        4,5 ✓7ᵗʰ **S48.911** Complete traumatic amputation of right shoulder and upper arm, level unspecified **NRS** ▽

        4,5 ✓7ᵗʰ **S48.912** Complete traumatic amputation of left shoulder and upper arm, level unspecified **NRS** ▽

        ✓7ᵗʰ **S48.919** Complete traumatic amputation of unspecified shoulder and upper arm, level unspecified ▽

    ✓6ᵗʰ **S48.92** Partial traumatic amputation of shoulder and upper arm, level unspecified

        4,5 ✓7ᵗʰ **S48.921** Partial traumatic amputation of right shoulder and upper arm, level unspecified **NRS** ▽

        4,5 ✓7ᵗʰ **S48.922** Partial traumatic amputation of left shoulder and upper arm, level unspecified **NRS** ▽

        ✓7ᵗʰ **S48.929** Partial traumatic amputation of unspecified shoulder and upper arm, level unspecified ▽

✓4ᵗʰ **S49** Other and unspecified injuries **of shoulder and upper arm**

    The appropriate 7th character is to be added to each code from subcategories S49.0 and S49.1.
    A   initial encounter for closed fracture
    D   subsequent encounter for fracture with routine healing
    G   subsequent encounter for fracture with delayed healing
    K   subsequent encounter for fracture with nonunion
    P   subsequent encounter for fracture with malunion
    S   sequela

    TIP: The term "improper alignment" is not synonymous with malunion or nonunion of a fracture when noted in provider documentation.

✓5ᵗʰ **S49.0** Physeal fracture of upper end of humerus

    ✓6ᵗʰ **S49.00** Unspecified physeal fracture of upper end of humerus

        1 ✓7ᵗʰ **S49.001** Unspecified physeal fracture of upper end of humerus, right arm ▽

        1 ✓7ᵗʰ **S49.002** Unspecified physeal fracture of upper end of humerus, left arm ▽

        ✓7ᵗʰ **S49.009** Unspecified physeal fracture of upper end of humerus, unspecified arm ▽

    ✓6ᵗʰ **S49.01** Salter-Harris Type I physeal fracture of upper end of humerus

        1 ✓7ᵗʰ **S49.011** Salter-Harris Type I physeal fracture of upper end of humerus, right arm

        1 ✓7ᵗʰ **S49.012** Salter-Harris Type I physeal fracture of upper end of humerus, left arm

        ✓7ᵗʰ **S49.019** Salter-Harris Type I physeal fracture of upper end of humerus, unspecified arm ▽

    ✓6ᵗʰ **S49.02** Salter-Harris Type II physeal fracture of upper end of humerus

        1 ✓7ᵗʰ **S49.021** Salter-Harris Type II physeal fracture of upper end of humerus, right arm

        1 ✓7ᵗʰ **S49.022** Salter-Harris Type II physeal fracture of upper end of humerus, left arm

        ✓7ᵗʰ **S49.029** Salter-Harris Type II physeal fracture of upper end of humerus, unspecified arm\ ▽

    ✓6ᵗʰ **S49.03** Salter-Harris Type III physeal fracture of upper end of humerus

        1 ✓7ᵗʰ **S49.031** Salter-Harris Type III physeal fracture of upper end of humerus, right arm

---

1 Case-mix diagnosis with 7th character indicating subsequent encounter.
4 Case-mix diagnosis with 7th character indicating initial or subsequent encounter.
5 NRS supply diagnosis with 7th character indicating initial or subsequent encounter.

☑ Additional Character Req   ✓x7ᵗʰ Placeholder Alert   Case-Mix Diagnosis   Manifestation   ▽ Unspecified Dx   **EXCLUDES 1** Not coded here   **EXCLUDES 2** Not included here

Chapter 19. Injury, Poisoning and Certain Other Consequences of External Causes

¹ √7ᵗʰ **S49.032** **Salter-Harris Type III physeal fracture of upper end of humerus, left arm**

√7ᵗʰ **S49.039** Salter-Harris Type III physeal fracture of upper end of humerus, unspecified arm ▽

√6ᵗʰ **S49.04** Salter-Harris Type IV physeal fracture of upper end of humerus

¹ √7ᵗʰ **S49.041** **Salter-Harris Type IV physeal fracture of upper end of humerus, right arm**

¹ √7ᵗʰ **S49.042** **Salter-Harris Type IV physeal fracture of upper end of humerus, left arm**

√7ᵗʰ **S49.049** Salter-Harris Type IV physeal fracture of upper end of humerus, unspecified arm ▽

√6ᵗʰ **S49.09** Other physeal fracture of upper end of humerus

¹ √7ᵗʰ **S49.091** **Other physeal fracture of upper end of humerus, right arm**

¹ √7ᵗʰ **S49.092** **Other physeal fracture of upper end of humerus, left arm**

√7ᵗʰ **S49.099** Other physeal fracture of upper end of humerus, unspecified arm ▽

√5ᵗʰ **S49.1** Physeal fracture of lower end of humerus

√6ᵗʰ **S49.10** Unspecified physeal fracture of lower end of humerus

¹ √7ᵗʰ **S49.101** **Unspecified physeal fracture of lower end of humerus, right arm** ▽

¹ √7ᵗʰ **S49.102** **Unspecified physeal fracture of lower end of humerus, left arm** ▽

√7ᵗʰ **S49.109** Unspecified physeal fracture of lower end of humerus, unspecified arm ▽

√6ᵗʰ **S49.11** Salter-Harris Type I physeal fracture of lower end of humerus

¹ √7ᵗʰ **S49.111** **Salter-Harris Type I physeal fracture of lower end of humerus, right arm**

¹ √7ᵗʰ **S49.112** **Salter-Harris Type I physeal fracture of lower end of humerus, left arm**

√7ᵗʰ **S49.119** Salter-Harris Type I physeal fracture of lower end of humerus, unspecified arm ▽

√6ᵗʰ **S49.12** Salter-Harris Type II physeal fracture of lower end of humerus

¹ √7ᵗʰ **S49.121** **Salter-Harris Type II physeal fracture of lower end of humerus, right arm**

¹ √7ᵗʰ **S49.122** **Salter-Harris Type II physeal fracture of lower end of humerus, left arm**

√7ᵗʰ **S49.129** Salter-Harris Type II physeal fracture of lower end of humerus, unspecified arm ▽

√6ᵗʰ **S49.13** Salter Harris Type III physeal fracture of lower end of humerus

¹ √7ᵗʰ **S49.131** **Salter-Harris Type III physeal fracture of lower end of humerus, right arm**

¹ √7ᵗʰ **S49.132** **Salter-Harris Type III physeal fracture of lower end of humerus, left arm**

√7ᵗʰ **S49.139** Salter-Harris Type III physeal fracture of lower end of humerus, unspecified arm ▽

√6ᵗʰ **S49.14** Salter-Harris Type IV physeal fracture of lower end of humerus

¹ √7ᵗʰ **S49.141** **Salter-Harris Type IV physeal fracture of lower end of humerus, right arm**

¹ √7ᵗʰ **S49.142** **Salter-Harris Type IV physeal fracture of lower end of humerus, left arm**

√7ᵗʰ **S49.149** Salter-Harris Type IV physeal fracture of lower end of humerus, unspecified arm ▽

√6ᵗʰ **S49.19** Other physeal fracture of lower end of humerus

¹ √7ᵗʰ **S49.191** **Other physeal fracture of lower end of humerus, right arm**

¹ √7ᵗʰ **S49.192** **Other physeal fracture of lower end of humerus, left arm**

√7ᵗʰ **S49.199** Other physeal fracture of lower end of humerus, unspecified arm ▽

√5ᵗʰ **S49.8** Other specified injuries of shoulder and upper arm

The appropriate 7th character is to be added to each code in subcategory S49.8.
A   initial encounter
D   subsequent encounter
S   sequela

√x7ᵗʰ **S49.80** Other specified injuries of shoulder and upper arm, unspecified arm ▽

√x7ᵗʰ **S49.81** Other specified injuries of right shoulder and upper arm

√x7ᵗʰ **S49.82** Other specified injuries of left shoulder and upper arm

√5ᵗʰ **S49.9** Unspecified injury of shoulder and upper arm

The appropriate 7th character is to be added to each code in subcategory S49.9.
A   initial encounter
D   subsequent encounter
S   sequela

√x7ᵗʰ **S49.90** Unspecified injury of shoulder and upper arm, unspecified arm ▽

√x7ᵗʰ **S49.91** Unspecified injury of right shoulder and upper arm ▽

√x7ᵗʰ **S49.92** Unspecified injury of left shoulder and upper arm ▽

Injuries to the elbow and forearm (S50-S59)

EXCLUDES 2   burns and corrosions (T20-T32)
       frostbite (T33-T34)
       injuries of wrist and hand (S60-S69)
       insect bite or sting, venomous (T63.4)

√4ᵗʰ **S50** **Superficial injury of elbow and forearm**

EXCLUDES 2   superficial injury of wrist and hand (S60.-)

The appropriate 7th character is to be added to each code from category S50.
A   initial encounter
D   subsequent encounter
S   sequela

√5ᵗʰ **S50.0** Contusion of elbow

√x7ᵗʰ **S50.00** Contusion of unspecified elbow ▽

√x7ᵗʰ **S50.01** Contusion of right elbow

√x7ᵗʰ **S50.02** Contusion of left elbow

√5ᵗʰ **S50.1** Contusion of forearm

√x7ᵗʰ **S50.10** Contusion of unspecified forearm ▽

√x7ᵗʰ **S50.11** Contusion of right forearm

√x7ᵗʰ **S50.12** Contusion of left forearm

√5ᵗʰ **S50.3** Other superficial injuries of elbow

√6ᵗʰ **S50.31** Abrasion of elbow

√7ᵗʰ **S50.311** Abrasion of right elbow

√7ᵗʰ **S50.312** Abrasion of left elbow

√7ᵗʰ **S50.319** Abrasion of unspecified elbow ▽

√6ᵗʰ **S50.32** Blister (nonthermal) of elbow

√7ᵗʰ **S50.321** Blister (nonthermal) of right elbow

√7ᵗʰ **S50.322** Blister (nonthermal) of left elbow

√7ᵗʰ **S50.329** Blister (nonthermal) of unspecified elbow ▽

√6ᵗʰ **S50.34** External constriction of elbow

√7ᵗʰ **S50.341** External constriction of right elbow

√7ᵗʰ **S50.342** External constriction of left elbow

√7ᵗʰ **S50.349** External constriction of unspecified elbow ▽

√6ᵗʰ **S50.35** Superficial foreign body of elbow
Splinter in the elbow

√7ᵗʰ **S50.351** Superficial foreign body of right elbow

√7ᵗʰ **S50.352** Superficial foreign body of left elbow

√7ᵗʰ **S50.359** Superficial foreign body of unspecified elbow ▽

√6ᵗʰ **S50.36** Insect bite (nonvenomous) of elbow

√7ᵗʰ **S50.361** Insect bite (nonvenomous) of right elbow

√7ᵗʰ **S50.362** Insect bite (nonvenomous) of left elbow

√7ᵗʰ **S50.369** Insect bite (nonvenomous) of unspecified elbow ▽

---

¹   Case-mix diagnosis with 7th character indicating subsequent encounter.

Ⓝ Newborn: 0   Ⓟ Pediatric: 0-17   Ⓜ Maternity: 12-55   Ⓐ Adult: 15-124   NRS Nonroutine supply Dx   NCDx Noncancer Dx   PDx Primary Dx   ▶◀ Revised Text   ● New Code   ▲ Revised Title

964   ICD-10-CM 2018

√6ᵗʰ **S50.37** Other **superficial** bite of elbow
> *EXCLUDES 1*   open bite of elbow (S51.Ø5)

    √7ᵗʰ **S50.371**   Other superficial bite of right elbow

    √7ᵗʰ **S50.372**   Other superficial bite of left elbow

    √7ᵗʰ **S50.379**   Other superficial bite of unspecified ▽
                   elbow

√5ᵗʰ **S50.8** **Other superficial injuries of** forearm

   √6ᵗʰ **S50.81** **Abrasion** of forearm

     √7ᵗʰ **S50.811**   Abrasion of right forearm

     √7ᵗʰ **S50.812**   Abrasion of left forearm

     √7ᵗʰ **S50.819**   Abrasion of unspecified forearm ▽

   √6ᵗʰ **S50.82** **Blister (nonthermal)** of forearm

     √7ᵗʰ **S50.821**   Blister (nonthermal) of right forearm

     √7ᵗʰ **S50.822**   Blister (nonthermal) of left forearm

     √7ᵗʰ **S50.829**   Blister (nonthermal) of unspecified ▽
                   forearm

   √6ᵗʰ **S50.84** **External constriction** of forearm

     √7ᵗʰ **S50.841**   External constriction of right forearm

     √7ᵗʰ **S50.842**   External constriction of left forearm

     √7ᵗʰ **S50.849**   External constriction of unspecified ▽
                   forearm

   √6ᵗʰ **S50.85** **Superficial** foreign body **of forearm**
             Splinter in the forearm

     √7ᵗʰ **S50.851**   Superficial foreign body of right forearm

     √7ᵗʰ **S50.852**   Superficial foreign body of left forearm

     √7ᵗʰ **S50.859**   Superficial foreign body of unspecified ▽
                   forearm

   √6ᵗʰ **S50.86** Insect bite (nonvenomous) of forearm

     √7ᵗʰ **S50.861**   Insect bite (nonvenomous) of right
                   forearm

     √7ᵗʰ **S50.862**   Insect bite (nonvenomous) of left forearm

     √7ᵗʰ **S50.869**   Insect bite (nonvenomous) of ▽
                   unspecified forearm

   √6ᵗʰ **S50.87** Other **superficial** bite of forearm
> *EXCLUDES 1*   open bite of forearm (S51.85)

     √7ᵗʰ **S50.871**   Other superficial bite of right forearm

     √7ᵗʰ **S50.872**   Other superficial bite of left forearm

     √7ᵗʰ **S50.879**   Other superficial bite of unspecified ▽
                   forearm

√5ᵗʰ **S50.9** **Unspecified superficial injury of elbow and forearm**

   √6ᵗʰ **S50.90** **Unspecified superficial injury of** elbow

     √7ᵗʰ **S50.901**   Unspecified superficial injury of right ▽
                   elbow

     √7ᵗʰ **S50.902**   Unspecified superficial injury of left ▽
                   elbow

     √7ᵗʰ **S50.909**   Unspecified superficial injury of ▽
                   unspecified elbow

   √6ᵗʰ **S50.91** **Unspecified superficial injury of** forearm

     √7ᵗʰ **S50.911**   Unspecified superficial injury of right ▽
                   forearm

     √7ᵗʰ **S50.912**   Unspecified superficial injury of left ▽
                   forearm

     √7ᵗʰ **S50.919**   Unspecified superficial injury of ▽
                   unspecified forearm

√4ᵗʰ **S51** **Open wound of elbow and forearm**
    Code also any associated wound infection
> *EXCLUDES 1*   open fracture of elbow and forearm (S52- with open fracture 7th
>   character)
>   traumatic amputation of elbow and forearm (S58.-)
>
> *EXCLUDES 2*   open wound of wrist and hand (S61.-)

> The appropriate 7th character is to be added to each code from
> category S51.
> A   initial encounter
> D   subsequent encounter
> S   sequela

√5ᵗʰ **S51.Ø** **Open wound of** elbow

   √6ᵗʰ **S51.ØØ** Unspecified **open wound of elbow**

     5 √7ᵗʰ **S51.ØØ1**   Unspecified open wound of right   NRS ▽
                   elbow
                   AHA: 2012, 4Q, 108

     5 √7ᵗʰ **S51.ØØ2**   Unspecified open wound of left   NRS
                   elbow

     √7ᵗʰ **S51.ØØ9**   Unspecified open wound of unspecified ▽
                   elbow
                   Open wound of elbow NOS

   √6ᵗʰ **S51.Ø1** Laceration without foreign body **of elbow**

     4,5 √7ᵗʰ **S51.Ø11**   **Laceration without foreign body of**   NRS
                   right elbow

     4,5 √7ᵗʰ **S51.Ø12**   **Laceration without foreign body of**   NRS
                   left elbow

     √7ᵗʰ **S51.Ø19**   Laceration without foreign body of ▽
                   unspecified elbow

   √6ᵗʰ **S51.Ø2** Laceration with foreign body **of elbow**

     4,5 √7ᵗʰ **S51.Ø21**   **Laceration with foreign body of** right   NRS
                   elbow

     4,5 √7ᵗʰ **S51.Ø22**   **Laceration with foreign body of** left   NRS
                   elbow

     √7ᵗʰ **S51.Ø29**   Laceration with foreign body of ▽
                   unspecified elbow

   √6ᵗʰ **S51.Ø3** Puncture wound without foreign body **of elbow**

     4,5 √7ᵗʰ **S51.Ø31**   **Puncture wound without foreign**   NRS
                   body of right **elbow**

     4,5 √7ᵗʰ **S51.Ø32**   **Puncture wound without foreign**   NRS
                   body of left **elbow**

     √7ᵗʰ **S51.Ø39**   Puncture wound without foreign body ▽
                   of unspecified elbow

   √6ᵗʰ **S51.Ø4** Puncture wound with foreign body **of elbow**

     4,5 √7ᵗʰ **S51.Ø41**   **Puncture wound with foreign body**   NRS
                   of right **elbow**

     4,5 √7ᵗʰ **S51.Ø42**   **Puncture wound with foreign body**   NRS
                   of left **elbow**

     √7ᵗʰ **S51.Ø49**   Puncture wound with foreign body of ▽
                   unspecified elbow

   √6ᵗʰ **S51.Ø5** Open bite **of elbow**
             Bite of elbow NOS
> *EXCLUDES 1*   superficial bite of elbow (S50.36, S50.37)

     4,5 √7ᵗʰ **S51.Ø51**   **Open bite, right elbow**   NRS

     4,5 √7ᵗʰ **S51.Ø52**   **Open bite, left elbow**   NRS

     √7ᵗʰ **S51.Ø59**   Open bite, unspecified elbow ▽

√5ᵗʰ **S51.8** **Open wound of** forearm
> *EXCLUDES 2*   open wound of elbow (S51.Ø-)

   √6ᵗʰ **S51.8Ø** Unspecified **open wound of forearm**
             AHA: 2016, 3Q, 24

     5 √7ᵗʰ **S51.8Ø1**   Unspecified open wound of right   NRS ▽
                   forearm

     5 √7ᵗʰ **S51.8Ø2**   Unspecified open wound of left   NRS ▽
                   forearm

     √7ᵗʰ **S51.8Ø9**   Unspecified open wound of ▽
                   unspecified forearm
                   Open wound of forearm NOS

   √6ᵗʰ **S51.81** Laceration without foreign body **of forearm**

     4,5 √7ᵗʰ **S51.811**   **Laceration without foreign body of**   NRS
                   right **forearm**

     4,5 √7ᵗʰ **S51.812**   **Laceration without foreign body of**   NRS
                   left **forearm**

     √7ᵗʰ **S51.819**   Laceration without foreign body of ▽
                   unspecified forearm

   √6ᵗʰ **S51.82** Laceration with foreign body **of forearm**

     4,5 √7ᵗʰ **S51.821**   **Laceration with foreign body of** right   NRS
                   forearm

     4,5 √7ᵗʰ **S51.822**   **Laceration with foreign body of** left   NRS
                   forearm

     √7ᵗʰ **S51.829**   Laceration with foreign body of ▽
                   unspecified forearm

   √6ᵗʰ **S51.83** Puncture wound without foreign body **of forearm**
             AHA: 2016, 3Q, 24

     4,5 √7ᵗʰ **S51.831**   **Puncture wound without foreign**   NRS
                   body of right **forearm**

     4,5 √7ᵗʰ **S51.832**   **Puncture wound without foreign**   NRS
                   body of left **forearm**

     √7ᵗʰ **S51.839**   Puncture wound without foreign ▽
                   body of unspecified forearm

---

4   Case-mix diagnosis with 7th character indicating initial or subsequent encounter.
5   NRS supply diagnosis with 7th character indicating initial or subsequent encounter.

☑ Additional Character Req   √7ᵗʰ Placeholder Alert   Case-Mix Diagnosis   Manifestation   ▽ Unspecified Dx   *EXCLUDES 1* Not coded here   *EXCLUDES 2* Not included here

Chapter 19. Injury, Poisoning and Certain Other Consequences of External Causes

✓6ᵗʰ **S51.84**   Puncture wound with foreign body **of forearm**
AHA: 2016, 3Q, 24

4,5 ✓7ᵗʰ **S51.841**   **Puncture wound with foreign body of right forearm**   NRS

4,5 ✓7ᵗʰ **S51.842**   **Puncture wound with foreign body of left forearm**   NRS

✓7ᵗʰ **S51.849**   **Puncture wound with foreign body of unspecified forearm**   ▽

✓6ᵗʰ **S51.85**   Open bite **of forearm**
Bite of forearm NOS
EXCLUDES 1   superficial bite of forearm (S50.86, S50.87)

4,5 ✓7ᵗʰ **S51.851**   **Open bite of right forearm**   NRS

4,5 ✓7ᵗʰ **S51.852**   **Open bite of left forearm**   NRS

✓7ᵗʰ **S51.859**   **Open bite of unspecified forearm**   ▽

✓4ᵗʰ **S52**   **Fracture of forearm**
NOTE   A fracture not indicated as displaced or nondisplaced should be coded to displaced.
A fracture not indicated as open or closed should be coded to closed.
The open fracture designations are based on the Gustilo open fracture classification.
EXCLUDES 1   traumatic amputation of forearm (S58.-)
EXCLUDES 2   fracture at wrist and hand level (S62.-)
AHA: 2016, 1Q, 33; 2015, 3Q, 37-39
TIP: The term "improper alignment" is not synonymous with malunion or nonunion of a fracture when noted in provider documentation.

The appropriate 7th character is to be added to all codes from category S52 [unless otherwise indicated].
A   initial encounter for closed fracture
B   initial encounter for open fracture type I or II
     initial encounter for open fracture NOS
C   initial encounter for open fracture type IIIA, IIIB, or IIIC
D   subsequent encounter for closed fracture with routine healing
E   subsequent encounter for open fracture type I or II with routine healing
F   subsequent encounter for open fracture type IIIA, IIIB, or IIIC with routine healing
G   subsequent encounter for closed fracture with delayed healing
H   subsequent encounter for open fracture type I or II with delayed healing
J   subsequent encounter for open fracture type IIIA, IIIB, or IIIC with delayed healing
K   subsequent encounter for closed fracture with nonunion
M   subsequent encounter for open fracture type I or II with nonunion
N   subsequent encounter for open fracture type IIIA, IIIB, or IIIC with nonunion
P   subsequent encounter for closed fracture with malunion
Q   subsequent encounter for open fracture type I or II with malunion
R   subsequent encounter for open fracture type IIIA, IIIB, or IIIC with malunion
S   sequela

✓5ᵗʰ **S52.0**   **Fracture of upper end of ulna**
Fracture of proximal end of ulna
EXCLUDES 2   fracture of elbow NOS (S42.40-)
fractures of shaft of ulna (S52.2-)

✓6ᵗʰ **S52.00**   Unspecified **fracture of upper end of ulna**

1 ✓7ᵗʰ **S52.001**   **Unspecified fracture of upper end of right ulna**   ▽

1 ✓7ᵗʰ **S52.002**   **Unspecified fracture of upper end of left ulna**   ▽

✓7ᵗʰ **S52.009**   **Unspecified fracture of upper end of unspecified ulna**   ▽

✓6ᵗʰ **S52.01**   Torus **fracture of upper end of ulna**

The appropriate 7th character is to be added to all codes in subcategory S52.01.
A   initial encounter for closed fracture
D   subsequent encounter for fracture with routine healing
G   subsequent encounter for fracture with delayed healing
K   subsequent encounter for fracture with nonunion
P   subsequent encounter for fracture with malunion
S   sequela

1 ✓7ᵗʰ **S52.011**   **Torus fracture of upper end of right ulna**

1 ✓7ᵗʰ **S52.012**   **Torus fracture of upper end of left ulna**

✓7ᵗʰ **S52.019**   **Torus fracture of upper end of unspecified ulna**   ▽

✓6ᵗʰ **S52.02**   Fracture of olecranon process without intraarticular extension **of ulna**

1 ✓7ᵗʰ **S52.021**   **Displaced fracture of olecranon process without intraarticular extension of right ulna**

1 ✓7ᵗʰ **S52.022**   **Displaced fracture of olecranon process without intraarticular extension of left ulna**

✓7ᵗʰ **S52.023**   **Displaced fracture of olecranon process without intraarticular extension of unspecified ulna**   ▽

1 ✓7ᵗʰ **S52.024**   **Nondisplaced fracture of olecranon process without intraarticular extension of right ulna**

1 ✓7ᵗʰ **S52.025**   **Nondisplaced fracture of olecranon process without intraarticular extension of left ulna**

✓7ᵗʰ **S52.026**   **Nondisplaced fracture of olecranon process without intraarticular extension of unspecified ulna**   ▽

✓6ᵗʰ **S52.03**   Fracture of olecranon process with intraarticular extension **of ulna**

1 ✓7ᵗʰ **S52.031**   **Displaced fracture of olecranon process with intraarticular extension of right ulna**

1 ✓7ᵗʰ **S52.032**   **Displaced fracture of olecranon process with intraarticular extension of left ulna**

✓7ᵗʰ **S52.033**   **Displaced fracture of olecranon process with intraarticular extension of unspecified ulna**   ▽

1 ✓7ᵗʰ **S52.034**   **Nondisplaced fracture of olecranon process with intraarticular extension of right ulna**

1 ✓7ᵗʰ **S52.035**   **Nondisplaced fracture of olecranon process with intraarticular extension of left ulna**

✓7ᵗʰ **S52.036**   **Nondisplaced fracture of olecranon process with intraarticular extension of unspecified ulna**   ▽

✓6ᵗʰ **S52.04**   Fracture of coronoid process **of ulna**

1 ✓7ᵗʰ **S52.041**   **Displaced fracture of coronoid process of right ulna**

1 ✓7ᵗʰ **S52.042**   **Displaced fracture of coronoid process of left ulna**

✓7ᵗʰ **S52.043**   **Displaced fracture of coronoid process of unspecified ulna**   ▽

1 ✓7ᵗʰ **S52.044**   **Nondisplaced fracture of coronoid process of right ulna**

1 ✓7ᵗʰ **S52.045**   **Nondisplaced fracture of coronoid process of left ulna**

✓7ᵗʰ **S52.046**   **Nondisplaced fracture of coronoid process of unspecified ulna**   ▽

✓6ᵗʰ **S52.09**   Other **fracture of upper end of ulna**

1 ✓7ᵗʰ **S52.091**   **Other fracture of upper end of right ulna**

1 ✓7ᵗʰ **S52.092**   **Other fracture of upper end of left ulna**

✓7ᵗʰ **S52.099**   **Other fracture of upper end of unspecified ulna**   ▽

---

1   Case-mix diagnosis with 7th character indicating subsequent encounter.
4   Case-mix diagnosis with 7th character indicating initial or subsequent encounter.
5   NRS supply diagnosis with 7th character indicating initial or subsequent encounter.

✓6ᵗʰ **S52.1 Fracture of** upper end of radius
Fracture of proximal end of radius
EXCLUDES 2   physeal fractures of upper end of radius (S59.2-)
fracture of shaft of radius (S52.3-)

✓6ᵗʰ **S52.10 Unspecified fracture of upper end of radius**
1 ✓7ᵗʰ **S52.101 Unspecified fracture of upper end of** right **radius** ▽
1 ✓7ᵗʰ **S52.102 Unspecified fracture of upper end of** left **radius** ▽
✓7ᵗʰ **S52.109 Unspecified fracture of upper end of unspecified radius** ▽

✓6ᵗʰ **S52.11 Torus fracture of upper end of radius**

The appropriate 7th character is to be added to all codes in subcategory S52.11.
A   initial encounter for closed fracture
D   subsequent encounter for fracture with routine healing
G   subsequent encounter for fracture with delayed healing
K   subsequent encounter for fracture with nonunion
P   subsequent encounter for fracture with malunion
S   sequela

1 ✓7ᵗʰ **S52.111 Torus fracture of upper end of** right **radius**
1 ✓7ᵗʰ **S52.112 Torus fracture of upper end of** left **radius**
✓7ᵗʰ **S52.119 Torus fracture of upper end of unspecified radius** ▽

✓6ᵗʰ **S52.12 Fracture of** head of radius
1 ✓7ᵗʰ **S52.121 Displaced fracture of head of** right **radius**
1 ✓7ᵗʰ **S52.122 Displaced fracture of head of** left **radius**
✓7ᵗʰ **S52.123 Displaced fracture of head of unspecified radius** ▽
1 ✓7ᵗʰ **S52.124 Nondisplaced fracture of head of** right **radius**
1 ✓7ᵗʰ **S52.125 Nondisplaced fracture of head of** left **radius**
✓7ᵗʰ **S52.126 Nondisplaced fracture of head of unspecified radius** ▽

✓6ᵗʰ **S52.13 Fracture of** neck of radius
1 ✓7ᵗʰ **S52.131 Displaced fracture of neck of** right **radius**
1 ✓7ᵗʰ **S52.132 Displaced fracture of neck of** left **radius**
✓7ᵗʰ **S52.133 Displaced fracture of neck of unspecified radius** ▽
1 ✓7ᵗʰ **S52.134 Nondisplaced fracture of neck of** right **radius**
1 ✓7ᵗʰ **S52.135 Nondisplaced fracture of neck of** left **radius**
✓7ᵗʰ **S52.136 Nondisplaced fracture of neck of unspecified radius** ▽

✓6ᵗʰ **S52.18 Other fracture of upper end of radius**
1 ✓7ᵗʰ **S52.181 Other fracture of upper end of** right **radius**
1 ✓7ᵗʰ **S52.182 Other fracture of upper end of** left **radius**
✓7ᵗʰ **S52.189 Other fracture of upper end of unspecified radius** ▽

✓5ᵗʰ **S52.2 Fracture of** shaft of ulna
✓6ᵗʰ **S52.20 Unspecified fracture of shaft of ulna**
Fracture of ulna NOS
1 ✓7ᵗʰ **S52.201 Unspecified fracture of shaft of** right **ulna** ▽
1 ✓7ᵗʰ **S52.202 Unspecified fracture of shaft of** left **ulna** ▽
✓7ᵗʰ **S52.209 Unspecified fracture of shaft of unspecified ulna** ▽

✓6ᵗʰ **S52.21 Greenstick fracture of shaft of ulna**

The appropriate 7th character is to be added to all codes in subcategory S52.21.
A   initial encounter for closed fracture
D   subsequent encounter for fracture with routine healing
G   subsequent encounter for fracture with delayed healing
K   subsequent encounter for fracture with nonunion
P   subsequent encounter for fracture with malunion
S   sequela

1 ✓7ᵗʰ **S52.211 Greenstick fracture of shaft of** right **ulna**
1 ✓7ᵗʰ **S52.212 Greenstick fracture of shaft of** left **ulna**
✓7ᵗʰ **S52.219 Greenstick fracture of shaft of unspecified ulna** ▽

✓6ᵗʰ **S52.22 Transverse fracture of shaft of ulna**
1 ✓7ᵗʰ **S52.221 Displaced transverse fracture of shaft of** right **ulna**
1 ✓7ᵗʰ **S52.222 Displaced transverse fracture of shaft of** left **ulna**
✓7ᵗʰ **S52.223 Displaced transverse fracture of shaft of unspecified ulna** ▽
1 ✓7ᵗʰ **S52.224 Nondisplaced transverse fracture of shaft of** right **ulna**
1 ✓7ᵗʰ **S52.225 Nondisplaced transverse fracture of shaft of** left **ulna**
✓7ᵗʰ **S52.226 Nondisplaced transverse fracture of shaft of unspecified ulna** ▽

✓6ᵗʰ **S52.23 Oblique fracture of shaft of ulna**
1 ✓7ᵗʰ **S52.231 Displaced oblique fracture of shaft of** right **ulna**
1 ✓7ᵗʰ **S52.232 Displaced oblique fracture of shaft of** left **ulna**
✓7ᵗʰ **S52.233 Displaced oblique fracture of shaft of unspecified ulna** ▽
1 ✓7ᵗʰ **S52.234 Nondisplaced oblique fracture of shaft of** right **ulna**
1 ✓7ᵗʰ **S52.235 Nondisplaced oblique fracture of shaft of** left **ulna**
✓7ᵗʰ **S52.236 Nondisplaced oblique fracture of shaft of unspecified ulna** ▽

✓6ᵗʰ **S52.24 Spiral fracture of shaft of ulna**
1 ✓7ᵗʰ **S52.241 Displaced spiral fracture of shaft of ulna,** right **arm**
1 ✓7ᵗʰ **S52.242 Displaced spiral fracture of shaft of ulna,** left **arm**
✓7ᵗʰ **S52.243 Displaced spiral fracture of shaft of ulna, unspecified arm** ▽
1 ✓7ᵗʰ **S52.244 Nondisplaced spiral fracture of shaft of ulna,** right **arm**
1 ✓7ᵗʰ **S52.245 Nondisplaced spiral fracture of shaft of ulna,** left **arm**
✓7ᵗʰ **S52.246 Nondisplaced spiral fracture of shaft of ulna, unspecified arm** ▽

✓6ᵗʰ **S52.25 Comminuted fracture of shaft of ulna**
1 ✓7ᵗʰ **S52.251 Displaced comminuted fracture of shaft of ulna,** right **arm**
1 ✓7ᵗʰ **S52.252 Displaced comminuted fracture of shaft of ulna,** left **arm**
✓7ᵗʰ **S52.253 Displaced comminuted fracture of shaft of ulna, unspecified arm** ▽
1 ✓7ᵗʰ **S52.254 Nondisplaced comminuted fracture of shaft of ulna,** right **arm**
1 ✓7ᵗʰ **S52.255 Nondisplaced comminuted fracture of shaft of ulna,** left **arm**
✓7ᵗʰ **S52.256 Nondisplaced comminuted fracture of shaft of ulna, unspecified arm** ▽

---

1   Case-mix diagnosis with 7th character indicating subsequent encounter.

✓6ᵗʰ S52.26 Segmental fracture of shaft of ulna

- **1 ✓7ᵗʰ S52.261** Displaced segmental fracture of shaft of ulna, right arm
- **1 ✓7ᵗʰ S52.262** Displaced segmental fracture of shaft of ulna, left arm
- **✓7ᵗʰ S52.263** Displaced segmental fracture of shaft of ulna, unspecified arm ▽
- **1 ✓7ᵗʰ S52.264** Nondisplaced segmental fracture of shaft of ulna, right arm
- **1 ✓7ᵗʰ S52.265** Nondisplaced segmental fracture of shaft of ulna, left arm
- **✓7ᵗʰ S52.266** Nondisplaced segmental fracture of shaft of ulna, unspecified arm ▽

✓6ᵗʰ S52.27 Monteggia's fracture of ulna
Fracture of upper shaft of ulna with dislocation of radial head

- **1 ✓7ᵗʰ S52.271** Monteggia's fracture of right ulna
- **1 ✓7ᵗʰ S52.272** Monteggia's fracture of left ulna
- **✓7ᵗʰ S52.279** Monteggia's fracture of unspecified ulna ▽

✓6ᵗʰ S52.28 Bent bone of ulna

- **1 ✓7ᵗʰ S52.281** Bent bone of right ulna
- **1 ✓7ᵗʰ S52.282** Bent bone of left ulna
- **✓7ᵗʰ S52.283** Bent bone of unspecified ulna ▽

✓6ᵗʰ S52.29 Other fracture of shaft of ulna

- **1 ✓7ᵗʰ S52.291** Other fracture of shaft of right ulna
- **1 ✓7ᵗʰ S52.292** Other fracture of shaft of left ulna
- **✓7ᵗʰ S52.299** Other fracture of shaft of unspecified ulna ▽

✓5ᵗʰ S52.3 Fracture of shaft of radius

✓6ᵗʰ S52.30 Unspecified fracture of shaft of radius

- **1 ✓7ᵗʰ S52.301** Unspecified fracture of shaft of right radius ▽
- **1 ✓7ᵗʰ S52.302** Unspecified fracture of shaft of left radius ▽
- **✓7ᵗʰ S52.309** Unspecified fracture of shaft of unspecified radius ▽

✓6ᵗʰ S52.31 Greenstick fracture of shaft of radius

> The appropriate 7th character is to be added to all codes in subcategory S52.31.
> A   initial encounter for closed fracture
> D   subsequent encounter for fracture with routine healing
> G   subsequent encounter for fracture with delayed healing
> K   subsequent encounter for fracture with nonunion
> P   subsequent encounter for fracture with malunion
> S   sequela

- **1 ✓7ᵗʰ S52.311** Greenstick fracture of shaft of radius, right arm
- **1 ✓7ᵗʰ S52.312** Greenstick fracture of shaft of radius, left arm
- **✓7ᵗʰ S52.319** Greenstick fracture of shaft of radius, unspecified arm ▽

✓6ᵗʰ S52.32 Transverse fracture of shaft of radius

- **1 ✓7ᵗʰ S52.321** Displaced transverse fracture of shaft of right radius
- **1 ✓7ᵗʰ S52.322** Displaced transverse fracture of shaft of left radius
- **✓7ᵗʰ S52.323** Displaced transverse fracture of shaft of unspecified radius ▽
- **1 ✓7ᵗʰ S52.324** Nondisplaced transverse fracture of shaft of right radius
- **1 ✓7ᵗʰ S52.325** Nondisplaced transverse fracture of shaft of left radius
- **✓7ᵗʰ S52.326** Nondisplaced transverse fracture of shaft of unspecified radius ▽

✓6ᵗʰ S52.33 Oblique fracture of shaft of radius

- **1 ✓7ᵗʰ S52.331** Displaced oblique fracture of shaft of right radius

1 ✓7ᵗʰ S52.332 Displaced oblique fracture of shaft of left radius

- **✓7ᵗʰ S52.333** Displaced oblique fracture of shaft of unspecified radius ▽
- **1 ✓7ᵗʰ S52.334** Nondisplaced oblique fracture of shaft of right radius
- **1 ✓7ᵗʰ S52.335** Nondisplaced oblique fracture of shaft of left radius
- **✓7ᵗʰ S52.336** Nondisplaced oblique fracture of shaft of unspecified radius ▽

✓6ᵗʰ S52.34 Spiral fracture of shaft of radius

- **1 ✓7ᵗʰ S52.341** Displaced spiral fracture of shaft of radius, right arm
- **1 ✓7ᵗʰ S52.342** Displaced spiral fracture of shaft of radius, left arm
- **✓7ᵗʰ S52.343** Displaced spiral fracture of shaft of radius, unspecified arm ▽
- **1 ✓7ᵗʰ S52.344** Nondisplaced spiral fracture of shaft of radius, right arm
- **1 ✓7ᵗʰ S52.345** Nondisplaced spiral fracture of shaft of radius, left arm
- **✓7ᵗʰ S52.346** Nondisplaced spiral fracture of shaft of radius, unspecified arm ▽

✓6ᵗʰ S52.35 Comminuted fracture of shaft of radius

- **1 ✓7ᵗʰ S52.351** Displaced comminuted fracture of shaft of radius, right arm
- **1 ✓7ᵗʰ S52.352** Displaced comminuted fracture of shaft of radius, left arm
- **✓7ᵗʰ S52.353** Displaced comminuted fracture of shaft of radius, unspecified arm ▽
- **1 ✓7ᵗʰ S52.354** Nondisplaced comminuted fracture of shaft of radius, right arm
- **1 ✓7ᵗʰ S52.355** Nondisplaced comminuted fracture of shaft of radius, left arm
- **✓7ᵗʰ S52.356** Nondisplaced comminuted fracture of shaft of radius, unspecified arm ▽

✓6ᵗʰ S52.36 Segmental fracture of shaft of radius

- **1 ✓7ᵗʰ S52.361** Displaced segmental fracture of shaft of radius, right arm
- **1 ✓7ᵗʰ S52.362** Displaced segmental fracture of shaft of radius, left arm
- **✓7ᵗʰ S52.363** Displaced segmental fracture of shaft of radius, unspecified arm ▽
- **1 ✓7ᵗʰ S52.364** Nondisplaced segmental fracture of shaft of radius, right arm
- **1 ✓7ᵗʰ S52.365** Nondisplaced segmental fracture of shaft of radius, left arm
- **✓7ᵗʰ S52.366** Nondisplaced segmental fracture of shaft of radius, unspecified arm ▽

✓6ᵗʰ S52.37 Galeazzi's fracture
Fracture of lower shaft of radius with radioulnar joint dislocation

- **1 ✓7ᵗʰ S52.371** Galeazzi's fracture of right radius
- **1 ✓7ᵗʰ S52.372** Galeazzi's fracture of left radius
- **✓7ᵗʰ S52.379** Galeazzi's fracture of unspecified radius ▽

✓6ᵗʰ S52.38 Bent bone of radius

- **1 ✓7ᵗʰ S52.381** Bent bone of right radius
- **1 ✓7ᵗʰ S52.382** Bent bone of left radius
- **✓7ᵗʰ S52.389** Bent bone of unspecified radius ▽

✓6ᵗʰ S52.39 Other fracture of shaft of radius

- **1 ✓7ᵗʰ S52.391** Other fracture of shaft of radius, right arm
- **1 ✓7ᵗʰ S52.392** Other fracture of shaft of radius, left arm
- **✓7ᵗʰ S52.399** Other fracture of shaft of radius, unspecified arm ▽

✓5ᵗʰ S52.5 Fracture of lower end of radius
Fracture of distal end of radius
EXCLUDES 2   physeal fractures of lower end of radius (S59.2-)
DEF: Fracture of distal end of radius above the wrist; most commonly caused by fall onto an outstretched hand.

✓6ᵗʰ S52.50 Unspecified fracture of the lower end of radius

- **1 ✓7ᵗʰ S52.501** Unspecified fracture of the lower end of right radius ▽

---

1   Case-mix diagnosis with 7th character indicating subsequent encounter.

Ⓝ Newborn: 0   Ⓟ Pediatric: 0-17   Ⓜ Maternity: 12-55   Ⓐ Adult: 15-124   **NRS** Nonroutine supply Dx   **NC Dx** Noncancer Dx   **PDx** Primary Dx   ▶◀ Revised Text   ● New Code   ▲ Revised Title

968   ICD-10-CM 2018

1 ✓7ᵗʰ **S52.502** **Unspecified fracture of the lower end of left radius** ▽

✓7ᵗʰ **S52.509** Unspecified fracture of the lower end of unspecified radius ▽

✓6ᵗʰ **S52.51** **Fracture of** radial styloid process

1 ✓7ᵗʰ **S52.511** Displaced **fracture of** right **radial styloid process**

1 ✓7ᵗʰ **S52.512** Displaced **fracture of** left **radial styloid process**

✓7ᵗʰ **S52.513** Displaced **fracture of unspecified radial styloid process** ▽

1 ✓7ᵗʰ **S52.514** Nondisplaced **fracture of** right **radial styloid process**

1 ✓7ᵗʰ **S52.515** Nondisplaced **fracture of** left **radial styloid process**

✓7ᵗʰ **S52.516** Nondisplaced **fracture of unspecified radial styloid process** ▽

✓6ᵗʰ **S52.52** Torus **fracture of lower end of radius**

The appropriate 7th character is to be added to all codes in subcategory S52.52.
A   initial encounter for closed fracture
D   subsequent encounter for fracture with routine healing
G   subsequent encounter for fracture with delayed healing
K   subsequent encounter for fracture with nonunion
P   subsequent encounter for fracture with malunion
S   sequela

1 ✓7ᵗʰ **S52.521** **Torus fracture of lower end of** right **radius**

1 ✓7ᵗʰ **S52.522** **Torus fracture of lower end of** left **radius**

✓7ᵗʰ **S52.529** **Torus fracture of lower end of unspecified radius** ▽

✓6ᵗʰ **S52.53** Colles' fracture
AHA: 2016, 2Q, 4

1 ✓7ᵗʰ **S52.531** **Colles' fracture of** right **radius**

1 ✓7ᵗʰ **S52.532** **Colles' fracture of** left **radius**

✓7ᵗʰ **S52.539** **Colles' fracture of unspecified radius** ▽

✓6ᵗʰ **S52.54** Smith's **fracture**

1 ✓7ᵗʰ **S52.541** **Smith's fracture of** right **radius**

1 ✓7ᵗʰ **S52.542** **Smith's fracture of** left **radius**

✓7ᵗʰ **S52.549** **Smith's fracture of unspecified radius** ▽

✓6ᵗʰ **S52.55** Other extraarticular **fracture of lower end of radius**

1 ✓7ᵗʰ **S52.551** **Other extraarticular fracture of lower end of** right **radius**

1 ✓7ᵗʰ **S52.552** **Other extraarticular fracture of lower end of** left **radius**

✓7ᵗʰ **S52.559** **Other extraarticular fracture of lower end of unspecified radius** ▽

✓6ᵗʰ **S52.56** Barton's **fracture**

1 ✓7ᵗʰ **S52.561** **Barton's fracture of** right **radius**

1 ✓7ᵗʰ **S52.562** **Barton's fracture of** left **radius**

✓7ᵗʰ **S52.569** **Barton's fracture of unspecified radius** ▽

✓6ᵗʰ **S52.57** Other intraarticular **fracture of lower end of radius**

1 ✓7ᵗʰ **S52.571** **Other intraarticular fracture of lower end of** right **radius**

1 ✓7ᵗʰ **S52.572** **Other intraarticular fracture of lower end of** left **radius**

✓7ᵗʰ **S52.579** **Other intraarticular fracture of lower end of unspecified radius** ▽

✓6ᵗʰ **S52.59** Other **fractures of lower end of radius**

1 ✓7ᵗʰ **S52.591** **Other fractures of lower end of** right **radius**

1 ✓7ᵗʰ **S52.592** **Other fractures of lower end of** left **radius**

✓7ᵗʰ **S52.599** **Other fractures of lower end of unspecified radius** ▽

✓5ᵗʰ **S52.6** Fracture of lower end of ulna

✓6ᵗʰ **S52.60** Unspecified **fracture of lower end of ulna**

1 ✓7ᵗʰ **S52.601** **Unspecified fracture of lower end of** right **ulna** ▽

1 ✓7ᵗʰ **S52.602** **Unspecified fracture of lower end of** left **ulna** ▽

✓7ᵗʰ **S52.609** Unspecified fracture of lower end of unspecified ulna ▽

✓6ᵗʰ **S52.61** **Fracture of ulna** styloid process

1 ✓7ᵗʰ **S52.611** Displaced **fracture of** right **ulna styloid process**

1 ✓7ᵗʰ **S52.612** Displaced **fracture of** left **ulna styloid process**

✓7ᵗʰ **S52.613** Displaced **fracture of unspecified ulna styloid process** ▽

1 ✓7ᵗʰ **S52.614** Nondisplaced **fracture of** right **ulna styloid process**

1 ✓7ᵗʰ **S52.615** Nondisplaced **fracture of** left **ulna styloid process**

✓7ᵗʰ **S52.616** Nondisplaced **fracture of unspecified ulna styloid process** ▽

✓6ᵗʰ **S52.62** Torus **fracture of lower end of ulna**

The appropriate 7th character is to be added to all codes in subcategory S52.62.
A   initial encounter for closed fracture
D   subsequent encounter for fracture with routine healing
G   subsequent encounter for fracture with delayed healing
K   subsequent encounter for fracture with nonunion
P   subsequent encounter for fracture with malunion
S   sequela

1 ✓7ᵗʰ **S52.621** **Torus fracture of lower end of** right **ulna**

1 ✓7ᵗʰ **S52.622** **Torus fracture of lower end of** left **ulna**

✓7ᵗʰ **S52.629** **Torus fracture of lower end of unspecified ulna** ▽

✓6ᵗʰ **S52.69** Other **fracture of lower end of ulna**

1 ✓7ᵗʰ **S52.691** **Other fracture of lower end of** right **ulna**

1 ✓7ᵗʰ **S52.692** **Other fracture of lower end of** left **ulna**

✓7ᵗʰ **S52.699** **Other fracture of lower end of unspecified ulna** ▽

✓5ᵗʰ **S52.9** Unspecified fracture of forearm

✓x7ᵗʰ **S52.90** Unspecified fracture of unspecified forearm ▽

1 ✓x7ᵗʰ **S52.91** **Unspecified fracture of** right **forearm** ▽

1 ✓x7ᵗʰ **S52.92** **Unspecified fracture of** left **forearm** ▽

✓4ᵗʰ **S53** **Dislocation and sprain of joints and ligaments of elbow**

    INCLUDES avulsion of joint or ligament of elbow
                laceration of cartilage, joint or ligament of elbow
                sprain of cartilage, joint or ligament of elbow
                traumatic hemarthrosis of joint or ligament of elbow
                traumatic rupture of joint or ligament of elbow
                traumatic subluxation of joint or ligament of elbow
                traumatic tear of joint or ligament of elbow

Code also any associated open wound

EXCLUDES 2 *strain of muscle, fascia and tendon at forearm level (S56.-)*

The appropriate 7th character is to be added to each code from category S53.
A   initial encounter
D   subsequent encounter
S   sequela

✓5ᵗʰ **S53.0** **Subluxation and dislocation of** radial head
     Dislocation of radiohumeral joint
     Subluxation of radiohumeral joint
     EXCLUDES 1 *Monteggia's fracture-dislocation (S52.27-)*

✓6ᵗʰ **S53.00** Unspecified **subluxation and dislocation of radial head**

1 ✓7ᵗʰ **S53.001** **Unspecified** subluxation **of** right **radial head** ▽

1 ✓7ᵗʰ **S53.002** **Unspecified** subluxation **of** left **radial head** ▽

---

1   Case-mix diagnosis with 7th character indicating subsequent encounter.

☑ Additional Character Req   ✓x7ᵗʰ Placeholder Alert   Case-Mix Diagnosis   Manifestation   ▽ Unspecified Dx   **EXCLUDES 1** Not coded here   **EXCLUDES 2** Not included here

ICD-10-CM 2018   969

Chapter 19. Injury, Poisoning and Certain Other Consequences of External Causes

S53.003–S53.32

√7ᵗʰ **S53.003** Unspecified subluxation of unspecified radial head ▽

1 √7ᵗʰ **S53.004** Unspecified dislocation of right radial head ▽

1 √7ᵗʰ **S53.005** Unspecified dislocation of left radial head ▽

√7ᵗʰ **S53.006** Unspecified dislocation of unspecified radial head ▽

√6ᵗʰ **S53.01** Anterior subluxation and dislocation of radial head
Anteriomedial subluxation and dislocation of radial head

1 √7ᵗʰ **S53.011** Anterior subluxation of right radial head

1 √7ᵗʰ **S53.012** Anterior subluxation of left radial head

√7ᵗʰ **S53.013** Anterior subluxation of unspecified radial head

1 √7ᵗʰ **S53.014** Anterior dislocation of right radial head

1 √7ᵗʰ **S53.015** Anterior dislocation of left radial head

√7ᵗʰ **S53.016** Anterior dislocation of unspecified radial head ▽

√6ᵗʰ **S53.02** Posterior subluxation and dislocation of radial head
Posteriolateral subluxation and dislocation of radial head

1 √7ᵗʰ **S53.021** Posterior subluxation of right radial head

1 √7ᵗʰ **S53.022** Posterior subluxation of left radial head

√7ᵗʰ **S53.023** Posterior subluxation of unspecified radial head ▽

1 √7ᵗʰ **S53.024** Posterior dislocation of right radial head

1 √7ᵗʰ **S53.025** Posterior dislocation of left radial head

√7ᵗʰ **S53.026** Posterior dislocation of unspecified radial head ▽

√6ᵗʰ **S53.03** Nursemaid's elbow

1 √7ᵗʰ **S53.031** Nursemaid's elbow, right elbow

1 √7ᵗʰ **S53.032** Nursemaid's elbow, left elbow

√7ᵗʰ **S53.033** Nursemaid's elbow, unspecified elbow ▽

√6ᵗʰ **S53.09** Other subluxation and dislocation of radial head

1 √7ᵗʰ **S53.091** Other subluxation of right radial head

1 √7ᵗʰ **S53.092** Other subluxation of left radial head

√7ᵗʰ **S53.093** Other subluxation of unspecified radial head ▽

1 √7ᵗʰ **S53.094** Other dislocation of right radial head

1 √7ᵗʰ **S53.095** Other dislocation of left radial head

√7ᵗʰ **S53.096** Other dislocation of unspecified radial head ▽

√5ᵗʰ **S53.1** Subluxation and dislocation of ulnohumeral joint
Subluxation and dislocation of elbow NOS
EXCLUDES 1 dislocation of radial head alone (S53.0-)

√6ᵗʰ **S53.10** Unspecified subluxation and dislocation of ulnohumeral joint

1 √7ᵗʰ **S53.101** Unspecified subluxation of right ulnohumeral joint ▽

1 √7ᵗʰ **S53.102** Unspecified subluxation of left ulnohumeral joint ▽

√7ᵗʰ **S53.103** Unspecified subluxation of unspecified ulnohumeral joint ▽

1 √7ᵗʰ **S53.104** Unspecified dislocation of right ulnohumeral joint ▽

1 √7ᵗʰ **S53.105** Unspecified dislocation of left ulnohumeral joint ▽

√7ᵗʰ **S53.106** Unspecified dislocation of unspecified ulnohumeral joint ▽

√6ᵗʰ **S53.11** Anterior subluxation and dislocation of ulnohumeral joint

1 √7ᵗʰ **S53.111** Anterior subluxation of right ulnohumeral joint

1 √7ᵗʰ **S53.112** Anterior subluxation of left ulnohumeral joint

√7ᵗʰ **S53.113** Anterior subluxation of unspecified ulnohumeral joint ▽

1 √7ᵗʰ **S53.114** Anterior dislocation of right ulnohumeral joint
AHA: 2012, 4Q, 108

1 √7ᵗʰ **S53.115** Anterior dislocation of left ulnohumeral joint

√7ᵗʰ **S53.116** Anterior dislocation of unspecified ulnohumeral joint ▽

√6ᵗʰ **S53.12** Posterior subluxation and dislocation of ulnohumeral joint

1 √7ᵗʰ **S53.121** Posterior subluxation of right ulnohumeral joint

1 √7ᵗʰ **S53.122** Posterior subluxation of left ulnohumeral joint

√7ᵗʰ **S53.123** Posterior subluxation of unspecified ulnohumeral joint ▽

1 √7ᵗʰ **S53.124** Posterior dislocation of right ulnohumeral joint

1 √7ᵗʰ **S53.125** Posterior dislocation of left ulnohumeral joint

√7ᵗʰ **S53.126** Posterior dislocation of unspecified ulnohumeral joint ▽

√6ᵗʰ **S53.13** Medial subluxation and dislocation of ulnohumeral joint

1 √7ᵗʰ **S53.131** Medial subluxation of right ulnohumeral joint

1 √7ᵗʰ **S53.132** Medial subluxation of left ulnohumeral joint

√7ᵗʰ **S53.133** Medial subluxation of unspecified ulnohumeral joint ▽

1 √7ᵗʰ **S53.134** Medial dislocation of right ulnohumeral joint

1 √7ᵗʰ **S53.135** Medial dislocation of left ulnohumeral joint

√7ᵗʰ **S53.136** Medial dislocation of unspecified ulnohumeral joint ▽

√6ᵗʰ **S53.14** Lateral subluxation and dislocation of ulnohumeral joint

1 √7ᵗʰ **S53.141** Lateral subluxation of right ulnohumeral joint

1 √7ᵗʰ **S53.142** Lateral subluxation of left ulnohumeral joint

√7ᵗʰ **S53.143** Lateral subluxation of unspecified ulnohumeral joint ▽

1 √7ᵗʰ **S53.144** Lateral dislocation of right ulnohumeral joint

1 √7ᵗʰ **S53.145** Lateral dislocation of left ulnohumeral joint

√7ᵗʰ **S53.146** Lateral dislocation of unspecified ulnohumeral joint ▽

√6ᵗʰ **S53.19** Other subluxation and dislocation of ulnohumeral joint

1 √7ᵗʰ **S53.191** Other subluxation of right ulnohumeral joint

1 √7ᵗʰ **S53.192** Other subluxation of left ulnohumeral joint

√7ᵗʰ **S53.193** Other subluxation of unspecified ulnohumeral joint ▽

1 √7ᵗʰ **S53.194** Other dislocation of right ulnohumeral joint

1 √7ᵗʰ **S53.195** Other dislocation of left ulnohumeral joint

√7ᵗʰ **S53.196** Other dislocation of unspecified ulnohumeral joint ▽

√5ᵗʰ **S53.2** Traumatic rupture of radial collateral ligament
EXCLUDES 1 sprain of radial collateral ligament NOS (S53.43-)

√x7ᵗʰ **S53.20** Traumatic rupture of unspecified radial collateral ligament ▽

√x7ᵗʰ **S53.21** Traumatic rupture of right radial collateral ligament

√x7ᵗʰ **S53.22** Traumatic rupture of left radial collateral ligament

√5ᵗʰ **S53.3** Traumatic rupture of ulnar collateral ligament
EXCLUDES 1 sprain of ulnar collateral ligament (S53.44-)

√x7ᵗʰ **S53.30** Traumatic rupture of unspecified ulnar collateral ligament ▽

√x7ᵗʰ **S53.31** Traumatic rupture of right ulnar collateral ligament

√x7ᵗʰ **S53.32** Traumatic rupture of left ulnar collateral ligament

---

1   Case-mix diagnosis with 7th character indicating subsequent encounter.

Ⓝ Newborn: 0 Ⓟ Pediatric: 0-17 Ⓜ Maternity: 12-55 Ⓐ Adult: 15-124 **NRS** Nonroutine supply Dx **NCDx** Noncancer Dx **PDx** Primary Dx ▶◀ Revised Text ● New Code ▲ Revised Title

970   ICD-10-CM 2018

✓5ᵗʰ **S53.4** **Sprain of** elbow
- EXCLUDES 2   *traumatic rupture of radial collateral ligament (S53.2-)*
              traumatic rupture of ulnar collateral ligament (S53.3-)
- ✓6ᵗʰ **S53.40** **Unspecified** sprain of elbow
  - ✓7ᵗʰ **S53.401** Unspecified sprain of right elbow ▽
  - ✓7ᵗʰ **S53.402** Unspecified sprain of left elbow ▽
  - ✓7ᵗʰ **S53.409** Unspecified sprain of unspecified elbow ▽
    - Sprain of elbow NOS
- ✓6ᵗʰ **S53.41** **Radiohumeral** (joint) sprain
  - ✓7ᵗʰ **S53.411** Radiohumeral (joint) sprain of right elbow
  - ✓7ᵗʰ **S53.412** Radiohumeral (joint) sprain of left elbow
  - ✓7ᵗʰ **S53.419** Radiohumeral (joint) sprain of unspecified elbow ▽
- ✓6ᵗʰ **S53.42** **Ulnohumeral** (joint) sprain
  - ✓7ᵗʰ **S53.421** Ulnohumeral (joint) sprain of right elbow
  - ✓7ᵗʰ **S53.422** Ulnohumeral (joint) sprain of left elbow
  - ✓7ᵗʰ **S53.429** Ulnohumeral (joint) sprain of unspecified elbow ▽
- ✓6ᵗʰ **S53.43** **Radial collateral ligament** sprain
  - ✓7ᵗʰ **S53.431** Radial collateral ligament sprain of right elbow
  - ✓7ᵗʰ **S53.432** Radial collateral ligament sprain of left elbow
  - ✓7ᵗʰ **S53.439** Radial collateral ligament sprain of unspecified elbow ▽
- ✓6ᵗʰ **S53.44** **Ulnar collateral ligament** sprain
  - ✓7ᵗʰ **S53.441** Ulnar collateral ligament sprain of right elbow
  - ✓7ᵗʰ **S53.442** Ulnar collateral ligament sprain of left elbow
  - ✓7ᵗʰ **S53.449** Ulnar collateral ligament sprain of unspecified elbow ▽
- ✓6ᵗʰ **S53.49** **Other** sprain of elbow
  - ✓7ᵗʰ **S53.491** Other sprain of right elbow
  - ✓7ᵗʰ **S53.492** Other sprain of left elbow
  - ✓7ᵗʰ **S53.499** Other sprain of unspecified elbow ▽

✓4ᵗʰ **S54** **Injury of nerves at forearm level**
- Code also any associated open wound (S51.-)
- EXCLUDES 2 *injury of nerves at wrist and hand level (S64.-)*

The appropriate 7th character is to be added to each code from category S54.
A   initial encounter
D   subsequent encounter
S   sequela

- ✓5ᵗʰ **S54.0** **Injury of** ulnar **nerve at forearm level**
  - Injury of ulnar nerve NOS
  - ✓x7ᵗʰ **S54.00** Injury of ulnar nerve at forearm level, unspecified arm ▽
  - 2 ✓x7ᵗʰ **S54.01** Injury of ulnar nerve at forearm level, right arm
  - 2 ✓x7ᵗʰ **S54.02** Injury of ulnar nerve at forearm level, left arm
- ✓5ᵗʰ **S54.1** **Injury of** median **nerve at forearm level**
  - Injury of median nerve NOS
  - ✓x7ᵗʰ **S54.10** Injury of median nerve at forearm level, unspecified arm ▽
  - 2 ✓x7ᵗʰ **S54.11** Injury of median nerve at forearm level, right arm
  - 2 ✓x7ᵗʰ **S54.12** Injury of median nerve at forearm level, left arm
- ✓5ᵗʰ **S54.2** **Injury of** radial **nerve at forearm level**
  - Injury of radial nerve NOS
  - ✓x7ᵗʰ **S54.20** Injury of radial nerve at forearm level, unspecified arm ▽
  - 2 ✓x7ᵗʰ **S54.21** Injury of radial nerve at forearm level, right arm
  - 2 ✓x7ᵗʰ **S54.22** Injury of radial nerve at forearm level, left arm
- ✓5ᵗʰ **S54.3** **Injury of** cutaneous sensory **nerve at forearm level**
  - ✓x7ᵗʰ **S54.30** Injury of cutaneous sensory nerve at forearm level, unspecified arm ▽
  - 2 ✓x7ᵗʰ **S54.31** Injury of cutaneous sensory nerve at forearm level, right arm
  - 2 ✓x7ᵗʰ **S54.32** Injury of cutaneous sensory nerve at forearm level, left arm

- ✓5ᵗʰ **S54.8** **Injury of** other **nerves at forearm level**
  - ✓6ᵗʰ **S54.8X** **Injury of other nerves at forearm level**
    - 2 ✓7ᵗʰ **S54.8X1** **Injury of other nerves at forearm level, right arm**
    - 2 ✓7ᵗʰ **S54.8X2** **Injury of other nerves at forearm level, left arm**
    - ✓7ᵗʰ **S54.8X9** Injury of other nerves at forearm level unspecified arm ▽
- ✓5ᵗʰ **S54.9** **Injury of** unspecified **nerve at forearm level**
  - ✓x7ᵗʰ **S54.90** Injury of unspecified nerve at forearm level, unspecified arm ▽
  - 2 ✓x7ᵗʰ **S54.91** Injury of unspecified nerve at forearm level, right arm ▽
  - 2 ✓x7ᵗʰ **S54.92** Injury of unspecified nerve at forearm level, left arm ▽

✓4ᵗʰ **S55** **Injury of blood vessels at forearm level**
- Code also any associated open wound (S51.-)
- EXCLUDES 2 *injury of blood vessels at wrist and hand level (S65.-)*
               injury of brachial vessels (S45.1-S45.2)

The appropriate 7th character is to be added to each code from category S55.
A   initial encounter
D   subsequent encounter
S   sequela

- ✓5ᵗʰ **S55.0** **Injury of** ulnar artery **at forearm level**
  - ✓6ᵗʰ **S55.00** **Unspecified** injury of ulnar artery at forearm level
    - ✓7ᵗʰ **S55.001** Unspecified injury of ulnar artery at forearm level, right arm ▽
    - ✓7ᵗʰ **S55.002** Unspecified injury of ulnar artery at forearm level, left arm ▽
    - ✓7ᵗʰ **S55.009** Unspecified injury of ulnar artery at forearm level, unspecified arm ▽
  - ✓6ᵗʰ **S55.01** **Laceration** of ulnar artery at forearm level
    - ✓7ᵗʰ **S55.011** Laceration of ulnar artery at forearm level, right arm
    - ✓7ᵗʰ **S55.012** Laceration of ulnar artery at forearm level, left arm
    - ✓7ᵗʰ **S55.019** Laceration of ulnar artery at forearm level, unspecified arm ▽
  - ✓6ᵗʰ **S55.09** **Other** specified injury of ulnar artery at forearm level
    - ✓7ᵗʰ **S55.091** Other specified injury of ulnar artery at forearm level, right arm
    - ✓7ᵗʰ **S55.092** Other specified injury of ulnar artery at forearm level, left arm
    - ✓7ᵗʰ **S55.099** Other specified injury of ulnar artery at forearm level, unspecified arm ▽
- ✓5ᵗʰ **S55.1** **Injury of** radial artery **at forearm level**
  - ✓6ᵗʰ **S55.10** **Unspecified** injury of radial artery at forearm level
    - ✓7ᵗʰ **S55.101** Unspecified injury of radial artery at forearm level, right arm ▽
    - ✓7ᵗʰ **S55.102** Unspecified injury of radial artery at forearm level, left arm ▽
    - ✓7ᵗʰ **S55.109** Unspecified injury of radial artery at forearm level, unspecified arm ▽
  - ✓6ᵗʰ **S55.11** **Laceration** of radial artery at forearm level
    - ✓7ᵗʰ **S55.111** Laceration of radial artery at forearm level, right arm
    - ✓7ᵗʰ **S55.112** Laceration of radial artery at forearm level, left arm
    - ✓7ᵗʰ **S55.119** Laceration of radial artery at forearm level, unspecified arm ▽
  - ✓6ᵗʰ **S55.19** **Other** specified injury of radial artery at forearm level
    - ✓7ᵗʰ **S55.191** Other specified injury of radial artery at forearm level, right arm
    - ✓7ᵗʰ **S55.192** Other specified injury of radial artery at forearm level, left arm
    - ✓7ᵗʰ **S55.199** Other specified injury of radial artery at forearm level, unspecified arm ▽

---

2   Case-mix diagnosis with 7th character indicating subsequent encounter or sequela.

✓ Additional Character Req   ✓x7ᵗʰ Placeholder Alert   Case-Mix Diagnosis   Manifestation   ▽ Unspecified Dx   EXCLUDES 1 Not coded here   EXCLUDES 2 Not included here

✓5th S55.2 Injury of vein at forearm level

  ✓6th S55.20 Unspecified injury of vein at forearm level

    ✓7th **S55.201 Unspecified injury of vein at forearm level, right arm** ▽

    ✓7th **S55.202 Unspecified injury of vein at forearm level, left arm** ▽

    ✓7th **S55.209 Unspecified injury of vein at forearm level, unspecified arm** ▽

  ✓6th S55.21 Laceration of vein at forearm level

    ✓7th **S55.211 Laceration of vein at forearm level, right arm**

    ✓7th **S55.212 Laceration of vein at forearm level, left arm**

    ✓7th **S55.219 Laceration of vein at forearm level, unspecified arm** ▽

  ✓6th S55.29 Other specified injury of vein at forearm level

    ✓7th **S55.291 Other specified injury of vein at forearm level, right arm**

    ✓7th **S55.292 Other specified injury of vein at forearm level, left arm**

    ✓7th **S55.299 Other specified injury of vein at forearm level, unspecified arm** ▽

✓5th S55.8 Injury of other blood vessels at forearm level

  ✓6th S55.80 Unspecified injury of other blood vessels at forearm level

    ✓7th **S55.801 Unspecified injury of other blood vessels at forearm level, right arm** ▽

    ✓7th **S55.802 Unspecified injury of other blood vessels at forearm level, left arm** ▽

    ✓7th **S55.809 Unspecified injury of other blood vessels at forearm level, unspecified arm** ▽

  ✓6th S55.81 Laceration of other blood vessels at forearm level

    ✓7th **S55.811 Laceration of other blood vessels at forearm level, right arm**

    ✓7th **S55.812 Laceration of other blood vessels at forearm level, left arm**

    ✓7th **S55.819 Laceration of other blood vessels at forearm level, unspecified arm** ▽

  ✓6th S55.89 Other specified injury of other blood vessels at forearm level

    ✓7th **S55.891 Other specified injury of other blood vessels at forearm level, right arm**

    ✓7th **S55.892 Other specified injury of other blood vessels at forearm level, left arm**

    ✓7th **S55.899 Other specified injury of other blood vessels at forearm level, unspecified arm** ▽

✓5th S55.9 Injury of unspecified blood vessel at forearm level

  ✓6th S55.90 Unspecified injury of unspecified blood vessel at forearm level

    ✓7th **S55.901 Unspecified injury of unspecified blood vessel at forearm level, right arm** ▽

    ✓7th **S55.902 Unspecified injury of unspecified blood vessel at forearm level, left arm** ▽

    ✓7th **S55.909 Unspecified injury of unspecified blood vessel at forearm level, unspecified arm** ▽

  ✓6th S55.91 Laceration of unspecified blood vessel at forearm level

    ✓7th **S55.911 Laceration of unspecified blood vessel at forearm level, right arm** ▽

    ✓7th **S55.912 Laceration of unspecified blood vessel at forearm level, left arm** ▽

    ✓7th **S55.919 Laceration of unspecified blood vessel at forearm level, unspecified arm** ▽

  ✓6th S55.99 Other specified injury of unspecified blood vessel at forearm level

    ✓7th **S55.991 Other specified injury of unspecified blood vessel at forearm level, right arm** ▽

    ✓7th **S55.992 Other specified injury of unspecified blood vessel at forearm level, left arm** ▽

    ✓7th **S55.999 Other specified injury of unspecified blood vessel at forearm level, unspecified arm** ▽

✓4th S56 Injury of muscle, fascia and tendon at forearm level

Code also any associated open wound (S51.-)

EXCLUDES 2 *injury of muscle, fascia and tendon at or below wrist (S66.-)*
     sprain of joints and ligaments of elbow (S53.4-)

TIP: Refer to the Muscle/Tendon table at the beginning of this chapter.

> The appropriate 7th character is to be added to each code from category S56.
> A   initial encounter
> D   subsequent encounter
> S   sequela

✓5th S56.0 Injury of flexor muscle, fascia and tendon of thumb at forearm level

  ✓6th S56.00 Unspecified injury of flexor muscle, fascia and tendon of thumb at forearm level

    ✓7th **S56.001 Unspecified injury of flexor muscle, fascia and tendon of right thumb at forearm level** ▽

    ✓7th **S56.002 Unspecified injury of flexor muscle, fascia and tendon of left thumb at forearm level** ▽

    ✓7th **S56.009 Unspecified injury of flexor muscle, fascia and tendon of unspecified thumb at forearm level** ▽

  ✓6th S56.01 Strain of flexor muscle, fascia and tendon of thumb at forearm level

    ✓7th **S56.011 Strain of flexor muscle, fascia and tendon of right thumb at forearm level**

    ✓7th **S56.012 Strain of flexor muscle, fascia and tendon of left thumb at forearm level**

    ✓7th **S56.019 Strain of flexor muscle, fascia and tendon of unspecified thumb at forearm level** ▽

  ✓6th S56.02 Laceration of flexor muscle, fascia and tendon of thumb at forearm level

    4,5 ✓7th **S56.021 Laceration of flexor muscle, fascia and tendon of right thumb at forearm level** NRS

    4,5 ✓7th **S56.022 Laceration of flexor muscle, fascia and tendon of left thumb at forearm level** NRS

    ✓7th **S56.029 Laceration of flexor muscle, fascia and tendon of unspecified thumb at forearm level** ▽

  ✓6th S56.09 Other injury of flexor muscle, fascia and tendon of thumb at forearm level

    ✓7th **S56.091 Other injury of flexor muscle, fascia and tendon of right thumb at forearm level**

    ✓7th **S56.092 Other injury of flexor muscle, fascia and tendon of left thumb at forearm level**

    ✓7th **S56.099 Other injury of flexor muscle, fascia and tendon of unspecified thumb at forearm level** ▽

✓5th S56.1 Injury of flexor muscle, fascia and tendon of other and unspecified finger at forearm level

  ✓6th S56.10 Unspecified injury of flexor muscle, fascia and tendon of other and unspecified finger at forearm level

    ✓7th **S56.101 Unspecified injury of flexor muscle, fascia and tendon of right index finger at forearm level** ▽

    ✓7th **S56.102 Unspecified injury of flexor muscle, fascia and tendon of left index finger at forearm level** ▽

    ✓7th **S56.103 Unspecified injury of flexor muscle, fascia and tendon of right middle finger at forearm level** ▽

    ✓7th **S56.104 Unspecified injury of flexor muscle, fascia and tendon of left middle finger at forearm level** ▽

---

4 Case-mix diagnosis with 7th character indicating initial or subsequent encounter.
5 NRS supply diagnosis with 7th character indicating initial or subsequent encounter.

Ⓝ Newborn: 0   Ⓟ Pediatric: 0-17   Ⓜ Maternity: 12-55   Ⓐ Adult: 15-124   NRS Nonroutine supply Dx   NCDx Noncancer Dx   PDx Primary Dx   ▶◀ Revised Text   ● New Code   ▲ Revised Title

972   ICD-10-CM 2018

✓7ᵗʰ **S56.105** Unspecified injury of flexor muscle, fascia and tendon of right ring finger at forearm level ▽

✓7ᵗʰ **S56.106** Unspecified injury of flexor muscle, fascia and tendon of left ring finger at forearm level ▽

✓7ᵗʰ **S56.107** Unspecified injury of flexor muscle, fascia and tendon of right little finger at forearm level ▽

✓7ᵗʰ **S56.108** Unspecified injury of flexor muscle, fascia and tendon of left little finger at forearm level ▽

✓7ᵗʰ **S56.109** Unspecified injury of flexor muscle, fascia and tendon of unspecified finger at forearm level ▽

✓6ᵗʰ **S56.11** Strain of flexor muscle, fascia and tendon of other and unspecified finger at forearm level

✓7ᵗʰ **S56.111** Strain of flexor muscle, fascia and tendon of right index finger at forearm level

✓7ᵗʰ **S56.112** Strain of flexor muscle, fascia and tendon of left index finger at forearm level

✓7ᵗʰ **S56.113** Strain of flexor muscle, fascia and tendon of right middle finger at forearm level

✓7ᵗʰ **S56.114** Strain of flexor muscle, fascia and tendon of left middle finger at forearm level

✓7ᵗʰ **S56.115** Strain of flexor muscle, fascia and tendon of right ring finger at forearm level

✓7ᵗʰ **S56.116** Strain of flexor muscle, fascia and tendon of left ring finger at forearm level

✓7ᵗʰ **S56.117** Strain of flexor muscle, fascia and tendon of right little finger at forearm level

✓7ᵗʰ **S56.118** Strain of flexor muscle, fascia and tendon of left little finger at forearm level

✓7ᵗʰ **S56.119** Strain of flexor muscle, fascia and tendon of finger of unspecified finger at forearm level ▽

✓6ᵗʰ **S56.12** Laceration of flexor muscle, fascia and tendon of other and unspecified finger at forearm level

4,5 ✓7ᵗʰ **S56.121** Laceration of flexor muscle, fascia and tendon of right index finger at forearm level NRS

4,5 ✓7ᵗʰ **S56.122** Laceration of flexor muscle, fascia and tendon of left index finger at forearm level NRS

4,5 ✓7ᵗʰ **S56.123** Laceration of flexor muscle, fascia and tendon of right middle finger at forearm level NRS

4,5 ✓7ᵗʰ **S56.124** Laceration of flexor muscle, fascia and tendon of left middle finger at forearm level NRS

4,5 ✓7ᵗʰ **S56.125** Laceration of flexor muscle, fascia and tendon of right ring finger at forearm level NRS

4,5 ✓7ᵗʰ **S56.126** Laceration of flexor muscle, fascia and tendon of left ring finger at forearm level NRS

4,5 ✓7ᵗʰ **S56.127** Laceration of flexor muscle, fascia and tendon of right little finger at forearm level NRS

4,5 ✓7ᵗʰ **S56.128** Laceration of flexor muscle, fascia and tendon of left little finger at forearm level NRS

✓7ᵗʰ **S56.129** Laceration of flexor muscle, fascia and tendon of unspecified finger at forearm level ▽

✓6ᵗʰ **S56.19** Other injury of flexor muscle, fascia and tendon of other and unspecified finger at forearm level

✓7ᵗʰ **S56.191** Other injury of flexor muscle, fascia and tendon of right index finger at forearm level

✓7ᵗʰ **S56.192** Other injury of flexor muscle, fascia and tendon of left index finger at forearm level

✓7ᵗʰ **S56.193** Other injury of flexor muscle, fascia and tendon of right middle finger at forearm level

✓7ᵗʰ **S56.194** Other injury of flexor muscle, fascia and tendon of left middle finger at forearm level

✓7ᵗʰ **S56.195** Other injury of flexor muscle, fascia and tendon of right ring finger at forearm level

✓7ᵗʰ **S56.196** Other injury of flexor muscle, fascia and tendon of left ring finger at forearm level

✓7ᵗʰ **S56.197** Other injury of flexor muscle, fascia and tendon of right little finger at forearm level

✓7ᵗʰ **S56.198** Other injury of flexor muscle, fascia and tendon of left little finger at forearm level

✓7ᵗʰ **S56.199** Other injury of flexor muscle, fascia and tendon of unspecified finger at forearm level ▽

✓5ᵗʰ **S56.2** Injury of other flexor muscle, fascia and tendon at forearm level

✓6ᵗʰ **S56.20** Unspecified injury of other flexor muscle, fascia and tendon at forearm level

✓7ᵗʰ **S56.201** Unspecified injury of other flexor muscle, fascia and tendon at forearm level, right arm ▽

✓7ᵗʰ **S56.202** Unspecified injury of other flexor muscle, fascia and tendon at forearm level, left arm ▽

✓7ᵗʰ **S56.209** Unspecified injury of other flexor muscle, fascia and tendon at forearm level, unspecified arm ▽

✓6ᵗʰ **S56.21** Strain of other flexor muscle, fascia and tendon at forearm level

✓7ᵗʰ **S56.211** Strain of other flexor muscle, fascia and tendon at forearm level, right arm

✓7ᵗʰ **S56.212** Strain of other flexor muscle, fascia and tendon at forearm level, left arm

✓7ᵗʰ **S56.219** Strain of other flexor muscle, fascia and tendon at forearm level, unspecified arm ▽

✓6ᵗʰ **S56.22** Laceration of other flexor muscle, fascia and tendon at forearm level

4,5 ✓7ᵗʰ **S56.221** Laceration of other flexor muscle, fascia and tendon at forearm level, right arm NRS

4,5 ✓7ᵗʰ **S56.222** Laceration of other flexor muscle, fascia and tendon at forearm level, left arm NRS

✓7ᵗʰ **S56.229** Laceration of other flexor muscle, fascia and tendon at forearm level, unspecified arm ▽

✓6ᵗʰ **S56.29** Other injury of other flexor muscle, fascia and tendon at forearm level

✓7ᵗʰ **S56.291** Other injury of other flexor muscle, fascia and tendon at forearm level, right arm

✓7ᵗʰ **S56.292** Other injury of other flexor muscle, fascia and tendon at forearm level, left arm

✓7ᵗʰ **S56.299** Other injury of other flexor muscle, fascia and tendon at forearm level, unspecified arm ▽

✓5ᵗʰ **S56.3** Injury of extensor or abductor muscles, fascia and tendons of thumb at forearm level

✓6ᵗʰ **S56.30** Unspecified injury of extensor or abductor muscles, fascia and tendons of thumb at forearm level

✓7ᵗʰ **S56.301** Unspecified injury of extensor or abductor muscles, fascia and tendons of right thumb at forearm level ▽

✓7ᵗʰ **S56.302** Unspecified injury of extensor or abductor muscles, fascia and tendons of left thumb at forearm level ▽

✓7ᵗʰ **S56.309** Unspecified injury of extensor or abductor muscles, fascia and tendons of unspecified thumb at forearm level ▽

---

4 Case-mix diagnosis with 7th character indicating initial or subsequent encounter.
5 NRS supply diagnosis with 7th character indicating initial or subsequent encounter.

☑ Additional Character Req ✓×7ᵗʰ Placeholder Alert Case-Mix Diagnosis Manifestation ▽ Unspecified Dx EXCLUDES 1 Not coded here EXCLUDES 2 Not included here

✓6ᵗʰ **S56.31** Strain of extensor or abductor muscles, fascia and tendons of thumb at forearm level

    ✓7ᵗʰ **S56.311** Strain of extensor or abductor muscles, fascia and tendons of right thumb at forearm level

    ✓7ᵗʰ **S56.312** Strain of extensor or abductor muscles, fascia and tendons of left thumb at forearm level

    ✓7ᵗʰ **S56.319** Strain of extensor or abductor muscles, fascia and tendons of unspecified thumb at forearm level ▽

✓6ᵗʰ **S56.32** Laceration of extensor or abductor muscles, fascia and tendons of thumb at forearm level

    4,5 ✓7ᵗʰ **S56.321** Laceration of extensor or abductor muscles, fascia and tendons of right thumb at forearm level **NRS**

    4,5 ✓7ᵗʰ **S56.322** Laceration of extensor or abductor muscles, fascia and tendons of left thumb at forearm level **NRS**

    ✓7ᵗʰ **S56.329** Laceration of extensor or abductor muscles, fascia and tendons of unspecified thumb at forearm level ▽

✓6ᵗʰ **S56.39** Other injury of extensor or abductor muscles, fascia and tendons of thumb at forearm level

    ✓7ᵗʰ **S56.391** Other injury of extensor or abductor muscles, fascia and tendons of right thumb at forearm level

    ✓7ᵗʰ **S56.392** Other injury of extensor or abductor muscles, fascia and tendons of left thumb at forearm level

    ✓7ᵗʰ **S56.399** Other injury of extensor or abductor muscles, fascia and tendons of unspecified thumb at forearm level ▽

✓5ᵗʰ **S56.4** Injury of extensor muscle, fascia and tendon of other and unspecified finger at forearm level

    ✓6ᵗʰ **S56.40** Unspecified injury of extensor muscle, fascia and tendon of other and unspecified finger at forearm level

      ✓7ᵗʰ **S56.401** Unspecified injury of extensor muscle, fascia and tendon of right index finger at forearm level ▽

      ✓7ᵗʰ **S56.402** Unspecified injury of extensor muscle, fascia and tendon of left index finger at forearm level ▽

      ✓7ᵗʰ **S56.403** Unspecified injury of extensor muscle, fascia and tendon of right middle finger at forearm level ▽

      ✓7ᵗʰ **S56.404** Unspecified injury of extensor muscle, fascia and tendon of left middle finger at forearm level ▽

      ✓7ᵗʰ **S56.405** Unspecified injury of extensor muscle, fascia and tendon of right ring finger at forearm level ▽

      ✓7ᵗʰ **S56.406** Unspecified injury of extensor muscle, fascia and tendon of left ring finger at forearm level ▽

      ✓7ᵗʰ **S56.407** Unspecified injury of extensor muscle, fascia and tendon of right little finger at forearm level ▽

      ✓7ᵗʰ **S56.408** Unspecified injury of extensor muscle, fascia and tendon of left little finger at forearm level ▽

      ✓7ᵗʰ **S56.409** Unspecified injury of extensor muscle, fascia and tendon of unspecified finger at forearm level ▽

    ✓6ᵗʰ **S56.41** Strain of extensor muscle, fascia and tendon of other and unspecified finger at forearm level

      ✓7ᵗʰ **S56.411** Strain of extensor muscle, fascia and tendon of right index finger at forearm level

      ✓7ᵗʰ **S56.412** Strain of extensor muscle, fascia and tendon of left index finger at forearm level

      ✓7ᵗʰ **S56.413** Strain of extensor muscle, fascia and tendon of right middle finger at forearm level

✓7ᵗʰ **S56.414** Strain of extensor muscle, fascia and tendon of left middle finger at forearm level

✓7ᵗʰ **S56.415** Strain of extensor muscle, fascia and tendon of right ring finger at forearm level

✓7ᵗʰ **S56.416** Strain of extensor muscle, fascia and tendon of left ring finger at forearm level

✓7ᵗʰ **S56.417** Strain of extensor muscle, fascia and tendon of right little finger at forearm level

✓7ᵗʰ **S56.418** Strain of extensor muscle, fascia and tendon of left little finger at forearm level

✓7ᵗʰ **S56.419** Strain of extensor muscle, fascia and tendon of finger, unspecified finger at forearm level ▽

✓6ᵗʰ **S56.42** Laceration of extensor muscle, fascia and tendon of other and unspecified finger at forearm level

    4,5 ✓7ᵗʰ **S56.421** Laceration of extensor muscle, fascia and tendon of right index finger at forearm level **NRS**

    4,5 ✓7ᵗʰ **S56.422** Laceration of extensor muscle, fascia and tendon of left index finger at forearm level **NRS**

    4,5 ✓7ᵗʰ **S56.423** Laceration of extensor muscle, fascia and tendon of right middle finger at forearm level **NRS**

    4,5 ✓7ᵗʰ **S56.424** Laceration of extensor muscle, fascia and tendon of left middle finger at forearm level **NRS**

    4,5 ✓7ᵗʰ **S56.425** Laceration of extensor muscle, fascia and tendon of right ring finger at forearm level **NRS**

    4,5 ✓7ᵗʰ **S56.426** Laceration of extensor muscle, fascia and tendon of left ring finger at forearm level **NRS**

    4,5 ✓7ᵗʰ **S56.427** Laceration of extensor muscle, fascia and tendon of right little finger at forearm level **NRS**

    4,5 ✓7ᵗʰ **S56.428** Laceration of extensor muscle, fascia and tendon of left little finger at forearm level **NRS**

    ✓7ᵗʰ **S56.429** Laceration of extensor muscle, fascia and tendon of unspecified finger at forearm level ▽

✓6ᵗʰ **S56.49** Other injury of extensor muscle, fascia and tendon of other and unspecified finger at forearm level

    ✓7ᵗʰ **S56.491** Other injury of extensor muscle, fascia and tendon of right index finger at forearm level

    ✓7ᵗʰ **S56.492** Other injury of extensor muscle, fascia and tendon of left index finger at forearm level

    ✓7ᵗʰ **S56.493** Other injury of extensor muscle, fascia and tendon of right middle finger at forearm level

    ✓7ᵗʰ **S56.494** Other injury of extensor muscle, fascia and tendon of left middle finger at forearm level

    ✓7ᵗʰ **S56.495** Other injury of extensor muscle, fascia and tendon of right ring finger at forearm level

    ✓7ᵗʰ **S56.496** Other injury of extensor muscle, fascia and tendon of left ring finger at forearm level

    ✓7ᵗʰ **S56.497** Other injury of extensor muscle, fascia and tendon of right little finger at forearm level

    ✓7ᵗʰ **S56.498** Other injury of extensor muscle, fascia and tendon of left little finger at forearm level

    ✓7ᵗʰ **S56.499** Other injury of extensor muscle, fascia and tendon of unspecified finger at forearm level ▽

---

4 Case-mix diagnosis with 7th character indicating initial or subsequent encounter.
5 NRS supply diagnosis with 7th character indicating initial or subsequent encounter.

Ⓝ Newborn: 0   Ⓟ Pediatric: 0-17   Ⓜ Maternity: 12-55   Ⓐ Adult: 15-124   **NRS** Nonroutine supply Dx   **NCDx** Noncancer Dx   **PDx** Primary Dx   ▶◀ Revised Text   ● New Code   ▲ Revised Title

974   ICD-10-CM 2018

✓5ᵗʰ **S56.5** Injury of other extensor muscle, fascia and tendon at forearm level

  ✓6ᵗʰ **S56.50** Unspecified injury of other extensor muscle, fascia and tendon at forearm level

    ✓7ᵗʰ **S56.501** Unspecified injury of other extensor muscle, fascia and tendon at forearm level, right arm ▽

    ✓7ᵗʰ **S56.502** Unspecified injury of other extensor muscle, fascia and tendon at forearm level, left arm ▽

    ✓7ᵗʰ **S56.509** Unspecified injury of other extensor muscle, fascia and tendon at forearm level, unspecified arm ▽

  ✓6ᵗʰ **S56.51** Strain of other extensor muscle, fascia and tendon at forearm level

    ✓7ᵗʰ **S56.511** Strain of other extensor muscle, fascia and tendon at forearm level, right arm

    ✓7ᵗʰ **S56.512** Strain of other extensor muscle, fascia and tendon at forearm level, left arm

    ✓7ᵗʰ **S56.519** Strain of other extensor muscle, fascia and tendon at forearm level, unspecified arm ▽

  ✓6ᵗʰ **S56.52** Laceration of other extensor muscle, fascia and tendon at forearm level

    4,5 ✓7ᵗʰ **S56.521** Laceration of other extensor muscle, fascia and tendon at forearm level, right arm `NRS`

    4,5 ✓7ᵗʰ **S56.522** Laceration of other extensor muscle, fascia and tendon at forearm level, left arm `NRS`

    ✓7ᵗʰ **S56.529** Laceration of other extensor muscle, fascia and tendon at forearm level, unspecified arm ▽

  ✓6ᵗʰ **S56.59** Other injury of other extensor muscle, fascia and tendon at forearm level

    ✓7ᵗʰ **S56.591** Other injury of other extensor muscle, fascia and tendon at forearm level, right arm

    ✓7ᵗʰ **S56.592** Other injury of other extensor muscle, fascia and tendon at forearm level, left arm

    ✓7ᵗʰ **S56.599** Other injury of other extensor muscle, fascia and tendon at forearm level, unspecified arm ▽

✓5ᵗʰ **S56.8** Injury of other muscles, fascia and tendons at forearm level

  ✓6ᵗʰ **S56.80** Unspecified injury of other muscles, fascia and tendons at forearm level

    ✓7ᵗʰ **S56.801** Unspecified injury of other muscles, fascia and tendons at forearm level, right arm ▽

    ✓7ᵗʰ **S56.802** Unspecified injury of other muscles, fascia and tendons at forearm level, left arm ▽

    ✓7ᵗʰ **S56.809** Unspecified injury of other muscles, fascia and tendons at forearm level, unspecified arm ▽

  ✓6ᵗʰ **S56.81** Strain of other muscles, fascia and tendons at forearm level

    ✓7ᵗʰ **S56.811** Strain of other muscles, fascia and tendons at forearm level, right arm

    ✓7ᵗʰ **S56.812** Strain of other muscles, fascia and tendons at forearm level, left arm

    ✓7ᵗʰ **S56.819** Strain of other muscles, fascia and tendons at forearm level, unspecified arm ▽

  ✓6ᵗʰ **S56.82** Laceration of other muscles, fascia and tendons at forearm level

    4,5 ✓7ᵗʰ **S56.821** Laceration of other muscles, fascia and tendons at forearm level, right arm `NRS`

    4,5 ✓7ᵗʰ **S56.822** Laceration of other muscles, fascia and tendons at forearm level, left arm `NRS`

    ✓7ᵗʰ **S56.829** Laceration of other muscles, fascia and tendons at forearm level, unspecified arm ▽

  ✓6ᵗʰ **S56.89** Other injury of other muscles, fascia and tendons at forearm level

    ✓7ᵗʰ **S56.891** Other injury of other muscles, fascia and tendons at forearm level, right arm

    ✓7ᵗʰ **S56.892** Other injury of other muscles, fascia and tendons at forearm level, left arm

    ✓7ᵗʰ **S56.899** Other injury of other muscles, fascia and tendons at forearm level, unspecified arm ▽

✓5ᵗʰ **S56.9** Injury of unspecified muscles, fascia and tendons at forearm level

  ✓6ᵗʰ **S56.90** Unspecified injury of unspecified muscles, fascia and tendons at forearm level ▽

    ✓7ᵗʰ **S56.901** Unspecified injury of unspecified muscles, fascia and tendons at forearm level, right arm ▽

    ✓7ᵗʰ **S56.902** Unspecified injury of unspecified muscles, fascia and tendons at forearm level, left arm ▽

    ✓7ᵗʰ **S56.909** Unspecified injury of unspecified muscles, fascia and tendons at forearm level, unspecified arm ▽

  ✓6ᵗʰ **S56.91** Strain of unspecified muscles, fascia and tendons at forearm level

    ✓7ᵗʰ **S56.911** Strain of unspecified muscles, fascia and tendons at forearm level, right arm ▽

    ✓7ᵗʰ **S56.912** Strain of unspecified muscles, fascia and tendons at forearm level, left arm ▽

    ✓7ᵗʰ **S56.919** Strain of unspecified muscles, fascia and tendons at forearm level, unspecified arm ▽

  ✓6ᵗʰ **S56.92** Laceration of unspecified muscles, fascia and tendons at forearm level

    4,5 ✓7ᵗʰ **S56.921** Laceration of unspecified muscles, fascia and tendons at forearm level, right arm `NRS` ▽

    4,5 ✓7ᵗʰ **S56.922** Laceration of unspecified muscles, fascia and tendons at forearm level, left arm `NRS` ▽

    ✓7ᵗʰ **S56.929** Laceration of unspecified muscles, fascia and tendons at forearm level, unspecified arm ▽

  ✓6ᵗʰ **S56.99** Other injury of unspecified muscles, fascia and tendons at forearm level

    ✓7ᵗʰ **S56.991** Other injury of unspecified muscles, fascia and tendons at forearm level, right arm ▽

    ✓7ᵗʰ **S56.992** Other injury of unspecified muscles, fascia and tendons at forearm level, left arm ▽

    ✓7ᵗʰ **S56.999** Other injury of unspecified muscles, fascia and tendons at forearm level, unspecified arm ▽

✓4ᵗʰ **S57** Crushing injury of elbow and forearm

Use additional code(s) for all associated injuries

EXCLUDES 2 crushing injury of wrist and hand (S67.-)

The appropriate 7th character is to be added to each code from category S57.
A   initial encounter
D   subsequent encounter
S   sequela

✓5ᵗʰ **S57.0** Crushing injury of elbow

  ✓x7ᵗʰ **S57.00** Crushing injury of unspecified elbow ▽

  1 ✓x7ᵗʰ **S57.01** Crushing injury of right elbow

  1 ✓x7ᵗʰ **S57.02** Crushing injury of left elbow

✓5ᵗʰ **S57.8** Crushing injury of forearm

  ✓x7ᵗʰ **S57.80** Crushing injury of unspecified forearm ▽

  1 ✓x7ᵗʰ **S57.81** Crushing injury of right forearm

  1 ✓x7ᵗʰ **S57.82** Crushing injury of left forearm

---

1 Case-mix diagnosis with 7th character indicating subsequent encounter.
4 Case-mix diagnosis with 7th character indicating initial or subsequent encounter.
5 NRS supply diagnosis with 7th character indicating initial or subsequent encounter.

☑ Additional Character Req   ✓x7ᵗʰ Placeholder Alert   Case-Mix Diagnosis   Manifestation   ▽ Unspecified Dx   *EXCLUDES 1* Not coded here   *EXCLUDES 2* Not included here

Chapter 19. Injury, Poisoning and Certain Other Consequences of External Causes

✓4ᵗʰ **S58** **Traumatic amputation** of elbow and forearm

An amputation not identified as partial or complete should be coded to complete.

EXCLUDES 1 *traumatic amputation of wrist and hand (S68.-)*

The appropriate 7th character is to be added to each code from category S58.
A   initial encounter
D   subsequent encounter
S   sequela

✓5ᵗʰ **S58.0** **Traumatic amputation at** elbow **level**

   ✓6ᵗʰ **S58.01** Complete **traumatic amputation at elbow level**

      4,5 ✓7ᵗʰ **S58.011** **Complete traumatic amputation at elbow level,** right **arm** NRS

      4,5 ✓7ᵗʰ **S58.012** **Complete traumatic amputation at elbow level,** left **arm** NRS

      ✓7ᵗʰ **S58.019** **Complete traumatic amputation at elbow level, unspecified arm** ▽

   ✓6ᵗʰ **S58.02** Partial **traumatic amputation at elbow level**

      4,5 ✓7ᵗʰ **S58.021** **Partial traumatic amputation at elbow level,** right **arm** NRS

      4,5 ✓7ᵗʰ **S58.022** **Partial traumatic amputation at elbow level,** left **arm** NRS

      ✓7ᵗʰ **S58.029** **Partial traumatic amputation at elbow level, unspecified arm** ▽

✓5ᵗʰ **S58.1** **Traumatic amputation at level** between elbow and wrist

   ✓6ᵗʰ **S58.11** Complete **traumatic amputation at level between elbow and wrist**

      4,5 ✓7ᵗʰ **S58.111** **Complete traumatic amputation at level between elbow and wrist,** right **arm** NRS

      4,5 ✓7ᵗʰ **S58.112** **Complete traumatic amputation at level between elbow and wrist,** left **arm** NRS

      ✓7ᵗʰ **S58.119** **Complete traumatic amputation at level between elbow and wrist, unspecified arm** ▽

   ✓6ᵗʰ **S58.12** Partial **traumatic amputation at level between elbow and wrist**

      4,5 ✓7ᵗʰ **S58.121** **Partial traumatic amputation at level between elbow and wrist,** right **arm** NRS

      4,5 ✓7ᵗʰ **S58.122** **Partial traumatic amputation at level between elbow and wrist,** left **arm** NRS

      ✓7ᵗʰ **S58.129** **Partial traumatic amputation at level between elbow and wrist, unspecified arm** ▽

✓5ᵗʰ **S58.9** **Traumatic amputation of** forearm, level unspecified

EXCLUDES 1 *traumatic amputation of wrist (S68.-)*

   ✓6ᵗʰ **S58.91** Complete **traumatic amputation of forearm, level unspecified**

      4 ✓7ᵗʰ **S58.911** **Complete traumatic amputation of** right **forearm, level unspecified** ▽

      4 ✓7ᵗʰ **S58.912** **Complete traumatic amputation of** left **forearm, level unspecified** ▽

      ✓7ᵗʰ **S58.919** **Complete traumatic amputation of unspecified forearm, level unspecified** ▽

   ✓6ᵗʰ **S58.92** Partial **traumatic amputation of forearm, level unspecified**

      4 ✓7ᵗʰ **S58.921** **Partial traumatic amputation of** right **forearm, level unspecified** ▽

      4 ✓7ᵗʰ **S58.922** **Partial traumatic amputation of** left **forearm, level unspecified** ▽

      ✓7ᵗʰ **S58.929** **Partial traumatic amputation of unspecified forearm, level unspecified** ▽

✓4ᵗʰ **S59** **Other and unspecified injuries** of elbow and forearm

EXCLUDES 2 *other and unspecified injuries of wrist and hand (S69.-)*
AHA: 2015, 3Q, 37-39
TIP: The term "improper alignment" is not synonymous with malunion or nonunion of a fracture when noted in provider documentation.

The appropriate 7th character is to be added to each code from subcategories S59.0, S59.1, and S59.2.
A   initial encounter for closed fracture
D   subsequent encounter for fracture with routine healing
G   subsequent encounter for fracture with delayed healing
K   subsequent encounter for fracture with nonunion
P   subsequent encounter for fracture with malunion
S   sequela

✓5ᵗʰ **S59.0** **Physeal fracture of** lower end of ulna

   ✓6ᵗʰ **S59.00** Unspecified **physeal fracture of lower end of ulna**

      1 ✓7ᵗʰ **S59.001** **Unspecified physeal fracture of lower end of ulna,** right **arm** ▽

      1 ✓7ᵗʰ **S59.002** **Unspecified physeal fracture of lower end of ulna,** left **arm** ▽

      ✓7ᵗʰ **S59.009** **Unspecified physeal fracture of lower end of ulna, unspecified arm** ▽

   ✓6ᵗʰ **S59.01** Salter-Harris Type I **physeal fracture of lower end of ulna**

      1 ✓7ᵗʰ **S59.011** **Salter-Harris Type I physeal fracture of lower end of ulna,** right **arm**

      1 ✓7ᵗʰ **S59.012** **Salter-Harris Type I physeal fracture of lower end of ulna,** left **arm**

      ✓7ᵗʰ **S59.019** **Salter-Harris Type I physeal fracture of lower end of ulna, unspecified arm** ▽

   ✓6ᵗʰ **S59.02** Salter-Harris Type II **physeal fracture of lower end of ulna**

      1 ✓7ᵗʰ **S59.021** **Salter-Harris Type II physeal fracture of lower end of ulna,** right **arm**

      1 ✓7ᵗʰ **S59.022** **Salter-Harris Type II physeal fracture of lower end of ulna,** left **arm**

      ✓7ᵗʰ **S59.029** **Salter-Harris Type II physeal fracture of lower end of ulna, unspecified arm** ▽

   ✓6ᵗʰ **S59.03** Salter-Harris Type III **physeal fracture of lower end of ulna**

      1 ✓7ᵗʰ **S59.031** **Salter-Harris Type III physeal fracture of lower end of ulna,** right **arm**

      1 ✓7ᵗʰ **S59.032** **Salter-Harris Type III physeal fracture of lower end of ulna,** left **arm**

      ✓7ᵗʰ **S59.039** **Salter-Harris Type III physeal fracture of lower end of ulna, unspecified arm** ▽

   ✓6ᵗʰ **S59.04** Salter-Harris Type IV **physeal fracture of lower end of ulna**

      1 ✓7ᵗʰ **S59.041** **Salter-Harris Type IV physeal fracture of lower end of ulna,** right **arm**

      1 ✓7ᵗʰ **S59.042** **Salter-Harris Type IV physeal fracture of lower end of ulna,** left **arm**

      ✓7ᵗʰ **S59.049** **Salter-Harris Type IV physeal fracture of lower end of ulna, unspecified arm** ▽

   ✓6ᵗʰ **S59.09** Other **physeal fracture of lower end of ulna**

      1 ✓7ᵗʰ **S59.091** **Other physeal fracture of lower end of ulna,** right **arm**

      1 ✓7ᵗʰ **S59.092** **Other physeal fracture of lower end of ulna,** left **arm**

      ✓7ᵗʰ **S59.099** **Other physeal fracture of lower end of ulna, unspecified arm** ▽

✓5ᵗʰ **S59.1** **Physeal fracture of** upper end of radius

   ✓6ᵗʰ **S59.10** Unspecified **physeal fracture of upper end of radius**

      1 ✓7ᵗʰ **S59.101** **Unspecified physeal fracture of upper end of radius,** right **arm** ▽

      1 ✓7ᵗʰ **S59.102** **Unspecified physeal fracture of upper end of radius,** left **arm** ▽

      ✓7ᵗʰ **S59.109** **Unspecified physeal fracture of upper end of radius, unspecified arm** ▽

   ✓6ᵗʰ **S59.11** Salter-Harris Type I **physeal fracture of upper end of radius**

      1 ✓7ᵗʰ **S59.111** **Salter-Harris Type I physeal fracture of upper end of radius,** right **arm**

---

1 Case-mix diagnosis with 7th character indicating subsequent encounter.
4 Case-mix diagnosis with 7th character indicating initial or subsequent encounter.
5 NRS supply diagnosis with 7th character indicating initial or subsequent encounter.

Ⓝ Newborn: 0   Ⓟ Pediatric: 0-17   Ⓜ Maternity: 12-55   Ⓐ Adult: 15-124   **NRS** Nonroutine supply Dx   **NC Dx** Noncancer Dx   **PDx** Primary Dx   ▶◀ Revised Text   ● New Code   ▲ Revised Title

976   ICD-10-CM 2018

1 ✓7ᵗʰ **S59.112** Salter-Harris Type I physeal fracture of upper end of radius, **left** arm

✓7ᵗʰ **S59.119** Salter-Harris Type I physeal fracture of ▽ upper end of radius, unspecified arm

✓6ᵗʰ **S59.12** Salter-Harris Type II physeal fracture of upper end of radius

1 ✓7ᵗʰ **S59.121** Salter-Harris Type II physeal fracture of upper end of radius, **right** arm

1 ✓7ᵗʰ **S59.122** Salter-Harris Type II physeal fracture of upper end of radius, **left** arm

✓7ᵗʰ **S59.129** Salter-Harris Type II physeal fracture ▽ of upper end of radius, unspecified arm

✓6ᵗʰ **S59.13** Salter-Harris Type III physeal fracture of upper end of radius

1 ✓7ᵗʰ **S59.131** Salter-Harris Type III physeal fracture of upper end of radius, **right** arm

1 ✓7ᵗʰ **S59.132** Salter-Harris Type III physeal fracture of upper end of radius, **left** arm

✓7ᵗʰ **S59.139** Salter-Harris Type III physeal fracture ▽ of upper end of radius, unspecified arm

✓6ᵗʰ **S59.14** Salter-Harris Type IV physeal fracture of upper end of radius

1 ✓7ᵗʰ **S59.141** Salter-Harris Type IV physeal fracture of upper end of radius, **right** arm

1 ✓7ᵗʰ **S59.142** Salter-Harris Type IV physeal fracture of upper end of radius, **left** arm

✓7ᵗʰ **S59.149** Salter-Harris Type IV physeal fracture ▽ of upper end of radius, unspecified arm

✓6ᵗʰ **S59.19** Other physeal fracture of upper end of radius

1 ✓7ᵗʰ **S59.191** Other physeal fracture of upper end of radius, **right** arm

1 ✓7ᵗʰ **S59.192** Other physeal fracture of upper end of radius, **left** arm

✓7ᵗʰ **S59.199** Other physeal fracture of upper end of ▽ radius, unspecified arm

✓5ᵗʰ **S59.2** Physeal fracture of lower end of radius

✓6ᵗʰ **S59.20** Unspecified physeal fracture of lower end of radius

1 ✓7ᵗʰ **S59.201** Unspecified physeal fracture of lower ▽ end of radius, **right** arm

1 ✓7ᵗʰ **S59.202** Unspecified physeal fracture of lower ▽ end of radius, **left** arm

✓7ᵗʰ **S59.209** Unspecified physeal fracture of lower ▽ end of radius, unspecified arm

✓6ᵗʰ **S59.21** Salter-Harris Type I physeal fracture of lower end of radius

1 ✓7ᵗʰ **S59.211** Salter-Harris Type I physeal fracture of lower end of radius, **right** arm

1 ✓7ᵗʰ **S59.212** Salter-Harris Type I physeal fracture of lower end of radius, **left** arm

✓7ᵗʰ **S59.219** Salter-Harris Type I physeal fracture of ▽ lower end of radius, unspecified arm

✓6ᵗʰ **S59.22** Salter-Harris Type II physeal fracture of lower end of radius

1 ✓7ᵗʰ **S59.221** Salter-Harris Type II physeal fracture of lower end of radius, **right** arm

1 ✓7ᵗʰ **S59.222** Salter-Harris Type II physeal fracture of lower end of radius, **left** arm

✓7ᵗʰ **S59.229** Salter-Harris Type II physeal fracture of ▽ lower end of radius, unspecified arm

✓6ᵗʰ **S59.23** Salter-Harris Type III physeal fracture of lower end of radius

1 ✓7ᵗʰ **S59.231** Salter-Harris Type III physeal fracture of lower end of radius, **right** arm

1 ✓7ᵗʰ **S59.232** Salter-Harris Type III physeal fracture of lower end of radius, **left** arm

✓7ᵗʰ **S59.239** Salter-Harris Type III physeal fracture ▽ of lower end of radius, unspecified arm

✓6ᵗʰ **S59.24** Salter-Harris Type IV physeal fracture of lower end of radius

1 ✓7ᵗʰ **S59.241** Salter-Harris Type IV physeal fracture of lower end of radius, **right** arm

1 ✓7ᵗʰ **S59.242** Salter-Harris Type IV physeal fracture of lower end of radius, **left** arm

✓7ᵗʰ **S59.249** Salter-Harris Type IV physeal fracture ▽ of lower end of radius, unspecified arm

✓6ᵗʰ **S59.29** Other physeal fracture of lower end of radius

1 ✓7ᵗʰ **S59.291** Other physeal fracture of lower end of radius, **right** arm

1 ✓7ᵗʰ **S59.292** Other physeal fracture of lower end of radius, **left** arm

✓7ᵗʰ **S59.299** Other physeal fracture of lower end of ▽ radius, unspecified arm

✓5ᵗʰ **S59.8** Other specified injuries of elbow and forearm

The appropriate 7th character is to be added to each code in subcategory S59.8.
A   initial encounter
D   subsequent encounter
S   sequela

✓6ᵗʰ **S59.80** Other specified injuries of elbow

✓7ᵗʰ **S59.801** Other specified injuries of **right** elbow

✓7ᵗʰ **S59.802** Other specified injuries of **left** elbow

✓7ᵗʰ **S59.809** Other specified injuries of unspecified ▽ elbow

✓6ᵗʰ **S59.81** Other specified injuries of forearm

✓7ᵗʰ **S59.811** Other specified injuries **right** forearm

✓7ᵗʰ **S59.812** Other specified injuries **left** forearm

✓7ᵗʰ **S59.819** Other specified injuries unspecified ▽ forearm

✓5ᵗʰ **S59.9** Unspecified injury of elbow and forearm

The appropriate 7th character is to be added to each code in subcategory S59.9.
A   initial encounter
D   subsequent encounter
S   sequela

✓6ᵗʰ **S59.90** Unspecified injury of elbow

✓7ᵗʰ **S59.901** Unspecified injury of **right** elbow ▽

✓7ᵗʰ **S59.902** Unspecified injury of **left** elbow ▽

✓7ᵗʰ **S59.909** Unspecified injury of unspecified elbow ▽

✓6ᵗʰ **S59.91** Unspecified injury of forearm

✓7ᵗʰ **S59.911** Unspecified injury of **right** forearm ▽

✓7ᵗʰ **S59.912** Unspecified injury of **left** forearm ▽

✓7ᵗʰ **S59.919** Unspecified injury of unspecified ▽ forearm

Injuries to the wrist, hand and fingers (S60-S69)

EXCLUDES 2 burns and corrosions (T20-T32)
frostbite (T33-T34)
insect bite or sting, venomous (T63.4)

✓4ᵗʰ **S60** Superficial injury of wrist, hand and fingers

The appropriate 7th character is to be added to each code from category S60.
A   initial encounter
D   subsequent encounter
S   sequela

✓5ᵗʰ **S60.0** Contusion of finger without damage to nail
EXCLUDES 1 contusion involving nail (matrix) (S60.1)

✓x7ᵗʰ **S60.00** Contusion of unspecified finger without damage ▽ to nail
Contusion of finger(s) NOS

✓6ᵗʰ **S60.01** Contusion of thumb without damage to nail

✓7ᵗʰ **S60.011** Contusion of **right** thumb without damage to nail

✓7ᵗʰ **S60.012** Contusion of **left** thumb without damage to nail

✓7ᵗʰ **S60.019** Contusion of unspecified thumb ▽ without damage to nail

✓6ᵗʰ **S60.02** Contusion of index finger without damage to nail

✓7ᵗʰ **S60.021** Contusion of **right** index finger without damage to nail

✓7ᵗʰ **S60.022** Contusion of **left** index finger without damage to nail

✓7ᵗʰ **S60.029** Contusion of unspecified index ▽ finger without damage to nail

---

1   Case-mix diagnosis with 7th character indicating subsequent encounter.

✓6ᵗʰ **S60.03** Contusion of middle finger without damage to nail
- ✓7ᵗʰ **S60.031** Contusion of right middle finger without damage to nail
- ✓7ᵗʰ **S60.032** Contusion of left middle finger without damage to nail
- ✓7ᵗʰ **S60.039** Contusion of unspecified middle finger without damage to nail ▽

✓6ᵗʰ **S60.04** Contusion of ring finger without damage to nail
- ✓7ᵗʰ **S60.041** Contusion of right ring finger without damage to nail
- ✓7ᵗʰ **S60.042** Contusion of left ring finger without damage to nail
- ✓7ᵗʰ **S60.049** Contusion of unspecified ring finger without damage to nail ▽

✓6ᵗʰ **S60.05** Contusion of little finger without damage to nail
- ✓7ᵗʰ **S60.051** Contusion of right little finger without damage to nail
- ✓7ᵗʰ **S60.052** Contusion of left little finger without damage to nail
- ✓7ᵗʰ **S60.059** Contusion of unspecified little finger without damage to nail ▽

✓5ᵗʰ **S60.1** Contusion of finger with damage to nail
- ✓ˣ7ᵗʰ **S60.10** Contusion of unspecified finger with damage to nail ▽

✓6ᵗʰ **S60.11** Contusion of thumb with damage to nail
- ✓7ᵗʰ **S60.111** Contusion of right thumb with damage to nail
- ✓7ᵗʰ **S60.112** Contusion of left thumb with damage to nail
- ✓7ᵗʰ **S60.119** Contusion of unspecified thumb with damage to nail ▽

✓6ᵗʰ **S60.12** Contusion of index finger with damage to nail
- ✓7ᵗʰ **S60.121** Contusion of right index finger with damage to nail
- ✓7ᵗʰ **S60.122** Contusion of left index finger with damage to nail
- ✓7ᵗʰ **S60.129** Contusion of unspecified index finger with damage to nail ▽

✓6ᵗʰ **S60.13** Contusion of middle finger with damage to nail
- ✓7ᵗʰ **S60.131** Contusion of right middle finger with damage to nail
- ✓7ᵗʰ **S60.132** Contusion of left middle finger with damage to nail
- ✓7ᵗʰ **S60.139** Contusion of unspecified middle finger with damage to nail ▽

✓6ᵗʰ **S60.14** Contusion of ring finger with damage to nail
- ✓7ᵗʰ **S60.141** Contusion of right ring finger with damage to nail
- ✓7ᵗʰ **S60.142** Contusion of left ring finger with damage to nail
- ✓7ᵗʰ **S60.149** Contusion of unspecified ring finger with damage to nail ▽

✓6ᵗʰ **S60.15** Contusion of little finger with damage to nail
- ✓7ᵗʰ **S60.151** Contusion of right little finger with damage to nail
- ✓7ᵗʰ **S60.152** Contusion of left little finger with damage to nail
- ✓7ᵗʰ **S60.159** Contusion of unspecified little finger with damage to nail ▽

✓5ᵗʰ **S60.2** Contusion of wrist and hand
- **EXCLUDES 2** contusion of fingers (S60.0-, S60.1-)

✓6ᵗʰ **S60.21** Contusion of wrist
- ✓7ᵗʰ **S60.211** Contusion of right wrist
- ✓7ᵗʰ **S60.212** Contusion of left wrist
- ✓7ᵗʰ **S60.219** Contusion of unspecified wrist ▽

✓6ᵗʰ **S60.22** Contusion of hand
- ✓7ᵗʰ **S60.221** Contusion of right hand
- ✓7ᵗʰ **S60.222** Contusion of left hand
- ✓7ᵗʰ **S60.229** Contusion of unspecified hand ▽

✓5ᵗʰ **S60.3** Other superficial injuries of thumb

✓6ᵗʰ **S60.31** Abrasion of thumb
- ✓7ᵗʰ **S60.311** Abrasion of right thumb
- ✓7ᵗʰ **S60.312** Abrasion of left thumb
- ✓7ᵗʰ **S60.319** Abrasion of unspecified thumb ▽

✓6ᵗʰ **S60.32** Blister (nonthermal) of thumb
- ✓7ᵗʰ **S60.321** Blister (nonthermal) of right thumb
- ✓7ᵗʰ **S60.322** Blister (nonthermal) of left thumb
- ✓7ᵗʰ **S60.329** Blister (nonthermal) of unspecified thumb ▽

✓6ᵗʰ **S60.34** External constriction of thumb
- Hair tourniquet syndrome of thumb
- Use additional cause code to identify the constricting item (W49.0-)
- ✓7ᵗʰ **S60.341** External constriction of right thumb
- ✓7ᵗʰ **S60.342** External constriction of left thumb
- ✓7ᵗʰ **S60.349** External constriction of unspecified thumb ▽

✓6ᵗʰ **S60.35** Superficial foreign body of thumb
- Splinter in the thumb
- ✓7ᵗʰ **S60.351** Superficial foreign body of right thumb
- ✓7ᵗʰ **S60.352** Superficial foreign body of left thumb
- ✓7ᵗʰ **S60.359** Superficial foreign body of unspecified thumb ▽

✓6ᵗʰ **S60.36** Insect bite (nonvenomous) of thumb
- ✓7ᵗʰ **S60.361** Insect bite (nonvenomous) of right thumb
- ✓7ᵗʰ **S60.362** Insect bite (nonvenomous) of left thumb
- ✓7ᵗʰ **S60.369** Insect bite (nonvenomous) of unspecified thumb ▽

✓6ᵗʰ **S60.37** Other superficial bite of thumb
- **EXCLUDES 1** open bite of thumb (S61.05-, S61.15-)
- ✓7ᵗʰ **S60.371** Other superficial bite of right thumb
- ✓7ᵗʰ **S60.372** Other superficial bite of left thumb
- ✓7ᵗʰ **S60.379** Other superficial bite of unspecified thumb ▽

✓6ᵗʰ **S60.39** Other superficial injuries of thumb
- ✓7ᵗʰ **S60.391** Other superficial injuries of right thumb
- ✓7ᵗʰ **S60.392** Other superficial injuries of left thumb
- ✓7ᵗʰ **S60.399** Other superficial injuries of unspecified thumb ▽

✓5ᵗʰ **S60.4** Other superficial injuries of other fingers

✓6ᵗʰ **S60.41** Abrasion of fingers
- ✓7ᵗʰ **S60.410** Abrasion of right index finger
- ✓7ᵗʰ **S60.411** Abrasion of left index finger
- ✓7ᵗʰ **S60.412** Abrasion of right middle finger
- ✓7ᵗʰ **S60.413** Abrasion of left middle finger
- ✓7ᵗʰ **S60.414** Abrasion of right ring finger
- ✓7ᵗʰ **S60.415** Abrasion of left ring finger
- ✓7ᵗʰ **S60.416** Abrasion of right little finger
- ✓7ᵗʰ **S60.417** Abrasion of left little finger
- ✓7ᵗʰ **S60.418** Abrasion of other finger
  - Abrasion of specified finger with unspecified laterality
- ✓7ᵗʰ **S60.419** Abrasion of unspecified finger ▽

✓6ᵗʰ **S60.42** Blister (nonthermal) of fingers
- ✓7ᵗʰ **S60.420** Blister (nonthermal) of right index finger
- ✓7ᵗʰ **S60.421** Blister (nonthermal) of left index finger
- ✓7ᵗʰ **S60.422** Blister (nonthermal) of right middle finger
- ✓7ᵗʰ **S60.423** Blister (nonthermal) of left middle finger
- ✓7ᵗʰ **S60.424** Blister (nonthermal) of right ring finger
- ✓7ᵗʰ **S60.425** Blister (nonthermal) of left ring finger
- ✓7ᵗʰ **S60.426** Blister (nonthermal) of right little finger
- ✓7ᵗʰ **S60.427** Blister (nonthermal) of left little finger
- ✓7ᵗʰ **S60.428** Blister (nonthermal) of other finger
  - Blister (nonthermal) of specified finger with unspecified laterality
- ✓7ᵗʰ **S60.429** Blister (nonthermal) of unspecified finger ▽

Ⓝ Newborn: 0　Ⓟ Pediatric: 0-17　Ⓜ Maternity: 12-55　Ⓐ Adult: 15-124　**NRS** Nonroutine supply Dx　**NC Dx** Noncancer Dx　**PDx** Primary Dx　▶◀ Revised Text　● New Code　▲ Revised Title

978　　　　　　　　　　　　　　　　　　　　　　　　　　　　　　　　　　ICD-10-CM 2018

☑6ᵗʰ **S60.44 External constriction of fingers**
Hair tourniquet syndrome of finger
Use additional cause code to identify the constricting item (W49.0-)

√7ᵗʰ **S60.440 External constriction of** right index **finger**

√7ᵗʰ **S60.441 External constriction of** left index **finger**

√7ᵗʰ **S60.442 External constriction of** right middle **finger**

√7ᵗʰ **S60.443 External constriction of** left middle **finger**

√7ᵗʰ **S60.444 External constriction of** right ring **finger**

√7ᵗʰ **S60.445 External constriction of** left ring **finger**

√7ᵗʰ **S60.446 External constriction of** right little **finger**

√7ᵗʰ **S60.447 External constriction of** left little **finger**

√7ᵗʰ **S60.448 External constriction of other finger**
External constriction of specified finger with unspecified laterality

√7ᵗʰ **S60.449 External constriction of unspecified finger** ▽

☑6ᵗʰ **S60.45 Superficial** foreign body **of fingers**
Splinter in the finger(s)

√7ᵗʰ **S60.450 Superficial foreign body of** right index **finger**

√7ᵗʰ **S60.451 Superficial foreign body of** left index **finger**

√7ᵗʰ **S60.452 Superficial foreign body of** right middle **finger**

√7ᵗʰ **S60.453 Superficial foreign body of** left middle **finger**

√7ᵗʰ **S60.454 Superficial foreign body of** right ring **finger**

√7ᵗʰ **S60.455 Superficial foreign body of** left ring **finger**

√7ᵗʰ **S60.456 Superficial foreign body of** right little **finger**

√7ᵗʰ **S60.457 Superficial foreign body of** left little **finger**

√7ᵗʰ **S60.458 Superficial foreign body of other finger**
Superficial foreign body of specified finger with unspecified laterality

√7ᵗʰ **S60.459 Superficial foreign body of unspecified finger** ▽

☑6ᵗʰ **S60.46 Insect bite (nonvenomous) of fingers**

√7ᵗʰ **S60.460 Insect bite (nonvenomous) of** right index **finger**

√7ᵗʰ **S60.461 Insect bite (nonvenomous) of** left index **finger**

√7ᵗʰ **S60.462 Insect bite (nonvenomous) of** right middle **finger**

√7ᵗʰ **S60.463 Insect bite (nonvenomous) of** left middle **finger**

√7ᵗʰ **S60.464 Insect bite (nonvenomous) of** right ring **finger**

√7ᵗʰ **S60.465 Insect bite (nonvenomous) of** left ring **finger**

√7ᵗʰ **S60.466 Insect bite (nonvenomous) of** right little **finger**

√7ᵗʰ **S60.467 Insect bite (nonvenomous) of** left little **finger**

√7ᵗʰ **S60.468 Insect bite (nonvenomous) of other finger**
Insect bite (nonvenomous) of specified finger with unspecified laterality

√7ᵗʰ **S60.469 Insect bite (nonvenomous) of unspecified finger** ▽

☑6ᵗʰ **S60.47 Other** superficial bite **of fingers**
EXCLUDES 1 open bite of fingers (S61.25-, S61.35-)

√7ᵗʰ **S60.470 Other superficial bite of** right index **finger**

√7ᵗʰ **S60.471 Other superficial bite of** left index **finger**

√7ᵗʰ **S60.472 Other superficial bite of** right middle **finger**

√7ᵗʰ **S60.473 Other superficial bite of** left middle **finger**

√7ᵗʰ **S60.474 Other superficial bite of** right ring **finger**

√7ᵗʰ **S60.475 Other superficial bite of** left ring **finger**

√7ᵗʰ **S60.476 Other superficial bite of** right little **finger**

√7ᵗʰ **S60.477 Other superficial bite of** left little **finger**

√7ᵗʰ **S60.478 Other superficial bite of other finger**
Other superficial bite of specified finger with unspecified laterality

√7ᵗʰ **S60.479 Other superficial bite of unspecified finger** ▽

☑5ᵗʰ **S60.5 Other superficial injuries of** hand
EXCLUDES 2 superficial injuries of fingers (S60.3-, S60.4-)

☑6ᵗʰ **S60.51 Abrasion of hand**

√7ᵗʰ **S60.511 Abrasion of** right **hand**

√7ᵗʰ **S60.512 Abrasion of** left **hand**

√7ᵗʰ **S60.519 Abrasion of unspecified hand** ▽

☑6ᵗʰ **S60.52 Blister (nonthermal) of hand**

√7ᵗʰ **S60.521 Blister (nonthermal) of** right **hand**

√7ᵗʰ **S60.522 Blister (nonthermal) of** left **hand**

√7ᵗʰ **S60.529 Blister (nonthermal) of unspecified hand** ▽

☑6ᵗʰ **S60.54 External constriction of hand**

√7ᵗʰ **S60.541 External constriction of** right **hand**

√7ᵗʰ **S60.542 External constriction of** left **hand**

√7ᵗʰ **S60.549 External constriction of unspecified hand** ▽

☑6ᵗʰ **S60.55 Superficial** foreign body **of hand**
Splinter in the hand

√7ᵗʰ **S60.551 Superficial foreign body of** right **hand**

√7ᵗʰ **S60.552 Superficial foreign body of** left **hand**

√7ᵗʰ **S60.559 Superficial foreign body of unspecified hand** ▽

☑6ᵗʰ **S60.56 Insect bite (nonvenomous) of hand**

√7ᵗʰ **S60.561 Insect bite (nonvenomous) of** right **hand**

√7ᵗʰ **S60.562 Insect bite (nonvenomous) of** left **hand**

√7ᵗʰ **S60.569 Insect bite (nonvenomous) of unspecified hand** ▽

☑6ᵗʰ **S60.57 Other** superficial bite **of hand**
EXCLUDES 1 open bite of hand (S61.45-)

√7ᵗʰ **S60.571 Other superficial bite of hand of** right **hand**

√7ᵗʰ **S60.572 Other superficial bite of hand of** left **hand**

√7ᵗʰ **S60.579 Other superficial bite of hand of unspecified hand** ▽

☑5ᵗʰ **S60.8 Other superficial injuries of** wrist

☑6ᵗʰ **S60.81 Abrasion of wrist**

√7ᵗʰ **S60.811 Abrasion of** right **wrist**

√7ᵗʰ **S60.812 Abrasion of** left **wrist**

√7ᵗʰ **S60.819 Abrasion of unspecified wrist** ▽

☑6ᵗʰ **S60.82 Blister (nonthermal) of wrist**

√7ᵗʰ **S60.821 Blister (nonthermal) of** right **wrist**

√7ᵗʰ **S60.822 Blister (nonthermal) of** left **wrist**

√7ᵗʰ **S60.829 Blister (nonthermal) of unspecified wrist** ▽

☑6ᵗʰ **S60.84 External constriction of wrist**

√7ᵗʰ **S60.841 External constriction of** right **wrist**

√7ᵗʰ **S60.842 External constriction of** left **wrist**

√7ᵗʰ **S60.849 External constriction of unspecified wrist** ▽

☑6ᵗʰ **S60.85 Superficial** foreign body **of wrist**
Splinter in the wrist

√7ᵗʰ **S60.851 Superficial foreign body of** right **wrist**

√7ᵗʰ **S60.852 Superficial foreign body of** left **wrist**

√7ᵗʰ **S60.859 Superficial foreign body of unspecified wrist** ▽

☑6ᵗʰ **S60.86 Insect bite (nonvenomous) of wrist**

√7ᵗʰ **S60.861 Insect bite (nonvenomous) of** right **wrist**

√7ᵗʰ **S60.862 Insect bite (nonvenomous) of** left **wrist**

√7ᵗʰ **S60.869 Insect bite (nonvenomous) of unspecified wrist** ▽

☑6ᵗʰ **S60.87 Other** superficial bite **of wrist**
EXCLUDES 1 open bite of wrist (S61.55)

√7ᵗʰ **S60.871 Other superficial bite of** right **wrist**

√7ᵗʰ **S60.872 Other superficial bite of** left **wrist**

☑ Additional Character Req   √x7ᵗʰ Placeholder Alert   Case-Mix Diagnosis   Manifestation   ▽ Unspecified Dx   EXCLUDES 1 Not coded here   EXCLUDES 2 Not included here

ICD-10-CM 2018   979

✓7ᵗʰ **S60.879** Other superficial bite of unspecified wrist ▽

✓5ᵗʰ **S60.9** Unspecified superficial injury of wrist, hand and fingers

  ✓6ᵗʰ **S60.91** Unspecified superficial injury of wrist

    ✓7ᵗʰ **S60.911** Unspecified superficial injury of right wrist ▽

    ✓7ᵗʰ **S60.912** Unspecified superficial injury of left wrist ▽

    ✓7ᵗʰ **S60.919** Unspecified superficial injury of unspecified wrist ▽

  ✓6ᵗʰ **S60.92** Unspecified superficial injury of hand

    ✓7ᵗʰ **S60.921** Unspecified superficial injury of right hand ▽

    ✓7ᵗʰ **S60.922** Unspecified superficial injury of left hand ▽

    ✓7ᵗʰ **S60.929** Unspecified superficial injury of unspecified hand ▽

  ✓6ᵗʰ **S60.93** Unspecified superficial injury of thumb

    ✓7ᵗʰ **S60.931** Unspecified superficial injury of right thumb ▽

    ✓7ᵗʰ **S60.932** Unspecified superficial injury of left thumb ▽

    ✓7ᵗʰ **S60.939** Unspecified superficial injury of unspecified thumb ▽

  ✓6ᵗʰ **S60.94** Unspecified superficial injury of other fingers

    ✓7ᵗʰ **S60.940** Unspecified superficial injury of right index finger ▽

    ✓7ᵗʰ **S60.941** Unspecified superficial injury of left index finger ▽

    ✓7ᵗʰ **S60.942** Unspecified superficial injury of right middle finger ▽

    ✓7ᵗʰ **S60.943** Unspecified superficial injury of left middle finger ▽

    ✓7ᵗʰ **S60.944** Unspecified superficial injury of right ring finger ▽

    ✓7ᵗʰ **S60.945** Unspecified superficial injury of left ring finger ▽

    ✓7ᵗʰ **S60.946** Unspecified superficial injury of right little finger ▽

    ✓7ᵗʰ **S60.947** Unspecified superficial injury of left little finger ▽

    ✓7ᵗʰ **S60.948** Unspecified superficial injury of other finger ▽
        Unspecified superficial injury of specified finger with unspecified laterality

    ✓7ᵗʰ **S60.949** Unspecified superficial injury of unspecified finger ▽

✓4ᵗʰ **S61** **Open wound of wrist, hand and fingers**
  Code also any associated wound infection
  EXCLUDES 1 open fracture of wrist, hand and finger (S62- with 7th character B)
    traumatic amputation of wrist and hand (S68.-)

  The appropriate 7th character is to be added to each code from category S61.
  A   initial encounter
  D   subsequent encounter
  S   sequela

✓5ᵗʰ **S61.0** Open wound of thumb without damage to nail
  EXCLUDES 1 open wound of thumb with damage to nail (S61.1-)

  ✓6ᵗʰ **S61.00** Unspecified open wound of thumb without damage to nail

    5 ✓7ᵗʰ **S61.001** Unspecified open wound of right thumb without damage to nail NRS ▽

    5 ✓7ᵗʰ **S61.002** Unspecified open wound of left thumb without damage to nail NRS ▽

    ✓7ᵗʰ **S61.009** Unspecified open wound of unspecified thumb without damage to nail ▽

  ✓6ᵗʰ **S61.01** Laceration without foreign body of thumb without damage to nail

    4,5 ✓7ᵗʰ **S61.011** Laceration without foreign body of right thumb without damage to nail NRS

4,5 ✓7ᵗʰ **S61.012** Laceration without foreign body of left thumb without damage to nail NRS

✓7ᵗʰ **S61.019** Laceration without foreign body of unspecified thumb without damage to nail ▽

✓6ᵗʰ **S61.02** Laceration with foreign body of thumb without damage to nail

  4,5 ✓7ᵗʰ **S61.021** Laceration with foreign body of right thumb without damage to nail NRS

  4,5 ✓7ᵗʰ **S61.022** Laceration with foreign body of left thumb without damage to nail NRS

  ✓7ᵗʰ **S61.029** Laceration with foreign body of unspecified thumb without damage to nail ▽

✓6ᵗʰ **S61.03** Puncture wound without foreign body of thumb without damage to nail

  4,5 ✓7ᵗʰ **S61.031** Puncture wound without foreign body of right thumb without damage to nail NRS

  4,5 ✓7ᵗʰ **S61.032** Puncture wound without foreign body of left thumb without damage to nail NRS

  ✓7ᵗʰ **S61.039** Puncture wound without foreign body of unspecified thumb without damage to nail ▽

✓6ᵗʰ **S61.04** Puncture wound with foreign body of thumb without damage to nail

  4,5 ✓7ᵗʰ **S61.041** Puncture wound with foreign body of right thumb without damage to nail NRS

  4,5 ✓7ᵗʰ **S61.042** Puncture wound with foreign body of left thumb without damage to nail NRS

  ✓7ᵗʰ **S61.049** Puncture wound with foreign body of unspecified thumb without damage to nail ▽

✓6ᵗʰ **S61.05** Open bite of thumb without damage to nail
  Bite of thumb NOS
  EXCLUDES 1 superficial bite of thumb (S60.36-, S60.37-)

  4,5 ✓7ᵗʰ **S61.051** Open bite of right thumb without damage to nail NRS

  4,5 ✓7ᵗʰ **S61.052** Open bite of left thumb without damage to nail NRS

  ✓7ᵗʰ **S61.059** Open bite of unspecified thumb without damage to nail ▽

✓5ᵗʰ **S61.1** Open wound of thumb with damage to nail

  ✓6ᵗʰ **S61.10** Unspecified open wound of thumb with damage to nail

    5 ✓7ᵗʰ **S61.101** Unspecified open wound of right thumb with damage to nail NRS ▽

    5 ✓7ᵗʰ **S61.102** Unspecified open wound of left thumb with damage to nail NRS ▽

    ✓7ᵗʰ **S61.109** Unspecified open wound of unspecified thumb with damage to nail ▽

  ✓6ᵗʰ **S61.11** Laceration without foreign body of thumb with damage to nail

    4,5 ✓7ᵗʰ **S61.111** Laceration without foreign body of right thumb with damage to nail NRS

    4,5 ✓7ᵗʰ **S61.112** Laceration without foreign body of left thumb with damage to nail NRS

    ✓7ᵗʰ **S61.119** Laceration without foreign body of unspecified thumb with damage to nail ▽

  ✓6ᵗʰ **S61.12** Laceration with foreign body of thumb with damage to nail

    4,5 ✓7ᵗʰ **S61.121** Laceration with foreign body of right thumb with damage to nail NRS

    4,5 ✓7ᵗʰ **S61.122** Laceration with foreign body of left thumb with damage to nail NRS

    ✓7ᵗʰ **S61.129** Laceration with foreign body of unspecified thumb with damage to nail ▽

  ✓6ᵗʰ **S61.13** Puncture wound without foreign body of thumb with damage to nail

    4,5 ✓7ᵗʰ **S61.131** Puncture wound without foreign body of right thumb with damage to nail NRS

---

4 Case-mix diagnosis with 7th character indicating initial or subsequent encounter.
5 NRS supply diagnosis with 7th character indicating initial or subsequent encounter.

4,5 ✓7ᵗʰ **S61.132 Puncture wound without foreign body of left thumb with damage to nail** NRS

✓7ᵗʰ **S61.139** Puncture wound without foreign body of unspecified thumb with damage to nail ▽

✓6ᵗʰ **S61.14** Puncture wound with foreign body of thumb with damage to nail

4,5 ✓7ᵗʰ **S61.141 Puncture wound with foreign body of right thumb with damage to nail** NRS

4,5 ✓7ᵗʰ **S61.142 Puncture wound with foreign body of left thumb with damage to nail** NRS

✓7ᵗʰ **S61.149** Puncture wound with foreign body of unspecified thumb with damage to nail ▽

✓6ᵗʰ **S61.15** Open bite of thumb with damage to nail
  Bite of thumb with damage to nail NOS
    EXCLUDES 1 superficial bite of thumb (S60.36-, S60.37-)

4,5 ✓7ᵗʰ **S61.151 Open bite of right thumb with damage to nail** NRS

4,5 ✓7ᵗʰ **S61.152 Open bite of left thumb with damage to nail** NRS

✓7ᵗʰ **S61.159** Open bite of unspecified thumb with damage to nail ▽

✓5ᵗʰ **S61.2 Open wound of other finger without damage to nail**
    EXCLUDES 1 open wound of finger involving nail (matrix) (S61.3-)
    EXCLUDES 2 open wound of thumb without damage to nail (S61.0-)

✓6ᵗʰ **S61.20** Unspecified open wound of other finger without damage to nail

5 ✓7ᵗʰ **S61.200** Unspecified open wound of right index finger without damage to nail NRS ▽

5 ✓7ᵗʰ **S61.201** Unspecified open wound of left index finger without damage to nail NRS ▽

5 ✓7ᵗʰ **S61.202** Unspecified open wound of right middle finger without damage to nail NRS ▽

5 ✓7ᵗʰ **S61.203** Unspecified open wound of left middle finger without damage to nail NRS ▽

5 ✓7ᵗʰ **S61.204** Unspecified open wound of right ring finger without damage to nail NRS ▽

5 ✓7ᵗʰ **S61.205** Unspecified open wound of left ring finger without damage to nail NRS ▽

5 ✓7ᵗʰ **S61.206** Unspecified open wound of right little finger without damage to nail NRS ▽

5 ✓7ᵗʰ **S61.207** Unspecified open wound of left little finger without damage to nail NRS ▽

5 ✓7ᵗʰ **S61.208** Unspecified open wound of other finger without damage to nail NRS ▽
    Unspecified open wound of specified finger with unspecified laterality without damage to nail

✓7ᵗʰ **S61.209** Unspecified open wound of unspecified finger without damage to nail ▽

✓6ᵗʰ **S61.21** Laceration without foreign body of finger without damage to nail

4,5 ✓7ᵗʰ **S61.210 Laceration without foreign body of right index finger without damage to nail** NRS

4,5 ✓7ᵗʰ **S61.211 Laceration without foreign body of left index finger without damage to nail** NRS

4,5 ✓7ᵗʰ **S61.212 Laceration without foreign body of right middle finger without damage to nail** NRS

4,5 ✓7ᵗʰ **S61.213 Laceration without foreign body of left middle finger without damage to nail** NRS

4,5 ✓7ᵗʰ **S61.214 Laceration without foreign body of right ring finger without damage to nail** NRS

4,5 ✓7ᵗʰ **S61.215 Laceration without foreign body of left ring finger without damage to nail** NRS

4,5 ✓7ᵗʰ **S61.216 Laceration without foreign body of right little finger without damage to nail** NRS

4,5 ✓7ᵗʰ **S61.217 Laceration without foreign body of left little finger without damage to nail** NRS

5 ✓7ᵗʰ **S61.218 Laceration without foreign body of other finger without damage to nail** NRS
    Laceration without foreign body of specified finger with unspecified laterality without damage to nail

✓7ᵗʰ **S61.219** Laceration without foreign body of unspecified finger without damage to nail ▽

✓6ᵗʰ **S61.22** Laceration with foreign body of finger without damage to nail

4,5 ✓7ᵗʰ **S61.220 Laceration with foreign body of right index finger without damage to nail** NRS

4,5 ✓7ᵗʰ **S61.221 Laceration with foreign body of left index finger without damage to nail** NRS

4,5 ✓7ᵗʰ **S61.222 Laceration with foreign body of right middle finger without damage to nail** NRS

4,5 ✓7ᵗʰ **S61.223 Laceration with foreign body of left middle finger without damage to nail** NRS

4,5 ✓7ᵗʰ **S61.224 Laceration with foreign body of right ring finger without damage to nail** NRS

4,5 ✓7ᵗʰ **S61.225 Laceration with foreign body of left ring finger without damage to nail** NRS

4,5 ✓7ᵗʰ **S61.226 Laceration with foreign body of right little finger without damage to nail** NRS

4,5 ✓7ᵗʰ **S61.227 Laceration with foreign body of left little finger without damage to nail** NRS

5 ✓7ᵗʰ **S61.228 Laceration with foreign body of other finger without damage to nail** NRS
    Laceration with foreign body of specified finger with unspecified laterality without damage to nail

✓7ᵗʰ **S61.229** Laceration with foreign body of unspecified finger without damage to nail ▽

✓6ᵗʰ **S61.23** Puncture wound without foreign body of finger without damage to nail

4,5 ✓7ᵗʰ **S61.230 Puncture wound without foreign body of right index finger without damage to nail** NRS

4,5 ✓7ᵗʰ **S61.231 Puncture wound without foreign body of left index finger without damage to nail** NRS

4,5 ✓7ᵗʰ **S61.232 Puncture wound without foreign body of right middle finger without damage to nail** NRS

4,5 ✓7ᵗʰ **S61.233 Puncture wound without foreign body of left middle finger without damage to nail** NRS

4,5 ✓7ᵗʰ **S61.234 Puncture wound without foreign body of right ring finger without damage to nail** NRS

4,5 ✓7ᵗʰ **S61.235 Puncture wound without foreign body of left ring finger without damage to nail** NRS

4,5 ✓7ᵗʰ **S61.236 Puncture wound without foreign body of right little finger without damage to nail** NRS

4,5 ✓7ᵗʰ **S61.237 Puncture wound without foreign body of left little finger without damage to nail** NRS

5 ✓7ᵗʰ **S61.238 Puncture wound without foreign body of other finger without damage to nail** NRS
    Puncture wound without foreign body of specified finger with unspecified laterality without damage to nail

✓7ᵗʰ **S61.239** Puncture wound without foreign body of unspecified finger without damage to nail ▽

✓6ᵗʰ **S61.24** Puncture wound with foreign body of finger without damage to nail

4,5 ✓7ᵗʰ **S61.240 Puncture wound with foreign body of right index finger without damage to nail** NRS

---

4 Case-mix diagnosis with 7th character indicating initial or subsequent encounter.
5 NRS supply diagnosis with 7th character indicating initial or subsequent encounter.

✓ Additional Character Req   ✓x7ᵗʰ Placeholder Alert   Case-Mix Diagnosis   Manifestation   ▽ Unspecified Dx   EXCLUDES 1 Not coded here   EXCLUDES 2 Not included here

4,5 ✓7ᵗʰ **S61.241** Puncture wound with foreign body of left index finger without damage to nail NRS

4,5 ✓7ᵗʰ **S61.242** Puncture wound with foreign body of right middle finger without damage to nail NRS

4,5 ✓7ᵗʰ **S61.243** Puncture wound with foreign body of left middle finger without damage to nail NRS

4,5 ✓7ᵗʰ **S61.244** Puncture wound with foreign body of right ring finger without damage to nail NRS

4,5 ✓7ᵗʰ **S61.245** Puncture wound with foreign body of left ring finger without damage to nail NRS

4,5 ✓7ᵗʰ **S61.246** Puncture wound with foreign body of right little finger without damage to nail NRS

4,5 ✓7ᵗʰ **S61.247** Puncture wound with foreign body of left little finger without damage to nail NRS

5 ✓7ᵗʰ **S61.248** Puncture wound with foreign body of other finger without damage to nail NRS
     Puncture wound with foreign body of specified finger with unspecified laterality without damage to nail

✓7ᵗʰ **S61.249** Puncture wound with foreign body of unspecified finger without damage to nail ▽

✓6ᵗʰ **S61.25** Open bite of finger without damage to nail
     Bite of finger without damage to nail NOS
     EXCLUDES 1 superficial bite of finger (S60.46-, S60.47-)

4,5 ✓7ᵗʰ **S61.250** Open bite of right index finger without damage to nail NRS

4,5 ✓7ᵗʰ **S61.251** Open bite of left index finger without damage to nail NRS

4,5 ✓7ᵗʰ **S61.252** Open bite of right middle finger without damage to nail NRS

4,5 ✓7ᵗʰ **S61.253** Open bite of left middle finger without damage to nail NRS

4,5 ✓7ᵗʰ **S61.254** Open bite of right ring finger without damage to nail NRS

4,5 ✓7ᵗʰ **S61.255** Open bite of left ring finger without damage to nail NRS

4,5 ✓7ᵗʰ **S61.256** Open bite of right little finger without damage to nail NRS

4,5 ✓7ᵗʰ **S61.257** Open bite of left little finger without damage to nail NRS

5 ✓7ᵗʰ **S61.258** Open bite of other finger without damage to nail NRS
     Open bite of specified finger with unspecified laterality without damage to nail

✓7ᵗʰ **S61.259** Open bite of unspecified finger without damage to nail ▽

✓5ᵗʰ **S61.3** Open wound of other finger with damage to nail

✓6ᵗʰ **S61.30** Unspecified open wound of finger with damage to nail

5 ✓7ᵗʰ **S61.300** Unspecified open wound of right index finger with damage to nail NRS ▽

5 ✓7ᵗʰ **S61.301** Unspecified open wound of left index finger with damage to nail NRS ▽

5 ✓7ᵗʰ **S61.302** Unspecified open wound of right middle finger with damage to nail NRS ▽

5 ✓7ᵗʰ **S61.303** Unspecified open wound of left middle finger with damage to nail NRS ▽

5 ✓7ᵗʰ **S61.304** Unspecified open wound of right ring finger with damage to nail NRS ▽

5 ✓7ᵗʰ **S61.305** Unspecified open wound of left ring finger with damage to nail NRS ▽

5 ✓7ᵗʰ **S61.306** Unspecified open wound of right little finger with damage to nail NRS ▽

5 ✓7ᵗʰ **S61.307** Unspecified open wound of left little finger with damage to nail NRS ▽

5 ✓7ᵗʰ **S61.308** Unspecified open wound of other finger with damage to nail NRS ▽
     Unspecified open wound of specified finger with unspecified laterality with damage to nail

✓7ᵗʰ **S61.309** Unspecified open wound of unspecified finger with damage to nail ▽

✓6ᵗʰ **S61.31** Laceration without foreign body of finger with damage to nail

4,5 ✓7ᵗʰ **S61.310** Laceration without foreign body of right index finger with damage to nail NRS

4,5 ✓7ᵗʰ **S61.311** Laceration without foreign body of left index finger with damage to nail NRS

4,5 ✓7ᵗʰ **S61.312** Laceration without foreign body of right middle finger with damage to nail NRS

4,5 ✓7ᵗʰ **S61.313** Laceration without foreign body of left middle finger with damage to nail NRS

4,5 ✓7ᵗʰ **S61.314** Laceration without foreign body of right ring finger with damage to nail NRS

4,5 ✓7ᵗʰ **S61.315** Laceration without foreign body of left ring finger with damage to nail NRS

4,5 ✓7ᵗʰ **S61.316** Laceration without foreign body of right little finger with damage to nail NRS

4,5 ✓7ᵗʰ **S61.317** Laceration without foreign body of left little finger with damage to nail NRS

5 ✓7ᵗʰ **S61.318** Laceration without foreign body of other finger with damage to nail NRS
     Laceration without foreign body of specified finger with unspecified laterality with damage to nail

✓7ᵗʰ **S61.319** Laceration without foreign body of unspecified finger with damage to nail ▽

✓6ᵗʰ **S61.32** Laceration with foreign body of finger with damage to nail

4,5 ✓7ᵗʰ **S61.320** Laceration with foreign body of right index finger with damage to nail NRS

4,5 ✓7ᵗʰ **S61.321** Laceration with foreign body of left index finger with damage to nail NRS

4,5 ✓7ᵗʰ **S61.322** Laceration with foreign body of right middle finger with damage to nail NRS

4,5 ✓7ᵗʰ **S61.323** Laceration with foreign body of left middle finger with damage to nail NRS

4,5 ✓7ᵗʰ **S61.324** Laceration with foreign body of right ring finger with damage to nail NRS

4,5 ✓7ᵗʰ **S61.325** Laceration with foreign body of left ring finger with damage to nail NRS

4,5 ✓7ᵗʰ **S61.326** Laceration with foreign body of right little finger with damage to nail NRS

4,5 ✓7ᵗʰ **S61.327** Laceration with foreign body of left little finger with damage to nail NRS

5 ✓7ᵗʰ **S61.328** Laceration with foreign body of other finger with damage to nail NRS
     Laceration with foreign body of specified finger with unspecified laterality with damage to nail

✓7ᵗʰ **S61.329** Laceration with foreign body of unspecified finger with damage to nail ▽

✓6ᵗʰ **S61.33** Puncture wound without foreign body of finger with damage to nail

4,5 ✓7ᵗʰ **S61.330** Puncture wound without foreign body of right index finger with damage to nail NRS

4,5 ✓7ᵗʰ **S61.331** Puncture wound without foreign body of left index finger with damage to nail NRS

4,5 ✓7ᵗʰ **S61.332** Puncture wound without foreign body of right middle finger with damage to nail NRS

4,5 ✓7ᵗʰ **S61.333** Puncture wound without foreign body of left middle finger with damage to nail NRS

4,5 ✓7ᵗʰ **S61.334** Puncture wound without foreign body of right ring finger with damage to nail NRS

4   Case-mix diagnosis with 7th character indicating initial or subsequent encounter.
5   NRS supply diagnosis with 7th character indicating initial or subsequent encounter.

Ⓝ Newborn: 0   Ⓟ Pediatric: 0-17   Ⓜ Maternity: 12-55   Ⓐ Adult: 15-124   NRS Nonroutine supply Dx   NC Dx Noncancer Dx   PDx Primary Dx   ▶◀ Revised Text   ● New Code   ▲ Revised Title

982   ICD-10-CM 2018

4,5 ✓7th **S61.335 Puncture wound without foreign body of left ring finger with damage to nail** NRS

4,5 ✓7th **S61.336 Puncture wound without foreign body of right little finger with damage to nail** NRS

4,5 ✓7th **S61.337 Puncture wound without foreign body of left little finger with damage to nail** NRS

5 ✓7th **S61.338 Puncture wound without foreign body of other finger with damage to nail** NRS
     Puncture wound without foreign body of specified finger with unspecified laterality with damage to nail

✓7th **S61.339 Puncture wound without foreign body of unspecified finger with damage to nail** ▽

✓6th **S61.34 Puncture wound with foreign body of finger with damage to nail**

4,5 ✓7th **S61.340 Puncture wound with foreign body of right index finger with damage to nail** NRS

4,5 ✓7th **S61.341 Puncture wound with foreign body of left index finger with damage to nail** NRS

4,5 ✓7th **S61.342 Puncture wound with foreign body of right middle finger with damage to nail** NRS

4,5 ✓7th **S61.343 Puncture wound with foreign body of left middle finger with damage to nail** NRS

4,5 ✓7th **S61.344 Puncture wound with foreign body of right ring finger with damage to nail** NRS

4,5 ✓7th **S61.345 Puncture wound with foreign body of left ring finger with damage to nail** NRS

4,5 ✓7th **S61.346 Puncture wound with foreign body of right little finger with damage to nail** NRS

4,5 ✓7th **S61.347 Puncture wound with foreign body of left little finger with damage to nail** NRS

5 ✓7th **S61.348 Puncture wound with foreign body of other finger with damage to nail** NRS
     Puncture wound with foreign body of specified finger with unspecified laterality with damage to nail

✓7th **S61.349 Puncture wound with foreign body of unspecified finger with damage to nail** ▽

✓6th **S61.35 Open bite of finger with damage to nail**
     Bite of finger with damage to nail NOS
     EXCLUDES 1 superficial bite of finger (S60.46-, S60.47-)

4,5 ✓7th **S61.350 Open bite of right index finger with damage to nail** NRS

4,5 ✓7th **S61.351 Open bite of left index finger with damage to nail** NRS

4,5 ✓7th **S61.352 Open bite of right middle finger with damage to nail** NRS

4,5 ✓7th **S61.353 Open bite of left middle finger with damage to nail** NRS

4,5 ✓7th **S61.354 Open bite of right ring finger with damage to nail** NRS

4,5 ✓7th **S61.355 Open bite of left ring finger with damage to nail** NRS

4,5 ✓7th **S61.356 Open bite of right little finger with damage to nail** NRS

4,5 ✓7th **S61.357 Open bite of left little finger with damage to nail** NRS

5 ✓7th **S61.358 Open bite of other finger with damage to nail** NRS
     Open bite of specified finger with unspecified laterality with damage to nail

✓7th **S61.359 Open bite of unspecified finger with damage to nail** ▽

✓5th **S61.4 Open wound of hand**

✓6th **S61.40 Unspecified open wound of hand**

5 ✓7th **S61.401 Unspecified open wound of right hand** NRS ▽

5 ✓7th **S61.402 Unspecified open wound of left hand** NRS ▽

✓7th **S61.409 Unspecified open wound of unspecified hand** ▽

✓6th **S61.41 Laceration without foreign body of hand**

4,5 ✓7th **S61.411 Laceration without foreign body of right hand** NRS

4,5 ✓7th **S61.412 Laceration without foreign body of left hand** NRS

✓7th **S61.419 Laceration without foreign body of unspecified hand** ▽

✓6th **S61.42 Laceration with foreign body of hand**

4,5 ✓7th **S61.421 Laceration with foreign body of right hand** NRS

4,5 ✓7th **S61.422 Laceration with foreign body of left hand** NRS

✓7th **S61.429 Laceration with foreign body of unspecified hand** ▽

✓6th **S61.43 Puncture wound without foreign body of hand**

4,5 ✓7th **S61.431 Puncture wound without foreign body of right hand** NRS

4,5 ✓7th **S61.432 Puncture wound without foreign body of left hand** NRS

✓7th **S61.439 Puncture wound without foreign body of unspecified hand** ▽

✓6th **S61.44 Puncture wound with foreign body of hand**

4,5 ✓7th **S61.441 Puncture wound with foreign body of right hand** NRS

4,5 ✓7th **S61.442 Puncture wound with foreign body of left hand** NRS

✓7th **S61.449 Puncture wound with foreign body of unspecified hand** ▽

✓6th **S61.45 Open bite of hand**
     Bite of hand NOS
     EXCLUDES 1 superficial bite of hand (S60.56-, S60.57-)

4,5 ✓7th **S61.451 Open bite of right hand** NRS

4,5 ✓7th **S61.452 Open bite of left hand** NRS

✓7th **S61.459 Open bite of unspecified hand** ▽

✓5th **S61.5 Open wound of wrist**

✓6th **S61.50 Unspecified open wound of wrist**

5 ✓7th **S61.501 Unspecified open wound of right wrist** NRS ▽

5 ✓7th **S61.502 Unspecified open wound of left wrist** NRS ▽

✓7th **S61.509 Unspecified open wound of unspecified wrist** ▽

✓6th **S61.51 Laceration without foreign body of wrist**

4,5 ✓7th **S61.511 Laceration without foreign body of right wrist** NRS

4,5 ✓7th **S61.512 Laceration without foreign body of left wrist** NRS

✓7th **S61.519 Laceration without foreign body of unspecified wrist** ▽

✓6th **S61.52 Laceration with foreign body of wrist**

4,5 ✓7th **S61.521 Laceration with foreign body of right wrist** NRS

4,5 ✓7th **S61.522 Laceration with foreign body of left wrist** NRS

✓7th **S61.529 Laceration with foreign body of unspecified wrist** ▽

✓6th **S61.53 Puncture wound without foreign body of wrist**

4,5 ✓7th **S61.531 Puncture wound without foreign body of right wrist** NRS

4,5 ✓7th **S61.532 Puncture wound without foreign body of left wrist** NRS

✓7th **S61.539 Puncture wound without foreign body of unspecified wrist** ▽

Case-mix diagnosis with 7th character indicating initial or subsequent encounter.
NRS supply diagnosis with 7th character indicating initial or subsequent encounter.

Additional Character Req   ✓x7th Placeholder Alert   Case-Mix Diagnosis   Manifestation   ▽ Unspecified Dx   *EXCLUDES 1* Not coded here   *EXCLUDES 2* Not included here

✓6ᵗʰ **S61.54** Puncture wound with foreign body of wrist

   4,5 ✓7ᵗʰ **S61.541** **Puncture wound with foreign body of right wrist** NRS

   4,5 ✓7ᵗʰ **S61.542** **Puncture wound with foreign body of left wrist** NRS

   ✓7ᵗʰ **S61.549** **Puncture wound with foreign body of unspecified wrist** ▽

✓6ᵗʰ **S61.55** Open bite of wrist
    Bite of wrist NOS
    EXCLUDES 1   superficial bite of wrist (S60.86-, S60.87-)

   4,5 ✓7ᵗʰ **S61.551** **Open bite of right wrist** NRS

   4,5 ✓7ᵗʰ **S61.552** **Open bite of left wrist** NRS

   ✓7ᵗʰ **S61.559** **Open bite of unspecified wrist** ▽

✓4ᵗʰ **S62** **Fracture at wrist and hand level**
    NOTE   A fracture not indicated as displaced or nondisplaced should be coded to displaced.
      A fracture not indicated as open or closed should be coded to closed.
    EXCLUDES 1   traumatic amputation of wrist and hand (S68.-)
    EXCLUDES 2   fracture of distal parts of ulna and radius (S52.-)
    AHA: 2015, 3Q, 37-39
    TIP: The term "improper alignment" is not synonymous with malunion or nonunion of a fracture when noted in provider documentation.

> The appropriate 7th character is to be added to each code from category S62.
> A   initial encounter for closed fracture
> B   initial encounter for open fracture
> D   subsequent encounter for fracture with routine healing
> G   subsequent encounter for fracture with delayed healing
> K   subsequent encounter for fracture with nonunion
> P   subsequent encounter for fracture with malunion
> S   sequela

✓5ᵗʰ **S62.0** **Fracture of** navicular **[scaphoid] bone of wrist**

  ✓6ᵗʰ **S62.00** Unspecified **fracture of navicular [scaphoid] bone of wrist**

   1 ✓7ᵗʰ **S62.001** **Unspecified fracture of navicular [scaphoid] bone of right wrist** ▽

   1 ✓7ᵗʰ **S62.002** **Unspecified fracture of navicular [scaphoid] bone of left wrist** ▽
      AHA: 2012, 4Q, 106

   ✓7ᵗʰ **S62.009** **Unspecified fracture of navicular [scaphoid] bone of unspecified wrist** ▽

  ✓6ᵗʰ **S62.01** Fracture of distal pole of navicular **[scaphoid] bone of wrist**
    Fracture of volar tuberosity of navicular [scaphoid] bone of wrist

   1 ✓7ᵗʰ **S62.011** **Displaced fracture of distal pole of navicular [scaphoid] bone of right wrist**

   1 ✓7ᵗʰ **S62.012** **Displaced fracture of distal pole of navicular [scaphoid] bone of left wrist**

   ✓7ᵗʰ **S62.013** **Displaced fracture of distal pole of navicular [scaphoid] bone of unspecified wrist** ▽

   1 ✓7ᵗʰ **S62.014** **Nondisplaced fracture of distal pole of navicular [scaphoid] bone of right wrist**

   1 ✓7ᵗʰ **S62.015** **Nondisplaced fracture of distal pole of navicular [scaphoid] bone of left wrist**

   ✓7ᵗʰ **S62.016** **Nondisplaced fracture of distal pole of navicular [scaphoid] bone of unspecified wrist** ▽

  ✓6ᵗʰ **S62.02** Fracture of middle third of navicular **[scaphoid] bone of wrist**

   1 ✓7ᵗʰ **S62.021** **Displaced fracture of middle third of navicular [scaphoid] bone of right wrist**

   1 ✓7ᵗʰ **S62.022** **Displaced fracture of middle third of navicular [scaphoid] bone of left wrist**

   ✓7ᵗʰ **S62.023** **Displaced fracture of middle third of navicular [scaphoid] bone of unspecified wrist** ▽

   1 ✓7ᵗʰ **S62.024** **Nondisplaced fracture of middle third of navicular [scaphoid] bone of right wrist**

   1 ✓7ᵗʰ **S62.025** **Nondisplaced fracture of middle third of navicular [scaphoid] bone of left wrist**

   ✓7ᵗʰ **S62.026** **Nondisplaced fracture of middle third of navicular [scaphoid] bone of unspecified wrist** ▽

  ✓6ᵗʰ **S62.03** **Fracture of** proximal third of navicular **[scaphoid] bone of wrist**

   1 ✓7ᵗʰ **S62.031** **Displaced fracture of proximal third of navicular [scaphoid] bone of right wrist**

   1 ✓7ᵗʰ **S62.032** **Displaced fracture of proximal third of navicular [scaphoid] bone of left wrist**

   ✓7ᵗʰ **S62.033** **Displaced fracture of proximal third of navicular [scaphoid] bone of unspecified wrist** ▽

   1 ✓7ᵗʰ **S62.034** **Nondisplaced fracture of proximal third of navicular [scaphoid] bone of right wrist**

   1 ✓7ᵗʰ **S62.035** **Nondisplaced fracture of proximal third of navicular [scaphoid] bone of left wrist**

   ✓7ᵗʰ **S62.036** **Nondisplaced fracture of proximal third of navicular [scaphoid] bone of unspecified wrist** ▽

✓5ᵗʰ **S62.1** **Fracture of other and unspecified** carpal **bone(s)**
    EXCLUDES 2   fracture of scaphoid of wrist (S62.0-)

  ✓6ᵗʰ **S62.10** **Fracture of** unspecified **carpal bone**
    Fracture of wrist NOS

   1 ✓7ᵗʰ **S62.101** **Fracture of unspecified carpal bone, right wrist** ▽

   1 ✓7ᵗʰ **S62.102** **Fracture of unspecified carpal bone, left wrist** ▽
      AHA: 2012, 4Q, 95

   ✓7ᵗʰ **S62.109** **Fracture of unspecified carpal bone, unspecified wrist** ▽

  ✓6ᵗʰ **S62.11** **Fracture of** triquetrum **[cuneiform] bone of wrist**

   1 ✓7ᵗʰ **S62.111** **Displaced fracture of triquetrum [cuneiform] bone, right wrist**

   1 ✓7ᵗʰ **S62.112** **Displaced fracture of triquetrum [cuneiform] bone, left wrist**

   ✓7ᵗʰ **S62.113** **Displaced fracture of triquetrum [cuneiform] bone, unspecified wrist** ▽

   1 ✓7ᵗʰ **S62.114** **Nondisplaced fracture of triquetrum [cuneiform] bone, right wrist**

   1 ✓7ᵗʰ **S62.115** **Nondisplaced fracture of triquetrum [cuneiform] bone, left wrist**

   ✓7ᵗʰ **S62.116** **Nondisplaced fracture of triquetrum [cuneiform] bone, unspecified wrist** ▽

  ✓6ᵗʰ **S62.12** **Fracture of** lunate **[semilunar]**

   1 ✓7ᵗʰ **S62.121** **Displaced fracture of lunate [semilunar], right wrist**

   1 ✓7ᵗʰ **S62.122** **Displaced fracture of lunate [semilunar], left wrist**

   ✓7ᵗʰ **S62.123** **Displaced fracture of lunate [semilunar], unspecified wrist** ▽

   1 ✓7ᵗʰ **S62.124** **Nondisplaced fracture of lunate [semilunar], right wrist**

   1 ✓7ᵗʰ **S62.125** **Nondisplaced fracture of lunate [semilunar], left wrist**

   ✓7ᵗʰ **S62.126** **Nondisplaced fracture of lunate [semilunar], unspecified wrist** ▽

  ✓6ᵗʰ **S62.13** **Fracture of** capitate **[os magnum] bone**

   1 ✓7ᵗʰ **S62.131** **Displaced fracture of capitate [os magnum] bone, right wrist**

   1 ✓7ᵗʰ **S62.132** **Displaced fracture of capitate [os magnum] bone, left wrist**

   ✓7ᵗʰ **S62.133** **Displaced fracture of capitate [os magnum] bone, unspecified wrist** ▽

   1 ✓7ᵗʰ **S62.134** **Nondisplaced fracture of capitate [os magnum] bone, right wrist**

   1 ✓7ᵗʰ **S62.135** **Nondisplaced fracture of capitate [os magnum] bone, left wrist**

   ✓7ᵗʰ **S62.136** **Nondisplaced fracture of capitate [os magnum] bone, unspecified wrist** ▽

  ✓6ᵗʰ **S62.14** **Fracture of** body of hamate **[unciform] bone**
    Fracture of hamate [unciform] bone NOS

   1 ✓7ᵗʰ **S62.141** **Displaced fracture of body of hamate [unciform] bone, right wrist**

---

1   Case-mix diagnosis with 7th character indicating subsequent encounter.
4   Case-mix diagnosis with 7th character indicating initial or subsequent encounter.
5   NRS supply diagnosis with 7th character indicating initial or subsequent encounter.

Ⓝ Newborn: 0   Ⓟ Pediatric: 0-17   Ⓜ Maternity: 12-55   Ⓐ Adult: 15-124   **NRS** Nonroutine supply Dx   **NC Dx** Noncancer Dx   **PD Dx** Primary Dx   ►◄ Revised Text   ● New Code   ▲ Revised Tit

[1] √7ᵗʰ **S62.142** Displaced fracture of body of hamate [unciform] bone, left wrist

√7ᵗʰ **S62.143** Displaced fracture of body of hamate [unciform] bone, unspecified wrist ▽

[1] √7ᵗʰ **S62.144** Nondisplaced fracture of body of hamate [unciform] bone, right wrist

[1] √7ᵗʰ **S62.145** Nondisplaced fracture of body of hamate [unciform] bone, left wrist

√7ᵗʰ **S62.146** Nondisplaced fracture of body of hamate [unciform] bone, unspecified wrist ▽

√6ᵗʰ **S62.15** Fracture of hook process of hamate [unciform] bone
Fracture of unciform process of hamate [unciform] bone

[1] √7ᵗʰ **S62.151** Displaced fracture of hook process of hamate [unciform] bone, right wrist

[1] √7ᵗʰ **S62.152** Displaced fracture of hook process of hamate [unciform] bone, left wrist

√7ᵗʰ **S62.153** Displaced fracture of hook process of hamate [unciform] bone, unspecified wrist ▽

[1] √7ᵗʰ **S62.154** Nondisplaced fracture of hook process of hamate [unciform] bone, right wrist

[1] √7ᵗʰ **S62.155** Nondisplaced fracture of hook process of hamate [unciform] bone, left wrist

√7ᵗʰ **S62.156** Nondisplaced fracture of hook process of hamate [unciform] bone, unspecified wrist ▽

√6ᵗʰ **S62.16** Fracture of pisiform

[1] √7ᵗʰ **S62.161** Displaced fracture of pisiform, right wrist

[1] √7ᵗʰ **S62.162** Displaced fracture of pisiform, left wrist

√7ᵗʰ **S62.163** Displaced fracture of pisiform, unspecified wrist ▽

[1] √7ᵗʰ **S62.164** Nondisplaced fracture of pisiform, right wrist

[1] √7ᵗʰ **S62.165** Nondisplaced fracture of pisiform, left wrist

√7ᵗʰ **S62.166** Nondisplaced fracture of pisiform, unspecified wrist ▽

√6ᵗʰ **S62.17** Fracture of trapezium [larger multangular]

[1] √7ᵗʰ **S62.171** Displaced fracture of trapezium [larger multangular], right wrist

[1] √7ᵗʰ **S62.172** Displaced fracture of trapezium [larger multangular], left wrist

√7ᵗʰ **S62.173** Displaced fracture of trapezium [larger multangular], unspecified wrist ▽

[1] √7ᵗʰ **S62.174** Nondisplaced fracture of trapezium [larger multangular], right wrist

[1] √7ᵗʰ **S62.175** Nondisplaced fracture of trapezium [larger multangular], left wrist

√7ᵗʰ **S62.176** Nondisplaced fracture of trapezium [larger multangular], unspecified wrist ▽

√6ᵗʰ **S62.18** Fracture of trapezoid [smaller multangular]

[1] √7ᵗʰ **S62.181** Displaced fracture of trapezoid [smaller multangular], right wrist

[1] √7ᵗʰ **S62.182** Displaced fracture of trapezoid [smaller multangular], left wrist

√7ᵗʰ **S62.183** Displaced fracture of trapezoid [smaller multangular], unspecified wrist ▽

[1] √7ᵗʰ **S62.184** Nondisplaced fracture of trapezoid [smaller multangular], right wrist

[1] √7ᵗʰ **S62.185** Nondisplaced fracture of trapezoid [smaller multangular], left wrist

√7ᵗʰ **S62.186** Nondisplaced fracture of trapezoid [smaller multangular], unspecified wrist ▽

√5ᵗʰ **S62.2** Fracture of first metacarpal bone

√6ᵗʰ **S62.20** Unspecified fracture of first metacarpal bone

[1] √7ᵗʰ **S62.201** Unspecified fracture of first metacarpal bone, right hand ▽

[1] √7ᵗʰ **S62.202** Unspecified fracture of first metacarpal bone, left hand ▽

√7ᵗʰ **S62.209** Unspecified fracture of first metacarpal bone, unspecified hand ▽

√6ᵗʰ **S62.21** Bennett's fracture

[1] √7ᵗʰ **S62.211** Bennett's fracture, right hand

[1] √7ᵗʰ **S62.212** Bennett's fracture, left hand

√7ᵗʰ **S62.213** Bennett's fracture, unspecified hand ▽

√6ᵗʰ **S62.22** Rolando's fracture

[1] √7ᵗʰ **S62.221** Displaced Rolando's fracture, right hand

[1] √7ᵗʰ **S62.222** Displaced Rolando's fracture, left hand

√7ᵗʰ **S62.223** Displaced Rolando's fracture, unspecified hand ▽

[1] √7ᵗʰ **S62.224** Nondisplaced Rolando's fracture, right hand

[1] √7ᵗʰ **S62.225** Nondisplaced Rolando's fracture, left hand

√7ᵗʰ **S62.226** Nondisplaced Rolando's fracture, unspecified hand ▽

√6ᵗʰ **S62.23** Other fracture of base of first metacarpal bone

[1] √7ᵗʰ **S62.231** Other displaced fracture of base of first metacarpal bone, right hand

[1] √7ᵗʰ **S62.232** Other displaced fracture of base of first metacarpal bone, left hand

√7ᵗʰ **S62.233** Other displaced fracture of base of first metacarpal bone, unspecified hand ▽

√7ᵗʰ **S62.234** Other nondisplaced fracture of base of first metacarpal bone, right hand

[1] √7ᵗʰ **S62.235** Other nondisplaced fracture of base of first metacarpal bone, left hand

√7ᵗʰ **S62.236** Other nondisplaced fracture of base of first metacarpal bone, unspecified hand ▽

√6ᵗʰ **S62.24** Fracture of shaft of first metacarpal bone

[1] √7ᵗʰ **S62.241** Displaced fracture of shaft of first metacarpal bone, right hand

[1] √7ᵗʰ **S62.242** Displaced fracture of shaft of first metacarpal bone, left hand

√7ᵗʰ **S62.243** Displaced fracture of shaft of first metacarpal bone, unspecified hand ▽

[1] √7ᵗʰ **S62.244** Nondisplaced fracture of shaft of first metacarpal bone, right hand

[1] √7ᵗʰ **S62.245** Nondisplaced fracture of shaft of first metacarpal bone, left hand

√7ᵗʰ **S62.246** Nondisplaced fracture of shaft of first metacarpal bone, unspecified hand ▽

√6ᵗʰ **S62.25** Fracture of neck of first metacarpal bone

[1] √7ᵗʰ **S62.251** Displaced fracture of neck of first metacarpal bone, right hand

[1] √7ᵗʰ **S62.252** Displaced fracture of neck of first metacarpal bone, left hand

√7ᵗʰ **S62.253** Displaced fracture of neck of first metacarpal bone, unspecified hand ▽

[1] √7ᵗʰ **S62.254** Nondisplaced fracture of neck of first metacarpal bone, right hand

[1] √7ᵗʰ **S62.255** Nondisplaced fracture of neck of first metacarpal bone, left hand

√7ᵗʰ **S62.256** Nondisplaced fracture of neck of first metacarpal bone, unspecified hand ▽

√6ᵗʰ **S62.29** Other fracture of first metacarpal bone

[1] √7ᵗʰ **S62.291** Other fracture of first metacarpal bone, right hand

[1] √7ᵗʰ **S62.292** Other fracture of first metacarpal bone, left hand

√7ᵗʰ **S62.299** Other fracture of first metacarpal bone, unspecified hand ▽

√5ᵗʰ **S62.3** Fracture of other and unspecified metacarpal bone
EXCLUDES 2   fracture of first metacarpal bone (S62.2-)

√6ᵗʰ **S62.30** Unspecified fracture of other metacarpal bone

[1] √7ᵗʰ **S62.300** Unspecified fracture of second metacarpal bone, right hand ▽

[1] √7ᵗʰ **S62.301** Unspecified fracture of second metacarpal bone, left hand ▽

[1] √7ᵗʰ **S62.302** Unspecified fracture of third metacarpal bone, right hand ▽

[1] √7ᵗʰ **S62.303** Unspecified fracture of third metacarpal bone, left hand ▽

[1] √7ᵗʰ **S62.304** Unspecified fracture of fourth metacarpal bone, right hand ▽

---

[1]   Case-mix diagnosis with 7th character indicating subsequent encounter.

☑ Additional Character Req   √x7ᵗʰ Placeholder Alert   Case-Mix Diagnosis   Manifestation   ▽ Unspecified Dx   *EXCLUDES 1* Not coded here   *EXCLUDES 2* Not included here

ICD-10-CM 2018   985

Chapter 19. Injury, Poisoning and Certain Other Consequences of External Causes

S62.305–S62.366

1 ✓7ᵗʰ **S62.305 Unspecified fracture of** fourth metacarpal bone, left hand ▽

1 ✓7ᵗʰ **S62.306 Unspecified fracture of** fifth metacarpal bone, right hand ▽

1 ✓7ᵗʰ **S62.307 Unspecified fracture of** fifth metacarpal bone, left hand ▽

✓7ᵗʰ **S62.308 Unspecified fracture of other metacarpal bone** ▽
     Unspecified fracture of specified metacarpal bone with unspecified laterality

✓7ᵗʰ **S62.309 Unspecified fracture of unspecified metacarpal bone** ▽

✓6ᵗʰ **S62.31** Displaced fracture of base of other metacarpal bone ▲

1 ✓7ᵗʰ **S62.310 Displaced fracture of base of** second metacarpal bone, right hand

1 ✓7ᵗʰ **S62.311 Displaced fracture of base of** second metacarpal bone, left hand

1 ✓7ᵗʰ **S62.312 Displaced fracture of base of** third metacarpal bone, right hand

1 ✓7ᵗʰ **S62.313 Displaced fracture of base of** third metacarpal bone, left hand

1 ✓7ᵗʰ **S62.314 Displaced fracture of base of** fourth metacarpal bone, right hand

1 ✓7ᵗʰ **S62.315 Displaced fracture of base of** fourth metacarpal bone, left hand

1 ✓7ᵗʰ **S62.316 Displaced fracture of base of** fifth metacarpal bone, right hand

1 ✓7ᵗʰ **S62.317 Displaced fracture of base of** fifth metacarpal bone, left hand

1 ✓7ᵗʰ **S62.318 Displaced fracture of base of other metacarpal bone**
     Displaced fracture of base of specified metacarpal bone with unspecified laterality

✓7ᵗʰ **S62.319 Displaced fracture of base of unspecified metacarpal bone** ▽

✓6ᵗʰ **S62.32** Displaced fracture of shaft of other metacarpal bone

1 ✓7ᵗʰ **S62.320 Displaced fracture of shaft of** second metacarpal bone, right hand

1 ✓7ᵗʰ **S62.321 Displaced fracture of shaft of** second metacarpal bone, left hand

1 ✓7ᵗʰ **S62.322 Displaced fracture of shaft of** third metacarpal bone, right hand

1 ✓7ᵗʰ **S62.323 Displaced fracture of shaft of** third metacarpal bone, left hand

1 ✓7ᵗʰ **S62.324 Displaced fracture of shaft of** fourth metacarpal bone, right hand

1 ✓7ᵗʰ **S62.325 Displaced fracture of shaft of** fourth metacarpal bone, left hand

1 ✓7ᵗʰ **S62.326 Displaced fracture of shaft of** fifth metacarpal bone, right hand

1 ✓7ᵗʰ **S62.327 Displaced fracture of shaft of** fifth metacarpal bone, left hand

1 ✓7ᵗʰ **S62.328 Displaced fracture of shaft of other metacarpal bone**
     Displaced fracture of shaft of specified metacarpal bone with unspecified laterality

1 ✓7ᵗʰ **S62.329 Displaced fracture of shaft of unspecified metacarpal bone** ▽

✓6ᵗʰ **S62.33** Displaced fracture of neck of other metacarpal bone

1 ✓7ᵗʰ **S62.330 Displaced fracture of neck of** second metacarpal bone, right hand

1 ✓7ᵗʰ **S62.331 Displaced fracture of neck of** second metacarpal bone, left hand

1 ✓7ᵗʰ **S62.332 Displaced fracture of neck of** third metacarpal bone, right hand

1 ✓7ᵗʰ **S62.333 Displaced fracture of neck of** third metacarpal bone, left hand

1 ✓7ᵗʰ **S62.334 Displaced fracture of neck of** fourth metacarpal bone, right hand

1 ✓7ᵗʰ **S62.335 Displaced fracture of neck of** fourth metacarpal bone, left hand

1 ✓7ᵗʰ **S62.336 Displaced fracture of neck of** fifth metacarpal bone, right hand

1 ✓7ᵗʰ **S62.337 Displaced fracture of neck of** fifth metacarpal bone, left hand

1 ✓7ᵗʰ **S62.338 Displaced fracture of neck of other metacarpal bone**
     Displaced fracture of neck of specified metacarpal bone with unspecified laterality

✓7ᵗʰ **S62.339 Displaced fracture of neck of unspecified metacarpal bone** ▽

✓6ᵗʰ **S62.34** Nondisplaced fracture of base of other metacarpal bone

1 ✓7ᵗʰ **S62.340 Nondisplaced fracture of base of** second metacarpal bone, right hand

1 ✓7ᵗʰ **S62.341 Nondisplaced fracture of base of** second metacarpal bone, left hand

1 ✓7ᵗʰ **S62.342 Nondisplaced fracture of base of** third metacarpal bone, right hand

1 ✓7ᵗʰ **S62.343 Nondisplaced fracture of base of** third metacarpal bone, left hand

1 ✓7ᵗʰ **S62.344 Nondisplaced fracture of base of** fourth metacarpal bone, right hand

1 ✓7ᵗʰ **S62.345 Nondisplaced fracture of base of** fourth metacarpal bone, left hand

1 ✓7ᵗʰ **S62.346 Nondisplaced fracture of base of** fifth metacarpal bone, right hand

1 ✓7ᵗʰ **S62.347 Nondisplaced fracture of base of** fifth metacarpal bone, left hand

1 ✓7ᵗʰ **S62.348 Nondisplaced fracture of base of other metacarpal bone**
     Nondisplaced fracture of base of specified metacarpal bone with unspecified laterality

✓7ᵗʰ **S62.349 Nondisplaced fracture of base of unspecified metacarpal bone** ▽

✓6ᵗʰ **S62.35** Nondisplaced fracture of shaft of other metacarpal bone

1 ✓7ᵗʰ **S62.350 Nondisplaced fracture of shaft of** second metacarpal bone, right hand

1 ✓7ᵗʰ **S62.351 Nondisplaced fracture of shaft of** second metacarpal bone, left hand

1 ✓7ᵗʰ **S62.352 Nondisplaced fracture of shaft of** third metacarpal bone, right hand

1 ✓7ᵗʰ **S62.353 Nondisplaced fracture of shaft of** third metacarpal bone, left hand

1 ✓7ᵗʰ **S62.354 Nondisplaced fracture of shaft of** fourth metacarpal bone, right hand

1 ✓7ᵗʰ **S62.355 Nondisplaced fracture of shaft of** fourth metacarpal bone, left hand

1 ✓7ᵗʰ **S62.356 Nondisplaced fracture of shaft of** fifth metacarpal bone, right hand

1 ✓7ᵗʰ **S62.357 Nondisplaced fracture of shaft of** fifth metacarpal bone, left hand

1 ✓7ᵗʰ **S62.358 Nondisplaced fracture of shaft of other metacarpal bone**
     Nondisplaced fracture of shaft of specified metacarpal bone with unspecified laterality

✓7ᵗʰ **S62.359 Nondisplaced fracture of shaft of unspecified metacarpal bone** ▽

✓6ᵗʰ **S62.36** Nondisplaced fracture of neck of other metacarpal bone

1 ✓7ᵗʰ **S62.360 Nondisplaced fracture of neck of** second metacarpal bone, right hand

1 ✓7ᵗʰ **S62.361 Nondisplaced fracture of neck of** second metacarpal bone, left hand

1 ✓7ᵗʰ **S62.362 Nondisplaced fracture of neck of** third metacarpal bone, right hand

1 ✓7ᵗʰ **S62.363 Nondisplaced fracture of neck of** third metacarpal bone, left hand

1 ✓7ᵗʰ **S62.364 Nondisplaced fracture of neck of** fourth metacarpal bone, right hand

1 ✓7ᵗʰ **S62.365 Nondisplaced fracture of neck of** fourth metacarpal bone, left hand

1 ✓7ᵗʰ **S62.366 Nondisplaced fracture of neck of** fifth metacarpal bone, right hand

---

1   Case-mix diagnosis with 7th character indicating subsequent encounter.

Ⓝ Newborn: 0   Ⓟ Pediatric: 0-17   Ⓜ Maternity: 12-55   Ⓐ Adult: 15-124   **NRS** Nonroutine supply Dx   **NC Dx** Noncancer Dx   **PDx** Primary Dx   ▶◀ Revised Text   ● New Code   ▲ Revised Title

986   ICD-10-CM 2018

1 ✓7ᵗʰ S62.367 **Nondisplaced fracture of neck of fifth metacarpal bone, left hand**

1 ✓7ᵗʰ S62.368 **Nondisplaced fracture of neck of other metacarpal bone**
    Nondisplaced fracture of neck of specified metacarpal bone with unspecified laterality

✓7ᵗʰ S62.369 **Nondisplaced fracture of neck of unspecified metacarpal bone** ▽

✓6ᵗʰ S62.39 **Other fracture of other metacarpal bone**

1 ✓7ᵗʰ S62.390 **Other fracture of second metacarpal bone, right hand**

1 ✓7ᵗʰ S62.391 **Other fracture of second metacarpal bone, left hand**

1 ✓7ᵗʰ S62.392 **Other fracture of third metacarpal bone, right hand**

1 ✓7ᵗʰ S62.393 **Other fracture of third metacarpal bone, left hand**

1 ✓7ᵗʰ S62.394 **Other fracture of fourth metacarpal bone, right hand**

1 ✓7ᵗʰ S62.395 **Other fracture of fourth metacarpal bone, left hand**

1 ✓7ᵗʰ S62.396 **Other fracture of fifth metacarpal bone, right hand**

1 ✓7ᵗʰ S62.397 **Other fracture of fifth metacarpal bone, left hand**

✓7ᵗʰ S62.398 **Other fracture of other metacarpal bone**
    Other fracture of specified metacarpal bone with unspecified laterality

✓7ᵗʰ S62.399 **Other fracture of unspecified metacarpal bone** ▽

✓5ᵗʰ S62.5 **Fracture of thumb**

✓6ᵗʰ S62.50 **Fracture of unspecified phalanx of thumb**

1 ✓7ᵗʰ S62.501 **Fracture of unspecified phalanx of right thumb** ▽

1 ✓7ᵗʰ S62.502 **Fracture of unspecified phalanx of left thumb** ▽

✓7ᵗʰ S62.509 **Fracture of unspecified phalanx of unspecified thumb** ▽

✓6ᵗʰ S62.51 **Fracture of proximal phalanx of thumb**

1 ✓7ᵗʰ S62.511 **Displaced fracture of proximal phalanx of right thumb** ▲

1 ✓7ᵗʰ S62.512 **Displaced fracture of proximal phalanx of left thumb** ▲

✓7ᵗʰ S62.513 **Displaced fracture of proximal phalanx of unspecified thumb** ▽ ▲

1 ✓7ᵗʰ S62.514 **Nondisplaced fracture of proximal phalanx of right thumb** ▲

1 ✓7ᵗʰ S62.515 **Nondisplaced fracture of proximal phalanx of left thumb** ▲

✓7ᵗʰ S62.516 **Nondisplaced fracture of proximal phalanx of unspecified thumb** ▽ ▲

✓6ᵗʰ S62.52 **Fracture of distal phalanx of thumb**

1 ✓7ᵗʰ S62.521 **Displaced fracture of distal phalanx of right thumb**

1 ✓7ᵗʰ S62.522 **Displaced fracture of distal phalanx of left thumb**

✓7ᵗʰ S62.523 **Displaced fracture of distal phalanx of unspecified thumb** ▽

1 ✓7ᵗʰ S62.524 **Nondisplaced fracture of distal phalanx of right thumb**

1 ✓7ᵗʰ S62.525 **Nondisplaced fracture of distal phalanx of left thumb**

✓7ᵗʰ S62.526 **Nondisplaced fracture of distal phalanx of unspecified thumb** ▽

✓5ᵗʰ S62.6 **Fracture of other and unspecified finger(s)**
    EXCLUDES 2   fracture of thumb (S62.5-)

✓6ᵗʰ S62.60 **Fracture of unspecified phalanx of finger**

1 ✓7ᵗʰ S62.600 **Fracture of unspecified phalanx of right index finger** ▽

1 ✓7ᵗʰ S62.601 **Fracture of unspecified phalanx of left index finger** ▽

1 ✓7ᵗʰ S62.602 **Fracture of unspecified phalanx of right middle finger** ▽

1 ✓7ᵗʰ S62.603 **Fracture of unspecified phalanx of left middle finger** ▽

1 ✓7ᵗʰ S62.604 **Fracture of unspecified phalanx of right ring finger** ▽

1 ✓7ᵗʰ S62.605 **Fracture of unspecified phalanx of left ring finger** ▽

1 ✓7ᵗʰ S62.606 **Fracture of unspecified phalanx of right little finger** ▽

1 ✓7ᵗʰ S62.607 **Fracture of unspecified phalanx of left little finger** ▽

1 ✓7ᵗʰ S62.608 **Fracture of unspecified phalanx of other finger** ▽
    Fracture of unspecified phalanx of specified finger with unspecified laterality

✓7ᵗʰ S62.609 **Fracture of unspecified phalanx of unspecified finger** ▽

✓6ᵗʰ S62.61 **Displaced fracture of proximal phalanx of finger**

1 ✓7ᵗʰ S62.610 **Displaced fracture of proximal phalanx of right index finger**

1 ✓7ᵗʰ S62.611 **Displaced fracture of proximal phalanx of left index finger**

1 ✓7ᵗʰ S62.612 **Displaced fracture of proximal phalanx of right middle finger**

1 ✓7ᵗʰ S62.613 **Displaced fracture of proximal phalanx of left middle finger**

1 ✓7ᵗʰ S62.614 **Displaced fracture of proximal phalanx of right ring finger**

1 ✓7ᵗʰ S62.615 **Displaced fracture of proximal phalanx of left ring finger**

1 ✓7ᵗʰ S62.616 **Displaced fracture of proximal phalanx of right little finger**

1 ✓7ᵗʰ S62.617 **Displaced fracture of proximal phalanx of left little finger**

1 ✓7ᵗʰ S62.618 **Displaced fracture of proximal phalanx of other finger**
    Displaced fracture of proximal phalanx of specified finger with unspecified laterality

✓7ᵗʰ S62.619 **Displaced fracture of proximal phalanx of unspecified finger** ▽

✓6ᵗʰ S62.62 **Displaced fracture of middle phalanx of finger**

1 ✓7ᵗʰ S62.620 **Displaced fracture of middle phalanx of right index finger**

1 ✓7ᵗʰ S62.621 **Displaced fracture of middle phalanx of left index finger**

1 ✓7ᵗʰ S62.622 **Displaced fracture of middle phalanx of right middle finger**

1 ✓7ᵗʰ S62.623 **Displaced fracture of middle phalanx of left middle finger**

1 ✓7ᵗʰ S62.624 **Displaced fracture of middle phalanx of right ring finger**

1 ✓7ᵗʰ S62.625 **Displaced fracture of middle phalanx of left ring finger**

1 ✓7ᵗʰ S62.626 **Displaced fracture of middle phalanx of right little finger**

1 ✓7ᵗʰ S62.627 **Displaced fracture of medial phalanx of left little finger**

1 ✓7ᵗʰ S62.628 **Displaced fracture of medial phalanx of other finger**
    Displaced fracture of medial phalanx of specified finger with unspecified laterality

✓7ᵗʰ S62.629 **Displaced fracture of medial phalanx of unspecified finger** ▽

✓6ᵗʰ S62.63 **Displaced fracture of distal phalanx of finger**

1 ✓7ᵗʰ S62.630 **Displaced fracture of distal phalanx of right index finger**

1 ✓7ᵗʰ S62.631 **Displaced fracture of distal phalanx of left index finger**

1 ✓7ᵗʰ S62.632 **Displaced fracture of distal phalanx of right middle finger**

1 ✓7ᵗʰ S62.633 **Displaced fracture of distal phalanx of left middle finger**

1 ✓7ᵗʰ S62.634 **Displaced fracture of distal phalanx of right ring finger**

---

1   Case-mix diagnosis with 7th character indicating subsequent encounter.

✅ Additional Character Req   ✓x7ᵗʰ Placeholder Alert   Case-Mix Diagnosis   Manifestation   ▽ Unspecified Dx   EXCLUDES 1 Not coded here   EXCLUDES 2 Not included here

1 ✓7ᵗʰ **S62.635** **Displaced fracture of distal phalanx of** left **ring** finger

1 ✓7ᵗʰ **S62.636** **Displaced fracture of distal phalanx of** right little **finger**

1 ✓7ᵗʰ **S62.637** **Displaced fracture of distal phalanx of** left little **finger**

1 ✓7ᵗʰ **S62.638** **Displaced fracture of distal phalanx of other finger**
   Displaced fracture of distal phalanx of specified finger with unspecified laterality

✓7ᵗʰ **S62.639** **Displaced fracture of distal phalanx of unspecified finger** ▽

✓6ᵗʰ **S62.64** Nondisplaced **fracture of** proximal phalanx **of finger**

1 ✓7ᵗʰ **S62.640** **Nondisplaced fracture of proximal phalanx of** right index **finger**

1 ✓7ᵗʰ **S62.641** **Nondisplaced fracture of proximal phalanx of** left index **finger**

1 ✓7ᵗʰ **S62.642** **Nondisplaced fracture of proximal phalanx of** right middle **finger**

1 ✓7ᵗʰ **S62.643** **Nondisplaced fracture of proximal phalanx of** left middle **finger**

1 ✓7ᵗʰ **S62.644** **Nondisplaced fracture of proximal phalanx of** right ring **finger**

1 ✓7ᵗʰ **S62.645** **Nondisplaced fracture of proximal phalanx of** left ring **finger**

1 ✓7ᵗʰ **S62.646** **Nondisplaced fracture of proximal phalanx of** right little **finger**

1 ✓7ᵗʰ **S62.647** **Nondisplaced fracture of proximal phalanx of** left little **finger**

1 ✓7ᵗʰ **S62.648** **Nondisplaced fracture of proximal phalanx of other finger**
   Nondisplaced fracture of proximal phalanx of specified finger with unspecified laterality

✓7ᵗʰ **S62.649** **Nondisplaced fracture of proximal phalanx of unspecified finger** ▽

▲ ✓6ᵗʰ **S62.65** Nondisplaced **fracture of** middle phalanx **of finger**

▲ 1 ✓7ᵗʰ **S62.650** **Nondisplaced fracture of middle phalanx of** right index **finger**

▲ 1 ✓7ᵗʰ **S62.651** **Nondisplaced fracture of middle phalanx of** left index **finger**

▲ 1 ✓7ᵗʰ **S62.652** **Nondisplaced fracture of middle phalanx of** right middle **finger**

▲ 1 ✓7ᵗʰ **S62.653** **Nondisplaced fracture of middle phalanx of** left middle **finger**

1 ✓7ᵗʰ **S62.654** **Nondisplaced fracture of medial phalanx of** right ring **finger**

1 ✓7ᵗʰ **S62.655** **Nondisplaced fracture of medial phalanx of** left ring **finger**

1 ✓7ᵗʰ **S62.656** **Nondisplaced fracture of medial phalanx of** right little **finger**

1 ✓7ᵗʰ **S62.657** **Nondisplaced fracture of medial phalanx of** left little **finger**

1 ✓7ᵗʰ **S62.658** **Nondisplaced fracture of medial phalanx of other finger**
   Nondisplaced fracture of medial phalanx of specified finger with unspecified laterality

✓7ᵗʰ **S62.659** **Nondisplaced fracture of medial phalanx of unspecified finger** ▽

✓6ᵗʰ **S62.66** Nondisplaced **fracture of** distal phalanx **of finger**

1 ✓7ᵗʰ **S62.660** **Nondisplaced fracture of distal phalanx of** right index **finger**

1 ✓7ᵗʰ **S62.661** **Nondisplaced fracture of distal phalanx of** left index **finger**

1 ✓7ᵗʰ **S62.662** **Nondisplaced fracture of distal phalanx of** right middle **finger**

1 ✓7ᵗʰ **S62.663** **Nondisplaced fracture of distal phalanx of** left middle **finger**

1 ✓7ᵗʰ **S62.664** **Nondisplaced fracture of distal phalanx of** right ring **finger**

1 ✓7ᵗʰ **S62.665** **Nondisplaced fracture of distal phalanx of** left ring **finger**

1 ✓7ᵗʰ **S62.666** **Nondisplaced fracture of distal phalanx of** right little **finger**

1 ✓7ᵗʰ **S62.667** **Nondisplaced fracture of distal phalanx of** left little **finger**

1 ✓7ᵗʰ **S62.668** **Nondisplaced fracture of distal phalanx of other finger**
   Nondisplaced fracture of distal phalanx of specified finger with unspecified laterality

✓7ᵗʰ **S62.669** **Nondisplaced fracture of distal phalanx of unspecified finger** ▽

✓5ᵗʰ **S62.9** **Unspecified fracture of wrist and hand**

✓x7ᵗʰ **S62.90** **Unspecified fracture of unspecified wrist and hand** ▽

1 ✓x7ᵗʰ **S62.91** **Unspecified fracture of** right **wrist and hand** ▽

1 ✓x7ᵗʰ **S62.92** **Unspecified fracture of** left **wrist and hand** ▽

✓4ᵗʰ **S63** **Dislocation and sprain of joints and ligaments at wrist and hand level**

INCLUDES   avulsion of joint or ligament at wrist and hand level
   laceration of cartilage, joint or ligament at wrist and hand level
   sprain of cartilage, joint or ligament at wrist and hand level
   traumatic hemarthrosis of joint or ligament at wrist and hand level
   traumatic rupture of joint or ligament at wrist and hand level
   traumatic subluxation of joint or ligament at wrist and hand level
   traumatic tear of joint or ligament at wrist and hand level

Code also any associated open wound

EXCLUDES 2   *strain of muscle, fascia and tendon of wrist and hand (S66.-)*

> The appropriate 7th character is to be added to each code from category S63.
> A   initial encounter
> D   subsequent encounter
> S   sequela

✓5ᵗʰ **S63.0** **Subluxation and dislocation of** wrist and hand joints

✓6ᵗʰ **S63.00** **Unspecified subluxation and dislocation of wrist and hand**
   Dislocation of carpal bone NOS
   Dislocation of distal end of radius NOS
   Subluxation of carpal bone NOS
   Subluxation of distal end of radius NOS

1 ✓7ᵗʰ **S63.001** **Unspecified** subluxation **of** right **wrist and hand** ▽

1 ✓7ᵗʰ **S63.002** **Unspecified** subluxation **of** left **wrist and hand** ▽

✓7ᵗʰ **S63.003** **Unspecified** subluxation **of unspecified wrist and hand** ▽

1 ✓7ᵗʰ **S63.004** **Unspecified** dislocation **of** right **wrist and hand** ▽

1 ✓7ᵗʰ **S63.005** **Unspecified** dislocation **of** left **wrist and hand** ▽

✓7ᵗʰ **S63.006** **Unspecified** dislocation **of unspecified wrist and hand** ▽

✓6ᵗʰ **S63.01** **Subluxation and dislocation of** distal radioulnar **joint**

1 ✓7ᵗʰ **S63.011** Subluxation **of distal radioulnar joint of** right **wrist**

1 ✓7ᵗʰ **S63.012** Subluxation **of distal radioulnar joint of** left **wrist**

✓7ᵗʰ **S63.013** Subluxation **of distal radioulnar joint of unspecified wrist** ▽

1 ✓7ᵗʰ **S63.014** Dislocation **of distal radioulnar joint of** right **wrist**

1 ✓7ᵗʰ **S63.015** Dislocation **of distal radioulnar joint of** left **wrist**

✓7ᵗʰ **S63.016** Dislocation **of distal radioulnar joint of unspecified wrist** ▽

✓6ᵗʰ **S63.02** **Subluxation and dislocation of** radiocarpal **joint**

1 ✓7ᵗʰ **S63.021** Subluxation **of radiocarpal joint of** right **wrist**

1 ✓7ᵗʰ **S63.022** Subluxation **of radiocarpal joint of** left **wrist**

✓7ᵗʰ **S63.023** Subluxation **of radiocarpal joint of unspecified wrist** ▽

1 ✓7ᵗʰ **S63.024** Dislocation **of radiocarpal joint of** right **wrist**

---

1   Case-mix diagnosis with 7th character indicating subsequent encounter.

N Newborn: 0   P Pediatric: 0-17   M Maternity: 12-55   A Adult: 15-124   NRS Nonroutine supply Dx   NCDx Noncancer Dx   PDx Primary Dx   ►◄ Revised Text   ● New Code   ▲ Revised Title

988   ICD-10-CM 2018

¹ ✓7ᵗʰ **S63.025** Dislocation of radiocarpal joint of left wrist

✓7ᵗʰ **S63.026** Dislocation of radiocarpal joint of unspecified wrist ▽

✓6ᵗʰ **S63.03** Subluxation and dislocation of midcarpal joint

¹ ✓7ᵗʰ **S63.031** Subluxation of midcarpal joint of right wrist

¹ ✓7ᵗʰ **S63.032** Subluxation of midcarpal joint of left wrist

✓7ᵗʰ **S63.033** Subluxation of midcarpal joint of unspecified wrist ▽

¹ ✓7ᵗʰ **S63.034** Dislocation of midcarpal joint of right wrist

¹ ✓7ᵗʰ **S63.035** Dislocation of midcarpal joint of left wrist

✓7ᵗʰ **S63.036** Dislocation of midcarpal joint of unspecified wrist ▽

✓6ᵗʰ **S63.04** Subluxation and dislocation of carpometacarpal joint of thumb
> EXCLUDES 2   interphalangeal subluxation and dislocation of thumb (S63.1-)

¹ ✓7ᵗʰ **S63.041** Subluxation of carpometacarpal joint of right thumb

¹ ✓7ᵗʰ **S63.042** Subluxation of carpometacarpal joint of left thumb

✓7ᵗʰ **S63.043** Subluxation of carpometacarpal joint of unspecified thumb ▽

¹ ✓7ᵗʰ **S63.044** Dislocation of carpometacarpal joint of right thumb

¹ ✓7ᵗʰ **S63.045** Dislocation of carpometacarpal joint of left thumb

✓7ᵗʰ **S63.046** Dislocation of carpometacarpal joint of unspecified thumb ▽

✓6ᵗʰ **S63.05** Subluxation and dislocation of other carpometacarpal joint ▲
> EXCLUDES 2   subluxation and dislocation of carpometacarpal joint of thumb (S63.04-) ▲ ▲

¹ ✓7ᵗʰ **S63.051** Subluxation of other carpometacarpal joint of right hand ▲

¹ ✓7ᵗʰ **S63.052** Subluxation of other carpometacarpal joint of left hand ▲

✓7ᵗʰ **S63.053** Subluxation of other carpometacarpal joint of unspecified hand ▽

¹ ✓7ᵗʰ **S63.054** Dislocation of other carpometacarpal joint of right hand ▲

¹ ✓7ᵗʰ **S63.055** Dislocation of other carpometacarpal joint of left hand ▲

✓7ᵗʰ **S63.056** Dislocation of other carpometacarpal joint of unspecified hand ▽

✓6ᵗʰ **S63.06** Subluxation and dislocation of metacarpal (bone), proximal end

¹ ✓7ᵗʰ **S63.061** Subluxation of metacarpal (bone), proximal end of right hand

¹ ✓7ᵗʰ **S63.062** Subluxation of metacarpal (bone), proximal end of left hand

✓7ᵗʰ **S63.063** Subluxation of metacarpal (bone), proximal end of unspecified hand ▽

¹ ✓7ᵗʰ **S63.064** Dislocation of metacarpal (bone), proximal end of right hand

¹ ✓7ᵗʰ **S63.065** Dislocation of metacarpal (bone), proximal end of left hand

✓7ᵗʰ **S63.066** Dislocation of metacarpal (bone), proximal end of unspecified hand ▽

✓6ᵗʰ **S63.07** Subluxation and dislocation of distal end of ulna

¹ ✓7ᵗʰ **S63.071** Subluxation of distal end of right ulna

¹ ✓7ᵗʰ **S63.072** Subluxation of distal end of left ulna

✓7ᵗʰ **S63.073** Subluxation of distal end of unspecified ulna ▽

¹ ✓7ᵗʰ **S63.074** Dislocation of distal end of right ulna

¹ ✓7ᵗʰ **S63.075** Dislocation of distal end of left ulna

✓7ᵗʰ **S63.076** Dislocation of distal end of unspecified ulna ▽

✓6ᵗʰ **S63.09** Other subluxation and dislocation of wrist and hand

¹ ✓7ᵗʰ **S63.091** Other subluxation of right wrist and hand

¹ ✓7ᵗʰ **S63.092** Other subluxation of left wrist and hand

✓7ᵗʰ **S63.093** Other subluxation of unspecified wrist and hand ▽

¹ ✓7ᵗʰ **S63.094** Other dislocation of right wrist and hand

¹ ✓7ᵗʰ **S63.095** Other dislocation of left wrist and hand

✓7ᵗʰ **S63.096** Other dislocation of unspecified wrist and hand ▽

✓5ᵗʰ **S63.1** Subluxation and dislocation of thumb

✓6ᵗʰ **S63.10** Unspecified subluxation and dislocation of thumb

✓7ᵗʰ **S63.101** Unspecified subluxation of right thumb ▽

✓7ᵗʰ **S63.102** Unspecified subluxation of left thumb ▽

✓7ᵗʰ **S63.103** Unspecified subluxation of unspecified thumb ▽

✓7ᵗʰ **S63.104** Unspecified dislocation of right thumb ▽

✓7ᵗʰ **S63.105** Unspecified dislocation of left thumb ▽

✓7ᵗʰ **S63.106** Unspecified dislocation of unspecified thumb ▽

✓6ᵗʰ **S63.11** Subluxation and dislocation of metacarpophalangeal joint of thumb

✓7ᵗʰ **S63.111** Subluxation of metacarpophalangeal joint of right thumb

✓7ᵗʰ **S63.112** Subluxation of metacarpophalangeal joint of left thumb

✓7ᵗʰ **S63.113** Subluxation of metacarpophalangeal joint of unspecified thumb ▽

✓7ᵗʰ **S63.114** Dislocation of metacarpophalangeal joint of right thumb

✓7ᵗʰ **S63.115** Dislocation of metacarpophalangeal joint of left thumb

✓7ᵗʰ **S63.116** Dislocation of metacarpophalangeal joint of unspecified thumb of thumb ▽

✓6ᵗʰ **S63.12** Subluxation and dislocation of interphalangeal joint of thumb

✓7ᵗʰ **S63.121** Subluxation of interphalangeal joint of right thumb

✓7ᵗʰ **S63.122** Subluxation of interphalangeal joint of left thumb

✓7ᵗʰ **S63.123** Subluxation of interphalangeal joint of unspecified thumb ▽

✓7ᵗʰ **S63.124** Dislocation of interphalangeal joint of right thumb

✓7ᵗʰ **S63.125** Dislocation of interphalangeal joint of left thumb

✓7ᵗʰ **S63.126** Dislocation of interphalangeal joint of unspecified thumb ▽

✓6ᵗʰ **S63.13** ~~Subluxation and dislocation of proximal interphalangeal joint of thumb~~

✓7ᵗʰ **S63.131** ~~Subluxation of proximal interphalangeal joint of right thumb~~

✓7ᵗʰ **S63.132** ~~Subluxation of proximal interphalangeal joint of left thumb~~

✓7ᵗʰ **S63.133** ~~Subluxation of proximal interphalangeal joint of unspecified thumb~~

✓7ᵗʰ **S63.134** ~~Dislocation of proximal interphalangeal joint of right thumb~~

✓7ᵗʰ **S63.135** ~~Dislocation of proximal interphalangeal joint of left thumb~~

✓7ᵗʰ **S63.136** ~~Dislocation of proximal interphalangeal joint of unspecified thumb~~

✓6ᵗʰ **S63.14** ~~Subluxation and dislocation of distal interphalangeal joint of thumb~~

✓7ᵗʰ **S63.141** ~~Subluxation of distal interphalangeal joint of right thumb~~

✓7ᵗʰ **S63.142** ~~Subluxation of distal interphalangeal joint of left thumb~~

✓7ᵗʰ **S63.143** ~~Subluxation of distal interphalangeal joint of unspecified thumb~~

✓7ᵗʰ **S63.144** ~~Dislocation of distal interphalangeal joint of right thumb~~

✓7ᵗʰ **S63.145** ~~Dislocation of distal interphalangeal joint of left thumb~~

✓7ᵗʰ **S63.146** ~~Dislocation of distal interphalangeal joint of unspecified thumb~~

---

¹ Case-mix diagnosis with 7th character indicating subsequent encounter.

✓ Additional Character Req   ✓x7ᵗʰ Placeholder Alert   Case-Mix Diagnosis   Manifestation   ▽ Unspecified Dx   EXCLUDES 1 Not coded here   EXCLUDES 2 Not included here

S63.2 Subluxation and dislocation of other finger(s)

> EXCLUDES 2   subluxation and dislocation of thumb (S63.1-)

√6ᵗʰ **S63.20 Unspecified subluxation of other finger**

√7ᵗʰ **S63.200** Unspecified subluxation of right index finger ▽

√7ᵗʰ **S63.201** Unspecified subluxation of left index finger ▽

√7ᵗʰ **S63.202** Unspecified subluxation of right middle finger ▽

√7ᵗʰ **S63.203** Unspecified subluxation of left middle finger ▽

√7ᵗʰ **S63.204** Unspecified subluxation of right ring finger ▽

√7ᵗʰ **S63.205** Unspecified subluxation of left ring finger ▽

√7ᵗʰ **S63.206** Unspecified subluxation of right little finger ▽

√7ᵗʰ **S63.207** Unspecified subluxation of left little finger ▽

√7ᵗʰ **S63.208** Unspecified subluxation of other finger ▽
> Unspecified subluxation of specified finger with unspecified laterality

√7ᵗʰ **S63.209** Unspecified subluxation of unspecified finger ▽

√6ᵗʰ **S63.21 Subluxation of metacarpophalangeal joint of finger**

√7ᵗʰ **S63.210** Subluxation of metacarpophalangeal joint of right index finger

√7ᵗʰ **S63.211** Subluxation of metacarpophalangeal joint of left index finger

√7ᵗʰ **S63.212** Subluxation of metacarpophalangeal joint of right middle finger

√7ᵗʰ **S63.213** Subluxation of metacarpophalangeal joint of left middle finger

√7ᵗʰ **S63.214** Subluxation of metacarpophalangeal joint of right ring finger

√7ᵗʰ **S63.215** Subluxation of metacarpophalangeal joint of left ring finger

√7ᵗʰ **S63.216** Subluxation of metacarpophalangeal joint of right little finger

√7ᵗʰ **S63.217** Subluxation of metacarpophalangeal joint of left little finger

√7ᵗʰ **S63.218** Subluxation of metacarpophalangeal joint of other finger
> Subluxation of metacarpophalangeal joint of specified finger with unspecified laterality

√7ᵗʰ **S63.219** Subluxation of metacarpophalangeal joint of unspecified finger ▽

√6ᵗʰ **S63.22 Subluxation of unspecified interphalangeal joint of finger**

√7ᵗʰ **S63.220** Subluxation of unspecified interphalangeal joint of right index finger ▽

√7ᵗʰ **S63.221** Subluxation of unspecified interphalangeal joint of left index finger ▽

√7ᵗʰ **S63.222** Subluxation of unspecified interphalangeal joint of right middle finger ▽

√7ᵗʰ **S63.223** Subluxation of unspecified interphalangeal joint of left middle finger ▽

√7ᵗʰ **S63.224** Subluxation of unspecified interphalangeal joint of right ring finger ▽

√7ᵗʰ **S63.225** Subluxation of unspecified interphalangeal joint of left ring finger ▽

√7ᵗʰ **S63.226** Subluxation of unspecified interphalangeal joint of right little finger ▽

√7ᵗʰ **S63.227** Subluxation of unspecified interphalangeal joint of left little finger ▽

√7ᵗʰ **S63.228** Subluxation of unspecified interphalangeal joint of other finger ▽
> Subluxation of unspecified interphalangeal joint of specified finger with unspecified laterality

√7ᵗʰ **S63.229** Subluxation of unspecified interphalangeal joint of unspecified finger ▽

√6ᵗʰ **S63.23 Subluxation of proximal interphalangeal joint of finger**

√7ᵗʰ **S63.230** Subluxation of proximal interphalangeal joint of right index finger

√7ᵗʰ **S63.231** Subluxation of proximal interphalangeal joint of left index finger

√7ᵗʰ **S63.232** Subluxation of proximal interphalangeal joint of right middle finger

√7ᵗʰ **S63.233** Subluxation of proximal interphalangeal joint of left middle finger

√7ᵗʰ **S63.234** Subluxation of proximal interphalangeal joint of right ring finger

√7ᵗʰ **S63.235** Subluxation of proximal interphalangeal joint of left ring finger

√7ᵗʰ **S63.236** Subluxation of proximal interphalangeal joint of right little finger

√7ᵗʰ **S63.237** Subluxation of proximal interphalangeal joint of left little finger

√7ᵗʰ **S63.238** Subluxation of proximal interphalangeal joint of other finger
> Subluxation of proximal interphalangeal joint of specified finger with unspecified laterality

√7ᵗʰ **S63.239** Subluxation of proximal interphalangeal joint of unspecified finger ▽

√6ᵗʰ **S63.24 Subluxation of distal interphalangeal joint of finger**

√7ᵗʰ **S63.240** Subluxation of distal interphalangeal joint of right index finger

√7ᵗʰ **S63.241** Subluxation of distal interphalangeal joint of left index finger

√7ᵗʰ **S63.242** Subluxation of distal interphalangeal joint of right middle finger

√7ᵗʰ **S63.243** Subluxation of distal interphalangeal joint of left middle finger

√7ᵗʰ **S63.244** Subluxation of distal interphalangeal joint of right ring finger

√7ᵗʰ **S63.245** Subluxation of distal interphalangeal joint of left ring finger

√7ᵗʰ **S63.246** Subluxation of distal interphalangeal joint of right little finger

√7ᵗʰ **S63.247** Subluxation of distal interphalangeal joint of left little finger

√7ᵗʰ **S63.248** Subluxation of distal interphalangeal joint of other finger
> Subluxation of distal interphalangeal joint of specified finger with unspecified laterality

√7ᵗʰ **S63.249** Subluxation of distal interphalangeal joint of unspecified finger ▽

√6ᵗʰ **S63.25 Unspecified dislocation of other finger**

√7ᵗʰ **S63.250** Unspecified dislocation of right index finger ▽

√7ᵗʰ **S63.251** Unspecified dislocation of left index finger ▽

√7ᵗʰ **S63.252** Unspecified dislocation of right middle finger ▽

√7ᵗʰ **S63.253** Unspecified dislocation of left middle finger ▽

√7ᵗʰ **S63.254** Unspecified dislocation of right ring finger ▽

√7ᵗʰ **S63.255** Unspecified dislocation of left ring finger ▽

√7ᵗʰ **S63.256** Unspecified dislocation of right little finger ▽

√7ᵗʰ **S63.257** Unspecified dislocation of left little finger ▽

√7ᵗʰ **S63.258** Unspecified dislocation of other finger ▽
> Unspecified dislocation of specified finger with unspecified laterality

√7ᵗʰ **S63.259** Unspecified dislocation of unspecified finger ▽
> ▶Unspecified dislocation of unspecified finger with unspecified laterality◀

√6ᵗʰ **S63.26 Dislocation of metacarpophalangeal joint of finger**

√7ᵗʰ **S63.260** Dislocation of metacarpophalangeal joint of right index finger

Ⓝ Newborn: 0   Ⓟ Pediatric: 0-17   Ⓜ Maternity: 12-55   Ⓐ Adult: 15-124   NRS Nonroutine supply Dx   NC Dx Noncancer Dx   PDx Primary Dx   ▶◀ Revised Text   ● New Code   ▲ Revised Title

990   ICD-10-CM 2018

√7ᵗʰ **S63.261** **Dislocation of metacarpophalangeal joint of** left index **finger**

√7ᵗʰ **S63.262** **Dislocation of metacarpophalangeal joint of** right middle **finger**

√7ᵗʰ **S63.263** **Dislocation of metacarpophalangeal joint of** left middle **finger**

√7ᵗʰ **S63.264** **Dislocation of metacarpophalangeal joint of** right ring **finger**

√7ᵗʰ **S63.265** **Dislocation of metacarpophalangeal joint of** left ring **finger**

√7ᵗʰ **S63.266** **Dislocation of metacarpophalangeal joint of** right little **finger**

√7ᵗʰ **S63.267** **Dislocation of metacarpophalangeal joint of** left little **finger**

√7ᵗʰ **S63.268** **Dislocation of metacarpophalangeal joint of other finger**
Dislocation of metacarpophalangeal joint of specified finger with unspecified laterality

√7ᵗʰ **S63.269** **Dislocation of metacarpophalangeal joint of unspecified finger** ▽

√6ᵗʰ **S63.27** **Dislocation of unspecified** interphalangeal joint **of finger**

√7ᵗʰ **S63.270** **Dislocation of unspecified inter-phalangeal joint of** right index **finger** ▽

√7ᵗʰ **S63.271** **Dislocation of unspecified inter-phalangeal joint of** left index **finger** ▽

√7ᵗʰ **S63.272** **Dislocation of unspecified inter-phalangeal joint of** right middle **finger** ▽

√7ᵗʰ **S63.273** **Dislocation of unspecified inter-phalangeal joint of** left middle **finger** ▽

√7ᵗʰ **S63.274** **Dislocation of unspecified inter-phalangeal joint of** right ring **finger** ▽

√7ᵗʰ **S63.275** **Dislocation of unspecified inter-phalangeal joint of** left ring **finger** ▽

√7ᵗʰ **S63.276** **Dislocation of unspecified inter-phalangeal joint of** right little **finger** ▽

√7ᵗʰ **S63.277** **Dislocation of unspecified inter-phalangeal joint of** left little **finger** ▽

√7ᵗʰ **S63.278** **Dislocation of unspecified inter-phalangeal joint of other finger** ▽
Dislocation of unspecified interphalangeal joint of specified finger with unspecified laterality

√7ᵗʰ **S63.279** **Dislocation of unspecified inter-phalangeal joint of unspecified finger** ▽
▶Dislocation of unspecified interphalangeal joint of unspecified finger without specified laterality◀

√6ᵗʰ **S63.28** **Dislocation of** proximal interphalangeal joint **of finger**

√7ᵗʰ **S63.280** **Dislocation of proximal interphalangeal joint of** right index **finger**

√7ᵗʰ **S63.281** **Dislocation of proximal interphalangeal joint of** left index **finger**

√7ᵗʰ **S63.282** **Dislocation of proximal interphalangeal joint of** right middle **finger**

√7ᵗʰ **S63.283** **Dislocation of proximal interphalangeal joint of** left middle **finger**

√7ᵗʰ **S63.284** **Dislocation of proximal interphalangeal joint of** right ring **finger**

√7ᵗʰ **S63.285** **Dislocation of proximal interphalangeal joint of** left ring **finger**

√7ᵗʰ **S63.286** **Dislocation of proximal interphalangeal joint of** right little **finger**

√7ᵗʰ **S63.287** **Dislocation of proximal interphalangeal joint of** left little **finger**

√7ᵗʰ **S63.288** **Dislocation of proximal interphalangeal joint of other finger**
Dislocation of proximal interphalangeal joint of specified finger with unspecified laterality

√7ᵗʰ **S63.289** **Dislocation of proximal inter-phalangeal joint of unspecified finger** ▽

√6ᵗʰ **S63.29** **Dislocation of** distal interphalangeal joint **of finger**

√7ᵗʰ **S63.290** **Dislocation of distal interphalangeal joint of** right index **finger**

√7ᵗʰ **S63.291** **Dislocation of distal interphalangeal joint of** left index **finger**

√7ᵗʰ **S63.292** **Dislocation of distal interphalangeal joint of** right middle **finger**

√7ᵗʰ **S63.293** **Dislocation of distal interphalangeal joint of** left middle **finger**

√7ᵗʰ **S63.294** **Dislocation of distal interphalangeal joint of** right ring **finger**

√7ᵗʰ **S63.295** **Dislocation of distal interphalangeal joint of** left ring **finger**

√7ᵗʰ **S63.296** **Dislocation of distal interphalangeal joint of** right little **finger**

√7ᵗʰ **S63.297** **Dislocation of distal interphalangeal joint of** left little **finger**

√7ᵗʰ **S63.298** **Dislocation of distal interphalangeal joint of other finger**
Dislocation of distal interphalangeal joint of specified finger with unspecified laterality

√7ᵗʰ **S63.299** **Dislocation of distal interphalangeal joint of unspecified finger** ▽

√5ᵗʰ **S63.3** **Traumatic rupture of** ligament of wrist

√6ᵗʰ **S63.30** **Traumatic rupture of** unspecified **ligament of wrist**

√7ᵗʰ **S63.301** **Traumatic rupture of unspecified ligament of** right **wrist** ▽

√7ᵗʰ **S63.302** **Traumatic rupture of unspecified ligament of** left **wrist** ▽

√7ᵗʰ **S63.309** **Traumatic rupture of unspecified ligament of unspecified wrist** ▽

√6ᵗʰ **S63.31** **Traumatic rupture of** collateral **ligament of wrist**

√7ᵗʰ **S63.311** **Traumatic rupture of collateral ligament of** right **wrist**

√7ᵗʰ **S63.312** **Traumatic rupture of collateral ligament of** left **wrist**

√7ᵗʰ **S63.319** **Traumatic rupture of collateral ligament of unspecified wrist** ▽

√6ᵗʰ **S63.32** **Traumatic rupture of** radiocarpal ligament

√7ᵗʰ **S63.321** **Traumatic rupture of** right **radiocarpal ligament**

√7ᵗʰ **S63.322** **Traumatic rupture of** left **radiocarpal ligament**

√7ᵗʰ **S63.329** **Traumatic rupture of unspecified radiocarpal ligament** ▽

√6ᵗʰ **S63.33** **Traumatic rupture of** ulnocarpal (palmar) ligament

√7ᵗʰ **S63.331** **Traumatic rupture of** right **ulnocarpal (palmar) ligament**

√7ᵗʰ **S63.332** **Traumatic rupture of** left **ulnocarpal (palmar) ligament**

√7ᵗʰ **S63.339** **Traumatic rupture of unspecified ulnocarpal (palmar) ligament** ▽

√6ᵗʰ **S63.39** **Traumatic rupture of** other ligament **of wrist**

√7ᵗʰ **S63.391** **Traumatic rupture of other ligament of** right **wrist**

√7ᵗʰ **S63.392** **Traumatic rupture of other ligament of** left **wrist**

√7ᵗʰ **S63.399** **Traumatic rupture of other ligament of** ▽ **unspecified wrist**

√5ᵗʰ **S63.4** **Traumatic rupture of ligament of finger at** metacarpophalangeal and interphalangeal joint(s)

√6ᵗʰ **S63.40** **Traumatic rupture of** unspecified ligament **of finger at metacarpophalangeal and interphalangeal joint**

√7ᵗʰ **S63.400** **Traumatic rupture of unspecified ligament of** right index **finger at metacarpophalangeal and interphalangeal joint** ▽

√7ᵗʰ **S63.401** **Traumatic rupture of unspecified ligament of** left index **finger at metacarpo-phalangeal and interphalangeal joint** ▽

☑ Additional Character Req   √x7ᵗʰ Placeholder Alert   Case-Mix Diagnosis   Manifestation   ▽ Unspecified Dx   **EXCLUDES 1** Not coded here   **EXCLUDES 2** Not included here

ICD-10-CM 2018   991

√7ᵗʰ **S63.402** Traumatic rupture of unspecified ligament of right middle finger at metacarpophalangeal and interphalangeal joint ▽

√7ᵗʰ **S63.403** Traumatic rupture of unspecified ligament of left middle finger at metacarpophalangeal and interphalangeal joint ▽

√7ᵗʰ **S63.404** Traumatic rupture of unspecified ligament of right ring finger at metacarpophalangeal and interphalangeal joint ▽

√7ᵗʰ **S63.405** Traumatic rupture of unspecified ligament of left ring finger at metacarpophalangeal and interphalangeal joint ▽

√7ᵗʰ **S63.406** Traumatic rupture of unspecified ligament of right little finger at metacarpophalangeal and interphalangeal joint ▽

√7ᵗʰ **S63.407** Traumatic rupture of unspecified ligament of left little finger at metacarpophalangeal and interphalangeal joint ▽

√7ᵗʰ **S63.408** Traumatic rupture of unspecified ligament of other finger at metacarpophalangeal and interphalangeal joint ▽
　　　Traumatic rupture of unspecified ligament of specified finger with unspecified laterality at metacarpophalangeal and interphalangeal joint

√7ᵗʰ **S63.409** Traumatic rupture of unspecified ligament of unspecified finger at metacarpophalangeal and interphalangeal joint ▽

√6ᵗʰ **S63.41** Traumatic rupture of collateral ligament of finger at metacarpophalangeal and interphalangeal joint

√7ᵗʰ **S63.410** Traumatic rupture of collateral ligament of right index finger at metacarpophalangeal and interphalangeal joint

√7ᵗʰ **S63.411** Traumatic rupture of collateral ligament of left index finger at metacarpophalangeal and interphalangeal joint

√7ᵗʰ **S63.412** Traumatic rupture of collateral ligament of right middle finger at metacarpophalangeal and interphalangeal joint

√7ᵗʰ **S63.413** Traumatic rupture of collateral ligament of left middle finger at metacarpophalangeal and interphalangeal joint

√7ᵗʰ **S63.414** Traumatic rupture of collateral ligament of right ring finger at metacarpophalangeal and interphalangeal joint

√7ᵗʰ **S63.415** Traumatic rupture of collateral ligament of left ring finger at metacarpophalangeal and interphalangeal joint

√7ᵗʰ **S63.416** Traumatic rupture of collateral ligament of right little finger at metacarpophalangeal and interphalangeal joint

√7ᵗʰ **S63.417** Traumatic rupture of collateral ligament of left little finger at metacarpophalangeal and interphalangeal joint

√7ᵗʰ **S63.418** Traumatic rupture of collateral ligament of other finger at metacarpophalangeal and interphalangeal joint
　　　Traumatic rupture of collateral ligament of specified finger with unspecified laterality at metacarpophalangeal and interphalangeal joint

√7ᵗʰ **S63.419** Traumatic rupture of collateral ligament of unspecified finger at metacarpophalangeal and interphalangeal joint ▽

√6ᵗʰ **S63.42** Traumatic rupture of palmar ligament of finger at metacarpophalangeal and interphalangeal joint

√7ᵗʰ **S63.420** Traumatic rupture of palmar ligament of right index finger at metacarpophalangeal and interphalangeal joint

√7ᵗʰ **S63.421** Traumatic rupture of palmar ligament of left index finger at metacarpophalangeal and interphalangeal joint

√7ᵗʰ **S63.422** Traumatic rupture of palmar ligament of right middle finger at metacarpophalangeal and interphalangeal joint

√7ᵗʰ **S63.423** Traumatic rupture of palmar ligament of left middle finger at metacarpophalangeal and interphalangeal joint

√7ᵗʰ **S63.424** Traumatic rupture of palmar ligament of right ring finger at metacarpophalangeal and interphalangeal joint

√7ᵗʰ **S63.425** Traumatic rupture of palmar ligament of left ring finger at metacarpophalangeal and interphalangeal joint

√7ᵗʰ **S63.426** Traumatic rupture of palmar ligament of right little finger at metacarpophalangeal and interphalangeal joint

√7ᵗʰ **S63.427** Traumatic rupture of palmar ligament of left little finger at metacarpophalangeal and interphalangeal joint

√7ᵗʰ **S63.428** Traumatic rupture of palmar ligament of other finger at metacarpophalangeal and interphalangeal joint
　　　Traumatic rupture of palmar ligament of specified finger with unspecified laterality at metacarpophalangeal and interphalangeal joint

√7ᵗʰ **S63.429** Traumatic rupture of palmar ligament of unspecified finger at metacarpophalangeal and interphalangeal joint ▽

√6ᵗʰ **S63.43** Traumatic rupture of volar plate of finger at metacarpophalangeal and interphalangeal joint

√7ᵗʰ **S63.430** Traumatic rupture of volar plate of right index finger at metacarpophalangeal and interphalangeal joint

√7ᵗʰ **S63.431** Traumatic rupture of volar plate of left index finger at metacarpophalangeal and interphalangeal joint

√7ᵗʰ **S63.432** Traumatic rupture of volar plate of right middle finger at metacarpophalangeal and interphalangeal joint

√7ᵗʰ **S63.433** Traumatic rupture of volar plate of left middle finger at metacarpophalangeal and interphalangeal joint

√7ᵗʰ **S63.434** Traumatic rupture of volar plate of right ring finger at metacarpophalangeal and interphalangeal joint

√7ᵗʰ **S63.435** Traumatic rupture of volar plate of left ring finger at metacarpophalangeal and interphalangeal joint

√7ᵗʰ **S63.436** Traumatic rupture of volar plate of right little finger at metacarpophalangeal and interphalangeal joint

√7ᵗʰ **S63.437** Traumatic rupture of volar plate of left little finger at metacarpophalangeal and interphalangeal joint

√7ᵗʰ **S63.438** Traumatic rupture of volar plate of other finger at metacarpophalangeal and interphalangeal joint
　　　Traumatic rupture of volar plate of specified finger with unspecified laterality at metacarpophalangeal and interphalangeal joint

√7ᵗʰ **S63.439** Traumatic rupture of volar plate of unspecified finger at metacarpophalangeal and interphalangeal joint ▽

√6ᵗʰ **S63.49** Traumatic rupture of other ligament of finger at metacarpophalangeal and interphalangeal joint

√7ᵗʰ **S63.490** Traumatic rupture of other ligament of right index finger at metacarpophalangeal and interphalangeal joint

√7ᵗʰ **S63.491** Traumatic rupture of other ligament of left index finger at metacarpophalangeal and interphalangeal joint

√7ᵗʰ **S63.492** Traumatic rupture of other ligament of right middle finger at metacarpophalangeal and interphalangeal joint

√7ᵗʰ **S63.493** Traumatic rupture of other ligament of left middle finger at metacarpophalangeal and interphalangeal joint

Ⓝ Newborn: 0   Ⓟ Pediatric: 0-17   Ⓜ Maternity: 12-55   Ⓐ Adult: 15-124   **NRS** Nonroutine supply Dx   **NCDx** Noncancer Dx   **PDx** Primary Dx   ▶◀ Revised Text   ● New Code   ▲ Revised Title

992   ICD-10-CM 2018

√7ᵗʰ **S63.494** Traumatic rupture of other ligament of right ring finger at metacarpophalangeal and interphalangeal joint

√7ᵗʰ **S63.495** Traumatic rupture of other ligament of left ring finger at metacarpophalangeal and interphalangeal joint

√7ᵗʰ **S63.496** Traumatic rupture of other ligament of right little finger at metacarpophalangeal and interphalangeal joint

√7ᵗʰ **S63.497** Traumatic rupture of other ligament of left little finger at metacarpophalangeal and interphalangeal joint

√7ᵗʰ **S63.498** Traumatic rupture of other ligament of other finger at metacarpophalangeal and interphalangeal joint
    Traumatic rupture of ligament of specified finger with unspecified laterality at metacarpophalangeal and interphalangeal joint

√7ᵗʰ **S63.499** Traumatic rupture of other ligament of unspecified finger at metacarpophalangeal and interphalangeal joint ▽

√5ᵗʰ **S63.5** Other and unspecified sprain of wrist

  √6ᵗʰ **S63.50** Unspecified sprain of wrist

    √7ᵗʰ **S63.501** Unspecified sprain of right wrist ▽

    √7ᵗʰ **S63.502** Unspecified sprain of left wrist ▽

    √7ᵗʰ **S63.509** Unspecified sprain of unspecified wrist ▽

  √6ᵗʰ **S63.51** Sprain of carpal (joint)

    √7ᵗʰ **S63.511** Sprain of carpal joint of right wrist

    √7ᵗʰ **S63.512** Sprain of carpal joint of left wrist

    √7ᵗʰ **S63.519** Sprain of carpal joint of unspecified wrist ▽

  √6ᵗʰ **S63.52** Sprain of radiocarpal joint
    EXCLUDES 1 traumatic rupture of radiocarpal ligament (S63.32-)

    √7ᵗʰ **S63.521** Sprain of radiocarpal joint of right wrist

    √7ᵗʰ **S63.522** Sprain of radiocarpal joint of left wrist

    √7ᵗʰ **S63.529** Sprain of radiocarpal joint of unspecified wrist ▽

  √6ᵗʰ **S63.59** Other specified sprain of wrist

    √7ᵗʰ **S63.591** Other specified sprain of right wrist

    √7ᵗʰ **S63.592** Other specified sprain of left wrist

    √7ᵗʰ **S63.599** Other specified sprain of unspecified wrist ▽

√5ᵗʰ **S63.6** Other and unspecified sprain of finger(s)
  EXCLUDES 1 traumatic rupture of ligament of finger at metacarpophalangeal and interphalangeal joint(s) (S63.4-)

  √6ᵗʰ **S63.60** Unspecified sprain of thumb

    √7ᵗʰ **S63.601** Unspecified sprain of right thumb ▽

    √7ᵗʰ **S63.602** Unspecified sprain of left thumb ▽

    √7ᵗʰ **S63.609** Unspecified sprain of unspecified thumb ▽

  √6ᵗʰ **S63.61** Unspecified sprain of other and unspecified finger(s)

    √7ᵗʰ **S63.610** Unspecified sprain of right index finger ▽

    √7ᵗʰ **S63.611** Unspecified sprain of left index finger ▽

    √7ᵗʰ **S63.612** Unspecified sprain of right middle finger ▽

    √7ᵗʰ **S63.613** Unspecified sprain of left middle finger ▽

    √7ᵗʰ **S63.614** Unspecified sprain of right ring finger ▽

    √7ᵗʰ **S63.615** Unspecified sprain of left ring finger ▽

    √7ᵗʰ **S63.616** Unspecified sprain of right little finger ▽

    √7ᵗʰ **S63.617** Unspecified sprain of left little finger ▽

    √7ᵗʰ **S63.618** Unspecified sprain of other finger ▽
      Unspecified sprain of specified finger with unspecified laterality

    √7ᵗʰ **S63.619** Unspecified sprain of unspecified finger ▽

  √6ᵗʰ **S63.62** Sprain of interphalangeal joint of thumb

    √7ᵗʰ **S63.621** Sprain of interphalangeal joint of right thumb

    √7ᵗʰ **S63.622** Sprain of interphalangeal joint of left thumb

√7ᵗʰ **S63.629** Sprain of interphalangeal joint of unspecified thumb ▽

√6ᵗʰ **S63.63** Sprain of interphalangeal joint of other and unspecified finger(s)

  √7ᵗʰ **S63.630** Sprain of interphalangeal joint of right index finger

  √7ᵗʰ **S63.631** Sprain of interphalangeal joint of left index finger

  √7ᵗʰ **S63.632** Sprain of interphalangeal joint of right middle finger

  √7ᵗʰ **S63.633** Sprain of interphalangeal joint of left middle finger

  √7ᵗʰ **S63.634** Sprain of interphalangeal joint of right ring finger

  √7ᵗʰ **S63.635** Sprain of interphalangeal joint of left ring finger

  √7ᵗʰ **S63.636** Sprain of interphalangeal joint of right little finger

  √7ᵗʰ **S63.637** Sprain of interphalangeal joint of left little finger

  √7ᵗʰ **S63.638** Sprain of interphalangeal joint of other finger

  √7ᵗʰ **S63.639** Sprain of interphalangeal joint of unspecified finger ▽

√6ᵗʰ **S63.64** Sprain of metacarpophalangeal joint of thumb

  √7ᵗʰ **S63.641** Sprain of metacarpophalangeal joint of right thumb

  √7ᵗʰ **S63.642** Sprain of metacarpophalangeal joint of left thumb

  √7ᵗʰ **S63.649** Sprain of metacarpophalangeal joint of unspecified thumb ▽

√6ᵗʰ **S63.65** Sprain of metacarpophalangeal joint of other and unspecified finger(s)

  √7ᵗʰ **S63.650** Sprain of metacarpophalangeal joint of right index finger

  √7ᵗʰ **S63.651** Sprain of metacarpophalangeal joint of left index finger

  √7ᵗʰ **S63.652** Sprain of metacarpophalangeal joint of right middle finger

  √7ᵗʰ **S63.653** Sprain of metacarpophalangeal joint of left middle finger

  √7ᵗʰ **S63.654** Sprain of metacarpophalangeal joint of right ring finger

  √7ᵗʰ **S63.655** Sprain of metacarpophalangeal joint of left ring finger

  √7ᵗʰ **S63.656** Sprain of metacarpophalangeal joint of right little finger

  √7ᵗʰ **S63.657** Sprain of metacarpophalangeal joint of left little finger

  √7ᵗʰ **S63.658** Sprain of metacarpophalangeal joint of other finger
    Sprain of metacarpophalangeal joint of specified finger with unspecified laterality

  √7ᵗʰ **S63.659** Sprain of metacarpophalangeal joint of unspecified finger ▽

√6ᵗʰ **S63.68** Other sprain of thumb

  √7ᵗʰ **S63.681** Other sprain of right thumb

  √7ᵗʰ **S63.682** Other sprain of left thumb

  √7ᵗʰ **S63.689** Other sprain of unspecified thumb ▽

√6ᵗʰ **S63.69** Other sprain of other and unspecified finger(s)

  √7ᵗʰ **S63.690** Other sprain of right index finger

  √7ᵗʰ **S63.691** Other sprain of left index finger

  √7ᵗʰ **S63.692** Other sprain of right middle finger

  √7ᵗʰ **S63.693** Other sprain of left middle finger

  √7ᵗʰ **S63.694** Other sprain of right ring finger

  √7ᵗʰ **S63.695** Other sprain of left ring finger

  √7ᵗʰ **S63.696** Other sprain of right little finger

  √7ᵗʰ **S63.697** Other sprain of left little finger

  √7ᵗʰ **S63.698** Other sprain of other finger
    Other sprain of specified finger with unspecified laterality

  √7ᵗʰ **S63.699** Other sprain of unspecified finger ▽

☑ Additional Character Req   √×7ᵗʰ Placeholder Alert   Case-Mix Diagnosis   Manifestation   ▽ Unspecified Dx   **EXCLUDES 1** Not coded here   **EXCLUDES 2** Not included here

ICD-10-CM 2018   993

Chapter 19. Injury, Poisoning and Certain Other Consequences of External Causes

S63.494-S63.699

✓5th **S63.8** Sprain of other part of wrist and hand
 ✓6th **S63.8X** Sprain of other part of wrist and hand
  ✓7th **S63.8X1** Sprain of other part of right wrist and hand
  ✓7th **S63.8X2** Sprain of other part of left wrist and hand
  ✓7th **S63.8X9** Sprain of other part of unspecified wrist and hand ▽

✓5th **S63.9** Sprain of unspecified part of wrist and hand
 ✓x7th **S63.90** Sprain of unspecified part of unspecified wrist and hand ▽
 ✓x7th **S63.91** Sprain of unspecified part of right wrist and hand ▽
 ✓x7th **S63.92** Sprain of unspecified part of left wrist and hand ▽

✓4th **S64** **Injury of nerves at wrist and hand level**
Code also any associated open wound (S61.-)

> The appropriate 7th character is to be added to each code from category S64.
> A initial encounter
> D subsequent encounter
> S sequela

✓5th **S64.0** Injury of ulnar nerve at wrist and hand level
 ✓x7th **S64.00** Injury of ulnar nerve at wrist and hand level of unspecified arm ▽
 2 ✓x7th **S64.01** Injury of ulnar nerve at wrist and hand level of right arm
 2 ✓x7th **S64.02** Injury of ulnar nerve at wrist and hand level of left arm

✓5th **S64.1** Injury of median nerve at wrist and hand level
 ✓x7th **S64.10** Injury of median nerve at wrist and hand level of unspecified arm ▽
 2 ✓x7th **S64.11** Injury of median nerve at wrist and hand level of right arm
 2 ✓x7th **S64.12** Injury of median nerve at wrist and hand level of left arm

✓5th **S64.2** Injury of radial nerve at wrist and hand level
 ✓x7th **S64.20** Injury of radial nerve at wrist and hand level of unspecified arm ▽
 2 ✓x7th **S64.21** Injury of radial nerve at wrist and hand level of right arm
 2 ✓x7th **S64.22** Injury of radial nerve at wrist and hand level of left arm

✓5th **S64.3** Injury of digital nerve of thumb
 ✓x7th **S64.30** Injury of digital nerve of unspecified thumb ▽
 2 ✓x7th **S64.31** Injury of digital nerve of right thumb
 2 ✓x7th **S64.32** Injury of digital nerve of left thumb

✓5th **S64.4** Injury of digital nerve of other and unspecified finger
 ✓x7th **S64.40** Injury of digital nerve of unspecified finger ▽
 ✓6th **S64.49** Injury of digital nerve of other finger
  2 ✓7th **S64.490** Injury of digital nerve of right index finger
  2 ✓7th **S64.491** Injury of digital nerve of left index finger
  2 ✓7th **S64.492** Injury of digital nerve of right middle finger
  2 ✓7th **S64.493** Injury of digital nerve of left middle finger
  2 ✓7th **S64.494** Injury of digital nerve of right ring finger
  2 ✓7th **S64.495** Injury of digital nerve of left ring finger
  2 ✓7th **S64.496** Injury of digital nerve of right little finger
  2 ✓7th **S64.497** Injury of digital nerve of left little finger
  2 ✓7th **S64.498** Injury of digital nerve of other finger
   Injury of digital nerve of specified finger with unspecified laterality

✓5th **S64.8** Injury of other nerves at wrist and hand level
 ✓6th **S64.8X** Injury of other nerves at wrist and hand level
  2 ✓7th **S64.8X1** Injury of other nerves at wrist and hand level of right arm
  2 ✓7th **S64.8X2** Injury of other nerves at wrist and hand level of left arm
  ✓7th **S64.8X9** Injury of other nerves at wrist and hand level of unspecified arm ▽

✓5th **S64.9** Injury of unspecified nerve at wrist and hand level
 ✓x7th **S64.90** Injury of unspecified nerve at wrist and hand level of unspecified arm ▽

2 ✓x7th **S64.91** Injury of unspecified nerve at wrist and hand level of right arm ▽
2 ✓x7th **S64.92** Injury of unspecified nerve at wrist and hand level of left arm ▽

✓4th **S65** **Injury of blood vessels at wrist and hand level**
Code also any associated open wound (S61.-)

> The appropriate 7th character is to be added to each code from category S65.
> A initial encounter
> D subsequent encounter
> S sequela

✓5th **S65.0** Injury of ulnar artery at wrist and hand level
 ✓6th **S65.00** Unspecified injury of ulnar artery at wrist and hand level
  ✓7th **S65.001** Unspecified injury of ulnar artery at wrist and hand level of right arm ▽
  ✓7th **S65.002** Unspecified injury of ulnar artery at wrist and hand level of left arm ▽
  ✓7th **S65.009** Unspecified injury of ulnar artery at wrist and hand level of unspecified arm ▽
 ✓6th **S65.01** Laceration of ulnar artery at wrist and hand level
  ✓7th **S65.011** Laceration of ulnar artery at wrist and hand level of right arm
  ✓7th **S65.012** Laceration of ulnar artery at wrist and hand level of left arm
  ✓7th **S65.019** Laceration of ulnar artery at wrist and hand level of unspecified arm ▽
 ✓6th **S65.09** Other specified injury of ulnar artery at wrist and hand level
  ✓7th **S65.091** Other specified injury of ulnar artery at wrist and hand level of right arm
  ✓7th **S65.092** Other specified injury of ulnar artery at wrist and hand level of left arm
  ✓7th **S65.099** Other specified injury of ulnar artery at wrist and hand level of unspecified arm ▽

✓5th **S65.1** Injury of radial artery at wrist and hand level
 ✓6th **S65.10** Unspecified injury of radial artery at wrist and hand level
  ✓7th **S65.101** Unspecified injury of radial artery at wrist and hand level of right arm ▽
  ✓7th **S65.102** Unspecified injury of radial artery at wrist and hand level of left arm ▽
  ✓7th **S65.109** Unspecified injury of radial artery at wrist and hand level of unspecified arm ▽
 ✓6th **S65.11** Laceration of radial artery at wrist and hand level
  ✓7th **S65.111** Laceration of radial artery at wrist and hand level of right arm
  ✓7th **S65.112** Laceration of radial artery at wrist and hand level of left arm
  ✓7th **S65.119** Laceration of radial artery at wrist and hand level of unspecified arm ▽
 ✓6th **S65.19** Other specified injury of radial artery at wrist and hand level
  ✓7th **S65.191** Other specified injury of radial artery at wrist and hand level of right arm
  ✓7th **S65.192** Other specified injury of radial artery at wrist and hand level of left arm
  ✓7th **S65.199** Other specified injury of radial artery at wrist and hand level of unspecified arm ▽

✓5th **S65.2** Injury of superficial palmar arch
 ✓6th **S65.20** Unspecified injury of superficial palmar arch
  ✓7th **S65.201** Unspecified injury of superficial palmar arch of right hand ▽
  ✓7th **S65.202** Unspecified injury of superficial palmar arch of left hand ▽
  ✓7th **S65.209** Unspecified injury of superficial palmar arch of unspecified hand ▽
 ✓6th **S65.21** Laceration of superficial palmar arch
  ✓7th **S65.211** Laceration of superficial palmar arch of right hand
  ✓7th **S65.212** Laceration of superficial palmar arch of left hand

---

2 Case-mix diagnosis with 7th character indicating subsequent encounter or sequela.

Ⓝ Newborn: 0 Ⓟ Pediatric: 0-17 Ⓜ Maternity: 12-55 Ⓐ Adult: 15-124 **NRS** Nonroutine supply Dx **NCDx** Noncancer Dx **PDx** Primary Dx ▶◀ Revised Text ● New Code ▲ Revised Title

994   ICD-10-CM 2018

✓7ᵗʰ **S65.219** Laceration of superficial palmar arch of unspecified hand ▽

✓6ᵗʰ **S65.29** Other specified injury of superficial palmar arch

✓7ᵗʰ **S65.291** Other specified injury of superficial palmar arch of right hand

✓7ᵗʰ **S65.292** Other specified injury of superficial palmar arch of left hand

✓7ᵗʰ **S65.299** Other specified injury of superficial palmar arch of unspecified hand

✓5ᵗʰ **S65.3** Injury of deep palmar arch

✓6ᵗʰ **S65.30** Unspecified injury of deep palmar arch

✓7ᵗʰ **S65.301** Unspecified injury of deep palmar arch of right hand ▽

✓7ᵗʰ **S65.302** Unspecified injury of deep palmar arch of left hand ▽

✓7ᵗʰ **S65.309** Unspecified injury of deep palmar arch of unspecified hand ▽

✓6ᵗʰ **S65.31** Laceration of deep palmar arch

✓7ᵗʰ **S65.311** Laceration of deep palmar arch of right hand

✓7ᵗʰ **S65.312** Laceration of deep palmar arch of left hand

✓7ᵗʰ **S65.319** Laceration of deep palmar arch of unspecified hand ▽

✓6ᵗʰ **S65.39** Other specified injury of deep palmar arch

✓7ᵗʰ **S65.391** Other specified injury of deep palmar arch of right hand

✓7ᵗʰ **S65.392** Other specified injury of deep palmar arch of left hand

✓7ᵗʰ **S65.399** Other specified injury of deep palmar arch of unspecified hand ▽

✓5ᵗʰ **S65.4** Injury of blood vessel of thumb

✓6ᵗʰ **S65.40** Unspecified injury of blood vessel of thumb

✓7ᵗʰ **S65.401** Unspecified injury of blood vessel of right thumb ▽

✓7ᵗʰ **S65.402** Unspecified injury of blood vessel of left thumb ▽

✓7ᵗʰ **S65.409** Unspecified injury of blood vessel of unspecified thumb ▽

✓6ᵗʰ **S65.41** Laceration of blood vessel of thumb

✓7ᵗʰ **S65.411** Laceration of blood vessel of right thumb

✓7ᵗʰ **S65.412** Laceration of blood vessel of left thumb

✓7ᵗʰ **S65.419** Laceration of blood vessel of unspecified thumb ▽

✓6ᵗʰ **S65.49** Other specified injury of blood vessel of thumb

✓7ᵗʰ **S65.491** Other specified injury of blood vessel of right thumb

✓7ᵗʰ **S65.492** Other specified injury of blood vessel of left thumb

✓7ᵗʰ **S65.499** Other specified injury of blood vessel of unspecified thumb ▽

✓5ᵗʰ **S65.5** Injury of blood vessel of other and unspecified finger

✓6ᵗʰ **S65.50** Unspecified injury of blood vessel of other and unspecified finger

✓7ᵗʰ **S65.500** Unspecified injury of blood vessel of right index finger ▽

✓7ᵗʰ **S65.501** Unspecified injury of blood vessel of left index finger ▽

✓7ᵗʰ **S65.502** Unspecified injury of blood vessel of right middle finger ▽

✓7ᵗʰ **S65.503** Unspecified injury of blood vessel of left middle finger ▽

✓7ᵗʰ **S65.504** Unspecified injury of blood vessel of right ring finger ▽

✓7ᵗʰ **S65.505** Unspecified injury of blood vessel of left ring finger ▽

✓7ᵗʰ **S65.506** Unspecified injury of blood vessel of right little finger ▽

✓7ᵗʰ **S65.507** Unspecified injury of blood vessel of left little finger ▽

✓7ᵗʰ **S65.508** Unspecified injury of blood vessel of other finger ▽
Unspecified injury of blood vessel of specified finger with unspecified laterality

✓7ᵗʰ **S65.509** Unspecified injury of blood vessel of unspecified finger ▽

✓6ᵗʰ **S65.51** Laceration of blood vessel of other and unspecified finger

✓7ᵗʰ **S65.510** Laceration of blood vessel of right index finger

✓7ᵗʰ **S65.511** Laceration of blood vessel of left index finger

✓7ᵗʰ **S65.512** Laceration of blood vessel of right middle finger

✓7ᵗʰ **S65.513** Laceration of blood vessel of left middle finger

✓7ᵗʰ **S65.514** Laceration of blood vessel of right ring finger

✓7ᵗʰ **S65.515** Laceration of blood vessel of left ring finger

✓7ᵗʰ **S65.516** Laceration of blood vessel of right little finger

✓7ᵗʰ **S65.517** Laceration of blood vessel of left little finger

✓7ᵗʰ **S65.518** Laceration of blood vessel of other finger
Laceration of blood vessel of specified finger with unspecified laterality

✓7ᵗʰ **S65.519** Laceration of blood vessel of unspecified finger ▽

✓6ᵗʰ **S65.59** Other specified injury of blood vessel of other and unspecified finger

✓7ᵗʰ **S65.590** Other specified injury of blood vessel of right index finger

✓7ᵗʰ **S65.591** Other specified injury of blood vessel of left index finger

✓7ᵗʰ **S65.592** Other specified injury of blood vessel of right middle finger

✓7ᵗʰ **S65.593** Other specified injury of blood vessel of left middle finger

✓7ᵗʰ **S65.594** Other specified injury of blood vessel of right ring finger

✓7ᵗʰ **S65.595** Other specified injury of blood vessel of left ring finger

✓7ᵗʰ **S65.596** Other specified injury of blood vessel of right little finger

✓7ᵗʰ **S65.597** Other specified injury of blood vessel of left little finger

✓7ᵗʰ **S65.598** Other specified injury of blood vessel of other finger
Other specified injury of blood vessel of specified finger with unspecified laterality

✓7ᵗʰ **S65.599** Other specified injury of blood vessel of unspecified finger ▽

✓5ᵗʰ **S65.8** Injury of other blood vessels at wrist and hand level

✓6ᵗʰ **S65.80** Unspecified injury of other blood vessels at wrist and hand level

✓7ᵗʰ **S65.801** Unspecified injury of other blood vessels at wrist and hand level of right arm ▽

✓7ᵗʰ **S65.802** Unspecified injury of other blood vessels at wrist and hand level of left arm ▽

✓7ᵗʰ **S65.809** Unspecified injury of other blood vessels at wrist and hand level of unspecified arm ▽

✓6ᵗʰ **S65.81** Laceration of other blood vessels at wrist and hand level

✓7ᵗʰ **S65.811** Laceration of other blood vessels at wrist and hand level of right arm

✓7ᵗʰ **S65.812** Laceration of other blood vessels at wrist and hand level of left arm

✓7ᵗʰ **S65.819** Laceration of other blood vessels at wrist and hand level of unspecified arm ▽

✓ Additional Character Req   ✓ₓ7ᵗʰ Placeholder Alert   Case-Mix Diagnosis   Manifestation   ▽ Unspecified Dx   **EXCLUDES 1** Not coded here   **EXCLUDES 2** Not included here

✓6ᵗʰ **S65.89** Other specified injury of other blood vessels at wrist and hand level

     ✓7ᵗʰ **S65.891** Other specified injury of other blood vessels at wrist and hand level of right arm

     ✓7ᵗʰ **S65.892** Other specified injury of other blood vessels at wrist and hand level of left arm

     ✓7ᵗʰ **S65.899** Other specified injury of other blood vessels at wrist and hand level of unspecified arm ▽

✓5ᵗʰ **S65.9** Injury of unspecified blood vessel at wrist and hand level

     ✓6ᵗʰ **S65.90** Unspecified injury of unspecified blood vessel at wrist and hand level

         ✓7ᵗʰ **S65.901** Unspecified injury of unspecified blood vessel at wrist and hand level of right arm ▽

         ✓7ᵗʰ **S65.902** Unspecified injury of unspecified blood vessel at wrist and hand level of left arm ▽

         ✓7ᵗʰ **S65.909** Unspecified injury of unspecified blood vessel at wrist and hand level of unspecified arm ▽

     ✓6ᵗʰ **S65.91** Laceration of unspecified blood vessel at wrist and hand level

         ✓7ᵗʰ **S65.911** Laceration of unspecified blood vessel at wrist and hand level of right arm ▽

         ✓7ᵗʰ **S65.912** Laceration of unspecified blood vessel at wrist and hand level of left arm ▽

         ✓7ᵗʰ **S65.919** Laceration of unspecified blood vessel at wrist and hand level of unspecified arm ▽

     ✓6ᵗʰ **S65.99** Other specified injury of unspecified blood vessel at wrist and hand level

         ✓7ᵗʰ **S65.991** Other specified injury of unspecified blood vessel at wrist and hand of right arm ▽

         ✓7ᵗʰ **S65.992** Other specified injury of unspecified blood vessel at wrist and hand of left arm ▽

         ✓7ᵗʰ **S65.999** Other specified injury of unspecified blood vessel at wrist and hand of unspecified arm ▽

✓4ᵗʰ **S66** **Injury of muscle, fascia and tendon at wrist and hand level**

     Code also any associated open wound (S61.-)

     EXCLUDES 2   *sprain of joints and ligaments of wrist and hand (S63.-)*

     TIP: Refer to the Muscle/Tendon table at the beginning of this chapter.

> The appropriate 7th character is to be added to each code from category S66.
> A   initial encounter
> D   subsequent encounter
> S   sequela

     ✓5ᵗʰ **S66.0** Injury of long flexor muscle, fascia and tendon of thumb at wrist and hand level

       ✓6ᵗʰ **S66.00** Unspecified injury of long flexor muscle, fascia and tendon of thumb at wrist and hand level

         ✓7ᵗʰ **S66.001** Unspecified injury of long flexor muscle, fascia and tendon of right thumb at wrist and hand level ▽

         ✓7ᵗʰ **S66.002** Unspecified injury of long flexor muscle, fascia and tendon of left thumb at wrist and hand level ▽

         ✓7ᵗʰ **S66.009** Unspecified injury of long flexor muscle, fascia and tendon of unspecified thumb at wrist and hand level ▽

       ✓6ᵗʰ **S66.01** Strain of long flexor muscle, fascia and tendon of thumb at wrist and hand level

         ✓7ᵗʰ **S66.011** Strain of long flexor muscle, fascia and tendon of right thumb at wrist and hand level

         ✓7ᵗʰ **S66.012** Strain of long flexor muscle, fascia and tendon of left thumb at wrist and hand level

         ✓7ᵗʰ **S66.019** Strain of long flexor muscle, fascia and tendon of unspecified thumb at wrist and hand level ▽

✓6ᵗʰ **S66.02** Laceration of long flexor muscle, fascia and tendon of thumb at wrist and hand level

     4,5 ✓7ᵗʰ **S66.021** Laceration of long flexor muscle, fascia and tendon of right thumb at wrist and hand level   NRS

     4,5 ✓7ᵗʰ **S66.022** Laceration of long flexor muscle, fascia and tendon of left thumb at wrist and hand level   NRS

     ✓7ᵗʰ **S66.029** Laceration of long flexor muscle, fascia and tendon of unspecified thumb at wrist and hand level ▽

✓6ᵗʰ **S66.09** Other specified injury of long flexor muscle, fascia and tendon of thumb at wrist and hand level

     ✓7ᵗʰ **S66.091** Other specified injury of long flexor muscle, fascia and tendon of right thumb at wrist and hand level

     ✓7ᵗʰ **S66.092** Other specified injury of long flexor muscle, fascia and tendon of left thumb at wrist and hand level

     ✓7ᵗʰ **S66.099** Other specified injury of long flexor muscle, fascia and tendon of unspecified thumb at wrist and hand level ▽

✓5ᵗʰ **S66.1** Injury of flexor muscle, fascia and tendon of other and unspecified finger at wrist and hand level

     EXCLUDES 2   *Injury of long flexor muscle, fascia and tendon of thumb at wrist and hand level (S66.0-)*

     ✓6ᵗʰ **S66.10** Unspecified injury of flexor muscle, fascia and tendon of other and unspecified finger at wrist and hand level

       ✓7ᵗʰ **S66.100** Unspecified injury of flexor muscle, fascia and tendon of right index finger at wrist and hand level ▽

       ✓7ᵗʰ **S66.101** Unspecified injury of flexor muscle, fascia and tendon of left index finger at wrist and hand level ▽

       ✓7ᵗʰ **S66.102** Unspecified injury of flexor muscle, fascia and tendon of right middle finger at wrist and hand level ▽

       ✓7ᵗʰ **S66.103** Unspecified injury of flexor muscle, fascia and tendon of left middle finger at wrist and hand level ▽

       ✓7ᵗʰ **S66.104** Unspecified injury of flexor muscle, fascia and tendon of right ring finger at wrist and hand level ▽

       ✓7ᵗʰ **S66.105** Unspecified injury of flexor muscle, fascia and tendon of left ring finger at wrist and hand level ▽

       ✓7ᵗʰ **S66.106** Unspecified injury of flexor muscle, fascia and tendon of right little finger at wrist and hand level ▽

       ✓7ᵗʰ **S66.107** Unspecified injury of flexor muscle, fascia and tendon of left little finger at wrist and hand level ▽

       ✓7ᵗʰ **S66.108** Unspecified injury of flexor muscle, fascia and tendon of other finger at wrist and hand level ▽

         Unspecified injury of flexor muscle, fascia and tendon of specified finger with unspecified laterality at wrist and hand level

       ✓7ᵗʰ **S66.109** Unspecified injury of flexor muscle, fascia and tendon of unspecified finger at wrist and hand level ▽

     ✓6ᵗʰ **S66.11** Strain of flexor muscle, fascia and tendon of other and unspecified finger at wrist and hand level

       ✓7ᵗʰ **S66.110** Strain of flexor muscle, fascia and tendon of right index finger at wrist and hand level

       ✓7ᵗʰ **S66.111** Strain of flexor muscle, fascia and tendon of left index finger at wrist and hand level

       ✓7ᵗʰ **S66.112** Strain of flexor muscle, fascia and tendon of right middle finger at wrist and hand level

       ✓7ᵗʰ **S66.113** Strain of flexor muscle, fascia and tendon of left middle finger at wrist and hand level

---

4   Case-mix diagnosis with 7th character indicating initial or subsequent encounter.
5   NRS supply diagnosis with 7th character indicating initial or subsequent encounter.

Ⓝ Newborn: 0   Ⓟ Pediatric: 0-17   Ⓜ Maternity: 12-55   Ⓐ Adult: 15-124   NRS Nonroutine supply Dx   NCDx Noncancer Dx   PDx Primary Dx   ▶◀ Revised Text   ● New Code   ▲ Revised Title

996   ICD-10-CM 2018

√7ᵗʰ **S66.114** Strain of flexor muscle, fascia and tendon of right ring finger at wrist and hand level

√7ᵗʰ **S66.115** Strain of flexor muscle, fascia and tendon of left ring finger at wrist and hand level

√7ᵗʰ **S66.116** Strain of flexor muscle, fascia and tendon of right little finger at wrist and hand level

√7ᵗʰ **S66.117** Strain of flexor muscle, fascia and tendon of left little finger at wrist and hand level

√7ᵗʰ **S66.118** Strain of flexor muscle, fascia and tendon of other finger at wrist and hand level

Strain of flexor muscle, fascia and tendon of specified finger with unspecified laterality at wrist and hand level

√7ᵗʰ **S66.119** Strain of flexor muscle, fascia and tendon of unspecified finger at wrist and hand level ▽

√6ᵗʰ **S66.12** Laceration of flexor muscle, fascia and tendon of other and unspecified finger at wrist and hand level

4,5 √7ᵗʰ **S66.120** Laceration of flexor muscle, fascia and tendon of right index finger at wrist and hand level   NRS

4,5 √7ᵗʰ **S66.121** Laceration of flexor muscle, fascia and tendon of left index finger at wrist and hand level   NRS

4,5 √7ᵗʰ **S66.122** Laceration of flexor muscle, fascia and tendon of right middle finger at wrist and hand level   NRS

4,5 √7ᵗʰ **S66.123** Laceration of flexor muscle, fascia and tendon of left middle finger at wrist and hand level   NRS

4,5 √7ᵗʰ **S66.124** Laceration of flexor muscle, fascia and tendon of right ring finger at wrist and hand level   NRS

4,5 √7ᵗʰ **S66.125** Laceration of flexor muscle, fascia and tendon of left ring finger at wrist and hand level   NRS

4,5 √7ᵗʰ **S66.126** Laceration of flexor muscle, fascia and tendon of right little finger at wrist and hand level   NRS

4,5 √7ᵗʰ **S66.127** Laceration of flexor muscle, fascia and tendon of left little finger at wrist and hand level   NRS

5 √7ᵗʰ **S66.128** Laceration of flexor muscle, fascia and tendon of other finger at wrist and hand level   NRS

Laceration of flexor muscle, fascia and tendon of specified finger with unspecified laterality at wrist and hand level

√7ᵗʰ **S66.129** Laceration of flexor muscle, fascia and tendon of unspecified finger at wrist and hand level ▽

√6ᵗʰ **S66.19** Other injury of flexor muscle, fascia and tendon of other and unspecified finger at wrist and hand level

√7ᵗʰ **S66.190** Other injury of flexor muscle, fascia and tendon of right index finger at wrist and hand level

√7ᵗʰ **S66.191** Other injury of flexor muscle, fascia and tendon of left index finger at wrist and hand level

√7ᵗʰ **S66.192** Other injury of flexor muscle, fascia and tendon of right middle finger at wrist and hand level

√7ᵗʰ **S66.193** Other injury of flexor muscle, fascia and tendon of left middle finger at wrist and hand level

√7ᵗʰ **S66.194** Other injury of flexor muscle, fascia and tendon of right ring finger at wrist and hand level

√7ᵗʰ **S66.195** Other injury of flexor muscle, fascia and tendon of left ring finger at wrist and hand level

√7ᵗʰ **S66.196** Other injury of flexor muscle, fascia and tendon of right little finger at wrist and hand level

√7ᵗʰ **S66.197** Other injury of flexor muscle, fascia and tendon of left little finger at wrist and hand level

√7ᵗʰ **S66.198** Other injury of flexor muscle, fascia and tendon of other finger at wrist and hand level

Other injury of flexor muscle, fascia and tendon of specified finger with unspecified laterality at wrist and hand level

√7ᵗʰ **S66.199** Other injury of flexor muscle, fascia and tendon of unspecified finger at wrist and hand level ▽

√5ᵗʰ **S66.2** Injury of extensor muscle, fascia and tendon of thumb at wrist and hand level

√6ᵗʰ **S66.20** Unspecified injury of extensor muscle, fascia and tendon of thumb at wrist and hand level

√7ᵗʰ **S66.201** Unspecified injury of extensor muscle, fascia and tendon of right thumb at wrist and hand level ▽

√7ᵗʰ **S66.202** Unspecified injury of extensor muscle, fascia and tendon of left thumb at wrist and hand level ▽

√7ᵗʰ **S66.209** Unspecified injury of extensor muscle, fascia and tendon of unspecified thumb at wrist and hand level ▽

√6ᵗʰ **S66.21** Strain of extensor muscle, fascia and tendon of thumb at wrist and hand level

√7ᵗʰ **S66.211** Strain of extensor muscle, fascia and tendon of right thumb at wrist and hand level

√7ᵗʰ **S66.212** Strain of extensor muscle, fascia and tendon of left thumb at wrist and hand level

√7ᵗʰ **S66.219** Strain of extensor muscle, fascia and tendon of unspecified thumb at wrist and hand level ▽

√6ᵗʰ **S66.22** Laceration of extensor muscle, fascia and tendon of thumb at wrist and hand level

4,5 √7ᵗʰ **S66.221** Laceration of extensor muscle, fascia and tendon of right thumb at wrist and hand level   NRS

4,5 √7ᵗʰ **S66.222** Laceration of extensor muscle, fascia and tendon of left thumb at wrist and hand level   NRS

√7ᵗʰ **S66.229** Laceration of extensor muscle, fascia and tendon of unspecified thumb at wrist and hand level ▽

√6ᵗʰ **S66.29** Other specified injury of extensor muscle, fascia and tendon of thumb at wrist and hand level

√7ᵗʰ **S66.291** Other specified injury of extensor muscle, fascia and tendon of right thumb at wrist and hand level

√7ᵗʰ **S66.292** Other specified injury of extensor muscle, fascia and tendon of left thumb at wrist and hand level

√7ᵗʰ **S66.299** Other specified injury of extensor muscle, fascia and tendon of unspecified thumb at wrist and hand level ▽

√5ᵗʰ **S66.3** Injury of extensor muscle, fascia and tendon of other and unspecified finger at wrist and hand level

> EXCLUDES 2   Injury of extensor muscle, fascia and tendon of thumb at wrist and hand level (S66.2-)

√6ᵗʰ **S66.30** Unspecified injury of extensor muscle, fascia and tendon of other and unspecified finger at wrist and hand level

√7ᵗʰ **S66.300** Unspecified injury of extensor muscle, fascia and tendon of right index finger at wrist and hand level ▽

√7ᵗʰ **S66.301** Unspecified injury of extensor muscle, fascia and tendon of left index finger at wrist and hand level ▽

√7ᵗʰ **S66.302** Unspecified injury of extensor muscle, fascia and tendon of right middle finger at wrist and hand level ▽

---

4   Case-mix diagnosis with 7th character indicating initial or subsequent encounter.
5   NRS supply diagnosis with 7th character indicating initial or subsequent encounter.

✓ Additional Character Req   √x7ᵗʰ Placeholder Alert   Case-Mix Diagnosis   Manifestation   ▽ Unspecified Dx   EXCLUDES 1 Not coded here   EXCLUDES 2 Not included here

√7ᵗʰ **S66.303** Unspecified injury of extensor muscle, fascia and tendon of left middle finger at wrist and hand level ▽

√7ᵗʰ **S66.304** Unspecified injury of extensor muscle, fascia and tendon of right ring finger at wrist and hand level ▽

√7ᵗʰ **S66.305** Unspecified injury of extensor muscle, fascia and tendon of left ring finger at wrist and hand level ▽

√7ᵗʰ **S66.306** Unspecified injury of extensor muscle, fascia and tendon of right little finger at wrist and hand level ▽

√7ᵗʰ **S66.307** Unspecified injury of extensor muscle, fascia and tendon of left little finger at wrist and hand level ▽

√7ᵗʰ **S66.308** Unspecified injury of extensor muscle, fascia and tendon of other finger at wrist and hand level ▽
　　Unspecified injury of extensor muscle, fascia and tendon of specified finger with unspecified laterality at wrist and hand level

√7ᵗʰ **S66.309** Unspecified injury of extensor muscle, fascia and tendon of unspecified finger at wrist and hand level ▽

√6ᵗʰ **S66.31** Strain of extensor muscle, fascia and tendon of other and unspecified finger at wrist and hand level

√7ᵗʰ **S66.310** Strain of extensor muscle, fascia and tendon of right index finger at wrist and hand level

√7ᵗʰ **S66.311** Strain of extensor muscle, fascia and tendon of left index finger at wrist and hand level

√7ᵗʰ **S66.312** Strain of extensor muscle, fascia and tendon of right middle finger at wrist and hand level

√7ᵗʰ **S66.313** Strain of extensor muscle, fascia and tendon of left middle finger at wrist and hand level

√7ᵗʰ **S66.314** Strain of extensor muscle, fascia and tendon of right ring finger at wrist and hand level

√7ᵗʰ **S66.315** Strain of extensor muscle, fascia and tendon of left ring finger at wrist and hand level

√7ᵗʰ **S66.316** Strain of extensor muscle, fascia and tendon of right little finger at wrist and hand level

√7ᵗʰ **S66.317** Strain of extensor muscle, fascia and tendon of left little finger at wrist and hand level

√7ᵗʰ **S66.318** Strain of extensor muscle, fascia and tendon of other finger at wrist and hand level
　　Strain of extensor muscle, fascia and tendon of specified finger with unspecified laterality at wrist and hand level

√7ᵗʰ **S66.319** Strain of extensor muscle, fascia and tendon of unspecified finger at wrist and hand level ▽

√6ᵗʰ **S66.32** Laceration of extensor muscle, fascia and tendon of other and unspecified finger at wrist and hand level

4,5 √7ᵗʰ **S66.320** Laceration of extensor muscle, fascia and tendon of right index finger at wrist and hand level **NRS**

4,5 √7ᵗʰ **S66.321** Laceration of extensor muscle, fascia and tendon of left index finger at wrist and hand level **NRS**

4,5 √7ᵗʰ **S66.322** Laceration of extensor muscle, fascia and tendon of right middle finger at wrist and hand level **NRS**

4,5 √7ᵗʰ **S66.323** Laceration of extensor muscle, fascia and tendon of left middle finger at wrist and hand level **NRS**

4,5 √7ᵗʰ **S66.324** Laceration of extensor muscle, fascia and tendon of right ring finger at wrist and hand level **NRS**

4,5 √7ᵗʰ **S66.325** Laceration of extensor muscle, fascia and tendon of left ring finger at wrist and hand level **NRS**

4,5 √7ᵗʰ **S66.326** Laceration of extensor muscle, fascia and tendon of right little finger at wrist and hand level **NRS**

4,5 √7ᵗʰ **S66.327** Laceration of extensor muscle, fascia and tendon of left little finger at wrist and hand level **NRS**

5 √7ᵗʰ **S66.328** Laceration of extensor muscle, fascia and tendon of other finger at wrist and hand level **NRS**
　　Laceration of extensor muscle, fascia and tendon of specified finger with unspecified laterality at wrist and hand level

√7ᵗʰ **S66.329** Laceration of extensor muscle, fascia and tendon of unspecified finger at wrist and hand level ▽

√6ᵗʰ **S66.39** Other injury of extensor muscle, fascia and tendon of other and unspecified finger at wrist and hand level

√7ᵗʰ **S66.390** Other injury of extensor muscle, fascia and tendon of right index finger at wrist and hand level

√7ᵗʰ **S66.391** Other injury of extensor muscle, fascia and tendon of left index finger at wrist and hand level

√7ᵗʰ **S66.392** Other injury of extensor muscle, fascia and tendon of right middle finger at wrist and hand level

√7ᵗʰ **S66.393** Other injury of extensor muscle, fascia and tendon of left middle finger at wrist and hand level

√7ᵗʰ **S66.394** Other injury of extensor muscle, fascia and tendon of right ring finger at wrist and hand level

√7ᵗʰ **S66.395** Other injury of extensor muscle, fascia and tendon of left ring finger at wrist and hand level

√7ᵗʰ **S66.396** Other injury of extensor muscle, fascia and tendon of right little finger at wrist and hand level

√7ᵗʰ **S66.397** Other injury of extensor muscle, fascia and tendon of left little finger at wrist and hand level

√7ᵗʰ **S66.398** Other injury of extensor muscle, fascia and tendon of other finger at wrist and hand level
　　Other injury of extensor muscle, fascia and tendon of specified finger with unspecified laterality at wrist and hand level

√7ᵗʰ **S66.399** Other injury of extensor muscle, fascia and tendon of unspecified finger at wrist and hand level ▽

√5ᵗʰ **S66.4** Injury of intrinsic muscle, fascia and tendon of thumb at wrist and hand level

√6ᵗʰ **S66.40** Unspecified injury of intrinsic muscle, fascia and tendon of thumb at wrist and hand level

√7ᵗʰ **S66.401** Unspecified injury of intrinsic muscle, fascia and tendon of right thumb at wrist and hand level ▽

√7ᵗʰ **S66.402** Unspecified injury of intrinsic muscle, fascia and tendon of left thumb at wrist and hand level ▽

√7ᵗʰ **S66.409** Unspecified injury of intrinsic muscle, fascia and tendon of unspecified thumb at wrist and hand level ▽

√6ᵗʰ **S66.41** Strain of intrinsic muscle, fascia and tendon of thumb at wrist and hand level

√7ᵗʰ **S66.411** Strain of intrinsic muscle, fascia and tendon of right thumb at wrist and hand level

---

4   Case-mix diagnosis with 7th character indicating initial or subsequent encounter.
5   NRS supply diagnosis with 7th character indicating initial or subsequent encounter.

Ⓝ Newborn: 0   Ⓟ Pediatric: 0-17   Ⓜ Maternity: 12-55   Ⓐ Adult: 15-124   **NRS** Nonroutine supply Dx   **NCDx** Noncancer Dx   **PDx** Primary Dx   ►◄ Revised Text   ● New Code   ▲ Revised Title

998   ICD-10-CM 2018

☑7ᵗʰ **S66.412** Strain of intrinsic muscle, fascia and tendon of left thumb at wrist and hand level

☑7ᵗʰ **S66.419** Strain of intrinsic muscle, fascia and tendon of unspecified thumb at wrist and hand level ▽

☑6ᵗʰ **S66.42** Laceration of intrinsic muscle, fascia and tendon of thumb at wrist and hand level

4,5 ☑7ᵗʰ **S66.421** Laceration of intrinsic muscle, fascia and tendon of right thumb at wrist and hand level NRS

4,5 ☑7ᵗʰ **S66.422** Laceration of intrinsic muscle, fascia and tendon of left thumb at wrist and hand level NRS

☑7ᵗʰ **S66.429** Laceration of intrinsic muscle, fascia and tendon of unspecified thumb at wrist and hand level ▽

☑6ᵗʰ **S66.49** Other specified injury of intrinsic muscle, fascia and tendon of thumb at wrist and hand level

☑7ᵗʰ **S66.491** Other specified injury of intrinsic muscle, fascia and tendon of right thumb at wrist and hand level

☑7ᵗʰ **S66.492** Other specified injury of intrinsic muscle, fascia and tendon of left thumb at wrist and hand level

☑7ᵗʰ **S66.499** Other specified injury of intrinsic muscle, fascia and tendon of unspecified thumb at wrist and hand level ▽

☑5ᵗʰ **S66.5** Injury of intrinsic muscle, fascia and tendon of other and unspecified finger at wrist and hand level
EXCLUDES 2 injury of intrinsic muscle, fascia and tendon of thumb at wrist and hand level (S66.4-)

☑6ᵗʰ **S66.50** Unspecified injury of intrinsic muscle, fascia and tendon of other and unspecified finger at wrist and hand level

☑7ᵗʰ **S66.500** Unspecified injury of intrinsic muscle, fascia and tendon of right index finger at wrist and hand level ▽

☑7ᵗʰ **S66.501** Unspecified injury of intrinsic muscle, fascia and tendon of left index finger at wrist and hand level ▽

☑7ᵗʰ **S66.502** Unspecified injury of intrinsic muscle, fascia and tendon of right middle finger at wrist and hand level ▽

☑7ᵗʰ **S66.503** Unspecified injury of intrinsic muscle, fascia and tendon of left middle finger at wrist and hand level ▽

☑7ᵗʰ **S66.504** Unspecified injury of intrinsic muscle, fascia and tendon of right ring finger at wrist and hand level ▽

☑7ᵗʰ **S66.505** Unspecified injury of intrinsic muscle, fascia and tendon of left ring finger at wrist and hand level ▽

☑7ᵗʰ **S66.506** Unspecified injury of intrinsic muscle, fascia and tendon of right little finger at wrist and hand level ▽

☑7ᵗʰ **S66.507** Unspecified injury of intrinsic muscle, fascia and tendon of left little finger at wrist and hand level ▽

☑7ᵗʰ **S66.508** Unspecified injury of intrinsic muscle, fascia and tendon of other finger at wrist and hand level ▽
Unspecified injury of intrinsic muscle, fascia and tendon of specified finger with unspecified laterality at wrist and hand level

☑7ᵗʰ **S66.509** Unspecified injury of intrinsic muscle, fascia and tendon of unspecified finger at wrist and hand level ▽

☑6ᵗʰ **S66.51** Strain of intrinsic muscle, fascia and tendon of other and unspecified finger at wrist and hand level

☑7ᵗʰ **S66.510** Strain of intrinsic muscle, fascia and tendon of right index finger at wrist and hand level

☑7ᵗʰ **S66.511** Strain of intrinsic muscle, fascia and tendon of left index finger at wrist and hand level

☑7ᵗʰ **S66.512** Strain of intrinsic muscle, fascia and tendon of right middle finger at wrist and hand level

☑7ᵗʰ **S66.513** Strain of intrinsic muscle, fascia and tendon of left middle finger at wrist and hand level

☑7ᵗʰ **S66.514** Strain of intrinsic muscle, fascia and tendon of right ring finger at wrist and hand level

☑7ᵗʰ **S66.515** Strain of intrinsic muscle, fascia and tendon of left ring finger at wrist and hand level

☑7ᵗʰ **S66.516** Strain of intrinsic muscle, fascia and tendon of right little finger at wrist and hand level

☑7ᵗʰ **S66.517** Strain of intrinsic muscle, fascia and tendon of left little finger at wrist and hand level

☑7ᵗʰ **S66.518** Strain of intrinsic muscle, fascia and tendon of other finger at wrist and hand level
Strain of intrinsic muscle, fascia and tendon of specified finger with unspecified laterality at wrist and hand level

☑7ᵗʰ **S66.519** Strain of intrinsic muscle, fascia and tendon of unspecified finger at wrist and hand level ▽

☑6ᵗʰ **S66.52** Laceration of intrinsic muscle, fascia and tendon of other and unspecified finger at wrist and hand level

4,5 ☑7ᵗʰ **S66.520** Laceration of intrinsic muscle, fascia and tendon of right index finger at wrist and hand level NRS

4,5 ☑7ᵗʰ **S66.521** Laceration of intrinsic muscle, fascia and tendon of left index finger at wrist and hand level NRS

4,5 ☑7ᵗʰ **S66.522** Laceration of intrinsic muscle, fascia and tendon of right middle finger at wrist and hand level NRS

4,5 ☑7ᵗʰ **S66.523** Laceration of intrinsic muscle, fascia and tendon of left middle finger at wrist and hand level NRS

4,5 ☑7ᵗʰ **S66.524** Laceration of intrinsic muscle, fascia and tendon of right ring finger at wrist and hand level NRS

4,5 ☑7ᵗʰ **S66.525** Laceration of intrinsic muscle, fascia and tendon of left ring finger at wrist and hand level NRS

4,5 ☑7ᵗʰ **S66.526** Laceration of intrinsic muscle, fascia and tendon of right little finger at wrist and hand level NRS

4,5 ☑7ᵗʰ **S66.527** Laceration of intrinsic muscle, fascia and tendon of left little finger at wrist and hand level NRS

5 ☑7ᵗʰ **S66.528** Laceration of intrinsic muscle, fascia and tendon of other finger at wrist and hand level NRS
Laceration of intrinsic muscle, fascia and tendon of specified finger with unspecified laterality at wrist and hand level

☑7ᵗʰ **S66.529** Laceration of intrinsic muscle, fascia and tendon of unspecified finger at wrist and hand level ▽

☑6ᵗʰ **S66.59** Other injury of intrinsic muscle, fascia and tendon of other and unspecified finger at wrist and hand level

☑7ᵗʰ **S66.590** Other injury of intrinsic muscle, fascia and tendon of right index finger at wrist and hand level

☑7ᵗʰ **S66.591** Other injury of intrinsic muscle, fascia and tendon of left index finger at wrist and hand level

☑7ᵗʰ **S66.592** Other injury of intrinsic muscle, fascia and tendon of right middle finger at wrist and hand level

☑7ᵗʰ **S66.593** Other injury of intrinsic muscle, fascia and tendon of left middle finger at wrist and hand level

---

4 Case-mix diagnosis with 7th character indicating initial or subsequent encounter.
5 NRS supply diagnosis with 7th character indicating initial or subsequent encounter.

☑ Additional Character Req   ☑x7ᵗʰ Placeholder Alert   Case-Mix Diagnosis   Manifestation   ▽ Unspecified Dx   EXCLUDES 1 Not coded here   EXCLUDES 2 Not included here

Chapter 19. Injury, Poisoning and Certain Other Consequences of External Causes

✓7ᵗʰ **S66.594** Other injury of intrinsic muscle, fascia and tendon of right ring finger at wrist and hand level

✓7ᵗʰ **S66.595** Other injury of intrinsic muscle, fascia and tendon of left ring finger at wrist and hand level

✓7ᵗʰ **S66.596** Other injury of intrinsic muscle, fascia and tendon of right little finger at wrist and hand level

✓7ᵗʰ **S66.597** Other injury of intrinsic muscle, fascia and tendon of left little finger at wrist and hand level

✓7ᵗʰ **S66.598** Other injury of intrinsic muscle, fascia and tendon of other finger at wrist and hand level

Other injury of intrinsic muscle, fascia and tendon of specified finger with unspecified laterality at wrist and hand level

✓7ᵗʰ **S66.599** Other injury of intrinsic muscle, fascia and tendon of unspecified finger at wrist and hand level ▽

✓5ᵗʰ **S66.8** Injury of other specified muscles, fascia and tendons at wrist and hand level

✓6ᵗʰ **S66.80** Unspecified injury of other specified muscles, fascia and tendons at wrist and hand level

✓7ᵗʰ **S66.801** Unspecified injury of other specified muscles, fascia and tendons at wrist and hand level, right hand ▽

✓7ᵗʰ **S66.802** Unspecified injury of other specified muscles, fascia and tendons at wrist and hand level, left hand ▽

✓7ᵗʰ **S66.809** Unspecified injury of other specified muscles, fascia and tendons at wrist and hand level, unspecified hand ▽

✓6ᵗʰ **S66.81** Strain of other specified muscles, fascia and tendons at wrist and hand level

✓7ᵗʰ **S66.811** Strain of other specified muscles, fascia and tendons at wrist and hand level, right hand

✓7ᵗʰ **S66.812** Strain of other specified muscles, fascia and tendons at wrist and hand level, left hand

✓7ᵗʰ **S66.819** Strain of other specified muscles, fascia and tendons at wrist and hand level, unspecified hand ▽

✓6ᵗʰ **S66.82** Laceration of other specified muscles, fascia and tendons at wrist and hand level

4,5 ✓7ᵗʰ **S66.821** Laceration of other specified muscles, fascia and tendons at wrist and hand level, right hand **NRS**

4,5 ✓7ᵗʰ **S66.822** Laceration of other specified muscles, fascia and tendons at wrist and hand level, left hand **NRS**

5 ✓7ᵗʰ **S66.829** Laceration of other specified muscles, fascia and tendons at wrist and hand level, unspecified hand **NRS** ▽

✓6ᵗʰ **S66.89** Other injury of other specified muscles, fascia and tendons at wrist and hand level

✓7ᵗʰ **S66.891** Other injury of other specified muscles, fascia and tendons at wrist and hand level, right hand

✓7ᵗʰ **S66.892** Other injury of other specified muscles, fascia and tendons at wrist and hand level, left hand

✓7ᵗʰ **S66.899** Other injury of other specified muscles, fascia and tendons at wrist and hand level, unspecified hand ▽

✓5ᵗʰ **S66.9** Injury of unspecified muscle, fascia and tendon at wrist and hand level

✓6ᵗʰ **S66.90** Unspecified injury of unspecified muscle, fascia and tendon at wrist and hand level

✓7ᵗʰ **S66.901** Unspecified injury of unspecified muscle, fascia and tendon at wrist and hand level, right hand ▽

✓7ᵗʰ **S66.902** Unspecified injury of unspecified muscle, fascia and tendon at wrist and hand level, left hand ▽

✓7ᵗʰ **S66.909** Unspecified injury of unspecified muscle, fascia and tendon at wrist and hand level, unspecified hand ▽

✓6ᵗʰ **S66.91** Strain of unspecified muscle, fascia and tendon at wrist and hand level

✓7ᵗʰ **S66.911** Strain of unspecified muscle, fascia and tendon at wrist and hand level, right hand ▽

✓7ᵗʰ **S66.912** Strain of unspecified muscle, fascia and tendon at wrist and hand level, left hand ▽

✓7ᵗʰ **S66.919** Strain of unspecified muscle, fascia and tendon at wrist and hand level, unspecified hand ▽

✓6ᵗʰ **S66.92** Laceration of unspecified muscle, fascia and tendon at wrist and hand level

4,5 ✓7ᵗʰ **S66.921** Laceration of unspecified muscle, fascia and tendon at wrist and hand level, right hand **NRS** ▽

4,5 ✓7ᵗʰ **S66.922** Laceration of unspecified muscle, fascia and tendon at wrist and hand level, left hand **NRS** ▽

✓7ᵗʰ **S66.929** Laceration of unspecified muscle, fascia and tendon at wrist and hand level, unspecified hand ▽

✓6ᵗʰ **S66.99** Other injury of unspecified muscle, fascia and tendon at wrist and hand level

✓7ᵗʰ **S66.991** Other injury of unspecified muscle, fascia and tendon at wrist and hand level, right hand ▽

✓7ᵗʰ **S66.992** Other injury of unspecified muscle, fascia and tendon at wrist and hand level, left hand ▽

✓7ᵗʰ **S66.999** Other injury of unspecified muscle, fascia and tendon at wrist and hand level, unspecified hand ▽

✓4ᵗʰ **S67** Crushing injury of wrist, hand and fingers

Use additional code for all associated injuries, such as:
fracture of wrist and hand (S62.-)
open wound of wrist and hand (S61.-)

The appropriate 7th character is to be added to each code from category S67.
A   initial encounter
D   subsequent encounter
S   sequela

✓5ᵗʰ **S67.0** Crushing injury of thumb

✓x7ᵗʰ **S67.00** Crushing injury of unspecified thumb ▽

1 ✓x7ᵗʰ **S67.01** Crushing injury of right thumb

1 ✓x7ᵗʰ **S67.02** Crushing injury of left thumb

✓5ᵗʰ **S67.1** Crushing injury of other and unspecified finger(s)

EXCLUDES 2   crushing injury of thumb (S67.0-)

✓x7ᵗʰ **S67.10** Crushing injury of unspecified finger(s) ▽

✓6ᵗʰ **S67.19** Crushing injury of other finger(s)

1 ✓7ᵗʰ **S67.190** Crushing injury of right index finger

1 ✓7ᵗʰ **S67.191** Crushing injury of left index finger

1 ✓7ᵗʰ **S67.192** Crushing injury of right middle finger

1 ✓7ᵗʰ **S67.193** Crushing injury of left middle finger

1 ✓7ᵗʰ **S67.194** Crushing injury of right ring finger

1 ✓7ᵗʰ **S67.195** Crushing injury of left ring finger

1 ✓7ᵗʰ **S67.196** Crushing injury of right little finger

1 ✓7ᵗʰ **S67.197** Crushing injury of left little finger

✓7ᵗʰ **S67.198** Crushing injury of other finger

Crushing injury of specified finger with unspecified laterality

---

1   Case-mix diagnosis with 7th character indicating subsequent encounter.
4   Case-mix diagnosis with 7th character indicating initial or subsequent encounter.
5   NRS supply diagnosis with 7th character indicating initial or subsequent encounter.

Ⓝ Newborn: 0   Ⓟ Pediatric: 0-17   Ⓜ Maternity: 12-55   Ⓐ Adult: 15-124   **NRS** Nonroutine supply Dx   **NC-Dx** Noncancer Dx   **PDx** Primary Dx   ▶◀ Revised Text   ● New Code   ▲ Revised Title

1000   ICD-10-CM 2018

√5ᵗʰ **S67.2** **Crushing injury of** hand
- EXCLUDES 2   crushing injury of fingers (S67.1-)
  - crushing injury of thumb (S67.0-)

√x7ᵗʰ **S67.20**   Crushing injury of unspecified hand ▽
1 √x7ᵗʰ **S67.21**   Crushing injury of right hand
1 √x7ᵗʰ **S67.22**   Crushing injury of left hand

√5ᵗʰ **S67.3** **Crushing injury of** wrist
√x7ᵗʰ **S67.30**   Crushing injury of unspecified wrist ▽
1 √x7ᵗʰ **S67.31**   Crushing injury of right wrist
1 √x7ᵗʰ **S67.32**   Crushing injury of left wrist

√5ᵗʰ **S67.4** **Crushing injury of** wrist and hand
- EXCLUDES 1   crushing injury of hand alone (S67.2-)
  - crushing injury of wrist alone (S67.3-)
- EXCLUDES 2   crushing injury of fingers (S67.1-)
  - crushing injury of thumb (S67.0-)

√x7ᵗʰ **S67.40**   Crushing injury of unspecified wrist and hand ▽
1 √x7ᵗʰ **S67.41**   Crushing injury of right wrist and hand
1 √x7ᵗʰ **S67.42**   Crushing injury of left wrist and hand

√5ᵗʰ **S67.9** **Crushing injury of** unspecified part(s) of wrist, hand and fingers
√x7ᵗʰ **S67.90**   Crushing injury of unspecified part(s) of unspecified wrist, hand and fingers ▽
1 √x7ᵗʰ **S67.91**   Crushing injury of unspecified part(s) of right wrist, hand and fingers ▽
1 √x7ᵗʰ **S67.92**   Crushing injury of unspecified part(s) of left wrist, hand and fingers ▽

√4ᵗʰ **S68** **Traumatic amputation of wrist, hand and fingers**
An amputation not identified as partial or complete should be coded to complete.

The appropriate 7th character is to be added to each code from category S68.
A   initial encounter
D   subsequent encounter
S   sequela

√5ᵗʰ **S68.0** **Traumatic** metacarpophalangeal amputation of thumb
Traumatic amputation of thumb NOS

√6ᵗʰ **S68.01**   Complete traumatic metacarpophalangeal amputation of thumb
4,5 √7ᵗʰ **S68.011**   Complete traumatic metacarpophalangeal amputation of right thumb NRS
4,5 √7ᵗʰ **S68.012**   Complete traumatic metacarpophalangeal amputation of left thumb NRS
√7ᵗʰ **S68.019**   Complete traumatic metacarpophalangeal amputation of unspecified thumb ▽

√6ᵗʰ **S68.02**   Partial traumatic metacarpophalangeal amputation of thumb
4,5 √7ᵗʰ **S68.021**   Partial traumatic metacarpophalangeal amputation of right thumb NRS
4,5 √7ᵗʰ **S68.022**   Partial traumatic metacarpophalangeal amputation of left thumb NRS
√7ᵗʰ **S68.029**   Partial traumatic metacarpophalangeal amputation of unspecified thumb ▽

√5ᵗʰ **S68.1** **Traumatic** metacarpophalangeal **amputation of** other and unspecified finger
Traumatic amputation of finger NOS
- EXCLUDES 2   traumatic metacarpophalangeal amputation of thumb (S68.0-)

√6ᵗʰ **S68.11**   Complete traumatic metacarpophalangeal amputation of other and unspecified finger
4,5 √7ᵗʰ **S68.110**   Complete traumatic metacarpophalangeal amputation of right index finger NRS
4,5 √7ᵗʰ **S68.111**   Complete traumatic metacarpophalangeal amputation of left index finger NRS
4,5 √7ᵗʰ **S68.112**   Complete traumatic metacarpophalangeal amputation of right middle finger NRS

4,5 √7ᵗʰ **S68.113**   Complete traumatic metacarpophalangeal amputation of left middle finger NRS
4,5 √7ᵗʰ **S68.114**   Complete traumatic metacarpophalangeal amputation of right ring finger NRS
4,5 √7ᵗʰ **S68.115**   Complete traumatic metacarpophalangeal amputation of left ring finger NRS
4,5 √7ᵗʰ **S68.116**   Complete traumatic metacarpophalangeal amputation of right little finger NRS
4,5 √7ᵗʰ **S68.117**   Complete traumatic metacarpophalangeal amputation of left little finger NRS
5 √7ᵗʰ **S68.118**   Complete traumatic metacarpophalangeal amputation of other finger NRS
Complete traumatic metacarpophalangeal amputation of specified finger with unspecified laterality
√7ᵗʰ **S68.119**   Complete traumatic metacarpophalangeal amputation of unspecified finger ▽

√6ᵗʰ **S68.12**   Partial traumatic metacarpophalangeal amputation of other and unspecified finger
4,5 √7ᵗʰ **S68.120**   Partial traumatic metacarpophalangeal amputation of right index finger NRS
4,5 √7ᵗʰ **S68.121**   Partial traumatic metacarpophalangeal amputation of left index finger NRS
4,5 √7ᵗʰ **S68.122**   Partial traumatic metacarpophalangeal amputation of right middle finger NRS
4,5 √7ᵗʰ **S68.123**   Partial traumatic metacarpophalangeal amputation of left middle finger NRS
4,5 √7ᵗʰ **S68.124**   Partial traumatic metacarpophalangeal amputation of right ring finger NRS
4,5 √7ᵗʰ **S68.125**   Partial traumatic metacarpophalangeal amputation of left ring finger NRS
4,5 √7ᵗʰ **S68.126**   Partial traumatic metacarpophalangeal amputation of right little finger NRS
4,5 √7ᵗʰ **S68.127**   Partial traumatic metacarpophalangeal amputation of left little finger NRS
5 √7ᵗʰ **S68.128**   Partial traumatic metacarpophalangeal amputation of other finger NRS
Partial traumatic metacarpophalangeal amputation of specified finger with unspecified laterality
√7ᵗʰ **S68.129**   Partial traumatic metacarpophalangeal amputation of unspecified finger ▽

√5ᵗʰ **S68.4** **Traumatic amputation of** hand at wrist level
Traumatic amputation of hand NOS
Traumatic amputation of wrist

√6ᵗʰ **S68.41**   Complete traumatic amputation of hand at wrist level
4,5 √7ᵗʰ **S68.411**   Complete traumatic amputation of right hand at wrist level NRS
4,5 √7ᵗʰ **S68.412**   Complete traumatic amputation of left hand at wrist level NRS
√7ᵗʰ **S68.419**   Complete traumatic amputation of unspecified hand at wrist level ▽

√6ᵗʰ **S68.42**   Partial traumatic amputation of hand at wrist level
4,5 √7ᵗʰ **S68.421**   Partial traumatic amputation of right hand at wrist level NRS
4,5 √7ᵗʰ **S68.422**   Partial traumatic amputation of left hand at wrist level NRS
√7ᵗʰ **S68.429**   Partial traumatic amputation of unspecified hand at wrist level ▽

√5ᵗʰ **S68.5** **Traumatic** transphalangeal **amputation of** thumb
Traumatic interphalangeal joint amputation of thumb

√6ᵗʰ **S68.51**   Complete traumatic transphalangeal amputation of thumb
4,5 √7ᵗʰ **S68.511**   Complete traumatic transphalangeal amputation of right thumb NRS
4,5 √7ᵗʰ **S68.512**   Complete traumatic transphalangeal amputation of left thumb NRS

---

1   Case-mix diagnosis with 7th character indicating subsequent encounter.
4   Case-mix diagnosis with 7th character indicating initial or subsequent encounter.
5   NRS supply diagnosis with 7th character indicating initial or subsequent encounter.

✓ Additional Character Req   √x7ᵗʰ Placeholder Alert   Case-Mix Diagnosis   Manifestation   ▽ Unspecified Dx   EXCLUDES 1 Not coded here   EXCLUDES 2 Not included here

Chapter 19. Injury, Poisoning and Certain Other Consequences of External Causes

√7th **S68.519** Complete traumatic transphalangeal amputation of unspecified thumb ▽

√6th **S68.52** Partial traumatic transphalangeal amputation of thumb

    4,5 √7th **S68.521** **Partial traumatic transphalangeal amputation of right thumb** NRS

    4,5 √7th **S68.522** **Partial traumatic transphalangeal amputation of left thumb** NRS

    √7th **S68.529** **Partial traumatic transphalangeal amputation of unspecified thumb** ▽

√5th **S68.6** Traumatic transphalangeal amputation of other and unspecified finger

√6th **S68.61** Complete traumatic transphalangeal amputation of other and unspecified finger(s)

    4,5 √7th **S68.610** **Complete traumatic transphalangeal amputation of right index finger** NRS

    4,5 √7th **S68.611** **Complete traumatic transphalangeal amputation of left index finger** NRS

    4,5 √7th **S68.612** **Complete traumatic transphalangeal amputation of right middle finger** NRS

    4,5 √7th **S68.613** **Complete traumatic transphalangeal amputation of left middle finger** NRS

    4,5 √7th **S68.614** **Complete traumatic transphalangeal amputation of right ring finger** NRS

    4,5 √7th **S68.615** **Complete traumatic transphalangeal amputation of left ring finger** NRS

    4,5 √7th **S68.616** **Complete traumatic transphalangeal amputation of right little finger** NRS

    4,5 √7th **S68.617** **Complete traumatic transphalangeal amputation of left little finger** NRS

    5 √7th **S68.618** **Complete traumatic transphalangeal amputation of other finger** NRS
       Complete traumatic transphalangeal amputation of specified finger with unspecified laterality

    √7th **S68.619** **Complete traumatic transphalangeal amputation of unspecified finger** ▽

√6th **S68.62** Partial traumatic transphalangeal amputation of other and unspecified finger

    4,5 √7th **S68.620** **Partial traumatic transphalangeal amputation of right index finger** NRS

    4,5 √7th **S68.621** **Partial traumatic transphalangeal amputation of left index finger** NRS

    4,5 √7th **S68.622** **Partial traumatic transphalangeal amputation of right middle finger** NRS

    4,5 √7th **S68.623** **Partial traumatic transphalangeal amputation of left middle finger** NRS

    4,5 √7th **S68.624** **Partial traumatic transphalangeal amputation of right ring finger** NRS

    4,5 √7th **S68.625** **Partial traumatic transphalangeal amputation of left ring finger** NRS

    4,5 √7th **S68.626** **Partial traumatic transphalangeal amputation of right little finger** NRS

    4,5 √7th **S68.627** **Partial traumatic transphalangeal amputation of left little finger** NRS

    5 √7th **S68.628** **Partial traumatic transphalangeal amputation of other finger** NRS
       Partial traumatic transphalangeal amputation of specified finger with unspecified laterality

    √7th **S68.629** **Partial traumatic transphalangeal amputation of unspecified finger** ▽

√5th **S68.7** Traumatic transmetacarpal amputation of hand

√6th **S68.71** Complete traumatic transmetacarpal amputation of hand

    4,5 √7th **S68.711** **Complete traumatic transmetacarpal amputation of right hand** NRS

    4,5 √7th **S68.712** **Complete traumatic transmetacarpal amputation of left hand** NRS

    √7th **S68.719** **Complete traumatic transmetacarpal amputation of unspecified hand** ▽

√6th **S68.72** Partial traumatic transmetacarpal amputation of hand

    4,5 √7th **S68.721** **Partial traumatic transmetacarpal amputation of right hand** NRS

    4,5 √7th **S68.722** **Partial traumatic transmetacarpal amputation of left hand** NRS

    √7th **S68.729** **Partial traumatic transmetacarpal amputation of unspecified hand** ▽

√4th **S69** **Other and unspecified injuries of wrist, hand and finger(s)**

The appropriate 7th character is to be added to each code from category S69.
A   initial encounter
D   subsequent encounter
S   sequela

√5th **S69.8** Other specified injuries of wrist, hand and finger(s)

    √x7th **S69.80** Other specified injuries of unspecified wrist, hand and finger(s) ▽

    √x7th **S69.81** Other specified injuries of right wrist, hand and finger(s)

    √x7th **S69.82** Other specified injuries of left wrist, hand and finger(s)

√5th **S69.9** Unspecified injury of wrist, hand and finger(s)

    √x7th **S69.90** Unspecified injury of unspecified wrist, hand and finger(s) ▽

    √x7th **S69.91** Unspecified injury of right wrist, hand and finger(s) ▽

    √x7th **S69.92** Unspecified injury of left wrist, hand and fingers ▽

Injuries to the hip and thigh (S70-S79)

EXCLUDES 2   burns and corrosions (T20-T32)
    frostbite (T33-T34)
    snake bite (T63.0-)
    venomous insect bite or sting (T63.4-)

√4th **S70** **Superficial injury of hip and thigh**

The appropriate 7th character is to be added to each code from category S70.
A   initial encounter
D   subsequent encounter
S   sequela

√5th **S70.0** Contusion of hip

    √x7th **S70.00** Contusion of unspecified hip ▽

    √x7th **S70.01** Contusion of right hip

    √x7th **S70.02** Contusion of left hip

√5th **S70.1** Contusion of thigh

    √x7th **S70.10** Contusion of unspecified thigh ▽

    √x7th **S70.11** Contusion of right thigh

    √x7th **S70.12** Contusion of left thigh

√5th **S70.2** Other superficial injuries of hip

    √6th **S70.21** Abrasion of hip

       √7th **S70.211** Abrasion, right hip

       √7th **S70.212** Abrasion, left hip

       √7th **S70.219** Abrasion, unspecified hip ▽

    √6th **S70.22** Blister (nonthermal) of hip

       √7th **S70.221** Blister (nonthermal), right hip

       √7th **S70.222** Blister (nonthermal), left hip

       √7th **S70.229** Blister (nonthermal), unspecified hip ▽

    √6th **S70.24** External constriction of hip

       √7th **S70.241** External constriction, right hip

       √7th **S70.242** External constriction, left hip

       √7th **S70.249** External constriction, unspecified hip ▽

    √6th **S70.25** Superficial foreign body of hip
       Splinter in the hip

       √7th **S70.251** Superficial foreign body, right hip

       √7th **S70.252** Superficial foreign body, left hip

       √7th **S70.259** Superficial foreign body, unspecified hip ▽

    √6th **S70.26** Insect bite (nonvenomous) of hip

       √7th **S70.261** Insect bite (nonvenomous), right hip

---

4   Case-mix diagnosis with 7th character indicating initial or subsequent encounter.
5   NRS supply diagnosis with 7th character indicating initial or subsequent encounter.

N Newborn: 0   P Pediatric: 0-17   M Maternity: 12-55   A Adult: 15-124   NRS Nonroutine supply Dx   NCDx Noncancer Dx   PDx Primary Dx   ▶◀ Revised Text   ● New Code   ▲ Revised Title

Chapter 19. Injury, Poisoning and Certain Other Consequences of External Causes

    √7th S70.262   Insect bite (nonvenomous), left hip

    √7th S70.269   Insect bite (nonvenomous), unspecified hip ▽

  √6th S70.27   Other superficial bite of hip
    EXCLUDES 1   open bite of hip (S71.05-)

    √7th S70.271   Other superficial bite of hip, right hip

    √7th S70.272   Other superficial bite of hip, left hip

    √7th S70.279   Other superficial bite of hip, unspecified hip ▽

√5th S70.3   **Other superficial injuries of** thigh

  √6th S70.31   Abrasion of thigh

    √7th S70.311   Abrasion, right thigh

    √7th S70.312   Abrasion, left thigh

    √7th S70.319   Abrasion, unspecified thigh ▽

  √6th S70.32   Blister (nonthermal) of thigh

    √7th S70.321   Blister (nonthermal), right thigh

    √7th S70.322   Blister (nonthermal), left thigh

    √7th S70.329   Blister (nonthermal), unspecified thigh ▽

  √6th S70.34   External constriction of thigh

    √7th S70.341   External constriction, right thigh

    √7th S70.342   External constriction, left thigh

    √7th S70.349   External constriction, unspecified thigh ▽

  √6th S70.35   Superficial foreign body of thigh
    Splinter in the thigh

    √7th S70.351   Superficial foreign body, right thigh

    √7th S70.352   Superficial foreign body, left thigh

    √7th S70.359   Superficial foreign body, unspecified thigh ▽

  √6th S70.36   Insect bite (nonvenomous) of thigh

    √7th S70.361   Insect bite (nonvenomous), right thigh

    √7th S70.362   Insect bite (nonvenomous), left thigh

    √7th S70.369   Insect bite (nonvenomous), unspecified thigh ▽

  √6th S70.37   Other superficial bite of thigh
    EXCLUDES 1   open bite of thigh (S71.15)

    √7th S70.371   Other superficial bite of right thigh

    √7th S70.372   Other superficial bite of left thigh

    √7th S70.379   Other superficial bite of unspecified thigh ▽

√5th S70.9   **Unspecified superficial injury of** hip and thigh

  √6th S70.91   Unspecified superficial injury of hip

    √7th S70.911   Unspecified superficial injury of right hip ▽

    √7th S70.912   Unspecified superficial injury of left hip ▽

    √7th S70.919   Unspecified superficial injury of unspecified hip ▽

  √6th S70.92   Unspecified superficial injury of thigh

    √7th S70.921   Unspecified superficial injury of right thigh ▽

    √7th S70.922   Unspecified superficial injury of left thigh ▽

    √7th S70.929   Unspecified superficial injury of unspecified thigh ▽

√4th **S71**   **Open wound of hip and thigh**
  Code also any associated wound infection
  EXCLUDES 1   open fracture of hip and thigh (S72.-)
            traumatic amputation of hip and thigh (S78.-)
  EXCLUDES 2   bite of venomous animal (T63.-)
            open wound of ankle, foot and toes (S91.-)
            open wound of knee and lower leg (S81.-)

> The appropriate 7th character is to be added to each code from category S71.
> A   initial encounter
> D   subsequent encounter
> S   sequela

√5th S71.0   **Open wound of** hip

  √6th S71.00   Unspecified open wound of hip

    5 √7th S71.001   Unspecified open wound, right hip   NRS ▽

    5 √7th S71.002   Unspecified open wound, left hip   NRS ▽

    √7th S71.009   Unspecified open wound, unspecified hip ▽

  √6th S71.01   Laceration without foreign body of hip

    4,5 √7th S71.011   Laceration without foreign body, right hip   NRS

    4,5 √7th S71.012   Laceration without foreign body, left hip   NRS

    √7th S71.019   Laceration without foreign body, unspecified hip ▽

  √6th S71.02   Laceration with foreign body of hip

    4,5 √7th S71.021   Laceration with foreign body, right hip NRS

    4,5 √7th S71.022   Laceration with foreign body, left hip NRS

    √7th S71.029   Laceration with foreign body, unspecified hip ▽

  √6th S71.03   Puncture wound without foreign body of hip

    4,5 √7th S71.031   Puncture wound without foreign body, right hip   NRS

    4,5 √7th S71.032   Puncture wound without foreign body, left hip   NRS

    √7th S71.039   Puncture wound without foreign body, unspecified hip ▽

  √6th S71.04   Puncture wound with foreign body of hip

    4,5 √7th S71.041   Puncture wound with foreign body, right hip   NRS

    4,5 √7th S71.042   Puncture wound with foreign body, left hip   NRS

    √7th S71.049   Puncture wound with foreign body, unspecified hip ▽

  √6th S71.05   Open bite of hip
    Bite of hip NOS
    EXCLUDES 1   superficial bite of hip (S70.26, S70.27)

    4,5 √7th S71.051   Open bite, right hip   NRS

    4,5 √7th S71.052   Open bite, left hip   NRS

    √7th S71.059   Open bite, unspecified hip ▽

√5th S71.1   **Open wound of** thigh

  √6th S71.10   Unspecified open wound of thigh
    AHA: 2016, 3Q, 24

    5 √7th S71.101   Unspecified open wound, right thigh   NRS ▽

    5 √7th S71.102   Unspecified open wound, left thigh   NRS ▽

    √7th S71.109   Unspecified open wound, unspecified thigh ▽

  √6th S71.11   Laceration without foreign body of thigh

    4,5 √7th S71.111   Laceration without foreign body, right thigh   NRS

    4,5 √7th S71.112   Laceration without foreign body, left thigh   NRS

    √7th S71.119   Laceration without foreign body, unspecified thigh ▽

  √6th S71.12   Laceration with foreign body of thigh

    4,5 √7th S71.121   Laceration with foreign body, right thigh   NRS

    4,5 √7th S71.122   Laceration with foreign body, left thigh   NRS

    √7th S71.129   Laceration with foreign body, unspecified thigh ▽

  √6th S71.13   Puncture wound without foreign body of thigh
    AHA: 2016, 3Q, 24

    4,5 √7th S71.131   Puncture wound without foreign body, right thigh   NRS

    4,5 √7th S71.132   Puncture wound without foreign body, left thigh   NRS

    √7th S71.139   Puncture wound without foreign body, unspecified thigh ▽

---

4   Case-mix diagnosis with 7th character indicating initial or subsequent encounter.
5   NRS supply diagnosis with 7th character indicating initial or subsequent encounter.

Chapter 19. Injury, Poisoning and Certain Other Consequences of External Causes

✓6ᵗʰ **S71.14** **Puncture wound with foreign body** of thigh
AHA: 2016, 3Q, 24

4,5 ✓7ᵗʰ **S71.141** **Puncture wound with foreign body, right thigh** NRS

4,5 ✓7ᵗʰ **S71.142** **Puncture wound with foreign body, left thigh** NRS

✓7ᵗʰ **S71.149** **Puncture wound with foreign body, unspecified thigh** ▽

✓6ᵗʰ **S71.15** **Open bite** of thigh
Bite of thigh NOS
EXCLUDES 1   superficial bite of thigh (S70.37-)

4,5 ✓7ᵗʰ **S71.151** **Open bite, right thigh** NRS
4,5 ✓7ᵗʰ **S71.152** **Open bite, left thigh** NRS
✓7ᵗʰ **S71.159** **Open bite, unspecified thigh** ▽

✓4ᵗʰ **S72** **Fracture of femur**
NOTE   A fracture not indicated as displaced or nondisplaced should be coded to displaced.
The open fracture designations are based on the Gustilo open fracture classification.
A fracture not indicated as open or closed should be coded to closed.
EXCLUDES 1   traumatic amputation of hip and thigh (S78.-)
EXCLUDES 2   fracture of lower leg and ankle (S82.-)
fracture of foot (S92.-)
periprosthetic fracture of prosthetic implant of hip ▶(M97.0-)◀
AHA: 2016, 1Q, 33; 2015, 3Q, 37-39; 2015, 1Q, 17; 2013, 4Q, 128
TIP: The term "improper alignment" is not synonymous with malunion or nonunion of a fracture when noted in provider documentation.

The appropriate 7th character is to be added to all codes from category S72 [unless otherwise indicated].
A   initial encounter for closed fracture
B   initial encounter for open fracture type I or II
    initial encounter for open fracture NOS
C   initial encounter for open fracture type IIIA, IIIB, or IIIC
D   subsequent encounter for closed fracture with routine healing
E   subsequent encounter for open fracture type I or II with routine healing
F   subsequent encounter for open fracture type IIIA, IIIB, or IIIC with routine healing
G   subsequent encounter for closed fracture with delayed healing
H   subsequent encounter for open fracture type I or II with delayed healing
J   subsequent encounter for open fracture type IIIA, IIIB, or IIIC with delayed healing
K   subsequent encounter for closed fracture with nonunion
M   subsequent encounter for open fracture type I or II with nonunion
N   subsequent encounter for open fracture type IIIA, IIIB, or IIIC with nonunion
P   subsequent encounter for closed fracture with malunion
Q   subsequent encounter for open fracture type I or II with malunion
R   subsequent encounter for open fracture type IIIA, IIIB, or IIIC with malunion
S   sequela

✓5ᵗʰ **S72.0** **Fracture of head and neck** of femur
EXCLUDES 2   physeal fracture of upper end of femur (S79.0-)
AHA: 2016, 3Q, 16

✓6ᵗʰ **S72.00** **Fracture of unspecified** part of neck of femur
Fracture of hip NOS   Fracture of neck of femur NOS

1 ✓7ᵗʰ **S72.001** **Fracture of unspecified part of neck of right femur** ▽

1 ✓7ᵗʰ **S72.002** **Fracture of unspecified part of neck of left femur** ▽

✓7ᵗʰ **S72.009** **Fracture of unspecified part of neck of unspecified femur** ▽

✓6ᵗʰ **S72.01** **Unspecified intracapsular fracture of femur**
Subcapital fracture of femur

1 ✓7ᵗʰ **S72.011** **Unspecified intracapsular fracture of right femur** ▽

1 ✓7ᵗʰ **S72.012** **Unspecified intracapsular fracture of left femur** ▽

✓7ᵗʰ **S72.019** **Unspecified intracapsular fracture of unspecified femur** ▽

✓6ᵗʰ **S72.02** **Fracture of epiphysis (separation) (upper)** of femur
Transepiphyseal fracture of femur
EXCLUDES 1   capital femoral epiphyseal fracture (pediatric) of femur (S79.01-)
Salter-Harris Type I physeal fracture of upper end of femur (S79.01-)

1 ✓7ᵗʰ **S72.021** **Displaced fracture of epiphysis (separation) (upper) of right femur**

1 ✓7ᵗʰ **S72.022** **Displaced fracture of epiphysis (separation) (upper) of left femur**

✓7ᵗʰ **S72.023** **Displaced fracture of epiphysis (separation) (upper) of unspecified femur** ▽

1 ✓7ᵗʰ **S72.024** **Nondisplaced fracture of epiphysis (separation) (upper) of right femur**

1 ✓7ᵗʰ **S72.025** **Nondisplaced fracture of epiphysis (separation) (upper) of left femur**

✓7ᵗʰ **S72.026** **Nondisplaced fracture of epiphysis (separation) (upper) of unspecified femur** ▽

✓6ᵗʰ **S72.03** **Midcervical fracture** of femur
Transcervical fracture of femur NOS

1 ✓7ᵗʰ **S72.031** **Displaced midcervical fracture of right femur**

1 ✓7ᵗʰ **S72.032** **Displaced midcervical fracture of left femur**

1 ✓7ᵗʰ **S72.033** **Displaced midcervical fracture of unspecified femur** ▽

1 ✓7ᵗʰ **S72.034** **Nondisplaced midcervical fracture of right femur**

1 ✓7ᵗʰ **S72.035** **Nondisplaced midcervical fracture of left femur**

✓7ᵗʰ **S72.036** **Nondisplaced midcervical fracture of unspecified femur** ▽

✓6ᵗʰ **S72.04** **Fracture of base of neck** of femur
Cervicotrochanteric fracture of femur

1 ✓7ᵗʰ **S72.041** **Displaced fracture of base of neck of right femur**

1 ✓7ᵗʰ **S72.042** **Displaced fracture of base of neck of left femur**

✓7ᵗʰ **S72.043** **Displaced fracture of base of neck of unspecified femur** ▽

1 ✓7ᵗʰ **S72.044** **Nondisplaced fracture of base of neck of right femur**

1 ✓7ᵗʰ **S72.045** **Nondisplaced fracture of base of neck of left femur**

✓7ᵗʰ **S72.046** **Nondisplaced fracture of base of neck of unspecified femur** ▽

✓6ᵗʰ **S72.05** **Unspecified fracture of head** of femur
Fracture of head of femur NOS

1 ✓7ᵗʰ **S72.051** **Unspecified fracture of head of right femur** ▽

1 ✓7ᵗʰ **S72.052** **Unspecified fracture of head of left femur** ▽

✓7ᵗʰ **S72.059** **Unspecified fracture of head of unspecified femur** ▽

✓6ᵗʰ **S72.06** **Articular fracture of head** of femur

1 ✓7ᵗʰ **S72.061** **Displaced articular fracture of head of right femur**

1 ✓7ᵗʰ **S72.062** **Displaced articular fracture of head of left femur**

✓7ᵗʰ **S72.063** **Displaced articular fracture of head of unspecified femur** ▽

1 ✓7ᵗʰ **S72.064** **Nondisplaced articular fracture of head of right femur**

1 ✓7ᵗʰ **S72.065** **Nondisplaced articular fracture of head of left femur**

✓7ᵗʰ **S72.066** **Nondisplaced articular fracture of head of unspecified femur** ▽

✓6ᵗʰ **S72.09** **Other fracture of head and neck** of femur

1 ✓7ᵗʰ **S72.091** **Other fracture of head and neck of right femur**

1 ✓7ᵗʰ **S72.092** **Other fracture of head and neck of left femur**

---

1   Case-mix diagnosis with 7th character indicating subsequent encounter.
4   Case-mix diagnosis with 7th character indicating initial or subsequent encounter.
5   NRS supply diagnosis with 7th character indicating initial or subsequent encounter.

Ⓝ Newborn: 0   Ⓟ Pediatric: 0-17   Ⓜ Maternity: 12-55   Ⓐ Adult: 15-124   NRS Nonroutine supply Dx   NC Dx Noncancer Dx   PDx Primary Dx   ▶◀ Revised Text   ● New Code   ▲ Revised Title

☑7ᵗʰ **S72.099** Other fracture of head and neck of unspecified femur ▽

☑6ᵗʰ **S72.1** Pertrochanteric fracture
AHA: 2016, 3Q, 16

☑6ᵗʰ **S72.10** Unspecified trochanteric fracture of femur
Fracture of trochanter NOS

1 ☑7ᵗʰ **S72.101** Unspecified trochanteric fracture of right femur ▽

1 ☑7ᵗʰ **S72.102** Unspecified trochanteric fracture of left femur ▽

☑7ᵗʰ **S72.109** Unspecified trochanteric fracture of unspecified femur ▽

☑6ᵗʰ **S72.11** Fracture of greater trochanter of femur

1 ☑7ᵗʰ **S72.111** Displaced fracture of greater trochanter of right femur

1 ☑7ᵗʰ **S72.112** Displaced fracture of greater trochanter of left femur

☑7ᵗʰ **S72.113** Displaced fracture of greater trochanter of unspecified femur ▽

1 ☑7ᵗʰ **S72.114** Nondisplaced fracture of greater trochanter of right femur

1 ☑7ᵗʰ **S72.115** Nondisplaced fracture of greater trochanter of left femur

☑7ᵗʰ **S72.116** Nondisplaced fracture of greater trochanter of unspecified femur ▽

☑6ᵗʰ **S72.12** Fracture of lesser trochanter of femur

1 ☑7ᵗʰ **S72.121** Displaced fracture of lesser trochanter of right femur

1 ☑7ᵗʰ **S72.122** Displaced fracture of lesser trochanter of left femur

☑7ᵗʰ **S72.123** Displaced fracture of lesser trochanter of unspecified femur ▽

1 ☑7ᵗʰ **S72.124** Nondisplaced fracture of lesser trochanter of right femur

1 ☑7ᵗʰ **S72.125** Nondisplaced fracture of lesser trochanter of left femur

☑7ᵗʰ **S72.126** Nondisplaced fracture of lesser trochanter of unspecified femur ▽

☑6ᵗʰ **S72.13** Apophyseal fracture of femur
EXCLUDES 1 chronic (nontraumatic) slipped upper femoral epiphysis (M93.0-)

1 ☑7ᵗʰ **S72.131** Displaced apophyseal fracture of right femur

1 ☑7ᵗʰ **S72.132** Displaced apophyseal fracture of left femur

☑7ᵗʰ **S72.133** Displaced apophyseal fracture of unspecified femur ▽

1 ☑7ᵗʰ **S72.134** Nondisplaced apophyseal fracture of right femur

1 ☑7ᵗʰ **S72.135** Nondisplaced apophyseal fracture of left femur

☑7ᵗʰ **S72.136** Nondisplaced apophyseal fracture of unspecified femur ▽

☑6ᵗʰ **S72.14** Intertrochanteric fracture of femur

1 ☑7ᵗʰ **S72.141** Displaced intertrochanteric fracture of right femur

1 ☑7ᵗʰ **S72.142** Displaced intertrochanteric fracture of left femur

☑7ᵗʰ **S72.143** Displaced intertrochanteric fracture of unspecified femur ▽

1 ☑7ᵗʰ **S72.144** Nondisplaced intertrochanteric fracture of right femur

1 ☑7ᵗʰ **S72.145** Nondisplaced intertrochanteric fracture of left femur

☑7ᵗʰ **S72.146** Nondisplaced intertrochanteric fracture of unspecified femur ▽

☑5ᵗʰ **S72.2** Subtrochanteric fracture of femur

1 ☑x7ᵗʰ **S72.21** Displaced subtrochanteric fracture of right femur

1 ☑x7ᵗʰ **S72.22** Displaced subtrochanteric fracture of left femur

☑x7ᵗʰ **S72.23** Displaced subtrochanteric fracture of unspecified femur ▽

1 ☑x7ᵗʰ **S72.24** Nondisplaced subtrochanteric fracture of right femur

1 ☑x7ᵗʰ **S72.25** Nondisplaced subtrochanteric fracture of left femur

☑x7ᵗʰ **S72.26** Nondisplaced subtrochanteric fracture of unspecified femur ▽

☑5ᵗʰ **S72.3** Fracture of shaft of femur

☑6ᵗʰ **S72.30** Unspecified fracture of shaft of femur

1 ☑7ᵗʰ **S72.301** Unspecified fracture of shaft of right femur

1 ☑7ᵗʰ **S72.302** Unspecified fracture of shaft of left femur ▽

☑7ᵗʰ **S72.309** Unspecified fracture of shaft of unspecified femur ▽

☑6ᵗʰ **S72.32** Transverse fracture of shaft of femur

1 ☑7ᵗʰ **S72.321** Displaced transverse fracture of shaft of right femur

1 ☑7ᵗʰ **S72.322** Displaced transverse fracture of shaft of left femur

☑7ᵗʰ **S72.323** Displaced transverse fracture of shaft of unspecified femur

1 ☑7ᵗʰ **S72.324** Nondisplaced transverse fracture of shaft of right femur

1 ☑7ᵗʰ **S72.325** Nondisplaced transverse fracture of shaft of left femur

☑7ᵗʰ **S72.326** Nondisplaced transverse fracture of shaft of unspecified femur ▽

☑6ᵗʰ **S72.33** Oblique fracture of shaft of femur

1 ☑7ᵗʰ **S72.331** Displaced oblique fracture of shaft of right femur

1 ☑7ᵗʰ **S72.332** Displaced oblique fracture of shaft of left femur

☑7ᵗʰ **S72.333** Displaced oblique fracture of shaft of unspecified femur ▽

1 ☑7ᵗʰ **S72.334** Nondisplaced oblique fracture of shaft of right femur

1 ☑7ᵗʰ **S72.335** Nondisplaced oblique fracture of shaft of left femur

☑7ᵗʰ **S72.336** Nondisplaced oblique fracture of shaft of unspecified femur ▽

☑6ᵗʰ **S72.34** Spiral fracture of shaft of femur

1 ☑7ᵗʰ **S72.341** Displaced spiral fracture of shaft of right femur

1 ☑7ᵗʰ **S72.342** Displaced spiral fracture of shaft of left femur

☑7ᵗʰ **S72.343** Displaced spiral fracture of shaft of unspecified femur ▽

1 ☑7ᵗʰ **S72.344** Nondisplaced spiral fracture of shaft of right femur

1 ☑7ᵗʰ **S72.345** Nondisplaced spiral fracture of shaft of left femur

☑7ᵗʰ **S72.346** Nondisplaced spiral fracture of shaft of unspecified femur ▽

☑6ᵗʰ **S72.35** Comminuted fracture of shaft of femur

1 ☑7ᵗʰ **S72.351** Displaced comminuted fracture of shaft of right femur

1 ☑7ᵗʰ **S72.352** Displaced comminuted fracture of shaft of left femur

☑7ᵗʰ **S72.353** Displaced comminuted fracture of shaft of unspecified femur ▽

1 ☑7ᵗʰ **S72.354** Nondisplaced comminuted fracture of shaft of right femur

1 ☑7ᵗʰ **S72.355** Nondisplaced comminuted fracture of shaft of left femur

☑7ᵗʰ **S72.356** Nondisplaced comminuted fracture of shaft of unspecified femur ▽

☑6ᵗʰ **S72.36** Segmental fracture of shaft of femur

1 ☑7ᵗʰ **S72.361** Displaced segmental fracture of shaft of right femur

1 ☑7ᵗʰ **S72.362** Displaced segmental fracture of shaft of left femur

☑7ᵗʰ **S72.363** Displaced segmental fracture of shaft of unspecified femur ▽

1 ☑7ᵗʰ **S72.364** Nondisplaced segmental fracture of shaft of right femur

1 ☑7ᵗʰ **S72.365** Nondisplaced segmental fracture of shaft of left femur

1 Case-mix diagnosis with 7th character indicating subsequent encounter.

√7ᵗʰ **S72.366** Nondisplaced segmental fracture of shaft of unspecified femur ▽

√6ᵗʰ **S72.39** Other fracture of shaft of femur

   1 √7ᵗʰ **S72.391** Other fracture of shaft of right femur

   1 √7ᵗʰ **S72.392** Other fracture of shaft of left femur

   √7ᵗʰ **S72.399** Other fracture of shaft of unspecified femur ▽

√5ᵗʰ **S72.4** Fracture of lower end of femur
Fracture of distal end of femur
   EXCLUDES 2   fracture of shaft of femur (S72.3-)
          physeal fracture of lower end of femur (S79.1-)

√6ᵗʰ **S72.40** Unspecified fracture of lower end of femur

   1 √7ᵗʰ **S72.401** Unspecified fracture of lower end of right femur ▽

   1 √7ᵗʰ **S72.402** Unspecified fracture of lower end of left femur ▽

   √7ᵗʰ **S72.409** Unspecified fracture of lower end of unspecified femur ▽

√6ᵗʰ **S72.41** Unspecified condyle fracture of lower end of femur
Condyle fracture of femur NOS

   1 √7ᵗʰ **S72.411** Displaced unspecified condyle fracture of lower end of right femur ▽

   1 √7ᵗʰ **S72.412** Displaced unspecified condyle fracture of lower end of left femur ▽

   √7ᵗʰ **S72.413** Displaced unspecified condyle fracture of lower end of unspecified femur ▽

   1 √7ᵗʰ **S72.414** Nondisplaced unspecified condyle fracture of lower end of right femur ▽

   1 √7ᵗʰ **S72.415** Nondisplaced unspecified condyle fracture of lower end of left femur ▽

   √7ᵗʰ **S72.416** Nondisplaced unspecified condyle fracture of lower end of unspecified femur ▽

√6ᵗʰ **S72.42** Fracture of lateral condyle of femur

   1 √7ᵗʰ **S72.421** Displaced fracture of lateral condyle of right femur

   1 √7ᵗʰ **S72.422** Displaced fracture of lateral condyle of left femur

   √7ᵗʰ **S72.423** Displaced fracture of lateral condyle of unspecified femur ▽

   1 √7ᵗʰ **S72.424** Nondisplaced fracture of lateral condyle of right femur

   1 √7ᵗʰ **S72.425** Nondisplaced fracture of lateral condyle of left femur

   √7ᵗʰ **S72.426** Nondisplaced fracture of lateral condyle of unspecified femur ▽

√6ᵗʰ **S72.43** Fracture of medial condyle of femur

   1 √7ᵗʰ **S72.431** Displaced fracture of medial condyle of right femur

   1 √7ᵗʰ **S72.432** Displaced fracture of medial condyle of left femur

   √7ᵗʰ **S72.433** Displaced fracture of medial condyle of unspecified femur ▽

   1 √7ᵗʰ **S72.434** Nondisplaced fracture of medial condyle of right femur

   1 √7ᵗʰ **S72.435** Nondisplaced fracture of medial condyle of left femur

   √7ᵗʰ **S72.436** Nondisplaced fracture of medial condyle of unspecified femur ▽

√6ᵗʰ **S72.44** Fracture of lower epiphysis (separation) of femur
   EXCLUDES 1   Salter-Harris Type I physeal fracture of lower end of femur (S79.11-)

   1 √7ᵗʰ **S72.441** Displaced fracture of lower epiphysis (separation) of right femur

   1 √7ᵗʰ **S72.442** Displaced fracture of lower epiphysis (separation) of left femur

   √7ᵗʰ **S72.443** Displaced fracture of lower epiphysis (separation) of unspecified femur ▽

   1 √7ᵗʰ **S72.444** Nondisplaced fracture of lower epiphysis (separation) of right femur

   1 √7ᵗʰ **S72.445** Nondisplaced fracture of lower epiphysis (separation) of left femur

   √7ᵗʰ **S72.446** Nondisplaced fracture of lower epiphysis (separation) of unspecified femur ▽

√6ᵗʰ **S72.45** Supracondylar fracture without intracondylar extension of lower end of femur
Supracondylar fracture of lower end of femur NOS
   EXCLUDES 1   supracondylar fracture with intracondylar extension of lower end of femur (S72.46-)

   1 √7ᵗʰ **S72.451** Displaced supracondylar fracture without intracondylar extension of lower end of right femur

   1 √7ᵗʰ **S72.452** Displaced supracondylar fracture without intracondylar extension of lower end of left femur

   √7ᵗʰ **S72.453** Displaced supracondylar fracture without intracondylar extension of lower end of unspecified femur ▽

   1 √7ᵗʰ **S72.454** Nondisplaced supracondylar fracture without intracondylar extension of lower end of right femur

   1 √7ᵗʰ **S72.455** Nondisplaced supracondylar fracture without intracondylar extension of lower end of left femur

   √7ᵗʰ **S72.456** Nondisplaced supracondylar fracture without intracondylar extension of lower end of unspecified femur ▽

√6ᵗʰ **S72.46** Supracondylar fracture with intracondylar extension of lower end of femur
   EXCLUDES 1   supracondylar fracture without intracondylar extension of lower end of femur (S72.45-)

   1 √7ᵗʰ **S72.461** Displaced supracondylar fracture with intracondylar extension of lower end of right femur

   1 √7ᵗʰ **S72.462** Displaced supracondylar fracture with intracondylar extension of lower end of left femur

   √7ᵗʰ **S72.463** Displaced supracondylar fracture with intracondylar extension of lower end of unspecified femur ▽

   1 √7ᵗʰ **S72.464** Nondisplaced supracondylar fracture with intracondylar extension of lower end of right femur

   1 √7ᵗʰ **S72.465** Nondisplaced supracondylar fracture with intracondylar extension of lower end of left femur

   √7ᵗʰ **S72.466** Nondisplaced supracondylar fracture with intracondylar extension of lower end of unspecified femur ▽

√6ᵗʰ **S72.47** Torus fracture of lower end of femur

> The appropriate 7th character is to be added to all codes in subcategory S72.47.
> A   initial encounter for closed fracture
> D   subsequent encounter for fracture with routine healing
> G   subsequent encounter for fracture with delayed healing
> K   subsequent encounter for fracture with nonunion
> P   subsequent encounter for fracture with malunion
> S   sequela

   1 √7ᵗʰ **S72.471** Torus fracture of lower end of right femur

   1 √7ᵗʰ **S72.472** Torus fracture of lower end of left femur

   √7ᵗʰ **S72.479** Torus fracture of lower end of unspecified femur ▽

√6ᵗʰ **S72.49** Other fracture of lower end of femur

   1 √7ᵗʰ **S72.491** Other fracture of lower end of right femur

   1 √7ᵗʰ **S72.492** Other fracture of lower end of left femur

   √7ᵗʰ **S72.499** Other fracture of lower end of unspecified femur ▽

√5ᵗʰ **S72.8** Other fracture of femur

√6ᵗʰ **S72.8X** Other fracture of femur

   1 √7ᵗʰ **S72.8X1** Other fracture of right femur

   1 √7ᵗʰ **S72.8X2** Other fracture of left femur

   √7ᵗʰ **S72.8X9** Other fracture of unspecified femur ▽

---

1   Case-mix diagnosis with 7th character indicating subsequent encounter.

Ⓝ Newborn: 0   Ⓟ Pediatric: 0-17   Ⓜ Maternity: 12-55   Ⓐ Adult: 15-124   **NRS** Nonroutine supply Dx   **NC Dx** Noncancer Dx   **PDx** Primary Dx   ▶◀ Revised Text   ● New Code   ▲ Revised Title

1006   ICD-10-CM 2018

✓5ᵗʰ S72.9 Unspecified fracture of femur
Fracture of thigh NOS
Fracture of upper leg NOS
EXCLUDES 1   fracture of hip NOS (S72.00-, S72.01-)

✓x7ᵗʰ **S72.90 Unspecified fracture of unspecified femur** ▽
AHA: 2012, 4Q, 93

¹ ✓x7ᵗʰ **S72.91 Unspecified fracture of right femur** ▽

¹ ✓x7ᵗʰ **S72.92 Unspecified fracture of left femur** ▽

✓4ᵗʰ S73 Dislocation and sprain of joint and ligaments of hip
INCLUDES   avulsion of joint or ligament of hip
laceration of cartilage, joint or ligament of hip
sprain of cartilage, joint or ligament of hip
traumatic hemarthrosis of joint or ligament of hip
traumatic rupture of joint or ligament of hip
traumatic subluxation of joint or ligament of hip
traumatic tear of joint or ligament of hip

Code also any associated open wound
EXCLUDES 2   strain of muscle, fascia and tendon of hip and thigh (S76.-)

The appropriate 7th character is to be added to each code from
category S73.
A   initial encounter
D   subsequent encounter
S   sequela

✓5ᵗʰ S73.0 Subluxation and dislocation of hip
EXCLUDES 2   dislocation and subluxation of hip prosthesis (T84.020,
T84.021)

✓6ᵗʰ S73.00 Unspecified subluxation and dislocation of hip
Dislocation of hip NOS
Subluxation of hip NOS

✓7ᵗʰ **S73.001 Unspecified subluxation of right hip** ▽

✓7ᵗʰ **S73.002 Unspecified subluxation of left hip** ▽

✓7ᵗʰ **S73.003 Unspecified subluxation of unspecified hip** ▽

✓7ᵗʰ **S73.004 Unspecified dislocation of right hip** ▽

¹ ✓7ᵗʰ **S73.005 Unspecified dislocation of left hip** ▽

✓7ᵗʰ **S73.006 Unspecified dislocation of unspecified hip** ▽

✓6ᵗʰ S73.01 Posterior subluxation and dislocation of hip

¹ ✓7ᵗʰ **S73.011 Posterior subluxation of right hip**

¹ ✓7ᵗʰ **S73.012 Posterior subluxation of left hip**

✓7ᵗʰ **S73.013 Posterior subluxation of unspecified hip** ▽

¹ ✓7ᵗʰ **S73.014 Posterior dislocation of right hip**

¹ ✓7ᵗʰ **S73.015 Posterior dislocation of left hip**

✓7ᵗʰ **S73.016 Posterior dislocation of unspecified hip** ▽

✓6ᵗʰ S73.02 Obturator subluxation and dislocation of hip

¹ ✓7ᵗʰ **S73.021 Obturator subluxation of right hip**

¹ ✓7ᵗʰ **S73.022 Obturator subluxation of left hip**

✓7ᵗʰ **S73.023 Obturator subluxation of unspecified hip** ▽

¹ ✓7ᵗʰ **S73.024 Obturator dislocation of right hip**

¹ ✓7ᵗʰ **S73.025 Obturator dislocation of left hip**

✓7ᵗʰ **S73.026 Obturator dislocation of unspecified hip** ▽

▲ **✓6ᵗʰ S73.03 Other anterior subluxation and dislocation of hip**

¹ ✓7ᵗʰ **S73.031 Other anterior subluxation of right hip**

¹ ✓7ᵗʰ **S73.032 Other anterior subluxation of left hip**

✓7ᵗʰ **S73.033 Other anterior subluxation of unspecified hip** ▽

¹ ✓7ᵗʰ **S73.034 Other anterior dislocation of right hip**

¹ ✓7ᵗʰ **S73.035 Other anterior dislocation of left hip**

✓7ᵗʰ **S73.036 Other anterior dislocation of unspecified hip** ▽

▲ **✓6ᵗʰ S73.04 Central subluxation and dislocation of hip**

¹ ✓7ᵗʰ **S73.041 Central subluxation of right hip**

¹ ✓7ᵗʰ **S73.042 Central subluxation of left hip**

✓7ᵗʰ **S73.043 Central subluxation of unspecified hip** ▽

¹ ✓7ᵗʰ **S73.044 Central dislocation of right hip**

¹ ✓7ᵗʰ **S73.045 Central dislocation of left hip**

✓7ᵗʰ **S73.046 Central dislocation of unspecified hip** ▽

✓5ᵗʰ S73.1 Sprain of hip
AHA: 2014, 4Q, 25

✓6ᵗʰ S73.10 Unspecified sprain of hip

✓7ᵗʰ **S73.101 Unspecified sprain of right hip** ▽

✓7ᵗʰ **S73.102 Unspecified sprain of left hip** ▽

✓7ᵗʰ **S73.109 Unspecified sprain of unspecified hip** ▽

✓6ᵗʰ S73.11 Iliofemoral ligament sprain of hip

✓7ᵗʰ **S73.111 Iliofemoral ligament sprain of right hip**

✓7ᵗʰ **S73.112 Iliofemoral ligament sprain of left hip**

✓7ᵗʰ **S73.119 Iliofemoral ligament sprain of unspecified hip**

✓6ᵗʰ S73.12 Ischiocapsular (ligament) sprain of hip

✓7ᵗʰ **S73.121 Ischiocapsular ligament sprain of right hip**

✓7ᵗʰ **S73.122 Ischiocapsular ligament sprain of left hip**

✓7ᵗʰ **S73.129 Ischiocapsular ligament sprain of unspecified hip** ▽

✓6ᵗʰ S73.19 Other sprain of hip

✓7ᵗʰ **S73.191 Other sprain of right hip**

✓7ᵗʰ **S73.192 Other sprain of left hip**

✓7ᵗʰ **S73.199 Other sprain of unspecified hip** ▽

✓4ᵗʰ S74 Injury of nerves at hip and thigh level
Code also any associated open wound (S71.-)
EXCLUDES 2   injury of nerves at ankle and foot level (S94.-)
injury of nerves at lower leg level (S84.-)

The appropriate 7th character is to be added to each code from
category S74.
A   initial encounter
D   subsequent encounter
S   sequela

✓5ᵗʰ S74.0 Injury of sciatic nerve at hip and thigh level

✓x7ᵗʰ **S74.00 Injury of sciatic nerve at hip and thigh level, unspecified leg** ▽

² ✓x7ᵗʰ **S74.01 Injury of sciatic nerve at hip and thigh level, right leg**

² ✓x7ᵗʰ **S74.02 Injury of sciatic nerve at hip and thigh level, left leg**

✓5ᵗʰ S74.1 Injury of femoral nerve at hip and thigh level

✓x7ᵗʰ **S74.10 Injury of femoral nerve at hip and thigh level, unspecified leg** ▽

² ✓x7ᵗʰ **S74.11 Injury of femoral nerve at hip and thigh level, right leg**

² ✓x7ᵗʰ **S74.12 Injury of femoral nerve at hip and thigh level, left leg**

✓5ᵗʰ S74.2 Injury of cutaneous sensory nerve at hip and thigh level

✓x7ᵗʰ **S74.20 Injury of cutaneous sensory nerve at hip and thigh level, unspecified leg** ▽

² ✓x7ᵗʰ **S74.21 Injury of cutaneous sensory nerve at hip and high level, right leg**

² ✓x7ᵗʰ **S74.22 Injury of cutaneous sensory nerve at hip and thigh level, left leg**

✓5ᵗʰ S74.8 Injury of other nerves at hip and thigh level

✓6ᵗʰ S74.8X Injury of other nerves at hip and thigh level

² ✓7ᵗʰ **S74.8X1 Injury of other nerves at hip and thigh level, right leg**

² ✓7ᵗʰ **S74.8X2 Injury of other nerves at hip and thigh level, left leg**

✓7ᵗʰ **S74.8X9 Injury of other nerves at hip and thigh level, unspecified leg** ▽

✓5ᵗʰ S74.9 Injury of unspecified nerve at hip and thigh level

✓x7ᵗʰ **S74.90 Injury of unspecified nerve at hip and thigh level, unspecified leg** ▽

² ✓x7ᵗʰ **S74.91 Injury of unspecified nerve at hip and thigh level, right leg** ▽

² ✓x7ᵗʰ **S74.92 Injury of unspecified nerve at hip and thigh level, left leg** ▽

---

¹ Case-mix diagnosis with 7th character indicating subsequent encounter.
² Case-mix diagnosis with 7th character indicating subsequent encounter or sequela.

Chapter 19. Injury, Poisoning and Certain Other Consequences of External Causes

☑4ᵗʰ S75 Injury of blood vessels at hip and thigh level

Code also any associated open wound (S71.-)

EXCLUDES 2   *injury of blood vessels at lower leg level (S85.-)*
injury of popliteal artery (S85.0)

The appropriate 7th character is to be added to each code from category S75.

A   initial encounter
D   subsequent encounter
S   sequela

☑5ᵗʰ S75.0 Injury of femoral artery

   ☑6ᵗʰ S75.00 Unspecified injury of femoral artery

     ☑7ᵗʰ **S75.001 Unspecified injury of femoral artery, right leg** ▽

     ☑7ᵗʰ **S75.002 Unspecified injury of femoral artery, left leg** ▽

     ☑7ᵗʰ **S75.009 Unspecified injury of femoral artery, unspecified leg** ▽

   ☑6ᵗʰ S75.01 Minor laceration of femoral artery

     Incomplete transection of femoral artery
     Laceration of femoral artery NOS
     Superficial laceration of femoral artery

     ☑7ᵗʰ **S75.011 Minor laceration of femoral artery, right leg**

     ☑7ᵗʰ **S75.012 Minor laceration of femoral artery, left leg**

     ☑7ᵗʰ **S75.019 Minor laceration of femoral artery, unspecified leg** ▽

   ☑6ᵗʰ S75.02 Major laceration of femoral artery

     Complete transection of femoral artery
     Traumatic rupture of femoral artery

     ☑7ᵗʰ **S75.021 Major laceration of femoral artery, right leg**

     ☑7ᵗʰ **S75.022 Major laceration of femoral artery, left leg**

     ☑7ᵗʰ **S75.029 Major laceration of femoral artery, unspecified leg** ▽

   ☑6ᵗʰ S75.09 Other specified injury of femoral artery

     ☑7ᵗʰ **S75.091 Other specified injury of femoral artery, right leg**

     ☑7ᵗʰ **S75.092 Other specified injury of femoral artery, left leg**

     ☑7ᵗʰ **S75.099 Other specified injury of femoral artery, unspecified leg** ▽

☑5ᵗʰ S75.1 Injury of femoral vein at hip and thigh level

   ☑6ᵗʰ S75.10 Unspecified injury of femoral vein at hip and thigh level

     ☑7ᵗʰ **S75.101 Unspecified injury of femoral vein at hip and thigh level, right leg** ▽

     ☑7ᵗʰ **S75.102 Unspecified injury of femoral vein at hip and thigh level, left leg** ▽

     ☑7ᵗʰ **S75.109 Unspecified injury of femoral vein at hip and thigh level, unspecified leg** ▽

   ☑6ᵗʰ S75.11 Minor laceration of femoral vein at hip and thigh level

     Incomplete transection of femoral vein at hip and thigh level
     Laceration of femoral vein at hip and thigh level NOS
     Superficial laceration of femoral vein at hip and thigh level

     ☑7ᵗʰ **S75.111 Minor laceration of femoral vein at hip and thigh level, right leg**

     ☑7ᵗʰ **S75.112 Minor laceration of femoral vein at hip and thigh level, left leg**

     ☑7ᵗʰ **S75.119 Minor laceration of femoral vein at hip and thigh level, unspecified leg** ▽

   ☑6ᵗʰ S75.12 Major laceration of femoral vein at hip and thigh level

     Complete transection of femoral vein at hip and thigh level
     Traumatic rupture of femoral vein at hip and thigh level

     ☑7ᵗʰ **S75.121 Major laceration of femoral vein at hip and thigh level, right leg**

     ☑7ᵗʰ **S75.122 Major laceration of femoral vein at hip and thigh level, left leg**

     ☑7ᵗʰ **S75.129 Major laceration of femoral vein at hip and thigh level, unspecified leg** ▽

   ☑6ᵗʰ S75.19 Other specified injury of femoral vein at hip and thigh level

     ☑7ᵗʰ **S75.191 Other specified injury of femoral vein at hip and thigh level, right leg**

     ☑7ᵗʰ **S75.192 Other specified injury of femoral vein at hip and thigh level, left leg**

     ☑7ᵗʰ **S75.199 Other specified injury of femoral vein at hip and thigh level, unspecified leg** ▽

☑5ᵗʰ S75.2 Injury of greater saphenous vein at hip and thigh level

EXCLUDES 1   *greater saphenous vein NOS (S85.3)*

   ☑6ᵗʰ S75.20 Unspecified injury of greater saphenous vein at hip and thigh level

     ☑7ᵗʰ **S75.201 Unspecified injury of greater saphenous vein at hip and thigh level, right leg** ▽

     ☑7ᵗʰ **S75.202 Unspecified injury of greater saphenous vein at hip and thigh level, left leg** ▽

     ☑7ᵗʰ **S75.209 Unspecified injury of greater saphenous vein at hip and thigh level, unspecified leg** ▽

   ☑6ᵗʰ S75.21 Minor laceration of greater saphenous vein at hip and thigh level

     Incomplete transection of greater saphenous vein at hip and thigh level
     Laceration of greater saphenous vein at hip and thigh level NOS
     Superficial laceration of greater saphenous vein at hip and thigh level

     ☑7ᵗʰ **S75.211 Minor laceration of greater saphenous vein at hip and thigh level, right leg**

     ☑7ᵗʰ **S75.212 Minor laceration of greater saphenous vein at hip and thigh level, left leg**

     ☑7ᵗʰ **S75.219 Minor laceration of greater saphenous vein at hip and thigh level, unspecified leg** ▽

   ☑6ᵗʰ S75.22 Major laceration of greater saphenous vein at hip and thigh level

     Complete transection of greater saphenous vein at hip and thigh level
     Traumatic rupture of greater saphenous vein at hip and thigh level

     ☑7ᵗʰ **S75.221 Major laceration of greater saphenous vein at hip and thigh level, right leg**

     ☑7ᵗʰ **S75.222 Major laceration of greater saphenous vein at hip and thigh level, left leg**

     ☑7ᵗʰ **S75.229 Major laceration of greater saphenous vein at hip and thigh level, unspecified leg** ▽

   ☑6ᵗʰ S75.29 Other specified injury of greater saphenous vein at hip and thigh level

     ☑7ᵗʰ **S75.291 Other specified injury of greater saphenous vein at hip and thigh level, right leg**

     ☑7ᵗʰ **S75.292 Other specified injury of greater saphenous vein at hip and thigh level, left leg**

     ☑7ᵗʰ **S75.299 Other specified injury of greater saphenous vein at hip and thigh level, unspecified leg** ▽

☑5ᵗʰ S75.8 Injury of other blood vessels at hip and thigh level

   ☑6ᵗʰ S75.80 Unspecified injury of other blood vessels at hip and thigh level

     ☑7ᵗʰ **S75.801 Unspecified injury of other blood vessels at hip and thigh level, right leg** ▽

     ☑7ᵗʰ **S75.802 Unspecified injury of other blood vessels at hip and thigh level, left leg** ▽

     ☑7ᵗʰ **S75.809 Unspecified injury of other blood vessels at hip and thigh level, unspecified leg** ▽

   ☑6ᵗʰ S75.81 Laceration of other blood vessels at hip and thigh level

     ☑7ᵗʰ **S75.811 Laceration of other blood vessels at hip and thigh level, right leg**

     ☑7ᵗʰ **S75.812 Laceration of other blood vessels at hip and thigh level, left leg**

     ☑7ᵗʰ **S75.819 Laceration of other blood vessels at hip and thigh level, unspecified leg** ▽

Ⓝ Newborn: 0   Ⓟ Pediatric: 0-17   Ⓜ Maternity: 12-55   Ⓐ Adult: 15-124   **NRS** Nonroutine supply Dx   **NCDx** Noncancer Dx   **PDx** Primary Dx   ▶◀ Revised Text   ● New Code   ▲ Revised Title

✓6th **S75.89** Other specified injury of other blood vessels at hip and thigh level

✓7th **S75.891** Other specified injury of other blood vessels at hip and thigh level, right leg

✓7th **S75.892** Other specified injury of other blood vessels at hip and thigh level, left leg

✓7th **S75.899** Other specified injury of other blood vessels at hip and thigh level, unspecified leg ▽

✓5th **S75.9** Injury of unspecified blood vessel at hip and thigh level

✓6th **S75.90** Unspecified injury of unspecified blood vessel at hip and thigh level

✓7th **S75.901** Unspecified injury of unspecified blood vessel at hip and thigh level, right leg ▽

✓7th **S75.902** Unspecified injury of unspecified blood vessel at hip and thigh level, left leg ▽

✓7th **S75.909** Unspecified injury of unspecified blood vessel at hip and thigh level, unspecified leg ▽

✓6th **S75.91** Laceration of unspecified blood vessel at hip and thigh level

✓7th **S75.911** Laceration of unspecified blood vessel at hip and thigh level, right leg ▽

✓7th **S75.912** Laceration of unspecified blood vessel at hip and thigh level, left leg ▽

✓7th **S75.919** Laceration of unspecified blood vessel at hip and thigh level, unspecified leg ▽

✓6th **S75.99** Other specified injury of unspecified blood vessel at hip and thigh level

✓7th **S75.991** Other specified injury of unspecified blood vessel at hip and thigh level, right leg ▽

✓7th **S75.992** Other specified injury of unspecified blood vessel at hip and thigh level, left leg ▽

✓7th **S75.999** Other specified injury of unspecified blood vessel at hip and thigh level, unspecified leg ▽

✓4th **S76** Injury of muscle, fascia and tendon at hip and thigh level

Code also any associated open wound (S71.-)

EXCLUDES 2 injury of muscle, fascia and tendon at lower leg level (S86)
sprain of joint and ligament of hip (S73.1)

TIP: Refer to the Muscle/Tendon table at the beginning of this chapter.

The appropriate 7th character is to be added to each code from category S76.
A initial encounter
D subsequent encounter
S sequela

✓5th **S76.0** Injury of muscle, fascia and tendon of hip

✓6th **S76.00** Unspecified injury of muscle, fascia and tendon of hip

✓7th **S76.001** Unspecified injury of muscle, fascia and tendon of right hip ▽

✓7th **S76.002** Unspecified injury of muscle, fascia and tendon of left hip ▽

✓7th **S76.009** Unspecified injury of muscle, fascia and tendon of unspecified hip ▽

✓6th **S76.01** Strain of muscle, fascia and tendon of hip

✓7th **S76.011** Strain of muscle, fascia and tendon of right hip

✓7th **S76.012** Strain of muscle, fascia and tendon of left hip

✓7th **S76.019** Strain of muscle, fascia and tendon of unspecified hip ▽

✓6th **S76.02** Laceration of muscle, fascia and tendon of hip

4,5 ✓7th **S76.021** Laceration of muscle, fascia and tendon of right hip NRS

4,5 ✓7th **S76.022** Laceration of muscle, fascia and tendon of left hip NRS

✓7th **S76.029** Laceration of muscle, fascia and tendon of unspecified hip ▽

✓6th **S76.09** Other specified injury of muscle, fascia and tendon of hip

✓7th **S76.091** Other specified injury of muscle, fascia and tendon of right hip

✓7th **S76.092** Other specified injury of muscle, fascia and tendon of left hip

✓7th **S76.099** Other specified injury of muscle, fascia and tendon of unspecified hip ▽

✓5th **S76.1** Injury of quadriceps muscle, fascia and tendon
Injury of patellar ligament (tendon)

✓6th **S76.10** Unspecified injury of quadriceps muscle, fascia and tendon

✓7th **S76.101** Unspecified injury of right quadriceps muscle, fascia and tendon ▽

✓7th **S76.102** Unspecified injury of left quadriceps muscle, fascia and tendon ▽

✓7th **S76.109** Unspecified injury of unspecified quadriceps muscle, fascia and tendon ▽

✓6th **S76.11** Strain of quadriceps muscle, fascia and tendon

✓7th **S76.111** Strain of right quadriceps muscle, fascia and tendon

✓7th **S76.112** Strain of left quadriceps muscle, fascia and tendon

✓7th **S76.119** Strain of unspecified quadriceps muscle, fascia and tendon ▽

✓6th **S76.12** Laceration of quadriceps muscle, fascia and tendon

4,5 ✓7th **S76.121** Laceration of right quadriceps muscle, fascia and tendon NRS

4,5 ✓7th **S76.122** Laceration of left quadriceps muscle, fascia and tendon NRS

✓7th **S76.129** Laceration of unspecified quadriceps muscle, fascia and tendon ▽

✓6th **S76.19** Other specified injury of quadriceps muscle, fascia and tendon

✓7th **S76.191** Other specified injury of right quadriceps muscle, fascia and tendon

✓7th **S76.192** Other specified injury of left quadriceps muscle, fascia and tendon

✓7th **S76.199** Other specified injury of unspecified quadriceps muscle, fascia and tendon ▽

✓5th **S76.2** Injury of adductor muscle, fascia and tendon of thigh

✓6th **S76.20** Unspecified injury of adductor muscle, fascia and tendon of thigh

✓7th **S76.201** Unspecified injury of adductor muscle, fascia and tendon of right thigh ▽

✓7th **S76.202** Unspecified injury of adductor muscle, fascia and tendon of left thigh ▽

✓7th **S76.209** Unspecified injury of adductor muscle, fascia and tendon of unspecified thigh ▽

✓6th **S76.21** Strain of adductor muscle, fascia and tendon of thigh

✓7th **S76.211** Strain of adductor muscle, fascia and tendon of right thigh

✓7th **S76.212** Strain of adductor muscle, fascia and tendon of left thigh

✓7th **S76.219** Strain of adductor muscle, fascia and tendon of unspecified thigh ▽

✓6th **S76.22** Laceration of adductor muscle, fascia and tendon of thigh

4,5 ✓7th **S76.221** Laceration of adductor muscle, fascia and tendon of right thigh NRS

4,5 ✓7th **S76.222** Laceration of adductor muscle, fascia and tendon of left thigh NRS

✓7th **S76.229** Laceration of adductor muscle, fascia and tendon of unspecified thigh ▽

✓6th **S76.29** Other injury of adductor muscle, fascia and tendon of thigh

✓7th **S76.291** Other injury of adductor muscle, fascia and tendon of right thigh

✓7th **S76.292** Other injury of adductor muscle, fascia and tendon of left thigh

✓7th **S76.299** Other injury of adductor muscle, fascia and tendon of unspecified thigh ▽

---

4 Case-mix diagnosis with 7th character indicating initial or subsequent encounter.
5 NRS supply diagnosis with 7th character indicating initial or subsequent encounter.

✓ Additional Character Req   ✓x7th Placeholder Alert   Case-Mix Diagnosis   Manifestation   ▽ Unspecified Dx   EXCLUDES 1 Not coded here   EXCLUDES 2 Not included here

✓5ᵗʰ **S76.3** Injury of muscle, fascia and tendon of the posterior muscle group at thigh level

  ✓6ᵗʰ **S76.30** Unspecified injury of muscle, fascia and tendon of the posterior muscle group at thigh level

    ✓7ᵗʰ **S76.301** Unspecified injury of muscle, fascia and tendon of the posterior muscle group at thigh level, right thigh ▽

    ✓7ᵗʰ **S76.302** Unspecified injury of muscle, fascia and tendon of the posterior muscle group at thigh level, left thigh ▽

    ✓7ᵗʰ **S76.309** Unspecified injury of muscle, fascia and tendon of the posterior muscle group at thigh level, unspecified thigh ▽

  ✓6ᵗʰ **S76.31** Strain of muscle, fascia and tendon of the posterior muscle group at thigh level

    ✓7ᵗʰ **S76.311** Strain of muscle, fascia and tendon of the posterior muscle group at thigh level, right thigh

    ✓7ᵗʰ **S76.312** Strain of muscle, fascia and tendon of the posterior muscle group at thigh level, left thigh

    ✓7ᵗʰ **S76.319** Strain of muscle, fascia and tendon of the posterior muscle group at thigh level, unspecified thigh ▽

  ✓6ᵗʰ **S76.32** Laceration of muscle, fascia and tendon of the posterior muscle group at thigh level

    4,5 ✓7ᵗʰ **S76.321** Laceration of muscle, fascia and tendon of the posterior muscle group at thigh level, right thigh   **NRS**

    4,5 ✓7ᵗʰ **S76.322** Laceration of muscle, fascia and tendon of the posterior muscle group at thigh level, left thigh   **NRS**

    ✓7ᵗʰ **S76.329** Laceration of muscle, fascia and tendon of the posterior muscle group at thigh level, unspecified thigh ▽

  ✓6ᵗʰ **S76.39** Other specified injury of muscle, fascia and tendon of the posterior muscle group at thigh level

    ✓7ᵗʰ **S76.391** Other specified injury of muscle, fascia and tendon of the posterior muscle group at thigh level, right thigh

    ✓7ᵗʰ **S76.392** Other specified injury of muscle, fascia and tendon of the posterior muscle group at thigh level, left thigh

    ✓7ᵗʰ **S76.399** Other specified injury of muscle, fascia and tendon of the posterior muscle group at thigh level, unspecified thigh ▽

✓5ᵗʰ **S76.8** Injury of other specified muscles, fascia and tendons at thigh level

  ✓6ᵗʰ **S76.80** Unspecified injury of other specified muscles, fascia and tendons at thigh level

    ✓7ᵗʰ **S76.801** Unspecified injury of other specified muscles, fascia and tendons at thigh level, right thigh ▽

    ✓7ᵗʰ **S76.802** Unspecified injury of other specified muscles, fascia and tendons at thigh level, left thigh ▽

    ✓7ᵗʰ **S76.809** Unspecified injury of other specified muscles, fascia and tendons at thigh level, unspecified thigh ▽

  ✓6ᵗʰ **S76.81** Strain of other specified muscles, fascia and tendons at thigh level

    ✓7ᵗʰ **S76.811** Strain of other specified muscles, fascia and tendons at thigh level, right thigh

    ✓7ᵗʰ **S76.812** Strain of other specified muscles, fascia and tendons at thigh level, left thigh

    ✓7ᵗʰ **S76.819** Strain of other specified muscles, fascia and tendons at thigh level, unspecified thigh ▽

  ✓6ᵗʰ **S76.82** Laceration of other specified muscles, fascia and tendons at thigh level

    4,5 ✓7ᵗʰ **S76.821** Laceration of other specified muscles, fascia and tendons at thigh level, right thigh   **NRS**

    4,5 ✓7ᵗʰ **S76.822** Laceration of other specified muscles, fascia and tendons at thigh level, left thigh   **NRS**

    ✓7ᵗʰ **S76.829** Laceration of other specified muscles, fascia and tendons at thigh level, unspecified thigh ▽

  ✓6ᵗʰ **S76.89** Other injury of other specified muscles, fascia and tendons at thigh level

    ✓7ᵗʰ **S76.891** Other injury of other specified muscles, fascia and tendons at thigh level, right thigh

    ✓7ᵗʰ **S76.892** Other injury of other specified muscles, fascia and tendons at thigh level, left thigh

    ✓7ᵗʰ **S76.899** Other injury of other specified muscles, fascia and tendons at thigh level, unspecified thigh ▽

✓5ᵗʰ **S76.9** Injury of unspecified muscles, fascia and tendons at thigh level

  ✓6ᵗʰ **S76.90** Unspecified injury of unspecified muscles, fascia and tendons at thigh level

    ✓7ᵗʰ **S76.901** Unspecified injury of unspecified muscles, fascia and tendons at thigh level, right thigh ▽

    ✓7ᵗʰ **S76.902** Unspecified injury of unspecified muscles, fascia and tendons at thigh level, left thigh ▽

    ✓7ᵗʰ **S76.909** Unspecified injury of unspecified muscles, fascia and tendons at thigh level, unspecified thigh ▽

  ✓6ᵗʰ **S76.91** Strain of unspecified muscles, fascia and tendons at thigh level

    ✓7ᵗʰ **S76.911** Strain of unspecified muscles, fascia and tendons at thigh level, right thigh ▽

    ✓7ᵗʰ **S76.912** Strain of unspecified muscles, fascia and tendons at thigh level, left thigh ▽

    ✓7ᵗʰ **S76.919** Strain of unspecified muscles, fascia and tendons at thigh level, unspecified thigh ▽

  ✓6ᵗʰ **S76.92** Laceration of unspecified muscles, fascia and tendons at thigh level

    4,5 ✓7ᵗʰ **S76.921** Laceration of unspecified muscles, fascia and tendons at thigh level, right thigh   **NRS** ▽

    4,5 ✓7ᵗʰ **S76.922** Laceration of unspecified muscles, fascia and tendons at thigh level, left thigh   **NRS** ▽

    ✓7ᵗʰ **S76.929** Laceration of unspecified muscles, fascia and tendons at thigh level, unspecified thigh ▽

  ✓6ᵗʰ **S76.99** Other specified injury of unspecified muscles, fascia and tendons at thigh level

    ✓7ᵗʰ **S76.991** Other specified injury of unspecified muscles, fascia and tendons at thigh level, right thigh ▽

    ✓7ᵗʰ **S76.992** Other specified injury of unspecified muscles, fascia and tendons at thigh level, left thigh ▽

    ✓7ᵗʰ **S76.999** Other specified injury of unspecified muscles, fascia and tendons at thigh level, unspecified thigh ▽

✓4ᵗʰ **S77** Crushing injury of hip and thigh

  Use additional code(s) for all associated injuries

  EXCLUDES 2   crushing injury of ankle and foot (S97.-)
                 crushing injury of lower leg (S87.-)

> The appropriate 7th character is to be added to each code from category S77.
> A   initial encounter
> D   subsequent encounter
> S   sequela

  ✓5ᵗʰ **S77.0** Crushing injury of hip

    ✓×7ᵗʰ **S77.00** Crushing injury of unspecified hip ▽

    1 ✓×7ᵗʰ **S77.01** Crushing injury of right hip

    1 ✓×7ᵗʰ **S77.02** Crushing injury of left hip

---

1   Case-mix diagnosis with 7th character indicating subsequent encounter.
4   Case-mix diagnosis with 7th character indicating initial or subsequent encounter.
5   NRS supply diagnosis with 7th character indicating initial or subsequent encounter.

N Newborn: 0   P Pediatric: 0-17   M Maternity: 12-55   A Adult: 15-124   **NRS** Nonroutine supply Dx   **NC Dx** Noncancer Dx   **PDx** Primary Dx   ▶◀ Revised Text   ● New Code   ▲ Revised Title

✓5ᵗʰ **S77.1**   Crushing injury of thigh

   ✓x7ᵗʰ **S77.10**   Crushing injury of unspecified thigh   ▽

   ¹ ✓x7ᵗʰ **S77.11**   **Crushing injury of right thigh**

   ¹ ✓x7ᵗʰ **S77.12**   **Crushing injury of left thigh**

✓5ᵗʰ **S77.2**   Crushing injury of hip with thigh

   ✓x7ᵗʰ **S77.20**   Crushing injury of unspecified hip with thigh   ▽

   ¹ ✓x7ᵗʰ **S77.21**   **Crushing injury of right hip with thigh**

   ¹ ✓x7ᵗʰ **S77.22**   **Crushing injury of left hip with thigh**

✓4ᵗʰ **S78**   **Traumatic amputation of hip and thigh**

   An amputation not identified as partial or complete should be coded to complete.

   EXCLUDES1   *traumatic amputation of knee (S88.0-)*

   The appropriate 7th character is to be added to each code from category S78.
   A   initial encounter
   D   subsequent encounter
   S   sequela

   ✓5ᵗʰ **S78.0**   Traumatic amputation at hip joint

     ✓6ᵗʰ **S78.01**   Complete traumatic amputation at hip joint

      ⁴,⁵ ✓7ᵗʰ **S78.011**   **Complete traumatic amputation at right hip joint**   NRS

      ⁴,⁵ ✓7ᵗʰ **S78.012**   **Complete traumatic amputation at left hip joint**   NRS

      ✓7ᵗʰ **S78.019**   Complete traumatic amputation at unspecified hip joint   NRS ▽

     ✓6ᵗʰ **S78.02**   Partial traumatic amputation at hip joint

      ⁴,⁵ ✓7ᵗʰ **S78.021**   **Partial traumatic amputation at right hip joint**   NRS

      ⁴,⁵ ✓7ᵗʰ **S78.022**   **Partial traumatic amputation at left hip joint**   NRS

      ✓7ᵗʰ **S78.029**   Partial traumatic amputation at unspecified hip joint   NRS ▽

   ✓5ᵗʰ **S78.1**   Traumatic amputation at level between hip and knee

     EXCLUDES1   *traumatic amputation of knee (S88.0-)*

     ✓6ᵗʰ **S78.11**   Complete traumatic amputation at level between hip and knee

      ⁴,⁵ ✓7ᵗʰ **S78.111**   **Complete traumatic amputation at level between right hip and knee**   NRS

      ⁴,⁵ ✓7ᵗʰ **S78.112**   **Complete traumatic amputation at level between left hip and knee**   NRS

      ✓7ᵗʰ **S78.119**   Complete traumatic amputation at level between unspecified hip and knee   ▽

     ✓6ᵗʰ **S78.12**   Partial traumatic amputation at level between hip and knee

      ⁴,⁵ ✓7ᵗʰ **S78.121**   **Partial traumatic amputation at level between right hip and knee**   NRS

      ⁴,⁵ ✓7ᵗʰ **S78.122**   **Partial traumatic amputation at level between left hip and knee**   NRS

      ✓7ᵗʰ **S78.129**   Partial traumatic amputation at level between unspecified hip and knee   ▽

   ✓5ᵗʰ **S78.9**   Traumatic amputation of hip and thigh, level unspecified

     ✓6ᵗʰ **S78.91**   Complete traumatic amputation of hip and thigh, level unspecified

      ⁴,⁵ ✓7ᵗʰ **S78.911**   **Complete traumatic amputation of right hip and thigh, level unspecified**   NRS ▽

      ⁴,⁵ ✓7ᵗʰ **S78.912**   **Complete traumatic amputation of left hip and thigh, level unspecified**   NRS ▽

      ⁵ ✓7ᵗʰ **S78.919**   Complete traumatic amputation of unspecified hip and thigh, level unspecified   NRS ▽

     ✓6ᵗʰ **S78.92**   Partial traumatic amputation of hip and thigh, level unspecified

      ⁴,⁵ ✓7ᵗʰ **S78.921**   **Partial traumatic amputation of right hip and thigh, level unspecified**   NRS ▽

      ⁴,⁵ ✓7ᵗʰ **S78.922**   **Partial traumatic amputation of left hip and thigh, level unspecified**   NRS ▽

      ✓7ᵗʰ **S78.929**   Partial traumatic amputation of unspecified hip and thigh, level unspecified   ▽

✓4ᵗʰ **S79**   **Other and unspecified injuries of hip and thigh**

   NOTE   A fracture not indicated as open or closed should be coded to closed.

   AHA: 2015, 3Q, 37-39

   TIP: The term "improper alignment" is not synonymous with malunion or nonunion of a fracture when noted in provider documentation.

   The appropriate 7th character is to be added to each code from subcategory S79.0 and S79.1
   A   initial encounter for closed fracture
   D   subsequent encounter for fracture with routine healing
   G   subsequent encounter for fracture with delayed healing
   K   subsequent encounter for fracture with nonunion
   P   subsequent encounter for fracture with malunion
   S   sequela

   ✓5ᵗʰ **S79.0**   Physeal fracture of upper end of femur

     EXCLUDES1   *apophyseal fracture of upper end of femur (S72.13-)*
     nontraumatic slipped upper femoral epiphysis (M93.0-)

     ✓6ᵗʰ **S79.00**   Unspecified physeal fracture of upper end of femur

      ¹ ✓7ᵗʰ **S79.001**   **Unspecified physeal fracture of upper end of right femur**   ▽

      ¹ ✓7ᵗʰ **S79.002**   **Unspecified physeal fracture of upper end of left femur**   ▽

      ✓7ᵗʰ **S79.009**   Unspecified physeal fracture of upper end of unspecified femur   ▽

     ✓6ᵗʰ **S79.01**   Salter-Harris Type I physeal fracture of upper end of femur

      Acute on chronic slipped capital femoral epiphysis (traumatic)
      Acute slipped capital femoral epiphysis (traumatic)
      Capital femoral epiphyseal fracture

      EXCLUDES1   *chronic slipped upper femoral epiphysis (nontraumatic) (M93.02-)*

      ¹ ✓7ᵗʰ **S79.011**   **Salter-Harris Type I physeal fracture of upper end of right femur**

      ¹ ✓7ᵗʰ **S79.012**   **Salter-Harris Type I physeal fracture of upper end of left femur**

      ✓7ᵗʰ **S79.019**   Salter-Harris Type I physeal fracture of upper end of unspecified femur   ▽

     ✓6ᵗʰ **S79.09**   Other physeal fracture of upper end of femur

      ¹ ✓7ᵗʰ **S79.091**   **Other physeal fracture of upper end of right femur**

      ¹ ✓7ᵗʰ **S79.092**   **Other physeal fracture of upper end of left femur**

      ✓7ᵗʰ **S79.099**   Other physeal fracture of upper end of unspecified femur   ▽

   ✓5ᵗʰ **S79.1**   Physeal fracture of lower end of femur

     ✓6ᵗʰ **S79.10**   Unspecified physeal fracture of lower end of femur

      ¹ ✓7ᵗʰ **S79.101**   **Unspecified physeal fracture of lower end of right femur**   ▽

      ¹ ✓7ᵗʰ **S79.102**   **Unspecified physeal fracture of lower end of left femur**   ▽

      ✓7ᵗʰ **S79.109**   Unspecified physeal fracture of lower end of unspecified femur   ▽

     ✓6ᵗʰ **S79.11**   Salter-Harris Type I physeal fracture of lower end of femur

      ¹ ✓7ᵗʰ **S79.111**   **Salter-Harris Type I physeal fracture of lower end of right femur**

      ¹ ✓7ᵗʰ **S79.112**   **Salter-Harris Type I physeal fracture of lower end of left femur**

      ✓7ᵗʰ **S79.119**   Salter-Harris Type I physeal fracture of lower end of unspecified femur   ▽

     ✓6ᵗʰ **S79.12**   Salter-Harris Type II physeal fracture of lower end of femur

      ¹ ✓7ᵗʰ **S79.121**   **Salter-Harris Type II physeal fracture of lower end of right femur**

      ¹ ✓7ᵗʰ **S79.122**   **Salter-Harris Type II physeal fracture of lower end of left femur**

      ✓7ᵗʰ **S79.129**   Salter-Harris Type II physeal fracture of lower end of unspecified femur   ▽

     ✓6ᵗʰ **S79.13**   Salter-Harris Type III physeal fracture of lower end of femur

      ¹ ✓7ᵗʰ **S79.131**   **Salter-Harris Type III physeal fracture of lower end of right femur**

---

1   Case-mix diagnosis with 7th character indicating subsequent encounter.
4   Case-mix diagnosis with 7th character indicating initial or subsequent encounter.
5   NRS supply diagnosis with 7th character indicating initial or subsequent encounter.

✓ Additional Character Req   ✓x7ᵗʰ Placeholder Alert   Case-Mix Diagnosis   Manifestation   ▽ Unspecified Dx   EXCLUDES1 Not coded here   EXCLUDES2 Not included here

1 √7ᵗʰ **S79.132** Salter-Harris Type III physeal fracture of lower end of left femur

√7ᵗʰ **S79.139** Salter-Harris Type III physeal fracture of lower end of unspecified femur ▽

√6ᵗʰ **S79.14** Salter-Harris Type IV physeal fracture of lower end of femur

1 √7ᵗʰ **S79.141** Salter-Harris Type IV physeal fracture of lower end of right femur

1 √7ᵗʰ **S79.142** Salter-Harris Type IV physeal fracture of lower end of left femur

√7ᵗʰ **S79.149** Salter-Harris Type IV physeal fracture of lower end of unspecified femur ▽

√6ᵗʰ **S79.19** Other physeal fracture of lower end of femur

1 √7ᵗʰ **S79.191** Other physeal fracture of lower end of right femur

1 √7ᵗʰ **S79.192** Other physeal fracture of lower end of left femur

√7ᵗʰ **S79.199** Other physeal fracture of lower end of unspecified femur ▽

√5ᵗʰ **S79.8** Other specified injuries of hip and thigh

> The appropriate 7th character is to be added to each code in subcategory S79.8.
> A   initial encounter
> D   subsequent encounter
> S   sequela

√6ᵗʰ **S79.81** Other specified injuries of hip

√7ᵗʰ **S79.811** Other specified injuries of right hip

√7ᵗʰ **S79.812** Other specified injuries of left hip

√7ᵗʰ **S79.819** Other specified injuries of unspecified hip ▽

√6ᵗʰ **S79.82** Other specified injuries of thigh

√7ᵗʰ **S79.821** Other specified injuries of right thigh

√7ᵗʰ **S79.822** Other specified injuries of left thigh

√7ᵗʰ **S79.829** Other specified injuries of unspecified thigh ▽

√5ᵗʰ **S79.9** Unspecified injury of hip and thigh

> The appropriate 7th character is to be added to each code in subcategory S79.9.
> A   initial encounter
> D   subsequent encounter
> S   sequela

√6ᵗʰ **S79.91** Unspecified injury of hip

√7ᵗʰ **S79.911** Unspecified injury of right hip ▽

√7ᵗʰ **S79.912** Unspecified injury of left hip ▽

√7ᵗʰ **S79.919** Unspecified injury of unspecified hip ▽

√6ᵗʰ **S79.92** Unspecified injury of thigh

√7ᵗʰ **S79.921** Unspecified injury of right thigh ▽

√7ᵗʰ **S79.922** Unspecified injury of left thigh ▽

√7ᵗʰ **S79.929** Unspecified injury of unspecified thigh ▽

Injuries to the knee and lower leg (S80-S89)

EXCLUDES 2   burns and corrosions (T20-T32)
> frostbite (T33-T34)
> injuries of ankle and foot, except fracture of ankle and malleolus (S90-S99)
> insect bite or sting, venomous (T63.4)

√4ᵗʰ **S80** Superficial injury of knee and lower leg

EXCLUDES 2   superficial injury of ankle and foot (S90.-)

> The appropriate 7th character is to be added to each code from category S80.
> A   initial encounter
> D   subsequent encounter
> S   sequela

√5ᵗʰ **S80.0** Contusion of knee

√×7ᵗʰ **S80.00** Contusion of unspecified knee ▽

√×7ᵗʰ **S80.01** Contusion of right knee

√×7ᵗʰ **S80.02** Contusion of left knee

√5ᵗʰ **S80.1** Contusion of lower leg

√×7ᵗʰ **S80.10** Contusion of unspecified lower leg ▽

√×7ᵗʰ **S80.11** Contusion of right lower leg

√×7ᵗʰ **S80.12** Contusion of left lower leg

√5ᵗʰ **S80.2** Other superficial injuries of knee

√6ᵗʰ **S80.21** Abrasion of knee

√7ᵗʰ **S80.211** Abrasion, right knee

√7ᵗʰ **S80.212** Abrasion, left knee

√7ᵗʰ **S80.219** Abrasion, unspecified knee ▽

√6ᵗʰ **S80.22** Blister (nonthermal) of knee

√7ᵗʰ **S80.221** Blister (nonthermal), right knee

√7ᵗʰ **S80.222** Blister (nonthermal), left knee

√7ᵗʰ **S80.229** Blister (nonthermal), unspecified knee ▽

√6ᵗʰ **S80.24** External constriction of knee

√7ᵗʰ **S80.241** External constriction, right knee

√7ᵗʰ **S80.242** External constriction, left knee

√7ᵗʰ **S80.249** External constriction, unspecified knee ▽

√6ᵗʰ **S80.25** Superficial foreign body of knee
Splinter in the knee

√7ᵗʰ **S80.251** Superficial foreign body, right knee

√7ᵗʰ **S80.252** Superficial foreign body, left knee

√7ᵗʰ **S80.259** Superficial foreign body, unspecified knee ▽

√6ᵗʰ **S80.26** Insect bite (nonvenomous) of knee

√7ᵗʰ **S80.261** Insect bite (nonvenomous), right knee

√7ᵗʰ **S80.262** Insect bite (nonvenomous), left knee

√7ᵗʰ **S80.269** Insect bite (nonvenomous), unspecified knee ▽

√6ᵗʰ **S80.27** Other superficial bite of knee
EXCLUDES 1   open bite of knee (S81.05-)

√7ᵗʰ **S80.271** Other superficial bite of right knee

√7ᵗʰ **S80.272** Other superficial bite of left knee

√7ᵗʰ **S80.279** Other superficial bite of unspecified knee ▽

√5ᵗʰ **S80.8** Other superficial injuries of lower leg

√6ᵗʰ **S80.81** Abrasion of lower leg

√7ᵗʰ **S80.811** Abrasion, right lower leg

√7ᵗʰ **S80.812** Abrasion, left lower leg

√7ᵗʰ **S80.819** Abrasion, unspecified lower leg ▽

√6ᵗʰ **S80.82** Blister (nonthermal) of lower leg

√7ᵗʰ **S80.821** Blister (nonthermal), right lower leg

√7ᵗʰ **S80.822** Blister (nonthermal), left lower leg

√7ᵗʰ **S80.829** Blister (nonthermal), unspecified lower leg ▽

√6ᵗʰ **S80.84** External constriction of lower leg

√7ᵗʰ **S80.841** External constriction, right lower leg

√7ᵗʰ **S80.842** External constriction, left lower leg

√7ᵗʰ **S80.849** External constriction, unspecified lower leg ▽

√6ᵗʰ **S80.85** Superficial foreign body of lower leg
Splinter in the lower leg

√7ᵗʰ **S80.851** Superficial foreign body, right lower leg

√7ᵗʰ **S80.852** Superficial foreign body, left lower leg

√7ᵗʰ **S80.859** Superficial foreign body, unspecified lower leg ▽

√6ᵗʰ **S80.86** Insect bite (nonvenomous) of lower leg

√7ᵗʰ **S80.861** Insect bite (nonvenomous), right lower leg

√7ᵗʰ **S80.862** Insect bite (nonvenomous), left lower leg

√7ᵗʰ **S80.869** Insect bite (nonvenomous), unspecified lower leg ▽

√6ᵗʰ **S80.87** Other superficial bite of lower leg
EXCLUDES 1   open bite of lower leg (S81.85-)

√7ᵗʰ **S80.871** Other superficial bite, right lower leg

√7ᵗʰ **S80.872** Other superficial bite, left lower leg

√7ᵗʰ **S80.879** Other superficial bite, unspecified lower leg ▽

√5ᵗʰ **S80.9** Unspecified superficial injury of knee and lower leg

√6ᵗʰ **S80.91** Unspecified superficial injury of knee

√7ᵗʰ **S80.911** Unspecified superficial injury of right knee ▽

---

1   Case-mix diagnosis with 7th character indicating subsequent encounter.

✓7ᵗʰ **S80.912** Unspecified superficial injury of left knee ▽

✓7ᵗʰ **S80.919** Unspecified superficial injury of unspecified knee ▽

✓6ᵗʰ **S80.92** Unspecified superficial injury of lower leg

  ✓7ᵗʰ **S80.921** Unspecified superficial injury of right lower leg ▽

  ✓7ᵗʰ **S80.922** Unspecified superficial injury of left lower leg ▽

  ✓7ᵗʰ **S80.929** Unspecified superficial injury of unspecified lower leg ▽

✓4ᵗʰ **S81** Open wound of knee and lower leg

Code also any associated wound infection

EXCLUDES 1   open fracture of knee and lower leg (S82.-)
        traumatic amputation of lower leg (S88.-)
EXCLUDES 2   open wound of ankle and foot (S91.-)

The appropriate 7th character is to be added to each code from category S81.
A   initial encounter
D   subsequent encounter
S   sequela

✓5ᵗʰ **S81.0** Open wound of knee

 ✓6ᵗʰ **S81.00** Unspecified open wound of knee

  5 ✓7ᵗʰ **S81.001** Unspecified open wound, right knee   NRS ▽

  5 ✓7ᵗʰ **S81.002** Unspecified open wound, left knee   NRS ▽

  ✓7ᵗʰ **S81.009** Unspecified open wound, unspecified knee ▽

 ✓6ᵗʰ **S81.01** Laceration without foreign body of knee

  4,5 ✓7ᵗʰ **S81.011** Laceration without foreign body, right knee NRS

  4,5 ✓7ᵗʰ **S81.012** Laceration without foreign body, left knee NRS

  ✓7ᵗʰ **S81.019** Laceration without foreign body, unspecified knee ▽

 ✓6ᵗʰ **S81.02** Laceration with foreign body of knee

  4,5 ✓7ᵗʰ **S81.021** Laceration with foreign body, right knee NRS

  4,5 ✓7ᵗʰ **S81.022** Laceration with foreign body, left knee NRS

  ✓7ᵗʰ **S81.029** Laceration with foreign body, unspecified knee ▽

 ✓6ᵗʰ **S81.03** Puncture wound without foreign body of knee

  4,5 ✓7ᵗʰ **S81.031** Puncture wound without foreign body, right knee NRS

  4,5 ✓7ᵗʰ **S81.032** Puncture wound without foreign body, left knee NRS

  ✓7ᵗʰ **S81.039** Puncture wound without foreign body, unspecified knee ▽

 ✓6ᵗʰ **S81.04** Puncture wound with foreign body of knee

  4,5 ✓7ᵗʰ **S81.041** Puncture wound with foreign body, right knee NRS

  4,5 ✓7ᵗʰ **S81.042** Puncture wound with foreign body, left knee NRS

  ✓7ᵗʰ **S81.049** Puncture wound with foreign body, unspecified knee ▽

 ✓6ᵗʰ **S81.05** Open bite of knee

Bite of knee NOS

EXCLUDES 1   superficial bite of knee (S80.27-)

  4,5 ✓7ᵗʰ **S81.051** Open bite, right knee NRS

  4,5 ✓7ᵗʰ **S81.052** Open bite, left knee NRS

  ✓7ᵗʰ **S81.059** Open bite, unspecified knee ▽

✓5ᵗʰ **S81.8** Open wound of lower leg

 ✓6ᵗʰ **S81.80** Unspecified open wound of lower leg
AHA: 2016, 3Q, 24

  5 ✓7ᵗʰ **S81.801** Unspecified open wound, right lower leg   NRS ▽

  5 ✓7ᵗʰ **S81.802** Unspecified open wound, left lower leg   NRS ▽

  ✓7ᵗʰ **S81.809** Unspecified open wound, unspecified lower leg ▽

 ✓6ᵗʰ **S81.81** Laceration without foreign body of lower leg

  4,5 ✓7ᵗʰ **S81.811** Laceration without foreign body, right NRS lower leg

  4,5 ✓7ᵗʰ **S81.812** Laceration without foreign body, left NRS lower leg

  ✓7ᵗʰ **S81.819** Laceration without foreign body, unspecified lower leg ▽

 ✓6ᵗʰ **S81.82** Laceration with foreign body of lower leg

  4,5 ✓7ᵗʰ **S81.821** Laceration with foreign body, right NRS lower leg

  4,5 ✓7ᵗʰ **S81.822** Laceration with foreign body, left NRS lower leg

  ✓7ᵗʰ **S81.829** Laceration with foreign body, unspecified lower leg ▽

 ✓6ᵗʰ **S81.83** Puncture wound without foreign body of lower leg
AHA: 2016, 3Q, 24

  4,5 ✓7ᵗʰ **S81.831** Puncture wound without foreign body, right lower leg NRS

  4,5 ✓7ᵗʰ **S81.832** Puncture wound without foreign body, left lower leg NRS

  ✓7ᵗʰ **S81.839** Puncture wound without foreign body, unspecified lower leg ▽

 ✓6ᵗʰ **S81.84** Puncture wound with foreign body of lower leg
AHA: 2016, 3Q, 24

  4,5 ✓7ᵗʰ **S81.841** Puncture wound with foreign body, right lower leg NRS

  4,5 ✓7ᵗʰ **S81.842** Puncture wound with foreign body, left lower leg NRS

  ✓7ᵗʰ **S81.849** Puncture wound with foreign body, unspecified lower leg ▽

 ✓6ᵗʰ **S81.85** Open bite of lower leg

Bite of lower leg NOS

EXCLUDES 1   superficial bite of lower leg (S80.86-, S80.87-)

  4,5 ✓7ᵗʰ **S81.851** Open bite, right lower leg NRS

  4,5 ✓7ᵗʰ **S81.852** Open bite, left lower leg NRS

  ✓7ᵗʰ **S81.859** Open bite, unspecified lower leg ▽

---

⁴   Case-mix diagnosis with 7th character indicating initial or subsequent encounter.
⁵   NRS supply diagnosis with 7th character indicating initial or subsequent encounter.

☑ Additional Character Req   ✓x7ᵗʰ Placeholder Alert   Case-Mix Diagnosis   Manifestation   ▽ Unspecified Dx   *EXCLUDES 1* Not coded here   *EXCLUDES 2* Not included here

√4ᵗʰ **S82 Fracture of lower leg, including ankle**

NOTE A fracture not indicated as displaced or nondisplaced should be coded to displaced.

A fracture not designated as open or closed should be coded to closed.

The open fracture designations are based on the Gustilo open fracture classification.

INCLUDES fracture of malleolus

EXCLUDES 1 *traumatic amputation of lower leg (S88.-)*

EXCLUDES 2 *fracture of foot, except ankle (S92.-)*
periprosthetic fracture of prosthetic implant of knee
►*(M97.0-)*◄

AHA: 2016, 1Q, 33; 2015, 3Q, 37-39

TIP: The term "improper alignment" is not synonymous with malunion or nonunion of a fracture when noted in provider documentation.

The appropriate 7th character is to be added to all codes from category S82 [unless otherwise indicated].

A	initial encounter for closed fracture
B	initial encounter for open fracture type I or II
	initial encounter for open fracture NOS
C	initial encounter for open fracture type IIIA, IIIB, or IIIC
D	subsequent encounter for closed fracture with routine healing
E	subsequent encounter for open fracture type I or II with routine healing
F	subsequent encounter for open fracture type IIIA, IIIB, or IIIC with routine healing
G	subsequent encounter for closed fracture with delayed healing
H	subsequent encounter for open fracture type I or II with delayed healing
J	subsequent encounter for open fracture type IIIA, IIIB or IIIC with delayed healing
K	subsequent encounter for closed fracture with nonunion
M	subsequent encounter for open fracture type I or II with nonunion
N	subsequent encounter for open fracture type IIIA, IIIB or IIIC with nonunion
P	subsequent encounter for closed fracture with malunion
Q	subsequent encounter for open fracture type I or II with malunion
R	subsequent encounter for open fracture type IIIA, IIIB or IIIC with malunion
S	sequela

√5ᵗʰ **S82.0 Fracture of patella**
Knee cap

√6ᵗʰ **S82.00 Unspecified fracture of patella**
- ¹ √7ᵗʰ **S82.001 Unspecified fracture of right patella** ▽
- ¹ √7ᵗʰ **S82.002 Unspecified fracture of left patella** ▽
- √7ᵗʰ **S82.009 Unspecified fracture of unspecified patella** ▽

√6ᵗʰ **S82.01 Osteochondral fracture of patella**
- ¹ √7ᵗʰ **S82.011 Displaced osteochondral fracture of right patella**
- ¹ √7ᵗʰ **S82.012 Displaced osteochondral fracture of left patella**
- √7ᵗʰ **S82.013 Displaced osteochondral fracture of unspecified patella** ▽
- ¹ √7ᵗʰ **S82.014 Nondisplaced osteochondral fracture of right patella**
- ¹ √7ᵗʰ **S82.015 Nondisplaced osteochondral fracture of left patella**
- √7ᵗʰ **S82.016 Nondisplaced osteochondral fracture of unspecified patella** ▽

√6ᵗʰ **S82.02 Longitudinal fracture of patella**
- ¹ √7ᵗʰ **S82.021 Displaced longitudinal fracture of right patella**
- ¹ √7ᵗʰ **S82.022 Displaced longitudinal fracture of left patella**
- √7ᵗʰ **S82.023 Displaced longitudinal fracture of unspecified patella** ▽
- ¹ √7ᵗʰ **S82.024 Nondisplaced longitudinal fracture of right patella**
- ¹ √7ᵗʰ **S82.025 Nondisplaced longitudinal fracture of left patella**
- √7ᵗʰ **S82.026 Nondisplaced longitudinal fracture of unspecified patella** ▽

√6ᵗʰ **S82.03 Transverse fracture of patella**
- ¹ √7ᵗʰ **S82.031 Displaced transverse fracture of right patella**
- ¹ √7ᵗʰ **S82.032 Displaced transverse fracture of left patella**
- √7ᵗʰ **S82.033 Displaced transverse fracture of unspecified patella** ▽
- ¹ √7ᵗʰ **S82.034 Nondisplaced transverse fracture of right patella**
- ¹ √7ᵗʰ **S82.035 Nondisplaced transverse fracture of left patella**
- √7ᵗʰ **S82.036 Nondisplaced transverse fracture of unspecified patella** ▽

√6ᵗʰ **S82.04 Comminuted fracture of patella**
- ¹ √7ᵗʰ **S82.041 Displaced comminuted fracture of right patella**
- ¹ √7ᵗʰ **S82.042 Displaced comminuted fracture of left patella**
- √7ᵗʰ **S82.043 Displaced comminuted fracture of unspecified patella** ▽
- ¹ √7ᵗʰ **S82.044 Nondisplaced comminuted fracture of right patella**
- ¹ √7ᵗʰ **S82.045 Nondisplaced comminuted fracture of left patella**
- √7ᵗʰ **S82.046 Nondisplaced comminuted fracture of unspecified patella** ▽

√6ᵗʰ **S82.09 Other fracture of patella**
- ¹ √7ᵗʰ **S82.091 Other fracture of right patella**
- ¹ √7ᵗʰ **S82.092 Other fracture of left patella**
- √7ᵗʰ **S82.099 Other fracture of unspecified patella** ▽

√5ᵗʰ **S82.1 Fracture of upper end of tibia**
Fracture of proximal end of tibia

EXCLUDES 2 *fracture of shaft of tibia (S82.2-)*
physeal fracture of upper end of tibia (S89.0-)

√6ᵗʰ **S82.10 Unspecified fracture of upper end of tibia**
- ¹ √7ᵗʰ **S82.101 Unspecified fracture of upper end of right tibia** ▽
- ¹ √7ᵗʰ **S82.102 Unspecified fracture of upper end of left tibia** ▽
- √7ᵗʰ **S82.109 Unspecified fracture of upper end of unspecified tibia** ▽

√6ᵗʰ **S82.11 Fracture of tibial spine**
- ¹ √7ᵗʰ **S82.111 Displaced fracture of right tibial spine**
- ¹ √7ᵗʰ **S82.112 Displaced fracture of left tibial spine**
- √7ᵗʰ **S82.113 Displaced fracture of unspecified tibial spine** ▽
- ¹ √7ᵗʰ **S82.114 Nondisplaced fracture of right tibial spine**
- ¹ √7ᵗʰ **S82.115 Nondisplaced fracture of left tibial spine**
- √7ᵗʰ **S82.116 Nondisplaced fracture of unspecified tibial spine** ▽

√6ᵗʰ **S82.12 Fracture of lateral condyle of tibia**
- ¹ √7ᵗʰ **S82.121 Displaced fracture of lateral condyle of right tibia**
- ¹ √7ᵗʰ **S82.122 Displaced fracture of lateral condyle of left tibia**
- √7ᵗʰ **S82.123 Displaced fracture of lateral condyle of unspecified tibia** ▽
- ¹ √7ᵗʰ **S82.124 Nondisplaced fracture of lateral condyle of right tibia**
- ¹ √7ᵗʰ **S82.125 Nondisplaced fracture of lateral condyle of left tibia**
- √7ᵗʰ **S82.126 Nondisplaced fracture of lateral condyle of unspecified tibia** ▽

√6ᵗʰ **S82.13 Fracture of medial condyle of tibia**
- ¹ √7ᵗʰ **S82.131 Displaced fracture of medial condyle of right tibia**
- ¹ √7ᵗʰ **S82.132 Displaced fracture of medial condyle of left tibia**
- √7ᵗʰ **S82.133 Displaced fracture of medial condyle of unspecified tibia** ▽
- ¹ √7ᵗʰ **S82.134 Nondisplaced fracture of medial condyle of right tibia**

---

¹ Case-mix diagnosis with 7th character indicating subsequent encounter.

N Newborn: 0   P Pediatric: 0-17   M Maternity: 12-55   A Adult: 15-124   NRS Nonroutine supply Dx   NCDx Noncancer Dx   PDx Primary Dx   ►◄ Revised Text   ● New Code   ▲ Revised Title

1014   ICD-10-CM 2018

1 ✓7ᵗʰ **S82.135** Nondisplaced **fracture of medial condyle of left tibia**

✓7ᵗʰ **S82.136** Nondisplaced **fracture of medial** ▽ condyle of unspecified tibia

✓6ᵗʰ **S82.14** Bicondylar **fracture of tibia**
    Fracture of tibial plateau NOS

1 ✓7ᵗʰ **S82.141** Displaced **bicondylar fracture of right tibia**

1 ✓7ᵗʰ **S82.142** Displaced **bicondylar fracture of left tibia**

✓7ᵗʰ **S82.143** Displaced **bicondylar fracture of unspecified tibia** ▽

1 ✓7ᵗʰ **S82.144** Nondisplaced **bicondylar fracture of right tibia**

1 ✓7ᵗʰ **S82.145** Nondisplaced **bicondylar fracture of left tibia**

✓7ᵗʰ **S82.146** Nondisplaced **bicondylar fracture of unspecified tibia** ▽

✓6ᵗʰ **S82.15** Fracture of tibial tuberosity

1 ✓7ᵗʰ **S82.151** Displaced **fracture of right tibial tuberosity**

1 ✓7ᵗʰ **S82.152** Displaced **fracture of left tibial tuberosity**

✓7ᵗʰ **S82.153** Displaced **fracture of unspecified tibial tuberosity** ▽

1 ✓7ᵗʰ **S82.154** Nondisplaced **fracture of right tibial tuberosity**

1 ✓7ᵗʰ **S82.155** Nondisplaced **fracture of left tibial tuberosity**

✓7ᵗʰ **S82.156** Nondisplaced **fracture of unspecified tibial tuberosity** ▽

✓6ᵗʰ **S82.16** Torus **fracture of upper end of tibia**

The appropriate 7th character is to be added to all codes in subcategory S82.16.
A   initial encounter for closed fracture
D   subsequent encounter for fracture with routine healing
G   subsequent encounter for fracture with delayed healing
K   subsequent encounter for fracture with nonunion
P   subsequent encounter for fracture with malunion
S   sequela

1 ✓7ᵗʰ **S82.161** Torus **fracture of upper end of right tibia**

1 ✓7ᵗʰ **S82.162** Torus **fracture of upper end of left tibia**

✓7ᵗʰ **S82.169** Torus **fracture of upper end of unspecified tibia** ▽

✓6ᵗʰ **S82.19** Other **fracture of upper end of tibia**

1 ✓7ᵗʰ **S82.191** Other **fracture of upper end of right tibia**

1 ✓7ᵗʰ **S82.192** Other **fracture of upper end of left tibia**

✓7ᵗʰ **S82.199** Other **fracture of upper end of unspecified tibia** ▽

✓5ᵗʰ **S82.2** Fracture of shaft of tibia

✓6ᵗʰ **S82.20** Unspecified **fracture of shaft of tibia**
    Fracture of tibia NOS

1 ✓7ᵗʰ **S82.201** Unspecified **fracture of shaft of right tibia** ▽

1 ✓7ᵗʰ **S82.202** Unspecified **fracture of shaft of left tibia** ▽

1 ✓7ᵗʰ **S82.209** Unspecified **fracture of shaft of unspecified tibia** ▽

✓6ᵗʰ **S82.22** Transverse **fracture of shaft of tibia**

1 ✓7ᵗʰ **S82.221** Displaced **transverse fracture of shaft of right tibia**

1 ✓7ᵗʰ **S82.222** Displaced **transverse fracture of shaft of left tibia**

✓7ᵗʰ **S82.223** Displaced **transverse fracture of shaft of unspecified tibia** ▽

1 ✓7ᵗʰ **S82.224** Nondisplaced **transverse fracture of shaft of right tibia**

1 ✓7ᵗʰ **S82.225** Nondisplaced **transverse fracture of shaft of left tibia**

✓7ᵗʰ **S82.226** Nondisplaced **transverse fracture of shaft of unspecified tibia** ▽

✓6ᵗʰ **S82.23** Oblique **fracture of shaft of tibia**

1 ✓7ᵗʰ **S82.231** Displaced **oblique fracture of shaft of right tibia**

1 ✓7ᵗʰ **S82.232** Displaced **oblique fracture of shaft of left tibia**

1 ✓7ᵗʰ **S82.233** Displaced **oblique fracture of shaft of unspecified tibia** ▽

1 ✓7ᵗʰ **S82.234** Nondisplaced **oblique fracture of shaft of right tibia**

1 ✓7ᵗʰ **S82.235** Nondisplaced **oblique fracture of shaft of left tibia**

✓7ᵗʰ **S82.236** Nondisplaced **oblique fracture of shaft of unspecified tibia** ▽

✓6ᵗʰ **S82.24** Spiral **fracture of shaft of tibia**
    Toddler fracture

1 ✓7ᵗʰ **S82.241** Displaced **spiral fracture of shaft of right tibia**

1 ✓7ᵗʰ **S82.242** Displaced **spiral fracture of shaft of left tibia**

✓7ᵗʰ **S82.243** Displaced **spiral fracture of shaft of unspecified tibia** ▽

1 ✓7ᵗʰ **S82.244** Nondisplaced **spiral fracture of shaft of right tibia**

1 ✓7ᵗʰ **S82.245** Nondisplaced **spiral fracture of shaft of left tibia**

✓7ᵗʰ **S82.246** Nondisplaced **spiral fracture of shaft of unspecified tibia** ▽

✓6ᵗʰ **S82.25** Comminuted **fracture of shaft of tibia**

1 ✓7ᵗʰ **S82.251** Displaced **comminuted fracture of shaft of right tibia**

1 ✓7ᵗʰ **S82.252** Displaced **comminuted fracture of shaft of left tibia**

✓7ᵗʰ **S82.253** Displaced **comminuted fracture of shaft of unspecified tibia** ▽

1 ✓7ᵗʰ **S82.254** Nondisplaced **comminuted fracture of shaft of right tibia**

1 ✓7ᵗʰ **S82.255** Nondisplaced **comminuted fracture of shaft of left tibia**

✓7ᵗʰ **S82.256** Nondisplaced **comminuted fracture of shaft of unspecified tibia** ▽

✓6ᵗʰ **S82.26** Segmental **fracture of shaft of tibia**

1 ✓7ᵗʰ **S82.261** Displaced **segmental fracture of shaft of right tibia**

1 ✓7ᵗʰ **S82.262** Displaced **segmental fracture of shaft of left tibia**

✓7ᵗʰ **S82.263** Displaced **segmental fracture of shaft of unspecified tibia** ▽

1 ✓7ᵗʰ **S82.264** Nondisplaced **segmental fracture of shaft of right tibia**

1 ✓7ᵗʰ **S82.265** Nondisplaced **segmental fracture of shaft of left tibia**

✓7ᵗʰ **S82.266** Nondisplaced **segmental fracture of shaft of unspecified tibia** ▽

✓6ᵗʰ **S82.29** Other **fracture of shaft of tibia**

1 ✓7ᵗʰ **S82.291** Other **fracture of shaft of right tibia**

1 ✓7ᵗʰ **S82.292** Other **fracture of shaft of left tibia**

✓7ᵗʰ **S82.299** Other **fracture of shaft of unspecified tibia** ▽

✓5ᵗʰ **S82.3** Fracture of lower end of tibia

    EXCLUDES 1   bimalleolar fracture of lower leg (S82.84-)
                  fracture of medial malleolus alone (S82.5-)
                  Maisonneuve's fracture (S82.86-)
                  pilon fracture of distal tibia (S82.87-)
                  trimalleolar fractures of lower leg (S82.85-)

✓6ᵗʰ **S82.30** Unspecified **fracture of lower end of tibia**

1 ✓7ᵗʰ **S82.301** Unspecified **fracture of lower end of right tibia** ▽

1 ✓7ᵗʰ **S82.302** Unspecified **fracture of lower end of left tibia** ▽

✓7ᵗʰ **S82.309** Unspecified **fracture of lower end of unspecified tibia** ▽

---

1   Case-mix diagnosis with 7th character indicating subsequent encounter.

✓ Additional Character Req   ✓ₓ7ᵗʰ Placeholder Alert   Case-Mix Diagnosis   Manifestation   ▽ Unspecified Dx   **EXCLUDES 1** Not coded here   **EXCLUDES 2** Not included here

ICD-10-CM 2018   **1015**

✓6ᵗʰ **S82.31** Torus **fracture of lower end of tibia**

> The appropriate 7th character is to be added to all codes in subcategory S82.31.
> A   initial encounter for closed fracture
> D   subsequent encounter for fracture with routine healing
> G   subsequent encounter for fracture with delayed healing
> K   subsequent encounter for fracture with nonunion
> P   subsequent encounter for fracture with malunion
> S   sequela

    1 ✓7ᵗʰ **S82.311** **Torus fracture of lower end of right tibia**
    1 ✓7ᵗʰ **S82.312** **Torus fracture of lower end of left tibia**
    ✓7ᵗʰ **S82.319** **Torus fracture of lower end of unspecified tibia** ▽

✓6ᵗʰ **S82.39** Other **fracture of lower end of tibia**
    AHA: 2015, 1Q, 25
    1 ✓7ᵗʰ **S82.391** **Other fracture of lower end of right tibia**
    1 ✓7ᵗʰ **S82.392** **Other fracture of lower end of left tibia**
    ✓7ᵗʰ **S82.399** **Other fracture of lower end of unspecified tibia** ▽

✓5ᵗʰ **S82.4** **Fracture of** shaft of fibula
    EXCLUDES 2   fracture of lateral malleolus alone (S82.6-)

    ✓6ᵗʰ **S82.40** Unspecified **fracture of shaft of fibula**
      1 ✓7ᵗʰ **S82.401** **Unspecified fracture of shaft of right fibula** ▽
      1 ✓7ᵗʰ **S82.402** **Unspecified fracture of shaft of left fibula** ▽
      ✓7ᵗʰ **S82.409** **Unspecified fracture of shaft of unspecified fibula** ▽

    ✓6ᵗʰ **S82.42** Transverse **fracture of shaft of fibula**
      1 ✓7ᵗʰ **S82.421** **Displaced transverse fracture of shaft of right fibula**
      1 ✓7ᵗʰ **S82.422** **Displaced transverse fracture of shaft of left fibula**
      ✓7ᵗʰ **S82.423** **Displaced transverse fracture of shaft of unspecified fibula** ▽
      1 ✓7ᵗʰ **S82.424** **Nondisplaced transverse fracture of shaft of right fibula**
      1 ✓7ᵗʰ **S82.425** **Nondisplaced transverse fracture of shaft of left fibula**
      ✓7ᵗʰ **S82.426** **Nondisplaced transverse fracture of shaft of unspecified fibula** ▽

    ✓6ᵗʰ **S82.43** Oblique **fracture of shaft of fibula**
      1 ✓7ᵗʰ **S82.431** **Displaced oblique fracture of shaft of right fibula**
      1 ✓7ᵗʰ **S82.432** **Displaced oblique fracture of shaft of left fibula**
      ✓7ᵗʰ **S82.433** **Displaced oblique fracture of shaft of unspecified fibula** ▽
      1 ✓7ᵗʰ **S82.434** **Nondisplaced oblique fracture of shaft of right fibula**
      1 ✓7ᵗʰ **S82.435** **Nondisplaced oblique fracture of shaft of left fibula**
      ✓7ᵗʰ **S82.436** **Nondisplaced oblique fracture of shaft of unspecified fibula** ▽

    ✓6ᵗʰ **S82.44** Spiral **fracture of shaft of fibula**
      1 ✓7ᵗʰ **S82.441** **Displaced spiral fracture of shaft of right fibula**
      1 ✓7ᵗʰ **S82.442** **Displaced spiral fracture of shaft of left fibula**
      ✓7ᵗʰ **S82.443** **Displaced spiral fracture of shaft of unspecified fibula** ▽
      1 ✓7ᵗʰ **S82.444** **Nondisplaced spiral fracture of shaft of right fibula**
      1 ✓7ᵗʰ **S82.445** **Nondisplaced spiral fracture of shaft of left fibula**
      ✓7ᵗʰ **S82.446** **Nondisplaced spiral fracture of shaft of unspecified fibula** ▽

✓6ᵗʰ **S82.45** Comminuted **fracture of shaft of fibula**
    1 ✓7ᵗʰ **S82.451** **Displaced comminuted fracture of shaft of right fibula**
    1 ✓7ᵗʰ **S82.452** **Displaced comminuted fracture of shaft of left fibula**
    ✓7ᵗʰ **S82.453** **Displaced comminuted fracture of shaft of unspecified fibula** ▽
    1 ✓7ᵗʰ **S82.454** **Nondisplaced comminuted fracture of shaft of right fibula**
    1 ✓7ᵗʰ **S82.455** **Nondisplaced comminuted fracture of shaft of left fibula**
    ✓7ᵗʰ **S82.456** **Nondisplaced comminuted fracture of shaft of unspecified fibula** ▽

✓6ᵗʰ **S82.46** Segmental **fracture of shaft of fibula**
    1 ✓7ᵗʰ **S82.461** **Displaced segmental fracture of shaft of right fibula**
    1 ✓7ᵗʰ **S82.462** **Displaced segmental fracture of shaft of left fibula**
    ✓7ᵗʰ **S82.463** **Displaced segmental fracture of shaft of unspecified fibula** ▽
    1 ✓7ᵗʰ **S82.464** **Nondisplaced segmental fracture of shaft of right fibula**
    1 ✓7ᵗʰ **S82.465** **Nondisplaced segmental fracture of shaft of left fibula**
    ✓7ᵗʰ **S82.466** **Nondisplaced segmental fracture of shaft of unspecified fibula** ▽

✓6ᵗʰ **S82.49** Other **fracture of shaft of fibula**
    1 ✓7ᵗʰ **S82.491** **Other fracture of shaft of right fibula**
    1 ✓7ᵗʰ **S82.492** **Other fracture of shaft of left fibula**
    ✓7ᵗʰ **S82.499** **Other fracture of shaft of unspecified fibula** ▽

✓5ᵗʰ **S82.5** **Fracture of** medial malleolus
    EXCLUDES 1   pilon fracture of distal tibia (S82.87-)
             Salter-Harris type III of lower end of tibia (S89.13-)
             Salter-Harris type IV of lower end of tibia (S89.14-)
    1 ✓x7ᵗʰ **S82.51** **Displaced fracture of medial malleolus of right tibia**
    1 ✓x7ᵗʰ **S82.52** **Displaced fracture of medial malleolus of left tibia**
    ✓x7ᵗʰ **S82.53** **Displaced fracture of medial malleolus of unspecified tibia** ▽
    1 ✓x7ᵗʰ **S82.54** **Nondisplaced fracture of medial malleolus of right tibia**
    1 ✓x7ᵗʰ **S82.55** **Nondisplaced fracture of medial malleolus of left tibia**
    ✓x7ᵗʰ **S82.56** **Nondisplaced fracture of medial malleolus of unspecified tibia** ▽

✓5ᵗʰ **S82.6** **Fracture of** lateral malleolus
    EXCLUDES 1   pilon fracture of distal tibia (S82.87-)
    1 ✓x7ᵗʰ **S82.61** **Displaced fracture of lateral malleolus of right fibula**
    1 ✓x7ᵗʰ **S82.62** **Displaced fracture of lateral malleolus of left fibula**
    ✓x7ᵗʰ **S82.63** **Displaced fracture of lateral malleolus of unspecified fibula** ▽
    1 ✓x7ᵗʰ **S82.64** **Nondisplaced fracture of lateral malleolus of right fibula**
    1 ✓x7ᵗʰ **S82.65** **Nondisplaced fracture of lateral malleolus of left fibula**
    ✓x7ᵗʰ **S82.66** **Nondisplaced fracture of lateral malleolus of unspecified fibula** ▽

✓5ᵗʰ **S82.8** **Other fractures of** lower leg
    ✓6ᵗʰ **S82.81** Torus **fracture of upper end of fibula**

> The appropriate 7th character is to be added to all codes in subcategory S82.81.
> A   initial encounter for closed fracture
> D   subsequent encounter for fracture with routine healing
> G   subsequent encounter for fracture with delayed healing
> K   subsequent encounter for fracture with nonunion
> P   subsequent encounter for fracture with malunion
> S   sequela

      1 ✓7ᵗʰ **S82.811** **Torus fracture of upper end of right fibula**
      1 ✓7ᵗʰ **S82.812** **Torus fracture of upper end of left fibula**

---

1   Case-mix diagnosis with 7th character indicating subsequent encounter.

Ⓝ Newborn: 0   Ⓟ Pediatric: 0-17   Ⓜ Maternity: 12-55   Ⓐ Adult: 15-124   **NRS** Nonroutine supply Dx   **NCDx** Noncancer Dx   **PDx** Primary Dx   ▶◀ Revised Text   ● New Code   ▲ Revised Title

1016   ICD-10-CM 2018

√7ᵗʰ **S82.819** Torus fracture of upper end of △
unspecified fibula

√6ᵗʰ **S82.82** Torus **fracture of** lower end of fibula

> The appropriate 7th character is to be added to all
> codes in subcategory S82.82.
> A   initial encounter for closed fracture
> D   subsequent encounter for fracture with
>   routine healing
> G   subsequent encounter for fracture with
>   delayed healing
> K   subsequent encounter for fracture with
>   nonunion
> P   subsequent encounter for fracture with
>   malunion
> S   sequela

¹ √7ᵗʰ **S82.821** Torus fracture of lower end of right fibula
¹ √7ᵗʰ **S82.822** Torus fracture of lower end of left fibula
√7ᵗʰ **S82.829** Torus fracture of lower end of △
unspecified fibula

√6ᵗʰ **S82.83** Other **fracture of** upper and lower end of fibula
     AHA: 2015, 1Q, 25
¹ √7ᵗʰ **S82.831** Other fracture of upper and lower end of
right fibula
¹ √7ᵗʰ **S82.832** Other fracture of upper and lower end of
left fibula
√7ᵗʰ **S82.839** Other fracture of upper and lower △
end of unspecified fibula

√6ᵗʰ **S82.84** Bimalleolar **fracture of lower leg**
¹ √7ᵗʰ **S82.841** Displaced **bimalleolar fracture of**
right **lower leg**
¹ √7ᵗʰ **S82.842** Displaced **bimalleolar fracture of**
left **lower leg**
√7ᵗʰ **S82.843** Displaced **bimalleolar fracture of** △
unspecified lower leg
¹ √7ᵗʰ **S82.844** Nondisplaced **bimalleolar fracture of**
right **lower leg**
¹ √7ᵗʰ **S82.845** Nondisplaced **bimalleolar fracture of**
left **lower leg**
√7ᵗʰ **S82.846** Nondisplaced **bimalleolar fracture of** △
unspecified lower leg

√6ᵗʰ **S82.85** Trimalleolar **fracture of lower leg**
¹ √7ᵗʰ **S82.851** Displaced **trimalleolar fracture of**
right **lower leg**
¹ √7ᵗʰ **S82.852** Displaced **trimalleolar fracture of**
left **lower leg**
√7ᵗʰ **S82.853** Displaced **trimalleolar fracture of** △
unspecified lower leg

Right Bimalleolar Fracture

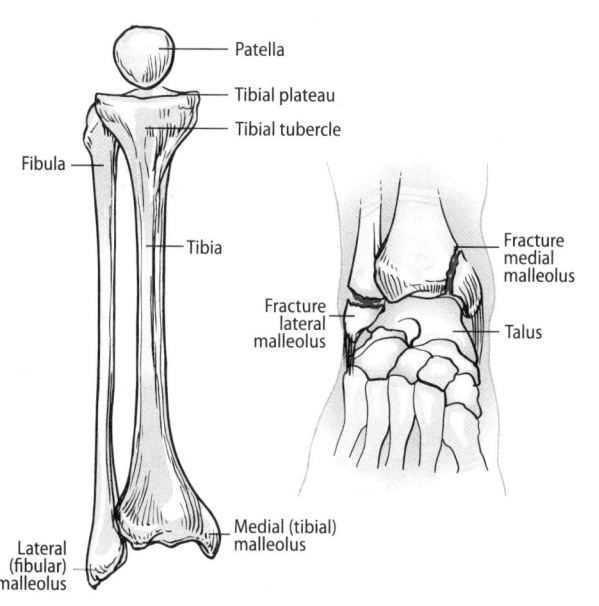

¹ √7ᵗʰ **S82.854** Nondisplaced **trimalleolar fracture of**
right **lower leg**
¹ √7ᵗʰ **S82.855** Nondisplaced **trimalleolar fracture of**
left **lower leg**
√7ᵗʰ **S82.856** Nondisplaced **trimalleolar fracture of** △
unspecified **lower leg**

√6ᵗʰ **S82.86** Maisonneuve's **fracture**
¹ √7ᵗʰ **S82.861** Displaced **Maisonneuve's fracture of**
right **leg**
¹ √7ᵗʰ **S82.862** Displaced **Maisonneuve's fracture of**
left **leg**
√7ᵗʰ **S82.863** Displaced **Maisonneuve's fracture of** △
unspecified leg
¹ √7ᵗʰ **S82.864** Nondisplaced **Maisonneuve's fracture of**
right **leg**
¹ √7ᵗʰ **S82.865** Nondisplaced **Maisonneuve's fracture of**
left **leg**
√7ᵗʰ **S82.866** Nondisplaced **Maisonneuve's fracture** △
of unspecified leg

√6ᵗʰ **S82.87** Pilon **fracture of tibia**
¹ √7ᵗʰ **S82.871** Displaced **pilon fracture of right tibia**
¹ √7ᵗʰ **S82.872** Displaced **pilon fracture of left tibia**
√7ᵗʰ **S82.873** Displaced **pilon fracture of** △
unspecified tibia
¹ √7ᵗʰ **S82.874** Nondisplaced **pilon fracture of right tibia**
¹ √7ᵗʰ **S82.875** Nondisplaced **pilon fracture of left tibia**
√7ᵗʰ **S82.876** Nondisplaced **pilon fracture of** △
unspecified tibia

√6ᵗʰ **S82.89** Other **fractures of lower leg**
     Fracture of ankle NOS
¹ √7ᵗʰ **S82.891** Other fracture of right **lower leg**
¹ √7ᵗʰ **S82.892** Other fracture of left **lower leg**
√7ᵗʰ **S82.899** Other fracture of unspecified lower leg △

√5ᵗʰ **S82.9** Unspecified **fracture of lower leg**
√×7ᵗʰ **S82.90** Unspecified fracture of unspecified lower leg △
¹ √×7ᵗʰ **S82.91** Unspecified fracture of right **lower leg** △
¹ √×7ᵗʰ **S82.92** Unspecified fracture of left **lower leg** △

√4ᵗʰ **S83** **Dislocation and sprain of joints and ligaments of knee**
   INCLUDES   avulsion of joint or ligament of knee
            laceration of cartilage, joint or ligament of knee
            sprain of cartilage, joint or ligament of knee
            traumatic hemarthrosis of joint or ligament of knee
            traumatic rupture of joint or ligament of knee
            traumatic subluxation of joint or ligament of knee
            traumatic tear of joint or ligament of knee
Code also any associated open wound
   EXCLUDES 1   derangement of patella (M22.0-M22.3)
            injury of patellar ligament (tendon) (S76.1-)
            internal derangement of knee (M23.-)
            old dislocation of knee (M24.36)
            pathological dislocation of knee (M24.36)
            recurrent dislocation of knee (M22.0)
   EXCLUDES 2   strain of muscle, fascia and tendon of lower leg (S86.-)

> The appropriate 7th character is to be added to each code from
> category S83.
> A   initial encounter
> D   subsequent encounter
> S   sequela

√5ᵗʰ **S83.0** **Subluxation and dislocation of** patella
√6ᵗʰ **S83.00** Unspecified **subluxation and dislocation of patella**
¹ √7ᵗʰ **S83.001** Unspecified **subluxation of right** △
patella
¹ √7ᵗʰ **S83.002** Unspecified **subluxation of left** △
patella
√7ᵗʰ **S83.003** Unspecified **subluxation of** △
unspecified patella
¹ √7ᵗʰ **S83.004** Unspecified **dislocation of right** △
patella
¹ √7ᵗʰ **S83.005** Unspecified **dislocation of left patella** △
√7ᵗʰ **S83.006** Unspecified **dislocation of** △
unspecified patella

---

¹   Case-mix diagnosis with 7th character indicating subsequent encounter.

☑ Additional Character Req   √×7ᵗʰ Placeholder Alert   Case-Mix Diagnosis   Manifestation   △ Unspecified Dx   EXCLUDES 1 Not coded here   EXCLUDES 2 Not included here

Labels in figure:
Patella
Tibial plateau
Tibial tubercle
Fibula
Tibia
Lateral (fibular) malleolus
Medial (tibial) malleolus
Fracture medial malleolus
Fracture lateral malleolus
Talus

✓6th **S83.01** Lateral subluxation and dislocation of patella
- 1 ✓7th **S83.011** Lateral subluxation of right patella
- 1 ✓7th **S83.012** Lateral subluxation of left patella
- ✓7th **S83.013** Lateral subluxation of unspecified patella ▽
- 1 ✓7th **S83.014** Lateral dislocation of right patella
- 1 ✓7th **S83.015** Lateral dislocation of left patella
- ✓7th **S83.016** Lateral dislocation of unspecified patella ▽

✓6th **S83.09** Other subluxation and dislocation of patella
- 1 ✓7th **S83.091** Other subluxation of right patella
- 1 ✓7th **S83.092** Other subluxation of left patella
- ✓7th **S83.093** Other subluxation of unspecified patella ▽
- 1 ✓7th **S83.094** Other dislocation of right patella
- 1 ✓7th **S83.095** Other dislocation of left patella
- ✓7th **S83.096** Other dislocation of unspecified patella ▽

✓5th **S83.1** Subluxation and dislocation of knee
> EXCLUDES 2   instability of knee prosthesis (T84.022, T84.023)

✓6th **S83.10** Unspecified subluxation and dislocation of knee
- 1 ✓7th **S83.101** Unspecified subluxation of right knee ▽
- 1 ✓7th **S83.102** Unspecified subluxation of left knee ▽
- ✓7th **S83.103** Unspecified subluxation of unspecified knee ▽
- 1 ✓7th **S83.104** Unspecified dislocation of right knee ▽
- 1 ✓7th **S83.105** Unspecified dislocation of left knee ▽
- ✓7th **S83.106** Unspecified dislocation of unspecified knee ▽

✓6th **S83.11** Anterior subluxation and dislocation of proximal end of tibia
> Posterior subluxation and dislocation of distal end of femur
- 1 ✓7th **S83.111** Anterior subluxation of proximal end of tibia, right knee
- 1 ✓7th **S83.112** Anterior subluxation of proximal end of tibia, left knee
- ✓7th **S83.113** Anterior subluxation of proximal end of tibia, unspecified knee ▽
- 1 ✓7th **S83.114** Anterior dislocation of proximal end of tibia, right knee
- 1 ✓7th **S83.115** Anterior dislocation of proximal end of tibia, left knee
- ✓7th **S83.116** Anterior dislocation of proximal end of tibia, unspecified knee ▽

✓6th **S83.12** Posterior subluxation and dislocation of proximal end of tibia
> Anterior dislocation of distal end of femur
- 1 ✓7th **S83.121** Posterior subluxation of proximal end of tibia, right knee
- 1 ✓7th **S83.122** Posterior subluxation of proximal end of tibia, left knee
- ✓7th **S83.123** Posterior subluxation of proximal end of tibia, unspecified knee ▽
- 1 ✓7th **S83.124** Posterior dislocation of proximal end of tibia, right knee
- 1 ✓7th **S83.125** Posterior dislocation of proximal end of tibia, left knee
- ✓7th **S83.126** Posterior dislocation of proximal end of tibia, unspecified knee ▽

✓6th **S83.13** Medial subluxation and dislocation of proximal end of tibia
- 1 ✓7th **S83.131** Medial subluxation of proximal end of tibia, right knee
- 1 ✓7th **S83.132** Medial subluxation of proximal end of tibia, left knee
- ✓7th **S83.133** Medial subluxation of proximal end of tibia, unspecified knee ▽
- 1 ✓7th **S83.134** Medial dislocation of proximal end of tibia, right knee
- 1 ✓7th **S83.135** Medial dislocation of proximal end of tibia, left knee

✓7th **S83.136** Medial dislocation of proximal end of tibia, unspecified knee ▽

✓6th **S83.14** Lateral subluxation and dislocation of proximal end of tibia
- 1 ✓7th **S83.141** Lateral subluxation of proximal end of tibia, right knee
- 1 ✓7th **S83.142** Lateral subluxation of proximal end of tibia, left knee
- ✓7th **S83.143** Lateral subluxation of proximal end of tibia, unspecified knee ▽
- 1 ✓7th **S83.144** Lateral dislocation of proximal end of tibia, right knee
- 1 ✓7th **S83.145** Lateral dislocation of proximal end of tibia, left knee
- ✓7th **S83.146** Lateral dislocation of proximal end of tibia, unspecified knee ▽

✓6th **S83.19** Other subluxation and dislocation of knee
- 1 ✓7th **S83.191** Other subluxation of right knee
- 1 ✓7th **S83.192** Other subluxation of left knee
- ✓7th **S83.193** Other subluxation of unspecified knee ▽
- 1 ✓7th **S83.194** Other dislocation of right knee
- 1 ✓7th **S83.195** Other dislocation of left knee
- ✓7th **S83.196** Other dislocation of unspecified knee ▽

✓5th **S83.2** Tear of meniscus, current injury
> EXCLUDES 1   old bucket-handle tear (M23.2)

✓6th **S83.20** Tear of unspecified meniscus, current injury
> Tear of meniscus of knee NOS
- 1 ✓7th **S83.200** Bucket-handle tear of unspecified meniscus, current injury, right knee ▽
- 1 ✓7th **S83.201** Bucket-handle tear of unspecified meniscus, current injury, left knee ▽
- ✓7th **S83.202** Bucket-handle tear of unspecified meniscus, current injury, unspecified knee ▽
- 1 ✓7th **S83.203** Other tear of unspecified meniscus, current injury, right knee ▽
- 1 ✓7th **S83.204** Other tear of unspecified meniscus, current injury, left knee ▽
- ✓7th **S83.205** Other tear of unspecified meniscus, current injury, unspecified knee ▽
- 1 ✓7th **S83.206** Unspecified tear of unspecified meniscus, current injury, right knee ▽
- 1 ✓7th **S83.207** Unspecified tear of unspecified meniscus, current injury, left knee ▽
- ✓7th **S83.209** Unspecified tear of unspecified meniscus, current injury, unspecified knee ▽

✓6th **S83.21** Bucket-handle tear of medial meniscus, current injury
- 1 ✓7th **S83.211** Bucket-handle tear of medial meniscus, current injury, right knee
- 1 ✓7th **S83.212** Bucket-handle tear of medial meniscus, current injury, left knee
- ✓7th **S83.219** Bucket-handle tear of medial meniscus, current injury, unspecified knee ▽

✓6th **S83.22** Peripheral tear of medial meniscus, current injury
- 1 ✓7th **S83.221** Peripheral tear of medial meniscus, current injury, right knee
- 1 ✓7th **S83.222** Peripheral tear of medial meniscus, current injury, left knee
- ✓7th **S83.229** Peripheral tear of medial meniscus, current injury, unspecified knee ▽

✓6th **S83.23** Complex tear of medial meniscus, current injury
- 1 ✓7th **S83.231** Complex tear of medial meniscus, current injury, right knee
- 1 ✓7th **S83.232** Complex tear of medial meniscus, current injury, left knee
- ✓7th **S83.239** Complex tear of medial meniscus, current injury, unspecified knee ▽

✓6th **S83.24** Other tear of medial meniscus, current injury
- 1 ✓7th **S83.241** Other tear of medial meniscus, current injury, right knee
- 1 ✓7th **S83.242** Other tear of medial meniscus, current injury, left knee

---

1   Case-mix diagnosis with 7th character indicating subsequent encounter.

N Newborn: 0   P Pediatric: 0-17   M Maternity: 12-55   A Adult: 15-124   NRS Nonroutine supply Dx   NC Dx Noncancer Dx   PDx Primary Dx   ►◄ Revised Text   ● New Code   ▲ Revised Title

1018   ICD-10-CM 2018

✓7ᵗʰ **S83.249** Other tear of medial meniscus, current injury, unspecified knee ▽

✓6ᵗʰ **S83.25** Bucket-handle tear of lateral meniscus, current injury

   1 ✓7ᵗʰ **S83.251** Bucket-handle tear of lateral meniscus, current injury, right knee

   1 ✓7ᵗʰ **S83.252** Bucket-handle tear of lateral meniscus, current injury, left knee

   ✓7ᵗʰ **S83.259** Bucket-handle tear of lateral meniscus, current injury, unspecified knee ▽

✓6ᵗʰ **S83.26** Peripheral tear of lateral meniscus, current injury

   1 ✓7ᵗʰ **S83.261** Peripheral tear of lateral meniscus, current injury, right knee

   1 ✓7ᵗʰ **S83.262** Peripheral tear of lateral meniscus, current injury, left knee

   ✓7ᵗʰ **S83.269** Peripheral tear of lateral meniscus, current injury, unspecified knee ▽

✓6ᵗʰ **S83.27** Complex tear of lateral meniscus, current injury

   1 ✓7ᵗʰ **S83.271** Complex tear of lateral meniscus, current injury, right knee

   1 ✓7ᵗʰ **S83.272** Complex tear of lateral meniscus, current injury, left knee

   ✓7ᵗʰ **S83.279** Complex tear of lateral meniscus, current injury, unspecified knee ▽

✓6ᵗʰ **S83.28** Other tear of lateral meniscus, current injury

   1 ✓7ᵗʰ **S83.281** Other tear of lateral meniscus, current injury, right knee

   1 ✓7ᵗʰ **S83.282** Other tear of lateral meniscus, current injury, left knee

   ✓7ᵗʰ **S83.289** Other tear of lateral meniscus, current injury, unspecified knee ▽

✓5ᵗʰ **S83.3** Tear of articular cartilage of knee, current

   ✓x7ᵗʰ **S83.30** Tear of articular cartilage of unspecified knee, current ▽

   1 ✓x7ᵗʰ **S83.31** Tear of articular cartilage of right knee, current

   1 ✓x7ᵗʰ **S83.32** Tear of articular cartilage of left knee, current

✓5ᵗʰ **S83.4** Sprain of collateral ligament of knee

   ✓6ᵗʰ **S83.40** Sprain of unspecified collateral ligament of knee

      ✓7ᵗʰ **S83.401** Sprain of unspecified collateral ligament of right knee ▽

      ✓7ᵗʰ **S83.402** Sprain of unspecified collateral ligament of left knee ▽

      ✓7ᵗʰ **S83.409** Sprain of unspecified collateral ligament of unspecified knee ▽

   ✓6ᵗʰ **S83.41** Sprain of medial collateral ligament of knee
      Sprain of tibial collateral ligament

      ✓7ᵗʰ **S83.411** Sprain of medial collateral ligament of right knee

      ✓7ᵗʰ **S83.412** Sprain of medial collateral ligament of left knee

      ✓7ᵗʰ **S83.419** Sprain of medial collateral ligament of unspecified knee ▽

   ✓6ᵗʰ **S83.42** Sprain of lateral collateral ligament of knee
      Sprain of fibular collateral ligament

      ✓7ᵗʰ **S83.421** Sprain of lateral collateral ligament of right knee

      ✓7ᵗʰ **S83.422** Sprain of lateral collateral ligament of left knee

      ✓7ᵗʰ **S83.429** Sprain of lateral collateral ligament of unspecified knee ▽

✓5ᵗʰ **S83.5** Sprain of cruciate ligament of knee
   AHA: 2016, 2Q, 3

   ✓6ᵗʰ **S83.50** Sprain of unspecified cruciate ligament of knee

      ✓7ᵗʰ **S83.501** Sprain of unspecified cruciate ligament of right knee ▽

      ✓7ᵗʰ **S83.502** Sprain of unspecified cruciate ligament of left knee ▽

      ✓7ᵗʰ **S83.509** Sprain of unspecified cruciate ligament of unspecified knee ▽

✓6ᵗʰ **S83.51** Sprain of anterior cruciate ligament of knee

   ✓7ᵗʰ **S83.511** Sprain of anterior cruciate ligament of right knee

   ✓7ᵗʰ **S83.512** Sprain of anterior cruciate ligament of left knee

   ✓7ᵗʰ **S83.519** Sprain of anterior cruciate ligament of unspecified knee ▽

✓6ᵗʰ **S83.52** Sprain of posterior cruciate ligament of knee

   ✓7ᵗʰ **S83.521** Sprain of posterior cruciate ligament of right knee

   ✓7ᵗʰ **S83.522** Sprain of posterior cruciate ligament of left knee

   ✓7ᵗʰ **S83.529** Sprain of posterior cruciate ligament of unspecified knee ▽

✓5ᵗʰ **S83.6** Sprain of the superior tibiofibular joint and ligament

   ✓x7ᵗʰ **S83.60** Sprain of the superior tibiofibular joint and ligament, unspecified knee ▽

   ✓x7ᵗʰ **S83.61** Sprain of the superior tibiofibular joint and ligament, right knee

   ✓x7ᵗʰ **S83.62** Sprain of the superior tibiofibular joint and ligament, left knee

✓5ᵗʰ **S83.8** Sprain of other specified parts of knee

   ✓6ᵗʰ **S83.8X** Sprain of other specified parts of knee

      ✓7ᵗʰ **S83.8X1** Sprain of other specified parts of right knee

      ✓7ᵗʰ **S83.8X2** Sprain of other specified parts of left knee

      ✓7ᵗʰ **S83.8X9** Sprain of other specified parts of unspecified knee ▽

✓5ᵗʰ **S83.9** Sprain of unspecified site of knee

   ✓x7ᵗʰ **S83.90** Sprain of unspecified site of unspecified knee ▽

   ✓x7ᵗʰ **S83.91** Sprain of unspecified site of right knee ▽

   ✓x7ᵗʰ **S83.92** Sprain of unspecified site of left knee ▽

✓4ᵗʰ **S84** **Injury of nerves at lower leg level**
   Code also any associated open wound (S81.-)
   EXCLUDES 2 injury of nerves at ankle and foot level (S94.-)

   The appropriate 7th character is to be added to each code from category S84.
   A   initial encounter
   D   subsequent encounter
   S   sequela

✓5ᵗʰ **S84.0** Injury of tibial nerve at lower leg level

   ✓x7ᵗʰ **S84.00** Injury of tibial nerve at lower leg level, unspecified leg ▽

   2 ✓x7ᵗʰ **S84.01** Injury of tibial nerve at lower leg level, right leg

   2 ✓x7ᵗʰ **S84.02** Injury of tibial nerve at lower leg level, left leg

✓5ᵗʰ **S84.1** Injury of peroneal nerve at lower leg level

   ✓x7ᵗʰ **S84.10** Injury of peroneal nerve at lower leg level, unspecified leg ▽

   2 ✓x7ᵗʰ **S84.11** Injury of peroneal nerve at lower leg level, right leg

   2 ✓x7ᵗʰ **S84.12** Injury of peroneal nerve at lower leg level, left leg

✓5ᵗʰ **S84.2** Injury of cutaneous sensory nerve at lower leg level

   ✓x7ᵗʰ **S84.20** Injury of cutaneous sensory nerve at lower leg level, unspecified leg ▽

   2 ✓x7ᵗʰ **S84.21** Injury of cutaneous sensory nerve at lower leg level, right leg

   2 ✓x7ᵗʰ **S84.22** Injury of cutaneous sensory nerve at lower leg level, left leg

✓5ᵗʰ **S84.8** Injury of other nerves at lower leg level

   ✓6ᵗʰ **S84.80** Injury of other nerves at lower leg level

      2 ✓7ᵗʰ **S84.801** Injury of other nerves at lower leg level, right leg

      2 ✓7ᵗʰ **S84.802** Injury of other nerves at lower leg level, left leg

      ✓7ᵗʰ **S84.809** Injury of other nerves at lower leg level, unspecified leg ▽

✓5ᵗʰ **S84.9** Injury of unspecified nerve at lower leg level

   ✓x7ᵗʰ **S84.90** Injury of unspecified nerve at lower leg level, unspecified leg ▽

   2 ✓x7ᵗʰ **S84.91** Injury of unspecified nerve at lower leg level, right leg ▽

---

1 Case-mix diagnosis with 7th character indicating subsequent encounter.
2 Case-mix diagnosis with 7th character indicating subsequent encounter or sequela.

☑ Additional Character Req   ✓x7ᵗʰ Placeholder Alert   Case-Mix Diagnosis   Manifestation   ▽ Unspecified Dx   *EXCLUDES 1* Not coded here   *EXCLUDES 2* Not included here

Chapter 19. Injury, Poisoning and Certain Other Consequences of External Causes

2 ✓x7ᵗʰ **S84.92** **Injury of unspecified nerve at lower leg level, left leg** ▽

✓4ᵗʰ **S85** **Injury of blood vessels at lower leg level**
    Code also any associated open wound (S81.-)
    EXCLUDES 2 *injury of blood vessels at ankle and foot level (S95.-)*

    The appropriate 7th character is to be added to each code from category S85.
    A   initial encounter
    D   subsequent encounter
    S   sequela

✓5ᵗʰ **S85.0** **Injury of popliteal artery**
    ✓6ᵗʰ **S85.00** **Unspecified injury of popliteal artery**
        ✓7ᵗʰ **S85.001** **Unspecified injury of popliteal artery, right leg** ▽
        ✓7ᵗʰ **S85.002** **Unspecified injury of popliteal artery, left leg** ▽
        ✓7ᵗʰ **S85.009** **Unspecified injury of popliteal artery, unspecified leg** ▽
    ✓6ᵗʰ **S85.01** **Laceration of popliteal artery**
        ✓7ᵗʰ **S85.011** **Laceration of popliteal artery, right leg**
        ✓7ᵗʰ **S85.012** **Laceration of popliteal artery, left leg**
        ✓7ᵗʰ **S85.019** **Laceration of popliteal artery, unspecified leg** ▽
    ✓6ᵗʰ **S85.09** **Other specified injury of popliteal artery**
        ✓7ᵗʰ **S85.091** **Other specified injury of popliteal artery, right leg**
        ✓7ᵗʰ **S85.092** **Other specified injury of popliteal artery, left leg**
        ✓7ᵗʰ **S85.099** **Other specified injury of popliteal artery, unspecified leg** ▽

✓5ᵗʰ **S85.1** **Injury of tibial artery**
    ✓6ᵗʰ **S85.10** **Unspecified injury of unspecified tibial artery**
            Injury of tibial artery NOS
        ✓7ᵗʰ **S85.101** **Unspecified injury of unspecified tibial artery, right leg** ▽
        ✓7ᵗʰ **S85.102** **Unspecified injury of unspecified tibial artery, left leg** ▽
        ✓7ᵗʰ **S85.109** **Unspecified injury of unspecified tibial artery, unspecified leg** ▽
    ✓6ᵗʰ **S85.11** **Laceration of unspecified tibial artery**
        ✓7ᵗʰ **S85.111** **Laceration of unspecified tibial artery, right leg** ▽
        ✓7ᵗʰ **S85.112** **Laceration of unspecified tibial artery, left leg** ▽
        ✓7ᵗʰ **S85.119** **Laceration of unspecified tibial artery, unspecified leg** ▽
    ✓6ᵗʰ **S85.12** **Other specified injury of unspecified tibial artery**
        ✓7ᵗʰ **S85.121** **Other specified injury of unspecified tibial artery, right leg** ▽
        ✓7ᵗʰ **S85.122** **Other specified injury of unspecified tibial artery, left leg** ▽
        ✓7ᵗʰ **S85.129** **Other specified injury of unspecified tibial artery, unspecified leg** ▽
    ✓6ᵗʰ **S85.13** **Unspecified injury of anterior tibial artery**
        ✓7ᵗʰ **S85.131** **Unspecified injury of anterior tibial artery, right leg** ▽
        ✓7ᵗʰ **S85.132** **Unspecified injury of anterior tibial artery, left leg** ▽
        ✓7ᵗʰ **S85.139** **Unspecified injury of anterior tibial artery, unspecified leg** ▽
    ✓6ᵗʰ **S85.14** **Laceration of anterior tibial artery**
        ✓7ᵗʰ **S85.141** **Laceration of anterior tibial artery, right leg**
        ✓7ᵗʰ **S85.142** **Laceration of anterior tibial artery, left leg**
        ✓7ᵗʰ **S85.149** **Laceration of anterior tibial artery, unspecified leg** ▽
    ✓6ᵗʰ **S85.15** **Other specified injury of anterior tibial artery**
        ✓7ᵗʰ **S85.151** **Other specified injury of anterior tibial artery, right leg**
        ✓7ᵗʰ **S85.152** **Other specified injury of anterior tibial artery, left leg**

        ✓7ᵗʰ **S85.159** **Other specified injury of anterior tibial artery, unspecified leg** ▽
    ✓6ᵗʰ **S85.16** **Unspecified injury of posterior tibial artery**
        ✓7ᵗʰ **S85.161** **Unspecified injury of posterior tibial artery, right leg** ▽
        ✓7ᵗʰ **S85.162** **Unspecified injury of posterior tibial artery, left leg** ▽
        ✓7ᵗʰ **S85.169** **Unspecified injury of posterior tibial artery, unspecified leg** ▽
    ✓6ᵗʰ **S85.17** **Laceration of posterior tibial artery**
        ✓7ᵗʰ **S85.171** **Laceration of posterior tibial artery, right leg**
        ✓7ᵗʰ **S85.172** **Laceration of posterior tibial artery, left leg**
        ✓7ᵗʰ **S85.179** **Laceration of posterior tibial artery, unspecified leg** ▽
    ✓6ᵗʰ **S85.18** **Other specified injury of posterior tibial artery**
        ✓7ᵗʰ **S85.181** **Other specified injury of posterior tibial artery, right leg**
        ✓7ᵗʰ **S85.182** **Other specified injury of posterior tibial artery, left leg**
        ✓7ᵗʰ **S85.189** **Other specified injury of posterior tibial artery, unspecified leg** ▽

✓5ᵗʰ **S85.2** **Injury of peroneal artery**
    ✓6ᵗʰ **S85.20** **Unspecified injury of peroneal artery**
        ✓7ᵗʰ **S85.201** **Unspecified injury of peroneal artery, right leg** ▽
        ✓7ᵗʰ **S85.202** **Unspecified injury of peroneal artery, left leg** ▽
        ✓7ᵗʰ **S85.209** **Unspecified injury of peroneal artery, unspecified leg** ▽
    ✓6ᵗʰ **S85.21** **Laceration of peroneal artery**
        ✓7ᵗʰ **S85.211** **Laceration of peroneal artery, right leg**
        ✓7ᵗʰ **S85.212** **Laceration of peroneal artery, left leg**
        ✓7ᵗʰ **S85.219** **Laceration of peroneal artery, unspecified leg** ▽
    ✓6ᵗʰ **S85.29** **Other specified injury of peroneal artery**
        ✓7ᵗʰ **S85.291** **Other specified injury of peroneal artery, right leg**
        ✓7ᵗʰ **S85.292** **Other specified injury of peroneal artery, left leg**
        ✓7ᵗʰ **S85.299** **Other specified injury of peroneal artery, unspecified leg** ▽

✓5ᵗʰ **S85.3** **Injury of greater saphenous vein at lower leg level**
            Injury of greater saphenous vein NOS
            Injury of saphenous vein NOS
    ✓6ᵗʰ **S85.30** **Unspecified injury of greater saphenous vein at lower leg level**
        ✓7ᵗʰ **S85.301** **Unspecified injury of greater saphenous vein at lower leg level, right leg** ▽
        ✓7ᵗʰ **S85.302** **Unspecified injury of greater saphenous vein at lower leg level, left leg** ▽
        ✓7ᵗʰ **S85.309** **Unspecified injury of greater saphenous vein at lower leg level, unspecified leg** ▽
    ✓6ᵗʰ **S85.31** **Laceration of greater saphenous vein at lower leg level**
        ✓7ᵗʰ **S85.311** **Laceration of greater saphenous vein at lower leg level, right leg**
        ✓7ᵗʰ **S85.312** **Laceration of greater saphenous vein at lower leg level, left leg**
        ✓7ᵗʰ **S85.319** **Laceration of greater saphenous vein at lower leg level, unspecified leg** ▽
    ✓6ᵗʰ **S85.39** **Other specified injury of greater saphenous vein at lower leg level**
        ✓7ᵗʰ **S85.391** **Other specified injury of greater saphenous vein at lower leg level, right leg**
        ✓7ᵗʰ **S85.392** **Other specified injury of greater saphenous vein at lower leg level, left leg**

2   Case-mix diagnosis with 7th character indicating subsequent encounter or sequela.

Ⓝ Newborn: 0   Ⓟ Pediatric: 0-17   Ⓜ Maternity: 12-55   Ⓐ Adult: 15-124   NRS Nonroutine supply Dx   NC Dx Noncancer Dx   PDx Primary Dx   ►◄ Revised Text   ● New Code   ▲ Revised Title

1020   ICD-10-CM 2018

√7ᵗʰ **S85.399** Other specified injury of greater saphenous vein at lower leg level, unspecified leg ▽

√5ᵗʰ **S85.4 Injury of** lesser saphenous vein at lower leg level

  √6ᵗʰ **S85.40** Unspecified injury of lesser saphenous vein at lower leg level

    √7ᵗʰ **S85.401** Unspecified injury of lesser saphenous vein at lower leg level, right leg ▽

    √7ᵗʰ **S85.402** Unspecified injury of lesser saphenous vein at lower leg level, left leg ▽

    √7ᵗʰ **S85.409** Unspecified injury of lesser saphenous vein at lower leg level, unspecified leg ▽

  √6ᵗʰ **S85.41** Laceration of lesser saphenous vein at lower leg level

    √7ᵗʰ **S85.411** Laceration of lesser saphenous vein at lower leg level, right leg

    √7ᵗʰ **S85.412** Laceration of lesser saphenous vein at lower leg level, left leg

    √7ᵗʰ **S85.419** Laceration of lesser saphenous vein at lower leg level, unspecified leg ▽

  √6ᵗʰ **S85.49** Other specified injury of lesser saphenous vein at lower leg level

    √7ᵗʰ **S85.491** Other specified injury of lesser saphenous vein at lower leg level, right leg

    √7ᵗʰ **S85.492** Other specified injury of lesser saphenous vein at lower leg level, left leg

    √7ᵗʰ **S85.499** Other specified injury of lesser saphenous vein at lower leg level, unspecified leg ▽

√5ᵗʰ **S85.5 Injury of** popliteal vein

  √6ᵗʰ **S85.50** Unspecified injury of popliteal vein

    √7ᵗʰ **S85.501** Unspecified injury of popliteal vein, right leg ▽

    √7ᵗʰ **S85.502** Unspecified injury of popliteal vein, left leg ▽

    √7ᵗʰ **S85.509** Unspecified injury of popliteal vein, unspecified leg ▽

  √6ᵗʰ **S85.51** Laceration of popliteal vein

    √7ᵗʰ **S85.511** Laceration of popliteal vein, right leg

    √7ᵗʰ **S85.512** Laceration of popliteal vein, left leg

    √7ᵗʰ **S85.519** Laceration of popliteal vein, unspecified leg ▽

  √6ᵗʰ **S85.59** Other specified injury of popliteal vein

    √7ᵗʰ **S85.591** Other specified injury of popliteal vein, right leg

    √7ᵗʰ **S85.592** Other specified injury of popliteal vein, left leg

    √7ᵗʰ **S85.599** Other specified injury of popliteal vein, unspecified leg ▽

√5ᵗʰ **S85.8 Injury of** other blood vessels at lower leg level

  √6ᵗʰ **S85.80** Unspecified injury of other blood vessels at lower leg level

    √7ᵗʰ **S85.801** Unspecified injury of other blood vessels at lower leg level, right leg ▽

    √7ᵗʰ **S85.802** Unspecified injury of other blood vessels at lower leg level, left leg ▽

    √7ᵗʰ **S85.809** Unspecified injury of other blood vessels at lower leg level, unspecified leg ▽

  √6ᵗʰ **S85.81** Laceration of other blood vessels at lower leg level

    √7ᵗʰ **S85.811** Laceration of other blood vessels at lower leg level, right leg

    √7ᵗʰ **S85.812** Laceration of other blood vessels at lower leg level, left leg

    √7ᵗʰ **S85.819** Laceration of other blood vessels at lower leg level, unspecified leg ▽

  √6ᵗʰ **S85.89** Other specified injury of other blood vessels at lower leg level

    √7ᵗʰ **S85.891** Other specified injury of other blood vessels at lower leg level, right leg

    √7ᵗʰ **S85.892** Other specified injury of other blood vessels at lower leg level, left leg

    √7ᵗʰ **S85.899** Other specified injury of other blood vessels at lower leg level, unspecified leg ▽

√5ᵗʰ **S85.9 Injury of** unspecified blood vessel at lower leg level

  √6ᵗʰ **S85.90** Unspecified injury of unspecified blood vessel at lower leg level

    √7ᵗʰ **S85.901** Unspecified injury of unspecified blood vessel at lower leg level, right leg ▽

    √7ᵗʰ **S85.902** Unspecified injury of unspecified blood vessel at lower leg level, left leg ▽

    √7ᵗʰ **S85.909** Unspecified injury of unspecified blood vessel at lower leg level, unspecified leg ▽

  √6ᵗʰ **S85.91** Laceration of unspecified blood vessel at lower leg level

    √7ᵗʰ **S85.911** Laceration of unspecified blood vessel at lower leg level, right leg ▽

    √7ᵗʰ **S85.912** Laceration of unspecified blood vessel at lower leg level, left leg ▽

    √7ᵗʰ **S85.919** Laceration of unspecified blood vessel at lower leg level, unspecified leg ▽

  √6ᵗʰ **S85.99** Other specified injury of unspecified blood vessel at lower leg level

    √7ᵗʰ **S85.991** Other specified injury of unspecified blood vessel at lower leg level, right leg ▽

    √7ᵗʰ **S85.992** Other specified injury of unspecified blood vessel at lower leg level, left leg ▽

    √7ᵗʰ **S85.999** Other specified injury of unspecified blood vessel at lower leg level, unspecified leg ▽

√4ᵗʰ **S86 Injury of muscle, fascia and tendon at lower leg level**

Code also any associated open wound (S81.-)

EXCLUDES 2   injury of muscle, fascia and tendon at ankle (S96.-)
injury of patellar ligament (tendon) (S76.1-)
sprain of joints and ligaments of knee (S83.-)

TIP: Refer to the Muscle/Tendon table at the beginning of this chapter.

> The appropriate 7th character is to be added to each code from category S86.
> A   initial encounter
> D   subsequent encounter
> S   sequela

√5ᵗʰ **S86.0 Injury of** Achilles tendon

  √6ᵗʰ **S86.00** Unspecified injury of Achilles tendon

    √7ᵗʰ **S86.001** Unspecified injury of right Achilles tendon ▽

    √7ᵗʰ **S86.002** Unspecified injury of left Achilles tendon ▽

    √7ᵗʰ **S86.009** Unspecified injury of unspecified Achilles tendon ▽

  √6ᵗʰ **S86.01** Strain of Achilles tendon

    √7ᵗʰ **S86.011** Strain of right Achilles tendon

    √7ᵗʰ **S86.012** Strain of left Achilles tendon

    √7ᵗʰ **S86.019** Strain of unspecified Achilles tendon ▽

  √6ᵗʰ **S86.02** Laceration of Achilles tendon

    4,5 √7ᵗʰ **S86.021** Laceration of right Achilles tendon   NRS

    4,5 √7ᵗʰ **S86.022** Laceration of left Achilles tendon   NRS

    √7ᵗʰ **S86.029** Laceration of unspecified Achilles tendon ▽

  √6ᵗʰ **S86.09** Other specified injury of Achilles tendon

    √7ᵗʰ **S86.091** Other specified injury of right Achilles tendon

    √7ᵗʰ **S86.092** Other specified injury of left Achilles tendon

    √7ᵗʰ **S86.099** Other specified injury of unspecified Achilles tendon ▽

---

4   Case-mix diagnosis with 7th character indicating initial or subsequent encounter.
5   NRS supply diagnosis with 7th character indicating initial or subsequent encounter.

☑ Additional Character Req   √×7ᵗʰ Placeholder Alert   Case-Mix Diagnosis   Manifestation   ▽ Unspecified Dx   *EXCLUDES 1* Not coded here   *EXCLUDES 2* Not included here

Chapter 19. Injury, Poisoning and Certain Other Consequences of External Causes *(side tab)*

S86.1–S86.809 *(side tab)*

✓5ᵗʰ **S86.1** Injury of other muscle(s) and tendon(s) of posterior muscle group at lower leg level

✓6ᵗʰ **S86.10** Unspecified injury of other muscle(s) and tendon(s) of posterior muscle group at lower leg level

✓7ᵗʰ **S86.101** Unspecified injury of other muscle(s) and tendon(s) of posterior muscle group at lower leg level, right leg ▽

✓7ᵗʰ **S86.102** Unspecified injury of other muscle(s) and tendon(s) of posterior muscle group at lower leg level, left leg ▽

✓7ᵗʰ **S86.109** Unspecified injury of other muscle(s) and tendon(s) of posterior muscle group at lower leg level, unspecified leg ▽

✓6ᵗʰ **S86.11** Strain of other muscle(s) and tendon(s) of posterior muscle group at lower leg level

✓7ᵗʰ **S86.111** Strain of other muscle(s) and tendon(s) of posterior muscle group at lower leg level, right leg

✓7ᵗʰ **S86.112** Strain of other muscle(s) and tendon(s) of posterior muscle group at lower leg level, left leg

✓7ᵗʰ **S86.119** Strain of other muscle(s) and tendon(s) of posterior muscle group at lower leg level, unspecified leg ▽

✓6ᵗʰ **S86.12** Laceration of other muscle(s) and tendon(s) of posterior muscle group at lower leg level

4,5 ✓7ᵗʰ **S86.121** Laceration of other muscle(s) and tendon(s) of posterior muscle group at lower leg level, right leg **NRS**

4,5 ✓7ᵗʰ **S86.122** Laceration of other muscle(s) and tendon(s) of posterior muscle group at lower leg level, left leg **NRS**

✓7ᵗʰ **S86.129** Laceration of other muscle(s) and tendon(s) of posterior muscle group at lower leg level, unspecified leg ▽

✓6ᵗʰ **S86.19** Other injury of other muscle(s) and tendon(s) of posterior muscle group at lower leg level

✓7ᵗʰ **S86.191** Other injury of other muscle(s) and tendon(s) of posterior muscle group at lower leg level, right leg

✓7ᵗʰ **S86.192** Other injury of other muscle(s) and tendon(s) of posterior muscle group at lower leg level, left leg

✓7ᵗʰ **S86.199** Other injury of other muscle(s) and tendon(s) of posterior muscle group at lower leg level, unspecified leg ▽

✓5ᵗʰ **S86.2** Injury of muscle(s) and tendon(s) of anterior muscle group at lower leg level

✓6ᵗʰ **S86.20** Unspecified injury of muscle(s) and tendon(s) of anterior muscle group at lower leg level

✓7ᵗʰ **S86.201** Unspecified injury of muscle(s) and tendon(s) of anterior muscle group at lower leg level, right leg ▽

✓7ᵗʰ **S86.202** Unspecified injury of muscle(s) and tendon(s) of anterior muscle group at lower leg level, left leg ▽

✓7ᵗʰ **S86.209** Unspecified injury of muscle(s) and tendon(s) of anterior muscle group at lower leg level, unspecified leg ▽

✓6ᵗʰ **S86.21** Strain of muscle(s) and tendon(s) of anterior muscle group at lower leg level

✓7ᵗʰ **S86.211** Strain of muscle(s) and tendon(s) of anterior muscle group at lower leg level, right leg

✓7ᵗʰ **S86.212** Strain of muscle(s) and tendon(s) of anterior muscle group at lower leg level, left leg

✓7ᵗʰ **S86.219** Strain of muscle(s) and tendon(s) of anterior muscle group at lower leg level, unspecified leg ▽

✓6ᵗʰ **S86.22** Laceration of muscle(s) and tendon(s) of anterior muscle group at lower leg level

4,5 ✓7ᵗʰ **S86.221** Laceration of muscle(s) and tendon(s) of anterior muscle group at lower leg level, right leg **NRS**

4,5 ✓7ᵗʰ **S86.222** Laceration of muscle(s) and tendon(s) of anterior muscle group at lower leg level, left leg **NRS**

✓7ᵗʰ **S86.229** Laceration of muscle(s) and tendon(s) of anterior muscle group at lower leg level, unspecified leg ▽

✓6ᵗʰ **S86.29** Other injury of muscle(s) and tendon(s) of anterior muscle group at lower leg level

✓7ᵗʰ **S86.291** Other injury of muscle(s) and tendon(s) of anterior muscle group at lower leg level, right leg

✓7ᵗʰ **S86.292** Other injury of muscle(s) and tendon(s) of anterior muscle group at lower leg level, left leg

✓7ᵗʰ **S86.299** Other injury of muscle(s) and tendon(s) of anterior muscle group at lower leg level, unspecified leg ▽

✓5ᵗʰ **S86.3** Injury of muscle(s) and tendon(s) of peroneal muscle group at lower leg level

✓6ᵗʰ **S86.30** Unspecified injury of muscle(s) and tendon(s) of peroneal muscle group at lower leg level

✓7ᵗʰ **S86.301** Unspecified injury of muscle(s) and tendon(s) of peroneal muscle group at lower leg level, right leg ▽

✓7ᵗʰ **S86.302** Unspecified injury of muscle(s) and tendon(s) of peroneal muscle group at lower leg level, left leg ▽

✓7ᵗʰ **S86.309** Unspecified injury of muscle(s) and tendon(s) of peroneal muscle group at lower leg level, unspecified leg ▽

✓6ᵗʰ **S86.31** Strain of muscle(s) and tendon(s) of peroneal muscle group at lower leg level

✓7ᵗʰ **S86.311** Strain of muscle(s) and tendon(s) of peroneal muscle group at lower leg level, right leg

✓7ᵗʰ **S86.312** Strain of muscle(s) and tendon(s) of peroneal muscle group at lower leg level, left leg

✓7ᵗʰ **S86.319** Strain of muscle(s) and tendon(s) of peroneal muscle group at lower leg level, unspecified leg ▽

✓6ᵗʰ **S86.32** Laceration of muscle(s) and tendon(s) of peroneal muscle group at lower leg level

4,5 ✓7ᵗʰ **S86.321** Laceration of muscle(s) and tendon(s) of peroneal muscle group at lower leg level, right leg **NRS**

4,5 ✓7ᵗʰ **S86.322** Laceration of muscle(s) and tendon(s) of peroneal muscle group at lower leg level, left leg **NRS**

✓7ᵗʰ **S86.329** Laceration of muscle(s) and tendon(s) of peroneal muscle group at lower leg level, unspecified leg ▽

✓6ᵗʰ **S86.39** Other injury of muscle(s) and tendon(s) of peroneal muscle group at lower leg level

✓7ᵗʰ **S86.391** Other injury of muscle(s) and tendon(s) of peroneal muscle group at lower leg level, right leg

✓7ᵗʰ **S86.392** Other injury of muscle(s) and tendon(s) of peroneal muscle group at lower leg level, left leg

✓7ᵗʰ **S86.399** Other injury of muscle(s) and tendon(s) of peroneal muscle group at lower leg level, unspecified leg ▽

✓5ᵗʰ **S86.8** Injury of other muscles and tendons at lower leg level

✓6ᵗʰ **S86.80** Unspecified injury of other muscles and tendons at lower leg level

✓7ᵗʰ **S86.801** Unspecified injury of other muscle(s) and tendon(s) at lower leg level, right leg ▽

✓7ᵗʰ **S86.802** Unspecified injury of other muscle(s) and tendon(s) at lower leg level, left leg ▽

✓7ᵗʰ **S86.809** Unspecified injury of other muscle(s) and tendon(s) at lower leg level, unspecified leg ▽

---

4 Case-mix diagnosis with 7th character indicating initial or subsequent encounter.
5 NRS supply diagnosis with 7th character indicating initial or subsequent encounter.

Ⓝ Newborn: 0   Ⓟ Pediatric: 0-17   Ⓜ Maternity: 12-55   Ⓐ Adult: 15-124   **NRS** Nonroutine supply Dx   **NCDx** Noncancer Dx   **PDx** Primary Dx   ►◄ Revised Text   ● New Code   ▲ Revised Title

✓6ᵗʰ **S86.81** Strain of other muscles and tendons at lower leg level

　✓7ᵗʰ **S86.811** Strain of other muscle(s) and tendon(s) at lower leg level, right leg

　✓7ᵗʰ **S86.812** Strain of other muscle(s) and tendon(s) at lower leg level, left leg

　✓7ᵗʰ **S86.819** Strain of other muscle(s) and tendon(s) at lower leg level, unspecified leg ▽

✓6ᵗʰ **S86.82** Laceration of other muscles and tendons at lower leg level

　4,5 ✓7ᵗʰ **S86.821** Laceration of other muscle(s) and tendon(s) at lower leg level, right leg **NRS**

　4,5 ✓7ᵗʰ **S86.822** Laceration of other muscle(s) and tendon(s) at lower leg level, left leg **NRS**

　✓7ᵗʰ **S86.829** Laceration of other muscle(s) and tendon(s) at lower leg level, unspecified leg ▽

✓6ᵗʰ **S86.89** Other injury of other muscles and tendons at lower leg level

　✓7ᵗʰ **S86.891** Other injury of other muscle(s) and tendon(s) at lower leg level, right leg

　✓7ᵗʰ **S86.892** Other injury of other muscle(s) and tendon(s) at lower leg level, left leg

　✓7ᵗʰ **S86.899** Other injury of other muscle(s) and tendon(s) at lower leg level, unspecified leg ▽

✓5ᵗʰ **S86.9** Injury of unspecified muscle and tendon at lower leg level

　✓6ᵗʰ **S86.90** Unspecified injury of unspecified muscle and tendon at lower leg level

　　✓7ᵗʰ **S86.901** Unspecified injury of unspecified muscle(s) and tendon(s) at lower leg level, right leg ▽

　　✓7ᵗʰ **S86.902** Unspecified injury of unspecified muscle(s) and tendon(s) at lower leg level, left leg ▽

　　✓7ᵗʰ **S86.909** Unspecified injury of unspecified muscle(s) and tendon(s) at lower leg level, unspecified leg ▽

　✓6ᵗʰ **S86.91** Strain of unspecified muscle and tendon at lower leg level

　　✓7ᵗʰ **S86.911** Strain of unspecified muscle(s) and tendon(s) at lower leg level, right leg ▽

　　✓7ᵗʰ **S86.912** Strain of unspecified muscle(s) and tendon(s) at lower leg level, left leg ▽

　　✓7ᵗʰ **S86.919** Strain of unspecified muscle(s) and tendon(s) at lower leg level, unspecified leg ▽

　✓6ᵗʰ **S86.92** Laceration of unspecified muscle and tendon at lower leg level

　　4,5 ✓7ᵗʰ **S86.921** Laceration of unspecified muscle(s) and tendon(s) at lower leg level, right leg **NRS** ▽

　　4,5 ✓7ᵗʰ **S86.922** Laceration of unspecified muscle(s) and tendon(s) at lower leg level, left leg **NRS** ▽

　　✓7ᵗʰ **S86.929** Laceration of unspecified muscle(s) and tendon(s) at lower leg level, unspecified leg ▽

　✓6ᵗʰ **S86.99** Other injury of unspecified muscle and tendon at lower leg level

　　✓7ᵗʰ **S86.991** Other injury of unspecified muscle(s) and tendon(s) at lower leg level, right leg ▽

　　✓7ᵗʰ **S86.992** Other injury of unspecified muscle(s) and tendon(s) at lower leg level, left leg ▽

　　✓7ᵗʰ **S86.999** Other injury of unspecified muscle(s) and tendon(s) at lower leg level, unspecified leg ▽

✓4ᵗʰ **S87** Crushing injury of lower leg

Use additional code(s) for all associated injuries

EXCLUDES 2 crushing injury of ankle and foot (S97.-)

The appropriate 7th character is to be added to each code from category S87.
A　initial encounter
D　subsequent encounter
S　sequela

✓5ᵗʰ **S87.0** Crushing injury of knee

　✓x7ᵗʰ **S87.00** Crushing injury of unspecified knee ▽

　1 ✓x7ᵗʰ **S87.01** Crushing injury of right knee

　1 ✓x7ᵗʰ **S87.02** Crushing injury of left knee

✓5ᵗʰ **S87.8** Crushing injury of lower leg

　✓x7ᵗʰ **S87.80** Crushing injury of unspecified lower leg ▽

　1 ✓x7ᵗʰ **S87.81** Crushing injury of right lower leg

　1 ✓x7ᵗʰ **S87.82** Crushing injury of left lower leg

✓4ᵗʰ **S88** Traumatic amputation of lower leg

An amputation not identified as partial or complete should be coded to complete.

EXCLUDES 1 traumatic amputation of ankle and foot (S98.-)

The appropriate 7th character is to be added to each code from category S88.
A　initial encounter
D　subsequent encounter
S　sequela

✓5ᵗʰ **S88.0** Traumatic amputation at knee level

　✓6ᵗʰ **S88.01** Complete traumatic amputation at knee level

　　4,5 ✓7ᵗʰ **S88.011** Complete traumatic amputation at knee level, right lower leg **NRS**

　　4,5 ✓7ᵗʰ **S88.012** Complete traumatic amputation at knee level, left lower leg **NRS**

　　✓7ᵗʰ **S88.019** Complete traumatic amputation at knee level, unspecified lower leg ▽

　✓6ᵗʰ **S88.02** Partial traumatic amputation at knee level

　　4,5 ✓7ᵗʰ **S88.021** Partial traumatic amputation at knee level, right lower leg **NRS**

　　4,5 ✓7ᵗʰ **S88.022** Partial traumatic amputation at knee level, left lower leg **NRS**

　　4 ✓7ᵗʰ **S88.029** Partial traumatic amputation at knee level, unspecified lower leg ▽

✓5ᵗʰ **S88.1** Traumatic amputation at level between knee and ankle

　✓6ᵗʰ **S88.11** Complete traumatic amputation at level between knee and ankle

　　4,5 ✓7ᵗʰ **S88.111** Complete traumatic amputation at level between knee and ankle, right lower leg **NRS**

　　4,5 ✓7ᵗʰ **S88.112** Complete traumatic amputation at level between knee and ankle, left lower leg **NRS**

　　✓7ᵗʰ **S88.119** Complete traumatic amputation at level between knee and ankle, unspecified lower leg ▽

　✓6ᵗʰ **S88.12** Partial traumatic amputation at level between knee and ankle

　　4,5 ✓7ᵗʰ **S88.121** Partial traumatic amputation at level between knee and ankle, right lower leg **NRS**

　　4,5 ✓7ᵗʰ **S88.122** Partial traumatic amputation at level between knee and ankle, left lower leg **NRS**

　　✓7ᵗʰ **S88.129** Partial traumatic amputation at level between knee and ankle, unspecified lower leg ▽

✓5ᵗʰ **S88.9** Traumatic amputation of lower leg, level unspecified

　✓6ᵗʰ **S88.91** Complete traumatic amputation of lower leg, level unspecified

　　4,5 ✓7ᵗʰ **S88.911** Complete traumatic amputation of right lower leg, level unspecified **NRS** ▽

　　4,5 ✓7ᵗʰ **S88.912** Complete traumatic amputation of left lower leg, level unspecified **NRS** ▽

---

1 Case-mix diagnosis with 7th character indicating subsequent encounter.
4 Case-mix diagnosis with 7th character indicating initial or subsequent encounter.
5 NRS supply diagnosis with 7th character indicating initial or subsequent encounter.

☑ Additional Character Req　　✓x7ᵗʰ Placeholder Alert　　Case-Mix Diagnosis　　Manifestation　　▽ Unspecified Dx　　**EXCLUDES 1** Not coded here　　**EXCLUDES 2** Not included here

✓7ᵗʰ **S88.919** Complete traumatic amputation of unspecified lower leg, level unspecified

✓6ᵗʰ **S88.92** Partial **traumatic amputation of lower leg, level unspecified**

4,5 ✓7ᵗʰ **S88.921** Partial traumatic amputation of right lower leg, level unspecified   NRS ▽

4,5 ✓7ᵗʰ **S88.922** Partial traumatic amputation of left lower leg, level unspecified   NRS ▽

✓7ᵗʰ **S88.929** Partial traumatic amputation of unspecified lower leg, level unspecified ▽

✓4ᵗʰ **S89** **Other and unspecified injuries of lower leg**

NOTE   A fracture not indicated as open or closed should be coded to closed.

EXCLUDES 2   *other and unspecified injuries of ankle and foot (S99.-)*

AHA: 2015, 3Q, 37-39

TIP: The term "improper alignment" is not synonymous with malunion or nonunion of a fracture when noted in provider documentation.

The appropriate 7th character is to be added to each code from subcategories S89.0, S89.1, S89.2, and S89.3.
A   initial encounter for closed fracture
D   subsequent encounter for fracture with routine healing
G   subsequent encounter for fracture with delayed healing
K   subsequent encounter for fracture with nonunion
P   subsequent encounter for fracture with malunion
S   sequela

✓5ᵗʰ **S89.0** **Physeal fracture of** upper end of tibia

✓6ᵗʰ **S89.00** **Unspecified physeal fracture of upper end of tibia**

1 ✓7ᵗʰ **S89.001** Unspecified physeal fracture of upper end of right tibia ▽

1 ✓7ᵗʰ **S89.002** Unspecified physeal fracture of upper end of left tibia ▽

✓7ᵗʰ **S89.009** Unspecified physeal fracture of upper end of unspecified tibia ▽

✓6ᵗʰ **S89.01** Salter-Harris Type I physeal fracture of upper end of tibia

1 ✓7ᵗʰ **S89.011** Salter-Harris Type I physeal fracture of upper end of right tibia

1 ✓7ᵗʰ **S89.012** Salter-Harris Type I physeal fracture of upper end of left tibia

✓7ᵗʰ **S89.019** Salter-Harris Type I physeal fracture of upper end of unspecified tibia ▽

✓6ᵗʰ **S89.02** Salter-Harris Type II physeal fracture of upper end of tibia

1 ✓7ᵗʰ **S89.021** Salter-Harris Type II physeal fracture of upper end of right tibia

1 ✓7ᵗʰ **S89.022** Salter-Harris Type II physeal fracture of upper end of left tibia

✓7ᵗʰ **S89.029** Salter-Harris Type II physeal fracture of upper end of unspecified tibia ▽

✓6ᵗʰ **S89.03** Salter-Harris Type III physeal fracture of upper end of tibia

1 ✓7ᵗʰ **S89.031** Salter-Harris Type III physeal fracture of upper end of right tibia

1 ✓7ᵗʰ **S89.032** Salter-Harris Type III physeal fracture of upper end of left tibia

✓7ᵗʰ **S89.039** Salter-Harris Type III physeal fracture of upper end of unspecified tibia ▽

✓6ᵗʰ **S89.04** Salter-Harris Type IV physeal fracture of upper end of tibia

1 ✓7ᵗʰ **S89.041** Salter-Harris Type IV physeal fracture of upper end of right tibia

1 ✓7ᵗʰ **S89.042** Salter-Harris Type IV physeal fracture of upper end of left tibia

✓7ᵗʰ **S89.049** Salter-Harris Type IV physeal fracture of upper end of unspecified tibia ▽

✓6ᵗʰ **S89.09** Other physeal fracture of upper end of tibia

1 ✓7ᵗʰ **S89.091** Other physeal fracture of upper end of right tibia

1 ✓7ᵗʰ **S89.092** Other physeal fracture of upper end of left tibia

✓7ᵗʰ **S89.099** Other physeal fracture of upper end of unspecified tibia ▽

✓5ᵗʰ **S89.1** **Physeal fracture of** lower end of tibia

✓6ᵗʰ **S89.10** Unspecified physeal fracture of lower end of tibia

1 ✓7ᵗʰ **S89.101** Unspecified physeal fracture of lower end of right tibia ▽

1 ✓7ᵗʰ **S89.102** Unspecified physeal fracture of lower end of left tibia ▽

1 ✓7ᵗʰ **S89.109** Unspecified physeal fracture of lower end of unspecified tibia ▽

✓6ᵗʰ **S89.11** Salter-Harris Type I physeal fracture of ower end of tibia

1 ✓7ᵗʰ **S89.111** Salter-Harris Type I physeal fracture of lower end of right tibia

1 ✓7ᵗʰ **S89.112** Salter-Harris Type I physeal fracture of lower end of left tibia

✓7ᵗʰ **S89.119** Salter-Harris Type I physeal fracture of lower end of unspecified tibia ▽

✓6ᵗʰ **S89.12** Salter-Harris Type II physeal fracture of lower end of tibia

1 ✓7ᵗʰ **S89.121** Salter-Harris Type II physeal fracture of lower end of right tibia

1 ✓7ᵗʰ **S89.122** Salter-Harris Type II physeal fracture of lower end of left tibia

✓7ᵗʰ **S89.129** Salter-Harris Type II physeal fracture of lower end of unspecified tibia ▽

✓6ᵗʰ **S89.13** Salter-Harris Type III physeal fracture of lower end of tibia

EXCLUDES 1   *fracture of medial malleolus (adult) (S82.5-)*

1 ✓7ᵗʰ **S89.131** Salter-Harris Type III physeal fracture of lower end of right tibia

1 ✓7ᵗʰ **S89.132** Salter-Harris Type III physeal fracture of lower end of left tibia

✓7ᵗʰ **S89.139** Salter-Harris Type III physeal fracture of lower end of unspecified tibia ▽

✓6ᵗʰ **S89.14** Salter-Harris Type IV physeal fracture of lower end of tibia

EXCLUDES 1   *fracture of medial malleolus (adult) (S82.5-)*

1 ✓7ᵗʰ **S89.141** Salter-Harris Type IV physeal fracture of lower end of right tibia

1 ✓7ᵗʰ **S89.142** Salter-Harris Type IV physeal fracture of lower end of left tibia

✓7ᵗʰ **S89.149** Salter-Harris Type IV physeal fracture of lower end of unspecified tibia ▽

✓6ᵗʰ **S89.19** Other physeal fracture of lower end of tibia

1 ✓7ᵗʰ **S89.191** Other physeal fracture of lower end of right tibia

1 ✓7ᵗʰ **S89.192** Other physeal fracture of lower end of left tibia

✓7ᵗʰ **S89.199** Other physeal fracture of lower end of unspecified tibia ▽

✓5ᵗʰ **S89.2** **Physeal fracture of** upper end of fibula

✓6ᵗʰ **S89.20** Unspecified physeal fracture of upper end of fibula

1 ✓7ᵗʰ **S89.201** Unspecified physeal fracture of upper end of right fibula ▽

1 ✓7ᵗʰ **S89.202** Unspecified physeal fracture of upper end of left fibula ▽

✓7ᵗʰ **S89.209** Unspecified physeal fracture of upper end of unspecified fibula ▽

✓6ᵗʰ **S89.21** Salter-Harris Type I physeal fracture of upper end of fibula

1 ✓7ᵗʰ **S89.211** Salter-Harris Type I physeal fracture of upper end of right fibula

1 ✓7ᵗʰ **S89.212** Salter-Harris Type I physeal fracture of upper end of left fibula

✓7ᵗʰ **S89.219** Salter-Harris Type I physeal fracture of upper end of unspecified fibula ▽

✓6ᵗʰ **S89.22** Salter-Harris Type II physeal fracture of upper end of fibula

1 ✓7ᵗʰ **S89.221** Salter-Harris Type II physeal fracture of upper end of right fibula

1 ✓7ᵗʰ **S89.222** Salter-Harris Type II physeal fracture of upper end of left fibula

---

1   Case-mix diagnosis with 7th character indicating subsequent encounter.
4   Case-mix diagnosis with 7th character indicating initial or subsequent encounter.
5   NRS supply diagnosis with 7th character indicating initial or subsequent encounter.

N Newborn: 0   P Pediatric: 0-17   M Maternity: 12-55   A Adult: 15-124   NRS Nonroutine supply Dx   NC Dx Noncancer Dx   PDx Primary Dx   ▶◀ Revised Text   ● New Code   ▲ Revised Title

✓7ᵗʰ **S89.229** Salter-Harris Type II physeal fracture of upper end of unspecified fibula ▽

✓6ᵗʰ **S89.29** Other physeal fracture of upper end of fibula

  ¹ ✓7ᵗʰ **S89.291** **Other physeal fracture of upper end of right fibula**

  ¹ ✓7ᵗʰ **S89.292** **Other physeal fracture of upper end of left fibula**

  ✓7ᵗʰ **S89.299** Other physeal fracture of upper end of unspecified fibula ▽

✓5ᵗʰ **S89.3** Physeal fracture of lower end of fibula

  ✓6ᵗʰ **S89.30** Unspecified physeal fracture of lower end of fibula

   ¹ ✓7ᵗʰ **S89.301** **Unspecified physeal fracture of lower end of right fibula** ▽

   ¹ ✓7ᵗʰ **S89.302** **Unspecified physeal fracture of lower end of left fibula** ▽

   ✓7ᵗʰ **S89.309** Unspecified physeal fracture of lower end of unspecified fibula ▽

  ✓6ᵗʰ **S89.31** Salter-Harris Type I physeal fracture of lower end of fibula

   ¹ ✓7ᵗʰ **S89.311** **Salter-Harris Type I physeal fracture of lower end of right fibula**

   ¹ ✓7ᵗʰ **S89.312** **Salter-Harris Type I physeal fracture of lower end of left fibula**

   ✓7ᵗʰ **S89.319** Salter-Harris Type I physeal fracture of lower end of unspecified fibula ▽

  ✓6ᵗʰ **S89.32** Salter-Harris Type II physeal fracture of lower end of fibula

   ¹ ✓7ᵗʰ **S89.321** **Salter-Harris Type II physeal fracture of lower end of right fibula**

   ¹ ✓7ᵗʰ **S89.322** **Salter-Harris Type II physeal fracture of lower end of left fibula**

   ✓7ᵗʰ **S89.329** Salter-Harris Type II physeal fracture of lower end of unspecified fibula ▽

  ✓6ᵗʰ **S89.39** Other physeal fracture of lower end of fibula

   ¹ ✓7ᵗʰ **S89.391** **Other physeal fracture of lower end of right fibula**

   ¹ ✓7ᵗʰ **S89.392** **Other physeal fracture of lower end of left fibula**

   ✓7ᵗʰ **S89.399** Other physeal fracture of lower end of unspecified fibula ▽

✓5ᵗʰ **S89.8** Other specified injuries of lower leg

> The appropriate 7th character is to be added to each code in subcategory S89.8.
> A   initial encounter
> D   subsequent encounter
> S   sequela

  ✓×7ᵗʰ **S89.80** Other specified injuries of unspecified lower leg ▽

  ✓×7ᵗʰ **S89.81** Other specified injuries of right lower leg

  ✓×7ᵗʰ **S89.82** Other specified injuries of left lower leg

✓5ᵗʰ **S89.9** Unspecified injury of lower leg

> The appropriate 7th character is to be added to each code in subcategory S89.9.
> A   initial encounter
> D   subsequent encounter
> S   sequela

  ✓×7ᵗʰ **S89.90** Unspecified injury of unspecified lower leg ▽

  ✓×7ᵗʰ **S89.91** Unspecified injury of right lower leg ▽

  ✓×7ᵗʰ **S89.92** Unspecified injury of left lower leg ▽

Injuries to the ankle and foot (S90-S99)

EXCLUDES 2   burns and corrosions (T20-T32)
          fracture of ankle and malleolus (S82.-)
          frostbite (T33-T34)
          insect bite or sting, venomous (T63.4)

✓4ᵗʰ **S90   Superficial injury of ankle, foot and toes**

> The appropriate 7th character is to be added to each code from category S90.
> A   initial encounter
> D   subsequent encounter
> S   sequela

✓5ᵗʰ **S90.0** Contusion of ankle

  ✓×7ᵗʰ **S90.00** Contusion of unspecified ankle ▽

  ✓×7ᵗʰ **S90.01** Contusion of right ankle

  ✓×7ᵗʰ **S90.02** Contusion of left ankle

✓5ᵗʰ **S90.1** Contusion of toe without damage to nail

  ✓6ᵗʰ **S90.11** Contusion of great toe without damage to nail

   ✓7ᵗʰ **S90.111** Contusion of right great toe without damage to nail

   ✓7ᵗʰ **S90.112** Contusion of left great toe without damage to nail

   ✓7ᵗʰ **S90.119** Contusion of unspecified great toe without damage to nail ▽

  ✓6ᵗʰ **S90.12** Contusion of lesser toe without damage to nail

   ✓7ᵗʰ **S90.121** Contusion of right lesser toe(s) without damage to nail

   ✓7ᵗʰ **S90.122** Contusion of left lesser toe(s) without damage to nail

   ✓7ᵗʰ **S90.129** Contusion of unspecified lesser toe(s) without damage to nail ▽
       Contusion of toe NOS

✓5ᵗʰ **S90.2** Contusion of toe with damage to nail

  ✓6ᵗʰ **S90.21** Contusion of great toe with damage to nail

   ✓7ᵗʰ **S90.211** Contusion of right great toe with damage to nail

   ✓7ᵗʰ **S90.212** Contusion of left great toe with damage to nail

   ✓7ᵗʰ **S90.219** Contusion of unspecified great toe with damage to nail ▽

  ✓6ᵗʰ **S90.22** Contusion of lesser toe with damage to nail

   ✓7ᵗʰ **S90.221** Contusion of right lesser toe(s) with damage to nail

   ✓7ᵗʰ **S90.222** Contusion of left lesser toe(s) with damage to nail

   ✓7ᵗʰ **S90.229** Contusion of unspecified lesser toe(s) with damage to nail ▽

✓5ᵗʰ **S90.3** Contusion of foot

  EXCLUDES 2   contusion of toes (S90.1-, S90.2-)

  ✓×7ᵗʰ **S90.30** Contusion of unspecified foot ▽
       Contusion of foot NOS

  ✓×7ᵗʰ **S90.31** Contusion of right foot

  ✓×7ᵗʰ **S90.32** Contusion of left foot

✓5ᵗʰ **S90.4** Other superficial injuries of toe

  ✓6ᵗʰ **S90.41** Abrasion of toe

   ✓7ᵗʰ **S90.411** Abrasion, right great toe

   ✓7ᵗʰ **S90.412** Abrasion, left great toe

   ✓7ᵗʰ **S90.413** Abrasion, unspecified great toe ▽

   ✓7ᵗʰ **S90.414** Abrasion, right lesser toe(s)

   ✓7ᵗʰ **S90.415** Abrasion, left lesser toe(s)

   ✓7ᵗʰ **S90.416** Abrasion, unspecified lesser toe(s) ▽

  ✓6ᵗʰ **S90.42** Blister (nonthermal) of toe

   ✓7ᵗʰ **S90.421** Blister (nonthermal), right great toe

   ✓7ᵗʰ **S90.422** Blister (nonthermal), left great toe

   ✓7ᵗʰ **S90.423** Blister (nonthermal), unspecified great toe ▽

   ✓7ᵗʰ **S90.424** Blister (nonthermal), right lesser toe(s)

   ✓7ᵗʰ **S90.425** Blister (nonthermal), left lesser toe(s)

   ✓7ᵗʰ **S90.426** Blister (nonthermal), unspecified lesser toe(s) ▽

---

¹ Case-mix diagnosis with 7th character indicating subsequent encounter.

☑ Additional Character Req   ✓×7ᵗʰ Placeholder Alert   Case-Mix Diagnosis   Manifestation   ▽ Unspecified Dx   *EXCLUDES 1* Not coded here   *EXCLUDES 2* Not included here

Chapter 19. Injury, Poisoning and Certain Other Consequences of External Causes

S90.44–S91.001

✓6ᵗʰ **S90.44** External constriction of toe
     Hair tourniquet syndrome of toe

     ✓7ᵗʰ **S90.441** External constriction, right great toe
     ✓7ᵗʰ **S90.442** External constriction, left great toe
     ✓7ᵗʰ **S90.443** External constriction, unspecified ▽ great toe
     ✓7ᵗʰ **S90.444** External constriction, right lesser toe(s)
     ✓7ᵗʰ **S90.445** External constriction, left lesser toe(s)
     ✓7ᵗʰ **S90.446** External constriction, unspecified ▽ lesser toe(s)

✓6ᵗʰ **S90.45** Superficial foreign body of toe
     Splinter in the toe

     ✓7ᵗʰ **S90.451** Superficial foreign body, right great toe
     ✓7ᵗʰ **S90.452** Superficial foreign body, left great toe
     ✓7ᵗʰ **S90.453** Superficial foreign body, unspecified ▽ great toe
     ✓7ᵗʰ **S90.454** Superficial foreign body, right lesser toe(s)
     ✓7ᵗʰ **S90.455** Superficial foreign body, left lesser toe(s)
     ✓7ᵗʰ **S90.456** Superficial foreign body, unspecified ▽ lesser toe(s)

✓6ᵗʰ **S90.46** Insect bite (nonvenomous) of toe

     ✓7ᵗʰ **S90.461** Insect bite (nonvenomous), right great toe
     ✓7ᵗʰ **S90.462** Insect bite (nonvenomous), left great toe
     ✓7ᵗʰ **S90.463** Insect bite (nonvenomous), ▽ unspecified great toe
     ✓7ᵗʰ **S90.464** Insect bite (nonvenomous), right lesser toe(s)
     ✓7ᵗʰ **S90.465** Insect bite (nonvenomous), left lesser toe(s)
     ✓7ᵗʰ **S90.466** Insect bite (nonvenomous), ▽ unspecified lesser toe(s)

✓6ᵗʰ **S90.47** Other superficial bite of toe
     EXCLUDES 1   *open bite of toe (S91.15-, S91.25-)*

     ✓7ᵗʰ **S90.471** Other superficial bite of right great toe
     ✓7ᵗʰ **S90.472** Other superficial bite of left great toe
     ✓7ᵗʰ **S90.473** Other superficial bite of unspecified ▽ great toe
     ✓7ᵗʰ **S90.474** Other superficial bite of right lesser toe(s)
     ✓7ᵗʰ **S90.475** Other superficial bite of left lesser toe(s)
     ✓7ᵗʰ **S90.476** Other superficial bite of unspecified ▽ lesser toe(s)

✓5ᵗʰ **S90.5** Other superficial injuries of ankle

✓6ᵗʰ **S90.51** Abrasion of ankle
     ✓7ᵗʰ **S90.511** Abrasion, right ankle
     ✓7ᵗʰ **S90.512** Abrasion, left ankle
     ✓7ᵗʰ **S90.519** Abrasion, unspecified ankle   ▽

✓6ᵗʰ **S90.52** Blister (nonthermal) of ankle
     ✓7ᵗʰ **S90.521** Blister (nonthermal), right ankle
     ✓7ᵗʰ **S90.522** Blister (nonthermal), left ankle
     ✓7ᵗʰ **S90.529** Blister (nonthermal), unspecified ankle ▽

✓6ᵗʰ **S90.54** External constriction of ankle
     ✓7ᵗʰ **S90.541** External constriction, right ankle
     ✓7ᵗʰ **S90.542** External constriction, left ankle
     ✓7ᵗʰ **S90.549** External constriction, unspecified ankle ▽

✓6ᵗʰ **S90.55** Superficial foreign body of ankle
     Splinter in the ankle

     ✓7ᵗʰ **S90.551** Superficial foreign body, right ankle
     ✓7ᵗʰ **S90.552** Superficial foreign body, left ankle
     ✓7ᵗʰ **S90.559** Superficial foreign body, unspecified ▽ ankle

✓6ᵗʰ **S90.56** Insect bite (nonvenomous) of ankle
     ✓7ᵗʰ **S90.561** Insect bite (nonvenomous), right ankle
     ✓7ᵗʰ **S90.562** Insect bite (nonvenomous), left ankle
     ✓7ᵗʰ **S90.569** Insect bite (nonvenomous), unspecified ▽ ankle

✓6ᵗʰ **S90.57** Other superficial bite of ankle
     EXCLUDES 1   *open bite of ankle (S91.05-)*

     ✓7ᵗʰ **S90.571** Other superficial bite of ankle, right ankle
     ✓7ᵗʰ **S90.572** Other superficial bite of ankle, left ankle

---

     ✓7ᵗʰ **S90.579** Other superficial bite of ankle,   ▽ unspecified ankle

✓5ᵗʰ **S90.8** Other superficial injuries of foot

✓6ᵗʰ **S90.81** Abrasion of foot
     ✓7ᵗʰ **S90.811** Abrasion, right foot
     ✓7ᵗʰ **S90.812** Abrasion, left foot
     ✓7ᵗʰ **S90.819** Abrasion, unspecified foot   ▽

✓6ᵗʰ **S90.82** Blister (nonthermal) of foot
     ✓7ᵗʰ **S90.821** Blister (nonthermal), right foot
     ✓7ᵗʰ **S90.822** Blister (nonthermal), left foot
     ✓7ᵗʰ **S90.829** Blister (nonthermal), unspecified foot ▽

✓6ᵗʰ **S90.84** External constriction of foot
     ✓7ᵗʰ **S90.841** External constriction, right foot
     ✓7ᵗʰ **S90.842** External constriction, left foot
     ✓7ᵗʰ **S90.849** External constriction, unspecified foot ▽

✓6ᵗʰ **S90.85** Superficial foreign body of foot
     Splinter in the foot

     ✓7ᵗʰ **S90.851** Superficial foreign body, right foot
     ✓7ᵗʰ **S90.852** Superficial foreign body, left foot
     ✓7ᵗʰ **S90.859** Superficial foreign body, unspecified ▽ foot

✓6ᵗʰ **S90.86** Insect bite (nonvenomous) of foot
     ✓7ᵗʰ **S90.861** Insect bite (nonvenomous), right foot
     ✓7ᵗʰ **S90.862** Insect bite (nonvenomous), left foot
     ✓7ᵗʰ **S90.869** Insect bite (nonvenomous),   ▽ unspecified foot

✓6ᵗʰ **S90.87** Other superficial bite of foot
     EXCLUDES 1   *open bite of foot (S91.35-)*

     ✓7ᵗʰ **S90.871** Other superficial bite of right foot
     ✓7ᵗʰ **S90.872** Other superficial bite of left foot
     ✓7ᵗʰ **S90.879** Other superficial bite of unspecified foot ▽

✓5ᵗʰ **S90.9** Unspecified superficial injury of ankle, foot and toe

✓6ᵗʰ **S90.91** Unspecified superficial injury of ankle
     ✓7ᵗʰ **S90.911** Unspecified superficial injury of right ▽ ankle
     ✓7ᵗʰ **S90.912** Unspecified superficial injury of left ankle ▽
     ✓7ᵗʰ **S90.919** Unspecified superficial injury of   ▽ unspecified ankle

✓6ᵗʰ **S90.92** Unspecified superficial injury of foot
     ✓7ᵗʰ **S90.921** Unspecified superficial injury of right ▽ foot
     ✓7ᵗʰ **S90.922** Unspecified superficial injury of left foot ▽
     ✓7ᵗʰ **S90.929** Unspecified superficial injury of   ▽ unspecified foot

✓6ᵗʰ **S90.93** Unspecified superficial injury of toes
     ✓7ᵗʰ **S90.931** Unspecified superficial injury of right ▽ great toe
     ✓7ᵗʰ **S90.932** Unspecified superficial injury of left ▽ great toe
     ✓7ᵗʰ **S90.933** Unspecified superficial injury of ▽ unspecified great toe
     ✓7ᵗʰ **S90.934** Unspecified superficial injury of right ▽ lesser toe(s)
     ✓7ᵗʰ **S90.935** Unspecified superficial injury of left ▽ lesser toe(s)
     ✓7ᵗʰ **S90.936** Unspecified superficial injury of ▽ unspecified lesser toe(s)

✓4ᵗʰ **S91** Open wound of ankle, foot and toes
     Code also any associated wound infection
     EXCLUDES 1   *open fracture of ankle, foot and toes (S92-with 7th character B)*
             traumatic amputation of ankle and foot (S98.-)

     The appropriate 7th character is to be added to each code from category S91.
     A   initial encounter
     D   subsequent encounter
     S   sequela

✓5ᵗʰ **S91.0** Open wound of ankle
     ✓6ᵗʰ **S91.00** Unspecified open wound of ankle
         ⁵ ✓7ᵗʰ **S91.001** Unspecified open wound, right   **NRS** ▽ ankle

---

⁵   NRS supply diagnosis with 7th character indicating initial or subsequent encounter.

Ⓝ Newborn: 0   Ⓟ Pediatric: 0-17   Ⓜ Maternity: 12-55   Ⓐ Adult: 15-124   **NRS** Nonroutine supply Dx   **NC Dx** Noncancer Dx   **PDx** Primary Dx   ▶◀ Revised Text   ● New Code   ▲ Revised Title

1026   ICD-10-CM 2018

5 ✓7ᵗʰ **S91.002** Unspecified open wound, left ankle NRS ▽

✓7ᵗʰ **S91.009** Unspecified open wound, unspecified ankle ▽

✓6ᵗʰ **S91.01** Laceration without foreign body of ankle

4,5 ✓7ᵗʰ **S91.011** **Laceration without foreign body, right ankle** NRS

4,5 ✓7ᵗʰ **S91.012** **Laceration without foreign body, left ankle** NRS

✓7ᵗʰ **S91.019** Laceration without foreign body, unspecified ankle ▽

✓6ᵗʰ **S91.02** Laceration with foreign body of ankle

4,5 ✓7ᵗʰ **S91.021** **Laceration with foreign body, right ankle** NRS

4,5 ✓7ᵗʰ **S91.022** **Laceration with foreign body, left ankle** NRS

✓7ᵗʰ **S91.029** Laceration with foreign body, unspecified ankle ▽

✓6ᵗʰ **S91.03** Puncture wound without foreign body of ankle

4,5 ✓7ᵗʰ **S91.031** **Puncture wound without foreign body, right ankle** NRS

4,5 ✓7ᵗʰ **S91.032** **Puncture wound without foreign body, left ankle** NRS

✓7ᵗʰ **S91.039** Puncture wound without foreign body, unspecified ankle ▽

✓6ᵗʰ **S91.04** Puncture wound with foreign body of ankle

4,5 ✓7ᵗʰ **S91.041** **Puncture wound with foreign body, right ankle** NRS

4,5e **S91.042** **Puncture wound with foreign body, left ankle** NRS

✓7ᵗʰ **S91.049** Puncture wound with foreign body, unspecified ankle ▽

✓6ᵗʰ **S91.05** Open bite of ankle

EXCLUDES 1 *superficial bite of ankle (S90.56-, S90.57-)*

4,5 ✓7ᵗʰ **S91.051** **Open bite, right ankle** NRS

4,5 ✓7ᵗʰ **S91.052** **Open bite, left ankle** NRS

✓7ᵗʰ **S91.059** Open bite, unspecified ankle ▽

✓5ᵗʰ **S91.1** Open wound of toe without damage to nail

✓6ᵗʰ **S91.10** Unspecified open wound of toe without damage to nail

5 ✓7ᵗʰ **S91.101** Unspecified open wound of right great toe without damage to nail NRS ▽

5 ✓7ᵗʰ **S91.102** Unspecified open wound of left great toe without damage to nail NRS ▽

5 ✓7ᵗʰ **S91.103** Unspecified open wound of unspecified great toe without damage to nail NRS ▽

5 ✓7ᵗʰ **S91.104** Unspecified open wound of right lesser toe(s) without damage to nail NRS ▽

5 ✓7ᵗʰ **S91.105** Unspecified open wound of left lesser toe(s) without damage to nail NRS ▽

✓7ᵗʰ **S91.106** Unspecified open wound of unspecified lesser toe(s) without damage to nail ▽

✓7ᵗʰ **S91.109** Unspecified open wound of unspecified toe(s) without damage to nail ▽

✓6ᵗʰ **S91.11** Laceration without foreign body of toe without damage to nail

4,5 ✓7ᵗʰ **S91.111** **Laceration without foreign body of right great toe without damage to nail** NRS

4,5 ✓7ᵗʰ **S91.112** **Laceration without foreign body of left great toe without damage to nail**

✓7ᵗʰ **S91.113** Laceration without foreign body of unspecified great toe without damage to nail ▽

4,5 ✓7ᵗʰ **S91.114** **Laceration without foreign body of right lesser toe(s) without damage to nail** NRS

4,5 ✓7ᵗʰ **S91.115** **Laceration without foreign body of left lesser toe(s) without damage to nail** NRS

✓7ᵗʰ **S91.116** Laceration without foreign body of unspecified lesser toe(s) without damage to nail ▽

✓7ᵗʰ **S91.119** Laceration without foreign body of unspecified toe without damage to nail ▽

✓6ᵗʰ **S91.12** Laceration with foreign body of toe without damage to nail

4,5 ✓7ᵗʰ **S91.121** **Laceration with foreign body of right great toe without damage to nail** NRS

4,5 ✓7ᵗʰ **S91.122** **Laceration with foreign body of left great toe without damage to nail** NRS

✓7ᵗʰ **S91.123** Laceration with foreign body of unspecified great toe without damage to nail ▽

4,5 ✓7ᵗʰ **S91.124** **Laceration with foreign body of right lesser toe(s) without damage to nail** NRS

4,5 ✓7ᵗʰ **S91.125** **Laceration with foreign body of left lesser toe(s) without damage to nail** NRS

✓7ᵗʰ **S91.126** Laceration with foreign body of unspecified lesser toe(s) without damage to nail ▽

✓7ᵗʰ **S91.129** Laceration with foreign body of unspecified toe(s) without damage to nail ▽

✓6ᵗʰ **S91.13** Puncture wound without foreign body of toe without damage to nail

4,5 ✓7ᵗʰ **S91.131** **Puncture wound without foreign body of right great toe without damage to nail** NRS

4,5 ✓7ᵗʰ **S91.132** **Puncture wound without foreign body of left great toe without damage to nail** NRS

✓7ᵗʰ **S91.133** Puncture wound without foreign body of unspecified great toe without damage to nail ▽

4,5 ✓7ᵗʰ **S91.134** **Puncture wound without foreign body of right lesser toe(s) without damage to nail** NRS

4,5 ✓7ᵗʰ **S91.135** **Puncture wound without foreign body of left lesser toe(s) without damage to nail** NRS

✓7ᵗʰ **S91.136** Puncture wound without foreign body of unspecified lesser toe(s) without damage to nail ▽

✓7ᵗʰ **S91.139** Puncture wound without foreign body of unspecified toe(s) without damage to nail ▽

✓6ᵗʰ **S91.14** Puncture wound with foreign body of toe without damage to nail

4,5 ✓7ᵗʰ **S91.141** **Puncture wound with foreign body of right great toe without damage to nail** NRS

4,5 ✓7ᵗʰ **S91.142** **Puncture wound with foreign body of left great toe without damage to nail** NRS

✓7ᵗʰ **S91.143** Puncture wound with foreign body of unspecified great toe without damage to nail ▽

4,5 ✓7ᵗʰ **S91.144** **Puncture wound with foreign body of right lesser toe(s) without damage to nail** NRS

4,5 ✓7ᵗʰ **S91.145** **Puncture wound with foreign body of left lesser toe(s) without damage to nail** NRS

✓7ᵗʰ **S91.146** Puncture wound with foreign body of unspecified lesser toe(s) without damage to nail ▽

5 ✓7ᵗʰ **S91.149** Puncture wound with foreign body of unspecified toe(s) without damage to nail NRS ▽

✓6ᵗʰ **S91.15** Open bite of toe without damage to nail

Bite of toe NOS

EXCLUDES 1 *superficial bite of toe (S90.46-, S90.47-)*

4,5 ✓7ᵗʰ **S91.151** **Open bite of right great toe without damage to nail** NRS

4,5 ✓7ᵗʰ **S91.152** **Open bite of left great toe without damage to nail** NRS

✓7ᵗʰ **S91.153** Open bite of unspecified great toe without damage to nail ▽

4,5 ✓7ᵗʰ **S91.154** **Open bite of right lesser toe(s) without damage to nail** NRS

---

4 Case-mix diagnosis with 7th character indicating initial or subsequent encounter.
5 NRS supply diagnosis with 7th character indicating initial or subsequent encounter.

✔ Additional Character Req   ✓x7ᵗʰ Placeholder Alert   Case-Mix Diagnosis   Manifestation   ▽ Unspecified Dx   EXCLUDES 1 Not coded here   EXCLUDES 2 Not included here

Chapter 19. Injury, Poisoning and Certain Other Consequences of External Causes

4,5 ✓7ᵗʰ **S91.155** **Open bite of left lesser toe(s) without damage to nail** NRS

✓7ᵗʰ **S91.156** Open bite of unspecified lesser toe(s) without damage to nail ▽

✓7ᵗʰ **S91.159** Open bite of unspecified toe(s) without damage to nail ▽

S91.2 Open wound **of toe** with damage to nail

✓6ᵗʰ **S91.20** Unspecified open wound of toe with damage to nail

5 ✓7ᵗʰ **S91.201** Unspecified open wound of right great toe with damage to nail NRS ▽

5 ✓7ᵗʰ **S91.202** Unspecified open wound of left great toe with damage to nail NRS ▽

✓7ᵗʰ **S91.203** Unspecified open wound of unspecified great toe with damage to nail ▽

5 ✓7ᵗʰ **S91.204** Unspecified open wound of right lesser toe(s) with damage to nail NRS ▽

5 ✓7ᵗʰ **S91.205** Unspecified open wound of left lesser toe(s) with damage to nail NRS ▽

✓7ᵗʰ **S91.206** Unspecified open wound of unspecified lesser toe(s) with damage to nail ▽

✓7ᵗʰ **S91.209** Unspecified open wound of unspecified toe(s) with damage to nail ▽

✓6ᵗʰ **S91.21** Laceration without foreign body of toe with damage to nail

4,5 ✓7ᵗʰ **S91.211** **Laceration without foreign body of right great toe with damage to nail** NRS

4,5 ✓7ᵗʰ **S91.212** **Laceration without foreign body of left great toe with damage to nail** NRS

✓7ᵗʰ **S91.213** Laceration without foreign body of unspecified great toe with damage to nail ▽

4,5 ✓7ᵗʰ **S91.214** **Laceration without foreign body of right lesser toe(s) with damage to nail** NRS

4,5 ✓7ᵗʰ **S91.215** **Laceration without foreign body of left lesser toe(s) with damage to nail** NRS

✓7ᵗʰ **S91.216** Laceration without foreign body of unspecified lesser toe(s) with damage to nail ▽

✓7ᵗʰ **S91.219** Laceration without foreign body of unspecified toe(s) with damage to nail ▽

✓6ᵗʰ **S91.22** Laceration with foreign body of toe with damage to nail

4,5 ✓7ᵗʰ **S91.221** **Laceration with foreign body of right great toe with damage to nail** NRS

4,5 ✓7ᵗʰ **S91.222** **Laceration with foreign body of left great toe with damage to nail** NRS

✓7ᵗʰ **S91.223** Laceration with foreign body of unspecified great toe with damage to nail ▽

4,5 ✓7ᵗʰ **S91.224** **Laceration with foreign body of right lesser toe(s) with damage to nail** NRS

4,5 ✓7ᵗʰ **S91.225** **Laceration with foreign body of left lesser toe(s) with damage to nail** NRS

✓7ᵗʰ **S91.226** Laceration with foreign body of unspecified lesser toe(s) with damage to nail ▽

✓7ᵗʰ **S91.229** Laceration with foreign body of unspecified toe(s) with damage to nail ▽

✓6ᵗʰ **S91.23** Puncture wound without foreign body of toe with damage to nail

4,5 ✓7ᵗʰ **S91.231** **Puncture wound without foreign body of right great toe with damage to nail** NRS

4,5 ✓7ᵗʰ **S91.232** **Puncture wound without foreign body of left great toe with damage to nail** NRS

✓7ᵗʰ **S91.233** Puncture wound without foreign body of unspecified great toe with damage to nail ▽

4,5 ✓7ᵗʰ **S91.234** **Puncture wound without foreign body of right lesser toe(s) with damage to nail** NRS

4,5 ✓7ᵗʰ **S91.235** **Puncture wound without foreign body of left lesser toe(s) with damage to nail** NRS

✓7ᵗʰ **S91.236** Puncture wound without foreign body of unspecified lesser toe(s) with damage to nail ▽

4 ✓7ᵗʰ **S91.239** **Puncture wound without foreign body of unspecified toe(s) with damage to nail** ▽

✓6ᵗʰ **S91.24** Puncture wound with foreign body of toe with damage to nail

4,5 ✓7ᵗʰ **S91.241** **Puncture wound with foreign body of right great toe with damage to nail** NRS

4,5 ✓7ᵗʰ **S91.242** **Puncture wound with foreign body of left great toe with damage to nail** NRS

✓7ᵗʰ **S91.243** Puncture wound with foreign body of unspecified great toe with damage to nail ▽

4,5 ✓7ᵗʰ **S91.244** **Puncture wound with foreign body of right lesser toe(s) with damage to nail** NRS

4,5 ✓7ᵗʰ **S91.245** **Puncture wound with foreign body of left lesser toe(s) with damage to nail** NRS

✓7ᵗʰ **S91.246** Puncture wound with foreign body of unspecified lesser toe(s) with damage to nail ▽

✓7ᵗʰ **S91.249** Puncture wound with foreign body of unspecified toe(s) with damage to nail ▽

✓6ᵗʰ **S91.25** Open bite of toe with damage to nail
Bite of toe with damage to nail NOS
  EXCLUDES 1   superficial bite of toe (S90.46-, S90.47-)

4,5 ✓7ᵗʰ **S91.251** **Open bite of right great toe with damage to nail** NRS

4,5 ✓7ᵗʰ **S91.252** **Open bite of left great toe with damage to nail** NRS

✓7ᵗʰ **S91.253** Open bite of unspecified great toe with damage to nail ▽

4,5 ✓7ᵗʰ **S91.254** **Open bite of right lesser toe(s) with damage to nail** NRS

4,5 ✓7ᵗʰ **S91.255** **Open bite of left lesser toe(s) with damage to nail** NRS

✓7ᵗʰ **S91.256** Open bite of unspecified lesser toe(s) with damage to nail ▽

✓7ᵗʰ **S91.259** Open bite of unspecified toe(s) with damage to nail ▽

✓5ᵗʰ **S91.3** Open wound **of foot**

✓6ᵗʰ **S91.30** Unspecified open wound of foot

5 ✓7ᵗʰ **S91.301** Unspecified open wound, right foot NRS ▽

5 ✓7ᵗʰ **S91.302** Unspecified open wound, left foot NRS ▽

✓7ᵗʰ **S91.309** Unspecified open wound, unspecified foot ▽

✓6ᵗʰ **S91.31** Laceration without foreign body of foot

4,5 ✓7ᵗʰ **S91.311** **Laceration without foreign body, right foot** NRS

4,5 ✓7ᵗʰ **S91.312** **Laceration without foreign body, left foot** NRS

✓7ᵗʰ **S91.319** Laceration without foreign body, unspecified foot ▽

✓6ᵗʰ **S91.32** Laceration with foreign body of foot

4,5 ✓7ᵗʰ **S91.321** **Laceration with foreign body, right foot** NRS

4,5 ✓7ᵗʰ **S91.322** **Laceration with foreign body, left foot** NRS

✓7ᵗʰ **S91.329** Laceration with foreign body, unspecified foot ▽

✓6ᵗʰ **S91.33** Puncture wound without foreign body of foot

4,5 ✓7ᵗʰ **S91.331** **Puncture wound without foreign body, right foot** NRS

4,5 ✓7ᵗʰ **S91.332** **Puncture wound without foreign body, left foot** NRS

✓7ᵗʰ **S91.339** Puncture wound without foreign body, unspecified foot ▽

✓6ᵗʰ **S91.34** Puncture wound with foreign body of foot

4,5 ✓7ᵗʰ **S91.341** **Puncture wound with foreign body, right foot** NRS

4,5 ✓7ᵗʰ **S91.342** **Puncture wound with foreign body, left foot** NRS

✓7ᵗʰ **S91.349** Puncture wound with foreign body, unspecified foot ▽

✓6ᵗʰ **S91.35** Open bite of foot
  EXCLUDES 1   superficial bite of foot (S90.86-, S90.87-)

4,5 ✓7ᵗʰ **S91.351** **Open bite, right foot** NRS

---

4   Case-mix diagnosis with 7th character indicating initial or subsequent encounter.
5   NRS supply diagnosis with 7th character indicating initial or subsequent encounter.

N Newborn: 0   P Pediatric: 0-17   M Maternity: 12-55   A Adult: 15-124   NRS Nonroutine supply Dx   NCDx Noncancer Dx   PDx Primary Dx   ►◄ Revised Text   ● New Code   ▲ Revised Title

1028   ICD-10-CM 2018

4,5 ✓7ᵗʰ **S91.352**   **Open bite, left** foot   NRS
   ✓7ᵗʰ **S91.359**   **Open bite, unspecified** foot   ▽

✓4ᵗʰ **S92** **Fracture of foot and toe, except ankle**
      NOTE   A fracture not indicated as displaced or nondisplaced should
                  be coded to displaced.
                  A fracture not indicated as open or closed should be coded
                  to closed.
   EXCLUDES 1 *traumatic amputation of ankle and foot (S98.-)*
   EXCLUDES 2 *fracture of ankle (S82.-)*
                  fracture of malleolus (S82.-)
   AHA: 2015, 3Q, 37-39
   TIP: The term "improper alignment" is not synonymous with malunion or
   nonunion of a fracture when noted in provider documentation.

   The appropriate 7th character is to be added to each code from
   category S92.
   A   initial encounter for closed fracture
   B   initial encounter for open fracture
   D   subsequent encounter for fracture with routine healing
   G   subsequent encounter for fracture with delayed healing
   K   subsequent encounter for fracture with nonunion
   P   subsequent encounter for fracture with malunion
   S   sequela

✓6ᵗʰ **S92.0** **Fracture of** calcaneus
      Heel bone
      Os calcis
      EXCLUDES 2 *physeal fracture of calcaneus (S99.0-)*

   ✓6ᵗʰ **S92.00** **Unspecified fracture of calcaneus**
      1 ✓7ᵗʰ **S92.001** **Unspecified fracture of right calcaneus**   ▽
      1 ✓7ᵗʰ **S92.002** **Unspecified fracture of left calcaneus**   ▽
        ✓7ᵗʰ **S92.009** **Unspecified fracture of unspecified**   ▽
                          calcaneus

   ✓6ᵗʰ **S92.01** **Fracture of** body of calcaneus
      1 ✓7ᵗʰ **S92.011** Displaced **fracture of body of right**
                          calcaneus
      1 ✓7ᵗʰ **S92.012** Displaced **fracture of body of left**
                          calcaneus
        ✓7ᵗʰ **S92.013** Displaced **fracture of body of**   ▽
                          unspecified calcaneus
      1 ✓7ᵗʰ **S92.014** Nondisplaced **fracture of body of right**
                          calcaneus
      1 ✓7ᵗʰ **S92.015** Nondisplaced **fracture of body of left**
                          calcaneus
        ✓7ᵗʰ **S92.016** Nondisplaced **fracture of body of**   ▽
                          unspecified calcaneus

   ✓6ᵗʰ **S92.02** **Fracture of** anterior process of calcaneus
      1 ✓7ᵗʰ **S92.021** Displaced **fracture of anterior process of**
                          right calcaneus
      1 ✓7ᵗʰ **S92.022** Displaced **fracture of anterior process of**
                          left calcaneus
        ✓7ᵗʰ **S92.023** Displaced **fracture of anterior process**   ▽
                          of unspecified calcaneus
      1 ✓7ᵗʰ **S92.024** Nondisplaced **fracture of anterior process**
                          of right calcaneus
      1 ✓7ᵗʰ **S92.025** Nondisplaced **fracture of anterior process**
                          of left calcaneus
        ✓7ᵗʰ **S92.026** Nondisplaced **fracture of anterior**   ▽
                          process of unspecified calcaneus

   ✓6ᵗʰ **S92.03** **Avulsion** fracture of tuberosity of calcaneus
      1 ✓7ᵗʰ **S92.031** Displaced **avulsion fracture of tuberosity**
                          of right calcaneus
      1 ✓7ᵗʰ **S92.032** Displaced **avulsion fracture of tuberosity**
                          of left calcaneus
        ✓7ᵗʰ **S92.033** Displaced **avulsion fracture of**   ▽
                          tuberosity of unspecified calcaneus
      1 ✓7ᵗʰ **S92.034** Nondisplaced **avulsion fracture of**
                          tuberosity of right calcaneus
      1 ✓7ᵗʰ **S92.035** Nondisplaced **avulsion fracture of**
                          tuberosity of left calcaneus
        ✓7ᵗʰ **S92.036** Nondisplaced **avulsion fracture of**   ▽
                          tuberosity of unspecified calcaneus

   ✓6ᵗʰ **S92.04** **Other** fracture of tuberosity of calcaneus
      1 ✓7ᵗʰ **S92.041** Displaced **other fracture of tuberosity of**
                          right calcaneus

---

      1 ✓7ᵗʰ **S92.042** Displaced **other fracture of tuberosity of**
                          left calcaneus
        ✓7ᵗʰ **S92.043** Displaced **other fracture of tuberosity**   ▽
                          of unspecified calcaneus
      1 ✓7ᵗʰ **S92.044** Nondisplaced **other fracture of tuberosity**
                          of right calcaneus
      1 ✓7ᵗʰ **S92.045** Nondisplaced **other fracture of tuberosity**
                          of left calcaneus
        ✓7ᵗʰ **S92.046** Nondisplaced **other fracture of**   ▽
                          tuberosity of unspecified calcaneus

   ✓6ᵗʰ **S92.05** **Other** extraarticular fracture of calcaneus
      1 ✓7ᵗʰ **S92.051** Displaced **other extraarticular fracture of**
                          right calcaneus
      1 ✓7ᵗʰ **S92.052** Displaced **other extraarticular fracture of**
                          left calcaneus
        ✓7ᵗʰ **S92.053** Displaced **other extraarticular fracture**   ▽
                          of unspecified calcaneus
      1 ✓7ᵗʰ **S92.054** Nondisplaced **other extraarticular fracture**
                          of right calcaneus
      1 ✓7ᵗʰ **S92.055** Nondisplaced **other extraarticular fracture**
                          of left calcaneus
        ✓7ᵗʰ **S92.056** Nondisplaced **other extraarticular**   ▽
                          fracture of unspecified calcaneus

   ✓6ᵗʰ **S92.06** **Intraarticular** fracture of calcaneus
      1 ✓7ᵗʰ **S92.061** Displaced **intraarticular fracture of right**
                          calcaneus
      1 ✓7ᵗʰ **S92.062** Displaced **intraarticular fracture of left**
                          calcaneus
        ✓7ᵗʰ **S92.063** Displaced **intraarticular fracture of**   ▽
                          unspecified calcaneus
      1 ✓7ᵗʰ **S92.064** Nondisplaced **intraarticular fracture of**
                          right calcaneus
      1 ✓7ᵗʰ **S92.065** Nondisplaced **intraarticular fracture of left**
                          calcaneus
        ✓7ᵗʰ **S92.066** Nondisplaced **intraarticular fracture**   ▽
                          of unspecified calcaneus

✓5ᵗʰ **S92.1** **Fracture of** talus
      Astragalus
   ✓6ᵗʰ **S92.10** **Unspecified** fracture of talus
      1 ✓7ᵗʰ **S92.101** **Unspecified fracture of right talus**   ▽
      1 ✓7ᵗʰ **S92.102** **Unspecified fracture of left talus**   ▽
        ✓7ᵗʰ **S92.109** **Unspecified fracture of unspecified**   ▽
                          talus

   ✓6ᵗʰ **S92.11** **Fracture of** neck of talus
      1 ✓7ᵗʰ **S92.111** Displaced **fracture of neck of right talus**
      1 ✓7ᵗʰ **S92.112** Displaced **fracture of neck of left talus**
        ✓7ᵗʰ **S92.113** Displaced **fracture of neck of**   ▽
                          unspecified talus
      1 ✓7ᵗʰ **S92.114** Nondisplaced **fracture of neck of right**
                          talus
      1 ✓7ᵗʰ **S92.115** Nondisplaced **fracture of neck of left talus**
        ✓7ᵗʰ **S92.116** Nondisplaced **fracture of neck of**   ▽
                          unspecified talus

   ✓6ᵗʰ **S92.12** **Fracture of** body of talus
      1 ✓7ᵗʰ **S92.121** Displaced **fracture of body of right talus**
      1 ✓7ᵗʰ **S92.122** Displaced **fracture of body of left talus**
        ✓7ᵗʰ **S92.123** Displaced **fracture of body of**   ▽
                          unspecified talus
      1 ✓7ᵗʰ **S92.124** Nondisplaced **fracture of body of right**
                          talus
      1 ✓7ᵗʰ **S92.125** Nondisplaced **fracture of body of left talus**
        ✓7ᵗʰ **S92.126** Nondisplaced **fracture of body of**   ▽
                          unspecified talus

   ✓6ᵗʰ **S92.13** **Fracture of** posterior process of talus
      1 ✓7ᵗʰ **S92.131** Displaced **fracture of posterior process of**
                          right talus
      1 ✓7ᵗʰ **S92.132** Displaced **fracture of posterior process of**
                          left talus
        ✓7ᵗʰ **S92.133** Displaced **fracture of posterior process**   ▽
                          of unspecified talus

---

1 Case-mix diagnosis with 7th character indicating subsequent encounter.
4 Case-mix diagnosis with 7th character indicating initial or subsequent encounter.
5 NRS supply diagnosis with 7th character indicating initial or subsequent encounter.

☑ Additional Character Req   ✓x7ᵗʰ Placeholder Alert   Case-Mix Diagnosis   Manifestation   ▽ Unspecified Dx   **EXCLUDES 1** Not coded here   **EXCLUDES 2** Not included here

ICD-10-CM 2018   **1029**

Chapter 19. Injury, Poisoning and Certain Other Consequences of External Causes

S92.134–S92.331

1 ✓7ᵗʰ **S92.134** Nondisplaced **fracture of posterior process of right talus**

1 ✓7ᵗʰ **S92.135** Nondisplaced **fracture of posterior process of left talus**

✓7ᵗʰ **S92.136** Nondisplaced **fracture of posterior process of unspecified talus** ▽

✓6ᵗʰ **S92.14** Dome **fracture of talus**
     EXCLUDES 1   *osteochondritis dissecans (M93.2)*

1 ✓7ᵗʰ **S92.141** Displaced **dome fracture of right talus**

1 ✓7ᵗʰ **S92.142** Displaced **dome fracture of left talus**

✓7ᵗʰ **S92.143** Displaced **dome fracture of unspecified talus** ▽

1 ✓7ᵗʰ **S92.144** Nondisplaced **dome fracture of right talus**

1 ✓7ᵗʰ **S92.145** Nondisplaced **dome fracture of left talus**

✓7ᵗʰ **S92.146** Nondisplaced **dome fracture of unspecified talus** ▽

✓6ᵗʰ **S92.15** Avulsion **fracture (chip fracture) of talus**

1 ✓7ᵗʰ **S92.151** Displaced **avulsion fracture (chip fracture) of right talus**

1 ✓7ᵗʰ **S92.152** Displaced **avulsion fracture (chip fracture) of left talus**

✓7ᵗʰ **S92.153** Displaced **avulsion fracture (chip fracture) of unspecified talus** ▽

1 ✓7ᵗʰ **S92.154** Nondisplaced **avulsion fracture (chip fracture) of right talus**

1 ✓7ᵗʰ **S92.155** Nondisplaced **avulsion fracture (chip fracture) of left talus**

✓7ᵗʰ **S92.156** Nondisplaced **avulsion fracture (chip fracture) of unspecified talus** ▽

✓6ᵗʰ **S92.19** Other **fracture of talus**

1 ✓7ᵗʰ **S92.191** **Other fracture of right talus**

1 ✓7ᵗʰ **S92.192** **Other fracture of left talus**

✓7ᵗʰ **S92.199** **Other fracture of unspecified talus** ▽

✓5ᵗʰ **S92.2** **Fracture of other and unspecified tarsal bone(s)**

✓6ᵗʰ **S92.20** Fracture of unspecified tarsal bone(s)

1 ✓7ᵗʰ **S92.201** **Fracture of unspecified tarsal bone(s) of right foot** ▽

1 ✓7ᵗʰ **S92.202** **Fracture of unspecified tarsal bone(s) of left foot** ▽

✓7ᵗʰ **S92.209** **Fracture of unspecified tarsal bone(s) of unspecified foot** ▽

✓6ᵗʰ **S92.21** Fracture of cuboid **bone**

1 ✓7ᵗʰ **S92.211** Displaced **fracture of cuboid bone of right foot**

1 ✓7ᵗʰ **S92.212** Displaced **fracture of cuboid bone of left foot**

✓7ᵗʰ **S92.213** Displaced **fracture of cuboid bone of unspecified foot** ▽

1 ✓7ᵗʰ **S92.214** Nondisplaced **fracture of cuboid bone of right foot**

1 ✓7ᵗʰ **S92.215** Nondisplaced **fracture of cuboid bone of left foot**

✓7ᵗʰ **S92.216** Nondisplaced **fracture of cuboid bone of unspecified foot** ▽

✓6ᵗʰ **S92.22** Fracture of lateral cuneiform

1 ✓7ᵗʰ **S92.221** Displaced **fracture of lateral cuneiform of right foot**

1 ✓7ᵗʰ **S92.222** Displaced **fracture of lateral cuneiform of left foot**

✓7ᵗʰ **S92.223** Displaced **fracture of lateral cuneiform of unspecified foot** ▽

1 ✓7ᵗʰ **S92.224** Nondisplaced **fracture of lateral cuneiform of right foot**

1 ✓7ᵗʰ **S92.225** Nondisplaced **fracture of lateral cuneiform of left foot**

✓7ᵗʰ **S92.226** Nondisplaced **fracture of lateral cuneiform of unspecified foot** ▽

✓6ᵗʰ **S92.23** Fracture of intermediate cuneiform

1 ✓7ᵗʰ **S92.231** Displaced **fracture of intermediate cuneiform of right foot**

1 ✓7ᵗʰ **S92.232** Displaced **fracture of intermediate cuneiform of left foot**

✓7ᵗʰ **S92.233** Displaced **fracture of intermediate cuneiform of unspecified foot** ▽

1 ✓7ᵗʰ **S92.234** Nondisplaced **fracture of intermediate cuneiform of right foot**

1 ✓7ᵗʰ **S92.235** Nondisplaced **fracture of intermediate cuneiform of left foot**

✓7ᵗʰ **S92.236** Nondisplaced **fracture of intermediate cuneiform of unspecified foot** ▽

✓6ᵗʰ **S92.24** Fracture of medial cuneiform

1 ✓7ᵗʰ **S92.241** Displaced **fracture of medial cuneiform of right foot**

1 ✓7ᵗʰ **S92.242** Displaced **fracture of medial cuneiform of left foot**

✓7ᵗʰ **S92.243** Displaced **fracture of medial cuneiform of unspecified foot** ▽

1 ✓7ᵗʰ **S92.244** Nondisplaced **fracture of medial cuneiform of right foot**

1 ✓7ᵗʰ **S92.245** Nondisplaced **fracture of medial cuneiform of left foot**

✓7ᵗʰ **S92.246** Nondisplaced **fracture of medial cuneiform of unspecified foot** ▽

✓6ᵗʰ **S92.25** Fracture of navicular [scaphoid] of foot

1 ✓7ᵗʰ **S92.251** Displaced **fracture of navicular [scaphoid] of right foot**

1 ✓7ᵗʰ **S92.252** Displaced **fracture of navicular [scaphoid] of left foot**

✓7ᵗʰ **S92.253** Displaced **fracture of navicular [scaphoid] of unspecified foot** ▽

1 ✓7ᵗʰ **S92.254** Nondisplaced **fracture of navicular [scaphoid] of right foot**

1 ✓7ᵗʰ **S92.255** Nondisplaced **fracture of navicular [scaphoid] of left foot**

✓7ᵗʰ **S92.256** Nondisplaced **fracture of navicular [scaphoid] of unspecified foot** ▽

✓5ᵗʰ **S92.3** **Fracture of metatarsal bone(s)**
     EXCLUDES 2   *physeal fracture of metatarsal (S99.1-)*

✓6ᵗʰ **S92.30** Fracture of unspecified metatarsal bone(s)

1 ✓7ᵗʰ **S92.301** **Fracture of unspecified metatarsal bone(s), right foot** ▽

1 ✓7ᵗʰ **S92.302** **Fracture of unspecified metatarsal bone(s), left foot** ▽

✓7ᵗʰ **S92.309** **Fracture of unspecified metatarsal bone(s), unspecified foot** ▽

✓6ᵗʰ **S92.31** Fracture of first metatarsal bone

1 ✓7ᵗʰ **S92.311** Displaced **fracture of first metatarsal bone, right foot**

1 ✓7ᵗʰ **S92.312** Displaced **fracture of first metatarsal bone, left foot**

✓7ᵗʰ **S92.313** Displaced **fracture of first metatarsal bone, unspecified foot** ▽

1 ✓7ᵗʰ **S92.314** Nondisplaced **fracture of first metatarsal bone, right foot**

1 ✓7ᵗʰ **S92.315** Nondisplaced **fracture of first metatarsal bone, left foot**

✓7ᵗʰ **S92.316** Nondisplaced **fracture of first metatarsal bone, unspecified foot** ▽

✓6ᵗʰ **S92.32** Fracture of second metatarsal bone

1 ✓7ᵗʰ **S92.321** Displaced **fracture of second metatarsal bone, right foot**
     1

✓7ᵗʰ **S92.322** Displaced **fracture of second metatarsal bone, left foot**

✓7ᵗʰ **S92.323** Displaced **fracture of second metatarsal bone, unspecified foot** ▽

1 ✓7ᵗʰ **S92.324** Nondisplaced **fracture of second metatarsal bone, right foot**

1 ✓7ᵗʰ **S92.325** Nondisplaced **fracture of second metatarsal bone, left foot**

✓7ᵗʰ **S92.326** Nondisplaced **fracture of second metatarsal bone, unspecified foot** ▽

✓6ᵗʰ **S92.33** Fracture of third metatarsal bone

1 ✓7ᵗʰ **S92.331** Displaced **fracture of third metatarsal bone, right foot**

---

1   Case-mix diagnosis with 7th character indicating subsequent encounter.

Ⓝ Newborn: 0   Ⓟ Pediatric: 0-17   Ⓜ Maternity: 12-55   Ⓐ Adult: 15-124   NRS Nonroutine supply Dx   NC Dx Noncancer Dx   PDx Primary Dx   ►◄ Revised Text   ● New Code   ▲ Revised Title

¹ ✓7ᵗʰ S92.332   Displaced fracture of third metatarsal bone, left foot

✓7ᵗʰ S92.333   Displaced fracture of third metatarsal bone, unspecified foot ▽

¹ ✓7ᵗʰ S92.334   Nondisplaced fracture of third metatarsal bone, right foot

¹ ✓7ᵗʰ S92.335   Nondisplaced fracture of third metatarsal bone, left foot

✓7ᵗʰ S92.336   Nondisplaced fracture of third metatarsal bone, unspecified foot ▽

✓6ᵗʰ S92.34   Fracture of fourth metatarsal bone

¹ ✓7ᵗʰ S92.341   Displaced fracture of fourth metatarsal bone, right foot

¹ ✓7ᵗʰ S92.342   Displaced fracture of fourth metatarsal bone, left foot

✓7ᵗʰ S92.343   Displaced fracture of fourth metatarsal bone, unspecified foot ▽

¹ ✓7ᵗʰ S92.344   Nondisplaced fracture of fourth metatarsal bone, right foot

¹ ✓7ᵗʰ S92.345   Nondisplaced fracture of fourth metatarsal bone, left foot

✓7ᵗʰ S92.346   Nondisplaced fracture of fourth metatarsal bone, unspecified foot ▽

✓6ᵗʰ S92.35   Fracture of fifth metatarsal bone

¹ ✓7ᵗʰ S92.351   Displaced fracture of fifth metatarsal bone, right foot

¹ ✓7ᵗʰ S92.352   Displaced fracture of fifth metatarsal bone, left foot

✓7ᵗʰ S92.353   Displaced fracture of fifth metatarsal bone, unspecified foot ▽

¹ ✓7ᵗʰ S92.354   Nondisplaced fracture of fifth metatarsal bone, right foot

¹ ✓7ᵗʰ S92.355   Nondisplaced fracture of fifth metatarsal bone, left foot

✓7ᵗʰ S92.356   Nondisplaced fracture of fifth metatarsal bone, unspecified foot ▽

✓5ᵗʰ S92.4   Fracture of great toe

EXCLUDES 2   physeal fracture of phalanx of toe (S99.2-)

✓6ᵗʰ S92.40   Unspecified fracture of great toe

✓7ᵗʰ S92.401   Displaced unspecified fracture of right great toe ▽

✓7ᵗʰ S92.402   Displaced unspecified fracture of left great toe ▽

✓7ᵗʰ S92.403   Displaced unspecified fracture of unspecified great toe ▽

✓7ᵗʰ S92.404   Nondisplaced unspecified fracture of right great toe ▽

✓7ᵗʰ S92.405   Nondisplaced unspecified fracture of left great toe ▽

✓7ᵗʰ S92.406   Nondisplaced unspecified fracture of unspecified great toe ▽

✓6ᵗʰ S92.41   Fracture of proximal phalanx of great toe

✓7ᵗʰ S92.411   Displaced fracture of proximal phalanx of right great toe

✓7ᵗʰ S92.412   Displaced fracture of proximal phalanx of left great toe

✓7ᵗʰ S92.413   Displaced fracture of proximal phalanx of unspecified great toe ▽

✓7ᵗʰ S92.414   Nondisplaced fracture of proximal phalanx of right great toe

✓7ᵗʰ S92.415   Nondisplaced fracture of proximal phalanx of left great toe

✓7ᵗʰ S92.416   Nondisplaced fracture of proximal phalanx of unspecified great toe ▽

✓6ᵗʰ S92.42   Fracture of distal phalanx of great toe

✓7ᵗʰ S92.421   Displaced fracture of distal phalanx of right great toe

✓7ᵗʰ S92.422   Displaced fracture of distal phalanx of left great toe

✓7ᵗʰ S92.423   Displaced fracture of distal phalanx of unspecified great toe ▽

✓7ᵗʰ S92.424   Nondisplaced fracture of distal phalanx of right great toe

✓7ᵗʰ S92.425   Nondisplaced fracture of distal phalanx of left great toe

✓7ᵗʰ S92.426   Nondisplaced fracture of distal phalanx of unspecified great toe ▽

✓6ᵗʰ S92.49   Other fracture of great toe

✓7ᵗʰ S92.491   Other fracture of right great toe

✓7ᵗʰ S92.492   Other fracture of left great toe

✓7ᵗʰ S92.499   Other fracture of unspecified great toe ▽

✓5ᵗʰ S92.5   Fracture of lesser toe(s)

EXCLUDES 2   physeal fracture of phalanx of toe (S99.2-)

✓6ᵗʰ S92.50   Unspecified fracture of lesser toe(s)

✓7ᵗʰ S92.501   Displaced unspecified fracture of right lesser toe(s) ▽

✓7ᵗʰ S92.502   Displaced unspecified fracture of left lesser toe(s) ▽

✓7ᵗʰ S92.503   Displaced unspecified fracture of unspecified lesser toe(s) ▽

✓7ᵗʰ S92.504   Nondisplaced unspecified fracture of right lesser toe(s) ▽

✓7ᵗʰ S92.505   Nondisplaced unspecified fracture of left lesser toe(s) ▽

✓7ᵗʰ S92.506   Nondisplaced unspecified fracture of unspecified lesser toe(s) ▽

✓6ᵗʰ S92.51   Fracture of proximal phalanx of lesser toe(s)

✓7ᵗʰ S92.511   Displaced fracture of proximal phalanx of right lesser toe(s)

✓7ᵗʰ S92.512   Displaced fracture of proximal phalanx of left lesser toe(s)

✓7ᵗʰ S92.513   Displaced fracture of proximal phalanx of unspecified lesser toe(s) ▽

✓7ᵗʰ S92.514   Nondisplaced fracture of proximal phalanx of right lesser toe(s)

✓7ᵗʰ S92.515   Nondisplaced fracture of proximal phalanx of left lesser toe(s)

✓7ᵗʰ S92.516   Nondisplaced fracture of proximal phalanx of unspecified lesser toe(s) ▽

✓6ᵗʰ S92.52   Fracture of middle phalanx of lesser toe(s)

✓7ᵗʰ S92.521   Displaced fracture of middle phalanx of right lesser toe(s)

✓7ᵗʰ S92.522   Displaced fracture of middle phalanx of left lesser toe(s)

✓7ᵗʰ S92.523   Displaced fracture of middle phalanx of unspecified lesser toe(s) ▽

✓7ᵗʰ S92.524   Nondisplaced fracture of middle phalanx of right lesser toe(s)

✓7ᵗʰ S92.525   Nondisplaced fracture of middle phalanx of left lesser toe(s)

✓7ᵗʰ S92.526   Nondisplaced fracture of middle phalanx of unspecified lesser toe(s) ▽

✓6ᵗʰ S92.53   Fracture of distal phalanx of lesser toe(s)

✓7ᵗʰ S92.531   Displaced fracture of distal phalanx of right lesser toe(s)

✓7ᵗʰ S92.532   Displaced fracture of distal phalanx of left lesser toe(s)

✓7ᵗʰ S92.533   Displaced fracture of distal phalanx of unspecified lesser toe(s) ▽

✓7ᵗʰ S92.534   Nondisplaced fracture of distal phalanx of right lesser toe(s)

✓7ᵗʰ S92.535   Nondisplaced fracture of distal phalanx of left lesser toe(s)

✓7ᵗʰ S92.536   Nondisplaced fracture of distal phalanx of unspecified lesser toe(s) ▽

✓6ᵗʰ S92.59   Other fracture of lesser toe(s)

✓7ᵗʰ S92.591   Other fracture of right lesser toe(s)

✓7ᵗʰ S92.592   Other fracture of left lesser toe(s)

✓7ᵗʰ S92.599   Other fracture of unspecified lesser toe(s) ▽

✓5ᵗʰ S92.8   Other fracture of foot, except ankle

✓6ᵗʰ S92.81   Other fracture of foot
Sesamoid fracture of foot

¹ ✓7ᵗʰ S92.811   Other fracture of right foot

¹ ✓7ᵗʰ S92.812   Other fracture of left foot

---

¹   Case-mix diagnosis with 7th character indicating subsequent encounter.

☑ Additional Character Req   ✓ₓ7ᵗʰ Placeholder Alert   Case-Mix Diagnosis   Manifestation   ▽ Unspecified Dx   EXCLUDES 1 Not coded here   EXCLUDES 2 Not included here

Chapter 19. Injury, Poisoning and Certain Other Consequences of External Causes

   ☑7ᵗʰ **S92.819**   Other fracture of unspecified foot ▽

☑5ᵗʰ **S92.9**   Unspecified fracture of foot and toe

   ☑6ᵗʰ **S92.90**   Unspecified fracture of foot

     1 ☑7ᵗʰ **S92.901**   **Unspecified fracture of right foot** ▽

     1 ☑7ᵗʰ **S92.902**   **Unspecified fracture of left foot** ▽

     ☑7ᵗʰ **S92.909**   Unspecified fracture of unspecified foot ▽

   ☑6ᵗʰ **S92.91**   Unspecified fracture of toe

     ☑7ᵗʰ **S92.911**   Unspecified fracture of right toe(s) ▽

     ☑7ᵗʰ **S92.912**   Unspecified fracture of left toe(s) ▽

     ☑7ᵗʰ **S92.919**   Unspecified fracture of unspecified toe(s) ▽

☑4ᵗʰ **S93**   **Dislocation and sprain of joints and ligaments at ankle, foot and toe level**

   INCLUDES   avulsion of joint or ligament of ankle, foot and toe
      laceration of cartilage, joint or ligament of ankle, foot and toe
      sprain of cartilage, joint or ligament of ankle, foot and toe
      traumatic hemarthrosis of joint or ligament of ankle, foot and toe
      traumatic rupture of joint or ligament of ankle, foot and toe
      traumatic subluxation of joint or ligament of ankle, foot and toe
      traumatic tear of joint or ligament of ankle, foot and toe

   Code also any associated open wound

   EXCLUDES 2   *strain of muscle and tendon of ankle and foot (S96.-)*

   The appropriate 7th character is to be added to each code from category S93.
   A   initial encounter
   D   subsequent encounter
   S   sequela

☑5ᵗʰ **S93.0**   **Subluxation and dislocation of ankle joint**
   Subluxation and dislocation of astragalus
   Subluxation and dislocation of fibula, lower end
   Subluxation and dislocation of talus
   Subluxation and dislocation of tibia, lower end

   1 ☑x7ᵗʰ **S93.01**   Subluxation of right ankle joint

   1 ☑x7ᵗʰ **S93.02**   Subluxation of left ankle joint

   ☑x7ᵗʰ **S93.03**   Subluxation of unspecified ankle joint ▽

   1 ☑x7ᵗʰ **S93.04**   Dislocation of right ankle joint

   1 ☑x7ᵗʰ **S93.05**   Dislocation of left ankle joint

   ☑x7ᵗʰ **S93.06**   Dislocation of unspecified ankle joint ▽

☑5ᵗʰ **S93.1**   **Subluxation and dislocation of toe**

   ☑6ᵗʰ **S93.10**   Unspecified subluxation and dislocation of toe
     Dislocation of toe NOS
     Subluxation of toe NOS

     1 ☑7ᵗʰ **S93.101**   **Unspecified subluxation of right toe(s)** ▽

     1 ☑7ᵗʰ **S93.102**   **Unspecified subluxation of left toe(s)** ▽

     ☑7ᵗʰ **S93.103**   Unspecified subluxation of unspecified toe(s) ▽

     1 ☑7ᵗʰ **S93.104**   **Unspecified dislocation of right toe(s)** ▽

     1 ☑7ᵗʰ **S93.105**   **Unspecified dislocation of left toe(s)** ▽

     ☑7ᵗʰ **S93.106**   Unspecified dislocation of unspecified toe(s) ▽

   ☑6ᵗʰ **S93.11**   Dislocation of interphalangeal joint

     1 ☑7ᵗʰ **S93.111**   **Dislocation of interphalangeal joint of right great toe**

     1 ☑7ᵗʰ **S93.112**   **Dislocation of interphalangeal joint of left great toe**

     ☑7ᵗʰ **S93.113**   Dislocation of interphalangeal joint of unspecified great toe ▽

     1 ☑7ᵗʰ **S93.114**   **Dislocation of interphalangeal joint of right lesser toe(s)**

     1 ☑7ᵗʰ **S93.115**   **Dislocation of interphalangeal joint of left lesser toe(s)**

     ☑7ᵗʰ **S93.116**   Dislocation of interphalangeal joint of unspecified lesser toe(s) ▽

     ☑7ᵗʰ **S93.119**   Dislocation of interphalangeal joint of unspecified toe(s) ▽

   ☑6ᵗʰ **S93.12**   Dislocation of metatarsophalangeal joint

     1 ☑7ᵗʰ **S93.121**   **Dislocation of metatarsophalangeal joint of right great toe**

     1 ☑7ᵗʰ **S93.122**   **Dislocation of metatarsophalangeal joint of left great toe**

     ☑7ᵗʰ **S93.123**   Dislocation of metatarsophalangeal joint of unspecified great toe ▽

     1 ☑7ᵗʰ **S93.124**   **Dislocation of metatarsophalangeal joint of right lesser toe(s)**

     1 ☑7ᵗʰ **S93.125**   **Dislocation of metatarsophalangeal joint of left lesser toe(s)**

     ☑7ᵗʰ **S93.126**   Dislocation of metatarsophalangeal joint of unspecified lesser toe(s) ▽

     ☑7ᵗʰ **S93.129**   Dislocation of metatarsophalangeal joint of unspecified toe(s) ▽

   ☑6ᵗʰ **S93.13**   Subluxation of interphalangeal joint

     1 ☑7ᵗʰ **S93.131**   **Subluxation of interphalangeal joint of right great toe**

     1 ☑7ᵗʰ **S93.132**   **Subluxation of interphalangeal joint of left great toe**

     ☑7ᵗʰ **S93.133**   Subluxation of interphalangeal joint of unspecified great toe ▽

     1 ☑7ᵗʰ **S93.134**   **Subluxation of interphalangeal joint of right lesser toe(s)**

     1 ☑7ᵗʰ **S93.135**   **Subluxation of interphalangeal joint of left lesser toe(s)**

     ☑7ᵗʰ **S93.136**   Subluxation of interphalangeal joint of unspecified lesser toe(s) ▽

     ☑7ᵗʰ **S93.139**   Subluxation of interphalangeal joint of unspecified toe(s) ▽

   ☑6ᵗʰ **S93.14**   Subluxation of metatarsophalangeal joint

     1 ☑7ᵗʰ **S93.141**   **Subluxation of metatarsophalangeal joint of right great toe**

     1 ☑7ᵗʰ **S93.142**   **Subluxation of metatarsophalangeal joint of left great toe**

     ☑7ᵗʰ **S93.143**   Subluxation of metatarsophalangeal joint of unspecified great toe ▽

     1 ☑7ᵗʰ **S93.144**   **Subluxation of metatarsophalangeal joint of right lesser toe(s)**

     1 ☑7ᵗʰ **S93.145**   **Subluxation of metatarsophalangeal joint of left lesser toe(s)**

     ☑7ᵗʰ **S93.146**   Subluxation of metatarsophalangeal joint of unspecified lesser toe(s) ▽

     ☑7ᵗʰ **S93.149**   Subluxation of metatarsophalangeal joint of unspecified toe(s) ▽

☑5ᵗʰ **S93.3**   **Subluxation and dislocation of foot**
   EXCLUDES 2   *dislocation of toe (S93.1-)*

   ☑6ᵗʰ **S93.30**   Unspecified subluxation and dislocation of foot
     Dislocation of foot NOS
     Subluxation of foot NOS

     1 ☑7ᵗʰ **S93.301**   **Unspecified subluxation of right foot** ▽

     1 ☑7ᵗʰ **S93.302**   **Unspecified subluxation of left foot** ▽

     ☑7ᵗʰ **S93.303**   Unspecified subluxation of unspecified foot ▽

     1 ☑7ᵗʰ **S93.304**   **Unspecified dislocation of right foot** ▽

     1 ☑7ᵗʰ **S93.305**   **Unspecified dislocation of left foot** ▽

     ☑7ᵗʰ **S93.306**   Unspecified dislocation of unspecified foot ▽

   ☑6ᵗʰ **S93.31**   Subluxation and dislocation of tarsal joint

     1 ☑7ᵗʰ **S93.311**   Subluxation of tarsal joint of right foot

     1 ☑7ᵗʰ **S93.312**   Subluxation of tarsal joint of left foot

     ☑7ᵗʰ **S93.313**   Subluxation of tarsal joint of unspecified foot ▽

     1 ☑7ᵗʰ **S93.314**   Dislocation of tarsal joint of right foot

     1 ☑7ᵗʰ **S93.315**   Dislocation of tarsal joint of left foot

     ☑7ᵗʰ **S93.316**   Dislocation of tarsal joint of unspecified foot ▽

   ☑6ᵗʰ **S93.32**   Subluxation and dislocation of tarsometatarsal joint

     1 ☑7ᵗʰ **S93.321**   Subluxation of tarsometatarsal joint of right foot

     1 ☑7ᵗʰ **S93.322**   Subluxation of tarsometatarsal joint of left foot

     ☑7ᵗʰ **S93.323**   Subluxation of tarsometatarsal joint of unspecified foot ▽

     1 ☑7ᵗʰ **S93.324**   Dislocation of tarsometatarsal joint of right foot

---

1   Case-mix diagnosis with 7th character indicating subsequent encounter.

N Newborn: 0   P Pediatric: 0-17   M Maternity: 12-55   A Adult: 15-124   NRS Nonroutine supply Dx   NCDx Noncancer Dx   PDx Primary Dx   ►◄ Revised Text   ● New Code   ▲ Revised Title

1032   ICD-10-CM 2018

1 ✓7ᵗʰ **S93.325** Dislocation of tarsometatarsal joint of left foot

✓7ᵗʰ **S93.326** Dislocation of tarsometatarsal joint of unspecified foot ▽

✓6ᵗʰ **S93.33** Other subluxation and dislocation of foot

     1 ✓7ᵗʰ **S93.331** Other subluxation of right foot

     1 ✓7ᵗʰ **S93.332** Other subluxation of left foot

     ✓7ᵗʰ **S93.333** Other subluxation of unspecified foot ▽

     1 ✓7ᵗʰ **S93.334** Other dislocation of right foot

     1 ✓7ᵗʰ **S93.335** Other dislocation of left foot

     ✓7ᵗʰ **S93.336** Other dislocation of unspecified foot ▽

✓5ᵗʰ **S93.4** Sprain of ankle

     EXCLUDES 2   injury of Achilles tendon (S86.0-)

   ✓6ᵗʰ **S93.40** Sprain of unspecified ligament of ankle
     Sprain of ankle NOS
     Sprained ankle NOS

     ✓7ᵗʰ **S93.401** Sprain of unspecified ligament of right ankle ▽

     ✓7ᵗʰ **S93.402** Sprain of unspecified ligament of left ankle ▽

     ✓7ᵗʰ **S93.409** Sprain of unspecified ligament of unspecified ankle ▽

   ✓6ᵗʰ **S93.41** Sprain of calcaneofibular ligament

     ✓7ᵗʰ **S93.411** Sprain of calcaneofibular ligament of right ankle

     ✓7ᵗʰ **S93.412** Sprain of calcaneofibular ligament of left ankle

     ✓7ᵗʰ **S93.419** Sprain of calcaneofibular ligament of unspecified ankle ▽

   ✓6ᵗʰ **S93.42** Sprain of deltoid ligament

     ✓7ᵗʰ **S93.421** Sprain of deltoid ligament of right ankle

     ✓7ᵗʰ **S93.422** Sprain of deltoid ligament of left ankle

     ✓7ᵗʰ **S93.429** Sprain of deltoid ligament of unspecified ankle ▽

   ✓6ᵗʰ **S93.43** Sprain of tibiofibular ligament

     ✓7ᵗʰ **S93.431** Sprain of tibiofibular ligament of right ankle

     ✓7ᵗʰ **S93.432** Sprain of tibiofibular ligament of left ankle

     ✓7ᵗʰ **S93.439** Sprain of tibiofibular ligament of unspecified ankle ▽

   ✓6ᵗʰ **S93.49** Sprain of other ligament of ankle
     Sprain of internal collateral ligament
     Sprain of talofibular ligament

     ✓7ᵗʰ **S93.491** Sprain of other ligament of right ankle

     ✓7ᵗʰ **S93.492** Sprain of other ligament of left ankle

     ✓7ᵗʰ **S93.499** Sprain of other ligament of unspecified ankle ▽

✓5ᵗʰ **S93.5** Sprain of toe

   ✓6ᵗʰ **S93.50** Unspecified sprain of toe

     ✓7ᵗʰ **S93.501** Unspecified sprain of right great toe ▽

     ✓7ᵗʰ **S93.502** Unspecified sprain of left great toe ▽

     ✓7ᵗʰ **S93.503** Unspecified sprain of unspecified great toe ▽

     ✓7ᵗʰ **S93.504** Unspecified sprain of right lesser toe(s) ▽

     ✓7ᵗʰ **S93.505** Unspecified sprain of left lesser toe(s) ▽

     ✓7ᵗʰ **S93.506** Unspecified sprain of unspecified lesser toe(s) ▽

     ✓7ᵗʰ **S93.509** Unspecified sprain of unspecified toe(s) ▽

   ✓6ᵗʰ **S93.51** Sprain of interphalangeal joint of toe

     ✓7ᵗʰ **S93.511** Sprain of interphalangeal joint of right great toe

     ✓7ᵗʰ **S93.512** Sprain of interphalangeal joint of left great toe

     ✓7ᵗʰ **S93.513** Sprain of interphalangeal joint of unspecified great toe ▽

     ✓7ᵗʰ **S93.514** Sprain of interphalangeal joint of right lesser toe(s)

     ✓7ᵗʰ **S93.515** Sprain of interphalangeal joint of left lesser toe(s)

     ✓7ᵗʰ **S93.516** Sprain of interphalangeal joint of unspecified lesser toe(s) ▽

     ✓7ᵗʰ **S93.519** Sprain of interphalangeal joint of unspecified toe(s) ▽

   ✓6ᵗʰ **S93.52** Sprain of metatarsophalangeal joint of toe

     ✓7ᵗʰ **S93.521** Sprain of metatarsophalangeal joint of right great toe

     ✓7ᵗʰ **S93.522** Sprain of metatarsophalangeal joint of left great toe

     ✓7ᵗʰ **S93.523** Sprain of metatarsophalangeal joint of unspecified great toe ▽

     ✓7ᵗʰ **S93.524** Sprain of metatarsophalangeal joint of right lesser toe(s)

     ✓7ᵗʰ **S93.525** Sprain of metatarsophalangeal joint of left lesser toe(s)

     ✓7ᵗʰ **S93.526** Sprain of metatarsophalangeal joint of unspecified lesser toe(s) ▽

     ✓7ᵗʰ **S93.529** Sprain of metatarsophalangeal joint of unspecified toe(s) ▽

✓5ᵗʰ **S93.6** Sprain of foot

     EXCLUDES 2   sprain of metatarsophalangeal joint of toe (S93.52-)
          sprain of toe (S93.5-)

   ✓6ᵗʰ **S93.60** Unspecified sprain of foot

     ✓7ᵗʰ **S93.601** Unspecified sprain of right foot ▽

     ✓7ᵗʰ **S93.602** Unspecified sprain of left foot ▽

     ✓7ᵗʰ **S93.609** Unspecified sprain of unspecified foot ▽

   ✓6ᵗʰ **S93.61** Sprain of tarsal ligament of foot

     ✓7ᵗʰ **S93.611** Sprain of tarsal ligament of right foot

     ✓7ᵗʰ **S93.612** Sprain of tarsal ligament of left foot

     ✓7ᵗʰ **S93.619** Sprain of tarsal ligament of unspecified foot ▽

   ✓6ᵗʰ **S93.62** Sprain of tarsometatarsal ligament of foot

     ✓7ᵗʰ **S93.621** Sprain of tarsometatarsal ligament of right foot

     ✓7ᵗʰ **S93.622** Sprain of tarsometatarsal ligament of left foot

     ✓7ᵗʰ **S93.629** Sprain of tarsometatarsal ligament of unspecified foot ▽

   ✓6ᵗʰ **S93.69** Other sprain of foot

     ✓7ᵗʰ **S93.691** Other sprain of right foot

     ✓7ᵗʰ **S93.692** Other sprain of left foot

     ✓7ᵗʰ **S93.699** Other sprain of unspecified foot ▽

✓4ᵗʰ **S94** Injury of nerves at ankle and foot level
     Code also any associated open wound (S91.-)

     The appropriate 7th character is to be added to each code from category S94.
     A   initial encounter
     D   subsequent encounter
     S   sequela

✓5ᵗʰ **S94.0** Injury of lateral plantar nerve

     ✓x7ᵗʰ **S94.00** Injury of lateral plantar nerve, unspecified leg ▽

   2 ✓x7ᵗʰ **S94.01** Injury of lateral plantar nerve, right leg

   2 ✓x7ᵗʰ **S94.02** Injury of lateral plantar nerve, left leg

✓5ᵗʰ **S94.1** Injury of medial plantar nerve

     ✓x7ᵗʰ **S94.10** Injury of medial plantar nerve, unspecified leg ▽

   2 ✓x7ᵗʰ **S94.11** Injury of medial plantar nerve, right leg

   2 ✓x7ᵗʰ **S94.12** Injury of medial plantar nerve, left leg

✓5ᵗʰ **S94.2** Injury of deep peroneal nerve at ankle and foot level
     Injury of terminal, lateral branch of deep peroneal nerve

     ✓x7ᵗʰ **S94.20** Injury of deep peroneal nerve at ankle and foot level, unspecified leg ▽

   2 ✓x7ᵗʰ **S94.21** Injury of deep peroneal nerve at ankle and foot level, right leg

   2 ✓x7ᵗʰ **S94.22** Injury of deep peroneal nerve at ankle and foot level, left leg

✓5ᵗʰ **S94.3** Injury of cutaneous sensory nerve at ankle and foot level

     ✓x7ᵗʰ **S94.30** Injury of cutaneous sensory nerve at ankle and foot level, unspecified leg ▽

   2 ✓x7ᵗʰ **S94.31** Injury of cutaneous sensory nerve at ankle and foot level, right leg

---

1   Case-mix diagnosis with 7th character indicating subsequent encounter.
2   Case-mix diagnosis with 7th character indicating subsequent encounter or sequela.

☑ Additional Character Req   ✓x7ᵗʰ Placeholder Alert   Case-Mix Diagnosis   Manifestation   ▽ Unspecified Dx   EXCLUDES 1 Not coded here   EXCLUDES 2 Not included here

Chapter 19. Injury, Poisoning and Certain Other Consequences of External Causes

2 ✓x7th **S94.32** **Injury of cutaneous sensory nerve at ankle and foot level, left leg**

✓5th **S94.8** Injury of other nerves at ankle and foot level

  ✓6th **S94.8X** Injury of other nerves at ankle and foot level

    2 ✓7th **S94.8X1** **Injury of other nerves at ankle and foot level, right leg**

    2 ✓7th **S94.8X2** **Injury of other nerves at ankle and foot level, left leg**

    ✓7th **S94.8X9** Injury of other nerves at ankle and foot ▽ level, unspecified leg

✓5th **S94.9** Injury of unspecified nerve at ankle and foot level

  ✓x7th **S94.90** Injury of unspecified nerve at ankle and foot ▽ level, unspecified leg

  1 ✓x7th **S94.91** **Injury of unspecified nerve at ankle and foot** ▽ **level, right leg**

  1 ✓x7th **S94.92** **Injury of unspecified nerve at ankle and foot** ▽ **level, left leg**

✓4th **S95** **Injury of blood vessels at ankle and foot level**
    Code also any associated open wound (S91.-)
    EXCLUDES 2 *injury of posterior tibial artery and vein (S85.1-, S85.8-)*

    The appropriate 7th character is to be added to each code from category S95.
    A   initial encounter
    D   subsequent encounter
    S   sequela

✓5th **S95.0** Injury of dorsal artery of foot

  ✓6th **S95.00** Unspecified injury of dorsal artery of foot

    ✓7th **S95.001** Unspecified injury of dorsal artery of ▽ right foot

    ✓7th **S95.002** Unspecified injury of dorsal artery of ▽ left foot

    ✓7th **S95.009** Unspecified injury of dorsal artery of ▽ unspecified foot

  ✓6th **S95.01** Laceration of dorsal artery of foot

    ✓7th **S95.011** Laceration of dorsal artery of right foot

    ✓7th **S95.012** Laceration of dorsal artery of left foot

    ✓7th **S95.019** Laceration of dorsal artery of ▽ unspecified foot

  ✓6th **S95.09** Other specified injury of dorsal artery of foot

    ✓7th **S95.091** Other specified injury of dorsal artery of right foot

    ✓7th **S95.092** Other specified injury of dorsal artery of left foot

    ✓7th **S95.099** Other specified injury of dorsal artery ▽ of unspecified foot

✓5th **S95.1** Injury of plantar artery of foot

  ✓6th **S95.10** Unspecified injury of plantar artery of foot

    ✓7th **S95.101** Unspecified injury of plantar artery of ▽ right foot

    ✓7th **S95.102** Unspecified injury of plantar artery of ▽ left foot

    ✓7th **S95.109** Unspecified injury of plantar artery of ▽ unspecified foot

  ✓6th **S95.11** Laceration of plantar artery of foot

    ✓7th **S95.111** Laceration of plantar artery of right foot

    ✓7th **S95.112** Laceration of plantar artery of left foot

    ✓7th **S95.119** Laceration of plantar artery of ▽ unspecified foot

  ✓6th **S95.19** Other specified injury of plantar artery of foot

    ✓7th **S95.191** Other specified injury of plantar artery of right foot

    ✓7th **S95.192** Other specified injury of plantar artery of left foot

    ✓7th **S95.199** Other specified injury of plantar artery ▽ of unspecified foot

✓5th **S95.2** Injury of dorsal vein of foot

  ✓6th **S95.20** Unspecified injury of dorsal vein of foot

    ✓7th **S95.201** Unspecified injury of dorsal vein of ▽ right foot

    ✓7th **S95.202** Unspecified injury of dorsal vein of ▽ left foot

    ✓7th **S95.209** Unspecified injury of dorsal vein of ▽ unspecified foot

  ✓6th **S95.21** Laceration of dorsal vein of foot

    ✓7th **S95.211** Laceration of dorsal vein of right foot

    ✓7th **S95.212** Laceration of dorsal vein of left foot

    ✓7th **S95.219** Laceration of dorsal vein of ▽ unspecified foot

  ✓6th **S95.29** Other specified injury of dorsal vein of foot

    ✓7th **S95.291** Other specified injury of dorsal vein of right foot

    ✓7th **S95.292** Other specified injury of dorsal vein of left foot

    ✓7th **S95.299** Other specified injury of dorsal vein of ▽ unspecified foot

✓5th **S95.8** Injury of other blood vessels at ankle and foot level

  ✓6th **S95.80** Unspecified injury of other blood vessels at ankle and foot level

    ✓7th **S95.801** Unspecified injury of other blood ▽ vessels at ankle and foot level, right leg

    ✓7th **S95.802** Unspecified injury of other blood ▽ vessels at ankle and foot level, left leg

    ✓7th **S95.809** Unspecified injury of other blood ▽ vessels at ankle and foot level, unspecified leg

  ✓6th **S95.81** Laceration of other blood vessels at ankle and foot level

    ✓7th **S95.811** Laceration of other blood vessels at ankle and foot level, right leg

    ✓7th **S95.812** Laceration of other blood vessels at ankle and foot level, left leg

    ✓7th **S95.819** Laceration of other blood vessels at ▽ ankle and foot level, unspecified leg

  ✓6th **S95.89** Other specified injury of other blood vessels at ankle and foot level

    ✓7th **S95.891** Other specified injury of other blood vessels at ankle and foot level, right leg

    ✓7th **S95.892** Other specified injury of other blood vessels at ankle and foot level, left leg

    ✓7th **S95.899** Other specified injury of other blood ▽ vessels at ankle and foot level, unspecified leg

✓5th **S95.9** Injury of unspecified blood vessel at ankle and foot level

  ✓6th **S95.90** Unspecified injury of unspecified blood vessel at ankle and foot level

    ✓7th **S95.901** Unspecified injury of unspecified blood ▽ vessel at ankle and foot level, right leg

    ✓7th **S95.902** Unspecified injury of unspecified blood ▽ vessel at ankle and foot level, left leg

    ✓7th **S95.909** Unspecified injury of unspecified blood ▽ vessel at ankle and foot level, unspecified leg

  ✓6th **S95.91** Laceration of unspecified blood vessel at ankle and foot level

    ✓7th **S95.911** Laceration of unspecified blood vessel ▽ at ankle and foot level, right leg

    ✓7th **S95.912** Laceration of unspecified blood vessel ▽ at ankle and foot level, left leg

    ✓7th **S95.919** Laceration of unspecified blood vessel ▽ at ankle and foot level, unspecified leg

  ✓6th **S95.99** Other specified injury of unspecified blood vessel at ankle and foot level

    ✓7th **S95.991** Other specified injury of unspecified ▽ blood vessel at ankle and foot level, right leg

    ✓7th **S95.992** Other specified injury of unspecified ▽ blood vessel at ankle and foot level, left leg

    ✓7th **S95.999** Other specified injury of unspecified ▽ blood vessel at ankle and foot level, unspecified leg

---

1 Case-mix diagnosis with 7th character indicating subsequent encounter.
2 Case-mix diagnosis with 7th character indicating subsequent encounter or sequela.

N Newborn: 0 P Pediatric: 0-17 M Maternity: 12-55 A Adult: 15-124 NRS Nonroutine supply Dx NCDx Noncancer Dx PDx Primary Dx ►◄ Revised Text ● New Code ▲ Revised Title

✓4ᵗʰ **S96 Injury of muscle and tendon at ankle and foot level**

Code also any associated open wound (S91.-)

EXCLUDES 2   *injury of Achilles tendon (S86.0-)*

      sprain of joints and ligaments of ankle and foot (S93.-)

TIP: Refer to the Muscle/Tendon table at the beginning of this chapter.

The appropriate 7th character is to be added to each code from category S96.

A   initial encounter

D   subsequent encounter

S   sequela

✓5ᵗʰ **S96.0 Injury of muscle and tendon of long flexor muscle of toe at ankle and foot level**

✓6ᵗʰ **S96.00 Unspecified injury of muscle and tendon of long flexor muscle of toe at ankle and foot level**

    ✓7ᵗʰ **S96.001** Unspecified injury of muscle and tendon of long flexor muscle of toe at ankle and foot level, right foot   ▽

    ✓7ᵗʰ **S96.002** Unspecified injury of muscle and tendon of long flexor muscle of toe at ankle and foot level, left foot   ▽

    ✓7ᵗʰ **S96.009** Unspecified injury of muscle and tendon of long flexor muscle of toe at ankle and foot level, unspecified foot   ▽

✓6ᵗʰ **S96.01 Strain of muscle and tendon of long flexor muscle of toe at ankle and foot level**

    ✓7ᵗʰ **S96.011** Strain of muscle and tendon of long flexor muscle of toe at ankle and foot level, right foot

    ✓7ᵗʰ **S96.012** Strain of muscle and tendon of long flexor muscle of toe at ankle and foot level, left foot

    ✓7ᵗʰ **S96.019** Strain of muscle and tendon of long flexor muscle of toe at ankle and foot level, unspecified foot   ▽

✓6ᵗʰ **S96.02 Laceration of muscle and tendon of long flexor muscle of toe at ankle and foot level**

    4,5 ✓7ᵗʰ **S96.021** Laceration of muscle and tendon of long flexor muscle of toe at ankle and foot level, right foot   NRS

    4,5 ✓7ᵗʰ **S96.022** Laceration of muscle and tendon of long flexor muscle of toe at ankle and foot level, left foot   NRS

    ✓7ᵗʰ **S96.029** Laceration of muscle and tendon of long flexor muscle of toe at ankle and foot level, unspecified foot   ▽

✓6ᵗʰ **S96.09 Other injury of muscle and tendon of long flexor muscle of toe at ankle and foot level**

    ✓7ᵗʰ **S96.091** Other injury of muscle and tendon of long flexor muscle of toe at ankle and foot level, right foot

    ✓7ᵗʰ **S96.092** Other injury of muscle and tendon of long flexor muscle of toe at ankle and foot level, left foot

    ✓7ᵗʰ **S96.099** Other injury of muscle and tendon of long flexor muscle of toe at ankle and foot level, unspecified foot   ▽

✓5ᵗʰ **S96.1 Injury of muscle and tendon of long extensor muscle of toe at ankle and foot level**

✓6ᵗʰ **S96.10 Unspecified injury of muscle and tendon of long extensor muscle of toe at ankle and foot level**

    ✓7ᵗʰ **S96.101** Unspecified injury of muscle and tendon of long extensor muscle of toe at ankle and foot level, right foot   ▽

    ✓7ᵗʰ **S96.102** Unspecified injury of muscle and tendon of long extensor muscle of toe at ankle and foot level, left foot   ▽

    ✓7ᵗʰ **S96.109** Unspecified injury of muscle and tendon of long extensor muscle of toe at ankle and foot level, unspecified foot   ▽

✓6ᵗʰ **S96.11 Strain of muscle and tendon of long extensor muscle of toe at ankle and foot level**

    ✓7ᵗʰ **S96.111** Strain of muscle and tendon of long extensor muscle of toe at ankle and foot level, right foot

    ✓7ᵗʰ **S96.112** Strain of muscle and tendon of long extensor muscle of toe at ankle and foot level, left foot

    ✓7ᵗʰ **S96.119** Strain of muscle and tendon of long extensor muscle of toe at ankle and foot level, unspecified foot   ▽

✓6ᵗʰ **S96.12 Laceration of muscle and tendon of long extensor muscle of toe at ankle and foot level**

    4,5 ✓7ᵗʰ **S96.121** Laceration of muscle and tendon of long extensor muscle of toe at ankle and foot level, right foot   NRS

    4,5 ✓7ᵗʰ **S96.122** Laceration of muscle and tendon of long extensor muscle of toe at ankle and foot level, left foot   NRS

    ✓7ᵗʰ **S96.129** Laceration of muscle and tendon of long extensor muscle of toe at ankle and foot level, unspecified foot   ▽

✓6ᵗʰ **S96.19 Other specified injury of muscle and tendon of long extensor muscle of toe at ankle and foot level**

    ✓7ᵗʰ **S96.191** Other specified injury of muscle and tendon of long extensor muscle of toe at ankle and foot level, right foot

    ✓7ᵗʰ **S96.192** Other specified injury of muscle and tendon of long extensor muscle of toe at ankle and foot level, left foot

    ✓7ᵗʰ **S96.199** Other specified injury of muscle and tendon of long extensor muscle of toe at ankle and foot level, unspecified foot   ▽

✓5ᵗʰ **S96.2 Injury of intrinsic muscle and tendon at ankle and foot level**

✓6ᵗʰ **S96.20 Unspecified injury of intrinsic muscle and tendon at ankle and foot level**

    ✓7ᵗʰ **S96.201** Unspecified injury of intrinsic muscle and tendon at ankle and foot level, right foot   ▽

    ✓7ᵗʰ **S96.202** Unspecified injury of intrinsic muscle and tendon at ankle and foot level, left foot   ▽

    ✓7ᵗʰ **S96.209** Unspecified injury of intrinsic muscle and tendon at ankle and foot level, unspecified foot   ▽

✓6ᵗʰ **S96.21 Strain of intrinsic muscle and tendon at ankle and foot level**

    ✓7ᵗʰ **S96.211** Strain of intrinsic muscle and tendon at ankle and foot level, right foot

    ✓7ᵗʰ **S96.212** Strain of intrinsic muscle and tendon at ankle and foot level, left foot

    ✓7ᵗʰ **S96.219** Strain of intrinsic muscle and tendon at ankle and foot level, unspecified foot   ▽

✓6ᵗʰ **S96.22 Laceration of intrinsic muscle and tendon at ankle and foot level**

    4,5 ✓7ᵗʰ **S96.221** Laceration of intrinsic muscle and tendon at ankle and foot level, right foot   NRS

    4,5 ✓7ᵗʰ **S96.222** Laceration of intrinsic muscle and tendon at ankle and foot level, left foot   NRS

    ✓7ᵗʰ **S96.229** Laceration of intrinsic muscle and tendon at ankle and foot level, unspecified foot   ▽

✓6ᵗʰ **S96.29 Other specified injury of intrinsic muscle and tendon at ankle and foot level**

    ✓7ᵗʰ **S96.291** Other specified injury of intrinsic muscle and tendon at ankle and foot level, right foot

    ✓7ᵗʰ **S96.292** Other specified injury of intrinsic muscle and tendon at ankle and foot level, left foot

    ✓7ᵗʰ **S96.299** Other specified injury of intrinsic muscle and tendon at ankle and foot level, unspecified foot   ▽

---

4   Case-mix diagnosis with 7th character indicating initial or subsequent encounter.

5   NRS supply diagnosis with 7th character indicating initial or subsequent encounter.

✓ Additional Character Req   ✓x7 Placeholder Alert   Case-Mix Diagnosis   Manifestation   ▽ Unspecified Dx   EXCLUDES 1 Not coded here   EXCLUDES 2 Not included here

Chapter 19. Injury, Poisoning and Certain Other Consequences of External Causes

✓5ᵗʰ S96.8 Injury of other specified **muscles and tendons at ankle and foot level**

✓6ᵗʰ S96.80 Unspecified **injury of other specified muscles and tendons at ankle and foot level**

   ✓7ᵗʰ S96.801 Unspecified injury of other specified muscles and tendons at ankle and foot level, **right** foot ▽

   ✓7ᵗʰ S96.802 Unspecified injury of other specified muscles and tendons at ankle and foot level, **left** foot ▽

   ✓7ᵗʰ S96.809 Unspecified injury of other specified muscles and tendons at ankle and foot level, unspecified foot ▽

✓6ᵗʰ S96.81 Strain **of other specified muscles and tendons at ankle and foot level**

   ✓7ᵗʰ S96.811 Strain of other specified muscles and tendons at ankle and foot level, **right** foot

   ✓7ᵗʰ S96.812 Strain of other specified muscles and tendons at ankle and foot level, **left** foot

   ✓7ᵗʰ S96.819 Strain of other specified muscles and tendons at ankle and foot level, unspecified foot ▽

✓6ᵗʰ S96.82 Laceration **of other specified muscles and tendons at ankle and foot level**

   4,5 **✓7ᵗʰ S96.821 Laceration of other specified muscles and tendons at ankle and foot level, right foot** NRS

   4,5 **✓7ᵗʰ S96.822 Laceration of other specified muscles and tendons at ankle and foot level, left foot** NRS

   ✓7ᵗʰ S96.829 Laceration of other specified muscles and tendons at ankle and foot level, unspecified foot ▽

✓6ᵗʰ S96.89 Other **specified injury of other specified muscles and tendons at ankle and foot level**

   ✓7ᵗʰ S96.891 Other specified injury of other specified muscles and tendons at ankle and foot level, **right** foot

   ✓7ᵗʰ S96.892 Other specified injury of other specified muscles and tendons at ankle and foot level, **left** foot

   ✓7ᵗʰ S96.899 Other specified injury of other specified muscles and tendons at ankle and foot level, unspecified foot ▽

✓5ᵗʰ S96.9 Injury of unspecified **muscle and tendon at ankle and foot level**

✓6ᵗʰ S96.90 Unspecified **injury of unspecified muscle and tendon at ankle and foot level**

   ✓7ᵗʰ S96.901 Unspecified injury of unspecified muscle and tendon at ankle and foot level, **right** foot ▽

   ✓7ᵗʰ S96.902 Unspecified injury of unspecified muscle and tendon at ankle and foot level, **left** foot ▽

   ✓7ᵗʰ S96.909 Unspecified injury of unspecified muscle and tendon at ankle and foot level, unspecified foot ▽

✓6ᵗʰ S96.91 Strain **of unspecified muscle and tendon at ankle and foot level**

   ✓7ᵗʰ S96.911 Strain of unspecified muscle and tendon at ankle and foot level, **right** foot ▽

   ✓7ᵗʰ S96.912 Strain of unspecified muscle and tendon at ankle and foot level, **left** foot ▽

   ✓7ᵗʰ S96.919 Strain of unspecified muscle and tendon at ankle and foot level, unspecified foot ▽

✓6ᵗʰ S96.92 Laceration **of unspecified muscle and tendon at ankle and foot level**

   4,5 **✓7ᵗʰ S96.921 Laceration of unspecified muscle and tendon at ankle and foot level, right foot** NRS ▽

   4,5 **✓7ᵗʰ S96.922 Laceration of unspecified muscle and tendon at ankle and foot level, left foot** NRS ▽

   ✓7ᵗʰ S96.929 Laceration of unspecified muscle and tendon at ankle and foot level, unspecified foot ▽

✓6ᵗʰ S96.99 Other **specified injury of unspecified muscle and tendon at ankle and foot level**

   ✓7ᵗʰ S96.991 Other specified injury of unspecified muscle and tendon at ankle and foot level, **right** foot ▽

   ✓7ᵗʰ S96.992 Other specified injury of unspecified muscle and tendon at ankle and foot level, **left** foot ▽

   ✓7ᵗʰ S96.999 Other specified injury of unspecified muscle and tendon at ankle and foot level, unspecified foot ▽

✓4ᵗʰ S97 Crushing injury of ankle and foot

Use additional code(s) for all associated injuries

The appropriate 7th character is to be added to each code from category S97.
A   initial encounter
D   subsequent encounter
S   sequela

✓5ᵗʰ S97.0 Crushing injury of ankle

   ✓x7ᵗʰ S97.00 Crushing injury of unspecified ankle ▽

   1 **✓x7ᵗʰ S97.01 Crushing injury of right ankle**

   1 **✓x7ᵗʰ S97.02 Crushing injury of left ankle**

✓5ᵗʰ S97.1 Crushing injury of toe

  ✓6ᵗʰ S97.10 Crushing injury of unspecified toe(s)

   ✓7ᵗʰ S97.101 Crushing injury of unspecified **right** toe(s) ▽

   ✓7ᵗʰ S97.102 Crushing injury of unspecified **left** toe(s) ▽

   ✓7ᵗʰ S97.109 Crushing injury of unspecified toe(s) ▽
      Crushing injury of toe NOS

  ✓6ᵗʰ S97.11 Crushing injury of great toe

   1 **✓7ᵗʰ S97.111 Crushing injury of right great toe**

   1 **✓7ᵗʰ S97.112 Crushing injury of left great toe**

   ✓7ᵗʰ S97.119 Crushing injury of unspecified great toe ▽

  ✓6ᵗʰ S97.12 Crushing injury of lesser toe(s)

   1 **✓7ᵗʰ S97.121 Crushing injury of right lesser toe(s)**

   1 **✓7ᵗʰ S97.122 Crushing injury of left lesser toe(s)**

   ✓7ᵗʰ S97.129 Crushing injury of unspecified lesser toe(s) ▽

✓5ᵗʰ S97.8 Crushing injury of foot

   ✓x7ᵗʰ S97.80 Crushing injury of unspecified foot ▽
      Crushing injury of foot NOS

   1 **✓x7ᵗʰ S97.81 Crushing injury of right foot**

   1 **✓x7ᵗʰ S97.82 Crushing injury of left foot**

✓4ᵗʰ S98 Traumatic amputation of ankle and foot

An amputation not identified as partial or complete should be coded to complete

The appropriate 7th character is to be added to each code from category S98.
A   initial encounter
D   subsequent encounter
S   sequela

✓5ᵗʰ S98.0 Traumatic amputation of foot at ankle level

  ✓6ᵗʰ S98.01 Complete **traumatic amputation of foot at ankle level**

   4,5 **✓7ᵗʰ S98.011 Complete traumatic amputation of right foot at ankle level** NRS

   4,5 **✓7ᵗʰ S98.012 Complete traumatic amputation of left foot at ankle level** NRS

   ✓7ᵗʰ S98.019 Complete traumatic amputation of unspecified foot at ankle level ▽

  ✓6ᵗʰ S98.02 Partial **traumatic amputation of foot at ankle level**

   4,5 **✓7ᵗʰ S98.021 Partial traumatic amputation of right foot at ankle level** NRS

   4,5 **✓7ᵗʰ S98.022 Partial traumatic amputation of left foot at ankle level** NRS

---

1 Case-mix diagnosis with 7th character indicating subsequent encounter.
4 Case-mix diagnosis with 7th character indicating initial or subsequent encounter.
5 NRS supply diagnosis with 7th character indicating initial or subsequent encounter.

N Newborn: 0   P Pediatric: 0-17   M Maternity: 12-55   A Adult: 15-124   NRS Nonroutine supply Dx   NCDx Noncancer Dx   PDx Primary Dx   ►◄ Revised Text   ● New Code   ▲ Revised Title

1036   ICD-10-CM 2018

✓7th **S98.029** Partial traumatic amputation of unspecified foot at ankle level ▽

✓5th **S98.1** Traumatic amputation of one toe

✓6th **S98.11** Complete traumatic amputation of great toe

4,5 ✓7th **S98.111** Complete traumatic amputation of right great toe `NRS`

4,5 ✓7th **S98.112** Complete traumatic amputation of left great toe `NRS`

✓7th **S98.119** Complete traumatic amputation of unspecified great toe ▽

✓6th **S98.12** Partial traumatic amputation of great toe

4,5 ✓7th **S98.121** Partial traumatic amputation of right great toe `NRS`

4,5 ✓7th **S98.122** Partial traumatic amputation of left great toe `NRS`

✓7th **S98.129** Partial traumatic amputation of unspecified great toe ▽

✓6th **S98.13** Complete traumatic amputation of one lesser toe
Traumatic amputation of toe NOS

4,5 ✓7th **S98.131** Complete traumatic amputation of one right lesser toe `NRS`

4,5 ✓7th **S98.132** Complete traumatic amputation of one left lesser toe `NRS`

✓7th **S98.139** Complete traumatic amputation of one unspecified lesser toe ▽

✓6th **S98.14** Partial traumatic amputation of one lesser toe

4,5 ✓7th **S98.141** Partial traumatic amputation of one right lesser toe `NRS`

4,5 ✓7th **S98.142** Partial traumatic amputation of one left lesser toe `NRS`

✓7th **S98.149** Partial traumatic amputation of one unspecified lesser toe ▽

✓5th **S98.2** Traumatic amputation of two or more lesser toes

✓6th **S98.21** Complete traumatic amputation of two or more lesser toes

4,5 ✓7th **S98.211** Complete traumatic amputation of two or more right lesser toes `NRS`

4,5 ✓7th **S98.212** Complete traumatic amputation of two or more left lesser toes `NRS`

✓7th **S98.219** Complete traumatic amputation of two or more unspecified lesser toes ▽

✓6th **S98.22** Partial traumatic amputation of two or more lesser toes

4,5 ✓7th **S98.221** Partial traumatic amputation of two or more right lesser toes `NRS`

4,5 ✓7th **S98.222** Partial traumatic amputation of two or more left lesser toes `NRS`

✓7th **S98.229** Partial traumatic amputation of two or more unspecified lesser toes ▽

✓5th **S98.3** Traumatic amputation of midfoot

✓6th **S98.31** Complete traumatic amputation of midfoot

4,5 ✓7th **S98.311** Complete traumatic amputation of right midfoot `NRS`

4,5 ✓7th **S98.312** Complete traumatic amputation of left midfoot `NRS`

✓7th **S98.319** Complete traumatic amputation of unspecified midfoot ▽

✓6th **S98.32** Partial traumatic amputation of midfoot

4,5 ✓7th **S98.321** Partial traumatic amputation of right midfoot `NRS`

4,5 ✓7th **S98.322** Partial traumatic amputation of left midfoot `NRS`

✓7th **S98.329** Partial traumatic amputation of unspecified midfoot ▽

✓5th **S98.9** Traumatic amputation of foot, level unspecified

✓6th **S98.91** Complete traumatic amputation of foot, level unspecified

4,5 ✓7th **S98.911** Complete traumatic amputation of right foot, level unspecified `NRS` ▽

4,5 ✓7th **S98.912** Complete traumatic amputation of left foot, level unspecified `NRS` ▽

✓7th **S98.919** Complete traumatic amputation of unspecified foot, level unspecified ▽

✓6th **S98.92** Partial traumatic amputation of foot, level unspecified

4,5 ✓7th **S98.921** Partial traumatic amputation of right foot, level unspecified `NRS` ▽

4,5 ✓7th **S98.922** Partial traumatic amputation of left foot, level unspecified `NRS` ▽

✓7th **S98.929** Partial traumatic amputation of unspecified foot, level unspecified ▽

✓4th **S99** Other and unspecified injuries of ankle and foot

TIP: The term "improper alignment" is not synonymous with malunion or nonunion of a fracture when noted in provider documentation.

✓5th **S99.0** Physeal fracture of calcaneus

The appropriate 7th character is to be added to each code from subcategories S99.0.
A initial encounter for closed fracture
B initial encounter for open fracture
D subsequent encounter for fracture with routine healing
G subsequent encounter for fracture with delayed healing
K subsequent encounter for fracture with nonunion
P subsequent encounter for fracture with malunion
S sequela

✓6th **S99.00** Unspecified physeal fracture of calcaneus

1 ✓7th **S99.001** Unspecified physeal fracture of right calcaneus ▽

1 ✓7th **S99.002** Unspecified physeal fracture of left calcaneus ▽

✓7th **S99.009** Unspecified physeal fracture of unspecified calcaneus ▽

✓6th **S99.01** Salter-Harris Type I physeal fracture of calcaneus

1 ✓7th **S99.011** Salter-Harris Type I physeal fracture of right calcaneus

1 ✓7th **S99.012** Salter-Harris Type I physeal fracture of left calcaneus

✓7th **S99.019** Salter-Harris Type I physeal fracture of unspecified calcaneus ▽

✓6th **S99.02** Salter-Harris Type II physeal fracture of calcaneus

1 ✓7th **S99.021** Salter-Harris Type II physeal fracture of right calcaneus

1 ✓7th **S99.022** Salter-Harris Type II physeal fracture of left calcaneus

✓7th **S99.029** Salter-Harris Type II physeal fracture of unspecified calcaneus ▽

✓6th **S99.03** Salter-Harris Type III physeal fracture of calcaneus

1 ✓7th **S99.031** Salter-Harris Type III physeal fracture of right calcaneus

1 ✓7th **S99.032** Salter-Harris Type III physeal fracture of left calcaneus

✓7th **S99.039** Salter-Harris Type III physeal fracture of unspecified calcaneus ▽

✓6th **S99.04** Salter-Harris Type IV physeal fracture of calcaneus

1 ✓7th **S99.041** Salter-Harris Type IV physeal fracture of right calcaneus

1 ✓7th **S99.042** Salter-Harris Type IV physeal fracture of left calcaneus

✓7th **S99.049** Salter-Harris Type IV physeal fracture of unspecified calcaneus ▽

✓6th **S99.09** Other physeal fracture of calcaneus

1 ✓7th **S99.091** Other physeal fracture of right calcaneus

1 ✓7th **S99.092** Other physeal fracture of left calcaneus

✓7th **S99.099** Other physeal fracture of unspecified calcaneus ▽

1 Case-mix diagnosis with 7th character indicating subsequent encounter.
4 Case-mix diagnosis with 7th character indicating initial or subsequent encounter.
5 NRS supply diagnosis with 7th character indicating initial or subsequent encounter.

✓ Additional Character Req ✓x7th Placeholder Alert Case-Mix Diagnosis Manifestation ▽ Unspecified Dx *EXCLUDES 1* Not coded here *EXCLUDES 2* Not included here

ICD-10-CM 2018

1037

✓5ᵗʰ **S99.1** **Physeal fracture of** metatarsal

> The appropriate 7th character is to be added to each code from subcategories S99.1.
> A   initial encounter for closed fracture
> B   initial encounter for open fracture
> D   subsequent encounter for fracture with routine healing
> G   subsequent encounter for fracture with delayed healing
> K   subsequent encounter for fracture with nonunion
> P   subsequent encounter for fracture with malunion
> S   sequela

  ✓6ᵗʰ **S99.10** Unspecified physeal fracture of metatarsal
    1 ✓7ᵗʰ **S99.101** **Unspecified physeal fracture of** right **metatarsal** ▽
    1 ✓7ᵗʰ **S99.102** **Unspecified physeal fracture of** left **metatarsal** ▽
    ✓7ᵗʰ **S99.109** **Unspecified physeal fracture of unspecified metatarsal** ▽

  ✓6ᵗʰ **S99.11** Salter-Harris Type I **physeal fracture of metatarsal**
    1 ✓7ᵗʰ **S99.111** **Salter-Harris Type I physeal fracture of** right **metatarsal**
    1 ✓7ᵗʰ **S99.112** **Salter-Harris Type I physeal fracture of** left **metatarsal**
    ✓7ᵗʰ **S99.119** **Salter-Harris Type I physeal fracture of unspecified metatarsal** ▽

  ✓6ᵗʰ **S99.12** Salter-Harris Type II **physeal fracture of metatarsal**
    1 ✓7ᵗʰ **S99.121** **Salter-Harris Type II physeal fracture of** right **metatarsal**
    1 ✓7ᵗʰ **S99.122** **Salter-Harris Type II physeal fracture of** left **metatarsal**
    ✓7ᵗʰ **S99.129** **Salter-Harris Type II physeal fracture of unspecified metatarsal** ▽

  ✓6ᵗʰ **S99.13** Salter-Harris Type III **physeal fracture of metatarsal**
    1 ✓7ᵗʰ **S99.131** **Salter-Harris Type III physeal fracture of** right **metatarsal**
    1 ✓7ᵗʰ **S99.132** **Salter-Harris Type III physeal fracture of** left **metatarsal**
    ✓7ᵗʰ **S99.139** **Salter-Harris Type III physeal fracture of unspecified metatarsal** ▽

  ✓6ᵗʰ **S99.14** Salter-Harris Type IV **physeal fracture of metatarsal**
    1 ✓7ᵗʰ **S99.141** **Salter-Harris Type IV physeal fracture of** right **metatarsal**
    1 ✓7ᵗʰ **S99.142** **Salter-Harris Type IV physeal fracture of** left **metatarsal**
    ✓7ᵗʰ **S99.149** **Salter-Harris Type IV physeal fracture of unspecified metatarsal** ▽

  ✓6ᵗʰ **S99.19** Other **physeal fracture of metatarsal**
    1 ✓7ᵗʰ **S99.191** **Other physeal fracture of** right **metatarsal**
    1 ✓7ᵗʰ **S99.192** **Other physeal fracture of** left **metatarsal**
    ✓7ᵗʰ **S99.199** **Other physeal fracture of unspecified metatarsal** ▽

✓5ᵗʰ **S99.2** **Physeal fracture of** phalanx of toe

> The appropriate 7th character is to be added to each code from subcategories S99.2.
> A   initial encounter for closed fracture
> B   initial encounter for open fracture
> D   subsequent encounter for fracture with routine healing
> G   subsequent encounter for fracture with delayed healing
> K   subsequent encounter for fracture with nonunion
> P   subsequent encounter for fracture with malunion
> S   sequela

  ✓6ᵗʰ **S99.20** Unspecified physeal fracture of phalanx of toe
    1 ✓7ᵗʰ **S99.201** **Unspecified physeal fracture of phalanx of** right **toe** ▽
    1 ✓7ᵗʰ **S99.202** **Unspecified physeal fracture of phalanx of** left **toe** ▽
    ✓7ᵗʰ **S99.209** **Unspecified physeal fracture of phalanx of unspecified toe** ▽

  ✓6ᵗʰ **S99.21** Salter-Harris Type I **physeal fracture of phalanx of toe**
    1 ✓7ᵗʰ **S99.211** **Salter-Harris Type I physeal fracture of phalanx of** right **toe**
    1 ✓7ᵗʰ **S99.212** **Salter-Harris Type I physeal fracture of phalanx of** left **toe**

    ✓7ᵗʰ **S99.219** **Salter-Harris Type I physeal fracture of phalanx of unspecified toe** ▽

  ✓6ᵗʰ **S99.22** Salter-Harris Type II **physeal fracture of phalanx of toe**
    1 ✓7ᵗʰ **S99.221** **Salter-Harris Type II physeal fracture of phalanx of** right **toe**
    1 ✓7ᵗʰ **S99.222** **Salter-Harris Type II physeal fracture of phalanx of** left **toe**
    ✓7ᵗʰ **S99.229** **Salter-Harris Type II physeal fracture of phalanx of unspecified toe** ▽

  ✓6ᵗʰ **S99.23** Salter-Harris Type III **physeal fracture of phalanx of toe**
    1 ✓7ᵗʰ **S99.231** **Salter-Harris Type III physeal fracture of phalanx of** right **toe**
    1 ✓7ᵗʰ **S99.232** **Salter-Harris Type III physeal fracture of phalanx of** left **toe**
    ✓7ᵗʰ **S99.239** **Salter-Harris Type III physeal fracture of phalanx of unspecified toe** ▽

  ✓6ᵗʰ **S99.24** Salter-Harris Type IV **physeal fracture of phalanx of toe**
    1 ✓7ᵗʰ **S99.241** **Salter-Harris Type IV physeal fracture of phalanx of** right **toe**
    1 ✓7ᵗʰ **S99.242** **Salter-Harris Type IV physeal fracture of phalanx of** left **toe**
    ✓7ᵗʰ **S99.249** **Salter-Harris Type IV physeal fracture of phalanx of unspecified toe** ▽

  ✓6ᵗʰ **S99.29** Other **physeal fracture of phalanx of toe**
    1 ✓7ᵗʰ **S99.291** **Other physeal fracture of phalanx of** right **toe**
    1 ✓7ᵗʰ **S99.292** **Other physeal fracture of phalanx of** left **toe**
    ✓7ᵗʰ **S99.299** **Other physeal fracture of phalanx of unspecified toe** ▽

✓5ᵗʰ **S99.8** Other **specified injuries of ankle and foot**

> The appropriate 7th character is to be added to each code from subcategory S99.8.
> A   initial encounter
> D   subsequent encounter
> S   sequela

  ✓6ᵗʰ **S99.81** Other specified injuries of ankle
    ✓7ᵗʰ **S99.811** Other specified injuries of right ankle
    ✓7ᵗʰ **S99.812** Other specified injuries of left ankle
    ✓7ᵗʰ **S99.819** Other specified injuries of unspecified ankle ▽

  ✓6ᵗʰ **S99.82** Other specified injuries of foot
    ✓7ᵗʰ **S99.821** Other specified injuries of right foot
    ✓7ᵗʰ **S99.822** Other specified injuries of left foot
    ✓7ᵗʰ **S99.829** Other specified injuries of unspecified foot ▽

✓5ᵗʰ **S99.9** Unspecified **injury of ankle and foot**

> The appropriate 7th character is to be added to each code from subcategory S99.9.
> A   initial encounter
> D   subsequent encounter
> S   sequela

  ✓6ᵗʰ **S99.91** Unspecified injury of ankle
    ✓7ᵗʰ **S99.911** Unspecified injury of right ankle ▽
    ✓7ᵗʰ **S99.912** Unspecified injury of left ankle ▽
    ✓7ᵗʰ **S99.919** Unspecified injury of unspecified ankle ▽

  ✓6ᵗʰ **S99.92** Unspecified injury of foot
    ✓7ᵗʰ **S99.921** Unspecified injury of right foot ▽
    ✓7ᵗʰ **S99.922** Unspecified injury of left foot ▽
    ✓7ᵗʰ **S99.929** Unspecified injury of unspecified foot ▽

---

1 Case-mix diagnosis with 7th character indicating subsequent encounter.

N Newborn: 0   P Pediatric: 0-17   M Maternity: 12-55   A Adult: 15-124   NRS Nonroutine supply Dx   NCDx Noncancer Dx   PDx Primary Dx   ▶◀ Revised Text   ● New Code   ▲ Revised Title

1038   ICD-10-CM 2018

Injury, Poisoning And Certain Other Consequences Of External Causes (T07-T88)

Injuries involving multiple body regions (T07)

EXCLUDES 1   *burns and corrosions (T20-T32)*
frostbite (T33-T34)
insect bite or sting, venomous (T63.4)
sunburn (L55.-)

✓x7ᵗʰ **T07**   **Unspecified multiple injuries**   ▽
      EXCLUDES 1   *injury NOS ▶(T14.90)◀*

> The appropriate 7th character is to be added to code T07.
> A   initial encounter
> D   subsequent encounter
> S   sequela

Injury of unspecified body region (T14)

✓4ᵗʰ **T14**   **Injury of unspecified body region**
      EXCLUDES 1   *multiple unspecified injuries (T07)*

> The appropriate 7th character is to be added to each code from category T14.
> A   initial encounter
> D   subsequent encounter
> S   sequela

    ✓x7ᵗʰ **T14.8**   **Other injury of unspecified body region**
      Abrasion NOS
      Contusion NOS
      Crush injury NOS
      Fracture NOS
      Skin injury NOS
      Vascular injury NOS
      ▶Wound NOS◀

    ✓5ᵗʰ **T14.9**   **Unspecified injury**

      ✓x7ᵗʰ **T14.90**   **Injury, unspecified**   ▽
        Injury NOS

      ✓x7ᵗʰ **T14.91**   **Suicide attempt**
        Attempted suicide NOS

Effects of foreign body entering through natural orifice (T15-T19)

EXCLUDES 2   *foreign body accidentally left in operation wound (T81.5-)*
foreign body in penetrating wound—See open wound by body region
residual foreign body in soft tissue (M79.5)
splinter, without open wound—See superficial injury by body region

✓4ᵗʰ **T15**   **Foreign body on external eye**
      EXCLUDES 2   *foreign body in penetrating wound of orbit and eye ball (S05.4-, S05.5-)*
open wound of eyelid and periocular area (S01.1-)
retained foreign body in eyelid (H02.8-)
retained (old) foreign body in penetrating wound of orbit and eye ball (H05.5-, H44.6-, H44.7-)
superficial foreign body of eyelid and periocular area (S00.25-)

> The appropriate 7th character is to be added to each code from category T15.
> A   initial encounter
> D   subsequent encounter
> S   sequela

    ✓5ᵗʰ **T15.0**   **Foreign body in cornea**

      ✓x7ᵗʰ **T15.00**   **Foreign body in cornea, unspecified eye**   ▽
      ✓x7ᵗʰ **T15.01**   **Foreign body in cornea, right eye**
      ✓x7ᵗʰ **T15.02**   **Foreign body in cornea, left eye**

    ✓5ᵗʰ **T15.1**   **Foreign body in conjunctival sac**

      ✓x7ᵗʰ **T15.10**   **Foreign body in conjunctival sac, unspecified eye**   ▽
      ✓x7ᵗʰ **T15.11**   **Foreign body in conjunctival sac, right eye**
      ✓x7ᵗʰ **T15.12**   **Foreign body in conjunctival sac, left eye**

    ✓5ᵗʰ **T15.8**   **Foreign body in other and multiple parts of external eye**
      Foreign body in lacrimal punctum

      ✓x7ᵗʰ **T15.80**   **Foreign body in other and multiple parts of external eye, unspecified eye**   ▽
      ✓x7ᵗʰ **T15.81**   **Foreign body in other and multiple parts of external eye, right eye**
      ✓x7ᵗʰ **T15.82**   **Foreign body in other and multiple parts of external eye, left eye**

    ✓5ᵗʰ **T15.9**   **Foreign body on external eye, part unspecified**

      ✓x7ᵗʰ **T15.90**   **Foreign body on external eye, part unspecified, unspecified eye**   ▽
      ✓x7ᵗʰ **T15.91**   **Foreign body on external eye, part unspecified, right eye**   ▽
      ✓x7ᵗʰ **T15.92**   **Foreign body on external eye, part unspecified, left eye**   ▽

✓4ᵗʰ **T16**   **Foreign body in ear**
      INCLUDES   foreign body in auditory canal

> The appropriate 7th character is to be added to each code from category T16.
> A   initial encounter
> D   subsequent encounter
> S   sequela

    ✓x7ᵗʰ **T16.1**   **Foreign body in right ear**
    ✓x7ᵗʰ **T16.2**   **Foreign body in left ear**
    ✓x7ᵗʰ **T16.9**   **Foreign body in ear, unspecified ear**   ▽

✓4ᵗʰ **T17**   **Foreign body in respiratory tract**

> The appropriate 7th character is to be added to each code from category T17.
> A   initial encounter
> D   subsequent encounter
> S   sequela

    ✓x7ᵗʰ **T17.0**   **Foreign body in nasal sinus**
    ✓x7ᵗʰ **T17.1**   **Foreign body in nostril**
      Foreign body in nose NOS

    ✓5ᵗʰ **T17.2**   **Foreign body in pharynx**
      Foreign body in nasopharynx
      Foreign body in throat NOS

      ✓6ᵗʰ **T17.20**   **Unspecified foreign body in pharynx**

        ✓7ᵗʰ **T17.200**   **Unspecified foreign body in pharynx causing asphyxiation**   ▽
        ✓7ᵗʰ **T17.208**   **Unspecified foreign body in pharynx causing other injury**   ▽

      ✓6ᵗʰ **T17.21**   **Gastric contents in pharynx**
        Aspiration of gastric contents into pharynx
        Vomitus in pharynx

        ✓7ᵗʰ **T17.210**   **Gastric contents in pharynx causing asphyxiation**
        ✓7ᵗʰ **T17.218**   **Gastric contents in pharynx causing other injury**

      ✓6ᵗʰ **T17.22**   **Food in pharynx**
        Bones in larynx
        Seeds in pharynx

        ✓7ᵗʰ **T17.220**   **Food in pharynx causing asphyxiation**
        ✓7ᵗʰ **T17.228**   **Food in pharynx causing other injury**

      ✓6ᵗʰ **T17.29**   **Other foreign object in pharynx**

        ✓7ᵗʰ **T17.290**   **Other foreign object in pharynx causing asphyxiation**
        ✓7ᵗʰ **T17.298**   **Other foreign object in pharynx causing other injury**

    ✓5ᵗʰ **T17.3**   **Foreign body in larynx**

      ✓6ᵗʰ **T17.30**   **Unspecified foreign body in larynx**

        ✓7ᵗʰ **T17.300**   **Unspecified foreign body in larynx causing asphyxiation**   ▽
        ✓7ᵗʰ **T17.308**   **Unspecified foreign body in larynx causing other injury**   ▽

      ✓6ᵗʰ **T17.31**   **Gastric contents in larynx**
        Aspiration of gastric contents into larynx
        Vomitus in larynx

        ✓7ᵗʰ **T17.310**   **Gastric contents in larynx causing asphyxiation**
        ✓7ᵗʰ **T17.318**   **Gastric contents in larynx causing other injury**

      ✓6ᵗʰ **T17.32**   **Food in larynx**
        Bones in pharynx
        Seeds in larynx

        ✓7ᵗʰ **T17.320**   **Food in larynx causing asphyxiation**
        ✓7ᵗʰ **T17.328**   **Food in larynx causing other injury**

✓ Additional Character Req   ✓x7ᵗʰ Placeholder Alert   Case-Mix Diagnosis   Manifestation   ▽ Unspecified Dx   **EXCLUDES 1** Not coded here   **EXCLUDES 2** Not included here

✓⁶ᵗʰ **T17.39** Other foreign object in larynx
- ✓⁷ᵗʰ **T17.390** Other foreign object in larynx causing asphyxiation
- ✓⁷ᵗʰ **T17.398** Other foreign object in larynx causing other injury

✓⁵ᵗʰ **T17.4** Foreign body in trachea

✓⁶ᵗʰ **T17.40** Unspecified foreign body in trachea
- ✓⁷ᵗʰ **T17.400** Unspecified foreign body in trachea causing asphyxiation ▽
- ✓⁷ᵗʰ **T17.408** Unspecified foreign body in trachea causing other injury ▽

✓⁶ᵗʰ **T17.41** Gastric contents in trachea
Aspiration of gastric contents into trachea
Vomitus in trachea
- ✓⁷ᵗʰ **T17.410** Gastric contents in trachea causing asphyxiation
- ✓⁷ᵗʰ **T17.418** Gastric contents in trachea causing other injury

✓⁶ᵗʰ **T17.42** Food in trachea
Bones in trachea
Seeds in trachea
- ✓⁷ᵗʰ **T17.420** Food in trachea causing asphyxiation
- ✓⁷ᵗʰ **T17.428** Food in trachea causing other injury

✓⁶ᵗʰ **T17.49** Other foreign object in trachea
- ✓⁷ᵗʰ **T17.490** Other foreign object in trachea causing asphyxiation
- ✓⁷ᵗʰ **T17.498** Other foreign object in trachea causing other injury

✓⁵ᵗʰ **T17.5** Foreign body in bronchus

✓⁶ᵗʰ **T17.50** Unspecified foreign body in bronchus
- ✓⁷ᵗʰ **T17.500** Unspecified foreign body in bronchus causing asphyxiation ▽
- ✓⁷ᵗʰ **T17.508** Unspecified foreign body in bronchus causing other injury ▽

✓⁶ᵗʰ **T17.51** Gastric contents in bronchus
Aspiration of gastric contents into bronchus
Vomitus in bronchus
- ✓⁷ᵗʰ **T17.510** Gastric contents in bronchus causing asphyxiation
- ✓⁷ᵗʰ **T17.518** Gastric contents in bronchus causing other injury

✓⁶ᵗʰ **T17.52** Food in bronchus
Bones in bronchus
Seeds in bronchus
- ✓⁷ᵗʰ **T17.520** Food in bronchus causing asphyxiation
- ✓⁷ᵗʰ **T17.528** Food in bronchus causing other injury

✓⁶ᵗʰ **T17.59** Other foreign object in bronchus
- ✓⁷ᵗʰ **T17.590** Other foreign object in bronchus causing asphyxiation
- ✓⁷ᵗʰ **T17.598** Other foreign object in bronchus causing other injury

✓⁵ᵗʰ **T17.8** Foreign body in other parts of respiratory tract
Foreign body in bronchioles
Foreign body in lung

✓⁶ᵗʰ **T17.80** Unspecified foreign body in other parts of respiratory tract
- ✓⁷ᵗʰ **T17.800** Unspecified foreign body in other parts of respiratory tract causing asphyxiation ▽
- ✓⁷ᵗʰ **T17.808** Unspecified foreign body in other parts of respiratory tract causing other injury ▽

✓⁶ᵗʰ **T17.81** Gastric contents in other parts of respiratory tract
Aspiration of gastric contents into other parts of respiratory tract
Vomitus in other parts of respiratory tract
- ✓⁷ᵗʰ **T17.810** Gastric contents in other parts of respiratory tract causing asphyxiation
- ✓⁷ᵗʰ **T17.818** Gastric contents in other parts of respiratory tract causing other injury

✓⁶ᵗʰ **T17.82** Food in other parts of respiratory tract
Bones in other parts of respiratory tract
Seeds in other parts of respiratory tract
- ✓⁷ᵗʰ **T17.820** Food in other parts of respiratory tract causing asphyxiation
- ✓⁷ᵗʰ **T17.828** Food in other parts of respiratory tract causing other injury

✓⁶ᵗʰ **T17.89** Other foreign object in other parts of respiratory tract
- ✓⁷ᵗʰ **T17.890** Other foreign object in other parts of respiratory tract causing asphyxiation
- ✓⁷ᵗʰ **T17.898** Other foreign object in other parts of respiratory tract causing other injury

✓⁵ᵗʰ **T17.9** Foreign body in respiratory tract, part unspecified

✓⁶ᵗʰ **T17.90** Unspecified foreign body in respiratory tract, part unspecified
- ✓⁷ᵗʰ **T17.900** Unspecified foreign body in respiratory tract, part unspecified causing asphyxiation ▽
- ✓⁷ᵗʰ **T17.908** Unspecified foreign body in respiratory tract, part unspecified causing other injury ▽

✓⁶ᵗʰ **T17.91** Gastric contents in respiratory tract, part unspecified
Aspiration of gastric contents into respiratory tract, part unspecified
Vomitus in trachea respiratory tract, part unspecified
- ✓⁷ᵗʰ **T17.910** Gastric contents in respiratory tract, part unspecified causing asphyxiation ▽
- ✓⁷ᵗʰ **T17.918** Gastric contents in respiratory tract, part unspecified causing other injury ▽

✓⁶ᵗʰ **T17.92** Food in respiratory tract, part unspecified
Bones in respiratory tract, part unspecified
Seeds in respiratory tract, part unspecified
- ✓⁷ᵗʰ **T17.920** Food in respiratory tract, part unspecified causing asphyxiation ▽
- ✓⁷ᵗʰ **T17.928** Food in respiratory tract, part unspecified causing other injury ▽

✓⁶ᵗʰ **T17.99** Other foreign object in respiratory tract, part unspecified
- ✓⁷ᵗʰ **T17.990** Other foreign object in respiratory tract, part unspecified in causing asphyxiation ▽
- ✓⁷ᵗʰ **T17.998** Other foreign object in respiratory tract, part unspecified causing other injury ▽

✓⁴ᵗʰ **T18** **Foreign body in alimentary tract**
EXCLUDES 2   foreign body in pharynx (T17.2-)

The appropriate 7th character is to be added to each code from category T18.
A   initial encounter
D   subsequent encounter
S   sequela

✓ˣ⁷ᵗʰ **T18.0** Foreign body in mouth

✓⁵ᵗʰ **T18.1** Foreign body in esophagus
EXCLUDES 2   foreign body in respiratory tract (T17.-)

✓⁶ᵗʰ **T18.10** Unspecified foreign body in esophagus
- ✓⁷ᵗʰ **T18.100** Unspecified foreign body in esophagus causing compression of trachea ▽
Unspecified foreign body in esophagus causing obstruction of respiration
- ✓⁷ᵗʰ **T18.108** Unspecified foreign body in esophagus causing other injury ▽

✓⁶ᵗʰ **T18.11** Gastric contents in esophagus
Vomitus in esophagus
- ✓⁷ᵗʰ **T18.110** Gastric contents in esophagus causing compression of trachea
Gastric contents in esophagus causing obstruction of respiration
- ✓⁷ᵗʰ **T18.118** Gastric contents in esophagus causing other injury

✓⁶ᵗʰ **T18.12** Food in esophagus
Bones in esophagus
Seeds in esophagus
- ✓⁷ᵗʰ **T18.120** Food in esophagus causing compression of trachea
Food in esophagus causing obstruction of respiration
- ✓⁷ᵗʰ **T18.128** Food in esophagus causing other injury

Ⓝ Newborn: 0   Ⓟ Pediatric: 0-17   Ⓜ Maternity: 12-55   Ⓐ Adult: 15-124   **NRS** Nonroutine supply Dx   **NCDx** Noncancer Dx   **PDx** Primary Dx   ►◄ Revised Text   ● New Code   ▲ Revised Title

1040   ICD-10-CM 2018

✓6ᵗʰ **T18.19** Other **foreign object in esophagus**
     AHA: 2015, 1Q, 23

   ✓7ᵗʰ **T18.190** Other **foreign object in esophagus** causing **compression of trachea**
     Other foreign body in esophagus causing obstruction of respiration

   ✓7ᵗʰ **T18.198** Other **foreign object in esophagus** causing **other injury**

✓x7ᵗʰ **T18.2** **Foreign body in** stomach

✓x7ᵗʰ **T18.3** **Foreign body in** small intestine

✓x7ᵗʰ **T18.4** **Foreign body in** colon

✓x7ᵗʰ **T18.5** **Foreign body in** anus and rectum
     Foreign body in rectosigmoid (junction)

✓x7ᵗʰ **T18.8** **Foreign body in other** parts **of alimentary tract**

✓x7ᵗʰ **T18.9** **Foreign body of alimentary tract, part unspecified** ▽
     Foreign body in digestive system NOS
     Swallowed foreign body NOS

✓4ᵗʰ **T19** **Foreign body in genitourinary tract**
   EXCLUDES 2 *complications due to implanted mesh (T83.7-)*
      mechanical complications of contraceptive device (intrauterine) (vaginal) (T83.3-)
      presence of contraceptive device (intrauterine) (vaginal) (Z97.5)

> The appropriate 7th character is to be added to each code from category T19.
> A   initial encounter
> D   subsequent encounter
> S   sequela

✓x7ᵗʰ **T19.0** **Foreign body in** urethra

✓x7ᵗʰ **T19.1** **Foreign body in** bladder

✓x7ᵗʰ **T19.2** **Foreign body in** vulva and vagina   ♀

✓x7ᵗʰ **T19.3** **Foreign body in** uterus   ♀

✓x7ᵗʰ **T19.4** **Foreign body in** penis   ♂

✓x7ᵗʰ **T19.8** **Foreign body in other parts of genitourinary tract**

✓x7ᵗʰ **T19.9** **Foreign body in genitourinary tract, part unspecified** ▽

Burns and corrosions (T20-T32)

INCLUDES   burns (thermal) from electrical heating appliances
      burns (thermal) from electricity
      burns (thermal) from flame
      burns (thermal) from friction
      burns (thermal) from hot air and hot gases
      burns (thermal) from hot objects
      burns (thermal) from lightning
      burns (thermal) from radiation
      chemical burn [corrosion] (external) (internal)
      scalds

EXCLUDES 2 *erythema [dermatitis] ab igne (L59.0)*
      radiation-related disorders of the skin and subcutaneous tissue (L55-L59)
      sunburn (L55.-)

AHA: 2016, 2Q, 4
TIP: Burn wound treatment is considered active care and reported with 7th character A.

Burns and corrosions of external body surface, specified by site (T20-T25)
INCLUDES   burns and corrosions of first degree [erythema]
      burns and corrosions of second degree [blisters] [epidermal loss]
      burns and corrosions of third degree [deep necrosis of underlying tissue] [full-thickness skin loss]

Use additional code from category T31 or T32 to identify extent of body surface involved

✓4ᵗʰ **T20** **Burn and corrosion of head, face, and neck**
   EXCLUDES 2 *burn and corrosion of ear drum (T28.41, T28.91)*
      burn and corrosion of eye and adnexa (T26.-)
      burn and corrosion of mouth and pharynx (T28.0)
   AHA: 2015, 1Q, 18-19

> The appropriate 7th character is to be added to each code from category T20.
> A   initial encounter
> D   subsequent encounter
> S   sequela

✓5ᵗʰ **T20.0** **Burn of** unspecified degree **of head, face, and neck**
   Use additional external cause code to identify the source, place and intent of the burn (X00-X19, X75-X77, X96-X98, Y92)

   ✓x7ᵗʰ **T20.00** **Burn of unspecified degree of head, face, and neck, unspecified site** ▽

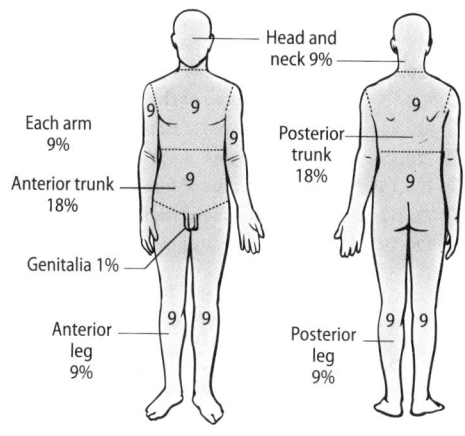

Rule of Nines Estimation of Total Body Surface Burned

Head and neck 9%
Each arm 9%
Anterior trunk 18%
Posterior trunk 18%
Genitalia 1%
Anterior leg 9%
Posterior leg 9%

✓6ᵗʰ **T20.01** **Burn of unspecified degree of** ear **[any part, except ear drum]**
   EXCLUDES 2 *burn of ear drum (T28.41-)*

   ✓7ᵗʰ **T20.011** **Burn of unspecified degree of** right ear **[any part, except ear drum]** ▽

   ✓7ᵗʰ **T20.012** **Burn of unspecified degree of** left ear **[any part, except ear drum]** ▽

   ✓7ᵗʰ **T20.019** **Burn of unspecified degree of unspecified ear [any part, except ear drum]** ▽

✓x7ᵗʰ **T20.02** **Burn of unspecified degree of** lip(s) ▽

✓x7ᵗʰ **T20.03** **Burn of unspecified degree of** chin ▽

✓x7ᵗʰ **T20.04** **Burn of unspecified degree of** nose (septum) ▽

✓x7ᵗʰ **T20.05** **Burn of unspecified degree of** scalp [any part] ▽

✓x7ᵗʰ **T20.06** **Burn of unspecified degree of** forehead and cheek ▽

✓x7ᵗʰ **T20.07** **Burn of unspecified degree of** neck ▽

✓x7ᵗʰ **T20.09** **Burn of unspecified degree of** multiple sites of head, face, and neck ▽

✓5ᵗʰ **T20.1** **Burn of** first degree **of head, face, and neck**
   Use additional external cause code to identify the source, place and intent of the burn (X00-X19, X75-X77, X96-X98, Y92)

   ✓x7ᵗʰ **T20.10** **Burn of first degree of head, face, and neck, unspecified site** ▽

   ✓6ᵗʰ **T20.11** **Burn of first degree of** ear **[any part, except ear drum]**
     EXCLUDES 2 *burn of ear drum (T28.41-)*

     ✓7ᵗʰ **T20.111** **Burn of first degree of** right ear **[any part, except ear drum]**

Degree of Burns

Epidermis
Dermis
Subcutaneous

Normal   First Degree Burn

Epidermis
Dermis
Subcutaneous

Second Degree Burn   Third Degree Burn

✓ Additional Character Req   ✓x7ᵗʰ Placeholder Alert   Case-Mix Diagnosis   Manifestation   ▽ Unspecified Dx   EXCLUDES 1 Not coded here   EXCLUDES 2 Not included here

ICD-10-CM 2018   1041

Chapter 19. Injury, Poisoning and Certain Other Consequences of External Causes

√7ᵗʰ **T20.112** **Burn of first degree of** left **ear [any part, except ear drum]**

√7ᵗʰ **T20.119** **Burn of first degree of unspecified ear [any part, except ear drum]** ▽

√x7ᵗʰ **T20.12** **Burn of first degree of** lip(s)

√x7ᵗʰ **T20.13** **Burn of first degree of** chin

√x7ᵗʰ **T20.14** **Burn of first degree of** nose (septum)

√x7ᵗʰ **T20.15** **Burn of first degree of** scalp [any part]

√x7ᵗʰ **T20.16** **Burn of first degree of** forehead and cheek

√x7ᵗʰ **T20.17** **Burn of first degree of** neck

√x7ᵗʰ **T20.19** **Burn of first degree of** multiple sites **of head, face, and neck**

√5ᵗʰ **T20.2** **Burn of** second degree **of head, face, and neck**
Use additional external cause code to identify the source, place and intent of the burn (X00-X19, X75-X77, X96-X98, Y92)

4,5 √7ᵗʰ **T20.20** **Burn of second degree of head, face, and neck, unspecified site** NRS ▽

√6ᵗʰ **T20.21** **Burn of second degree of** ear **[any part, except ear drum]**
EXCLUDES 2 *burn of ear drum (T28.41-)*

4,5 √7ᵗʰ **T20.211** **Burn of second degree of** right **ear [any part, except ear drum]** NRS

4,5 √7ᵗʰ **T20.212** **Burn of second degree of** left **ear [any part, except ear drum]** NRS

√7ᵗʰ **T20.219** **Burn of second degree of unspecified ear [any part, except ear drum]** ▽

4,5 √x7ᵗʰ **T20.22** **Burn of second degree of** lip(s) NRS

4,5 √x7ᵗʰ **T20.23** **Burn of second degree of** chin NRS

4,5 √x7ᵗʰ **T20.24** **Burn of second degree of** nose (septum) NRS

4,5 √x7ᵗʰ **T20.25** **Burn of second degree of** scalp [any part] NRS

4,5 √x7ᵗʰ **T20.26** **Burn of second degree of** forehead and cheek NRS

4,5 √x7ᵗʰ **T20.27** **Burn of second degree of** neck NRS

4,5 √x7ᵗʰ **T20.29** **Burn of second degree of** multiple sites **of head, face, and neck** NRS

√5ᵗʰ **T20.3** **Burn of** third degree **of head, face, and neck**
Use additional external cause code to identify the source, place and intent of the burn (X00-X19, X75-X77, X96-X98, Y92)

4,5 √7ᵗʰ **T20.30** **Burn of third degree of head, face, and neck, unspecified site** NRS ▽

√6ᵗʰ **T20.31** **Burn of third degree of** ear **[any part, except ear drum]**
EXCLUDES 2 *burn of ear drum (T28.41-)*
AHA: 2015, 1Q, 18

4,5 √7ᵗʰ **T20.311** **Burn of third degree of** right **ear [any part, except ear drum]** NRS

4,5 √7ᵗʰ **T20.312** **Burn of third degree of** left **ear [any part, except ear drum]** NRS

√7ᵗʰ **T20.319** **Burn of third degree of unspecified ear [any part, except ear drum]** ▽

4,5 √x7ᵗʰ **T20.32** **Burn of third degree of** lip(s) NRS

4,5 √x7ᵗʰ **T20.33** **Burn of third degree of** chin NRS

4,5 √x7ᵗʰ **T20.34** **Burn of third degree of** nose (septum) NRS

4,5 √x7ᵗʰ **T20.35** **Burn of third degree of** scalp [any part] NRS

4,5 √x7ᵗʰ **T20.36** **Burn of third degree of** forehead and cheek NRS

4,5 √x7ᵗʰ **T20.37** **Burn of third degree of** neck NRS

4,5 √x7ᵗʰ **T20.39** **Burn of third degree of** multiple sites **of head, face, and neck** NRS

√5ᵗʰ **T20.4** **Corrosion of** unspecified degree **of head, face, and neck**
Code first (T51-T65) to identify chemical and intent
Use additional external cause code to identify place (Y92)

√x7ᵗʰ **T20.40** **Corrosion of unspecified degree of head, face, and neck, unspecified site** ▽

√6ᵗʰ **T20.41** **Corrosion of unspecified degree of** ear **[any part, except ear drum]**
EXCLUDES 2 *corrosion of ear drum (T28.91-)*

√7ᵗʰ **T20.411** **Corrosion of unspecified degree of** right **ear [any part, except ear drum]** ▽

√7ᵗʰ **T20.412** **Corrosion of unspecified degree of** left **ear [any part, except ear drum]** ▽

√7ᵗʰ **T20.419** **Corrosion of unspecified degree of unspecified ear [any part, except ear drum]** ▽

√x7ᵗʰ **T20.42** **Corrosion of unspecified degree of** lip(s) ▽

√x7ᵗʰ **T20.43** **Corrosion of unspecified degree of** chin ▽

√x7ᵗʰ **T20.44** **Corrosion of unspecified degree of** nose (septum) ▽

√x7ᵗʰ **T20.45** **Corrosion of unspecified degree of** scalp [any part] ▽

√x7ᵗʰ **T20.46** **Corrosion of unspecified degree of** forehead and cheek ▽

√x7ᵗʰ **T20.47** **Corrosion of unspecified degree of** neck ▽

√x7ᵗʰ **T20.49** **Corrosion of unspecified degree of** multiple sites **of head, face, and neck** ▽

√5ᵗʰ **T20.5** **Corrosion of** first degree **of head, face, and neck**
Code first (T51-T65) to identify chemical and intent
Use additional external cause code to identify place (Y92)

√x7ᵗʰ **T20.50** **Corrosion of first degree of head, face, and neck, unspecified site** ▽

√6ᵗʰ **T20.51** **Corrosion of first degree of** ear **[any part, except ear drum]**
EXCLUDES 2 *corrosion of ear drum (T28.91-)*

√7ᵗʰ **T20.511** **Corrosion of first degree of** right **ear [any part, except ear drum]**

√7ᵗʰ **T20.512** **Corrosion of first degree of** left **ear [any part, except ear drum]**

√7ᵗʰ **T20.519** **Corrosion of first degree of unspecified ear [any part, except ear drum]** ▽

√x7ᵗʰ **T20.52** **Corrosion of first degree of** lip(s)

√x7ᵗʰ **T20.53** **Corrosion of first degree of** chin

√x7ᵗʰ **T20.54** **Corrosion of first degree of** nose (septum)

√x7ᵗʰ **T20.55** **Corrosion of first degree of** scalp [any part]

√x7ᵗʰ **T20.56** **Corrosion of first degree of** forehead and cheek

√x7ᵗʰ **T20.57** **Corrosion of first degree of** neck

√x7ᵗʰ **T20.59** **Corrosion of first degree of** multiple sites **of head, face, and neck**

√5ᵗʰ **T20.6** **Corrosion of** second degree **of head, face, and neck**
Code first (T51-T65) to identify chemical and intent
Use additional external cause code to identify place (Y92)

4,5 √x7ᵗʰ **T20.60** **Corrosion of second degree of head, face, and neck, unspecified site** NRS ▽

√6ᵗʰ **T20.61** **Corrosion of second degree of** ear **[any part, except ear drum]**
EXCLUDES 2 *corrosion of ear drum (T28.91-)*

4,5 √7ᵗʰ **T20.611** **Corrosion of second degree of** right **ear [any part, except ear drum]** NRS

4,5 √7ᵗʰ **T20.612** **Corrosion of second degree of** left **ear [any part, except ear drum]** NRS

√7ᵗʰ **T20.619** **Corrosion of second degree of unspecified ear [any part, except ear drum]** ▽

4,5 √x7ᵗʰ **T20.62** **Corrosion of second degree of** lip(s) NRS

4,5 √x7ᵗʰ **T20.63** **Corrosion of second degree of** chin NRS

4,5 √x7ᵗʰ **T20.64** **Corrosion of second degree of** nose (septum) NRS

4,5 √x7ᵗʰ **T20.65** **Corrosion of second degree of** scalp [any part] NRS

4,5 √x7ᵗʰ **T20.66** **Corrosion of second degree of** forehead and cheek NRS

4,5 √x7ᵗʰ **T20.67** **Corrosion of second degree of** neck NRS

4,5 √x7ᵗʰ **T20.69** **Corrosion of second degree of** multiple sites **of head, face, and neck** NRS

√5ᵗʰ **T20.7** **Corrosion of** third degree **of head, face, and neck**
Code first (T51-T65) to identify chemical and intent
Use additional external cause code to identify place (Y92)

5 √x7ᵗʰ **T20.70** **Corrosion of third degree of head, face, and neck, unspecified site** NRS ▽

√6ᵗʰ **T20.71** **Corrosion of third degree of** ear **[any part, except ear drum]**
EXCLUDES 2 *corrosion of ear drum (T28.91-)*

4,5 √7ᵗʰ **T20.711** **Corrosion of third degree of** right **ear [any part, except ear drum]** NRS

4,5 √7ᵗʰ **T20.712** **Corrosion of third degree of** left **ear [any part, except ear drum]** NRS

√7ᵗʰ **T20.719** **Corrosion of third degree of unspecified ear [any part, except ear drum]** ▽

---

4   Case-mix diagnosis with 7th character indicating initial or subsequent encounter.
5   NRS supply diagnosis with 7th character indicating initial or subsequent encounter.

N Newborn: 0   P Pediatric: 0-17   M Maternity: 12-55   A Adult: 15-124   NRS Nonroutine supply Dx   NC Dx Noncancer Dx   PDx Primary Dx   ▶◀ Revised Text   ● New Code   ▲ Revised Title

1042   ICD-10-CM 2018

4,5 √x7ᵗʰ **T20.72** **Corrosion of third degree of** lip(s) NRS
4,5 √x7ᵗʰ **T20.73** **Corrosion of third degree of** chin NRS
4,5 √x7ᵗʰ **T20.74** **Corrosion of third degree of** nose (septum) NRS
4,5 √x7ᵗʰ **T20.75** **Corrosion of third degree of** scalp [any part] NRS
4,5 √x7ᵗʰ **T20.76** **Corrosion of third degree of** forehead and cheek NRS
4,5 √x7ᵗʰ **T20.77** **Corrosion of third degree of** neck NRS
4,5 √x7ᵗʰ **T20.79** **Corrosion of third degree of** multiple sites of head, face, and neck NRS

✓4ᵗʰ **T21** **Burn and corrosion of trunk**
   INCLUDES   burns and corrosion of hip region
   EXCLUDES 2   burns and corrosion of axilla (T22.- with fifth character 4)
     burns and corrosion of scapular region (T22.- with fifth character 6)
     burns and corrosion of shoulder (T22.- with fifth character 5)

The appropriate 7th character is to be added to each code from category T21.
A   initial encounter
D   subsequent encounter
S   sequela

✓5ᵗʰ **T21.0** **Burn of** unspecified degree **of trunk**
Use additional external cause code to identify the source, place and intent of the burn (X00-X19, X75-X77, X96-X98, Y92)

√x7ᵗʰ **T21.00** **Burn of unspecified degree of trunk, unspecified site** ▽
√x7ᵗʰ **T21.01** **Burn of unspecified degree of** chest wall ▽
  Burn of unspecified degree of breast
√x7ᵗʰ **T21.02** **Burn of unspecified degree of** abdominal wall ▽
  Burn of unspecified degree of flank
  Burn of unspecified degree of groin
√x7ᵗʰ **T21.03** **Burn of unspecified degree of** upper back ▽
  Burn of unspecified degree of interscapular region
√x7ᵗʰ **T21.04** **Burn of unspecified degree of** lower back ▽
√x7ᵗʰ **T21.05** **Burn of unspecified degree of** buttock ▽
  Burn of unspecified degree of anus
√x7ᵗʰ **T21.06** **Burn of unspecified degree of** male genital region ♂▽
  Burn of unspecified degree of penis
  Burn of unspecified degree of scrotum
  Burn of unspecified degree of testis
√x7ᵗʰ **T21.07** **Burn of unspecified degree of** female genital region ♀▽
  Burn of unspecified degree of labium (majus) (minus)
  Burn of unspecified degree of perineum
  Burn of unspecified degree of vulva
   EXCLUDES 2   burn of vagina (T28.3)
√x7ᵗʰ **T21.09** **Burn of unspecified degree of other site of trunk** ▽

✓5ᵗʰ **T21.1** **Burn of** first degree **of trunk**
Use additional external cause code to identify the source, place and intent of the burn (X00-X19, X75-X77, X96-X98, Y92)

√x7ᵗʰ **T21.10** **Burn of first degree of trunk, unspecified site** ▽
√x7ᵗʰ **T21.11** **Burn of first degree of** chest wall
  Burn of first degree of breast
√x7ᵗʰ **T21.12** **Burn of first degree of** abdominal wall
  Burn of first degree of flank
  Burn of first degree of groin
√x7ᵗʰ **T21.13** **Burn of first degree of** upper back
  Burn of first degree of interscapular region
√x7ᵗʰ **T21.14** **Burn of first degree of** lower back
√x7ᵗʰ **T21.15** **Burn of first degree of** buttock
  Burn of first degree of anus
√x7ᵗʰ **T21.16** **Burn of first degree of** male genital region ♂
  Burn of first degree of penis
  Burn of first degree of scrotum
  Burn of first degree of testis
√x7ᵗʰ **T21.17** **Burn of first degree of** female genital region ♀
  Burn of first degree of labium (majus) (minus)
  Burn of first degree of perineum
  Burn of first degree of vulva
   EXCLUDES 2   burn of vagina (T28.3)
√x7ᵗʰ **T21.19** **Burn of first degree of other site of trunk**

✓5ᵗʰ **T21.2** **Burn of** second degree **of trunk**
Use additional external cause code to identify the source, place and intent of the burn (X00-X19, X75-X77, X96-X98, Y92)

√x7ᵗʰ **T21.20** **Burn of second degree of trunk, unspecified site** ▽
4,5 √x7ᵗʰ **T21.21** **Burn of second degree of** chest wall NRS
  Burn of second degree of breast
4,5 √x7ᵗʰ **T21.22** **Burn of second degree of** abdominal wall NRS
  Burn of second degree of flank
  Burn of second degree of groin
4,5 √x7ᵗʰ **T21.23** **Burn of second degree of** upper back NRS
  Burn of second degree of interscapular region
4,5 √x7ᵗʰ **T21.24** **Burn of second degree of** lower back NRS
4,5 √x7ᵗʰ **T21.25** **Burn of second degree of** buttock NRS
  Burn of second degree of anus
4,5 √x7ᵗʰ **T21.26** **Burn of second degree of** male genital region NRS♂
  Burn of second degree of penis
  Burn of second degree of scrotum
  Burn of second degree of testis
4,5 √x7ᵗʰ **T21.27** **Burn of second degree of** female genital region NRS♀
  Burn of second degree of labium (majus) (minus)
  Burn of second degree of perineum
  Burn of second degree of vulva
   EXCLUDES 2   burn of vagina (T28.3)
4,5 √x7ᵗʰ **T21.29** **Burn of second degree of other site of trunk** NRS

✓5ᵗʰ **T21.3** **Burn of** third degree **of trunk**
Use additional external cause code to identify the source, place and intent of the burn (X00-X19, X75-X77, X96-X98, Y92)

4,5 √x7ᵗʰ **T21.30** **Burn of third degree of trunk, unspecified site** ▽
4,5 √x7ᵗʰ **T21.31** **Burn of third degree of** chest wall NRS
  Burn of third degree of breast
  AHA: 2016, 2Q, 5
4,5 √x7ᵗʰ **T21.32** **Burn of third degree of** abdominal wall NRS
  Burn of third degree of flank
  Burn of third degree of groin
4,5 √x7ᵗʰ **T21.33** **Burn of third degree of** upper back NRS
  Burn of third degree of interscapular region
4,5 √x7ᵗʰ **T21.34** **Burn of third degree of** lower back NRS
4,5 √x7ᵗʰ **T21.35** **Burn of third degree of** buttock NRS
  Burn of third degree of anus
4,5 √x7ᵗʰ **T21.36** **Burn of third degree of** male genital region NRS♂
  Burn of third degree of penis
  Burn of third degree of scrotum
  Burn of third degree of testis
4,5 √x7ᵗʰ **T21.37** **Burn of third degree of** female genital region NRS♀
  Burn of third degree of labium (majus) (minus)
  Burn of third degree of perineum
  Burn of third degree of vulva
   EXCLUDES 2   burn of vagina (T28.3)
4,5 √x7ᵗʰ **T21.39** **Burn of third degree of other site of trunk** NRS

✓5ᵗʰ **T21.4** **Corrosion of** unspecified degree **of trunk**
Code first (T51-T65) to identify chemical and intent
Use additional external cause code to identify place (Y92)

√x7ᵗʰ **T21.40** **Corrosion of unspecified degree of trunk, unspecified site** ▽
√x7ᵗʰ **T21.41** **Corrosion of unspecified degree of** chest wall ▽
  Corrosion of unspecified degree of breast
√x7ᵗʰ **T21.42** **Corrosion of unspecified degree of** abdominal wall ▽
  Corrosion of unspecified degree of flank
  Corrosion of unspecified degree of groin
√x7ᵗʰ **T21.43** **Corrosion of unspecified degree of** upper back ▽
  Corrosion of unspecified degree of interscapular region
√x7ᵗʰ **T21.44** **Corrosion of unspecified degree of** lower back ▽
√x7ᵗʰ **T21.45** **Corrosion of unspecified degree of** buttock ▽
  Corrosion of unspecified degree of anus
√x7ᵗʰ **T21.46** **Corrosion of unspecified degree of** male genital region ♂▽
  Corrosion of unspecified degree of penis
  Corrosion of unspecified degree of scrotum
  Corrosion of unspecified degree of testis

4   Case-mix diagnosis with 7th character indicating initial or subsequent encounter.
5   NRS supply diagnosis with 7th character indicating initial or subsequent encounter.

✓ Additional Character Req   √x7ᵗʰ Placeholder Alert   Case-Mix Diagnosis   Manifestation   ▽ Unspecified Dx   EXCLUDES 1 Not coded here   EXCLUDES 2 Not included here
ICD-10-CM 2018   1043

√x7th **T21.47** **Corrosion of unspecified degree of female** ♀▽
genital region
Corrosion of unspecified degree of labium (majus)
(minus)
Corrosion of unspecified degree of perineum
Corrosion of unspecified degree of vulva
EXCLUDES 2 *corrosion of vagina (T28.8)*

√x7th **T21.49** **Corrosion of unspecified degree of other site of** ▽
trunk

√5th **T21.5** **Corrosion of first degree of trunk**
Code first (T51-T65) to identify chemical and intent
Use additional external cause code to identify place (Y92)

√x7th **T21.50** **Corrosion of first degree of trunk, unspecified site** ▽

√x7th **T21.51** **Corrosion of first degree of chest wall**
Corrosion of first degree of breast

√x7th **T21.52** **Corrosion of first degree of abdominal wall**
Corrosion of first degree of flank
Corrosion of first degree of groin

√x7th **T21.53** **Corrosion of first degree of upper back**
Corrosion of first degree of interscapular region

√x7th **T21.54** **Corrosion of first degree of lower back**

√x7th **T21.55** **Corrosion of first degree of buttock**
Corrosion of first degree of anus

√x7th **T21.56** **Corrosion of first degree of male genital region** ♂
Corrosion of first degree of penis
Corrosion of first degree of scrotum
Corrosion of first degree of testis

√x7th **T21.57** **Corrosion of first degree of female genital region** ♀
Corrosion of first degree of labium (majus) (minus)
Corrosion of first degree of perineum
Corrosion of first degree of vulva
EXCLUDES 2 *corrosion of vagina (T28.8)*

√x7th **T21.59** **Corrosion of first degree of other site of trunk**

√5th **T21.6** **Corrosion of second degree of trunk**
Code first (T51-T65) to identify chemical and intent
Use additional external cause code to identify place (Y92)

√x7th **T21.60** **Corrosion of second degree of trunk,** ▽
unspecified site

4,5 √x7th **T21.61** **Corrosion of second degree of chest wall** NRS
Corrosion of second degree of breast

4,5 √x7th **T21.62** **Corrosion of second degree of abdominal wall** NRS
Corrosion of second degree of flank
Corrosion of second degree of groin

4,5 √x7th **T21.63** **Corrosion of second degree of upper back** NRS
Corrosion of second degree of interscapular region

4,5 √x7th **T21.64** **Corrosion of second degree of lower back** NRS

4,5 √x7th **T21.65** **Corrosion of second degree of buttock** NRS
Corrosion of second degree of anus

4,5 √x7th **T21.66** **Corrosion of second degree of male genital** NRS♂
region
Corrosion of second degree of penis
Corrosion of second degree of scrotum
Corrosion of second degree of testis

4,5 √x7th **T21.67** **Corrosion of second degree of female genital** NRS♀
region
Corrosion of second degree of labium (majus) (minus)
Corrosion of second degree of perineum
Corrosion of second degree of vulva
EXCLUDES 2 *corrosion of vagina (T28.8)*

4,5 √x7th **T21.69** **Corrosion of second degree of other site** NRS
of trunk

√5th **T21.7** **Corrosion of third degree of trunk**
Code first (T51-T65) to identify chemical and intent
Use additional external cause code to identify place (Y92)

4 √x7th **T21.70** **Corrosion of third degree of trunk,** ▽
unspecified site

4,5 √x7th **T21.71** **Corrosion of third degree of chest wall** NRS
Corrosion of third degree of breast

4,5 √x7th **T21.72** **Corrosion of third degree of abdominal wall** NRS
Corrosion of third degree of flank
Corrosion of third degree of groin

4,5 √x7th **T21.73** **Corrosion of third degree of upper back** NRS
Corrosion of third degree of interscapular region

4,5 √x7th **T21.74** **Corrosion of third degree of lower back** NRS

4,5 √x7th **T21.75** **Corrosion of third degree of buttock** NRS
Corrosion of third degree of anus

4,5 √x7th **T21.76** **Corrosion of third degree of male genital** NRS♂
region
Corrosion of third degree of penis
Corrosion of third degree of scrotum
Corrosion of third degree of testis

4,5 √x7th **T21.77** **Corrosion of third degree of female genital** NRS♀
region
Corrosion of third degree of labium (majus) (minus)
Corrosion of third degree of perineum
Corrosion of third degree of vulva
EXCLUDES 2 *corrosion of vagina (T28.8)*

4,5 √x7th **T21.79** **Corrosion of third degree of other site of trunk** NRS

√4th **T22** **Burn and corrosion of shoulder and upper limb, except wrist and**
hand
EXCLUDES 2 *burn and corrosion of interscapular region (T21.-)*
burn and corrosion of wrist and hand (T23.-)

The appropriate 7th character is to be added to each code from
category T22.
A   initial encounter
D   subsequent encounter
S   sequela

√5th **T22.0** **Burn of unspecified degree of shoulder and upper limb,**
except wrist and hand
Use additional external cause code to identify the source, place
and intent of the burn (X00-X19, X75-X77, X96-X98, Y92)

√x7th **T22.00** **Burn of unspecified degree of shoulder and** ▽
upper limb, except wrist and hand, unspecified site

√6th **T22.01** **Burn of unspecified degree of forearm**

√7th **T22.011** **Burn of unspecified degree of right** ▽
forearm

√7th **T22.012** **Burn of unspecified degree of left** ▽
forearm

√7th **T22.019** **Burn of unspecified degree of** ▽
unspecified forearm

√6th **T22.02** **Burn of unspecified degree of elbow**

√7th **T22.021** **Burn of unspecified degree of right** ▽
elbow

√7th **T22.022** **Burn of unspecified degree of left** ▽
elbow

√7th **T22.029** **Burn of unspecified degree of** ▽
unspecified elbow

√6th **T22.03** **Burn of unspecified degree of upper arm**

√7th **T22.031** **Burn of unspecified degree of right** ▽
upper arm

√7th **T22.032** **Burn of unspecified degree of left** ▽
upper arm

√7th **T22.039** **Burn of unspecified degree of** ▽
unspecified upper arm

√6th **T22.04** **Burn of unspecified degree of axilla**

√7th **T22.041** **Burn of unspecified degree of right** ▽
axilla

√7th **T22.042** **Burn of unspecified degree of left** ▽
axilla

√7th **T22.049** **Burn of unspecified degree of** ▽
unspecified axilla

√6th **T22.05** **Burn of unspecified degree of shoulder**

√7th **T22.051** **Burn of unspecified degree of right** ▽
shoulder

√7th **T22.052** **Burn of unspecified degree of left** ▽
shoulder

√7th **T22.059** **Burn of unspecified degree of** ▽
unspecified shoulder

√6th **T22.06** **Burn of unspecified degree of scapular region**

√7th **T22.061** **Burn of unspecified degree of right** ▽
scapular region

√7th **T22.062** **Burn of unspecified degree of left** ▽
scapular region

√7th **T22.069** **Burn of unspecified degree of** ▽
unspecified scapular region

---

4 Case-mix diagnosis with 7th character indicating initial or subsequent encounter.
5 NRS supply diagnosis with 7th character indicating initial or subsequent encounter.

N Newborn: 0 P Pediatric: 0-17 M Maternity: 12-55 A Adult: 15-124 NRS Nonroutine supply Dx NC Dx Noncancer Dx PDx Primary Dx ►◄ Revised Text ● New Code ▲ Revised Title

1044   ICD-10-CM 2018

√6th **T22.09** Burn of unspecified degree of multiple sites of shoulder and upper limb, except wrist and hand

    √7th **T22.091** Burn of unspecified degree of multiple sites of right shoulder and upper limb, except wrist and hand ▽

    √7th **T22.092** Burn of unspecified degree of multiple sites of left shoulder and upper limb, except wrist and hand ▽

    √7th **T22.099** Burn of unspecified degree of multiple sites of unspecified shoulder and upper limb, except wrist and hand ▽

√5th **T22.1** Burn of first degree of shoulder and upper limb, except wrist and hand

    Use additional external cause code to identify the source, place and intent of the burn (X00-X19, X75-X77, X96-X98, Y92)

√x7th **T22.10** Burn of first degree of shoulder and upper limb, except wrist and hand, unspecified site ▽

√6th **T22.11** Burn of first degree of forearm

    √7th **T22.111** Burn of first degree of right forearm

    √7th **T22.112** Burn of first degree of left forearm

    √7th **T22.119** Burn of first degree of unspecified forearm ▽

√6th **T22.12** Burn of first degree of elbow

    √7th **T22.121** Burn of first degree of right elbow

    √7th **T22.122** Burn of first degree of left elbow

    √7th **T22.129** Burn of first degree of unspecified elbow ▽

√6th **T22.13** Burn of first degree of upper arm

    √7th **T22.131** Burn of first degree of right upper arm

    √7th **T22.132** Burn of first degree of left upper arm

    √7th **T22.139** Burn of first degree of unspecified upper arm ▽

√6th **T22.14** Burn of first degree of axilla

    √7th **T22.141** Burn of first degree of right axilla

    √7th **T22.142** Burn of first degree of left axilla

    √7th **T22.149** Burn of first degree of unspecified axilla ▽

√6th **T22.15** Burn of first degree of shoulder

    √7th **T22.151** Burn of first degree of right shoulder

    √7th **T22.152** Burn of first degree of left shoulder

    √7th **T22.159** Burn of first degree of unspecified shoulder ▽

√6th **T22.16** Burn of first degree of scapular region

    √7th **T22.161** Burn of first degree of right scapular region

    √7th **T22.162** Burn of first degree of left scapular region

    √7th **T22.169** Burn of first degree of unspecified scapular region ▽

√6th **T22.19** Burn of first degree of multiple sites of shoulder and upper limb, except wrist and hand

    √7th **T22.191** Burn of first degree of multiple sites of right shoulder and upper limb, except wrist and hand

    √7th **T22.192** Burn of first degree of multiple sites of left shoulder and upper limb, except wrist and hand

    √7th **T22.199** Burn of first degree of multiple sites of unspecified shoulder and upper limb, except wrist and hand ▽

√5th **T22.2** Burn of second degree of shoulder and upper limb, except wrist and hand

    Use additional external cause code to identify the source, place and intent of the burn (X00-X19, X75-X77, X96-X98, Y92)

√x7th **T22.20** Burn of second degree of shoulder and upper limb, except wrist and hand, unspecified site ▽

√6th **T22.21** Burn of second degree of forearm

    4,5 √7th **T22.211** **Burn of second degree of right forearm** NRS

    4,5 √7th **T22.212** **Burn of second degree of left forearm** NRS

    √7th **T22.219** Burn of second degree of unspecified forearm ▽

√6th **T22.22** Burn of second degree of elbow

    4,5 √7th **T22.221** **Burn of second degree of right elbow** NRS

    4,5 √7th **T22.222** **Burn of second degree of left elbow** NRS

    √7th **T22.229** Burn of second degree of unspecified elbow ▽

√6th **T22.23** Burn of second degree of upper arm

    4,5 √7th **T22.231** **Burn of second degree of right upper arm** NRS

    4,5 √7th **T22.232** **Burn of second degree of left upper arm** NRS

    √7th **T22.239** Burn of second degree of unspecified upper arm ▽

√6th **T22.24** Burn of second degree of axilla

    4,5 √7th **T22.241** **Burn of second degree of right axilla** NRS

    4,5 √7th **T22.242** **Burn of second degree of left axilla** NRS

    √7th **T22.249** Burn of second degree of unspecified axilla ▽

√6th **T22.25** Burn of second degree of shoulder

    4,5 √7th **T22.251** **Burn of second degree of right shoulder** NRS

    4,5 √7th **T22.252** **Burn of second degree of left shoulder** NRS

    √7th **T22.259** Burn of second degree of unspecified shoulder ▽

√6th **T22.26** Burn of second degree of scapular region

    4,5 √7th **T22.261** **Burn of second degree of right scapular region** NRS

    4,5 √7th **T22.262** **Burn of second degree of left scapular region** NRS

    √7th **T22.269** Burn of second degree of unspecified scapular region ▽

√6th **T22.29** Burn of second degree of multiple sites of shoulder and upper limb, except wrist and hand

    4,5 √7th **T22.291** **Burn of second degree of multiple sites of right shoulder and upper limb, except wrist and hand** NRS

    4,5 √7th **T22.292** **Burn of second degree of multiple sites of left shoulder and upper limb, except wrist and hand** NRS

    √7th **T22.299** Burn of second degree of multiple sites of unspecified shoulder and upper limb, except wrist and hand ▽

√5th **T22.3** Burn of third degree of shoulder and upper limb, except wrist and hand

    Use additional external cause code to identify the source, place and intent of the burn (X00-X19, X75-X77, X96-X98, Y92)

5 √x7th **T22.30** Burn of third degree of shoulder and upper limb, except wrist and hand, unspecified site NRS ▽

√6th **T22.31** Burn of third degree of forearm

    4,5 √7th **T22.311** **Burn of third degree of right forearm** NRS

    4,5 √7th **T22.312** **Burn of third degree of left forearm** NRS

    √7th **T22.319** Burn of third degree of unspecified forearm ▽

√6th **T22.32** Burn of third degree of elbow

    4,5 √7th **T22.321** **Burn of third degree of right elbow** NRS

    4,5 √7th **T22.322** **Burn of third degree of left elbow** NRS

    √7th **T22.329** Burn of third degree of unspecified elbow ▽

√6th **T22.33** Burn of third degree of upper arm

    4,5 √7th **T22.331** **Burn of third degree of right upper arm** NRS

    4,5 √7th **T22.332** **Burn of third degree of left upper arm** NRS

    √7th **T22.339** Burn of third degree of unspecified upper arm ▽

√6th **T22.34** Burn of third degree of axilla

    4,5 √7th **T22.341** **Burn of third degree of right axilla** NRS

    4,5 √7th **T22.342** **Burn of third degree of left axilla** NRS

    √7th **T22.349** Burn of third degree of unspecified axilla ▽

√6th **T22.35** Burn of third degree of shoulder

    4,5 √7th **T22.351** **Burn of third degree of right shoulder** NRS

    4,5 √7th **T22.352** **Burn of third degree of left shoulder** NRS

---

4   Case-mix diagnosis with 7th character indicating initial or subsequent encounter.
5   NRS supply diagnosis with 7th character indicating initial or subsequent encounter.

☑ Additional Character Req   √x7th Placeholder Alert   Case-Mix Diagnosis   Manifestation   ▽ Unspecified Dx   EXCLUDES 1 Not coded here   EXCLUDES 2 Not included here

☑7th **T22.359** **Burn of third degree of unspecified shoulder** ▽

☑6th **T22.36** **Burn of third degree of** scapular region

    4,5 ☑7th **T22.361** **Burn of third degree of** right **scapular region** NRS

    4,5 ☑7th **T22.362** **Burn of third degree of** left **scapular region** NRS

    ☑7th **T22.369** **Burn of third degree of unspecified scapular region** ▽

☑6th **T22.39** **Burn of third degree of** multiple sites **of shoulder and upper limb, except wrist and hand**

    4,5 ☑7th **T22.391** **Burn of third degree of multiple sites of** right **shoulder and upper limb, except wrist and hand** NRS

    4,5 ☑7th **T22.392** **Burn of third degree of multiple sites of** left **shoulder and upper limb, except wrist and hand** NRS

    ☑7th **T22.399** **Burn of third degree of multiple sites of unspecified shoulder and upper limb, except wrist and hand** ▽

☑5th **T22.4** **Corrosion of** unspecified degree **of shoulder and upper limb, except wrist and hand**

    Code first (T51-T65) to identify chemical and intent
    Use additional external cause code to identify place (Y92)

    ☑x7th **T22.40** **Corrosion of unspecified degree of shoulder and upper limb, except wrist and hand, unspecified site** ▽

    ☑6th **T22.41** **Corrosion of unspecified degree of** forearm

      ☑7th **T22.411** **Corrosion of unspecified degree of** right **forearm** ▽

      ☑7th **T22.412** **Corrosion of unspecified degree of** left **forearm** ▽

      ☑7th **T22.419** **Corrosion of unspecified degree of unspecified forearm** ▽

    ☑6th **T22.42** **Corrosion of unspecified degree of** elbow

      ☑7th **T22.421** **Corrosion of unspecified degree of** right **elbow** ▽

      ☑7th **T22.422** **Corrosion of unspecified degree of** left **elbow** ▽

      ☑7th **T22.429** **Corrosion of unspecified degree of unspecified elbow** ▽

    ☑6th **T22.43** **Corrosion of unspecified degree of** upper arm

      ☑7th **T22.431** **Corrosion of unspecified degree of** right **upper arm** ▽

      ☑7th **T22.432** **Corrosion of unspecified degree of** left **upper arm** ▽

      ☑7th **T22.439** **Corrosion of unspecified degree of unspecified upper arm** ▽

    ☑6th **T22.44** **Corrosion of unspecified degree of** axilla

      ☑7th **T22.441** **Corrosion of unspecified degree of** right **axilla** ▽

      ☑7th **T22.442** **Corrosion of unspecified degree of** left **axilla** ▽

      ☑7th **T22.449** **Corrosion of unspecified degree of unspecified axilla** ▽

    ☑6th **T22.45** **Corrosion of unspecified degree of** shoulder

      ☑7th **T22.451** **Corrosion of unspecified degree of** right **shoulder** ▽

      ☑7th **T22.452** **Corrosion of unspecified degree of** left **shoulder** ▽

      ☑7th **T22.459** **Corrosion of unspecified degree of unspecified shoulder** ▽

    ☑6th **T22.46** **Corrosion of unspecified degree of** scapular region

      ☑7th **T22.461** **Corrosion of unspecified degree of** right **scapular region** ▽

      ☑7th **T22.462** **Corrosion of unspecified degree of** left **scapular region** ▽

      ☑7th **T22.469** **Corrosion of unspecified degree of unspecified scapular region** ▽

    ☑6th **T22.49** **Corrosion of unspecified degree of** multiple sites **of shoulder and upper limb, except wrist and hand**

      ☑7th **T22.491** **Corrosion of unspecified degree of multiple sites of** right **shoulder and upper limb, except wrist and hand** ▽

      ☑7th **T22.492** **Corrosion of unspecified degree of multiple sites of** left **shoulder and upper limb, except wrist and hand** ▽

      ☑7th **T22.499** **Corrosion of unspecified degree of multiple sites of unspecified shoulder and upper limb, except wrist and hand** ▽

☑5th **T22.5** **Corrosion of** first degree **of shoulder and upper limb, except wrist and hand**

    Code first (T51-T65) to identify chemical and intent
    Use additional external cause code to identify place (Y92)

    ☑x7th **T22.50** **Corrosion of first degree of shoulder and upper limb, except wrist and hand unspecified site** ▽

    ☑6th **T22.51** **Corrosion of first degree of** forearm

      ☑7th **T22.511** **Corrosion of first degree of** right **forearm**

      ☑7th **T22.512** **Corrosion of first degree of** left **forearm**

      ☑7th **T22.519** **Corrosion of first degree of unspecified forearm** ▽

    ☑6th **T22.52** **Corrosion of first degree of** elbow

      ☑7th **T22.521** **Corrosion of first degree of** right **elbow**

      ☑7th **T22.522** **Corrosion of first degree of** left **elbow**

      ☑7th **T22.529** **Corrosion of first degree of unspecified elbow** ▽

    ☑6th **T22.53** **Corrosion of first degree of** upper arm

      ☑7th **T22.531** **Corrosion of first degree of** right **upper arm**

      ☑7th **T22.532** **Corrosion of first degree of** left **upper arm**

      ☑7th **T22.539** **Corrosion of first degree of unspecified upper arm** ▽

    ☑6th **T22.54** **Corrosion of first degree of** axilla

      ☑7th **T22.541** **Corrosion of first degree of** right **axilla**

      ☑7th **T22.542** **Corrosion of first degree of** left **axilla**

      ☑7th **T22.549** **Corrosion of first degree of unspecified axilla** ▽

    ☑6th **T22.55** **Corrosion of first degree of** shoulder

      ☑7th **T22.551** **Corrosion of first degree of** right **shoulder**

      ☑7th **T22.552** **Corrosion of first degree of** left **shoulder**

      ☑7th **T22.559** **Corrosion of first degree of unspecified shoulder** ▽

    ☑6th **T22.56** **Corrosion of first degree of** scapular region

      ☑7th **T22.561** **Corrosion of first degree of** right **scapular region**

      ☑7th **T22.562** **Corrosion of first degree of** left **scapular region**

      ☑7th **T22.569** **Corrosion of first degree of unspecified scapular region** ▽

    ☑6th **T22.59** **Corrosion of first degree of** multiple sites **of shoulder and upper limb, except wrist and hand**

      ☑7th **T22.591** **Corrosion of first degree of multiple sites of** right **shoulder and upper limb, except wrist and hand**

      ☑7th **T22.592** **Corrosion of first degree of multiple sites of** left **shoulder and upper limb, except wrist and hand**

      ☑7th **T22.599** **Corrosion of first degree of multiple sites of unspecified shoulder and upper limb, except wrist and hand** ▽

☑5th **T22.6** **Corrosion of** second degree **of shoulder and upper limb, except wrist and hand**

    Code first (T51-T65) to identify chemical and intent
    Use additional external cause code to identify place (Y92)

    ☑x7th **T22.60** **Corrosion of second degree of shoulder and upper limb, except wrist and hand, unspecified site** ▽

    ☑6th **T22.61** **Corrosion of second degree of** forearm

      4,5 ☑7th **T22.611** **Corrosion of second degree of** right **forearm** NRS

      4,5 ☑7th **T22.612** **Corrosion of second degree of** left **forearm** NRS

      ☑7th **T22.619** **Corrosion of second degree of unspecified forearm** ▽

    ☑6th **T22.62** **Corrosion of second degree of** elbow

      4,5 ☑7th **T22.621** **Corrosion of second degree of** right **elbow** NRS

---

4 Case-mix diagnosis with 7th character indicating initial or subsequent encounter.
5 NRS supply diagnosis with 7th character indicating initial or subsequent encounter.

N Newborn: 0   P Pediatric: 0-17   M Maternity: 12-55   A Adult: 15-124   NRS Nonroutine supply Dx   NCDx Noncancer Dx   PDx Primary Dx   ►◄ Revised Text   ● New Code   ▲ Revised Title

4,5 ✓7ᵗʰ **T22.622** **Corrosion of second degree of** left **elbow** NRS

✓7ᵗʰ **T22.629** **Corrosion of second degree of unspecified elbow** ▽

✓6ᵗʰ **T22.63** Corrosion of second degree of upper arm

4,5 ✓7ᵗʰ **T22.631** **Corrosion of second degree of** right **upper arm** NRS

4,5 ✓7ᵗʰ **T22.632** **Corrosion of second degree of** left **upper arm** NRS

✓7ᵗʰ **T22.639** **Corrosion of second degree of unspecified upper arm** ▽

✓6ᵗʰ **T22.64** Corrosion of second degree of axilla

4,5 ✓7ᵗʰ **T22.641** **Corrosion of second degree of** right **axilla** NRS

4,5 ✓7ᵗʰ **T22.642** **Corrosion of second degree of** left **axilla** NRS

✓7ᵗʰ **T22.649** **Corrosion of second degree of unspecified axilla** ▽

✓6ᵗʰ **T22.65** Corrosion of second degree of shoulder

4,5 ✓7ᵗʰ **T22.651** **Corrosion of second degree of** right **shoulder** NRS

4,5 ✓7ᵗʰ **T22.652** **Corrosion of second degree of** left **shoulder** NRS

✓7ᵗʰ **T22.659** **Corrosion of second degree of unspecified shoulder** ▽

✓6ᵗʰ **T22.66** Corrosion of second degree of scapular region

4,5 ✓7ᵗʰ **T22.661** **Corrosion of second degree of** right **scapular region** NRS

4,5 ✓7ᵗʰ **T22.662** **Corrosion of second degree of** left **scapular region** NRS

✓7ᵗʰ **T22.669** **Corrosion of second degree of unspecified scapular region** ▽

✓6ᵗʰ **T22.69** Corrosion of second degree of multiple sites of shoulder and upper limb, except wrist and hand

4,5 ✓7ᵗʰ **T22.691** **Corrosion of second degree of multiple sites of** right **shoulder and upper limb, except wrist and hand** NRS

4,5 ✓7ᵗʰ **T22.692** **Corrosion of second degree of multiple sites of** left **shoulder and upper limb, except wrist and hand** NRS

✓7ᵗʰ **T22.699** **Corrosion of second degree of multiple sites of unspecified shoulder and upper limb, except wrist and hand** ▽

✓5ᵗʰ **T22.7** Corrosion of third degree of shoulder and upper limb, except wrist and hand

Code first (T51-T65) to identify chemical and intent
Use additional external cause code to identify place (Y92)

✓x7ᵗʰ **T22.70** **Corrosion of third degree of shoulder and upper limb, except wrist and hand, unspecified site** ▽

✓6ᵗʰ **T22.71** Corrosion of third degree of forearm

4,5 ✓7ᵗʰ **T22.711** **Corrosion of third degree of** right **forearm** NRS

4,5 ✓7ᵗʰ **T22.712** **Corrosion of third degree of** left **forearm** NRS

✓7ᵗʰ **T22.719** **Corrosion of third degree of unspecified forearm** ▽

✓6ᵗʰ **T22.72** Corrosion of third degree of elbow

4,5 ✓7ᵗʰ **T22.721** **Corrosion of third degree of** right **elbow** NRS

4,5 ✓7ᵗʰ **T22.722** **Corrosion of third degree of** left **elbow** NRS

✓7ᵗʰ **T22.729** **Corrosion of third degree of unspecified elbow** ▽

✓6ᵗʰ **T22.73** Corrosion of third degree of upper arm

4,5 ✓7ᵗʰ **T22.731** **Corrosion of third degree of** right **upper arm** NRS

4,5 ✓7ᵗʰ **T22.732** **Corrosion of third degree of** left **upper arm** NRS

✓7ᵗʰ **T22.739** **Corrosion of third degree of unspecified upper arm** ▽

✓6ᵗʰ **T22.74** Corrosion of third degree of axilla

4,5 ✓7ᵗʰ **T22.741** **Corrosion of third degree of** right **axilla** NRS

4,5 ✓7ᵗʰ **T22.742** **Corrosion of third degree of** left **axilla** NRS

✓7ᵗʰ **T22.749** **Corrosion of third degree of unspecified axilla** ▽

✓6ᵗʰ **T22.75** Corrosion of third degree of shoulder

4,5 ✓7ᵗʰ **T22.751** **Corrosion of third degree of** right **shoulder** NRS

4,5 ✓7ᵗʰ **T22.752** **Corrosion of third degree of** left **shoulder** NRS

✓7ᵗʰ **T22.759** **Corrosion of third degree of unspecified shoulder** ▽

✓6ᵗʰ **T22.76** Corrosion of third degree of scapular region

4,5 ✓7ᵗʰ **T22.761** **Corrosion of third degree of** right **scapular region** NRS

4,5 ✓7ᵗʰ **T22.762** **Corrosion of third degree of** left **scapular region** NRS

✓7ᵗʰ **T22.769** **Corrosion of third degree of unspecified scapular region** ▽

✓6ᵗʰ **T22.79** Corrosion of third degree of multiple sites of shoulder and upper limb, except wrist and hand

4,5 ✓7ᵗʰ **T22.791** **Corrosion of third degree of multiple sites of** right **shoulder and upper limb, except wrist and hand** NRS

4,5 ✓7ᵗʰ **T22.792** **Corrosion of third degree of multiple sites of** left **shoulder and upper limb, except wrist and hand** NRS

✓7ᵗʰ **T22.799** **Corrosion of third degree of multiple sites of unspecified shoulder and upper limb, except wrist and hand** ▽

✓4ᵗʰ **T23** **Burn and corrosion of wrist and hand**
AHA: 2015, 1Q, 19

The appropriate 7th character is to be added to each code from category T23.
A   initial encounter
D   subsequent encounter
S   sequela

✓5ᵗʰ **T23.0** **Burn of** unspecified degree **of wrist and hand**
Use additional external cause code to identify the source, place and intent of the burn (X00-X19, X75-X77, X96-X98, Y92)

✓6ᵗʰ **T23.00** Burn of unspecified degree of hand, unspecified site

✓7ᵗʰ **T23.001** **Burn of unspecified degree of** right **hand, unspecified site** ▽

✓7ᵗʰ **T23.002** **Burn of unspecified degree of** left **hand, unspecified site** ▽

✓7ᵗʰ **T23.009** **Burn of unspecified degree of unspecified hand, unspecified site** ▽

✓6ᵗʰ **T23.01** Burn of unspecified degree of thumb (nail)

✓7ᵗʰ **T23.011** **Burn of unspecified degree of** right **thumb (nail)** ▽

✓7ᵗʰ **T23.012** **Burn of unspecified degree of** left **thumb (nail)** ▽

✓7ᵗʰ **T23.019** **Burn of unspecified degree of unspecified thumb (nail)** ▽

✓6ᵗʰ **T23.02** Burn of unspecified degree of single finger (nail) except thumb

✓7ᵗʰ **T23.021** **Burn of unspecified degree of single** right **finger (nail) except thumb** ▽

✓7ᵗʰ **T23.022** **Burn of unspecified degree of single** left **finger (nail) except thumb** ▽

✓7ᵗʰ **T23.029** **Burn of unspecified degree of unspecified single finger (nail) except thumb** ▽

✓6ᵗʰ **T23.03** Burn of unspecified degree of multiple fingers (nail), not including thumb

✓7ᵗʰ **T23.031** **Burn of unspecified degree of multiple** right **fingers (nail), not including thumb** ▽

✓7ᵗʰ **T23.032** **Burn of unspecified degree of multiple** left **fingers (nail), not including thumb** ▽

✓7ᵗʰ **T23.039** **Burn of unspecified degree of unspecified multiple fingers (nail), not including thumb** ▽

---

4 Case-mix diagnosis with 7th character indicating initial or subsequent encounter.
5 NRS supply diagnosis with 7th character indicating initial or subsequent encounter.

☑ Additional Character Req   ✓x7ᵗʰ Placeholder Alert   Case-Mix Diagnosis   Manifestation   ▽ Unspecified Dx   **EXCLUDES 1** Not coded here   **EXCLUDES 2** Not included here

√6ᵗʰ **T23.04 Burn of unspecified degree of** multiple fingers **(nail), including thumb**

    √7ᵗʰ **T23.041** Burn of unspecified degree of multiple right fingers (nail), including thumb ▽

    √7ᵗʰ **T23.042** Burn of unspecified degree of multiple left fingers (nail), including thumb ▽

    √7ᵗʰ **T23.049** Burn of unspecified degree of unspecified multiple fingers (nail), including thumb ▽

√6ᵗʰ **T23.05 Burn of unspecified degree of** palm

    √7ᵗʰ **T23.051** Burn of unspecified degree of right palm ▽

    √7ᵗʰ **T23.052** Burn of unspecified degree of left palm ▽

    √7ᵗʰ **T23.059** Burn of unspecified degree of unspecified palm ▽

√6ᵗʰ **T23.06 Burn of unspecified degree of** back of hand

    √7ᵗʰ **T23.061** Burn of unspecified degree of back of right hand ▽

    √7ᵗʰ **T23.062** Burn of unspecified degree of back of left hand ▽

    √7ᵗʰ **T23.069** Burn of unspecified degree of back of unspecified hand ▽

√6ᵗʰ **T23.07 Burn of unspecified degree of** wrist

    √7ᵗʰ **T23.071** Burn of unspecified degree of right wrist ▽

    √7ᵗʰ **T23.072** Burn of unspecified degree of left wrist ▽

    √7ᵗʰ **T23.079** Burn of unspecified degree of unspecified wrist ▽

√6ᵗʰ **T23.09 Burn of unspecified degree of** multiple sites **of wrist and hand**

    √7ᵗʰ **T23.091** Burn of unspecified degree of multiple sites of right wrist and hand ▽

    √7ᵗʰ **T23.092** Burn of unspecified degree of multiple sites of left wrist and hand ▽

    √7ᵗʰ **T23.099** Burn of unspecified degree of multiple sites of unspecified wrist and hand ▽

√5ᵗʰ **T23.1 Burn of** first degree **of wrist and hand**
Use additional external cause code to identify the source, place and intent of the burn (X00-X19, X75-X77, X96-X98, Y92)

    √6ᵗʰ **T23.10 Burn of first degree of hand,** unspecified site

      √7ᵗʰ **T23.101** Burn of first degree of right hand, unspecified site ▽

      √7ᵗʰ **T23.102** Burn of first degree of left hand, unspecified site ▽

      √7ᵗʰ **T23.109** Burn of first degree of unspecified hand, unspecified site ▽

    √6ᵗʰ **T23.11 Burn of first degree of** thumb (nail)

      √7ᵗʰ **T23.111** Burn of first degree of right thumb (nail)

      √7ᵗʰ **T23.112** Burn of first degree of left thumb (nail)

      √7ᵗʰ **T23.119** Burn of first degree of unspecified thumb (nail) ▽

    √6ᵗʰ **T23.12 Burn of first degree of** single finger **(nail) except thumb**

      √7ᵗʰ **T23.121** Burn of first degree of single right finger (nail) except thumb

      √7ᵗʰ **T23.122** Burn of first degree of single left finger (nail) except thumb

      √7ᵗʰ **T23.129** Burn of first degree of unspecified single finger (nail) except thumb ▽

    √6ᵗʰ **T23.13 Burn of first degree of** multiple fingers **(nail),** not including thumb

      √7ᵗʰ **T23.131** Burn of first degree of multiple right fingers (nail), not including thumb

      √7ᵗʰ **T23.132** Burn of first degree of multiple left fingers (nail), not including thumb

      √7ᵗʰ **T23.139** Burn of first degree of unspecified multiple fingers (nail), not including thumb ▽

√6ᵗʰ **T23.14 Burn of first degree of** multiple fingers **(nail), including thumb**

    √7ᵗʰ **T23.141** Burn of first degree of multiple right fingers (nail), including thumb

    √7ᵗʰ **T23.142** Burn of first degree of multiple left fingers (nail), including thumb

    √7ᵗʰ **T23.149** Burn of first degree of unspecified multiple fingers (nail), including thumb ▽

√6ᵗʰ **T23.15 Burn of first degree of** palm

    √7ᵗʰ **T23.151** Burn of first degree of right palm

    √7ᵗʰ **T23.152** Burn of first degree of left palm

    √7ᵗʰ **T23.159** Burn of first degree of unspecified palm ▽

√6ᵗʰ **T23.16 Burn of first degree of** back of hand

    √7ᵗʰ **T23.161** Burn of first degree of back of right hand

    √7ᵗʰ **T23.162** Burn of first degree of back of left hand

    √7ᵗʰ **T23.169** Burn of first degree of back of unspecified hand ▽

√6ᵗʰ **T23.17 Burn of first degree of** wrist

    √7ᵗʰ **T23.171** Burn of first degree of right wrist

    √7ᵗʰ **T23.172** Burn of first degree of left wrist

    √7ᵗʰ **T23.179** Burn of first degree of unspecified wrist ▽

√6ᵗʰ **T23.19 Burn of first degree of** multiple sites **of wrist and hand**

    √7ᵗʰ **T23.191** Burn of first degree of multiple sites of right wrist and hand

    √7ᵗʰ **T23.192** Burn of first degree of multiple sites of left wrist and hand

    √7ᵗʰ **T23.199** Burn of first degree of multiple sites of unspecified wrist and hand ▽

√5ᵗʰ **T23.2 Burn of** second degree **of wrist and hand**
Use additional external cause code to identify the source, place and intent of the burn (X00-X19, X75-X77, X96-X98, Y92)

    √6ᵗʰ **T23.20 Burn of second degree of hand,** unspecified site

      4,5 √7ᵗʰ **T23.201** Burn of second degree of right hand, unspecified site ⟨NRS⟩ ▽

      4,5 √7ᵗʰ **T23.202** Burn of second degree of left hand, unspecified site ⟨NRS⟩ ▽

      √7ᵗʰ **T23.209** Burn of second degree of unspecified hand, unspecified site ▽

    √6ᵗʰ **T23.21 Burn of second degree of** thumb (nail)

      4,5 √7ᵗʰ **T23.211** Burn of second degree of right thumb (nail) ⟨NRS⟩

      4,5 √7ᵗʰ **T23.212** Burn of second degree of left thumb (nail) ⟨NRS⟩

      √7ᵗʰ **T23.219** Burn of second degree of unspecified thumb (nail) ▽

    √6ᵗʰ **T23.22 Burn of second degree of** single finger **(nail) except thumb**

      4,5 √7ᵗʰ **T23.221** Burn of second degree of single right finger (nail) except thumb ⟨NRS⟩

      4,5 √7ᵗʰ **T23.222** Burn of second degree of single left finger (nail) except thumb ⟨NRS⟩

      √7ᵗʰ **T23.229** Burn of second degree of unspecified single finger (nail) except thumb ▽

    √6ᵗʰ **T23.23 Burn of second degree of** multiple fingers **(nail),** not including thumb

      4,5 √7ᵗʰ **T23.231** Burn of second degree of multiple right fingers (nail), not including thumb ⟨NRS⟩

      4,5 √7ᵗʰ **T23.232** Burn of second degree of multiple left fingers (nail), not including thumb ⟨NRS⟩

      √7ᵗʰ **T23.239** Burn of second degree of unspecified multiple fingers (nail), not including thumb ▽

    √6ᵗʰ **T23.24 Burn of second degree of** multiple fingers **(nail),** including thumb

      4,5 √7ᵗʰ **T23.241** Burn of second degree of multiple right fingers (nail), including thumb ⟨NRS⟩

      4,5 √7ᵗʰ **T23.242** Burn of second degree of multiple left fingers (nail), including thumb ⟨NRS⟩

      √7ᵗʰ **T23.249** Burn of second degree of unspecified multiple fingers (nail), including thumb ▽

---

4   Case-mix diagnosis with 7th character indicating initial or subsequent encounter.
5   NRS supply diagnosis with 7th character indicating initial or subsequent encounter.

Ⓝ Newborn: 0   Ⓟ Pediatric: 0-17   Ⓜ Maternity: 12-55   Ⓐ Adult: 15-124   ⟨NRS⟩ Nonroutine supply Dx   ⟨NC Dx⟩ Noncancer Dx   ⟨PDx⟩ Primary Dx   ►◄ Revised Text   ● New Code   ▲ Revised Title

√6ᵗʰ **T23.25** Burn of second degree of palm

4,5 √7ᵗʰ T23.251   Burn of second degree of right palm   NRS

4,5 √7ᵗʰ T23.252   Burn of second degree of left palm   NRS

√7ᵗʰ T23.259   Burn of second degree of unspecified palm   ▽

√6ᵗʰ **T23.26** Burn of second degree of back of hand

4,5 √7ᵗʰ T23.261   Burn of second degree of back of right hand   NRS

4,5 √7ᵗʰ T23.262   Burn of second degree of back of left hand   NRS

√7ᵗʰ T23.269   Burn of second degree of back of unspecified hand   ▽

√6ᵗʰ **T23.27** Burn of second degree of wrist

4,5 √7ᵗʰ T23.271   Burn of second degree of right wrist   NRS

4,5 √7ᵗʰ T23.272   Burn of second degree of left wrist   NRS

√7ᵗʰ T23.279   Burn of second degree of unspecified wrist   ▽

√6ᵗʰ **T23.29** Burn of second degree of multiple sites of wrist and hand

4,5 √7ᵗʰ T23.291   Burn of second degree of multiple sites of right wrist and hand   NRS

4,5 √7ᵗʰ T23.292   Burn of second degree of multiple sites of left wrist and hand   NRS

√7ᵗʰ T23.299   Burn of second degree of multiple sites of unspecified wrist and hand   ▽

√5ᵗʰ **T23.3** Burn of third degree of wrist and hand

Use additional external cause code to identify the source, place and intent of the burn (X00-X19, X75-X77, X96-X98, Y92)

√6ᵗʰ **T23.30** Burn of third degree of hand, unspecified site

AHA: 2016, 2Q, 5

4,5 √7ᵗʰ T23.301   Burn of third degree of right hand, unspecified site   NRS ▽

4,5 √7ᵗʰ T23.302   Burn of third degree of left hand, unspecified site   NRS ▽

√7ᵗʰ T23.309   Burn of third degree of unspecified hand, unspecified site   ▽

√6ᵗʰ **T23.31** Burn of third degree of thumb (nail)

4,5 √7ᵗʰ T23.311   Burn of third degree of right thumb (nail)   NRS

4,5 √7ᵗʰ T23.312   Burn of third degree of left thumb (nail)   NRS

√7ᵗʰ T23.319   Burn of third degree of unspecified thumb (nail)   ▽

√6ᵗʰ **T23.32** Burn of third degree of single finger (nail) except thumb

4,5 √7ᵗʰ T23.321   Burn of third degree of single right finger (nail) except thumb   NRS

4,5 √7ᵗʰ T23.322   Burn of third degree of single left finger (nail) except thumb   NRS

√7ᵗʰ T23.329   Burn of third degree of unspecified single finger (nail) except thumb   ▽

√6ᵗʰ **T23.33** Burn of third degree of multiple fingers (nail), not including thumb

4,5 √7ᵗʰ T23.331   Burn of third degree of multiple right fingers (nail), not including thumb   NRS

4,5 √7ᵗʰ T23.332   Burn of third degree of multiple left fingers (nail), not including thumb   NRS

√7ᵗʰ T23.339   Burn of third degree of unspecified multiple fingers (nail), not including thumb   ▽

√6ᵗʰ **T23.34** Burn of third degree of multiple fingers (nail), including thumb

4,5 √7ᵗʰ T23.341   Burn of third degree of multiple right fingers (nail), including thumb   NRS

4,5 √7ᵗʰ T23.342   Burn of third degree of multiple left fingers (nail), including thumb   NRS

√7ᵗʰ T23.349   Burn of third degree of unspecified multiple fingers (nail), including thumb   ▽

√6ᵗʰ **T23.35** Burn of third degree of palm

4,5 √7ᵗʰ T23.351   Burn of third degree of right palm   NRS

4,5 √7ᵗʰ T23.352   Burn of third degree of left palm   NRS

√7ᵗʰ T23.359   Burn of third degree of unspecified palm   ▽

√6ᵗʰ **T23.36** Burn of third degree of back of hand

4,5 √7ᵗʰ T23.361   Burn of third degree of back of right hand   NRS

4,5 √7ᵗʰ T23.362   Burn of third degree of back of left hand   NRS

√7ᵗʰ T23.369   Burn of third degree of back of unspecified hand   ▽

√6ᵗʰ **T23.37** Burn of third degree of wrist

4,5 √7ᵗʰ T23.371   Burn of third degree of right wrist   NRS

4,5 √7ᵗʰ T23.372   Burn of third degree of left wrist   NRS

√7ᵗʰ T23.379   Burn of third degree of unspecified wrist   ▽

√6ᵗʰ **T23.39** Burn of third degree of multiple sites of wrist and hand

4,5 √7ᵗʰ T23.391   Burn of third degree of multiple sites of right wrist and hand   NRS

4,5 √7ᵗʰ T23.392   Burn of third degree of multiple sites of left wrist and hand   NRS

√7ᵗʰ T23.399   Burn of third degree of multiple sites of unspecified wrist and hand   ▽

√5ᵗʰ **T23.4** Corrosion of unspecified degree of wrist and hand

Code first (T51-T65) to identify chemical and intent

Use additional external cause code to identify place (Y92)

√6ᵗʰ **T23.40** Corrosion of unspecified degree of hand, unspecified site

√7ᵗʰ T23.401   Corrosion of unspecified degree of right hand, unspecified site   ▽

√7ᵗʰ T23.402   Corrosion of unspecified degree of left hand, unspecified site   ▽

√7ᵗʰ T23.409   Corrosion of unspecified degree of unspecified hand, unspecified site   ▽

√6ᵗʰ **T23.41** Corrosion of unspecified degree of thumb (nail)

√7ᵗʰ T23.411   Corrosion of unspecified degree of right thumb (nail)   ▽

√7ᵗʰ T23.412   Corrosion of unspecified degree of left thumb (nail)   ▽

√7ᵗʰ T23.419   Corrosion of unspecified degree of unspecified thumb (nail)   ▽

√6ᵗʰ **T23.42** Corrosion of unspecified degree of single finger (nail) except thumb

√7ᵗʰ T23.421   Corrosion of unspecified degree of single right finger (nail) except thumb   ▽

√7ᵗʰ T23.422   Corrosion of unspecified degree of single left finger (nail) except thumb   ▽

√7ᵗʰ T23.429   Corrosion of unspecified degree of unspecified single finger (nail) except thumb   ▽

√6ᵗʰ **T23.43** Corrosion of unspecified degree of multiple fingers (nail), not including thumb

√7ᵗʰ T23.431   Corrosion of unspecified degree of multiple right fingers (nail), not including thumb   ▽

√7ᵗʰ T23.432   Corrosion of unspecified degree of multiple left fingers (nail), not including thumb   ▽

√7ᵗʰ T23.439   Corrosion of unspecified degree of unspecified multiple fingers (nail), not including thumb   ▽

√6ᵗʰ **T23.44** Corrosion of unspecified degree of multiple fingers (nail), including thumb

√7ᵗʰ T23.441   Corrosion of unspecified degree of multiple right fingers (nail), including thumb   ▽

√7ᵗʰ T23.442   Corrosion of unspecified degree of multiple left fingers (nail), including thumb   ▽

√7ᵗʰ T23.449   Corrosion of unspecified degree of unspecified multiple fingers (nail), including thumb   ▽

---

4   Case-mix diagnosis with 7th character indicating initial or subsequent encounter.

5   NRS supply diagnosis with 7th character indicating initial or subsequent encounter.

☑ Additional Character Req   √x7ᵗʰ Placeholder Alert   Case-Mix Diagnosis   Manifestation   ▽ Unspecified Dx   **EXCLUDES 1** Not coded here   **EXCLUDES 2** Not included here

√6ᵗʰ T23.45 Corrosion of unspecified degree of palm
- √7ᵗʰ T23.451 Corrosion of unspecified degree of right palm ▽
- √7ᵗʰ T23.452 Corrosion of unspecified degree of left palm ▽
- √7ᵗʰ T23.459 Corrosion of unspecified degree of unspecified palm ▽

√6ᵗʰ T23.46 Corrosion of unspecified degree of back of hand
- √7ᵗʰ T23.461 Corrosion of unspecified degree of back of right hand ▽
- √7ᵗʰ T23.462 Corrosion of unspecified degree of back of left hand ▽
- √7ᵗʰ T23.469 Corrosion of unspecified degree of back of unspecified hand ▽

√6ᵗʰ T23.47 Corrosion of unspecified degree of wrist
- √7ᵗʰ T23.471 Corrosion of unspecified degree of right wrist ▽
- √7ᵗʰ T23.472 Corrosion of unspecified degree of left wrist ▽
- √7ᵗʰ T23.479 Corrosion of unspecified degree of unspecified wrist ▽

√6ᵗʰ T23.49 Corrosion of unspecified degree of multiple sites of wrist and hand
- √7ᵗʰ T23.491 Corrosion of unspecified degree of multiple sites of right wrist and hand ▽
- √7ᵗʰ T23.492 Corrosion of unspecified degree of multiple sites of left wrist and hand ▽
- √7ᵗʰ T23.499 Corrosion of unspecified degree of multiple sites of unspecified wrist and hand ▽

√5ᵗʰ T23.5 Corrosion of first degree of wrist and hand
Code first (T51-T65) to identify chemical and intent
Use additional external cause code to identify place (Y92)

√6ᵗʰ T23.50 Corrosion of first degree of hand, unspecified site
- √7ᵗʰ T23.501 Corrosion of first degree of right hand, unspecified site ▽
- √7ᵗʰ T23.502 Corrosion of first degree of left hand, unspecified site ▽
- √7ᵗʰ T23.509 Corrosion of first degree of unspecified hand, unspecified site ▽

√6ᵗʰ T23.51 Corrosion of first degree of thumb (nail)
- √7ᵗʰ T23.511 Corrosion of first degree of right thumb (nail)
- √7ᵗʰ T23.512 Corrosion of first degree of left thumb (nail)
- √7ᵗʰ T23.519 Corrosion of first degree of unspecified thumb (nail) ▽

√6ᵗʰ T23.52 Corrosion of first degree of single finger (nail) except thumb
- √7ᵗʰ T23.521 Corrosion of first degree of single right finger (nail) except thumb
- √7ᵗʰ T23.522 Corrosion of first degree of single left finger (nail) except thumb
- √7ᵗʰ T23.529 Corrosion of first degree of unspecified single finger (nail) except thumb ▽

√6ᵗʰ T23.53 Corrosion of first degree of multiple fingers (nail), not including thumb
- √7ᵗʰ T23.531 Corrosion of first degree of multiple right fingers (nail), not including thumb
- √7ᵗʰ T23.532 Corrosion of first degree of multiple left fingers (nail), not including thumb
- √7ᵗʰ T23.539 Corrosion of first degree of unspecified multiple fingers (nail), not including thumb ▽

√6ᵗʰ T23.54 Corrosion of first degree of multiple fingers (nail), including thumb
- √7ᵗʰ T23.541 Corrosion of first degree of multiple right fingers (nail), including thumb
- √7ᵗʰ T23.542 Corrosion of first degree of multiple left fingers (nail), including thumb
- √7ᵗʰ T23.549 Corrosion of first degree of unspecified multiple fingers (nail), including thumb ▽

√6ᵗʰ T23.55 Corrosion of first degree of palm
- √7ᵗʰ T23.551 Corrosion of first degree of right palm
- √7ᵗʰ T23.552 Corrosion of first degree of left palm
- √7ᵗʰ T23.559 Corrosion of first degree of unspecified palm ▽

√6ᵗʰ T23.56 Corrosion of first degree of back of hand
- √7ᵗʰ T23.561 Corrosion of first degree of back of right hand
- √7ᵗʰ T23.562 Corrosion of first degree of back of left hand
- √7ᵗʰ T23.569 Corrosion of first degree of back of unspecified hand ▽

√6ᵗʰ T23.57 Corrosion of first degree of wrist
- √7ᵗʰ T23.571 Corrosion of first degree of right wrist
- √7ᵗʰ T23.572 Corrosion of first degree of left wrist
- √7ᵗʰ T23.579 Corrosion of first degree of unspecified wrist ▽

√6ᵗʰ T23.59 Corrosion of first degree of multiple sites of wrist and hand
- √7ᵗʰ T23.591 Corrosion of first degree of multiple sites of right wrist and hand
- √7ᵗʰ T23.592 Corrosion of first degree of multiple sites of left wrist and hand
- √7ᵗʰ T23.599 Corrosion of first degree of multiple sites of unspecified wrist and hand ▽

√5ᵗʰ T23.6 Corrosion of second degree of wrist and hand
Code first (T51-T65) to identify chemical and intent
Use additional external cause code to identify place (Y92)

√6ᵗʰ T23.60 Corrosion of second degree of hand, unspecified site
- 4,5 √7ᵗʰ T23.601 Corrosion of second degree of right hand, unspecified site   NRS ▽
- 4,5 √7ᵗʰ T23.602 Corrosion of second degree of left hand, unspecified site   NRS ▽
- √7ᵗʰ T23.609 Corrosion of second degree of unspecified hand, unspecified site ▽

√6ᵗʰ T23.61 Corrosion of second degree of thumb (nail)
- 4,5 √7ᵗʰ T23.611 Corrosion of second degree of right thumb (nail)   NRS
- 4,5 √7ᵗʰ T23.612 Corrosion of second degree of left thumb (nail)   NRS
- √7ᵗʰ T23.619 Corrosion of second degree of unspecified thumb (nail) ▽

√6ᵗʰ T23.62 Corrosion of second degree of single finger (nail) except thumb
- 4,5 √7ᵗʰ T23.621 Corrosion of second degree of single right finger (nail) except thumb   NRS
- 4,5 √7ᵗʰ T23.622 Corrosion of second degree of single left finger (nail) except thumb   NRS
- √7ᵗʰ T23.629 Corrosion of second degree of unspecified single finger (nail) except thumb ▽

√6ᵗʰ T23.63 Corrosion of second degree of multiple fingers (nail), not including thumb
- 4,5 √7ᵗʰ T23.631 Corrosion of second degree of multiple right fingers (nail), not including thumb   NRS
- 4,5 √7ᵗʰ T23.632 Corrosion of second degree of multiple left fingers (nail), not including thumb   NRS
- √7ᵗʰ T23.639 Corrosion of second degree of unspecified multiple fingers (nail), not including thumb ▽

√6ᵗʰ T23.64 Corrosion of second degree of multiple fingers (nail), including thumb
- 4,5 √7ᵗʰ T23.641 Corrosion of second degree of multiple right fingers (nail), including thumb   NRS
- 4,5 √7ᵗʰ T23.642 Corrosion of second degree of multiple left fingers (nail), including thumb   NRS
- √7ᵗʰ T23.649 Corrosion of second degree of unspecified multiple fingers (nail), including thumb ▽

---

4   Case-mix diagnosis with 7th character indicating initial or subsequent encounter.
5   NRS supply diagnosis with 7th character indicating initial or subsequent encounter.

Ⓝ Newborn: 0   Ⓟ Pediatric: 0-17   Ⓜ Maternity: 12-55   Ⓐ Adult: 15-124   NRS Nonroutine supply Dx   NCDx Noncancer Dx   PDx Primary Dx   ►◄ Revised Text   ● New Code   ▲ Revised Title

1050   ICD-10-CM 2018

√6ᵗʰ **T23.65** Corrosion of second degree of palm

    4,5 √7ᵗʰ **T23.651** **Corrosion of second degree of right palm** NRS

    4,5 √7ᵗʰ **T23.652** **Corrosion of second degree of left palm** NRS

    √7ᵗʰ **T23.659** Corrosion of second degree of unspecified palm ▽

√6ᵗʰ **T23.66** Corrosion of second degree of back of hand

    4,5 √7ᵗʰ **T23.661** **Corrosion of second degree back of right hand** NRS

    4,5 √7ᵗʰ **T23.662** **Corrosion of second degree back of left hand** NRS

    √7ᵗʰ **T23.669** Corrosion of second degree back of unspecified hand ▽

√6ᵗʰ **T23.67** Corrosion of second degree of wrist

    4,5 √7ᵗʰ **T23.671** **Corrosion of second degree of right wrist** NRS

    4,5 √7ᵗʰ **T23.672** **Corrosion of second degree of left wrist** NRS

    √7ᵗʰ **T23.679** Corrosion of second degree of unspecified wrist ▽

√6ᵗʰ **T23.69** Corrosion of second degree of multiple sites of wrist and hand

    4,5 √7ᵗʰ **T23.691** **Corrosion of second degree of multiple sites of right wrist and hand** NRS

    4,5 √7ᵗʰ **T23.692** **Corrosion of second degree of multiple sites of left wrist and hand** NRS

    √7ᵗʰ **T23.699** Corrosion of second degree of multiple sites of unspecified wrist and hand ▽

√5ᵗʰ **T23.7** **Corrosion of** third degree **of wrist and hand**
     Code first (T51-T65) to identify chemical and intent
     Use additional external cause code to identify place (Y92)

√6ᵗʰ **T23.70** Corrosion of third degree of hand, unspecified site

    4,5 √7ᵗʰ **T23.701** **Corrosion of third degree of right hand, unspecified site** NRS ▽

    4,5 √7ᵗʰ **T23.702** **Corrosion of third degree of left hand, unspecified site** NRS ▽

    √7ᵗʰ **T23.709** Corrosion of third degree of unspecified hand, unspecified site ▽

√6ᵗʰ **T23.71** Corrosion of third degree of thumb (nail)

    4,5 √7ᵗʰ **T23.711** **Corrosion of third degree of right thumb (nail)** NRS

    4,5 √7ᵗʰ **T23.712** **Corrosion of third degree of left thumb (nail)** NRS

    √7ᵗʰ **T23.719** Corrosion of third degree of unspecified thumb (nail) ▽

√6ᵗʰ **T23.72** Corrosion of third degree of single finger (nail) except thumb

    4,5 √7ᵗʰ **T23.721** **Corrosion of third degree of single right finger (nail) except thumb** NRS

    4,5 √7ᵗʰ **T23.722** **Corrosion of third degree of single left finger (nail) except thumb** NRS

    √7ᵗʰ **T23.729** Corrosion of third degree of unspecified single finger (nail) except thumb ▽

√6ᵗʰ **T23.73** Corrosion of third degree of multiple fingers (nail), not including thumb

    4,5 √7ᵗʰ **T23.731** **Corrosion of third degree of multiple right fingers (nail), not including thumb** NRS

    4,5 √7ᵗʰ **T23.732** **Corrosion of third degree of multiple left fingers (nail), not including thumb** NRS

    √7ᵗʰ **T23.739** Corrosion of third degree of unspecified multiple fingers (nail), not including thumb ▽

√6ᵗʰ **T23.74** Corrosion of third degree of multiple fingers (nail), including thumb

    4,5 √7ᵗʰ **T23.741** **Corrosion of third degree of multiple right fingers (nail), including thumb** NRS

    4,5 √7ᵗʰ **T23.742** **Corrosion of third degree of multiple left fingers (nail), including thumb** NRS

    √7ᵗʰ **T23.749** Corrosion of third degree of unspecified multiple fingers (nail), including thumb ▽

√6ᵗʰ **T23.75** Corrosion of third degree of palm

    4,5 √7ᵗʰ **T23.751** **Corrosion of third degree of right palm** NRS

    4,5 √7ᵗʰ **T23.752** **Corrosion of third degree of left palm** NRS

    √7ᵗʰ **T23.759** Corrosion of third degree of unspecified palm ▽

√6ᵗʰ **T23.76** Corrosion of third degree of back of hand

    4,5 √7ᵗʰ **T23.761** **Corrosion of third degree of back of right hand** NRS

    4,5 √7ᵗʰ **T23.762** **Corrosion of third degree of back of left hand** NRS

    √7ᵗʰ **T23.769** Corrosion of third degree back of unspecified hand ▽

√6ᵗʰ **T23.77** Corrosion of third degree of wrist

    4,5 √7ᵗʰ **T23.771** **Corrosion of third degree of right wrist** NRS

    4,5 √7ᵗʰ **T23.772** **Corrosion of third degree of left wrist** NRS

    √7ᵗʰ **T23.779** Corrosion of third degree of unspecified wrist ▽

√6ᵗʰ **T23.79** Corrosion of third degree of multiple sites of wrist and hand

    4,5 √7ᵗʰ **T23.791** **Corrosion of third degree of multiple sites of right wrist and hand** NRS

    4,5 √7ᵗʰ **T23.792** **Corrosion of third degree of multiple sites of left wrist and hand** NRS

    √7ᵗʰ **T23.799** Corrosion of third degree of multiple sites of unspecified wrist and hand ▽

√4ᵗʰ **T24** **Burn and corrosion of lower limb, except ankle and foot**
    EXCLUDES 2   *burn and corrosion of ankle and foot (T25.-)*
               burn and corrosion of hip region (T21.-)

> The appropriate 7th character is to be added to each code from category T24.
> A   initial encounter
> D   subsequent encounter
> S   sequela

√5ᵗʰ **T24.0** **Burn of** unspecified degree **of lower limb, except ankle and foot**
     Use additional external cause code to identify the source, place and intent of the burn (X00-X19, X75-X77, X96-X98, Y92)

√6ᵗʰ **T24.00** Burn of unspecified degree of unspecified site of lower limb, except ankle and foot

    √7ᵗʰ **T24.001** Burn of unspecified degree of unspecified site of right lower limb, except ankle and foot ▽

    √7ᵗʰ **T24.002** Burn of unspecified degree of unspecified site of left lower limb, except ankle and foot ▽

    √7ᵗʰ **T24.009** Burn of unspecified degree of unspecified site of unspecified lower limb, except ankle and foot ▽

√6ᵗʰ **T24.01** Burn of unspecified degree of thigh

    √7ᵗʰ **T24.011** Burn of unspecified degree of right thigh ▽

    √7ᵗʰ **T24.012** Burn of unspecified degree of left thigh ▽

    √7ᵗʰ **T24.019** Burn of unspecified degree of unspecified thigh ▽

√6ᵗʰ **T24.02** Burn of unspecified degree of knee

    √7ᵗʰ **T24.021** Burn of unspecified degree of right knee ▽

    √7ᵗʰ **T24.022** Burn of unspecified degree of left knee ▽

    √7ᵗʰ **T24.029** Burn of unspecified degree of unspecified knee ▽

√6ᵗʰ **T24.03** Burn of unspecified degree of lower leg

    √7ᵗʰ **T24.031** Burn of unspecified degree of right lower leg ▽

    √7ᵗʰ **T24.032** Burn of unspecified degree of left lower leg ▽

    √7ᵗʰ **T24.039** Burn of unspecified degree of unspecified lower lege ▽

---

4   Case-mix diagnosis with 7th character indicating initial or subsequent encounter.
5   NRS supply diagnosis with 7th character indicating initial or subsequent encounter.

☑ Additional Character Req   √x7ᵗʰ Placeholder Alert   Case-Mix Diagnosis   Manifestation   ▽ Unspecified Dx   EXCLUDES 1 Not coded here   EXCLUDES 2 Not included here

✓6th **T24.09**   Burn of unspecified degree of multiple sites of lower limb, except ankle and foot

     ✓7th **T24.091**   Burn of unspecified degree of multiple sites of right lower limb, except ankle and foot ▽

     ✓7th **T24.092**   Burn of unspecified degree of multiple sites of left lower limb, except ankle and foot ▽

     ✓7th **T24.099**   Burn of unspecified degree of multiple sites of unspecified lower limb, except ankle and foot ▽

✓5th **T24.1**   Burn of first degree of lower limb, except ankle and foot

     Use additional external cause code to identify the source, place and intent of the burn (X00-X19, X75-X77, X96-X98, Y92)

     ✓6th **T24.10**   Burn of first degree of unspecified site of lower limb, except ankle and foot

       ✓7th **T24.101**   Burn of first degree of unspecified site of right lower limb, except ankle and foot ▽

       ✓7th **T24.102**   Burn of first degree of unspecified site of left lower limb, except ankle and foot ▽

       ✓7th **T24.109**   Burn of first degree of unspecified site of unspecified lower limb, except ankle and foot ▽

     ✓6th **T24.11**   Burn of first degree of thigh

       ✓7th **T24.111**   Burn of first degree of right thigh

       ✓7th **T24.112**   Burn of first degree of left thigh

       ✓7th **T24.119**   Burn of first degree of unspecified thigh ▽

     ✓6th **T24.12**   Burn of first degree of knee

       ✓7th **T24.121**   Burn of first degree of right knee

       ✓7th **T24.122**   Burn of first degree of left knee

       ✓7th **T24.129**   Burn of first degree of unspecified knee ▽

     ✓6th **T24.13**   Burn of first degree of lower leg

       ✓7th **T24.131**   Burn of first degree of right lower leg

       ✓7th **T24.132**   Burn of first degree of left lower leg

       ✓7th **T24.139**   Burn of first degree of unspecified lower leg ▽

     ✓6th **T24.19**   Burn of first degree of multiple sites of lower limb, except ankle and foot

       ✓7th **T24.191**   Burn of first degree of multiple sites of right lower limb, except ankle and foot

       ✓7th **T24.192**   Burn of first degree of multiple sites of left lower limb, except ankle and foot

       ✓7th **T24.199**   Burn of first degree of multiple sites of unspecified lower limb, except ankle and foot ▽

✓5th **T24.2**   Burn of second degree of lower limb, except ankle and foot

     Use additional external cause code to identify the source, place and intent of the burn (X00-X19, X75-X77, X96-X98, Y92)

     ✓6th **T24.20**   Burn of second degree of unspecified site of lower limb, except ankle and foot

       4,5 ✓7th **T24.201**   Burn of second degree of unspecified site of right lower limb, except ankle and foot NRS ▽

       4,5 ✓7th **T24.202**   Burn of second degree of unspecified site of left lower limb, except ankle and foot NRS ▽

       ✓7th **T24.209**   Burn of second degree of unspecified site of unspecified lower limb, except ankle and foot ▽

     ✓6th **T24.21**   Burn of second degree of thigh

       4,5 ✓7th **T24.211**   Burn of second degree of right thigh NRS

       4,5 ✓7th **T24.212**   Burn of second degree of left thigh NRS

       ✓7th **T24.219**   Burn of second degree of unspecified thigh ▽

     ✓6th **T24.22**   Burn of second degree of knee

       4,5 ✓7th **T24.221**   Burn of second degree of right knee NRS

       4,5 ✓7th **T24.222**   Burn of second degree of left knee

       ✓7th **T24.229**   Burn of second degree of unspecified knee NRS ▽

✓6th **T24.23**   Burn of second degree of lower leg

     4,5 ✓7th **T24.231**   Burn of second degree of right lower leg NRS

     4,5 ✓7th **T24.232**   Burn of second degree of left lower leg NRS

     ✓7th **T24.239**   Burn of second degree of unspecified lower leg ▽

✓6th **T24.29**   Burn of second degree of multiple sites of lower limb, except ankle and foot

     4,5 ✓7th **T24.291**   Burn of second degree of multiple sites of right lower limb, except ankle and foot NRS

     4,5 ✓7th **T24.292**   Burn of second degree of multiple sites of left lower limb, except ankle and foot NRS

     ✓7th **T24.299**   Burn of second degree of multiple sites of unspecified lower limb, except ankle and foot ▽

✓5th **T24.3**   Burn of third degree of lower limb, except ankle and foot

     Use additional external cause code to identify the source, place and intent of the burn (X00-X19, X75-X77, X96-X98, Y92)

     ✓6th **T24.30**   Burn of third degree of unspecified site of lower limb, except ankle and foot

       4,5 ✓7th **T24.301**   Burn of third degree of unspecified site of right lower limb, except ankle and foot NRS ▽

       4,5 ✓7th **T24.302**   Burn of third degree of unspecified site of left lower limb, except ankle and foot NRS ▽

       ✓7th **T24.309**   Burn of third degree of unspecified site of unspecified lower limb, except ankle and foot ▽

     ✓6th **T24.31**   Burn of third degree of thigh

       4,5 ✓7th **T24.311**   Burn of third degree of right thigh NRS

       4,5 ✓7th **T24.312**   Burn of third degree of left thigh NRS

       ✓7th **T24.319**   Burn of third degree of unspecified thigh ▽

     ✓6th **T24.32**   Burn of third degree of knee

       4,5 ✓7th **T24.321**   Burn of third degree of right knee NRS

       4,5 ✓7th **T24.322**   Burn of third degree of left knee NRS

       ✓7th **T24.329**   Burn of third degree of unspecified knee ▽

     ✓6th **T24.33**   Burn of third degree of lower leg

       4,5 ✓7th **T24.331**   Burn of third degree of right lower leg NRS

       4,5 ✓7th **T24.332**   Burn of third degree of left lower leg NRS

       ✓7th **T24.339**   Burn of third degree of unspecified lower leg ▽

     ✓6th **T24.39**   Burn of third degree of multiple sites of lower limb, except ankle and foot

       AHA: 2016, 2Q, 4

       4,5 ✓7th **T24.391**   Burn of third degree of multiple sites of right lower limb, except ankle and foot NRS

       4,5 ✓7th **T24.392**   Burn of third degree of multiple sites of left lower limb, except ankle and foot NRS

       ✓7th **T24.399**   Burn of third degree of multiple sites of unspecified lower limb, except ankle and foot ▽

✓5th **T24.4**   Corrosion of unspecified degree of lower limb, except ankle and foot

     Code first (T51-T65) to identify chemical and intent

     Use additional external cause code to identify place (Y92)

     ✓6th **T24.40**   Corrosion of unspecified degree of unspecified site of lower limb, except ankle and foot

       ✓7th **T24.401**   Corrosion of unspecified degree of unspecified site of right lower limb, except ankle and foot ▽

       ✓7th **T24.402**   Corrosion of unspecified degree of unspecified site of left lower limb, except ankle and foot ▽

       ✓7th **T24.409**   Corrosion of unspecified degree of unspecified site of unspecified lower limb, except ankle and foot ▽

---

4   Case-mix diagnosis with 7th character indicating initial or subsequent encounter.

5   NRS supply diagnosis with 7th character indicating initial or subsequent encounter.

☑6ᵗʰ **T24.41** Corrosion of unspecified degree of thigh

     ☑7ᵗʰ **T24.411** Corrosion of unspecified degree of right thigh ▽

     ☑7ᵗʰ **T24.412** Corrosion of unspecified degree of left thigh ▽

     ☑7ᵗʰ **T24.419** Corrosion of unspecified degree of unspecified thigh ▽

☑6ᵗʰ **T24.42** Corrosion of unspecified degree of knee

     ☑7ᵗʰ **T24.421** Corrosion of unspecified degree of right knee ▽

     ☑7ᵗʰ **T24.422** Corrosion of unspecified degree of left knee ▽

     ☑7ᵗʰ **T24.429** Corrosion of unspecified degree of unspecified knee ▽

☑6ᵗʰ **T24.43** Corrosion of unspecified degree of lower leg

     ☑7ᵗʰ **T24.431** Corrosion of unspecified degree of right lower leg ▽

     ☑7ᵗʰ **T24.432** Corrosion of unspecified degree of left lower leg ▽

     ☑7ᵗʰ **T24.439** Corrosion of unspecified degree of unspecified lower leg ▽

☑6ᵗʰ **T24.49** Corrosion of unspecified degree of multiple sites of lower limb, except ankle and foot

     ☑7ᵗʰ **T24.491** Corrosion of unspecified degree of multiple sites of right lower limb, except ankle and foot ▽

     ☑7ᵗʰ **T24.492** Corrosion of unspecified degree of multiple sites of left lower limb, except ankle and foot ▽

     ☑7ᵗʰ **T24.499** Corrosion of unspecified degree of multiple sites of unspecified lower limb, except ankle and foot ▽

☑5ᵗʰ **T24.5** Corrosion of first degree of lower limb, except ankle and foot

     Code first (T51-T65) to identify chemical and intent

     Use additional external cause code to identify place (Y92)

   ☑6ᵗʰ **T24.50** Corrosion of first degree of unspecified site of lower limb, except ankle and foot

     ☑7ᵗʰ **T24.501** Corrosion of first degree of unspecified site of right lower limb, except ankle and foot ▽

     ☑7ᵗʰ **T24.502** Corrosion of first degree of unspecified site of left lower limb, except ankle and foot ▽

     ☑7ᵗʰ **T24.509** Corrosion of first degree of unspecified site of unspecified lower limb, except ankle and foot ▽

   ☑6ᵗʰ **T24.51** Corrosion of first degree of thigh

     ☑7ᵗʰ **T24.511** Corrosion of first degree of right thigh

     ☑7ᵗʰ **T24.512** Corrosion of first degree of left thigh

     ☑7ᵗʰ **T24.519** Corrosion of first degree of unspecified thigh ▽

   ☑6ᵗʰ **T24.52** Corrosion of first degree of knee

     ☑7ᵗʰ **T24.521** Corrosion of first degree of right knee

     ☑7ᵗʰ **T24.522** Corrosion of first degree of left knee

     ☑7ᵗʰ **T24.529** Corrosion of first degree of unspecified knee ▽

   ☑6ᵗʰ **T24.53** Corrosion of first degree of lower leg

     ☑7ᵗʰ **T24.531** Corrosion of first degree of right lower leg

     ☑7ᵗʰ **T24.532** Corrosion of first degree of left lower leg

     ☑7ᵗʰ **T24.539** Corrosion of first degree of unspecified lower leg ▽

   ☑6ᵗʰ **T24.59** Corrosion of first degree of multiple sites of lower limb, except ankle and foot

     ☑7ᵗʰ **T24.591** Corrosion of first degree of multiple sites of right lower limb, except ankle and foot

     ☑7ᵗʰ **T24.592** Corrosion of first degree of multiple sites of left lower limb, except ankle and foot

     ☑7ᵗʰ **T24.599** Corrosion of first degree of multiple sites of unspecified lower limb, except ankle and foot ▽

☑5ᵗʰ **T24.6** Corrosion of second degree of lower limb, except ankle and foot

     Code first (T51-T65) to identify chemical and intent

     Use additional external cause code to identify place (Y92)

   ☑6ᵗʰ **T24.60** Corrosion of second degree of unspecified site of lower limb, except ankle and foot

     4,5 ☑7ᵗʰ **T24.601** Corrosion of second degree of unspecified site of right lower limb, except ankle and foot   NRS ▽

     4,5 ☑7ᵗʰ **T24.602** Corrosion of second degree of unspecified site of left lower limb, except ankle and foot   NRS ▽

     ☑7ᵗʰ **T24.609** Corrosion of second degree of unspecified site of unspecified lower limb, except ankle and foot ▽

   ☑6ᵗʰ **T24.61** Corrosion of second degree of thigh

     4,5 ☑7ᵗʰ **T24.611** Corrosion of second degree of right thigh   NRS

     4,5 ☑7ᵗʰ **T24.612** Corrosion of second degree of left thigh   NRS

     ☑7ᵗʰ **T24.619** Corrosion of second degree of unspecified thigh ▽

   ☑6ᵗʰ **T24.62** Corrosion of second degree of knee

     4,5 ☑7ᵗʰ **T24.621** Corrosion of second degree of right knee   NRS

     4,5 ☑7ᵗʰ **T24.622** Corrosion of second degree of left knee   NRS

     ☑7ᵗʰ **T24.629** Corrosion of second degree of unspecified knee ▽

   ☑6ᵗʰ **T24.63** Corrosion of second degree of lower leg

     4,5 ☑7ᵗʰ **T24.631** Corrosion of second degree of right lower leg   NRS

     4,5 ☑7ᵗʰ **T24.632** Corrosion of second degree of left lower leg   NRS

     ☑7ᵗʰ **T24.639** Corrosion of second degree of unspecified lower leg ▽

   ☑6ᵗʰ **T24.69** Corrosion of second degree of multiple sites of lower limb, except ankle and foot

     4,5 ☑7ᵗʰ **T24.691** Corrosion of second degree of multiple sites of right lower limb, except ankle and foot   NRS

     4,5 ☑7ᵗʰ **T24.692** Corrosion of second degree of multiple sites of left lower limb, except ankle and foot   NRS

     ☑7ᵗʰ **T24.699** Corrosion of second degree of multiple sites of unspecified lower limb, except ankle and foot ▽

☑5ᵗʰ **T24.7** Corrosion of third degree of lower limb, except ankle and foot

     Code first (T51-T65) to identify chemical and intent

     Use additional external cause code to identify place (Y92)

   ☑6ᵗʰ **T24.70** Corrosion of third degree of unspecified site of lower limb, except ankle and foot

     4,5 ☑7ᵗʰ **T24.701** Corrosion of third degree of unspecified site of right lower limb, except ankle and foot   NRS ▽

     4,5 ☑7ᵗʰ **T24.702** Corrosion of third degree of unspecified site of left lower limb, except ankle and foot   NRS ▽

     ☑7ᵗʰ **T24.709** Corrosion of third degree of unspecified site of unspecified lower limb, except ankle and foot ▽

   ☑6ᵗʰ **T24.71** Corrosion of third degree of thigh

     4,5 ☑7ᵗʰ **T24.711** Corrosion of third degree of right thigh   NRS

     4,5 ☑7ᵗʰ **T24.712** Corrosion of third degree of left thigh   NRS

     ☑7ᵗʰ **T24.719** Corrosion of third degree of unspecified thigh ▽

   ☑6ᵗʰ **T24.72** Corrosion of third degree of knee

     4,5 ☑7ᵗʰ **T24.721** Corrosion of third degree of right knee   NRS

     4,5 ☑7ᵗʰ **T24.722** Corrosion of third degree of left knee   NRS

     ☑7ᵗʰ **T24.729** Corrosion of third degree of unspecified knee ▽

---

⁴ Case-mix diagnosis with 7th character indicating initial or subsequent encounter.
⁵ NRS supply diagnosis with 7th character indicating initial or subsequent encounter.

☑ Additional Character Req   ☑×7ᵗʰ Placeholder Alert   Case-Mix Diagnosis   Manifestation   ▽ Unspecified Dx   **EXCLUDES 1** Not coded here   **EXCLUDES 2** Not included here

ICD-10-CM 2018   **1053**

✓6ᵗʰ **T24.73** Corrosion of third degree of lower leg

4,5 ✓7ᵗʰ **T24.731** **Corrosion of third degree of right lower leg** NRS

4,5 ✓7ᵗʰ **T24.732** **Corrosion of third degree of left lower leg** NRS

✓7ᵗʰ **T24.739** Corrosion of third degree of unspecified lower leg ▽

✓6ᵗʰ **T24.79** Corrosion of third degree of multiple sites of lower limb, except ankle and foot

4,5 ✓7ᵗʰ **T24.791** **Corrosion of third degree of multiple sites of right lower limb, except ankle and foot** NRS

4,5 ✓7ᵗʰ **T24.792** **Corrosion of third degree of multiple sites of left lower limb, except ankle and foot** NRS

✓7ᵗʰ **T24.799** Corrosion of third degree of multiple sites of unspecified lower limb, except ankle and foot ▽

✓4ᵗʰ **T25** **Burn and corrosion of ankle and foot**

The appropriate 7th character is to be added to each code from category T25.
A   initial encounter
D   subsequent encounter
S   sequela

✓5ᵗʰ **T25.0** **Burn of unspecified degree of ankle and foot**
Use additional external cause code to identify the source, place and intent of the burn (X00-X19, X75-X77, X96-X98, Y92)

✓6ᵗʰ **T25.01** **Burn of unspecified degree of ankle**

✓7ᵗʰ **T25.011** Burn of unspecified degree of right ankle ▽

✓7ᵗʰ **T25.012** Burn of unspecified degree of left ankle ▽

✓7ᵗʰ **T25.019** Burn of unspecified degree of unspecified ankle ▽

✓6ᵗʰ **T25.02** **Burn of unspecified degree of foot**
EXCLUDES 2 burn of unspecified degree of toe(s) (nail) (T25.03-)

✓7ᵗʰ **T25.021** Burn of unspecified degree of right foot ▽

✓7ᵗʰ **T25.022** Burn of unspecified degree of left foot ▽

✓7ᵗʰ **T25.029** Burn of unspecified degree of unspecified foot ▽

✓6ᵗʰ **T25.03** **Burn of unspecified degree of toe(s) (nail)**

✓7ᵗʰ **T25.031** Burn of unspecified degree of right toe(s) (nail) ▽

✓7ᵗʰ **T25.032** Burn of unspecified degree of left toe(s) (nail) ▽

✓7ᵗʰ **T25.039** Burn of unspecified degree of unspecified toe(s) (nail) ▽

✓6ᵗʰ **T25.09** **Burn of unspecified degree of multiple sites of ankle and foot**

✓7ᵗʰ **T25.091** Burn of unspecified degree of multiple sites of right ankle and foot ▽

✓7ᵗʰ **T25.092** Burn of unspecified degree of multiple sites of left ankle and foot ▽

✓7ᵗʰ **T25.099** Burn of unspecified degree of multiple sites of unspecified ankle and foot ▽

✓5ᵗʰ **T25.1** **Burn of first degree of ankle and foot**
Use additional external cause code to identify the source, place and intent of the burn (X00-X19, X75-X77, X96-X98, Y92)

✓6ᵗʰ **T25.11** **Burn of first degree of ankle**

✓7ᵗʰ **T25.111** Burn of first degree of right ankle

✓7ᵗʰ **T25.112** Burn of first degree of left ankle

✓7ᵗʰ **T25.119** Burn of first degree of unspecified ankle ▽

✓6ᵗʰ **T25.12** **Burn of first degree of foot**
EXCLUDES 2 burn of first degree of toe(s) (nail) (T25.13-)

✓7ᵗʰ **T25.121** Burn of first degree of right foot

✓7ᵗʰ **T25.122** Burn of first degree of left foot

✓7ᵗʰ **T25.129** Burn of first degree of unspecified foot ▽

✓6ᵗʰ **T25.13** **Burn of first degree of toe(s) (nail)**

✓7ᵗʰ **T25.131** Burn of first degree of right toe(s) (nail)

✓7ᵗʰ **T25.132** Burn of first degree of left toe(s) (nail)

✓7ᵗʰ **T25.139** Burn of first degree of unspecified toe(s) (nail) ▽

✓6ᵗʰ **T25.19** **Burn of first degree of multiple sites of ankle and foot**

✓7ᵗʰ **T25.191** Burn of first degree of multiple sites of right ankle and foot

✓7ᵗʰ **T25.192** Burn of first degree of multiple sites of left ankle and foot

✓7ᵗʰ **T25.199** Burn of first degree of multiple sites of unspecified ankle and foot ▽

✓5ᵗʰ **T25.2** **Burn of second degree of ankle and foot**
Use additional external cause code to identify the source, place and intent of the burn (X00-X19, X75-X77, X96-X98, Y92)

✓6ᵗʰ **T25.21** **Burn of second degree of ankle**

4,5 ✓7ᵗʰ **T25.211** **Burn of second degree of right ankle** NRS

4,5 ✓7ᵗʰ **T25.212** **Burn of second degree of left ankle** NRS

✓7ᵗʰ **T25.219** Burn of second degree of unspecified ankle ▽

✓6ᵗʰ **T25.22** **Burn of second degree of foot**
EXCLUDES 2 burn of second degree of toe(s) (nail) (T25.23-)

4,5 ✓7ᵗʰ **T25.221** **Burn of second degree of right foot** NRS

4,5 ✓7ᵗʰ **T25.222** **Burn of second degree of left foot** NRS

✓7ᵗʰ **T25.229** Burn of second degree of unspecified foot ▽

✓6ᵗʰ **T25.23** **Burn of second degree of toe(s) (nail)**

4,5 ✓7ᵗʰ **T25.231** **Burn of second degree of right toe(s) (nail)** NRS

4,5 ✓7ᵗʰ **T25.232** **Burn of second degree of left toe(s) (nail)** NRS

✓7ᵗʰ **T25.239** Burn of second degree of unspecified toe(s) (nail) ▽

✓6ᵗʰ **T25.29** **Burn of second degree of multiple sites of ankle and foot**

4,5 ✓7ᵗʰ **T25.291** **Burn of second degree of multiple sites of right ankle and foot** NRS

4,5 ✓7ᵗʰ **T25.292** **Burn of second degree of multiple sites of left ankle and foot** NRS

✓7ᵗʰ **T25.299** Burn of second degree of multiple sites of unspecified ankle and foot ▽

✓5ᵗʰ **T25.3** **Burn of third degree of ankle and foot**
Use additional external cause code to identify the source, place and intent of the burn (X00-X19, X75-X77, X96-X98, Y92)

✓6ᵗʰ **T25.31** **Burn of third degree of ankle**

4,5 ✓7ᵗʰ **T25.311** **Burn of third degree of right ankle** NRS

4,5 ✓7ᵗʰ **T25.312** **Burn of third degree of left ankle** NRS

✓7ᵗʰ **T25.319** Burn of third degree of unspecified ankle ▽

✓6ᵗʰ **T25.32** **Burn of third degree of foot**
EXCLUDES 2 burn of third degree of toe(s) (nail) (T25.33-)

4,5 ✓7ᵗʰ **T25.321** **Burn of third degree of right foot** NRS

4,5 ✓7ᵗʰ **T25.322** **Burn of third degree of left foot** NRS

✓7ᵗʰ **T25.329** Burn of third degree of unspecified foot NRS ▽

✓6ᵗʰ **T25.33** **Burn of third degree of toe(s) (nail)**

4,5 ✓7ᵗʰ **T25.331** **Burn of third degree of right toe(s) (nail)** NRS

4,5 ✓7ᵗʰ **T25.332** **Burn of third degree of left toe(s) (nail)** NRS

✓7ᵗʰ **T25.339** Burn of third degree of unspecified toe(s) (nail) ▽

✓6ᵗʰ **T25.39** **Burn of third degree of multiple sites of ankle and foot**

4,5 ✓7ᵗʰ **T25.391** **Burn of third degree of multiple sites of right ankle and foot** NRS

4,5 ✓7ᵗʰ **T25.392** **Burn of third degree of multiple sites of left ankle and foot** NRS

✓7ᵗʰ **T25.399** Burn of third degree of multiple sites of unspecified ankle and foot ▽

---

4   Case-mix diagnosis with 7th character indicating initial or subsequent encounter.
5   NRS supply diagnosis with 7th character indicating initial or subsequent encounter.

N Newborn: 0   P Pediatric: 0-17   M Maternity: 12-55   A Adult: 15-124   NRS Nonroutine supply Dx   NC Dx Noncancer Dx   PDx Primary Dx   ▶◀ Revised Text   ● New Code   ▲ Revised Title

1054   ICD-10-CM 2018

√5ᵗʰ **T25.4** **Corrosion of** unspecified degree **of ankle and foot**
　Code first (T51-T65) to identify chemical and intent
　Use additional external cause code to identify place (Y92)

√6ᵗʰ **T25.41** **Corrosion of unspecified degree of** ankle

√7ᵗʰ **T25.411** **Corrosion of unspecified degree of** right **ankle** ▽

√7ᵗʰ **T25.412** **Corrosion of unspecified degree of** left **ankle** ▽

√7ᵗʰ **T25.419** **Corrosion of unspecified degree of unspecified ankle** ▽

√6ᵗʰ **T25.42** **Corrosion of unspecified degree of** foot
　EXCLUDES 2　corrosion of unspecified degree of toe(s) (nail) (T25.43-)

√7ᵗʰ **T25.421** **Corrosion of unspecified degree of** right **foot** ▽

√7ᵗʰ **T25.422** **Corrosion of unspecified degree of** left **foot** ▽

√7ᵗʰ **T25.429** **Corrosion of unspecified degree of unspecified foot** ▽

√6ᵗʰ **T25.43** **Corrosion of unspecified degree of** toe(s) (nail)

√7ᵗʰ **T25.431** **Corrosion of unspecified degree of** right **toe(s) (nail)** ▽

√7ᵗʰ **T25.432** **Corrosion of unspecified degree of** left **toe(s) (nail)** ▽

√7ᵗʰ **T25.439** **Corrosion of unspecified degree of unspecified toe(s) (nail)** ▽

√6ᵗʰ **T25.49** **Corrosion of unspecified degree of** multiple sites **of ankle and foot**

√7ᵗʰ **T25.491** **Corrosion of unspecified degree of multiple sites of** right **ankle and foot** ▽

√7ᵗʰ **T25.492** **Corrosion of unspecified degree of multiple sites of** left **ankle and foot** ▽

√7ᵗʰ **T25.499** **Corrosion of unspecified degree of multiple sites of unspecified ankle and foot** ▽

√5ᵗʰ **T25.5** **Corrosion of** first degree **of ankle and foot**
　Code first (T51-T65) to identify chemical and intent
　Use additional external cause code to identify place (Y92)

√6ᵗʰ **T25.51** **Corrosion of first degree of** ankle

√7ᵗʰ **T25.511** **Corrosion of first degree of** right **ankle**

√7ᵗʰ **T25.512** **Corrosion of first degree of** left **ankle**

√7ᵗʰ **T25.519** **Corrosion of first degree of unspecified ankle** ▽

√6ᵗʰ **T25.52** **Corrosion of first degree of** foot
　EXCLUDES 2　corrosion of first degree of toe(s) (nail) (T25.53-)

√7ᵗʰ **T25.521** **Corrosion of first degree of** right **foot**

√7ᵗʰ **T25.522** **Corrosion of first degree of** left **foot**

√7ᵗʰ **T25.529** **Corrosion of first degree of unspecified foot** ▽

√6ᵗʰ **T25.53** **Corrosion of first degree of** toe(s) (nail)

√7ᵗʰ **T25.531** **Corrosion of first degree of** right **toe(s) (nail)**

√7ᵗʰ **T25.532** **Corrosion of first degree of** left **toe(s) (nail)**

√7ᵗʰ **T25.539** **Corrosion of first degree of unspecified toe(s) (nail)** ▽

√6ᵗʰ **T25.59** **Corrosion of first degree of** multiple sites **of ankle and foot**

√7ᵗʰ **T25.591** **Corrosion of first degree of multiple sites of** right **ankle and foot**

√7ᵗʰ **T25.592** **Corrosion of first degree of multiple sites of** left **ankle and foot**

√7ᵗʰ **T25.599** **Corrosion of first degree of multiple sites of unspecified ankle and foot** ▽

√5ᵗʰ **T25.6** **Corrosion of** second degree **of ankle and foot**
　Code first (T51-T65) to identify chemical and intent
　Use additional external cause code to identify place (Y92)

√6ᵗʰ **T25.61** **Corrosion of second degree of** ankle

4,5 √7ᵗʰ **T25.611** **Corrosion of second degree of** right **ankle** NRS

4,5 √7ᵗʰ **T25.612** **Corrosion of second degree of** left **ankle** NRS

√7ᵗʰ **T25.619** **Corrosion of second degree of unspecified ankle** ▽

√6ᵗʰ **T25.62** **Corrosion of second degree of** foot
　EXCLUDES 2　corrosion of second degree of toe(s) (nail) (T25.63-)

4,5 √7ᵗʰ **T25.621** **Corrosion of second degree of** right **foot** NRS

4,5 √7ᵗʰ **T25.622** **Corrosion of second degree of** left **foot** NRS

√7ᵗʰ **T25.629** **Corrosion of second degree of unspecified foot** ▽

√6ᵗʰ **T25.63** **Corrosion of second degree of** toe(s) (nail)

4,5 √7ᵗʰ **T25.631** **Corrosion of second degree of** right **toe(s) (nail)** NRS

4,5 √7ᵗʰ **T25.632** **Corrosion of second degree of** left **toe(s) (nail)** NRS

√7ᵗʰ **T25.639** **Corrosion of second degree of unspecified toe(s) (nail)** ▽

√6ᵗʰ **T25.69** **Corrosion of second degree of** multiple sites **of ankle and foot**

4,5 √7ᵗʰ **T25.691** **Corrosion of second degree of** right **ankle and foot** NRS

4,5 √7ᵗʰ **T25.692** **Corrosion of second degree of** left **ankle and foot** NRS

√7ᵗʰ **T25.699** **Corrosion of second degree of unspecified ankle and foot** ▽

√5ᵗʰ **T25.7** **Corrosion of** third degree **of ankle and foot**
　Code first (T51-T65) to identify chemical and intent
　Use additional external cause code to identify place (Y92)

√6ᵗʰ **T25.71** **Corrosion of third degree of** ankle

4,5 √7ᵗʰ **T25.711** **Corrosion of third degree of** right **ankle** NRS

4,5 √7ᵗʰ **T25.712** **Corrosion of third degree of** left **ankle** NRS

√7ᵗʰ **T25.719** **Corrosion of third degree of unspecified ankle** ▽

√6ᵗʰ **T25.72** **Corrosion of third degree of** foot
　EXCLUDES 2　corrosion of third degree of toe(s) (nail) (T25.73-)

4,5 √7ᵗʰ **T25.721** **Corrosion of third degree of** right **foot** NRS

4,5 √7ᵗʰ **T25.722** **Corrosion of third degree of** left **foot** NRS

√7ᵗʰ **T25.729** **Corrosion of third degree of unspecified foot** ▽

√6ᵗʰ **T25.73** **Corrosion of third degree of** toe(s) (nail)

4,5 √7ᵗʰ **T25.731** **Corrosion of third degree of** right **toe(s) (nail)** NRS

4,5 √7ᵗʰ **T25.732** **Corrosion of third degree of** left **toe(s) (nail)** NRS

√7ᵗʰ **T25.739** **Corrosion of third degree of unspecified toe(s) (nail)** ▽

√6ᵗʰ **T25.79** **Corrosion of third degree of** multiple sites **of ankle and foot**

4,5 √7ᵗʰ **T25.791** **Corrosion of third degree of multiple sites of** right **ankle and foot** NRS

4,5 √7ᵗʰ **T25.792** **Corrosion of third degree of multiple sites of** left **ankle and foot** NRS

√7ᵗʰ **T25.799** **Corrosion of third degree of multiple sites of unspecified ankle and foot** ▽

4　Case-mix diagnosis with 7th character indicating initial or subsequent encounter.
5　NRS supply diagnosis with 7th character indicating initial or subsequent encounter.

☑ Additional Character Req　　√x7ᵗʰ Placeholder Alert　　Case-Mix Diagnosis　　Manifestation　　▽ Unspecified Dx　　EXCLUDES 1 Not coded here　　EXCLUDES 2 Not included here

Burns and corrosions confined to eye and internal organs (T26-T28)

✓4ᵗʰ T26   Burn and corrosion confined to eye and adnexa

> The appropriate 7th character is to be added to each code from category T26.
> A   initial encounter
> D   subsequent encounter
> S   sequela

✓5ᵗʰ T26.0   Burn of eyelid and periocular area
Use additional external cause code to identify the source, place and intent of the burn (X00-X19, X75-X77, X96-X98, Y92)

    ✓x7ᵗʰ   **T26.00**   Burn of unspecified eyelid and periocular area   ▽

    ✓x7ᵗʰ   **T26.01**   Burn of right eyelid and periocular area

    ✓x7ᵗʰ   **T26.02**   Burn of left eyelid and periocular area

✓5ᵗʰ T26.1   Burn of cornea and conjunctival sac
Use additional external cause code to identify the source, place and intent of the burn (X00-X19, X75-X77, X96-X98, Y92)

    ✓x7ᵗʰ   **T26.10**   Burn of cornea and conjunctival sac, unspecified eye   ▽

    ✓x7ᵗʰ   **T26.11**   Burn of cornea and conjunctival sac, right eye

    ✓x7ᵗʰ   **T26.12**   Burn of cornea and conjunctival sac, left eye

✓5ᵗʰ T26.2   Burn with resulting rupture and destruction of eyeball
Use additional external cause code to identify the source, place and intent of the burn (X00-X19, X75-X77, X96-X98, Y92)

    ✓x7ᵗʰ   **T26.20**   Burn with resulting rupture and destruction of unspecified eyeball   ▽

   4,5   ✓x7ᵗʰ   **T26.21**   Burn with resulting rupture and destruction of right eyeball   `NRS`

   4,5   ✓x7ᵗʰ   **T26.22**   Burn with resulting rupture and destruction of left eyeball   `NRS`

✓5ᵗʰ T26.3   Burns of other specified parts of eye and adnexa
Use additional external cause code to identify the source, place and intent of the burn (X00-X19, X75-X77, X96-X98, Y92)

    ✓x7ᵗʰ   **T26.30**   Burns of other specified parts of unspecified eye and adnexa   ▽

    ✓x7ᵗʰ   **T26.31**   Burns of other specified parts of right eye and adnexa

    ✓x7ᵗʰ   **T26.32**   Burns of other specified parts of left eye and adnexa

✓5ᵗʰ T26.4   Burn of eye and adnexa, part unspecified
Use additional external cause code to identify the source, place and intent of the burn (X00-X19, X75-X77, X96-X98, Y92)

    ✓x7ᵗʰ   **T26.40**   Burn of unspecified eye and adnexa, part unspecified   ▽

    ✓x7ᵗʰ   **T26.41**   Burn of right eye and adnexa, part unspecified   ▽

    ✓x7ᵗʰ   **T26.42**   Burn of left eye and adnexa, part unspecified   ▽

✓5ᵗʰ T26.5   Corrosion of eyelid and periocular area
Code first (T51-T65) to identify chemical and intent
Use additional external cause code to identify place (Y92)

    ✓x7ᵗʰ   **T26.50**   Corrosion of unspecified eyelid and periocular area   ▽

    ✓x7ᵗʰ   **T26.51**   Corrosion of right eyelid and periocular area

    ✓x7ᵗʰ   **T26.52**   Corrosion of left eyelid and periocular area

✓5ᵗʰ T26.6   Corrosion of cornea and conjunctival sac
Code first (T51-T65) to identify chemical and intent
Use additional external cause code to identify place (Y92)

    ✓x7ᵗʰ   **T26.60**   Corrosion of cornea and conjunctival sac, unspecified eye   ▽

    ✓x7ᵗʰ   **T26.61**   Corrosion of cornea and conjunctival sac, right eye

    ✓x7ᵗʰ   **T26.62**   Corrosion of cornea and conjunctival sac, left eye

✓5ᵗʰ T26.7   Corrosion with resulting rupture and destruction of eyeball
Code first (T51-T65) to identify chemical and intent
Use additional external cause code to identify place (Y92)

    ✓x7ᵗʰ   **T26.70**   Corrosion with resulting rupture and destruction of unspecified eyeball   ▽

    ✓x7ᵗʰ   **T26.71**   Corrosion with resulting rupture and destruction of right eyeball

    ✓x7ᵗʰ   **T26.72**   Corrosion with resulting rupture and destruction of left eyeball

---

    ✓5ᵗʰ   **T26.8**   Corrosions of other specified parts of eye and adnexa
Code first (T51-T65) to identify chemical and intent
Use additional external cause code to identify place (Y92)

    ✓x7ᵗʰ   **T26.80**   Corrosions of other specified parts of unspecified eye and adnexa   ▽

    ✓x7ᵗʰ   **T26.81**   Corrosions of other specified parts of right eye and adnexa

    ✓x7ᵗʰ   **T26.82**   Corrosions of other specified parts of left eye and adnexa

    ✓5ᵗʰ   **T26.9**   Corrosion of eye and adnexa, part unspecified
Code first (T51-T65) to identify chemical and intent
Use additional external cause code to identify place (Y92)

    ✓x7ᵗʰ   **T26.90**   Corrosion of unspecified eye and adnexa, part unspecified   ▽

    ✓x7ᵗʰ   **T26.91**   Corrosion of right eye and adnexa, part unspecified   ▽

    ✓x7ᵗʰ   **T26.92**   Corrosion of left eye and adnexa, part unspecified ▽

✓4ᵗʰ T27   Burn and corrosion of respiratory tract

Use additional external cause code to identify the source and intent of the burn (X00-X19, X75-X77, X96-X98)
Use additional external cause code to identify place (Y92)

> The appropriate 7th character is to be added to each code from category T27.
> A   initial encounter
> D   subsequent encounter
> S   sequela

    ✓x7ᵗʰ   **T27.0**   Burn of larynx and trachea

    ✓x7ᵗʰ   **T27.1**   Burn involving larynx and trachea with lung

    ✓x7ᵗʰ   **T27.2**   Burn of other parts of respiratory tract
        Burn of thoracic cavity

    ✓x7ᵗʰ   **T27.3**   Burn of respiratory tract, part unspecified   ▽
        ~~Code first (T51-T65) to identify chemical and intent for codes T27.4-T27.7~~

    ✓x7ᵗʰ   **T27.4**   Corrosion of larynx and trachea
        ▶Code first (T51-T65) to identify chemical and intent◀

    ✓x7ᵗʰ   **T27.5**   Corrosion involving larynx and trachea with lung

    ✓x7ᵗʰ   **T27.6**   Corrosion of other parts of respiratory tract
        ▶Code first (T51-T65) to identify chemical and intent◀

    ✓x7ᵗʰ   **T27.7**   Corrosion of respiratory tract, part unspecified   ▽
        ▶Code first (T51-T65) to identify chemical and intent◀

✓4ᵗʰ T28   Burn and corrosion of other internal organs

Use additional external cause code to identify the source and intent of the burn (X00- X19, X75-X77, X96-X98)
Use additional external cause code to identify place (Y92)

> The appropriate 7th character is to be added to each code from category T28.
> A   initial encounter
> D   subsequent encounter
> S   sequela

    ✓x7ᵗʰ   **T28.0**   Burn of mouth and pharynx

    ✓x7ᵗʰ   **T28.1**   Burn of esophagus

    ✓x7ᵗʰ   **T28.2**   Burn of other parts of alimentary tract

    ✓x7ᵗʰ   **T28.3**   Burn of internal genitourinary organs

    ✓5ᵗʰ   **T28.4**   Burns of other and unspecified internal organs
        ▶Code first (T51-T65) to identify chemical and intent◀

       ✓x7ᵗʰ   **T28.40**   Burn of unspecified internal organ   ▽

       ✓6ᵗʰ   **T28.41**   Burn of ear drum

          ✓7ᵗʰ   **T28.411**   Burn of right ear drum

          ✓7ᵗʰ   **T28.412**   Burn of left ear drum

          ✓7ᵗʰ   **T28.419**   Burn of unspecified ear drum   ▽

       ✓x7ᵗʰ   **T28.49**   Burn of other internal organ
          ~~Code first (T51-T65) to identify chemical and intent for T28.5-T28.9~~

    ✓x7ᵗʰ   **T28.5**   Corrosion of mouth and pharynx
        ▶Code first (T51-T65) to identify chemical and intent◀

    ✓x7ᵗʰ   **T28.6**   Corrosion of esophagus
        ▶Code first (T51-T65) to identify chemical and intent◀

    ✓x7ᵗʰ   **T28.7**   Corrosion of other parts of alimentary tract
        ▶Code first (T51-T65) to identify chemical and intent◀

---

4   Case-mix diagnosis with 7th character indicating initial or subsequent encounter.
5   NRS supply diagnosis with 7th character indicating initial or subsequent encounter.

Ⓝ Newborn: 0   Ⓟ Pediatric: 0-17   Ⓜ Maternity: 12-55   Ⓐ Adult: 15-124   `NRS` Nonroutine supply Dx   `NCDx` Noncancer Dx   `PDx` Primary Dx   ▶◀ Revised Text   ● New Code   ▲ Revised Title

1056   ICD-10-CM 2018

✓x7ᵗʰ **T28.8**   **Corrosion of internal** genitourinary organs
▶Code first (T51-T65) to identify chemical and intent◀

✓5ᵗʰ **T28.9**   **Corrosions of other and unspecified internal organs**
▶Code first (T51-T65) to identify chemical and intent◀

    ✓x7ᵗʰ **T28.90**   **Corrosions of unspecified internal organs**   ▽

    ✓6ᵗʰ **T28.91**   **Corrosions of** ear drum

       ✓7ᵗʰ **T28.911**   **Corrosions of** right **ear drum**

       ✓7ᵗʰ **T28.912**   **Corrosions of** left **ear drum**

       ✓7ᵗʰ **T28.919**   **Corrosions of unspecified ear drum**   ▽

    ✓x7ᵗʰ **T28.99**   **Corrosions of other internal organs**

Burns and corrosions of multiple and unspecified body regions (T30-T32)

✓4ᵗʰ **T30**   **Burn and corrosion, body region unspecified**

    T30.0   Burn **of unspecified body region, unspecified degree**   ▽
This code is not for inpatient use. Code to specified site and degree of burns.
Burn NOS
Multiple burns NOS

    T30.4   Corrosion **of unspecified body region, unspecified degree**   ▽
This code is not for inpatient use. Code to specified site and degree of corrosion.
Corrosion NOS
Multiple corrosion NOS

✓4ᵗʰ **T31**   **Burns classified according to** extent of body surface involved
NOTE   This category is to be used as the primary code only when the site of the burn is unspecified. It should be used as a supplementary code with categories T20-T25 when the site is specified.

    T31.0   **Burns involving** less than 10% **of body surface**   NRS

    ✓5ᵗʰ **T31.1**   **Burns involving** 10-19% **of body surface**

      T31.10   **Burns involving 10-19% of body surface with**   NRS
0% to 9% third degree **burns**
Burns involving 10-19% of body surface NOS

      T31.11   **Burns involving 10-19% of body surface with**   NRS
10-19% third degree **burns**

    ✓5ᵗʰ **T31.2**   **Burns involving** 20-29% **of body surface**

      T31.20   **Burns involving 20-29% of body surface with**   NRS
0% to 9% third degree **burns**
Burns involving 20-29% of body surface NOS

      T31.21   **Burns involving 20-29% of body surface with**   NRS
10-19% third degree **burns**

      T31.22   **Burns involving 20-29% of body surface with**   NRS
20-29% third degree **burns**

    ✓5ᵗʰ **T31.3**   **Burns involving** 30-39% **of body surface**

      T31.30   **Burns involving 30-39% of body surface with**   NRS
0% to 9% third degree **burns**
Burns involving 30-39% of body surface NOS

      T31.31   **Burns involving 30-39% of body surface with**   NRS
10-19% third degree **burns**

      T31.32   **Burns involving 30-39% of body surface with**   NRS
20-29% third degree **burns**

      T31.33   **Burns involving 30-39% of body surface with**   NRS
30-39% third degree **burns**

    ✓5ᵗʰ **T31.4**   **Burns involving** 40-49% **of body surface**

      T31.40   **Burns involving 40-49% of body surface with**   NRS
0% to 9% third degree **burns**
Burns involving 40-49% of body surface NOS

      T31.41   **Burns involving 40-49% of body surface with**   NRS
10-19% third degree **burns**

      T31.42   **Burns involving 40-49% of body surface with**   NRS
20-29% third degree **burns**

      T31.43   **Burns involving 40-49% of body surface with**   NRS
30-39% third degree **burns**

      T31.44   **Burns involving 40-49% of body surface with**   NRS
40-49% third degree **burns**

    ✓5ᵗʰ **T31.5**   **Burns involving** 50-59% o+f **body surface**

      T31.50   **Burns involving 50-59% of body surface with**   NRS
0% to 9% third degree **burns**
Burns involving 50-59% of body surface NOS

      T31.51   **Burns involving 50-59% of body surface with**   NRS
10-19% third degree **burns**

      T31.52   **Burns involving 50-59% of body surface with**   NRS
20-29% third degree **burns**

      T31.53   **Burns involving 50-59% of body surface with**   NRS
30-39% third degree **burns**

      T31.54   **Burns involving 50-59% of body surface with**   NRS
40-49% third degree **burns**

      T31.55   **Burns involving 50-59% of body surface with**   NRS
50-59% third degree **burns**

    ✓5ᵗʰ **T31.6**   **Burns involving** 60-69% **of body surface**

      T31.60   **Burns involving 60-69% of body surface with**   NRS
0% to 9% third degree **burns**
Burns involving 60-69% of body surface NOS

      T31.61   **Burns involving 60-69% of body surface with**   NRS
10-19% third degree **burns**

      T31.62   **Burns involving 60-69% of body surface with**   NRS
20-29% third degree **burns**

      T31.63   **Burns involving 60-69% of body surface with**   NRS
30-39% third degree **burns**

      T31.64   **Burns involving 60-69% of body surface with**   NRS
40-49% third degree **burns**

      T31.65   **Burns involving 60-69% of body surface with**   NRS
50-59% third degree **burns**

      T31.66   **Burns involving 60-69% of body surface with**   NRS
60-69% third degree **burns**

    ✓5ᵗʰ **T31.7**   **Burns involving** 70-79% **of body surface**

      T31.70   **Burns involving 70-79% of body surface with**   NRS
0% to 9% third degree **burns**
Burns involving 70-79% of body surface NOS

      T31.71   **Burns involving 70-79% of body surface with**   NRS
10-19% third degree **burns**

      T31.72   **Burns involving 70-79% of body surface with**   NRS
20-29% third degree **burns**

      T31.73   **Burns involving 70-79% of body surface with**   NRS
30-39% third degree **burns**

      T31.74   **Burns involving 70-79% of body surface with**   NRS
40-49% third degree **burns**

      T31.75   **Burns involving 70-79% of body surface with**   NRS
50-59% third degree **burns**

      T31.76   **Burns involving 70-79% of body surface with**   NRS
60-69% third degree **burns**

      T31.77   **Burns involving 70-79% of body surface with**   NRS
70-79% third degree **burns**

    ✓5ᵗʰ **T31.8**   **Burns involving** 80-89% **of body surface**

      T31.80   **Burns involving 80-89% of body surface with**   NRS
0% to 9% third degree **burns**
Burns involving 80-89% of body surface NOS

      T31.81   **Burns involving 80-89% of body surface with**   NRS
10-19% third degree **burns**

      T31.82   **Burns involving 80-89% of body surface with**   NRS
20-29% third degree **burns**

      T31.83   **Burns involving 80-89% of body surface with**   NRS
30-39% third degree **burns**

      T31.84   **Burns involving 80-89% of body surface with**   NRS
40-49% third degree **burns**

      T31.85   **Burns involving 80-89% of body surface with**   NRS
50-59% third degree **burns**

      T31.86   **Burns involving 80-89% of body surface with**   NRS
60-69% third degree **burns**

      T31.87   **Burns involving 80-89% of body surface with**   NRS
70-79% third degree **burns**

      T31.88   **Burns involving 80-89% of body surface with**   NRS
80-89% third degree **burns**

    ✓5ᵗʰ **T31.9**   **Burns involving** 90% or more **of body surface**

      T31.90   **Burns involving 90% or more of body surface**   NRS
with 0% to 9% third degree **burns**
Burns involving 90% or more of body surface NOS

      T31.91   **Burns involving 90% or more of body surface**   NRS
with 10-19% third degree **burns**

      T31.92   **Burns involving 90% or more of body surface**   NRS
with 20-29% third degree **burns**

      T31.93   **Burns involving 90% or more of body surface**   NRS
with 30-39% third degree **burns**

      T31.94   **Burns involving 90% or more of body surface**   NRS
with 40-49% third degree **burns**

      T31.95   **Burns involving 90% or more of body surface**   NRS
with 50-59% third degree **burns**

      T31.96   **Burns involving 90% or more of body surface**   NRS
with 60-69% third degree **burns**

✓ Additional Character Req   ✓x7ᵗʰ Placeholder Alert   Case-Mix Diagnosis   Manifestation   ▽ Unspecified Dx   **EXCLUDES 1** Not coded here   **EXCLUDES 2** Not included here

T31.97   Burns involving 90% or more of body surface with 70-79% third degree **burns**   NRS

T31.98   Burns involving 90% or more of body surface with 80-89% third degree **burns**   NRS

T31.99   Burns involving 90% or more of body surface with 90% or more third degree **burns**   NRS

✓4th **T32**   Corrosions **classified** according to extent of body surface involved

> NOTE   This category is to be used as the primary code only when the site of the corrosion is unspecified. It may be used as a supplementary code with categories T20-T25 when the site is specified.

T32.0   Corrosions involving less than 10% of body surface   NRS

✓5th **T32.1**   Corrosions involving 10-19% of body surface

    T32.10   Corrosions involving 10-19% of body surface with 0% to 9% third degree **corrosion**   NRS
       Corrosions involving 10-19% of body surface NOS

    T32.11   Corrosions involving 10-19% of body surface with 10-19% third degree **corrosion**   NRS

✓5th **T32.2**   Corrosions involving 20-29% of body surface

    T32.20   Corrosions involving 20-29% of body surface with 0% to 9% third degree **corrosion**   NRS

    T32.21   Corrosions involving 20-29% of body surface with 10-19% third degree **corrosion**   NRS

    T32.22   Corrosions involving 20-29% of body surface with 20-29% third degree **corrosion**   NRS

✓5th **T32.3**   Corrosions involving 30-39% of body surface

    T32.30   Corrosions involving 30-39% of body surface with 0% to 9% third degree **corrosion**   NRS

    T32.31   Corrosions involving 30-39% of body surface with 10-19% third degree **corrosion**   NRS

    T32.32   Corrosions involving 30-39% of body surface with 20-29% third degree **corrosion**   NRS

    T32.33   Corrosions involving 30-39% of body surface with 30-39% third degree **corrosion**   NRS

✓5th **T32.4**   Corrosions involving 40-49% of body surface

    T32.40   Corrosions involving 40-49% of body surface with 0% to 9% third degree **corrosion**   NRS

    T32.41   Corrosions involving 40-49% of body surface with 10-19% third degree **corrosion**   NRS

    T32.42   Corrosions involving 40-49% of body surface with 20-29% third degree **corrosion**   NRS

    T32.43   Corrosions involving 40-49% of body surface with 30-39% third degree **corrosion**   NRS

    T32.44   Corrosions involving 40-49% of body surface with 40-49% third degree **corrosion**   NRS

✓5th **T32.5**   Corrosions involving 50-59% of body surface

    T32.50   Corrosions involving 50-59% of body surface with 0% to 9% third degree **corrosion**   NRS

    T32.51   Corrosions involving 50-59% of body surface with 10-19% third degree **corrosion**   NRS

    T32.52   Corrosions involving 50-59% of body surface with 20-29% third degree **corrosion**   NRS

    T32.53   Corrosions involving 50-59% of body surface with 30-39% third degree **corrosion**   NRS

    T32.54   Corrosions involving 50-59% of body surface with 40-49% third degree **corrosion**   NRS

    T32.55   Corrosions involving 50-59% of body surface with 50-59% third degree **corrosion**   NRS

✓5th **T32.6**   Corrosions involving 60-69% of body surface

    T32.60   Corrosions involving 60-69% of body surface with 0% to 9% third degree **corrosion**   NRS

    T32.61   Corrosions involving 60-69% of body surface with 10-19% third degree **corrosion**   NRS

    T32.62   Corrosions involving 60-69% of body surface with 20-29% third degree **corrosion**   NRS

    T32.63   Corrosions involving 60-69% of body surface with 30-39% third degree **corrosion**   NRS

    T32.64   Corrosions involving 60-69% of body surface with 40-49% third degree **corrosion**   NRS

    T32.65   Corrosions involving 60-69% of body surface with 50-59% third degree **corrosion**   NRS

    T32.66   Corrosions involving 60-69% of body surface with 60-69% third degree **corrosion**   NRS

✓5th **T32.7**   Corrosions involving 70-79% of body surface

    T32.70   Corrosions involving 70-79% of body surface with 0% to 9% third degree **corrosion**   NRS

    T32.71   Corrosions involving 70-79% of body surface with 10-19% third degree **corrosion**   NRS

    T32.72   Corrosions involving 70-79% of body surface with 20-29% third degree **corrosion**   NRS

    T32.73   Corrosions involving 70-79% of body surface with 30-39% third degree **corrosion**   NRS

    T32.74   Corrosions involving 70-79% of body surface with 40-49% third degree **corrosion**   NRS

    T32.75   Corrosions involving 70-79% of body surface with 50-59% third degree **corrosion**   NRS

    T32.76   Corrosions involving 70-79% of body surface with 60-69% third degree **corrosion**   NRS

    T32.77   Corrosions involving 70-79% of body surface with 70-79% third degree **corrosion**   NRS

✓5th **T32.8**   Corrosions involving 80-89% of body surface

    T32.80   Corrosions involving 80-89% of body surface with 0% to 9% third degree **corrosion**   NRS

    T32.81   Corrosions involving 80-89% of body surface with 10-19% third degree **corrosion**   NRS

    T32.82   Corrosions involving 80-89% of body surface with 20-29% third degree **corrosion**   NRS

    T32.83   Corrosions involving 80-89% of body surface with 30-39% third degree **corrosion**   NRS

    T32.84   Corrosions involving 80-89% of body surface with 40-49% third degree **corrosion**   NRS

    T32.85   Corrosions involving 80-89% of body surface with 50-59% third degree **corrosion**   NRS

    T32.86   Corrosions involving 80-89% of body surface with 60-69% third degree **corrosion**   NRS

    T32.87   Corrosions involving 80-89% of body surface with 70-79% third degree **corrosion**   NRS

    T32.88   Corrosions involving 80-89% of body surface with 80-89% third degree **corrosion**   NRS

✓5th **T32.9**   Corrosions involving 90% or more of body surface

    T32.90   Corrosions involving 90% or more of body surface with 0% to 9% third degree **corrosion**   NRS

    T32.91   Corrosions involving 90% or more of body surface with 10-19% third degree **corrosion**   NRS

    T32.92   Corrosions involving 90% or more of body surface with 20-29% third degree **corrosion**   NRS

    T32.93   Corrosions involving 90% or more of body surface with 30-39% third degree **corrosion**   NRS

    T32.94   Corrosions involving 90% or more of body surface with 40-49% third degree **corrosion**   NRS

    T32.95   Corrosions involving 90% or more of body surface with 50-59% third degree **corrosion**   NRS

    T32.96   Corrosions involving 90% or more of body surface with 60-69% third degree **corrosion**   NRS

    T32.97   Corrosions involving 90% or more of body surface with 70-79% third degree **corrosion**   NRS

    T32.98   Corrosions involving 90% or more of body surface with 80-89% third degree **corrosion**   NRS

    T32.99   Corrosions involving 90% or more of body surface with 90% or more third degree **corrosion**   NRS

Frostbite (T33-T34)

EXCLUDES 2   *hypothermia and other effects of reduced temperature (T68, T69-)*

✓4th **T33**   Superficial **frostbite**

> INCLUDES   frostbite with partial thickness skin loss

> The appropriate 7th character is to be added to each code from category T33.
> A   initial encounter
> D   subsequent encounter
> S   sequela

✓5th **T33.0**   Superficial frostbite of head

    ✓6th **T33.01**   Superficial frostbite of ear

       ✓7th **T33.011**   Superficial frostbite of right ear

       ✓7th **T33.012**   Superficial frostbite of left ear

       ✓7th **T33.019**   Superficial frostbite of unspecified ear ▽

    ✓x7th **T33.02**   Superficial frostbite of nose

    ✓x7th **T33.09**   Superficial frostbite of other part of head

---

N Newborn: 0   P Pediatric: 0-17   M Maternity: 12-55   A Adult: 15-124   NRS Nonroutine supply Dx   NCDx Noncancer Dx   PDx Primary Dx   ►◄ Revised Text   ● New Code   ▲ Revised Title

1058   ICD-10-CM 2018

√x7ᵗʰ **T33.1** Superficial frostbite of neck

√x7ᵗʰ **T33.2** Superficial frostbite of thorax

√x7ᵗʰ **T33.3** Superficial frostbite of abdominal wall, lower back and pelvis

√5ᵗʰ **T33.4** Superficial frostbite of arm
> *EXCLUDES 2*   superficial frostbite of wrist and hand (T33.5-)

    √x7ᵗʰ **T33.40** Superficial frostbite of unspecified arm   ▽

    √x7ᵗʰ **T33.41** Superficial frostbite of right arm

    √x7ᵗʰ **T33.42** Superficial frostbite of left arm

√5ᵗʰ **T33.5** Superficial frostbite of wrist, hand, and fingers

    √6ᵗʰ **T33.51** Superficial frostbite of wrist

      √7ᵗʰ **T33.511** Superficial frostbite of right wrist

      √7ᵗʰ **T33.512** Superficial frostbite of left wrist

      √7ᵗʰ **T33.519** Superficial frostbite of unspecified   ▽
                       wrist

    √6ᵗʰ **T33.52** Superficial frostbite of hand
> *EXCLUDES 2*   superficial frostbite of fingers (T33.53-)

      √7ᵗʰ **T33.521** Superficial frostbite of right hand

      √7ᵗʰ **T33.522** Superficial frostbite of left hand

      √7ᵗʰ **T33.529** Superficial frostbite of unspecified   ▽
                       hand

    √6ᵗʰ **T33.53** Superficial frostbite of finger(s)

      √7ᵗʰ **T33.531** Superficial frostbite of right finger(s)

      √7ᵗʰ **T33.532** Superficial frostbite of left finger(s)

      √7ᵗʰ **T33.539** Superficial frostbite of unspecified   ▽
                       finger(s)

√5ᵗʰ **T33.6** Superficial frostbite of hip and thigh

    √x7ᵗʰ **T33.60** Superficial frostbite of unspecified hip and thigh   ▽

    √x7ᵗʰ **T33.61** Superficial frostbite of right hip and thigh

    √x7ᵗʰ **T33.62** Superficial frostbite of left hip and thigh

√5ᵗʰ **T33.7** Superficial frostbite of knee and lower leg
> *EXCLUDES 2*   superficial frostbite of ankle and foot (T33.8-)

    √x7ᵗʰ **T33.70** Superficial frostbite of unspecified knee and   ▽
                  lower leg

    √x7ᵗʰ **T33.71** Superficial frostbite of right knee and lower leg

    √x7ᵗʰ **T33.72** Superficial frostbite of left knee and lower leg

√5ᵗʰ **T33.8** Superficial frostbite of ankle, foot, and toe(s)

    √6ᵗʰ **T33.81** Superficial frostbite of ankle

      √7ᵗʰ **T33.811** Superficial frostbite of right ankle

      √7ᵗʰ **T33.812** Superficial frostbite of left ankle

      √7ᵗʰ **T33.819** Superficial frostbite of unspecified   ▽
                       ankle

    √6ᵗʰ **T33.82** Superficial frostbite of foot

      √7ᵗʰ **T33.821** Superficial frostbite of right foot

      √7ᵗʰ **T33.822** Superficial frostbite of left foot

      √7ᵗʰ **T33.829** Superficial frostbite of unspecified foot ▽

    √6ᵗʰ **T33.83** Superficial frostbite of toe(s)

      √7ᵗʰ **T33.831** Superficial frostbite of right toe(s)

      √7ᵗʰ **T33.832** Superficial frostbite of left toe(s)

      √7ᵗʰ **T33.839** Superficial frostbite of unspecified   ▽
                       toe(s)

√5ᵗʰ **T33.9** Superficial frostbite of other and unspecified sites

    √x7ᵗʰ **T33.90** Superficial frostbite of unspecified sites   ▽
                  Superficial frostbite NOS

    √x7ᵗʰ **T33.99** Superficial frostbite of other sites
                  Superficial frostbite of leg NOS
                  Superficial frostbite of trunk NOS

√4ᵗʰ **T34** **Frostbite with tissue necrosis**

> The appropriate 7th character is to be added to each code from category T34.
> A   initial encounter
> D   subsequent encounter
> S   sequela

√5ᵗʰ **T34.0** Frostbite with tissue necrosis of head

    √6ᵗʰ **T34.01** Frostbite with tissue necrosis of ear

      √7ᵗʰ **T34.011** Frostbite with tissue necrosis of right ear

      √7ᵗʰ **T34.012** Frostbite with tissue necrosis of left ear

      √7ᵗʰ **T34.019** Frostbite with tissue necrosis of   ▽
                       unspecified ear

√x7ᵗʰ **T34.02** Frostbite with tissue necrosis of nose

√x7ᵗʰ **T34.09** Frostbite with tissue necrosis of other part of head

√x7ᵗʰ **T34.1** Frostbite with tissue necrosis of neck

√x7ᵗʰ **T34.2** Frostbite with tissue necrosis of thorax

√x7ᵗʰ **T34.3** Frostbite with tissue necrosis of abdominal wall, lower back and pelvis

√5ᵗʰ **T34.4** Frostbite with tissue necrosis of arm
> *EXCLUDES 2*   frostbite with tissue necrosis of wrist and hand (T34.5-)

    √x7ᵗʰ **T34.40** Frostbite with tissue necrosis of unspecified arm   ▽

    √x7ᵗʰ **T34.41** Frostbite with tissue necrosis of right arm

    √x7ᵗʰ **T34.42** Frostbite with tissue necrosis of left arm

√5ᵗʰ **T34.5** Frostbite with tissue necrosis of wrist, hand, and finger(s)

    √6ᵗʰ **T34.51** Frostbite with tissue necrosis of wrist

      √7ᵗʰ **T34.511** Frostbite with tissue necrosis of right wrist

      √7ᵗʰ **T34.512** Frostbite with tissue necrosis of left wrist

      √7ᵗʰ **T34.519** Frostbite with tissue necrosis of   ▽
                       unspecified wrist

    √6ᵗʰ **T34.52** Frostbite with tissue necrosis of hand
> *EXCLUDES 2*   frostbite with tissue necrosis of finger(s) (T34.53-)

      √7ᵗʰ **T34.521** Frostbite with tissue necrosis of right
                       hand

      √7ᵗʰ **T34.522** Frostbite with tissue necrosis of left hand

      √7ᵗʰ **T34.529** Frostbite with tissue necrosis of   ▽
                       unspecified hand

    √6ᵗʰ **T34.53** Frostbite with tissue necrosis of finger(s)

      √7ᵗʰ **T34.531** Frostbite with tissue necrosis of right
                       finger(s)

      √7ᵗʰ **T34.532** Frostbite with tissue necrosis of left
                       finger(s)

      √7ᵗʰ **T34.539** Frostbite with tissue necrosis of   ▽
                       unspecified finger(s)

√5ᵗʰ **T34.6** Frostbite with tissue necrosis of hip and thigh

    √x7ᵗʰ **T34.60** Frostbite with tissue necrosis of unspecified hip   ▽
                  and thigh

    √x7ᵗʰ **T34.61** Frostbite with tissue necrosis of right hip and thigh

    √x7ᵗʰ **T34.62** Frostbite with tissue necrosis of left hip and thigh

√5ᵗʰ **T34.7** Frostbite with tissue necrosis of knee and lower leg
> *EXCLUDES 2*   frostbite with tissue necrosis of ankle and foot (T34.8-)

    √x7ᵗʰ **T34.70** Frostbite with tissue necrosis of unspecified   ▽
                  knee and lower leg

    √x7ᵗʰ **T34.71** Frostbite with tissue necrosis of right knee and
                  lower leg

    √x7ᵗʰ **T34.72** Frostbite with tissue necrosis of left knee and lower
                  leg

√5ᵗʰ **T34.8** Frostbite with tissue necrosis of ankle, foot, and toe(s)

    √6ᵗʰ **T34.81** Frostbite with tissue necrosis of ankle

      √7ᵗʰ **T34.811** Frostbite with tissue necrosis of right
                       ankle

      √7ᵗʰ **T34.812** Frostbite with tissue necrosis of left ankle

      √7ᵗʰ **T34.819** Frostbite with tissue necrosis of   ▽
                       unspecified ankle

    √6ᵗʰ **T34.82** Frostbite with tissue necrosis of foot

      √7ᵗʰ **T34.821** Frostbite with tissue necrosis of right foot

      √7ᵗʰ **T34.822** Frostbite with tissue necrosis of left foot

      √7ᵗʰ **T34.829** Frostbite with tissue necrosis of   ▽
                       unspecified foot

    √6ᵗʰ **T34.83** Frostbite with tissue necrosis of toe(s)

      √7ᵗʰ **T34.831** Frostbite with tissue necrosis of right
                       toe(s)

      √7ᵗʰ **T34.832** Frostbite with tissue necrosis of left toe(s)

      √7ᵗʰ **T34.839** Frostbite with tissue necrosis of   ▽
                       unspecified toe(s)

√5ᵗʰ **T34.9** Frostbite with tissue necrosis of other and unspecified sites

    √x7ᵗʰ **T34.90** Frostbite with tissue necrosis of unspecified sites ▽
                  Frostbite with tissue necrosis NOS

    √x7ᵗʰ **T34.99** Frostbite with tissue necrosis of other sites
                  Frostbite with tissue necrosis of leg NOS
                  Frostbite with tissue necrosis of trunk NOS

☑ Additional Character Req   √x7ᵗʰ Placeholder Alert   Case-Mix Diagnosis   Manifestation   ▽ Unspecified Dx   *EXCLUDES 1* Not coded here   *EXCLUDES 2* Not included here

Poisoning by, adverse effects of and underdosing of drugs, medicaments and biological substances (T36-T50)

INCLUDES   adverse effect of correct substance properly administered
poisoning by overdose of substance
poisoning by wrong substance given or taken in error
underdosing by (inadvertently) (deliberately) taking less substance than prescribed or instructed

Code first, for adverse effects, the nature of the adverse effect, such as:
adverse effect NOS (T88.7)
aspirin gastritis (K29.-)
blood disorders (D56-D76)
contact dermatitis (L23-L25)
dermatitis due to substances taken internally (L27.-)
nephropathy (N14.0-N14.2)

NOTE   The drug giving rise to the adverse effect should be identified by use of codes from categories T36-T50 with fifth or sixth character 5.

Use additional code(s) to specify:
manifestations of poisoning
underdosing or failure in dosage during medical and surgical care (Y63.6, Y63.8-Y63.9)
underdosing of medication regimen (Z91.12-, Z91.13-)

EXCLUDES 1   *toxic reaction to local anesthesia in pregnancy (O29.3-)*
EXCLUDES 2   *abuse and dependence of psychoactive substances (F10-F19)*
abuse of non-dependence-producing substances (F55.-)
drug reaction and poisoning affecting newborn (P00-P96)
pathological drug intoxication (inebriation) (F10-F19)

AHA: 2016, 2Q, 8; 2015, 3Q, 22
TIP: When the intent of a poisoning is not specified, the intent should be coded as accidental.
TIP: Assign any condition resulting from a poisoning, toxic effect, or adverse effect, followed by the appropriate code from categories T36-T50 while the resulting effects of the poisoning, toxic effect, or adverse effect remains unresolved and requires treatment.

√4ᵗʰ T36   Poisoning by, adverse effect of and underdosing of systemic antibiotics

    EXCLUDES 1   *antineoplastic antibiotics (T45.1-)*
       locally applied antibiotic NEC (T49.0)
       topically used antibiotic for ear, nose and throat (T49.6)
       topically used antibiotic for eye (T49.5)

> The appropriate 7th character is to be added to each code from category T36.
> A   initial encounter
> D   subsequent encounter
> S   sequela

√5ᵗʰ T36.0   Poisoning by, adverse effect of and underdosing of penicillins

   √6ᵗʰ T36.0X   Poisoning by, adverse effect of and underdosing of penicillins

     √7ᵗʰ T36.0X1   Poisoning by penicillins, accidental (unintentional)
        Poisoning by penicillins NOS

     √7ᵗʰ T36.0X2   Poisoning by penicillins, intentional self-harm

     √7ᵗʰ T36.0X3   Poisoning by penicillins, assault

     √7ᵗʰ T36.0X4   Poisoning by penicillins, undetermined

     √7ᵗʰ T36.0X5   Adverse effect of penicillins

     √7ᵗʰ T36.0X6   Underdosing of penicillins

√5ᵗʰ T36.1   Poisoning by, adverse effect of and underdosing of cephalosporins and other beta-lactam antibiotics

   √6ᵗʰ T36.1X   Poisoning by, adverse effect of and underdosing of cephalosporins and other beta-lactam antibiotics

     √7ᵗʰ T36.1X1   Poisoning by cephalosporins and other beta-lactam antibiotics, accidental (unintentional)
        Poisoning by cephalosporins and other beta-lactam antibiotics NOS

     √7ᵗʰ T36.1X2   Poisoning by cephalosporins and other beta-lactam antibiotics, intentional self-harm

     √7ᵗʰ T36.1X3   Poisoning by cephalosporins and other beta-lactam antibiotics, assault

     √7ᵗʰ T36.1X4   Poisoning by cephalosporins and other beta-lactam antibiotics, undetermined

     √7ᵗʰ T36.1X5   Adverse effect of cephalosporins and other beta-lactam antibiotics

     √7ᵗʰ T36.1X6   Underdosing of cephalosporins and other beta-lactam antibiotics

√5ᵗʰ T36.2   Poisoning by, adverse effect of and underdosing of chloramphenicol group

   √6ᵗʰ T36.2X   Poisoning by, adverse effect of and underdosing of chloramphenicol group

     √7ᵗʰ T36.2X1   Poisoning by chloramphenicol group, accidental (unintentional)
        Poisoning by chloramphenicol group NOS

     √7ᵗʰ T36.2X2   Poisoning by chloramphenicol group, intentional self-harm

     √7ᵗʰ T36.2X3   Poisoning by chloramphenicol group, assault

     √7ᵗʰ T36.2X4   Poisoning by chloramphenicol group, undetermined

     √7ᵗʰ T36.2X5   Adverse effect of chloramphenicol group

     √7ᵗʰ T36.2X6   Underdosing of chloramphenicol group

√5ᵗʰ T36.3   Poisoning by, adverse effect of and underdosing of macrolides

   √6ᵗʰ T36.3X   Poisoning by, adverse effect of and underdosing of macrolides

     √7ᵗʰ T36.3X1   Poisoning by macrolides, accidental (unintentional)
        Poisoning by macrolides NOS

     √7ᵗʰ T36.3X2   Poisoning by macrolides, intentional self-harm

     √7ᵗʰ T36.3X3   Poisoning by macrolides, assault

     √7ᵗʰ T36.3X4   Poisoning by macrolides, undetermined

     √7ᵗʰ T36.3X5   Adverse effect of macrolides

     √7ᵗʰ T36.3X6   Underdosing of macrolides

√5ᵗʰ T36.4   Poisoning by, adverse effect of and underdosing of tetracyclines

   √6ᵗʰ T36.4X   Poisoning by, adverse effect of and underdosing of tetracyclines

     √7ᵗʰ T36.4X1   Poisoning by tetracyclines, accidental (unintentional)
        Poisoning by tetracyclines NOS

     √7ᵗʰ T36.4X2   Poisoning by tetracyclines, intentional self-harm

     √7ᵗʰ T36.4X3   Poisoning by tetracyclines, assault

     √7ᵗʰ T36.4X4   Poisoning by tetracyclines, undetermined

     √7ᵗʰ T36.4X5   Adverse effect of tetracyclines

     √7ᵗʰ T36.4X6   Underdosing of tetracyclines

√5ᵗʰ T36.5   Poisoning by, adverse effect of and underdosing of aminoglycosides
     Poisoning by, adverse effect of and underdosing of streptomycin

   √6ᵗʰ T36.5X   Poisoning by, adverse effect of and underdosing of aminoglycosides

     √7ᵗʰ T36.5X1   Poisoning by aminoglycosides, accidental (unintentional)
        Poisoning by aminoglycosides NOS

     √7ᵗʰ T36.5X2   Poisoning by aminoglycosides, intentional self-harm

     √7ᵗʰ T36.5X3   Poisoning by aminoglycosides, assault

     √7ᵗʰ T36.5X4   Poisoning by aminoglycosides, undetermined

     √7ᵗʰ T36.5X5   Adverse effect of aminoglycosides

     √7ᵗʰ T36.5X6   Underdosing of aminoglycosides

√5ᵗʰ T36.6   Poisoning by, adverse effect of and underdosing of rifampicins

   √6ᵗʰ T36.6X   Poisoning by, adverse effect of and underdosing of rifampicins

     √7ᵗʰ T36.6X1   Poisoning by rifampicins, accidental (unintentional)
        Poisoning by rifampicins NOS

     √7ᵗʰ T36.6X2   Poisoning by rifampicins, intentional self-harm

     √7ᵗʰ T36.6X3   Poisoning by rifampicins, assault

     √7ᵗʰ T36.6X4   Poisoning by rifampicins, undetermined

     √7ᵗʰ T36.6X5   Adverse effect of rifampicins

     √7ᵗʰ T36.6X6   Underdosing of rifampicins

✓5ᵗʰ **T36.7** **Poisoning by, adverse effect of and underdosing of antifungal antibiotics, systemically used**

　✓6ᵗʰ **T36.7X** **Poisoning by, adverse effect of and underdosing of antifungal antibiotics, systemically used**

　　✓7ᵗʰ **T36.7X1** **Poisoning by antifungal antibiotics, systemically used, accidental (unintentional)**
　　　　　　　Poisoning by antifungal antibiotics, systemically used NOS

　　✓7ᵗʰ **T36.7X2** **Poisoning by antifungal antibiotics, systemically used, intentional self-harm**

　　✓7ᵗʰ **T36.7X3** **Poisoning by antifungal antibiotics, systemically used, assault**

　　✓7ᵗʰ **T36.7X4** **Poisoning by antifungal antibiotics, systemically used, undetermined**

　　✓7ᵗʰ **T36.7X5** **Adverse effect of antifungal antibiotics, systemically used**

　　✓7ᵗʰ **T36.7X6** **Underdosing of antifungal antibiotics, systemically used**

✓5ᵗʰ **T36.8** **Poisoning by, adverse effect of and underdosing of other systemic antibiotics**

　✓6ᵗʰ **T36.8X** **Poisoning by, adverse effect of and underdosing of other systemic antibiotics**
　　　　　　AHA: 2017, 1Q, 39

　　✓7ᵗʰ **T36.8X1** **Poisoning by other systemic antibiotics, accidental (unintentional)**
　　　　　　　Poisoning by other systemic antibiotics NOS

　　✓7ᵗʰ **T36.8X2** **Poisoning by other systemic antibiotics, intentional self-harm**

　　✓7ᵗʰ **T36.8X3** **Poisoning by other systemic antibiotics, assault**

　　✓7ᵗʰ **T36.8X4** **Poisoning by other systemic antibiotics, undetermined**

　　✓7ᵗʰ **T36.8X5** **Adverse effect of other systemic antibiotics**

　　✓7ᵗʰ **T36.8X6** **Underdosing of other systemic antibiotics**

✓5ᵗʰ **T36.9** **Poisoning by, adverse effect of and underdosing of unspecified systemic antibiotic**

　✓×7ᵗʰ **T36.91** **Poisoning by unspecified systemic antibiotic, accidental (unintentional)** ▽
　　　　　　Poisoning by systemic antibiotic NOS

　✓×7ᵗʰ **T36.92** **Poisoning by unspecified systemic antibiotic, intentional self-harm** ▽

　✓×7ᵗʰ **T36.93** **Poisoning by unspecified systemic antibiotic, assault** ▽

　✓×7ᵗʰ **T36.94** **Poisoning by unspecified systemic antibiotic, undetermined** ▽

　✓×7ᵗʰ **T36.95** **Adverse effect of unspecified systemic antibiotic** ▽

　✓×7ᵗʰ **T36.96** **Underdosing of unspecified systemic antibiotic** ▽

✓4ᵗʰ **T37** **Poisoning by, adverse effect of and underdosing of other systemic anti- infectives and antiparasitics**
　　　EXCLUDES 1　_anti-infectives topically used for ear, nose and throat (T49.6-)_
　　　　　　anti-infectives topically used for eye (T49.5-)
　　　　　　locally applied anti-infectives NEC (T49.0-)

　The appropriate 7th character is to be added to each code from category T37.
　A　initial encounter
　D　subsequent encounter
　S　sequela

✓5ᵗʰ **T37.0** **Poisoning by, adverse effect of and underdosing of sulfonamides**

　✓6ᵗʰ **T37.0X** **Poisoning by, adverse effect of and underdosing of sulfonamides**

　　✓7ᵗʰ **T37.0X1** **Poisoning by sulfonamides, accidental (unintentional)**
　　　　　　　Poisoning by sulfonamides NOS

　　✓7ᵗʰ **T37.0X2** **Poisoning by sulfonamides, intentional self-harm**

　　✓7ᵗʰ **T37.0X3** **Poisoning by sulfonamides, assault**

　　✓7ᵗʰ **T37.0X4** **Poisoning by sulfonamides, undetermined**

　　✓7ᵗʰ **T37.0X5** **Adverse effect of sulfonamides**

　　✓7ᵗʰ **T37.0X6** **Underdosing of sulfonamides**

✓5ᵗʰ **T37.1** **Poisoning by, adverse effect of and underdosing of antimycobacterial drugs**
　　　EXCLUDES 1　_rifampicins (T36.6-)_
　　　　　　streptomycin (T36.5-)

　✓6ᵗʰ **T37.1X** **Poisoning by, adverse effect of and underdosing of antimycobacterial drugs**

　　✓7ᵗʰ **T37.1X1** **Poisoning by antimycobacterial drugs, accidental (unintentional)**
　　　　　　　Poisoning by antimycobacterial drugs NOS

　　✓7ᵗʰ **T37.1X2** **Poisoning by antimycobacterial drugs, intentional self-harm**

　　✓7ᵗʰ **T37.1X3** **Poisoning by antimycobacterial drugs, assault**

　　✓7ᵗʰ **T37.1X4** **Poisoning by antimycobacterial drugs, undetermined**

　　✓7ᵗʰ **T37.1X5** **Adverse effect of antimycobacterial drugs**

　　✓7ᵗʰ **T37.1X6** **Underdosing of antimycobacterial drugs**

✓5ᵗʰ **T37.2** **Poisoning by, adverse effect of and underdosing of antimalarials and drugs acting on other blood protozoa**
　　　EXCLUDES 1　_hydroxyquinoline derivatives (T37.8-)_

　✓6ᵗʰ **T37.2X** **Poisoning by, adverse effect of and underdosing of antimalarials and drugs acting on other blood protozoa**

　　✓7ᵗʰ **T37.2X1** **Poisoning by antimalarials and drugs acting on other blood protozoa, accidental (unintentional)**
　　　　　　　Poisoning by antimalarials and drugs acting on other blood protozoa NOS

　　✓7ᵗʰ **T37.2X2** **Poisoning by antimalarials and drugs acting on other blood protozoa, intentional self-harm**

　　✓7ᵗʰ **T37.2X3** **Poisoning by antimalarials and drugs acting on other blood protozoa, assault**

　　✓7ᵗʰ **T37.2X4** **Poisoning by antimalarials and drugs acting on other blood protozoa, undetermined**

　　✓7ᵗʰ **T37.2X5** **Adverse effect of antimalarials and drugs acting on other blood protozoa**

　　✓7ᵗʰ **T37.2X6** **Underdosing of antimalarials and drugs acting on other blood protozoa**

✓5ᵗʰ **T37.3** **Poisoning by, adverse effect of and underdosing of other antiprotozoal drugs**

　✓6ᵗʰ **T37.3X** **Poisoning by, adverse effect of and underdosing of other antiprotozoal drugs**

　　✓7ᵗʰ **T37.3X1** **Poisoning by other antiprotozoal drugs, accidental (unintentional)**
　　　　　　　Poisoning by other antiprotozoal drugs NOS

　　✓7ᵗʰ **T37.3X2** **Poisoning by other antiprotozoal drugs, intentional self-harm**

　　✓7ᵗʰ **T37.3X3** **Poisoning by other antiprotozoal drugs, assault**

　　✓7ᵗʰ **T37.3X4** **Poisoning by other antiprotozoal drugs, undetermined**

　　✓7ᵗʰ **T37.3X5** **Adverse effect of other antiprotozoal drugs**

　　✓7ᵗʰ **T37.3X6** **Underdosing of other antiprotozoal drugs**

✓5ᵗʰ **T37.4** **Poisoning by, adverse effect of and underdosing of anthelminthics**

　✓6ᵗʰ **T37.4X** **Poisoning by, adverse effect of and underdosing of anthelminthics**

　　✓7ᵗʰ **T37.4X1** **Poisoning by anthelminthics, accidental (unintentional)**
　　　　　　　Poisoning by anthelminthics NOS

　　✓7ᵗʰ **T37.4X2** **Poisoning by anthelminthics, intentional self-harm**

　　✓7ᵗʰ **T37.4X3** **Poisoning by anthelminthics, assault**

　　✓7ᵗʰ **T37.4X4** **Poisoning by anthelminthics, undetermined**

　　✓7ᵗʰ **T37.4X5** **Adverse effect of anthelminthics**

　　✓7ᵗʰ **T37.4X6** **Underdosing of anthelminthics**

✓ Additional Character Req　✓×7ᵗʰ Placeholder Alert　Case-Mix Diagnosis　Manifestation　▽ Unspecified Dx　_EXCLUDES 1_ Not coded here　_EXCLUDES 2_ Not included here

ICD-10-CM 2018

1061

✓5ᵗʰ **T37.5** **Poisoning by, adverse effect of and underdosing of antiviral drugs**
   EXCLUDES 1   amantadine (T42.8-)
              cytarabine (T45.1-)

   ✓6ᵗʰ **T37.5X** **Poisoning by, adverse effect of and underdosing of antiviral drugs**

     ✓7ᵗʰ **T37.5X1** **Poisoning by antiviral drugs, accidental (unintentional)**
            Poisoning by antiviral drugs NOS

     ✓7ᵗʰ **T37.5X2** **Poisoning by antiviral drugs, intentional self-harm**

     ✓7ᵗʰ **T37.5X3** **Poisoning by antiviral drugs, assault**

     ✓7ᵗʰ **T37.5X4** **Poisoning by antiviral drugs, undetermined**

     ✓7ᵗʰ **T37.5X5** **Adverse effect of antiviral drugs**

     ✓7ᵗʰ **T37.5X6** **Underdosing of antiviral drugs**

✓5ᵗʰ **T37.8** **Poisoning by, adverse effect of and underdosing of other specified systemic anti-infectives and antiparasitics**
     Poisoning by, adverse effect of and underdosing of hydroxyquinoline derivatives
   EXCLUDES 1   antimalarial drugs (T37.2-)

   ✓6ᵗʰ **T37.8X** **Poisoning by, adverse effect of and underdosing of other specified systemic anti-infectives and antiparasitics**

     ✓7ᵗʰ **T37.8X1** **Poisoning by other specified systemic anti-infectives and antiparasitics, accidental (unintentional)**
            Poisoning by other specified systemic anti-infectives and antiparasitics NOS

     ✓7ᵗʰ **T37.8X2** **Poisoning by other specified systemic anti-infectives and antiparasitics, intentional self-harm**

     ✓7ᵗʰ **T37.8X3** **Poisoning by other specified systemic anti-infectives and antiparasitics, assault**

     ✓7ᵗʰ **T37.8X4** **Poisoning by other specified systemic anti-infectives and antiparasitics, undetermined**

     ✓7ᵗʰ **T37.8X5** **Adverse effect of other specified systemic anti-infectives and antiparasitics**

     ✓7ᵗʰ **T37.8X6** **Underdosing of other specified systemic anti-infectives and antiparasitics**

✓5ᵗʰ **T37.9** **Poisoning by, adverse effect of and underdosing of unspecified systemic anti-infective and antiparasitics**

   ✓x7ᵗʰ **T37.91** **Poisoning by unspecified systemic anti-infective and antiparasitics, accidental (unintentional)** ▽
     Poisoning by, adverse effect of and underdosing of systemic anti-infective and antiparasitics NOS

   ✓x7ᵗʰ **T37.92** **Poisoning by unspecified systemic anti-infective and antiparasitics, intentional self-harm** ▽

   ✓x7ᵗʰ **T37.93** **Poisoning by unspecified systemic anti-infective and antiparasitics, assault** ▽

   ✓x7ᵗʰ **T37.94** **Poisoning by unspecified systemic anti-infective and antiparasitics, undetermined** ▽

   ✓x7ᵗʰ **T37.95** **Adverse effect of unspecified systemic anti-infective and antiparasitic** ▽

   ✓x7ᵗʰ **T37.96** **Underdosing of unspecified systemic anti-infectives and antiparasitics** ▽

✓4ᵗʰ **T38** **Poisoning by, adverse effect of and underdosing of hormones and their synthetic substitutes and antagonists, not elsewhere classified**
   EXCLUDES 1   mineralocorticoids and their antagonists (T50.0-)
              oxytocic hormones (T48.0-)
              parathyroid hormones and derivatives (T50.9-)

> The appropriate 7th character is to be added to each code from category T38.
> A   initial encounter
> D   subsequent encounter
> S   sequela

   ✓5ᵗʰ **T38.0** **Poisoning by, adverse effect of and underdosing of glucocorticoids and synthetic analogues**
     EXCLUDES 1   glucocorticoids, topically used (T49.-)

     ✓6ᵗʰ **T38.0X** **Poisoning by, adverse effect of and underdosing of glucocorticoids and synthetic analogues**

     ✓7ᵗʰ **T38.0X1** **Poisoning by glucocorticoids and synthetic analogues, accidental (unintentional)**
            Poisoning by glucocorticoids and synthetic analogues NOS

     ✓7ᵗʰ **T38.0X2** **Poisoning by glucocorticoids and synthetic analogues, intentional self-harm**

     ✓7ᵗʰ **T38.0X3** **Poisoning by glucocorticoids and synthetic analogues, assault**

     ✓7ᵗʰ **T38.0X4** **Poisoning by glucocorticoids and synthetic analogues, undetermined**

     ✓7ᵗʰ **T38.0X5** **Adverse effect of glucocorticoids and synthetic analogues**

     ✓7ᵗʰ **T38.0X6** **Underdosing of glucocorticoids and synthetic analogues**

   ✓5ᵗʰ **T38.1** **Poisoning by, adverse effect of and underdosing of thyroid hormones and substitutes**

     ✓6ᵗʰ **T38.1X** **Poisoning by, adverse effect of and underdosing of thyroid hormones and substitutes**

     ✓7ᵗʰ **T38.1X1** **Poisoning by thyroid hormones and substitutes, accidental (unintentional)**
            Poisoning by thyroid hormones and substitutes NOS

     ✓7ᵗʰ **T38.1X2** **Poisoning by thyroid hormones and substitutes, intentional self-harm**

     ✓7ᵗʰ **T38.1X3** **Poisoning by thyroid hormones and substitutes, assault**

     ✓7ᵗʰ **T38.1X4** **Poisoning by thyroid hormones and substitutes, undetermined**

     ✓7ᵗʰ **T38.1X5** **Adverse effect of thyroid hormones and substitutes**

     ✓7ᵗʰ **T38.1X6** **Underdosing of thyroid hormones and substitutes**

   ✓5ᵗʰ **T38.2** **Poisoning by, adverse effect of and underdosing of antithyroid drugs**

     ✓6ᵗʰ **T38.2X** **Poisoning by, adverse effect of and underdosing of antithyroid drugs**

     ✓7ᵗʰ **T38.2X1** **Poisoning by antithyroid drugs, accidental (unintentional)**
            Poisoning by antithyroid drugs NOS

     ✓7ᵗʰ **T38.2X2** **Poisoning by antithyroid drugs, intentional self-harm**

     ✓7ᵗʰ **T38.2X3** **Poisoning by antithyroid drugs, assault**

     ✓7ᵗʰ **T38.2X4** **Poisoning by antithyroid drugs, undetermined**

     ✓7ᵗʰ **T38.2X5** **Adverse effect of antithyroid drugs**

     ✓7ᵗʰ **T38.2X6** **Underdosing of antithyroid drugs**

   ✓5ᵗʰ **T38.3** **Poisoning by, adverse effect of and underdosing of insulin and oral hypoglycemic [antidiabetic] drugs**

     ✓6ᵗʰ **T38.3X** **Poisoning by, adverse effect of and underdosing of insulin and oral hypoglycemic [antidiabetic] drugs**

     ✓7ᵗʰ **T38.3X1** **Poisoning by insulin and oral hypoglycemic [antidiabetic] drugs, accidental (unintentional)**
            Poisoning by insulin and oral hypoglycemic [antidiabetic] drugs NOS

     ✓7ᵗʰ **T38.3X2** **Poisoning by insulin and oral hypoglycemic [antidiabetic] drugs, intentional self-harm**

     ✓7ᵗʰ **T38.3X3** **Poisoning by insulin and oral hypoglycemic [antidiabetic] drugs, assault**

     ✓7ᵗʰ **T38.3X4** **Poisoning by insulin and oral hypoglycemic [antidiabetic] drugs, undetermined**

     ✓7ᵗʰ **T38.3X5** **Adverse effect of insulin and oral hypoglycemic [antidiabetic] drugs**

     ✓7ᵗʰ **T38.3X6** **Underdosing of insulin and oral hypoglycemic [antidiabetic] drugs**

   ✓5ᵗʰ **T38.4** **Poisoning by, adverse effect of and underdosing of oral contraceptives**
     Poisoning by, adverse effect of and underdosing of multiple- and single-ingredient oral contraceptive preparations

     ✓6ᵗʰ **T38.4X** **Poisoning by, adverse effect of and underdosing of oral contraceptives**

     ✓7ᵗʰ **T38.4X1** **Poisoning by oral contraceptives, accidental (unintentional)**
            Poisoning by oral contraceptives NOS

✓7th **T38.4X2** Poisoning by oral contraceptives, intentional self-harm

✓7th **T38.4X3** Poisoning by oral contraceptives, assault

✓7th **T38.4X4** Poisoning by oral contraceptives, undetermined

✓7th **T38.4X5** Adverse effect of oral contraceptives

✓7th **T38.4X6** Underdosing of oral contraceptives

✓5th **T38.5** Poisoning by, adverse effect of and underdosing of other estrogens and progestogens

Poisoning by, adverse effect of and underdosing of estrogens and progestogens mixtures and substitutes

  ✓6th **T38.5X** Poisoning by, adverse effect of and underdosing of other estrogens and progestogens

    ✓7th **T38.5X1** Poisoning by other estrogens and progestogens, accidental (unintentional)

Poisoning by other estrogens and progestogens NOS

    ✓7th **T38.5X2** Poisoning by other estrogens and progestogens, intentional self-harm

    ✓7th **T38.5X3** Poisoning by other estrogens and progestogens, assault

    ✓7th **T38.5X4** Poisoning by other estrogens and progestogens, undetermined

    ✓7th **T38.5X5** Adverse effect of other estrogens and progestogens

    ✓7th **T38.5X6** Underdosing of other estrogens and progestogens

✓5th **T38.6** Poisoning by, adverse effect of and underdosing of antigonadotrophins, antiestrogens, antiandrogens, not elsewhere classified

Poisoning by, adverse effect of and underdosing of tamoxifen

  ✓6th **T38.6X** Poisoning by, adverse effect of and underdosing of antigonadotrophins, antiestrogens, antiandrogens, not elsewhere classified

    ✓7th **T38.6X1** Poisoning by antigonadotrophins, antiestrogens, antiandrogens, not elsewhere classified, accidental (unintentional)

Poisoning by antigonadotrophins, antiestrogens, antiandrogens, not elsewhere classified NOS

    ✓7th **T38.6X2** Poisoning by antigonadotrophins, antiestrogens, antiandrogens, not elsewhere classified, intentional self-harm

    ✓7th **T38.6X3** Poisoning by antigonadotrophins, antiestrogens, antiandrogens, not elsewhere classified, assault

    ✓7th **T38.6X4** Poisoning by antigonadotrophins, antiestrogens, antiandrogens, not elsewhere classified, undetermined

    ✓7th **T38.6X5** Adverse effect of antigonadotrophins, antiestrogens, antiandrogens, not elsewhere classified

    ✓7th **T38.6X6** Underdosing of antigonadotrophins, antiestrogens, antiandrogens, not elsewhere classified

✓5th **T38.7** Poisoning by, adverse effect of and underdosing of androgens and anabolic congeners

  ✓6th **T38.7X** Poisoning by, adverse effect of and underdosing of androgens and anabolic congeners

    ✓7th **T38.7X1** Poisoning by androgens and anabolic congeners, accidental (unintentional)

Poisoning by androgens and anabolic congeners NOS

    ✓7th **T38.7X2** Poisoning by androgens and anabolic congeners, intentional self-harm

    ✓7th **T38.7X3** Poisoning by androgens and anabolic congeners, assault

    ✓7th **T38.7X4** Poisoning by androgens and anabolic congeners, undetermined

    ✓7th **T38.7X5** Adverse effect of androgens and anabolic congeners

    ✓7th **T38.7X6** Underdosing of androgens and anabolic congeners

✓5th **T38.8** Poisoning by, adverse effect of and underdosing of other and unspecified hormones and synthetic substitutes

  ✓6th **T38.80** Poisoning by, adverse effect of and underdosing of unspecified hormones and synthetic substitutes

    ✓7th **T38.801** Poisoning by unspecified hormones and synthetic substitutes, accidental (unintentional) ▽

Poisoning by unspecified hormones and synthetic substitutes NOS

    ✓7th **T38.802** Poisoning by unspecified hormones and synthetic substitutes, intentional self-harm ▽

    ✓7th **T38.803** Poisoning by unspecified hormones and synthetic substitutes, assault ▽

    ✓7th **T38.804** Poisoning by unspecified hormones and synthetic substitutes, undetermined ▽

    ✓7th **T38.805** Adverse effect of unspecified hormones and synthetic substitutes ▽

    ✓7th **T38.806** Underdosing of unspecified hormones and synthetic substitutes ▽

  ✓6th **T38.81** Poisoning by, adverse effect of and underdosing of anterior pituitary [adenohypophyseal] hormones

    ✓7th **T38.811** Poisoning by anterior pituitary [adenohypophyseal] hormones, accidental (unintentional)

Poisoning by anterior pituitary [adenohypophyseal] hormones NOS

    ✓7th **T38.812** Poisoning by anterior pituitary [adenohypophyseal] hormones, intentional self-harm

    ✓7th **T38.813** Poisoning by anterior pituitary [adenohypophyseal] hormones, assault

    ✓7th **T38.814** Poisoning by anterior pituitary [adenohypophyseal] hormones, undetermined

    ✓7th **T38.815** Adverse effect of anterior pituitary [adenohypophyseal] hormones

    ✓7th **T38.816** Underdosing of anterior pituitary [adenohypophyseal] hormones

  ✓6th **T38.89** Poisoning by, adverse effect of and underdosing of other hormones and synthetic substitutes

    ✓7th **T38.891** Poisoning by other hormones and synthetic substitutes, accidental (unintentional)

Poisoning by other hormones and synthetic substitutes NOS

    ✓7th **T38.892** Poisoning by other hormones and synthetic substitutes, intentional self-harm

    ✓7th **T38.893** Poisoning by other hormones and synthetic substitutes, assault

    ✓7th **T38.894** Poisoning by other hormones and synthetic substitutes, undetermined

    ✓7th **T38.895** Adverse effect of other hormones and synthetic substitutes

    ✓7th **T38.896** Underdosing of other hormones and synthetic substitutes

✓5th **T38.9** Poisoning by, adverse effect of and underdosing of other and unspecified hormone antagonists

  ✓6th **T38.90** Poisoning by, adverse effect of and underdosing of unspecified hormone antagonists

    ✓7th **T38.901** Poisoning by unspecified hormone antagonists, accidental (unintentional) ▽

Poisoning by unspecified hormone antagonists NOS

    ✓7th **T38.902** Poisoning by unspecified hormone antagonists, intentional self-harm ▽

    ✓7th **T38.903** Poisoning by unspecified hormone antagonists, assault ▽

    ✓7th **T38.904** Poisoning by unspecified hormone antagonists, undetermined ▽

    ✓7th **T38.905** Adverse effect of unspecified hormone antagonists ▽

    ✓7th **T38.906** Underdosing of unspecified hormone antagonists ▽

✓ Additional Character Req   ✓x7th Placeholder Alert   Case-Mix Diagnosis   Manifestation   ▽ Unspecified Dx   EXCLUDES 1 Not coded here   EXCLUDES 2 Not included here

ICD-10-CM 2018   1063

☑6ᵗʰ T38.99 Poisoning by, adverse effect of and underdosing of other hormone antagonists

    ☑7ᵗʰ **T38.991 Poisoning by other hormone antagonists, accidental (unintentional)**
        Poisoning by other hormone antagonists NOS

    ☑7ᵗʰ **T38.992 Poisoning by other hormone antagonists, intentional self-harm**

    ☑7ᵗʰ **T38.993 Poisoning by other hormone antagonists, assault**

    ☑7ᵗʰ **T38.994 Poisoning by other hormone antagonists, undetermined**

    ☑7ᵗʰ **T38.995 Adverse effect of other hormone antagonists**

    ☑7ᵗʰ **T38.996 Underdosing of other hormone antagonists**

☑4ᵗʰ T39 Poisoning by, adverse effect of and underdosing of nonopioid analgesics, antipyretics and antirheumatics

> The appropriate 7th character is to be added to each code from category T39.
> A   initial encounter
> D   subsequent encounter
> S   sequela

☑5ᵗʰ T39.0 Poisoning by, adverse effect of and underdosing of salicylates

    ☑6ᵗʰ T39.01 Poisoning by, adverse effect of and underdosing of aspirin
        Poisoning by, adverse effect of and underdosing of acetylsalicylic acid

        ☑7ᵗʰ **T39.011 Poisoning by aspirin, accidental (unintentional)**

        ☑7ᵗʰ **T39.012 Poisoning by aspirin, intentional self-harm**

        ☑7ᵗʰ **T39.013 Poisoning by aspirin, assault**

        ☑7ᵗʰ **T39.014 Poisoning by aspirin, undetermined**

        ☑7ᵗʰ **T39.015 Adverse effect of aspirin**
            AHA: 2016, 1Q, 15

        ☑7ᵗʰ **T39.016 Underdosing of aspirin**

    ☑6ᵗʰ T39.09 Poisoning by, adverse effect of and underdosing of other salicylates

        ☑7ᵗʰ **T39.091 Poisoning by salicylates, accidental (unintentional)**
            Poisoning by salicylates NOS

        ☑7ᵗʰ **T39.092 Poisoning by salicylates, intentional self-harm**

        ☑7ᵗʰ **T39.093 Poisoning by salicylates, assault**

        ☑7ᵗʰ **T39.094 Poisoning by salicylates, undetermined**

        ☑7ᵗʰ **T39.095 Adverse effect of salicylates**

        ☑7ᵗʰ **T39.096 Underdosing of salicylates**

☑5ᵗʰ T39.1 Poisoning by, adverse effect of and underdosing of 4-Aminophenol derivatives

    ☑6ᵗʰ T39.1X Poisoning by, adverse effect of and underdosing of 4-Aminophenol derivatives

        ☑7ᵗʰ **T39.1X1 Poisoning by 4-Aminophenol derivatives, accidental (unintentional)**
            Poisoning by 4-Aminophenol derivatives NOS

        ☑7ᵗʰ **T39.1X2 Poisoning by 4-Aminophenol derivatives, intentional self-harm**

        ☑7ᵗʰ **T39.1X3 Poisoning by 4-Aminophenol derivatives, assault**

        ☑7ᵗʰ **T39.1X4 Poisoning by 4-Aminophenol derivatives, undetermined**

        ☑7ᵗʰ **T39.1X5 Adverse effect of 4-Aminophenol derivatives**

        ☑7ᵗʰ **T39.1X6 Underdosing of 4-Aminophenol derivatives**

☑5ᵗʰ T39.2 Poisoning by, adverse effect of and underdosing of pyrazolone derivatives

    ☑6ᵗʰ T39.2X Poisoning by, adverse effect of and underdosing of pyrazolone derivatives

        ☑7ᵗʰ **T39.2X1 Poisoning by pyrazolone derivatives, accidental (unintentional)**
            Poisoning by pyrazolone derivatives NOS

        ☑7ᵗʰ **T39.2X2 Poisoning by pyrazolone derivatives, intentional self-harm**

        ☑7ᵗʰ **T39.2X3 Poisoning by pyrazolone derivatives, assault**

        ☑7ᵗʰ **T39.2X4 Poisoning by pyrazolone derivatives, undetermined**

        ☑7ᵗʰ **T39.2X5 Adverse effect of pyrazolone derivatives**

        ☑7ᵗʰ **T39.2X6 Underdosing of pyrazolone derivatives**

☑5ᵗʰ T39.3 Poisoning by, adverse effect of and underdosing of other nonsteroidal anti-inflammatory drugs [NSAID]

    ☑6ᵗʰ T39.31 Poisoning by, adverse effect of and underdosing of propionic acid derivatives
        Poisoning by, adverse effect of and underdosing of fenoprofen
        Poisoning by, adverse effect of and underdosing of flurbiprofen
        Poisoning by, adverse effect of and underdosing of ibuprofen
        Poisoning by, adverse effect of and underdosing of ketoprofen
        Poisoning by, adverse effect of and underdosing of naproxen
        Poisoning by, adverse effect of and underdosing of oxaprozin

        ☑7ᵗʰ **T39.311 Poisoning by propionic acid derivatives, accidental (unintentional)**

        ☑7ᵗʰ **T39.312 Poisoning by propionic acid derivatives, intentional self-harm**

        ☑7ᵗʰ **T39.313 Poisoning by propionic acid derivatives, assault**

        ☑7ᵗʰ **T39.314 Poisoning by propionic acid derivatives, undetermined**

        ☑7ᵗʰ **T39.315 Adverse effect of propionic acid derivatives**

        ☑7ᵗʰ **T39.316 Underdosing of propionic acid derivatives**

    ☑6ᵗʰ T39.39 Poisoning by, adverse effect of and underdosing of other nonsteroidal anti-inflammatory drugs [NSAID]

        ☑7ᵗʰ **T39.391 Poisoning by other nonsteroidal anti-inflammatory drugs [NSAID], accidental (unintentional)**
            Poisoning by other nonsteroidal anti-inflammatory drugs NOS

        ☑7ᵗʰ **T39.392 Poisoning by other nonsteroidal anti-inflammatory drugs [NSAID], intentional self-harm**

        ☑7ᵗʰ **T39.393 Poisoning by other nonsteroidal anti-inflammatory drugs [NSAID], assault**

        ☑7ᵗʰ **T39.394 Poisoning by other nonsteroidal anti-inflammatory drugs [NSAID], undetermined**

        ☑7ᵗʰ **T39.395 Adverse effect of other nonsteroidal anti-inflammatory drugs [NSAID]**

        ☑7ᵗʰ **T39.396 Underdosing of other nonsteroidal anti-inflammatory drugs [NSAID]**

☑5ᵗʰ T39.4 Poisoning by, adverse effect of and underdosing of antirheumatics, not elsewhere classified

> **EXCLUDES 1**   poisoning by, adverse effect of and underdosing of glucocorticoids (T38.0-)
> poisoning by, adverse effect of and underdosing of salicylates (T39.0-)

    ☑6ᵗʰ T39.4X Poisoning by, adverse effect of and underdosing of antirheumatics, not elsewhere classified

        ☑7ᵗʰ **T39.4X1 Poisoning by antirheumatics, not elsewhere classified, accidental (unintentional)**
            Poisoning by antirheumatics, not elsewhere classified NOS

        ☑7ᵗʰ **T39.4X2 Poisoning by antirheumatics, not elsewhere classified, intentional self-harm**

        ☑7ᵗʰ **T39.4X3 Poisoning by antirheumatics, not elsewhere classified, assault**

        ☑7ᵗʰ **T39.4X4 Poisoning by antirheumatics, not elsewhere classified, undetermined**

        ☑7ᵗʰ **T39.4X5 Adverse effect of antirheumatics, not elsewhere classified**

        ☑7ᵗʰ **T39.4X6 Underdosing of antirheumatics, not elsewhere classified**

Ⓝ Newborn: 0   Ⓟ Pediatric: 0-17   Ⓜ Maternity: 12-55   Ⓐ Adult: 15-124   **NRS** Nonroutine supply Dx   **NC Dx** Noncancer Dx   **PDx** Primary Dx   ►◄ Revised Text   ● New Code   ▲ Revised Title

1064   ICD-10-CM 2018

☑5ᵗʰ **T39.8** **Poisoning by, adverse effect of and underdosing of other nonopioid analgesics and antipyretics, not elsewhere classified**

  ☑6ᵗʰ **T39.8X** **Poisoning by, adverse effect of and underdosing of** other nonopioid analgesics and antipyretics, **not elsewhere classified**

    ☑7ᵗʰ **T39.8X1** **Poisoning by other nonopioid analgesics and antipyretics, not elsewhere classified,** accidental (unintentional)
      Poisoning by other nonopioid analgesics and antipyretics, not elsewhere classified NOS

    ☑7ᵗʰ **T39.8X2** **Poisoning by other nonopioid analgesics and antipyretics, not elsewhere classified,** intentional self-harm

    ☑7ᵗʰ **T39.8X3** **Poisoning by other nonopioid analgesics and antipyretics, not elsewhere classified,** assault

    ☑7ᵗʰ **T39.8X4** **Poisoning by other nonopioid analgesics and antipyretics, not elsewhere classified,** undetermined

    ☑7ᵗʰ **T39.8X5** Adverse effect **of other nonopioid analgesics and antipyretics, not elsewhere classified**

    ☑7ᵗʰ **T39.8X6** Underdosing **of other nonopioid analgesics and antipyretics, not elsewhere classified**

☑5ᵗʰ **T39.9** **Poisoning by, adverse effect of and underdosing of** unspecified nonopioid analgesic, antipyretic and antirheumatic

  ☑x7ᵗʰ **T39.91** **Poisoning by unspecified nonopioid analgesic, antipyretic and antirheumatic,** accidental (unintentional)   ▽
    Poisoning by nonopioid analgesic, antipyretic and antirheumatic NOS

  ☑x7ᵗʰ **T39.92** **Poisoning by unspecified nonopioid analgesic, antipyretic and antirheumatic,** intentional self-harm   ▽

  ☑x7ᵗʰ **T39.93** **Poisoning by unspecified nonopioid analgesic, antipyretic and antirheumatic,** assault   ▽

  ☑x7ᵗʰ **T39.94** **Poisoning by unspecified nonopioid analgesic, antipyretic and antirheumatic,** undetermined   ▽

  ☑x7ᵗʰ **T39.95** Adverse effect **of unspecified nonopioid analgesic, antipyretic and antirheumatic**   ▽

  ☑x7ᵗʰ **T39.96** Underdosing **of unspecified nonopioid analgesic, antipyretic and antirheumatic**   ▽

☑4ᵗʰ **T40** **Poisoning by, adverse effect of and underdosing of narcotics and psychodysleptics [hallucinogens]**

  EXCLUDES 2 *drug dependence and related mental and behavioral disorders due to psychoactive substance use (F10-F19-)*

  The appropriate 7th character is to be added to each code from category T40.
  A   initial encounter
  D   subsequent encounter
  S   sequela

☑5ᵗʰ **T40.0** **Poisoning by, adverse effect of and underdosing of opium**

  ☑6ᵗʰ **T40.0X** **Poisoning by, adverse effect of and underdosing of** opium

    ☑7ᵗʰ **T40.0X1** **Poisoning by opium,** accidental (unintentional)
      Poisoning by opium NOS

    ☑7ᵗʰ **T40.0X2** **Poisoning by opium,** intentional self-harm

    ☑7ᵗʰ **T40.0X3** **Poisoning by opium,** assault

    ☑7ᵗʰ **T40.0X4** **Poisoning by opium,** undetermined

    ☑7ᵗʰ **T40.0X5** Adverse effect **of opium**

    ☑7ᵗʰ **T40.0X6** Underdosing **of opium**

☑5ᵗʰ **T40.1** **Poisoning by and adverse effect of** heroin

  ☑6ᵗʰ **T40.1X** **Poisoning by and adverse effect of heroin**

    ☑7ᵗʰ **T40.1X1** **Poisoning by heroin,** accidental (unintentional)
      Poisoning by heroin NOS

    ☑7ᵗʰ **T40.1X2** **Poisoning by heroin,** intentional self-harm

    ☑7ᵗʰ **T40.1X3** **Poisoning by heroin,** assault

    ☑7ᵗʰ **T40.1X4** **Poisoning by heroin,** undetermined

☑5ᵗʰ **T40.2** **Poisoning by, adverse effect of and underdosing of other opioids**

  ☑6ᵗʰ **T40.2X** **Poisoning by, adverse effect of and underdosing of** other opioids

    ☑7ᵗʰ **T40.2X1** **Poisoning by other opioids,** accidental (unintentional)
      Poisoning by other opioids NOS

    ☑7ᵗʰ **T40.2X2** **Poisoning by other opioids,** intentional self-harm

    ☑7ᵗʰ **T40.2X3** **Poisoning by other opioids,** assault
    ☑7ᵗʰ **T40.2X4** **Poisoning by other opioids,** undetermined
    ☑7ᵗʰ **T40.2X5** Adverse effect **of other opioids**
    ☑7ᵗʰ **T40.2X6** Underdosing **of other opioids**

☑5ᵗʰ **T40.3** **Poisoning by, adverse effect of and underdosing of methadone**

  ☑6ᵗʰ **T40.3X** **Poisoning by, adverse effect of and underdosing of** methadone

    ☑7ᵗʰ **T40.3X1** **Poisoning by methadone,** accidental (unintentional)
      Poisoning by methadone NOS

    ☑7ᵗʰ **T40.3X2** **Poisoning by methadone,** intentional self-harm

    ☑7ᵗʰ **T40.3X3** **Poisoning by methadone,** assault
    ☑7ᵗʰ **T40.3X4** **Poisoning by methadone,** undetermined
    ☑7ᵗʰ **T40.3X5** Adverse effect **of methadone**
    ☑7ᵗʰ **T40.3X6** Underdosing **of methadone**

☑5ᵗʰ **T40.4** **Poisoning by, adverse effect of and underdosing of other synthetic narcotics**

  ☑6ᵗʰ **T40.4X** **Poisoning by, adverse effect of and underdosing of** other synthetic narcotics

    ☑7ᵗʰ **T40.4X1** **Poisoning by other synthetic narcotics,** accidental (unintentional)
      Poisoning by other synthetic narcotics NOS

    ☑7ᵗʰ **T40.4X2** **Poisoning by other synthetic narcotics,** intentional self-harm

    ☑7ᵗʰ **T40.4X3** **Poisoning by other synthetic narcotics,** assault

    ☑7ᵗʰ **T40.4X4** **Poisoning by other synthetic narcotics,** undetermined

    ☑7ᵗʰ **T40.4X5** Adverse effect **of other synthetic narcotics**
    ☑7ᵗʰ **T40.4X6** Underdosing **of other synthetic narcotics**

☑5ᵗʰ **T40.5** **Poisoning by, adverse effect of and underdosing of cocaine**

  ☑6ᵗʰ **T40.5X** **Poisoning by, adverse effect of and underdosing of** cocaine

    ☑7ᵗʰ **T40.5X1** **Poisoning by cocaine,** accidental (unintentional)
      Poisoning by cocaine NOS
      AHA: 2016, 2Q, 8

    ☑7ᵗʰ **T40.5X2** **Poisoning by cocaine,** intentional self-harm

    ☑7ᵗʰ **T40.5X3** **Poisoning by cocaine,** assault
    ☑7ᵗʰ **T40.5X4** **Poisoning by cocaine,** undetermined
    ☑7ᵗʰ **T40.5X5** Adverse effect **of cocaine**
    ☑7ᵗʰ **T40.5X6** Underdosing **of cocaine**

☑5ᵗʰ **T40.6** **Poisoning by, adverse effect of and underdosing of other and unspecified narcotics**

  ☑6ᵗʰ **T40.60** **Poisoning by, adverse effect of and underdosing of** unspecified narcotics

    ☑7ᵗʰ **T40.601** **Poisoning by unspecified narcotics,** accidental (unintentional)   ▽
      Poisoning by narcotics NOS

    ☑7ᵗʰ **T40.602** **Poisoning by unspecified narcotics,** intentional self-harm   ▽

    ☑7ᵗʰ **T40.603** **Poisoning by unspecified narcotics,** assault   ▽

    ☑7ᵗʰ **T40.604** **Poisoning by unspecified narcotics,** undetermined   ▽

    ☑7ᵗʰ **T40.605** Adverse effect **of unspecified narcotics**   ▽
    ☑7ᵗʰ **T40.606** Underdosing **of unspecified narcotics**   ▽

  ☑6ᵗʰ **T40.69** **Poisoning by, adverse effect of and underdosing of** other narcotics

    ☑7ᵗʰ **T40.691** **Poisoning by other narcotics,** accidental (unintentional)
      Poisoning by other narcotics NOS

☑ Additional Character Req   ☑x7ᵗʰ Placeholder Alert   Case-Mix Diagnosis   Manifestation   ▽ Unspecified Dx   EXCLUDES 1 Not coded here   EXCLUDES 2 Not included here

ICD-10-CM 2018   1065

✓7ᵗʰ **T40.692** **Poisoning by other narcotics,** intentional self-harm

✓7ᵗʰ **T40.693** **Poisoning by other narcotics,** assault

✓7ᵗʰ **T40.694** **Poisoning by other narcotics,** undetermined

✓7ᵗʰ **T40.695** Adverse effect **of other narcotics**

✓7ᵗʰ **T40.696** Underdosing **of other narcotics**

✓5ᵗʰ **T40.7** **Poisoning by, adverse effect of and underdosing of cannabis (derivatives)**

    ✓6ᵗʰ **T40.7X** **Poisoning by, adverse effect of and underdosing of** cannabis (derivatives)

      ✓7ᵗʰ **T40.7X1** **Poisoning by cannabis (derivatives),** accidental (unintentional)
        Poisoning by cannabis NOS

      ✓7ᵗʰ **T40.7X2** **Poisoning by cannabis (derivatives),** intentional self-harm

      ✓7ᵗʰ **T40.7X3** **Poisoning by cannabis (derivatives),** assault

      ✓7ᵗʰ **T40.7X4** **Poisoning by cannabis (derivatives),** undetermined

      ✓7ᵗʰ **T40.7X5** Adverse effect **of cannabis (derivatives)**

      ✓7ᵗʰ **T40.7X6** Underdosing **of cannabis (derivatives)**

✓5ᵗʰ **T40.8** **Poisoning by and adverse effect of** lysergide [LSD]

    ✓6ᵗʰ **T40.8X** **Poisoning by and adverse effect of lysergide [LSD]**

      ✓7ᵗʰ **T40.8X1** **Poisoning by lysergide [LSD],** accidental (unintentional)
        Poisoning by lysergide [LSD]NOS

      ✓7ᵗʰ **T40.8X2** **Poisoning by lysergide [LSD],** intentional self-harm

      ✓7ᵗʰ **T40.8X3** **Poisoning by lysergide [LSD],** assault

      ✓7ᵗʰ **T40.8X4** **Poisoning by lysergide [LSD],** undetermined

✓5ᵗʰ **T40.9** **Poisoning by, adverse effect of and underdosing of other and unspecified psychodysleptics [hallucinogens]**

    ✓6ᵗʰ **T40.90** **Poisoning by, adverse effect of and underdosing of** unspecified psychodysleptics [hallucinogens]

      ✓7ᵗʰ **T40.901** **Poisoning by unspecified psychodysleptics [hallucinogens],** accidental (unintentional) ▽

      ✓7ᵗʰ **T40.902** **Poisoning by unspecified psychodysleptics [hallucinogens],** intentional self-harm ▽

      ✓7ᵗʰ **T40.903** **Poisoning by unspecified psychodysleptics [hallucinogens],** assault ▽

      ✓7ᵗʰ **T40.904** **Poisoning by unspecified psychodysleptics [hallucinogens],** undetermined ▽

      ✓7ᵗʰ **T40.905** Adverse effect **of unspecified psychodysleptics [hallucinogens]** ▽

      ✓7ᵗʰ **T40.906** Underdosing **of unspecified psychodysleptics** ▽

    ✓6ᵗʰ **T40.99** **Poisoning by, adverse effect of and underdosing of** other psychodysleptics [hallucinogens]

      ✓7ᵗʰ **T40.991** **Poisoning by other psychodysleptics [hallucinogens],** accidental (unintentional)
        Poisoning by other psychodysleptics [hallucinogens] NOS

      ✓7ᵗʰ **T40.992** **Poisoning by other psychodysleptics [hallucinogens],** intentional self-harm

      ✓7ᵗʰ **T40.993** **Poisoning by other psychodysleptics [hallucinogens],** assault

      ✓7ᵗʰ **T40.994** **Poisoning by other psychodysleptics [hallucinogens],** undetermined

      ✓7ᵗʰ **T40.995** Adverse effect **of other psychodysleptics [hallucinogens]**

      ✓7ᵗʰ **T40.996** Underdosing **of other psychodysleptics**

✓4ᵗʰ **T41** **Poisoning by, adverse effect of and underdosing of anesthetics and therapeutic gases**

    EXCLUDES 1 *benzodiazepines (T42.4-)*
      cocaine (T40.5-)
      complications of anesthesia during labor and delivery (O74.-)
      complications of anesthesia during pregnancy (O29.-)
      complications of anesthesia during the puerperium (O89.-)
      opioids (T40.0-T40.2-)

> The appropriate 7th character is to be added to each code from category T41.
> A   initial encounter
> D   subsequent encounter
> S   sequela

✓5ᵗʰ **T41.0** **Poisoning by, adverse effect of and underdosing of inhaled anesthetics**

    EXCLUDES 1 *oxygen (T41.5-)*

    ✓6ᵗʰ **T41.0X** **Poisoning by, adverse effect of and underdosing of** inhaled anesthetics

      ✓7ᵗʰ **T41.0X1** **Poisoning by inhaled anesthetics,** accidental (unintentional)
        Poisoning by inhaled anesthetics NOS

      ✓7ᵗʰ **T41.0X2** **Poisoning by inhaled anesthetics,** intentional self-harm

      ✓7ᵗʰ **T41.0X3** **Poisoning by inhaled anesthetics,** assault

      ✓7ᵗʰ **T41.0X4** **Poisoning by inhaled anesthetics,** undetermined

      ✓7ᵗʰ **T41.0X5** Adverse effect **of inhaled anesthetics**

      ✓7ᵗʰ **T41.0X6** Underdosing **of inhaled anesthetics**

✓5ᵗʰ **T41.1** **Poisoning by, adverse effect of and underdosing of intravenous anesthetics**
    Poisoning by, adverse effect of and underdosing of thiobarbiturates

    ✓6ᵗʰ **T41.1X** **Poisoning by, adverse effect of and underdosing of** intravenous anesthetics

      ✓7ᵗʰ **T41.1X1** **Poisoning by intravenous anesthetics,** accidental (unintentional)
        Poisoning by intravenous anesthetics NOS

      ✓7ᵗʰ **T41.1X2** **Poisoning by intravenous anesthetics,** intentional self-harm

      ✓7ᵗʰ **T41.1X3** **Poisoning by intravenous anesthetics,** assault

      ✓7ᵗʰ **T41.1X4** **Poisoning by intravenous anesthetics,** undetermined

      ✓7ᵗʰ **T41.1X5** Adverse effect **of intravenous anesthetics**

      ✓7ᵗʰ **T41.1X6** Underdosing **of intravenous anesthetics**

✓5ᵗʰ **T41.2** **Poisoning by, adverse effect of and underdosing of other and unspecified general anesthetics**

    ✓6ᵗʰ **T41.20** **Poisoning by, adverse effect of and underdosing of** unspecified general anesthetics

      ✓7ᵗʰ **T41.201** **Poisoning by unspecified general anesthetics,** accidental (unintentional) ▽
        Poisoning by general anesthetics NOS

      ✓7ᵗʰ **T41.202** **Poisoning by unspecified general anesthetics,** intentional self-harm ▽

      ✓7ᵗʰ **T41.203** **Poisoning by unspecified general anesthetics,** assault ▽

      ✓7ᵗʰ **T41.204** **Poisoning by unspecified general anesthetics,** undetermined ▽

      ✓7ᵗʰ **T41.205** Adverse effect **of unspecified general anesthetics** ▽

      ✓7ᵗʰ **T41.206** Underdosing **of unspecified general anesthetics** ▽

    ✓6ᵗʰ **T41.29** **Poisoning by, adverse effect of and underdosing of** other general anesthetics

      ✓7ᵗʰ **T41.291** **Poisoning by other general anesthetics,** accidental (unintentional)
        Poisoning by other general anesthetics NOS

      ✓7ᵗʰ **T41.292** **Poisoning by other general anesthetics,** intentional self-harm

      ✓7ᵗʰ **T41.293** **Poisoning by other general anesthetics,** assault

      ✓7ᵗʰ **T41.294** **Poisoning by other general anesthetics,** undetermined

      ✓7ᵗʰ **T41.295** Adverse effect **of other general anesthetics**

Ⓝ Newborn: 0   Ⓟ Pediatric: 0-17   Ⓜ Maternity: 12-55   Ⓐ Adult: 15-124   NRS Nonroutine supply Dx   NCDx Noncancer Dx   PDx Primary Dx   ▶◀ Revised Text   ● New Code   ▲ Revised Title

1066   ICD-10-CM 2018

✓7ᵗʰ **T41.296** Underdosing of other general anesthetics

✓5ᵗʰ **T41.3** Poisoning by, adverse effect of and underdosing of local anesthetics
> Cocaine (topical)
>
> EXCLUDES 2   poisoning by cocaine used as a central nervous system stimulant (T40.5X1-T40.5X4)

✓6ᵗʰ **T41.3X** Poisoning by, adverse effect of and underdosing of local anesthetics

✓7ᵗʰ **T41.3X1** Poisoning by local anesthetics, accidental (unintentional)
> Poisoning by local anesthetics NOS

✓7ᵗʰ **T41.3X2** Poisoning by local anesthetics, intentional self-harm

✓7ᵗʰ **T41.3X3** Poisoning by local anesthetics, assault

✓7ᵗʰ **T41.3X4** Poisoning by local anesthetics, undetermined

✓7ᵗʰ **T41.3X5** Adverse effect of local anesthetics

✓7ᵗʰ **T41.3X6** Underdosing of local anesthetics

✓5ᵗʰ **T41.4** Poisoning by, adverse effect of and underdosing of unspecified anesthetic

✓x7ᵗʰ **T41.41** Poisoning by unspecified anesthetic, accidental (unintentional) ▽
> Poisoning by anesthetic NOS

✓x7ᵗʰ **T41.42** Poisoning by unspecified anesthetic, intentional self-harm ▽

✓x7ᵗʰ **T41.43** Poisoning by unspecified anesthetic, assault ▽

✓x7ᵗʰ **T41.44** Poisoning by unspecified anesthetic, undetermined ▽

✓x7ᵗʰ **T41.45** Adverse effect of unspecified anesthetic ▽

✓x7ᵗʰ **T41.46** Underdosing of unspecified anesthetics ▽

✓5ᵗʰ **T41.5** Poisoning by, adverse effect of and underdosing of therapeutic gases

✓6ᵗʰ **T41.5X** Poisoning by, adverse effect of and underdosing of therapeutic gases

✓7ᵗʰ **T41.5X1** Poisoning by therapeutic gases, accidental (unintentional)
> Poisoning by therapeutic gases NOS

✓7ᵗʰ **T41.5X2** Poisoning by therapeutic gases, intentional self-harm

✓7ᵗʰ **T41.5X3** Poisoning by therapeutic gases, assault

✓7ᵗʰ **T41.5X4** Poisoning by therapeutic gases, undetermined

✓7ᵗʰ **T41.5X5** Adverse effect of therapeutic gases

✓7ᵗʰ **T41.5X6** Underdosing of therapeutic gases

✓4ᵗʰ **T42** Poisoning by, adverse effect of and underdosing of antiepileptic, sedative- hypnotic and antiparkinsonism drugs
> EXCLUDES 2   drug dependence and related mental and behavioral disorders due to psychoactive substance use (F10.- -F19.-)

> The appropriate 7th character is to be added to each code from category T42.
> A   initial encounter
> D   subsequent encounter
> S   sequela

✓5ᵗʰ **T42.0** Poisoning by, adverse effect of and underdosing of hydantoin derivatives

✓6ᵗʰ **T42.0X** Poisoning by, adverse effect of and underdosing of hydantoin derivatives

✓7ᵗʰ **T42.0X1** Poisoning by hydantoin derivatives, accidental (unintentional)
> Poisoning by hydantoin derivatives NOS

✓7ᵗʰ **T42.0X2** Poisoning by hydantoin derivatives, intentional self-harm

✓7ᵗʰ **T42.0X3** Poisoning by hydantoin derivatives, assault

✓7ᵗʰ **T42.0X4** Poisoning by hydantoin derivatives, undetermined

✓7ᵗʰ **T42.0X5** Adverse effect of hydantoin derivatives

✓7ᵗʰ **T42.0X6** Underdosing of hydantoin derivatives

✓5ᵗʰ **T42.1** Poisoning by, adverse effect of and underdosing of iminostilbenes
> Poisoning by, adverse effect of and underdosing of carbamazepine

✓6ᵗʰ **T42.1X** Poisoning by, adverse effect of and underdosing of iminostilbenes

✓7ᵗʰ **T42.1X1** Poisoning by iminostilbenes, accidental (unintentional)
> Poisoning by iminostilbenes NOS

✓7ᵗʰ **T42.1X2** Poisoning by iminostilbenes, intentional self-harm

✓7ᵗʰ **T42.1X3** Poisoning by iminostilbenes, assault

✓7ᵗʰ **T42.1X4** Poisoning by iminostilbenes, undetermined

✓7ᵗʰ **T42.1X5** Adverse effect of iminostilbenes

✓7ᵗʰ **T42.1X6** Underdosing of iminostilbenes

✓6ᵗʰ **T42.2** Poisoning by, adverse effect of and underdosing of succinimides and oxazolidinediones

✓6ᵗʰ **T42.2X** Poisoning by, adverse effect of and underdosing of succinimides and oxazolidinediones

✓7ᵗʰ **T42.2X1** Poisoning by succinimides and oxazolidinediones, accidental (unintentional)
> Poisoning by succinimides and oxazolidinediones NOS

✓7ᵗʰ **T42.2X2** Poisoning by succinimides and oxazolidinediones, intentional self-harm

✓7ᵗʰ **T42.2X3** Poisoning by succinimides and oxazolidinediones, assault

✓7ᵗʰ **T42.2X4** Poisoning by succinimides and oxazolidinediones, undetermined

✓7ᵗʰ **T42.2X5** Adverse effect of succinimides and oxazolidinediones

✓7ᵗʰ **T42.2X6** Underdosing of succinimides and oxazolidinediones

✓5ᵗʰ **T42.3** Poisoning by, adverse effect of and underdosing of barbiturates
> EXCLUDES 1   poisoning by, adverse effect of and underdosing of thiobarbiturates (T41.1-)

✓6ᵗʰ **T42.3X** Poisoning by, adverse effect of and underdosing of barbiturates

✓7ᵗʰ **T42.3X1** Poisoning by barbiturates, accidental (unintentional)
> Poisoning by barbiturates NOS

✓7ᵗʰ **T42.3X2** Poisoning by barbiturates, intentional self-harm

✓7ᵗʰ **T42.3X3** Poisoning by barbiturates, assault

✓7ᵗʰ **T42.3X4** Poisoning by barbiturates, undetermined

✓7ᵗʰ **T42.3X5** Adverse effect of barbiturates

✓7ᵗʰ **T42.3X6** Underdosing of barbiturates

✓5ᵗʰ **T42.4** Poisoning by, adverse effect of and underdosing of benzodiazepines

✓6ᵗʰ **T42.4X** Poisoning by, adverse effect of and underdosing of benzodiazepines

✓7ᵗʰ **T42.4X1** Poisoning by benzodiazepines, accidental (unintentional)
> Poisoning by benzodiazepines NOS

✓7ᵗʰ **T42.4X2** Poisoning by benzodiazepines, intentional self-harm

✓7ᵗʰ **T42.4X3** Poisoning by benzodiazepines, assault

✓7ᵗʰ **T42.4X4** Poisoning by benzodiazepines, undetermined

✓7ᵗʰ **T42.4X5** Adverse effect of benzodiazepines

✓7ᵗʰ **T42.4X6** Underdosing of benzodiazepines

✓5ᵗʰ **T42.5** Poisoning by, adverse effect of and underdosing of mixed antiepileptics

✓6ᵗʰ **T42.5X** Poisoning by, adverse effect of and underdosing of antiepileptics

✓7ᵗʰ **T42.5X1** Poisoning by mixed antiepileptics, accidental (unintentional)
> Poisoning by mixed antiepileptics NOS

✓7ᵗʰ **T42.5X2** Poisoning by mixed antiepileptics, intentional self-harm

✓7ᵗʰ **T42.5X3** Poisoning by mixed antiepileptics, assault

✓ Additional Character Req   ✓x7ᵗʰ Placeholder Alert   Case-Mix Diagnosis   Manifestation   ▽ Unspecified Dx   EXCLUDES 1 Not coded here   EXCLUDES 2 Not included here

√7ᵗʰ **T42.5X4** **Poisoning by mixed antiepileptics,** undetermined

√7ᵗʰ **T42.5X5** Adverse effect **of mixed antiepileptics**

√7ᵗʰ **T42.5X6** Underdosing **of mixed antiepileptics**

√5ᵗʰ **T42.6** **Poisoning by, adverse effect of and underdosing of other antiepileptic and sedative-hypnotic drugs**

Poisoning by, adverse effect of and underdosing of methaqualone

Poisoning by, adverse effect of and underdosing of valproic acid

EXCLUDES 1   *poisoning by, adverse effect of and underdosing of carbamazepine (T42.1-)*

√6ᵗʰ **T42.6X** **Poisoning by, adverse effect of and underdosing of** other antiepileptic and sedative-hypnotic **drugs**

√7ᵗʰ **T42.6X1** **Poisoning by other antiepileptic and sedative-hypnotic drugs,** accidental (unintentional)

Poisoning by other antiepileptic and sedative-hypnotic drugs NOS

√7ᵗʰ **T42.6X2** **Poisoning by other antiepileptic and sedative-hypnotic drugs,** intentional self-harm

√7ᵗʰ **T42.6X3** **Poisoning by other antiepileptic and sedative-hypnotic drugs,** assault

√7ᵗʰ **T42.6X4** **Poisoning by other antiepileptic and sedative-hypnotic drugs,** undetermined

√7ᵗʰ **T42.6X5** Adverse effect **of other antiepileptic and sedative-hypnotic drugs**

√7ᵗʰ **T42.6X6** Underdosing **of other antiepileptic and sedative-hypnotic drugs**

√5ᵗʰ **T42.7** **Poisoning by, adverse effect of and underdosing of** unspecified antiepileptic and sedative-hypnotic **drugs**

√x 7ᵗʰ **T42.71** **Poisoning by unspecified antiepileptic and sedative-hypnotic drugs,** accidental (unintentional) ▽

Poisoning by antiepileptic and sedative-hypnotic drugs NOS

√x 7ᵗʰ **T42.72** **Poisoning by unspecified antiepileptic and sedative-hypnotic drugs,** intentional self-harm ▽

√x 7ᵗʰ **T42.73** **Poisoning by unspecified antiepileptic and sedative-hypnotic drugs,** assault ▽

√x 7ᵗʰ **T42.74** **Poisoning by unspecified antiepileptic and sedative-hypnotic drugs,** undetermined ▽

√x 7ᵗʰ **T42.75** Adverse effect **of unspecified antiepileptic and sedative-hypnotic drugs** ▽

√x 7ᵗʰ **T42.76** Underdosing **of unspecified antiepileptic and sedative-hypnotic drugs** ▽

√5ᵗʰ **T42.8** **Poisoning by, adverse effect of and underdosing of antiparkinsonism drugs and other central muscle-tone depressants**

Poisoning by, adverse effect of and underdosing of amantadine

√6ᵗʰ **T42.8X** **Poisoning by, adverse effect of and underdosing of** antiparkinsonism drugs and other central muscle-tone depressants

√7ᵗʰ **T42.8X1** **Poisoning by antiparkinsonism drugs and other central muscle-tone depressants,** accidental (unintentional)

Poisoning by antiparkinsonism drugs and other central muscle-tone depressants NOS

√7ᵗʰ **T42.8X2** **Poisoning by antiparkinsonism drugs and other central muscle-tone depressants,** intentional self-harm

√7ᵗʰ **T42.8X3** **Poisoning by antiparkinsonism drugs and other central muscle-tone depressants,** assault

√7ᵗʰ **T42.8X4** **Poisoning by antiparkinsonism drugs and other central muscle-tone depressants,** undetermined

√7ᵗʰ **T42.8X5** Adverse effect **of antiparkinsonism drugs and other central muscle-tone depressants**

√7ᵗʰ **T42.8X6** Underdosing **of antiparkinsonism drugs and other central muscle-tone depressants**

√4ᵗʰ **T43** **Poisoning by, adverse effect of and underdosing of psychotropic drugs, not elsewhere classified**

EXCLUDES 1   *appetite depressants (T5Ø.5-)*
barbiturates (T42.3-)
benzodiazepines (T42.4-)
methaqualone (T42.6-)
psychodysleptics [hallucinogens] (T4Ø.7-T4Ø.9-)

EXCLUDES 2   *drug dependence and related mental and behavioral disorders due to psychoactive substance use (F1Ø.- -F19.-)*

The appropriate 7th character is to be added to each code from category T43.
A   initial encounter
D   subsequent encounter
S   sequela

√5ᵗʰ **T43.Ø** **Poisoning by, adverse effect of and underdosing of tricyclic and tetracyclic antidepressants**

√6ᵗʰ **T43.Ø1** **Poisoning by, adverse effect of and underdosing of** tricyclic antidepressants

√7ᵗʰ **T43.Ø11** **Poisoning by tricyclic antidepressants,** accidental (unintentional)

Poisoning by tricyclic antidepressants NOS

√7ᵗʰ **T43.Ø12** **Poisoning by tricyclic antidepressants,** intentional self-harm

√7ᵗʰ **T43.Ø13** **Poisoning by tricyclic antidepressants,** assault

√7ᵗʰ **T43.Ø14** **Poisoning by tricyclic antidepressants,** undetermined

√7ᵗʰ **T43.Ø15** Adverse effect **of tricyclic antidepressants**

√7ᵗʰ **T43.Ø16** Underdosing **of tricyclic antidepressants**

√6ᵗʰ **T43.Ø2** **Poisoning by, adverse effect of and underdosing of** tetracyclic antidepressants

√7ᵗʰ **T43.Ø21** **Poisoning by tetracyclic antidepressants,** accidental (unintentional)

Poisoning by tetracyclic antidepressants NOS

√7ᵗʰ **T43.Ø22** **Poisoning by tetracyclic antidepressants,** intentional self-harm

√7ᵗʰ **T43.Ø23** **Poisoning by tetracyclic antidepressants,** assault

√7ᵗʰ **T43.Ø24** **Poisoning by tetracyclic antidepressants,** undetermined

√7ᵗʰ **T43.Ø25** Adverse effect **of tetracyclic antidepressants**

√7ᵗʰ **T43.Ø26** Underdosing **of tetracyclic antidepressants**

√5ᵗʰ **T43.1** **Poisoning by, adverse effect of and underdosing of monoamine-oxidase-inhibitor antidepressants**

√6ᵗʰ **T43.1X** **Poisoning by, adverse effect of and underdosing of** monoamine-oxidase-inhibitor antidepressants

√7ᵗʰ **T43.1X1** **Poisoning by monoamine-oxidase-inhibitor antidepressants,** accidental (unintentional)

Poisoning by monoamine-oxidase-inhibitor antidepressants NOS

√7ᵗʰ **T43.1X2** **Poisoning by monoamine-oxidase-inhibitor antidepressants,** intentional self-harm

√7ᵗʰ **T43.1X3** **Poisoning by monoamine-oxidase-inhibitor antidepressants,** assault

√7ᵗʰ **T43.1X4** **Poisoning by monoamine-oxidase-inhibitor antidepressants,** undetermined

√7ᵗʰ **T43.1X5** Adverse effect **of monoamine-oxidase-inhibitor antidepressants**

√7ᵗʰ **T43.1X6** Underdosing **of monoamine-oxidase-inhibitor antidepressants**

√5ᵗʰ **T43.2** **Poisoning by, adverse effect of and underdosing of other and unspecified antidepressants**

√6ᵗʰ **T43.2Ø** **Poisoning by, adverse effect of and underdosing of** unspecified antidepressants

√7ᵗʰ **T43.2Ø1** **Poisoning by unspecified anti-depressants,** accidental (unintentional) ▽

Poisoning by antidepressants NOS

√7ᵗʰ **T43.2Ø2** **Poisoning by unspecified anti-depressants,** intentional self-harm ▽

√7ᵗʰ **T43.2Ø3** **Poisoning by unspecified anti-depressants,** assault ▽

Ⓝ Newborn: 0   Ⓟ Pediatric: 0-17   Ⓜ Maternity: 12-55   Ⓐ Adult: 15-124   **NRS** Nonroutine supply Dx   **NCDx** Noncancer Dx   **PDx** Primary Dx   ▶◀ Revised Text   ● New Code   ▲ Revised Title

✓7ᵗʰ **T43.204** Poisoning by unspecified antidepressants, **undetermined** ▽

✓7ᵗʰ **T43.205** **Adverse effect** of unspecified antidepressants ▽
> ▶Antidepressant discontinuation syndrome◀

✓7ᵗʰ **T43.206** **Underdosing** of unspecified antidepressants ▽

✓6ᵗʰ **T43.21** Poisoning by, adverse effect of and underdosing of selective serotonin and norepinephrine reuptake inhibitors
> Poisoning by, adverse effect of and underdosing of SSNRI antidepressants

✓7ᵗʰ **T43.211** **Poisoning by selective serotonin and norepinephrine reuptake inhibitors, accidental (unintentional)**

✓7ᵗʰ **T43.212** **Poisoning by selective serotonin and norepinephrine reuptake inhibitors, intentional self-harm**

✓7ᵗʰ **T43.213** **Poisoning by selective serotonin and norepinephrine reuptake inhibitors, assault**

✓7ᵗʰ **T43.214** **Poisoning by selective serotonin and norepinephrine reuptake inhibitors, undetermined**

✓7ᵗʰ **T43.215** **Adverse effect** of selective serotonin and norepinephrine reuptake inhibitors

✓7ᵗʰ **T43.216** **Underdosing** of selective serotonin and norepinephrine reuptake inhibitors

✓6ᵗʰ **T43.22** Poisoning by, adverse effect of and underdosing of selective serotonin reuptake inhibitors
> Poisoning by, adverse effect of and underdosing of SSRI antidepressants

✓7ᵗʰ **T43.221** **Poisoning by selective serotonin reuptake inhibitors, accidental (unintentional)**

✓7ᵗʰ **T43.222** **Poisoning by selective serotonin reuptake inhibitors, intentional self-harm**

✓7ᵗʰ **T43.223** **Poisoning by selective serotonin reuptake inhibitors, assault**

✓7ᵗʰ **T43.224** **Poisoning by selective serotonin reuptake inhibitors, undetermined**

✓7ᵗʰ **T43.225** **Adverse effect** of selective serotonin reuptake inhibitors

✓7ᵗʰ **T43.226** **Underdosing** of selective serotonin reuptake inhibitors

✓6ᵗʰ **T43.29** Poisoning by, adverse effect of and underdosing of other antidepressants

✓7ᵗʰ **T43.291** **Poisoning by other antidepressants, accidental (unintentional)**
> Poisoning by other antidepressants NOS

✓7ᵗʰ **T43.292** **Poisoning by other antidepressants, intentional self-harm**

✓7ᵗʰ **T43.293** **Poisoning by other antidepressants, assault**

✓7ᵗʰ **T43.294** **Poisoning by other antidepressants, undetermined**

✓7ᵗʰ **T43.295** **Adverse effect** of other antidepressants

✓7ᵗʰ **T43.296** **Underdosing** of other antidepressants

✓5ᵗʰ **T43.3** Poisoning by, adverse effect of and underdosing of phenothiazine antipsychotics and neuroleptics

✓6ᵗʰ **T43.3X** Poisoning by, adverse effect of and underdosing of phenothiazine antipsychotics and neuroleptics

✓7ᵗʰ **T43.3X1** **Poisoning by phenothiazine antipsychotics and neuroleptics, accidental (unintentional)**
> Poisoning by phenothiazine antipsychotics and neuroleptics NOS

✓7ᵗʰ **T43.3X2** **Poisoning by phenothiazine antipsychotics and neuroleptics, intentional self-harm**

✓7ᵗʰ **T43.3X3** **Poisoning by phenothiazine antipsychotics and neuroleptics, assault**

✓7ᵗʰ **T43.3X4** **Poisoning by phenothiazine antipsychotics and neuroleptics, undetermined**

✓7ᵗʰ **T43.3X5** **Adverse effect** of phenothiazine antipsychotics and neuroleptics

✓7ᵗʰ **T43.3X6** **Underdosing** of phenothiazine antipsychotics and neuroleptics

✓5ᵗʰ **T43.4** Poisoning by, adverse effect of and underdosing of butyrophenone and thiothixene neuroleptics

✓6ᵗʰ **T43.4X** Poisoning by, adverse effect of and underdosing of butyrophenone and thiothixene neuroleptics

✓7ᵗʰ **T43.4X1** **Poisoning by butyrophenone and thiothixene neuroleptics, accidental (unintentional)**
> Poisoning by butyrophenone and thiothixene neuroleptics NOS

✓7ᵗʰ **T43.4X2** **Poisoning by butyrophenone and thiothixene neuroleptics, intentional self-harm**

✓7ᵗʰ **T43.4X3** **Poisoning by butyrophenone and thiothixene neuroleptics, assault**

✓7ᵗʰ **T43.4X4** **Poisoning by butyrophenone and thiothixene neuroleptics, undetermined**

✓7ᵗʰ **T43.4X5** **Adverse effect** of butyrophenone and thiothixene neuroleptics

✓7ᵗʰ **T43.4X6** **Underdosing** of butyrophenone and thiothixene neuroleptics

✓5ᵗʰ **T43.5** Poisoning by, adverse effect of and underdosing of other and unspecified antipsychotics and neuroleptics
> **EXCLUDES 1** poisoning by, adverse effect of and underdosing of rauwolfia (T46.5-)

✓6ᵗʰ **T43.50** Poisoning by, adverse effect of and underdosing of unspecified antipsychotics and neuroleptics

✓7ᵗʰ **T43.501** **Poisoning by unspecified antipsychotics and neuroleptics, accidental (unintentional)** ▽
> Poisoning by antipsychotics and neuroleptics NOS

✓7ᵗʰ **T43.502** **Poisoning by unspecified antipsychotics and neuroleptics, intentional self-harm** ▽

✓7ᵗʰ **T43.503** **Poisoning by unspecified antipsychotics and neuroleptics, assault** ▽

✓7ᵗʰ **T43.504** **Poisoning by unspecified antipsychotics and neuroleptics, undetermined** ▽

✓7ᵗʰ **T43.505** **Adverse effect** of unspecified antipsychotics and neuroleptics ▽

✓7ᵗʰ **T43.506** **Underdosing** of unspecified antipsychotics and neuroleptics ▽

✓6ᵗʰ **T43.59** Poisoning by, adverse effect of and underdosing of other antipsychotics and neuroleptics
> **AHA:** 2017, 1Q, 40

✓7ᵗʰ **T43.591** **Poisoning by other antipsychotics and neuroleptics, accidental (unintentional)**
> Poisoning by other antipsychotics and neuroleptics NOS

✓7ᵗʰ **T43.592** **Poisoning by other antipsychotics and neuroleptics, intentional self-harm**

✓7ᵗʰ **T43.593** **Poisoning by other antipsychotics and neuroleptics, assault**

✓7ᵗʰ **T43.594** **Poisoning by other antipsychotics and neuroleptics, undetermined**

✓7ᵗʰ **T43.595** **Adverse effect** of other antipsychotics and neuroleptics

✓7ᵗʰ **T43.596** **Underdosing** of other antipsychotics and neuroleptics

✓5ᵗʰ **T43.6** Poisoning by, adverse effect of and underdosing of psychostimulants
> **EXCLUDES 1** poisoning by, adverse effect of and underdosing of cocaine (T40.5-)

✓6ᵗʰ **T43.60** Poisoning by, adverse effect of and underdosing of unspecified psychostimulant

✓7ᵗʰ **T43.601** **Poisoning by unspecified psychostimulants, accidental (unintentional)** ▽
> Poisoning by psychostimulants NOS

✓7ᵗʰ **T43.602** **Poisoning by unspecified psychostimulants, intentional self-harm** ▽

✓7ᵗʰ **T43.603** **Poisoning by unspecified psychostimulants, assault** ▽

✓ Additional Character Req   ✓7ᵗʰ Placeholder Alert   Case-Mix Diagnosis   Manifestation   ▽ Unspecified Dx   **EXCLUDES 1** Not coded here   **EXCLUDES 2** Not included here

ICD-10-CM 2018   **1069**

Chapter 19. Injury, Poisoning and Certain Other Consequences of External Causes

☑7ᵗʰ **T43.604** **Poisoning by unspecified psychostimulants,** undetermined ▽

☑7ᵗʰ **T43.605** Adverse effect **of unspecified psychostimulants** ▽

☑7ᵗʰ **T43.606** Underdosing **of unspecified psychostimulants** ▽

☑6ᵗʰ **T43.61** **Poisoning by, adverse effect of and underdosing of** caffeine

☑7ᵗʰ **T43.611** **Poisoning by caffeine,** accidental (unintentional)
Poisoning by caffeine NOS

☑7ᵗʰ **T43.612** **Poisoning by caffeine,** intentional self-harm

☑7ᵗʰ **T43.613** **Poisoning by caffeine,** assault

☑7ᵗʰ **T43.614** **Poisoning by caffeine,** undetermined

☑7ᵗʰ **T43.615** Adverse effect **of caffeine**

☑7ᵗʰ **T43.616** Underdosing **of caffeine**

☑6ᵗʰ **T43.62** **Poisoning by, adverse effect of and underdosing of** amphetamines
Poisoning by, adverse effect of and underdosing of methamphetamines

☑7ᵗʰ **T43.621** **Poisoning by amphetamines,** accidental (unintentional)
Poisoning by amphetamines NOS

☑7ᵗʰ **T43.622** **Poisoning by amphetamines,** intentional self-harm

☑7ᵗʰ **T43.623** **Poisoning by amphetamines,** assault

☑7ᵗʰ **T43.624** **Poisoning by amphetamines,** undetermined

☑7ᵗʰ **T43.625** Adverse effect **of amphetamines**

☑7ᵗʰ **T43.626** Underdosing **of amphetamines**

☑6ᵗʰ **T43.63** **Poisoning by, adverse effect of and underdosing of** methylphenidate

☑7ᵗʰ **T43.631** **Poisoning by methylphenidate,** accidental (unintentional)
Poisoning by methylphenidate NOS

☑7ᵗʰ **T43.632** **Poisoning by methylphenidate,** intentional self-harm

☑7ᵗʰ **T43.633** **Poisoning by methylphenidate,** assault

☑7ᵗʰ **T43.634** **Poisoning by methylphenidate,** undetermined

☑7ᵗʰ **T43.635** Adverse effect **of methylphenidate**

☑7ᵗʰ **T43.636** Underdosing **of methylphenidate**

☑6ᵗʰ **T43.69** **Poisoning by, adverse effect of and underdosing of** other psychostimulants

☑7ᵗʰ **T43.691** **Poisoning by other psychostimulants,** accidental (unintentional)
Poisoning by other psychostimulants NOS

☑7ᵗʰ **T43.692** **Poisoning by other psychostimulants,** intentional self-harm

☑7ᵗʰ **T43.693** **Poisoning by other psychostimulants,** assault

☑7ᵗʰ **T43.694** **Poisoning by other psychostimulants,** undetermined

☑7ᵗʰ **T43.695** Adverse effect **of other psychostimulants**

☑7ᵗʰ **T43.696** Underdosing **of other psychostimulants**

☑5ᵗʰ **T43.8** **Poisoning by, adverse effect of and underdosing of other psychotropic drugs**

☑6ᵗʰ **T43.8X** **Poisoning by, adverse effect of and underdosing of** other psychotropic **drugs**

☑7ᵗʰ **T43.8X1** **Poisoning by other psychotropic drugs,** accidental (unintentional)
Poisoning by other psychotropic drugs NOS

☑7ᵗʰ **T43.8X2** **Poisoning by other psychotropic drugs,** intentional self-harm

☑7ᵗʰ **T43.8X3** **Poisoning by other psychotropic drugs,** assault

☑7ᵗʰ **T43.8X4** **Poisoning by other psychotropic drugs,** undetermined

☑7ᵗʰ **T43.8X5** Adverse effect **of other psychotropic drugs**

☑7ᵗʰ **T43.8X6** Underdosing **of other psychotropic drugs**

☑5ᵗʰ **T43.9** **Poisoning by, adverse effect of and underdosing of** unspecified psychotropic **drug**

☑x7ᵗʰ **T43.91** **Poisoning by unspecified psychotropic drug,** accidental (unintentional) ▽
Poisoning by psychotropic drug NOS

☑x7ᵗʰ **T43.92** **Poisoning by unspecified psychotropic drug,** intentional self-harm ▽

☑x7ᵗʰ **T43.93** **Poisoning by unspecified psychotropic drug,** assault ▽

☑x7ᵗʰ **T43.94** **Poisoning by unspecified psychotropic drug,** undetermined ▽

☑x7ᵗʰ **T43.95** Adverse effect **of unspecified psychotropic drug** ▽

☑x7ᵗʰ **T43.96** Underdosing **of unspecified psychotropic drug** ▽

☑4ᵗʰ **T44** **Poisoning by, adverse effect of and underdosing of drugs primarily affecting the autonomic nervous system**

> The appropriate 7th character is to be added to each code from category T44.
> A   initial encounter
> D   subsequent encounter
> S   sequela

☑5ᵗʰ **T44.0** **Poisoning by, adverse effect of and underdosing of anticholinesterase agents**

☑6ᵗʰ **T44.0X** **Poisoning by, adverse effect of and underdosing of** anticholinesterase agents

☑7ᵗʰ **T44.0X1** **Poisoning by anticholinesterase agents,** accidental (unintentional)
Poisoning by anticholinesterase agents NOS

☑7ᵗʰ **T44.0X2** **Poisoning by anticholinesterase agents,** intentional self-harm

☑7ᵗʰ **T44.0X3** **Poisoning by anticholinesterase agents,** assault

☑7ᵗʰ **T44.0X4** **Poisoning by anticholinesterase agents,** undetermined

☑7ᵗʰ **T44.0X5** Adverse effect **of anticholinesterase agents**

☑7ᵗʰ **T44.0X6** Underdosing **of anticholinesterase agents**

☑5ᵗʰ **T44.1** **Poisoning by, adverse effect of and underdosing of other parasympathomimetics [cholinergics]**

☑6ᵗʰ **T44.1X** **Poisoning by, adverse effect of and underdosing of** other parasympathomimetics [cholinergics]

☑7ᵗʰ **T44.1X1** **Poisoning by other parasympathomimetics [cholinergics],** accidental (unintentional)
Poisoning by other parasympathomimetics [cholinergics] NOS

☑7ᵗʰ **T44.1X2** **Poisoning by other parasympathomimetics [cholinergics],** intentional self-harm

☑7ᵗʰ **T44.1X3** **Poisoning by other parasympathomimetics [cholinergics],** assault

☑7ᵗʰ **T44.1X4** **Poisoning by other parasympathomimetics [cholinergics],** undetermined

☑7ᵗʰ **T44.1X5** Adverse effect **of other parasympathomimetics [cholinergics]**

☑7ᵗʰ **T44.1X6** Underdosing **of other parasympathomimetics**

☑5ᵗʰ **T44.2** **Poisoning by, adverse effect of and underdosing of ganglionic blocking drugs**

☑6ᵗʰ **T44.2X** **Poisoning by, adverse effect of and underdosing of** ganglionic blocking drugs

☑7ᵗʰ **T44.2X1** **Poisoning by ganglionic blocking drugs,** accidental (unintentional)
Poisoning by ganglionic blocking drugs NOS

☑7ᵗʰ **T44.2X2** **Poisoning by ganglionic blocking drugs,** intentional self-harm

☑7ᵗʰ **T44.2X3** **Poisoning by ganglionic blocking drugs,** assault

☑7ᵗʰ **T44.2X4** **Poisoning by ganglionic blocking drugs,** undetermined

☑7ᵗʰ **T44.2X5** Adverse effect **of ganglionic blocking drugs**

☑7ᵗʰ **T44.2X6** Underdosing **of ganglionic blocking drugs**

Ⓝ Newborn: 0   Ⓟ Pediatric: 0-17   Ⓜ Maternity: 12-55   Ⓐ Adult: 15-124   NRS Nonroutine supply Dx   NCDx Noncancer Dx   PDx Primary Dx   ▶◀ Revised Text   ● New Code   ▲ Revised Title

1070   ICD-10-CM 2018

✓5ᵗʰ **T44.3** **Poisoning by, adverse effect of and underdosing of other parasympatholytics [anticholinergics and antimuscarinics] and spasmolytics**
Poisoning by, adverse effect of and underdosing of papaverine

✓6ᵗʰ **T44.3X** **Poisoning by, adverse effect of and underdosing of other parasympatholytics [anticholinergics and antimuscarinics] and spasmolytics**

✓7ᵗʰ **T44.3X1** **Poisoning by other parasympatholytics [anticholinergics and antimuscarinics] and spasmolytics, accidental (unintentional)**
Poisoning by other parasympatholytics [anticholinergics and antimuscarinics] and spasmolytics NOS

✓7ᵗʰ **T44.3X2** **Poisoning by other parasympatholytics [anticholinergics and antimuscarinics] and spasmolytics, intentional self-harm**

✓7ᵗʰ **T44.3X3** **Poisoning by other parasympatholytics [anticholinergics and antimuscarinics] and spasmolytics, assault**

✓7ᵗʰ **T44.3X4** **Poisoning by other parasympatholytics [anticholinergics and antimuscarinics] and spasmolytics, undetermined**

✓7ᵗʰ **T44.3X5** **Adverse effect of other parasympatholytics [anticholinergics and antimuscarinics] and spasmolytics**

✓7ᵗʰ **T44.3X6** **Underdosing of other parasympatholytics [anticholinergics and antimuscarinics] and spasmolytics**

✓5ᵗʰ **T44.4** **Poisoning by, adverse effect of and underdosing of predominantly alpha-adrenoreceptor agonists**
Poisoning by, adverse effect of and underdosing of metaraminol

✓6ᵗʰ **T44.4X** **Poisoning by, adverse effect of and underdosing of predominantly alpha-adrenoreceptor agonists**

✓7ᵗʰ **T44.4X1** **Poisoning by predominantly alpha-adrenoreceptor agonists, accidental (unintentional)**
Poisoning by predominantly alpha-adrenoreceptor agonists NOS

✓7ᵗʰ **T44.4X2** **Poisoning by predominantly alpha-adrenoreceptor agonists, intentional self-harm**

✓7ᵗʰ **T44.4X3** **Poisoning by predominantly alpha-adrenoreceptor agonists, assault**

✓7ᵗʰ **T44.4X4** **Poisoning by predominantly alpha-adrenoreceptor agonists, undetermined**

✓7ᵗʰ **T44.4X5** **Adverse effect of predominantly alpha-adrenoreceptor agonists**

✓7ᵗʰ **T44.4X6** **Underdosing of predominantly alpha-adrenoreceptor agonists**

✓5ᵗʰ **T44.5** **Poisoning by, adverse effect of and underdosing of predominantly beta-adrenoreceptor agonists**
EXCLUDES 1 *poisoning by, adverse effect of and underdosing of beta-adrenoreceptor agonists used in asthma therapy (T48.6-)*

✓6ᵗʰ **T44.5X** **Poisoning by, adverse effect of and underdosing of predominantly beta-adrenoreceptor agonists**

✓7ᵗʰ **T44.5X1** **Poisoning by predominantly beta-adrenoreceptor agonists, accidental (unintentional)**
Poisoning by predominantly beta-adrenoreceptor agonists NOS

✓7ᵗʰ **T44.5X2** **Poisoning by predominantly beta-adrenoreceptor agonists, intentional self-harm**

✓7ᵗʰ **T44.5X3** **Poisoning by predominantly beta-adrenoreceptor agonists, assault**

✓7ᵗʰ **T44.5X4** **Poisoning by predominantly beta-adrenoreceptor agonists, undetermined**

✓7ᵗʰ **T44.5X5** **Adverse effect of predominantly beta-adrenoreceptor agonists**

✓7ᵗʰ **T44.5X6** **Underdosing of predominantly beta-adrenoreceptor agonists**

✓5ᵗʰ **T44.6** **Poisoning by, adverse effect of and underdosing of alpha-adrenoreceptor antagonists**
EXCLUDES 1 *poisoning by, adverse effect of and underdosing of ergot alkaloids (T48.0)*

✓6ᵗʰ **T44.6X** **Poisoning by, adverse effect of and underdosing of alpha-adrenoreceptor antagonists**

✓7ᵗʰ **T44.6X1** **Poisoning by alpha-adrenoreceptor antagonists, accidental (unintentional)**
Poisoning by alpha-adrenoreceptor antagonists NOS

✓7ᵗʰ **T44.6X2** **Poisoning by alpha-adrenoreceptor antagonists, intentional self-harm**

✓7ᵗʰ **T44.6X3** **Poisoning by alpha-adrenoreceptor antagonists, assault**

✓7ᵗʰ **T44.6X4** **Poisoning by alpha-adrenoreceptor antagonists, undetermined**

✓7ᵗʰ **T44.6X5** **Adverse effect of alpha-adrenoreceptor antagonists**

✓7ᵗʰ **T44.6X6** **Underdosing of alpha-adrenoreceptor antagonists**

✓5ᵗʰ **T44.7** **Poisoning by, adverse effect of and underdosing of beta-adrenoreceptor antagonists**

✓6ᵗʰ **T44.7X** **Poisoning by, adverse effect of and underdosing of beta-adrenoreceptor antagonists**

✓7ᵗʰ **T44.7X1** **Poisoning by beta-adrenoreceptor antagonists, accidental (unintentional)**
Poisoning by beta-adrenoreceptor antagonists NOS

✓7ᵗʰ **T44.7X2** **Poisoning by beta-adrenoreceptor antagonists, intentional self-harm**

✓7ᵗʰ **T44.7X3** **Poisoning by beta-adrenoreceptor antagonists, assault**

✓7ᵗʰ **T44.7X4** **Poisoning by beta-adrenoreceptor antagonists, undetermined**

✓7ᵗʰ **T44.7X5** **Adverse effect of beta-adrenoreceptor antagonists**

✓7ᵗʰ **T44.7X6** **Underdosing of beta-adrenoreceptor antagonists**

✓5ᵗʰ **T44.8** **Poisoning by, adverse effect of and underdosing of centrally-acting and adrenergic-neuron- blocking agents**
EXCLUDES 1 *poisoning by, adverse effect of and underdosing of clonidine (T46.5)*
poisoning by, adverse effect of and underdosing of guanethidine (T46.5)

✓6ᵗʰ **T44.8X** **Poisoning by, adverse effect of and underdosing of centrally-acting and adrenergic-neuron-blocking agents**

✓7ᵗʰ **T44.8X1** **Poisoning by centrally-acting and adrenergic-neuron-blocking agents, accidental (unintentional)**
Poisoning by centrally-acting and adrenergic-neuron-blocking agents NOS

✓7ᵗʰ **T44.8X2** **Poisoning by centrally-acting and adrenergic-neuron-blocking agents, intentional self-harm**

✓7ᵗʰ **T44.8X3** **Poisoning by centrally-acting and adrenergic-neuron-blocking agents, assault**

✓7ᵗʰ **T44.8X4** **Poisoning by centrally-acting and adrenergic-neuron-blocking agents, undetermined**

✓7ᵗʰ **T44.8X5** **Adverse effect of centrally-acting and adrenergic-neuron-blocking agents**

✓7ᵗʰ **T44.8X6** **Underdosing of centrally-acting and adrenergic-neuron-blocking agents**

✓ Additional Character Req   ✓ˣ7ᵗʰ Placeholder Alert   Case-Mix Diagnosis   Manifestation   ▽ Unspecified Dx   **EXCLUDES 1** Not coded here   **EXCLUDES 2** Not included here

ICD-10-CM 2018   1071

✓5ᵗʰ **T44.9** **Poisoning by, adverse effect of and underdosing of other and unspecified drugs** primarily affecting the autonomic nervous system
     Poisoning by, adverse effect of and underdosing of drug stimulating both alpha and beta-adrenoreceptors

   ✓6ᵗʰ **T44.90** **Poisoning by, adverse effect of and underdosing of** unspecified **drugs primarily affecting the autonomic nervous system**

     ✓7ᵗʰ **T44.901** **Poisoning by unspecified drugs primarily affecting the autonomic nervous system,** accidental **(unintentional)** ▽
       Poisoning by unspecified drugs primarily affecting the autonomic nervous system NOS

     ✓7ᵗʰ **T44.902** **Poisoning by unspecified drugs primarily affecting the autonomic nervous system,** intentional self-harm ▽

     ✓7ᵗʰ **T44.903** **Poisoning by unspecified drugs primarily affecting the autonomic nervous system,** assault ▽

     ✓7ᵗʰ **T44.904** **Poisoning by unspecified drugs primarily affecting the autonomic nervous system,** undetermined ▽

     ✓7ᵗʰ **T44.905** Adverse effect **of unspecified drugs primarily affecting the autonomic nervous system** ▽

     ✓7ᵗʰ **T44.906** Underdosing **of unspecified drugs primarily affecting the autonomic nervous system** ▽

   ✓6ᵗʰ **T44.99** **Poisoning by, adverse effect of and underdosing of** other **drugs primarily affecting the autonomic nervous system**

     ✓7ᵗʰ **T44.991** **Poisoning by other drug primarily affecting the autonomic nervous system,** accidental **(unintentional)**
       Poisoning by other drugs primarily affecting the autonomic nervous system NOS

     ✓7ᵗʰ **T44.992** **Poisoning by other drug primarily affecting the autonomic nervous system,** intentional self-harm

     ✓7ᵗʰ **T44.993** **Poisoning by other drug primarily affecting the autonomic nervous system,** assault

     ✓7ᵗʰ **T44.994** **Poisoning by other drug primarily affecting the autonomic nervous system,** undetermined

     ✓7ᵗʰ **T44.995** Adverse effect **of other drug primarily affecting the autonomic nervous system**

     ✓7ᵗʰ **T44.996** Underdosing **of other drug primarily affecting the autonomic nervous system**

✓4ᵗʰ **T45** **Poisoning by, adverse effect of and underdosing of primarily systemic and hematological agents, not elsewhere classified**

   The appropriate 7th character is to be added to each code from category T45.
   A   initial encounter
   D   subsequent encounter
   S   sequela

   ✓5ᵗʰ **T45.0** **Poisoning by, adverse effect of and underdosing of antiallergic and antiemetic drugs**
     EXCLUDES 1 *poisoning by, adverse effect of and underdosing of phenothiazine-based neuroleptics (T43.3)*

   ✓6ᵗʰ **T45.0X** **Poisoning by, adverse effect of and underdosing of antiallergic and antiemetic drugs**

     ✓7ᵗʰ **T45.0X1** **Poisoning by antiallergic and antiemetic drugs,** accidental **(unintentional)**
       Poisoning by antiallergic and antiemetic drugs NOS

     ✓7ᵗʰ **T45.0X2** **Poisoning by antiallergic and antiemetic drugs,** intentional self-harm

     ✓7ᵗʰ **T45.0X3** **Poisoning by antiallergic and antiemetic drugs,** assault

     ✓7ᵗʰ **T45.0X4** **Poisoning by antiallergic and antiemetic drugs,** undetermined

     ✓7ᵗʰ **T45.0X5** Adverse effect **of antiallergic and antiemetic drugs**

     ✓7ᵗʰ **T45.0X6** Underdosing **of antiallergic and antiemetic drugs**

   ✓5ᵗʰ **T45.1** **Poisoning by, adverse effect of and underdosing of antineoplastic and immunosuppressive drugs**
     EXCLUDES 1 *poisoning by, adverse effect of and underdosing of tamoxifen (T38.6)*
     AHA: 2014, 4Q, 22

   ✓6ᵗʰ **T45.1X** **Poisoning by, adverse effect of and underdosing of** antineoplastic and immunosuppressive **drugs**

     ✓7ᵗʰ **T45.1X1** **Poisoning by antineoplastic and immunosuppressive drugs,** accidental **(unintentional)**
       Poisoning by antineoplastic and immunosuppressive drugs NOS

     ✓7ᵗʰ **T45.1X2** **Poisoning by antineoplastic and immunosuppressive drugs,** intentional self-harm

     ✓7ᵗʰ **T45.1X3** **Poisoning by antineoplastic and immunosuppressive drugs,** assault

     ✓7ᵗʰ **T45.1X4** **Poisoning by antineoplastic and immunosuppressive drugs,** undetermined

     ✓7ᵗʰ **T45.1X5** Adverse effect **of antineoplastic and immunosuppressive drugs**

     ✓7ᵗʰ **T45.1X6** Underdosing **of antineoplastic and immunosuppressive drugs**

   ✓5ᵗʰ **T45.2** **Poisoning by, adverse effect of and underdosing of vitamins**
     EXCLUDES 2 *poisoning by, adverse effect of and underdosing of iron (T45.4)*
     poisoning by, adverse effect of and underdosing of nicotinic acid (derivatives) (T46.7)
     poisoning by, adverse effect of and underdosing of vitamin K (T45.7)

   ✓6ᵗʰ **T45.2X** **Poisoning by, adverse effect of and underdosing of** vitamins

     ✓7ᵗʰ **T45.2X1** **Poisoning by vitamins,** accidental **(unintentional)**
       Poisoning by vitamins NOS

     ✓7ᵗʰ **T45.2X2** **Poisoning by vitamins,** intentional self-harm

     ✓7ᵗʰ **T45.2X3** **Poisoning by vitamins,** assault

     ✓7ᵗʰ **T45.2X4** **Poisoning by vitamins,** undetermined

     ✓7ᵗʰ **T45.2X5** Adverse effect **of vitamins**

     ✓7ᵗʰ **T45.2X6** Underdosing **of vitamins**
       EXCLUDES 1 *vitamin deficiencies (E50-E56)*

   ✓5ᵗʰ **T45.3** **Poisoning by, adverse effect of and underdosing of enzymes**

   ✓6ᵗʰ **T45.3X** **Poisoning by, adverse effect of and underdosing of** enzymes

     ✓7ᵗʰ **T45.3X1** **Poisoning by enzymes,** accidental **(unintentional)**
       Poisoning by enzymes NOS

     ✓7ᵗʰ **T45.3X2** **Poisoning by enzymes,** intentional self-harm

     ✓7ᵗʰ **T45.3X3** **Poisoning by enzymes,** assault

     ✓7ᵗʰ **T45.3X4** **Poisoning by enzymes,** undetermined

     ✓7ᵗʰ **T45.3X5** Adverse effect **of enzymes**

     ✓7ᵗʰ **T45.3X6** Underdosing **of enzymes**

   ✓5ᵗʰ **T45.4** **Poisoning by, adverse effect of and underdosing of iron and its compounds**

   ✓6ᵗʰ **T45.4X** **Poisoning by, adverse effect of and underdosing of** iron **and its compounds**

     T45.4X1 **Poisoning by iron and its compounds,** accidental **(unintentional)**
       Poisoning by iron and its compounds NOS

     ✓7ᵗʰ **T45.4X2** **Poisoning by iron and its compounds,** intentional self-harm

     ✓7ᵗʰ **T45.4X3** **Poisoning by iron and its compounds,** assault

     ✓7ᵗʰ **T45.4X4** **Poisoning by iron and its compounds,** undetermined

     ✓7ᵗʰ **T45.4X5** Adverse effect **of iron and its compounds**

     ✓7ᵗʰ **T45.4X6** Underdosing **of iron and its compounds**
       EXCLUDES 1 *iron deficiency (E61.1)*

Ⓝ Newborn: 0   Ⓟ Pediatric: 0-17   Ⓜ Maternity: 12-55   Ⓐ Adult: 15-124   **NRS** Nonroutine supply Dx   **NC Dx** Noncancer Dx   **PDx** Primary Dx   ▶◀ Revised Text   ● New Code   ▲ Revised Title

1072   ICD-10-CM 2018

✓5ᵗʰ T45.5 Poisoning by, adverse effect of and underdosing of anticoagulants and antithrombotic drugs

✓6ᵗʰ T45.51 Poisoning by, adverse effect of and underdosing of anticoagulants

✓7ᵗʰ T45.511 Poisoning by anticoagulants, accidental (unintentional)
Poisoning by anticoagulants NOS

✓7ᵗʰ T45.512 Poisoning by anticoagulants, intentional self-harm

✓7ᵗʰ T45.513 Poisoning by anticoagulants, assault

✓7ᵗʰ T45.514 Poisoning by anticoagulants, undetermined

✓7ᵗʰ T45.515 Adverse effect of anticoagulants
AHA: 2016, 1Q, 14; 2013, 2Q, 34

✓7ᵗʰ T45.516 Underdosing of anticoagulants

✓6ᵗʰ T45.52 Poisoning by, adverse effect of and underdosing of antithrombotic drugs
Poisoning by, adverse effect of and underdosing of antiplatelet drugs
EXCLUDES 2 poisoning by, adverse effect of and underdosing of aspirin (T39.01-)
poisoning by, adverse effect of and underdosing of acetylsalicylic acid (T39.01-)

✓7ᵗʰ T45.521 Poisoning by antithrombotic drugs, accidental (unintentional)
Poisoning by antithrombotic drug NOS

✓7ᵗʰ T45.522 Poisoning by antithrombotic drugs, intentional self-harm

✓7ᵗʰ T45.523 Poisoning by antithrombotic drugs, assault

✓7ᵗʰ T45.524 Poisoning by antithrombotic drugs, undetermined

✓7ᵗʰ T45.525 Adverse effect of antithrombotic drugs
AHA: 2016, 1Q, 15

✓7ᵗʰ T45.526 Underdosing of antithrombotic drugs

✓5ᵗʰ T45.6 Poisoning by, adverse effect of and underdosing of fibrinolysis-affecting drugs

✓6ᵗʰ T45.60 Poisoning by, adverse effect of and underdosing of unspecified fibrinolysis-affecting drugs

✓7ᵗʰ T45.601 Poisoning by unspecified fibrinolysis-affecting drugs, accidental (unintentional) ▽
Poisoning by fibrinolysis-affecting drug NOS

✓7ᵗʰ T45.602 Poisoning by unspecified fibrinolysis-affecting drugs, intentional self-harm ▽

✓7ᵗʰ T45.603 Poisoning by unspecified fibrinolysis-affecting drugs, assault ▽

✓7ᵗʰ T45.604 Poisoning by unspecified fibrinolysis-affecting drugs, undetermined ▽

✓7ᵗʰ T45.605 Adverse effect of unspecified fibrinolysis- affecting drugs ▽

✓7ᵗʰ T45.606 Underdosing of unspecified fibrinolysis- affecting drugs ▽

✓6ᵗʰ T45.61 Poisoning by, adverse effect of and underdosing of thrombolytic drugs

✓7ᵗʰ T45.611 Poisoning by thrombolytic drug, accidental (unintentional)
Poisoning by thrombolytic drug NOS

✓7ᵗʰ T45.612 Poisoning by thrombolytic drug, intentional self-harm

✓7ᵗʰ T45.613 Poisoning by thrombolytic drug, assault

✓7ᵗʰ T45.614 Poisoning by thrombolytic drug, undetermined

✓7ᵗʰ T45.615 Adverse effect of thrombolytic drugs
AHA: 2017, 2Q, 9

✓7ᵗʰ T45.616 Underdosing of thrombolytic drugs

✓6ᵗʰ T45.62 Poisoning by, adverse effect of and underdosing of hemostatic drugs

✓7ᵗʰ T45.621 Poisoning by hemostatic drug, accidental (unintentional)
Poisoning by hemostatic drug NOS

✓7ᵗʰ T45.622 Poisoning by hemostatic drug, intentional self-harm

✓7ᵗʰ T45.623 Poisoning by hemostatic drug, assault

✓7ᵗʰ T45.624 Poisoning by hemostatic drug, undetermined

✓7ᵗʰ T45.625 Adverse effect of hemostatic drug

✓7ᵗʰ T45.626 Underdosing of hemostatic drugs

✓6ᵗʰ T45.69 Poisoning by, adverse effect of and underdosing of other fibrinolysis-affecting drugs

✓7ᵗʰ T45.691 Poisoning by other fibrinolysis-affecting drugs, accidental (unintentional)
Poisoning by other fibrinolysis-affecting drug NOS

✓7ᵗʰ T45.692 Poisoning by other fibrinolysis-affecting drugs, intentional self-harm

✓7ᵗʰ T45.693 Poisoning by other fibrinolysis-affecting drugs, assault

✓7ᵗʰ T45.694 Poisoning by other fibrinolysis-affecting drugs, undetermined

✓7ᵗʰ T45.695 Adverse effect of other fibrinolysis-affecting drugs

✓7ᵗʰ T45.696 Underdosing of other fibrinolysis-affecting drugs

✓5ᵗʰ T45.7 Poisoning by, adverse effect of and underdosing of anticoagulant antagonists, vitamin K and other coagulants

✓6ᵗʰ T45.7X Poisoning by, adverse effect of and underdosing of anticoagulant antagonists, vitamin K and other coagulants

✓7ᵗʰ T45.7X1 Poisoning by anticoagulant antagonists, vitamin K and other coagulants, accidental (unintentional)
Poisoning by anticoagulant antagonists, vitamin K and other coagulants NOS

✓7ᵗʰ T45.7X2 Poisoning by anticoagulant antagonists, vitamin K and other coagulants, intentional self-harm

✓7ᵗʰ T45.7X3 Poisoning by anticoagulant antagonists, vitamin K and other coagulants, assault

✓7ᵗʰ T45.7X4 Poisoning by anticoagulant antagonists, vitamin K and other coagulants, undetermined

✓7ᵗʰ T45.7X5 Adverse effect of anticoagulant antagonists, vitamin K and other coagulants

✓7ᵗʰ T45.7X6 Underdosing of anticoagulant antagonist, vitamin K and other coagulants
EXCLUDES 1 vitamin K deficiency (E56.1)

✓5ᵗʰ T45.8 Poisoning by, adverse effect of and underdosing of other primarily systemic and hematological agents
Poisoning by, adverse effect of and underdosing of liver preparations and other antianemic agents
Poisoning by, adverse effect of and underdosing of natural blood and blood products
Poisoning by, adverse effect of and underdosing of plasma substitute
EXCLUDES 2 poisoning by, adverse effect of and underdosing of immunoglobulin (T50.Z1)
poisoning by, adverse effect of and underdosing of iron (T45.4)
transfusion reactions (T80.-)

✓6ᵗʰ T45.8X Poisoning by, adverse effect of and underdosing of other primarily systemic and hematological agents

✓7ᵗʰ T45.8X1 Poisoning by other primarily systemic and hematological agents, accidental (unintentional)
Poisoning by other primarily systemic and hematological agents NOS

✓7ᵗʰ T45.8X2 Poisoning by other primarily systemic and hematological agents, intentional self-harm

✓7ᵗʰ T45.8X3 Poisoning by other primarily systemic and hematological agents, assault

✓7ᵗʰ T45.8X4 Poisoning by other primarily systemic and hematological agents, undetermined

✓7ᵗʰ T45.8X5 Adverse effect of other primarily systemic and hematological agents

✓7ᵗʰ T45.8X6 Underdosing of other primarily systemic and hematological agents

✓5ᵗʰ T45.9 Poisoning by, adverse effect of and underdosing of unspecified primarily systemic and hematological agent

✓x7ᵗʰ T45.91 Poisoning by unspecified primarily systemic and hematological agent, accidental (unintentional) ▽
Poisoning by primarily systemic and hematological agent NOS

✓ Additional Character Req   ✓x7ᵗʰ Placeholder Alert   Case-Mix Diagnosis   Manifestation   ▽ Unspecified Dx   EXCLUDES 1 Not coded here   EXCLUDES 2 Not included here

✓7th **T45.92 Poisoning by unspecified primarily systemic and hematological agent, intentional self-harm** ▽

✓x7th **T45.93 Poisoning by unspecified primarily systemic and hematological agent, assault** ▽

✓x7th **T45.94 Poisoning by unspecified primarily systemic and hematological agent, undetermined** ▽

✓x7th **T45.95 Adverse effect of unspecified primarily systemic and hematological agent** ▽

✓x7th **T45.96 Underdosing of unspecified primarily systemic and hematological agent** ▽

✓4th **T46 Poisoning by, adverse effect of and underdosing of agents primarily affecting the cardiovascular system**

> EXCLUDES 1　*poisoning by, adverse effect of and underdosing of metaraminol (T44.4)*

> The appropriate 7th character is to be added to each code from category T46.
> A　initial encounter
> D　subsequent encounter
> S　sequela

✓5th **T46.0 Poisoning by, adverse effect of and underdosing of cardiac-stimulant glycosides and drugs of similar action**

✓6th **T46.0X Poisoning by, adverse effect of and underdosing of cardiac-stimulant glycosides and drugs of similar action**

✓7th **T46.0X1 Poisoning by cardiac-stimulant glycosides and drugs of similar action, accidental (unintentional)**
　　Poisoning by cardiac-stimulant glycosides and drugs of similar action NOS

✓7th **T46.0X2 Poisoning by cardiac-stimulant glycosides and drugs of similar action, intentional self-harm**

✓7th **T46.0X3 Poisoning by cardiac-stimulant glycosides and drugs of similar action, assault**

✓7th **T46.0X4 Poisoning by cardiac-stimulant glycosides and drugs of similar action, undetermined**

✓7th **T46.0X5 Adverse effect of cardiac-stimulant glycosides and drugs of similar action**

✓7th **T46.0X6 Underdosing of cardiac-stimulant glycosides and drugs of similar action**

✓5th **T46.1 Poisoning by, adverse effect of and underdosing of calcium-channel blockers**

✓6th **T46.1X Poisoning by, adverse effect of and underdosing of calcium-channel blockers**

✓7th **T46.1X1 Poisoning by calcium-channel blockers, accidental (unintentional)**
　　Poisoning by calcium-channel blockers NOS

✓7th **T46.1X2 Poisoning by calcium-channel blockers, intentional self-harm**

✓7th **T46.1X3 Poisoning by calcium-channel blockers, assault**

✓7th **T46.1X4 Poisoning by calcium-channel blockers, undetermined**

✓7th **T46.1X5 Adverse effect of calcium-channel blockers**

✓7th **T46.1X6 Underdosing of calcium-channel blockers**

✓5th **T46.2 Poisoning by, adverse effect of and underdosing of other antidysrhythmic drugs, not elsewhere classified**

> EXCLUDES 1　*poisoning by, adverse effect of and underdosing of beta-adrenoreceptor antagonists (T44.7-)*

✓6th **T46.2X Poisoning by, adverse effect of and underdosing of other antidysrhythmic drugs**

✓7th **T46.2X1 Poisoning by other antidysrhythmic drugs, accidental (unintentional)**
　　Poisoning by other antidysrhythmic drugs NOS

✓7th **T46.2X2 Poisoning by other antidysrhythmic drugs, intentional self-harm**

✓7th **T46.2X3 Poisoning by other antidysrhythmic drugs, assault**

✓7th **T46.2X4 Poisoning by other antidysrhythmic drugs, undetermined**

✓7th **T46.2X5 Adverse effect of other antidysrhythmic drugs**

✓7th **T46.2X6 Underdosing of other antidysrhythmic drugs**

✓5th **T46.3 Poisoning by, adverse effect of and underdosing of coronary vasodilators**
　　Poisoning by, adverse effect of and underdosing of dipyridamole

> EXCLUDES 1　*poisoning by, adverse effect of and underdosing of calcium-channel blockers (T46.1)*

✓6th **T46.3X Poisoning by, adverse effect of and underdosing of coronary vasodilators**

✓7th **T46.3X1 Poisoning by coronary vasodilators, accidental (unintentional)**
　　Poisoning by coronary vasodilators NOS

✓7th **T46.3X2 Poisoning by coronary vasodilators, intentional self-harm**

✓7th **T46.3X3 Poisoning by coronary vasodilators, assault**

✓7th **T46.3X4 Poisoning by coronary vasodilators, undetermined**

✓7th **T46.3X5 Adverse effect of coronary vasodilators**

✓7th **T46.3X6 Underdosing of coronary vasodilators**

✓5th **T46.4 Poisoning by, adverse effect of and underdosing of angiotensin-converting-enzyme inhibitors**

✓6th **T46.4X Poisoning by, adverse effect of and underdosing of angiotensin-converting-enzyme inhibitors**

✓7th **T46.4X1 Poisoning by angiotensin-converting-enzyme inhibitors, accidental (unintentional)**
　　Poisoning by angiotensin-converting-enzyme inhibitors NOS

✓7th **T46.4X2 Poisoning by angiotensin-converting-enzyme inhibitors, intentional self-harm**

✓7th **T46.4X3 Poisoning by angiotensin-converting-enzyme inhibitors, assault**

✓7th **T46.4X4 Poisoning by angiotensin-converting-enzyme inhibitors, undetermined**

✓7th **T46.4X5 Adverse effect of angiotensin-converting-enzyme inhibitors**

✓7th **T46.4X6 Underdosing of angiotensin-converting-enzyme inhibitors**

✓5th **T46.5 Poisoning by, adverse effect of and underdosing of other antihypertensive drugs**

> EXCLUDES 2　*poisoning by, adverse effect of and underdosing of beta-adrenoreceptor antagonists (T44.7)*
> *poisoning by, adverse effect of and underdosing of calcium-channel blockers (T46.1)*
> *poisoning by, adverse effect of and underdosing of diuretics (T50.0-T50.2)*

✓6th **T46.5X Poisoning by, adverse effect of and underdosing of other antihypertensive drugs**

✓7th **T46.5X1 Poisoning by other antihypertensive drugs, accidental (unintentional)**
　　Poisoning by other antihypertensive drugs NOS

✓7th **T46.5X2 Poisoning by other antihypertensive drugs, intentional self-harm**

✓7th **T46.5X3 Poisoning by other antihypertensive drugs, assault**

✓7th **T46.5X4 Poisoning by other antihypertensive drugs, undetermined**

✓7th **T46.5X5 Adverse effect of other antihypertensive drugs**

✓7th **T46.5X6 Underdosing of other antihypertensive drugs**

✓5th **T46.6 Poisoning by, adverse effect of and underdosing of antihyperlipidemic and antiarteriosclerotic drugs**

✓6th **T46.6X Poisoning by, adverse effect of and underdosing of antihyperlipidemic and antiarteriosclerotic drugs**

✓7th **T46.6X1 Poisoning by antihyperlipidemic and antiarteriosclerotic drugs, accidental (unintentional)**
　　Poisoning by antihyperlipidemic and antiarteriosclerotic drugs NOS

✓7th **T46.6X2 Poisoning by antihyperlipidemic and antiarteriosclerotic drugs, intentional self-harm**

✓7ᵗʰ **T46.6X3** **Poisoning by antihyperlipidemic and antiarteriosclerotic drugs,** assault

✓7ᵗʰ **T46.6X4** **Poisoning by antihyperlipidemic and antiarteriosclerotic drugs,** undetermined

✓7ᵗʰ **T46.6X5** Adverse effect **of antihyperlipidemic and antiarteriosclerotic drugs**

✓7ᵗʰ **T46.6X6** Underdosing **of antihyperlipidemic and antiarteriosclerotic drugs**

✓5ᵗʰ **T46.7** **Poisoning by, adverse effect of and underdosing of peripheral vasodilators**
     Poisoning by, adverse effect of and underdosing of nicotinic acid (derivatives)

     EXCLUDES 1   poisoning by, adverse effect of and underdosing of papaverine (T44.3)

   ✓6ᵗʰ **T46.7X** **Poisoning by, adverse effect of and underdosing of** peripheral vasodilators

     ✓7ᵗʰ **T46.7X1** **Poisoning by peripheral vasodilators,** accidental **(unintentional)**
       Poisoning by peripheral vasodilators NOS

     ✓7ᵗʰ **T46.7X2** **Poisoning by peripheral vasodilators,** intentional self-harm

     ✓7ᵗʰ **T46.7X3** **Poisoning by peripheral vasodilators,** assault

     ✓7ᵗʰ **T46.7X4** **Poisoning by peripheral vasodilators,** undetermined

     ✓7ᵗʰ **T46.7X5** Adverse effect **of peripheral vasodilators**

     ✓7ᵗʰ **T46.7X6** Underdosing **of peripheral vasodilators**

✓5ᵗʰ **T46.8** **Poisoning by, adverse effect of and underdosing of antivaricose drugs, including sclerosing agents**

   ✓6ᵗʰ **T46.8X** **Poisoning by, adverse effect of and underdosing of** antivaricose **drugs, including sclerosing agents**

     ✓7ᵗʰ **T46.8X1** **Poisoning by antivaricose drugs, including sclerosing agents,** accidental **(unintentional)**
       Poisoning by antivaricose drugs, including sclerosing agents NOS

     ✓7ᵗʰ **T46.8X2** **Poisoning by antivaricose drugs, including sclerosing agents,** intentional self-harm

     ✓7ᵗʰ **T46.8X3** **Poisoning by antivaricose drugs, including sclerosing agents,** assault

     ✓7ᵗʰ **T46.8X4** **Poisoning by antivaricose drugs, including sclerosing agents,** undetermined

     ✓7ᵗʰ **T46.8X5** Adverse effect **of antivaricose drugs, including sclerosing agents**

     ✓7ᵗʰ **T46.8X6** Underdosing **of antivaricose drugs, including sclerosing agents**

✓5ᵗʰ **T46.9** **Poisoning by, adverse effect of and underdosing of other and unspecified** agents primarily affecting the cardiovascular system

   ✓6ᵗʰ **T46.90** **Poisoning by, adverse effect of and underdosing of** unspecified **agents primarily affecting the cardiovascular system**

     ✓7ᵗʰ **T46.901** **Poisoning by unspecified agents primarily affecting the cardiovascular system,** accidental **(unintentional)** ▽

     ✓7ᵗʰ **T46.902** **Poisoning by unspecified agents primarily affecting the cardiovascular system,** intentional self-harm ▽

     ✓7ᵗʰ **T46.903** **Poisoning by unspecified agents primarily affecting the cardiovascular system,** assault ▽

     ✓7ᵗʰ **T46.904** **Poisoning by unspecified agents primarily affecting the cardiovascular system,** undetermined ▽

     ✓7ᵗʰ **T46.905** Adverse effect **of unspecified agents primarily affecting the cardiovascular system** ▽

     ✓7ᵗʰ **T46.906** Underdosing **of unspecified agents primarily affecting the cardiovascular system** ▽

   ✓6ᵗʰ **T46.99** **Poisoning by, adverse effect of and underdosing of** other **agents primarily affecting the cardiovascular system**

     ✓7ᵗʰ **T46.991** **Poisoning by other agents primarily affecting the cardiovascular system,** accidental **(unintentional)**

✓7ᵗʰ **T46.992** **Poisoning by other agents primarily affecting the cardiovascular system,** intentional self-harm

✓7ᵗʰ **T46.993** **Poisoning by other agents primarily affecting the cardiovascular system,** assault

✓7ᵗʰ **T46.994** **Poisoning by other agents primarily affecting the cardiovascular system,** undetermined

✓7ᵗʰ **T46.995** Adverse effect **of other agents primarily affecting the cardiovascular system**

✓7ᵗʰ **T46.996** Underdosing **of other agents primarily affecting the cardiovascular system**

✓4ᵗʰ **T47** **Poisoning by, adverse effect of and underdosing of agents primarily affecting the gastrointestinal system**

> The appropriate 7th character is to be added to each code from category T47.
> A   initial encounter
> D   subsequent encounter
> S   sequela

✓5ᵗʰ **T47.0** **Poisoning by, adverse effect of and underdosing of histamine H2-receptor blockers**

   ✓6ᵗʰ **T47.0X** **Poisoning by, adverse effect of and underdosing of** histamine H2-receptor blockers

     ✓7ᵗʰ **T47.0X1** **Poisoning by histamine H2-receptor blockers,** accidental **(unintentional)**
       Poisoning by histamine H2-receptor blockers NOS

     ✓7ᵗʰ **T47.0X2** **Poisoning by histamine H2-receptor blockers,** intentional self-harm

     ✓7ᵗʰ **T47.0X3** **Poisoning by histamine H2-receptor blockers,** assault

     ✓7ᵗʰ **T47.0X4** **Poisoning by histamine H2-receptor blockers,** undetermined

     ✓7ᵗʰ **T47.0X5** Adverse effect **of histamine H2-receptor blockers**

     ✓7ᵗʰ **T47.0X6** Underdosing **of histamine H2-receptor blockers**

✓5ᵗʰ **T47.1** **Poisoning by, adverse effect of and underdosing of other antacids and anti-gastric-secretion drugs**

   ✓6ᵗʰ **T47.1X** **Poisoning by, adverse effect of and underdosing of** other antacids and anti-gastric-secretion **drugs**

     ✓7ᵗʰ **T47.1X1** **Poisoning by other antacids and anti-gastric-secretion drugs,** accidental **(unintentional)**
       Poisoning by other antacids and anti-gastric-secretion drugs NOS

     ✓7ᵗʰ **T47.1X2** **Poisoning by other antacids and anti-gastric-secretion drugs,** intentional self-harm

     ✓7ᵗʰ **T47.1X3** **Poisoning by other antacids and anti-gastric-secretion drugs,** assault

     ✓7ᵗʰ **T47.1X4** **Poisoning by other antacids and anti-gastric-secretion drugs,** undetermined

     ✓7ᵗʰ **T47.1X5** Adverse effect **of other antacids and anti-gastric-secretion drugs**

     ✓7ᵗʰ **T47.1X6** Underdosing **of other antacids and anti-gastric-secretion drugs**

✓5ᵗʰ **T47.2** **Poisoning by, adverse effect of and underdosing of stimulant laxatives**

   ✓6ᵗʰ **T47.2X** **Poisoning by, adverse effect of and underdosing of** stimulant laxatives

     ✓7ᵗʰ **T47.2X1** **Poisoning by stimulant laxatives,** accidental **(unintentional)**
       Poisoning by stimulant laxatives NOS

     ✓7ᵗʰ **T47.2X2** **Poisoning by stimulant laxatives,** intentional self-harm

     ✓7ᵗʰ **T47.2X3** **Poisoning by stimulant laxatives,** assault

     ✓7ᵗʰ **T47.2X4** **Poisoning by stimulant laxatives,** undetermined

     ✓7ᵗʰ **T47.2X5** Adverse effect **of stimulant laxatives**

     ✓7ᵗʰ **T47.2X6** Underdosing **of stimulant laxatives**

✓ Additional Character Req   ✓x7ᵗʰ Placeholder Alert   Case-Mix Diagnosis   Manifestation   ▽ Unspecified Dx   *EXCLUDES 1* Not coded here   *EXCLUDES 2* Not included here

☑5ᵗʰ T47.3 Poisoning by, adverse effect of and underdosing of saline and osmotic laxatives

    ☑6ᵗʰ T47.3X Poisoning by and adverse effect of saline and osmotic laxatives

        ☑7ᵗʰ T47.3X1 Poisoning by saline and osmotic laxatives, accidental (unintentional)
             Poisoning by saline and osmotic laxatives NOS

        ☑7ᵗʰ T47.3X2 Poisoning by saline and osmotic laxatives, intentional self-harm

        ☑7ᵗʰ T47.3X3 Poisoning by saline and osmotic laxatives, assault

        ☑7ᵗʰ T47.3X4 Poisoning by saline and osmotic laxatives, undetermined

        ☑7ᵗʰ T47.3X5 Adverse effect **of saline and osmotic laxatives**

        ☑7ᵗʰ T47.3X6 Underdosing **of saline and osmotic laxatives**

☑5ᵗʰ T47.4 Poisoning by, adverse effect of and underdosing of other laxatives

    ☑6ᵗʰ T47.4X Poisoning by, adverse effect of and underdosing of other laxatives

        ☑7ᵗʰ T47.4X1 Poisoning by other laxatives, accidental (unintentional)
             Poisoning by other laxatives NOS

        ☑7ᵗʰ T47.4X2 Poisoning by other laxatives, intentional self-harm

        ☑7ᵗʰ T47.4X3 Poisoning by other laxatives, assault

        ☑7ᵗʰ T47.4X4 Poisoning by other laxatives, undetermined

        ☑7ᵗʰ T47.4X5 Adverse effect **of other laxatives**

        ☑7ᵗʰ T47.4X6 Underdosing **of other laxatives**

☑5ᵗʰ T47.5 Poisoning by, adverse effect of and underdosing of digestants

    ☑6ᵗʰ T47.5X Poisoning by, adverse effect of and underdosing of digestants

        ☑7ᵗʰ T47.5X1 Poisoning by digestants, accidental (unintentional)
             Poisoning by digestants NOS

        ☑7ᵗʰ T47.5X2 Poisoning by digestants, intentional self-harm

        ☑7ᵗʰ T47.5X3 Poisoning by digestants, assault

        ☑7ᵗʰ T47.5X4 Poisoning by digestants, undetermined

        ☑7ᵗʰ T47.5X5 Adverse effect **of digestants**

        ☑7ᵗʰ T47.5X6 Underdosing **of digestants**

☑5ᵗʰ T47.6 Poisoning by, adverse effect of and underdosing of antidiarrheal drugs

        EXCLUDES 2 *poisoning by, adverse effect of and underdosing of systemic antibiotics and other anti-infectives (T36-T37)*

    ☑6ᵗʰ T47.6X Poisoning by, adverse effect of and underdosing of antidiarrheal **drugs**

        ☑7ᵗʰ T47.6X1 Poisoning by antidiarrheal drugs, accidental (unintentional)
             Poisoning by antidiarrheal drugs NOS

        ☑7ᵗʰ T47.6X2 Poisoning by antidiarrheal drugs, intentional self-harm

        ☑7ᵗʰ T47.6X3 Poisoning by antidiarrheal drugs, assault

        ☑7ᵗʰ T47.6X4 Poisoning by antidiarrheal drugs, undetermined

        ☑7ᵗʰ T47.6X5 Adverse effect **of antidiarrheal drugs**

        ☑7ᵗʰ T47.6X6 Underdosing **of antidiarrheal drugs**

☑5ᵗʰ T47.7 Poisoning by, adverse effect of and underdosing of emetics

    ☑6ᵗʰ T47.7X Poisoning by, adverse effect of and underdosing of emetics

        ☑7ᵗʰ T47.7X1 Poisoning by emetics, accidental (unintentional)
             Poisoning by emetics NOS

        ☑7ᵗʰ T47.7X2 Poisoning by emetics, intentional self-harm

        ☑7ᵗʰ T47.7X3 Poisoning by emetics, assault

        ☑7ᵗʰ T47.7X4 Poisoning by emetics, undetermined

        ☑7ᵗʰ T47.7X5 Adverse effect **of emetics**

        ☑7ᵗʰ T47.7X6 Underdosing **of emetics**

☑5ᵗʰ T47.8 Poisoning by, adverse effect of and underdosing of other agents primarily affecting gastrointestinal system

    ☑6ᵗʰ T47.8X Poisoning by, adverse effect of and underdosing of other **agents primarily affecting gastrointestinal system**

        ☑7ᵗʰ T47.8X1 Poisoning by other agents primarily affecting gastrointestinal system, accidental (unintentional)
             Poisoning by other agents primarily affecting gastrointestinal system NOS

        ☑7ᵗʰ T47.8X2 Poisoning by other agents primarily affecting gastrointestinal system, intentional self-harm

        ☑7ᵗʰ T47.8X3 Poisoning by other agents primarily affecting gastrointestinal system, assault

        ☑7ᵗʰ T47.8X4 Poisoning by other agents primarily affecting gastrointestinal system, undetermined

        ☑7ᵗʰ T47.8X5 Adverse effect **of other agents primarily affecting gastrointestinal system**

        ☑7ᵗʰ T47.8X6 Underdosing **of other agents primarily affecting gastrointestinal system**

☑5ᵗʰ T47.9 Poisoning by, adverse effect of and underdosing of unspecified **agents primarily affecting the gastrointestinal system**

    ☑x7ᵗʰ T47.91 Poisoning by unspecified agents primarily affecting the gastrointestinal system, accidental (unintentional) ▽▽
         Poisoning by agents primarily affecting the gastrointestinal system NOS

    ☑x7ᵗʰ T47.92 Poisoning by unspecified agents primarily affecting the gastrointestinal system, intentional self-harm ▽

    ☑x7ᵗʰ T47.93 Poisoning by unspecified agents primarily affecting the gastrointestinal system, assault ▽▽

    ☑x7ᵗʰ T47.94 Poisoning by unspecified agents primarily affecting the gastrointestinal system, undetermined ▽

    ☑x7ᵗʰ T47.95 Adverse effect **of unspecified agents primarily affecting the gastrointestinal system** ▽

    ☑x7ᵗʰ T47.96 Underdosing **of unspecified agents primarily affecting the gastrointestinal system** ▽

☑4ᵗʰ T48 Poisoning by, adverse effect of and underdosing of agents primarily acting on smooth and skeletal muscles and the respiratory system

> The appropriate 7th character is to be added to each code from category T48.
> A   initial encounter
> D   subsequent encounter
> S   sequela

☑5ᵗʰ T48.0 Poisoning by, adverse effect of and underdosing of oxytocic drugs

        EXCLUDES 1 *poisoning by, adverse effect of and underdosing of estrogens, progestogens and antagonists (T38.4-T38.6)*

    ☑6ᵗʰ T48.0X Poisoning by, adverse effect of and underdosing of oxytocic **drugs**

        ☑7ᵗʰ T48.0X1 Poisoning by oxytocic drugs, accidental (unintentional)
             Poisoning by oxytocic drugs NOS

        ☑7ᵗʰ T48.0X2 Poisoning by oxytocic drugs, intentional self-harm

        ☑7ᵗʰ T48.0X3 Poisoning by oxytocic drugs, assault

        ☑7ᵗʰ T48.0X4 Poisoning by oxytocic drugs, undetermined

        ☑7ᵗʰ T48.0X5 Adverse effect **of oxytocic drugs**

        ☑7ᵗʰ T48.0X6 Underdosing **of oxytocic drugs**

☑5ᵗʰ T48.1 Poisoning by, adverse effect of and underdosing of skeletal muscle relaxants [neuromuscular blocking agents]

    ☑6ᵗʰ T48.1X Poisoning by, adverse effect of and underdosing of skeletal muscle relaxants **[neuromuscular blocking agents]**

        ☑7ᵗʰ T48.1X1 Poisoning by skeletal muscle relaxants [neuromuscular blocking agents], accidental (unintentional)
             Poisoning by skeletal muscle relaxants [neuromuscular blocking agents] NOS

Ⓝ Newborn: 0   Ⓟ Pediatric: 0-17   Ⓜ Maternity: 12-55   Ⓐ Adult: 15-124   **NRS** Nonroutine supply Dx   **NCDx** Noncancer Dx   **PDx** Primary Dx   ▶◀ Revised Text   ● New Code   ▲ Revised Title

1076   ICD-10-CM 2018

√7ᵗʰ **T48.1X2** **Poisoning by skeletal muscle relaxants [neuromuscular blocking agents], intentional self-harm**

√7ᵗʰ **T48.1X3** **Poisoning by skeletal muscle relaxants [neuromuscular blocking agents], assault**

√7ᵗʰ **T48.1X4** **Poisoning by skeletal muscle relaxants [neuromuscular blocking agents], undetermined**

√7ᵗʰ **T48.1X5** **Adverse effect of skeletal muscle relaxants [neuromuscular blocking agents]**

√7ᵗʰ **T48.1X6** **Underdosing of skeletal muscle relaxants [neuromuscular blocking agents]**

√5ᵗʰ **T48.2** **Poisoning by, adverse effect of and underdosing of other and unspecified drugs acting on muscles**

√6ᵗʰ **T48.20** **Poisoning by, adverse effect of and underdosing of unspecified drugs acting on muscles**

√7ᵗʰ **T48.201** **Poisoning by unspecified drugs acting on muscles, accidental (unintentional)** ▽
Poisoning by unspecified drugs acting on muscles NOS

√7ᵗʰ **T48.202** **Poisoning by unspecified drugs acting on muscles, intentional self-harm** ▽

√7ᵗʰ **T48.203** **Poisoning by unspecified drugs acting on muscles, assault** ▽

√7ᵗʰ **T48.204** **Poisoning by unspecified drugs acting on muscles, undetermined** ▽

√7ᵗʰ **T48.205** **Adverse effect of unspecified drugs acting on muscles** ▽

√7ᵗʰ **T48.206** **Underdosing of unspecified drugs acting on muscles** ▽

√6ᵗʰ **T48.29** **Poisoning by, adverse effect of and underdosing of other drugs acting on muscles**

√7ᵗʰ **T48.291** **Poisoning by other drugs acting on muscles, accidental (unintentional)**
Poisoning by other drugs acting on muscles NOS

√7ᵗʰ **T48.292** **Poisoning by other drugs acting on muscles, intentional self-harm**

√7ᵗʰ **T48.293** **Poisoning by other drugs acting on muscles, assault**

√7ᵗʰ **T48.294** **Poisoning by other drugs acting on muscles, undetermined**

√7ᵗʰ **T48.295** **Adverse effect of other drugs acting on muscles**

√7ᵗʰ **T48.296** **Underdosing of other drugs acting on muscles**

√5ᵗʰ **T48.3** **Poisoning by, adverse effect of and underdosing of antitussives**

√6ᵗʰ **T48.3X** **Poisoning by, adverse effect of and underdosing of antitussives**

√7ᵗʰ **T48.3X1** **Poisoning by antitussives, accidental (unintentional)**
Poisoning by antitussives NOS

√7ᵗʰ **T48.3X2** **Poisoning by antitussives, intentional self-harm**

√7ᵗʰ **T48.3X3** **Poisoning by antitussives, assault** ·

√7ᵗʰ **T48.3X4** **Poisoning by antitussives, undetermined**

√7ᵗʰ **T48.3X5** **Adverse effect of antitussives**

√7ᵗʰ **T48.3X6** **Underdosing of antitussives**

√5ᵗʰ **T48.4** **Poisoning by, adverse effect of and underdosing of expectorants**

√6ᵗʰ **T48.4X** **Poisoning by, adverse effect of and underdosing of expectorants**

√7ᵗʰ **T48.4X1** **Poisoning by expectorants, accidental (unintentional)**
Poisoning by expectorants NOS

√7ᵗʰ **T48.4X2** **Poisoning by expectorants, intentional self-harm**

√7ᵗʰ **T48.4X3** **Poisoning by expectorants, assault**

√7ᵗʰ **T48.4X4** **Poisoning by expectorants, undetermined**

√7ᵗʰ **T48.4X5** **Adverse effect of expectorants**

√7ᵗʰ **T48.4X6** **Underdosing of expectorants**

√5ᵗʰ **T48.5** **Poisoning by, adverse effect of and underdosing of other anti-common-cold drugs**
Poisoning by, adverse effect of and underdosing of decongestants

EXCLUDES 2   *poisoning by, adverse effect of and underdosing of antipyretics, NEC (T39.9-)*
poisoning by, adverse effect of and underdosing of non-steroidal antiinflammatory drugs (T39.3-)
poisoning by, adverse effect of and underdosing of salicylates (T39.0-)

√6ᵗʰ **T48.5X** **Poisoning by, adverse effect of and underdosing of other anti-common-cold drugs**

√7ᵗʰ **T48.5X1** **Poisoning by other anti-common-cold drugs, accidental (unintentional)**
Poisoning by other anti-common-cold drugs NOS

√7ᵗʰ **T48.5X2** **Poisoning by other anti-common-cold drugs, intentional self-harm**

√7ᵗʰ **T48.5X3** **Poisoning by other anti-common-cold drugs, assault**

√7ᵗʰ **T48.5X4** **Poisoning by other anti-common-cold drugs, undetermined**

√7ᵗʰ **T48.5X5** **Adverse effect of other anti-common-cold drugs**

√7ᵗʰ **T48.5X6** **Underdosing of other anti-common-cold drugs**

√5ᵗʰ **T48.6** **Poisoning by, adverse effect of and underdosing of antiasthmatics, not elsewhere classified**
Poisoning by, adverse effect of and underdosing of beta-adrenoreceptor agonists used in asthma therapy

EXCLUDES 1   *poisoning by, adverse effect of and underdosing of anterior pituitary [adenohypophyseal] hormones (T38.8)*
poisoning by, adverse effect of and underdosing of beta-adrenoreceptor agonists not used in asthma therapy (T44.5)

√6ᵗʰ **T48.6X** **Poisoning by, adverse effect of and underdosing of antiasthmatics**

√7ᵗʰ **T48.6X1** **Poisoning by antiasthmatics, accidental (unintentional)**
Poisoning by antiasthmatics NOS

√7ᵗʰ **T48.6X2** **Poisoning by antiasthmatics, intentional self-harm**

√7ᵗʰ **T48.6X3** **Poisoning by antiasthmatics, assault**

√7ᵗʰ **T48.6X4** **Poisoning by antiasthmatics, undetermined**

√7ᵗʰ **T48.6X5** **Adverse effect of antiasthmatics**

√7ᵗʰ **T48.6X6** **Underdosing of antiasthmatics**

√5ᵗʰ **T48.9** **Poisoning by, adverse effect of and underdosing of other and unspecified agents primarily acting on the respiratory system**

√6ᵗʰ **T48.90** **Poisoning by, adverse effect of and underdosing of unspecified agents primarily acting on the respiratory system**

√7ᵗʰ **T48.901** **Poisoning by unspecified agents primarily acting on the respiratory system, accidental (unintentional)** ▽

√7ᵗʰ **T48.902** **Poisoning by unspecified agents primarily acting on the respiratory system, intentional self-harm** ▽

√7ᵗʰ **T48.903** **Poisoning by unspecified agents primarily acting on the respiratory system, assault** ▽

√7ᵗʰ **T48.904** **Poisoning by unspecified agents primarily acting on the respiratory system, undetermined** ▽

√7ᵗʰ **T48.905** **Adverse effect of unspecified agents primarily acting on the respiratory system** ▽

√7ᵗʰ **T48.906** **Underdosing of unspecified agents primarily acting on the respiratory system** ▽

√6ᵗʰ **T48.99** **Poisoning by, adverse effect of and underdosing of other agents primarily acting on the respiratory system**

√7ᵗʰ **T48.991** **Poisoning by other agents primarily acting on the respiratory system, accidental (unintentional)**

√7ᵗʰ **T48.992** **Poisoning by other agents primarily acting on the respiratory system, intentional self-harm**

☑ Additional Character Req   √x7ᵗʰ Placeholder Alert   Case-Mix Diagnosis   Manifestation   ▽ Unspecified Dx   EXCLUDES 1 Not coded here   EXCLUDES 2 Not included here

ICD-10-CM 2018   **1077**

Chapter 19. Injury, Poisoning and Certain Other Consequences of External Causes

T48.1X2–T48.992

✓7ᵗʰ **T48.993** **Poisoning by other agents primarily acting on the respiratory system,** assault

✓7ᵗʰ **T48.994** **Poisoning by other agents primarily acting on the respiratory system,** undetermined

✓7ᵗʰ **T48.995** Adverse effect **of other agents primarily acting on the respiratory system**

✓7ᵗʰ **T48.996** Underdosing **of other agents primarily acting on the respiratory system**

✓4ᵗʰ **T49** **Poisoning by, adverse effect of and underdosing of topical agents primarily affecting skin and mucous membrane and by ophthalmological, otorhinolaryngological and dental drugs**

INCLUDES   poisoning by, adverse effect of and underdosing of glucocorticoids, topically used

> The appropriate 7th character is to be added to each code from category T49.
> A   initial encounter
> D   subsequent encounter
> S   sequela

✓5ᵗʰ **T49.0** **Poisoning by, adverse effect of and underdosing of local antifungal, anti-infective and anti-inflammatory drugs**

✓6ᵗʰ **T49.0X** **Poisoning by, adverse effect of and underdosing of** local antifungal, anti-infective and anti-inflammatory **drugs**

✓7ᵗʰ **T49.0X1** **Poisoning by local antifungal, anti-infective and anti-inflammatory drugs,** accidental **(unintentional)**
Poisoning by local antifungal, anti-infective and anti-inflammatory drugs NOS

✓7ᵗʰ **T49.0X2** **Poisoning by local antifungal, anti-infective and anti-inflammatory drugs,** intentional self-harm

✓7ᵗʰ **T49.0X3** **Poisoning by local antifungal, anti-infective and anti-inflammatory drugs,** assault

✓7ᵗʰ **T49.0X4** **Poisoning by local antifungal, anti-infective and anti-inflammatory drugs,** undetermined

✓7ᵗʰ **T49.0X5** Adverse effect **of local antifungal, anti-infective and anti-inflammatory drugs**

✓7ᵗʰ **T49.0X6** Underdosing **of local antifungal, anti-infective and anti-inflammatory drugs**

✓5ᵗʰ **T49.1** **Poisoning by, adverse effect of and underdosing of antipruritics**

✓6ᵗʰ **T49.1X** **Poisoning by, adverse effect of and underdosing of** antipruritics

✓7ᵗʰ **T49.1X1** **Poisoning by antipruritics,** accidental **(unintentional)**
Poisoning by antipruritics NOS

✓7ᵗʰ **T49.1X2** **Poisoning by antipruritics,** intentional self-harm

✓7ᵗʰ **T49.1X3** **Poisoning by antipruritics,** assault

✓7ᵗʰ **T49.1X4** **Poisoning by antipruritics,** undetermined

✓7ᵗʰ **T49.1X5** Adverse effect **of antipruritics**

✓7ᵗʰ **T49.1X6** Underdosing **of antipruritics**

✓5ᵗʰ **T49.2** **Poisoning by, adverse effect of and underdosing of local astringents and local detergents**

✓6ᵗʰ **T49.2X** **Poisoning by, adverse effect of and underdosing of** local astringents and local detergents

✓7ᵗʰ **T49.2X1** **Poisoning by local astringents and local detergents,** accidental **(unintentional)**
Poisoning by local astringents and local detergents NOS

✓7ᵗʰ **T49.2X2** **Poisoning by local astringents and local detergents,** intentional self-harm

✓7ᵗʰ **T49.2X3** **Poisoning by local astringents and local detergents,** assault

✓7ᵗʰ **T49.2X4** **Poisoning by local astringents and local detergents,** undetermined

✓7ᵗʰ **T49.2X5** Adverse effect **of local astringents and local detergents**

✓7ᵗʰ **T49.2X6** Underdosing **of local astringents and local detergents**

✓5ᵗʰ **T49.3** **Poisoning by, adverse effect of and underdosing of emollients, demulcents and protectants**

✓6ᵗʰ **T49.3X** **Poisoning by, adverse effect of and underdosing of** emollients, demulcents and protectants

✓7ᵗʰ **T49.3X1** **Poisoning by emollients, demulcents and protectants,** accidental **(unintentional)**
Poisoning by emollients, demulcents and protectants NOS

✓7ᵗʰ **T49.3X2** **Poisoning by emollients, demulcents and protectants,** intentional self-harm

✓7ᵗʰ **T49.3X3** **Poisoning by emollients, demulcents and protectants,** assault

✓7ᵗʰ **T49.3X4** **Poisoning by emollients, demulcents and protectants,** undetermined

✓7ᵗʰ **T49.3X5** Adverse effect **of emollients, demulcents and protectants**

✓7ᵗʰ **T49.3X6** Underdosing **of emollients, demulcents and protectants**

✓5ᵗʰ **T49.4** **Poisoning by, adverse effect of and underdosing of keratolytics, keratoplastics, and other hair treatment drugs and preparations**

✓6ᵗʰ **T49.4X** **Poisoning by, adverse effect of and underdosing of** keratolytics, keratoplastics, and other hair treatment drugs and preparations

✓7ᵗʰ **T49.4X1** **Poisoning by keratolytics, keratoplastics, and other hair treatment drugs and preparations,** accidental **(unintentional)**
Poisoning by keratolytics, keratoplastics, and other hair treatment drugs and preparations NOS

✓7ᵗʰ **T49.4X2** **Poisoning by keratolytics, keratoplastics, and other hair treatment drugs and preparations,** intentional self-harm

✓7ᵗʰ **T49.4X3** **Poisoning by keratolytics, keratoplastics, and other hair treatment drugs and preparations,** assault

✓7ᵗʰ **T49.4X4** **Poisoning by keratolytics, keratoplastics, and other hair treatment drugs and preparations,** undetermined

✓7ᵗʰ **T49.4X5** Adverse effect **of keratolytics, keratoplastics, and other hair treatment drugs and preparations**

✓7ᵗʰ **T49.4X6** Underdosing **of keratolytics, keratoplastics, and other hair treatment drugs and preparations**

✓5ᵗʰ **T49.5** **Poisoning by, adverse effect of and underdosing of ophthalmological drugs and preparations**

✓6ᵗʰ **T49.5X** **Poisoning by, adverse effect of and underdosing of** ophthalmological **drugs and preparations**

✓7ᵗʰ **T49.5X1** **Poisoning by ophthalmological drugs and preparations,** accidental **(unintentional)**
Poisoning by ophthalmological drugs and preparations NOS

✓7ᵗʰ **T49.5X2** **Poisoning by ophthalmological drugs and preparations,** intentional self-harm

✓7ᵗʰ **T49.5X3** **Poisoning by ophthalmological drugs and preparations,** assault

✓7ᵗʰ **T49.5X4** **Poisoning by ophthalmological drugs and preparations,** undetermined

✓7ᵗʰ **T49.5X5** Adverse effect **of ophthalmological drugs and preparations**

✓7ᵗʰ **T49.5X6** Underdosing **of ophthalmological drugs and preparations**

✓5ᵗʰ **T49.6** **Poisoning by, adverse effect of and underdosing of otorhinolaryngological drugs and preparations**

✓6ᵗʰ **T49.6X** **Poisoning by, adverse effect of and underdosing of** otorhinolaryngological **drugs and preparations**

✓7ᵗʰ **T49.6X1** **Poisoning by otorhinolaryngological drugs and preparations,** accidental **(unintentional)**
Poisoning by otorhinolaryngological drugs and preparations NOS

✓7ᵗʰ **T49.6X2** **Poisoning by otorhinolaryngological drugs and preparations,** intentional self-harm

✓7ᵗʰ **T49.6X3** **Poisoning by otorhinolaryngological drugs and preparations,** assault

---

N Newborn: 0   P Pediatric: 0-17   M Maternity: 12-55   A Adult: 15-124   NRS Nonroutine supply Dx   NC Dx Noncancer Dx   PDx Primary Dx   ►◄ Revised Text   ● New Code   ▲ Revised Title

1078   ICD-10-CM 2018

☑7ᵗʰ **T49.6X4** Poisoning by otorhinolaryngological drugs and preparations, undetermined

☑7ᵗʰ **T49.6X5** Adverse effect of otorhinolaryngological drugs and preparations

☑7ᵗʰ **T49.6X6** Underdosing of otorhinolaryngological drugs and preparations

☑5ᵗʰ **T49.7** Poisoning by, adverse effect of and underdosing of dental drugs, topically applied

☑6ᵗʰ **T49.7X** Poisoning by, adverse effect of and underdosing of dental drugs, topically applied

☑7ᵗʰ **T49.7X1** Poisoning by dental drugs, topically applied, accidental (unintentional)
Poisoning by dental drugs, topically applied NOS

☑7ᵗʰ **T49.7X2** Poisoning by dental drugs, topically applied, intentional self-harm

☑7ᵗʰ **T49.7X3** Poisoning by dental drugs, topically applied, assault

☑7ᵗʰ **T49.7X4** Poisoning by dental drugs, topically applied, undetermined

☑7ᵗʰ **T49.7X5** Adverse effect of dental drugs, topically applied

☑7ᵗʰ **T49.7X6** Underdosing of dental drugs, topically applied

☑5ᵗʰ **T49.8** Poisoning by, adverse effect of and underdosing of other topical agents
Poisoning by, adverse effect of and underdosing of spermicides

☑6ᵗʰ **T49.8X** Poisoning by, adverse effect of and underdosing of other topical agents

☑7ᵗʰ **T49.8X1** Poisoning by other topical agents, accidental (unintentional)
Poisoning by other topical agents NOS

☑7ᵗʰ **T49.8X2** Poisoning by other topical agents, intentional self-harm

☑7ᵗʰ **T49.8X3** Poisoning by other topical agents, assault

☑7ᵗʰ **T49.8X4** Poisoning by other topical agents, undetermined

☑7ᵗʰ **T49.8X5** Adverse effect of other topical agents

☑7ᵗʰ **T49.8X6** Underdosing of other topical agents

☑5ᵗʰ **T49.9** Poisoning by, adverse effect of and underdosing of unspecified topical agent

☑x7ᵗʰ **T49.91** Poisoning by unspecified topical agent, accidental (unintentional) ▽

☑x7ᵗʰ **T49.92** Poisoning by unspecified topical agent, intentional self-harm ▽

☑x7ᵗʰ **T49.93** Poisoning by unspecified topical agent, assault ▽

☑x7ᵗʰ **T49.94** Poisoning by unspecified topical agent, undetermined ▽

☑x7ᵗʰ **T49.95** Adverse effect of unspecified topical agent ▽

☑x7ᵗʰ **T49.96** Underdosing of unspecified topical agent ▽

☑4ᵗʰ **T50** Poisoning by, adverse effect of and underdosing of diuretics and other and unspecified drugs, medicaments and biological substances

The appropriate 7th character is to be added to each code from category T50.
A   initial encounter
D   subsequent encounter
S   sequela

☑5ᵗʰ **T50.0** Poisoning by, adverse effect of and underdosing of mineralocorticoids and their antagonists

☑6ᵗʰ **T50.0X** Poisoning by, adverse effect of and underdosing of mineralocorticoids and their antagonists

☑7ᵗʰ **T50.0X1** Poisoning by mineralocorticoids and their antagonists, accidental (unintentional)
Poisoning by mineralocorticoids and their antagonists NOS

☑7ᵗʰ **T50.0X2** Poisoning by mineralocorticoids and their antagonists, intentional self-harm

☑7ᵗʰ **T50.0X3** Poisoning by mineralocorticoids and their antagonists, assault

☑7ᵗʰ **T50.0X4** Poisoning by mineralocorticoids and their antagonists, undetermined

☑7ᵗʰ **T50.0X5** Adverse effect of mineralocorticoids and their antagonists

☑7ᵗʰ **T50.0X6** Underdosing of mineralocorticoids and their antagonists

☑5ᵗʰ **T50.1** Poisoning by, adverse effect of and underdosing of loop [high-ceiling] diuretics

☑6ᵗʰ **T50.1X** Poisoning by, adverse effect of and underdosing of loop [high-ceiling] diuretics

☑7ᵗʰ **T50.1X1** Poisoning by loop [high-ceiling] diuretics, accidental (unintentional)
Poisoning by loop [high-ceiling] diuretics NOS

☑7ᵗʰ **T50.1X2** Poisoning by loop [high-ceiling] diuretics, intentional self-harm

☑7ᵗʰ **T50.1X3** Poisoning by loop [high-ceiling] diuretics, assault

☑7ᵗʰ **T50.1X4** Poisoning by loop [high-ceiling] diuretics, undetermined

☑7ᵗʰ **T50.1X5** Adverse effect of loop [high-ceiling] diuretics

☑7ᵗʰ **T50.1X6** Underdosing of loop [high-ceiling] diuretics

☑5ᵗʰ **T50.2** Poisoning by, adverse effect of and underdosing of carbonic-anhydrase inhibitors, benzothiadiazides and other diuretics
Poisoning by, adverse effect of and underdosing of acetazolamide

☑6ᵗʰ **T50.2X** Poisoning by, adverse effect of and underdosing of carbonic-anhydrase inhibitors, benzothiadiazides and other diuretics

☑7ᵗʰ **T50.2X1** Poisoning by carbonic-anhydrase inhibitors, benzothiadiazides and other diuretics, accidental (unintentional)
Poisoning by carbonic-anhydrase inhibitors, benzothiadiazides and other diuretics NOS

☑7ᵗʰ **T50.2X2** Poisoning by carbonic-anhydrase inhibitors, benzothiadiazides and other diuretics, intentional self-harm

☑7ᵗʰ **T50.2X3** Poisoning by carbonic-anhydrase inhibitors, benzothiadiazides and other diuretics, assault

☑7ᵗʰ **T50.2X4** Poisoning by carbonic-anhydrase inhibitors, benzothiadiazides and other diuretics, undetermined

☑7ᵗʰ **T50.2X5** Adverse effect of carbonic-anhydrase inhibitors, benzothiadiazides and other diuretics

☑7ᵗʰ **T50.2X6** Underdosing of carbonic-anhydrase inhibitors, benzothiadiazides and other diuretics

☑5ᵗʰ **T50.3** Poisoning by, adverse effect of and underdosing of electrolytic, caloric and water-balance agents
Poisoning by, adverse effect of and underdosing of oral rehydration salts

☑6ᵗʰ **T50.3X** Poisoning by, adverse effect of and underdosing of electrolytic, caloric and water-balance agents

☑7ᵗʰ **T50.3X1** Poisoning by electrolytic, caloric and water-balance agents, accidental (unintentional)
Poisoning by electrolytic, caloric and water-balance agents NOS

☑7ᵗʰ **T50.3X2** Poisoning by electrolytic, caloric and water-balance agents, intentional self-harm

☑7ᵗʰ **T50.3X3** Poisoning by electrolytic, caloric and water-balance agents, assault

☑7ᵗʰ **T50.3X4** Poisoning by electrolytic, caloric and water-balance agents, undetermined

☑7ᵗʰ **T50.3X5** Adverse effect of electrolytic, caloric and water-balance agents

☑7ᵗʰ **T50.3X6** Underdosing of electrolytic, caloric and water-balance agents

☑ Additional Character Req   ☑x7ᵗʰ Placeholder Alert   Case-Mix Diagnosis   Manifestation   ▽ Unspecified Dx   **EXCLUDES 1** Not coded here   **EXCLUDES 2** Not included here

ICD-10-CM 2018   1079

√5ᵗʰ **T50.4 Poisoning by, adverse effect of and underdosing of drugs affecting uric acid metabolism**

     √6ᵗʰ **T50.4X Poisoning by, adverse effect of and underdosing of drugs** affecting uric acid metabolism

         √7ᵗʰ **T50.4X1 Poisoning by drugs affecting uric acid metabolism, accidental (unintentional)**
                 Poisoning by drugs affecting uric acid metabolism NOS

         √7ᵗʰ **T50.4X2 Poisoning by drugs affecting uric acid metabolism, intentional self-harm**

         √7ᵗʰ **T50.4X3 Poisoning by drugs affecting uric acid metabolism, assault**

         √7ᵗʰ **T50.4X4 Poisoning by drugs affecting uric acid metabolism, undetermined**

         √7ᵗʰ **T50.4X5 Adverse effect of drugs affecting uric acid metabolism**

         √7ᵗʰ **T50.4X6 Underdosing of drugs affecting uric acid metabolism**

√5ᵗʰ **T50.5 Poisoning by, adverse effect of and underdosing of appetite depressants**

     √6ᵗʰ **T50.5X Poisoning by, adverse effect of and underdosing of appetite depressants**

         √7ᵗʰ **T50.5X1 Poisoning by appetite depressants, accidental (unintentional)**
                 Poisoning by appetite depressants NOS

         √7ᵗʰ **T50.5X2 Poisoning by appetite depressants, intentional self-harm**

         √7ᵗʰ **T50.5X3 Poisoning by appetite depressants, assault**

         √7ᵗʰ **T50.5X4 Poisoning by appetite depressants, undetermined**

         √7ᵗʰ **T50.5X5 Adverse effect of appetite depressants**

         √7ᵗʰ **T50.5X6 Underdosing of appetite depressants**

√5ᵗʰ **T50.6 Poisoning by, adverse effect of and underdosing of antidotes and chelating agents**
       Poisoning by, adverse effect of and underdosing of alcohol deterrents

     √6ᵗʰ **T50.6X Poisoning by, adverse effect of and underdosing of antidotes and chelating agents**

         √7ᵗʰ **T50.6X1 Poisoning by antidotes and chelating agents, accidental (unintentional)**
                 Poisoning by antidotes and chelating agents NOS

         √7ᵗʰ **T50.6X2 Poisoning by antidotes and chelating agents, intentional self-harm**

         √7ᵗʰ **T50.6X3 Poisoning by antidotes and chelating agents, assault**

         √7ᵗʰ **T50.6X4 Poisoning by antidotes and chelating agents, undetermined**

         √7ᵗʰ **T50.6X5 Adverse effect of antidotes and chelating agents**

         √7ᵗʰ **T50.6X6 Underdosing of antidotes and chelating agents**

√5ᵗʰ **T50.7 Poisoning by, adverse effect of and underdosing of analeptics and opioid receptor antagonists**

     √6ᵗʰ **T50.7X Poisoning by, adverse effect of and underdosing of analeptics and opioid receptor antagonists**

         √7ᵗʰ **T50.7X1 Poisoning by analeptics and opioid receptor antagonists, accidental (unintentional)**
                 Poisoning by analeptics and opioid receptor antagonists NOS

         √7ᵗʰ **T50.7X2 Poisoning by analeptics and opioid receptor antagonists, intentional self-harm**

         √7ᵗʰ **T50.7X3 Poisoning by analeptics and opioid receptor antagonists, assault**

         √7ᵗʰ **T50.7X4 Poisoning by analeptics and opioid receptor antagonists, undetermined**

         √7ᵗʰ **T50.7X5 Adverse effect of analeptics and opioid receptor antagonists**

         √7ᵗʰ **T50.7X6 Underdosing of analeptics and opioid receptor antagonists**

√5ᵗʰ **T50.8 Poisoning by, adverse effect of and underdosing of diagnostic agents**

     √6ᵗʰ **T50.8X Poisoning by, adverse effect of and underdosing of diagnostic agents**

         √7ᵗʰ **T50.8X1 Poisoning by diagnostic agents, accidental (unintentional)**
                 Poisoning by diagnostic agents NOS

         √7ᵗʰ **T50.8X2 Poisoning by diagnostic agents, intentional self-harm**

         √7ᵗʰ **T50.8X3 Poisoning by diagnostic agents, assault**

         √7ᵗʰ **T50.8X4 Poisoning by diagnostic agents, undetermined**

         √7ᵗʰ **T50.8X5 Adverse effect of diagnostic agents**

         √7ᵗʰ **T50.8X6 Underdosing of diagnostic agents**

√5ᵗʰ **T50.A Poisoning by, adverse effect of and underdosing of bacterial vaccines**

     √6ᵗʰ **T50.A1 Poisoning by, adverse effect of and underdosing of pertussis vaccine, including combinations with a pertussis component**

         √7ᵗʰ **T50.A11 Poisoning by pertussis vaccine, including combinations with a pertussis component, accidental (unintentional)**

         √7ᵗʰ **T50.A12 Poisoning by pertussis vaccine, including combinations with a pertussis component, intentional self-harm**

         √7ᵗʰ **T50.A13 Poisoning by pertussis vaccine, including combinations with a pertussis component, assault**

         √7ᵗʰ **T50.A14 Poisoning by pertussis vaccine, including combinations with a pertussis component, undetermined**

         √7ᵗʰ **T50.A15 Adverse effect of pertussis vaccine, including combinations with a pertussis component**

         √7ᵗʰ **T50.A16 Underdosing of pertussis vaccine, including combinations with a pertussis component**

     √6ᵗʰ **T50.A2 Poisoning by, adverse effect of and underdosing of mixed bacterial vaccines without a pertussis component**

         √7ᵗʰ **T50.A21 Poisoning by mixed bacterial vaccines without a pertussis component, accidental (unintentional)**

         √7ᵗʰ **T50.A22 Poisoning by mixed bacterial vaccines without a pertussis component, intentional self-harm**

         √7ᵗʰ **T50.A23 Poisoning by mixed bacterial vaccines without a pertussis component, assault**

         √7ᵗʰ **T50.A24 Poisoning by mixed bacterial vaccines without a pertussis component, undetermined**

         √7ᵗʰ **T50.A25 Adverse effect of mixed bacterial vaccines without a pertussis component**

         √7ᵗʰ **T50.A26 Underdosing of mixed bacterial vaccines without a pertussis component**

     √6ᵗʰ **T50.A9 Poisoning by, adverse effect of and underdosing of other bacterial vaccines**

         √7ᵗʰ **T50.A91 Poisoning by other bacterial vaccines, accidental (unintentional)**

         √7ᵗʰ **T50.A92 Poisoning by other bacterial vaccines, intentional self-harm**

         √7ᵗʰ **T50.A93 Poisoning by other bacterial vaccines, assault**

         √7ᵗʰ **T50.A94 Poisoning by other bacterial vaccines, undetermined**

         √7ᵗʰ **T50.A95 Adverse effect of other bacterial vaccines**

         √7ᵗʰ **T50.A96 Underdosing of other bacterial vaccines**

√5ᵗʰ **T50.B Poisoning by, adverse effect of and underdosing of viral vaccines**

     √6ᵗʰ **T50.B1 Poisoning by, adverse effect of and underdosing of smallpox vaccines**

         √7ᵗʰ **T50.B11 Poisoning by smallpox vaccines, accidental (unintentional)**

         √7ᵗʰ **T50.B12 Poisoning by smallpox vaccines, intentional self-harm**

         √7ᵗʰ **T50.B13 Poisoning by smallpox vaccines, assault**

√7ᵗʰ **T50.B14** Poisoning by smallpox vaccines, undetermined

√7ᵗʰ **T50.B15** Adverse effect of smallpox vaccines

√7ᵗʰ **T50.B16** Underdosing of smallpox vaccines

√6ᵗʰ **T50.B9** Poisoning by, adverse effect of and underdosing of other viral vaccines

√7ᵗʰ **T50.B91** Poisoning by other viral vaccines, accidental (unintentional)

√7ᵗʰ **T50.B92** Poisoning by other viral vaccines, intentional self-harm

√7ᵗʰ **T50.B93** Poisoning by other viral vaccines, assault

√7ᵗʰ **T50.B94** Poisoning by other viral vaccines, undetermined

√7ᵗʰ **T50.B95** Adverse effect of other viral vaccines

√7ᵗʰ **T50.B96** Underdosing of other viral vaccines

√5ᵗʰ **T50.Z** Poisoning by, adverse effect of and underdosing of other vaccines and biological substances

√6ᵗʰ **T50.Z1** Poisoning by, adverse effect of and underdosing of immunoglobulin

√7ᵗʰ **T50.Z11** Poisoning by immunoglobulin, accidental (unintentional)

√7ᵗʰ **T50.Z12** Poisoning by immunoglobulin, intentional self-harm

√7ᵗʰ **T50.Z13** Poisoning by immunoglobulin, assault

√7ᵗʰ **T50.Z14** Poisoning by immunoglobulin, undetermined

√7ᵗʰ **T50.Z15** Adverse effect of immunoglobulin

√7ᵗʰ **T50.Z16** Underdosing of immunoglobulin

√6ᵗʰ **T50.Z9** Poisoning by, adverse effect of and underdosing of other vaccines and biological substances

√7ᵗʰ **T50.Z91** Poisoning by other vaccines and biological substances, accidental (unintentional)

√7ᵗʰ **T50.Z92** Poisoning by other vaccines and biological substances, intentional self-harm

√7ᵗʰ **T50.Z93** Poisoning by other vaccines and biological substances, assault

√7ᵗʰ **T50.Z94** Poisoning by other vaccines and biological substances, undetermined

√7ᵗʰ **T50.Z95** Adverse effect of other vaccines and biological substances

√7ᵗʰ **T50.Z96** Underdosing of other vaccines and biological substances

√5ᵗʰ **T50.9** Poisoning by, adverse effect of and underdosing of other and unspecified drugs, medicaments and biological substances
AHA: 2016, 1Q, 38; 2015, 1Q, 21

√6ᵗʰ **T50.90** Poisoning by, adverse effect of and underdosing of unspecified drugs, medicaments and biological substances

√7ᵗʰ **T50.901** Poisoning by unspecified drugs, medicaments and biological substances, accidental (unintentional) ▽

√7ᵗʰ **T50.902** Poisoning by unspecified drugs, medicaments and biological substances, intentional self-harm ▽

√7ᵗʰ **T50.903** Poisoning by unspecified drugs, medicaments and biological substances, assault ▽

√7ᵗʰ **T50.904** Poisoning by unspecified drugs, medicaments and biological substances, undetermined ▽

√7ᵗʰ **T50.905** Adverse effect of unspecified drugs, medicaments and biological substances ▽

√7ᵗʰ **T50.906** Underdosing of unspecified drugs, medicaments and biological substances ▽

√6ᵗʰ **T50.99** Poisoning by, adverse effect of and underdosing of other drugs, medicaments and biological substances

√7ᵗʰ **T50.991** Poisoning by other drugs, medicaments and biological substances, accidental (unintentional)

√7ᵗʰ **T50.992** Poisoning by other drugs, medicaments and biological substances, intentional self-harm

√7ᵗʰ **T50.993** Poisoning by other drugs, medicaments and biological substances, assault

√7ᵗʰ **T50.994** Poisoning by other drugs, medicaments and biological substances, undetermined

√7ᵗʰ **T50.995** Adverse effect of other drugs, medicaments and biological substances

√7ᵗʰ **T50.996** Underdosing of other drugs, medicaments and biological substances

Toxic effects of substances chiefly nonmedicinal as to source (T51-T65)

NOTE When no intent is indicated code to accidental. Undetermined intent is only for use when there is specific documentation in the record that the intent of the toxic effect cannot be determined.

Use additional code(s) for all associated manifestations of toxic effect, such as:
personal history of foreign body fully removed (Z87.821)
respiratory conditions due to external agents (J60-J70)
to identify any retained foreign body, if applicable (Z18.-)

EXCLUDES 1 contact with and (suspected) exposure to toxic substances (Z77.-)
AHA: 2017, 1Q, 39-40
TIP: Assign any condition resulting from a poisoning, toxic effect, or adverse effect, followed by the appropriate code from categories T51–T65 while the resulting effects of the poisoning, toxic effect, or adverse effect remain unresolved and require treatment.

√4ᵗʰ **T51** **Toxic effect of alcohol**

The appropriate 7th character is to be added to each code from category T51.
A   initial encounter
D   subsequent encounter
S   sequela

√5ᵗʰ **T51.0** **Toxic effect of ethanol**
Toxic effect of ethyl alcohol
EXCLUDES 2 acute alcohol intoxication or 'hangover' effects (F10.129, F10.229, F10.929)
drunkenness (F10.129, F10.229, F10.929)
pathological alcohol intoxication (F10.129, F10.229, F10.929)

√6ᵗʰ **T51.0X** **Toxic effect of ethanol**

√7ᵗʰ **T51.0X1** Toxic effect of ethanol, accidental (unintentional)
Toxic effect of ethanol NOS

√7ᵗʰ **T51.0X2** Toxic effect of ethanol, intentional self-harm

√7ᵗʰ **T51.0X3** Toxic effect of ethanol, assault

√7ᵗʰ **T51.0X4** Toxic effect of ethanol, undetermined

√5ᵗʰ **T51.1** **Toxic effect of methanol**
Toxic effect of methyl alcohol

√6ᵗʰ **T51.1X** **Toxic effect of methanol**

√7ᵗʰ **T51.1X1** Toxic effect of methanol, accidental (unintentional)
Toxic effect of methanol NOS

√7ᵗʰ **T51.1X2** Toxic effect of methanol, intentional self-harm

√7ᵗʰ **T51.1X3** Toxic effect of methanol, assault

√7ᵗʰ **T51.1X4** Toxic effect of methanol, undetermined

√5ᵗʰ **T51.2** **Toxic effect of 2-Propanol**
Toxic effect of isopropyl alcohol

√6ᵗʰ **T51.2X** **Toxic effect of 2-Propanol**

√7ᵗʰ **T51.2X1** Toxic effect of 2-Propanol, accidental (unintentional)
Toxic effect of 2-Propanol NOS

√7ᵗʰ **T51.2X2** Toxic effect of 2-Propanol, intentional self-harm

√7ᵗʰ **T51.2X3** Toxic effect of 2-Propanol, assault

√7ᵗʰ **T51.2X4** Toxic effect of 2-Propanol, undetermined

√5ᵗʰ **T51.3** **Toxic effect of fusel oil**
Toxic effect of amyl alcohol
Toxic effect of butyl [1-butanol] alcohol
Toxic effect of propyl [1-propanol] alcohol

√6ᵗʰ **T51.3X** **Toxic effect of fusel oil**

√7ᵗʰ **T51.3X1** Toxic effect of fusel oil, accidental (unintentional)
Toxic effect of fusel oil NOS

√7ᵗʰ **T51.3X2** Toxic effect of fusel oil, intentional self-harm

√7ᵗʰ **T51.3X3** Toxic effect of fusel oil, assault

√7ᵗʰ **T51.3X4** Toxic effect of fusel oil, undetermined

✓5ᵗʰ **T51.8**   **Toxic effect of other alcohols**

    ✓6ᵗʰ **T51.8X**   **Toxic effect of** other alcohols

       ✓7ᵗʰ **T51.8X1**   **Toxic effect of other alcohols, accidental (unintentional)**
              Toxic effect of other alcohols NOS

       ✓7ᵗʰ **T51.8X2**   **Toxic effect of other alcohols, intentional self-harm**

       ✓7ᵗʰ **T51.8X3**   **Toxic effect of other alcohols, assault**

       ✓7ᵗʰ **T51.8X4**   **Toxic effect of other alcohols, undetermined**

✓5ᵗʰ **T51.9**   **Toxic effect of** unspecified **alcohol**

    ✓x7ᵗʰ **T51.91**   **Toxic effect of unspecified alcohol, accidental (unintentional)** ▽

    ✓x7ᵗʰ **T51.92**   **Toxic effect of unspecified alcohol, intentional self-harm** ▽

    ✓x7ᵗʰ **T51.93**   **Toxic effect of unspecified alcohol, assault** ▽

    ✓x7ᵗʰ **T51.94**   **Toxic effect of unspecified alcohol, undetermined** ▽

✓4ᵗʰ **T52**   **Toxic effect of organic solvents**

    EXCLUDES 1   *halogen derivatives of aliphatic and aromatic hydrocarbons (T53.-)*

    The appropriate 7th character is to be added to each code from category T52.
    A   initial encounter
    D   subsequent encounter
    S   sequela

    ✓5ᵗʰ **T52.0**   **Toxic effects of petroleum products**
       Toxic effects of ether petroleum
       Toxic effects of gasoline [petrol]
       Toxic effects of kerosene [paraffin oil]
       Toxic effects of naphtha petroleum
       Toxic effects of paraffin wax
       Toxic effects of spirit petroleum

       ✓6ᵗʰ **T52.0X**   **Toxic effects of** petroleum products

          ✓7ᵗʰ **T52.0X1**   **Toxic effect of petroleum products, accidental (unintentional)**
               Toxic effects of petroleum products NOS

          ✓7ᵗʰ **T52.0X2**   **Toxic effect of petroleum products, intentional self-harm**

          ✓7ᵗʰ **T52.0X3**   **Toxic effect of petroleum products, assault**

          ✓7ᵗʰ **T52.0X4**   **Toxic effect of petroleum products, undetermined**

    ✓5ᵗʰ **T52.1**   **Toxic effects of benzene**

       EXCLUDES 1   *homologues of benzene (T52.2)*
                 nitroderivatives and aminoderivatives of benzene and its homologues (T65.3)

       ✓6ᵗʰ **T52.1X**   **Toxic effects of** benzene

          ✓7ᵗʰ **T52.1X1**   **Toxic effect of benzene, accidental (unintentional)**
               Toxic effect of benzene NOS

          ✓7ᵗʰ **T52.1X2**   **Toxic effect of benzene, intentional self-harm**

          ✓7ᵗʰ **T52.1X3**   **Toxic effect of benzene, assault**

          ✓7ᵗʰ **T52.1X4**   **Toxic effect of benzene, undetermined**

    ✓5ᵗʰ **T52.2**   **Toxic effects of homologues of benzene**
       Toxic effects of toluene [methylbenzene]
       Toxic effects of xylene [dimethylbenzene]

       ✓6ᵗʰ **T52.2X**   **Toxic effects of** homologues of benzene

          ✓7ᵗʰ **T52.2X1**   **Toxic effect of homologues of benzene, accidental (unintentional)**
               Toxic effects of homologues of benzene NOS

          ✓7ᵗʰ **T52.2X2**   **Toxic effect of homologues of benzene, intentional self-harm**

          ✓7ᵗʰ **T52.2X3**   **Toxic effect of homologues of benzene, assault**

          ✓7ᵗʰ **T52.2X4**   **Toxic effect of homologues of benzene, undetermined**

    ✓5ᵗʰ **T52.3**   **Toxic effects of glycols**

       ✓6ᵗʰ **T52.3X**   **Toxic effects of** glycols

          ✓7ᵗʰ **T52.3X1**   **Toxic effect of glycols, accidental (unintentional)**
               Toxic effect of glycols NOS

          ✓7ᵗʰ **T52.3X2**   **Toxic effect of glycols, intentional self-harm**

          ✓7ᵗʰ **T52.3X3**   **Toxic effect of glycols, assault**

          ✓7ᵗʰ **T52.3X4**   **Toxic effect of glycols, undetermined**

✓5ᵗʰ **T52.4**   **Toxic effects of ketones**

    ✓6ᵗʰ **T52.4X**   **Toxic effects of** ketones

       ✓7ᵗʰ **T52.4X1**   **Toxic effect of ketones, accidental (unintentional)**
              Toxic effects of ketones NOS

       ✓7ᵗʰ **T52.4X2**   **Toxic effect of ketones, intentional self-harm**

       ✓7ᵗʰ **T52.4X3**   **Toxic effect of ketones, assault**

       ✓7ᵗʰ **T52.4X4**   **Toxic effect of ketones, undetermined**

✓5ᵗʰ **T52.8**   **Toxic effects of other organic solvents**

    ✓6ᵗʰ **T52.8X**   **Toxic effects of** other organic solvents

       ✓7ᵗʰ **T52.8X1**   **Toxic effect of other organic solvents, accidental (unintentional)**
              Toxic effects of other organic solvents NOS

       ✓7ᵗʰ **T52.8X2**   **Toxic effect of other organic solvents, intentional self-harm**

       ✓7ᵗʰ **T52.8X3**   **Toxic effect of other organic solvents, assault**

       ✓7ᵗʰ **T52.8X4**   **Toxic effect of other organic solvents, undetermined**

✓5ᵗʰ **T52.9**   **Toxic effects of** unspecified **organic solvent**

    ✓x7ᵗʰ **T52.91**   **Toxic effect of unspecified organic solvent, accidental (unintentional)** ▽

    ✓x7ᵗʰ **T52.92**   **Toxic effect of unspecified organic solvent, intentional self-harm** ▽

    ✓x7ᵗʰ **T52.93**   **Toxic effect of unspecified organic solvent, assault** ▽

    ✓x7ᵗʰ **T52.94**   **Toxic effect of unspecified organic solvent, undetermined** ▽

✓4ᵗʰ **T53**   **Toxic effect of halogen derivatives of aliphatic and aromatic hydrocarbons**

    The appropriate 7th character is to be added to each code from category T53.
    A   initial encounter
    D   subsequent encounter
    S   sequela

    ✓5ᵗʰ **T53.0**   **Toxic effects of carbon tetrachloride**
       Toxic effects of tetrachloromethane

       ✓6ᵗʰ **T53.0X**   **Toxic effects of** carbon tetrachloride

          ✓7ᵗʰ **T53.0X1**   **Toxic effect of carbon tetrachloride, accidental (unintentional)**
               Toxic effects of carbon tetrachloride NOS

          ✓7ᵗʰ **T53.0X2**   **Toxic effect of carbon tetrachloride, intentional self-harm**

          ✓7ᵗʰ **T53.0X3**   **Toxic effect of carbon tetrachloride, assault**

          ✓7ᵗʰ **T53.0X4**   **Toxic effect of carbon tetrachloride, undetermined**

    ✓5ᵗʰ **T53.1**   **Toxic effects of chloroform**
       Toxic effects of trichloromethane

       ✓6ᵗʰ **T53.1X**   **Toxic effects of** chloroform

          ✓7ᵗʰ **T53.1X1**   **Toxic effect of chloroform, accidental (unintentional)**
               Toxic effects of chloroform NOS

          ✓7ᵗʰ **T53.1X2**   **Toxic effect of chloroform, intentional self-harm**

          ✓7ᵗʰ **T53.1X3**   **Toxic effect of chloroform, assault**

          ✓7ᵗʰ **T53.1X4**   **Toxic effect of chloroform, undetermined**

    ✓5ᵗʰ **T53.2**   **Toxic effects of trichloroethylene**
       Toxic effects of trichloroethene

       ✓6ᵗʰ **T53.2X**   **Toxic effects of** trichloroethylene

          ✓7ᵗʰ **T53.2X1**   **Toxic effect of trichloroethylene, accidental (unintentional)**
               Toxic effects of trichloroethylene NOS

          ✓7ᵗʰ **T53.2X2**   **Toxic effect of trichloroethylene, intentional self-harm**

          ✓7ᵗʰ **T53.2X3**   **Toxic effect of trichloroethylene, assault**

          ✓7ᵗʰ **T53.2X4**   **Toxic effect of trichloroethylene, undetermined**

Ⓝ Newborn: 0   Ⓟ Pediatric: 0-17   Ⓜ Maternity: 12-55   Ⓐ Adult: 15-124   **NRS** Nonroutine supply Dx   **NCDx** Noncancer Dx   **PDx** Primary Dx   ►◄ Revised Text   ● New Code   ▲ Revised Title

1082   ICD-10-CM 2018

✓5ᵗʰ **T53.3** **Toxic effects of tetrachloroethylene**
Toxic effects of perchloroethylene
Toxic effect of tetrachloroethene

  ✓6ᵗʰ **T53.3X** **Toxic effects of** tetrachloroethylene

    ✓7ᵗʰ **T53.3X1** **Toxic effect of tetrachloroethylene, accidental (unintentional)**
Toxic effects of tetrachloroethylene NOS

    ✓7ᵗʰ **T53.3X2** **Toxic effect of tetrachloroethylene, intentional self-harm**

    ✓7ᵗʰ **T53.3X3** **Toxic effect of tetrachloroethylene, assault**

    ✓7ᵗʰ **T53.3X4** **Toxic effect of tetrachloroethylene, undetermined**

✓5ᵗʰ **T53.4** **Toxic effects of dichloromethane**
Toxic effects of methylene chloride

  ✓6ᵗʰ **T53.4X** **Toxic effects of** dichloromethane

    ✓7ᵗʰ **T53.4X1** **Toxic effect of dichloromethane, accidental (unintentional)**
Toxic effects of dichloromethane NOS

    ✓7ᵗʰ **T53.4X2** **Toxic effect of dichloromethane, intentional self-harm**

    ✓7ᵗʰ **T53.4X3** **Toxic effect of dichloromethane, assault**

    ✓7ᵗʰ **T53.4X4** **Toxic effect of dichloromethane, undetermined**

✓5ᵗʰ **T53.5** **Toxic effects of chlorofluorocarbons**

  ✓6ᵗʰ **T53.5X** **Toxic effects of** chlorofluorocarbons

    ✓7ᵗʰ **T53.5X1** **Toxic effect of chlorofluorocarbons, accidental (unintentional)**
Toxic effects of chlorofluorocarbons NOS

    ✓7ᵗʰ **T53.5X2** **Toxic effect of chlorofluorocarbons, intentional self-harm**

    ✓7ᵗʰ **T53.5X3** **Toxic effect of chlorofluorocarbons, assault**

    ✓7ᵗʰ **T53.5X4** **Toxic effect of chlorofluorocarbons, undetermined**

✓5ᵗʰ **T53.6** **Toxic effects of other halogen derivatives of aliphatic hydrocarbons**

  ✓6ᵗʰ **T53.6X** **Toxic effects of other** halogen derivatives of aliphatic hydrocarbons

    ✓7ᵗʰ **T53.6X1** **Toxic effect of other halogen derivatives of aliphatic hydrocarbons, accidental (unintentional)**
Toxic effects of other halogen derivatives of aliphatic hydrocarbons NOS

    ✓7ᵗʰ **T53.6X2** **Toxic effect of other halogen derivatives of aliphatic hydrocarbons, intentional self-harm**

    ✓7ᵗʰ **T53.6X3** **Toxic effect of other halogen derivatives of aliphatic hydrocarbons, assault**

    ✓7ᵗʰ **T53.6X4** **Toxic effect of other halogen derivatives of aliphatic hydrocarbons, undetermined**

✓5ᵗʰ **T53.7** **Toxic effects of other halogen derivatives of aromatic hydrocarbons**

  ✓6ᵗʰ **T53.7X** **Toxic effects of other** halogen derivatives of aromatic hydrocarbons

    ✓7ᵗʰ **T53.7X1** **Toxic effect of other halogen derivatives of aromatic hydrocarbons, accidental (unintentional)**
Toxic effects of other halogen derivatives of aromatic hydrocarbons NOS

    ✓7ᵗʰ **T53.7X2** **Toxic effect of other halogen derivatives of aromatic hydrocarbons, intentional self-harm**

    ✓7ᵗʰ **T53.7X3** **Toxic effect of other halogen derivatives of aromatic hydrocarbons, assault**

    ✓7ᵗʰ **T53.7X4** **Toxic effect of other halogen derivatives of aromatic hydrocarbons, undetermined**

✓5ᵗʰ **T53.9** **Toxic effects of** unspecified halogen derivatives of aliphatic and aromatic hydrocarbons

  ✓x7ᵗʰ **T53.91** **Toxic effect of unspecified halogen derivatives of aliphatic and aromatic hydrocarbons, accidental (unintentional)** ▽

  ✓x7ᵗʰ **T53.92** **Toxic effect of unspecified halogen derivatives of aliphatic and aromatic hydrocarbons, intentional self-harm** ▽

  ✓x7ᵗʰ **T53.93** **Toxic effect of unspecified halogen derivatives of aliphatic and aromatic hydrocarbons, assault** ▽

  ✓x7ᵗʰ **T53.94** **Toxic effect of unspecified halogen derivatives of aliphatic and aromatic hydrocarbons, undetermined** ▽

✓4ᵗʰ **T54** **Toxic effect of corrosive substances**

> The appropriate 7th character is to be added to each code from category T54.
> A   initial encounter
> D   subsequent encounter
> S   sequela

✓5ᵗʰ **T54.0** **Toxic effects of phenol and phenol homologues**

  ✓6ᵗʰ **T54.0X** **Toxic effects of** phenol and phenol homologues

    ✓7ᵗʰ **T54.0X1** **Toxic effect of phenol and phenol homologues, accidental (unintentional)**
Toxic effects of phenol and phenol homologues NOS

    ✓7ᵗʰ **T54.0X2** **Toxic effect of phenol and phenol homologues, intentional self-harm**

    ✓7ᵗʰ **T54.0X3** **Toxic effect of phenol and phenol homologues, assault**

    ✓7ᵗʰ **T54.0X4** **Toxic effect of phenol and phenol homologues, undetermined**

✓5ᵗʰ **T54.1** **Toxic effects of other corrosive organic compounds**

  ✓6ᵗʰ **T54.1X** **Toxic effects of** other corrosive organic compounds

    ✓7ᵗʰ **T54.1X1** **Toxic effect of other corrosive organic compounds, accidental (unintentional)**
Toxic effects of other corrosive organic compounds NOS

    ✓7ᵗʰ **T54.1X2** **Toxic effect of other corrosive organic compounds, intentional self-harm**

    ✓7ᵗʰ **T54.1X3** **Toxic effect of other corrosive organic compounds, assault**

    ✓7ᵗʰ **T54.1X4** **Toxic effect of other corrosive organic compounds, undetermined**

✓5ᵗʰ **T54.2** **Toxic effects of corrosive acids and acid-like substances**
Toxic effects of hydrochloric acid
Toxic effects of sulfuric acid

  ✓6ᵗʰ **T54.2X** **Toxic effects of corrosive** acids and acid-like substances

    ✓7ᵗʰ **T54.2X1** **Toxic effect of corrosive acids and acid-like substances, accidental (unintentional)**
Toxic effects of corrosive acids and acid-like substances NOS

    ✓7ᵗʰ **T54.2X2** **Toxic effect of corrosive acids and acid-like substances, intentional self-harm**

    ✓7ᵗʰ **T54.2X3** **Toxic effect of corrosive acids and acid-like substances, assault**

    ✓7ᵗʰ **T54.2X4** **Toxic effect of corrosive acids and acid-like substances, undetermined**

✓5ᵗʰ **T54.3** **Toxic effects of corrosive alkalis and alkali-like substances**
Toxic effects of potassium hydroxide
Toxic effects of sodium hydroxide

  ✓6ᵗʰ **T54.3X** **Toxic effects of corrosive** alkalis and alkali-like substances

    ✓7ᵗʰ **T54.3X1** **Toxic effect of corrosive alkalis and alkali-like substances, accidental (unintentional)**
Toxic effects of corrosive alkalis and alkali-like substances NOS

    ✓7ᵗʰ **T54.3X2** **Toxic effect of corrosive alkalis and alkali-like substances, intentional self-harm**

    ✓7ᵗʰ **T54.3X3** **Toxic effect of corrosive alkalis and alkali-like substances, assault**

    ✓7ᵗʰ **T54.3X4** **Toxic effect of corrosive alkalis and alkali-like substances, undetermined**

✓5ᵗʰ **T54.9** **Toxic effects of** unspecified corrosive substance

  ✓x7ᵗʰ **T54.91** **Toxic effect of unspecified corrosive substance, accidental (unintentional)** ▽

  ✓x7ᵗʰ **T54.92** **Toxic effect of unspecified corrosive substance, intentional self-harm** ▽

  ✓x7ᵗʰ **T54.93** **Toxic effect of unspecified corrosive substance, assault** ▽

  ✓x7ᵗʰ **T54.94** **Toxic effect of unspecified corrosive substance, undetermined** ▽

✓ Additional Character Req   ✓x7ᵗʰ Placeholder Alert   Case-Mix Diagnosis   Manifestation   ▽ Unspecified Dx   **EXCLUDES 1** Not coded here   **EXCLUDES 2** Not included here

ICD-10-CM 2018   **1083**

Chapter 19. Injury, Poisoning and Certain Other Consequences of External Causes

✓4ᵗʰ **T55** **Toxic effect of soaps and detergents**

> The appropriate 7th character is to be added to each code from category T55.
> A   initial encounter
> D   subsequent encounter
> S   sequela

✓5ᵗʰ **T55.0** **Toxic effect of soaps**

  ✓6ᵗʰ **T55.0X** **Toxic effect of soaps**

    ✓7ᵗʰ **T55.0X1** **Toxic effect of soaps, accidental (unintentional)**
      Toxic effect of soaps NOS

    ✓7ᵗʰ **T55.0X2** **Toxic effect of soaps, intentional self-harm**

    ✓7ᵗʰ **T55.0X3** **Toxic effect of soaps, assault**

    ✓7ᵗʰ **T55.0X4** **Toxic effect of soaps, undetermined**

✓5ᵗʰ **T55.1** **Toxic effect of detergents**

  ✓6ᵗʰ **T55.1X** **Toxic effect of detergents**

    ✓7ᵗʰ **T55.1X1** **Toxic effect of detergents, accidental (unintentional)**
      Toxic effect of detergents NOS

    ✓7ᵗʰ **T55.1X2** **Toxic effect of detergents, intentional self-harm**

    ✓7ᵗʰ **T55.1X3** **Toxic effect of detergents, assault**

    ✓7ᵗʰ **T55.1X4** **Toxic effect of detergents, undetermined**

✓4ᵗʰ **T56** **Toxic effect of metals**

> **INCLUDES** toxic effects of fumes and vapors of metals
> toxic effects of metals from all sources, except medicinal substances
>
> Use additional code to identify any retained metal foreign body, if applicable (Z18.0-, T18.1-)
>
> **EXCLUDES 1** *arsenic and its compounds (T57.0)*
> *manganese and its compounds (T57.2)*

> The appropriate 7th character is to be added to each code from category T56.
> A   initial encounter
> D   subsequent encounter
> S   sequela

✓5ᵗʰ **T56.0** **Toxic effects of lead and its compounds**

  ✓6ᵗʰ **T56.0X** **Toxic effects of lead and its compounds**

    ✓7ᵗʰ **T56.0X1** **Toxic effect of lead and its compounds, accidental (unintentional)**
      Toxic effects of lead and its compounds NOS

    ✓7ᵗʰ **T56.0X2** **Toxic effect of lead and its compounds, intentional self-harm**

    ✓7ᵗʰ **T56.0X3** **Toxic effect of lead and its compounds, assault**

    ✓7ᵗʰ **T56.0X4** **Toxic effect of lead and its compounds, undetermined**

✓5ᵗʰ **T56.1** **Toxic effects of mercury and its compounds**

  ✓6ᵗʰ **T56.1X** **Toxic effects of mercury and its compounds**

    ✓7ᵗʰ **T56.1X1** **Toxic effect of mercury and its compounds, accidental (unintentional)**
      Toxic effects of mercury and its compounds NOS

    ✓7ᵗʰ **T56.1X2** **Toxic effect of mercury and its compounds, intentional self-harm**

    ✓7ᵗʰ **T56.1X3** **Toxic effect of mercury and its compounds, assault**

    ✓7ᵗʰ **T56.1X4** **Toxic effect of mercury and its compounds, undetermined**

✓5ᵗʰ **T56.2** **Toxic effects of chromium and its compounds**

  ✓6ᵗʰ **T56.2X** **Toxic effects of chromium and its compounds**

    ✓7ᵗʰ **T56.2X1** **Toxic effect of chromium and its compounds, accidental (unintentional)**
      Toxic effects of chromium and its compounds NOS

    ✓7ᵗʰ **T56.2X2** **Toxic effect of chromium and its compounds, intentional self-harm**

    ✓7ᵗʰ **T56.2X3** **Toxic effect of chromium and its compounds, assault**

    ✓7ᵗʰ **T56.2X4** **Toxic effect of chromium and its compounds, undetermined**

✓5ᵗʰ **T56.3** **Toxic effects of cadmium and its compounds**

  ✓6ᵗʰ **T56.3X** **Toxic effects of cadmium and its compounds**

    ✓7ᵗʰ **T56.3X1** **Toxic effect of cadmium and its compounds, accidental (unintentional)**
      Toxic effects of cadmium and its compounds NOS

    ✓7ᵗʰ **T56.3X2** **Toxic effect of cadmium and its compounds, intentional self-harm**

    ✓7ᵗʰ **T56.3X3** **Toxic effect of cadmium and its compounds, assault**

    ✓7ᵗʰ **T56.3X4** **Toxic effect of cadmium and its compounds, undetermined**

✓5ᵗʰ **T56.4** **Toxic effects of copper and its compounds**

  ✓6ᵗʰ **T56.4X** **Toxic effects of copper and its compounds**

    ✓7ᵗʰ **T56.4X1** **Toxic effect of copper and its compounds, accidental (unintentional)**
      Toxic effects of copper and its compounds NOS

    ✓7ᵗʰ **T56.4X2** **Toxic effect of copper and its compounds, intentional self-harm**

    ✓7ᵗʰ **T56.4X3** **Toxic effect of copper and its compounds, assault**

    ✓7ᵗʰ **T56.4X4** **Toxic effect of copper and its compounds, undetermined**

✓5ᵗʰ **T56.5** **Toxic effects of zinc and its compounds**

  ✓6ᵗʰ **T56.5X** **Toxic effects of zinc and its compounds**

    ✓7ᵗʰ **T56.5X1** **Toxic effect of zinc and its compounds, accidental (unintentional)**
      Toxic effects of zinc and its compounds NOS

    ✓7ᵗʰ **T56.5X2** **Toxic effect of zinc and its compounds, intentional self-harm**

    ✓7ᵗʰ **T56.5X3** **Toxic effect of zinc and its compounds, assault**

    ✓7ᵗʰ **T56.5X4** **Toxic effect of zinc and its compounds, undetermined**

✓5ᵗʰ **T56.6** **Toxic effects of tin and its compounds**

  ✓6ᵗʰ **T56.6X** **Toxic effects of tin and its compounds**

    ✓7ᵗʰ **T56.6X1** **Toxic effect of tin and its compounds, accidental (unintentional)**
      Toxic effect of tin and its compounds NOS

    ✓7ᵗʰ **T56.6X2** **Toxic effect of tin and its compounds, intentional self-harm**

    ✓7ᵗʰ **T56.6X3** **Toxic effect of tin and its compounds, assault**

    ✓7ᵗʰ **T56.6X4** **Toxic effect of tin and its compounds, undetermined**

✓5ᵗʰ **T56.7** **Toxic effects of beryllium and its compounds**

  ✓6ᵗʰ **T56.7X** **Toxic effects of beryllium and its compounds**

    ✓7ᵗʰ **T56.7X1** **Toxic effect of beryllium and its compounds, accidental (unintentional)**
      Toxic effects of beryllium and its compounds NOS

    ✓7ᵗʰ **T56.7X2** **Toxic effect of beryllium and its compounds, intentional self-harm**

    ✓7ᵗʰ **T56.7X3** **Toxic effect of beryllium and its compounds, assault**

    ✓7ᵗʰ **T56.7X4** **Toxic effect of beryllium and its compounds, undetermined**

✓5ᵗʰ **T56.8** **Toxic effects of other metals**

  ✓6ᵗʰ **T56.81** **Toxic effect of thallium**

    ✓7ᵗʰ **T56.811** **Toxic effect of thallium, accidental (unintentional)**
      Toxic effect of thallium NOS

    ✓7ᵗʰ **T56.812** **Toxic effect of thallium, intentional self-harm**

    ✓7ᵗʰ **T56.813** **Toxic effect of thallium, assault**

    ✓7ᵗʰ **T56.814** **Toxic effect of thallium, undetermined**

  ✓6ᵗʰ **T56.89** **Toxic effects of other metals**

    ✓7ᵗʰ **T56.891** **Toxic effect of other metals, accidental (unintentional)**
      Toxic effect of other metals NOS

    ✓7ᵗʰ **T56.892** **Toxic effect of other metals, intentional self-harm**

    ✓7ᵗʰ **T56.893** **Toxic effect of other metals, assault**

Ⓝ Newborn: 0 Ⓟ Pediatric: 0-17 Ⓜ Maternity: 12-55 Ⓐ Adult: 15-124 **NRS** Nonroutine supply Dx **NC Dx** Noncancer Dx **PDx** Primary Dx ►◄ Revised Text ● New Code ▲ Revised Title

1084   ICD-10-CM 2018

✓7ᵗʰ **T56.894 Toxic effect of other metals,** undetermined

✓5ᵗʰ **T56.9 Toxic effects of** unspecified metal

   ✓x7ᵗʰ **T56.91 Toxic effect of unspecified metal,** accidental **(unintentional)** ▽

   ✓x7ᵗʰ **T56.92 Toxic effect of unspecified metal,** intentional **self-harm** ▽

   ✓x7ᵗʰ **T56.93 Toxic effect of unspecified metal,** assault ▽

   ✓x7ᵗʰ **T56.94 Toxic effect of unspecified metal,** undetermined ▽

✓4ᵗʰ **T57 Toxic effect of other inorganic substances**

> The appropriate 7th character is to be added to each code from category T57.
> A   initial encounter
> D   subsequent encounter
> S   sequela

✓5ᵗʰ **T57.0 Toxic effect of arsenic and its compounds**

  ✓6ᵗʰ **T57.0X Toxic effect of** arsenic **and its compounds**

    ✓7ᵗʰ **T57.0X1 Toxic effect of arsenic and its compounds,** accidental **(unintentional)**
      Toxic effect of arsenic and its compounds NOS

    ✓7ᵗʰ **T57.0X2 Toxic effect of arsenic and its compounds,** intentional self-harm

    ✓7ᵗʰ **T57.0X3 Toxic effect of arsenic and its compounds,** assault

    ✓7ᵗʰ **T57.0X4 Toxic effect of arsenic and its compounds,** undetermined

✓5ᵗʰ **T57.1 Toxic effect of phosphorus and its compounds**
   EXCLUDES 1 *organophosphate insecticides (T60.0)*

  ✓6ᵗʰ **T57.1X Toxic effect of** phosphorus **and its compounds**

    ✓7ᵗʰ **T57.1X1 Toxic effect of phosphorus and its compounds,** accidental **(unintentional)**
      Toxic effect of phosphorus and its compounds NOS

    ✓7ᵗʰ **T57.1X2 Toxic effect of phosphorus and its compounds,** intentional self-harm

    ✓7ᵗʰ **T57.1X3 Toxic effect of phosphorus and its compounds,** assault

    ✓7ᵗʰ **T57.1X4 Toxic effect of phosphorus and its compounds,** undetermined

✓5ᵗʰ **T57.2 Toxic effect of manganese and its compounds**

  ✓6ᵗʰ **T57.2X Toxic effect of** manganese **and its compounds**

    ✓7ᵗʰ **T57.2X1 Toxic effect of** manganese **and its compounds,** accidental **(unintentional)**
      Toxic effect of manganese and its compounds NOS

    ✓7ᵗʰ **T57.2X2 Toxic effect of manganese and its compounds,** intentional self-harm

    ✓7ᵗʰ **T57.2X3 Toxic effect of manganese and its compounds,** assault

    ✓7ᵗʰ **T57.2X4 Toxic effect of manganese and its compounds,** undetermined

✓5ᵗʰ **T57.3 Toxic effect of hydrogen cyanide**

  ✓6ᵗʰ **T57.3X Toxic effect of** hydrogen cyanide

    ✓7ᵗʰ **T57.3X1 Toxic effect of hydrogen cyanide,** accidental **(unintentional)**
      Toxic effect of hydrogen cyanide NOS

    ✓7ᵗʰ **T57.3X2 Toxic effect of hydrogen cyanide,** intentional self-harm

    ✓7ᵗʰ **T57.3X3 Toxic effect of hydrogen cyanide,** assault

    ✓7ᵗʰ **T57.3X4 Toxic effect of hydrogen cyanide,** undetermined

✓5ᵗʰ **T57.8 Toxic effect of other specified inorganic substances**

  ✓6ᵗʰ **T57.8X Toxic effect of** other **specified** inorganic substances

    ✓7ᵗʰ **T57.8X1 Toxic effect of other specified inorganic substances,** accidental **(unintentional)**
      Toxic effect of other specified inorganic substances NOS

    ✓7ᵗʰ **T57.8X2 Toxic effect of other specified inorganic substances,** intentional self-harm

    ✓7ᵗʰ **T57.8X3 Toxic effect of other specified inorganic substances,** assault

    ✓7ᵗʰ **T57.8X4 Toxic effect of other specified inorganic substances,** undetermined

✓5ᵗʰ **T57.9 Toxic effect of** unspecified inorganic substance

   ✓x7ᵗʰ **T57.91 Toxic effect of unspecified inorganic substance,** accidental **(unintentional)** ▽

   ✓x7ᵗʰ **T57.92 Toxic effect of unspecified inorganic substance,** intentional self-harm ▽

   ✓x7ᵗʰ **T57.93 Toxic effect of unspecified inorganic substance,** assault ▽

   ✓x7ᵗʰ **T57.94 Toxic effect of unspecified inorganic substance,** undetermined ▽

✓4ᵗʰ **T58 Toxic effect of carbon monoxide**
   INCLUDES   asphyxiation from carbon monoxide
        toxic effect of carbon monoxide from all sources

> The appropriate 7th character is to be added to each code from category T58.
> A   initial encounter
> D   subsequent encounter
> S   sequela

✓5ᵗʰ **T58.0 Toxic effect of carbon monoxide** from motor vehicle exhaust
  Toxic effect of exhaust gas from gas engine
  Toxic effect of exhaust gas from motor pump

   ✓x7ᵗʰ **T58.01 Toxic effect of carbon monoxide from motor vehicle exhaust,** accidental **(unintentional)**

   ✓x7ᵗʰ **T58.02 Toxic effect of carbon monoxide from motor vehicle exhaust,** intentional self-harm

   ✓x7ᵗʰ **T58.03 Toxic effect of carbon monoxide from motor vehicle exhaust,** assault

   ✓x7ᵗʰ **T58.04 Toxic effect of carbon monoxide from motor vehicle exhaust,** undetermined

✓5ᵗʰ **T58.1 Toxic effect of carbon monoxide** from utility gas
  Toxic effect of acetylene
  Toxic effect of gas NOS used for lighting, heating, cooking
  Toxic effect of water gas

   ✓x7ᵗʰ **T58.11 Toxic effect of carbon monoxide from utility gas,** accidental **(unintentional)**

   ✓x7ᵗʰ **T58.12 Toxic effect of carbon monoxide from utility gas,** intentional self-harm

   ✓x7ᵗʰ **T58.13 Toxic effect of carbon monoxide from utility gas,** assault

   ✓x7ᵗʰ **T58.14 Toxic effect of carbon monoxide from utility gas,** undetermined

✓5ᵗʰ **T58.2 Toxic effect of carbon monoxide** from incomplete combustion of other domestic fuels
  Toxic effect of carbon monoxide from incomplete combustion of coal, coke, kerosene, wood

  ✓6ᵗʰ **T58.2X Toxic effect of carbon monoxide from incomplete combustion of other domestic fuels**

    ✓7ᵗʰ **T58.2X1 Toxic effect of carbon monoxide from incomplete combustion of other domestic fuels,** accidental **(unintentional)**

    ✓7ᵗʰ **T58.2X2 Toxic effect of carbon monoxide from incomplete combustion of other domestic fuels,** intentional self-harm

    ✓7ᵗʰ **T58.2X3 Toxic effect of carbon monoxide from incomplete combustion of other domestic fuels,** assault

    ✓7ᵗʰ **T58.2X4 Toxic effect of carbon monoxide from incomplete combustion of other domestic fuels,** undetermined

✓5ᵗʰ **T58.8 Toxic effect of carbon monoxide** from other source
  Toxic effect of carbon monoxide from blast furnace gas
  Toxic effect of carbon monoxide from fuels in industrial use
  Toxic effect of carbon monoxide from kiln vapor

  ✓6ᵗʰ **T58.8X Toxic effect of carbon monoxide from other source**

    ✓7ᵗʰ **T58.8X1 Toxic effect of carbon monoxide from other source,** accidental **(unintentional)**

    ✓7ᵗʰ **T58.8X2 Toxic effect of carbon monoxide from other source,** intentional self-harm

    ✓7ᵗʰ **T58.8X3 Toxic effect of carbon monoxide from other source,** assault

    ✓7ᵗʰ **T58.8X4 Toxic effect of carbon monoxide from other source,** undetermined

✓5ᵗʰ **T58.9 Toxic effect of carbon monoxide** from unspecified source

   ✓x7ᵗʰ **T58.91 Toxic effect of carbon monoxide from unspecified source,** accidental **(unintentional)** ▽

✓ Additional Character Req   ✓x7ᵗʰ Placeholder Alert   Case-Mix Diagnosis   Manifestation   ▽ Unspecified Dx   EXCLUDES 1 Not coded here   EXCLUDES 2 Not included here

√x7ᵗʰ **T58.92** **Toxic effect of carbon monoxide from unspecified source,** intentional self-harm ▽

√x7ᵗʰ **T58.93** **Toxic effect of carbon monoxide from unspecified source,** assault ▽

√x7ᵗʰ **T58.94** **Toxic effect of carbon monoxide from unspecified source,** undetermined ▽

√4ᵗʰ **T59** **Toxic effect of other gases, fumes and vapors**
   INCLUDES   aerosol propellants
   EXCLUDES 1   *chlorofluorocarbons (T53.5)*

The appropriate 7th character is to be added to each code from category T59.
A   initial encounter
D   subsequent encounter
S   sequela

√5ᵗʰ **T59.0** **Toxic effect of nitrogen oxides**
   √6ᵗʰ **T59.0X** **Toxic effect of** nitrogen oxides
     √7ᵗʰ **T59.0X1** **Toxic effect of nitrogen oxides,** accidental (unintentional)
       Toxic effect of nitrogen oxides NOS
     √7ᵗʰ **T59.0X2** **Toxic effect of nitrogen oxides,** intentional self-harm
     √7ᵗʰ **T59.0X3** **Toxic effect of nitrogen oxides,** assault
     √7ᵗʰ **T59.0X4** **Toxic effect of nitrogen oxides,** undetermined

√5ᵗʰ **T59.1** **Toxic effect of sulfur dioxide**
   √6ᵗʰ **T59.1X** **Toxic effect of** sulfur dioxide
     √7ᵗʰ **T59.1X1** **Toxic effect of sulfur dioxide,** accidental (unintentional)
       Toxic effect of sulfur dioxide NOS
     √7ᵗʰ **T59.1X2** **Toxic effect of sulfur dioxide,** intentional self-harm
     √7ᵗʰ **T59.1X3** **Toxic effect of sulfur dioxide,** assault
     √7ᵗʰ **T59.1X4** **Toxic effect of sulfur dioxide,** undetermined

√5ᵗʰ **T59.2** **Toxic effect of formaldehyde**
   √6ᵗʰ **T59.2X** **Toxic effect of** formaldehyde
     √7ᵗʰ **T59.2X1** **Toxic effect of formaldehyde,** accidental (unintentional)
       Toxic effect of formaldehyde NOS
     √7ᵗʰ **T59.2X2** **Toxic effect of formaldehyde,** intentional self-harm
     √7ᵗʰ **T59.2X3** **Toxic effect of formaldehyde,** assault
     √7ᵗʰ **T59.2X4** **Toxic effect of formaldehyde,** undetermined

√5ᵗʰ **T59.3** **Toxic effect of lacrimogenic gas**
   Toxic effect of tear gas
   √6ᵗʰ **T59.3X** **Toxic effect of** lacrimogenic gas
     √7ᵗʰ **T59.3X1** **Toxic effect of lacrimogenic gas,** accidental (unintentional)
       Toxic effect of lacrimogenic gas NOS
     √7ᵗʰ **T59.3X2** **Toxic effect of lacrimogenic gas,** intentional self-harm
     √7ᵗʰ **T59.3X3** **Toxic effect of lacrimogenic gas,** assault
     √7ᵗʰ **T59.3X4** **Toxic effect of lacrimogenic gas,** undetermined

√5ᵗʰ **T59.4** **Toxic effect of chlorine gas**
   √6ᵗʰ **T59.4X** **Toxic effect of** chlorine gas
     √7ᵗʰ **T59.4X1** **Toxic effect of chlorine gas,** accidental (unintentional)
       Toxic effect of chlorine gas NOS
     √7ᵗʰ **T59.4X2** **Toxic effect of chlorine gas,** intentional self-harm
     √7ᵗʰ **T59.4X3** **Toxic effect of chlorine gas,** assault
     √7ᵗʰ **T59.4X4** **Toxic effect of chlorine gas,** undetermined

√5ᵗʰ **T59.5** **Toxic effect of fluorine gas and hydrogen fluoride**
   √6ᵗʰ **T59.5X** **Toxic effect of** fluorine gas **and** hydrogen fluoride
     √7ᵗʰ **T59.5X1** **Toxic effect of fluorine gas and hydrogen fluoride,** accidental (unintentional)
       Toxic effect of fluorine gas and hydrogen fluoride NOS
     √7ᵗʰ **T59.5X2** **Toxic effect of fluorine gas and hydrogen fluoride,** intentional self-harm

√7ᵗʰ **T59.5X3** **Toxic effect of fluorine gas and hydrogen fluoride,** assault

√7ᵗʰ **T59.5X4** **Toxic effect of fluorine gas and hydrogen fluoride,** undetermined

√5ᵗʰ **T59.6** **Toxic effect of hydrogen sulfide**
   √6ᵗʰ **T59.6X** **Toxic effect of** hydrogen sulfide
     √7ᵗʰ **T59.6X1** **Toxic effect of hydrogen sulfide,** accidental (unintentional)
       Toxic effect of hydrogen sulfide NOS
     √7ᵗʰ **T59.6X2** **Toxic effect of hydrogen sulfide,** intentional self-harm
     √7ᵗʰ **T59.6X3** **Toxic effect of hydrogen sulfide,** assault
     √7ᵗʰ **T59.6X4** **Toxic effect of hydrogen sulfide,** undetermined

√5ᵗʰ **T59.7** **Toxic effect of carbon dioxide**
   √6ᵗʰ **T59.7X** **Toxic effect of** carbon dioxide
     √7ᵗʰ **T59.7X1** **Toxic effect of carbon dioxide,** accidental (unintentional)
       Toxic effect of carbon dioxide NOS
     √7ᵗʰ **T59.7X2** **Toxic effect of carbon dioxide,** intentional self-harm
     √7ᵗʰ **T59.7X3** **Toxic effect of carbon dioxide,** assault
     √7ᵗʰ **T59.7X4** **Toxic effect of carbon dioxide,** undetermined

√5ᵗʰ **T59.8** **Toxic effect of** other **specified gases, fumes and vapors**
   √6ᵗʰ **T59.81** **Toxic effect of** smoke
     Smoke inhalation
     EXCLUDES 2   *toxic effect of cigarette (tobacco) smoke (T65.22-)*
     √7ᵗʰ **T59.811** **Toxic effect of smoke,** accidental (unintentional)
       Toxic effect of smoke NOS
       AHA: 2013, 4Q, 121
     √7ᵗʰ **T59.812** **Toxic effect of smoke,** intentional self-harm
     √7ᵗʰ **T59.813** **Toxic effect of smoke,** assault
     √7ᵗʰ **T59.814** **Toxic effect of smoke,** undetermined
   √6ᵗʰ **T59.89** **Toxic effect of** other **specified gases, fumes and vapors**
     √7ᵗʰ **T59.891** **Toxic effect of other specified gases, fumes and vapors,** accidental (unintentional)
     √7ᵗʰ **T59.892** **Toxic effect of other specified gases, fumes and vapors,** intentional self-harm
     √7ᵗʰ **T59.893** **Toxic effect of other specified gases, fumes and vapors,** assault
     √7ᵗʰ **T59.894** **Toxic effect of other specified gases, fumes and vapors,** undetermined

√5ᵗʰ **T59.9** **Toxic effect of** unspecified **gases, fumes and vapors**
   √x7ᵗʰ **T59.91** **Toxic effect of unspecified gases, fumes and vapors,** accidental (unintentional) ▽
   √x7ᵗʰ **T59.92** **Toxic effect of unspecified gases, fumes and vapors,** intentional self-harm ▽
   √x7ᵗʰ **T59.93** **Toxic effect of unspecified gases, fumes and vapors,** assault ▽
   √x7ᵗʰ **T59.94** **Toxic effect of unspecified gases, fumes and vapors,** undetermined ▽

√4ᵗʰ **T60** **Toxic effect of pesticides**
   INCLUDES   toxic effect of wood preservatives

The appropriate 7th character is to be added to each code from category T60.
A   initial encounter
D   subsequent encounter
S   sequela

√5ᵗʰ **T60.0** **Toxic effect of organophosphate and carbamate insecticides**
   √6ᵗʰ **T60.0X** **Toxic effect of** organophosphate and carbamate insecticides
     √7ᵗʰ **T60.0X1** **Toxic effect of organophosphate and carbamate insecticides,** accidental (unintentional)
       Toxic effect of organophosphate and carbamate insecticides NOS
     √7ᵗʰ **T60.0X2** **Toxic effect of organophosphate and carbamate insecticides,** intentional self-harm

N Newborn: 0   P Pediatric: 0-17   M Maternity: 12-55   A Adult: 15-124   NRS Nonroutine supply Dx   NCDx Noncancer Dx   PDx Primary Dx   ▶◀ Revised Text   ● New Code   ▲ Revised Title

1086   ICD-10-CM 2018

✓7ᵗʰ **T60.0X3** **Toxic effect of organophosphate and carbamate insecticides,** assault

✓7ᵗʰ **T60.0X4** **Toxic effect of organophosphate and carbamate insecticides,** undetermined

✓5ᵗʰ **T60.1** **Toxic effect of halogenated insecticides**
  EXCLUDES 1   *chlorinated hydrocarbon (T53.-)*

  ✓6ᵗʰ **T60.1X** **Toxic effect of** halogenated insecticides

  ✓7ᵗʰ **T60.1X1** **Toxic effect of halogenated insecticides, accidental (unintentional)**
       Toxic effect of halogenated insecticides NOS

  ✓7ᵗʰ **T60.1X2** **Toxic effect of halogenated insecticides,** intentional self-harm

  ✓7ᵗʰ **T60.1X3** **Toxic effect of halogenated insecticides,** assault

  ✓7ᵗʰ **T60.1X4** **Toxic effect of halogenated insecticides,** undetermined

✓5ᵗʰ **T60.2** **Toxic effect of other insecticides**

  ✓6ᵗʰ **T60.2X** **Toxic effect of** other insecticides

  ✓7ᵗʰ **T60.2X1** **Toxic effect of other insecticides, accidental (unintentional)**
       Toxic effect of other insecticides NOS

  ✓7ᵗʰ **T60.2X2** **Toxic effect of other insecticides,** intentional self-harm

  ✓7ᵗʰ **T60.2X3** **Toxic effect of other insecticides,** assault

  ✓7ᵗʰ **T60.2X4** **Toxic effect of other insecticides,** undetermined

✓5ᵗʰ **T60.3** **Toxic effect of herbicides and fungicides**

  ✓6ᵗʰ **T60.3X** **Toxic effect of** herbicides and fungicides

  ✓7ᵗʰ **T60.3X1** **Toxic effect of herbicides and fungicides, accidental (unintentional)**
       Toxic effect of herbicides and fungicides NOS

  ✓7ᵗʰ **T60.3X2** **Toxic effect of herbicides and fungicides,** intentional self-harm

  ✓7ᵗʰ **T60.3X3** **Toxic effect of herbicides and fungicides,** assault

  ✓7ᵗʰ **T60.3X4** **Toxic effect of herbicides and fungicides,** undetermined

✓5ᵗʰ **T60.4** **Toxic effect of rodenticides**
  EXCLUDES 1   *strychnine and its salts (T65.1)*
            thallium (T56.81-)

  ✓6ᵗʰ **T60.4X** **Toxic effect of** rodenticides

  ✓7ᵗʰ **T60.4X1** **Toxic effect of rodenticides,** accidental (unintentional)
       Toxic effect of rodenticides NOS

  ✓7ᵗʰ **T60.4X2** **Toxic effect of rodenticides,** intentional self-harm

  ✓7ᵗʰ **T60.4X3** **Toxic effect of rodenticides,** assault

  ✓7ᵗʰ **T60.4X4** **Toxic effect of rodenticides,** undetermined

✓5ᵗʰ **T60.8** **Toxic effect of other pesticides**

  ✓6ᵗʰ **T60.8X** **Toxic effect of** other pesticides

  ✓7ᵗʰ **T60.8X1** **Toxic effect of other pesticides,** accidental (unintentional)
       Toxic effect of other pesticides NOS

  ✓7ᵗʰ **T60.8X2** **Toxic effect of other pesticides,** intentional self-harm

  ✓7ᵗʰ **T60.8X3** **Toxic effect of other pesticides,** assault

  ✓7ᵗʰ **T60.8X4** **Toxic effect of other pesticides,** undetermined

✓5ᵗʰ **T60.9** **Toxic effect of** unspecified pesticide

  ✓x7ᵗʰ **T60.91** **Toxic effect of unspecified pesticide,** accidental (unintentional)   ▽

  ✓x7ᵗʰ **T60.92** **Toxic effect of unspecified pesticide,** intentional self-harm   ▽

  ✓x7ᵗʰ **T60.93** **Toxic effect of unspecified pesticide,** assault   ▽

  ✓x7ᵗʰ **T60.94** **Toxic effect of unspecified pesticide,** undetermined   ▽

✓4ᵗʰ **T61** **Toxic effect of noxious substances eaten as seafood**
  EXCLUDES 1   *allergic reaction to food, such as:*
       anaphylactic reaction or shock due to adverse food reaction (T78.0-)
       bacterial foodborne intoxications (A05.-)
       dermatitis (L23.6, L25.4, L27.2)
       food protein-induced enterocolitis syndrome (K52.21)
       food protein-induced enteropathy (K52.22)
       gastroenteritis (noninfective) (K52.29)
     toxic effect of aflatoxin and other mycotoxins (T64)
     toxic effect of cyanides (T65.0-)
     toxic effect of harmful algae bloom (T65.82-)
     toxic effect of hydrogen cyanide (T57.3-)
     toxic effect of mercury (T56.1-)
     toxic effect of red tide (T65.82-)

  > The appropriate 7th character is to be added to each code from category T61.
  > A   initial encounter
  > D   subsequent encounter
  > S   sequela

✓5ᵗʰ **T61.0** Ciguatera fish poisoning

  ✓x7ᵗʰ **T61.01** **Ciguatera fish poisoning,** accidental (unintentional)

  ✓x7ᵗʰ **T61.02** **Ciguatera fish poisoning,** intentional self-harm

  ✓x7ᵗʰ **T61.03** **Ciguatera fish poisoning,** assault

  ✓x7ᵗʰ **T61.04** **Ciguatera fish poisoning,** undetermined

✓5ᵗʰ **T61.1** Scombroid fish poisoning
       Histamine-like syndrome

  ✓x7ᵗʰ **T61.11** **Scombroid fish poisoning,** accidental (unintentional)

  ✓x7ᵗʰ **T61.12** **Scombroid fish poisoning,** intentional self-harm

  ✓x7ᵗʰ **T61.13** **Scombroid fish poisoning,** assault

  ✓x7ᵗʰ **T61.14** **Scombroid fish poisoning,** undetermined

✓5ᵗʰ **T61.7** Other fish and shellfish poisoning

  ✓6ᵗʰ **T61.77** **Other** fish **poisoning**

  ✓7ᵗʰ **T61.771** **Other fish poisoning,** accidental (unintentional)

  ✓7ᵗʰ **T61.772** **Other fish poisoning,** intentional self-harm

  ✓7ᵗʰ **T61.773** **Other fish poisoning,** assault

  ✓7ᵗʰ **T61.774** **Other fish poisoning,** undetermined

  ✓6ᵗʰ **T61.78** **Other** shellfish **poisoning**

  ✓7ᵗʰ **T61.781** **Other shellfish poisoning,** accidental (unintentional)

  ✓7ᵗʰ **T61.782** **Other shellfish poisoning,** intentional self-harm

  ✓7ᵗʰ **T61.783** **Other shellfish poisoning,** assault

  ✓7ᵗʰ **T61.784** **Other shellfish poisoning,** undetermined

✓5ᵗʰ **T61.8** **Toxic effect of other seafood**

  ✓6ᵗʰ **T61.8X** **Toxic effect of** other seafood

  ✓7ᵗʰ **T61.8X1** **Toxic effect of other seafood,** accidental (unintentional)

  ✓7ᵗʰ **T61.8X2** **Toxic effect of other seafood,** intentional self-harm

  ✓7ᵗʰ **T61.8X3** **Toxic effect of other seafood,** assault

  ✓7ᵗʰ **T61.8X4** **Toxic effect of other seafood,** undetermined

✓5ᵗʰ **T61.9** **Toxic effect of** unspecified seafood

  ✓x7ᵗʰ **T61.91** **Toxic effect of unspecified seafood,** accidental (unintentional)   ▽

  ✓x7ᵗʰ **T61.92** **Toxic effect of unspecified seafood,** intentional self-harm   ▽

  ✓x7ᵗʰ **T61.93** **Toxic effect of unspecified seafood,** assault   ▽

  ✓x7ᵗʰ **T61.94** **Toxic effect of unspecified seafood,** undetermined   ▽

☑ Additional Character Req   ✓x7ᵗʰ Placeholder Alert   Case-Mix Diagnosis   Manifestation   ▽ Unspecified Dx   EXCLUDES 1 Not coded here   EXCLUDES 2 Not included here

ICD-10-CM 2018   **1087**

T60.0X3–T61.94

✓4ᵗʰ **T62 Toxic effect of other noxious substances eaten as food**

EXCLUDES 1   allergic reaction to food, such as:
    anaphylactic shock (reaction) due to adverse food reaction (T78.0-)
    bacterial food borne intoxications (A05.-)
    dermatitis (L23.6, L25.4, L27.2)
    food protein-induced enterocolitis syndrome (K52.21)
    food protein-induced enteropathy (K52.22)
    gastroenteritis (noninfective) (K52.29)
    toxic effect of aflatoxin and other mycotoxins (T64)
    toxic effect of cyanides (T65.0-)
    toxic effect of hydrogen cyanide (T57.3-)
    toxic effect of mercury (T56.1-)

The appropriate 7th character is to be added to each code from category T62.
A   initial encounter
D   subsequent encounter
S   sequela

✓5ᵗʰ **T62.0 Toxic effect of ingested mushrooms**

   ✓6ᵗʰ **T62.0X Toxic effect of** ingested mushrooms

     ✓7ᵗʰ **T62.0X1 Toxic effect of ingested mushrooms, accidental (unintentional)**
       Toxic effect of ingested mushrooms NOS

     ✓7ᵗʰ **T62.0X2 Toxic effect of ingested mushrooms, intentional self-harm**

     ✓7ᵗʰ **T62.0X3 Toxic effect of ingested mushrooms, assault**

     ✓7ᵗʰ **T62.0X4 Toxic effect of ingested mushrooms, undetermined**

✓5ᵗʰ **T62.1 Toxic effect of ingested berries**

   ✓6ᵗʰ **T62.1X Toxic effect of** ingested berries

     ✓7ᵗʰ **T62.1X1 Toxic effect of ingested berries, accidental (unintentional)**
       Toxic effect of ingested berries NOS

     ✓7ᵗʰ **T62.1X2 Toxic effect of ingested berries, intentional self-harm**

     ✓7ᵗʰ **T62.1X3 Toxic effect of ingested berries, assault**

     ✓7ᵗʰ **T62.1X4 Toxic effect of ingested berries, undetermined**

✓5ᵗʰ **T62.2 Toxic effect of other ingested (parts of) plant(s)**

   ✓6ᵗʰ **T62.2X Toxic effect of** other ingested (parts of) plant(s)

     ✓7ᵗʰ **T62.2X1 Toxic effect of other ingested (parts of) plant(s), accidental (unintentional)**
       Toxic effect of other ingested (parts of) plant(s) NOS

     ✓7ᵗʰ **T62.2X2 Toxic effect of other ingested (parts of) plant(s), intentional self-harm**

     ✓7ᵗʰ **T62.2X3 Toxic effect of other ingested (parts of) plant(s), assault**

     ✓7ᵗʰ **T62.2X4 Toxic effect of other ingested (parts of) plant(s), undetermined**

✓5ᵗʰ **T62.8 Toxic effect of other specified noxious substances eaten as food**

   ✓6ᵗʰ **T62.8X Toxic effect of** other specified noxious substances eaten as food

     ✓7ᵗʰ **T62.8X1 Toxic effect of other specified noxious substances eaten as food, accidental (unintentional)**
       Toxic effect of other specified noxious substances eaten as food NOS

     ✓7ᵗʰ **T62.8X2 Toxic effect of other specified noxious substances eaten as food, intentional self-harm**

     ✓7ᵗʰ **T62.8X3 Toxic effect of other specified noxious substances eaten as food, assault**

     ✓7ᵗʰ **T62.8X4 Toxic effect of other specified noxious substances eaten as food, undetermined**

✓5ᵗʰ **T62.9 Toxic effect of** unspecified **noxious substance eaten as food**

   ✓×7ᵗʰ **T62.91 Toxic effect of unspecified noxious substance eaten as food, accidental (unintentional)**
     Toxic effect of unspecified noxious substance eaten as food NOS

   ✓×7ᵗʰ **T62.92 Toxic effect of unspecified noxious substance eaten as food, intentional self-harm**

   ✓×7ᵗʰ **T62.93 Toxic effect of unspecified noxious substance eaten as food, assault**

   ✓×7ᵗʰ **T62.94 Toxic effect of unspecified noxious substance eaten as food, undetermined**

✓4ᵗʰ **T63 Toxic effect of contact with venomous animals and plants**

INCLUDES   bite or touch of venomous animal
    pricked or stuck by thorn or leaf

EXCLUDES 2   ingestion of toxic animal or plant (T61.-, T62.-)

The appropriate 7th character is to be added to each code from category T63.
A   initial encounter
D   subsequent encounter
S   sequela

✓5ᵗʰ **T63.0 Toxic effect of** snake venom

   ✓6ᵗʰ **T63.00 Toxic effect of** unspecified **snake venom**

     ✓7ᵗʰ **T63.001 Toxic effect of unspecified snake venom, accidental (unintentional)**
       Toxic effect of unspecified snake venom NOS

     ✓7ᵗʰ **T63.002 Toxic effect of unspecified snake venom, intentional self-harm**

     ✓7ᵗʰ **T63.003 Toxic effect of unspecified snake venom, assault**

     ✓7ᵗʰ **T63.004 Toxic effect of unspecified snake venom, undetermined**

   ✓6ᵗʰ **T63.01 Toxic effect of** rattlesnake **venom**

     ✓7ᵗʰ **T63.011 Toxic effect of rattlesnake venom, accidental (unintentional)**
       Toxic effect of rattlesnake venom NOS

     ✓7ᵗʰ **T63.012 Toxic effect of rattlesnake venom, intentional self-harm**

     ✓7ᵗʰ **T63.013 Toxic effect of rattlesnake venom, assault**

     ✓7ᵗʰ **T63.014 Toxic effect of rattlesnake venom, undetermined**

   ✓6ᵗʰ **T63.02 Toxic effect of** coral snake **venom**

     ✓7ᵗʰ **T63.021 Toxic effect of coral snake venom, accidental (unintentional)**
       Toxic effect of coral snake venom NOS

     ✓7ᵗʰ **T63.022 Toxic effect of coral snake venom, intentional self-harm**

     ✓7ᵗʰ **T63.023 Toxic effect of coral snake venom, assault**

     ✓7ᵗʰ **T63.024 Toxic effect of coral snake venom, undetermined**

   ✓6ᵗʰ **T63.03 Toxic effect of** taipan **venom**

     ✓7ᵗʰ **T63.031 Toxic effect of taipan venom, accidental (unintentional)**
       Toxic effect of taipan venom NOS

     ✓7ᵗʰ **T63.032 Toxic effect of taipan venom, intentional self-harm**

     ✓7ᵗʰ **T63.033 Toxic effect of taipan venom, assault**

     ✓7ᵗʰ **T63.034 Toxic effect of taipan venom, undetermined**

   ✓6ᵗʰ **T63.04 Toxic effect of** cobra **venom**

     ✓7ᵗʰ **T63.041 Toxic effect of cobra venom, accidental (unintentional)**
       Toxic effect of cobra venom NOS

     ✓7ᵗʰ **T63.042 Toxic effect of cobra venom, intentional self-harm**

     ✓7ᵗʰ **T63.043 Toxic effect of cobra venom, assault**

     ✓7ᵗʰ **T63.044 Toxic effect of cobra venom, undetermined**

   ✓6ᵗʰ **T63.06 Toxic effect of venom of** other North and South American snake

     ✓7ᵗʰ **T63.061 Toxic effect of venom of other North and South American snake, accidental (unintentional)**
       Toxic effect of venom of other North and South American snake NOS

     ✓7ᵗʰ **T63.062 Toxic effect of venom of other North and South American snake, intentional self-harm**

     ✓7ᵗʰ **T63.063 Toxic effect of venom of other North and South American snake, assault**

     ✓7ᵗʰ **T63.064 Toxic effect of venom of other North and South American snake, undetermined**

☑6ᵗʰ **T63.07** Toxic effect of venom of other Australian snake

  ☑7ᵗʰ **T63.071** Toxic effect of venom of other Australian snake, accidental (unintentional)
    Toxic effect of venom of other Australian snake NOS

  ☑7ᵗʰ **T63.072** Toxic effect of venom of other Australian snake, intentional self-harm

  ☑7ᵗʰ **T63.073** Toxic effect of venom of other Australian snake, assault

  ☑7ᵗʰ **T63.074** Toxic effect of venom of other Australian snake, undetermined

☑6ᵗʰ **T63.08** Toxic effect of venom of other African and Asian snake

  ☑7ᵗʰ **T63.081** Toxic effect of venom of other African and Asian snake, accidental (unintentional)
    Toxic effect of venom of other African and Asian snake NOS

  ☑7ᵗʰ **T63.082** Toxic effect of venom of other African and Asian snake, intentional self-harm

  ☑7ᵗʰ **T63.083** Toxic effect of venom of other African and Asian snake, assault

  ☑7ᵗʰ **T63.084** Toxic effect of venom of other African and Asian snake, undetermined

☑6ᵗʰ **T63.09** Toxic effect of venom of other snake

  ☑7ᵗʰ **T63.091** Toxic effect of venom of other snake, accidental (unintentional)
    Toxic effect of venom of other snake NOS

  ☑7ᵗʰ **T63.092** Toxic effect of venom of other snake, intentional self-harm

  ☑7ᵗʰ **T63.093** Toxic effect of venom of other snake, assault

  ☑7ᵗʰ **T63.094** Toxic effect of venom of other snake, undetermined

☑5ᵗʰ **T63.1** Toxic effect of venom of other reptiles

☑6ᵗʰ **T63.11** Toxic effect of venom of gila monster

  ☑7ᵗʰ **T63.111** Toxic effect of venom of gila monster, accidental (unintentional)
    Toxic effect of venom of gila monster NOS

  ☑7ᵗʰ **T63.112** Toxic effect of venom of gila monster, intentional self-harm

  ☑7ᵗʰ **T63.113** Toxic effect of venom of gila monster, assault

  ☑7ᵗʰ **T63.114** Toxic effect of venom of gila monster, undetermined

☑6ᵗʰ **T63.12** Toxic effect of venom of other venomous lizard

  ☑7ᵗʰ **T63.121** Toxic effect of venom of other venomous lizard, accidental (unintentional)
    Toxic effect of venom of other venomous lizard NOS

  ☑7ᵗʰ **T63.122** Toxic effect of venom of other venomous lizard, intentional self-harm

  ☑7ᵗʰ **T63.123** Toxic effect of venom of other venomous lizard, assault

  ☑7ᵗʰ **T63.124** Toxic effect of venom of other venomous lizard, undetermined

☑6ᵗʰ **T63.19** Toxic effect of venom of other reptiles

  ☑7ᵗʰ **T63.191** Toxic effect of venom of other reptiles, accidental (unintentional)
    Toxic effect of venom of other reptiles NOS

  ☑7ᵗʰ **T63.192** Toxic effect of venom of other reptiles, intentional self-harm

  ☑7ᵗʰ **T63.193** Toxic effect of venom of other reptiles, assault

  ☑7ᵗʰ **T63.194** Toxic effect of venom of other reptiles, undetermined

☑5ᵗʰ **T63.2** Toxic effect of venom of scorpion

☑6ᵗʰ **T63.2X** Toxic effect of venom of scorpion

  ☑7ᵗʰ **T63.2X1** Toxic effect of venom of scorpion, accidental (unintentional)
    Toxic effect of venom of scorpion NOS

  ☑7ᵗʰ **T63.2X2** Toxic effect of venom of scorpion, intentional self-harm

  ☑7ᵗʰ **T63.2X3** Toxic effect of venom of scorpion, assault

  ☑7ᵗʰ **T63.2X4** Toxic effect of venom of scorpion, undetermined

☑5ᵗʰ **T63.3** Toxic effect of venom of spider

☑6ᵗʰ **T63.30** Toxic effect of unspecified spider venom

  ☑7ᵗʰ **T63.301** Toxic effect of unspecified spider venom, accidental (unintentional) ▽

  ☑7ᵗʰ **T63.302** Toxic effect of unspecified spider venom, intentional self-harm ▽

  ☑7ᵗʰ **T63.303** Toxic effect of unspecified spider venom, assault ▽

  ☑7ᵗʰ **T63.304** Toxic effect of unspecified spider venom, undetermined ▽

☑6ᵗʰ **T63.31** Toxic effect of venom of black widow spider

  ☑7ᵗʰ **T63.311** Toxic effect of venom of black widow spider, accidental (unintentional)

  ☑7ᵗʰ **T63.312** Toxic effect of venom of black widow spider, intentional self-harm

  ☑7ᵗʰ **T63.313** Toxic effect of venom of black widow spider, assault

  ☑7ᵗʰ **T63.314** Toxic effect of venom of black widow spider, undetermined

☑6ᵗʰ **T63.32** Toxic effect of venom of tarantula

  ☑7ᵗʰ **T63.321** Toxic effect of venom of tarantula, accidental (unintentional)

  ☑7ᵗʰ **T63.322** Toxic effect of venom of tarantula, intentional self-harm

  ☑7ᵗʰ **T63.323** Toxic effect of venom of tarantula, assault

  ☑7ᵗʰ **T63.324** Toxic effect of venom of tarantula, undetermined

☑6ᵗʰ **T63.33** Toxic effect of venom of brown recluse spider

  ☑7ᵗʰ **T63.331** Toxic effect of venom of brown recluse spider, accidental (unintentional)

  ☑7ᵗʰ **T63.332** Toxic effect of venom of brown recluse spider, intentional self-harm

  ☑7ᵗʰ **T63.333** Toxic effect of venom of brown recluse spider, assault

  ☑7ᵗʰ **T63.334** Toxic effect of venom of brown recluse spider, undetermined

☑6ᵗʰ **T63.39** Toxic effect of venom of other spider

  ☑7ᵗʰ **T63.391** Toxic effect of venom of other spider, accidental (unintentional)

  ☑7ᵗʰ **T63.392** Toxic effect of venom of other spider, intentional self-harm

  ☑7ᵗʰ **T63.393** Toxic effect of venom of other spider, assault

  ☑7ᵗʰ **T63.394** Toxic effect of venom of other spider, undetermined

☑5ᵗʰ **T63.4** Toxic effect of venom of other arthropods

☑6ᵗʰ **T63.41** Toxic effect of venom of centipedes and venomous millipedes

  ☑7ᵗʰ **T63.411** Toxic effect of venom of centipedes and venomous millipedes, accidental (unintentional)

  ☑7ᵗʰ **T63.412** Toxic effect of venom of centipedes and venomous millipedes, intentional self-harm

  ☑7ᵗʰ **T63.413** Toxic effect of venom of centipedes and venomous millipedes, assault

  ☑7ᵗʰ **T63.414** Toxic effect of venom of centipedes and venomous millipedes, undetermined

☑6ᵗʰ **T63.42** Toxic effect of venom of ants

  ☑7ᵗʰ **T63.421** Toxic effect of venom of ants, accidental (unintentional)

  ☑7ᵗʰ **T63.422** Toxic effect of venom of ants, intentional self-harm

  ☑7ᵗʰ **T63.423** Toxic effect of venom of ants, assault

  ☑7ᵗʰ **T63.424** Toxic effect of venom of ants, undetermined

☑6ᵗʰ **T63.43** Toxic effect of venom of caterpillars

  ☑7ᵗʰ **T63.431** Toxic effect of venom of caterpillars, accidental (unintentional)

  ☑7ᵗʰ **T63.432** Toxic effect of venom of caterpillars, intentional self-harm

  ☑7ᵗʰ **T63.433** Toxic effect of venom of caterpillars, assault

☑ Additional Character Req   ☑x7ᵗʰ Placeholder Alert   Case-Mix Diagnosis   Manifestation   ▽ Unspecified Dx   EXCLUDES 1 Not coded here   EXCLUDES 2 Not included here

ICD-10-CM 2018   1089

Chapter 19. Injury, Poisoning and Certain Other Consequences of External Causes

√7ᵗʰ **T63.434** Toxic effect of venom of caterpillars, undetermined

√6ᵗʰ **T63.44** Toxic effect of venom of bees
- √7ᵗʰ **T63.441** Toxic effect of venom of bees, accidental (unintentional)
- √7ᵗʰ **T63.442** Toxic effect of venom of bees, intentional self-harm
- √7ᵗʰ **T63.443** Toxic effect of venom of bees, assault
- √7ᵗʰ **T63.444** Toxic effect of venom of bees, undetermined

√6ᵗʰ **T63.45** Toxic effect of venom of hornets
- √7ᵗʰ **T63.451** Toxic effect of venom of hornets, accidental (unintentional)
- √7ᵗʰ **T63.452** Toxic effect of venom of hornets, intentional self-harm
- √7ᵗʰ **T63.453** Toxic effect of venom of hornets, assault
- √7ᵗʰ **T63.454** Toxic effect of venom of hornets, undetermined

√6ᵗʰ **T63.46** Toxic effect of venom of wasps
Toxic effect of yellow jacket
- √7ᵗʰ **T63.461** Toxic effect of venom of wasps, accidental (unintentional)
- √7ᵗʰ **T63.462** Toxic effect of venom of wasps, intentional self-harm
- √7ᵗʰ **T63.463** Toxic effect of venom of wasps, assault
- √7ᵗʰ **T63.464** Toxic effect of venom of wasps, undetermined

√6ᵗʰ **T63.48** Toxic effect of venom of other arthropod
- √7ᵗʰ **T63.481** Toxic effect of venom of other arthropod, accidental (unintentional)
- √7ᵗʰ **T63.482** Toxic effect of venom of other arthropod, intentional self-harm
- √7ᵗʰ **T63.483** Toxic effect of venom of other arthropod, assault
- √7ᵗʰ **T63.484** Toxic effect of venom of other arthropod, undetermined

√5ᵗʰ **T63.5** Toxic effect of contact with venomous fish
    EXCLUDES 2 poisoning by ingestion of fish (T61.-)

√6ᵗʰ **T63.51** Toxic effect of contact with stingray
- √7ᵗʰ **T63.511** Toxic effect of contact with stingray, accidental (unintentional)
- √7ᵗʰ **T63.512** Toxic effect of contact with stingray, intentional self-harm
- √7ᵗʰ **T63.513** Toxic effect of contact with stingray, assault
- √7ᵗʰ **T63.514** Toxic effect of contact with stingray, undetermined

√6ᵗʰ **T63.59** Toxic effect of contact with other venomous fish
- √7ᵗʰ **T63.591** Toxic effect of contact with other venomous fish, accidental (unintentional)
- √7ᵗʰ **T63.592** Toxic effect of contact with other venomous fish, intentional self-harm
- √7ᵗʰ **T63.593** Toxic effect of contact with other venomous fish, assault
- √7ᵗʰ **T63.594** Toxic effect of contact with other venomous fish, undetermined

√5ᵗʰ **T63.6** Toxic effect of contact with other venomous marine animals
    EXCLUDES 1 sea-snake venom (T63.09)
    EXCLUDES 2 poisoning by ingestion of shellfish (T61.78-)

√6ᵗʰ **T63.61** Toxic effect of contact with Portugese Man-o-war
Toxic effect of contact with bluebottle
- √7ᵗʰ **T63.611** Toxic effect of contact with Portugese Man-o-war, accidental (unintentional)
- √7ᵗʰ **T63.612** Toxic effect of contact with Portugese Man-o-war, intentional self-harm
- √7ᵗʰ **T63.613** Toxic effect of contact with Portugese Man-o-war, assault
- √7ᵗʰ **T63.614** Toxic effect of contact with Portugese Man-o-war, undetermined

√6ᵗʰ **T63.62** Toxic effect of contact with other jellyfish
- √7ᵗʰ **T63.621** Toxic effect of contact with other jellyfish, accidental (unintentional)
- √7ᵗʰ **T63.622** Toxic effect of contact with other jellyfish, intentional self-harm
- √7ᵗʰ **T63.623** Toxic effect of contact with other jellyfish, assault
- √7ᵗʰ **T63.624** Toxic effect of contact with other jellyfish, undetermined

√6ᵗʰ **T63.63** Toxic effect of contact with sea anemone
- √7ᵗʰ **T63.631** Toxic effect of contact with sea anemone, accidental (unintentional)
- √7ᵗʰ **T63.632** Toxic effect of contact with sea anemone, intentional self-harm
- √7ᵗʰ **T63.633** Toxic effect of contact with sea anemone, assault
- √7ᵗʰ **T63.634** Toxic effect of contact with sea anemone, undetermined

√6ᵗʰ **T63.69** Toxic effect of contact with other venomous marine animals
- √7ᵗʰ **T63.691** Toxic effect of contact with other venomous marine animals, accidental (unintentional)
- √7ᵗʰ **T63.692** Toxic effect of contact with other venomous marine animals, intentional self-harm
- √7ᵗʰ **T63.693** Toxic effect of contact with other venomous marine animals, assault
- √7ᵗʰ **T63.694** Toxic effect of contact with other venomous marine animals, undetermined

√5ᵗʰ **T63.7** Toxic effect of contact with venomous plant

√6ᵗʰ **T63.71** Toxic effect of contact with venomous marine plant
- √7ᵗʰ **T63.711** Toxic effect of contact with venomous marine plant, accidental (unintentional)
- √7ᵗʰ **T63.712** Toxic effect of contact with venomous marine plant, intentional self-harm
- √7ᵗʰ **T63.713** Toxic effect of contact with venomous marine plant, assault
- √7ᵗʰ **T63.714** Toxic effect of contact with venomous marine plant, undetermined

√6ᵗʰ **T63.79** Toxic effect of contact with other venomous plant
- √7ᵗʰ **T63.791** Toxic effect of contact with other venomous plant, accidental (unintentional)
- √7ᵗʰ **T63.792** Toxic effect of contact with other venomous plant, intentional self-harm
- √7ᵗʰ **T63.793** Toxic effect of contact with other venomous plant, assault
- √7ᵗʰ **T63.794** Toxic effect of contact with other venomous plant, undetermined

√5ᵗʰ **T63.8** Toxic effect of contact with other venomous animals

√6ᵗʰ **T63.81** Toxic effect of contact with venomous frog
    EXCLUDES 1 contact with nonvenomous frog (W62.0)
- √7ᵗʰ **T63.811** Toxic effect of contact with venomous frog, accidental (unintentional)
- √7ᵗʰ **T63.812** Toxic effect of contact with venomous frog, intentional self-harm
- √7ᵗʰ **T63.813** Toxic effect of contact with venomous frog, assault
- √7ᵗʰ **T63.814** Toxic effect of contact with venomous frog, undetermined

√6ᵗʰ **T63.82** Toxic effect of contact with venomous toad
    EXCLUDES 1 contact with nonvenomous toad (W62.1)
- √7ᵗʰ **T63.821** Toxic effect of contact with venomous toad, accidental (unintentional)
- √7ᵗʰ **T63.822** Toxic effect of contact with venomous toad, intentional self-harm
- √7ᵗʰ **T63.823** Toxic effect of contact with venomous toad, assault
- √7ᵗʰ **T63.824** Toxic effect of contact with venomous toad, undetermined

√6ᵗʰ **T63.83** Toxic effect of contact with other venomous amphibian
    EXCLUDES 1 contact with nonvenomous amphibian (W62.9)
- √7ᵗʰ **T63.831** Toxic effect of contact with other venomous amphibian, accidental (unintentional)

N Newborn: 0   P Pediatric: 0-17   M Maternity: 12-55   A Adult: 15-124   **NRS** Nonroutine supply Dx   **NC Dx** Noncancer Dx   **PD x** Primary Dx   ►◄ Revised Text   ● New Code   ▲ Revised Title

☑7ᵗʰ **T63.832** Toxic effect of contact with other venomous amphibian, intentional self-harm

☑7ᵗʰ **T63.833** Toxic effect of contact with other venomous amphibian, assault

☑7ᵗʰ **T63.834** Toxic effect of contact with other venomous amphibian, undetermined

☑6ᵗʰ **T63.89** Toxic effect of contact with other venomous animals

☑7ᵗʰ **T63.891** Toxic effect of contact with other venomous animals, accidental (unintentional)

☑7ᵗʰ **T63.892** Toxic effect of contact with other venomous animals, intentional self-harm

☑7ᵗʰ **T63.893** Toxic effect of contact with other venomous animals, assault

☑7ᵗʰ **T63.894** Toxic effect of contact with other venomous animals, undetermined

☑5ᵗʰ **T63.9** Toxic effect of contact with unspecified venomous animal

☑x7ᵗʰ **T63.91** Toxic effect of contact with unspecified venomous animal, accidental (unintentional) ▽

☑x7ᵗʰ **T63.92** Toxic effect of contact with unspecified venomous animal, intentional self-harm ▽

☑x7ᵗʰ **T63.93** Toxic effect of contact with unspecified venomous animal, assault ▽

☑x7ᵗʰ **T63.94** Toxic effect of contact with unspecified venomous animal, undetermined ▽

☑4ᵗʰ **T64** Toxic effect of aflatoxin and other mycotoxin food contaminants

> The appropriate 7th character is to be added to each code from category T64.
> A   initial encounter
> D   subsequent encounter
> S   sequela

☑5ᵗʰ **T64.0** Toxic effect of aflatoxin

☑x7ᵗʰ **T64.01** Toxic effect of aflatoxin, accidental (unintentional)

☑x7ᵗʰ **T64.02** Toxic effect of aflatoxin, intentional self-harm

☑x7ᵗʰ **T64.03** Toxic effect of aflatoxin, assault

☑x7ᵗʰ **T64.04** Toxic effect of aflatoxin, undetermined

☑5ᵗʰ **T64.8** Toxic effect of other mycotoxin food contaminants

☑x7ᵗʰ **T64.81** Toxic effect of other mycotoxin food contaminants, accidental (unintentional)

☑x7ᵗʰ **T64.82** Toxic effect of other mycotoxin food contaminants, intentional self-harm

☑x7ᵗʰ **T64.83** Toxic effect of other mycotoxin food contaminants, assault

☑x7ᵗʰ **T64.84** Toxic effect of other mycotoxin food contaminants, undetermined

☑4ᵗʰ **T65** Toxic effect of other and unspecified substances

> The appropriate 7th character is to be added to each code from category T65.
> A   initial encounter
> D   subsequent encounter
> S   sequela

☑5ᵗʰ **T65.0** Toxic effect of cyanides

EXCLUDES 1   hydrogen cyanide (T57.3-)

☑6ᵗʰ **T65.0X** Toxic effect of cyanides

☑7ᵗʰ **T65.0X1** Toxic effect of cyanides, accidental (unintentional)
Toxic effect of cyanides NOS

☑7ᵗʰ **T65.0X2** Toxic effect of cyanides, intentional self-harm

☑7ᵗʰ **T65.0X3** Toxic effect of cyanides, assault

☑7ᵗʰ **T65.0X4** Toxic effect of cyanides, undetermined

☑5ᵗʰ **T65.1** Toxic effect of strychnine and its salts

☑6ᵗʰ **T65.1X** Toxic effect of strychnine and its salts

☑7ᵗʰ **T65.1X1** Toxic effect of strychnine and its salts, accidental (unintentional)
Toxic effect of strychnine and its salts NOS

☑7ᵗʰ **T65.1X2** Toxic effect of strychnine and its salts, intentional self-harm

☑7ᵗʰ **T65.1X3** Toxic effect of strychnine and its salts, assault

☑7ᵗʰ **T65.1X4** Toxic effect of strychnine and its salts, undetermined

☑5ᵗʰ **T65.2** Toxic effect of tobacco and nicotine
EXCLUDES 2   nicotine dependence (F17.-)

☑6ᵗʰ **T65.21** Toxic effect of chewing tobacco

☑7ᵗʰ **T65.211** Toxic effect of chewing tobacco, accidental (unintentional)
Toxic effect of chewing tobacco NOS

☑7ᵗʰ **T65.212** Toxic effect of chewing tobacco, intentional self-harm

☑7ᵗʰ **T65.213** Toxic effect of chewing tobacco, assault

☑7ᵗʰ **T65.214** Toxic effect of chewing tobacco, undetermined

☑6ᵗʰ **T65.22** Toxic effect of tobacco cigarettes
Toxic effect of tobacco smoke
Use additional code for exposure to second hand tobacco smoke (Z57.31, Z77.22)

☑7ᵗʰ **T65.221** Toxic effect of tobacco cigarettes, accidental (unintentional)
Toxic effect of tobacco cigarettes NOS

☑7ᵗʰ **T65.222** Toxic effect of tobacco cigarettes, intentional self-harm

☑7ᵗʰ **T65.223** Toxic effect of tobacco cigarettes, assault

☑7ᵗʰ **T65.224** Toxic effect of tobacco cigarettes, undetermined

☑6ᵗʰ **T65.29** Toxic effect of other tobacco and nicotine

☑7ᵗʰ **T65.291** Toxic effect of other tobacco and nicotine, accidental (unintentional)
Toxic effect of other tobacco and nicotine NOS

☑7ᵗʰ **T65.292** Toxic effect of other tobacco and nicotine, intentional self-harm

☑7ᵗʰ **T65.293** Toxic effect of other tobacco and nicotine, assault

☑7ᵗʰ **T65.294** Toxic effect of other tobacco and nicotine, undetermined

☑5ᵗʰ **T65.3** Toxic effect of nitroderivatives and aminoderivatives of benzene and its homologues
Toxic effect of anilin [benzenamine]
Toxic effect of nitrobenzene
Toxic effect of trinitrotoluene

☑6ᵗʰ **T65.3X** Toxic effect of nitroderivatives and aminoderivatives of benzene and its homologues

☑7ᵗʰ **T65.3X1** Toxic effect of nitroderivatives and aminoderivatives of benzene and its homologues, accidental (unintentional)
Toxic effect of nitroderivatives and aminoderivatives of benzene and its homologues NOS

☑7ᵗʰ **T65.3X2** Toxic effect of nitroderivatives and aminoderivatives of benzene and its homologues, intentional self-harm

☑7ᵗʰ **T65.3X3** Toxic effect of nitroderivatives and aminoderivatives of benzene and its homologues, assault

☑7ᵗʰ **T65.3X4** Toxic effect of nitroderivatives and aminoderivatives of benzene and its homologues, undetermined

☑5ᵗʰ **T65.4** Toxic effect of carbon disulfide

☑6ᵗʰ **T65.4X** Toxic effect of carbon disulfide

☑7ᵗʰ **T65.4X1** Toxic effect of carbon disulfide, accidental (unintentional)
Toxic effect of carbon disulfide NOS

☑7ᵗʰ **T65.4X2** Toxic effect of carbon disulfide, intentional self-harm

☑7ᵗʰ **T65.4X3** Toxic effect of carbon disulfide, assault

☑7ᵗʰ **T65.4X4** Toxic effect of carbon disulfide, undetermined

☑5ᵗʰ **T65.5** Toxic effect of nitroglycerin and other nitric acids and esters
Toxic effect of 1,2,3-Propanetriol trinitrate

☑6ᵗʰ **T65.5X** Toxic effect of nitroglycerin and other nitric acids and esters

☑7ᵗʰ **T65.5X1** Toxic effect of nitroglycerin and other nitric acids and esters, accidental (unintentional)
Toxic effect of nitroglycerin and other nitric acids and esters NOS

☑ Additional Character Req   ☑x7ᵗʰ Placeholder Alert   Case-Mix Diagnosis   Manifestation   ▽ Unspecified Dx   EXCLUDES 1 Not coded here   EXCLUDES 2 Not included here

✓7th **T65.5X2** **Toxic effect of nitroglycerin and other nitric acids and esters,** intentional self-harm

✓7th **T65.5X3** **Toxic effect of nitroglycerin and other nitric acids and esters,** assault

✓7th **T65.5X4** **Toxic effect of nitroglycerin and other nitric acids and esters,** undetermined

✓5th **T65.6** **Toxic effect of** paints and dyes, **not elsewhere classified**

  ✓6th **T65.6X** **Toxic effect of paints and dyes, not elsewhere classified**

    ✓7th **T65.6X1** **Toxic effect of paints and dyes, not elsewhere classified,** accidental (unintentional)
        Toxic effect of paints and dyes NOS

    ✓7th **T65.6X2** **Toxic effect of paints and dyes, not elsewhere classified,** intentional self-harm

    ✓7th **T65.6X3** **Toxic effect of paints and dyes, not elsewhere classified,** assault

    ✓7th **T65.6X4** **Toxic effect of paints and dyes, not elsewhere classified,** undetermined

✓5th **T65.8** **Toxic effect of** other specified substances

  ✓6th **T65.81** **Toxic effect of** latex

    ✓7th **T65.811** **Toxic effect of latex,** accidental (unintentional)
        Toxic effect of latex NOS

    ✓7th **T65.812** **Toxic effect of latex,** intentional self-harm

    ✓7th **T65.813** **Toxic effect of latex,** assault

    ✓7th **T65.814** **Toxic effect of latex,** undetermined

  ✓6th **T65.82** **Toxic effect of harmful** algae and algae toxins
    Toxic effect of (harmful) algae bloom NOS
    Toxic effect of blue-green algae bloom
    Toxic effect of brown tide
    Toxic effect of cyanobacteria bloom
    Toxic effect of Florida red tide
    Toxic effect of pfiesteria piscicida
    Toxic effect of red tide

    ✓7th **T65.821** **Toxic effect of harmful algae and algae toxins,** accidental (unintentional)
        Toxic effect of harmful algae and algae toxins NOS

    ✓7th **T65.822** **Toxic effect of harmful algae and algae toxins,** intentional self-harm

    ✓7th **T65.823** **Toxic effect of harmful algae and algae toxins,** assault

    ✓7th **T65.824** **Toxic effect of harmful algae and algae toxins,** undetermined

  ✓6th **T65.83** **Toxic effect of** fiberglass

    ✓7th **T65.831** **Toxic effect of fiberglass,** accidental (unintentional)
        Toxic effect of fiberglass NOS

    ✓7th **T65.832** **Toxic effect of fiberglass,** intentional self-harm

    ✓7th **T65.833** **Toxic effect of fiberglass,** assault

    ✓7th **T65.834** **Toxic effect of fiberglass,** undetermined

  ✓6th **T65.89** **Toxic effect of** other **specified substances**

    ✓7th **T65.891** **Toxic effect of other specified substances,** accidental (unintentional)
        Toxic effect of other specified substances NOS

    ✓7th **T65.892** **Toxic effect of other specified substances,** intentional self-harm

    ✓7th **T65.893** **Toxic effect of other specified substances,** assault

    ✓7th **T65.894** **Toxic effect of other specified substances,** undetermined

✓5th **T65.9** **Toxic effect of** unspecified **substance**

  ✓x7th **T65.91** **Toxic effect of unspecified substance,** accidental (unintentional)   ▽
    Poisoning NOS

  ✓x7th **T65.92** **Toxic effect of unspecified substance,** intentional self-harm   ▽

  ✓x7th **T65.93** **Toxic effect of unspecified substance,** assault   ▽

  ✓x7th **T65.94** **Toxic effect of unspecified substance,** undetermined

Other and unspecified effects of external causes (T66-T78)

✓x7th **T66** **Radiation sickness, unspecified**   ▽
  EXCLUDES 1   specified adverse effects of radiation, such as:
        burns (T20-T31)
        leukemia (C91-C95)
        radiation gastroenteritis and colitis (K52.0)
        radiation pneumonitis (J70.0)
        radiation related disorders of the skin and subcutaneous tissue (L55-L59)
        radiation sunburn (L55.-)

The appropriate 7th character is to be added to code T66.
A   initial encounter
D   subsequent encounter
S   sequela

✓4th **T67** **Effects of heat and light**
  EXCLUDES 1   erythema [dermatitis] ab igne (L59.0)
        malignant hyperpyrexia due to anesthesia (T88.3)
        radiation-related disorders of the skin and subcutaneous tissue (L55-L59)
  EXCLUDES 2   burns (T20-T31)
        sunburn (L55.-)
        sweat disorder due to heat (L74-L75)

The appropriate 7th character is to be added to each code from category T67.
A   initial encounter
D   subsequent encounter
S   sequela

  ✓x7th **T67.0** **Heatstroke and sunstroke**
    Heat apoplexy
    Heat pyrexia
    Siriasis
    Thermoplegia
    Use additional code(s) to identify any associated complications of heatstroke, such as:
        coma and stupor (R40.-)
        systemic inflammatory response syndrome (R65.1-)
    DEF: Headache, vertigo, cramps, and elevated body temperature due to prolonged exposure to high environmental temperatures; requires emergency intervention.

  ✓x7th **T67.1** **Heat** syncope
    Heat collapse

  ✓x7th **T67.2** **Heat** cramp

  ✓x7th **T67.3** **Heat exhaustion, anhydrotic**
    Heat prostration due to water depletion
    EXCLUDES 1   heat exhaustion due to salt depletion (T67.4)

  ✓x7th **T67.4** **Heat exhaustion due to salt depletion**
    Heat prostration due to salt (and water) depletion

  ✓x7th **T67.5** **Heat exhaustion, unspecified**   ▽
    Heat prostration NOS

  ✓x7th **T67.6** **Heat** fatigue, transient

  ✓x7th **T67.7** **Heat** edema

  ✓x7th **T67.8** **Other effects of heat and light**

  ✓x7th **T67.9** **Effect of heat and light, unspecified**   ▽

✓x7th **T68** **Hypothermia**
  Accidental hypothermia
  Hypothermia NOS
  Use additional code to identify source of exposure:
    exposure to excessive cold of man-made origin (W93)
    exposure to excessive cold of natural origin (X31)
  EXCLUDES 1   hypothermia following anesthesia (T88.51)
        hypothermia not associated with low environmental temperature (R68.0)
        hypothermia of newborn (P80.-)
  EXCLUDES 2   frostbite (T33-T34)

The appropriate 7th character is to be added to code T68.
A   initial encounter
D   subsequent encounter
S   sequela

☑4ᵗʰ **T69**   **Other effects of reduced temperature**
Use additional code to identify source of exposure:
exposure to excessive cold of man-made origin (W93)
exposure to excessive cold of natural origin (X31)
EXCLUDES 2   frostbite (T33-T34)

The appropriate 7th character is to be added to each code from category T69.
A   initial encounter
D   subsequent encounter
S   sequela

☑5ᵗʰ **T69.0**   **Immersion hand and foot**
   ☑6ᵗʰ **T69.01**   **Immersion** hand
     ☑7ᵗʰ **T69.011**   **Immersion hand, right hand**
     ☑7ᵗʰ **T69.012**   **Immersion hand, left hand**
     ☑7ᵗʰ **T69.019**   **Immersion hand, unspecified hand** ▽
   ☑6ᵗʰ **T69.02**   **Immersion** foot
     Trench foot
     ☑7ᵗʰ **T69.021**   **Immersion foot, right foot**
     ☑7ᵗʰ **T69.022**   **Immersion foot, left foot**
     ☑7ᵗʰ **T69.029**   **Immersion foot, unspecified foot** ▽

☑x7ᵗʰ **T69.1**   **Chilblains**
DEF: Red, swollen, itchy skin primarily affecting the fingers and toes, nose and ears, and legs; follows damp-cold exposure; can also be associated with pruritus and a burning feeling.

☑x7ᵗʰ **T69.8**   **Other specified effects of reduced temperature**

☑x7ᵗʰ **T69.9**   **Effect of reduced temperature, unspecified** ▽

☑4ᵗʰ **T70**   **Effects of air pressure and water pressure**

The appropriate 7th character is to be added to each code from category T70.
A   initial encounter
D   subsequent encounter
S   sequela

☑x7ᵗʰ **T70.0**   **Otitic barotrauma**
Aero-otitis media
Effects of change in ambient atmospheric pressure or water pressure on ears

☑x7ᵗʰ **T70.1**   **Sinus barotrauma**
Aerosinusitis
Effects of change in ambient atmospheric pressure on sinuses

☑5ᵗʰ **T70.2**   **Other and unspecified effects of high altitude**
EXCLUDES 2   polycythemia due to high altitude (D75.1)
   ☑x7ᵗʰ **T70.20**   **Unspecified effects of high altitude** ▽
   ☑x7ᵗʰ **T70.29**   **Other effects of high altitude**
     Alpine sickness   Hypobaropathy
     Anoxia due to high altitude   Mountain sickness
     Barotrauma NOS

☑x7ᵗʰ **T70.3**   **Caisson disease [decompression sickness]**
Compressed-air disease
Diver's palsy or paralysis
DEF: Rapid reduction in air pressure while breathing compressed air; symptoms include skin lesions, joint pains, and respiratory and neurological problems.

☑x7ᵗʰ **T70.4**   **Effects of high-pressure fluids**
Hydraulic jet injection (industrial)
Pneumatic jet injection (industrial)
Traumatic jet injection (industrial)

☑x7ᵗʰ **T70.8**   **Other effects of air pressure and water pressure**

☑x7ᵗʰ **T70.9**   **Effect of air pressure and water pressure, unspecified** ▽

☑4ᵗʰ **T71**   **Asphyxiation**
Mechanical suffocationTraumatic suffocation
EXCLUDES 1   acute respiratory distress (syndrome) (J80)
anoxia due to high altitude (T70.2)
asphyxia NOS (R09.01)
asphyxia from carbon monoxide (T58.-)
asphyxia from inhalation of food or foreign body (T17.-)
asphyxia from other gases, fumes and vapors (T59.-)
respiratory distress (syndrome) in newborn (P22.-)

The appropriate 7th character is to be added to each code from category T71.
A   initial encounter
D   subsequent encounter
S   sequela

☑5ᵗʰ **T71.1**   **Asphyxiation due to mechanical threat to breathing**
Suffocation due to mechanical threat to breathing

   ☑6ᵗʰ **T71.11**   **Asphyxiation due to smothering under pillow**
     ☑7ᵗʰ **T71.111**   **Asphyxiation due to smothering under pillow, accidental**
       Asphyxiation due to smothering under pillow NOS
     ☑7ᵗʰ **T71.112**   **Asphyxiation due to smothering under pillow, intentional self-harm**
     ☑7ᵗʰ **T71.113**   **Asphyxiation due to smothering under pillow, assault**
     ☑7ᵗʰ **T71.114**   **Asphyxiation due to smothering under pillow, undetermined**

   ☑6ᵗʰ **T71.12**   **Asphyxiation due to plastic bag**
     ☑7ᵗʰ **T71.121**   **Asphyxiation due to plastic bag, accidental**
       Asphyxiation due to plastic bag NOS
     ☑7ᵗʰ **T71.122**   **Asphyxiation due to plastic bag, intentional self-harm**
     ☑7ᵗʰ **T71.123**   **Asphyxiation due to plastic bag, assault**
     ☑7ᵗʰ **T71.124**   **Asphyxiation due to plastic bag, undetermined**

   ☑6ᵗʰ **T71.13**   **Asphyxiation due to being trapped in bed linens**
     ☑7ᵗʰ **T71.131**   **Asphyxiation due to being trapped in bed linens, accidental**
       Asphyxiation due to being trapped in bed linens NOS
     ☑7ᵗʰ **T71.132**   **Asphyxiation due to being trapped in bed linens, intentional self-harm**
     ☑7ᵗʰ **T71.133**   **Asphyxiation due to being trapped in bed linens, assault**
     ☑7ᵗʰ **T71.134**   **Asphyxiation due to being trapped in bed linens, undetermined**

   ☑6ᵗʰ **T71.14**   **Asphyxiation due to smothering under another person's body (in bed)**
     ☑7ᵗʰ **T71.141**   **Asphyxiation due to smothering under another person's body (in bed), accidental**
       Asphyxiation due to smothering under another person's body (in bed) NOS
     ☑7ᵗʰ **T71.143**   **Asphyxiation due to smothering under another person's body (in bed), assault**
     ☑7ᵗʰ **T71.144**   **Asphyxiation due to smothering under another person's body (in bed), undetermined**

   ☑6ᵗʰ **T71.15**   **Asphyxiation due to smothering in furniture**
     ☑7ᵗʰ **T71.151**   **Asphyxiation due to smothering in furniture, accidental**
       Asphyxiation due to smothering in furniture NOS
     ☑7ᵗʰ **T71.152**   **Asphyxiation due to smothering in furniture, intentional self-harm**
     ☑7ᵗʰ **T71.153**   **Asphyxiation due to smothering in furniture, assault**
     ☑7ᵗʰ **T71.154**   **Asphyxiation due to smothering in furniture, undetermined**

   ☑6ᵗʰ **T71.16**   **Asphyxiation due to hanging**
     Hanging by window shade cord
     Use additional code for any associated injuries, such as:
       crushing injury of neck (S17.-)
       fracture of cervical vertebrae (S12.0-S12.2-)
       open wound of neck (S11.-)
     ☑7ᵗʰ **T71.161**   **Asphyxiation due to hanging, accidental**
       Asphyxiation due to hanging NOS
       Hanging NOS
     ☑7ᵗʰ **T71.162**   **Asphyxiation due to hanging, intentional self-harm**
     ☑7ᵗʰ **T71.163**   **Asphyxiation due to hanging, assault**
     ☑7ᵗʰ **T71.164**   **Asphyxiation due to hanging, undetermined**

   ☑6ᵗʰ **T71.19**   **Asphyxiation due to mechanical threat to breathing due to other causes**
     ☑7ᵗʰ **T71.191**   **Asphyxiation due to mechanical threat to breathing due to other causes, accidental**
       Asphyxiation due to other causes NOS
     ☑7ᵗʰ **T71.192**   **Asphyxiation due to mechanical threat to breathing due to other causes, intentional self-harm**

☑ Additional Character Req   ☑x7ᵗʰ Placeholder Alert   Case-Mix Diagnosis   Manifestation   ▽ Unspecified Dx   EXCLUDES 1 Not coded here   EXCLUDES 2 Not included here

Chapter 19. Injury, Poisoning and Certain Other Consequences of External Causes

✓7th **T71.193** Asphyxiation due to mechanical threat to breathing due to other causes, assault

✓7th **T71.194** Asphyxiation due to mechanical threat to breathing due to other causes, undetermined

✓5th **T71.2** Asphyxiation due to systemic oxygen deficiency due to low oxygen content in ambient air
     Suffocation due to systemic oxygen deficiency due to low oxygen content in ambient air

✓x7th **T71.20** Asphyxiation due to systemic oxygen deficiency due to low oxygen content in ambient air due to unspecified cause ▽

✓x7th **T71.21** Asphyxiation due to cave-in or falling earth
     Use additional code for any associated cataclysm (X34-X38)

✓6th **T71.22** Asphyxiation due to being trapped in a car trunk

     ✓7th **T71.221** Asphyxiation due to being trapped in a car trunk, accidental

     ✓7th **T71.222** Asphyxiation due to being trapped in a car trunk, intentional self-harm

     ✓7th **T71.223** Asphyxiation due to being trapped in a car trunk, assault

     ✓7th **T71.224** Asphyxiation due to being trapped in a car trunk, undetermined

✓6th **T71.23** Asphyxiation due to being trapped in a (discarded) refrigerator

     ✓7th **T71.231** Asphyxiation due to being trapped in a (discarded) refrigerator, accidental

     ✓7th **T71.232** Asphyxiation due to being trapped in a (discarded) refrigerator, intentional self-harm

     ✓7th **T71.233** Asphyxiation due to being trapped in a (discarded) refrigerator, assault

     ✓7th **T71.234** Asphyxiation due to being trapped in a (discarded) refrigerator, undetermined

✓x7th **T71.29** Asphyxiation due to being trapped in other low oxygen environment

✓x7th **T71.9** Asphyxiation due to unspecified cause ▽
     Suffocation (by strangulation) due to unspecified cause
     Suffocation NOS
     Systemic oxygen deficiency due to low oxygen content in ambient air due to unspecified cause
     Systemic oxygen deficiency due to mechanical threat to breathing due to unspecified cause
     Traumatic asphyxia NOS

✓4th **T73** Effects of other deprivation

> The appropriate 7th character is to be added to each code from category T73.
> A   initial encounter
> D   subsequent encounter
> S   sequela

✓x7th **T73.0** Starvation
     Deprivation of food

✓x7th **T73.1** Deprivation of water

✓x7th **T73.2** Exhaustion due to exposure

✓x7th **T73.3** Exhaustion due to excessive exertion
     Exhaustion due to overexertion

✓x7th **T73.8** Other effects of deprivation

✓x7th **T73.9** Effect of deprivation, unspecified ▽

✓4th **T74** Adult and child abuse, neglect and other maltreatment, confirmed
     Use additional code, if applicable, to identify any associated current injury
     Use additional external cause code to identify perpetrator, if known (Y07.-)
     EXCLUDES 1   abuse and maltreatment in pregnancy (O9A.3-, O9A.4-, O9A.5-)
                   adult and child maltreatment, suspected (T76.-)

> The appropriate 7th character is to be added to each code from category T74.
> A   initial encounter
> D   subsequent encounter
> S   sequela

✓5th **T74.0** Neglect or abandonment, confirmed

     ✓x7th **T74.01** Adult neglect or abandonment, confirmed 🅐

     ✓x7th **T74.02** Child neglect or abandonment, confirmed 🅟

✓5th **T74.1** Physical abuse, confirmed
     EXCLUDES 2   sexual abuse (T74.2-)

     ✓x7th **T74.11** Adult physical abuse, confirmed 🅐

     ✓x7th **T74.12** Child physical abuse, confirmed 🅟
           EXCLUDES 2   shaken infant syndrome (T74.4)

✓5th **T74.2** Sexual abuse, confirmed
     Rape, confirmed
     Sexual assault, confirmed

     ✓x7th **T74.21** Adult sexual abuse, confirmed 🅐

     ✓x7th **T74.22** Child sexual abuse, confirmed 🅟

✓5th **T74.3** Psychological abuse, confirmed

     ✓x7th **T74.31** Adult psychological abuse, confirmed 🅐

     ✓x7th **T74.32** Child psychological abuse, confirmed 🅟

✓x7th **T74.4** Shaken infant syndrome 🅟

✓5th **T74.9** Unspecified maltreatment, confirmed

     ✓x7th **T74.91** Unspecified adult maltreatment, confirmed 🅐▽

     ✓x7th **T74.92** Unspecified child maltreatment, confirmed 🅟▽

✓4th **T75** Other and unspecified effects of other external causes
     EXCLUDES 1   adverse effects NEC (T78.-)
     EXCLUDES 2   burns (electric) (T20-T31)

> The appropriate 7th character is to be added to each code from category T75.
> A   initial encounter
> D   subsequent encounter
> S   sequela

✓5th **T75.0** Effects of lightning
     Struck by lightning

     ✓x7th **T75.00** Unspecified effects of lightning ▽
           Struck by lightning NOS

     ✓x7th **T75.01** Shock due to being struck by lightning

     ✓x7th **T75.09** Other effects of lightning
           Use additional code for other effects of lightning

✓x7th **T75.1** Unspecified effects of drowning and nonfatal submersion ▽
     Immersion
     EXCLUDES 1   specified effects of drowning—code to effects

✓5th **T75.2** Effects of vibration

     ✓x7th **T75.20** Unspecified effects of vibration ▽

     ✓x7th **T75.21** Pneumatic hammer syndrome

     ✓x7th **T75.22** Traumatic vasospastic syndrome

     ✓x7th **T75.23** Vertigo from infrasound
           EXCLUDES 1   vertigo NOS (R42)

     ✓x7th **T75.29** Other effects of vibration

✓x7th **T75.3** Motion sickness
     Airsickness
     Seasickness
     Travel sickness
     Use additional external cause code to identify vehicle or type of motion (Y92.81-, Y93.5-)

✓x7th **T75.4** Electrocution
     Shock from electric current
     Shock from electroshock gun (taser)

✓5th **T75.8** Other specified effects of external causes

     ✓x7th **T75.81** Effects of abnormal gravitation [G] forces

     ✓x7th **T75.82** Effects of weightlessness

     ✓x7th **T75.89** Other specified effects of external causes

🅝 Newborn: 0   🅟 Pediatric: 0-17   🅜 Maternity: 12-55   🅐 Adult: 15-124   **NRS** Nonroutine supply Dx   **NCDx** Noncancer Dx   **PDx** Primary Dx   ▶◀ Revised Text   ● New Code   ▲ Revised Title

1094   ICD-10-CM 2018

☑4ᵗʰ **T76** **Adult and child abuse, neglect and other maltreatment, suspected**

> Use additional code, if applicable, to identify any associated current injury
>
> **EXCLUDES1**   adult and child maltreatment, confirmed (T74.-)
> suspected abuse and maltreatment in pregnancy (O9A.3-, O9A.4-, O9A.5-)
> suspected adult physical abuse, ruled out (Z04.71)
> suspected adult sexual abuse, ruled out (Z04.41)
> suspected child physical abuse, ruled out (Z04.72)
> suspected child sexual abuse, ruled out (Z04.42)

> The appropriate 7th character is to be added to each code from category T76.
> A   initial encounter
> D   subsequent encounter
> S   sequela

✓5ᵗʰ **T76.0** **Neglect or abandonment, suspected**

   ✓x7ᵗʰ **T76.01**   **Adult** neglect or abandonment, suspected   🅰

   ✓x7ᵗʰ **T76.02**   **Child** neglect or abandonment, suspected   🅿

✓5ᵗʰ **T76.1** **Physical abuse, suspected**

   ✓x7ᵗʰ **T76.11**   **Adult** physical abuse, suspected   🅰

   ✓x7ᵗʰ **T76.12**   **Child** physical abuse, suspected   🅿

✓5ᵗʰ **T76.2** **Sexual abuse, suspected**
> Rape, suspected
> ~~Sexual abuse, suspected~~
> **EXCLUDES1**   alleged abuse, ruled out (Z04.7)

   ✓x7ᵗʰ **T76.21**   **Adult** sexual abuse, suspected   🅰

   ✓x7ᵗʰ **T76.22**   **Child** sexual abuse, suspected   🅿

✓5ᵗʰ **T76.3** **Psychological abuse, suspected**

   ✓x7ᵗʰ **T76.31**   **Adult** psychological abuse, suspected   🅰

   ✓x7ᵗʰ **T76.32**   **Child** psychological abuse, suspected   🅿

✓5ᵗʰ **T76.9** **Unspecified maltreatment, suspected**

   ✓x7ᵗʰ **T76.91**   **Unspecified adult** maltreatment, suspected   🅰▽

   ✓x7ᵗʰ **T76.92**   **Unspecified child** maltreatment, suspected   🅿▽

☑4ᵗʰ **T78** **Adverse effects, not elsewhere classified**

> **EXCLUDES2**   complications of surgical and medical care NEC (T80-T88)
> **TIP:** Do not assign to indicate previous, resolved allergic reactions or the presence of drug and other allergies; use a code from category Z88 Allergy status to drugs, medicaments and biological substances, to report status only.

> The appropriate 7th character is to be added to each code from category T78.
> A   initial encounter
> D   subsequent encounter
> S   sequela

✓5ᵗʰ **T78.0** **Anaphylactic reaction due to food**
> Anaphylactic reaction due to adverse food reaction
> Anaphylactic shock or reaction due to nonpoisonous foods
> Anaphylactoid reaction due to food

   ✓x7ᵗʰ **T78.00**   **Anaphylactic reaction due to unspecified food**   ▽

   ✓x7ᵗʰ **T78.01**   **Anaphylactic reaction due to** peanuts

   ✓x7ᵗʰ **T78.02**   **Anaphylactic reaction due to** shellfish (crustaceans)

   ✓x7ᵗʰ **T78.03**   **Anaphylactic reaction due to** other fish

   ✓x7ᵗʰ **T78.04**   **Anaphylactic reaction due to** fruits and vegetables

   ✓x7ᵗʰ **T78.05**   **Anaphylactic reaction due to** tree nuts and seeds
>   **EXCLUDES2**   anaphylactic reaction due to peanuts (T78.01)

   ✓x7ᵗʰ **T78.06**   **Anaphylactic reaction due to** food additives

   ✓x7ᵗʰ **T78.07**   **Anaphylactic reaction due to** milk and dairy products

   ✓x7ᵗʰ **T78.08**   **Anaphylactic reaction due to** eggs

   ✓x7ᵗʰ **T78.09**   **Anaphylactic reaction due to other** food products

---

✓x7ᵗʰ **T78.1** **Other adverse food reactions, not elsewhere classified**
> Use additional code to identify the type of reaction, if applicable
> **EXCLUDES1**   anaphylactic reaction or shock due to adverse food reaction (T78.0-)
> anaphylactic reaction due to food (T78.0-)
> bacterial food borne intoxications (A05.-)
> **EXCLUDES2**   allergic and dietetic gastroenteritis and colitis (K52.29)
> allergic rhinitis due to food (J30.5)
> dermatitis due to food in contact with skin (L23.6, L24.6, L25.4)
> dermatitis due to ingested food (L27.2)
> food protein-induced enterocolitis syndrome (K52.21)
> food protein-induced enteropathy (K52.22)

✓x7ᵗʰ **T78.2** **Anaphylactic shock, unspecified**   ▽
> Allergic shock
> Anaphylactic reaction
> Anaphylaxis
> **EXCLUDES1**   anaphylactic reaction or shock due to adverse effect of correct medicinal substance properly administered (T88.6)
> anaphylactic reaction or shock due to adverse food reaction (T78.0-)
> anaphylactic reaction or shock due to serum (T80.5-)

✓x7ᵗʰ **T78.3** **Angioneurotic edema**
> Allergic angioedema
> Quincke's edema
> Giant urticaria
> **EXCLUDES1**   serum urticaria (T80.6-)
> urticaria (L50.-)

✓5ᵗʰ **T78.4** **Other and unspecified allergy**
> **EXCLUDES1**   specified types of allergic reaction such as:
> allergic diarrhea (K52.29)
> allergic gastroenteritis and colitis (K52.29)
> dermatitis (L23-L25, L27-)
> food protein-induced enterocolitis syndrome (K52.21)
> food protein-induced enteropathy (K52.22)
> hay fever (J30.1)

   ✓x7ᵗʰ **T78.40**   **Allergy, unspecified**   ▽
> Allergic reaction NOS
> Hypersensitivity NOS

   ✓x7ᵗʰ **T78.41**   **Arthus phenomenon**
> Arthus reaction

   ✓x7ᵗʰ **T78.49**   **Other allergy**

✓x7ᵗʰ **T78.8** **Other adverse effects, not elsewhere classified**

Certain early complications of trauma (T79)

☑4ᵗʰ **T79** **Certain early complications of trauma, not elsewhere classified**

> **EXCLUDES2**   acute respiratory distress syndrome (J80)
> complications occurring during or following medical procedures (T80-T88)
> complications of surgical and medical care NEC (T80-T88)
> newborn respiratory distress syndrome (P22.0)

> The appropriate 7th character is to be added to each code from category T79.
> A   initial encounter
> D   subsequent encounter
> S   sequela

✓x7ᵗʰ **T79.0** **Air embolism (traumatic)**
> **EXCLUDES1**   air embolism complicating abortion or ectopic or molar pregnancy (O00-O07, O08.2)
> air embolism complicating pregnancy, childbirth and the puerperium (O88.0)
> air embolism following infusion, transfusion, and therapeutic injection (T80.0)
> air embolism following procedure NEC (T81.7-)
> **DEF:** Arterial or venous obstruction due to introduction of air bubbles into the blood vessels following surgery or trauma.

✓x7ᵗʰ **T79.1** **Fat embolism (traumatic)**
> **EXCLUDES1**   fat embolism complicating:
> abortion or ectopic or molar pregnancy (O00-O07, O08.2)
> pregnancy, childbirth and the puerperium (O88.8)
> **DEF:** Arterial blockage due to the entrance of fat into the circulatory system after fracture of large bones or administration of corticosteroids.

✓x7ᵗʰ **T79.2** **Traumatic secondary and recurrent hemorrhage and seroma**

☑ Additional Character Req   ✓x7ᵗʰ Placeholder Alert   Case-Mix Diagnosis   Manifestation   ▽ Unspecified Dx   **EXCLUDES1** Not coded here   **EXCLUDES2** Not included here

ICD-10-CM 2018   **1095**

Chapter 19. Injury, Poisoning and Certain Other Consequences of External Causes

✓x 7ᵗʰ **T79.4 Traumatic shock**
Shock (immediate) (delayed) following injury
EXCLUDES 1   *anaphylactic shock due to adverse food reaction (T78.0-)*
anaphylactic shock due to correct medicinal substance properly administered (T88.6)
anaphylactic shock due to serum (T80.5-)
anaphylactic shock NOS (T78.2)
anesthetic shock (T88.2)
electric shock (T75.4)
nontraumatic shock NEC (R57.-)
obstetric shock (O75.1)
postprocedural shock (T81.1-)
septic shock (R65.21)
shock complicating abortion or ectopic or molar pregnancy (O00-O07, O08.3)
shock due to lightning (T75.01)
shock NOS (R57.9)

✓x 7ᵗʰ **T79.5 Traumatic anuria**
Crush syndrome
Renal failure following crushing

✓x 7ᵗʰ **T79.6 Traumatic ischemia of muscle**
Traumatic rhabdomyolysis
Volkmann's ischemic contracture
EXCLUDES 2   *anterior tibial syndrome (M76.8)*
compartment syndrome (traumatic) (T79.A-)
nontraumatic ischemia of muscle (M62.2-)

✓x 7ᵗʰ **T79.7 Traumatic subcutaneous emphysema**
EXCLUDES 1   *emphysema NOS (J43)*
emphysema (subcutaneous) resulting from a procedure (T81.82)

✓ 5ᵗʰ **T79.A Traumatic compartment syndrome**
EXCLUDES 1   *fibromyalgia (M79.7)*
nontraumatic compartment syndrome (M79.A-)
traumatic ischemic infarction of muscle (T79.6)
DEF: Compression of nerves and blood vessels within an enclosed muscle space due to previous trauma, which leads to impaired blood flow and muscle and nerve damage.

   ✓x 7ᵗʰ **T79.A0 Compartment syndrome, unspecified** ▽
Compartment syndrome NOS

   ✓ 6ᵗʰ **T79.A1 Traumatic compartment syndrome of upper extremity**
Traumatic compartment syndrome of shoulder, arm, forearm, wrist, hand, and fingers

     ✓ 7ᵗʰ **T79.A11 Traumatic compartment syndrome of right upper extremity**

     ✓ 7ᵗʰ **T79.A12 Traumatic compartment syndrome of left upper extremity**

     ✓ 7ᵗʰ **T79.A19 Traumatic compartment syndrome of unspecified upper extremity** ▽

   ✓ 6ᵗʰ **T79.A2 Traumatic compartment syndrome of lower extremity**
Traumatic compartment syndrome of hip, buttock, thigh, leg, foot, and toes

     ✓ 7ᵗʰ **T79.A21 Traumatic compartment syndrome of right lower extremity**

     ✓ 7ᵗʰ **T79.A22 Traumatic compartment syndrome of left lower extremity**

     ✓ 7ᵗʰ **T79.A29 Traumatic compartment syndrome of unspecified lower extremity** ▽

   ✓x 7ᵗʰ **T79.A3 Traumatic compartment syndrome of abdomen**

   ✓x 7ᵗʰ **T79.A9 Traumatic compartment syndrome of other sites**

✓x 7ᵗʰ **T79.8 Other early complications of trauma**

✓x 7ᵗʰ **T79.9 Unspecified early complication of trauma** ▽

Complications of surgical and medical care, not elsewhere classified (T80-T88)

Use additional code for adverse effect, if applicable, to identify drug (T36-T50 with fifth or sixth character 5)
Use additional code(s) to identify the specified condition resulting from the complication
Use additional code to identify devices involved and details of circumstances (Y62-Y82)

EXCLUDES 2   *any encounters with medical care for postprocedural conditions in which no complications are present, such as:*
     artificial opening status (Z93.-)
     closure of external stoma (Z43.-)
     fitting and adjustment of external prosthetic device (Z44.-)
burns and corrosions from local applications and irradiation (T20-T32)
complications of surgical procedures during pregnancy, childbirth and the puerperium (O00-O9A)
mechanical complication of respirator [ventilator] (J95.850)
poisoning and toxic effects of drugs and chemicals (T36-T65 with fifth or sixth character 1-4 or 6)
postprocedural fever (R50.82)
specified complications classified elsewhere, such as:
     cerebrospinal fluid leak from spinal puncture (G97.0)
     colostomy malfunction (K94.0-)
     disorders of fluid and electrolyte imbalance (E86-E87)
     functional disturbances following cardiac surgery (I97.0-I97.1)
     intraoperative and postprocedural complications of specified body systems (D78.-, E36.-, E89.-, G97.3-, G97.4, H59.3-, H59.-, H95.2-, H95.3, I97.4-, I97.5, J95.6-, J95.7, K91.6-, L76-, M96-, N99.-)
     ostomy complications (J95.0-, K94-, N99.5-)
     postgastric surgery syndromes (K91.1)
     postlaminectomy syndrome NEC (M96.1)
     postmastectomy lymphedema syndrome (I97.2)
     postsurgical blind-loop syndrome (K91.2)
     ventilator associated pneumonia (J95.851)

AHA: 2015, 1Q, 15

✓ 4ᵗʰ **T80 Complications following infusion, transfusion and therapeutic injection**
INCLUDES   complications following perfusion
EXCLUDES 2   *bone marrow transplant rejection (T86.01)*
febrile nonhemolytic transfusion reaction (R50.84)
fluid overload due to transfusion (E87.71)
posttransfusion purpura (D69.51)
transfusion associated circulatory overload (TACO) (E87.71)
transfusion (red blood cell) associated hemochromatosis (E83.111)
transfusion related acute lung injury (TRALI) (J95.84)

> The appropriate 7th character is to be added to each code from category T80.
> A   initial encounter
> D   subsequent encounter
> S   sequela

   ✓x 7ᵗʰ **T80.0 Air embolism following infusion, transfusion and therapeutic injection**

   ✓x 7ᵗʰ **T80.1 Vascular complications following infusion, transfusion and therapeutic injection**
Use additional code to identify the vascular complication
EXCLUDES 2   *extravasation of vesicant agent (T80.81-)*
infiltration of vesicant agent (T80.81-)
postprocedural vascular complications (T81.7-)
vascular complications specified as due to prosthetic devices, implants and grafts (T82.8-, T83.8-, T84.8-, T85.8-)

   ✓ 5ᵗʰ **T80.2 Infections following infusion, transfusion and therapeutic injection**
Use additional code to identify the specific infection, such as: sepsis (A41.9)
Use additional code (R65.2-) to identify severe sepsis, if applicable
EXCLUDES 2   *infections specified as due to prosthetic devices, implants and grafts (T82.6-T82.7, T83.5-T83.6, T84.5-T84.7, T85.7)*
postprocedural infections (T81.4-)

     ✓ 6ᵗʰ **T80.21 Infection due to central venous catheter**
Infection due to pulmonary artery catheter (Swan-Ganz catheter)
TIP: Provider documentation needs to support that an existing, unresolved infection is directly linked to the central venous catheter.

Ⓝ Newborn: 0   Ⓟ Pediatric: 0-17   Ⓜ Maternity: 12-55   Ⓐ Adult: 15-124   **NRS** Nonroutine supply Dx   **NC Dx** Noncancer Dx   **PDx** Primary Dx   ▶◀ Revised Text   ● New Code   ▲ Revised Title

1096   ICD-10-CM 2018

✔️7ᵗʰ **T80.211** Bloodstream infection **due to central venous catheter**

    Catheter-related bloodstream infection (CRBSI) NOS

    Central line-associated bloodstream infection (CLABSI)

    Bloodstream infection due to Hickman catheter

    Bloodstream infection due to peripherally inserted central catheter (PICC)

    Bloodstream infection due to portacath (port-a-cath)

    Bloodstream infection due to pulmonary artery catheter

    Bloodstream infection due to triple lumen catheter

    Bloodstream infection due to umbilical venous catheter

✔️7ᵗʰ **T80.212** Local infection **due to central venous catheter**

    Exit or insertion site infection

    Local infection due to Hickman catheter

    Local infection due to peripherally inserted central catheter (PICC)

    Local infection due to portacath (port-a-cath)

    Local infection due to pulmonary artery catheter

    Local infection due to triple lumen catheter

    Local infection due to umbilical venous catheter

    Port or reservoir infection

    Tunnel infection

✔️7ᵗʰ **T80.218** **Other infection due to central venous catheter**

    Other central line-associated infection

    Other infection due to Hickman catheter

    Other infection due to peripherally inserted central catheter (PICC)

    Other infection due to portacath (port-a-cath)

    Other infection due to pulmonary artery catheter

    Other infection due to triple lumen catheter

    Other infection due to umbilical venous catheter

✔️7ᵗʰ **T80.219** **Unspecified infection due to central venous catheter** ▽

    Central line-associated infection NOS

    Unspecified infection due to Hickman catheter

    Unspecified infection due to peripherally inserted central catheter (PICC)

    Unspecified infection due to portacath (port-a-cath)

    Unspecified infection due to pulmonary artery catheter

    Unspecified infection due to triple lumen catheter

    Unspecified infection due to umbilical venous catheter

✔️x7ᵗʰ **T80.22** **Acute infection following transfusion, infusion, or injection of blood and blood products**

✔️x7ᵗʰ **T80.29** **Infection following other infusion, transfusion and therapeutic injection**

✔️5ᵗʰ **T80.3** ABO incompatibility **reaction due to transfusion of blood or blood products**

    EXCLUDES 1 *minor blood group antigens reactions (Duffy) (E) (K(ell)) (Kidd) (Lewis) (M) (N) (P) (S) (T80.A)*

✔️x7ᵗʰ **T80.30** **ABO incompatibility reaction due to transfusion of blood or blood products, unspecified** ▽

    ABO incompatibility blood transfusion NOS

    Reaction to ABO incompatibility from transfusion NOS

✔️6ᵗʰ **T80.31** **ABO incompatibility** with hemolytic transfusion reaction

✔️7ᵗʰ **T80.310** **ABO incompatibility with** acute **hemolytic transfusion reaction**

    ABO incompatibility with hemolytic transfusion reaction less than 24 hours after transfusion

    Acute hemolytic transfusion reaction (AHTR) due to ABO incompatibility

✔️7ᵗʰ **T80.311** **ABO incompatibility with** delayed **hemolytic transfusion reaction**

    ABO incompatibility with hemolytic transfusion reaction 24 hours or more after transfusion

    Delayed hemolytic transfusion reaction (DHTR) due to ABO incompatibility

✔️7ᵗʰ **T80.319** **ABO incompatibility with hemolytic transfusion reaction, unspecified** ▽

    ABO incompatibility with hemolytic transfusion reaction at unspecified time after transfusion

    Hemolytic transfusion reaction (HTR) due to ABO incompatibility NOS

✔️x7ᵗʰ **T80.39** **Other ABO incompatibility reaction due to transfusion of blood or blood products**

    Delayed serologic transfusion reaction (DSTR) from ABO incompatibility

    Other ABO incompatible blood transfusion

    Other reaction to ABO incompatible blood transfusion

✔️5ᵗʰ **T80.4** Rh incompatibility **reaction due to transfusion of blood or blood products**

    Reaction due to incompatibility of Rh antigens (C) (c) (D) (E) (e)

✔️x7ᵗʰ **T80.40** **Rh incompatibility reaction due to transfusion of blood or blood products, unspecified** ▽

    Reaction due to Rh factor in transfusion NOS

    Rh incompatible blood transfusion NOS

✔️6ᵗʰ **T80.41** **Rh incompatibility** with hemolytic transfusion reaction

✔️7ᵗʰ **T80.410** **Rh incompatibility with** acute **hemolytic transfusion reaction**

    Acute hemolytic transfusion reaction (AHTR) due to Rh incompatibility

    Rh incompatibility with hemolytic transfusion reaction less than 24 hours after transfusion

✔️7ᵗʰ **T80.411** **Rh incompatibility with** delayed **hemolytic transfusion reaction**

    Delayed hemolytic transfusion reaction (DHTR) due to Rh incompatibility

    Rh incompatibility with hemolytic transfusion reaction 24 hours or more after transfusion

✔️7ᵗʰ **T80.419** **Rh incompatibility with hemolytic transfusion reaction, unspecified** ▽

    Hemolytic transfusion reaction (HTR) due to Rh incompatibility NOS

    Rh incompatibility with hemolytic transfusion reaction at unspecified time after transfusion

✔️x7ᵗʰ **T80.49** **Other Rh incompatibility reaction due to transfusion of blood or blood products**

    Delayed serologic transfusion reaction (DSTR) from Rh incompatibility

    Other reaction to Rh incompatible blood transfusion

✔️5ᵗʰ **T80.A** Non-ABO incompatibility **reaction due to transfusion of blood or blood products**

    Reaction due to incompatibility of minor antigens (Duffy) (Kell) (Kidd) (Lewis) (M) (N) (P) (S)

✔️x7ᵗʰ **T80.A0** **Non-ABO incompatibility reaction due to transfusion of blood or blood products, unspecified** ▽

    Non-ABO antigen incompatibility reaction from transfusion NOS

✔️6ᵗʰ **T80.A1** **Non-ABO incompatibility** with hemolytic transfusion reaction

✔️7ᵗʰ **T80.A10** **Non-ABO incompatibility with** acute **hemolytic transfusion reaction**

    Acute hemolytic transfusion reaction (AHTR) due to non-ABO incompatibility

    Non-ABO incompatibility with hemolytic transfusion reaction less than 24 hours after transfusion

✔️7ᵗʰ **T80.A11** **Non-ABO incompatibility with** delayed **hemolytic transfusion reaction**

    Delayed hemolytic transfusion reaction (DHTR) due to non-ABO incompatibility

    Non-ABO incompatibility with hemolytic transfusion reaction 24 or more hours after transfusion

---

✔️ Additional Character Req   ✔️x7ᵗʰ Placeholder Alert   Case-Mix Diagnosis   Manifestation   ▽ Unspecified Dx   **EXCLUDES 1** Not coded here   **EXCLUDES 2** Not included here

√7ᵗʰ **T80.A19** **Non-ABO incompatibility with hemolytic transfusion reaction, unspecified** ▽

Hemolytic transfusion reaction (HTR) due to non-ABO incompatibility NOS

Non-ABO incompatibility with hemolytic transfusion reaction at unspecified time after transfusion

√x7ᵗʰ **T80.A9** **Other non-ABO incompatibility reaction due to transfusion of blood or blood products**

Delayed serologic transfusion reaction (DSTR) from non-ABO incompatibility

Other reaction to non-ABO incompatible blood transfusion

√5ᵗʰ **T80.5** **Anaphylactic reaction due to serum**

Allergic shock due to serum

Anaphylactic shock due to serum

Anaphylactoid reaction due to serum

Anaphylaxis due to serum

EXCLUDES 1 *ABO incompatibility reaction due to transfusion of blood or blood products (T80.3-)*

allergic reaction or shock NOS (T78.2)

anaphylactic reaction or shock NOS (T78.2)

anaphylactic reaction or shock due to adverse effect of correct medicinal substance properly administered (T88.6)

other serum reaction (T80.6-)

DEF: Life-threatening hypersensitivity to foreign serum; causes respiratory distress, vascular collapse, and shock.

√x7ᵗʰ **T80.51** **Anaphylactic reaction due to** administration of blood and blood products

√x7ᵗʰ **T80.52** **Anaphylactic reaction due to** vaccination

√x7ᵗʰ **T80.59** **Anaphylactic reaction due to other** serum

√5ᵗʰ **T80.6** **Other serum reactions**

Intoxication by serum

Protein sickness

Serum rash

Serum sickness

Serum urticaria

EXCLUDES 2 *serum hepatitis (B16-B19)*

DEF: Serum sickness: Hypersensitivity to foreign serum; causes fever, hives, swelling, and lymphadenopathy.

√x7ᵗʰ **T80.61** **Other serum reaction** due to administration of blood and blood products

√x7ᵗʰ **T80.62** **Other serum reaction** due to vaccination

√x7ᵗʰ **T80.69** **Other serum reaction due to other** serum

▶Code also, if applicable, arthropathy in hypersensitivity reactions classified elsewhere (M36.4)◀

√5ᵗʰ **T80.8** **Other complications following infusion, transfusion and therapeutic injection**

√6ᵗʰ **T80.81** **Extravasation of vesicant agent**

Infiltration of vesicant agent

√7ᵗʰ **T80.810** **Extravasation of vesicant antineoplastic chemotherapy**

Infiltration of vesicant antineoplastic chemotherapy

√7ᵗʰ **T80.818** **Extravasation of other vesicant agent**

Infiltration of other vesicant agent

√x7ᵗʰ **T80.89** **Other complications following infusion, transfusion and therapeutic injection**

Delayed serologic transfusion reaction (DSTR), unspecified incompatibility

Use additional code to identify graft-versus-host reaction, if applicable, (D89.81-)

√5ᵗʰ **T80.9** **Unspecified complication following infusion, transfusion and therapeutic injection**

√x7ᵗʰ **T80.90** **Unspecified complication** following infusion and therapeutic injection ▽

√6ᵗʰ **T80.91** **Hemolytic transfusion reaction, unspecified incompatibility**

EXCLUDES 1 *ABO incompatibility with hemolytic transfusion reaction (T80.31-)*

Non-ABO incompatibility with hemolytic transfusion reaction (T80.A1-)

Rh incompatibility with hemolytic transfusion reaction (T80.41-)

√7ᵗʰ **T80.910** **Acute hemolytic transfusion reaction, unspecified incompatibility** ▽

√7ᵗʰ **T80.911** **Delayed hemolytic transfusion reaction, unspecified incompatibility** ▽

√7ᵗʰ **T80.919** **Hemolytic transfusion reaction, unspecified incompatibility, unspecified as acute or delayed** ▽

Hemolytic transfusion reaction NOS

√x7ᵗʰ **T80.92** **Unspecified transfusion reaction** ▽

Transfusion reaction NOS

√4ᵗʰ **T81** **Complications of procedures, not elsewhere classified**

Use additional code for adverse effect, if applicable, to identify drug (T36-T50 with fifth or sixth character 5)

EXCLUDES 2 *complications following immunization (T88.0-T88.1)*

complications following infusion, transfusion and therapeutic injection (T80.-)

complications of transplanted organs and tissue (T86.-)

specified complications classified elsewhere, such as:

complication of prosthetic devices, implants and grafts (T82-T85)

dermatitis due to drugs and medicaments (L23.3, L24.4, L25.1, L27.0-L27.1)

endosseous dental implant failure (M27.6-)

floppy iris syndrome (IFIS) (intraoperative) (H21.81)

intraoperative and postprocedural complications of specific body system (D78.-, E36.-, E89.-, G97.3-, G97.4, H59.3-, H59.-, H95.2-, H95.3, I97.4-, I97.5, J95, K91.-, L76.-, M96.-, N99.-)

ostomy complications (J95.0-, K94.-, N99.5-)

plateau iris syndrome (post-iridectomy) (postprocedural) (H21.82)

poisoning and toxic effects of drugs and chemicals (T36-T65 with fifth or sixth character 1-4 or 6)

> The appropriate 7th character is to be added to each code from category T81.
> A   initial encounter
> D   subsequent encounter
> S   sequela

√5ᵗʰ **T81.1** **Postprocedural shock**

Shock during or resulting from a procedure, not elsewhere classified

EXCLUDES 1 *anaphylactic shock due to correct substance properly administered (T88.6*

anaphylactic shock due to serum (T80.5-)

anaphylactic shock NOS (T78.2)

anesthetic shock (T88.2)

electric shock (T75.4)

obstetric shock (O75.1)

septic shock (R65.21)

shock following abortion or ectopic or molar pregnancy (O00-O07, O08.3)

traumatic shock (T79.4)

√x7ᵗʰ **T81.10** **Postprocedural shock unspecified** ▽

Collapse NOS during or resulting from a procedure, not elsewhere classified

Postprocedural failure of peripheral circulation

Postprocedural shock NOS

√x7ᵗʰ **T81.11** **Postprocedural** cardiogenic **shock**

√x7ᵗʰ **T81.12** **Postprocedural** septic **shock**

Postprocedural endotoxic shock resulting from a procedure, not elsewhere classified

Postprocedural gram-negative shock resulting from a procedure, not elsewhere classified

Code first underlying infection

Use additional code, to identify any associated acute organ dysfunction, if applicable

√x7ᵗʰ **T81.19** **Other postprocedural shock**

Postprocedural hypovolemic shock

Ⓝ Newborn: 0   Ⓟ Pediatric: 0-17   Ⓜ Maternity: 12-55   Ⓐ Adult: 15-124   **NRS** Nonroutine supply Dx   **NCDx** Noncancer Dx   **PDx** Primary Dx   ▶◀ Revised Text   ● New Code   ▲ Revised Title

1098   ICD-10-CM 2018

✓5ᵗʰ **T81.3 Disruption of wound, not elsewhere classified**
Disruption of any suture materials or other closure methods

> *EXCLUDES 1*   *breakdown (mechanical) of permanent sutures (T85.612)*
> *displacement of permanent sutures (T85.622)*
> *disruption of cesarean delivery wound (O90.0)*
> *disruption of perineal obstetric wound (O90.1)*
> *mechanical complication of permanent sutures NEC (T85.692)*

AHA: 2014, 1Q, 23

4,5 ✓x7ᵗʰ **T81.30 Disruption of wound, unspecified**   NRS ▽
Disruption of wound NOS

4,5 ✓x7ᵗʰ **T81.31 Disruption of external operation (surgical)**   NRS
wound, not elsewhere classified
Dehiscence of operation wound NOS
Disruption of operation wound NOS
Disruption or dehiscence of closure of cornea
Disruption or dehiscence of closure of mucosa
Disruption or dehiscence of closure of skin and
subcutaneous tissue
Full-thickness skin disruption or dehiscence
Superficial disruption or dehiscence of operation
wound

> *EXCLUDES 1*   *dehiscence of amputation stump (T87.81)*

4,5 ✓x7ᵗʰ **T81.32 Disruption of internal operation (surgical)**   NRS
wound, not elsewhere classified
Deep disruption or dehiscence of operation wound
NOS
Disruption or dehiscence of closure of internal organ
or other internal tissue
Disruption or dehiscence of closure of muscle or
muscle flap
Disruption or dehiscence of closure of ribs or rib cage
Disruption or dehiscence of closure of skull or
craniotomy
Disruption or dehiscence of closure of sternum or
sternotomy
Disruption or dehiscence of closure of tendon or
ligament
Disruption or dehiscence of closure of superficial or
muscular fascia

4,5 ✓x7ᵗʰ **T81.33 Disruption of traumatic injury wound repair**   NRS
Disruption or dehiscence of closure of traumatic
laceration (external) (internal)

4,5 ✓x7ᵗʰ **T81.4 Infection following a procedure**   NRS
Intra-abdominal abscess following a procedure
Postprocedural infection, not elsewhere classified
Sepsis following a procedure
Stitch abscess following a procedure
Subphrenic abscess following a procedure
Wound abscess following a procedure
Use additional code to identify infection
Use additional code (R65.2-) to identify severe sepsis, if
applicable

> *EXCLUDES 1*   *obstetric surgical wound infection (O86.0)*
> *postprocedural fever NOS (R50.82)*
> *postprocedural retroperitoneal abscess (K68.11)*
> *EXCLUDES 2*   *bleb associated endophthalmitis (H59.4-)*
> *infection due to infusion, transfusion and therapeutic*
> *injection (T80.2-)*
> *infection due to prosthetic devices, implants and grafts*
> *(T82.6-T82.7, T83.5-T83.6, T84.5-T84.7, T85.7)*

AHA: 2014, 1Q, 23

✓5ᵗʰ **T81.5 Complications of foreign body accidentally left in body**
following procedure
AHA: 2014, 4Q, 24

✓6ᵗʰ **T81.50 Unspecified complication of foreign body**
accidentally left in body following procedure

✓7ᵗʰ **T81.500 Unspecified complication of foreign**   ▽
body accidentally left in body following
surgical operation

✓7ᵗʰ **T81.501 Unspecified complication of foreign**   ▽
body accidentally left in body following
infusion or transfusion

✓7ᵗʰ **T81.502 Unspecified complication of foreign**   ▽
body accidentally left in body following
kidney dialysis

✓7ᵗʰ **T81.503 Unspecified complication of foreign**   ▽
body accidentally left in body following
injection or immunization

✓7ᵗʰ **T81.504 Unspecified complication of foreign**   ▽
body accidentally left in body following
endoscopic examination

✓7ᵗʰ **T81.505 Unspecified complication of foreign**   ▽
body accidentally left in body following
heart catheterization

✓7ᵗʰ **T81.506 Unspecified complication of foreign**   ▽
body accidentally left in body following
aspiration, puncture or other
catheterization

✓7ᵗʰ **T81.507 Unspecified complication of foreign**   ▽
body accidentally left in body following
removal of catheter or packing

✓7ᵗʰ **T81.508 Unspecified complication of foreign**   ▽
body accidentally left in body following
other procedure

✓7ᵗʰ **T81.509 Unspecified complication of foreign**   ▽
body accidentally left in body following
unspecified procedure

✓6ᵗʰ **T81.51 Adhesions due to foreign body accidentally left in**
body following procedure

1,6 ✓7ᵗʰ **T81.510 Adhesions due to foreign body**   NRS
accidentally left in body following
surgical operation

1,6 ✓7ᵗʰ **T81.511 Adhesions due to foreign body**   NRS
accidentally left in body following
infusion or transfusion

1,6 ✓7ᵗʰ **T81.512 Adhesions due to foreign body**   NRS
accidentally left in body following
kidney dialysis

1,6 ✓7ᵗʰ **T81.513 Adhesions due to foreign body**   NRS
accidentally left in body following
injection or immunization

1,6 ✓7ᵗʰ **T81.514 Adhesions due to foreign body**   NRS
accidentally left in body following
endoscopic examination

1,6 ✓7ᵗʰ **T81.515 Adhesions due to foreign body**   NRS
accidentally left in body following
heart catheterization

1,6 ✓7ᵗʰ **T81.516 Adhesions due to foreign body**   NRS
accidentally left in body following
aspiration, puncture or other
catheterization

1,6 ✓7ᵗʰ **T81.517 Adhesions due to foreign body**   NRS
accidentally left in body following
removal of catheter or packing

1,6 ✓7ᵗʰ **T81.518 Adhesions due to foreign body**   NRS
accidentally left in body following
other procedure

1,6 ✓7ᵗʰ **T81.519 Adhesions due to foreign body**   NRS ▽
accidentally left in body following
unspecified procedure

✓6ᵗʰ **T81.52 Obstruction due to foreign body accidentally left in**
body following procedure

1,6 ✓7ᵗʰ **T81.520 Obstruction due to foreign body**   NRS
accidentally left in body following
surgical operation

1,6 ✓7ᵗʰ **T81.521 Obstruction due to foreign body**   NRS
accidentally left in body following
infusion or transfusion

1,6 ✓7ᵗʰ **T81.522 Obstruction due to foreign body**   NRS
accidentally left in body following
kidney dialysis

1,6 ✓7ᵗʰ **T81.523 Obstruction due to foreign body**   NRS
accidentally left in body following
injection or immunization

1,6 ✓7ᵗʰ **T81.524 Obstruction due to foreign body**   NRS
accidentally left in body following
endoscopic examination

1,6 ✓7ᵗʰ **T81.525 Obstruction due to foreign body**   NRS
accidentally left in body following
heart catheterization

---

1 Case-mix diagnosis with 7th character indicating subsequent encounter.
4 Case-mix diagnosis with 7th character indicating initial or subsequent encounter.
5 NRS supply diagnosis with 7th character indicating initial or subsequent encounter.
6 NRS supply diagnosis with 7th character indicating subsequent encounter.

✓ Additional Character Req   ✓x7ᵗʰ Placeholder Alert   Case-Mix Diagnosis   Manifestation   ▽ Unspecified Dx   *EXCLUDES 1* Not coded here   *EXCLUDES 2* Not included here

ICD-10-CM 2018   **1099**

Chapter 19. Injury, Poisoning and Certain Other Consequences of External Causes

1, 6 ✓7ᵗʰ **T81.526 Obstruction due to foreign body accidentally left in body following aspiration, puncture or other catheterization** NRS

1, 6 ✓7ᵗʰ **T81.527 Obstruction due to foreign body accidentally left in body following removal of catheter or packing** NRS

1, 6 ✓7ᵗʰ **T81.528 Obstruction due to foreign body accidentally left in body following other procedure** NRS

1, 6 ✓7ᵗʰ **T81.529 Obstruction due to foreign body accidentally left in body following unspecified procedure** NRS ▽

✓6ᵗʰ **T81.53 Perforation due to foreign body accidentally left in body following procedure**

1, 6 ✓7ᵗʰ **T81.530 Perforation due to foreign body accidentally left in body following surgical operation** NRS

1, 6 ✓7ᵗʰ **T81.531 Perforation due to foreign body accidentally left in body following infusion or transfusion** NRS

1, 6 ✓7ᵗʰ **T81.532 Perforation due to foreign body accidentally left in body following kidney dialysis** NRS

1, 6 ✓7ᵗʰ **T81.533 Perforation due to foreign body accidentally left in body following injection or immunization** NRS

1, 6 ✓7ᵗʰ **T81.534 Perforation due to foreign body accidentally left in body following endoscopic examination** NRS

1, 6 ✓7ᵗʰ **T81.535 Perforation due to foreign body accidentally left in body following heart catheterization** NRS

1, 6 ✓7ᵗʰ **T81.536 Perforation due to foreign body accidentally left in body following aspiration, puncture or other catheterization** NRS

1, 6 ✓7ᵗʰ **T81.537 Perforation due to foreign body accidentally left in body following removal of catheter or packing** NRS

1, 6 ✓7ᵗʰ **T81.538 Perforation due to foreign body accidentally left in body following other procedure** NRS

1, 6 ✓7ᵗʰ **T81.539 Perforation due to foreign body accidentally left in body following unspecified procedure** NRS ▽

✓6ᵗʰ **T81.59 Other complications of foreign body accidentally left in body following procedure**
> EXCLUDES 2   *obstruction or perforation due to prosthetic devices and implants intentionally left in body (T82.0-T82.5, T83.0-T83.4, T83.7, T84.0-T84.4, T85.0-T85.6)*

4,5 ✓7ᵗʰ **T81.590 Other complications of foreign body accidentally left in body following surgical operation** NRS

4,5 ✓7ᵗʰ **T81.591 Other complications of foreign body accidentally left in body following infusion or transfusion** NRS

4,5 ✓7ᵗʰ **T81.592 Other complications of foreign body accidentally left in body following kidney dialysis** NRS

4,5 ✓7ᵗʰ **T81.593 Other complications of foreign body accidentally left in body following injection or immunization** NRS

4,5 ✓7ᵗʰ **T81.594 Other complications of foreign body accidentally left in body following endoscopic examination** NRS

4,5 ✓7ᵗʰ **T81.595 Other complications of foreign body accidentally left in body following heart catheterization** NRS

4,5 ✓7ᵗʰ **T81.596 Other complications of foreign body accidentally left in body following aspiration, puncture or other catheterization** NRS

4,5 ✓7ᵗʰ **T81.597 Other complications of foreign body accidentally left in body following removal of catheter or packing** NRS

4,5 ✓7ᵗʰ **T81.598 Other complications of foreign body accidentally left in body following other procedure** NRS

4,5 ✓7ᵗʰ **T81.599 Other complications of foreign body accidentally left in body following unspecified procedure** NRS ▽

✓5ᵗʰ **T81.6 Acute reaction to foreign substance accidentally left during a procedure**
> EXCLUDES 2   *complications of foreign body accidentally left in body cavity or operation wound following procedure (T81.5-)*

✓x7ᵗʰ **T81.60 Unspecified acute reaction to foreign substance accidentally left during a procedure** ▽

✓x7ᵗʰ **T81.61 Aseptic peritonitis due to foreign substance accidentally left during a procedure**
    Chemical peritonitis

✓x7ᵗʰ **T81.69 Other acute reaction to foreign substance accidentally left during a procedure**

✓5ᵗʰ **T81.7 Vascular complications following a procedure, not elsewhere classified**
    Air embolism following procedure NEC
    Phlebitis or thrombophlebitis resulting from a procedure
> EXCLUDES 1   *embolism complicating abortion or ectopic or molar pregnancy (O00-O07, O08.2)*
> *embolism complicating pregnancy, childbirth and the puerperium (O88.-)*
> *traumatic embolism (T79.0)*
> EXCLUDES 2   *embolism due to prosthetic devices, implants and grafts (T82.8-, T83.81, T84.8-, T85.81-)*
> *embolism following infusion, transfusion and therapeutic injection (T80.0)*

✓6ᵗʰ **T81.71 Complication of artery following a procedure, not elsewhere classified**

✓7ᵗʰ **T81.710 Complication of mesenteric artery following a procedure, not elsewhere classified**

✓7ᵗʰ **T81.711 Complication of renal artery following a procedure, not elsewhere classified**

✓7ᵗʰ **T81.718 Complication of other artery following a procedure, not elsewhere classified**

✓7ᵗʰ **T81.719 Complication of unspecified artery following a procedure, not elsewhere classified** ▽

✓x7ᵗʰ **T81.72 Complication of vein following a procedure, not elsewhere classified**

✓5ᵗʰ **T81.8 Other complications of procedures, not elsewhere classified**
> EXCLUDES 2   *hypothermia following anesthesia (T88.51)*
> *malignant hyperpyrexia due to anesthesia (T88.3)*

✓x7ᵗʰ **T81.81 Complication of inhalation therapy**

✓x7ᵗʰ **T81.82 Emphysema (subcutaneous) resulting from a procedure**

4,5 ✓x7ᵗʰ **T81.83 Persistent postprocedural fistula** NRS

✓x7ᵗʰ **T81.89 Other complications of procedures, not elsewhere classified**
    Use additional code to specify complication, such as:
      postprocedural delirium (F05)
    AHA: 2014, 1Q, 23

✓x7ᵗʰ **T81.9 Unspecified complication of procedure** ▽

---

1   Case-mix diagnosis with 7th character indicating subsequent encounter.
4   Case-mix diagnosis with 7th character indicating initial or subsequent encounter.
5   NRS supply diagnosis with 7th character indicating initial or subsequent encounter.
6   NRS supply diagnosis with 7th character indicating subsequent encounter.

N Newborn: 0   P Pediatric: 0-17   M Maternity: 12-55   A Adult: 15-124   NRS Nonroutine supply Dx   NC Dx Noncancer Dx   PDx Primary Dx   ▶◀ Revised Text   ● New Code   ▲ Revised Title

✓4ᵗʰ T82 Complications of cardiac and vascular prosthetic devices, implants and grafts

> **EXCLUDES 2** *failure and rejection of transplanted organs and tissue (T86.-)*

> The appropriate 7th character is to be added to each code from category T82.
> A   initial encounter
> D   subsequent encounter
> S   sequela

✓5ᵗʰ T82.Ø Mechanical complication of heart valve prosthesis
Mechanical complication of artificial heart valve
> **EXCLUDES 1** *mechanical complication of biological heart valve graft (T82.22-)*

✓x7ᵗʰ T82.Ø1 Breakdown **(mechanical) of heart valve prosthesis**

✓x7ᵗʰ T82.Ø2 Displacement **of heart valve prosthesis**
Malposition of heart valve prosthesis

✓x7ᵗʰ T82.Ø3 Leakage **of heart valve prosthesis**

✓x7ᵗʰ T82.Ø9 Other mechanical complication of heart valve prosthesis
Obstruction (mechanical) of heart valve prosthesis
Perforation of heart valve prosthesis
Protrusion of heart valve prosthesis

✓5ᵗʰ T82.1 Mechanical complication of cardiac electronic device

✓6ᵗʰ T82.11 Breakdown **(mechanical) of cardiac electronic device**

✓7ᵗʰ T82.11Ø Breakdown (mechanical) of cardiac electrode

✓7ᵗʰ T82.111 Breakdown (mechanical) of cardiac pulse generator (battery)

✓7ᵗʰ T82.118 Breakdown (mechanical) of other cardiac electronic device

✓7ᵗʰ T82.119 Breakdown (mechanical) of unspecified cardiac electronic device ▽

✓6ᵗʰ T82.12 Displacement **of cardiac electronic device**
Malposition of cardiac electronic device

✓7ᵗʰ T82.12Ø Displacement of cardiac electrode

✓7ᵗʰ T82.121 Displacement of cardiac pulse generator (battery)

✓7ᵗʰ T82.128 Displacement of other cardiac electronic device

✓7ᵗʰ T82.129 Displacement of unspecified cardiac electronic device ▽

✓6ᵗʰ T82.19 Other **mechanical complication of cardiac electronic device**
Leakage of cardiac electronic device
Obstruction of cardiac electronic device
Perforation of cardiac electronic device
Protrusion of cardiac electronic device

✓7ᵗʰ T82.19Ø Other mechanical complication of cardiac electrode

✓7ᵗʰ T82.191 Other mechanical complication of cardiac pulse generator (battery)

✓7ᵗʰ T82.198 Other mechanical complication of other cardiac electronic device

✓7ᵗʰ T82.199 Other mechanical complication of unspecified cardiac device ▽

✓5ᵗʰ T82.2 Mechanical complication of coronary artery bypass graft **and** biological heart valve graft
> **EXCLUDES 1** *mechanical complication of artificial heart valve prosthesis (T82.Ø-)*

✓6ᵗʰ T82.21 Mechanical complication of coronary artery bypass graft

✓7ᵗʰ T82.211 Breakdown **(mechanical) of coronary artery bypass graft**

✓7ᵗʰ T82.212 Displacement **of coronary artery bypass graft**
Malposition of coronary artery bypass graft

✓7ᵗʰ T82.213 Leakage **of coronary artery bypass graft**

✓7ᵗʰ T82.218 Other mechanical complication of coronary artery bypass graft
Obstruction, mechanical of coronary artery bypass graft
Perforation of coronary artery bypass graft
Protrusion of coronary artery bypass graft

✓6ᵗʰ T82.22 Mechanical complication of biological heart valve graft

✓7ᵗʰ T82.221 Breakdown **(mechanical) of biological heart valve graft**

✓7ᵗʰ T82.222 Displacement **of biological heart valve graft**
Malposition of biological heart valve graft

✓7ᵗʰ T82.223 Leakage **of biological heart valve graft**

✓7ᵗʰ T82.228 Other mechanical complication of biological heart valve graft
Obstruction of biological heart valve graft
Perforation of biological heart valve graft
Protrusion of biological heart valve graft

✓5ᵗʰ T82.3 Mechanical complication of other vascular grafts

✓6ᵗʰ T82.31 Breakdown **(mechanical) of other vascular grafts**

✓7ᵗʰ T82.31Ø Breakdown (mechanical) of aortic (bifurcation) graft (replacement)

✓7ᵗʰ T82.311 Breakdown (mechanical) of carotid arterial graft (bypass)

✓7ᵗʰ T82.312 Breakdown (mechanical) of femoral arterial graft (bypass)

✓7ᵗʰ T82.318 Breakdown (mechanical) of other vascular grafts

✓7ᵗʰ T82.319 Breakdown (mechanical) of unspecified ▽ **vascular grafts**

✓6ᵗʰ T82.32 Displacement **of other vascular grafts**
Malposition of other vascular grafts

✓7ᵗʰ T82.32Ø Displacement of aortic (bifurcation) graft (replacement)

✓7ᵗʰ T82.321 Displacement of carotid arterial graft (bypass)

✓7ᵗʰ T82.322 Displacement of femoral arterial graft (bypass)

✓7ᵗʰ T82.328 Displacement of other vascular grafts

✓7ᵗʰ T82.329 Displacement of unspecified vascular ▽ **grafts**

✓6ᵗʰ T82.33 Leakage **of other vascular grafts**

✓7ᵗʰ T82.33Ø Leakage of aortic (bifurcation) graft (replacement)

✓7ᵗʰ T82.331 Leakage of carotid arterial graft (bypass)

✓7ᵗʰ T82.332 Leakage of femoral arterial graft (bypass)

✓7ᵗʰ T82.338 Leakage of other vascular grafts

✓7ᵗʰ T82.339 Leakage of unspecified vascular graft ▽

✓6ᵗʰ T82.39 Other **mechanical complication of other vascular grafts**
Obstruction (mechanical) of other vascular grafts
Perforation of other vascular grafts
Protrusion of other vascular grafts

✓7ᵗʰ T82.39Ø Other mechanical complication of aortic (bifurcation) graft (replacement)

✓7ᵗʰ T82.391 Other mechanical complication of carotid arterial graft (bypass)

✓7ᵗʰ T82.392 Other mechanical complication of femoral arterial graft (bypass)

✓7ᵗʰ T82.398 Other mechanical complication of other vascular grafts

✓7ᵗʰ T82.399 Other mechanical complication of unspecified vascular grafts ▽

✓5ᵗʰ T82.4 Mechanical complication of vascular dialysis catheter
Mechanical complication of hemodialysis catheter
> **EXCLUDES 1** *mechanical complication of intraperitoneal dialysis catheter (T85.62)*

✓x7ᵗʰ T82.41 Breakdown **(mechanical) of vascular dialysis catheter**

✓x7ᵗʰ T82.42 Displacement **of vascular dialysis catheter**
Malposition of vascular dialysis catheter

✓x7ᵗʰ T82.43 Leakage **of vascular dialysis catheter**

✓x7ᵗʰ T82.49 Other complication of vascular dialysis catheter
Obstruction (mechanical) of vascular dialysis catheter
Perforation of vascular dialysis catheter
Protrusion of vascular dialysis catheter

✓5ᵗʰ T82.5 Mechanical complication of other cardiac and vascular devices and implants
> **EXCLUDES 2** *mechanical complication of epidural and subdural infusion catheter (T85.61)*

✓6ᵗʰ T82.51 Breakdown **(mechanical) of other cardiac and vascular devices and implants**

✓7ᵗʰ T82.51Ø Breakdown (mechanical) of surgically created arteriovenous fistula

---

Chapter 19. Injury, Poisoning and Certain Other Consequences of External Causes

T82.511–T83.Ø12

√7ᵗʰ **T82.511** **Breakdown (mechanical) of** surgically created arteriovenous shunt

√7ᵗʰ **T82.512** **Breakdown (mechanical) of** artificial heart

√7ᵗʰ **T82.513** **Breakdown (mechanical) of** balloon (counterpulsation) device

√7ᵗʰ **T82.514** **Breakdown (mechanical) of** infusion catheter

√7ᵗʰ **T82.515** **Breakdown (mechanical) of** umbrella device

√7ᵗʰ **T82.518** **Breakdown (mechanical) of other cardiac and vascular devices and implants**

√7ᵗʰ **T82.519** **Breakdown (mechanical) of unspecified** ▽ **cardiac and vascular devices and implants**

√6ᵗʰ **T82.52** **Displacement of other cardiac and vascular devices and implants**
   Malposition of other cardiac and vascular devices and implants

√7ᵗʰ **T82.52Ø** **Displacement of** surgically created arteriovenous fistula

√7ᵗʰ **T82.521** **Displacement of** surgically created arteriovenous shunt

√7ᵗʰ **T82.522** **Displacement of** artificial heart

√7ᵗʰ **T82.523** **Displacement of** balloon (counterpulsation) device

√7ᵗʰ **T82.524** **Displacement of** infusion catheter

√7ᵗʰ **T82.525** **Displacement of** umbrella device

√7ᵗʰ **T82.528** **Displacement of other cardiac and vascular devices and implants**

√7ᵗʰ **T82.529** **Displacement of unspecified cardiac** ▽ **and vascular devices and implants**

√6ᵗʰ **T82.53** **Leakage of other cardiac and vascular devices and implants**

√7ᵗʰ **T82.53Ø** **Leakage of** surgically created arteriovenous fistula

√7ᵗʰ **T82.531** **Leakage of** surgically created arteriovenous shunt

√7ᵗʰ **T82.532** **Leakage of** artificial heart

√7ᵗʰ **T82.533** **Leakage of** balloon (counterpulsation) device

√7ᵗʰ **T82.534** **Leakage of** infusion catheter

√7ᵗʰ **T82.535** **Leakage of** umbrella device

√7ᵗʰ **T82.538** **Leakage of other cardiac and vascular devices and implants**

√7ᵗʰ **T82.539** **Leakage of unspecified cardiac and** ▽ **vascular devices and implants**

√6ᵗʰ **T82.59** **Other mechanical complication of other cardiac and vascular devices and implants**
   Obstruction (mechanical) of other cardiac and vascular devices and implants
   Perforation of other cardiac and vascular devices and implants
   Protrusion of other cardiac and vascular devices and implants

√7ᵗʰ **T82.59Ø** **Other mechanical complication of** surgically created arteriovenous fistula

√7ᵗʰ **T82.591** **Other mechanical complication of** surgically created arteriovenous shunt

√7ᵗʰ **T82.592** **Other mechanical complication of** artificial heart

√7ᵗʰ **T82.593** **Other mechanical complication of** balloon (counterpulsation) device

√7ᵗʰ **T82.594** **Other mechanical complication of** infusion catheter

√7ᵗʰ **T82.595** **Other mechanical complication of** umbrella device

√7ᵗʰ **T82.598** **Other mechanical complication of other cardiac and vascular devices and implants**

√7ᵗʰ **T82.599** **Other mechanical complication of** ▽ **unspecified cardiac and vascular devices and implants**

√x7ᵗʰ **T82.6** **Infection and inflammatory reaction due to** cardiac valve prosthesis
   Use additional code to identify infection

√x7ᵗʰ **T82.7** **Infection and inflammatory reaction due to** other cardiac and vascular devices, implants and grafts
   Use additional code to identify infection

√5ᵗʰ **T82.8** **Other specified complications** of cardiac and vascular prosthetic devices, implants and grafts

√6ᵗʰ **T82.81** **Embolism** due to cardiac and vascular prosthetic devices, implants and grafts

√7ᵗʰ **T82.817** **Embolism due to** cardiac prosthetic devices, implants and grafts

√7ᵗʰ **T82.818** **Embolism due to** vascular prosthetic devices, implants and grafts

√6ᵗʰ **T82.82** **Fibrosis** due to cardiac and vascular prosthetic devices, implants and grafts

√7ᵗʰ **T82.827** **Fibrosis due to** cardiac prosthetic devices, implants and grafts

√7ᵗʰ **T82.828** **Fibrosis due to** vascular prosthetic devices, implants and grafts

√6ᵗʰ **T82.83** **Hemorrhage** due to cardiac and vascular prosthetic devices, implants and grafts

√7ᵗʰ **T82.837** **Hemorrhage due to** cardiac prosthetic devices, implants and grafts

√7ᵗʰ **T82.838** **Hemorrhage due to** vascular prosthetic devices, implants and grafts

√6ᵗʰ **T82.84** **Pain** due to cardiac and vascular prosthetic devices, implants and grafts

√7ᵗʰ **T82.847** **Pain due to** cardiac prosthetic devices, implants and grafts

√7ᵗʰ **T82.848** **Pain due to** vascular prosthetic devices, implants and grafts

√6ᵗʰ **T82.85** **Stenosis** due to cardiac and vascular prosthetic devices, implants and grafts

√7ᵗʰ **T82.855** **Stenosis of** coronary artery stent
   In-stent stenosis (restenosis) of coronary artery stent
   Restenosis of coronary artery stent

√7ᵗʰ **T82.856** **Stenosis of** peripheral vascular stent
   In-stent stenosis (restenosis) of peripheral vascular stent
   Restenosis of peripheral vascular stent

√7ᵗʰ **T82.857** **Stenosis of other** cardiac prosthetic devices, implants and grafts

√7ᵗʰ **T82.858** **Stenosis of other** vascular prosthetic devices, implants and grafts

√6ᵗʰ **T82.86** **Thrombosis** of cardiac and vascular prosthetic devices, implants and grafts

√7ᵗʰ **T82.867** **Thrombosis due to** cardiac prosthetic devices, implants and grafts

√7ᵗʰ **T82.868** **Thrombosis due to** vascular prosthetic devices, implants and grafts

√6ᵗʰ **T82.89** **Other** specified complication of cardiac and vascular prosthetic devices, implants and grafts

√7ᵗʰ **T82.897** **Other specified complication of** cardiac prosthetic devices, implants and grafts

√7ᵗʰ **T82.898** **Other specified complication of** vascular prosthetic devices, implants and grafts

√x7ᵗʰ **T82.9** **Unspecified complication of cardiac and vascular** ▽ **prosthetic device, implant and graft**

√4ᵗʰ **T83** **Complications of genitourinary prosthetic devices, implants and grafts**
   EXCLUDES 2   *failure and rejection of transplanted organs and tissue (T86.-)*
   TIP: Use to report treatment for a urinary device complication; do not assign a code from category Z46.6 Encounter for fitting and adjustment of urinary device, when a complication of the urinary device is the focus of treatment.

   The appropriate 7th character is to be added to each code from category T83.
   A   initial encounter
   D   subsequent encounter
   S   sequela

√5ᵗʰ **T83.Ø** **Mechanical complication of** urinary catheter
   EXCLUDES 2   *complications of stoma of urinary tract (N99.5-)*

√6ᵗʰ **T83.Ø1** **Breakdown** (mechanical) of urinary catheter

√7ᵗʰ **T83.Ø1Ø** **Breakdown (mechanical) of** cystostomy catheter

√7ᵗʰ **T83.Ø11** **Breakdown (mechanical) of** indwelling urethral catheter

√7ᵗʰ **T83.Ø12** **Breakdown (mechanical) of** nephrostomy catheter

Ⓝ Newborn: 0   Ⓟ Pediatric: 0-17   Ⓜ Maternity: 12-55   Ⓐ Adult: 15-124   **NRS** Nonroutine supply Dx   **NCDx** Noncancer Dx   **PDx** Primary Dx   ▶◀ Revised Text   ● New Code   ▲ Revised Title

1102   ICD-10-CM 2018

✓7ᵗʰ **T83.018** **Breakdown (mechanical) of** other **urinary catheter**
Breakdown (mechanical) of Hopkins catheter
Breakdown (mechanical) of ileostomy catheter
Breakdown (mechanical) urostomy catheter

✓6ᵗʰ **T83.02** **Displacement of urinary catheter**
Malposition of urinary catheter

✓7ᵗʰ **T83.020** **Displacement of** cystostomy **catheter**

✓7ᵗʰ **T83.021** **Displacement of** indwelling urethral **catheter**

✓7ᵗʰ **T83.022** **Displacement of** nephrostomy **catheter**

✓7ᵗʰ **T83.028** **Displacement of** other **urinary catheter**
Displacement of Hopkins catheter
Displacement of ileostomy catheter
Displacement of urostomy catheter

✓6ᵗʰ **T83.03** Leakage **of urinary catheter**

✓7ᵗʰ **T83.030** **Leakage of** cystostomy **catheter**

✓7ᵗʰ **T83.031** **Leakage of** indwelling urethral **catheter**

✓7ᵗʰ **T83.032** **Leakage of** nephrostomy **catheter**

✓7ᵗʰ **T83.038** **Leakage of** other **urinary catheter**
Leakage of Hopkins catheter
Leakage of ileostomy catheter
Leakage of urostomy catheter

✓6ᵗʰ **T83.09** Other **mechanical complication of urinary catheter**
Obstruction (mechanical) of urinary catheter
Perforation of urinary catheter
Protrusion of urinary catheter

✓7ᵗʰ **T83.090** **Other mechanical complication of** cystostomy **catheter**

✓7ᵗʰ **T83.091** **Other mechanical complication of** indwelling urethral **catheter**

✓7ᵗʰ **T83.092** **Other mechanical complication of** nephrostomy **catheter**

✓7ᵗʰ **T83.098** **Other mechanical complication of** other **urinary catheter**
Other mechanical complication of Hopkins catheter
Other mechanical complication of ileostomy catheter
Other mechanical complication of urostomy catheter

✓5ᵗʰ **T83.1** **Mechanical complication of** other urinary devices and implants

✓6ᵗʰ **T83.11** Breakdown **(mechanical) of other urinary devices and implants**

✓7ᵗʰ **T83.110** **Breakdown (mechanical) of urinary** electronic stimulator device
EXCLUDES 2 *breakdown (mechanical) of electrode (lead) for sacral nerve neurostimulator (T85.111)*
breakdown (mechanical) of implanted electronic sacral neurostimulator, pulse generator or receiver (T85.113)

✓7ᵗʰ **T83.111** **Breakdown (mechanical) of** implanted urinary sphincter

✓7ᵗʰ **T83.112** **Breakdown (mechanical) of** indwelling ureteral stent

✓7ᵗʰ **T83.113** **Breakdown (mechanical) of** other urinary stents
Breakdown (mechanical) of ileal conduit stent
Breakdown (mechanical) of nephroureteral stent

✓7ᵗʰ **T83.118** **Breakdown (mechanical) of** other **urinary devices and implants**

✓6ᵗʰ **T83.12** Displacement **of other urinary devices and implants**
Malposition of other urinary devices and implants

✓7ᵗʰ **T83.120** **Displacement of urinary** electronic stimulator device
EXCLUDES 2 *displacement of electrode (lead) for sacral nerve neurostimulator (T85.121)*
displacement of implanted electronic sacral neurostimulator, pulse generator or receiver (T85.123)

✓7ᵗʰ **T83.121** **Displacement of** implanted urinary sphincter

✓7ᵗʰ **T83.122** **Displacement of** indwelling ureteral stent

✓7ᵗʰ **T83.123** **Displacement of** other urinary stents
Displacement of ileal conduit stent
Displacement of nephroureteral stent

✓7ᵗʰ **T83.128** **Displacement of** other **urinary devices and implants**

✓6ᵗʰ **T83.19** Other **mechanical complication of other urinary devices and implants**
Leakage of other urinary devices and implants
Obstruction (mechanical) of other urinary devices and implants
Perforation of other urinary devices and implants
Protrusion of other urinary devices and implants

✓7ᵗʰ **T83.190** **Other mechanical complication of urinary** electronic stimulator device
EXCLUDES 2 *other mechanical complication of electrode (lead) for sacral nerve neurostimulator (T85.191)*
other mechanical complication of implanted electronic sacral neurostimulator, pulse generator or receiver (T85.193)

✓7ᵗʰ **T83.191** **Other mechanical complication of** implanted urinary sphincter

✓7ᵗʰ **T83.192** **Other mechanical complication of** indwelling ureteral stent

✓7ᵗʰ **T83.193** **Other mechanical complication of** other urinary stent
Other mechanical complication of ileal conduit stent
Other mechanical complication of nephroureteral stent

✓7ᵗʰ **T83.198** **Other mechanical complication of** other urinary devices and implants

✓5ᵗʰ **T83.2** **Mechanical complication of** graft of urinary organ

✓x7ᵗʰ **T83.21** Breakdown **(mechanical) of graft of urinary organ**

✓x7ᵗʰ **T83.22** Displacement **of graft of urinary organ**
Malposition of graft of urinary organ

✓x7ᵗʰ **T83.23** Leakage **of graft of urinary organ**

✓x7ᵗʰ **T83.24** Erosion **of graft of urinary organ**

✓x7ᵗʰ **T83.25** Exposure **of graft of urinary organ**

✓x7ᵗʰ **T83.29** Other **mechanical complication of graft of urinary organ**
Obstruction (mechanical) of graft of urinary organ
Perforation of graft of urinary organ
Protrusion of graft of urinary organ

✓5ᵗʰ **T83.3** **Mechanical complication of** intrauterine contraceptive device

✓x7ᵗʰ **T83.31** Breakdown **(mechanical) of intrauterine contraceptive device** ♀

✓x7ᵗʰ **T83.32** Displacement **of intrauterine contraceptive device** ♀
Malposition of intrauterine contraceptive device
Missing string of intrauterine contraceptive device

✓x7ᵗʰ **T83.39** Other **mechanical complication of intrauterine contraceptive device** ♀
Leakage of intrauterine contraceptive device
Obstruction (mechanical) of intrauterine contraceptive device
Perforation of intrauterine contraceptive device
Protrusion of intrauterine contraceptive device

Chapter 19. Injury, Poisoning and Certain Other Consequences of External Causes

T83.018–T83.39

✓5ᵗʰ **T83.4 Mechanical complication of** other prosthetic devices, implants and grafts of genital tract

✓6ᵗʰ **T83.41 Breakdown (mechanical) of** other prosthetic devices, implants and grafts of genital tract

✓7ᵗʰ **T83.410 Breakdown (mechanical) of** implanted penile prosthesis ♂
Breakdown (mechanical) of penile prosthesis cylinder
Breakdown (mechanical) of penile prosthesis pump
Breakdown (mechanical) of penile prosthesis reservoir

✓7ᵗʰ **T83.411 Breakdown (mechanical) of** implanted testicular prosthesis

✓7ᵗʰ **T83.418 Breakdown (mechanical) of other** prosthetic devices, implants and grafts of genital tract

✓6ᵗʰ **T83.42 Displacement of** other prosthetic devices, implants and grafts of genital tract
Malposition of other prosthetic devices, implants and grafts of genital tract

✓7ᵗʰ **T83.420 Displacement of** implanted penile prosthesis ♂
Displacement of penile prosthesis cylinder
Displacement of penile prosthesis pump
Displacement of penile prosthesis reservoir

✓7ᵗʰ **T83.421 Displacement of** implanted testicular prosthesis

✓7ᵗʰ **T83.428 Displacement of other** prosthetic devices, implants and grafts of genital tract

✓6ᵗʰ **T83.49 Other mechanical complication of other prosthetic devices, implants and grafts of genital tract**
Leakage of other prosthetic devices, implants and grafts of genital tract
Obstruction, mechanical of other prosthetic devices, implants and grafts of genital tract
Perforation of other prosthetic devices, implants and grafts of genital tract
Protrusion of other prosthetic devices, implants and grafts of genital tract

✓7ᵗʰ **T83.490 Other mechanical complication of** implanted penile prosthesis ♂
Other mechanical complication of penile prosthesis cylinder
Other mechanical complication of penile prosthesis pump
Other mechanical complication of penile prosthesis reservoir

✓7ᵗʰ **T83.491 Other mechanical complication of** implanted testicular prosthesis

✓7ᵗʰ **T83.498 Other mechanical complication of other** prosthetic devices, implants and grafts of genital tract

✓5ᵗʰ **T83.5 Infection and inflammatory reaction due to prosthetic device, implant and graft in** urinary system
Use additional code to identify infection

✓6ᵗʰ **T83.51 Infection and inflammatory reaction due to** urinary catheter
EXCLUDES 2 complications of stoma of urinary tract (N99.5-)

✓7ᵗʰ **T83.510 Infection and inflammatory reaction due to** cystostomy catheter

✓7ᵗʰ **T83.511 Infection and inflammatory reaction due to** indwelling urethral catheter

✓7ᵗʰ **T83.512 Infection and inflammatory reaction due to** nephrostomy catheter

✓7ᵗʰ **T83.518 Infection and inflammatory reaction due to other** urinary catheter
Infection and inflammatory reaction due to Hopkins catheter
Infection and inflammatory reaction due to ileostomy catheter
Infection and inflammatory reaction due to urostomy catheter

✓6ᵗʰ **T83.59 Infection and inflammatory reaction due to** prosthetic device, implant and graft in urinary system

✓7ᵗʰ **T83.590 Infection and inflammatory reaction due to implanted urinary** neurostimulation device
EXCLUDES 2 infection and inflammatory reaction due to electrode lead of sacral nerve neurostimulator (T85.732)
infection and inflammatory reaction due to pulse generator or receiver of sacral nerve neurostimulator (T85.734)

✓7ᵗʰ **T83.591 Infection and inflammatory reaction due to** implanted urinary sphincter

✓7ᵗʰ **T83.592 Infection and inflammatory reaction due to** indwelling ureteral stent

✓7ᵗʰ **T83.593 Infection and inflammatory reaction due to** other urinary stents
Infection and inflammatory reaction due to ileal conduit stents
Infection and inflammatory reaction due to nephroureteral stent

✓7ᵗʰ **T83.598 Infection and inflammatory reaction due to** other prosthetic device, implant and graft in urinary system

✓5ᵗʰ **T83.6 Infection and inflammatory reaction due to prosthetic device, implant and graft in** genital tract
Use additional code to identify infection

✓x7ᵗʰ **T83.61 Infection and inflammatory reaction due to implanted** penile prosthesis
Infection and inflammatory reaction due to penile prosthesis cylinder
Infection and inflammatory reaction due to penile prosthesis pump
Infection and inflammatory reaction due to penile prosthesis reservoir

✓x7ᵗʰ **T83.62 Infection and inflammatory reaction due to implanted** testicular prosthesis

✓x7ᵗʰ **T83.69 Infection and inflammatory reaction due to other prosthetic device, implant and graft in genital tract**

✓5ᵗʰ **T83.7 Complications due to** implanted mesh and other prosthetic materials

✓6ᵗʰ **T83.71 Erosion of implanted mesh and other prosthetic materials to surrounding organ or tissue**

✓7ᵗʰ **T83.711 Erosion of implanted vaginal mesh to surrounding organ or tissue** ♀
Erosion of implanted vaginal mesh into pelvic floor muscles

✓7ᵗʰ **T83.712 Erosion of implanted urethral mesh to surrounding organ or tissue**
Erosion of implanted female urethral sling
Erosion of implanted male urethral sling
Erosion of implanted urethral mesh into pelvic floor muscles

✓7ᵗʰ **T83.713 Erosion of implanted urethral bulking agent to surrounding organ or tissue**

✓7ᵗʰ **T83.714 Erosion of implanted ureteral bulking agent to surrounding organ or tissue**

✓7ᵗʰ **T83.718 Erosion of other implanted mesh to organ or tissue**

✓7ᵗʰ **T83.719 Erosion of other prosthetic materials to surrounding organ or tissue**

✓6ᵗʰ **T83.72 Exposure of implanted mesh and other prosthetic materials into surrounding organ or tissue**
Extrusion of implanted mesh

✓7ᵗʰ **T83.721 Exposure of implanted vaginal mesh into vagina** ♀
Exposure of implanted vaginal mesh through vaginal wall

✓7ᵗʰ **T83.722 Exposure of implanted urethral mesh into urethra**
Exposure of implanted female urethral sling
Exposure of implanted male urethral sling
Exposure of implanted urethral mesh through urethral wall

✓7ᵗʰ **T83.723 Exposure of implanted urethral bulking agent into urethra**

√7ᵗʰ **T83.724** **Exposure of implanted** ureteral bulking agent **into** ureter

√7ᵗʰ **T83.728** **Exposure of** other implanted mesh **into** organ or tissue

√7ᵗʰ **T83.729** **Exposure of** other prosthetic materials into organ or tissue

√x7ᵗʰ **T83.79** **Other specified complications due to other genitourinary prosthetic materials**

√5ᵗʰ **T83.8** **Other specified complications of** genitourinary prosthetic devices, implants and grafts

√x7ᵗʰ **T83.81** **Embolism** due to genitourinary prosthetic devices, implants and grafts

√x7ᵗʰ **T83.82** **Fibrosis** due to genitourinary prosthetic devices, implants and grafts

√x7ᵗʰ **T83.83** **Hemorrhage** due to genitourinary prosthetic devices, implants and grafts

√x7ᵗʰ **T83.84** **Pain** due to genitourinary prosthetic devices, implants and grafts

√x7ᵗʰ **T83.85** **Stenosis** due to genitourinary prosthetic devices, implants and grafts

√x7ᵗʰ **T83.86** **Thrombosis** due to genitourinary prosthetic devices, implants and grafts

√x7ᵗʰ **T83.89** **Other specified complication of genitourinary prosthetic devices, implants and grafts**

√x7ᵗʰ **T83.9** **Unspecified complication of genitourinary prosthetic device, implant and graft** ▽

√4ᵗʰ **T84** **Complications of internal orthopedic prosthetic devices, implants and grafts**

EXCLUDES 2 *failure and rejection of transplanted organs and tissues (T86.-)*
fracture of bone following insertion of orthopedic implant, joint prosthesis or bone plate (M96.6)

The appropriate 7th character is to be added to each code from category T84.
A   initial encounter
D   subsequent encounter
S   sequela

√5ᵗʰ **T84.0** **Mechanical complication of** internal joint prosthesis

√6ᵗʰ **T84.01** **Broken** internal joint prosthesis
Breakage (fracture) of prosthetic joint
Broken prosthetic joint implant
EXCLUDES 1 *periprosthetic joint implant fracture ►(M97-)◄*

√7ᵗʰ **T84.010** **Broken internal** right hip **prosthesis**

√7ᵗʰ **T84.011** **Broken internal** left hip **prosthesis**

√7ᵗʰ **T84.012** **Broken internal** right knee **prosthesis**

√7ᵗʰ **T84.013** **Broken internal** left knee **prosthesis**

√7ᵗʰ **T84.018** **Broken internal joint prosthesis, other site**
Use additional code to identify the joint (Z96.6-)

√7ᵗʰ **T84.019** **Broken internal joint prosthesis, unspecified site** ▽

√6ᵗʰ **T84.02** **Dislocation** of internal joint prosthesis
Instability of internal joint prosthesis
Subluxation of internal joint prosthesis

√7ᵗʰ **T84.020** **Dislocation of internal** right hip **prosthesis**

√7ᵗʰ **T84.021** **Dislocation of internal** left hip **prosthesis**

√7ᵗʰ **T84.022** **Instability** of internal right knee **prosthesis**

√7ᵗʰ **T84.023** **Instability** of internal left knee **prosthesis**

√7ᵗʰ **T84.028** **Dislocation of other internal joint prosthesis**
Use additional code to identify the joint (Z96.6-)

√7ᵗʰ **T84.029** **Dislocation of unspecified internal joint prosthesis** ▽

√6ᵗʰ **T84.03** **Mechanical loosening** of internal prosthetic joint
Aseptic loosening of internal prosthetic joint

√7ᵗʰ **T84.030** **Mechanical loosening of internal** right hip **prosthetic joint**

√7ᵗʰ **T84.031** **Mechanical loosening of internal** left hip **prosthetic joint**

√7ᵗʰ **T84.032** **Mechanical loosening of internal** right knee **prosthetic joint**

√7ᵗʰ **T84.033** **Mechanical loosening of internal** left knee **prosthetic joint**

√7ᵗʰ **T84.038** **Mechanical loosening of other internal prosthetic joint**
Use additional code to identify the joint (Z96.6-)

√7ᵗʰ **T84.039** **Mechanical loosening of unspecified internal prosthetic joint** ▽

√6ᵗʰ **T84.05** **Periprosthetic osteolysis** of internal prosthetic joint
Use additional code to identify major osseous defect, if applicable (M89.7-)

√7ᵗʰ **T84.050** **Periprosthetic osteolysis of internal prosthetic** right hip joint

√7ᵗʰ **T84.051** **Periprosthetic osteolysis of internal prosthetic** left hip joint

√7ᵗʰ **T84.052** **Periprosthetic osteolysis of internal prosthetic** right knee joint

√7ᵗʰ **T84.053** **Periprosthetic osteolysis of internal prosthetic** left knee joint

√7ᵗʰ **T84.058** **Periprosthetic osteolysis of other internal prosthetic joint**
Use additional code to identify the joint (Z96.6-)

√7ᵗʰ **T84.059** **Periprosthetic osteolysis of unspecified internal prosthetic joint** ▽

√6ᵗʰ **T84.06** **Wear of articular bearing surface** of internal prosthetic joint

√7ᵗʰ **T84.060** **Wear of articular bearing surface of internal prosthetic** right hip joint

√7ᵗʰ **T84.061** **Wear of articular bearing surface of internal prosthetic** left hip joint

√7ᵗʰ **T84.062** **Wear of articular bearing surface of internal prosthetic** right knee joint

√7ᵗʰ **T84.063** **Wear of articular bearing surface of internal prosthetic** left knee joint

√7ᵗʰ **T84.068** **Wear of articular bearing surface of other internal prosthetic joint**
Use additional code to identify the joint (Z96.6-)

√7ᵗʰ **T84.069** **Wear of articular bearing surface of unspecified internal prosthetic joint** ▽

√6ᵗʰ **T84.09** **Other mechanical complication of internal joint prosthesis**
Prosthetic joint implant failure NOS

√7ᵗʰ **T84.090** **Other mechanical complication of internal** right hip **prosthesis**

√7ᵗʰ **T84.091** **Other mechanical complication of internal** left hip **prosthesis**

√7ᵗʰ **T84.092** **Other mechanical complication of internal** right knee **prosthesis**

√7ᵗʰ **T84.093** **Other mechanical complication of internal** left knee **prosthesis**

√7ᵗʰ **T84.098** **Other mechanical complication of other internal joint prosthesis**
Use additional code to identify the joint (Z96.6-)

√7ᵗʰ **T84.099** **Other mechanical complication of unspecified internal joint prosthesis** ▽

√5ᵗʰ **T84.1** **Mechanical complication of** internal fixation device **of bones of** limb

EXCLUDES 2 *mechanical complication of internal fixation device of bones of feet (T84.2-)*
mechanical complication of internal fixation device of bones of fingers (T84.2-)
mechanical complication of internal fixation device of bones of hands (T84.2-)
mechanical complication of internal fixation device of bones of toes (T84.2-)

√6ᵗʰ **T84.11** **Breakdown (mechanical)** of internal fixation device of bones of limb

√7ᵗʰ **T84.110** **Breakdown (mechanical) of internal fixation device of** right humerus

√7ᵗʰ **T84.111** **Breakdown (mechanical) of internal fixation device of** left humerus

√7ᵗʰ **T84.112** **Breakdown (mechanical) of internal fixation device of bone of** right forearm

√7ᵗʰ **T84.113** **Breakdown (mechanical) of internal fixation device of bone of** left forearm

---

☑ Additional Character Req   √x7ᵗʰ Placeholder Alert   Case-Mix Diagnosis   Manifestation   ▽ Unspecified Dx   **EXCLUDES 1** Not coded here   **EXCLUDES 2** Not included here

✓7ᵗʰ **T84.114** **Breakdown (mechanical) of internal fixation device of** right femur

✓7ᵗʰ **T84.115** **Breakdown (mechanical) of internal fixation device of** left femur

✓7ᵗʰ **T84.116** **Breakdown (mechanical) of internal fixation device of bone of** right lower leg

✓7ᵗʰ **T84.117** **Breakdown (mechanical) of internal fixation device of bone of** left lower leg

✓7ᵗʰ **T84.119** **Breakdown (mechanical) of internal fixation device of unspecified bone of limb** ▽

✓6ᵗʰ **T84.12** **Displacement of internal fixation device of bones of limb**
Malposition of internal fixation device of bones of limb

✓7ᵗʰ **T84.120** **Displacement of internal fixation device of** right humerus

✓7ᵗʰ **T84.121** **Displacement of internal fixation device of** left humerus

✓7ᵗʰ **T84.122** **Displacement of internal fixation device of bone of** right forearm

✓7ᵗʰ **T84.123** **Displacement of internal fixation device of bone of** left forearm

✓7ᵗʰ **T84.124** **Displacement of internal fixation device of** right femur

✓7ᵗʰ **T84.125** **Displacement of internal fixation device of** left femur

✓7ᵗʰ **T84.126** **Displacement of internal fixation device of bone of** right lower leg

✓7ᵗʰ **T84.127** **Displacement of internal fixation device of bone of** left lower leg

✓7ᵗʰ **T84.129** **Displacement of internal fixation device of unspecified bone of limb** ▽

✓6ᵗʰ **T84.19** **Other mechanical complication of internal fixation device of bones of limb**
Obstruction (mechanical) of internal fixation device of bones of limb
Perforation of internal fixation device of bones of limb
Protrusion of internal fixation device of bones of limb

✓7ᵗʰ **T84.190** **Other mechanical complication of internal fixation device of** right humerus

✓7ᵗʰ **T84.191** **Other mechanical complication of internal fixation device of** left humerus

✓7ᵗʰ **T84.192** **Other mechanical complication of internal fixation device of bone of** right forearm

✓7ᵗʰ **T84.193** **Other mechanical complication of internal fixation device of bone of** left forearm

✓7ᵗʰ **T84.194** **Other mechanical complication of internal fixation device of** right femur

✓7ᵗʰ **T84.195** **Other mechanical complication of internal fixation device of** left femur

✓7ᵗʰ **T84.196** **Other mechanical complication of internal fixation device of bone of** right lower leg

✓7ᵗʰ **T84.197** **Other mechanical complication of internal fixation device of bone of** left lower leg

✓7ᵗʰ **T84.199** **Other mechanical complication of internal fixation device of unspecified bone of limb** ▽

✓5ᵗʰ **T84.2** **Mechanical complication of** internal fixation device **of** other bones

✓6ᵗʰ **T84.21** **Breakdown (mechanical) of internal fixation device of other bones**

✓7ᵗʰ **T84.210** **Breakdown (mechanical) of internal fixation device of bones of** hand and fingers

✓7ᵗʰ **T84.213** **Breakdown (mechanical) of internal fixation device of bones of** foot and toes

✓7ᵗʰ **T84.216** **Breakdown (mechanical) of internal fixation device of** vertebrae

✓7ᵗʰ **T84.218** **Breakdown (mechanical) of internal fixation device of other bones**

✓6ᵗʰ **T84.22** **Displacement of internal fixation device of other bones**
Malposition of internal fixation device of other bones

✓7ᵗʰ **T84.220** **Displacement of internal fixation device of bones of** hand and fingers

✓7ᵗʰ **T84.223** **Displacement of internal fixation device of bones of** foot and toes

✓7ᵗʰ **T84.226** **Displacement of internal fixation device of** vertebrae

✓7ᵗʰ **T84.228** **Displacement of internal fixation device of other bones**

✓6ᵗʰ **T84.29** **Other** mechanical complication of internal fixation device of other bones
Obstruction (mechanical) of internal fixation device of other bones
Perforation of internal fixation device of other bones
Protrusion of internal fixation device of other bones

✓7ᵗʰ **T84.290** **Other mechanical complication of internal fixation device of bones of** hand and fingers

✓7ᵗʰ **T84.293** **Other mechanical complication of internal fixation device of bones of** foot and toes

✓7ᵗʰ **T84.296** **Other mechanical complication of internal fixation device of** vertebrae

✓7ᵗʰ **T84.298** **Other mechanical complication of internal fixation device of other bones**

✓5ᵗʰ **T84.3** **Mechanical complication of** other bone devices, implants and grafts
EXCLUDES 2   other complications of bone graft (T86.83-)

✓6ᵗʰ **T84.31** **Breakdown (mechanical) of other bone devices, implants and grafts**

✓7ᵗʰ **T84.310** **Breakdown (mechanical) of** electronic bone stimulator

✓7ᵗʰ **T84.318** **Breakdown (mechanical) of other bone devices, implants and grafts**

✓6ᵗʰ **T84.32** **Displacement of other bone devices, implants and grafts**
Malposition of other bone devices, implants and grafts

✓7ᵗʰ **T84.320** **Displacement of** electronic bone stimulator

✓7ᵗʰ **T84.328** **Displacement of other bone devices, implants and grafts**
AHA: 2014, 4Q, 28

✓6ᵗʰ **T84.39** **Other** mechanical complication of other bone devices, implants and grafts
Obstruction (mechanical) of other bone devices, implants and grafts
Perforation of other bone devices, implants and grafts
Protrusion of other bone devices, implants and grafts

✓7ᵗʰ **T84.390** **Other mechanical complication of** electronic bone stimulator

✓7ᵗʰ **T84.398** **Other mechanical complication of other bone devices, implants and grafts**

✓5ᵗʰ **T84.4** **Mechanical complication of** other internal orthopedic devices, implants and grafts

✓6ᵗʰ **T84.41** **Breakdown (mechanical) of other internal orthopedic devices, implants and grafts**

✓7ᵗʰ **T84.410** **Breakdown (mechanical) of** muscle and tendon graft

✓7ᵗʰ **T84.418** **Breakdown (mechanical) of other internal orthopedic devices, implants and grafts**

✓6ᵗʰ **T84.42** **Displacement of other internal orthopedic devices, implants and grafts**
Malposition of other internal orthopedic devices, implants and grafts

✓7ᵗʰ **T84.420** **Displacement of** muscle and tendon graft

✓7ᵗʰ **T84.428** **Displacement of other internal orthopedic devices, implants and grafts**

✓6ᵗʰ **T84.49** **Other** mechanical complication of other internal orthopedic devices, implants and grafts
Mechanical complication of other internal orthopedic devices, implants and grafts NOS
Obstruction (mechanical) of other internal orthopedic devices, implants and grafts
Perforation of other internal orthopedic devices, implants and grafts
Protrusion of other internal orthopedic devices, implants and grafts

✓7ᵗʰ **T84.490** **Other mechanical complication of** muscle and tendon graft

✓7ᵗʰ **T84.498** **Other mechanical complication of other internal orthopedic devices, implants and grafts**

Ⓝ Newborn: 0   ⓅPediatric: 0-17   Ⓜ Maternity: 12-55   Ⓐ Adult: 15-124   **NRS** Nonroutine supply Dx   **NCDx** Noncancer Dx   **PDx** Primary Dx   ▶◀ Revised Text   ● New Code   ▲ Revised Title

1106   ICD-10-CM 2018

√5ʰ T84.5 Infection and inflammatory reaction due to internal joint prosthesis
Use additional code to identify infection
AHA: 2015, 1Q, 16

　√x7ʰ T84.5Ø Infection and inflammatory reaction due to unspecified internal joint prosthesis ▽

　√x7ʰ T84.51 Infection and inflammatory reaction due to internal right hip **prosthesis**

　√x7ʰ T84.52 Infection and inflammatory reaction due to internal left hip **prosthesis**

　√x7ʰ T84.53 Infection and inflammatory reaction due to internal right knee **prosthesis**

　√x7ʰ T84.54 Infection and inflammatory reaction due to internal left knee **prosthesis**

　√x7ʰ T84.59 Infection and inflammatory reaction due to other internal joint prosthesis

√5ʰ T84.6 Infection and inflammatory reaction due to internal fixation device
Use additional code to identify infection

　√x7ʰ T84.6Ø Infection and inflammatory reaction due to internal fixation device of unspecified site ▽

　√6ʰ T84.61 Infection and inflammatory reaction due to internal fixation device of arm

　　√7ʰ T84.61Ø Infection and inflammatory reaction due to internal fixation device of right humerus

　　√7ʰ T84.611 Infection and inflammatory reaction due to internal fixation device of left humerus

　　√7ʰ T84.612 Infection and inflammatory reaction due to internal fixation device of right radius

　　√7ʰ T84.613 Infection and inflammatory reaction due to internal fixation device of left radius

　　√7ʰ T84.614 Infection and inflammatory reaction due to internal fixation device of right ulna

　　√7ʰ T84.615 Infection and inflammatory reaction due to internal fixation device of left ulna

　　√7ʰ T84.619 Infection and inflammatory reaction due to internal fixation device of unspecified bone **of arm** ▽

　√6ʰ T84.62 Infection and inflammatory reaction due to internal fixation device of leg

　　√7ʰ T84.62Ø Infection and inflammatory reaction due to internal fixation device of right femur

　　√7ʰ T84.621 Infection and inflammatory reaction due to internal fixation device of left femur

　　√7ʰ T84.622 Infection and inflammatory reaction due to internal fixation device of right tibia

　　√7ʰ T84.623 Infection and inflammatory reaction due to internal fixation device of left tibia

　　√7ʰ T84.624 Infection and inflammatory reaction due to internal fixation device of right fibula

　　√7ʰ T84.625 Infection and inflammatory reaction due to internal fixation device of left fibula

　　√7ʰ T84.629 Infection and inflammatory reaction due to internal fixation device of unspecified bone **of leg** ▽

　√x7ʰ T84.63 Infection and inflammatory reaction due to internal fixation device of spine

　√x7ʰ T84.69 Infection and inflammatory reaction due to internal fixation device of other site

√x7ʰ T84.7 Infection and inflammatory reaction due to other internal orthopedic prosthetic devices, implants and grafts
Use additional code to identify infection

√5ʰ T84.8 Other specified complications of internal orthopedic prosthetic devices, implants and grafts

　√x7ʰ T84.81 Embolism **due to internal orthopedic prosthetic devices, implants and grafts**

　√x7ʰ T84.82 Fibrosis **due to internal orthopedic prosthetic devices, implants and grafts**

　√x7ʰ T84.83 Hemorrhage **due to internal orthopedic prosthetic devices, implants and grafts**

√x7ʰ T84.84 Pain **due to internal orthopedic prosthetic devices, implants and grafts**

√x7ʰ T84.85 Stenosis **due to internal orthopedic prosthetic devices, implants and grafts**

√x7ʰ T84.86 Thrombosis **due to internal orthopedic prosthetic devices, implants and grafts**

√x7ʰ T84.89 Other specified complication of internal orthopedic prosthetic devices, implants and grafts

√x7ʰ T84.9 Unspecified complication of internal orthopedic prosthetic device, implant and graft ▽

√4ʰ T85 Complications of other internal prosthetic devices, implants and grafts
EXCLUDES 2　*failure and rejection of transplanted organs and tissue (T86.-)*

　The appropriate 7th character is to be added to each code from category T85.
　A　　initial encounter
　D　　subsequent encounter
　S　　sequela

√5ʰ T85.Ø Mechanical complication of ventricular intracranial (communicating) shunt

　√x7ʰ T85.Ø1 Breakdown (mechanical) of ventricular intracranial (communicating) shunt

　√x7ʰ T85.Ø2 Displacement **of ventricular intracranial (communicating) shunt**
　　Malposition of ventricular intracranial (communicating) shunt

　√x7ʰ T85.Ø3 Leakage **of ventricular intracranial (communicating) shunt**

　√x7ʰ T85.Ø9 Other mechanical complication of ventricular intracranial (communicating) shunt
　　Obstruction (mechanical) of ventricular intracranial (communicating) shunt
　　Perforation of ventricular intracranial (communicating) shunt
　　Protrusion of ventricular intracranial (communicating) shunt

√5ʰ T85.1 Mechanical complication of implanted electronic stimulator **of** nervous system

　√6ʰ T85.11 Breakdown (mechanical) of implanted electronic stimulator of nervous system

　　√7ʰ T85.11Ø Breakdown (mechanical) of implanted electronic neurostimulator of brain electrode (lead)

　　√7ʰ T85.111 Breakdown (mechanical) of implanted electronic neurostimulator of peripheral nerve electrode (lead)
　　　Breakdown of electrode (lead) for cranial nerve neurostimulators
　　　Breakdown of electrode (lead) for gastric neurostimulator
　　　Breakdown of electrode (lead) for sacral nerve neurostimulator
　　　Breakdown of electrode (lead) for vagal nerve neurostimulators

　　√7ʰ T85.112 Breakdown (mechanical) of implanted electronic neurostimulator of spinal cord electrode (lead)

　　√7ʰ T85.113 Breakdown (mechanical) of implanted electronic neurostimulator, generator
　　　Breakdown (mechanical) of implanted electronic neurostimuator generator, brain, peripheral, gastric, spinal
　　　Breakdown (mechanical) of implanted electronic sacral neurostimulator, pulse generator or receiver

　　√7ʰ T85.118 Breakdown (mechanical) of other implanted electronic stimulator of nervous system

　√6ʰ T85.12 Displacement **of implanted electronic stimulator of nervous system**
　　Malposition of implanted electronic stimulator of nervous system

　　√7ʰ T85.12Ø Displacement of implanted electronic neurostimulator of brain electrode (lead)

√7ᵗʰ **T85.121　Displacement of implanted electronic neurostimulator** of peripheral nerve electrode (lead)
Displacement of electrode (lead) for cranial nerve neurostimulators
Displacement of electrode (lead) for gastric neurostimulator
Displacement of electrode (lead) for sacral nerve neurostimulator
Displacement of electrode (lead) for vagal nerve neurostimulators

√7ᵗʰ **T85.122　Displacement of implanted electronic neurostimulator** of spinal cord electrode (lead)

√7ᵗʰ **T85.123　Displacement of implanted electronic neurostimulator,** generator
Displacement of implanted electronic neurostimulator generator, brain, peripheral, gastric, spinal
Displacement of implanted electronic sacral neurostimulator, pulse generator or receiver

√7ᵗʰ **T85.128　Displacement of other implanted electronic stimulator of** nervous system

√6ᵗʰ **T85.19　Other mechanical complication of implanted electronic stimulator of nervous system**
Leakage of implanted electronic stimulator of nervous system
Obstruction (mechanical) of implanted electronic stimulator of nervous system
Perforation of implanted electronic stimulator of nervous system
Protrusion of implanted electronic stimulator of nervous system

√7ᵗʰ **T85.190　Other mechanical complication of implanted electronic neurostimulator** of brain electrode (lead)

√7ᵗʰ **T85.191　Other mechanical complication of implanted electronic neurostimulator** of peripheral nerve electrode (lead)
Other mechanical complication of electrode (lead) for cranial nerve neurostimulators
Other mechanical complication of electrode (lead) for gastric neurostimulator
Other mechanical complication of electrode (lead) for sacral nerve neurostimulator
Other mechanical complication of electrode (lead) for vagal nerve neurostimulators

√7ᵗʰ **T85.192　Other mechanical complication of implanted electronic neurostimulator** of spinal cord electrode (lead)

√7ᵗʰ **T85.193　Other mechanical complication of implanted electronic neurostimulator,** generator
Other mechanical complication of implanted electronic neurostimulator generator, brain, peripheral, gastric, spinal
Other mechanical complication of implanted electronic sacral neurostimulator, pulse generator or receiver

√7ᵗʰ **T85.199　Other mechanical complication of other implanted electronic stimulator of nervous system**

√5ᵗʰ **T85.2　Mechanical complication of** intraocular lens

√×7ᵗʰ **T85.21　Breakdown (mechanical) of intraocular lens**

√×7ᵗʰ **T85.22　Displacement of intraocular lens**
Malposition of intraocular lens

√×7ᵗʰ **T85.29　Other mechanical complication of intraocular lens**
Obstruction (mechanical) of intraocular lens
Perforation of intraocular lens
Protrusion of intraocular lens

√5ᵗʰ **T85.3　Mechanical complication of** other ocular prosthetic devices, implants and grafts
EXCLUDES 2　other complications of corneal graft (T86.84-)

√6ᵗʰ **T85.31　Breakdown (mechanical) of other ocular prosthetic devices, implants and grafts**

√7ᵗʰ **T85.310　Breakdown (mechanical) of prosthetic orbit of** right eye

√7ᵗʰ **T85.311　Breakdown (mechanical) of prosthetic orbit of** left eye

√7ᵗʰ **T85.318　Breakdown (mechanical) of other ocular prosthetic devices, implants and grafts**

√6ᵗʰ **T85.32　Displacement of other ocular prosthetic devices, implants and grafts**
Malposition of other ocular prosthetic devices, implants and grafts

√7ᵗʰ **T85.320　Displacement of prosthetic orbit of** right eye

√7ᵗʰ **T85.321　Displacement of prosthetic orbit of** left eye

√7ᵗʰ **T85.328　Displacement of other ocular prosthetic devices, implants and grafts**

√6ᵗʰ **T85.39　Other mechanical complication of other ocular prosthetic devices, implants and grafts**
Obstruction (mechanical) of other ocular prosthetic devices, implants and grafts
Perforation of other ocular prosthetic devices, implants and grafts
Protrusion of other ocular prosthetic devices, implants and grafts

√7ᵗʰ **T85.390　Other mechanical complication of prosthetic orbit of** right eye

√7ᵗʰ **T85.391　Other mechanical complication of prosthetic orbit of** left eye

√7ᵗʰ **T85.398　Other mechanical complication of other ocular prosthetic devices, implants and grafts**

√5ᵗʰ **T85.4　Mechanical complication of** breast prosthesis and implant

√×7ᵗʰ **T85.41　Breakdown (mechanical) of breast prosthesis and implant**

√×7ᵗʰ **T85.42　Displacement of breast prosthesis and implant**
Malposition of breast prosthesis and implant

√×7ᵗʰ **T85.43　Leakage of breast prosthesis and implant**

√×7ᵗʰ **T85.44　Capsular contracture of breast implant**

√×7ᵗʰ **T85.49　Other mechanical complication of breast prosthesis and implant**
Obstruction (mechanical) of breast prosthesis and implant
Perforation of breast prosthesis and implant
Protrusion of breast prosthesis and implant

√5ᵗʰ **T85.5　Mechanical complication of** gastrointestinal prosthetic devices, implants and grafts

√6ᵗʰ **T85.51　Breakdown (mechanical) of gastrointestinal prosthetic devices, implants and grafts**

√7ᵗʰ **T85.510　Breakdown (mechanical) of** bile duct prosthesis

√7ᵗʰ **T85.511　Breakdown (mechanical) of** esophageal anti-reflux device

√7ᵗʰ **T85.518　Breakdown (mechanical) of other gastrointestinal prosthetic devices, implants and grafts**

√6ᵗʰ **T85.52　Displacement of gastrointestinal prosthetic devices, implants and grafts**
Malposition of gastrointestinal prosthetic devices, implants and grafts

√7ᵗʰ **T85.520　Displacement of** bile duct prosthesis

√7ᵗʰ **T85.521　Displacement of** esophageal anti-reflux device

√7ᵗʰ **T85.528　Displacement of other gastrointestinal prosthetic devices, implants and grafts**

N Newborn: 0　　P Pediatric: 0-17　　M Maternity: 12-55　　A Adult: 15-124　　NRS Nonroutine supply Dx　　NC Dx Noncancer Dx　　PD Dx Primary Dx　　▶◀ Revised Text　　● New Code　　▲ Revised Title

1108　　　　　　　　　　　　　　　　　　　　　　　　　　　　　　　　　　　ICD-10-CM 2018

✓6ᵗʰ **T85.59** Other mechanical complication of gastrointestinal prosthetic devices, implants and grafts

Obstruction, mechanical of gastrointestinal prosthetic devices, implants and grafts

Perforation of gastrointestinal prosthetic devices, implants and grafts

Protrusion of gastrointestinal prosthetic devices, implants and grafts

    ✓7ᵗʰ **T85.590** Other mechanical complication of bile duct prosthesis

    ✓7ᵗʰ **T85.591** Other mechanical complication of esophageal anti-reflux device

    ✓7ᵗʰ **T85.598** Other mechanical complication of other gastrointestinal prosthetic devices, implants and grafts

✓5ᵗʰ **T85.6** Mechanical complication of other specified internal and external prosthetic devices, implants and grafts

    ✓6ᵗʰ **T85.61** Breakdown (mechanical) of other specified internal prosthetic devices, implants and grafts

      ✓7ᵗʰ **T85.610** Breakdown (mechanical) of cranial or spinal infusion catheter

Breakdown (mechanical) of epidural infusion catheter

Breakdown (mechanical) of intrathecal infusion catheter

Breakdown (mechanical) of subarachnoid infusion catheter

Breakdown (mechanical) of subdural infusion catheter

      ✓7ᵗʰ **T85.611** Breakdown (mechanical) of intraperitoneal dialysis catheter

EXCLUDES 1   *mechanical complication of vascular dialysis catheter (T82.4-)*

      ✓7ᵗʰ **T85.612** Breakdown (mechanical) of permanent sutures

EXCLUDES 1   *mechanical complication of permanent (wire) suture used in bone repair (T84.1-T84.2)*

      ✓7ᵗʰ **T85.613** Breakdown (mechanical) of artificial skin graft and decellularized allodermis

Failure of artificial skin graft and decellularized allodermis

Non-adherence of artificial skin graft and decellularized allodermis

Poor incorporation of artificial skin graft and decellularized allodermis

Shearing of artificial skin graft and decellularized allodermis

      ✓7ᵗʰ **T85.614** Breakdown (mechanical) of insulin pump

      ✓7ᵗʰ **T85.615** Breakdown (mechanical) of other nervous system device, implant or graft

Breakdown (mechanical) of intrathecal infusion pump

      ✓7ᵗʰ **T85.618** Breakdown (mechanical) of other specified internal prosthetic devices, implants and grafts

    ✓6ᵗʰ **T85.62** Displacement of other specified internal prosthetic devices, implants and grafts

Malposition of other specified internal prosthetic devices, implants and grafts

      ✓7ᵗʰ **T85.620** Displacement of cranial or spinal infusion catheter

Displacement of epidural infusion catheter

Displacement of intrathecal infusion catheter

Displacement of subarachnoid infusion catheter

Displacement of subdural infusion catheterx

      ✓7ᵗʰ **T85.621** Displacement of intraperitoneal dialysis catheter

EXCLUDES 1   *mechanical complication of vascular dialysis catheter (T82.4-)*

      ✓7ᵗʰ **T85.622** Displacement of permanent sutures

EXCLUDES 1   *mechanical complication of permanent (wire) suture used in bone repair (T84.1-T84.2)*

      ✓7ᵗʰ **T85.623** Displacement of artificial skin graft and decellularized allodermis

Dislodgement of artificial skin graft and decellularized allodermis

~~Displacement of artificial skin graft and decellularized allodermis~~

      ✓7ᵗʰ **T85.624** Displacement of insulin pump

      ✓7ᵗʰ **T85.625** Displacement of other nervous system device, implant or graft

Displacement of intrathecal infusion pump

      ✓7ᵗʰ **T85.628** Displacement of other specified internal prosthetic devices, implants and grafts

    ✓6ᵗʰ **T85.63** Leakage of other specified internal prosthetic devices, implants and grafts

      ✓7ᵗʰ **T85.630** Leakage of cranial or spinal infusion catheter

Leakage of epidural infusion catheter

Leakage of intrathecal infusion catheter infusion catheter

Leakage of subdural infusion catheter

Leakage of subarachnoid infusion catheter

      ✓7ᵗʰ **T85.631** Leakage of intraperitoneal dialysis catheter

EXCLUDES 1   *mechanical complication of vascular dialysis catheter (T82.4)*

      ✓7ᵗʰ **T85.633** Leakage of insulin pump

      ✓7ᵗʰ **T85.635** Leakage of other nervous system device, implant or graft

Leakage of intrathecal infusion pump

      ✓7ᵗʰ **T85.638** Leakage of other specified internal prosthetic devices, implants and grafts

    ✓6ᵗʰ **T85.69** Other mechanical complication of other specified internal prosthetic devices, implants and grafts

Obstruction, mechanical of other specified internal prosthetic devices, implants and grafts

Perforation of other specified internal prosthetic devices, implants and grafts

Protrusion of other specified internal prosthetic devices, implants and grafts

      ✓7ᵗʰ **T85.690** Other mechanical complication of cranial or spinal infusion catheter

Other mechanical complication of epidural infusion catheter

Other mechanical complication of intrathecal infusion catheter

Other mechanical complication of subarachnoid infusion catheter

Other mechanical complication of subdural infusion catheter

      ✓7ᵗʰ **T85.691** Other mechanical complication of intraperitoneal dialysis catheter

EXCLUDES 1   *mechanical complication of vascular dialysis catheter (T82.4)*

      ✓7ᵗʰ **T85.692** Other mechanical complication of permanent sutures

EXCLUDES 1   *mechanical complication of permanent (wire) suture used in bone repair (T84.1-T84.2)*

      ✓7ᵗʰ **T85.693** Other mechanical complication of artificial skin graft and decellularized allodermis

      ✓7ᵗʰ **T85.694** Other mechanical complication of insulin pump

      ✓7ᵗʰ **T85.695** Other mechanical complication of other nervous system device, implant or graft

Other mechanical complication of intrathecal infusion pump

      ✓7ᵗʰ **T85.698** Other mechanical complication of other specified internal prosthetic devices, implants and grafts

Mechanical complication of nonabsorbable surgical material NOS

✓5ᵗʰ **T85.7** Infection and inflammatory reaction due to other internal prosthetic devices, implants and grafts

Use additional code to identify infection

    ✓x7ᵗʰ **T85.71** Infection and inflammatory reaction due to peritoneal dialysis catheter

---

✓ Additional Character Req   ✓x7ᵗʰ Placeholder Alert   Case-Mix Diagnosis   Manifestation   ▽ Unspecified Dx   *EXCLUDES 1* Not coded here   *EXCLUDES 2* Not included here

ICD-10-CM 2018   **1109**

√7th **T85.72** Infection and inflammatory reaction due to insulin pump

√6th **T85.73** Infection and inflammatory reaction due to nervous system devices, implants and graft

  √7th **T85.730** Infection and inflammatory reaction due to ventricular intracranial (communicating) shunt

  √7th **T85.731** Infection and inflammatory reaction due to implanted electronic neurostimulator of brain, electrode (lead)

  √7th **T85.732** Infection and inflammatory reaction due to implanted electronic neurostimulator of peripheral nerve, electrode (lead)
Infection and inflammatory reaction due to electrode (lead) for cranial nerve neurostimulators
Infection and inflammatory reaction due to electrode (lead) for gastric neurostimulator
Infection and inflammatory reaction due to electrode (lead) for sacral nerve neurostimulator
Infection and inflammatory reaction due to electrode (lead) for vagal nerve neurostimulators

  √7th **T85.733** Infection and inflammatory reaction due to implanted electronic neurostimulator of spinal cord, electrode (lead)

  √7th **T85.734** Infection and inflammatory reaction due to implanted electronic neurostimulator, generator
Generator pocket infection

  √7th **T85.735** Infection and inflammatory reaction due to cranial or spinal infusion catheter
Infection and inflammatory reaction due to epidural catheter
Infection and inflammatory reaction due to intrathecal infusion catheter
Infection and inflammatory reaction due to subarachnoid catheter
Infection and inflammatory reaction due to subdural catheter

  √7th **T85.738** Infection and inflammatory reaction due to other nervous system device, implant or graft
Infection and inflammatory reaction due to intrathecal infusion pump

√x7th **T85.79** Infection and inflammatory reaction due to other internal prosthetic devices, implants and grafts

√5th **T85.8** Other specified complications of internal prosthetic devices, implants and grafts, not elsewhere classified

√6th **T85.81** Embolism due to internal prosthetic devices, implants and grafts, not elsewhere classified

  √7th **T85.810** Embolism due to nervous system prosthetic devices, implants and grafts

  √7th **T85.818** Embolism due to other internal prosthetic devices, implants and grafts

√6th **T85.82** Fibrosis due to internal prosthetic devices, implants and grafts, not elsewhere classified

  √7th **T85.820** Fibrosis due to nervous system prosthetic devices, implants and grafts

  √7th **T85.828** Fibrosis due to other internal prosthetic devices, implants and grafts

√6th **T85.83** Hemorrhage due to internal prosthetic devices, implants and grafts, not elsewhere classified

  √7th **T85.830** Hemorrhage due to nervous system prosthetic devices, implants and grafts

  √7th **T85.838** Hemorrhage due to other internal prosthetic devices, implants and grafts

√6th **T85.84** Pain due to internal prosthetic devices, implants and grafts, not elsewhere classified

  √7th **T85.840** Pain due to nervous system prosthetic devices, implants and grafts

  √7th **T85.848** Pain due to other internal prosthetic devices, implants and grafts

√6th **T85.85** Stenosis due to internal prosthetic devices, implants and grafts, not elsewhere classified

  √7th **T85.850** Stenosis due to nervous system prosthetic devices, implants and grafts

  √7th **T85.858** Stenosis due to other internal prosthetic devices, implants and grafts

√6th **T85.86** Thrombosis due to internal prosthetic devices, implants and grafts, not elsewhere classified

  √7th **T85.860** Thrombosis due to nervous system prosthetic devices, implants and grafts

  √7th **T85.868** Thrombosis due to other internal prosthetic devices, implants and grafts

√6th **T85.89** Other specified complication of internal prosthetic devices, implants and grafts, not elsewhere classified
Erosion or breakdown of subcutaneous device pocket

  √7th **T85.890** Other specified complication of nervous system prosthetic devices, implants and grafts

  √7th **T85.898** Other specified complication of other internal prosthetic devices, implants and grafts

√x7th **T85.9** Unspecified complication of internal prosthetic device, implant and graft
Complication of internal prosthetic device, implant and graft NOS

√4th **T86** Complications of transplanted organs and tissue
Use additional code to identify other transplant complications, such as:
graft-versus-host disease (D89.81-)
malignancy associated with organ transplant (C80.2)
post-transplant lymphoproliferative disorders (PTLD) (D47.Z1)
TIP: A nonmalignancy associated complication in a transplanted organ should be directly indicated in provider documentation.

√5th **T86.0** Complications of bone marrow transplant
T86.00 Unspecified complication of bone marrow transplant
T86.01 Bone marrow transplant rejection
T86.02 Bone marrow transplant failure
T86.03 Bone marrow transplant infection
T86.09 Other complications of bone marrow transplant

√5th **T86.1** Complications of kidney transplant
T86.10 Unspecified complication of kidney transplant
T86.11 Kidney transplant rejection
T86.12 Kidney transplant failure
  AHA: 2013, 1Q, 24
T86.13 Kidney transplant infection
Use additional code to specify infection
T86.19 Other complication of kidney transplant

√5th **T86.2** Complications of heart transplant
EXCLUDES 1 complication of:
artificial heart device (T82.5)
heart-lung transplant (T86.3)
T86.20 Unspecified complication of heart transplant
T86.21 Heart transplant rejection
T86.22 Heart transplant failure
T86.23 Heart transplant infection
Use additional code to specify infection
√6th **T86.29** Other complications of heart transplant
T86.290 Cardiac allograft vasculopathy
EXCLUDES 1 atherosclerosis of coronary arteries (I25.75-, I25.76-, I25.81-)
T86.298 Other complications of heart transplant

√5th **T86.3** Complications of heart-lung transplant
T86.30 Unspecified complication of heart-lung transplant
T86.31 Heart-lung transplant rejection
T86.32 Heart-lung transplant failure
T86.33 Heart-lung transplant infection
Use additional code to specify infection
T86.39 Other complications of heart-lung transplant

√5th **T86.4** Complications of liver transplant
T86.40 Unspecified complication of liver transplant
T86.41 Liver transplant rejection
T86.42 Liver transplant failure
T86.43 Liver transplant infection
Use additional code to identify infection, such as:
cytomegalovirus (CMV) infection (B25.-)
T86.49 Other complications of liver transplant

T86.5   **Complications of** stem cell **transplant**
Complications from stem cells from peripheral blood
Complications from stem cells from umbilical cord

✓5ᵗʰ T86.8   **Complications of other transplanted organs and tissues**

✓6ᵗʰ T86.81   **Complications of** lung **transplant**
EXCLUDES 1 *complication of heart-lung transplant (T86.3-)*
T86.810   **Lung transplant** rejection
T86.811   **Lung transplant** failure
T86.812   **Lung transplant** infection
Use additional code to specify infection
T86.818   **Other complications of lung transplant**
T86.819   **Unspecified complication of lung**   ▽
transplant

✓6ᵗʰ T86.82   **Complications of** skin graft **(allograft) (autograft)**
EXCLUDES 2 *complication of artificial skin graft (T85.693)*
T86.820   **Skin graft (allograft)** rejection
T86.821   **Skin graft (allograft) (autograft)** failure
T86.822   **Skin graft (allograft) (autograft)** infection
Use additional code to specify infection
T86.828   **Other complications of skin graft**
(allograft) (autograft)
T86.829   **Unspecified complication of skin graft**   ▽
(allograft) (autograft)

✓6ᵗʰ T86.83   **Complications of** bone graft
EXCLUDES 2 *mechanical complications of bone graft (T84.3-)*
T86.830   **Bone graft** rejection
T86.831   **Bone graft** failure
T86.832   **Bone graft** infection
Use additional code to specify infection
T86.838   **Other complications of bone graft**
T86.839   **Unspecified complication of bone graft** ▽

✓6ᵗʰ T86.84   **Complications of** corneal **transplant**
EXCLUDES 2 *mechanical complications of corneal graft (T85.3-)*
T86.840   **Corneal transplant** rejection
T86.841   **Corneal transplant** failure
T86.842   **Corneal transplant** infection
Use additional code to specify infection
T86.848   **Other complications of corneal transplant**
T86.849   **Unspecified complication of corneal**   ▽
transplant

✓6ᵗʰ T86.85   **Complication of** intestine **transplant**
T86.850   **Intestine transplant** rejection
T86.851   **Intestine transplant** failure
T86.852   **Intestine transplant** infection
Use additional code to specify infection
T86.858   **Other complications of intestine**
transplant
T86.859   **Unspecified complication of intestine**   ▽
transplant

✓6ᵗʰ T86.89   **Complications of other transplanted tissue**
Transplant failure or rejection of pancreas
T86.890   **Other transplanted tissue** rejection
T86.891   **Other transplanted tissue** failure
T86.892   **Other transplanted tissue** infection
Use additional code to specify infection
T86.898   **Other complications of other transplanted**
tissue
T86.899   **Unspecified complication of other**   ▽
transplanted tissue

✓5ᵗʰ T86.9   **Complication of unspecified transplanted organ and tissue**
T86.90   **Unspecified complication of unspecified**   ▽
transplanted organ and tissue
T86.91   **Unspecified transplanted organ and tissue**   ▽
rejection
T86.92   **Unspecified transplanted organ and tissue**   ▽
failure
T86.93   **Unspecified transplanted organ and tissue**   ▽
infection
Use additional code to specify infection
T86.99   **Other complications of unspecified transplanted** ▽
organ and tissue

✓4ᵗʰ **T87   Complications peculiar to reattachment and amputation**

✓5ᵗʰ T87.0   **Complications of reattached (part of) upper extremity**
✓6ᵗʰ T87.0X   **Complications of reattached (part of)** upper
extremity
T87.0X1   **Complications of reattached (part of)** right
upper extremity
T87.0X2   **Complications of reattached (part of)** left
upper extremity
T87.0X9   **Complications of reattached (part of)**   ▽
unspecified upper extremity

✓5ᵗʰ T87.1   **Complications of reattached (part of) lower extremity**
✓6ᵗʰ T87.1X   **Complications of reattached (part of)** lower
extremity
T87.1X1   **Complications of reattached (part of)** right
lower extremity
T87.1X2   **Complications of reattached (part of)** left
lower extremity
T87.1X9   **Complications of reattached (part of)**   ▽
unspecified lower extremity

T87.2   **Complications of other reattached body part**

✓5ᵗʰ T87.3   **Neuroma of amputation stump**
DEF: Non-neoplastic tumor generated at the proximal end of
severed, partially transected, or injured nerve following
amputation.
T87.30   **Neuroma of amputation stump, unspecified**   ▽
extremity
T87.31   **Neuroma of amputation stump,** right upper
extremity
T87.32   **Neuroma of amputation stump,** left upper **extremity**
T87.33   **Neuroma of amputation stump,** right lower
extremity
T87.34   **Neuroma of amputation stump,** left lower **extremity**

✓5ᵗʰ T87.4   **Infection of amputation stump**
T87.40   **Infection of amputation stump, unspecified**   ▽
extremity
T87.41   **Infection of amputation stump,** right upper
extremity
T87.42   **Infection of amputation stump,** left upper **extremity**
T87.43   **Infection of amputation stump,** right lower
extremity
T87.44   **Infection of amputation stump,** left lower **extremity**

✓5ᵗʰ T87.5   **Necrosis of amputation stump**
T87.50   **Necrosis of amputation stump, unspecified**   ▽
extremity
T87.51   **Necrosis of amputation stump,** right upper
extremity
T87.52   **Necrosis of amputation stump,** left upper **extremity**
T87.53   **Necrosis of amputation stump,** right lower **extremity**
T87.54   **Necrosis of amputation stump,** left lower **extremity**

✓5ᵗʰ T87.8   **Other complications of amputation stump**
TIP: An ulcer (such as pressure ulcer, diabetic ulcer, or other) is
generally not considered a complication of the amputation stump.
Code the ulcer by site and etiology.
T87.81   **Dehiscence of amputation stump**
T87.89   **Other complications of amputation stump**
Amputation stump contracture
Amputation stump contracture of next proximal joint
Amputation stump flexion
Amputation stump edema
Amputation stump hematoma
EXCLUDES 2 *phantom limb syndrome (G54.6-G54.7)*

T87.9   **Unspecified complications of amputation stump** ▽

Chapter 19. Injury, Poisoning and Certain Other Consequences of External Causes

☑4ᵗʰ **T88** **Other complications of surgical and medical care, not elsewhere classified**

> EXCLUDES 2   complication following infusion, transfusion and therapeutic injection (T80.-)
> complication following procedure NEC (T81.-)
> complications of anesthesia in labor and delivery (O74.-)
> complications of anesthesia in pregnancy (O29.-)
> complications of anesthesia in puerperium (O89.-)
> complications of devices, implants and grafts (T82-T85)
> complications of obstetric surgery and procedure (O75.4)
> dermatitis due to drugs and medicaments (L23.3, L24.4, L25.1, L27.0-L27.1)
> poisoning and toxic effects of drugs and chemicals (T36-T65 with fifth or sixth character 1-4 or 6)
> specified complications classified elsewhere

> The appropriate 7th character is to be added to each code from category T88.
> A   initial encounter
> D   subsequent encounter
> S   sequela

☑x7ᵗʰ **T88.0** **Infection following immunization**
> Sepsis following immunization

☑x7ᵗʰ **T88.1** **Other complications following immunization, not elsewhere classified**
> Generalized vaccinia
> Rash following immunization
> EXCLUDES 1   vaccinia not from vaccine (B08.011)
> EXCLUDES 2   anaphylactic shock due to serum (T80.5-)
> other serum reactions (T80.6-)
> postimmunization arthropathy (M02.2)
> postimmunization encephalitis (G04.02)
> postimmunization fever (R50.83)

☑x7ᵗʰ **T88.2** **Shock due to anesthesia**
> Use additional code for adverse effect, if applicable, to identify drug (T41.- with fifth or sixth character 5)
> EXCLUDES 1   complications of anesthesia (in):
> labor and delivery (O74.-)
> postprocedural shock NOS (T81.1-)
> pregnancy (O29.-)
> puerperium (O89.-)

☑x7ᵗʰ **T88.3** **Malignant hyperthermia due to anesthesia**
> Use additional code for adverse effect, if applicable, to identify drug (T41.- with fifth or sixth character 5)

☑x7ᵗʰ **T88.4** **Failed or difficult intubation**

☑5ᵗʰ **T88.5** **Other complications of anesthesia**
> Use additional code for adverse effect, if applicable, to identify drug (T41.- with fifth or sixth character 5)

☑x7ᵗʰ **T88.51** **Hypothermia following anesthesia**

☑x7ᵗʰ **T88.52** **Failed moderate sedation during procedure**
> Failed conscious sedation during procedure
> EXCLUDES 2   personal history of failed moderate sedation (Z92.83)

☑x7ᵗʰ **T88.53** **Unintended awareness under general anesthesia during procedure**
> EXCLUDES 2   personal history of unintended awareness under general anesthesia (Z92.84)

☑x7ᵗʰ **T88.59** **Other complications of anesthesia**

☑x7ᵗʰ **T88.6** **Anaphylactic reaction due to adverse effect of correct drug or medicament properly administered**
> Anaphylactic shock due to adverse effect of correct drug or medicament properly administered
> Anaphylactoid reaction NOS
> Use additional code for adverse effect, if applicable, to identify drug (T36-T50 with fifth or sixth character 5)
> EXCLUDES 1   anaphylactic reaction due to serum (T80.5-)
> anaphylactic shock or reaction due to adverse food reaction (T78.0-)

☑x7ᵗʰ **T88.7** **Unspecified adverse effect of drug or medicament** ▽
> Drug hypersensitivity NOS
> Drug reaction NOS
> Use additional code for adverse effect, if applicable, to identify drug (T36-T50 with fifth or sixth character 5)
> EXCLUDES 1   specified adverse effects of drugs and medicaments (A00-R94 and T80-T88.6, T88.8)

☑x7ᵗʰ **T88.8** **Other specified complications of surgical and medical care, not elsewhere classified**
> Use additional code to identify the complication

☑x7ᵗʰ **T88.9** **Complication of surgical and medical care, unspecified** ▽

Ⓝ Newborn: 0   Ⓟ Pediatric: 0-17   Ⓜ Maternity: 12-55   Ⓐ Adult: 15-124   **NRS** Nonroutine supply Dx   **NC Dx** Noncancer Dx   **PDx** Primary Dx   ▶◀ Revised Text   ● New Code   ▲ Revised Title

1112   ICD-10-CM 2018

Chapter 20. External Causes of Morbidity (V00–Y99)

Chapter Specific Guidelines with Coding Examples

The chapter specific guidelines from the ICD-10-CM Official Guidelines for Coding and Reporting have been provided below. Along with these guidelines are coding examples, contained in the shaded boxes, that have been developed to help illustrate the coding and/or sequencing guidance found in these guidelines.

The external causes of morbidity codes should never be sequenced as the first-listed or principal diagnosis.

External cause codes are intended to provide data for injury research and evaluation of injury prevention strategies. These codes capture how the injury or health condition happened (cause), the intent (unintentional or accidental; or intentional, such as suicide or assault), the place where the event occurred, the activity of the patient at the time of the event, and the person's status (e.g., civilian, military).

There is no national requirement for mandatory ICD-10-CM external cause code reporting. Unless a provider is subject to a state-based external cause code reporting mandate or these codes are required by a particular payer, reporting of ICD-10-CM codes in Chapter 20, External Causes of Morbidity, is not required. In the absence of a mandatory reporting requirement, providers are encouraged to voluntarily report external cause codes, as they provide valuable data for injury research and evaluation of injury prevention strategies.

a. General external cause coding guidelines

1) Used with any code in the range of A00.0–T88.9, Z00–Z99

An external cause code may be used with any code in the range of A00.0–T88.9, Z00-Z99, classification that **represents** a health condition due to an external cause. Though they are most applicable to injuries, they are also valid for use with such things as infections or diseases due to an external source, and other health conditions, such as a heart attack that occurs during strenuous physical activity.

> Patient has bilateral sensorineural hearing loss due to history of exposure to loud noise over 100 dB for a period of greater than 10 years as a sound technician for a band.
>
> **H90.3**   **Sensorineural hearing loss, bilateral**
>
> **W42.9XXS**   **Exposure to other noise, sequela**
>
> *Explanation:* The hearing loss is due to noise exposure. An external cause code identifies the noise as the cause. The seventh character S is used in this case as the hearing loss is a residual effect of the exposure.

2) External cause code used for length of treatment

Assign the external cause code, with the appropriate 7th character (initial encounter, subsequent encounter or sequela) for each encounter for which the injury or condition is being treated.

Most categories in chapter 20 have a 7th character requirement for each applicable code. Most categories in this chapter have three 7th character values: A, initial encounter, D, subsequent encounter and S, sequela. While the patient may be seen by a new or different provider over the course of treatment for an injury or condition, assignment of the 7th character for external cause should match the 7th character of the code assigned for the associated injury or condition for the encounter.

3) Use the full range of external cause codes

Use the full range of external cause codes to completely describe the cause, the intent, the place of occurrence, and if applicable, the activity of the patient at the time of the event, and the patient's status, for all injuries, and other health conditions due to an external cause.

4) Assign as many external cause codes as necessary

Assign as many external cause codes as necessary to fully explain each cause. If only one external code can be recorded, assign the code most related to the principal diagnosis.

5) The selection of the appropriate external cause code

The selection of the appropriate external cause code is guided by the Alphabetic Index of External Causes and by Inclusion and Exclusion notes in the Tabular List.

6) External cause code can never be a principal diagnosis

An external cause code can never be a principal (first-listed) diagnosis.

7) Combination external cause codes

Certain of the external cause codes are combination codes that identify sequential events that result in an injury, such as a fall which results in striking against an object. The injury may be due to either event or both.

The combination external cause code used should correspond to the sequence of events regardless of which caused the most serious injury.

> An 86-year-old patient fell and hit his head against the nightstand. He went to the local ER and returned the same day with a diagnosis of scalp contusion.
>
> **S00.03XD**   **Contusion of scalp, subsequent encounter**
>
> **W01.190D**   **Fall on same level from slipping, tripping, and stumbling with subsequent striking against furniture, subsequent encounter**
>
> *Explanation:* Combination external cause codes identify sequential events that result in an injury, such as a fall resulting in striking against an object. The injury may be due to either or both events.

8) No external cause code needed in certain circumstances

No external cause code from Chapter 20 is needed if the external cause and intent are included in a code from another chapter (e.g. T36.0X1-Poisoning by penicillins, accidental (unintentional)).

b. Place of occurrence guideline

Codes from category Y92, Place of occurrence of the external cause, are secondary codes for use after other external cause codes to identify the location of the patient at the time of injury or other condition.

Generally, a place of occurrence code is assigned only once, at the initial encounter for treatment. However, in the rare instance that a new injury occurs during hospitalization, an additional place of occurrence code may be assigned. No 7th characters are used for Y92.

Do not use place of occurrence code Y92.9 if the place is not stated or is not applicable.

c. Activity code

Assign a code from category Y93, Activity code, to describe the activity of the patient at the time the injury or other health condition occurred.

An activity code is used only once, at the initial encounter for treatment. Only one code from Y93 should be recorded on a medical record.

The activity codes are not applicable to poisonings, adverse effects, misadventures or sequela.

Do not assign Y93.9, Unspecified activity, if the activity is not stated.

A code from category Y93 is appropriate for use with external cause and intent codes if identifying the activity provides additional information about the event.

d. Place of occurrence, activity, and status codes used with other external cause code

When applicable, place of occurrence, activity, and external cause status codes are sequenced after the main external cause code(s). Regardless of the number of external cause codes assigned, there should be only one place of occurrence code, one activity code, and one external cause status code assigned to an encounter. However, in the rare instance that a new injury occurs during hospitalization, an additional place of occurrence code may be assigned.

e. If the reporting format limits the number of external cause codes

If the reporting format limits the number of external cause codes that can be used in reporting clinical data, report the code for the cause/intent most related to the principal diagnosis. If the format permits, capture of additional external cause codes, the cause/intent, including medical misadventures, of the additional events should be reported rather than the codes for place, activity, or external status.

f. Multiple external cause coding guidelines

More than one external cause code is required to fully describe the external cause of an illness or injury. The assignment of external cause codes should be sequenced in the following priority:

If two or more events cause separate injuries, an external cause code should be assigned for each cause. The first-listed external cause code will be selected in the following order:

External codes for child and adult abuse take priority over all other external cause codes.

See Section I.C.19., Child and Adult abuse guidelines.

External cause codes for terrorism events take priority over all other external cause codes except child and adult abuse.

External cause codes for cataclysmic events take priority over all other external cause codes except child and adult abuse and terrorism.

External cause codes for transport accidents take priority over all other external cause codes except cataclysmic events, child and adult abuse and terrorism.

Activity and external cause status codes are assigned following all causal (intent) external cause codes.

The first-listed external cause code should correspond to the cause of the most serious diagnosis due to an assault, accident, or self-harm, following the order of hierarchy listed above.

A 70-year-old male was cleaning his basement and accidentally discharged a handgun, resulting in a gunshot wound to his left foot. As he was attempting to go up his stairs to seek help, he fell backwards and sustained a left hip fracture. The GSW is currently being treated with a wound VAC.

S91.332A	Puncture wound without foreign body, left foot, initial encounter
W32.0XXA	Accidental handgun discharge, initial encounter
S72.002D	Fracture of unspecified part of neck of left femur, subsequent encounter for closed fracture with routine healing
W10.8XXD	Fall (on) (from) other stairs and steps, subsequent encounter

Explanation: If one or more events cause separate injuries, each injury and the appropriate external cause code should be assigned. The left foot wound requires active treatment with a VAC dressing and should be coded with seventh character A.

---

g. Child and adult abuse guideline

Adult and child abuse, neglect and maltreatment are classified as assault. Any of the assault codes may be used to indicate the external cause of any injury resulting from the confirmed abuse.

For confirmed cases of abuse, neglect and maltreatment, when the perpetrator is known, a code from Y07, Perpetrator of maltreatment and neglect, should accompany any other assault codes.

See Section I.C.19. Adult and child abuse, neglect and other maltreatment

h. Unknown or undetermined intent guideline

If the intent (accident, self-harm, assault) of the cause of an injury or other condition is unknown or unspecified, code the intent as accidental intent. All transport accident categories assume accidental intent.

1) Use of undetermined intent

External cause codes for events of undetermined intent are only for use if the documentation in the record specifies that the intent cannot be determined.

i. Sequelae (late effects) of external cause guidelines

1) Sequelae external cause codes

Sequela are reported using the external cause code with the 7th character "S" for sequela. These codes should be used with any report of a late effect or sequela resulting from a previous injury.

See Section I.B.10 Sequela (Late Effects)

A patient is in a persistent vegetative state resulting from traumatic brain injury 1 year ago that was sustained in a diving accident in which his head hit the diving board.

R40.3	Persistent vegetative state
S06.9X9S	Unspecified intracranial injury with loss of consciousness of unspecified duration, sequela
W21.4XXS	Striking against diving board, sequela

Explanation: The persistent vegetative state is identified as a result of the intracranial injury and should be coded first, followed by the injury code with seventh character S to identify the sequelae condition. An external cause code also using seventh character S may be assigned if the cause of the injury is known.

---

2) Sequela external cause code with a related current injury

A sequela external cause code should never be used with a related current nature of injury code.

3) Use of sequela external cause codes for subsequent visits

Use a late effect external cause code for subsequent visits when a late effect of the initial injury is being treated. Do not use a late effect external cause code for subsequent visits for follow-up care (e.g., to assess healing, to receive rehabilitative therapy) of the injury when no late effect of the injury has been documented.

j. Terrorism guidelines

1) Cause of injury identified by the Federal Government (FBI) as terrorism

When the cause of an injury is identified by the Federal Government (FBI) as terrorism, the first-listed external cause code should be a code from category Y38, Terrorism. The definition of terrorism employed by the FBI is found at the inclusion note at the beginning of category Y38. Use additional code for place of occurrence (Y92.-). More than one Y38 code may be assigned if the injury is the result of more than one mechanism of terrorism.

2) Cause of an injury is suspected to be the result of terrorism

When the cause of an injury is suspected to be the result of terrorism a code from category Y38 should not be assigned. Suspected cases should be classified as assault.

3) Code Y38.9, Terrorism, secondary effects

Assign code Y38.9, Terrorism, secondary effects, for conditions occurring subsequent to the terrorist event. This code should not be assigned for conditions that are due to the initial terrorist act.

It is acceptable to assign code Y38.9 with another code from Y38 if there is an injury due to the initial terrorist event and an injury that is a subsequent result of the terrorist event.

k. External cause status

A code from category Y99, External cause status, should be assigned whenever any other external cause code is assigned for an encounter, including an Activity code, except for the events noted below. Assign a code from category Y99, External cause status, to indicate the work status of the person at the time the event occurred. The status code indicates whether the event occurred during military activity, whether a non-military person was at work, whether an individual including a student or volunteer was involved in a non-work activity at the time of the causal event.

A code from Y99, External cause status, should be assigned, when applicable, with other external cause codes, such as transport accidents and falls. The external cause status codes are not applicable to poisonings, adverse effects, misadventures or late effects.

Do not assign a code from category Y99 if no other external cause codes (cause, activity) are applicable for the encounter.

An external cause status code is used only once, at the initial encounter for treatment. Only one code from Y99 should be recorded on a medical record.

Do not assign code Y99.9, Unspecified external cause status, if the status is not stated.

Chapter 20. External Causes of Morbidity (V00-Y99)

NOTE This chapter permits the classification of environmental events and circumstances as the cause of injury, and other adverse effects. Where a code from this section is applicable, it is intended that it shall be used secondary to a code from another chapter of the Classification indicating the nature of the condition. Most often, the condition will be classifiable to Chapter 19, Injury, poisoning and certain other consequences of external causes (S00-T88). Other conditions that may be stated to be due to external causes are classified in Chapters I to XVIII. For these conditions, codes from Chapter 20 should be used to provide additional information as to the cause of the condition.

This chapter contains the following blocks:

V00-X58	Accidents
V00-V99	Transport accidents
V00-V09	Pedestrian injured in transport accident
V10-V19	Pedal cycle rider injured in transport accident
V20-V29	Motorcycle rider injured in transport accident
V30-V39	Occupant of three-wheeled motor vehicle injured in transport accident
V40-V49	Car occupant injured in transport accident
V50-V59	Occupant of pick-up truck or van injured in transport accident
V60-V69	Occupant of heavy transport vehicle injured in transport accident
V70-V79	Bus occupant injured in transport accident
V80-V89	Other land transport accidents
V90-V94	Water transport accidents
V95-V97	Air and space transport accidents
V98-V99	Other and unspecified transport accidents
W00-X58	Other external causes of accidental injury
W00-W19	Slipping, tripping, stumbling and falls
W20-W49	Exposure to inanimate mechanical forces
W50-W64	Exposure to animate mechanical forces
W65-W74	Accidental non-transport drowning and submersion
W85-W99	Exposure to electric current, radiation and extreme ambient air temperature and pressure
X00-X08	Exposure to smoke, fire and flames
X10-X19	Contact with heat and hot substances
X30-X39	Exposure to forces of nature
~~X50~~	~~Overexertion and strenuous or repetitive movements~~
X52-X58	Accidental exposure to other specified factors
X71-X83	Intentional self-harm
X92-Y09	Assault
Y21-Y33	Event of undetermined intent
Y35-Y38	Legal intervention, operations of war, military operations, and terrorism
Y62-Y84	Complications of medical and surgical care
Y62-Y69	Misadventures to patients during surgical and medical care
Y70-Y82	Medical devices associated with adverse incidents in diagnostic and therapeutic use
Y83-Y84	Surgical and other medical procedures as the cause of abnormal reaction of the patient, or of later complication, without mention of misadventure at the time of the procedure
Y90-Y99	Supplementary factors related to causes of morbidity classified elsewhere

Accidents (V00-X58)

Transport accidents (V00-V99)

NOTE This section is structured in 12 groups. Those relating to land transport accidents (V00-V89) reflect the victim's mode of transport and are subdivided to identify the victim's 'counterpart' or the type of event. The vehicle of which the injured person is an occupant is identified in the first two characters since it is seen as the most important factor to identify for prevention purposes. A transport accident is one in which the vehicle involved must be moving or running or in use for transport purposes at the time of the accident.

Use additional code to identify:
    airbag injury (W22.1)
    type of street or road (Y92.4-)
    use of cellular telephone and other electronic equipment at the time of the transport accident (Y93.C-)

EXCLUDES 1 *agricultural vehicles in stationary use or maintenance (W31.-)*
    assault by crashing of motor vehicle (Y03.-)
    automobile or motor cycle in stationary use or maintenance—code to type of accident
    crashing of motor vehicle, undetermined intent (Y32)
    intentional self-harm by crashing of motor vehicle (X82)
EXCLUDES 2 *transport accidents due to cataclysm (X34-X38)*

NOTE Definitions related to transport accidents:
(a) A transport accident (V00-V99) is any accident involving a device designed primarily for, or used at the time primarily for, conveying persons or good from one place to another.
(b) A public highway [trafficway] or street is the entire width between property lines (or other boundary lines) of land open to the public as a matter of right or custom for purposes of moving persons or property from one place to another. A roadway is that part of the public highway designed, improved and customarily used for vehicular traffic.
(c) A traffic accident is any vehicle accident occurring on the public highway [i.e. originating on, terminating on, or involving a vehicle partially on the highway]. A vehicle accident is assumed to have occurred on the public highway unless another place is specified, except in the case of accidents involving only off-road motor vehicles, which are classified as nontraffic accidents unless the contrary is stated.
(d) A nontraffic accident is any vehicle accident that occurs entirely in any place other than a public highway.
(e) A pedestrian is any person involved in an accident who was not at the time of the accident riding in or on a motor vehicle, railway train, streetcar or animal-drawn or other vehicle, or on a pedal cycle or animal. This includes, a person changing a tire, working on a parked car, or a person on foot. It also includes the user of a pedestrian conveyance such as a babystroller, ice-skates, skis, sled, roller skates, a skateboard, nonmotorized or motorized wheelchair, motorized mobility scooter, or nonmotorized scooter.
(f) A driver is an occupant of a transport vehicle who is operating or intending to operate it.
(g) A passenger is any occupant of a transport vehicle other than the driver, except a person traveling on the outside of the vehicle.
(h) A person on the outside of a vehicle is any person being transported by a vehicle but not occupying the space normally reserved for the driver or passengers, or the space intended for the transport of property. This includes a person travelling on the bodywork, bumper, fender, roof, running board or step of a vehicle, as well as, hanging on the outside of the vehicle.
(i) A pedal cycle is any land transport vehicle operated solely by nonmotorized pedals including a bicycle or tricycle.
(j) A pedal cyclist is any person riding a pedal cycle or in a sidecar or trailer attached to a pedal cycle.
(k) A motorcycle is a two-wheeled motor vehicle with one or two riding saddles and sometimes with a third wheel for the support of a sidecar. The sidecar is considered part of the motorcycle. This includes a moped, motor scooter, or motorized bicycle.
(l) A motorcycle rider is any person riding a motorcycle or in a sidecar or trailer attached to the motorcycle.
(m) A three-wheeled motor vehicle is a motorized tricycle designed primarily for on-road use. This includes a motor-driven tricycle, a motorized rickshaw, or a three-wheeled motor car.
(n) A car [automobile] is a four-wheeled motor vehicle designed primarily for carrying up to 7 persons. A trailer being towed by the car is considered part of the car. It does not include a van or minivan - see definition (o).
(o) A pick-up truck or van is a four or six-wheeled motor vehicle designed for carrying passengers as well as property or cargo weighing less than the local limit for classification as a heavy goods vehicle, and not requiring a special driver's license. This includes a minivan and a sport-utility vehicle (SUV).
(p) A heavy transport vehicle is a motor vehicle designed primarily for carrying property, meeting local criteria for classification as a heavy goods vehicle in terms of weight and requiring a special driver's license.
(q) A bus (coach) is a motor vehicle designed or adapted primarily for carrying more than 10 passengers, and requiring a special driver's license.
(r) A railway train or railway vehicle is any device, with or without freight or passenger cars couple to it, designed for traffic on a railway track. This includes subterranean (subways) or elevated trains.
(s) A streetcar, is a device designed and used primarily for transporting passengers within a municipality, running on rails, usually subject to normal traffic control signals, and operated principally on a right-of-way that forms part of the roadway. This includes a tram or trolley that runs on rails. A trailer being towed by a streetcar is considered part of the streetcar.
(t) A special vehicle mainly used on industrial premises is a motor vehicle designed primarily for use within the buildings and premises of industrial or commercial establishments. This includes battery-powered airport passenger vehicles or baggage/mail trucks, forklifts, coal-cars in a coal mine, logging cars and trucks used in mines or quarries.

✅ Additional Character Req   ✔x7ᵗʰ Placeholder Alert   Case-Mix Diagnosis   Manifestation   ▽ Unspecified Dx   **EXCLUDES 1** Not coded here   **EXCLUDES 2** Not included here

ICD-10-CM 2018   **1115**

(u) A special vehicle mainly used in agriculture is a motor vehicle designed specifically for use in farming and agriculture (horticulture), to work the land, tend and harvest crops and transport materials on the farm. This includes harvesters, farm machinery and tractor and trailers.

(v) A special construction vehicle is a motor vehicle designed specifically for use on construction and demolition sites. This includes bulldozers, diggers, earth levellers, dump trucks. backhoes, front-end loaders, pavers, and mechanical shovels.

(w) A special all-terrain vehicle is a motor vehicle of special design to enable it to negotiate over rough or soft terrain, snow or sand. Examples of special design are high construction, special wheels and tires, tracks, and support on a cushion of air. This includes snow mobiles, All-terrain vehicles (ATV), and dune buggies. It does not include passenger vehicle designated as Sport Utility Vehicles. (SUV)

(x) A watercraft is any device designed for transporting passengers or goods on water. This includes motor or sailboats, ships, and hovercraft.

(y) An aircraft is any device for transporting passengers or goods in the air. This includes hot-air balloons, gliders, helicopters and airplanes.

(z) A military vehicle is any motorized vehicle operating on a public roadway owned by the military and being operated by a member of the military

Pedestrian injured in transport accident (V00-V09)

INCLUDES   person changing tire on transport vehicle
person examining engine of vehicle broken down in (on side of) road

EXCLUDES 1   *fall due to non-transport collision with other person (W03)*
pedestrian on foot falling (slipping) on ice and snow (W00.-)
struck or bumped by another person (W51)

> The appropriate 7th character is to be added to each code from categories V00-V09.
> A   initial encounter
> D   subsequent encounter
> S   sequela

✓4ᵗʰ **V00**   **Pedestrian conveyance accident**

Use additional place of occurrence and activity external cause codes, if known (Y92-, Y93-)

EXCLUDES 1   *collision with another person without fall (W51)*
fall due to person on foot colliding with another person on foot (W03)
fall from non-moving wheelchair, nonmotorized scooter and motorized mobility scooter without collision (W05.-)
pedestrian (conveyance) collision with other land transport vehicle (V01-V09)
pedestrian on foot falling (slipping) on ice and snow (W00.-)

✓5ᵗʰ **V00.0**   **Pedestrian on foot injured in collision with pedestrian conveyance**

   ✓x 7ᵗʰ **V00.01**   **Pedestrian on foot injured in collision with roller-skater**

   ✓x 7ᵗʰ **V00.02**   **Pedestrian on foot injured in collision with skateboarder**

   ✓x 7ᵗʰ **V00.09**   **Pedestrian on foot injured in collision with other pedestrian conveyance**

✓5ᵗʰ **V00.1**   **Rolling-type pedestrian conveyance accident**

   EXCLUDES 1   *accident with babystroller (V00.82-)*
accident with motorized mobility scooter (V00.83-)
accident with wheelchair (powered) (V00.81-)

   ✓6ᵗʰ **V00.11**   **In-line roller-skate accident**

     ✓7ᵗʰ **V00.111**   **Fall from in-line roller-skates**

     ✓7ᵗʰ **V00.112**   **In-line roller-skater colliding with stationary object**

     ✓7ᵗʰ **V00.118**   **Other in-line roller-skate accident**
       EXCLUDES 1   *roller-skater collision with other land transport vehicle (V01-V09 with 5th character 1)*

   ✓6ᵗʰ **V00.12**   **Non-in- line roller-skate accident**

     ✓7ᵗʰ **V00.121**   **Fall from non-in-line roller-skates**

     ✓7ᵗʰ **V00.122**   **Non-in-line roller-skater colliding with stationary object**

     ✓7ᵗʰ **V00.128**   **Other non-in-line roller-skating accident**
       EXCLUDES 1   *roller-skater collision with other land transport vehicle (V01-V09 with 5th character 1)*

   ✓6ᵗʰ **V00.13**   **Skateboard accident**

     ✓7ᵗʰ **V00.131**   **Fall from skateboard**

     ✓7ᵗʰ **V00.132**   **Skateboarder colliding with stationary object**

     ✓7ᵗʰ **V00.138**   **Other skateboard accident**
       EXCLUDES 1   *skateboarder collision with other land transport vehicle (V01-V09 with 5th character 2)*

   ✓6ᵗʰ **V00.14**   **Scooter (nonmotorized) accident**
     EXCLUDES 1   *motorscooter accident (V20-V29)*

     ✓7ᵗʰ **V00.141**   **Fall from scooter (nonmotorized)**

     ✓7ᵗʰ **V00.142**   **Scooter (nonmotorized) colliding with stationary object**

     ✓7ᵗʰ **V00.148**   **Other scooter (nonmotorized) accident**
       EXCLUDES 1   *scooter (nonmotorized) collision with other land transport vehicle (V01-V09 with fifth character 9)*

   ✓6ᵗʰ **V00.15**   **Heelies accident**
     Rolling shoe
     Wheeled shoe
     Wheelies accident

     ✓7ᵗʰ **V00.151**   **Fall from heelies**

     ✓7ᵗʰ **V00.152**   **Heelies colliding with stationary object**

     ✓7ᵗʰ **V00.158**   **Other heelies accident**

   ✓6ᵗʰ **V00.18**   **Accident on other rolling-type pedestrian conveyance**

     ✓7ᵗʰ **V00.181**   **Fall from other rolling-type pedestrian conveyance**

     ✓7ᵗʰ **V00.182**   **Pedestrian on other rolling-type pedestrian conveyance colliding with stationary object**

     ✓7ᵗʰ **V00.188**   **Other accident on other rolling-type pedestrian conveyance**

✓5ᵗʰ **V00.2**   **Gliding-type pedestrian conveyance accident**

   ✓6ᵗʰ **V00.21**   **Ice-skates accident**

     ✓7ᵗʰ **V00.211**   **Fall from ice-skates**

     ✓7ᵗʰ **V00.212**   **Ice-skater colliding with stationary object**

     ✓7ᵗʰ **V00.218**   **Other ice-skates accident**
       EXCLUDES 1   *ice-skater collision with other land transport vehicle (V01-V09 with 5th digit 9)*

   ✓6ᵗʰ **V00.22**   **Sled accident**

     ✓7ᵗʰ **V00.221**   **Fall from sled**

     ✓7ᵗʰ **V00.222**   **Sledder colliding with stationary object**

     ✓7ᵗʰ **V00.228**   **Other sled accident**
       EXCLUDES 1   *sled collision with other land transport vehicle (V01-V09 with 5th digit 9)*

   ✓6ᵗʰ **V00.28**   **Other gliding-type pedestrian conveyance accident**

     ✓7ᵗʰ **V00.281**   **Fall from other gliding-type pedestrian conveyance**

     ✓7ᵗʰ **V00.282**   **Pedestrian on other gliding-type pedestrian conveyance colliding with stationary object**

     ✓7ᵗʰ **V00.288**   **Other accident on other gliding-type pedestrian conveyance**
       EXCLUDES 1   *gliding-type pedestrian conveyance collision with other land transport vehicle (V01-V09 with 5th digit 9)*

✓5ᵗʰ **V00.3**   **Flat-bottomed pedestrian conveyance accident**

   ✓6ᵗʰ **V00.31**   **Snowboard accident**

     ✓7ᵗʰ **V00.311**   **Fall from snowboard**

     ✓7ᵗʰ **V00.312**   **Snowboarder colliding with stationary object**

     ✓7ᵗʰ **V00.318**   **Other snowboard accident**
       EXCLUDES 1   *snowboarder collision with other land transport vehicle (V01-V09 with 5th digit 9)*

   ✓6ᵗʰ **V00.32**   **Snow-ski accident**

     ✓7ᵗʰ **V00.321**   **Fall from snow-skis**

     ✓7ᵗʰ **V00.322**   **Snow-skier colliding with stationary object**

Ⓝ Newborn: 0   Ⓟ Pediatric: 0-17   Ⓜ Maternity: 12-55   Ⓐ Adult: 15-124   NRS Nonroutine supply Dx   NCDx Noncancer Dx   PDx Primary Dx   ▶◀ Revised Text   ● New Code   ▲ Revised Title

1116   ICD-10-CM 2018

✓7th **V00.328** Other snow-ski accident
> EXCLUDES 1   *snow-skier collision with other land transport vehicle (V01-V09 with 5th digit 9)*

✓6th **V00.38** Other flat-bottomed pedestrian conveyance accident

     ✓7th **V00.381** Fall from other flat-bottomed pedestrian conveyance

     ✓7th **V00.382** Pedestrian on other flat-bottomed pedestrian conveyance colliding with stationary object

     ✓7th **V00.388** Other accident on other flat-bottomed pedestrian conveyance

✓5th **V00.8** Accident on other pedestrian conveyance

   ✓6th **V00.81** Accident with wheelchair (powered)

     ✓7th **V00.811** Fall from moving wheelchair (powered)
> EXCLUDES 1   *fall from non-moving wheelchair (W05.0)*

     ✓7th **V00.812** Wheelchair (powered) colliding with stationary object

     ✓7th **V00.818** Other accident with wheelchair (powered)

   ✓6th **V00.82** Accident with babystroller

     ✓7th **V00.821** Fall from babystroller

     ✓7th **V00.822** Babystroller colliding with stationary object

     ✓7th **V00.828** Other accident with babystroller

   ✓6th **V00.83** Accident with motorized mobility scooter

     ✓7th **V00.831** Fall from motorized mobility scooter
> EXCLUDES 1   *fall from non-moving motorized mobility scooter (W05.2)*

     ✓7th **V00.832** Motorized mobility scooter colliding with stationary object

     ✓7th **V00.838** Other accident with motorized mobility scooter

   ✓6th **V00.89** Accident on other pedestrian conveyance

     ✓7th **V00.891** Fall from other pedestrian conveyance

     ✓7th **V00.892** Pedestrian on other pedestrian conveyance colliding with stationary object

     ✓7th **V00.898** Other accident on other pedestrian conveyance
> EXCLUDES 1   *other pedestrian (conveyance) collision with other land transport vehicle (V01-V09 with 5th digit 9)*

✓4th **V01** Pedestrian injured in collision with pedal cycle

   ✓5th **V01.0** Pedestrian injured in collision with pedal cycle in nontraffic accident

     ✓x7th **V01.00** Pedestrian on foot injured in collision with pedal cycle in nontraffic accident
> Pedestrian NOS injured in collision with pedal cycle in nontraffic accident

     ✓x7th **V01.01** Pedestrian on roller-skates injured in collision with pedal cycle in nontraffic accident

     ✓x7th **V01.02** Pedestrian on skateboard injured in collision with pedal cycle in nontraffic accident

     ✓x7th **V01.09** Pedestrian with other conveyance injured in collision with pedal cycle in nontraffic accident
> Pedestrian with babystroller injured in collision with pedal cycle in nontraffic accident
> Pedestrian on ice-skates injured in collision with pedal cycle in nontraffic accident
> Pedestrian on nonmotorized scooter injured in collision with pedal cycle in nontraffic accident
> Pedestrian on sled injured in collision with pedal cycle in nontraffic accident
> Pedestrian on snowboard injured in collision with pedal cycle in nontraffic accident
> Pedestrian on snow-skis injured in collision with pedal cycle in nontraffic accident
> Pedestrian in wheelchair (powered) injured in collision with pedal cycle in nontraffic accident
> Pedestrian in motorized mobility scooter injured in collision with pedal cycle in nontraffic accident

   ✓5th **V01.1** Pedestrian injured in collision with pedal cycle in traffic accident

     ✓x7th **V01.10** Pedestrian on foot injured in collision with pedal cycle in traffic accident
> Pedestrian NOS injured in collision with pedal cycle in traffic accident

     ✓x7th **V01.11** Pedestrian on roller-skates injured in collision with pedal cycle in traffic accident

     ✓x7th **V01.12** Pedestrian on skateboard injured in collision with pedal cycle in traffic accident

     ✓x7th **V01.19** Pedestrian with other conveyance injured in collision with pedal cycle in traffic accident
> Pedestrian with babystroller injured in collision with pedal cycle in traffic accident
> Pedestrian on ice-skates injured in collision with pedal cycle in traffic accident
> Pedestrian on nonmotorized scooter injured in collision with pedal cycle in traffic accident
> Pedestrian on sled injured in collision with pedal cycle in traffic accident
> Pedestrian on snowboard injured in collision with pedal cycle in traffic accident
> Pedestrian on snow-skis injured in collision with pedal cycle in traffic accident
> Pedestrian in wheelchair (powered) injured in collision with pedal cycle in traffic accident
> Pedestrian in motorized mobility scooter injured in collision with pedal cycle in traffic accident

   ✓5th **V01.9** Pedestrian injured in collision with pedal cycle, unspecified whether traffic or nontraffic accident

     ✓x7th **V01.90** Pedestrian on foot injured in collision with pedal cycle, unspecified whether traffic or nontraffic accident ▽
> Pedestrian NOS injured in collision with pedal cycle, unspecified whether traffic or nontraffic accident

     ✓x7th **V01.91** Pedestrian on roller-skates injured in collision with pedal cycle, unspecified whether traffic or nontraffic accident ▽

     ✓x7th **V01.92** Pedestrian on skateboard injured in collision with pedal cycle, unspecified whether traffic or nontraffic accident ▽

     ✓x7th **V01.99** Pedestrian with other conveyance injured in collision with pedal cycle, unspecified whether traffic or nontraffic accident ▽
> Pedestrian with babystroller injured in collision with pedal cycle, unspecified whether traffic or nontraffic accident
> Pedestrian on ice-skates injured in collision with pedal cycle unspecified, whether traffic or nontraffic accident
> Pedestrian on nonmotorized scooter injured in collision with pedal cycle, unspecified whether traffic or nontraffic accident
> Pedestrian on sled injured in collision with pedal cycle unspecified, whether traffic or nontraffic accident
> Pedestrian on snowboard injured in collision with pedal cycle, unspecified whether traffic or nontraffic accident
> Pedestrian on snow-skis injured in collision with pedal cycle, unspecified whether traffic or nontraffic accident
> Pedestrian in wheelchair (powered) injured in collision with pedal cycle, unspecified whether traffic or nontraffic accident
> Pedestrian in motorized mobility scooter injured in collision with pedal cycle, unspecified whether traffic or nontraffic accident

✓4th **V02** Pedestrian injured in collision with two- or three-wheeled motor vehicle

   ✓5th **V02.0** Pedestrian injured in collision with two- or three-wheeled motor vehicle in nontraffic accident

     ✓x7th **V02.00** Pedestrian on foot injured in collision with two- or three-wheeled motor vehicle in nontraffic accident
> Pedestrian NOS injured in collision with two- or three-wheeled motor vehicle in nontraffic accident

     ✓x7th **V02.01** Pedestrian on roller-skates injured in collision with two- or three-wheeled motor vehicle in nontraffic accident

---

✓ Additional Character Req   ✓x7th Placeholder Alert   Case-Mix Diagnosis   Manifestation   ▽ Unspecified Dx   EXCLUDES 1 Not coded here   EXCLUDES 2 Not included here

☑x7th **V02.02** **Pedestrian on skateboard injured in collision with two- or three-wheeled motor vehicle in nontraffic accident**

☑x7th **V02.09** **Pedestrian with other conveyance injured in collision with two- or three-wheeled motor vehicle in nontraffic accident**
   Pedestrian with babystroller injured in collision with two- or three-wheeled motor vehicle in nontraffic accident
   Pedestrian on ice-skates injured in collision with two- or three-wheeled motor vehicle in nontraffic accident
   Pedestrian on nonmotorized scooter injured in collision with two- or three-wheeled motor vehicle in nontraffic accident
   Pedestrian on sled injured in collision with two- or three-wheeled motor vehicle in nontraffic accident
   Pedestrian on snowboard injured in collision with two- or three-wheeled motor vehicle in nontraffic accident
   Pedestrian on snow-skis injured in collision with two- or three-wheeled motor vehicle in nontraffic accident
   Pedestrian in wheelchair (powered) injured in collision with two- or three-wheeled motor vehicle in nontraffic accident
   Pedestrian in motorized mobility scooter injured in collision with two- or three-wheeled motor vehicle in nontraffic accident

☑5th **V02.1** **Pedestrian injured in collision with two- or three-wheeled motor vehicle in traffic accident**

☑x7th **V02.10** **Pedestrian on foot injured in collision with two- or three-wheeled motor vehicle in traffic accident**
   Pedestrian NOS injured in collision with two- or three-wheeled motor vehicle in traffic accident

☑x7th **V02.11** **Pedestrian on roller-skates injured in collision with two- or three-wheeled motor vehicle in traffic accident**

☑x7th **V02.12** **Pedestrian on skateboard injured in collision with two- or three-wheeled motor vehicle in traffic accident**

☑x7th **V02.19** **Pedestrian with other conveyance injured in collision with two- or three-wheeled motor vehicle in traffic accident**
   Pedestrian with babystroller injured in collision with two- or three-wheeled motor vehicle in traffic accident
   Pedestrian on ice-skates injured in collision with two- or three-wheeled motor vehicle in traffic accident
   Pedestrian on nonmotorized scooter injured in collision with two- or three-wheeled motor vehicle in traffic accident
   Pedestrian on sled injured in collision with two- or three-wheeled motor vehicle in traffic accident
   Pedestrian on snowboard injured in collision with two- or three-wheeled motor vehicle in traffic accident
   Pedestrian on snow-skis injured in collision with two- or three-wheeled motor vehicle in traffic accident
   Pedestrian in wheelchair (powered) injured in collision with two- or three-wheeled motor vehicle in traffic accident
   Pedestrian in motorized mobility scooter injured in collision with two- or three-wheeled motor vehicle in traffic accident

☑5th **V02.9** **Pedestrian injured in collision with two- or three-wheeled motor vehicle, unspecified whether traffic or nontraffic accident**

☑x7th **V02.90** **Pedestrian on foot injured in collision with two- or three-wheeled motor vehicle, unspecified whether traffic or nontraffic accident** ▽
   Pedestrian NOS injured in collision with two- or three-wheeled motor vehicle, unspecified whether traffic or nontraffic accident

☑x7th **V02.91** **Pedestrian on roller-skates injured in collision with two- or three-wheeled motor vehicle, unspecified whether traffic or nontraffic accident** ▽

☑x7th **V02.92** **Pedestrian on skateboard injured in collision with two- or three-wheeled motor vehicle, unspecified whether traffic or nontraffic accident** ▽

☑x7th **V02.99** **Pedestrian with other conveyance injured in collision with two- or three-wheeled motor vehicle, unspecified whether traffic or nontraffic accident** ▽
   Pedestrian with babystroller injured in collision with two- or three-wheeled motor vehicle, unspecified whether traffic or nontraffic accident
   Pedestrian on ice-skates injured in collision with two- or three-wheeled motor vehicle, unspecified whether traffic or nontraffic accident
   Pedestrian on nonmotorized scooter injured in collision with two- or three-wheeled motor vehicle, unspecified whether traffic or nontraffic accident
   Pedestrian on sled injured in collision with two- or three-wheeled motor vehicle, unspecified whether traffic or nontraffic accident
   Pedestrian on snowboard injured in collision with two- or three-wheeled motor vehicle, unspecified whether traffic or nontraffic accident
   Pedestrian on snow-skis injured in collision with two- or three-wheeled motor vehicle, unspecified whether traffic or nontraffic accident
   Pedestrian in wheelchair (powered) injured in collision with two- or three-wheeled motor vehicle, unspecified whether traffic or nontraffic accident
   Pedestrian in motorized mobility scooter injured in collision with two- or three-wheeled motor vehicle, unspecified whether traffic or nontraffic accident

☑4th **V03** **Pedestrian injured in collision with car, pick-up truck or van**

☑5th **V03.0** **Pedestrian injured in collision with car, pick-up truck or van in nontraffic accident**

☑x7th **V03.00** **Pedestrian on foot injured in collision with car, pick-up truck or van in nontraffic accident**
   Pedestrian NOS injured in collision with car, pick-up truck or van in nontraffic accident

☑x7th **V03.01** **Pedestrian on roller-skates injured in collision with car, pick-up truck or van in nontraffic accident**

☑x7th **V03.02** **Pedestrian on skateboard injured in collision with car, pick-up truck or van in nontraffic accident**

☑x7th **V03.09** **Pedestrian with other conveyance injured in collision with car, pick-up truck or van in nontraffic accident**
   Pedestrian with babystroller injured in collision with car, pick-up truck or van in nontraffic accident
   Pedestrian on ice-skates injured in collision with car, pick-up truck or van in nontraffic accident
   Pedestrian on nonmotorized scooter injured in collision with car, pick-up truck or van in nontraffic accident
   Pedestrian on sled injured in collision with car, pick-up truck or van in nontraffic accident
   Pedestrian on snowboard injured in collision with car, pick-up truck or van in nontraffic accident
   Pedestrian on snow-skis injured in collision with car, pick-up truck or van in nontraffic accident
   Pedestrian in wheelchair (powered) injured in collision with car, pick-up truck or van in nontraffic accident
   Pedestrian in motorized mobility scooter injured in collision with car, pick-up truck or van in nontraffic accident

☑5th **V03.1** **Pedestrian injured in collision with car, pick-up truck or van in traffic accident**

☑x7th **V03.10** **Pedestrian on foot injured in collision with car, pick-up truck or van in traffic accident**
   Pedestrian NOS injured in collision with car, pick-up truck or van in traffic accident

☑x7th **V03.11** **Pedestrian on roller-skates injured in collision with car, pick-up truck or van in traffic accident**

☑x7th **V03.12** **Pedestrian on skateboard injured in collision with car, pick-up truck or van in traffic accident**

✓x7ᵗʰ **V03.19 Pedestrian with other** conveyance **injured in collision with car, pick-up truck or van in traffic accident**

> Pedestrian with babystroller injured in collision with car, pick-up truck or van in traffic accident
> Pedestrian on ice-skates injured in collision with car, pick-up truck or van in traffic accident
> Pedestrian on nonmotorized scooter injured in collision with car, pick-up truck or van in traffic accident
> Pedestrian on sled injured in collision with car, pick-up truck or van in traffic accident
> Pedestrian on snowboard injured in collision with car, pick-up truck or van in traffic accident
> Pedestrian on snow-skis injured in collision with car, pick-up truck or van in traffic accident
> Pedestrian in wheelchair (powered) injured in collision with car, pick-up truck or van in traffic accident
> Pedestrian in motorized mobility scooter injured in collision with car, pick-up truck or van in traffic accident

✓5ᵗʰ **V03.9 Pedestrian injured in collision with car, pick-up truck or van, unspecified whether traffic or nontraffic accident**

     ✓x7ᵗʰ **V03.90 Pedestrian** on foot **injured in collision with car, pick-up truck or van, unspecified whether traffic or nontraffic accident** ▽

> Pedestrian NOS injured in collision with car, pick-up truck or van, unspecified whether traffic or nontraffic accident

     ✓x7ᵗʰ **V03.91 Pedestrian** on roller-skates **injured in collision with car, pick-up truck or van, unspecified whether traffic or nontraffic accident** ▽

     ✓x7ᵗʰ **V03.92 Pedestrian** on skateboard **injured in collision with car, pick-up truck or van, unspecified whether traffic or nontraffic accident** ▽

     ✓x7ᵗʰ **V03.99 Pedestrian with other** conveyance **injured in collision with car, pick-up truck or van, unspecified whether traffic or nontraffic accident** ▽

> Pedestrian with babystroller injured in collision with car, pick-up truck or van, unspecified whether traffic or nontraffic accident
> Pedestrian on ice-skates injured in collision with car, pick-up truck or van, unspecified whether traffic or nontraffic accident
> Pedestrian on nonmotorized scooter injured in collision with car, pick-up truck or van, unspecified whether traffic or nontraffic accident
> Pedestrian on sled injured in collision with car, pick-up truck or van in nontraffic accident
> Pedestrian on snowboard injured in collision with car, pick-up truck or van, unspecified whether traffic or nontraffic accident
> Pedestrian on snow-skis injured in collision with car, pick-up truck or van, unspecified whether traffic or nontraffic accident
> Pedestrian in wheelchair (powered) injured in collision with car, pick-up truck or van, unspecified whether traffic or nontraffic accident
> Pedestrian in motorized mobility scooter injured in collision with car, pick-up truck or van, unspecified whether traffic or nontraffic accident

✓4ᵗʰ **V04 Pedestrian injured in collision with heavy transport vehicle or bus**

> **EXCLUDES 1** *pedestrian injured in collision with military vehicle (V09.01, V09.21)*

✓5ᵗʰ **V04.0 Pedestrian injured in collision with heavy transport vehicle or bus** in nontraffic accident

     ✓x7ᵗʰ **V04.00 Pedestrian** on foot **injured in collision with heavy transport vehicle or bus in nontraffic accident**

> Pedestrian NOS injured in collision with heavy transport vehicle or bus in nontraffic accident

     ✓x7ᵗʰ **V04.01 Pedestrian** on roller-skates **injured in collision with heavy transport vehicle or bus in nontraffic accident**

     ✓x7ᵗʰ **V04.02 Pedestrian** on skateboard **injured in collision with heavy transport vehicle or bus in nontraffic accident**

✓x7ᵗʰ **V04.09 Pedestrian with other** conveyance **injured in collision with heavy transport vehicle or bus in nontraffic accident**

> Pedestrian with babystroller injured in collision with heavy transport vehicle or bus in nontraffic accident
> Pedestrian on ice-skates injured in collision with heavy transport vehicle or bus in nontraffic accident
> Pedestrian on nonmotorized scooter injured in collision with heavy transport vehicle or bus in nontraffic accident
> Pedestrian on sled injured in collision with heavy transport vehicle or bus in nontraffic accident
> Pedestrian on snowboard injured in collision with heavy transport vehicle or bus in nontraffic accident
> Pedestrian on snow-skis injured in collision with heavy transport vehicle or bus in nontraffic accident
> Pedestrian in wheelchair (powered) injured in collision with heavy transport vehicle or bus in nontraffic accident
> Pedestrian in motorized mobility scooter injured in collision with heavy transport vehicle or bus in nontraffic accident

✓5ᵗʰ **V04.1 Pedestrian injured in collision with heavy transport vehicle or bus** in traffic accident

     ✓x7ᵗʰ **V04.10 Pedestrian** on foot **injured in collision with heavy transport vehicle or bus in traffic accident**

> Pedestrian NOS injured in collision with heavy transport vehicle or bus in traffic accident

     ✓x7ᵗʰ **V04.11 Pedestrian** on roller-skates **injured in collision with heavy transport vehicle or bus in traffic accident**

     ✓x7ᵗʰ **V04.12 Pedestrian** on skateboard **injured in collision with heavy transport vehicle or bus in traffic accident**

     ✓x7ᵗʰ **V04.19 Pedestrian with other** conveyance **injured in collision with heavy transport vehicle or bus in traffic accident**

> Pedestrian with babystroller injured in collision with heavy transport vehicle or bus in traffic accident
> Pedestrian on ice-skates injured in collision with heavy transport vehicle or bus in traffic accident
> Pedestrian on nonmotorized scooter injured in collision with heavy transport vehicle or bus in traffic accident
> Pedestrian on sled injured in collision with heavy transport vehicle or bus in traffic accident
> Pedestrian on snowboard injured in collision with heavy transport vehicle or bus in traffic accident
> Pedestrian on snow-skis injured in collision with heavy transport vehicle or bus in traffic accident
> Pedestrian in wheelchair (powered) injured in collision with heavy transport vehicle or bus in traffic accident
> Pedestrian in motorized mobility scooter injured in collision with heavy transport vehicle or bus in traffic accident

✓5ᵗʰ **V04.9 Pedestrian injured in collision with heavy transport vehicle or bus,** unspecified whether traffic or nontraffic accident

     ✓x7ᵗʰ **V04.90 Pedestrian** on foot **injured in collision with heavy transport vehicle or bus, unspecified whether traffic or nontraffic accident** ▽

> Pedestrian NOS injured in collision with heavy transport vehicle or bus, unspecified whether traffic or nontraffic accident

     ✓x7ᵗʰ **V04.91 Pedestrian** on roller-skates **injured in collision with heavy transport vehicle or bus, unspecified whether traffic or nontraffic accident** ▽

     ✓x7ᵗʰ **V04.92 Pedestrian** on skateboard **injured in collision with heavy transport vehicle or bus, unspecified whether traffic or nontraffic accident** ▽

✓ Additional Character Req   ✓x7ᵗʰ Placeholder Alert   Case-Mix Diagnosis   Manifestation   ▽ Unspecified Dx   **EXCLUDES 1** Not coded here   **EXCLUDES 2** Not included here

ICD-10-CM 2018   1119

√x7ᵗʰ **V04.99 Pedestrian with other** conveyance **injured in collision with heavy transport vehicle or bus, unspecified whether traffic or nontraffic accident** ▽

Pedestrian with babystroller injured in collision with heavy transport vehicle or bus, unspecified whether traffic or nontraffic accident

Pedestrian on ice-skates injured in collision with heavy transport vehicle or bus, unspecified whether traffic or nontraffic accident

Pedestrian on nonmotorized scooter injured in collision with heavy transport vehicle or bus, unspecified whether traffic or nontraffic accident

Pedestrian on sled injured in collision with heavy transport vehicle or bus, unspecified whether traffic or nontraffic accident

Pedestrian on snowboard injured in collision with heavy transport vehicle or bus, unspecified whether traffic or nontraffic accident

Pedestrian on snow-skis injured in collision with heavy transport vehicle or bus, unspecified whether traffic or nontraffic accident

Pedestrian in wheelchair (powered) injured in collision with heavy transport vehicle or bus, unspecified whether traffic or nontraffic accident

Pedestrian in motorized mobility scooter injured in collision with heavy transport vehicle or bus, unspecified whether traffic or nontraffic accident

√4ᵗʰ **V05 Pedestrian injured in collision with railway train or railway vehicle**

√5ᵗʰ **V05.0 Pedestrian injured in collision with railway train or railway vehicle** in nontraffic accident

√x7ᵗʰ **V05.00 Pedestrian on foot injured in collision with railway train or railway vehicle in nontraffic accident**

Pedestrian NOS injured in collision with railway train or railway vehicle in nontraffic accident

√x7ᵗʰ **V05.01 Pedestrian on roller-skates injured in collision with railway train or railway vehicle in nontraffic accident**

√x7ᵗʰ **V05.02 Pedestrian on skateboard injured in collision with railway train or railway vehicle in nontraffic accident**

√x7ᵗʰ **V05.09 Pedestrian with other** conveyance **injured in collision with railway train or railway vehicle in nontraffic accident**

Pedestrian with babystroller injured in collision with railway train or railway vehicle in nontraffic accident

Pedestrian on ice-skates injured in collision with railway train or railway vehicle in nontraffic accident

Pedestrian on nonmotorized scooter injured in collision with railway train or railway vehicle in nontraffic accident

Pedestrian on sled injured in collision with railway train or railway vehicle in nontraffic accident

Pedestrian on snowboard injured in collision with railway train or railway vehicle in nontraffic accident

Pedestrian on snow-skis injured in collision with railway train or railway vehicle in nontraffic accident

Pedestrian in wheelchair (powered) injured in collision with railway train or railway vehicle in nontraffic accident

Pedestrian in motorized mobility scooter injured in collision with railway train or railway vehicle in nontraffic accident

√5ᵗʰ **V05.1 Pedestrian injured in collision with railway train or railway vehicle** in traffic accident

√x7ᵗʰ **V05.10 Pedestrian on foot injured in collision with railway train or railway vehicle in traffic accident**

Pedestrian NOS injured in collision with railway train or railway vehicle in traffic accident

√x7ᵗʰ **V05.11 Pedestrian on roller-skates injured in collision with railway train or railway vehicle in traffic accident**

√x7ᵗʰ **V05.12 Pedestrian on skateboard injured in collision with railway train or railway vehicle in traffic accident**

√x7ᵗʰ **V05.19 Pedestrian with other** conveyance **injured in collision with railway train or railway vehicle in traffic accident**

Pedestrian with babystroller injured in collision with railway train or railway vehicle in traffic accident

Pedestrian on ice-skates injured in collision with railway train or railway vehicle in traffic accident

Pedestrian on nonmotorized scooter injured in collision with railway train or railway vehicle in traffic accident

Pedestrian on sled injured in collision with railway train or railway vehicle in traffic accident

Pedestrian on snowboard injured in collision with railway train or railway vehicle in traffic accident

Pedestrian on snow-skis injured in collision with railway train or railway vehicle in traffic accident

Pedestrian in wheelchair (powered) injured in collision with railway train or railway vehicle in traffic accident

Pedestrian in motorized mobility scooter injured in collision with railway train or railway vehicle in traffic accident

√5ᵗʰ **V05.9 Pedestrian injured in collision with railway train or railway vehicle,** unspecified whether traffic or nontraffic accident

√x7ᵗʰ **V05.90 Pedestrian on foot injured in collision with railway train or railway vehicle, unspecified whether traffic or nontraffic accident** ▽

Pedestrian NOS injured in collision with railway train or railway vehicle, unspecified whether traffic or nontraffic accident

√x7ᵗʰ **V05.91 Pedestrian on roller-skates injured in collision with railway train or railway vehicle, unspecified whether traffic or nontraffic accident** ▽

√x7ᵗʰ **V05.92 Pedestrian on skateboard injured in collision with railway train or railway vehicle, unspecified whether traffic or nontraffic accident** ▽

√x7ᵗʰ **V05.99 Pedestrian with other** conveyance **injured in collision with railway train or railway vehicle, unspecified whether traffic or nontraffic accident** ▽

Pedestrian with babystroller injured in collision with railway train or railway vehicle, unspecified whether traffic or nontraffic

Pedestrian on ice-skates injured in collision with railway train or railway vehicle, unspecified whether traffic or nontraffic

Pedestrian on nonmotorized scooter injured in collision with railway train or railway vehicle, unspecified whether traffic or nontraffic

Pedestrian on sled injured in collision with railway train or railway vehicle, unspecified whether traffic or nontraffic

Pedestrian on snowboard injured in collision with railway train or railway vehicle, unspecified whether traffic or nontraffic

Pedestrian on snow-skis injured in collision with railway train or railway vehicle, unspecified whether traffic or nontraffic

Pedestrian in wheelchair (powered) injured in collision with railway train or railway vehicle, unspecified whether traffic or nontraffic

Pedestrian in motorized mobility scooter injured in collision with railway train or railway vehicle, unspecified whether traffic or nontraffic

√4ᵗʰ **V06 Pedestrian injured in collision with other nonmotor vehicle**

INCLUDES   collision with animal-drawn vehicle, animal being ridden, nonpowered streetcar

EXCLUDES 1   pedestrian injured in collision with pedestrian conveyance (V00.0-)

√5ᵗʰ **V06.0 Pedestrian injured in collision with other nonmotor vehicle in** nontraffic accident

√x7ᵗʰ **V06.00 Pedestrian on foot injured in collision with other nonmotor vehicle in nontraffic accident**

Pedestrian NOS injured in collision with other nonmotor vehicle in nontraffic accident

√x7ᵗʰ **V06.01 Pedestrian on roller-skates injured in collision with other nonmotor vehicle in nontraffic accident**

√x7ᵗʰ **V06.02 Pedestrian on skateboard injured in collision with other nonmotor vehicle in nontraffic accident**

N Newborn: 0   P Pediatric: 0-17   M Maternity: 12-55   A Adult: 15-124   NRS Nonroutine supply Dx   NCDx Noncancer Dx   PDx Primary Dx   ▶◀ Revised Text   ● New Code   ▲ Revised Title

√x7ᵗʰ **V06.09** **Pedestrian with other** conveyance **injured in collision with other nonmotor vehicle in nontraffic accident**

Pedestrian with babystroller injured in collision with other nonmotor vehicle in nontraffic accident

Pedestrian on ice-skates injured in collision with other nonmotor vehicle in nontraffic accident

Pedestrian on nonmotorized scooter injured in collision with other nonmotor vehicle in nontraffic accident

Pedestrian on sled injured in collision with other nonmotor vehicle in nontraffic accident

Pedestrian on snowboard injured in collision with other nonmotor vehicle in nontraffic accident

Pedestrian on snow-skis injured in collision with other nonmotor vehicle in nontraffic accident

Pedestrian in wheelchair (powered) injured in collision with other nonmotor vehicle in nontraffic accident

Pedestrian in motorized mobility scooter injured in collision with other nonmotor vehicle in nontraffic accident

√5ᵗʰ **V06.1** **Pedestrian injured in collision with other nonmotor vehicle** in traffic accident

√x7ᵗʰ **V06.10** **Pedestrian** on foot **injured in collision with other nonmotor vehicle in traffic accident**

Pedestrian NOS injured in collision with other nonmotor vehicle in traffic accident

√x7ᵗʰ **V06.11** **Pedestrian** on roller-skates **injured in collision with other nonmotor vehicle in traffic accident**

√x7ᵗʰ **V06.12** **Pedestrian** on skateboard **injured in collision with other nonmotor vehicle in traffic accident**

√x7ᵗʰ **V06.19** **Pedestrian with other** conveyance **injured in collision with other nonmotor vehicle in traffic accident**

Pedestrian with babystroller injured in collision with other nonmotor vehicle in nontraffic accident

Pedestrian on ice-skates injured in collision with other nonmotor vehicle in traffic accident

Pedestrian on nonmotorized scooter injured in collision with other nonmotor vehicle in traffic accident

Pedestrian on sled injured in collision with other nonmotor vehicle in traffic accident

Pedestrian on snowboard injured in collision with other nonmotor vehicle in traffic accident

Pedestrian on snow-skis injured in collision with other nonmotor vehicle in traffic accident

Pedestrian in wheelchair (powered) injured in collision with other nonmotor vehicle in traffic accident

Pedestrian in motorized mobility scooter injured in collision with other nonmotor vehicle in traffic accident

√5ᵗʰ **V06.9** **Pedestrian injured in collision with other nonmotor vehicle, unspecified whether traffic or nontraffic accident**

√x7ᵗʰ **V06.90** **Pedestrian** on foot **injured in collision with other** ▽ **nonmotor vehicle, unspecified whether traffic or nontraffic accident**

Pedestrian NOS injured in collision with other nonmotor vehicle, unspecified whether traffic or nontraffic accident

√x7ᵗʰ **V06.91** **Pedestrian** on roller-skates **injured in collision** ▽ **with other nonmotor vehicle, unspecified whether traffic or nontraffic accident**

√x7ᵗʰ **V06.92** **Pedestrian** on skateboard **injured in collision** ▽ **with other nonmotor vehicle, unspecified whether traffic or nontraffic accident**

√x7ᵗʰ **V06.99** **Pedestrian with other** conveyance **injured in** ▽ **collision with other nonmotor vehicle, unspecified whether traffic or nontraffic accident**

Pedestrian with babystroller injured in collision with other nonmotor vehicle, unspecified whether traffic or nontraffic accident

Pedestrian on ice-skates injured in collision with other nonmotor vehicle, unspecified whether traffic or nontraffic accident

Pedestrian on nonmotorized scooter injured in collision with other nonmotor vehicle, unspecified whether traffic or nontraffic accident

Pedestrian on sled injured in collision with other nonmotor vehicle, unspecified whether traffic or nontraffic accident

Pedestrian on snowboard injured in collision with other nonmotor vehicle, unspecified whether traffic or nontraffic accident

Pedestrian on snow-skis injured in collision with other nonmotor vehicle, unspecified whether traffic or nontraffic accident

Pedestrian in wheelchair (powered) injured in collision with other nonmotor vehicle, unspecified whether traffic or nontraffic accident

Pedestrian in motorized mobility scooter injured in collision with other nonmotor vehicle, unspecified whether traffic or nontraffic accident

√4ᵗʰ **V09** **Pedestrian injured in other and unspecified transport accidents**

√5ᵗʰ **V09.0** **Pedestrian injured in** nontraffic **accident involving** other **and unspecified motor vehicles**

√x7ᵗʰ **V09.00** **Pedestrian injured in nontraffic accident** ▽ **involving unspecified motor vehicles**

√x7ᵗʰ **V09.01** **Pedestrian injured in nontraffic accident involving** military **vehicle**

√x7ᵗʰ **V09.09** **Pedestrian injured in nontraffic accident involving other motor vehicles**

Pedestrian injured in nontraffic accident by special vehicle

√x7ᵗʰ **V09.1** **Pedestrian injured in unspecified** nontraffic **accident** ▽

√5ᵗʰ **V09.2** **Pedestrian injured in** traffic accident **involving other and unspecified motor vehicles**

√x7ᵗʰ **V09.20** **Pedestrian injured in traffic accident involving** ▽ **unspecified motor vehicles**

√x7ᵗʰ **V09.21** **Pedestrian injured in traffic accident involving** military vehicle

√x7ᵗʰ **V09.29** **Pedestrian injured in traffic accident involving other motor vehicles**

√x7ᵗʰ **V09.3** **Pedestrian injured in unspecified** traffic **accident** ▽

√x7ᵗʰ **V09.9** **Pedestrian injured in unspecified** transport **accident** ▽

Pedal cycle rider injured in transport accident (V10-V19)

INCLUDES any non-motorized vehicle, excluding an animal-drawn vehicle, or a sidecar or trailer attached to the pedal cycle

EXCLUDES 2 rupture of pedal cycle tire (W37.0)

> The appropriate 7th character is to be added to each code from categories V10-V19.
> A   initial encounter
> D   subsequent encounter
> S   sequela

√4ᵗʰ **V10** **Pedal cycle rider injured in collision with pedestrian or animal**

EXCLUDES 1 pedal cycle rider collision with animal-drawn vehicle or animal being ridden (V16.-)

√x7ᵗʰ **V10.0** **Pedal cycle** driver **injured in collision with pedestrian or animal** in nontraffic accident

√x7ᵗʰ **V10.1** **Pedal cycle** passenger **injured in collision with pedestrian or animal** in nontraffic accident

√x7ᵗʰ **V10.2** **Unspecified pedal cyclist injured in collision with** ▽ **pedestrian or animal** in nontraffic accident

√x7ᵗʰ **V10.3** Person boarding or alighting **a pedal cycle injured in colli** **with pedestrian or animal**

√x7ᵗʰ **V10.4** **Pedal cycle** driver **injured in collision with pedest animal** in traffic accident

√x7ᵗʰ **V10.5** **Pedal cycle** passenger **injured in collisi animal** in traffic accident

√x7ᵗʰ **V10.9** **Unspecified pedal cyclist injured pedestrian or animal** in traffi

√4ᵗʰ **V11 Pedal cycle rider injured in collision with other pedal cycle**

√x7ᵗʰ **V11.0** Pedal cycle driver injured in collision with other pedal cycle in nontraffic accident

√x7ᵗʰ **V11.1** Pedal cycle passenger injured in collision with other pedal cycle in nontraffic accident

√x7ᵗʰ **V11.2** Unspecified pedal cyclist injured in collision with other pedal cycle in nontraffic accident ▽

√x7ᵗʰ **V11.3** Person boarding or alighting a pedal cycle injured in collision with other pedal cycle

√x7ᵗʰ **V11.4** Pedal cycle driver injured in collision with other pedal cycle in traffic accident

√x7ᵗʰ **V11.5** Pedal cycle passenger injured in collision with other pedal cycle in traffic accident

√x7ᵗʰ **V11.9** Unspecified pedal cyclist injured in collision with other pedal cycle in traffic accident ▽

√4ᵗʰ **V12 Pedal cycle rider injured in collision with two- or three-wheeled motor vehicle**

√x7ᵗʰ **V12.0** Pedal cycle driver injured in collision with two- or three-wheeled motor vehicle in nontraffic accident

√x7ᵗʰ **V12.1** Pedal cycle passenger injured in collision with two- or three-wheeled motor vehicle in nontraffic accident

√x7ᵗʰ **V12.2** Unspecified pedal cyclist injured in collision with two- or three-wheeled motor vehicle in nontraffic accident ▽

√x7ᵗʰ **V12.3** Person boarding or alighting a pedal cycle injured in collision with two- or three-wheeled motor vehicle

√x7ᵗʰ **V12.4** Pedal cycle driver injured in collision with two- or three-wheeled motor vehicle in traffic accident

√x7ᵗʰ **V12.5** Pedal cycle passenger injured in collision with two- or three-wheeled motor vehicle in traffic accident

√x7ᵗʰ **V12.9** Unspecified pedal cyclist injured in collision with two- or three-wheeled motor vehicle in traffic accident ▽

√4ᵗʰ **V13 Pedal cycle rider injured in collision with car, pick-up truck or van**

√x7ᵗʰ **V13.0** Pedal cycle driver injured in collision with car, pick-up truck or van in nontraffic accident

√x7ᵗʰ **V13.1** Pedal cycle passenger injured in collision with car, pick-up truck or van in nontraffic accident

√x7ᵗʰ **V13.2** Unspecified pedal cyclist injured in collision with car, pick-up truck or van in nontraffic accident ▽

√x7ᵗʰ **V13.3** Person boarding or alighting a pedal cycle injured in collision with car, pick-up truck or van

√x7ᵗʰ **V13.4** Pedal cycle driver injured in collision with car, pick-up truck or van in traffic accident

√x7ᵗʰ **V13.5** Pedal cycle passenger injured in collision with car, pick-up truck or van in traffic accident

√x7ᵗʰ **V13.9** Unspecified pedal cyclist injured in collision with car, pick-up truck or van in traffic accident ▽

√4ᵗʰ **V14 Pedal cycle rider injured in collision with heavy transport vehicle or bus**

> **EXCLUDES 1** *pedal cycle rider injured in collision with military vehicle (V19.81)*

√x7ᵗʰ **V14.0** Pedal cycle driver injured in collision with heavy transport vehicle or bus in nontraffic accident

√x7ᵗʰ **V14.1** Pedal cycle passenger injured in collision with heavy transport vehicle or bus in nontraffic accident

√x7ᵗʰ **V14.2** Unspecified pedal cyclist injured in collision with heavy transport ~~vehicle or bus~~ in nontraffic accident ▽

√x7ᵗʰ **V14.3** ~~...ghting~~ a pedal cycle injured in collision ~~...icle or bus~~

~~...ed in collision with heavy transport ...cident~~

~~...ed in collision with heavy ...affic accident~~

~~...ed in collision with heavy ▽ ...ffic accident~~

~~...with railway train or railway~~

~~...ion with railway train or ...nt~~

~~...lision with railway train or~~

~~...llision with railway ▽ ...cident~~

√x7ᵗʰ **V15.3** Person boarding or alighting a pedal cycle injured in collision with railway train or railway vehicle

√x7ᵗʰ **V15.4** Pedal cycle driver injured in collision with railway train or railway vehicle in traffic accident

√x7ᵗʰ **V15.5** Pedal cycle passenger injured in collision with railway train or railway vehicle in traffic accident

√x7ᵗʰ **V15.9** Unspecified pedal cyclist injured in collision with railway train or railway vehicle in traffic accident ▽

√4ᵗʰ **V16 Pedal cycle rider injured in collision with other nonmotor vehicle**

> **INCLUDES** collision with animal-drawn vehicle, animal being ridden, streetcar

√x7ᵗʰ **V16.0** Pedal cycle driver injured in collision with other nonmotor vehicle in nontraffic accident

√x7ᵗʰ **V16.1** Pedal cycle passenger injured in collision with other nonmotor vehicle in nontraffic accident

√x7ᵗʰ **V16.2** Unspecified pedal cyclist injured in collision with other nonmotor vehicle in nontraffic accident ▽

√x7ᵗʰ **V16.3** Person boarding or alighting a pedal cycle injured in collision with other nonmotor vehicle in nontraffic accident

√x7ᵗʰ **V16.4** Pedal cycle driver injured in collision with other nonmotor vehicle in traffic accident

√x7ᵗʰ **V16.5** Pedal cycle passenger injured in collision with other nonmotor vehicle in traffic accident

√x7ᵗʰ **V16.9** Unspecified pedal cyclist injured in collision with other nonmotor vehicle in traffic accident ▽

√4ᵗʰ **V17 Pedal cycle rider injured in collision with fixed or stationary object**

√x7ᵗʰ **V17.0** Pedal cycle driver injured in collision with fixed or stationary object in nontraffic accident

√x7ᵗʰ **V17.1** Pedal cycle passenger injured in collision with fixed or stationary object in nontraffic accident

√x7ᵗʰ **V17.2** Unspecified pedal cyclist injured in collision with fixed or stationary object in nontraffic accident ▽

√x7ᵗʰ **V17.3** Person boarding or alighting a pedal cycle injured in collision with fixed or stationary object

√x7ᵗʰ **V17.4** Pedal cycle driver injured in collision with fixed or stationary object in traffic accident

√x7ᵗʰ **V17.5** Pedal cycle passenger injured in collision with fixed or stationary object in traffic accident

√x7ᵗʰ **V17.9** Unspecified pedal cyclist injured in collision with fixed or stationary object in traffic accident ▽

√4ᵗʰ **V18 Pedal cycle rider injured in noncollision transport accident**

> **INCLUDES** fall or thrown from pedal cycle (without antecedent collision)
> overturning pedal cycle NOS
> overturning pedal cycle without collision

√x7ᵗʰ **V18.0** Pedal cycle driver injured in noncollision transport accident in nontraffic accident

√x7ᵗʰ **V18.1** Pedal cycle passenger injured in noncollision transport accident in nontraffic accident

√x7ᵗʰ **V18.2** Unspecified pedal cyclist injured in noncollision transport accident in nontraffic accident ▽

√x7ᵗʰ **V18.3** Person boarding or alighting a pedal cycle injured in noncollision transport accident

√x7ᵗʰ **V18.4** Pedal cycle driver injured in noncollision transport accident in traffic accident

√x7ᵗʰ **V18.5** Pedal cycle passenger injured in noncollision transport accident in traffic accident

√x7ᵗʰ **V18.9** Unspecified pedal cyclist injured in noncollision transport accident in traffic accident ▽

√4ᵗʰ **V19 Pedal cycle rider injured in other and unspecified transport accidents**

√5ᵗʰ **V19.0** Pedal cycle driver injured in collision with other and unspecified motor vehicles in nontraffic accident

√x7ᵗʰ **V19.00** Pedal cycle driver injured in collision with unspecified motor vehicles in nontraffic accident ▽

√x7ᵗʰ **V19.09** Pedal cycle driver injured in collision with other motor vehicles in nontraffic accident

√5ᵗʰ **V19.1** Pedal cycle passenger injured in collision with other and unspecified motor vehicles in nontraffic accident

√x7ᵗʰ **V19.10** Pedal cycle passenger injured in collision with unspecified motor vehicles in nontraffic accident ▽

√x7ᵗʰ **V19.19** Pedal cycle passenger injured in collision with other motor vehicles in nontraffic accident

NRS Nonroutine supply Dx   **NC Dx** Noncancer Dx   **PDx** Primary Dx   ▶◀ Revised Text   ● New Code   ▲ Revised Title

☑5ᵗʰ **V19.2** Unspecified pedal cyclist injured in collision with other and unspecified motor vehicles in nontraffic accident

    ☑x7ᵗʰ **V19.20** Unspecified pedal cyclist injured in collision with ▽ unspecified motor vehicles in nontraffic accident
Pedal cycle collision NOS, nontraffic

    ☑x7ᵗʰ **V19.29** Unspecified pedal cyclist injured in collision with ▽ other motor vehicles in nontraffic accident

☑x7ᵗʰ **V19.3** Pedal cyclist (driver) (passenger) injured in unspecified ▽ nontraffic accident
Pedal cycle accident NOS, nontraffic
Pedal cyclist injured in nontraffic accident NOS

☑5ᵗʰ **V19.4** Pedal cycle driver injured in collision with other and unspecified motor vehicles in traffic accident

    ☑x7ᵗʰ **V19.40** Pedal cycle driver injured in collision with ▽ unspecified motor vehicles in traffic accident

    ☑x7ᵗʰ **V19.49** Pedal cycle driver injured in collision with other motor vehicles in traffic accident

☑5ᵗʰ **V19.5** Pedal cycle passenger injured in collision with other and unspecified motor vehicles in traffic accident

    ☑x7ᵗʰ **V19.50** Pedal cycle passenger injured in collision with ▽ unspecified motor vehicles in traffic accident

    ☑x7ᵗʰ **V19.59** Pedal cycle passenger injured in collision with other motor vehicles in traffic accident

☑5ᵗʰ **V19.6** Unspecified pedal cyclist injured in collision with other and unspecified motor vehicles in traffic accident

    ☑x7ᵗʰ **V19.60** Unspecified pedal cyclist injured in collision ▽ with unspecified motor vehicles in traffic accident
Pedal cycle collision NOS (traffic)

    ☑x7ᵗʰ **V19.69** Unspecified pedal cyclist injured in collision ▽ with other motor vehicles in traffic accident

☑5ᵗʰ **V19.8** Pedal cyclist (driver) (passenger) injured in other specified transport accidents

    ☑x7ᵗʰ **V19.81** Pedal cyclist (driver) (passenger) injured in transport accident with military vehicle

    ☑x7ᵗʰ **V19.88** Pedal cyclist (driver) (passenger) injured in other specified transport accidents

☑x7ᵗʰ **V19.9** Pedal cyclist (driver) (passenger) injured in unspecified ▽ traffic accident
Pedal cycle accident NOS

Motorcycle rider injured in transport accident (V20-V29)

INCLUDES   moped
motorcycle with sidecar
motorized bicycle
motor scooter

EXCLUDES 1   three-wheeled motor vehicle (V30-V39)

The appropriate 7th character is to be added to each code from categories V20-V29.
A   initial encounter
D   subsequent encounter
S   sequela

☑4ᵗʰ **V20** Motorcycle rider injured in collision with pedestrian or animal

    EXCLUDES 1   motorcycle rider collision with animal-drawn vehicle or animal being ridden (V26.-)

    ☑x7ᵗʰ **V20.0** Motorcycle driver injured in collision with pedestrian or animal in nontraffic accident

    ☑x7ᵗʰ **V20.1** Motorcycle passenger injured in collision with pedestrian or animal in nontraffic accident

    ☑x7ᵗʰ **V20.2** Unspecified motorcycle rider injured in collision with ▽ pedestrian or animal in nontraffic accident

    ☑x7ᵗʰ **V20.3** Person boarding or alighting a motorcycle injured in collision with pedestrian or animal

    ☑x7ᵗʰ **V20.4** Motorcycle driver injured in collision with pedestrian or animal in traffic accident

    ☑x7ᵗʰ **V20.5** Motorcycle passenger injured in collision with pedestrian or animal in traffic accident

    ☑x7ᵗʰ **V20.9** Unspecified motorcycle rider injured in collision with ▽ pedestrian or animal in traffic accident

☑4ᵗʰ **V21** Motorcycle rider injured in collision with pedal cycle

    ☑x7ᵗʰ **V21.0** Motorcycle driver injured in collision with pedal cycle in nontraffic accident

    ☑x7ᵗʰ **V21.1** Motorcycle passenger injured in collision with pedal cycle in nontraffic accident

    ☑x7ᵗʰ **V21.2** Unspecified motorcycle rider injured in collision with ▽ pedal cycle in nontraffic accident

    ☑x7ᵗʰ **V21.3** Person boarding or alighting a motorcycle injured in collision with pedal cycle

    ☑x7ᵗʰ **V21.4** Motorcycle driver injured in collision with pedal cycle in traffic accident

    ☑x7ᵗʰ **V21.5** Motorcycle passenger injured in collision with pedal cycle in traffic accident

    ☑x7ᵗʰ **V21.9** Unspecified motorcycle rider injured in collision with ▽ pedal cycle in traffic accident

☑4ᵗʰ **V22** Motorcycle rider injured in collision with two- or three-wheeled motor vehicle

    ☑x7ᵗʰ **V22.0** Motorcycle driver injured in collision with two- or three-wheeled motor vehicle in nontraffic accident

    ☑x7ᵗʰ **V22.1** Motorcycle passenger injured in collision with two- or three-wheeled motor vehicle in nontraffic accident

    ☑x7ᵗʰ **V22.2** Unspecified motorcycle rider injured in collision with ▽ two- or three-wheeled motor vehicle in nontraffic accident

    ☑x7ᵗʰ **V22.3** Person boarding or alighting a motorcycle injured in collision with two- or three-wheeled motor vehicle

    ☑x7ᵗʰ **V22.4** Motorcycle driver injured in collision with two- or three-wheeled motor vehicle in traffic accident

    ☑x7ᵗʰ **V22.5** Motorcycle passenger injured in collision with two- or three-wheeled motor vehicle in traffic accident

    ☑x7ᵗʰ **V22.9** Unspecified motorcycle rider injured in collision with ▽ two- or three-wheeled motor vehicle in traffic accident

☑4ᵗʰ **V23** Motorcycle rider injured in collision with car, pick-up truck or van

    ☑x7ᵗʰ **V23.0** Motorcycle driver injured in collision with car, pick-up truck or van in nontraffic accident

    ☑x7ᵗʰ **V23.1** Motorcycle passenger injured in collision with car, pick-up truck or van in nontraffic accident

    ☑x7ᵗʰ **V23.2** Unspecified motorcycle rider injured in collision with car, ▽ pick-up truck or van in nontraffic accident

    ☑x7ᵗʰ **V23.3** Person boarding or alighting a motorcycle injured in collision with car, pick-up truck or van

    ☑x7ᵗʰ **V23.4** Motorcycle driver injured in collision with car, pick-up truck or van in traffic accident

    ☑x7ᵗʰ **V23.5** Motorcycle passenger injured in collision with car, pick-up truck or van in traffic accident

    ☑x7ᵗʰ **V23.9** Unspecified motorcycle rider injured in collision with car, ▽ pick-up truck or van in traffic accident

☑4ᵗʰ **V24** Motorcycle rider injured in collision with heavy transport vehicle or bus

    EXCLUDES 1   motorcycle rider injured in collision with military vehicle (V29.81)

    ☑x7ᵗʰ **V24.0** Motorcycle driver injured in collision with heavy transport vehicle or bus in nontraffic accident

    ☑x7ᵗʰ **V24.1** Motorcycle passenger injured in collision with heavy transport vehicle or bus in nontraffic accident

    ☑x7ᵗʰ **V24.2** Unspecified motorcycle rider injured in collision with ▽ heavy transport vehicle or bus in nontraffic accident

    ☑x7ᵗʰ **V24.3** Person boarding or alighting a motorcycle injured in collision with heavy transport vehicle or bus

    ☑x7ᵗʰ **V24.4** Motorcycle driver injured in collision with heavy transport vehicle or bus in traffic accident

    ☑x7ᵗʰ **V24.5** Motorcycle passenger injured in collision with heavy transport vehicle or bus in traffic accident

    ☑x7ᵗʰ **V24.9** Unspecified motorcycle rider injured in collision with ▽ heavy transport vehicle or bus in traffic accident

☑4ᵗʰ **V25** Motorcycle rider injured in collision with railway train or railway vehicle

    ☑x7ᵗʰ **V25.0** Motorcycle driver injured in collision with railway train or railway vehicle in nontraffic accident

    ☑x7ᵗʰ **V25.1** Motorcycle passenger injured in collision with railway t[rain or] railway vehicle in nontraffic accident

    ☑x7ᵗʰ **V25.2** Unspecified motorcycle rider injured in collisio[n with] railway train or railway vehicle in nontraffi[c]

    ☑x7ᵗʰ **V25.3** Person boarding or alighting a motor[cycle] with railway train or railway vehic[le]

    ☑x7ᵗʰ **V25.4** Motorcycle driver injured in co[llision] railway vehicle in traffic ac[cident]

Chapter 20. External Causes of Morbidity

√x7ᵗʰ **V25.5** Motorcycle passenger injured in collision with railway train or railway vehicle in traffic accident

√x7ᵗʰ **V25.9** Unspecified motorcycle rider injured in collision with railway train or railway vehicle in traffic accident ▽

√4ᵗʰ **V26** Motorcycle rider injured in collision with other nonmotor vehicle
     INCLUDES   collision with animal-drawn vehicle, animal being ridden, streetcar

√x7ᵗʰ **V26.0** Motorcycle driver injured in collision with other nonmotor vehicle in nontraffic accident

√x7ᵗʰ **V26.1** Motorcycle passenger injured in collision with other nonmotor vehicle in nontraffic accident

√x7ᵗʰ **V26.2** Unspecified motorcycle rider injured in collision with other nonmotor vehicle in nontraffic accident ▽

√x7ᵗʰ **V26.3** Person boarding or alighting a motorcycle injured in collision with other nonmotor vehicle

√x7ᵗʰ **V26.4** Motorcycle driver injured in collision with other nonmotor vehicle in traffic accident

√x7ᵗʰ **V26.5** Motorcycle passenger injured in collision with other nonmotor vehicle in traffic accident

√x7ᵗʰ **V26.9** Unspecified motorcycle rider injured in collision with other nonmotor vehicle in traffic accident ▽

√4ᵗʰ **V27** Motorcycle rider injured in collision with fixed or stationary object

√x7ᵗʰ **V27.0** Motorcycle driver injured in collision with fixed or stationary object in nontraffic accident

√x7ᵗʰ **V27.1** Motorcycle passenger injured in collision with fixed or stationary object in nontraffic accident

√x7ᵗʰ **V27.2** Unspecified motorcycle rider injured in collision with fixed or stationary object in nontraffic accident ▽

√x7ᵗʰ **V27.3** Person boarding or alighting a motorcycle injured in collision with fixed or stationary object

√x7ᵗʰ **V27.4** Motorcycle driver injured in collision with fixed or stationary object in traffic accident

√x7ᵗʰ **V27.5** Motorcycle passenger injured in collision with fixed or stationary object in traffic accident

√x7ᵗʰ **V27.9** Unspecified motorcycle rider injured in collision with fixed or stationary object in traffic accident ▽

√4ᵗʰ **V28** Motorcycle rider injured in noncollision transport accident
     INCLUDES   fall or thrown from motorcycle (without antecedent collision)
               overturning motorcycle NOS
               overturning motorcycle without collision

√x7ᵗʰ **V28.0** Motorcycle driver injured in noncollision transport accident in nontraffic accident

√x7ᵗʰ **V28.1** Motorcycle passenger injured in noncollision transport accident in nontraffic accident

√x7ᵗʰ **V28.2** Unspecified motorcycle rider injured in noncollision transport accident in nontraffic accident ▽

√x7ᵗʰ **V28.3** Person boarding or alighting a motorcycle injured in noncollision transport accident

√x7ᵗʰ **V28.4** Motorcycle driver injured in noncollision transport accident in traffic accident

√x7ᵗʰ **V28.5** Motorcycle passenger injured in noncollision transport accident in traffic accident

√x7ᵗʰ **V28.9** Unspecified motorcycle rider injured in noncollision transport accident in traffic accident ▽

√4ᵗʰ **V29** Motorcycle rider injured in other and unspecified transport accidents

√5ᵗʰ **V29.0** [obscured] injured in collision with other and [obscured] les in nontraffic accident

√5ᵗʰ **V29.2** Unspecified motorcycle rider injured in collision with other and unspecified motor vehicles in nontraffic accident

√x7ᵗʰ **V29.20** Unspecified motorcycle rider injured in collision with unspecified motor vehicles in nontraffic accident ▽
         Motorcycle collision NOS, nontraffic

√x7ᵗʰ **V29.29** Unspecified motorcycle rider injured in collision with other motor vehicles in nontraffic accident ▽

√x7ᵗʰ **V29.3** Motorcycle rider (driver) (passenger) injured in unspecified nontraffic accident ▽
         Motorcycle accident NOS, nontraffic
         Motorcycle rider injured in nontraffic accident NOS

√5ᵗʰ **V29.4** Motorcycle driver injured in collision with other and unspecified motor vehicles in traffic accident

√x7ᵗʰ **V29.40** Motorcycle driver injured in collision with unspecified motor vehicles in traffic accident ▽

√x7ᵗʰ **V29.49** Motorcycle driver injured in collision with other motor vehicles in traffic accident

√5ᵗʰ **V29.5** Motorcycle passenger injured in collision with other and unspecified motor vehicles in traffic accident

√x7ᵗʰ **V29.50** Motorcycle passenger injured in collision with unspecified motor vehicles in traffic accident ▽

√x7ᵗʰ **V29.59** Motorcycle passenger injured in collision with other motor vehicles in traffic accident

√5ᵗʰ **V29.6** Unspecified motorcycle rider injured in collision with other and unspecified motor vehicles in traffic accident

√x7ᵗʰ **V29.60** Unspecified motorcycle rider injured in collision with unspecified motor vehicles in traffic accident ▽
         Motorcycle collision NOS (traffic)

√x7ᵗʰ **V29.69** Unspecified motorcycle rider injured in collision with other motor vehicles in traffic accident ▽

√5ᵗʰ **V29.8** Motorcycle rider (driver) (passenger) injured in other specified transport accidents

√x7ᵗʰ **V29.81** Motorcycle rider (driver) (passenger) injured in transport accident with military vehicle

√x7ᵗʰ **V29.88** Motorcycle rider (driver) (passenger) injured in other specified transport accidents

√x7ᵗʰ **V29.9** Motorcycle rider (driver) (passenger) injured in unspecified traffic accident ▽
         Motorcycle accident NOS

Occupant of three-wheeled motor vehicle injured in transport accident (V30-V39)

     INCLUDES   motorized tricycle
               motorized rickshaw
               three-wheeled motor car
     EXCLUDES 1   all-terrain vehicles (V86.-)
               motorcycle with sidecar (V20-V29)
               vehicle designed primarily for off-road use (V86.-)

> The appropriate 7th character is to be added to each code from categories V30-V39.
> A   initial encounter
> D   subsequent encounter
> S   sequela

√4ᵗʰ **V30** Occupant of three-wheeled motor vehicle injured in collision with pedestrian or animal
     EXCLUDES 1   three-wheeled motor vehicle collision with animal-drawn vehicle or animal being ridden (V36.-)

√x7ᵗʰ **V30.0** Driver of three-wheeled motor vehicle injured in collision with pedestrian or animal in nontraffic accident

√x7ᵗʰ **V30.1** Passenger in three-wheeled motor vehicle injured in collision with pedestrian or animal in nontraffic accident

√x7ᵗʰ **V30.2** Person on outside of three-wheeled motor vehicle injured in collision with pedestrian or animal in nontraffic accident

√x7ᵗʰ **V30.3** Unspecified occupant of three-wheeled motor vehicle injured in collision with pedestrian or animal in nontraffic accident ▽

√x7ᵗʰ **V30.4** Person boarding or alighting a three-wheeled motor vehicle injured in collision with pedestrian or animal

√x7ᵗʰ **V30.5** Driver of three-wheeled motor vehicle injured in collision with pedestrian or animal in traffic accident

√x7ᵗʰ **V30.6** Passenger in three-wheeled motor vehicle injured in collision with pedestrian or animal in traffic accident

√x7ᵗʰ **V30.7** Person on outside of three-wheeled motor vehicle injured in collision with pedestrian or animal in traffic accident

√x7ᵗʰ **V30.9** Unspecified occupant of three-wheeled motor vehicle injured in collision with pedestrian or animal in traffic accident ▽

√4ᵗʰ **V31** Occupant of three-wheeled motor vehicle injured in collision with pedal cycle

√x7ᵗʰ **V31.0** Driver of three-wheeled motor vehicle injured in collision with pedal cycle in nontraffic accident

√x7ᵗʰ **V31.1** Passenger in three-wheeled motor vehicle injured in collision with pedal cycle in nontraffic accident

√x7ᵗʰ **V31.2** Person on outside of three-wheeled motor vehicle injured in collision with pedal cycle in nontraffic accident

√x7ᵗʰ **V31.3** Unspecified occupant of three-wheeled motor vehicle injured in collision with pedal cycle in nontraffic accident ▽

√x7ᵗʰ **V31.4** Person boarding or alighting a three-wheeled motor vehicle injured in collision with pedal cycle

√x7ᵗʰ **V31.5** Driver of three-wheeled motor vehicle injured in collision with pedal cycle in traffic accident

√x7ᵗʰ **V31.6** Passenger in three-wheeled motor vehicle injured in collision with pedal cycle in traffic accident

√x7ᵗʰ **V31.7** Person on outside of three-wheeled motor vehicle injured in collision with pedal cycle in traffic accident

√x7ᵗʰ **V31.9** Unspecified occupant of three-wheeled motor vehicle injured in collision with pedal cycle in traffic accident ▽

√4ᵗʰ **V32** Occupant of three-wheeled motor vehicle injured in collision with two- or three-wheeled motor vehicle

√x7ᵗʰ **V32.0** Driver of three-wheeled motor vehicle injured in collision with two- or three-wheeled motor vehicle in nontraffic accident

√x7ᵗʰ **V32.1** Passenger in three-wheeled motor vehicle injured in collision with two- or three-wheeled motor vehicle in nontraffic accident

√x7ᵗʰ **V32.2** Person on outside of three-wheeled motor vehicle injured in collision with two- or three-wheeled motor vehicle in nontraffic accident

√x7ᵗʰ **V32.3** Unspecified occupant of three-wheeled motor vehicle injured in collision with two- or three-wheeled motor vehicle in nontraffic accident ▽

√x7ᵗʰ **V32.4** Person boarding or alighting a three-wheeled motor vehicle injured in collision with two- or three-wheeled motor vehicle

√x7ᵗʰ **V32.5** Driver of three-wheeled motor vehicle injured in collision with two- or three-wheeled motor vehicle in traffic accident

√x7ᵗʰ **V32.6** Passenger in three-wheeled motor vehicle injured in collision with two- or three-wheeled motor vehicle in traffic accident

√x7ᵗʰ **V32.7** Person on outside of three-wheeled motor vehicle injured in collision with two- or three-wheeled motor vehicle in traffic accident

√x7ᵗʰ **V32.9** Unspecified occupant of three-wheeled motor vehicle injured in collision with two- or three-wheeled motor vehicle in traffic accident ▽

√4ᵗʰ **V33** Occupant of three-wheeled motor vehicle injured in collision with car, pick-up truck or van

√x7ᵗʰ **V33.0** Driver of three-wheeled motor vehicle injured in collision with car, pick-up truck or van in nontraffic accident

√x7ᵗʰ **V33.1** Passenger in three-wheeled motor vehicle injured in collision with car, pick-up truck or van in nontraffic accident

√x7ᵗʰ **V33.2** Person on outside of three-wheeled motor vehicle injured in collision with car, pick-up truck or van in nontraffic accident

√x7ᵗʰ **V33.3** Unspecified occupant of three-wheeled motor vehicle injured in collision with car, pick-up truck or van in nontraffic accident ▽

√x7ᵗʰ **V33.4** Person boarding or alighting a three-wheeled motor vehicle injured in collision with car, pick-up truck or van

√x7ᵗʰ **V33.5** Driver of three-wheeled motor vehicle injured in collision with car, pick-up truck or van in traffic accident

√x7ᵗʰ **V33.6** Passenger in three-wheeled motor vehicle injured in collision with car, pick-up truck or van in traffic accident

√x7ᵗʰ **V33.7** Person on outside of three-wheeled motor vehicle injured in collision with car, pick-up truck or van in traffic accident

√x7ᵗʰ **V33.9** Unspecified occupant of three-wheeled motor vehicle injured in collision with car, pick-up truck or van in traffic accident ▽

√4ᵗʰ **V34** Occupant of three-wheeled motor vehicle injured in collision with heavy transport vehicle or bus

EXCLUDES 1 occupant of three-wheeled motor vehicle injured in collision with military vehicle (V39.81)

√x7ᵗʰ **V34.0** Driver of three-wheeled motor vehicle injured in collision with heavy transport vehicle or bus in nontraffic accident

√x7ᵗʰ **V34.1** Passenger in three-wheeled motor vehicle injured in collision with heavy transport vehicle or bus in nontraffic accident

√x7ᵗʰ **V34.2** Person on outside of three-wheeled motor vehicle injured in collision with heavy transport vehicle or bus in nontraffic accident

√x7ᵗʰ **V34.3** Unspecified occupant of three-wheeled motor vehicle injured in collision with heavy transport vehicle or bus in nontraffic accident ▽

√x7ᵗʰ **V34.4** Person boarding or alighting a three-wheeled motor vehicle injured in collision with heavy transport vehicle or bus

√x7ᵗʰ **V34.5** Driver of three-wheeled motor vehicle injured in collision with heavy transport vehicle or bus in traffic accident

√x7ᵗʰ **V34.6** Passenger in three-wheeled motor vehicle injured in collision with heavy transport vehicle or bus in traffic accident

√x7ᵗʰ **V34.7** Person on outside of three-wheeled motor vehicle injured in collision with heavy transport vehicle or bus in traffic accident

√x7ᵗʰ **V34.9** Unspecified occupant of three-wheeled motor vehicle injured in collision with heavy transport vehicle or bus in traffic accident ▽

√4ᵗʰ **V35** Occupant of three-wheeled motor vehicle injured in collision with railway train or railway vehicle

√x7ᵗʰ **V35.0** Driver of three-wheeled motor vehicle injured in collision with railway train or railway vehicle in nontraffic accident

√x7ᵗʰ **V35.1** Passenger in three-wheeled motor vehicle injured in collision with railway train or railway vehicle in nontraffic accident

√x7ᵗʰ **V35.2** Person on outside of three-wheeled motor vehicle injured in collision with railway train or railway vehicle in nontraffic accident

√x7ᵗʰ **V35.3** Unspecified occupant of three-wheeled motor vehicle injured in collision with railway train or railway vehicle in nontraffic accident ▽

√x7ᵗʰ **V35.4** Person boarding or alighting a three-wheeled motor vehicle injured in collision with railway train or railway vehicle

√x7ᵗʰ **V35.5** Driver of three-wheeled motor vehicle injured in collision with railway train or railway vehicle in traffic accident

√x7ᵗʰ **V35.6** Passenger in three-wheeled motor vehicle injured in collision with railway train or railway vehicle in traffic accident

√x7ᵗʰ **V35.7** Person on outside of three-wheeled motor vehicle injured in collision with railway train or railway vehicle in traffic accident

√x7ᵗʰ **V35.9** Unspecified occupant of three-wheeled motor vehicle injured in collision with railway train or railway vehicle in traffic accident ▽

√4ᵗʰ **V36** Occupant of three-wheeled motor vehicle injured in collision with other nonmotor vehicle

INCLUDES collision with animal-drawn vehicle, animal being ridden, streetcar

√x7ᵗʰ **V36.0** Driver of three-wheeled motor vehicle injured in collision with other nonmotor vehicle in nontraffic accident

√x7ᵗʰ **V36.1** Passenger in three-wheeled motor vehicle injured in collision with other nonmotor vehicle in nontraffic accident

√x7ᵗʰ **V36.2** Person on outside of three-wheeled motor vehicle injured in collision with other nonmotor vehicle in nontraffic accident

√x7ᵗʰ **V36.3** Unspecified occupant of three-wheeled motor vehicle injured in collision with other nonmotor vehicle in nontraffic accident ▽

√x7ᵗʰ **V36.4** Person boarding or alighting a three-wheeled motor vehicle injured in collision with other nonmotor vehicle

√x7ᵗʰ **V36.5** Driver of three-wheeled motor vehicle injured in collision with other nonmotor vehicle in traffic accident

√x7ᵗʰ **V36.6** Passenger in three-wheeled motor vehicle injured in collision with other nonmotor vehicle in traffic accident

√x7ᵗʰ **V36.7** Person on outside of three-wheeled motor vehicle injured in collision with other nonmotor vehicle in traffic accident

√x7ᵗʰ **V36.9** Unspecified occupant of three-wheeled motor vehicle injured in collision with other nonmotor vehicle in traffic accident

Chapter 20. External Causes of Morbidity

√4ᵗʰ **V37 Occupant of three-wheeled motor vehicle injured in collision with fixed or stationary object**

√x7ᵗʰ **V37.0** Driver of three-wheeled motor vehicle injured in collision with fixed or stationary object in nontraffic accident

√x7ᵗʰ **V37.1** Passenger in three-wheeled motor vehicle injured in collision with fixed or stationary object in nontraffic accident

√x7ᵗʰ **V37.2** Person on outside of three-wheeled motor vehicle injured in collision with fixed or stationary object in nontraffic accident

√x7ᵗʰ **V37.3** Unspecified occupant of three-wheeled motor vehicle injured in collision with fixed or stationary object in nontraffic accident ▽

√x7ᵗʰ **V37.4** Person boarding or alighting a three-wheeled motor vehicle injured in collision with fixed or stationary object

√x7ᵗʰ **V37.5** Driver of three-wheeled motor vehicle injured in collision with fixed or stationary object in traffic accident

√x7ᵗʰ **V37.6** Passenger in three-wheeled motor vehicle injured in collision with fixed or stationary object in traffic accident

√x7ᵗʰ **V37.7** Person on outside of three-wheeled motor vehicle injured in collision with fixed or stationary object in traffic accident

√x7ᵗʰ **V37.9** Unspecified occupant of three-wheeled motor vehicle injured in collision with fixed or stationary object in traffic accident ▽

√4ᵗʰ **V38 Occupant of three-wheeled motor vehicle injured in noncollision transport accident**

INCLUDES fall or thrown from three-wheeled motor vehicle
overturning of three-wheeled motor vehicle NOS
overturning of three-wheeled motor vehicle without collision

√x7ᵗʰ **V38.0** Driver of three-wheeled motor vehicle injured in noncollision transport accident in nontraffic accident

√x7ᵗʰ **V38.1** Passenger in three-wheeled motor vehicle injured in noncollision transport accident in nontraffic accident

√x7ᵗʰ **V38.2** Person on outside of three-wheeled motor vehicle injured in noncollision transport accident in nontraffic accident

√x7ᵗʰ **V38.3** Unspecified occupant of three-wheeled motor vehicle injured in noncollision transport accident in nontraffic accident ▽

√x7ᵗʰ **V38.4** Person boarding or alighting a three-wheeled motor vehicle injured in noncollision transport accident

√x7ᵗʰ **V38.5** Driver of three-wheeled motor vehicle injured in noncollision transport accident in traffic accident

√x7ᵗʰ **V38.6** Passenger in three-wheeled motor vehicle injured in noncollision transport accident in traffic accident

√x7ᵗʰ **V38.7** Person on outside of three-wheeled motor vehicle injured in noncollision transport accident in traffic accident

√x7ᵗʰ **V38.9** Unspecified occupant of three-wheeled motor vehicle injured in noncollision transport accident in traffic accident ▽

√4ᵗʰ **V39 Occupant of three-wheeled motor vehicle injured in other and unspecified transport accidents**

√5ᵗʰ **V39.0** Driver of three-wheeled motor vehicle injured in collision with other and unspecified motor vehicles in nontraffic accident

√x7ᵗʰ **V39.00** Driver of three-wheeled motor vehicle injured in collision with unspecified motor vehicles in nontraffic accident ▽

√x7ᵗʰ **V39.09** Driver of three-wheeled motor vehicle injured in collision with other motor vehicles in nontraffic accident

√5ᵗʰ **V39.1** Passenger in [three-wheeled] motor vehicle injured in collision with [...specified] motor vehicles in nontraffic

√x7ᵗʰ **V39.29** Unspecified occupant of three-wheeled motor vehicle injured in collision with other motor vehicles in nontraffic accident ▽

√x7ᵗʰ **V39.3** Occupant (driver) (passenger) of three-wheeled motor vehicle injured in unspecified nontraffic accident ▽

Accident NOS involving three-wheeled motor vehicle, nontraffic
Occupant of three-wheeled motor vehicle injured in nontraffic accident NOS

√5ᵗʰ **V39.4** Driver of three-wheeled motor vehicle injured in collision with other and unspecified motor vehicles in traffic accident

√x7ᵗʰ **V39.40** Driver of three-wheeled motor vehicle injured in collision with unspecified motor vehicles in traffic accident ▽

√x7ᵗʰ **V39.49** Driver of three-wheeled motor vehicle injured in collision with other motor vehicles in traffic accident

√5ᵗʰ **V39.5** Passenger in three-wheeled motor vehicle injured in collision with other and unspecified motor vehicles in traffic accident

√x7ᵗʰ **V39.50** Passenger in three-wheeled motor vehicle injured in collision with unspecified motor vehicles in traffic accident ▽

√x7ᵗʰ **V39.59** Passenger in three-wheeled motor vehicle injured in collision with other motor vehicles in traffic accident

√5ᵗʰ **V39.6** Unspecified occupant of three-wheeled motor vehicle injured in collision with other and unspecified motor vehicles in traffic accident

√x7ᵗʰ **V39.60** Unspecified occupant of three-wheeled motor vehicle injured in collision with unspecified motor vehicles in traffic accident ▽

Collision NOS involving three-wheeled motor vehicle (traffic)

√x7ᵗʰ **V39.69** Unspecified occupant of three-wheeled motor vehicle injured in collision with other motor vehicles in traffic accident ▽

√5ᵗʰ **V39.8** Occupant (driver) (passenger) of three-wheeled motor vehicle injured in other specified transport accidents

√x7ᵗʰ **V39.81** Occupant (driver) (passenger) of three-wheeled motor vehicle injured in transport accident with military vehicle

√x7ᵗʰ **V39.89** Occupant (driver) (passenger) of three-wheeled motor vehicle injured in other specified transport accidents

√x7ᵗʰ **V39.9** Occupant (driver) (passenger) of three-wheeled motor vehicle injured in unspecified traffic accident ▽

Accident NOS involving three-wheeled motor vehicle

Car occupant injured in transport accident (V40-V49)

INCLUDES a four-wheeled motor vehicle designed primarily for carrying passengers
automobile (pulling a trailer or camper)

EXCLUDES 1 bus (V50-V59)
minibus (V50-V59)
minivan (V50-V59)
motorcoach (V70-V79)
pick-up truck (V50-V59)
sport utility vehicle (SUV) (V50-V59)

The appropriate 7th character is to be added to each code from categories V40-V49.
A initial encounter
D subsequent encounter
S sequela

√4ᵗʰ **V40 Car occupant injured in collision with pedestrian or animal**

EXCLUDES 1 car collision with animal-drawn vehicle or animal being ridden (V46.-)

√x7ᵗʰ **V40.0** Car driver injured in collision with pedestrian or animal in nontraffic accident

√x7ᵗʰ **V40.1** Car passenger injured in collision with pedestrian or animal in nontraffic accident

√x7ᵗʰ **V40.2** Person on outside of car injured in collision with pedestrian or animal in nontraffic accident

√x7ᵗʰ **V40.3** Unspecified car occupant injured in collision with pedestrian or animal in nontraffic accident ▽

√x7ᵗʰ **V40.4** Person boarding or alighting a car injured in collision with pedestrian or animal

√x7ᵗʰ **V40.5** Car driver injured in collision with pedestrian or animal in traffic accident

√x7ᵗʰ **V40.6** Car passenger injured in collision with pedestrian or animal in traffic accident

√x7ᵗʰ **V40.7** Person on outside of car injured in collision with pedestrian or animal in traffic accident

√x7ᵗʰ **V40.9** Unspecified car occupant injured in collision with pedestrian or animal in traffic accident ▽

☑4ᵗʰ **V41 Car occupant injured in collision with pedal cycle**

√x7ᵗʰ **V41.0** Car driver injured in collision with pedal cycle in nontraffic accident

√x7ᵗʰ **V41.1** Car passenger injured in collision with pedal cycle in nontraffic accident

√x7ᵗʰ **V41.2** Person on outside of car injured in collision with pedal cycle in nontraffic accident

√x7ᵗʰ **V41.3** Unspecified car occupant injured in collision with pedal cycle in nontraffic accident ▽

√x7ᵗʰ **V41.4** Person boarding or alighting a car injured in collision with pedal cycle

√x7ᵗʰ **V41.5** Car driver injured in collision with pedal cycle in traffic accident

√x7ᵗʰ **V41.6** Car passenger injured in collision with pedal cycle in traffic accident

√x7ᵗʰ **V41.7** Person on outside of car injured in collision with pedal cycle in traffic accident

√x7ᵗʰ **V41.9** Unspecified car occupant injured in collision with pedal cycle in traffic accident ▽

☑4ᵗʰ **V42 Car occupant injured in collision with two- or three-wheeled motor vehicle**

√x7ᵗʰ **V42.0** Car driver injured in collision with two- or three-wheeled motor vehicle in nontraffic accident

√x7ᵗʰ **V42.1** Car passenger injured in collision with two- or three-wheeled motor vehicle in nontraffic accident

√x7ᵗʰ **V42.2** Person on outside of car injured in collision with two- or three-wheeled motor vehicle in nontraffic accident

√x7ᵗʰ **V42.3** Unspecified car occupant injured in collision with two- or three-wheeled motor vehicle in nontraffic accident ▽

√x7ᵗʰ **V42.4** Person boarding or alighting a car injured in collision with two- or three-wheeled motor vehicle

√x7ᵗʰ **V42.5** Car driver injured in collision with two- or three-wheeled motor vehicle in traffic accident

√x7ᵗʰ **V42.6** Car passenger injured in collision with two- or three-wheeled motor vehicle in traffic accident

√x7ᵗʰ **V42.7** Person on outside of car injured in collision with two- or three-wheeled motor vehicle in traffic accident

√x7ᵗʰ **V42.9** Unspecified car occupant injured in collision with two- or three-wheeled motor vehicle in traffic accident ▽

☑4ᵗʰ **V43 Car occupant injured in collision with car, pick-up truck or van**

√5ᵗʰ **V43.0** Car driver injured in collision with car, pick-up truck or van in nontraffic accident

√x7ᵗʰ **V43.01** Car driver injured in collision with sport utility vehicle in nontraffic accident

√x7ᵗʰ **V43.02** Car driver injured in collision with other type car in nontraffic accident

√x7ᵗʰ **V43.03** Car driver injured in collision with pick-up truck in nontraffic accident

√x7ᵗʰ **V43.04** Car driver injured in collision with van in nontraffic accident

√5ᵗʰ **V43.1** Car passenger injured in collision with car, pick-up truck or van in nontraffic accident

√x7ᵗʰ **V43.11** Car passenger injured in collision with sport utility vehicle in nontraffic accident

√x7ᵗʰ **V43.12** Car passenger injured in collision with other type car in nontraffic accident

√x7ᵗʰ **V43.13** Car passenger injured in collision with pick-up in nontraffic accident

√x7ᵗʰ **V43.14** Car passenger injured in collision with van in nontraffic accident

√5ᵗʰ **V43.2** Person on outside of car injured in collision with car, pick-up truck or van in nontraffic accident

√x7ᵗʰ **V43.21** Person on outside of car injured in collision with sport utility vehicle in nontraffic accident

√x7ᵗʰ **V43.22** Person on outside of car injured in collision with other type car in nontraffic accident

√x7ᵗʰ **V43.23** Person on outside of car injured in collision with pick-up truck in nontraffic accident

√x7ᵗʰ **V43.24** Person on outside of car injured in collision with van in nontraffic accident

√5ᵗʰ **V43.3** Unspecified car occupant injured in collision with car, pick-up truck or van in nontraffic accident

√x7ᵗʰ **V43.31** Unspecified car occupant injured in collision with sport utility vehicle in nontraffic accident ▽

√x7ᵗʰ **V43.32** Unspecified car occupant injured in collision with other type car in nontraffic accident ▽

√x7ᵗʰ **V43.33** Unspecified car occupant injured in collision with pick-up truck in nontraffic accident ▽

√x7ᵗʰ **V43.34** Unspecified car occupant injured in collision with van in nontraffic accident ▽

√5ᵗʰ **V43.4** Person boarding or alighting a car injured in collision with car, pick-up truck or van

√x7ᵗʰ **V43.41** Person boarding or alighting a car injured in collision with sport utility vehicle

√x7ᵗʰ **V43.42** Person boarding or alighting a car injured in collision with other type car

√x7ᵗʰ **V43.43** Person boarding or alighting a car injured in collision with pick-up truck

√x7ᵗʰ **V43.44** Person boarding or alighting a car injured in collision with van

√5ᵗʰ **V43.5** Car driver injured in collision with car, pick-up truck or van in traffic accident

√x7ᵗʰ **V43.51** Car driver injured in collision with sport utility vehicle in traffic accident

√x7ᵗʰ **V43.52** Car driver injured in collision with other type car in traffic accident

√x7ᵗʰ **V43.53** Car driver injured in collision with pick-up truck in traffic accident

√x7ᵗʰ **V43.54** Car driver injured in collision with van in traffic accident

√5ᵗʰ **V43.6** Car passenger injured in collision with car, pick-up truck or van in traffic accident

√x7ᵗʰ **V43.61** Car passenger injured in collision with sport utility vehicle in traffic accident

√x7ᵗʰ **V43.62** Car passenger injured in collision with other type car in traffic accident

√x7ᵗʰ **V43.63** Car passenger injured in collision with pick-up truck in traffic accident

√x7ᵗʰ **V43.64** Car passenger injured in collision with van in traffic accident

√5ᵗʰ **V43.7** Person on outside of car injured in collision with car, pick-up truck or van in traffic accident

√x7ᵗʰ **V43.71** Person on outside of car injured in collision with sport utility vehicle in traffic accident

√x7ᵗʰ **V43.72** Person on outside of car injured in collision with other type car in traffic accident

√x7ᵗʰ **V43.73** Person on outside of car injured in collision with pick-up truck in traffic accident

√x7ᵗʰ **V43.74** Person on outside of car injured in collision with van in traffic accident

√5ᵗʰ **V43.9** Unspecified car occupant injured in collision with car, pick-up truck or van in traffic accident

√x7ᵗʰ **V43.91** Unspecified car occupant injured in collision with sport utility vehicle in traffic accident ▽

√x7ᵗʰ **V43.92** Unspecified car occupant injured in collision with other type car in traffic accident ▽

√x7ᵗʰ **V43.93** Unspecified car occupant injured in collision with pick-up truck in traffic accident ▽

√x7ᵗʰ **V43.94** Unspecified car occupant injured in collision with van in traffic accident ▽

☑4ᵗʰ **V44 Car occupant injured in collision with heavy transport vehicle or bus**

EXCLUDES 1 car occupant injured in collision with military vehicle

√x7ᵗʰ **V44.0** Car driver injured in collision with heavy transport vehicle or bus in nontraffic accident

√x7ᵗʰ **V44.1** Car passenger injured in collision with heavy transport vehicle or bus in nontraffic accident

√x7ᵗʰ **V44.2** Person on outside of car injured in collision with heavy transport vehicle or bus in traffic accident

√x7ᵗʰ **V44.3** Unspecified car occupant injured in collision with heavy ▽
transport vehicle or bus in nontraffic accident

√x7ᵗʰ **V44.4** Person boarding or alighting a car injured in collision with
heavy transport vehicle or bus

√x7ᵗʰ **V44.5** Car driver injured in collision with heavy transport vehicle or
bus in traffic accident

√x7ᵗʰ **V44.6** Car passenger injured in collision with heavy transport
vehicle or bus in traffic accident

√x7ᵗʰ **V44.7** Person on outside of car injured in collision with heavy
transport vehicle or bus in traffic accident

√x7ᵗʰ **V44.9** Unspecified car occupant injured in collision with heavy ▽
transport vehicle or bus in traffic accident

√4ᵗʰ **V45** Car occupant injured in collision with railway train or railway
vehicle

√x7ᵗʰ **V45.0** Car driver injured in collision with railway train or railway
vehicle in nontraffic accident

√x7ᵗʰ **V45.1** Car passenger injured in collision with railway train or railway
vehicle in nontraffic accident

√x7ᵗʰ **V45.2** Person on outside of car injured in collision with railway train
or railway vehicle in nontraffic accident

√x7ᵗʰ **V45.3** Unspecified car occupant injured in collision with railway ▽
train or railway vehicle in nontraffic accident

√x7ᵗʰ **V45.4** Person boarding or alighting a car injured in collision with
railway train or railway vehicle

√x7ᵗʰ **V45.5** Car driver injured in collision with railway train or railway
vehicle in traffic accident

√x7ᵗʰ **V45.6** Car passenger injured in collision with railway train or railway
vehicle in traffic accident

√x7ᵗʰ **V45.7** Person on outside of car injured in collision with railway train
or railway vehicle in traffic accident

√x7ᵗʰ **V45.9** Unspecified car occupant injured in collision with railway ▽
train or railway vehicle in traffic accident

√4ᵗʰ **V46** Car occupant injured in collision with other nonmotor vehicle
INCLUDES collision with animal-drawn vehicle, animal being ridden,
streetcar

√x7ᵗʰ **V46.0** Car driver injured in collision with other nonmotor vehicle in
nontraffic accident

√x7ᵗʰ **V46.1** Car passenger injured in collision with other nonmotor
vehicle in nontraffic accident

√x7ᵗʰ **V46.2** Person on outside of car injured in collision with other
nonmotor vehicle in nontraffic accident

√x7ᵗʰ **V46.3** Unspecified car occupant injured in collision with other ▽
nonmotor vehicle in nontraffic accident

√x7ᵗʰ **V46.4** Person boarding or alighting a car injured in collision with
other nonmotor vehicle

√x7ᵗʰ **V46.5** Car driver injured in collision with other nonmotor vehicle in
traffic accident

√x7ᵗʰ **V46.6** Car passenger injured in collision with other nonmotor
vehicle in traffic accident

√x7ᵗʰ **V46.7** Person on outside of car injured in collision with other
nonmotor vehicle in traffic accident

√x7ᵗʰ **V46.9** Unspecified car occupant injured in collision with other ▽
nonmotor vehicle in traffic accident

√4ᵗʰ **V47** Car occupant injured in collision with fixed or stationary object

√x7ᵗʰ **V47.0** Car driver injured in collision with fixed or stationary object in
nontraffic accide...

√x7ᵗʰ **V47.1** Car p... in collision with fixed or stationary
...dent

...injured in collision with fixed or
...ffic accident

...jured in collision with fixed or
...fic accident

...a car injured in collision with

...th fixed or stationary object in

...with fixed or stationary

...collision with fixed or

...llision with fixed or

√4ᵗʰ **V48** Car occupant injured in noncollision transport accident
INCLUDES overturning car NOS
overturning car without collision

√x7ᵗʰ **V48.0** Car driver injured in noncollision transport accident in
nontraffic accident

√x7ᵗʰ **V48.1** Car passenger injured in noncollision transport accident in
nontraffic accident

√x7ᵗʰ **V48.2** Person on outside of car injured in noncollision transport
accident in nontraffic accident

√x7ᵗʰ **V48.3** Unspecified car occupant injured in noncollision ▽
transport accident in nontraffic accident

√x7ᵗʰ **V48.4** Person boarding or alighting a car injured in noncollision
transport accident

√x7ᵗʰ **V48.5** Car driver injured in noncollision transport accident in traffic
accident

√x7ᵗʰ **V48.6** Car passenger injured in noncollision transport accident in
traffic accident

√x7ᵗʰ **V48.7** Person on outside of car injured in noncollision transport
accident in traffic accident

√x7ᵗʰ **V48.9** Unspecified car occupant injured in noncollision ▽
transport accident in traffic accident

√4ᵗʰ **V49** Car occupant injured in other and unspecified transport
accidents

√5ᵗʰ **V49.0** Driver injured in collision with other and unspecified motor
vehicles in nontraffic accident

√x7ᵗʰ **V49.00** Driver injured in collision with unspecified ▽
motor vehicles in nontraffic accident

√x7ᵗʰ **V49.09** Driver injured in collision with other motor vehicles
in nontraffic accident

√5ᵗʰ **V49.1** Passenger injured in collision with other and unspecified
motor vehicles in nontraffic accident

√x7ᵗʰ **V49.10** Passenger injured in collision with unspecified ▽
motor vehicles in nontraffic accident

√x7ᵗʰ **V49.19** Passenger injured in collision with other motor
vehicles in nontraffic accident

√5ᵗʰ **V49.2** Unspecified car occupant injured in collision with other and
unspecified motor vehicles in nontraffic accident

√x7ᵗʰ **V49.20** Unspecified car occupant injured in collision with ▽
unspecified motor vehicles in nontraffic accident
Car collision NOS, nontraffic

√x7ᵗʰ **V49.29** Unspecified car occupant injured in collision with ▽
other motor vehicles in nontraffic accident

√x7ᵗʰ **V49.3** Car occupant (driver) (passenger) injured in unspecified ▽
nontraffic accident
Car accident NOS, nontraffic
Car occupant injured in nontraffic accident NOS

√5ᵗʰ **V49.4** Driver injured in collision with other and unspecified motor
vehicles in traffic accident

√x7ᵗʰ **V49.40** Driver injured in collision with unspecified ▽
motor vehicles in traffic accident

√x7ᵗʰ **V49.49** Driver injured in collision with other motor vehicles
in traffic accident

√5ᵗʰ **V49.5** Passenger injured in collision with other and unspecified
motor vehicles in traffic accident

√x7ᵗʰ **V49.50** Passenger injured in collision with unspecified ▽
motor vehicles in traffic accident

√x7ᵗʰ **V49.59** Passenger injured in collision with other motor
vehicles in traffic accident

√5ᵗʰ **V49.6** Unspecified car occupant injured in collision with other and
unspecified motor vehicles in traffic accident

√x7ᵗʰ **V49.60** Unspecified car occupant injured in collision ▽
with unspecified motor vehicles in traffic accident
Car collision NOS (traffic)

√x7ᵗʰ **V49.69** Unspecified car occupant injured in collision with ▽
other motor vehicles in traffic accident

√5ᵗʰ **V49.8** Car occupant (driver) (passenger) injured in other specified
transport accidents

√x7ᵗʰ **V49.81** Car occupant (driver) (passenger) injured in
transport accident with military vehicle

√x7ᵗʰ **V49.88** Car occupant (driver) (passenger) injured in other
specified transport accidents

√x7ᵗʰ **V49.9** Car occupant (driver) (passenger) injured in unspecified ▽
traffic accident
Car accident NOS

Occupant of pick-up truck or van injured in transport accident (V50-V59)

INCLUDES   a four or six wheel motor vehicle designed primarily for carrying passengers and property but weighing less than the local limit for classification as a heavy goods vehicle
      minibus
      minivan
      sport utility vehicle (SUV)
      truck
      van

EXCLUDES 1   *heavy transport vehicle (V60-V69)*

> The appropriate 7th character is to be added to each code from categories V50-V59.
> A   initial encounter
> D   subsequent encounter
> S   sequela

✓4ᵗʰ V50 Occupant of pick-up truck or van injured in collision with pedestrian or animal

     EXCLUDES 1   *pick-up truck or van collision with animal-drawn vehicle or animal being ridden (V56.-)*

   ✓x7ᵗʰ **V50.0** Driver of pick-up truck or van injured in collision with pedestrian or animal in nontraffic accident

   ✓x7ᵗʰ **V50.1** Passenger in pick-up truck or van injured in collision with pedestrian or animal in nontraffic accident

   ✓x7ᵗʰ **V50.2** Person on outside of pick-up truck or van injured in collision with pedestrian or animal in nontraffic accident

   ✓x7ᵗʰ **V50.3** Unspecified occupant of pick-up truck or van injured in collision with pedestrian or animal in nontraffic accident   ▽

   ✓x7ᵗʰ **V50.4** Person boarding or alighting a pick-up truck or van injured in collision with pedestrian or animal

   ✓x7ᵗʰ **V50.5** Driver of pick-up truck or van injured in collision with pedestrian or animal in traffic accident

   ✓x7ᵗʰ **V50.6** Passenger in pick-up truck or van injured in collision with pedestrian or animal in traffic accident

   ✓x7ᵗʰ **V50.7** Person on outside of pick-up truck or van injured in collision with pedestrian or animal in traffic accident

   ✓x7ᵗʰ **V50.9** Unspecified occupant of pick-up truck or van injured in collision with pedestrian or animal in traffic accident   ▽

✓4ᵗʰ V51 Occupant of pick-up truck or van injured in collision with pedal cycle

   ✓x7ᵗʰ **V51.0** Driver of pick-up truck or van injured in collision with pedal cycle in nontraffic accident

   ✓x7ᵗʰ **V51.1** Passenger in pick-up truck or van injured in collision with pedal cycle in nontraffic accident

   ✓x7ᵗʰ **V51.2** Person on outside of pick-up truck or van injured in collision with pedal cycle in nontraffic accident

   ✓x7ᵗʰ **V51.3** Unspecified occupant of pick-up truck or van injured in collision with pedal cycle in nontraffic accident   ▽

   ✓x7ᵗʰ **V51.4** Person boarding or alighting a pick-up truck or van injured in collision with pedal cycle

   ✓x7ᵗʰ **V51.5** Driver of pick-up truck or van injured in collision with pedal cycle in traffic accident

   ✓x7ᵗʰ **V51.6** Passenger in pick-up truck or van injured in collision with pedal cycle in traffic accident

   ✓x7ᵗʰ **V51.7** Person on outside of pick-up truck or van injured in collision with pedal cycle in traffic accident

   ✓x7ᵗʰ **V51.9** Unspecified occupant of pick-up truck or van injured in collision with pedal cycle in traffic accident   ▽

✓4ᵗʰ V52 Occupant of pick-up truck or van injured in collision with two- or three-wheeled motor vehicle

   ✓x7ᵗʰ **V52.0** Driver of pick-up truck or van injured in collision with two- or three-wheeled motor vehicle in nontraffic accident

   ✓x7ᵗʰ **V52.1** Passenger in pick-up truck or van injured in collision with two- or three-wheeled motor vehicle in nontraffic accident

   ✓x7ᵗʰ **V52.2** Person on outside of pick-up truck or van injured in collision with two- or three-wheeled motor vehicle in nontraffic accident

   ✓x7ᵗʰ **V52.3** Unspecified occupant of pick-up truck or van injured in collision with two- or three-wheeled motor vehicle in nontraffic accident   ▽

   ✓x7ᵗʰ **V52.4** Person boarding or alighting a pick-up truck or van injured in collision with two- or three-wheeled motor vehicle

   ✓x7ᵗʰ **V52.5** Driver of pick-up truck or van injured in collision with two- or three-wheeled motor vehicle in traffic accident

   ✓x7ᵗʰ **V52.6** Passenger in pick-up truck or van injured in collision with two- or three-wheeled motor vehicle in traffic accident

   ✓x7ᵗʰ **V52.7** Person on outside of pick-up truck or van injured in collision with two- or three-wheeled motor vehicle in traffic accident

   ✓x7ᵗʰ **V52.9** Unspecified occupant of pick-up truck or van injured in collision with two- or three-wheeled motor vehicle in traffic accident   ▽

✓4ᵗʰ V53 Occupant of pick-up truck or van injured in collision with car, pick-up truck or van

   ✓x7ᵗʰ **V53.0** Driver of pick-up truck or van injured in collision with car, pick-up truck or van in nontraffic accident

   ✓x7ᵗʰ **V53.1** Passenger in pick-up truck or van injured in collision with car, pick-up truck or van in nontraffic accident

   ✓x7ᵗʰ **V53.2** Person on outside of pick-up truck or van injured in collision with car, pick-up truck or van in nontraffic accident

   ✓x7ᵗʰ **V53.3** Unspecified occupant of pick-up truck or van injured in collision with car, pick-up truck or van in nontraffic accident   ▽

   ✓x7ᵗʰ **V53.4** Person boarding or alighting a pick-up truck or van injured in collision with car, pick-up truck or van

   ✓x7ᵗʰ **V53.5** Driver of pick-up truck or van injured in collision with car, pick-up truck or van in traffic accident

   ✓x7ᵗʰ **V53.6** Passenger in pick-up truck or van injured in collision with car, pick-up truck or van in traffic accident

   ✓x7ᵗʰ **V53.7** Person on outside of pick-up truck or van injured in collision with car, pick-up truck or van in traffic accident

   ✓x7ᵗʰ **V53.9** Unspecified occupant of pick-up truck or van injured in collision with car, pick-up truck or van in traffic accident   ▽

✓4ᵗʰ V54 Occupant of pick-up truck or van injured in collision with heavy transport vehicle or bus

     EXCLUDES 1   *occupant of pick-up truck or van injured in collision with military vehicle (V59.81)*

   ✓x7ᵗʰ **V54.0** Driver of pick-up truck or van injured in collision with heavy transport vehicle or bus in nontraffic accident

   ✓x7ᵗʰ **V54.1** Passenger in pick-up truck or van injured in collision with heavy transport vehicle or bus in nontraffic accident

   ✓x7ᵗʰ **V54.2** Person on outside of pick-up truck or van injured in collision with heavy transport vehicle or bus in nontraffic accident

   ✓x7ᵗʰ **V54.3** Unspecified occupant of pick-up truck or van injured in collision with heavy transport vehicle or bus in nontraffic accident   ▽

   ✓x7ᵗʰ **V54.4** Person boarding or alighting a pick-up truck or van injured in collision with heavy transport vehicle or bus

   ✓x7ᵗʰ **V54.5** Driver of pick-up truck or van injured in collision with heavy transport vehicle or bus in traffic accident

   ✓x7ᵗʰ **V54.6** Passenger in pick-up truck or van injured in collision with heavy transport vehicle or bus in traffic accident

   ✓x7ᵗʰ **V54.7** Person on outside of pick-up truck or van injured in collision with heavy transport vehicle or bus in traffic accident

   ✓x7ᵗʰ **V54.9** Unspecified occupant of pick-up truck or van injured in collision with heavy transport vehicle or bus in traffic accident   ▽

✓4ᵗʰ V55 Occupant of pick-up truck or van injured in collision with railway train or railway vehicle

   ✓x7ᵗʰ **V55.0** Driver of pick-up truck or van injured in collision with railway train or railway vehicle in nontraffic accident

   ✓x7ᵗʰ **V55.1** Passenger in pick-up truck or van injured in collision with railway train or railway vehicle in nontraffic accident

   ✓x7ᵗʰ **V55.2** Person on outside of pick-up truck or van injured in collision with railway train or railway vehicle in nontraffic accident

   ✓x7ᵗʰ **V55.3** Unspecified occupant of pick-up truck or van injured in collision with railway train or railway vehicle in nontraffic accident   ▽

   ✓x7ᵗʰ **V55.4** Person boarding or alighting a pick-up truck or van injured in collision with railway train or railway vehicle

   ✓x7ᵗʰ **V55.5** Driver of pick-up truck or van injured in collision with railway train or railway vehicle in traffic accident

   ✓x7ᵗʰ **V55.6** Passenger in pick-up truck or van injured in collision with railway train or railway vehicle in traffic accident

   ✓x7ᵗʰ **V55.7** Person on outside of pick-up truck or van injured in collision with railway train or railway vehicle in traffic accident

   ✓x7ᵗʰ **V55.9** Unspecified occupant of pick-up truck or van injured in collision with railway train or railway vehicle in traffic accident   ▽

✓ Additional Character Req   ✓x7ᵗʰ Placeholder Alert   Case-Mix Diagnosis   Manifestation   ▽ Unspecified Dx   **EXCLUDES 1** Not coded here   **EXCLUDES 2** Not included here

✓4ᵗʰ **V56** **Occupant of pick-up truck or van injured in collision with other nonmotor vehicle**
INCLUDES   collision with animal-drawn vehicle, animal being ridden, streetcar

✓x7ᵗʰ **V56.0** Driver of pick-up truck or van injured in collision with other nonmotor vehicle in nontraffic accident

✓x7ᵗʰ **V56.1** Passenger in pick-up truck or van injured in collision with other nonmotor vehicle in nontraffic accident

✓x7ᵗʰ **V56.2** Person on outside of pick-up truck or van injured in collision with other nonmotor vehicle in nontraffic accident

✓x7ᵗʰ **V56.3** Unspecified occupant of pick-up truck or van injured in collision with other nonmotor vehicle in nontraffic accident ▽

✓x7ᵗʰ **V56.4** Person boarding or alighting a pick-up truck or van injured in collision with other nonmotor vehicle

✓x7ᵗʰ **V56.5** Driver of pick-up truck or van injured in collision with other nonmotor vehicle in traffic accident

✓x7ᵗʰ **V56.6** Passenger in pick-up truck or van injured in collision with other nonmotor vehicle in traffic accident

✓x7ᵗʰ **V56.7** Person on outside of pick-up truck or van injured in collision with other nonmotor vehicle in traffic accident

✓x7ᵗʰ **V56.9** Unspecified occupant of pick-up truck or van injured in collision with other nonmotor vehicle in traffic accident ▽

✓4ᵗʰ **V57** **Occupant of pick-up truck or van injured in collision with fixed or stationary object**

✓x7ᵗʰ **V57.0** Driver of pick-up truck or van injured in collision with fixed or stationary object in nontraffic accident

✓x7ᵗʰ **V57.1** Passenger in pick-up truck or van injured in collision with fixed or stationary object in nontraffic accident

✓x7ᵗʰ **V57.2** Person on outside of pick-up truck or van injured in collision with fixed or stationary object in nontraffic accident

✓x7ᵗʰ **V57.3** Unspecified occupant of pick-up truck or van injured in collision with fixed or stationary object in nontraffic accident ▽

✓x7ᵗʰ **V57.4** Person boarding or alighting a pick-up truck or van injured in collision with fixed or stationary object

✓x7ᵗʰ **V57.5** Driver of pick-up truck or van injured in collision with fixed or stationary object in traffic accident

✓x7ᵗʰ **V57.6** Passenger in pick-up truck or van injured in collision with fixed or stationary object in traffic accident

✓x7ᵗʰ **V57.7** Person on outside of pick-up truck or van injured in collision with fixed or stationary object in traffic accident

✓x7ᵗʰ **V57.9** Unspecified occupant of pick-up truck or van injured in collision with fixed or stationary object in traffic accident ▽

✓4ᵗʰ **V58** **Occupant of pick-up truck or van injured in noncollision transport accident**
INCLUDES   overturning pick-up truck or van NOS
overturning pick-up truck or van without collision

✓x7ᵗʰ **V58.0** Driver of pick-up truck or van injured in noncollision transport accident in nontraffic accident

✓x7ᵗʰ **V58.1** Passenger in pick-up truck or van injured in noncollision transport accident in nontraffic accident

✓x7ᵗʰ **V58.2** Person on outside of pick-up truck or van injured in noncollision transport accident in nontraffic accident

✓x7ᵗʰ **V58.3** Unspecified occupant of pick-up truck or van injured in noncollision transport accident in nontraffic accident ▽

✓x7ᵗʰ **V58.4** Person boarding or alighting a pick-up truck or van injured in noncollision transport accident

✓x7ᵗʰ **V58.5** Driver of pick-up truck or van injured in noncollision transport accident in traffic accident

✓x7ᵗʰ **V58.6** Passenger in pick-up truck or van injured in noncollision transport accident in traffic accident

✓x7ᵗʰ **V58.7** Person on outside of pick-up truck or van injured in noncollision transport accident in traffic accident

✓x7ᵗʰ **V58.9** Unspecified occupant of pick-up truck or van injured in noncollision transport accident in traffic accident ▽

✓4ᵗʰ **V59** **Occupant of pick-up truck or van injured in other and unspecified transport accidents**

✓5ᵗʰ **V59.0** Driver of pick-up truck or van injured in collision with other and unspecified motor vehicles in nontraffic accident

✓x7ᵗʰ **V59.00** Driver of pick-up truck or van injured in collision with unspecified motor vehicles in nontraffic accident ▽

✓x7ᵗʰ **V59.09** Driver of pick-up truck or van injured in collision with other motor vehicles in nontraffic accident

✓5ᵗʰ **V59.1** Passenger in pick-up truck or van injured in collision with other and unspecified motor vehicles in nontraffic accident

✓x7ᵗʰ **V59.10** Passenger in pick-up truck or van injured in collision with unspecified motor vehicles in nontraffic accident ▽

✓x7ᵗʰ **V59.19** Passenger in pick-up truck or van injured in collision with other motor vehicles in nontraffic accident

✓5ᵗʰ **V59.2** Unspecified occupant of pick-up truck or van injured in collision with other and unspecified motor vehicles in nontraffic accident

✓x7ᵗʰ **V59.20** Unspecified occupant of pick-up truck or van injured in collision with unspecified motor vehicles in nontraffic accident ▽
Collision NOS involving pick-up truck or van, nontraffic

✓x7ᵗʰ **V59.29** Unspecified occupant of pick-up truck or van injured in collision with other motor vehicles in nontraffic accident ▽

✓x7ᵗʰ **V59.3** Occupant (driver) (passenger) of pick-up truck or van injured in unspecified nontraffic accident ▽
Accident NOS involving pick-up truck or van, nontraffic
Occupant of pick-up truck or van injured in nontraffic accident NOS

✓5ᵗʰ **V59.4** Driver of pick-up truck or van injured in collision with other and unspecified motor vehicles in traffic accident

✓x7ᵗʰ **V59.40** Driver of pick-up truck or van injured in collision with unspecified motor vehicles in traffic accident ▽

✓x7ᵗʰ **V59.49** Driver of pick-up truck or van injured in collision with other motor vehicles in traffic accident

✓5ᵗʰ **V59.5** Passenger in pick-up truck or van injured in collision with other and unspecified motor vehicles in traffic accident

✓x7ᵗʰ **V59.50** Passenger in pick-up truck or van injured in collision with unspecified motor vehicles in traffic accident ▽

✓x7ᵗʰ **V59.59** Passenger in pick-up truck or van injured in collision with other motor vehicles in traffic accident

✓5ᵗʰ **V59.6** Unspecified occupant of pick-up truck or van injured in collision with other and unspecified motor vehicles in traffic accident

✓x7ᵗʰ **V59.60** Unspecified occupant of pick-up truck or van injured in collision with unspecified motor vehicles in traffic accident ▽
Collision NOS involving pick-up truck or van (traffic)

✓x7ᵗʰ **V59.69** Unspecified occupant of pick-up truck or van injured in collision with other motor vehicles in traffic accident ▽

✓5ᵗʰ **V59.8** Occupant (driver) (passenger) of pick-up truck or van injured in other specified transport accidents

✓x7ᵗʰ **V59.81** Occupant (driver) (passenger) of pick-up truck or van injured in transport accident with military vehicle

✓x7ᵗʰ **V59.88** Occupant (driver) (passenger) of pick-up truck or van injured in other specified transport accidents

✓x7ᵗʰ **V59.9** Occupant (driver) (passenger) of pick-up truck or van injured in unspecified traffic accident ▽
Accident NOS involving pick-up truck or van

Occupant of heavy transport vehicle injured in transport accident (V60-V69)

INCLUDES   18 wheeler
armored car
panel truck
EXCLUDES1   *bus*
motorcoach

The appropriate 7th character is to be added to each code from categories V60-V69.
A   initial encounter
D   subsequent encounter
S   sequela

✓4ᵗʰ **V60** **Occupant of heavy transport vehicle injured in collision with pedestrian or animal**
EXCLUDES1   *heavy transport vehicle collision with animal-drawn vehicle or animal being ridden (V66.-)*

✓x7ᵗʰ **V60.0** Driver of heavy transport vehicle injured in collision with pedestrian or animal in nontraffic accident

✓x7ᵗʰ **V60.1** Passenger in heavy transport vehicle injured in collision with pedestrian or animal in nontraffic accident

---

Ⓝ Newborn: 0   Ⓟ Pediatric: 0-17   Ⓜ Maternity: 12-55   Ⓐ Adult: 15-124   NRS Nonroutine supply Dx   NCDx Noncancer Dx   PDx Primary Dx   ▶◀ Revised Text   ● New Code   ▲ Revised Title

✓x7ᵗʰ V60.2 Person on outside of heavy transport vehicle injured in collision with pedestrian or animal in nontraffic accident

✓x7ᵗʰ V60.3 Unspecified occupant of heavy transport vehicle injured in collision with pedestrian or animal in nontraffic accident ▽

✓x7ᵗʰ V60.4 Person boarding or alighting a heavy transport vehicle injured in collision with pedestrian or animal

✓x7ᵗʰ V60.5 Driver of heavy transport vehicle injured in collision with pedestrian or animal in traffic accident

✓x7ᵗʰ V60.6 Passenger in heavy transport vehicle injured in collision with pedestrian or animal in traffic accident

✓x7ᵗʰ V60.7 Person on outside of heavy transport vehicle injured in collision with pedestrian or animal in traffic accident

✓x7ᵗʰ V60.9 Unspecified occupant of heavy transport vehicle injured in collision with pedestrian or animal in traffic accident ▽

✓4ᵗʰ V61 Occupant of heavy transport vehicle injured in collision with pedal cycle

✓x7ᵗʰ V61.0 Driver of heavy transport vehicle injured in collision with pedal cycle in nontraffic accident

✓x7ᵗʰ V61.1 Passenger in heavy transport vehicle injured in collision with pedal cycle in nontraffic accident

✓x7ᵗʰ V61.2 Person on outside of heavy transport vehicle injured in collision with pedal cycle in nontraffic accident

✓x7ᵗʰ V61.3 Unspecified occupant of heavy transport vehicle injured in collision with pedal cycle in nontraffic accident ▽

✓x7ᵗʰ V61.4 Person boarding or alighting a heavy transport vehicle injured in collision with pedal cycle while boarding or alighting

✓x7ᵗʰ V61.5 Driver of heavy transport vehicle injured in collision with pedal cycle in traffic accident

✓x7ᵗʰ V61.6 Passenger in heavy transport vehicle injured in collision with pedal cycle in traffic accident

✓x7ᵗʰ V61.7 Person on outside of heavy transport vehicle injured in collision with pedal cycle in traffic accident

✓x7ᵗʰ V61.9 Unspecified occupant of heavy transport vehicle injured in collision with pedal cycle in traffic accident ▽

✓4ᵗʰ V62 Occupant of heavy transport vehicle injured in collision with two- or three-wheeled motor vehicle

✓x7ᵗʰ V62.0 Driver of heavy transport vehicle injured in collision with two- or three-wheeled motor vehicle in nontraffic accident

✓x7ᵗʰ V62.1 Passenger in heavy transport vehicle injured in collision with two- or three-wheeled motor vehicle in nontraffic accident

✓x7ᵗʰ V62.2 Person on outside of heavy transport vehicle injured in collision with two- or three-wheeled motor vehicle in nontraffic accident

✓x7ᵗʰ V62.3 Unspecified occupant of heavy transport vehicle injured in collision with two- or three-wheeled motor vehicle in nontraffic accident ▽

✓x7ᵗʰ V62.4 Person boarding or alighting a heavy transport vehicle injured in collision with two- or three-wheeled motor vehicle

✓x7ᵗʰ V62.5 Driver of heavy transport vehicle injured in collision with two- or three-wheeled motor vehicle in traffic accident

✓x7ᵗʰ V62.6 Passenger in heavy transport vehicle injured in collision with two- or three-wheeled motor vehicle in traffic accident

✓x7ᵗʰ V62.7 Person on outside of heavy transport vehicle injured in collision with two- or three-wheeled motor vehicle in traffic accident

✓x7ᵗʰ V62.9 Unspecified occupant of heavy transport vehicle injured in collision with two- or three-wheeled motor vehicle in traffic accident ▽

✓4ᵗʰ V63 Occupant of heavy transport vehicle injured in collision with car, pick-up truck or van

✓x7ᵗʰ V63.0 Driver of heavy transport vehicle injured in collision with car, pick-up truck or van in nontraffic accident

✓x7ᵗʰ V63.1 Passenger in heavy transport vehicle injured in collision with car, pick-up truck or van in nontraffic accident

✓x7ᵗʰ V63.2 Person on outside of heavy transport vehicle injured in collision with car, pick-up truck or van in nontraffic accident

✓x7ᵗʰ V63.3 Unspecified occupant of heavy transport vehicle injured in collision with car, pick-up truck or van in nontraffic accident ▽

✓x7ᵗʰ V63.4 Person boarding or alighting a heavy transport vehicle injured in collision with car, pick-up truck or van

✓x7ᵗʰ V63.5 Driver of heavy transport vehicle injured in collision with car, pick-up truck or van in traffic accident

✓x7ᵗʰ V63.6 Passenger in heavy transport vehicle injured in collision with car, pick-up truck or van in traffic accident

✓x7ᵗʰ V63.7 Person on outside of heavy transport vehicle injured in collision with car, pick-up truck or van in traffic accident

✓x7ᵗʰ V63.9 Unspecified occupant of heavy transport vehicle injured in collision with car, pick-up truck or van in traffic accident ▽

✓4ᵗʰ V64 Occupant of heavy transport vehicle injured in collision with heavy transport vehicle or bus
> **EXCLUDES 1** occupant of heavy transport vehicle injured in collision with military vehicle (V69.81)

✓x7ᵗʰ V64.0 Driver of heavy transport vehicle injured in collision with heavy transport vehicle or bus in nontraffic accident

✓x7ᵗʰ V64.1 Passenger in heavy transport vehicle injured in collision with heavy transport vehicle or bus in nontraffic accident

✓x7ᵗʰ V64.2 Person on outside of heavy transport vehicle injured in collision with heavy transport vehicle or bus in nontraffic accident

✓x7ᵗʰ V64.3 Unspecified occupant of heavy transport vehicle injured in collision with heavy transport vehicle or bus in nontraffic accident ▽

✓x7ᵗʰ V64.4 Person boarding or alighting a heavy transport vehicle injured in collision with heavy transport vehicle or bus while boarding or alighting

✓x7ᵗʰ V64.5 Driver of heavy transport vehicle injured in collision with heavy transport vehicle or bus in traffic accident

✓x7ᵗʰ V64.6 Passenger in heavy transport vehicle injured in collision with heavy transport vehicle or bus in traffic accident

✓x7ᵗʰ V64.7 Person on outside of heavy transport vehicle injured in collision with heavy transport vehicle or bus in traffic accident

✓x7ᵗʰ V64.9 Unspecified occupant of heavy transport vehicle injured in collision with heavy transport vehicle or bus in traffic accident ▽

✓4ᵗʰ V65 Occupant of heavy transport vehicle injured in collision with railway train or railway vehicle

✓x7ᵗʰ V65.0 Driver of heavy transport vehicle injured in collision with railway train or railway vehicle in nontraffic accident

✓x7ᵗʰ V65.1 Passenger in heavy transport vehicle injured in collision with railway train or railway vehicle in nontraffic accident

✓x7ᵗʰ V65.2 Person on outside of heavy transport vehicle injured in collision with railway train or railway vehicle in nontraffic accident

✓x7ᵗʰ V65.3 Unspecified occupant of heavy transport vehicle injured in collision with railway train or railway vehicle in nontraffic accident ▽

✓x7ᵗʰ V65.4 Person boarding or alighting a heavy transport vehicle injured in collision with railway train or railway vehicle

✓x7ᵗʰ V65.5 Driver of heavy transport vehicle injured in collision with railway train or railway vehicle in traffic accident

✓x7ᵗʰ V65.6 Passenger in heavy transport vehicle injured in collision with railway train or railway vehicle in traffic accident

✓x7ᵗʰ V65.7 Person on outside of heavy transport vehicle injured in collision with railway train or railway vehicle in traffic accident

✓x7ᵗʰ V65.9 Unspecified occupant of heavy transport vehicle injured in collision with railway train or railway vehicle in traffic accident ▽

✓4ᵗʰ V66 Occupant of heavy transport vehicle injured in collision with other nonmotor vehicle
> **INCLUDES** collision with animal-drawn vehicle, animal being ridden, streetcar

✓x7ᵗʰ V66.0 Driver of heavy transport vehicle injured in collision with other nonmotor vehicle in nontraffic accident

✓x7ᵗʰ V66.1 Passenger in heavy transport vehicle injured in collision with other nonmotor vehicle in nontraffic accident

✓x7ᵗʰ V66.2 Person on outside of heavy transport vehicle injured in collision with other nonmotor vehicle in nontraffic accident

✓x7ᵗʰ V66.3 Unspecified occupant of heavy transport vehicle injured in collision with other nonmotor vehicle in nontraffic accident ▽

✓x7ᵗʰ V66.4 Person boarding or alighting a heavy transport vehicle injured in collision with other nonmotor vehicle

✓x7ᵗʰ V66.5 Driver of heavy transport vehicle injured in collision with other nonmotor vehicle in traffic accident

✓x7ᵗʰ V66.6 Passenger in heavy transport vehicle injured in collision with other nonmotor vehicle in traffic accident

---

✓ Additional Character Req   ✓x7ᵗʰ Placeholder Alert   Case-Mix Diagnosis   Manifestation   ▽ Unspecified Dx   EXCLUDES 1 Not coded here   EXCLUDES 2 Not included here

ICD-10-CM 2018   1131

Chapter 20. External Causes of Morbidity

√x7ᵗʰ **V66.7** Person on outside of heavy transport vehicle injured in collision with other nonmotor vehicle in traffic accident

√x7ᵗʰ **V66.9** Unspecified occupant of heavy transport vehicle injured in ▽ collision with other nonmotor vehicle in traffic accident

√4ᵗʰ **V67 Occupant of heavy transport vehicle injured in collision with fixed or stationary object**

√x7ᵗʰ **V67.0** Driver of heavy transport vehicle injured in collision with fixed or stationary object in nontraffic accident

√x7ᵗʰ **V67.1** Passenger in heavy transport vehicle injured in collision with fixed or stationary object in nontraffic accident

√x7ᵗʰ **V67.2** Person on outside of heavy transport vehicle injured in collision with fixed or stationary object in nontraffic accident

√x7ᵗʰ **V67.3** Unspecified occupant of heavy transport vehicle injured in ▽ collision with fixed or stationary object in nontraffic accident

√x7ᵗʰ **V67.4** Person boarding or alighting a heavy transport vehicle injured in collision with fixed or stationary object

√x7ᵗʰ **V67.5** Driver of heavy transport vehicle injured in collision with fixed or stationary object in traffic accident

√x7ᵗʰ **V67.6** Passenger in heavy transport vehicle injured in collision with fixed or stationary object in traffic accident

√x7ᵗʰ **V67.7** Person on outside of heavy transport vehicle injured in collision with fixed or stationary object in traffic accident

√x7ᵗʰ **V67.9** Unspecified occupant of heavy transport vehicle injured in ▽ collision with fixed or stationary object in traffic accident

√4ᵗʰ **V68 Occupant of heavy transport vehicle injured in noncollision transport accident**

INCLUDES   overturning heavy transport vehicle NOS
overturning heavy transport vehicle without collision

√x7ᵗʰ **V68.0** Driver of heavy transport vehicle injured in noncollision transport accident in nontraffic accident

√x7ᵗʰ **V68.1** Passenger in heavy transport vehicle injured in noncollision transport accident in nontraffic accident

√x7ᵗʰ **V68.2** Person on outside of heavy transport vehicle injured in noncollision transport accident in nontraffic accident

√x7ᵗʰ **V68.3** Unspecified occupant of heavy transport vehicle injured in ▽ noncollision transport accident in nontraffic accident

√x7ᵗʰ **V68.4** Person boarding or alighting a heavy transport vehicle injured in noncollision transport accident

√x7ᵗʰ **V68.5** Driver of heavy transport vehicle injured in noncollision transport accident in traffic accident

√x7ᵗʰ **V68.6** Passenger in heavy transport vehicle injured in noncollision transport accident in traffic accident

√x7ᵗʰ **V68.7** Person on outside of heavy transport vehicle injured in noncollision transport accident in traffic accident

√x7ᵗʰ **V68.9** Unspecified occupant of heavy transport vehicle injured in ▽ noncollision transport accident in traffic accident

√4ᵗʰ **V69 Occupant of heavy transport vehicle injured in other and unspecified transport accidents**

√5ᵗʰ **V69.0** Driver of heavy transport vehicle injured in collision with other and unspecified motor vehicles in nontraffic accident

√x7ᵗʰ **V69.00** Driver of heavy transport vehicle injured in ▽ collision with unspecified motor vehicles in nontraffic accident

√x7ᵗʰ **V69.09** Driver of heavy transport vehicle injured in collision with other motor vehicles in nontraffic accident

√5ᵗʰ **V69.1** Passenger in heavy transport vehicle injured in collision with other and unspecified motor vehicles in nontraffic accident

√x7ᵗʰ **V69.10** Passenger in heavy transport vehicle injured ▽ in collision with unspecified motor vehicles in nontraffic accident

√x7ᵗʰ **V69.19** Passenger in heavy transport vehicle injured in collision with other motor vehicles in nontraffic accident

√5ᵗʰ **V69.2** Unspecified occupant of heavy transport vehicle injured in collision with other and unspecified motor vehicles in nontraffic accident

√x7ᵗʰ **V69.20** Unspecified occupant of heavy transport vehicle ▽ injured in collision with unspecified motor vehicles in nontraffic accident

Collision NOS involving heavy transport vehicle, nontraffic

√x7ᵗʰ **V69.29** Unspecified occupant of heavy transport vehicle ▽ injured in collision with other motor vehicles in nontraffic accident

√x7ᵗʰ **V69.3** Occupant (driver) (passenger) of heavy transport vehicle ▽ injured in unspecified nontraffic accident

Accident NOS involving heavy transport vehicle, nontraffic
Occupant of heavy transport vehicle injured in nontraffic accident NOS

√5ᵗʰ **V69.4** Driver of heavy transport vehicle injured in collision with other and unspecified motor vehicles in traffic accident

√x7ᵗʰ **V69.40** Driver of heavy transport vehicle injured in ▽ collision with unspecified motor vehicles in traffic accident

√x7ᵗʰ **V69.49** Driver of heavy transport vehicle injured in collision with other motor vehicles in traffic accident

√5ᵗʰ **V69.5** Passenger in heavy transport vehicle injured in collision with other and unspecified motor vehicles in traffic accident

√x7ᵗʰ **V69.50** Passenger in heavy transport vehicle injured in ▽ collision with unspecified motor vehicles in traffic accident

√x7ᵗʰ **V69.59** Passenger in heavy transport vehicle injured in collision with other motor vehicles in traffic accident

√5ᵗʰ **V69.6** Unspecified occupant of heavy transport vehicle injured in collision with other and unspecified motor vehicles in traffic accident

√x7ᵗʰ **V69.60** Unspecified occupant of heavy transport vehicle ▽ injured in collision with unspecified motor vehicles in traffic accident

Collision NOS involving heavy transport vehicle (traffic)

√x7ᵗʰ **V69.69** Unspecified occupant of heavy transport vehicle ▽ injured in collision with other motor vehicles in traffic accident

√5ᵗʰ **V69.8** Occupant (driver) (passenger) of heavy transport vehicle injured in other specified transport accidents

√x7ᵗʰ **V69.81** Occupant (driver) (passenger) of heavy transport vehicle injured in transport accidents with military vehicle

√x7ᵗʰ **V69.88** Occupant (driver) (passenger) of heavy transport vehicle injured in other specified transport accidents

√x7ᵗʰ **V69.9** Occupant (driver) (passenger) of heavy transport vehicle ▽ injured in unspecified traffic accident

Accident NOS involving heavy transport vehicle

Bus occupant injured in transport accident (V70-V79)

INCLUDES   motorcoach
EXCLUDES 1   minibus (V50-V59)

The appropriate 7th character is to be added to each code from categories V70-V79.
A   initial encounter
D   subsequent encounter
S   sequela

√4ᵗʰ **V70 Bus occupant injured in collision with pedestrian or animal**

EXCLUDES 1   bus collision with animal-drawn vehicle or animal being ridden (V76.-)

√x7ᵗʰ **V70.0** Driver of bus injured in collision with pedestrian or animal in nontraffic accident

√x7ᵗʰ **V70.1** Passenger on bus injured in collision with pedestrian or animal in nontraffic accident

√x7ᵗʰ **V70.2** Person on outside of bus injured in collision with pedestrian or animal in nontraffic accident

√x7ᵗʰ **V70.3** Unspecified occupant of bus injured in collision with ▽ pedestrian or animal in nontraffic accident

√x7ᵗʰ **V70.4** Person boarding or alighting from bus injured in collision with pedestrian or animal

√x7ᵗʰ **V70.5** Driver of bus injured in collision with pedestrian or animal in traffic accident

√x7ᵗʰ **V70.6** Passenger on bus injured in collision with pedestrian or animal in traffic accident

√x7ᵗʰ **V70.7** Person on outside of bus injured in collision with pedestrian or animal in traffic accident

√x7ᵗʰ **V70.9** Unspecified occupant of bus injured in collision with ▽ pedestrian or animal in traffic accident

√4ᵗʰ **V71 Bus occupant injured in collision with pedal cycle**

√x7ᵗʰ **V71.0** Driver of bus injured in collision with pedal cycle in nontraffic accident

√x7ᵗʰ **V71.1** Passenger on bus injured in collision with pedal cycle in nontraffic accident

---

Ⓝ Newborn: 0   Ⓟ Pediatric: 0-17   Ⓜ Maternity: 12-55   Ⓐ Adult: 15-124   **NRS** Nonroutine supply Dx   **NCDx** Noncancer Dx   **PDx** Primary Dx   ▶◀ Revised Text   ● New Code   ▲ Revised Title

1132   ICD-10-CM 2018

√x7ᵗʰ **V71.2** Person on outside of bus injured in collision with pedal cycle in nontraffic accident

√x7ᵗʰ **V71.3** Unspecified occupant of bus injured in collision with pedal ▽ cycle in nontraffic accident

√x7ᵗʰ **V71.4** Person boarding or alighting from bus injured in collision with pedal cycle

√x7ᵗʰ **V71.5** Driver of bus injured in collision with pedal cycle in traffic accident

√x7ᵗʰ **V71.6** Passenger on bus injured in collision with pedal cycle in traffic accident

√x7ᵗʰ **V71.7** Person on outside of bus injured in collision with pedal cycle in traffic accident

√x7ᵗʰ **V71.9** Unspecified occupant of bus injured in collision with pedal ▽ cycle in traffic accident

✓4ᵗʰ **V72** Bus occupant injured in collision with two- or three-wheeled motor vehicle

√x7ᵗʰ **V72.0** Driver of bus injured in collision with two- or three-wheeled motor vehicle in nontraffic accident

√x7ᵗʰ **V72.1** Passenger on bus injured in collision with two- or three-wheeled motor vehicle in nontraffic accident

√x7ᵗʰ **V72.2** Person on outside of bus injured in collision with two- or three-wheeled motor vehicle in nontraffic accident

√x7ᵗʰ **V72.3** Unspecified occupant of bus injured in collision with two- ▽ or three-wheeled motor vehicle in nontraffic accident

√x7ᵗʰ **V72.4** Person boarding or alighting from bus injured in collision with two- or three-wheeled motor vehicle

√x7ᵗʰ **V72.5** Driver of bus injured in collision with two- or three-wheeled motor vehicle in traffic accident

√x7ᵗʰ **V72.6** Passenger on bus injured in collision with two- or three-wheeled motor vehicle in traffic accident

√x7ᵗʰ **V72.7** Person on outside of bus injured in collision with two- or three-wheeled motor vehicle in traffic accident

√x7ᵗʰ **V72.9** Unspecified occupant of bus injured in collision with two- ▽ or three-wheeled motor vehicle in traffic accident

✓4ᵗʰ **V73** Bus occupant injured in collision with car, pick-up truck or van

√x7ᵗʰ **V73.0** Driver of bus injured in collision with car, pick-up truck or van in nontraffic accident

√x7ᵗʰ **V73.1** Passenger on bus injured in collision with car, pick-up truck or van in nontraffic accident

√x7ᵗʰ **V73.2** Person on outside of bus injured in collision with car, pick-up truck or van in nontraffic accident

√x7ᵗʰ **V73.3** Unspecified occupant of bus injured in collision with car, ▽ pick-up truck or van in nontraffic accident

√x7ᵗʰ **V73.4** Person boarding or alighting from bus injured in collision with car, pick-up truck or van

√x7ᵗʰ **V73.5** Driver of bus injured in collision with car, pick-up truck or van in traffic accident

√x7ᵗʰ **V73.6** Passenger on bus injured in collision with car, pick-up truck or van in traffic accident

√x7ᵗʰ **V73.7** Person on outside of bus injured in collision with car, pick-up truck or van in traffic accident

√x7ᵗʰ **V73.9** Unspecified occupant of bus injured in collision with car, ▽ pick-up truck or van in traffic accident

✓4ᵗʰ **V74** Bus occupant injured in collision with heavy transport vehicle or bus

EXCLUDES 1   bus occupant injured in collision with military vehicle (V79.81)

√x7ᵗʰ **V74.0** Driver of bus injured in collision with heavy transport vehicle or bus in nontraffic accident

√x7ᵗʰ **V74.1** Passenger on bus injured in collision with heavy transport vehicle or bus in nontraffic accident

√x7ᵗʰ **V74.2** Person on outside of bus injured in collision with heavy transport vehicle or bus in nontraffic accident

√x7ᵗʰ **V74.3** Unspecified occupant of bus injured in collision with ▽ heavy transport vehicle or bus in nontraffic accident

√x7ᵗʰ **V74.4** Person boarding or alighting from bus injured in collision with heavy transport vehicle or bus

√x7ᵗʰ **V74.5** Driver of bus injured in collision with heavy transport vehicle or bus in traffic accident

√x7ᵗʰ **V74.6** Passenger on bus injured in collision with heavy transport vehicle or bus in traffic accident

√x7ᵗʰ **V74.7** Person on outside of bus injured in collision with heavy transport vehicle or bus in traffic accident

√x7ᵗʰ **V74.9** Unspecified occupant of bus injured in collision with ▽ heavy transport vehicle or bus in traffic accident

✓4ᵗʰ **V75** Bus occupant injured in collision with railway train or railway vehicle

√x7ᵗʰ **V75.0** Driver of bus injured in collision with railway train or railway vehicle in nontraffic accident

√x7ᵗʰ **V75.1** Passenger on bus injured in collision with railway train or railway vehicle in nontraffic accident

√x7ᵗʰ **V75.2** Person on outside of bus injured in collision with railway train or railway vehicle in nontraffic accident

√x7ᵗʰ **V75.3** Unspecified occupant of bus injured in collision with ▽ railway train or railway vehicle in nontraffic accident

√x7ᵗʰ **V75.4** Person boarding or alighting from bus injured in collision with railway train or railway vehicle

√x7ᵗʰ **V75.5** Driver of bus injured in collision with railway train or railway vehicle in traffic accident

√x7ᵗʰ **V75.6** Passenger on bus injured in collision with railway train or railway vehicle in traffic accident

√x7ᵗʰ **V75.7** Person on outside of bus injured in collision with railway train or railway vehicle in traffic accident

√x7ᵗʰ **V75.9** Unspecified occupant of bus injured in collision with ▽ railway train or railway vehicle in traffic accident

✓4ᵗʰ **V76** Bus occupant injured in collision with other nonmotor vehicle

INCLUDES   collision with animal-drawn vehicle, animal being ridden, streetcar

√x7ᵗʰ **V76.0** Driver of bus injured in collision with other nonmotor vehicle in nontraffic accident

√x7ᵗʰ **V76.1** Passenger on bus injured in collision with other nonmotor vehicle in nontraffic accident

√x7ᵗʰ **V76.2** Person on outside of bus injured in collision with other nonmotor vehicle in nontraffic accident

√x7ᵗʰ **V76.3** Unspecified occupant of bus injured in collision with ▽ other nonmotor vehicle in nontraffic accident

√x7ᵗʰ **V76.4** Person boarding or alighting from bus injured in collision with other nonmotor vehicle

√x7ᵗʰ **V76.5** Driver of bus injured in collision with other nonmotor vehicle in traffic accident

√x7ᵗʰ **V76.6** Passenger on bus injured in collision with other nonmotor vehicle in traffic accident

√x7ᵗʰ **V76.7** Person on outside of bus injured in collision with other nonmotor vehicle in traffic accident

√x7ᵗʰ **V76.9** Unspecified occupant of bus injured in collision with ▽ other nonmotor vehicle in traffic accident

✓4ᵗʰ **V77** Bus occupant injured in collision with fixed or stationary object

√x7ᵗʰ **V77.0** Driver of bus injured in collision with fixed or stationary object in nontraffic accident

√x7ᵗʰ **V77.1** Passenger on bus injured in collision with fixed or stationary object in nontraffic accident

√x7ᵗʰ **V77.2** Person on outside of bus injured in collision with fixed or stationary object in nontraffic accident

√x7ᵗʰ **V77.3** Unspecified occupant of bus injured in collision with fixed ▽ or stationary object in nontraffic accident

√x7ᵗʰ **V77.4** Person boarding or alighting from bus injured in collision with fixed or stationary object

√x7ᵗʰ **V77.5** Driver of bus injured in collision with fixed or stationary object in traffic accident

√x7ᵗʰ **V77.6** Passenger on bus injured in collision with fixed or stationary object in traffic accident

√x7ᵗʰ **V77.7** Person on outside of bus injured in collision with fixed or stationary object in traffic accident

√x7ᵗʰ **V77.9** Unspecified occupant of bus injured in collision with fixed ▽ or stationary object in traffic accident

✓4ᵗʰ **V78** Bus occupant injured in noncollision transport accident

INCLUDES   overturning bus NOS
overturning bus without collision

√x7ᵗʰ **V78.0** Driver of bus injured in noncollision transport accident in nontraffic accident

√x7ᵗʰ **V78.1** Passenger on bus injured in noncollision transport accident in nontraffic accident

√x7ᵗʰ **V78.2** Person on outside of bus injured in noncollision transport accident in nontraffic accident

√x7ᵗʰ **V78.3** Unspecified occupant of bus injured in noncollision ▽ transport accident in nontraffic accident

---

✓ Additional Character Req   √x7ᵗʰ Placeholder Alert   Case-Mix Diagnosis   Manifestation   ▽ Unspecified Dx   EXCLUDES 1 Not coded here   EXCLUDES 2 Not included here

Chapter 20. External Causes of Morbidity

√x7ᵗʰ **V78.4** Person boarding or alighting from bus injured in noncollision transport accident

√x7ᵗʰ **V78.5** Driver of bus injured in noncollision transport accident in traffic accident

√x7ᵗʰ **V78.6** Passenger on bus injured in noncollision transport accident in traffic accident

√x7ᵗʰ **V78.7** Person on outside of bus injured in noncollision transport accident in traffic accident

√x7ᵗʰ **V78.9** Unspecified occupant of bus injured in noncollision transport accident in traffic accident

√4ᵗʰ **V79 Bus occupant injured in other and unspecified transport accidents**

√5ᵗʰ **V79.0** Driver of bus injured in collision with other and unspecified motor vehicles in nontraffic accident

     √x7ᵗʰ **V79.00** Driver of bus injured in collision with unspecified motor vehicles in nontraffic accident ▽

     √x7ᵗʰ **V79.09** Driver of bus injured in collision with other motor vehicles in nontraffic accident

√5ᵗʰ **V79.1** Passenger on bus injured in collision with other and unspecified motor vehicles in nontraffic accident

     √x7ᵗʰ **V79.10** Passenger on bus injured in collision with unspecified motor vehicles in nontraffic accident ▽

     √x7ᵗʰ **V79.19** Passenger on bus injured in collision with other motor vehicles in nontraffic accident

√5ᵗʰ **V79.2** Unspecified bus occupant injured in collision with other and unspecified motor vehicles in nontraffic accident

     √x7ᵗʰ **V79.20** Unspecified bus occupant injured in collision with unspecified motor vehicles in nontraffic accident ▽
         Bus collision NOS, nontraffic

     √x7ᵗʰ **V79.29** Unspecified bus occupant injured in collision with other motor vehicles in nontraffic accident ▽

√x7ᵗʰ **V79.3** Bus occupant (driver) (passenger) injured in unspecified nontraffic accident ▽
     Bus accident NOS, nontraffic
     Bus occupant injured in nontraffic accident NOS

√5ᵗʰ **V79.4** Driver of bus injured in collision with other and unspecified motor vehicles in traffic accident

     √x7ᵗʰ **V79.40** Driver of bus injured in collision with unspecified motor vehicles in traffic accident ▽

     √x7ᵗʰ **V79.49** Driver of bus injured in collision with other motor vehicles in traffic accident

√5ᵗʰ **V79.5** Passenger on bus injured in collision with other and unspecified motor vehicles in traffic accident

     √x7ᵗʰ **V79.50** Passenger on bus injured in collision with unspecified motor vehicles in traffic accident ▽

     √x7ᵗʰ **V79.59** Passenger on bus injured in collision with other motor vehicles in traffic accident

√5ᵗʰ **V79.6** Unspecified bus occupant injured in collision with other and unspecified motor vehicles in traffic accident

     √x7ᵗʰ **V79.60** Unspecified bus occupant injured in collision with unspecified motor vehicles in traffic accident ▽
         Bus collision NOS (traffic)

     √x7ᵗʰ **V79.69** Unspecified bus occupant injured in collision with other motor vehicles in traffic accident ▽

√5ᵗʰ **V79.8** Bus occupant (driver) (passenger) injured in other specified transport accidents

     √x7ᵗʰ **V79.81** Bus occupant (driver) (passenger) injured in transport accidents with military vehicle

     √x7ᵗʰ **V79.88** Bus occupant (driver) (passenger) injured in other specified transport accidents

√x7ᵗʰ **V79.9** Bus occupant (driver) (passenger) injured in unspecified traffic accident ▽
     Bus accident NOS

Other land transport accidents (V80-V89)

The appropriate 7th character is to be added to each code from categories V80-V89.
A   initial encounter
D   subsequent encounter
S   sequela

√4ᵗʰ **V80 Animal-rider or occupant of animal-drawn vehicle injured in transport accident**

√5ᵗʰ **V80.0** Animal-rider or occupant of animal drawn vehicle injured by fall from or being thrown from animal or animal-drawn vehicle in noncollision accident

     √6ᵗʰ **V80.01** Animal-rider injured by fall from or being thrown from animal in noncollision accident

         √7ᵗʰ **V80.010** Animal-rider injured by fall from or being thrown from horse in noncollision accident

         √7ᵗʰ **V80.018** Animal-rider injured by fall from or being thrown from other animal in noncollision accident

     √x7ᵗʰ **V80.02** Occupant of animal-drawn vehicle injured by fall from or being thrown from animal-drawn vehicle in noncollision accident
         Overturning animal-drawn vehicle NOS
         Overturning animal-drawn vehicle without collision

√5ᵗʰ **V80.1** Animal-rider or occupant of animal-drawn vehicle injured in collision with pedestrian or animal
     EXCLUDES 1   animal-rider or animal-drawn vehicle collision with animal-drawn vehicle or animal being ridden (V80.7)

     √x7ᵗʰ **V80.11** Animal-rider injured in collision with pedestrian or animal

     √x7ᵗʰ **V80.12** Occupant of animal-drawn vehicle injured in collision with pedestrian or animal

√5ᵗʰ **V80.2** Animal-rider or occupant of animal-drawn vehicle injured in collision with pedal cycle

     √x7ᵗʰ **V80.21** Animal-rider injured in collision with pedal cycle

     √x7ᵗʰ **V80.22** Occupant of animal-drawn vehicle injured in collision with pedal cycle

√5ᵗʰ **V80.3** Animal-rider or occupant of animal-drawn vehicle injured in collision with two- or three-wheeled motor vehicle

     √x7ᵗʰ **V80.31** Animal-rider injured in collision with two- or three-wheeled motor vehicle

     √x7ᵗʰ **V80.32** Occupant of animal-drawn vehicle injured in collision with two- or three-wheeled motor vehicle

√5ᵗʰ **V80.4** Animal-rider or occupant of animal-drawn vehicle injured in collision with car, pick-up truck, van, heavy transport vehicle or bus
     EXCLUDES 1   animal-rider injured in collision with military vehicle (V80.910)
         occupant of animal-drawn vehicle injured in collision with military vehicle (V80.920)

     √x7ᵗʰ **V80.41** Animal-rider injured in collision with car, pick-up truck, van, heavy transport vehicle or bus

     √x7ᵗʰ **V80.42** Occupant of animal-drawn vehicle injured in collision with car, pick-up truck, van, heavy transport vehicle or bus

√5ᵗʰ **V80.5** Animal-rider or occupant of animal-drawn vehicle injured in collision with other specified motor vehicle

     √x7ᵗʰ **V80.51** Animal-rider injured in collision with other specified motor vehicle

     √x7ᵗʰ **V80.52** Occupant of animal-drawn vehicle injured in collision with other specified motor vehicle

√5ᵗʰ **V80.6** Animal-rider or occupant of animal-drawn vehicle injured in collision with railway train or railway vehicle

     √x7ᵗʰ **V80.61** Animal-rider injured in collision with railway train or railway vehicle

     √x7ᵗʰ **V80.62** Occupant of animal-drawn vehicle injured in collision with railway train or railway vehicle

√5ᵗʰ **V80.7** Animal-rider or occupant of animal-drawn vehicle injured in collision with other nonmotor vehicles

     √6ᵗʰ **V80.71** Animal-rider or occupant of animal-drawn vehicle injured in collision with animal being ridden

         √7ᵗʰ **V80.710** Animal-rider injured in collision with other animal being ridden

N Newborn: 0   P Pediatric: 0-17   M Maternity: 12-55   A Adult: 15-124   NRS Nonroutine supply Dx   NC Dx Noncancer Dx   PD₁ Primary Dx   ▶◀ Revised Text   ● New Code   ▲ Revised Title

1134   ICD-10-CM 2018

☑7ᵗʰ **V80.711** Occupant of animal-drawn vehicle injured in collision with animal being ridden

☑6ᵗʰ **V80.72** Animal-rider or occupant of animal-drawn vehicle injured in collision with other animal-drawn vehicle

☑7ᵗʰ **V80.720** Animal-rider injured in collision with animal-drawn vehicle

☑7ᵗʰ **V80.721** Occupant of animal-drawn vehicle injured in collision with other animal-drawn vehicle

☑6ᵗʰ **V80.73** Animal-rider or occupant of animal-drawn vehicle injured in collision with streetcar

☑7ᵗʰ **V80.730** Animal-rider injured in collision with streetcar

☑7ᵗʰ **V80.731** Occupant of animal-drawn vehicle injured in collision with streetcar

☑6ᵗʰ **V80.79** Animal-rider or occupant of animal-drawn vehicle injured in collision with other nonmotor vehicles

☑7ᵗʰ **V80.790** Animal-rider injured in collision with other nonmotor vehicles

☑7ᵗʰ **V80.791** Occupant of animal-drawn vehicle injured in collision with other nonmotor vehicles

☑5ᵗʰ **V80.8** Animal-rider or occupant of animal-drawn vehicle injured in collision with fixed or stationary object

☑7ᵗʰ **V80.81** Animal-rider injured in collision with fixed or stationary object

☑7ᵗʰ **V80.82** Occupant of animal-drawn vehicle injured in collision with fixed or stationary object

☑5ᵗʰ **V80.9** Animal-rider or occupant of animal-drawn vehicle injured in other and unspecified transport accidents

☑6ᵗʰ **V80.91** Animal-rider injured in other and unspecified transport accidents

☑7ᵗʰ **V80.910** Animal-rider injured in transport accident with military vehicle

☑7ᵗʰ **V80.918** Animal-rider injured in other transport accident

☑7ᵗʰ **V80.919** Animal-rider injured in unspecified transport accident ▽
Animal rider accident NOS

☑6ᵗʰ **V80.92** Occupant of animal-drawn vehicle injured in other and unspecified transport accidents

☑7ᵗʰ **V80.920** Occupant of animal-drawn vehicle injured in transport accident with military vehicle

☑7ᵗʰ **V80.928** Occupant of animal-drawn vehicle injured in other transport accident

☑7ᵗʰ **V80.929** Occupant of animal-drawn vehicle injured in unspecified transport accident ▽
Animal-drawn vehicle accident NOS

☑4ᵗʰ **V81** Occupant of railway train or railway vehicle injured in transport accident

INCLUDES   derailment of railway train or railway vehicle
person on outside of train

EXCLUDES 1   streetcar (V82.-)

☑x7ᵗʰ **V81.0** Occupant of railway train or railway vehicle injured in collision with motor vehicle in nontraffic accident

EXCLUDES 1   occupant of railway train or railway vehicle injured due to collision with military vehicle (V81.83)

☑x7ᵗʰ **V81.1** Occupant of railway train or railway vehicle injured in collision with motor vehicle in traffic accident

EXCLUDES 1   occupant of railway train or railway vehicle injured due to collision with military vehicle (V81.83)

☑x7ᵗʰ **V81.2** Occupant of railway train or railway vehicle injured in collision with or hit by rolling stock

☑x7ᵗʰ **V81.3** Occupant of railway train or railway vehicle injured in collision with other object
Railway collision NOS

☑x7ᵗʰ **V81.4** Person injured while boarding or alighting from railway train or railway vehicle

☑x7ᵗʰ **V81.5** Occupant of railway train or railway vehicle injured by fall in railway train or railway vehicle

☑x7ᵗʰ **V81.6** Occupant of railway train or railway vehicle injured by fall from railway train or railway vehicle

☑x7ᵗʰ **V81.7** Occupant of railway train or railway vehicle injured in derailment without antecedent collision

☑5ᵗʰ **V81.8** Occupant of railway train or railway vehicle injured in other specified railway accidents

☑x7ᵗʰ **V81.81** Occupant of railway train or railway vehicle injured due to explosion or fire on train

☑x7ᵗʰ **V81.82** Occupant of railway train or railway vehicle injured due to object falling onto train
Occupant of railway train or railway vehicle injured due to falling earth onto train
Occupant of railway train or railway vehicle injured due to falling rocks onto train
Occupant of railway train or railway vehicle injured due to falling snow onto train
Occupant of railway train or railway vehicle injured due to falling trees onto train

☑x7ᵗʰ **V81.83** Occupant of railway train or railway vehicle injured due to collision with military vehicle

☑x7ᵗʰ **V81.89** Occupant of railway train or railway vehicle injured due to other specified railway accident

☑x7ᵗʰ **V81.9** Occupant of railway train or railway vehicle injured in unspecified railway accident ▽
Railway accident NOS

☑4ᵗʰ **V82** Occupant of powered streetcar injured in transport accident

INCLUDES   interurban electric car
person on outside of streetcar
tram (car)
trolley (car)

EXCLUDES 1   bus (V70-V79)
motorcoach (V70-V79)
nonpowered streetcar (V76.-)
train (V81.-)

☑x7ᵗʰ **V82.0** Occupant of streetcar injured in collision with motor vehicle in nontraffic accident

☑x7ᵗʰ **V82.1** Occupant of streetcar injured in collision with motor vehicle in traffic accident

☑x7ᵗʰ **V82.2** Occupant of streetcar injured in collision with or hit by rolling stock

☑x7ᵗʰ **V82.3** Occupant of streetcar injured in collision with other object

EXCLUDES 1   collision with animal-drawn vehicle or animal being ridden (V82.8)

☑x7ᵗʰ **V82.4** Person injured while boarding or alighting from streetcar

☑x7ᵗʰ **V82.5** Occupant of streetcar injured by fall in streetcar

EXCLUDES 1   fall in streetcar:
while boarding or alighting (V82.4)
with antecedent collision (V82.0-V82.3)

☑x7ᵗʰ **V82.6** Occupant of streetcar injured by fall from streetcar

EXCLUDES 1   fall from streetcar:
while boarding or alighting (V82.4)
with antecedent collision (V82.0-V82.3)

☑x7ᵗʰ **V82.7** Occupant of streetcar injured in derailment without antecedent collision

EXCLUDES 1   occupant of streetcar injured in derailment with antecedent collision (V82.0-V82.3)

☑x7ᵗʰ **V82.8** Occupant of streetcar injured in other specified transport accidents
Streetcar collision with military vehicle
Streetcar collision with train or nonmotor vehicles

☑x7ᵗʰ **V82.9** Occupant of streetcar injured in unspecified traffic accident ▽
Streetcar accident NOS

☑4ᵗʰ **V83** Occupant of special vehicle mainly used on industrial premises injured in transport accident

INCLUDES   battery-powered airport passenger vehicle
battery-powered truck (baggage) (mail)
coal-car in mine
forklift (truck)
logging car
self-propelled industrial truck
station baggage truck (powered)
tram, truck, or tub (powered) in mine or quarry

EXCLUDES 1   special construction vehicles (V85.-)
special industrial vehicle in stationary use or maintenance (W31.-)

☑x7ᵗʰ **V83.0** Driver of special industrial vehicle injured in traffic accident

☑x7ᵗʰ **V83.1** Passenger of special industrial vehicle injured in traffic accident

☑x7ᵗʰ **V83.2** Person on outside of special industrial vehicle injured in traffic accident

---

☑ Additional Character Req   ☑x7ᵗʰ Placeholder Alert   Case-Mix Diagnosis   Manifestation   ▽ Unspecified Dx   EXCLUDES 1 Not coded here   EXCLUDES 2 Not included here

Chapter 20. External Causes of Morbidity

V83.3–V86.36

√x7ᵗʰ **V83.3 Unspecified occupant of special industrial vehicle injured in traffic accident** ▽

√x7ᵗʰ **V83.4 Person injured while** boarding or alighting **from special industrial vehicle**

√x7ᵗʰ **V83.5 Driver of special industrial vehicle injured** in nontraffic accident

√x7ᵗʰ **V83.6 Passenger of special industrial vehicle injured** in nontraffic accident

√x7ᵗʰ **V83.7 Person on outside of special industrial vehicle injured in** nontraffic accident

√x7ᵗʰ **V83.9 Unspecified occupant of special industrial vehicle injured** in nontraffic accident ▽
Special-industrial-vehicle accident NOS

√4ᵗʰ **V84 Occupant of special vehicle mainly used in agriculture injured in transport accident**
INCLUDES   self-propelled farm machinery
           tractor (and trailer)
EXCLUDES 1   animal-powered farm machinery accident (W30.8-)
           contact with combine harvester (W30.0)
           special agricultural vehicle in stationary use or maintenance (W30.-)

√x7ᵗʰ **V84.0 Driver** of special agricultural vehicle injured **in traffic accident**

√x7ᵗʰ **V84.1 Passenger** of special agricultural vehicle injured **in traffic accident**

√x7ᵗʰ **V84.2 Person on outside** of special agricultural vehicle injured **in** traffic accident

√x7ᵗʰ **V84.3 Unspecified occupant** of special agricultural vehicle injured **in traffic accident** ▽

√x7ᵗʰ **V84.4 Person injured while** boarding or alighting **from special agricultural vehicle**

√x7ᵗʰ **V84.5 Driver** of special agricultural vehicle injured **in nontraffic accident**

√x7ᵗʰ **V84.6 Passenger** of special agricultural vehicle injured **in nontraffic accident**

√x7ᵗʰ **V84.7 Person on outside** of special agricultural vehicle injured **in** nontraffic accident

√x7ᵗʰ **V84.9 Unspecified occupant** of special agricultural vehicle **injured in** nontraffic accident ▽
Special-agricultural vehicle accident NOS

√4ᵗʰ **V85 Occupant of special construction vehicle injured in transport accident**
INCLUDES   bulldozer
           digger
           dump truck
           earth-leveller
           mechanical shovel
           road-roller
EXCLUDES 1   special industrial vehicle (V83.-)
           special construction vehicle in stationary use or maintenance (W31.-)

√x7ᵗʰ **V85.0 Driver** of special construction vehicle injured **in traffic accident**

√x7ᵗʰ **V85.1 Passenger** of special construction vehicle injured **in traffic accident**

√x7ᵗʰ **V85.2 Person on outside** of special construction vehicle injured **in** traffic accident

√x7ᵗʰ **V85.3 Unspecified occupant** of special construction vehicle **injured** in traffic accident ▽

√x7ᵗʰ **V85.4 Person injured while** boarding or alighting **from special construction vehicle**

√x7ᵗʰ **V85.5 Driver of special construction vehicle injured** in nontraffic accident

√x7ᵗʰ **V85.6 Passenger** of special construction vehicle injured in nontraffic accident

√x7ᵗʰ **V85.7 Person on outside** of special construction vehicle injured **in** nontraffic accident

√x7ᵗʰ **V85.9 Unspecified occupant** of special construction vehicle **injured** in nontraffic accident ▽
Special-construction-vehicle accident NOS

√4ᵗʰ **V86 Occupant of special all-terrain or other off-road motor vehicle, injured in transport accident**
EXCLUDES 1   special all-terrain vehicle in stationary use or maintenance (W31.-)
           sport-utility vehicle (V50-V59)
           three-wheeled motor vehicle designed for on-road use (V30-V39)

√5ᵗʰ **V86.0 Driver** of special all-terrain or other off-road motor vehicle injured **in traffic accident**

√x7ᵗʰ **V86.01 Driver of** ambulance **or** fire engine **injured in traffic accident**

√x7ᵗʰ **V86.02 Driver of** snowmobile **injured in traffic accident**

√x7ᵗʰ **V86.03 Driver of** dune buggy **injured in traffic accident**

√x7ᵗʰ **V86.04 Driver of** military vehicle **injured in traffic accident**

● √x7ᵗʰ **V86.05 Driver of** 3- or 4- wheeled all-terrain vehicle (ATV) **injured in traffic accident**

● √x7ᵗʰ **V86.06 Driver of** dirt bike or motor/cross bike **injured in traffic accident**

√x7ᵗʰ **V86.09 Driver of other special all-terrain or other off-road motor vehicle injured in traffic accident**
Driver of dirt bike injured in traffic accident
Driver of go cart injured in traffic accident
Driver of golf cart injured in traffic accident

√5ᵗʰ **V86.1 Passenger** of special all-terrain or other off-road motor vehicle injured **in traffic accident**

√x7ᵗʰ **V86.11 Passenger of** ambulance **or** fire engine **injured in traffic accident**

√x7ᵗʰ **V86.12 Passenger of** snowmobile **injured in traffic accident**

√x7ᵗʰ **V86.13 Passenger of** dune buggy **injured in traffic accident**

√x7ᵗʰ **V86.14 Passenger of** military vehicle **injured in traffic accident**

● √x7ᵗʰ **V86.15 Passenger of** 3- or 4- wheeled all-terrain vehicle (ATV) **injured in traffic accident**

● √x7ᵗʰ **V86.16 Passenger of** dirt bike or motor/cross bike **injured in traffic accident**

√x7ᵗʰ **V86.19 Passenger of other special all-terrain or other off-road motor vehicle injured in traffic accident**
Passenger of dirt bike injured in traffic accident
Passenger of go cart injured in traffic accident
Passenger of golf cart injured in traffic accident

√5ᵗʰ **V86.2 Person on outside** of special all-terrain or other off-road motor vehicle injured **in traffic accident**

√x7ᵗʰ **V86.21 Person on outside of** ambulance **or** fire engine **injured in traffic accident**

√x7ᵗʰ **V86.22 Person on outside of** snowmobile **injured in traffic accident**

√x7ᵗʰ **V86.23 Person on outside of** dune buggy **injured in traffic accident**

√x7ᵗʰ **V86.24 Person on outside of** military vehicle **injured in traffic accident**

● √x7ᵗʰ **V86.25 Person on outside of** 3- or 4- wheeled all-terrain vehicle (ATV) **injured in traffic accident**

● √x7ᵗʰ **V86.26 Person on outside of** dirt bike or motor/cross bike **injured in traffic accident**

√x7ᵗʰ **V86.29 Person on outside of other special all-terrain or other off-road motor vehicle injured in traffic accident**
Person on outside of dirt bike injured in traffic accident
Person on outside of go cart in traffic accident
Person on outside of golf cart injured in traffic accident

√5ᵗʰ **V86.3 Unspecified occupant** of special all-terrain or other off-road motor vehicle injured **in traffic accident**

√x7ᵗʰ **V86.31 Unspecified occupant of** ambulance **or** fire engine **injured in traffic accident** ▽

√x7ᵗʰ **V86.32 Unspecified occupant of** snowmobile **injured in traffic accident** ▽

√x7ᵗʰ **V86.33 Unspecified occupant of** dune buggy **injured in traffic accident** ▽

√x7ᵗʰ **V86.34 Unspecified occupant of** military vehicle **injured in traffic accident** ▽

● √x7ᵗʰ **V86.35 Unspecified occupant of** 3- or 4- wheeled all-terrain vehicle (ATV) **injured in traffic accident** ▽

● √x7ᵗʰ **V86.36 Unspecified occupant of** dirt bike or motor/cross bike **injured in traffic accident** ▽

N Newborn: 0   P Pediatric: 0-17   M Maternity: 12-55   A Adult: 15-124   NRS Nonroutine supply Dx   NCDx Noncancer Dx   PDx Primary Dx   ►◄ Revised Text   ● New Code   ▲ Revised Title

1136   ICD-10-CM 2018

✓x7ᵗʰ V86.39 Unspecified occupant of other special all-terrain or other off-road motor vehicle injured in traffic accident ▽

     Unspecified occupant of dirt bike injured in traffic accident

     Unspecified occupant of go cart injured in traffic accident

     Unspecified occupant of golf cart injured in traffic accident

✓5ᵗʰ V86.4 Person injured while boarding or alighting **from special all-terrain or other off-road motor vehicle**

✓x7ᵗʰ V86.41 Person injured while boarding or alighting from ambulance **or** fire engine

✓x7ᵗʰ V86.42 Person injured while boarding or alighting from snowmobile

✓x7ᵗʰ V86.43 Person injured while boarding or alighting from dune buggy

✓x7ᵗʰ V86.44 Person injured while boarding or alighting from military vehicle

● **✓x7ᵗʰ V86.45 Person injured while boarding or alighting from a** 3- or 4- wheeled all-terrain vehicle (ATV)

● **✓x7ᵗʰ V86.46 Person injured while boarding or alighting from a** dirt bike or motor/cross bike

✓x7ᵗʰ V86.49 Person injured while boarding or alighting from other special all-terrain or other off-road motor vehicle

     Person injured while boarding or alighting from dirt bike

     Person injured while boarding or alighting from go cart

     Person injured while boarding or alighting from golf cart

✓5ᵗʰ V86.5 Driver **of special all-terrain or other off-road motor vehicle injured** in nontraffic accident

✓x7ᵗʰ V86.51 Driver of ambulance or fire engine **injured in nontraffic accident**

✓x7ᵗʰ V86.52 Driver of snowmobile **injured in nontraffic accident**

✓x7ᵗʰ V86.53 Driver of dune buggy **injured in nontraffic accident**

✓x7ᵗʰ V86.54 Driver of military vehicle **injured in nontraffic accident**

● **✓x7ᵗʰ V86.55 Driver of** 3- or 4- wheeled all-terrain vehicle (ATV) **injured in nontraffic accident**

● **✓x7ᵗʰ V86.56 Driver of** dirt bike or motor/cross bike **injured in nontraffic accident**

✓x7ᵗʰ V86.59 Driver of other special all-terrain or other off-road motor vehicle injured in nontraffic accident

     Driver of dirt bike injured in nontraffic accident

     Driver of go cart injured in nontraffic accident

     Driver of golf cart injured in nontraffic accident

✓5ᵗʰ V86.6 Passenger **of special all-terrain or other off-road motor vehicle injured** in nontraffic accident

✓x7ᵗʰ V86.61 Passenger of ambulance or fire engine **injured in nontraffic accident**

✓x7ᵗʰ V86.62 Passenger of snowmobile **injured in nontraffic accident**

✓x7ᵗʰ V86.63 Passenger of dune buggy **injured in nontraffic accident**

✓x7ᵗʰ V86.64 Passenger of military vehicle **injured in nontraffic accident**

● **✓x7ᵗʰ V86.65 Passenger of** 3- or 4- wheeled all-terrain vehicle (ATV) **injured in nontraffic accident**

● **✓x7ᵗʰ V86.66 Passenger of** dirt bike or motor/cross bike **injured in nontraffic accident**

✓x7ᵗʰ V86.69 Passenger of other special all-terrain or other off-road motor vehicle injured in nontraffic accident

     Passenger of dirt bike injured in nontraffic accident

     Passenger of go cart injured in nontraffic accident

     Passenger of golf cart injured in nontraffic accident

✓5ᵗʰ V86.7 Person on outside **of special all-terrain or other off-road motor vehicle injured** in nontraffic accident

✓x7ᵗʰ V86.71 Person on outside of ambulance or fire engine **injured in nontraffic accident**

✓x7ᵗʰ V86.72 Person on outside of snowmobile **injured in nontraffic accident**

✓x7ᵗʰ V86.73 Person on outside of dune buggy **injured in nontraffic accident**

✓x7ᵗʰ V86.74 Person on outside of military **vehicle injured in nontraffic accident**

● **✓x7ᵗʰ V86.75 Person on outside of** 3- or 4- wheeled all-terrain vehicle (ATV) **injured in nontraffic accident**

● **✓x7ᵗʰ V86.76 Person on outside of** dirt bike or motor/cross bike **injured in nontraffic accident**

✓x7ᵗʰ V86.79 Person on outside of other special all-terrain or other off-road motor vehicles injured in nontraffic accident

     Person on outside of dirt bike injured in nontraffic accident

     Person on outside of go cart injured in nontraffic accident

     Person on outside of golf cart injured in nontraffic accident

✓5ᵗʰ V86.9 Unspecified occupant **of special all-terrain or other off-road motor vehicle injured** in nontraffic accident

✓x7ᵗʰ V86.91 Unspecified occupant of ambulance or fire engine **injured in nontraffic accident** ▽

✓x7ᵗʰ V86.92 Unspecified occupant of snowmobile **injured in nontraffic accident** ▽

✓x7ᵗʰ V86.93 Unspecified occupant of dune buggy **injured in nontraffic accident** ▽

✓x7ᵗʰ V86.94 Unspecified occupant of military vehicle **injured in nontraffic accident** ▽

● **✓x7ᵗʰ V86.95 Unspecified occupant of** 3- or 4- wheeled all-terrain vehicle (ATV) **injured in nontraffic accident** ▽

● **✓x7ᵗʰ V86.96 Unspecified occupant of** dirt bike or motor/cross bike **injured in nontraffic accident** ▽

✓x7ᵗʰ V86.99 Unspecified occupant of other special all-terrain or other off-road motor vehicle injured in nontraffic accident ▽

     ~~All-terrain motor-vehicle accident NOS~~

     Off-road motor-vehicle accident NOS

     Other motor-vehicle accident NOS

     ~~Unspecified occupant of dirt bike injured in nontraffic accident~~

     Unspecified occupant of go cart injured in nontraffic accident

     Unspecified occupant of golf cart injured in nontraffic accident

✓4ᵗʰ V87 Traffic accident of specified type but victim's mode of transport unknown

     EXCLUDES 1 *collision involving:*
         pedal cycle (V10-V19)
         pedestrian (V01-V09)

✓x7ᵗʰ V87.0 Person injured in collision between car and two- or three-wheeled powered vehicle **(traffic)**

✓x7ᵗʰ V87.1 Person injured in collision between other motor vehicle and two- or three-wheeled motor vehicle **(traffic)**

✓x7ᵗʰ V87.2 Person injured in collision between car and pick-up truck or van **(traffic)**

✓x7ᵗʰ V87.3 Person injured in collision between car and bus **(traffic)**

✓x7ᵗʰ V87.4 Person injured in collision between car and heavy transport vehicle **(traffic)**

✓x7ᵗʰ V87.5 Person injured in collision between heavy transport vehicle and bus **(traffic)**

✓x7ᵗʰ V87.6 Person injured in collision between railway train or railway vehicle and car **(traffic)**

✓x7ᵗʰ V87.7 Person injured in collision between other specified motor vehicles **(traffic)**

✓x7ᵗʰ V87.8 Person injured in other specified noncollision transport accidents **involving** motor vehicle **(traffic)**

✓x7ᵗʰ V87.9 Person injured in other specified (collision)(noncollision) transport accidents **involving** nonmotor vehicle **(traffic)**

✓4ᵗʰ V88 Nontraffic accident of specified type but victim's mode of transport unknown

     EXCLUDES 1 *collision involving:*
         pedal cycle (V10-V19)
         pedestrian (V01-V09)

✓x7ᵗʰ V88.0 Person injured in collision between car and two- or three-wheeled motor vehicle, **nontraffic**

✓x7ᵗʰ V88.1 Person injured in collision between other motor vehicle and two- or three-wheeled motor vehicle, **nontraffic**

✓x7ᵗʰ V88.2 Person injured in collision between car and pick-up truck or van, **nontraffic**

☑ Additional Character Req   ✓x7ᵗʰ Placeholder Alert   Case-Mix Diagnosis   Manifestation   ▽ Unspecified Dx   **EXCLUDES 1** Not coded here   **EXCLUDES 2** Not included here

ICD-10-CM 2018   1137

√x7ᵗʰ **V88.3** **Person injured in collision between** car and bus, **nontraffic**

√x7ᵗʰ **V88.4** **Person injured in collision between** car and heavy transport vehicle, **nontraffic**

√x7ᵗʰ **V88.5** **Person injured in collision between** heavy transport vehicle and bus, **nontraffic**

√x7ᵗʰ **V88.6** **Person injured in collision between** railway train or railway vehicle and car, **nontraffic**

√x7ᵗʰ **V88.7** **Person injured in collision between other** specified motor vehicle, **nontraffic**

√x7ᵗʰ **V88.8** **Person injured in other** specified noncollision transport accidents **involving** motor vehicle, **nontraffic**

√x7ᵗʰ **V88.9** **Person injured in** other specified (collision)(noncollision) transport accidents **involving** nonmotor vehicle, **nontraffic**

√4ᵗʰ **V89 Motor- or nonmotor-vehicle accident, type of vehicle unspecified**

√x7ᵗʰ **V89.0** **Person injured in unspecified** motor-vehicle **accident,** nontraffic ▽
Motor-vehicle accident NOS, nontraffic

√x7ᵗʰ **V89.1** **Person injured in unspecified** nonmotor-vehicle **accident,** nontraffic ▽
Nonmotor-vehicle accident NOS (nontraffic)

√x7ᵗʰ **V89.2** **Person injured in unspecified** motor-vehicle **accident,** traffic ▽
Motor-vehicle accident [MVA] NOS
Road (traffic) accident [RTA] NOS

√x7ᵗʰ **V89.3** **Person injured in unspecified** nonmotor-vehicle **accident,** traffic ▽
Nonmotor-vehicle traffic accident NOS

√x7ᵗʰ **V89.9** **Person injured in unspecified** vehicle accident ▽
Collision NOS

Water transport accidents (V90-V94)

The appropriate 7th character is to be added to each code from categories V90-V94.
A   initial encounter
D   subsequent encounter
S   sequela

√4ᵗʰ **V90 Drowning and submersion due to accident to watercraft**
EXCLUDES 1   civilian water transport accident involving military watercraft (V94.81-)
fall into water not from watercraft (W16.-)
military watercraft accident in military or war operations (Y36.0-, Y37.0-)
water-transport-related drowning or submersion without accident to watercraft (V92.-)

√5ᵗʰ **V90.0** **Drowning and submersion due to** watercraft overturning

√x7ᵗʰ **V90.00** **Drowning and submersion due to** merchant ship overturning

√x7ᵗʰ **V90.01** **Drowning and submersion due to** passenger ship overturning
Drowning and submersion due to Ferry-boat overturning
Drowning and submersion due to Liner overturning

√x7ᵗʰ **V90.02** **Drowning and submersion due to** fishing boat overturning

√x7ᵗʰ **V90.03** **Drowning and submersion due to other** powered watercraft overturning
Drowning and submersion due to Hovercraft (on open water) overturning
Drowning and submersion due to Jet ski overturning

√x7ᵗʰ **V90.04** **Drowning and submersion due to** sailboat overturning

√x7ᵗʰ **V90.05** **Drowning and submersion due to** canoe or kayak overturning

√x7ᵗʰ **V90.06** **Drowning and submersion due to (nonpowered)** inflatable craft **overturning**

√x7ᵗʰ **V90.08** **Drowning and submersion due to other** unpowered watercraft overturning
Drowning and submersion due to windsurfer overturning

√x7ᵗʰ **V90.09** **Drowning and submersion due to unspecified** watercraft overturning ▽
Drowning and submersion due to boat NOS overturning
Drowning and submersion due to ship NOS overturning
Drowning and submersion due to watercraft NOS overturning

√5ᵗʰ **V90.1** **Drowning and submersion due to** watercraft sinking

√x7ᵗʰ **V90.10** **Drowning and submersion due to** merchant ship sinking

√x7ᵗʰ **V90.11** **Drowning and submersion due to** passenger ship sinking
Drowning and submersion due to Ferry-boat sinking
Drowning and submersion due to Liner sinking

√x7ᵗʰ **V90.12** **Drowning and submersion due to** fishing boat sinking

√x7ᵗʰ **V90.13** **Drowning and submersion due to other** powered watercraft sinking
Drowning and submersion due to Hovercraft (on open water) sinking
Drowning and submersion due to Jet ski sinking

√x7ᵗʰ **V90.14** **Drowning and submersion due to** sailboat sinking

√x7ᵗʰ **V90.15** **Drowning and submersion due to** canoe or kayak sinking

√x7ᵗʰ **V90.16** **Drowning and submersion due to (nonpowered)** inflatable craft **sinking**

√x7ᵗʰ **V90.18** **Drowning and submersion due to other** unpowered watercraft sinking

√x7ᵗʰ **V90.19** **Drowning and submersion due to unspecified** watercraft sinking ▽
Drowning and submersion due to boat NOS sinking
Drowning and submersion due to ship NOS sinking
Drowning and submersion due to watercraft NOS sinking

√5ᵗʰ **V90.2** **Drowning and submersion due to** falling or jumping from burning watercraft

√x7ᵗʰ **V90.20** **Drowning and submersion due to falling or jumping from burning** merchant ship

√x7ᵗʰ **V90.21** **Drowning and submersion due to falling or jumping from burning** passenger ship
Drowning and submersion due to falling or jumping from burning Ferry-boat
Drowning and submersion due to falling or jumping from burning Liner

√x7ᵗʰ **V90.22** **Drowning and submersion due to falling or jumping from burning** fishing boat

√x7ᵗʰ **V90.23** **Drowning and submersion due to falling or jumping from other burning** powered **watercraft**
Drowning and submersion due to falling and jumping from burning Hovercraft (on open water)
Drowning and submersion due to falling and jumping from burning Jet ski

√x7ᵗʰ **V90.24** **Drowning and submersion due to falling or jumping from burning** sailboat

√x7ᵗʰ **V90.25** **Drowning and submersion due to falling or jumping from burning** canoe or kayak

√x7ᵗʰ **V90.26** **Drowning and submersion due to falling or jumping from burning (nonpowered)** inflatable craft

√x7ᵗʰ **V90.27** **Drowning and submersion due to falling or jumping from burning** water-skis

√x7ᵗʰ **V90.28** **Drowning and submersion due to falling or jumping from other burning** unpowered **watercraft**
Drowning and submersion due to falling and jumping from burning surf-board
Drowning and submersion due to falling and jumping from burning windsurfer

√x7ᵗʰ **V90.29** **Drowning and submersion due to falling or jumping from unspecified burning watercraft** ▽
Drowning and submersion due to falling or jumping from burning boat NOS
Drowning and submersion due to falling or jumping from burning ship NOS
Drowning and submersion due to falling or jumping from burning watercraft NOS

√5ᵗʰ **V90.3** **Drowning and submersion due to** falling or jumping from crushed watercraft

√x7ᵗʰ **V90.30** **Drowning and submersion due to falling or jumping from crushed** merchant ship

√x7ᵗʰ **V90.31** **Drowning and submersion due to falling or jumping from crushed** passenger ship
Drowning and submersion due to falling and jumping from crushed Ferry boat
Drowning and submersion due to falling and jumping from crushed Liner

Ⓝ Newborn: 0   Ⓟ Pediatric: 0-17   Ⓜ Maternity: 12-55   Ⓐ Adult: 15-124   **NRS** Nonroutine supply Dx   **NC Dx** Noncancer Dx   **PDx** Primary Dx   ▶◀ Revised Text   ● New Code   ▲ Revised Title

√x7th **V90.32** **Drowning and submersion due to falling or jumping from crushed** fishing boat

√x7th **V90.33** **Drowning and submersion due to falling or jumping from other crushed** powered **watercraft**
Drowning and submersion due to falling and jumping from crushed Hovercraft
Drowning and submersion due to falling and jumping from crushed Jet ski

√x7th **V90.34** **Drowning and submersion due to falling or jumping from crushed** sailboat

√x7th **V90.35** **Drowning and submersion due to falling or jumping from crushed** canoe or kayak

√x7th **V90.36** **Drowning and submersion due to falling or jumping from crushed (nonpowered)** inflatable craft

√x7th **V90.37** **Drowning and submersion due to falling or jumping from crushed** water-skis

√x7th **V90.38** **Drowning and submersion due to falling or jumping from other crushed** unpowered **watercraft**
Drowning and submersion due to falling and jumping from crushed surf-board
Drowning and submersion due to falling and jumping from crushed windsurfer

√x7th **V90.39** **Drowning and submersion due to falling or jumping from crushed unspecified watercraft** ▽
Drowning and submersion due to falling and jumping from crushed boat NOS
Drowning and submersion due to falling and jumping from crushed ship NOS
Drowning and submersion due to falling and jumping from crushed watercraft NOS

√5th **V90.8** **Drowning and submersion due to** other accident to watercraft

√x7th **V90.80** **Drowning and submersion due to other accident to** merchant ship

√x7th **V90.81** **Drowning and submersion due to other accident to** passenger ship
Drowning and submersion due to other accident to Ferry-boat
Drowning and submersion due to other accident to Liner

√x7th **V90.82** **Drowning and submersion due to other accident to** fishing boat

√x7th **V90.83** **Drowning and submersion due to other accident to other** powered **watercraft**
Drowning and submersion due to other accident to Hovercraft (on open water)
Drowning and submersion due to other accident to Jet ski

√x7th **V90.84** **Drowning and submersion due to other accident to** sailboat

√x7th **V90.85** **Drowning and submersion due to other accident to** canoe or kayak

√x7th **V90.86** **Drowning and submersion due to other accident to (nonpowered)** inflatable craft

√x7th **V90.87** **Drowning and submersion due to other accident to** water-skis

√x7th **V90.88** **Drowning and submersion due to other accident to other** unpowered **watercraft**
Drowning and submersion due to other accident to surf-board
Drowning and submersion due to other accident to windsurfer

√x7th **V90.89** **Drowning and submersion due to other accident to unspecified watercraft** ▽
Drowning and submersion due to other accident to boat NOS
Drowning and submersion due to other accident to ship NOS
Drowning and submersion due to other accident to watercraft NOS

√4th **V91** **Other injury due to accident to watercraft**
INCLUDES   any injury except drowning and submersion as a result of an accident to watercraft
EXCLUDES 1   civilian water transport accident involving military watercraft (V94.81-)
military watercraft accident in military or war operations (Y36, Y37.-)
EXCLUDES 2   drowning and submersion due to accident to watercraft (V90.-)

√5th **V91.0** **Burn due to watercraft on fire**
EXCLUDES 1   burn from localized fire or explosion on board ship without accident to watercraft (V93.-)

√x7th **V91.00** **Burn due to** merchant ship **on fire**

√x7th **V91.01** **Burn due to** passenger ship **on fire**
Burn due to Ferry-boat on fire
Burn due to Liner on fire

√x7th **V91.02** **Burn due to** fishing boat **on fire**

√x7th **V91.03** **Burn due to other** powered **watercraft on fire**
Burn due to Hovercraft (on open water) on fire
Burn due to Jet ski on fire

√x7th **V91.04** **Burn due to** sailboat **on fire**

√x7th **V91.05** **Burn due to** canoe or kayak **on fire**

√x7th **V91.06** **Burn due to (nonpowered)** inflatable craft **on fire**

√x7th **V91.07** **Burn due to** water-skis **on fire**

√x7th **V91.08** **Burn due to other** unpowered **watercraft on fire**

√x7th **V91.09** **Burn due to unspecified watercraft on fire** ▽
Burn due to boat NOS on fire
Burn due to ship NOS on fire
Burn due to watercraft NOS on fire

√5th **V91.1** **Crushed between watercraft and other watercraft or other object due to collision**
Crushed by lifeboat after abandoning ship in a collision
NOTE   Select the specified type of watercraft that the victim was on at the time of the collision

√x7th **V91.10** **Crushed between** merchant ship **and other watercraft or other object due to collision**

√x7th **V91.11** **Crushed between** passenger ship **and other watercraft or other object due to collision**
Crushed between Ferry-boat and other watercraft or other object due to collision
Crushed between Liner and other watercraft or other object due to collision

√x7th **V91.12** **Crushed between** fishing boat **and other watercraft or other object due to collision**

√x7th **V91.13** **Crushed between other** powered **watercraft and other watercraft or other object due to collision**
Crushed between Hovercraft (on open water) and other watercraft or other object due to collision
Crushed between Jet ski and other watercraft or other object due to collision

√x7th **V91.14** **Crushed between** sailboat **and other watercraft or other object due to collision**

√x7th **V91.15** **Crushed between** canoe or kayak **and other watercraft or other object due to collision**

√x7th **V91.16** **Crushed between (nonpowered)** inflatable craft **and other watercraft or other object due to collision**

√x7th **V91.18** **Crushed between other** unpowered **watercraft and other watercraft or other object due to collision**
Crushed between surfboard and other watercraft or other object due to collision
Crushed between windsurfer and other watercraft or other object due to collision

√x7th **V91.19** **Crushed between unspecified watercraft and other watercraft or other object due to collision** ▽
Crushed between boat NOS and other watercraft or other object due to collision
Crushed between ship NOS and other watercraft or other object due to collision
Crushed between watercraft NOS and other watercraft or other object due to collision

---

√5ᵗʰ **V91.2** **Fall due to collision between watercraft and other watercraft or other object**
Fall while remaining on watercraft after collision
NOTE Select the specified type of watercraft that the victim was on at the time of the collision.
EXCLUDES 1 *crushed between watercraft and other watercraft and other object due to collision (V91.1-)*
drowning and submersion due to falling from crushed watercraft (V90.3-)

√x 7ᵗʰ **V91.20** **Fall due to collision between merchant ship and other watercraft or other object**

√x 7ᵗʰ **V91.21** **Fall due to collision between passenger ship and other watercraft or other object**
Fall due to collision between Ferry-boat and other watercraft or other object
Fall due to collision between Liner and other watercraft or other object

√x 7ᵗʰ **V91.22** **Fall due to collision between fishing boat and other watercraft or other object**

√x 7ᵗʰ **V91.23** **Fall due to collision between other powered watercraft and other watercraft or other object**
Fall due to collision between Hovercraft (on open water) and other watercraft or other object
Fall due to collision between Jet ski and other watercraft or other object

√x 7ᵗʰ **V91.24** **Fall due to collision between sailboat and other watercraft or other object**

√x 7ᵗʰ **V91.25** **Fall due to collision between canoe or kayak and other watercraft or other object**

√x 7ᵗʰ **V91.26** **Fall due to collision between (nonpowered) inflatable craft and other watercraft or other object**

√x 7ᵗʰ **V91.29** **Fall due to collision between unspecified** ▽ **watercraft and other watercraft or other object**
Fall due to collision between boat NOS and other watercraft or other object
Fall due to collision between ship NOS and other watercraft or other object
Fall due to collision between watercraft NOS and other watercraft or other object

√5ᵗʰ **V91.3** **Hit or struck by falling object due to accident to watercraft**
Hit or struck by falling object (part of damaged watercraft or other object) after falling or jumping from damaged watercraft
EXCLUDES 2 *drowning or submersion due to fall or jumping from damaged watercraft (V90.2-, V90.3-)*

√x 7ᵗʰ **V91.30** **Hit or struck by falling object due to accident to merchant ship**

√x 7ᵗʰ **V91.31** **Hit or struck by falling object due to accident to passenger ship**
Hit or struck by falling object due to accident to Ferry-boat
Hit or struck by falling object due to accident to Liner

√x 7ᵗʰ **V91.32** **Hit or struck by falling object due to accident to fishing boat**

√x 7ᵗʰ **V91.33** **Hit or struck by falling object due to accident to other powered watercraft**
Hit or struck by falling object due to accident to Hovercraft (on open water)
Hit or struck by falling object due to accident to Jet ski

√x 7ᵗʰ **V91.34** **Hit or struck by falling object due to accident to sailboat**

√x 7ᵗʰ **V91.35** **Hit or struck by falling object due to accident to canoe or kayak**

√x 7ᵗʰ **V91.36** **Hit or struck by falling object due to accident to (nonpowered) inflatable craft**

√x 7ᵗʰ **V91.37** **Hit or struck by falling object due to accident to water-skis**
Hit by water-skis after jumping off of waterskis

√x 7ᵗʰ **V91.38** **Hit or struck by falling object due to accident to other unpowered watercraft**
Hit or struck by surf-board after falling off damaged surf-board
Hit or struck by object after falling off damaged windsurfer

√x 7ᵗʰ **V91.39** **Hit or struck by falling object due to accident to** ▽ **unspecified watercraft**
Hit or struck by falling object due to accident to boat NOS
Hit or struck by falling object due to accident to ship NOS
Hit or struck by falling object due to accident to watercraft NOS

√5ᵗʰ **V91.8** **Other injury due to other accident to watercraft**

√x 7ᵗʰ **V91.80** **Other injury due to other accident to merchant ship**

√x 7ᵗʰ **V91.81** **Other injury due to other accident to passenger ship**
Other injury due to other accident to Ferry-boat
Other injury due to other accident to Liner

√x 7ᵗʰ **V91.82** **Other injury due to other accident to fishing boat**

√x 7ᵗʰ **V91.83** **Other injury due to other accident to other powered watercraft**
Other injury due to other accident to Hovercraft (on open water)
Other injury due to other accident to Jet ski

√x 7ᵗʰ **V91.84** **Other injury due to other accident to sailboat**

√x 7ᵗʰ **V91.85** **Other injury due to other accident to canoe or kayak**

√x 7ᵗʰ **V91.86** **Other injury due to other accident to (nonpowered) inflatable craft**

√x 7ᵗʰ **V91.87** **Other injury due to other accident to water-skis**

√x 7ᵗʰ **V91.88** **Other injury due to other accident to other unpowered watercraft**
Other injury due to other accident to surf-board
Other injury due to other accident to windsurfer

√x 7ᵗʰ **V91.89** **Other injury due to other accident to unspecified** ▽ **watercraft**
Other injury due to other accident to boat NOS
Other injury due to other accident to ship NOS
Other injury due to other accident to watercraft NOS

√4ᵗʰ **V92** **Drowning and submersion due to accident on board watercraft, without accident to watercraft**
EXCLUDES 1 *civilian water transport accident involving military watercraft (V94.81-)*
drowning or submersion due to accident to watercraft (V90-V91)
drowning or submersion of diver who voluntarily jumps from boat not involved in an accident (W16.711, W16.721)
fall into water without watercraft (W16.-)
military watercraft accident in military or war operations (Y36, Y37)

√5ᵗʰ **V92.0** **Drowning and submersion due to fall off watercraft**
Drowning and submersion due to fall from gangplank of watercraft
Drowning and submersion due to fall overboard watercraft
EXCLUDES 2 *hitting head on object or bottom of body of water due to fall from watercraft (V94.0-)*

√x 7ᵗʰ **V92.00** **Drowning and submersion due to fall off merchant ship**

√x 7ᵗʰ **V92.01** **Drowning and submersion due to fall off passenger ship**
Drowning and submersion due to fall off Ferry-boat
Drowning and submersion due to fall off Liner

√x 7ᵗʰ **V92.02** **Drowning and submersion due to fall off fishing boat**

√x 7ᵗʰ **V92.03** **Drowning and submersion due to fall off other powered watercraft**
Drowning and submersion due to fall off Hovercraft (on open water)
Drowning and submersion due to fall off Jet ski

√x 7ᵗʰ **V92.04** **Drowning and submersion due to fall off sailboat**

√x 7ᵗʰ **V92.05** **Drowning and submersion due to fall off canoe or kayak**

√x 7ᵗʰ **V92.06** **Drowning and submersion due to fall off (nonpowered) inflatable craft**

√x 7ᵗʰ **V92.07** **Drowning and submersion due to fall off water-skis**
EXCLUDES 1 *drowning and submersion due to falling off burning water-skis (V90.27)*
drowning and submersion due to falling off crushed water-skis (V90.37)
hit by boat while water-skiing NOS (V94.X)

Ⓝ Newborn: 0   Ⓟ Pediatric: 0-17   Ⓜ Maternity: 12-55   Ⓐ Adult: 15-124   **NRS** Nonroutine supply Dx   **NCDx** Noncancer Dx   **PDx** Primary Dx   ▶◀ Revised Text   ● New Code   ▲ Revised Title

1140   ICD-10-CM 2018

✓x7ᵗʰ V92.08 Drowning and submersion due to fall off other unpowered watercraft
    Drowning and submersion due to fall off surf-board
    Drowning and submersion due to fall off windsurfer
    EXCLUDES 1   *drowning and submersion due to fall off burning unpowered watercraft (V90.28)*
              drowning and submersion due to fall off crushed unpowered watercraft (V90.38)
              drowning and submersion due to fall off damaged unpowered watercraft (V90.88)
              drowning and submersion due to rider of nonpowered watercraft being hit by other watercraft (V94.-)
              other injury due to rider of nonpowered watercraft being hit by other watercraft (V94.-)

✓x7ᵗʰ V92.09 Drowning and submersion due to fall off unspecified watercraft   ▽
    Drowning and submersion due to fall off boat NOS
    Drowning and submersion due to fall off ship
    Drowning and submersion due to fall off watercraft NOS

✓5ᵗʰ V92.1 Drowning and submersion due to being thrown overboard by motion of watercraft
    EXCLUDES 1   *drowning and submersion due to fall off surf-board (V92.08)*
              drowning and submersion due to fall off water-skis (V92.07)
              drowning and submersion due to fall off windsurfer (V92.08)

✓x7ᵗʰ V92.10 Drowning and submersion due to being thrown overboard by motion of merchant ship

✓x7ᵗʰ V92.11 Drowning and submersion due to being thrown overboard by motion of passenger ship
    Drowning and submersion due to being thrown overboard by motion of Ferry-boat
    Drowning and submersion due to being thrown overboard by motion of Liner

✓x7ᵗʰ V92.12 Drowning and submersion due to being thrown overboard by motion of fishing boat

✓x7ᵗʰ V92.13 Drowning and submersion due to being thrown overboard by motion of other powered watercraft
    Drowning and submersion due to being thrown overboard by motion of Hovercraft

✓x7ᵗʰ V92.14 Drowning and submersion due to being thrown overboard by motion of sailboat

✓x7ᵗʰ V92.15 Drowning and submersion due to being thrown overboard by motion of canoe or kayak

✓x7ᵗʰ V92.16 Drowning and submersion due to being thrown overboard by motion of (nonpowered) inflatable craft

✓x7ᵗʰ V92.19 Drowning and submersion due to being thrown overboard by motion of unspecified watercraft   ▽
    Drowning and submersion due to being thrown overboard by motion of boat NOS
    Drowning and submersion due to being thrown overboard by motion of ship NOS
    Drowning and submersion due to being thrown overboard by motion of watercraft NOS

✓5ᵗʰ V92.2 Drowning and submersion due to being washed overboard from watercraft
    Code first any associated cataclysm (X37.0-)

✓x7ᵗʰ V92.20 Drowning and submersion due to being washed overboard from merchant ship

✓x7ᵗʰ V92.21 Drowning and submersion due to being washed overboard from passenger ship
    Drowning and submersion due to being washed overboard from Ferry-boat
    Drowning and submersion due to being washed overboard from Liner

✓x7ᵗʰ V92.22 Drowning and submersion due to being washed overboard from fishing boat

✓x7ᵗʰ V92.23 Drowning and submersion due to being washed overboard from other powered watercraft
    Drowning and submersion due to being washed overboard from Hovercraft (on open water)
    Drowning and submersion due to being washed overboard from Jet ski

✓x7ᵗʰ V92.24 Drowning and submersion due to being washed overboard from sailboat

✓x7ᵗʰ V92.25 Drowning and submersion due to being washed overboard from canoe or kayak

✓x7ᵗʰ V92.26 Drowning and submersion due to being washed overboard from (nonpowered) inflatable craft

✓x7ᵗʰ V92.27 Drowning and submersion due to being washed overboard from water-skis
    EXCLUDES 1   *drowning and submersion due to fall off water-skis (V92.07)*

✓x7ᵗʰ V92.28 Drowning and submersion due to being washed overboard from other unpowered watercraft
    Drowning and submersion due to being washed overboard from surf-board
    Drowning and submersion due to being washed overboard from windsurfer

✓x7ᵗʰ V92.29 Drowning and submersion due to being washed overboard from unspecified watercraft   ▽
    Drowning and submersion due to being washed overboard from boat NOS
    Drowning and submersion due to being washed overboard from ship NOS
    Drowning and submersion due to being washed overboard from watercraft NOS

✓4ᵗʰ V93 Other injury due to accident on board watercraft, without accident to watercraft
    EXCLUDES 1   *civilian water transport accident involving military watercraft (V94.81-)*
              other injury due to accident to watercraft (V91.-)
              military watercraft accident in military or war operations (Y36, Y37.-)
    EXCLUDES 2   *drowning and submersion due to accident on board watercraft, without accident to watercraft (V92.-)*

✓5ᵗʰ V93.0 Burn due to localized fire on board watercraft
    EXCLUDES 1   *burn due to watercraft on fire (V91.0-)*

✓x7ᵗʰ V93.00 Burn due to localized fire on board merchant vessel

✓x7ᵗʰ V93.01 Burn due to localized fire on board passenger vessel
    Burn due to localized fire on board Ferry-boat
    Burn due to localized fire on board Liner

✓x7ᵗʰ V93.02 Burn due to localized fire on board fishing boat

✓x7ᵗʰ V93.03 Burn due to localized fire on board other powered watercraft
    Burn due to localized fire on board Hovercraft
    Burn due to localized fire on board Jet ski

✓x7ᵗʰ V93.04 Burn due to localized fire on board sailboat

✓x7ᵗʰ V93.09 Burn due to localized fire on board unspecified watercraft   ▽
    Burn due to localized fire on board boat NOS
    Burn due to localized fire on board ship NOS
    Burn due to localized fire on board watercraft NOS

✓5ᵗʰ V93.1 Other burn on board watercraft
    Burn due to source other than fire on board watercraft
    EXCLUDES 1   *burn due to watercraft on fire (V91.0-)*

✓x7ᵗʰ V93.10 Other burn on board merchant vessel

✓x7ᵗʰ V93.11 Other burn on board passenger vessel
    Other burn on board Ferry-boat
    Other burn on board Liner

✓x7ᵗʰ V93.12 Other burn on board fishing boat

✓x7ᵗʰ V93.13 Other burn on board other powered watercraft
    Other burn on board Hovercraft
    Other burn on board Jet ski

✓x7ᵗʰ V93.14 Other burn on board sailboat

✓x7ᵗʰ V93.19 Other burn on board unspecified watercraft   ▽
    Other burn on board boat NOS
    Other burn on board ship NOS
    Other burn on board watercraft NOS

✓5ᵗʰ V93.2 Heat exposure on board watercraft
    EXCLUDES 1   *exposure to man-made heat not aboard watercraft (W92)*
              exposure to natural heat while on board watercraft (X30)
              exposure to sunlight while on board watercraft (X32)
    EXCLUDES 2   *burn due to fire on board watercraft (V93.0-)*

✓x7ᵗʰ V93.20 Heat exposure on board merchant ship

✓x7ᵗʰ V93.21 Heat exposure on board passenger ship
    Heat exposure on board Ferry-boat
    Heat exposure on board Liner

✓x7ᵗʰ V93.22 Heat exposure on board fishing boat

✓ Additional Character Req   ✓x7ᵗʰ Placeholder Alert   Case-Mix Diagnosis   Manifestation   ▽ Unspecified Dx   *EXCLUDES 1* Not coded here   *EXCLUDES 2* Not included here

√x7ᵗʰ **V93.23** **Heat exposure on board other** powered **watercraft**
Heat exposure on board hovercraft

√x7ᵗʰ **V93.24** **Heat exposure on board** sailboat

√x7ᵗʰ **V93.29** **Heat exposure on board unspecified watercraft** ▽
Heat exposure on board boat NOS
Heat exposure on board ship NOS
Heat exposure on board watercraft NOS

✓5ᵗʰ **V93.3** **Fall on board watercraft**
EXCLUDES 1   *fall due to collision of watercraft (V91.2-)*

√x7ᵗʰ **V93.30** **Fall on board** merchant ship

√x7ᵗʰ **V93.31** **Fall on board** passenger ship
Fall on board Ferry-boat
Fall on board Liner

√x7ᵗʰ **V93.32** **Fall on board** fishing boat

√x7ᵗʰ **V93.33** **Fall on board other** powered **watercraft**
Fall on board Hovercraft (on open water)
Fall on board Jet ski

√x7ᵗʰ **V93.34** **Fall on board** sailboat

√x7ᵗʰ **V93.35** **Fall on board** canoe or kayak

√x7ᵗʰ **V93.36** **Fall on board (nonpowered)** inflatable craft

√x7ᵗʰ **V93.38** **Fall on board other** unpowered **watercraft**

√x7ᵗʰ **V93.39** **Fall on board unspecified watercraft** ▽
Fall on board boat NOS
Fall on board ship NOS
Fall on board watercraft NOS

✓5ᵗʰ **V93.4** **Struck by falling object on board watercraft**
Hit by falling object on board watercraft
EXCLUDES 1   *struck by falling object due to accident to watercraft (V91.3)*

√x7ᵗʰ **V93.40** **Struck by falling object on** merchant ship

√x7ᵗʰ **V93.41** **Struck by falling object on** passenger ship
Struck by falling object on Ferry-boat
Struck by falling object on Liner

√x7ᵗʰ **V93.42** **Struck by falling object on** fishing boat

√x7ᵗʰ **V93.43** **Struck by falling object on other** powered **watercraft**
Struck by falling object on Hovercraft

√x7ᵗʰ **V93.44** **Struck by falling object on** sailboat

√x7ᵗʰ **V93.48** **Struck by falling object on other** unpowered **watercraft**

√x7ᵗʰ **V93.49** **Struck by falling object on unspecified watercraft** ▽

✓5ᵗʰ **V93.5** **Explosion on board watercraft**
Boiler explosion on steamship
EXCLUDES 2   *fire on board watercraft (V93.0-)*

√x7ᵗʰ **V93.50** **Explosion on board** merchant ship

√x7ᵗʰ **V93.51** **Explosion on board** passenger ship
Explosion on board Ferry-boat
Explosion on board Liner

√x7ᵗʰ **V93.52** **Explosion on board** fishing boat

√x7ᵗʰ **V93.53** **Explosion on board other** powered **watercraft**
Explosion on board Hovercraft
Explosion on board Jet ski

√x7ᵗʰ **V93.54** **Explosion on board** sailboat

√x7ᵗʰ **V93.59** **Explosion on board unspecified watercraft** ▽
Explosion on board boat NOS
Explosion on board ship NOS
Explosion on board watercraft NOS

✓5ᵗʰ **V93.6** **Machinery accident on board watercraft**
EXCLUDES 1   *machinery explosion on board watercraft (V93.4-)*
machinery fire on board watercraft (V93.0-)

√x7ᵗʰ **V93.60** **Machinery accident on board** merchant ship

√x7ᵗʰ **V93.61** **Machinery accident on board** passenger ship
Machinery accident on board Ferry-boat
Machinery accident on board Liner

√x7ᵗʰ **V93.62** **Machinery accident on board** fishing boat

√x7ᵗʰ **V93.63** **Machinery accident on board other** powered **watercraft**
Machinery accident on board Hovercraft

√x7ᵗʰ **V93.64** **Machinery accident on board** sailboat

√x7ᵗʰ **V93.69** **Machinery accident on board unspecified** ▽ **watercraft**
Machinery accident on board boat NOS
Machinery accident on board ship NOS
Machinery accident on board watercraft NOS

✓5ᵗʰ **V93.8** **Other injury due to other accident on board watercraft**
Accidental poisoning by gases or fumes on watercraft

√x7ᵗʰ **V93.80** **Other injury due to other accident on board** merchant ship

√x7ᵗʰ **V93.81** **Other injury due to other accident on board** passenger ship
Other injury due to other accident on board Ferry-boat
Other injury due to other accident on board Liner

√x7ᵗʰ **V93.82** **Other injury due to other accident on board** fishing boat

√x7ᵗʰ **V93.83** **Other injury due to other accident on board other** powered **watercraft**
Other injury due to other accident on board Hovercraft
Other injury due to other accident on board Jet ski

√x7ᵗʰ **V93.84** **Other injury due to other accident on board** sailboat

√x7ᵗʰ **V93.85** **Other injury due to other accident on board** canoe or kayak

√x7ᵗʰ **V93.86** **Other injury due to other accident on board (nonpowered)** inflatable craft

√x7ᵗʰ **V93.87** **Other injury due to other accident on board** water-skis
Hit or struck by object while waterskiing

√x7ᵗʰ **V93.88** **Other injury due to other accident on board other** unpowered **watercraft**
Hit or struck by object while surfing
Hit or struck by object while on board windsurfer

√x7ᵗʰ **V93.89** **Other injury due to other accident on board** ▽ **unspecified watercraft**
Other injury due to other accident on board boat NOS
Other injury due to other accident on board ship NOS
Other injury due to other accident on board watercraft NOS

✓4ᵗʰ **V94** **Other and unspecified water transport accidents**
EXCLUDES 1   *military watercraft accidents in military or war operations (Y36, Y37)*

√x7ᵗʰ **V94.0** **Hitting object or bottom of body of water due to fall from watercraft**
EXCLUDES 2   *drowning and submersion due to fall from watercraft (V92.0-)*

✓5ᵗʰ **V94.1** **Bather struck by watercraft**
Swimmer hit by watercraft

√x7ᵗʰ **V94.11** **Bather struck by** powered **watercraft**

√x7ᵗʰ **V94.12** **Bather struck by** nonpowered **watercraft**

✓5ᵗʰ **V94.2** **Rider of nonpowered watercraft struck by other watercraft**

√x7ᵗʰ **V94.21** **Rider of nonpowered watercraft struck by other** nonpowered **watercraft**
Canoer hit by other nonpowered watercraft
Surfer hit by other nonpowered watercraft
Windsurfer hit by other nonpowered watercraft

√x7ᵗʰ **V94.22** **Rider of nonpowered watercraft struck by** powered **watercraft**
Canoer hit by motorboat
Surfer hit by motorboat
Windsurfer hit by motorboat

✓5ᵗʰ **V94.3** **Injury to rider of (inflatable) watercraft being pulled behind other watercraft**

√x7ᵗʰ **V94.31** **Injury to rider of (inflatable)** recreational **watercraft being pulled behind other watercraft**
Injury to rider of inner-tube pulled behind motor boat

√x7ᵗʰ **V94.32** **Injury to rider of** non-recreational **watercraft being pulled behind other watercraft**
Injury to occupant of dingy being pulled behind boat or ship
Injury to occupant of life-raft being pulled behind boat or ship

√x7ᵗʰ **V94.4** **Injury to barefoot water-skier**
Injury to person being pulled behind boat or ship

✓5ᵗʰ **V94.8** **Other water transport accident**

✓6ᵗʰ **V94.81** **Water transport accident involving military watercraft**

√7ᵗʰ **V94.810** **Civilian watercraft involved in water transport accident with military watercraft**
Passenger on civilian watercraft injured due to accident with military watercraft

---

Ⓝ Newborn: 0   Ⓟ Pediatric: 0-17   Ⓜ Maternity: 12-55   Ⓐ Adult: 15-124   **NRS** Nonroutine supply Dx   **NCDx** Noncancer Dx   **PDx** Primary Dx   ▶◀ Revised Text   ● New Code   ▲ Revised Title

✔7ᵗʰ **V94.811** Civilian in water injured by military watercraft

✔7ᵗʰ **V94.818** Other water transport accident involving military watercraft

✔x7ᵗʰ **V94.89** Other water transport accident

✔x7ᵗʰ **V94.9** Unspecified water transport accident ▽
Water transport accident NOS

Air and space transport accidents (V95-V97)

EXCLUDES 1   *military aircraft accidents in military or war operations (Y36, Y37)*

The appropriate 7th character is to be added to each code from categories V95-V97.
A   initial encounter
D   subsequent encounter
S   sequela

✔4ᵗʰ **V95** **Accident to powered aircraft causing injury to occupant**

✔5ᵗʰ **V95.0** Helicopter accident injuring occupant

✔x7ᵗʰ **V95.00** Unspecified helicopter accident injuring occupant ▽

✔x7ᵗʰ **V95.01** Helicopter crash injuring occupant

✔x7ᵗʰ **V95.02** Forced landing of helicopter injuring occupant

✔x7ᵗʰ **V95.03** Helicopter collision injuring occupant
Helicopter collision with any object, fixed, movable or moving

✔x7ᵗʰ **V95.04** Helicopter fire injuring occupant

✔x7ᵗʰ **V95.05** Helicopter explosion injuring occupant

✔x7ᵗʰ **V95.09** Other helicopter accident injuring occupant

✔5ᵗʰ **V95.1** Ultralight, microlight or powered-glider accident injuring occupant

✔x7ᵗʰ **V95.10** Unspecified ultralight, microlight or powered-glider accident injuring occupant ▽

✔x7ᵗʰ **V95.11** Ultralight, microlight or powered-glider crash injuring occupant

✔x7ᵗʰ **V95.12** Forced landing of ultralight, microlight or powered-glider injuring occupant

✔x7ᵗʰ **V95.13** Ultralight, microlight or powered-glider collision injuring occupant
Ultralight, microlight or powered-glider collision with any object, fixed, movable or moving

✔x7ᵗʰ **V95.14** Ultralight, microlight or powered-glider fire injuring occupant

✔x7ᵗʰ **V95.15** Ultralight, microlight or powered-glider explosion injuring occupant

✔x7ᵗʰ **V95.19** Other ultralight, microlight or powered-glider accident injuring occupant

✔5ᵗʰ **V95.2** Other private fixed-wing aircraft accident injuring occupant

✔x7ᵗʰ **V95.20** Unspecified accident to other private fixed-wing aircraft, injuring occupant ▽

✔x7ᵗʰ **V95.21** Other private fixed-wing aircraft crash injuring occupant

✔x7ᵗʰ **V95.22** Forced landing of other private fixed-wing aircraft injuring occupant

✔x7ᵗʰ **V95.23** Other private fixed-wing aircraft collision injuring occupant
Other private fixed-wing aircraft collision with any object, fixed, movable or moving

✔x7ᵗʰ **V95.24** Other private fixed-wing aircraft fire injuring occupant

✔x7ᵗʰ **V95.25** Other private fixed-wing aircraft explosion injuring occupant

✔x7ᵗʰ **V95.29** Other accident to other private fixed-wing aircraft injuring occupant

✔5ᵗʰ **V95.3** Commercial fixed-wing aircraft accident injuring occupant

✔x7ᵗʰ **V95.30** Unspecified accident to commercial fixed-wing aircraft injuring occupant ▽

✔x7ᵗʰ **V95.31** Commercial fixed-wing aircraft crash injuring occupant

✔x7ᵗʰ **V95.32** Forced landing of commercial fixed-wing aircraft injuring occupant

✔x7ᵗʰ **V95.33** Commercial fixed-wing aircraft collision injuring occupant
Commercial fixed-wing aircraft collision with any object, fixed, movable or moving

✔x7ᵗʰ **V95.34** Commercial fixed-wing aircraft fire injuring occupant

✔x7ᵗʰ **V95.35** Commercial fixed-wing aircraft explosion injuring occupant

✔x7ᵗʰ **V95.39** Other accident to commercial fixed-wing aircraft injuring occupant

✔5ᵗʰ **V95.4** Spacecraft accident injuring occupant

✔x7ᵗʰ **V95.40** Unspecified spacecraft accident injuring occupant ▽

✔x7ᵗʰ **V95.41** Spacecraft crash injuring occupant

✔x7ᵗʰ **V95.42** Forced landing of spacecraft injuring occupant

✔x7ᵗʰ **V95.43** Spacecraft collision injuring occupant
Spacecraft collision with any object, fixed, moveable or moving

✔x7ᵗʰ **V95.44** Spacecraft fire injuring occupant

✔x7ᵗʰ **V95.45** Spacecraft explosion injuring occupant

✔x7ᵗʰ **V95.49** Other spacecraft accident injuring occupant

✔x7ᵗʰ **V95.8** Other powered aircraft accidents injuring occupant

✔x7ᵗʰ **V95.9** Unspecified aircraft accident injuring occupant ▽
Aircraft accident NOS
Air transport accident NOS

✔4ᵗʰ **V96** **Accident to nonpowered aircraft causing injury to occupant**

✔5ᵗʰ **V96.0** Balloon accident injuring occupant

✔x7ᵗʰ **V96.00** Unspecified balloon accident injuring occupant ▽

✔x7ᵗʰ **V96.01** Balloon crash injuring occupant

✔x7ᵗʰ **V96.02** Forced landing of balloon injuring occupant

✔x7ᵗʰ **V96.03** Balloon collision injuring occupant
Balloon collision with any object, fixed, moveable or moving

✔x7ᵗʰ **V96.04** Balloon fire injuring occupant

✔x7ᵗʰ **V96.05** Balloon explosion injuring occupant

✔x7ᵗʰ **V96.09** Other balloon accident injuring occupant

✔5ᵗʰ **V96.1** Hang-glider accident injuring occupant

✔x7ᵗʰ **V96.10** Unspecified hang-glider accident injuring occupant ▽

✔x7ᵗʰ **V96.11** Hang-glider crash injuring occupant

✔x7ᵗʰ **V96.12** Forced landing of hang-glider injuring occupant

✔x7ᵗʰ **V96.13** Hang-glider collision injuring occupant
Hang-glider collision with any object, fixed, moveable or moving

✔x7ᵗʰ **V96.14** Hang-glider fire injuring occupant

✔x7ᵗʰ **V96.15** Hang-glider explosion injuring occupant

✔x7ᵗʰ **V96.19** Other hang-glider accident injuring occupant

✔5ᵗʰ **V96.2** Glider (nonpowered) accident injuring occupant

✔x7ᵗʰ **V96.20** Unspecified glider (nonpowered) accident injuring occupant ▽

✔x7ᵗʰ **V96.21** Glider (nonpowered) crash injuring occupant

✔x7ᵗʰ **V96.22** Forced landing of glider (nonpowered) injuring occupant

✔x7ᵗʰ **V96.23** Glider (nonpowered) collision injuring occupant
Glider (nonpowered) collision with any object, fixed, moveable or moving

✔x7ᵗʰ **V96.24** Glider (nonpowered) fire injuring occupant

✔x7ᵗʰ **V96.25** Glider (nonpowered) explosion injuring occupant

✔x7ᵗʰ **V96.29** Other glider (nonpowered) accident injuring occupant

✔x7ᵗʰ **V96.8** Other nonpowered-aircraft accidents injuring occupant
Kite carrying a person accident injuring occupant

✔x7ᵗʰ **V96.9** Unspecified nonpowered-aircraft accident injuring occupant ▽
Nonpowered-aircraft accident NOS

✔4ᵗʰ **V97** **Other specified air transport accidents**

✔x7ᵗʰ **V97.0** Occupant of aircraft injured in other specified air transport accidents
Fall in, on or from aircraft in air transport accident
EXCLUDES 1   *accident while boarding or alighting aircraft (V97.1)*

✔x7ᵗʰ **V97.1** Person injured while boarding or alighting from aircraft

✔5ᵗʰ **V97.2** Parachutist accident

✔x7ᵗʰ **V97.21** Parachutist entangled in object
Parachutist landing in tree

✔x7ᵗʰ **V97.22** Parachutist injured on landing

☑ Additional Character Req   ✔x7ᵗʰ Placeholder Alert   Case-Mix Diagnosis   Manifestation   ▽ Unspecified Dx   *EXCLUDES 1* Not coded here   *EXCLUDES 2* Not included here

ICD-10-CM 2018   1143

✓x7ᵗʰ **V97.29 Other parachutist accident**

✓5ᵗʰ **V97.3 Person on ground injured in air transport accident**

✓x7ᵗʰ **V97.31 Hit by object falling from aircraft**
Hit by crashing aircraft
Injured by aircraft hitting house
Injured by aircraft hitting car

✓x7ᵗʰ **V97.32 Injured by rotating propeller**

✓x7ᵗʰ **V97.33 Sucked into jet engine**

✓x7ᵗʰ **V97.39 Other injury to person on ground due to air transport accident**

✓5ᵗʰ **V97.8 Other air transport accidents, not elsewhere classified**

> EXCLUDES 1   *aircraft accident NOS (V95.9)*
> *exposure to changes in air pressure during ascent or descent (W94.-)*

✓6ᵗʰ **V97.81 Air transport accident involving military aircraft**

✓7ᵗʰ **V97.810 Civilian aircraft involved in air transport accident with military aircraft**
Passenger in civilian aircraft injured due to accident with military aircraft

✓7ᵗʰ **V97.811 Civilian injured by military aircraft**

✓7ᵗʰ **V97.818 Other air transport accident involving military aircraft**

✓x7ᵗʰ **V97.89 Other air transport accidents, not elsewhere classified**
Injury from machinery on aircraft

Other and unspecified transport accidents (V98-V99)

> EXCLUDES 1   *vehicle accident, type of vehicle unspecified (V89.-)*

The appropriate 7th character is to be added to each code from categories V98-V99.
A   initial encounter
D   subsequent encounter
S   sequela

✓4ᵗʰ **V98 Other specified transport accidents**

✓x7ᵗʰ **V98.0 Accident to, on or involving cable-car, not on rails**
Caught or dragged by cable-car, not on rails
Fall or jump from cable-car, not on rails
Object thrown from or in cable-car, not on rails

✓x7ᵗʰ **V98.1 Accident to, on or involving land-yacht**

✓x7ᵗʰ **V98.2 Accident to, on or involving ice yacht**

✓x7ᵗʰ **V98.3 Accident to, on or involving ski lift**
Accident to, on or involving ski chair-lift
Accident to, on or involving ski-lift with gondola

✓x7ᵗʰ **V98.8 Other specified transport accidents**

✓x7ᵗʰ **V99 Unspecified transport accident** ▽

OTHER EXTERNAL CAUSES OF ACCIDENTAL INJURY (W00-X58)

Slipping, tripping, stumbling and falls (W00-W19)

> EXCLUDES 1   *assault involving a fall (Y01-Y02)*
> *fall from animal (V80.-)*
> *fall (in) (from) machinery (in operation) (W28-W31)*
> *fall (in) (from) transport vehicle (V01-V99)*
> *intentional self-harm involving a fall (X80-X81)*

> EXCLUDES 2   *at risk for fall (history of fall) (Z91.81)*
> *fall (in) (from) burning building (X00.-)*
> *fall into fire ▶(X00-X04, X08)◀*

The appropriate 7th character is to be added to each code from category W00-W19.
A   initial encounter
D   subsequent encounter
S   sequela

✓4ᵗʰ **W00 Fall due to ice and snow**

> INCLUDES   pedestrian on foot falling (slipping) on ice and snow

> EXCLUDES 1   *fall on (from) ice and snow involving pedestrian conveyance (V00.-)*
> *fall from stairs and steps not due to ice and snow (W10.-)*

> AHA: 2016, 2Q, 4

✓x7ᵗʰ **W00.0 Fall on same level due to ice and snow**

✓x7ᵗʰ **W00.1 Fall from stairs and steps due to ice and snow**

✓x7ᵗʰ **W00.2 Other fall from one level to another due to ice and snow**

✓x7ᵗʰ **W00.9 Unspecified fall due to ice and snow** ▽

✓4ᵗʰ **W01 Fall on same level from slipping, tripping and stumbling**

> INCLUDES   fall on moving sidewalk

> EXCLUDES 1   *fall due to bumping (striking) against object (W18.0-)*
> *fall in shower or bathtub (W18.2-)*
> *fall on same level NOS (W18.30)*
> *fall on same level from slipping, tripping and stumbling due to ice or snow (W00.0)*
> *fall off or from toilet (W18.1-)*
> *slipping, tripping and stumbling NOS (W18.40)*
> *slipping, tripping and stumbling without falling (W18.4-)*

✓x7ᵗʰ **W01.0 Fall on same level from slipping, tripping and stumbling without subsequent striking against object**
Falling over animal

✓5ᵗʰ **W01.1 Fall on same level from slipping, tripping and stumbling with subsequent striking against object**

✓x7ᵗʰ **W01.10 Fall on same level from slipping, tripping and stumbling with subsequent striking against unspecified object** ▽

✓6ᵗʰ **W01.11 Fall on same level from slipping, tripping and stumbling with subsequent striking against sharp object**

✓7ᵗʰ **W01.110 Fall on same level from slipping, tripping and stumbling with subsequent striking against sharp glass**

✓7ᵗʰ **W01.111 Fall on same level from slipping, tripping and stumbling with subsequent striking against power tool or machine**

✓7ᵗʰ **W01.118 Fall on same level from slipping, tripping and stumbling with subsequent striking against other sharp object**

✓7ᵗʰ **W01.119 Fall on same level from slipping, tripping and stumbling with subsequent striking against unspecified sharp object** ▽

✓6ᵗʰ **W01.19 Fall on same level from slipping, tripping and stumbling with subsequent striking against other object**

✓7ᵗʰ **W01.190 Fall on same level from slipping, tripping and stumbling with subsequent striking against furniture**

✓7ᵗʰ **W01.198 Fall on same level from slipping, tripping and stumbling with subsequent striking against other object**

✓x7ᵗʰ **W03 Other fall on same level due to collision with another person**
Fall due to non-transport collision with other person

> EXCLUDES 1   *collision with another person without fall (W51)*
> *crushed or pushed by a crowd or human stampede (W52)*
> *fall involving pedestrian conveyance (V00-V09)*
> *fall due to ice or snow (W00)*
> *fall on same level NOS (W18.30)*

> AHA: 2012, 4Q, 108

✓x7ᵗʰ **W04 Fall while being carried or supported by other persons**
Accidentally dropped while being carried

✓4ᵗʰ **W05 Fall from non-moving wheelchair, nonmotorized scooter and motorized mobility scooter**

> EXCLUDES 1   *fall from moving wheelchair (powered) (V00.811)*
> *fall from moving motorized mobility scooter (V00.831)*
> *fall from nonmotorized scooter (V00.141)*

✓x7ᵗʰ **W05.0 Fall from non-moving wheelchair**

✓x7ᵗʰ **W05.1 Fall from non-moving nonmotorized scooter**

✓x7ᵗʰ **W05.2 Fall from non-moving motorized mobility scooter**

✓x7ᵗʰ **W06 Fall from bed**

✓x7ᵗʰ **W07 Fall from chair**

✓x7ᵗʰ **W08 Fall from other furniture**

✓4ᵗʰ **W09 Fall on and from playground equipment**

> EXCLUDES 1   *fall involving recreational machinery (W31)*

✓x7ᵗʰ **W09.0 Fall on or from playground slide**

✓x7ᵗʰ **W09.1 Fall from playground swing**

✓x7ᵗʰ **W09.2 Fall on or from jungle gym**

✓x7ᵗʰ **W09.8 Fall on or from other playground equipment**

✓4ᵗʰ **W10 Fall on and from stairs and steps**

> EXCLUDES 1   *Fall from stairs and steps due to ice and snow (W00.1)*

✓x7ᵗʰ **W10.0 Fall (on)(from) escalator**

✓x7ᵗʰ **W10.1 Fall (on)(from) sidewalk curb**

✓x7ᵗʰ **W10.2 Fall (on)(from) incline**
Fall (on) (from) ramp

Ⓝ Newborn: 0   Ⓟ Pediatric: 0-17   Ⓜ Maternity: 12-55   Ⓐ Adult: 15-124   NRS Nonroutine supply Dx   NCDx Noncancer Dx   PDx Primary Dx   ▶◀ Revised Text   ● New Code   ▲ Revised Title

Chapter 20. External Causes of Morbidity

- ✓x7ᵗʰ **W10.8** Fall (on) (from) other stairs and steps
- ✓x7ᵗʰ **W10.9** Fall (on) (from) unspecified stairs and steps ▽

✓x7ᵗʰ **W11 Fall on and from ladder**

✓x7ᵗʰ **W12 Fall on and from scaffolding**

✓4ᵗʰ **W13 Fall from, out of or through building or structure**

- ✓x7ᵗʰ **W13.0 Fall from, out of or through balcony**
  Fall from, out of or through railing

- ✓x7ᵗʰ **W13.1 Fall from, out of or through bridge**

- ✓x7ᵗʰ **W13.2 Fall from, out of or through roof**

- ✓x7ᵗʰ **W13.3 Fall through floor**

- ✓x7ᵗʰ **W13.4 Fall from, out of or through window**
  - EXCLUDES 2   *fall with subsequent striking against sharp glass (W01.110)*

- ✓x7ᵗʰ **W13.8 Fall from, out of or through other building or structure**
  Fall from, out of or through viaduct
  Fall from, out of or through wall
  Fall from, out of or through flag-pole

- ✓x7ᵗʰ **W13.9 Fall from, out of or through building, not otherwise specified** ▽
  - EXCLUDES 1   *collapse of a building or structure (W20.-)*
    fall or jump from burning building or structure (X00.-)

✓x7ᵗʰ **W14 Fall from tree**

✓x7ᵗʰ **W15 Fall from cliff**

✓4ᵗʰ **W16 Fall, jump or diving into water**
- EXCLUDES 1   *accidental non-watercraft drowning and submersion not involving fall (W65-W74)*
  effects of air pressure from diving (W94.-)
  fall into water from watercraft (V90-V94)
  hitting an object or against bottom when falling from watercraft (V94.0)
- EXCLUDES 2   *striking or hitting diving board (W21.4)*

- ✓5ᵗʰ **W16.0 Fall into swimming pool**
  Fall into swimming pool NOS
  - EXCLUDES 1   *fall into empty swimming pool (W17.3)*

  - ✓6ᵗʰ **W16.01 Fall into swimming pool** striking water surface
    - ✓7ᵗʰ **W16.011 Fall into swimming pool striking water surface causing** drowning **and submersion**
      - EXCLUDES 1   *drowning and submersion while in swimming pool without fall (W67)*
    - ✓7ᵗʰ **W16.012 Fall into swimming pool striking water surface causing other injury**

  - ✓6ᵗʰ **W16.02 Fall into swimming pool** striking bottom
    - ✓7ᵗʰ **W16.021 Fall into swimming pool striking bottom causing** drowning **and submersion**
      - EXCLUDES 1   *drowning and submersion while in swimming pool without fall (W67)*
    - ✓7ᵗʰ **W16.022 Fall into swimming pool striking bottom causing other injury**

  - ✓6ᵗʰ **W16.03 Fall into swimming pool** striking wall
    - ✓7ᵗʰ **W16.031 Fall into swimming pool striking wall causing** drowning **and submersion**
      - EXCLUDES 1   *drowning and submersion while in swimming pool without fall (W67)*
    - ✓7ᵗʰ **W16.032 Fall into swimming pool striking wall causing other injury**

- ✓5ᵗʰ **W16.1 Fall into natural body of water**
  Fall into lake
  Fall into open sea
  Fall into river
  Fall into stream

  - ✓6ᵗʰ **W16.11 Fall into natural body of water** striking water surface
    - ✓7ᵗʰ **W16.111 Fall into natural body of water striking water surface causing** drowning **and submersion**
      - EXCLUDES 1   *drowning and submersion while in natural body of water without fall (W69)*
    - ✓7ᵗʰ **W16.112 Fall into natural body of water striking water surface causing other injury**

- ✓6ᵗʰ **W16.12 Fall into natural body of water** striking bottom
  - ✓7ᵗʰ **W16.121 Fall into natural body of water striking bottom causing** drowning **and submersion**
    - EXCLUDES 1   *drowning and submersion while in natural body of water without fall (W69)*
  - ✓7ᵗʰ **W16.122 Fall into natural body of water striking bottom causing other injury**

- ✓6ᵗʰ **W16.13 Fall into natural body of water** striking side
  - ✓7ᵗʰ **W16.131 Fall into natural body of water striking side causing** drowning **and submersion**
    - EXCLUDES 1   *drowning and submersion while in natural body of water without fall (W69)*
  - ✓7ᵗʰ **W16.132 Fall into natural body of water striking side causing other injury**

- ✓5ᵗʰ **W16.2 Fall in (into) filled bathtub or bucket of water**
  - ✓6ᵗʰ **W16.21 Fall in (into)** filled bathtub
    - EXCLUDES 1   *fall into empty bathtub (W18.2)*
    - ✓7ᵗʰ **W16.211 Fall in (into) filled bathtub causing** drowning **and submersion**
      - EXCLUDES 1   *drowning and submersion while in filled bathtub without fall (W65)*
    - ✓7ᵗʰ **W16.212 Fall in (into) filled bathtub causing other injury**

  - ✓6ᵗʰ **W16.22 Fall in (into)** bucket of water
    - ✓7ᵗʰ **W16.221 Fall in (into) bucket of water causing** drowning **and submersion**
    - ✓7ᵗʰ **W16.222 Fall in (into) bucket of water causing other injury**

- ✓5ᵗʰ **W16.3 Fall into other water**
  Fall into fountain
  Fall into reservoir

  - ✓6ᵗʰ **W16.31 Fall into other water** striking water surface
    - ✓7ᵗʰ **W16.311 Fall into other water striking water surface causing** drowning **and submersion**
      - EXCLUDES 1   *drowning and submersion while in other water without fall (W73)*
    - ✓7ᵗʰ **W16.312 Fall into other water striking water surface causing other injury**

  - ✓6ᵗʰ **W16.32 Fall into other water** striking bottom
    - ✓7ᵗʰ **W16.321 Fall into other water striking bottom causing** drowning **and submersion**
      - EXCLUDES 1   *drowning and submersion while in other water without fall (W73)*
    - ✓7ᵗʰ **W16.322 Fall into other water striking bottom causing other injury**

  - ✓6ᵗʰ **W16.33 Fall into other water** striking wall
    - ✓7ᵗʰ **W16.331 Fall into other water striking wall causing** drowning **and submersion**
      - EXCLUDES 1   *drowning and submersion while in other water without fall (W73)*
    - ✓7ᵗʰ **W16.332 Fall into other water striking wall causing other injury**

- ✓5ᵗʰ **W16.4 Fall into unspecified water**
  - ✓x7ᵗʰ **W16.41 Fall into unspecified water causing drowning and submersion** ▽
  - ✓x7ᵗʰ **W16.42 Fall into unspecified water causing other injury** ▽

- ✓5ᵗʰ **W16.5 Jumping or diving into swimming pool**
  - ✓6ᵗʰ **W16.51 Jumping or diving into swimming pool** striking water surface
    - ✓7ᵗʰ **W16.511 Jumping or diving into swimming pool striking water surface causing** drowning **and submersion**
      - EXCLUDES 1   *drowning and submersion while in swimming pool without jumping or diving (W67)*
    - ✓7ᵗʰ **W16.512 Jumping or diving into swimming pool striking water surface causing other injury**

✓ Additional Character Req   ✓x7ᵗʰ Placeholder Alert   Case-Mix Diagnosis   Manifestation   ▽ Unspecified Dx   EXCLUDES 1 Not coded here   EXCLUDES 2 Not included here

ICD-10-CM 2018   1145

✓6ᵗʰ **W16.52 Jumping or diving into swimming pool** striking bottom

✓7ᵗʰ **W16.521 Jumping or diving into swimming pool striking bottom causing** drowning **and submersion**
EXCLUDES 1 *drowning and submersion while in swimming pool without jumping or diving (W67)*

✓7ᵗʰ **W16.522 Jumping or diving into swimming pool striking bottom causing other injury**

✓6ᵗʰ **W16.53 Jumping or diving into swimming pool** striking wall

✓7ᵗʰ **W16.531 Jumping or diving into swimming pool striking wall causing** drowning **and submersion**
EXCLUDES 1 *drowning and submersion while in swimming pool without jumping or diving (W67)*

✓7ᵗʰ **W16.532 Jumping or diving into swimming pool striking wall causing other injury**

✓5ᵗʰ **W16.6 Jumping or diving into** natural body of water
Jumping or diving into lake
Jumping or diving into open sea
Jumping or diving into river
Jumping or diving into stream

✓6ᵗʰ **W16.61 Jumping or diving into natural body of water** striking water surface

✓7ᵗʰ **W16.611 Jumping or diving into natural body of water striking water surface causing** drowning **and submersion**
EXCLUDES 1 *drowning and submersion while in natural body of water without jumping or diving (W69)*

✓7ᵗʰ **W16.612 Jumping or diving into natural body of water striking water surface causing other injury**

✓6ᵗʰ **W16.62 Jumping or diving into natural body of water** striking bottom

✓7ᵗʰ **W16.621 Jumping or diving into natural body of water striking bottom causing** drowning **and submersion**
EXCLUDES 1 *drowning and submersion while in natural body of water without jumping or diving (W69)*

✓7ᵗʰ **W16.622 Jumping or diving into natural body of water striking bottom causing other injury**

✓5ᵗʰ **W16.7 Jumping or diving** from boat
EXCLUDES 1 *fall from boat into water—see watercraft accident (V90-V94)*

✓6ᵗʰ **W16.71 Jumping or diving from boat** striking water surface

✓7ᵗʰ **W16.711 Jumping or diving from boat striking water surface causing** drowning **and submersion**

✓7ᵗʰ **W16.712 Jumping or diving from boat striking water surface causing other injury**

✓6ᵗʰ **W16.72 Jumping or diving from boat** striking bottom

✓7ᵗʰ **W16.721 Jumping or diving from boat striking bottom causing** drowning **and submersion**

✓7ᵗʰ **W16.722 Jumping or diving from boat striking bottom causing other injury**

✓5ᵗʰ **W16.8 Jumping or diving** into other water
Jumping or diving into fountain
Jumping or diving into reservoir

✓6ᵗʰ **W16.81 Jumping or diving into other water** striking water surface

✓7ᵗʰ **W16.811 Jumping or diving into other water striking water surface causing** drowning **and submersion**
EXCLUDES 1 *drowning and submersion while in other water without jumping or diving (W73)*

✓7ᵗʰ **W16.812 Jumping or diving into other water striking water surface causing other injury**

✓6ᵗʰ **W16.82 Jumping or diving into other water** striking bottom

✓7ᵗʰ **W16.821 Jumping or diving into other water striking bottom causing** drowning **and submersion**
EXCLUDES 1 *drowning and submersion while in other water without jumping or diving (W73)*

✓7ᵗʰ **W16.822 Jumping or diving into other water striking bottom causing other injury**

✓6ᵗʰ **W16.83 Jumping or diving into other water** striking wall

✓7ᵗʰ **W16.831 Jumping or diving into other water striking wall causing** drowning **and submersion**
EXCLUDES 1 *drowning and submersion while in other water without jumping or diving (W73)*

✓7ᵗʰ **W16.832 Jumping or diving into other water striking wall causing other injury**

✓5ᵗʰ **W16.9 Jumping or diving into** unspecified water

✓ₓ7ᵗʰ **W16.91 Jumping or diving into unspecified water causing** ▽ drowning **and submersion**

✓ₓ7ᵗʰ **W16.92 Jumping or diving into unspecified water causing** ▽ **other injury**

✓4ᵗʰ **W17 Other fall from one level to another**

✓ₓ7ᵗʰ **W17.0 Fall into well**

✓ₓ7ᵗʰ **W17.1 Fall into storm drain or manhole**

✓ₓ7ᵗʰ **W17.2 Fall into hole**
Fall into pit

✓ₓ7ᵗʰ **W17.3 Fall into empty swimming pool**
EXCLUDES 1 *fall into filled swimming pool (W16.0-)*

✓ₓ7ᵗʰ **W17.4 Fall from dock**

✓5ᵗʰ **W17.8 Other fall from one level to another**

✓ₓ7ᵗʰ **W17.81 Fall down embankment (hill)**

✓ₓ7ᵗʰ **W17.82 Fall from (out of) grocery cart**
Fall due to grocery cart tipping over

✓ₓ7ᵗʰ **W17.89 Other fall from one level to another**
Fall from cherry picker
Fall from lifting device
Fall from mobile elevated work platform [MEWP]
Fall from sky lift
AHA: 2015, 2Q, 6

✓4ᵗʰ **W18 Other slipping, tripping and stumbling and falls**

✓5ᵗʰ **W18.0 Fall due to bumping against object**
Striking against object with subsequent fall
EXCLUDES 1 *fall on same level due to slipping, tripping, or stumbling with subsequent striking against object (W01.1-)*

✓ₓ7ᵗʰ **W18.00 Striking against unspecified object with** ▽ **subsequent fall**

✓ₓ7ᵗʰ **W18.01 Striking against** sports equipment **with subsequent fall**

✓ₓ7ᵗʰ **W18.02 Striking against** glass **with subsequent fall**

✓ₓ7ᵗʰ **W18.09 Striking against other object with subsequent fall**

✓5ᵗʰ **W18.1 Fall from or off toilet**

✓ₓ7ᵗʰ **W18.11 Fall from or off toilet** without subsequent striking **against object**
Fall from (off) toilet NOS

✓ₓ7ᵗʰ **W18.12 Fall from or off toilet** with subsequent striking **against object**

✓ₓ7ᵗʰ **W18.2 Fall in (into) shower or empty bathtub**
EXCLUDES 1 *fall in full bathtub causing drowning or submersion (W16.21-)*

✓5ᵗʰ **W18.3 Other and unspecified fall on same level**

✓ₓ7ᵗʰ **W18.30 Fall on same level, unspecified** ▽

✓ₓ7ᵗʰ **W18.31 Fall on same level due to stepping on an object**
Fall on same level due to stepping on an animal
EXCLUDES 1 *slipping, tripping and stumbling without fall due to stepping on animal (W18.41)*

✓ₓ7ᵗʰ **W18.39 Other fall on same level**

✓5ᵗʰ **W18.4 Slipping, tripping and stumbling without falling**
EXCLUDES 1 *collision with another person without fall (W51)*

✓ₓ7ᵗʰ **W18.40 Slipping, tripping and stumbling without falling,** ▽ **unspecified**

✓x7th **W18.41 Slipping, tripping and stumbling without falling due to** stepping on object
Slipping, tripping and stumbling without falling due to stepping on animal
EXCLUDES 1 *slipping, tripping and stumbling with fall due to stepping on animal (W18.31)*

✓x7th **W18.42 Slipping, tripping and stumbling without falling due to** stepping into hole or opening

✓x7th **W18.43 Slipping, tripping and stumbling without falling due to** stepping from one level to another

✓x7th **W18.49 Other slipping, tripping and stumbling without falling**

✓x7th **W19 Unspecified fall** ▽
Accidental fall NOS
AHA: 2012, 4Q, 95

Exposure to inanimate mechanical forces (W20-W49)

EXCLUDES 1 *assault (X92-Y09)*
contact or collision with animals or persons (W50-W64)
exposure to inanimate mechanical forces involving military or war operations (Y36.-, Y37.-)
intentional self-harm (X71-X83)

The appropriate 7th character is to be added to each code from categories W20-W49.
A   initial encounter
D   subsequent encounter
S   sequela

✓4th **W20 Struck by thrown, projected or falling object**
Code first any associated:
cataclysm (X34-X39)
lightning strike (T75.00)
EXCLUDES 1 *falling object in machinery accident (W24, W28-W31)*
falling object in transport accident (V01-V99)
object set in motion by explosion (W35-W40)
object set in motion by firearm (W32-W34)
struck by thrown sports equipment (W21.-)

✓x7th **W20.0 Struck by falling object in cave-in**
EXCLUDES 2 *asphyxiation due to cave-in (T71.21)*

✓x7th **W20.1 Struck by object due to collapse of building**
EXCLUDES 1 *struck by object due to collapse of burning building (X00.2, X02.2)*

✓x7th **W20.8 Other cause of strike by thrown, projected or falling object**
EXCLUDES 1 *struck by thrown sports equipment (W21.-)*

✓4th **W21 Striking against or struck by sports equipment**
EXCLUDES 1 *assault with sports equipment (Y08.0-)*
striking against or struck by sports equipment with subsequent fall (W18.01)

✓5th **W21.0 Struck by** hit **or** thrown ball
✓x7th **W21.00 Struck by hit or thrown ball, unspecified type** ▽
✓x7th **W21.01 Struck by** football
✓x7th **W21.02 Struck by** soccer ball
✓x7th **W21.03 Struck by** baseball
✓x7th **W21.04 Struck by** golf ball
✓x7th **W21.05 Struck by** basketball
✓x7th **W21.06 Struck by** volleyball
✓x7th **W21.07 Struck by** softball
✓x7th **W21.09 Struck by other hit or thrown ball**

✓5th **W21.1 Struck by** bat, racquet **or** club
✓x7th **W21.11 Struck by** baseball bat
✓x7th **W21.12 Struck by** tennis racquet
✓x7th **W21.13 Struck by** golf club
✓x7th **W21.19 Struck by other bat, racquet or club**

✓5th **W21.2 Struck by** hockey stick **or** puck
✓6th **W21.21 Struck by** hockey stick
✓7th **W21.210 Struck by** ice hockey stick
✓7th **W21.211 Struck by** field hockey stick
✓6th **W21.22 Struck by** hockey puck
✓7th **W21.220 Struck by** ice hockey puck
✓7th **W21.221 Struck by** field hockey puck

✓5th **W21.3 Struck by sports** foot wear
✓x7th **W21.31 Struck by** shoe cleats
Stepped on by shoe cleats

✓x7th **W21.32 Struck by skate** blades
Skated over by skate blades
✓x7th **W21.39 Struck by other sports foot wear**

✓x7th **W21.4 Striking against** diving board
Use additional code for subsequent falling into water, if applicable (W16.-)

✓5th **W21.8 Striking against or struck by** other sports equipment
✓x7th **W21.81 Striking against or struck by** football helmet
✓x7th **W21.89 Striking against or struck by other sports equipment**

✓x7th **W21.9 Striking against or struck by unspecified sports equipment** ▽

✓4th **W22 Striking against or struck by other objects**
EXCLUDES 1 *striking against or struck by object with subsequent fall (W18.09)*

✓5th **W22.0 Striking against** stationary object
EXCLUDES 1 *striking against stationary sports equipment (W21.8)*
✓x7th **W22.01 Walked into** wall
✓x7th **W22.02 Walked into** lamppost
✓x7th **W22.03 Walked into** furniture
✓6th **W22.04 Striking against wall of** swimming pool
✓7th **W22.041 Striking against wall of swimming pool causing** drowning **and submersion**
EXCLUDES 1 *drowning and submersion while swimming without striking against wall (W67)*
✓7th **W22.042 Striking against wall of swimming pool causing other injury**
✓x7th **W22.09 Striking against other** stationary object

✓5th **W22.1 Striking against or struck by** automobile airbag
✓x7th **W22.10 Striking against or struck by unspecified automobile airbag** ▽
✓x7th **W22.11 Striking against or struck by** driver side **automobile airbag**
✓x7th **W22.12 Striking against or struck by** front passenger side **automobile airbag**
✓x7th **W22.19 Striking against or struck by other automobile airbag**

✓x7th **W22.8 Striking against or struck by other objects**
Striking against or struck by object NOS
EXCLUDES 1 *struck by thrown, projected or falling object (W20.-)*

✓4th **W23 Caught, crushed, jammed or pinched in or between objects**
EXCLUDES 1 *injury caused by cutting or piercing instruments (W25-W27)*
injury caused by firearms malfunction (W32.1, W33.1-, W34.1-)
injury caused by lifting and transmission devices (W24.-)
injury caused by machinery (W28-W31)
injury caused by nonpowered hand tools (W27.-)
injury caused by transport vehicle being used as a means of transportation (V01-V99)
injury caused by struck by thrown, projected or falling object (W20.-)

✓x7th **W23.0 Caught, crushed, jammed, or pinched between** moving objects
✓x7th **W23.1 Caught, crushed, jammed, or pinched between** stationary objects

✓4th **W24 Contact with lifting and transmission devices, not elsewhere classified**
EXCLUDES 1 *transport accidents (V01-V99)*
✓x7th **W24.0 Contact with lifting devices, not elsewhere classified**
Contact with chain hoist
Contact with drive belt
Contact with pulley (block)
✓x7th **W24.1 Contact with transmission devices, not elsewhere classified**
Contact with transmission belt or cable

✓x7th **W25 Contact with sharp glass**
Code first any associated:
injury due to flying glass from explosion or firearm discharge (W32-W40)
transport accident (V00-V99)
EXCLUDES 1 *fall on same level due to slipping, tripping and stumbling with subsequent striking against sharp glass (W01.10)*
striking against sharp glass with subsequent fall (W18.02)
EXCLUDES 2 *glass embedded in skin (W45)*

✓ Additional Character Req   ✓x7th Placeholder Alert   Case-Mix Diagnosis   Manifestation   ▽ Unspecified Dx   **EXCLUDES 1** Not coded here   **EXCLUDES 2** Not included here

Chapter 20. External Causes of Morbidity *(side margin)*

W26–W31.9 *(side margin)*

☑4th **W26 Contact with other sharp objects**
> EXCLUDES 2   *sharp object(s) embedded in skin (W45)*

☑x7th **W26.0 Contact with knife**
> EXCLUDES 1   *contact with electric knife (W29.1)*

☑x7th **W26.1 Contact with sword or dagger**

☑x7th **W26.2 Contact with edge of stiff paper**
> Paper cut

☑x7th **W26.8 Contact with other sharp object(s), not elsewhere classified**
> Contact with tin can lid

☑x7th **W26.9 Contact with unspecified sharp object(s)** ▽

☑4th **W27 Contact with nonpowered hand tool**

☑x7th **W27.0 Contact with workbench tool**
> Contact with auger   Contact with handsaw
> Contact with axe   Contact with screwdriver
> Contact with chisel

☑x7th **W27.1 Contact with garden tool**
> Contact with hoe
> Contact with nonpowered lawn mower
> Contact with pitchfork
> Contact with rake

☑x7th **W27.2 Contact with scissors**

☑x7th **W27.3 Contact with needle (sewing)**
> EXCLUDES 1   *contact with hypodermic needle (W46.-)*

☑x7th **W27.4 Contact with kitchen utensil**
> Contact with fork
> Contact with ice-pick
> Contact with can-opener NOS

☑x7th **W27.5 Contact with paper-cutter**

☑x7th **W27.8 Contact with other nonpowered hand tool**
> Contact with nonpowered sewing machine
> Contact with shovel

☑x7th **W28 Contact with powered lawn mower**
> Powered lawn mower (commercial) (residential)
> EXCLUDES 1   *contact with nonpowered lawn mower (W27.1)*
> EXCLUDES 2   *exposure to electric current (W86.-)*

☑4th **W29 Contact with other powered hand tools and household machinery**
> EXCLUDES 1   *contact with commercial machinery (W31.82)*
> *contact with hot household appliance (X15)*
> *contact with nonpowered hand tool (W27.-)*
> *exposure to electric current (W86)*

☑x7th **W29.0 Contact with powered kitchen appliance**
> Contact with blender
> Contact with can-opener
> Contact with garbage disposal
> Contact with mixer

☑x7th **W29.1 Contact with electric knife**

☑x7th **W29.2 Contact with other powered household machinery**
> Contact with electric fan
> Contact with powered dryer (clothes) (powered) (spin)
> Contact with washing-machine
> Contact with sewing machine

☑x7th **W29.3 Contact with powered garden and outdoor hand tools and machinery**
> Contact with chainsaw
> Contact with edger
> Contact with garden cultivator (tiller)
> Contact with hedge trimmer
> Contact with other powered garden tool
> EXCLUDES 1   *contact with powered lawn mower (W28)*

☑x7th **W29.4 Contact with nail gun**

▲ ☑x7th **W29.8 Contact with other powered hand tools and household machinery**
> Contact with do-it-yourself tool NOS

☑4th **W30 Contact with agricultural machinery**
> INCLUDES   animal-powered farm machine
> EXCLUDES 1   *agricultural transport vehicle accident (V01-V99)*
> *explosion of grain store (W40.8)*
> *exposure to electric current (W86.-)*

☑x7th **W30.0 Contact with combine harvester**
> Contact with reaper
> Contact with thresher

☑x7th **W30.1 Contact with power take-off devices (PTO)**

☑x7th **W30.2 Contact with hay derrick**

☑x7th **W30.3 Contact with grain storage elevator**
> EXCLUDES 1   *explosion of grain store (W40.8)*

☑5th **W30.8 Contact with other specified agricultural machinery**

☑x7th **W30.81 Contact with agricultural transport vehicle in stationary use**
> Contact with agricultural transport vehicle under repair, not on public roadway
> EXCLUDES 1   *agricultural transport vehicle accident (V01-V99)*

☑x7th **W30.89 Contact with other specified agricultural machinery**

☑x7th **W30.9 Contact with unspecified agricultural machinery** ▽
> Contact with farm machinery NOS

☑4th **W31 Contact with other and unspecified machinery**
> EXCLUDES 1   *contact with agricultural machinery (W30.-)*
> *contact with machinery in transport under own power or being towed by a vehicle (V01-V99)*
> *exposure to electric current (W86)*

☑x7th **W31.0 Contact with mining and earth-drilling machinery**
> Contact with bore or drill (land) (seabed)
> Contact with shaft hoist
> Contact with shaft lift
> Contact with undercutter

☑x7th **W31.1 Contact with metalworking machines**
> Contact with abrasive wheel
> Contact with forging machine
> Contact with lathe
> Contact with mechanical shears
> Contact with metal drilling machine
> Contact with milling machine
> Contact with power press
> Contact with rolling-mill
> Contact with metal sawing machine

☑x7th **W31.2 Contact with powered woodworking and forming machines**
> Contact with band saw
> Contact with bench saw
> Contact with circular saw
> Contact with molding machine
> Contact with overhead plane
> Contact with powered saw
> Contact with radial saw
> Contact with sander
> EXCLUDES 1   *nonpowered woodworking tools (W27.0)*

☑x7th **W31.3 Contact with prime movers**
> Contact with gas turbine
> Contact with internal combustion engine
> Contact with steam engine
> Contact with water driven turbine

☑5th **W31.8 Contact with other specified machinery**

☑x7th **W31.81 Contact with recreational machinery**
> Contact with roller coaster

☑x7th **W31.82 Contact with other commercial machinery**
> Contact with commercial electric fan
> Contact with commercial kitchen appliances
> Contact with commercial powered dryer (clothes) (powered) (spin)
> Contact with commercial washing-machine
> Contact with commercial sewing machine
> EXCLUDES 1   *contact with household machinery (W29.-)*
> *contact with powered lawn mower (W28)*

☑x7th **W31.83 Contact with special construction vehicle in stationary use**
> Contact with special construction vehicle under repair, not on public roadway
> EXCLUDES 1   *special construction vehicle accident (V01-V99)*

☑x7th **W31.89 Contact with other specified machinery**

☑x7th **W31.9 Contact with unspecified machinery** ▽
> Contact with machinery NOS

N Newborn: 0   P Pediatric: 0-17   M Maternity: 12-55   A Adult: 15-124   NRS Nonroutine supply Dx   NCDx Noncancer Dx   PDx Primary Dx   ►◄ Revised Text   ● New Code   ▲ Revised Title

1148   ICD-10-CM 2018

✓4ᵗʰ W32 Accidental handgun discharge and malfunction

INCLUDES   accidental discharge and malfunction of gun for single hand use
accidental discharge and malfunction of pistol
accidental discharge and malfunction of revolver
handgun discharge and malfunction NOS

EXCLUDES 1   accidental airgun discharge and malfunction (W34.010, W34.110)
accidental BB gun discharge and malfunction (W34.010, W34.110)
accidental pellet gun discharge and malfunction (W34.010, W34.110)
accidental shotgun discharge and malfunction (W33.01, W33.11)
assault by handgun discharge (X93)
handgun discharge involving legal intervention (Y35.0-)
handgun discharge involving military or war operations (Y36.4-)
intentional self-harm by handgun discharge (X72)
Very pistol discharge and malfunction (W34.09, W34.19)

✓x7ᵗʰ W32.0 Accidental handgun discharge

✓x7ᵗʰ W32.1 Accidental handgun malfunction
Injury due to explosion of handgun (parts)
Injury due to malfunction of mechanism or component of handgun
Injury due to recoil of handgun
Powder burn from handgun

✓4ᵗʰ W33 Accidental rifle, shotgun and larger firearm discharge and malfunction

INCLUDES   rifle, shotgun and larger firearm discharge and malfunction NOS

EXCLUDES 1   accidental airgun discharge and malfunction (W34.010, W34.110)
accidental BB gun discharge and malfunction (W34.010, W34.110)
accidental handgun discharge and malfunction (W32.-)
accidental pellet gun discharge and malfunction (W34.010, W34.110)
assault by rifle, shotgun and larger firearm discharge (X94)
firearm discharge involving legal intervention (Y35.0-)
firearm discharge involving military or war operations (Y36.4-)
intentional self-harm by rifle, shotgun and larger firearm discharge (X73)

✓5ᵗʰ W33.0 Accidental rifle, shotgun and larger firearm discharge

✓x7ᵗʰ W33.00 Accidental discharge of unspecified larger firearm ▽
Discharge of unspecified larger firearm NOS

✓x7ᵗʰ W33.01 Accidental discharge of shotgun
Discharge of shotgun NOS

✓x7ᵗʰ W33.02 Accidental discharge of hunting rifle
Discharge of hunting rifle NOS

✓x7ᵗʰ W33.03 Accidental discharge of machine gun
Discharge of machine gun NOS

✓x7ᵗʰ W33.09 Accidental discharge of other larger firearm
Discharge of other larger firearm NOS

✓5ᵗʰ W33.1 Accidental rifle, shotgun and larger firearm malfunction
Injury due to explosion of rifle, shotgun and larger firearm (parts)
Injury due to malfunction of mechanism or component of rifle, shotgun and larger firearm
Injury due to piercing, cutting, crushing or pinching due to (by) slide trigger mechanism, scope or other gun part
Injury due to recoil of rifle, shotgun and larger firearm
Powder burn from rifle, shotgun and larger firearm

✓x7ᵗʰ W33.10 Accidental malfunction of unspecified larger firearm ▽
Malfunction of unspecified larger firearm NOS

✓x7ᵗʰ W33.11 Accidental malfunction of shotgun
Malfunction of shotgun NOS

✓x7ᵗʰ W33.12 Accidental malfunction of hunting rifle
Malfunction of hunting rifle NOS

✓x7ᵗʰ W33.13 Accidental malfunction of machine gun
Malfunction of machine gun NOS

✓x7ᵗʰ W33.19 Accidental malfunction of other larger firearm
Malfunction of other larger firearm NOS

✓4ᵗʰ W34 Accidental discharge and malfunction from other and unspecified firearms and guns

✓5ᵗʰ W34.0 Accidental discharge from other and unspecified firearms and guns

✓x7ᵗʰ W34.00 Accidental discharge from unspecified firearms or gun ▽
Discharge from firearm NOS
Gunshot wound NOS
Shot NOS

✓6ᵗʰ W34.01 Accidental discharge of gas, air or spring-operated guns

✓7ᵗʰ W34.010 Accidental discharge of airgun
Accidental discharge of BB gun
Accidental discharge of pellet gun

✓7ᵗʰ W34.011 Accidental discharge of paintball gun
Accidental injury due to paintball discharge

✓7ᵗʰ W34.018 Accidental discharge of other gas, air or spring-operated gun

✓x7ᵗʰ W34.09 Accidental discharge from other specified firearms
Accidental discharge from Very pistol [flare]

✓5ᵗʰ W34.1 Accidental malfunction from other and unspecified firearms and guns

✓x7ᵗʰ W34.10 Accidental malfunction from unspecified firearms ▽ or gun
Firearm malfunction NOS

✓6ᵗʰ W34.11 Accidental malfunction of gas, air or spring-operated guns

✓7ᵗʰ W34.110 Accidental malfunction of airgun
Accidental malfunction of BB gun
Accidental malfunction of pellet gun

✓7ᵗʰ W34.111 Accidental malfunction of paintball gun
Accidental injury due to paintball gun malfunction

✓7ᵗʰ W34.118 Accidental malfunction of other gas, air or spring-operated gun

✓x7ᵗʰ W34.19 Accidental malfunction from other specified firearms
Accidental malfunction from Very pistol [flare]

✓x7ᵗʰ W35 Explosion and rupture of boiler
EXCLUDES 1   explosion and rupture of boiler on watercraft (V93.4)

✓4ᵗʰ W36 Explosion and rupture of gas cylinder
✓x7ᵗʰ W36.1 Explosion and rupture of aerosol can
✓x7ᵗʰ W36.2 Explosion and rupture of air tank
✓x7ᵗʰ W36.3 Explosion and rupture of pressurized-gas tank
✓x7ᵗʰ W36.8 Explosion and rupture of other gas cylinder
✓x7ᵗʰ W36.9 Explosion and rupture of unspecified gas cylinder   ▽

✓4ᵗʰ W37 Explosion and rupture of pressurized tire, pipe or hose
✓x7ᵗʰ W37.0 Explosion of bicycle tire
✓x7ᵗʰ W37.8 Explosion and rupture of other pressurized tire, pipe or hose

✓x7ᵗʰ W38 Explosion and rupture of other specified pressurized devices

✓x7ᵗʰ W39 Discharge of firework

✓4ᵗʰ W40 Explosion of other materials
EXCLUDES 1   assault by explosive material (X96)
explosion involving legal intervention (Y35.1-)
explosion involving military or war operations (Y36.0-, Y36.2-)
intentional self-harm by explosive material (X75)

✓x7ᵗʰ W40.0 Explosion of blasting material
Explosion of blasting cap
Explosion of detonator
Explosion of dynamite
Explosion of explosive (any) used in blasting operations

✓x7ᵗʰ W40.1 Explosion of explosive gases
Explosion of acetylene
Explosion of butane
Explosion of coal gas
Explosion in mine NOS
Explosion of explosive gas
Explosion of fire damp
Explosion of gasoline fumes
Explosion of methane
Explosion of propane

✓ Additional Character Req   ✓x7ᵗʰ Placeholder Alert   Case-Mix Diagnosis   Manifestation   ▽ Unspecified Dx   **EXCLUDES 1** Not coded here   **EXCLUDES 2** Not included here

ICD-10-CM 2018   1149

√x7ᵗʰ W40.8 Explosion of other specified explosive materials
Explosion in dump NOS
Explosion in factory NOS
Explosion in grain store
Explosion in munitions
EXCLUDES 1   *explosion involving legal intervention (Y35.1-)*
explosion involving military or war operations (Y36.0-, Y36.2-)

√x7ᵗʰ W40.9 Explosion of unspecified explosive materials ▽
Explosion NOS

√4ᵗʰ W42 Exposure to noise

√x7ᵗʰ W42.0 Exposure to supersonic waves

√x7ᵗʰ W42.9 Exposure to other noise
Exposure to sound waves NOS

√4ᵗʰ W45 Foreign body or object entering through skin
INCLUDES   foreign body or object embedded in skin
nail embedded in skin
EXCLUDES 2   *contact with hand tools (nonpowered) (powered) (W27-W29)*
contact with other sharp object(s) (W26.-)
contact with sharp glass (W25.-)
struck by objects (W20-W22)

√x7ᵗʰ W45.0 Nail entering through skin

√x7ᵗʰ W45.8 Other foreign body or object entering through skin
Splinter in skin NOS

√4ᵗʰ W46 Contact with hypodermic needle

√x7ᵗʰ W46.0 Contact with hypodermic needle
Hypodermic needle stick NOS

√x7ᵗʰ W46.1 Contact with contaminated hypodermic needle

√4ᵗʰ W49 Exposure to other inanimate mechanical forces
INCLUDES   exposure to abnormal gravitational [G] forces
exposure to inanimate mechanical forces NEC
EXCLUDES 1   *exposure to inanimate mechanical forces involving military or war operations (Y36.-, Y37.-)*

√5ᵗʰ W49.0 Item causing external constriction

√x7ᵗʰ W49.01 Hair causing external constriction

√x7ᵗʰ W49.02 String or thread causing external constriction

√x7ᵗʰ W49.03 Rubber band causing external constriction

√x7ᵗʰ W49.04 Ring or other jewelry causing external constriction

√x7ᵗʰ W49.09 Other specified item causing external constriction

√x7ᵗʰ W49.9 Exposure to other inanimate mechanical forces

Exposure to animate mechanical forces (W50-W64)
EXCLUDES 1   *toxic effect of contact with venomous animals and plants (T63.-)*

The appropriate 7th character is to be added to each code from categories W50-W64.
A   initial encounter
D   subsequent encounter
S   sequela

√4ᵗʰ W50 Accidental hit, strike, kick, twist, bite or scratch by another person
INCLUDES   hit, strike, kick, twist, bite, or scratch by another person NOS
EXCLUDES 1   *assault by bodily force (Y04)*
struck by objects (W20-W22)

√x7ᵗʰ W50.0 Accidental hit or strike by another person
Hit or strike by another person NOS

√x7ᵗʰ W50.1 Accidental kick by another person
Kick by another person NOS

√x7ᵗʰ W50.2 Accidental twist by another person
Twist by another person NOS

√x7ᵗʰ W50.3 Accidental bite by another person
Human bite
Bite by another person NOS

√x7ᵗʰ W50.4 Accidental scratch by another person
Scratch by another person NOS

√x7ᵗʰ W51 Accidental striking against or bumped into by another person
EXCLUDES 1   *assault by striking against or bumping into by another person (Y04.2)*
fall due to collision with another person (W03)

√x7ᵗʰ W52 Crushed, pushed or stepped on by crowd or human stampede
Crushed, pushed or stepped on by crowd or human stampede with or without fall

√4ᵗʰ W53 Contact with rodent
INCLUDES   contact with saliva, feces or urine of rodent

√5ᵗʰ W53.0 Contact with mouse

√x7ᵗʰ W53.01 Bitten by mouse

√x7ᵗʰ W53.09 Other contact with mouse

√5ᵗʰ W53.1 Contact with rat

√x7ᵗʰ W53.11 Bitten by rat

√x7ᵗʰ W53.19 Other contact with rat

√5ᵗʰ W53.2 Contact with squirrel

√x7ᵗʰ W53.21 Bitten by squirrel

√x7ᵗʰ W53.29 Other contact with squirrel

√5ᵗʰ W53.8 Contact with other rodent

√x7ᵗʰ W53.81 Bitten by other rodent

√x7ᵗʰ W53.89 Other contact with other rodent

√4ᵗʰ W54 Contact with dog
INCLUDES   contact with saliva, feces or urine of dog

√x7ᵗʰ W54.0 Bitten by dog

√x7ᵗʰ W54.1 Struck by dog
Knocked over by dog

√x7ᵗʰ W54.8 Other contact with dog

√4ᵗʰ W55 Contact with other mammals
INCLUDES   contact with saliva, feces or urine of mammal
EXCLUDES 1   *animal being ridden—see transport accidents*
bitten or struck by dog (W54)
bitten or struck by rodent (W53.-)
contact with marine mammals (W56.-)

√5ᵗʰ W55.0 Contact with cat

√x7ᵗʰ W55.01 Bitten by cat

√x7ᵗʰ W55.03 Scratched by cat

√x7ᵗʰ W55.09 Other contact with cat

√5ᵗʰ W55.1 Contact with horse

√x7ᵗʰ W55.11 Bitten by horse

√x7ᵗʰ W55.12 Struck by horse

√x7ᵗʰ W55.19 Other contact with horse

√5ᵗʰ W55.2 Contact with cow
Contact with bull

√x7ᵗʰ W55.21 Bitten by cow

√x7ᵗʰ W55.22 Struck by cow
Gored by bull

√x7ᵗʰ W55.29 Other contact with cow

√5ᵗʰ W55.3 Contact with other hoof stock
Contact with goats
Contact with sheep

√x7ᵗʰ W55.31 Bitten by other hoof stock

√x7ᵗʰ W55.32 Struck by other hoof stock
Gored by goat
Gored by ram

√x7ᵗʰ W55.39 Other contact with other hoof stock

√5ᵗʰ W55.4 Contact with pig

√x7ᵗʰ W55.41 Bitten by pig

√x7ᵗʰ W55.42 Struck by pig

√x7ᵗʰ W55.49 Other contact with pig

√5ᵗʰ W55.5 Contact with raccoon

√x7ᵗʰ W55.51 Bitten by raccoon

√x7ᵗʰ W55.52 Struck by raccoon

√x7ᵗʰ W55.59 Other contact with raccoon

√5ᵗʰ W55.8 Contact with other mammals

√x7ᵗʰ W55.81 Bitten by other mammals

√x7ᵗʰ W55.82 Struck by other mammals

√x7ᵗʰ W55.89 Other contact with other mammals

√4ᵗʰ W56 Contact with nonvenomous marine animal
EXCLUDES 1   *contact with venomous marine animal (T63.-)*

√5ᵗʰ W56.0 Contact with dolphin

√x7ᵗʰ W56.01 Bitten by dolphin

√x7ᵗʰ W56.02 Struck by dolphin

√x7ᵗʰ W56.09 Other contact with dolphin

N Newborn: 0   P Pediatric: 0-17   M Maternity: 12-55   A Adult: 15-124   NRS Nonroutine supply Dx   NCDx Noncancer Dx   PDx Primary Dx   ►◄ Revised Text   ● New Code   ▲ Revised Title

1150   ICD-10-CM 2018

✓5th **W56.1 Contact with** sea lion

  ✓x7th **W56.11** Bitten **by sea lion**

  ✓x7th **W56.12** Struck **by sea lion**

  ✓x7th **W56.19 Other contact with sea lion**

✓5th **W56.2 Contact with** orca

  Contact with killer whale

  ✓x7th **W56.21** Bitten **by orca**

  ✓x7th **W56.22** Struck **by orca**

  ✓x7th **W56.29 Other contact with orca**

✓5th **W56.3 Contact with** other marine mammals

  ✓x7th **W56.31** Bitten **by other marine mammals**

  ✓x7th **W56.32** Struck **by other marine mammals**

  ✓x7th **W56.39 Other contact with other marine mammals**

✓5th **W56.4 Contact with** shark

  ✓x7th **W56.41** Bitten **by shark**

  ✓x7th **W56.42** Struck **by shark**

  ✓x7th **W56.49 Other contact with shark**

✓5th **W56.5 Contact with other** fish

  ✓x7th **W56.51** Bitten **by other fish**

  ✓x7th **W56.52** Struck **by other fish**

  ✓x7th **W56.59 Other contact with other fish**

✓5th **W56.8 Contact with** other **nonvenomous marine animals**

  ✓x7th **W56.81** Bitten **by other nonvenomous marine animals**

  ✓x7th **W56.82** Struck **by other nonvenomous marine animals**

  ✓x7th **W56.89 Other contact with other nonvenomous animals**

✓x7th **W57 Bitten or stung by nonvenomous insect and other nonvenomous arthropods**

  EXCLUDES 1 *contact with venomous insects and arthropods (T63.2-, T63.3-, T63.4-)*

✓4th **W58 Contact with crocodile or alligator**

✓5th **W58.0 Contact with** alligator

  ✓x7th **W58.01** Bitten **by alligator**

  ✓x7th **W58.02** Struck **by alligator**

  ✓x7th **W58.03** Crushed **by alligator**

  ✓x7th **W58.09 Other contact with alligator**

✓5th **W58.1 Contact with** crocodile

  ✓x7th **W58.11** Bitten **by crocodile**

  ✓x7th **W58.12** Struck **by crocodile**

  ✓x7th **W58.13** Crushed **by crocodile**

  ✓x7th **W58.19 Other contact with crocodile**

✓4th **W59 Contact with other nonvenomous reptiles**

  EXCLUDES 1 *contact with venomous reptile (T63.0-, T63.1-)*

✓5th **W59.0 Contact with nonvenomous** lizards

  ✓x7th **W59.01** Bitten **by nonvenomous lizards**

  ✓x7th **W59.02** Struck **by nonvenomous lizards**

  ✓x7th **W59.09 Other contact with nonvenomous lizards**

    Exposure to nonvenomous lizards

✓5th **W59.1 Contact with nonvenomous** snakes

  ✓x7th **W59.11** Bitten **by nonvenomous snake**

  ✓x7th **W59.12** Struck **by nonvenomous snake**

  ✓x7th **W59.13** Crushed **by nonvenomous snake**

  ✓x7th **W59.19 Other contact with nonvenomous snake**

✓5th **W59.2 Contact with** turtles

  EXCLUDES 1 *contact with tortoises (W59.8-)*

  ✓x7th **W59.21** Bitten **by turtle**

  ✓x7th **W59.22** Struck **by turtle**

  ✓x7th **W59.29 Other contact with turtle**

    Exposure to turtles

✓5th **W59.8 Contact with** other **nonvenomous reptiles**

  ✓x7th **W59.81** Bitten **by other nonvenomous reptiles**

  ✓x7th **W59.82** Struck **by other nonvenomous reptiles**

  ✓x7th **W59.83** Crushed **by other nonvenomous reptiles**

  ✓x7th **W59.89 Other contact with other nonvenomous reptiles**

✓x7th **W60 Contact with nonvenomous plant thorns and spines and sharp leaves**

  EXCLUDES 1 *contact with venomous plants (T63.7-)*

✓4th **W61 Contact with birds (domestic) (wild)**

  INCLUDES contact with excreta of birds

✓5th **W61.0 Contact with** parrot

  ✓x7th **W61.01** Bitten **by parrot**

  ✓x7th **W61.02** Struck **by parrot**

  ✓x7th **W61.09 Other contact with parrot**

    Exposure to parrots

✓5th **W61.1 Contact with** macaw

  ✓x7th **W61.11** Bitten **by macaw**

  ✓x7th **W61.12** Struck **by macaw**

  ✓x7th **W61.19 Other contact with macaw**

    Exposure to macaws

✓5th **W61.2 Contact with other** psittacines

  ✓x7th **W61.21** Bitten **by other psittacines**

  ✓x7th **W61.22** Struck **by other psittacines**

  ✓x7th **W61.29 Other contact with other psittacines**

    Exposure to other psittacines

✓6th **W61.3 Contact with** chicken

  ✓x7th **W61.32** Struck **by chicken**

  ✓x7th **W61.33** Pecked **by chicken**

  ✓x7th **W61.39 Other contact with chicken**

    Exposure to chickens

✓5th **W61.4 Contact with** turkey

  ✓x7th **W61.42** Struck **by turkey**

  ✓x7th **W61.43** Pecked **by turkey**

  ✓x7th **W61.49 Other contact with turkey**

✓5th **W61.5 Contact with** goose

  ✓x7th **W61.51** Bitten **by goose**

  ✓x7th **W61.52** Struck **by goose**

  ✓x7th **W61.59 Other contact with goose**

✓5th **W61.6 Contact with** duck

  ✓x7th **W61.61** Bitten **by duck**

  ✓x7th **W61.62** Struck **by duck**

  ✓x7th **W61.69 Other contact with duck**

✓5th **W61.9 Contact with** other **birds**

  ✓x7th **W61.91** Bitten **by other birds**

  ✓x7th **W61.92** Struck **by other birds**

  ✓x7th **W61.99 Other contact with other birds**

    Contact with bird NOS

✓4th **W62 Contact with nonvenomous amphibians**

  EXCLUDES 1 *contact with venomous amphibians (T63.81-R63.83)*

✓x7th **W62.0 Contact with nonvenomous** frogs

✓x7th **W62.1 Contact with nonvenomous** toads

✓x7th **W62.9 Contact with other nonvenomous** amphibians

✓x7th **W64 Exposure to other animate mechanical forces**

  INCLUDES exposure to nonvenomous animal NOS

  EXCLUDES 1 *contact with venomous animal (T63.-)*

Accidental non-transport drowning and submersion (W65-W74)

  EXCLUDES 1 *accidental drowning and submersion due to fall into water (W16.-)*
    accidental drowning and submersion due to water transport accident (V90.-, V92.-)

  EXCLUDES 2 *accidental drowning and submersion due to cataclysm (X34-X39)*

The appropriate 7th character is to be added to each code from categories W65-W74.
A   initial encounter
D   subsequent encounter
S   sequela

✓x7th **W65 Accidental drowning and submersion while in** bath-tub

  EXCLUDES 1 *accidental drowning and submersion due to fall in (into) bathtub (W16.211)*

✓x7th **W67 Accidental drowning and submersion while in** swimming-pool

  EXCLUDES 1 *accidental drowning and submersion due to fall into swimming pool (W16.011, W16.021, W16.031)*
    accidental drowning and submersion due to striking into wall of swimming pool (W22.041)

✓ Additional Character Req   ✓x7th Placeholder Alert   Case-Mix Diagnosis   Manifestation   ∇ Unspecified Dx   EXCLUDES 1 Not coded here   EXCLUDES 2 Not included here

ICD-10-CM 2018   1151

Chapter 20. External Causes of Morbidity *(left margin, vertical)*

W69–X01.4 *(left margin, vertical)*

☑x7ᵗʰ **W69 Accidental drowning and submersion while in** natural water
     Accidental drowning and submersion while in lake
     Accidental drowning and submersion while in open sea
     Accidental drowning and submersion while in river
     Accidental drowning and submersion while in stream
     EXCLUDES 1   accidental drowning and submersion due to fall into natural
               body of water (W16.111, W16.121, W16.131)

☑x7ᵗʰ **W73 Other specified cause of accidental non-transport drowning and submersion**
     Accidental drowning and submersion while in quenching tank
     Accidental drowning and submersion while in reservoir
     EXCLUDES 1   accidental drowning and submersion due to fall into other
               water (W16.311, W16.321, W16.331)

☑x7ᵗʰ **W74 Unspecified cause of accidental drowning and submersion**   ▽
     Drowning NOS

Exposure to electric current, radiation and extreme ambient air temperature and pressure (W85–W99)

EXCLUDES 1   exposure to:
     failure in dosage of radiation or temperature during surgical and
        medical care (Y63.2-Y63.5)
     lightning (T75.0-)
     natural cold (X31)
     natural heat (X30)
     natural radiation NOS (X39)
     radiological procedure and radiotherapy (Y84.2)
     sunlight (X32)

> The appropriate 7th character is to be added to each code from categories W85-W99.
> A   initial encounter
> D   subsequent encounter
> S   sequela

☑x7ᵗʰ **W85 Exposure to electric transmission lines**
     Broken power line

☑4ᵗʰ **W86 Exposure to other specified electric current**

   ☑x7ᵗʰ **W86.0 Exposure to domestic wiring and appliances**

   ☑x7ᵗʰ **W86.1 Exposure to industrial wiring, appliances and electrical machinery**
       Exposure to conductors
       Exposure to control apparatus
       Exposure to electrical equipment and machinery
       Exposure to transformers

   ☑x7ᵗʰ **W86.8 Exposure to other electric current**
       Exposure to wiring and appliances in or on farm (not farmhouse)
       Exposure to wiring and appliances outdoors
       Exposure to wiring and appliances in or on public building
       Exposure to wiring and appliances in or on residential
         institutions
       Exposure to wiring and appliances in or on schools

☑4ᵗʰ **W88 Exposure to ionizing radiation**
     EXCLUDES 1   exposure to sunlight (X32)

   ☑x7ᵗʰ **W88.0 Exposure to** X-rays

   ☑x7ᵗʰ **W88.1 Exposure to** radioactive isotopes

   ☑x7ᵗʰ **W88.8 Exposure to other ionizing radiation**

☑4ᵗʰ **W89 Exposure to man-made visible and ultraviolet light**
     INCLUDES   exposure to welding light (arc)
     EXCLUDES 1   exposure to sunlight (X32)

   ☑x7ᵗʰ **W89.0 Exposure to** welding light **(arc)**

   ☑x7ᵗʰ **W89.1 Exposure to** tanning bed

   ☑x7ᵗʰ **W89.8 Exposure to other man-made visible and ultraviolet light**

   ☑x7ᵗʰ **W89.9 Exposure to unspecified man-made visible and ultraviolet**   ▽
        light

☑4ᵗʰ **W90 Exposure to other nonionizing radiation**
     EXCLUDES 1   exposure to sunlight (X32)

   ☑x7ᵗʰ **W90.0 Exposure to** radiofrequency

   ☑x7ᵗʰ **W90.1 Exposure to** infrared radiation

   ☑x7ᵗʰ **W90.2 Exposure to** laser radiation

   ☑x7ᵗʰ **W90.8 Exposure to other nonionizing radiation**

☑x7ᵗʰ **W92 Exposure to excessive heat of man-made origin**

☑4ᵗʰ **W93 Exposure to excessive cold of man-made origin**

   ☑5ᵗʰ **W93.0 Contact with or inhalation of** dry ice

     ☑x7ᵗʰ **W93.01 Contact with dry ice**

     ☑x7ᵗʰ **W93.02 Inhalation of dry ice**

   ☑5ᵗʰ **W93.1 Contact with or inhalation of** liquid air

     ☑x7ᵗʰ **W93.11 Contact with liquid air**
         Contact with liquid hydrogen
         Contact with liquid nitrogen

     ☑x7ᵗʰ **W93.12 Inhalation of liquid air**
         Inhalation of liquid hydrogen
         Inhalation of liquid nitrogen

   ☑x7ᵗʰ **W93.2 Prolonged exposure in deep freeze unit or refrigerator**

   ☑x7ᵗʰ **W93.8 Exposure to other excessive cold of man-made origin**

☑4ᵗʰ **W94 Exposure to high and low air pressure and changes in air pressure**

   ☑x7ᵗʰ **W94.0 Exposure to prolonged high air pressure**

   ☑5ᵗʰ **W94.1 Exposure to prolonged low air pressure**

     ☑x7ᵗʰ **W94.11 Exposure to residence or prolonged visit at high altitude**

     ☑x7ᵗʰ **W94.12 Exposure to other prolonged low air pressure**

   ☑5ᵗʰ **W94.2 Exposure to rapid changes in air pressure during** ascent

     ☑x7ᵗʰ **W94.21 Exposure to reduction in atmospheric pressure while surfacing from** deep-water diving

     ☑x7ᵗʰ **W94.22 Exposure to reduction in atmospheric pressure while surfacing from** underground

     ☑x7ᵗʰ **W94.23 Exposure to sudden change in air pressure in** aircraft **during ascent**

     ☑x7ᵗʰ **W94.29 Exposure to other rapid changes in air pressure during ascent**

   ☑5ᵗʰ **W94.3 Exposure to rapid changes in air pressure during** descent

     ☑x7ᵗʰ **W94.31 Exposure to sudden change in air pressure in** aircraft **during descent**

     ☑x7ᵗʰ **W94.32 Exposure to high air pressure from rapid descent in** water

     ☑x7ᵗʰ **W94.39 Exposure to other rapid changes in air pressure during descent**

☑x7ᵗʰ **W99 Exposure to other man-made environmental factors**

Exposure to smoke, fire and flames (X00–X08)

EXCLUDES 1   arson (X97)
EXCLUDES 2   explosions (W35-W40)
           lightning (T75.0-)
           transport accident (V01-V99)

> The appropriate 7th character is to be added to each code from categories X00-X08.
> A   initial encounter
> D   subsequent encounter
> S   sequela

☑4ᵗʰ **X00 Exposure to** uncontrolled fire **in building or structure**
     INCLUDES   conflagration in building or structure
     Code first any associated cataclysm
     EXCLUDES 2   exposure to ignition or melting of nightwear (X05)
           exposure to ignition or melting of other clothing and apparel
            (X06.-)
           exposure to other specified smoke, fire and flames (X08.-)
     AHA: 2016, 2Q, 5

   ☑x7ᵗʰ **X00.0 Exposure to** flames **in uncontrolled fire in building or structure**

   ☑x7ᵗʰ **X00.1 Exposure to** smoke **in uncontrolled fire in building or structure**

   ☑x7ᵗʰ **X00.2 Injury due to collapse of burning building or structure in uncontrolled fire**
       EXCLUDES 1   injury due to collapse of building not on fire (W20.1)

   ☑x7ᵗʰ **X00.3 Fall from burning building or structure in uncontrolled fire**

   ☑x7ᵗʰ **X00.4 Hit by object from burning building or structure in uncontrolled fire**

   ☑x7ᵗʰ **X00.5 Jump from burning building or structure in uncontrolled fire**

   ☑x7ᵗʰ **X00.8 Other exposure to uncontrolled fire in building or structure**

☑4ᵗʰ **X01 Exposure to uncontrolled fire, not in building or structure**
     INCLUDES   exposure to forest fire

   ☑x7ᵗʰ **X01.0 Exposure to** flames **in uncontrolled fire, not in building or structure**

   ☑x7ᵗʰ **X01.1 Exposure to** smoke **in uncontrolled fire, not in building or structure**

   ☑x7ᵗʰ **X01.3 Fall due to uncontrolled fire, not in building or structure**

   ☑x7ᵗʰ **X01.4 Hit by object due to uncontrolled fire, not in building or structure**

Ⓝ Newborn: 0   Ⓟ Pediatric: 0-17   Ⓜ Maternity: 12-55   Ⓐ Adult: 15-124   **NRS** Nonroutine supply Dx   **NCDx** Noncancer Dx   **PDx** Primary Dx   ▶◀ Revised Text   ● New Code   ▲ Revised Title

1152   ICD-10-CM 2018

✓x7ᵗʰ **X01.8 Other exposure to uncontrolled fire, not in building or structure**

✓4ᵗʰ **X02 Exposure to** controlled fire **in building or structure**
   [INCLUDES] exposure to fire in fireplace
          exposure to fire in stove

✓x7ᵗʰ **X02.0 Exposure to** flames **in controlled fire in building or structure**

✓x7ᵗʰ **X02.1 Exposure to** smoke **in controlled fire in building or structure**

✓x7ᵗʰ **X02.2 Injury due to collapse of burning building or structure in controlled fire**
   [EXCLUDES1] injury due to collapse of building not on fire (W20.1)

✓x7ᵗʰ **X02.3 Fall from burning building or structure in controlled fire**

✓x7ᵗʰ **X02.4 Hit by object from burning building or structure in controlled fire**

✓x7ᵗʰ **X02.5 Jump from burning building or structure in controlled fire**

✓x7ᵗʰ **X02.8 Other exposure to controlled fire in building or structure**

✓4ᵗʰ **X03 Exposure to** controlled fire, **not in building or structure**
   [INCLUDES] exposure to bon fire
          exposure to camp-fire
          exposure to trash fire

✓x7ᵗʰ **X03.0 Exposure to** flames **in controlled fire, not in building or structure**

✓x7ᵗʰ **X03.1 Exposure to** smoke **in controlled fire, not in building or structure**

✓x7ᵗʰ **X03.3 Fall due to controlled fire, not in building or structure**

✓x7ᵗʰ **X03.4 Hit by object due to controlled fire, not in building or structure**

✓x7ᵗʰ **X03.8 Other exposure to controlled fire, not in building or structure**

✓x7ᵗʰ **X04 Exposure to ignition of highly flammable material**
   Exposure to ignition of gasoline
   Exposure to ignition of kerosene
   Exposure to ignition of petrol
   [EXCLUDES2] exposure to ignition or melting of nightwear (X05)
         exposure to ignition or melting of other clothing and apparel (X06)
   AHA: 2016, 2Q, 4

✓x7ᵗʰ **X05 Exposure to ignition or melting of nightwear**
   [EXCLUDES2] exposure to uncontrolled fire in building or structure (X00.-)
         exposure to uncontrolled fire, not in building or structure (X01.-)
         exposure to controlled fire in building or structure (X02.-)
         exposure to controlled fire, not in building or structure (X03.-)
         exposure to ignition of highly flammable materials (X04.-)

✓4ᵗʰ **X06 Exposure to ignition or melting of other clothing and apparel**
   [EXCLUDES2] exposure to uncontrolled fire in building or structure (X00.-)
         exposure to uncontrolled fire, not in building or structure (X01.-)
         exposure to controlled fire in building or structure (X02.-)
         exposure to controlled fire, not in building or structure (X03.-)
         exposure to ignition of highly flammable materials (X04.-)

✓x7ᵗʰ **X06.0 Exposure to ignition of plastic jewelry**

✓x7ᵗʰ **X06.1 Exposure to melting of plastic jewelry**

✓x7ᵗʰ **X06.2 Exposure to ignition of other clothing and apparel**

✓x7ᵗʰ **X06.3 Exposure to melting of other clothing and apparel**

✓4ᵗʰ **X08 Exposure to other specified smoke, fire and flames**

✓5ᵗʰ **X08.0 Exposure to** bed **fire**
   Exposure to mattress fire

✓x7ᵗʰ **X08.00 Exposure to bed fire due to unspecified burning material** ▽

✓x7ᵗʰ **X08.01 Exposure to bed fire due to** burning cigarette

✓x7ᵗʰ **X08.09 Exposure to bed fire due to other burning material**

✓5ᵗʰ **X08.1 Exposure to** sofa **fire**

✓x7ᵗʰ **X08.10 Exposure to sofa fire due to unspecified burning material** ▽

✓x7ᵗʰ **X08.11 Exposure to sofa fire due to** burning cigarette

✓x7ᵗʰ **X08.19 Exposure to sofa fire due to other burning material**

✓5ᵗʰ **X08.2 Exposure to** other furniture **fire**

✓x7ᵗʰ **X08.20 Exposure to other furniture fire due to unspecified burning material** ▽

✓x7ᵗʰ **X08.21 Exposure to other furniture fire due to** burning cigarette

✓x7ᵗʰ **X08.29 Exposure to other furniture fire due to other burning material**

✓x7ᵗʰ **X08.8 Exposure to other specified smoke, fire and flames**

Contact with heat and hot substances (X10-X19)
   [EXCLUDES1] exposure to excessive natural heat (X30)
         exposure to fire and flames ▶(X00-X08)◀

The appropriate 7th character is to be added to each code from categories X10-X19.
A   initial encounter
D   subsequent encounter
S   sequela

✓4ᵗʰ **X10 Contact with hot drinks, food, fats and cooking oils**

✓x7ᵗʰ **X10.0 Contact with hot** drinks

✓x7ᵗʰ **X10.1 Contact with hot** food

✓x7ᵗʰ **X10.2 Contact with** fats and cooking oils

✓4ᵗʰ **X11 Contact with hot tap-water**
   [INCLUDES] contact with boiling tap-water
         contact with boiling water NOS
   [EXCLUDES1] contact with water heated on stove (X12)

✓x7ᵗʰ **X11.0 Contact with hot water in bath or tub**
   [EXCLUDES1] contact with running hot water in bath or tub (X11.1)

✓x7ᵗʰ **X11.1 Contact with** running **hot water**
   Contact with hot water running out of hose
   Contact with hot water running out of tap

✓x7ᵗʰ **X11.8 Contact with other hot tap-water**
   Contact with hot water in bucket
   Contact with hot tap-water NOS

✓x7ᵗʰ **X12 Contact with other hot fluids**
   Contact with water heated on stove
   [EXCLUDES1] hot (liquid) metals (X18)

✓4ᵗʰ **X13 Contact with steam and other hot vapors**

✓x7ᵗʰ **X13.0 Inhalation of steam and other hot vapors**

✓x7ᵗʰ **X13.1 Other contact with steam and other hot vapors**

✓4ᵗʰ **X14 Contact with hot air and other hot gases**

✓x7ᵗʰ **X14.0 Inhalation of hot air and gases**

✓x7ᵗʰ **X14.1 Other contact with hot air and other hot gases**

✓4ᵗʰ **X15 Contact with hot household appliances**
   [EXCLUDES1] contact with heating appliances (X16)
         contact with powered household appliances (W29.-)
         exposure to controlled fire in building or structure due to household appliance (X02.8)
         exposure to household appliances electrical current (W86.0)

✓x7ᵗʰ **X15.0 Contact with hot** stove **(kitchen)**

✓x7ᵗʰ **X15.1 Contact with hot** toaster

✓x7ᵗʰ **X15.2 Contact with** hotplate

✓x7ᵗʰ **X15.3 Contact with hot** saucepan or skillet

✓x7ᵗʰ **X15.8 Contact with other hot household appliances**
   Contact with cooker   Contact with light bulbs
   Contact with kettle

✓x7ᵗʰ **X16 Contact with hot heating appliances, radiators and pipes**
   [EXCLUDES1] contact with powered appliances (W29.-)
         exposure to controlled fire in building or structure due to appliance (X02.8)
         exposure to industrial appliances electrical current (W86.1)

✓x7ᵗʰ **X17 Contact with hot engines, machinery and tools**
   [EXCLUDES1] contact with hot heating appliances, radiators and pipes (X16)
         contact with hot household appliances (X15)

✓x7ᵗʰ **X18 Contact with other hot metals**
   Contact with liquid metal

✓x7ᵗʰ **X19 Contact with other heat and hot substances**
   [EXCLUDES1] objects that are not normally hot, e.g., an object made hot by a house fire ▶(X00-X08)◀

✓ Additional Character Req   ✓x7ᵗʰ Placeholder Alert   Case-Mix Diagnosis   Manifestation   ▽ Unspecified Dx   [EXCLUDES1] Not coded here   [EXCLUDES2] Not included here
ICD-10-CM 2018   1153

X01.8–X19

Chapter 20. External Causes of Morbidity *(side margin)*

X30–X71.9 *(side margin, bottom)*

Exposure to forces of nature (X30-X39)

The appropriate 7th character is to be added to each code from categories X30-X39.
A   initial encounter
D   subsequent encounter
S   sequela

√x7ᵗʰ **X30** **Exposure to excessive** natural heat
   Exposure to excessive heat as the cause of sunstroke
   Exposure to heat NOS
   EXCLUDES 1   excessive heat of man-made origin (W92)
              exposure to man-made radiation (W89)
              exposure to sunlight (X32)
              exposure to tanning bed (W89)

√x7ᵗʰ **X31** **Exposure to excessive** natural cold
   Excessive cold as the cause of chilblains NOS
   Excessive cold as the cause of immersion foot or hand
   Exposure to cold NOS
   Exposure to weather conditions
   EXCLUDES 1   cold of man-made origin (W93.-)
              contact with or inhalation of dry ice (W93.-)
              contact with or inhalation of liquefied gas (W93.-)

√x7ᵗʰ **X32** **Exposure to sunlight**
   EXCLUDES 1   man-made radiation (tanning bed) (W89)
   EXCLUDES 2   ▶radiation-related disorders of the skin and subcutaneous tissue
              (L55-L59)◄

√x7ᵗʰ **X34** **Earthquake**
   EXCLUDES 2   tidal wave (tsunami) due to earthquake (X37.41)

√x7ᵗʰ **X35** **Volcanic eruption**
   EXCLUDES 2   tidal wave (tsunami) due to volcanic eruption (X37.41)

√4ᵗʰ **X36** **Avalanche, landslide and other earth movements**
   INCLUDES   victim of mudslide of cataclysmic nature
   EXCLUDES 1   earthquake (X34)
   EXCLUDES 2   transport accident involving collision with avalanche or
              landslide not in motion (V01-V99)

√x7ᵗʰ **X36.0** **Collapse of dam or man-made structure causing earth movement**

√x7ᵗʰ **X36.1** **Avalanche, landslide, or mudslide**

√4ᵗʰ **X37** **Cataclysmic storm**

√x7ᵗʰ **X37.0** **Hurricane**
   Storm surge
   Typhoon

√x7ᵗʰ **X37.1** **Tornado**
   Cyclone
   Twister

√x7ᵗʰ **X37.2** **Blizzard (snow)(ice)**

√x7ᵗʰ **X37.3** **Dust storm**

√5ᵗʰ **X37.4** **Tidalwave**

√x7ᵗʰ **X37.41** **Tidal wave due to** earthquake **or** volcanic eruption
   Tidal wave NOS
   Tsunami

√x7ᵗʰ **X37.42** **Tidal wave due to** storm

√x7ᵗʰ **X37.43** **Tidal wave due to** landslide

√x7ᵗʰ **X37.8** **Other cataclysmic storms**
   Cloudburst
   Torrential rain
   EXCLUDES 2   flood (X38)

√x7ᵗʰ **X37.9** **Unspecified cataclysmic storm**   ▽
   Storm NOS
   EXCLUDES 1   collapse of dam or man-made structure causing earth
              movement (X39.0)

√x7ᵗʰ **X38** **Flood**
   Flood arising from remote storm
   Flood of cataclysmic nature arising from melting snow
   Flood resulting directly from storm
   EXCLUDES 1   collapse of dam or man-made structure causing earth
              movement (X39.0)
              tidal wave NOS (X37.41)
              tidal wave caused by storm (X37.2)

√4ᵗʰ **X39** **Exposure to other forces of nature**

√5ᵗʰ **X39.0** **Exposure to natural radiation**
   EXCLUDES 1   contact with and (suspected) exposure to radon and
              other naturally occuring radiation (Z77.123)
              exposure to man-made radiation (W88-W90)
              exposure to sunlight (X32)

√x7ᵗʰ **X39.01** **Exposure to radon**

√x7ᵗʰ **X39.08** **Exposure to other natural radiation**

√x7ᵗʰ **X39.8** **Other exposure to forces of nature**

Overexertion and strenuous or repetitive movements (X50)

√4ᵗʰ **X50** **Overexertion and strenuous or repetitive movements**

The appropriate 7th character is to be added to each code from category X50.
A   initial encounter
D   subsequent encounter
S   sequela

√x7ᵗʰ **X50.0** **Overexertion from strenuous movement or load**
   Lifting heavy objects
   Lifting weights

√x7ᵗʰ **X50.1** **Overexertion from prolonged static or awkward postures**
   Prolonged bending
   Prolonged kneeling
   Prolonged reaching
   Prolonged sitting
   Prolonged standing
   Prolonged twisting
   Static bending
   Static kneeling
   Static reaching
   Static sitting
   Static standing
   Static twisting

√x7ᵗʰ **X50.3** **Overexertion from repetitive movements**
   Use of hand as hammer
   EXCLUDES 2   overuse from prolonged static or awkward postures
              (X50.1)

√x7ᵗʰ **X50.9** **Other and unspecified overexertion or strenuous**   ▽
   movements or postures
   Contact pressure
   Contact stress

Accidental exposure to other specified factors (X52-X58)

The appropriate 7th character is to be added to each code from categories X52, X58.
A   initial encounter
D   subsequent encounter
S   sequela

√x7ᵗʰ **X52** **Prolonged stay in weightless environment**
   Weightlessness in spacecraft (simulator)

√x7ᵗʰ **X58** **Exposure to other specified factors**
   Accident NOS
   Exposure NOS

Intentional self-harm (X71-X83)

Purposely self-inflicted injury
Suicide (attempted)

The appropriate 7th character is to be added to each code from categories X71-X83.
A   initial encounter
D   subsequent encounter
S   sequela

√4ᵗʰ **X71** **Intentional self-harm by drowning and submersion**

√x7ᵗʰ **X71.0** **Intentional self-harm by drowning and submersion while in** bathtub

√x7ᵗʰ **X71.1** **Intentional self-harm by drowning and submersion while in** swimming pool

√x7ᵗʰ **X71.2** **Intentional self-harm by drowning and submersion** after jump into swimming pool

√x7ᵗʰ **X71.3** **Intentional self-harm by drowning and submersion in** natural water

√x7ᵗʰ **X71.8** **Other intentional self-harm by drowning and submersion**

√x7ᵗʰ **X71.9** **Intentional self-harm by drowning and submersion,**   ▽
   unspecified

Ⓝ Newborn: 0   Ⓟ Pediatric: 0-17   Ⓜ Maternity: 12-55   Ⓐ Adult: 15-124   NRS Nonroutine supply Dx   NC Dx Noncancer Dx   PDx Primary Dx   ▶◄ Revised Text   ● New Code   ▲ Revised Title

1154   ICD-10-CM 2018

✓x7th X72 Intentional self-harm by handgun discharge
Intentional self-harm by gun for single hand use
Intentional self-harm by pistol
Intentional self-harm by revolver
EXCLUDES 1 *Very pistol (X74.8)*

✓4th X73 Intentional self-harm by rifle, shotgun and larger firearm discharge
EXCLUDES 1 *airgun (X74.01)*
✓x7th X73.0 Intentional self-harm by shotgun discharge
✓x7th X73.1 Intentional self-harm by hunting rifle discharge
✓x7th X73.2 Intentional self-harm by machine gun discharge
✓x7th X73.8 Intentional self-harm by other larger firearm discharge
✓x7th X73.9 Intentional self-harm by unspecified larger firearm discharge ▽

✓4th X74 Intentional self-harm by other and unspecified firearm and gun discharge
✓5th X74.0 Intentional self-harm by gas, air or spring-operated guns
✓x7th X74.01 Intentional self-harm by airgun
Intentional self-harm by BB gun discharge
Intentional self-harm by pellet gun discharge
✓x7th X74.02 Intentional self-harm by paintball gun
✓x7th X74.09 Intentional self-harm by other gas, air or spring-operated gun
✓x7th X74.8 Intentional self-harm by other firearm discharge
Intentional self-harm by Very pistol [flare] discharge
✓x7th X74.9 Intentional self-harm by unspecified firearm discharge ▽

✓x7th X75 Intentional self-harm by explosive material
✓x7th X76 Intentional self-harm by smoke, fire and flames

✓4th X77 Intentional self-harm by steam, hot vapors and hot objects
✓x7th X77.0 Intentional self-harm by steam or hot vapors
✓x7th X77.1 Intentional self-harm by hot tap water
✓x7th X77.2 Intentional self-harm by other hot fluids
✓x7th X77.3 Intentional self-harm by hot household appliances
✓x7th X77.8 Intentional self-harm by other hot objects
✓x7th X77.9 Intentional self-harm by unspecified hot objects ▽

✓4th X78 Intentional self-harm by sharp object
✓x7th X78.0 Intentional self-harm by sharp glass
✓x7th X78.1 Intentional self-harm by knife
✓x7th X78.2 Intentional self-harm by sword or dagger
✓x7th X78.8 Intentional self-harm by other sharp object
✓x7th X78.9 Intentional self-harm by unspecified sharp object ▽

✓x7th X79 Intentional self-harm by blunt object
✓x7th X80 Intentional self-harm by jumping from a high place
Intentional fall from one level to another

✓4th X81 Intentional self-harm by jumping or lying in front of moving object
✓x7th X81.0 Intentional self-harm by jumping or lying in front of motor vehicle
✓x7th X81.1 Intentional self-harm by jumping or lying in front of (subway) train
✓x7th X81.8 Intentional self-harm by jumping or lying in front of other moving object

✓4th X82 Intentional self-harm by crashing of motor vehicle
✓x7th X82.0 Intentional collision of motor vehicle with other motor vehicle
✓x7th X82.1 Intentional collision of motor vehicle with train
✓x7th X82.2 Intentional collision of motor vehicle with tree
✓x7th X82.8 Other intentional self-harm by crashing of motor vehicle

✓4th X83 Intentional self-harm by other specified means
EXCLUDES 1 *intentional self-harm by poisoning or contact with toxic substance—see Table of Drugs and Chemicals*
✓x7th X83.0 Intentional self-harm by crashing of aircraft
✓x7th X83.1 Intentional self-harm by electrocution
✓x7th X83.2 Intentional self-harm by exposure to extremes of cold
✓x7th X83.8 Intentional self-harm by other specified means

Assault (X92-Y09)

INCLUDES homicide
injuries inflicted by another person with intent to injure or kill, by any means
EXCLUDES 1 *injuries due to legal intervention (Y35.-)*
injuries due to operations of war (Y36.-)
injuries due to terrorism (Y38.-)

The appropriate 7th character is to be added to each code from categories X92-Y04 and Y08.
A   initial encounter
D   subsequent encounter
S   sequela

✓4th X92 Assault by drowning and submersion
✓x7th X92.0 Assault by drowning and submersion while in bathtub
✓x7th X92.1 Assault by drowning and submersion while in swimming pool
✓x7th X92.2 Assault by drowning and submersion after push into swimming pool
✓x7th X92.3 Assault by drowning and submersion in natural water
✓x7th X92.8 Other assault by drowning and submersion
✓x7th X92.9 Assault by drowning and submersion, unspecified ▽

✓x7th X93 Assault by handgun discharge
Assault by discharge of gun for single hand use
Assault by discharge of pistol
Assault by discharge of revolver
EXCLUDES 1 *Very pistol (X95.8)*

✓4th X94 Assault by rifle, shotgun and larger firearm discharge
EXCLUDES 1 *airgun (X95.01)*
✓x7th X94.0 Assault by shotgun
✓x7th X94.1 Assault by hunting rifle
✓x7th X94.2 Assault by machine gun
✓x7th X94.8 Assault by other larger firearm discharge
✓x7th X94.9 Assault by unspecified larger firearm discharge ▽

✓4th X95 Assault by other and unspecified firearm and gun discharge
✓5th X95.0 Assault by gas, air or spring-operated guns
✓x7th X95.01 Assault by airgun discharge
Assault by BB gun discharge
Assault by pellet gun discharge
✓x7th X95.02 Assault by paintball gun discharge
✓x7th X95.09 Assault by other gas, air or spring-operated gun
✓x7th X95.8 Assault by other firearm discharge
Assault by Very pistol [flare] discharge
✓x7th X95.9 Assault by unspecified firearm discharge ▽

✓4th X96 Assault by explosive material
EXCLUDES 1 *incendiary device (X97)*
terrorism involving explosive material (Y38.2-)
✓x7th X96.0 Assault by antipersonnel bomb
EXCLUDES 1 *antipersonnel bomb use in military or war (Y36.2-)*
✓x7th X96.1 Assault by gasoline bomb
✓x7th X96.2 Assault by letter bomb
✓x7th X96.3 Assault by fertilizer bomb
✓x7th X96.4 Assault by pipe bomb
✓x7th X96.8 Assault by other specified explosive
✓x7th X96.9 Assault by unspecified explosive ▽

✓x7th X97 Assault by smoke, fire and flames
Assault by arson
Assault by cigarettes
Assault by incendiary device

✓4th X98 Assault by steam, hot vapors and hot objects
✓x7th X98.0 Assault by steam or hot vapors
✓x7th X98.1 Assault by hot tap water
✓x7th X98.2 Assault by hot fluids
✓x7th X98.3 Assault by hot household appliances
✓x7th X98.8 Assault by other hot objects
✓x7th X98.9 Assault by unspecified hot objects ▽

✓4th X99 Assault by sharp object
EXCLUDES 1 *assault by strike by sports equipment (Y08.0-)*
✓x7th X99.0 Assault by sharp glass
✓x7th X99.1 Assault by knife
✓x7th X99.2 Assault by sword or dagger

✓ Additional Character Req   ✓x7th Placeholder Alert   Case-Mix Diagnosis   Manifestation   ▽ Unspecified Dx   EXCLUDES 1 Not coded here   EXCLUDES 2 Not included here

Chapter 20. External Causes of Morbidity

√x7ᵗʰ **X99.8 Assault by other sharp object**

√x7ᵗʰ **X99.9 Assault by unspecified sharp object** ▽
Assault by stabbing NOS

√x7ᵗʰ **Y00 Assault by blunt object**
EXCLUDES1 assault by strike by sports equipment (Y08.0-)

√x7ᵗʰ **Y01 Assault by pushing from high place**

√4ᵗʰ **Y02 Assault by pushing or placing victim in front of moving object**

√x7ᵗʰ **Y02.0 Assault by pushing or placing victim in front of motor vehicle**

√x7ᵗʰ **Y02.1 Assault by pushing or placing victim in front of (subway) train**

√x7ᵗʰ **Y02.8 Assault by pushing or placing victim in front of other moving object**

√4ᵗʰ **Y03 Assault by crashing of motor vehicle**

√x7ᵗʰ **Y03.0 Assault by being hit or run over by motor vehicle**

√x7ᵗʰ **Y03.8 Other assault by crashing of motor vehicle**

√4ᵗʰ **Y04 Assault by bodily force**
EXCLUDES1 assault by:
submersion (X92.-)
use of weapon (X93-X95, X99, Y00)

√x7ᵗʰ **Y04.0 Assault by unarmed brawl or fight**

√x7ᵗʰ **Y04.1 Assault by human bite**

√x7ᵗʰ **Y04.2 Assault by strike against or bumped into by another person**

√x7ᵗʰ **Y04.8 Assault by other bodily force**
Assault by bodily force NOS

√4ᵗʰ **Y07 Perpetrator of assault, maltreatment and neglect**
NOTE   Codes from this category are for use only in cases of confirmed abuse (T74.-)
Selection of the correct perpetrator code is based on the relationship between the perpetrator and the victim
INCLUDES   perpetrator of abandonment
perpetrator of emotional neglect
perpetrator of mental cruelty
perpetrator of physical abuse
perpetrator of physical neglect
perpetrator of sexual abuse
perpetrator of torture

√5ᵗʰ **Y07.0 Spouse or partner, perpetrator of maltreatment and neglect**
Spouse or partner, perpetrator of maltreatment and neglect against spouse or partner

Y07.01 Husband, perpetrator of maltreatment and neglect

Y07.02 Wife, perpetrator of maltreatment and neglect

Y07.03 Male partner, perpetrator of maltreatment and neglect

Y07.04 Female partner, perpetrator of maltreatment and neglect

√5ᵗʰ **Y07.1 Parent (adoptive) (biological), perpetrator of maltreatment and neglect**

Y07.11 Biological father, perpetrator of maltreatment and neglect

Y07.12 Biological mother, perpetrator of maltreatment and neglect

Y07.13 Adoptive father, perpetrator of maltreatment and neglect

Y07.14 Adoptive mother, perpetrator of maltreatment and neglect

√5ᵗʰ **Y07.4 Other family member, perpetrator of maltreatment and neglect**

√6ᵗʰ **Y07.41 Sibling, perpetrator of maltreatment and neglect**
EXCLUDES1 stepsibling, perpetrator of maltreatment and neglect (Y07.435, Y07.436)

Y07.410 Brother, perpetrator of maltreatment and neglect

Y07.411 Sister, perpetrator of maltreatment and neglect

√6ᵗʰ **Y07.42 Foster parent, perpetrator of maltreatment and neglect**

Y07.420 Foster father, perpetrator of maltreatment and neglect

Y07.421 Foster mother, perpetrator of maltreatment and neglect

√6ᵗʰ **Y07.43 Stepparent or stepsibling, perpetrator of maltreatment and neglect**

Y07.430 Stepfather, perpetrator of maltreatment and neglect

Y07.432 Male friend of parent (co-residing in household), perpetrator of maltreatment and neglect

Y07.433 Stepmother, perpetrator of maltreatment and neglect

Y07.434 Female friend of parent (co-residing in household), perpetrator of maltreatment and neglect

Y07.435 Stepbrother, perpetrator or maltreatment and neglect

Y07.436 Stepsister, perpetrator of maltreatment and neglect

√6ᵗʰ **Y07.49 Other family member, perpetrator of maltreatment and neglect**

Y07.490 Male cousin, perpetrator of maltreatment and neglect

Y07.491 Female cousin, perpetrator of maltreatment and neglect

Y07.499 Other family member, perpetrator of maltreatment and neglect

√5ᵗʰ **Y07.5 Non-family member, perpetrator of maltreatment and neglect**

Y07.50 Unspecified non-family member, perpetrator of maltreatment and neglect ▽

√6ᵗʰ **Y07.51 Daycare provider, perpetrator of maltreatment and neglect**

Y07.510 At-home childcare provider, perpetrator of maltreatment and neglect

Y07.511 Daycare center childcare provider, perpetrator of maltreatment and neglect

Y07.512 At-home adultcare provider, perpetrator of maltreatment and neglect

Y07.513 Adultcare center provider, perpetrator of maltreatment and neglect

Y07.519 Unspecified daycare provider, perpetrator of maltreatment and neglect ▽

√6ᵗʰ **Y07.52 Healthcare provider, perpetrator of maltreatment and neglect**

Y07.521 Mental health provider, perpetrator of maltreatment and neglect

Y07.528 Other therapist or healthcare provider, perpetrator of maltreatment and neglect
Nurse, perpetrator of maltreatment and neglect
Occupational therapist, perpetrator of maltreatment and neglect
Physical therapist, perpetrator of maltreatment and neglect
Speech therapist, perpetrator of maltreatment and neglect

Y07.529 Unspecified healthcare provider, perpetrator of maltreatment and neglect ▽

Y07.53 Teacher or instructor, perpetrator of maltreatment and neglect
Coach, perpetrator of maltreatment and neglect

Y07.59 Other non-family member, perpetrator of maltreatment and neglect

Y07.9 Unspecified perpetrator of maltreatment and neglect ▽

√4ᵗʰ **Y08 Assault by other specified means**

√5ᵗʰ **Y08.0 Assault by strike by sport equipment**

√x7ᵗʰ **Y08.01 Assault by strike by hockey stick**

√x7ᵗʰ **Y08.02 Assault by strike by baseball bat**

√x7ᵗʰ **Y08.09 Assault by strike by other specified type of sport equipment**

√5ᵗʰ **Y08.8 Assault by other specified means**

√x7ᵗʰ **Y08.81 Assault by crashing of aircraft**

√x7ᵗʰ **Y08.89 Assault by other specified means**

Y09 Assault by unspecified means ▽
Assassination (attempted) NOS
Homicide (attempted) NOS
Manslaughter (attempted) NOS
Murder (attempted) NOS

N Newborn: 0   P Pediatric: 0-17   M Maternity: 12-55   A Adult: 15-124   NRS Nonroutine supply Dx   NCDx Noncancer Dx   PDx Primary Dx   ►◄ Revised Text   ● New Code   ▲ Revised Title

1156   ICD-10-CM 2018

Event of undetermined intent (Y21-Y33)

Undetermined intent is only for use when there is specific documentation in the record that the intent of the injury cannot be determined. If no such documentation is present, code to accidental (unintentional)

The appropriate 7th character is to be added to each code from category Y21-Y33.
A   initial encounter
D   subsequent encounter
S   sequela

Y21 Drowning and submersion, undetermined intent

Y21.0 Drowning and submersion while in bathtub, **undetermined intent**

Y21.1 Drowning and submersion after fall into bathtub, **undetermined intent**

Y21.2 Drowning and submersion while in swimming pool, **undetermined intent**

Y21.3 Drowning and submersion after fall into swimming pool, **undetermined intent**

Y21.4 Drowning and submersion in natural water, **undetermined intent**

Y21.8 Other drowning and submersion, undetermined intent

Y21.9 Unspecified drowning and submersion, undetermined intent ▽

Y22 Handgun discharge, undetermined intent
Discharge of gun for single hand use, undetermined intent
Discharge of pistol, undetermined intent
Discharge of revolver, undetermined intent
EXCLUDES 2   Very pistol (Y24.8)

Y23 Rifle, shotgun and larger firearm discharge, undetermined intent
EXCLUDES 2   airgun (Y24.0)

Y23.0 Shotgun discharge, undetermined intent

Y23.1 Hunting rifle discharge, undetermined intent

Y23.2 Military firearm discharge, undetermined intent

Y23.3 Machine gun discharge, undetermined intent

Y23.8 Other larger firearm discharge, undetermined intent

Y23.9 Unspecified larger firearm discharge, undetermined intent ▽

Y24 Other and unspecified firearm discharge, undetermined intent

Y24.0 Airgun discharge, undetermined intent
BB gun discharge, undetermined intent
Pellet gun discharge, undetermined intent

Y24.8 Other firearm discharge, undetermined intent
Paintball gun discharge, undetermined intent
Very pistol [flare] discharge, undetermined intent

Y24.9 Unspecified firearm discharge, undetermined intent ▽

Y25 Contact with explosive material, undetermined intent

Y26 Exposure to smoke, fire and flames, undetermined intent

Y27 Contact with steam, hot vapors and hot objects, undetermined intent

Y27.0 Contact with steam and hot vapors, undetermined intent

Y27.1 Contact with hot tap water, undetermined intent

Y27.2 Contact with hot fluids, undetermined intent

Y27.3 Contact with hot household appliance, undetermined intent

Y27.8 Contact with other hot objects, undetermined intent

Y27.9 Contact with unspecified sharp object, undetermined intent ▽

Y28 Contact with sharp object, undetermined intent

Y28.0 Contact with sharp glass, undetermined intent

Y28.1 Contact with knife, undetermined intent

Y28.2 Contact with sword or dagger, undetermined intent

Y28.8 Contact with other sharp object, undetermined intent

Y28.9 Contact with unspecified hot objects, undetermined intent ▽

Y29 Contact with blunt object, undetermined intent

Y30 Falling, jumping or pushed from a high place, undetermined intent
Victim falling from one level to another, undetermined intent

Y31 Falling, lying or running before or into moving object, undetermined intent

Y32 Crashing of motor vehicle, undetermined intent

Y33 Other specified events, undetermined intent

Legal intervention, operations of war, military operations, and terrorism (Y35-Y38)

The appropriate 7th character is to be added to each code from categories Y35-Y38.
A   initial encounter
D   subsequent encounter
S   sequela

Y35 Legal intervention
INCLUDES   any injury sustained as a result of an encounter with any law enforcement official, serving in any capacity at the time of the encounter, whether on-duty or off-duty. Includes: injury to law enforcement official, suspect and bystander

Y35.0 Legal intervention involving firearm discharge

Y35.00 Legal intervention involving unspecified firearm discharge
Legal intervention involving gunshot wound
Legal intervention involving shot NOS

Y35.001 Legal intervention involving unspecified firearm discharge, law enforcement official injured ▽

Y35.002 Legal intervention involving unspecified firearm discharge, bystander injured ▽

Y35.003 Legal intervention involving unspecified firearm discharge, suspect injured ▽

Y35.01 Legal intervention involving injury by machine gun

Y35.011 Legal intervention involving injury by machine gun, law enforcement official injured

Y35.012 Legal intervention involving injury by machine gun, bystander injured

Y35.013 Legal intervention involving injury by machine gun, suspect injured

Y35.02 Legal intervention involving injury by handgun

Y35.021 Legal intervention involving injury by handgun, law enforcement official injured

Y35.022 Legal intervention involving injury by handgun, bystander injured

Y35.023 Legal intervention involving injury by handgun, suspect injured

Y35.03 Legal intervention involving injury by rifle pellet

Y35.031 Legal intervention involving injury by rifle pellet, law enforcement official injured

Y35.032 Legal intervention involving injury by rifle pellet, bystander injured

Y35.033 Legal intervention involving injury by rifle pellet, suspect injured

Y35.04 Legal intervention involving injury by rubber bullet

Y35.041 Legal intervention involving injury by rubber bullet, law enforcement official injured

Y35.042 Legal intervention involving injury by rubber bullet, bystander injured

Y35.043 Legal intervention involving injury by rubber bullet, suspect injured

Y35.09 Legal intervention involving other firearm discharge

Y35.091 Legal intervention involving other firearm discharge, law enforcement official injured

Y35.092 Legal intervention involving other firearm discharge, bystander injured

Y35.093 Legal intervention involving other firearm discharge, suspect injured

Y35.1 Legal intervention involving explosives

Y35.10 Legal intervention involving unspecified explosives

Y35.101 Legal intervention involving unspecified explosives, law enforcement official injured ▽

☑ Additional Character Req   Placeholder Alert   Case-Mix Diagnosis   Manifestation   ▽ Unspecified Dx   *EXCLUDES 1* Not coded here   *EXCLUDES 2* Not included here

√7th **Y35.102** **Legal intervention involving unspecified explosives, bystander injured** ▽

√7th **Y35.103** **Legal intervention involving unspecified explosives, suspect injured**

√6th **Y35.11** **Legal intervention involving injury by dynamite**

√7th **Y35.111** **Legal intervention involving injury by dynamite, law enforcement official injured**

√7th **Y35.112** **Legal intervention involving injury by dynamite, bystander injured**

√7th **Y35.113** **Legal intervention involving injury by dynamite, suspect injured**

√6th **Y35.12** **Legal intervention involving injury by explosive shell**

√7th **Y35.121** **Legal intervention involving injury by explosive shell, law enforcement official injured**

√7th **Y35.122** **Legal intervention involving injury by explosive shell, bystander injured**

√7th **Y35.123** **Legal intervention involving injury by explosive shell, suspect injured**

√6th **Y35.19** **Legal intervention involving other explosives**
Legal intervention involving injury by grenade
Legal intervention involving injury by mortar bomb

√7th **Y35.191** **Legal intervention involving other explosives, law enforcement official injured**

√7th **Y35.192** **Legal intervention involving other explosives, bystander injured**

√7th **Y35.193** **Legal intervention involving other explosives, suspect injured**

√5th **Y35.2** **Legal intervention involving gas**
Legal intervention involving asphyxiation by gas
Legal intervention involving poisoning by gas

√6th **Y35.20** **Legal intervention involving unspecified gas**

√7th **Y35.201** **Legal intervention involving unspecified gas, law enforcement official injured** ▽

√7th **Y35.202** **Legal intervention involving unspecified gas, bystander injured** ▽

√7th **Y35.203** **Legal intervention involving unspecified gas, suspect injured** ▽

√6th **Y35.21** **Legal intervention involving injury by tear gas**

√7th **Y35.211** **Legal intervention involving injury by tear gas, law enforcement official injured**

√7th **Y35.212** **Legal intervention involving injury by tear gas, bystander injured**

√7th **Y35.213** **Legal intervention involving injury by tear gas, suspect injured**

√6th **Y35.29** **Legal intervention involving other gas**

√7th **Y35.291** **Legal intervention involving other gas, law enforcement official injured**

√7th **Y35.292** **Legal intervention involving other gas, bystander injured**

√7th **Y35.293** **Legal intervention involving other gas, suspect injured**

√5th **Y35.3** **Legal intervention involving blunt objects**
Legal intervention involving being hit or struck by blunt object

√6th **Y35.30** **Legal intervention involving unspecified blunt objects**

√7th **Y35.301** **Legal intervention involving unspecified blunt objects, law enforcement official injured** ▽

√7th **Y35.302** **Legal intervention involving unspecified blunt objects, bystander injured** ▽

√7th **Y35.303** **Legal intervention involving unspecified blunt objects, suspect injured** ▽

√6th **Y35.31** **Legal intervention involving baton**

√7th **Y35.311** **Legal intervention involving baton, law enforcement official injured**

√7th **Y35.312** **Legal intervention involving baton, bystander injured**

√7th **Y35.313** **Legal intervention involving baton, suspect injured**

√6th **Y35.39** **Legal intervention involving other blunt objects**

√7th **Y35.391** **Legal intervention involving other blunt objects, law enforcement official injured**

√7th **Y35.392** **Legal intervention involving other blunt objects, bystander injured**

√7th **Y35.393** **Legal intervention involving other blunt objects, suspect injured**

√5th **Y35.4** **Legal intervention involving sharp objects**
Legal intervention involving being cut by sharp objects
Legal intervention involving being stabbed by sharp objects

√6th **Y35.40** **Legal intervention involving unspecified sharp objects**

√7th **Y35.401** **Legal intervention involving unspecified sharp objects, law enforcement official injured** ▽

√7th **Y35.402** **Legal intervention involving unspecified sharp objects, bystander injured** ▽

√7th **Y35.403** **Legal intervention involving unspecified sharp objects, suspect injured** ▽

√6th **Y35.41** **Legal intervention involving bayonet**

√7th **Y35.411** **Legal intervention involving bayonet, law enforcement official injured**

√7th **Y35.412** **Legal intervention involving bayonet, bystander injured**

√7th **Y35.413** **Legal intervention involving bayonet, suspect injured**

√6th **Y35.49** **Legal intervention involving other sharp objects**

√7th **Y35.491** **Legal intervention involving other sharp objects, law enforcement official injured**

√7th **Y35.492** **Legal intervention involving other sharp objects, bystander injured**

√7th **Y35.493** **Legal intervention involving other sharp objects, suspect injured**

√5th **Y35.8** **Legal intervention involving other specified means**

√6th **Y35.81** **Legal intervention involving manhandling**

√7th **Y35.811** **Legal intervention involving manhandling, law enforcement official injured**

√7th **Y35.812** **Legal intervention involving manhandling, bystander injured**

√7th **Y35.813** **Legal intervention involving manhandling, suspect injured**

√6th **Y35.89** **Legal intervention involving other specified means**

√7th **Y35.891** **Legal intervention involving other specified means, law enforcement official injured**

√7th **Y35.892** **Legal intervention involving other specified means, bystander injured**

√7th **Y35.893** **Legal intervention involving other specified means, suspect injured**

√5th **Y35.9** **Legal intervention, means unspecified**

√x7th **Y35.91** **Legal intervention, means unspecified, law enforcement official injured** ▽

√x7th **Y35.92** **Legal intervention, means unspecified, bystander injured** ▽

√x7th **Y35.93** **Legal intervention, means unspecified, suspect injured** ▽

√4th **Y36** **Operations of war**
INCLUDES injuries to military personnel and civilians caused by war, civil insurrection, and peacekeeping missions
EXCLUDES 1 injury to military personnel occurring during peacetime military operations (Y37.-)
military vehicles involved in transport accidents with non-military vehicle during peacetime (V09.01, V09.21, V19.81, V29.81, V39.81, V49.81, V59.81, V69.81, V79.81)
AHA: 2014, 3Q, 4

√5th **Y36.0** **War operations involving explosion of marine weapons**

√6th **Y36.00** **War operations involving explosion of unspecified marine weapon**
War operations involving underwater blast NOS

√7th **Y36.000** **War operations involving explosion of unspecified marine weapon, military personnel** ▽

☑7ᵗʰ **Y36.001** **War operations involving explosion of unspecified marine weapon,** civilian ▽

☑6ᵗʰ **Y36.01** **War operations involving explosion of** depth-charge

   ☑7ᵗʰ **Y36.010** **War operations involving explosion of depth-charge,** military personnel

   ☑7ᵗʰ **Y36.011** **War operations involving explosion of depth-charge,** civilian

☑6ᵗʰ **Y36.02** **War operations involving explosion of** marine mine
   War operations involving explosion of marine mine, at sea or in harbor

   ☑7ᵗʰ **Y36.020** **War operations involving explosion of marine mine,** military personnel

   ☑7ᵗʰ **Y36.021** **War operations involving explosion of marine mine,** civilian

☑6ᵗʰ **Y36.03** **War operations involving explosion of** sea-based artillery shell

   ☑7ᵗʰ **Y36.030** **War operations involving explosion of sea-based artillery shell,** military personnel

   ☑7ᵗʰ **Y36.031** **War operations involving explosion of sea-based artillery shell,** civilian

☑6ᵗʰ **Y36.04** **War operations involving explosion of** torpedo

   ☑7ᵗʰ **Y36.040** **War operations involving explosion of torpedo,** military personnel

   ☑7ᵗʰ **Y36.041** **War operations involving explosion of torpedo,** civilian

☑6ᵗʰ **Y36.05** **War operations involving** accidental detonation of onboard marine weapons

   ☑7ᵗʰ **Y36.050** **War operations involving accidental detonation of onboard marine weapons,** military personnel

   ☑7ᵗʰ **Y36.051** **War operations involving accidental detonation of onboard marine weapons,** civilian

☑6ᵗʰ **Y36.09** **War operations involving explosion of** other marine weapons

   ☑7ᵗʰ **Y36.090** **War operations involving explosion of other marine weapons,** military personnel

   ☑7ᵗʰ **Y36.091** **War operations involving explosion of other marine weapons,** civilian

☑5ᵗʰ **Y36.1** **War operations involving** destruction of aircraft

☑6ᵗʰ **Y36.10** **War operations involving** unspecified destruction of aircraft

   ☑7ᵗʰ **Y36.100** **War operations involving unspecified destruction of aircraft,** military personnel ▽

   ☑7ᵗʰ **Y36.101** **War operations involving unspecified destruction of aircraft,** civilian ▽

☑6ᵗʰ **Y36.11** **War operations involving destruction of aircraft due to** enemy fire or explosives
   War operations involving destruction of aircraft due to air to air missile
   War operations involving destruction of aircraft due to explosive placed on aircraft
   War operations involving destruction of aircraft due to rocket propelled grenade [RPG]
   War operations involving destruction of aircraft due to small arms fire
   War operations involving destruction of aircraft due to surface to air missile

   ☑7ᵗʰ **Y36.110** **War operations involving destruction of aircraft due to enemy fire or explosives,** military personnel

   ☑7ᵗʰ **Y36.111** **War operations involving destruction of aircraft due to enemy fire or explosives,** civilian

☑6ᵗʰ **Y36.12** **War operations involving destruction of aircraft due to** collision with other aircraft

   ☑7ᵗʰ **Y36.120** **War operations involving destruction of aircraft due to collision with other aircraft,** military personnel

   ☑7ᵗʰ **Y36.121** **War operations involving destruction of aircraft due to collision with other aircraft,** civilian

☑6ᵗʰ **Y36.13** **War operations involving destruction of aircraft due to** onboard fire

   ☑7ᵗʰ **Y36.130** **War operations involving destruction of aircraft due to onboard fire,** military personnel

   ☑7ᵗʰ **Y36.131** **War operations involving destruction of aircraft due to onboard fire,** civilian

☑6ᵗʰ **Y36.14** **War operations involving destruction of aircraft due to** accidental detonation of onboard munitions and explosives

   ☑7ᵗʰ **Y36.140** **War operations involving destruction of aircraft due to accidental detonation of onboard munitions and explosives,** military personnel

   ☑7ᵗʰ **Y36.141** **War operations involving destruction of aircraft due to accidental detonation of onboard munitions and explosives,** civilian

☑6ᵗʰ **Y36.19** **War operations involving** other destruction of aircraft

   ☑7ᵗʰ **Y36.190** **War operations involving other destruction of aircraft,** military personnel

   ☑7ᵗʰ **Y36.191** **War operations involving other destruction of aircraft,** civilian

☑5ᵗʰ **Y36.2** **War operations involving** other explosions and fragments

   EXCLUDES 1 *war operations involving explosion of aircraft (Y36.1-)*
     war operations involving explosion of marine weapons (Y36.0-)
     war operations involving explosion of nuclear weapons (Y36.5-)
     war operations involving explosion occurring after cessation of hostilities (Y36.8-)

☑6ᵗʰ **Y36.20** **War operations involving** unspecified explosion and fragments
   War operations involving air blast NOS
   War operations involving blast NOS
   War operations involving blast fragments NOS
   War operations involving blast wave NOS
   War operations involving blast wind NOS
   War operations involving explosion NOS
   War operations involving explosion of bomb NOS

   ☑7ᵗʰ **Y36.200** **War operations involving unspecified explosion and fragments,** military personnel ▽

   ☑7ᵗʰ **Y36.201** **War operations involving unspecified explosion and fragments,** civilian ▽

☑6ᵗʰ **Y36.21** **War operations involving explosion of** aerial bomb

   ☑7ᵗʰ **Y36.210** **War operations involving explosion of aerial bomb,** military personnel

   ☑7ᵗʰ **Y36.211** **War operations involving explosion of aerial bomb,** civilian

☑6ᵗʰ **Y36.22** **War operations involving explosion of** guided missile

   ☑7ᵗʰ **Y36.220** **War operations involving explosion of guided missile,** military personnel

   ☑7ᵗʰ **Y36.221** **War operations involving explosion of guided missile,** civilian

☑6ᵗʰ **Y36.23** **War operations involving explosion of** improvised explosive device [IED]
   War operations involving explosion of person-borne improvised explosive device [IED]
   War operations involving explosion of vehicle-borne improvised explosive device [IED]
   War operations involving explosion of roadside improvised explosive device [IED]

   ☑7ᵗʰ **Y36.230** **War operations involving explosion of improvised explosive device [IED],** military personnel

   ☑7ᵗʰ **Y36.231** **War operations involving explosion of improvised explosive device [IED],** civilian

☑6ᵗʰ **Y36.24** **War operations involving explosion due to** accidental detonation and discharge of own munitions or munitions launch device

   ☑7ᵗʰ **Y36.240** **War operations involving explosion due to accidental detonation and discharge of own munitions or munitions launch device,** military personnel

☑ Additional Character Req   ☑x7ᵗʰ Placeholder Alert   Case-Mix Diagnosis   Manifestation   ▽ Unspecified Dx   EXCLUDES 1 Not coded here   EXCLUDES 2 Not included here

ICD-10-CM 2018   1159

Chapter 20. External Causes of Morbidity

✓7ᵗʰ **Y36.241** **War operations involving explosion due to accidental detonation and discharge of own munitions or munitions launch device,** civilian

✓6ᵗʰ **Y36.25** **War operations involving** fragments from munitions

  ✓7ᵗʰ **Y36.250** **War operations involving fragments from munitions,** military personnel

  ✓7ᵗʰ **Y36.251** **War operations involving fragments from munitions,** civilian

✓6ᵗʰ **Y36.26** **War operations involving fragments of** improvised explosive device [IED]

    War operations involving fragments of person-borne improvised explosive device [IED]

    War operations involving fragments of vehicle-borne improvised explosive device [IED]

    War operations involving fragments of roadside improvised explosive device [IED]

  ✓7ᵗʰ **Y36.260** **War operations involving fragments of improvised explosive device [IED],** military personnel

  ✓7ᵗʰ **Y36.261** **War operations involving fragments of improvised explosive device [IED],** civilian

✓6ᵗʰ **Y36.27** **War operations involving** fragments from weapons

  ✓7ᵗʰ **Y36.270** **War operations involving fragments from weapons,** military personnel

  ✓7ᵗʰ **Y36.271** **War operations involving fragments from weapons,** civilian

✓6ᵗʰ **Y36.29** **War operations involving** other explosions and fragments

    War operations involving explosion of grenade

    War operations involving explosions of land mine

    War operations involving shrapnel NOS

  ✓7ᵗʰ **Y36.290** **War operations involving other explosions and fragments,** military personnel

  ✓7ᵗʰ **Y36.291** **War operations involving other explosions and fragments,** civilian

✓5ᵗʰ **Y36.3** **War operations involving** fires, conflagrations and hot substances

    War operations involving smoke, fumes, and heat from fires, conflagrations and hot substances

    EXCLUDES 1   *war operations involving fires and conflagrations aboard military aircraft (Y36.1-)*

             war operations involving fires and conflagrations aboard military watercraft (Y36.0-)

             war operations involving fires and conflagrations caused indirectly by conventional weapons (Y36.2-)

             war operations involving fires and thermal effects of nuclear weapons (Y36.53-)

✓6ᵗʰ **Y36.30** **War operations involving** unspecified **fire, conflagration and hot substance**

  ✓7ᵗʰ **Y36.300** **War operations involving unspecified fire, conflagration and hot substance,** military personnel ▽

  ✓7ᵗʰ **Y36.301** **War operations involving unspecified fire, conflagration and hot substance,** civilian ▽

✓6ᵗʰ **Y36.31** **War operations involving** gasoline bomb

    War operations involving incendiary bomb

    War operations involving petrol bomb

  ✓7ᵗʰ **Y36.310** **War operations involving gasoline bomb,** military personnel

  ✓7ᵗʰ **Y36.311** **War operations involving gasoline bomb,** civilian

✓6ᵗʰ **Y36.32** **War operations involving** incendiary bullet

  ✓7ᵗʰ **Y36.320** **War operations involving incendiary bullet,** military personnel

  ✓7ᵗʰ **Y36.321** **War operations involving incendiary bullet,** civilian

✓6ᵗʰ **Y36.33** **War operations involving** flamethrower

  ✓7ᵗʰ **Y36.330** **War operations involving flamethrower,** military personnel

  ✓7ᵗʰ **Y36.331** **War operations involving flamethrower,** civilian

✓6ᵗʰ **Y36.39** **War operations involving other fires,** conflagrations and hot substances

  ✓7ᵗʰ **Y36.390** **War operations involving other fires, conflagrations and hot substances,** military personnel

  ✓7ᵗʰ **Y36.391** **War operations involving other fires, conflagrations and hot substances,** civilian

✓5ᵗʰ **Y36.4** **War operations involving firearm discharge and other forms of conventional warfare**

✓6ᵗʰ **Y36.41** **War operations involving** rubber bullets

  ✓7ᵗʰ **Y36.410** **War operations involving rubber bullets,** military personnel

  ✓7ᵗʰ **Y36.411** **War operations involving rubber bullets,** civilian

✓6ᵗʰ **Y36.42** **War operations involving** firearms pellets

  ✓7ᵗʰ **Y36.420** **War operations involving firearms pellets,** military personnel

  ✓7ᵗʰ **Y36.421** **War operations involving firearms pellets,** civilian

✓6ᵗʰ **Y36.43** **War operations involving** other **firearms discharge**

    War operations involving bullets NOS

    EXCLUDES 1   *war operations involving munitions fragments (Y36.25-)*

             war operations involving incendiary bullets (Y36.32-)

  ✓7ᵗʰ **Y36.430** **War operations involving other firearms discharge,** military personnel

  ✓7ᵗʰ **Y36.431** **War operations involving other firearms discharge,** civilian

✓6ᵗʰ **Y36.44** **War operations involving** unarmed hand to hand combat

    EXCLUDES 1   *war operations involving combat using blunt or piercing object (Y36.45-)*

             war operations involving intentional restriction of air and airway (Y36.46-)

             war operations involving unintentional restriction of air and airway (Y36.47-)

  ✓7ᵗʰ **Y36.440** **War operations involving unarmed hand to hand combat,** military personnel

  ✓7ᵗʰ **Y36.441** **War operations involving unarmed hand to hand combat,** civilian

✓6ᵗʰ **Y36.45** **War operations involving combat using blunt or** piercing object

  ✓7ᵗʰ **Y36.450** **War operations involving combat using blunt or piercing object,** military personnel

  ✓7ᵗʰ **Y36.451** **War operations involving combat using blunt or piercing object,** civilian

✓6ᵗʰ **Y36.46** **War operations involving** intentional restriction of air and airway

  ✓7ᵗʰ **Y36.460** **War operations involving intentional restriction of air and airway,** military personnel

  ✓7ᵗʰ **Y36.461** **War operations involving intentional restriction of air and airway,** civilian

✓6ᵗʰ **Y36.47** **War operations involving** unintentional restriction of air and airway

  ✓7ᵗʰ **Y36.470** **War operations involving unintentional restriction of air and airway,** military personnel

  ✓7ᵗʰ **Y36.471** **War operations involving unintentional restriction of air and airway,** civilian

✓6ᵗʰ **Y36.49** **War operations involving** other **forms of** conventional warfare

  ✓7ᵗʰ **Y36.490** **War operations involving other forms of conventional warfare,** military personnel

  ✓7ᵗʰ **Y36.491** **War operations involving other forms of conventional warfare,** civilian

✓5ᵗʰ **Y36.5** **War operations involving** nuclear weapons

    War operations involving dirty bomb NOS

✓6ᵗʰ **Y36.50** **War operations involving** unspecified **effect of nuclear weapon**

  ✓7ᵗʰ **Y36.500** **War operations involving unspecified effect of nuclear weapon,** military personnel ▽

Ⓝ Newborn: 0   Ⓟ Pediatric: 0-17   Ⓜ Maternity: 12-55   Ⓐ Adult: 15-124   **NRS** Nonroutine supply Dx   **NCDx** Noncancer Dx   **PDx** Primary Dx   ▶◀ Revised Text   ● New Code   ▲ Revised Title

✓7ᵗʰ Y36.5Ø1   War operations involving unspecified △ effect of nuclear weapon, **civilian**

✓6ᵗʰ Y36.51   War operations involving **direct blast** effect of nuclear weapon
     War operations involving blast pressure of nuclear weapon

     ✓7ᵗʰ Y36.51Ø   War operations involving direct blast effect of nuclear weapon, **military personnel**

     ✓7ᵗʰ Y36.511   War operations involving direct blast effect of nuclear weapon, **civilian**

✓6ᵗʰ Y36.52   War operations involving **indirect blast** effect of nuclear weapon
     War operations involving being thrown by blast of nuclear weapon
     War operations involving being struck or crushed by blast debris of nuclear weapon

     ✓7ᵗʰ Y36.52Ø   War operations involving indirect blast effect of nuclear weapon, **military personnel**

     ✓7ᵗʰ Y36.521   War operations involving indirect blast effect of nuclear weapon, **civilian**

✓6ᵗʰ Y36.53   War operations involving **thermal radiation** effect of nuclear weapon
     War operations involving direct heat from nuclear weapon
     War operation involving fireball effects from nuclear weapon

     ✓7ᵗʰ Y36.53Ø   War operations involving thermal radiation effect of nuclear weapon, **military personnel**

     ✓7ᵗʰ Y36.531   War operations involving thermal radiation effect of nuclear weapon, **civilian**

✓6ᵗʰ Y36.54   War operation involving **nuclear radiation** effects of nuclear weapon
     War operation involving acute radiation exposure from nuclear weapon
     War operation involving exposure to immediate ionizing radiation from nuclear weapon
     War operation involving fallout exposure from nuclear weapon
     War operation involving secondary effects of nuclear weapons

     ✓7ᵗʰ Y36.54Ø   War operation involving nuclear radiation effects of nuclear weapon, **military personnel**

     ✓7ᵗʰ Y36.541   War operation involving nuclear radiation effects of nuclear weapon, **civilian**

✓6ᵗʰ Y36.59   War operation involving **other** effects of nuclear weapons

     ✓7ᵗʰ Y36.59Ø   War operation involving other effects of nuclear weapons, **military personnel**

     ✓7ᵗʰ Y36.591   War operation involving other effects of nuclear weapons, **civilian**

✓5ᵗʰ Y36.6   War operations involving biological weapons

     ✓6ᵗʰ Y36.6X   War operations involving **biological weapons**

         ✓7ᵗʰ Y36.6XØ   War operations involving biological weapons, **military personnel**

         ✓7ᵗʰ Y36.6X1   War operations involving biological weapons, **civilian**

✓5ᵗʰ Y36.7   War operations involving chemical weapons and other forms of unconventional warfare
     EXCLUDES 1   war operations involving incendiary devices (Y36.3-, Y36.5-)

     ✓6ᵗʰ Y36.7X   War operations involving **chemical weapons** and **other** forms of **unconventional warfare**

         ✓7ᵗʰ Y36.7XØ   War operations involving chemical weapons and other forms of unconventional warfare, **military personnel**

         ✓7ᵗʰ Y36.7X1   War operations involving chemical weapons and other forms of unconventional warfare, **civilian**

✓5ᵗʰ Y36.8   War operations occurring **after cessation of hostilities**
     War operations classifiable to categories Y36.Ø-Y36.8 but occurring after cessation of hostilities

     ✓6ᵗʰ Y36.81   Explosion of **mine** placed during war operations but exploding after cessation of hostilities

         ✓7ᵗʰ Y36.81Ø   Explosion of mine placed during war operations but exploding after cessation of hostilities, **military personnel**

         ✓7ᵗʰ Y36.811   Explosion of mine placed during war operations but exploding after cessation of hostilities, **civilian**

     ✓6ᵗʰ Y36.82   Explosion of **bomb** placed during war operations but exploding after cessation of hostilities

         ✓7ᵗʰ Y36.82Ø   Explosion of bomb placed during war operations but exploding after cessation of hostilities, **military personnel**

         ✓7ᵗʰ Y36.821   Explosion of bomb placed during war operations but exploding after cessation of hostilities, **civilian**

     ✓6ᵗʰ Y36.88   **Other** war operations occurring after cessation of hostilities

         ✓7ᵗʰ Y36.88Ø   Other war operations occurring after cessation of hostilities, **military personnel**

         ✓7ᵗʰ Y36.881   Other war operations occurring after cessation of hostilities, **civilian**

     ✓6ᵗʰ Y36.89   **Unspecified** war operations occurring after cessation of hostilities

         ✓7ᵗʰ Y36.89Ø   Unspecified war operations occurring after cessation of hostilities, **military personnel** △

         ✓7ᵗʰ Y36.891   Unspecified war operations occurring after cessation of hostilities, **civilian** △

✓5ᵗʰ Y36.9   Other and unspecified war operations

     ✓x7ᵗʰ Y36.9Ø   War operations, unspecified △

     ✓x7ᵗʰ Y36.91   War operations involving unspecified **weapon of mass destruction [WMD]** △

     ✓x7ᵗʰ Y36.92   War operations involving **friendly fire**

✓4ᵗʰ Y37   **Military operations**
     INCLUDES   injuries to military personnel and civilians occurring during peacetime on military property and during routine military exercises and operations
     EXCLUDES 1   military aircraft involved in aircraft accident with civilian aircraft (V97.81-)
         military vehicles involved in transport accident with civilian vehicle (VØ9.Ø1, VØ9.21, V19.81, V29.81, V39.81, V49.81, V59.81, V69.81, V79.81)
         military watercraft involved in water transport accident with civilian watercraft (V94.81-)
         war operations (Y36.-)

✓5ᵗʰ Y37.Ø   Military operations involving **explosion of marine weapons**

     ✓6ᵗʰ Y37.ØØ   Military operations involving explosion of **unspecified** marine weapon
         Military operations involving underwater blast NOS

         ✓7ᵗʰ Y37.ØØØ   Military operations involving explosion of unspecified marine weapon, **military personnel** △

         ✓7ᵗʰ Y37.ØØ1   Military operations involving explosion of unspecified marine weapon, **civilian** △

     ✓6ᵗʰ Y37.Ø1   Military operations involving explosion of **depth-charge**

         ✓7ᵗʰ Y37.Ø1Ø   Military operations involving explosion of depth-charge, **military personnel**

         ✓7ᵗʰ Y37.Ø11   Military operations involving explosion of depth-charge, **civilian**

     ✓6ᵗʰ Y37.Ø2   Military operations involving explosion of **marine mine**
         Military operations involving explosion of marine mine, at sea or in harbor

         ✓7ᵗʰ Y37.Ø2Ø   Military operations involving explosion of marine mine, **military personnel**

         ✓7ᵗʰ Y37.Ø21   Military operations involving explosion of marine mine, **civilian**

     ✓6ᵗʰ Y37.Ø3   Military operations involving explosion of **sea-based artillery shell**

         ✓7ᵗʰ Y37.Ø3Ø   Military operations involving explosion of sea-based artillery shell, **military personnel**

✓ Additional Character Req   ✓x7ᵗʰ Placeholder Alert   Case-Mix Diagnosis   Manifestation   △ Unspecified Dx   **EXCLUDES 1** Not coded here   **EXCLUDES 2** Not included here

ICD-10-CM 2018   1161

Chapter 20. External Causes of Morbidity

Y37.031–Y37.260

√7ᵗʰ **Y37.031** **Military operations involving explosion of sea-based artillery shell,** civilian

√6ᵗʰ **Y37.04** **Military operations involving explosion of** torpedo

√7ᵗʰ **Y37.040** **Military operations involving explosion of torpedo,** military personnel

√7ᵗʰ **Y37.041** **Military operations involving explosion of torpedo,** civilian

√6ᵗʰ **Y37.05** **Military operations involving accidental detonation of** onboard marine weapons

√7ᵗʰ **Y37.050** **Military operations involving accidental detonation of onboard marine weapons,** military personnel

√7ᵗʰ **Y37.051** **Military operations involving accidental detonation of onboard marine weapons,** civilian

√6ᵗʰ **Y37.09** **Military operations involving explosion of** other marine weapons

√7ᵗʰ **Y37.090** **Military operations involving explosion of other marine weapons,** military personnel

√7ᵗʰ **Y37.091** **Military operations involving explosion of other marine weapons,** civilian

√5ᵗʰ **Y37.1** **Military operations involving** destruction of aircraft

√6ᵗʰ **Y37.10** **Military operations involving** unspecified destruction of aircraft

√7ᵗʰ **Y37.100** **Military operations involving unspecified destruction of aircraft,** military personnel ▽

√7ᵗʰ **Y37.101** **Military operations involving unspecified destruction of aircraft,** civilian ▽

√6ᵗʰ **Y37.11** **Military operations involving destruction of aircraft** due to enemy fire or explosives
Military operations involving destruction of aircraft due to air to air missile
Military operations involving destruction of aircraft due to explosive placed on aircraft
Military operations involving destruction of aircraft due to rocket propelled grenade [RPG]
Military operations involving destruction of aircraft due to small arms fire
Military operations involving destruction of aircraft due to surface to air missile

√7ᵗʰ **Y37.110** **Military operations involving destruction of aircraft due to enemy fire or explosives,** military personnel

√7ᵗʰ **Y37.111** **Military operations involving destruction of aircraft due to enemy fire or explosives,** civilian

√6ᵗʰ **Y37.12** **Military operations involving destruction of aircraft** due to collision with other aircraft

√7ᵗʰ **Y37.120** **Military operations involving destruction of aircraft due to collision with other aircraft,** military personnel

√7ᵗʰ **Y37.121** **Military operations involving destruction of aircraft due to collision with other aircraft,** civilian

√6ᵗʰ **Y37.13** **Military operations involving destruction of aircraft** due to onboard fire

√7ᵗʰ **Y37.130** **Military operations involving destruction of aircraft due to onboard fire,** military personnel

√7ᵗʰ **Y37.131** **Military operations involving destruction of aircraft due to onboard fire,** civilian

√6ᵗʰ **Y37.14** **Military operations involving destruction of aircraft due to** accidental detonation of onboard munitions and explosives

√7ᵗʰ **Y37.140** **Military operations involving destruction of aircraft due to accidental detonation of onboard munitions and explosives,** military personnel

√7ᵗʰ **Y37.141** **Military operations involving destruction of aircraft due to accidental detonation of onboard munitions and explosives,** civilian

√6ᵗʰ **Y37.19** **Military operations involving other** destruction of aircraft

√7ᵗʰ **Y37.190** **Military operations involving other destruction of aircraft,** military personnel

√7ᵗʰ **Y37.191** **Military operations involving other destruction of aircraft,** civilian

√5ᵗʰ **Y37.2** **Military operations involving** other explosions and fragments
EXCLUDES 1 *military operations involving explosion of aircraft (Y37.1-)*
military operations involving explosion of marine weapons (Y37.0-)
military operations involving explosion of nuclear weapons (Y37.5-)

√6ᵗʰ **Y37.20** **Military operations involving** unspecified **explosion and fragments**
Military operations involving air blast NOS
Military operations involving blast NOS
Military operations involving blast fragments NOS
Military operations involving blast wave NOS
Military operations involving blast wind NOS
Military operations involving explosion NOS
Military operations involving explosion of bomb NOS

√7ᵗʰ **Y37.200** **Military operations involving unspecified explosion and fragments,** military personnel ▽

√7ᵗʰ **Y37.201** **Military operations involving unspecified explosion and fragments,** civilian ▽

√6ᵗʰ **Y37.21** **Military operations involving explosion of** aerial bomb

√7ᵗʰ **Y37.210** **Military operations involving explosion of aerial bomb,** military personnel

√7ᵗʰ **Y37.211** **Military operations involving explosion of aerial bomb,** civilian

√6ᵗʰ **Y37.22** **Military operations involving explosion of** guided missile

√7ᵗʰ **Y37.220** **Military operations involving explosion of guided missile,** military personnel

√7ᵗʰ **Y37.221** **Military operations involving explosion of guided missile,** civilian

√6ᵗʰ **Y37.23** **Military operations involving explosion of** improvised explosive device [IED]
Military operations involving explosion of person-borne improvised explosive device [IED]
Military operations involving explosion of vehicle-borne improvised explosive device [IED]
Military operations involving explosion of roadside improvised explosive device [IED]

√7ᵗʰ **Y37.230** **Military operations involving explosion of improvised explosive device [IED],** military personnel

√7ᵗʰ **Y37.231** **Military operations involving explosion of improvised explosive device [IED],** civilian

√6ᵗʰ **Y37.24** **Military operations involving explosion** due to accidental detonation and discharge of own munitions or munitions launch device

√7ᵗʰ **Y37.240** **Military operations involving explosion due to accidental detonation and discharge of own munitions or munitions launch device,** military personnel

√7ᵗʰ **Y37.241** **Military operations involving explosion due to accidental detonation and discharge of own munitions or munitions launch device,** civilian

√6ᵗʰ **Y37.25** **Military operations involving** fragments from munitions

√7ᵗʰ **Y37.250** **Military operations involving fragments from munitions,** military personnel

√7ᵗʰ **Y37.251** **Military operations involving fragments from munitions,** civilian

√6ᵗʰ **Y37.26** **Military operations involving fragments of** improvised explosive device [IED]
Military operations involving fragments of person-borne improvised explosive device [IED]
Military operations involving fragments of vehicle-borne improvised explosive device [IED]
Military operations involving fragments of roadside improvised explosive device [IED]

√7ᵗʰ **Y37.260** **Military operations involving fragments of improvised explosive device [IED],** military personnel

✓7ᵗʰ **Y37.261 Military operations involving fragments of improvised explosive device [IED],** civilian

✓6ᵗʰ **Y37.27 Military operations involving fragments from** weapons

    ✓7ᵗʰ **Y37.270 Military operations involving fragments from weapons,** military personnel

    ✓7ᵗʰ **Y37.271 Military operations involving fragments from weapons,** civilian

✓6ᵗʰ **Y37.29 Military operations involving** other **explosions and fragments**

    Military operations involving explosion of grenade
    Military operations involving explosions of land mine
    Military operations involving shrapnel NOS

    ✓7ᵗʰ **Y37.290 Military operations involving other explosions and fragments,** military personnel

    ✓7ᵗʰ **Y37.291 Military operations involving other explosions and fragments,** civilian

✓5ᵗʰ **Y37.3 Military operations involving** fires, conflagrations and hot substances

    Military operations involving smoke, fumes, and heat from fires, conflagrations and hot substances

    EXCLUDES 1 *military operations involving fires and conflagrations aboard military aircraft (Y37.1-)*
    military operations involving fires and conflagrations aboard military watercraft (Y37.0-)
    military operations involving fires and conflagrations caused indirectly by conventional weapons (Y37.2-)
    military operations involving fires and thermal effects of nuclear weapons (Y36.53-)

✓6ᵗʰ **Y37.30 Military operations involving** unspecified **fire, conflagration and hot substance**

    ✓7ᵗʰ **Y37.300 Military operations involving unspecified fire, conflagration and hot substance,** military personnel ▽

    ✓7ᵗʰ **Y37.301 Military operations involving unspecified fire, conflagration and hot substance,** civilian ▽

✓6ᵗʰ **Y37.31 Military operations involving** gasoline bomb

    Military operations involving incendiary bomb
    Military operations involving petrol bomb

    ✓7ᵗʰ **Y37.310 Military operations involving gasoline bomb,** military personnel

    ✓7ᵗʰ **Y37.311 Military operations involving gasoline bomb,** civilian

✓6ᵗʰ **Y37.32 Military operations involving** incendiary bullet

    ✓7ᵗʰ **Y37.320 Military operations involving incendiary bullet,** military personnel

    ✓7ᵗʰ **Y37.321 Military operations involving incendiary bullet,** civilian

✓6ᵗʰ **Y37.33 Military operations involving** flamethrower

    ✓7ᵗʰ **Y37.330 Military operations involving flamethrower,** military personnel

    ✓7ᵗʰ **Y37.331 Military operations involving flamethrower,** civilian

✓6ᵗʰ **Y37.39 Military operations involving** other **fires, conflagrations and hot substances**

    ✓7ᵗʰ **Y37.390 Military operations involving other fires, conflagrations and hot substances,** military personnel

    ✓7ᵗʰ **Y37.391 Military operations involving other fires, conflagrations and hot substances,** civilian

✓5ᵗʰ **Y37.4 Military operations involving firearm discharge and other forms of conventional warfare**

✓6ᵗʰ **Y37.41 Military operations involving** rubber bullets

    ✓7ᵗʰ **Y37.410 Military operations involving rubber bullets,** military personnel

    ✓7ᵗʰ **Y37.411 Military operations involving rubber bullets,** civilian

✓6ᵗʰ **Y37.42 Military operations involving** firearms pellets

    ✓7ᵗʰ **Y37.420 Military operations involving firearms pellets,** military personnel

    ✓7ᵗʰ **Y37.421 Military operations involving firearms pellets,** civilian

✓6ᵗʰ **Y37.43 Military operations involving** other firearms discharge

    Military operations involving bullets NOS

    EXCLUDES 1 *military operations involving munitions fragments (Y37.25-)*
    military operations involving incendiary bullets (Y37.32-)

    ✓7ᵗʰ **Y37.430 Military operations involving other firearms discharge,** military personnel

    ✓7ᵗʰ **Y37.431 Military operations involving other firearms discharge,** civilian

✓6ᵗʰ **Y37.44 Military operations involving** unarmed hand to hand combat

    EXCLUDES 1 *military operations involving combat using blunt or piercing object (Y37.45-)*
    military operations involving intentional restriction of air and airway (Y37.46-)
    military operations involving unintentional restriction of air and airway (Y37.47-)

    ✓7ᵗʰ **Y37.440 Military operations involving unarmed hand to hand combat,** military personnel

    ✓7ᵗʰ **Y37.441 Military operations involving unarmed hand to hand combat,** civilian

✓6ᵗʰ **Y37.45 Military operations involving** combat using blunt or piercing object

    ✓7ᵗʰ **Y37.450 Military operations involving combat using blunt or piercing object,** military personnel

    ✓7ᵗʰ **Y37.451 Military operations involving combat using blunt or piercing object,** civilian

✓6ᵗʰ **Y37.46 Military operations involving** intentional restriction of air and airway

    ✓7ᵗʰ **Y37.460 Military operations involving intentional restriction of air and airway,** military personnel

    ✓7ᵗʰ **Y37.461 Military operations involving intentional restriction of air and airway,** civilian

✓6ᵗʰ **Y37.47 Military operations involving** unintentional restriction of air and airway

    ✓7ᵗʰ **Y37.470 Military operations involving unintentional restriction of air and airway,** military personnel

    ✓7ᵗʰ **Y37.471 Military operations involving unintentional restriction of air and airway,** civilian

✓6ᵗʰ **Y37.49 Military operations involving** other **forms of conventional warfare**

    ✓7ᵗʰ **Y37.490 Military operations involving other forms of conventional warfare,** military personnel

    ✓7ᵗʰ **Y37.491 Military operations involving other forms of conventional warfare,** civilian

✓5ᵗʰ **Y37.5 Military operations involving** nuclear weapons

    Military operation involving dirty bomb NOS

✓6ᵗʰ **Y37.50 Military operations involving** unspecified effect **of nuclear weapon**

    ✓7ᵗʰ **Y37.500 Military operations involving unspecified effect of nuclear weapon,** military personnel ▽

    ✓7ᵗʰ **Y37.501 Military operations involving unspecified effect of nuclear weapon,** civilian ▽

✓6ᵗʰ **Y37.51 Military operations involving** direct blast effect **of nuclear weapon**

    Military operations involving blast pressure of nuclear weapon

    ✓7ᵗʰ **Y37.510 Military operations involving direct blast effect of nuclear weapon,** military personnel

    ✓7ᵗʰ **Y37.511 Military operations involving direct blast effect of nuclear weapon,** civilian

✓ Additional Character Req   ✓x7ᵗʰ Placeholder Alert   Case-Mix Diagnosis   Manifestation   ▽ Unspecified Dx   **EXCLUDES 1** Not coded here   **EXCLUDES 2** Not included here

ICD-10-CM 2018   1163

Chapter 20. External Causes of Morbidity

✓6ᵗʰ Y37.52 Military operations involving indirect blast effect of nuclear weapon

Military operations involving being thrown by blast of nuclear weapon

Military operations involving being struck or crushed by blast debris of nuclear weapon

   ✓7ᵗʰ Y37.520 Military operations involving indirect blast effect of nuclear weapon, military personnel

   ✓7ᵗʰ Y37.521 Military operations involving indirect blast effect of nuclear weapon, civilian

✓6ᵗʰ Y37.53 Military operations involving thermal radiation effect of nuclear weapon

Military operations involving direct heat from nuclear weapon

Military operation involving fireball effects from nuclear weapon

   ✓7ᵗʰ Y37.530 Military operations involving thermal radiation effect of nuclear weapon, military personnel

   ✓7ᵗʰ Y37.531 Military operations involving thermal radiation effect of nuclear weapon, civilian

✓6ᵗʰ Y37.54 Military operation involving nuclear radiation effects of nuclear weapon

Military operation involving acute radiation exposure from nuclear weapon

Military operation involving exposure to immediate ionizing radiation from nuclear weapon

Military operation involving fallout exposure from nuclear weapon

Military operation involving secondary effects of nuclear weapons

   ✓7ᵗʰ Y37.540 Military operation involving nuclear radiation effects of nuclear weapon, military personnel

   ✓7ᵗʰ Y37.541 Military operation involving nuclear radiation effects of nuclear weapon, civilian

✓6ᵗʰ Y37.59 Military operation involving other effects of nuclear weapons

   ✓7ᵗʰ Y37.590 Military operation involving other effects of nuclear weapons, military personnel

   ✓7ᵗʰ Y37.591 Military operation involving other effects of nuclear weapons, civilian

✓5ᵗʰ Y37.6 Military operations involving biological weapons

  ✓6ᵗʰ Y37.6X Military operations involving biological weapons

   ✓7ᵗʰ Y37.6X0 Military operations involving biological weapons, military personnel

   ✓7ᵗʰ Y37.6X1 Military operations involving biological weapons, civilian

✓5ᵗʰ Y37.7 Military operations involving chemical weapons and other forms of unconventional warfare

  EXCLUDES 1 *military operations involving incendiary devices (Y36.3-, Y36.5-)*

  ✓6ᵗʰ Y37.7X Military operations involving chemical weapons and other forms of unconventional warfare

   ✓7ᵗʰ Y37.7X0 Military operations involving chemical weapons and other forms of unconventional warfare, military personnel

   ✓7ᵗʰ Y37.7X1 Military operations involving chemical weapons and other forms of unconventional warfare, civilian

✓5ᵗʰ Y37.9 Other and unspecified military operations

  ✓x7ᵗʰ Y37.90 Military operations, unspecified ▽

  ✓x7ᵗʰ Y37.91 Military operations involving unspecified weapon of mass destruction [WMD] ▽

  ✓x7ᵗʰ Y37.92 Military operations involving friendly fire

✓4ᵗʰ Y38 Terrorism

These codes are for use to identify injuries resulting from the unlawful use of force or violence against persons or property to intimidate or coerce a Government, the civilian population, or any segment thereof, in furtherance of political or social objective.

Use additional code for place of occurrence (Y92.-)

✓5ᵗʰ Y38.0 Terrorism involving explosion of marine weapons

Terrorism involving depth-charge

Terrorism involving marine mine

Terrorism involving mine NOS, at sea or in harbor

Terrorism involving sea-based artillery shell

Terrorism involving torpedo

Terrorism involving underwater blast

  ✓6ᵗʰ Y38.0X Terrorism involving explosion of marine weapons

   ✓7ᵗʰ Y38.0X1 Terrorism involving explosion of marine weapons, public safety official injured

   ✓7ᵗʰ Y38.0X2 Terrorism involving explosion of marine weapons, civilian injured

   ✓7ᵗʰ Y38.0X3 Terrorism involving explosion of marine weapons, terrorist injured

✓5ᵗʰ Y38.1 Terrorism involving destruction of aircraft

Terrorism involving aircraft burned

Terrorism involving aircraft exploded

Terrorism involving aircraft being shot down

Terrorism involving aircraft used as a weapon

  ✓6ᵗʰ Y38.1X Terrorism involving destruction of aircraft

   ✓7ᵗʰ Y38.1X1 Terrorism involving destruction of aircraft, public safety official injured

   ✓7ᵗʰ Y38.1X2 Terrorism involving destruction of aircraft, civilian injured

   ✓7ᵗʰ Y38.1X3 Terrorism involving destruction of aircraft, terrorist injured

✓5ᵗʰ Y38.2 Terrorism involving other explosions and fragments

Terrorism involving antipersonnel (fragments) bomb

Terrorism involving blast NOS

Terrorism involving explosion NOS

Terrorism involving explosion of breech block

Terrorism involving explosion of cannon block

Terrorism involving explosion (fragments) of artillery shell

Terrorism involving explosion (fragments) of bomb

Terrorism involving explosion (fragments) of grenade

Terrorism involving explosion (fragments) of guided missile

Terrorism involving explosion (fragments) of land mine

Terrorism involving explosion of mortar bomb

Terrorism involving explosion of munitions

Terrorism involving explosion (fragments) of rocket

Terrorism involving explosion (fragments) of shell

Terrorism involving shrapnel

Terrorism involving mine NOS, on land

  EXCLUDES 1 *terrorism involving explosion of nuclear weapon (Y38.5)*

            terrorism involving suicide bomber (Y38.81)

  ✓6ᵗʰ Y38.2X Terrorism involving other explosions and fragments

   ✓7ᵗʰ Y38.2X1 Terrorism involving other explosions and fragments, public safety official injured

   ✓7ᵗʰ Y38.2X2 Terrorism involving other explosions and fragments, civilian injured

   ✓7ᵗʰ Y38.2X3 Terrorism involving other explosions and fragments, terrorist injured

✓5ᵗʰ Y38.3 Terrorism involving fires, conflagration and hot substances

Terrorism involving conflagration NOS

Terrorism involving fire NOS

Terrorism involving petrol bomb

  EXCLUDES 1 *terrorism involving fire or heat of nuclear weapon (Y38.5)*

  ✓6ᵗʰ Y38.3X Terrorism involving fires, conflagration and hot substances

   ✓7ᵗʰ Y38.3X1 Terrorism involving fires, conflagration and hot substances, public safety official injured

   ✓7ᵗʰ Y38.3X2 Terrorism involving fires, conflagration and hot substances, civilian injured

   ✓7ᵗʰ Y38.3X3 Terrorism involving fires, conflagration and hot substances, terrorist injured

Ⓝ Newborn: 0   Ⓟ Pediatric: 0-17   Ⓜ Maternity: 12-55   Ⓐ Adult: 15-124   **NRS** Nonroutine supply Dx   **NCDx** Noncancer Dx   **PDx** Primary Dx   ▶◀ Revised Text   ● New Code   ▲ Revised Title

1164   ICD-10-CM 2018

✓5ᵗʰ Y38.4 Terrorism involving firearms
Terrorism involving carbine bullet
Terrorism involving machine gun bullet
Terrorism involving pellets (shotgun)
Terrorism involving pistol bullet
Terrorism involving rifle bullet
Terrorism involving rubber (rifle) bullet

✓6ᵗʰ Y38.4X Terrorism involving firearms

  ✓7ᵗʰ Y38.4X1 Terrorism involving firearms, public safety official injured

  ✓7ᵗʰ Y38.4X2 Terrorism involving firearms, civilian injured

  ✓7ᵗʰ Y38.4X3 Terrorism involving firearms, terrorist injured

✓5ᵗʰ Y38.5 Terrorism involving nuclear weapons
Terrorism involving blast effects of nuclear weapon
Terrorism involving exposure to ionizing radiation from nuclear weapon
Terrorism involving fireball effect of nuclear weapon
Terrorism involving heat from nuclear weapon

✓6ᵗʰ Y38.5X Terrorism involving nuclear weapons

  ✓7ᵗʰ Y38.5X1 Terrorism involving nuclear weapons, public safety official injured

  ✓7ᵗʰ Y38.5X2 Terrorism involving nuclear weapons, civilian injured

  ✓7ᵗʰ Y38.5X3 Terrorism involving nuclear weapons, terrorist injured

✓5ᵗʰ Y38.6 Terrorism involving biological weapons
Terrorism involving anthrax
Terrorism involving cholera
Terrorism involving smallpox

✓6ᵗʰ Y38.6X Terrorism involving biological weapons

  ✓7ᵗʰ Y38.6X1 Terrorism involving biological weapons, public safety official injured

  ✓7ᵗʰ Y38.6X2 Terrorism involving biological weapons, civilian injured

  ✓7ᵗʰ Y38.6X3 Terrorism involving biological weapons, terrorist injured

✓5ᵗʰ Y38.7 Terrorism involving chemical weapons
Terrorism involving gases, fumes, chemicals
Terrorism involving hydrogen cyanide
Terrorism involving phosgene
Terrorism involving sarin

✓6ᵗʰ Y38.7X Terrorism involving chemical weapons

  ✓7ᵗʰ Y38.7X1 Terrorism involving chemical weapons, public safety official injured

  ✓7ᵗʰ Y38.7X2 Terrorism involving chemical weapons, civilian injured

  ✓7ᵗʰ Y38.7X3 Terrorism involving chemical weapons, terrorist injured

✓5ᵗʰ Y38.8 Terrorism involving other and unspecified means

  ✓x7ᵗʰ Y38.80 Terrorism involving unspecified means ▽
Terrorism NOS

  ✓6ᵗʰ Y38.81 Terrorism involving suicide bomber

    ✓7ᵗʰ Y38.811 Terrorism involving suicide bomber, public safety official injured

    ✓7ᵗʰ Y38.812 Terrorism involving suicide bomber, civilian injured

  ✓6ᵗʰ Y38.89 Terrorism involving other means
Terrorism involving drowning and submersion
Terrorism involving lasers
Terrorism involving piercing or stabbing instruments

    ✓7ᵗʰ Y38.891 Terrorism involving other means, public safety official injured

    ✓7ᵗʰ Y38.892 Terrorism involving other means, civilian injured

    ✓7ᵗʰ Y38.893 Terrorism involving other means, terrorist injured

✓5ᵗʰ Y38.9 Terrorism, secondary effects
NOTE This code is for use to identify injuries occurring subsequent to a terrorist attack, not those that are due to the initial terrorist attack.

✓6ᵗʰ Y38.9X Terrorism, secondary effects

  ✓7ᵗʰ Y38.9X1 Terrorism, secondary effects, public safety official injured

  ✓7ᵗʰ Y38.9X2 Terrorism, secondary effects, civilian injured

Complications of medical and surgical care (Y62-Y84)

INCLUDES complications of medical devices
surgical and medical procedures as the cause of abnormal reaction of the patient, or of later complication, without mention of misadventure at the time of the procedure

Misadventures to patients during surgical and medical care (Y62-Y69)

EXCLUDES 1 surgical and medical procedures as the cause of abnormal reaction of the patient, without mention of misadventure at the time of the procedure (Y83-Y84)
EXCLUDES 2 breakdown or malfunctioning of medical device (during procedure) (after implantation) (ongoing use) (Y70-Y82)

✓4ᵗʰ Y62 Failure of sterile precautions during surgical and medical care
  Y62.0 Failure of sterile precautions during surgical operation
  Y62.1 Failure of sterile precautions during infusion or transfusion
  Y62.2 Failure of sterile precautions during kidney dialysis and other perfusion
  Y62.3 Failure of sterile precautions during injection or immunization
  Y62.4 Failure of sterile precautions during endoscopic examination
  Y62.5 Failure of sterile precautions during heart catheterization
  Y62.6 Failure of sterile precautions during aspiration, puncture and other catheterization
  Y62.8 Failure of sterile precautions during other surgical and medical care
  Y62.9 Failure of sterile precautions during unspecified surgical and medical care ▽

✓4ᵗʰ Y63 Failure in dosage during surgical and medical care
EXCLUDES 2 accidental overdose of drug or wrong drug given in error (T36-T50)
  Y63.0 Excessive amount of blood or other fluid given during transfusion or infusion
  Y63.1 Incorrect dilution of fluid used during infusion
  Y63.2 Overdose of radiation given during therapy
  Y63.3 Inadvertent exposure of patient to radiation during medical care
  Y63.4 Failure in dosage in electroshock or insulin-shock therapy
  Y63.5 Inappropriate temperature in local application and packing
  Y63.6 Underdosing and nonadministration of necessary drug, medicament or biological substance
  Y63.8 Failure in dosage during other surgical and medical care
  Y63.9 Failure in dosage during unspecified surgical and medical care ▽

✓4ᵗʰ Y64 Contaminated medical or biological substances
  Y64.0 Contaminated medical or biological substance, transfused or infused
  Y64.1 Contaminated medical or biological substance, injected or used for immunization
  Y64.8 Contaminated medical or biological substance administered by other means
  Y64.9 Contaminated medical or biological substance administered by unspecified means ▽
Administered contaminated medical or biological substance NOS

✓4ᵗʰ Y65 Other misadventures during surgical and medical care
  Y65.0 Mismatched blood in transfusion
  Y65.1 Wrong fluid used in infusion
  Y65.2 Failure in suture or ligature during surgical operation
  Y65.3 Endotracheal tube wrongly placed during anesthetic procedure
  Y65.4 Failure to introduce or to remove other tube or instrument
  ✓5ᵗʰ Y65.5 Performance of wrong procedure (operation)
    Y65.51 Performance of wrong procedure (operation) on correct patient
Wrong device implanted into correct surgical site
EXCLUDES 1 performance of correct procedure (operation) on wrong side or body part (Y65.53)

✓ Additional Character Req ✓x7ᵗʰ Placeholder Alert Case-Mix Diagnosis Manifestation ▽ Unspecified Dx EXCLUDES 1 Not coded here EXCLUDES 2 Not included here

ICD-10-CM 2018   1165

Chapter 20. External Causes of Morbidity

Y65.52 Performance of procedure (operation) on patient not scheduled for surgery
Performance of procedure (operation) intended for another patient
Performance of procedure (operation) on wrong patient

Y65.53 Performance of correct procedure (operation) on wrong side or body part
Performance of correct procedure (operation) on wrong side
Performance of correct procedure (operation) on wrong site

Y65.8 Other specified misadventures **during surgical and medical care**

Y66 Nonadministration of surgical and medical care
Premature cessation of surgical and medical care
> **EXCLUDES 1**   DNR status (Z66)
> palliative care (Z51.5)

Y69 Unspecified misadventure during surgical and medical care ▽

Medical devices associated with adverse incidents in diagnostic and therapeutic use (Y70-Y82)

> **INCLUDES**   breakdown or malfunction of medical devices (during use) (after implantation) (ongoing use)

> **EXCLUDES 2**   breakdown or malfunctioning of medical device (after implantation) (during procedure) (ongoing use) (Y70-Y82)
> later complications following use of medical devices without breakdown or malfunctioning of device (Y83-Y84)
> misadventure to patients during surgical and medical care, classifiable to (Y62-Y69)
> surgical and other medical procedures as the cause of abnormal reaction of the patient, or of later complication, without mention of misadventure at the time of the procedure (Y83-Y84)

✓4ᵗʰ Y70 Anesthesiology devices associated with adverse incidents

Y70.0 Diagnostic and monitoring **anesthesiology devices associated with adverse incidents**

Y70.1 Therapeutic (nonsurgical) and rehabilitative **anesthesiology devices associated with adverse incidents**

Y70.2 Prosthetic and other implants, **materials and accessory anesthesiology devices associated with adverse incidents**

Y70.3 Surgical instruments, materials **and anesthesiology devices (including sutures) associated with adverse incidents**

Y70.8 Miscellaneous anesthesiology devices associated with adverse incidents, not elsewhere classified

✓4ᵗʰ Y71 Cardiovascular devices associated with adverse incidents

Y71.0 Diagnostic and monitoring **cardiovascular devices associated with adverse incidents**

Y71.1 Therapeutic (nonsurgical) and rehabilitative **cardiovascular devices associated with adverse incidents**

Y71.2 Prosthetic and other implants, **materials and accessory cardiovascular devices associated with adverse incidents**

Y71.3 Surgical instruments, materials **and cardiovascular devices (including sutures) associated with adverse incidents**

Y71.8 Miscellaneous cardiovascular devices associated with adverse incidents, not elsewhere classified

✓4ᵗʰ Y72 Otorhinolaryngological devices associated with adverse incidents

Y72.0 Diagnostic and monitoring **otorhinolaryngological devices associated with adverse incidents**

Y72.1 Therapeutic (nonsurgical) and rehabilitative **otorhinolaryngological devices associated with adverse incidents**

Y72.2 Prosthetic and other implants, **materials and accessory otorhinolaryngological devices associated with adverse incidents**

Y72.3 Surgical instruments, materials **and otorhinolaryngological devices (including sutures) associated with adverse incidents**

Y72.8 Miscellaneous otorhinolaryngological devices associated with adverse incidents, not elsewhere classified

✓4ᵗʰ Y73 Gastroenterology and urology devices associated with adverse incidents

Y73.0 Diagnostic and monitoring **gastroenterology and urology devices associated with adverse incidents**

Y73.1 Therapeutic (nonsurgical) and rehabilitative **gastroenterology and urology devices associated with adverse incidents**

Y73.2 Prosthetic and other implants, **materials and accessory gastroenterology and urology devices associated with adverse incidents**

Y73.3 Surgical instruments, materials **and gastroenterology and urology devices (including sutures) associated with adverse incidents**

Y73.8 Miscellaneous gastroenterology and urology devices associated with adverse incidents, not elsewhere classified

✓4ᵗʰ Y74 General hospital and personal-use devices associated with adverse incidents

Y74.0 Diagnostic and monitoring **general hospital and personal-use devices associated with adverse incidents**

Y74.1 Therapeutic (nonsurgical) and rehabilitative **general hospital and personal-use devices associated with adverse incidents**

Y74.2 Prosthetic and other implants, **materials and accessory general hospital and personal-use devices associated with adverse incidents**

Y74.3 Surgical instruments, materials **and general hospital and personal-use devices (including sutures) associated with adverse incidents**

Y74.8 Miscellaneous general hospital and personal-use devices associated with adverse incidents, not elsewhere classified

✓4ᵗʰ Y75 Neurological devices associated with adverse incidents

Y75.0 Diagnostic and monitoring **neurological devices associated with adverse incidents**

Y75.1 Therapeutic (nonsurgical) and rehabilitative **neurological devices associated with adverse incidents**

Y75.2 Prosthetic and other implants, **materials and neurological devices associated with adverse incidents**

Y75.3 Surgical instruments, materials **and neurological devices (including sutures) associated with adverse incidents**

Y75.8 Miscellaneous neurological devices associated with adverse incidents, not elsewhere classified

✓4ᵗʰ Y76 Obstetric and gynecological devices associated with adverse incidents

Y76.0 Diagnostic and monitoring **obstetric and gynecological devices associated with adverse incidents** ♀

Y76.1 Therapeutic (nonsurgical) and rehabilitative **obstetric and gynecological devices associated with adverse incidents** ♀

Y76.2 Prosthetic and other implants, **materials and accessory obstetric and gynecological devices associated with adverse incidents** ♀

Y76.3 Surgical instruments, materials **and obstetric and gynecological devices (including sutures) associated with adverse incidents** ♀

Y76.8 Miscellaneous obstetric and gynecological devices associated with adverse incidents, not elsewhere classified ♀

✓4ᵗʰ Y77 Ophthalmic devices associated with adverse incidents

Y77.0 Diagnostic and monitoring **ophthalmic devices associated with adverse incidents**

Y77.1 Therapeutic (nonsurgical) and rehabilitative **ophthalmic devices associated with adverse incidents**

Y77.2 Prosthetic and other implants, **materials and accessory ophthalmic devices associated with adverse incidents**

Y77.3 Surgical instruments, materials **and ophthalmic devices (including sutures) associated with adverse incidents**

Y77.8 Miscellaneous ophthalmic devices associated with adverse incidents, not elsewhere classified

✓4ᵗʰ Y78 Radiological devices associated with adverse incidents

Y78.0 Diagnostic and monitoring **radiological devices associated with adverse incidents**

Y78.1 Therapeutic (nonsurgical) and rehabilitative **radiological devices associated with adverse incidents**

Y78.2 Prosthetic and other implants, **materials and accessory radiological devices associated with adverse incidents**

Y78.3 Surgical instruments, materials **and radiological devices (including sutures) associated with adverse incidents**

Y78.8 Miscellaneous radiological devices associated with adverse incidents, not elsewhere classified

✓4ᵗʰ Y79 Orthopedic devices associated with adverse incidents

Y79.0 Diagnostic and monitoring **orthopedic devices associated with adverse incidents**

Y79.1 Therapeutic (nonsurgical) and rehabilitative **orthopedic devices associated with adverse incidents**

Y79.2 Prosthetic and other implants, **materials and accessory orthopedic devices associated with adverse incidents**

Ⓝ Newborn: 0   Ⓟ Pediatric: 0-17   Ⓜ Maternity: 12-55   Ⓐ Adult: 15-124   **NRS** Nonroutine supply Dx   **NCDx** Noncancer Dx   **PDx** Primary Dx   ▶◀ Revised Text   ● New Code   ▲ Revised Title

1166   ICD-10-CM 2018

Y79.3   Surgical instruments, materials and orthopedic devices (including sutures) associated with adverse incidents

Y79.8   Miscellaneous orthopedic devices associated with adverse incidents, not elsewhere classified

✓4ᵗʰ **Y80**   Physical medicine devices associated with adverse incidents

Y80.0   Diagnostic and monitoring physical medicine devices associated with adverse incidents

Y80.1   Therapeutic (nonsurgical) and rehabilitative physical medicine devices associated with adverse incidents

Y80.2   Prosthetic and other implants, materials and accessory physical medicine devices associated with adverse incidents

Y80.3   Surgical instruments, materials and physical medicine devices (including sutures) associated with adverse incidents

Y80.8   Miscellaneous physical medicine devices associated with adverse incidents, not elsewhere classified

✓4ᵗʰ **Y81**   General- and plastic-surgery devices associated with adverse incidents

Y81.0   Diagnostic and monitoring general- and plastic-surgery devices associated with adverse incidents

Y81.1   Therapeutic (nonsurgical) and rehabilitative general- and plastic-surgery devices associated with adverse incidents

Y81.2   Prosthetic and other implants, materials and accessory general- and plastic-surgery devices associated with adverse incidents

Y81.3   Surgical instruments, materials and general- and plastic-surgery devices (including sutures) associated with adverse incidents

Y81.8   Miscellaneous general- and plastic-surgery devices associated with adverse incidents, not elsewhere classified

✓4ᵗʰ **Y82**   Other and unspecified medical devices associated with adverse incidents

Y82.8   Other medical devices associated with adverse incidents

Y82.9   Unspecified medical devices associated with adverse incidents   ▽

Surgical and other medical procedures as the cause of abnormal reaction of the patient, or of later complication, without mention of misadventure at the time of the procedure (Y83-Y84)

EXCLUDES 1   misadventures to patients during surgical and medical care, classifiable to (Y62-Y69)

EXCLUDES 2   breakdown or malfunctioning of medical device (after implantation) (during procedure) (ongoing use) (Y70-Y82)

✓4ᵗʰ **Y83**   Surgical operation and other surgical procedures as the cause of abnormal reaction of the patient, or of later complication, without mention of misadventure at the time of the procedure

Y83.0   Surgical operation with transplant of whole organ as the cause of abnormal reaction of the patient, or of later complication, without mention of misadventure at the time of the procedure

Y83.1   Surgical operation with implant of artificial internal device as the cause of abnormal reaction of the patient, or of later complication, without mention of misadventure at the time of the procedure

Y83.2   Surgical operation with anastomosis, bypass or graft as the cause of abnormal reaction of the patient, or of later complication, without mention of misadventure at the time of the procedure

Y83.3   Surgical operation with formation of external stoma as the cause of abnormal reaction of the patient, or of later complication, without mention of misadventure at the time of the procedure

Y83.4   Other reconstructive surgery as the cause of abnormal reaction of the patient, or of later complication, without mention of misadventure at the time of the procedure

Y83.5   Amputation of limb(s) as the cause of abnormal reaction of the patient, or of later complication, without mention of misadventure at the time of the procedure

Y83.6   Removal of other organ (partial) (total) as the cause of abnormal reaction of the patient, or of later complication, without mention of misadventure at the time of the procedure

Y83.8   Other surgical procedures as the cause of abnormal reaction of the patient, or of later complication, without mention of misadventure at the time of the procedure

Y83.9   Surgical procedure, unspecified as the cause of abnormal reaction of the patient, or of later complication, without mention of misadventure at the time of the procedure   ▽

✓4ᵗʰ **Y84**   Other medical procedures as the cause of abnormal reaction of the patient, or of later complication, without mention of misadventure at the time of the procedure

Y84.0   Cardiac catheterization as the cause of abnormal reaction of the patient, or of later complication, without mention of misadventure at the time of the procedure

Y84.1   Kidney dialysis as the cause of abnormal reaction of the patient, or of later complication, without mention of misadventure at the time of the procedure

Y84.2   Radiological procedure and radiotherapy as the cause of abnormal reaction of the patient, or of later complication, without mention of misadventure at the time of the procedure
AHA: 2017, 1Q, 33

Y84.3   Shock therapy as the cause of abnormal reaction of the patient, or of later complication, without mention of misadventure at the time of the procedure

Y84.4   Aspiration of fluid as the cause of abnormal reaction of the patient, or of later complication, without mention of misadventure at the time of the procedure

Y84.5   Insertion of gastric or duodenal sound as the cause of abnormal reaction of the patient, or of later complication, without mention of misadventure at the time of the procedure

Y84.6   Urinary catheterization as the cause of abnormal reaction of the patient, or of later complication, without mention of misadventure at the time of the procedure

Y84.7   Blood-sampling as the cause of abnormal reaction of the patient, or of later complication, without mention of misadventure at the time of the procedure

Y84.8   Other medical procedures as the cause of abnormal reaction of the patient, or of later complication, without mention of misadventure at the time of the procedure
AHA: 2014, 4Q, 24

Y84.9   Medical procedure, unspecified as the cause of abnormal reaction of the patient, or of later complication, without mention of misadventure at the time of the procedure   ▽

Supplementary factors related to causes of morbidity classified elsewhere (Y90-Y99)

NOTE   These categories may be used to provide supplementary information concerning causes of morbidity. They are not to be used for single-condition coding.

✓4ᵗʰ **Y90**   Evidence of alcohol involvement determined by blood alcohol level

Code first any associated alcohol related disorders (F10)

Y90.0   Blood alcohol level of less than 20 mg/100 ml

Y90.1   Blood alcohol level of 20-39 mg/100 ml

Y90.2   Blood alcohol level of 40-59 mg/100 ml

Y90.3   Blood alcohol level of 60-79 mg/100 ml

Y90.4   Blood alcohol level of 80-99 mg/100 ml

Y90.5   Blood alcohol level of 100-119 mg/100 ml

Y90.6   Blood alcohol level of 120-199 mg/100 ml

Y90.7   Blood alcohol level of 200-239 mg/100 ml

Y90.8   Blood alcohol level of 240 mg/100 ml or more

Y90.9   Presence of alcohol in blood, level not specified   ▽

✓4ᵗʰ **Y92**   Place of occurrence of the external cause

The following category is for use, when relevant, to identify the place of occurrence of the external cause. Use in conjunction with an activity code.

Place of occurrence should be recorded only at the initial encounter for treatment

✓5ᵗʰ   Y92.0   Non-institutional (private) residence as the place of occurrence of the external cause

EXCLUDES 1   abandoned or derelict house (Y92.89)
home under construction but not yet occupied (Y92.6-)
institutional place of residence (Y92.1-)

✓6ᵗʰ   Y92.00   Unspecified non-institutional (private) residence as the place of occurrence of the external cause

Y92.000   Kitchen of unspecified non-institutional ▽ (private) residence as the place of occurrence of the external cause

Y92.001   Dining room of unspecified   ▽ non-institutional (private) residence as the place of occurrence of the external cause

✔ Additional Character Req   ✔x7ᵗʰ Placeholder Alert   Case-Mix Diagnosis   Manifestation   ▽ Unspecified Dx   *EXCLUDES 1* Not coded here   *EXCLUDES 2* Not included here

ICD-10-CM 2018   **1167**

Chapter 20. External Causes of Morbidity (side tab)

Y92.002–Y92.111 (side tab)

Y92.002 Bathroom of unspecified non-institutional (private) residence ▽
single-family (private) house as the place of occurrence of the external cause

Y92.003 Bedroom of unspecified non-institutional (private) residence as the place of occurrence of the external cause ▽

Y92.007 Garden or yard of unspecified non-institutional (private) residence as the place of occurrence of the external cause ▽

Y92.008 Other place in unspecified non-institutional (private) residence as the place of occurrence of the external cause ▽

Y92.009 Unspecified place in unspecified non-institutional (private) residence as the place of occurrence of the external cause ▽
Home (NOS) as the place of occurrence of the external cause

✓6ᵗʰ **Y92.01** Single-family non-institutional (private) house as the place of occurrence of the external cause
Farmhouse as the place of occurrence of the external cause
EXCLUDES 1　barn (Y92.71)
chicken coop or hen house (Y92.72)
farm field (Y92.73)
orchard (Y92.74)
single family mobile home or trailer (Y92.02-)
slaughter house (Y92.86)

Y92.010 Kitchen of single-family (private) house as the place of occurrence of the external cause

Y92.011 Dining room of single-family (private) house as the place of occurrence of the external cause

Y92.012 Bathroom of single-family (private) house as the place of occurrence of the external cause

Y92.013 Bedroom of single-family (private) house as the place of occurrence of the external cause

Y92.014 Private driveway to single-family (private) house as the place of occurrence of the external cause

Y92.015 Private garage of single-family (private) house as the place of occurrence of the external cause

Y92.016 Swimming-pool in single-family (private) house or garden as the place of occurrence of the external cause

Y92.017 Garden or yard in single-family (private) house as the place of occurrence of the external cause

Y92.018 Other place in single-family (private) house as the place of occurrence of the external cause

Y92.019 Unspecified place in single-family (private) house as the place of occurrence of the external cause ▽

✓6ᵗʰ **Y92.02** Mobile home as the place of occurrence of the external cause

Y92.020 Kitchen in mobile home as the place of occurrence of the external cause

Y92.021 Dining room in mobile home as the place of occurrence of the external cause

Y92.022 Bathroom in mobile home as the place of occurrence of the external cause

Y92.023 Bedroom in mobile home as the place of occurrence of the external cause

Y92.024 Driveway of mobile home as the place of occurrence of the external cause

Y92.025 Garage of mobile home as the place of occurrence of the external cause

Y92.026 Swimming-pool of mobile home as the place of occurrence of the external cause

Y92.027 Garden or yard of mobile home as the place of occurrence of the external cause

Y92.028 Other place in mobile home as the place of occurrence of the external cause

Y92.029 Unspecified place in mobile home as the place of occurrence of the external cause ▽

✓6ᵗʰ **Y92.03** Apartment as the place of occurrence of the external cause
Condominium as the place of occurrence of the external cause
Co-op apartment as the place of occurrence of the external cause

Y92.030 Kitchen in apartment as the place of occurrence of the external cause

Y92.031 Bathroom in apartment as the place of occurrence of the external cause

Y92.032 Bedroom in apartment as the place of occurrence of the external cause

Y92.038 Other place in apartment as the place of occurrence of the external cause

Y92.039 Unspecified place in apartment as the place of occurrence of the external cause ▽

✓6ᵗʰ **Y92.04** Boarding-house as the place of occurrence of the external cause

Y92.040 Kitchen in boarding-house as the place of occurrence of the external cause

Y92.041 Bathroom in boarding-house as the place of occurrence of the external cause

Y92.042 Bedroom in boarding-house as the place of occurrence of the external cause

Y92.043 Driveway of boarding-house as the place of occurrence of the external cause

Y92.044 Garage of boarding-house as the place of occurrence of the external cause

Y92.045 Swimming-pool of boarding-house as the place of occurrence of the external cause

Y92.046 Garden or yard of boarding-house as the place of occurrence of the external cause

Y92.048 Other place in boarding-house as the place of occurrence of the external cause

Y92.049 Unspecified place in boarding-house as the place of occurrence of the external cause ▽

✓6ᵗʰ **Y92.09** Other non-institutional residence as the place of occurrence of the external cause
AHA: 2017, 2Q, 10

Y92.090 Kitchen in other non-institutional residence as the place of occurrence of the external cause

Y92.091 Bathroom in other non-institutional residence as the place of occurrence of the external cause

Y92.092 Bedroom in other non-institutional residence as the place of occurrence of the external cause

Y92.093 Driveway of other non-institutional residence as the place of occurrence of the external cause

Y92.094 Garage of other non-institutional residence as the place of occurrence of the external cause

Y92.095 Swimming-pool of other non-institutional residence as the place of occurrence of the external cause

Y92.096 Garden or yard of other non-institutional residence as the place of occurrence of the external cause

Y92.098 Other place in other non-institutional residence as the place of occurrence of the external cause

Y92.099 Unspecified place in other non-institutional residence as the place of occurrence of the external cause ▽

✓5ᵗʰ **Y92.1** Institutional (nonprivate) residence as the place of occurrence of the external cause

Y92.10 Unspecified residential institution as the place of occurrence of the external cause ▽

✓6ᵗʰ **Y92.11** Children's home and orphanage as the place of occurrence of the external cause

Y92.110 Kitchen in children's home and orphanage as the place of occurrence of the external cause

Y92.111 Bathroom in children's home and orphanage as the place of occurrence of the external cause

N Newborn: 0　P Pediatric: 0-17　M Maternity: 12-55　A Adult: 15-124　NRS Nonroutine supply Dx　NCDx Noncancer Dx　PDx Primary Dx　▶◀ Revised Text　● New Code　▲ Revised Title

1168　　　　　　　　　　　　　　　　　　　　　　　　　　　　　　　　　　　　　ICD-10-CM 2018

Y92.112   Bedroom in children's home and orphanage as the place of occurrence of the external cause

Y92.113   Driveway of children's home and orphanage as the place of occurrence of the external cause

Y92.114   Garage of children's home and orphanage as the place of occurrence of the external cause

Y92.115   Swimming-pool of children's home and orphanage as the place of occurrence of the external cause

Y92.116   Garden or yard of children's home and orphanage as the place of occurrence of the external cause

Y92.118   Other place in children's home and orphanage as the place of occurrence of the external cause

Y92.119   Unspecified place in children's home and orphanage as the place of occurrence of the external cause   ▽

✓6ᵗʰ **Y92.12**   Nursing home as the place of occurrence of the external cause
Home for the sick as the place of occurrence of the external cause
Hospice as the place of occurrence of the external cause
AHA: 2017, 2Q, 10

Y92.120   Kitchen in nursing home as the place of occurrence of the external cause

Y92.121   Bathroom in nursing home as the place of occurrence of the external cause

Y92.122   Bedroom in nursing home as the place of occurrence of the external cause

Y92.123   Driveway of nursing home as the place of occurrence of the external cause

Y92.124   Garage of nursing home as the place of occurrence of the external cause

Y92.125   Swimming-pool of nursing home as the place of occurrence of the external cause

Y92.126   Garden or yard of nursing home as the place of occurrence of the external cause

Y92.128   Other place in nursing home as the place of occurrence of the external cause

Y92.129   Unspecified place in nursing home as the place of occurrence of the external cause   ▽

✓6ᵗʰ **Y92.13**   Military base as the place of occurrence of the external cause
EXCLUDES 1   military training grounds (Y92.83)

Y92.130   Kitchen on military base as the place of occurrence of the external cause

Y92.131   Mess hall on military base as the place of occurrence of the external cause

Y92.133   Barracks on military base as the place of occurrence of the external cause

Y92.135   Garage on military base as the place of occurrence of the external cause

Y92.136   Swimming-pool on military base as the place of occurrence of the external cause

Y92.137   Garden or yard on military base as the place of occurrence of the external cause

Y92.138   Other place on military base as the place of occurrence of the external cause

Y92.139   Unspecified place military base as the place of occurrence of the external cause   ▽

✓6ᵗʰ **Y92.14**   Prison as the place of occurrence of the external cause

Y92.140   Kitchen in prison as the place of occurrence of the external cause

Y92.141   Dining room in prison as the place of occurrence of the external cause

Y92.142   Bathroom in prison as the place of occurrence of the external cause

Y92.143   Cell of prison as the place of occurrence of the external cause

Y92.146   Swimming-pool of prison as the place of occurrence of the external cause

Y92.147   Courtyard of prison as the place of occurrence of the external cause

Y92.148   Other place in prison as the place of occurrence of the external cause

Y92.149   Unspecified place in prison as the place of occurrence of the external cause   ▽

✓6ᵗʰ **Y92.15**   Reform school as the place of occurrence of the external cause

Y92.150   Kitchen in reform school as the place of occurrence of the external cause

Y92.151   Dining room in reform school as the place of occurrence of the external cause

Y92.152   Bathroom in reform school as the place of occurrence of the external cause

Y92.153   Bedroom in reform school as the place of occurrence of the external cause

Y92.154   Driveway of reform school as the place of occurrence of the external cause

Y92.155   Garage of reform school as the place of occurrence of the external cause

Y92.156   Swimming-pool of reform school as the place of occurrence of the external cause

Y92.157   Garden or yard of reform school as the place of occurrence of the external cause

Y92.158   Other place in reform school as the place of occurrence of the external cause

Y92.159   Unspecified place in reform school as the place of occurrence of the external cause   ▽

✓6ᵗʰ **Y92.16**   School dormitory as the place of occurrence of the external cause
EXCLUDES 1   reform school as the place of occurrence of the external cause (Y92.15-)
school buildings and grounds as the place of occurrence of the external cause (Y92.2-)
school sports and athletic areas as the place of occurrence of the external cause (Y92.3-)

Y92.160   Kitchen in school dormitory as the place of occurrence of the external cause

Y92.161   Dining room in school dormitory as the place of occurrence of the external cause

Y92.162   Bathroom in school dormitory as the place of occurrence of the external cause

Y92.163   Bedroom in school dormitory as the place of occurrence of the external cause

Y92.168   Other place in school dormitory as the place of occurrence of the external cause

Y92.169   Unspecified place in school dormitory as the place of occurrence of the external cause   ▽

✓6ᵗʰ **Y92.19**   Other specified residential institution as the place of occurrence of the external cause
AHA: 2017, 2Q, 10

Y92.190   Kitchen in other specified residential institution as the place of occurrence of the external cause

Y92.191   Dining room in other specified residential institution as the place of occurrence of the external cause

Y92.192   Bathroom in other specified residential institution as the place of occurrence of the external cause

Y92.193   Bedroom in other specified residential institution as the place of occurrence of the external cause

Y92.194   Driveway of other specified residential institution as the place of occurrence of the external cause

Y92.195   Garage of other specified residential institution as the place of occurrence of the external cause

Y92.196   Pool of other specified residential institution as the place of occurrence of the external cause

Y92.197   Garden or yard of other specified residential institution as the place of occurrence of the external cause

Y92.198   Other place in other specified residential institution as the place of occurrence of the external cause

---

✓ Additional Character Req   ✓x7ᵗʰ Placeholder Alert   Case-Mix Diagnosis   Manifestation   ▽ Unspecified Dx   EXCLUDES 1 Not coded here   EXCLUDES 2 Not included here

ICD-10-CM 2018   1169

Chapter 20. External Causes of Morbidity

Y92.199   **Unspecified place in other specified residential institution as the place of occurrence of the external cause**   ▽

✓5ᵗʰ **Y92.2**   **School, other institution and public administrative area as the place of occurrence of the external cause**
Building and adjacent grounds used by the general public or by a particular group of the public

> *EXCLUDES 1*   *building under construction as the place of occurrence of the external cause (Y92.6)*
> *residential institution as the place of occurrence of the external cause (Y92.1)*
> *school dormitory as the place of occurrence of the external cause (Y92.16-)*
> *sports and athletics area of schools as the place of occurrence of the external cause (Y92.3-)*

✓6ᵗʰ **Y92.21**   **School (private) (public) (state) as the place of occurrence of the external cause**

    Y92.210   **Daycare center as the place of occurrence of the external cause**

    Y92.211   **Elementary school as the place of occurrence of the external cause**
       Kindergarten as the place of occurrence of the external cause

    Y92.212   **Middle school as the place of occurrence of the external cause**

    Y92.213   **High school as the place of occurrence of the external cause**
       AHA: 2012, 4Q, 108

    Y92.214   **College as the place of occurrence of the external cause**
       University as the place of occurrence of the external cause

    Y92.215   **Trade school as the place of occurrence of the external cause**

    Y92.218   **Other school as the place of occurrence of the external cause**

    Y92.219   **Unspecified school as the place of occurrence of the external cause**   ▽

Y92.22   **Religious institution as the place of occurrence of the external cause**
    Church as the place of occurrence of the external cause
    Mosque as the place of occurrence of the external cause
    Synagogue as the place of occurrence of the external cause

✓6ᵗʰ **Y92.23**   **Hospital as the place of occurrence of the external cause**

> *EXCLUDES 1*   *ambulatory (outpatient) health services establishments (Y92.53-)*
> *home for the sick as the place of occurrence of the external cause (Y92.12-)*
> *hospice as the place of occurrence of the external cause (Y92.12-)*
> *nursing home as the place of occurrence of the external cause (Y92.12-)*

    Y92.230   **Patient room in hospital as the place of occurrence of the external cause**

    Y92.231   **Patient bathroom in hospital as the place of occurrence of the external cause**

    Y92.232   **Corridor of hospital as the place of occurrence of the external cause**

    Y92.233   **Cafeteria of hospital as the place of occurrence of the external cause**

    Y92.234   **Operating room of hospital as the place of occurrence of the external cause**

    Y92.238   **Other place in hospital as the place of occurrence of the external cause**

    Y92.239   **Unspecified place in hospital as the place of occurrence of the external cause**   ▽

✓6ᵗʰ **Y92.24**   **Public administrative building as the place of occurrence of the external cause**

    Y92.240   **Courthouse as the place of occurrence of the external cause**

    Y92.241   **Library as the place of occurrence of the external cause**

    Y92.242   **Post office as the place of occurrence of the external cause**

    Y92.243   **City hall as the place of occurrence of the external cause**

    Y92.248   **Other public administrative building as the place of occurrence of the external cause**

✓6ᵗʰ **Y92.25**   **Cultural building as the place of occurrence of the external cause**

    Y92.250   **Art Gallery as the place of occurrence of the external cause**

    Y92.251   **Museum as the place of occurrence of the external cause**

    Y92.252   **Music hall as the place of occurrence of the external cause**

    Y92.253   **Opera house as the place of occurrence of the external cause**

    Y92.254   **Theater (live) as the place of occurrence of the external cause**

    Y92.258   **Other cultural public building as the place of occurrence of the external cause**

Y92.26   **Movie house or cinema as the place of occurrence of the external cause**

Y92.29   **Other specified public building as the place of occurrence of the external cause**
    Assembly hall as the place of occurrence of the external cause
    Clubhouse as the place of occurrence of the external cause

✓5ᵗʰ **Y92.3**   **Sports and athletics area as the place of occurrence of the external cause**

✓6ᵗʰ **Y92.31**   **Athletic court as the place of occurrence of the external cause**

> *EXCLUDES 1*   *tennis court in private home or garden (Y92.09)*

    Y92.310   **Basketball court as the place of occurrence of the external cause**

    Y92.311   **Squash court as the place of occurrence of the external cause**

    Y92.312   **Tennis court as the place of occurrence of the external cause**

    Y92.318   **Other athletic court as the place of occurrence of the external cause**

✓6ᵗʰ **Y92.32**   **Athletic field as the place of occurrence of the external cause**

    Y92.320   **Baseball field as the place of occurrence of the external cause**

    Y92.321   **Football field as the place of occurrence of the external cause**

    Y92.322   **Soccer field as the place of occurrence of the external cause**

    Y92.328   **Other athletic field as the place of occurrence of the external cause**
       Cricket field as the place of occurrence of the external cause
       Hockey field as the place of occurrence of the external cause

✓6ᵗʰ **Y92.33**   **Skating rink as the place of occurrence of the external cause**

    Y92.330   **Ice skating rink (indoor) (outdoor) as the place of occurrence of the external cause**

    Y92.331   **Roller skating rink as the place of occurrence of the external cause**

Y92.34   **Swimming pool (public) as the place of occurrence of the external cause**

> *EXCLUDES 1*   *swimming pool in private home or garden (Y92.016)*

Y92.39   **Other specified sports and athletic area as the place of occurrence of the external cause**
    Golf-course as the place of occurrence of the external cause
    Gymnasium as the place of occurrence of the external cause
    Riding-school as the place of occurrence of the external cause
    Stadium as the place of occurrence of the external cause

Ⓝ Newborn: 0   Ⓟ Pediatric: 0-17   Ⓜ Maternity: 12-55   Ⓐ Adult: 15-124   **NRS** Nonroutine supply Dx   **NC Dx** Noncancer Dx   **PDx** Primary Dx   ▶◀ Revised Text   ● New Code   ▲ Revised Title

1170   ICD-10-CM 2018

✓5ᵗʰ **Y92.4** **Street, highway and other paved roadways as the place of occurrence of the external cause**

> *EXCLUDES 1*   *private driveway of residence (Y92.014, Y92.024, Y92.043, Y92.093, Y92.113, Y92.123, Y92.154, Y92.194)*

✓6ᵗʰ **Y92.41** **Street and highway as the place of occurrence of the external cause**

Y92.410 **Unspecified street and highway as the ▽ place of occurrence of the external cause**
> Road NOS as the place of occurrence of the external cause

Y92.411 **Interstate highway as the place of occurrence of the external cause**
> Freeway as the place of occurrence of the external cause
> Motorway as the place of occurrence of the external cause

Y92.412 **Parkway as the place of occurrence of the external cause**

Y92.413 **State road as the place of occurrence of the external cause**

Y92.414 **Local residential or business street as the place of occurrence of the external cause**

Y92.415 **Exit ramp or entrance ramp of street or highway as the place of occurrence of the external cause**

✓6ᵗʰ **Y92.48** **Other paved roadways as the place of occurrence of the external cause**

Y92.480 **Sidewalk as the place of occurrence of the external cause**

Y92.481 **Parking lot as the place of occurrence of the external cause**

Y92.482 **Bike path as the place of occurrence of the external cause**

Y92.488 **Other paved roadways as the place of occurrence of the external cause**

✓5ᵗʰ **Y92.5** **Trade and service area as the place of occurrence of the external cause**

> *EXCLUDES 1*   *garage in private home (Y92.015)*
> *schools and other public administration buildings (Y92.2-)*

✓6ᵗʰ **Y92.51** **Private commercial establishments as the place of occurrence of the external cause**

Y92.510 **Bank as the place of occurrence of the external cause**

Y92.511 **Restaurant or café as the place of occurrence of the external cause**

Y92.512 **Supermarket, store or market as the place of occurrence of the external cause**

Y92.513 **Shop (commercial) as the place of occurrence of the external cause**

✓6ᵗʰ **Y92.52** **Service areas as the place of occurrence of the external cause**

Y92.520 **Airport as the place of occurrence of the external cause**

Y92.521 **Bus station as the place of occurrence of the external cause**

Y92.522 **Railway station as the place of occurrence of the external cause**

Y92.523 **Highway rest stop as the place of occurrence of the external cause**

Y92.524 **Gas station as the place of occurrence of the external cause**
> Petroleum station as the place of occurrence of the external cause
> Service station as the place of occurrence of the external cause

✓6ᵗʰ **Y92.53** **Ambulatory health services establishments as the place of occurrence of the external cause**

Y92.530 **Ambulatory surgery center as the place of occurrence of the external cause**
> Outpatient surgery center, including that connected with a hospital as the place of occurrence of the external cause
> Same day surgery center, including that connected with a hospital as the place of occurrence of the external cause

Y92.531 **Health care provider office as the place of occurrence of the external cause**
> Physician office as the place of occurrence of the external cause

Y92.532 **Urgent care center as the place of occurrence of the external cause**

Y92.538 **Other ambulatory health services establishments as the place of occurrence of the external cause**

Y92.59 **Other trade areas as the place of occurrence of the external cause**
> Office building as the place of occurrence of the external cause
> Casino as the place of occurrence of the external cause
> Garage (commercial) as the place of occurrence of the external cause
> Hotel as the place of occurrence of the external cause
> Radio or television station as the place of occurrence of the external cause
> Shopping mall as the place of occurrence of the external cause
> Warehouse as the place of occurrence of the external cause

✓5ᵗʰ **Y92.6** **Industrial and construction area as the place of occurrence of the external cause**

Y92.61 **Building [any] under construction as the place of occurrence of the external cause**

Y92.62 **Dock or shipyard as the place of occurrence of the external cause**
> Dockyard as the place of occurrence of the external cause
> Dry dock as the place of occurrence of the external cause
> Shipyard as the place of occurrence of the external cause

Y92.63 **Factory as the place of occurrence of the external cause**
> Factory building as the place of occurrence of the external cause
> Factory premises as the place of occurrence of the external cause
> Industrial yard as the place of occurrence of the external cause

Y92.64 **Mine or pit as the place of occurrence of the external cause**
> Mine as the place of occurrence of the external cause

Y92.65 **Oil rig as the place of occurrence of the external cause**
> Pit (coal) (gravel) (sand) as the place of occurrence of the external cause

Y92.69 **Other specified industrial and construction area as the place of occurrence of the external cause**
> Gasworks as the place of occurrence of the external cause
> Power-station (coal) (nuclear) (oil) as the place of occurrence of the external cause
> Tunnel under construction as the place of occurrence of the external cause
> Workshop as the place of occurrence of the external cause

✓5ᵗʰ **Y92.7** **Farm as the place of occurrence of the external cause**
> Ranch as the place of occurrence of the external cause
> *EXCLUDES 1*   *farmhouse and home premises of farm (Y92.01-)*

Y92.71 **Barn as the place of occurrence of the external cause**

Y92.72 **Chicken coop as the place of occurrence of the external cause**
> Hen house as the place of occurrence of the external cause

Y92.73 **Farm field as the place of occurrence of the external cause**

Y92.74 **Orchard as the place of occurrence of the external cause**

Y92.79 **Other farm location as the place of occurrence of the external cause**

✓5ᵗʰ **Y92.8** **Other places as the place of occurrence of the external cause**

✓6ᵗʰ **Y92.81** **Transport vehicle as the place of occurrence of the external cause**
> *EXCLUDES 1*   *transport accidents (V00-V99)*

Y92.810 **Car as the place of occurrence of the external cause**

✓ Additional Character Req   ✓x7ᵗʰ Placeholder Alert   Case-Mix Diagnosis   Manifestation   ▽ Unspecified Dx   *EXCLUDES 1* Not coded here   *EXCLUDES 2* Not included here

ICD-10-CM 2018   1171

Y92.811 Bus as the place of occurrence of the external cause

Y92.812 Truck as the place of occurrence of the external cause

Y92.813 Airplane as the place of occurrence of the external cause

Y92.814 Boat as the place of occurrence of the external cause

Y92.815 Train as the place of occurrence of the external cause

Y92.816 Subway car as the place of occurrence of the external cause

Y92.818 Other transport vehicle as the place of occurrence of the external cause

✓6ᵗʰ **Y92.82** Wilderness area

Y92.820 Desert as the place of occurrence of the external cause

Y92.821 Forest as the place of occurrence of the external cause

Y92.828 Other wilderness area as the place of occurrence of the external cause

Swamp as the place of occurrence of the external cause

Mountain as the place of occurrence of the external cause

Marsh as the place of occurrence of the external cause

Prairie as the place of occurrence of the external cause

✓6ᵗʰ **Y92.83** Recreation area as the place of occurrence of the external cause

Y92.830 Public park as the place of occurrence of the external cause

Y92.831 Amusement park as the place of occurrence of the external cause

Y92.832 Beach as the place of occurrence of the external cause

Seashore as the place of occurrence of the external cause

Y92.833 Campsite as the place of occurrence of the external cause

Y92.834 Zoological garden (Zoo) as the place of occurrence of the external cause

Y92.838 Other recreation area as the place of occurrence of the external cause

Y92.84 Military training ground as the place of occurrence of the external cause

Y92.85 Railroad track as the place of occurrence of the external cause

Y92.86 Slaughter house as the place of occurrence of the external cause

Y92.89 Other specified places as the place of occurrence of the external cause

Derelict house as the place of occurrence of the external cause

Y92.9 Unspecified place or not applicable ▽

✓4ᵗʰ **Y93** **Activity codes**

NOTE   Category Y93 is provided for use to indicate the activity of the person seeking healthcare for an injury or health condition, such as a heart attack while shoveling snow, which resulted from, or was contributed to, by the activity. These codes are appropriate for use for both acute injuries, such as those from chapter 19, and conditions that are due to the long-term, cumulative effects of an activity, such as those from chapter 13. They are also appropriate for use with external cause codes for cause and intent if identifying the activity provides additional information on the event. These codes should be used in conjunction with codes for external cause status (Y99) and place of occurrence (Y92).

This section contains the following broad activity categories:

Y93.0   Activities involving walking and running
Y93.1   Activities involving water and water craft
Y93.2   Activities involving ice and snow
Y93.3   Activities involving climbing, rappelling, and jumping off
Y93.4   Activities involving dancing and other rhythmic movement
Y93.5   Activities involving other sports and athletics played individually
Y93.6   Activities involving other sports and athletics played as a team or group
Y93.7   Activities involving other specified sports and athletics
Y93.A   Activities involving other cardiorespiratory exercise
Y93.B   Activities involving other muscle strengthening exercises
Y93.C   Activities involving computer technology and electronic devices
Y93.D   Activities involving arts and handcrafts
Y93.E   Activities involving personal hygiene and interior property and clothing maintenance
Y93.F   Activities involving caregiving
Y93.G   Activities involving food preparation, cooking and grilling
Y93.H   Activities involving exterior property and land maintenance, building and construction
Y93.I   Activities involving roller coasters and other types of external motion
Y93.J   Activities involving playing musical instrument
Y93.K   Activities involving animal care
Y93.8   Activities, other specified
Y93.9   Activity, unspecified

✓5ᵗʰ **Y93.0** **Activities involving walking and running**

EXCLUDES 1   *activity, walking an animal (Y93.K1)*
activity, walking or running on a treadmill (Y93.A1)

Y93.01 **Activity, walking, marching and hiking**
Activity, walking, marching and hiking on level or elevated terrain
EXCLUDES 1   *activity, mountain climbing (Y93.31)*

Y93.02 **Activity, running**

✓5ᵗʰ **Y93.1** **Activities involving water and water craft**

EXCLUDES 1   *activities involving ice (Y93.2-)*

Y93.11 **Activity, swimming**

Y93.12 **Activity, springboard and platform diving**

Y93.13 **Activity, water polo**

Y93.14 **Activity, water aerobics and water exercise**

Y93.15 **Activity, underwater diving and snorkeling**
Activity, SCUBA diving

Y93.16 **Activity, rowing, canoeing, kayaking, rafting and tubing**
Activity, canoeing, kayaking, rafting and tubing in calm and turbulent water

Y93.17 **Activity, water skiing and wake boarding**

Y93.18 **Activity, surfing, windsurfing and boogie boarding**
Activity, water sliding

Y93.19 **Activity, other involving water and watercraft**
Activity involving water NOS
Activity, parasailing
Activity, water survival training and testing

✓5ᵗʰ **Y93.2** **Activities involving ice and snow**

EXCLUDES 1   *activity, shoveling ice and snow (Y93.H1)*

Y93.21 **Activity, ice skating**
Activity, figure skating (singles) (pairs)
Activity, ice dancing
EXCLUDES 1   *activity, ice hockey (Y93.22)*

Y93.22 **Activity, ice hockey**

Y93.23 **Activity, snow (alpine) (downhill) skiing, snow boarding, sledding, tobogganing and snow tubing**
EXCLUDES 1   *activity, cross country skiing (Y93.24)*

Y93.24 **Activity, cross country skiing**
Activity, nordic skiing

Ⓝ Newborn: 0   Ⓟ Pediatric: 0-17   Ⓜ Maternity: 12-55   Ⓐ Adult: 15-124   NRS Nonroutine supply Dx   NCDx Noncancer Dx   PDx Primary Dx   ▶◀ Revised Text   ● New Code   ▲ Revised Title

1172   ICD-10-CM 2018

Y93.29   **Activity, other involving** ice and snow
       Activity involving ice and snow NOS

✓5ᵗʰ **Y93.3**   **Activities involving climbing, rappelling and jumping off**
     EXCLUDES 1   *activity, hiking on level or elevated terrain (Y93.01)*
           activity, jumping rope (Y93.56)
           activity, trampoline jumping (Y93.44)

Y93.31   **Activity, mountain climbing, rock climbing and wall
climbing**

Y93.32   **Activity, rappelling**

Y93.33   **Activity, BASE jumping**
       Activity, Building, Antenna, Span, Earth jumping

Y93.34   **Activity, bungee jumping**

Y93.35   **Activity, hang gliding**

Y93.39   **Activity, other involving climbing, rappelling and
jumping off**

✓5ᵗʰ **Y93.4**   **Activities involving dancing and other rhythmic movement**
     EXCLUDES 1   *activity, martial arts (Y93.75)*

Y93.41   **Activity, dancing**
       AHA: 2012, 4Q, 108

Y93.42   **Activity, yoga**

Y93.43   **Activity, gymnastics**
       Activity, rhythmic gymnastics
       EXCLUDES 1   *activity, trampolining (Y93.44)*

Y93.44   **Activity, trampolining**

Y93.45   **Activity, cheerleading**

Y93.49   **Activity, other involving dancing and other rhythmic
movements**

✓5ᵗʰ **Y93.5**   **Activities involving other sports and athletics played
individually**
     EXCLUDES 1   *activity, dancing (Y93.41)*
           activity, gymnastic (Y93.43)
           activity, trampolining (Y93.44)
           activity, yoga (Y93.42)

Y93.51   **Activity, roller skating (inline) and skateboarding**

Y93.52   **Activity, horseback riding**

Y93.53   **Activity, golf**

Y93.54   **Activity, bowling**

Y93.55   **Activity, bike riding**

Y93.56   **Activity, jumping rope**

Y93.57   **Activity, non-running track and field events**
       EXCLUDES 1   *activity, running (any form) (Y93.02)*

Y93.59   **Activity, other involving other sports and athletics
played individually**
       EXCLUDES 1   *activities involving climbing, rappelling, and
jumping (Y93.3-)*
           activities involving ice and snow (Y93.2-)
           *activities involving walking and running
(Y93.0-)*
           *activities involving water and watercraft
(Y93.1-)*

✓5ᵗʰ **Y93.6**   **Activities involving other sports and athletics played as a
team or group**
     EXCLUDES 1   *activity, ice hockey (Y93.22)*
           activity, water polo (Y93.13)

Y93.61   **Activity, American tackle football**
       Activity, football NOS

Y93.62   **Activity, American flag or touch football**

Y93.63   **Activity, rugby**

Y93.64   **Activity, baseball**
       Activity, softball

Y93.65   **Activity, lacrosse and field hockey**

Y93.66   **Activity, soccer**

Y93.67   **Activity, basketball**

Y93.68   **Activity, volleyball (beach) (court)**

Y93.6A   **Activity, physical games generally associated
with school recess, summer camp and children**
       Activity, capture the flag
       Activity, dodge ball
       Activity, four square
       Activity, kickball

Y93.69   **Activity, other involving other sports and athletics
played as a team or group**
       Activity, cricket

✓5ᵗʰ **Y93.7**   **Activities involving other specified sports and athletics**

Y93.71   **Activity, boxing**

Y93.72   **Activity, wrestling**

Y93.73   **Activity, racquet and hand sports**
       Activity, handball
       Activity, racquetball
       Activity, squash
       Activity, tennis

Y93.74   **Activity, frisbee**
       Activity, ultimate frisbee

Y93.75   **Activity, martial arts**
       Activity, combatives

Y93.79   **Activity, other specified sports and athletics**
       EXCLUDES 1   *sports and athletics activities specified in
categories Y93.0-Y93.6*

✓5ᵗʰ **Y93.A**   **Activities involving other cardiorespiratory exercise**
       Activities involving physical training

Y93.A1   **Activity, exercise machines primarily for
cardiorespiratory conditioning**
       Activity, elliptical and stepper machines
       Activity, stationary bike
       Activity, treadmill

Y93.A2   **Activity, calisthenics**
       Activity, jumping jacks
       Activity, warm up and cool down

Y93.A3   **Activity, aerobic and step exercise**

Y93.A4   **Activity, circuit training**

Y93.A5   **Activity, obstacle course**
       Activity, challenge course
       Activity, confidence course

Y93.A6   **Activity, grass drills**
       Activity, guerilla drills

Y93.A9   **Activity, other involving cardiorespiratory exercise**
       EXCLUDES 1   *activities involving cardiorespiratory exercise
specified in categories Y93.0-Y93.7*

✓5ᵗʰ **Y93.B**   **Activities involving other muscle strengthening exercises**

Y93.B1   **Activity, exercise machines primarily for muscle
strengthening**

Y93.B2   **Activity, push-ups, pull-ups, sit-ups**

Y93.B3   **Activity, free weights**
       Activity, barbells
       Activity, dumbbells

Y93.B4   **Activity, pilates**

Y93.B9   **Activity, other involving muscle strengthening
exercises**
       EXCLUDES 1   *activities involving muscle strengthening
specified in categories Y93.0-Y93.A*

✓5ᵗʰ **Y93.C**   **Activities involving computer technology and electronic
devices**
     EXCLUDES 1   *activity, electronic musical keyboard or instruments
(Y93.J-)*

Y93.C1   **Activity, computer keyboarding**
       Activity, electronic game playing using keyboard or
other stationary device

Y93.C2   **Activity, hand held interactive electronic device**
       Activity, cellular telephone and communication device
       Activity, electronic game playing using interactive
device
       EXCLUDES 1   *activity, electronic game playing using
keyboard or other stationary device
(Y93.C1)*

Y93.C9   **Activity, other involving computer technology and
electronic devices**

✓5ᵗʰ **Y93.D**   **Activities involving arts and handcrafts**
     EXCLUDES 1   *activities involving playing musical instrument (Y93.J-)*

Y93.D1   **Activity, knitting and crocheting**

Y93.D2   **Activity, sewing**

Y93.D3   **Activity, furniture building and finishing**
       Activity, furniture repair

Y93.D9   **Activity, other involving arts and handcrafts**

✓5ᵗʰ **Y93.E**   **Activities involving personal hygiene and interior property
and clothing maintenance**
     EXCLUDES 1   *activities involving cooking and grilling (Y93.G-)*
           *activities involving exterior property and land
maintenance, building and construction (Y93.H-)*
           activities involving caregiving (Y93.F-)
           activity, dishwashing (Y93.G1)
           activity, food preparation (Y93.G1)
           activity, gardening (Y93.H2)

Y93.E1   **Activity, personal bathing and showering**

Y93.E2   **Activity, laundry**

✓ Additional Character Req   ✓x7ᵗʰ Placeholder Alert   Case-Mix Diagnosis   Manifestation   ▽ Unspecified Dx   EXCLUDES 1 Not coded here   EXCLUDES 2 Not included here

Y93.E3   **Activity,** vacuuming

Y93.E4   **Activity,** ironing

Y93.E5   **Activity,** floor mopping and cleaning

Y93.E6   **Activity,** residential relocation
Activity, packing up and unpacking involved in moving to a new residence

Y93.E8   **Activity, other** personal hygiene

Y93.E9   **Activity, other** interior property and clothing maintenance

✓5ᵗʰ Y93.F   **Activities involving** caregiving
Activity involving the provider of caregiving

Y93.F1   **Activity, caregiving,** bathing

Y93.F2   **Activity, caregiving,** lifting

Y93.F9   **Activity, other caregiving**

✓5ᵗʰ Y93.G   **Activities involving food preparation, cooking and grilling**

Y93.G1   **Activity, food** preparation and clean up
Activity, dishwashing

Y93.G2   **Activity,** grilling and smoking food

Y93.G3   **Activity,** cooking and baking
Activity, use of stove, oven and microwave oven

Y93.G9   **Activity, other involving cooking and grilling**

✓5ᵗʰ Y93.H   **Activities involving exterior property and land maintenance, building and construction**

Y93.H1   **Activity,** digging, shoveling and raking
Activity, dirt digging
Activity, raking leaves
Activity, snow shoveling

Y93.H2   **Activity,** gardening and landscaping
Activity, pruning, trimming shrubs, weeding

Y93.H3   **Activity,** building and construction

Y93.H9   **Activity, other involving exterior property and land maintenance, building and construction**

✓5ᵗʰ Y93.I   **Activities involving roller coasters and other types of external motion**

Y93.I1   **Activity,** rollercoaster riding

Y93.I9   **Activity, other involving external motion**

✓5ᵗʰ Y93.J   **Activities involving** playing musical instrument
Activity involving playing electric musical instrument

Y93.J1   **Activity,** piano playing
Activity, musical keyboard (electronic) playing

Y93.J2   **Activity,** drum and other percussion instrument playing

Y93.J3   **Activity,** string instrument playing

Y93.J4   **Activity,** winds and brass instrument playing

✓5ᵗʰ Y93.K   **Activities involving** animal care
EXCLUDES 1   *activity, horseback riding (Y93.52)*

Y93.K1   **Activity,** walking an animal

Y93.K2   **Activity,** milking an animal

Y93.K3   **Activity,** grooming and shearing an animal

Y93.K9   **Activity, other involving animal care**

✓5ᵗʰ Y93.8   **Activities, other specified**

Y93.81   **Activity,** refereeing a sports activity

Y93.82   **Activity,** spectator at an event

Y93.83   **Activity,** rough housing and horseplay

Y93.84   **Activity,** sleeping

Y93.85   **Activity,** choking game
Activity, blackout game
Activity, fainting game
Activity, pass out game

Y93.89   **Activity, other specified**

Y93.9   **Activity, unspecified**   ▽

Y95   **Nosocomial condition**
AHA: 2013, 4Q, 119

✓4ᵗʰ Y99   **External cause status**
NOTE   A single code from category Y99 should be used in conjunction with the external cause code(s) assigned to a record to indicate the status of the person at the time the event occurred.

Y99.0   **Civilian** activity done for income or pay
Civilian activity done for financial or other compensation
EXCLUDES 1   *military activity (Y99.1)*
volunteer activity (Y99.2)

Y99.1   **Military** activity
EXCLUDES 1   *activity of off duty military personnel (Y99.8)*

Y99.2   **Volunteer** activity
EXCLUDES 1   *activity of child or other family member assisting in compensated work of other family member (Y99.8)*

Y99.8   **Other external cause status**
Activity NEC
Activity of child or other family member assisting in compensated work of other family member
Hobby not done for income
Leisure activity
Off-duty activity of military personnel
Recreation or sport not for income or while a student
Student activity
EXCLUDES 1   *civilian activity done for income or compensation (Y99.0)*
military activity (Y99.1)
AHA: 2012, 4Q, 108

Y99.9   **Unspecified external cause status**   ▽

Ⓝ Newborn: 0   Ⓟ Pediatric: 0-17   Ⓜ Maternity: 12-55   Ⓐ Adult: 15-124   **NRS** Nonroutine supply Dx   **NCDx** Noncancer Dx   **PDx** Primary Dx   ▶◀ Revised Text   ● New Code   ▲ Revised Title

1174   ICD-10-CM 2018

Chapter 21. Factors Influencing Health Status and Contact with Health Services (Z00–Z99)

Chapter Specific Guidelines with Coding Examples

The chapter specific guidelines from the ICD-10-CM Official Guidelines for Coding and Reporting have been provided below. Along with these guidelines are coding examples, contained in the shaded boxes, that have been developed to help illustrate the coding and/or sequencing guidance found in these guidelines.

Note: The chapter specific guidelines provide additional information about the use of Z codes for specified encounters.

a. Use of Z codes in any healthcare setting

Z codes are for use in any healthcare setting. Z codes may be used as either a first-listed (principal diagnosis code in the inpatient setting) or secondary code, depending on the circumstances of the encounter. Certain Z codes may only be used as first-listed or principal diagnosis.

> Patient with middle lobe lung cancer admitted for observation and discontinuation of chemotherapy
>
> **Z51.11**   **Encounter for antineoplastic chemotherapy**
>
> **C34.2**   **Malignant neoplasm of middle lobe, bronchus or lung**
>
> *Explanation:* A Z code can be used as first-listed in this situation based on guidelines in this chapter as well as chapter 2, "Neoplasms."

b. Z Codes indicate a reason for an encounter

Z codes are not procedure codes. A corresponding procedure code must accompany a Z code to describe any procedure performed.

c. Categories of Z codes

1) Contact/exposure

Category Z20 indicates contact with, and suspected exposure to, communicable diseases. These codes are for patients who do not show any sign or symptom of a disease but are suspected to have been exposed to it by close personal contact with an infected individual or are in an area where a disease is epidemic.

Category Z77, Other contact with and (suspected) exposures hazardous to health, indicates contact with and suspected exposures hazardous to health.

Contact/exposure codes may be used as a first-listed code to explain an encounter for testing, or, more commonly, as a secondary code to identify a potential risk.

2) Inoculations and vaccinations

Code Z23 is for encounters for inoculations and vaccinations. It indicates that a patient is being seen to receive a prophylactic inoculation against a disease. Procedure codes are required to identify the actual administration of the injection and the type(s) of immunizations given. Code Z23 may be used as a secondary code if the inoculation is given as a routine part of preventive health care, such as a well-baby visit.

3) Status

Status codes indicate that a patient is either a carrier of a disease or has the sequelae or residual of a past disease or condition. This includes such things as the presence of prosthetic or mechanical devices resulting from past treatment. A status code is informative, because the status may affect the course of treatment and its outcome. A status code is distinct from a history code. The history code indicates that the patient no longer has the condition.

A status code should not be used with a diagnosis code from one of the body system chapters, if the diagnosis code includes the information provided by the status code. For example, code Z94.1, Heart transplant status, should not be used with a code from subcategory T86.2, Complications of heart transplant. The status code does not provide additional information. The complication code indicates that the patient is a heart transplant patient.

For encounters for weaning from a mechanical ventilator, assign a code from subcategory J96.1, Chronic respiratory failure, followed by code Z99.11, Dependence on respirator [ventilator] status.

The status Z codes/categories are:

Z14   Genetic carrier

       Genetic carrier status indicates that a person carries a gene, associated with a particular disease, which may be passed to

offspring who may develop that disease. The person does not have the disease and is not at risk of developing the disease.

Z15   Genetic susceptibility to disease

       Genetic susceptibility indicates that a person has a gene that increases the risk of that person developing the disease.

       Codes from category Z15 should not be used as principal or first-listed codes. If the patient has the condition to which he/she is susceptible, and that condition is the reason for the encounter, the code for the current condition should be sequenced first. If the patient is being seen for follow-up after completed treatment for this condition, and the condition no longer exists, a follow-up code should be sequenced first, followed by the appropriate personal history and genetic susceptibility codes. If the purpose of the encounter is genetic counseling associated with procreative management, code Z31.5, Encounter for genetic counseling, should be assigned as the first-listed code, followed by a code from category Z15. Additional codes should be assigned for any applicable family or personal history.

Z16   Resistance to antimicrobial drugs

       This code indicates that a patient has a condition that is resistant to antimicrobial drug treatment. Sequence the infection code first.

Z17   Estrogen receptor status

Z18   Retained foreign body fragments

Z19   Hormone sensitivity malignancy status

Z21   Asymptomatic HIV infection status

       This code indicates that a patient has tested positive for HIV but has manifested no signs or symptoms of the disease.

Z22   Carrier of infectious disease

       Carrier status indicates that a person harbors the specific organisms of a disease without manifest symptoms and is capable of transmitting the infection.

Z28.3   Underimmunization status

Z33.1   Pregnant state, incidental

       This code is a secondary code only for use when the pregnancy is in no way complicating the reason for visit. Otherwise, a code from the obstetric chapter is required.

Z66   Do not resuscitate

       This code may be used when it is documented by the provider that a patient is on do not resuscitate status at any time during the stay.

Z67   Blood type

Z68   Body mass index (BMI)

       As with all other secondary diagnosis codes, the BMI codes should only be assigned when they meet the definition of a reportable diagnosis (see Section III, Reporting Additional Diagnoses).

Z74.01   Bed confinement status

Z76.82   Awaiting organ transplant status

Z78   Other specified health status

       Code Z78.1, Physical restraint status, may be used when it is documented by the provider that a patient has been put in restraints during the current encounter. Please note that this code should not be reported when it is documented by the provider that a patient is temporarily restrained during a procedure.

Z79   Long-term (current) drug therapy

       Codes from this category indicate a patient's continuous use of a prescribed drug (including such things as aspirin therapy) for the long-term treatment of a condition or for prophylactic use. It is not for use for patients who have addictions to drugs. This subcategory is not for use of medications for detoxification or maintenance programs to prevent withdrawal symptoms in patients with drug dependence (e.g., methadone maintenance for opiate dependence). Assign the appropriate code for the drug dependence instead.

       Assign a code from Z79 if the patient is receiving a medication for an extended period as a prophylactic measure (such as for the prevention of deep vein thrombosis) or as treatment of a chronic condition (such as arthritis) or a disease requiring a lengthy course of treatment (such as cancer). Do not assign a code from category Z79 for medication being administered for a brief period of time to treat an acute illness or injury (such as a course of antibiotics to treat acute bronchitis).

Z88   Allergy status to drugs, medicaments and biological substances

Except: Z88.9, Allergy status to unspecified drugs, medicaments and biological substances status

Z89   Acquired absence of limb

Z9Ø   Acquired absence of organs, not elsewhere classified

Z91.Ø-   Allergy status, other than to drugs and biological substances

Z92.82   Status post administration of tPA (rtPA) in a different facility within the last 24 hours prior to admission to a current facility

Assign code Z92.82, Status post administration of tPA (rtPA) in a different facility within the last 24 hours prior to admission to current facility, as a secondary diagnosis when a patient is received by transfer into a facility and documentation indicates they were administered tissue plasminogen activator (tPA) within the last 24 hours prior to admission to the current facility.

This guideline applies even if the patient is still receiving the tPA at the time they are received into the current facility.

The appropriate code for the condition for which the tPA was administered (such as cerebrovascular disease or myocardial infarction) should be assigned first.

Code Z92.82 is only applicable to the receiving facility record and not to the transferring facility record.

Z93   Artificial opening status

Z94   Transplanted organ and tissue status

Z95   Presence of cardiac and vascular implants and grafts

Z96   Presence of other functional implants

Z97   Presence of other devices

Z98   Other postprocedural states

Assign code Z98.85, Transplanted organ removal status, to indicate that a transplanted organ has been previously removed. This code should not be assigned for the encounter in which the transplanted organ is removed. The complication necessitating removal of the transplant organ should be assigned for that encounter.

See section I.C19. for information on the coding of organ transplant complications.

Z99   Dependence on enabling machines and devices, not elsewhere classified

Note: Categories Z89-Z9Ø and Z93-Z99 are for use only if there are no complications or malfunctions of the organ or tissue replaced, the amputation site or the equipment on which the patient is dependent..

4) History (of)

There are two types of history Z codes, personal and family. Personal history codes explain a patient's past medical condition that no longer exists and is not receiving any treatment, but that has the potential for recurrence, and therefore may require continued monitoring.

Patient with a history of bladder cancer underwent a cystectomy 6 months ago with ileal conduit formation, for which she requires assistance and instruction to manage. No further treatment for the neoplasm has been provided. The patient has been experiencing frequent episodes of pyelonephritis since the surgery. It is noted in the preadmission provider H&P that antibiotic therapy was discontinued 3 days ago.

Z85.51   **Personal history of malignant neoplasm of bladder**

Z87.44Ø   **Personal history of urinary (tract) infections**

Z43.6   **Encounter for attention to other artificial openings of urinary tract**

Explanation: Since the malignancy has been excised with no further treatment noted, code Z85 should be assigned to report the personal history of malignancy. The antibiotic treatment for pyelonephritis has been discontinued, and it is not appropriate to code the infection as active. Instead Z87.44Ø should be assigned to report that the patient has a significant history of urinary infection. Code Z43.6 captures the presence of and the care needed to manage the ileal conduit.

Family history codes are for use when a patient has a family member(s) who has had a particular disease that causes the patient to be at higher risk of also contracting the disease.

Personal history codes may be used in conjunction with follow-up codes and family history codes may be used in conjunction with screening codes to explain the need for a test or procedure. History codes are also acceptable on any medical record regardless of the reason for visit. A history of an illness, even if no longer present, is important information that may alter the type of treatment ordered.

The history Z code categories are:

Z8Ø   Family history of primary malignant neoplasm

Z81   Family history of mental and behavioral disorders

Z82   Family history of certain disabilities and chronic diseases (leading to disablement)

Z83   Family history of other specific disorders

Z84   Family history of other conditions

Z85   Personal history of malignant neoplasm

Z86   Personal history of certain other diseases

Z87   Personal history of other diseases and conditions

Z91.4-   Personal history of psychological trauma, not elsewhere classified

Z91.5   Personal history of self-harm

Z91.81   **History of falling**

Z91.82   **Personal history of military deployment**

Z92   Personal history of medical treatment

Except: Z92.Ø, Personal history of contraception

Except: Z92.82, Status post administration of tPA (rtPA) in a different facility within the last 24 hours prior to admission to a current facility

5) Screening

Screening is the testing for disease or disease precursors in seemingly well individuals so that early detection and treatment can be provided for those who test positive for the disease (e.g., screening mammogram).

The testing of a person to rule out or confirm a suspected diagnosis because the patient has some sign or symptom is a diagnostic examination, not a screening. In these cases, the sign or symptom is used to explain the reason for the test.

A screening code may be a first-listed code if the reason for the visit is specifically the screening exam. It may also be used as an additional code if the screening is done during an office visit for other health problems. A screening code is not necessary if the screening is inherent to a routine examination, such as a pap smear done during a routine pelvic examination.

Should a condition be discovered during the screening then the code for the condition may be assigned as an additional diagnosis.

The Z code indicates that a screening exam is planned. A procedure code is required to confirm that the screening was performed.

The screening Z codes/categories:

Z11   Encounter for screening for infectious and parasitic diseases

Z12   Encounter for screening for malignant neoplasms

Z13   Encounter for screening for other diseases and disorders

Except: Z13.9, Encounter for screening, unspecified

Z36   Encounter for antenatal screening for mother

6) Observation

There are three observation Z code categories. They are for use in very limited circumstances when a person is being observed for a suspected condition that is ruled out. The observation codes are not for use if an injury or illness or any signs or symptoms related to the suspected condition are present. In such cases the diagnosis/symptom code is used with the corresponding external cause code.

The observation codes are to be used as principal diagnosis only. The only exception to this is when the principal diagnosis is required to be a code from category Z38, Liveborn infants according to place of birth and type of delivery. Then a code from category Z05, Encounter for observation and evaluation of newborn for suspected diseases and conditions ruled out, is sequenced after the Z38 code. Additional codes may be used in addition to the observation code but only if they are unrelated to the suspected condition being observed.

Codes from subcategory Z03.7, Encounter for suspected maternal and fetal conditions ruled out, may either be used as a first-listed or as an additional code assignment depending on the case. They are for use in very limited circumstances on a maternal record when an encounter is for a suspected maternal or fetal condition that is ruled out during that encounter (for example, a maternal or fetal condition may be suspected due to an abnormal test result). These codes should not be used when the condition is confirmed. In those cases, the confirmed condition should be coded. In addition, these codes are not for use if an illness or any signs or symptoms related to the suspected condition or problem are present. In such cases the diagnosis/symptom code is used.

Additional codes may be used in addition to the code from subcategory Z03.7, but only if they are unrelated to the suspected condition being evaluated.

Codes from subcategory Z03.7 may not be used for encounters for antenatal screening of mother. *See Section I.C.21. Screening.*

For encounters for suspected fetal condition that are inconclusive following testing and evaluation, assign the appropriate code from category O35, O36, O40 or O41.

The observation Z code categories:

Z03	Encounter for medical observation for suspected diseases and conditions ruled out
Z04	Encounter for examination and observation for other reasons
	Except: Z04.9, Encounter for examination and observation for unspecified reason
Z05	Encounter for observation and evaluation of newborn for suspected diseases and conditions ruled out

7) Aftercare

Aftercare visit codes cover situations when the initial treatment of a disease has been performed and the patient requires continued care during the healing or recovery phase, or for the long-term consequences of the disease. The aftercare Z code should not be used if treatment is directed at a current, acute disease. The diagnosis code is to be used in these cases. Exceptions to this rule are codes Z51.0, Encounter for antineoplastic radiation therapy, and codes from subcategory Z51.1, Encounter for antineoplastic chemotherapy and immunotherapy. These codes are to be first-listed, followed by the diagnosis code when a patient's encounter is solely to receive radiation therapy, chemotherapy, or immunotherapy for the treatment of a neoplasm. If the reason for the encounter is more than one type of antineoplastic therapy, code Z51.0 and a code from subcategory Z51.1 may be assigned together, in which case one of these codes would be reported as a secondary diagnosis.

The aftercare Z codes should also not be used for aftercare for injuries. For aftercare of an injury, assign the acute injury code with the appropriate 7th character (for subsequent encounter).

The aftercare codes are generally first-listed to explain the specific reason for the encounter. An aftercare code may be used as an additional code when some type of aftercare is provided in addition to the reason for admission and no diagnosis code is applicable. An example of this would be the closure of a colostomy during an encounter for treatment of another condition.

Aftercare codes should be used in conjunction with other aftercare codes or diagnosis codes to provide better detail on the specifics of an aftercare encounter visit, unless otherwise directed by the classification. Should a patient receive multiple types of antineoplastic therapy during the same encounter, code Z51.0, Encounter for antineoplastic radiation therapy, and codes from subcategory Z51.1, Encounter for antineoplastic chemotherapy and immunotherapy, may be used together on a record. The sequencing of multiple aftercare codes depends on the circumstances of the encounter.

Certain aftercare Z code categories need a secondary diagnosis code to describe the resolving condition or sequelae. For others, the condition is included in the code title.

Additional Z code aftercare category terms include fitting and adjustment, and attention to artificial openings.

Status Z codes may be used with aftercare Z codes to indicate the nature of the aftercare. For example code Z95.1, Presence of aortocoronary bypass graft, may be used with code Z48.812, Encounter for surgical aftercare following surgery on the circulatory system, to indicate the surgery for which the aftercare is being performed. A status code should not be used when the aftercare code indicates the type of status, such as using Z43.0, Encounter for attention to tracheostomy, with Z93.0, Tracheostomy status.

The aftercare Z category/codes:

Z42	Encounter for plastic and reconstructive surgery following medical procedure or healed injury
Z43	Encounter for attention to artificial openings
Z44	Encounter for fitting and adjustment of external prosthetic device
Z45	Encounter for adjustment and management of implanted device
Z46	Encounter for fitting and adjustment of other devices
Z47	Orthopedic aftercare
Z48	Encounter for other postprocedural aftercare
Z49	Encounter for care involving renal dialysis
Z51	Encounter for other aftercare and medical care

> Patient admitted post right total knee replacement for physical therapy
>
> **Z47.1**   **Aftercare following joint replacement surgery**
>
> **Z96.651**   **Presence of right artificial knee joint**
>
> *Explanation:* An elective joint replacement, that is one done by choice and not to correct a fracture or other injury, should reported by the post-acute care provider by using code Z47.1. Guidelines for the assignment of Z47.1 include instructions to "use additional code to identify the joint."

8) Follow-up

The follow-up codes are used to explain continuing surveillance following completed treatment of a disease, condition, or injury. They imply that the condition has been fully treated and no longer exists. They should not be confused with aftercare codes, or injury codes with a 7th character for subsequent encounter, that explain ongoing care of a healing condition or its sequelae. Follow-up codes may be used in conjunction with history codes to provide the full picture of the healed condition and its treatment. The follow-up code is sequenced first, followed by the history code.

A follow-up code may be used to explain multiple visits. Should a condition be found to have recurred on the follow-up visit, then the diagnosis code for the condition should be assigned in place of the follow-up code.

The follow-up Z code categories:

Z08	Encounter for follow-up examination after completed treatment for malignant neoplasm
Z09	Encounter for follow-up examination after completed treatment for conditions other than malignant neoplasm
Z39	Encounter for maternal postpartum care and examination

9) Donor

Codes in category Z52, Donors of organs and tissues, are used for living individuals who are donating blood or other body tissue. These codes are only for individuals donating for others, not for self-donations. They are not used to identify cadaveric donations.

10) Counseling

Counseling Z codes are used when a patient or family member receives assistance in the aftermath of an illness or injury, or when support is required in coping with family or social problems.

The counseling Z codes/categories:

Z30.0-	Encounter for general counseling and advice on contraception
Z31.5	Encounter for **procreative** genetic counseling
Z31.6-	Encounter for general counseling and advice on procreation
Z32.2	Encounter for childbirth instruction
Z32.3	Encounter for childcare instruction
Z69	Encounter for mental health services for victim and perpetrator of abuse
Z70	Counseling related to sexual attitude, behavior and orientation
Z71	Persons encountering health services for other counseling and medical advice, not elsewhere classified
Z76.81	Expectant mother prebirth pediatrician visit

11) Encounters for obstetrical and reproductive services

See Section I.C.15. Pregnancy, Childbirth, and the Puerperium, for further instruction on the use of these codes.

Z codes for pregnancy are for use in those circumstances when none of the problems or complications included in the codes from the Obstetrics chapter exist (a routine prenatal visit or postpartum care). Codes in category Z34, Encounter for supervision of normal pregnancy, are always first-listed and are not to be used with any other code from the OB chapter.

Codes in category Z3A, Weeks of gestation, may be assigned to provide additional information about the pregnancy. Category Z3A codes should not be assigned for pregnancies with abortive outcomes (categories O00–O08), elective termination of pregnancy (code **Z33.2**), nor for postpartum conditions, as category Z3A is not applicable to these conditions. The date of the admission should be used to determine weeks of gestation for inpatient admissions that encompass more than one gestational week.

The outcome of delivery, category Z37, should be included on all maternal delivery records. It is always a secondary code. Codes in category Z37 should not be used on the newborn record.

Z codes for family planning (contraceptive) or procreative management and counseling should be included on an obstetric record either during the pregnancy or the postpartum stage, if applicable.

Z codes/categories for obstetrical and reproductive services:

Z30	Encounter for contraceptive management
Z31	Encounter for procreative management
Z32.2	Encounter for childbirth instruction
Z32.3	Encounter for childcare instruction
Z33	Pregnant state
Z34	Encounter for supervision of normal pregnancy
Z36	Encounter for antenatal screening of mother
Z3A	Weeks of gestation
Z37	Outcome of delivery
Z39	Encounter for maternal postpartum care and examination
Z76.81	Expectant mother prebirth pediatrician visit

12) Newborns and infants

See Section I.C.16. Newborn (Perinatal) Guidelines, for further instruction on the use of these codes.

Newborn Z codes/categories:

Z76.1	Encounter for health supervision and care of foundling
Z00.1-	Encounter for routine child health examination
Z38	Liveborn infants according to place of birth and type of delivery

13) Routine and administrative examinations

The Z codes allow for the description of encounters for routine examinations, such as, a general check-up, or, examinations for administrative purposes, such as, a pre-employment physical. The codes are not to be used if the examination is for diagnosis of a suspected condition or for treatment purposes. In such cases the diagnosis code is used. During a routine exam, should a diagnosis or condition be discovered, it should be coded as an additional code. Pre-existing and chronic conditions and history codes may also be included as additional codes as long as the examination is for administrative purposes and not focused on any particular condition.

Some of the codes for routine health examinations distinguish between "with" and "without" abnormal findings. Code assignment depends on the information that is known at the time the encounter is being coded. For example, if no abnormal findings were found during the examination, but the encounter is being coded before test results are back, it is acceptable to assign the code for "without abnormal findings." When assigning a code for "with abnormal findings," additional code(s) should be assigned to identify the specific abnormal finding(s).

Pre-operative examination and pre-procedural laboratory examination Z codes are for use only in those situations when a patient is being cleared for a procedure or surgery and no treatment is given.

The Z codes/categories for routine and administrative examinations:

Z00	Encounter for general examination without complaint, suspected or reported diagnosis
Z01	Encounter for other special examination without complaint, suspected or reported diagnosis
Z02	Encounter for administrative examination
	Except: Z02.9, Encounter for administrative examinations, unspecified
Z32.0-	Encounter for pregnancy test

14) Miscellaneous Z codes

The miscellaneous Z codes capture a number of other health care encounters that do not fall into one of the other categories. Certain of these codes identify the reason for the encounter; others are for use as additional codes that provide useful information on circumstances that may affect a patient's care and treatment.

Patient has Asperger's syndrome and wanders.

F84.5   **Asperger's syndrome**

Z91.83   **Wandering in diseases classified elsewhere**

Explanation: Code Z91.83 is a miscellaneous Z code that provides additional insight into this patient's Asperger's diagnosis. Care provided to an Asperger's patient who wanders or elopes may be different than for an Asperger's patient who does not wander.

Prophylactic organ removal

For encounters specifically for prophylactic removal of an organ (such as prophylactic removal of breasts due to a genetic susceptibility to cancer or a family history of cancer), the principal or first-listed code should be a code from category Z40, Encounter for prophylactic surgery, followed by the appropriate codes to identify the associated risk factor (such as genetic susceptibility or family history).

If the patient has a malignancy of one site and is having prophylactic removal at another site to prevent either a new primary malignancy or metastatic disease, a code for the malignancy should also be assigned in addition to a code from subcategory Z40.0, Encounter for prophylactic surgery for risk factors related to malignant neoplasms. A Z40.0 code should not be assigned if the patient is having organ removal for treatment of a malignancy, such as the removal of the testes for the treatment of prostate cancer.

Miscellaneous Z codes/categories:

Z28	Immunization not carried out
	Except: Z28.3, Underimmunization status
Z29	Encounter for other prophylactic measures
Z40	Encounter for prophylactic surgery
Z41	Encounter for procedures for purposes other than remedying health state
	Except: Z41.9, Encounter for procedure for purposes other than remedying health state, unspecified
Z53	Persons encountering health services for specific procedures and treatment, not carried out
Z55	Problems related to education and literacy
Z56	Problems related to employment and unemployment
Z57	Occupational exposure to risk factors
Z58	Problems related to physical environment
Z59	Problems related to housing and economic circumstances
Z60	Problems related to social environment
Z62	Problems related to upbringing
Z63	Other problems related to primary support group, including family circumstances
Z64	Problems related to certain psychosocial circumstances
Z65	Problems related to other psychosocial circumstances
Z72	Problems related to lifestyle
	Note: These codes should be assigned only when the documentation specifies that the patient has an associated problem
Z73	Problems related to life management difficulty
Z74	Problems related to care provider dependency
	Except: Z74.01, Bed confinement status
Z75	Problems related to medical facilities and other health care
Z76.0	Encounter for issue of repeat prescription
Z76.3	Healthy person accompanying sick person
Z76.4	Other boarder to healthcare facility
Z76.5	Malingerer [conscious simulation]
Z91.1-	Patient's noncompliance with medical treatment and regimen
Z91.83	Wandering in diseases classified elsewhere
Z91.84-	**Oral health risk factors**
Z91.89	Other specified personal risk factors, not elsewhere classified

15) Nonspecific Z codes

Certain Z codes are so non-specific, or potentially redundant with other codes in the classification, that there can be little justification for their use in the inpatient setting. Their use in the outpatient setting should be limited to those instances when there is no further documentation to permit more precise coding. Otherwise, any sign or symptom or any other reason for visit that is captured in another code should be used.

Nonspecific Z codes/categories:

Z02.9	Encounter for administrative examinations, unspecified
Z04.9	Encounter for examination and observation for unspecified reason
Z13.9	Encounter for screening, unspecified
Z41.9	Encounter for procedure for purposes other than remedying health state, unspecified
Z52.9	Donor of unspecified organ or tissue
Z86.59	Personal history of other mental and behavioral disorders
Z88.9	Allergy status to unspecified drugs, medicaments and biological substances status
Z92.0	Personal history of contraception

16) Z codes that may only be principal/first-listed diagnosis

The following Z codes/categories may only be reported as the principal/first-listed diagnosis, except when there are multiple encounters on the same day and the medical records for the encounters are combined:

Z00	Encounter for general examination without complaint, suspected or reported diagnosis
	Except: Z00.6
Z01	Encounter for other special examination without complaint, suspected or reported diagnosis
Z02	Encounter for administrative examination
Z03	Encounter for medical observation for suspected diseases and conditions ruled out
Z04	Encounter for examination and observation for other reasons
Z33.2	Encounter for elective termination of pregnancy
Z31.81	Encounter for male factor infertility in female patient
Z31.82	Encounter for Rh incompatibility status
Z31.83	Encounter for assisted reproductive fertility procedure cycle
Z31.84	Encounter for fertility preservation procedure
Z34	Encounter for supervision of normal pregnancy
Z39	Encounter for maternal postpartum care and examination
Z38	Liveborn infants according to place of birth and type of delivery
Z40	**Encounter for prophylactic surgery**
Z42	Encounter for plastic and reconstructive surgery following medical procedure or healed injury
Z51.0	Encounter for antineoplastic radiation therapy
Z51.1-	Encounter for antineoplastic chemotherapy and immunotherapy
Z52	Donors of organs and tissues
	Except: Z52.9, Donor of unspecified organ or tissue
Z76.1	Encounter for health supervision and care of foundling
Z76.2	Encounter for health supervision and care of other healthy infant and child
Z99.12	Encounter for respirator [ventilator] dependence during power failure

Chapter 21. Factors Influencing Health Status and Contact With Health Services (Z00-Z99)

NOTE   Z codes represent reasons for encounters. A corresponding procedure code must accompany a Z code if a procedure is performed. Categories Z00-Z99 are provided for occasions when circumstances other than a disease, injury or external cause classifiable to categories A00-Y89 are recorded as "diagnoses" or "problems". This can arise in two main ways:

(a) When a person who may or may not be sick encounters the health services for some specific purpose, such as to receive limited care or service for a current condition, to donate an organ or tissue, to receive prophylactic vaccination (immunization), or to discuss a problem which is in itself not a disease or injury.

(b) When some circumstance or problem is present which influences the person's health status but is not in itself a current illness or injury.

This chapter contains the following blocks:

Z00-Z13   Persons encountering health services for examinations
Z14-Z15   Genetic carrier and genetic susceptibility to disease
Z16   Resistance to antimicrobial drugs
Z17   Estrogen receptor status
Z18   Retained foreign body fragments
~~Z19~~   ~~Hormone sensitivity malignancy status~~
Z20-Z29   Persons with potential health hazards related to communicable diseases
Z30-Z39   Persons encountering health services in circumstances related to reproduction
Z40-Z53   Encounters for other specific health care
Z55-Z65   Persons with potential health hazards related to socioeconomic and psychosocial circumstances
Z66   Do not resuscitate status
Z67   Blood type
Z68   Body mass index (BMI)
Z69-Z76   Persons encountering health services in other circumstances
Z77-Z99   Persons with potential health hazards related to family and personal history and certain conditions influencing health status

Persons encountering health services for examinations (Z00-Z13)

NOTE   Nonspecific abnormal findings disclosed at the time of these examinations are classified to categories R70-R94.
EXCLUDES 1   *examinations related to pregnancy and reproduction (Z30-Z36, Z39-)*

√4ᵗʰ **Z00**   **Encounter for general examination without complaint, suspected or reported diagnosis**
    EXCLUDES 1   *encounter for examination for administrative purposes (Z02.-)*
    EXCLUDES 2   *encounter for pre-procedural examinations (Z01.81-)*
        special screening examinations (Z11-Z13)

√5ᵗʰ **Z00.0**   **Encounter for general adult medical examination**
    Encounter for adult periodic examination (annual) (physical) and any associated laboratory and radiologic examinations
    EXCLUDES 1   *encounter for examination of sign or symptom—code to sign or symptom*
        general health check-up of infant or child (Z00.12-)

    Z00.00   **Encounter for general adult medical** PDx A
        examination without abnormal findings
        Encounter for adult health check-up NOS
        AHA: 2016, 1Q, 36

    Z00.01   **Encounter for general adult medical** PDx A
        examination with abnormal findings
        Use additional code to identify abnormal findings
        AHA: 2016, 1Q, 35-36

√5ᵗʰ **Z00.1**   **Encounter for newborn, infant and child health examinations**

    √6ᵗʰ **Z00.11**   **Newborn health examination**
        Health check for child under 29 days old
        Use additional code to identify any abnormal findings
        EXCLUDES 1   *health check for child over 28 days old (Z00.12-)*

        Z00.110   **Health examination for newborn** PDx N
            under 8 days old
            Health check for newborn under 8 days old

        Z00.111   **Health examination for newborn** PDx N
            8 to 28 days old
            Health check for newborn 8 to 28 days old
            Newborn weight check

√6ᵗʰ **Z00.12**   **Encounter for routine child health examination**
    Encounter for development testing of infant or child
    Health check (routine) for child over 28 days old
    EXCLUDES 1   *health check for child under 29 days old (Z00.11-)*
        health supervision of foundling or other healthy infant or child (Z76.1-Z76.2)
        newborn health examination (Z00.11-)

    Z00.121   **Encounter for routine child health** PDx P
        examination with abnormal findings
        Use additional code to identify abnormal findings
        AHA: 2016, 1Q, 34-35

    Z00.129   **Encounter for routine child health** PDx P
        examination without abnormal findings
        Encounter for routine child health examination NOS
        AHA: 2016, 1Q, 34

Z00.2   **Encounter for examination for period of rapid growth** PDx P
    in childhood

Z00.3   **Encounter for examination for adolescent** PDx P
    development state
    Encounter for puberty development state

Z00.5   **Encounter for examination for potential donor of organ** PDx
    and tissue

Z00.6   **Encounter for examination for normal comparison and control in clinical research program**
    Examination of participant or control in clinical research program

√5ᵗʰ **Z00.7**   **Encounter for examination for period of delayed growth in childhood**

    Z00.70   **Encounter for examination for period of** PDx P
        delayed growth in childhood without abnormal findings

    Z00.71   **Encounter for examination for period of** PDx P
        delayed growth in childhood with abnormal findings
        Use additional code to identify abnormal findings

Z00.8   **Encounter for other general examination** PDx
    Encounter for health examination in population surveys

√4ᵗʰ **Z01**   **Encounter for other special examination without complaint, suspected or reported diagnosis**
    INCLUDES   routine examination of specific system
    NOTE   Codes from category Z01 represent the reason for the encounter. A separate procedure code is required to identify any examinations or procedures performed.
    EXCLUDES 1   *encounter for examination for administrative purposes (Z02.-)*
        encounter for examination for suspected conditions, proven not to exist (Z03.-)
        encounter for laboratory and radiologic examinations as a component of general medical examinations (Z00.0-)
        encounter for laboratory, radiologic and imaging examinations for sign(s) and symptom(s)—code to the sign(s) or symptom(s)
    EXCLUDES 2   *screening examinations (Z11-Z13)*

√5ᵗʰ **Z01.0**   **Encounter for examination of eyes and vision**
    EXCLUDES 1   *examination for driving license (Z02.4)*

    Z01.00   **Encounter for examination of eyes and vision** PDx
        without abnormal findings
        Encounter for examination of eyes and vision NOS

    Z01.01   **Encounter for examination of eyes and vision** PDx
        with abnormal findings
        Use additional code to identify abnormal findings

√5ᵗʰ **Z01.1**   **Encounter for examination of ears and hearing**

    Z01.10   **Encounter for examination of ears and hearing** PDx
        without abnormal findings
        Encounter for examination of ears and hearing NOS
        AHA: 2016, 4Q, 24

    √6ᵗʰ **Z01.11**   **Encounter for examination of ears and hearing with abnormal findings**
        AHA: 2016, 3Q, 17-18

        Z01.110   **Encounter for hearing examination** PDx
            following failed hearing screening

        Z01.118   **Encounter for examination of ears** PDx
            and hearing with other abnormal findings
            Use additional code to identify abnormal findings

    Z01.12   **Encounter for hearing conservation and** PDx
        treatment

N Newborn: 0   P Pediatric: 0-17   M Maternity: 12-55   A Adult: 15-124   **NRS** Nonroutine supply Dx   **NCDx** Noncancer Dx   **PDx** Primary Dx   ▶◀ Revised Text   ● New Code   ▲ Revised Title

1180   ICD-10-CM 2018

☑5ᵗʰ **Z01.2** **Encounter for** dental examination and cleaning

    Z01.20 **Encounter for dental examination and** PDx
        cleaning without abnormal findings
        Encounter for dental examination and cleaning NOS

    Z01.21 **Encounter for dental examination and cleaning** PDx
        with abnormal findings
        Use additional code to identify abnormal findings

☑5ᵗʰ **Z01.3** **Encounter for examination of** blood pressure

    Z01.30 **Encounter for examination of blood pressure** PDx
        without abnormal findings
        Encounter for examination of blood pressure NOS

    Z01.31 **Encounter for examination of blood pressure** PDx
        with abnormal findings
        Use additional code to identify abnormal findings

☑5ᵗʰ **Z01.4** **Encounter for** gynecological examination

    EXCLUDES 2   pregnancy examination or test (Z32.0-)
           routine examination for contraceptive maintenance
           (Z30.4-)

   ☑6ᵗʰ **Z01.41** **Encounter for** routine gynecological examination
        Encounter for general gynecological examination with
           or without cervical smear
        Encounter for gynecological examination (general)
           (routine) NOS
        Encounter for pelvic examination (annual) (periodic)
        Use additional code:
           for screening for human papillomavirus, if
              applicable, (Z11.51)
           for screening vaginal pap smear, if applicable
              (Z12.72)
           to identify acquired absence of uterus, if applicable
              (Z90.71-)
        EXCLUDES 1   gynecologic examination status-post
                 hysterectomy for malignant condition
                 (Z08)
                 screening cervical pap smear not a part of a
                 routine gynecological examination
                 (Z12.4)

        Z01.411 **Encounter for gynecological** PDx ♀
            examination (general) (routine) with
            abnormal findings
            Use additional code to identify abnormal
              findings

        Z01.419 **Encounter for gynecological** PDx ♀
            examination (general) (routine) without
            abnormal findings

    Z01.42 **Encounter for** cervical smear to confirm PDx ♀
        findings **of recent normal smear following initial**
        abnormal smear

☑5ᵗʰ **Z01.8** **Encounter for** other specified special examinations

   ☑6ᵗʰ **Z01.81** **Encounter for** preprocedural examinations
        Encounter for preoperative examinations
        Encounter for radiological and imaging examinations
           as part of preprocedural examination

        Z01.810 **Encounter for preprocedural** PDx
            cardiovascular examination

        Z01.811 **Encounter for preprocedural** PDx
            respiratory examination

        Z01.812 **Encounter for preprocedural** PDx
            laboratory examination
            Blood and urine tests prior to treatment or
              procedure

        Z01.818 **Encounter for other preprocedural** PDx
            examination
            Encounter for preprocedural examination
              NOS
            Encounter for examinations prior to
              antineoplastic chemotherapy

    Z01.82 **Encounter for** allergy testing PDx
        EXCLUDES 1   encounter for antibody response
                examination (Z01.84)

    Z01.83 **Encounter for** blood typing PDx
        Encounter for Rh typing

    Z01.84 **Encounter for** antibody response examination PDx
        Encounter for immunity status testing
        EXCLUDES 1   encounter for allergy testing (Z01.82)

    Z01.89 **Encounter for other specified special** PDx
        examinations

☑4ᵗʰ **Z02** **Encounter for** administrative examination

    Z02.0 **Encounter for examination for** admission to educational PDx
        institution
        Encounter for examination for admission to preschool
           (education)
        Encounter for examination for re-admission to school following
           illness or medical treatment

    Z02.1 **Encounter for** pre-employment examination PDx

    Z02.2 **Encounter for examination for** admission to residential PDx
        institution
        EXCLUDES 1   examination for admission to prison (Z02.89)

    Z02.3 **Encounter for examination for** recruitment to armed PDx
        forces

    Z02.4 **Encounter for examination for** driving license PDx

    Z02.5 **Encounter for examination for** participation in sport PDx
        EXCLUDES 1   blood-alcohol and blood-drug test (Z02.83)

    Z02.6 **Encounter for examination for** insurance purposes PDx

  ☑5ᵗʰ **Z02.7** **Encounter for** issue of medical certificate
        EXCLUDES 1   encounter for general medical examination (Z00-Z01,
                Z02.0-Z02.6, Z02.8-Z02.9)

        Z02.71 **Encounter for** disability determination PDx
            Encounter for issue of medical certificate of incapacity
            Encounter for issue of medical certificate of invalidity

        Z02.79 **Encounter for issue of other medical certificate** PDx

  ☑5ᵗʰ **Z02.8** **Encounter for** other administrative examinations

        Z02.81 **Encounter for** paternity testing PDx

        Z02.82 **Encounter for** adoption services PDx

        Z02.83 **Encounter for** blood-alcohol and blood-drug PDx
            test
            Use additional code for findings of alcohol or drugs in
              blood (R78.-)

        Z02.89 **Encounter for other administrative** PDx
            examinations
            Encounter for examination for admission to prison
            Encounter for examination for admission to summer
              camp
            Encounter for immigration examination
            Encounter for naturalization examination
            Encounter for premarital examination
            EXCLUDES 1   health supervision of foundling or other
                   healthy infant or child (Z76.1-Z76.2)

    Z02.9 **Encounter for administrative examinations, unspecified** PDx ▽

☑4ᵗʰ **Z03** **Encounter for** medical observation **for suspected diseases and conditions ruled out**
    NOTE   This category is to be used when a person without a
        diagnosis is suspected of having an abnormal condition,
        without signs or symptoms, which requires study, but after
        examination and observation, is ruled out. This category is
        also for use for administrative and legal observation status.
    EXCLUDES 1   contact with and (suspected) exposures hazardous to health
           (Z77.-)
       ▶encounter for observation and evaluation of newborn for
          suspected diseases and conditions ruled out (Z05.0-)◀
       ~~newborn observation for suspected condition, ruled out~~
          ~~(P00-P04)~~
       person with feared complaint in whom no diagnosis is made
          (Z71.1)
       signs or symptoms under study—code to signs or symptoms

    Z03.6 **Encounter for observation for suspected** toxic effect PDx
    from ingested substance **ruled out**
        Encounter for observation for suspected adverse effect from
           drug
        Encounter for observation for suspected poisoning

  ☑5ᵗʰ **Z03.7** **Encounter for suspected** maternal and fetal conditions **ruled out**
        Encounter for suspected maternal and fetal conditions not
           found
        EXCLUDES 1   known or suspected fetal anomalies affecting
                 management of mother, not ruled out (O26-,
                 O35-, O36-, O40-, O41-)

        Z03.71 **Encounter for suspected problem with** PDx M ♀
            amniotic cavity and membrane ruled out
            Encounter for suspected oligohydramnios ruled out
            Encounter for suspected polyhydramnios ruled out

        Z03.72 **Encounter for suspected** placental PDx M ♀
            problem ruled out

        Z03.73 **Encounter for suspected** fetal anomaly PDx M ♀
            ruled out

☑ Additional Character Req   ✓x7ᵗʰ Placeholder Alert   Case-Mix Diagnosis   Manifestation   ▽ Unspecified Dx   *EXCLUDES 1* Not coded here   *EXCLUDES 2* Not included here

ICD-10-CM 2018   **1181**

Z03.74   Encounter for suspected problem with fetal growth ruled out   PDx M ♀

Z03.75   Encounter for suspected cervical shortening ruled out   PDx M ♀

Z03.79   Encounter for other suspected maternal and fetal conditions ruled out   PDx M ♀

✓5ᵗʰ **Z03.8**   **Encounter for observation for other suspected diseases and conditions ruled out**

✓6ᵗʰ **Z03.81**   **Encounter for observation for suspected exposure to biological agents ruled out**

Z03.810   Encounter for observation for suspected exposure to anthrax ruled out   PDx

Z03.818   Encounter for observation for suspected exposure to other biological agents ruled out   PDx

Z03.89   Encounter for observation for other suspected diseases and conditions ruled out   PDx

✓4ᵗʰ **Z04**   **Encounter for examination and observation for other reasons**
> **INCLUDES**   encounter for examination for medicolegal reasons
> This category is to be used when a person without a diagnosis is suspected of having an abnormal condition, without signs or symptoms, which requires study, but after examination and observation, is ruled-out. This category is also for use for administrative and legal observation status.

Z04.1   **Encounter for examination and observation following transport accident**   PDx
> **EXCLUDES 1**   *encounter for examination and observation following work accident (Z04.2)*

Z04.2   **Encounter for examination and observation following work accident**   PDx

Z04.3   **Encounter for examination and observation following other accident**   PDx

✓5ᵗʰ **Z04.4**   **Encounter for examination and observation following alleged rape**
> Encounter for examination and observation of victim following alleged rape
> Encounter for examination and observation of victim following alleged sexual abuse

Z04.41   **Encounter for examination and observation following alleged adult rape**   PDx A
> Suspected adult rape, ruled out
> Suspected adult sexual abuse, ruled out

Z04.42   **Encounter for examination and observation following alleged child rape**   PDx P
> Suspected child rape, ruled out
> Suspected child sexual abuse, ruled out

Z04.6   **Encounter for general psychiatric examination, requested by authority**   PDx

✓5ᵗʰ **Z04.7**   **Encounter for examination and observation following alleged physical abuse**

Z04.71   **Encounter for examination and observation following alleged adult physical abuse**   PDx A
> Suspected adult physical abuse, ruled out
> **EXCLUDES 1**   *confirmed case of adult physical abuse (T74.-)*
> *encounter for examination and observation following alleged adult sexual abuse (Z04.41)*
> *suspected case of adult physical abuse, not ruled out (T76.-)*

Z04.72   **Encounter for examination and observation following alleged child physical abuse**   PDx P
> Suspected child physical abuse, ruled out
> **EXCLUDES 1**   *confirmed case of child physical abuse (T74.-)*
> *encounter for examination and observation following alleged child sexual abuse (Z04.42)*
> *suspected case of child physical abuse, not ruled out (T76.-)*

Z04.8   **Encounter for examination and observation for other specified reasons**   PDx
> Encounter for examination and observation for request for expert evidence

Z04.9   **Encounter for examination and observation for unspecified reason**   PDx ▽
> Encounter for observation NOS

✓4ᵗʰ **Z05**   **Encounter for observation of newborn for suspected diseases and conditions ruled out**
> ►This category is to be used for newborns, within the neonatal period (the first 28 days of life), who are suspected of having an abnormal condition, but without signs or symptoms, and which, after examination and observation, is ruled out.◄
> **EXCLUDES 2**   *newborn observation for suspected condition, related to exposure from the mother or birth process (P00–P04)*

Z05.0   **Observation and evaluation of newborn for suspected cardiac condition ruled out**

Z05.1   **Observation and evaluation of newborn for suspected infectious condition ruled out**

Z05.2   **Observation and evaluation of newborn for suspected neurological condition ruled out**

Z05.3   **Observation and evaluation of newborn for suspected respiratory condition ruled out**

✓5ᵗʰ **Z05.4**   **Observation and evaluation of newborn for suspected genetic, metabolic or immunologic condition ruled out**

Z05.41   **Observation and evaluation of newborn for suspected genetic condition ruled out**

Z05.42   **Observation and evaluation of newborn for suspected metabolic condition ruled out**

Z05.43   **Observation and evaluation of newborn for suspected immunologic condition ruled out**

Z05.5   **Observation and evaluation of newborn for suspected gastrointestinal condition ruled out**

Z05.6   **Observation and evaluation of newborn for suspected genitourinary condition ruled out**

✓5ᵗʰ **Z05.7**   **Observation and evaluation of newborn for suspected skin, subcutaneous, musculoskeletal and connective tissue condition ruled out**

Z05.71   **Observation and evaluation of newborn for suspected skin and subcutaneous tissue condition ruled out**

Z05.72   **Observation and evaluation of newborn for suspected musculoskeletal condition ruled out**

Z05.73   **Observation and evaluation of newborn for suspected connective tissue condition ruled out**

Z05.8   **Observation and evaluation of newborn for other specified suspected condition ruled out**

Z05.9   **Observation and evaluation of newborn for unspecified suspected condition ruled out**   ▽

Z08   **Encounter for follow-up examination after completed treatment for malignant neoplasm**
> Medical surveillance following completed treatment
> Use additional code to identify any acquired absence of organs (Z90.-)
> Use additional code to identify the personal history of malignant neoplasm (Z85.-)
> **EXCLUDES 1**   *aftercare following medical care (Z43–Z49, Z51)*

Z09   **Encounter for follow-up examination after completed treatment for conditions other than malignant neoplasm**
> Medical surveillance following completed treatment
> Use additional code to identify any applicable history of disease code (Z86-. Z87-)
> **EXCLUDES 1**   *aftercare following medical care (Z43–Z49, Z51)*
> *surveillance of contraception (Z30.4-)*
> *surveillance of prosthetic and other medical devices (Z44–Z46)*
> **AHA:** 2017, 1Q, 9; 2015, 1Q, 8

✓4ᵗʰ **Z11**   **Encounter for screening for infectious and parasitic diseases**
> Screening is the testing for disease or disease precursors in asymptomatic individuals so that early detection and treatment can be provided for those who test positive for the disease.
> **EXCLUDES 1**   *encounter for diagnostic examination—code to sign or symptom*

Z11.0   **Encounter for screening for intestinal infectious diseases**

Z11.1   **Encounter for screening for respiratory tuberculosis**

Z11.2   **Encounter for screening for other bacterial diseases**

Z11.3   **Encounter for screening for infections with a predominantly sexual mode of transmission**
> **EXCLUDES 2**   *encounter for screening for human immunodeficiency virus [HIV] (Z11.4)*
> *encounter for screening for human papillomavirus (Z11.51)*

Z11.4   **Encounter for screening for human immunodeficiency virus [HIV]**

N Newborn: 0   P Pediatric: 0-17   M Maternity: 12-55   A Adult: 15-124   **NRS** Nonroutine supply Dx   **NC Dx** Noncancer Dx   **PDx** Primary Dx   ►◄ Revised Text   ● New Code   ▲ Revised Title

1182   ICD-10-CM 2018

✓5ᵗʰ **Z11.5 Encounter for screening for** other viral **diseases**

> EXCLUDES 2 *encounter for screening for viral intestinal disease (Z11.0)*

Z11.51 Encounter for screening for human papillomavirus (HPV)

Z11.59 Encounter for screening for other viral **diseases**

Z11.6 Encounter for screening for other protozoal diseases and helminthiases

> EXCLUDES 2 *encounter for screening for protozoal intestinal disease (Z11.0)*

Z11.8 Encounter for screening for other infectious and parasitic diseases

> Encounter for screening for chlamydia
> Encounter for screening for rickettsial
> Encounter for screening for spirochetal
> Encounter for screening for mycoses

Z11.9 Encounter for screening for infectious and parasitic ▽ **diseases, unspecified**

✓4ᵗʰ **Z12 Encounter for** screening **for** malignant neoplasms

> Screening is the testing for disease or disease precursors in asymptomatic individuals so that early detection and treatment can be provided for those who test positive for the disease.
> Use additional code to identify any family history of malignant neoplasm (Z80.-)

> EXCLUDES 1 *encounter for diagnostic examination—code to sign or symptom*

Z12.0 Encounter for screening for malignant neoplasm of stomach

✓5ᵗʰ **Z12.1 Encounter for screening for malignant neoplasm of** intestinal tract

> AHA: 2017, 1Q, 8, 9

Z12.10 Encounter for screening for malignant neoplasm ▽ **of intestinal tract, unspecified**

Z12.11 Encounter for screening for malignant neoplasm of colon

> Encounter for screening colonoscopy NOS

Z12.12 Encounter for screening for malignant neoplasm of rectum

Z12.13 Encounter for screening for malignant neoplasm of small intestine

Z12.2 Encounter for screening for malignant neoplasm of respiratory organs

✓5ᵗʰ **Z12.3 Encounter for screening for malignant neoplasm of** breast

Z12.31 Encounter for screening mammogram **for malignant neoplasm of breast**

> EXCLUDES 1 *inconclusive mammogram (R92.2)*
> AHA: 2015, 1Q, 24

Z12.39 Encounter for other screening for malignant neoplasm of breast

Z12.4 Encounter for screening for malignant neoplasm of cervix ♀

> Encounter for screening pap smear for malignant neoplasm of cervix

> EXCLUDES 1 *when screening is part of general gynecological examination (Z01.4-)*

> EXCLUDES 2 *encounter for screening for human papillomavirus (Z11.51)*

Z12.5 Encounter for screening for malignant neoplasm of prostate ♂

Z12.6 Encounter for screening for malignant neoplasm of bladder

✓5ᵗʰ **Z12.7 Encounter for screening for malignant neoplasm of** other genitourinary organs

Z12.71 Encounter for screening for malignant neoplasm ♂ **of** testis

Z12.72 Encounter for screening for malignant neoplasm ♀ **of** vagina

> Vaginal pap smear status-post hysterectomy for non-malignant condition
> Use additional code to identify acquired absence of uterus (Z90.71-)

> EXCLUDES 1 *vaginal pap smear status-post hysterectomy for malignant conditions (Z08)*

Z12.73 Encounter for screening for malignant neoplasm ♀ **of** ovary

Z12.79 Encounter for screening for malignant neoplasm of other genitourinary organs

✓5ᵗʰ **Z12.8 Encounter for screening for malignant neoplasm of** other sites

Z12.81 Encounter for screening for malignant neoplasm of oral cavity

Z12.82 Encounter for screening for malignant neoplasm of nervous system

Z12.83 Encounter for screening for malignant neoplasm of skin

Z12.89 Encounter for screening for malignant neoplasm of other sites

Z12.9 Encounter for screening for malignant neoplasm, site ▽ **unspecified**

✓4ᵗʰ **Z13 Encounter for screening for** other diseases and disorders

> Screening is the testing for disease or disease precursors in asymptomatic individuals so that early detection and treatment can be provided for those who test positive for the disease.

> EXCLUDES 1 *encounter for diagnostic examination—code to sign or symptom*

Z13.0 Encounter for screening for diseases of the blood and blood-forming organs **and certain disorders involving the immune mechanism**

Z13.1 Encounter for screening for diabetes mellitus

✓5ᵗʰ **Z13.2 Encounter for screening for nutritional, metabolic and other endocrine disorders**

Z13.21 Encounter for screening for nutritional **disorder**

✓6ᵗʰ **Z13.22 Encounter for screening for** metabolic **disorder**

Z13.220 Encounter for screening for lipoid disorders

> Encounter for screening for cholesterol level
> Encounter for screening for hypercholesterolemia
> Encounter for screening for hyperlipidemia

Z13.228 Encounter for screening for other metabolic disorders

Z13.29 Encounter for screening for other suspected endocrine disorder

> EXCLUDES 1 *encounter for screening for diabetes mellitus (Z13.1)*

Z13.4 Encounter for screening for certain developmental 🅟 **disorders in** childhood

> Encounter for screening for developmental handicaps in early childhood

> EXCLUDES 1 *routine development testing of infant or child (Z00.1-)*

Z13.5 Encounter for screening for eye and ear **disorders**

> EXCLUDES 2 *encounter for general hearing examination (Z01.1-)*
> *encounter for general vision examination (Z01.0-)*
> AHA: 2016, 3Q, 17

Z13.6 Encounter for screening for cardiovascular **disorders**

✓5ᵗʰ **Z13.7 Encounter for screening for** genetic **and** chromosomal **anomalies**

> EXCLUDES 1 *genetic testing for procreative management (Z31.4-)*

Z13.71 Encounter for nonprocreative screening for genetic disease carrier status

Z13.79 Encounter for other screening for genetic and chromosomal anomalies

✓5ᵗʰ **Z13.8 Encounter for screening for** other **specified diseases and disorders**

> EXCLUDES 2 *screening for malignant neoplasms (Z12.-)*

✓6ᵗʰ **Z13.81 Encounter for screening for** digestive system **disorders**

Z13.810 Encounter for screening for upper gastrointestinal **disorder**

Z13.811 Encounter for screening for lower gastrointestinal **disorder**

> EXCLUDES 1 *encounter for screening for intestinal infectious disease (Z11.0)*

Z13.818 Encounter for screening for other digestive system disorders

✓6ᵗʰ **Z13.82 Encounter for screening for** musculoskeletal **disorder**

Z13.820 Encounter for screening for osteoporosis

Z13.828 Encounter for screening for other musculoskeletal disorder

---

☑ Additional Character Req ✓x7ᵗʰ Placeholder Alert Case-Mix Diagnosis Manifestation ▽ Unspecified Dx EXCLUDES 1 Not coded here EXCLUDES 2 Not included here

ICD-10-CM 2018 **1183**

Z13.83   **Encounter for screening for respiratory disorder NEC**
> EXCLUDES 1   *encounter for screening for respiratory tuberculosis (Z11.1)*

Z13.84   **Encounter for screening for dental disorders**

√6th **Z13.85**   **Encounter for screening for nervous system disorders**

     Z13.850   **Encounter for screening for traumatic brain injury**

     Z13.858   **Encounter for screening for other nervous system disorders**

Z13.88   **Encounter for screening for disorder due to exposure to contaminants**
> EXCLUDES 1   *those exposed to contaminants without suspected disorders (Z57-Z77-)*

Z13.89   **Encounter for screening for other disorder**
> Encounter for screening for genitourinary disorders

Z13.9   **Encounter for screening, unspecified**   ▽

Genetic carrier and genetic susceptibility to disease (Z14-Z15)

√4th **Z14**   **Genetic carrier**
> **DEF:** Individuals carrying a gene mutation associated with a certain disease who typically do not develop the disease but are able to pass mutated gene to offspring.

√5th **Z14.0**   **Hemophilia A carrier**

     Z14.01   **Asymptomatic hemophilia A carrier**

     Z14.02   **Symptomatic hemophilia A carrier**

Z14.1   **Cystic fibrosis carrier**

Z14.8   **Genetic carrier of other disease**

√4th **Z15**   **Genetic susceptibility to disease**
> INCLUDES   confirmed abnormal gene
>
> Use additional code, if applicable, for any associated family history of the disease (Z80-Z84)
>
> EXCLUDES 1   *chromosomal anomalies (Q90-Q99)*

√5th **Z15.0**   **Genetic susceptibility to malignant neoplasm**
> Code first, if applicable, any current malignant neoplasm (C00-C75, C81-C96)
>
> Use additional code, if applicable, for any personal history of malignant neoplasm (Z85.-)

     Z15.01   **Genetic susceptibility to malignant neoplasm of breast**
> **TIP:** May be assigned in addition to a code for aftercare following prophylactic mastectomy.

     Z15.02   **Genetic susceptibility to malignant neoplasm of ovary**   ♀

     Z15.03   **Genetic susceptibility to malignant neoplasm of prostate**   ♂

     Z15.04   **Genetic susceptibility to malignant neoplasm of endometrium**   ♀

     Z15.09   **Genetic susceptibility to other malignant neoplasm**

√5th **Z15.8**   **Genetic susceptibility to other disease**

     Z15.81   **Genetic susceptibility to multiple endocrine neoplasia [MEN]**
> EXCLUDES 1   *multiple endocrine neoplasia [MEN] syndromes (E31.2-)*

     Z15.89   **Genetic susceptibility to other disease**

Resistance to antimicrobial drugs (Z16)

√4th **Z16**   **Resistance to antimicrobial drugs**
> NOTE   The codes in this category are provided for use as additional codes to identify the resistance and non-responsiveness of a condition to antimicrobial drugs.
>
> Code first the infection
>
> EXCLUDES 1   *Methicillin resistant Staphylococcus aureus infection (A49.02)*
> ~~Methicillin resistant Staphylococcus aureus infection in diseases classified elsewhere (B95.62)~~
> *Methicillin resistant Staphylococcus aureus pneumonia (J15.212)*
> *sepsis due to Methicillin resistant Staphylococcus aureus (A41.02)*

√5th **Z16.1**   **Resistance to beta lactam antibiotics**

     Z16.10   **Resistance to unspecified beta lactam antibiotics**   ▽

     Z16.11   **Resistance to penicillins**
> Resistance to amoxicillin
> Resistance to ampicillin

     Z16.12   **Extended spectrum beta lactamase (ESBL) resistance**
> EXCLUDES 2   ►*Methicillin resistant Staphylococcus aureus infection in diseases classified elsewhere (B95.62)*◄

     Z16.19   **Resistance to other specified beta lactam antibiotics**
> Resistance to cephalosporins

√5th **Z16.2**   **Resistance to other antibiotics**

     Z16.20   **Resistance to unspecified antibiotic**   ▽
> Resistance to antibiotics NOS

     Z16.21   **Resistance to vancomycin**

     Z16.22   **Resistance to vancomycin related antibiotics**

     Z16.23   **Resistance to quinolones and fluoroquinolones**

     Z16.24   **Resistance to multiple antibiotics**

     Z16.29   **Resistance to other single specified antibiotic**
> Resistance to aminoglycosides
> Resistance to macrolides
> Resistance to sulfonamides
> Resistance to tetracyclines

√5th **Z16.3**   **Resistance to other antimicrobial drugs**
> EXCLUDES 1   *resistance to antibiotics (Z16.1-, Z16.2-)*

     Z16.30   **Resistance to unspecified antimicrobial drugs**   ▽
> Drug resistance NOS

     Z16.31   **Resistance to antiparasitic drug(s)**
> Resistance to quinine and related compounds

     Z16.32   **Resistance to antifungal drug(s)**

     Z16.33   **Resistance to antiviral drug(s)**

√6th   **Z16.34**   **Resistance to antimycobacterial drug(s)**
> Resistance to tuberculostatics

     Z16.341   **Resistance to single antimycobacterial drug**
> Resistance to antimycobacterial drug NOS

     Z16.342   **Resistance to multiple antimycobacterial drugs**

     Z16.35   **Resistance to multiple antimicrobial drugs**
> EXCLUDES 1   *resistance to multiple antibiotics only (Z16.24)*

     Z16.39   **Resistance to other specified antimicrobial drug**

Estrogen receptor status (Z17)

√4th **Z17**   **Estrogen receptor status**
> Code first malignant neoplasm of breast (C50.-)

Z17.0   **Estrogen receptor positive status [ER+]**

Z17.1   **Estrogen receptor negative status [ER-]**

Retained foreign body fragment (Z18)

√4th **Z18**   **Retained foreign body fragments**
> INCLUDES   embedded fragment (status)
> embedded splinter (status)
> retained foreign body status
>
> EXCLUDES 1   *artificial joint prosthesis status (Z96.6-)*
> *foreign body accidentally left during a procedure (T81.5-)*
> *foreign body entering through orifice (T15-T19)*
> *in situ cardiac device (Z95.-)*
> *organ or tissue replaced by means other than transplant (Z96.-, Z97.-)*
> *organ or tissue replaced by transplant (Z94.-)*
> *personal history of retained foreign body fully removed (Z87.821)*
> *superficial foreign body (non-embedded splinter)—code to superficial foreign body, by site*
>
> **DEF:** Embedded or retained fragment, splinter, or foreign body; natural or synthetic; can cause infection.

√5th **Z18.0**   **Retained radioactive fragments**

     Z18.01   **Retained depleted uranium fragments**

     Z18.09   **Other retained radioactive fragments**
> Other retained depleted isotope fragments
> Retained nontherapeutic radioactive fragments

√5th **Z18.1**   **Retained metal fragments**
> EXCLUDES 1   *retained radioactive metal fragments (Z18.01-Z18.09)*

     Z18.10   **Retained metal fragments, unspecified**   ▽
> Retained metal fragment NOS

     Z18.11   **Retained magnetic metal fragments**

     Z18.12   **Retained nonmagnetic metal fragments**

N Newborn: 0   P Pediatric: 0-17   M Maternity: 12-55   A Adult: 15-124   NRS Nonroutine supply Dx   NCDx Noncancer Dx   PDx Primary Dx   ►◄ Revised Text   ● New Code   ▲ Revised Title

1184   ICD-10-CM 2018

Z18.2   Retained plastic fragments
Acrylics fragments
Diethylhexylphthalates fragments
Isocyanate fragments

✅5ᵗʰ **Z18.3   Retained organic fragments**

Z18.31   Retained animal quills or spines

Z18.32   Retained tooth

Z18.33   Retained wood fragments

Z18.39   Other retained organic fragments

✅5ᵗʰ **Z18.8   Other specified retained foreign body**

Z18.81   Retained glass fragments

Z18.83   Retained stone or crystalline fragments
Retained concrete or cement fragments

Z18.89   Other specified retained foreign body fragments

Z18.9   Retained foreign body fragments, unspecified material   ▽

Hormone sensitivity malignancy status (Z19)

✅4ᵗʰ **Z19   Hormone sensitivity malignancy status**
Code first malignant neoplasm — see Table of Neoplasms, by site, malignant

Z19.1   Hormone sensitive malignancy status

Z19.2   Hormone resistant malignancy status
Castrate resistant prostate malignancy status

Persons with potential health hazards related to communicable diseases (Z20-Z29)

✅4ᵗʰ **Z20   Contact with and (suspected) exposure to communicable diseases**
EXCLUDES 1   carrier of infectious disease (Z22.-)
diagnosed current infectious or parasitic disease—see Alphabetic Index
EXCLUDES 2   personal history of infectious and parasitic diseases (Z86.1-)

✅5ᵗʰ **Z20.0   Contact with and (suspected) exposure to intestinal infectious diseases**

Z20.01   Contact with and (suspected) exposure to intestinal infectious diseases due to Escherichia coli (E. coli)

Z20.09   Contact with and (suspected) exposure to other intestinal infectious diseases

Z20.1   Contact with and (suspected) exposure to tuberculosis

Z20.2   Contact with and (suspected) exposure to infections with a predominantly sexual mode of transmission

Z20.3   Contact with and (suspected) exposure to rabies

Z20.4   Contact with and (suspected) exposure to rubella

Z20.5   Contact with and (suspected) exposure to viral hepatitis

Z20.6   Contact with and (suspected) exposure to human immunodeficiency virus [HIV]
EXCLUDES 1   asymptomatic human immunodeficiency virus [HIV] HIV infection status (Z21)

Z20.7   Contact with and (suspected) exposure to pediculosis, acariasis and other infestations

✅5ᵗʰ **Z20.8   Contact with and (suspected) exposure to other communicable diseases**

✅6ᵗʰ **Z20.81   Contact with and (suspected) exposure to other bacterial communicable diseases**

Z20.810   Contact with and (suspected) exposure to anthrax

Z20.811   Contact with and (suspected) exposure to meningococcus

Z20.818   Contact with and (suspected) exposure to other bacterial communicable diseases

✅6ᵗʰ **Z20.82   Contact with and (suspected) exposure to other viral communicable diseases**

Z20.820   Contact with and (suspected) exposure to varicella

Z20.828   Contact with and (suspected) exposure to other viral communicable diseases

Z20.89   Contact with and (suspected) exposure to other communicable diseases

Z20.9   Contact with and (suspected) exposure to unspecified communicable disease   ▽

Z21   Asymptomatic human immunodeficiency virus [HIV] infection status
HIV positive NOS
Code first human immunodeficiency virus [HIV] disease complicating pregnancy, childbirth and the puerperium, if applicable (O98.7-)
EXCLUDES 1   acquired immunodeficiency syndrome (B20)
contact with human immunodeficiency virus [HIV] (Z20.6)
exposure to human immunodeficiency virus [HIV] (Z20.6)
human immunodeficiency virus [HIV] disease (B20)
inconclusive laboratory evidence of human immunodeficiency virus [HIV] (R75)
DEF: Phase of human immunodeficiency virus (HIV) infection with no clinical symptoms; may last for 10 years or more.

✅4ᵗʰ **Z22   Carrier of infectious disease**
INCLUDES   colonization status
suspected carrier
EXCLUDES 2   carrier of viral hepatitis (B18.-)

Z22.0   Carrier of typhoid

Z22.1   Carrier of other intestinal infectious diseases

Z22.2   Carrier of diphtheria

✅5ᵗʰ **Z22.3   Carrier of other specified bacterial diseases**

Z22.31   Carrier of bacterial disease due to meningococci

✅6ᵗʰ **Z22.32   Carrier of bacterial disease due to staphylococci**

Z22.321   Carrier or suspected carrier of Methicillin susceptible Staphylococcus aureus
MSSA colonization

Z22.322   Carrier or suspected carrier of Methicillin resistant Staphylococcus aureus
MRSA colonization

✅6ᵗʰ **Z22.33   Carrier of bacterial disease due to streptococci**

Z22.330   Carrier of Group B streptococcus
EXCLUDES 1   carrier of streptococcus group B (GBS) complicating pregnancy, childbirth and the puerperium (O99.82-)

Z22.338   Carrier of other streptococcus

Z22.39   Carrier of other specified bacterial diseases

Z22.4   Carrier of infections with a predominantly sexual mode of transmission

Z22.6   Carrier of human T-lymphotropic virus type-1 [HTLV-1] infection

Z22.8   Carrier of other infectious diseases

Z22.9   Carrier of infectious disease, unspecified   ▽

Z23   Encounter for immunization
Code first any routine childhood examination
NOTE   Procedure codes are required to identify the types of immunizations given

✅4ᵗʰ **Z28   Immunization not carried out and underimmunization status**
INCLUDES   vaccination not carried out

✅5ᵗʰ **Z28.0   Immunization not carried out because of contraindication**

Z28.01   Immunization not carried out because of acute illness of patient

Z28.02   Immunization not carried out because of chronic illness or condition of patient

Z28.03   Immunization not carried out because of immune compromised state of patient

Z28.04   Immunization not carried out because of patient allergy to vaccine or component

Z28.09   Immunization not carried out because of other contraindication

Z28.1   Immunization not carried out because of patient decision for reasons of belief or group pressure
Immunization not carried out because of religious belief

✅5ᵗʰ **Z28.2   Immunization not carried out because of patient decision for other and unspecified reason**

Z28.20   Immunization not carried out because of patient decision for unspecified reason   ▽

Z28.21   Immunization not carried out because of patient refusal

Z28.29   Immunization not carried out because of patient decision for other reason

Z28.3   Underimmunization status
Delinquent immunization status
Lapsed immunization schedule status

✅ Additional Character Req   ✅ˣ7ᵗʰ Placeholder Alert   Case-Mix Diagnosis   Manifestation   ▽ Unspecified Dx   *EXCLUDES 1* Not coded here   *EXCLUDES 2* Not included here

ICD-10-CM 2018   1185

Chapter 21. Factors Influencing Health Status and Contact with Health Services

Z28.8–Z31.61

✓5ᵗʰ **Z28.8 Immunization not carried out for other reason**

   Z28.81 Immunization not carried out due to patient having had the disease

   Z28.82 Immunization not carried out because of caregiver refusal
     Immunization not carried out because of guardian refusal
     Immunization not carried out because of parent refusal
     EXCLUDES 1 *immunization not carried out because of caregiver refusal because of religious belief (Z28.1)*

   Z28.89 Immunization not carried out for other reason

  Z28.9 Immunization not carried out for unspecified reason ▽

✓4ᵗʰ **Z29 Encounter for other prophylactic measures**
  EXCLUDES 1 *desensitization to allergens (Z51.6)*
     prophylactic surgery (Z40.-)

✓5ᵗʰ **Z29.1 Encounter for prophylactic immunotherapy**
  Encounter for administration of immunoglobulin

   Z29.11 Encounter for prophylactic immunotherapy for respiratory syncytial virus (RSV)

   Z29.12 Encounter for prophylactic antivenin

   Z29.13 Encounter for prophylactic Rho(D) immune globulin

   Z29.14 Encounter for prophylactic rabies immune globin

  Z29.3 Encounter for prophylactic fluoride **administration**

  Z29.8 Encounter for other **specified prophylactic measures**

  Z29.9 Encounter for prophylactic measures, unspecified ▽

Persons encountering health services in circumstances related to reproduction (Z30-Z39)

✓4ᵗʰ **Z30 Encounter for contraceptive management**
  DEF: Contraceptive management to prevent pregnancy; methods include oral medications, intrauterine devices, and surgical procedures for males and females (sterilization).

✓5ᵗʰ **Z30.0 Encounter for general counseling and advice on** contraception

✓6ᵗʰ **Z30.01 Encounter for** initial prescription **of contraceptives**
     EXCLUDES 1 *encounter for surveillance of contraceptives (Z30.4-)*

    Z30.011 Encounter for initial prescription **of contraceptive pills** ♀

    Z30.012 Encounter for prescription of emergency **contraception** ♀
      Encounter for postcoital contraception

    Z30.013 Encounter for initial prescription of injectable **contraceptive** ♀

    Z30.014 Encounter for initial prescription of intrauterine **contraceptive device** ♀
      EXCLUDES 1 *encounter for insertion of intrauterine contraceptive device (Z30.430, Z30.432)*

    Z30.015 Encounter for initial prescription of vaginal ring hormonal **contraceptive**

    Z30.016 Encounter for initial prescription of transdermal patch hormonal **contraceptive device**

    Z30.017 Encounter for initial prescription of implantable subdermal **contraceptive**

    Z30.018 Encounter for initial prescription of other **contraceptives** ♀
      Encounter for initial prescription of barrier contraception
      Encounter for initial prescription of diaphragm

    Z30.019 Encounter for initial prescription of contraceptives, unspecified ♀▽

   Z30.02 Counseling and instruction in natural family planning **to avoid pregnancy**

   Z30.09 Encounter for other general counseling and advice on contraception
    Encounter for family planning advice NOS

  Z30.2 Encounter for sterilization

✓5ᵗʰ **Z30.4 Encounter for** surveillance of contraceptives

  Z30.40 Encounter for surveillance of contraceptives, unspecified ▽

  Z30.41 Encounter for surveillance of contraceptive pills ♀
    Encounter for repeat prescription for contraceptive pill

  Z30.42 Encounter for surveillance of injectable **contraceptive** ♀

✓6ᵗʰ **Z30.43 Encounter for surveillance of** intrauterine **contraceptive device**

    Z30.430 Encounter for insertion **of intrauterine contraceptive device** ♀

    Z30.431 Encounter for routine checking **of intrauterine contraceptive device** ♀

    Z30.432 Encounter for removal **of intrauterine contraceptive device** ♀

    Z30.433 Encounter for removal and reinsertion **of intrauterine contraceptive device**
      Encounter for replacement of intrauterine contraceptive device

  Z30.44 Encounter for surveillance of vaginal ring hormonal **contraceptive device** ♀

  Z30.45 Encounter for surveillance of transdermal patch hormonal **contraceptive device** ♀

  Z30.46 Encounter for surveillance of implantable subdermal **contraceptive** ♀
    Encounter for checking, reinsertion or removal of implantable subdermal contraceptive

  Z30.49 Encounter for surveillance of other contraceptives ♀
    Encounter for surveillance of barrier contraception
    Encounter for surveillance of diaphragm

 Z30.8 Encounter for other contraceptive management
  Encounter for postvasectomy sperm count
  Encounter for routine examination for contraceptive maintenance
  EXCLUDES 1 *sperm count following sterilization reversal (Z31.42)*
     sperm count for fertility testing (Z31.41)

 Z30.9 Encounter for contraceptive management, unspecified ▽

✓4ᵗʰ **Z31 Encounter for procreative management**
  EXCLUDES 1 *complications associated with artificial fertilization (N98.-)*
     female infertility (N97.-)
     male infertility (N46.-)

 Z31.0 Encounter for reversal of previous sterilization

✓5ᵗʰ **Z31.4 Encounter for** procreative investigation and testing
  EXCLUDES 1 *postvasectomy sperm count (Z30.8)*

  Z31.41 Encounter for fertility testing
    Encounter for fallopian tube patency testing
    Encounter for sperm count for fertility testing

  Z31.42 Aftercare **following** sterilization reversal
    Sperm count following sterilization reversal

✓6ᵗʰ **Z31.43 Encounter for genetic testing of** female **for procreative management**
    Use additional code for recurrent pregnancy loss, if applicable (N96, O26.2-)
    EXCLUDES 1 *nonprocreative genetic testing (Z13.7-)*

    Z31.430 Encounter of female for testing for genetic disease carrier status **for procreative management** ♀

    Z31.438 Encounter for other genetic testing of female for procreative management ♀

✓6ᵗʰ **Z31.44 Encounter for genetic testing of** male **for procreative management**
    EXCLUDES 1 *nonprocreative genetic testing (Z13.7-)*

    Z31.440 Encounter of male for testing for genetic disease carrier status **for procreative management** ♂

    Z31.441 Encounter for testing of male partner of patient with recurrent pregnancy loss Ⓐ♂

    Z31.448 Encounter for other genetic testing of male for procreative management Ⓐ♂

  Z31.49 Encounter for other procreative investigation and testing

▲ **Z31.5 Encounter for procreative genetic counseling**

✓5ᵗʰ **Z31.6 Encounter for general counseling and advice on procreation**

  Z31.61 Procreative counseling and advice using natural family planning

Ⓝ Newborn: 0   Ⓟ Pediatric: 0-17   Ⓜ Maternity: 12-55   Ⓐ Adult: 15-124   **NRS** Nonroutine supply Dx   **NC Dx** Noncancer Dx   **PDx** Primary Dx   ▶◀ Revised Text   ● New Code   ▲ Revised Title

1186   ICD-10-CM 2018

Z31.62 Encounter for fertility preservation counseling
Encounter for fertility preservation counseling prior to cancer therapy
Encounter for fertility preservation counseling prior to surgical removal of gonads

Z31.69 Encounter for other general counseling and advice on procreation

Z31.7 Encounter for procreative management and counseling for gestational carrier
EXCLUDES 1 pregnant state, gestational carrier (Z33.3)

✓5th **Z31.8 Encounter for other procreative management**

Z31.81 Encounter for male factor infertility in female patient ♀

Z31.82 Encounter for Rh incompatibility status ♀
AHA: 2015, 3Q, 40; 2014, 4Q, 17

Z31.83 Encounter for assisted reproductive fertility procedure cycle ♀
Patient undergoing in vitro fertilization cycle
Use additional code to identify the type of infertility
EXCLUDES 1 pre-cycle diagnosis and testing—code to reason for encounter

Z31.84 Encounter for fertility preservation procedure
Encounter for fertility preservation procedure prior to cancer therapy
Encounter for fertility preservation procedure prior to surgical removal of gonads

Z31.89 Encounter for other procreative management

Z31.9 Encounter for procreative management, unspecified ▽

✓4th **Z32 Encounter for pregnancy test and childbirth and childcare instruction**

✓5th **Z32.0 Encounter for pregnancy test**

Z32.00 Encounter for pregnancy test, result unknown ♀
Encounter for pregnancy test NOS

Z32.01 Encounter for pregnancy test, result positive ♀

Z32.02 Encounter for pregnancy test, result negative ♀

Z32.2 Encounter for childbirth instruction

Z32.3 Encounter for childcare instruction
Encounter for prenatal or postpartum childcare instruction

✓4th **Z33 Pregnant state**

Z33.1 Pregnant state, incidental ♀
Pregnant state NOS
EXCLUDES 1 complications of pregnancy (O00-O9A)
pregnant state, gestational carrier (Z33.3)

Z33.2 Encounter for elective termination of pregnancy ♀
EXCLUDES 1 early fetal death with retention of dead fetus (O02.1)
late fetal death (O36.4)
spontaneous abortion (O03)

Z33.3 Pregnant state, gestational carrier ♀
EXCLUDES 1 encounter for procreative management and counseling for gestational carrier (Z31.7)

✓4th **Z34 Encounter for supervision of normal pregnancy**
EXCLUDES 1 any complication of pregnancy (O00-O9A)
encounter for pregnancy test (Z32.0-)
encounter for supervision of high risk pregnancy (O09.-)
AHA: 2014, 4Q, 17

✓5th **Z34.0 Encounter for supervision of normal first pregnancy**

Z34.00 Encounter for supervision of normal first pregnancy, unspecified trimester ♀ ▽

Z34.01 Encounter for supervision of normal first pregnancy, first trimester ♀

Z34.02 Encounter for supervision of normal first pregnancy, second trimester ♀

Z34.03 Encounter for supervision of normal first pregnancy, third trimester ♀

✓5th **Z34.8 Encounter for supervision of other normal pregnancy**

Z34.80 Encounter for supervision of other normal pregnancy, unspecified trimester ♀ ▽

Z34.81 Encounter for supervision of other normal pregnancy, first trimester ♀

Z34.82 Encounter for supervision of other normal pregnancy, second trimester ♀

Z34.83 Encounter for supervision of other normal pregnancy, third trimester ♀

✓5th **Z34.9 Encounter for supervision of normal pregnancy, unspecified**

Z34.90 Encounter for supervision of normal pregnancy, unspecified, unspecified trimester ♀ ▽

Z34.91 Encounter for supervision of normal pregnancy, unspecified, first trimester ♀

Z34.92 Encounter for supervision of normal pregnancy, unspecified, second trimester ♀

Z34.93 Encounter for supervision of normal pregnancy, unspecified, third trimester ♀

✓4th **Z36 Encounter for antenatal screening of mother**
INCLUDES ► encounter for placental sample (taken vaginally)
screening is the testing for disease or disease precursors in asymptomatic individuals so that early detection and treatment can be provided for those who test positive for the disease ◄
EXCLUDES 1 abnormal findings on antenatal screening of mother (O28.-)
diagnostic examination—code to sign or symptom
encounter for suspected maternal and fetal conditions ruled out (Z03.7-)
suspected fetal condition affecting management of pregnancy—code to condition in Chapter 15
EXCLUDES 2 ► abnormal findings on antenatal screening of mother (O28.-) ◄
genetic counseling and testing (Z31.43-, Z31.5)
routine prenatal care (Z34)

Z36.0 Encounter for antenatal screening for chromosomal anomalies

Z36.1 Encounter for antenatal screening for raised alphafetoprotein level
Encounter for antenatal screening for elevated maternal serum alphafetoprotein level

Z36.2 Encounter for other antenatal screening follow-up
Non-visualized anatomy on a previous scan

Z36.3 Encounter for antenatal screening for malformations
Screening for a suspected anomaly

Z36.4 Encounter for antenatal screening for fetal growth retardation
Intrauterine growth restriction (IUGR)/small-for-dates

Z36.5 Encounter for antenatal screening for isoimmunization

✓5th **Z36.8 Encounter for other antenatal screening**

Z36.81 Encounter for antenatal screening for hydrops fetalis

Z36.82 Encounter for antenatal screening for nuchal translucency

Z36.83 Encounter for fetal screening for congenital cardiac abnormalities

Z36.84 Encounter for antenatal screening for fetal lung maturity

Z36.85 Encounter for antenatal screening for Streptococcus B

Z36.86 Encounter for antenatal screening for cervical length
Screening for risk of pre-term labor

Z36.87 Encounter for antenatal screening for uncertain dates

Z36.88 Encounter for antenatal screening for fetal macrosomia
Screening for large-for-dates

Z36.89 Encounter for other specified antenatal screening

Z36.8A Encounter for antenatal screening for other genetic defects

Z36.9 Encounter for antenatal screening, unspecified ▽

✓4th **Z3A Weeks of gestation**
NOTE Codes from category Z3A are for use, only on the maternal record, to indicate the weeks of gestation of the pregnancy, if known.
Code first complications of pregnancy, childbirth and the puerperium ►(O09-O9A)◄
AHA: 2016, 2Q, 34; 2014, 3Q, 17; 2014, 2Q, 9; 2013, 2Q, 33

✓5th **Z3A.0 Weeks of gestation of pregnancy, unspecified or less than 10 weeks**

Z3A.00 Weeks of gestation of pregnancy not specified ♀

Z3A.01 Less than 8 weeks gestation of pregnancy ♀

Z3A.08 8 weeks gestation of pregnancy ♀

Z3A.09 9 weeks gestation of pregnancy ♀

✓5th **Z3A.1 Weeks of gestation of pregnancy, weeks 10-19**

Z3A.10 10 weeks gestation of pregnancy ♀

Z3A.11 11 weeks gestation of pregnancy ♀

Z3A.12 12 weeks gestation of pregnancy ♀

Z3A.13 13 weeks gestation of pregnancy ♀

Z3A.14 14 weeks gestation of pregnancy ♀

Z3A.15 15 weeks **gestation of pregnancy** Ⓜ♀
Z3A.16 16 weeks **gestation of pregnancy** Ⓜ♀
Z3A.17 17 weeks **gestation of pregnancy** Ⓜ♀
Z3A.18 18 weeks **gestation of pregnancy** Ⓜ♀
Z3A.19 19 weeks **gestation of pregnancy** Ⓜ♀

✓5ᵗʰ **Z3A.2 Weeks of gestation of pregnancy, weeks 20-29**
Z3A.20 20 weeks **gestation of pregnancy** Ⓜ♀
Z3A.21 21 weeks **gestation of pregnancy** Ⓜ♀
Z3A.22 22 weeks **gestation of pregnancy** Ⓜ♀
Z3A.23 23 weeks **gestation of pregnancy** Ⓜ♀
Z3A.24 24 weeks **gestation of pregnancy** Ⓜ♀
Z3A.25 25 weeks **gestation of pregnancy** Ⓜ♀
Z3A.26 26 weeks **gestation of pregnancy** Ⓜ♀
Z3A.27 27 weeks **gestation of pregnancy** Ⓜ♀
Z3A.28 28 weeks **gestation of pregnancy** Ⓜ♀
Z3A.29 29 weeks **gestation of pregnancy** Ⓜ♀

✓5ᵗʰ **Z3A.3 Weeks of gestation of pregnancy, weeks 30-39**
Z3A.30 30 weeks **gestation of pregnancy** Ⓜ♀
Z3A.31 31 weeks **gestation of pregnancy** Ⓜ♀
Z3A.32 32 weeks **gestation of pregnancy** Ⓜ♀
Z3A.33 33 weeks **gestation of pregnancy** Ⓜ♀
Z3A.34 34 weeks **gestation of pregnancy** Ⓜ♀
Z3A.35 35 weeks **gestation of pregnancy** Ⓜ♀
Z3A.36 36 weeks **gestation of pregnancy** Ⓜ♀
Z3A.37 37 weeks **gestation of pregnancy** Ⓜ♀
Z3A.38 38 weeks **gestation of pregnancy** Ⓜ♀
Z3A.39 39 weeks **gestation of pregnancy** Ⓜ♀

✓5ᵗʰ **Z3A.4 Weeks of gestation of pregnancy, weeks 40 or greater**
AHA: 2014, 4Q, 23
Z3A.40 40 weeks **gestation of pregnancy** Ⓜ♀
Z3A.41 41 weeks **gestation of pregnancy** Ⓜ♀
Z3A.42 42 weeks **gestation of pregnancy** Ⓜ♀
Z3A.49 Greater than 42 weeks **gestation of pregnancy** Ⓜ♀

✓4ᵗʰ **Z37 Outcome of delivery**
This category is intended for use as an additional code to identify the outcome of delivery on the mother's record. It is not for use on the newborn record.
EXCLUDES 1 stillbirth (P95)
Z37.0 Single live birth Ⓜ♀
AHA: 2016, 2Q, 34; 2014, 2Q, 9
Z37.1 Single stillbirth Ⓜ♀
Z37.2 Twins, both liveborn Ⓜ♀
Z37.3 Twins, one liveborn and one stillborn Ⓜ♀
Z37.4 Twins, both stillborn Ⓜ♀
✓5ᵗʰ **Z37.5 Other multiple births, all liveborn**
Z37.50 Multiple births, unspecified, all liveborn Ⓜ♀▽
Z37.51 Triplets, all liveborn Ⓜ♀
Z37.52 Quadruplets, all liveborn Ⓜ♀
Z37.53 Quintuplets, all liveborn Ⓜ♀
Z37.54 Sextuplets, all liveborn Ⓜ♀
Z37.59 Other multiple births, all liveborn Ⓜ♀
✓5ᵗʰ **Z37.6 Other multiple births, some liveborn**
Z37.60 Multiple births, unspecified, some liveborn Ⓜ♀▽
Z37.61 Triplets, some liveborn Ⓜ♀
Z37.62 Quadruplets, some liveborn Ⓜ♀
Z37.63 Quintuplets, some liveborn Ⓜ♀
Z37.64 Sextuplets, some liveborn Ⓜ♀
Z37.69 Other multiple births, some liveborn Ⓜ♀
Z37.7 Other multiple births, all stillborn Ⓜ♀
Z37.9 Outcome of delivery, unspecified Ⓜ♀▽
Multiple birth NOS
Single birth NOS

✓4ᵗʰ **Z38 Liveborn infants according to place of birth and type of delivery**
This category is for use as the principal code on the initial record of a newborn baby. It is to be used for the initial birth record only. It is not to be used on the mother's record.
AHA: 2017, 2Q, 5-7; 2016, 3Q, 18; 2015, 2Q, 15
✓5ᵗʰ **Z38.0 Single liveborn infant, born in hospital**
Single liveborn infant, born in birthing center or other health care facility
Z38.00 Single liveborn infant, delivered vaginally PDx Ⓝ

Z38.01 Single liveborn infant, delivered by cesarean PDx Ⓝ
Z38.1 Single liveborn infant, born outside hospital PDx Ⓝ
Z38.2 Single liveborn infant, unspecified as to place of birth PDx Ⓝ▽
Single liveborn infant NOS
✓5ᵗʰ **Z38.3 Twin liveborn infant, born in hospital**
Z38.30 Twin liveborn infant, delivered vaginally PDx Ⓝ
Z38.31 Twin liveborn infant, delivered by cesarean PDx Ⓝ
Z38.4 Twin liveborn infant, born outside hospital PDx Ⓝ
Z38.5 Twin liveborn infant, unspecified as to place of birth PDx Ⓝ▽
✓5ᵗʰ **Z38.6 Other multiple liveborn infant, born in hospital**
Z38.61 Triplet liveborn infant, delivered vaginally PDx Ⓝ
Z38.62 Triplet liveborn infant, delivered by cesarean PDx Ⓝ
Z38.63 Quadruplet liveborn infant, delivered vaginally PDx Ⓝ
Z38.64 Quadruplet liveborn infant, delivered by cesarean PDx Ⓝ
Z38.65 Quintuplet liveborn infant, delivered vaginally PDx Ⓝ
Z38.66 Quintuplet liveborn infant, delivered by cesarean PDx Ⓝ
Z38.68 Other multiple liveborn infant, delivered vaginally PDx Ⓝ
Z38.69 Other multiple liveborn infant, delivered by cesarean PDx Ⓝ
Z38.7 Other multiple liveborn infant, born outside hospital PDx Ⓝ
Z38.8 Other multiple liveborn infant, unspecified as to place of birth PDx Ⓝ▽

✓4ᵗʰ **Z39 Encounter for maternal postpartum care and examination**
Z39.0 Encounter for care and examination of mother immediately after delivery PDx Ⓜ♀
Care and observation in uncomplicated cases when the delivery occurs outside a healthcare facility
EXCLUDES 1 care for postpartum complication—see Alphabetic index
Z39.1 Encounter for care and examination of lactating mother PDx Ⓜ♀
Encounter for supervision of lactation
EXCLUDES 1 disorders of lactation (O92.-)
Z39.2 Encounter for routine postpartum follow-up PDx Ⓜ♀

Encounters for other specific health care (Z40-Z53)

Categories Z40-Z53 are intended for use to indicate a reason for care. They may be used for patients who have already been treated for a disease or injury, but who are receiving aftercare or prophylactic care, or care to consolidate the treatment, or to deal with a residual state.
EXCLUDES 2 follow-up examination for medical surveillance after treatment (Z08-Z09)

✓4ᵗʰ **Z40 Encounter for prophylactic surgery**
EXCLUDES 1 organ donations (Z52.-)
therapeutic organ removal—code to condition
✓5ᵗʰ **Z40.0 Encounter for prophylactic surgery for risk factors related to malignant neoplasms**
Admission for prophylactic organ removal
Use additional code to identify risk factor
Z40.00 Encounter for prophylactic removal of unspecified organ ▽
Z40.01 Encounter for prophylactic removal of breast
TIP: Use during the surgical encounter for removal of the breast; do not assign to indicate aftercare of prophylactic breast removal.
▲ Z40.02 Encounter for prophylactic removal of ovary(s) ♀
▶Encounter for prophylactic removal of ovary(s) and fallopian tube(s)◀
● Z40.03 Encounter for prophylactic removal of fallopian tube(s)
Z40.09 Encounter for prophylactic removal of other organ
Z40.8 Encounter for other prophylactic surgery
Z40.9 Encounter for prophylactic surgery, unspecified ▽

✓4ᵗʰ Z41   Encounter for procedures for purposes other than remedying health state

Z41.1   Encounter for cosmetic surgery
Encounter for cosmetic breast implant
Encounter for cosmetic procedure
EXCLUDES 1   *encounter for plastic and reconstructive surgery following medical procedure or healed injury (Z42.-)*
encounter for post-mastectomy breast implantation (Z42.1)

Z41.2   Encounter for routine and ritual male circumcision   ♂

Z41.3   Encounter for ear piercing

Z41.8   Encounter for other procedures for purposes other than remedying health state

Z41.9   Encounter for procedure for purposes other than   ▽
remedying health state, unspecified

✓4ᵗʰ Z42   Encounter for plastic and reconstructive surgery following medical procedure or healed injury
EXCLUDES 1   *encounter for cosmetic plastic surgery (Z41.1)*
encounter for plastic surgery for treatment of current injury—code to relevent injury

Z42.1   Encounter for breast reconstruction following   PDx A
mastectomy
EXCLUDES 1   *deformity and disproportion of reconstructed breast (N65.1-)*

Z42.8   Encounter for other plastic and reconstructive surgery   PDx
following medical procedure or healed injury
AHA: 2017, 1Q, 42

✓4ᵗʰ Z43   Encounter for attention to artificial openings
INCLUDES   closure of artificial openings
passage of sounds or bougies through artificial openings
reforming artificial openings
removal of catheter from artificial openings
toilet or cleansing of artificial openings
EXCLUDES 1   ~~artificial opening status only, without need for care (Z93.-)~~
complications of external stoma (J95.0-, K94.-, N99.5-)
EXCLUDES 2   *fitting and adjustment of prosthetic and other devices (Z44-Z46)*
TIP: Use only for routine care of the artificial opening.

Z43.0   Encounter for attention to tracheostomy   NRS

Z43.1   Encounter for attention to gastrostomy
EXCLUDES 2   ▶*artificial opening status only, without need for care (Z93.-)*◀

Z43.2   Encounter for attention to ileostomy

Z43.3   Encounter for attention to colostomy

Z43.4   Encounter for attention to other artificial openings of
digestive tract

Z43.5   Encounter for attention to cystostomy   NRS

Z43.6   Encounter for attention to other artificial openings   NRS
of urinary tract
Encounter for attention to nephrostomy
Encounter for attention to ureterostomy
Encounter for attention to urethrostomy

Z43.7   Encounter for attention to artificial vagina

Z43.8   Encounter for attention to other artificial openings

Z43.9   Encounter for attention to unspecified artificial opening   ▽

✓4ᵗʰ Z44   Encounter for fitting and adjustment of external prosthetic device
INCLUDES   removal or replacement of external prosthetic device
EXCLUDES 1   *malfunction or other complications of device—see Alphabetical Index*
presence of prosthetic device (Z97.-)

✓5ᵗʰ Z44.0   Encounter for fitting and adjustment of artificial arm

✓6ᵗʰ Z44.00   Encounter for fitting and adjustment of unspecified
artificial arm

Z44.001   Encounter for fitting and adjustment   ▽
of unspecified right **artificial arm**

Z44.002   Encounter for fitting and adjustment   ▽
of unspecified left **artificial arm**

Z44.009   Encounter for fitting and adjustment of ▽
unspecified artificial arm, unspecified arm

✓6ᵗʰ Z44.01   Encounter for fitting and adjustment of complete
artificial arm

**Z44.011   Encounter for fitting and adjustment of
complete** right **artificial arm**

**Z44.012   Encounter for fitting and adjustment of
complete** left **artificial arm**

Z44.019   Encounter for fitting and adjustment of ▽
complete artificial arm, unspecified arm

✓6ᵗʰ Z44.02   Encounter for fitting and adjustment of partial
artificial arm

**Z44.021   Encounter for fitting and adjustment of
partial artificial** right **arm**

**Z44.022   Encounter for fitting and adjustment of
partial artificial** left **arm**

Z44.029   Encounter for fitting and adjustment of ▽
partial artificial arm, unspecified arm

✓5ᵗʰ Z44.1   Encounter for fitting and adjustment of artificial leg

✓6ᵗʰ Z44.10   Encounter for fitting and adjustment of unspecified
artificial leg

Z44.101   Encounter for fitting and adjustment of ▽
unspecified right **artificial leg**

Z44.102   Encounter for fitting and adjustment of ▽
unspecified left **artificial leg**

Z44.109   Encounter for fitting and adjustment of ▽
unspecified artificial leg, unspecified leg

✓6ᵗʰ Z44.11   Encounter for fitting and adjustment of complete
artificial leg

**Z44.111   Encounter for fitting and adjustment of
complete** right **artificial leg**

**Z44.112   Encounter for fitting and adjustment of
complete** left **artificial leg**

Z44.119   Encounter for fitting and adjustment of ▽
complete artificial leg, unspecified leg

✓6ᵗʰ Z44.12   Encounter for fitting and adjustment of partial
artificial leg

**Z44.121   Encounter for fitting and adjustment of
partial artificial** right **leg**

**Z44.122   Encounter for fitting and adjustment of
partial artificial** left **leg**

Z44.129   Encounter for fitting and adjustment ▽
of partial artificial leg, unspecified leg

✓5ᵗʰ Z44.2   Encounter for fitting and adjustment of artificial eye
EXCLUDES 1   *mechanical complication of ocular prosthesis (T85.3)*

Z44.20   Encounter for fitting and adjustment of artificial ▽
eye, unspecified

**Z44.21   Encounter for fitting and adjustment of artificial
right eye**

Z44.22   Encounter for fitting and adjustment of artificial left
eye

✓5ᵗʰ Z44.3   Encounter for fitting and adjustment of external breast
prosthesis
EXCLUDES 1   *complications of breast implant (T85.4-)*
encounter for adjustment or removal of breast implant (Z45.81-)
encounter for initial breast implant insertion for cosmetic breast augmentation (Z41.1)
encounter for breast reconstruction following mastectomy (Z42.1)

Z44.30   Encounter for fitting and adjustment of external ▽
breast prosthesis, unspecified breast

**Z44.31   Encounter for fitting and adjustment of external
right breast prosthesis**

Z44.32   Encounter for fitting and adjustment of external
left **breast prosthesis**

**Z44.8   Encounter for fitting and adjustment of other external
prosthetic devices**

Z44.9   Encounter for fitting and adjustment of unspecified ▽
external prosthetic device

✓ Additional Character Req   ✓ₓ7ᵗʰ Placeholder Alert   Case-Mix Diagnosis   Manifestation   ▽ Unspecified Dx   *EXCLUDES 1* Not coded here   *EXCLUDES 2* Not included here

ICD-10-CM 2018   **1189**

✓4ᵗʰ **Z45　Encounter for adjustment and management of implanted device**
　INCLUDES　removal or replacement of implanted device
　EXCLUDES1　malfunction or other complications of device – see Alphabetical Index
　　　~~presence of prosthetic and other devices (Z95-Z97)~~
　EXCLUDES2　encounter for fitting and adjustment of non-implanted device (Z46.-)

✓5ᵗʰ **Z45.0　Encounter for adjustment and management of cardiac device**
　　TIP: Do not assign to indicate the presence of a pacemaker; these codes are reserved for indicating services provided to adjust the pacemaker rate, battery, and other management of the device, which generally are not performed by post-acute care providers.

　✓6ᵗʰ **Z45.01　Encounter for adjustment and management of cardiac pacemaker**
　　　Encounter for adjustment and management of cardiac resynchronization therapy pacemaker (CRT-P)
　　　EXCLUDES1　encounter for adjustment and management of automatic implantable cardiac defibrillator with synchronous cardiac pacemaker (Z45.02)

　　Z45.010　Encounter for checking and testing of cardiac pacemaker pulse generator [battery]
　　　Encounter for replacing cardiac pacemaker pulse generator [battery]

　　Z45.018　Encounter for adjustment and management of other part of cardiac pacemaker
　　　EXCLUDES2　▶presence of prosthetic and other devices (Z95-Z97)◀

　Z45.02　Encounter for adjustment and management of automatic implantable cardiac defibrillator
　　Encounter for adjustment and management of automatic implantable cardiac defibrillator with synchronous cardiac pacemaker
　　Encounter for adjustment and management of cardiac resynchronization therapy defibrillator (CRT-D)

　Z45.09　Encounter for adjustment and management of other cardiac device

Z45.1　Encounter for adjustment and management of infusion pump

Z45.2　Encounter for adjustment and management of vascular access device
　Encounter for adjustment and management of vascular catheters
　EXCLUDES1　encounter for adjustment and management of renal dialysis catheter (Z49.01)

✓5ᵗʰ **Z45.3　Encounter for adjustment and management of implanted devices of the special senses**

　Z45.31　Encounter for adjustment and management of implanted visual substitution device

　✓6ᵗʰ **Z45.32　Encounter for adjustment and management of implanted hearing device**
　　　EXCLUDES1　encounter for fitting and adjustment of hearing aide (Z46.1)

　　Z45.320　Encounter for adjustment and management of bone conduction device

　　Z45.321　Encounter for adjustment and management of cochlear device

　　Z45.328　Encounter for adjustment and management of other implanted hearing device

✓5ᵗʰ **Z45.4　Encounter for adjustment and management of implanted nervous system device**

　Z45.41　Encounter for adjustment and management of cerebrospinal fluid drainage device
　　Encounter for adjustment and management of cerebral ventricular (communicating) shunt

　Z45.42　Encounter for adjustment and management of neuropacemaker (brain) (peripheral nerve) (spinal cord)

　Z45.49　Encounter for adjustment and management of other implanted nervous system device
　　AHA: 2014, 3Q, 19

✓5ᵗʰ **Z45.8　Encounter for adjustment and management of other implanted devices**

　✓6ᵗʰ **Z45.81　Encounter for adjustment or removal of breast implant**
　　　Encounter for elective implant exchange (different material) (different size)
　　　Encounter removal of tissue expander without synchronous insertion of permanent implant
　　　EXCLUDES1　complications of breast implant (T85.4-)
　　　　encounter for initial breast implant insertion for cosmetic breast augmentation (Z41.1)
　　　　encounter for breast reconstruction following mastectomy (Z42.1)

　　Z45.811　Encounter for adjustment or removal of right breast implant

　　Z45.812　Encounter for adjustment or removal of left breast implant

　　Z45.819　Encounter for adjustment or removal of unspecified breast implant　▽

　Z45.82　Encounter for adjustment or removal of myringotomy device (stent) (tube)

　Z45.89　Encounter for adjustment and management of other implanted devices
　　AHA: 2014, 4Q, 26-28

Z45.9　Encounter for adjustment and management of unspecified implanted device　▽

✓4ᵗʰ **Z46　Encounter for fitting and adjustment of other devices**
　INCLUDES　removal or replacement of other device
　EXCLUDES1　malfunction or other complications of device—see Alphabetical Index
　EXCLUDES2　encounter for fitting and management of implanted devices (Z45.-)
　　　issue of repeat prescription only (Z76.0)
　　　presence of prosthetic and other devices (Z95-Z97)

Z46.0　Encounter for fitting and adjustment of spectacles and contact lenses

Z46.1　Encounter for fitting and adjustment of hearing aid
　EXCLUDES1　encounter for adjustment and management of implanted hearing device (Z45.32-)

Z46.2　Encounter for fitting and adjustment of other devices related to nervous system and special senses
　EXCLUDES2　encounter for adjustment and management of implanted nervous system device (Z45.4-)
　　　encounter for adjustment and management of implanted visual substitution device (Z45.31)

Z46.3　Encounter for fitting and adjustment of dental prosthetic device
　Encounter for fitting and adjustment of dentures

Z46.4　Encounter for fitting and adjustment of orthodontic device

✓5ᵗʰ **Z46.5　Encounter for fitting and adjustment of other gastrointestinal appliance and device**
　EXCLUDES1　encounter for attention to artificial openings of digestive tract (Z43.1-Z43.4)

　Z46.51　Encounter for fitting and adjustment of gastric lap band

　Z46.59　Encounter for fitting and adjustment of other gastrointestinal appliance and device

Z46.6　Encounter for fitting and adjustment of urinary device
　EXCLUDES2　attention to artificial openings of urinary tract (Z43.5, Z43.6)

✓5ᵗʰ **Z46.8　Encounter for fitting and adjustment of other specified devices**

　Z46.81　Encounter for fitting and adjustment of insulin pump
　　Encounter for insulin pump instruction and training
　　Encounter for insulin pump titration

　Z46.82　Encounter for fitting and adjustment of non-vascular catheter

　Z46.89　Encounter for fitting and adjustment of other specified devices
　　Encounter for fitting and adjustment of wheelchair

Z46.9　Encounter for fitting and adjustment of unspecified device　▽

✓4ᵗʰ **Z47　Orthopedic aftercare**
　EXCLUDES1　aftercare for healing fracture—code to fracture with 7th character D

　Z47.1　Aftercare following joint replacement surgery
　　Use additional code to identify the joint (Z96.6-)

Z47.2   **Encounter for removal of** internal fixation device

> *EXCLUDES 1*   *encounter for adjustment of internal fixation device for fracture treatment—code to fracture with appropriate 7th character*
> *encounter for removal of external fixation device—code to fracture with 7th character D*
> *infection or inflammatory reaction to internal fixation device (T84.6-)*
> *mechanical complication of internal fixation device (T84.1-)*

✓5ᵗʰ **Z47.3**   **Aftercare following explantation of** joint prosthesis

Aftercare following explantation of joint prosthesis, staged procedure

Encounter for joint prosthesis insertion following prior explantation of joint prosthesis

AHA: 2015, 1Q, 16

TIP: Do not assign when a complication necessitating joint prosthesis explantation remains active or unresolved. When the complication remains, even in the presence of explantation of the prosthesis, assign the appropriate complication code.

Z47.31   **Aftercare following explantation of** shoulder **joint prosthesis**

> *EXCLUDES 1*   *acquired absence of shoulder joint following prior explantation of shoulder joint prosthesis (Z89.23-)*
> *shoulder joint prosthesis explantation status (Z89.23-)*

Z47.32   **Aftercare following explantation of** hip **joint prosthesis**

> *EXCLUDES 1*   *acquired absence of hip joint following prior explantation of hip joint prosthesis (Z89.62-)*
> *hip joint prosthesis explantation status (Z89.62-)*

Z47.33   **Aftercare following explantation of** knee **joint prosthesis**

> *EXCLUDES 1*   *acquired absence of knee joint following prior explantation of knee prosthesis (Z89.52-)*
> *knee joint prosthesis explantation status (Z89.52-)*

✓5ᵗʰ **Z47.8**   **Encounter for** other **orthopedic aftercare**

Z47.81   **Encounter for orthopedic aftercare** following surgical amputation

Use additional code to identify the limb amputated (Z89.-)

Z47.82   **Encounter for orthopedic aftercare** following scoliosis surgery

Z47.89   **Encounter for other orthopedic aftercare**

AHA: 2015, 1Q, 8

✓4ᵗʰ **Z48**   **Encounter for other postprocedural aftercare**

> *EXCLUDES 1*   *encounter for follow-up examination after completed treatment (Z08-Z09)*
> ▶*encounter for aftercare following injury – code to Injury, by site, with appropriate 7th character for subsequent encounter*◀

> *EXCLUDES 2*   *encounter for attention to artificial openings (Z43.-)*
> *encounter for fitting and adjustment of prosthetic and other devices (Z44-Z46)*

AHA: 2015, 4Q, 38; 2015, 1Q, 6-7

✓5ᵗʰ **Z48.0**   **Encounter for** attention to dressings, sutures and drains

> *EXCLUDES 1*   *encounter for planned postprocedural wound closure (Z48.1)*

Z48.00   **Encounter for change or removal of** nonsurgical wound dressing

Encounter for change or removal of wound dressing NOS

Z48.01   **Encounter for change or removal of** surgical wound dressing

Z48.02   **Encounter for removal of** sutures

Encounter for removal of staples

Z48.03   **Encounter for change or removal of** drains

Z48.1   **Encounter for planned** postprocedural **wound closure**

> *EXCLUDES 1*   *encounter for attention to dressings and sutures (Z48.0-)*

✓5ᵗʰ **Z48.2**   **Encounter for aftercare following** organ transplant

Z48.21   **Encounter for aftercare following** heart **transplant**

Z48.22   **Encounter for aftercare following** kidney **transplant**

Z48.23   **Encounter for aftercare following** liver **transplant**

Z48.24   **Encounter for aftercare following** lung **transplant**

✓6ᵗʰ **Z48.28**   **Encounter for aftercare following** multiple **organ transplant**

Z48.280   **Encounter for aftercare following** heart-lung **transplant**

Z48.288   **Encounter for aftercare following** multiple **organ transplant**

✓6ᵗʰ **Z48.29**   **Encounter for aftercare following** other **organ transplant**

Z48.290   **Encounter for aftercare following** bone marrow **transplant**

Z48.298   **Encounter for aftercare following other organ transplant**

Z48.3   **Aftercare following** surgery for neoplasm

Use additional code to identify the neoplasm

✓5ᵗʰ **Z48.8**   **Encounter for other specified postprocedural aftercare**

✓6ᵗʰ **Z48.81**   **Encounter for surgical aftercare following** surgery on specified body systems

These codes identify the body system requiring aftercare. They are for use in conjunction with other aftercare codes to fully explain the aftercare encounter. The condition treated should also be coded if still present.

> *EXCLUDES 1*   *aftercare for injury—code the injury with 7th character D*
> *aftercare following surgery for neoplasm (Z48.3)*

> *EXCLUDES 2*   *aftercare following organ transplant (Z48.2-)*
> *orthopedic aftercare (Z47.-)*

AHA: 2015, 4Q, 38

Z48.810   **Encounter for surgical aftercare following surgery on the** sense organs

Z48.811   **Encounter for surgical aftercare following surgery on the** nervous system

> *EXCLUDES 2*   *encounter for surgical aftercare following surgery on the sense organs (Z48.810)*

Z48.812   **Encounter for surgical aftercare following surgery on the** circulatory system

AHA: 2012, 4Q, 96

Z48.813   **Encounter for surgical aftercare following surgery on the** respiratory system

Z48.814   **Encounter for surgical aftercare following surgery on the** teeth or oral cavity

Z48.815   **Encounter for surgical aftercare following surgery on the** digestive system

Z48.816   **Encounter for surgical aftercare following surgery on the** genitourinary system

> *EXCLUDES 1*   *encounter for aftercare following sterilization reversal (Z31.42)*

Z48.817   **Encounter for surgical aftercare following surgery on the** skin and subcutaneous tissue

Z48.89   **Encounter for other specified surgical aftercare**

✓4ᵗʰ **Z49**   **Encounter for care involving renal dialysis**

Code also associated end stage renal disease (N18.6)

✓5ᵗʰ **Z49.0**   Preparatory care **for renal dialysis**

Encounter for dialysis instruction and training

Z49.01   **Encounter for fitting and adjustment of** extracorporeal dialysis catheter

Removal or replacement of renal dialysis catheter

Toilet or cleansing of renal dialysis catheter

Z49.02   **Encounter for fitting and adjustment of** peritoneal dialysis catheter

✓5ᵗʰ **Z49.3**   **Encounter for** adequacy testing for dialysis

Z49.31   **Encounter for adequacy testing for** hemodialysis

Z49.32   **Encounter for adequacy testing for** peritoneal dialysis

Encounter for peritoneal equilibration test

✓4ᵗʰ **Z51**   **Encounter for other aftercare and medical care**

Code also condition requiring care

> *EXCLUDES 1*   *follow-up examination after treatment (Z08-Z09)*

Z51.0   **Encounter for antineoplastic** radiation therapy   `PDx`

✓5ᵗʰ **Z51.1**   **Encounter for antineoplastic chemotherapy and immunotherapy**

> *EXCLUDES 2*   *encounter for chemotherapy and immunotherapy for nonneoplastic condition—code to condition*

✓ Additional Character Req   ✓ˣ7ᵗʰ Placeholder Alert   Case-Mix Diagnosis   Manifestation   ▽ Unspecified Dx   *EXCLUDES 1* Not coded here   *EXCLUDES 2* Not included here

Z51.11 Encounter for antineoplastic chemotherapy [PDx]
   AHA: 2015, 3Q, 19

Z51.12 Encounter for antineoplastic immunotherapy [PDx]

Z51.5 Encounter for palliative care
   AHA: 2017, 1Q, 48
   TIP: Post-acute providers may assign as a primary diagnosis if the purpose of the admission is for palliative care.

Z51.6 Encounter for desensitization to allergens

✓5ᵗʰ **Z51.8 Encounter for** other **specified aftercare**
   EXCLUDES1 holiday relief care (Z75.5)

   Z51.81 Encounter for therapeutic drug level **monitoring**
      Code also any long-term (current) drug therapy (Z79.-)
      EXCLUDES1 encounter for blood-drug test for administrative or medicolegal reasons (Z02.83)
      DEF: Drug monitoring: Measurement of the level of a specific drug in the body or measurement of a specific function to assess effectiveness of a drug.

   Z51.89 Encounter for other specified aftercare
      AHA: 2012, 4Q, 95-97

✓4ᵗʰ **Z52 Donors of organs and tissues**
   INCLUDES autologous and other living donors
   EXCLUDES1 cadaveric donor—omit code examination of potential donor (Z00.5)
   AHA: 2012, 4Q, 99

✓5ᵗʰ **Z52.0 Blood** donor

   ✓6ᵗʰ **Z52.00** Unspecified **blood donor**
      Z52.000 Unspecified donor, whole **blood** [PDx] ▽
      Z52.001 Unspecified donor, stem cells [PDx] ▽
      Z52.008 Unspecified donor, other blood [PDx] ▽

   ✓6ᵗʰ **Z52.01** Autologous **blood donor**
      Z52.010 Autologous donor, whole **blood** [PDx]
      Z52.011 Autologous donor, stem cells [PDx]
      Z52.018 Autologous donor, other blood [PDx]

   ✓6ᵗʰ **Z52.09** Other **blood donor**
      Volunteer donor
      Z52.090 Other blood donor, whole **blood** [PDx]
      Z52.091 Other blood donor, stem cells [PDx]
      Z52.098 Other blood donor, other blood [PDx]

✓5ᵗʰ **Z52.1** Skin **donor**
   Z52.10 Skin donor, unspecified [PDx] ▽
   Z52.11 Skin donor, autologous [PDx]
   Z52.19 Skin donor, other [PDx]

✓5ᵗʰ **Z52.2 Bone** donor
   Z52.20 Bone donor, unspecified [PDx] ▽
   Z52.21 Bone donor, autologous [PDx]
   Z52.29 Bone donor, other [PDx]

Z52.3 Bone marrow donor [PDx]
Z52.4 Kidney **donor** [PDx]
Z52.5 Cornea **donor** [PDx]
Z52.6 Liver **donor** [PDx]

✓5ᵗʰ **Z52.8 Donor of** other **specified organs or tissues**

   ✓6ᵗʰ **Z52.81** Egg (Oocyte) **donor**
      Z52.810 Egg (Oocyte) donor under age 35, anonymous **recipient** [PDx] ♀
         Egg donor under age 35 NOS
      Z52.811 Egg (Oocyte) donor under age 35, designated **recipient** [PDx] ♀
      Z52.812 Egg (Oocyte) donor age 35 and over, anonymous **recipient** [PDx] ♀
         Egg donor age 35 and over NOS
      Z52.813 Egg (Oocyte) donor age 35 and over, designated **recipient** [PDx] ♀
      Z52.819 Egg (Oocyte) donor, unspecified [PDx] ♀ ▽

   Z52.89 Donor of other specified organs or tissues [PDx]

Z52.9 Donor of unspecified organ or tissue ▽
   Donor NOS

✓4ᵗʰ **Z53 Persons encountering health services for specific procedures and treatment, not carried out**

   ✓5ᵗʰ **Z53.0 Procedure and treatment not carried out because of** contraindication

      Z53.01 Procedure and treatment not carried out due to patient smoking

   Z53.09 Procedure and treatment not carried out because of other contraindication

   Z53.1 Procedure and treatment not carried out because of patient's decision for reasons of belief and group pressure

   ✓5ᵗʰ **Z53.2 Procedure and treatment not carried out because of patient's decision for** other and unspecified **reasons**

      Z53.20 Procedure and treatment not carried out because of patient's decision for unspecified reasons ▽

      Z53.21 Procedure and treatment not carried out due to patient leaving prior to being seen by health care provider

      Z53.29 Procedure and treatment not carried out because of patient's decision for other reasons

   ✓5ᵗʰ **Z53.3 Procedure converted to open procedure**

      Z53.31 Laparoscopic **surgical procedure converted to open procedure**

      Z53.32 Thoracoscopic **surgical procedure converted to open procedure**

      Z53.33 Arthroscopic **surgical procedure converted to open procedure**

      Z53.39 Other specified **procedure converted to open procedure**

   Z53.8 Procedure and treatment not carried out for other reasons

   Z53.9 Procedure and treatment not carried out, unspecified reason ▽

Persons with potential health hazards related to socioeconomic and psychosocial circumstances (Z55-Z65)

✓4ᵗʰ **Z55 Problems related to education and literacy**
   EXCLUDES1 disorders of psychological development (F80-F89)

   Z55.0 Illiteracy and low-level literacy
   Z55.1 Schooling unavailable and unattainable
   Z55.2 Failed school examinations
   Z55.3 Underachievement in school
   Z55.4 Educational maladjustment and discord with teachers and classmates
   Z55.8 Other problems related to education and literacy
      Problems related to inadequate teaching
   Z55.9 Problems related to education and literacy, unspecified ▽
      Academic problems NOS

✓4ᵗʰ **Z56 Problems related to employment and unemployment**
   EXCLUDES2 occupational exposure to risk factors (Z57.-) problems related to housing and economic circumstances (Z59.-)

   Z56.0 Unemployment, unspecified ▽
   Z56.1 Change of job [A]
   Z56.2 Threat of job loss
   Z56.3 Stressful work schedule
   Z56.4 Discord with boss and workmates
   Z56.5 Uncongenial work environment
      Difficult conditions at work
   Z56.6 Other physical and mental strain related to work
   ✓5ᵗʰ **Z56.8 Other problems related to employment**
      Z56.81 Sexual harassment on the job
      Z56.82 Military deployment status
         Individual (civilian or military) currently deployed in theater or in support of military war, peacekeeping and humanitarian operations
      Z56.89 Other problems related to employment
   Z56.9 Unspecified problems related to employment ▽
      Occupational problems NOS

✓4ᵗʰ **Z57 Occupational exposure to risk factors**
   Z57.0 Occupational exposure to noise
   Z57.1 Occupational exposure to radiation
   Z57.2 Occupational exposure to dust
   ✓5ᵗʰ **Z57.3 Occupational exposure to** other air contaminants
      Z57.31 Occupational exposure to environmental tobacco smoke
         EXCLUDES2 exposure to environmental tobacco smoke (Z77.22)
      Z57.39 Occupational exposure to other air contaminants

N Newborn: 0 P Pediatric: 0-17 M Maternity: 12-55 A Adult: 15-124 NRS Nonroutine supply Dx NCDx Noncancer Dx PDx Primary Dx ▶◀ Revised Text ● New Code ▲ Revised Title

1192   ICD-10-CM 2018

Z57.4 Occupational exposure to toxic agents in agriculture
Occupational exposure to solids, liquids, gases or vapors in agriculture

Z57.5 Occupational exposure to toxic agents in other industries
Occupational exposure to solids, liquids, gases or vapors in other industries

Z57.6 Occupational exposure to extreme temperature

Z57.7 Occupational exposure to vibration

Z57.8 Occupational exposure to other risk factors

Z57.9 Occupational exposure to unspecified risk factor ▽

✓4ᵗʰ **Z59 Problems related to housing and economic circumstances**
EXCLUDES 2 problems related to upbringing (Z62.-)

Z59.0 Homelessness

Z59.1 Inadequate housing
Lack of heating
Restriction of space
Technical defects in home preventing adequate care
Unsatisfactory surroundings
EXCLUDES 1 problems related to the natural and physical environment (Z77.1-)

Z59.2 Discord with neighbors, lodgers and landlord

Z59.3 Problems related to living in residential institution
Boarding-school resident
EXCLUDES 1 institutional upbringing (Z62.2)

Z59.4 Lack of adequate food and safe drinking water
Inadequate drinking water supply
EXCLUDES 1 effects of hunger (T73.0)
inappropriate diet or eating habits (Z72.4)
malnutrition (E40-E46)

Z59.5 Extreme poverty

Z59.6 Low income

Z59.7 Insufficient social insurance and welfare support

Z59.8 Other problems related to housing and economic circumstances
Foreclosure on loan
Isolated dwelling
Problems with creditors

Z59.9 Problem related to housing and economic circumstances, unspecified ▽

✓4ᵗʰ **Z60 Problems related to social environment**

Z60.0 Problems of adjustment to life-cycle transitions
Empty nest syndrome
Phase of life problem
Problem with adjustment to retirement [pension]

Z60.2 Problems related to living alone

Z60.3 Acculturation difficulty
Problem with migration
Problem with social transplantation
DEF: A problem in adapting to a different culture or environment not based on any coexisting mental disorder.

Z60.4 Social exclusion and rejection
Exclusion and rejection on the basis of personal characteristics, such as unusual physical appearance, illness or behavior.
EXCLUDES 1 target of adverse discrimination such as for racial or religious reasons (Z60.5)

Z60.5 Target of (perceived) adverse discrimination and persecution
EXCLUDES 1 social exclusion and rejection (Z60.4)

Z60.8 Other problems related to social environment

Z60.9 Problem related to social environment, unspecified ▽

✓4ᵗʰ **Z62 Problems related to upbringing**
INCLUDES current and past negative life events in childhood
current and past problems of a child related to upbringing
EXCLUDES 2 maltreatment syndrome (T74.-)
problems related to housing and economic circumstances (Z59.-)

Z62.0 Inadequate parental supervision and control

Z62.1 Parental overprotection

✓5ᵗʰ **Z62.2 Upbringing away from parents**
EXCLUDES 1 problems with boarding school (Z59.3)

Z62.21 Child in welfare custody ℗
Child in care of non-parental family member
Child in foster care
EXCLUDES 2 problem for parent due to child in welfare custody (Z63.5)

Z62.22 Institutional upbringing
Child living in orphanage or group home

Z62.29 Other upbringing away from parents

Z62.3 Hostility towards and scapegoating of child ℗

Z62.6 Inappropriate (excessive) parental pressure

✓5ᵗʰ **Z62.8 Other specified problems related to upbringing**

✓6ᵗʰ **Z62.81 Personal history of abuse in childhood**

Z62.810 Personal history of physical and sexual **abuse in childhood**
EXCLUDES 1 current child physical abuse (T74.12, T76.12)
current child sexual abuse (T74.22, T76.22)

Z62.811 Personal history of psychological abuse **in childhood**
EXCLUDES 1 current child psychological abuse (T74.32, T76.32)

Z62.812 Personal history of neglect **in childhood**
EXCLUDES 1 current child neglect (T74.02, T76.02)

Z62.819 Personal history of unspecified abuse in childhood ▽
EXCLUDES 1 current child abuse NOS (T74.92, T76.92)

✓6ᵗʰ **Z62.82 Parent-child conflict**

Z62.820 Parent-biological **child conflict**
Parent-child problem NOS

Z62.821 Parent-adopted **child conflict**

Z62.822 Parent-foster **child conflict**

✓6ᵗʰ **Z62.89 Other specified problems related to upbringing**

Z62.890 Parent-child estrangement NEC

Z62.891 Sibling rivalry

Z62.898 Other specified problems related to upbringing

Z62.9 Problem related to upbringing, unspecified ▽

✓4ᵗʰ **Z63 Other problems related to primary support group, including family circumstances**
EXCLUDES 2 maltreatment syndrome (T74, T76)
parent-child problems (Z62.-)
problems related to negative life events in childhood (Z62.-)
problems related to upbringing (Z62.-)

Z63.0 Problems in relationship with spouse or partner
▶Relationship distress with spouse or intimate partner◀
EXCLUDES 1 counseling for spousal or partner abuse problems (Z69.1)
counseling related to sexual attitude, behavior, and orientation (Z70.-)

Z63.1 Problems in relationship with in-laws

✓5ᵗʰ **Z63.3 Absence of family member**
EXCLUDES 1 absence of family member due to disappearance and death (Z63.4)
absence of family member due to separation and divorce (Z63.5)

Z63.31 Absence of family member due to military deployment
Individual or family affected by other family member being on military deployment
EXCLUDES 1 family disruption due to return of family member from military deployment (Z63.71)

Z63.32 Other absence of family member

Z63.4 Disappearance and death of family member
Assumed death of family member
Bereavement
AHA: 2014, 1Q, 25

Z63.5 Disruption of family by separation and divorce
Marital estrangement

Z63.6 Dependent relative needing care at home

✓5ᵗʰ **Z63.7 Other stressful life events affecting family and household**

Z63.71 Stress on family due to return of family member from military deployment
Individual or family affected by family member having returned from military deployment (current or past conflict)

Z63.72 Alcoholism and drug addiction in family

Chapter 21. Factors Influencing Health Status and Contact with Health Services

Z63.79 **Other stressful life events affecting family and household**
Anxiety (normal) about sick person in family
Health problems within family
Ill or disturbed family member
Isolated family

Z63.8 **Other specified problems related to primary support group**
Family discord NOS
Family estrangement NOS
High expressed emotional level within family
Inadequate family support NOS
Inadequate or distorted communication within family

Z63.9 **Problem related to primary support group, unspecified** ▽
Relationship disorder NOS

✓4ᵗʰ **Z64** **Problems related to certain psycho social circumstances**

Z64.0 **Problems related to unwanted pregnancy** ♀

Z64.1 **Problems related to multiparity** ♀

Z64.4 **Discord with counselors**
Discord with probation officer
Discord with social worker

✓4ᵗʰ **Z65** **Problems related to other psychosocial circumstances**

Z65.0 **Conviction in civil and criminal proceedings without imprisonment**

Z65.1 **Imprisonment and other incarceration**

Z65.2 **Problems related to release from prison**

Z65.3 **Problems related to other legal circumstances**
Arrest
Child custody or support proceedings
Litigation
Prosecution

Z65.4 **Victim of crime and terrorism**
Victim of torture

Z65.5 **Exposure to disaster, war and other hostilities**
EXCLUDES 1　*target of perceived discrimination or persecution (Z60.5)*

Z65.8 **Other specified problems related to psychosocial circumstances**
▶Religious or spiritual problem◀

Z65.9 **Problem related to unspecified psychosocial circumstances** ▽

Do not resuscitate status (Z66)

Z66 **Do not resuscitate**
DNR status
DEF: Medical order written by a physician that instructs others not to perform cardiopulmonary resuscitation (CPR), intubation, or advanced life support (ACLS); prevents unnecessary invasive treatment to prolong life should breathing stop or cardiac arrest occur.

Blood type (Z67)

✓4ᵗʰ **Z67** **Blood type**
AHA: 2015, 3Q, 40

✓5ᵗʰ **Z67.1** Type A blood

Z67.10 Type A blood, Rh positive
Z67.11 Type A blood, Rh negative

✓5ᵗʰ **Z67.2** Type B blood

Z67.20 Type B blood, Rh positive
Z67.21 Type B blood, Rh negative

✓5ᵗʰ **Z67.3** Type AB blood

Z67.30 Type AB blood, Rh positive
Z67.31 Type AB blood, Rh negative

✓5ᵗʰ **Z67.4** Type O blood

Z67.40 Type O blood, Rh positive
Z67.41 Type O blood, Rh negative

✓5ᵗʰ **Z67.9** Unspecified blood type

Z67.90 Unspecified blood type, Rh positive ▽
Z67.91 Unspecified blood type, Rh negative ▽

Blood Types

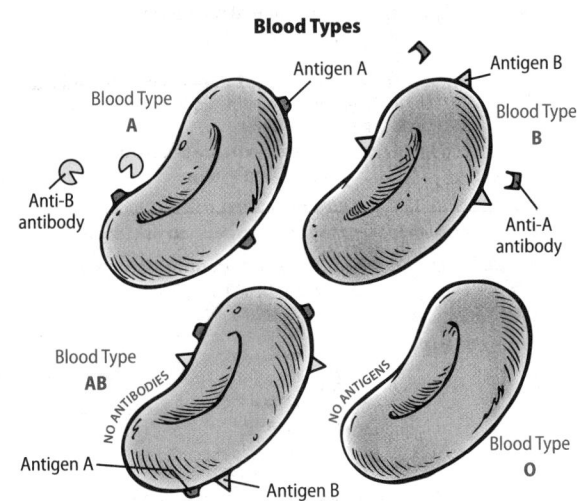

Body mass index [BMI] (Z68)

✓4ᵗʰ **Z68** **Body mass index [BMI]**
Kilograms per meters squared
NOTE　BMI adult codes are for use for persons 21 years of age or older.
BMI pediatric codes are for use for persons 2-20 years of age. These percentiles are based on the growth charts published by the Centers for Disease Control and Prevention (CDC).
AHA: 2017, 1Q, 39
DEF: Index used to help determine whether an individual is underweight, a healthy weight, overweight, or obese.
TIP: BMI may be assigned as a secondary diagnosis based on documentation of clinicians other than the diagnosing provider when a diagnosis of overweight or obesity has been documented by the diagnosing provider.

▲ **Z68.1** **Body mass index [BMI] 19.9 or less, adult** 🅰

✓5ᵗʰ **Z68.2** **Body mass index [BMI] 20-29, adult**
Z68.20 Body mass index [BMI] 20.0-20.9, adult 🅰
Z68.21 Body mass index [BMI] 21.0-21.9, adult 🅰
Z68.22 Body mass index [BMI] 22.0-22.9, adult 🅰
Z68.23 Body mass index [BMI] 23.0-23.9, adult 🅰
Z68.24 Body mass index [BMI] 24.0-24.9, adult 🅰
Z68.25 Body mass index [BMI] 25.0-25.9, adult 🅰
Z68.26 Body mass index [BMI] 26.0-26.9, adult 🅰
Z68.27 Body mass index [BMI] 27.0-27.9, adult 🅰
Z68.28 Body mass index [BMI] 28.0-28.9, adult 🅰
Z68.29 Body mass index [BMI] 29.0-29.9, adult 🅰

✓5ᵗʰ **Z68.3** **Body mass index [BMI] 30-39, adult**
Z68.30 Body mass index [BMI] 30.0-30.9, adult 🅰
Z68.31 Body mass index [BMI] 31.0-31.9, adult 🅰
Z68.32 Body mass index [BMI] 32.0-32.9, adult 🅰
Z68.33 Body mass index [BMI] 33.0-33.9, adult 🅰
Z68.34 Body mass index [BMI] 34.0-34.9, adult 🅰
Z68.35 Body mass index [BMI] 35.0-35.9, adult 🅰
Z68.36 Body mass index [BMI] 36.0-36.9, adult 🅰
Z68.37 Body mass index [BMI] 37.0-37.9, adult 🅰
Z68.38 Body mass index [BMI] 38.0-38.9, adult 🅰
Z68.39 Body mass index [BMI] 39.0-39.9, adult 🅰

✓5ᵗʰ **Z68.4** **Body mass index [BMI] 40 or greater, adult**
Z68.41 Body mass index [BMI] 40.0-44.9, adult 🅰
Z68.42 Body mass index [BMI] 45.0-49.9, adult 🅰
Z68.43 Body mass index [BMI] 50-59.9, adult 🅰
Z68.44 Body mass index [BMI] 60.0-69.9, adult 🅰
Z68.45 Body mass index [BMI] 70 or greater, adult 🅰

✓5ᵗʰ **Z68.5** **Body mass index [BMI] pediatric**
Z68.51 Body mass index [BMI] pediatric, less than 5th percentile for age
Z68.52 Body mass index [BMI] pediatric, 5th to less than 85th percentile for age
Z68.53 Body mass index [BMI] pediatric, 85th percentile to less than 95th percentile for age
Z68.54 Body mass index [BMI] pediatric, greater than or equal to 95th percentile for age

Ⓝ Newborn: 0　Ⓟ Pediatric: 0-17　Ⓜ Maternity: 12-55　🅰 Adult: 15-124　NRS Nonroutine supply Dx　NCDx Noncancer Dx　PDx Primary Dx　▶◀ Revised Text　● New Code　▲ Revised Title

1194　　　ICD-10-CM 2018

Persons encountering health services in other circumstances (Z69-Z76)

✓4ᵗʰ Z69 Encounter for mental health services for victim and perpetrator of abuse
INCLUDES counseling for victims and perpetrators of abuse

✓5ᵗʰ Z69.0 Encounter for mental health services for child abuse problems

✓6ᵗʰ Z69.01 Encounter for mental health services for parental child abuse

Z69.010 Encounter for mental health services for victim of parental child abuse P
▶Encounter for mental health services for victim of child abuse by parent
Encounter for mental health services for victim of child neglect by parent
Encounter for mental health services for victim of child psychological abuse by parent
Encounter for mental health services for victim of child sexual abuse by parent◀

Z69.011 Encounter for mental health services for perpetrator of parental child abuse
▶Encounter for mental health services for perpetrator of parental child neglect
Encounter for mental health services for perpetrator of parental child psychological abuse
Encounter for mental health services for perpetrator of parental child sexual abuse◀
EXCLUDES 1 encounter for mental health services for non-parental child abuse (Z69.02-)

✓6ᵗʰ Z69.02 Encounter for mental health services for non-parental child abuse

Z69.020 Encounter for mental health services for victim of non-parental child abuse P
▶Encounter for mental health services for victim of non-parental child neglect
Encounter for mental health services for victim of non-parental child psychological abuse
Encounter for mental health services for victim of non-parental child sexual abuse◀

Z69.021 Encounter for mental health services for perpetrator of non-parental child abuse
▶Encounter for mental health services for perpetrator of non-parental child neglect
Encounter for mental health services for perpetrator of non-parental child psychological abuse
Encounter for mental health services for perpetrator of non-parental child sexual abuse◀

✓5ᵗʰ Z69.1 Encounter for mental health services for spousal or partner abuse problems

Z69.11 Encounter for mental health services for victim of spousal or partner abuse
▶Encounter for mental health services for victim of spouse or partner neglect
Encounter for mental health services for victim of spouse or partner psychological abuse
Encounter for mental health services for victim of spouse or partner violence, physical◀

Z69.12 Encounter for mental health services for perpetrator of spousal or partner abuse
▶Encounter for mental health services for perpetrator of spouse or partner neglect
Encounter for mental health services for perpetrator of spouse or partner psychological abuse
Encounter for mental health services for perpetrator of spouse or partner violence, physical
Encounter for mental health services for perpetrator of spouse or partner violence, sexual◀

✓5ᵗʰ Z69.8 Encounter for mental health services for victim or perpetrator of other abuse

Z69.81 Encounter for mental health services for victim of other abuse
▶Encounter for mental health services for perpetrator of non-spousal adult abuse
Encounter for mental health services for victim of non-spousal adult abuse
Encounter for mental health services for victim of spouse or partner violence, sexual◀
Encounter for rape victim counseling

Z69.82 Encounter for mental health services for perpetrator of other abuse

✓4ᵗʰ Z70 Counseling related to sexual attitude, behavior and orientation
INCLUDES encounter for mental health services for sexual attitude, behavior and orientation
EXCLUDES 2 contraceptive or procreative counseling (Z30-Z31)

Z70.0 Counseling related to sexual attitude

Z70.1 Counseling related to patient's sexual behavior and orientation
Patient concerned regarding impotence
Patient concerned regarding non-responsiveness
Patient concerned regarding promiscuity
Patient concerned regarding sexual orientation

Z70.2 Counseling related to sexual behavior and orientation of third party
Advice sought regarding sexual behavior and orientation of child
Advice sought regarding sexual behavior and orientation of partner
Advice sought regarding sexual behavior and orientation of spouse

Z70.3 Counseling related to combined concerns regarding sexual attitude, behavior and orientation

Z70.8 Other sex counseling
Encounter for sex education

Z70.9 Sex counseling, unspecified ▽

✓4ᵗʰ Z71 Persons encountering health services for other counseling and medical advice, not elsewhere classified
EXCLUDES 2 contraceptive or procreation counseling (Z30-Z31)
sex counseling (Z70.-)

Z71.0 Person encountering health services to consult on behalf of another person
Person encountering health services to seek advice or treatment for non-attending third party
EXCLUDES 2 anxiety (normal) about sick person in family (Z63.7)
expectant (adoptive) parent(s) pre-birth pediatrician visit (Z76.81)

Z71.1 Person with feared health complaint in whom no diagnosis is made
Person encountering health services with feared condition which was not demonstrated
Person encountering health services in which problem was normal state
"Worried well"
EXCLUDES 1 medical observation for suspected diseases and conditions proven not to exist (Z03.-)

Z71.2 Person consulting for explanation of examination or test findings

Z71.3 Dietary counseling and surveillance
Use additional code for any associated underlying medical condition
Use additional code to identify body mass index (BMI), if known (Z68.-)

✓5ᵗʰ Z71.4 Alcohol abuse counseling and surveillance
Use additional code for alcohol abuse or dependence (F10.-)

Z71.41 Alcohol abuse counseling and surveillance of alcoholic

Z71.42 Counseling for family member of alcoholic
Counseling for significant other, partner, or friend of alcoholic

✓5ᵗʰ Z71.5 Drug abuse counseling and surveillance
Use additional code for drug abuse or dependence (F11-F16, F18-F19)

Z71.51 Drug abuse counseling and surveillance of drug abuser

Z71.52 Counseling for family member of drug abuser
Counseling for significant other, partner, or friend of drug abuser

Chapter 21. Factors Influencing Health Status and Contact with Health Services

Z71.6   Tobacco abuse counseling
Use additional code for nicotine dependence (F17.-)

Z71.7   Human immunodeficiency virus [HIV] counseling

✓5ᵗʰ **Z71.8   Other specified counseling**
EXCLUDES 2   counseling for contraception (Z30.0-)
~~counseling for genetics (Z31.5)~~
~~counseling for procreative management (Z31.6-)~~

●   **Z71.81   Spiritual or religious counseling**

●   **Z71.82   Exercise counseling**

   Z71.83   Encounter for nonprocreative genetic counseling
EXCLUDES 1   counseling for procreative genetics (Z31.5)
counseling for procreative management (Z31.6)

   Z71.89   Other specified counseling

Z71.9   Counseling, unspecified ▽
Encounter for medical advice NOS

✓4ᵗʰ **Z72   Problems related to lifestyle**
EXCLUDES 2   problems related to life-management difficulty (Z73.-)
problems related to socioeconomic and psychosocial circumstances (Z55-Z65)

Z72.0   Tobacco use
Tobacco use NOS
EXCLUDES 1   history of tobacco dependence (Z87.891)
nicotine dependence (F17.2-)
tobacco dependence (F17.2-)
tobacco use during pregnancy (O99.33-)

Z72.3   Lack of physical exercise

Z72.4   Inappropriate diet and eating habits
EXCLUDES 1   behavioral eating disorders of infancy or childhood (F98.2- F98.3)
eating disorders (F50.-)
lack of adequate food (Z59.4)
malnutrition and other nutritional deficiencies (E40-E64)

✓5ᵗʰ **Z72.5   High risk sexual behavior**
Promiscuity
EXCLUDES 1   paraphilias (F65)

   Z72.51   High risk heterosexual behavior

   Z72.52   High risk homosexual behavior

   Z72.53   High risk bisexual behavior

Z72.6   Gambling and betting
EXCLUDES 1   compulsive or pathological gambling (F63.0)

✓5ᵗʰ **Z72.8   Other problems related to lifestyle**

✓6ᵗʰ   **Z72.81   Antisocial behavior**
EXCLUDES 1   conduct disorders (F91.-)

     Z72.810   Child and adolescent antisocial behavior P
Antisocial behavior (child) (adolescent) without manifest psychiatric disorder
Delinquency NOS
Group delinquency
Offenses in the context of gang membership
Stealing in company with others
Truancy from school

     Z72.811   Adult antisocial behavior A
Adult antisocial behavior without manifest psychiatric disorder

✓6ᵗʰ   **Z72.82   Problems related to sleep**

     Z72.820   Sleep deprivation
Lack of adequate sleep
EXCLUDES 1   insomnia (G47.0-)

     Z72.821   Inadequate sleep hygiene
Bad sleep habits
Irregular sleep habits
Unhealthy sleep wake schedule
EXCLUDES 1   insomnia (F51.0-, G47.0-)

   Z72.89   Other problems related to lifestyle
Self-damaging behavior

Z72.9   Problem related to lifestyle, unspecified ▽

✓4ᵗʰ **Z73   Problems related to life management difficulty**
EXCLUDES 2   problems related to socioeconomic and psychosocial circumstances (Z55-Z65)
DEF: State of emotional, mental, and physical exhaustion; causing difficulties in managing personal, school, or work circumstances; usually due to prolonged stress; poor interpersonal relationship skills, or parenting skills.

Z73.0   Burn-out

Z73.1   Type A behavior pattern

Z73.2   Lack of relaxation and leisure

Z73.3   Stress, not elsewhere classified
Physical and mental strain NOS
EXCLUDES 1   stress related to employment or unemployment (Z56.-)

Z73.4   Inadequate social skills, not elsewhere classified

Z73.5   Social role conflict, not elsewhere classified

Z73.6   Limitation of activities due to disability
EXCLUDES 1   care-provider dependency (Z74.-)

✓5ᵗʰ **Z73.8   Other problems related to life management difficulty**

✓6ᵗʰ   **Z73.81   Behavioral insomnia of childhood**
DEF: Behaviors on the part of the child or caregivers that cause negative compliance with a child's sleep schedule; results in lack of adequate sleep.

     Z73.810   Behavioral insomnia of childhood, sleep-onset association type P

     Z73.811   Behavioral insomnia of childhood, limit setting type P

     Z73.812   Behavioral insomnia of childhood, combined type P

     Z73.819   Behavioral insomnia of childhood, unspecified type P ▽

   Z73.82   Dual sensory impairment

   Z73.89   Other problems related to life management difficulty

Z73.9   Problem related to life management difficulty, unspecified ▽

✓4ᵗʰ **Z74   Problems related to care provider dependency**
EXCLUDES 2   dependence on enabling machines or devices NEC (Z99.-)

✓5ᵗʰ **Z74.0   Reduced mobility**

   Z74.01   Bed confinement status
Bedridden

   Z74.09   Other reduced mobility
Chair ridden
Reduced mobility NOS
EXCLUDES 2   wheelchair dependence (Z99.3)

Z74.1   Need for assistance with personal care

Z74.2   Need for assistance at home and no other household member able to render care

Z74.3   Need for continuous supervision

Z74.8   Other problems related to care provider dependency

Z74.9   Problem related to care provider dependency, unspecified ▽

✓4ᵗʰ **Z75   Problems related to medical facilities and other health care**

Z75.0   Medical services not available in home
EXCLUDES 1   no other household member able to render care (Z74.2)

Z75.1   Person awaiting admission to adequate facility elsewhere

Z75.2   Other waiting period for investigation and treatment

Z75.3   Unavailability and inaccessibility of health-care facilities
EXCLUDES 1   bed unavailable (Z75.1)

Z75.4   Unavailability and inaccessibility of other helping agencies

Z75.5   Holiday relief care

Z75.8   Other problems related to medical facilities and other health care

Z75.9   Unspecified problem related to medical facilities and other health care ▽

✓4ᵗʰ **Z76   Persons encountering health services in other circumstances**

Z76.0   Encounter for issue of repeat prescription
Encounter for issue of repeat prescription for appliance
Encounter for issue of repeat prescription for medicaments
Encounter for issue of repeat prescription for spectacles
EXCLUDES 2   issue of medical certificate (Z02.7)
repeat prescription for contraceptive (Z30.4-)

Z76.1   Encounter for health supervision and care of foundling PDx

---

N Newborn: 0   P Pediatric: 0-17   M Maternity: 12-55   A Adult: 15-124   NRS Nonroutine supply Dx   NCDx Noncancer Dx   PDx Primary Dx   ▶◀ Revised Text   ● New Code   ▲ Revised Title

1196   ICD-10-CM 2018

Z76.2 Encounter for health supervision and care of other healthy infant and child PDx P
Encounter for medical or nursing care or supervision of healthy infant under circumstances such as adverse socioeconomic conditions at home
Encounter for medical or nursing care or supervision of healthy infant under circumstances such as awaiting foster or adoptive placement
Encounter for medical or nursing care or supervision of healthy infant under circumstances such as maternal illness
Encounter for medical or nursing care or supervision of healthy infant under circumstances such as number of children at home preventing or interfering with normal care

Z76.3 Healthy person accompanying sick person

Z76.4 Other boarder to healthcare facility
EXCLUDES 1 homelessness (Z59.0)

Z76.5 Malingerer [conscious simulation]
Person feigning illness (with obvious motivation)
EXCLUDES 1 factitious disorder (F68.1-)
peregrinating patient (F68.1-)
DEF: Act of intentionally exaggerating an illness or disability in order to receive personal gain; or to avoid punishment or responsibility.

✓5ᵗʰ Z76.8 Persons encountering health services in other specified circumstances

Z76.81 Expectant parent(s) prebirth pediatrician visit
Pre-adoption pediatrician visit for adoptive parent(s)

Z76.82 Awaiting organ transplant status
Patient waiting for organ availability

Z76.89 Persons encountering health services in other specified circumstances
Persons encountering health services NOS
AHA: 2014, 2Q, 10

Persons with potential health hazards related to family and personal history and certain conditions influencing health status (Z77-Z99)

Code also any follow-up examination (Z08-Z09)

✓4ᵗʰ Z77 Other contact with and (suspected) exposures hazardous to health
INCLUDES contact with and (suspected) exposures to potential hazards to health
EXCLUDES 2 contact with and (suspected) exposure to communicable diseases (Z20.-)
exposure to (parental) (environmental) tobacco smoke in the perinatal period (P96.81)
newborn affected by noxious substances transmitted via placenta or breast milk (P04.-)
occupational exposure to risk factors (Z57.-)
retained foreign body (Z18.-)
retained foreign body fully removed (Z87.821)
toxic effects of substances chiefly nonmedicinal as to source (T51-T65)

✓5ᵗʰ Z77.0 Contact with and (suspected) exposure to hazardous, chiefly nonmedicinal, chemicals

✓6ᵗʰ Z77.01 Contact with and (suspected) exposure to hazardous metals

Z77.010 Contact with and (suspected) exposure to arsenic

Z77.011 Contact with and (suspected) exposure to lead

Z77.012 Contact with and (suspected) exposure to uranium
EXCLUDES 1 retained depleted uranium fragments (Z18.01)

Z77.018 Contact with and (suspected) exposure to other hazardous metals
Contact with and (suspected) exposure to chromium compounds
Contact with and (suspected) exposure to nickel dust

✓6ᵗʰ Z77.02 Contact with and (suspected) exposure to hazardous aromatic compounds

Z77.020 Contact with and (suspected) exposure to aromatic amines

Z77.021 Contact with and (suspected) exposure to benzene

Z77.028 Contact with and (suspected) exposure to other hazardous aromatic compounds
Aromatic dyes NOS
Polycyclic aromatic hydrocarbons

✓6ᵗʰ Z77.09 Contact with and (suspected) exposure to other hazardous, chiefly nonmedicinal, chemicals

Z77.090 Contact with and (suspected) exposure to asbestos

Z77.098 Contact with and (suspected) exposure to other hazardous, chiefly nonmedicinal, chemicals
Dyes NOS

✓5ᵗʰ Z77.1 Contact with and (suspected) exposure to environmental pollution and hazards in the physical environment

✓6ᵗʰ Z77.11 Contact with and (suspected) exposure to environmental pollution

Z77.110 Contact with and (suspected) exposure to air pollution

Z77.111 Contact with and (suspected) exposure to water pollution

Z77.112 Contact with and (suspected) exposure to soil pollution

Z77.118 Contact with and (suspected) exposure to other environmental pollution

✓6ᵗʰ Z77.12 Contact with and (suspected) exposure to hazards in the physical environment

Z77.120 Contact with and (suspected) exposure to mold (toxic)

Z77.121 Contact with and (suspected) exposure to harmful algae and algae toxins
Contact with and (suspected) exposure to (harmful) algae bloom NOS
Contact with and (suspected) exposure to blue-green algae bloom
Contact with and (suspected) exposure to brown tide
Contact with and (suspected) exposure to cyanobacteria bloom
Contact with and (suspected) exposure to Florida red tide
Contact with and (suspected) exposure to pfiesteria piscicida
Contact with and (suspected) exposure to red tide

Z77.122 Contact with and (suspected) exposure to noise

Z77.123 Contact with and (suspected) exposure to radon and other naturally occuring radiation
EXCLUDES 2 radiation exposure as the cause of a confirmed condition (W88-W90, X39.0-)
radiation sickness NOS (T66)

Z77.128 Contact with and (suspected) exposure to other hazards in the physical environment

✓5ᵗʰ Z77.2 Contact with and (suspected) exposure to other hazardous substances

Z77.21 Contact with and (suspected) exposure to potentially hazardous body fluids

Z77.22 Contact with and (suspected) exposure to environmental tobacco smoke (acute) (chronic)
Exposure to second hand tobacco smoke (acute) (chronic)
Passive smoking (acute) (chronic)
EXCLUDES 1 nicotine dependence (F17.-)
tobacco use (Z72.0)
EXCLUDES 2 occupational exposure to environmental tobacco smoke (Z57.31)

Z77.29 Contact with and (suspected) exposure to other hazardous substances
AHA: 2016, 2Q, 33

Z77.9 Other contact with and (suspected) exposures hazardous to health

✓4ᵗʰ Z78 Other specified health status
EXCLUDES 2 asymptomatic human immunodeficiency virus [HIV] infection status (Z21)
postprocedural status (Z93- Z99)
sex reassignment status (Z87.890)

Z78.0 Asymptomatic menopausal state A ♀
Menopausal state NOS
Postmenopausal status NOS
EXCLUDES 2 symptomatic menopausal state (N95.1)

✓ Additional Character Req   ✓x7ᵗʰ Placeholder Alert   Case-Mix Diagnosis   Manifestation   ∇ Unspecified Dx   EXCLUDES 1 Not coded here   EXCLUDES 2 Not included here

ICD-10-CM 2018   1197

Chapter 21. Factors Influencing Health Status and Contact with Health Services

Z78.1   **Physical restraint status**
> EXCLUDES 1   *physical restraint due to a procedure - omit code*
> **DEF:** Application of mechanical restraining devices or manual restraints; used to limit physical mobility of a patient.

Z78.9   **Other specified health status**

✓4th **Z79**   **Long term (current) drug therapy**
> INCLUDES   long term (current) drug use for prophylactic purposes
> Code also any therapeutic drug level monitoring (Z51.81)
> EXCLUDES 2   *drug abuse and dependence (F11-F19)*
> *drug use complicating pregnancy, childbirth, and the puerperium (O99.32-)*
> *long term (current) use of oral antidiabetic drugs (Z79.84)*
> *long term (current) use of oral hypoglycemic drugs (Z79.84)*
> **TIP:** Do not assign when the focus of an encounter is due to the adverse effect or poisoning of a drug; use in the absence of current, unresolved complications.

✓5th **Z79.0**   **Long term (current) use of anticoagulants and antithrombotics/antiplatelets**
> EXCLUDES 2   *long term (current) use of aspirin (Z79.82)*

    Z79.01   **Long term (current) use of** anticoagulants

    Z79.02   **Long term (current) use of** antithrombotics/antiplatelets

Z79.1   **Long term (current) use of** non-steroidal anti-inflammatories **(NSAID)**
> EXCLUDES 2   *long term (current) use of aspirin (Z79.82)*

Z79.2   **Long term (current) use of** antibiotics

Z79.3   **Long term (current) use of** hormonal contraceptives
> Long term (current) use of birth control pill or patch

Z79.4   **Long term (current) use of** insulin

✓5th **Z79.5**   **Long term (current) use of** steroids

    Z79.51   **Long term (current) use of** inhaled steroids

    Z79.52   **Long term (current) use of** systemic steroids

✓5th **Z79.8**   **Other long term (current) drug therapy**

✓6th **Z79.81**   **Long term (current) use of agents affecting estrogen receptors and estrogen levels**
> Code first, if applicable:
> malignant neoplasm of breast (C50.-)
> malignant neoplasm of prostate (C61)
> Use additional code, if applicable, to identify:
> estrogen receptor positive status (Z17.0)
> family history of breast cancer (Z80.3)
> genetic susceptibility to malignant neoplasm (cancer) (Z15.0-)
> personal history of breast cancer (Z85.3)
> personal history of prostate cancer (Z85.46)
> postmenopausal status (Z78.0)
> EXCLUDES 1 ►hormone replacement therapy◄ (Z79.890)

    Z79.810   **Long term (current) use of selective estrogen receptor modulators (SERMs)**
> Long term (current) use of raloxifene (Evista)
> Long term (current) use of tamoxifen (Nolvadex)
> Long term (current) use of toremifene (Fareston)

    Z79.811   **Long term (current) use of** aromatase **inhibitors**
> Long term (current) use of anastrozole (Arimidex)
> Long term (current) use of exemestane (Aromasin)
> Long term (current) use of letrozole (Femara)

    Z79.818   **Long term (current) use of other agents affecting estrogen receptors and estrogen levels**
> Long term (current) use of estrogen receptor downregulators
> Long term (current) use of fulvestrant (Faslodex)
> Long term (current) use of gonadotropin-releasing hormone (GnRH) agonist
> Long term (current) use of goserelin acetate (Zoladex)
> Long term (current) use of leuprolide acetate (leuprorelin) (Lupron)
> Long term (current) use of megestrol acetate (Megace)

    Z79.82   **Long term (current) use of** aspirin

    Z79.83   **Long term (current) use of** bisphosphonates

Z79.84   **Long term (current) use of** oral hypoglycemic drugs
> Long term (current) use of oral antidiabetic drugs
> EXCLUDES 2   *long term (current) use of insulin (Z79.4)*

✓6th **Z79.89**   **Other long term (current) drug therapy**

    Z79.890   **Hormone replacement therapy**

    Z79.891   **Long term (current) use of** opiate analgesic
> Long term (current) use of methadone for pain management
> EXCLUDES 1   *methadone use NOS (F11.9-)*
> *use of methadone for treatment of heroin addiction (F11.2-)*

    Z79.899   **Other long term (current) drug therapy**
> AHA: 2015, 4Q, 34; 2015, 3Q, 21

✓4th **Z80**   **Family history of primary malignant neoplasm**

Z80.0   **Family history of malignant neoplasm of** digestive organs
> Conditions classifiable to C15-C26

Z80.1   **Family history of malignant neoplasm of** trachea, bronchus and lung
> Conditions classifiable to C33-C34

Z80.2   **Family history of malignant neoplasm of other** respiratory and intrathoracic organs
> Conditions classifiable to C30-C32, C37-C39

Z80.3   **Family history of malignant neoplasm of** breast
> Conditions classifiable to C50-

✓5th **Z80.4**   **Family history of malignant neoplasm of genital organs**
> Conditions classifiable to C51-C63

    Z80.41   **Family history of malignant neoplasm of** ovary

    Z80.42   **Family history of malignant neoplasm of** prostate

    Z80.43   **Family history of malignant neoplasm of** testis

    Z80.49   **Family history of malignant neoplasm of other genital organs**

✓5th **Z80.5**   **Family history of malignant neoplasm of urinary tract**
> Conditions classifiable to C64-C68

    Z80.51   **Family history of malignant neoplasm of** kidney

    Z80.52   **Family history of malignant neoplasm of** bladder

    Z80.59   **Family history of malignant neoplasm of other urinary tract organ**

Z80.6   **Family history of** leukemia
> Conditions classifiable to C91-C95

Z80.7   **Family history of other malignant neoplasms of** lymphoid, hematopoietic and related tissues
> Conditions classifiable to C81-C90, C96-

Z80.8   **Family history of malignant neoplasm of other** organs or systems
> Conditions classifiable to C00-C14, C40-C49, C69-C79

Z80.9   **Family history of malignant neoplasm, unspecified**
> Conditions classifiable to C80.1

✓4th **Z81**   **Family history of mental and behavioral disorders**

Z81.0   **Family history of** intellectual disabilities
> Conditions classifiable to F70-F79

Z81.1   **Family history of** alcohol abuse and dependence
> Conditions classifiable to F10-

Z81.2   **Family history of** tobacco abuse and dependence
> Conditions classifiable to F17-

Z81.3   **Family history of other** psychoactive substance abuse and dependence
> Conditions classifiable to F11-F16, F18-F19

Z81.4   **Family history of other** substance abuse and dependence
> Conditions classifiable to F55

Z81.8   **Family history of other** mental and behavioral **disorders**
> Conditions classifiable elsewhere in F01-F99

✓4th **Z82**   **Family history of certain disabilities and chronic diseases (leading to disablement)**

Z82.0   **Family history of** epilepsy and other diseases of the nervous system
> Conditions classifiable to G00-G99

Z82.1   **Family history of** blindness and visual loss
> Conditions classifiable to H54-

Z82.2   **Family history of** deafness and hearing loss
> Conditions classifiable to H90-H91

Z82.3   **Family history of** stroke
> Conditions classifiable to I60-I64

N Newborn: 0   P Pediatric: 0-17   M Maternity: 12-55   A Adult: 15-124   NRS Nonroutine supply Dx   NC Dx Noncancer Dx   PDx Primary Dx   ►◄ Revised Text   ● New Code   ▲ Revised Title

1198   ICD-10-CM 2018

✓5ᵗʰ Z82.4 **Family history of ischemic heart disease and other diseases of the circulatory system**
Conditions classifiable to I00-I52, I65-I99

    Z82.41 **Family history of** sudden cardiac death

    Z82.49 **Family history of** ischemic heart disease **and other diseases of the circulatory system**

Z82.5 **Family history of** asthma **and other chronic lower respiratory diseases**
Conditions classifiable to J40-J47
> EXCLUDES 2   *family history of other diseases of the respiratory system (Z83.6)*

✓5ᵗʰ Z82.6 **Family history of arthritis and other diseases of the musculoskeletal system and connective tissue**
Conditions classifiable to M00-M99

    Z82.61 **Family history of** arthritis

    Z82.62 **Family history of** osteoporosis

    Z82.69 **Family history of other diseases of the musculoskeletal system and connective tissue**

✓5ᵗʰ Z82.7 **Family history of congenital malformations, deformations and chromosomal abnormalities**
Conditions classifiable to Q00-Q99

    Z82.71 **Family history of** polycystic kidney

    Z82.79 **Family history of other congenital malformations, deformations and chromosomal abnormalities**

Z82.8 **Family history of** other disabilities and chronic diseases leading to disablement, **not elsewhere classified**

✓4ᵗʰ Z83 **Family history of other specific disorders**
> EXCLUDES 2   *contact with and (suspected) exposure to communicable disease in the family (Z20.-)*

Z83.0 **Family history of** human immunodeficiency virus [HIV] disease
Conditions classifiable to B20

Z83.1 **Family history of other** infectious and parasitic diseases
Conditions classifiable to A00-B19, B25-B94, B99

Z83.2 **Family history of diseases of the** blood and blood-forming organs **and certain disorders involving the immune mechanism**
Conditions classifiable to D50-D89

Z83.3 **Family history of** diabetes mellitus
Conditions classifiable to E08-E13

✓5ᵗʰ Z83.4 **Family history of other endocrine, nutritional and metabolic diseases**
Conditions classifiable to E00-E07, E15-E88

    Z83.41 **Family history of** multiple endocrine neoplasia [MEN] syndrome

    Z83.42 **Family history of** familial hypercholesterolemia

    Z83.49 **Family history of other endocrine, nutritional and metabolic diseases**

✓5ᵗʰ Z83.5 **Family history of eye and ear disorders**

    ✓6ᵗʰ Z83.51 **Family history of** eye **disorders**
Conditions classifiable to H00-H53, H55-H59
> EXCLUDES 2   *family history of blindness and visual loss (Z82.1)*

        Z83.511 **Family history of** glaucoma

        Z83.518 **Family history of other specified eye disorder**

    Z83.52 **Family history of** ear **disorders**
Conditions classifiable to H60-H83, H92-H95
> EXCLUDES 2   *family history of deafness and hearing loss (Z82.2)*

Z83.6 **Family history of other diseases of the** respiratory system
Conditions classifiable to J00-J39, J60-J99
> EXCLUDES 2   *family history of asthma and other chronic lower respiratory diseases (Z82.5)*

✓5ᵗʰ Z83.7 **Family history of diseases of the digestive system**
Conditions classifiable to K00-K93

    Z83.71 **Family history of** colonic polyps
> EXCLUDES 1   ~~family history of malignant neoplasm of digestive organs (Z80.0)~~
> EXCLUDES 2   ▶*family history of malignant neoplasm of digestive organs (Z80.0)*◀

    Z83.79 **Family history of other diseases of the digestive system**

✓4ᵗʰ Z84 **Family history of other conditions**

    Z84.0 **Family history of diseases of the** skin and subcutaneous tissue
Conditions classifiable to L00-L99

    Z84.1 **Family history of disorders of** kidney and ureter
Conditions classifiable to N00-N29

    Z84.2 **Family history of other diseases of the** genitourinary system
Conditions classifiable to N30-N99

    Z84.3 **Family history of** consanguinity

    ✓5ᵗʰ Z84.8 **Family history of other specified conditions**

        Z84.81 **Family history of carrier of** genetic disease

        Z84.82 **Family history of** sudden infant death syndrome
Family history of SIDS

        Z84.89 **Family history of other specified conditions**

✓4ᵗʰ Z85 **Personal history of malignant neoplasm**
Code first any follow-up examination after treatment of malignant neoplasm (Z08)
Use additional code to identify:
alcohol use and dependence (F10.-)
exposure to environmental tobacco smoke (Z77.22)
history of tobacco dependence (Z87.891)
occupational exposure to environmental tobacco smoke (Z57.31)
tobacco dependence (F17.-)
tobacco use (Z72.0)
> EXCLUDES 2   *personal history of benign neoplasm (Z86.01-)*
> *personal history of carcinoma-in-situ (Z86.00-)*

    ✓5ᵗʰ Z85.0 **Personal history of malignant neoplasm of** digestive organs
AHA: 2017, 1Q, 9

        Z85.00 **Personal history of malignant neoplasm of unspecified digestive organ**   ▽

        Z85.01 **Personal history of malignant neoplasm of** esophagus
Conditions classifiable to C15

    ✓6ᵗʰ Z85.02 **Personal history of malignant neoplasm of** stomach

        Z85.020 **Personal history of malignant** carcinoid tumor **of stomach**
Conditions classifiable to C7A.092

        Z85.028 **Personal history of other malignant neoplasm of stomach**
Conditions classifiable to C16

    ✓6ᵗʰ Z85.03 **Personal history of malignant neoplasm of** large intestine

        Z85.030 **Personal history of** malignant carcinoid tumor **of large intestine**
Conditions classifiable to C7A.022-C7A.025, C7A.029

        Z85.038 **Personal history of other malignant neoplasm of large intestine**
Conditions classifiable to C18

    ✓6ᵗʰ Z85.04 **Personal history of malignant neoplasm of** rectum, rectosigmoid junction, and anus

        Z85.040 **Personal history of malignant** carcinoid tumor **of rectum**
Conditions classifiable to C7A.026

        Z85.048 **Personal history of other malignant neoplasm of rectum, rectosigmoid junction, and anus**
Conditions classifiable to C19-C21

        Z85.05 **Personal history of malignant neoplasm of** liver
Conditions classifiable to C22

    ✓6ᵗʰ Z85.06 **Personal history of malignant neoplasm of** small intestine

        Z85.060 **Personal history of malignant** carcinoid tumor **of small intestine**
Conditions classifiable to C7A.01-

        Z85.068 **Personal history of other malignant neoplasm of small intestine**
Conditions classifiable to C17

        Z85.07 **Personal history of malignant neoplasm of** pancreas
Conditions classifiable to C25

        Z85.09 **Personal history of malignant neoplasm of other digestive organs**

✓5ᵗʰ **Z85.1** **Personal history of malignant neoplasm of** trachea, bronchus and lung

   ✓6ᵗʰ **Z85.11** **Personal history of malignant neoplasm of** bronchus and lung

      Z85.110 **Personal history of malignant** carcinoid tumor **of bronchus and lung**
         Conditions classifiable to C7A.090

      Z85.118 **Personal history of other malignant neoplasm of bronchus and lung**
         Conditions classifiable to C34

   Z85.12 **Personal history of malignant neoplasm of** trachea
      Conditions classifiable to C33

✓5ᵗʰ **Z85.2** **Personal history of malignant neoplasm of other** respiratory and intrathoracic organs

   Z85.20 **Personal history of malignant neoplasm of unspecified respiratory organ** ▽

   Z85.21 **Personal history of malignant neoplasm of** larynx
      Conditions classifiable to C32

   Z85.22 **Personal history of malignant neoplasm of** nasal cavities, middle ear, and accessory sinuses
      Conditions classifiable to C30-C31

   ✓6ᵗʰ **Z85.23** **Personal history of malignant neoplasm of** thymus

      Z85.230 **Personal history of malignant** carcinoid tumor **of thymus**
         Conditions classifiable to C7A.091

      Z85.238 **Personal history of other malignant neoplasm of thymus**
         Conditions classifiable to C37

   Z85.29 **Personal history of malignant neoplasm of other respiratory and intrathoracic organs**

Z85.3 **Personal history of malignant neoplasm of** breast
   Conditions classifiable to C50.-

✓5ᵗʰ **Z85.4** **Personal history of malignant neoplasm of** genital organs
   Conditions classifiable to C51-C63

   Z85.40 **Personal history of malignant neoplasm of unspecified** female **genital organ** ♀▽

   Z85.41 **Personal history of malignant neoplasm of** cervix uteri ♀

   Z85.42 **Personal history of malignant neoplasm of other parts of uterus** ♀

   Z85.43 **Personal history of malignant neoplasm of** ovary ♀

   Z85.44 **Personal history of malignant neoplasm of other** female **genital organs** ♀

   Z85.45 **Personal history of malignant neoplasm of unspecified** male **genital organ** ♂▽

   Z85.46 **Personal history of malignant neoplasm of** prostate ♂

   Z85.47 **Personal history of malignant neoplasm of** testis ♂

   Z85.48 **Personal history of malignant neoplasm of** epididymis ♂

   Z85.49 **Personal history of malignant neoplasm of other** male **genital organs** ♂

✓5ᵗʰ **Z85.5** **Personal history of malignant neoplasm of** urinary tract
   Conditions classifiable to C64-C68

   Z85.50 **Personal history of malignant neoplasm of unspecified urinary tract organ** ▽

   Z85.51 **Personal history of malignant neoplasm of** bladder

   ✓6ᵗʰ **Z85.52** **Personal history of malignant neoplasm of** kidney
      EXCLUDES 1 *personal history of malignant neoplasm of renal pelvis (Z85.53)*

      Z85.520 **Personal history of malignant** carcinoid tumor **of kidney**
         Conditions classifiable to C7A.093

      Z85.528 **Personal history of other malignant neoplasm of kidney**
         Conditions classifiable to C64

   Z85.53 **Personal history of malignant neoplasm of** renal pelvis

   Z85.54 **Personal history of malignant neoplasm of** ureter

   Z85.59 **Personal history of malignant neoplasm of other urinary tract organ**

Z85.6 **Personal history of** leukemia
   Conditions classifiable to C91-C95
      EXCLUDES 1 *leukemia in remission C91.0-C95.9 with 5th character 1*

✓5ᵗʰ **Z85.7** **Personal history of other malignant neoplasms of lymphoid, hematopoietic and related tissues**

   Z85.71 **Personal history of** Hodgkin lymphoma
      Conditions classifiable to C81

   Z85.72 **Personal history of** non-Hodgkin lymphomas
      Conditions classifiable to C82-C85

   Z85.79 **Personal history of other malignant neoplasms of lymphoid, hematopoietic and related tissues**
      Conditions classifiable to C88-C90, C96
      EXCLUDES 1 *multiple myeloma in remission (C90.01)*
         plasma cell leukemia in remission (C90.11)
         plasmacytoma in remission (C90.21)

✓5ᵗʰ **Z85.8** **Personal history of malignant neoplasms of other organs and systems**
   Conditions classifiable to C00-C14, C40-C49, C69-C75, C7A.098, C76-C79

   ✓6ᵗʰ **Z85.81** **Personal history of malignant neoplasm of** lip, oral cavity, and pharynx

      Z85.810 **Personal history of malignant neoplasm of** tongue

      Z85.818 **Personal history of malignant neoplasm of other sites of** lip, oral cavity, and pharynx

      Z85.819 **Personal history of malignant neoplasm of unspecified site of** lip, oral cavity, and pharynx ▽

   ✓6ᵗʰ **Z85.82** **Personal history of malignant neoplasm of** skin

      Z85.820 **Personal history of malignant** melanoma **of skin**
         Conditions classifiable to C43

      Z85.821 **Personal history of** Merkel cell carcinoma
         Conditions classifiable to C4A

      Z85.828 **Personal history of other malignant neoplasm of skin**
         Conditions classifiable to C44

   ✓6ᵗʰ **Z85.83** **Personal history of malignant neoplasm of** bone and soft tissue

      Z85.830 **Personal history of malignant neoplasm of** bone

      Z85.831 **Personal history of malignant neoplasm of** soft tissue
         EXCLUDES 2 *personal history of malignant neoplasm of skin (Z85.82-)*

   ✓6ᵗʰ **Z85.84** **Personal history of malignant neoplasm of** eye and nervous tissue

      Z85.840 **Personal history of malignant neoplasm of** eye

      Z85.841 **Personal history of malignant neoplasm of** brain

      Z85.848 **Personal history of malignant neoplasm of other parts of nervous tissue**

   ✓6ᵗʰ **Z85.85** **Personal history of malignant neoplasm of** endocrine glands

      Z85.850 **Personal history of malignant neoplasm of** thyroid

      Z85.858 **Personal history of malignant neoplasm of other endocrine glands**

   Z85.89 **Personal history of malignant neoplasm of other organs and systems**

   Z85.9 **Personal history of malignant neoplasm, unspecified** ▽
      Conditions classifiable to C7A.00, C80.1

✓4ᵗʰ **Z86** **Personal history of certain other diseases**
   Code first any follow-up examination after treatment (Z09)

   ✓5ᵗʰ **Z86.0** **Personal history of in-situ and benign neoplasms and neoplasms of uncertain behavior**
      EXCLUDES 2 *personal history of malignant neoplasms (Z85.-)*
      AHA: 2017, 1Q, 9

      ✓6ᵗʰ **Z86.00** **Personal history of** in-situ neoplasm
         Conditions classifiable to D00-D09

         Z86.000 **Personal history of in-situ neoplasm of breast**

         Z86.001 **Personal history of in-situ neoplasm of** cervix uteri ♀
            Personal history of cervical intraepithelial neoplasia III [CIN III]

N Newborn: 0 P Pediatric: 0-17 M Maternity: 12-55 A Adult: 15-124 NRS Nonroutine supply Dx NC Dx Noncancer Dx PD Dx Primary Dx ▶◀ Revised Text ● New Code ▲ Revised Title

1200   ICD-10-CM 2018

Z86.008   **Personal history of in-situ neoplasm of other site**
Personal history of vaginal intraepithelial neoplasia III [VAIN III]
Personal history of vulvar intraepithelial neoplasia III [VIN III]

✓6ᵗʰ **Z86.01**   **Personal history of benign neoplasm**

Z86.010   **Personal history of colonic polyps**
AHA: 2017, 1Q, 14

Z86.011   **Personal history of benign neoplasm of the brain**

Z86.012   **Personal history of benign carcinoid tumor**

Z86.018   **Personal history of other benign neoplasm**
AHA: 2017, 1Q, 14

Z86.03   **Personal history of neoplasm of uncertain behavior**

✓5ᵗʰ **Z86.1**   **Personal history of infectious and parasitic diseases**
Conditions classifiable to A00-B89, B99
EXCLUDES 1   *personal history of infectious diseases specific to a body system*
sequelae of infectious and parasitic diseases (B90-B94)

Z86.11   **Personal history of tuberculosis**

Z86.12   **Personal history of poliomyelitis**

Z86.13   **Personal history of malaria**

Z86.14   **Personal history of Methicillin resistant Staphylococcus aureus infection**
Personal history of MRSA infection

Z86.19   **Personal history of other infectious and parasitic diseases**

Z86.2   **Personal history of diseases of the blood and blood-forming organs and certain disorders involving the immune mechanism**
Conditions classifiable to D50-D89

✓5ᵗʰ **Z86.3**   **Personal history of endocrine, nutritional and metabolic diseases**
Conditions classifiable to E00-E88

Z86.31   **Personal history of diabetic foot ulcer**
EXCLUDES 2   *current diabetic foot ulcer (E08.621, E09.621, E10.621, E11.621, E13.621)*

Z86.32   **Personal history of gestational diabetes**   ♀
Personal history of conditions classifiable to O24.4-
EXCLUDES 1   *gestational diabetes mellitus in current pregnancy (O24.4-)*

Z86.39   **Personal history of other endocrine, nutritional and metabolic disease**

✓5ᵗʰ **Z86.5**   **Personal history of mental and behavioral disorders**
Conditions classifiable to F40-F59

Z86.51   **Personal history of combat and operational stress reaction**   Ⓐ

Z86.59   **Personal history of other mental and behavioral disorders**

✓5ᵗʰ **Z86.6**   **Personal history of diseases of the nervous system and sense organs**
Conditions classifiable to G00-G99, H00-H95
EXCLUDES 2   *personal history of anaphylactic shock (Z87.892)*

Z86.61   **Personal history of infections of the central nervous system**
Personal history of encephalitis
Personal history of meningitis

Z86.69   **Personal history of other diseases of the nervous system and sense organs**

✓5ᵗʰ **Z86.7**   **Personal history of diseases of the circulatory system**
Conditions classifiable to I00-I99
EXCLUDES 2   *old myocardial infarction (I25.2)*
personal history of anaphylactic shock (Z87.892)
postmyocardial infarction syndrome (I24.1)

✓6ᵗʰ **Z86.71**   **Personal history of venous thrombosis and embolism**

Z86.711   **Personal history of pulmonary embolism**

Z86.718   **Personal history of other venous thrombosis and embolism**

Z86.72   **Personal history of thrombophlebitis**

Z86.73   **Personal history of transient ischemic attack (TIA), and cerebral infarction without residual deficits**
Personal history of prolonged reversible ischemic neurological deficit (PRIND)
Personal history of stroke NOS without residual deficits
EXCLUDES 1   *personal history of traumatic brain injury (Z87.820)*
sequelae of cerebrovascular disease (I69.-)
AHA: 2012, 4Q, 92

Z86.74   **Personal history of sudden cardiac arrest**
Personal history of sudden cardiac death successfully resuscitated

Z86.79   **Personal history of other diseases of the circulatory system**

✓4ᵗʰ **Z87**   **Personal history of other diseases and conditions**
Code first any follow-up examination after treatment (Z09)

✓5ᵗʰ **Z87.0**   **Personal history of diseases of the respiratory system**
Conditions classifiable to J00-J99

Z87.01   **Personal history of pneumonia (recurrent)**

Z87.09   **Personal history of other diseases of the respiratory system**

✓5ᵗʰ **Z87.1**   **Personal history of diseases of the digestive system**
Conditions classifiable to K00-K93

Z87.11   **Personal history of peptic ulcer disease**

Z87.19   **Personal history of other diseases of the digestive system**
AHA: 2017, 1Q, 14

Z87.2   **Personal history of diseases of the skin and subcutaneous tissue**
Conditions classifiable to L00-L99
EXCLUDES 2   *personal history of diabetic foot ulcer (Z86.31)*

✓5ᵗʰ **Z87.3**   **Personal history of diseases of the musculoskeletal system and connective tissue**
Conditions classifiable to M00-M99
EXCLUDES 2   *personal history of (healed) traumatic fracture (Z87.81)*

✓6ᵗʰ **Z87.31**   **Personal history of (healed) nontraumatic fracture**

Z87.310   **Personal history of (healed) osteoporosis fracture**
Personal history of (healed) fragility fracture
Personal history of (healed) collapsed vertebra due to osteoporosis
TIP: Assign to indicate history of osteoporosis fractures that have resolved, even when a code from category M80 indicating current osteoporosis fracture is assigned.

Z87.311   **Personal history of (healed) other pathological fracture**
Personal history of (healed) collapsed vertebra NOS
EXCLUDES 2   *personal history of osteoporosis fracture (Z87.310)*

Z87.312   **Personal history of (healed) stress fracture**
Personal history of (healed) fatigue fracture

Z87.39   **Personal history of other diseases of the musculoskeletal system and connective tissue**

✓5ᵗʰ **Z87.4**   **Personal history of diseases of genitourinary system**
Conditions classifiable to N00-N99

✓6ᵗʰ **Z87.41**   **Personal history of dysplasia of the female genital tract**
EXCLUDES 1   *personal history of intraepithelial neoplasia III of female genital tract ▶(Z86.001, Z86.008)◀*
personal history of malignant neoplasm of female genital tract (Z85.40-Z85.44)

Z87.410   **Personal history of cervical dysplasia**   ♀

Z87.411   **Personal history of vaginal dysplasia**   ♀

Z87.412   **Personal history of vulvar dysplasia**   ♀

Z87.42   **Personal history of other diseases of the female genital tract**   ♀

✓6ᵗʰ **Z87.43**   **Personal history of diseases of the male genital organs**

Z87.430   **Personal history of prostatic dysplasia**   ♂
EXCLUDES 1   *personal history of malignant neoplasm of prostate (Z85.46)*

Z87.438   **Personal history of other diseases of male genital organs**   ♂

☑ Additional Character Req   ✓x7ᵗʰ Placeholder Alert   Case-Mix Diagnosis   Manifestation   ▽ Unspecified Dx   EXCLUDES 1 Not coded here   EXCLUDES 2 Not included here

✓6ᵗʰ **Z87.44 Personal history of diseases of the urinary system**
> EXCLUDES 1 *personal history of malignant neoplasm of cervix uteri (Z85.41)*

Z87.440 Personal history of urinary (tract) infections

Z87.441 Personal history of nephrotic syndrome

Z87.442 Personal history of urinary calculi
Personal history of kidney stones

Z87.448 Personal history of other diseases of urinary system

✓5ᵗʰ **Z87.5 Personal history of complications of pregnancy, childbirth and the puerperium**
Conditions classifiable to O00-O9A
> EXCLUDES 2 *recurrent pregnancy loss (N96)*

Z87.51 Personal history of pre-term labor ♀
> EXCLUDES 1 *current pregnancy with history of pre-term labor (O09.21-)*

Z87.59 Personal history of other complications of pregnancy, childbirth and the puerperium ♀
Personal history of trophoblastic disease

✓5ᵗʰ **Z87.7 Personal history of (corrected) congenital malformations**
Conditions classifiable to Q00-Q89 that have been repaired or corrected
> EXCLUDES 1 *congenital malformations that have been partially corrected or repaired but which still require medical treatment—code to condition*
> EXCLUDES 2 *other postprocedural states (Z98.-)*
> *personal history of medical treatment (Z92.-)*
> *presence of cardiac and vascular implants and grafts (Z95.-)*
> *presence of other devices (Z97.-)*
> *presence of other functional implants (Z96.-)*
> *transplanted organ and tissue status (Z94.-)*

✓6ᵗʰ **Z87.71 Personal history of (corrected) congenital malformations of genitourinary system**

Z87.710 Personal history of (corrected) hypospadias ♂

Z87.718 Personal history of other specified (corrected) congenital malformations of genitourinary system

✓6ᵗʰ **Z87.72 Personal history of (corrected) congenital malformations of nervous system and sense organs**

Z87.720 Personal history of (corrected) congenital malformations of eye

Z87.721 Personal history of (corrected) congenital malformations of ear

Z87.728 Personal history of other specified (corrected) congenital malformations of nervous system and sense organs

✓6ᵗʰ **Z87.73 Personal history of (corrected) congenital malformations of digestive system**

Z87.730 Personal history of (corrected) cleft lip and palate

Z87.738 Personal history of other specified (corrected) congenital malformations of digestive system

Z87.74 Personal history of (corrected) congenital malformations of heart and circulatory system

Z87.75 Personal history of (corrected) congenital malformations of respiratory system

Z87.76 Personal history of (corrected) congenital malformations of integument, limbs and musculoskeletal system

✓6ᵗʰ **Z87.79 Personal history of other (corrected) congenital malformations**

Z87.790 Personal history of (corrected) congenital malformations of face and neck

Z87.798 Personal history of other (corrected) congenital malformations

✓5ᵗʰ **Z87.8 Personal history of other specified conditions**
> EXCLUDES 2 *personal history of self harm (Z91.5)*

Z87.81 Personal history of (healed) traumatic fracture
> EXCLUDES 2 *personal history of (healed) nontraumatic fracture (Z87.31-)*

✓6ᵗʰ **Z87.82 Personal history of other (healed) physical injury and trauma**
Conditions classifiable to S00-T88, except traumatic fractures

Z87.820 Personal history of traumatic brain injury
> EXCLUDES 1 *personal history of transient ischemic attack (TIA), and cerebral infarction without residual deficits (Z86.73)*

Z87.821 Personal history of retained foreign body fully removed

Z87.828 Personal history of other (healed) physical injury and trauma

✓6ᵗʰ **Z87.89 Personal history of other specified conditions**

Z87.890 Personal history of sex reassignment

Z87.891 Personal history of nicotine dependence
> EXCLUDES 1 *current nicotine dependence (F17.2-)*
AHA: 2017, 2Q, 27

Z87.892 Personal history of anaphylaxis
Code also allergy status such as:
allergy status to drugs, medicaments and biological substances (Z88.-)
allergy status, other than to drugs and biological substances (Z91.0-)

Z87.898 Personal history of other specified conditions
AHA: 2013, 1Q, 21

✓4ᵗʰ **Z88 Allergy status to drugs, medicaments and biological substances**
> EXCLUDES 2 *allergy status, other than to drugs and biological substances (Z91.0-)*
AHA: 2015, 3Q, 23

Z88.0 Allergy status to penicillin

Z88.1 Allergy status to other antibiotic agents status

Z88.2 Allergy status to sulfonamides status

Z88.3 Allergy status to other anti-infective agents status

Z88.4 Allergy status to anesthetic agent status

Z88.5 Allergy status to narcotic agent status

Z88.6 Allergy status to analgesic agent status

Z88.7 Allergy status to serum and vaccine status

Z88.8 Allergy status to other drugs, medicaments and biological substances status

Z88.9 Allergy status to unspecified drugs, medicaments and biological substances status ▽

✓4ᵗʰ **Z89 Acquired absence of limb**
> INCLUDES amputation status
> postprocedural loss of limb
> post-traumatic loss of limb
> EXCLUDES 1 *acquired deformities of limbs (M20-M21)*
> *congenital absence of limbs (Q71-Q73)*

✓5ᵗʰ **Z89.0 Acquired absence of thumb and other finger(s)**

✓6ᵗʰ **Z89.01 Acquired absence of thumb**

Z89.011 Acquired absence of right thumb

Z89.012 Acquired absence of left thumb

Z89.019 Acquired absence of unspecified thumb ▽

✓6ᵗʰ **Z89.02 Acquired absence of other finger(s)**
> EXCLUDES 2 *acquired absence of thumb (Z89.01-)*

Z89.021 Acquired absence of right finger(s)

Z89.022 Acquired absence of left finger(s)

Z89.029 Acquired absence of unspecified finger(s) ▽

✓5ᵗʰ **Z89.1 Acquired absence of hand and wrist**

✓6ᵗʰ **Z89.11 Acquired absence of hand**

Z89.111 Acquired absence of right hand

Z89.112 Acquired absence of left hand

Z89.119 Acquired absence of unspecified hand ▽

✓6ᵗʰ **Z89.12 Acquired absence of wrist**
Disarticulation at wrist

Z89.121 Acquired absence of right wrist

Z89.122 Acquired absence of left wrist

Z89.129 Acquired absence of unspecified wrist ▽

✓5ᵗʰ **Z89.2 Acquired absence of upper limb above wrist**

✓6ᵗʰ **Z89.20 Acquired absence of upper limb, unspecified level**

Z89.201 Acquired absence of right upper limb, unspecified level ▽

N Newborn: 0   P Pediatric: 0-17   M Maternity: 12-55   A Adult: 15-124   **NRS** Nonroutine supply Dx   **NC Dx** Noncancer Dx   **PDx** Primary Dx   ►◄ Revised Text   ● New Code   ▲ Revised Title

1202   ICD-10-CM 2018

Z89.202　Acquired absence of left upper limb, unspecified level ▽

Z89.209　Acquired absence of unspecified upper limb, unspecified level ▽
　　　　　Acquired absence of arm NOS

✓6ᵗʰ **Z89.21**　Acquired absence of upper limb below elbow

Z89.211　Acquired absence of right upper limb below elbow

Z89.212　Acquired absence of left upper limb below elbow

Z89.219　Acquired absence of unspecified upper limb below elbow ▽

✓6ᵗʰ **Z89.22**　Acquired absence of upper limb above elbow
　　　　　Disarticulation at elbow

Z89.221　Acquired absence of right upper limb above elbow

Z89.222　Acquired absence of left upper limb above elbow

Z89.229　Acquired absence of unspecified upper limb above elbow ▽

✓6ᵗʰ **Z89.23**　Acquired absence of shoulder
　　　　　Acquired absence of shoulder joint following explantation of shoulder joint prosthesis, with or without presence of antibiotic-impregnated cement spacer

Z89.231　Acquired absence of right shoulder

Z89.232　Acquired absence of left shoulder

Z89.239　Acquired absence of unspecified shoulder ▽

✓5ᵗʰ **Z89.4**　Acquired absence of toe(s), foot, and ankle

✓6ᵗʰ **Z89.41**　Acquired absence of great toe

Z89.411　Acquired absence of right great toe

Z89.412　Acquired absence of left great toe

Z89.419　Acquired absence of unspecified great toe ▽

✓6ᵗʰ **Z89.42**　Acquired absence of other toe(s)
　　　　　EXCLUDES 2　acquired absence of great toe (Z89.41-)

Z89.421　Acquired absence of other right toe(s)

Z89.422　Acquired absence of other left toe(s)

Z89.429　Acquired absence of other toe(s), unspecified side ▽

✓6ᵗʰ **Z89.43**　Acquired absence of foot

Z89.431　Acquired absence of right foot

Z89.432　Acquired absence of left foot

Z89.439　Acquired absence of unspecified foot ▽

✓6ᵗʰ **Z89.44**　Acquired absence of ankle
　　　　　Disarticulation of ankle

Z89.441　Acquired absence of right ankle

Z89.442　Acquired absence of left ankle

Z89.449　Acquired absence of unspecified ankle ▽

✓5ᵗʰ **Z89.5**　Acquired absence of leg below knee

✓6ᵗʰ **Z89.51**　Acquired absence of leg below knee

Z89.511　Acquired absence of right leg below knee

Z89.512　Acquired absence of left leg below knee

Z89.519　Acquired absence of unspecified leg below knee ▽

✓6ᵗʰ **Z89.52**　Acquired absence of knee
　　　　　Acquired absence of knee joint following explantation of knee joint prosthesis, with or without presence of antibiotic-impregnated cement spacer

Z89.521　Acquired absence of right knee

Z89.522　Acquired absence of left knee

Z89.529　Acquired absence of unspecified knee ▽

✓5ᵗʰ **Z89.6**　Acquired absence of leg above knee

✓6ᵗʰ **Z89.61**　Acquired absence of leg above knee
　　　　　Acquired absence of leg NOS　Disarticulation at knee

Z89.611　Acquired absence of right leg above knee

Z89.612　Acquired absence of left leg above knee

Z89.619　Acquired absence of unspecified leg above knee ▽

✓6ᵗʰ **Z89.62**　Acquired absence of hip
　　　　　Acquired absence of hip joint following explantation of hip joint prosthesis, with or without presence of antibiotic-impregnated cement spacer
　　　　　Disarticulation at hip

Z89.621　Acquired absence of right hip joint

Z89.622　Acquired absence of left hip joint

Z89.629　Acquired absence of unspecified hip joint ▽

Z89.9　Acquired absence of limb, unspecified ▽

✓4ᵗʰ **Z90**　**Acquired absence of organs, not elsewhere classified**
　　　INCLUDES　postprocedural or post-traumatic loss of body part NEC
　　　EXCLUDES 1　congenital absence—see Alphabetical Index
　　　EXCLUDES 2　postprocedural absence of endocrine glands (E89.-)

✓5ᵗʰ **Z90.0**　Acquired absence of part of head and neck

Z90.01　Acquired absence of eye

Z90.02　Acquired absence of larynx

Z90.09　Acquired absence of other part of head and neck
　　　　　Acquired absence of nose
　　　　　EXCLUDES 2　teeth (K08.1)

✓5ᵗʰ **Z90.1**　Acquired absence of breast and nipple

Z90.10　Acquired absence of unspecified breast and nipple ▽

Z90.11　Acquired absence of right breast and nipple

Z90.12　Acquired absence of left breast and nipple

Z90.13　Acquired absence of bilateral breasts and nipples

Z90.2　Acquired absence of lung [part of]

Z90.3　Acquired absence of stomach [part of]

✓5ᵗʰ **Z90.4**　Acquired absence of other specified parts of digestive tract

✓6ᵗʰ **Z90.41**　Acquired absence of pancreas
　　　　　Code also exocrine pancreatic insufficiency (K86.81)
　　　　　Use additional code to identify any associated:
　　　　　insulin use (Z79.4)
　　　　　diabetes mellitus, postpancreatectomy (E13.-)

Z90.410　Acquired total absence of pancreas
　　　　　Acquired absence of pancreas NOS

Z90.411　Acquired partial absence of pancreas

Z90.49　Acquired absence of other specified parts of digestive tract

Z90.5　Acquired absence of kidney

Z90.6　Acquired absence of other parts of urinary tract
　　　　　Acquired absence of bladder

✓5ᵗʰ **Z90.7**　Acquired absence of genital organ(s)
　　　EXCLUDES 1　personal history of sex reassignment (Z87.890)
　　　EXCLUDES 2　female genital mutilation status (N90.81-)

✓6ᵗʰ **Z90.71**　Acquired absence of cervix and uterus

Z90.710　Acquired absence of both cervix and uterus ♀
　　　　　Acquired absence of uterus NOS
　　　　　Status post total hysterectomy

Z90.711　Acquired absence of uterus with remaining cervical stump ♀
　　　　　Status post partial hysterectomy with remaining cervical stump

Z90.712　Acquired absence of cervix with remaining uterus ♀

✓6ᵗʰ **Z90.72**　Acquired absence of ovaries

Z90.721　Acquired absence of ovaries, unilateral ♀

Z90.722　Acquired absence of ovaries, bilateral ♀

Z90.79　Acquired absence of other genital organ(s)

✓5ᵗʰ **Z90.8**　Acquired absence of other organs

Z90.81　Acquired absence of spleen

Z90.89　Acquired absence of other organs

☑ Additional Character Req　　✓x7ᵗʰ Placeholder Alert　　Case-Mix Diagnosis　　Manifestation　　▽ Unspecified Dx　　**EXCLUDES 1** Not coded here　　**EXCLUDES 2** Not included here

Chapter 21. Factors Influencing Health Status and Contact with Health Services

✓4th Z91   Personal risk factors, not elsewhere classified

> *EXCLUDES 2*   contact with and (suspected) exposures hazardous to health (Z77.-)
>
> exposure to pollution and other problems related to physical environment (Z77.1-)
>
> ▶female genital mutilation status (N90.81-)◀
>
> personal history of physical injury and trauma (Z87.81, Z87.82-)
>
> occupational exposure to risk factors (Z57.-)

✓5th Z91.0   Allergy status, other than to drugs and biological substances

> *EXCLUDES 2*   allergy status to drugs, medicaments, and biological substances (Z88.-)

  ✓6th Z91.01   Food allergy status

> *EXCLUDES 2*   food additives allergy status (Z91.02)

    Z91.010   Allergy to peanuts

    Z91.011   Allergy to milk products

> *EXCLUDES 1*   lactose intolerance (E73.-)

    Z91.012   Allergy to eggs

    Z91.013   Allergy to seafood

> Allergy to shellfish
>
> Allergy to octopus or squid ink

    Z91.018   Allergy to other foods

> Allergy to nuts other than peanuts

  Z91.02   Food additives allergy status

  ✓6th Z91.03   Insect allergy status

    Z91.030   Bee allergy status

    Z91.038   Other insect allergy status

  ✓6th Z91.04   Nonmedicinal substance allergy status

    Z91.040   Latex allergy status

> Latex sensitivity status

    Z91.041   Radiographic dye allergy status

> Allergy status to contrast media used for diagnostic X-ray procedure

    Z91.048   Other nonmedicinal substance allergy status

  Z91.09   Other allergy status, other than to drugs and biological substances

✓5th Z91.1   Patient's noncompliance with medical treatment and regimen

  Z91.11   Patient's noncompliance with dietary regimen

  ✓6th Z91.12   Patient's intentional underdosing of medication regimen

> Code first underdosing of medication (T36-T50) with fifth or sixth character 6
>
> *EXCLUDES 1*   adverse effect of prescribed drug taken as directed—code to adverse effect
>
> poisoning (overdose)—code to poisoning

    Z91.120   Patient's intentional underdosing of medication regimen due to financial hardship

    Z91.128   Patient's intentional underdosing of medication regimen for other reason

  ✓6th Z91.13   Patient's unintentional underdosing of medication regimen

> Code first underdosing of medication (T36-T50) with fifth or sixth character 6
>
> *EXCLUDES 1*   adverse effect of prescribed drug taken as directed—code to adverse effect
>
> poisoning (overdose)—code to poisoning

    Z91.130   Patient's unintentional underdosing of medication regimen due to age-related debility

    Z91.138   Patient's unintentional underdosing of medication regimen for other reason

  Z91.14   Patient's other noncompliance with medication regimen

> Patient's underdosing of medication NOS

  Z91.15   Patient's noncompliance with renal dialysis

  Z91.19   Patient's noncompliance with other medical treatment and regimen

> ▶Nonadherence to medical treatment◀

✓5th Z91.4   Personal history of psychological trauma, not elsewhere classified

  ✓6th Z91.41   Personal history of adult abuse

> *EXCLUDES 2*   personal history of abuse in childhood (Z62.81-)

    Z91.410   Personal history of adult physical and sexual abuse 🅰

> *EXCLUDES 1*   current adult physical abuse (T74.11, T76.11)
>
> current adult sexual abuse (T74.21, T76.11)

    Z91.411   Personal history of adult psychological abuse 🅰

    Z91.412   Personal history of adult neglect 🅰

> *EXCLUDES 1*   current adult neglect (T74.01, T76.01)

    Z91.419   Personal history of unspecified adult abuse 🅰▽

  Z91.49   Other personal history of psychological trauma, not elsewhere classified

Z91.5   Personal history of self-harm

> Personal history of parasuicide
>
> Personal history of self-poisoning
>
> Personal history of suicide attempt

✓5th Z91.8   Other specified personal risk factors, not elsewhere classified

  Z91.81   History of falling

> At risk for falling

  Z91.82   Personal history of military deployment 🅰

> Individual (civilian or military) with past history of military war, peacekeeping and humanitarian deployment (current or past conflict)
>
> Returned from military deployment

  Z91.83   *Wandering in diseases classified elsewhere*

> Code first underlying disorder such as:
>
> Alzheimer's disease (G30.-)
>
> autism or pervasive developmental disorder (F84.-)
>
> intellectual disabilities (F70-F79)
>
> unspecified dementia with behavioral disturbance (F03.9-)

  ✓6th Z91.84   Oral health risk factors

    Z91.841   Risk for dental caries, low

    Z91.842   Risk for dental caries, moderate

    Z91.843   Risk for dental caries, high

    Z91.849   Unspecified risk for dental caries ▽

  Z91.89   Other specified personal risk factors, not elsewhere classified

> **AHA:** 2017, 1Q, 45

✓4th Z92   Personal history of medical treatment

> *EXCLUDES 2*   postprocedural states (Z98.-)

Z92.0   Personal history of contraception

> *EXCLUDES 1*   counseling or management of current contraceptive practices (Z30.-)
>
> long term (current) use of contraception (Z79.3)
>
> presence of (intrauterine) contraceptive device (Z97.5)

✓5th Z92.2   Personal history of drug therapy

> *EXCLUDES 2*   long term (current) drug therapy (Z79.-)

  Z92.21   Personal history of antineoplastic chemotherapy

  Z92.22   Personal history of monoclonal drug therapy

  Z92.23   Personal history of estrogen therapy

  ✓6th Z92.24   Personal history of steroid therapy

    Z92.240   Personal history of inhaled steroid therapy

    Z92.241   Personal history of systemic steroid therapy

> Personal history of steroid therapy NOS

  Z92.25   Personal history of immunosupression therapy

> *EXCLUDES 2*   personal history of steroid therapy (Z92.24)

  Z92.29   Personal history of other drug therapy

Z92.3   Personal history of irradiation

> Personal history of exposure to therapeutic radiation
>
> *EXCLUDES 1*   exposure to radiation in the physical environment (Z77.12)
>
> occupational exposure to radiation (Z57.1)

✓5th Z92.8   Personal history of other medical treatment

  Z92.81   Personal history of extracorporeal membrane oxygenation (ECMO)

Ⓝ Newborn: 0   Ⓟ Pediatric: 0-17   Ⓜ Maternity: 12-55   🅰 Adult: 15-124   **NRS** Nonroutine supply Dx   **NC Dx** Noncancer Dx   **PDx** Primary Dx   ▶◀ Revised Text   ● New Code   ▲ Revised Title

Chapter 21. Factors Influencing Health Status and Contact with Health Services   Z92.82–Z96.641

Z92.82 **Status post administration of tPA (rtPA) in a different facility within the last 24 hours prior to admission to current facility**
Code first condition requiring tPA administration, such as:
acute cerebral infarction (I63.-)
acute myocardial infarction (I21-, I22-)
AHA: 2013, 4Q, 124

Z92.83 **Personal history of failed moderate sedation**
Personal history of failed conscious sedation
EXCLUDES 2 *failed moderate sedation during procedure (T88.52)*

Z92.84 **Personal history of unintended awareness under general anesthesia**
EXCLUDES 2 *unintended awareness under general anesthesia during procedure (T88.53)*

Z92.89 **Personal history of other medical treatment**

✓4th **Z93** **Artificial opening status**
EXCLUDES 1 *artificial openings requiring attention or management (Z43.-)*
complications of external stoma (J95.0-, K94.-, N99.5-)

Z93.0 **Tracheostomy status**
AHA: 2013, 4Q, 129

Z93.1 **Gastrostomy status**

Z93.2 **Ileostomy status**

Z93.3 **Colostomy status**

Z93.4 **Other artificial openings of gastrointestinal tract status**

✓5th **Z93.5** **Cystostomy status**

Z93.50 **Unspecified cystostomy status** ▽

Z93.51 **Cutaneous-vesicostomy status**

Z93.52 **Appendico-vesicostomy status**

Z93.59 **Other cystostomy status**

Z93.6 **Other artificial openings of urinary tract status**
Nephrostomy status   Ureterostomy status
Urethrostomy status

Z93.8 **Other artificial opening status**

Z93.9 **Artificial opening status, unspecified** ▽

✓4th **Z94** **Transplanted organ and tissue status**
INCLUDES organ or tissue replaced by heterogenous or homogenous transplant
EXCLUDES 1 *complications of transplanted organ or tissue—see Alphabetical Index*
EXCLUDES 2 *presence of vascular grafts (Z95.-)*

Z94.0 **Kidney transplant status**

Z94.1 **Heart transplant status**
EXCLUDES 1 *artificial heart status (Z95.812)*
heart-valve replacement status (Z95.2-Z95.4)

Z94.2 **Lung transplant status**

Z94.3 **Heart and lungs transplant status**

Z94.4 **Liver transplant status**

Z94.5 **Skin transplant status**
Autogenous skin transplant status

Z94.6 **Bone transplant status**

Z94.7 **Corneal transplant status**

✓5th **Z94.8** **Other transplanted organ and tissue status**

Z94.81 **Bone marrow transplant status**

Z94.82 **Intestine transplant status**

Z94.83 **Pancreas transplant status**

Z94.84 **Stem cells transplant status**

Z94.89 **Other transplanted organ and tissue status**

Z94.9 **Transplanted organ and tissue status, unspecified** ▽

✓4th **Z95** **Presence of cardiac and vascular implants and grafts**
EXCLUDES 1 ~~complications of cardiac and vascular devices, implants and grafts (T82.-)~~
EXCLUDES 2 ▶complications of cardiac and vascular devices, implants and grafts (T82.-)◀

Z95.0 **Presence of cardiac pacemaker**
Presence of cardiac resynchronization therapy (CRT-P) pacemaker
EXCLUDES 1 *adjustment or management of cardiac device (Z45.0-)*
adjustment or management of cardiac pacemaker (Z45.0)
presence of automatic (implantable) cardiac defibrillator with synchronous cardiac pacemaker (Z95.810)

Z95.1 **Presence of aortocoronary bypass graft**
Presence of coronary artery bypass graft

Z95.2 **Presence of prosthetic heart valve**
Presence of heart valve NOS

Z95.3 **Presence of xenogenic heart valve**

Z95.4 **Presence of other heart-valve replacement**

Z95.5 **Presence of coronary angioplasty implant and graft**
EXCLUDES 1 *coronary angioplasty status without implant and graft (Z98.61)*

✓5th **Z95.8** **Presence of other cardiac and vascular implants and grafts**

✓6th **Z95.81** **Presence of other cardiac implants and grafts**

Z95.810 **Presence of automatic (implantable) cardiac defibrillator**
Presence of automatic (implantable) cardiac defibrillator with synchronous cardiac pacemaker
Presence of cardiac resynchronization therapy defibrillator (CRT-D)
Presence of cardioverter-defibrillator (ICD)

Z95.811 **Presence of heart assist device**

Z95.812 **Presence of fully implantable artificial heart**

Z95.818 **Presence of other cardiac implants and grafts**

✓6th **Z95.82** **Presence of other vascular implants and grafts**

Z95.820 **Peripheral vascular angioplasty status with implants and grafts**
EXCLUDES 1 *peripheral vascular angioplasty without implant and graft (Z98.62)*

Z95.828 **Presence of other vascular implants and grafts**
Presence of intravascular prosthesis NEC

Z95.9 **Presence of cardiac and vascular implant and graft, unspecified** ▽

✓4th **Z96** **Presence of other functional implants**
EXCLUDES 2 *complications of internal prosthetic devices, implants and grafts (T82-T85)*
fitting and adjustment of prosthetic and other devices (Z44-Z46)

Z96.0 **Presence of urogenital implants**

Z96.1 **Presence of intraocular lens**
Presence of pseudophakia

✓5th **Z96.2** **Presence of otological and audiological implants**

Z96.20 **Presence of otological and audiological implant, unspecified** ▽

Z96.21 **Cochlear implant status**

Z96.22 **Myringotomy tube(s) status**

Z96.29 **Presence of other otological and audiological implants**
Presence of bone-conduction hearing device
Presence of eustachian tube stent
Stapes replacement

Z96.3 **Presence of artificial larynx**

✓5th **Z96.4** **Presence of endocrine implants**

Z96.41 **Presence of insulin pump (external) (internal)**

Z96.49 **Presence of other endocrine implants**

Z96.5 **Presence of tooth-root and mandibular implants**

✓5th **Z96.6** **Presence of orthopedic joint implants**

Z96.60 **Presence of unspecified orthopedic joint implant** ▽

✓6th **Z96.61** **Presence of artificial shoulder joint**

Z96.611 **Presence of right artificial shoulder joint**

Z96.612 **Presence of left artificial shoulder joint**

Z96.619 **Presence of unspecified artificial shoulder joint** ▽

✓6th **Z96.62** **Presence of artificial elbow joint**

Z96.621 **Presence of right artificial elbow joint**

Z96.622 **Presence of left artificial elbow joint**

Z96.629 **Presence of unspecified artificial elbow joint** ▽

✓6th **Z96.63** **Presence of artificial wrist joint**

Z96.631 **Presence of right artificial wrist joint**

Z96.632 **Presence of left artificial wrist joint**

Z96.639 **Presence of unspecified artificial wrist joint** ▽

✓6th **Z96.64** **Presence of artificial hip joint**
Hip-joint replacement (partial) (total)

Z96.641 **Presence of right artificial hip joint**

Chapter 21. Factors Influencing Health Status and Contact with Health Services

Z96.642 **Presence of** left **artificial hip joint**

Z96.643 **Presence of artificial hip joint,** bilateral

Z96.649 **Presence of unspecified artificial hip** ▽
joint

✓6ᵗʰ Z96.65 **Presence of** artificial knee joint

Z96.651 **Presence of** right **artificial knee joint**

Z96.652 **Presence of** left **artificial knee joint**

Z96.653 **Presence of artificial knee joint,** bilateral

Z96.659 **Presence of unspecified artificial knee** ▽
joint

✓6ᵗʰ Z96.66 **Presence of** artificial ankle joint

Z96.661 **Presence of** right **artificial ankle joint**

Z96.662 **Presence of** left **artificial ankle joint**

Z96.669 **Presence of unspecified artificial ankle** ▽
joint

✓6ᵗʰ Z96.69 **Presence of** other orthopedic joint **implants**

Z96.691 **Finger-joint replacement of** right **hand**

Z96.692 **Finger-joint replacement of** left **hand**

Z96.693 **Finger-joint replacement,** bilateral

Z96.698 **Presence of other orthopedic joint**
implants

Z96.7 **Presence of other bone and tendon implants**
Presence of skull plate

✓5ᵗʰ Z96.8 **Presence of other specified functional implants**

Z96.81 **Presence of artificial skin**

Z96.89 **Presence of other specified functional implants**

Z96.9 **Presence of functional implant, unspecified** ▽

✓4ᵗʰ Z97 **Presence of other devices**

EXCLUDES 1 *complications of internal prosthetic devices, implants and grafts*
(T82-T85)
fitting and adjustment of prosthetic and other devices (Z44-Z46)

EXCLUDES 2 *presence of cerebrospinal fluid drainage device (Z98.2)*

Z97.0 **Presence of** artificial eye

✓5ᵗʰ Z97.1 **Presence of** artificial limb (complete) (partial)

Z97.10 **Presence of artificial limb (complete) (partial),** ▽
unspecified

Z97.11 **Presence of artificial** right **arm (complete) (partial)**

Z97.12 **Presence of artificial** left **arm (complete) (partial)**

Z97.13 **Presence of artificial** right **leg (complete) (partial)**

Z97.14 **Presence of artificial** left **leg (complete) (partial)**

Z97.15 **Presence of artificial arms, bilateral (complete)**
(partial)

Z97.16 **Presence of artificial legs, bilateral (complete)**
(partial)

Z97.2 **Presence of** dental prosthetic device **(complete) (partial)**
Presence of dentures (complete) (partial)

Z97.3 **Presence of** spectacles and contact lenses

Z97.4 **Presence of** external hearing-aid

Z97.5 **Presence of (intrauterine)** contraceptive device   ♀

EXCLUDES 1 *checking, reinsertion or removal of implantable*
subdermal contraceptive (Z30.46)
checking, reinsertion or removal of intrauterine
contraceptive device (Z30.43-)

Z97.8 **Presence of other specified devices**

✓4ᵗʰ Z98 **Other postprocedural states**

EXCLUDES 2 *aftercare (Z43-Z49, Z51)*
follow-up medical care (Z08- Z09)
postprocedural complication—see Alphabetical Index

Z98.0 **Intestinal bypass and anastomosis status**

EXCLUDES 2 *bariatric surgery status (Z98.84)*
gastric bypass status (Z98.84)
obesity surgery status (Z98.84)

Z98.1 **Arthrodesis status**

Z98.2 **Presence of cerebrospinal fluid drainage device**
Presence of CSF shunt

Z98.3 **Post therapeutic collapse of lung status**
Code first underlying disease

✓5ᵗʰ Z98.4 **Cataract extraction status**
Use additional code to identify intraocular lens implant status
(Z96.1)

EXCLUDES 1 *aphakia (H27.0)*

Z98.41 **Cataract extraction status,** right **eye**

Z98.42 **Cataract extraction status,** left **eye**

Z98.49 **Cataract extraction status, unspecified eye** ▽

✓5ᵗʰ Z98.5 **Sterilization status**

EXCLUDES 1 *female infertility (N97.-)*
male infertility (N46.-)

Z98.51 **Tubal ligation status**   ♀

Z98.52 **Vasectomy status**   Ⓐ♂

✓5ᵗʰ Z98.6 **Angioplasty status**

Z98.61 **Coronary angioplasty status**

EXCLUDES 1 *coronary angioplasty status with implant*
and graft (Z95.5)

Z98.62 **Peripheral vascular angioplasty status**

EXCLUDES 1 *peripheral vascular angioplasty status with*
implant and graft (Z95.820)

✓5ᵗʰ Z98.8 **Other specified postprocedural states**

✓6ᵗʰ Z98.81 **Dental procedure status**

Z98.810 **Dental sealant status**

Z98.811 **Dental restoration status**
Dental crown status
Dental fillings status

Z98.818 **Other dental procedure status**

Z98.82 **Breast implant status**

EXCLUDES 1 *breast implant removal status (Z98.86)*

Z98.83 **Filtering (vitreous) bleb after glaucoma surgery**
status

EXCLUDES 1 *inflammation (infection) of postprocedural*
bleb (H59.4-)

Z98.84 **Bariatric surgery status**
Gastric banding status
Gastric bypass status for obesity
Obesity surgery status

EXCLUDES 1 *bariatric surgery status complicating*
pregnancy, childbirth, or the
puerperium (O99.84)

EXCLUDES 2 *intestinal bypass and anastomosis status*
(Z98.0)

Z98.85 **Transplanted organ removal status**
Transplanted organ previously removed due to
complication, failure, rejection or infection

EXCLUDES 1 *encounter for removal of transplanted*
organ—code to complication of
transplanted organ (T86.-)

Z98.86 **Personal history of breast implant removal**

✓6ᵗʰ Z98.87 **Personal history of in** utero **procedure**

Z98.870 **Personal history of in utero procedure**   ♀
during pregnancy

EXCLUDES 2 *complications from in utero*
procedure for current
pregnancy (O35.7)
supervision of current pregnancy
with history of in utero pro-
cedure during previous preg-
nancy (O09.82-)

Z98.871 **Personal history of in utero procedure**
while a fetus

✓6ᵗʰ Z98.89 **Other specified postprocedural states**

Z98.890 **Other specified postprocedural states**
Personal history of surgery, not elsewhere
classified

Z98.891 **History of uterine scar from previous**
surgery

EXCLUDES 1 *maternal care due to uterine scar*
from previous surgery
(O34.2-)

Ⓝ Newborn: 0   Ⓟ Pediatric: 0-17   Ⓜ Maternity: 12-55   Ⓐ Adult: 15-124   **NRS** Nonroutine supply Dx   **NC Dx** Noncancer Dx   **PDx** Primary Dx   ▶◀ Revised Text   ● New Code   ▲ Revised Title

1206   ICD-10-CM 2018

✓4ᵗʰ Z99   Dependence on enabling machines and devices, not elsewhere classified
     EXCLUDES 1   *cardiac pacemaker status (Z95.0)*

Z99.0   Dependence on aspirator

✓5ᵗʰ Z99.1   Dependence on respirator
     Dependence on ventilator

     Z99.11   Dependence on respirator [ventilator] status
         AHA: 2015, 1Q, 21

     Z99.12   Encounter for respirator [ventilator]   **PDx**
         dependence during power failure
         EXCLUDES 1   *mechanical complication of respirator [ventilator] (J95.850)*

Z99.2   Dependence on renal dialysis
     Hemodialysis status
     Peritoneal dialysis status
     Presence of arteriovenous shunt for dialysis
     Renal dialysis status NOS
     EXCLUDES 1   *encounter for fitting and adjustment of dialysis catheter (Z49.0-)*
     EXCLUDES 2   *noncompliance with renal dialysis (Z91.15)*
     AHA: 2016, 1Q, 12; 2013, 4Q, 125

Z99.3   Dependence on wheelchair
     Wheelchair confinement status
     Code first cause of dependence, such as:
         muscular dystrophy (G71.0)
         obesity (E66.-)

✓5ᵗʰ Z99.8   Dependence on other enabling machines and devices

     Z99.81   Dependence on supplemental oxygen
         Dependence on long-term oxygen
         AHA: 2013, 4Q, 129

     Z99.89   Dependence on other enabling machines and devices
         Dependence on machine or device NOS

✓ Additional Character Req   ✓x7ᵗʰ Placeholder Alert   Case-Mix Diagnosis   Manifestation   ∇ Unspecified Dx   **EXCLUDES 1** Not coded here   **EXCLUDES 2** Not included here

Appendixes

Appendix A: 10 Steps to Correct Coding

Follow the 10 steps below to correctly code encounters for health care services.

Step 1: Identify the reason for the visit or encounter (i.e., a sign, symptom, diagnosis and/or condition).

The medical record documentation should accurately reflect the patient's condition, using terminology that includes specific diagnoses and symptoms or clearly states the reasons for the encounter.

Choosing the main term that best describes the reason chiefly responsible for the service provided is the most important step in coding. If symptoms are present and documented but a definitive diagnosis has not been determined, code the symptoms. **For outpatient cases, do not code conditions that are referred to as "rule out," "suspected," "probable," or "questionable."** Diagnoses often are not established at the time of the initial encounter/visit and may require two or more visits to be established. Code only what is documented in the available records and only to the highest degree of certainty known at the time of the patient's visit, unless it is an inpatient medical record, in which case uncertain diagnoses may be reported if documented at the time of discharge.

Step 2: After selecting the reason for the encounter, always consult the alphabetic index before verifying code selection in the tabular section.

The most critical rule is to begin code selection in the *alphabetic index*. Never turn first to the tabular list. The index provides cross-references, essential and nonessential modifiers, and inclusion terms not found in the tabular list. To prevent coding errors, always use both the alphabetic index (to identify a code) and the tabular list (to verify a code), as the index does not include the important instructional notes found in the tabular list. An added benefit of using the tabular list, which groups like things together, is that while looking at one code in the list, a coder might see a more specific one that would have been missed had the coder relied solely on the alphabetic index. Additionally, many of the codes require a fourth, fifth, sixth, or seventh, character to be valid, and many of these characters can be found only in the tabular list.

Step 3: Locate the main term entry.

The alphabetic index is a listing of conditions, which may be expressed as nouns or eponyms, with critical use of adjectives. Some conditions known by several names have multiple main entries. Reasons for encounters may be located under general terms such as admission, encounter, and examination. Other general terms such as history of, status post, or presence (of) are used to locate factors influencing health.

Step 4: Read cross-references listed with the main term or the subterm.

Cross-references such as *"see"* and *"see also"* are identified by italicized type and should always be checked to ensure that all alternative terms are researched.

Step 5: Review entries for modifiers.

Nonessential modifiers are the terms in parentheses following the main term entry. These parenthetical terms are supplementary words or explanatory information that may or may not appear in the diagnostic statement and do not affect code selection. The subterms listed under the main term are essential modifiers that do affect coding assignment. Each line of indent represents a more specific code entry. The nonessential modifiers apply to the subterms following a main term except when they are mutually exclusive, in which case the subterm takes precedence. For example, if "acute" is listed as a nonessential modifier but there is a subentry for "chronic," then the nonessential modifier of "acute" does not apply.

Step 6: Interpret abbreviations, cross-references, default codes, additional characters, and brackets.

The abbreviation NEC (not elsewhere classified) that follows some main terms or subterms indicates that there is no specific code for the condition even though the medical documentation may be very specific. The code next to the main term is called the default code. It represents the condition most commonly associated with the main term or the unspecified code for the main term. Additional characters may be required to construct the code; the tabular list must be referenced to determine what those specific characters should be. The alphabetic index uses brackets [ ] to enclose manifestation codes that can be used only as secondary codes to the underlying condition code immediately preceding it. Both codes must be reported in this multiple-coding situation.

Step 7: Choose a potential code and locate it in the tabular list.

The coder must follow any Includes, Excludes 1 and Excludes 2 notes, and other instructional notes, such as "Code first" and "Use additional code," listed in the tabular list for the chapter, category, subcategory, and subclassification level of code selection that direct the coder to use a different or additional code. Any codes in the tabular range, A00.0- through T88.9-, may be used to identify the diagnostic reason for the encounter. The tabular list encompasses many codes describing disease and injury classifications (e.g., infectious and parasitic diseases, neoplasms, symptoms, nervous and circulatory system etc.).

Codes that describe symptoms and signs, as opposed to definitive diagnoses, should be used for reporting purposes when an established diagnosis has not been made (confirmed) by the physician. Chapter 18 of the ICD-10-CM code book, "Symptoms, Signs, and Abnormal Clinical and Laboratory Findings, Not Elsewhere Classified" (codes R00.--R99), contains many, but not all, codes for symptoms.

ICD-10-CM classifies encounters with health care providers for circumstances other than a disease or injury using codes in chapter 21, "Factors Influencing Health Status and Contact with Health Services" (codes Z00–Z99). Circumstances other than a disease or injury often are recorded as chiefly responsible for the encounter.

Step 8: Determine whether the code is at the highest level of specificity.

A code is invalid if it has not been coded to the full number of characters (greatest level of specificity) required. Codes in ICD-10-CM can contain from three up to seven alphanumeric characters. A three-character code is to be used only if the category is not further subdivided into four-, five-, six-, or seven- character codes. Placeholder character X is used both to allow for future expansion and as a placeholder for empty characters in a code that requires a seventh character but has no fourth, fifth, or sixth character. Certain categories require seventh characters that apply to all codes in that category. Always check the category level for applicable seventh characters for that category.

Step 9: Assign the code.

Having reviewed all relevant information concerning the possible code choices, assign the code that most completely describes the condition.

Repeat steps one through nine for all additional documented conditions that meet the following criteria:

- Conditions that currently exist at the time of the visit

- Conditions that require or affect patient care, treatment, or management

Step 10: Sequence codes correctly

Sequencing is the order in which the codes are listed on the claim. List first the ICD-10-CM code for the diagnosis, condition, problem, or other reason for the encounter/visit, which is shown in the medical record to be chiefly responsible for the services provided. List additional codes that describe any coexisting conditions. Follow the official coding guidelines (see section II, "Selection of Principal Diagnosis"; section III, "Reporting Additional Diagnoses"; and section IV, "Diagnostic Coding and Reporting Guidelines for Outpatient Services") on proper sequencing of codes.

Coding Examples

Diagnosis: Anorexia

Step 1: The reason for the encounter was the condition, anorexia.

Step 2: Consult the alphabetic index.

Step 3: Locate the main term "Anorexia."

Step 4: There are no cross-references to check.

Step 5: Note that there are two possible subterms (essential modifiers), "hysterical" and "nervosa," neither of which is documented in this instance and therefore cannot be used in code selection. The code listed next to the main term is called the default code selection.

Step 6: There are no abbreviations, cross-references, additional character icons, or brackets.

Step 7: Turn to code R63.0 in the tabular list and read the instructional notes. In this case the Excludes 1 note indicates that anorexia nervosa and loss of appetite determined to be of nonorganic origin should be coded to a code from chapter 5. The diagnostic statement does not indicate nonorganic origin.

Step 8: There is no further division of the category past the fourth character subcategory. Therefore, the subcategory code level is the highest level of specificity.

Step 9: The default code, R63.0 Anorexia, is the correct code selection.

Step 10: Since anorexia is listed as the chief reason for the health care encounter, the first-listed, or principal, diagnosis is R63.0. Note that this is a chapter 18 symptom code but can be assigned since the provider did not establish a more definitive diagnosis.

Diagnosis: Acute bronchitis

Step 1: The reason for the encounter was the condition, acute bronchitis.

Step 2: Consult the alphabetic index.

Step 3: Locate the main term "Bronchitis."

Step 4: There are cross-references to interpret.

Step 5: Review entries for modifiers. Since "acute" is not listed as a nonessential modifier, read past the "with" modifier until you find the subterm "acute or subacute" with a nonessential modifier of "with bronchospasm or obstruction," code J20.9.

Step 6: There are no abbreviations, cross-references, additional character icons, or brackets.

Step 7: Since there are no more appropriate subterms, turn to code J20.9 in the tabular list. The Includes note under category J20 does refer to other alternative terms for acute bronchitis. Note that the inclusion term list is not exhaustive but is only a representative selection of diagnoses that are included in the subcategory. The Excludes 1 note refers bronchitis and tracheobronchitis NOS to category J40. There are several Excludes 2 notes that, if applicable, can be coded in addition to this code.

Step 8: Note that the subcategories included in J20 represent acute bronchitis due to various infectious organisms that would be selected if identified in the documentation. In this case, the organism was not identified and there is no further division of the category past the fourth character subcategory. Therefore, the subcategory code level is the highest level of specificity.

Step 9: Assign code J20.9 Acute bronchitis, unspecified.

Step 10: Repeat steps 1-9 for any additional code assignments.

Diagnosis: Infectious diarrhea

Step 1: The reason for the encounter was the condition, infectious diarrhea.

Step 2: Consult the alphabetic index.

Step 3: Locate the main term "Diarrhea" in the alphabetic index.

Step 4: There are no cross-references to check.

Step 5: Review entries for modifiers. Note that the nonessential modifiers (in parentheses) after the main term do not include the term "infectious," which means that the coder should search the subterms for the term "infectious." The subterm "infectious" refers to code A09.

Step 6: There are no abbreviations, cross-references, additional character icons, or brackets.

Step 7: Locate code A09 in the tabular list, and read all instructional notes under the main category and subcategories. The Includes notes does not list the term "infectious diarrhea" under code A09; however, as instructed by the alphabetic index, you should code the condition to A09. The ICD-10-CM code book implies that infectious diarrhea is the same as infectious gastroenteritis, enteritis, and colitis.

Step 8: There is no further division of the category past the third-character category level. Therefore, the category code level is the highest level of specificity. The final code assignment would be A09.

Step 9: Assign code A09 Infectious gastroenteritis and colitis, unspecified.

Step 10: Since infectious diarrhea is listed as the chief reason for the health care encounter, the first-listed, or principal, diagnosis is A09.

Diagnosis: Decubitus ulcer of right elbow with skin loss and necrosis of subcutaneous tissue

Step 1: The reason for the encounter was the condition, decubitus ulcer.

Step 2: Consult the alphabetic index.

Step 3: Locate the main term "Ulcer" in the alphabetic index.

Step 4: There are no cross-references to check.

Step 5: This entry does not have any important nonessential modifiers; however, there are other terms such as ulcerated, ulcerating, etc., that are included as main terms. Locate the subterm "decubitus" and note that there is an italicized cross-reference to "see Ulcer, pressure, by site." Go to the subterm "pressure" and locate "elbow," which refers to code L89.0-.

Step 6: Note that the code L89.0 is followed by a dash and an additional character icon, which indicate that more characters are required. From here, the tabular list can be consulted at code L89.0-.

Step 7: Locate code L89.0 in the tabular list, and check the category level L89 for any instructional, Includes, and Excludes 1 and 2 notes. Note that "decubitus" is an Includes note under L89 Pressure ulcer. Excludes 2 notes indicate that if this were documented as a diabetic pressure ulcer, it would be necessary to use a code from chapter 4.

Step 8: Read through the subcategory codes under L89.0 and note that the fifth character describes laterality. Locate the right elbow at subcategory L89.01. See that an additional sixth character is now needed to complete the code. The sixth character specifies the stage of the ulcer, which can be determined either by the specific documentation of the stage (e.g., stage 1, stage 2) or in this case, a description that matches one of the Includes notes that follow each stage code. For example, the description in this case of "skin loss and necrosis of the subcutaneous tissue" matches the Includes notes under L89.013 Pressure ulcer of right elbow, stage 3.

Step 9: Assign code L89.013 Pressure ulcer of right elbow, stage 3.

Step 10: Since the decubitus ulcer is listed as the chief reason for the health care encounter, the first-listed, or principal, diagnosis is L89.013. However, according to the Code first instructional note at the L89 category level, gangrene would be sequenced before the pressure ulcer if it were documented.

Diagnosis: First visit for bimalleolar fracture of the right ankle due to trauma

Step 1: The reason for the encounter was the condition, bimalleolar fracture of the right ankle.

Step 2: Consult the alphabetic index.

Step 3: Locate the main term "Fracture" in the alphabetic index.

Step 4: Note that the first main term for Fracture is pathological with cross-reference to "see also Fracture, traumatic." Locate the main term "Fracture, traumatic."

Step 5: Review entries for nonessential modifiers. Locate the subterms "ankle," "bimalleolar." Note that "displaced" is a nonessential modifier following "bimalleolar," indicating that S82.84- is the default code unless the fracture is specified as nondisplaced.

Step 6: Note that code S82.84- is followed by a dash and an additional character icon, both of which indicate that more characters are required. From here, the tabular list can be consulted at code S82.84.

Step 7: Locate code S82.84 Bimalleolar fracture of lower leg, in the tabular list and check the category level S82 for any instructional, Includes, and Excludes 1 and 2 notes. See the instructional notes indicating that fractures not specified as displaced or nondisplaced default to displaced, and fractures not designated as open or closed default to closed. See also the list of appropriate seventh characters to be added to all codes from category S82.

Step 8: Read through the subcategory codes under S82.84, and note that the sixth character specifies displaced or nondisplaced and laterality. Locate the displaced bimalleolar fracture of the right lower leg at code S82.841. See that an additional seventh character is still needed to complete the code. The seventh character specifies the type of encounter and whether the fracture is open or closed. Use character A listed in the box at the category level to describe initial encounter, closed fracture.

Step 9: Assign code S82.841A Displaced bimalleolar fracture of right lower leg, initial encounter for closed fracture.

Step 10: Since this is an injury code, code additionally any external cause, place of occurrence, and activity codes, with the injury (fracture) sequenced first.

Code	Description
A09	Infectious gastroenteritis and colitis, unspecified
A33	Tetanus neonatorum
A34	Obstetrical tetanus
A35	Other tetanus
A46	Erysipelas
A55	Chlamydial lymphogranuloma (venereum)
A57	Chancroid
A58	Granuloma inguinale
A64	Unspecified sexually transmitted disease
A65	Nonvenereal syphilis
A70	Chlamydia psittaci infections
A78	Q fever
A86	Unspecified viral encephalitis
A89	Unspecified viral infection of central nervous system
A90	Dengue fever [classical dengue]
A91	Dengue hemorrhagic fever
A94	Unspecified arthropod-borne viral fever
A99	Unspecified viral hemorrhagic fever
B03	Smallpox
B04	Monkeypox
B09	Unspecified viral infection characterized by skin and mucous membrane lesions
B20	Human immunodeficiency virus [HIV] disease
B49	Unspecified mycosis
B54	Unspecified malaria
B59	Pneumocystosis
B64	Unspecified protozoal disease
B72	Dracunculiasis
B75	Trichinellosis
B79	Trichuriasis
B80	Enterobiasis
B86	Scabies
B89	Unspecified parasitic disease
B91	Sequelae of poliomyelitis
B92	Sequelae of leprosy
C01	Malignant neoplasm of base of tongue
C07	Malignant neoplasm of parotid gland
C12	Malignant neoplasm of pyriform sinus
C19	Malignant neoplasm of rectosigmoid junction
C20	Malignant neoplasm of rectum
C23	Malignant neoplasm of gallbladder
C33	Malignant neoplasm of trachea
C37	Malignant neoplasm of thymus
C52	Malignant neoplasm of vagina
C55	Malignant neoplasm of uterus, part unspecified
C58	Malignant neoplasm of placenta
C61	Malignant neoplasm of prostate
C73	Malignant neoplasm of thyroid gland
D34	Benign neoplasm of thyroid gland
D45	Polycythemia vera
D62	Acute posthemorrhagic anemia
D65	Disseminated intravascular coagulation [defibrination syndrome]
D66	Hereditary factor VIII deficiency
D67	Hereditary factor IX deficiency
D71	Functional disorders of polymorphonuclear neutrophils
D77	Other disorders of blood and blood-forming organs in diseases classified elsewhere
E02	Subclinical iodine-deficiency hypothyroidism
E15	Nondiabetic hypoglycemic coma
E35	Disorders of endocrine glands in diseases classified elsewhere
E40	Kwashiorkor
E41	Nutritional marasmus
E42	Marasmic kwashiorkor
E43	Unspecified severe protein-calorie malnutrition
E45	Retarded development following protein-calorie malnutrition
E46	Unspecified protein-calorie malnutrition
E52	Niacin deficiency [pellagra]
E54	Ascorbic acid deficiency
E58	Dietary calcium deficiency
E59	Dietary selenium deficiency
E60	Dietary zinc deficiency
E65	Localized adiposity
E68	Sequelae of hyperalimentation
F04	Amnestic disorder due to known physiological condition
F05	Delirium due to known physiological condition
F09	Unspecified mental disorder due to known physiological condition
F21	Schizotypal disorder
F22	Delusional disorders
F23	Brief psychotic disorder
F24	Shared psychotic disorder
F28	Other psychotic disorder not due to a substance or known physiological condition
F29	Unspecified psychosis not due to a substance or known physiological condition
F39	Unspecified mood [affective] disorder
F53	Puerperal psychosis
F54	Psychological and behavioral factors associated with disorders or diseases classified elsewhere
F59	Unspecified behavioral syndromes associated with physiological disturbances and physical factors
F66	Other sexual disorders
F69	Unspecified disorder of adult personality and behavior
F70	Mild intellectual disabilities
F71	Moderate intellectual disabilities
F72	Severe intellectual disabilities
F73	Profound intellectual disabilities
F78	Other intellectual disabilities
F79	Unspecified intellectual disabilities
F82	Specific developmental disorder of motor function
F88	Other disorders of psychological development
F89	Unspecified disorder of psychological development
F99	Mental disorder, not otherwise specified
G01	Meningitis in bacterial diseases classified elsewhere
G02	Meningitis in other infectious and parasitic diseases classified elsewhere
G07	Intracranial and intraspinal abscess and granuloma in diseases classified elsewhere
G08	Intracranial and intraspinal phlebitis and thrombophlebitis
G09	Sequelae of inflammatory diseases of central nervous system
G10	Huntington's disease
G14	Postpolio syndrome
G20	Parkinson's disease
G26	Extrapyramidal and movement disorders in diseases classified elsewhere
G35	Multiple sclerosis
G53	Cranial nerve disorders in diseases classified elsewhere
G55	Nerve root and plexus compressions in diseases classified elsewhere
G59	Mononeuropathy in diseases classified elsewhere
G63	Polyneuropathy in diseases classified elsewhere
G64	Other disorders of peripheral nervous system
G92	Toxic encephalopathy
G94	Other disorders of brain in diseases classified elsewhere
H22	Disorders of iris and ciliary body in diseases classified elsewhere
H28	Cataract in diseases classified elsewhere
H32	Chorioretinal disorders in diseases classified elsewhere
H36	Retinal disorders in diseases classified elsewhere
H42	Glaucoma in diseases classified elsewhere
I00	Rheumatic fever without heart involvement
I10	Essential (primary) hypertension
I32	Pericarditis in diseases classified elsewhere
I38	Endocarditis, valve unspecified
I39	Endocarditis and heart valve disorders in diseases classified elsewhere
I41	Myocarditis in diseases classified elsewhere
I43	Cardiomyopathy in diseases classified elsewhere
I52	Other heart disorders in diseases classified elsewhere

I76	Septic arterial embolism
I81	Portal vein thrombosis
I96	Gangrene, not elsewhere classified
J00	Acute nasopharyngitis (common cold)
J13	Pneumonia due to Streptococcus pneumoniae
J14	Pneumonia due to Hemophilus influenzae
J17	Pneumonia in diseases classified elsewhere
J22	Unspecified acute lower respiratory infection
J36	Peritonsillar abscess
J40	Bronchitis, not specified as acute or chronic
J42	Unspecified chronic bronchitis
J60	Coalworker's pneumoconiosis
J61	Pneumoconiosis due to asbestos and other mineral fibers
J64	Unspecified pneumoconiosis
J65	Pneumoconiosis associated with tuberculosis
J80	Acute respiratory distress syndrome
J82	Pulmonary eosinophilia, not elsewhere classified
J90	Pleural effusion, not elsewhere classified
J99	Respiratory disorders in diseases classified elsewhere
K23	Disorders of esophagus in diseases classified elsewhere
K30	Functional dyspepsia
K36	Other appendicitis
K37	Unspecified appendicitis
K67	Disorders of peritoneum in infectious diseases classified elsewhere
K77	Liver disorders in diseases classified elsewhere
K87	Disorders of gallbladder, biliary tract and pancreas in diseases classified elsewhere
L00	Staphylococcal scalded skin syndrome
L14	Bullous disorders in diseases classified elsewhere
L22	Diaper dermatitis
L26	Exfoliative dermatitis
L42	Pityriasis rosea
L45	Papulosquamous disorders in diseases classified elsewhere
L52	Erythema nodosum
L54	Erythema in diseases classified elsewhere
L62	Nail disorders in diseases classified elsewhere
L80	Vitiligo
L83	Acanthosis nigricans
L84	Corns and callosities
L86	Keratoderma in diseases classified elsewhere
L88	Pyoderma gangrenosum
L99	Other disorders of skin and subcutaneous tissue in diseases classified elsewhere
N08	Glomerular disorders in diseases classified elsewhere
N10	Acute tubulo-interstitial nephritis
N12	Tubulo-interstitial nephritis, not specified as acute or chronic
N16	Renal tubulo-interstitial disorders in diseases classified elsewhere
N19	Unspecified kidney failure
N22	Calculus of urinary tract in diseases classified elsewhere
N23	Unspecified renal colic
N29	Other disorders of kidney and ureter in diseases classified elsewhere
N33	Bladder disorders in diseases classified elsewhere
N37	Urethral disorders in diseases classified elsewhere
N51	Disorders of male genital organs in diseases classified elsewhere
N62	Hypertrophy of breast
N72	Inflammatory disease of cervix uteri
N74	Female pelvic inflammatory disorders in diseases classified elsewhere
N86	Erosion and ectropion of cervix uteri
N96	Recurrent pregnancy loss
O68	Labor and delivery complicated by abnormality of fetal acid-base balance
O76	Abnormality in fetal heart rate and rhythm complicating labor and delivery
O80	Encounter for full-term uncomplicated delivery
O82	Encounter for cesarean delivery without indication
O85	Puerperal sepsis
O94	Sequelae of complication of pregnancy, childbirth, and the puerperium
P09	Abnormal findings on neonatal screening
P53	Hemorrhagic disease of newborn
P60	Disseminated intravascular coagulation of newborn
P84	Other problems with newborn

P90	Convulsions of newborn
P95	Stillbirth
Q02	Microcephaly
R05	Cough
R12	Heartburn
R17	Unspecified jaundice
R21	Rash and other nonspecific skin eruption
R32	Unspecified urinary incontinence
R34	Anuria and oliguria
R37	Sexual dysfunction, unspecified
R42	Dizziness and giddiness
R51	Headache
R52	Pain, unspecified
R54	Age-related physical debility
R55	Syncope and collapse
R58	Hemorrhage, not elsewhere classified
R61	Generalized hyperhidrosis
R64	Cachexia
R69	Illness, unspecified
R75	Inconclusive laboratory evidence of human immunodeficiency virus [HIV]
R81	Glycosuria
R99	Ill-defined and unknown cause of mortality
Y09	Assault by unspecified means
Y66	Nonadministration of surgical and medical care
Y69	Unspecified misadventure during surgical and medical care
Y95	Nosocomial condition
Z08	Encounter for follow-up examination after completed treatment for malignant neoplasm
Z09	Encounter for follow-up examination after completed treatment for conditions other than malignant neoplasm
Z21	Asymptomatic human immunodeficiency virus [HIV] infection status
Z23	Encounter for immunization
Z66	Do not resuscitate

This section enables the coder to quickly review drugs, drug actions, and indications that are often associated with overlooked or undocumented diagnoses. The coder should review the patient's medication record and know what condition the physician is treating with the prescribed medication based on documentation in the medical record. When documentation is lacking, the coder can reference this section to locate the drug, determine the drug action, confirm drug indications, and when necessary query the physician.

Drug	Z Code	Drug Action	Indications
Abilify [aripiprazole]		Antipsychotic	Depression, bipolar disorder, schizophrenia, autism symptoms
Acarbose [acarbose]	Z79.84	Blood glucose regulator	Diabetes mellitus
Accupril [quinapril hydrochloride]		ACE inhibitor; antihypertensive	Congestive heart failure; essential hypertension
Acetaminophen with codeine [acetaminophen/codeine phosphate]	Z79.891	Analgesic, general; analgesic-narcotic	Pain, moderate to severe
Actemra [tocilizumab]		Antirheumatic	Rheumatoid arthritis
Actimmune [interferon gamma-1b]	Z79.899	Antineoplastic interferons; antiviral interferons	Chronic granulomatous disease; malignant osteopetrosis
Activella [estradiol/norethindrone acetate]	Z79.890	Estrogen therapy	Menopause symptoms; vaginal and vulvar atrophy; osteoporosis prevention
Actonel [risedronate sodium]	Z79.83	Electrolytic and renal agent; bone resorption inhibitor	Decrease in bone loss in multiple myeloma patients; Paget's disease; hyperparathyroidism; osteoporosis
Actoplus Met [metformin hydrochloride/pioglitazone hydrochloride]	Z79.84	Blood glucose regulator	Diabetes mellitus
Actos [pioglitazone hydrochloride]	Z79.84	Blood glucose regulator	Diabetes mellitus
Adalat CC [nifedipine]		Calcium channel blocker	Vasospastic angina; chronic stable angina; essential hypertension
Advair [fluticasone propionate/salmeterol xinafoate]	Z79.51	Corticosteroids--inhaled; antiasthmatic	Prophylaxis and treatment of asthma and COPD
Advil [ibuprofen]	Z79.1	Nonsteroidal anti-inflammatory drug (NSAID)	Pain or fever relief
Aerospan [flunisolide]	Z79.51	Corticosteroids--inhaled; antiasthmatic	Prophylaxis and treatment of asthma
Afrezza [human insulin recombinant]	Z79.4	Blood glucose regulator	Diabetes mellitus
Aggrastat [tirofiban hydrochloride]	Z79.02	Antithrombotic platelet aggregation inhibitor	Unstable angina or heart attacks
Aggrenox [aspirin/dipyridamole]	Z79.02	Antithrombotic platelet aggregation inhibitor	Lessening of the chance of heart attack or stroke
Akne-Mycin [erythromycin]	Z79.2	Antibacterial	Severe acne treatment
Aldactone [spironolactone]		Cardiovascular agent; antihypertensive agent; diuretic; electrolytic and renal agent	Severe heart failure; ascites associated with cirrhosis; hypokalemia
Aleve [naproxen sodium]	Z79.1	Nonsteroidal anti-inflammatory drug (NSAID)	Reduction of temporary aches and pains
Allegra [fexofenadine hydrochloride]		Antihistamine	Seasonal allergic rhinitis
Allopurinol [allopurinol]		Antigout	Gouty arthritis, renal calculus, hyperuricemia, hyperuricemia secondary to leukemia, hyperuricemia secondary to lymphoma
Alora [estradiol]	Z79.890	Estrogen therapy	Menopause symptoms
Alphagan P [brimonidine tartrate]		Antiglaucoma agent (ophthalmic) antihypertensive, ocular	Open angle glaucoma or another condition in which pressure in the eye is too high (ocular hypertension)
Alprazolam [alprazolam]		Antianxiety; sedative/hypnotic	
Altabax [retapamulin]	Z79.2	Antibacterial	Skin infections
Altace [ramipril]		ACE inhibitor; antihypertensive	Congestive heart failure, essential hypertension
Altavera [ethinyl estradiol/levonorgestrel]	Z79.3	Contraceptive	Contraception
Alvesco [ciclesonide]	Z79.51	Corticosteroids--inhaled; antiasthmatic	Prophylaxis and treatment of asthma
Alyacen [ethinyl estradiol/norethindrone]	Z79.3	Contraceptive	Contraception
Amaryl [glimepiride]	Z79.84	Blood glucose regulator	Diabetes mellitus
Ambien [zolpidem tartrate]		Sedative/hypnotic	Insomnia
A-Methapred [methylprednisolone sodium succinate]	Z79.52	Corticosteroids	Severe inflammation

Drug	Z Code	Drug Action	Indications
Amikacin [amikacin sulfate]		Aminoglycoside antibiotic	Active in treatment of gram-negative bacterial infections such as *Pseudomonas, Escherichia coli (E. coli), Proteus, Klebsiella-Enterobacter-Serratia*
Aminophylline [aminophylline]		Bronchodilator, pulmonary vasodilator, smooth muscle relaxant	Relief and/or prevention of symptoms from asthma and reversible bronchospasms in bronchitis and emphysema
Amitriptyline hydrochloride [amitriptyline hydrochloride]		Anorexiant/CNS stimulant; antidepressant	Depression
Amoxicillin [amoxicillin]	Z79.2	Penicillin	Effective for infections with a broad spectrum of bactericidal activity against many gram-positive and gram-negative micro-organisms; otitis media, gonorrhea, skin, respiratory, gastrointestinal, and genitourinary infections
Ampicillin [ampicillin sodium]	Z79.2	Antibacterial	Bacterial infections
Amrix [cyclobenzaprine hydrochloride]		Muscle relaxant	Adjunct to rest and physical therapy for muscle spasms
Anaprox [naproxen sodium]	Z79.1	Nonsteroidal anti-inflammatory drug (NSAID)	Pain, inflammation, or fever relief
Anastrozole [anastrozole]	Z79.811	Aromatase inhibitor	Postmenopausal breast cancer
Ancef [cefazolin sodium]	Z79.2	Semisynthetic cephalosporin antibiotic	Respiratory tract infections due to *Streptococcus pneumoniae, Klebsiella species, Haemophilus influenzae (H. influenzae), Staphylococcus aureus,* and group A betahemolytic streptococci; urinary tract infections due to *E. coli, Proteus mirabilis, Klebsiella* species and some strains of *Enterobacter* and enterococci; skin and skin structure infections, biliary tract infections, bone and joint infections, genital infections, septicemia, and endocarditis
Angeliq [drospirenone/estradiol]	Z79.890	Estrogen therapy	Menopause symptoms
Angiomax [bivalirudin]	Z79.02	Antithrombotic platelet aggregation inhibitor	Prevention of blood clots
Antabuse [disulfiram]		Alcohol treatment	Alcoholism
Antineoplastic/chemotherapy	Z79.899	Antineoplastic	Cancer
Anzemet [dolasetron mesylate]		Antiemetic/antinauseant	Management of nausea/vomiting following surgery or from effects of chemotherapy or cancer
Apidra [insulin glulisine recombinant]	Z79.4	Blood glucose regulator	Diabetes mellitus
Aranelle [ethinyl estradiol/norethindrone]	Z79.3	Contraceptive	Contraception; acne
Aranesp [darbepoetin alfa]		Erythropoiesis-stimulating agent (ESA)	Lower than normal blood cell count (anemia) from disorders such as CKD and neoplasms
Argatroban [argatroban]	Z79.02	Antithrombotic platelet aggregation inhibitor	Prophylaxis and treatment of venous thrombosis in thrombocytopenia patients
Aricept [donepezil hydrochloride]		Acetylcholine sterase inhibitor	Symptoms of mild to moderate Alzheimer's disease; can improve thinking ability in some patients
Arimidex [anastrozole]	Z79.811	Aromatase inhibitor	Postmenopausal breast cancer
Aristospan [triamcinolone hexacetonide]	Z79.52	Corticosteroids	Severe inflammation
Arixtra [fondaparinux sodium]	Z79.01	Anticoagulant	Venous thrombosis and pulmonary embolism
Arnuity Ellipta [fluticasone furoate]	Z79.51	Corticosteroids--inhaled; antiasthmatic	Prophylaxis and treatment of asthma
Aromasin [exemestane]	Z79.811	Aromatase inhibitor	Postmenopausal breast cancer
Arthrotec [diclofenac sodium/misoprostol]	Z79.1	Analgesic	Arthritis in patients who may develop stomach ulcers from taking nonsteroidal anti-inflammatory drugs (NSAIDs) alone; used to help relieve some symptoms of arthritis, such as inflammation, swelling, stiffness, and joint pain
Ashlyna [ethinyl estradiol/levonorgestrel]	Z79.3	Contraceptive	Contraception
Asmanex [mometasone furoate]	Z79.51	Corticosteroids--inhaled; antiasthmatic	Prophylaxis and treatment of asthma
Astagraf XL [tacrolimus]	Z79.899	Immunosuppressant	Prophylaxis of organ transplant rejection
Astramorph [morphine sulfate]	Z79.891	Narcotic analgesic	Pain
Atelvia [risedronate sodium]	Z79.83	Bisphosphonates	Prevention of thinning of the bones (osteoporosis)
Atenolol [atenolol]		Antianginal; antihypertensive; beta blocker	Chronic stable angina pectoris; essential hypertension; reduces cardiovascular mortality in those with definite or suspected acute myocardial infarction
Ativan [lorazepam]		Antianxiety; sedative/hypnotic	Anxiety disorder associated with depressive symptoms; controls tension, agitation, irritability, and insomnia
Atrovent [ipratropium bromide]		Antiasthmatic/bronchodilator	Chronic bronchitis, emphysema; bronchial asthma

Appendix C: Pharmacology List 2018

Drug	Z Code	Drug Action	Indications
Augmentin [amoxicillin/clavulanate potassium]	Z79.2	Antibacterial	Middle ear, lower respiratory, sinus, skin and skin structures, and urinary tract infections
Avandia [rosiglitazone maleate]	Z79.84	Blood glucose regulator	Diabetes mellitus
Avapro [irbesartan]		Antihypertensive	Hypertension
Aviane [ethinyl estradiol/levonorgestrel]	Z79.3	Contraceptive	Contraception
Avonex [interferon beta-1a]	Z79.899	Antiviral interferon	Relapsing multiple sclerosis
Axid AR [nizatidine]		Histamine H2-receptor antagonist	Acid/peptic disorder; gastroesophageal reflux; duodenal, gastric, and peptic ulcers
Aygestin [norethindrone acetate]	Z79.3	Contraceptive	Contraception; menstrual disorders
Azactam [aztreonam]	Z79.2	Antibacterial	Severe or life-threatening bacterial infections
Azithromycin [azithromycin]	Z79.2	Antibacterial	Treatment of bacterial infections
Bactrim [sulfamethoxazole/trimethoprim]	Z79.2	Antibacterial	Urinary tract infections, acute otitis media, acute exacerbation of chronic bronchitis, shigellosis, and *Pneumocystis carinii*
Bactroban [mupirocin]	Z79.2	Dermatologic; topical anti-infective	Topical treatment of impetigo
Balziva [ethinyl estradiol/norethindrone]	Z79.3	Contraceptive	Contraception
Basaglar [insulin glargine]	Z79.4	Blood glucose regulator	Diabetes mellitus
Bayer [acetylsalicylic acid]	Z79.82	Aspirin	Prophylaxis and treatment of heart attacks, angina, or strokes; reduction of fever, pain, and inflammation
Beconase AQ [beclomethasone dipropionate monohydrate]		Corticosteroids; antiasthmatic	Bronchial asthma, prevention of nasal polyps, perennial allergies, seasonal allergies, and vasomotor rhinitis
Bekyree [desogestrel/ethinyl estradiol]	Z79.3	Contraceptive	Contraception
Betoptic [betaxolol hydrochloride]		Cardioselective beta-adrenergic receptor blocking agent	Lowering of intraocular pressure; also used for treatment of ocular hypertension and chronic open-angle glaucoma
Beyaz [drospirenone/ethinyl estradiol/levomefolate calcium]	Z79.3	Contraceptive	Contraception; acne
Biaxin [clarithromycin]		Macrolide	Acid/peptic disorder or ulcer, acute exacerbation chronic bronchitis, HIV, lower and upper respiratory tract infections, sinus infection, prophylaxis mycobacterium avium complex, pharyngitis, pneumonia, tonsillitis
Binosto [alendronate sodium]	Z79.83	Bisphosphonates	Prevention of thinning of the bones (osteoporosis)
Boniva [ibandronate sodium]	Z79.83	Bisphosphonates	Prevention of thinning of the bones (osteoporosis)
Brevicon [ethinyl estradiol/norethindrone]	Z79.3	Contraceptive	Contraception; acne
Briellyn [ethinyl estradiol/norethindrone]	Z79.3	Contraceptive	Contraception
Brilinta [ticagrelor]	Z79.02	Antithrombotic platelet aggregation inhibitor	Unstable angina or heart attacks and prevention of blood clots
Bufferin [acetylsalicylic acid]	Z79.82	Aspirin	Prophylaxis and treatment of heart attacks, angina or strokes; reduction of fever, pain, and inflammation
Buprenex [buprenorphine hydrochloride]	Z79.891	Narcotic analgesic	Moderate to severe pain
Buprenorphine HCl [buprenorphine hydrochloride]	Z79.891	Narcotic analgesic	Moderate to severe pain
Buspirone [buspirone hydrochloride]		Antianxiety agent	Generalized anxiety disorder
Butorphanol Tartrate [butorphanol tartrate]		Narcotic analgesic	Moderate to severe postsurgical pain
Butrans [buprenorphine]	Z79.891	Narcotic analgesic	Chronic pain
Calan [verapamil hydrochloride]		Antianginal; antiarrhythmic, antiarthritic, antihypertensive, calcium channel blocker	Angina pectoris at rest and chronic stable, arrhythmia, atrial fibrillation, atrial flutter, paroxysmal supraventricular tachycardia, ventricular arrhythmia, essential hypertension
Caldolor [ibuprofen]	Z79.1	Nonsteroidal anti-inflammatory drug (NSAID)	Pain or fever relief
Cambia [diclofenac potassium]	Z79.1	Nonsteroidal anti-inflammatory drug (NSAID)	Migraine headaches
Camila [norethindrone]	Z79.3	Contraceptive	Contraception; menstrual disorders
Cardizem CD [diltiazem hydrochloride]		Antianginal, antiarrhythmic, antihypertensive, channel blocker, coronary vasodilator	Chronic stable angina, atrial fibrillation, atrial flutter, essential hypertension, paroxysmal supraventricular tachycardia
Cardura [doxazosin mesylate]		Antihypertensive	Benign prostatic hyperplasia, essential hypertension

Drug	Z Code	Drug Action	Indications
Catapres [clonidine hydrochloride]		Antihypertensive	Hypertension
Cefprozil [cefprozil]		Antibiotic: second generation cephalosporins	Acute exacerbation and chronic bronchitis, lower and upper respiratory tract infections, pharyngitis, tonsillitis
Ceftin [cefuroxime axetil]		Antibiotic: second generation cephalosporins	Acute exacerbation and chronic bronchitis, middle ear infection, sexually transmitted gonorrhea infection, upper respiratory tract infection, urinary tract infection, pharyngitis, tonsillitis
Ceftriaxone [ceftriaxone sodium]	Z79.2	Antibacterial	Bacterial infections
Celebrex [celecoxib]	Z79.1	Antirheumatic, nonsteroidal anti-inflammatory	Relief of some symptoms caused by arthritis, such as inflammation, swelling, stiffness, and joint pain
Celestone Soluspan [betamethasone acetate/ betamethasone sodium phosphate]	Z79.52	Corticosteroids; antiasthmatic	Asthma; severe inflammation
Celexa [citalopram hydrobromide]		Antidepressant	Depression
Cellcept [mycophenolate mofetil]	Z79.899	Immunosuppressant	Prophylaxis of organ transplant rejection
Centany [mupirocin]	Z79.2	Antibacterial	Topical treatment of skin infections
Cephalexin [cephalexin]	Z79.2	Antibacterial	Bacterial infections
Chantix [varenicline tartrate]		Smoking cessation aid	Nicotine addiction, smoking
Cipro [ciprofloxacin hydrochloride]	Z79.2	Anti-infective; quinolone	Cystitis, infectious diarrhea, gonorrhea, bone and joint infection, gastrointestinal tract infection, lower and upper respiratory tract infections, sinus infection, urinary tract infection, nosocomial pneumonia, chronic prostatitis
Ciprofloxacin [ciprofloxacin]	Z79.2	Antibacterial	Bacterial infections
Clarithromycin [clarithromycin]	Z79.2	Antibacterial	Skin and respiratory bacterial infections
Claritin [loratadine]		Antihistamine	Seasonal allergic rhinitis, chronic idiopathic urticaria
Cleocin [clindamycin phosphate]	Z79.2	Antibacterial	Bacterial infections
Climara [estradiol]	Z79.890	Estrogen therapy	Osteoporosis prevention and menopausal symptoms; vaginal and vulvar atrophy; hypoestrogenism; ovarian failure
Clindamycin [clindamycin phosphate]	Z79.2	Antibacterial	Bacterial infections
Clonazepam [clonazepam]		Anticonvulsant	Absence, akinetic, and myoclonic epilepsy, Lennox-Gastaut syndrome
Clonidine [clonidine hydrochloride]		Antihypertensive	Hypertension
Clopidogrel bisulfate [clopidogrel bisulfate]	Z79.02	Antithrombotic platelet aggregation inhibitor	Treatment of unstable angina or heart attacks and prevention of blood clots
Codeine [codeine sulfate]	Z79.891	Narcotic analgesic	Mild to moderate pain
Cogentin [benztropine mesylate]		Antiparkinsonism	Parkinson's disease
Colace [docusate sodium]		Gastrointestinal agent; laxative, stool softener	Constipation
Colocort [hydrocortisone]	Z79.52	Corticosteroids	Inflammation of the colon
CombiPatch [ethinyl estradiol/norethindrone acetate]	Z79.890	Estrogen therapy	Menopause symptoms; vaginal and vulvar atrophy; osteoporosis prevention
Combivent [ipratropium bromide/albuterol sulfate]		Antiasthmatic/bronchodilator	Chronic bronchitis, emphysema; bronchial asthma
Compro [prochlorperazine]		Antiemetic, antipsychotic	Nausea, vomiting, and manic phase of bipolar syndrome or schizophrenia
Cortef [hydrocortisone]	Z79.52	Corticosteroids	Severe inflammation
Cortenema [hydrocortisone]	Z79.52	Corticosteroids	Inflammation of the colon
Cortifoam [hydrocortisone acetate]	Z79.52	Corticosteroids	Colon and rectum inflammation
Cortisone acetate [cortisone acetate]	Z79.52	Corticosteroids	Inflammation
Cortisporin [hydrocortisone acetate/neomycin sulfate/polymyxin B sulfate]		Topical anti-infective, topical steroid	Dermatosis
Coumadin [warfarin sodium]	Z79.01	Anticoagulant	Prophylaxis and treatment of venous thrombosis, treatment of atrial fibrillation with embolization (pulmonary embolism), arrhythmias, myocardial infarction, and stroke prevention
Cozaar [losartan potassium]		Antihypertensive	Essential hypertension
Crestor [rosuvastatin calcium]		HMG-CoA reductase inhibitor (statin)	Hypercholesterolemia, hyperlipidemia, hyperproteinemia
Crixivan [indinavir sulfate]		HIV inhibitor	HIV, asymptomatic HIV
Cryselle [ethinyl estradiol/norgestrel]	Z79.3	Contraceptive	Contraception

Drug	Z Code	Drug Action	Indications
Cyclafem [ethinyl estradiol/norethindrone]	Z79.3	Contraceptive	Contraception
Cyclessa [desogestrel/ethinyl estradiol]	Z79.3	Contraceptive	Contraception
Cyclosporine [cyclosporine]	Z79.899	Immunosuppressant	Prophylaxis of organ transplant rejection
Cytomel [liothyronine sodium]		Thyroid hormone	Treatment of hypothyroidism or prevention of euthyroid goiters
Daptomycin [daptomycin]	Z79.2	Antibacterial	Skin and underlying tissue bacterial infections
Dasetta [ethinyl estradiol/norethindrone]	Z79.3	Contraceptive	Contraception
Daypro [oxaprozin]	Z79.1	Nonsteroidal anti-inflammatory drug (NSAID)	Osteoarthritis and rheumatoid arthritis
Daysee [ethinyl estradiol/levonorgestrel]	Z79.3	Contraceptive	Contraception
Delestrogen [estradiol valerate]	Z79.890	Estrogen therapy	Menopause symptoms
Demerol [meperidine hydrochloride]	Z79.891	Narcotic analgesic	Moderate to severe pain
Depakote [divalproex sodium]		Anticonvulsant	Bipolar affective disorder; complex absence, complex partial, and mixed pattern epilepsy; migraine headache
Depo-Medrol [methylprednisolone acetate]	Z79.52	Corticosteroids	Arthritis and joint disorders
Depo-Provera [medroxyprogesterone acetate]	Z79.3, Z79.890	Antineoplastic; contraceptive; progestin	Amenorrhea; carcinoma, endometrium, adjunct; carcinoma, renal; contraception; hemorrhage
Depo-SubQ Provera [medroxyprogesterone acetate]	Z79.3	Contraceptive	Contraception; menstrual disorder pain
Desogen [desogestrel/ethinyl estradiol]	Z79.3	Contraceptive; estrogen/progestin	Contraception
Detrol [tolterodine tartrate]		Muscarinic receptor antagonist	Overactive bladders in patients with urinary frequency, urgency, or urge incontinence
Dexamethasone Intensol [dexamethasone]	Z79.52	Corticosteroids	Arthritis; allergic disorders; breathing disorders; lupus
Didronel [etidronate disodium]	Z79.83	Bisphosphonates	Paget's disease and irregular bone growth
Dificid [fidaxomicin]	Z79.2	Antibacterial	*Clostridium difficile*
Diflucan [fluconazole]		Antifungal agent	Oropharyngeal and esophageal candidiasis and cryptococcal meningitis in AIDS patients
Digoxin [digoxin]		Cardiotonic glycoside	Heart failure, atrial flutter, atrial fibrillation, and supraventricular tachycardia
Dilantin [phenytoin sodium]		Anticonvulsant	Control of grand mal and psychomotor seizures
Dilaudid [hydromorphone hydrochloride]	Z79.891	Narcotic analgesic	Moderate to severe pain
Diovan [valsartan]		ACE inhibitor	Essential hypertension
Divigel [estradiol]	Z79.890	Estrogen therapy	Menopause symptoms
Dolophine HCl [methadone hydrochloride]	Z79.891	Narcotic analgesic	Pain; treatment of opoid addiction
Doxycycline [doxycycline]	Z79.2	Antibacterial	Treatment of bacterial infections; acne
Duavee [bazedoxifene acetate/conjugated estrogens]	Z79.890	Estrogen therapy	Treatment of menopause symptoms; osteoporosis prevention
Duetact [glimepiride/pioglitazone hydrochloride]	Z79.84	Blood glucose regulator	Diabetes mellitus
Duexis [famotidine/ibuprofen]	Z79.1	Nonsteroidal anti-inflammatory drug (NSAID)	Symptomatic treatment of osteoarthritis and rheumatoid arthritis; reduction of risk of ulcers
Dulera [formoterol fumarate/mometasone furoate]	Z79.51	Corticosteroids -inhaled; antiasthmatic	Prophylaxis and treatment of asthma
Duragesic [fentanyl]	Z79.891	Narcotic analgesic	Chronic pain
Duramorph [morphine sulfate]	Z79.891	Narcotic analgesic	Moderate to severe pain
Dyloject [diclofenac sodium]	Z79.1	Nonsteroidal anti-inflammatory drug (NSAID)	Pain relief
Dynacin [minocycline hydrochloride]	Z79.2	Antibacterial	Severe acne treatment
E.E.S. [erythromycin ethylsuccinate]	Z79.2	Antibacterial	Bacterial infections
Ecotrin [acetylsalicylic acid]	Z79.82	Aspirin	Prophylaxis and treatment of heart attacks, angina or strokes; reduction of fever, pain and inflammation
Effexor XR [venlafaxine hydrochloride]		Antidepressant	Depression

Drug	Z Code	Drug Action	Indications
Effient [prasugrel hydrochloride]	Z79.02	Antithrombotic platelet aggregation inhibitor	Lessening of the chance of heart attack or stroke
Elestrin [estradiol]	Z79.890	Estrogen therapy	Menopause symptoms
Eligard [leuprolide acetate]	Z79.818	Agents affecting estrogen receptors and estrogen levels	Endometriosis; uterine fibroids; symptoms of prostate cancer
Elinest [norgestrel/ethinyl estradiol]	Z79.3	Contraceptive	Contraception
Eliquis [apixaban]	Z79.01	Anticoagulant	Venous thrombosis
Embeda [morphine sulfate/naltrexone hydrochloride]	Z79.891	Narcotic analgesic	Moderate to severe pain
Emoquette [ethinyl estradiol/desogestrel]	Z79.3	Contraceptive	Contraception
Enjuvia [conjugated synthetic b estrogens]	Z79.890	Estrogen therapy	Osteoporosis prevention and to treat menopausal symptoms; vaginal and vulvar atrophy; hypoestrogenism; ovarian failure
Enpresse [ethinyl estradiol/levonorgestrel]	Z79.3	Contraceptive	Contraception
Enskyce [desogestrel/ethinyl estradiol]	Z79.3	Contraceptive	Contraception
Entocort EC [budesonide]	Z79.52	Corticosteroids	Crohn's disease; ulcerative colitis
Envarsus XR [tacrolimus]	Z79.899	Immunosuppressant	Prophylaxis of organ transplant rejection
Epinephrine [epinephrine]		Bronchodilator, cardiotonic	Most commonly, relief of respiratory distress due to bronchospasm and restoration of cardiac rhythm in cardiac arrest
Epivir, Epivir-HBV [lamivudine]		HIV and HBV inhibitor	HIV, hepatitis B (HBV), asymptomatic HIV
Errin [norethindrone]	Z79.3	Contraceptive	Contraception
Ertapenem [ertapenem sodium]	Z79.2	Antibacterial	Stomach, urinary tract, pelvis, skin and lung infections
ERYC [erythromycin]	Z79.2	Antibacterial	Lower respiratory tract infections
Erygel [erythromycin]	Z79.2	Antibacterial	Treatment of bacterial infections; rheumatic fever attacks
EryPed [erythromycin ethylsuccinate]	Z79.2	Antibacterial	Treatment of bacterial infections; rheumatic fever attacks
Ery-Tab [erythromycin]	Z79.2	Acne product; macrolide; ocular anti-infective; topical anti-infective	Acne vulgaris, intestinal amebiasis, infectious conjunctivitis, diphtheria, endocarditis, prevention, treatment of erythrasma infections: endocervical, gynecologic, lower and upper respiratory tract, ophthalmic, and rectal; skin and skin structures, and urethral; Legionnaires' disease, pelvic inflammatory disease, pertussis, pneumonia, rheumatic fever, prophylaxis, syphilis
Erythrocin [erythromycin lactobionate]	Z79.2	Antibacterial	Bacterial infections
Erythromycin [erythromycin]	Z79.2	Antibacterial	Respiratory tract infections
Estarylla [ethinyl estradiol/norgestimate]	Z79.3	Contraceptive	Contraception
Estrace [estradiol]	Z79.890	Estrogen therapy	Vaginal cream used to treat vaginal and vulvar atrophy
Estraderm [estradiol]	Z79.890	Estrogen therapy	Osteoporosis prevention and to treat menopausal symptoms, vaginal and vulvar atrophy, hypoestrogenism, ovarian failure
Estrasorb [estradiol hemihydrate]	Z79.890	Estrogen therapy	Menopause symptoms
EstroGel [estradiol]	Z79.890	Estrogen therapy	Menopause symptoms
Estrostep Fe [ethinyl estradiol/norethindrone acetate]	Z79.3	Contraceptive	Contraception
Evista [raloxifene hydrochloride]	Z79.810	Estrogen receptor modulator, selective osteoporosis prophylactic	Prevention of thinning of the bones (osteoporosis) only in postmenopausal women
Exalgo [hydromorphone hydrochloride]	Z79.891	Narcotic analgesic	Moderate to severe pain
Exemestane [exemestane]	Z79.811	Aromatase inhibitor	Postmenopausal breast cancer
Factive [gemifloxacin mesylate]	Z79.2	Antibacterial	Bacterial lung infections
Falmina [ethinyl estradiol/levonorgestrel]	Z79.3	Contraceptive	Contraception
Fareston [toremifene citrate]	Z79.810	Selective estrogen receptor modulator (SERM)	Metastatic breast cancer in postmenopausal women
Faslodex [fulvestrant]	Z79.818	Agents affecting estrogen receptors and estrogen levels	Metastatic breast cancer in postmenopausal women
Feldene [piroxicam]	Z79.1	Nonsteroidal anti-inflammatory drug (NSAID)	Treatment of pain and inflammation due to arthritis
Femara [letrozole]	Z79.811	Aromatase inhibitor	Postmenopausal breast cancer
Femcon Fe [ethinyl estradiol/norethindrone]	Z79.3	Contraceptive	Contraception; acne

Appendix C: Pharmacology List 2018

Drug	Z Code	Drug Action	Indications
Femhrt [ethinyl estradiol/norethindrone acetate]	Z79.3, Z79.89Ø	Contraceptive; estrogen therapy	Contraception; menopause symptoms; osteoporosis prevention
Femring [estradiol acetate]	Z79.89Ø	Estrogen therapy	Osteoporosis prevention and to treat menopausal symptoms; hypoestrogenism; ovarian failure
Femtrace [estradiol acetate]	Z79.89Ø	Estrogen therapy	Menopause symptoms
Fentanyl [fentanyl]	Z79.891	Narcotic analgesic	Postprocedural or chronic pain
Fentora [fentanyl citrate]	Z79.891	Narcotic analgesic	Breakthrough cancer pain
Fioricet with codeine [acetaminophen/butalbital/caffeine/codeine phosphate]	Z79.891	Narcotic analgesic	Tension headaches
Flagyl [metronidazole]	Z79.2	Antibacterial	Treatment of bacterial infections
Flavoxate hydrochloride [flavoxate hydrochloride]		Urinary tract spasmolytic	Relief of dysuria, urgency, nocturia, suprapubic pain, frequency, and incontinence associated with cystitis, prostatitis, urethritis, and urethrocystitis/urethrotrigonitis
Flomax [tamsulosin hydrochloride]		Alpha-adrenergic blocker, benign prostatic hypertrophy therapy agent	Signs and symptoms of benign enlargement of the prostate (benign prostatic hyperplasia, or BPH)
Flonase [fluticasone propionate]		Corticosteroid-inhalation/nasal; topical steroid	Corticosteroid-responsive dermatosis; perennial allergic and seasonal allergic rhinitis
Flovent HFA [fluticasone propionate]	Z79.51	Corticosteroid-inhaled/nasal; topical steroid	Corticosteroid-responsive dermatosis, perennial allergic and seasonal allergic rhinitis
Fortamet [metformin hydrochloride]	Z79.84	Blood glucose regulator	Diabetes mellitus
Fortaz [ceftazidime]	Z79.2	Antibacterial	Pneumonia and lower respiratory infections
Fosamax [alendronate sodium]	Z79.83	Calcium metabolism	Osteoporosis; Paget's disease
Fosinopril sodium [fosinopril sodium]		ACE inhibitor; antihypertensive	Essential hypertension
Fragmin [dalteparin sodium]	Z79.Ø1	Anticoagulant	Prophylaxis and treatment of blood clots
Fulvestrant [fulvestrant]	Z79.818	Agents affecting estrogen receptors and estrogen levels	Treatment of metastatic breast cancer in postmenopausal women
Gengraf [cyclosporine]	Z79.899	Immunosuppressant	Prophylaxis of organ transplant rejection
Gentamicin sulfate [gentamicin sulfate]	Z79.2	Antibacterial	Severe bacterial infections
Gildagia [ethinyl estradiol/norethindrone]	Z79.3	Contraceptive	Contraception
Gildess [ethinyl estradiol/norethindrone acetate]	Z79.3	Contraceptive	Contraception
Glimepiride [glimepiride]	Z79.84	Blood glucose regulator	Diabetes mellitus
Glucophage [metformin hydrochloride]	Z79.84	Blood glucose regulator	Diabetes mellitus
Glucotrol [glipizide]	Z79.84	Oral blood-glucose-lowering agent	Diabetes mellitus
Glucovance [glyburide/metformin hydrochloride]	Z79.84	Blood glucose regulator	Diabetes mellitus
Glumetza [metformin hydrochloride]	Z79.84	Blood glucose regulator	Diabetes mellitus
Glyburide (micronized) [glyburide]	Z79.84	Blood glucose regulator	Diabetes mellitus
Heparin sodium [heparin sodium]	Z79.Ø1	Anticoagulant	Prophylaxis and treatment of venous thrombosis, pulmonary embolism; prevention of cerebral thrombosis, and treatment of consumptive coagulopathies
Humalog [insulin lispro recombinant]	Z79.4	Blood glucose regulator	Diabetes mellitus
Humulin [insulin recombinant]	Z79.4	Blood glucose regulator	Diabetes mellitus
Hydrochlorothiazide [hydrochlorothiazide]		Diuretic, antihypertensive	Management of hypertension and in adjunctive therapy for edema associated with congestive heart failure, hepatic cirrhosis, corticosteroid, and estrogen therapy
Hydrocodone [acetaminophen/hydrocodone bitartrate]	Z79.891	Narcotic analgesic	Moderate to severe pain
Hydrocodone bitartrate and acetaminophen [acetaminophen/hydrocodone bitartrate]	Z79.891	Analgesic, general; analgesic-narcotic; antitussive/expectorant	Pain, moderate to severe
Hydrocortisone [hydrocortisone]	Z79.52	Corticosteroids	Addison's disease; arthritis; immune disorders; allergies; breathing problems
Hydromorphone HCl [hydromorphone hydrochloride]	Z79.891	Narcotic analgesic	Moderate to severe pain
Hyzaar [hydrochlorothiazide/ losartan potassium]		Antihypertensive	Hypertension

Drug	Z Code	Drug Action	Indications
Ibuprofen [ibuprofen]	Z79.1	Nonsteroidal anti-inflammatory drug (NSAID)	Pain or fever relief
Imitrex [sumatriptan succinate]		Antimigraine	Migraine headache
Imuran [azathioprine]	Z79.899	Immunosuppressant	Rheumatoid arthritis
Inderal [propranolol hydrochloride]		Beta-adrenergic blocking agent	Management of hypertension, long-term management of angina pectoris due to coronary atherosclerosis, cardiac arrhythmias
Indocin [indomethacin]	Z79.1	Nonsteroidal anti-inflammatory drug (NSAID)	Treatment of pain and inflammation
Integrilin [eptifibatide]	Z79.02	Antithrombotic platelet aggregation inhibitor	Treatment of unstable angina or heart attacks and prevention of blood clots
Intron [interferon alfa 2-b]	Z79.899	Antineoplastic interferons; antiviral interferons	Cancer; hepatitis
Introvale [levonorgestrel/ethinyl estradiol]	Z79.3	Contraceptive	Contraception
Invanz [ertapeneum sodium]	Z79.2	Antibacterial	Stomach, urinary tract, pelvis, skin and lung infections
Invokamet [canagliflozin/metformin hydrochloride]	Z79.84	Blood glucose regulator	Diabetes mellitus
Iprivask [desirudin recombinant]	Z79.02	Antithrombotic platelet aggregation inhibitor	Prophylaxis and treatment of venous thrombosis and pulmonary embolism
Isoniazid [isoniazid]	Z79.2	Antibacterial	Prophylaxis and treatment of tuberculosis
Isordil [isosorbide dinitrate]		Smooth muscle relaxant	Acute anginal attacks
Isuprel [isoproterenol hydrochloride]		Adrenergic agent	Bronchodilator for asthma, chronic pulmonary emphysema, bronchitis, and other conditions accompanied by bronchospasm; can be used in cardiogenic shock cases
Jantoven [warfarin sodium]	Z79.01	Anticoagulant	Prophylaxis and treatment of venous thrombosis, pulmonary embolism; prevention of cerebral thrombosis, and treatment of consumptive coagulopathies
Janumet [metformin hydrochloride/sitagliptin phosphate]	Z79.84	Blood glucose regulator	Diabetes mellitus
Januvia [sitagliptin phosphate]	Z79.84	Blood glucose regulator	Diabetes mellitus
Jencycla [norethindrone]	Z79.3	Contraceptive	Contraception
Jentadueto [linagliptin/metformin hydrochloride]]	Z79.84	Blood glucose regulator	Diabetes mellitus
Junel [ethinyl estradiol/norethindrone acetate]	Z79.3	Contraceptive	Contraception
Kadian [morphine sulfate]	Z79.891	Narcotic analgesic	Moderate to severe pain
Kariva [desogestrel/ethinyl estradiol]	Z79.3	Contraceptive	Contraception
Kazano [alogliptin benzoate/metformin hydrochloride]	Z79.84	Blood glucose regulator	Diabetes mellitus
Keflex [cephalexin]	Z79.2	Antibacterial	Bone, middle ear, skin and skin structures, upper respiratory tract and urinary tract infections; acute prostatitis
Kefzol [cefazolin sodium]	Z79.2	Antibacterial	Skin, ear, urinary tract, and upper respiratory bacterial infections
Kelnor [ethynodiol diacetate/ethinyl estradiol]	Z79.3	Contraceptive	Contraception
Kenalog [triamcinolone acetonide]	Z79.52	Corticosteroids	Eczema; allergic reactions; psoriasis
Kimidess [ethinyl estradiol/desogestrel]	Z79.3	Contraceptive	Contraception
Klaron [sulfacetamide sodium]	Z79.2	Antibacterial	Acne
Klonopin [clonazepam]		Anticonvulsant, anxiolytic - benzodiazepine	Epilepsy, seizures, panic disorder
Klor-Con [potassium chloride]		Replaces potassium and maintains potassium level	Hypokalemia
Kombiglyze [metformin hydrochloride/saxagliptin hydrochloride]	Z79.84	Blood glucose regulator	Diabetes mellitus
K-Tab [potassium chloride]		Replaces potassium and maintains potassium level	Hypokalemia
Kurvelo [ethinyl estradiol/levonorgestrel]	Z79.3	Contraceptive	Contraception; menstrual disorders
Lamisil [terbinafine hydrochloride]		Antifungal	*Tinea cruris* (jock itch), *T. pedis* (athlete's foot), *T. corporis* (ringworm)
Lanoxin [digoxin]		Cardiotonic glycoside	Congestive heart failure

Drug	Z Code	Drug Action	Indications
Lantus [insulin glargine recombinant]	Z79.4	Blood glucose regulator	Diabetes mellitus
Larin [ethinyl estradiol/norethindrone acetate]	Z79.3	Contraceptive	Contraception
Lasix [furosemide]		Antihypertensive; diuretic	Management of edema associated with congestive heart failure, renal disease, including nephrotic syndrome and hypertension
Lescol [fluvastatin sodium]		HMG-CoA reductase inhibitor (statin)	Hypercholesterolemia; hyperlipidemia; hyperlipoproteinemia
Lessina [ethinyl estradiol/levonorgestrel]	Z79.3	Contraceptive	Contraception
Letrozole [letrozole]	Z79.811	Aromatase inhibitor	Postmenopausal breast cancer
Levaquin [levofloxacin]	Z79.2	Fluoroquinolone antibacterial	Acute exacerbation chronic bronchitis; cellulitis; furuncle; impetigo; infections of the lower and upper respiratory tracts, sinus, skin and skin structures, and urinary tract; pneumonia, community-acquired; pyoderma
Levemir [insulin detemir recombinant]	Z79.4	Blood glucose regulator	Diabetes mellitus
Levonest [levonorgestrel/ethinyl estradiol]	Z79.3	Contraceptive	Contraception; menstrual disorders; acne
Levora [levonorgestrel/ethinyl estradiol]	Z79.3	Contraceptive	Contraception
Levothroid [levothyroxine sodium]		Thyroid hormone	Treatment of hypothyroidism
Levoxyl [levothyroxine sodium]		Synthetic thyroid hormone	Euthyroid goiter; hypothyroidism
Lexapro [escitalopram oxalate]		Antidepressant—selective serotonin reuptake inhibitor (SSRI)	Depression, anxiety
Librium [chlordiazepoxide hydrochloride]		Antianxiety agent	Acute withdrawal symptoms, especially from alcohol, or for other anxiety-producing conditions
Lidocaine hydrochloride [lidocaine hydrochloride]		Antiarrhythmic	Management of ventricular arrhythmias or during cardiac manipulation, such as cardiac surgery
Liletta [levonorgestrel]	Z79.3	Contraceptive	Intrauterine device for contraception
Lincocin [lincocin hydrochloride]	Z79.2	Antibacterial	Serious bacterial infections
Lipitor [atorvastatin calcium]		HMG-CoA reductase inhibitor (statin)	Hypercholesterolemia, hyperlipidemia, hyperproteinemia
Lithium [lithium carbonate]		Antimanic	Control of manic episodes in bipolar disorders
Lo Loestrin Fe [ethinyl estradiol/norethindrone acetate]	Z79.3	Contraceptive	Contraception
Lo Minastrin Fe [ethinyl estradiol/norethindrone acetate]	Z79.3	Contraceptive	Contraception
Loestrin [ethinyl estradiol/norethindrone acetate]	Z79.3	Contraceptive	Contraception
Lomotil [diphenoxylate hydrochloride/atropine sulfate]		Antidiarrheal	Treatment of symptoms of chronic and functional diarrhea
Lopid [gemfibrozil]		Lipid regulating agent	Hypercholesterolemia, hyperlipidemia, hyperlipoproteinemia, hypertriglyceridemia
Lopressor [metoprolol tartrate]		Antihypertensive, betablocker antianginal; antihypertensive; betablocker	Essential hypertension therapy, angina pectoris, and myocardial infarction
Lorazepam [lorazepam]		Antianxiety; sedative/hypnotic	Anxiety disorder associated with depressive symptoms; controls tension, agitation, irritability, and insomnia
Loryna [drospirenone/ethinyl estradiol]	Z79.3	Contraceptive	Contraception
LoSeasonique [ethinyl estradiol/levonorgestrel]	Z79.3	Contraceptive	Contraception
Lotensin [benazepril hydrochloride]		ACE inhibitor; antihypertensive	Essential hypertension
Lotrel [amlodipine besylate/benazepril hydrochloride]		Antihypertensive	Hypertension
Lotrisone [clotrimazole/ betamethasone dipropionate]		Antifungal-corticosteroid	Relief of redness, swelling, itching, and other discomfort of fungus infections
Lovastatin [lovastatin]		HMG-CoA reductase inhibitor (statin)	Hypercholesterolemia; hyperlipidemia; hyperlipoproteinemia
Lovenox [enoxaparin sodium]	Z79.01	Anticoagulant	Prophylaxis and treatment of venous thrombosis and pulmonary embolism
Low-Ogestrel [norgestrel/ethinyl estradiol]	Z79.3	Contraceptive	Contraception
Lupron [leuprolide acetate]	Z79.818	Agents affecting estrogen receptors and estrogen levels	Treatment of metastatic breast cancer in postmenopausal women; prostate cancer symptoms
Macrobid [nitrofuantoin]	Z79.2	Antibacterial	Bacterial urinary tract infections
Macrodantin [nitrofurantoin]		Antibacterial	Urinary tract infection; prophylaxis

Drug	Z Code	Drug Action	Indications
Marlissa [ethinyl estradiol/levonorgestrel]	Z79.3	Contraceptive	Contraception
Maxipime [cefepime hydrochloride]	Z79.2	Antibacterial	Treatment of bacterial infections
Meclizine hydrochloride [meclizine hydrochloride]		Antihistamine	Management of nausea and vomiting, and dizziness associated with motion sickness
Medrol [methylprednisolone]	Z79.52	Glucocorticoid; anti-inflammatory	Acute/chronic adrenal insufficiency, congenital adrenal hyperplasia, adrenal insufficiency secondary to pituitary insufficiency; nonendocrine disorders, including arthritis, rheumatic carditis, bronchial asthma, cerebral edema, and allergic, collagen, intestinal tract, liver, ocular, renal, and skin diseases
Mefoxin [cefoxitin sodium]	Z79.2	Antibacterial	Bacterial infections
Megace ES [megestrol acetate]	Z79.818	Agents affecting estrogen receptors and estrogen levels	Endometrial or advanced breast cancers; weight loss due to AIDS
Menest [esteriefied estrogens]	Z79.890	Estrogen therapy	Menopause symptoms; ovarian failure
Menostar [estradiol]	Z79.890	Estrogen therapy	Menopause symptoms; osteoporosis prevention
Mepron [atovaquone]	Z79.2	Antibacterial	Pneumonia
Merrem [meropenem]	Z79.2	Antibacterial	Bacterial infections of skin or stomach; bacterial meningitis
Metformin [metformin hydrochloride]	Z79.84	Blood glucose regulator	Diabetes mellitus
Methadone HCl [methadone hydrochloride]	Z79.891	Narcotic analgesic	Pain; treatment of opioid addiction
Methadose [methadone hydrochloride]	Z79.891	Narcotic analgesic	Acute and chronic pain
Methergine [methylergonovine maleate]		Oxytocic agent	Routine management of postpartum hemorrhage after delivery of placenta
Methylprednisolone [methylprednisolone]	Z79.52	Corticosteroids	Inflammatory disorders
Metro [metronidazole]	Z79.2	Antibacterial	Bacterial infections
Metronidazole [metronidazole]	Z79.2	Antibacterial	Bacterial infections
Miacalcin [calcitonin salmon]		Calcitonin; a peptide hormone	Hypercalcemia, osteoporosis, postmenopausal symptoms, Paget's disease
Microgestin [ethinyl estradiol/norethindrone acetate]	Z79.3	Contraceptive	Contraception
Micronor [norethindrone]	Z79.3	Contraceptive	Contraception
Minastrin [ethinyl estradiol/norethindrone acetate]	Z79.3	Contraceptive	Contraception
Minivelle [estradiol]	Z79.890	Estrogen therapy	Menopause symptoms; osteoporosis prevention
Minocin [minocycline hydrochloride]	Z79.2	Antibacterial	Bacterial infections; acne
Mirena [levonorgestrel]	Z79.3	Contraceptive	Intrauterine device for contraception; menstrual disorders
Mobic [meloxicam]	Z79.1	Nonsteroidal anti-inflammatory drug (NSAID)	Pain and inflammation due to osteoarthritis and rheumatoid arthritis
Modicon [ethinyl estradiol/norethindrone]	Z79.3	Contraceptive	Contraception
Monoclonal antibodies	Z79.899	Monoclonal antibodies	Cancer; prophylaxis of organ transplant rejection
Monodox [doxycycline]	Z79.2	Antibacterial	Bacterial infections; acne
Monoket [isosorbide mononitrate]		Antianginal; coronary vasodilator, nitrate	Angina pectoris
Mono-Linyah [norgestimate/ethinyl estradiol]	Z79.3	Contraceptive	Contraception; menstrual disorders; acne
Monurol [fosfomycin tromethamine]	Z79.2	Antibacterial	Bacterial bladder infections
Morphine [morphine sulfate]	Z79.891	Narcotic analgesic	Moderate to severe pain
Motrin [ibuprofen]	Z79.1	Analgesic, general; analgesic, non-narcotic; antiarthritic; antigout; antipyretic; NSAID	Osteoarthritis and rheumatoid arthritis, dysmenorrhea, fever; pain, mild to moderate
Moxatag [amoxicillin]	Z79.2	Antibacterial	Bacterial tonsillitis and pharyngitis
MS Contin [morphine sulfate]	Z79.891	Narcotic analgesic	Moderate to severe pain
Multaq [dronedarone hydrochloride]		Cardiac rhythm regulator	Treatment of patients with recent episodes of atrial fibrillation or atrial flutter
Mycobutin [rifabutin]	Z79.2	Antibacterial	Mycobacterium avium complex (MAC) prophylactic
Myzilra [ethinyl estradiol/levonorgestrel]	Z79.3	Contraceptive	Contraception
Nabumetone [nabumetone]	Z79.1	Non-steroidal anti-inflammatory drug (NSAID)	Osteoarthritis and rheumatoid arthritis

Drug	Z Code	Drug Action	Indications
Nalfon [fenoprofen calcium]	Z79.1	Nonsteroidal anti-inflammatory drug (NSAID)	Pain or inflammation relief
Naprelan [naproxen sodium]	Z79.1	Nonsteroidal anti-inflammatory drug (NSAID)	Pain or inflammation relief
Naprosyn [naproxen]	Z79.1	Anti-inflammatory analgesic, general; analgesic, non-narcotic; antiarthritic; antigout; NSAID	Rheumatoid, gouty arthritis and osteoarthritis; ankylosing spondylitis; bursitis; dysmenorrhea; pain, mild to moderate; tendonitis
Natazia [estradiol valerate/dienogest]	Z79.3	Contraceptive	Contraception; menstrual disorders
Nebupent [pentamidine isethionate]	Z79.2	Antibacterial	Serious bacterial lung infection in high-risk patients with HIV
Nefazodone hydrochloride [nefazodone hydrochloride]		Antidepressant	Depression
Nembutal sodium [pentobarbital sodium]		Sedative; hypnotic	Adjunct medication in diagnostic procedures or for emergency use with convulsive disorders
NeoProfen [ibuprofen lysine]	Z79.1	Nonsteroidal anti-inflammatory drug (NSAID)	Pain or fever relief
Neoral [cyclosporine]	Z79.899	Immunosuppressant	Prophylaxis of organ transplant rejection
Neurontin [gabapentin]		Anticonvulsant	Epilepsy, partial
Nexium [esomeprazole magnesium]		Proton pump inhibitor	Gastroesophageal reflux disease (GERD), erosive esophagitis
Nexplanon [etonogestrel]	Z79.3	Contraceptive	Implantable contraception
Nitrofurantoin [nitrofurantoin]	Z79.2	Antibacterial	Bacterial urinary tract infections
Nitropress [sodium nitroprusside]		Vasodilator	Potent, rapid action in reducing blood pressure in hypertensive crisis or for controlling bleeding during anesthesia by producing controlled hypotension
Nitrostat [nitroglycerin]		Muscle relaxant antianginal; antihypertensive; coronary vasodilator	Prophylaxis and treatment of angina pectoris; heart failure associated with myocardial infarction; hypertension, perioperative; surgery, adjunct
Norco [acetaminophen/hydrocodone bitartrate]	Z79.891	Narcotic analgesic	Moderate to severe pain
Norinyl [mestranol/norethisterone]	Z79.3	Contraceptive	Contraception
Norpace [disopyramide phosphate]		Antiarrhythmic	Coronary artery disease, for prevention, recurrence, and control of unifocal, multifocal, and paired PVCs
Nor-QD [norethindrone]	Z79.3	Contraceptive	Contraception
Nortrel [ethinyl estradiol/norethindrone]	Z79.3	Contraceptive	Contraception
Norvasc [amlodipine besylate]		Calcium channel blocker	Hypertension, chronic stable angina, and vasospastic angina
Novolin [insulin recombinant]	Z79.4	Blood glucose regulator	Diabetes mellitus
NovoLog [insulin recombinant]	Z79.4	Blood glucose regulator	Diabetes mellitus
Nucynta [tapentadol hydrochloride]	Z79.891	Narcotic analgesic	Moderate to severe pain
NuvaRing [etonogestrel/ethinyl estradiol]	Z79.3	Contraceptive	Vaginal ring for contraception
Ogestrel [norgestrel/ethinyl estradiol]	Z79.3	Contraceptive	Contraception
Onglyza [saxagliptin hydrochloride]	Z79.84	Blood glucose regulator	Diabetes mellitus
Opana [oxymorphone hydrochloride]	Z79.891	Narcotic analgesic	Moderate to severe pain
Oracea [doxycycline]	Z79.2	Antibacterial	Rosacea
Orapred ODT [prednisolone sodium phosphate]	Z79.52	Corticosteroids	Inflammatory disorders
Orbactiv [oritavancin diphosphate]	Z79.2	Antibacterial	Bacterial skin infections
Orphenadrine citrate [orphenadrine citrate]		Muscle relaxant	Acute spasms, tension, and post-trauma cases
Orsythia [ethinyl estradiol/levonorgestrel]	Z79.3	Contraceptive	Contraception
Ortho Cyclen [ethinyl estradiol/norgestimate]	Z79.3	Contraceptive	Contraception
Ortho-Novum [norethindrone/ethinyl estradiol]	Z79.3	Contraceptive	Contraception
Ortho-Tri-Cyclen [ethinyl estradiol/norgestimate]	Z79.3	Contraceptive	Contraception
Oseni [alogliptin benzoate/pioglitazone hydrochloride]	Z79.84	Blood glucose regulator	Diabetes mellitus

Drug	Z Code	Drug Action	Indications
Osphena [ospemifene]	Z79.810, Z79.890	Selective estrogen receptor modulator (SERM)	Postmenopausal dyspareunia due to vaginal atrophy; osteoporosis prevention and treatment of menopause symptoms
Oxazepam [oxazepam]		Antianxiety agent	Anxiety, tension, and alcohol withdrawal
Oxycodone HCl [oxycodone hydrochloride]	Z79.891	Narcotic analgesic	Moderate to severe pain
OxyContin [oxycodone hydrochloride]	Z79.891	Narcotic analgesic	Moderate to severe pain
Pavabid [papaverine hydrochloride]		Vasodilator	Relief of cerebral and peripheral ischemia
Paxil [paroxetine hydrochloride]		Antidepressant	Anxiety with panic disorder and depression; obsessive-compulsive disorder
PCE [erythromycin]	Z79.2	Antibacterial	Bacterial infections
PediaPred [prednisolone sodium phosphate]	Z79.52	Corticosteroids	Inflammatory disorders
Pegintron [peginterferon alfa-2b]	Z79.899	Antiviral interferon	Hepatitis C
Penicillin-VK [penicillin V potassium]	Z79.2	Natural penicillin	Chorea prevention; endocarditis prevention, secondary to tooth extraction; erysipelas; infections of the skin and skin structures, upper respiratory tract; rheumatic fever, prophylaxis; scarlet fever; Vincent's gingivitis; Vincent's pharyngitis
Pentam [pentamidine isethionate]	Z79.2	Antibacterial	Serious bacterial lung infections
Pepcid [famotidine]		Histamine H2-receptor inhibitor	Acid/peptic disorder; adenoma, secretory; gastroesophageal reflux; duodenal and gastric ulcer; Zollinger-Ellison syndrome
Percocet [oxycodone hydrochloride/acetaminophen]	Z79.891	Analgesic, general; analgesic-narcotic	Pain, moderate to severe
Persantine [dipyridamole]	Z79.02	Platelet inhibitor	Therapy for chronic angina pectoris, preventing clots post heart valve surgery
Pfizerpen [penicillin g potassium]	Z79.2	Antibacterial	Severe bacterial infections
Phenobarbital [phenobarbital sodium]		Barbiturate	Grand mal epilepsy
Philith [ethinyl estradiol/norethindrone]	Z79.3	Contraceptive	Contraception
Pimtrea [desogestrel/ethinyl estradiol]	Z79.3	Contraceptive	Contraception
Pirmella [ethinyl estradiol/norethindrone]	Z79.3	Contraceptive	Contraception
Pitocin [oxytocin]		Synthetic oxytocin	Induction or stimulation of labor at term
Plan B One-Step [levonorgestrel]	Z79.3	Contraceptive	Contraception
Plasmanate [plasma, plasma protein fraction]		Blood volume expander	Hypovolemic shock, burn patients, and hemorrhages when whole blood is unavailable
Plavix [clopidogrel bisulfate]	Z79.02	Antithrombotic platelet aggregation inhibitor	Lessening of the chance of heart attack or stroke
Ponstel [mefenamic acid]	Z79.1	Nonsteroidal anti-inflammatory drug (NSAID)	Pain
Portia [ethinyl estradiol/levonorgestrel]	Z79.3	Contraceptive	Contraception
Pradaxa [dabigatran etexilate mesylate]	Z79.01	Anticoagulant	Prophylaxis and treatment of blood clots in patients with atrial fibrillation
Prandimet [metformin hydrochloride/repaglinide]	Z79.84	Blood glucose regulator	Diabetes mellitus
Prandin [repaglinide]	Z79.84	Blood glucose regulator	Diabetes mellitus
Pravachol [pravastatin sodium]		HMG-CoA reductase inhibitor (statin)	Hypercholesterolemia, hyperlipidemia, hyperlipoproteinemia
Precose [acarbose]	Z79.84	Blood glucose regulator	Diabetes mellitus
Prednisolone [prednisolone]	Z79.52	Corticosteroids	Inflammatory disorders
Prednisone [prednisone]	Z79.52	Adrenocorticoid, corticosteroid	Used for its immunosuppressant effects and for relief of inflammations; used in arthritis, polymyositis and other systemic diseases
Pregnyl [chorionic gonadotropin]		Gonadotropic hormone	Prepubertal cryptorchidism, hypogonadism, corpus luteum insufficiency and infertility
Prelone [prednisolone]	Z79.52	Corticosteroids; antiasthmatic	Inflammatory disorders
Premarin [conjugated estrogens]	Z79.890	Antineoplastic; estrogen	Vasomotor symptoms associated with menopause; atrophic vaginitis; kraurosis vulvae, female hypogonadism; primary ovarian failure
Prempro [conjugated estrogens/medroxyprogesterone acetate]	Z79.890	Estrogen/progestin	Menopause, osteoporosis, atrophic vaginitis

Drug	Z Code	Drug Action	Indications
Prevacid [lansoprazole]		Proton pump inhibitor (PPI)	Acid/peptic disorder, erosive esophagitis, duodenal ulcer, Zollinger-Ellison syndrome
Previfem [ethinyl estradiol/norgestimate]	Z79.3	Contraceptive	Contraception
Priftin [rifapentine]	Z79.2	Antibacterial	Prophylaxis and treatment of tuberculosis
Prilosec [omeprazole magnesium]		Proton pump inhibitor	Acid/peptic disorder; endocrine adenoma; erosive esophagitis; systemic mastocytosis; gastroesophageal reflux; duodenal, peptic and gastric ulcer; Zollinger-Ellison syndrome
Primaxin [cilastatin sodium/imipenem]	Z79.2	Antibacterial	Skin, stomach, female reproductive organs or lower respiratory tract infections
Prinivil [lisinopril]		Synthetic peptide derivative, long-acting angiotensin converting enzyme inhibitor	Congestive heart failure, essential hypertension
Procardia [nifedipine]		Antianginal agent; calcium channel blocker	Management of vasospastic angina and chronic stable angina, essential hypertension
Prograf [tacrolimus]	Z79.899	Immunosuppressant	Prophylaxis of organ transplant rejection
Promethazine hydrochloride [promethazine hydrochloride]		Anesthesia, adjunct to; antiemetic; antihistamine; antitussive/expectorant; sedative/hypnotic; vertigo/motion sickness/vomiting	Anesthesia; adjunct; angioedema; conjunctivitis; dermographism; hypersensitivity, motion sickness; pain; perennial, seasonal, and allergic rhinitis; sedation, obstetrical; urticaria
Protonix [pantoprazole]		Proton pump inhibitor (PPI)	Short-term treatment and maintenance therapy of erosive esophagitis associated with gastroesophageal reflux disease (GERD)
Protopic [tacrolimus]	Z79.899	Immunosuppressant	Atomic dermatitis (eczema)
Proventil-HFA [albuterol sulfate]		Antiasthmatic/bronchodilator	Asthma
Provera [medroxyprogesterone acetate]	Z79.3, Z79.890	Antineoplastic; contraceptive; progestin	Amenorrhea; carcinoma, endometrium, adjunct; carcinoma, renal; contraception; hemorrhage
Prozac [fluoxetine hydrochloride]		Serotonin reuptake inhibitor	Bulimia nervosa; depression; obsessive-compulsive disorder
Pulmicort [budesonide]	Z79.51	Corticosteroids -inhaled; antiasthmatic	Prophylaxis and treatment of asthma
Qnasl [beclomethasone dipropionate]		Corticosteroid	Perennial allergies, seasonal allergies, and vasomotor rhinitis
Qtern [dapagliflozin propanediol/saxagliptin hydrochloride]	Z79.84	Blood glucose regulator	Diabetes mellitus
Quartette [levonorgestrel/ethinyl estradiol]	Z79.3	Contraceptive	Contraception
Quasense [ethinyl estradiol/levonorgestrel]	Z79.3	Contraceptive	Contraception
Quinidine gluconate [quinidine gluconate]		Antiarrhythmic	Management of cardiac arrhythmias
Qvar [beclomethasone dipropionate]	Z79.51	Corticosteroids -inhaled; antiasthmatic	Prevention and control of symptoms related to asthma
Raloxifene [raloxifene hydrochloride]	Z79.810	Selective estrogen receptor modulator (SERM)	Prevention of thinning of the bones (osteoporosis) only in postmenopausal women
Rapamune [sirolimus]	Z79.899	Immunosuppressant	Prophylaxis of organ transplant rejection
Rayos [prednisone]	Z79.52	Corticosteroids; antiasthmatic	Arthritis, blood disorders, allergies, asthma
Rebif [interferon beta-1a]	Z79.899	Antiviral interferon	Relapsing multiple sclerosis
Reclast [zoledronic acid]	Z79.83	Bisphosphonates	Prevention of thinning of the bones (osteoporosis); Paget's disease; bone cancer
Repaglinide [repaglinide]	Z79.84	Blood glucose regulator	Diabetes mellitus
Reprexain [hydrocodone bitartrate/ibuprofen]	Z79.891	Opioid analgesic/Nonsteroidal anti-inflammatory drug (NSAID)	Pain, inflammation, or fever relief
Restoril [temazepam]		Sedative/hypnotic	Insomnia
Retrovir [zidovudine]		Antiretroviral agent	Indicated in symptomatic HIV infection
Rifadin [rifampin]	Z79.2	Antibacterial	Prophylaxis and treatment of tuberculosis
Rimactane [rifampin]	Z79.2	Antibacterial	Prophylaxis and treatment of tuberculosis
Riomet [metformin hydrochloride]	Z79.84	Blood glucose regulator	Diabetes mellitus
Risperdal [risperidone]		Antipsychotic/antimanic	Schizophrenia; bipolar I disorder
Ritalin [methylphenidate hydrochloride]		Central nervous system (CNS) stimulant	Treatment of depression and hyperkinetic activity in children
Roxicet [oxycodone hydrochloride/acetaminophen]	Z79.891	Analgesic, general; analgesic-narcotic	Pain, moderate to severe
Roxicodone [oxycodone hydrochloride]	Z79.891	Narcotic analgesic	Pain relief

Drug	Z Code	Drug Action	Indications
Ryzodeg [insulin aspart/insulin degludec]	Z79.4	Blood glucose regulator	Diabetes mellitus
Sabril [vigabatrin]		Anticonvulsant	Refractory complex partial seizures
Safyral [drospirenone/ethinyl estradiol/levomefolate calcium]	Z79.3	Contraceptive	Contraception
Sandimmune [cyclosporine]	Z79.899	Immunosuppressant	Prophylaxis of organ transplant rejection
Savaysa [edoxaban tosylate]	Z79.Ø1	Anticoagulant	Prophylaxis and treatment of venous thrombosis, pulmonary embolism; prevention of blood clots due to atrial fibrillation
Seasonale [levonorgestrel/ethinyl estradiol]	Z79.3	Contraceptive	Contraception
Seasonique [ethinyl estradiol/levonorgestrel]	Z79.3	Contraceptive	Contraception
Septra [sulfamethoxazole trimethoprim]	Z79.2	Antibacterial	Treatment of urinary tract infections, acute otitis media, acute exacerbations of chronic bronchitis, and shigellosis
Serevent [salmeterol xinafoate]		Bronchodilator	Asthma
Seromycin [cycloserine]	Z79.2	Antibacterial	Tuberculosis; urinary tract infections
Setlakin [ethinyl estradiol/levonorgestrel]	Z79.3	Contraceptive	Contraception
Simulect [basiliximab]	Z79.899	Immunosuppressant	Prophylaxis of organ transplant rejection
Sinemet [carbidopa/levodopa]		Antiparkinsonian	Parkinson's disease
Singulair [montelukast sodium]		Antiasthmatic, leukotriene receptor antagonist	Treatment of mild to moderate asthma to decrease the symptoms of asthma and the number of acute asthma attacks
Sirolimus [sirolimus]	Z79.899	Immunosuppressant	Prophylaxis of organ transplant rejection
Sitagliptin [sitagliptin/metformin hydrochloride]	Z79.84	Blood glucose regulator	Diabetes mellitus
Sivextro [tedizolid phosphate]	Z79.2	Antibacterial	Skin infections including MRSA
Skyla [levonorgestrel]	Z79.3	Contraceptive	Intrauterine device for contraception
Solodyn [minocycline hydrochloride]	Z79.2	Antibacterial	Bacterial infections
Soltamox [tamoxifen citrate]	Z79.81Ø	Selective estrogen receptor modulator (SERM)	Breast cancer
Solu-Cortef [hydrocortisone sodium succinate]	Z79.52	Corticosteroids; antiasthmatic	Asthma; severe inflammation; allergic reactions
Solu-Medrol [methylprednisolone sodium succinate]	Z79.52	Adrenocorticosteroid	Anti-inflammatory and antiallergenic for shock and ulcerative colitis
Sprintec [norgestimate/ethinyl estradiol]	Z79.3	Contraceptive	Contraception
Streptomycin sulfate [streptomycin sulfate]	Z79.2	Antibacterial	Severe bacterial infections
Sublimaze [fentanyl citrate]	Z79.891	Narcotic analgesic	Pain relief
Supprelin LA [histrelin acetate]	Z79.818	Agents affecting estrogen receptors and estrogen levels	Precocious puberty; prostate cancer symptoms
Suprax [cefixime]	Z79.2	Antibacterial	Bacterial infections
Syeda [drospirenone/ethinyl estradiol]	Z79.3	Contraceptive	Contraception
Sylatron [peginterferon alfa-2b]	Z79.899	Antineoplastic interferons; antiviral interferons	Prevention of recurrent malignant melanoma
Symbicort [budesonide/formoterol fumarate dihydrate]	Z79.51	Corticosteroids -inhaled; antiasthmatic	Prophylaxis and treatment of asthma and COPD
Synarel [nafarelin acetate]	Z79.818	Agents affecting estrogen receptors and estrogen levels	Endometriosis symptoms; precocious puberty
Synercid [dalfopristin/quinupristin]	Z79.2	Antibacterial	Severe blood infections
Synjardy [empagliflozin/metformin hydrochloride]	Z79.84	Blood glucose regulator	Diabetes mellitus
Synthroid [levothyroxine sodium]		Thyroid hormone	Treatment of hypothyroidism
Tacrolimus [tacrolimus]	Z79.899	Immunosuppressant	Prophylaxis of organ transplant rejection
Tagamet HB [cimetidine]		Acid reducer	Treatment of active duodenal ulcer, short-term treatment of active, benign gastric ulcer, and treatment of pathological hypersecretory conditions
Tamoxifen [tamoxifen citrate]	Z79.81Ø	Selective estrogen receptor modulator (SERM)	Metastatic breast cancer in postmenopausal women
Tazicef [ceftazidime]	Z79.2	Antibacterial	Confirmed or suspected bacterial infections

Drug	Z Code	Drug Action	Indications
Teflaro [ceftaroline fosamil]	Z79.2	Antibacterial	Bacterial skin infections; pneumonia
Tegretol [carbamazepine]		Anticonvulsant; analgesic	Epilepsy, especially with complex symptomatology; specific analgesic for trigeminal neuralgia
Tenormin [atenolol]		Antianginal; antihypertensive; beta blocker	Treatment of hypertension; lowering blood pressure lowers the risk of fatal and nonfatal cardiovascular events, primarily strokes and myocardial infarctions
Terazosin hydrochloride [terazosin hydrochloride]		Alpha-blocker; antihypertensive; diuretic	Benign prostatic hypertrophy; essential hypertension
Tetracycline HCl [tetracycline hydrochloride]	Z79.2	Antibacterial	Bacterial infections
Tiazac [diltiazem hydrochloride]		Antianginal, antiarrhythmic, antihypertensive, channel blocker, coronary vasodilator	Chronic stable angina, atrial fibrillation, atrial flutter, essential hypertension, paroxysmal supraventricular tachycardia
Tivorbex [indomethacin]	Z79.1	Nonsteroidal anti-inflammatory drug (NSAID)	Pain, inflammation and joint stiffness
Tobradex [tobramycin/dexamethasone]		Aminoglycoside ocular anti-infective; anti-inflammatory	Infectious conjunctivitis; dermatosis, corticosteroid-responsive with secondary infection; foreign body in eye; corneal inflammation; uveitis
Tobramycin [dexamethasone/tobramycin]	Z79.2	Antibacterial	Bacterial eye infections
Toprol-XL [metoprolol succinate]		Antianginal antihypertensive beta blocker	Angina pectoris, essential hypertension
Toremifene [toremifene citrate]	Z79.810	Selective estrogen receptor modulator (SERM)	Metastatic breast cancer in postmenopausal women
Torisel [temsirolimus]	Z79.899	Antineoplastic	Renal cell carcinoma
Toujeo Solostar [insulin glargine recombinant]	Z79.4	Blood glucose regulator	Diabetes mellitus
Trazodone hydrochloride [trazodone hydrochloride]		Antidepressant	Depression
Trelstar [triptorelin pamoate]	Z79.818	Agents affecting estrogen receptors and estrogen levels	Prophylaxis of chemo-induced menopause; prostate cancer symptoms
Tresiba [insulin degludec]	Z79.4	Blood glucose regulator	Diabetes mellitus
Triamterene and hydrochlorothiazide [triamterene/ hydrochlorothiazide]		Antihypertensive, diuretic	Edema; essential hypertension
Tri-Estarylla [ethinyl estradiol/norgestimate]	Z79.3	Contraceptive	Contraception; acne
Tri-Legest [ethinyl estradiol/norethindrone acetate]	Z79.3	Contraceptive	Contraception
Tri-Linyah [ethinyl estradiol/norgestimate]	Z79.3	Contraceptive	Contraception
Tri-Lo-Estarylla [ethinyl estradiol/norgestimate]	Z79.3	Contraceptive	Contraception
Tri-Lo-Sprintec [ethinyl estradiol/norgestimate]	Z79.3	Contraceptive	Contraception
Trimethoprim [trimethoprim]	Z79.2	Antibacterial	Acute exacerbation chronic bronchitis; travelers' diarrhea; infections of the middle and lower respiratory tracts, and urinary tract; pneumonia, pneumocystis; shigellosis
Tri-Norinyl [ethinyl estradiol/norethindrone]	Z79.3	Contraceptive	Contraception
Tri-Previfem [ethinyl estradiol/norgestimate]	Z79.3	Contraceptive	Contraception
Tri-Sprintec [ethinyl estradiol/norgestimate]	Z79.3	Contraceptive	Contraception; acne
Trivora [ethinyl estradiol/ levonorgestrel]	Z79.3	Contraceptive	Contraception
Tygacil [tigecycline]	Z79.2	Antibacterial	Bacterial skin or digestive system infections; pneumonia
Tylenol with codeine [acetaminophen/codeine phosphate]	Z79.891	Narcotic analgesic	Pain and cough
Ultram [tramadol hydrochloride]	Z79.891	Analgesic, non-narcotic (opiate, narcotic-like)	Pain, moderate to moderately severe
Unasyn [ampicillin sodium/sulbactam sodium]	Z79.2	Antibacterial	Bacterial infections
Vagifem [estradiol]	Z79.890	Estrogen therapy	Menopause symptoms

Drug	Z Code	Drug Action	Indications
Valium [diazepam]		Antianxiety, muscle relaxant, anticonvulsant	Anxiety, tension, withdrawal from alcohol, muscle spasms and anticonvulsant therapy; epilepsy, generalized tonic-clonic; status epilepticus; stiff-man syndrome; tetanus
Vancocin HCl [vancomycin hydrochloride]	Z79.2	Antibacterial	Serious bacterial infections
Vancomycin HCl [vancomycin hydrochloride]	Z79.2	Antibacterial	Serious bacterial infections
Vantas [histrelin acetate]	Z79.818	Agents affecting estrogen receptors and estrogen levels	Prostate cancer symptoms; breast cancer; endometriosis
Vasotec [enalaprilat maleate]		ACE inhibitor; antihypertensive	Congestive heart failure; essential hypertension
Velivet [desogestrel/ethinyl estradiol]	Z79.3	Contraceptive	Contraception
Ventolin HFA [albuterol sulfate]		Antiasthmatic/bronchodilator	Asthma
Verapamil HCL [verapamil hydrochloride]		Antianginal, antiarrhythmic, antiarthritic, antihypertensive, calcium channel blocker	Angina pectoris, chronic stable angina, atrial fibrillation, atrial flutter, paroxysmal supraventricular tachycardia, ventricular arrhythmia, essential hypertension
Viagra [sildenafil citrate]		Phosphodiesterase-5 (PDE5) inhibitor	Erectile dysfunction
Vibativ [telavancin hydrochloride]	Z79.2	Antibacterial	Pneumonia; severe bacterial skin infections
Vibramycin [doxycycline calcium]	Z79.2	Antibacterial	Bacterial infections
Vicoprofen [hydrocodone bitartrate/ibuprofen]	Z79.891	Opioid analgesic/ Nonsteroidal anti-inflammatory drug (NSAID)	Pain, inflammation, or fever relief
Victoza [liraglutide (rDNA) injection]		Glucagon-like peptide-1 (GLP-1) receptor agonist	Diabetes mellitus
Vienva [ethinyl estradiol/levonorgestrel]	Z79.3	Contraceptive	Contraception
Viorele [desogestrel/ethinyl estradiol]	Z79.3	Contraceptive	Contraception
Virazole [ribavirin]		Antiviral	Respiratory syncytial virus (RSV)
Vistaril [hydroxyzine pamoate]		Antianxiety agent, antiemetic	Treatment of nausea and vomiting, for reducing narcotic requirement in surgery and as tranquilizer for tension, anxiety, or agitation states
Vivelle [estradiol]	Z79.89Ø	Estrogen therapy	Menopause symptoms; osteoporosis prevention
Voltaren [diclofenac sodium]	Z79.1	Nonsteroidal anti-inflammatory drug (NSAID)	Treatment of pain, inflammation, and joint stiffness due to arthritis
Warfarin [warfarin sodium]	Z79.Ø1	Anticoagulant	Prophylaxis and treatment of venous thrombosis, treatment of atrial fibrillation with embolization (pulmonary embolism), arrhythmias, myocardial infarction, and stroke prevention
Wellbutrin SR, Wellbutrin XL [bupropion hydrochloride]		Antidepressant; CNS	Depression; smoking cessation
Wera [ethinyl estradiol/norethindrone]	Z79.3	Contraceptive	Contraception
Xalatan [latanoprost]		Prostaglandin F2α analogue	Glaucoma, open-angle; ocular hypertension
Xanax, Xanax XR [alprazolam]		Antianxiety; sedative/hypnotic	Anxiety disorders with panic disorder and depression
Xarelto [rivaraxaban]	Z79.Ø1	Anticoagulant	Prophylaxis and treatment of venous thrombosis, pulmonary embolism; prevention of blood clots due to atrial fibrillation
Xifaxan [rifaximin]	Z79.2	Antibacterial	*E. coli* diarrhea
Xigduo [dapagliflozin propanediol/metformin hydrochloride]	Z79.84	Blood glucose regulator	Diabetes mellitus
Xigris [drotrecogin alfa]		Biologic response modifier	Severe sepsis
Yasmin [drospirenone/ethinyl estradiol]	Z79.3	Contraceptive	Contraception
Yaz [drospirenone/ethinyl estradiol]	Z79.3	Contraceptive	Contraception; menstrual disorders
Zantac [ranitidine hydrochloride]		Histamine H2-receptors inhibitor	Acid/peptic disorder, erosive esophagitis, gastrointestinal hypersecretion, mastocytosis, gastroesophageal reflux, peptic ulcer, Zollinger-Ellison syndrome
Zerbaxa [ceftolozane sulfate/tazobactam sodium]	Z79.2	Antibacterial	Complicated urinary tract and intra-abdominal infections
Zestoretic [lisinopril/hydrochlorothiazide]		ACE inhibitor; antihypertensive	Congestive heart failure; essential hypertension
Zestril [lisinopril]		ACE inhibitor; antihypertensive	Congestive heart failure; essential hypertension
Ziac [bisoprolol fumarate/ hydrochlorothiazide]		Antihypertensive	Essential hypertension
Zinacef [cefuroxime sodium]	Z79.2	Antibacterial	Bacterial infections

Drug	Z Code	Drug Action	Indications
Zipsor [diclofenac potassium]	Z79.1	Nonsteroidal anti-inflammatory drug (NSAID)	Pain and inflammation relief
Zithromax [azithromycin]	Z79.2	Macrolide	Infections of the cervix, lower respiratory tract, skin and skin structures, urethra, nongonococcal; mycobacterium avium complex; pharyngitis, streptococcal pneumonia; tonsillitis
Zmax [azithromycin]	Z79.2	Antibacterial	Pneumonia; sinusitis
Zocor [simvastatin]		HMG-CoA reductase inhibitor (statin)	Hypercholesterolemia, hyperlipidemia, hyperlipoproteinemia, hypertriglyceridemia
Zoladex [goserelin acetate]	Z79.818	Agents affecting estrogen receptors and estrogen levels	Prostate cancer symptoms and advanced breast cancer
Zoloft [sertraline hydrochloride]		Antidepressant	Anxiety with panic disorder and depression; obsessive-compulsive disorder
Zometa [zoledronic acid]	Z79.83	Bisphosphonates	Multiple myeloma; Paget's disease
Zorvolex [diclofenac]	Z79.1	Nonsteroidal anti-inflammatory drug (NSAID)	Pain, inflammation or fever relief
Zosyn [piperacillin sodium/tazobactam sodium]	Z79.2	Antibacterial	Bacterial infections
Zovia [ethynodiol diacetate/ethinyl estradiol]	Z79.3	Contraceptive	Contraception
Zovirax [acyclovir]		Antiviral	Genital herpes and herpes zoster infections
Zyloprim [allopurinol]		Antigout	Gouty arthritis, renal calculus, hyperuricemia, hyperuricemia secondary to leukemia, hyperuricemia secondary to lymphoma
Zyprexa [olanzapine]		Antipsychotic/antimanic	Psychotic disorders; schizophrenia
Zyrtec [cetirizine hydrochloride]		Antihistamine	Perennial allergic and seasonal allergic rhinitis; chronic urticaria
Zyvox [linezolid]	Z79.2	Antibacterial	Serious bacterial infections

Appendix D: Z Codes for Long-Term Drug Use with Associated Drugs

Z79.01	**Long term (current) use of anticoagulants**		Clindamycin	**Z79.3**	**Long term (current) use of hormonal contraceptives**

Z79.01 Long term (current) use of anticoagulants
- Arixtra
- Coumadin
- Eliquis
- Fragmin
- Heparin
- Jantoven
- Lovenox
- Pradaxa
- Savaysa
- Warfarin
- Xarelto

Z79.02 Long term (current) use of antithrombotics/antiplatelets
- Aggrastat
- Aggrenox
- Angiomax
- Argatroban
- Brilinta
- Clopidogrel bisulfate
- Effient
- Integrilin
- Iprivask
- Persantine
- Plavix

Z79.1 Long term (current) use of non-steroidal anti-inflammatories (NSAID)
- Advil
- Aleve
- Anaprox
- Arthrotec
- Caldolor
- Cambia
- Celebrex
- Daypro
- Duexis
- Dyloject
- Feldene
- Ibuprofen
- Indocin
- Mobic
- Motrin
- Nabumetone
- Nalfon
- Naprelan
- Naprosyn
- NeoProfen
- Ponstel
- Tivorbex
- Voltaren
- Zipsor
- Zorvolex

Z79.2 Long term (current) use of antibiotics
- Akne-Mycin
- Altabax
- Amoxicillin
- Ampicillin
- Ancef
- Augmentin
- Azactam
- Azithromycin
- Bactrim
- Bactroban
- Ceftriaxone
- Centany
- Cephalexin
- Cipro
- Ciprofloxacin
- Clarithromycin
- Cleocin
- Clindamycin
- Daptomycin
- Dificid
- Doxycycline
- Dynacin
- E.E.S.
- Ertapenem
- ERYC
- Erygel
- EryPed
- Ery-Tab
- Erythrocin
- Erythromycin
- Factive
- Flagyl
- Fortaz
- Gentamicin sulfate
- Invanz
- Isoniazid
- Keflex
- Kefzol
- Klaron
- Levaquin
- Lincocin
- Macrobid
- Maxipime
- Mefoxin
- Mepron
- Merrem
- Metro
- Metronidazole
- Minocin
- Monodox
- Monurol
- Moxatag
- Mycobutin
- Nebupent
- Nitrofurantoin
- Oracea
- Orbactiv
- PCE
- Penicillin-VK
- Pentam
- Pfizerpen
- Priftin
- Primaxin
- Rifadin
- Rimactane
- Septra
- Seromycin
- Sivextro
- Solodyn
- Streptomycin sulfate
- Suprax
- Synercid
- Tazicef
- Teflaro
- Tetracycline HCl
- Tobramycin
- Trimethoprim
- Tygacil
- Unasyn
- Vancocin HCl
- Vancomycin HCl
- Vibativ
- Vibramycin
- Xifaxan
- Zerbaxa
- Zinacef
- Zithromax
- Zmax
- Zosyn
- Zyvox

Z79.3 Long term (current) use of hormonal contraceptives
- Altavera
- Alyacen
- Aranelle
- Ashlyna
- Aviane
- Aygestin
- Balziva
- Bekyree
- Beyaz
- Brevicon
- Briellyn
- Camila
- Cryselle
- Cyclafem
- Cyclessa
- Dasetta
- Daysee
- Depo-Provera
- Depo-SubQ Provera
- Desogen
- Elinest
- Emoquette
- Enpresse
- Enskyce
- Errin
- Estarylla
- Estrostep Fe
- Falmina
- Femcon Fe
- Femhrt
- Gildagia
- Gildess
- Introvale
- Jencycla
- Junel
- Kariva
- Kelnor
- Kimidess
- Kurvelo
- Larin
- Lessina
- Levonest
- Levora
- Liletta
- Lo Loestrin Fe
- Lo Minastrin Fe
- Loestrin
- Loryna
- LoSeasonique
- Low-Ogestrel
- Marlissa
- Microgestin
- Micronor
- Minastrin
- Mirena
- Modicon
- Mono-Linyah
- Myzilra
- Natazia
- Nexplanon
- Norinyl
- Nor-QD
- Nortrel
- NuvaRing
- Ogestrel
- Orsythia
- Ortho Cyclen
- Ortho-Novum
- Ortho-Tri-Cyclen
- Philith
- Pimtrea

Pirmella
Plan B One-Step
Portia
Previfem
Provera
Quartette
Quasense
Safyral
Seasonale
Seasonique
Setlakin
Skyla
Sprintec
Syeda
Tri-Estarylla
Tri-Legest
Tri-Linyah
Tri-Lo-Estarylla
Tri-Lo-Sprintec
Tri-Norinyl
Tri-Previfem
Tri-Sprintec
Trivora
Velivet
Vienva
Viorele
Wera
Yasmin
Yaz
Zovia

Z79.4   Long term (current) use of insulin
Afrezza
Apidra
Basaglar
Humalog
Humulin
Lantus
Levemir
Novolin
NovoLog
Ryzodeg
Toujeo Solostar
Tresiba

Z79.51   Long term (current) use of inhaled steroids
Advair
Aerospan
Alvesco
Arnuity Ellipta
Asmanex
Dulera
Flovent
Pulmicort
Qvar
Symbicort

Z79.52   Long term (current) use of systemic steroids
A-Methapred
Aristospan
Celestone Soluspan
Colocort
Cortef
Cortenema
Cortifoam
Cortisone acetate
Depo-Medrol
Dexamethasone Intensol
Entocort EC
Hydrocortisone
Kenalog
Medrol
Methylprednisolone
Orapred ODT
PediaPred
Prednisolone
Prednisone

Prelone
Rayos
Solu-Cortef
Solu-Medrol

Z79.810   Long term (current) use of selective estrogen receptor modulators (SERMs)
Evista
Fareston
Osphena
Raloxifene
Soltamox
Tamoxifen
Toremifene

Z79.811   Long term (current) use of aromatase inhibitors
Anastrozole
Arimidex
Aromasin
Exemestane
Femara
Letrozole

Z79.818   Long term (current) use of other agents affecting estrogen receptors and estrogen levels
Eligard
Faslodex
Fulvestrant
Lupron
Megace ES
Supprelin LA
Synarel
Trelstar
Vantas
Zoladex

Z79.82   Long term (current) use of aspirin
Bayer
Bufferin
Ecotrin

Z79.83   Long term (current) use of bisphosphonates
Actonel
Atelvia
Binosto
Boniva
Didronel
Fosamax
Reclast
Zometa

Z79.84   Long term (current) use of oral hypoglycemic drugs
Acarbose
Actoplus Met
Actos
Amaryl
Avandia
Duetact
Fortamet
Glimepiride
Glucophage
Glucotrol
Glucovance
Glumetza
Glyburide
Invokamet
Janumet
Januvia
Jentadueto
Kazano
Kombiglyze
Metformin
Onglyza
Oseni
PrandiMet
Prandin
Precose

Qtern
Repaglinide
Riomet
Sitagliptin
Synjardy
Xigduo

Z79.890   Hormone replacement therapy
Activella
Alora
Angeliq
Climara
CombiPatch
Delestrogen
Divigel
Duavee
Elestrin
Enjuvia
Estrace
Estraderm
Estrasorb
EstroGel
Femhrt
Femring
Femtrace
Menest
Menostar
Minivelle
Osphena
Premarin
Prempro
Provera
Vagifem
Vivelle

Z79.891   Long term (current) use of opiate analgesic
Acetaminophen with codeine
Astramorph
Buprenex
Buprenorphine HCl
Butrans
Codeine
Demerol
Dilaudid
Dolophine HCl
Duragesic
Duramorph
Embeda
Exalgo
Fentanyl
Fentora
Fioricet with codeine
Hydrocodone
Hydrocodone bitartrate and acetaminophen
Hydromorphone HCl
Kadian
Methadone HCl
Methadose
Morphine
MS Contin
Norco
Nucynta
Opana
Oxycodone HCl
OxyContin
Percocet
Reprexain
Roxicet
Roxicodone
Sublimaze
Tylenol with codeine
Ultram
Vicoprofen

Z79.899 Other long term (current) drug therapy
    Actimmune
    Antineoplastic/chemotherapy
    Astagraf XL
    Avonex
    Cellcept
    Cyclosporine
    Envarsus XR
    Gengraf
    Imuran
    Intron
    Monoclonal antibodies
    Neoral
    Pegintron
    Prograf
    Protopic
    Rapamune
    Rebif
    Sandimmune
    Simulect
    Sirolimus
    Sylatron
    Tacrolimus
    Torisel

Z79.899 Other long term (current) drug therapy

Z00.00	Z01.419	Z02.9	Z31.84	Z38.62	Z52.090
Z00.01	Z01.42	Z03.6	Z33.2	Z38.63	Z52.091
Z00.110	Z01.810	Z03.71	Z34.00	Z38.64	Z52.098
Z00.111	Z01.811	Z03.72	Z34.01	Z38.65	Z52.10
Z00.121	Z01.812	Z03.73	Z34.02	Z38.66	Z52.11
Z00.129	Z01.818	Z03.74	Z34.03	Z38.68	Z52.19
Z00.2	Z01.82	Z03.75	Z34.80	Z38.69	Z52.20
Z00.3	Z01.83	Z03.79	Z34.81	Z38.7	Z52.21
Z00.5	Z01.84	Z03.810	Z34.82	Z38.8	Z52.29
Z00.70	Z01.89	Z03.818	Z34.83	Z39.0	Z52.3
Z00.71	Z02.0	Z03.89	Z34.90	Z39.1	Z52.4
Z00.8	Z02.1	Z04.1	Z34.91	Z39.2	Z52.5
Z01.00	Z02.2	Z04.2	Z34.92	Z42.1	Z52.6
Z01.01	Z02.3	Z04.3	Z34.93	Z42.8	Z52.810
Z01.10	Z02.4	Z04.41	Z38.00	Z51.0	Z52.811
Z01.110	Z02.5	Z04.42	Z38.01	Z51.11	Z52.812
Z01.118	Z02.6	Z04.6	Z38.1	Z51.12	Z52.813
Z01.12	Z02.71	Z04.71	Z38.2	Z52.000	Z52.819
Z01.20	Z02.79	Z04.72	Z38.30	Z52.001	Z52.89
Z01.21	Z02.81	Z04.8	Z38.31	Z52.008	Z76.1
Z01.30	Z02.82	Z04.9	Z38.4	Z52.010	Z76.2
Z01.31	Z02.83	Z31.81	Z38.5	Z52.011	Z99.12
Z01.411	Z02.89	Z31.83	Z38.61	Z52.018	

Appendix F: Qualifications for Medicare Coverage of Home Health Services

The criteria that must be met by the patient to qualify for Medicare coverage of home health services are specified in the following sections of the Medicare Benefit Policy Manual (Pub. 100-02), Chapter 7 - Home Health Services.

Conditions to be Met for Coverage of Home Health Services

Medicare covers HHA services when the following criteria are met:

1. The person to whom the services are provided is an eligible Medicare beneficiary;
2. The HHA that is providing the services to the beneficiary has in effect a valid agreement to participate in the Medicare program;
3. The beneficiary qualifies for coverage of home health services as described in §30;
4. The services for which payment is claimed are covered as described in §§40 and 50;
5. Medicare is the appropriate payer; and
6. The services for which payment is claimed are not otherwise excluded from payment.

Reasonable and Necessary Services

Background: In enacting the Medicare program, Congress recognized that the physician would play an important role in determining utilization of services. The law requires that payment can be made only if a physician certifies the need for services and establishes a plan of care. The Secretary is responsible for ensuring that Medicare covers the claimed services, including determining whether they are "reasonable and necessary."

The Medicare contractor's decision on whether care is reasonable and necessary is based on information reflected in the home health plan of care, the OASIS as required by 42 CFR 484.55 or a medical record of the individual patient. Medicare does not deny coverage solely on the basis of the reviewer's general inferences about patients with similar diagnoses or on data related to utilization generally, but bases it upon objective clinical evidence regarding the patient's individual need for care.

Coverage of skilled nursing care or therapy to perform a maintenance program does not turn on presence or absence of a patient's potential for improvement from nursing care or therapy, but rather on the patient's need for skilled care. Skilled care may be necessary to improve a patient's current condition, to maintain the patient's current condition, or to prevent or slow further deterioration of the patient's condition.

Impact of Other Available Caregivers and Other Available Coverage on Medicare Coverage of Home Health Services

Where the Medicare criteria for coverage of home health services are met, patients are entitled by law to coverage of reasonable and necessary home health services. Therefore, a patient is entitled to have the costs of reasonable and necessary services reimbursed by Medicare without regard to whether there is someone available to furnish the services. However, where a family member or other person is or will be providing services that adequately meet the patient's needs, it would not be reasonable and necessary for HHA personnel to furnish such services. Ordinarily it can be presumed that there is no able and willing person in the home to provide the services being rendered by the HHA unless the patient or family indicates otherwise and objects to the provision of the services by the HHA, or unless the HHA has first hand knowledge to the contrary.

Similarly, a patient is entitled to reasonable and necessary Medicare home health services even if the patient would qualify for institutional care (e.g., hospital care or skilled nursing facility care) and Medicare payment should be made for reasonable and necessary home health services where the patient is also receiving supplemental services that do not meet Medicare's definition of skilled nursing care or home health aide services.

Example 1: A patient who lives with an adult daughter and otherwise qualifies for Medicare coverage of home health services, requires the assistance of a home health aide for bathing and assistance with an exercise program to improve endurance. The daughter is unwilling to bathe her elderly father and assist him with the exercise program. Home health aide services would be reasonable and necessary.

Example 2: A patient who is being discharged from a hospital with a diagnosis of osteomyelitis and requires continuation of the I.V. antibiotic therapy that was begun in the hospital was found to meet the criteria for Medicare coverage of skilled nursing facility services. If the patient also meets the qualifying criteria for coverage of home health services, payment may be made for the reasonable and necessary home health services the patient needs, notwithstanding the availability of coverage in a skilled nursing facility.

Example 3: A patient who needs skilled nursing care on an intermittent basis also hires a licensed practical (vocational) nurse to provide nighttime assistance while family members sleep. The care provided by the nurse, as respite to the family members, does not require the skills of a licensed nurse (as defined in §40.1) and therefore has no impact on the beneficiary's eligibility for Medicare payment of home health services even though another third party insurer may pay for that nursing care.

Use of Utilization Screens and "Rules of Thumb"

Medicare recognizes that determinations of whether home health services are reasonable and necessary must be based on an assessment of each beneficiary's individual care needs. Therefore, denial of services based on numerical utilization screens, diagnostic screens, diagnosis or specific treatment norms is not appropriate.

Conditions Patient Must Meet to Qualify for Coverage of Home Health Services

To qualify for the Medicare home health benefit a Medicare beneficiary must meet the following requirements:

- Be confined to the home;
- Under the care of a physician;
- Receiving services under a plan of care established and periodically reviewed by a physician;
- Be in need of skilled nursing care on an intermittent basis or physical therapy or speech-language pathology; or
- Have a continuing need for occupational therapy.

For purposes of benefit eligibility, "intermittent" means skilled nursing care that is either provided or needed on fewer than seven days each week or less than eight hours of each day for periods of 21 days or less with extensions in exceptional circumstances when the need for additional care is finite and predictable.

A patient must meet each of the criteria specified in this section. Patients who meet each of these criteria are eligible to have payment made on their behalf for services discussed in §§40 and 50.

Confined to the Home

For a patient to be eligible to receive covered home health services under both Part A and Part B, the law requires that a physician certify in all cases that the patient is confined to his/her home. For purposes of the statute, an individual shall be considered "confined to the home" (homebound) if the following two criteria are met:

1. Criteria-One:

   The patient must either:

   - Because of illness or injury, need the aid of supportive devices such as crutches, canes, wheelchairs, and walkers; the use of special transportation; or the assistance of another person in order to leave their place of residence

   OR

   - Have a condition such that leaving his or her home is medically contraindicated.

   - If the patient meets one of the Criteria-One conditions, then the patient must ALSO meet two additional requirements defined in Criteria-Two below.

2. Criteria-Two:

   - There must exist a normal inability to leave home;

   AND

   - Leaving home must require a considerable and taxing effort.

To clarify, in determining whether the patient meets criterion two of the homebound definition, the clinician needs to take into account the illness or injury for which the patient met criterion one and consider the illness or injury in the context of the patient's overall condition. The clinician is not required to include standardized phrases reflecting the patient's condition (e.g., repeating the words "taxing effort to leave the home") in the patient's chart, nor are such phrases sufficient, by themselves, to demonstrate that criterion two has been met. For example, longitudinal clinical information about the patient's health status is typically needed to sufficiently demonstrate a normal inability to leave the home and that leaving home requires a considerable and taxing effort. Such clinical information about the patient's overall health status may include, but is not limited to, such factors as the patient's diagnosis, duration of the patient's condition, clinical course (worsening or improvement), prognosis, nature and extent of functional limitations, other therapeutic interventions and results, etc.

If the patient does in fact leave the home, the patient may nevertheless be considered homebound if the absences from the home are infrequent or for periods of relatively short duration, or are attributable to the need to receive health care treatment. Absences attributable to the need to receive health care treatment include, but are not limited to:

- Attendance at adult day centers to receive medical care;
- Ongoing receipt of outpatient kidney dialysis; or
- The receipt of outpatient chemotherapy or radiation therapy.

Any absence of an individual from the home attributable to the need to receive health care treatment, including regular absences for the purpose of participating in therapeutic, psychosocial, or medical treatment in an adult day-care program that is licensed or certified by a State, or accredited to furnish adult day-care services in a State, shall not disqualify an individual from being considered to be confined to his home. Any other absence of an individual from the home shall not so disqualify an individual if the absence is of an infrequent or of relatively short duration. For purposes of the preceding sentence, any absence for the purpose of attending a religious service shall be deemed to be an absence of infrequent or short duration. It is expected that in most instances, absences from the home that occur will be for the purpose of receiving health care treatment. However, occasional absences from the home for nonmedical purposes, e.g., an occasional trip to the barber, a walk around the block or a drive, attendance at a family reunion, funeral, graduation, or other infrequent or unique event would not necessitate a finding that the patient is not homebound if the absences are undertaken on an infrequent basis or are of relatively short duration and do not indicate that the patient has the capacity to obtain the health care provided outside rather than in the home.

Some examples of homebound patients that illustrate the factors used to determine whether a homebound condition exists are listed below.

- A patient paralyzed from a stroke who is confined to a wheelchair or requires the aid of crutches in order to walk.
- A patient who is blind or senile and requires the assistance of another person in leaving their place of residence.
- A patient who has lost the use of their upper extremities and, therefore, is unable to open doors, use handrails on stairways, etc., and requires the assistance of another individual to leave their place of residence.
- A patient in the late stages of ALS or neurodegenerative disabilities. In determining whether the patient has the general inability to leave the home and leaves the home only infrequently or for periods of short duration, it is necessary (as is the case in determining whether skilled nursing services are intermittent) to look at the patient's condition over a period of time rather than for short periods within the home health stay. For example, a patient may leave the home (meeting both criteria listed above) more frequently during a short period when the patient has multiple appointments with health care professionals and medical tests in 1 week. So long as the patient's overall condition and experience is such that he or she meets these qualifications, he or she should be considered confined to the home.
- A patient who has just returned from a hospital stay involving surgery, who may be suffering from resultant weakness and pain because of the surgery and; therefore, their actions may be restricted by their physician to certain specified and limited activities (such as getting out of bed only for a specified period of time, walking stairs only once a day, etc.).
  - A patient with arteriosclerotic heart disease of such severity that they must avoid all stress and physical activity.
  - A patient with a psychiatric illness that is manifested in part by a refusal to leave home or is of such a nature that it would not be considered safe for the patient to leave home unattended, even if they have no physical limitations.

- The aged person who does not often travel from home because of feebleness and insecurity brought on by advanced age would not be considered confined to the home for purposes of receiving home health services unless they meet one of the above conditions.

Although a patient must be confined to the home to be eligible for covered home health services, some services cannot be provided at the patient's residence because equipment is required that cannot be made available there. If the services required by an individual involve the use of such equipment, the HHA may make arrangements with a hospital, SNF, or a rehabilitation center to provide these services on an outpatient basis. (See §50.6.) However, even in these situations, for the services to be covered as home health services the patient must be considered confined to home and meet both criteria listed above.

Place of Residence

A patient's residence is wherever he/she makes his/her home. This may be his/her own dwelling, an apartment, a relative's home, a home for the aged, or some other type of institution. However, an institution may not be considered a patient's home if the institution meets the requirements of §§1861(e)(1) or 1819(a)(1) of the Act. Included in this group are hospitals and skilled nursing facilities. as well as most nursing facilities under Medicaid. (See the Medicare State Operations Manual, §2166.)

Thus, if a patient is in an institution or distinct part of an institution identified above, the patient is not entitled to have payment made for home health services under either Part A or Part B since these institutions may not be considered his/her residence. When a patient remains in a participating SNF following his/her discharge from active care, the facility may not be considered his/her residence for purposes of home health coverage.

A patient may have more than one home, and the Medicare rules do not prohibit a patient from having one or more places of residence. A patient, under a Medicare home health plan of care, who resides in more than one place of residence during an episode of Medicare covered home health services will not disqualify the patient's homebound status for purposes of eligibility. For example, a person may reside in a principal home and also a second vacation home, mobile home, or the home of a caretaker relative. The fact that the patient must transit from one residence to the other is not in itself an indication that the patient is not homebound. The requirements of homebound must be met at each location (e.g., considerable taxing effort etc).

A – Assisted Living Facilities, Group Homes, and Personal Care Homes
An individual may be "confined to the home" for purposes of Medicare coverage of home health services if he or she resides in an institution that is not primarily engaged in providing to inpatients:

- Diagnostic and therapeutic services for medical diagnosis;
- Treatment;
- Care of injured, disabled or sick persons;
- Rehabilitation services or other skilled services needed to maintain a patient's current condition or to prevent or slow further deterioration; or
- Skilled nursing care or related services for patients who require medical or nursing care

If it is determined that the assisted living facility (also called personal care homes, group homes, etc.) in which the individuals reside are not primarily engaged in providing the above services, then Medicare will cover reasonable and necessary home health care furnished to these individuals.

If it is determined that the services furnished by the home health agency are duplicative of services furnished by an assisted living facility (also called personal care homes, group homes, etc.) when provision of such care is required of the facility under State licensure requirements, claims for such services should be denied under §1862(a)(1)(A) of the Act. Section 1862(a)(1)(A) excludes services that are not necessary for the diagnosis or treatment of illness or injury or to improve the functioning of a malformed body member from Medicare coverage. Services to people who already have access to appropriate care from a willing caregiver would not be considered reasonable and necessary to the treatment of the individual's illness or injury.

Medicare coverage would not be an optional substitute for the services that a facility that is required to provide by law to its patients or where the services are included in the base contract of the facility. An individual's choice to reside in such a facility is also a choice to accept the services it holds itself out as offering to its patients.

B – Day Care Centers and Patient's Place of Residence
The current statutory definition of homebound or confined does not imply that Medicare coverage has been expanded to include adult day care services.

The law does not permit an HHA to furnish a Medicare covered billable visit to a patient under a home health plan of care outside his or her home, except in those limited circumstances where the patient needs to use medical equipment that is too cumbersome to bring to the home. Section 1861(m) of the Act stipulates that home health services provided to a patient be provided to the patient on a visiting basis in a place of residence used as the individual's home. A licensed/certified day care center does not meet the definition of a place of residence.

C – State Licensure/Certification of Day Care Facilities
Per section 1861(m) of the Act, an adult day care center must be either licensed or certified by the State or accredited by a private accrediting body. State licensure or certification as an adult day care facility must be based on State interpretations of its process. For example, several States do not license adult day care facilities as a whole, but do certify some entities as Medicaid certified centers for purposes of providing adult day care under the Medicaid home and community based waiver program. It is the responsibility of the State to determine the necessary criteria for "State certification" in such a situation. A State could determine that Medicaid certification is an acceptable standard and consider its Medicaid certified adult day care facilities to be "State certified." On the other hand, a State could determine Medicaid certification to be insufficient and require other conditions to be met before the adult day care facility is considered "State certified."

D – Determination of the Therapeutic, Medical or Psychosocial Treatment of the Patient at the Day Care Facility
It is not the obligation of the HHA to determine whether the adult day care facility is providing psychosocial treatment, but only to assure that the adult day care center is licensed/certified by the State or accrediting body. The intent of the law, in extending the homebound exception status to attendance at such adult day care facilities, recognizes that they ordinarily furnish psychosocial services.

Services Are Provided Under a Plan of Care Established and Approved by a Physician

The HHA must be acting upon a physician plan of care that meets the requirements of this section for HHA services to be covered. The plan of care must contain all pertinent diagnoses, including the patient's mental status, the types of services, supplies, and equipment required, the frequency of visits to be made, prognosis, rehabilitation potential, functional limitations, activities permitted, nutritional requirements, all medications and treatments, safety measures to protect against injury, instructions for timely discharge or referral, and any additional items the HHA or physician choose to include.

If the plan of care includes a course of treatment for therapy services: the course of therapy treatment must be established by the physician after any needed consultation with the qualified therapist; the plan must include measurable therapy treatment goals which pertain directly to the patient's illness or injury, and the patient's resultant impairments; the plan must include the expected duration of therapy services; and the plan must describe a course of treatment which is consistent with the qualified therapist's assessment of the patient's function.

The orders on the plan of care must specify the type of services to be provided to the patient, both with respect to the professional who will provide them and the nature of the individual services, as well as the frequency of the services.

Example 1: SN x 7/wk x 1 wk; 3/wk x 4 wk; 2/wk x 3 wk, (skilled nursing visits seven times per week for one week; three times per week for four weeks; and two times per week for three weeks) for skilled observation and evaluation of the surgical site, for teaching sterile dressing changes and to perform sterile dressing changes. The sterile change consists of (detail of procedure).

Orders for care may indicate a specific range in the frequency of visits to ensure that the most appropriate level of service is provided during the 60-day episode to home health patients. When a range of visits is ordered, the upper limit of the range is considered the specific frequency.

Example 2: SN x 2-4/wk x 4 wk; 1-2/wk x 4 wk for skilled observation and evaluation of the surgical site.

Orders for services to be furnished "as needed" or "PRN" must be accompanied by a description of the patient's medical signs and symptoms that would occasion a visit and a specific limit on the number of those visits to be made under the order before an additional physician order would have to be obtained.

The physician who signs the plan of care must be qualified to sign the physician certification as described in 42 CFR 424.22.

A – Initial Percentage Payment
If a physician signed plan of care is not available at the beginning of the episode, the HHA may submit a RAP for the initial percentage payment based on physician verbal orders OR a referral prescribing detailed orders for the services to be rendered that is signed and dated by the physician. If the RAP submission is based on physician verbal orders, the verbal order must be recorded in the plan of care, include a description of the patient's condition and the services to be provided by the home health agency, include an attestation (relating to the physician's orders and the date received per 42 CFR 409.43), and the plan of care is copied and immediately submitted to the physician. A billable visit must be rendered prior to the submission of a RAP.

B – Final Percentage Payment
The plan of care must be signed and dated by a physician as described who meets the certification and recertification requirements of 42 CFR 424.22 and before the claim for each episode for services is submitted for the final percentage payment. Any changes in the plan of care must be signed and dated by a physician.

Verbal Orders

When services are furnished based on a physician's oral order, the orders may be accepted and put in writing by personnel authorized to do so by applicable State and Federal laws and regulations, as well as by the HHA's internal policies. The orders must be signed and dated with the date of receipt by the registered nurse or qualified therapist (i.e., physical therapist, speech-language pathologist, occupational therapist, or medical social worker) responsible for furnishing or supervising the ordered services. The orders may be signed by the supervising registered nurse or qualified therapist after the services have been rendered, as long as HHA personnel who receive the oral orders notify that nurse or therapist before the service is rendered. Thus, the rendering of a service that is based on an oral order would not be delayed pending signature of the supervising nurse or therapist. Oral orders must be countersigned and dated by the physician before the HHA bills for the care in the same way as the plan of care.

Services that are provided from the beginning of the 60-day episode certification period based on a request for anticipated payment and before the physician signs the plan of care are considered to be provided under a plan of care established and approved by the physician where there is an oral order for the care prior to rendering the services which is documented in the medical record and where the services are included in a signed plan of care.

Services that are provided in the subsequent 60-day episode certification period are considered to be provided under the subsequent plan of care where there is an oral order before the services provided in the subsequent period are furnished and the order is reflected in the medical record. However, services that are provided after the expiration of a plan of care, but before the acquisition of an oral order or a signed plan of care, cannot be considered to be provided under a plan of care.

Example 1: The patient is under a plan of care in which the physician orders I.V. medication administration every two weeks. The last day covered by the initial plan of care is July 31. The patient's next I.V. medication administration is scheduled for August 5, and the physician signs the plan of care for the new period on August 1. The I.V. medication administration on August 5 is provided under a plan of care established and approved by the physician. The episode begins on the 61st day regardless of the date of the first covered visit.

Example 2: The HHA acquires an oral order for I.V. medication administration for a patient to be performed on August 1. The HHA provides the I.V. medication administration August 1 and evaluates the patient's need for continued care. The physician signs the plan of care for the I.V. medication administration on August 15. The visit is covered since it is considered provided under a plan of care established and approved by the physician, and the HHA had acquired an oral order prior to the delivery of services.

Example 3: The patient is under a plan of care in which the physician orders I.V. medication administration every two weeks. The last day covered by the plan of care is July 31. The patient's next I.V. medication administration is scheduled for August 5, and the physician does not sign the plan of care until August 6. The HHA acquires an oral order for the I.V. medication administration before the August 5 visit, and therefore the visit is considered to be provided under a plan of care established and approved by the physician. The episode begins on the 61st day regardless of the date of the first covered visit.

Any increase in the frequency of services or addition of new services during a certification period must be authorized by a physician by way of a written or oral order prior to the provision of the increased or additional services.

The plan of care must be reviewed and signed by the physician who established the plan of care, in consultation with HHA professional personnel, at least every 60 days. Each review of a patient's plan of care must contain the signature of the physician and the date of review.

The plan of care or oral order may be transmitted by facsimile machine. The HHA is not required to have the original signature on file. However, the HHA is responsible for obtaining original signatures if an issue surfaces that would require verification of an original signature.

HHAs that maintain patient records by computer rather than hard copy may use electronic signatures. However, all such entries must be appropriately authenticated and dated. Authentication must include signatures, written initials, or computer secure entry by a unique identifier of a primary author who has reviewed and approved the entry. The HHA must have safeguards to prevent unauthorized access to the records and a process for reconstruction of the records in the event of a system breakdown.

The plan of care is considered to be terminated if the patient does not receive at least one covered skilled nursing, physical therapy, speech-language pathology service, or occupational therapy visit in a 60-day period since these are qualifying services for the home health benefit. An exception is if the physician documents that the interval without such care is appropriate to the treatment of the patient's illness or injury.

Once patient eligibility has been confirmed and the plan of care contains physician orders for the qualifying service as well as other Medicare covered home health services, the qualifying service does not have to be rendered prior to the other Medicare covered home health services ordered in the plan of care. The sequence of visits performed by the disciplines must be dictated by the individual patient's plan of care. For example, for an eligible patient in an initial 60-day episode that has both physical therapy and occupational therapy orders in the plan of care, the sequence of the delivery of the type of therapy is irrelevant as long as the need for the qualifying service is established prior to the delivery of other Medicare covered services and the qualifying discipline provides a billable visit prior to transfer or discharge in accordance with 42 CFR 409.43(f).

Dependent services provided after the final qualifying skilled service are not covered under the home health benefit, except when the dependent service was not followed by a qualifying skilled service due to unexpected inpatient admission or death of the patient or due to some other unanticipated event.

Under the Care of a Physician
The patient must be under the care of a physician who is qualified to sign the physician certification and plan of care in accordance with 42 CFR 424.22.

A patient is expected to be under the care of the physician who signs the plan of care. It is expected, but not required for coverage, that in most instances, the physician who certifies the patient's eligibility for Medicare home health services, in accordance with §30.5 below, will be the same physician who establishes and signs the plan of care.

Needs Skilled Nursing Care on an Intermittent Basis (Other than Solely Venipuncture for the Purposes of Obtaining a Blood Sample) or Physical Therapy or Speech-Language Pathology Services or Has Continued Need for Occupational Therapy
The patient must need one of the following types of skilled services:

1. Skilled nursing care that is
   - Reasonable and necessary as defined in §40.1;
   - Needed on an "intermittent" based as defined in §40.1.3; and
   - Not solely needed for venipuncture for the purposes of obtaining blood sample as defined in §40.1.2.13; or
2. Physical therapy as defined in §40.2.2; or
3. Speech-language pathology services as defined in §40.2.3; or
4. Have a continuing need for occupational therapy as defined in §§40.2.4.

The patient has a continued need for occupational therapy when:

1. The services which the patient requires meet the definition of "occupational therapy" services of §40.2.4, and
2. The patient's eligibility for home health services has been established by virtue of a prior need for skilled nursing care (other than solely venipuncture for the purposes of obtaining a blood sample), speech-language pathology services, or physical therapy in the current or prior certification period.
   Example: A patient who is recovering from a cerebrovascular accident (CVA) has an initial plan of care that called for physical therapy, speech-language pathology services, occupational therapy, and home health aide services. In

the next certification period, the physician orders only occupational therapy and home health aide services because the patient no longer needs the skills of a physical therapist or a speech-language pathologist, but needs the services provided by the occupational therapist. The patient's need for occupational therapy qualifies him for home health services, including home health aide services (presuming that all other qualifying criteria are met), because in the prior certification period the beneficiary's eligibility for home health services was established by virtue of prior needs for physical therapy and speech-language pathology, and occupational therapy was initiated while the patient still required physical therapy and/or speech language-pathology.

Physician Certification
The HHA must be acting upon a plan of care as described in §30.2, and a physician certification or recertification that meets the requirements of this section for HHA services to be covered.

A certification (versus recertification) is considered to be any time that a Start of Care OASIS is completed to initiate care. In such instances, a physician must certify (attest) that:

1. The home health services are or were needed because the patient is or was confined to the home as defined in §30.1.1;
2. The patient needs or needed skilled nursing services on an intermittent basis (other than solely venipuncture for the purposes of obtaining a blood sample), or physical therapy, or speech-language pathology services. Where a patient's sole skilled service need is for skilled oversight of unskilled services (management and evaluation of the care plan as defined in §40.1.2.2), the physician must include a brief narrative describing the clinical justification of this need as part of the certification, or as a signed addendum to the certification;
3. A plan of care has been established and is periodically reviewed by a physician;
4. The services are or were furnished while the patient is or was under the care of a physician;
5. For episodes with starts of care beginning January 1, 2011 and later, in accordance with §30.5.1.1 below, a face-to-face encounter occurred no more than 90 days prior to or within 30 days after the start of the home health care, was related to the primary reason the patient requires home health services, and was performed by an allowed provider type. The certifying physician must also document the date of the encounter.

Example Certification Statement:

> I certify that this patient is confined to his/her home and needs intermittent skilled nursing care, physical therapy and/or speech therapy or continues to need occupational therapy. The patient is under my care, and I have authorized services on this plan of care and will periodically review the plan. The patient had a face-to-face encounter with an allowed provider type on 11/01/2016 and the encounter was related to the primary reason for home health care.
>
> Physician's Signature and Date Signed: John Doe, MD 11/05/2016
>
> Physician's Name and Address
>
> John Doe, MD
> 2121 Washington Pkwy
> Suite 220
> Washington, DC 20000
>
> *Note: This represents one example of a valid certification statement. Certification statements can be included in varying forms or formats as long as the content requirements (#1-5 above) for the certification are met.*

If the patient is starting home health directly after discharge from an acute/post-acute care setting where the physician, with privileges, that cared for the patient in that setting is certifying the patient's eligibility for the home health benefit, but will not be following the patient after discharge, then the certifying physician must identify the community physician who will be following the patient after discharge. One of the criteria that must be met for a patient to be considered eligible for the home health benefit is that the patient must be under the care of a physician (number 4 listed above). Otherwise, the certification is not valid.

The certification must be complete prior to when an HHA bills Medicare for reimbursement; however, physicians should complete the certification when the plan of care is established, or as soon as possible thereafter. This is longstanding CMS policy as referenced in Pub 100-01, Medicare General Information, Eligibility, and Entitlement Manual, chapter 4, section 30.1. It is not acceptable for HHAs to wait until the end of a 60-day episode of care to obtain a completed certification/recertification.

Face-to-Face Encounter

Allowed provider types:

1. As part of the certification of patient eligibility for the Medicare home health benefit, a face-to-face encounter with the patient must be performed by the certifying physician himself or herself, a physician that cared for the patient in the acute or post-acute care facility (with privileges who cared for the patient in an acute or post-acute care facility from which the patient was directly admitted to home health) or an allowed non-physician practitioner (NPP). NPPs who are allowed to perform the encounter are:

   – A nurse practitioner or a clinical nurse specialist working in accordance with State law and in collaboration with the certifying physician or in collaboration with an acute or post-acute care physician, with privileges, who cared for the patient in the acute or post-acute care facility from which the patient was directly admitted to home health;

   – A certified nurse midwife, as authorized by State law, under the supervision of the certifying physician or under the supervision of an acute or post-acute care physician with privileges who cared for the patient in the acute or post-acute care facility from which the patient was directly admitted to home health;

   – A physician assistant under the supervision of the certifying physician or under the supervision of an acute or post-acute care physician with privileges who cared for the patient in the acute or post-acute care facility from which the patient was directly admitted to home health.

2. Timeframe Requirements:

   The encounter must occur no more than 90 days prior to the home health start of care date or within 30 days after the start of care. In situations when a physician orders home health care for the patient based on a new condition that was not evident during a visit within the 90 days prior to start of care, the certifying physician or an allowed NPP must see the patient again within 30 days after admission. Specifically, if a patient saw the certifying physician or NPP within the 90 days prior to start of care, another encounter would be needed if the patient's condition had changed to the extent that standards of practice would indicate that the physician or a non-physician practitioner should examine the patient in order to establish an effective treatment plan.

3. Exceptional Circumstances:

   When a home health patient dies shortly after admission, before the face-to-face encounter occurs, if the contractor determines a good faith effort existed on the part of the HHA to facilitate/coordinate the encounter and if all other certification requirements are met, the certification is deemed to be complete.

4. Telehealth

   The face-to-face encounter can be performed via a telehealth service, in an approved originating site. An originating site is considered to be the location of an eligible Medicare beneficiary at the time the service being furnished via a telecommunications system occurs. Medicare beneficiaries are eligible for telehealth services only if they are presented from an originating site located in a rural health professional shortage area or in a county outside of a Metropolitan Statistical Area.

   Entities that participate in a Federal telemedicine demonstration project approved by (or receiving funding from) the Secretary of the Department of Health and Human Services as of December 31, 2000, qualify as originating sites regardless of geographic location.

   The originating sites authorized by law are: the office of a physician or practitioner; hospitals; Critical Access Hospitals (CAH); Rural Health Clinics (RHC); Federally Qualified Health Centers (FQHC); Hospital-based or CAH-based Renal Dialysis Centers (including satellites); Skilled Nursing Facilities (SNF); and Community Mental Health Centers (CMHC).

Supporting Documentation Requirements

As of January 1, 2015, documentation in the certifying physician's medical records and/or the acute/post-acute care facility's medical records (if the patient was directly admitted to home health) will be used as the basis upon which patient eligibility for the Medicare home health benefit will be determined. Documentation from the certifying physician's medical records and/or the acute/post-acute care facility's medical records used to support the certification of home health eligibility must be provided, upon request, to the home health agency, review entities, and/or the Centers for Medicare and Medicaid Services (CMS). In turn, an HHA must be able to provide, upon request, the supporting documentation that substantiates the eligibility for the Medicare home health benefit to review entities and/or CMS. If the documentation used as the basis for the certification of eligibility is not sufficient to demonstrate that the patient is or was eligible to receive services under the Medicare home health benefit, payment will not be rendered for home health services provided.

The certifying physician and/or the acute/post-acute care facility medical record for the patient must contain information that justifies the referral for Medicare home health services. This includes documentation that substantiates the patient's:

- Need for the skilled services; and

- Homebound status;

The certifying physician and/or the acute/post-acute care facility medical record (if the patient was directly admitted to home health) for the patient must contain the actual clinical note for the face-to-face encounter visit that demonstrates that the encounter:

- Occurred within the required timeframe;

- Was related to the primary reason the patient requires home health services; and

- Was performed by an allowed provider type.

This information can be found most often in clinical and progress notes and discharge summaries. While the face-to-face encounter must be related to the primary reason for home health services, the patient's skilled need and homebound status can be substantiated through an examination of all submitted medical record documentation from the certifying physician, acute/post-acute care facility, and/or HHA (see below). The synthesis of progress notes, diagnostic findings, medications, nursing notes, etc., help to create a longitudinal clinical picture of the patient's health status.

- Information from the HHA, such as the plan of care required per 42 CFR §409.43 and the initial and/or comprehensive assessment of the patient, can be incorporated into the certifying physician's medical record for the patient and used to support the patient's homebound status and need for skilled care. However, this information must be corroborated by other medical record entries in the certifying physician's and/or the acute/post-acute care facility's medical record for the patient. This means that the appropriately incorporated HHA information, along with the certifying physician's and/or the acute/post-acute care facility's medical record, creates a clinically consistent picture that the patient is eligible for Medicare home health services.

- The certifying physician demonstrates the incorporation of the HHA information into his/her medical record for the patient by signing and dating the material. Once incorporated, the documentation from the HHA, in conjunction with the certifying physician and/or acute/post-acute care facility documentation must substantiate the patient's eligibility for home health services.

At the end of the 60-day episode, a decision must be made whether or not to recertify the patient for a subsequent 60-day episode. An eligible beneficiary who qualifies for a subsequent 60-day episode would start the subsequent 60-day episode on day 61. Under HH PPS, the plan of care must be reviewed and signed by the physician every 60 days unless one of the following occurs:

- A beneficiary transfers to another HHA;

- A discharge and return to the same HHA during the 60-day episode.

The physician must include an estimate of how much longer the skilled services will be required and must certify that:

- The home health services are or were needed because the patient is or was confined to the home;

- The patient needs or needed skilled nursing services on an intermittent basis (other than solely venipuncture for the purposes of obtaining a blood sample), or physical therapy, or speech-language pathology services; or continues to need occupational therapy after the need for skilled nursing care, physical therapy, or speech-language pathology services ceased. Where a patient's sole skilled service need is for skilled oversight of unskilled services the physician must include a brief narrative describing the clinical justification of this need as part of the recertification, or as a signed addendum to the recertification;

- A plan of care has been established and is periodically reviewed by a physician; and

- The services are or were furnished while the patient is or was under the care of a physician.

Medicare does not limit the number of continuous episode recertifications for beneficiaries who continue to be eligible for the home health benefit. The physician certification may cover a period less than but not greater than 60 days.

See §10.4 for counting initial and subsequent 60-day episodes and recertifications. See §10.5 for recertifications for split percentage payments.

The physician who signs the certification or recertification must be permitted to do so by 42 CFR 424.22.

Appendix F: Qualifications for Medicare Coverage of Home Health Services (vertical sidebar)

Physician Billing for Certification and Recertification

Physician certification/recertification claims are Part B physician claims paid for under the Physician Fee Schedule. These claims are billed using HCPCS codes G0180 (certification) or G0179 (recertification). The descriptions of these two codes indicate that they are used to bill for certification or recertification of patient eligibility "for Medicare-covered home health services under a home health plan of care (patient not present), including contacts with the HHA and review of reports of patient status required by physicians to affirm the initial implementation of the plan of care that meets patient's needs, per certification period." As noted above, these codes are for physician certification or recertification for Medicare-covered home health services. If there are no Medicare-covered home health services, these codes should not be billed or paid. As such, physician claims for certification/recertification of eligibility for home health services will not be covered if the HHA claim itself was noncovered because the certification/recertification of eligibility was not complete or because there was insufficient documentation to support that the patient was eligible for the Medicare home health benefit.

Covered Services Under a Qualifying Home Health Plan of Care

Section 1861(m)of the Act governs the Medicare home health services that may be provided to eligible beneficiaries by or under arrangements made by a participating home health agency (HHA). Section 1861(m) describes home health services as

- Part-time or intermittent skilled nursing care (other than solely venipuncture for the purposes of obtaining a blood sample);
- Part-time or intermittent home health aide services;
- Physical therapy;
- Speech-language pathology;
- Occupational therapy;
- Medical social services;
- Medical supplies (including catheters, catheter supplies, ostomy bags, supplies related to ostomy care, and a covered osteoporosis drug (as defined in §1861(kk) of the Act), but excluding other drugs and biologicals);

- Durable medical equipment while under the plan of care established by physician;
- Medical services provided by an intern or resident-in-training under an approved teaching program of the hospital in the case of an HHA which is affiliated or under common control with a hospital; and
- Services at hospitals, skilled nursing facilities, or rehabilitation centers when they involve equipment too cumbersome to bring to the home.

Quality Reporting

Medicare home health regulations require HHAs to submit OASIS assessments and Home Health Care Consumer Assessment of Healthcare Providers and Systems (HHCAHPS) Survey data to meet quality reporting requirements. CMS provides quality measure data to HHAs via the Certification and Survey Provider Enhanced Reports (CASPER) which are available on the CMS Health Care Quality Improvement System (QIES).

CY 2012 and CY 2013 HH PPS used measures derived from Medicare claims data to measure HH quality. In the CY 2014 HH PPS final rule, CMS added two claims-based measures to the HH QRP. These claims-based measures are: (1) Rehospitalization during the first 30 days of HH; and (2) Emergency Department Use without Hospital Readmission during the first 30 days of HH. While regulations state that for 2007 and each subsequent year, in the case of a home health agency that does not submit data to the Secretary in accordance with subclause (II) with respect to such a year, the home health market basket percentage increase applicable under such clause for such year shall be reduced by 2 percentage points. This "pay-for-reporting" requirement was implemented on January 1, 2007. But the quantity of OASIS assessments each HHA must submit to meet this requirement has never been proposed and finalized through rulemaking or through the subregulatory process.

The CY 2016 final rule established a minimum threshold for submission of OASIS assessments for purposes of quality reporting compliance, a policy for the adoption of changes to measures that occur in-between rulemaking cycles as a result of the NQF process, and submission dates for the HHCAHPS Survey moving forward through CY 2018.

Appendix G: Overview of the Home Health Prospective Payment System

Section 4603 of the Balanced Budget Act of 1997, as amended by section 5101 of the Omnibus Consolidated and Emergency Supplemental Appropriations Act for Fiscal Year 1999 required the implementation of a prospective payment system for home health agencies, consolidated billing requirements, and a number of other related changes. The prospective payment system replaced the retrospective reasonable-cost-based system used by Medicare for the payment of home health services under Part A and Part B.

I. Home Health Prospective Payment System (HH PPS)

The unit of payment under home health PPS is a national 60-day episode rate with applicable adjustments. The episodes, rate, and adjustments to the rates are detailed in the following sections.

10.1 – National 60-Day Episode Rate

A – Services Included: The law requires the 60-day episode to include all covered home health services, including medical supplies, paid on a reasonable cost basis. That means the 60-day episode rate includes costs for the six home health disciplines and the costs for routine and nonroutine medical supplies. The six home health disciplines included in the 60-day episode rate are:

1. Skilled nursing services
2. Home health aide services;
3. Physical therapy;
4. Speech-language pathology services;
5. Occupational therapy services; and
6. Medical social services.

The 60-day episode rate also includes amounts for:

1. Nonroutine medical supplies and therapies that could have been unbundled to part B prior to HH PPS. See §10.12.C for those services;

B – Excluded Services: The law specifically excludes durable medical equipment (DME) from the 60-day episode rate and consolidated billing requirements. DME continues to be paid on the fee schedule outside of the HH PPS rate.

The osteoporosis drug (injectable calcitonin), which is covered where a woman is postmenopausal and has a bone fracture. This drug is also excluded from the 60-day episode rate but must be billed by the home health agency (HHA) while a patient is under a home health plan of care since the law requires consolidated billing of osteoporosis drugs. The osteoporosis drug continues to be paid on a reasonable cost basis.

10.2 – Adjustments to the 60-Day Episode Rates

A – Case-Mix Adjustment: A case-mix methodology adjusts payment rates based on characteristics of the patient and his/her corresponding resource needs (e.g., diagnosis, clinical factors, functional factors, service needs). The 60-day episode rates are adjusted by case-mix methodology based on data elements from the Outcome and Assessment Information Set (OASIS). The data elements of the case-mix adjustment methodology are organized into three dimensions to capture clinical severity factors, functional severity factors, and service utilization factors influencing case mix. In the clinical, functional, and service utilization dimensions, each data element is assigned a score value. The scores are summed to determine the patient's case-mix group.

B - Labor Adjustments: The labor portion of the 60-day episode rates is adjusted to reflect the wage index based on the site of service of the beneficiary. The beneficiary's location is the determining factor for the labor adjustment. The HH PPS rates are adjusted by the pre-floor and pre-reclassified hospital wage index. The hospital wage index is adjusted to account for the geographic reclassification of hospitals in accordance with §§1886(d)(8)(B) and 1886(d)(10) of the Social Security Act (the Act.) According to the law, geographic reclassification only applies to hospitals. Additionally, the hospital wage index has specific floors that are required by law. Because these reclassifications and floors do not apply to HHAs, the home health rates are adjusted by the pre-floor and pre-reclassified hospital wage index. NOTE: The pre-floor and pre-reclassified hospital wage index varies slightly from the numbers published in the Medicare inpatient hospital PPS regulation that reflects the floor and reclassification adjustments. The wage indices published in the home health final rule and subsequent annual updates reflect the most recent available pre-floor and pre-reclassified hospital wage index available at the time of publication.

Calendar Year (CY) 2017 Wage Index Changes

On February 28, 2013, OMB issued Bulletin No. 13-01, announcing revisions to the delineations of MSAs, Micropolitan Statistical Areas, and CBSAs, and guidance on uses of the delineation of these areas. This bulletin is available online at http://www.whitehouse.gov/sites/default/files/omb/bulletins/2013/b-13-01.pdf. This bulletin states that it "provides the delineations of all Metropolitan Statistical Areas, Metropolitan Divisions, Micropolitan Statistical Areas, Combined Statistical Areas, and New England City and Town Areas in the United States and Puerto Rico based on the standards published on June 28, 2010, in the Federal Register (75 FR 37246-37252) and Census Bureau data."

In the CY 2015 HH PPS final rule (79 FR 66085 through 66087), we finalized changes to the HH PPS wage index based on the OMB delineations, as described in OMB Bulletin No. 13-01. In CY 2015, we included a one-year transition to those delineations by using a blended wage index for CY 2015. The CY 2016 HH PPS wage index was fully based on the revised OMB delineations adopted in CY 2015.

The OMB's most recent update to the geographic area delineations was published on July 15, 2015 in OBM bulletin 15-01. This bulletin is available online at https://www.whitehouse.gov/sites/default/files/omb/bulletins/2015/15-01.pdf. The revisions to the delineations that affect the HH PPS are changes to CBSA titles and the addition of CBSA 21420, Enid, Oklahoma. CBSA 21420 encompasses Garfield County, Oklahoma.

The CY 2017 wage index is available on the CMS Web site at http://www.cms.gov/Medicare/Medicare-Fee-for-Service-Payment/HomeHealth PPS/Home-Health-Prospective-Payment-System-Regulations-and-Notices.html.

10.3 – Continuous 60-Day Episode Recertification

Home Health PPS permits continuous episode recertifications for patients who continue to be eligible for the home health benefit. Medicare does not limit the number of continuous episode recertifications for beneficiaries who continue to be eligible for the home health benefit.

10.4 – Counting 60-Day Episodes

A – Initial Episodes: The "From" date for the initial certification must match the start of care (SOC) date, which is the first billable visit date for the 60-day episode. The "To" date is up to and including the last day of the episode which is not the first day of the subsequent episode. The "To" date can be up to, but never exceed a total of 60 days that includes the SOC date plus 59 days.

B – Subsequent Episodes: If a patient continues to be eligible for the home health benefit, the HH PPS permits continuous episode recertifications. At the end of the 60-day episode, a decision must be made whether or not to recertify the patient for a subsequent 60-day episode. An eligible beneficiary who qualifies for a subsequent 60-day episode would start the subsequent 60-day episode on day 61. The "From" date for the first subsequent episode is day 61 up to including day 120. The "To" date for the subsequent episode in this example can be up to, but never exceed a total of 60 days that includes day 61 plus 59 days. Note that the certification or recertification visit can be done during a prior episode. The Medicare Conditions of Participation require that the recertification assessment be done during the last 5 days of the previous episode (days 56-60).

10.5 – Split Percentage Payment Approach to the 60-Day Episode

In order to ensure adequate cash flow to HHAs, the HH PPS has set forth a split percentage payment approach to the 60-day episode. The split percentage occurs through the request for anticipated payment (RAP) at the start of the episode and the final claim at the end of the episode. For initial episodes, there will be a 60/40 split percentage payment. An initial percentage payment of 60 percent of the episode will be paid at the beginning of the episode and a final percentage payment of 40 percent will be paid at the end of the episode, unless there is an applicable adjustment. For all subsequent episodes for beneficiaries who receive continuous home health care, the episodes will be paid at a 50/50-percentage payment split.

Appendix G: Overview of the Home Health Prospective Payment System

10.6 – Physician Signature Requirements for the Split Percentage Payments

A – Initial Percentage Payment: If a physician-signed plan of care is not available at the beginning of the episode, the HHA may submit a RAP for the initial percentage payment based on physician verbal orders or a referral prescribing detailed orders for the services to be rendered that is signed and dated by the physician. If the RAP submission is based on a physician's verbal orders, the verbal order must be recorded in the plan of care, include a description of the patient's condition and the services to be provided by the home health agency, and include an attestation (relating to the physician's orders and the date received per Code of Federal Regulation (CFR) 42 CFR 409.43). The plan of care is copied and immediately submitted to the physician. A billable visit must be rendered prior to the submission of a RAP.

The CMS has the authority to reduce or disapprove requests for anticipated payments in situations when protecting Medicare program integrity warrants this action. Since the request for anticipated payment is based on verbal orders and is not a Medicare claim for purposes of the Act (although it is a claim for purposes of Federal, civil, criminal, and administrative law enforcement authorities, including but not limited to the Civil Monetary Penalties Law, Civil False Claims Act, and the Criminal False Claims Act), the request for anticipated payment will be canceled and recovered unless the claim is submitted within the greater of 60 days from the end of the episode or 60 days from the issuance of the request for anticipated payment.

B – Final Percentage Payment: The plan of care must be signed and dated by a physician who meets the certification and recertification requirements of 42 CFR 424.22 before the claim for each episode for services is submitted for the final percentage payment. Any changes in the plan of care must be signed and dated by a physician.

10.7 – Low Utilization Payment Adjustment (LUPA)

An episode with four or fewer visits is paid the national per visit amount by discipline adjusted by the appropriate wage index based on the site of service of the beneficiary. Such episodes of four or fewer visits are paid the wage-adjusted per visit amount for each of the visits rendered instead of the full episode amount. The national per visit amounts by discipline (skilled nursing, home health aide, physical therapy, speech-language pathology, occupational therapy, and medical social services) are updated annually by the applicable market basket for each visit type and published annually. LUPA payment rates are not case mix adjusted.

An additional low-utilization payment adjustment will be made for LUPA episodes which are either the only episode or the initial episode in a sequence of adjacent episodes. A sequence of adjacent episodes is defined as a series of claims with no more than 60 days between the end of one episode and the beginning of the next episode (except for episodes that have been PEP-adjusted). And note the additional payment for such LUPA episodes will be updated annually by the home health market basket percentage increase. As with the other components of the LUPA methodology, this increase for situations where a LUPA is the only episode or the initial episode in a sequence of adjacent episodes will be wage-adjusted.

10.8 – Partial Episode Payment (PEP) Adjustment

A – PEP Adjustment Criteria: The PEP adjustment accounts for key intervening events in a patient's care defined as:

- A beneficiary-elected transfer; or
- A discharge and return to the same HHA during the 60-day episode.

The intervening event defined as the beneficiary-elected transfer or discharge and return to the same HHA during the 60-day episode warrants a new 60-day episode for purposes of payment. A start of care OASIS assessment and physician certification of the new plan of care are required. When a new 60-day episode begins due to the intervening event of the beneficiary-elected transfer or discharge and return to the same HHA during the 60-day episode, the original 60-day episode is proportionally adjusted to reflect the length of time the beneficiary remained under the agency's care prior to the intervening event. Home health agencies have the option to discharge the patient within the scope of their own operating policies. An HHA discharging a patient as a result of hospital (skilled nursing facility (SNF) or rehab facility) admission with the patient returning to home health services at the same HHA during the 60-day episode will not be recognized by Medicare as a discharge for billing and payment purposes, and thus a Partial Episode Payment (PEP) adjustment would not apply. An intervening hospital (SNF or rehab facility) stay will result in a full 60-day episode spanning the start of care date prior to the hospital admission, through and including the days of the hospital admission, and ending 59 days after the original start of care date.

B – Methodology Used to Calculate PEP Adjustment: The PEP adjustment for the original 60-day episode is calculated to reflect the length of time the beneficiary remained under the care of the original HHA based on the first billable visit date through and including the last billable visit date. The PEP adjustment is calculated by determining the actual days served by the original HHA (first billable visit date through and including last billable visit date as a proportion of 60 multiplied by the original 60-day episode payment).

The current PEP adjustment system of proportional payments based on billable visit dates continues to be the payment methodology for PEP episodes. CMS will continue to research the nature of HHA resource use during and following PEP episodes, as well as explore alternative methodologies for payment adjustment.

C – Application of Therapy Threshold to PEP Adjusted Episode: The therapy threshold item included in the case-mix methodology used in HH PPS is not combined or prorated across episodes. Each episode whether full or proportionately adjusted, is subject to the therapy threshold for purposes of case-mix adjusting the payment for that individual patient's resource needs.

D – Common Ownership Exception to PEP Adjustment: If an HHA has a significant ownership as defined in 42 CFR 424.22, then the PEP adjustment would not apply in those situations of beneficiary-elected transfer. Those situations would be considered services provided under arrangement on behalf of the originating HHA by the receiving HHA with the ownership interest until the end of the episode. The common ownership exception to the transfer PEP adjustment does not apply if the beneficiary moved out of their Metropolitan Statistical Area (MSA) or non-MSA during the 60-day episode before the transfer to the receiving HHA.

E – Beneficiary-Elected Transfer Verification: In order for a receiving HHA to accept a beneficiary-elected transfer, the receiving HHA must document that the beneficiary has been informed that the initial HHA will no longer receive Medicare payment on behalf of the patient and will no longer provide Medicare covered services to the patient after the date of the patient's elected transfer in accordance with current patient rights requirements at 42 CFR 484.10(e). The receiving HHA must also document in the record that it accessed the Medicare contractor's inquiry system to determine whether or not the patient was under an established home health plan of care and it must contact the initial HHA on the effective date of transfer. In the rare circumstance of a dispute between HHAs, the Medicare contractor is responsible for working with both HHAs to resolve the dispute. If the receiving HHA can provide documentation of its notice of patient rights on Medicare payment liability provided to the patient upon transfer and its contact of the initial HHA of the transfer date, then the initial HHA will be ineligible for payment for the period of overlap in addition to the appropriate PEP adjustment. If the receiving HHA cannot provide the appropriate documentation, the receiving HHA's RAP and/or final claim will be cancelled, and full episode payment will be provided to the initial HHA. For the receiving HHA to properly document that it contacted the initial HHA on the effective date of transfer it must maintain similar information as the initial HHA, including the same basic beneficiary information, personnel contacted, dates and times. The initial HHA must also properly document that it was contacted and it accepted the transfer. Where it disputes a transfer, the initial HHA must call its Medicare contractor to resolve the dispute. The Medicare contractor is responsible for working with both HHAs to resolve the dispute.

10.9 – Outlier Payments

When cases experience an unusually high level of services in a 60-day period, Medicare systems will provide additional or "outlier" payments to the case-mix and wage-adjusted episode payment. Outlier payments can result from medically necessary high utilization in any or all home health service disciplines. The CMS makes outlier payments when the cost of care exceeds a threshold dollar amount. The outlier threshold for each case-mix group is the episode payment amount for that group or the PEP adjustment amount for the episode, plus a fixed dollar loss amount, which is the same for all case-mix groups. The outlier payment is a proportion of the amount of imputed costs beyond the threshold. The CMS calculates the imputed cost for each episode by multiplying the national per visit amount of each discipline by the number of visits in the discipline and computing the total imputed cost for all disciplines. If the imputed cost for the episode is greater than the sum of the case-mix and wage-adjusted episode payment plus the fixed dollar loss amount (the outlier threshold), a set percentage (the loss sharing ratio) of the difference between the imputed amount and outlier threshold will be paid to the HHA as a wage-adjusted outlier payment in addition to the episode payment. The amount of the outlier payment is determined as follows:

1. Calculate the case-mix and wage-adjusted episode payment (including non-routine supplies (NRS));
2. Add the wage-adjusted fixed dollar loss amount. The sum of steps 1 and 2 is the outlier threshold for the episode;

3. Calculate the wage-adjusted imputed cost of the episode by first multiplying the total number of visits for each home health discipline by the national per visit amounts, and wage-adjusting those amounts. Sum the per discipline wage-adjusted imputed amounts to yield the total wage-adjusted imputed cost for the episode;

4. Subtract the total imputed costs for the episode (total from Step 3) from the sum of the case-mix and wage-adjusted episode payment and the wage-adjusted fixed dollar loss amount (sum of Steps 1 and 2 outlier threshold);

5. Multiply the difference by the loss sharing ratio; and

6. That total amount is the outlier payment for the episode.

For episodes ending on or after January 1, 2017, units considered for outlier payment are subject to a limit of 32 units (8 hours), summed across the six disciplines of care, per date of service.

Effective January 1, 2010, an outlier cap precludes any HHA from receiving more than 10 percent of their total home health payment in outliers.

10.10 – Discharge Issues

A – Hospice Election Mid-Episode: If a patient elects hospice before the end of the episode and there was no PEP or LUPA adjustment, the HHA will receive a full episode payment. HH PPS does not change the current rules that permit a hospice patient to receive home health services for a condition unrelated to the terminal illness and related conditions. Consistent with all episodes in which a patient receives four or fewer visits, the episode with four or fewer visits in which a patient elects hospice would be paid at the low utilization payment adjusted amount.

B – Patient's Death: The documented event of a patient's death would result in a full episode payment, unless the death occurred in a low utilization payment adjusted episode. Consistent with all episodes in which a patient receives four or fewer visits, if the patient's death occurred during an episode with four or fewer visits, the episode would be paid at the low utilization payment adjusted amount. In the event of a patient's death during an adjusted episode, the total adjusted episode would constitute the full episode payment.

C – Patient is No Longer Eligible for Home Health: (e.g., no longer homebound, no skilled need): If the patient is discharged because he or she is no longer eligible for the Medicare home health benefit and has received more than four visits, then the HHA would receive full episode payment. However, if the patient becomes subsequently eligible for the Medicare home health benefit during the same 60-day episode and later transferred to another HHA or returned to the same HHA, then this would result in a PEP adjustment.

D – Discharge Due to Patient Refusal of Services or is a Documented Safety Threat, Abuse Threat or is Noncompliant: If the patient is discharged because he or she refuses services or becomes a documented safety, abuse, or noncompliance discharge and has received more than four visits, then the HHA would receive full episode payment unless the patient becomes subsequently eligible for the Medicare home health benefit during the same 60-day episode and later transferred to another HHA or returned to the same HHA, then this would result in a PEP adjustment.

E – Patient Enrolls in Managed Care Eligible Mid-Episode: If a patient's enrollment in a Medicare Advantage (MA) plan becomes effective mid episode, the 60-day episode payment will be made proportionally adjusted with a PEP adjustment since the patient is receiving coverage under the MA. Beginning with the effective date of enrollment, the MA will receive a capitation payment for covered services.

F – Submission of Final Claims Prior to the End of the 60-day Episode: The claim may be submitted upon discharge before the end of the 60-day episode. However, subsequent adjustments to any payments based on the claim may be made due to an intervening event resulting in a PEP adjustment or other adjustment.

G – Patient Discharge and Financial Responsibility for Part B Bundled Medical Supplies and Services: As discussed in detail under §10.11, below, the law governing the Medicare HH PPS requires the HHA to provide all bundled home health services (except DME) either directly or under arrangement while a patient is under a home health plan of care during an open episode. The HHA is responsible for providing all covered home health services (except DME) either directly or under arrangement while a patient is under a home health plan of care during an open episode. Once the patient is discharged, the HHA is no longer responsible for providing home health services including the bundled Part B medical supplies and therapy services.

H – Discharge Issues Associated with Inpatient Admission Overlapping Into Subsequent Episodes: If a patient is admitted to an inpatient facility and

the inpatient stay overlaps into what would have been the subsequent episode and there is no recertification assessment of the patient, then the new certification begins with the new start of care date after inpatient discharge. If a patient is admitted to an inpatient facility and the inpatient stay overlaps into what would have been the subsequent episode and there was a recertification assessment of the patient during days 56-60 and the patient returns home from the inpatient stay on day 61, if the home health resource group (HHRG) remains the same then the second episode of care would be considered continuous and thus be considered a recertification. If the HHRG is different, this would result in a new start of care OASIS and thus be considered a new certification and begins with the new start of care date after inpatient discharge. If a patient is admitted to an inpatient facility and the inpatient stay overlaps into what would have been the subsequent episode and there was a recertification assessment of the patient during days 56-60 and the patient returns home from the inpatient stay after day 61 then a new certification begins with the new start of care date after inpatient discharge.

10.11 – Consolidated Billing

For individuals under a home health plan of care, payment for all services and supplies, with the exception of the osteoporosis drugs and DME, is included in the HH PPS base payment rates. HHAs must provide the covered home health services (except DME) either directly or under arrangement, and must bill for such covered home health services. Payment must be made to the HHA.

A - Home Health Services Subject to Consolidated Billing Requirements: The home health services included in the consolidated billing governing HH PPS are:

- Part-time or intermittent skilled nursing services;
- Part-time or intermittent home health aide services;
- Physical therapy;
- Speech-language pathology services;
- Occupational therapy;
- Medical social services;
- Routine and nonroutine medical supplies;
- Covered osteoporosis drug as defined in §1861(kk) of the Act, but excluding other drugs and biologicals;
- Medical services provided by an intern or resident-in-training of the program of the hospital in the case of an HHA that is affiliated or under common control with a hospital with an approved teaching program; and
- Home health services defined in §1861(m) provided under arrangement at hospitals, SNFs, or rehabilitation centers when they involve equipment too cumbersome to bring to the home or are furnished while the patient is at the facility to receive such services.

B - Medical Supplies: The law requires all medical supplies (routine and nonroutine) bundled to the agency while the patient is under a home health plan of care. The agency that establishes the episode is the only entity that can bill and receive payment for medical supplies during an episode for a patient under a home health plan of care. Both routine and nonroutine medical supplies are included in the base rates for every Medicare home health patient regardless of whether or not the patient requires medical supplies during the episode. Due to the consolidated billing requirements, CMS provided additional amounts in the base rates for those nonroutine medical supplies that have a duplicate Part B code that could have been unbundled to Part B prior to HH PPS. See §§50.4 for detailed discussion of medical supplies.

Medical supplies used by the patient, provider, or other practitioners under arrangement on behalf of the agency (other than physicians) are subject to consolidated billing and bundled to the HHA episodic payment rate. Once a patient is discharged from home health and not under a home health plan of care, the HHA is not responsible for medical supplies.

DME, including supplies covered as DME, are paid separately from the HH PPS rates and are excluded from the consolidated billing requirements governing the HH PPS. The determining factor is the medical classification of the supply, not the diagnosis of the patient. For example, infusion therapy will continue to be covered under the DME benefit separately paid from the PPS rate and excluded from the consolidated billing requirements governing the HH PPS. The DME supplies that are currently covered and paid in accordance with the DME fee schedule as category SU are billed under the DME benefit and not included in the bundled HHA episodic payment rate. The HHAs are not required to do consolidated billing of SU supplies.

The osteoporosis drug (injectable calcitonin) is included in consolidated billing under the home health benefit. However, payment is not bundled into the episodic payment rate. The HHAs must bill for osteoporosis drugs in accordance with billing instructions. Payment is in addition to the episodic payment rate.

C - Relationship between Consolidated Billing Requirements and Part B Supplies and Part B Therapies Included in the Baseline Rates That Could Have Been Unbundled Prior to HH PPS That No Longer Can Be Unbundled: The HHA is responsible for the services provided under arrangement on their behalf by other entities. Covered home health services at §1861(m) of the Act (except DME) are included in the baseline HH PPS rates and subject to the consolidated billing requirements while the patient is under a plan of care of the HHA. The time the services are bundled is while the patient is under a home health plan of care.

Physician services or nurse practitioner services paid under the physician fee schedule payments are not recognized as a home health services included in the PPS rate. Supplies incident to a physician service or related to a physician service billed to the Medicare contractor are not subject to the consolidated billing requirements. The physician would not be acting as a supplier billing the DME Medicare contractor in this situation.

Therapies (physical therapy, occupational therapy, and speech-language pathology services) are covered home health services that are included in the baseline rates and subject to the consolidated billing requirements. In addition to therapies that had been paid on a cost basis under home health, CMS has included in the rates additional amounts for Part B therapies that could have been unbundled prior to PPS. These therapies are subject to the consolidated billing requirements. There are revenue center codes that reflect the ranges of outpatient physical therapy, occupational therapy, and speech-language pathology services and Healthcare Common Procedure Coding System (HCPCS) codes that reflect physician supplier codes that are physical therapy, occupational therapy, and speech-language pathology services by code definition and are subject to the consolidated billing requirements. Therefore, the above-mentioned therapies must be provided directly or under arrangement on behalf of the HHA while a patient is under a home health plan of care and cannot be separately billed to Part B during an open 60-day episode.

D - Freedom of Choice Issues: A beneficiary exercises his or her freedom of choice for the services under the home health benefit listed in §1861(m) of the Act, including medical supplies, but excluding DME covered as a home health service by choosing the HHA. Once a home health patient chooses a particular HHA, he or she has clearly exercised freedom of choice with respect to all items and services included within the scope of the Medicare home health benefit (except DME). The HHA's consolidated billing role supersedes all other billing situations the beneficiary may wish to establish for home health services covered under the scope of the Medicare home health benefit during the certified episode.

E - Knowledge of Services Arranged for on Behalf of the HHA: The consolidated billing requirements governing HH PPS require that the HHA provide all covered home health services (except DME) either directly or under arrangement while a patient is under a home health plan of care. Providing services either directly or under arrangement requires knowledge of the services provided during the episode. In addition, in accordance with current Medicare conditions of participation and Medicare coverage guidelines governing home health, the patient's plan of care must reflect the physician ordered services that the HHA provides either directly or under arrangement. An HHA would not be responsible for payment in the situation in which they have no prior knowledge (unaware of physicians orders) of the services provided by an entity during an episode to a patient who is under their home health plan of care. An HHA is responsible for payment in the situation in which services are provided to a patient by another entity, under arrangement with the HHA, during an episode in which the patient is under the HHA's home health plan of care. However, it is in the best interest of future business relationships to discuss the situation with any entity that seeks payment from the HHA during an episode in an effort to resolve any misunderstanding and avoid such situations in the future.

10.12 – Change of Ownership Relationship to Episodes Under PPS

A - Change of Ownership with Assignment: When there is a change of ownership and the new owner accepts assignment of the existing provider agreement, the new owner is subject to all the terms and conditions under which the existing agreement was issued. The provider number remains the same if the new HHA owner accepts assignment of the existing provider agreement. As long as the new owner complies with the regulations governing home health PPS, billing and payment for episodes with applicable adjustments for existing patients under an established plan of care will continue on schedule through the change in ownership with assignment. The episode would be uninterrupted spanning the date of sale. The former owner is required to file a terminating cost report.

Instructions regarding when a cost report is filed are in the Provider Reimbursement Manual, §1500.

B - Change of Ownership without Assignment: When there is a change of ownership, and the new owner does not take the assignment of the existing provider agreement, the provider agreement and provider number of the former owner is terminated. The former owner will receive partial episode payment adjusted payments in accordance with the methodology set forth in the Medicare Claims Processing Manual, Chapter 10, "Home Health Agency Billing," §40.2, and 42 CFR 484.235, based on the last billable visit date for existing patients under a home health plan of care ending on or before the date of sale. The former owner is required to file a terminating cost report. The new owner cannot bill Medicare for payment until the effective date of the Medicare approval. The new HHA will not be able to participate in the Medicare program without going through the same process as any new provider, which includes an initial survey. Once the new owner is Medicare-approved, the HHA may start a new episode for purposes of payment, OASIS assessment, and certification of the home health plan of care for all new patients in accordance with the regulations governing home health PPS, effective with the date of the new provider certification.

C - Change of Ownership – Mergers: The merger of a provider corporation into another corporation constitutes a change of ownership. For information on specific procedures, refer to the State Operations Manual.

II. Basis of Medicare Prospective Payment Systems and Case-Mix

There are multiple prospective payment systems (PPS) for Medicare for different provider types. Before 1997, prospective payment was a term specifically applied to inpatient hospital services. In 1997, with passage of the Balanced Budget Act, prospective payment systems were mandated for other provider groups/bill types:

- Skilled nursing facilities;
- Outpatient hospital services;
- Home health agencies;
- Rehabilitation hospitals; and
- Others.

While there are commonalities among these systems, there are also variations in how each system operates and in the payment units for these systems. HH PPS is the only system with the 60-day episode as the payment unit.

The term prospective payment for Medicare does not imply a system where payment is made before services are delivered, or where payment levels are determined prior to the providing of care. With HH PPS, at least one service must be delivered before billing can occur. For HH PPS, a significant portion for the 60-day episode unit of payment is made at the beginning of the episode with as little as one visit delivered. HH PPS also means a shift of the basis of payment from payment tied to a claim or distinct revenue or procedural code, to an episode.

Case-mix is an underlying concept in prospective payment. With the creation of inpatient hospital PPS, the first Medicare PPS, there was a recognition that the differing characteristics of hospitals, such as teaching status or number of beds, contributed to substantial cost differences, but that even more cost impact was linked to the characteristics of the patient populations of the hospitals. Other Medicare PPS systems, where research is applied to adjust payments for patients requiring more complex or costly care, use this concept of case-mix complexity, meaning that patient characteristics affect the complexity, and therefore, cost of care. HH PPS considers a patient's clinical and functional condition, as well as service demands, in determining case-mix for home health care.

For individual Medicare inpatient acute care hospital bills, DRGs are produced by an electronic stream of claim information, which includes data elements such as procedure and diagnoses, through Grouper software that reads these pertinent elements on the claim and groups services into appropriate DRGs. DRGs are then priced by a separate Pricer software module at the A/B MAC (A). Processing for HH PPS is built on this model, using home health resources groups (HHRGs), instead of DRGs. In HH PPS, 60-day episode payments are case-mix adjusted using elements of the patient assessment.

Since 1999, HHAs have been required by Medicare to assess potential patients, and reassess existing patients, incorporating the OASIS (Outcome and Assessment Information Set) tool as part of the assessment process. The total case-mix adjusted episode payment is based on elements of the OASIS data set including the therapy visits provided over the course of the episode. The number of therapy visits projected at the start of the episode, entered in OASIS, will be confirmed by the visit information submitted on the claim for the episode. Though therapy visits are adjusted only with receipt of the claim at the end of the episode, both split percentage payments made for the episode are case-mix adjusted based on Grouper software run by the HHAs, often incorporated in the HAVEN software supporting OASIS. Pricer software run by the A/B MAC (HHH) processing home health claims performs pricing including wage index adjustment on both episode split percentage payments.

III. HHA PPS Framework—How the System Works

Calendar Year (CY) 2017 Changes

As required by section 3131(a) of the Affordable Care Act, and finalized in the CY 2014 HH PPS final rule (78 FR 77256, December 2, 2013), CMS implemented the final year of the 4-year phase-in of the rebasing adjustments to the national, standardized 60-day episode payment amount, the national per-visit rates and the NRS conversion factor in section III.C.3. The rebasing adjustments for CY 2017 will reduce the national, standardized 60-day episode payment amount by $80.95, increase the national per-visit payment amounts by 3.5 percent of the national per-visit payment amounts in CY 2010 with the increases ranging from $1.79 for home health aide services to $6.34 for medical social services, and reduce the NRS conversion factor by 2.82 percent. In addition, in section III.C.3 of the rule, CMS implemented a reduction to the national, standardized 60-day episode payment rate in CY 2017 of 0.97 percent to account for estimated case-mix growth unrelated to increases in patient acuity (that is, nominal case-mix growth) between CY 2012 and CY 2014. This reduction was finalized in the CY 2016 HH PPS final rule (80 FR 68624). Section III.A of the rule discusses CMS efforts to monitor for potential impacts due to the rebasing adjustments mandated by section 3131(a) of the Affordable Care Act.

In the CY 2015 HH PPS final rule (79 FR 66072), CMS finalized its proposal to recalibrate the case-mix weights every year with more current data. In section III.B of the rule, CMS recalibrated the HH PPS case-mix weights, using the most current cost and utilization data available, in a budget neutral manner. In section III.C.1 of the rule, CMS updated the payment rates under the HH PPS by the home health payment update percentage of 2.5 percent (using the 2010-based Home Health Agency (HHA) market basket update of 2.8 percent, minus 0.3 percentage point for productivity), as required by section 1895(b)(3)(B)(vi)(I) of the Act, and in section III.C.2 of the rule, CMS updated the CY 2017 home health wage index using more current hospital wage data. In section III.D, CMS finalized a change to the current methodology used to estimate the cost of an episode of care to determine whether the episode of care would receive an outlier payment. The methodology change includes calculating the cost of an episode of care using a cost-per-unit calculation, which takes into account visit length, rather than the current methodology that uses a cost-per-visit calculation. In section III.E of this rule, as a result of the Consolidated Appropriations Act, 2016 (Pub. L. 114-113), CMS implemented changes in payment for furnishing Negative Pressure Wound Therapy (NPWT) using a disposable device for a patient under a home health plan of care for which payment is otherwise made under the HH PPS.

In section III.F of the final rule, CMS provide an update on recent research and analysis pertaining to the home health study required by section 3131(d) of the Affordable Care Act. Finally, in section III.G of the rule, CMS provided an update a process for grouping the HH PPS claim centrally during claims processing.

In section IV of the CY2017 Final Rule, CMS finalized changes to the HHVBP Model that was implemented January 1, 2016. We are finalizing: the removal of the definition of "starter set"; a revised definition for "benchmark"; calculation of benchmarks and achievement thresholds at the state level; a minimum requirement of eight HHAs in a cohort; an increased timeframe for submitting New Measure data; removal of four measures from the set of applicable measures; an annual reporting period and submission date for one of the New Measures; and an appeals process that includes a recalculation and reconsideration process. CMS also provided an update on the progress towards developing public reporting of performance under the HHVBP Model.

This final rule also included updates to the Home Health Quality Reporting Program in section V, including removing six quality measures, adopting four new quality measures, mentioning future measures under consideration, following a calendar year schedule for measure and data submission requirements, and aligning quarterly reporting timeframes and quarterly review and correction periods.

A. Submission of Request for Anticipated Payment (RAP)

The HHA can submit a Request for Anticipated Payment, or RAP, to Medicare when all of the four following conditions are met.

- After the OASIS assessment is complete, locked or export ready, or there is an agency-wide internal policy establishing the OASIS data is finalized for transmission to the national assessment system;

- Once a physician's verbal orders for home care have been received and documented;

- A plan of care has been established and sent to the physician; and

- The first service visit under that plan has been delivered.

An episode will be opened on CWF with the receipt and processing of the RAP. RAPs, or in special cases claims, must be submitted for initial HH PPS episodes, subsequent HH PPS episodes, or in transfer situations to start a new HH PPS episode when another episode is already open at a different agency. HHAs should submit the RAP as soon as possible after care begins in order to assure being established as the primary HHA for the beneficiary.

RAPs are submitted using TOB 0322. RAPs must include the information output by Grouper for HH PPS in addition to other claim elements. While Medicare requires very limited information on RAPs, HHAs have the option of reporting service lines in addition to the Medicare requirements, either to meet the requirements of other payers, or to generate a charge for billing software. In the latter case, HHAs may report a single service line showing an amount equal to the expected payment amount to aid balancing in accounts receivable systems. Medicare will not use charges on a RAP to determine payment or for later data collection.

The HH Pricer software will determine the first of the two HH PPS split percentage payments for the episode, which is made in response to the RAP.

Case-mix is an underlying concept in prospective payment. With the creation of inpatient hospital PPS, the first Medicare PPS, there was a recognition that the differing characteristics of hospitals, such as teaching status or number of beds, contributed to substantial cost differences, but that even more cost impact was linked to the characteristics of the patient populations of the hospitals. Other Medicare PPS systems, where research is applied to adjust payments for patients requiring more complex or costly care, use this concept of case-mix complexity, meaning that patient characteristics affect the complexity, and therefore, cost of care. HH PPS considers a patient's clinical and functional condition, as well as service demands, in determining case-mix for home health care.

For individual Medicare inpatient acute care hospital bills, DRGs are produced by an electronic stream of claim information, which includes data elements such as procedure and diagnoses, through Grouper software that reads these pertinent elements on the claim and groups services into appropriate DRGs. DRGs are then priced by a separate Pricer software module at the A/B MAC (A). Processing for HH PPS is built on this model, using home health resources groups (HHRGs), instead of DRGs. In HH PPS, 60-day episode payments are case-mix adjusted using elements of the patient assessment.

Since 1999, HHAs have been required by Medicare to assess potential patients, and reassess existing patients, incorporating the OASIS (Outcome and Assessment Information Set) tool as part of the assessment process. The total case-mix adjusted episode payment is based on elements of the OASIS data set including the therapy visits provided over the course of the episode. The number of therapy visits projected at the start of the episode, entered in OASIS, will be confirmed by the visit information submitted on the claim for the episode. Though therapy visits are adjusted only with receipt of the claim at the end of the episode, both split percentage payments made for the episode are case-mix adjusted based on Grouper software run by the HHAs, often incorporated in the HAVEN software supporting OASIS. Pricer software run by the A/B MAC (HHH) processing home health claims performs pricing including wage index adjustment on both episode split percentage payments.

The HHA submits a RAP to their A/B MAC (HHH) to request the initial split percentage payment for an HH PPS episode. The RAP may be submitted after receiving verbal orders and delivering at least one service to the beneficiary. Though they are submitted on standard institutional claim formats, the RAP is not considered a Medicare home health claim and is not subject to many of the stipulations applied to claims in regulations. (NOTE: RAPs may be considered claims for purposes of other Federal laws and regulations.) In particular, RAPs are not subject to the payment floor, are not subject to interest payment if delayed in processing, and do not have appeal rights. Appeal rights for the episode are attached to claims submitted at the end of the episode.

In addition to a split percentage payment (see §10.1.6), RAPs may be paid zero percent if:

- Medicare is the secondary payer (see §30.10), or
- a provider has lost the privilege of receiving RAP payment, or
- the beneficiary is enrolled in a Medicare Advantage plan.

B. Payment, Claim Adjustments and Cancellations

A number of conditions can cause the episode payment or the RAP to be adjusted or cancelled.

The HHA must cancel a RAP sent in error. RAPs cannot be adjusted. They may be rebilled with appropriate information after cancellation. Type of bill 0328 is used for a cancel transaction, for both claims and RAPs.

Claims may be cancelled by HHAs or adjusted. Adjustments (TOB 0327) are used to correct information which may change payment. A cancellation is needed to change the beneficiary HICN or the HHA's provider number, if originally submitted incorrectly.

Adjustment claims may also be used to change information on a previously submitted claim (TOB 0327), which may also change payment. RAPs can only be canceled, not adjusted, but may be re-billed after cancellation.

Transfer Situations—Payment Effects

Transfer describes when a single beneficiary chooses to change HHAs during the same 60-day period. By law under the HH PPS system, beneficiaries must be able to transfer among HHAs, and episode payments must be pro-rated to reflect these changes. To accommodate this requirement, HHAs submit a RAP with a transfer indicator in the condition code field on the institutional claim when an episode may already be open for the same beneficiary at another HHA. In order for a receiving (new) HHA to accept a beneficiary elected transfer, the receiving HHA must document that the beneficiary has been informed that the initial HHA will no longer receive Medicare payment on behalf of the patient and will no longer provide Medicare covered services to the patient after the date of the patient's elected transfer in accordance with current patient rights requirements at 42 CFR 484.10(e). The receiving HHA must also document in its records that it accessed the Medicare inquiry system to determine whether or not the patient was under an established home health plan of care and contacted the initial HHA on the effective date of transfer.

In such cases, the previously open episode will be automatically closed in Medicare claims processing systems as of the date services began at the HHA the beneficiary transferred to, as reported in the RAP; and the new episode for the "transfer to" agency will begin on that same date. Payment will be pro-rated for the shortened episode of the "transferred from" agency, adjusted to a period less than 60 days either according to the claim closing the episode from that agency or according to the RAP from the "transfer to" agency. Note that HHAs may not submit RAPs opening episodes when anticipating a transfer if actual services have yet to be delivered.

In rare cases, a beneficiary may elect to transfer between HHAs and their admission date at the "transfer to" HHA may fall on the day immediately following the end of an episode at the "transferred from" agency. The "transferred from" agency may not have submitted a RAP for the new episode of continuous care, so the "transfer to" HHA may not see a record of an open episode when they access the Medicare inquiry system. They will likely see the record of the immediately adjacent episode and should provide the same notifications to the beneficiary as in any other

Discharge and Readmission Situation Under HH PPS—Payment Effects

Under HH PPS, HHAs may discharge beneficiaries before the 60-day episode has closed if all treatment goals of the plan of care have been met, or if the beneficiary ends care by transferring to another home health agency. Cases may occur in which an HHA has discharged a beneficiary during a 60-day episode, but the beneficiary is readmitted to the same agency in the same 60 days. Since no portion of the 60-day episode can be paid twice, the payment for the first episode must be pro-rated to reflect the shortened period (see §10.1.15). A new episode can be opened by the HHA. Medicare systems will allow this in cases where the CMS certification number (CCN) on the new RAP matches the CCN on the prior episode. The next episode will begin the date the first service is supplied under readmission (setting a new 60-day "clock").

Note that beneficiaries do not have to be discharged within the episode period because of admissions to other types of health care providers (i.e., hospitals, skilled nursing facilities), but HHAs may choose to discharge in such cases. If an agency chooses not to discharge and the patient returns to the agency in the same 60-day

period, the same episode continues. However, if an agency chooses to discharge, based on an expectation that the beneficiary will not return, the agency should recognize that if the beneficiary does return to them in the same 60-day period, the discharge is not recognized for Medicare payment purposes. All the HH services provided in the complete 60-day episode, both before and after the inpatient stay, should be billed on one claim.

When discharging, full episode payment would still be made unless the beneficiary received more home care later in the same 60-day period. Discharge should be made at the end of the 60-day episode period in all cases if the beneficiary has not returned to the HHA, and is not expected to return for treatment under any existing plan of care.

Adjustments of Episode Payment—Special Submission Case: "No-RAP" LUPAs

Normally, there will be two percentage payments (initial and final) paid for an HH PPS episode, the first paid in response to a RAP, and the last in response to a claim. However, there will be some cases in which a HHA knows that an episode will be four visits or less even before the episode begins or before the RAP is submitted, and therefore the episode will be paid a per-visit-based LUPA payment instead of an episode payment. In such cases and only in such cases, the HHA may choose not to submit a RAP, foregoing the initial percentage payment that otherwise would later likely be largely recouped. Physician orders must be signed when these claims are submitted. If a HHA later needs to add visits to the claim, so that the claim will have more than four visits and no longer be a LUPA, the claim should be adjusted and the full episode payment based on the HIPPS code will be made.

Adjustments of Episode Payment–Validation of HIPPS Codes

Recoding Based on OASIS-calculated HIPPS Codes

The HIPPS code calculated based on the OASIS assessment for an episode is reported on the HH RAP and claim. HHAs may calculate the HIPPS code using CMS-provided Grouper software or with their own software that recreates CMS grouping logic. When the OASIS assessment is submitted to the Medicare quality system, the HIPPS code is independently calculated using the CMS-provided Grouper program.

When processing the claim for an episode, Medicare systems compare the provider-submitted HIPPS code with the HIPPS code calculated based on the assessment information in the quality system. If the codes do not match, the OASIS-calculated HIPPS code is used for payment.

Medicare systems display the OASIS-calculated HIPPS code in Direct Data Entry (DDE) in a field named "RETURN-HIPPS1." When the OASIS-calculated HIPPS code is used for payment, the code in this field will match the code on the electronic remittance advice. In other cases, the HIPPS code in this field will match what the HHA submitted on their claim.

The OASIS-calculated HIPPS code may be re-coded further by Medicare systems. The OASIS-calculated HIPPS code will be sent to the HH PPS Pricer program which may change the code based on changes in therapy services (see section 10.1.19.1) or whether the claim is for an early or later episode (see section 10.1.19.2). In this case, the Pricer re-coded HIPPS code will be used for payment and will continue to be recorded in the APC-HIPPS field. This code will match the code on the electronic remittance advice. HHAs will be able to recognize this case because there will be three HIPPS codes on the claim record in DDE:

Field in DDE	DDE Map	Represents
HCPC	MAP171E	HHA-submitted HIPPS code
RETURN-HIPPS1	MAP171E	OASIS-calculated HIPPS code
APC-HIPPS	MAP171A	Pricer re-coded HIPPS code

The OASIS-calculated HIPPS code may also be re-coded by medical reviewers, based on their review of the documentation supporting the claim. In this case, the HIPPS code determined by medical review will be used for payment and will be recorded in the APC-HIPPS field. This code will match the code on the electronic remittance advice.

Submission of an OASIS assessment is a condition of payment for HH episodes of care. OASIS reporting regulations require the OASIS to be transmitted within 30 days of completing the assessment of the beneficiary. In most cases, this 30 day period will have elapsed by the time a 60 day episode of HH services is completed and the final claim for that episode is submitted to Medicare. If the OASIS assessment is not found in the quality system upon receipt of a final claim for an HH episode and the receipt date of the claim is more than 30 days after the assessment completion date, Medicare systems will deny the HH claim.

The contractor shall use the following remittance advice messages and associated codes when denying claims under this policy. This CARC/RARC combination is compliant with CAQH CORE Business Scenario Three.

Group Code: CO
CARC: 272
RARC: N/A
MSN: 41.17

Insufficient Documentation

The Comprehensive Error Rate Testing (CERT) program, calculates the Medicare Fee-for-Service (FFS) improper payment rate. For the FY 2013 report period (reflecting claims processed between July 2011 and June 2012), the national Medicare FFS improper payment rate was calculated to be 10.1 percent. For that same report period, the improper payment rate for home health services was 17.3 percent, representing a projected improper payment amount of approximately $3 billion. The improper payments identified by the CERT program represent instances in which a health care provider fails to comply with the Medicare coverage and billing requirements and are not necessarily a result of fraudulent activity.

The majority of home health improper payments were due to "insufficient documentation" errors. "Insufficient documentation" errors occur when the medical documentation submitted is inadequate to support payment for the services billed or when a specific documentation element that is required (as described above) is missing. Most "insufficient documentation" errors for home health occurred when the narrative portion of the face-to-face encounter documentation did not sufficiently describe how the clinical findings from the encounter supported the beneficiary's homebound status and need for skilled services.

Certification Requirements: Supporting Documentation

Documentation in the certifying physician's medical records and/or the acute/post-acute care facility's medical records (if the patient was directly admitted to home health) shall be used as the basis for certification of home health eligibility. If the documentation used as the basis for the certification of eligibility is not sufficient to demonstrate that the patient is or was eligible to receive services under the Medicare home health benefit, payment will not be rendered for home health services provided.

According to the regulations at 42 CFR 424.22(c), Certifying physicians and acute/post-acute care facilities must provide, upon request, the medical record documentation that supports the certification of patient eligibility for the Medicare home health benefit to the home health agency, review entities, and/or CMS. Certifying physicians who show patterns of non-compliance with this requirement, including those physicians whose records are inadequate or incomplete for this purpose, may be subject to increased reviews, such as provider-specific probe reviews.

Information from the HHA, such as the patient's comprehensive assessment, can be incorporated into the certifying physician's and/or the acute/post-acute care facility's medical record for the patient.

- Information from the HHA must be corroborated by other medical record entries and align with the time period in which services were rendered.
- The certifying physician must review and sign off on anything incorporated into the patient's medical record that is used to support the certification of patient eligibility (that is, agree with the material by signing and dating the entry).

The certifying physician's and/or the acute/post-acute care facility's medical record for the patient must contain information that justifies the referral for Medicare home health services. This includes documentation that substantiates the patient's:

1. Need for the skilled services; and
2. Homebound status.

The certifying physician's and/or the acute/post-acute care facility's medical record for the patient must contain the actual clinical note for the face-to-face encounter visit that demonstrates that the encounter:

1. Occurred within the required timeframe;
2. Was related to the primary reason the patient requires home health services; and
3. Was performed by an allowed provider type.

This information can be found most often in, but is not limited to, clinical and progress notes and discharge summaries.

Appendix H: OASIS Diagnosis Guidance

The following tables are "Instructions for Completing the OASIS Diagnosis Items," found in the OASIS-C2 Guidance Manual, January 2017, chapter 3, section C—Diagnosis "OASIS Item Guidance Patient History & Diagnoses."

Chapter 3 contains item-by-item guidance for all OASIS items.

Included here are *only* the items which pertain to assigning an ICD-10-CM diagnosis code.

Item Number	Item Description
M1011	List of each Inpatient Diagnosis and ICD-10-CM code at the level of highest specificity for only those conditions actively treated during an inpatient stay and having a discharge date within the last 14 days.
M1017	Diagnoses requiring medical or treatment regimen change within the last 14 days.
M1021	Primary Diagnosis, ICD-10-CM and symptom control rating.
M1023	Other Diagnoses, ICD-10-CM and symptom control rating.
M1025	Optional Diagnoses and ICD-10-CM codes.

For each item, guidance is provided on the following topics:

ITEM INTENT: Describes the rationale for collecting the information, in the context of outcome and process quality measurement, care planning, outcome risk adjustment, or prospective payment rate adjustment.

TIME POINTS: Describes when the information is to be collected during the patient's home health episode of care.

RESPONSE-SPECIFIC INSTRUCTIONS: Describes how the clinician should decide which of the possible responses should apply. These instructions may not always provide definitive guidance for selecting responses in every case, because clinical judgment is often required to determine the most accurate response to a specific item.

DATA SOURCES/RESOURCES: Describes the potential sources of information that should be accessed during the assessment to determine the most accurate response to this specific item. May include other clinicians, administrative records, online guidance regarding coding or other assessment guidelines, or standards promulgated by professional or accrediting organizations.

M1011

Item Intent	Time Points	Response-specific Instructions	Data Sources/resources
Identifies diagnosis(es) for which patient was actively receiving treatment in an inpatient facility within the past 14 days. This list of diagnoses is intended to include only those diagnoses that required active treatment during the inpatient stay and may or may not correspond with the hospital admitting diagnosis.	Start of care Resumption of care Follow-up	• "Actively treated" should be defined as receiving something more than the regularly scheduled medications and treatments necessary to maintain or treat an existing condition. • The term "past 14 days" is the two-week period immediately preceding the Start/Resumption of Care date (or for Follow-Up, the M0090 Date Assessment Completed). This means that for purposes of counting the 14-day period, the date of Start of Care date is day 0 and the day immediately prior to the Start of Care date is day 1. For example, if the patient's SOC date is August 20, any diagnoses related to inpatient stays with discharges falling on or after August 6 and prior to the HHA admission would be reported. • If a diagnosis was not treated during an inpatient admission, it should not be listed. (Example: The patient has a long-standing diagnosis of "osteoarthritis," but was treated during hospitalization only for "peptic ulcer disease." Do not list "osteoarthritis" as an inpatient diagnosis.) • No surgical codes. List the underlying diagnosis that was surgically treated. If a joint replacement was done for osteoarthritis, list the disease, not the procedure. • No V, W, X, Y, or Z codes. List the underlying diagnosis. • It is not necessary to fill in every line (a–f) if the patient had fewer than six inpatient diagnoses. • Select "NA" at follow-up if the patient was not discharged from an inpatient facility within the past 14 days.	• Patient/caregiver interview • Referral information (may include inpatient facility discharge summary, physician history and physical, progress notes, etc.) • Physician • The current ICD-10-CM List of Codes and Descriptions and the ICD-10-CM Official Guidelines for Coding and Reporting should be the source for coding.

M1017

Item Intent	Time Points	Response-specific Instructions	Data Sources/resources
Identifies if any change has occurred to the patient's treatment regimen, health care services, or medications within the past 14 days. The purpose of this question is to help identify the patient's recent history by identifying new diagnoses or diagnoses that have exacerbated over the past 2 weeks.	Start of care Resumption of care	• No surgical codes—list the underlying diagnosis. • No V, W, X, Y, or Z codes—list the appropriate diagnosis. • A diagnosis reported in M1011 – Inpatient Diagnosis may also be reported in M1017 if within the 14 days prior to the SOC/ROC date the condition was new or exacerbated, required changes in the treatment regimen, AND the patient was discharged from an inpatient facility where the condition was actively treated. • Mark "NA" if no medical or treatment regimen changes were made within the past 14 days OR all changes in the medical or treatment regimen were made because a diagnosis improved. • The term "past 14 days" is the two-week period immediately preceding the start/resumption of care. This means that for purposes of counting the 14-day period, the date of Start of Care date is day 0 and the day immediately prior to the date of admission is day 1. For example, if the patient's SOC date is August 20, any diagnoses requiring medical or treatment regimen change on or after August 6 and prior to the HHA admission would be reported.	• Patient/caregiver interview • Physician • Physician orders • Referral information • The current ICD-10-CM List of Codes and Descriptions and the ICD-10-CM Official Guidelines for Coding and Reporting should be the source for coding.

M1021, M1023 and M1025 have specific instructions related to reporting diagnoses in the various columns on the form and are as follows.

Diagnoses, Symptom Control, and Optional Diagnoses

List each diagnosis for which the patient is receiving home care in Column 1, and enter its ICD-10-CM code at the level of highest specificity in Column 2 (diagnosis codes only—no surgical or procedure codes allowed). Diagnoses are listed in the order that best reflects the seriousness of each condition and supports the disciplines and services provided. Rate the degree of symptom control for each condition in Column 2. ICD-10-C M sequencing requirements must be followed if multiple coding is indicated for any diagnoses. If a Z-code is reported in Column 2 in place of a diagnosis that is no longer active (a resolved condition), then optional item M1025 (Optional Diagnoses—Columns 3 and 4) may be completed. Diagnoses reported in M1025 will not impact payment.

Code each row according to the following directions for each column.

Column 1: Enter the description of the diagnosis. Sequencing of diagnoses should reflect the seriousness of each condition and support the disciplines and services provided.

Column 2: Enter the ICD-10-CM code for the condition described in Column 1 - no surgical or procedure codes allowed. Codes must be entered at the level of highest specificity and ICD-10-CM coding rules and sequencing requirements must be followed. Note that external cause codes (ICD-10-CM codes beginning with V, W, X, or Y) may not be reported in M1021 (Primary Diagnosis) but may be reported in M1023 (Secondary Diagnoses). Also note that when a Z-code is reported in Column 2, the code for the underlying condition can often be entered in Column 2, as long as it is an active on-going condition impacting home health care.

Rate the degree of symptom control for the condition listed in Column 1. Do not assign a symptom control rating if the diagnosis is a V, W, X, Y or Z-code. Choose one value that represents the degree of symptom control appropriate for each diagnosis using the following scale:

    0—Asymptomatic, no treatment needed at this time

    1—Symptoms well controlled with current therapy

    2—Symptoms controlled with difficulty, affecting daily functioning; patient needs ongoing monitoring

    3—Symptoms poorly controlled; patient needs frequent adjustment in treatment and dose monitoring

    4—Symptoms poorly controlled; history of re-hospitalizations

Note that the rating for symptom control in Column 2 should not be used to determine the sequencing of the diagnoses listed in Column 1. These are separate items and sequencing may not coincide.

Column 3: (OPTIONAL) There is no requirement that HHAs enter a diagnosis code in M1025 (Columns 3 and 4). Diagnoses reported in M1025 will not impact payment.

Agencies may choose to report an underlying condition in M1025 (Columns 3 and 4) when:

• a Z-code is reported in Column 2 AND

• the underlying condition for the Z-code in Column 2 is a resolved condition. An example of a resolved condition is uterine cancer that is no longer being treated following a hysterectomy.

Column 4: (OPTIONAL) If a Z-code is reported in M1021/M1023 (Column 2) and the agency chooses to report a resolved underlying condition that requires multiple diagnosis codes under ICD-10-CM coding guidelines, enter the diagnosis descriptions and the ICD-10-CM codes in the same row in Columns 3 and 4. For example, if the resolved condition is a manifestation code, record the diagnosis description and ICD-10-CM code for the underlying condition in Column 3 of that row and the diagnosis description and ICD-10-CM code for the manifestation in Column 4 of that row. Otherwise, leave Column 4 blank in that row.

M1021

Item Intent	Time Points	Response-specific Instructions	Data Sources/resources
The intent of this item is to accurately report and code the patient's primary home health diagnosis and document the degree of symptom control for that diagnosis. The patient's primary home health diagnosis is defined as the chief reason the patient is receiving home care and the diagnosis most related to the current home health Plan of Care.	Start of care Resumption of care Follow-up	• HHA clinicians and coders must comply with the ICD-10-CM Official Guidelines for Coding and Reporting when assigning primary diagnoses to the OASIS item M1021. See Chapter 5 for link. - The ICD-10-CM is a morbidity classification published by the United States for classifying diagnoses and reason for care in all health care settings. The ICD-10-CM is based on the ICD-10, the international classification of disease published by the World Health Organization (WHO). - The ICD-10-CM Official Guidelines for Coding and Reporting were developed by the Centers for Medicare & Medicaid Services (CMS) and the National Center for Health Statistics (NCHS). These guidelines are a set of rules that have been developed to accompany and complement the official conventions and instructions provided within the ICD-10-CM itself and should be used as a companion document to the official version of the ICD-10-CM List of Codes and Descriptions. - Adherence to the ICD-10-CM Official Guidelines for Coding and Reporting when assigning ICD-10-CM diagnosis codes is required under the Health Insurance Portability and Accountability Act (HIPAA). It is expected that each agency will ensure that diagnoses and ICD-10-CM codes reported in the OASIS data set meet these guidelines. • Identifying the patient's Primary Home Health Diagnoses - The assessing clinician is expected to complete the patient's comprehensive assessment and understand the patient's overall medical condition and care needs before selecting and assigning diagnoses. - The determination of the patient's primary home health diagnoses must be made by the assessing clinician based on the findings of the assessment, information in the medical record, and input from the physician. - As noted in the Item Intent, the patient's primary diagnosis is defined as the chief reason the patient is receiving home care and the diagnosis most related to the current home health Plan of Care. The primary diagnosis may or may not relate to the patient's most recent hospital stay, but must relate to the skilled services (skilled nursing, physical therapy, occupational therapy, and speech language pathology) rendered by the HHA. - As noted in the Item Intent, the secondary diagnoses include coexisting conditions actively addressed in the patient's Plan of Care, and any comorbid conditions having the potential to affect the patient's responsiveness to treatment and rehabilitative prognosis. The secondary diagnoses may or may not be related to a patient's recent hospital stay, but must have the potential to impact the skilled services provided by the HHA. - When determining secondary diagnoses, the assessing clinician should consider diagnoses that are actively addressed in the Plan of Care as well as diagnoses that affect the patient's responsiveness to treatment and rehabilitative prognosis, even if the condition is not the focus of any home health treatment itself. - Diagnoses may change during the course of the home health stay due to a change in the patient's health status or a change in the focus of home health care. At each required OASIS time point, the clinician must assess the patient's clinical status and determine the primary diagnosis based on patient status and treatment plan at the time of the assessment. - Only current medical diagnoses should be reported as primary diagnosis in M1021. Diagnoses should be excluded if they are resolved or do not have the potential to impact the skilled services provided by the HHA. An example of a resolved condition is cholecystitis following a cholecystectomy.	• Patient/caregiver interview • Physician • Physician orders • Referral information • Current medication list • The current ICD-10-CM List of Codes and Descriptions and the ICD-10-CM Official Guidelines for Coding and Reporting should be the source for coding (see Chapter 5 for link). • For degree of symptom control, data sources may include patient/caregiver interview, physician, physical assessment, and review of past health history.

M1021 (Continued)

Item Intent	Time Points	Response-specific Instructions	Data Sources/resources

		- In addition to following the ICD-10-CM Official Guidelines for Coding and Reporting, selection of home health diagnoses must be performed in compliance with Medicare's rules and regulations for coverage and payment to ensure provider compliance with Section 1862(a)(1)(A) of the Social Security Act. Section 1862(a)(1)(A) excludes provider services from Medicare coverage and payment that "are not reasonable and necessary for diagnosis or treatment of illness or injury or to improve the functioning of a malformed body member."
		• Reporting Primary Diagnosis in M1021
		  - At each required OASIS time point, the assessing clinician should enter the patient's current primary diagnosis in Column 1 of M1021. Complete Column 1 from top to bottom, leaving any blank entries at the bottom.
		• Reporting ICD-10-CM Codes in Column 2 of M1021
		  - The assessing clinician can enter the actual numeric ICD-10-CM codes for each diagnosis listed in Column 1 and 2 of M1021, once the assessment is completed and the diagnosis is entered in Column 1. Alternatively, a coding specialist in the agency may enter the actual numeric ICD-10-CM codes in Column 2, as long as the assessing clinician has determined the primary diagnosis in Column 1.
		  - The correct process for selecting an ICD-10-CM code using the Alphabetic Index and the Tabular List is described in the ICD-10-CM Official Guidelines for Coding and Reporting. Follow the official conventions and instructions provided within the ICD-10-CM List of Codes and Descriptions and the Official Guidelines to code each row in Column 2.
		  - Each ICD-10-CM code must be entered at its highest level of specificity (diagnosis codes only - no surgical or procedure codes allowed).
		  - ICD-10-CM does not allow external cause codes (ICD-10-CM codes beginning with V, W, X, or Y) to be reported in M1021 (Primary Diagnosis) but they may be reported in M1023 (Secondary Diagnoses).
		  - Also note that when a Z-code is reported in Column 2, the code for the underlying condition may be entered in Column 2, as long as it is a current on-going condition that has a potential to impact the skilled services provided by the HHA. See the ICD-10-CM Official Guidelines for Coding and Reporting for complete instructions on code assignment and sequencing related to the use of Z-codes and use of multiple coding for a single condition (such as manifestation/etiology pairs).
		• Reporting the Symptom Control Rating in Column 2 of M1021
		  - At each required time point, the assessing clinician should record the symptom control rating for the primary diagnosis in column 2 of M1021.
		  - Assessing degree of symptom control includes review of presenting signs and symptoms, type and number of medications, frequency of treatment readjustments, and frequency of contact with health care provider. Inquire about the degree to which each condition limits daily activities. Assess the patient to determine if symptoms are controlled by current treatments. Clarify which diagnoses/symptoms have been poorly controlled in the recent past.
		  - Choose one value that represents the degree of symptom control appropriate for the diagnosis using the scale provided in the M1021 instructions.	

Appendix H: OASIS Diagnosis Guidance

M1023

Item Intent	Time Points	Response-specific Instructions	Data Sources/resources

The intent of this item is to accurately report and code the patient's secondary home health diagnoses and document the degree of symptom control for each diagnosis. Secondary diagnoses are comorbid conditions that exist at the time of the assessment, that are actively addressed in the patient's Plan of Care, or that have the potential to affect the patient's responsiveness to treatment and rehabilitative prognosis.	Start of care
	Resumption of care
	Follow-up
		• HHA clinicians and coders must comply with the ICD-10-CM Official Guidelines for Coding and Reporting when assigning secondary diagnoses to the OASIS items M1023. See Chapter 5 for link.
		
		  - The ICD-10-CM is a morbidity classification published by the United States for classifying diagnoses and reason for care in all health care settings. The ICD-10-CM is based on the ICD-10, the international classification of disease published by the World Health Organization (WHO).
		  - The ICD-10-CM Official Guidelines for Coding and Reporting were developed by the Centers for Medicare & Medicaid Services (CMS) and the National Center for Health Statistics (NCHS). These guidelines are a set of rules that have been developed to accompany and complement the official conventions and instructions provided within the ICD-10-CM itself and should be used as a companion document to the official version of the ICD-10-CM List of Codes and Descriptions.
		  - Adherence to the ICD-10-CM Official Guidelines for Coding and Reporting when assigning ICD-10-CM diagnosis codes is required under the Health Insurance Portability and Accountability Act (HIPAA). It is expected that each agency will ensure that diagnoses and ICD-10-CM codes reported in the OASIS data set meet these guidelines.
		• Identifying the patient's Secondary Home Health Diagnoses
		
		  - The assessing clinician is expected to complete the patient's comprehensive assessment and understand the patient's overall medical condition and care needs before selecting and assigning diagnoses.
		  - The determination of the patient's secondary home health diagnoses must be made by the assessing clinician based on the findings of the assessment, information in the medical record, and input from the physician.
		  - As noted in the Item Intent, the secondary diagnoses include coexisting conditions actively addressed in the patient's Plan of Care, and any comorbid conditions having the potential to affect the patient's responsiveness to treatment and rehabilitative prognosis. The secondary diagnoses may or may not be related to a patient's recent hospital stay, but must have the potential to impact the skilled services provided by the HHA.
		  - When determining secondary diagnoses, the assessing clinician should consider diagnoses that are actively addressed in the Plan of Care as well as diagnoses that affect the patient's responsiveness to treatment and rehabilitative prognosis, even if the condition is not the focus of any home health treatment itself.
		  - Diagnoses may change during the course of the home health stay due to a change in the patient's health status or a change in the focus of home health care. At each required OASIS time point, the clinician must assess the patient's clinical status and determine the secondary diagnoses based on patient status and treatment plan at the time of the assessment.
		  - Only current medical diagnoses should be reported as secondary diagnoses in M1023. Diagnoses should be excluded if they are resolved or do not have the potential to impact the skilled services provided by the HHA. An example of a resolved condition is cholecystitis following a cholecystectomy.
		  - In addition to following the ICD-10-CM Official Guidelines for Coding and Reporting, selection of home health diagnoses must be performed in compliance with Medicare's rules and regulations for coverage and payment to ensure provider compliance with Section 1862(a)(1)(A) of the Social Security Act. Section 1862(a)(1)(A) excludes provider services from Medicare coverage and payment that "are not reasonable and necessary for diagnosis or treatment of illness or injury or to improve the functioning of a malformed body member."
			• Patient/caregiver interview
			• Physician
			• Physician orders
			• Referral information
			• Current medication list
			• The current ICD-10-CM List of Codes and Descriptions and the ICD-10-CM Official Guidelines for Coding and Reporting should be the source for coding.
			• For degree of symptom control, data sources may include patient/caregiver interview, physician, physical assessment, and review of past health history.

M1023 (Continued)

Item Intent	Time Points	Response-specific Instructions	Data Sources/resources

		• Reporting Secondary Diagnoses in M1023
		
		  - At each required OASIS time point, the assessing clinician should enter the patient's current secondary diagnoses in Column 1 of M1023. Complete Column 1 from top to bottom, leaving any blank entries at the bottom.
		  - The order that secondary diagnoses are entered should be determined by the degree that they impact the patient's health and need for home health care, rather than the degree of symptom control. For example, if a patient is receiving home health care for Type 2 diabetes that is "controlled with difficulty," this diagnosis would be listed above a diagnosis of a fungal infection of a toenail that is receiving treatment, even if the fungal infection is "poorly controlled."
		• Reporting ICD-10-CM Codes in Column 2 of M1023
		
		  - The assessing clinician can enter the actual numeric ICD-10-CM codes for each diagnosis listed in Column 1 and 2 of M1023, once the assessment is completed and the diagnosis is entered in Column 1. Alternatively, a coding specialist in the agency may enter the actual numeric ICD-10-CM codes in Column 2, as long as the assessing clinician has determined the secondary diagnoses in Column 1.
		  - The correct process for selecting an ICD-10-CM code using the Alphabetic Index and the Tabular List is described in the ICD-10-CM Official Guidelines for Coding and Reporting. Follow the official conventions and instructions provided within the ICD-10-CM List of Codes and Descriptions and the Official Guidelines to code each row in Column 2.
		  - Each ICD-10-CM code must be entered at its highest level of specificity (diagnosis codes only - no surgical or procedure codes allowed).
		  - ICD-10-CM does not allow external cause codes (ICD-10-CM codes beginning with V, W, X, or Y) to be reported in M1021 (Primary Diagnosis) but they may be reported in M1023 (Secondary Diagnoses).
		  - Also note that when a Z-code is reported in Column 2, the code for the underlying condition may be entered in Column 2, as long as it is a current on-going condition that has a potential to impact the skilled services provided by the HHA. See the ICD-10-CM Official Guidelines for Coding and Reporting for complete instructions on code assignment and sequencing related to the use of Z-codes and use of multiple coding for a single condition (such as manifestation/etiology pairs).
		• Reporting the Symptom Control Rating in Column 2 of M1023
		
		  - At each required time point, the assessing clinician should record the symptom control ratings for each secondary diagnosis in column 2 of M1023.
		  - Assessing degree of symptom control includes review of presenting signs and symptoms, type and number of medications, frequency of treatment readjustments, and frequency of contact with health care provider. Inquire about the degree to which each condition limits daily activities. Assess the patient to determine if symptoms are controlled by current treatments. Clarify which diagnoses/symptoms have been poorly controlled in the recent past.
		  - Choose one value that represents the degree of symptom control appropriate for each diagnosis using the scale provided in the M1023 instructions.	

M1025 (Optional)

Item Intent	Time Points	Response-specific Instructions	Data Sources/resources

The intent of this item is to provide the agency with the option of documenting a resolved underlying condition in Columns 3 and 4, if a Z-code is reported as a primary or secondary diagnosis in Columns 1 and 2, and the underlying condition is no longer active.	Start of care
	Resumption of care
		• Optional
		  - If a Z-code is reported in Column 2 and the underlying condition for the Z-code is resolved, then the resolved condition may be reported in Columns 3 and 4 at the agency's discretion.
		  - If an agency chooses to report a diagnosis in Columns 3 and 4, then the instructions that accompany items M1021/M1023/M1025 in the OASIS-C2 data set should be followed to code each row in Column 3 and/or 4. If a diagnosis and ICD-10-CM code is entered in Columns 3 and/or 4, it must be placed in the same row as the corresponding Z-code. Note that external cause codes (ICD-10-CM codes beginning with V, W, X, or Y) may not be reported in M1025.
		• Refer to the ICD-10-CM Official Guidelines for Coding and Reporting for instructions on multiple coding for a single condition (such as manifestation/etiology pairs).
			• Patient/caregiver interview
			• Physician
			• Physician orders
			• Referral information
			• Current medication list
			• The current ICD-10-CM List of Codes and Descriptions and the ICD-10-CM Official Guidelines for Coding and Reporting should be the source for coding.
			• For degree of symptom control, data sources may include patient/caregiver interview, physician, physical assessment, and review of past health history.

Appendix I: Case-Mix Adjustment Variables and Scores

The Home Health Resource Group (HHRG) classification system measures three dimensions of case mix: clinical dimension, functional scores, and services utilization dimension. The table below contains the current 45 diagnosis categories in the clinical dimension measurements, and the six measurements currently designated as the functional scores. The source for this information is the January 2017 Home Health Prospective Payment System (HH PPS) Grouper software v6117, update effective January 1, 2017.

Note: An updated version of the home health prospective payment system (HH PPS) Grouper software was not available at the time this book was printed and therefore this appendix does not reflect any fiscal 2018 code changes. Updated versions of the software can be found at https://www.cms.gov/Medicare/Medicare-Fee-for-Service-Payment/HomeHealthPPS/CaseMixGrouperSoftware.html.

Case-Mix Adjustment Variables and Scores

	Episode number within sequence of adjacent episodes	1 or 2	1 or 2	3+	3+
	Therapy visits	0-13	14+	0-13	14+
	EQUATION:	1	2	3	4
CLINICAL DIMENSION					
1	Primary or Other Diagnosis = Blindness/low vision	0	0	0	0
2	Primary or Other Diagnosis = Blood disorders	0	2	0	0
3	Primary or Other Diagnosis = Cancer, selected benign neoplasms	0	5	0	5
4	Primary Diagnosis = Diabetes	0	4	0	2
5	Other Diagnosis = Diabetes	1	0	0	0
6	Primary or Other Diagnosis = Dysphagia **AND** Primary or Other Diagnosis = Neuro 3 - Stroke	2	18	2	12
7	Primary or Other Diagnosis = Dysphagia **AND** M1030 (Therapy at home) = 3 (Enteral)	2	6	0	6
8	Primary or Other Diagnosis = Gastrointestinal disorders	0	0	0	0
9	Primary or Other Diagnosis = Gastrointestinal disorders **AND** M1630 (ostomy)= 1 or 2	0	7	0	0
10	Primary or Other Diagnosis = Gastrointestinal disorders **AND** Primary or Other Diagnosis = Neuro 1 - Brain disorders and paralysis, **OR** Neuro 2 - Peripheral neurological disorders, **OR** Neuro 3 - Stroke, **OR** Neuro 4 - Multiple sclerosis	0	0	0	0
11	Primary or Other Diagnosis = Heart Disease **OR** Hypertension	1	2	0	2
12	Primary Diagnosis = Neuro 1 - Brain disorders and paralysis	2	12	7	12
13	Primary or Other Diagnosis = Neuro 1 - Brain disorders and paralysis **AND** M1840 (Toilet transfer) = 2 or more	0	3	0	3
14	Primary or Other Diagnosis = Neuro 1 - Brain disorders and paralysis **OR** Neuro 2 - Peripheral neurological disorders **AND** M1810 or M1820 (Dressing upper or lower body)= 1, 2, or 3	2	3	1	3
15	Primary or Other Diagnosis = Neuro 3 - Stroke	3	12	2	5
16	Primary or Other Diagnosis = Neuro 3 - Stroke **AND** M1810 or M1820 (Dressing upper or lower body)= 1, 2, or 3	0	0	0	0
17	Primary or Other Diagnosis = Neuro 3 - Stroke **AND** M1860 (Ambulation) = 4 or more	0	0	0	0
18	Primary or Other Diagnosis = Neuro 4 - Multiple Sclerosis **AND AT LEAST ONE OF THE FOLLOWING:** M1830 (bathing) = 2 or more **OR** M1840 (Toilet transferring) = 2 or more **OR** M1850 (Transferring) = 2 or more **OR** M1860 (Ambulation) = 4 or more	3	7	6	11
19	Primary or Other Diagnosis = Ortho 1 - Leg disorders or gait disorders **AND** M1324 (most problematic pressure ulcer stage)= 1, 2, 3 or 4	8	1	7	0

Case-Mix Adjustment Variables and Scores

20	Primary or Other Diagnosis = Ortho 1 - Leg **OR** Ortho 2 - Other orthopaedic disorders **AND** M1030 (Therapy at home) = 1 (IV/Infusion) or 2 (Parenteral)	3	0	3	4
21	Primary or Other Diagnosis = Psych 1 – Affective and other psychoses, depression	0	0	0	0
22	Primary or Other Diagnosis = Psych 2 - Degenerative and other organic psychiatric disorders	0	0	0	0
23	Primary or Other Diagnosis = Pulmonary disorders	0	0	0	1
24	Primary or Other Diagnosis = Pulmonary disorders **AND** M1860 (Ambulation) = 1 or more	0	1	0	0
25	Primary Diagnosis = Skin 1 -Traumatic wounds, burns, and post-operative complications	4	20	7	18
26	Other Diagnosis = Skin 1 - Traumatic wounds, burns, post-operative complications	7	15	8	15
27	Primary or Other Diagnosis = Skin 1 -Traumatic wounds, burns, and post-operative complications **OR** Skin 2 – Ulcers and other skin conditions **AND** M1030 (Therapy at home) = 1 (IV/Infusion) or 2 (Parenteral)	3	0	0	0
28	Primary or Other Diagnosis = Skin 2 - Ulcers and other skin conditions	2	17	8	17
29	Primary or Other Diagnosis = Tracheostomy	4	17	4	17
30	Primary or Other Diagnosis = Urostomy/Cystostomy	0	18	0	13
31	M1030 (Therapy at home) = 1 (IV/Infusion) or 2 (Parenteral)	0	17	6	17
32	M1030 (Therapy at home) = 3 (Enteral)	0	16	0	9
33	M1200 (Vision) = 1 or more	0	0	0	0
34	M1242 (Pain)= 3 or 4	3	0	2	0
35	M1311 = Two or more pressure ulcers at stage 3 or 4	5	10	5	10
36	M1324 (Most problematic pressure ulcer stage)= 1 or 2	4	19	7	16
37	M1324 (Most problematic pressure ulcer stage)= 3 or 4	9	32	11	26
38	M1334 (Stasis ulcer status)= 2	4	15	8	15
39	M1334 (Stasis ulcer status)= 3	7	17	10	17
40	M1342 (Surgical wound status)= 2	2	7	5	11
41	M1342 (Surgical wound status)= 3	0	6	4	9
42	M1400 (Dyspnea) = 2, 3, or 4	0	0	0	0
43	M1620 (Bowel Incontinence) = 2 to 5	0	4	0	3
44	M1630 (Ostomy)= 1 or 2	4	12	2	8
45	M2030 (Injectable Drug Use) = 0, 1, 2, or 3	0	0	0	0
FUNCTIONAL DIMENSION					
46	M1810 or M1820 (Dressing upper or lower body)= 1, 2, or 3	1	0	1	0
47	M1830 (Bathing) = 2 or more	6	5	5	2
48	M1840 (Toilet transferring) = 2 or more	1	2	0	0
49	M1850 (Transferring) = 2 or more	3	1	2	0
50	M1860 (Ambulation) = 1, 2, or 3	7	0	4	0
51	M1860 (Ambulation) = 4 or more	8	9	6	8

Appendix J: Case-Mix Groups

Diagnosis codes considered to be case-mix codes are conditions recognized and used by the Home Health Prospective Payment System (HH PPS) for scoring when recorded as primary and/or secondary codes on the OASIS form. Each case-mix diagnosis code is assigned to one of 22 diagnosis groups. This resource lists each diagnosis group along with the case-mix codes that fall into that group. This information is taken from the January 2017 HH PPS Grouper software files v6117, effective January 1, 2017.

Note: An updated version of the home health prospective payment system (HH PPS) Grouper software was not available at the time this book was printed and therefore this appendix does not reflect any fiscal 2018 code changes. Updated versions of the software can be found at https://www.cms.gov/Medicare/Medicare-Fee-for-Service-Payment/HomeHealthPPS/CaseMixGrouperSoftware.html.

A three-character code followed by an asterisk indicates a code range and that all codes in that category are included. All codes should be reported to the highest level of specificity.

Manifestation codes are represented in ***italic bold***. The underlying disease or condition code must be sequenced first. ICD-10-CM guidelines pertaining to multiple coding and sequencing of diagnosis codes apply to OASIS diagnosis items.

For official ICD-10-CM coding guidance, please refer to the ICD-10-CM Official Guidelines for Coding and Reporting 2018 located in the introduction section of this code book.

01 Blindness and low vision	D69.59	C26*	C4A.61	C44.619	C50.112
Currently there are no ICD-10-CM codes included in this case-mix group.	D69.6	C30*	C4A.62	C44.622	C50.121
	D69.8	C31*	C4A.71	C44.629	C50.122
	D69.9	C32*	C4A.72	C44.692	C50.211
	D70*	C33	C4A.8	C44.699	C50.212
	D71	C34*	C4A.9	C44.702	C50.221
	D72*	C37	C44.00	C44.709	C50.222
02 Blood disorders	D73*	C38*	C44.01	C44.712	C50.311
D47.3	D74*	C39*	C44.02	C44.719	C50.312
D47.4	D75*	C40.01	C44.09	C44.722	C50.321
D51*	D76*	C40.02	C44.102	C44.729	C50.322
D52*	*D77*	C40.11	C44.109	C44.792	C50.411
D53*	D89.2	C40.12	C44.112	C44.799	C50.412
D55*	I88*	C40.21	C44.119	C44.80	C50.421
D56.0		C40.22	C44.122	C44.81	C50.422
D56.1	**03 Cancer and selected benign neoplasms**	C40.31	C44.129	C44.82	C50.511
D56.2		C40.32	C44.192	C44.89	C50.512
D56.3		C40.81	C44.199	C45*	C50.521
D56.4	C00.0	C40.82	C44.202	C46*	C50.522
D56.5	C00.1	C40.91	C44.209	C47.0	C50.611
D56.8	C00.3	C40.92	C44.212	C47.11	C50.612
D57.02	C00.4	C41.0	C44.219	C47.12	C50.621
D57.1	C00.8	C41.1	C44.222	C47.21	C50.622
D57.20	C01	C41.2	C44.229	C47.22	C50.811
D57.212	C02*	C41.3	C44.292	C47.3	C50.812
D57.40	C03.0	C41.4	C44.299	C47.4	C50.821
D57.412	C03.1	C43.0	C44.301	C47.5	C50.822
D57.80	C04*	C43.11	C44.309	C47.6	C50.911
D57.812	C05*	C43.12	C44.311	C47.8	C50.912
D58*	C06.0	C43.21	C44.319	C47.9	C50.921
D59*	C06.1	C43.22	C44.321	C48*	C50.922
D60*	C06.2	C43.31	C44.329	C49.0	C51*
D61*	C06.80	C43.39	C44.391	C49.11	C52
D64.0	C06.89	C43.4	C44.399	C49.12	C53*
D64.2	C07	C43.51	C44.40	C49.21	C54*
D64.3	C08*	C43.52	C44.41	C49.22	C55
D64.4	C09*	C43.59	C44.42	C49.3	C56*
D64.81	C10*	C43.61	C44.49	C49.4	C57*
D64.89	C11*	C43.62	C44.500	C49.5	C58
D64.9	C12	C43.71	C44.501	C49.6	C60*
D68.51	C13*	C43.72	C44.509	C49.8	C61
D68.52	C14*	C43.8	C44.510	C49.9	C62*
D68.59	C15*	C4A.0	C44.511	C49.A1	C63.00
D68.61	C16*	C4A.11	C44.519	C49.A2	C63.01
D68.62	C17*	C4A.12	C44.520	C49.A3	C63.02
D68.69	C18*	C4A.21	C44.521	C49.A4	C63.10
D69.0	C19	C4A.22	C44.529	C49.A5	C63.11
D69.1	C20	C4A.31	C44.590	C49.A9	C63.12
D69.2	C21*	C4A.39	C44.591	C50.011	C63.2
D69.3	C22*	C4A.4	C44.599	C50.012	C63.7
D69.41	C23	C4A.51	C44.602	C50.021	C63.8
D69.42	C24*	C4A.52	C44.609	C50.022	C64*
D69.49	C25*	C4A.59	C44.612	C50.111	

03 Cancer and selected benign neoplasms (continued)

C65*	C79.70	D01.0	E09.33*	E11.630	A06.3
C66*	C79.71	D01.1	E09.34*	E11.638	A06.4
C67*	C79.72	D01.2	E09.35*	E11.649	A06.81
C68*	C79.81	D01.3	E09.36	E11.65	A06.82
C69.01	C79.82	D01.40	E09.37*	E11.69	A06.89
C69.02	C79.89	D01.49	E09.40	E11.8	A06.9
C69.11	C80.0	D01.5	E09.41	E11.9	A07*
C69.12	C80.2	D02.0	E09.42	E13.10	A08*
C69.21	C81*	D02.1	E09.43	E13.21	A09
C69.22	C82*	D02.20	E09.621	E13.22	B25.1
C69.31	C83*	D02.21	E10.10	E13.29	K20*
C69.32	C84*	D02.22	E10.21	E13.31*	K21*
C69.40	C85*	D02.3	E10.22	E13.32*	K22.0
C69.41	C86*	D03.0	E10.29	E13.33*	K22.10
C69.42	C88.2	D03.11	E10.31*	E13.34*	K22.4
C69.51	C88.3	D03.12	E10.32*	E13.35*	K22.5
C69.52	C88.4	D03.21	E10.33*	E13.36	K22.70
C69.61	C88.8	D03.22	E10.34*	E13.39	K22.710
C69.62	C88.9	D03.39	E10.35*	E13.40	K22.711
C69.81	C90*	D03.4	E10.36	E13.41	K22.719
C69.82	C91*	D03.51	E10.37*	E13.42	K22.8
C69.91	C92*	D03.52	E10.39	E13.43	K22.9
C69.92	C93.00	D03.59	E10.40	E13.44	*K23*
C72.20	C93.01	D03.61	E10.41	E13.49	K25.3
C72.21	C93.02	D03.62	E10.42	E13.51	K25.7
C72.22	C93.10	D03.71	E10.43	E13.52	K25.9
C72.30	C93.11	D03.72	E10.44	E13.59	K26.3
C72.31	C93.12	D03.8	E10.49	E13.610	K26.7
C72.32	C93.30	D04.0	E10.51	E13.618	K26.9
C72.40	C93.31	D04.11	E10.52	E13.620	K27.3
C72.41	C93.32	D04.12	E10.59	E13.621	K27.7
C72.42	C93.Z0	D04.21	E10.610	E13.622	K27.9
C72.50	C93.Z1	D04.22	E10.618	E13.628	K28.7
C72.59	C93.90	D04.39	E10.620	E13.630	K28.9
C72.9	C93.91	D04.4	E10.621	E13.638	K29.00
C73	C93.92	D04.5	E10.622	E13.649	K29.20
C74*	C94.00	D04.61	E10.628	E13.65	K29.30
C75*	C94.01	D04.62	E10.630	E13.69	K29.40
C7A*	C94.02	D04.71	E10.638	E13.8	K29.50
C7B*	C94.20	D04.72	E10.649	E13.9	K29.60
C76.0	C94.21	D04.8	E10.65		K29.70
C76.1	C94.22	D05.01	E10.69	**05 Dysphagia**	K29.80
C76.2	C94.30	D05.02	E10.8	R13*	K29.90
C76.3	C94.31	D05.11	E10.9		K31.3
C76.41	C94.32	D05.12	E11.21	**06 Gait abnormality**	K31.4
C76.42	C94.80	D05.81	E11.22	R26.0	K31.819
C76.51	C94.81	D05.82	E11.29	R26.1	K31.83
C76.52	C94.82	D05.91	E11.31*	R26.81	K31.89
C76.8	C95*	D05.92	E11.32*	R26.89	K38.2
C77*	C96.0	D06*	E11.33*		K38.8
C78*	C96.4	D07*	E11.34*	**07 Gastrointestinal disorders**	K38.9
C79.00	C96.A	D09.0	E11.35*	A01.00	K50.00
C79.01	C96.Z	D09.21	E11.36	A01.09	K50.011
C79.02	C96.9	D09.22	E11.37*	A01.1	K50.014
C79.10	D00*	D09.3	E11.39	A01.2	K50.018
C79.11		D09.8	E11.40	A01.3	K50.019
C79.19		D16.01	E11.41	A01.4	K50.10
C79.2		D16.02	E11.42	A02.0	K50.118
C79.31		D16.11	E11.43	A02.20	K50.119
C79.32		D16.12	E11.44	A02.25	K50.80
C79.40		D16.21	E11.49	A02.29	K50.814
C79.49		D16.22	E11.51	A02.8	K50.818
C79.51		D16.31	E11.52	A02.9	K50.819
C79.52		D16.32	E11.59	A03*	K50.90
C79.60		D16.4	E11.610	A04*	K50.918
C79.61		D16.5	E11.618	A05*	K50.919
C79.62		D16.6	E11.620	A06.0	K51.00
		D16.7	E11.621	A06.1	K51.20
		D16.8	E11.622	A06.2	
		D33.3	E11.628		
		D33.7			

04 Diabetes
E08.31
E08.32
E08.33
E08.34
E08.35
E08.40
E08.41
E08.42
E08.43
E08.44
E08.621
E08.622
E09.31*
E09.32*

07 Gastrointestinal disorders (continued)	K76.9	I21.3	10 Neuro 1 – Brain disorders and paralysis	G12.9	S06.311[D,S]
K51.218	*K77*	I21.4	A01.01	G31.81	S06.312[D,S]
K51.219	K80.10	I22*	A02.21	G31.82	S06.313[D,S]
K51.30	K80.12	I24*	A06.6	*G32.0*	S06.314[D,S]
K51.319	K80.18	I25.10	A17*	G37.4	S06.315[D,S]
K51.40	K80.20	I25.110	A81*	G82*	S06.316[D,S]
K51.418	K80.30	I25.111	A85.0	G83.5	S06.319[D,S]
K51.419	K80.32	I25.118	A85.1	G83.81	S06.320[D,S]
K51.50	K80.34	I25.119	A85.8	G83.82	S06.321[D,S]
K51.518	K80.36	I25.3	A86	G83.83	S06.322[D,S]
K51.519	K80.40	I25.41	A87*	G83.84	S06.323[D,S]
K51.80	K80.42	I25.42	A88.0	G83.89	S06.324[D,S]
K51.818	K80.44	I25.5	A88.8	G92	S06.325[D,S]
K51.819	K80.46	I25.6	A89	G93.0	S06.326[D,S]
K51.90	K80.50	I25.700	B45.1	G93.1	S06.329[D,S]
K51.918	K80.60	I25.701	C70.1	G93.2	S06.330[D,S]
K51.919	K80.64	I25.708	C71*	G93.40	S06.331[D,S]
K52*	K80.70	I25.709	C72.0	G93.41	S06.332[D,S]
K55.1	K80.80	I25.710	C72.1	G93.49	S06.333[D,S]
K55.20	K81.1	I25.711	D32.0	G93.5	S06.334[D,S]
K55.8	K81.9	I25.718	D32.1	G93.81	S06.335[D,S]
K55.9	K82.4	I25.719	D33.0	G93.89	S06.336[D,S]
K56.41	K82.8	I25.720	D33.1	G95.0	S06.339[D,S]
K56.49	K82.9	I25.721	D33.2	G95.11	S06.340[D,S]
K57.10	K83.4	I25.728	D33.4	G95.19	S06.341[D,S]
K57.12	K83.5	I25.729	E03.5	G95.81	S06.342[D,S]
K57.30	K83.8	I25.730	E75.00	G95.89	S06.343[D,S]
K57.32	K83.9	I25.731	E75.01	*G99.2*	S06.344[D,S]
K57.50	K86*	I25.738	E75.02	I67.3	S06.345[D,S]
K57.52	K90.0	I25.739	E75.09	Q05*	S06.346[D,S]
K57.90	K90.1	I25.750	E75.10	Q07.00	S06.349[D,S]
K57.92	K90.2	I25.751	E75.11	Q07.01	S06.350[D,S]
K58*	K90.3	I25.758	E75.19	Q07.02	S06.351[D,S]
K59.1	K90.4	I25.759	E75.23	Q07.03	S06.352[D,S]
K59.2	K90.89	I25.760	E75.25	R40.2*	S06.353[D,S]
K59.3*	K90.9	I25.761	E75.29	R40.3	S06.354[D,S]
K59.8	K91.0	I25.768	E75.4	S04.02XS	S06.355[D,S]
K62.6	K91.1	I25.769	F84.2	S04.031S	S06.356[D,S]
K62.7	K91.2	I25.790	G00*	S04.032S	S06.359[D,S]
K62.82	K91.5	I25.791	*G01*	S04.041S	S06.360[D,S]
K62.89	K91.850	I25.798	*G02*	S04.042S	S06.361[D,S]
K62.9	K91.858	I25.799	G03*	S04.30XS	S06.362[D,S]
K63.0	K91.89	I25.810	G04.00	S06.0X0S	S06.363[D,S]
K63.3	K92.89	I25.811	G04.01	S06.0X1S	S06.364[D,S]
K63.89	K94.02	I25.812	G04.1	S06.0X9S	S06.365[D,S]
K65.4	K94.03	I25.82	G04.2	S06.1X0[D,S]	S06.366[D,S]
K66.0	K94.09	I25.83	G04.30	S06.1X1[D,S]	S06.367D
K66.8	K94.12	I25.89	G04.31	S06.1X2[D,S]	S06.368D
K67	K94.13	I50.1	G04.81	S06.1X3[D,S]	S06.369[D,S]
K68.9	K94.19	I50.20	G04.89	S06.1X4[D,S]	S06.370[D,S]
K70*	K94.22	I50.21	G04.90	S06.1X5[D,S]	S06.371[D,S]
K72.10	K94.23	I50.22	G04.91	S06.1X6[D,S]	S06.372[D,S]
K72.11	K94.29	I50.23	*G05.3*	S06.1X9[D,S]	S06.373[D,S]
K72.90	K94.32	I50.30	*G05.4*	S06.2X0[D,S]	S06.374[D,S]
K72.91	K94.33	I50.31	G06.0	S06.2X1[D,S]	S06.375[D,S]
K73*	K94.39	I50.32	G06.1	S06.2X2[D,S]	S06.376[D,S]
K74*	N99.4	I50.33	G06.2	S06.2X3[D,S]	S06.377D
K75.2	R11.13	I50.40	*G07*	S06.2X4[D,S]	S06.379[D,S]
K75.3	R18.8	I50.41	G08	S06.2X5[D,S]	S06.380[D,S]
K75.4		I50.42	G09	S06.2X6[D,S]	S06.381[D,S]
K75.81	**08 Heart Disease**	I50.43	G11.4	S06.2X9[D,S]	S06.382[D,S]
K75.89	A01.02	I50.9	G12.0	S06.300[D,S]	S06.383[D,S]
K75.9	I20.0		G12.1	S06.301[D,S]	S06.384[D,S]
K76.0	I21.01	**09 Hypertension**	G12.20	S06.302[D,S]	S06.385[D,S]
K76.1	I21.02	I11*	G12.21	S06.303[D,S]	S06.386[D,S]
K76.5	I21.09	I12*	G12.22	S06.304[D,S]	S06.389[D,S]
K76.6	I21.11	I13*	G12.29	S06.305[D,S]	S06.4X0[D,S]
K76.7	I21.19	I15*	G12.8	S06.306[D,S]	S06.4X1[D,S]
K76.89	I21.21			S06.309[D,S]	S06.4X2[D,S]
	I21.29			S06.310[D,S]	S06.4X3[D,S]

10 Neuro 1 – Brain disorders and paralysis (continued)

S06.4X4[D,S]	S14.116[D,S]	S24.4XX[D,S]	G52*	I02.9	S44.01X[D,S]
S06.4X5[D,S]	S14.117[D,S]	S34.01X[D,S]	*G53*	M05.411	S44.02X[D,S]
S06.4X6[D,S]	S14.118[D,S]	S34.02X[D,S]	G54.0	M05.412	S44.11X[D,S]
S06.4X9[D,S]	S14.119[D,S]	S34.101[D,S]	G54.1	M05.421	S44.12X[D,S]
S06.5X0[D,S]	S14.121[D,S]	S34.102[D,S]	G54.5	M05.422	S44.21X[D,S]
S06.5X1[D,S]	S14.122[D,S]	S34.103[D,S]	G57.21	M05.431	S44.22X[D,S]
S06.5X2[D,S]	S14.123[D,S]	S34.104[D,S]	G57.22	M05.432	S44.31X[D,S]
S06.5X3[D,S]	S14.124[D,S]	S34.105[D,S]	G57.23	M05.441	S44.32X[D,S]
S06.5X4[D,S]	S14.125[D,S]	S34.109[D,S]	G58.7	M05.442	S44.41X[D,S]
S06.5X5[D,S]	S14.126[D,S]	S34.111[D,S]	G58.8	M05.451	S44.42X[D,S]
S06.5X6[D,S]	S14.127[D,S]	S34.112[D,S]	G58.9	M05.452	S44.51X[D,S]
S06.5X9[D,S]	S14.128[D,S]	S34.113[D,S]	G60*	M05.461	S44.52X[D,S]
S06.6X0[D,S]	S14.129[D,S]	S34.114[D,S]	G61.0	M05.462	S44.8X1[D,S]
S06.6X1[D,S]	S14.131[D,S]	S34.115[D,S]	G61.1	M05.471	S44.8X2[D,S]
S06.6X2[D,S]	S14.132[D,S]	S34.119[D,S]	G61.81	M05.472	S44.91X[D,S]
S06.6X3[D,S]	S14.133[D,S]	S34.121[D,S]	G61.89	M05.49	S44.92X[D,S]
S06.6X4[D,S]	S14.134[D,S]	S34.122[D,S]	G62.0	M05.511	S54.01X[D,S]
S06.6X5[D,S]	S14.135[D,S]	S34.123[D,S]	G62.1	M05.512	S54.02X[D,S]
S06.6X6[D,S]	S14.136[D,S]	S34.124[D,S]	G62.2	M05.521	S54.11X[D,S]
S06.6X9[D,S]	S14.137[D,S]	S34.125[D,S]	G62.81	M05.522	S54.12X[D,S]
S06.810[D,S]	S14.138[D,S]	S34.129[D,S]	G62.82	M05.531	S54.21X[D,S]
S06.811[D,S]	S14.139[D,S]	S34.131[D,S]	G62.89	M05.532	S54.22X[D,S]
S06.812[D,S]	S14.141[D,S]	S34.132[D,S]	*G63*	M05.541	S54.31X[D,S]
S06.813[D,S]	S14.142[D,S]	S34.139[D,S]	G64	M05.542	S54.32X[D,S]
S06.814[D,S]	S14.143[D,S]	S34.21X[D,S]	G70.00	M05.551	S54.8X1[D,S]
S06.815[D,S]	S14.144[D,S]	S34.22X[D,S]	G70.01	M05.552	S54.8X2[D,S]
S06.816[D,S]	S14.145[D,S]	S34.3XX[D,S]	G70.1	M05.561	S54.91X[D,S]
S06.819[D,S]	S14.146[D,S]	S34.4XXS	G71.0	M05.562	S54.92X[D,S]
S06.820[D,S]	S14.147[D,S]	S34.5XX[D,S]	G71.2	M05.571	S64.01X[D,S]
S06.821[D,S]	S14.148[D,S]	S74.01XS	G71.3	M05.572	S64.02X[D,S]
S06.822[D,S]	S14.149[D,S]	S74.02XS	G71.8	M05.59	S64.11X[D,S]
S06.823[D,S]	S14.151[D,S]	S74.11XS	G72.0	M33.02	S64.12X[D,S]
S06.824[D,S]	S14.152[D,S]	S74.12XS	G72.1	M33.12	S64.21X[D,S]
S06.825[D,S]	S14.153[D,S]	S94.21XS	G72.2	M33.22	S64.22X[D,S]
S06.826[D,S]	S14.154[D,S]	S94.22XS	G72.3	M33.92	S64.31X[D,S]
S06.829[D,S]	S14.155[D,S]		G72.41	M34.82	S64.32X[D,S]
S06.890[D,S]	S14.156[D,S]		G72.49	M34.83	S64.490[D,S]
S06.891[D,S]	S14.157[D,S]	**11 Neuro 2 –**	G72.81	M35.03	S64.491S[D,S]
S06.892[D,S]	S14.158[D,S]	**Peripheral**	G72.89	S04.011[D,S]	S64.492[D,S]
S06.893[D,S]	S14.159[D,S]	**neurological disorders**	*G73.3*	S04.012[D,S]	S64.493[D,S]
S06.894[D,S]	S14.2XX[D,S]	A52.15	*G73.7*	S04.11X[D,S]	S64.494[D,S]
S06.895[D,S]	S14.3XXS	B91	G80*	S04.12X[D,S]	S64.495[D,S]
S06.896[D,S]	S14.5XX[D,S]	E09.44	G83.0	S04.21X[D,S]	S64.496[D,S]
S06.899[D,S]	S24.0XX[A,D,S]	G10	G90.01	S04.22X[D,S]	S64.497[D,S]
S06.9X0[D,S]	S24.101[D,S]	G11.0	G90.09	S04.31X[D,S]	S64.498[D,S]
S06.9X1[D,S]	S24.102[D,S]	G11.1	G90.2	S04.32X[D,S]	S64.8X1[D,S]
S06.9X2[D,S]	S24.103[D,S]	G11.2	G90.3	S04.41X[D,S]	S64.8X2[D,S]
S06.9X3[D,S]	S24.104[D,S]	G11.3	G90.50	S04.42X[D,S]	S64.91X[D,S]
S06.9X4[D,S]	S24.109[D,S]	G11.8	G90.511	S04.51X[D,S]	S64.92X[D,S]
S06.9X5[D,S]	S24.111[D,S]	*G13.0*	G90.512	S04.52X[D,S]	S74.01XD
S06.9X6[D,S]	S24.112[D,S]	*G13.1*	G90.513	S04.61X[D,S]	S74.02XD
S06.9X9[D,S]	S24.113[D,S]	G14	G90.521	S04.62X[D,S]	S74.11XD
S14.0XX[D,S]	S24.114[D,S]	G20	G90.522	S04.71X[D,S]	S74.12XD
S14.101[D,S]	S24.119[D,S]	G21*	G90.523	S04.72X[D,S]	S74.21X[D,S]
S14.102[D,S]	S24.131[D,S]	G23*	G90.59	S04.811[D,S]	S74.22X[D,S]
S14.103[D,S]	S24.132[D,S]	G24*	G90.8	S04.812[D,S]	S74.8X1[D,S]
S14.104[D,S]	S24.133[D,S]	G25.0	G90.9	S04.891[D,S]	S74.8X2[D,S]
S14.105[D,S]	S24.134[D,S]	G25.1	G90.511	S04.892[D,S]	S74.91X[D,S]
S14.106[D,S]	S24.139[D,S]	G25.2	*G99.0*	S04.9XX[D,S]	S74.92X[D,S]
S14.107[D,S]	S24.141[D,S]	G25.3	H81.01	S14.3XXD	S84.01X[D,S]
S14.108[D,S]	S24.142[D,S]	G25.4	H81.02	S14.4XX[D,S]	S84.02X[D,S]
S14.109[D,S]	S24.143[D,S]	G25.5	H81.03	S14.8XX[D,S]	S84.11X[D,S]
S14.111[D,S]	S24.144[D,S]	G25.61	H81.41	S14.9XX[D,S]	S84.12X[D,S]
S14.112[D,S]	S24.149[D,S]	G25.69	H81.42	S24.3XX[D,S]	S84.21X[D,S]
S14.113[D,S]	S24.151[D,S]	G25.70	H81.43	S24.8XX[D,S]	S84.22X[D,S]
S14.114[D,S]	S24.152[D,S]	G25.71	H81.49	S24.9XX[D,S]	S84.801[D,S]
S14.115[D,S]	S24.153[D,S]	G25.79	H83.01	S34.4XXD	S84.802[D,S]
	S24.154[D,S]	G25.82	H83.02	S34.6XX[D,S]	S84.91X[D,S]
	S24.159[D,S]	G25.89	H83.03	S34.8XX[D,S]	S84.92X[D,S]
	S24.2XX[D,S]	G25.9	H83.09	S34.9XX[D,S]	S94.01X[D,S]
		G32.89	I02.0		

11 Neuro 2 – Peripheral neurological disorders (continued)

S94.02X[D,S]
S94.11X[D,S]
S94.12X[D,S]
S94.31X[D,S]
S94.32X[D,S]
S94.8X1[D,S]
S94.8X2[D,S]
S94.91X[D,S]
S94.92X[D,S]

12 Neuro 3 – Stroke

G81.01
G81.02
G81.03
G81.04
G81.11
G81.12
G81.13
G81.14
G81.91
G81.92
G81.93
G81.94
G83.11
G83.12
G83.13
G83.14
G83.21
G83.22
G83.23
G83.24
G83.4
I69.00
I69.01*
I69.020
I69.021
I69.022
I69.023
I69.028
I69.031
I69.032
I69.033
I69.034
I69.039
I69.041
I69.042
I69.043
I69.044
I69.051
I69.052
I69.053
I69.054
I69.061
I69.062
I69.063
I69.064
I69.065
I69.090
I69.091
I69.092
I69.093
I69.098
I69.10
I69.11*
I69.120
I69.121

I69.122
I69.123
I69.128
I69.131
I69.132
I69.133
I69.134
I69.139
I69.141
I69.142
I69.143
I69.144
I69.151
I69.152
I69.153
I69.154
I69.161
I69.162
I69.163
I69.164
I69.165
I69.190
I69.191
I69.192
I69.193
I69.198
I69.20
I69.21*
I69.220
I69.221
I69.222
I69.223
I69.228
I69.231
I69.232
I69.233
I69.234
I69.241
I69.242
I69.243
I69.244
I69.251
I69.252
I69.253
I69.254
I69.261
I69.262
I69.263
I69.264
I69.265
I69.290
I69.291
I69.292
I69.293
I69.298
I69.30
I69.31*
I69.320
I69.321
I69.322
I69.323
I69.328
I69.331
I69.332
I69.333
I69.334
I69.341
I69.342
I69.343
I69.344

I69.351
I69.352
I69.353
I69.354
I69.361
I69.362
I69.363
I69.364
I69.365
I69.390
I69.391
I69.392
I69.393
I69.398
I69.80
I69.81*
I69.820
I69.821
I69.822
I69.823
I69.828
I69.831
I69.832
I69.833
I69.834
I69.841
I69.842
I69.843
I69.844
I69.851
I69.852
I69.853
I69.854
I69.861
I69.862
I69.863
I69.864
I69.865
I69.890
I69.891
I69.892
I69.893
I69.898
I69.90
I69.91*
I69.920
I69.921
I69.922
I69.923
I69.928
I69.931
I69.932
I69.933
I69.934
I69.941
I69.942
I69.943
I69.944
I69.951
I69.952
I69.953
I69.954
I69.961
I69.962
I69.963
I69.964
I69.965
I69.990
I69.991
I69.992

I69.993
I69.998
R41.4

13 Neuro 4 – Multiple sclerosis

G35
G36*
G37.0
G37.1
G37.2
G37.3
G37.5
G37.8
G37.9

14 Ortho 1 – Leg disorders

M00.051
M00.052
M00.061
M00.062
M00.071
M00.072
M00.151
M00.152
M00.161
M00.162
M00.171
M00.172
M00.251
M00.252
M00.261
M00.262
M00.271
M00.272
M00.851
M00.852
M00.861
M00.862
M00.871
M00.872
M01.X51
M01.X52
M01.X61
M01.X62
M01.X71
M01.X72
M02.051
M02.052
M02.061
M02.062
M02.071
M02.072
M02.151
M02.152
M02.161
M02.162
M02.171
M02.172
M02.251
M02.252
M02.261
M02.262
M02.271
M02.272
M02.351
M02.352
M02.361
M02.362

M02.371
M02.372
M02.851
M02.852
M02.861
M02.862
M02.871
M02.872
M07.651
M07.652
M07.661
M07.662
M07.671
M07.672
M07.679
M11.051
M11.052
M11.061
M11.062
M11.071
M11.072
M11.151
M11.152
M11.161
M11.162
M11.171
M11.172
M11.251
M11.252
M11.261
M11.262
M11.271
M11.272
M11.851
M11.852
M11.861
M11.862
M11.871
M11.872
M12.151
M12.152
M12.161
M12.162
M12.171
M12.172
M12.251
M12.252
M12.261
M12.262
M12.271
M12.272
M12.351
M12.352
M12.361
M12.362
M12.371
M12.372
M12.451
M12.452
M12.461
M12.462
M12.471
M12.472
M12.551
M12.552
M12.561
M12.562
M12.571
M12.572
M12.851

M12.852
M12.861
M12.862
M12.871
M12.872
M13.851
M13.852
M13.861
M13.862
M13.871
M13.872
M14.651
M14.652
M14.661
M14.662
M14.671
M14.672
M14.851
M14.852
M14.861
M14.862
M14.871
M14.872
M22.01
M22.02
M22.11
M22.12
M22.2X1
M22.2X2
M22.3X1
M22.3X2
M22.41
M22.42
M22.8X1
M22.8X2
M22.91
M22.92
M23.000
M23.001
M23.003
M23.004
M23.006
M23.007
M23.011
M23.012
M23.021
M23.022
M23.031
M23.032
M23.041
M23.042
M23.051
M23.052
M23.061
M23.062
M23.200
M23.201
M23.203
M23.204
M23.206
M23.207
M23.211
M23.212
M23.221
M23.222
M23.231
M23.232
M23.241

14 Ortho 1 – Leg disorders (continued)

M23.242	M24.471	M61.461	M84.751[D,G,K,P,S]	M89.451	S32.482[D,G,K]
M23.251	M24.472	M61.462	M84.752[D,G,K,P,S]	M89.452	S32.484[D,G,K]
M23.252	M24.474	M61.471	M84.754[D,G,K,P,S]	M89.461	S32.485[D,G,K]
M23.261	M24.475	M61.472	M84.755[D,G,K,P,S]	M89.462	S32.491[D,G,K]
M23.262	M24.477	M61.551	M84.757[D,G,K,P,S]	M89.471	S32.492[D,G,K]
M23.300	M24.478	M61.552	M84.758[D,G,K,P,S]	M89.472	S32.501[D,G,K]
M23.301	M24.551	M61.561	M86.051	M89.651	S32.502[D,G,K]
M23.303	M24.552	M61.562	M86.052	M89.652	S32.511[D,G,K]
M23.304	M24.561	M61.571	M86.061	M89.661	S32.512[D,G,K]
M23.306	M24.562	M61.572	M86.062	M89.662	S32.591[D,G,K]
M23.307	M24.571	M66.251	M86.071	M89.671	S32.592[D,G,K]
M23.311	M24.572	M66.252	M86.072	M89.672	S32.601[D,G,K]
M23.312	M24.574	M66.261	M86.151	*M90.551*	S32.602[D,G,K]
M23.321	M24.575	M66.262	M86.152	*M90.552*	S32.611[D,G,K]
M23.322	M24.651	M66.271	M86.161	*M90.561*	S32.612[D,G,K]
M23.331	M24.652	M66.272	M86.162	*M90.562*	S32.614[D,G,K]
M23.332	M24.661	M66.361	M86.171	*M90.571*	S32.615[D,G,K]
M23.341	M24.662	M66.362	M86.172	*M90.572*	S32.691[D,G,K]
M23.342	M24.671	M66.371	M86.251	*M90.651*	S32.692[D,G,K]
M23.351	M24.672	M66.372	M86.252	*M90.652*	S32.810[D,G,K]
M23.352	M24.674	M66.861	M86.261	*M90.661*	S32.811[D,G,K]
M23.361	M24.675	M66.862	M86.262	*M90.662*	S32.82X[D,G,K]
M23.362	M25.051	M66.871	M86.271	*M90.671*	S32.89X[D,G,K]
M23.41	M25.052	M66.872	M86.272	*M90.672*	S32.9XX[D,G,K]
M23.42	M25.061	M80.051[D,G,K,P]	M86.351	*M90.851*	S72.001[D,E,F,G,H, J,K,M,N,P,Q,R]
M23.51	M25.062	M80.052[D,G,K,P]	M86.352	*M90.852*	S72.002[D,E,F,G,H, J,K,M,N,P,Q,R]
M23.52	M25.071	M80.061[D,G,K,P]	M86.361	*M90.861*	S72.011[D,E,F,G,H, J,K,M,N,P,Q,R]
M23.601	M25.072	M80.062[D,G,K,P]	M86.362	*M90.862*	S72.012[D,E,F,G,H, J,K,M,N,P,Q,R]
M23.602	M25.074	M80.071[D,G,K,P]	M86.371	*M90.871*	S72.021[D,E,F,G,H, J,K,M,N,P,Q,R]
M23.611	M25.075	M80.072[D,G,K,P]	M86.372	*M90.872*	S72.022[D,E,F,G,H, J,K,M,N,P,Q,R]
M23.612	M60.051	M80.851[D,G,K,P]	M86.451	Q68.6	S72.024[D,E,F,G,H, J,K,M,N,P,Q,R]
M23.621	M60.052	M80.852[D,G,K,P]	M86.452	S32.301[D,G,K]	S72.025[D,E,F,G,H, J,K,M,N,P,Q,R]
M23.622	M60.061	M80.861[D,G,K,P]	M86.461	S32.302[D,G,K]	S72.031[D,E,F,G,H, J,K,M,N,P,Q,R]
M23.631	M60.062	M80.862[D,G,K,P]	M86.462	S32.311[D,G,K]	S72.032[D,E,F,G,H, J,K,M,N,P,Q,R]
M23.632	M60.070	M80.871[D,G,K,P]	M86.471	S32.312[D,G,K]	S72.034[D,E,F,G,H, J,K,M,N,P,Q,R]
M23.641	M60.071	M80.872[D,G,K,P]	M86.472	S32.314[D,G,K]	S72.035[D,E,F,G,H, J,K,M,N,P,Q,R]
M23.642	M60.073	M84.451[D,G,K,P]	M86.551	S32.315[D,G,K]	S72.041[D,E,F,G,H, J,K,M,N,P,Q,R]
M23.671	M60.074	M84.452[D,G,K,P]	M86.552	S32.391[D,G,K]	S72.042[D,E,F,G,H, J,K,M,N,P,Q,R]
M23.672	M60.076	M84.461[D,G,K,P]	M86.561	S32.392[D,G,K]	S72.044[D,E,F,G,H, J,K,M,N,P,Q,R]
M23.8X1	M60.077	M84.462[D,G,K,P]	M86.562	S32.401[D,G,K]	S72.045[D,E,F,G,H, J,K,M,N,P,Q,R]
M23.8X2	M61.051	M84.463[D,G,K,P]	M86.571	S32.402[D,G,K]	S72.051[D,E,F,G,H, J,K,M,N,P,Q,R]
M23.91	M61.052	M84.464[D,G,K,P]	M86.572	S32.411[D,G,K]	S72.052[D,E,F,G,H, J,K,M,N,P,Q,R]
M23.92	M61.061	M84.471[D,G,K,P]	M86.651	S32.412[D,G,K]	S72.061[D,E,F,G,H, J,K,M,N,P,Q,R]
M24.051	M61.062	M84.472[D,G,K,P]	M86.652	S32.414[D,G,K]	S72.062[D,E,F,G,H, J,K,M,N,P,Q,R]
M24.052	M61.071	M84.474[D,G,K,P]	M86.661	S32.415[D,G,K]	S72.064[D,E,F,G,H, J,K,M,N,P,Q,R]
M24.071	M61.072	M84.475[D,G,K,P]	M86.662	S32.421[D,G,K]	S72.065[D,E,F,G,H, J,K,M,N,P,Q,R]
M24.072	M61.151	M84.477[D,G,K,P]	M86.671	S32.422[D,G,K]	S72.091[D,E,F,G,H, J,K,M,N,P,Q,R]
M24.074	M61.152	M84.478[D,G,K,P]	M86.672	S32.424[D,G,K]	S72.092[D,E,F,G,H, J,K,M,N,P,Q,R]
M24.075	M61.161	M84.550[D,G,K,P]	M86.8X5	S32.425[D,G,K]	
M24.08	M61.162	M84.551[D,G,K,P]	M86.8X6	S32.431[D,G,K]	
M24.151	M61.171	M84.552[D,G,K,P]	M86.8X7	S32.432[D,G,K]	
M24.152	M61.172	M84.561[G,K,P] (per CMS)	M87.051	S32.434[D,G,K]	
M24.171	M61.174	M84.562[D,G,K,P]	M87.052	S32.435[D,G,K]	
M24.172	M61.175	M84.563[D,G,K,P]	M87.150	S32.441[D,G,K]	
M24.174	M61.177	M84.564[D,G,K,P]	M87.151	S32.442[D,G,K]	
M24.175	M61.178	M84.571[D,G,K,P]	M87.152	S32.444[D,G,K]	
M24.351	M61.251	M84.572[D,G,K,P]	M87.251	S32.445[D,G,K]	
M24.352	M61.252	M84.574[D,G,K,P]	M87.252	S32.451[D,G,K]	
M24.361	M61.261	M84.575[D,G,K,P]	M87.350	S32.452[D,G,K]	
M24.362	M61.262	M84.650[D,G,K,P]	M87.351	S32.454[D,G,K]	
M24.371	M61.271	M84.651[D,G,K,P]	M87.352	S32.455[D,G,K]	
M24.372	M61.272	M84.652[D,G,K,P]	M87.850	S32.461[D,G,K]	
M24.374	M61.351	M84.661[D,G,K,P]	M87.851	S32.462[D,G,K]	
M24.375	M61.352	M84.662[D,G,K,P]	M87.852	S32.464[D,G,K]	
M24.451	M61.361	M84.663[D,G,K,P]	M88.851	S32.465[D,G,K]	
M24.452	M61.362	M84.664[D,G,K,P]	M88.852	S32.471[D,G,K]	
M24.461	M61.371	M84.671[D,G,K,P]	M88.861	S32.472[D,G,K]	
M24.462	M61.372	M84.672[D,G,K,P]	M88.862	S32.474[D,G,K]	
	M61.451	M84.674[D,G,K,P]	M88.871	S32.475[D,G,K]	
	M61.452	M84.675[D,G,K,P]	M88.872	S32.481[D,G,K]	

14 Ortho 1 – Leg disorders (continued)

S72.101[D,E,F,G,H,J,K,M,N,P,Q,R]
S72.102[D,E,F,G,H,J,K,M,N,P,Q,R]
S72.111[D,E,F,G,H,J,K,M,N,P,Q,R]
S72.112[D,E,F,G,H,J,K,M,N,P,Q,R]
S72.114[D,E,F,G,H,J,K,M,N,P,Q,R]
S72.115[D,E,F,G,H,J,K,M,N,P,Q,R]
S72.121[D,E,F,G,H,J,K,M,N,P,Q,R]
S72.122[D,E,F,G,H,J,K,M,N,P,Q,R]
S72.124[D,E,F,G,H,J,K,M,N,P,Q,R]
S72.125[D,E,F,G,H,J,K,M,N,P,Q,R]
S72.131[D,E,F,G,H,J,K,M,N,P,Q,R]
S72.132[D,E,F,G,H,J,K,M,N,P,Q,R]
S72.134[D,E,F,G,H,J,K,M,N,P,Q,R]
S72.135[D,E,F,G,H,J,K,M,N,P,Q,R]
S72.141[D,E,F,G,H,J,K,M,N,P,Q,R]
S72.142[D,E,F,G,H,J,K,M,N,P,Q,R]
S72.144[D,E,F,G,H,J,K,M,N,P,Q,R]
S72.145[D,E,F,G,H,J,K,M,N,P,Q,R]
S72.21X[D,E,F,G,H,J,K,M,N,P,Q,R]
S72.22X[D,E,F,G,H,J,K,M,N,P,Q,R]
S72.24X[D,E,F,G,H,J,K,M,N,P,Q,R]
S72.25X[D,E,F,G,H,J,K,M,N,P,Q,R]
S72.301[D,E,F,G,H,J,K,M,N,P,Q,R]
S72.302[D,E,F,G,H,J,K,M,N,P,Q,R]
S72.321[D,E,F,G,H,J,K,M,N,P,Q,R]
S72.322[D,E,F,G,H,J,K,M,N,P,Q,R]
S72.324[D,E,F,G,H,J,K,M,N,P,Q,R]
S72.325[D,E,F,G,H,J,K,M,N,P,Q,R]
S72.331[D,E,F,G,H,J,K,M,N,P,Q,R]
S72.332[D,E,F,G,H,J,K,M,N,P,Q,R]
S72.334[D,E,F,G,H,J,K,M,N,P,Q,R]
S72.335[D,E,F,G,H,J,K,M,N,P,Q,R]
S72.341[D,E,F,G,H,J,K,M,N,P,Q,R]
S72.342[D,E,F,G,H,J,K,M,N,P,Q,R]
S72.344[D,E,F,G,H,J,K,M,N,P,Q,R]

S72.345[D,E,F,G,H,J,K,M,N,P,Q,R]
S72.351[D,E,F,G,H,J,K,M,N,P,Q,R]
S72.352[D,E,F,G,H,J,K,M,N,P,Q,R]
S72.354[D,E,F,G,H,J,K,M,N,P,Q,R]
S72.355[D,E,F,G,H,J,K,M,N,P,Q,R]
S72.361[D,E,F,G,H,J,K,M,N,P,Q,R]
S72.362[D,E,F,G,H,J,K,M,N,P,Q,R]
S72.364[D,E,F,G,H,J,K,M,N,P,Q,R]
S72.365[D,E,F,G,H,J,K,M,N,P,Q,R]
S72.391[D,E,F,G,H,J,K,M,N,P,Q,R]
S72.392[D,E,F,G,H,J,K,M,N,P,Q,R]
S72.401[E,F,H,J,M,N,Q,R]
S72.402[E,F,H,J,M,N,Q,R]
S72.411[E,F,H,J,M,N,Q,R]
S72.412[E,F,H,J,M,N,Q,R]
S72.414[E,F,H,J,M,N,Q,R]
S72.415[E,F,H,J,M,N,Q,R]
S72.421[E,F,H,J,M,N,Q,R]
S72.422[E,F,H,J,M,N,Q,R]
S72.424[E,F,H,J,M,N,Q,R]
S72.425[E,F,H,J,M,N,Q,R]
S72.431[E,F,H,J,M,N,Q,R]
S72.432[E,F,H,J,M,N,Q,R]
S72.434[E,F,H,J,M,N,Q,R]
S72.435[E,F,H,J,M,N,Q,R]
S72.441[E,F,H,J,M,N,Q,R]
S72.442[E,F,H,J,M,N,Q,R]
S72.444[E,F,H,J,M,N,Q,R]
S72.445[E,F,H,J,M,N,Q,R]
S72.451[D,E,F,G,H,J,K,M,N,P,Q,R]
S72.452[D,E,F,G,H,J,K,M,N,P,Q,R]
S72.454[D,E,F,G,H,J,K,M,N,P,Q,R]
S72.455[D,E,F,G,H,J,K,M,N,P,Q,R]
S72.461[D,E,F,G,H,J,K,M,N,P,Q,R]
S72.462[D,E,F,G,H,J,K,M,N,P,Q,R]
S72.464[D,E,F,G,H,J,K,M,N,P,Q,R]
S72.465[D,E,F,G,H,J,K,M,N,P,Q,R]
S72.471[D,G,K,P]
S72.472[D,G,K,P]
S72.491[D,E,F,G,H,J,K,M,N,P,Q,R]
S72.492[D,E,F,G,H,J,K,M,N,P,Q,R]
S72.8X1[D,E,F,G,H,J,K,M,N,P,Q,R]
S72.8X2[D,E,F,G,H,J,K,M,N,P,Q,R]
S72.91X[D,E,F,G,H,J,K,M,N,P,Q,R]
S72.92X[D,E,F,G,H,J,K,M,N,P,Q,R]
S73.005D
S73.011D

S73.012D
S73.014D
S73.015D
S73.021D
S73.022D
S73.024D
S73.025D
S73.031D
S73.032D
S73.034D
S73.035D
S73.041D
S73.042D
S73.044D
S73.045D
S77.01XD
S77.02XD
S77.11XD
S77.12XD
S77.21XD
S77.22XD
S78.011[A,D]
S78.012[A,D]
S78.021[A,D]
S78.022[A,D]
S78.111[A,D]
S78.112[A,D]
S78.121[A,D]
S78.122[A,D]
S78.911[A,D]
S78.912[A,D]
S78.921[A,D]
S78.922[A,D]
S79.001[D,G,K,P]
S79.002[D,G,K,P]
S79.011[D,G,K,P]
S79.012[D,G,K,P]
S79.091[D,G,K,P]
S79.092[D,G,K,P]
S79.101[D,G,K,P]
S79.102[D,G,K,P]
S79.111[D,G,K,P]
S79.112[D,G,K,P]
S79.121[D,G,K,P]
S79.122[D,G,K,P]
S79.131[D,G,K,P]
S79.132[D,G,K,P]
S79.141[D,G,K,P]
S79.142[D,G,K,P]
S79.191[D,G,K,P]
S79.192[D,G,K,P]
S82.001[D,E,F,G,H,J,K,M,N,P,Q,R]
S82.002[D,E,F,G,H,J,K,M,N,P,Q,R]
S82.011[D,E,F,G,H,J,K,M,N,P,Q,R]
S82.012[D,E,F,G,H,J,K,M,N,P,Q,R]
S82.014[D,E,F,G,H,J,K,M,N,P,Q,R]
S82.015[D,E,F,G,H,J,K,M,N,P,Q,R]
S82.021[D,E,F,G,H,J,K,M,N,P,Q,R]
S82.022[D,E,F,G,H,J,K,M,N,P,Q,R]
S82.024[D,E,F,G,H,J,K,M,N,P,Q,R]
S82.025[D,E,F,G,H,J,K,M,N,P,Q,R]

S82.031[D,E,F,G,H,J,K,M,N,P,Q,R]
S82.032[D,E,F,G,H,J,K,M,N,P,Q,R]
S82.034[D,E,F,G,H,J,K,M,N,P,Q,R]
S82.035[D,E,F,G,H,J,K,M,N,P,Q,R]
S82.041[D,E,F,G,H,J,K,M,N,P,Q,R]
S82.042[D,E,F,G,H,J,K,M,N,P,Q,R]
S82.044[D,E,F,G,H,J,K,M,N,P,Q,R]
S82.045[D,E,F,G,H,J,K,M,N,P,Q,R]
S82.091[D,E,F,G,H,J,K,M,N,P,Q,R]
S82.092[D,E,F,G,H,J,K,M,N,P,Q,R]
S82.101[D,E,F,G,H,J,K,M,N,P,Q,R]
S82.102[D,E,F,G,H,J,K,M,N,P,Q,R]
S82.111[D,E,F,G,H,J,K,M,N,P,Q,R]
S82.112[D,E,F,G,H,J,K,M,N,P,Q,R]
S82.114[D,E,F,G,H,J,K,M,N,P,Q,R]
S82.115[D,E,F,G,H,J,K,M,N,P,Q,R]
S82.121[D,E,F,G,H,J,K,M,N,P,Q,R]
S82.122[D,E,F,G,H,J,K,M,N,P,Q,R]
S82.124[D,E,F,G,H,J,K,M,N,P,Q,R]
S82.125[D,E,F,G,H,J,K,M,N,P,Q,R]
S82.131[D,E,F,G,H,J,K,M,N,P,Q,R]
S82.132[D,E,F,G,H,J,K,M,N,P,Q,R]
S82.134[D,E,F,G,H,J,K,M,N,P,Q,R]
S82.135[D,E,F,G,H,J,K,M,N,P,Q,R]
S82.141[D,E,F,G,H,J,K,M,N,P,Q,R]
S82.142[D,E,F,G,H,J,K,M,N,P,Q,R]
S82.144[D,E,F,G,H,J,K,M,N,P,Q,R]
S82.145[D,E,F,G,H,J,K,M,N,P,Q,R]
S82.151[D,E,F,G,H,J,K,M,N,P,Q,R]
S82.152[D,E,F,G,H,J,K,M,N,P,Q,R]
S82.154[D,E,F,G,H,J,K,M,N,P,Q,R]
S82.155[D,E,F,G,H,J,K,M,N,P,Q,R]
S82.161[D,G,K,P]
S82.162[D,G,K,P]
S82.191[D,E,F,G,H,J,K,M,N,P,Q,R]
S82.192[D,E,F,G,H,J,K,M,N,P,Q,R]
S82.201[D,E,F,G,H,J,K,M,N,P,Q,R]

S82.202[D,E,F,G,H,J,K,M,N,P,Q,R]
S82.209[E,F,H,J,M,N,Q,R]
S82.221[D,E,F,G,H,J,K,M,N,P,Q,R]
S82.222[D,E,F,G,H,J,K,M,N,P,Q,R]
S82.224[D,E,F,G,H,J,K,M,N,P,Q,R]
S82.225[D,E,F,G,H,J,K,M,N,P,Q,R]
S82.231[D,E,F,G,H,J,K,M,N,P,Q,R]
S82.232[D,E,F,G,H,J,K,M,N,P,Q,R]
S82.234[D,E,F,G,H,J,K,M,N,P,Q,R]
S82.235[D,E,F,G,H,J,K,M,N,P,Q,R]
S82.241[D,E,F,G,H,J,K,M,N,P,Q,R]
S82.242[D,E,F,G,H,J,K,M,N,P,Q,R]
S82.244[D,E,F,G,H,J,K,M,N,P,Q,R]
S82.245[D,E,F,G,H,J,K,M,N,P,Q,R]
S82.251[D,E,F,G,H,J,K,M,N,P,Q,R]
S82.252[D,E,F,G,H,J,K,M,N,P,Q,R]
S82.254[D,E,F,G,H,J,K,M,N,P,Q,R]
S82.255[D,E,F,G,H,J,K,M,N,P,Q,R]
S82.261[D,E,F,G,H,J,K,M,N,P,Q,R]
S82.262[D,E,F,G,H,J,K,M,N,P,Q,R]
S82.264[D,E,F,G,H,J,K,M,N,P,Q,R]
S82.265[D,E,F,G,H,J,K,M,N,P,Q,R]
S82.291[D,E,F,G,H,J,K,M,N,P,Q,R]
S82.292[D,E,F,G,H,J,K,M,N,P,Q,R]
S82.301[D,E,F,G,H,J,K,M,N,P,Q,R]
S82.302[D,E,F,G,H,J,K,M,N,P,Q,R]
S82.311[D,G,K,P]
S82.312[D,G,K,P]
S82.391[D,E,F,G,H,J,K,M,N,P,Q,R]
S82.392[D,E,F,G,H,J,K,M,N,P,Q,R]
S82.401[D,E,F,G,H,J,K,M,N,P,Q,R]
S82.402[D,E,F,G,H,J,K,M,N,P,Q,R]
S82.421[D,E,F,G,H,J,K,M,N,P,Q,R]
S82.422[D,E,F,G,H,J,K,M,N,P,Q,R]
S82.424[D,E,F,G,H,J,K,M,N,P,Q,R]
S82.425[D,E,F,G,H,J,K,M,N,P,Q,R]
S82.431[D,E,F,G,H,J,K,M,N,P,Q,R]
S82.432[D,E,F,G,H,J,K,M,N,P,Q,R]

S82.434[D,E,F,G,H,J,K,M,N,P,Q,R]
S82.435[D,E,F,G,H,J,K,M,N,P,Q,R]
S82.441[D,E,F,G,H,J,K,M,N,P,Q,R]
S82.442[D,E,F,G,H,J,K,M,N,P,Q,R]
S82.444[D,E,F,G,H,J,K,M,N,P,Q,R]
S82.445[D,E,F,G,H,J,K,M,N,P,Q,R]
S82.451[D,E,F,G,H,J,K,M,N,P,Q,R]
S82.452[D,E,F,G,H,J,K,M,N,P,Q,R]
S82.454[D,E,F,G,H,J,K,M,N,P,Q,R]
S82.455[D,E,F,G,H,J,K,M,N,P,Q,R]
S82.461[D,E,F,G,H,J,K,M,N,P,Q,R]
S82.462[D,E,F,G,H,J,K,M,N,P,Q,R]
S82.464[D,E,F,G,H,J,K,M,N,P,Q,R]
S82.465[D,E,F,G,H,J,K,M,N,P,Q,R]
S82.491[D,E,F,G,H,J,K,M,N,P,Q,R]
S82.492[D,E,F,G,H,J,K,M,N,P,Q,R]
S82.51X[D,E,F,G,H,J,K,M,N,P,Q,R]
S82.52X[D,E,F,G,H,J,K,M,N,P,Q,R]
S82.54X[D,E,F,G,H,J,K,M,N,P,Q,R]
S82.55X[D,E,F,G,H,J,K,M,N,P,Q,R]
S82.61X[D,E,F,G,H,J,K,M,N,P,Q,R]
S82.62X[D,E,F,G,H,J,K,M,N,P,Q,R]
S82.64X[D,E,F,G,H,J,K,M,N,P,Q,R]
S82.65X[D,E,F,G,H,J,K,M,N,P,Q,R]
S82.811[D,G,K,P]
S82.812[D,G,K,P]
S82.821[D,G,K,P]
S82.822[D,G,K,P]
S82.831[D,E,F,G,H,J,K,M,N,P,Q,R]
S82.832[D,E,F,G,H,J,K,M,N,P,Q,R]
S82.841[D,E,F,G,H,J,K,M,N,P,Q,R]
S82.842[D,E,F,G,H,J,K,M,N,P,Q,R]
S82.844[D,E,F,G,H,J,K,M,N,P,Q,R]
S82.845[D,E,F,G,H,J,K,M,N,P,Q,R]
S82.851[D,E,F,G,H,J,K,M,N,P,Q,R]
S82.852[D,E,F,G,H,J,K,M,N,P,Q,R]
S82.854[D,E,F,G,H,J,K,M,N,P,Q,R]
S82.855[D,E,F,G,H,J,K,M,N,P,Q,R]

14 Ortho 1 – Leg disorders (continued)

S82.861[D,E,F,G,H, J,K,M,N,P,Q,R]	S83.222D	S89.322[D,G,K,P]	S92.245[D,G,K,P]	S99.232[D,G,K,P]	M02.011
S82.862[D,E,F,G,H, J,K,M,N,P,Q,R]	S83.231D	S89.391[D,G,K,P]	S92.251[D,G,K,P]	S99.241[D,G,K,P]	M02.012
	S83.232D	S89.392[D,G,K,P]	S92.252[D,G,K,P]	S99.242[D,G,K,P]	M02.021
S82.864[D,E,F,G,H, J,K,M,N,P,Q,R]	S83.241D	S92.001[D,G,K,P]	S92.254[D,G,K,P]	S99.291[D,G,K,P]	M02.022
	S83.242D	S92.002[D,G,K,P]	S92.255[D,G,K,P]	S99.292[D,G,K,P]	M02.031
S82.865[D,E,F,G,H, J,K,M,N,P,Q,R]	S83.251D	S92.011[D,G,K,P]	S92.301[D,G,K,P]		M02.032
	S83.252D	S92.012[D,G,K,P]	S92.302[D,G,K,P]	**15 Ortho 2 – Other**	M02.041
S82.871[D,E,F,G,H, J,K,M,N,P,Q,R]	S83.261D	S92.014[D,G,K,P]	S92.311[D,G,K,P]	**orthopedic disorders**	M02.042
	S83.262D	S92.015[D,G,K,P]	S92.312[D,G,K,P]	A01.04	M02.08
S82.872[D,E,F,G,H, J,K,M,N,P,Q,R]	S83.271D	S92.021[D,G,K,P]	S92.314[D,G,K,P]	A01.05	M02.09
	S83.272D	S92.022[D,G,K,P]	S92.315[D,G,K,P]	A02.23	M02.111
S82.874[D,E,F,G,H, J,K,M,N,P,Q,R]	S83.281D	S92.024[D,G,K,P]	S92.321[D,G,K,P]	A02.24	M02.112
	S83.282D	S92.025[D,G,K,P]	S92.322[D,G,K,P]	A18.01	M02.121
S82.875[D,E,F,G,H, J,K,M,N,P,Q,R]	S83.31XD	S92.031[D,G,K,P]	S92.324[D,G,K,P]	A18.02	M02.122
	S83.32XD	S92.032[D,G,K,P]	S92.325[D,G,K,P]	A18.03	M02.131
S82.891[D,E,F,G,H, J,K,M,N,P,Q,R]	S87.01XD	S92.034[D,G,K,P]	S92.331[D,G,K,P]	A52.16	M02.132
	S87.02XD	S92.035[D,G,K,P]	S92.332[D,G,K,P]	*E08.610*	M02.141
S82.892[D,E,F,G,H, J,K,M,N,P,Q,R]	S87.81XD	S92.041[D,G,K,P]	S92.334[D,G,K,P]	*E08.618*	M02.142
	S87.82XD	S92.042[D,G,K,P]	S92.335[D,G,K,P]	E09.610	M02.18
S82.91X[D,E,F,G,H, J,K,M,N,P,Q,R]	S88.011[A,D]	S92.044[D,G,K,P]	S92.341[D,G,K,P]	E09.618	M02.19
	S88.012[A,D]	S92.045[D,G,K,P]	S92.342[D,G,K,P]	M00.011	M02.211
S82.92X[D,E,F,G,H, J,K,M,N,P,Q,R]	S88.021[A,D]	S92.051[D,G,K,P]	S92.344[D,G,K,P]	M00.012	M02.212
	S88.022[A,D]	S92.052[D,G,K,P]	S92.345[D,G,K,P]	M00.021	M02.221
S83.001D	S88.029[A,D]	S92.054[D,G,K,P]	S92.351[D,G,K,P]	M00.022	M02.222
S83.002D	S88.111[A,D]	S92.055[D,G,K,P]	S92.352[D,G,K,P]	M00.031	M02.231
S83.004D	S88.112[A,D]	S92.061[D,G,K,P]	S92.354[D,G,K,P]	M00.032	M02.232
S83.005D	S88.121[A,D]	S92.062[D,G,K,P]	S92.355[D,G,K,P]	M00.041	M02.241
S83.011D	S88.122[A,D]	S92.064[D,G,K,P]	S92.811[D,G,K,P]	M00.042	M02.242
S83.012D	S88.911[A,D]	S92.065[D,G,K,P]	S92.812[D,G,K,P]	M00.08	M02.28
S83.014D	S88.912[A,D]	S92.101[D,G,K,P]	S92.901[D,G,K,P]	M00.09	M02.29
S83.015D	S88.921[A,D]	S92.102[D,G,K,P]	S92.902[D,G,K,P]	M00.111	M02.311
S83.091D	S88.922[A,D]	S92.111[D,G,K,P]	S97.01XD	M00.112	M02.312
S83.092D	S89.001[D,G,K,P]	S92.112[D,G,K,P]	S97.02XD	M00.121	M02.321
S83.094D	S89.002[D,G,K,P]	S92.114[D,G,K,P]	S97.111D	M00.122	M02.322
S83.095D	S89.011[D,G,K,P]	S92.115[D,G,K,P]	S97.112D	M00.131	M02.331
S83.101D	S89.012[D,G,K,P]	S92.121[D,G,K,P]	S97.121D	M00.132	M02.332
S83.102D	S89.021[D,G,K,P]	S92.122[D,G,K,P]	S97.122D	M00.141	M02.341
S83.104D	S89.022[D,G,K,P]	S92.124[D,G,K,P]	S97.81XD	M00.142	M02.342
S83.105D	S89.031[D,G,K,P]	S92.125[D,G,K,P]	S97.82XD	M00.18	M02.38
S83.111D	S89.032[D,G,K,P]	S92.131[D,G,K,P]	S99.001[D,G,K,P]	M00.19	M02.39
S83.112D	S89.041[D,G,K,P]	S92.132[D,G,K,P]	S99.002[D,G,K,P]	M00.211	*M02.811*
S83.114D	S89.042[D,G,K,P]	S92.134[D,G,K,P]	S99.011[D,G,K,P]	M00.212	*M02.812*
S83.115D	S89.091[D,G,K,P]	S92.135[D,G,K,P]	S99.012[D,G,K,P]	M00.221	*M02.821*
S83.121D	S89.092[D,G,K,P]	S92.141[D,G,K,P]	S99.021[D,G,K,P]	M00.222	*M02.822*
S83.122D	S89.101[D,G,K,P]	S92.142[D,G,K,P]	S99.022[D,G,K,P]	M00.231	*M02.831*
S83.124D	S89.102[D,G,K,P]	S92.144[D,G,K,P]	S99.031[D,G,K,P]	M00.232	*M02.832*
S83.125D	S89.109[D,G,K,P]	S92.145[D,G,K,P]	S99.032[D,G,K,P]	M00.241	*M02.841*
S83.131D	S89.111[D,G,K,P]	S92.151[D,G,K,P]	S99.041[D,G,K,P]	M00.242	*M02.842*
S83.132D	S89.112[D,G,K,P]	S92.152[D,G,K,P]	S99.042[D,G,K,P]	M00.28	*M02.88*
S83.134D	S89.121[D,G,K,P]	S92.154[D,G,K,P]	S99.091[D,G,K,P]	M00.29	*M02.89*
S83.135D	S89.122[D,G,K,P]	S92.155[D,G,K,P]	S99.092[D,G,K,P]	M00.811	*M02.9*
S83.141D	S89.131[D,G,K,P]	S92.191[D,G,K,P]	S99.101[D,G,K,P]	M00.812	M05.011
S83.142D	S89.132[D,G,K,P]	S92.192[D,G,K,P]	S99.102[D,G,K,P]	M00.821	M05.012
S83.144D	S89.141[D,G,K,P]	S92.201[D,G,K,P]	S99.111[D,G,K,P]	M00.822	M05.021
S83.145D	S89.142[D,G,K,P]	S92.202[D,G,K,P]	S99.112[D,G,K,P]	M00.831	M05.022
S83.191D	S89.191[D,G,K,P]	S92.211[D,G,K,P]	S99.121[D,G,K,P]	M00.832	M05.031
S83.192D	S89.192[D,G,K,P]	S92.212[D,G,K,P]	S99.122[D,G,K,P]	M00.841	M05.032
S83.194D	S89.201[D,G,K,P]	S92.214[D,G,K,P]	S99.131[D,G,K,P]	M00.842	M05.041
S83.195D	S89.202[D,G,K,P]	S92.215[D,G,K,P]	S99.132[D,G,K,P]	M00.88	M05.042
S83.200D	S89.211[D,G,K,P]	S92.221[D,G,K,P]	S99.141[D,G,K,P]	M00.89	M05.051
S83.201D	S89.212[D,G,K,P]	S92.222[D,G,K,P]	S99.142[D,G,K,P]	*M01.X11*	M05.052
S83.203D	S89.221[D,G,K,P]	S92.224[D,G,K,P]	S99.191[D,G,K,P]	*M01.X12*	M05.061
S83.204D	S89.222[D,G,K,P]	S92.225[D,G,K,P]	S99.192[D,G,K,P]	*M01.X21*	M05.062
S83.206D	S89.291[D,G,K,P]	S92.231[D,G,K,P]	S99.201[D,G,K,P]	*M01.X22*	M05.071
S83.207D	S89.292[D,G,K,P]	S92.232[D,G,K,P]	S99.202[D,G,K,P]	*M01.X31*	M05.072
S83.211D	S89.301[D,G,K,P]	S92.234[D,G,K,P]	S99.211[D,G,K,P]	*M01.X32*	M05.09
S83.212D	S89.302[D,G,K,P]	S92.235[D,G,K,P]	S99.212[D,G,K,P]	*M01.X41*	M05.111
S83.221D	S89.311[D,G,K,P]	S92.241[D,G,K,P]	S99.221[D,G,K,P]	*M01.X42*	M05.112
	S89.312[D,G,K,P]	S92.242[D,G,K,P]	S99.222[D,G,K,P]	*M01.X8*	M05.121
	S89.321[D,G,K,P]	S92.244[D,G,K,P]	S99.231[D,G,K,P]	*M01.X9*	M05.122

15 Ortho 2 – Other orthopedic disorders (continued)

M05.131	M05.762	M06.812	M08.462	M11.831	M12.58
M05.132	M05.771	M06.821	M08.471	M11.832	M12.59
M05.141	M05.772	M06.822	M08.472	M11.841	M12.811
M05.142	M05.79	M06.831	M08.48	M11.842	M12.812
M05.151	M05.811	M06.832	M08.811	M11.88	M12.821
M05.152	M05.812	M06.841	M08.812	M11.89	M12.822
M05.161	M05.821	M06.842	M08.821	M12.011	M12.831
M05.162	M05.822	M06.851	M08.822	M12.012	M12.832
M05.171	M05.831	M06.852	M08.831	M12.021	M12.841
M05.172	M05.832	M06.861	M08.832	M12.022	M12.842
M05.19	M05.841	M06.862	M08.841	M12.031	M12.88
M05.211	M05.842	M06.871	M08.842	M12.032	M12.89
M05.212	M05.851	M06.872	M08.851	M12.041	M13.811
M05.221	M05.852	M06.88	M08.852	M12.042	M13.812
M05.222	M05.861	M06.89	M08.861	M12.051	M13.821
M05.231	M05.862	M07.611	M08.862	M12.052	M13.822
M05.232	M05.871	M07.612	M08.871	M12.061	M13.831
M05.241	M05.872	M07.621	M08.872	M12.062	M13.832
M05.242	M05.89	M07.622	M08.88	M12.071	M13.841
M05.251	M06.011	M07.631	M08.89	M12.072	M13.842
M05.252	M06.012	M07.632	M08.911	M12.08	M13.88
M05.261	M06.021	M07.641	M08.912	M12.09	M13.89
M05.262	M06.022	M07.642	M08.921	M12.111	M14.611
M05.271	M06.031	M07.68	M08.922	M12.112	M14.612
M05.272	M06.032	M07.69	M08.931	M12.121	M14.621
M05.29	M06.041	M08.011	M08.932	M12.122	M14.622
M05.311	M06.042	M08.012	M08.941	M12.131	M14.631
M05.312	M06.051	M08.021	M08.942	M12.132	M14.632
M05.321	M06.052	M08.022	M08.951	M12.141	M14.641
M05.322	M06.061	M08.031	M08.952	M12.142	M14.642
M05.331	M06.062	M08.032	M08.961	M12.18	M14.68
M05.332	M06.071	M08.041	M08.962	M12.19	M14.69
M05.341	M06.072	M08.042	M08.971	M12.211	*M14.811*
M05.342	M06.08	M08.051	M08.972	M12.212	*M14.812*
M05.351	M06.09	M08.052	M08.98	M12.221	*M14.821*
M05.352	M06.1	M08.061	M08.99	M12.222	*M14.822*
M05.361	M06.211	M08.062	M11.011	M12.231	*M14.831*
M05.362	M06.212	M08.071	M11.012	M12.232	*M14.832*
M05.371	M06.221	M08.072	M11.021	M12.241	*M14.841*
M05.372	M06.222	M08.08	M11.022	M12.242	*M14.842*
M05.39	M06.231	M08.09	M11.031	M12.28	*M14.88*
M05.611	M06.232	M08.1	M11.032	M12.29	*M14.89*
M05.612	M06.241	M08.211	M11.041	M12.311	M16.0
M05.621	M06.242	M08.212	M11.042	M12.312	M16.11
M05.622	M06.251	M08.221	M11.08	M12.321	M16.12
M05.631	M06.252	M08.222	M11.09	M12.322	M16.2
M05.632	M06.261	M08.231	M11.111	M12.331	M16.31
M05.641	M06.262	M08.232	M11.112	M12.332	M16.32
M05.642	M06.271	M08.241	M11.121	M12.341	M16.4
M05.651	M06.272	M08.242	M11.122	M12.342	M16.51
M05.652	M06.28	M08.251	M11.131	M12.38	M16.52
M05.661	M06.29	M08.252	M11.132	M12.39	M16.6
M05.662	M06.311	M08.261	M11.141	M12.411	M16.7
M05.671	M06.312	M08.262	M11.142	M12.412	M17.0
M05.672	M06.321	M08.271	M11.18	M12.421	M17.11
M05.69	M06.322	M08.272	M11.19	M12.422	M17.12
M05.711	M06.331	M08.28	M11.211	M12.431	M17.2
M05.712	M06.332	M08.29	M11.212	M12.432	M17.31
M05.721	M06.341	M08.3	M11.221	M12.441	M17.32
M05.722	M06.342	M08.411	M11.222	M12.442	M17.4
M05.731	M06.351	M08.412	M11.231	M12.48	M17.5
M05.732	M06.352	M08.421	M11.232	M12.49	M24.011
M05.741	M06.361	M08.422	M11.241	M12.511	M24.012
M05.742	M06.362	M08.431	M11.242	M12.512	M24.021
M05.751	M06.371	M08.432	M11.28	M12.521	M24.022
M05.752	M06.372	M08.441	M11.29	M12.522	M24.031
M05.761	M06.38	M08.442	M11.811	M12.531	M24.032
	M06.39	M08.451	M11.812	M12.532	M24.111
	M06.4	M08.452	M11.821	M12.541	M24.112
	M06.811	M08.461	M11.822	M12.542	M24.121

Appendix J: Case-Mix Groups

15 Ortho 2 – Other orthopedic disorders (continued)					
M24.122	M42.16	M46.52	M47.898	*M49.85*	M60.021
M24.131	M42.17	M46.53	M47.899	*M49.86*	M60.022
M24.132	M42.18	M46.54	M47.9	*M49.87*	M60.031
M24.141	M42.19	M46.55	M48.00	*M49.88*	M60.032
M24.142	M42.9	M46.56	M48.01	*M49.89*	M60.041
M24.311	M43.27	M46.57	M48.02	M50.00	M60.042
M24.312	M43.28	M46.58	M48.03	M50.01	M60.044
M24.321	M43.3	M46.59	M48.04	M50.02	M60.045
M24.322	M43.4	M46.80	M48.05	M50.03	M60.08
M24.331	M43.5X2	M46.81	M48.07	M50.10	M60.09
M24.332	M43.5X3	M46.82	M48.08	M50.11	M61.011
M24.341	M43.5X4	M46.83	M48.10	M50.12	M61.012
M24.342	M43.5X5	M46.84	M48.11	M50.13	M61.021
M24.411	M43.5X6	M46.85	M48.12	M50.20	M61.022
M24.412	M43.5X7	M46.86	M48.13	M50.21	M61.031
M24.421	M43.5X8	M46.87	M48.14	M50.22	M61.032
M24.422	M43.5X9	M46.88	M48.15	M50.23	M61.041
M24.431	M43.6	M46.89	M48.16	M50.30	M61.042
M24.432	M45.0	M46.90	M48.17	M50.31	M61.08
M24.441	M45.1	M46.91	M48.18	M50.32	M61.09
M24.442	M45.2	M46.92	M48.19	M50.33	M61.111
M24.511	M45.3	M46.93	M48.20	M50.80	M61.112
M24.512	M45.4	M46.94	M48.21	M50.81	M61.121
M24.521	M45.5	M46.95	M48.22	M50.82	M61.122
M24.522	M45.6	M46.96	M48.23	M50.83	M61.131
M24.531	M45.7	M46.97	M48.24	M50.90	M61.132
M24.532	M45.8	M46.98	M48.25	M50.91	M61.141
M24.541	M45.9	M46.99	M48.26	M50.92	M61.142
M24.542	M46.00	M47.011	M48.27	M50.93	M61.144
M24.611	M46.01	M47.012	M48.30	M51.04	M61.145
M24.612	M46.02	M47.013	M48.31	M51.05	M61.18
M24.621	M46.03	M47.014	M48.32	M51.06	M61.19
M24.622	M46.04	M47.015	M48.33	M51.14	M61.211
M24.631	M46.05	M47.016	M48.34	M51.15	M61.212
M24.632	M46.06	M47.019	M48.35	M51.16	M61.221
M24.641	M46.07	M47.021	M48.36	M51.17	M61.222
M24.642	M46.08	M47.022	M48.37	M51.24	M61.231
M25.011	M46.09	M47.029	M48.38	M51.25	M61.232
M25.012	M46.1	M47.10	M48.50XD	M51.26	M61.241
M25.021	M46.20	M47.11	M48.50XG	M51.27	M61.242
M25.022	M46.21	M47.12	M48.51XD	M51.34	M61.28
M25.031	M46.22	M47.13	M48.51XG	M51.35	M61.29
M25.032	M46.23	M47.14	M48.52XD	M51.36	M61.311
M25.041	M46.24	M47.15	M48.52XG	M51.37	M61.312
M25.042	M46.25	M47.16	M48.53XD	M51.84	M61.321
M25.08	M46.26	M47.20	M48.53XG	M51.85	M61.322
M25.78	M46.27	M47.21	M48.54XD	M51.86	M61.331
M35.3	M46.28	M47.22	M48.54XG	M51.87	M61.332
M36.1	M46.30	M47.23	M48.55XD	M51.9	M61.341
M36.2	M46.31	M47.24	M48.55XG	M53.0	M61.342
M36.3	M46.32	M47.25	M48.56XD	M53.1	M61.38
M36.4	M46.33	M47.26	M48.56XG	M53.2X7	M61.39
M42.00	M46.34	M47.27	M48.57XD	M53.2X8	M61.411
M42.01	M46.35	M47.28	M48.57XG	M53.3	M61.412
M42.02	M46.36	M47.811	M48.58XD	M53.86	M61.421
M42.03	M46.37	M47.812	M48.58XG	M53.87	M61.422
M42.04	M46.38	M47.813	M48.8X1	M53.88	M61.431
M42.05	M46.39	M47.814	M48.8X2	M54.11	M61.432
M42.06	M46.40	M47.815	M48.8X3	M54.12	M61.441
M42.07	M46.41	M47.816	M48.8X4	M54.13	M61.442
M42.08	M46.42	M47.817	M48.8X5	M54.14	M61.48
M42.09	M46.43	M47.818	M48.8X6	M54.15	M61.49
M42.11	M46.44	M47.819	M48.8X7	M54.16	M61.511
M42.12	M46.45	M47.891	M48.8X8	M54.17	M61.512
M42.13	M46.46	M47.892	M48.8X9	M54.31	M61.521
M42.14	M46.47	M47.893	M48.9	M54.32	M61.522
M42.15	M46.48	M47.894	*M49.81*	M54.41	M61.531
	M46.49	M47.895	*M49.82*	M54.42	M61.532
	M46.50	M47.896	*M49.83*	M60.011	M61.541
	M46.51	M47.897	*M49.84*	M60.012	M61.542

15 Ortho 2 – Other orthopedic disorders (continued)					
M61.58	M84.641[D,G,K,P]	M86.642	*M90.89*	M93.842	M99.64
M61.59	M84.642[D,G,K,P]	M86.68	M91.0	M93.851	M99.65
M66.211	M84.68X[D,G,K,P]	M86.69	M91.11	M93.852	M99.66
M66.212	M86.011	M86.8X0	M91.12	M93.861	M99.67
M66.811	M86.012	M86.8X1	M91.21	M93.862	M99.68
M66.812	M86.021	M86.8X2	M91.22	M93.871	M99.69
M67.88	M86.022	M86.8X3	M91.31	M93.872	M99.70
M72.0	M86.031	M86.8X4	M91.32	M93.88	M99.71
M75.01	M86.032	M86.8X8	M91.41	M93.89	M99.72
M75.02	M86.041	M88.0	M91.42	M93.911	M99.73
M75.111	M86.042	M88.1	M91.81	M93.912	M99.74
M75.112	M86.08	M88.811	M91.82	M93.921	M99.75
M75.21	M86.09	M88.812	M91.91	M93.922	M99.76
M75.22	M86.111	M88.821	M91.92	M93.931	M99.77
M75.31	M86.112	M88.822	M92.01	M93.932	M99.78
M75.32	M86.121	M88.831	M92.02	M93.941	M99.79
M75.51	M86.122	M88.832	M92.11	M93.942	S02.0XX[D,G,K]
M75.52	M86.131	M88.841	M92.12	M93.951	S02.101[D,G,K]
M80.011[D,G,K,P]	M86.132	M88.842	M92.201	M93.952	S02.102[D,G,K]
M80.012[D,G,K,P]	M86.141	M88.88	M92.202	M93.961	S02.113[D,G,K]
M80.021[D,G,K,P]	M86.142	M88.89	M92.211	M93.962	S02.119[D,G,K]
M80.022[D,G,K,P]	M86.18	M89.411	M92.212	M93.971	S02.11A[D,G,K]
M80.031[D,G,K,P]	M86.19	M89.412	M92.221	M93.972	S02.11B[D,G,K]
M80.032[D,G,K,P]	M86.211	M89.421	M92.222	M93.98	S02.11C[D,G,K]
M80.041[D,G,K,P]	M86.212	M89.422	M92.291	M93.99	S02.11D[D,G,K]
M80.042[D,G,K,P]	M86.221	M89.431	M92.292	M96.1	S02.11E[D,G,K]
M80.08X[D,G,K,P]	M86.222	M89.432	M92.31	M99.20	S02.11F[D,G,K]
M80.811[D,G,K,P]	M86.231	M89.441	M92.32	M99.21	S02.11G[D,G,K]
M80.812[D,G,K,P]	M86.232	M89.442	M92.41	M99.22	S02.11H[D,G,K]
M80.821[D,G,K,P]	M86.241	M89.48	M92.42	M99.23	S02.19X[D,G,K]
M80.822[D,G,K,P]	M86.242	M89.49	M92.51	M99.24	S02.2XX[D,G,K]
M80.831[D,G,K,P]	M86.28	M89.611	M92.52	M99.25	S02.31X[D,G,K]
M80.832[D,G,K,P]	M86.29	M89.612	M92.61	M99.26	S02.32X[D,G,K]
M80.841[D,G,K,P]	M86.311	M89.621	M92.62	M99.27	S02.40A[D,G,K]
M80.842[D,G,K,P]	M86.312	M89.622	M92.70	M99.28	S02.40B[D,G,K]
M80.88X[D,G,K,P]	M86.321	M89.631	M92.71	M99.29	S02.40C[D,G,K]
M84.411[D,G,K,P]	M86.322	M89.632	M92.72	M99.30	S02.40D[D,G,K]
M84.412[D,G,K,P]	M86.331	M89.641	M92.8	M99.31	S02.40E[D,G,K]
M84.421[D,G,K,P]	M86.332	M89.642	M93.001	M99.32	S02.40F[D,G,K]
M84.422[D,G,K,P]	M86.341	M89.68	M93.002	M99.33	S02.411[D,G,K]
M84.431[D,G,K,P]	M86.342	M89.69	M93.011	M99.34	S02.412[D,G,K]
M84.432[D,G,K,P]	M86.38	*M90.511*	M93.012	M99.35	S02.413[D,G,K]
M84.433[D,G,K,P]	M86.39	*M90.512*	M93.021	M99.36	S02.42X[D,G,K]
M84.434[D,G,K,P]	M86.411	*M90.521*	M93.022	M99.37	S02.601[D,G,K]
M84.441[D,G,K,P]	M86.412	*M90.522*	M93.031	M99.38	S02.602[D,G,K]
M84.442[D,G,K,P]	M86.421	*M90.531*	M93.032	M99.39	S02.609[D,G,K]
M84.454[D,G,K,P]	M86.422	*M90.532*	M93.1	M99.40	S02.611[D,G,K]
M84.48X[D,G,K,P]	M86.431	*M90.541*	M93.211	M99.41	S02.612[D,G,K]
M84.511[D,G,K,P]	M86.432	*M90.542*	M93.212	M99.42	S02.620[D,G,K]
M84.512[D,G,K,P]	M86.441	*M90.58*	M93.221	M99.43	S02.621[D,G,K]
M84.521[D,G,K,P]	M86.442	*M90.59*	M93.222	M99.44	S02.622[D,G,K]
M84.522[D,G,K,P]	M86.48	*M90.611*	M93.231	M99.45	S02.631[D,G,K]
M84.531[D,G,K,P]	M86.49	*M90.612*	M93.232	M99.46	S02.632[D,G,K]
M84.532[D,G,K,P]	M86.511	*M90.621*	M93.241	M99.47	S02.641[D,G,K]
M84.533[D,G,K,P]	M86.512	*M90.622*	M93.242	M99.48	S02.642[D,G,K]
M84.534[D,G,K,P]	M86.521	*M90.631*	M93.251	M99.49	S02.651[D,G,K]
M84.541[D,G,K,P]	M86.522	*M90.632*	M93.252	M99.50	S02.652[D,G,K]
M84.542[D,G,K,P]	M86.531	*M90.641*	M93.261	M99.51	S02.66X[D,G,K]
M84.58X[D,G,K,P]	M86.532	*M90.642*	M93.262	M99.52	S02.671[D,G,K]
M84.611[D,G,K,P]	M86.541	*M90.68*	M93.271	M99.53	S02.672[D,G,K]
M84.612[D,G,K,P]	M86.542	*M90.69*	M93.272	M99.54	S02.69X[D,G,K]
M84.621[D,G,K,P]	M86.58	*M90.811*	M93.28	M99.55	S02.81X[D,G,K]
M84.622[D,G,K,P]	M86.59	*M90.812*	M93.29	M99.56	S02.82X[D,G,K]
M84.631[D,G,K,P]	M86.611	*M90.821*	M93.811	M99.57	S02.91X[D,G,K]
M84.632[D,G,K,P]	M86.612	*M90.822*	M93.812	M99.58	S02.92X[D,G,K]
M84.633[D,G,K,P]	M86.621	*M90.831*	M93.821	M99.59	S12.000[D,G,K]
M84.634[D,G,K,P]	M86.622	*M90.832*	M93.822	M99.60	S12.001[D,G,K]
	M86.631	*M90.841*	M93.831	M99.61	S12.01X[D,G,K]
	M86.632	*M90.842*	M93.832	M99.62	S12.02X[D,G,K]
	M86.641	*M90.88*	M93.841	M99.63	S12.030[D,G,K]

Appendix J: Case-Mix Groups

15 Ortho 2 – Other orthopedic disorders (continued)

S12.031[D,G,K]	S13.8XX[A,D]	S32.012[D,G,K]	S42.124[D,G,K,P]	S42.401[D,G,K,P]	S43.151D
S12.040[D,G,K]	S13.9XX[A,D]	S32.018[D,G,K]	S42.125[D,G,K,P]	S42.402[D,G,K,P]	S43.152D
S12.041[D,G,K]	S16.1XX[A,D]	S32.019[D,G,K]	S42.131[D,G,K,P]	S42.411[D,G,K,P]	S43.301D
S12.090[D,G,K]	S22.000[D,G,K]	S32.020[D,G,K]	S42.132[D,G,K,P]	S42.412[D,G,K,P]	S43.302D
S12.091[D,G,K]	S22.001[D,G,K]	S32.021[D,G,K]	S42.134[D,G,K,P]	S42.414[D,G,K,P]	S43.304D
S12.100[D,G,K]	S22.002[D,G,K]	S32.022[D,G,K]	S42.135[D,G,K,P]	S42.415[D,G,K,P]	S43.305D
S12.101[D,G,K]	S22.008[D,G,K]	S32.028[D,G,K]	S42.141[D,G,K,P]	S42.421[D,G,K,P]	S43.311D
S12.110[D,G,K]	S22.009[D,G,K]	S32.029[D,G,K]	S42.142[D,G,K,P]	S42.422[D,G,K,P]	S43.312D
S12.111[D,G,K]	S22.010[D,G,K]	S32.030[D,G,K]	S42.144[D,G,K,P]	S42.424[D,G,K,P]	S43.314D
S12.112[D,G,K]	S22.011[D,G,K]	S32.031[D,G,K]	S42.145[D,G,K,P]	S42.425[D,G,K,P]	S43.315D
S12.120[D,G,K]	S22.012[D,G,K]	S32.032[D,G,K]	S42.151[D,G,K,P]	S42.431[D,G,K,P]	S43.391D
S12.121[D,G,K]	S22.018[D,G,K]	S32.038[D,G,K]	S42.152[D,G,K,P]	S42.432[D,G,K,P]	S43.392D
S12.130[D,G,K]	S22.019[D,G,K]	S32.039[D,G,K]	S42.154[D,G,K,P]	S42.434[D,G,K,P]	S43.394D
S12.131[D,G,K]	S22.020[D,G,K]	S32.040[D,G,K]	S42.155[D,G,K,P]	S42.435[D,G,K,P]	S43.395D
S12.14X[D,G,K]	S22.021[D,G,K]	S32.041[D,G,K]	S42.191[D,G,K,P]	S42.441[D,G,K,P]	S49.001[D,G,K,P]
S12.150[D,G,K]	S22.022[D,G,K]	S32.042[D,G,K]	S42.192[D,G,K,P]	S42.442[D,G,K,P]	S49.002[D,G,K,P]
S12.151[D,G,K]	S22.028[D,G,K]	S32.048[D,G,K]	S42.201[D,G,K,P]	S42.444[D,G,K,P]	S49.011[D,G,K,P]
S12.190[D,G,K]	S22.029[D,G,K]	S32.049[D,G,K]	S42.202[D,G,K,P]	S42.445[D,G,K,P]	S49.012[D,G,K,P]
S12.191[D,G,K]	S22.030[D,G,K]	S32.050[D,G,K]	S42.211[D,G,K,P]	S42.447[D,G,K,P]	S49.021[D,G,K,P]
S12.200[D,G,K]	S22.031[D,G,K]	S32.051[D,G,K]	S42.212[D,G,K,P]	S42.448[D,G,K,P]	S49.022[D,G,K,P]
S12.201[D,G,K]	S22.032[D,G,K]	S32.052[D,G,K]	S42.214[D,G,K,P]	S42.451[D,G,K,P]	S49.031[D,G,K,P]
S12.230[D,G,K]	S22.038[D,G,K]	S32.058[D,G,K]	S42.215[D,G,K,P]	S42.452[D,G,K,P]	S49.032[D,G,K,P]
S12.231[D,G,K]	S22.039[D,G,K]	S32.059[D,G,K]	S42.221[D,G,K,P]	S42.454[D,G,K,P]	S49.041[D,G,K,P]
S12.24X[D,G,K]	S22.040[D,G,K]	S32.10X[D,G,K]	S42.222[D,G,K,P]	S42.455[D,G,K,P]	S49.042[D,G,K,P]
S12.250[D,G,K]	S22.041[D,G,K]	S32.110[D,G,K]	S42.224[D,G,K,P]	S42.461[D,G,K,P]	S49.091[D,G,K,P]
S12.251[D,G,K]	S22.042[D,G,K]	S32.111[D,G,K]	S42.225[D,G,K,P]	S42.462[D,G,K,P]	S49.092[D,G,K,P]
S12.290[D,G,K]	S22.048[D,G,K]	S32.112[D,G,K]	S42.231[D,G,K,P]	S42.464[D,G,K,P]	S49.101[D,G,K,P]
S12.291[D,G,K]	S22.049[D,G,K]	S32.119[D,G,K]	S42.232[D,G,K,P]	S42.465[D,G,K,P]	S49.102[D,G,K,P]
S12.300[D,G,K]	S22.050[D,G,K]	S32.120[D,G,K]	S42.241[D,G,K,P]	S42.471[D,G,K,P]	S49.111[D,G,K,P]
S12.301[D,G,K]	S22.051[D,G,K]	S32.121[D,G,K]	S42.242[D,G,K,P]	S42.472[D,G,K,P]	S49.112[D,G,K,P]
S12.330[D,G,K]	S22.052[D,G,K]	S32.122[D,G,K]	S42.251[D,G,K,P]	S42.474[D,G,K,P]	S49.121[D,G,K,P]
S12.331[D,G,K]	S22.058[D,G,K]	S32.129[D,G,K]	S42.252[D,G,K,P]	S42.475[D,G,K,P]	S49.122[D,G,K,P]
S12.34X[D,G,K]	S22.059[D,G,K]	S32.130[D,G,K]	S42.254[D,G,K,P]	S42.481[D,G,K,P]	S49.131[D,G,K,P]
S12.350[D,G,K]	S22.060[D,G,K]	S32.131[D,G,K]	S42.255[D,G,K,P]	S42.482[D,G,K,P]	S49.132[D,G,K,P]
S12.351[D,G,K]	S22.061[D,G,K]	S32.132[D,G,K]	S42.261[D,G,K,P]	S42.491[D,G,K,P]	S49.141[D,G,K,P]
S12.390[D,G,K]	S22.062[D,G,K]	S32.139[D,G,K]	S42.262[D,G,K,P]	S42.492[D,G,K,P]	S49.142[D,G,K,P]
S12.391[D,G,K]	S22.068[D,G,K]	S32.14X[D,G,K]	S42.264[D,G,K,P]	S42.494[D,G,K,P]	S49.191[D,G,K,P]
S12.400[D,G,K]	S22.069[D,G,K]	S32.15X[D,G,K]	S42.265[D,G,K,P]	S42.495[D,G,K,P]	S49.192[D,G,K,P]
S12.401[D,G,K]	S22.070[D,G,K]	S32.16X[D,G,K]	S42.271[D,G,K,P]	S42.91X[D,G,K,P]	S52.001[D,E,F,G,H,
J,K,M,N,P,Q,R]
S12.430[D,G,K]	S22.071[D,G,K]	S32.17X[D,G,K]	S42.272[D,G,K,P]	S42.92X[D,G,K,P]	S52.002[D,E,F,G,H,
J,K,M,N,P,Q,R]
S12.431[D,G,K]	S22.072[D,G,K]	S32.19X[D,G,K]	S42.291[D,G,K,P]	S43.001D	S52.011[D,G,K,P]
S12.44X[D,G,K]	S22.078[D,G,K]	S32.2XX[D,G,K]	S42.292[D,G,K,P]	S43.002D	S52.012[D,G,K,P]
S12.450[D,G,K]	S22.079[D,G,K]	S33.5XX[A,D]	S42.294[D,G,K,P]	S43.004D	S52.021[D,E,F,G,H,
J,K,M,N,P,Q,R]
S12.451[D,G,K]	S22.080[D,G,K]	S33.6XX[A,D]	S42.295[D,G,K,P]	S43.005D	S52.022[D,E,F,G,H,
J,K,M,N,P,Q,R]
S12.490[D,G,K]	S22.081[D,G,K]	S33.8XX[A,D]	S42.301[D,G,K,P]	S43.011D	S52.024[D,E,F,G,H,
J,K,M,N,P,Q,R]
S12.491[D,G,K]	S22.082[D,G,K]	S33.9XX[A,D]	S42.302[D,G,K,P]	S43.012D	S52.025[D,E,F,G,H,
J,K,M,N,P,Q,R]
S12.500[D,G,K]	S22.088[D,G,K]	S42.001[D,G,K,P]	S42.311[D,G,K,P]	S43.014D	S52.031[D,E,F,G,H,
J,K,M,N,P,Q,R]
S12.501[D,G,K]	S22.089[D,G,K]	S42.002[D,G,K,P]	S42.312[D,G,K,P]	S43.015D	S52.032[D,E,F,G,H,
J,K,M,N,P,Q,R]
S12.530[D,G,K]	S22.20X[D,G,K]	S42.011[D,G,K,P]	S42.321[D,G,K,P]	S43.021D	S52.034[D,E,F,G,H,
J,K,M,N,P,Q,R]
S12.531[D,G,K]	S22.21X[D,G,K]	S42.012[D,G,K,P]	S42.322[D,G,K,P]	S43.022D	S52.035[D,E,F,G,H,
J,K,M,N,P,Q,R]
S12.54X[D,G,K]	S22.22X[D,G,K]	S42.014[D,G,K,P]	S42.324[D,G,K,P]	S43.024D	S52.041[D,E,F,G,H,
J,K,M,N,P,Q,R]
S12.550[D,G,K]	S22.23X[D,G,K]	S42.015[D,G,K,P]	S42.325[D,G,K,P]	S43.025D	S52.042[D,E,F,G,H,
J,K,M,N,P,Q,R]
S12.551[D,G,K]	S22.24X[D,G,K]	S42.017[D,G,K,P]	S42.331[D,G,K,P]	S43.031D	S52.044[D,E,F,G,H,
J,K,M,N,P,Q,R]
S12.590[D,G,K]	S22.31X[D,G,K]	S42.018[D,G,K,P]	S42.332[D,G,K,P]	S43.032D	S52.045[D,E,F,G,H,
J,K,M,N,P,Q,R]
S12.591[D,G,K]	S22.32X[D,G,K]	S42.021[D,G,K,P]	S42.334[D,G,K,P]	S43.034D	S52.091[D,E,F,G,H,
J,K,M,N,P,Q,R]
S12.600[D,G,K]	S22.41X[D,G,K]	S42.022[D,G,K,P]	S42.335[D,G,K,P]	S43.035D	
S12.601[D,G,K]	S22.42X[D,G,K]	S42.024[D,G,K,P]	S42.341[D,G,K,P]	S43.081D	
S12.630[D,G,K]	S22.43X[D,G,K]	S42.025[D,G,K,P]	S42.342[D,G,K,P]	S43.082D	
S12.631[D,G,K]	S22.5XX[D,G,K]	S42.031[D,G,K,P]	S42.344[D,G,K,P]	S43.084D	
S12.64X[D,G,K]	S22.9XX[D,G,K]	S42.032[D,G,K,P]	S42.345[D,G,K,P]	S43.085D	
S12.650[D,G,K]	S23.3XX[A,D]	S42.034[D,G,K,P]	S42.351[D,G,K,P]	S43.101D	
S12.651[D,G,K]	S23.8XX[A,D]	S42.035[D,G,K,P]	S42.352[D,G,K,P]	S43.102D	
S12.690[D,G,K]	S23.9XX[A,D]	S42.101[D,G,K,P]	S42.354[D,G,K,P]	S43.111D	
S12.691[D,G,K]	S32.000[D,G,K]	S42.102[D,G,K,P]	S42.355[D,G,K,P]	S43.112D	
S12.8XXD	S32.001[D,G,K]	S42.111[D,G,K,P]	S42.361[D,G,K,P]	S43.121D	
S12.9XXD	S32.002[D,G,K]	S42.112[D,G,K,P]	S42.362[D,G,K,P]	S43.122D	
S13.4XX[A,D]	S32.008[D,G,K]	S42.114[D,G,K,P]	S42.364[D,G,K,P]	S43.131D	
	S32.009[D,G,K]	S42.115[D,G,K,P]	S42.365[D,G,K,P]	S43.132D	
	S32.010[D,G,K]	S42.121[D,G,K,P]	S42.391[D,G,K,P]	S43.141D	
	S32.011[D,G,K]	S42.122[D,G,K,P]	S42.392[D,G,K,P]	S43.142D	

15 Ortho 2 – Other orthopedic disorders (continued)

S52.092[D,E,F,G,H,
   J,K,M,N,P,Q,R]
S52.101[D,E,F,G,H,
   J,K,M,N,P,Q,R]
S52.102[D,E,F,G,H,
   J,K,M,N,P,Q,R]
S52.111[D,G,K,P]
S52.112[D,G,K,P]
S52.121[D,E,F,G,H,
   J,K,M,N,P,Q,R]
S52.122[D,E,F,G,H,
   J,K,M,N,P,Q,R]
S52.124[D,E,F,G,H,
   J,K,M,N,P,Q,R]
S52.125[D,E,F,G,H,
   J,K,M,N,P,Q,R]
S52.131[D,E,F,G,H,
   J,K,M,N,P,Q,R]
S52.132[D,E,F,G,H,
   J,K,M,N,P,Q,R]
S52.134[D,E,F,G,H,
   J,K,M,N,P,Q,R]
S52.135[D,E,F,G,H,
   J,K,M,N,P,Q,R]
S52.181[D,E,F,G,H,
   J,K,M,N,P,Q,R]
S52.182[D,E,F,G,H,
   J,K,M,N,P,Q,R]
S52.201[D,E,F,G,H,
   J,K,M,N,P,Q,R]
S52.202[D,E,F,G,H,
   J,K,M,N,P,Q,R]
S52.211[D,G,K,P]
S52.212[D,G,K,P]
S52.221[D,E,F,G,H,
   J,K,M,N,P,Q,R]
S52.222[D,E,F,G,H,
   J,K,M,N,P,Q,R]
S52.224[D,E,F,G,H,
   J,K,M,N,P,Q,R]
S52.225[D,E,F,G,H,
   J,K,M,N,P,Q,R]
S52.231[D,E,F,G,H,
   J,K,M,N,P,Q,R]
S52.232[D,E,F,G,H,
   J,K,M,N,P,Q,R]
S52.234[D,E,F,G,H,J,K,M,
   N,P,Q,R]
S52.235[D,E,F,G,H,
   J,K,M,N,P,Q,R]
S52.241[D,E,F,G,H,
   J,K,M,N,P,Q,R]
S52.242[D,E,F,G,H,
   J,K,M,N,P,Q,R]
S52.244[D,E,F,G,H,
   J,K,M,N,P,Q,R]
S52.245[D,E,F,G,H,J,K,M,
   N,P,Q,R]
S52.251[D,E,F,G,H,
   J,K,M,N,P,Q,R]
S52.252[D,E,F,G,H,
   J,K,M,N,P,Q,R]
S52.254[D,E,F,G,H,
   J,K,M,N,P,Q,R]
S52.255[D,E,F,G,H,
   J,K,M,N,P,Q,R]
S52.261[D,E,F,G,H,
   J,K,M,N,P,Q,R]
S52.262[D,E,F,G,H,
   J,K,M,N,P,Q,R]

S52.264[D,E,F,G,H,
   J,K,M,N,P,Q,R]
S52.265[D,E,F,G,H,
   J,K,M,N,P,Q,R]
S52.271[D,E,F,G,H,
   J,K,M,N,P,Q,R]
S52.272[D,E,F,G,H,
   J,K,M,N,P,Q,R]
S52.281[D,E,F,G,H,
   J,K,M,N,P,Q,R]
S52.282[D,E,F,G,H,
   J,K,M,N,P,Q,R]
S52.291[D,E,F,G,H,
   J,K,M,N,P,Q,R]
S52.292[D,E,F,G,H,
   J,K,M,N,P,Q,R]
S52.301[D,E,F,G,H,
   J,K,M,N,P,Q,R]
S52.302[D,E,F,G,H,
   J,K,M,N,P,Q,R]
S52.311[D,G,K,P]
S52.312[D,G,K,P]
S52.321[D,E,F,G,H,
   J,K,M,N,P,Q,R]
S52.322[D,E,F,G,H,
   J,K,M,N,P,Q,R]
S52.324[D,E,F,G,H,
   J,K,M,N,P,Q,R]
S52.325[D,E,F,G,H,
   J,K,M,N,P,Q,R]
S52.331[D,E,F,G,H,
   J,K,M,N,P,Q,R]
S52.332[D,E,F,G,H,
   J,K,M,N,P,Q,R]
S52.334[D,E,F,G,H,
   J,K,M,N,P,Q,R]
S52.335[D,E,F,G,H,
   J,K,M,N,P,Q,R]
S52.341[D,E,F,G,H,
   J,K,M,N,P,Q,R]
S52.342[D,E,F,G,H,
   J,K,M,N,P,Q,R]
S52.344[D,E,F,G,H,J,K,M,
   N,P,Q,R]
S52.345[D,E,F,G,H,
   J,K,M,N,P,Q,R]
S52.351[D,E,F,G,H,
   J,K,M,N,P,Q,R]
S52.352[D,E,F,G,H,
   J,K,M,N,P,Q,R]
S52.354[D,E,F,G,H,
   J,K,M,N,P,Q,R]
S52.355[D,E,F,G,H,
   J,K,M,N,P,Q,R]
S52.361[D,E,F,G,H,
   J,K,M,N,P,Q,R]
S52.362[D,E,F,G,H,
   J,K,M,N,P,Q,R]
S52.364[D,E,F,G,H,
   J,K,M,N,P,Q,R]
S52.365[D,E,F,G,H,
   J,K,M,N,P,Q,R]
S52.371[D,E,F,G,H,
   J,K,M,N,P,Q,R]
S52.372[D,E,F,G,H,
   J,K,M,N,P,Q,R]
S52.381[D,E,F,G,H,
   J,K,M,N,P,Q,R]
S52.382[D,E,F,G,H,
   J,K,M,N,P,Q,R]
S52.391[D,E,F,G,H,
   J,K,M,N,P,Q,R]

S52.392[D,E,F,G,H,
   J,K,M,N,P,Q,R]
S52.501[D,E,F,G,H,J,K,M,
   N,P,Q,R]
S52.502[D,E,F,G,H,
   J,K,M,N,P,Q,R]
S52.511[E,F,G,H,J,K,M,N,
   P,Q,R]
S52.512[D,E,F,G,H,J,K,M,
   N,P,Q,R]
S52.514[D,E,F,G,H,J,K,M,
   N,P,Q,R]
S52.515[D,E,F,G,H,J,K,M,
   N,P,Q,R]
S52.521[D,G,K,P]
S52.522[D,G,K,P]
S52.531[D,E,F,G,H,
   J,K,M,N,P,Q,R]
S52.532[D,E,F,G,H,
   J,K,M,N,P,Q,R]
S52.541[D,E,F,G,H,
   J,K,M,N,P,Q,R]
S52.542[D,E,F,G,H,
   J,K,M,N,P,Q,R]
S52.551[D,E,F,G,H,
   J,K,M,N,P,Q,R]
S52.552[D,E,F,G,H,
   J,K,M,N,P,Q,R]
S52.561[D,E,F,G,H,
   J,K,M,N,P,Q,R]
S52.562[D,E,F,G,H,
   J,K,M,N,P,Q,R]
S52.571[D,E,F,G,H,
   J,K,M,N,P,Q,R]
S52.572[D,E,F,G,H,
   J,K,M,N,P,Q,R]
S52.591[D,E,F,G,H,
   J,K,M,N,P,Q,R]
S52.592[D,E,F,G,H,
   J,K,M,N,P,Q,R]
S52.601[D,E,F,G,H,
   J,K,M,N,P,Q,R]
S52.602[D,E,F,G,H,
   J,K,M,N,P,Q,R]
S52.611[D,E,F,G,H,
   J,K,M,N,P,Q,R]
S52.612[D,E,F,G,H,
   J,K,M,N,P,Q,R]
S52.614[D,E,F,G,H,
   J,K,M,N,P,Q,R]
S52.615[D,E,F,G,H,
   J,K,M,N,P,Q,R]
S52.621[D,G,K,P]
S52.622[D,G,K,P]
S52.691[D,E,F,G,H,
   J,K,M,N,P,Q,R]
S52.692[D,E,F,G,H,
   J,K,M,N,P,Q,R]
S52.91X[D,E,F,G,H,
   J,K,M,N,P,Q,R]
S52.92X[D,E,F,G,H,
   J,K,M,N,P,Q,R]
S53.001D
S53.002D
S53.004D
S53.005D
S53.011D
S53.012D
S53.014D
S53.015D
S53.021D
S53.022D

S53.024D
S53.025D
S53.031D
S53.032D
S53.091D
S53.092D
S53.094D
S53.095D
S53.101D
S53.102D
S53.104D
S53.105D
S53.111D
S53.112D
S53.114D
S53.115D
S53.121D
S53.122D
S53.124D
S53.125D
S53.131D
S53.132D
S53.134D
S53.135D
S53.141D
S53.142D
S53.144D
S53.145D
S53.191D
S53.192D
S53.194D
S53.195D
S59.001[D,G,K,P]
S59.002[D,G,K,P]
S59.011[D,G,K,P]
S59.012[D,G,K,P]
S59.021[D,G,K,P]
S59.022[D,G,K,P]
S59.031[D,G,K,P]
S59.032[D,G,K,P]
S59.041[D,G,K,P]
S59.042[D,G,K,P]
S59.091[D,G,K,P]
S59.092[D,G,K,P]
S59.101[D,G,K,P]
S59.102[D,G,K,P]
S59.111[D,G,K,P]
S59.112[D,G,K,P]
S59.121[D,G,K,P]
S59.122[D,G,K,P]
S59.131[D,G,K,P]
S59.132[D,G,K,P]
S59.141[D,G,K,P]
S59.142[D,G,K,P]
S59.191[D,G,K,P]
S59.192[D,G,K,P]
S59.201[D,G,K,P]
S59.202[D,G,K,P]
S59.211[D,G,K,P]
S59.212[D,G,K,P]
S59.221[D,G,K,P]
S59.222[D,G,K,P]
S59.231[D,G,K,P]
S59.232[D,G,K,P]
S59.241[D,G,K,P]
S59.242[D,G,K,P]
S59.291[D,G,K,P]
S59.292[D,G,K,P]
S62.001[D,G,K,P]
S62.002[D,G,K,P]

S62.011[D,G,K,P]
S62.012[D,G,K,P]
S62.014[D,G,K,P]
S62.015[D,G,K,P]
S62.021[D,G,K,P]
S62.022[D,G,K,P]
S62.024[D,G,K,P]
S62.025[D,G,K,P]
S62.031[D,G,K,P]
S62.032[D,G,K,P]
S62.034[D,G,K,P]
S62.035[D,G,K,P]
S62.101[D,G,K,P]
S62.102[D,G,K,P]
S62.111[D,G,K,P]
S62.112[D,G,K,P]
S62.114[D,G,K,P]
S62.115[D,G,K,P]
S62.121[D,G,K,P]
S62.122[D,G,K,P]
S62.124[D,G,K,P]
S62.125[D,G,K,P]
S62.131[D,G,K,P]
S62.132[D,G,K,P]
S62.134[D,G,K,P]
S62.135[D,G,K,P]
S62.141[D,G,K,P]
S62.142[D,G,K,P]
S62.144[D,G,K,P]
S62.145[D,G,K,P]
S62.151[D,G,K,P]
S62.152[D,G,K,P]
S62.154[D,G,K,P]
S62.155[D,G,K,P]
S62.161[D,G,K,P]
S62.162[D,G,K,P]
S62.164[D,G,K,P]
S62.165[D,G,K,P]
S62.171[D,G,K,P]
S62.172[D,G,K,P]
S62.174[D,G,K,P]
S62.175[D,G,K,P]
S62.181[D,G,K,P]
S62.182[D,G,K,P]
S62.184[D,G,K,P]
S62.185[D,G,K,P]
S62.201[D,G,K,P]
S62.202[D,G,K,P]
S62.211[D,G,K,P]
S62.212[D,G,K,P]
S62.221[D,G,K,P]
S62.222[D,G,K,P]
S62.224[D,G,K,P]
S62.225[D,G,K,P]
S62.231[D,G,K,P]
S62.232[D,G,K,P]
S62.234[D,G,K,P]
S62.235[D,G,K,P]
S62.241[D,G,K,P]
S62.242[D,G,K,P]
S62.244[D,G,K,P]
S62.245[D,G,K,P]
S62.251[D,G,K,P]
S62.252[D,G,K,P]
S62.254[D,G,K,P]
S62.255[D,G,K,P]
S62.291[D,G,K,P]
S62.292[D,G,K,P]
S62.300[D,G,K,P]
S62.301[D,G,K,P]

S62.302[D,G,K,P]
S62.303[D,G,K,P]
S62.304[D,G,K,P]
S62.305[D,G,K,P]
S62.306[D,G,K,P]
S62.307[D,G,K,P]
S62.310[D,G,K,P]
S62.311[D,G,K,P]
S62.312[D,G,K,P]
S62.313[D,G,K,P]
S62.314[D,G,K,P]
S62.315[D,G,K,P]
S62.316[D,G,K,P]
S62.317[D,G,K,P]
S62.318[G,K,P] (per CMS)
S62.320[D,G,K,P]
S62.321[D,G,K,P]
S62.322[D,G,K,P]
S62.323[D,G,K,P]
S62.324[D,G,K,P]
S62.325[D,G,K,P]
S62.326[D,G,K,P]
S62.327[D,G,K,P]
S62.328[D,G,K,P]
S62.329D
S62.330[D,G,K,P]
S62.331[D,G,K,P]
S62.332[D,G,K,P]
S62.333[D,G,K,P]
S62.334[D,G,K,P]
S62.335[D,G,K,P]
S62.336[D,G,K,P]
S62.337[D,G,K,P]
S62.338[D,G,K,P]
S62.340[D,G,K,P]
S62.341[D,G,K,P]
S62.342[D,G,K,P]
S62.343[D,G,K,P]
S62.344[D,G,K,P]
S62.345[D,G,K,P]
S62.346[D,G,K,P]
S62.347[D,G,K,P]
S62.348[D,G,K,P]
S62.350[D,G,K,P]
S62.351[D,G,K,P]
S62.352[D,G,K,P]
S62.353[D,G,K,P]
S62.354[D,G,K,P]
S62.355[D,G,K,P]
S62.356[D,G,K,P]
S62.357[D,G,K,P]
S62.358[D,G,K,P]
S62.360[D,G,K,P]
S62.361[D,G,K,P]
S62.362[D,G,K,P]
S62.363[D,G,K,P]
S62.364[D,G,K,P]
S62.365[D,G,K,P]
S62.366[D,G,K,P]
S62.367[D,G,K,P]
S62.368[D,G,K,P]
S62.390[D,G,K,P]
S62.391[D,G,K,P]
S62.392[D,G,K,P]
S62.393[D,G,K,P]
S62.394[D,G,K,P]
S62.395[D,G,K,P]
S62.396[D,G,K,P]
S62.397[D,G,K,P]
S62.501[D,G,K,P]

15 Ortho 2 – Other orthopedic disorders (continued)

S62.502[D,G,K,P]
S62.511[D,G,K,P]
S62.512[D,G,K,P]
S62.514[D,G,K,P]
S62.515[D,G,K,P]
S62.521[D,G,K,P]
S62.522[D,G,K,P]
S62.524[D,G,K,P]
S62.525[D,G,K,P]
S62.600[D,G,K,P]
S62.601[D,G,K,P]
S62.602[D,G,K,P]
S62.603[D,G,K,P]
S62.604[D,G,K,P]
S62.605[D,G,K,P]
S62.606[D,G,K,P]
S62.607[D,G,K,P]
S62.608[G,K,P] (per CMS)
S62.610[D,G,K,P]
S62.611[D,G,K,P]
S62.612[D,G,K,P]
S62.613[D,G,K,P]
S62.614[D,G,K,P]
S62.615[D,G,K,P]
S62.616[D,G,K,P]
S62.617[D,G,K,P]
S62.618[D,G,K,P]
S62.620[D,G,K,P]
S62.621[D,G,K,P]
S62.622[D,G,K,P]
S62.623[D,G,K,P]
S62.624[D,G,K,P]
S62.625[D,G,K,P]
S62.626[D,G,K,P]
S62.627[D,G,K,P]
S62.628[D,G,K,P]
S62.630[D,G,K,P]
S62.631[D,G,K,P]
S62.632[D,G,K,P]
S62.633[D,G,K,P]
S62.634[D,G,K,P]
S62.635[D,G,K,P]
S62.636[D,G,K,P]
S62.637[D,G,K,P]
S62.638[D,G,K,P]
S62.640[D,G,K,P]
S62.641[D,G,K,P]
S62.642[D,G,K,P]
S62.643[D,G,K,P]
S62.644[D,G,K,P]
S62.645[D,G,K,P]
S62.646[D,G,K,P]
S62.647[D,G,K,P]
S62.648[D,G,K,P]
S62.650[D,G,K,P]
S62.651[D,G,K,P]
S62.652[D,G,K,P]
S62.653[D,G,K,P]
S62.654[D,G,K,P]
S62.655[D,G,K,P]
S62.656[D,G,K,P]
S62.657[D,G,K,P]
S62.658[D,G,K,P]
S62.660[D,G,K,P]
S62.661[D,G,K,P]
S62.662[D,G,K,P]
S62.663[D,G,K,P]

S62.664[D,G,K,P]
S62.665[D,G,K,P]
S62.666[D,G,K,P]
S62.667[D,G,K,P]
S62.668[D,G,K,P]
S62.91X[D,G,K,P]
S62.92X[D,G,K,P]
S63.001D
S63.002D
S63.004D
S63.005D
S63.011D
S63.012D
S63.014D
S63.015D
S63.021D
S63.022D
S63.024D
S63.025D
S63.031D
S63.032D
S63.034D
S63.035D
S63.041D
S63.042D
S63.044D
S63.045D
S63.051D
S63.052D
S63.054D
S63.055D
S63.061D
S63.062D
S63.064D
S63.065D
S63.071D
S63.072D
S63.074D
S63.075D
S63.091D
S63.092D
S63.094D
S63.095D
S93.01XD
S93.02XD
S93.04XD
S93.05XD
S93.101D
S93.102D
S93.104D
S93.105D
S93.111D
S93.112D
S93.114D
S93.115D
S93.121D
S93.122D
S93.124D
S93.125D
S93.131D
S93.132D
S93.134D
S93.135D
S93.141D
S93.142D
S93.144D
S93.145D
S93.301D
S93.302D
S93.304D

S93.305D
S93.311D
S93.312D
S93.314D
S93.315D
S93.321D
S93.322D
S93.324D
S93.325D
S93.331D
S93.332D
S93.334D
S93.335D

16 Psych 1 – Affective and other psychoses, depression

Currently there are no ICD-10-CM codes included in this case-mix group.

17 Psych 2 – Degenerative and other organic psychiatric disorders

Currently there are no ICD-10-CM codes included in this case-mix group.

18 Pulmonary disorders

J41*
J43*
J44*

19 Skin 1 – Traumatic wounds, burns and postoperative complications

K68.11
S01.01X[A,D]
S01.02X[A,D]
S01.03X[A,D]
S01.04X[A,D]
S01.05X[A,D]
S01.111[A,D]
S01.112[A,D]
S01.121[A,D]
S01.122[A,D]
S01.131[A,D]
S01.132[A,D]
S01.141[A,D]
S01.142[A,D]
S01.151[A,D]
S01.152[A,D]
S01.21X[A,D]
S01.22X[A,D]
S01.23X[A,D]
S01.24X[A,D]
S01.25X[A,D]
S01.311[A,D]
S01.312[A,D]
S01.321[A,D]
S01.322[A,D]
S01.331[A,D]
S01.332[A,D]
S01.341[A,D]
S01.342[A,D]
S01.351[A,D]
S01.352[A,D]

S01.401[A,D]
S01.402[A,D]
S01.411[A,D]
S01.412[A,D]
S01.421[A,D]
S01.422[A,D]
S01.431[A,D]
S01.432[A,D]
S01.441[A,D]
S01.442[A,D]
S01.451[A,D]
S01.452[A,D]
S01.511[A,D]
S01.512[A,D]
S01.521[A,D]
S01.522[A,D]
S01.531[A,D]
S01.532[A,D]
S01.541[A,D]
S01.542[A,D]
S01.551[A,D]
S01.552[A,D]
S01.81X[A,D]
S01.82X[A,D]
S01.83X[A,D]
S01.84X[A,D]
S01.85X[A,D]
S05.41XD
S05.42XD
S08.0XX[A,D]
S08.111[A,D]
S08.112[A,D]
S08.121[A,D]
S08.122[A,D]
S08.811[A,D]
S08.812[A,D]
S08.89X[A,D]
S09.12X[A,D]
S09.21XD
S09.22XD
S09.301D
S09.302D
S09.311[A,D]
S09.312[A,D]
S09.313[A,D]
S09.391D
S09.392D
S09.8XX[A,D]
S11.011D
S11.012D
S11.013D
S11.014D
S11.015D
S11.021D
S11.022D
S11.023D
S11.024D
S11.025D
S11.031D
S11.032D
S11.033D
S11.034D
S11.035D
S11.11XD
S11.12XD
S11.13XD
S11.14XD
S11.15XD
S11.21XD
S11.22XD

S11.23XD
S11.24XD
S11.25XD
S11.81X[A,D]
S11.82X[A,D]
S11.83X[A,D]
S11.84X[A,D]
S11.85X[A,D]
S11.89X[A,D]
S11.91X[A,D]
S11.92X[A,D]
S11.93X[A,D]
S11.94X[A,D]
S11.95X[A,D]
S16.2XX[A,D]
S21.011[A,D]
S21.012[A,D]
S21.021[A,D]
S21.022[A,D]
S21.031[A,D]
S21.032[A,D]
S21.041[A,D]
S21.042[A,D]
S21.051[A,D]
S21.052[A,D]
S21.131[A,D]
S21.132[A,D]
S21.141[A,D]
S21.142[A,D]
S21.151[A,D]
S21.152[A,D]
S21.211[A,D]
S21.212[A,D]
S21.221[A,D]
S21.222[A,D]
S21.231[A,D]
S21.232[A,D]
S21.241[A,D]
S21.242[A,D]
S21.251[A,D]
S21.252[A,D]
S21.91X[A,D]
S21.93X[A,D]
S28.1XXD
S28.211D
S28.212D
S28.221D
S28.222D
S29.021[A,D]
S29.022[A,D]
S29.029[A,D]
S31.010[A,D]
S31.020[A,D]
S31.030[A,D]
S31.040[A,D]
S31.050[A,D]
S31.110[A,D]
S31.111[A,D]
S31.112[A,D]
S31.113[A,D]
S31.114[A,D]
S31.115[A,D]
S31.120[A,D]
S31.121[A,D]
S31.122[A,D]
S31.123[A,D]

S31.124[A,D]
S31.125[A,D]
S31.130[A,D]
S31.131[A,D]
S31.132[A,D]
S31.133[A,D]
S31.134[A,D]
S31.135[A,D]
S31.140[A,D]
S31.141[A,D]
S31.142[A,D]
S31.143[A,D]
S31.144[A,D]
S31.145[A,D]
S31.150[A,D]
S31.151[A,D]
S31.152[A,D]
S31.153[A,D]
S31.154[A,D]
S31.155[A,D]
S31.21X[A,D]
S31.22X[A,D]
S31.23X[A,D]
S31.24X[A,D]
S31.25X[A,D]
S31.31X[A,D]
S31.32X[A,D]
S31.33X[A,D]
S31.34X[A,D]
S31.35X[A,D]
S31.41X[A,D]
S31.42X[A,D]
S31.43X[A,D]
S31.44X[A,D]
S31.45X[A,D]
S31.511[A,D]
S31.512[A,D]
S31.521[A,D]
S31.522[A,D]
S31.531[A,D]
S31.532[A,D]
S31.541[A,D]
S31.542[A,D]
S31.551[A,D]
S31.552[A,D]
S31.811[A,D]
S31.812[A,D]
S31.813[A,D]
S31.814[A,D]
S31.815[A,D]
S31.821[A,D]
S31.822[A,D]
S31.823[A,D]
S31.824[A,D]
S31.825[A,D]
S31.831[A,D]
S31.832[A,D]
S31.833[A,D]
S31.834[A,D]
S31.835[A,D]
S38.211D
S38.212D
S38.221D
S38.222D
S38.231D
S38.232D
S38.3XXD
S39.021[A,D]
S39.022[A,D]
S39.023[A,D]

19 Skin 1 – Traumatic wounds, burns and postoperative complications (continued)

S41.011[A,D]	S51.842[A,D]	S61.213[A,D]	S61.351[A,D]	S67.197D	S71.122[A,D]
S41.012[A,D]	S51.851[A,D]	S61.214[A,D]	S61.352[A,D]	S67.21XD	S71.131[A,D]
S41.021[A,D]	S51.852[A,D]	S61.215[A,D]	S61.353[A,D]	S67.22XD	S71.132[A,D]
S41.022[A,D]	S56.021[A,D]	S61.216[A,D]	S61.354[A,D]	S67.31XD	S71.141[A,D]
S41.031[A,D]	S56.022[A,D]	S61.217[A,D]	S61.355[A,D]	S67.32XD	S71.142[A,D]
S41.032[A,D]	S56.121[A,D]	S61.220[A,D]	S61.356[A,D]	S67.41XD	S71.151[A,D]
S41.039[A,D]	S56.122[A,D]	S61.221[A,D]	S61.357[A,D]	S67.42XD	S71.152[A,D]
S41.041[A,D]	S56.123[A,D]	S61.222[A,D]	S61.411[A,D]	S67.91XD	S76.021[A,D]
S41.042[A,D]	S56.124[A,D]	S61.223[A,D]	S61.412[A,D]	S67.92XD	S76.022[A,D]
S41.051[A,D]	S56.125[A,D]	S61.224[A,D]	S61.421[A,D]	S68.011[A,D]	S76.121[A,D]
S41.052[A,D]	S56.126[A,D]	S61.225[A,D]	S61.422[A,D]	S68.012[A,D]	S76.122[A,D]
S41.111[A,D]	S56.127[A,D]	S61.226[A,D]	S61.431[A,D]	S68.021[A,D]	S76.221[A,D]
S41.112[A,D]	S56.128[A,D]	S61.227[A,D]	S61.432[A,D]	S68.022[A,D]	S76.222[A,D]
S41.121[A,D]	S56.221[A,D]	S61.230[A,D]	S61.441[A,D]	S68.110[A,D]	S76.321[A,D]
S41.122[A,D]	S56.222[A,D]	S61.231[A,D]	S61.442[A,D]	S68.111[A,D]	S76.322[A,D]
S41.131[A,D]	S56.321[A,D]	S61.232[A,D]	S61.451[A,D]	S68.112[A,D]	S76.821[A,D]
S41.132[A,D]	S56.322[A,D]	S61.233[A,D]	S61.452[A,D]	S68.113[A,D]	S76.822[A,D]
S41.139[A,D]	S56.421[A,D]	S61.234[A,D]	S61.511[A,D]	S68.114[A,D]	S76.921[A,D]
S41.141[A,D]	S56.422[A,D]	S61.235[A,D]	S61.512[A,D]	S68.115[A,D]	S76.922[A,D]
S41.142[A,D]	S56.423[A,D]	S61.236[A,D]	S61.521[A,D]	S68.116[A,D]	S81.011[A,D]
S41.151[A,D]	S56.424[A,D]	S61.237[A,D]	S61.522[A,D]	S68.117[A,D]	S81.012[A,D]
S41.152[A,D]	S56.425[A,D]	S61.240[A,D]	S61.531[A,D]	S68.120[A,D]	S81.021[A,D]
S46.021[A,D]	S56.426[A,D]	S61.241[A,D]	S61.532[A,D]	S68.121[A,D]	S81.022[A,D]
S46.022[A,D]	S56.427[A,D]	S61.242[A,D]	S61.541[A,D]	S68.122[A,D]	S81.031[A,D]
S46.121[A,D]	S56.428[A,D]	S61.243[A,D]	S61.542[A,D]	S68.123[A,D]	S81.032[A,D]
S46.122[A,D]	S56.521[A,D]	S61.244[A,D]	S61.551[A,D]	S68.124[A,D]	S81.041[A,D]
S46.221[A,D]	S56.522[A,D]	S61.245[A,D]	S61.552[A,D]	S68.125[A,D]	S81.042[A,D]
S46.222[A,D]	S56.821[A,D]	S61.246[A,D]	S66.021[A,D]	S68.126[A,D]	S81.051[A,D]
S46.321[A,D]	S56.822[A,D]	S61.247[A,D]	S66.022[A,D]	S68.127[A,D]	S81.052[A,D]
S46.322[A,D]	S56.921[A,D]	S61.250[A,D]	S66.120[A,D]	S68.411[A,D]	S81.811[A,D]
S46.821[A,D]	S56.922[A,D]	S61.251[A,D]	S66.121[A,D]	S68.412[A,D]	S81.812[A,D]
S46.822[A,D]	S57.01XD	S61.252[A,D]	S66.122[A,D]	S68.421[A,D]	S81.821[A,D]
S46.921[A,D]	S57.02XD	S61.253[A,D]	S66.123[A,D]	S68.422[A,D]	S81.822[A,D]
S46.922[A,D]	S57.81XD	S61.254[A,D]	S66.124[A,D]	S68.511[A,D]	S81.831[A,D]
S47.1XX[A,D]	S57.82XD	S61.255[A,D]	S66.125[A,D]	S68.512[A,D]	S81.832[A,D]
S47.2XX[A,D]	S58.011[A,D]	S61.256[A,D]	S66.126[A,D]	S68.521[A,D]	S81.841[A,D]
S48.011[A,D]	S58.012[A,D]	S61.257[A,D]	S66.127[A,D]	S68.522[A,D]	S81.842[A,D]
S48.012[A,D]	S58.021[A,D]	S61.310[A,D]	S66.221[A,D]	S68.610[A,D]	S81.851[A,D]
S48.021[A,D]	S58.022[A,D]	S61.311[A,D]	S66.222[A,D]	S68.611[A,D]	S81.852[A,D]
S48.022[A,D]	S58.111[A,D]	S61.312[A,D]	S66.320[A,D]	S68.612[A,D]	S86.021[A,D]
S48.111[A,D]	S58.112[A,D]	S61.313[A,D]	S66.321[A,D]	S68.613[A,D]	S86.022[A,D]
S48.112[A,D]	S58.121[A,D]	S61.314[A,D]	S66.322[A,D]	S68.614[A,D]	S86.121[A,D]
S48.121[A,D]	S58.122[A,D]	S61.315[A,D]	S66.323[A,D]	S68.615[A,D]	S86.122[A,D]
S48.122[A,D]	S58.911[A,D]	S61.316[A,D]	S66.324[A,D]	S68.616[A,D]	S86.221[A,D]
S48.911[A,D]	S58.912[A,D]	S61.317[A,D]	S66.325[A,D]	S68.617[A,D]	S86.222[A,D]
S48.912[A,D]	S58.921[A,D]	S61.320[A,D]	S66.326[A,D]	S68.620[A,D]	S86.321[A,D]
S48.921[A,D]	S58.922[A,D]	S61.321[A,D]	S66.327[A,D]	S68.621[A,D]	S86.322[A,D]
S48.922[A,D]	S61.011[A,D]	S61.322[A,D]	S66.421[A,D]	S68.622[A,D]	S86.821[A,D]
S51.011[A,D]	S61.012[A,D]	S61.323[A,D]	S66.422[A,D]	S68.623[A,D]	S86.822[A,D]
S51.012[A,D]	S61.021[A,D]	S61.324[A,D]	S66.520[A,D]	S68.624[A,D]	S86.921[A,D]
S51.021[A,D]	S61.022[A,D]	S61.325[A,D]	S66.521[A,D]	S68.625[A,D]	S86.922[A,D]
S51.022[A,D]	S61.031[A,D]	S61.326[A,D]	S66.522[A,D]	S68.626[A,D]	S91.011[A,D]
S51.031[A,D]	S61.032[A,D]	S61.327[A,D]	S66.523[A,D]	S68.627[A,D]	S91.012[A,D]
S51.032[A,D]	S61.041[A,D]	S61.330[A,D]	S66.524[A,D]	S68.711[A,D]	S91.021[A,D]
S51.041[A,D]	S61.042[A,D]	S61.331[A,D]	S66.525[A,D]	S68.712[A,D]	S91.022[A,D]
S51.042[A,D]	S61.051[A,D]	S61.332[A,D]	S66.526[A,D]	S68.721[A,D]	S91.031[A,D]
S51.051[A,D]	S61.052[A,D]	S61.333[A,D]	S66.527[A,D]	S68.722[A,D]	S91.032[A,D]
S51.052[A,D]	S61.111[A,D]	S61.334[A,D]	S66.821[A,D]	S71.011[A,D]	S91.041[A,D]
S51.811[A,D]	S61.112[A,D]	S61.335[A,D]	S66.822[A,D]	S71.012[A,D]	S91.042[A,D]
S51.812[A,D]	S61.121[A,D]	S61.336[A,D]	S66.921[A,D]	S71.021[A,D]	S91.051[A,D]
S51.821[A,D]	S61.122[A,D]	S61.337[A,D]	S66.922[A,D]	S71.022[A,D]	S91.052[A,D]
S51.822[A,D]	S61.131[A,D]	S61.340[A,D]	S67.01XD	S71.031[A,D]	S91.111[A,D]
S51.831[A,D]	S61.132[A,D]	S61.341[A,D]	S67.02XD	S71.032[A,D]	S91.112[A,D]
S51.832[A,D]	S61.141[A,D]	S61.342[A,D]	S67.190D	S71.041[A,D]	S91.114[A,D]
S51.841[A,D]	S61.142[A,D]	S61.343[A,D]	S67.191D	S71.042[A,D]	S91.115[A,D]
	S61.151[A,D]	S61.344[A,D]	S67.192D	S71.051[A,D]	S91.121[A,D]
	S61.152[A,D]	S61.345[A,D]	S67.193D	S71.052[A,D]	S91.122[A,D]
	S61.210[A,D]	S61.346[A,D]	S67.194D	S71.111[A,D]	S91.124[A,D]
	S61.211[A,D]	S61.347[A,D]	S67.195D	S71.112[A,D]	S91.125[A,D]
	S61.212[A,D]	S61.350[A,D]	S67.196D	S71.121[A,D]	S91.131[A,D]

19 Skin 1 – Traumatic wounds, burns and postoperative complications (continued)					
S91.132[A,D]	S98.142[A,D]	T21.62X[A,D]	T22.791[A,D]	T23.771[A,D]	T25.721[A,D]
S91.134[A,D]	S98.211[A,D]	T21.63X[A,D]	T22.792[A,D]	T23.772[A,D]	T25.722[A,D]
S91.135[A,D]	S98.212[A,D]	T21.64X[A,D]	T23.201[A,D]	T23.791[A,D]	T25.731[A,D]
S91.141[A,D]	S98.221[A,D]	T21.65X[A,D]	T23.202[A,D]	T23.792[A,D]	T25.732[A,D]
S91.142[A,D]	S98.222[A,D]	T21.66X[A,D]	T23.211[A,D]	T24.201[A,D]	T25.791[A,D]
S91.144[A,D]	S98.311[A,D]	T21.67X[A,D]	T23.212[A,D]	T24.202[A,D]	T25.792[A,D]
S91.145[A,D]	S98.312[A,D]	T21.69X[A,D]	T23.221[A,D]	T24.211[A,D]	T26.21X[A,D]
S91.151[A,D]	S98.321[A,D]	T21.70X[A,D]	T23.222[A,D]	T24.212[A,D]	T26.22X[A,D]
S91.152[A,D]	S98.322[A,D]	T21.71X[A,D]	T23.231[A,D]	T24.221[A,D]	T31.10
S91.154[A,D]	S98.911[A,D]	T21.72X[A,D]	T23.232[A,D]	T24.222[A,D]	T31.11
S91.155[A,D]	S98.912[A,D]	T21.73X[A,D]	T23.241[A,D]	T24.231[A,D]	T31.20
S91.211[A,D]	S98.921[A,D]	T21.74X[A,D]	T23.242[A,D]	T24.232[A,D]	T31.21
S91.212[A,D]	S98.922[A,D]	T21.75X[A,D]	T23.251[A,D]	T24.291[A,D]	T31.22
S91.214[A,D]	T20.20X[A,D]	T21.76X[A,D]	T23.252[A,D]	T24.292[A,D]	T31.30
S91.215[A,D]	T20.211[A,D]	T21.77X[A,D]	T23.261[A,D]	T24.301[A,D]	T31.31
S91.221[A,D]	T20.212[A,D]	T21.79X[A,D]	T23.262[A,D]	T24.302[A,D]	T31.32
S91.222[A,D]	T20.22X[A,D]	T22.211[A,D]	T23.271[A,D]	T24.311[A,D]	T31.33
S91.224[A,D]	T20.23X[A,D]	T22.212[A,D]	T23.272[A,D]	T24.312[A,D]	T31.40
S91.225[A,D]	T20.24X[A,D]	T22.221[A,D]	T23.291[A,D]	T24.321[A,D]	T31.41
S91.231[A,D]	T20.25X[A,D]	T22.222[A,D]	T23.292[A,D]	T24.322[A,D]	T31.42
S91.232[A,D]	T20.26X[A,D]	T22.231[A,D]	T23.301[A,D]	T24.331[A,D]	T31.43
S91.234[A,D]	T20.27X[A,D]	T22.232[A,D]	T23.302[A,D]	T24.332[A,D]	T31.44
S91.235[A,D]	T20.29X[A,D]	T22.241[A,D]	T23.311[A,D]	T24.391[A,D]	T31.50
S91.239[A,D]	T20.30X[A,D]	T22.242[A,D]	T23.312[A,D]	T24.392[A,D]	T31.51
S91.241[A,D]	T20.311[A,D]	T22.251[A,D]	T23.321[A,D]	T24.601[A,D]	T31.52
S91.242[A,D]	T20.312[A,D]	T22.252[A,D]	T23.322[A,D]	T24.602[A,D]	T31.53
S91.244[A,D]	T20.32X[A,D]	T22.261[A,D]	T23.331[A,D]	T24.611[A,D]	T31.54
S91.245[A,D]	T20.33X[A,D]	T22.262[A,D]	T23.332[A,D]	T24.612[A,D]	T31.55
S91.251[A,D]	T20.34X[A,D]	T22.291[A,D]	T23.341[A,D]	T24.621[A,D]	T31.60
S91.252[A,D]	T20.35X[A,D]	T22.292[A,D]	T23.342[A,D]	T24.622[A,D]	T31.61
S91.254[A,D]	T20.36X[A,D]	T22.311[A,D]	T23.351[A,D]	T24.631[A,D]	T31.62
S91.255[A,D]	T20.37X[A,D]	T22.312[A,D]	T23.352[A,D]	T24.632[A,D]	T31.63
S91.311[A,D]	T20.39X[A,D]	T22.321[A,D]	T23.361[A,D]	T24.691[A,D]	T31.64
S91.312[A,D]	T20.60X[A,D]	T22.322[A,D]	T23.362[A,D]	T24.692[A,D]	T31.65
S91.321[A,D]	T20.611[A,D]	T22.331[A,D]	T23.371[A,D]	T24.701[A,D]	T31.66
S91.322[A,D]	T20.612[A,D]	T22.332[A,D]	T23.372[A,D]	T24.702[A,D]	T31.70
S91.331[A,D]	T20.62X[A,D]	T22.341[A,D]	T23.391[A,D]	T24.711[A,D]	T31.71
S91.332[A,D]	T20.63X[A,D]	T22.342[A,D]	T23.392[A,D]	T24.712[A,D]	T31.72
S91.341[A,D]	T20.64X[A,D]	T22.351[A,D]	T23.601[A,D]	T24.721[A,D]	T31.73
S91.342[A,D]	T20.65X[A,D]	T22.352[A,D]	T23.602[A,D]	T24.722[A,D]	T31.74
S91.351[A,D]	T20.66X[A,D]	T22.361[A,D]	T23.611[A,D]	T24.731[A,D]	T31.75
S91.352[A,D]	T20.67X[A,D]	T22.362[A,D]	T23.612[A,D]	T24.732[A,D]	T31.76
S94.21XD	T20.69X[A,D]	T22.391[A,D]	T23.621[A,D]	T24.791[A,D]	T31.77
S94.22XD	T20.711[A,D]	T22.392[A,D]	T23.622[A,D]	T24.792[A,D]	T31.80
S96.021[A,D]	T20.712[A,D]	T22.611[A,D]	T23.631[A,D]	T25.211[A,D]	T31.81
S96.022[A,D]	T20.72X[A,D]	T22.612[A,D]	T23.632[A,D]	T25.212[A,D]	T31.82
S96.121[A,D]	T20.73X[A,D]	T22.621[A,D]	T23.641[A,D]	T25.221[A,D]	T31.83
S96.122[A,D]	T20.74X[A,D]	T22.622[A,D]	T23.642[A,D]	T25.222[A,D]	T31.84
S96.221[A,D]	T20.75X[A,D]	T22.631[A,D]	T23.651[A,D]	T25.231[A,D]	T31.85
S96.222[A,D]	T20.76X[A,D]	T22.632[A,D]	T23.652[A,D]	T25.232[A,D]	T31.86
S96.821[A,D]	T20.77X[A,D]	T22.641[A,D]	T23.661[A,D]	T25.291[A,D]	T31.87
S96.822[A,D]	T20.79X[A,D]	T22.642[A,D]	T23.662[A,D]	T25.292[A,D]	T31.88
S96.921[A,D]	T21.21X[A,D]	T22.651[A,D]	T23.671[A,D]	T25.311[A,D]	T31.90
S96.922[A,D]	T21.22X[A,D]	T22.652[A,D]	T23.672[A,D]	T25.312[A,D]	T31.91
S98.011[A,D]	T21.23X[A,D]	T22.661[A,D]	T23.691[A,D]	T25.321[A,D]	T31.92
S98.012[A,D]	T21.24X[A,D]	T22.662[A,D]	T23.692[A,D]	T25.322[A,D]	T31.93
S98.021[A,D]	T21.25X[A,D]	T22.691[A,D]	T23.701[A,D]	T25.331[A,D]	T31.94
S98.022[A,D]	T21.26X[A,D]	T22.692[A,D]	T23.702[A,D]	T25.332[A,D]	T31.95
S98.111[A,D]	T21.27X[A,D]	T22.711[A,D]	T23.711[A,D]	T25.391[A,D]	T31.96
S98.112[A,D]	T21.29X[A,D]	T22.712[A,D]	T23.712[A,D]	T25.392[A,D]	T31.97
S98.121[A,D]	T21.30X[A,D]	T22.721[A,D]	T23.721[A,D]	T25.611[A,D]	T31.98
S98.122[A,D]	T21.31X[A,D]	T22.722[A,D]	T23.722[A,D]	T25.612[A,D]	T31.99
S98.131[A,D]	T21.32X[A,D]	T22.731[A,D]	T23.731[A,D]	T25.621[A,D]	T32.10
S98.132[A,D]	T21.33X[A,D]	T22.732[A,D]	T23.732[A,D]	T25.622[A,D]	T32.11
S98.141[A,D]	T21.34X[A,D]	T22.741[A,D]	T23.741[A,D]	T25.631[A,D]	T32.20
	T21.35X[A,D]	T22.742[A,D]	T23.742[A,D]	T25.632[A,D]	T32.21
	T21.36X[A,D]	T22.751[A,D]	T23.751[A,D]	T25.691[A,D]	T32.22
	T21.37X[A,D]	T22.752[A,D]	T23.752[A,D]	T25.692[A,D]	T32.30
	T21.39X[A,D]	T22.761[A,D]	T23.761[A,D]	T25.711[A,D]	T32.31
	T21.61X[A,D]	T22.762[A,D]	T23.762[A,D]	T25.712[A,D]	T32.32

19 Skin 1 – Traumatic wounds, burns and postoperative complications (continued)

20 Skin 2 – Ulcers and other skin conditions

T32.33	T81.524D	I70.432	K60*	L03.022	L97.224
T32.40	T81.525D	I70.433	K61*	L03.031	L97.229
T32.41	T81.526D	I70.434	L02.01	L03.032	L97.311
T32.42	T81.527D	I70.435	L02.02	L03.041	L97.312
T32.43	T81.528D	I70.438	L02.03	L03.042	L97.313
T32.44	T81.529D	I70.441	L02.11	L03.111	L97.314
T32.50	T81.530D	I70.442	L02.12	L03.112	L97.319
T32.51	T81.531D	I70.443	L02.13	L03.113	L97.321
T32.52	T81.532D	I70.444	L02.211	L03.114	L97.322
T32.53	T81.533D	I70.445	L02.212	L03.115	L97.323
T32.54	T81.534D	I70.448	L02.213	L03.116	L97.324
T32.55	T81.535D	I70.45	L02.214	L03.121	L97.329
T32.60	T81.536D	I70.461	L02.215	L03.122	L97.411
T32.61	T81.537D	I70.462	L02.216	L03.123	L97.412
T32.62	T81.538D	I70.463	L02.221	L03.124	L97.413
T32.63	T81.539D	I70.468	L02.222	L03.125	L97.414
T32.64	T81.590[A,D]	I70.531	L02.223	L03.126	L97.419
T32.65	T81.591[A,D]	I70.532	L02.224	L03.211	L97.421
T32.66	T81.592[A,D]	I70.533	L02.225	L03.212	L97.422
T32.70	T81.593[A,D]	I70.534	L02.226	L03.221	L97.423
T32.71	T81.594[A,D]	I70.535	L02.231	L03.222	L97.424
T32.72	T81.595[A,D]	I70.538	L02.232	L03.311	L97.429
T32.73	T81.596[A,D]	I70.541	L02.233	L03.312	L97.501
T32.74	T81.597[A,D]	I70.542	L02.234	L03.313	L97.502
T32.75	T81.598[A,D]	I70.543	L02.235	L03.314	L97.503
T32.76	T81.599[A,D]	I70.544	L02.236	L03.315	L97.504
T32.77	T81.83X[A,D]	I70.545	L02.31	L03.316	L97.509
T32.80		I70.548	L02.32	L03.317	L97.511
T32.81	**20 Skin 2 – Ulcers and**	I70.55	L02.33	L03.321	L97.512
T32.82	**other skin conditions**	I70.561	L02.411	L03.322	L97.513
T32.83	A06.7	I70.562	L02.412	L03.323	L97.514
T32.84	B78.1	I70.563	L02.413	L03.324	L97.519
T32.85	E08.52	I70.568	L02.414	L03.325	L97.521
T32.86	E09.52	I70.631	L02.415	L03.326	L97.522
T32.87	E09.622	I70.632	L02.416	L03.327	L97.523
T32.88	I70.231	I70.633	L02.421	L03.329	L97.524
T32.90	I70.232	I70.634	L02.422	L03.811	L97.529
T32.91	I70.233	I70.635	L02.423	L03.818	L97.801
T32.92	I70.234	I70.638	L02.424	L03.891	L97.802
T32.93	I70.235	I70.641	L02.425	L03.898	L97.803
T32.94	I70.238	I70.642	L02.426	L04.0	L97.804
T32.95	I70.241	I70.643	L02.431	L04.1	L97.809
T32.96	I70.242	I70.644	L02.432	L04.2	L97.811
T32.97	I70.243	I70.645	L02.433	L04.3	L97.812
T32.98	I70.244	I70.648	L02.434	L04.8	L97.813
T32.99	I70.245	I70.65	L02.435	L05*	L97.814
T81.30X[A,D]	I70.248	I70.661	L02.436	L08.0	L97.819
T81.31X[A,D]	I70.25	I70.662	L02.511	L08.81	L97.821
T81.32X[A,D]	I70.261	I70.663	L02.512	L08.89	L97.822
T81.33X[A,D]	I70.262	I70.668	L02.521	L08.9	L97.823
T81.4XX[A,D]	I70.263	I70.731	L02.522	L88	L97.824
T81.510D	I70.268	I70.732	L02.531	L92.8	L97.829
T81.511D	I70.331	I70.733	L02.532	L97.111	L97.911
T81.512D	I70.332	I70.734	L02.611	L97.112	L97.912
T81.513D	I70.333	I70.735	L02.612	L97.113	L97.913
T81.514D	I70.334	I70.738	L02.621	L97.114	L97.914
T81.515D	I70.335	I70.741	L02.622	L97.119	L97.919
T81.516D	I70.338	I70.742	L02.631	L97.121	L97.921
T81.517D	I70.341	I70.743	L02.632	L97.122	L97.922
T81.518D	I70.342	I70.744	L02.811	L97.123	L97.923
T81.519D	I70.343	I70.745	L02.818	L97.124	L97.924
T81.520D	I70.344	I70.748	L02.821	L97.129	L97.929
T81.521D	I70.345	I70.75	L02.828	L97.211	L98.0
T81.522D	I70.348	I70.761	L02.831	L97.212	L98.3
T81.523D	I70.35	I70.762	L02.838	L97.213	L98.411
	I70.361	I70.763	L02.92	L97.214	L98.412
	I70.362	I70.768	L02.93	L97.219	L98.413
	I70.363	I73.01	L03.011	L97.221	L98.414
	I70.368	I96	L03.012	L97.222	L98.419
	I70.431	K12.2	L03.021*	L97.223	L98.421

20 Skin 2 – Ulcers and other skin conditions (continued)	21 Tracheostomy care	22 Urostomy/ cystostomy care			
L98.422	Z43.0	Z43.5			
L98.423		Z43.6			
L98.424					
L98.429					
L98.491					
L98.492					
L98.493					
L98.494					
L98.499					
20 Skin 2 – Ulcers and	21 Tracheostomy care	22 Urostomy/ cystostomy care			

Appendix K: NRS Case-Mix Adjustment Variables and Scores

The nonroutine supply case-mix adjustment is based upon a six-group severity level approach. The severity level is determined by primary/secondary diagnosis combinations. Each level is assigned a score. The table below provides the condition variables and the scores. Note: points are additive. However points may not be given for the same line item in the table more than once. Points are not assigned for a secondary diagnosis if points are already assigned for a primary diagnosis from the same diagnosis/condition group. Refer to the resource titled "Diagnosis Categories for Nonroutine Supplies Case-Mix Adjustment" for definitions of the diagnosis/condition groups. The source for this information is the January 2017 Home Health Prospective Payment System (HH PPS) Grouper software v6117; update effective January 1, 2017.

Note: An updated version of the home health prospective payment system (HH PPS) Grouper software was not available at the time this book was printed and therefore this appendix does not reflect any fiscal 2018 code changes. Updated versions of the software can be found at https://www.cms.gov/Medicare/Medicare-Fee-for-Service-Payment/HomeHealthPPS/CaseMixGrouperSoftware.html.

Item	Description	Points
SELECTED SKIN CONDITIONS:		
1	Primary diagnosis = Anal fissure, fistula, and abscess	15
2	Other diagnosis = Anal fissure, fistula, and abscess	13
3	Primary diagnosis = Cellulitis and abscess	14
4	Other diagnosis = Cellulitis and abscess	8
5	Primary diagnosis = Diabetic ulcers	20
6	Primary diagnosis = Gangrene	11
7	Other diagnosis = Gangrene	8
8	Primary diagnosis = Malignant neoplasms of skin	15
9	Other diagnosis = Malignant neoplasms of skin	4
10	Primary or Other diagnosis = Non-pressure and non-stasis ulcers	13
11	Primary diagnosis = Other infections of skin and subcutaneous tissue	16
12	Other diagnosis = Other infections of skin and subcutaneous tissue	7
13	Primary diagnosis = Postoperative complications	23
14	Other diagnosis = Postoperative complications	15
15	Primary diagnosis = Traumatic wounds, burns and post-operative complications	19
16	Other diagnosis = Traumatic wounds, burns and post-operative complications	8
17	Primary or other diagnosis = V code, Cystostomy care	16
18	Primary or other diagnosis = V code, Tracheostomy care	23
19	Primary or other diagnosis = V code, Urostomy care	24
20	OASIS M1322 = 1 or 2 pressure ulcers, stage 1	4
21	OASIS M1322 = 3+ pressure ulcers, stage 1	6
22	OASIS M1311 = 1 pressure ulcer, stage 2	14
23	OASIS M1311 = 2 pressure ulcers, stage 2	22
24	OASIS M1311 = 3 pressure ulcers, stage 2	29
25	OASIS M1311 = 4+ pressure ulcers, stage 2	35
26	OASIS M1311 = 1 pressure ulcer, stage 3	29
27	OASIS M1311 = 2 pressure ulcers, stage 3	41
28	OASIS M1311 = 3 pressure ulcers, stage 3	46
29	OASIS M1311 = 4+ pressure ulcers, stage 3	58
30	OASIS M1311 = 1 pressure ulcer, stage 4	48
31	OASIS M1311 = 2 pressure ulcers, stage 4	67
32	OASIS M1311 = 3+ pressure ulcers, stage 4	75
33	OASIS M1311e = 1 (unobserved pressure ulcer(s))	17
34	OASIS M1332 = 2 (2 stasis ulcers)	6
35	OASIS M1332 = 3 (3 stasis ulcers)	12
36	OASIS M1332 = 4 (4+ stasis ulcers)	21
37	OASIS M1330 = 1 (unobservable stasis ulcers)	9
38	OASIS M1334 = 1 (status of most problematic stasis ulcer: fully granulating)	6
39	OASIS M1334 = 2 (status of most problematic stasis ulcer: early/partial granulation)	25
40	OASIS M1334 = 3 (status of most problematic stasis ulcer: not healing)	36
41	OASIS M1342 = 2 (status of most problematic surgical wound: early/partial granulation)	4
42	OASIS M1342 = 3 (status of most problematic surgical wound: not healing)	14

Appendix K: NRS Case-Mix Adjustment Variables and Scores

Item	Description	Points
OTHER CLINICAL FACTORS		
43	OASIS M1630 = 1 (ostomy not related to inpt stay/no regimen change)	27
44	OASIS M1630 = 2 (ostomy related to inpt stay/regimen change)	45
45	Any 'Selected Skin Conditions' (rows 1–42 above) **AND** M1630 = 1 (ostomy not related to inpt stay/no regimen change)	14
46	Any 'Selected Skin Conditions' (rows 1–42 above) **AND** M1630 = 2 (ostomy related to inpt stay/regimen change)	11
47	OASIS M1030 (Therapy at home) = 1 (IV/infusion)	5
48	OASIS M1610 = 2 (patient requires urinary catheter)	9
49	OASIS M1620 = 4 or 5 (bowel incontinence, daily or >daily)	10

Appendix L: Diagnosis Categories for Nonroutine Supplies Case-Mix Adjustment

The home health prospective payment system (HH PPS) provides for a case-mix adjustment for nonroutine supplies when reported appropriately with a code value in the fifth position of the HIPPS code, a valid HCPCS code for the supply with revenue code 27X (excluding 274) or 623, and a valid ICD-10-CM code, included below, on the OASIS instrument. All diagnosis code assignments must follow ICD-10-CM official coding guidelines. The data source for this information is the January 2017 HH PPS Grouper software v6117 update, effective January 1, 2017.

Note: An updated version of the home health prospective payment system (HH PPS) Grouper software was not available at the time this book was printed and therefore this appendix does not reflect any fiscal 2018 code changes. Updated versions of the software can be found at https://www.cms.gov/Medicare/Medicare-Fee-for-Service-Payment/HomeHealthPPS/CaseMixGrouperSoftware.html.

A code followed by an asterisk indicates a code range and that all codes in that category or subcategory are included. All codes should be reported to the highest level of specificity.

01 Anal fissure, fistula and abscess
K50.014
K50.114
K50.814
K50.914
K60*
K61*

02 Cellulitis and abscess
B43.1
K12.2
L02.01
L02.11
L02.211
L02.212
L02.213
L02.214
L02.215
L02.216
L02.219
L02.31
L02.411
L02.412
L02.413
L02.414
L02.415
L02.416
L02.511
L02.512
L02.611
L02.612
L02.811
L02.818
L03.011
L03.012
L03.021
L03.022
L03.031
L03.032
L03.041
L03.042
L03.111
L03.112
L03.113
L03.114
L03.115
L03.116
L03.121
L03.122
L03.123
L03.124
L03.125
L03.126
L03.2*

L03.3*
L03.8*
L98.3

03 Diabetic ulcers
E08.621
E08.622
E09.621
E09.622
E10.621
E10.622
E11.621
E11.622
E13.621
E13.622

04 Gangrene
E08.52
E09.52
E10.52
E11.52
E13.52
I70.261
I70.262
I70.263
I70.268
I70.361
I70.362
I70.363
I70.368
I70.461
I70.462
I70.463
I70.468
I70.561
I70.562
I70.563
I70.568
I70.661
I70.662
I70.663
I70.668
I70.761
I70.762
I70.763
I70.768
I73.01
I96

05 Malignant neoplasms of skin
C43*
C44*
C46.0
C4A*

C7B.1
C82.6*
C82.8*
C82.9*
C83.00
C83.01
C83.02
C83.03
C83.04
C83.05
C84.0*
C84.1*
C84.A*
D03.0
D03.11
D03.12
D03.21
D03.22
D03.39
D03.4
D03.5*
D03.61
D03.62
D03.71
D03.72
D03.8
D04*

06 Non-pressure and non-stasis ulcers (other than diabetic)
I70.231
I70.232
I70.233
I70.234
I70.235
I70.238
I70.241
I70.242
I70.243
I70.244
I70.245
I70.248
I70.249
I70.25
I70.331
I70.332
I70.333
I70.334
I70.335
I70.338
I70.341
I70.342
I70.343
I70.344

I70.345
I70.348
I70.35
I70.431
I70.432
I70.433
I70.434
I70.435
I70.438
I70.441
I70.442
I70.443
I70.444
I70.445
I70.448
I70.45
I70.531
I70.532
I70.533
I70.534
I70.535
I70.538
I70.541
I70.542
I70.543
I70.544
I70.545
I70.548
I70.55
I70.631
I70.632
I70.633
I70.634
I70.635
I70.638
I70.641
I70.642
I70.643
I70.644
I70.645
I70.648
I70.65
I70.731
I70.732
I70.733
I70.734
I70.735
I70.738
I70.741
I70.742
I70.743
I70.744
I70.745
I70.748
I70.75

L97.111
L97.112
L97.113
L97.114
L97.119
L97.121
L97.122
L97.123
L97.124
L97.129
L97.211
L97.212
L97.213
L97.214
L97.219
L97.221
L97.222
L97.223
L97.224
L97.229
L97.311
L97.312
L97.313
L97.314
L97.319
L97.321
L97.322
L97.323
L97.324
L97.329
L97.411
L97.412
L97.413
L97.414
L97.419
L97.421
L97.422
L97.423
L97.424
L97.429
L97.511
L97.512
L97.513
L97.514
L97.519
L97.521
L97.522
L97.523
L97.524
L97.529
L97.811
L97.812
L97.813
L97.814
L97.819

L97.821
L97.822
L97.823
L97.824
L97.829
L97.901
L97.902
L97.903
L97.904
L97.909
L97.911
L97.912
L97.913
L97.914
L97.919
L97.921
L97.922
L97.923
L97.924
L97.929
L98.411
L98.412
L98.413
L98.414
L98.419
L98.421
L98.422
L98.423
L98.424
L98.429
L98.491
L98.492
L98.493
L98.494
L98.499

07 Other infections of skin and subcutaneous tissue
A22.0
A26.0
A50.06
A50.07
B35.1
B35.2
B35.3
B35.4
B35.5
B35.6
B35.8
B35.9
B36*
B37.2
B38.3
B40.3

07 Other infections of skin and subcutaneous tissue (continued)	L98.0	S01.142[A,D]	S09.392[A,D]	S21.201[A,D]	S31.33X[A,D]
		S01.151[A,D]	S09.8XX[A,D]	S21.202[A,D]	S31.34X[A,D]
	08 Postoperative complications	S01.152[A,D]	S11.011D	S21.211[A,D]	S31.35X[A,D]
B43.0		S01.20X[A,D]	S11.012D	S21.212[A,D]	S31.40X[A,D]
B43.2	E89.810	S01.21X[A,D]	S11.013D	S21.221[A,D]	S31.41X[A,D]
B43.8	E89.811	S01.22X[A,D]	S11.014D	S21.222[A,D]	S31.42X[A,D]
B43.9	E89.820	S01.23X[A,D]	S11.015D	S21.231[A,D]	S31.43X[A,D]
B45.2	E89.821	S01.24X[A,D]	S11.019D	S21.232[A,D]	S31.44X[A,D]
B46.3	T81.510D	S01.25X[A,D]	S11.021D	S21.241[A,D]	S31.45X[A,D]
B47*	T81.511D	S01.301[A,D]	S11.022D	S21.242[A,D]	S31.501[A,D]
B48.0	T81.512D	S01.302[A,D]	S11.023D	S21.251[A,D]	S31.502[A,D]
B65.3	T81.513D	S01.311[A,D]	S11.024D	S21.252[A,D]	S31.511[A,D]
B78.1	T81.514D	S01.312[A,D]	S11.025D	S28.1XX[A,D]	S31.512[A,D]
L02.02	T81.515D	S01.321[A,D]	S11.029D	S28.211[A,D]	S31.521[A,D]
L02.03	T81.516D	S01.322[A,D]	S11.031D	S28.212[A,D]	S31.522[A,D]
L02.12	T81.517D	S01.331[A,D]	S11.032D	S28.221[A,D]	S31.531[A,D]
L02.13	T81.518D	S01.332[A,D]	S11.033D	S28.222[A,D]	S31.532[A,D]
L02.221	T81.519D	S01.341[A,D]	S11.034D	S29.021[A,D]	S31.541[A,D]
L02.222	T81.520D	S01.342[A,D]	S11.035D	S29.022[A,D]	S31.542[A,D]
L02.223	T81.521D	S01.351[A,D]	S11.039D	S31.000[A,D]	S31.551[A,D]
L02.224	T81.522D	S01.352[A,D]	S11.10XD	S31.010[A,D]	S31.552[A,D]
L02.225	T81.523D	S01.401[A,D]	S11.11XD	S31.020[A,D]	S31.811[A,D]
L02.226	T81.524D	S01.402[A,D]	S11.12XD	S31.030[A,D]	S31.812[A,D]
L02.231	T81.525D	S01.411[A,D]	S11.13XD	S31.040[A,D]	S31.813[A,D]
L02.232	T81.526D	S01.412[A,D]	S11.14XD	S31.050[A,D]	S31.814[A,D]
L02.233	T81.527D	S01.421[A,D]	S11.15XD	S31.100[A,D]	S31.815[A,D]
L02.234	T81.528D	S01.422[A,D]	S11.20XD	S31.101[A,D]	S31.819[A,D]
L02.235	T81.529D	S01.431[A,D]	S11.21XD	S31.102[A,D]	S31.821[A,D]
L02.236	T81.530D	S01.432[A,D]	S11.22XD	S31.103[A,D]	S31.822[A,D]
L02.32	T81.531D	S01.441[A,D]	S11.23XD	S31.104[A,D]	S31.823[A,D]
L02.33	T81.532D	S01.442[A,D]	S11.24XD	S31.105[A,D]	S31.824[A,D]
L02.421	T81.533D	S01.451[A,D]	S11.25XD	S31.110[A,D]	S31.825[A,D]
L02.422	T81.534D	S01.452[A,D]	S11.80X[A,D]	S31.111[A,D]	S31.829[A,D]
L02.423	T81.535D	S01.501[A,D]	S11.81X[A,D]	S31.112[A,D]	S31.831[A,D]
L02.424	T81.536D	S01.502[A,D]	S11.82X[A,D]	S31.113[A,D]	S31.832[A,D]
L02.425	T81.537D	S01.511[A,D]	S11.83X[A,D]	S31.114[A,D]	S31.833[A,D]
L02.426	T81.538D	S01.512[A,D]	S11.84X[A,D]	S31.115[A,D]	S31.834[A,D]
L02.431	T81.539D	S01.521[A,D]	S11.85X[A,D]	S31.120[A,D]	S31.835[A,D]
L02.432	T81.590[A,D]	S01.522[A,D]	S11.89X[A,D]	S31.121[A,D]	S31.839[A,D]
L02.433	T81.591[A,D]	S01.531[A,D]	S11.90X[A,D]	S31.122[A,D]	S38.211[A,D]
L02.434	T81.592[A,D]	S01.532[A,D]	S11.91X[A,D]	S31.123[A,D]	S38.212[A,D]
L02.435	T81.593[A,D]	S01.541[A,D]	S11.92X[A,D]	S31.124[A,D]	S38.221[A,D]
L02.436	T81.594[A,D]	S01.542[A,D]	S11.93X[A,D]	S31.125[A,D]	S38.222[A,D]
L02.521	T81.595[A,D]	S01.551[A,D]	S11.94X[A,D]	S31.130[A,D]	S38.231[A,D]
L02.522	T81.596[A,D]	S01.552[A,D]	S11.95X[A,D]	S31.131[A,D]	S38.232[A,D]
L02.531	T81.597[A,D]	S01.80X[A,D]	S16.2XX[A,D]	S31.132[A,D]	S38.3XX[A,D]
L02.532	T81.598[A,D]	S01.81X[A,D]	S21.001[A,D]	S31.133[A,D]	S39.021[A,D]
L02.621	T81.599[A,D]	S01.82X[A,D]	S21.002[A,D]	S31.134[A,D]	S39.022[A,D]
L02.622	T81.83X[A,D]	S01.83X[A,D]	S21.011[A,D]	S31.135[A,D]	S39.023[A,D]
L02.631		S01.84X[A,D]	S21.012[A,D]	S31.140[A,D]	S41.001[A,D]
L02.632	**09 Traumatic wounds, burns and postoperative complications**	S01.85X[A,D]	S21.021[A,D]	S31.141[A,D]	S41.002[A,D]
L02.821		S05.41XD	S21.022[A,D]	S31.142[A,D]	S41.009[A,D]
L02.828		S05.42XD	S21.031[A,D]	S31.143[A,D]	S41.011[A,D]
L02.831		S08.0XX[A,D]	S21.032[A,D]	S31.144[A,D]	S41.012[A,D]
L02.838	K68.11	S08.111[A,D]	S21.041[A,D]	S31.145[A,D]	S41.021[A,D]
L04.0	S01.00X[A,D]	S08.112[A,D]	S21.042[A,D]	S31.150[A,D]	S41.022[A,D]
L04.1	S01.01X[A,D]	S08.121[A,D]	S21.051[A,D]	S31.151[A,D]	S41.031[A,D]
L04.2	S01.02X[A,D]	S08.122[A,D]	S21.052[A,D]	S31.152[A,D]	S41.032[A,D]
L04.3	S01.03X[A,D]	S08.811[A,D]	S21.101[A,D]	S31.153[A,D]	S41.041[A,D]
L04.8	S01.04X[A,D]	S08.812[A,D]	S21.102[A,D]	S31.154[A,D]	S41.042[A,D]
L05.01	S01.05X[A,D]	S08.89X[A,D]	S21.111[A,D]	S31.155[A,D]	S41.051[A,D]
L05.02	S01.101[A,D]	S09.12XD	S21.112[A,D]	S31.20X[A,D]	S41.052[A,D]
L05.91	S01.102[A,D]	S09.21XD	S21.121[A,D]	S31.21X[A,D]	S41.101[A,D]
L05.92	S01.111[A,D]	S09.22XD	S21.122[A,D]	S31.22X[A,D]	S41.102[A,D]
L08.0	S01.112[A,D]	S09.301[A,D]	S21.131[A,D]	S31.23X[A,D]	S41.109[A,D]
L08.8*	S01.121[A,D]	S09.302[A,D]	S21.132[A,D]	S31.24X[A,D]	S41.111[A,D]
L08.9	S01.122[A,D]	S09.311[A,D]	S21.141[A,D]	S31.25X[A,D]	S41.112[A,D]
L88.	S01.131[A,D]	S09.312[A,D]	S21.142[A,D]	S31.30X[A,D]	S41.121[A,D]
L92.8	S01.132[A,D]	S09.313[A,D]	S21.151[A,D]	S31.31X[A,D]	S41.122[A,D]
	S01.141[A,D]	S09.391[A,D]	S21.152[A,D]	S31.32X[A,D]	S41.131[A,D]

09 Traumatic wounds, burns and postoperative complications (continued)

S41.132[A,D]	S56.222[A,D]	S61.223[A,D]	S61.341[A,D]	S66.525[A,D]	S71.042[A,D]
S41.141[A,D]	S56.321[A,D]	S61.224[A,D]	S61.342[A,D]	S66.526[A,D]	S71.051[A,D]
S41.142[A,D]	S56.322[A,D]	S61.225[A,D]	S61.343[A,D]	S66.527[A,D]	S71.052[A,D]
S41.151[A,D]	S56.421[A,D]	S61.226[A,D]	S61.344[A,D]	S66.528[A,D]	S71.101[A,D]
S41.152[A,D]	S56.422[A,D]	S61.227[A,D]	S61.345[A,D]	S66.821[A,D]	S71.102[A,D]
S41.159[A,D]	S56.423[A,D]	S61.228[A,D]	S61.346[A,D]	S66.822[A,D]	S71.111[A,D]
S46.021[A,D]	S56.424[A,D]	S61.230[A,D]	S61.347[A,D]	S66.829[A,D]	S71.112[A,D]
S46.022[A,D]	S56.425[A,D]	S61.231[A,D]	S61.348[A,D]	S66.921[A,D]	S71.121[A,D]
S46.121[A,D]	S56.426[A,D]	S61.232[A,D]	S61.350[A,D]	S66.922[A,D]	S71.122[A,D]
S46.122[A,D]	S56.427[A,D]	S61.233[A,D]	S61.351[A,D]	S68.011[A,D]	S71.131[A,D]
S46.221[A,D]	S56.428[A,D]	S61.234[A,D]	S61.352[A,D]	S68.012[A,D]	S71.132[A,D]
S46.222[A,D]	S56.521[A,D]	S61.235[A,D]	S61.353[A,D]	S68.021[A,D]	S71.141[A,D]
S46.321[A,D]	S56.522[A,D]	S61.236[A,D]	S61.354[A,D]	S68.022[A,D]	S71.142[A,D]
S46.322[A,D]	S56.821[A,D]	S61.237[A,D]	S61.355[A,D]	S68.110[A,D]	S71.151[A,D]
S46.821[A,D]	S56.822[A,D]	S61.238[A,D]	S61.356[A,D]	S68.111[A,D]	S71.152[A,D]
S46.822[A,D]	S56.921[A,D]	S61.240[A,D]	S61.357[A,D]	S68.112[A,D]	S76.021[A,D]
S46.921[A,D]	S56.922[A,D]	S61.241[A,D]	S61.358[A,D]	S68.113[A,D]	S76.022[A,D]
S46.922[A,D]	S58.011[A,D]	S61.242[A,D]	S61.401[A,D]	S68.114[A,D]	S76.121[A,D]
S48.011[A,D]	S58.012[A,D]	S61.243[A,D]	S61.402[A,D]	S68.115[A,D]	S76.122[A,D]
S48.012[A,D]	S58.021[A,D]	S61.244[A,D]	S61.411[A,D]	S68.116[A,D]	S76.221[A,D]
S48.021[A,D]	S58.022[A,D]	S61.245[A,D]	S61.412[A,D]	S68.117[A,D]	S76.222[A,D]
S48.022[A,D]	S58.111[A,D]	S61.246[A,D]	S61.421[A,D]	S68.118[A,D]	S76.321[A,D]
S48.111[A,D]	S58.112[A,D]	S61.247[A,D]	S61.422[A,D]	S68.120[A,D]	S76.322[A,D]
S48.112[A,D]	S58.121[A,D]	S61.248[A,D]	S61.431[A,D]	S68.121[A,D]	S76.821[A,D]
S48.121[A,D]	S58.122[A,D]	S61.250[A,D]	S61.432[A,D]	S68.122[A,D]	S76.822[A,D]
S48.122[A,D]	S61.001[A,D]	S61.251[A,D]	S61.441[A,D]	S68.123[A,D]	S76.921[A,D]
S48.911[A,D]	S61.002[A,D]	S61.252[A,D]	S61.442[A,D]	S68.124[A,D]	S76.922[A,D]
S48.912[A,D]	S61.011[A,D]	S61.253[A,D]	S61.451[A,D]	S68.125[A,D]	S78.011[A,D]
S48.921[A,D]	S61.012[A,D]	S61.254[A,D]	S61.452[A,D]	S68.126[A,D]	S78.012[A,D]
S48.922[A,D]	S61.021[A,D]	S61.255[A,D]	S61.501[A,D]	S68.127[A,D]	S78.019[A,D]
S51.001[A,D]	S61.022[A,D]	S61.256[A,D]	S61.502[A,D]	S68.128[A,D]	S78.021[A,D]
S51.002[A,D]	S61.031[A,D]	S61.257[A,D]	S61.511[A,D]	S68.411[A,D]	S78.022[A,D]
S51.011[A,D]	S61.032[A,D]	S61.258[A,D]	S61.512[A,D]	S68.412[A,D]	S78.029[A,D]
S51.012[A,D]	S61.041[A,D]	S61.300[A,D]	S61.521[A,D]	S68.421[A,D]	S78.111[A,D]
S51.021[A,D]	S61.042[A,D]	S61.301[A,D]	S61.522[A,D]	S68.422[A,D]	S78.112[A,D]
S51.022[A,D]	S61.051[A,D]	S61.302[A,D]	S61.531[A,D]	S68.511[A,D]	S78.121[A,D]
S51.031[A,D]	S61.052[A,D]	S61.303[A,D]	S61.532[A,D]	S68.512[A,D]	S78.122[A,D]
S51.032[A,D]	S61.101[A,D]	S61.304[A,D]	S61.541[A,D]	S68.521[A,D]	S78.911[A,D]
S51.041[A,D]	S61.102[A,D]	S61.305[A,D]	S61.542[A,D]	S68.522[A,D]	S78.912[A,D]
S51.042[A,D]	S61.111[A,D]	S61.306[A,D]	S61.551[A,D]	S68.610[A,D]	S78.919[A,D]
S51.051[A,D]	S61.112[A,D]	S61.307[A,D]	S61.552[A,D]	S68.611[A,D]	S78.921[A,D]
S51.052[A,D]	S61.121[A,D]	S61.308[A,D]	S66.021[A,D]	S68.612[A,D]	S78.922[A,D]
S51.801[A,D]	S61.122[A,D]	S61.310[A,D]	S66.022[A,D]	S68.613[A,D]	S81.001[A,D]
S51.802[A,D]	S61.131[A,D]	S61.311[A,D]	S66.120[A,D]	S68.614[A,D]	S81.002[A,D]
S51.811[A,D]	S61.132[A,D]	S61.312[A,D]	S66.121[A,D]	S68.615[A,D]	S81.011[A,D]
S51.812[A,D]	S61.141[A,D]	S61.313[A,D]	S66.122[A,D]	S68.616[A,D]	S81.012[A,D]
S51.821[A,D]	S61.142[A,D]	S61.314[A,D]	S66.123[A,D]	S68.617[A,D]	S81.021[A,D]
S51.822[A,D]	S61.151[A,D]	S61.315[A,D]	S66.124[A,D]	S68.618[A,D]	S81.022[A,D]
S51.831[A,D]	S61.152[A,D]	S61.316[A,D]	S66.125[A,D]	S68.620[A,D]	S81.031[A,D]
S51.832[A,D]	S61.200[A,D]	S61.317[A,D]	S66.126[A,D]	S68.621[A,D]	S81.032[A,D]
S51.841[A,D]	S61.201[A,D]	S61.318[A,D]	S66.127[A,D]	S68.622[A,D]	S81.041[A,D]
S51.842[A,D]	S61.202[A,D]	S61.320[A,D]	S66.128[A,D]	S68.623[A,D]	S81.042[A,D]
S51.851[A,D]	S61.203[A,D]	S61.321[A,D]	S66.221[A,D]	S68.624[A,D]	S81.051[A,D]
S51.852[A,D]	S61.204[A,D]	S61.322[A,D]	S66.222[A,D]	S68.625[A,D]	S81.052[A,D]
S56.021[A,D]	S61.205[A,D]	S61.323[A,D]	S66.320[A,D]	S68.626[A,D]	S81.801[A,D]
S56.022[A,D]	S61.206[A,D]	S61.324[A,D]	S66.321[A,D]	S68.627[A,D]	S81.802[A,D]
S56.121[A,D]	S61.207[A,D]	S61.325[A,D]	S66.322[A,D]	S68.628[A,D]	S81.811[A,D]
S56.122[A,D]	S61.208[A,D]	S61.326[A,D]	S66.323[A,D]	S68.711[A,D]	S81.812[A,D]
S56.123[A,D]	S61.210[A,D]	S61.327[A,D]	S66.324[A,D]	S68.712[A,D]	S81.821[A,D]
S56.124[A,D]	S61.211[A,D]	S61.328[A,D]	S66.325[A,D]	S68.721[A,D]	S81.822[A,D]
S56.125[A,D]	S61.212[A,D]	S61.330[A,D]	S66.326[A,D]	S68.722[A,D]	S81.831[A,D]
S56.126[A,D]	S61.213[A,D]	S61.331[A,D]	S66.327[A,D]	S71.001[A,D]	S81.832[A,D]
S56.127[A,D]	S61.214[A,D]	S61.332[A,D]	S66.328[A,D]	S71.002[A,D]	S81.841[A,D]
S56.128[A,D]	S61.215[A,D]	S61.333[A,D]	S66.421[A,D]	S71.011[A,D]	S81.842[A,D]
S56.221[A,D]	S61.216[A,D]	S61.334[A,D]	S66.422[A,D]	S71.012[A,D]	S81.851[A,D]
	S61.217[A,D]	S61.335[A,D]	S66.520[A,D]	S71.021[A,D]	S81.852[A,D]
	S61.218[A,D]	S61.336[A,D]	S66.521[A,D]	S71.022[A,D]	S86.021[A,D]
	S61.220[A,D]	S61.337[A,D]	S66.522[A,D]	S71.031[A,D]	S86.022[A,D]
	S61.221[A,D]	S61.338[A,D]	S66.523[A,D]	S71.032[A,D]	S86.121[A,D]
	S61.222[A,D]	S61.340[A,D]	S66.524[A,D]	S71.041[A,D]	S86.122[A,D]
					S86.221[A,D]

09 Traumatic wounds, burns and postoperative complications (continued)

S86.222[A,D]	S91.222[A,D]	T20.30X[A,D]	T22.252[A,D]	T23.322[A,D]	T24.611[A,D]
S86.321[A,D]	S91.224[A,D]	T20.311[A,D]	T22.261[A,D]	T23.331[A,D]	T24.612[A,D]
S86.322[A,D]	S91.225[A,D]	T20.312[A,D]	T22.262[A,D]	T23.332[A,D]	T24.621[A,D]
S86.821[A,D]	S91.231[A,D]	T20.32X[A,D]	T22.291[A,D]	T23.341[A,D]	T24.622[A,D]
S86.822[A,D]	S91.232[A,D]	T20.33X[A,D]	T22.292[A,D]	T23.342[A,D]	T24.631[A,D]
S86.921[A,D]	S91.234[A,D]	T20.34X[A,D]	T22.30X[A,D]	T23.351[A,D]	T24.632[A,D]
S86.922[A,D]	S91.235[A,D]	T20.35X[A,D]	T22.311[A,D]	T23.352[A,D]	T24.691[A,D]
S88.011[A,D]	S91.241[A,D]	T20.36X[A,D]	T22.312[A,D]	T23.361[A,D]	T24.692[A,D]
S88.012[A,D]	S91.242[A,D]	T20.37X[A,D]	T22.321[A,D]	T23.362[A,D]	T24.701[A,D]
S88.021[A,D]	S91.244[A,D]	T20.39X[A,D]	T22.322[A,D]	T23.371[A,D]	T24.702[A,D]
S88.022[A,D]	S91.245[A,D]	T20.60X[A,D]	T22.331[A,D]	T23.372[A,D]	T24.711[A,D]
S88.111[A,D]	S91.251[A,D]	T20.611[A,D]	T22.332[A,D]	T23.391[A,D]	T24.712[A,D]
S88.112[A,D]	S91.252[A,D]	T20.612[A,D]	T22.341[A,D]	T23.392[A,D]	T24.721[A,D]
S88.121[A,D]	S91.254[A,D]	T20.62X[A,D]	T22.342[A,D]	T23.601[A,D]	T24.722[A,D]
S88.122[A,D]	S91.255[A,D]	T20.63X[A,D]	T22.351[A,D]	T23.602[A,D]	T24.731[A,D]
S88.911[A,D]	S91.301[A,D]	T20.64X[A,D]	T22.352[A,D]	T23.611[A,D]	T24.732[A,D]
S88.912[A,D]	S91.302[A,D]	T20.65X[A,D]	T22.361[A,D]	T23.612[A,D]	T24.791[A,D]
S88.921[A,D]	S91.311[A,D]	T20.66X[A,D]	T22.362[A,D]	T23.621[A,D]	T24.792[A,D]
S88.922[A,D]	S91.312[A,D]	T20.67X[A,D]	T22.391[A,D]	T23.622[A,D]	T25.211[A,D]
S91.001[A,D]	S91.321[A,D]	T20.69X[A,D]	T22.392[A,D]	T23.631[A,D]	T25.212[A,D]
S91.002[A,D]	S91.322[A,D]	T20.70X[A,D]	T22.611[A,D]	T23.632[A,D]	T25.221[A,D]
S91.011[A,D]	S91.331[A,D]	T20.711[A,D]	T22.612[A,D]	T23.641[A,D]	T25.222[A,D]
S91.012[A,D]	S91.332[A,D]	T20.712[A,D]	T22.621[A,D]	T23.642[A,D]	T25.231[A,D]
S91.021[A,D]	S91.341[A,D]	T20.72X[A,D]	T22.622[A,D]	T23.651[A,D]	T25.232[A,D]
S91.022[A,D]	S91.342[A,D]	T20.73X[A,D]	T22.631[A,D]	T23.652[A,D]	T25.291[A,D]
S91.031[A,D]	S91.351[A,D]	T20.74X[A,D]	T22.632[A,D]	T23.661[A,D]	T25.292[A,D]
S91.032[A,D]	S91.352[A,D]	T20.75X[A,D]	T22.641[A,D]	T23.662[A,D]	T25.311[A,D]
S91.041[A,D]	S96.021[A,D]	T20.76X[A,D]	T22.642[A,D]	T23.671[A,D]	T25.312[A,D]
S91.042[A,D]	S96.022[A,D]	T20.77X[A,D]	T22.651[A,D]	T23.672[A,D]	T25.321[A,D]
S91.051[A,D]	S96.121[A,D]	T20.79X[A,D]	T22.652[A,D]	T23.691[A,D]	T25.322[A,D]
S91.052[A,D]	S96.122[A,D]	T21.21X[A,D]	T22.661[A,D]	T23.692[A,D]	T25.329[A,D]
S91.101[A,D]	S96.221[A,D]	T21.22X[A,D]	T22.662[A,D]	T23.701[A,D]	T25.331[A,D]
S91.102[A,D]	S96.222[A,D]	T21.23X[A,D]	T22.691[A,D]	T23.702[A,D]	T25.332[A,D]
S91.103[A,D]	S96.821[A,D]	T21.24X[A,D]	T22.692[A,D]	T23.711[A,D]	T25.391[A,D]
S91.104[A,D]	S96.822[A,D]	T21.25X[A,D]	T22.711[A,D]	T23.712[A,D]	T25.392[A,D]
S91.105[A,D]	S96.921[A,D]	T21.26X[A,D]	T22.712[A,D]	T23.721[A,D]	T25.611[A,D]
S91.111[A,D]	S96.922[A,D]	T21.27X[A,D]	T22.721[A,D]	T23.722[A,D]	T25.612[A,D]
S91.112[A,D]	S98.011[A,D]	T21.29X[A,D]	T22.722[A,D]	T23.731[A,D]	T25.621[A,D]
S91.114[A,D]	S98.012[A,D]	T21.31X[A,D]	T22.731[A,D]	T23.732[A,D]	T25.622[A,D]
S91.115[A,D]	S98.021[A,D]	T21.32X[A,D]	T22.732[A,D]	T23.741[A,D]	T25.631[A,D]
S91.121[A,D]	S98.022[A,D]	T21.33X[A,D]	T22.741[A,D]	T23.742[A,D]	T25.632[A,D]
S91.122[A,D]	S98.111[A,D]	T21.34X[A,D]	T22.742[A,D]	T23.751[A,D]	T25.691[A,D]
S91.124[A,D]	S98.112[A,D]	T21.35X[A,D]	T22.751[A,D]	T23.752[A,D]	T25.692[A,D]
S91.125[A,D]	S98.121[A,D]	T21.36X[A,D]	T22.752[A,D]	T23.761[A,D]	T25.711[A,D]
S91.131[A,D]	S98.122[A,D]	T21.37X[A,D]	T22.761[A,D]	T23.762[A,D]	T25.712[A,D]
S91.132[A,D]	S98.131[A,D]	T21.39X[A,D]	T22.762[A,D]	T23.771[A,D]	T25.721[A,D]
S91.134[A,D]	S98.132[A,D]	T21.61X[A,D]	T22.791[A,D]	T23.772[A,D]	T25.722[A,D]
S91.135[A,D]	S98.141[A,D]	T21.62X[A,D]	T22.792[A,D]	T23.791[A,D]	T25.731[A,D]
S91.141[A,D]	S98.142[A,D]	T21.63X[A,D]	T23.201[A,D]	T23.792[A,D]	T25.732[A,D]
S91.142[A,D]	S98.211[A,D]	T21.64X[A,D]	T23.202[A,D]	T24.201[A,D]	T25.791[A,D]
S91.144[A,D]	S98.212[A,D]	T21.65X[A,D]	T23.211[A,D]	T24.202[A,D]	T25.792[A,D]
S91.145[A,D]	S98.221[A,D]	T21.66X[A,D]	T23.212[A,D]	T24.211[A,D]	T26.21X[A,D]
S91.149[A,D]	S98.222[A,D]	T21.67X[A,D]	T23.221[A,D]	T24.212[A,D]	T26.22X[A,D]
S91.151[A,D]	S98.311[A,D]	T21.69X[A,D]	T23.222[A,D]	T24.221[A,D]	T31*
S91.152[A,D]	S98.312[A,D]	T21.71X[A,D]	T23.231[A,D]	T24.229[A,D]	T32*
S91.154[A,D]	S98.321[A,D]	T21.72X[A,D]	T23.232[A,D]	T24.231[A,D]	T81.30X[A,D]
S91.155[A,D]	S98.322[A,D]	T21.73X[A,D]	T23.241[A,D]	T24.232[A,D]	T81.31X[A,D]
S91.201[A,D]	S98.911[A,D]	T21.74X[A,D]	T23.242[A,D]	T24.291[A,D]	T81.32X[A,D]
S91.202[A,D]	S98.912[A,D]	T21.75X[A,D]	T23.251[A,D]	T24.292[A,D]	T81.33X[A,D]
S91.204[A,D]	S98.921[A,D]	T21.76X[A,D]	T23.252[A,D]	T24.301[A,D]	T81.4XX[A,D]
S91.205[A,D]	S98.922[A,D]	T21.77X[A,D]	T23.261[A,D]	T24.302[A,D]	
S91.211[A,D]	T20.20X[A,D]	T21.79X[A,D]	T23.262[A,D]	T24.311[A,D]	**10 Cystotomy care**
S91.212[A,D]	T20.211[A,D]	T22.211[A,D]	T23.271[A,D]	T24.312[A,D]	Z43.5
S91.214[A,D]	T20.212[A,D]	T22.212[A,D]	T23.272[A,D]	T24.321[A,D]	
S91.215[A,D]	T20.22X[A,D]	T22.221[A,D]	T23.291[A,D]	T24.322[A,D]	**11 Tracheostomy care**
S91.221[A,D]	T20.23X[A,D]	T22.222[A,D]	T23.292[A,D]	T24.331[A,D]	Z43.0
	T20.24X[A,D]	T22.231[A,D]	T23.301[A,D]	T24.332[A,D]	
	T20.25X[A,D]	T22.232[A,D]	T23.302[A,D]	T24.391[A,D]	**12 Urostomy care**
	T20.26X[A,D]	T22.241[A,D]	T23.311[A,D]	T24.392[A,D]	Z43.6
	T20.27X[A,D]	T22.242[A,D]	T23.312[A,D]	T24.601[A,D]	
	T20.29X[A,D]	T22.251[A,D]	T23.321[A,D]	T24.602[A,D]	

Appendix M: Valid Diagnosis/Etiology Pairings List

The home health prospective payment system (HH PPS) provides clinical dimension assignment and/or nonroutine supply (NRS) adjustments for valid etiology and manifestation code pairs that are entered in the payment diagnosis field. This section contains a complete list of these valid diagnosis/etiology pairs. The data source for this information is the January 2017 HH PPS Grouper software v6117 update, effective January 1, 2017.

Note: An updated version of the home health prospective payment system (HH PPS) Grouper software was not available at the time this book was printed and therefore this appendix does not reflect any fiscal 2018 code changes. Updated versions of the software can be found at https://www.cms.gov/Medicare/Medicare-Fee-for-Service-Payment/HomeHealthPPS/CaseMixGrouperSoftware.html.

D75.81	C50.011, C50.012, C50.019, C50.021, C50.022, C50.029, C50.111, C50.112, C50.119, C50.121, C50.122, C50.129, C50.211, C50.212, C50.219, C50.221, C50.222, C50.229, C50.311, C50.312, C50.319, C50.321, C50.322, C50.329, C50.411, C50.412, C50.419, C50.421, C50.422, C50.429, C50.511, C50.512, C50.519, C50.521, C50.522, C50.529, C50.611, C50.612, C50.619, C50.621, C50.622, C50.629, C50.811, C50.812, C50.819, C50.821, C50.822, C50.829, C50.911, C50.912, C50.919, C50.921, C50.922, C50.929
D77	A50.01, A50.02, A50.03, A50.04, A50.05, A50.06, A50.07, A50.08, A50.09, B50.0, B50.8, B50.9, B51.0, B51.8, B51.9, B52.0, B52.8, B52.9, B53.0, B53.1, B53.8, B54, B65.0, B65.1, B65.2, B65.3, B65.8, B65.9, B67.0, B67.1, B67.2, B67.31, B67.32, B67.39, B67.4, B67.5, B67.61, B67.69, B67.7, B67.8, B67.90, B67.99, E54, E85.0, E85.1, E85.2, E85.3, E85.4, E85.9
E08.311, E08.319, E08.3211, E08.3212, E08.3213, E08.3219, E08.3291, E08.3292, E08.3293, E08.3299, E08.3311, E08.3312, E08.3313, E08.3319, E08.3391, E08.3392, E08.3393, E08.3399, E08.3411, E08.3412, E08.3413, E08.3419, E08.3491, E08.3492, E08.3493, E08.3499, E08.3511, E08.3512, E08.3513, E08.3519, E08.3521, E08.3522, E08.3523, E08.3529, E08.3531, E08.3532, E08.3533, E08.3539, E08.3541, E08.3542, E08.3543, E08.3549, E08.3551, E08.3552, E08.3553, E08.3559, E08.3591, E08.3592, E08.3593, E08.3599, E08.40, E08.41, E08.42, E08.43, E08.44, E08.52, E08.610, E08.618, E08.621, E08.622	C00.0, C00.1, C00.2, C00.3, C00.4, C00.5, C00.6, C00.8, C00.9, C01, C02.0, C02.1, C02.2, C02.3, C02.4, C02.8, C02.9, C03.0, C03.1, C03.9, C04.0, C04.1, C04.8, C04.9, C05.0, C05.1, C05.2, C05.8, C05.9, C06.0, C06.1, C06.2, C06.80, C06.89, C06.9, C07, C08.0, C08.1, C08.9, C09.0, C09.1, C09.8, C09.9, C10.0, C10.1, C10.2, C10.3, C10.4, C10.8, C10.9, C11.0, C11.1, C11.2, C11.3, C11.8, C11.9, C12, C13.0, C13.1, C13.2, C13.8, C13.9, C14.0, C14.2, C14.8, C15.3, C15.4, C15.5, C15.8, C15.9, C16.0, C16.1, C16.2, C16.3, C16.4, C16.5, C16.6, C16.8, C16.9, C17.0, C17.1, C17.2, C17.3, C17.8, C17.9, C18.0, C18.1, C18.2, C18.3, C18.4, C18.5, C18.6, C18.7, C18.8, C18.9, C19, C20, C21.0, C21.1, C21.2, C21.8, C22.0, C22.1, C22.2, C22.3, C22.4, C22.7, C22.8, C22.9, C23, C24.0, C24.1, C24.8, C24.9, C25.0, C25.1, C25.2, C25.3, C25.4, C25.7, C25.8, C25.9, C26.0, C26.1, C26.9, C30.0, C30.1, C31.0, C31.1, C31.2, C31.3, C31.8, C31.9, C32.0, C32.1, C32.2, C32.3, C32.8, C32.9, C33, C34.00, C34.01, C34.02, C34.10, C34.11, C34.12, C34.2, C34.30, C34.31, C34.32, C34.80, C34.81, C34.82, C34.90, C34.91, C34.92, C37, C38.0, C38.1, C38.2, C38.3, C38.4, C38.8, C39.0, C39.9, C40.00, C40.01, C40.02, C40.10, C40.11, C40.12, C40.20, C40.21, C40.22, C40.30, C40.31, C40.32, C40.80, C40.81, C40.82, C40.90, C40.91, C40.92, C41.0, C41.1, C41.2, C41.3, C41.4, C41.9, C43.0, C43.10, C43.11, C43.12, C43.20, C43.21, C43.22, C43.30, C43.31, C43.39, C43.4, C43.51, C43.52, C43.59, C43.60, C43.61, C43.62, C43.70, C43.71, C43.72, C43.8, C43.9, C44.00, C44.01, C44.02, C44.09, C44.101, C44.102, C44.109, C44.111, C44.112, C44.119, C44.121, C44.122, C44.129, C44.191, C44.192, C44.199, C44.201, C44.202, C44.209, C44.211, C44.212, C44.219, C44.221, C44.222, C44.229, C44.291, C44.292, C44.299, C44.300, C44.301, C44.309, C44.310, C44.311, C44.319, C44.320, C44.321, C44.329, C44.390, C44.391, C44.399, C44.40, C44.41, C44.42, C44.49, C44.500, C44.501, C44.509, C44.510, C44.511, C44.519, C44.520, C44.521, C44.529, C44.590, C44.591, C44.599, C44.601, C44.602, C44.609, C44.611, C44.612, C44.619, C44.621, C44.622, C44.629, C44.691, C44.692, C44.699, C44.701, C44.702, C44.709, C44.711, C44.712, C44.719, C44.721, C44.722, C44.729, C44.791, C44.792, C44.799, C44.80, C44.81, C44.82, C44.89, C44.90, C44.91, C44.92, C44.99, C45.0, C45.1, C45.2, C45.7, C45.9, C46.0, C46.1, C46.2, C46.3, C46.4, C46.50, C46.51, C46.52, C46.7, C46.9, C47.0, C47.10, C47.11, C47.12, C47.20, C47.21, C47.22, C47.3, C47.4, C47.5, C47.6, C47.8, C47.9, C48.0, C48.1, C48.2, C48.8, C49.0, C49.10, C49.11, C49.12, C49.20, C49.21, C49.22, C49.3, C49.4, C49.5, C49.6, C49.8, C49.9, C49.A0, C49.A1, C49.A2, C49.A3, C49.A4, C49.A5, C49.A9, C4A.0, C4A.10, C4A.11, C4A.12, C4A.20, C4A.21, C4A.22, C4A.30, C4A.31, C4A.39, C4A.4, C4A.51, C4A.52, C4A.59, C4A.60, C4A.61, C4A.62, C4A.70, C4A.71, C4A.72, C4A.8, C4A.9, C50.011, C50.012, C50.019, C50.021, C50.022, C50.029, C50.111, C50.112, C50.119, C50.121, C50.122, C50.129, C50.211, C50.212, C50.219, C50.221, C50.222, C50.229, C50.311, C50.312, C50.319, C50.321, C50.322, C50.329, C50.411, C50.412, C50.419, C50.421, C50.422, C50.429, C50.511, C50.512, C50.519, C50.521, C50.522, C50.529, C50.611, C50.612, C50.619, C50.621, C50.622, C50.629, C50.811, C50.812, C50.819, C50.821, C50.822, C50.829, C50.911, C50.912, C50.919, C50.921, C50.922, C50.929, C51.0, C51.1, C51.2, C51.8, C51.9, C52, C53.0, C53.1, C53.8, C53.9, C54.0, C54.1, C54.2, C54.3, C54.8, C54.9, C55, C56.1, C56.2, C56.9, C57.00, C57.01, C57.02, C57.10, C57.11, C57.12, C57.20, C57.21, C57.22, C57.3, C57.4, C57.7, C57.8, C57.9, C58, C60.0, C60.1, C60.2, C60.8, C60.9, C61, C62.00, C62.01, C62.02, C62.10, C62.11, C62.12, C62.90, C62.91, C62.92, C63.00, C63.01, C63.02, C63.10, C63.11, C63.12, C63.2, C63.7, C63.8, C63.9, C64.1, C64.2, C64.9, C65.1, C65.2, C65.9, C66.1, C66.2, C66.9, C67.0, C67.1, C67.2, C67.3, C67.4, C67.5, C67.6, C67.7, C67.8, C67.9, C68.0, C68.1, C68.8, C68.9, C69.00, C69.01, C69.02, C69.10, C69.11, C69.12, C69.21, C69.22, C69.30, C69.31, C69.32, C69.40, C69.41, C69.42, C69.50, C69.51, C69.52, C69.60, C69.61, C69.62, C69.80, C69.81, C69.82, C69.90, C69.91, C69.92, C70.0, C70.1, C70.9, C71.0, C71.1, C71.2, C71.3, C71.4, C71.5, C71.6, C71.7, C71.8, C71.9, C72.0, C72.1, C72.20, C72.21, C72.22, C72.30, C72.31, C72.32, C72.40, C72.41, C72.42, C72.50, C72.59, C72.9, C73, C74.00, C74.01, C74.02, C74.10, C74.11, C74.12, C74.90, C74.91, C74.92, C75.0, C75.1, C75.2, C75.3, C75.4, C75.5, C75.8, C75.9, C76.0, C76.1, C76.2, C76.3, C76.40, C76.41, C76.42, C76.50, C76.51, C76.52, C76.8, C77.0, C77.1, C77.2, C77.3, C77.4, C77.5, C77.8, C77.9, C78.00, C78.01, C78.02, C78.1, C78.2, C78.30, C78.39, C78.4, C78.5, C78.6, C78.7, C78.80, C78.89, C79.00, C79.01, C79.02, C79.10, C79.11, C79.19, C79.2, C79.31, C79.32, C79.40, C79.49, C79.51, C79.52, C79.60, C79.61, C79.62, C79.70, C79.71, C79.72, C79.81, C79.82, C79.89, C79.9, C7A.00, C7A.010, C7A.011, C7A.012, C7A.019, C7A.020, C7A.021, C7A.022, C7A.023, C7A.024, C7A.025, C7A.026, C7A.029, C7A.090, C7A.091, C7A.092, C7A.093, C7A.094, C7A.095, C7A.096, C7A.098, C7A.1, C7A.8, C7B.00, C7B.01, C7B.02, C7B.03, C7B.04, C7B.09, C7B.1, C7B.8, C80.0, C80.1, C80.2, C81.00, C81.01, C81.02, C81.03, C81.04, C81.05, C81.06, C81.07, C81.08, C81.09, C81.10, C81.11, C81.12, C81.13, C81.14, C81.15, C81.16, C81.17, C81.18, C81.19, C81.20, C81.21, C81.22, C81.23, C81.24, C81.25, C81.26, C81.27, C81.28, C81.29, C81.30, C81.31, C81.32, C81.33, C81.34, C81.35, C81.36, C81.37, C81.38, C81.39, C81.40, C81.41, C81.42, C81.43, C81.44, C81.45, C81.46, C81.47, C81.48, C81.49, C81.70, C81.71, C81.72, C81.73, C81.74, C81.75, C81.76, C81.77, C81.78, C81.79, C81.90, C81.91, C81.92, C81.93, C81.94, C81.95, C81.96, C81.97, C81.98, C81.99, C82.00, C82.01, C82.02, C82.03, C82.04, C82.05, C82.06, C82.07, C82.08, C82.09, C82.10, C82.11, C82.12, C82.13, C82.14, C82.15, C82.16, C82.17, C82.18, C82.19, C82.20, C82.21, C82.22, C82.23, C82.24, C82.25, C82.26, C82.27, C82.28, C82.29, C82.30, C82.31, C82.32, C82.33, C82.34, C82.35, C82.36, C82.37, C82.38, C82.39, C82.40, C82.41, C82.42, C82.43, C82.44, C82.45, C82.46, C82.47, C82.48, C82.49, C82.50, C82.51, C82.52, C82.53, C82.54, C82.55, C82.56, C82.57, C82.58, C82.59, C82.60, C82.61, C82.62, C82.63, C82.64, C82.65, C82.66, C82.67, C82.68, C82.69, C82.80, C82.81, C82.82, C82.83, C82.84, C82.85, C82.86, C82.87, C82.88, C82.89, C82.90, C82.91, C82.92, C82.93, C82.94, C82.95, C82.96, C82.97, C82.98, C82.99, C83.00, C83.01, C83.02, C83.03, C83.04, C83.05, C83.06, C83.07, C83.08, C83.09, C83.10, C83.11, C83.12, C83.13, C83.14, C83.15, C83.16, C83.17, C83.18, C83.19, C83.30, C83.31, C83.32, C83.33, C83.34, C83.35, C83.36, C83.37, C83.38, C83.39, C83.50, C83.51, C83.52, C83.53, C83.54, C83.55, C83.56, C83.57, C83.58, C83.59, C83.70, C83.71, C83.72, C83.73, C83.74, C83.75, C83.76, C83.77, C83.78, C83.79, C83.80, C83.81, C83.82, C83.83, C83.84, C83.85, C83.86, C83.87, C83.88, C83.89, C83.90, C83.91, C83.92, C83.93, C83.94, C83.95, C83.96, C83.97, C83.98, C83.99, C84.00, C84.01, C84.02, C84.03, C84.04, C84.05, C84.06, C84.07, C84.08, C84.09, C84.10, C84.11, C84.12, C84.13, C84.14, C84.15, C84.16, C84.17, C84.18, C84.19, C84.40, C84.41, C84.42, C84.43, C84.44, C84.45, C84.46, C84.47, C84.48, C84.49, C84.60, C84.61, C84.62, C84.63, C84.64, C84.65, C84.66, C84.67, C84.68, C84.69, C84.70, C84.71, C84.72, C84.73, C84.74, C84.75, C84.76, C84.77, C84.78, C84.79, C84.90, C84.91, C84.92, C84.93, C84.94, C84.95, C84.96, C84.99, C84.A0, C84.A1, C84.A2, C84.A3, C84.A4, C84.A5, C84.A6, C84.A7, C84.A8, C84.A9, C84.Z0, C84.Z1, C84.Z2, C84.Z3, C84.Z4, C84.Z5, C84.Z6, C84.Z7, C84.Z8, C84.Z9, C85.10, C85.11, C85.12, C85.13, C85.14, C85.15, C85.16, C85.17, C85.18, C85.19, C85.20, C85.21, C85.22, C85.23, C85.24, C85.25, C85.26, C85.27, C85.28, C85.29, C85.80, C85.81, C85.82, C85.83, C85.84, C85.85, C85.86, C85.87, C85.88, C85.89, C85.90, C85.91, C85.92, C85.93, C85.94, C85.95,

E08.311, E08.319, E08.3211, E08.3212, E08.3213, E08.3219, E08.3291, E08.3292, E08.3293, E08.3299, E08.3311, E08.3312, E08.3313, E08.3319, E08.3391, E08.3392, E08.3393, E08.3399, E08.3411, E08.3412, E08.3413, E08.3419, E08.3491, E08.3492, E08.3493, E08.3499, E08.3511, E08.3512, E08.3513, E08.3519, E08.3521, E08.3522, E08.3523, E08.3529, E08.3531, E08.3532, E08.3533, E08.3539, E08.3541, E08.3542, E08.3543, E08.3549, E08.3551, E08.3552, E08.3553, E08.3559, E08.3591, E08.3592, E08.3593, E08.3599, E08.40, E08.41, E08.42, E08.43, E08.44, E08.52, E08.610, E08.618, E08.621, E08.622 (continued)	C85.96, C85.97, C85.98, C85.99, C86.0, C86.1, C86.2, C86.3, C86.4, C86.5, C86.6, C88.0, C88.2, C88.3, C88.4, C88.8, C88.9, C90.00, C90.01, C90.02, C90.10, C90.11, C90.12, C90.20, C90.21, C90.22, C90.30, C90.31, C90.32, C91.00, C91.01, C91.02, C91.10, C91.11, C91.12, C91.30, C91.31, C91.32, C91.40, C91.41, C91.42, C91.50, C91.51, C91.52, C91.60, C91.61, C91.62, C91.90, C91.91, C91.92, C91.A0, C91.A1, C91.A2, C91.Z0, C91.Z1, C91.Z2, C92.00, C92.01, C92.02, C92.10, C92.11, C92.12, C92.20, C92.21, C92.22, C92.30, C92.31, C92.32, C92.40, C92.41, C92.42, C92.50, C92.51, C92.52, C92.60, C92.61, C92.62, C92.90, C92.91, C92.92, C92.A0, C92.A1, C92.A2, C92.Z0, C92.Z1, C92.Z2, C93.00, C93.01, C93.02, C93.10, C93.11, C93.12, C93.30, C93.31, C93.32, C93.90, C93.91, C93.92, C93.Z0, C93.Z1, C93.Z2, C94.00, C94.01, C94.02, C94.20, C94.21, C94.22, C94.30, C94.31, C94.32, C94.40, C94.41, C94.42, C94.6, C94.80, C94.81, C94.82, C95.00, C95.01, C95.02, C95.10, C95.11, C95.12, C95.90, C95.91, C95.92, C96.0, C96.4, C96.5, C96.6, C96.9, C96.A, C96.Z, E24.0, F24.1, E24.2, E24.3, E24.4, E24.8, E24.9, E40, E41, E42, E43, E44.0, E44.1, E45, E46, E84.0, E84.11, E84.19, E84.8, E84.9, K85.00, K85.01, K85.02, K85.10, K85.11, K85.12, K85.20, K85.21, K85.22, K85.30, K85.31, K85.32, K85.80, K85.81, K85.82, K85.90, K85.91, K85.92, K86.0, K86.1, K86.2, K86.3, K86.81, K86.89, K86.9, P35.0
G01	A01.00, A01.01, A01.02, A01.03, A01.04, A01.05, A01.09, A20.0, A20.1, A20.2, A20.3, A20.7, A20.8, A20.9, A21.0, A21.1, A21.2, A21.3, A21.7, A21.8, A21.9, A22.0, A22.1, A22.2, A22.7, A22.8, A22.9, A23.0, A23.1, A23.2, A23.3, A23.8, A23.9, A24.0, A24.1, A24.2, A24.3, A24.9, A25.0, A25.1, A25.9, A26.0, A26.7, A26.8, A26.9, A28.0, A28.2, A28.8, A28.9, A32.0, A32.11, A32.12, A32.7, A32.81, A32.82, A32.89, A32.9, A36.0, A36.1, A36.2, A36.3, A36.81, A36.82, A36.83, A36.84, A36.85, A36.86, A36.89, A36.9, A37.00, A37.01, A37.10, A37.11, A37.80, A37.81, A37.90, A37.91, A38.0, A38.1, A38.8, A38.9, A40.0, A40.1, A40.3, A40.8, A40.9, A41.01, A41.02, A41.1, A41.2, A41.3, A41.4, A41.50, A41.51, A41.52, A41.53, A41.59, A41.81, A41.89, A41.9, A42.7, A42.81, A42.82, A42.89, A43.8, A48.0, A48.2, A48.3, A48.4, A48.51, A48.52, A48.8, A49.01, A49.02, A49.1, A49.2, A49.3, A49.8, A49.9, B95.0, B95.1, B95.2, B95.3, B95.4, B95.5, B95.61, B95.62, B95.7, B95.8, B96.0, B96.1, B96.20, B96.21, B96.22, B96.23, B96.29, B96.3, B96.4, B96.5, B96.6, B96.7, B96.81, B96.82, B96.89, J02.0, J03.00, J03.01, J20.0, J20.1, J20.2, K90.81, M00.10, M00.111, M00.112, M00.119, M00.121, M00.122, M00.129, M00.131, M00.132, M00.139, M00.141, M00.142, M00.149, M00.151, M00.152, M00.159, M00.161, M00.162, M00.169, M00.171, M00.172, M00.179, M00.18, M00.19, M60.009
G02	A80.0, A80.1, A80.2, A80.30, A80.39, A80.4, A80.9
G05.3, G05.4	A80.0, A80.1, A80.2, A80.30, A80.39, A80.4, A80.9, B75, H66.001, H66.002, H66.003, H66.004, H66.005, H66.006, H66.007, H66.009, H66.011, H66.012, H66.013, H66.014, H66.015, H66.016, H66.017, H66.019, H66.10, H66.11, H66.12, H66.13, H66.20, H66.21, H66.22, H66.23, H66.3X1, H66.3X2, H66.3X3, H66.3X9, H66.40, H66.41, H66.42, H66.43
G07	B65.0, B65.1, B65.2, B65.3, B65.8, B65.9
G13.0, G13.1	C00.0, C00.1, C00.2, C00.3, C00.4, C00.5, C00.6, C00.8, C00.9, C01, C02.0, C02.1, C02.2, C02.3, C02.4, C02.8, C02.9, C03.0, C03.1, C03.9, C04.0, C04.1, C04.8, C04.9, C05.0, C05.1, C05.2, C05.8, C05.9, C06.0, C06.1, C06.2, C06.80, C06.89, C06.9, C07, C08.0, C08.1, C08.9, C09.0, C09.1, C09.8, C09.9, C10.0, C10.1, C10.2, C10.3, C10.4, C10.8, C10.9, C11.0, C11.1, C11.2, C11.3, C11.8, C11.9, C12, C13.0, C13.1, C13.2, C13.8, C13.9, C14.0, C14.2, C14.8, C15.3, C15.4, C15.5, C15.8, C15.9, C16.0, C16.1, C16.2, C16.3, C16.4, C16.5, C16.6, C16.8, C16.9, C17.0, C17.1, C17.2, C17.3, C17.8, C17.9, C18.0, C18.1, C18.2, C18.3, C18.4, C18.5, C18.6, C18.7, C18.8, C18.9, C19, C20, C21.0, C21.1, C21.2, C21.8, C22.0, C22.1, C22.2, C22.3, C22.4, C22.7, C22.8, C22.9, C23, C24.0, C24.1, C24.8, C24.9, C25.0, C25.1, C25.2, C25.3, C25.4, C25.7, C25.8, C25.9, C26.0, C26.1, C26.9, C30.0, C30.1, C31.0, C31.1, C31.2, C31.3, C31.8, C31.9, C32.0, C32.1, C32.2, C32.3, C32.8, C32.9, C33, C34.00, C34.01, C34.02, C34.10, C34.11, C34.12, C34.2, C34.30, C34.31, C34.32, C34.80, C34.81, C34.82, C34.90, C34.91, C34.92, C37, C38.0, C38.1, C38.2, C38.3, C38.4, C38.8, C39.0, C39.9, C40.00, C40.01, C40.02, C40.10, C40.11, C40.12, C40.20, C40.21, C40.22, C40.30, C40.31, C40.32, C40.80, C40.81, C40.82, C40.90, C40.91, C40.92, C41.0, C41.1, C41.2, C41.3, C41.4, C41.9, C43.0, C43.10, C43.11, C43.12, C43.20, C43.21, C43.22, C43.30, C43.31, C43.39, C43.4, C43.51, C43.52, C43.59, C43.60, C43.61, C43.62, C43.70, C43.71, C43.72, C43.8, C43.9, C45.0, C45.1, C45.2, C45.7, C45.9, C46.0, C46.1, C46.2, C46.3, C46.4, C46.50, C46.51, C46.52, C46.7, C46.9, C47.0, C47.10, C47.11, C47.12, C47.20, C47.21, C47.22, C47.3, C47.4, C47.5, C47.6, C47.8, C47.9, C48.0, C48.1, C48.2, C48.8, C49.0, C49.10, C49.11, C49.12, C49.20, C49.21, C49.22, C49.3, C49.4, C49.5, C49.6, C49.8, C49.9, C49.A0, C49.A1, C49.A2, C49.A3, C49.A4, C49.A5, C49.A9, C4A.0, C4A.10, C4A.11, C4A.12, C4A.20, C4A.21, C4A.22, C4A.30, C4A.31, C4A.39, C4A.4, C4A.51, C4A.52, C4A.59, C4A.60, C4A.61, C4A.62, C4A.70, C4A.71, C4A.72, C4A.8, C4A.9, C50.011, C50.012, C50.019, C50.021, C50.022, C50.029, C50.111, C50.112, C50.119, C50.121, C50.122, C50.129, C50.211, C50.212, C50.219, C50.221, C50.222, C50.229, C50.311, C50.312, C50.319, C50.321, C50.322, C50.329, C50.411, C50.412, C50.419, C50.421, C50.422, C50.429, C50.511, C50.512, C50.519, C50.521, C50.522, C50.529, C50.611, C50.612, C50.619, C50.621, C50.622, C50.629, C50.811, C50.812, C50.819, C50.821, C50.822, C50.829, C50.911, C50.912, C50.919, C50.921, C50.922, C50.929, C51.0, C51.1, C51.2, C51.8, C51.9, C52, C53.0, C53.1, C53.8, C53.9, C54.0, C54.1, C54.2, C54.3, C54.8, C54.9, C55, C56.1, C56.2, C56.9, C57.00, C57.01, C57.02, C57.10, C57.11, C57.12, C57.20, C57.21, C57.22, C57.3, C57.4, C57.7, C57.8, C57.9, C58, C60.0, C60.1, C60.2, C60.8, C60.9, C61, C62.00, C62.01, C62.02, C62.10, C62.11, C62.12, C62.90, C62.91, C62.92, C63.00, C63.01, C63.02, C63.10, C63.11, C63.12, C63.2, C63.7, C63.8, C63.9, C64.1, C64.2, C64.9, C65.1, C65.2, C65.9, C66.1, C66.2, C66.9, C67.0, C67.1, C67.2, C67.3, C67.4, C67.5, C67.6, C67.7, C67.8, C67.9, C68.0, C68.1, C68.8, C68.9, C69.00, C69.01, C69.02, C69.10, C69.11, C69.12, C69.20, C69.21, C69.22, C69.30, C69.31, C69.32, C69.40, C69.41, C69.42, C69.50, C69.51, C69.52, C69.60, C69.61, C69.62, C69.80, C69.81, C69.82, C69.90, C69.91, C69.92, C70.0, C70.1, C70.9, C71.0, C71.1, C71.2, C71.3, C71.4, C71.5, C71.6, C71.7, C71.8, C71.9, C72.0, C72.1, C72.20, C72.21, C72.22, C72.30, C72.31, C72.32, C72.40, C72.41, C72.42, C72.50, C72.59, C72.9, C73, C74.00, C74.01, C74.02, C74.10, C74.11, C74.12, C74.90, C74.91, C74.92, C75.0, C75.1, C75.2, C75.3, C75.4, C75.5, C75.8, C75.9, C76.0, C76.1, C76.2, C76.3, C76.40, C76.41, C76.42, C76.50, C76.51, C76.52, C76.8, C77.0, C77.1, C77.2, C77.3, C77.4, C77.5, C77.8, C77.9, C78.00, C78.01, C78.02, C78.1, C78.2, C78.30, C78.39, C78.4, C78.5, C78.6, C78.7, C78.80, C78.89, C79.00, C79.01, C79.02, C79.10, C79.11, C79.19, C79.2, C79.31, C79.32, C79.40, C79.49, C79.51, C79.52, C79.60, C79.61, C79.62, C79.70, C79.71, C79.72, C79.81, C79.82, C79.89, C79.9, C7A.00, C7A.010, C7A.011, C7A.012,

G13.0, G13.1 (continued)	C7A.019, C7A.020, C7A.021, C7A.022, C7A.023, C7A.024, C7A.025, C7A.026, C7A.029, C7A.090, C7A.091, C7A.092, C7A.093, C7A.094, C7A.095, C7A.096, C7A.098, C7A.1, C7A.8, C7B.00, C7B.01, C7B.02, C7B.04, C7B.09, C7B.1, C7B.8, C80.0, C80.1, C80.2, C81.00, C81.01, C81.02, C81.03, C81.04, C81.05, C81.06, C81.07, C81.08, C81.09, C81.10, C81.11, C81.12, C81.13, C81.14, C81.15, C81.16, C81.17, C81.18, C81.19, C81.20, C81.21, C81.22, C81.23, C81.24, C81.25, C81.26, C81.27, C81.28, C81.29, C81.30, C81.31, C81.32, C81.33, C81.34, C81.35, C81.36, C81.37, C81.38, C81.39, C81.40, C81.41, C81.42, C81.43, C81.44, C81.45, C81.46, C81.47, C81.48, C81.49, C81.70, C81.71, C81.72, C81.73, C81.74, C81.75, C81.76, C81.77, C81.78, C81.79, C81.90, C81.91, C81.92, C81.93, C81.94, C81.95, C81.96, C81.97, C81.98, C81.99, C82.00, C82.01, C82.02, C82.03, C82.04, C82.05, C82.06, C82.07, C82.08, C82.09, C82.10, C82.11, C82.12, C82.13, C82.14, C82.15, C82.16, C82.17, C82.18, C82.19, C82.20, C82.21, C82.22, C82.23, C82.24, C82.25, C82.26, C82.27, C82.28, C82.29, C82.30, C82.31, C82.32, C82.33, C82.34, C82.35, C82.36, C82.37, C82.38, C82.39, C82.40, C82.41, C82.42, C82.43, C82.44, C82.45, C82.46, C82.47, C82.48, C82.49, C82.50, C82.51, C82.52, C82.53, C82.54, C82.55, C82.56, C82.57, C82.58, C82.59, C82.60, C82.61, C82.62, C82.63, C82.64, C82.65, C82.66, C82.67, C82.68, C82.69, C82.80, C82.81, C82.82, C82.83, C82.84, C82.85, C82.86, C82.87, C82.88, C82.89, C82.90, C82.91, C82.92, C82.93, C82.94, C82.95, C82.96, C82.97, C82.98, C82.99, C83.00, C83.01, C83.02, C83.03, C83.04, C83.05, C83.06, C83.07, C83.08, C83.09, C83.10, C83.11, C83.12, C83.13, C83.14, C83.15, C83.16, C83.17, C83.18, C83.19, C83.30, C83.31, C83.32, C83.33, C83.34, C83.35, C83.36, C83.37, C83.38, C83.39, C83.50, C83.51, C83.52, C83.53, C83.54, C83.55, C83.56, C83.57, C83.58, C83.59, C83.70, C83.71, C83.72, C83.73, C83.74, C83.75, C83.76, C83.77, C83.78, C83.79, C83.80, C83.81, C83.82, C83.83, C83.84, C83.85, C83.86, C83.87, C83.88, C83.89, C83.90, C83.91, C83.92, C83.93, C83.94, C83.95, C83.96, C83.97, C83.98, C83.99, C84.00, C84.01, C84.02, C84.03, C84.04, C84.05, C84.06, C84.07, C84.08, C84.09, C84.10, C84.11, C84.12, C84.13, C84.14, C84.15, C84.16, C84.17, C84.18, C84.19, C84.40, C84.41, C84.42, C84.43, C84.44, C84.45, C84.46, C84.47, C84.48, C84.49, C84.60, C84.61, C84.62, C84.63, C84.64, C84.65, C84.66, C84.67, C84.68, C84.69, C84.70, C84.71, C84.72, C84.73, C84.74, C84.75, C84.76, C84.77, C84.78, C84.79, C84.90, C84.91, C84.92, C84.93, C84.94, C84.95, C84.96, C84.97, C84.98, C84.99, C84.A0, C84.A1, C84.A2, C84.A3, C84.A4, C84.A5, C84.A6, C84.A7, C84.A8, C84.A9, C84.Z0, C84.Z1, C84.Z2, C84.Z3, C84.Z4, C84.Z5, C84.Z6, C84.Z7, C84.Z8, C84.Z9, C85.10, C85.11, C85.12, C85.13, C85.14, C85.15, C85.16, C85.17, C85.18, C85.19, C85.20, C85.21, C85.22, C85.23, C85.24, C85.25, C85.26, C85.27, C85.28, C85.29, C85.80, C85.81, C85.82, C85.83, C85.84, C85.85, C85.86, C85.87, C85.88, C85.89, C85.90, C85.91, C85.92, C85.93, C85.94, C85.95, C85.96, C85.97, C85.98, C85.99, C86.0, C86.1, C86.2, C86.3, C86.4, C86.5, C86.6, C88.0, C88.2, C88.3, C88.4, C88.8, C88.9, C90.00, C90.01, C90.02, C90.10, C90.11, C90.12, C90.20, C90.21, C90.22, C90.30, C90.31, C90.32, C91.00, C91.01, C91.02, C91.10, C91.11, C91.12, C91.30, C91.31, C91.32, C91.40, C91.41, C91.42, C91.50, C91.51, C91.52, C91.60, C91.61, C91.62, C91.90, C91.91, C91.92, C91.A0, C91.A1, C91.A2, C91.Z0, C91.Z1, C91.Z2, C92.00, C92.01, C92.02, C92.10, C92.11, C92.12, C92.20, C92.21, C92.22, C92.30, C92.31, C92.32, C92.40, C92.41, C92.42, C92.50, C92.51, C92.52, C92.60, C92.61, C92.62, C92.90, C92.91, C92.92, C92.A0, C92.A1, C92.A2, C92.Z0, C92.Z1, C92.Z2, C93.00, C93.01, C93.02, C93.10, C93.11, C93.12, C93.30, C93.31, C93.32, C93.90, C93.91, C93.92, C93.Z0, C93.Z1, C94.00, C94.01, C94.02, C94.20, C94.21, C94.22, C94.30, C94.31, C94.32, C94.40, C94.41, C94.42, C94.6, C94.80, C94.81, C94.82, C95.00, C95.01, C95.02, C95.10, C95.11, C95.12, C95.90, C95.91, C95.92, C96.0, C96.4, C96.5, C96.6, C96.9, C96.A, C96.Z, D00.00, D00.01, D00.02, D00.03, D00.04, D00.05, D00.06, D00.07, D00.08, D00.1, D00.2, D01.0, D01.1, D01.2, D01.3, D01.40, D01.49, D01.5, D01.7, D01.9, D02.0, D02.1, D02.20, D02.21, D02.22, D02.3, D02.4, D03.0, D03.10, D03.11, D03.12, D03.20, D03.21, D03.22, D03.30, D03.39, D03.4, D03.51, D03.52, D03.59, D03.60, D03.61, D03.62, D03.70, D03.71, D03.72, D03.8, D03.9, D04.0, D04.10, D04.11, D04.12, D04.20, D04.21, D04.22, D04.30, D04.39, D04.4, D04.5, D04.60, D04.61, D04.62, D04.70, D04.71, D04.72, D04.8, D04.9, D05.00, D05.01, D05.02, D05.10, D05.11, D05.12, D05.80, D05.81, D05.82, D05.90, D05.91, D05.92, D06.0, D06.1, D06.7, D06.9, D07.0, D07.1, D07.2, D07.30, D07.39, D07.4, D07.5, D07.60, D07.61, D07.69, D09.0, D09.10, D09.19, D09.20, D09.21, D09.22, D09.3, D09.8, D09.9, D10.0, D10.1, D10.2, D10.30, D10.39, D10.4, D10.5, D10.6, D10.7, D10.9, D11.0, D11.7, D11.9, D12.0, D12.1, D12.2, D12.3, D12.4, D12.5, D12.6, D12.7, D12.8, D12.9, D13.0, D13.1, D13.2, D13.30, D13.39, D13.4, D13.5, D13.6, D13.7, D13.9, D14.0, D14.1, D14.2, D14.30, D14.31, D14.32, D14.4, D15.0, D15.1, D15.2, D15.7, D15.9, D16.00, D16.01, D16.02, D16.10, D16.11, D16.12, D16.20, D16.21, D16.22, D16.30, D16.31, D16.32, D16.4, D16.5, D16.6, D16.7, D16.8, D16.9, D17.0, D17.1, D17.20, D17.21, D17.22, D17.23, D17.24, D17.30, D17.39, D17.4, D17.5, D17.6, D17.9, D18.00, D18.01, D18.02, D18.03, D18.09, D18.1, D19.0, D19.1, D19.7, D19.9, D20.0, D20.1, D21.0, D21.10, D21.11, D21.12, D21.20, D21.21, D21.22, D21.3, D21.4, D21.5, D21.6, D21.9, D22.0, D22.10, D22.11, D22.12, D22.20, D22.21, D22.22, D22.30, D22.39, D22.4, D22.5, D22.60, D22.61, D22.62, D22.70, D22.71, D22.72, D22.9, D23.0, D23.10, D23.11, D23.12, D23.20, D23.21, D23.22, D23.30, D23.39, D23.4, D23.5, D23.60, D23.61, D23.62, D23.70, D23.71, D23.72, D23.9, D24.1, D24.2, D24.9, D25.0, D25.1, D25.2, D25.9, D26.0, D26.1, D26.7, D26.9, D27.0, D27.1, D27.9, D28.0, D28.1, D28.2, D28.7, D28.9, D29.0, D29.1, D29.20, D29.21, D29.22, D29.30, D29.31, D29.32, D29.4, D29.8, D29.9, D30.00, D30.01, D30.02, D30.10, D30.11, D30.12, D30.20, D30.21, D30.22, D30.3, D30.4, D30.8, D30.9, D31.00, D31.01, D31.02, D31.10, D31.11, D31.12, D31.20, D31.21, D31.22, D31.30, D31.31, D31.32, D31.40, D31.41, D31.42, D31.50, D31.51, D31.52, D31.60, D31.61, D31.62, D31.90, D31.91, D31.92, D32.0, D32.1, D32.9, D33.0, D33.1, D33.2, D33.3, D33.4, D33.7, D33.9, D34, D35.00, D35.01, D35.02, D35.1, D35.2, D35.3, D35.4, D35.5, D35.6, D35.7, D35.9, D36.0, D36.10, D36.11, D36.12, D36.13, D36.14, D36.15, D36.16, D36.17, D36.7, D36.9, D37.01, D37.02, D37.030, D37.031, D37.032, D37.039, D37.04, D37.05, D37.09, D37.1, D37.2, D37.3, D37.4, D37.5, D37.6, D37.8, D37.9, D38.0, D38.1, D38.2, D38.3, D38.4, D38.5, D38.6, D39.0, D39.10, D39.11, D39.12, D39.2, D39.8, D39.9, D3A.00, D3A.010, D3A.011, D3A.012, D3A.019, D3A.020, D3A.021, D3A.022, D3A.023, D3A.024, D3A.025, D3A.026, D3A.029, D3A.090, D3A.091, D3A.092, D3A.093, D3A.094, D3A.095, D3A.096, D3A.098, D3A.8, D40.0, D40.10, D40.11, D40.12, D40.8, D40.9, D41.00, D41.01, D41.02, D41.10, D41.11, D41.12, D41.20, D41.21, D41.22, D41.3, D41.4, D41.8, D41.9, D42.0, D42.1, D42.9, D43.0, D43.1, D43.2, D43.3, D43.4, D43.8, D43.9, D44.0, D44.10, D44.11, D44.12, D44.2, D44.3, D44.4, D44.5, D44.6, D44.7, D44.9, D45, D46.0, D46.1, D46.20, D46.21, D46.22, D46.4, D46.9, D46.A, D46.B, D46.C, D46.Z, D47.1, D47.2, D47.3, D47.4, D47.9, D47.Z1, D47.Z2, D47.Z9, D48.0, D48.1, D48.2, D48.3, D48.4, D48.5, D48.60, D48.61, D48.62, D48.7, D48.9
G32.0	D51.0, D51.3, D51.9, E53.8

| G32.89 | C00.0, C00.1, C00.2, C00.3, C00.4, C00.5, C00.6, C00.8, C00.9, C01, C02.0, C02.1, C02.2, C02.3, C02.4, C02.8, C02.9, C03.0, C03.1, C03.9, C04.0, C04.1, C04.8, C04.9, C05.0, C05.1, C05.2, C05.8, C05.9, C06.0, C06.1, C06.2, C06.80, C06.89, C06.9, C07, C08.0, C08.1, C08.9, C09.0, C09.1, C09.8, C09.9, C10.0, C10.1, C10.2, C10.3, C10.4, C10.8, C10.9, C11.0, C11.1, C11.2, C11.3, C11.8, C11.9, C12, C13.0, C13.1, C13.2, C13.8, C13.9, C14.0, C14.2, C14.8, C15.3, C15.4, C15.5, C15.8, C15.9, C16.0, C16.1, C16.2, C16.3, C16.4, C16.5, C16.6, C16.8, C16.9, C17.0, C17.1, C17.2, C17.3, C17.8, C17.9, C18.0, C18.1, C18.2, C18.3, C18.4, C18.5, C18.6, C18.7, C18.8, C18.9, C19, C20, C21.0, C21.1, C21.2, C21.8, C22.0, C22.1, C22.2, C22.3, C22.4, C22.7, C22.8, C22.9, C23, C24.0, C24.1, C24.8, C24.9, C25.0, C25.1, C25.2, C25.3, C25.4, C25.7, C25.8, C25.9, C26.0, C26.1, C26.9, C30.0, C30.1, C31.0, C31.2, C31.3, C31.8, C31.9, C32.0, C32.1, C32.2, C32.3, C32.8, C32.9, C33, C34.00, C34.01, C34.02, C34.10, C34.11, C34.12, C34.2, C34.30, C34.31, C34.32, C34.80, C34.81, C34.82, C34.90, C34.91, C34.92, C37, C38.0, C38.1, C38.2, C38.3, C38.4, C38.8, C39.0, C39.9, C40.00, C40.01, C40.02, C40.10, C40.11, C40.12, C40.20, C40.21, C40.22, C40.30, C40.31, C40.32, C40.80, C40.81, C40.82, C40.90, C40.91, C40.92, C41.0, C41.1, C41.2, C41.3, C41.4, C41.9, C43.0, C43.10, C43.11, C43.12, C43.20, C43.21, C43.22, C43.30, C43.31, C43.39, C43.4, C43.51, C43.52, C43.59, C43.60, C43.61, C43.62, C43.70, C43.71, C43.72, C43.8, C43.9, C45.0, C45.1, C45.2, C45.7, C45.9, C46.0, C46.1, C46.2, C46.3, C46.4, C46.50, C46.51, C46.52, C46.7, C46.9, C47.0, C47.10, C47.11, C47.12, C47.20, C47.21, C47.22, C47.3, C47.4, C47.5, C47.6, C47.8, C47.9, C48.0, C48.1, C48.2, C48.8, C49.00, C49.10, C49.20, C49.21, C49.3, C49.4, C49.5, C49.6, C49.8, C49.9, C49.A0, C49.A1, C49.A2, C49.A3, C49.A4, C49.A5, C49.A9, C4A.0, C4A.10, C4A.11, C4A.12, C4A.20, C4A.21, C4A.22, C4A.30, C4A.31, C4A.39, C4A.4, C4A.51, C4A.52, C4A.59, C4A.60, C4A.61, C4A.62, C4A.70, C4A.71, C4A.72, C4A.8, C4A.9, C50.011, C50.012, C50.019, C50.021, C50.022, C50.029, C50.111, C50.112, C50.119, C50.121, C50.122, C50.129, C50.211, C50.212, C50.219, C50.221, C50.222, C50.229, C50.311, C50.312, C50.319, C50.321, C50.322, C50.329, C50.411, C50.412, C50.419, C50.421, C50.422, C50.429, C50.511, C50.512, C50.519, C50.521, C50.522, C50.529, C50.611, C50.612, C50.619, C50.621, C50.622, C50.629, C50.811, C50.812, C50.819, C50.821, C50.822, C50.829, C50.911, C50.912, C50.919, C50.921, C50.922, C50.929, C51.0, C51.1, C51.2, C51.8, C51.9, C52, C53.0, C53.1, C53.8, C53.9, C54.0, C54.1, C54.2, C54.3, C54.8, C54.9, C55, C56.1, C56.2, C56.9, C57.00, C57.01, C57.02, C57.10, C57.11, C57.12, C57.20, C57.21, C57.22, C57.3, C57.4, C57.7, C57.8, C57.9, C58, C60.0, C60.1, C60.2, C60.8, C60.9, C61, C62.00, C62.01, C62.02, C62.10, C62.11, C62.12, C62.90, C62.91, C62.92, C63.00, C63.01, C63.02, C63.10, C63.11, C63.12, C63.2, C63.7, C63.8, C63.9, C64.1, C64.2, C64.9, C65.1, C65.2, C65.9, C66.1, C66.2, C66.9, C67.0, C67.1, C67.2, C67.3, C67.4, C67.5, C67.6, C67.7, C67.8, C67.9, C68.0, C68.1, C68.8, C68.9, C69.00, C69.01, C69.02, C69.10, C69.11, C69.12, C69.20, C69.21, C69.22, C69.30, C69.31, C69.32, C69.40, C69.41, C69.42, C69.50, C69.51, C69.52, C69.60, C69.61, C69.62, C69.80, C69.81, C69.82, C69.90, C69.91, C69.92, C70.0, C70.1, C70.9, C71.0, C71.1, C71.2, C71.3, C71.4, C71.5, C71.6, C71.7, C71.8, C71.9, C72.0, C72.1, C72.20, C72.21, C72.22, C72.30, C72.31, C72.32, C72.40, C72.41, C72.42, C72.50, C72.59, C72.9, C73, C74.00, C74.01, C74.02, C74.10, C74.11, C74.12, C74.90, C74.91, C74.92, C75.0, C75.1, C75.2, C75.3, C75.4, C75.5, C75.8, C75.9, C76.0, C76.1, C76.2, C76.3, C76.40, C76.41, C76.42, C76.50, C76.51, C76.52, C76.8, C77.0, C77.1, C77.2, C77.3, C77.4, C77.5, C77.8, C77.9, C78.00, C78.01, C78.02, C78.1, C78.2, C78.30, C78.39, C78.4, C78.5, C78.6, C78.7, C78.80, C78.89, C79.00, C79.01, C79.02, C79.10, C79.11, C79.19, C79.2, C79.31, C79.32, C79.40, C79.49, C79.51, C79.52, C79.60, C79.61, C79.62, C79.70, C79.71, C79.72, C79.81, C79.82, C79.89, C79.9, C7A.00, C7A.010, C7A.011, C7A.012, C7A.019, C7A.020, C7A.021, C7A.022, C7A.023, C7A.024, C7A.025, C7A.026, C7A.029, C7A.090, C7A.091, C7A.092, C7A.093, C7A.094, C7A.095, C7A.096, C7A.098, C7A.1, C7A.8, C7B.00, C7B.01, C7B.02, C7B.03, C7B.04, C7B.09, C7B.1, C7B.8, C80.0, C80.1, C80.2, C81.00, C81.01, C81.02, C81.03, C81.04, C81.05, C81.06, C81.07, C81.08, C81.09, C81.10, C81.11, C81.12, C81.13, C81.14, C81.15, C81.16, C81.17, C81.18, C81.19, C81.20, C81.21, C81.22, C81.23, C81.24, C81.25, C81.26, C81.27, C81.28, C81.29, C81.30, C81.31, C81.32, C81.33, C81.34, C81.35, C81.36, C81.37, C81.38, C81.39, C81.40, C81.41, C81.42, C81.43, C81.44, C81.45, C81.46, C81.47, C81.48, C81.49, C81.70, C81.71, C81.72, C81.73, C81.74, C81.75, C81.76, C81.77, C81.78, C81.79, C81.90, C81.91, C81.92, C81.93, C81.94, C81.95, C81.96, C81.97, C81.98, C81.99, C82.00, C82.01, C82.02, C82.03, C82.04, C82.05, C82.06, C82.07, C82.08, C82.09, C82.10, C82.11, C82.12, C82.13, C82.14, C82.15, C82.16, C82.17, C82.18, C82.19, C82.20, C82.21, C82.22, C82.23, C82.24, C82.25, C82.26, C82.27, C82.28, C82.29, C82.30, C82.31, C82.32, C82.33, C82.34, C82.35, C82.36, C82.37, C82.38, C82.39, C82.40, C82.41, C82.42, C82.43, C82.44, C82.45, C82.46, C82.47, C82.48, C82.49, C82.50, C82.51, C82.52, C82.53, C82.54, C82.55, C82.56, C82.57, C82.58, C82.59, C82.60, C82.61, C82.62, C82.63, C82.64, C82.65, C82.66, C82.67, C82.68, C82.69, C82.80, C82.81, C82.82, C82.83, C82.84, C82.85, C82.86, C82.87, C82.88, C82.89, C82.91, C82.92, C82.93, C82.94, C82.95, C82.96, C82.97, C82.98, C82.99, C83.00, C83.01, C83.02, C83.03, C83.04, C83.05, C83.06, C83.07, C83.08, C83.09, C83.10, C83.11, C83.12, C83.13, C83.14, C83.15, C83.16, C83.17, C83.18, C83.19, C83.30, C83.31, C83.32, C83.33, C83.34, C83.35, C83.36, C83.37, C83.38, C83.39, C83.50, C83.51, C83.52, C83.53, C83.54, C83.55, C83.56, C83.57, C83.58, C83.59, C83.70, C83.71, C83.72, C83.73, C83.74, C83.75, C83.76, C83.77, C83.78, C83.79, C83.80, C83.81, C83.82, C83.83, C83.84, C83.85, C83.86, C83.87, C83.88, C83.89, C83.90, C83.91, C83.92, C83.93, C83.94, C83.95, C83.96, C83.97, C83.98, C83.99, C84.00, C84.01, C84.02, C84.03, C84.04, C84.05, C84.06, C84.07, C84.08, C84.09, C84.10, C84.11, C84.12, C84.13, C84.14, C84.15, C84.16, C84.17, C84.18, C84.19, C84.40, C84.41, C84.42, C84.43, C84.44, C84.45, C84.46, C84.47, C84.48, C84.49, C84.60, C84.61, C84.62, C84.63, C84.64, C84.65, C84.66, C84.67, C84.68, C84.69, C84.70, C84.71, C84.72, C84.73, C84.74, C84.75, C84.76, C84.77, C84.78, C84.79, C84.90, C84.91, C84.92, C84.93, C84.94, C84.95, C84.96, C84.97, C84.98, C84.99, C84.A0, C84.A1, C84.A2, C84.A3, C84.A4, C84.A5, C84.A6, C84.A7, C84.A8, C84.A9, C84.Z0, C84.Z1, C84.Z2, C84.Z3, C84.Z4, C84.Z5, C84.Z6, C84.Z7, C84.Z8, C84.Z9, C85.10, C85.11, C85.12, C85.13, C85.14, C85.15, C85.16, C85.17, C85.18, C85.19, C85.20, C85.21, C85.22, C85.23, C85.24, C85.25, C85.26, C85.27, C85.28, C85.29, C85.80, C85.81, C85.82, C85.83, C85.84, C85.85, C85.86, C85.87, C85.88, C85.89, C85.90, C85.91, C85.92, C85.93, C85.94, C85.95, C85.96, C85.97, C85.98, C85.99, C86.0, C86.1, C86.2, C86.3, C86.4, C86.5, C86.6, C88.0, C88.2, C88.3, C88.4, C88.8, C88.9, C90.00, C90.01, C90.02, C90.10, C90.11, C90.12, C90.20, C90.21, C90.22, C90.30, C90.31, C90.32, C91.00, C91.01, C91.02, C91.10, C91.11, C91.12, C91.30, C91.31, C91.32, C91.40, C91.41, C91.42, C91.50, C91.51, C91.52, C91.60, C91.61, C91.62, C91.90, C91.91, C91.92, C91.A0, C91.A1, C91.A2, C91.Z0, C91.Z1, C91.Z2, C92.00, C92.01, C92.02, C92.10, C92.11, C92.12, C92.20, C92.21, C92.22, C92.30, C92.31, C92.32, C92.40, C92.41, C92.42, C92.50, C92.51, C92.52, C92.60, C92.61, C92.62, C92.90, C92.91, C92.92, C92.A0, C92.A1, C92.A2, C92.Z0, C92.Z1, C92.Z2, C93.00, C93.01, C93.02, C93.10, C93.11, C93.12, C93.30, C93.31, C93.32, C93.90, C93.91, C93.92, C93.Z0, C93.Z1, C94.00, C94.01, C94.02, C94.20, C94.21, C94.22, C94.30, C94.31, C94.32, C94.40, C94.41, C94.42, C94.6, C94.80, C94.81, C94.82, C95.00, C95.01, C95.02, C95.10, C95.11, C95.12, C95.90, C95.91, C95.92, C96.0, C96.4, C96.5, C96.6, C96.9, C96.A, C96.Z, D00.00, D00.01, D00.02, D00.03, D00.04, D00.05, D00.06, D00.07, D00.08, D00.1, D00.2, D01.0, D01.1, D01.2, D01.3, D01.40, D01.49, D01.5, D01.7, D01.9, D02.0, D02.1, D02.20, D02.21, D02.22, D02.3, D02.4, D03.0, D03.10, D03.11, D03.12, D03.20, D03.21, D03.22, D03.30, D03.39, D03.4, D03.51, D03.52, D03.59, D03.60, D03.61, D03.62, D03.70, D03.71, D03.72, D03.8, D03.9, D04.0, D04.10, D04.11, D04.12, D04.20, D04.21, D04.22, D04.30, D04.39, D04.4, D04.5, D04.60, D04.61, D04.62, D04.70, D04.71, D04.72, D04.8, D04.9, D05.00, D05.01, D05.02, D05.10, D05.11, D05.12, D05.80, D05.81, D05.82, D05.90, D05.91, D05.92, D06.0, D06.1, D06.7, D06.9, D07.0, D07.1, D07.2, D07.30, D07.39, D07.4, D07.5, D07.60, D07.61, D07.69, D09.0, D09.10, D09.19, D09.20, D09.21, D09.22, D09.3, D09.8, D09.9, D10.0, D10.1, D10.2, D10.30, D10.39, D10.4, D10.5, D10.6, D10.7, D10.9, D11.0, D11.7, D11.9, D12.0, D12.1, D12.2, D12.3, D12.4, D12.5, D12.6, D12.7, D12.8, D12.9, D13.0, D13.1, D13.2, D13.30, D13.39, D13.4, D13.5, D13.6, D13.7, D13.9, D14.0, D14.1, D14.2, D14.30, D14.31, D14.32, D14.4, D15.0, D15.1, D15.2, D15.7, D15.9, D16.00, D16.01, D16.02, D16.10, D16.11, D16.21, D16.22, D16.31, D16.32, D16.4, D16.5, D16.6, D16.7, D16.8, D16.9, D17.0, D17.1, D17.20, D17.21, D17.22, D17.23, D17.24, D17.30, D17.39, D17.4, D17.5, D17.6, D17.9, D18.00, D18.01, D18.02, D18.03, D18.09, D18.1, D19.0, D19.1, D19.7, D19.9, D20.0, D20.1, D21.0, D21.10, D21.11, D21.12, D21.20, D21.21, D21.22, D21.3, D21.4, D21.5, D21.6, D21.9, D22.0, D22.10, D22.11, D22.12, D22.20, D22.21, D22.22, D22.30, D22.39, D22.4, D22.5, D22.60, D22.61, D22.62, D22.70, D22.71, D22.72, D22.9, D23.0, D23.10, D23.11, D23.12, D23.20, D23.21, D23.22, D23.30, D23.39, D23.4, D23.5, D23.60, D23.61, D23.62, D23.70, D23.71, D23.72, D23.9, D24.1, D24.2, D24.9, D25.0, D25.1, D25.2, D25.9, D26.0, D26.1, D26.7, D26.9, D27.0, D27.1, D27.9, D28.0, D28.1, D28.2, D28.7, D28.9, D29.0, D29.1, D29.20, D29.21, D29.22, D29.30, D29.31, D29.32, D29.4, D29.8, D29.9, D30.00, D30.01, D30.02, D30.10, D30.11, D30.12, D30.20, D30.21, D30.22, D30.3, D30.4, D30.8, D30.9, D31.00, D31.01, D31.02, D31.10, D31.11, D31.12, D31.20, D31.21, D31.22, D31.30, D31.31, D31.32, D31.40, D31.41, D31.42, D31.50, D31.51, D31.52, D31.60, D31.61, D31.62, D31.90, D31.91, |

G32.89 (continued)	D31.92, D32.0, D32.1, D32.9, D33.0, D33.1, D33.2, D33.3, D33.4, D33.7, D33.9, D34, D35.00, D35.01, D35.02, D35.1, D35.2, D35.3, D35.4, D35.5, D35.6, D35.7, D35.9, D36.0, D36.10, D36.11, D36.12, D36.13, D36.14, D36.15, D36.16, D36.17, D36.7, D36.9, D37.01, D37.02, D37.030, D37.031, D37.032, D37.039, D37.04, D37.05, D37.09, D37.1, D37.2, D37.3, D37.4, D37.5, D37.6, D37.8, D37.9, D38.0, D38.1, D38.2, D38.3, D38.4, D38.5, D38.6, D39.0, D39.10, D39.11, D39.12, D39.2, D39.8, D39.9, D3A.00, D3A.010, D3A.011, D3A.012, D3A.019, D3A.020, D3A.021, D3A.022, D3A.023, D3A.024, D3A.025, D3A.026, D3A.090, D3A.091, D3A.092, D3A.093, D3A.094, D3A.095, D3A.096, D3A.098, D3A.8, D40.0, D40.10, D40.11, D40.12, D40.8, D40.9, D41.00, D41.01, D41.02, D41.10, D41.11, D41.12, D41.20, D41.21, D41.22, D41.3, D41.4, D41.8, D41.9, D42.0, D42.1, D42.9, D43.0, D43.1, D43.2, D43.3, D43.4, D43.8, D43.9, D44.0, D44.10, D44.11, D44.12, D44.2, D44.3, D44.4, D44.5, D44.6, D44.7, D44.9, D45, D46.0, D46.1, D46.20, D46.21, D46.22, D46.4, D46.9, D46.A, D46.B, D46.C, D46.Z, D47.1, D47.2, D47.3, D47.4, D47.9, D47.Z1, D47.Z2, D47.Z9, D48.0, D48.1, D48.2, D48.3, D48.4, D48.5, D48.60, D48.61, D48.62, D48.7, D48.9, E00.0, E00.1, E00.2, E00.9, E03.0, E03.1, E03.2, E03.3, E03.4, E03.5, E03.8, E03.9, E52, E53.0, E53.1, E53.8, E53.9, E85.0, E85.1, E85.2, E85.3, E85.4, E85.9
G53	C00.0, C00.1, C00.2, C00.3, C00.4, C00.5, C00.6, C00.8, C00.9, C01, C02.0, C02.1, C02.2, C02.3, C02.4, C02.8, C02.9, C03.0, C03.1, C03.9, C04.0, C04.1, C04.8, C04.9, C05.0, C05.1, C05.2, C05.8, C05.9, C06.0, C06.1, C06.2, C06.80, C06.89, C06.9, C07, C08.0, C08.1, C08.9, C09.0, C09.1, C09.8, C09.9, C10.0, C10.1, C10.2, C10.3, C10.4, C10.8, C10.9, C11.0, C11.1, C11.2, C11.3, C11.8, C11.9, C12, C13.0, C13.1, C13.2, C13.8, C13.9, C14.0, C14.2, C14.8, C15.3, C15.4, C15.5, C15.8, C15.9, C16.0, C16.1, C16.2, C16.3, C16.4, C16.5, C16.6, C16.8, C16.9, C17.0, C17.1, C17.2, C17.3, C17.8, C17.9, C18.0, C18.1, C18.2, C18.3, C18.4, C18.5, C18.6, C18.7, C18.8, C18.9, C19, C20, C21.0, C21.1, C21.2, C21.8, C22.0, C22.1, C22.2, C22.3, C22.4, C22.7, C22.8, C22.9, C23, C24.0, C24.1, C24.8, C24.9, C25.0, C25.1, C25.2, C25.3, C25.4, C25.7, C25.8, C25.9, C26.0, C26.1, C26.9, C30.0, C30.1, C31.0, C31.1, C31.2, C31.3, C31.8, C31.9, C32.0, C32.1, C32.2, C32.3, C32.8, C32.9, C33, C34.00, C34.01, C34.02, C34.10, C34.11, C34.12, C34.2, C34.30, C34.31, C34.32, C34.80, C34.81, C34.82, C34.90, C34.91, C34.92, C37, C38.0, C38.1, C38.2, C38.3, C38.4, C38.8, C39.0, C39.9, C40.00, C40.01, C40.02, C40.10, C40.11, C40.12, C40.20, C40.21, C40.22, C40.30, C40.31, C40.32, C40.80, C40.81, C40.82, C40.90, C40.91, C40.92, C41.0, C41.1, C41.2, C41.3, C41.4, C41.9, C43.0, C43.10, C43.11, C43.12, C43.20, C43.21, C43.22, C43.30, C43.31, C43.39, C43.4, C43.51, C43.52, C43.59, C43.60, C43.61, C43.62, C43.70, C43.71, C43.72, C43.8, C43.9, C44.00, C44.01, C44.02, C44.09, C44.101, C44.102, C44.109, C44.111, C44.112, C44.119, C44.121, C44.122, C44.129, C44.191, C44.192, C44.199, C44.201, C44.202, C44.209, C44.211, C44.212, C44.219, C44.221, C44.222, C44.229, C44.291, C44.292, C44.299, C44.300, C44.301, C44.309, C44.310, C44.311, C44.319, C44.320, C44.321, C44.329, C44.390, C44.391, C44.399, C44.40, C44.41, C44.42, C44.49, C44.500, C44.501, C44.509, C44.510, C44.511, C44.519, C44.520, C44.521, C44.529, C44.590, C44.591, C44.599, C44.601, C44.602, C44.609, C44.611, C44.612, C44.619, C44.621, C44.622, C44.629, C44.691, C44.692, C44.699, C44.701, C44.702, C44.709, C44.711, C44.712, C44.719, C44.721, C44.722, C44.729, C44.791, C44.792, C44.799, C44.80, C44.81, C44.82, C44.89, C44.90, C44.91, C44.92, C44.99, C45.0, C45.1, C45.2, C45.7, C45.9, C46.0, C46.1, C46.2, C46.3, C46.4, C46.50, C46.51, C46.52, C46.7, C46.9, C47.0, C47.10, C47.11, C47.12, C47.20, C47.21, C47.22, C47.3, C47.4, C47.5, C47.6, C47.8, C47.9, C48.0, C48.1, C48.2, C48.8, C49.0, C49.10, C49.11, C49.12, C49.20, C49.21, C49.22, C49.3, C49.4, C49.5, C49.6, C49.8, C49.9, C49.A0, C49.A1, C49.A2, C49.A3, C49.A4, C49.A5, C49.A9, C4A.0, C4A.10, C4A.11, C4A.12, C4A.20, C4A.21, C4A.22, C4A.30, C4A.31, C4A.39, C4A.4, C4A.51, C4A.52, C4A.59, C4A.60, C4A.61, C4A.62, C4A.70, C4A.71, C4A.72, C4A.8, C4A.9, C50.011, C50.012, C50.019, C50.021, C50.022, C50.029, C50.111, C50.112, C50.119, C50.121, C50.122, C50.129, C50.211, C50.212, C50.219, C50.221, C50.222, C50.229, C50.311, C50.312, C50.319, C50.321, C50.322, C50.329, C50.411, C50.412, C50.419, C50.421, C50.422, C50.429, C50.511, C50.512, C50.519, C50.521, C50.522, C50.529, C50.611, C50.612, C50.619, C50.621, C50.622, C50.629, C50.811, C50.812, C50.819, C50.821, C50.822, C50.829, C50.911, C50.912, C50.919, C50.921, C50.922, C50.929, C51.0, C51.1, C51.2, C51.8, C51.9, C52, C53.0, C53.1, C53.8, C53.9, C54.0, C54.1, C54.2, C54.3, C54.8, C54.9, C55, C56.1, C56.2, C56.9, C57.00, C57.01, C57.02, C57.10, C57.11, C57.12, C57.20, C57.21, C57.22, C57.3, C57.4, C57.7, C57.8, C57.9, C58, C60.0, C60.1, C60.2, C60.8, C60.9, C61, C62.00, C62.01, C62.02, C62.10, C62.11, C62.12, C62.90, C62.91, C62.92, C63.00, C63.01, C63.02, C63.10, C63.11, C63.12, C63.2, C63.7, C63.8, C63.9, C64.1, C64.2, C64.9, C65.1, C65.2, C65.9, C66.1, C66.2, C66.9, C67.0, C67.1, C67.2, C67.3, C67.4, C67.5, C67.6, C67.7, C67.8, C67.9, C68.0, C68.1, C68.8, C68.9, C69.00, C69.01, C69.02, C69.10, C69.11, C69.12, C69.20, C69.21, C69.22, C69.30, C69.31, C69.32, C69.40, C69.41, C69.42, C69.50, C69.51, C69.52, C69.60, C69.61, C69.62, C69.80, C69.81, C69.82, C69.90, C69.91, C69.92, C70.0, C70.1, C70.9, C71.0, C71.1, C71.2, C71.3, C71.4, C71.5, C71.6, C71.7, C71.8, C71.9, C72.0, C72.1, C72.20, C72.21, C72.22, C72.30, C72.31, C72.32, C72.40, C72.41, C72.42, C72.59, C72.9, C73, C74.00, C74.01, C74.02, C74.10, C74.11, C74.12, C74.90, C74.91, C74.92, C75.0, C75.1, C75.2, C75.3, C75.4, C75.5, C75.8, C75.9, C76.0, C76.1, C76.2, C76.3, C76.40, C76.41, C76.42, C76.50, C76.51, C76.52, C76.8, C77.0, C77.1, C77.2, C77.3, C77.4, C77.5, C77.8, C77.9, C78.00, C78.01, C78.02, C78.1, C78.2, C78.30, C78.39, C78.4, C78.5, C78.6, C78.7, C78.80, C78.89, C79.00, C79.01, C79.02, C79.10, C79.11, C79.19, C79.2, C79.31, C79.32, C79.40, C79.49, C79.51, C79.52, C79.60, C79.61, C79.62, C79.70, C79.71, C79.72, C79.81, C79.82, C79.89, C79.9, C7A.00, C7A.010, C7A.011, C7A.012, C7A.019, C7A.020, C7A.021, C7A.022, C7A.023, C7A.024, C7A.025, C7A.026, C7A.029, C7A.090, C7A.091, C7A.092, C7A.093, C7A.094, C7A.095, C7A.096, C7A.098, C7A.1, C7A.8, C7B.00, C7B.01, C7B.02, C7B.03, C7B.04, C7B.09, C7B.1, C7B.8, C80.0, C80.1, C80.2, C81.00, C81.01, C81.02, C81.03, C81.04, C81.05, C81.06, C81.07, C81.08, C81.09, C81.10, C81.11, C81.12, C81.13, C81.14, C81.15, C81.16, C81.17, C81.18, C81.19, C81.20, C81.21, C81.22, C81.23, C81.24, C81.25, C81.26, C81.27, C81.28, C81.29, C81.30, C81.31, C81.32, C81.33, C81.34, C81.35, C81.36, C81.37, C81.38, C81.39, C81.40, C81.41, C81.42, C81.43, C81.44, C81.45, C81.46, C81.47, C81.48, C81.49, C81.70, C81.71, C81.72, C81.73, C81.74, C81.75, C81.76, C81.77, C81.78, C81.79, C81.90, C81.91, C81.92, C81.93, C81.94, C81.95, C81.96, C81.97, C81.98, C81.99, C82.00, C82.01, C82.02, C82.03, C82.04, C82.05, C82.06, C82.07, C82.08, C82.09, C82.10, C82.11, C82.12, C82.13, C82.14, C82.15, C82.16, C82.17, C82.18, C82.19, C82.20, C82.21, C82.22, C82.23, C82.24, C82.25, C82.26, C82.27, C82.28, C82.29, C82.30, C82.31, C82.32, C82.33, C82.34, C82.35, C82.36, C82.37, C82.38, C82.39, C82.40, C82.41, C82.42, C82.43, C82.44, C82.45, C82.46, C82.47, C82.48, C82.49, C82.50, C82.51, C82.52, C82.53, C82.54, C82.55, C82.56, C82.57, C82.58, C82.59, C82.60, C82.61, C82.62, C82.63, C82.64, C82.65, C82.66, C82.67, C82.68, C82.69, C82.80, C82.81, C82.82, C82.83, C82.84, C82.85, C82.86, C82.87, C82.88, C82.89, C82.90, C82.91, C82.92, C82.93, C82.94, C82.95, C82.96, C82.97, C82.98, C82.99, C83.00, C83.01, C83.02, C83.03, C83.04, C83.05, C83.06, C83.07, C83.08, C83.09, C83.10, C83.11, C83.12, C83.13, C83.14, C83.15, C83.16, C83.17, C83.18, C83.19, C83.30, C83.31, C83.32, C83.33, C83.34, C83.35, C83.36, C83.37, C83.38, C83.39, C83.50, C83.51, C83.52, C83.53, C83.54, C83.55, C83.56, C83.57, C83.58, C83.59, C83.70, C83.71, C83.72, C83.73, C83.74, C83.75, C83.76, C83.77, C83.78, C83.79, C83.80, C83.81, C83.82, C83.83, C83.84, C83.85, C83.86, C83.87, C83.88, C83.89, C83.90, C83.91, C83.92, C83.93, C83.94, C83.95, C83.96, C83.97, C83.98, C83.99, C84.00, C84.01, C84.02, C84.03, C84.04, C84.05, C84.06, C84.07, C84.08, C84.09, C84.10, C84.11, C84.12, C84.13, C84.14, C84.15, C84.16, C84.17, C84.18, C84.19, C84.40, C84.41, C84.42, C84.43, C84.44, C84.45, C84.46, C84.47, C84.48, C84.49, C84.60, C84.61, C84.62, C84.63, C84.64, C84.65, C84.66, C84.67, C84.68, C84.69, C84.70, C84.71, C84.72, C84.73, C84.74, C84.75, C84.76, C84.77, C84.78, C84.79, C84.90, C84.91, C84.92, C84.93, C84.94, C84.95, C84.96, C84.97, C84.98, C84.99, C84.A0, C84.A1, C84.A2, C84.A3, C84.A4, C84.A5, C84.A6, C84.A7, C84.A8, C84.A9, C84.Z0, C84.Z1, C84.Z2, C84.Z3, C84.Z4, C84.Z5, C84.Z6, C84.Z7, C84.Z8, C84.Z9, C85.10, C85.11, C85.12, C85.13, C85.14, C85.15, C85.16, C85.17, C85.18, C85.19, C85.20, C85.21, C85.22, C85.23, C85.24, C85.25, C85.26, C85.27, C85.28, C85.29, C85.80, C85.81, C85.82, C85.83, C85.84, C85.85, C85.86, C85.87, C85.88, C85.89, C85.90, C85.91, C85.92, C85.93, C85.94, C85.95, C85.96, C85.97, C85.98, C85.99, C86.0, C86.1, C86.2, C86.3, C86.4, C86.5, C86.6, C88.0, C88.2, C88.3, C88.4, C88.8, C88.9, C90.00, C90.01, C90.02, C90.10, C90.11, C90.12, C90.20, C90.21, C90.22, C90.30, C90.31, C90.32, C91.00, C91.01, C91.02, C91.10, C91.11, C91.12, C91.30, C91.31, C91.32, C91.40, C91.41, C91.42, C91.50, C91.51, C91.52, C91.60, C91.61, C91.62, C91.90, C91.91, C91.92, C91.A0, C91.A1, C91.A2, C91.Z0, C91.Z1, C91.Z2, C92.00, C92.01, C92.02, C92.10, C92.11, C92.12, C92.20, C92.21, C92.22, C92.30, C92.31, C92.32, C92.40, C92.41,

G53 (continued)	C92.42, C92.50, C92.51, C92.52, C92.60, C92.61, C92.62, C92.90, C92.91, C92.92, C92.A0, C92.A1, C92.A2, C92.Z0, C92.Z1, C92.Z2, C93.00, C93.01, C93.02, C93.10, C93.11, C93.12, C93.30, C93.31, C93.32, C93.90, C93.91, C93.92, C93.Z0, C93.Z1, C93.Z2, C94.00, C94.01, C94.02, C94.20, C94.21, C94.22, C94.30, C94.31, C94.32, C94.40, C94.41, C94.42, C94.6, C94.80, C94.81, C94.82, C95.00, C95.01, C95.02, C95.10, C95.11, C95.12, C95.90, C95.91, C95.92, C96.0, C96.4, C96.5, C96.6, C96.9, C96.A, C96.Z, D00.00, D00.01, D00.02, D00.03, D00.04, D00.05, D00.06, D00.07, D00.08, D00.1, D00.2, D01.0, D01.1, D01.2, D01.3, D01.40, D01.49, D01.5, D01.7, D01.9, D02.0, D02.1, D02.20, D02.21, D02.22, D02.3, D02.4, D03.0, D03.10, D03.11, D03.12, D03.20, D03.21, D03.22, D03.30, D03.39, D03.4, D03.51, D03.52, D03.59, D03.60, D03.61, D03.62, D03.70, D03.71, D03.72, D03.8, D03.9, D04.0, D04.10, D04.11, D04.12, D04.20, D04.21, D04.22, D04.30, D04.39, D04.4, D04.5, D04.60, D04.61, D04.62, D04.70, D04.71, D04.72, D04.8, D04.9, D05.00, D05.01, D05.02, D05.10, D05.11, D05.12, D05.80, D05.81, D05.82, D05.90, D05.91, D05.92, D06.0, D06.1, D06.7, D06.9, D07.0, D07.1, D07.2, D07.30, D07.39, D07.4, D07.5, D07.60, D07.61, D07.69, D09.0, D09.10, D09.19, D09.20, D09.21, D09.22, D09.3, D09.8, D09.9, D10.0, D10.1, D10.2, D10.30, D10.39, D10.4, D10.5, D10.6, D10.7, D10.9, D11.0, D11.7, D11.9, D12.0, D12.1, D12.2, D12.3, D12.4, D12.5, D12.6, D12.7, D12.8, D12.9, D13.0, D13.1, D13.2, D13.30, D13.39, D13.4, D13.5, D13.6, D13.7, D13.9, D14.0, D14.1, D14.2, D14.4, D15.0, D15.1, D15.2, D15.7, D15.9, D16.00, D16.01, D16.02, D16.10, D16.11, D16.12, D16.20, D16.21, D16.22, D16.30, D16.31, D16.32, D16.4, D16.5, D16.6, D16.7, D16.8, D16.9, D17.0, D17.1, D17.20, D17.21, D17.22, D17.23, D17.24, D17.30, D17.39, D17.4, D17.5, D17.6, D17.71, D17.72, D17.79, D17.9, D18.00, D18.01, D18.02, D18.03, D18.09, D18.1, D19.0, D19.1, D19.7, D19.9, D20.0, D20.1, D21.0, D21.10, D21.11, D21.12, D21.20, D21.21, D21.22, D21.3, D21.4, D21.5, D21.6, D21.9, D22.0, D22.10, D22.11, D22.12, D22.20, D22.21, D22.22, D22.30, D22.39, D22.4, D22.5, D22.60, D22.61, D22.62, D22.70, D22.71, D22.72, D22.9, D23.0, D23.10, D23.11, D23.12, D23.20, D23.21, D23.22, D23.30, D23.39, D23.4, D23.5, D23.60, D23.61, D23.62, D23.70, D23.71, D23.72, D23.9, D24.1, D24.2, D24.9, D25.0, D25.1, D25.2, D25.9, D26.0, D26.1, D26.7, D26.9, D27.0, D27.1, D27.9, D28.0, D28.1, D28.2, D28.7, D28.9, D29.0, D29.1, D29.20, D29.22, D29.30, D29.31, D29.32, D29.4, D29.8, D29.9, D30.00, D30.01, D30.02, D30.10, D30.12, D30.20, D30.21, D30.22, D30.3, D30.4, D30.8, D30.9, D31.00, D31.01, D31.02, D31.10, D31.11, D31.12, D31.20, D31.21, D31.22, D31.30, D31.31, D31.32, D31.40, D31.41, D31.42, D31.50, D31.51, D31.52, D31.60, D31.61, D31.62, D31.90, D31.91, D31.92, D32.0, D32.1, D32.9, D33.0, D33.1, D33.2, D33.3, D33.4, D33.7, D33.9, D34, D35.00, D35.01, D35.02, D35.1, D35.2, D35.3, D35.4, D35.5, D35.6, D35.7, D35.9, D36.0, D36.10, D36.11, D36.12, D36.13, D36.14, D36.15, D36.16, D36.17, D36.7, D36.9, D37.01, D37.02, D37.030, D37.031, D37.032, D37.039, D37.04, D37.05, D37.09, D37.1, D37.2, D37.3, D37.4, D37.5, D37.6, D37.8, D37.9, D38.0, D38.1, D38.2, D38.3, D38.4, D38.5, D38.6, D39.0, D39.10, D39.11, D39.12, D39.2, D39.8, D39.9, D3A.00, D3A.010, D3A.011, D3A.012, D3A.019, D3A.020, D3A.021, D3A.022, D3A.023, D3A.024, D3A.025, D3A.026, D3A.090, D3A.091, D3A.092, D3A.093, D3A.094, D3A.095, D3A.096, D3A.8, D40.0, D40.10, D40.11, D40.8, D40.9, D41.00, D41.01, D41.02, D41.10, D41.11, D41.12, D41.20, D41.21, D41.22, D41.3, D41.4, D41.8, D41.9, D42.0, D42.1, D42.9, D43.0, D43.1, D43.2, D43.3, D43.4, D43.8, D43.9, D44.0, D44.10, D44.11, D44.12, D44.2, D44.3, D44.4, D44.5, D44.6, D44.7, D44.9, D45, D46.0, D46.1, D46.20, D46.21, D46.22, D46.4, D46.9, D46.A, D46.B, D46.C, D46.Z, D47.1, D47.2, D47.3, D47.4, D47.9, D47.Z1, D47.Z2, D47.Z9, D48.0, D48.1, D48.2, D48.3, D48.4, D48.5, D48.60, D48.61, D48.62, D48.7, D48.9, D49.0, D49.1, D49.2, D49.3, D49.4, D49.511, D49.512, D49.519, D49.59, D49.6, D49.7, D49.81, D49.89, D49.9
G63	C00.0, C00.1, C00.2, C00.3, C00.4, C00.5, C00.6, C00.8, C00.9, C01, C02.0, C02.1, C02.2, C02.3, C02.4, C02.8, C02.9, C03.0, C03.1, C03.9, C04.0, C04.1, C04.8, C04.9, C05.0, C05.1, C05.2, C05.8, C05.9, C06.0, C06.1, C06.2, C06.80, C06.89, C06.9, C07, C08.0, C08.1, C08.9, C09.0, C09.1, C09.8, C09.9, C10.0, C10.1, C10.2, C10.3, C10.4, C10.8, C10.9, C11.0, C11.1, C11.2, C11.3, C11.8, C11.9, C12, C13.0, C13.1, C13.2, C13.8, C13.9, C14.0, C14.2, C14.8, C15.3, C15.4, C15.5, C15.8, C15.9, C16.0, C16.1, C16.2, C16.3, C16.4, C16.5, C16.6, C16.9, C17.0, C17.1, C17.2, C17.3, C17.8, C17.9, C18.0, C18.1, C18.2, C18.3, C18.4, C18.5, C18.6, C18.7, C18.8, C18.9, C19, C20, C21.0, C21.1, C21.2, C21.8, C22.0, C22.1, C22.2, C22.3, C22.4, C22.7, C22.8, C22.9, C23, C24.0, C24.1, C24.8, C24.9, C25.0, C25.1, C25.2, C25.3, C25.4, C25.7, C25.8, C25.9, C26.0, C26.1, C26.9, C30.0, C30.1, C31.0, C31.1, C31.2, C31.3, C31.8, C31.9, C32.0, C32.1, C32.2, C32.3, C32.8, C32.9, C33, C34.00, C34.01, C34.02, C34.10, C34.11, C34.12, C34.2, C34.30, C34.31, C34.32, C34.80, C34.81, C34.82, C34.90, C34.91, C34.92, C37, C38.0, C38.1, C38.2, C38.3, C38.4, C38.8, C39.0, C39.9, C40.00, C40.01, C40.02, C40.10, C40.11, C40.12, C40.20, C40.21, C40.22, C40.30, C40.31, C40.32, C40.80, C40.81, C40.82, C40.90, C40.91, C40.92, C41.0, C41.1, C41.2, C41.3, C41.4, C41.9, C43.0, C43.10, C43.11, C43.12, C43.20, C43.21, C43.22, C43.30, C43.31, C43.39, C43.4, C43.51, C43.52, C43.59, C43.60, C43.61, C43.62, C43.70, C43.71, C43.72, C43.8, C43.9, C45.0, C45.1, C45.2, C45.7, C45.9, C46.0, C46.1, C46.2, C46.3, C46.4, C46.50, C46.51, C46.52, C46.7, C46.9, C47.0, C47.10, C47.11, C47.12, C47.20, C47.21, C47.22, C47.3, C47.4, C47.5, C47.6, C47.8, C47.9, C48.0, C48.1, C48.2, C48.8, C49.0, C49.10, C49.11, C49.12, C49.20, C49.21, C49.22, C49.3, C49.4, C49.5, C49.6, C49.8, C49.9, C49.A0, C49.A1, C49.A2, C49.A3, C49.A4, C49.A5, C49.A9, C4A.0, C4A.10, C4A.11, C4A.12, C4A.20, C4A.21, C4A.22, C4A.30, C4A.31, C4A.39, C4A.4, C4A.51, C4A.52, C4A.59, C4A.60, C4A.61, C4A.62, C4A.70, C4A.71, C4A.72, C4A.8, C4A.9, C50.011, C50.012, C50.019, C50.021, C50.022, C50.029, C50.111, C50.112, C50.119, C50.121, C50.122, C50.129, C50.211, C50.212, C50.219, C50.221, C50.222, C50.229, C50.311, C50.312, C50.319, C50.321, C50.322, C50.329, C50.411, C50.412, C50.419, C50.421, C50.422, C50.429, C50.511, C50.512, C50.519, C50.521, C50.522, C50.529, C50.611, C50.612, C50.619, C50.621, C50.622, C50.629, C50.811, C50.812, C50.819, C50.821, C50.822, C50.829, C50.911, C50.912, C50.919, C50.921, C50.922, C50.929, C51.0, C51.1, C51.2, C51.8, C51.9, C52, C53.0, C53.1, C53.8, C53.9, C54.0, C54.1, C54.2, C54.3, C54.8, C54.9, C55, C56.1, C56.2, C56.9, C57.00, C57.01, C57.02, C57.10, C57.11, C57.12, C57.20, C57.21, C57.22, C57.3, C57.4, C57.7, C57.8, C57.9, C58, C60.0, C60.1, C60.2, C60.8, C60.9, C61, C62.00, C62.01, C62.02, C62.10, C62.11, C62.12, C62.90, C62.91, C62.92, C63.00, C63.01, C63.02, C63.10, C63.11, C63.12, C63.2, C63.7, C63.8, C63.9, C64.1, C64.2, C64.9, C65.1, C65.2, C65.9, C66.1, C66.2, C66.9, C67.0, C67.1, C67.2, C67.3, C67.4, C67.5, C67.6, C67.7, C67.8, C67.9, C68.0, C68.1, C68.8, C68.9, C69.00, C69.01, C69.02, C69.10, C69.11, C69.12, C69.20, C69.21, C69.22, C69.30, C69.31, C69.32, C69.40, C69.41, C69.42, C69.50, C69.51, C69.52, C69.60, C69.61, C69.62, C69.80, C69.81, C69.82, C69.90, C69.91, C69.92, C70.0, C70.1, C70.9, C71.0, C71.1, C71.2, C71.3, C71.4, C71.5, C71.6, C71.7, C71.8, C71.9, C72.0, C72.1, C72.20, C72.21, C72.22, C72.30, C72.31, C72.32, C72.40, C72.41, C72.42, C72.50, C72.59, C72.9, C73, C74.00, C74.01, C74.02, C74.10, C74.11, C74.12, C74.90, C74.91, C74.92, C75.0, C75.1, C75.2, C75.3, C75.4, C75.5, C75.8, C75.9, C76.0, C76.1, C76.2, C76.3, C76.40, C76.41, C76.42, C76.50, C76.51, C76.52, C76.8, C77.0, C77.1, C77.2, C77.3, C77.4, C77.5, C77.8, C77.9, C78.00, C78.01, C78.02, C78.1, C78.2, C78.30, C78.39, C78.4, C78.5, C78.6, C78.7, C78.80, C78.89, C79.00, C79.01, C79.02, C79.10, C79.11, C79.19, C79.2, C79.31, C79.32, C79.40, C79.49, C79.51, C79.52, C79.60, C79.61, C79.62, C79.70, C79.71, C79.72, C79.81, C79.82, C79.89, C79.9, C7A.00, C7A.010, C7A.011, C7A.012, C7A.019, C7A.020, C7A.021, C7A.022, C7A.023, C7A.024, C7A.025, C7A.026, C7A.029, C7A.090, C7A.091, C7A.092, C7A.093, C7A.094, C7A.095, C7A.096, C7A.098, C7A.1, C7A.8, C7B.00, C7B.01, C7B.02, C7B.03, C7B.04, C7B.09, C7B.1, C7B.8, C80.0, C80.1, C80.2, C81.00, C81.01, C81.02, C81.03, C81.04, C81.05, C81.06, C81.07, C81.08, C81.09, C81.10, C81.11, C81.12, C81.13, C81.14, C81.15, C81.16, C81.17, C81.18, C81.19, C81.20, C81.21, C81.22, C81.23, C81.24, C81.25, C81.26, C81.27, C81.28, C81.29, C81.30, C81.31, C81.32, C81.33, C81.34, C81.35, C81.36, C81.37, C81.38, C81.39, C81.40, C81.41, C81.42, C81.43, C81.44, C81.45, C81.46, C81.47, C81.48, C81.49, C81.70, C81.71, C81.72, C81.73, C81.74, C81.75, C81.76, C81.77, C81.78, C81.79, C81.90, C81.91, C81.92, C81.93, C81.94, C81.95, C81.96, C81.97, C81.98, C81.99, C82.00, C82.01, C82.02, C82.03, C82.04, C82.05, C82.06, C82.07, C82.08, C82.09, C82.10, C82.11, C82.12, C82.13, C82.14, C82.15, C82.16, C82.17, C82.18, C82.19, C82.20, C82.21, C82.22, C82.23, C82.24, C82.25, C82.26, C82.27, C82.28, C82.29, C82.30, C82.31, C82.32, C82.33, C82.34, C82.35, C82.36, C82.37, C82.38, C82.39, C82.40, C82.41, C82.42, C82.43, C82.44, C82.45, C82.46, C82.47, C82.48, C82.49, C82.50, C82.51, C82.52, C82.53, C82.54, C82.55, C82.56, C82.57, C82.58, C82.59, C82.60, C82.61, C82.62, C82.63, C82.64, C82.65, C82.66, C82.67, C82.68, C82.69, C82.80, C82.81, C82.82, C82.83, C82.84, C82.85, C82.86, C82.87, C82.88, C82.89, C82.90, C82.91, C82.92, C82.93, C82.94, C82.95, C82.96, C82.97, C82.98, C82.99, C83.00, C83.01, C83.02, C83.03, C83.04, C83.05, C83.06, C83.07, C83.08, C83.09, C83.10, C83.11, C83.12, C83.13, C83.14, C83.15, C83.16, C83.17, C83.18, C83.19, C83.30, C83.31, C83.32, C83.33, C83.34, C83.35, C83.36, C83.37, C83.38, C83.39, C83.50, C83.51, C83.52, C83.53, C83.54, C83.55, C83.56, C83.57, C83.58, C83.59, C83.70, C83.71, C83.72, C83.73,

G63 (continued)	C83.74, C83.75, C83.76, C83.77, C83.78, C83.79, C83.80, C83.81, C83.82, C83.83, C83.84, C83.85, C83.86, C83.87, C83.88, C83.89, C83.90, C83.91, C83.92, C83.93, C83.94, C83.95, C83.96, C83.97, C83.98, C83.99, C84.00, C84.01, C84.02, C84.03, C84.04, C84.05, C84.06, C84.07, C84.08, C84.09, C84.10, C84.11, C84.12, C84.13, C84.14, C84.15, C84.16, C84.17, C84.18, C84.19, C84.40, C84.41, C84.42, C84.43, C84.44, C84.45, C84.46, C84.47, C84.48, C84.49, C84.60, C84.61, C84.62, C84.63, C84.64, C84.65, C84.66, C84.67, C84.68, C84.69, C84.70, C84.71, C84.72, C84.73, C84.74, C84.75, C84.76, C84.77, C84.78, C84.79, C84.90, C84.91, C84.92, C84.93, C84.94, C84.95, C84.96, C84.97, C84.98, C84.99, C84.A0, C84.A1, C84.A2, C84.A3, C84.A4, C84.A5, C84.A6, C84.A7, C84.A8, C84.A9, C84.Z0, C84.Z1, C84.Z2, C84.Z3, C84.Z4, C84.Z5, C84.Z6, C84.Z7, C84.Z8, C84.Z9, C85.10, C85.11, C85.12, C85.13, C85.14, C85.15, C85.16, C85.17, C85.18, C85.19, C85.20, C85.21, C85.22, C85.23, C85.24, C85.25, C85.26, C85.27, C85.28, C85.29, C85.80, C85.81, C85.82, C85.83, C85.84, C85.85, C85.86, C85.87, C85.88, C85.89, C85.90, C85.91, C85.92, C85.93, C85.94, C85.95, C85.96, C85.97, C85.98, C85.99, C86.0, C86.1, C86.2, C86.3, C86.4, C86.5, C86.6, C88.0, C88.2, C88.3, C88.4, C88.8, C88.9, C90.00, C90.01, C90.02, C90.10, C90.11, C90.12, C90.20, C90.21, C90.22, C90.30, C90.31, C90.32, C91.00, C91.01, C91.02, C91.10, C91.11, C91.12, C91.30, C91.31, C91.32, C91.40, C91.41, C91.42, C91.50, C91.51, C91.52, C91.60, C91.61, C91.62, C91.90, C91.91, C91.92, C91.A0, C91.A1, C91.A2, C91.Z0, C91.Z1, C91.Z2, C92.00, C92.01, C92.02, C92.10, C92.11, C92.12, C92.20, C92.21, C92.22, C92.30, C92.31, C92.32, C92.40, C92.41, C92.42, C92.50, C92.51, C92.52, C92.60, C92.61, C92.62, C92.90, C92.91, C92.92, C92.A0, C92.A1, C92.A2, C92.Z0, C92.Z1, C92.Z2, C93.00, C93.01, C93.02, C93.10, C93.11, C93.12, C93.30, C93.31, C93.32, C93.90, C93.91, C93.92, C93.Z0, C93.Z1, C94.00, C94.01, C94.02, C94.20, C94.21, C94.22, C94.30, C94.31, C94.32, C94.40, C94.41, C94.42, C94.6, C94.80, C94.81, C94.82, C95.00, C95.01, C95.02, C95.10, C95.11, C95.12, C95.90, C95.91, C95.92, C96.0, C96.4, C96.5, C96.6, C96.9, C96.A, C96.Z, D00.00, D00.01, D00.02, D00.03, D00.04, D00.05, D00.06, D00.07, D00.08, D00.1, D00.2, D01.0, D01.1, D01.2, D01.3, D01.40, D01.49, D01.5, D01.7, D01.9, D02.0, D02.1, D02.20, D02.21, D02.22, D02.3, D02.4, D03.0, D03.10, D03.11, D03.12, D03.20, D03.21, D03.22, D03.30, D03.39, D03.4, D03.51, D03.52, D03.59, D03.60, D03.61, D03.62, D03.70, D03.71, D03.72, D03.8, D03.9, D04.0, D04.10, D04.11, D04.12, D04.20, D04.21, D04.22, D04.30, D04.39, D04.4, D04.5, D04.60, D04.61, D04.62, D04.70, D04.71, D04.72, D04.8, D04.9, D05.00, D05.01, D05.02, D05.10, D05.11, D05.12, D05.80, D05.81, D05.82, D05.90, D05.91, D05.92, D06.0, D06.1, D06.7, D06.9, D07.0, D07.1, D07.2, D07.30, D07.39, D07.4, D07.5, D07.60, D07.61, D07.69, D09.0, D09.10, D09.19, D09.20, D09.21, D09.22, D09.3, D09.8, D09.9, D10.0, D10.1, D10.2, D10.30, D10.39, D10.4, D10.5, D10.6, D10.7, D10.9, D11.0, D11.7, D11.9, D12.0, D12.1, D12.2, D12.3, D12.4, D12.5, D12.6, D12.7, D12.8, D12.9, D13.0, D13.1, D13.2, D13.30, D13.39, D13.4, D13.5, D13.6, D13.7, D13.9, D14.0, D14.1, D14.2, D14.30, D14.31, D14.32, D14.4, D15.0, D15.1, D15.2, D15.7, D15.9, D16.00, D16.01, D16.02, D16.10, D16.11, D16.12, D16.20, D16.21, D16.22, D16.30, D16.31, D16.32, D16.4, D16.5, D16.6, D16.7, D16.8, D16.9, D17.0, D17.1, D17.20, D17.21, D17.22, D17.23, D17.24, D17.30, D17.39, D17.4, D17.5, D17.6, D17.9, D18.00, D18.01, D18.02, D18.03, D18.09, D18.1, D19.0, D19.1, D19.7, D19.9, D20.0, D20.1, D21.0, D21.10, D21.11, D21.12, D21.20, D21.21, D21.22, D21.3, D21.4, D21.5, D21.6, D21.9, D22.0, D22.10, D22.11, D22.12, D22.20, D22.21, D22.22, D22.30, D22.39, D22.4, D22.5, D22.60, D22.61, D22.62, D22.70, D22.71, D22.72, D22.9, D23.0, D23.10, D23.11, D23.12, D23.20, D23.21, D23.22, D23.30, D23.39, D23.4, D23.5, D23.60, D23.61, D23.62, D23.70, D23.71, D23.72, D23.9, D24.1, D24.2, D24.9, D25.0, D25.1, D25.2, D25.9, D26.0, D26.1, D26.7, D26.9, D27.0, D27.1, D27.9, D28.0, D28.1, D28.2, D28.7, D28.9, D29.0, D29.1, D29.20, D29.21, D29.22, D29.30, D29.31, D29.32, D29.4, D29.8, D29.9, D30.00, D30.01, D30.02, D30.10, D30.11, D30.12, D30.20, D30.21, D30.22, D30.3, D30.4, D30.8, D30.9, D31.00, D31.01, D31.02, D31.10, D31.11, D31.12, D31.20, D31.21, D31.22, D31.30, D31.31, D31.32, D31.40, D31.41, D31.42, D31.50, D31.51, D31.52, D31.60, D31.61, D31.62, D31.90, D31.91, D31.92, D32.0, D32.1, D32.9, D33.0, D33.1, D33.2, D33.3, D33.4, D33.7, D33.9, D34, D35.00, D35.01, D35.02, D35.1, D35.2, D35.3, D35.4, D35.5, D35.6, D35.7, D35.9, D36.0, D36.10, D36.11, D36.12, D36.13, D36.14, D36.15, D36.16, D36.17, D36.7, D36.9, D37.01, D37.02, D37.030, D37.031, D37.032, D37.039, D37.04, D37.05, D37.09, D37.1, D37.2, D37.3, D37.4, D37.5, D37.6, D37.8, D37.9, D38.0, D38.1, D38.2, D38.3, D38.4, D38.5, D38.6, D39.0, D39.10, D39.11, D39.12, D39.2, D39.8, D39.9, D3A.00, D3A.010, D3A.011, D3A.012, D3A.019, D3A.020, D3A.021, D3A.022, D3A.023, D3A.024, D3A.025, D3A.026, D3A.029, D3A.090, D3A.091, D3A.092, D3A.093, D3A.094, D3A.095, D3A.096, D3A.098, D3A.8, D40.0, D40.10, D40.11, D40.12, D40.8, D40.9, D41.00, D41.01, D41.02, D41.10, D41.11, D41.12, D41.20, D41.21, D41.22, D41.3, D41.4, D41.8, D41.9, D42.0, D42.1, D42.9, D43.0, D43.1, D43.2, D43.3, D43.4, D43.8, D43.9, D44.0, D44.10, D44.11, D44.12, D44.2, D44.3, D44.4, D44.5, D44.6, D44.7, D44.9, D45, D46.0, D46.1, D46.20, D46.21, D46.22, D46.4, D46.9, D46.A, D46.B, D46.C, D46.Z, D47.1, D47.2, D47.3, D47.4, D47.9, D47.Z1, D47.Z2, D47.Z9, D48.0, D48.1, D48.2, D48.3, D48.4, D48.5, D48.60, D48.61, D48.62, D48.7, D48.9, E00.0, E00.1, E00.2, E00.9, E01.0, E01.1, E01.2, E01.8, E02, E03.0, E03.1, E03.2, E03.3, E03.4, E03.5, E03.8, E03.9, E04.0, E04.1, E04.2, E04.8, E04.9, E05.00, E05.01, E05.10, E05.11, E05.20, E05.21, E05.30, E05.31, E05.40, E05.41, E05.80, E05.81, E05.90, E05.91, E06.0, E06.1, E06.2, E06.3, E06.4, E06.5, E06.9, E07.0, E07.1, E07.81, E07.89, E07.9, E15, E16.0, E16.1, E16.2, E16.3, E16.4, E16.8, E16.9, E20.0, E20.1, E20.8, E20.9, E21.0, E21.1, E21.2, E21.3, E21.4, E21.5, E22.0, E22.1, E22.2, E22.8, E22.9, E23.0, E23.1, E23.2, E23.3, E23.6, E23.7, E24.0, E24.1, E24.2, E24.3, E24.4, E24.8, E24.9, E25.0, E25.8, E25.9, E26.01, E26.02, E26.09, E26.1, E26.81, E26.89, E26.9, E27.0, E27.1, E27.2, E27.3, E27.40, E27.49, E27.5, E27.8, E27.9, E28.0, E28.1, E28.2, E28.310, E28.319, E28.39, E28.8, E28.9, E29.0, E29.1, E29.8, E29.9, E30.0, E30.1, E30.8, E30.9, E31.0, E31.1, E31.20, E31.21, E31.22, E31.23, E31.8, E31.9, E32.0, E32.1, E32.8, E32.9, E34.0, E34.1, E34.2, E34.3, E34.4, E34.50, E34.51, E34.52, E34.8, E34.9, E40, E41, E42, E43, E44.0, E44.1, E45, E46, E50.0, E50.1, E50.2, E50.3, E50.4, E50.5, E50.6, E50.7, E50.8, E50.9, E51.11, E51.12, E51.2, E51.8, E51.9, E52, E53.0, E53.1, E53.8, E53.9, E54, E55.0, E55.9, E56.0, E56.1, E56.8, E56.9, E58, E59, E60, E61.0, E61.1, E61.2, E61.3, E61.4, E61.5, E61.6, E61.7, E61.8, E61.9, E63.0, E63.1, E63.8, E63.9, E64.0, E64.1, E64.2, E64.3, E64.8, E64.9, E70.0, E70.1, E70.20, E70.21, E70.29, E70.30, E70.310, E70.311, E70.318, E70.319, E70.320, E70.321, E70.328, E70.329, E70.330, E70.331, E70.338, E70.339, E70.39, E70.40, E70.41, E70.49, E70.5, E70.8, E70.9, E71.0, E71.110, E71.111, E71.118, E71.120, E71.121, E71.128, E71.19, E71.2, E71.30, E71.310, E71.311, E71.312, E71.313, E71.314, E71.318, E71.32, E71.39, E71.40, E71.41, E71.42, E71.43, E71.440, E71.448, E71.50, E71.510, E71.511, E71.518, E71.520, E71.521, E71.522, E71.528, E71.529, E71.53, E71.540, E71.541, E71.542, E71.548, E72.00, E72.01, E72.02, E72.03, E72.04, E72.09, E72.10, E72.11, E72.12, E72.19, E72.20, E72.21, E72.22, E72.23, E72.29, E72.3, E72.4, E72.50, E72.51, E72.52, E72.53, E72.59, E72.8, E72.9, E73.0, E73.1, E73.8, E73.9, E74.00, E74.01, E74.02, E74.03, E74.04, E74.09, E74.10, E74.11, E74.12, E74.19, E74.20, E74.21, E74.29, E74.31, E74.39, E74.4, E74.8, E74.9, E75.00, E75.01, E75.02, E75.09, E75.10, E75.11, E75.19, E75.21, E75.22, E75.23, E75.240, E75.241, E75.242, E75.243, E75.248, E75.249, E75.25, E75.29, E75.3, E75.4, E75.5, E75.6, E76.01, E76.02, E76.03, E76.1, E76.210, E76.211, E76.219, E76.22, E76.29, E76.3, E76.8, E76.9, E77.0, E77.1, E77.8, E77.9, E78.00, E78.01, E78.1, E78.2, E78.3, E78.4, E78.5, E78.6, E78.70, E78.71, E78.72, E78.79, E78.81, E78.89, E78.9, E79.0, E79.1, E79.2, E79.8, E79.9, E80.0, E80.1, E80.20, E80.21, E80.29, E80.3, E80.4, E80.5, E80.6, E80.7, E83.00, E83.01, E83.09, E83.10, E83.19, E83.2, E83.30, E83.31, E83.32, E83.39, E83.40, E83.41, E83.42, E83.49, E83.50, E83.51, E83.52, E83.59, E83.81, E83.89, E83.9, E84.0, E84.11, E84.19, E84.8, E84.9, E85.0, E85.1, E85.2, E85.3, E85.4, E85.9, E86.0, E86.1, E86.9, E87.0, E87.1, E87.2, E87.3, E87.4, E87.5, E87.6, E87.8, E88.01, E88.09, E88.1, E88.2, E88.3, E88.40, E88.41, E88.42, E88.49, E88.81, E88.89, E88.9
G73.3	C00.0, C00.1, C00.2, C00.3, C00.4, C00.5, C00.6, C00.8, C00.9, C01, C02.0, C02.1, C02.2, C02.3, C02.4, C02.8, C02.9, C03.0, C03.1, C03.9, C04.0, C04.1, C04.8, C04.9, C05.0, C05.1, C05.2, C05.8, C05.9, C06.0, C06.1, C06.2, C06.80, C06.89, C06.9, C07, C08.0, C08.1, C08.9, C09.0, C09.1, C09.8, C09.9, C10.0, C10.1, C10.2, C10.3, C10.4, C10.8, C10.9, C11.0, C11.1, C11.2, C11.3, C11.8, C11.9, C12, C13.0, C13.1, C13.2, C13.8, C13.9, C14.0, C14.2, C14.8, C15.3, C15.4, C15.5, C15.8, C15.9, C16.0, C16.1, C16.2, C16.3, C16.4, C16.5, C16.6, C16.8, C16.9, C17.0, C17.1, C17.2, C17.3, C17.8, C17.9, C18.0, C18.1, C18.2, C18.3, C18.4, C18.5, C18.6, C18.7, C18.8, C18.9, C19, C20, C21.0, C21.1, C21.2, C21.8, C22.0, C22.1, C22.2, C22.3, C22.4, C22.7, C22.8, C22.9, C23, C24.0, C24.1, C24.8, C24.9, C25.0, C25.1, C25.2, C25.3, C25.4, C25.7, C25.8, C25.9, C26.0, C26.1, C26.9, C30.0, C30.1, C31.0, C31.1, C31.2, C31.3, C31.8, C31.9, C32.0, C32.1, C32.2, C32.3, C32.8, C32.9, C33, C34.00, C34.01, C34.02, C34.10, C34.11, C34.12, C34.2, C34.30, C34.31, C34.32, C34.80, C34.81, C34.82, C34.90, C34.91, C34.92, C37, C38.0, C38.1, C38.2, C38.3, C38.4, C38.8, C39.0, C39.9, C40.00, C40.01, C40.02, C40.10, C40.11, C40.12, C40.20, C40.21, C40.22, C40.30, C40.31, C40.32, C40.80, C40.81, C40.82, C40.90, C40.91, C40.92, C41.0, C41.1, C41.2, C41.3, C41.4, C41.9, C43.0, C43.10, C43.11, C43.12, C43.20, C43.21, C43.22, C43.30, C43.31, C43.39, C43.4, C43.51, C43.52, C43.59, C43.60, C43.61, C43.62, C43.70, C43.71, C43.72, C43.8, C43.9, C45.0, C45.1, C45.2, C45.7,

| G73.3 (continued) | C45.9, C46.0, C46.1, C46.2, C46.3, C46.4, C46.50, C46.51, C46.52, C46.7, C46.9, C47.0, C47.10, C47.11, C47.12, C47.20, C47.21, C47.22, C47.3, C47.4, C47.5, C47.6, C47.8, C47.9, C48.0, C48.1, C48.2, C48.8, C49.0, C49.10, C49.11, C49.12, C49.20, C49.21, C49.22, C49.3, C49.4, C49.5, C49.6, C49.8, C49.9, C49.A0, C49.A1, C49.A2, C49.A3, C49.A4, C49.A5, C49.A9, C4A.0, C4A.10, C4A.11, C4A.12, C4A.20, C4A.21, C4A.22, C4A.30, C4A.31, C4A.39, C4A.4, C4A.51, C4A.52, C4A.59, C4A.60, C4A.61, C4A.62, C4A.70, C4A.71, C4A.72, C4A.8, C4A.9, C50.011, C50.012, C50.019, C50.021, C50.022, C50.029, C50.111, C50.112, C50.119, C50.121, C50.122, C50.129, C50.211, C50.212, C50.219, C50.221, C50.222, C50.229, C50.311, C50.312, C50.319, C50.321, C50.322, C50.329, C50.411, C50.412, C50.419, C50.421, C50.422, C50.429, C50.511, C50.512, C50.519, C50.521, C50.522, C50.529, C50.611, C50.612, C50.619, C50.621, C50.622, C50.629, C50.811, C50.812, C50.819, C50.821, C50.822, C50.829, C50.911, C50.912, C50.919, C50.921, C50.922, C50.929, C51.0, C51.1, C51.2, C51.8, C51.9, C52, C53.0, C53.1, C53.8, C53.9, C54.0, C54.1, C54.2, C54.3, C54.8, C54.9, C55, C56.1, C56.2, C56.9, C57.00, C57.01, C57.02, C57.10, C57.11, C57.12, C57.20, C57.21, C57.22, C57.3, C57.4, C57.7, C57.8, C57.9, C58, C60.0, C60.1, C60.2, C60.8, C60.9, C61, C62.00, C62.01, C62.02, C62.10, C62.11, C62.12, C62.90, C62.91, C62.92, C63.00, C63.01, C63.02, C63.10, C63.11, C63.12, C63.2, C63.7, C63.8, C63.9, C64.1, C64.2, C64.9, C65.1, C65.2, C65.9, C66.1, C66.2, C66.9, C67.0, C67.1, C67.2, C67.3, C67.4, C67.5, C67.6, C67.7, C67.8, C67.9, C68.0, C68.1, C68.8, C68.9, C69.00, C69.01, C69.02, C69.10, C69.11, C69.12, C69.20, C69.21, C69.22, C69.30, C69.31, C69.32, C69.40, C69.41, C69.42, C69.50, C69.51, C69.52, C69.60, C69.61, C69.62, C69.80, C69.81, C69.82, C69.90, C69.91, C69.92, C70.0, C70.1, C70.9, C71.0, C71.1, C71.2, C71.3, C71.4, C71.5, C71.6, C71.7, C71.8, C71.9, C72.0, C72.1, C72.20, C72.21, C72.22, C72.30, C72.31, C72.32, C72.40, C72.41, C72.42, C72.50, C72.59, C72.9, C73, C74.00, C74.01, C74.02, C74.10, C74.11, C74.12, C74.90, C74.91, C74.92, C75.0, C75.1, C75.2, C75.3, C75.4, C75.5, C75.8, C75.9, C76.0, C76.1, C76.2, C76.3, C76.40, C76.41, C76.42, C76.50, C76.51, C76.52, C76.8, C77.0, C77.1, C77.2, C77.3, C77.4, C77.5, C77.8, C77.9, C78.00, C78.01, C78.02, C78.1, C78.2, C78.30, C78.39, C78.4, C78.5, C78.6, C78.7, C78.80, C78.89, C79.00, C79.01, C79.02, C79.10, C79.11, C79.19, C79.2, C79.31, C79.32, C79.40, C79.49, C79.51, C79.52, C79.60, C79.61, C79.62, C79.70, C79.71, C79.72, C79.81, C79.82, C79.89, C79.9, C7A.00, C7A.010, C7A.011, C7A.012, C7A.019, C7A.020, C7A.021, C7A.022, C7A.023, C7A.024, C7A.025, C7A.026, C7A.029, C7A.090, C7A.091, C7A.092, C7A.093, C7A.094, C7A.095, C7A.096, C7A.098, C7A.1, C7A.8, C7B.00, C7B.01, C7B.02, C7B.03, C7B.04, C7B.09, C7B.1, C7B.8, C80.0, C80.1, C80.2, C81.00, C81.01, C81.02, C81.03, C81.04, C81.05, C81.06, C81.07, C81.08, C81.09, C81.10, C81.11, C81.12, C81.13, C81.14, C81.15, C81.16, C81.17, C81.18, C81.19, C81.20, C81.21, C81.22, C81.23, C81.24, C81.25, C81.26, C81.27, C81.28, C81.29, C81.30, C81.31, C81.32, C81.33, C81.34, C81.35, C81.36, C81.37, C81.38, C81.39, C81.40, C81.41, C81.42, C81.43, C81.44, C81.45, C81.46, C81.47, C81.48, C81.49, C81.70, C81.71, C81.72, C81.73, C81.74, C81.75, C81.76, C81.77, C81.78, C81.79, C81.90, C81.91, C81.92, C81.93, C81.94, C81.95, C81.96, C81.97, C81.98, C81.99, C82.00, C82.01, C82.02, C82.03, C82.04, C82.05, C82.06, C82.07, C82.08, C82.09, C82.10, C82.11, C82.12, C82.13, C82.14, C82.15, C82.16, C82.17, C82.18, C82.19, C82.20, C82.21, C82.22, C82.23, C82.24, C82.25, C82.26, C82.27, C82.28, C82.29, C82.30, C82.31, C82.33, C82.34, C82.35, C82.36, C82.37, C82.38, C82.39, C82.40, C82.41, C82.42, C82.43, C82.44, C82.45, C82.46, C82.47, C82.48, C82.49, C82.50, C82.51, C82.52, C82.53, C82.54, C82.55, C82.56, C82.57, C82.58, C82.59, C82.60, C82.61, C82.62, C82.63, C82.64, C82.65, C82.66, C82.67, C82.68, C82.69, C82.80, C82.81, C82.82, C82.83, C82.84, C82.85, C82.86, C82.87, C82.88, C82.89, C82.90, C82.91, C82.92, C82.93, C82.94, C82.95, C82.96, C82.97, C82.98, C82.99, C83.00, C83.01, C83.02, C83.03, C83.04, C83.05, C83.06, C83.07, C83.08, C83.09, C83.10, C83.11, C83.12, C83.13, C83.14, C83.15, C83.16, C83.17, C83.18, C83.19, C83.30, C83.31, C83.32, C83.33, C83.34, C83.35, C83.36, C83.37, C83.38, C83.39, C83.50, C83.51, C83.52, C83.53, C83.54, C83.55, C83.56, C83.57, C83.58, C83.59, C83.70, C83.71, C83.72, C83.73, C83.74, C83.75, C83.76, C83.77, C83.78, C83.79, C83.80, C83.81, C83.82, C83.83, C83.84, C83.85, C83.86, C83.87, C83.88, C83.89, C83.90, C83.91, C83.92, C83.93, C83.94, C83.95, C83.96, C83.97, C83.98, C83.99, C84.00, C84.01, C84.02, C84.03, C84.04, C84.05, C84.06, C84.07, C84.08, C84.09, C84.10, C84.11, C84.12, C84.13, C84.14, C84.15, C84.16, C84.17, C84.18, C84.19, C84.40, C84.41, C84.42, C84.43, C84.44, C84.45, C84.46, C84.47, C84.48, C84.49, C84.60, C84.61, C84.62, C84.63, C84.64, C84.65, C84.66, C84.67, C84.68, C84.69, C84.70, C84.71, C84.72, C84.73, C84.74, C84.75, C84.76, C84.77, C84.78, C84.79, C84.90, C84.91, C84.92, C84.93, C84.94, C84.95, C84.96, C84.97, C84.98, C84.99, C84.A0, C84.A1, C84.A2, C84.A3, C84.A4, C84.A5, C84.A6, C84.A7, C84.A8, C84.A9, C84.Z0, C84.Z1, C84.Z2, C84.Z3, C84.Z4, C84.Z5, C84.Z6, C84.Z7, C84.Z8, C84.Z9, C85.10, C85.11, C85.12, C85.13, C85.14, C85.15, C85.16, C85.17, C85.18, C85.19, C85.20, C85.21, C85.22, C85.23, C85.24, C85.25, C85.26, C85.27, C85.28, C85.29, C85.80, C85.81, C85.82, C85.83, C85.84, C85.85, C85.86, C85.87, C85.88, C85.89, C85.90, C85.91, C85.92, C85.93, C85.94, C85.95, C85.96, C85.97, C85.98, C85.99, C86.0, C86.1, C86.2, C86.3, C86.4, C86.5, C86.6, C88.0, C88.2, C88.3, C88.4, C88.8, C88.9, C90.00, C90.01, C90.02, C90.10, C90.11, C90.12, C90.20, C90.21, C90.22, C90.30, C90.31, C90.32, C91.00, C91.01, C91.02, C91.10, C91.11, C91.12, C91.30, C91.31, C91.32, C91.40, C91.41, C91.42, C91.50, C91.51, C91.52, C91.60, C91.61, C91.62, C91.90, C91.91, C91.92, C91.A0, C91.A1, C91.A2, C91.Z0, C91.Z1, C91.Z2, C92.00, C92.01, C92.02, C92.10, C92.11, C92.12, C92.20, C92.21, C92.22, C92.30, C92.31, C92.32, C92.40, C92.41, C92.42, C92.50, C92.51, C92.52, C92.60, C92.61, C92.62, C92.90, C92.91, C92.92, C92.A0, C92.A1, C92.A2, C92.Z0, C92.Z1, C92.Z2, C93.00, C93.01, C93.02, C93.10, C93.11, C93.12, C93.30, C93.31, C93.32, C93.90, C93.91, C93.92, C93.Z0, C93.Z1, C94.00, C94.01, C94.02, C94.20, C94.21, C94.22, C94.30, C94.31, C94.32, C94.40, C94.41, C94.42, C94.6, C94.80, C94.81, C94.82, C95.00, C95.01, C95.02, C95.10, C95.11, C95.12, C95.90, C95.91, C95.92, C96.0, C96.4, C96.5, C96.6, C96.9, C96.A, C96.Z, D00.00, D00.01, D00.02, D00.03, D00.04, D00.05, D00.06, D00.07, D00.08, D00.1, D00.2, D01.0, D01.1, D01.2, D01.3, D01.40, D01.49, D01.5, D01.7, D01.9, D02.0, D02.1, D02.20, D02.21, D02.22, D02.3, D02.4, D03.0, D03.10, D03.11, D03.12, D03.20, D03.21, D03.22, D03.30, D03.39, D03.4, D03.51, D03.52, D03.59, D03.60, D03.61, D03.62, D03.70, D03.71, D03.72, D03.8, D03.9, D04.0, D04.10, D04.11, D04.12, D04.20, D04.21, D04.22, D04.30, D04.39, D04.4, D04.5, D04.60, D04.61, D04.62, D04.70, D04.71, D04.72, D04.8, D04.9, D05.00, D05.01, D05.02, D05.10, D05.11, D05.12, D05.80, D05.81, D05.82, D05.90, D05.91, D05.92, D06.0, D06.1, D06.7, D06.9, D07.0, D07.1, D07.2, D07.30, D07.39, D07.4, D07.5, D07.60, D07.61, D07.69, D09.0, D09.10, D09.19, D09.20, D09.21, D09.22, D09.3, D09.8, D09.9, D10.0, D10.1, D10.2, D10.30, D10.39, D10.4, D10.5, D10.6, D10.7, D10.9, D11.0, D11.7, D11.9, D12.0, D12.1, D12.2, D12.3, D12.4, D12.5, D12.6, D12.7, D12.8, D12.9, D13.0, D13.1, D13.2, D13.30, D13.39, D13.4, D13.5, D13.6, D13.7, D13.9, D14.0, D14.1, D14.2, D14.30, D14.31, D14.32, D14.4, D15.0, D15.1, D15.2, D15.7, D15.9, D16.00, D16.01, D16.02, D16.10, D16.11, D16.12, D16.20, D16.21, D16.22, D16.30, D16.31, D16.32, D16.4, D16.5, D16.6, D16.7, D16.8, D16.9, D17.0, D17.1, D17.20, D17.21, D17.22, D17.23, D17.24, D17.30, D17.39, D17.4, D17.5, D17.6, D17.9, D18.00, D18.01, D18.02, D18.03, D18.09, D18.1, D19.0, D19.1, D19.7, D19.9, D20.0, D20.1, D21.0, D21.10, D21.11, D21.12, D21.20, D21.21, D21.22, D21.3, D21.4, D21.5, D21.6, D21.9, D22.0, D22.10, D22.11, D22.12, D22.20, D22.21, D22.22, D22.30, D22.39, D22.4, D22.5, D22.60, D22.61, D22.62, D22.70, D22.71, D22.72, D22.9, D23.0, D23.10, D23.11, D23.20, D23.21, D23.22, D23.30, D23.39, D23.4, D23.5, D23.60, D23.61, D23.62, D23.70, D23.71, D23.72, D23.9, D24.1, D24.2, D24.9, D25.0, D25.1, D25.2, D25.9, D26.0, D26.1, D26.7, D26.9, D27.0, D27.1, D27.9, D28.0, D28.1, D28.2, D28.7, D28.9, D29.0, D29.1, D29.20, D29.21, D29.22, D29.30, D29.31, D29.32, D29.4, D29.8, D29.9, D30.00, D30.01, D30.02, D30.10, D30.11, D30.12, D30.20, D30.21, D30.22, D30.3, D30.4, D30.8, D30.9, D31.00, D31.01, D31.02, D31.10, D31.11, D31.12, D31.20, D31.21, D31.22, D31.30, D31.31, D31.32, D31.40, D31.41, D31.42, D31.50, D31.51, D31.52, D31.60, D31.61, D31.62, D31.90, D31.91, D31.92, D32.0, D32.1, D32.9, D33.0, D33.1, D33.2, D33.3, D33.4, D33.7, D33.9, D34, D35.00, D35.01, D35.02, D35.1, D35.2, D35.3, D35.4, D35.5, D35.6, D35.7, D35.9, D36.0, D36.10, D36.11, D36.12, D36.13, D36.14, D36.15, D36.16, D36.17, D36.7, D36.9, D37.01, D37.02, D37.030, D37.031, D37.032, D37.039, D37.04, D37.05, D37.09, D37.1, D37.2, D37.3, D37.4, D37.5, D37.6, D37.8, D37.9, D38.0, D38.1, D38.2, D38.3, D38.4, D38.5, D38.6, D39.0, D39.10, D39.11, D39.12, D39.2, D39.8, D39.9, D3A.00, D3A.010, D3A.011, D3A.012, D3A.019, D3A.020, D3A.021, D3A.022, D3A.023, D3A.024, D3A.025, D3A.026, D3A.029, D3A.090, D3A.091, D3A.092, D3A.093, D3A.094, D3A.095, D3A.096, D3A.098, D3A.8, D40.0, D40.10, D40.11, D40.12, D40.8, D40.9, D41.00, D41.01, D41.02, D41.10, D41.11, D41.12, D41.20, D41.21, D41.22, D41.3, D41.4, D41.8, D41.9, D42.0, D42.1, D42.9, D43.0, D43.1, D43.2, D43.3, D43.4, D43.8, D43.9, D44.0, D44.10, D44.11, D44.12, D44.2, D44.3, D44.4, D44.5, D44.6, D44.7, D44.9, D45, D46.0, D46.1, D46.20, D46.21, D46.22, D46.4, D46.9, D46.A, D46.B, D46.C, D46.Z, D47.1, D47.2, D47.3, D47.4, D47.9, D47.Z1, D47.Z2, D47.Z9, D48.0, D48.1, D48.2, D48.3, D48.4, D48.5, D48.60, D48.61, D48.62, D48.7, D48.9, D49.0, D49.1, D49.2, D49.3, D49.4, D49.511, D49.512, D49.519, D49.59, D49.6, D49.7, D49.81, D49.89, E05.00, E05.01, E05.10, E05.11, |

G73.3 (continued)	E05.20, E05.21, E05.30, E05.31, E05.40, E05.41, E05.80, E05.81, E05.90, E05.91, E20.0, E20.1, E20.8, E20.9, E21.0, E21.3, E74.00, E74.01, E74.02, E74.03, E74.04, E74.09, E75.00, E75.01, E75.02, E75.09, E75.10, E75.11, E75.19, E75.21, E75.22, E75.23, E75.240, E75.241, E75.242, E75.243, E75.248, E75.249, E75.25, E75.29, E75.3, E75.4, E75.5, E75.6
G99.0	E05.00, E05.01, E05.10, E05.11, E05.20, E05.21, E05.30, E05.31, E05.40, E05.41, E05.80, E05.81, E05.90, E05.91, E85.0, E85.1, E85.2, E85.3, E85.4, E85.9, M10.00, M10.011, M10.012, M10.019, M10.021, M10.022, M10.029, M10.031, M10.032, M10.039, M10.041, M10.042, M10.049, M10.051, M10.052, M10.059, M10.061, M10.062, M10.069, M10.071, M10.072, M10.079, M10.08, M10.09, M10.10, M10.111, M10.112, M10.119, M10.121, M10.122, M10.129, M10.131, M10.132, M10.139, M10.141, M10.142, M10.149, M10.151, M10.152, M10.159, M10.161, M10.162, M10.169, M10.171, M10.172, M10.179, M10.18, M10.19, M10.20, M10.211, M10.212, M10.219, M10.221, M10.222, M10.229, M10.231, M10.232, M10.239, M10.241, M10.242, M10.249, M10.251, M10.252, M10.259, M10.261, M10.262, M10.269, M10.271, M10.272, M10.279, M10.28, M10.30, M10.311, M10.312, M10.319, M10.321, M10.322, M10.329, M10.331, M10.332, M10.339, M10.341, M10.342, M10.349, M10.351, M10.352, M10.359, M10.361, M10.362, M10.369, M10.371, M10.372, M10.379, M10.38, M10.39, M10.40, M10.411, M10.412, M10.419, M10.421, M10.422, M10.429, M10.431, M10.432, M10.439, M10.441, M10.442, M10.449, M10.451, M10.452, M10.459, M10.461, M10.462, M10.469, M10.471, M10.472, M10.479, M10.48, M10.49, M10.9, M1A.00X0, M1A.00X1, M1A.0110, M1A.0111, M1A.0120, M1A.0121, M1A.0190, M1A.0191, M1A.0210, M1A.0211, M1A.0220, M1A.0221, M1A.0290, M1A.0291, M1A.0310, M1A.0311, M1A.0320, M1A.0321, M1A.0390, M1A.0391, M1A.0410, M1A.0411, M1A.0420, M1A.0421, M1A.0490, M1A.0491, M1A.0510, M1A.0511, M1A.0520, M1A.0521, M1A.0590, M1A.0591, M1A.0610, M1A.0611, M1A.0620, M1A.0621, M1A.0690, M1A.0691, M1A.0710, M1A.0711, M1A.0720, M1A.0721, M1A.0790, M1A.0791, M1A.08X0, M1A.08X1, M1A.09X0, M1A.09X1, M1A.10X0, M1A.10X1, M1A.1110, M1A.1111, M1A.1120, M1A.1121, M1A.1190, M1A.1191, M1A.1210, M1A.1211, M1A.1220, M1A.1221, M1A.1290, M1A.1291, M1A.1310, M1A.1311, M1A.1320, M1A.1321, M1A.1390, M1A.1391, M1A.1410, M1A.1411, M1A.1420, M1A.1421, M1A.1490, M1A.1491, M1A.1510, M1A.1511, M1A.1520, M1A.1521, M1A.1590, M1A.1591, M1A.1610, M1A.1611, M1A.1620, M1A.1621, M1A.1690, M1A.1691, M1A.1710, M1A.1711, M1A.1720, M1A.1721, M1A.1790, M1A.1791, M1A.18X0, M1A.18X1, M1A.19X0, M1A.19X1, M1A.20X0, M1A.20X1, M1A.2110, M1A.2111, M1A.2120, M1A.2121, M1A.2190, M1A.2191, M1A.2210, M1A.2211, M1A.2220, M1A.2221, M1A.2290, M1A.2291, M1A.2310, M1A.2311, M1A.2320, M1A.2321, M1A.2390, M1A.2391, M1A.2410, M1A.2411, M1A.2420, M1A.2421, M1A.2490, M1A.2491, M1A.2510, M1A.2511, M1A.2520, M1A.2521, M1A.2590, M1A.2591, M1A.2610, M1A.2611, M1A.2620, M1A.2621, M1A.2690, M1A.2691, M1A.2710, M1A.2711, M1A.2720, M1A.2721, M1A.2790, M1A.2791, M1A.28X0, M1A.28X1, M1A.29X0, M1A.29X1, M1A.30X0, M1A.30X1, M1A.3110, M1A.3111, M1A.3120, M1A.3121, M1A.3190, M1A.3191, M1A.3210, M1A.3211, M1A.3220, M1A.3221, M1A.3290, M1A.3291, M1A.3310, M1A.3311, M1A.3320, M1A.3321, M1A.3390, M1A.3391, M1A.3410, M1A.3411, M1A.3420, M1A.3421, M1A.3490, M1A.3491, M1A.3510, M1A.3511, M1A.3520, M1A.3521, M1A.3590, M1A.3591, M1A.3610, M1A.3611, M1A.3620, M1A.3621, M1A.3690, M1A.3691, M1A.3710, M1A.3711, M1A.3720, M1A.3721, M1A.3790, M1A.3791, M1A.38X0, M1A.38X1, M1A.39X0, M1A.39X1, M1A.40X0, M1A.40X1, M1A.4110, M1A.4111, M1A.4120, M1A.4121, M1A.4190, M1A.4191, M1A.4210, M1A.4211, M1A.4220, M1A.4221, M1A.4290, M1A.4291, M1A.4310, M1A.4311, M1A.4320, M1A.4321, M1A.4390, M1A.4391, M1A.4410, M1A.4411, M1A.4420, M1A.4421, M1A.4490, M1A.4491, M1A.4510, M1A.4511, M1A.4520, M1A.4521, M1A.4590, M1A.4591, M1A.4610, M1A.4611, M1A.4620, M1A.4621, M1A.4690, M1A.4691, M1A.4710, M1A.4711, M1A.4720, M1A.4721, M1A.4790, M1A.4791, M1A.48X0, M1A.48X1, M1A.49X0, M1A.49X1, M1A.9XX0, M1A.9XX1
G99.2	C00.0, C00.1, C00.2, C00.3, C00.4, C00.5, C00.6, C00.8, C00.9, C01, C02.0, C02.1, C02.2, C02.3, C02.4, C02.8, C02.9, C03.0, C03.1, C03.9, C04.0, C04.1, C04.8, C04.9, C05.0, C05.1, C05.2, C05.8, C05.9, C06.0, C06.1, C06.2, C06.80, C06.89, C06.9, C07, C08.0, C08.1, C08.9, C09.0, C09.1, C09.8, C09.9, C10.0, C10.1, C10.2, C10.3, C10.4, C10.8, C10.9, C11.0, C11.1, C11.2, C11.3, C11.8, C11.9, C12, C13.0, C13.1, C13.2, C13.8, C13.9, C14.0, C14.2, C14.8, C15.3, C15.4, C15.5, C15.8, C15.9, C16.0, C16.1, C16.2, C16.3, C16.4, C16.5, C16.6, C16.8, C16.9, C17.0, C17.1, C17.2, C17.3, C17.8, C17.9, C18.0, C18.1, C18.2, C18.3, C18.4, C18.5, C18.6, C18.7, C18.8, C18.9, C19, C20, C21.0, C21.1, C21.2, C21.8, C22.0, C22.1, C22.2, C22.3, C22.4, C22.7, C22.8, C22.9, C23, C24.0, C24.1, C24.8, C24.9, C25.0, C25.1, C25.2, C25.3, C25.4, C25.7, C25.8, C25.9, C26.0, C26.1, C26.9, C30.0, C30.1, C31.0, C31.1, C31.2, C31.3, C31.8, C31.9, C32.0, C32.1, C32.2, C32.3, C32.8, C32.9, C33, C34.00, C34.01, C34.02, C34.10, C34.11, C34.12, C34.2, C34.30, C34.31, C34.32, C34.80, C34.81, C34.82, C34.90, C34.91, C34.92, C37, C38.0, C38.1, C38.2, C38.3, C38.4, C38.8, C39.0, C39.9, C40.00, C40.01, C40.02, C40.10, C40.11, C40.12, C40.20, C40.21, C40.22, C40.30, C40.31, C40.32, C40.80, C40.81, C40.82, C40.90, C40.91, C40.92, C41.0, C41.1, C41.2, C41.3, C41.4, C41.9, C43.0, C43.10, C43.11, C43.12, C43.20, C43.21, C43.22, C43.30, C43.31, C43.39, C43.4, C43.51, C43.52, C43.59, C43.60, C43.61, C43.62, C43.70, C43.71, C43.72, C43.8, C43.9, C45.0, C45.1, C45.2, C45.7, C45.9, C46.0, C46.1, C46.2, C46.3, C46.4, C46.50, C46.51, C46.52, C46.7, C46.9, C47.0, C47.10, C47.11, C47.12, C47.20, C47.21, C47.22, C47.3, C47.4, C47.5, C47.6, C47.8, C47.9, C48.0, C48.1, C48.2, C48.8, C49.0, C49.10, C49.11, C49.12, C49.20, C49.21, C49.22, C49.3, C49.4, C49.5, C49.6, C49.8, C49.9, C49.A0, C49.A1, C49.A2, C49.A3, C49.A4, C49.A5, C49.A9, C4A.0, C4A.10, C4A.11, C4A.12, C4A.20, C4A.21, C4A.22, C4A.30, C4A.31, C4A.39, C4A.51, C4A.52, C4A.59, C4A.60, C4A.61, C4A.62, C4A.70, C4A.71, C4A.72, C4A.8, C4A.9, C50.011, C50.012, C50.019, C50.021, C50.022, C50.029, C50.111, C50.112, C50.119, C50.121, C50.122, C50.129, C50.211, C50.212, C50.219, C50.221, C50.222, C50.229, C50.311, C50.312, C50.319, C50.321, C50.322, C50.329, C50.411, C50.412, C50.419, C50.421, C50.422, C50.429, C50.511, C50.512, C50.519, C50.521, C50.522, C50.529, C50.611, C50.612, C50.619, C50.621, C50.622, C50.629, C50.811, C50.812, C50.819, C50.821, C50.822, C50.829, C50.911, C50.912, C50.919, C50.921, C50.922, C50.929, C51.0, C51.1, C51.2, C51.8, C51.9, C52, C53.0, C53.1, C53.8, C53.9, C54.0, C54.1, C54.2, C54.3, C54.8, C54.9, C55, C56.1, C56.2, C56.9, C57.00, C57.01, C57.02, C57.10, C57.11, C57.12, C57.20, C57.21, C57.22, C57.3, C57.4, C57.7, C57.8, C57.9, C58, C60.0, C60.1, C60.2, C60.8, C60.9, C61, C62.00, C62.01, C62.02, C62.10, C62.11, C62.12, C62.90, C62.91, C62.92, C63.00, C63.01, C63.02, C63.10, C63.11, C63.12, C63.7, C63.8, C63.9, C64.1, C64.2, C64.9, C65.1, C65.2, C65.9, C66.1, C66.2, C66.9, C67.0, C67.1, C67.2, C67.3, C67.4, C67.5, C67.6, C67.7, C67.8, C67.9, C68.0, C68.1, C68.8, C68.9, C69.00, C69.01, C69.02, C69.10, C69.11, C69.12, C69.20, C69.21, C69.22, C69.30, C69.31, C69.32, C69.40, C69.41, C69.42, C69.50, C69.51, C69.52, C69.60, C69.61, C69.62, C69.80, C69.81, C69.82, C69.90, C69.91, C69.92, C70.0, C70.1, C70.9, C71.0, C71.1, C71.2, C71.3, C71.4, C71.5, C71.6, C71.7, C71.8, C71.9, C72.0, C72.1, C72.20, C72.21, C72.22, C72.30, C72.31, C72.32, C72.40, C72.41, C72.42, C72.50, C72.59, C72.9, C73, C74.00, C74.01, C74.02, C74.10, C74.11, C74.12, C74.90, C74.91, C74.92, C75.0, C75.1, C75.2, C75.3, C75.4, C75.5, C75.8, C75.9, C76.0, C76.1, C76.2, C76.3, C76.40, C76.41, C76.42, C76.50, C76.51, C76.52, C76.8, C77.0, C77.1, C77.2, C77.3, C77.4, C77.5, C77.8, C77.9, C78.00, C78.01, C78.02, C78.1, C78.2, C78.30, C78.39, C78.4, C78.5, C78.6, C78.7, C78.80, C78.89, C79.00, C79.01, C79.02, C79.10, C79.11, C79.19, C79.2, C79.31, C79.32, C79.40, C79.49, C79.51, C79.52, C79.60, C79.61, C79.62, C79.70, C79.71, C79.72, C79.81, C79.82, C79.89, C79.9, C7A.00, C7A.010, C7A.011, C7A.012, C7A.019, C7A.020, C7A.021, C7A.022, C7A.023, C7A.024, C7A.025, C7A.026, C7A.029, C7A.090, C7A.091, C7A.092, C7A.093, C7A.094, C7A.095, C7A.096, C7A.098, C7A.1, C7A.8, C7B.00, C7B.01, C7B.02, C7B.03, C7B.04, C7B.09, C7B.1, C7B.8, C80.0, C80.1, C80.2, C81.00, C81.01, C81.02, C81.03, C81.04, C81.05, C81.06, C81.07, C81.08, C81.09, C81.10, C81.11, C81.12, C81.13, C81.14, C81.15, C81.16, C81.17, C81.18, C81.19, C81.20, C81.21, C81.22, C81.23, C81.24, C81.25, C81.26, C81.27, C81.28, C81.29, C81.30, C81.31, C81.32, C81.33, C81.34, C81.35, C81.36, C81.37, C81.38, C81.39, C81.40, C81.41, C81.42, C81.43, C81.44, C81.45, C81.46, C81.47, C81.48, C81.49, C81.70, C81.71, C81.72, C81.73, C81.74, C81.75, C81.76, C81.77, C81.78, C81.79, C81.90, C81.91, C81.92, C81.93, C81.94, C81.95, C81.96, C81.97, C81.98, C81.99, C82.00, C82.01, C82.02, C82.03, C82.05, C82.06, C82.07, C82.08, C82.09, C82.10, C82.11, C82.12, C82.13, C82.14, C82.15, C82.16, C82.17, C82.18, C82.19, C82.20, C82.21, C82.22, C82.23, C82.24, C82.25, C82.26, C82.27, C82.28, C82.29, C82.30, C82.31, C82.32, C82.33, C82.34, C82.35, C82.36, C82.37, C82.38, C82.39, C82.40, C82.41, C82.42, C82.43, C82.44, C82.45, C82.46, C82.47, C82.48, C82.49, C82.50, C82.51, C82.52, C82.53, C82.54, C82.55, C82.56, C82.57, C82.58, C82.59, C82.60, C82.61, C82.62, C82.63, C82.64, C82.65, C82.66, C82.67, C82.68, C82.69, C82.80, C82.81, C82.82, C82.83, C82.84, C82.85, C82.86, C82.87, C82.88, C82.89, C82.90, C82.91, C82.92, C82.93, C82.94, C82.95, C82.96, C82.97, C82.98, C82.99, C83.00, C83.01, C83.02, C83.03, C83.04, C83.05, C83.06, C83.07, C83.08, C83.09, C83.10,

G99.2 (continued)	C83.11, C83.12, C83.13, C83.14, C83.15, C83.16, C83.17, C83.18, C83.19, C83.30, C83.31, C83.32, C83.33, C83.34, C83.35, C83.36, C83.37, C83.38, C83.39, C83.50, C83.51, C83.52, C83.53, C83.54, C83.55, C83.56, C83.57, C83.58, C83.59, C83.70, C83.71, C83.72, C83.73, C83.74, C83.75, C83.76, C83.77, C83.78, C83.79, C83.80, C83.81, C83.82, C83.83, C83.84, C83.85, C83.86, C83.87, C83.88, C83.89, C83.90, C83.91, C83.92, C83.93, C83.94, C83.95, C83.96, C83.97, C83.98, C83.99, C84.00, C84.01, C84.02, C84.03, C84.04, C84.05, C84.06, C84.07, C84.08, C84.09, C84.10, C84.11, C84.12, C84.13, C84.14, C84.15, C84.16, C84.17, C84.18, C84.19, C84.40, C84.41, C84.42, C84.43, C84.44, C84.45, C84.46, C84.47, C84.48, C84.49, C84.60, C84.61, C84.62, C84.63, C84.64, C84.65, C84.66, C84.67, C84.68, C84.69, C84.70, C84.71, C84.72, C84.73, C84.74, C84.75, C84.76, C84.77, C84.78, C84.79, C84.90, C84.91, C84.92, C84.93, C84.94, C84.95, C84.96, C84.97, C84.98, C84.99, C84.A0, C84.A1, C84.A2, C84.A3, C84.A4, C84.A5, C84.A6, C84.A7, C84.A8, C84.A9, C84.Z0, C84.Z1, C84.Z2, C84.Z3, C84.Z4, C84.Z5, C84.Z6, C84.Z7, C84.Z8, C84.Z9, C85.10, C85.11, C85.12, C85.13, C85.14, C85.15, C85.16, C85.17, C85.18, C85.19, C85.20, C85.21, C85.22, C85.23, C85.24, C85.25, C85.26, C85.27, C85.28, C85.29, C85.80, C85.81, C85.82, C85.83, C85.84, C85.85, C85.86, C85.87, C85.88, C85.89, C85.90, C85.91, C85.92, C85.93, C85.94, C85.95, C85.96, C85.97, C85.98, C85.99, C86.0, C86.1, C86.2, C86.3, C86.4, C86.5, C86.6, C88.0, C88.2, C88.3, C88.4, C88.8, C88.9, C90.00, C90.01, C90.02, C90.10, C90.11, C90.12, C90.20, C90.21, C90.22, C90.30, C90.31, C90.32, C91.00, C91.01, C91.02, C91.10, C91.11, C91.12, C91.30, C91.31, C91.32, C91.40, C91.41, C91.42, C91.50, C91.51, C91.52, C91.60, C91.61, C91.62, C91.90, C91.91, C91.92, C91.A0, C91.A1, C91.A2, C91.Z0, C91.Z1, C91.Z2, C92.00, C92.01, C92.02, C92.10, C92.11, C92.12, C92.21, C92.22, C92.30, C92.31, C92.32, C92.40, C92.41, C92.42, C92.50, C92.51, C92.52, C92.60, C92.61, C92.62, C92.90, C92.91, C92.92, C92.A0, C92.A1, C92.A2, C92.Z0, C92.Z1, C92.Z2, C93.00, C93.01, C93.02, C93.10, C93.11, C93.12, C93.30, C93.31, C93.32, C93.90, C93.91, C93.92, C93.Z0, C93.Z1, C94.00, C94.01, C94.02, C94.20, C94.21, C94.22, C94.30, C94.31, C94.32, C94.40, C94.41, C94.42, C94.6, C94.80, C94.81, C94.82, C95.00, C95.01, C95.02, C95.10, C95.11, C95.12, C95.90, C95.91, C95.92, C96.0, C96.4, C96.5, C96.6, C96.9, C96.A, C96.Z, D00.00, D00.01, D00.02, D00.03, D00.04, D00.05, D00.06, D00.07, D00.08, D00.1, D00.2, D01.0, D01.1, D01.2, D01.3, D01.40, D01.49, D01.5, D01.7, D01.9, D02.0, D02.1, D02.20, D02.21, D02.22, D02.3, D02.4, D03.0, D03.10, D03.11, D03.12, D03.20, D03.21, D03.22, D03.30, D03.39, D03.4, D03.51, D03.52, D03.59, D03.60, D03.61, D03.62, D03.70, D03.71, D03.72, D03.8, D03.9, D04.0, D04.10, D04.11, D04.12, D04.21, D04.22, D04.30, D04.39, D04.4, D04.5, D04.60, D04.61, D04.62, D04.70, D04.71, D04.72, D04.8, D04.9, D05.00, D05.01, D05.02, D05.10, D05.11, D05.12, D05.80, D05.81, D05.82, D05.90, D05.91, D05.92, D06.0, D06.1, D06.7, D06.9, D07.0, D07.1, D07.2, D07.30, D07.39, D07.4, D07.5, D07.60, D07.61, D07.69, D09.0, D09.10, D09.19, D09.20, D09.21, D09.22, D09.3, D09.8, D09.9, D10.0, D10.1, D10.2, D10.30, D10.39, D10.4, D10.5, D10.6, D10.7, D10.9, D11.0, D11.7, D11.9, D12.0, D12.1, D12.2, D12.3, D12.4, D12.5, D12.6, D12.7, D12.8, D12.9, D13.0, D13.1, D13.2, D13.30, D13.39, D13.4, D13.5, D13.6, D13.7, D13.9, D14.0, D14.1, D14.2, D14.30, D14.31, D14.32, D14.4, D15.0, D15.1, D15.2, D15.7, D15.9, D16.00, D16.01, D16.02, D16.10, D16.11, D16.12, D16.20, D16.21, D16.22, D16.30, D16.31, D16.32, D16.4, D16.5, D16.6, D16.7, D16.8, D16.9, D17.0, D17.1, D17.20, D17.21, D17.22, D17.23, D17.24, D17.30, D17.39, D17.4, D17.5, D17.6, D17.7, D17.9, D18.00, D18.01, D18.02, D18.03, D18.09, D18.1, D19.0, D19.1, D19.7, D19.9, D20.0, D20.1, D21.0, D21.10, D21.11, D21.12, D21.20, D21.21, D21.22, D21.3, D21.4, D21.5, D21.6, D21.9, D22.0, D22.10, D22.11, D22.12, D22.20, D22.21, D22.22, D22.30, D22.39, D22.4, D22.5, D22.60, D22.61, D22.62, D22.70, D22.71, D22.72, D22.9, D23.0, D23.10, D23.11, D23.12, D23.20, D23.21, D23.22, D23.30, D23.39, D23.4, D23.5, D23.60, D23.61, D23.62, D23.70, D23.71, D23.72, D23.9, D24.1, D24.2, D24.9, D25.0, D25.1, D25.2, D25.9, D26.0, D26.1, D26.7, D26.9, D27.0, D27.1, D27.9, D28.0, D28.1, D28.2, D28.7, D28.9, D29.0, D29.1, D29.20, D29.21, D29.22, D29.30, D29.31, D29.32, D29.4, D29.8, D29.9, D30.00, D30.01, D30.02, D30.10, D30.11, D30.12, D30.20, D30.21, D30.22, D30.3, D30.4, D30.8, D30.9, D31.00, D31.01, D31.02, D31.10, D31.11, D31.12, D31.20, D31.21, D31.22, D31.30, D31.31, D31.32, D31.40, D31.41, D31.42, D31.50, D31.51, D31.52, D31.60, D31.61, D31.62, D31.90, D31.91, D31.92, D32.0, D32.1, D32.9, D33.0, D33.1, D33.2, D33.3, D33.4, D33.7, D33.9, D34, D35.00, D35.01, D35.02, D35.1, D35.2, D35.3, D35.4, D35.5, D35.6, D35.7, D35.9, D36.0, D36.10, D36.11, D36.12, D36.13, D36.14, D36.15, D36.16, D36.17, D36.7, D36.9, D37.01, D37.02, D37.030, D37.031, D37.032, D37.039, D37.04, D37.05, D37.09, D37.1, D37.2, D37.3, D37.4, D37.5, D37.6, D37.8, D37.9, D38.0, D38.1, D38.2, D38.3, D38.4, D38.5, D38.6, D39.0, D39.10, D39.11, D39.12, D39.2, D39.8, D39.9, D3A.00, D3A.010, D3A.011, D3A.012, D3A.019, D3A.020, D3A.021, D3A.022, D3A.023, D3A.024, D3A.025, D3A.026, D3A.029, D3A.090, D3A.091, D3A.092, D3A.093, D3A.094, D3A.095, D3A.096, D3A.098, D3A.8, D40.0, D40.10, D40.11, D40.12, D40.8, D40.9, D41.00, D41.01, D41.02, D41.10, D41.11, D41.12, D41.20, D41.21, D41.22, D41.3, D41.4, D41.8, D41.9, D42.0, D42.1, D42.9, D43.0, D43.1, D43.2, D43.3, D43.4, D43.8, D43.9, D44.0, D44.10, D44.11, D44.12, D44.2, D44.3, D44.4, D44.5, D44.6, D44.7, D44.9, D45, D46.0, D46.1, D46.20, D46.21, D46.22, D46.4, D46.9, D46.A, D46.B, D46.C, D46.Z, D47.1, D47.2, D47.3, D47.4, D47.9, D47.Z1, D47.Z2, D47.Z9, D48.0, D48.1, D48.2, D48.3, D48.4, D48.5, D48.60, D48.61, D48.62, D48.7, D48.9
I96*	A34, A48.0, E03.4, E07.89, E35, H18.40, I50.9, I70.261, I70.262, I70.263, I70.268, I70.269, I89.1, J02.0, J02.8, J02.9, J03.00, J03.01, J03.80, J03.81, J03.90, J03.91, J04.0, J05.0, J39.0, J85.0, J85.1, J85.2, K04.1, K05.5, K06.1, K06.2, K06.8, K12.2, K14.0, K81.0, M27.3, N30.80, N30.81, N44.1, N44.2, N44.8, N45.1, N45.2, N45.3, N48.21, N48.22, N48.29, N49.1, N49.2, N49.3, N49.8, N49.9, N50.3, N53.12, N53.8, N53.9, N70.91, N70.92, N70.93, N71.9, N76.0, N76.1, N76.2, N76.3, O08.0, O08.82, O85, O86.12, O86.81, O86.89 * Manifestation code I96 (Gangrene) is not eligible for case-mix points when paired with one of the listed etiology codes.
K23	A50.51, A50.52, A50.53, A50.54, A50.55, A50.56, A50.57, A50.59
K67	A50.01, A50.02, A50.03, A50.04, A50.05, A50.06, A50.07, A50.08, A50.09, B65.0, B65.1, B65.2, B65.3, B65.8, B65.9, B66.0, B66.1, B66.2, B66.3, B66.4, B66.5, B66.8, B66.9, B67.0, B67.1, B67.2, B67.31, B67.32, B67.39, B67.4, B67.5, B67.61, B67.69, B67.7, B67.8, B67.90, B67.99, B68.0, B68.1, B68.9, B69.0, B69.1, B69.81, B69.89, B69.9, B70.0, B70.1, B71.0, B71.1, B71.8, B71.9, B72, B73.00, B73.01, B73.02, B73.09, B73.1, B74.0, B74.1, B74.2, B74.3, B74.4, B74.8, B74.9, B75, B76.0, B76.1, B76.8, B76.9, B77.0, B77.81, B77.89, B77.9, B78.0, B78.1, B78.7, B78.9, B79, B80, B81.0, B81.1, B81.2, B81.3, B81.4, B81.8, B82.0, B82.9, B83.0, B83.1, B83.2, B83.3, B83.4, B83.8, B83.9
K77	A50.01, A50.02, A50.03, A50.04, A50.05, A50.06, A50.07, A50.08, A50.09, A50.51, A50.52, A50.53, A50.54, A50.55, A50.56, A50.57, A50.59, B65.0, B65.1, B65.2, B65.3, B65.8, B65.9, P37.1
M01.X11, M01.X12, M01.X21, M01.X22, M01.X31, M01.X32, M01.X41, M01.X42, M01.X51, M01.X52, M01.X61, M01.X62, M01.X71, M01.X72, M01.X8, M01.X9	A01.1, A01.2, A01.3, A01.4, A30.0, A30.1, A30.2, A30.3, A30.4, A30.5, A30.8, A30.9, A92.1, B35.0, B35.1, B35.2, B35.3, B35.4, B35.5, B35.6, B35.8, B35.9, B36.0, B36.1, B36.2, B36.3, B36.8, B36.9, B37.0, B37.1, B37.2, B37.3, B37.41, B37.42, B37.49, B37.5, B37.6, B37.7, B37.81, B37.82, B37.83, B37.84, B37.89, B37.9, B38.0, B38.1, B38.2, B38.3, B38.4, B38.7, B38.81, B38.89, B38.9, B39.0, B39.1, B39.2, B39.3, B39.4, B39.5, B39.9, B40.0, B40.1, B40.2, B40.3, B40.7, B40.81, B40.89, B40.9, B41.0, B41.7, B41.8, B41.9, B42.0, B42.1, B42.7, B42.81, B42.82, B42.89, B42.9, B43.0, B43.1, B43.2, B43.8, B43.9, B44.0, B44.1, B44.2, B44.7, B44.89, B44.9, B45.0, B45.1, B45.2, B45.3, B45.7, B45.8, B45.9, B46.0, B46.1, B46.2, B46.3, B46.4, B46.5, B46.8, B46.9, B47.0, B47.1, B47.9, B48.0, B48.1, B48.2, B48.3, B48.4, B48.8, B49
M02.811, M02.812, M02.821, M02.822, M02.831, M02.832, M02.841, M02.842, M02.851, M02.852, M02.861, M02.862, M02.871, M02.872, M02.88, M02.89	A04.6, A50.51, A50.52, A50.53, A50.54, A50.55, A50.56, A50.57, A50.59, B15.0, B15.9, B16.0, B16.1, B16.2, B16.9, B17.0, B17.10, B17.11, B17.2, B17.8, B17.9, B18.0, B18.1, B18.2, B18.8, B18.9, B19.0, B19.10, B19.11, B19.20, B19.21, B19.9, I33.0

M02.9	A04.6, A50.52, A50.53, A50.54, A50.55, A50.56, A50.57, A50.59, B15.0, B15.9, B16.0, B16.1, B16.2, B16.9, B17.0, B17.10, B17.11, B17.2, B17.8, B17.9, B18.0, B18.1, B18.2, B18.8, B18.9, B19.0, B19.10, B19.11, B19.20, B19.21, B19.9, I33.0
M14.811, M14.812, M14.821, M14.822, M14.831, M14.832, M14.841, M14.842, M14.851, M14.852, M14.861, M14.862, M14.871, M14.872, M14.88, M14.89	D57.00, D57.01, D57.02, D57.1, D57.20, D57.211, D57.212, D57.219, D57.3, D57.40, D57.411, D57.412, D57.419, D57.80, D57.811, D57.812, D57.819, E00.0, E00.1, E00.2, E00.9, E01.0, E01.1, E01.2, E01.8, E02, E03.0, E03.1, E03.2, E03.3, E03.4, E03.5, E03.8, E03.9, E05.00, E05.01, E05.10, E05.11, E05.20, E05.21, E05.30, E05.31, E05.40, E05.41, E05.80, E05.81, E05.90, E05.91, E21.0, E21.1, E21.2, E21.3, E21.4, E21.5, E83.10, E83.19, E85.0, E85.1, E85.2, E85.3, E85.4, E85.9, K90.81, K90.89, L51.0, L51.1, L51.2, L51.3, L51.8, L51.9, L52
M36.1	C90.00, C90.01, C90.02, C90.10, C90.11, C90.12, C90.20, C90.21, C90.22, C90.30, C90.31, C90.32, C91.00, C91.01, C91.02, C91.10, C91.11, C91.12, C91.30, C91.31, C91.32, C91.40, C91.41, C91.42, C91.50, C91.51, C91.52, C91.60, C91.61, C91.62, C91.90, C91.91, C91.92, C91.A0, C91.A1, C91.A2, C91.Z0, C91.Z1, C91.Z2, C92.00, C92.01, C92.02, C92.10, C92.11, C92.12, C92.20, C92.21, C92.22, C92.30, C92.31, C92.40, C92.41, C92.42, C92.50, C92.51, C92.52, C92.60, C92.61, C92.62, C92.90, C92.91, C92.92, C92.A0, C92.A1, C92.A2, C92.Z0, C92.Z1, C92.Z2, C93.00, C93.01, C93.02, C93.10, C93.11, C93.12, C93.30, C93.31, C93.32, C93.90, C93.91, C93.92, C93.Z0, C93.Z1, C93.Z2, C94.00, C94.01, C94.02, C94.20, C94.21, C94.22, C94.30, C94.31, C94.32, C94.40, C94.41, C94.42, C94.6, C94.80, C94.81, C94.82, C95.00, C95.01, C95.02, C95.10, C95.11, C95.12, C95.90, C95.91, C95.92, C96.A
M36.2	D66, D67, D68.0, D68.1
M36.3	C90.00, C90.01, C90.02, C90.12, C90.22, C90.32, C91.00, C91.01, C91.02, C91.10, C91.11, C91.12, C91.30, C91.31, C91.32, C91.50, C91.51, C91.52, C91.60, C91.61, C91.62, C91.90, C91.91, C91.92, C91.A0, C91.A1, C91.A2, C91.Z0, C91.Z1, C91.Z2, C92.00, C92.01, C92.02, C92.10, C92.11, C92.12, C92.20, C92.21, C92.22, C92.30, C92.31, C92.32, C92.40, C92.41, C92.42, C92.50, C92.51, C92.52, C92.60, C92.61, C92.62, C92.90, C92.91, C92.92, C92.A0, C92.A1, C92.A2, C92.Z0, C92.Z1, C92.Z2, C93.00, C93.01, C93.02, C93.10, C93.11, C93.12, C93.30, C93.31, C93.32, C93.90, C93.91, C93.92, C93.Z0, C93.Z1, C93.Z2, C94.00, C94.01, C94.02, C94.20, C94.21, C94.22, C94.30, C94.31, C94.32, C94.80, C94.81, C94.82, C95.00, C95.01, C95.02, C95.10, C95.11, C95.12, C95.90, C95.91, C95.92, C96.A, D45, D56.0, D56.1, D56.2, D56.3, D56.4, D56.5, D56.8, D56.9, D57.00, D57.01, D57.02, D57.1, D57.20, D57.211, D57.212, D57.219, D57.3, D57.40, D57.411, D57.412, D57.419, D57.80, D57.811, D57.812, D57.819, D58.2
M36.4	D69.0, T80.61XA, T80.61XD, T80.61XS, T80.62XA, T80.62XD, T80.62XS, T80.69XA, T80.69XD, T80.69XS
M49.81, M49.82, M48.83, M49.84, M48.85, M49.86, M49.87, M49.88, M49.89	A00.0, A00.1, A00.9, A01.00, A01.01, A01.02, A01.03, A01.04, A01.05, A01.09, A01.1, A01.2, A01.3, A01.4, A02.0, A02.1, A02.20, A02.21, A02.22, A02.23, A02.24, A02.25, A02.29, A02.8, A02.9, A03.0, A03.1, A03.2, A03.3, A03.8, A03.9, A04.0, A04.1, A04.2, A04.3, A04.4, A04.5, A04.6, A04.8, A04.9, A23.0, A23.1, A23.2, A23.3, A23.8, A23.9, E21.0, G60.0
M90.511, M90.512, M90.521, M90.522, M90.531, M90.532, M90.541, M90.542, M90.551, M90.552, M90.561, M90.562, M90.571, M90.572, M90.58, M90.59	D50.0, D50.1, D50.8, D50.9, D51.0, D51.1, D51.2, D51.3, D51.8, D51.9, D52.0, D52.1, D52.8, D52.9, D53.0, D53.1, D53.2, D53.8, D53.9, D55.0, D55.1, D55.2, D55.3, D55.8, D55.9, D56.0, D56.1, D56.2, D56.3, D56.4, D56.8, D56.9, D57.00, D57.01, D57.02, D57.1, D57.20, D57.211, D57.212, D57.219, D57.3, D57.40, D57.411, D57.412, D57.419, D57.80, D57.811, D57.812, D57.819, D58.0, D58.1, D58.2, D58.8, D58.9, D59.0, D59.1, D59.2, D59.3, D59.4, D59.5, D59.6, D59.8, D59.9, D60.0, D60.1, D60.8, D60.9, D61.01, D61.09, D61.1, D61.2, D61.3, D61.82, D61.89, D61.9, D62, D64.0, D64.2, D64.3, D64.4, D64.81, D64.89, D64.9, T70.3XXA, T70.3XXD, T70.3XXS
M90.611, M90.612, M90.621, M90.622, M90.631, M90.632, M90.641, M90.642, M90.651, M90.652, M90.661, M90.662, M90.671, M90.672, M90.68, M90.69	C40.00, C40.01, C40.02, C40.10, C40.11, C40.12, C40.20, C40.21, C40.22, C40.30, C40.31, C40.32, C40.80, C40.81, C40.82, C40.90, C40.91, C40.92, C41.0, C41.1, C41.2, C41.3, C41.4, C41.9
M90.811, M90.812, M90.821, M90.822, M90.831, M90.832, M90.841, M90.842, M90.851, M90.852, M90.861, M90.862, M90.871, M90.872, M90.88, M90.89	E55.0, E83.30, E83.31, E83.32, E83.39

Appendix N: Hospice Criteria for Medicare Coverage of Noncancer Hospice Care

Coverage of Hospice Services Under Hospital Insurance

CMS Manual Publication Number 100-04, *Medicare Claims Processing Manual*, Chapter 11

CMS Manual Publication 100-2, *Medicare Benefits Policy Manual*, Chapter 9

Requirements – General

Hospice care is a benefit under the hospital insurance program. To be eligible to elect hospice care under Medicare, an individual must be entitled to Part A of Medicare and be certified as being terminally ill. An individual is considered to be terminally ill if the medical prognosis is that the individual's life expectancy is six months or less if the illness runs its normal course. Only care provided by (or under arrangements made by) a Medicare certified hospice is covered under the Medicare hospice benefit.

The hospice admits a patient only on the recommendation of the medical director in consultation with, or with input from, the patient's attending physician (if any).

In reaching a decision to certify that the patient is terminally ill, the hospice medical director must consider at least the following information:

1. Diagnosis of the terminal condition of the patient.
2. Other health conditions, whether related or unrelated to the terminal condition.
3. Current clinically relevant information supporting all diagnoses.

Section §1814(a)(7) of the Social Security Act (the Act) specifies that certification of terminal illness for hospice benefits shall be based on the clinical judgment of the hospice medical director or physician member of the interdisciplinary group (IDG) and the individual's attending physician, if he/she has one, regarding the normal course of the individual's illness. No one other than a medical doctor or doctor of osteopathy can certify or re-certify a terminal illness. Predicting of life expectancy is not always exact. The fact that a beneficiary lives longer than expected in itself is not cause to terminate benefits. "Attending physician" is further defined in section 20.1 and 40.1.3.1.

An individual (or his authorized representative) must elect hospice care to receive it. An individual may elect to receive Medicare coverage for an unlimited number of election periods of hospice care. The periods consist of two 90-day periods, and an unlimited number of 60-day periods. If the individual (or authorized representative) elects to receive hospice care, he or she must file an election statement with a particular hospice. Hospices obtain election statements from the individual and file a Notice of Election with the A/B MAC (HHH), which transmits them to the Common Working File (CWF) in electronic format. Once the initial election is processed, CWF maintains the beneficiary in hospice status until a final claim indicates a discharge (alive or due to death) or until an election termination is received.

For the duration of the election of hospice care, an individual must waive all rights to Medicare payments for the following services:

- Hospice care provided by a hospice other than the hospice designated by the individual (unless provided under arrangements made by the designated hospice); and

- Any Medicare services that are related to the treatment of the terminal condition for which hospice care was elected or a related condition or services that are equivalent to hospice care, except for services provided by:

  1. The designated hospice (either directly or under arrangement);
  2. Another hospice under arrangements made by the designated hospice; or
  3. The individual's attending physician, who may be a nurse practitioner (NP), if that physician or nurse practitioner is not an employee of the designated hospice or receiving compensation from the hospice for those services.

Medicare services for a condition completely unrelated to the terminal condition for which hospice was elected remain available to the patient if he or she is eligible for such care.

Noncancer Hospice Care Eligibility Criteria

Medicare coverage of hospice care depends upon a physician's certification of an individual's prognosis of a life expectancy of six months or less if the terminal illness runs its normal course. Recognizing that determination of life expectancy during the course of a terminal illness is difficult, the following policies were originally developed by the Medicare home health and hospice administrative contractors (HHH MACs) and are included in the resource for guidance only. These medical criteria form a reasonable approach to the determination of prognosis for certain noncancer diagnoses and were found not to be in conflict with any existing CMS national coverage rules and/or regulations. However, some patients may not meet the criteria, yet still be appropriate for hospice care, because of other comorbidities or rapid decline. Coverage for these patients may be approved on an individual consideration basis.

The criteria in each of these policies are considered to be the most accurate parameters to determine Medicare coverage for these specific noncancer diagnoses. As of May 2016, there were four HHH areas handled by three HHH MACs.

Hospice Election

Each hospice designs and prints its election statement. The election statement must include the following items of information:

- Identification of the particular hospice that will provide care to the individual;

- The individual's or representative's (as applicable) acknowledgment that the individual has been given a full understanding of hospice care, particularly the palliative rather than curative nature of treatment;

- The individual's or representative's (as applicable) acknowledgment that the individual understands that certain Medicare services are waived by the election;

- The effective date of the election, which may be the first day of hospice care or a later date, but may be no earlier than the date of the election statement. An individual may not designate an effective date that is retroactive;

- The individual's designated attending physician (if any). Information identifying the attending physician recorded on the election statement should provide enough detail so that it is clear which physician or Nurse Practitioner (NP) was designated as the attending physician. This information should include, but is not limited to, the attending physician's full name, office address, NPI number, or any other detailed information to clearly identify the attending physician.

- The individual's acknowledgment that the designated attending physician was the individual's or representative's choice.

- The signature of the individual or representative.

An election to receive hospice care will be considered to continue through the initial election period and through the subsequent election periods without a break in care as long as the individual:

1. Remains in the care of a hospice;
2. Does not revoke the election; and
3. Is not discharged from the hospice.

For Medicare payment purposes, an election for Medicare hospice care must be made on or after the date that the hospice provider is Medicare-certified. As with any election, the hospice must fulfill all other admission requirements, such as certification or recertification, any required face-to-face encounters, or Conditions of Participation (CoP) assessments. See also Pub. 100-04, Medicare Claims Processing Manual, chapter 11, section 20.1.1.

An individual may change, once in each election period, the designation of the particular hospice from which he or she elects to receive hospice care. The change of the designated hospice is not considered a revocation of the election, but is a transfer. To change the designation of hospice programs, the individual must file, with the hospice from which he or she has received care and with the newly designated hospice, a signed statement that includes the following information:

- the name of the hospice from which the individual has received care,
- the name of the hospice from which they plan to receive care, and
- the date the change is to be effective.

As described in Pub. 100-04, Medicare Claims Processing Manual, chapter 11, section 20.1.1, when a hospice patient transfers to a new hospice, the receiving hospice must file a new Notice of Election; however, the benefit period dates are unaffected. The receiving hospice must complete all assessments required by the hospice conditions of participation as described in 42 CFR 418.54. Because the benefit period does not change in a transfer situation, if the patient is in the third or later benefit period and transfers hospices, a face-to-face encounter is not required if the receiving hospice can verify that the originating hospice had the encounter.

A change of ownership of a hospice is not considered a change in the patient's designation of a hospice and requires no action on the patient's part.

Medicare beneficiaries enrolled in managed care plans may elect hospice benefits. Federal regulations require that the Medicare contractor assigned the hospice specialty workload maintain payment responsibility for hospice services and may pay for other claims if that contractor is the geographically assigned Medicare contractor for the managed care enrollees who elect hospice; for specifics, see regulations at 42 CFR 417, Subpart P, 417.585, Special Rules: Hospice Care (b), and 42 CFR 417.531 Hospice Care Services (b). Institutional claims for services not related to the terminal illness would otherwise be the responsibility of another geographically assigned Medicare contractor.

Managed care enrollees who have elected hospice may revoke hospice election at any time, but claims will continue to be paid by fee-for-service contractors as if the beneficiary were a fee-for-service beneficiary until the first day of the month following the month in which hospice was revoked. As specified above, by regulation, the duration of payment responsibility by fee-for-service contractors extends through the remainder of the month in which hospice is revoked by hospice beneficiaries.

Part I. Decline in clinical status guidelines

Patients will be considered to have a life expectancy of six months or less if there is documented evidence of decline in clinical status based on the guidelines listed below. Since determination of decline presumes assessment of the patient's status over time, it is essential that both baseline and follow-up determinations be reported where appropriate. Baseline data may be established on admission to hospice or by using existing information from records. Other clinical variables not on this list may support a six-month or less life expectancy. These should be documented in the clinical record.

These changes in clinical variables apply to patients whose decline is not considered to be reversible. They are examples of findings that generally connote a poor prognosis. However, some are clearly more predictive of a poor prognosis than others; significant ongoing weight loss is a strong predictor, while decreased functional status is less so.

Progression of disease as documented by worsening clinical status, symptoms, signs and laboratory results.

1. Clinical Status

   a. Recurrent or intractable infections such as pneumonia, sepsis or upper urinary tract. National Government Services (NGS) adds: or pyelonephritis in place of upper urinary tract)

   b. Progressive inanition as documented by:

      1) Weight loss (NGS states weight loss of at least 10% body weight in the prior six months) not due to reversible causes such as depression or use of diuretics

      2) Decreasing anthropomorphic measurements (mid-arm circumference, abdominal girth), not due to reversible causes such as depression or use of diuretics

      3) Decreasing serum albumin or cholesterol

      4) Dysphagia leading to recurrent aspiration and/or inadequate oral intake documented by decreasing food portion consumption

2. Symptoms

   a. Dyspnea with increasing respiratory rate

   b. Cough, intractable

   c. Nausea/vomiting poorly responsive to treatment

   d. Diarrhea, intractable

   e. Pain requiring increasing doses of major analgesics more than briefly

3. Signs

   a. Decline in systolic blood pressure to below 90 or progressive postural hypotension

   b. Ascites

   c. Venous, arterial or lymphatic obstruction due to local progression or metastatic disease

   d. Edema

   e. Pleural/pericardial effusion

   f. Weakness

   g. Change in level of consciousness

4. Laboratory (When available. Lab testing is not required to establish hospice eligibility.)

   a. Increasing pCO_2 or decreasing pO_2 or decreasing SaO_2

   b. Increasing calcium, creatinine or liver function studies

   c. Increasing tumor markers (e.g. CEA, PSA)

   d. Progressively decreasing or increasing serum sodium or increasing serum potassium

5. Decline in Karnofsky Performance Status (KPS) or Palliative Performance Score (PPS) (from <70% is stated by CGS)

6. Progressive decline in Functional Assessment Staging (FAST) for dementia (from ≥ 7A on the FAST)

7. Progression to dependence on assistance with additional activities of daily living. See Part II, Section B

8. Progressive stage 3-4 pressure ulcers in spite of optimal care

9. Increasing emergency room visits, hospitalizations, or physician's visits related to hospice primary diagnosis

Part II. Non-disease specific baseline guidelines (both of these should be met)

A. Physiologic impairment of functional status as demonstrated by: Karnofsky Performance Status (KPS) or Palliative Performance Score (PPS) < 70%. Note that two of the disease specific guidelines (HIV Disease, Stroke and Coma) establish a lower qualifying KPS or PPS.

B. Dependence on assistance for two or more activities of daily living (ADLs)

   1. Ambulation

   2. Continence

   3. Transfer

   4. Dressing

   5. Feeding

   6. Bathing

Part III. Co-morbidities

Although not the primary hospice diagnosis, the presence of disease such as the following, the severity of which is likely to contribute to a life expectancy of six months or less, should be considered in determining hospice eligibility.

   A. Chronic obstructive pulmonary disease

   B. Congestive heart failure

   C. Ischemic heart disease

   D. Diabetes mellitus

   E. Neurologic disease (CVA, ALS, MS, Parkinson's)

   F. Renal failure

   G. Liver Disease

   H. Neoplasia

   I. Acquired immune deficiency syndrome

   J. Dementia

(NGS adds: Refractory severe autoimmune disease [e.g., lupus or rheumatoid arthritis])

Hospice HIV Disease

34566 Palmetto GBA (PGBA)

Indications and limitations of coverage and/or medical necessity:

Patients will be considered to be in the terminal stage of their illness (life expectancy of six months or less) if they meet the following criteria (1 and 2 must be present; factors from 3 will add supporting documentation):

1. CD4+ Count < 25 cells/mcL (2 or more assays at least one month apart) or persistent viral load > l00,000 copies/ml, plus one of the following:

   - CNS lymphoma
   - Untreated, or not responsive to treatment, wasting (loss of 33% lean body mass)
   - Mycobacterium avium complex (MAC) bacteremia, untreated, unresponsive to treatment, or treatment refused
   - Progressive multifocal leukoencephalopathy
   - Systemic lymphoma, with advanced HIV disease and partial response to chemotherapy
   - Visceral Kaposi's sarcoma unresponsive to therapy
   - Renal failure in the absence of dialysis
   - Cryptosporidium infection
   - Toxoplasmosis, unresponsive to therapy

2. Decreased performance status, as measured by the KarnofskyPerformance Status (KPS) scale, of less than or equal to 50%

3. Documentation of the following factors will support eligibility for hospice care:

   - Chronic persistent diarrhea for one year
   - Persistent serum albumin <2.5
   - Concomitant, active substance abuse
   - Age > 50 years
   - Absence of antiretroviral, chemotherapeutic and prophylactic drug therapy related specifically to HIV disease
   - Advanced AIDS dementia complex
   - Toxoplasmosis
   - Congestive heart failure, symptomatic at rest
   - Advanced liver disease

ICD-10-CM codes that support medical necessity

B20 Human immunodeficiency virus (HIV) disease

ICD-10 codes that do not support medical necessity

R75 Inconclusive laboratory evidence of human immunodeficiency virus (HIV)

Z20.5 Contact with and (suspected) exposure to viral hepatitis

Z20.6 Contact with and (suspected) exposure to human immunodeficiency virus (HIV)

Z20.828 Contact with and (suspected) exposure to other viral communicable diseases

Z21 Asymptomatic human immunodeficiency virus (HIV) infection status

Hospice Cardiopulmonary Conditions and Heart Disease

A5354, L34548-Palmetto GBA, L34538—CGS Administrators, LLC, L3393—National Government Services, Inc.

Indications and limitations of coverage and/or medical necessity:

Palmetto Criteria:

Cardiopulmonary conditions are associated with impairments, activity limitations, and disability. Their impact on any given individual depends on the individual's over-all health status. Health status includes measures of functioning, physical illness, mental wellbeing, as well as environmental factors, such as the availability of palliative care services. The objective of this policy is to present a framework for identifying, documenting, and communicating the unique health care needs of individuals with cardiopulmonary conditions and thus promote the over-all goal of the appropriate care for every person, every time.

Cardiopulmonary conditions may support a prognosis of six months or less under many clinical scenarios. Medicare rules and regulations addressing hospice services require the documentation of sufficient "clinical information and other documentation" to support the certification of individuals as having a terminal illness with a life expectancy of 6 or fewer months, if the illness runs its normal course. The identification of specific structural/functional impairments, together with any relevant activity limitations, should serve as the basis for palliative interventions and care-planning. Use of the International Classification of Functioning, Disability and Health (ICF) to help identify and document the unique service needs of individuals with cardiopulmonary conditions is suggested, but not required.

The health status changes associated with cardiopulmonary conditions can be characterized using categories contained in the ICF. The ICF contains domains (e.g., structures of cardiovascular and respiratory systems, functions of the cardiovascular and respiratory system, communication, mobility, and self-care) that allow for a comprehensive description of an individual's health status and service needs. Information addressing relevant ICF categories, defined within each of these domains, should form the core of the clinical record and be incorporated into the care plan, as appropriate.

Additionally the care plan may be impacted by relevant secondary and/or comorbid conditions. Secondary conditions are directly related to a primary condition. In the case of cardiopulmonary conditions, examples of secondary conditions could include delirium, pneumonia, stasis ulcers and pressure ulcers. Comorbid conditions affecting beneficiaries with cardiopulmonary conditions are, by definition, distinct from the primary condition itself. An example of a comorbid condition would be End Stage Renal Disease (ESRD).

The important roles of secondary and comorbid conditions are described below in order to facilitate their recognition and assist providers in documenting their impact. The identification and documentation of relevant secondary and comorbid conditions, together with the identification and description of associated structural/functional impairments, activity limitations, and environmental factors would help establish hospice eligibility and maintain a beneficiary-centered plan of care.

Secondary Conditions:

Cardiopulmonary conditions may be complicated by secondary conditions. The significance of a given secondary condition is best described by defining the structural/functional impairments—together with any limitation in activity and restriction in participation—related to the secondary condition. The occurrence of secondary conditions in beneficiaries with cardiopulmonary conditions results from the presence of impairments in such body functions as heart/respiratory rate and rhythm, contraction force of ventricular muscles, blood supply to the heart, sleep functions, and depth of respiration. These impairments contribute to the increased incidence of secondary conditions such as delirium, pneumonia, stasis ulcers and pressure ulcers observed in Medicare beneficiaries with cardiopulmonary conditions. Secondary conditions themselves may be associated with a new set of structural/functional impairments that may or may not respond/be amenable to treatment.

Ultimately, in order to support a hospice plan of care, the combined effects of the primary cardiopulmonary condition and any identified secondary condition(s) should be such that most beneficiaries with the identified impairments would have a prognosis of six months or less.

Comorbid Conditions:

The significance of a given comorbid condition is best described by defining the structural/functional impairments—together with any limitation in activity and restriction in participation—related to the comorbid condition. For example a beneficiary with a primary cardiopulmonary condition and ESRD could have specific ESRD-related impairments of water, mineral and electrolyte balance functions coexisting with the cardiopulmonary impairments associated with the primary cardiopulmonary condition (e.g., Aortic Stenosis, Chronic Obstructive Pulmonary Disease, or Heart Failure).

Ultimately, in order to support a hospice plan of care, the combined effects of the primary cardiopulmonary condition and any identified comorbid condition(s) should be such that most beneficiaries with the identified impairments would have a prognosis of six months or less.

The documentation of structural/functional impairments and activity limitations facilitate the selection of the most appropriate intervention strategies (palliative/hospice versus long-term disease management) and provide objective criteria for determining the effects of such interventions. The documentation of these variables is thus essential in the determination of reasonable and necessary Medicare Hospice Services.

CGS Criteria:

Patients will be considered to be in the terminal stage of heart disease (life expectancy of six months or less) if they meet the following criteria. (1 and 2 should be present. Factors from 3 will add supporting documentation.):

1. At the time of initial certification or recertification for hospice, the patient is or has been already optimally treated for heart disease or is not a candidate for a surgical procedure or has declined a procedure. (Optimally treated means that patients who are not on vasodilators have a medical reason for refusing these drugs, e.g., hypotension or renal disease.)
2. The patient is classified as New York Heart Association (NYHA) Class IV and may have significant symptoms of heart failure or angina at rest. (Class IV patients with heart disease have an inability to carry on any physical activity without discomfort. Symptoms of heart failure or of the anginal syndrome may be present even at rest. If any physical activity is undertaken, discomfort is increased.) Significant congestive heart failure may be documented by an ejection fraction of ≤20%, but is not required if not already available.

Documentation of the following factors will support but is not required to establish eligibility for hospice care:

*   Treatment resistant symptomatic supraventricular or ventricular arrhythmias;
*   History of cardiac arrest or resuscitation;
*   History of unexplained syncope;
*   Brain embolism of cardiac origin;
*   Concomitant HIV disease.

Stages of Heart Failure (HF)

[ACC/AHA Guidelines for the Evaluation and Management of Chronic Heart Failure in the Adult: Executive Summary A Report of the American College of Cardiology/American Heart Association Task Force on Practice Guidelines (Committee to Revise the 1995 Guidelines for the Evaluation and Management of Heart Failure)]

Stage A
Patients at high risk of developing HF because of the presence of conditions that are strongly associated with the development of HF. Such patients have no identified structural or functional abnormalities of the pericardium, myocardium, or cardiac valves and have never shown signs or symptoms of HF.

Example: Systemic hypertension; coronary artery disease; diabetes mellitus; history of cardiotoxic drug therapy or alcohol abuse; personal history of rheumatic fever; family history of cardiomyopathy.

Stage B
Patients who have developed structural heart disease that is strongly associated with the development of HF but who have never shown signs or symptoms of HF.

Example: Left ventricular hypertrophy or fibrosis; left ventricular dilatation or hypocontractility; asymptomatic valvular heart disease; previous myocardial infarction.

Stage C
Patients who have current or prior symptoms of HF associated with underlying structural heart disease.

Example: Dyspnea or fatigue due to left ventricular systolic dysfunction; asymptomatic patients who are undergoing treatment for prior symptoms of HF.

Stage D
Patients with advanced structural heart disease and marked symptoms of HF at rest despite maximal medical therapy and who require specialized interventions.

Example: Patients who are frequently hospitalized for HF or cannot be safely discharged from the hospital; patients in the hospital awaiting heart transplantation; patients at home receiving continuous intravenous support for symptom relief or being supported with a mechanical circulatory assist device; patients in a hospice setting for management of HF.

NYHA Functional Classification for Congestive Heart Failure
The New York Heart Association (NYHA) Functional Classification provides a simple way of classifying heart disease (originally cardiac failure). It places patients in one of four categories, based on how much they are limited during physical activity:

Class I: patients with no limitation of activities; they suffer no symptoms from ordinary activities.

Class II: patients with slight, mild limitation of activity; they are comfortable with rest or with mild exertion.

Class III: patients with marked limitation of activity; they are comfortable only at rest.

Class IV: patients who should be at complete rest, confined to bed or chair; any physical activity brings on discomfort and symptoms occur at rest.

Hospice Stroke and Coma

L32015, CGS Administrators, LLC(CGS); L25678, National Government Services (NGS)

Indications and limitations of coverage and/or medical necessity: Patients will be considered to be in the terminal stage of stroke or coma (life expectancy of six months or less) if they meet the following criteria.

Stroke:

1. Poor functional status with Karnofsky score 40% or less;
2. Inability to maintain hydration and caloric intake with one of the following:
    *   Weight loss > 10% in the last 6 months or > 7.5% in the last 3 months
    *   Serum albumin < 2.5 gm/dl
    *   Current history of pulmonary aspiration not responsive to speech language pathology intervention; Sequential calorie counts documenting inadequate caloric/fluid intake
    *   Dysphagia severe enough to prevent patient from continuing fluids/foods necessary to sustain life and patient does not receive artificial nutrition and hydration

Coma (any etiology):

1. Comatose patients with any three of the following on day three of coma:
    *   Abnormal brain stem response
    *   Absent verbal response
    *   Absent withdrawal response to pain
    *   Serum creatinine >1.5 mg/dl

Documentation of the following factors will support eligibility for hospice care:

1. Documentation of medical complications, in the context of progressive clinical decline, within the previous 12 months, which support a terminal prognosis:
    *   Aspiration pneumonia
    *   Upper urinary tract infection (pyelonephritis)
    *   Sepsis
    *   Refractory stage 3-4 decubitus ulcers
    *   Fever recurrent after antibiotics

Documentation of diagnostic imaging factors which support poor prognosis after stroke include:

A. For non-traumatic hemorrhagic stroke:
    *   Large-volume hemorrhage on CT:
        – Infratentorial: ≥20 ml.
        – Supratentorial: ≥50 ml.
    *   Ventricular extension of hemorrhage.
    *   Surface area of involvement of hemorrhage ≥30% of cerebrum.
    *   Midline shift ≥1.5 cm.
    *   Obstructive hydrocephalus in patient who declines, or is not a candidate for, ventriculoperitoneal shunt.

B. For thrombotic/embolic stroke:
    *   Large anterior infarcts with both cortical and subcortical involvement.
    *   Large bihemispheric infarcts.

Appendix N: Hospice Criteria for Medicare Coverage of Noncancer Hospice Care

- Basilar artery occlusion.
- Bilateral vertebral artery occlusion.

ICD-10-CM codes that support medical necessity:

I60.00–I60.9	Nontraumatic subarachnoid hemorrhage
I61.0–I61.9	Nontraumatic intercerebral hemorrhage
I62.00–I62.9	Other and unspecified nontraumatic intracranial hemorrhage
I63.00–I63.9	Cerebral infarction due to occlusion and stenosis of cerebral and precerebral arteries
I65.01–I65.9	Occlusion and stenosis of precerebral arteries not resulting in cerebral infarction
I66.01–I66.9	Occlusion and stenosis of cerebral arteries not resulting in cerebral infarction
R40.20–R40.244	Coma

Hospice Alzheimer's Disease and Related Disorders

L34538—CGS Administrators, LLC, L3393—National Government Services, Inc, L34567—Palmetto GBA

The following criteria based on the FAST scale is from the PGBA local coverage determination.

The Reisberg Functional Assessment Staging (FAST) Scale has been used for many years to describe Medicare beneficiaries with Alzheimer's disease and a prognosis of six months or less. The FAST Scale is a 16-item scale designed to parallel the progressive activity limitations associated with Alzheimer's disease. Stage 7 identifies the threshold of activity limitation that would support a six-month prognosis. The FAST Scale does not address the impact of comorbid and secondary conditions. These two variables are thus considered separately by this policy.

FAST Scale Items:
Stage #1: (1) normal adult — No difficulty, either subjectively or objectively

Stage #2: (2) normal older adult — Complains of forgetting location of objects; subjective work difficulties

Stage #3: (3) early Alzheimer's disease — Decreased job functioning evident to coworkers; difficulty in traveling to new locations

Stage #4: (4) mild Alzheimer's — Decreased ability to perform complex tasks (e.g., planning dinner for guests; handling finances)

Stage #5: (5) moderate Alzheimer's — Requires assistance in choosing proper clothing

Stage #6: (6) moderately severe Alzheimer's — Decreased ability to dress, bathe, and toilet independently:

- Sub-stage 6a: Difficulty putting clothing on properly
- Sub-stage 6b: Unable to bathe properly; may develop fear of bathing
- Sub-stage 6c: Inability to handle mechanics of toileting (i.e., forgets to flush, does not wipe properly)
- Sub-stage 6d: Urinary incontinence
- Sub-stage 6e: Fecal incontinence

Stage #7: (7) severe Alzheimer's — Loss of speech, locomotion, and consciousness:

- Sub-stage 7a: Ability to speak limited (1 to 5 words a day)
- Sub-stage 7b: All intelligible vocabulary lost
- Sub-stage 7c: Non-ambulatory
- Sub-stage 7d: Unable to sit up independently
- Sub-stage 7e: Unable to smile
- Sub-stage 7f: Unable to hold head up

Comorbid Conditions:
The significance of a given comorbid condition is best described by defining the structural/functional impairments - together with any limitation in activity - related to the comorbid condition. For example, a beneficiary with Alzheimer's disease and clinically significant CHD or COPD would have specific impairments of cardiorespiratory function (e.g., dyspnea, orthopnea, wheezing, chest pain) which may or may not respond/be amenable to treatment. The identified impairments in cardiorespiratory function would be associated with both specific structural impairments of the coronary arteries or bronchial tree and may be associated with activity limitations (e.g., mobility, self-care). Ultimately, the combined effects of the

Alzheimer's disease (stage 7 or beyond) and any comorbid condition should be such that most beneficiaries with Alzheimer's disease and similar impairments would have a prognosis of six months or less.

Secondary Conditions:
Alzheimer's disease may be complicated by secondary conditions. The significance of a given secondary condition is best described by defining the structural/functional impairments - together with any limitation in activity related to the secondary condition. The occurrence of secondary conditions in beneficiaries with Alzheimer's disease is facilitated by the presence of impairments in such body functions as mental functioning and movement functions. Such functional impairments contribute to the increased incidence of secondary conditions such as delirium and pressure ulcers observed in Medicare beneficiaries with Alzheimer's Disease. Secondary conditions themselves may be associated with a new set of structural/functional impairments that may or may not respond/be amenable to treatment. Ultimately, the combined effects of the Alzheimer's disease (stage 7 or beyond) and any secondary condition should be such that most beneficiaries with Alzheimer's disease and similar impairments would have a prognosis of six months or less.

The documentation of structural/functional impairments and activity limitations facilitate the selection of intervention strategies (palliative vs. curative) and provide objective criteria for determining the effects of such interventions. The documentation of these variables is thus essential in the determination of reasonable and necessary Medicare Hospice Services.

For beneficiaries with Alzheimer's disease to be eligible for hospice the individual should have a FAST level of greater than or equal to 7 and specific comorbid or secondary conditions meeting the above criteria.

ICD-10-CM codes that support medical necessity:

F03.90–F03.91	Unspecified dementia
G30.0–G30.9	Alzheimer's disease
G31.01	Pick's disease
G31.1	Senile degeneration of brain, not elsewhere classified
G31.85	Corticobasal degeneration

The following criteria are from the CGS and NGS local coverage determinations.

Patients will be considered to be in the terminal stage of dementia (life expectancy of six months or less) if they meet the following criteria. This section is specific for Alzheimer's disease and related disorders.

1. Patients with dementia should show all the following characteristics:

   a. Stage seven or beyond according to the Functional Assessment Staging Scale;

   b. Unable to ambulate without assistance;

   c. Unable to dress without assistance;

   d. Unable to bathe without assistance;

   e. Urinary and fecal incontinence, intermittent or constant;

   f. No consistently meaningful verbal communication: stereotypical phrases only or the ability to speak is limited to six or fewer intelligible words.

2. Patients should have had one of the following within the past 12 months:

   a. Aspiration pneumonia;

   b. Pyelonephritis or other upper urinary tract infection;

   c. Septicemia;

   d. Decubitus ulcers, multiple, stage 3-4;

   e. Fever, recurrent after antibiotics;

   f. Inability to maintain sufficient fluid and calorie intake with 10% weight loss during the previous six months or serum albumin < 2.5 gm/dl.

Hospice Amyotrophic Lateral Sclerosis (ALS) and Neurological Conditions

34547—Palmetto GBA, L33393—National Government Services, L34538—CGS Administrators, LLC

Indications and limitations of coverage and/or medical necessity:

General Considerations:

1. ALS tends to progress in a linear fashion over time. Thus the overall rate of decline in each patient is fairly constant and predictable, unlike many other non-cancer diseases.

2. However, no single variable deteriorates at a uniform rate in all patients. Therefore, multiple clinical parameters are required to judge the progression of ALS.

3. Although ALS usually presents in a localized anatomical area, the location of initial presentation does not correlate with survival time. By the time patients become end-stage, muscle denervation has become widespread, affecting all areas of the body, and initial predominance patterns do not persist.

4. Progression of disease differs markedly from patient to patient. Some patients decline rapidly and die quickly; others progress more slowly. For this reason, the history of the rate of progression in individual patients is important to obtain to predict prognosis.

5. In end-stage ALS, two factors are critical in determining prognosis: ability to breathe, and to a lesser extent ability to swallow. The former can be managed by artificial ventilation, and the latter by gastrostomy or other artificial feeding, unless the patient has recurrent aspiration pneumonia. While not necessarily a contraindication to hospice care, the decision to institute either artificial ventilation or artificial feeding will significantly alter six month prognosis.

6. Examination by a neurologist within three months of assessment for hospice is advised, both to confirm the diagnosis and to assist with prognosis.

CGS specifics:

Patients will be considered to be in the terminal stage of ALS (life expectancy of six months or less) if they meet the following criteria: (Must fulfill 1, 2, or 3.)

1. The patient must demonstrate critically impaired breathing capacity.

   a. Critically impaired breathing capacity as demonstrated by all the following characteristics occurring within the 12 months preceding initial hospice certification:

      – Vital capacity (VC) less than 30% of normal
      – Significant dyspnea at rest
      – Requiring supplemental oxygen at rest
      – Patient declines invasive artificial ventilation.

2. Patient must demonstrate both rapid progression of ALS and critical nutritional impairment.

   a. Rapid progression of ALS as demonstrated by all the following characteristics occurring within the 12 months preceding initial hospice certification:

      – Progression from independent ambulation to wheelchair or bed-bound status;
      – Progression from normal to barely intelligible or unintelligible speech
      – Progression from normal to pureed diet;
      – Progression from independence in most or all activities of daily living (ADLs) to needing major assistance by caretaker in all ADLs.

   b. Critical nutritional impairment as demonstrated by all the following characteristics occurring within the 12 months preceding initial hospice certification:

      – Oral intake of nutrients and fluids insufficient to sustain life;
      – Continuing weight loss;
      – Dehydration or hypovolemia;
      – Absence of artificial feeding methods.

3. Patient must demonstrate both rapid progression of ALS and life-threatening complications

   a. Rapid progression of ALS, see 2.a. above.

   b. Life-threatening complications as demonstrated by one of the following characteristics occurring within the 12 months preceding initial hospice certification:

      – Recurrent aspiration pneumonia (with or without tube feedings);
      – Upper urinary tract infection, e.g., pyelonephritis;
      – Sepsis;
      – Recurrent fever after antibiotic therapy.;
      – Stage 3 or 4 decubitus ulcer(s).

NGS specifics:

Patients are considered eligible for Hospice care if they do not elect tracheostomy and invasive ventilation and display evidence of critically impaired respiratory function (with or without use of NIPPV) and/or severe nutritional insufficiency (with or without use of a gastrostomy tube).

Critically impaired respiratory function is as defined by:

1. FVC < 40% predicted (seated or supine) and 2 or more of the following symptoms and/or signs:

   Dyspnea at rest

   Orthopnea

   Use of accessory respiratory musculature

   Paradoxical abdominal motion

   Respiratory rate > 20

   Reduced speech/vocal volume

   Weakened cough

   Symptoms of sleep disordered breathing

   Frequent awakening

   Daytime somnolence / excessive daytime sleepiness

   Unexplained headaches

   Unexplained confusion

   Unexplained anxiety

   Unexplained nausea

2. If unable to perform the FVC test, patients meet this criterion if they manifest 3 or more of the above symptoms/signs.

Severe nutritional insufficiency is defined as:

   Dysphagia with progressive weight loss of at least 5% of body weight with or without election for gastrostomy tube insertion.

   These revised criteria rely less on the measured FVC, and as such reflect the reality that not all patients with ALS can or will undertake regular pulmonary function tests.

Hospice Liver Disease

L34544—Palmetto GBA, L33393—National Government Services, L34538—CGS Administrators, LLC

Indications and limitations of coverage and/or medical necessity:

Patients will be considered to be in the terminal stage of liver disease (life expectancy of six months or less) if they meet the following criteria: (1 and 2 must be present, factors from 3 will lend supporting documentation.)

1. The patient should show both a and b:

   a. Prothrombin time prolonged more than 5 seconds over control, or International Normalized Ration (INR) >1.5;

   b. Serum albumin < 2.5 gm/dl.

2. End stage liver disease is present and the patient shows at least one of the following:

   a. Ascites, refractory to treatment or patient noncompliant;

   b. Spontaneous bacterial peritonitis;

   c. Hepatorenal syndrome (elevated creatinine and BUN with oliguria (< 400 ml/day) and urine sodium concentration <10 mEq/l);

   d. Hepatic encephalopathy, refractory to treatment, or patient noncompliant;

   e. Recurrent variceal bleeding, despite intensive therapy.

3. Documentation of the following factors will support eligibility for hospice care:

   a. Progressive malnutrition

   b. Muscle wasting with reduced strength and endurance

   c. Continued active alcoholism (>80 gm ethanol/day)

d. Hepatocellular carcinoma

e. HBsAg (Hepatitis B) positivity

f. Hepatitis C refractory to interferon treatment.

Patients awaiting liver transplant who otherwise fit the above criteria may be certified for the Medicare hospice benefit, but if a donor organ is procured, the patient must be discharged from hospice.

ICD-10-CM codes that support medical necessity:

C22.0	Liver cell carcinoma
C22.2	Hepatoblastoma
C22.3–C22.7	Sarcoma of liver
C22.8	Malignant neoplasm of liver, primary, unspecified as to type
K70.2	Alcoholic fibrosis and sclerosis of liver
K70.30–K70.31	Alcoholic cirrhosis of liver
K70.41	Alcoholic hepatic failure with coma
K71.0–K71.9	Toxic liver disease
K72.01	Acute and subacute hepatic failure with coma
K72.11	Chronic hepatic failure with coma
K72.91	Hepatic failure, unspecified with coma
K74.0	Hepatic fibrosis
K73.0–K73.9	Chronic hepatitis not elsewhere classified
K74.3–K74.5	Biliary cirrhosis
K74.60–K74.69	Other and unspecified cirrhosis of liver
K75.2–K75.4	Hepatitis
K75.81	Nonalcoholic steatohepatitis (NASH)
K76.4	Peliosis hepatis
K76.7	Hepatorenal syndrome
K76.81	Hepatopulmonary syndrome

Hospice Renal Disease

L34559—Palmetto GBA, L33393—National Government Services, L34538—CGS Administrators, LLC

Indications and limitations of coverage and/or medical necessity:

Patients will be considered to be in the terminal stage of renal disease (life expectancy of six months or less) if they meet the following criteria:

CGS criteria:

Acute renal failure (1, 2, and 3 must be present; factors from 4 will lend supporting documentation):

1. The patient is not seeking dialysis or renal transplant;

2. Creatinine clearance <10 cc/min (<15 cc/min. for diabetes); based on measurement or calculation; or <15cc/min (<20cc/min for diabetics) with comorbidity of congestive heart failure;

3. Serum creatinine >8.0 mg/dl (>6.0 mg/dl for diabetes)

4. Comorbid conditions:

    • Mechanical ventilation;

    • Malignancy (other organ system);

    • Chronic lung disease;

    • Advanced cardiac disease;

    • Advanced liver disease;

    • Sepsis;

    • Immunosuppression/AIDS;

    • Albumin < 3.5 gm/dl;

    • Cachexia;

    • Platelet count < 25,000;

    • Disseminated intravascular coagulation;

    • Gastrointestinal bleeding.

Chronic renal failure (1, 2, and 3 must be present; factors from 4 will lend supporting documentation):

1. The patient is not seeking dialysis or renal transplant or is discontinuing dialysis;

2. Creatinine clearance <10 cc/min (<15 cc/min for diabetics) based on measurement or calculation; or < 15cc/min (< 20cc/min for diabetics) with co-morbidity of congestive heart failure

3. Serum creatinine > 8.0 mg/dl (> 6.0 mg/dl for diabetes);

4. Signs and symptoms of renal failure:

    • Uremia;

    • Oliguria (< 400 cc/24 hours);

    • Intractable hyperkalemia (> 7.0) not responsive to treatment;

    • Uremic pericarditis;

    • Hepatorenal syndrome;

    • Intractable fluid overload, not responsive to treatment.

NGS criteria:

Patients will be considered to be in the terminal stage of renal disease (life expectancy of six months or less) if they meet the following criteria:

Acute Renal Failure (1 and either 2, 3 or 4 should be present. Factors from 5 will lend supporting documentation.)

1. The patient is not seeking dialysis or renal transplant, or is discontinuing dialysis. As with any other condition, an individual with renal disease is eligible for the Hospice benefit if that individual has a prognosis of six months or less, if the illness runs its normal course. There is no regulation precluding patients on dialysis from electing Hospice care. However, the continuation of dialysis will significantly alter a patient's prognosis, and thus potentially impact that individual's eligibility.

    When an individual elects Hospice care for end stage renal disease (ESRD) or for a condition to which the need for dialysis is related, the Hospice agency is financially responsible for the dialysis. In such cases, there is no additional reimbursement beyond the per diem rate. The only situation in which a beneficiary may access both the Hospice benefit and the ESRD benefit is when the need for dialysis is not related to the patient's terminal illness.

2. Creatinine clearance <10 cc/min (<15 cc/min. for diabetics); or <15cc/min (<20cc/min for diabetics) with comorbidity of congestive heart failure.

3. Serum creatinine > 8.0 mg/dl (>6.0 mg/dl for diabetics).

4. Estimated glomerular filtration rate (GFR) <10 ml/min.

5. Comorbid conditions:

    a. Mechanical ventilation;

    b. Malignancy (other organ system);

    c. Chronic lung disease;

    d. Advanced cardiac disease;

    e. Advanced liver disease;

    f. Immunosuppression/AIDS;

    g. Albumin < 3.5 gm/dl;

    h. Platelet count < 25,000;

    i. Disseminated intravascular coagulation;

    j. Gastrointestinal bleeding.

Chronic Kidney Disease (1 and either 2, 3 or 4 should be present. Factors from 5 will lend supporting documentation.)

1. The patient is not seeking dialysis or renal transplant, or is discontinuing dialysis; As with any other condition, an individual with renal disease is eligible for the Hospice benefit if that individual has a prognosis of six months or less, if the illness runs its normal course. There is no regulation precluding patients on dialysis from electing Hospice care. However, the continuation of dialysis will significantly alter a patient's prognosis, and thus potentially impact that individual's eligibility.

When an individual elects hospice care for end stage renal disease (ESRD) or for a condition to which the need for dialysis is related, the Hospice agency is financially responsible for the dialysis. In such cases, there is no additional reimbursement beyond the per diem rate. The only situation in which a beneficiary may access both the Hospice benefit and the ESRD benefit is when the need for dialysis is not related to the patient's terminal illness.

2. Creatinine clearance <10 cc/min (<15 cc/min for diabetics); or <15cc/min (<20cc/min for diabetics) with comorbidity of congestive heart failure.

3. Serum creatinine >8.0 mg/dl (>6.0 mg/dl for diabetics).

4. Signs and symptoms of renal failure:

   a. Uremia;

   b. Oliguria (<400 cc/24 hours);

   c. Intractable hyperkalemia (> 7.0) not responsive to treatment;

   d. Uremic pericarditis;

   e. Hepatorenal syndrome;

   f. Intractable fluid overload, not responsive to treatment.

5. Estimated glomerular filtration rate (GFR) <10 ml/min.

Indications and/or limitations of coverage:

Palmetto Criteria

End stage renal disease (ESRD) may support a prognosis of six months or less under many clinical scenarios. The identification of specific structural/functional impairments, together with any relevant activity limitations, should serve as the basis for palliative interventions and care planning. The structural and functional impairments associated with a primary diagnosis of ESRD are often complicated by comorbid and/or secondary conditions. Comorbid conditions affecting beneficiaries with ESRD are by definition distinct from the ESRD itself—examples include vascular disease manifested as coronary heart disease (CHD), peripheral vascular disease (PVD), and vascular dementia. Secondary conditions, on the other hand, are directly related to a primary condition. In the case of ESRD, examples include secondary hyperparathyroidism, calciphylaxis, nephrogenic systemic fibrosis, electrolyte abnormalities and anorexia. The important roles of comorbid and secondary conditions are described below in order to facilitate their recognition and assist providers in documenting their impact. Use of the International Classification of Functioning, Disability and Health (ICF) is suggested, but not required.

For beneficiaries with ESRD the identification of relevant comorbid and secondary conditions, together with the identification and description of associated structural/functional impairments, activity limitations, and environmental factors would help establish hospice eligibility and maintain a beneficiary-centered plan of care.

Secondary Conditions:

ESRD may be complicated by secondary conditions. The significance of a given secondary condition is best described by defining the structural/functional impairments—together with any limitation in activity—related to the secondary condition. The occurrence of secondary conditions in beneficiaries with ESRD is facilitated by the presence of impairments in such body functions as urinary excretory function, water, mineral and electrolyte function, and endocrine gland functions. Such functional impairments contribute to the increased incidence of secondary conditions such as hyperkalemia, fluid overload, and secondary hyperparathyroidism observed in Medicare beneficiaries with ESRD. Secondary conditions themselves may be associated with a new set of structural/functional impairments that may or may not respond/be amenable to treatment. Ultimately, the combined effects of the ESRD and any secondary condition should be such that most beneficiaries with ESRD and similar impairments would have a prognosis of six months or less.

Comorbid Conditions:

The significance of a given comorbid condition is best described by defining the structural/functional impairments—together with any limitation in activity—related to the comorbid condition. For example, a beneficiary with ESRD and clinically significant CHD would have specific impairments of cardiovascular structure/function (e.g., narrowing of coronary arteries, dyspnea, orthopnea, chest pain) which may or may not respond/be amenable to treatment. The identified impairments in cardiovascular structure/function may be associated with activity limitations (e.g., mobility, self-care). Ultimately, the combined effects of the ESRD and any comorbid condition should be such that most beneficiaries with ESRD and similar impairments would have a prognosis of six months or less.

The documentation of structural/functional impairments and activity limitations facilitates the selection of intervention strategies (palliative vs. long-term disease management/curative) and provides objective criteria for determining the effects of such interventions. The documentation of these variables is thus essential in the determination of reasonable and necessary Medicare Hospice Services.

ICD-10-CM codes that support medical necessity:

I12.Ø	Hypertensive chronic kidney disease with stage 5 chronic kidney disease or end stage renal disease
N17.Ø	Acute kidney failure with tubular necrosis
N17.1	Acute kidney failure with acute cortical necrosis
N17.2	Acute kidney failure with medullary necrosis
N17.8	Other acute kidney failure
N17.9	Acute kidney failure, unspecified
N18.6	End stage renal disease
N19	Unspecified kidney failure

Hospice Pulmonary Disease

L33393—National Government Services, L34538—CGS Administrators, LLC

Indications and/or limitations of coverage:

Patients will be considered to be in the terminal stage of pulmonary disease (life expectancy of six months or less) if they meet the following criteria. The criteria refer to patients with various forms of advanced pulmonary disease who eventually follow a final common pathway for end stage pulmonary disease. (1 and 2 should be present. Documentation of 3, 4, and 5, will lend supporting documentation.):

1. Severe chronic lung disease as documented by both a and b:

   a. Disabling dyspnea at rest, poorly or unresponsive to bronchodilators, resulting in decreased functional capacity, e.g., bed to chair existence, fatigue, and cough: (Documentation of Forced Expiratory Volume in One Second (FEV1), after bronchodilator, less than 30% of predicted is objective evidence for disabling dyspnea, but is not necessary to obtain.)

   b. Progression of end stage pulmonary disease, as evidenced by increasing visits to the emergency department or hospitalizations for pulmonary infections and/or respiratory failure or increasing physician home visits prior to initial certification. (Documentation of serial decrease of FEV1>40 ml/year is objective evidence for disease progression, but is not necessary to obtain.)

2. Hypoxemia at rest on room air, as evidenced by pO2 =55 mmHg; or oxygen saturation =88%, determined either by arterial blood gases or oxygen saturation monitors; (These values may be obtained from recent hospital records.) OR Hypercapnia, as evidenced by pCO2 =50 mmHg. (This value may be obtained from recent [within 3 months] hospital records.)

3. Right heart failure (RHF) secondary to pulmonary disease (Cor pulmonale) (e.g., not secondary to left heart disease or valvulopathy).

4. Unintentional progressive weight loss of greater than 10% of body weight over the preceding six months.

5. Resting tachycardia >100/min.

Hospice the Adult Failure to Thrive Syndrome

L34558—Palmetto GBA.

Indications and/or limitations of coverage and medical necessity:

The adult failure to thrive syndrome is characterized by unexplained weight loss, malnutrition and disability. The syndrome has been associated with multiple primary conditions (e.g., infections and malignancies), but always includes two defining clinical elements, namely nutritional impairment and disability. The nutritional impairment and disability associated with the adult failure to thrive syndrome may be severe enough to have an impact on the patient's short-term survival.

The adult failure to thrive syndrome may manifest as an irreversible progression in the patient's nutritional impairment/disability despite a trial of therapy (i.e., treatment intended to affect the primary condition responsible for the patient's clinical presentation). The presence of comorbid conditions may hasten the patient's clinical progression and as such should be identified and addressed. This hospice policy addresses those cases where reversible causes of severe nutritional impairment and disability (i.e., the adult failure to thrive syndrome) have been excluded.

The Medicare Hospice Benefit is predicated upon physician-certification that an individual entitled to Part A of Medicare is terminally ill. An individual is considered to be terminally ill if the individual has a medical prognosis that his or her life expectancy is six months or less if the terminal illness runs its normal course. The medical criteria listed below would support a terminal prognosis for individuals with the adult failure to thrive syndrome. Medical criteria 1 and 2 are important indicators of nutritional and functional status respectively, and would thus support a terminal prognosis if met.

1. The nutritional impairment associated with the adult failure to thrive syndrome should be severe enough to impact a beneficiary's weight. It is expected that the Body Mass Index (BMI) of beneficiaries electing the Medicare Hospice Benefit for the adult failure to thrive syndrome will be below 22 kg/m 2 and that the patient is either declining enteral/parenteral nutritional support or has not responded to such nutritional support, despite an adequate caloric intake.

    BMI (kg/m 2) = 703 x (weight in pounds) divided by (height in inches) 2

2. The disability associated with the adult failure to thrive syndrome should be such that the individual is significantly disabled. Significant disability would be demonstrated by a Karnofsky or Palliative Performance Scale value less than or equal to 40%.

Both the beneficiary's BMI and level of disability should be determined using measurements/observations made within six months (180 days) of the most recent certification/recertification date. If enteral nutritional support has been instituted prior to the election of the Hospice Medicare Benefit and will be continued, the BMI and level of disability should be determined using measurements/observations made at the time of the initial certification and at each subsequent recertification.

At the time of recertification recumbent measurement(s) (anthropometry) such as mid-arm muscle area in cm 2 may be substituted for BMI with documentation as to why a BMI could not be measured. This information will be subject to review on a case by case basis.

In the event a beneficiary presenting with a nutritional impairment and disability does not meet the medical criteria listed above, but is still thought to be eligible for the Medicare Hospice Benefit, an alternate diagnosis that best describes the clinical circumstances of the individual beneficiary should be selected (e.g. R63.4 "abnormal loss of weight" and R64 "Cachexia").

ICD-10 Codes That Support Medical Necessity:

M62.84	Sarcopenia
R62.51	Failure to thrive (child)
R62.7	Adult failure to thrive
R63.4	Abnormal weight loss
R64	Cachexia

Source of Information
Social Security Act, Sections, 1102, 1812 (a)(4)and (d);1813 (a) (4); 1814 (a)(7) and (l); 1862 (a)(1),(6), and (9); 1861 (dd), 1871

42 CFR Part 418

CMS Manual Publication 100-2, Medicare Benefits Policy Chapter 9 Coverage of Hospice Services under Hospital Insurance, §10 Requirements

CMS Manual Publication 100-3, Medicare National Coverage Determinations

CMS Medicare Coverage Database:

http://www.cms.hhs.gov/mcd/search.asp? Search: Local Coverage, policies (LMRP/LCD); Final policies only Geographic area: all states Coverage topics: Hospice

Appendix O: Hospice Diagnosis and Quality Reporting Guidance

Highlights of the 2017 Hospice Final Rule

FY 2017 Hospice Wage Index and Rate Update

The hospice wage index is used to adjust payment rates for hospice agencies under the Medicare program to reflect local differences in area wage levels, based on the location where services are furnished. The hospice wage index utilizes the wage adjustment factors used by the Secretary for purposes of section 1886(d)(3)(E) of the Act for hospital wage adjustments. Our regulations at §418.306(c) require each labor market to be established using the most current hospital wage data available, including any changes made by the Office of Management and Budget (OMB) to the Metropolitan Statistical Areas (MSAs) definitions.

CMS used the previous FY's hospital wage index data to calculate the hospice wage index values. For FY 2017, the hospice wage index will be based on the FY 2016 pre-floor, prereclassified hospital wage index. This means that the hospital wage data used for the hospice wage index is not adjusted to take into account any geographic reclassification of hospitals including those in accordance with section 1886(d)(8)(B) or 1886(d)(10) of the Act. The appropriate wage index value is applied to the labor portion of the payment rate based on the geographic area in which the beneficiary resides when receiving RHC or CHC. The appropriate wage index value is applied to the labor portion of the payment rate based on the geographic location of the facility for beneficiaries receiving GIP or Inpatient Respite Care (IRC).

As described in the August 8, 1997 Hospice Wage Index final rule (62 FR 42860), the pre-floor and pre-reclassified hospital wage index is used as the raw wage index for the hospice benefit. These raw wage index values are then subject to application of the hospice floor to compute the hospice wage index used to determine payments to hospices. Pre-floor, prereclassified hospital wage index values below 0.8 are adjusted by a 15 percent increase subject to a maximum wage index value of 0.8. For example, if County A has a pre-floor, pre-reclassified hospital wage index value of 0.3994, we would multiply 0.3994 by 1.15, which equals 0.4593. Since 0.4593 is not greater than 0.8, then County A's hospice wage index would be 0.4593. In another example, if County B has a pre-floor, pre-reclassified hospital wage index value of 0.7440, we would multiply 0.7440 by 1.15 which equals 0.8556. Because 0.8556 is greater than 0.8, County B's hospice wage index would be 0.8.

OMB has published subsequent bulletins regarding CBSA changes. On February 28, 2013, OMB issued OMB Bulletin No. 13-01, announcing revisions to the delineation of MSAs, Micropolitan Statistical Areas, and Combined Statistical Areas, and guidance on uses of the delineation in these areas. A copy of this bulletin is available online at:

http://www.whitehouse.gov/sites/default/files/omb/bulletins/2013/b-13-01.pdf. This bulletin states that it "provides the delineations of all Metropolitan Statistical Areas, Metropolitan Divisions, Micropolitan Statistical Areas, Combined Statistical Areas, and New England City and Town Areas in the United States and Puerto Rico based on the standards published on June 28, 2010, in the Federal Register (75 FR 37246 through 37252) and Census Bureau data."

In the FY 2016 Hospice Wage Index final rule (80 FR 47178), CMS adopted the OMB's new area delineations using a 1-year transition. In the FY 2016 Hospice Wage Index and Payment Rate Update final rule (80 FR 47178), CMS stated that beginning October 1, 2016, the wage index for all hospice payments would be fully based on the new OMB delineations.

For FY 2017, the updated wage data are for hospital cost reporting periods beginning on or after October 1, 2011 and before October 1, 2012 (FY 2012 cost report data).

The wage index applicable for FY 2017 is available on the CMS Web site at http://www.cms.gov/Medicare/Medicare-Fee-for-Service-Payment/Hospice/index.html. As of FY 2012, the wage index values applicable for the upcoming fiscal year and subsequent fiscal years are no longer published in the Federal Register (77 FR 44242). The hospice wage index for FY 2017 will be effective October 1, 2016 through September 30, 2017.

Hospice Payment Update Percentage

Section 4441(a) of the Balanced Budget Act of 1997 (BBA) amended section 1814(i)(1)(C)(ii)(VI) of the Act to establish updates to hospice rates for FYs 1998 through 2002.

Hospice rates were to be updated by a factor equal to the inpatient hospital market basket index set out under section 1886(b)(3)(B)(iii) of the Act, minus 1 percentage point. Payment rates for FYs since 2002 have been updated according to section

1814(i)(1)(C)(ii)(VII) of the Act, which states that the update to the payment rates for subsequent FYs must be the inpatient market basket percentage for that FY. The Act requires CMS to use the inpatient hospital market basket to determine the hospice payment rate update. In addition, section 3401(g) of the Affordable Care Act mandates that, starting with FY 2013 (and in subsequent FYs), the hospice payment update percentage will be annually reduced by changes in economy-wide productivity as specified in section 1886(b)(3)(B)(xi)(II) of the Act. The statute defines the productivity adjustment to be equal to the 10-year moving average of changes in annual economy-wide private nonfarm business multifactor productivity (MFP) (as projected by the Secretary for the 10-year period ending with the applicable FY, year, cost reporting period, or other annual period) (the "MFP adjustment"). A complete description of the MFP projection methodology is available on CMS's website at: http://www.cms.gov/Research-Statistics-Data-and-Systems/Statistics-Trends-and-Reports/MedicareProgramRatesStats/MarketBasketResearch.html.

In addition to the MFP adjustment, section 3401(g) of the Affordable Care Act also mandates that in FY 2013 through FY 2019, the hospice payment update percentage will be reduced by an additional 0.3 percentage point (although for FY 2014 to FY 2019, the potential 0.3 percentage point reduction is subject to suspension under conditions specified in section 1814(i)(1)(C)(v) of the Act). The hospice payment update percentage for FY 2017 is based on the estimated inpatient hospital market basket update of 2.7 percent (based on IHS Global Insight, Inc.'s second quarter 2016 forecast with historical data through the first quarter of 2016).

Due to the requirements at sections 1886(b)(3)(B)(xi)(II) and 1814(i)(1)(C)(v) of the Act, the estimated inpatient hospital market basket update for FY 2017 of 2.7 percent must be reduced by a MFP adjustment as mandated by Affordable Care Act (currently estimated to be 0.3 percentage point for FY 2017). The estimated inpatient hospital market basket update for FY 2017 is reduced further by 0.3 percentage point, as mandated by the Affordable Care Act. In effect, the hospice payment update percentage for FY 2017 is 2.1 percent.

Currently, the labor portion of the hospice payment rates is as follows: for RHC, 68.71 percent; for CHC, 68.71 percent; for General Inpatient Care, 64.01 percent; and for Respite Care, 54.13 percent. The non-labor portion is equal to 100 percent minus the labor portion for each level of care. Therefore, the non-labor portion of the payment rates is as follows: for RHC, 31.29 percent; for CHC, 31.29 percent; for General Inpatient Care, 35.99 percent; and for Respite Care, 45.87 percent.

Based on IHS Global Insight, Inc.'s updated forecast, the hospice payment update percentage for FY 2017 will be 2.1 percent for hospices that submit the required quality data and 0.1 percent for hospices that do not submit the required quality data.

FY 2017 Hospice Payment Rates

There are four payment categories that are distinguished by the location and intensity of the services provided. The base payments are adjusted for geographic differences in wages by multiplying the labor share, which varies by category, of each base rate by the applicable hospice wage index. A hospice is paid the RHC rate for each day the beneficiary is enrolled in hospice, unless the hospice provides continuous home care, IRC, or general inpatient care. CHC is provided during a period of patient crisis to maintain the person at home; IRC is short-term care to allow the usual caregiver to rest and be relieved from caregiving; and General Inpatient Care (GIP) is to treat symptoms that cannot be managed in another setting.

As discussed in the FY 2016 Hospice Wage Index and Payment Rate Update final rule (80 FR 47172), CMS implemented two different RHC payment rates, one RHC rate for the first 60 days and a second RHC rate for days 61 and beyond. In addition, in the final rule, we adopted a Service Intensity Add-on (SIA) payment, when direct patient care is provided by a RN or social worker during the last 7 days of the beneficiary's life. The SIA payment is equal to the CHC hourly rate multiplied by the hours of nursing or social work provided (up to 4 hours total) that occurred on the day of service. In order to maintain budget neutrality, as required under section 1814(i)(6)(D)(ii) of the Act, the new RHC rates were adjusted by a SIA budget neutrality factor.

As discussed in the FY 2016 Hospice Wage Index and Payment Rate Update final rule (80 FR 47177), CMS will continue to make the SIA payments budget neutral through an annual determination of the SIA budget neutrality factor (SBNF), which will then be applied to the RHC payment rates. The SBNF will be calculated for each FY using the most current and complete FY utilization data available at the time of rulemaking. For FY 2017, the budget neutrality adjustment that applies to days 1

Appendix O: Hospice Diagnosis and Quality Reporting Guidance

through 60 is calculated to be 1.0000. The budget neutrality adjustment that applies to days 61 and beyond is calculated to be 0.9999.

For FY 2017, CMS applied a wage index standardization factor to the FY 2017 hospice payment rates in order to ensure overall budget neutrality when updating the hospice wage index with more recent hospital wage data. Wage index standardization factors are applied in other payment settings such as under home health Prospective Payment System (PPS), IRF PPS, and SNF PPS. Applying a wage index standardization factor to hospice payments will eliminate the aggregate effect of annual variations in hospital wage data. CMS believed that adopting a hospice wage index standardization factor will provide a safeguard to the Medicare program as well as to hospices because it will mitigate fluctuations in the wage index by ensuring that wage index updates and revisions are implemented in a budget neutral manner. To calculate the wage index standardization factor, CMS simulated total payments using the FY 2017 hospice wage index and compared it to our simulation of total payments using the FY 2016 hospice wage index. By dividing payments for each level of care using the FY 2017 wage index by payments for each level of care using the FY 2016 wage index, CMS obtain a wage index standardization factor for each level of care (RHC days 1-60, RHC days 61+, CHC, IRC, and GIP).

Lastly, the hospice payment rates for hospices that submit the required quality data will be increased by the full FY 2017 hospice payment update percentage of 2.1 percent as discussed in section III.C.3 of this final rule. The FY 2017 RHC rates are shown in Table 11. The FY 2017 payment rates for CHC, IRC, and GIP are shown in Table 12.

Table 11: FY 2017 Hospice RHC Payment Rates]

CODE	DESCRIPTION	FY 2017 PAYMENT RATE	SNBF	WAGE INDEX STANDARDIZATION FACTOR	FY 2017 HOSPICE PAYMENT UPDATE PERCENTAGE	FY 2017 PAYMENTRATES
651	Routine Home Care (days 1-60)	$186.84	X 1.0000	X 0.9989	X 1.021	$190.55
651	Routine Home Care (days 61+)	$146.83	X 0.9995	X 1.021	X 1.021	$149.82

Table 12: FY 2017 Hospice CHC, IRC, and GIP Payment Rates

CODE	DESCRIPTION	FY 2016 PAYMENT RATES	INDEX STANDARDIZATION FACTOR	HOSPICE PAYMENT UPDATE PERCENTAGE	FY 2017 PAYMENTRATES
652	Continuous Home Care Full Rate= 24 hours of care $40.19 = FY 2017 hourly Rate	$944.79	X 1.0000	X 1.021	$964.63
655	Inpatient Respite Care	$167.45	X 1.0000	X 1.021	$170.97
656	General Inpatient Care	$720.11	X 0.0006	X 1.021	$734.94

Sections 1814(i)(5)(A) through (C) of the Act required that hospices begin submitting quality data, based on measures to be specified by the Secretary. In the FY 2012 Hospice Wage Index final rule (76 FR 47320 through 47324), CMS implemented a Hospice Quality Reporting Program (HQRP), as required by section 3004 of the Affordable Care Act. Hospices were required to begin collecting quality data in October 2012, and submit that quality data in 2013. Section 1814(i)(5)(A)(i) of the Act requires that beginning with FY 2014 and for each subsequent FY, the Secretary shall reduce the market basket update by 2 percentage points for any hospice that does not comply with the quality data submission requirements with respect to that FY.

Hospice Cap Amount for FY 2017

As discussed in the FY 2016 Hospice Wage Index and Payment Rate Update final rule (80 FR 47183), CMS implemented changes mandated by the Improving Medicare Post-Acute Care Transformation Act of 2014 (IMPACT Act). Specifically, for accounting years that end after September 30, 2016 and before October 1, 2025, the hospice cap is updated by the hospice payment update percentage rather than using the consumer price index for urban consumers (CPI–U). As required by section 1814(i)(2)(B)(ii) of the Act, the hospice cap amount for the 2016 cap year, starting on November 1, 2015 and ending on October 31, 2016, is equal to the 2015

cap amount ($27,382.63) updated by the FY 2016 hospice payment update percentage of 1.6 percent. As such, the 2016 cap amount is $27,820.75.

In the FY 2016 Hospice Wage Index and Payment Rate Update final rule (80 FR 47142), CMS finalized aligning the cap accounting year with the federal FY beginning in 2017. Therefore, the 2017 cap year will start on October 1, 2016 and end on September 30, 2017. Table 26 in the FY 2016 Hospice Wage Index and Payment Rate Update final rule (80 FR 47185) outlines the timeframes for counting beneficiaries and payments during the 2017 transition year. The hospice cap amount for the 2017 cap year will be $28,404.99, which is equal to the 2016 cap amount ($27,820.75) updated by the FY 2017 hospice payment update percentage of 2.1 percent.

Proposed Updates to the Hospice Quality Reporting Program (HQRP)

For the purpose of streamlining the rulemaking process, CMS finalized it's policy in the FY 2016 Hospice Wage Index final rule (80 FR 47187) that when CMS adopted measures for the HQRP beginning with a payment determination year, these measures would automatically be adopted for all subsequent years' payment determinations, unless CMS proposed to remove, suspend, or replace the measures. Quality measures would be considered for removal by CMS for reasons including, but not limited to:

- Measure performance among hospices was so high and unvarying that meaningful distinction in improvements in performance could no longer be made;

- Performance or improvement on a measure did not result in better patient outcomes;

- A measure did not align with current clinical guidelines or practice;

- A more broadly applicable measure (across settings, populations, or conditions) for the particular topic was available;

- A measure that was more proximal in time to desired patient outcomes for the particular topic was available;

- A measure that was more strongly associated with desired patient outcomes for the particular topic was available; or

- Collection or public reporting of a measure led to negative unintended consequences.

For any such removal, the public would be given an opportunity to comment through the annual rulemaking process. However, if there were reason to believe continued collection of a measure raised potential safety concerns, CMS would take immediate action to remove the measure from the HQRP and not wait for the annual rulemaking cycle. The measures would be promptly removed, and CMS would immediately notify hospices and the public of such a decision through the usual CMS HQRP communication channels, including postings and announcements on the CMS HQRP Web site, Medicare Learning Network (MLN) eNews communications, national provider association calls, and announcements on Open Door Forums and Special Open Door Forums.

Previously Adopted Quality Measures for FY 2017 and FY 2018 Payment Determination

As stated in the CY 2013 HH PPS final rule (77 FR 67068 through 67133), CMS expanded the set of required measures to include additional measures endorsed by NQF. CMS also stated that to support the standardized collection and calculation of quality measures by CMS, collection of the needed data elements would require a standardized data collection instrument. In response, CMS developed, tested, and implemented a hospice patient-level item set, the HIS. Hospices are required to submit a HIS-Admission record and a HIS-Discharge record for each patient admission to hospice since July 1, 2014. In developing the standardized HIS, CMS considered comments offered in response to the CY 2013 HH PPS proposed rule (77 FR 41548 through 41573), and in the FY 2014 Hospice Wage Index final rule (78 FR 48257), and in compliance with section 1814(i)(5)(C) of the Act, CMS finalized the specific collection of data items that support the following 6 NQF-endorsed measures and 1 modified measure for hospice:

- NQF #1617 Patients Treated with an Opioid who are Given a Bowel Regimen,

- NQF #1634 Pain Screening,

- NQF #1637 Pain Assessment,

- NQF #1638 Dyspnea Treatment,

- NQF #1639 Dyspnea Screening,

- NQF #1641 Treatment Preferences,

- NQF #1647 Beliefs/Values Addressed (if desired by the patient) (modified).

To achieve a comprehensive set of hospice quality measures available for widespread use for quality improvement and informed decision making, and to carry out it's commitment to develop a quality reporting program for hospices that uses standardized methods to collect data needed to calculate quality measures, CMS finalized the HIS effective July 1, 2014 (78 FR 48258).

To meet the quality reporting requirements for hospices for the FY 2016 payment determination and each subsequent year, CMS required regular and ongoing electronic submission of the HIS data for each patient admission to hospice after July 1, 2014, regardless of payer or patient age (78 FR 48234 through 48258). CMS finalized a requirement in the FY 2014 Hospice Wage Index final rule (78 FR 48258) that hospice providers collect data on all patients to ensure that all patients regardless of payer or patient age are receiving the same care and that provider metrics measure performance across the spectrum of patients.

New Quality Measures for the FY 2019 Payment Determination and Subsequent Years

CMS proposed two new quality measures for the HRQP for the FY 2019 payment determination and subsequent years: Hospice Visits when Death is Imminent Measure Pair, and Hospice and Palliative Care Composite Process Measure-Comprehensive Assessment at Admission.

Proposed Quality Measure 1: Hospice Visits when Death is Imminent Measure Pair

This measure set addresses whether a hospice patient and their caregivers' needs were addressed by the hospice staff during the last days of life. This measure is specified as a set of 2 measures. Measure 1 assesses the percentage of patients receiving at least 1 visit from registered nurses, physicians, nurse practitioners, or physician assistants in the last 3 days of life. Measure 2 assesses the percentage of patients receiving at least 2 visits from medical social workers, chaplains or spiritual counselors, licensed practical nurses, or hospice aides in the last 7 days of life. Measure 1 addresses case management and clinical care, while Measure 2 gives providers the flexibility to provide individualized care that is in line with the patient, family, and caregiver's preferences and goals for care and contributing to the overall well-being of the individual and others important in their life.

The last week of life is typically the period in the terminal illness trajectory with the highest symptom burden. Particularly during the last few days before death, patients experience myriad physical and emotional symptoms, necessitating close care and attention from the integrated hospice team. Hospice responsiveness during times of patient and caregiver need is an important aspect of care for hospice consumers. In addition, clinician visits to patients at the end of life have been demonstrated to be associated with improved outcomes such as decreased risk of hospitalization, emergency room visits, hospital deaths, decreased distress for caregivers, and higher satisfaction with care.

This quality measure set will fill a gap by addressing hospice care provided at the end of life. No current HQRP measures address care beyond the hospice initial and comprehensive assessment period, nor do any current HQRP measures relate to the assessment of hospice staff visits to patients and caregivers in the last week of life.

Proposed Quality Measure 2: Hospice and Palliative Care Composite Process Measure—

Comprehensive Assessment at Admission

The Hospice and Palliative Care Composite Process Measure—

Comprehensive Assessment at Admission is a composite measure that assesses whether a comprehensive patient assessment is completed at hospice admission by evaluating the number of individual care processes completed upon admission for each hospice patient stay. A composite measure, as defined by the NQF, is a combination of two or more component measures, each of which individually reflects quality of care, fashioned into a single performance measure with a single score. For more information on composite measure definitions, guiding principles, and measure evaluation criteria, we refer readers to the NQF Composite Performance Measure Evaluation Guidance Publication available at https://www.qualityforum.org/Publications/2013/04/Composite_Performance_Measure_Evaluation_Guidance.aspx. A total of 7 individual care processes will be captured in this composite measure, which include the 6 NQF-endorsed quality measures and 1 modified NQF-endorsed quality measure currently implemented in the HQRP. Thus, the Hospice and Palliative Care Composite Process Measure will use the current HQRP quality measures as its components. These individual component measures address care processes around hospice admission that are clinically recommended or required in the hospice CoPs.23 This measure calculates the percentage of patients who received all care processes at admission. To calculate this measure, the individual components of the composite measure are assessed separately for each patient and then aggregated into one score for each hospice.

This composite quality measure for comprehensive assessment at admission addresses high priority aspects of quality hospice care as identified by both leading hospice stakeholders and beneficiaries receiving hospice services. The NCP for Quality Palliative Care Clinical Practice Guidelines for Quality Palliative Care established 8 core palliative care domains, and this composite measure captures 4 of those domains. The 4 domains captured by this composite measure are the Structure and Process of Care Domain; the Physical Aspects of Care Domain; the Spiritual, Religious, and Existential Aspects of Care Domain, and the Ethical and Legal Aspects of Care Domain. The NCP guidelines placed equal weight on both the physical and psychosocial domains, emphasizing a comprehensive approach to patient care.

The literature indicates that health care providers' practice is responsive to quality measures reported. CMS feels this research, while not specific to hospices, reasonably predicts the effect of measures on hospice provider behavior. Collecting information about the total number of care processes conducted for each patient will incentivize hospices to conduct all desirable care processes for each patient and provide services that will address their care needs and improve quality during the time he or she is receiving hospice care.

Additionally, creating a composite quality measure for comprehensive assessment at admission will provide consumers and providers with a single measure regarding the overall quality and completeness of assessment of patient needs at hospice admission, which can then be used to meaningfully and easily compare quality across hospice providers and increase transparency.

Hospice Medicare Care Choices Model

Effective January 1, 2016, hospices that apply for and are selected to participate in the Medicare Care Choices Model (MCCM) will provide services available under the Medicare hospice benefit for routine home care and in-home respite levels of care that cannot be separately billed under Medicare Parts A, B, and D. The MCCM will last for five years. It is to be funded using the Medicare Part A Trust Fund. MCCM will consist of up to 171 participating hospices with up to 71 participating in the first year and up to 70 additional hospices entering in year three. The number may decrease when a hospice chooses to no longer participate or it has been removed from the Model. CMS expects that the target number of patients will be 150,000 over the life of the Model. The Model expects to lower expenditures related to emergency department visits, ambulance services, acute care hospital stays, and diagnostic tests and procedures. A patient would be considered eligible if he/she meets all of the following criteria:

- Medicare Part A has been primary for at least 24 continuous months and the patient is currently enrolled in Part B.
- The patient is not enrolled in a Medicare managed care organization.
- The patient has a diagnosis as indicated by certain ICD-10-CM codes for certain types of cancer, congestive heart failure (CHF), human immunodeficiency virus (HIV), and chronic obstructive pulmonary disease (COPD).
- The patient has had at least two hospitalizations in the last 12 months, which were related to his/her MCCM qualifying diagnosis.
- The patient has had at least three office visits with his/her Medicare enrolled health care provider (defined as primary care or specialist provider) within the last 12 months, which were related to his/her MCCM qualifying diagnosis.
- The patient meets hospice eligibility and admission criteria as stated in 42 CFR §418.20, Eligibility requirements, and §418.25, Admission to hospice care.
- The patient has not elected the Medicare or Medicaid hospice benefit within the last 30 days prior to their participation in the MCCM.

A patient who leaves the Model for any reason would not be eligible to return to the Model at a later date.

Services are provided in the home based on the patient's care needs. CMS does not expect to see claims in the Medicare or Medicaid claims systems for home health services that should be provided by the hospice. CMS understands that there may be occasions where necessary home health services require the use of a home health agency that possesses the required skill level. The claims systems will be monitored specifically for use of services provided by home health agencies. MCCM participating hospices will be expected to provide documentation of each use of services by a home health agency for Model patients.

- Participating hospices should submit a MCCM-specific notice of election (NOE) on TOB 081A and 082A. Hospices should submit demonstration code 73 in FL 63 (or equivalent), "Treatment Authorization Code Occurrence." Code 27 Date of hospice certification or recertification, is not required on

Appendix O: Hospice Diagnosis and Quality Reporting Guidance

MCCM-specific notice of election (NOEs). Do not report occurrence code 27 and demo code 73 on the same NOE.

- Eligible hospices may bill once per calendar month per patient. Hospices will be paid the full $400 per-beneficiary-per-month (PBPM) for each eligible patient enrolled in the MCCM for 15 or more days and $200 PBPM for each eligible patient enrolled in the MCCM for less than 15 days. The hospice must provide at least one service in a calendar month with the exception of the month of discharge which will be paid $400 PBPM. The PBPM fee would be the total payment for those services for Model patients. The PBPM fee has no beneficiary coinsurance or deductible. Claims will be paid according to dates of service. Participating hospices will receive payment if they were on the list of approved participating hospices at the time services were rendered.

- Report the following revenue codes and associated HCPCS codes on the MCCM claim:

  G0299 and G0300 (revenue code 0551)

  G0155 (revenue code 0561 or 0569)

  G0156 (revenue code 0571)

  G9473, G9474, G9475, G9476, G9477, G9478, G9479, and G9480 (revenue code 0659)

- Providers and suppliers furnishing curative services to patients participating in the MCCM will be able to continue to bill Medicare (i.e., Parts A, B, and D) for the reasonable and necessary services they furnish. Total Medicare and Medicaid expenditures for qualifying patients are expected to be reduced as the result of key aspects of the MCCM, which include pain and symptom management, incorporation of patient-centered goals into the plan of care, care coordination, case management, and shared decision making provided by the MCCM participating hospice.

- While participating in the MCCM, patients would remain subject to any relevant cost-sharing requirements incurred as a result of curative care treatments. Providers furnishing curative services should continue to bill Medicare as they normally would. Other practitioners will be eligible to bill chronic care management services for the same patient during the same month.

Illustrations

Chapter 3. Diseases of the Blood and Blood-forming Organs and Certain Disorders Involving the Immune Mechanism (D5Ø–D89)

Red Blood Cells

White Blood Cell

Platelet

Coagulation

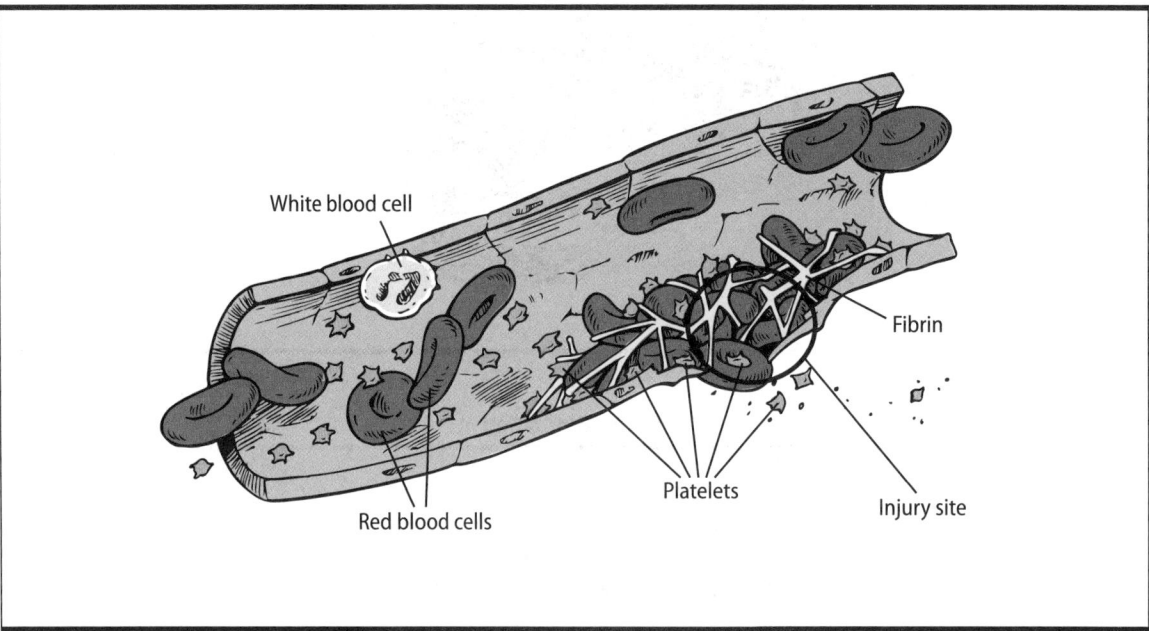

Spleen Anatomical Location and External Structures

Spleen Interior Structures

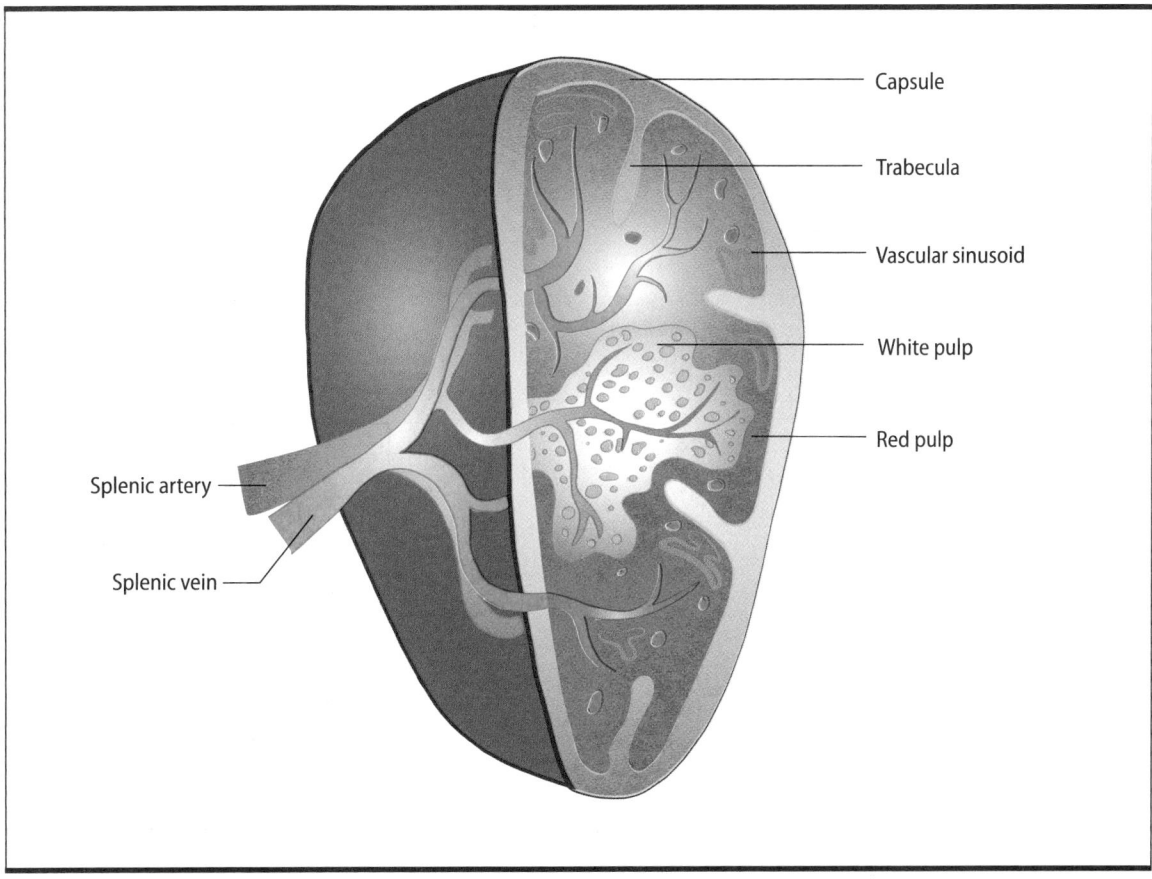

Chapter 4. Endocrine, Nutritional and Metabolic Diseases (E00–E89)

Endocrine System

Thyroid

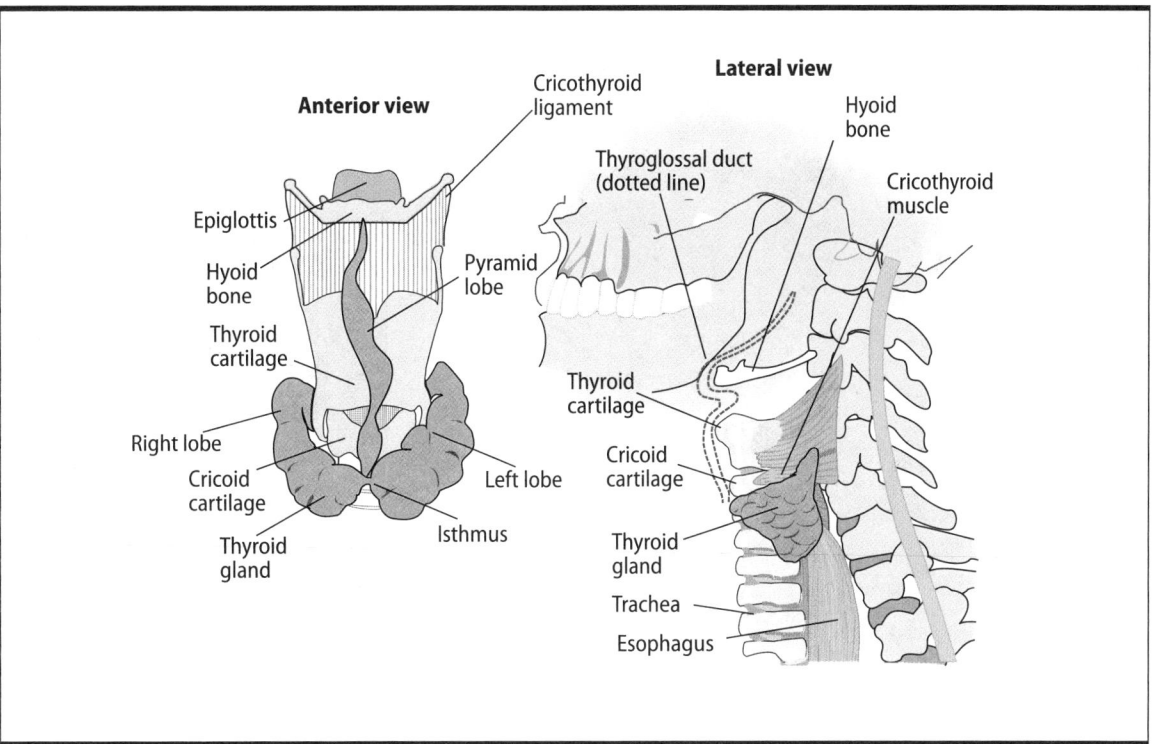

Anterior view

- Cricothyroid ligament
- Epiglottis
- Hyoid bone
- Thyroid cartilage
- Pyramid lobe
- Right lobe
- Cricoid cartilage
- Left lobe
- Thyroid gland
- Isthmus

Lateral view

- Hyoid bone
- Thyroglossal duct (dotted line)
- Cricothyroid muscle
- Thyroid cartilage
- Cricoid cartilage
- Thyroid gland
- Trachea
- Esophagus

Thyroid and Parathyroid Glands

Posterior view

- Epiglottis
- Pharynx
- Thyroid gland
- Parathyroid gland

Pancreas

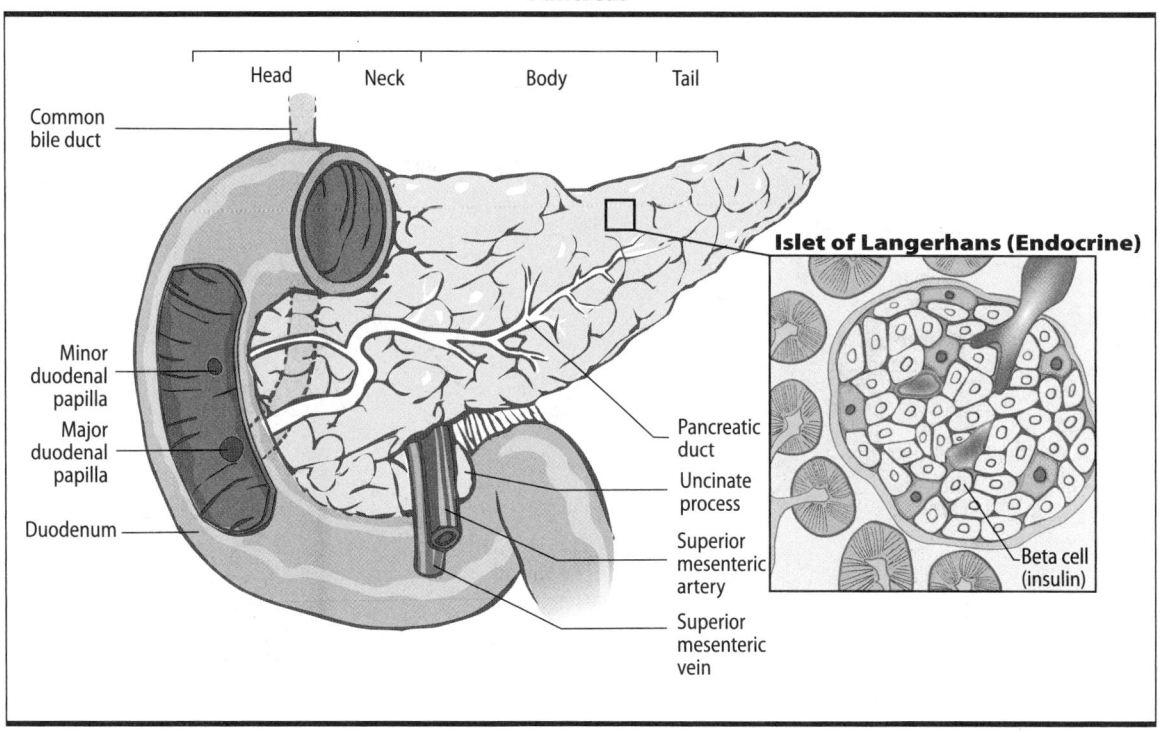

Anatomy of the Adrenal Gland

Structure of an Ovary

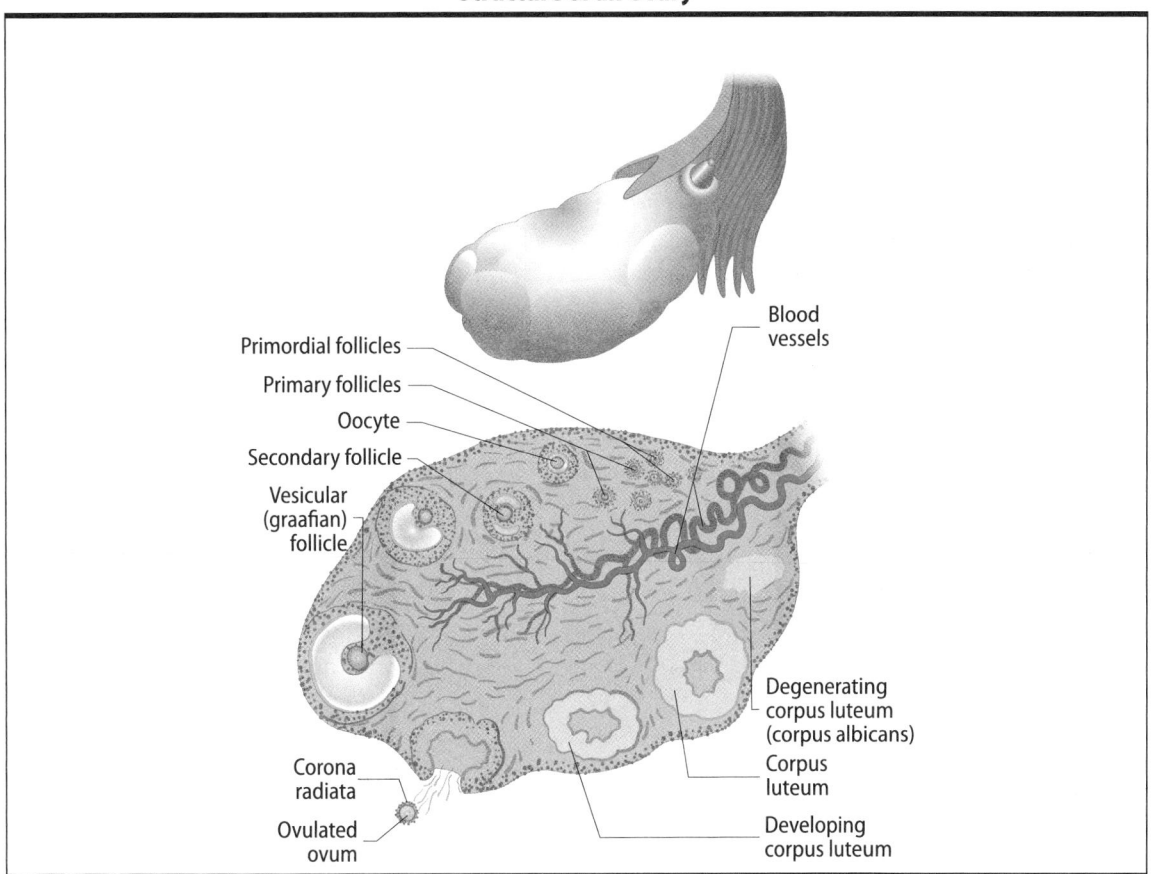

Primordial follicles
Primary follicles
Oocyte
Secondary follicle
Vesicular (graafian) follicle
Blood vessels
Degenerating corpus luteum (corpus albicans)
Corpus luteum
Developing corpus luteum
Corona radiata
Ovulated ovum

Testis and Associated Structures

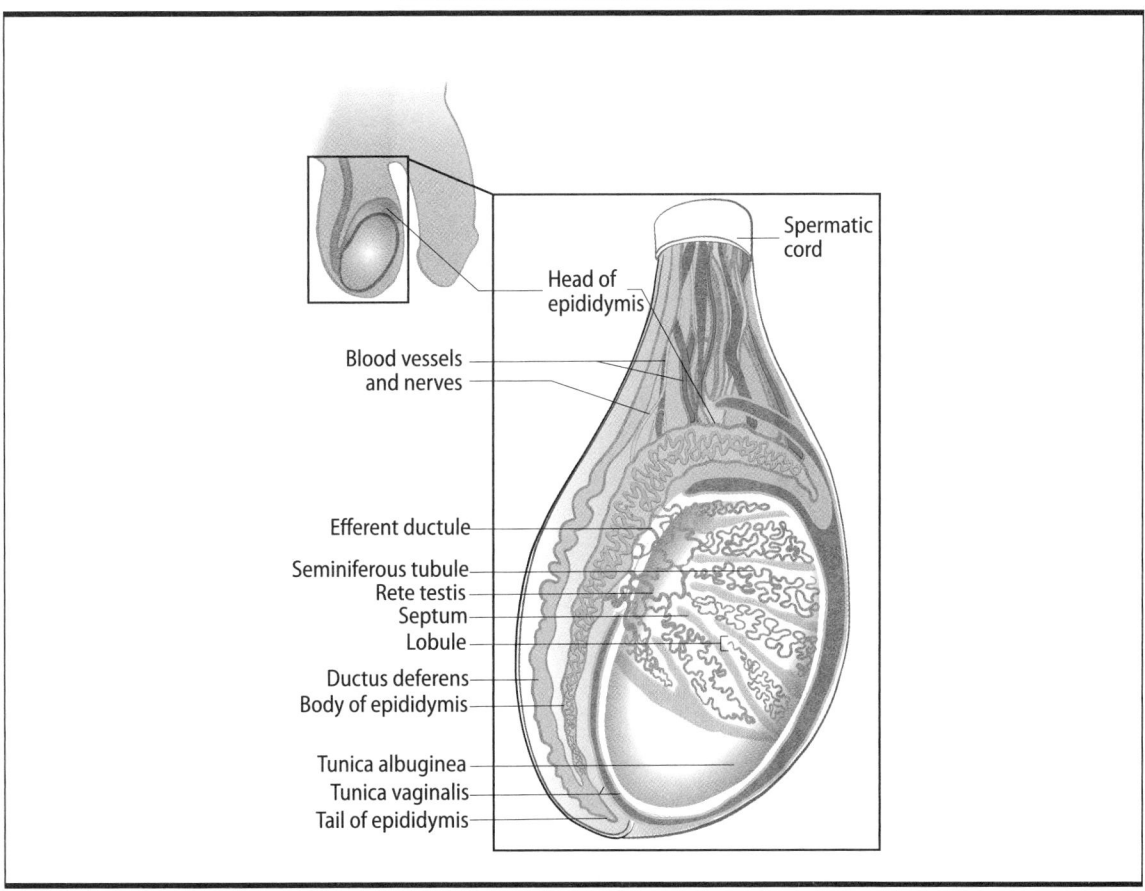

Spermatic cord
Head of epididymis
Blood vessels and nerves
Efferent ductule
Seminiferous tubule
Rete testis
Septum
Lobule
Ductus deferens
Body of epididymis
Tunica albuginea
Tunica vaginalis
Tail of epididymis

Thymus

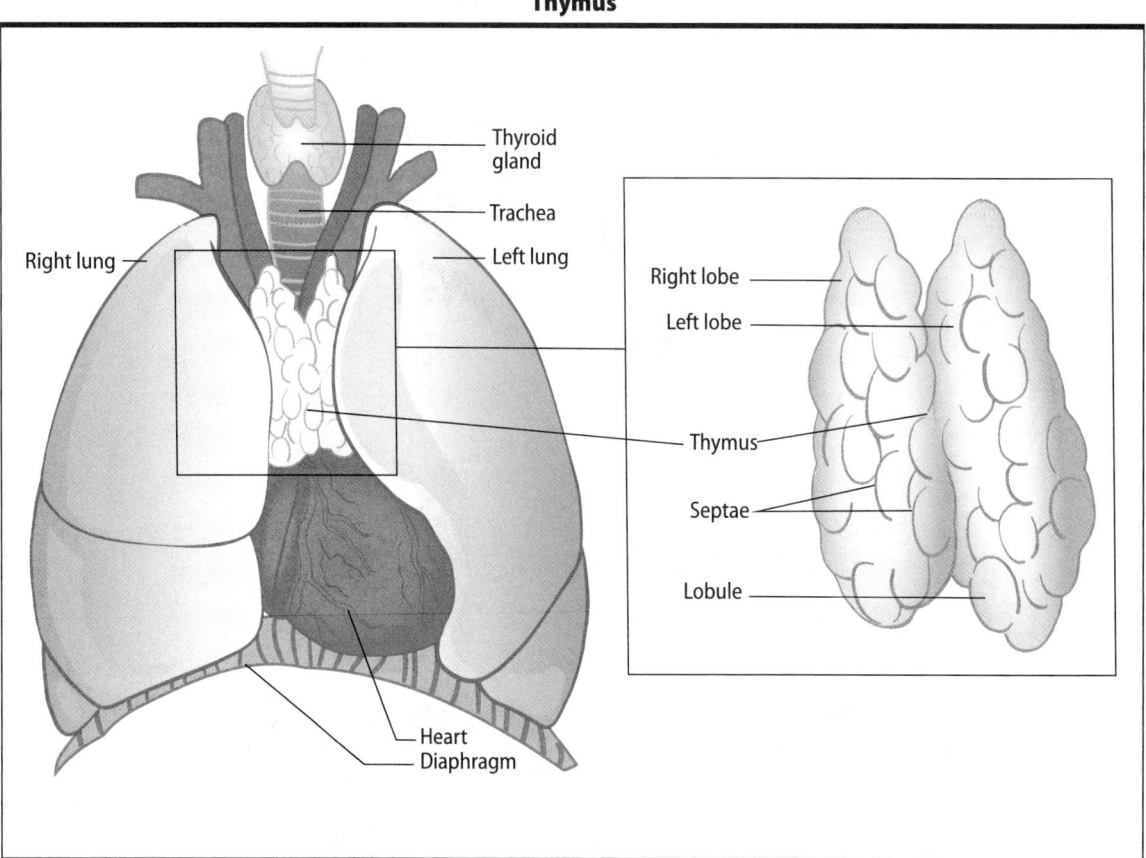

Chapter 6. Diseases of the Nervous System (G00–G99)

Brain

Cranial Nerves

Peripheral Nervous System

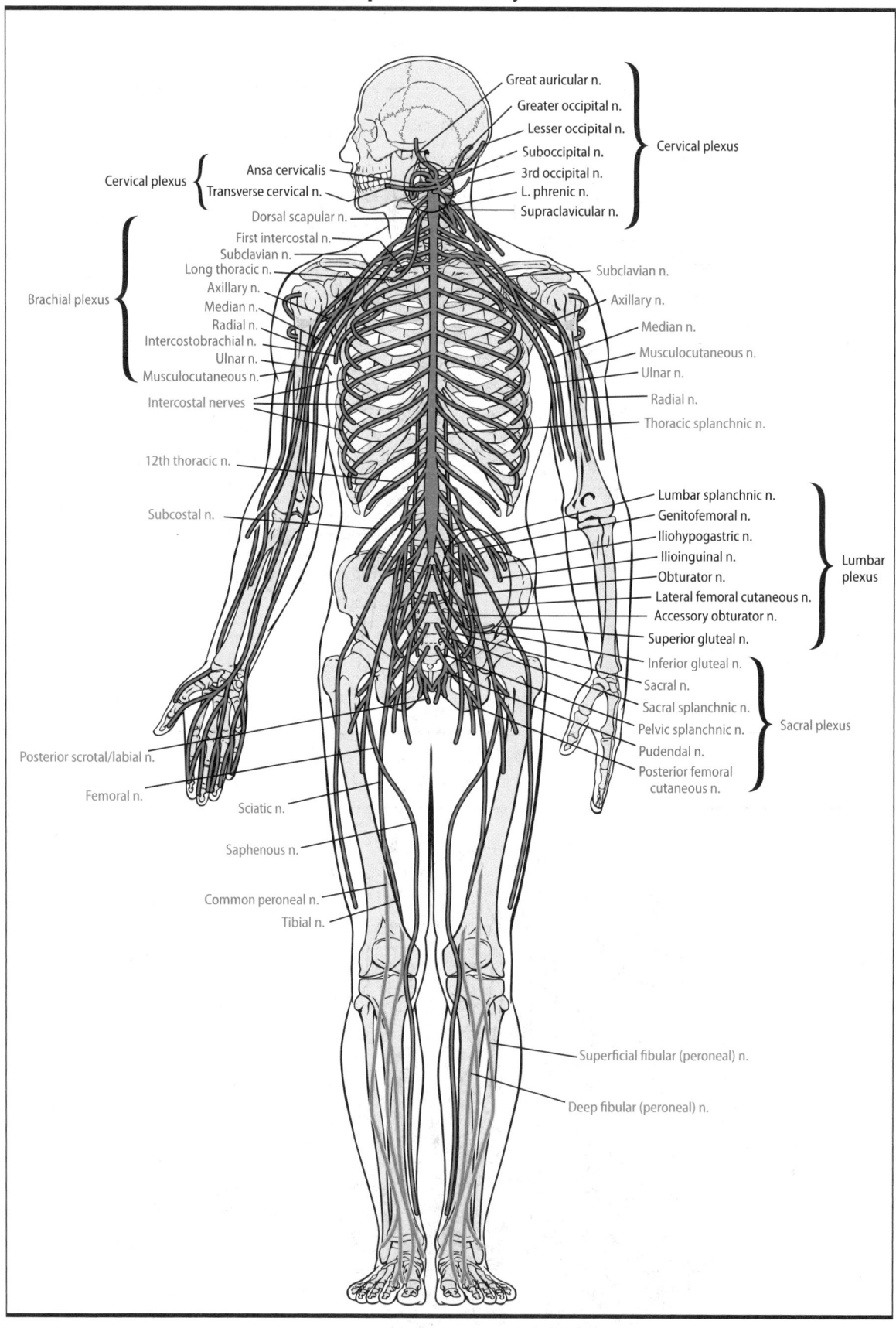

Spinal Cord and Spinal Nerves

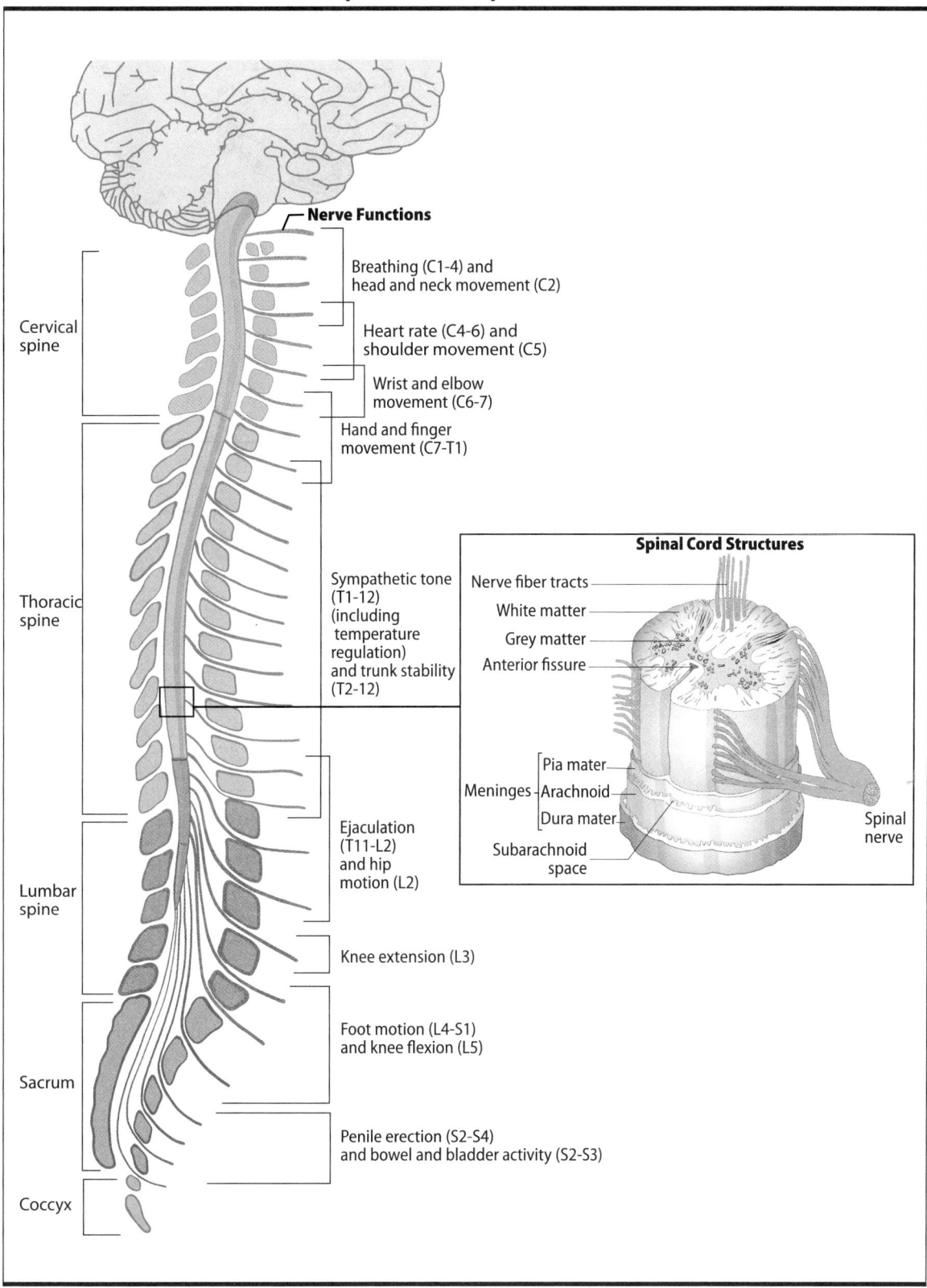

Nerve Functions

Breathing (C1-4) and
head and neck movement (C2)

Heart rate (C4-6) and
shoulder movement (C5)

Wrist and elbow
movement (C6-7)

Hand and finger
movement (C7-T1)

Sympathetic tone
(T1-12)
(including
temperature
regulation)
and trunk stability
(T2-12)

Ejaculation
(T11-L2)
and hip
motion (L2)

Knee extension (L3)

Foot motion (L4-S1)
and knee flexion (L5)

Penile erection (S2-S4)
and bowel and bladder activity (S2-S3)

Cervical
spine

Thoracic
spine

Lumbar
spine

Sacrum

Coccyx

Spinal Cord Structures

Nerve fiber tracts
White matter
Grey matter
Anterior fissure

Meninges — Pia mater
Arachnoid
Dura mater

Subarachnoid
space

Spinal
nerve

Nerve Cell

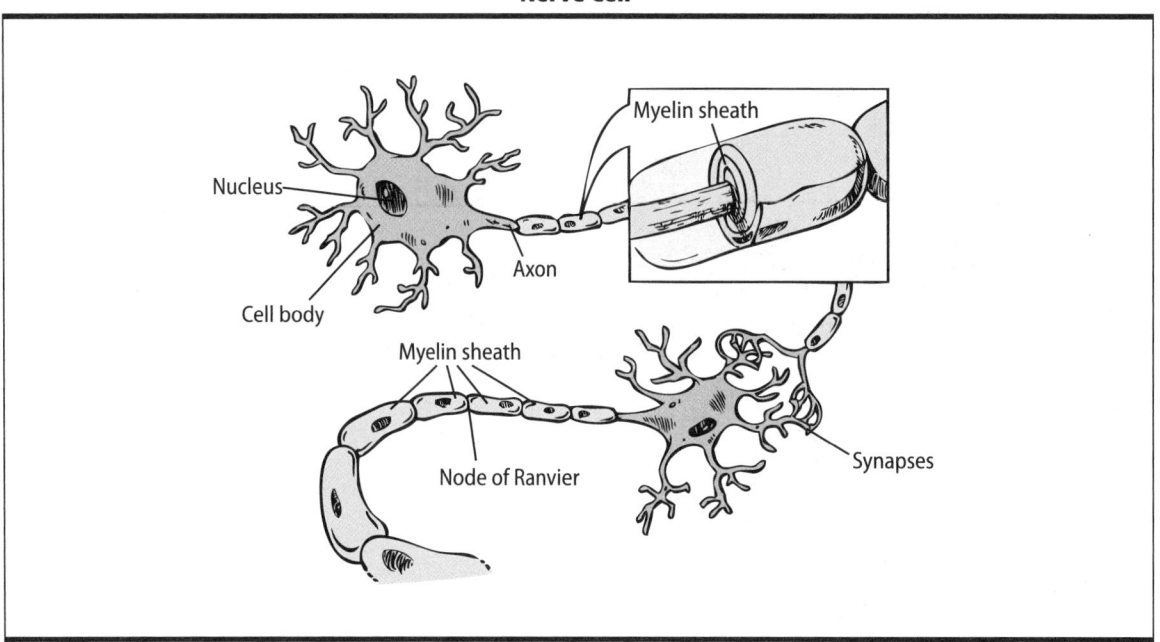

Chapter 7. Diseases of the Eye and Adnexa (HØØ–H59)

Eye

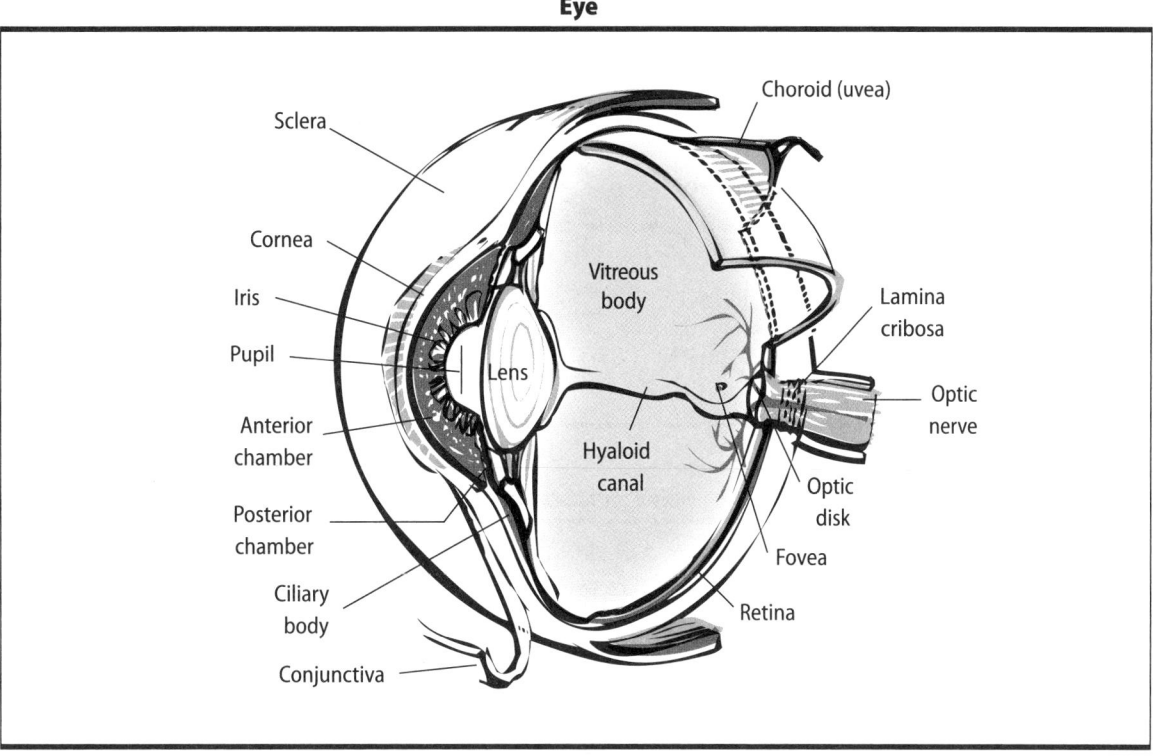

Posterior Pole of Globe/Flow of Aqueous Humor

Lacrimal System

Eye Musculature

Eyelid Structures

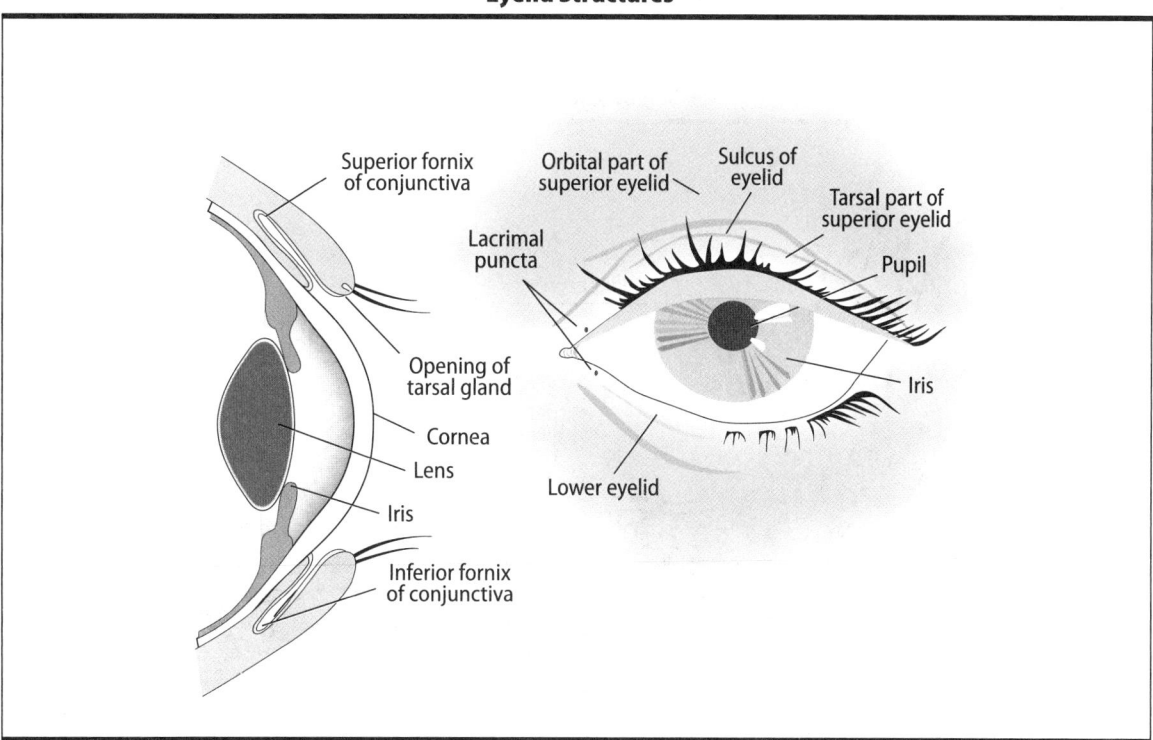

Chapter 8. Diseases of the Ear and Mastoid Process (H6Ø–H95)

Ear Anatomy

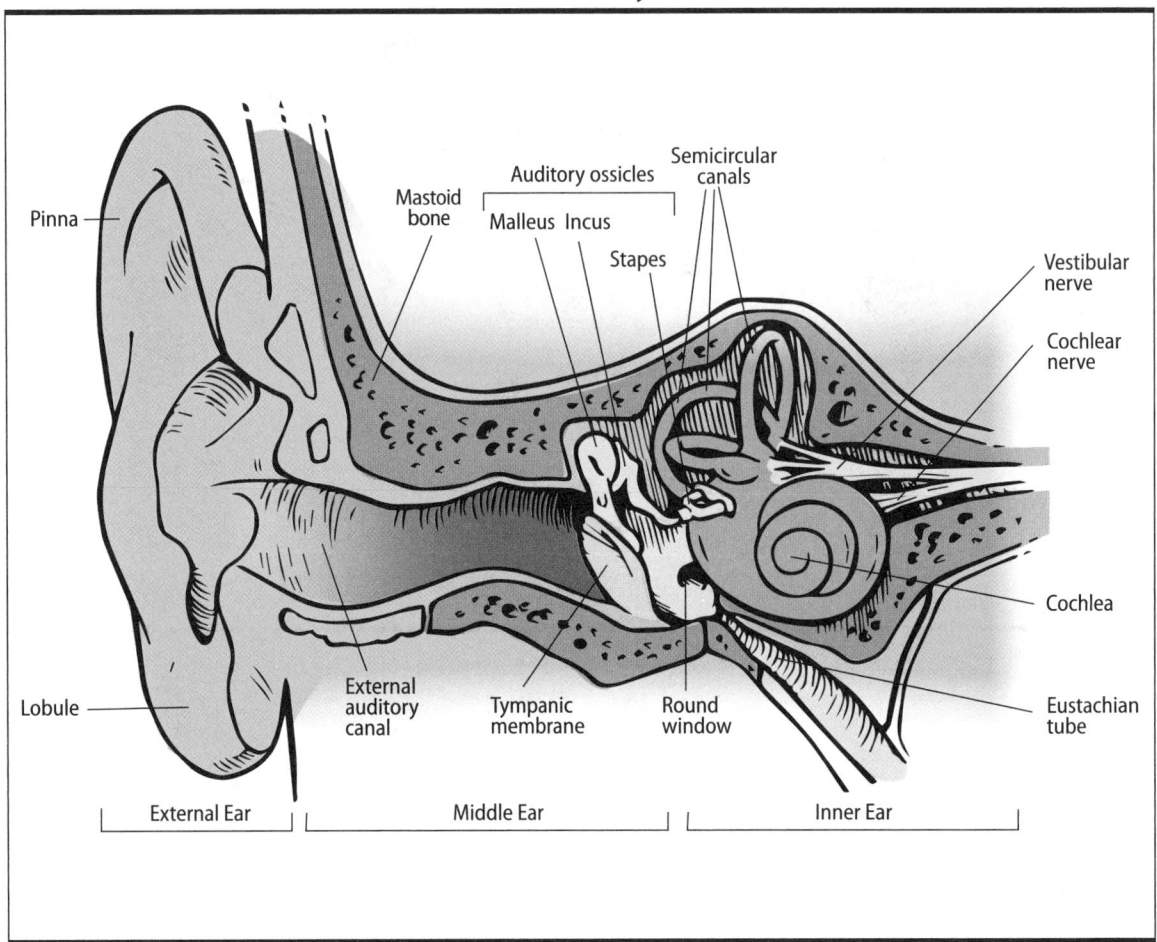

Chapter 9. Diseases of the Circulatory System (I00–I99)

Anatomy of the Heart

Superior vena cava

Aortic valve

Right atrium

Tricuspid valve

Right ventricle

Inferior vena cava

Aorta

Pulmonary artery

Pulmonary vein

Pulmonary valve

Left atrium

Mitral valve

Chorda tendinae

Left ventricle

Heart Cross Section

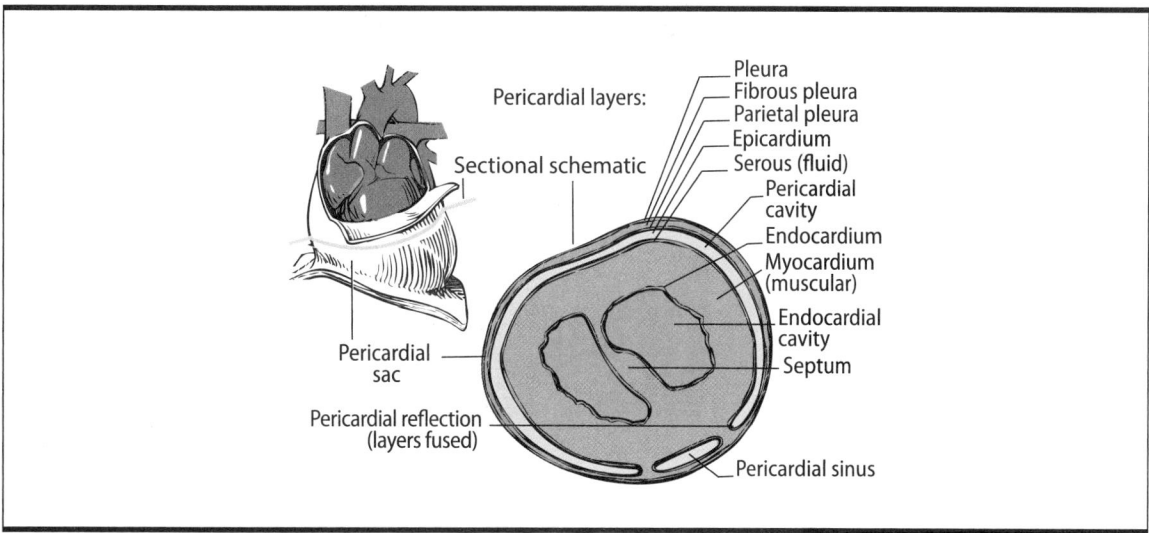

Pericardial layers:

Sectional schematic

Pleura
Fibrous pleura
Parietal pleura
Epicardium
Serous (fluid)
Pericardial cavity
Endocardium
Myocardium (muscular)
Endocardial cavity
Septum

Pericardial sac

Pericardial reflection (layers fused)

Pericardial sinus

Heart Valves

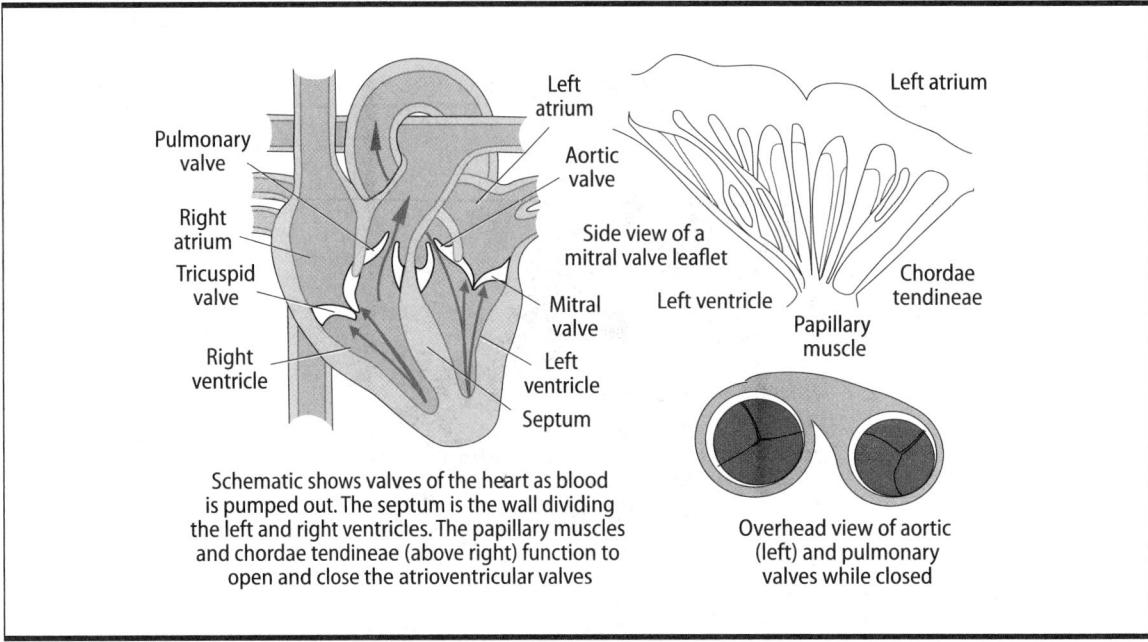

Schematic shows valves of the heart as blood is pumped out. The septum is the wall dividing the left and right ventricles. The papillary muscles and chordae tendineae (above right) function to open and close the atrioventricular valves

Overhead view of aortic (left) and pulmonary valves while closed

Heart Conduction System

Sinoatrial node (pacemaker)

Atrioventricular node

Atrioventricular bundle (of His)

Right bundle branch

Purkinje fibers

Left bundle branch

Coronary Arteries

Arteries

Veins

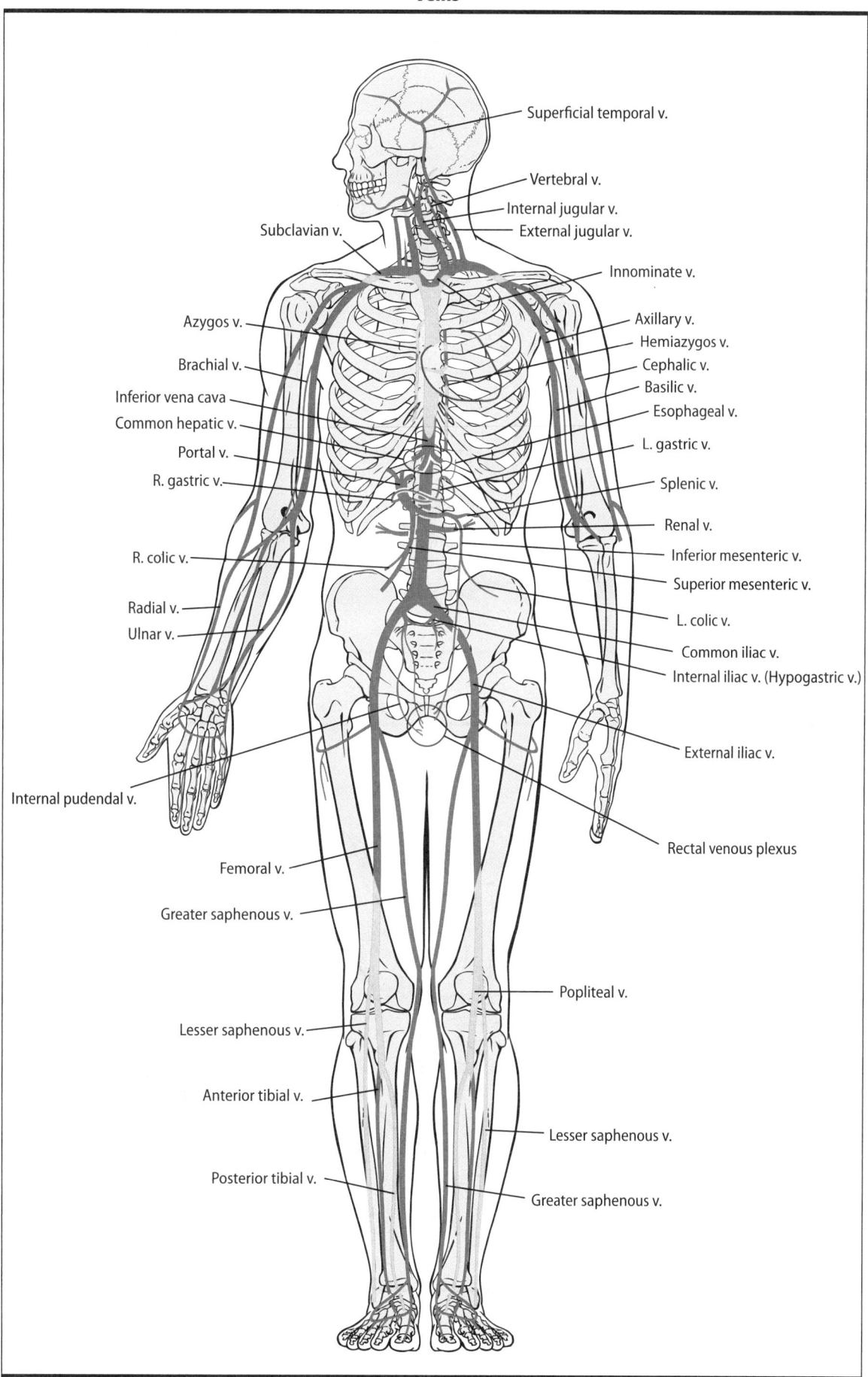

Internal Carotid and Vertebral Arteries and Branches

Side View

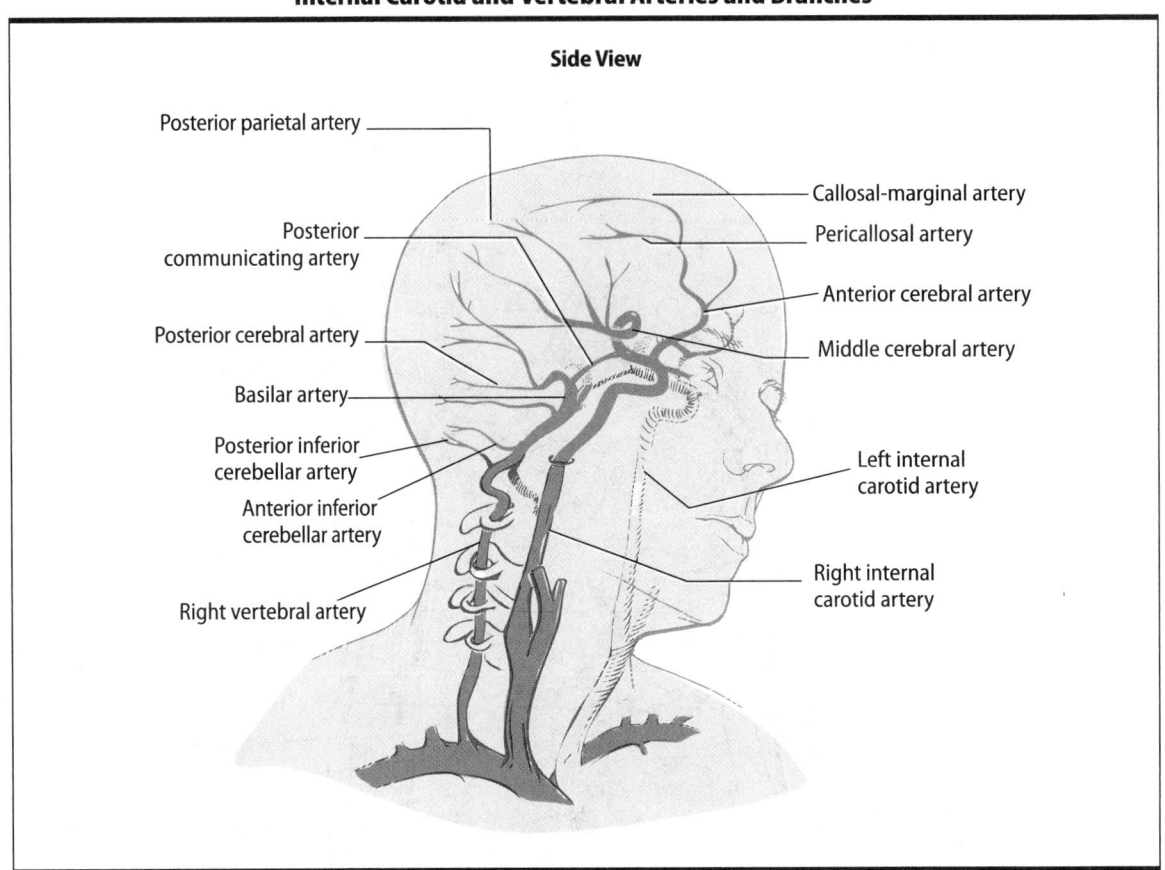

External Carotid Artery and Branches

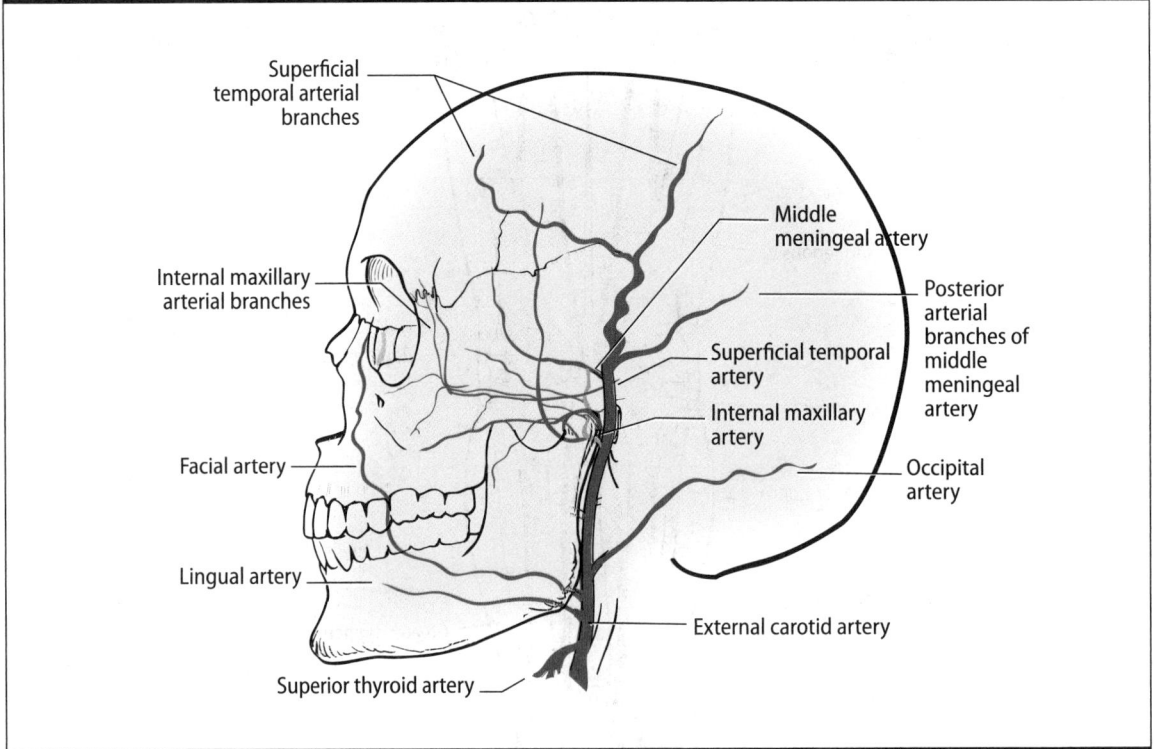

Branches of Abdominal Aorta

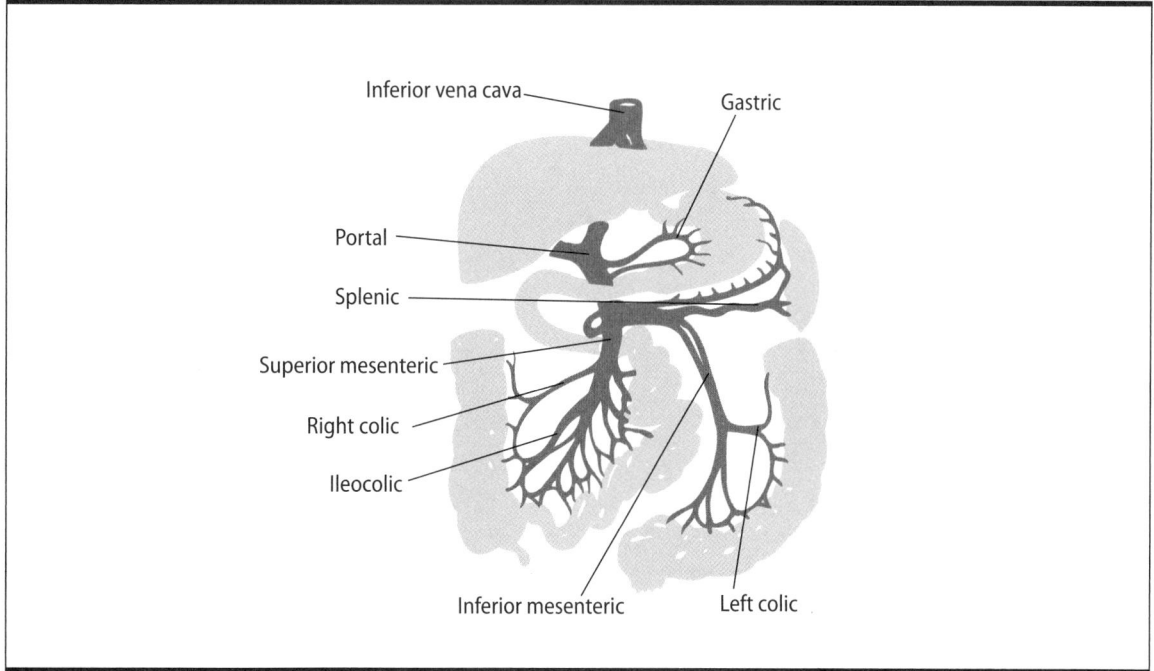

Portal Venous Circulation

Lymphatic System

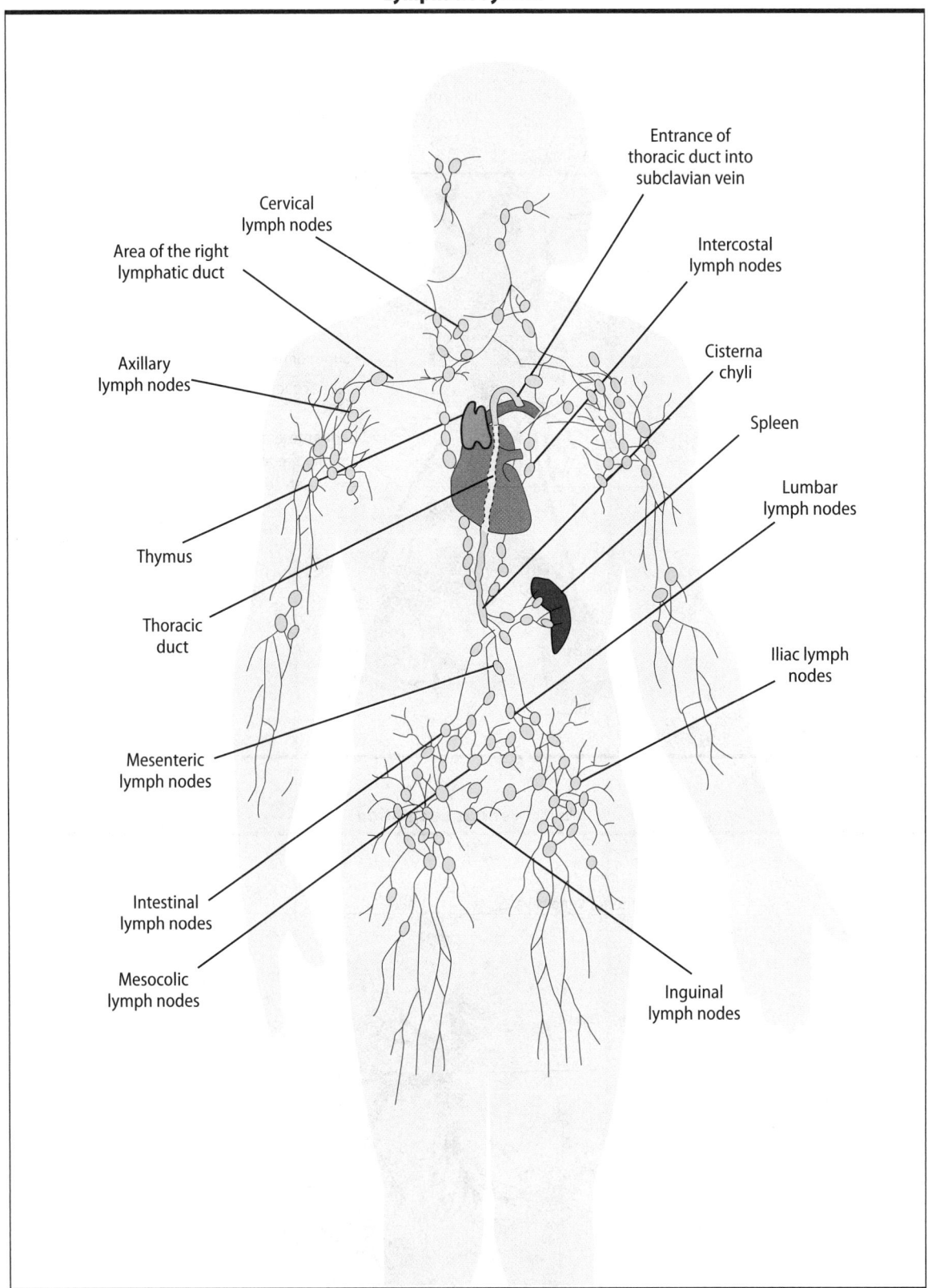

Axillary Lymph Nodes

Parasternal nodes

Sternum

Clavicle

Deltoid muscle

Brachialis muscle

Lateral nodes

Subscapular nodes

Pectoral nodes

Axillary lymph nodes

Central nodes

Latissimus dorsi muscle

Rectus abdominis muscle

Lymphatic System of Head and Neck

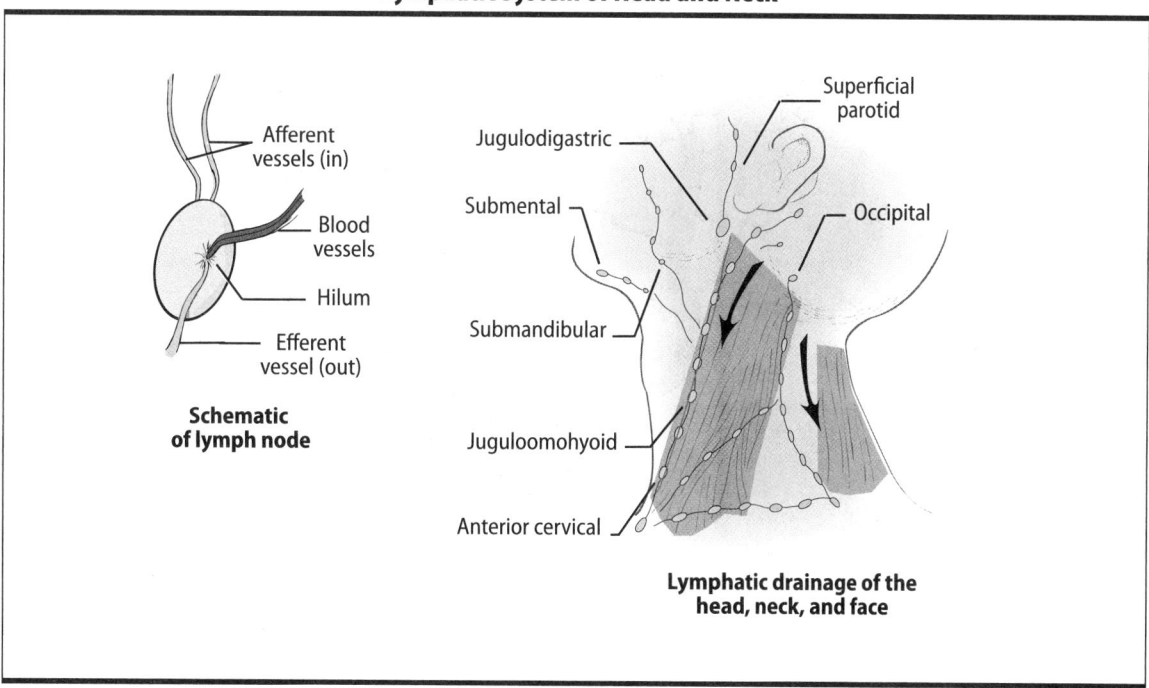

Afferent vessels (in)

Blood vessels

Hilum

Efferent vessel (out)

Schematic of lymph node

Jugulodigastric

Superficial parotid

Submental

Occipital

Submandibular

Juguloomohyoid

Anterior cervical

Lymphatic drainage of the head, neck, and face

Lymphatic Capillaries

Schematic of lymphatic capillaries

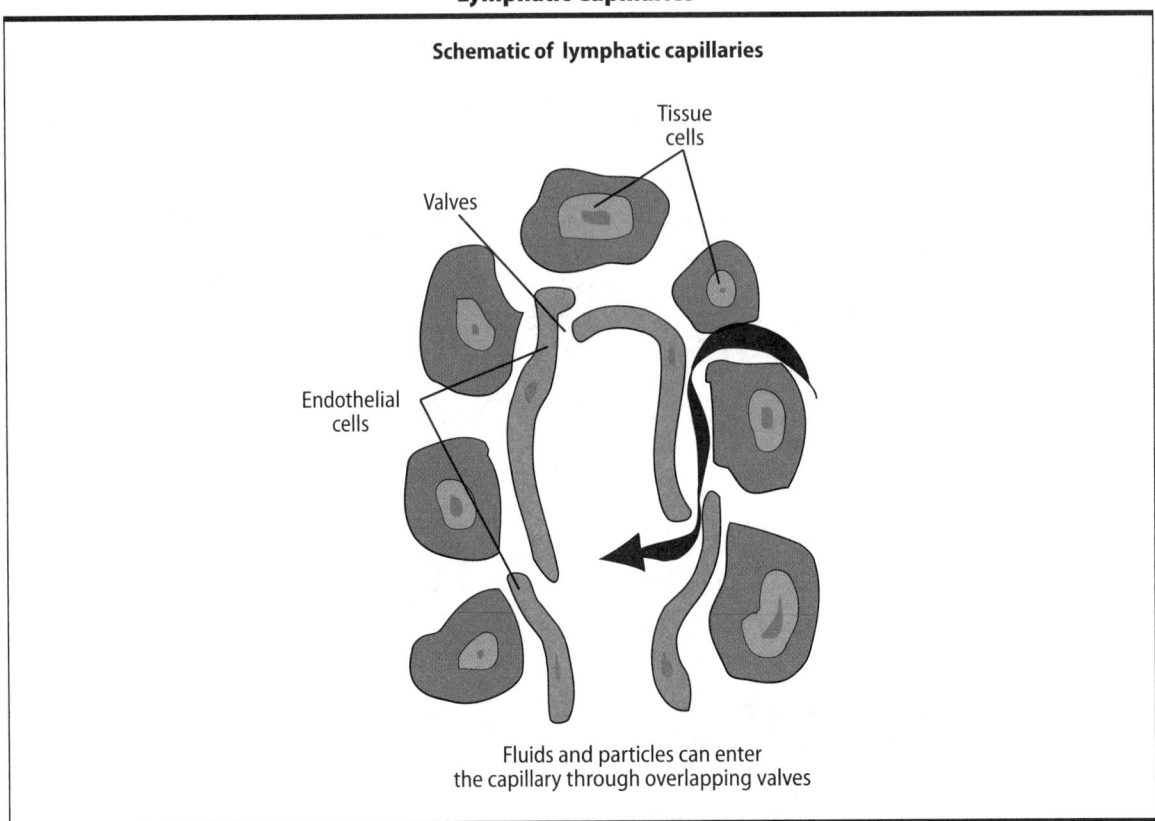

Tissue cells

Valves

Endothelial cells

Fluids and particles can enter
the capillary through overlapping valves

Lymphatic Drainage

Lymphatic drainage of the colon follows blood supply

Middle colic nodes

Paracolic nodes

Left colic nodes

Ascending colon

Cecum

Rectum

Chapter 10. Diseases of the Respiratory System (JØØ–J99)

Respiratory System

Upper Respiratory System

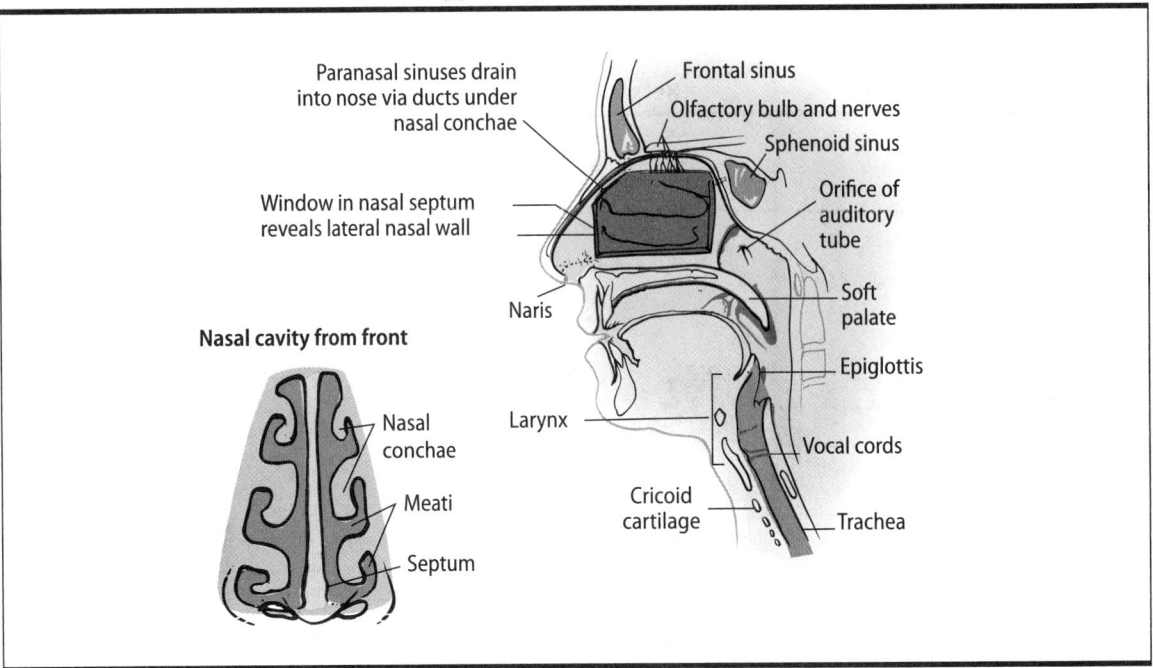

Paranasal sinuses drain into nose via ducts under nasal conchae

Window in nasal septum reveals lateral nasal wall

Nasal cavity from front

Nasal conchae

Meati

Septum

Frontal sinus

Olfactory bulb and nerves

Sphenoid sinus

Orifice of auditory tube

Soft palate

Naris

Epiglottis

Larynx

Vocal cords

Cricoid cartilage

Trachea

Lower Respiratory System

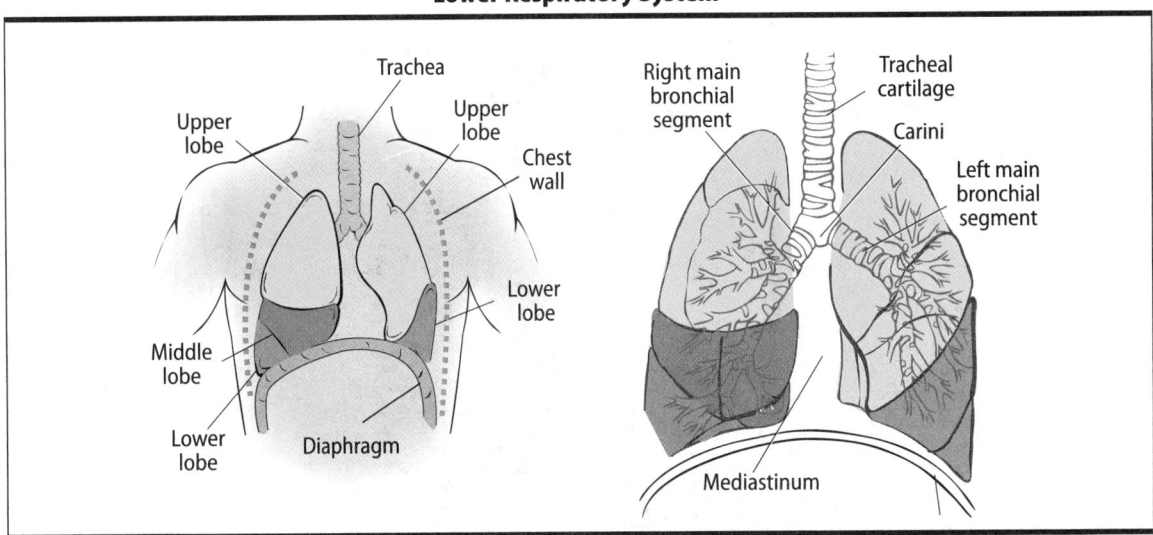

Trachea

Upper lobe

Upper lobe

Chest wall

Middle lobe

Lower lobe

Lower lobe

Diaphragm

Right main bronchial segment

Tracheal cartilage

Carini

Left main bronchial segment

Mediastinum

Paranasal Sinuses

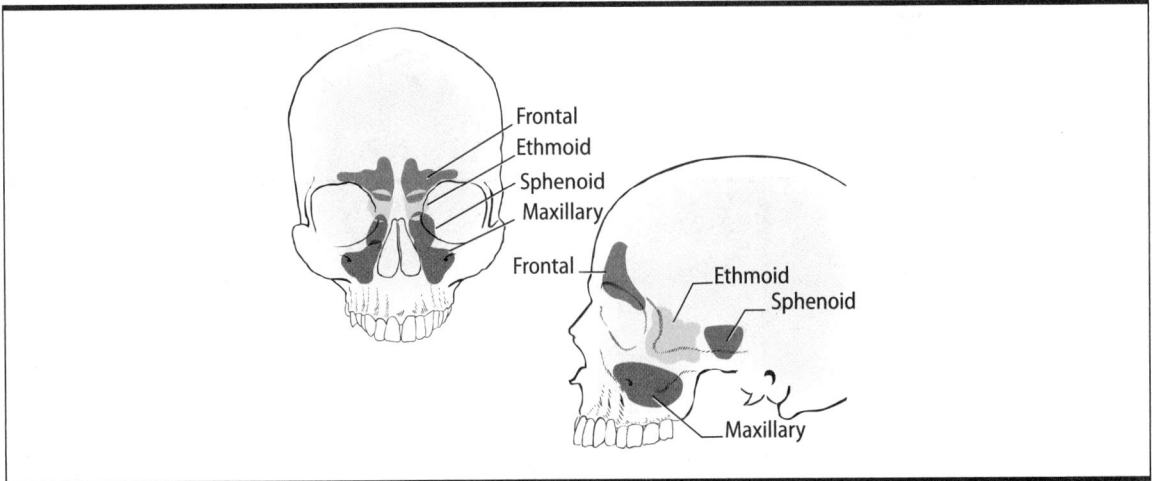

Frontal
Ethmoid
Sphenoid
Maxillary

Frontal

Ethmoid

Sphenoid

Maxillary

Lung Segments

Alveoli

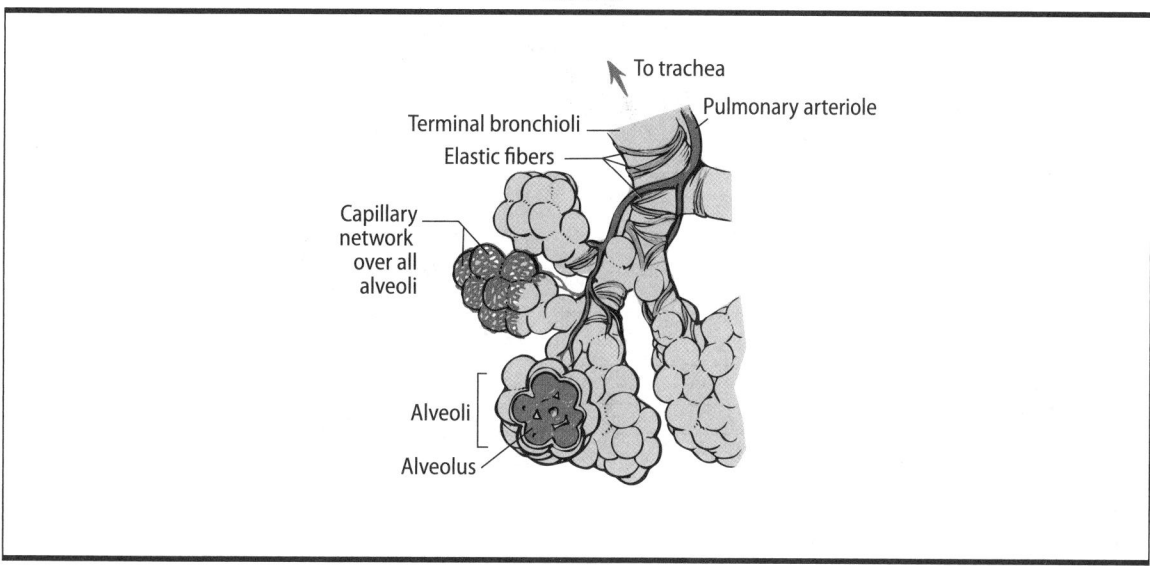

Chapter 11. Diseases of the Digestive System (KØØ–K95)

Digestive System

Omentum and Mesentery

Peritoneum and Retroperitoneum

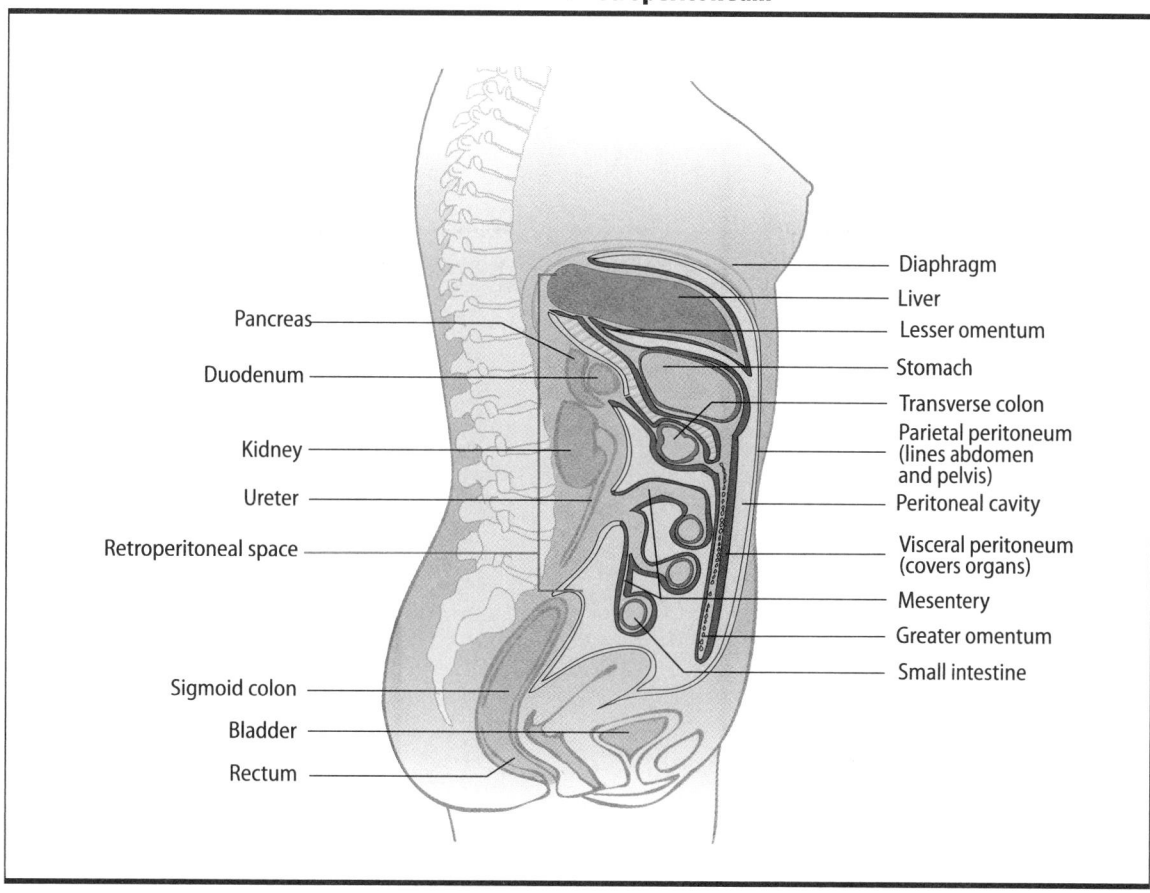

Chapter 12. Diseases of the Skin and Subcutaneous Tissue (L00–L99)

Nail Anatomy

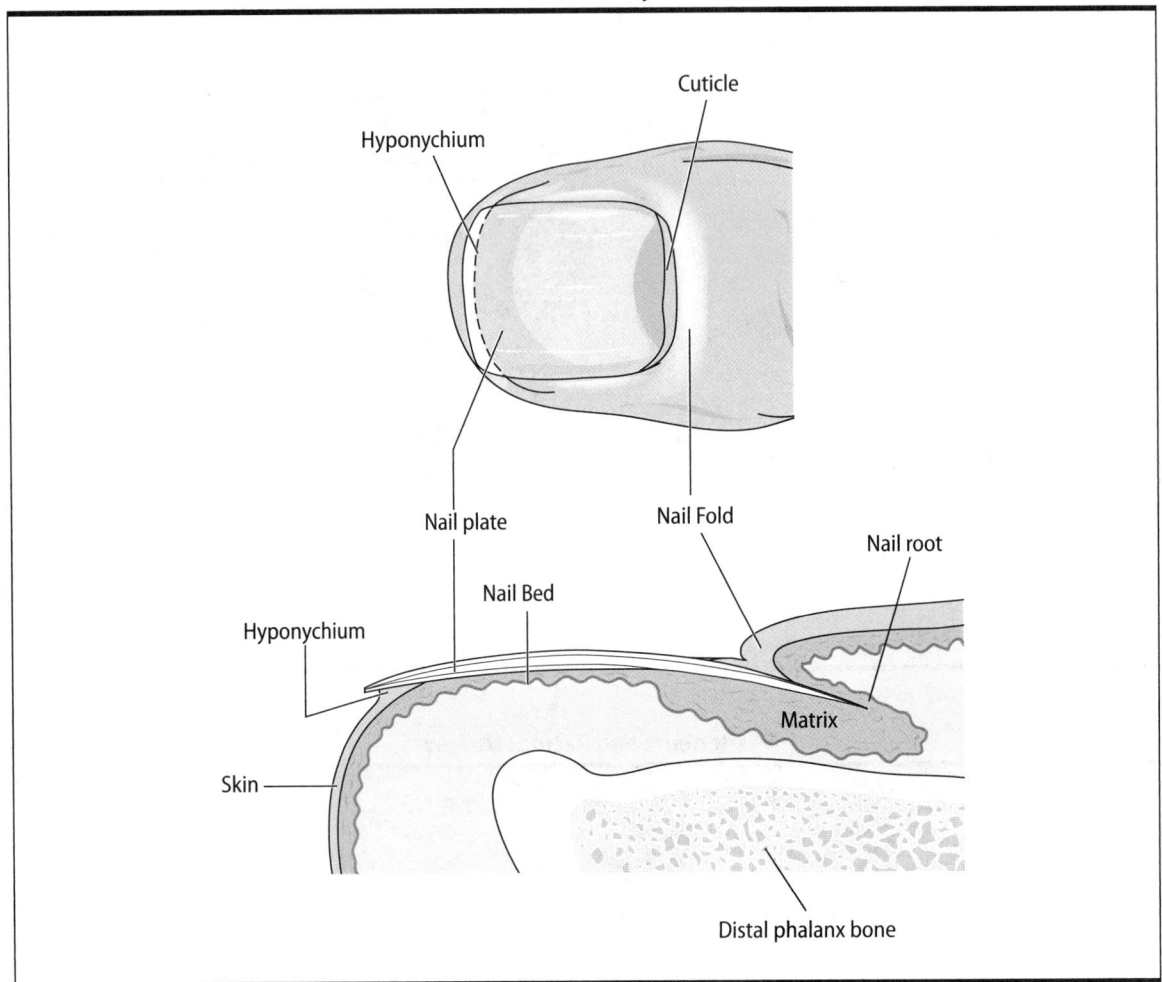

Skin and Subcutaneous Tissue

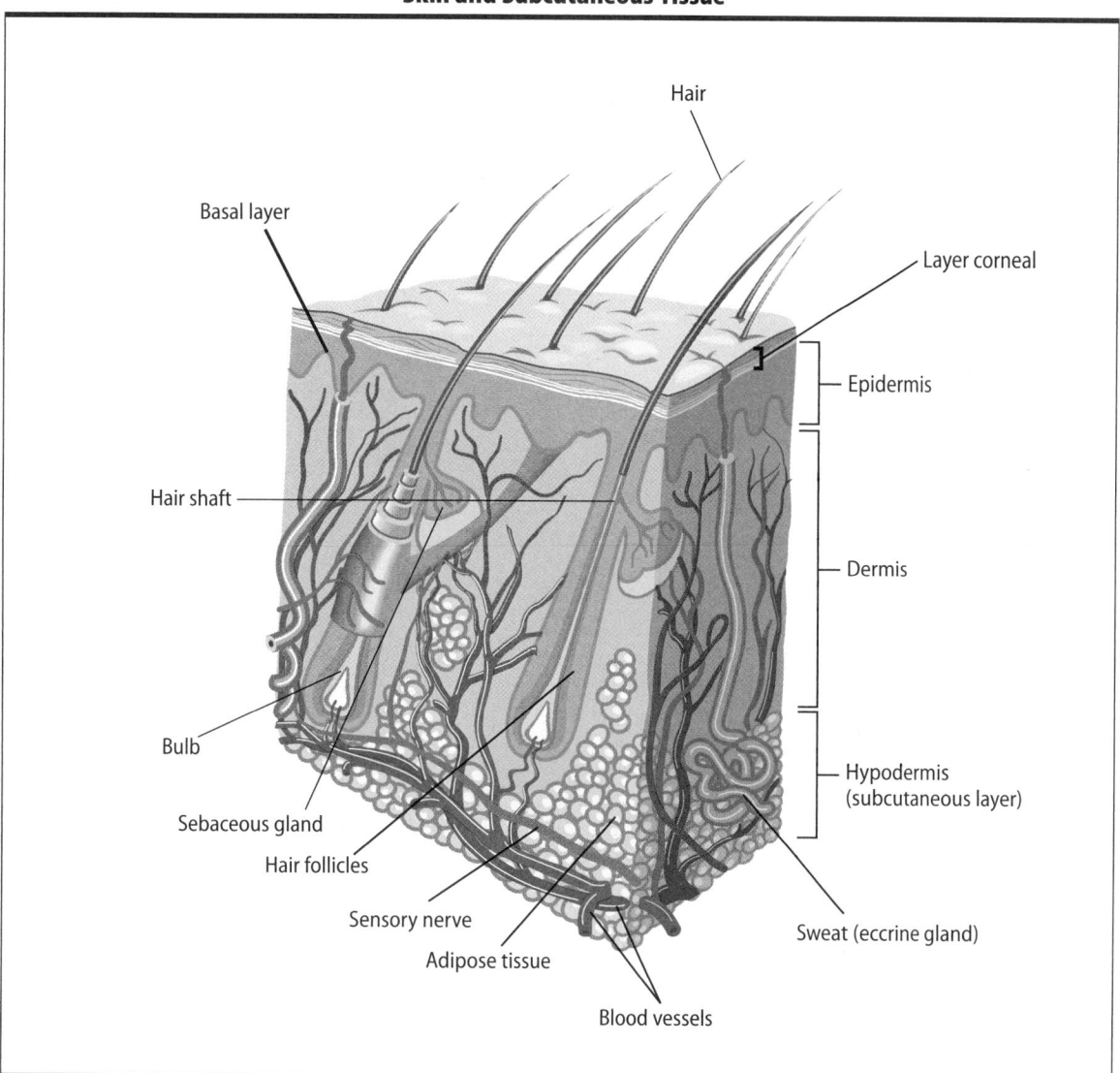

Chapter 13. Diseases of the Musculoskeletal System and Connective Tissue (MØØ–M99)

Bones and Joints

Shoulder Anterior View

Shoulder Posterior View

Elbow Anterior View

Elbow Posterior View

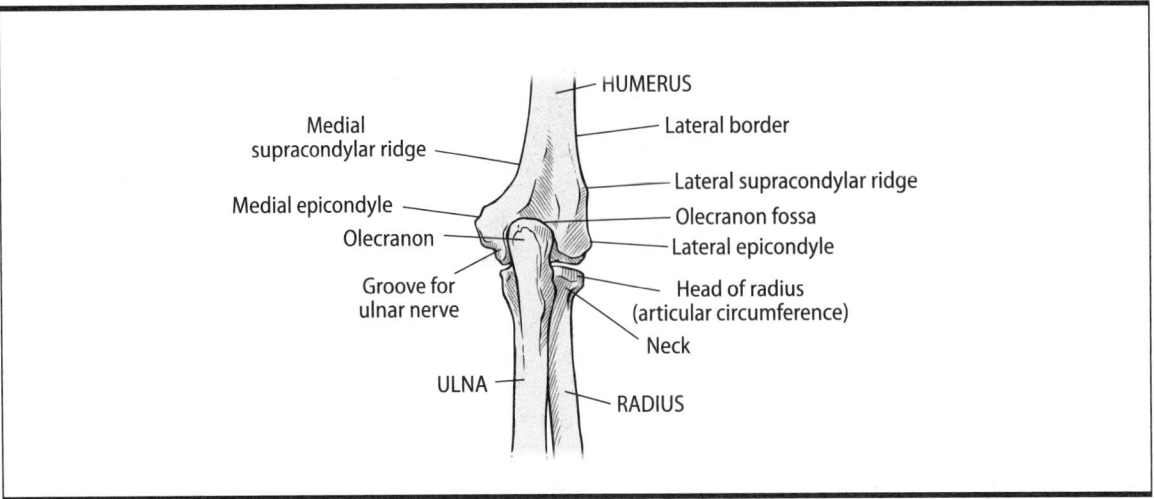

HUMERUS

Medial supracondylar ridge

Lateral border

Lateral supracondylar ridge

Medial epicondyle

Olecranon fossa

Olecranon

Lateral epicondyle

Groove for ulnar nerve

Head of radius (articular circumference)

Neck

ULNA

RADIUS

Hand

Phalanges (digits)

Distal phalanx

Middle phalanx

Proximal phalanx

Interphalangeal joints

Distal phalanx (thumb)

Metacarpophalangeal joint

Metacarpals

Proximal phalanx (thumb)

Carpometacarpal joint

Hamate

Pisiform

Carpals

Trapezium

Trapezoid

Scaphoid

Triquetral   Lunate   Cuboid

5   4   3   2   1

Hip Anterior View

Hip Posterior View

Knee Anterior View

Knee Posterior View

Foot

Muscles

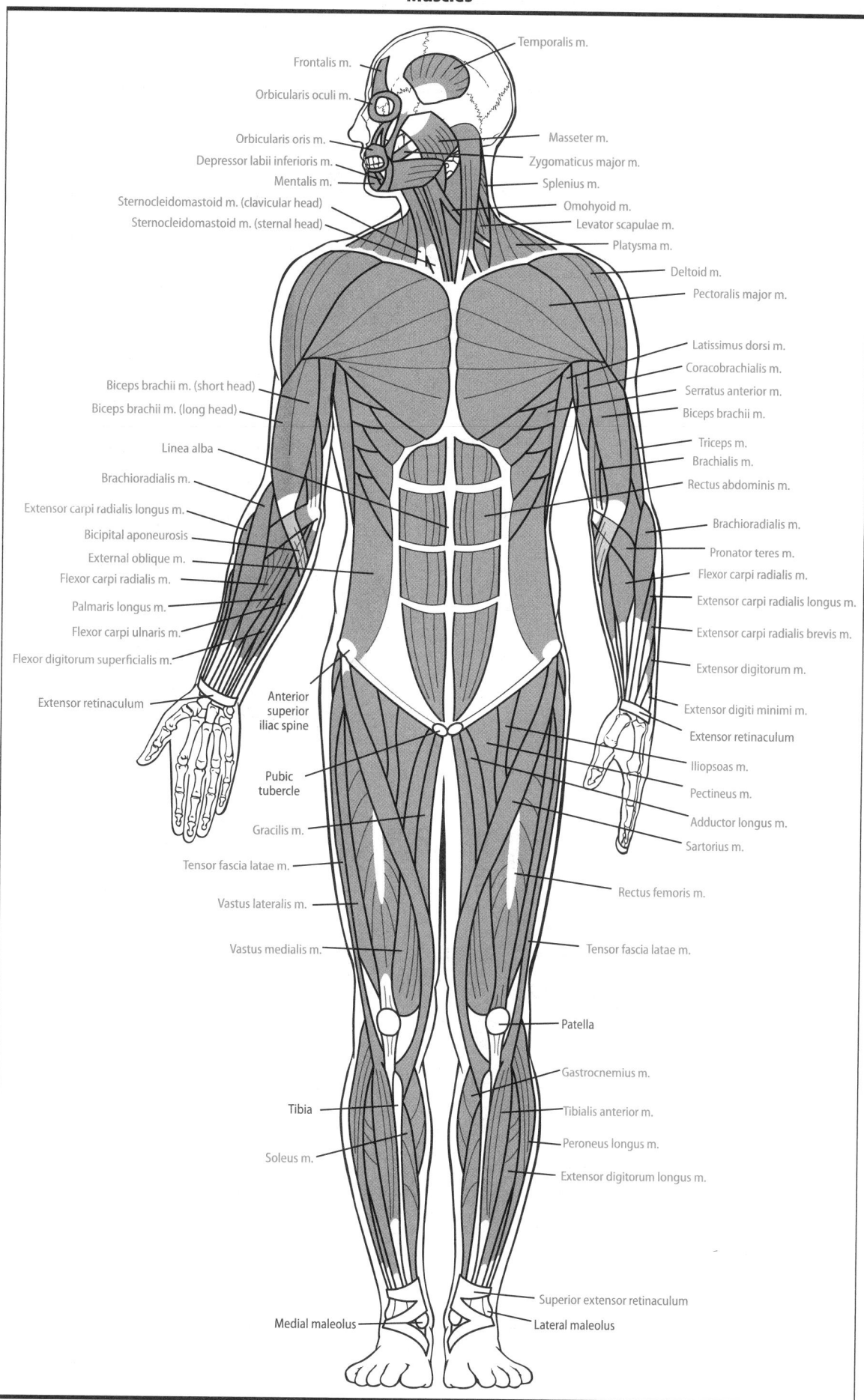

Chapter 14. Diseases of the Genitourinary System (NØØ–N99)

Urinary System

Male Genitourinary System

Female Internal Genitalia

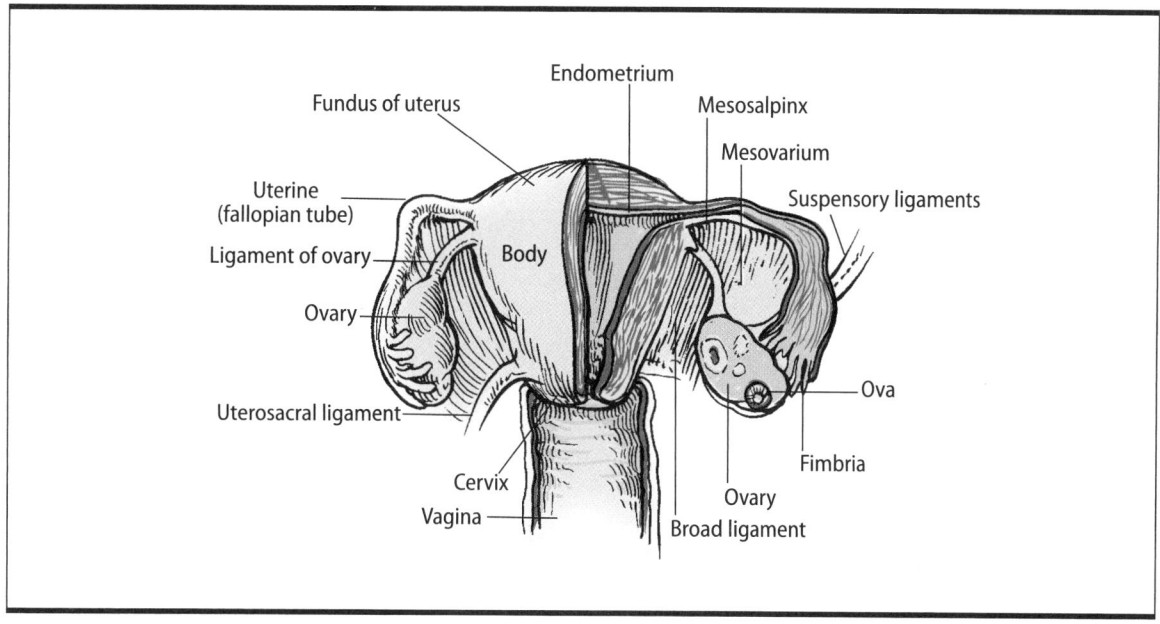

Female Genitourinary Tract Lateral View

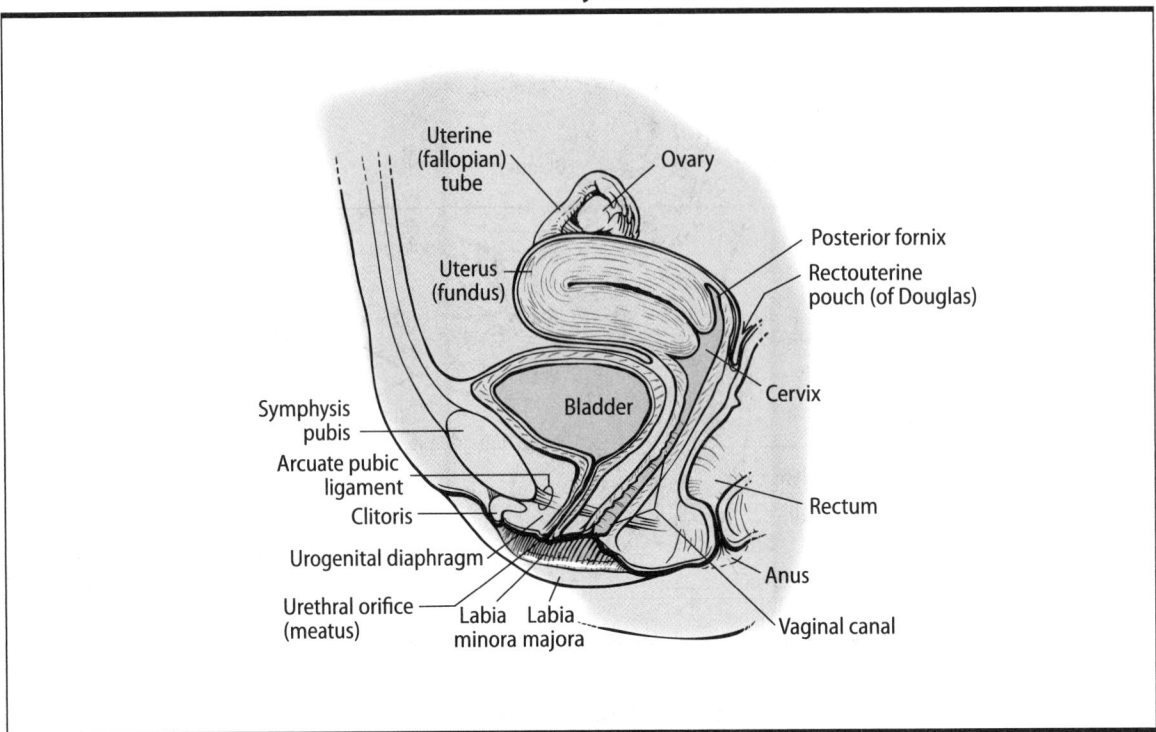

Chapter 15. Pregnancy, Childbirth and the Puerperium (O0Ø–O9A)

Term Pregnancy – Single Gestation

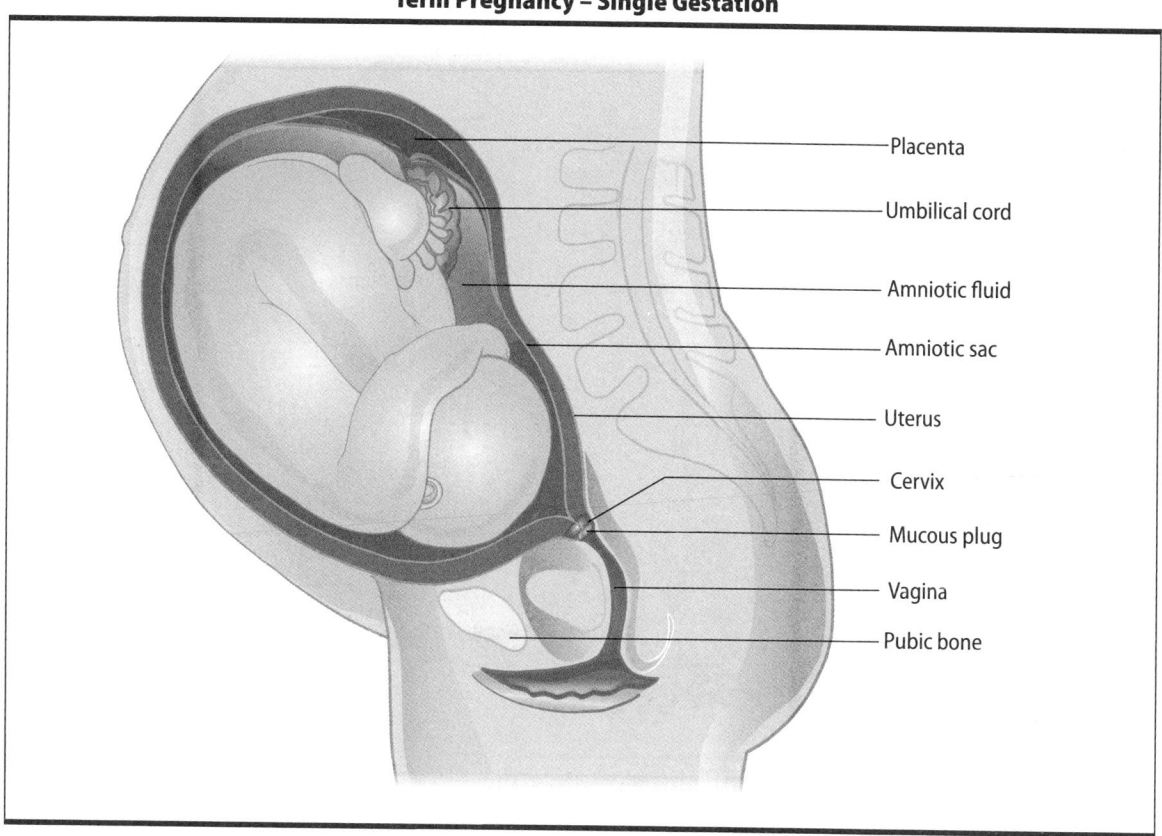

- Placenta
- Umbilical cord
- Amniotic fluid
- Amniotic sac
- Uterus
- Cervix
- Mucous plug
- Vagina
- Pubic bone

Twin Gestation–Dichorionic–Diamniotic (DI-DI)

- 2 Chorionic sacs
- 2 Amniotic sacs
- 2 Fetuses
- 2 Umbilical cords
- 2 Placentas

Twin Gestation–Monochorionic–Diamniotic (MO-DI)

1 Chorionic sac

2 Amniotic sacs

2 Fetuses

2 Umbilical cords

1 Placenta

Twin Gestation–Monochorionic–Monoamniotic (MO-MO)

1 Chorionic sac

1 Amniotic sac

2 Fetuses

2 Umbilical cords

1 Placenta

Chapter 19. Injury, Poisoning and Certain Other Consequences of External Causes (S00–T88)

Types of Fractures

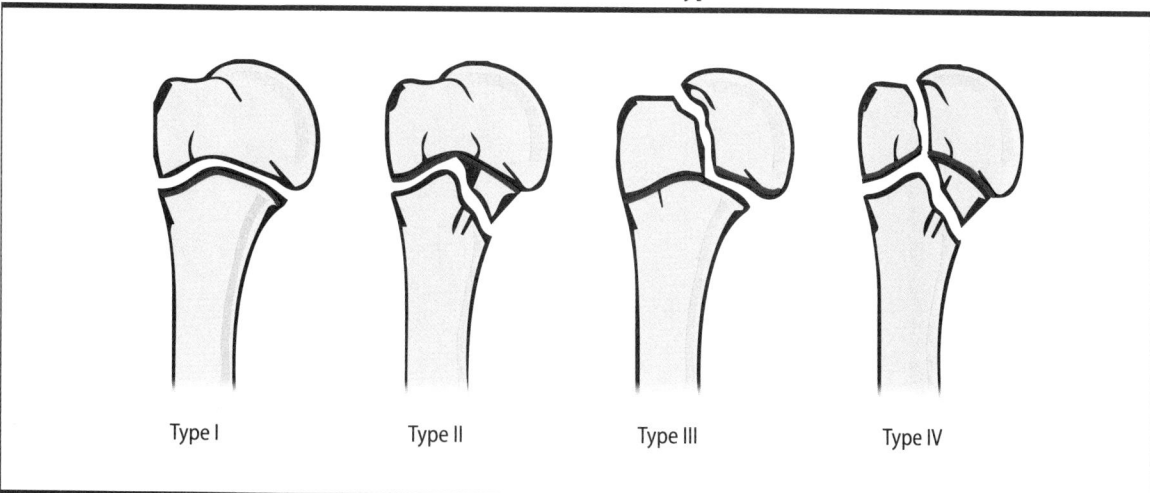

| Normal | Transverse | Open/Compound | Oblique | Oblique displaced |

| Comminuted | Segmental | Avulsed | Spiral | Greenstick |

Salter-Harris Fracture Types

| Type I | Type II | Type III | Type IV |

Notes

Notes